STEDMAN
Dicionário Médico

27ª Edição

Ilustrado em Cores

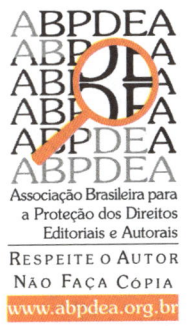

ABPDEA
Associação Brasileira para
a Proteção dos Direitos
Editoriais e Autorais
RESPEITE O AUTOR
NÃO FAÇA CÓPIA
www.abpdea.org.br

STEDMAN
Dicionário Médico

27ª Edição

Ilustrado em Cores

**Esta obra é uma tradução de
Stedman's Medical Dictionary**

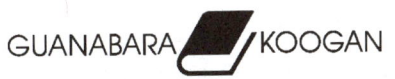

NOTA DA EDITORA: A área da saúde é um campo em constante mudança. As normas de segurança padronizadas precisam ser obedecidas; contudo, à medida que as novas pesquisas ampliam nossos conhecimentos, tornam-se necessárias e adequadas modificações terapêuticas e medicamentosas. Os editores, os consultores e os colaboradores desta obra verificaram cuidadosamente os nomes genéricos e comerciais dos medicamentos mencionados, bem como conferiram os dados referentes à posologia, de modo que as informações fossem acuradas e de acordo com os padrões aceitos por ocasião da publicação. Todavia, os leitores devem prestar atenção às informações fornecidas pelos fabricantes, a fim de se certificarem de que as doses preconizadas ou as contra-indicações não sofreram modificações. Isso é importante, sobretudo em relação a substâncias novas ou prescritas com pouca freqüência. Os editores, os consultores e os colaboradores não podem ser responsabilizados pelo uso impróprio ou pela aplicação incorreta do produto apresentado nesta obra.

No interesse de difusão da cultura e do conhecimento, os editores, os consultores e os colaboradores envidaram o máximo esforço para localizar os detentores dos direitos autorais de qualquer material utilizado, dispondo-se a possíveis acertos posteriores caso, inadvertidamente, a identificação de algum deles tenha sido omitida.

Stedman's Medical Dictionary
Copyright © 2000 Lippincott Williams & Wilkins
351 West Camden Street
Baltimore, Maryland 21201–2436 USA
Published by arrangement with Lippincott, Williams & Wilkins, Inc., USA

Copyright © by William Wood and Company: 1911, 1st ed.; 1912, 2nd ed.; 1914, 3rd ed.; 1916, 4th ed.; 1918, 5th ed.; 1920, 6th ed.; 1922, 7th ed.; 1924, 8th ed.; 1926, 9th ed.; 1928, 10th ed.; 1930, 11th ed.

Copyright © by Williams & Wilkins: 1933, 12th ed.; 1935, 13th ed.; 1939, 14th ed.; 1942, 15th ed.; 1946, 16th ed.; 1949, 17th ed.; 1953, 18th ed.; 1957, 19th ed.; 1961, 20th ed.; 1966, 21st ed.; 1972, 22nd ed.; 1976, 23rd ed.; 1982, 24th ed.; 1990, 25th ed.; 1995, 26th ed.

Direitos exclusivos para a língua portuguesa
Copyright © 2003 by
EDITORA GUANABARA KOOGAN S.A.
Travessa do Ouvidor, 11
Rio de Janeiro, RJ — CEP 20040-040
Tel.: 21–2221-9621
Fax: 21–2221-3202
www.editoraguanabara.com.br

Reservados todos os direitos. É proibida a duplicação
ou reprodução deste volume, no todo ou em parte,
sob quaisquer formas ou por quaisquer meios
(eletrônico, mecânico, gravação, fotocópia,
distribuição na Web ou outros),
sem permissão expressa da Editora.

Traduzido por

Claudia Coana

Cláudia Lúcia Caetano de Araújo

José Eduardo Ferreira de Figueiredo

Liane Oliveira Mufarrej Barbosa

Patricia Lydie Voeux

Sob a Supervisão de

Maria de Fátima Azevedo
Clínica Geral.
Formada pela Faculdade de Ciências Médicas da UERJ.
Pós-Graduação pela Sociedade Brasileira de Medicina Interna
(Hospital da Santa Casa da Misericórdia do Rio de Janeiro).
Médica Concursada do INAMPS.
Médica Concursada do Município do Rio de Janeiro.
Médica do Trabalho (FPGMCC–UNIRIO)

CONTEÚDO

Prefácio ix

Consultores xiii

Colaboradores xvi

Créditos das Ilustrações xvii

Fontes das Ilustrações xviii

Índice das Ilustrações xxii

Índice dos Quadros xxvii

Termos de Alta Importância Nesta Edição xxviii

Como Usar Este Dicionário xxix

Localizador de Gêneros LG1

Localizador de Subentradas LS1

Vocabulário de A a Z 1

Índice das Pranchas Anatômicas IPA1

Pranchas Anatômicas Coloridas A1

Pranchas de Técnicas de Imagens e Posicionamento Anatômico B1

Pranchas Clínicas e Microscópicas C1

Conteúdo dos Apêndices 1785

Glossário Português/Inglês 1870

PREFÁCIO

Seja bem-vindo à 27.ª edição do *Stedman/Dicionário Médico*. Esta edição continua a longa tradição de um dicionário médico abrangente, atual e acurado a serviço dos médicos e profissionais de saúde.

O *Stedman/Dicionário Médico* é o sucessor do primeiro dicionário médico norte-americano, *A New Dictionary of Medical Science and Literature*, do Dr. Robley Dunglison, publicado pela primeira vez em 1833. Esse dicionário manteve-se ao longo dos anos até a 23.ª edição (última), editada pelo Dr. Thomas Lathrop Stedman, em 1903. Cinco anos depois, o Dr. Stedman escreveu uma versão atualizada do dicionário de Dunglison que foi publicada em 1911. Essa versão recebeu o título *A Practical Medical Dictionary*, agora conhecido como *Stedman*.

Embora o *Stedman* seja rico em tradição, na Lippincott Williams & Wilkins utilizamos bancos de dados para a edição e revisão do léxico. Graças a esse banco de dados, conseguimos atingir um nível de acurácia e atualização que não seria possível na época do Dr. Stedman. Hoje em dia, o conteúdo do dicionário é mais consistente e mais acurado do que nunca. Nosso banco de dados também permitiu que produzíssemos o *Stedman's Electronic Medical Dictionary* para aqueles que desejam a prontidão e a conveniência do acesso digital às nossas referências médicas.

Novo nesta edição

Esta edição do *Stedman* foi meticulosamente revista por consultores de 52 especialidades médicas. As revisões de genética, bacteriologia, anatomia patológica e medicina laboratorial foram especialmente cuidadosas. Os termos de medicina veterinária foram revisados e deu-se ênfase à terminologia relevante para a medicina humana.

Editor de Termos Novos O Dr. Thomas Filardo cria a função de Editor de Termos Novos nesta edição. Como generalista, tem ele uma visão holística do dicionário e sugeriu a inclusão de termos novos para os consultores especialistas. Além disso, julgou o mérito dos termos sugeridos pelos consultores, buscando referências mais consistentes, completas e corretas.

Novas Especialidades Temos novos consultores em Oncologia, Pediatria, Pneumologia e Medicina de Emergência, que nada mais são que o reflexo da importância cada vez maior dessas especialidades.

Terminologia Anatômica Durante muitos anos, a Federative Committee on Anatomical Terminology (Comissão Federativa da Terminologia Anatômica) trabalhou para mudar a nomenclatura anatômica oficial da *Nomina Anatomica* [NA] para a *Terminologia Anatomica* [TA]. Os termos anatômicos em inglês e a TA em latim desta Comissão oficial foram aprovados pela International Federation of Associations of Anatomists.

Por ocasião da impressão desta obra, a Comissão já tinha completado a revisão da terminologia de Anatomia Patológica e Neuroanatomia, mas ainda estava trabalhando na da Embriologia, Citologia e Histologia. Esta edição do *Stedman*, portanto, utiliza a TA para os termos de Anatomia Patológica e Neuroanatomia, mas conserva a nomenclatura da NA para os termos de Embriologia, Citologia e Histologia. O leitor poderá observar que não deixamos de apresentar os termos em latim da *Nomina Anatomica*; apenas não são mais designados como NA.

Como fizemos na 26.ª edição, arrolamos as definições anatômicas onde é mais provável que os leitores irão procurá-las — nas traduções em inglês dos termos em latim.

Localizador de Gêneros Para encontrar a designação binomial e a definição de um microrganismo (exceto vírus) no *Stedman*, é preciso procurar o nome do gênero. Todavia, em grande parte da literatura médica, o gênero de um termo binomial é abreviado, mesmo na primeira referência, e nunca é identificado. Os leitores que não conhecerem o nome do gênero terão problemas para encontrar uma definição nos dicionários.

Nosso novo *Localizador de Gêneros* soluciona esse problema. Todos os termos binomiais têm referências cruzadas com os nomes das espécies. Por exemplo, para identificar *P. falciparum*, procure no *Localizador de Gêneros* a palavra "falciparum" e encontrará *Plasmodium*. A seguir, procure no dicionário a palavra *Plasmodium*, que é uma entrada principal, e encontrará a definição.

Como não se abrevia o nome dos gêneros de vírus, os vírus não são incluídos no *Localizador de Gêneros*.

Pranchas Anatômicas Em um dos apêndices deste dicionário (A1 – A27), você encontrará as pranchas anatômicas coloridas. Preparadas a partir de revisões da obra *Anatomia Orientada para a Clínica* do Dr. Keith Moore (4.ª edição), essas pranchas apresentam todas as artérias, veias, nervos e músculos do corpo humano, juntamente com informações relevantes, e obedecem à nomenclatura da *Terminologia Anatomica*.

O Projeto Gráfico Nosso propósito foi utilizar imagens e quadros que expandissem e elucidassem o significado dos verbetes apresentados neste dicionário. Para isso, nossos consultores e editores, sob a orientação do Diretor de Arte Jonathan Dimes, revisaram todas as imagens, de modo a preservar a clareza, a acurácia científica e a forma atualizada. O resultado consiste em mais de 1.050 ilustrações coloridas, fotografias e quadros.

Nesta edição, existem pranchas anatômicas coloridas e imagens diagnósticas que totalizam 64 páginas do dicionário. O atlas anatômico — acompanhado do índice — (32 páginas) é de referência rápida e tem como base o *adam.com*, o renomado *software* de educação médica. Um índice completo precede estas ilustrações.

Estamos orgulhosos por apresentar mais de 400 ilustrações criadas pelo famoso artista Neil O. Hardy. A excepcional carreira do Sr. Hardy (50 anos de trabalho) foi reconhecida por numerosos prêmios, inclusive o Lifetime Achievement Award da Association of Medical Illustrators.

Na seção A a Z existem mais de 700 ilustrações, muitas das quais com imagens múltiplas para ajudar o leitor a compreender melhor determinado assunto. Um símbolo ao lado do vocábulo — uma letra "I" branca dentro de um quadrado azul (🅘) — indica que para aquele verbete existe uma ilustração, na mesma página ou nas pranchas.

O leitor conseguirá encontrar facilmente qualquer imagem se utilizar o Índice das Ilustrações logo adiante. Basta procurar o termo ou expressão no Índice das Ilustrações para descobrir o número da página da ilustração referente.

A Tradição

Sim, nós acrescentamos muitas novidades ao *Stedman* para torná-lo mais acessível, informativo e abrangente; contudo, mantivemos as características que sempre foram úteis para os nossos leitores e nos diferenciaram de outros dicionários médicos.

Termos de Alta Importância Na 26.ª edição, introduzimos os "termos de alta importância". São conceitos que afetaram tão profundamente a prática da medicina que justificam mais que a definição padrão. O Dr. John Dirckx, internista e consultor de Etimologia, escreveu os termos de alta importância desta edição. Com a ajuda de nossos consultores, o Dr. Dirckx identificou 131 termos de alta importância, 51 deles expandidos por ele e revisados com cuidado a partir da edição anterior. Os restantes são novos. Esses termos aparecem na seção A–Z desta obra, realçados por linhas horizontais azuis.

Localizador de Subentradas Continuamos publicando uma longa lista de expressões ou múltiplos termos (subentradas). O objetivo dessa lista é identificar onde está a definição do verbete principal dessas expressões ou múltiplos termos — este é o principal desafio em um dicionário organizado em um formato de entradas principais e subentradas como o *Stedman*. As definições que envolvem "cochlear", por exemplo, não aparecem todas em "cochlear". Na verdade, aparecem como subentradas de outras entradas principais, como:

aqueduct; area; canal; canaliculus; duct; implant; joint; labyrinth; nerve; nucleus; part; prosthesis; recess; root; window.

Para obter mais informações sobre como utilizar o *Localizador de Subentradas*, procure a página LS1, que é a seção imediatamente anterior à seção A–Z.

Subentradas Fáceis de Encontrar Continuamos a nossa prática de colocar cada subentrada em uma nova linha para ajudar o leitor a identificar facilmente as informações necessárias.

Referências Cruzadas em Azul Muitas entradas ou subentradas não têm definições; elas são sinônimas de termos principais (preferíveis) que direcionarão o leitor para onde está a definição. Imprimimos todos esses sinônimos em azul, para que o leitor, procurando a definição deste vocábulo (em azul), encontre a explicação de sentido das entradas ou subentradas.

As Formas Combinantes Cerca de 1.200 partes combinantes em grego e em latim formam cerca de 90% da linguagem médica; portanto, o conhecimento desses elementos ajuda o leitor a compreender mais profundamente o significado dos vocábulos. Nós assinalamos esses sufixos, prefixos e outras formas combinantes com o símbolo universal de reciclagem ♻ nas margens da seção A–Z, e os arrolamos na página 1786.

Indexadores de Página Cada página apresenta um indexador verde com as duas primeiras letras do último vocábulo dessa página. Consideramos isso um marcador estratégico porque permite aos leitores descobrir rapidamente onde estão localizados sempre que abrirem este dicionário. É outra característica que ajuda os leitores a encontrar prontamente o que desejam.

Dicionário Funcional O *Stedman* é um dicionário funcional, um registro do idioma vivo, e as palavras estão grafadas com separação silábica, pronúncia e definição como são realmente usadas. Cada dicionário contém vocábulos, segundo os padrões filológicos, com erros de formação, de pronúncia e de separação silábica. Um dicionário pode sugerir padrões, mas não impô-los. Assim sendo, o *Stedman* é um parâmetro para aqueles que desejam falar e escrever o mais corretamente possível e adquirir novas palavras com maior acurácia.

Agradecimentos

A edição de uma obra como o *Stedman* é uma proeza imensa para ser atribuída a uma única pessoa. Uma equipe de consultores, editores, artistas, revisores e especialistas em bancos de dados é responsável por este livro. Nós da Lippincott Williams & Wilkins somos gratos, em primeiro lugar e sempre, aos consultores das especialidades médicas por terem escrito e revisado mais de 100.000 vocábulos deste dicionário.

Somos gratas especialmente ao Dr. Dirckx e ao Dr. Filardo, que, além do contrato de trabalho, colaboraram com toda sorte de assuntos, desde o emprego de termos e a grafia até a importância de uma ilustração.

Desejamos expressar nossos agradecimentos especiais a nossa Managing Editor, Barbara Werner, e a nossa Chief Online Editor, Barbara Ferretti, por terem nos presenteado com seu talento, diligência, dedicação e bom humor durante a realização das inumeráveis tarefas que lhes foram atribuídas nesta edição do *Stedman*.

Não poderíamos deixar de expressar nosso reconhecimento a outro grande grupo — os usuários do *Stedman* —, cujos comentários, sugestões, acréscimos e correções influenciam bastante as nossas edições. Agradecemos de coração a participação de todos vocês e pedimos que continuem a nos prestigiar para que possamos tornar nossos livros cada vez melhores.

Por fim, um tributo especial para Joan D. Caldwell, ex-Vice-Presidente e Editora da Lippincott Williams & Wilkins. Durante a última década do século XX, Joan conduziu os trabalhos de publicação do *Stedman* com argúcia e bom humor. Ela chamou a atenção de um número sem precedentes de profissionais de saúde e leigos para o *Stedman* e estabeleceu um padrão de desenvolvimento dos livros focalizado no usuário que até hoje só foi atingido por poucos editores. A ela agradecemos por nos ter mostrado o caminho.

Maureen Barlow Pugh
Senior Managing Editor
Lippincott Williams & Wilkins
Baltimore, Maryland

CONSULTORES

R. Donald Allison, PhD — *Bioquímica*
Associate Scientist, Department of Biochemistry and Molecular Biology, University of Florida College of Medicine, Gainesville, FL

Douglas R. Bacon, MD, MA — *Biografia e Epônimos*
Associate Professor and Vice Chairman for Education, Department of Anesthesiology, State University of New York at Buffalo; Chief of Anesthesiology Service, Buffalo VA Medical Center, Buffalo, NY

John Bennett, MD — *Micologia*
Head, Clinical Mycology Section, Laboratory of Clinical Investigation, National Institute of Allergy and Infectious Diseases, Bethesda, MD

David A. Bloom, MD — *Urologia e Cirurgia Urológica*
Chief, Pediatric Urology, Professor of Surgery, The University of Michigan & Mott Children's Hospital, Ann Arbor, MI

Alfred Jay Bollet, MD — *Medicina Interna*
Clinical Professor of Medicine, Yale University School of Medicine, New Haven, CT

David G. Bostwick, MD — *Patologia*
Consultant and Professor of Pathology and Urology, Mayo Clinic and Mayo Medical School, Rochester, MN

Michael J. Burridge, BVM&S, MPVM, PhD — *Medicina Veterinária*
Professor, Department of Pathobiology, College of Veterinary Medicine, University of Florida, Gainesville, FL

Philip M. Buttaravoli, MD, FACEP — *Medicina de Emergência*
Medical Director, Emergency Department, Palm Beach Gardens Medical Center, Palm Beach Gardens, FL

Patricia Charache, MD — *Bacteriologia*
Professor of Pathology, Medicine, and Oncology, Departments of Pathology and Medicine, Johns Hopkins Medical Institutions, Baltimore, MD

Barbara A. Conley, MD — *Oncologia*
Senior Investigator, Clinical Investigations Branch, Cancer Therapy Evaluation Program, National Cancer Institute, Rockville, MD

Arthur F. Dalley II, PhD — *Anatomia Macroscópica*
Professor of Cell Biology, Director of Gross Anatomy, Department of Cell Biology, Vanderbilt University School of Medicine, Nashville, TN; President, American Association of Clinical Anatomists

John A. Day, Jr., MD, FCCP — *Doença Pulmonar*
Assistant Professor of Medicine, University of Massachusetts Medical School, Attending Physician, Division of Pulmonary and Critical Care, St. Vincent Hospital and University of Massachusetts Memorial Health Care, Worcester, MA

John H. Dirckx, MD — *Etimologias e Termos de Alta Importância*
Director, University of Dayton Health Center, Dayton, OH

Thomas W. Filardo, M.D. — *Editor de Termos Novos*
Physician-Consultant, Evendale, OH

Clair A. Francomano, MD — *Genética*
Clinical Director, National Human Genome Research Institute, National Institutes of Health, Bethesda, MD

Paul J. Friedman, MD — *Radiologia*
Professor of Radiology and Chief of Thoracic Radiology, School of Medicine, University of California, San Diego, CA

Lynne S. Garcia, MS, MT(ASCP), CLS(NCA), F(AAM) — *Medicina Tropical/Parasitologia*
Department of Pathology and Laboratory Medicine, UCLA Medical Center, Los Angeles, CA

Steven I. Gutman, MD, MBA — *Patologia, Hematologia e Medicina Laboratorial/Corantes e Procedimentos*
Director, Division of Clinical Laboratory Devices, Division of Clinical Laboratory Devices, Food and Drug Administration, Rockville, MD

Duane E. Haines, PhD — *Neuroanatomia*
Professor of Anatomy, Chairman, Department of Anatomy, The University of Mississippi Medical Center, Jackson, MS

David E. Hall, MD — *Pediatria*
Clinical Associate Professor of Pediatrics, Emory University School of Medicine, Childrens Healthcare of Atlanta at Scottish Rite, Atlanta, GA

Iain Kalfas, MD — Neurocirurgia
Department of Neurosurgery, Cleveland Clinic Foundation, Cleveland, OH

John B. Kerrison, MD — Oftalmologia
Assistant Chief of Service, Wilmer Eye Institute, Johns Hopkins Hospital, Baltimore, MD

John M. Last, MD, FRACP, FRCPC — Estatísticas e Epidemiologia em Medicina
Professor Emeritus, Department of Epidemiology and Community Medicine, University of Ottawa, Ottawa, Ontario, Canada

Stanley S. Lefkowitz, PhD — Imunologia e Virologia
Professor, Department of Microbiology and Immunology, Texas Tech University Health Sciences Center, Lubbock, TX

David N. Menton, PhD — Histologia
Associate Professor of Anatomy, Washington University School of Medicine, St. Louis, MO

Edward D. Miller, MD — Anestesiologia
The Frances Watt Baker, M.D., and Lenox D. Baker, Jr., M.D., Dean of the Medical Faculty, Chief Executive Officer, Johns Hopkins Medicine, Johns Hopkins School of Medicine, Baltimore, MD

John B. Mulliken, MD — Cirurgia Plástica e Reconstrutora
Associate Professor of Surgery, Harvard Medical School; Director, Craniofacial Centre, Children's Hospital, Boston, MA

Martin L. Nusynowitz, MD — Medicina Nuclear
Professor, Radiology, Internal Medicine, and Pathology, University of Texas Medical Branch at Galveston, Galveston, TX

J. Patrick O'Leary, MD — Cirurgia Geral
The Isidore Cohn, Jr., Professor and Chairman of Surgery, Louisiana State University Medical School, New Orleans, LA

Sharon T. Phelan, MD — Obstetrícia e Ginecologia
Associate Professor, Department of Obstetrics and Gynecology, University of Alabama at Birmingham, Birmingham, AL

Ronald B. Ponn, MD — Cirurgia Torácica
Assistant Clinical Professor and Associate Section Chief of Cardiothoracic Surgery, Yale University School of Medicine and Yale-New Haven Hospital, New Haven, CT

Richard Prayson, MD — Neuropatologia
Department of Anatomic Pathology, The Cleveland Clinic Foundation, Cleveland, OH

Arthur Raines, PhD — Farmacologia e Toxicologia
Professor Emeritus of Pharmacology and Neurology, Department of Pharmacology, Georgetown University Medical Center, Washington, DC

George S. Schuster, DDS, MS, PhD — Odontologia
Ione and Arthur Merritt Professor, Chairman, Department of Oral Biology and Maxillofacial Pathology, Medical College of Georgia, School of Dentistry, Augusta, GA

Sheldon M. Schuster, PhD — Biotecnologia
Professor, Biochemistry and Molecular Biology, Program Director, Biotechnology Program, University of Florida, Gainesville, FL

James B. Snow, Jr., M.D., FACS — Otorrinolaringologia
Former Director, National Institute on Deafness and Other Communication Disorders, National Institutes of Health, Bethesda, MD; Professor Emeritus of Otorhinolaryngology, University of Pennsylvania School of Medicine, Philadelphia, PA

David H. Spodick, MD, DSc — Cardiologia
Professor of Medicine, University of Massachusetts Medical School; Lecturer in Medicine, Tufts University School of Medicine; Lecturer in Medicine, Boston University School of Medicine; Director of Clinical Cardiology and Director of Cardiovascular Fellowship Training, St. Vincent Hospital, Worcester, MA

Kathleen K. Sulik, PhD — Embriologia
Professor, Department of Cell Biology and Anatomy, University of North Carolina, Chapel Hill, NC

Asa J. Wilbourn, MD — Neurologia
Director, EMG Laboratory, The Cleveland Clinic Foundation, Clinical Professor of Neurology, Case-Western Reserve University School of Medicine, Cleveland, OH

Colin Wood, MD — Dermatologia
Professor Emeritus of Pathology, University of Maryland School of Medicine, Baltimore, MD

Douglas D. Woodruff, MD — **Psiquiatria/Psicologia**
Private Practice, Baltimore, MD

David B. Young, PhD — **Fisiologia**
Professor, Physiology and Biophysics, University of Mississippi Medical Center, Jackson, MS

Joseph D. Zuckerman, MD — **Ortopedia**
Walter A. L. Thompson Professor of Orthopaedic Surgery, New York University School of Medicine; Chairman, NYU-Hospital for Joint Diseases, Department of Orthopaedic Surgery, New York, NY

COLABORADORES

Janine Denis Cook, PhD, Department of Medical and Research Technology, University of Maryland School of Medicine. Contributing Editor, Apêndice de Valores de Referência em Laboratório

Show-Hong Duh, PhD, DABCC, Department of Pathology, University of Maryland School of Medicine. Contributing Editor, Apêndice de Valores de Referência em Laboratório

Doris L. Lefkowitz, PhD, Associate Professor, Department of Biological Sciences, Texas Tech University, Lubbock, TX. Contributing Editor, Imunologia

John B. Imboden, MD, Associate Professor of Psychiatry, Johns Hopkins University School of Medicine, Baltimore, MD. Contributing Editor, Psiquiatria

Nicola Ho, MD, Fellow, Medical Genetics Branch, National Human Genome Research Institute, National Institutes of Health, Bethesda, MD. Contributing Editor, Genética

Ivan Damjanov, MD, PhD, Professor, Department of Pathology, The University of Kansas School of Medicine, Kansas City, KS. Contributing Editor, Patologia

Linda A. Smith, PhD, CLS(NCA), Associate Professor and Graduate Program Director, Department of Clinical Laboratory Science, University of Texas Health Science Center, San Antonio, TX. Contributing Editor, Apêndice de Grupos Sangüíneos

CRÉDITOS DAS ILUSTRAÇÕES

As ilustrações desta edição do *Stedman/Dicionário Médico* foram criadas ou adaptadas pelos seguintes profissionais (ver em Fontes das Ilustrações as origens das adaptações):

Todo o projeto gráfico do suplemento de anatomia provém de **imagery © 1999 adam.com**™. Todos os direitos reservados.

Mary Anna Barratt-Dimes, Parkton, MD. 20, 36, 82, 90, 142, 151, 192, 274, 313, 334, 388, 391, 392, 404, 437, 512, 585, 713 (hemoglobina), 718, 726, 733, 738, 740, 781, 783, 796, 846, 862, 971, 1090, 1183, 1262, 1336, 1350, 1360, 1391, 1409, 1572, 1655, 1656, 1658, 1659, 1692 (timpanografia), 1721 (vasopressina), 1738, 1762

Kathryn Born, Arlington, TX. 1297 (exame da próstata)

Michael Budowick, Munich, Germany. 113

Susan Caldwell, Pikesville, MD, criou todos os quadros na seção A–Z deste livro.

Robert Demarest, Hawthorne, NJ. 1132

Duckwall Productions, Baltimore, MD. 738, 1140

Neil O. Hardy. Westport, CT. 2, 4, 9, 19, 47, 49, 53, 54, 62, 70, 72, 75, 86, 107, 120, 121, 123, 130, 141, 147, 152, 161, 163, 169, 170, 179, 183, 186, 187, 188, 198, 207, 220, 225, 230, 231 (queimaduras), 235, 237, 241, 244, 247, 249, 250, 260, 263, 265, 269, 273, 295, 313, 314, 315 (circulação sistêmica), 318, 325, 332, 339, 340, 341, 354, 367, 368, 388, 395, 411, 412, 413, 422, 428, 439, 445, 466, 473, 475, 480, 483, 484, 487, 497, 499 (retrator abdominal), 509, 511, 515, 516, 532, 540, 541, 548, 550, 565, 584, 595, 598, 603, 605, 607, 608, 610, 612, 617, 618, 619, 624, 631, 632, 633, 643, 646, 650, 651, 660, 665, 668, 676, 681, 688, 690, 692, 695, 708, 712 (hemodiálise), 715, 716, 722, 745, 746, 757, 762, 768, 776, 777, 786, 788, 800, 803, 804, 806, 814, 817, 823, 831, 834, 840, 844, 847, 860, 866, 871, 874, 887, 905, 913, 917, 920, 924, 934, 943 (manobra de Heimlich), 950 (massagem), 951, 954, 969, 970, 996 (mitose), 1001, 1006, 1007, 1030, 1045 (miopia), 1050, 1051, 1052, 1058, 1062, 1063, 1068, 1075, 1076, 1086, 1107, 1108, 1109, 1111, 1118 (olfação), 1130, 1131, 1132 (órgãos femininos e masculinos), 1139 (ossículo), 1143, 1144, 1148, 1155, 1157, 1158, 1159, 1161, 1186, 1196, 1197, 1202, 1208, 1235, 1236, 1239, 1240, 1246, 1255, 1259, 1265, 1278, 1280, 1288, 1297 (próstata), 1318, 1320, 1325, 1330, 1370, 1382, 1383, 1386, 1387, 1390, 1423, 1449, 1454, 1462, 1464, 1465, 1467, 1468, 1473, 1482, 1486, 1489, 1490, 1491, 1492, 1493, 1495, 1509, 1511, 1514, 1546, 1548, 1551, 1582, 1587, 1588, 1591, 1596, 1601, 1631, 1639, 1642 (dente), 1644, 1648, 1649 (traquéia), 1650, 1651, 1653, 1659, 1665, 1689, 1691, 1692 (gêmeos monozigóticos), 1694, 1701, 1708, 1714, 1716, 1719, 1721 (vasectomia), 1724, 1731, 1737, 1739, 1742, 1752, 1758, 1763, 1773, B8 (broncoscopia), B9 (laparoscopia), B11, B14, B15

Timothy Hengst, Thousand Oaks, CA. 56

Siri Mills, Munich, Germany. 702, 1193, 1675, 1678

Michael Schenk, Jackson, MS. 5, 78, 241, 242, 255, 432, 600, 722, 796, 1067, 1231, 1401

Mikki Senkarik, San Antonio, TX. 69, 134, 163, 167, 251, 338, 472, 499 (colocação dos eletrodos do ECG), 606, 769, 943 (manobra de Leopold), 949 (máscara unidirecional), 1153, 1522, 1742, 1783, B1, B2, B3, B8 (esofagoduodenoscopia), B9 (toracoscopia), B10 (colonoscopia)

Larry Ward, Salt Lake City, UT. 557, 678, 702, 949 (máscara de oxigênio), 950 (massa retal), 1123, 1319, 1520, 1641

FONTES DAS ILUSTRAÇÕES

Cortesia de Acuson Computed Sonography Corporation. Mountain View, CA. 1905. B11

Cortesia de Advanced Technology Laboratory. Bothell, WA. B11 (ultra-sonografia obstétrica)

Retirado de Agur AMR and Lee M. *Grant's Atlas of Anatomy* (9th ed.). Baltimore: Williams & Wilkins, 1991. 341

Cortesia de American Academy of Dermatology. Schamburg, IL. C8 (bolha, mácula, nódulo, pápula, placa, pústula, tumor, vesícula, vergão), C9 (hemangioma senil, crosta, equimose, erosão, fissura, quelóide, escama, telangiectasia, úlcera)

Cortesia de American Cancer Society, Inc. Atlanta, GA. C12 (melanoma maligno)

Cortesia de American Society of Clinical Pathologists Journal. Chicago, IL. C16 (*Giardia lamblia*)

Cortesia de American Society of Microbiology. Washington, DC. 718

Adaptado de *Application Manual: Cytokines/Chemokine Manual*, PharMingen Corporation, San Diego, CA. 1998. 402, 403

Retirado de Ballenger JJ & Snow JB. *Otorhinolaryngology: Head and Neck Surgery* (15th ed.). Baltimore: Williams & Wilkins, 1996. 194, 223, 473

Cortesia de Baschat A, MD. Center for Advanced Fetal Care, University of Maryland School of Medicine. Baltimore, MD. C11 (fluxo Doppler, coração fetal)

Retirado de Bear MF, Connors BW, Paradiso MA. *Neuroscience: Exploring the Brain.* Baltimore: Williams & Wilkins, 1996. 738

Cortesia de Bennett J, PhD. National Institutes of Health. Bethesda, MD. 207, C1 (corante metenamina-prata), C7 (hifas de *Aspergillus*, histoplasmose, micetoma), C15 (RM de cérebro normal)

Retirado de Bickley LS, MD. *Bates' Guide to Physical Examination and History Taking* (7th ed.). Philadelphia: Lippincott Williams & Wilkins, 1999. C8 (vitiligo), C15 (síndrome de Down, baqueteamento, cianose, icterícia, paralisia do nervo facial, sinal de Babinski, manchas de Brushfield)

Retirado de Brant WE & Helms CA. *Fundamentals of Diagnostic Radiology* (2nd ed.). Baltimore: Williams & Wilkins, 1999. 223, 381, 462, 519, 596, 605, 632, 748, 1444, 1457, B11 (carcinoma de ovário, fenda labial), B13 (mesotelioma), B14 (bronquiectasia, mamografia no câncer de mama, mamografia normal, mamografia, TC de fígado)

Adaptado de Braunwald E, Fauci AS, Isselbacher KJ, Kasper DL, Hauser SL, Longo DL, Jameson JL. *Harrison's Principles of Medicine* [livro em CD-ROM] (14th ed.). New York: McGraw-Hill Companies, 1998. 34, 258, 518, 1498

Cortesia de Brinkley W, PhD. Baylor College of Medicine, Houston, TX. 285

Cortesia de Bristow RE, MD. Johns Hopkins School of Medicine. Baltimore, MD. B9 (biopsia por laparoscopia, pelve normal)

Burtis CA, Ashwood ER, Aldrich JE. *Tietz Fundamentals of Clinical Chemistry* (4th ed.). Philadelphia: WB Saunders Company, 1996. 753, 763, 938

Cortesia de Caughman WF, DDS, Fazier KB, DDS, Haywood VB, DMD. Carbamide peroxide whitening of nonvital single discolored teeth: case reports. *Quintessance International*, 30: 155–161, 1999. B7 (dentes maxilares clareados)

Cortesia de Cavallucci D, CDA, EFDA, RDH. Harcum College, Bryn Mawr, PA. 599

Adaptado de Chaffee EE, RN, MN & Greisheimer, MD, PhD. *Basic Physiology and Anatomy* (3rd ed.). Philadelphia: JB Lippincott Company, 1974. 107, 169, 244, 273, 313, 363, 411, 484, 548, 619, 643, 855, 860, 913, 1014, 1076, 1278, 1467, 1509, 1567, 1588, 1650

Cortesia de Chai T, MD, & Sklar G, MD. University of Maryland School of Medicine. Baltimore, MD. B9 (tumor de bexiga à cistoscopia, cateter em ureteres)

Cortesia de College of American Pathologists, Chicago, IL. C16 (cilindro granular, ácido úrico, cristais hialinos)

Adaptado de Collier L & Mahy BWJ. *Topley & Wilson's Microbiology and Microbial Infections* (9th ed.) Vol. 1. London: Arnold Publications, 1998. 1121

Retirado de Daffner RH. *Clinical Radiology: The Essentials* (2nd ed.). Baltimore: Williams & Wilkins, 1998. 1306, B11 (placenta prévia), B12 (radiografia), B13 (pneumonia por *P. carinii*, edema pulmonar), B14 (hematoma cerebral, carcinoma pulmonar), B15 (RM do cérebro – esclerose múltipla, hérnia de núcleo pulposo), C13 (metástases nodulares), C14 (carcinoma de mama, carcinoma de colo, carcinoma de próstata, tumor de Ewing)

Retirado de Damjanov I, MD. *Histopathology: A Color Atlas and Textbook.* Baltimore: Williams & Wilkins, 1996. C13 (ceratose actínica, carcinoma de células escamosas, doença de Bowen, glioblastoma, lipossarcoma, linfoma, melanoma nodular, neuroblastoma, retinoblastoma, teratoma, adenoma hipofisário, tumor de Wilms)

Retirado de Danzi JT, Landma S. *Case Atlas of Gastroenterology*. Baltimore: Williams & Wilkins, 1995. B8 (esôfago de Barrett, pólipo gástrico)

Adaptado de Danforth N, MD & Scott JR, MD. *Danforth's Obstetrics and Gynecology* (8th ed.). Philadelphia: Lippincott Williams & Wilkins, 1999. 1183

Retirado de Davis RL, MD, Robertson DM, MD, MSC, FRCDC. *Textbook of Neuropathology* (3rd ed.). Baltimore: Williams & Wilkins, 1997. 195

Cortesia de Day JA, MD. University of Massachusetts School of Medicine, Boston, MA. B12 (SARA, colapso lobar), B13 (doença pulmonar intersticial)

Cortesia de Dirckx JH, MD. University of Dayton Health Center, Dayton, OH, 1021. 1581

Cortesia de Dura Pharmaceuticals, San Diego, CA. B9 (colangiografia intra-operatória)

Fadem B & Simring S. *High-Yield Psychiatry*. Baltimore: Lippincott Williams & Wilkins, 1998. Quadros — ansiedade, ansiolíticos, antidepressivos, fármacos para mania, antipsicóticos, desenvolvimento da criança normal, transtornos mentais, transtornos do humor, sono

Retirado de Feinsilver SH & Fein A. *Textbook of Bronchoscopy*. Baltimore: Williams & Wilkins, 1995. B8 (brônquio, carina, traquéia, cordas vocais)

Retirado de Fuller J, RN, PhD & Schaller-Ayers J, RNC, MNSc, PhD. *A Nursing Approach* (2nd ed.), 1994. 557, 565, 678, 702, 950, 1012, 1319, 1551, 1641, 1653

Adaptado de Garcia LS & Bruckner DA. *Diagnostic Medical Parasitology* (3rd ed.). Washington DC: ASM Press, 1997. 349

Retirado de Gartner LP & Hiatt JL. *Color Atlas of Histology* (2nd ed.). Baltimore: Williams & Wilkins, 1994. 346, 1418, C2 (basófilo, eosinófilo, monócito, neutrófilo)

Cortesia de General Electric Medical Systems. Milwaukee, WI. B15 (ressonância magnética, menisco roto do joelho), B16 (cintigrafia pulmonar, tomografia por emissão de pósitrons)

Retirado de Georgiade NG, Riefkohl R, Levine LS. Georgiade, GS. *Plastic, Maxillofacial and Reconstructive Surgery* (3rd ed.). Baltimore: Williams & Wilkins, 1996. 607, 608

Retirado de Goodheart HP, MD. *A Photoguide of Common Skin Disorders: Diagnosis and Management*. Baltimore: Lippincott Williams & Wilkins: 1999. C4 (foliculite, púrpura de Henoch-Schönlein), C5 (molusco contagioso), C8 (acantose nigricante, cisto pilomatricoma, dermatomiosite), C9 (escoriação, liquenificação), C11 (erupção cutânea fármaco-induzida, eritema multiforme, eritema nodoso, síndrome de Stevens-Johnson), C12 (neurofibromatose), C15 (exoftalmia, mixedema)

Retirado de Halstead CL, Blozis GG, Drinnan AJ, Gier RE. *Physical Evaluation of Dental Patient*. St. Louis: CV Mosby Company, 1982. 1642

Cortesia de Hawke M, MD. Toronto, Canada. B5 (colesteatoma, membrana timpânica normal, timpanosclerose)

Cortesia de Haywood VB, DMD. School of Dentistry, Medical College of Georgia, Augusta, GA. B7 (clareamento vital)

Cortesia de Haywood VB, DMD. Extended bleaching of tetracycline-stained teeth: a case report. *Contemporary Esthetics and Restorative Practice*. Jamesburg, NJ: Dental Learning Systems Co., Inc. 1 (1): 14-17, 1997. B7 (dentes manchados por tetraciclina)

Cortesia de Hoag Memorial Presbyterian Hospital. Newport Beach, CA. B16 (cintigrafia óssea)

Adaptado de Kapikian AZ. *Journal of the American Medical Association*. Chicago, IL: American Medical Association, 1993. Vol. 269:627. 1751

Retirado de Kini SR. *Color Atlas of Differential Diagnosis in Exfoliative and Aspiration Cytopathology*. Baltimore: Williams & Wilkins, 1998. 1118, C13 (ependimomas)

Retirado de Koneman EW, Allen SD, Janda WM, Schreckenberger PC, Winn WC, Jr. *Color Atlas and Textbook of Diagnostic Microbiology* (4th & 5th eds.). Philadelphia: Lippincott, 1992 & 1997. C1 (corante metenamina de prata, *Chlamydia*, *Clostridium tetani*, *Escherichia coli*, coloração hematoxilina-eosina, tecido acinar pancreático benigno, corante ácido periódico de Schiff, corante de Papanicolaou, *Streptococcus pneumoniae*, coloração de Warthin-Starry), C4 (*Pseudomonas*), C5 (vírus influenza A), C6 (ovo de *A. lumbricoides*, parasitas da malária, ovos de oxiúro), C7 (*Candida albicans, Alternaria (Penicillium), Isospora belli, Microsporum gypseum*)

Retirado de Kuby J. *Immunology* (3rd ed.). New York: WH Freeman Company, 1997. 34, 154, 780, 783, 784

Cortesia de Last JM, MD. University of Ottawa, Ontario, Canada. 945

Retirado de Lee RG, Foerster J, Lukens J, Paraskevas F, Greer JP, Rodgers GM. *Wintrobe's Clinical Hematology* (10th ed.). Vol. 1. Baltimore: Williams & Wilkins, 1998. C2 (mielócito neutrofílico), C3 (reticulócito)

Cortesia de Life Art. The Life Art Professional Collection–Surgery Collection. 290, 961, 996

Adaptado de Male D, Roitt I, Brostoff J. *Immunology: An Illustrated Outline.* (5th ed.). London: CV Mosby Company, 1998. 348, 948, 1000

Adaptado de Martin FN. *Introduction to Audiology* (5th ed.). Englewood Cliffs, NJ: Prentice Hall, 1994. 1691-1692

Retirado de McArdle WD, Katch FL, & Katch VL. *Essentials of Exercise Physiology.* Philadelphia: Lea & Febiger, 1994. 1705

Retirado de McClatchey K. *Clinical Laboratory Medicine.* Baltimore: Williams & Wilkins, 1994. 398, C2 (eritroblastos), C3 (corpúsculo de Heinz), C4 (célula bacteriana, gonococos), C5 (linfoma de Burkitt), C16 (aspirado de medula óssea, cilindro céreo, cristais de cistina, cristais de oxalato de cálcio, hemácias, leucócitos, sonda cromossomial integral)

Cortesia de McKenzie SB, Clare N, Burns C, Larson L, Metz J. *Textbook of Hematology* (2nd ed.). Baltimore: Williams & Wilkins, 1996. 308, 1256, 1617, C1 (coloração de Wright-Giemsa), C2 (megacarioblasto, promielócito), C3 (anemias aplásica, hemolítica, microcítica, falciforme); anisocitose, pontilhado basofílico, macrocitose, microcitose, poiquilocitose, reticulócitos, esferocitose)

Copyright de Mediclip: The Complete Medical Image Source. Clinical Images OB/GYN. 1709

Adaptado de Melnick JL, Adelberg EA, Brooks GF, Jawetz E, Morse SA, Butel JS. *Jawetz Melnick and Adelberg's Medical Microbiology* (21st ed.). New York, NY: McGraw Hill, 1998. 281, 724, 1750

Retirado de Mims C, Playfair J, Roitt I, Wakelin D, R Williams. *Medical Microbiology* (2nd ed.). London: CV Mosby Company, 1998. 1755

Retirado de Ming SC & Goldman H. *Pathology of the Gastrointestinal Tract* (2nd ed.). Baltimore: Williams & Wilkins, 1998. C12 (tumor benigno de estômago, tumor maligno de estroma, carcinoma ulcerativo)

Cortesia de Mission Hospital Regional Medical Center. Mission Viego, CA. B8 (gastrite, varizes esofágicas), B10 (polipectomia colônica), B11 (ultra-sonografia)

Retirado de Moore KL, PhD, FRSM, FIAC & Dalley AF II, PhD. *Clinically Oriented Anatomy* (4th ed.). Baltimore: Lippincott Williams & Wilkins, 1999. Material: quadros de artérias, músculos, nervos e veias (usados nos apêndices)

Adaptado de *Morbidity and Mortality Weekly Report Series.* Atlanta: Centers for Disease Control and Prevention, 1991. Vol 40 RR03. 1332

Retirado de Naeim F. *Pathology of Bone Marrow* (2nd ed.). Baltimore: Williams & Wilkins, 1998. C1 (coloração azul da Prússia)

Retirado de Neville BW, Damm DD, White DK. *Color Atlas of Clinical Oral Pathology* (2nd ed.). Baltimore: Williams & Wilkins, 1998. 35, 614, C10 (ameloblastoma, ulcerações aftosas, câncer de língua, *Candida albicans,* queilite, doença de Behçet, herpangina, estomatite herpética, leucoplaquia, leucoplaquia pilosa oral, fossetas labiais, mucocele, grânulos de Fordyce, estomatite)

Cortesia de Newport Diagnostic Center, Newport Beach, CA. B16 (PET de cérebro normal e na doença de Alzheimer)

Cortesia de Olympus America, Inc., Melville, NY. B9 (toracoscopia), B10 (colonoscópio)

Cortesia de Orange Coast College, Costa Mesa, CA. 528

Cortesia de Peroukta R, MD. Cockeysville, MD. B14 (artroscopia, enxerto de LCA, menisco normal, laceração de menisco)

Cortesia de Philips Medical Systems. Shelton, CT. B14 (tomografia computadorizada)

Retirado de Pillitteri A, PhD, RN, PNP. *Maternal & Child Health Nursing: Care of the Childbearing & Childrearing Family* (3rd ed.). Philadelphia: Lippincott Williams & Wilkins, 1998. 69, 251, 412, 943, 1783

Cortesia de Potter, B, DDS. School of Dentistry, Medical College of Georgia, Augusta, GA. B6 (radiografia cefalométrica, radiografia, implante em endósteo, dentição mista, radiotransparência, cárie recorrente, canal radicular, terceiro molar que não irrompeu)

Retirado de Rassner G. traduzido por WHC Burgdorf. *Atlas of Dermatology* (3rd ed.). Philadelphia: Lea & Febiger, 1994. 16, 230, 231, 491, 503, 724, 921, 1081, 1171, 1192, 1427, 1719, C4 (impetigo), C6 (elefantíase), C8 (síndrome de Peutz-Jeghers), C9 (hemangioma), C11 (dermatite de contato alérgica, dermatite herpetiforme, erupção cutânea polimórfica a exposição à luz, fotodermatite, radiodermatite), C12 (angiossarcoma, doença de Bowen, ceratose actínica, melanoma lentiginoso maligno, granuloma piogênico, ceratoses seborréicas), C15 (doença de Paget)

Retirado de Roche Lexikon Medizin (3rd ed.). Munich, Germany: Urban & Schwarzenberg, 1993. 3, 7, 14, 22, 23, 35, 73, 87, 113, 119, 120, 121, 135, 142, 163, 224, 255, 267, 299, 311, 315, 316, 373, 392, 456, 457, 503, 504, 524, 525, 540, 600, 601, 620, 621, 649, 684, 702, 716, 740, 783, 795, 851, 855, 860, 923, 936, 942, 960, 1039, 1044, 1053, 1054, 1073, 1081, 1128, 1139, 1193, 1208, 1217, 1219, 1234, 1252, 1263, 1266, 1307, 1315, 1323, 1360, 1389, 1394, 1426, 1433, 1466, 1487, 1491, 1492, 1609, 1648, 1649, 1675, 1678, 1772, 1777, 1783, 1784, B4 (blefarite, coloboma da íris, hifema, laceração de retina), B8 (carcinoma de laringe), B10 (colite ulcerativa, diverticulose), B15 (meningioma), B16 (captação tireóidea, cintigrafia hepática), C2 (células sangüíneas, linfócitos), C3 (eritrócitos na anemia perniciosa), C4 (estafilococos, estreptococos, *Mycobacterium tuberculosis*), C5 (HIV, herpes zoster, hepatite B), C9 (rosácea), C12 (neurofibromatose, ceratoacantoma), C16 (*ferning* do muco cervical)

Adaptado de Rosdahl Bunker C, RN, BSN, MA. *Textbook of Basic Nursing* (7th ed.). Philadelphia: Lippincott Williams & Wilkins, 1999. 56, 803

Cortesia de Ross MH. *Histology: A Text and Atlas* (3rd ed.). Baltimore: Williams & Wilkins, 1995. 276, 835, 1074

Retirado de Sanders CV, Nesbitt LT, Jr. *The Skin and Infection: A Color Atlas and Text.* Baltimore: Williams & Wilkins, 1995. 1053, 1054, C4 (doença de Lyme, erisipela, lepra lepromatosa, estafilococos, estreptococos), C5 (eritema infeccioso, hepatite B, hepatite C, herpes genital, mononucleose infecciosa, varicela hemorrágica, verruga plantar), C6 (larva migrans cutânea, pediculose do couro cabeludo, pediculose do púbis, escabiose), C7 (*Cryptococcus*, tinha da cabeça, tinha do pé, tinha versicolor), C10 (língua em morango), C12 (sarcoma de Kaposi)

Cortesia de Scheie Eye Institute. Philadelphia, PA. B4 (retina glaucomatosa, papiledema, retina normal, descolamento de retina, retinopatia diabética, retinopatia hipertensiva)

Cortesia de Schuster GS, DDS, PhD. School of Dentistry, Medical College of Georgia, Augusta, GA. B6 (cartão dentário)

Retirado de Seshan SV, D'Agati V, Appel GA, Churg, J. *Renal Disease: Classification and Atlas of Tubulo-interstitial and Vascular Diseases.* Baltimore: Williams & Wilkins, 1998. 145, 456, 457

Cortesia de Sheen, G, DDS, MS. School of Dentistry, Medical College of Georgia, Augusta, GA. B7 (restauração, jaquetas, diastema de resina, ponte ligada a resina, coroas de porcelana)

Adaptado de Skarin AT, Dorfman DM: Non-Hodgkin's lymphoma: current classification and management. *CA: A Cancer Journal for Clinicians.* Baltimore: Williams & Wilkins, 1997. Vol. 47 No 6. 930

Cortesia de Skin Cancer Foundation. New York, NY. C12 (carcinoma basocelular, carcinoma de células escamosas)

Retirado de Smeltzer SC & Bare BG. *Brunner & Suddarth's Textbook of Medical Surgical-Nursing* (8th ed.). Philadelphia: JB Lippincott Company, 1996. 134, 167, 220, 334, 338, 472, 499, 606, 769, 1153, 1155, 1271, 1319, 1423, 1482, 1522, 1659, 1742, B8 (broncoscopia com fibra óptica, esofagoduodenoscópio), B9 (laparoscopia, toracoscopia), B10 (colonoscopia), B11 (ultra-sonografia), B14 (radiografia), B15 (RM)

Stites DP, Terr AI, Parslow TG. *Basic and Clinical Medical Immunology* (8th ed.). New York, NY: McGraw Hill, 1994. 782

Adaptado de Suddarth Smith, D. *Lippincott's Manual of Nursing Practice* (5th ed.). Philadelphia: JB Lippincott Company, 1991. 413, 540, 1197, 1520, 1591

Retirado de Sun T. *Parasitic Disorders* (2nd ed.). Baltimore: Williams & Wilkins, 1998. 396, 530, 479, C6 (Acanthamoeba, elefantíase, *Giardia lamblia*, ovos de *Taenia*, *Trichomonas hominis*)

Retirado de Sun T, Tenenbaum MJ, Greenspan J. *Journal of Infectious Disease.* Chicago, IL: University of Chicago Press, 1993. Vol 238; 248. C6 (*Babesia*)

Cortesia de Temple University Hospital. Philadelphia, PA. B8 (broncoscopia)

Cortesia de Underwood L, MD & Underwood RD, MD. Mission Viejo, CA. C4 (sífilis), C9 (petéquia)

Cortesia de Wang F, MD. Orange, CA. B16 (cintigrafias de ventilação e perfusão)

Cortesia de Welch Allyn, Inc. Skaneateles Falls, NY. B4 (exame oftalmológico, oftalmoscópio), B5 (exostose, corpo estranho, otomicose, otite externa, otite média, otoscópio, otoscopia, perfuração), C11 (rinite alérgica, pólipos nasais)

Retirado de Wilcox RB. *High-Yield Biochemistry.* Baltimore: Lippincott Williams & Wilkins, 1999. 393, 1357, 1655, 1656

Retirado de Willis MC. *Medical Terminology: The Language of Health Care.* Baltimore: Williams & Wilkins, 1996. 877, 1254, 1396

Retirado de Yochum TR & Rowe LJ. *Essentials of Skeletal Radiology* (2nd ed.). Baltimore: Williams & Wilkins, 1996. 561, 1045, 1046

Cortesia de Zucker-Franklin D, PhD. New York University Medical Center, New York, NY. C2 (monócito), C3 (reticulócito)

ÍNDICE DAS ILUSTRAÇÕES

Os Índices das Ilustrações e dos Quadros são uma forma rápida de os leitores encontrarem qualquer imagem neste livro. O número da página ao lado de cada termo indica onde os leitores poderão encontrar uma ilustração daquele termo.

Os termos seguidos pela letra "A" e acompanhados de um número de página indicam que a imagem pode ser encontrada no conjunto A das pranchas coloridas, que é o atlas de anatomia com 32 páginas. Os termos seguidos pela letra "B" e acompanhados de um número de página indicam que a imagem pode ser encontrada no conjunto B das pranchas coloridas. Esse segundo bloco contém imagens diagnósticas e posicionamento anatômico. Já os termos seguidos pela letra "C" e acompanhados de um número de página são encontrados no conjunto C das pranchas coloridas, a seção sobre doenças e anormalidades.

Para encontrar a definição do termo ilustrado, simplesmente procure a palavra em negrito. Os leitores conseguirão identificar se um termo na seção A–Z for ilustrado — seja na ilustração próxima ao termo seja nas pranchas coloridas — caso esteja acompanhado pelo símbolo (🛈).

abdomen 2
abduction versus **adduction** B2
spherical **aberration** 3
alveolar **abscess** 4
perirectal **abscess** 5
Acanthamoeba C6
acanthosis nigricans C8
acarid 7
accommodation of the eye 9, 565
pancreatic **acinar** tissue C1
acne conglobata 14
acrodermatitis chronica atrophicans 16
acupuncture 19
adaptation 20
null-cell **adenoma** 22
pituitary **adenoma** C13
müllerian adenosarcoma 23
oral lesion associated with **AIDS** 35
albinism 36
Alternaria C7
pulmonary **alveolus** 47
Amanita muscaria and *phalloides* 47
ameba 49
ameloblastoma C10
amniocentesis 53
amnion 54
amputation 56
anastomosis 62
anatomy of **head** and **neck** A5, A6
aplastic **anemia** C3
hemolytic **anemia** C3
microcytic hypochromatic **anemia** C3
pernicious **anemia** C3
sickle cell **anemia** C3
regional **anesthesia** 69
aneurysm 70
angina pectoris 72
fluorescein **angiography** 73

renal **angiography** 73
cherry **angioma** C9
percutaneous transluminal **angioplasty** 75
angiosarcoma C12
venous **angle** 78
anisocytosis C3
anoxia 82
anterior versus **posterior** B1
antibody 86
monoclonal **antibody** 87
HL-A **antigen** 90
aphthous ulcerations C10
reflex **arc** 107
ARDS (radiograph) B12
cardiac **arrest** 113
arteries of head and neck A4
arteries of lower limb A20
arteries of thorax and abdomen A10
arteries of upper limb A16
major **arteries** of the body 130
arteriography 119
arteriole 119
temporal **arteritis** 120
artery structure 121
coronary **artery** 123
arthroplasty 134
arthroscopy B10
arthrosis 135
Ascaris lumbricoides C6
aspergilloma 139, C7
Aspergillus hyphae C7
asthma 141
astigmatism 142
atherosclerosis 145
atom 146
esophageal **atresia** 147
noise-induced **audiogram** 150
pure tone **audiogram** 151
mediate **auscultation** 152

auscultation points A11
Babesia C6
Bacillus 161
bacterial cell C4
bacteriophage 163
bandage 167
baroreceptor 169
blood-brain **barrier** 170
basophil C2
biceps 179
biopsy 183
laparoscopic **biopsy** B9
bite 186
urinary **bladder** 187
blastoderm 188
blastula 188
blepharitis angularis B4
blood C2
blood components 192
foreign **body** 194, B5
Heinz **body** C3
Lewy **body** 195
bone 198
brain 207, A7, B15, B16
breast 220
resin-bonded **bridge** B7
bronchiectasis 223
cystic **bronchiectasis** (CT scan) B14
bronchiolitis 224
bronchoscope B8
bronchoscopy B8
bronchus B8
segmental **bronchi** 225
Brugia malayi C6
bulla C8
burn 230
second-degree **burn** 231
coronary **bypass** 235
caduceus 237
callus 241
bomb **calorimeter** 241
human **calorimeter** 242
gamma **camera** 242
Haversian **canal** 244

Candida albicans 247, C7
candidiasis C10
capillary 249
interphalangeal **capsule** 250
caput succedaneum 251
types of **carcinoma** 255
carcinoma of breast B14, C14
carcinoma of prostate C14
carcinoma of tongue B10
basal cell **carcinoma** C12
bronchogenic **carcinoma** 255
colon **carcinoma** C14
esophageal **carcinoma** C12
laryngeal **carcinoma** B8
lung **carcinoma** (CT scan) B14
ovarian **carcinoma** (sonogram) B11
prostatic **carcinoma** C14
squamous cell **carcinoma** C10, C12, C13
ulcerative squamous cell **carcinoma** C12
dental **caries** 260
carina of trachea B8
cartilages of the nose 263
granular **cast** C16
hyaline **cast** C16
urinary **cast** 265, C16
waxy **cast** C16
cataract 267
cystoscopic view of **catheter** in ureter B9
Foley **catheter** 269
caudad versus **cephalad** B1
pleural **cavity** B9
cell 273
antigen-presenting **cell** 274
bacterial **cell** C4
development of blood **cells** C2
goblet **cells** 276

ÍNDICE DAS ILUSTRAÇÕES

red blood **cells** in urine C16
white blood **cells** in urine C16
centriole 285
counting **chamber** 290
dental numbering **chart** B6
cheilitis exfoliativa C10
optic **chiasm** 295
Chlamydia trachomatis C1
intraoperative **cholangiography** B9
percutaneous transhepatic **cholangiography** 299
cholecystectomy C4
cholelithiasis 301
cholesteatoma B5
chromosome 309
Philadelphia **chromosome** 308
cilia 311
circadian rhythm 313
circle of Willis 313
fetal **circulation** 314
systemic **circulation** 315
liver **cirrhosis** 316
anastomosis **clamp** 318
Clostridium tetani C1
blood **clot** 325
digital **clubbing** 326, C15
cochlea 332
coenzyme 334
ulcerative **colitis** B10
lobar **collapse** B12
coloboma B4
colon 338
colonoscope 339, B10
colonoscopy B10
colostomy 340
vertebral **column** 341
juxtaglomerular **complex** 346
Ranke **complex** B13
fecal **concentration** procedures 349
condyloma acuminatum C5
conization 354
successive **contrast** 359
spinal **cord** 363
corpuscle 367
cerebral **cortex** 368
coxa 373
porcelain **crowns** B7
crus of diaphragm 381
crust C9
Cryptococcus C7
spinal **curvature** 388
dose-response **curve** 388
cyanosis C15
cardiac **cycle** 391
menstrual **cycle** 392
tricarboxylic acid **cycle** 393
cyst C8
apical periodontal **cyst** 395
hydatid **cyst** 396
pericardial **cyst** (radiograph) B12

cystine crystals C16
cystinosis 398
cystoscopy B9
cytotoxicity 404
radiolucent **decay** B6
recurrent **decay** B6
decubitus positions B3
decussation 411
atrial septal **defects** 412
defibrillation 413
dentistry 421, B6, B7
esthetic **dentistry** (vital bleaching) 421, B7
dentition 422
mixed **dentition** B6
acute allergic **dermatitis** C11
contact **dermatitis** C11
dermatitis herpetiformis C11
dermatome 428
dermatomyositis C8
retinal **detachment** B4
milestones of **development** 432
Venn **diagram** 437
diaphragm 439
diarrhea C16
digestion 445
Alzheimer **disease** 452, B16
Behçet **disease** C10
Bowen **disease** C12, C13
Fabry **disease** 456
Fahr **disease** 457
interstitial lung **disease** B13
Lyme **disease** C4
Paget **disease** C15
Scheuermann **disease** 462
silicosis **disease** B12
herniated **disk** 466
dislocation 466
distal versus **proximal** B1
distribution of common skin disorders 472
diverticulosis 473, B10
diverticulum 473
pharyngoesophageal **diverticulum** 474
DNA 475
doppler, sonography B11
Dracunculus medinensis 479
postural **drainage** 480
cochlear **duct** 483
cystic **duct** B9
nasolacrimal **duct** 484
thoracic **duct** 484
duodenum 486
dura mater 487
dyshidrosis 491
ear 497
ecchymosis C9

ECG lead placement 499
echocardiogram B11
echocardiography 500, B11
eczema herpeticum 503
angioneurotic **edema** 503
pulmonary **edema** B13
Compton **effect** 504
electrocardiography 509
electroencephalography 511
electropherogram 512
electroretinography 513
elephantiasis C6
embolism 515
embryo 516
panlobular **emphysema** 519
endangiitis 524
vegetative **endocarditis** 525
endocrine system 525
barium **enema** 528
Entamoeba histolytica 530
enterostomy 532
eosinophil C2
ependymoma C13
episcleritis 540
episiotomy 540
epithelium types 541
ciliated **epithelium** 541
erosion C9
polymorphous light **eruption** C11
urticarial drug **eruption** C11
erysipelas C4
erythema infectiosum C5
erythema multiforma minor C11
erythema nodosum C11
erythroblast C2
erythrocyte 548, C3
Escherichia coli C1
esophagoduodenoscope B8
esophagus 550
Barrett **esophagus** B8
eversion versus **inversion** B2
ear **examination** B5
eye **examination** B4
pelvic **examination** 557
excoriation C9
exophthalmos C14
exostosis 561, B5
extension versus **flexion** 179, B2
eye 565
ferning of cervical mucus C16
fetus 583
fever 585
fibroid 595
cystic **fibrosis** 596
filaria 598
dental **film** 599
mallet **finger** 600
fingerprint 601
fissure C9

fissures of lung 603
tracheoesophageal **fistula** 605
vesicovaginal **fistula** 605
internal **fixation** 606
bone **flap** 607
skin **flap** 608
embryonic **flexures** 610
liver **fluke** 612
fluorosis 614
vocal **fold** 617, B8
follicle 618
folliculitis C4
fontanelle 619
foot deformities 620
interatrial **foramen** primum 621
obstetrical **forceps** 624
foxglove 631
fracture types 632
blow-out **fracture** 632
Le Fort **fracture** 633
normal **fundus** B4
gallbladder 643
spinal **ganglion** 646
gastritis 649, B8
gastroenterostomy 650
gastrula 651
Giardia lamblia C6, C16
types of **glands** 660
acinous **gland** 660
glaucoma 665, C12
glaucomatous B4
glioblastoma multiforma C13
glomerulus 668
goiter 676
goniometer 678
gonococci C4
graft 681
anterior cruciate ligament **graft** B10
pyogenic **granuloma** C12
Wegener **granulomatosis** 684
growth 688
gustation 690
gyrus 692
hair 695
hearing impairment 702
heart 702, A27
fetal **heart** (sonogram) B11
cavernous **hemangioma** C9
epidural **hematoma** (CT scan) B14
subdural **hematoma** 708
hemodialysis 712
hemoglobin 713
hemopericardium 715
cerebral **hemorrhage** 716
hemothorax 717
hepatitis B 718, C5
hepatitis C C5

xxiii

hiatal **hernia** 722
inguinal **hernia** 722
herpangina C10
genital **herpes** C5
herpes simplex 724
herpes zoster C5
heteroduplex 726
histoplasmosis C7
HIV 733
homunculus 738
hypophysial **hormone** 738
horopter 740
hydrocele 745
hydrocephalus 746
fetal **hydrops** 748
hyperopia 757
hyphema 762, B4
hypodontia 764
hypospadias 768
hypothalamus 769
ileocolostomy 776
ileostomy 777
magnetic resonance **imaging** B15
cell-mediated **immunity** 781
humoral **immunity** 781
immunoelectrophoresis 783
rocket **immunoelectrophoresis** 783
immunofluorescence of *Chlamydia trachomatis* C1
immunoglobulin 783
impetigo C4
cochlear **implant** 786
dental **implants** 786, B6
incision 788
Zahn **infarct** 795
myocardial **infarction** 796
intracranial **infection** 796
influenza A virus C5
metered-dose **inhaler** 800
mendelian **inheritance** 801
injection 803
spinal cord **injury** 803
innervation of hand and wrist 804
Insecta 806
intestine 814
intubation 817
islets of Langerhans 823
Isospora belli B7
jaundice C15
types of **joints** 831
temporomandibular **joint** 834
intercellular **junction** 835
karyotype 838
keloid C9
keratoacanthoma C12
keratoconus 840
penetrating **keratoplasty** 841
actinic **keratoses** C12, C13

seborrheic **keratoses** C12
kidney 844
kidney anomalies 844
kinin 846
knee 847
osseous **labyrinth** 851
basal **lamina** of cochlea duct 855
LAO (left anterior oblique) position B3
laparoscopy B9
larva migrans C6
larynx 860
laser 860
lateral position B3
lateral versus **medial** B2
Bowditch **law** 862
germ **layers** 866
leech 871
intraocular **lens** implant 874
lentigo maligna melanoma C12
lepromatous **leprosy** C4
lesions 877
granulocytic **leukemia** 879
leukocytes C16
leukoplakia 35, C10
lichenification C9
cruciate **ligament** 887
cleft **lip** 905, B11
liposarcoma C13
extracorporal shock wave **lithotripsy** 910
CT scan of lacerated **liver** B14
lobules of liver 913
louse 917
arteries of **lower** limb A20
arteries of **upper** limb A16
LPO (left posterior oblique) position B3
lung 920
lupus erythematosus 921
lymphadenography 923
lymph node 924
lymphocyte C2
lymphoma C13, C14
Burkitt **lymphoma** C5
heart-lung **machine** 934
macrocytosis C3
macule C8
bull's eye **maculopathy** 936
malaria B6
mammogram of normal breast B14
mammogram of breast with cancer B14
mammography B14
mandible 942
Heimlich **maneuver** 943
Leopold **maneuver** 943
choroplethic and spot **map** 945

bone **marrow** aspirate C16
oxygen **mask** 949
lung **mass** C10, C11
rectal **mass** 950
closed chest **massage** 950
mastication 951
Mastigophora 951
skinfold **measurement** 954
medulloblastoma 960
megakaryoblast C2
meiosis 961
malignant **melanoma** C12
nodular **melanoma** C13
normal tympanic **membrane** B5
meningioma 968, B15
meningocele 969
meninx 970
normal knee **meniscus** B10
trimming of a torn knee **meniscus** B10
menstruation 971
mesothelioma B13
liver **metastases** C14
microcytosis C3
Microsporum gypseum C7
mitochondrion 996
mitosis 996
impacted **molar** 998
unerupted third **molar** B6
molluscum contagiosum C5
electronic fetal **monitor** 1001
monocyte C2
infectious **mononucleosis** C5
morula 1006
mouth 1007
MRI of knee with torn meniscus B15
mucocele C10
murmur 1012
skeletal **muscle** structure 1014
musculature 1030
musculature of back A14
musculature of head and neck A3
musculature of lower limb A22
musculature of thorax and abdomen A12
musculature of thorax and upper limb A18
mycetoma C7
Mycobacterium tuberculosis C4
mycosis fungoides 1039
neutrophilic **myelocyte** C2
myoma (of uterus) 1044
myopia 1045
myositis ossificans 1046
myxedema C14
nail 1050
nasopharynx 1051

Necator americanus 1052
toxic epidural **necrolysis** 1053
hepatic **necrosis** 1054
neoplasia B12, B13
nephrolithiasis 1058
nephron 1059
cranial **nerves** 1062
facial **nerve** 1063
spinal **nerve** 1067
trigeminal **nerve** 1068
nerves of lower limb A21
nerves of upper limb A17
neurinoma 1073
neuroblastoma C13
neuroepithelium 1074
neurofibromatosis C12
neuroglia 1075
neuron 1076
neuron types 1077
neutrophil C2
nevus flammeus 1081
nevus sebaceus 1081
Heberden **nodes** 1086
nodule C8
nomogram 1090
herniated **nucleus** pulposus (MRI scan) B15
nutrient absorption 1107
total parenteral **nutrition** 1108
nystagmus 1109
obesity 1111
oblique position B3
obstruction 1112
olfaction 1118
oligodendroglioma 1118
onychopathy 1123
operon 1127
ophthalmoscope B4
ophthalmoscopy 1128, B4
orbit 1130
organelles 1132
internal female reproductive **organs** 1131
internal male reproductive **organs** 1132
auditory **ossicles** 1139
endochondral **ossification** 1139
osteoarthritis 1140
osteoporosis 1143
otitis externa 1144, B5
otitis media 1145, B5
otomycosis B5
otoscope B5
otoscopy B5
ovulation 1148
calcium **oxalate** crystal C16
nasal **packing** 1153
chest **pain** 1155
liver **palpation** 1157
Bell **palsy** C14

pancreas 1158
pancreatoduodenectomy 1159
circumvallate **papillae** 1161
papilledema B4
papilloma of skin 1162
papule C8
paronychia 1171
partogram 1183
patch C8
somatic and visceral reflex **pathways** 1186
pediculosis capitis C6
laparoscopic view of **pelvis** 557, B9
pemphigus vulgaris 1192
penis 1193
bimanual **percussion** 1196
perforation of tympanic membrane B5
pericardiocentesis 1197
periosteum 1202
petechia C9
phagocytosis 1208
phalanges of the fingers 1208
phlebography 1217
phonocardiography 1219
acute **photodermatitis** C11
pinch and grasp patterns 1231
pinworm C6
commissural lip **pits** C10
placenta 1234
placenta previa 1235, B11
anatomical **planes** 1236, B1
plaque C8
plasmid 1239
Plasmodium malariae 1240, C6
lumbosacral **plexus** 1246
pneumatosis cystoides intestinalis 1252
Pneumocystis carinii **pneumonia** B13
bacterial **pneumonia** B13
lobar **pneumonia** 1254
pneumothorax 1255, B13
poikilocytes 1256
poikilocytosis C3
poison ivy (*Toxicodendron*) 1259
polycythemia vera 1262
polymer 1263
polyp 1265
gastric **polyp** B8
nasal **polyps** C11
colon **polypectomy** B10
multiple intestinal **polyposis** 1266
anatomic **positioning** B1, B2, B3
positions on the operating table 1271

fetal development during **pregnancy** 1278
ectopic **pregnancy** 1278
breech **presentation** B11
fetal **presentation** 1280
whole chromosome **probe** C16
vertebral **process** 1288
radiographic **projections** 1293
promyelocyte C2
pronate versus **supinate** B2
prone position B3
prostate 1297
prostate examination 1297
proximal versus **distal** B1
pseudocyst 1306
pseudoisochromatic plate 1307
pseudomonas C4
pterygium 1315
Pthirus pubis C6
ptosis 1316
peripheral **pulses** 1318
pulsimeter 1319
lumbar **puncture** 1320
purpura fulminans C9
Henoch-Schönlein **purpura** C4
pustule C8
pyelography 1323
renal **pyramid** 1325
quadrants 1330
radiodermatitis C11
radiograph B6
cephalometric **radiograph** B6
cyst **radiograph** B6
panoramic **radiograph** B6
plain chest **radiography** B12
radioimmunoassay 1336
RAO (right anterior oblique) position B3
radiology B12, B13, B14
RAST test 1350
polymerase chain **reaction** 1357
receptive field 1360
deep tendon **reflex** 1370
respiration 1382
mouth-to-mouth **respiration** 1383
dental **restoration** B7
restoration replacement B7
post **retention** B6
reticulocytes C2, C3
endoplasmic **reticulum** 1386
retina B4
layers of the **retina** 1387
retinitis pigmentosa 1388

retinoblastoma C13
nonproliferative diabetic **retinopathy** B4
hypertensive **retinopathy** B4
retinoscopy 1389
abdominal **retractor** 1390
retroflexion of uterus 1390
retrovirus 1391
allergic **rhinitis** C11
rhinophyma 1394
rhythm 1396
rigidity 1401
rosacea C9
rouleaux formation 548, C3
RPO (right posterior oblique) position B3
Ogino-Knaus **rule** 1409
sarcoidosis 1417
Ewing **sarcoma** B12
Kaposi **sarcoma** 35, C12
sarcomere 1418
scabies C6
scale C9
bone **scan** B16
bone density **scan** B16
computed tomography **scan** B14
brain **scan** B16
liver **scan** B16
lung **scan** B16
myocardial perfusion **scan** B16
PET **scan** B16
ventilation-perfusion **scan** B16
Schistosoma mansoni 1423
scintiphotography 1426
scleroderma 1427
multiple **sclerosis** in brain (MRI scan) B15
bronchopulmonary **segments** 1433
upper GI **series** 1444
synovial tendon **sheath** 1449
Babinski **sign** 1454, C15
banana and lemon **signs** 1457
silicosis B12
dural cranial **sinus** 1462
paranasal **sinus** 1462
receptor **site** 1464
skeleton A8, A9, A13
skeleton of head and neck A2
skeleton of lower limb A19
skeleton of upper limb A15
skin 1465
skull 1466
Pap **smear** 1467
poisonous **snakes** 1468
somite 1473
sonogram of fetus B11
sonography B11
obstetrical **sonography** B11
speculum 1481

spermatogenesis 1482
spermatozoon 1482
spherocytosis C3
spina bifida 1486
sleep **spindle** 1487
Spirochaeta 1489
closed-circuit **spirometry** 1489
spleen 1490
splenomegaly 1491
airplane **splint** 1492
spondylolisthesis 1493
Brushfield **spots** C15
Fordyce **spots** C10
sprain 1495
Gram **stain** of *Clostridium* tetani C1
Gram **stain** of *Escherichia* coli C1
Gram **stain** of *Streptococcus* pneumoniae C1
hematoxylin and eosin **stain** of liver section C1
Papanicolaou **stain** C1
periodic acid-Schiff **stain** C1
Prussian blue **stain** C1
methenamine silver **stain** C1
Warthin-Starry silver **stain** C1
Wright-Giemsa **stain** C1
Ziehl-Neelsen **stain** 1504
staphylococci C4
pyloric **stenosis** 1509
vascular **stent** 1509
sternum 1511
basophilic **stippling** C3
stomach 1514
contact **stomatitis** C10
recurrent herpetic **stomatitis** C10
stomatocytosis 1514
strabismus 1515
streptococci C4
Streptococcus pneumoniae C1
stress response 1520
stripping of the saphenous vein 1522
stromal tumor C12
supine position B3
suture 1546
swallow 1548
synapse 1551
Behçet **syndrome** C10
carpal tunnel **syndrome** 1556
Down **syndrome** C15
mucocutaneous lymph node **syndrome** (Kawasaki disease) 1567

Peutz-Jeghers **syndrome** C8
sick sinus **syndrome** 1572
Stevens-Johnson
   syndrome C11
syphilis C4
Bethesda **system** 1581
digestive **system** A24
hepatic portal **system** 1582
lymphatic **system** A25
mononuclear phagocyte
   system 1583
respiratory **system** A23
male and female urogenital
   systems A26
Taenia C6
Taenia saginata 1587
talipes cavus 1588
cardiac **tamponade** 1588
meniscal **tears** 1591, B10
retinal **tear** B4
Hutchinson **teeth** 1643
bleached maxillary **teeth** B7
telangiectasia C9
tendons and ligaments of
   lower leg 1596
teratoma C13
Bárány caloric **test** 1601
Rorschach **test** 1609
thalassemia 1617
endoscopic **thoracoscopy** B9
thoracoscopic view of
   thoracic wall B9
thorax A18
thrombosis 1631
tinea capitis C7

tinea corporis (ringworm)
   C7
tinea pedis C7
tinea versicolor C7
hammer **toe** 1639
computed **tomography** B14
positron emission
   tomography (PET) B16
hairy **tongue** (glossotrichia)
   C10
strawberry **tongue**
   (scarlatina) C10
Schiötz **tonometer** 1641
tooth 1642
torsion of spermatic
   cord 1644
torus palatinus B10
trachea B8
tracheostomy 1648
trachoma 1649
corticospinal **tract** 1650
rubrospinal **tract** 1651
urinary **tract** 1653
Bryant **traction** 1653
reverse **transcriptase** 1655
transcription 1656
translocation trisomy 1658
transplantation and
   protheses 1659
heart **transplantation** 1659
active **transport** 1659
Trichinella C6
Trichinella spiralis 1665
Trichomonas hominis C6
sympathetic **trunk** 1675

uterine **tube** 1678
miliary **tuberculosis** B13
*mycobacterium
   tuberculosis* C4
tumor C8
benign **tumor** B12
benign **tumor** of stomach C12
bladder **tumor** B9
Ewing **tumor** C14
malignant stromal **tumor** C12
Wilms **tumor** C13
carpal **tunnel** 1689
monozygotic **twins** 1691
tympanogram 1692
tympanosclerosis B5
ulcer C9
decubitus **ulcer** 1694
aphthous **ulcerations** C10
Doppler **ultrasonography**
   1696, B11
thyroid **uptake** B16
open **urachus** 1701
uric acid crystals C16
urine 1705
intravenous **urography** 1706
uterus (changes during
   pregnancy) 1708
developmental anomalies of
   the **uterus** 1709
vagotomy 1714
heart **valves** 1716
venous **valve** 1717
varicella (chicken pox) C5
esophageal **varices** B8
varicosis 1719

vasectomy 1721
vasopressin 1721
vectorcardiogram 1723
major **veins** of body 1724
superficial **veins** of hand
   and forearm 1731
veneer hypoplasty B7
venom 1737
alveolar and dead space
   ventilation 1738
ventricles of the brain 1739
ventriculography C9
external cephalic
   version 1742
internal podalic **version**
   1742
vesicle C8
vitiligo C8
AIDS **virus** C5
human immunodeficiency
   virus (HIV) 1752
vision 1758
expiratory reserve **volume**
   1762
respiratory minute **volume**
   1762
vulvar 1763
palmar **wart** C5
wheal C8
worm 1772
wound healing 1773
yeast 1777
zosteriform 1783
Z-plasty 1783
Zygomycetes 1784

ÍNDICE DOS QUADROS

chromosome **aberrations** 2
aerosol therapy 28
AIDS 34
food **allergies** 42
antibiotic groups 85
autoimmune diseases in humans (**autoantibody**) 154
classification of **bacteria** 162
average **birth** measurements 185
ABO **blood** group 192
muscles used in **breathing** 221
etiologic classification of **cardiomyopathies** 258
T-helper subsets (**cell**) 281
chromosome (set) 308
Angle **classification** of malocclusion 319
coagulopathy 330
genetic **code** 333
complement **components** 348
minimal alveolar **concentration** (MAC) 350
cytokine 402, 403
diagnosis of **cytomegalovirus** (CMV) 404
deafness due to developmental dysplasia of the cochlea 408

dermatitis division into types 426
motor, social, verbal and cognitive **development** of the normal child 433
diabetes mellitus (DM): etiological classification 436
electroencephalogram 511
lipoprotein **electrophoresis** 512
types of **emphysema** 518
major digestive **enzymes** 534
accommodation of **eye** 565
development of the **fetus** 584
nerve **fiber** 592
human cerebrospinal **fluid** 612
types of **glycogenosis** 674
hepatitis antigens and the corresponding antibodies 719
classification of human **herpesviruses** 724
histamine 731
hydronephrosis (causes) 748
hypercalcemia 753
hypocalcemia 763
systemic **hypoxia** 771
nonspecific host defenses (**immunity**) 780

primary **immunodeficiency** disorders 782
hypersensitivity reactions (**immunoreaction**) 784
insulin (metabolic effects) 808
interferon 810
common **lasers** used in medicine 861
Head **lines** 900
plasma **lipoproteins** 908
lochia 915
lymphocytes 928
lymphoma 930
maldigestion or **malabsorption** 938
tumor **markers** 948
milk 994
adhesion **molecule** 1000
muscles of the eye 1018
neoplasia 1057
nonprotein **nitrogen** 1084
oncogene 1121
etiology of **osteomalacia** 1142
acute **pancreatitis** 1158
blood **plasma** 1238
precancer 1276
intracardial **pressure** 1282
units of **pressure** 1281
plasma **proteins** 1301, 1302
psychopharmacology 1313
puberty 1316

rabies postexposure prophylaxis guide 1332
rating of perceived exertion (RPE) 1351
β-adrenergic **receptors** 1360
reflexes 1366-1367
Glasgow coma **scale** 1420
Apgar **score** 1429
sensation 1439
sphingolipidoses 1485
Ann Arbor **staging** system 1498
TNM **staging** 1498
Down **syndrome** 1559
autonomic nervous **system** 1580
taxonomy 1591
coatings of the **tongue** 1640
classification of conjoined **twins** 1690
urine 1705
viral embryopathy 1749
DNA-containing tumor **viruses** 1750
acute gastroenteritis **viruses** 1751
major group **viruses** (DNA/RNA) 1755
oncogenic **viruses** 1754
vitamins and minerals 1759
causes of **vomiting** 1763

TERMOS DE ALTA IMPORTÂNCIA NESTA EDIÇÃO

activator, tissue plasminogen
AIDS
angioplasty, percutaneous transluminal coronary
antibody, monoclonal
antigen, prostate-specific
antileukotriene
antioxidant
apnea, obstructive sleep
apoptosis
asthma, bronchial
atherosclerosis
carcinoma
carcinoma, breast
carcinoma, prostate
care, end-of-life
care, managed
Chlamydia pneumoniae
ciguatera
CLIA
cloning
cocaine
colposcopy
complex, histocompatibility
cytogenetics
cytokine
dehydroepiandrosterone (DHEA)
depression, major
diabetes mellitus
diabetes, gestational
Diagnostic and Statistical Manual of Mental Disorders
diet, low fat

directive, advance
disease, Alzheimer
disease, cat-scratch
disease, Creutzfeldt-Jakob
disease, gastroesophageal reflux
disease, Lyme
ehrlichiosis
encephalopathy, bovine spongiform
excision, loop
fasciitis, necrotizing
fever, rheumatic
fingerprinting, DNA
flunitrazepam
fluoroquinolone
folic acid
Framingham Heart Study
gene, BRCA1, BRCA2
gene, tumor suppressor
Ginkgo biloba
Helicobacter pylori
hepatitis
herpesvirus 8
HMO
homocysteine
hospitalist
Human Genome Project
γ-hydroxybutyrate
hypertension
immunotherapy
infarction, myocardial
inhibitor, α-glucosidase
inhibitor, HMG CoA reductase

inhibitor, protease
insulin, lispro
interferon
knife, gamma
laparoscopy
leptin
leukoplakia, hairy
lipoprotein
lipoprotein (a)
load, viral
mammography
medicine, alternative
melatonin
meningitis, meningococcal
mouse, knockout
nephropathy, diabetic
neuropathy, diabetic
nicotine
nitric oxide
nurse practitioner
obesity
oncogene
osteoporosis
parvovirus B19
pill, morning after
prion
probe
psychopharmacology
radiation, background
radical, free
raloxifene
reaction, polymerase chain
resistance, drug
resistance, insulin
retinopathy, diabetic retrovirus

risks, radiation
schizophrenia
smallpox
stroke
suicide, physician-assisted
syndrome, fragile X
syndrome, premenstrual
syndrome, shaken baby
syndrome, sudden infant death
system, Bethesda
system, cytochrome P-450
tamoxifen citrate
telomerase
Terminologia Anatomica
test, stress
testing, genetic
therapy, gene
therapy, estrogen replacement
therapy, thrombolytic
tobacco
tomography, positron emission
trabeculoplasty, laser
trial, clinical
tuberculosis
ultrasonography, Doppler
universal precautions
virus, Ebola
virus, human papilloma
wellness
workaholic
wort, St. John's

COMO USAR ESTE DICIONÁRIO

ORGANIZAÇÃO DO VOCABULÁRIO xxx
   Formato das Entradas Principais e Subentradas xxx
      Palavras compostas xxx
      Termos químicos e substâncias nomeados por expressões xxx
   Dicas para Encontrar Termos Múltiplos ou Subentradas xxx

ALFABETAÇÃO xxxi
   Entradas Principais xxxi
   Exceções xxxi
   Subentradas xxxi
   Grafia xxxi
      Grafias alternativas xxxii
      Diferenças entre a grafia britânica e a norte-americana xxxii
      Sobrenomes xxxii

ORGANIZAÇÃO DAS ENTRADAS E DAS REFERÊNCIAS CRUZADAS xxxii
   Entradas Principais xxxii
      Entradas principais com definição xxxii
      Sinônimos xxxiii
      Nomes sistemáticos xxxiii
   Subentradas xxxiii
   Referências Cruzadas xxxiii
   Epônimos xxxiv
   Abreviaturas e Símbolos xxxiv

PRONÚNCIA xxxv
   Convenções xxxv
   Código de Pronúncia xxxv
      Vogais xxxv
      Consoantes xxxv

ETIMOLOGIA MÉDICA xxxvi
   Organização xxxvi
   Prefixos e Sufixos xxxvi

ABREVIATURAS E SÍMBOLOS USADOS NESTE DICIONÁRIO xxxvii

ORGANIZAÇÃO DO VOCABULÁRIO

Formato das Entradas Principais e Subentradas

O *Stedman/Dicionário Médico* tem uma organização diferente daquela dos dicionários gerais. Os dois tipos primários de entrada são as entradas principais e as subentradas. Uma entrada principal se constitui de um termo principal, ou expressão, abaixo do qual estão agrupadas as subentradas ou termos e locuções referentes. As entradas principais aparecem em negrito, sendo seguidas pela pronúncia entre parênteses. As subentradas são agrupadas de forma alfabética sob sua entrada principal orientadora. Por exemplo:

entrada principal → **groove** (groov) [TA]. Sulco; uma depressão ou fenda alongada e estreita, localizada sobre qualquer superfície. VER TAMBÉM sulcus.
subentrada → **alveolobuccal g.**, s. alveolobucal; a metade superior e inferior do vestíbulo bucal...

Para localizar uma subentrada, o leitor precisa procurar a entrada principal:

Para encontrar	**Procurar em**
myocardial infarction	infarction
hemorrhagic fever	fever
Q fever	
carcinoid tumor	
giant cell tumor of bone	tumor
Wilms tumor	

Verbos, adjetivos, advérbios, formas combinantes, prefixos, abreviaturas e símbolos seguem as regras gerais de indexação e, portanto, são localizados como entradas principais.

Palavras compostas, que geralmente são escritas juntas como uma palavra ou hifenizadas, são localizadas como entradas principais em vez de subentradas. Por exemplo, a palavra "aftercontraction" está localizada na letra "A" em vez de ser uma subentrada de "contraction"; "self-hypnosis" está localizada na letra "S" e não é uma subentrada de hypnosis.

Termos químicos e substâncias nomeados por expressões estão, geralmente, localizados como entradas principais pelo primeiro termo em inglês, a menos que haja um elemento principal como um substantivo, que seja considerado um tipo ou espécie. Por exemplo:

Para encontrar	**Procurar em**
adrenergic blocking agent (um tipo de agente)	agent
Agent Orange (um composto específico)	Agent Orange
bile acid (um tipo de ácido)	acid
acid red (um corante que não é ácido nem vermelho)	acid red
ribonucleic acid (uma molécula em vez de um ácido)	ribonucleic acid

Dicas para Encontrar Termos Múltiplos ou Subentradas

- Procurar em *Localizador de Subentradas* na página LS1, imediatamente antes da seção A–Z
- Para encontrar espécies, procurar em *Localizador de Gêneros*, na página LG1, imediatamente antes do *Localizador de Subentradas*
- Procurar a ordem alfabética dos vocábulos específicos que formam o termo múltiplo ou subentrada
- Procurar em outra entrada principal que seja semelhante ao termo que você está procurando
- Procurar nas referências cruzadas

Para encontrar	**Procurar em**
a surgical procedure	operation
	technique
	method
a disease	syndrome
	disease

ALFABETAÇÃO

Entradas Principais

As entradas principais são colocadas em ordem alfabética, letra por letra, em vez de palavra por palavra como em um catálogo telefônico:

blood	cross
blood bank	crossbreed
bloodletting	cross-cylinder
blood purple	crossing-over of genes
bloodstream	cross-matching
blood vessel	crossway

Expressões preposicionadas, sobretudo as em latim, são levadas em conta na alfabetação:

Para encontrar	**Procurar**
ante cibum	na letra A
in vitro	na letra I

As letras gregas e as formas configuracionais escritas por extenso também são levadas em conta na alfabetação:

Para encontrar	**Procurar**
α-naphthylurea	na letra N
alpha-blocker	na letra A
L-dopa	na letra D
levodopa	na letra L

Nomes próprios (primeira letra maiúscula) precedem as palavras em letras minúsculas (nomes comuns):

Streptococcus	aparece antes de streptococcus
Down	aparece antes de down

Exceções

Para colocar os vocábulos em ordem alfabética, este dicionário desprezou o seguinte: preposições, conjunções, artigos, apóstrofos de formas possessivas, espaços, pontuação, letras gregas (p. ex., α, β, γ), algarismos, caracteres de configuração (p. ex., D-, +, −) e formas em itálico (p. ex., *p-, N-, cis-*), seja como prefixos ou como componentes em termos químicos compostos.

Subentradas

As subentradas são colocadas em ordem alfabética, letra por letra, seguindo as mesmas regras apresentadas para as entradas principais, mas com algumas diferenças importantes.

Nas subentradas (bem como nas definições de entradas principais e subentradas), a entrada principal orientadora é representada por sua letra inicial, quando se tratar do singular; e pelo acréscimo de um apóstrofo e "s", quando se tratar de um plural regular; ou pela forma escrita, se for um plural irregular de uma palavra em latim. Por exemplo:

crest	**gyrus**
gluteal c.	angular g.
c. of greater tubercle	gyri breves insulae
inguinal c.	central gyri
c.'s of nail bed	g. dentales
nasal c.	short gyri of insula
c. of neck rib	gyri temporalis transversi

Seja qual for a forma, a palavra da entrada principal não é incluída na ordem alfabética das subentradas. Preposições, conjunções, artigos e formas possessivas também não são incluídos na ordem alfabética.

Grafia

Para a ordenação alfabética, não se levam em conta espaços, pontuação, letras gregas, algarismos, caracteres de configuração e formas em itálico.

As *grafias alternativas*, sobretudo aquelas de formas combinantes, são apresentadas como entradas principais com referências cruzadas para as outras grafias:

> **cu·ret.** Cureta. VER curette.
>
> **hem-, hema-.** hem-, hema-. Sangue. VER TAMBÉM hemat-, hemato-, hemo-. [G. *haima*]
>
> **kyto-.** VER cyto-.

As grafias antigas ou desatualizadas também são apresentadas como entradas principais com referências cruzadas para as grafias atuais:

> **oari-, oario-.** Formas combinantes obsoletas para indicar um ovário. VER oo-, oophor-, ovario-. [G. *ōarion*, um pequeno ovo, dim. de *ōon*, ovo]
>
> **pleio-.** Pleio-; grafia alternativa raramente usada para pleo-.

As *diferenças entre a grafia britânica e a norte-americana*, sobretudo aquelas no início ou perto do início de uma palavra, são apresentadas como entradas principais (prefixos) com referências cruzadas da grafia britânica para a norte-americana:

> **ae-.** No caso de palavras que começam assim e não são encontradas aqui, ver em e-.
>
> **oe-.** Para as palavras assim iniciadas e não encontradas aqui, ver e-.

A grafia britânica pode modificar a localização alfabética de algumas entradas de palavras:

	Britânica	**Norte-americana**
ae* para e	*ae*tiology	*e*tiology
	f*ae*ces	f*e*ces
oe para e	c*oe*liac	c*e*liac
	*oe*dema	*e*dema
	diarrh*oe*a	diarrh*e*a
our para or	tum*our*	tum*or*
re para er	fib*re*	fib*er*

Os *sobrenomes*, usados como entradas principais biográficas que fazem referência cruzada com epônimos associados, também são colocados em ordem alfabética segundo suas grafias mais utilizadas. Os usuários devem lembrar que existem variações na grafia, como "a/ae", "o/oe", "u/ue" e "Mac/Mc". No caso de nomes próprios que comecem com prefixos, como "Van", "van der", "von", "de", que podem ser empregados com ou sem o prefixo, as entradas principais que fazem referência cruzada direcionam o usuário para a localização apropriada. Seja qual for a forma de um sobrenome (p. ex., "Crohn", "Bence Jones", "d'Herelle", "von Willebrand", "Loeffler" ou "Löffler"), o nome é colocado em ordem alfabética, letra por letra, como é escrito.

ORGANIZAÇÃO DAS ENTRADAS E DAS REFERÊNCIAS CRUZADAS

A definição é fornecida apenas em um local para dois ou mais sinônimos. As entradas dos outros sinônimos apresentam referências cruzadas para o termo que oferece a definição. Esse sistema também é utilizado para termos obsoletos, para variações de grafia ou quando existe uma preferência ditada para seu uso. A prática de colocar uma definição apenas em um verbete serve para focalizar toda a informação sobre um termo em um único lugar, em vez de ser estritamente um indicador de preferência. Isso também evita a duplicação de definições que ampliaria o tamanho do *Stedman*.

Entradas Principais

As **entradas principais com definição** são, em geral, apresentadas da seguinte maneira: (1) entrada em negrito seguida por sua abreviatura ou símbolo (se houver) entre parênteses, (2) pronúncia entre parênteses, (3) a definição em si e (4) a origem do verbete entre colchetes.

> **elec·tro·car·di·o·gram (ECG, EKG)** (ē - lek - trō - kar′dē - ō - gram). Eletrocardiograma; registro gráfico das correntes de ação integradas do coração obtido com o eletrocardiógrafo, apresentado como modificações da voltagem com o passar do tempo. [electro- + G. *kardia*, coração, + *gramma*, desenho]

---

*"Ae" no radical "aero-" é aceito para os dois usos, como em "aerosol", "anaerobe" e outros termos derivados do G. *aer*, que significa ar. "Aeroplane"/"airplane" é uma exceção conhecida.

Se for utilizada em sua própria definição, a entrada principal é abreviada com a sua primeira letra ou com a abreviatura aceita, p. ex., "o" para "osso", "DNA" para "ácido desoxirribonucleico", "Hb" para "hemoglobina".

Os números em negrito seguidos por um ponto enumeram as múltiplas definições, mas sua seqüência numérica não indica necessariamente grau de importância, nem preferência:

> **mes·o·car·dia** (mez′ō-kar′dē-ă). Mesocardia. **1.** Posição atípica do coração em uma posição central no tórax, como no início da vida embrionária. **2.** Mesocárdios; plural de mesocardium. [meso- + G. *kardia*, coração]

Os ***sinônimos*** aparecem após o final da definição de um termo e são precedidos pela abreviatura "SIN". Um algarismo entre parênteses após um termo sinônimo indica o número da definição do termo do qual a entrada principal em negrito é sinônimo. Se uma entrada ou entrada principal for seguida por um sinônimo e não houver outra definição (o sinônimo aparece em azul), o leitor tem de procurar esse sinônimo para encontrar a definição.

> **ne·phrop·a·thy** (ne-frop′ă-thē). Nefropatia. Qualquer doença do rim. SIN nephropathia, nephrosis (1). [nephro- + G. *pathos*, sofrimento]
> **analgesic n.**, n. por analgésicos. SIN analgesic *nephritis.*

Os ***nomes sistemáticos*** de termos genéricos ou comuns de substâncias químicas ou drogas/fármacos aparecem no início da definição, juntamente com a fórmula molecular:

> **ac·e·tone** (as′e-tōn). Acetona; líquido incolor, volátil e inflamável; quantidades extremamente pequenas são ... SIN dimethyl ketone
>
> **as·pi·rin** (as′pi-rin). Nome comercial do ácido acetilsalicílico; um agente analgésico, antipirético e antiinflamatório amplamente utilizado; também usado como agente antiplaquetário. SIN acetylsalicylic acid.

Subentradas

As subentradas com definições são organizadas de forma bastante semelhante às entradas principais, como já foi descrito. A pronúncia e a origem do verbete são fornecidas quando as palavras principais que compõem a subentrada não são apresentadas como entradas principais no vocabulário, como no seguinte exemplo:

> **fo·lie**
> **f. à deux** (ă-du), transtorno psicótico compartilhado; distúrbios mentais idênticos ou semelhantes, tais como uma fixação paranóide, geralmente afetando dois membros da mesma família que vivem juntos. SIN shared psychotic disorder. [Fr. dois]

Na definição, a entrada principal, sempre que utilizada, é abreviada com a sua primeira letra ou com a abreviatura aceita, como um recurso para poupar espaço, p. ex., "o" para "osso", "DNA" para "ácido desoxirribonucleico", "Hb" para "hemoglobina".

Os algarismos em negrito e entre parênteses enumeram as definições múltiplas, mas sua seqüência numérica não indica necessariamente grau de importância, nem preferência:

> **age**
> **developmental a.**, i. do desenvolvimento; (**1**) idade fetal; idade calculada pelo desenvolvimento anatômico desde a nidação; (**2**) (**DA**), idade de um indivíduo calculada pelo grau de maturação anatômica, fisiológica, mental e emocional.

Referências Cruzadas

As referências cruzadas podem referir-se a entradas principais ou subentradas ou, ainda, remeter à definição de uma entrada principal ou subentrada. Podem direcionar o usuário para uma entrada com definição ou para uma entrada com informações correlatas ou adicionais. O *Stedman* emprega os seguintes tipos de referências cruzadas:

Sinônimo Uma palavra com o mesmo significado do termo da entrada. Quando é fornecido sem uma definição, um sinônimo aparece em azul após "SIN". Por exemplo:

> **boil** (boyl). Furúnculo. SIN furuncle [A. S. *byl*, uma inchação]

Quando o sinônimo importante é uma expressão ou locução localizada como uma subentrada, a entrada principal orientadora aparecerá em itálico, como no seguinte exemplo:

> **can·dle·pow·er** (kan′dl-pow′er). Vela (unidade de intensidade luminosa); potência em velas; intensidade luminosa expressa em candelas. SIN luminous *intensity*

Quando o sinônimo faz referência cruzada de uma subentrada para outra subentrada, sob a mesma entrada principal, a entrada principal é abreviada, como no seguinte exemplo:

>**cal·cu·lus**
>   **arthritic c.,** c. artrítico. SIN gouty *tophus.*
>   **biliary c.,** c. biliar. SIN gallstone.
>   **dendritic c.,** c. dendrítico. SIN staghorn c.

VER
Orienta o leitor para um termo com significado semelhante ao da entrada.

VER TAMBÉM
Orienta o leitor para um termo com informações adicionais sobre a entrada.

Cf. (L. *confer,* comparar) e q.v. (L. *quod vide*, queira ver)
Orienta o leitor para informações comparativas ou correlatas, embora com uma relação menos direta que a referência VER TAMBÉM.

Termo obsoleto para
O termo não é mais amplamente utilizado. Encaminha o leitor para o termo em voga.

Epônimos

Epônimos são termos designativos de nomes próprios e de locais. Uma breve biografia aparece ao lado do nome próprio, juntamente com uma referência cruzada.

>**Hoffmann,** Johann, neurologista alemão, 1857–1919. VER H. muscular *atrophy, phenomenon, reflex, sign;* Werdnig-H. *disease;* Werdnig-Hoffmann muscular *atrophy.*
>
>**Sylvius,** Le Böe, Franciscus (François), médico, anatomista e fisiologista holandês, 1614–1672. VER sylvian *angle;* sylvian *aqueduct;* sylvian *fissure;* sylvian *line;* sylvian *point;* sylvian *valve;* sylvian *ventricle; fossa* of S.; *vallecula* sylvii.
>
>**Wilms,** Max. cirurgião alemão, 1867–1918. VER W. *tumor.*

Refletindo a tendência observada nas publicações atuais, esta edição do *Stedman* não fez uso da forma possessiva dos epônimos.

Abreviaturas e Símbolos

As abreviaturas e os símbolos, bem como acrônimos e outras formas contratas, são incluídos no vocabulário quando de uso aceito (em vez de criações *ad hoc*). Estão localizados como entradas principais, geralmente com referência cruzada para os termos grafados, nos quais são citados entre parênteses e em negrito, imediatamente após a entrada em negrito:

>**Cyt** Símbolo de cytosine (citosina).
>
>**cy·to·sine (Cyt)** (sī′tō-sēn). Citosina; uma pirimidina ...
>
>**PET** Abreviatura de positron emission *tomography* (tomografia por emissão de pósitrons).
>
>**to·mog·ra·phy**
>   **positron emission t. (PET),** t. por emissão de pósitrons: criação de ...
>
>**stat.** Abreviatura do L. *statim,* imediatamente.
>
>**sta·tim** (stā′tim). Imediatamente. [L.]

Alguns símbolos e abreviaturas são auto-explicativos ou vêm definidos de forma mais apropriada em suas entradas em vez de na entrada para os termos grafados:

>**b.i.d.** Abreviatura do L. *bis in die*, duas vezes ao dia.
>
>**FUO** Abreviatura de fever of unknown origin (febre de origem indeterminada).
>
>**PUVA** Acrônimo para administração oral de *p*soraleno e subseqüente exposição à luz ultravioleta de comprimento de onda longo (*uv-a*); usado no tratamento da psoríase.
>
>Q_{CO_2}, Símbolo para os microlitros nas CPTP (condições padrões de temperatura e pressão, tempo seco) de CO_2 produzidos por miligrama de tecido por hora.

As abreviaturas podem aparecer com ou sem ponto. Algumas convenções de nomenclatura eliminaram o ponto de determinados tipos de abreviaturas. O uso geral de ponto na maioria das abreviaturas está declinando progressivamente, mas, em alguns casos, o ponto é mantido para evitar confusão.

PRONÚNCIA

Convenções

A grafia fonética para a pronúncia dos termos em inglês é apresentada entre parênteses, imediatamente após a entrada em negrito. A pronúncia é apresentada apenas após a entrada principal, exceto quando seria redundante porque a grafia fonética é igual à da entrada principal. A pronúncia não é fornecida nas subentradas, exceto para palavras em latim, quando um apóstrofo (´) indica a sílaba tônica.

O sistema fonético usado é básico e segue apenas algumas convenções:

- Utilizam-se duas marcas diacríticas: mácron (¯) para vogais longas e bráquia (˘) para vogais breves.
- As sílabas tônicas principais são seguidas por um apóstrofo (´). Monossílabos não têm indicação de tonicidade.
- Outras sílabas são separadas por pontos.

O código de pronúncia a seguir fornece exemplos e sons de consoantes e de vogais encontrados no sistema fonético. Não se tentou acomodar os sons indistintos comuns da fala ou as variações regionais dos sons da fala. Observe que uma vogal com uma marca breve (˘) é usada para o som indefinido de vogal de schwa (ə). A pronúncia original de palavras estrangeiras é o mais aproximada possível.

Código de Pronúncia

Vogais

ā	day, care, gauge
a	mat, damage
ă	about, para
ah	father
aw	fall, cause, raw
ē	be, equal, ear
ĕ	taken, genesis
e	term, learn
ī	pie
ĭ	pit, sieve, build
ō	note, for, so
o	not, oncology, ought
oo	food
ow	cow, out
oy	troy, void
ū	unit, curable
ŭ	cut

Consoantes

b	bad
ch	child
d	dog
dh	this, smooth
f	fit
g	got
h	hit
j	jade
k	kept
ks	tax
kw	quit
l	law
m	me
n	no
ng	ring
p	pan
r	rot
s	so, miss
sh	should
t	ten
th	thin, with
v	very
w	we
y	yes
z	zero
zh	azure, measure

Em algumas palavras, o som inicial não é o da(s) primeira(s) letra(s) ou a(s) primeira(s) letra(s) não é(são) pronunciada(s) ou tem(têm) um som diferente, como nos seguintes exemplos:

aerobe (ar′ob)	gnathic (nath′ik)	oedipism (ed′i-pizm)	pneumonia (nu-mo′ne-a)	ptosis (to′sis)
eimuria (ime′re-a)	knuckle (nuk-l)	phthalein (thal′e-in)	psychology (si-kol′o-je)	xanthoma (zan-tho′ma)

ETIMOLOGIA MÉDICA

Organização

A origem ou etimologia de um verbete (ou entrada) em negrito é fornecida entre colchetes [ ] ao final da entrada. As derivações são, necessariamente, sucintas e o mais simples possível para facilitar a memorização e promover a associação com os termos derivados. As informações fornecidas têm três componentes básicos: (1) a abreviatura do idioma a que pertencem o(s) termo(s) original(is); (2) em itálico, o(s) termo(s) original(is) do(s) qual(is) deriva a palavra; e (3) a significação do(s) termo(s). No caso de verbos em grego e latim, utiliza-se a primeira pessoa do singular do presente, e não o infinitivo, para o reconhecimento mais fácil da raiz da palavra; todavia, a significação é fornecida no infinitivo:

>**diph·the·ria** (dif - thē - r'ē - ā). Difteria; doença infecciosa específica... [G. *diphthera*, couro]
>
>**graph** (graf). Gráfico. **1.** Uma linha ou um traçado... [G. *graphō*, escrever]
>
>**un·ion** (ūn'yŭn). União. **1.** Junção ou amalgamação... [L. *unus*, um]

Quando a entrada em negrito tem o mesmo ou quase o mesmo significado e/ou grafia da(s) palavra(s) da(s) qual(is) se originou, a forma redundante não é incluída na derivação, como nos seguintes exemplos:

>**idea** (ī - dē'ā). Idéia; qualquer imagem ou conceito mental. [G. forma, aparência, fr. *idein*, ter visto, fr. obs. *eidō*, ver]
>
>**lo·cus**, pl. **lo·ci** (lō'kŭs, lō'sī). **1.** Um lugar; geralmente, um ... [L.]

Muitas vezes, as derivações incluem componentes adicionais, sobretudo quando envolvem locuções ou expressões ou mesmo mais de uma palavra de origens diferentes. Um verbo em grego ou latim pode ser hifenizado para indicar que a segunda parte da palavra existe como um verbo simples com o mesmo ou quase o mesmo significado, modificado pelo acréscimo de um prefixo com valor de adjetivo ou de advérbio. Se o verbo simples sofre uma modificação quando se torna parte de um verbo composto, essa modificação também é mostrada:

>**ap·o·crine** (ap'ō - krin). Apócrino; denotando um mecanismo de secreção glandular em que a porção apical das células secretoras é desprendida e incorporada na secreção. VER TAMBÉM apocrine *gland*. [G. *apo - krinō*, separar]
>
>**com·po·nent** (kom - pō'nent). Componente; elemento que forma uma parte do todo. [L. *compono*, pp. *-positus*, colocar junto]

Quando as palavras provêm de idiomas diferentes, a identificação do idioma de cada palavra com as respectivas significações é fornecida. Quando as palavras provêm do mesmo idioma, este é mencionado apenas para a primeira palavra:

>**ap·i·cec·to·my** (ap - i - sek'tō - mē). Apicectomia. **1.** Abertura e exenteração das células aéreas... [L. *apex*, extremidade ou cume + G. *ektomē*, excisão]
>
>**gon·e·cyst, gon·e·cys·tis** (gon'ē - sist, gon - ē - sis'tis). Glândula seminal... [G. *gonē*, semente, + *kystis*, bexiga]

Prefixos e Sufixos

As formas combinantes usadas como prefixos ou nas palavras derivadas são arroladas no vocabulário como entradas principais em negrito, com suas próprias derivações entre colchetes e definições completas. Elas são precedidas pelo símbolo de reciclagem (♻). Quando as formas combinantes aparecem em derivações entre colchetes de outras entradas em negrito, que se seguem alfabeticamente no vocabulário, não são fornecidos nem seu idioma de origem nem sua significação:

>♻ **neur-, neuri-, neuro-.** Neur-, neuri-, neuro-. Nervo, tecido nervoso, sistema nervoso. [G. *neuron*]
>
>**neu·ral·gia** (neo - ral'jē - ā). Neuralgia. Dor intensa, de caráter pulsátil ou em punhalada no trajeto ou na distribuição de um nervo. SIN neurodynia (neurodinia). [neur- + G. *algos*, dor]

As formas combinantes usadas como sufixos e terminações também são apresentadas como entradas principais em negrito, com suas próprias derivações entre colchetes e definições completas. Quando usadas em derivações entre colchetes de outras entradas em negrito, o idioma de origem é mencionado (apenas se for diferente da palavra precedente) e fornecida a significação:

> △ **-osis,** pl. **-oses.** Sufixo que significa um processo, condição ou estado geralmente anormal ou enfermo… [G.]
>
> **hal·i·to·sis** (hal - i - tō′sis). Halitose; hálito com cheiro desagradável. SIN fetor oris, ozostomia, stomatodysodia. [L. *halitus*, respiração, + G. *-osis*, condição]

ABREVIATURAS E SÍMBOLOS USADOS NESTE DICIONÁRIO

As abreviaturas e os símbolos abaixo são usados nas derivações e definições de entradas ao longo do dicionário. Devem ser diferenciados das abreviaturas e símbolos apresentados como entradas no vocabulário ou que acompanham os termos soletrados que eles representam, como visto acima.

A.A.A.	Alto Alemão Antigo	*i. e.*	L. *id est*, isto é
acc.	acusativo	I.M.	inglês médio
adj.	adjetivo	Ind.	índio, indígena
Áfr. Ocid.	África Ocidental	Ind. Am.	indígena norte-americano
Al.	alemão	Ing.	inglês
Ar.	árabe	Isl.	islandês
A.S.	anglo-saxão	It.	italiano
Br.	britânico	Jap.	japonês
c., ca	L. *circa*, cerca de	L.	Latim
car.	caráter	L. A.	Latim antigo
cf.	L. *confer*, comparar	L. Med., L. Mediev.	Latim medieval
Ch.	chinês	L. Mod.	Latim moderno
C.I. (I.C.)	Colour Index (Índice de Corantes)	masc.	masculino
dial.	dialeto	mit.	mitológico
dim.	diminutivo	N.A.	*Nomina Anatomica*
EC	Enzyme Commission (Comissão de Enzimas)	neut., ntr.	neutro
		N.G.	Nova Guiné
Esc.	escandinavo	obs.	obsoleto
Esc. ant.	escandinavo antigo	p.	particípio
Esp.	espanhol	p. ex.,	por exemplo
etim.	etimologia	p. pas.	particípio passado
EUA	Estados Unidos da América	p. pr.	particípio presente
fem.	feminino	Pers.	persa
Fr.	francês	Pg.	português
Fr. ant.	francês antigo	pl.	plural
fut.	futuro	priv.	exclusivo, negativo
G.	grego	*q.v.*	L. *quod vide*, queira ver
Gael.	gaélico	Sansc.	sânscrito
gen.	genitivo	sing.	singular
Hind.	hindu	Su.	sueco
Hol.	holandês	T.A.	*Terminologia Anatomica*
I. ant.	inglês antigo		

Nos dados biográficos, o sinal* indica o ano de nascimento, quando não é fornecido o ano do óbito, e † indica o ano de morte quando não é fornecido o ano de nascimento.

STEDMAN
Dicionário Médico

27ª Edição

Ilustrado em Cores

STEDMAN

LOCALIZADOR DE GÊNEROS

As páginas a seguir (LG1-LG5) contêm uma lista do gênero das espécies de A a Z. Estes termos estão dispostos em ordem alfabética de acordo com o nome da espécie. O *Localizador de Gêneros* deve ser utilizado quando se quer saber a definição de uma espécie mas não se conhece seu gênero. Se você deseja encontrar a definição de "B. abortus", por exemplo, procure pelo termo "abortus" no *Localizador de Gêneros* e você verá a palavra "Brucella". Vá então para "Brucella", no vocabulário de A a Z do dicionário, e você encontrará a definição de "Brucella abortus". O *Localizador de Gêneros* funciona também como uma referência rápida quando se quer apenas saber a grafia correta do gênero de uma espécie.

A

abortus: Brucella
abscessus: Mycobacterium
aceti: Turbatrix
acidophilum: Thermoplasma
acidophilus: Lactobacillus
acidovorans: Pseudomonas
acnes: Corynebacterium; Propionibacterium
aconitus: Anopheles
actinoides: Thysanosoma
actinomycetemcomitans: Actinobacillus; Haemophilus
aegypti: Aedes
aegyptius: Haemophilus
aerofaciens: Eubacterium
aerogenes: Enterobacter; Pasteurella; Peptococcus
aeruginosa: Pseudomonas
aethiopica: Leishmania
aethiopicum: Plasmodium
africae: Rickettsia
africana: Actinomadura; Taenia
afzelii: Borrelia
agalactiae: Streptococcus
ajacis: Delphinium
akamushi: Leptotrombidium; Trombicula
akari: Rickettsia
albicans: Candida
albimanus: Anopheles
albitarsus: Anopheles
albopictus: Aedes; Dermacentor
album: Veratrum
albus: Streptomyces
alcalescens subsp. alcalescens: Veillonella
alcalescens subsp. dispar: Veillonella
alcalesens: Veillonella
alcalifaciens: Providencia
alfreddugesi: Trombicula
alginolyticus: Vibrio
amalonatica: Citrobacter; Levinea
ambiguus: Passalurus
americana: Cochliomyia
americanum: Amblyomma
amycolatum: Corynebacterium
anaerobius: Peptostreptococcus
anatipestifer: Moraxella
anatolicum: Hyalomma
anatolicum anatolicum: Hyalomma
andersoni: Dermacentor
anginosus: Streptococcus
anitrata: Lingelsheimia
annua: Artemisia
annularis: Anopheles
annulipes: Anopheles
anomalus: Hoplopsyllus
anserina: Borrelia
anseris: Amidostomum
anthracis: Bacillus
anthropophaga: Cordylobia
aphrophilus: Haemophilus
apiospermum: Monosporium; Scedosporium
apiostomum: Oesophagostomum
aquasalis: Anopheles
aquatile: Flavobacterium
arabiensis: Anopheles
argentipes: Phlebotomus
armata: Taenia
armillatus: Armillifer; Porocephalus
asaccharolytica: Porphyromonas
asaccharolyticus: Peptostreptococcus
asini: Strongylus
asteroides: Nocardia
atlanticus: Aedes
atypica: Veillonella
audouinii: Microsporum
aureus: Staphylococcus
austeni: Culicoides
australiensis: Bipolaris
australis: Rickettsia
avium: Mycobacterium; Trypanosoma
avium-intracellulare complex: Mycobacterium
axanthum: Acholeplasma
axei: Trichostrongylus
aztecus: Anopheles

B

bacilliformis: Bartonella
bacteriovorus: Bdellovibrio
balabacensis: Anopheles
balatus: Acarus
bancrofti: Wuchereria
barbirostris: Anopheles
bellator: Anopheles
belli: Isospora
berghei: Plasmodium
bieneusi: Enterocytozoon
bifermentans: Clostridium
bifidum: Bifidobacterium
bigemina: Isospora
biloba: Ginkgo
bisonis: Cooperia
bivia: Prevotella
bivius: Bacteroides
botulinum: Clostridium
bovihominis: Sarcocystis
bovis: Actinomyces; Cysticercus; Mycobacterium; Streptococcus
boydii: Allescheria; Pseudallescheria; Shigella
bozemanii: Legionella
brasiliensis: Nocardia; Paracoccidioides
brazilianum: Plasmodium
braziliense: Ancylostoma
braziliensis: Leishmania
braziliensis braziliensis: Leishmania
braziliensis guyanensis: Leishmania
braziliensis panamensis: Leishmania
breve: Flavobacterium; Gymnodinium
brevicaeca: Heterophyes
brevicaudum: Oesophagostomum
brevis: Bacillus; Lactobacillus
bronchialis: Cyathostoma
bronchiseptica: Bordetella
brucei: Trypanosoma
brucei brucei: Trypanosoma
brucei gambiense: Trypanosoma
brucei rhodesiense: Trypanosoma
brumpti: Oesophagostomum
brunnipes: Anopheles
buccale: Mycoplasma
buccalis: Amoeba; Entamoeba; Leptotrichia; Trichomonas
buchneri: Lactobacillus
bulgaricus: Lactobacillus
burgdorferi: Borrelia
burgdorferi sensu lato: Borrelia
burgdorferi sensu stricto: Borrelia
burnetii: Coxiella; Rickettsia
buski: Fasciolopsis
bütschlii: Iodamoeba
butyricum: Clostridium
butzleri: Arcobacter

C

caballus: Aedes
cadaveris: Clostridium
caesar: Lucilia
cajennense: Amblyomma
calcitrans: Stomoxys
calcoaceticus: Acinetobacter
californiensis: Thelazia
callipaeda: Thelazia
campestris: Anopheles
canicularis: Anthomyia
canimorsus: Capnocytophaga
caninum: Ancylostoma; Dipylidium
canis: Brucella; Ehrlichia; Isospora; Microsporum; Rickettsia; Toxocara
canis, var. distortum: Microsporum
canium: Neospora
cantonensis: Angiostrongylus
capillaris: Muellerius
capillatus: Solenopotes
capillosus: Bacteroides
capitatus: Blastoschizomyces
capricola: Trichostrongylus
capsulatum: Histoplasma
carateum: Treponema
carinii: Pneumocystis
carnis: Clostridium
carrionii: Cladosporium
casei: Lactobacillus; Philopia; Piophila
catanella: Gonyaulax
catarrhalis: Branhamella; Moraxella; Neisseria
catenaformis: Lactobacillus
cati: Notoedres
caucasica: Borrelia
caudatus: Bodo
caviae: Neisseria; Nocardia
cayetanensis: Cyclospora
cellulosae: Cysticercus
cepacia: Burkholderia; Pseudomonas
cerebralis: Coenurus
cereus: Bacillus
cervi: Setaria
ceylanicum: Ancylostoma
ceylonica: Haemadipsa
chaffeensis: Ehrlichia
chattoni: Entamoeba
chauvoei: Clostridium
chelonae: Mycobacterium
chelonae subsp. abscessus: Mycobacterium
cheopis: Pulex
chinensis: Phlebotomus
cholerae: Vibrio
cinaedi: Helicobacter
cinnabarina: Haemaphysalis
circulans: Bacillus
cladosporioides: Cladosporium
clavatus: Aspergillus
cloacae: Enterobacter

Localizador de Gêneros

LG1

cochlearium: Clostridium
coli: Amoeba; Balantidium; Campylobacter; Entamoeba; Escherichia
colubriformis: Trichostrongylus
columbianum: Oesophagostomum
combesi: Eubacterium
concentricum: Trichophyton
concinna: Haemaphysalis
concisus: Campylobacter
conglomeratus: Micrococcus
congolense: Trypanosoma
congolensis: Dermatophilus
conjunctivae: Dirofilaria
conorii: Rickettsia
constellatus: Peptococcus; Streptococcus
contortum: Eubacterium
cookei: Ixodes
cordatum: Diphyllobothrium
cordatus: Bothriocephalus
coriaceus: Ornithodoros
corneum: Nosema
coronata: Entomophthora
corrodens: Bacteroides; Eikenella
corticale: Cryptostroma
corymbosa: Rivea
costaricensis: Angiostrongylus; Morerastrongylus
crassicollis: Taenia
crispatum: Eubacterium
crispatus: Lactobacillus
crocidurae: Borrelia
crucians: Anopheles
cruzi: Anopheles; Schizotrypanum; Trypanosoma
culicifacies: Anopheles
culicis: Agamomermis
cuniculi: Encephalitozoon; Treponema
curcas: Jatropha
curticei: Cooperia
curvatus: Lactobacillus
cyaniventris: Dermatobia
cynomolgi: Plasmodium

D

dammini: Ixodes
damnosum: Simulium
darlingi: Anopheles
dassonvillei: Nocardiopsis
davtiani: Teladorsagia
delbrueckii: Lactobacillus
deliensis: Trombicula
demarquayi: Mansonella
demerariensis: Taenia
deminutus: Ternidens
dendriticum: Diphyllobothrium
denitrificans: Listeria
dentalis: Amoeba
dentata: Taenia
dentatum: Oesophagostomum
dentatus: Stephanurus
denticola: Prevotella; Treponema
dentium: Bifidobacterium
dentocariosa: Rothia
dentrificans: Jonesia
dermatitidis: Blastomyces
destruens: Hyphomyces
difficile: Clostridium
diminuta: Hymenolepis; Pseudomonas
dimorphon: Trypanosoma
diphtheriae: Corynebacterium
disiens: Bacteroides; Prevotella
dispar: Entamoeba
distasonis: Bacteroides
divergens: Babesia
diversus: Citrobacter; Levinea
doloresi: Gnathostoma
donovani: Leishmania
donovani archibaldi: Leishmania
donovani chagasi: Leishmania
donovani donovani: Leishmania
donovani infantum: Leishmania
dorsalis: Aedes
ducreyi: Haemophilus
dumoffii: Legionella
duodenale: Ancylostoma
durans: Streptococcus
duttonii: Borrelia
dysenteriae: Amoeba; Shigella

E

echidninus: Laelaps
edentatus: Strongylus
elegans: Cunninghamella
enterica subsp. choleraesuis: Salmonella
enterica subsp. enteritidis: Salmonella
enterica subsp. paratyphi A: Salmonella
enterica subsp. paratyphi B: Salmonella
enterica subsp. typhi: Salmonella
enterica subsp. typhimurium: Salmonella
enterocolitica: Yersinia
epidermidis: Staphylococcus
equi: Corynebacterium; Ehrlichia; Ehrlichia; Rhodococcus
equina: Setaria; Taenia
equinum: Trichophyton; Trypanosoma
equinus: Strongylus
equiperdum: Trypanosoma
equorum: Ascaris; Parascaris
erraticus: Ornithodoros
escomelis: Trypanosoma
esculenta: Gyromitra; Helvella
evansi: Trypanosoma
evolutus: Peptostreptococcus

F

faecalis: Enterococcus; Streptococcus
faecium: Enterococcus
falciparum: Plasmodium
fallax: Clostridium
farcinica: Nocardia
fasciatus: Pulex
faucium: Mycoplasma
feeleii: Legionella
felineus: Opisthorchis
felis: Isospora
fennelliae: Helicobacter
fermentans: Mycoplasma
fermentum: Lactobacillus
ferrugineum: Microsporum
fetus: Campylobacter; Vibrio
fetus subsp. jejuni: Campylobacter
fieldingi: Cooperia
filamentosum: Eubacterium
flava: Neisseria
flavescens: Neisseria
flavirostris: Anopheles
flaviscutellata: Lutzomyia
flaviscutellatus: Phlebotomus
flavus: Aspergillus
flexneri: Shigella
fluorescens: Pseudomonas
fluvialis: Vibrio
fluviatilis: Anopheles
foetidus: Peptostreptococcus
foetus: Trichomonas
folliculorum: Acarus; Demodex
fortuitum: Mycobacterium
fragilis: Bacteroides; Dientamoeba
frederikseni: Yersinia
freeborni: Anopheles
freudenreichii: Propionibacterium
freundii: Citrobacter; Escherichia
fulvum: Microsporum
fumigatus: Aspergillus
funestus: Anopheles
furcosus: Bacteroides
furens: Culicoides
furfur: Malassezia
furnissii: Vibrio
furunculosa: Leishmania
fusiformis: Sarcocystis

G

gallinacea: Echidnophaga
gallinae: Acarus; Dermanyssus; Microsporum
gallinarum: Trichomonas
gambiae: Anopheles
gambiense: Trypanosoma
garinii: Borrelia
genitalis: Treponema
genitalium: Mycoplasma
georgianum: Oesophagostomum
gibsonii: Nocardia; Streptomyces
gigantica: Fasciola
gingivalis: Entamoeba
glabrata: Candida
glandulifera: Jatropha
glucuronolyticum: Corynebacterium
gondii: Toxoplasma
gonorrhoeae: Neisseria
gormanii: Legionella
gracilis: Euglena
granularum: Acholeplasma; Mycoplasma
granulomatis: Calymmatobacterium
granulosis: Noguchia
granulosus: Echinococcus
grayi: Listeria
gypseum: Microsporum

H

haematobium: Schistosoma
haemolysans: Neisseria
haemolyticum: Arcanobacterium; Clostridium; Corynebacterium
haemolyticus: Haemophilus; Staphylococcus
hartmanni: Entamoeba
hawaiiensis: Bipolaris
hebraeum: Amblyomma
heilmannii: Helicobacter
hellum: Encephalitozoon
hemipterus: Cimex
hemolyticus: Bacillus
henselae: Bartonella
heparinolytica: Prevotella
hepatica: Capillaria; Fasciola
hermsi: Ornithodoros
hermsii: Borrelia
heterophyes: Heterophyes
hians: Diphyllobothrium
hinshawii: Arizona
hinzii: Bordetella
hirudinaceus: Macracanthorhynchus
hispanica: Borrelia
hispidum: Gnathostoma
histolytica: Amoeba; Entamoeba
histolyticum: Clostridium
histolyticus: Bacillus
hofmannii: Corynebacterium
hollisae: Vibrio
holmesii: Bordetella
hominis: Blastocystis; Cardiobacterium; Dermatobia; Gastrodiscoides; Gastrodiscus; Mycoplasma; Octomitus; Sarcocystis; Staphylococcus; Taenia; Trichomonas; Trypanosoma
hominivorax: Cochliomyia
honei: Rickettsia
hordei: Acarus
houghtoni: Diphyllobothrium
hydatigena: Taenia
hydrophila: Aeromonas
hyodysenteriae: Treponema
hyointestinalis: Campylobacter

I

ignotum: Trypanosoma

illustris: Lucilia
ilocanum: Echinostoma
immitis: Dirofilaria
inconstans: Proteus
indologenes: Kingella
inflatum: Scedosporium
influenzae: Haemophilus
infundibulum: Choanotaenia
innominatum: Clostridium
inornata: Culiseta
insidiosa: Erysipelothrix
insidiosum: Pythium
intercalatum: Schistosoma
intermedia: Prevotella;
 Yersinia
intermedius: Lutzomyia;
 Peptostreptococcus;
 Streptococcus
interrogans: Leptospira
intestinale: Encephalitozoon
intestinalis: Giardia; Lamblia
intracellulare:
 Mycobacterium
invicta: Solenopsis
irritans: Pulex; Siphona
israelii: Actinomyces

J

japonica: Rickettsia; Scopolia
japonicum: Schistosoma
jeanselmei: Exophiala
jeikeium: Corynebacterium
jejuni: Campylobacter
jensenii: Lactobacillus;
 Propionibacterium
jeyporiensis: Anopheles

K

kansasii: Mycobacterium
karwari: Anopheles
katsuradai: Heterophyes
kellicotti: Paragonimus
kingae: Kingella; Moraxella
knowlesi: Plasmodium
kochi: Plasmodium
koseri: Citrobacter
kristensenii: Yersinia
kweiyangensis: Anopheles

L

labranchiae: Anopheles
lactis: Streptococcus
lacunata: Moraxella
lahorensis: Ornithodoros
laidlawii: Acholeplasma;
 Mycoplasma
lamblia: Giardia
lanceolata: Hymenolepis
lari: Campylobacter
laryngeus:
 Mammomonogamus
latina: Actinomadura
latum: Diphyllobothrium
latus: Bothriocephalus;
 Dibothriocephalus
latyschewii: Borrelia
leachi: Haemaphysalis
lectularia: Acanthia
lectularius: Cimex

lentum: Eubacterium
leonina: Toxascaris
leprae: Mycobacterium
lesteri: Anopheles
leucocelaenus: Aedes
leucosphyrus: Anopheles
lewisi: Trypanosoma
lignieresii: Actinobacillus
lilacinus: Paecilomyces
limosum: Eubacterium
lindemanni: Sarcocystis
linguloides: Diphyllobothrium
loboi: Loboa
longbeachae: Legionella
longior: Tyroglyphus
longipalpis: Lutzomyia;
 Phlebotomus
longispicularis:
 Trichostrongylus
longispiculata: Nematodirella
lova: Dracunculus
lumbricoides: Ascaris
lupi: Spirocerca
lurida: Nocardia
luteola: Auchmeromyia
luteus: Micrococcus

M

macrorchis: Prosthogonimus
mactans: Latrodectus
maculatum: Amblyomma
maculatus: Anopheles
maculipennis: Anopheles
madagascariensis:
 Inermicapsifer; Taenia
madurae: Nocardia
magnus: Peptostreptococcus
major: Leishmania;
 Phlebotomus
majus: Habronema
malariae: Plasmodium
malayanum: Echinostoma
malayensis: Schistosoma
malayi: Brugia; Wuchereria
malaysiensis: Angiostrongylus
mallei: Burkholderia;
 Pseudomonas
malonatica: Levinea
maltophilia: Pseudomonas;
 Stenotrophomonas;
 Xanthomonas
mangiferae: Nattrassia
mansoni: Bothriocephalus;
 Diphyllobothrium;
 Oxyspirura; Schistosoma;
 Spirometra
mansonoides:
 Bothriocephalus;
 Diphyllobothrium;
 Spirometra
marcescens: Serratia
marginatum: Hyalomma
marginatus: Dermacentor
marianum: Mycobacterium
marinum: Mycobacterium
marshalli: Marshallagia
matruchotii: Corynebacterium
mattheei: Schistosoma
maydis: Ustilago
mazzottii: Borrelia
medinensis: Dracunculus

mediterranei: Nocardia
megastoma: Habronema
megaterium: Bacillus
megninii: Trichophyton
mekongi: Schistosoma
melanimon: Aedes
melaninogenica: Prevotella
melaninogenicus: Bacteroides
melanura: Culiseta
melitensis: Brucella
melophagium: Trypanosoma
meningisepticum:
 Flavobacterium
meningitidis: Neisseria
mentagrophytes:
 Trichophyton
mesenteroides: Leuconostoc
messeae: Anopheles
metel: Datura
metschnikovii: Vibrio
mexicana: Leishmania
mexicana amazonensis:
 Leishmania
mexicana garnhami:
 Leishmania
mexicana mexicana:
 Leishmania
mexicana pifanoi: Leishmania
mexicana venezuelensis:
 Leishmania
micdadei: Legionella
micros: Peptostreptococcus
microstoma: Habronema
microti: Babesia;
 Mycobacterium
miescheriana: Sarcocystis
milleri: Streptococcus
milnei: Culicoides
mimicus: Vibrio
minima: Taenia
minimus: Anopheles
minus: Spirillum
minutissimum:
 Corynebacterium
minutum: Eubacterium
mirabilis: Proteus
mitchellae: Aedes
mitis: Streptococcus
mobilis: Klebsiella
moniliforme: Eubacterium
moniliformis: Streptobacillus
monocytogenes: Listeria
morbillorum: Gemella;
 Peptostreptococcus;
 Streptococcus
morganii: Morganella; Proteus
morsitans: Glossina
mortiferum: Fusobacterium
moshkovskii: Entamoeba
moubata complex:
 Ornithodoros
mucosum: Treponema
multiceps: Multiceps
multiformis: Haverhillia
multilocularis: Echinococcus
multipapillosa: Parafilaria
multocida: Pasteurella
muscae: Habronema
muscaria: Amanita
mutans: Streptococcus
mystax: Toxocara

N

naeslundii: Actinomyces
nana: Hymenolepis
nana, var. fraterna:
 Hymenolepis
nanum: Microsporum
neavei: Simulium
necrophorum: Fusobacterium
neoformans: Cryptococcus
nidulans: Aspergillus
niger: Aspergillus;
 Peptococcus
nigrescens: Mermis
nigrificans: Clostridium;
 Desulfotomaculum
nigripalpus: Culex
nigromaculis: Aedes
nihonkaiense:
 Diphyllobothrium
nilotica: Limnatis
nipponicum: Gnathostoma
nodosus: Bacteroides;
 Dichelobacter
noguchi: Phlebotomus
nonliquefaciens: Moraxella
nova: Nocardia
novyi: Clostridium
nucleatum: Fusobacterium

O

obermeieri: Spirochaeta
occidentalis: Dermacentor
ochraceum: Simulium
oculi: Dracunculus
odontolyticus: Actinomyces
oedematiens: Clostridium
oncophora: Cooperia
orale: Mycoplasma
oralis: Bacteroides; Prevotella
orbiculare: Pityrosporum
orcini: Diphyllobothrium
orientalis: Nocardia;
 Phlebotomus
orientalis subsp. lurida:
 Amycolatopsis
oris: Bacteroides; Prevotella
osloensis: Moraxella
otitidiscaviarum: Nocardia
ovale: Pityrosporum;
 Plasmodium
ovalis: Malassezia
ovatum: Loxotrema
ovis: Taenia;
 Tetratrichomonas;
 Trichomonas
oxytoca: Klebsiella
ozaenae: Klebsiella
ozzardi: Mansonella

P

pachydermatis: Malassezia
pacificum: Diphyllobothrium
pacificus: Ixodes
paleopneumoniae:
 Peptostreptococcus
pallidipes: Glossina
pallidum: Treponema
palpalis: Glossina

papatasii: Phlebotomus
pappilipes: Ornithodoros
parabotulinum: Clostridium
parahaemolyticus:
    Haemophilus; Vibrio
parainfluenzae: Haemophilus
parapertussis: Bordetella
parapsilosis: Candida
paraputrificum: Clostridium
paratropicalis: Haemophilus
paratuberculosis:
    Mycobacterium
parkeri: Borrelia;
    Ornithodoros
parva var. crescens:
    Emmonsia
parva var. parva: Emmonsia
parvula: Veillonella
parvula subsp. atypica:
    Veillonella
parvula subsp. parvula:
    Veillonella
parvula subsp. rodentium:
    Veillonella
parvulus: Peptostreptococcus
parvum: Chrysosporium;
    Corynebacterium;
    Cryptosporidium;
    Eubacterium
pectinata: Cooperia
pelliertieri: Actinomadura
penetrans: Pulex; Sarcopsylla;
    Tunga
perfoliata: Anoplocephala
perfringens: Clostridium
perniciosus: Phlebotomus
persarum: Dracunculus
persica: Borrelia
persicolor: Microsporum
perstans: Mansonella
persulcatus: Ixodes
pertenue: Treponema
pertussis: Bordetella
peruensis: Lutzomyia
peruviana: Leishmania
pestis: Pasteurella; Yersinia
phagocytophila: Ehrlichia
phalloides: Amanita
pharyngis: Mycoplasma
phenylpyruvica: Moraxella
philippina: Taenia
philippinensis: Capillaria
phlebotomum: Bunostomum
phlei: Mycobacterium
phosphoreum:
    Photobacterium
physalis: Physalia
pifanoi: Leishmania
pilulifera: Euphorbia
pipiens: Culex
piscicida: Flavobacterium;
    Pseudomonas
pisiformis: Taenia
plagarumbelli:
    Peptostreptococcus
plantarum: Lactobacillus
plebeius: Vaginulus
plicatilis: Spirochaeta
pneumoniae: Chlamydia;
    Klebsiella; Mycoplasma;
    Streptococcus

pneumoniae subsp. ozaenae:
    Klebsiella
pneumophila: Legionella
pneumosintes: Bacteroides
poeciloides: Eubacterium
polecki: Entamoeba
polymyxa: Bacillus
polynesiensis: Aedes
praeacuta: Tissierella
praeacutus: Bacteroides
procyonis: Baylisascaris
productus: Peptostreptococcus
prolificans: Scedosporium
prolixus: Rhodnius
propionica: Arachnia
propionicus:
    Propionibacterium
proteus: Amoeba
prowazekii: Rickettsia
prunifolium: Viburnum
pseudoalcaligenes:
    Pseudomonas
pseudodiphtheriticum:
    Corynebacterium
pseudomallei: Burkholderia;
    Pseudomonas
pseudopunctipennis:
    Anopheles
pseudospiralis.: Trichinella
pseudotortuosum:
    Eubacterium
pseudotuberculosis:
    Pasteurella; Yersinia
psittaci: Chlamydia; Rickettsia
pteronyssinus:
    Dermatophagoides
pulchrum: Gongylonema
pumilis: Bacillus
punctata: Cooperia
punjatensis: Ceratophyllus
purpureus: Rhinoestrus
putredinis: Bacteroides
putrefaciens: Alteromonas;
    Pseudomonas
putrescentiae: Tyrophagus
putridus: Peptostreptococcus
pylori: Campylobacter;
    Helicobacter
pyogenes: Streptococcus
pyogenes albus:
    Staphylococcus
pyogenes aureus:
    Staphylococcus
pyriformis: Tetrahymena

Q

quadrilobata: Taenia
quadrimaculatus: Anopheles
quadrispinulatum:
    Oesophagostomum
quadrumanus: Chiropsalmus
quartum: Eubacterium
quinquecirrha: Chrysaora
quinquefasciatus: Culex
quintana: Bartonella
quintum: Eubacterium

R

radiatum: Oesophagostomum
radiatus: Strongylus

ramosum: Clostridium
rangeli: Trypanosoma
ratellina: Grisonella
rathouisi: Fasciolopsis
reconditum: Dipetalonema
rectale: Eubacterium
recurrentis: Borrelia
redikorzevi: Ixodes
reflexus: Argas
regina: Phormia
renale: Dioctophyma
restuans: Culex
reticulatus: Dermacentor
rettgeri: Proteus; Providencia
rhinaria: Linguatula
rhinoscleromatis: Klebsiella
rhizoglypticus hyacinthi:
    Acarus
rhodesiense: Trypanosoma
rhusiopathiae: Erysipelothrix
richteri: Solenopsis
ricinus: Ixodes
rickettsii: Rickettsia
ringeri: Paragonimus
risticii: Ehrlichia
rivolta: Isospora
rodentium: Veillonella
romeroi: Pyrenochaeta
rosati: Neotestudina
rosea: Vinca
rubrocoerulea var. praecox:
    Ipomoea
rubrum: Trichophyton
rudis: Ornithodoros
rugglesi: Simulium

S

saginata: Taenia
sagitta: Dipus
sakazakii: Enterobacter
salinarius: Culex
salivarium: Mycoplasma
salivarius: Lactobacillus;
    Streptococcus
salmincola: Nanophyetus;
    Troglotrema
saltans: Bodo
sanguineus: Rhipicephalus
sanguis: Streptococcus
sapiens: Homo
saprophyticus:
    Staphylococcus
sardinae: Eimeria
savigni: Ornithodoros
scabei: Acarus
scabiei: Sarcoptes
scapularis: Ixodes
schneideri: Elaeophora
schoenleinii: Trichophyton
scoticum: Diphyllobothrium
scrofulaceum: Mycobacterium
seeberi: Rhinosporidium
segnis: Haemophilus
sennetsu: Ehrlichia; Rickettsia
seoi: Gymnophalloides
septicum: Clostridium
septique: Vibrion
sergenti: Phlebotomus
serialis: Coenurus; Multiceps
sericata: Lucilia; Phaenicia
serotina: Prunus

serrata: Linguatula
serraticeps: Pulex
sexalatus: Physocephalus
shigelloides: Plesiomonas
siamense: Gnathostoma
sibirica: Rickettsia
sicca: Neisseria
simiae: Trypanosoma
simii: Trichophyton
simulans: Staphylococcus
sinensis: Clonorchis;
    Opisthorchis
sinuatum: Entoloma
slovaca: Rickettsia
smegmatis: Mycobacterium
solium: Taenia
sollicitans: Aedes
somaliensis: Streptomyces
sonnei: Shigella
sordellii: Clostridium
spatulata: Cooperia
sphaericus: Bacillus
sphenoides: Clostridium
spicifera: Bipolaris
spiniger: Heterodoxus
spinigera: Haemaphysalis
spinigerum: Gnathostoma
spinipalpis: Ixodes
spiralis: Acuaria; Trichinella
splanchnicus: Bacteroides
sporogenes: Clostridium
sputorum: Campylobacter;
    Vibrio
stegomyiae: Myxococcidium
stephanostomum:
    Oesophagostomum
stephensi: Anopheles
stilesi: Stephanofilaria
stramonium: Datura
streptocerca: Dipetalonema;
    Mansonella
striatum: Corynebacterium
strongylina: Ascarops
stuartii: Providencia
studeri: Bertiella
stutzeri: Pseudomonas
subflava: Neisseria
subtilis: Bacillus
suihominis: Sarcocystis
suis: Balantidium; Brucella;
    Isospora; Trichomonas;
    Trichuris; Trypanosoma
sundaicus: Anopheles
superpictus: Anopheles

T

taeniaeformis: Hydatigera;
    Taenia
taeniorhynchus: Aedes
talaje: Alectorobius
talajé: Ornithodoros
tarsalis: Culex
tenax: Trichomonas
tenella: Sarcocystis
tenue: Eubacterium
tenuis: Trichostrongylus
terreus: Aspergillus
tertium: Clostridium
tetani: Clostridium
tetraptera: Aspiculuris

theileri: Trypanosoma
thermosaccharolyticum: Clostridium
thetaiotamicron: Bacteroides
tholozani: Ornithodoros
thuringiensis: Bacillus
tonsurans: Trichophyton
tortuosum: Eubacterium
toruloidea: Hendersonula
trachomatis: Chlamydia
transvalensis: Nocardia
triatomae: Trypanosoma
trichiura: Trichuris
trichodectis: Cryptocystis
trichodes: Lactobacillus
trigonocephalum: Bunostomum
triseriatus: Aedes
tritici: Pyemotes
trivittatus: Aedes
tropica: Leishmania
tropicalis: Candida
tropica major: Leishmania
tropica mexicana: Leishmania
tsutsugamushi: Orientia; Rickettsia
tubaeforme: Ancylostoma
tuberculosis: Mycobacterium
tucumana: Mansonella
tularensis: Francisella; Pasteurella
turicata: Ornithodoros
turicatae: Borrelia
typhi: Rickettsia; Salmonella
typhosa: Salmonella

U

ugandense: Trypanosoma
ulcerans: Mycobacterium
urealyticum: Ureaplasma
urens: Jatropha
ureolyticus: Bacteroides
urinarius: Bodo

V

vaccae: Mycobacterium
vaginalis: Gardnerella; Trichomonas
vanbreuseghemi: Microsporum
variabilis: Dermacentor
varians: Micrococcus
variegatum: Amblyomma; Hyalomma
variegatus: Aedes
vasiformis: Saksenaea
venezuelensis: Borrelia; Ornithodoros
ventricosus: Haemodipsus; Pediculoides; Strongylus
ventriculi: Sarcina
venulosum: Oesophagostomum
verrucarum: Phlebotomus
verrucosum: Trichophyton
verrucosus: Ornithodoros
versicolor: Ipomoea
vesicularis: Pseudomonas
vexans: Aedes
violaceum: Cardiobacterium; Chromobacterium; Trichophyton
virginiana: Prunus
viridans: Streptococcus
viride: Veratrum
viridis: Euglena
viscosus: Actinomyces
vitrinus: Trichostrongylus
vitulorum: Neoascaris
vivax: Plasmodium; Trypanosoma
viverrini: Opisthorchis
vivipara: Probstymayria
vogeli: Echinococcus
volutans: Spirillum
volvulus: Onchocerca
vulgaris: Proteus; Strongylus
vulnificus: Vibrio
vulpis: Crenosoma; Trichuris

W

wadsworthii: Legionella
watsoni: Cladorchis
welchii: Clostridium
werneckii: Cladosporium; Exophiala
westermani: Paragonimus
whippelii: Tropheryma
winthemi: Margaropus

X

xenopi: Mycobacterium
xerosis: Corynebacterium
(Xylohypha) bantianum: Cladosporium

Z

zeae: Ustilago
zoohelcum: Weeksella

LOCALIZADOR DE SUBENTRADAS

As páginas a seguir (LS1 – LS122) contêm uma lista de múltiplos termos (ou subentradas) de A a Z. Estes termos estão dispostos em ordem alfabética a partir de sua(s) primeira(s) palavra(s). O *Localizador de Subentradas* deve ser utilizado quando se quer saber a definição de uma subentrada, mas não se conhece a palavra principal que a forma. Se você deseja encontrar a definição de "Sinal de Aaron", por exemplo, procure por "Aaron" no *Localizador de Subentradas* e você verá a palavra "sign". Vá então para "sign", no vocabulário de A a Z do dicionário, e você encontrará a definição de "Aaron sign". O *Localizador de Subentradas* funciona também como uma referência rápida quando se quer apenas saber a grafia correta de um termo.

A

α′: hemolysis
α: fetoprotein; granules; helix; hemolysin; thalassemia; thalassemia intermedia
A: bands; bile; cells; chain; disks; fibers; wave
A1: segment of anterior cerebral artery
A2: segment of anterior cerebral artery
α₁-: antitrypsin; lipoprotein
A₂: thalassemia
A-: DNA; strabismus
α-: keto acid dehydrogenase
aaa: disease
Aagenaes: syndrome
Aaron: sign
Aarskog-Scott: syndrome
abacterial thrombotic: endocarditis
Abadie: sign of tabes dorsalis
abapical: pole
abarticular: gout
Abbe: flap
Abbé: condenser
Abbott: artery; stain for spores; tube
ABC: leads
A.B.C.: process
abdominal: angina; aorta; apoplexy; aura; ballottement; canal; cavity; dropsy; fibromatosis; fissure; fistula; guarding; hernia; hysterectomy; hysteropexy; hysterotomy; lymph nodes; migraine; myomectomy; nephrectomy; ostium of uterine tube; pad; part of aorta; part of esophagus; part of pectoralis major (muscle); part of peripheral autonomic plexuses and ganglia; part of thoracic duct; part of ureter; pool; pregnancy; pressure; pulse; reflexes; regions; respiration; ring; sac; salpingectomy; salpingo-oophorectomy; salpingotomy; section; testis; typhoid; zones
abdominal aortic (nervous): plexus
abdominal external oblique: muscle
abdominal internal oblique: muscle
abdominal muscle deficiency: syndrome
abdominocardiac: reflex
abdominojugular: reflux
abdominopelvic: cavity
abdominopelvic splanchnic: nerves
abdominoperineal: resection
abdominothoracic: arch
abdominovaginal: hysterectomy
abducens: eminence; nerve; nucleus
abducent: nerve [CN VI]
abductor: muscle; muscle of great toe; muscle of little finger; muscle of little toe
abductor digiti minimi: muscle of foot; muscle of hand
abductor hallucis: muscle
abductor pollicis brevis: muscle
abductor pollicis longus: muscle
abductor spasmodic: dysphonia
Abegg: rule
Abell-Kendall: method
Abelson murine leukemia: virus
Abernethy: fascia
aberrant: artery; bundles; complex; ducts; ductules; ganglion; goiter; hemoglobin; regeneration
aberrant bile: ducts
aberrant obturator: artery
aberrant ventricular: conduction
abnormal: cleavage of cardiac valve; correspondence; occlusion
abnormal ST: segment
ABO: antigens; factors
ABO hemolytic: disease of the newborn
aborted: systole
aborted ectopic: pregnancy
abortion: rate
abortive: neurofibromatosis; transduction
abortus: bacillus
abraded: wound
Abrahams: sign
Abrams heart: reflex
abrasive: strip
abscopal: effect
absence: seizure
absent: state
absolute: agraphia; alcohol; dehydration; glaucoma; hemianopia; humidity; hydration; hyperopia; leukocytosis; oils; pressure; scale; scotoma; system of units; temperature; threshold; unit; viscosity; zero
absolute cell: increase
absolute intensity threshold: acuity
absolute refractory: period
absolute terminal innervation: ratio
absorbable gelatin: film; sponge
absorbable surgical: suture
absorbancy: index
absorbed: dose
absorbent: cotton; points; system; vessels
absorption: band; cell; chromatography; coefficient; collapse; fever; lines; spectrum
absorptive: cells of intestine
abstinence: symptoms; syndrome
abstract: intelligence; thinking
a-c: interval
Acanthamoeba: medium
acanthocytosis with: chorea
acapnial: alkalosis
acarine: dermatosis
accelerated: conduction; eruption; hypertension; reaction; rejection
accelerator: factor; fibers; globulin; nerves
acceptor: RNA; site
acceptor splicing: site
access: opening
accessory: adrenal; atrium; auricles; branch of middle meningeal artery; breast; canal; cartilage; cell; chromosome; flocculus; gland; ligaments; lymph nodes; molecules; nerve [CN XI]; nipple; nuclei of optic tract; organs; organs of the eye; pancreas; placenta; portion of spinal accessory nerve; process of lumbar vertebra; root of tooth; sign; spleen; structures; symptom; thyroid; tragus; tubercle
accessory cephalic: vein
accessory cuneate: nucleus
accessory flexor: muscle of foot
accessory hemiazygos: vein
accessory lacrimal: glands
accessory meningeal: artery; branch; branch of middle meningeal artery
accessory nasal: cartilages
accessory nerve: lymph nodes; trunk
accessory obturator: artery
accessory olivary: nuclei
accessory pancreatic: duct
accessory parotid: gland
accessory phrenic: nerves
accessory plantar: ligaments
accessory quadrate: cartilage
accessory saphenous: vein
accessory suprarenal: glands
accessory thyroid: gland
accessory vertebral: vein
accessory visual: apparatus; structures
accessory volar: ligaments
accident: neurosis
accidental: abortion; host; hypothermia; image; murmur; myiasis; parasite; symptom
acclimating: fever
accolé: forms

accommodation: phosphene; reflex
accommodative: asthenopia; convergence; insufficiency; strabismus
accommodative convergence-accommodation: ratio
accompanying: vein; vein of hypoglossal nerve
accoucheur: hand
accretion: lines
accretionary: growth
accumulation: analysis; disease
acentric: chromosome; fragment
acephalgic: migraine
acetabular: artery; branch; fossa; labrum; lip; margin; notch
acetate replacement: factor
acetic: fermentation; solution
acetone: body; chloroform; compound; fixative; test
acetone-insoluble: antigen
aceto-orcein: stain
acetosoluble: albumin
acetyl: value
acetyl-activating: enzyme
Achard: syndrome
Achard-Thiers: syndrome
Achenbach: syndrome
achievement: age; motive; quotient; test
Achilles: bursa; reflex; tendon
achlorhydric: anemia
acholuric: jaundice
achondroplastic: dwarfism
achrestic: anemia
achromatic: apparatus; lens; objective; threshold; vision
acid: agglutination; alcohol; carboxypeptidase; cell; deoxyribonuclease; dextran; dextrin; dyspepsia; fuchsin; gland; indigestion; intoxication; maltase; oxide; phosphatase; radical; reaction; rigor; salt; seromucoid; stain; sulfate; tartrate; tide; wave
α_1-**acid:** glycoprotein
acid-ash: diet
acid-base: balance; equilibrium
acid etch cemented: splint
acid-etched: restoration
acidic: amino acid; dyes
acidified serum: test
acidophil: adenoma; cell; granule
acidophilic: leukocyte
acidophilus: milk
acid perfusion: test
acid phosphatase: test for semen

acid reflux: test
acinar: carcinoma; cell
acinar cell: tumor
acinic cell: adenocarcinoma; carcinoma
acinotubular: gland
acinous: cell; gland
ackee: poisoning
acne: keloid
acorn-tipped: catheter
Acosta: disease
acoustic: agraphia; aphasia; area; cell; crest; enhancement; impedance; lemniscus; lens; meatus; nerve; neurilemoma; neurinoma; neuroma; papilla; pressure; radiation; reflex; schwannoma; shadow; spots; striae; teeth; tetanus; tolerance; tubercle; tumor; vesicle
acoustical: surround
acousticofacial: ganglion
acousticopalpebral: reflex
acoustic reference: level
acoustic stimulation: test
acquired: agammaglobulinemia; character; cuticle; drives; hyperlipoproteinemia; hypogammaglobulinemia; ichthyosis; immunity; leukoderma; leukopathia; megacolon; methemoglobinemia; nevus; pellicle; reflex; sensitivity; toxoplasmosis in adults; trichoepithelioma
acquired centric: relation
acquired eccentric: relation
acquired epileptic: aphasia
acquired hemolytic: anemia; icterus
acquired immunodeficiency: syndrome
acquired tufted: angioma
acral lentiginous: melanoma
Acrel: ganglion
acrid: poison
acridine: dyes
acrocentric: chromosome
acrodynic: erythema
acrofacial: dysostosis; syndrome
acromegalic: gigantism
acromelic: dwarfism
acromesomelic: dwarfism
acromial: anastomosis of the thoracoacromial artery; angle; artery; branch of suprascapular artery; branch of thoracoacromial artery; end of clavicle; extremity of clavicle; facet of clavicle;

part of deltoid (muscle); plexus; process; reflex
acromial arterial: network
acromial articular: facies of clavicle; surface of clavicle
acromioclavicular: disk; joint; ligament
acromion: presentation
acromiothoracic: artery
acroparesthesia: syndrome
acrosomal: cap; granule; vesicle
acrylic: resin
acrylic resin: base; tooth; tray
ACTH-producing: adenoma
ACTH stimulation: test
actin: filament
actinic: cheilitis; conjunctivitis; dermatitis; granuloma; keratitis; keratosis; porokeratosis; prurigo; ray; reticuloid
actinide: elements
actinium: emanation
actinomycotic: appendicitis
action: current; potential; tremor
activated: acetaldehyde; amino acid; atom; carboxylic acid; charcoal; choline; fatty acid; glucose; hydrogen; macrophage; resin; sludge; state
activated clotting: time
activated partial thromboplastin: time
activated sludge: method
activation: analysis
active: acetate; aldehyde; anaphylaxis; carbon dioxide; caries; center; congestion; electrode; formaldehyde; formate; formyl; glycoaldehyde; hyperemia; immunity; immunization; inflammation; labor; methionine; methyl; movement; mutant; placebo; principle; prophylaxis; psychoanalysis; pyruvate; repressor; site; splint; succinate; sulfate; transport; treatment; vasoconstriction; vasodilation
active length-tension: curve
activities of daily living: scale
activity: coefficient
actual: cautery
acupuncture: anesthesia
acute: abdomen; abscess; alcoholism; angle; appendicitis; ataxia; chalazion; cholecystitis; chorea; delirium; glaucoma; glomerulonephritis; goiter; histoplasmosis;

inflammation; malaria; mania; nephritis; nephrosis; pyelonephritis; rejection; rhinitis; rickets; schizophrenia; trypanosomiasis; urticaria
acute adrenocortical: insufficiency
acute African sleeping: sickness
acute anterior: poliomyelitis
acute ascending: paralysis
acute bacterial: endocarditis
acute brachial: radiculitis
acute bulbar: poliomyelitis
acute catarrhal: conjunctivitis
acute cellular: rejection
acute compression: triad
acute contagious: conjunctivitis
acute crescentic: glomerulonephritis
acute cutaneous: leishmaniasis
acute decubitus: ulcer
acute disseminated: encephalomyelitis
acute epidemic: conjunctivitis; leukoencephalitis
acute febrile neutrophilic: dermatosis
acute fibrinous: pericarditis
acute follicular: conjunctivitis
acute fulminating: meningococcemia
acute fulminating meningococcal: septicemia
acute hallucinatory: paranoia
acute hemorrhagic: conjunctivitis; encephalitis; glomerulonephritis; leukoencephalitis; pancreatitis
acute idiopathic: polyneuritis
acute inclusion body: encephalitis
acute infectious nonbacterial: gastroenteritis
acute inflammatory: polyneuropathy
acute inflammatory demyelinating: polyradiculoneuropathy
acute intermittent: porphyria
acute interstitial: nephritis; pneumonia; pneumonitis
acute invasive: aspergillosis
acute isolated: myocarditis
acute lobar: nephrosis
acute massive liver: necrosis
acute motor axonal: neuropathy
acute multifocal placoid pigment: epitheliopathy

acute necrotizing: encephalitis; myelitis
acute necrotizing hemorrhagic: encephalomyelitis; leukoencephalitis
acute necrotizing ulcerative: gingivitis
acute organic brain: syndrome
acute parenchymatous: hepatitis
acute phase: protein; reactants; reaction; response
acute poststreptococcal: glomerulonephritis
acute primary hemorrhagic: meningoencephalitis
acute promyelocytic: leukemia
acute pulmonary: alveolitis
acute radiation: syndrome
acute recurrent: rhabdomyolysis
acute reflex bone: atrophy
acute respiratory distress: syndrome
acute retinal: necrosis
acute rheumatic: arthritis
acute scalp: cellulitis
acute schizophrenic: episode
acute sensory motor axonal: neuropathy
acute situational: reaction
acute splenic: tumor
acute stress: reaction
acute transverse: myelitis
acute vascular: purpura
acute viral: conjunctivitis
acute yellow: atrophy of the liver
acyclic: compound
acyl-activating: enzyme
acyl carrier: protein
acylmercaptan: bond
Adair-Koshland-Némethy-Filmer: model
adamantine: membrane
Adams-Stokes: disease; syncope; syndrome
adansonian: classification
adaptation: diseases; syndrome of Selye
adaptive: behavior; enzyme; hypertrophy
adaptive behavior: scales
adaptor: hypothesis
addictive: drug
Addis: count; test
Addison: anemia; disease
Addison-Biermer: disease
Addison clinical: planes
addisonian: anemia; crisis; syndrome
addition: compound; mutation
addition-deletion: mutation

additive: effect; model
addressin: ligands
adductor: canal; compartment of thigh; hiatus; muscle; muscle of great toe; muscle of thumb; reflex; tubercle of femur
adductor brevis: muscle
adductor hallucis: muscle
adductor longus: muscle
adductor magnus: muscle
adductor minimus: muscle
adductor pollicis: muscle
adductor spasmodic: dysphonia
Aden: fever; ulcer
adeno-associated: virus
adenoid: facies; tissue; tumor
adenoidal-pharyngeal-conjunctival: virus
adenoid cystic: carcinoma
adenomatoid: tumor
adenomatoid odontogenic: tumor
adenomatous: goiter; hyperplasia; polyp; polyposis coli
adenosatellite: virus
adenosquamous: carcinoma
adequal: cleavage
adequate: stimulus
adherence: syndrome
adherent: leukoma; pericardium; placenta
adhering: junctions
adhesion: dyspepsia; molecules; phenomenon; test
adhesive: arachnoiditis; atelectasis; bandage; capsulitis; inflammation; otitis; pericarditis; peritonitis; phlebitis; pleurisy; tape; vaginitis
adhesive absorbent: dressing
Adie: pupil; syndrome
adipokinetic: hormone
adipose: capsule; cell; degeneration; folds of the pleura; fossae; infiltration; tissue; tumor
adiposogenital: degeneration; dystrophy; syndrome
adjacent: angle
adjustable: articulator
adjustable axis: face-bow
adjustable occlusal: pivot
adjustment: disorders
adjuvant: chemotherapy; vaccine
Adler: test
adlerian: psychoanalysis; psychology
admaxillary: gland
adnexal: adenoma; carcinoma
adolescent: albuminuria; crisis; medicine

adolescent round: back
adoptive: immunity; immunotherapy
ADP: ribosylation
adrenal: androgen; apoplexy; body; capsule; cortex; crisis; gland; hermaphroditism; hypertension; leukodystrophy; rest; virilism
adrenal androgen-stimulating: hormone
adrenal cortex: injection
adrenal cortical: carcinoma; syndrome
adrenaline: reversal
adrenal virilizing: syndrome
adrenal weight: factor
α-**adrenergic:** receptors
β-**adrenergic:** receptors
adrenergic: amine; blockade; fibers; neurotransmitter; receptors
β-**adrenergic blocking:** agent
α-**adrenergic blocking:** agent
adrenergic blocking: agent
adrenergic neuronal blocking: agent
β-**adrenergic receptor blocking:** agent
α-**adrenoceptor:** antagonist
adrenocortical: adenoma; hormones; insufficiency
adrenocorticotropic: hormone; peptide
adrenocorticotropic releasing: factor
adrenogenital: syndrome
adrenomedullary: hormones
adrenomimetic: amine
β-**adrenoreceptor:** antagonist
adrenotropic: hormone
Adson: forceps; maneuver; test
adsorption: chromatography; theory of narcosis
adult: hypophosphatasia; medulloepithelioma; rickets; tuberculosis
adult foveomacular retinal: dystrophy
adult lactase: deficiency
adult-onset: diabetes
adult pseudohypertrophic muscular: dystrophy
adult respiratory distress: syndrome
adult T-cell: leukemia; lymphoma
advance: directive
advanced multiple-beam equalization: radiography
advancement: flap
adventitial: cell; neuritis
adventitious: albuminuria; bursa; cyst

adventitious breath: sounds
adverse: reaction
adversive: movement
adynamic: ileus
A-E: amputation
Aeby: plane
aerial: mycelium; sickness
aerobic: dehydrogenase; respiration
aerodynamic: theory
aerogenic: tuberculosis
aerosol: generator
aerospace: medicine
aestivoautumnal: fever
AFA: fixative
affect: displacement; hunger; memory; spasms
affective: disorders; personality; psychosis; tone
afferent: fibers; lymphatic; nerve; vessel
afferent glomerular: arteriole
afferent loop: syndrome
affinity: antibody; chromatography; column
afibrillar: cementum
AFORMED: phenomenon
African: histoplasmosis; trypanosomiasis
African endomyocardial: fibrosis
African furuncular: myiasis
African hemorrhagic: fever
African horse sickness: virus
African sleeping: sickness
African tick: fever
African tick-bite: fever
afterloading: radiation; screw
afunctional: occlusion
A/G: ratio
Ag-AS: stain
agene: process
age-related macular: degeneration
age-specific: rate
agglutinating: antibody
agglutination: test
agglutinative: thrombus
aggregate: anaphylaxis; glands
aggregated lymphatic: follicles of small intestine; follicles of vermiform appendix; nodules
aggregated lymphoid: nodules; nodules of small intestine
aggressive: angiomyxoma; instinct
aggressive infantile: fibromatosis
agitated: depression
aglossia-adactylia: syndrome
agminate: glands
agnogenic myeloid: metaplasia

agonal: clot; infection; leukocytosis; rhythm; thrombus
agranular: cortex; leukocyte
agranular endoplasmic: reticulum
agranulocytic: angina
AH: interval
AH conduction: time
Ahumada-Del Castillo: syndrome
Aicardi: syndrome
AIDS: dementia
AIDS dementia: complex
AIDS-related: complex; virus
air: bladder; bronchogram; cells; cells of auditory tube; conduction; dose; embolism; pollution; sac; sickness; splint; syringe; thermometer; tube; vesicles
air-bone: gap
airborne: infection
airbrasive: technique
air-conditioner: lung
air contrast: enema
air contrast barium: enema
air-gap: radiography; technique
airplane: splint
airport: malaria
air-slaked: lime
airspace-filling: pattern
airway: pattern; resistance
airway pressure release: ventilation
Airy: disk
A-K: amputation
Akabane: virus
akamushi: disease
Åkerlund: deformity
akinetic: mutism; seizure
ala central: lobule
alactic oxygen: debt
Alagille: syndrome
Åland Island: albinism
Alanson: amputation
alar: artery of nose; chest; folds of intrapatellar synovial fold; lamina of neural tube; ligaments; part of nasalis muscle; plate of neural tube; process; spine
alarm: reaction
alaryngeal: speech
Albarran: glands; test
Albarran y Dominguez: tubules
albedo: retinae
Albers-Schönberg: disease
Albert: disease; stain; suture
Albini: nodules
albino: rats
Albinus: muscle
Albrecht: bone
Albright: disease; syndrome

Albright hereditary: osteodystrophy
albumin-globulin: ratio
albuminized: iron
albuminocytologic: dissociation
albuminoid: degeneration
albuminous: cell; gland; swelling
albuminuric: retinitis
Alcock: canal
alcohol: addiction; diuresis
alcohol amnestic: syndrome
alcohol-glycerin: fixative
alcoholic: cardiomyopathy; cirrhosis; deterioration; extract; fermentation; hyalin; myocardiopathy; pneumonia; polyneuropathy; psychoses; tincture
alcoholic hyaline: bodies
alcoholic withdrawal: tremor
alcohol withdrawal: delirium
aldehyde: fuchsin; reaction
Alder: anomaly; bodies
aldol: condensation
aldosterone: antagonist
Aldrich: syndrome
alecithal: ovum
Aleppo: boil
aleukemic: leukemia; myelosis
Aleutian mink disease: virus
Alexander: disease; hearing impairment; law
alexin: unit
Alezzandrini: syndrome
algid: malaria; stage
algid pernicious: fever
algoid: cell
Alice in Wonderland: syndrome
alicyclic: compounds
alignment: curve; mark
alimentary: apparatus; canal; diabetes; glycosuria; hyperinsulinism; lipemia; osteopathy; pentosuria; system; tract
alimentary tract: smear
aliphatic: compound
alisphenoid: cartilage
alizarin: indicator
alkali: metal; reserve; therapy
alkali denaturation: test
alkali earth: metal
alkaline: earths; phosphatase; reaction; RNase; tide; toluidine blue O; water; wave
alkaline-ash: diet
alkaline earth: elements
alkaline milk: drip
alkaline reflux: gastritis
alkylating: agent
allantoenteric: diverticulum

allantoic: bladder; cyst; diverticulum; fluid; sac; stalk; vesicle
allantoid: membrane
allantoidoangiopagous: twins
allelic: exclusion; gene
Allen: test
Allen-Doisy: test; unit
Allen-Masters: syndrome
allergenic: extract
allergic: angiitis; conjunctivitis; coryza; eczema; extract; granulomatosis; inflammation; purpura; reaction; rhinitis
allergic bronchopulmonary: aspergillosis
allergic contact: dermatitis
allergic granulomatous: angiitis
Allgrove: syndrome
allied: reflexes
alligator: forceps; skin
Allis: forceps
all or none: law
allogeneic: antigen; graft; inhibition
allograft: rejection
allomeric: function
allopathic: keratoplasty
allosteric: enzyme; site
allotypic: determinants; marker
alloxan: diabetes
Almeida: disease
Almén: test for blood
Alpers: disease
Alpha: tests
alpha: alcoholism; angle; blocking; cells of anterior lobe of hypophysis; cells of pancreas; error; fibers; granule; particle; radiation; ray; rhythm; substance; units; wave
alpha-: oxidation
alpha methyl: dopa
Alpine: scurvy
Alport: syndrome
Alström: syndrome
ALT:AST: ratio
Altemeier: operation
alterative: inflammation
altercursive: intubation
alternate: hemianesthesia
alternate binaural loudness balance: test
alternate cover: test
alternate day: strabismus
alternating: current; hemiplegia; mydriasis; pulse; strabismus; tremor
alternating light: test

alternative: hypothesis; inheritance; medicine; splicing; tremor
altitude: chamber; disease; erythremia; sickness
altitudinal: hemianopia
Altmann: fixative; granule; theory
Altmann anilin-acid fuchsin: stain
Altmann-Gersh: method
Alu: sequences
alu: family
alu-equivalent: family
alum: whey
aluminum: penicillin
alveolar: abscess; adenocarcinoma; air; angle; arch of mandible; arch of maxilla; atrophy; body; bone; border; canals of maxilla; cell; crest; duct; foramina of maxilla; gas; gingiva; gland; index; macrophage; mucosa; osteitis; part of mandible; pattern; periosteum; point; pores; process of maxilla; ridge; sac; septum; ventilation; yokes
alveolar-arterial oxygen: difference
alveolar cell: carcinoma
alveolar dead: space
alveolar duct: emphysema
alveolar gas: equation
alveolar hydatid: cyst
alveolar soft part: sarcoma
alveolar supporting: bone
alveolobuccal: groove; sulcus
alveolocapillary: block; membrane
alveolodental: canals; ligament; membrane
alveololabial: groove; sulcus
alveololingual: groove; sulcus
alveolonasal: line
Alzheimer: dementia; disease; sclerosis
Alzheimer type I: astrocyte
Alzheimer type II: astrocyte
Am: antigens
amacrine: cell
Amadori: rearrangement
amalgam: carrier; matrix; strip; tattoo
amaranth: solution
amaurotic: mydriasis; nystagmus; pupil
amaurotic cat: eye
amber: codon; mutant; mutation; suppressor
Amberg lateral sinus: line
ambient: cistern
ambiguous: genitalia

ambiguous atrioventricular: connections
ambiguous external: genitalia
ambiguus: nucleus
amblyogenic: period
amboceptor: unit
Amboyna: button
Ambu: bag
ambulant: edema; erysipelas; plague
ambulatory: anesthesia; automatism; schizophrenia; surgery; typhoid
amebic: abscess; colitis; dysentery; granuloma; vaginitis
ameboid: cell; movement
amelanotic: melanoma
ameloblastic: fibroma; fibrosarcoma; layer; odontoma; sarcoma
ameloblastic adenomatoid: tumor
ameloblastomatous: craniopharyngioma
amelodental: junction
amenorrhea-galactorrhea: syndrome
American: leishmaniasis; tarantula; trypanosomiasis
American Law Institute: rule
American Sign: Language
Ames: assay; test
amide: oximes
amino: sugars
amino-: terminal
amino acid: activation; analysis; reagent
amino acid activating: enzyme
4-aminobutyrate: pathway
p-aminohippurate: clearance
δ-aminolevulinate dehydratase: porphyria
Ammon: fissure; horn; prominence
ammonia: assimilation; detoxication; fixation; rash
ammoniacal: urine
ammoniated: mercuric chloride; mercury; tincture
amnemonic: agraphia
amnestic: aphasia; syndrome
amniocardiac: vesicle
amnioembryonic: junction
amniogenic: cells
amnion: ring
amnionic: adhesions; amputation; band; cavity; corpuscle; duct; ectoderm; fluid; fold; raphe; sac
amnionic fluid: embolism; index; syndrome
amorphous: fraction of adrenal cortex; hydroxyapatite; phosphorus; silicon
amorphous insulin zinc: suspension
amorphous selenium: plate
AMPA: receptor
Ampère: postulate
amphibolic: fistula
amphiprotic: solvent
amphophil: granule
amphoric: rale; resonance; respiration; voice
amphoric voice: sound
amphoteric: electrolyte; element; reaction
amphotropic: virus
amplifier: host
amplitude of: accommodation; convergence
ampullar: abortion; pregnancy
ampullary: aneurysm; crest; crest (of semicircular ducts); crura of semicircular ducts; cupula; folds of uterine tube; groove; sulcus; type of renal pelvis
ampullary membranous: limbs of semicircular ducts
amputating: ulcer
amputation: knife; neuroma
Amsel: criteria
Amsler: chart; grid; test
Amsterdam: syndrome
Amussat: valve; valvula
amygdaloclaustral: area
amygdaloid: body; complex; fossa; nucleus; tubercle
amygdalopiriform transition: area
amylaceous: corpuscle
amylase-creatinine clearance: ratio
amylic: fermentation
amylogenic: body
amyloid: angiopathy; bodies of the prostate; degeneration; kidney; nephrosis; protein; tumor
amyotrophic lateral: sclerosis
AN: interval
anabiotic: cell
anabolic: steroid
anaclitic: depression; psychotherapy
anacrotic: limb; pulse
anaerobic: cellulitis; dehydrogenase; pneumonia; respiration
anagen: effluvium
anal: atresia; canal; cleft; columns; crypts; cushions; ducts; erotism; fascia; fissure; fistula; gland; membrane; orifice; pecten; phase; pit; plate; reflex; region; sinuses; triangle; valves; verge
analeptic: enema
analgesic: cuirass; nephritis; nephropathy
anal skin: tag
anal transitional: zone
analytic: chemistry; psychiatry; study; therapy
analytical: psychology; sensitivity; specificity
analyzing: rod
anamnestic: reaction; response
anaphase: lag
anaphylactic: antibody; intoxication; reaction; shock
anaphylactoid: crisis; purpura; shock
anaplastic: astrocytoma; carcinoma; cell; oligodendroglioma
anaplastic large cell: lymphoma
anaplerotic: reaction
anarthritic rheumatoid: disease
anastomosing: fibers; vessel
anastomotic: branch; branch of middle meningeal artery with lacrimal artery; stricture; ulcer; veins; vessel
anatomic: airway; pathology; position; rigidity; sphincter; tooth; tubercle; wart
anatomical: age; conjugate; crown; element; neck of humerus; root
anatomical internal: os of uterus
anatomic dead: space
anatrophic: nephrotomy
anchor: splint
anchorage: dependence
anchoring: fibrils; villus
ancillary: ports
anconal: fossa
anconeus: muscle
ancylostoma: dermatitis
Andernach: ossicles
Anders: disease
Andersch: ganglion; nerve
Andersen: disease
Anderson: splint
Anderson-Collip: test
Anderson and Goldberger: test
Andes: virus
Andral: decubitus
androgen: unit
androgen binding: protein
androgenic: alopecia; hormone; zone
androgen insensitivity: syndrome
androgen resistance: syndromes
android: obesity; pelvis
anechoic: chamber
Anel: method
anemic: anoxia; halo; hypoxia; infarct; murmur
anergic: leishmaniasis
aneroid: manometer
anesthesia: machine; record
anesthetic: circuit; depth; ether; gas; index; leprosy; shock; vapor
anestrous: ovulation
aneurysm: needle
aneurysmal: bruit; cough; murmur; sac; varix
aneurysmal bone: cyst
angel: wing
Angelman: syndrome
Angelucci: syndrome
Anger: camera
anginose: scarlatina
angioblastic: cells; cyst
angiodysgenetic: myelomalacia
angiofollicular mediastinal lymph node: hyperplasia
angiogenesis: factor
angiography: catheter
angioid: streaks
angioimmunoblastic: lymphadenopathy with dysproteinemia
angiolithic: degeneration; sarcoma
angiolymphoid: hyperplasia with eosinophilia
angioneurotic: edema
angioosteohypertrophy: syndrome
angiopathic: neurasthenia
angiopathic hemolytic: anemia
angioplasty: balloon
angiotensin: receptor
angiotensin-converting: enzyme
angiotensin-converting enzyme: inhibitors
angiotensin receptor: blockers
Angle: classification of malocclusion
angle: recession
angle of: convergence
angle-closure: glaucoma
Ångström: law; scale; unit
angular: acceleration; aldehyde; aperture; artery; cheilitis; conjunctivitis; convolution; curvature; gyrus; incisure; methyl; notch; spine; stomatitis; vein
anhepatic: jaundice
anhepatogenous: jaundice

anhidrotic ectodermal: dysplasia
anhydrous: alcohol; chloral; lanolin
anicteric: hepatitis; leptospirosis
anicteric virus: hepatitis
aniline: fuchsin
animal: charcoal; dextran; force; graft; magnetism; model; pole; psychology; soap; starch; toxin; viruses; wax
animal protein: factor
anion: gap
anion-exchange: resin
anionic: detergents
anionic neutrophil-activating: peptide
anisometropic: amblyopia
anisotropic: disks; lipid
Anitschkow: cell; myocyte
ankle: bone; clonus; jerk; joint; reflex; region
ankle-foot: orthosis
ankyloglossia superior: syndrome
ankylosed: tooth
ankylosing: hyperostosis; spondylitis
annealing: lamp; tray
annectent: gyrus
annihilation: radiation
annulate: lamellae
annuloaortic: ectasia
annuloplasty: ring
annulospiral: ending; organ
anococcygeal: body; ligament; nerve
anocutaneous: line
anodal: current
anodal closure: contraction
anodal opening: contraction
anode: rays
anogenital: band; raphe
anomalous: complex; conduction; trichromatism; uterus; viscosity
anomalous atrioventricular: excitation
anomalous mitral: arcade
anomalous pulmonary venous: connections, total or partial
anomalous retinal: correspondence
anomeric: carbon
anomic: aphasia
anonymous: veins
anorectal: angle; flexure; junction; lymph nodes; spasm; syndrome
anorectoperineal: muscles
anosognosic: epilepsy; seizures
anospinal: center

anovular: menstruation
anovular ovarian: follicle
anovulational: menstruation
anovulatory: cycle
anoxemia: test
anoxic: anoxia
ANP: receptors
ANP clearance: receptors
Anrep: effect; phenomenon
anserine: bursa; bursitis
ansiform: lobule
ansoparamedian: fissure
antagonistic: muscles; reflexes
antalgic: gait
antebrachial: fascia
antebrachial flexor: retinaculum
antecedent: sign
antecubital: space
antegonial: notch
antegrade: block; cardioplegia; conduction; cystography; pyelography; urography
antemortem: clot; thrombus
antenatal: diagnosis
anterior: aphasia; arch of atlas; asynclitism; belly of digastric muscle; border; border of body of pancreas; border of eyelids; border of fibula; border of lung; border of pancreas; border of radius; border of testis; border of tibia; border of ulna; branch; branch of the renal artery; canaliculus of chorda tympani; cells; centriole; chamber of eyeball; choroiditis; column; column of medulla oblongata; commissure; commissure of the larynx; compartment of arm; compartment of forearm; compartment of leg; compartment of thigh; component of force; crus of stapes; curvature; cusp of left atrioventricular valve; cusp of mitral valve; cusp of right atrioventricular valve; cusp of tricuspid valve; divisions of (trunks of) brachial plexus; embryotoxon; epithelium of cornea; extremity of caudate nucleus; extremity of spleen; fascicle of palatopharyngeus (muscle); fasciculus proprius; fontanelle; fovea; funiculus; guide; horn; layer of rectus sheath; layer of thoracolumbar fascia; ligament of fibular head; ligament of Helmholtz; ligament of malleus; limb of internal capsule; limb of stapes; lip of external os of uterus; lip of uterine os; lobe of hypophysis; margin; mediastinoscopy; mediastinotomy; mediastinum; megalophthalmos; naris; neuropore; notch of auricle; notch of cerebellum; notch of ear; nuclei of thalamus; nucleus; nucleus; nucleus of trapezoid body; occlusion; part; part of anterior commissure of brain; part of diaphragmatic surface of liver; part of fornix of vagina; part of pons; part of tongue; pillar of fauces; pillar of fornix; pituitary; pole of eyeball; pole of lens; portion of left medial segment IV of liver; process of malleus; pyramid; rami of cervical nerves; rami of lumbar nerves; rami of sacral nerves; rami of thoracic nerves; ramus of lateral sulcus of cerebrum; ramus of spinal nerve; recess; recess of tympanic membrane; region of arm; region of elbow; region of forearm; region of knee; region of leg; region of neck; region of thigh; region of wrist; rhinoscopy; rhizotomy; root of spinal nerve; scleritis; sclerotomy; segment; sinuses; staphyloma; surface; surface of arm; surface of cornea; surface of elbow; surface of eyelids; surface of forearm; surface of iris; surface of kidney; surface of leg; surface of lens; surface of lower limb; surface of maxilla; surface of patella; surface of petrous part of temporal bone; surface of prostate; surface of radius; surface of suprarenal gland; surface of thigh; surface of ulna; surface of uterus; symblepharon; synechia; thoracotomy; tooth; triangle of neck; tubercle of atlas; tubercle of cervical vertebrae; tubercle of thalamus; urethra; urethritis; uveitis; vein of septum pellucidum; vitrectomy; wall of middle ear; wall of stomach; wall of tympanic cavity; wall of vagina
anterior abdominal cutaneous: branch of intercostal nerve
anterior acoustic: stria
anterior ampullary: nerve
anterior amygdaloid: area
anterior antebrachial: nerve; region
anterior apprehension: test
anterior articular: surface of dens
anterior atlanto-occipital: membrane
anterior auricular: branches of superficial temporal artery; groove; muscle; nerves; vein
anterior axillary: fold; line; lymph nodes
anterior basal: branch; branch of superior basal vein (of right and left inferior pulmonary veins); vein
anterior basal (bronchopulmonary): segment [S VIII]
anterior basal segmental: artery
anterior brachial: region
anterior (bronchopulmonary): segment [S III]
anterior cardiac: veins
anterior carpal: region
anterior cecal: artery
anterior central: convolution; gyrus
anterior cerebellar: notch
anterior cerebral: artery; veins
anterior cervical: lymph nodes; region
anterior cervical intertransversarii: muscles
anterior cervical intertransverse: muscles
anterior chamber: trabecula
anterior chamber cleavage: syndrome
anterior choroidal: artery
anterior ciliary: arteries; veins
anterior circumflex humeral: artery; vein
anterior clear: space
anterior clinoid: process
anterior communicating: artery
anterior condyloid: canal of occipital bone; foramen
anterior conjunctival: artery
anterior corneal: dystrophy
anterior coronary periarterial: plexus

anterior corticospinal: tract
anterior costotransverse: ligament
anterior cranial: base; fossa
anterior cruciate: ligament
anterior crural: nerve; region
anterior cubital: region
anterior cutaneous: branches of femoral nerve; branches of intercostal nerves; branch of iliohypogastric nerve; nerves of abdomen
anterior deep cervical: lymph nodes
anterior elastic: layer
anterior ethmoidal: artery; cells; nerve
anterior ethmoidal air: cells
anterior external arcuate: fibers
anterior facial: height; vein
anterior femoral cutaneous: nerves
anterior focal: point
anterior gastric: branches of anterior vagal trunk
anterior glandular: branch of superior thyroid artery
anterior gray: column; commissure
anterior ground: bundle
anterior horn: cell
anterior humeral circumflex: artery
anterior hypothalamic: area; nucleus; region
anterior inferior cerebellar: artery
anterior inferior iliac: spine
anterior inferior renal: segment
anterior inferior segmental: artery of kidney
anterior intercondylar: area of tibia
anterior intercostal: arteries; branches of internal thoracic artery; veins
anterior intermediate: groove; sulcus
anterior interosseous: artery; nerve
anterior interpositus: nucleus
anterior interventricular: artery; branch of left coronary artery; groove; sulcus
anterior intestinal: portal
anterior intraoccipital: joint; synchondrosis
anterior jugular: lymph nodes; vein
anterior junction: line
anterior knee: region
anterior labial: arteries; branches of deep external pudendal artery; commissure; nerves; veins
anterior lacrimal: crest
anterior lateral malleolar: artery
anterior lateral nasal: branches of anterior ethmoidal artery
anterior/lateral/posterior glandular: branches of superior thyroid artery
anterior and lateral thoracic: regions
anterior limiting: lamina; layer of cornea; ring
anterior lingual: gland
anterior longitudinal: ligament
anterior lunate: lobule
anterior medial malleolar: artery
anterior median: fissure of medulla oblongata; fissure of spinal cord; line
anterior mediastinal: arteries; lymph nodes
anterior medullary: velum
anterior meningeal: artery; branch (of anterior ethmoidal artery)
anterior meniscofemoral: ligament
anterior myocardial: infarction
anterior nasal: spine; spine of maxilla
anterior ocular: segment
anterior olfactory: nucleus
anterior palatine: arch; foramen
anterior palpebral: margin
anterior paracentral: gyrus
anterior parietal: artery
anterior parolfactory: sulcus
anterior pectoral cutaneous: branch of intercostal nerves
anterior pelvic: exenteration
anterior perforated: substance
anterior perforating: arteries
anterior periventricular: nucleus
anterior peroneal: artery
anterior piriform: gyrus
anterior pituitary: gonadotropin
anterior pituitary-like: hormone
anterior pontomesencephalic: vein
(anterior and posterior) radicular: arteries
(anterior and posterior) superior pancreaticoduodenal: artery
(anterior and posterior) vestibular: veins
anterior primary: division
anterior pyramidal: fasciculus; tract
anterior quadrigeminal: body
anterior raphespinal: tract
anterior rectus: muscle of head
anterior sacrococcygeal: ligament
anterior sacroiliac: ligaments
anterior sacrosciatic: ligament
anterior scalene: muscle
anterior scrotal: branch of deep external pudendal artery; nerves; veins
anterior segmental: artery
anterior semicircular: canals
anterior septal: branches of anterior ethmoidal artery
anterior serratus: muscle
anterior spinal: artery
anterior spinocerebellar: tract
anterior spinothalamic: tract
anterior sternoclavicular: ligament
anterior superficial cervical: lymph nodes
anterior superior alveolar: arteries; branches of infraorbital nerve; nerves
anterior superior dental: arteries
anterior superior iliac: spine
anterior superior renal: segment
anterior superior segmental: artery of kidney
anterior supraclavicular: nerve
anterior talar articular: surface of calcaneus
anterior talofibular: ligament
anterior talotibial: ligament
anterior tarsal tendinous: sheaths
anterior tegmental: decussation
anterior temporal: artery; branch
anterior thalamic: radiation; tubercle
anterior tibial: artery; bursa; lymph node; muscle; nerve; node; veins
anterior tibial compartment: syndrome
anterior tibial recurrent: artery
anterior tibiofibular: ligament
anterior tibiotalar: ligament; part of deltoid ligament; part of medial ligament of ankle joint
anterior transverse temporal: gyrus
anterior trigeminothalamic: tract
anterior tympanic: artery
anterior urethral: valve
anterior vertebral: vein
anterior vestibular: artery
anterior white: commissure
anterodorsal: nucleus of thalamus
anterofacial: dysplasia
anterograde: amnesia; block; conduction; memory
anteroinferior: surface of pancreas
anteroinferior myocardial: infarction
anterolateral: column of spinal cord; cordotomy; fontanelle; groove; sulcus; surface of arytenoid cartilage; surface of (shaft of) humerus; system; tract; tractotomy
anterolateral central: arteries
anterolateral myocardial: infarction
anterolateral striate: arteries
anterolateral thalamostriate: arteries
anteromedial: nucleus; nucleus of thalamus; surface of shaft of humerus
anteromedial central: arteries; branches
anteromedial frontal: branch of callosomarginal artery
anteromedial intermuscular: septum
anteromedial thalamostriate: arteries
anteromedian: groove
anteroposterior: diameter of the pelvic inlet; projection
anteroseptal myocardial: infarction
anterosuperior: surface of body of pancreas
anteroventral: nucleus of thalamus
anthracotic: tuberculosis
anthrax: septicemia; toxin
anthropoid: pelvis
anthroponotic cutaneous: leishmaniasis
antialopecia: factor
antianemic: factor; principle
antiangiogenesis: factor
antianxiety: agent
anti–basement membrane: antibody; glomerulonephritis; nephritis
antiberiberi: factor; vitamin

antibiotic: enterocolitis; sensitivity
antibiotic sensitivity: test
anti–black-tongue: factor
antibody: excess
antibody-combining: site
antibody deficiency: disease; syndrome
antibody-dependent cell-mediated: cytotoxicity
anticardiolipin: antibodies
anticoagulant: therapy
anticoding: strand
anticomplementary: factor; serum
anti-D: immunoglobulin
antidermatitis: factor
antidiuretic: hormone
antidyskinetic: agent
antiepithelial: serum
antifoaming: agents
anti-G: suit
antigen: excess; interferon; peptides; unit
antigen-antibody: complex; reaction
antigen-binding: site
antigenic: competition; complex; determinant; drift; shift
antigen-presenting: cells
antigen-responsive: cell
antigen-sensitive: cell
antiglobulin: test
antigravity: muscles
antihemophilic: factor A; factor B; globulin; globulin A; globulin B; plasma
antihemorrhagic: factor; vitamin
antihuman: globulin
antihuman globulin: test
antiidiotype: antibody; autoantibody
anti–kidney serum: nephritis
antilymphocyte: globulin; serum
anti-MAG: antibody
antimicrobial: spectrum
anti-Monson: curve
anti-müllerian: hormone
antineuritic: factor; vitamin
antineutrophil cytoplasmic: antibodies; antibody
antinuclear: antibody; factor
antiparallel: strand
antipellagra: factor
antipernicious anemia: factor
antiphospholipid: antibodies
antipodal: cone
anti-Pr cold: autoagglutinin
antipsychotic: agent
antirabies: serum
antirachitic: vitamins
antireflection: coating
antireticular cytotoxic: serum

antiscorbutic: vitamin
antisense: DNA; RNA; strand; therapy
antiseptic: dressing
antiserum: anaphylaxis
antisocial: personality
antisocial personality: disorder
antisterility: factor; vitamin
antitermination: protein
antithrombin: test
antithyroglobulin: antibody
antitoxic: serum
antitoxin: rash; unit
antitragicus: muscle
antitragohelicine: fissure
antitrypsin: deficiency
α₁-antitrypsin: deficiency
α₁-antitrypsin deficiency: panniculitis
antitryptic: index
antitumor: enzyme; protein
antivenene: unit
antiviral: immunity; protein
Anton: syndrome
Antoni type A: neurilemoma
Antoni type B: neurilemoma
antral: follicle; lavage; pouch; sphincter
Antyllus: method
anular: band; cartilage; cataract; ligament; ligament of radius; ligament of stapes; ligaments of trachea; lipid; pancreas; part of fibrous digital sheath of digits of hand and foot; placenta; plexus; pulley; scleritis; scotoma; sphincter; staphyloma; stricture; synechia; syphilid
anvil: sound
anxiety: disorders; dream; hysteria; neurosis; reaction; syndrome
anxiety tension: state
anxious: delirium
aortic: aneurysm; arch; arches; area (of auscultation); atresia; bifurcation; bodies; bulb; coarctation; dissection; dwarfism; facies; foramen; glomera; hiatus; impression of left lung; incompetence; insufficiency; isthmus; knob; knuckle; murmur; nerve; nipple; notch; opening; orifice; ostium; reflex; regurgitation; sac; sinus; spindle; stenosis; sulcus; valve; vestibule; window
aortic arch: syndrome
aortic body: tumor
aortic lymphatic: plexus
aortico-left ventricular: tunnel

aorticopulmonary: window
aorticorenal: ganglia
aortic-pulmonic: window
aortic septal: defect
aortic sinus: aneurysm
aortoannular: ectasia
aortocoronary: bypass
aortoiliac: bypass
aortoiliac occlusive: disease
aortopulmonary: septum; window
aortorenal: bypass
AP: projection
APACHE: score
apallic: state; syndrome
apathetic: thyrotoxicosis
apatite: calculus
A-pattern: esotropia; exotropia; strabismus
A-P-C: virus
APC: compound
ape: fissure; hand
aperiodic: biopolymer
aperiosteal: amputation
Apert: hirsutism; syndrome
aperture: diaphragm
apex: beat; impulse; pneumonia
apex anterior: angulation
apex posterior: angulation
Apgar: score
aphakic: eye; glaucoma
aphonic: pectoriloquy
aphthous: stomatitis
apical: abscess; angle; area; branch of inferior lobar branch of right pulmonary artery; branch of right superior pulmonary vein; cap; complex; dendrite; foramen of tooth; gland; granuloma; infarction; infection; ligament of dens; periodontitis; process; space; vein
apical-aortic: conduit
apical axillary: lymph nodes
apical (bronchopulmonary): segment [S I]
apical dental: foramen
apical ectodermal: ridge
apical lordotic: projection
apical periodontal: abscess; cyst
apical segmental: artery; artery of superior lobar artery of right lung
apicoposterior: artery; branch of left superior pulmonary vein; vein
apicoposterior (bronchopulmonary): segment [SI + SII]
aplanatic: lens
aplastic: anemia; lymph
apnea-hypopnea: index

apneic: oxygenation; pause
apneustic: breathing
apochromatic: lens; objective
apocrine: adenoma; carcinoma; chromhidrosis; gland; hidrocystoma; metaplasia; miliaria
apocrine sweat: glands
apolar: bond; cell; interaction
aponeurogenic: ptosis
aponeurotic: fibroma; reflex
apophysary: point
apophysial: fracture
apoplectic: cyst; retinitis
apothecaries: weight
apparent: leukonychia; viscosity
appendiceal: abscess
appendicular: artery; colic; lymph nodes; muscle; skeleton; vein
apperceptive: mass
appetite: juice
appetitive: behavior
applanation: tonometer
apple jelly: nodules
applied: anatomy; anthropology; chemistry
appliqué: forms
apposition: suture
appositional: growth
approach-approach: conflict
approach-avoidance: conflict
approximal: surface of tooth
approximation: suture
Apt: test
aptitude: test
APUD: cells
apyretic: typhoid
aquagenic: pruritus
aqueduct: veil
aqueductal: intubation
aqueous: chambers; flare; humor; phase; solution; vaccine; vein
aqueous influx: phenomenon
aquo-: ion
arachnoid: cyst; foramen; granulations; membrane; trabecula; villi
arachnoidal: granulations
arachnoidea: mater cranialis; mater encephali
Aran-Duchenne: disease
Arantius: ligament; nodule; ventricle
arborescent: cataract
arborization: block
arc: perimeter
arc-flash: conjunctivitis
arch: bar; form; length; wire
archaic-paralogical: thinking
arched: crest
archenteric: canal
arch length: deficiency
arch-loop-whorl: system

arciform: arteries; veins of kidney
arcon: articulator
arcuate: arteries of kidney; artery (of foot) (inconstant); crest; crest of arytenoid cartilage; eminence; fasciculus; fibers; fibers of cerebrum; line; line of ilium; line of rectus sheath; nucleus; nucleus of thalamus; scotoma; uterus; veins of kidney; zone
arcuate popliteal: ligament
arcuate pubic: ligament
ardent: fever; spirits
areolar: choroiditis; choroidopathy; glands; tissue; tubercles
areolar venous: plexus
argentaffin: cells; granules
Argentinean hemorrhagic: fever
Argentine hemorrhagic fever: virus
arginine: oxytocin; vasopressin; vasotocin
argininosuccinic: aciduria
arginosuccinate lyase: deficiency
argon: laser
Argyll Robertson: pupil
argyrophilic: cells; fibers
Arias-Stella: effect; phenomenon; reaction
aristotelian: method
Aristotle: anomaly
arithmetic: mean
Arlt: operation; sinus
arm: bone; phenomenon
Armanni-Ebstein: change; kidney
armed: macrophage; rostellum
Armitage-Doll: model
armor: heart
armored: heart
Army Alpha: tests
Army Beta: tests
Army General Classification: Test
Arndt: law
Arndt-Gottron: syndrome
Arneth: classification; count; formula; index; stages
Arnold: bodies; bundle; canal; ganglion; nerve; tract
Arnold-Chiari: deformity; malformation; syndrome
aromatase: inhibitors
aromatic: bitters; castor oil; compound; series; water
aromatic ammonia: spirit
arousal: function; reaction
arrector: muscle of hair
arrector pili: muscles
arrest: signal

arrest of active phase: dystocia
arrest of descent: dystocia
arrested: tuberculosis
arrested dental: caries
Arrhenius: doctrine; equation; law
Arrhenius-Madsen: theory
arrow: poison
arrow point: tracing
Arruga: forceps
arsenic: pigmentation
arsenical: keratosis; polyneuropathy
arseniureted: hydrogen
arterial: arcades; arches of colon; arches of ileum; arches of jejunum; arch of lower eyelid; arch of upper eyelid; blood; bulb; canal; capillary; circle of cerebrum; cone; duct; flap; forceps; grooves; hyperemia; hypotension; ligament; line; murmur; nephrosclerosis; plexus; sclerosis; segments of kidney; spider; tension; transfusion; vein; wave
arterial switch: operation
arterial thoracic outlet: syndrome
arteriocapillary: sclerosis
arteriococcygeal: gland
arteriolar: nephrosclerosis; network; sclerosis
arteriolosclerotic: kidney
arteriolovenular: anastomosis; bridge
arteriosclerotic: aneurysm; gangrene; kidney; retinopathy
arteriovenous: anastomosis; aneurysm; fistula; nicking; shunt
arteriovenous carbon dioxide: difference
arteriovenous oxygen: difference
arthritic: atrophy; calculus
arthritic general: pseudoparalysis
arthrodial: articulation; cartilage; joint
Arthus: phenomenon; reaction
articular: branches; capsule; cartilage; cavity; chondrocalcinosis; circumference of head of radius; circumference of head of ulna; corpuscles; crepitus; crescent; crest; disk; disk of acromioclavicular joint; disk of distal radioulnar joint; disk of sternoclavicular joint; disk of

temporomandibular joint; eminence of temporal bone; facet; facet of head of fibula; facet of head of rib; facet of lateral malleolus; facet of medial malleolus; facet of radial head; facet of tubercle of rib; fossa of temporal bone; fracture; gout; labrum; lamella; leprosy; lip; margin; meniscus; muscle; muscle of elbow; muscle of knee; nerve; network; pit of head of radius; process; rheumatism; sensibility; surface; surface of acromion; surface of arytenoid cartilage; surface of mandibular fossa of temporal bone; surface on calcaneus for cuboid bone; surface of patella; tubercle of temporal bone
articularis cubiti: muscle
articularis genus: muscle
articular vascular: circle; network; network of elbow; network of knee; plexus
articulated: skeleton
articulating: paper
articulation: disorders
artificial: anatomy; ankylosis; crown; dentition; eye; fever; heart; insemination; intelligence; kidney; melanin; pacemaker; pneumothorax; pupil; radioactivity; respiration; selection; sphincter; stone; tears; ventilation
artificial active: immunity
artificial Carlsbad: salt
artificial Kissingen: salt
artificial membrane: rupture
artificial passive: immunity
artificial Vichy: salt
artistic: anatomy
arycorniculate: synchondrosis
aryepiglottic: fold; muscle; part of oblique arytenoid muscle
arylated: alkyl
arylsulfatase A: deficiency
arylsulfatase B: deficiency
arytenoepiglottidean: fold
arytenoid: cartilage; dislocation; glands; subluxation; swelling
arytenoidal articular: surface of cricoid
asbestos: bodies; corn; liner; wart
ascending: aorta; artery; branch; branch of the inferior mesenteric artery;

branch of superficial cervical artery; cholangitis; colon; current; degeneration; myelitis; neuritis; paralysis; part of aorta; part of duodenum; part of trapezius (muscle); process; pyelonephritis; ramus of lateral sulcus of cerebrum
ascending cervical: artery
ascending frontal: convolution; gyrus
ascending lumbar: vein
ascending palatine: artery
ascending parietal: convolution; gyrus
ascending pharyngeal: artery; plexus
ascertainment: bias
Ascher: syndrome
Ascher aqueous influx: phenomenon
Aschheim-Zondek: test
Aschner: phenomenon; reflex
Aschner-Dagnini: reflex
Aschoff: bodies; cell; nodules
Ascoli: reaction; test
ascorbate-cyanide: test
Aselli: gland; pancreas
aseptic: fever; necrosis; surgery
asexual: dwarfism; generation; reproduction
Ashby: method
ashen: tuber; tubercle; wing
Asherman: syndrome
ash-leaf: macule
Ashman: phenomenon
ashy: dermatosis
asialoglycoprotein: receptor
Asian: influenza
Asiatic: cholera; schistosomiasis
asiderotic: anemia
Askanazy: cell
Ask-Upmark: kidney
Asperger: disorder
aspermatogenic: sterility
aspheric: lens
asphyxiating thoracic: chondrodystrophy; dysplasia; dystrophy
aspirating: needle
aspiration: biopsy; pneumonia
asplenia: syndrome
Assam: fever
assassin: bug
assertive: conditioning; training
Assézat: triangle
assident: sign; symptom
assimilation: pelvis; sacrum
assist-control: ventilation
assisted: circulation; respiration; ventilation
assisted cephalic: delivery

assisted reproductive: technology
assistive: movement
Assmann tuberculous: infiltrate
associated: antagonist; movements
association: areas; constant; cortex; fibers; mechanism; neurosis; system; test; time; tract
associative: aphasia; reaction; strength
assortative: mating
astacoid: rash
astatic: seizure
asteroid: body; hyalosis
asthenic: personality
asthenic personality: disorder
asthma: crystals
asthmatic: bronchitis
asthmatoid: wheeze
astigmatic: dial; lens
Astler-Coller: classification
astral: fibers
astroglia: cell
Astwood: test
asymmetric: chondrodystrophy; disulfide
asymmetric fetal growth: restriction
asymmetric motor: neuropathy
asymptomatic: neurosyphilis
asynchronous pulse: generator
A/T: cloning
atactic: abasia; agraphia
atavistic: epiphysis
ataxia telangiectasia: syndrome
ataxic: aphasia; breathing; dysarthria; gait; paramyotonia; paraplegia
atelectatic: rale
ateliotic: dwarfism
atheromatous: degeneration; embolism; plaque
atherosclerotic: aneurysm
athlete's: foot; heart
athletic: heart
atlantic: part of vertebral artery
atlantoaxial: joint
atlanto-occipital: articulation; joint; membrane
atmospheric: pressure
atomic: core; heat; number; theory; volume; weight
atomic absorption: spectrophotometry
atomic mass: unit
atomistic: psychology
atonic: bladder; dyspepsia; ectropion; entropion; epiphora; seizure; ulcer

atopic: allergy; asthma; cataract; dermatitis; eczema; keratoconjunctivitis; reagin
ATP: citrate (*pro-3S*)-lyase; cobalamin adenoxyltransferase
atrabiliary: capsule
atraumatic: needle; suture
atresic: teratosis
atretic: corpus luteum
atretic ovarian: follicle
atrial: appendage; arteries; auricle; auricula; bigeminy; branches; capture; complex; diastole; dissociation; echo; extrasystole; fibrillation; flutter; gallop; kick; myxoma; septostomy; sound; standstill; systole; tachycardia
atrial anastomotic: branch of circumflex branch of left coronary artery
atrial capture: beat
atrial chaotic: tachycardia
atrial fusion: beat
atrial natriuretic: factor; peptide
atrial septal: defect
atrial synchronous pulse: generator
atrial transport: function
atrial triggered pulse: generator
atrial ventricular canal: defect
atrial-well: technique
atriosystolic: murmur
atrioventricular: band; block; bundle; canal; conduction; connections; dissociation; extrasystole; gradient; groove; interval; node; septum; sulcus; valves
atrioventricular canal: cushions
atrioventricular junctional: bigeminy; rhythm; tachycardia
atrioventricular nodal: branch
atrophic: arthritis; excavation; gastritis; glossitis; heterochromia; inflammation; kidney; pharyngitis; rhinitis; thrombosis; vaginitis
atropine: test
attached: craniotomy; gingiva
attached cranial: section
attachment: apparatus
attack: rate
attending: physician; staff; surgeon
attention: span
attention deficit: disorder

attention deficit hyperactivity: disorder
attenuated: tuberculosis; vaccine; virus
attenuation: compensation
attitudinal: reflexes
attraction: sphere
attributable: risk
atypical: achromatopsia; fibroxanthoma; gingivitis; lipoma; measles; mycobacteria; pneumonia; pseudocholinesterase
atypical absence: seizure
atypical antipsychotic: agent
atypical endometrial: hyperplasia
atypical facial: neuralgia
atypical glandular: cells of undetermined significance
atypical melanocytic: hyperplasia
atypical squamous: cells of undetermined significance
atypical trigeminal: neuralgia
atypical verrucous: endocarditis
Au: antigen
Aub-DuBois: table
Aubert: phenomenon
audiogenic: seizure
auditory: agnosia; alternans; aphasia; area; aura; canal; capsule; cortex; fatigue; feedback; field; ganglion; hairs; hallucination; hyperesthesia; lemniscus; localization; nerve; neuropathy; nucleus; organ; ossicles; pathway; pits; placodes; process; prosthesis; reflex; striae; strings; teeth; threshold; tract; tube; vesicle
auditory brainstem: response
auditory oculogyric: reflex
auditory receptor: cells
Auenbrugger: sign
Auer: bodies; rods
Auerbach: ganglia; plexus
Aufrecht: sign
Auger: electron
augmentation: mammaplasty
augmented: lead
augmented histamine: test
augmentor: fibers; nerves
Aujeszky disease: virus
aural: myiasis; vertigo
auramine O fluorescent: stain
auricular: appendage; appendectomy; appendix; arc; branch of occipital artery; branch of posterior auricular artery; branch of vagus nerve; canaliculus; cartilage; complex;

extrasystole; fissure; ganglion; index; ligaments; muscles; notch; point; reflex; standstill; surface of ilium; surface of sacrum; systole; tachycardia; triangle; tubercle; veins
auricularis anterior: muscle
auricularis posterior: muscle
auricularis superior: muscle
auriculoinfraorbital: plane
auriculopalpebral: reflex
auriculopressor: reflex
auriculotemporal: nerve
auriculotemporal nerve: syndrome
auriculoventricular: groove; interval
auropalpebral: reflex
Aus: antigen
auscultatory: triangle
auscultatory: alternans; gap; percussion; sound
Auspitz: sign
aussage: test
Austin Flint: murmur; phenomenon
Australia: antigen
Australian bat: Lyssavirus
Australian Q: fever
Australian tick: typhus
Australian X: disease; encephalitis
Australian X disease: virus
autacoid: substance
authoritarian: personality
authority: figure
autistic: disorder; parasite
autochthonous: ideas; malaria; parasite
autocrine: hypothesis
autoerythrocyte: sensitization
autoerythrocyte sensitization: syndrome
autogeneic: graft
autogenous: control; keratoplasty; union; vaccine
autohemolysis: test
autoimmune: disease; thyroiditis
autoimmune hemolytic: anemia
autoimmune neonatal: thrombocytopenia
autokinetic: effect
autologous: graft; protein
autolytic: enzyme
automated differential leukocyte: counter
automated lamellar: keratectomy
automatic: audiometer; audiometry; beat; condenser; contraction; epilepsy; plugger

automatic auditory brainstem: response
automatic gain: control
automotor: seizure
autonomic: division of nervous system; epilepsy; ganglia; imbalance; nerve; part; part of peripheral nervous system; plexuses; seizure
autonomic motor: neuron
autonomic nerve: fibers
autonomic nervous: system
autonomic neurogenic: bladder
autonomic (visceral motor): nuclei
autonomous: psychotherapy
autoparenchymatous: metaplasia
autophagic: vacuole
autoplastic: graft
autopolymer: resin
autoscopic: phenomenon
autoserum: therapy
autosomal: gene
autumn: fever
auxanographic: method
auxetic: growth
auxiliary: abutment
auxotrophic: mutant; strains
AV: difference; interval; junction
A-V: valves
available arch: length
avalanche: conduction
avascular: necrosis
Avellis: syndrome
average flow: rate
average pulse: magnitude
aversion: therapy
aversive: behavior; conditioning; control; stimulus; training
avian: sarcoma
avian encephalomyelitis: virus
avian influenza: virus
avian lymphomatosis: virus
avian neurolymphomatosis: virus
avian pneumoencephalitis: virus
avian viral arthritis: virus
aviation: medicine
aviator's: disease
avidity: antibody
AV junctional: rhythm; tachycardia
Avogadro: constant; hypothesis; law; number; postulate
avoidance: conditioning; training
avoidance-avoidance: conflict

avoidant: disorder of adolescence; disorder of childhood; personality
avoidant personality: disorder
A-V strabismus: syndrome
avulsed: wound
avulsion: fracture
axial: ametropia; aneurysm; angle; cataract; current; filament; hyperopia; illumination; muscle; myopia; neuritis; plane; plate; point; projection; section; skeleton; surfaces; view; walls of the pulp chambers
axial pattern: flap
axilla: thermometer
axillary: anesthesia; arch; artery; cavity; fascia; fold; fossa; glands; hairs; line; lymph nodes; nerve; plexus; region; sheath; space; thermometer; thoracotomy; triangle; vein
axillary arch: muscle
axillary lymphatic: plexus
axillary sweat: glands
axiolabiolingual: plane
axiomesiodistal: plane
axis: corpuscle; cylinder; deviation; ligament of malleus; shift; traction
axis-traction: forceps
axoaxonic: synapse
axodendritic: synapse
axon: degeneration; hillock; reflex; terminals
axonal: degeneration; polyneuropathy; process
axonal terminal: boutons
axon loss: polyneuropathy
axoplasmic: transport
axosomatic: synapse
Ayala: index; quotient
Ayerza: disease; syndrome
Ayre: brush
azin: dyes
azo: dyes; itch
azocarmine: dyes
Azorean: disease
azotemic: retinitis
azotobacter: nuclease
Aztec: ear
azure: lunula of nails
azurophil: granule
azygoesophageal: recess
azygos: artery of vagina; fissure; lobe of right lung; vein

B

β_1-: lipoprotein
β_2-: microglobulin

β: corynebacteriophage; hemolysin; hemolysis; phage; thalassemia
β_{1C}: globulin
B: bile; cell; chain; fibers; lymphocyte; virus; wave
B19: virus
B_T: factor
B-: DNA
β-: microglobulin
β-δ: thalassemia
Babbitt: metal
Babcock: tube
Babès: nodes
Babinski: phenomenon; reflex; sign; syndrome
baby: tooth
baby bottle: syndrome
Baccelli: sign
Bachman: test
Bachmann: bundle
Bachman-Pettit: test
bacillary: angiomatosis; dysentery; layer
Bacillus anthracis: toxin
bacillus Calmette-Guérin: vaccine
back: cross; mutation; pressure; tooth
back-action: plugger
backboard: splint
back of foot: reflex
background: level; radiation
back table: procedure
back vertex: power
backward: curvature
backward heart: failure
backwash: ileitis
Bacon: anoscope
bacterial: allergy; antagonism; capsule; cast; cystitis; encephalitis; endarteritis; endocarditis; growth; hemolysin; interference; peliosis; pericarditis; photosynthesis; plaque; pneumonia; toxin; translocation; vaginosis; vegetations; virus
bacterial food: poisoning
bacteriocin: factors
bacteriocinogenic: plasmids
bacteriogenic: agglutination
bacteriolytic: serum
bacteriophage: immunity; plaque; resistance; typing
bacteriostatic: agent
bacteriotropic: substance
Baehr-Lohlein: lesion
Baelz: disease
Baer: law; vesicle
Baermann: concentration
Baeyer: theory
bag of: waters
bag: ventilation
Baggenstoss: change

Bagolini: test
Baillarger: bands; lines
Bailliart: ophthalmodynamometer
Bainbridge: reflex
baked: tongue
Baker: cyst
baker: eczema; itch
Baker acid: hematein
Baker pyridine: extraction
baking: soda
Balamuth aqueous egg yolk infusion: medium
balance: theory
balanced: anesthesia; articulation; bite; diet; occlusion; polymorphism; translocation
balancing: contact; side
balancing occlusal: surface
balancing side: condyle
balanic: hypospadias
balanitic: epispadias
balantidial: dysentery
Balbani: ring
bald: tongue
Baldy: operation
Balint: syndrome
Balkan: beam; frame; nephropathy; splint
Ball: operation
ball: thrombus; valve; variance
Ballance: sign
ballerina-foot: pattern
balloon: atrioseptostomy; catheter; cell; septostomy; sickness
balloon cell: nevus
balloon counter: pulsation
ballooning: degeneration
balloon-tip: catheter
ballpoint pen: technique
ball and socket: abutment; joint
ball-valve: thrombus
ball valve: action
Baló: disease
Baltic myoclonus: disease
Bamberger: albuminuria; disease; sign
Bamberger-Marie: disease; syndrome
Bamberger-Pins-Ewart: sign
bamboo: hair; spine
banana: sign
bancroftian: filariasis
band: cell; centrifugation; neutrophil
bandage contact: lens
bandbox: resonance
Bandl: ring
bandpass: filter
band-shaped: keratopathy
Bang: disease
Bankart: lesion
Bannister: disease

Bannwarth: syndrome
Banti: disease; syndrome
bar: clasp
Bárány: sign
Bárány caloric: test
Barbados: leg
barbed: broach
barber: itch
barber pilonidal: sinus
bar clasp: arm
Barclay-Baron: disease
bar clip: attachments
Barcoo: rot; vomit
Barcroft-Warburg: apparatus; technique
Bardet-Biedl: syndrome
Bardinet: ligament
bare: area of liver; area of stomach
bare lymphocyte: syndrome
barium: enema
bar joint: denture
Barkan: membrane; operation
Barkman: reflex
Barkow: ligaments
Barlow: disease; maneuver; syndrome; test
Barmah Forest: virus
Barnes: curve; zone
barometric: pressure
baroreceptor: nerve
Barraquer: disease; method
Barr chromatin: body
Barré: sign
barrel: chest; distortion
barrel-shaped: thorax
Barrett: epithelium; esophagus; metaplasia; syndrome
barrier: contraceptive
bar-sleeve: attachments
Bart: syndrome
Barth: hernia; syndrome
Bartholin: abscess; anus; cyst; cystectomy; duct; gland
Barton: bandage; forceps; fracture
Bartonella: anemia
Bartter: syndrome
Baruch: law
baryta: water
basal: age; anesthesia; body; bone; cell; cistern; corpuscle; crest of cochlear duct; diet; encephalocele; ganglia; gland; granule; lamina; lamina of choroid; lamina of ciliary body; lamina of cochlear duct; lamina of neural tube; lamina of semicircular duct; layer; layer of choroid; layer of ciliary body; membrane of semicircular duct; metabolism; nuclei; nucleus of Ganser; part; part of left and right inferior pulmonary arteries; part of occipital bone; plate of neural tube; ridge; rod; seat; sphincter; striations; substantia; surface; tuberculosis; vein; vein of Rosenthal
basal body: temperature
basal cell: adenoma; carcinoma; epithelioma; hyperplasia; layer; nevus; papilloma
basal cell nevus: syndrome
basal joint: reflex
basal laminar: drusen
basal linear: drusen
basal metabolic: rate
basaloid: carcinoma; cell
basal seat: area
basal skull: fracture
basal squamous cell: carcinoma
basal tentorial: branch of internal carotid artery
Basan: syndrome
base: composition; deficit; excess; hospital; increase at low levels; line; material; metal; pair; plate; projection; units; view
baseball: finger
Basedow: disease; goiter; pseudoparaplegia
baseline: tonus; variability of fetal heart rate
baseline fetal heart: rate
basement: lamina; membrane
baseplate: wax
basibregmatic: axis
basic: amino acid; diet; dyes; esotropia; exotropia; fuchsin; oxide; personality; proteins; reaction; salt; stain
basic electrical: rhythm
basic fuchsin-methylene blue: stain
basic personality: type
basicranial: axis; flexure
basifacial: axis
basilar: angle; apophysis; artery; bone; cartilage; cell; crest of cochlear duct; fibrocartilage; impression; index; invagination; lamina; leptomeningitis; membrane of cochlear duct; meningitis; migraine; papilla; part of occipital bone; part of pons; parts; process; process of occipital bone; prognathism; sinus; sulcus; vertebra
basilar pontine: sulcus
basilar venous: plexus
basilic: vein
basinasal: line
basioccipital: bone
basipharyngeal: canal
basisphenoid: bone
basivertebral: veins
basket: cell; nucleus
basolateral amygdaloid: nucleus
basomedial amygdaloid: nucleus
basophil: adenoma; cell of anterior lobe of hypophysis; granule; substance
basophilic: degeneration; leukemia; leukocyte; leukocytosis; leukopenia; substance
basosquamous: carcinoma
Bassen-Kornzweig: syndrome
Bassini: herniorrhaphy; operation
Bassler: sign
Bassora: gum
Bastedo: sign
bat: ear
batch: analyzer; culture
bath: itch; pruritus
bathing trunk: nevus
Batista: procedure
Batson: plexus
Batten: disease
Batten-Mayou: disease
battered child: syndrome
battered spouse: syndrome
Battey: bacillus
Battista: operation
Battle: sign
battle: fatigue
battledore: placenta
Baudelocque: diameter; operation
Baudelocque uterine: circle
Bauer: syndrome
Bauer chromic acid leucofuchsin: stain
Bauer-Kirby: test
Bauhin: gland; valve
Baumé: scale
Baumès: symptom
Baumgarten: glands; veins
bauxite: pneumoconiosis
Bayes: theorem
Bayesian: hypothesis
Bayley: Scales of Infant Development
bayonet: apposition; forceps; hair
Bayou: virus
Bazett: formula
Bazex: syndrome
Bazin: disease
B6 bronchus: sign
B cell: co-receptor; receptors
B cell differentiating: factor
B cell differentiation/growth: factors
B cell stimulatory: factor 2
BCG: vaccine
B-E: amputation
Be[a]: antigens
beaded: hair
beak: sign
beaked: pelvis
beaker: cell
Beale: cell
bearing-down: pain
beat-to-beat: variability of fetal heart rate
Beau: lines
Bechterew: band; disease; nucleus; sign
Bechterew-Mendel: reflex
Beck: method; triad
Becker: antigen; disease; nevus; stain for spirochetes
Becker muscular: dystrophy
Becker-type tardive muscular: dystrophy
Beckmann: apparatus
Beckwith-Wiedemann: syndrome
Béclard: anastomosis; hernia; triangle
Becquerel: rays
bed: rest; sore
Bednar: aphthae; tumor
bedside: radiography
bee: toxin
beechwood: sugar
Beer: knife; law
beer: heart
Beer-Lambert: law
beet: sugar
beet-: tongue
Beevor: sign
Begg light wire differential force: technique
Béguez César: disease
behavior: chain; disorder; modification; reflex; therapy
behavioral: epidemic; genetics; health; manifestation; medicine; pathogen; psychology
behavioral observation: audiometry
behavioristic: psychology
Behçet: disease; syndrome
behind-the-ear: hearing aid
Behr: disease; syndrome
Behring: law
BEI: test
Békésy: audiometer; audiometry
Belgian Congo: anemia
Bell: law; muscle; palsy; phenomenon; spasm
bell: sound; stage
belladonna: extract; tincture
bell clapper: deformity
Bellini: ducts; ligament
Bell-Magendie: law
bellmetal: resonance
bellows: murmur

Bell respiratory: nerve
bell-shaped: crown
Belsey: fundoplication; procedure
Belsey Mark: operation
belt: test
Bence Jones: albumin; cylinders; myeloma; proteins; proteinuria; reaction
bench: testing
Bender gestalt: test
Bender Visual Motor Gestalt: test
bending: fracture
Benedek: reflex
Benedict: solution; test for glucose
Benedict-Hopkins-Cole: reagent
Benedict-Roth: apparatus; calorimeter
Benedikt: syndrome
benign: albuminuria; cementoblastoma; dyskeratosis; fructosuria; glycosuria; hypertension; lymphadenosis; lymphocytoma cutis; lymphoma of the rectum; mesothelioma; mesothelioma of genital tract; myoclonus of infancy; nephrosclerosis; stupor; tumor
benign bone: aneurysm
benign childhood: epilepsy with centrotemporal spikes
benign coital: cephalalgia
benign congenital: hypotonia
benign dry: pleurisy
benign essential: tremor
benign exertional: headache
benign familial: chorea; icterus
benign familial chronic: pemphigus
benign giant lymph node: hyperplasia
benign infantile: myoclonus
benign inoculation: lymphoreticulosis; reticulosis
benign juvenile: melanoma
benign lymphoepithelial: lesion
benign migratory: glossitis
benign monoclonal: gammopathy
benign mucosal: pemphigoid
benign myalgic: encephalomyelitis
benign neonatal: convulsions
benign paroxysmal: peritonitis; torticollis of infancy
benign paroxysmal positional: vertigo
benign positional: vertigo
benign prostatic: hyperplasia; hypertrophy
benign rheumatoid: nodules
benign tertian: fever; malaria
Bennett: angle; fracture; movement
Bennhold Congo red: stain
Bensley specific: granules
bentiromide: test
bentonite flocculation: test
benzene: nucleus; ring
benzidine: test
benzoinated: lard
benzyl: penicillin
Beradinelli: syndrome
Bérard: aneurysm
Berardinelli: syndrome
Béraud: valve
Berg: stain
Berger: cells; disease; rhythm; space
Berger focal: glomerulonephritis
Bergman: sign
Bergmann: cords; fibers
Bergmeister: papilla
beriberi: heart
Berkefeld: filter
Berlin: edema
berloque: dermatitis
Bernard: canal; duct; puncture
Bernard-Cannon: homeostasis
Bernard-Horner: syndrome
Bernard-Sergent: syndrome
Bernard-Soulier: disease; syndrome
Bernays: sponge
Bernhardt: disease; formula
Bernhardt-Roth: syndrome
Bernheim: syndrome
Bernoulli: distribution; effect; law; principle; theorem
Bernstein: test
Berry: ligaments
berry: aneurysm; cell
Berson: test
Berthelot: reaction
Berthollet: law
Bertin: bones; columns; ligament; ossicles
beryllium: granuloma
Besnier: prurigo
Besnier-Boeck-Schaumann: disease; syndrome
Best: disease
best: frequency
Best carmine: stain
Beta: tests
beta: alcoholism; angle; cell of anterior lobe of hypophysis; cell of pancreas; error; fibers; granule; particle; radiation; ray; rhythm; wave
beta-: oxidation
beta-oxidation-condensation: theory
betel: cancer
Bethesda: classification; system; unit
Betke-Kleihauer: test
Bettendorff: test
betula: oil
Betz: cells
Beuren: syndrome
Bevan-Lewis: cells
bevelled: anastomosis
Bezold: abscess; ganglion
Bezold-Jarisch: reflex
BH: interval
Bi: antigen
Bial: test
Bianchi: nodule
biauricular: axis
biaxial: joint
bi bi: reaction
bicameral: abscess
bicanalicular: sphincter
BICAP: cautery
biceps: muscle of arm; muscle of thigh; reflex
biceps brachii: muscle
biceps femoris: muscle; reflex
Bichat: canal; fat-pad; fissure; fossa; ligament; membrane; protuberance; tunic
bicipital: aponeurosis; fascia; groove; rib; ridges; tuberosity
bicipitoradial: bursa
Bickel: ring
biclonal: gammopathy; peak
biconcave: lens
bicondylar: articulation; joint
biconvex: lens
bicornate: uterus
bicoudate: catheter
bicuspid: tooth; valve
bidirectional: replication
bidirectional ventricular: tachycardia
bidiscoidal: placenta
Biebl: loop
Biederman: sign
Bielschowsky: disease; sign; stain
Biemond: syndrome
Bier: amputation; hyperemia; method
Biermer: anemia; disease
Biernacki: sign
Biesiadecki: fossa
bifid: epiglottis; penis; rib; thumb; tongue; uterus; uvula
bifidus: factor
bifocal: lens; spectacles
biforate: uterus
bifoveal: fixation
bifurcate: ligament
bifurcated: ligament
bifurcation: lymph nodes
big: ACTH
Bigelow: ligament; septum
bigeminal: bodies; pregnancy; pulse; rhythm
bilaminar: blastoderm
bilateral: hermaphroditism; left-sidedness; pleurisy; synchrony
bilateral medial orbital: ecchymoses
Bile: antigen
bile: capillary; cyst; duct; gastritis; papilla; peritonitis; pigments; salts; thrombus
bile: acids; alcohol
bile acid tolerance: test
bi-leaflet: valve
bile esculin: test
bile pigment: hemoglobin
bile salt: agar
bile solubility: test
bilharzial: appendicitis; dysentery; granuloma
biliaropancreatic: ampulla
biliary: atresia; calculus; canaliculus; cirrhosis; colic; duct; ductules; dyskinesia; fistula; glands; steatorrhea; xanthomatosis
bilious: headache; pneumonia; typhoid of Griesinger; vomit
bilious remittent: fever; malaria
bilirubin: encephalopathy
Bill: maneuver
Billings: method
billowing mitral valve: syndrome
Billroth: cords; operation I; operation II; venae cavernosae
Billroth I: anastomosis
Billroth II: anastomosis
bilocular: joint; stomach
bilocular femoral: hernia
bimalleolar: fracture
bimanual: palpation; percussion; version
bimaxillary: protrusion
bimaxillary dentoalveolar: protrusion
bimaxillary protrusive: occlusion
binangle: chisel
binary: combination; complex; digit; fission; nomenclature; process
binasal: hemianopia
binaural: stethoscope
binaural alternate loudness balance: test
binding: constant; energy
Binet: age; scale; test

Binet-Simon: scale
Bing: reflex
Bingham: flow; model; plastic
binocular: fixation; heterochromia; loupe; microscope; ophthalmoscope; parallax; rivalry; vision
binomial: distribution
Binswanger: disease; encephalopathy
biochemical: genetics; metastasis; modulation; pharmacology; profile
biochemical oxygen: demand
bioelectric: potential
biogenetic: law
biogenic: amines
biologic: assay; chemistry; control; evolution; half-life; hemolysis; immunotherapy; psychiatry; time; valve
biological: coefficient; sampling; vector
biological standard: unit
biologic response: modifier
biomedical: engineering; model
biometrical: school
Biondi-Heidenhain: stain
biophysical: profile
biopsy: needle
biopsychosocial: model
biorbital: angle
Biot: breathing; respiration; sign
Biot breathing: sign
biotic: community; factors; potential
biotinidase: deficiency
biparietal: diameter
bipartite: uterus; vagina
bipedicle: flap
bipennate: muscle
biphasic: insulin; response
biplane: angiography
bipolar: cautery; cell; disorder; lead; neuron; psychosis; taxis; version.
Birbeck: granule
Birch-Hirschfeld: stain
Bird: sign
bird: face; unit
bird-breeder's: disease; lung
birdseed: agar
bird shot: retinochoroiditis
bird's nest: filter
birth: canal; control; defect; fracture; palsy; rate; trauma; weight
birthing: center
Bischof: myelotomy
biscuit: bite
bisferious: pulse
Bishop: score; sphygmoscope
Biskra: boil; button

bismuth: line
bite: analysis; fork; gauge; plane; rim
bitemporal: hemianopia
bitewing: film; radiograph
bithermal caloric: test
biting: louse; pressure; strength
Bitot: spots
bitter: orange peel; orange peel, dried; orange peel, fresh; orange peel oil; peptides; principles; tonic; water
bitter almond: oil
Bittner: agent; virus
Bittner milk: factor
Bittorf: reaction
biundulant: meningoencephalitis
biuret: reaction; reagent; test
bivalent: antibody; chromosome
bivalent gas gangrene: antitoxin
bivalve: speculum
biventer: lobule
biventral: lobule
Bixler type: hypertelorism
Bizzozero: corpuscle
Bizzozero red: cells
Bjerrum: scotoma; screen; sign
Björk-Shiley: valve
Björnstad: syndrome
B-K: amputation
BK: virus
Black: classification; formula
black: box; cataract; death; eye; fever; heel; lead; line; lung; measles; mustard; piedra; plague; sickness; spore; tarantula; tongue; urine; vomit
Black Creek Canal: virus
black currant: rash
black-dot: ringworm
black hairy: tongue
black imported fire: ant
blackwater: fever
bladder: calculus; compliance; ear; reflex; schistosomiasis; stone
blade: bone
Blagden: law
Blainville: ears
Blalock: shunt
Blalock-Hanlon: operation
Blalock-Taussig: operation; shunt
bland: diet; embolism; infarct
Blandin: gland
blanket: suture
Blasius: duct
blast: cell; crisis; injury

blastodermic: disk; layers; vesicle
blastomycetic: dermatitis
blastoporic: canal
Blatin: syndrome
bleached: wax
bleaching: powder
blear: eye
bleary: eye
bleeding: polyp; time
blending: inheritance
blighted: ovum
blind: boil; enema; fistula; foramen of frontal bone; foramen of the tongue; gut; headache; passage; spot; study; test
blinding: disease; glare
blind loop: syndrome
blind nasotracheal: intubation
blink: reflex; response
blister: agent
blistering: collodion
blistering distal: dactylitis
Bloch: reaction
Bloch-Sulzberger: disease; syndrome
block: anesthesia; vertebrae
block design: test
blocked: aerogastria; reading frame
blocking: activity; agent; antibody
Blocq: disease
Blom-Singer: valve
blood: agar; albumin; blister; calculus; capillary; cast; cell; circulation; clot; corpuscle; count; crisis; crystals; cyst; disk; dyscrasia; gases; group; island; islet; lymph; mole; motes; pH; plasma; plastid; plate; poisoning; pressure; serum; spots; substitute; sugar; tumor; type; vessel
blood-air: barrier
blood-aqueous: barrier
blood-brain: barrier
blood-cerebrospinal fluid: barrier
blood gas: analysis
blood group: agglutinins; agglutinogens; antibodies; antigen; antiserums; substance; systems
blood group-specific: substances A and B
bloodless: amputation; decerebration; operation; phlebotomy
blood plasma: fractions
blood pool: imaging
blood-testis: barrier
blood-thymus: barrier
blood urea: nitrogen

blood-vascular: system
blood volume: nomogram
Bloom: syndrome
Blount: disease
Blount-Barber: disease
blowout: pipette
blow-out: fracture
blubber: finger
blue: atrophy; baby; cataract; dextran; disease; edema; fever; line; nevus; ointment; pus; sclera; spot; vision
blueberry muffin: baby
blue cone: monochromatism
blue diaper: syndrome
blue dome: cyst
blue dot: sign
blue-green: algae; bacteria; bacterium
blue pus: bacillus
blue rubber-bleb: nevi
blue toe: syndrome
bluetongue: virus
Blumberg: sign
Blumenau: nucleus
Blumenbach: clivus
Blumer: shelf
blunt duct: adenosis
blunted: affect
blunt-end: ligation
blunt-ended: DNA
boat: conformation; form
boat-shaped: abdomen
Bochdalek: foramen; ganglion; gap; muscle; valve
Bock: ganglion; nerve
Bockhart: impetigo
Bodansky: unit
Bödecker: index
Bodian copper-PROTARGOL: stain
body: cavity; image; language; mechanics; plethysmograph; schema; stalk
body dysmorphic: disorder
body mass: index
body righting: reflexes
body-weight: ratio
Boeck: disease; sarcoid
Boeck and Drbohlav Locke-egg-serum: medium
Boehmer: hematoxylin
Boerhaave: syndrome
Bogros: space
Bogros serous: membrane
Bohn: nodules
Bohr: atom; effect; equation; magneton; theory
boiling: point
Boley: gauge
Bolivian hemorrhagic: fever
Bolivian hemorrhagic fever: virus
Boll: cells
Bollinger: granules
Bolognini: symptom

bolster: finger
bolus: dressing
bomb: calorimeter
Bombay: phenomenon; trait
bone: abscess; ache; age; block; canaliculus; cell; charcoal; chips; conduction; corpuscle; cyst; density; flap; forceps; graft; infarct; island; marrow; matrix; phosphate; plate; resorption; salt; sclerosis; sensibility; tissue; wax
bone block: fusion
bone Gla: protein
bone marrow: dose; embolism; transplantation
Bonhoeffer: sign
Bonnet: capsule
Bonnet-Dechaume-Blanc: syndrome
Bonney: test
Bonnier: syndrome
Bonwill: triangle
bony: ampullae of semicircular canals; ankylosis; crepitus; heart; labyrinth; limbs of semicircular canals; palate; part of external acoustic meatus; part of nasal septum; part of pharyngotympanic (auditory) tube; part of skeletal system
bony nasal: septum
bony semicircular: canals
Böök: syndrome
booster: dose; response
BOR: syndrome
Bordeaux: mixture
border: cells; molding; movements; seal
borderline: case; hypertension; leprosy; personality
borderline ovarian: tumor
borderline personality: disorder
border tissue: movements
Bordet and Gengou: reaction
Bordet-Gengou: bacillus; phenomenon
Bordet-Gengou potato blood: agar
Börjeson-Forssman-Lehmann: syndrome
Born: method of wax plate reconstruction
Borna disease: virus
Bornholm: disease
Bornholm disease: virus
Borrel blue: stain
Borst-Jadassohn type intraepidermal: epithelioma
bosch: yaws
Bosin: disease

Boston: exanthema; opium
Botallo: duct; foramen; ligament
bothropic: antitoxin
Bothrops: antitoxin
botryoid: sarcoma
botryoid odontogenic: cyst
Böttcher: canal; cells; crystals; ganglion; space
botulinum: antitoxin
botulinus: toxin
botulism: antitoxin
Bouchard: disease
Bouchut: tube
Bouffardi white: mycetoma
Bouillaud: disease
Bouin: fixative
bound: water
boundary: lamina
bouquet: fever
Bourgery: ligament
Bourneville: disease
Bourneville-Pringle: disease
boutonneuse: fever
boutonnière: deformity
bovine: antitoxin; brucellosis; colloid; ketosis; rhinoviruses
bovine leukemia: virus
bovine leukosis: virus
bovine papular stomatitis: virus
bovine serum: albumin
bovine spongiform: encephalopathy
bovine virus diarrhea: virus
bow-: leg
Bowditch: effect; law
bowel: bypass; movement; sounds
bowel bypass: syndrome
Bowen: disease
Bowenoid: cells
bowenoid: papulosis
Bowen precancerous: dermatosis
Bowie: stain
Bowles type: stethoscope
Bowman: capsule; disks; gland; layer; membrane; muscle; probe; space; theory
Bowman-Birk: inhibitor
box: jelly
boxer's: ear; fracture
boxing: wax
Boyd communicating perforation: veins
Boyden: meal; sphincter
Boyer: bursa; cyst
Boyle: law
Bozeman: operation; position
Bozeman-Fritsch: catheter
Bozzolo: sign
BP: fistula
Braasch: bulb; catheter
brachial: anesthesia; artery; fascia; gland; lymph nodes;

muscle; neuritis; plexitis; plexus; veins
brachial autonomic: plexus
brachial birth: palsy
brachialis: muscle
brachial plexus: injury; neuropathy
brachiocephalic: arteritis; lymph nodes
brachiocephalic (arterial): trunk
brachioradial: muscle; reflex
brachioradialis: muscle
Bracht: maneuver
Bracht-Wächter: lesion
brachypellic: pelvis
Bradbury-Eggleston: syndrome
Bradford: frame
bradykinetic: analysis
bradykinin-potentiating: peptide
bradytachycardia: syndrome
Brailsford-Morquio: disease
Brain: reflex
brain: attack; box; cicatrix; concussion; congestion; contusion; death; edema; laceration; lipid; mantle; murmur; potential; sand; stem; sugar; swelling; wave
brain-heart infusion: agar
brainstem: glioma; hemorrhage
brainstem auditory evoked: potential
brainstem evoked: response
brain wave: complex; cycle
branch: migration
branched: calculus
branched chain: ketoaciduria; ketonuria
brancher deficiency: glycogenosis
brancher glycogen storage: disease
branchial: apparatus; arches; cartilages; clefts; cyst; fissure; fistula; groove; mesoderm; pouches
branchial cleft: cyst
branchial efferent: column
branching: enzyme; factor; type of renal pelvis
branchiomeric: muscles
branchiomotor: nuclei
branchiootorenal: dysplasia; syndrome
Brandt-Andrews: maneuver
brandy: nose
Branham: sign
branny: desquamation; tetter
Brasdor: method
brass founder's: ague; fever
brassy: body; cough
BRAT: diet

Braun: anastomosis
Braune: canal; muscle; valve
brawny: arm; edema; scleritis
Braxton Hicks: contraction; sign; version
Brazelton Neonatal Behavioral Assessment: Scale
Brazil: wax
Brazilian: blastomycosis; pemphigus
Brazilian hemorrhagic: fever
Brazilian purpuric: fever
Brazilian spotted: fever
BRCA1: gene
BRCA2: gene
BrDu-: banding
bread: pill
bread-and-butter: pericardium
break: shock
breakbone: fever
breakoff: phenomenon
breast: bone; pang; pump
breath: analysis; sounds; test
breath-holding: test
breathing: bag; reserve
Breda: disease
breech: delivery; extraction; presentation
bregmatic: fontanelle
bregmatolambdoid: arc
bregmocardiac: reflex
Brenner: tumor
Breschet: bones; canals; hiatus; sinus; vein
Brescia-Cimino: fistula
Breslow: thickness
Breus: mole
Brewer: infarcts
brewers': yeast
brickdust: deposit
Bricker: operation
brickmaker's: anemia
bridge: corpuscle
bridging hepatic: necrosis
bridle: stricture; suture
brief: psychotherapy
Brigg: test
Bright: disease
brightness difference: threshold
Brill: disease
Brill-Symmers: disease
Brill-Zinsser: disease
Brimacombe: fragment
Brinell hardness: number
Briquet: ataxia; disease; syndrome
Brissaud: disease; infantilism; reflex
Brissaud-Marie: syndrome
bristle: cell
British: gum
British thermal: unit
brittle: bones; diabetes

broad: fascia; ligament of the uterus; spectrum
Broadbent: law; sign
broad beta: disease
broadest: muscle of back
broad-spectrum: antibiotic
Broca: angles; aphasia; area; center; field; fissure; formula; pouch
Broca basilar: angle
Broca diagonal: band
Broca facial: angle
Broca parolfactory: area
Broca visual: plane
Brock: operation; syndrome
Brockenbrough: sign
Brocq: disease
Brödel bloodless: line
Brodie: abscess; bursa; disease; fluid; knee; ligament
Brodmann: areas
Broesike: fossa
bromide: acne
bromine: water
bromphenol: test
Brompton: cocktail
bromsulphalein: test
bronchial: adenoma; arteries; arteriography; asthma; atresia; branches of thoracic aorta; breathing; bud; calculus; fremitus; glands; mucosa; pneumonia; polyp; respiration; stenosis; tubes; veins; voice
bronchial breath: sounds
bronchial mucous gland: adenoma
bronchic: cells
bronchiolar: adenocarcinoma; carcinoma
bronchiolar exocrine: cell
bronchioloalveolar: adenocarcinoma
bronchiolo-alveolar: carcinoma
bronchitic: asthma
bronchoalveolar: carcinoma; fluid; lavage
broncho-aortic: constriction
bronchobiliary: fistula
bronchocavitary: fistula
bronchoesophageal: fistula; muscle
bronchoesophageus: muscle
bronchogenic: carcinoma; cyst
bronchomediastinal (lymphatic): trunk
bronchopleural: fistula
bronchopleural-cutaneous: fistula
bronchopulmonary: dysplasia; lymph nodes; segment; sequestration; spirochetosis
bronchoscopic: brush; smear
bronchovesicular: respiration
bronchovesicular breath: sounds
bronchus-associated lymphoid: tissue
Brønsted: acid; base; theory
bronze: diabetes
bronze baby: syndrome
bronzed: diabetes; disease; skin
brood: capsules; cell
Brooke: ileostomy; tumor
brother: complex
Broviac: catheter
brow: presentation
Brown: syndrome
brown: atrophy; edema; fat; induration of the lung; layer; lung; pellicle; striae; tumor
brown adipose: tissue
Brown-Adson: forceps
Brown-Brenn: stain
brownian: motion; movement
brownian-Zsigmondy: movement
Browning: vein
Brown-Séquard: paralysis; syndrome
Bruce: protocol
brucella strain 19: vaccine
Bruch: glands; membrane
Bruck: disease
Brücke: muscle; tunic
Brücke-Bartley: phenomenon
Brudzinski: sign
Brug: filariasis
Brugsch: syndrome
Brumpt white: mycetoma
Brunn: membrane; nest; reaction
Brunner: glands
Bruns: ataxia; nystagmus
Brunschwig: operation
brush: biopsy; border; burn; catheter
brush burn: abrasion
Brushfield: spots
Brushfield-Wyatt: disease
brush heap: structure
Bruton: agammaglobulinemia
Bryant: traction; triangle
BSP: test
bubble gum: dermatitis
bubbling: rale
bubonic: plague
buccal: angles; artery; branches of facial nerve; caries; cavity; curve; digestion; embrasure; fat-pad; flange; gingiva; glands; lymph node; nerve; occlusion; pit; region; root of tooth; smear; surface; tablet; vestibule
buccinator: crest; muscle; nerve; node
buccocervical: ridge
buccogingival: ridge
buccolingual: diameter; dimension; relation
bucconasal: membrane
bucconeural: duct
bucco-occlusal: angle
buccopharyngeal: fascia; membrane; part of superior pharyngeal constrictor
Büchner: extract; funnel
Buchwald: atrophy
Buck: extension; fascia; traction
buck: tooth
bucket-handle: incision; tear
buckled: aorta
buckled innominate: artery
buckthorn: polyneuropathy
Bucky: diaphragm
bud: fission; stage
Budd: syndrome
Budd-Chiari: syndrome
Budde: process
buddeized: milk
Budge: center
Budin obstetrical: joint
Buerger: disease
buffalo: hump; neck; type
buffer: capacity; index; pair; value; value of the blood
buffered crystalline: penicillin G
buffy: coat
buffy coat: concentration
bulbar: apoplexy; conjunctiva; myelitis; palsy; paralysis; pulse; ridge; septum
bulbar corticonuclear: fibers
bulbocavernosus: muscle; reflex
bulboid: corpuscles
bulbomimic: reflex
bulboreticulospinal: tract
bulbosacral: system
bulbospongiosus: muscle
bulbourethral: gland
bulbous: bougie
bulboventricular: loop; ridge
bulging eye: disease
bulk: modulus
bulky: disease; lymphadenopathy
bull: neck
bulldog: forceps; head
bullet: bubo; forceps
bullous: edema; edema vesicae; emphysema; impetigo of newborn; keratopathy; myringitis; pemphigoid; syphilid
bullous congenital ichthyosiform: erythroderma
bull's-eye: maculopathy
Bumke: pupil
bundle: bone
bundle-branch: block
Bunnell: suture
Bunsen-Roscoe: law
Bunsen solubility: coefficient
Bunyamwera: fever; virus
bunyavirus: encephalitis
buoyant: density
bur: drill
Burchard-Liebermann: reaction
Burdach: column; fasciculus; nucleus; tract
Burdwan: fever
Burger: triangle
Bürger-Grütz: disease; syndrome
Burgundy: pitch
buried: flap; penis; suture
Burkitt: lymphoma
Burlew: disk; wheel
burner: syndrome
Burnett: syndrome
burning: tongue
burning drops: sign
burning foot: syndrome
burning mouth: syndrome
burning tongue: syndrome
burning vulva: syndrome
Burn and Rand: theory
Burns: ligament; space
Burns falciform: process
burnt: alum
Burow: solution; triangle; vein
burr: cell
burrowing: hairs
bursal: abscess; cyst; synovitis
Burton: line
Buruli: ulcer
Bury: disease
Busacca: nodules
Buschke: disease
Buschke-Löwenstein: tumor
Buschke-Ollendorf: syndrome
bush: yaws
Busquet: disease
butanol-extractable: iodine
butanol-extractable iodine: test
butter: stools
butterfly: eruption; fragment; lung; patch; pattern; rash; vertebra
button: suture
buttonhole: iridectomy; stenosis
buttress: plate
buyo cheek: cancer
Buzzard: maneuver
Bwamba: fever; virus
By: antigen

Byars: flap
Byler: disease
by-product: material
bystander: lysis
Byzantine arch: palate

C

C: bile; cell; chain; factors; fibers; gene; terminus; value; wave
C1: esterase
CA: virus
CA-125: antigen
CA-15-3: antigen
CA-19-9: antigen
CAAT: box
cabbage: goiter
Cabot-Locke: murmur
Cabot ring: bodies
cacao: butter
cachectic: diarrhea; edema; endocarditis; fever; pallor
cadaveric: rigidity; spasm
caddis: worm
caeruleun: nucleus
caerulospinal: tract
cafe: coronary
café au lait: spots
Caffey: disease; syndrome
Caffey-Kempe: syndrome
Caffey-Silverman: syndrome
Cagot: ear
Cain: complex
caisson: disease; sickness
Cajal: cell
Cajal astrocyte: stain
cake: alum; kidney
caked: breast
Calabar: swelling
calabash: curare
calcaneal: anastomosis; apophysitis; arteries; bone; branches; gait; petechiae; process of cuboid; region; sulcus; tendon; tuber; tubercle; tuberosity
calcaneal arterial: network
calcaneal articular: surface of talus
calcaneocuboid: joint; ligament
calcaneofibular: ligament
calcaneonavicular: ligament
calcaneotibial: ligament
calcareous: conjunctivitis; corpuscles; degeneration; infiltration; metastasis; pancreatitis
calcarine: artery; branch of medial occipital artery; fasciculus; fissure; spur; sulcus
calcic: water
calcific: bursitis; pancreatitis
calcification: lines of Retzius

calcific nodular aortic: stenosis
calcified: cartilage
calcifying epithelial odontogenic: tumor
calcifying and keratinizing odontogenic: cyst
calcifying odontogenic: cyst
calcined: magnesia
calcinuric: diabetes
calcitonin gene-related: peptide
calcium: antagonist; gout; pump; rigor; sign; tungstate
calcium channel: blocker
calcium channel-blocking: agent
calcium pyrophosphate deposition: disease
calculated mean: organism
calculated serum: osmolality
Caldani: ligament
Caldwell: projection; view
Caldwell-Luc: operation
Caldwell-Moloy: classification
calf: bone; pump
calibration: curve; interval
caliceal: diverticulum
caliciform: cell
California: encephalitis; virus
California psychological inventory: test
caliper: micrometer
Calkins: sign
Callahan: method
Callander: amputation
Call-Exner: bodies
Callison: fluid
callosal: convolution; gyrus; sulcus
callosomarginal: artery; fissure; sulcus
Calmette: test
Calmette-Guérin: bacillus; vaccine
calomel: electrode
Calori: bursa
caloric: nystagmus; test; value
calorigenic: action
Calot: triangle
calvarial: hook
Calvé-Perthes: disease
calyciform: ending
cambium: layer
CAMP: factor; test
camp: fever; hospital
Campbell: ligament; sound
Camper: chiasm; fascia; ligament; line; plane
camphorated: menthol; phenol
cAMP receptor: protein
camptomelic: dwarfism; syndrome

Canada: balsam; snakeroot; turpentine
canalicular: adenoma; ducts; sphincter
Canavan: disease; sclerosis
Canavan-van Bogaert-Bertrand: disease
cancellous: bone; tissue
cancer: bodies; family
cancer antigen 125: test
cane: sugar
canicola: fever
canine: adenovirus 1; amebiasis; carcinoma 1; eminence; fossa; leishmaniasis; prominence; spasm; tooth
canine distemper: virus
canities: poliosis
canker: sores
Cannizzaro: reaction
Cannon: theory
Cannon: point; ring
cannon: wave
cannon: sound
cannonball: pulse
Cannon-Bard: theory
Cantelli: sign
cantering: rhythm
canthal: hypertelorism
cantharidal: collodion
cantharis: camphor
canthomeatal: plane
cantilever: beam; bridge
Cantor: tube
caoutchouc: pelvis
cap: splint; stage
capeline: bandage
Capgras: phenomenon; syndrome
Capillaria: granuloma
capillary: angioma; arteriole; attraction; bed; circulation; drainage; fracture; fragility; hemangioma; hemangioma of infancy; lake; lamina of choroid; loop; nevus; pulse; vein; vessel
capillary fragility: test
capillary permeability: factor
capillary resistance: test
capillary zone: electrophoresis
Capim: viruses
capital: operation
capitate: bone
capitular: joint
Caplan: nodules; syndrome
capon: unit
capon-comb: unit
capped: uterus
capping: proteins
Capps: reflex
capsular: advancement; antigen; branches of intrarenal arteries; branches of renal artery; cataract;

cirrhosis of liver; ligament; space
capsular flap: pyeloplasty
capsular precipitation: reaction
capsule: cell; forceps
capsulolenticular: cataract
capture-recapture: method
Capuron: points
caput: epididymis
car: sickness
Carabelli: tubercle
Caraparu: virus
carbacrylamine: resins
carbamino: compound
carbamylcholine: chloride
carbohydrate: loading; metabolism
carbohydrate-induced: hyperlipemia
carbohydrate utilization: test
carbol: fuchsin
carbol-fuchsin: paint
carbol-thionin: stain
carbon: autotrophy
carbonated: water
carbonate dehydratase: inhibitor
carbon dioxide: acidosis; content; cycle; electrode; elimination
carbon dioxide combining: power
carbon dioxide-free: water
carbon disulfide: poisoning
carbonic: anhydrase
carbonic acid: gas
carbonic anhydrase: inhibitor
carbonic anhydrase II deficiency: syndrome
carbon monoxide: hemoglobin; poisoning
carbonmonoxy: myoglobin
carboxy: terminal
carboxylic acid: ester
carboxymethyl: cellulose
carcinoembryonic: antigen
carcinoid: flush; syndrome; tumor
carcinomatous: encephalomyelopathy; implants; myelopathy; myopathy; neuromyopathy; pericarditis
Carden: amputation
cardiac: accident; albuminuria; alternation; aneurysm; antrum; arrest; arrhythmia; asthma; catheter; cirrhosis; competence; contractility; cycle; decompression; diuretic; dropsy; dyspnea; dysrhythmia; edema; failure; ganglia; gating; gland; glands; glands of esophagus;

glands of stomach;
glycosides; heterotaxia;
histiocyte; hormone;
impression of diaphragmatic
surface of liver; impression
on lung; impulse;
incompetence; index;
infarction; insufficiency;
jelly; liver; lung; mapping;
massage; monitor; murmur;
muscle; neurosis; notch;
notch of left lung; opening;
orifice; output; part of
stomach; polyp; prominence;
reserve; segment; shock;
skeleton; souffle; sound;
standstill; syncope;
tamponade; telemetry; tube;
veins
cardiac depressor: reflex
cardiac fibrous: skeleton
cardiac lymphatic: ring
cardiac muscle: tissue; wrap
cardiac (nervous): plexus
cardiac valve: prosthesis
cardiac valvular:
incompetence
cardial: notch; orifice; part of stomach
cardinal: ligament; points; symptom; veins
cardinal ocular: movements
cardioarterial: interval
cardiodiaphragmatic: angle
cardioesophageal: junction; relaxation
cardiofacial: syndrome
cardiogenic: plate; shock
cardiohepatic: angle; triangle
cardioid: condenser
cardiophrenic: angle
cardioplegic: arrest
cardiopulmonary: arrest;
bypass; murmur;
resuscitation; transplantation
cardiopulmonary splanchnic:
nerves
cardiorespiratory: murmur
cardiothoracic: ratio
cardiotoxic: myolysis
cardiovascular: radiology;
syphilis; system
Carey Coombs: murmur
carinal: lymph nodes
carinate: abdomen
Carlen: tube
Carman: sign
Carmody-Batson: operation
carnassial: tooth
carnauba: wax
carneous: degeneration; mole
Carnett: sign
Carney: complex
carnitine: deficiency
Carnoy: fixative
Caroli: disease; syndrome

β-carotene-cleavage: enzyme
caroticoclinoid: ligament
caroticotympanic: arteries (of
internal carotid artery);
canaliculi; nerves
carotid: arteries; body; branch
of glossopharyngeal nerve
(CN IX); bruit; bulb; canal;
duct; endarterectomy;
foramen; ganglion; groove;
pulse; sheath; shudder;
sinus; sulcus; triangle;
tubercle; wall of middle ear;
wall of tympanic cavity
carotid body: tumor
carotid-cavernous: fistula
carotid sinus: branch; nerve;
reflex; syncope; syndrome;
test
carp: mouth
carpal: arches; artery; bones;
canal; groove; joints; tunnel
carpal articular: surface of radius
carpal tendinous: sheaths
carpal tunnel: syndrome
Carpenter: syndrome
Carpentier-Edwards: valve
carpometacarpal: joints; joint
of thumb; ligaments (dorsal
and palmar)
carpopedal: spasm
Carrel: treatment
Carrel-Lindbergh: pump
carrier: cell; electrophoresis;
screening; state; strain
Carrington: disease
Carrión: disease
Carr-Price: reaction; test
Carr-Purcell: experiment
carrying: angle; capacity
Carter black: mycetoma
cartesian: nomogram
cartilage: bone; capsule; cell;
knife; lacuna; matrix; space
cartilage-hair: hypoplasia
cartilaginous: articulation;
joint; neurocranium; part of
external acoustic meatus;
part of nasal septum; part of
pharyngotympanic (auditory)
tube; part of skeletal system;
septum; tissue;
viscerocranium
Carus: circle; curve
Carvallo: sign
Casal: necklace
cascade: stomach
case: management
case control: study
case fatality: rate; ratio
caseous: abscess;
degeneration; necrosis;
osteitis; pneumonia; tubercle
Casoni: antigen
Casoni intradermal: test

Casoni skin: test
Casselberry: position
Casser: fontanelle
Casser perforated: muscle
cassette: mutagenesis
cassia: cinnamon
Castellani: bronchitis; paint
Castellani-Low: sign
Castile: soap
casting: flask; ring; wax
Castle intrinsic: factor
Castleman: disease
castration: anxiety; cells; complex
cat: unit
catabolite: repression
catabolite gene: activator
catabolite (gene) activator: protein
catacrotic: pulse
catadicrotic: pulse
catalatic: reaction
catalytic: antibody; center
catamenial: pneumothorax
cataract: lens; needle; spoon
cataract-oligophrenia: syndrome
catarrhal: asthma; fever;
gastritis; inflammation;
ophthalmia
catastrophe: theory
catastrophic: reaction
catatonic: dementia;
excitement; pupil; rigidity;
schizophrenia; stupor
catatropic: image
cat-bite: disease; fever
catchment: area
catechol: estrogen
categorical: trait
caterpillar: cell; dermatitis; rash
caterpillar-hair: ophthalmia
catgut: suture
catheter: embolus; fever;
gauge; guide
catheter coiling: sign
cathodal closure: contraction
cathodal duration: tetanus
cathodal opening: clonus; contraction
cathode: rays
cathode ray: oscilloscope; tube
cation-anion: difference
cation-exchange: resin
cationic: detergents
catscratch: disease; fever
cat's cry: syndrome
cat's-eye: pupil; syndrome
Cattell Infant Intelligence: Scale
Catu: virus
cauda: epididymis
cauda equina: syndrome

caudal: anesthesia; canal;
flexure; ligament;
neuropore; retinaculum;
sheath; vertebrae
caudal neurosecretory: system
caudal pancreatic: artery
caudal pharyngeal: complex
caudal pontine reticular: nucleus
caudal transtentorial: herniation
caudal transverse: fissure
caudate: branches of left
branch of portal vein; lobe;
nucleus; process
caudolenticular gray: bridges
cauliflower: ear
causal: additivity;
independence; treatment
caustic: alkali; potash; soda
cautery: conization; knife
caval: fold; opening of
diaphragm; valve
cavalry: bone
cave: sickness
cavernous: angioma; arteries;
bodies of anal canal; body
of clitoris; body of penis;
branch of cavernous part of
internal carotid artery;
groove; hemangioma;
lymphangiectasis; nerves of
clitoris; nerves of penis; part
of internal carotid artery;
plexus of clitoris; plexus of
penis; rale; resonance;
respiration; rhonchus; sinus;
space; spaces of corpora
cavernosa; spaces of
corpus spongiosum; tissue;
transformation of portal
vein; veins of penis; voice
cavernous nervous: plexus
cavernous sinus: branch of
internal carotid artery;
syndrome
cavernous (vascular): plexus of conchae
cavernous voice: sound
caviar: lesion
cavity: liner; margin;
preparation; wall
cavity line: angle
cavity preparation: base; form
cavopulmonary: anastomosis; shunt
cavosurface: angle; bevel
Cazenave: vitiligo
CB: lead
C-banding: stain
C carbohydrate: antigen
CD4/CD8: count
CDE: antigens
cDNA: clone; library

ceasmic: teratosis
cecal: arteries; folds; foramen of frontal bone; foramen of the tongue; hernia; recess; volvulus
Cecil: urethroplasty
cecocentral: scotoma
Ceelen-Gellerstedt: syndrome
Celestin: tube
celiac: artery; axis; branches of posterior vagal trunk; branches of vagus nerve; disease; ganglia; lymph nodes; plexus; rickets; sprue; syndrome
celiac (arterial): trunk
celiac (lymphatic): plexus
celiac (nervous): plexus
celiacoduodenal: part of suspensory muscle (ligament) of duodenum
celiac plexus: reflex
celiotomy: incision
cell: body; bridges; center; culture; cycle; determination; fusion; hybridization; inclusions; line; marker; matrix; membrane; nest; organelle; plate; sap; strain; transformation; wall
cell adhesion: molecule
cell-bound: antibody
cell-mediated: immunity; reaction
cell surface: marker
cellular: biology; biophysics; cartilage; embolism; immunodeficiency with abnormal immunoglobulin synthesis; infiltration; mosaicism; pathology; polyp; spill; tenacity; tumor
cellular blue: nevus
cellular immune: theory
cellular immunity deficiency: syndrome
cellulitic: phlegmasia
celluloid: strip
cellulose tape: technique
cell wall–defective: bacteria
CELO: virus
celomic: bay
celomic metaplasia: theory of endometriosis
Celsius: scale
Celsus: kerion; vitiligo
cement: base; corpuscle; disease; line
cemental: caries
cementing: substance
cementodentinal: junction
cementoenamel: junction
cementoossifying: fibroma
cementum: hyperplasia
centigrade: scale

centimeter-gram-second: system; unit
central: amputation; apnea; apparatus; artery; artery of retina; bearing; body; bone; bone of ankle; bradycardia; callus; canal; canals of cochlea; canal of spinal cord; canal of the vitreous; cataract; chromatolysis; complex; deafness; dogma; ganglioneuroma; gyri; illumination; implantation; incisor; inhibition; lacteal; lobule; lobule of cerebellum; necrosis; neuritis; nucleus; osteitis; paralysis; part of lateral ventricle; pit; placenta previa; pneumonia; scotoma; spindle; sulcus; sulcus of insula; tendon of diaphragm; tendon of perineum; veins of liver; vein of suprarenal gland; vision
central amygdaloid: nucleus
central angiospastic: retinitis; retinopathy
central areolar choroidal: atrophy; dystrophy; sclerosis
central axillary: lymph nodes
central-bearing: device; point
central-bearing tracing: device
central cloudy corneal: dystrophy of François
central cord: syndrome
central core: disease
central crystalline corneal: dystrophy of Snyder
Central European tick-borne: fever
Central European tick-borne encephalitis: virus
central excitatory: state
central fibrous: body
central gray: substance
centralization: phenomenon
central lateral: nucleus of thalamus
central and lateral intermediate: substances
central limit: theorem
central mesenteric: lymph nodes
central nervous: system
central ossifying: fibroma
central palmar: space
central pontine: myelinolysis
central retinal: artery; fovea; vein
central serous: choroidopathy; retinopathy
central sulcal: artery
central superior mesenteric: lymph nodes

central tegmental: fasciculus; tract
central terminal: electrode
central thalamic: radiation
central transactional: core
central type: neurofibromatosis
central venous: catheter; pressure
centrencephalic: epilepsy
centriacinar: emphysema
centric: contact; fusion; occlusion; position
centric jaw: relation
centrifugal: casting; current; nerve
centrifugal fast: analyzer
centrilobular: emphysema
centripetal: current; nerve
centroacinar: cell
centrofacial: lentiginosis
centrolecithal: egg; ovum
centromedian: nucleus
centromere banding: stain
centromeric: index
centronuclear: myopathy
cephalic: angle; curve; flexure; index; pole; presentation; replacement; tetanus; triangle; vein; vein of forearm; version
cephalic arterial: rami
cephalocaudal: axis
cephalomedullary: angle
cephalometric: analysis; radiograph; tracing
cephalo-oculocutaneous: telangiectasia
cephalo-orbital: index
cephalopalpebral: reflex
cephalopelvic: disproportion
cephalorrhachidian: index
cephalotrigeminal: angiomatosis
ceramide lactoside: lipidosis
ceramo-metal: casting
ceratocricoid: ligament; muscle
ceratoglossus: muscle
ceratopharyngeal: part of middle constrictor muscle of pharynx; part of middle pharyngeal constrictor (muscle) of pharynx
cercopithecrine: herpesvirus
cerebellar: arteries; astrocytoma; ataxia; atrophy; cortex; cyst; falx; fissures; fossa; frenulum; gait; nuclei; pyramid; rigidity; speech; sulci; syndrome; tentorium; tonsil; veins
cerebellohypothalamic: fibers
cerebellomedullary: cistern
cerebellomedullary malformation: syndrome

cerebelloolivary: fibers
cerebellopontile: angle
cerebellopontine: angle; cisternography; recess
cerebellopontine angle: syndrome; tumor
cerebellorubral: tract
cerebellospinal: fibers
cerebellothalamic: tract
cerebral: angiography; anthrax; aqueduct; arteries; arteriography; calculus; cladosporiosis; compression; cortex; death; decompression; decortication; diataxia; dominance; dysplasia; edema; falx; fissures; flexure; gigantism; gyri; hemisphere; hemorrhage; hernia; index; lacuna; layer of retina; lipidosis; lobes; localization; malaria; palsy; part of arachnoid; part of dura mater; part of internal carotid artery; peduncle; porosis; rheumatism; sinuses; sphingolipidosis; sulci; surface; tetanus; thrombosis; trigone; tuberculosis; veins; ventricles; vesicle; vomiting
cerebral amyloid: angiopathy
cerebral arterial: circle
cerebrohepatorenal: syndrome
cerebroretinal: angiomatosis
cerebroside: lipidosis; lipoidosis
cerebrospinal: axis; fever; fluid; index; meningitis; nematodiasis; pressure; system
cerebrospinal fluid: otorrhea; rhinorrhea
cerebrotendinous: xanthomatosis
cerebrovascular: accident; disease
Cerenkov: radiation
ceroid: lipofuscinosis
certified: milk
certified pasteurized: milk
certified reference: material
certified registered: nurse anesthetist
cerulean: cataract
ceruminous: glands
cervical: amputation; anchorage; anesthesia; auricle; branch of facial nerve; canal; cap; diverticulum; duct; dysplasia; enlargement; enlargement of spinal cord; fibrositis; flexure; glands;

glands of uterus; hydrocele;
hygroma; hyperesthesia;
ligament of uterus; line;
loop; lordosis; margin;
margin of tooth; myelogram;
myositis; myospasm; nerves
[C1–C8]; nystagmus;
orthosis; part of esophagus;
part of internal carotid
artery; part of spinal cord;
part of thoracic duct; part of
vertebral artery; patagium;
pleura; plexus; pregnancy;
rib; segments of spinal cord
[C1–C8]; sinus; smear;
spondylosis; triangle; vein;
vertebrae [C1–C7]; vesicle;
zone; zone of tooth
cervical aortic: knuckle
cervical compression:
 syndrome
cervical disk: syndrome
cervical fusion: syndrome
cervical iliocostal: muscle
cervical interspinal: muscle
cervical interspinales:
 muscles
cervical intraepithelial:
 neoplasia
cervical longissimus: muscle
cervical rib: syndrome
cervical rib and band:
 syndrome
cervical rotator: muscles
cervical splanchnic: nerves
cervical tension: syndrome
cervicoaxillary: canal
cervicocolumbar: phenomenon
cervicooculoacoustic:
 syndrome
cervicothoracic: ganglion;
 orthosis; transition
cervicovaginal: artery
cesarean: hysterectomy;
 operation; section
Cestan-Chenais: syndrome
C1 esterase: inhibitor
Ceylon: cinnamon; moss
CF: antibody; lead; test
C group: viruses
Chaddock: reflex; sign
Chadwick: sign
Chagas: disease
Chagas-Cruz: disease
chagasic: myocardiopathy
Chagres: virus
chain: ganglia; reaction; reflex
α chain: disease
chain-compensated:
 spirometer
chair: form
chalice: cell
challenge: diet
chalybeate: water
Chamberlain: line; procedure
Chamberlen: forceps

Champy: fixative
Chance: fracture
chancriform: pyoderma;
 syndrome
chancroidal: bubo
chandelier: sign
Chandler: syndrome
change: blindness
Chantemesse: reaction
chaos: theory
chaotic: heart; rhythm
character: analysis; disorder;
 neurosis
characteristic: curve;
 emission; frequency;
 radiation
characterizing: group
Charcot: arteries; disease;
 gait; joint; syndrome; triad;
 vertigo
Charcot-Böttcher:
 crystalloids
Charcot-Bouchard: aneurysm
Charcot intermittent: fever
Charcot-Leyden: crystals
Charcot-Marie-Tooth:
 disease
Charcot-Neumann: crystals
Charcot-Robin: crystals
Charcot-Weiss-Baker:
 syndrome
Chargaff: rule
CHARGE: association;
 syndrome
charge: nurse
charge transfer: complex;
 system
Charles: law
Charlouis: disease
Charnley hip: arthroplasty
Charrière: scale
Charters: method
Chassaignac: space; tubercle
Chauffard: syndrome
Chaussier: areola; line; sign
Chayes: method
Cheadle: disease
Cheatle: slit
check: ligaments of eyeball,
 medial and lateral; ligaments
 of medial and lateral rectus
 muscles; ligaments of
 odontoid
Chédiak-Higashi: disease;
 syndrome
**Chédiak-Steinbrinck-
 Higashi:** anomaly;
 syndrome
cheek: bone; muscle; tooth
cheese: maggot
cheese worker's: lung
cheesy: abscess; pus
chemical: antidote; attraction;
 burn; cautery; ceptor;
 complexity; conjunctivitis;
 depilatory; dermatitis;

diabetes; energy; equation;
evolution; formula; kinetics;
knife; modification; peeling;
peritonitis; pneumonia;
potential; pregnancy;
prophylaxis; ray; repair;
sampling; senses; shift;
solution; sympathectomy;
taxonomy; thyroidectomy
chemically cured: resin
chemical shift: artifact
chemiosmotic: theory
chemotherapeutic: index
Cheney: syndrome
cherry: angioma
cherry-red: spot
cherry-red spot myoclonus:
 syndrome
cherubic: facies
chest: index; leads; radiology;
 wall
Chevalier-Jackson: dilator
chevron: incision
chewing: cycle; force
Cheyne-Stokes: psychosis;
 respiration
chi: sequence; structure
Chian: turpentine
Chiari: disease; net; syndrome
Chiari-Budd: syndrome
Chiari-Frommel: syndrome
Chiari II: syndrome
chiasma: syndrome
chiasmatic: cistern; groove;
 sulcus
Chicago: disease
chicken: breast
**chicken embryo lethal
 orphan:** virus
chicken fat: clot
chickenpox: immunoglobulin;
 virus
chickenpox immune: globulin
 (human)
Chick-Martin: test
chiclero: ulcer
chief: agglutinin; artery of
 thumb; cell; cell of corpus
 pineale; cell of parathyroid
 gland; cell of stomach;
 complaint
Chievitz: layer; organ
chikungunya: virus
Chilaiditi: syndrome
chilblain: lupus; lupus
 erythematosus
CHILD: syndrome
child: abuse; psychiatry;
 psychology
childbearing: age
childbed: fever
childhood: epilepsy with
 occipital paroxysms;
 hypophosphatasia;
 schizophrenia; tuberculosis
childhood absence: epilepsy

childhood muscular:
 dystrophy
childhood type: tuberculosis
Chilean: saltpeter
chimeric: antibodies; molecule
chimney sweep's: cancer
chimpanzee coryza: agent
chin: cap; jerk; muscle; reflex
Chinese: cinnamon; ginger;
 wax
Chinese restaurant:
 syndrome
chip: syringe
chiral: crystal
chi-square: distribution; test
chloride: shift
chlorinated: lime; paraffin
chlorine: acne; water
chlorohemin: crystals
chloropercha: method
chlorophyll: unit
chloroprocaine: penicillin O
chlorotic: anemia
chlorotriazine: dyes
choanal: atresia; polyp
chocolate: agar; cyst
Chodzko: reflex
choked: disk
cholangiolitic: hepatitis
cholangitic: abscess
cholecystoduodenal: fistula
choledoch: duct
choledochal: cyst; sphincter
choledochoduodenal: junction
cholera: agar; bacillus; toxin;
 vaccine
choleraic: diarrhea
cholera-red: reaction
choleric: jaundice
cholestatic: hepatitis; jaundice
cholestatic hepatosis: icterus
 gravidarum
cholesterinized: antigen
cholesterol: cleft; embolism;
 granuloma
cholesterol ester storage:
 disease
cholesterol ester transport:
 proteins
cholesteryl ester storage:
 disease
cholestyramine: resin
cholinergic: agent; blockade;
 fibers; neurotransmitter;
 receptors; urticaria
cholinesterase: inhibitor
chondrification: center
chondrin: ball
chondrodystrophic: dwarfism
chondroectodermal: dysplasia
chondroglossus: muscle
chondroid: syringoma; tissue
chondromyxoid: fibroma
chondropharyngeal: part of
 middle constrictor muscle of
 pharynx; part of middle

pharyngeal constrictor
(muscle) of pharynx
chondroxiphoid: ligament
Chopart: amputation; joint
chorda: saliva
choreic: movement
chorioallantoic: graft;
membrane; placenta
chorioamnionic: placenta
choriocapillary: layer
chorionic: ectoderm;
gonadotropin; plate; sac;
villi
chorionic gonadotropic:
hormone
chorionic gonadotropin: unit
chorionic growth: hormone-
prolactin
chorionic villus: biopsy
choroid: blood vessels;
branches; enlargement;
fissure; glomus; line;
membrane; plexus; plexus of
fourth ventricle; plexus of
lateral ventricle; plexus of
third ventricle; skein; vein;
veins of eye
choroidal: fissure;
neovascularization; ring
choroidal vascular: atrophy
choroplethic: map
Chotzen: syndrome
Chr^a: antigens
Christchurch: chromosome
Christensen-Krabbe: disease
Christian: disease; syndrome
Christison: formula
Christmas: disease; factor
chromaffin: body; cell;
reaction; system; tissue;
tumor
chromate: stain for lead
chromatic: aberration;
apparatus; audition; fiber;
granule; spectrum; vision
chromatin: body; network;
nucleolus; particles
chromatography: paper
chrome: alum; ulcer
chrome alum hematoxylin-
phloxine: stain
chrome-cobalt: alloys
chromic: catgut
chromic phosphate P 32
colloidal: suspension
chromidial: apparatus; net;
substance
chromophil: granule;
substance
chromophobe: adenoma; cells
of anterior lobe of
hypophysis; granules
chromosomal: deletion; gap;
region; RNA; syndrome;
trait

chromosomal instability:
syndromes
chromosome: aberration;
band; map; mapping;
mosaicism; pair; satellite
chronic: abscess; alcoholism;
anaphylaxis; appendicitis;
ataxia; bronchitis;
cholecystitis; conjunctivitis;
eczema; glaucoma;
glomerulonephritis;
hepatitis; histoplasmosis;
inflammation; malaria;
nephritis; pancreatitis;
pleurisy; pneumonia;
pyelonephritis; rejection;
rheumatism; rhinitis; shock;
soroche; tamponade;
trypanosomiasis; ulcer;
urticaria; vertigo
chronic absorptive: arthritis
chronic acholuric: jaundice
chronic actinic: keratopathy
chronic active: hepatitis;
inflammation
chronic active liver: disease
chronic adrenocortical:
insufficiency
chronic African sleeping:
sickness
chronic allograft: rejection
chronic anterior:
poliomyelitis
chronic atrophic:
polychondritis; thyroiditis;
vulvitis
chronic bacillary: diarrhea
chronic bullous: dermatosis of
childhood
chronic cicatrizing: enteritis
chronic constrictive:
pericarditis
chronic cutaneous:
leishmaniasis
chronic cystic: mastitis
chronic desquamative:
gingivitis
chronic diffuse sclerosing:
osteomyelitis
chronic discoid: lupus
erythematosus
chronic endemic: fluorosis
chronic eosinophilic:
pneumonia
chronic familial: icterus;
jaundice; polyneuritis
chronic fibrosing: alveolitis;
pancreatitis
chronic fibrous: thyroiditis
chronic focal sclerosing:
osteomyelitis
chronic follicular:
conjunctivitis
chronic granulocytic:
leukemia

chronic granulomatous:
disease
chronic hemorrhagic villous:
synovitis
chronic hypertensive: disease
chronic hypertrophic:
vulvitis
chronic hyperventilation:
syndrome
chronic idiopathic: jaundice;
xanthomatosis
chronic inflammatory
demyelinating:
polyneuropathy
chronic interstitial: hepatitis;
salpingitis
chronic lymphadenoid:
thyroiditis
chronic lymphocytic:
lymphoma; thyroiditis
chronic mediastinal:
histoplasmosis
chronic mountain: sickness
chronic myelocytic: leukemia
chronic myelogenous:
leukemia
chronic myeloid: leukemia
chronic necrotizing:
aspergillosis
chronic nonleukemic:
myelosis
chronic obstructive
pulmonary: disease
chronic persistent: hepatitis
chronic persisting: hepatitis
chronic posterior: laryngitis
chronic progressive: chorea
chronic progressive external:
ophthalmoplegia
chronic progressive
syphilitic:
meningoencephalitis
chronic relapsing: pancreatitis
chronic subglottic: laryngitis
chronic ulcerative: proctitis
chronologic: age
Churg-Strauss: syndrome
Chvostek: sign
chyle: cistern; corpuscle; cyst;
fistula; peritonitis; vessel
chyliform: ascites
chylomicron retention:
disease
chylous: arthritis; ascites;
hydrothorax; urine
chymotropic: pigment
α-chymotrypsin-induced:
glaucoma
Ciaccio: glands; stain
Cianca: syndrome
cicatricial: alopecia;
conjunctivitis; ectropion;
entropion; horn
cicatrization: atelectasis
cigarette: drain
cigarette-paper: scars

ciliary: blepharitis; body;
border of iris; canals;
cartilage; crown; disk;
dyskinesis; folds; ganglion;
glands; ligament; margin of
iris; movement; muscle; part
of retina; poliosis; process;
ring; staphyloma; wreath;
zone; zonule
ciliary ganglionic: plexus
ciliated: epithelium
ciliospinal: center; reflex
cinchona: bark
cinematic: amputation
cineplastic: amputation
cingular: branch of
callosomarginal artery
cingulate: convolution; gyrus;
herniation; sulcus
cingulum: rest
circadian: rhythm
Circe: effect
circinate: retinitis; retinopathy
circle absorption: anesthesia
circular: amputation; bandage;
dichroism; fibers; folds of
small intestine; layer of
detrusor (muscle) of urinary
bladder; layer of muscle
coat of small intestine; layer
of muscular coat; layers of
muscular tunics; layer of
tympanic membrane;
reaction; sinus; sulcus of
insula; sulcus of Reil
circulation: time
circulatory: arrest; collapse;
system
circumalveolar: fixation
circumanal: glands
circumduction: gait
circumferential: cartilage;
clasp; fibrocartilage;
implantation; lamella; wiring
circumferential clasp: arm
circumferential pontine:
branches of pontine arteries
circumflex: branch of left
coronary artery; branch of
posterior tibial artery; nerve;
veins
circumflex femoral: arteries
circumflex fibular: artery;
branch (of posterior tibial
artery)
circumflex humeral: arteries
circumflex iliac: arteries
circumflex peroneal: branch
of posterior tibial artery
circumflex scapular: artery;
vein
circummandibular: fixation
circumscribed: craniomalacia;
myxedema; peritonitis;
pyocephalus

circumscribed posterior: keratoconus
circumsporozoite: protein
circumvallate: papillae
circumventricular: organs
circumzygomatic: fixation; wiring
circus: movement; rhythm
cirsoid: aneurysm; varix
cis: configuration
cis: phase
13-*cis*-: retinoic acid
***cis*-acting:** locus; protein
cisternal: puncture
***cis/trans*:** test
citrate: intoxication
citrate-cleavage: enzyme
citrated: calcium carbimide
citric acid: cycle
citrovorum: factor
Civatte: bodies; disease
Civinini: canal; ligament; process
CL: lead
Clado: anastomosis; band; ligament; point
Clagett: procedure for empyema
Claisen: condensation
clamp: forceps
clamshell: incision; thoracotomy
clang: association
Clapton: line
Clara: cell
Clark: electrode; level
Clarke: cells; column; nucleus
Clarke-Hadfield: syndrome
Clark weight: rule
clasp: arm; bar; guideline
clasping: reflex
clasp-knife: effect; rigidity; spasticity
class: switching
class I: antigens; molecule
classic: hemophilia; migraine
classical: conditioning; genetics
classical cesarean: section
classic cervical rib: syndrome
classic choroidal: neovascularization
classifiable: character
class II: antigens; molecule
class III: antigens
clastic: anatomy
clathrate: crystal
Clauberg: test; unit
Claude: syndrome
Claudius: cells; fossa
claustral: layer
clavate: papillae
clavicular: branch of thoracoacromial artery; facet; head of pectoralis major muscle; notch of sternum; part of deltoid (muscle); part of pectoralis major (muscle); percussion
clavicular articular: facet of acromion
clavipectoral: fascia; triangle
claw: foot; hand
Claybrook: sign
clay shoveler's: fracture
clean intermittent bladder: catheterization
cleansing: cream
clear: cell; layer of epidermis
clear cell: acanthoma; adenocarcinoma; carcinoma; carcinoma of kidney; carcinoma of salivary glands; hidradenoma
clearing: factors; medium
clear liquid: diet
cleavage: cavity; cell; division; lines; product; site; spindle
cleaved: cell
cleft: hand; lip; nose; palate; spine; tongue
cleidocranial: dysostosis; dysplasia
Cleland: nomenclature; reagent
clenched fist: sign
clerical: spectacles
Clevenger: fissure
click: syndrome
clicking: rale; tinnitus
client-centered: therapy
climacteric: syndrome
climatic: bubo; keratopathy
climatic droplike: keratopathy
climbing: fibers
clinical: anatomy; burden; chemistry; crown; depression; diagnosis; epidemiology; eruption; fitness; genetics; indicator; lethal; medicine; nurse specialist; path; pathology; pharmacologist; pharmacology; pharmacy; psychology; recording; root of tooth; sensitivity; spectrometry; spectroscopy; thermometer; trial
clinical end: point
clinical practice: guidelines
clinoid: process
clip: forceps
clipped: speech
clitoral: recession
clivus: branches of cerebral part of internal carotid artery
cloacal: exstrophy; membrane; plate; theory
cloacogenic: carcinoma
clomiphene: test
clonal: aging; expansion
clonal deletion: theory
clonal selection: theory
clonic: convulsion; seizure
clonidine growth hormone stimulation: test
cloning: vector
clonogenic: assay; cell
Cloquet: canal; hernia; septum; space
close: bite
closed: anesthesia; bite; circle; comedo; dislocation; drainage; fracture; hospital; laparoscopy; reading frame; reduction of fractures; surgery; system
closed-angle: glaucoma
closed chain: compound
closed chest: massage
closed circuit: method
closed head: injury
closed loop: obstruction
closed skull: fracture
closing: contraction; membranes; snap; volume
clostridial: myonecrosis
***Clostridium perfringens*:** enterotoxin
***Clostridium perfringens* alpha:** toxin
***Clostridium perfringens* beta:** toxin
***Clostridium perfringens* epsilon:** toxin
***Clostridium perfringens* iota:** toxin
closure: principle
clot retraction: time
clotting: factor; time
clouding of: consciousness
Cloudman: melanoma
cloudy: swelling; urine
cloverleaf: model; skull
cloverleaf skull: syndrome
club: foot; hair; hand; moss
clubbed: digit; fingers; penis
clue: cell
cluster: analysis; headache; sample
cluster of differentiation (CD): antigen
Clutton: joints
CO_2: narcosis
coagulation: factor; necrosis; time; vitamin
coal tar: naphtha
coal worker's: pneumoconiosis
coaptation: splint; suture
coarctate: retina
coarse: dispersion; tremor
coated: pit; tongue; vesicle
Coats: disease
Cobb: method; syndrome
cobbler's: suture
cobra: hemotoxin; toxin
cobra venom: cofactor; factor
cocarde: reaction
coccidioidal: granuloma
coccidioidin: test
coccygeal: body; bone; cornu; dimple; fistula; foveola; ganglion; gland; horn; joint; ligament; muscle; nerve [Co]; part of spinal cord; plexus; segment of spinal cord [Co]; sinus; vertebrae [Co1–Co4]; whorl
coccygeus: muscle
Cochin China: diarrhea
cochlear: aqueduct; area; branch of labyrinthine artery; branch of vestibulocochlear artery; canal; canaliculus; cupula; drill-out; duct; dysplasia; ganglion; implant; joint; labyrinth; nerve; nuclei; part of vestibulocochlear nerve; potential; prosthesis; recess; root of VIII nerve; window
cochlear hair: cells
cochleariform: process
cochleo-orbicular: reflex
cochleopalpebral: reflex
cochleopupillary: reflex
cochleostapedial: reflex
Cochrane: collaboration
Cockayne: disease; syndrome
Cockett communicating perforating: veins
cockscomb: ulcer
coconut: sound
codeine: phosphate; sulfate
codfish: vertebrae
coding: sequence; strand
Codman: triangle; tumor
codominant: allele; gene; inheritance; trait
Coe: virus
coelomic: metaplasia
coenzyme: factor
coffee-ground: vomit
Coffey: suspension
Coffin-Lowry: syndrome
Coffin-Siris: syndrome
Cogan: dystrophy; syndrome
Cogan-Reese: syndrome
cognitive: development; dissonance; psychology; therapy
cognitive dissonance: theory
cognitive laterality: quotient
cogwheel: phenomenon; respiration; rigidity
cogwheel ocular: movements
cohesive: gold
Cohnheim: area; field
cohort: study
coil: gland
coiled: artery of the uterus
coin: lesion of lungs; test

coincidental: evolution
cointegrate: structure
coital: headache
Coiter: muscle
cold: abscess; agglutination; agglutinin; allergy; antibody; autoagglutinin; autoantibody; cautery; chain; cream; erythema; gangrene; hemolysin; light; nodule; pack; snare; sore; stage; ulcer; urticaria; virus
cold agglutinin: syndrome
cold bend: test
cold-blooded: animal
cold cure: resin
cold hemagglutinin: disease
cold knife: conization
cold pressor: test
cold-reactive: antibody
cold-rigor: point
cold-sensitive: enzyme; mutant
Cole-Cecil: murmur
colic: arteries; branch of ileocolic artery; impression on liver; impression of spleen; intussusception; lymph nodes; sphincter; surface of spleen; teniae; veins
coliform: bacilli
collagen: disease; fiber; fibrils; helix; implantation; injection
collagenous: colitis; pneumoconiosis
collapse: therapy
collapsing: pulse
collar: bone; incision
collar-button: abscess
collared: flagellate
collar-stud: chalazion
collateral: artery; branches of posterior intercostal arteries 3–11; branch of intercostal nerves; circulation; eminence; fissure; hyperemia; inheritance; ligament; sulcus; trigone; vessel
collateral digital: artery
collective: unconscious
Colles: fascia; fracture; ligament; space
Collet-Sicard: syndrome
collicular: artery
Collier: sign; tract
collier: lung
Collier tucked lid: sign
colliquative: albuminuria; degeneration; diarrhea; necrosis; sweat
Collis: gastroplasty
Collis-Belsey: fundoplication; procedure
collision: tumor

Collis-Nissen: fundoplication
collodion: baby
colloid: acne; adenoma; bath; bodies; cancer; carcinoma; corpuscle; cyst; degeneration; goiter; system; theory of narcosis
colloidal: dispersion; gel; metal; silicon dioxide; silver iodide; solution
colloidal gold: reaction; test
colloidal radioactive: gold
colobomatous: microphthalmia
colocutaneous: fistula
coloileal: fistula
colon: bacillus
colon cutoff: sign
colonic: diverticula; fistula; smear
colony-forming: unit
colony-stimulating: factors
color: aberration; agnosia; blindness; constancy; hearing; radical; scotoma; sense; spectrum; taste
Colorado tick: fever
Colorado tick fever: virus
color-contrast: microscope
colored: vision
colorimetric: titration
colorimetric caries susceptibility: test
colostomy: bag
colostrum: corpuscle
colovaginal: fistula
colovesical: fistula
Columbia Mental Maturity: Scale
Columbia S. K.: virus
column: cells; chromatography
columnar: epithelium; layer
coma: aberration; cast; scale; vigil
combat: exhaustion; neurosis
comb-growth: test
combination: beat; chemotherapy; restoration
combination oral: contraceptive
combined: glaucoma; immunodeficiency; methods; pregnancy; sclerosis; version
combined fat- and carbohydrate-induced: hyperlipemia
combined immunodeficiency: syndrome
combined system: disease
combining: weight
comblike: septum
combustion: equivalent
Comby: sign
comet: sign
comet tail: sign

comfort: zone
comitant: artery of median nerve; strabismus
comma: bacillus; bundle of Schultze; tract of Schultze
command: hallucination
commando: operation; procedure
commemorative: sign
commensal: parasite
comminuted: fracture
comminuted skull: fracture
commissural: cell; cheilitis; fibers; myelotomy
commisural: pits
common: antigen; baldness; crus of semicircular ducts; migraine; opsonin; salt; wart
common basal: vein
common bile: duct
common cardinal: veins
common carotid: artery; plexus
common carotid nervous: plexus
common cochlear: artery
common cold: virus
common facial: vein
common fibular: nerve
common flexor: sheath (of hand)
common hepatic: artery; duct
common iliac: artery; lymph nodes; vein
common interosseous: artery
common membranous: limb of membranous semicircular ducts; limb of semicircular ducts
common modiolar: vein
common palmar digital: artery; nerves
common peroneal: nerve
common peroneal tendon: sheath
common plantar digital: artery; nerves
common tendinous: ring of extraocular muscles
common variable: immunodeficiency
communicable: disease
communicating: artery; branch; branch of anterior interosseous nerve with ulnar nerve; branch of chorda tympani to lingual nerve; branch of chorda tympani with lingual nerve; branches of auriculotemporal nerve with facial nerve; branches of lingual nerve with hypoglossal nerve; branches of spinal nerves; branches of sympathetic trunk; branch of facial nerve with glossopharyngeal nerve; branch of facial nerve with tympanic plexus; branch of fibular artery; branch of glossopharyngeal nerve with auricular branch of vagus nerve; branch of intermediate nerve with tympanic plexus; branch of internal laryngeal nerve with recurrent laryngeal nerve; branch of lacrimal nerve with zygomatic nerve; branch of median nerve with ulnar nerve; branch of nasociliary nerve with ciliary ganglion; branch of otic ganglion to auriculotemporal nerve; branch of otic ganglion to chorda tympani; branch of otic ganglion with chorda tympani; branch of otic ganglion with medial pterygoid nerve; branch of otic ganglion with meningeal branch of mandibular nerve; branch of peroneal artery; branch of radial nerve with ulnar nerve; branch of superficial radial nerve with ulnar nerve; branch of superior laryngeal nerve with recurrent laryngeal nerve; branch of tympanic plexus with auricular branch of vagus nerve; hematoma; hydrocele; hydrocephalus; junction; rami of sympathetic trunk
community: dentistry; medicine; nurse; psychiatry; psychology
community-acquired: pneumonia
community health: nurse
compact: bone; substance
companion: artery to sciatic nerve; lymph nodes of accessory nerve; vein; veins
comparative: anatomy; medicine; pathology; physiology; psychology
comparator: microscope
compartment: syndrome
compensated: acidosis; alkalosis; glaucoma
compensated metabolic: alkalosis
compensated respiratory: acidosis; alkalosis
compensating: curve; emphysema; ocular
compensation: neurosis

compensatory: circulation; hypertrophy; hypertrophy of the heart; pause; polycythemia
competing: risk
competitive: antagonist; inhibition
competitive binding: assay
competitor: DNA
complement: factor I; fixation; system; unit
complemental: air
complementarity determining: regions
complementary: air; colors; DNA; hypertrophy; medicine; role; strand; structures
complement binding: assay
complement chemotactic: factor
complement-fixation: reaction; test
complement-fixing: antibody
complete: abortion; achromatopsia; antibody; antigen; ascertainment; blood count; carcinogen; cataract; cleavage; denture; disinfectant; fistula; hemianopia; hernia; iridoplegia; mastoidectomy; medium; metamorphosis; tetanus; transduction
complete androgen insensitivity: syndrome
complete atrioventricular: dissociation
complete AV: block
complete denture: impression
completely in the canal: hearing aid
complete posterior laryngeal: cleft
complex: fracture; joint; locus; odontoma; sound
complex endometrial: hyperplasia
complex febrile: convulsion
complex learning: processes
complex motor: seizure
complex partial: seizure
complex pleural: effusion
complex precipitated: epilepsy
complicated: cataract; migraine
component: management
composite: flap; graft; joint; resin
composite dental: cement
compound: aneurysm; articulation; caries; character; cyst; dislocation; eye; fracture; gland; heterozygote; joint; lens; lipids; microscope; nevus; odontoma; pregnancy; presentation; protein; restoration
compound action: potential
compound granule: cell
compound hyperopic: astigmatism
compound myopic: astigmatism
compound skull: fracture
comprehensive medical: care
compressed: sponge; tablet; yeast
compressible cavernous: bodies
compression: anesthesia; cyanosis; molding; neuropathy; paralysis; plate; plating; retinopathy; syndrome; thrombosis
compressive: myelopathy; nystagmus; strength
compressor urethra: muscle
Compton: effect; scatter
compulsive: idea; neurosis; personality
computed: perimetry; radiography; tomography
computer: model; simulation
computerized axial: tomography
Concato: disease
concave: lens; mirror
concavoconcave: lens
concavoconvex: lens
concealed: conduction; hemorrhage; hernia; penis
concentrated human red blood: corpuscle
concentration: gradient
concentric: fibroma; hypertrophy; lamella
concept: formation
concerted: evolution; model
conchal: cartilage; crest; crest of body of maxilla; crest of palatine bone
conchoidal: bodies
concomitant: immunity; strabismus; symptom
concordance: rate
concordant: alternans; alternation
concordant atrioventricular: connections
concordant changes: electrocardiogram
concrete: oils; operations; seborrhea; thinking
concurrent: disinfection; validity
concussion: cataract; myelitis
condensation: compound
condensed: milk
condensing: enzyme; osteitis
conditional: probability
conditional-lethal: mutant
conditionally lethal: mutant
conditioned: avitaminosis; hemolysis; insomnia; reflex; response; stimulus
conditioning: therapy
conduct: disorder
conducting: airway; system of heart
conduction: analgesia; anesthesia; aphasia; block
conductive: hearing impairment; heat
condylar: articulation; axis; canal; fossa; guidance; guide; joint; process of mandible
condylar emissary: vein
condylar guidance: inclination
condylar hinge: position
condyle: cord; path
condyloid: canal; process
cone: cell of retina; degeneration; disks; dystrophy; fiber; granule; vision
cone-rod retinal: dystrophy
confidence: interval
confluent: articulation; smallpox
confluent and reticulate: papillomatosis
confocal: microscope
conformational: map
confrontation: method
confusion: colors
congelation: urticaria
congenic: strain
congenital: afibrinogenemia; amputation; anemia; aplasia of thymus; baldness; bronchiectasis; cataract; choreoathetosis; conus; dysphagocytosis; elephantiasis; epulis of newborn; fibrosis of the extraocular muscles; glaucoma; hydrocele; hydrocephalus; hypophosphatasia; hypothyroidism; lymphedema; megacolon; methemoglobinemia; myxedema; nevus; nystagmus; pancytopenia; paramyotonia; pneumonia; stridor; syphilis; torticollis; toxoplasmosis; valve
congenital adrenal: hyperplasia
congenital aplastic: anemia
congenital atonic: pseudoparalysis
congenital cerebellar: atrophy
congenital cerebral: aneurysm
congenital diaphragmatic: hernia
congenital dyserythropoietic: anemia
congenital dysplastic: angiectasia; angiomatosis
congenital ectodermal: defect; dysplasia
congenital erythropoietic: porphyria
congenital facial: diplegia
congenital generalized: fibromatosis
congenital heart: block
congenital hemolytic: anemia; icterus; jaundice
congenital hereditary endothelial: dystrophy
congenital hip: dysplasia
congenital hypoplastic: anemia
congenital ichthyosiform: erythroderma
congenital lobar: emphysema
congenital microvillus: atrophy
congenital nonregenerative: anemia
congenital pulmonary arteriovenous: fistula
congenital pyloric: stenosis
congenital rubella: syndrome
congenital sebaceous: hyperplasia
congenital selective glucose and galactose: malabsorption
congenital spastic: paraplegia
congenital sutural: alopecia
congenital total: lipodystrophy
congenital virilizing adrenal: hyperplasia
congestive: cardiomyopathy; cirrhosis; splenomegaly
congestive heart: failure
Congolian red: fever
congophilic: angiopathy
Congo red: paper
congruent: points
congruous: hemianopia
conic: papillae
conical: catheter; cornea; lobules of epididymis; papillae
conjoined: anastomosis; tendon; twins
conjoined asymmetrical: twins
conjoined equal: twins
conjoined symmetrical: twins
conjoined unequal: twins
conjoint: tendon; therapy
conjugal: cancer

conjugate: acid; axis; deviation of the eyes; diameter of pelvic inlet; diameter of pelvic outlet; division; foci; foramen; gaze; movement of eyes; nystagmus; point
conjugate acid-base: pair
conjugated: antigen; bilirubin; compound; estrogen; hapten; protein
conjugated double: bonds
conjugative: plasmid
conjunctival: arteries; cul-de-sac; fornix; glands; layer of bulb; layer of eyelids; reflex; ring; sac; varix; veins
Conn: syndrome
connecting: cartilage; stalk; tubule
connective: tissue; tumor
connective-tissue: disease
connective tissue: cell; group
connector: bar
Connell: suture
conoid: ligament; process; tubercle (of clavicle)
Conradi: disease; line
Conradi-Hünermann: disease; syndrome
consecutive: amputation; aneurysm; angiitis; esotropia
consensual: reaction; validation
consensual light: reflex
conservative: replication; treatment
consistency: principle
consolidation: chemotherapy
consonating: rale
constancy: phenomenon
constant: coupling; region
constant field: equation
constant infusion: pump
constitutional: cause; formula; hirsutism; psychology; reaction; symptom; thrombopathy; ulcer
constitutional hepatic: dysfunction
constitutive: enzyme; heterochromatin
constriction: hyperemia; ring
constrictive: bronchiolitis; endocarditis; pericarditis
construct: validity
constructional: agraphia; apraxia
consulting: staff
consumption: coagulopathy
contact: allergy; area; catalysis; ceptor; cheilitis; dermatitis; hypersensitivity; hysteroscope; illumination; inhibition; lens; point; surface of tooth

contagious: disease; ecthyma
contagious ecthyma (pustular dermatitis): virus of sheep
contagious pustular: dermatitis
contagious pustular stomatitis: virus
contained disk: herniation
content: analysis; validity
contig: map
contingency: table
continued: fever
continuous: arrhythmia; beam; capillary; clasp; culture; eruption; murmur; phase; spectrum; suture; tremor; variable; variation
continuous ambulatory peritoneal: dialysis
continuous bar: retainer
continuous epidural: anesthesia
continuous flow: analyzer
continuous interleaved: sampling
continuous loop: wiring
continuous otoacoustic: emission
continuous passive: motion
continuous positive airway: pressure
continuous positive pressure: ventilation
continuous random: variable
continuous spinal: anesthesia
continuous wave: laser
contour: lines of Owen
contraceptive: device; sponge
contracted: foot; kidney; pelvis
contractile: stricture; vacuole
contraction: band
contraction band: necrosis
contraction stress: test
contractual: psychiatry; psychotherapy
contractural: diathesis
contracture: deformity
contralateral: hemiplegia; reflex; sign
contralateral routing of: signals
contrast: agent; bath; echocardiography; enema; enhancement; material; medium; sensitivity; stain
contrast sensitivity: testing
contrasuppressor: cells
contrecoup: injury of brain
control: animal; experiment; gene; group; syringe
controlled: respiration; substance; ventilation
controlled mechanical: ventilation
control release: suture

convalescent: carrier; serum
convective: heat
convenience: form
conventional: animal; signs; thoracoplasty; tomography
convergence: excess; insufficiency; nucleus of Perlia
convergence-retraction: nystagmus
convergent: evolution; squint; strabismus
converging: meniscus
conversion: disorder; electron; hysteria; neurosis; reaction
conversion hysteria: neurosis
conversive: heat
convex: lens; mirror
convexoconcave: lens
convexoconvex: lens
convoluted: bone; gland; part of kidney lobule; tubule of kidney
convoluted seminiferous: tubule
convulsant: threshold
convulsive: seizure; state; therapy; tic
cooing: murmur
Cooke: speculum
cooled-knife: method
Cooley: anemia
Coolidge: tube
coolie: itch
Coombs: murmur; serum; test
Cooper: fascia; hernia; herniotome; ligaments
cooperative: enzyme
cooperativity: model
Cooper-Rand artificial: larynx
coordinate covalent: bond
Cope: clamp
copia: elements
copolymer: resin
copper: cataract; colic; nose; protein
copper phosphate: cement
copper sulfate: method
Coppet: law
copra: itch
coracoacromial: arch; ligament
coracobrachial: bursa; muscle
coracobrachialis: muscle
coracoclavicular: ligament
coracohumeral: ligament
coracoid: process; tuberosity
coral: calculus
coralliform: cataract
cord: blood; hydrocele
cordate: pelvis
cordiform: uterus
cordy: pulse
core: particle; pneumonia
Cori: cycle; disease; ester

corkscrew: vessels
corn: ergot; sugar
corneal: astigmatism; corpuscles; decompensation; dystrophy; ectasia; facet; graft; layer of epidermis; lens; limbus; margin; pannus; reflex; space; spot; staphyloma; transplantation; trepanation; vertex
corneal endothelial: polymorphism
Cornelia de Lange: syndrome
corneocyte: envelope
corneoscleral: junction; part of trabecular tissue of sclera
Corner: tampon
Corner-Allen: test; unit
corniculate: cartilage; tubercle
corniculopharyngeal: ligament
cornified: layer of nail
cornmeal: agar
cornoid: lamella
cornual: pregnancy
coronal: epispadias; hypospadias; plane; pulp; section; suture
coronary: angiography; arteriosclerosis; arteritis; artery; atherectomy; cataract; endarterectomy; failure; groove; insufficiency; ligament of knee; ligament of liver; node; occlusion; plexus; sinus; steal; sulcus; tendon; thrombosis; valve; vein
coronary artery: aneurysm; bypass
coronary care: unit
coronary nodal: rhythm
coronary ostial: stenosis
coronary perfusion: pressure
coronary-prone: behavior
coronary sinus: rhythm
coronoid: fossa of humerus; process; process of the mandible; process of the ulna
corpora lutea: cyst
corpus: epididymis
corpuscular: lymph; radiation
corpus luteum: hematoma
corpus luteum deficiency: syndrome
corpus luteum hormone: unit
corralin: yellow
corrected: dextrocardia; transposition of the great vessels
corrective emotional: experience
correlation: coefficient
correlational: method
correlative: differentiation

Correra: line
Corrigan: disease; pulse; sign
corrosion: preparation
corrosive: sublimate; ulcer
corrugator: muscle
corrugator cutis: muscle of anus
corrugator supercilii: muscle
Corti: arch; canal; cells; ganglion; membrane; organ; pillars; rods; tunnel
Corti auditory: teeth
cortical: apraxia; arches of kidney; arteries; audiometry; blindness; bone; cataract; convexity; deafness; dysgenesis; dysplasia; epilepsy; hormones; implantation; lobules of kidney; osteitis; part; part of middle cerebral artery; sensibility; substance
cortical amygdaloid: nucleus
cortical radiate: arteries
corticobasal: degeneration
corticobulbar: fibers; tract
corticomesencephalic: fibers
corticonuclear: fibers
corticopontine: fibers; tract
corticoreticular: fibers
corticorubral: fibers
corticospinal: fibers; tract
corticosteroid-binding: globulin; protein
corticosteroid-induced: glaucoma
corticothalamic: fibers
corticotropic: hormone
corticotropin-releasing: factor; hormone
Corvisart: facies
corymbose: syphilid
coryneform: bacteria
cosmetic: dermatitis; surgery
cosmic: rays
costal: angle; arch; cartilage; chondritis; facets; fringe; groove; line of pleural reflection; margin; notches; part of diaphragm; part of parietal pleura; pit of transverse process; pleura; pleurisy; process; respiration; surface; surface of lung; surface of scapula; tuberosity
costal arch: reflex
Costen: syndrome
costimulatory: molecule
costoaxillary: vein
costocervical: artery
costocervical (arterial): trunk
costochondral: joints; junctions; syndrome
costoclavicular: ligament; line; syndrome

costocolic: ligament
costodiaphragmatic: recess
costomediastinal: recess; sinus
costopectoral: reflex
costophrenic: angle; sulcus
costophrenic septal: lines
costotransverse: foramen; joint; ligament
costovertebral: angle; joints
costoxiphoid: angle; ligament
cot: death
Cotard: syndrome
Cotte: operation
Cotton: effect
cotton-dust: asthma
cotton-fiber: embolism
cotton-mill: fever
cotton-root: bark
cotton-wool: patches; spots
Cotunnius: aqueduct; canal; liquid; space
cotyledonary: placenta
cotyloid: cavity; joint; ligament; notch
couching: needle
cough: fracture; reflex
Coumel: tachycardia
Councilman: body
counseling: psychology
count: density
counter: transference
counter-: shock
countercurrent: distribution; mechanism
counting: chamber
coup: injury of brain
coupled: beats; pulse; rhythm
coupling: defect; factors; interval; phase
Cournand: dip
Courvoisier: gallbladder; law; sign
Couvelaire: uterus
covalent: modification
cove: plane
cover: glass; test
covert: sensitization
cover-uncover: test
cow: face; kidney
Cowden: disease
Cowdry type A inclusion: bodies
Cowdry type B inclusion: bodies
CO_2-withdrawal seizure: test
cowl: muscle
Cowling: rule
cow milk: anemia
Cowper: cyst; gland; ligament
cowpox: virus
coxal: bone
coxitic: scoliosis
coxsackie: encephalitis; virus
CR: lead
crab: hand; yaws

Crabtree: effect
crack: cocaine
cracked: heel
cracked-pot: resonance; sound
crackling: jaw; rale
cradle: cap
Crafoord: clamp
Cramer wire: splint
Crampton: line; muscle; test
Crandall: syndrome
cranial: arachnoid mater; arteritis; base; bones; capacity; cavity; dura mater; flexure; fontanelles; index; nerves; neuropore; part of parasympathetic part of autonomic division of nervous system; root of accessory nerve; sinuses; sutures; synchondroses; vault; vertebra
(cranial) extradural: space
cranial pia: mater
cranial synovial: joints
craniocardiac: reflex
craniocarpotarsal: dysplasia; dystrophy
craniocervical: part of peripheral autonomic plexuses and ganglia
craniodiaphysial: dysplasia
craniofacial: angle; appliance; axis; dysostosis; fixation; surgery
craniofacial dysjunction: fracture
craniofacial suspension: wiring
craniometaphysial: dysplasia
craniometric: points
craniopharyngeal: canal; duct
craniosacral: division of autonomic nervous system
craniosacral nervous: system
craniospinal sensory: ganglia
crater: arc
cravat: bandage
C-reactive: protein
cream of: tartar
crease: wound
creatine kinase: isoenzymes
creatinine: clearance; coefficient
creative: thinking
Credé: maneuvers; methods
creep: recovery
creeping: eruption; myiasis; thrombosis; ulcer
cremaster: muscle
cremasteric: artery; fascia; reflex
creola: bodies
crepitant: rale
crescendo: angina; murmur; sleep
crescent: cell; sign

crescentic: lobules of the cerebellum
CREST: syndrome
Cresylecht violet: stain
Creutzfeldt-Jakob: disease
crevicular: epithelium; fluid
crib: death
cribriform: area of the renal papilla; fascia; foramina; hymen; plate of ethmoid bone
cribrous: lamina
Crichton-Browne: sign
cricoarytenoid: articulation; joint; ligament
cricoarytenoid articular: capsule
cricoesophageal: tendon
cricoid: cartilage
cricoid split: operation
cricopharyngeal: achalasia; ligament; myotomy; part of inferior constrictor (muscle) of pharynx
cricopharyngeus: muscle
cricosantorinian: ligament
cricothyroid: artery; articulation; branch of superior thyroid artery; joint; membrane; muscle
cricothyroid articular: capsule
cricotracheal: ligament; membrane
cricovocal: membrane
cri-du-chat: syndrome
Crigler-Najjar: disease; syndrome
Crile: clamp
Crimean: fever
Crimean-Congo hemorrhagic: fever
Crimean-Congo hemorrhagic fever: virus
criminal: abortion; anthropology; hygiene; insanity; irresponsibility; psychology
crisis: intervention
crisscross: heart
criterion-related: validity
critical: angle; illumination; limit; organ; pathway; period; pH; point; pressure; rate; temperature
critical care: unit
critical flicker fusion: frequency
critical illness: polyneuropathy
critical micelle: concentration
crocodile: tears
crocodile tears: syndrome
Crocq: disease
Crohn: disease
Cronkhite-Canada: syndrome

Crooke: granules
Crooke hyaline: change; degeneration
Crookes: glass
Crookes-Hittorf: tube
Crosby: capsule
cross: agglutination; birth; circulation; flap; hybridization; infection; mating; section; tolerance
cross-: reaction
crossbite: tooth
cross-cultural: psychiatry
cross-cut: bur
crossed: anesthesia; aphasia; cylinders; diplopia; embolism; eyes; fixation; hemianesthesia; hemianopia; hemiplegia; immunoelectrophoresis; jerk; laterality; paralysis; reflex; reflex of pelvis
crossed adductor: jerk; reflex
crossed extension: reflex
crossed knee: jerk; reflex
crossed pyramidal: tract
crossed renal: ectopia
crossed spino-adductor: reflex
crossed testicular: ectopia
cross-level: bias
cross-linked: polymer; resin
cross-over: study
cross-reacting: agglutinin; antibody; material
cross-sectional: echocardiography; method; study
cross-table lateral: projection
crotalaria: poisoning
Crotalus: antitoxin; toxin
croup-associated: virus
croupous: bronchitis; laryngitis; lymph; membrane
Crouzon: disease; syndrome
crowding: phenomenon
Crowe-Davis mouth: gag
Crow-Fukase: syndrome
crowing: inspiration
crown: cavity; flask; glass; pulp; tubercle
crown-heel: length
crown-rump: length
crucial: bandage; ligament
cruciate: anastomosis; eminence; ligament of the atlas; ligament of leg; ligaments of knee; muscle
cruciform: eminence; ligament of atlas; loops; part of fibrous digital sheath; part of fibrous sheath; pulley
crude: calcium sulfide; death rate; drug; urine

crural: arch; fascia; fossa; hernia; ring; septum; sheath; triangle
crural interosseous: nerve
crush: kidney; syndrome
crusted: ringworm; scabies; tetter
crutch: palsy; paralysis
Cruveilhier: disease; fascia; fossa; joint; ligaments; plexus
Cruveilhier-Baumgarten: disease; murmur; sign; syndrome
Cruz: trypanosomiasis
cry: reflex
crypt: abscesses
cryptogenic: cirrhosis; epilepsy; infection; pyemia; septicemia
cryptogenic fibrosing: alveolitis
cryptophthalmus: syndrome
cryptorchid: testis
crystal: rash; structure
crystalline: capsule; cataract; digitalin; interface; lens
crystalline insulin zinc: suspension
crystallized: trypsin
crystal violet: vaccine
Csillag: disease
"C" sliding: osteotomy
CT: number; pelvimetry; unit
Cuban: itch
cube: pessary
cubic: centimeter; niter
cubital: anastomosis; bone; fossa; joint; lymph nodes; nerve
cubital tunnel: syndrome
cuboid: bone
cuboidal: carcinoma; epithelium
cuboidal articular: surface of calcaneus
cuboideonavicular: joint; ligaments
cuboidodigital: reflex
cued: speech
cuirass: respirator; ventilator
cul-de-sac: smear
Cullen: sign
Culp: pyeloplasty
cultivated: yeast
cultural: anthropology; shock
culture: medium
Culver: root
Cummer: classification; guideline
Cumulative: Index Medicus
cumulative: action; dose; effect
cumulative trauma: disorders
cuneate: fasciculus; funiculus; nucleus; tubercle

cuneiform: bone; cartilage; cataract; lobe; nucleus; part of vomer; tubercle
cuneocerebellar: fibers; tract
cuneocuboid: joint; ligaments
cuneocuboid interosseous: ligament
cuneometatarsal: joints
cuneometatarsal interosseous: ligaments
cuneonavicular: articulation; joint; ligaments
cuneospinal: fibers
cup biopsy: forceps
Cupid's: bow
cupping: glass
cupular: cecum of the cochlear duct; part of epitympanic recess
cupular blind: sac
cupuliform: cataract
curative: dose
curb: tenotomy
curd: soap
curdy: pus
curlicue: ureter
Curling: ulcer
currant jelly: clot; stool; thrombus
current of: injury
Curschmann: spirals
curvature: aberration; hyperopia; myopia
Cushing: basophilism; disease; disease of the omentum; effect; phenomenon; response; suture; syndrome; syndrome medicamentosus
Cushing pituitary: basophilism
cusp: angle; height
cuspal: interference
cuspid: tooth
cuspless: tooth
cutaneomeningospinal: angiomatosis
cutaneomucouveal: syndrome
cutaneous: absorption; albinism; ancylostomiasis; anthrax; apoplexy; blastomycosis; branch of anterior branch of obturator nerve; branch of mixed nerve; branch of obturator nerve; diphtheria; emphysema; gangrene; glands; hemorrhoids; horn; larva migrans; layer of tympanic membrane; leishmaniasis; lupus erythematosus; meningioma; muscle; nerve; pseudolymphoma; reflex; schistosomiasis japonica; test; tuberculosis;

ureterostomy; vasculitis; vein
cutaneous cervical: nerve
cutaneous focal: mucinosis
cutaneous graft versus host: reaction
cutaneous leishmaniasis: granuloma
cutaneous loop: ureterostomy
cutaneous pupil: reflex
cutaneous tuberculin: test
cuticular: drusen
cutireaction: test
cutis: plate
cutting: edge; forceps; needle; teeth
cuttlefish: disk
cuvette: oximeter
Cuvier: ducts; veins
cyanide: poisoning
cyanide-nitroprusside: test
cyanobacteriumlike: bodies
cyanogenic: glycoside
cyanose: tardive
cyanotic: asphyxia; atrophy; atrophy of the liver; induration
cycle length: alternans
cycle-specific: agent
cyclic: adenylic acid; albuminuria; compound; esotropia; guanosine 3′,5′-monophosphate; neutropenia; nucleotide; peptide; phosphate; phosphoric acid; strabismus; uridine 3′,5′-monophosphate; vomiting
cyclopian: eye
cyclothymic: disorder; personality
cyclothymic personality: disorder
cylinder: retinoscopy
cylindrical: bronchiectasis; epithelium; joint; lens
cylindroid: aneurysm
cylindromatous: carcinoma
Cyon: nerve
cysteine: hydrolases
cystic: acne; artery; bronchiectasis; carcinoma; diathesis; disease of the breast; disease of renal medulla; duct; fibrosis; goiter; hygroma; hyperplasia; hyperplasia of the breast; kidney; lung; lymphangiectasis; lymph node; mole; node; polyp; veins
cystic adenomatoid: malformation
cystic duct: cholangiography
cysticercus: disease
cystic gall: duct

cystic medial: necrosis
cystic papillomatous: craniopharyngioma
cystine: bridge; calculus
cystine storage: disease
cystinotic: leukocyte
cystoduodenal: ligament
cystohepatic: triangle
cystoid: maculopathy
cystoid macular: edema
cystoscopic: urography
cythemolytic: icterus
cytochrome: system
cytochrome P-450: system
cytocrine: secretion
cytogenetic: map
cytogenic: reproduction
cytoid: bodies
cytokeratin: filaments
cytologic: examination; screening; smear; specimen
cytologic filter: preparation
cytomegalic: cells
cytomegalic inclusion: disease
cytomegalovirus: disease
cytopathic: effect
cytopathogenic: virus
cytophagic histiocytic: panniculitis
cytophil: group
cytophilic: antibody
cytoplasmic: bridges; inheritance; matrix
cytoplasmic inclusion: bodies
cytoreductive: therapy
cytostatic: chemotherapy
cytotonic: enterotoxin
cytotoxic: cell; chemotherapy; reaction
cytotrophoblastic: cells; shell
cytotropic: antibody
cytotropic antibody: test
Czapek-Dox: medium
Czapek solution: agar
Czerny: suture
Czerny-Lembert: suture

D

D: antigen; cell; enzyme; loop; wave
D-: 3-hydroxybutyric acid dehydrogenase; proline reductase
Daae: disease
Da Fano: stain
daily: dose
Dakin: fluid; solution
Dakin-Carrel: treatment
Dale: reaction
Dale-Feldberg: law
Dalen-Fuchs: nodules
Dalrymple: sign
Dalton: law
Dalton-Henry: law
Dam: unit

Damus-Kaye-Stancel: procedure
Damus-Stancel-Kaye: anastomosis
Dana: operation
Dance: sign
dancing: chorea
Dandy: operation
dandy: fever
Dandy-Walker: syndrome
Dane: particles; stain
Danforth: sign
Danielssen: disease
Danielssen-Boeck: disease
Danubian endemic familial: nephropathy
Danysz: phenomenon
DAPI: stain
DA pregnancy: test
dapsone: neuropathy
d'Arcet: metal
Darier: disease; sign
dark: adaptation; cells; reaction
dark-adapted: eye
dark-field: condenser; illumination; microscope
dark-ground: illumination
Darling: disease
d'Arsonval: current; galvanometer
dartoic: tissue
dartos: fascia; muscle
darwinian: ear; evolution; reflex; theory; tubercle
date: boil; fever
datum: plane
Datura: poisoning
Daubenton: angle; line; plane
daughter: cell; colony; cyst; isotope; star
Davidoff: cells
Davidson: syringe
Daviel: operation; spoon
Davies: disease
Davis: graft
Davis battery model of: transduction
Davis interlocking: sound
dawn: phenomenon
Dawson: encephalitis
Day: test
day: blindness; hospital; residue; sight
dazzling: glare
D-dimer: test
dead: fingers; nerve; pulp; space; tooth; tracts
dead arm: syndrome
dead-end: host
dead fetus: syndrome
dead-in-bed: syndrome
deadly: agaric; nightshade
deamidizing: enzymes
deaminating: enzymes
Dean fluorosis: index

death: instinct; rate; trance
Deaver: incision; method
DeBakey: classification; forceps
de Bordeau: theory
debrancher: deficiency
debranching: enzymes; factors
debranching deficiency limit: dextrinosis
Debré: phenomenon
Debré-Sémélaigne: syndrome
debulking: operation
decapacitation: factor
decarboxylated: dopa
decay: constant; theory
decentered: lens
decerebrate: rigidity; state
decidual: cast; cell; endometritis; fissure; reaction
deciduate: placenta
deciduous: dentition; membrane; skin; tooth
decision: analysis
declamping: phenomenon; shock
de Clerambault: syndrome
decomposition of: movement
decompression: chamber; disease; operations; sickness
decorticate: rigidity; state
decoy: cell
decremental: conduction
decubital: gangrene
decubitus: film; radiograph; ulcer
de-emetinized: ipecacuanha
deep: artery of arm; artery of clitoris; artery of penis; artery of thigh; artery of tongue; bite; branch; branch of the lateral plantar nerve; branch of the medial circumflex femoral artery; branch of the medial plantar artery; branch of radial nerve; branch of the superior gluteal artery; branch of the transverse cervical artery; branch of the ulnar nerve; cell; cortex; fascia; fascia of arm; fascia of forearm; fascia of leg; fascia of neck; fascia of penis; fascia of thigh; head of flexor pollicis brevis; lamina; layer; layer of levator palpebrae superioris; layer of temporal fascia; muscles of back; part of anterior compartment of forearm; part of external anal sphincter; part of flexor retinaculum; part of masseter (muscle); part of palpebral part of orbicularis

oculi (muscle); part of parotid gland; part of posterior (flexor) compartment of leg; percussion; reflex; scleritis; sensibility; veins of clitoris; veins of penis; vein of thigh
deep abdominal: reflexes
deep anterior cervical: lymph nodes
deep auricular: artery
deep brachial: artery
deep cardiac: plexus
deep cerebral: veins
(deep) cervical: fascia
deep cervical: artery; vein
deep circumflex iliac: artery; vein
deep crural: arch
deep dorsal: vein of clitoris; vein of penis
deep dorsal sacrococcygeal: ligament
deep epigastric: artery; vein
deep facial: vein
deep femoral: vein
deep fibular: nerve
deep flexor: muscle of fingers
deep gray: layer of superior colliculus
deep hypothermic: arrest
deep infrapatellar: bursa
deep inguinal: lymph nodes; ring
deep lateral cervical: lymph nodes
deep lingual: artery; vein
deep lymph: vessel
deep middle cerebral: vein
deep palmar: branch of ulnar artery
deep palmar (arterial): arch
deep palmar venous: arch
deep parotid: lymph nodes
deep perineal: fascia; pouch; space
deep peroneal: nerve
deep petrosal: nerve
deep plantar: artery; branch of dorsalis pedis artery
deep posterior sacrococcygeal: ligament
deep punctate: keratitis
deep temporal: artery; nerves; veins
deep tendon: reflex
deep transitional: gyrus
deep transverse: muscle of perineum
deep transverse metacarpal: ligament
deep transverse metatarsal: ligament
deep transverse perineal: muscle

deep white: layer of superior colliculus; layer [TA] of superior colliculus
deer-fly: disease; fever
Deetjen: bodies
def caries: index
defective: bacteriophage; organism; phage; probacteriophage; prophage; virus
defective interfering: particle
defense: mechanism; reflex
defensive: circle; medicine
deferent: canal; duct
deferential: artery
deferential (nervous): plexus
deferred: shock
defervescent: stage
deficiency: anemia; disease; mutant; symptom
definitive: callus; host; lysosomes; method; prosthesis
deflective occlusal: contact
degenerative: arthritis; chorea; index; inflammation; myopia
degenerative joint: disease
degloving: injury
deglutition: apnea; pneumonia; reflex; syncope
Degos: acanthoma; disease; syndrome
degree of: kindred
Dehio: test
dehydrated: alcohol
dehydration: fever
dehydrocholate: test
deionized: water
deiterospinal: tract
Deiters: cells; nucleus
Deiters terminal: frames
déjà vu: phenomenon
Dejerine: disease; reflex; sign
Dejerine hand: phenomenon
Dejerine-Klumpke: palsy; syndrome
Dejerine-Roussy: syndrome
Dejerine-Sottas: disease
Delafield: hematoxylin
de Lange: syndrome
delayed: allergy; coma after hypoxia; conduction; dentition; eruption; flap; graft; hypersensitivity; puberty; reaction; reflex; sensation; suture
delayed reaction: experiment
Delbet: sign
Del Castillo: syndrome
deletion: mutation
Delhi: sore
delimiting: keratotomy
delphian: node
delta: agent; alcoholism; antigen; bilirubin; cell of anterior lobe of hypophysis; cell of pancreas; fibers; granule; hepatitis; rhythm; virus; wave
deltoid: branch; crest; eminence; impression; ligament; muscle; region; tubercle (of spine of scapula); tuberosity (of humerus)
deltoideopectoral: triangle; trigone
deltopectoral: flap; triangle
delusional: disorder
demand: pacemaker
demand pulse: generator
demarcation: current; line of retina; potential
Demarquay: sign
dematiaceous: fungi
demigauntlet: bandage
demilune: body
demodectic: acariasis; blepharitis; mange
Demoivre: formula
demonstration: ophthalmoscope
De Morgan: spots
de Morsier: syndrome
de Musset: sign
demyelinated: myelitis
demyelinating: disease; encephalopathy; polyneuropathy
denaturation: temperature of DNA
denatured: alcohol; protein
dendriform: keratitis
dendritic: calculus; cataract; cell; depolarization; process; spines; thorns
dendritic corneal: ulcer
dengue: fever; virus
dengue hemorrhagic: fever
dengue shock: syndrome
Denis Browne: pouch; splint
Denman spontaneous: evolution
Dennie: line
Dennie-Morgan: fold
Denonvilliers: aponeurosis; ligament
dense: bodies
dense-deposit: disease
density: gradient
density gradient: centrifugation
dental: abscess; anatomy; anesthesia; ankylosis; apparatus; arch; articulation; biomechanics; biophysics; branches; bulb; calculus; canals; caps; caries; cast; cement; cord; crest; crypt; curing; cuticle; drill; dysfunction; engineering; fistula; floss; follicle; forceps; formula; furnace; geriatrics; germ; granuloma; groove; hygienist; impaction; implants; index; jurisprudence; lamina; ledge; lever; lymph; material; neck; nerve; orthopedics; osteoma; papilla; pathology; plaque; polyp; process; prophylaxis; prosthesis; prosthetics; pulp; pump; rami; ridge; sac; sealant; senescence; shelf; surgeon; syringe; tubercle; tubules; ulcer; wedge
dentary: center
dentate: fascia; fissure; fracture; gyrus; ligament of spinal cord; line; nucleus of cerebellum; suture
dentatorubral: fibers
dentatorubral cerebellar: atrophy with polymyoclonus
dentatothalamic: fibers; tract
denticulate: hymen; ligament
dentigerous: cyst
dentin: bridge; dysplasia; globule
dentinal: canals; fibers; fluid; papilla; pulp; sheath; tubules
dentinocemental: junction
dentinoenamel: junction
dentoalveolar: joint
dentogingival: lamina
denture: base; border; brush; characterization; edge; esthetics; flange; flask; foundation; hyperplasia; packing; prognosis; retention; space; stability
denture basal: surface
denture-bearing: area
denture foundation: area; surface
denture impression: surface
denture occlusal: surface
denture polished: surface
denture sore: mouth
denture-supporting: area; structures
Denucé: ligament
denumerable: character
Denver: classification; shunt
Denver Developmental Screening: Test
Denys-Drash: syndrome
Denys-Leclef: phenomenon
deodorized: opium
deoxy: sugar
dependent: beat; drainage; edema; personality; variable
dependent personality: disorder
depersonalization: disorder; syndrome
de Pezzer: catheter
depletion: response
depletional: hyponatremia
depolarizing: block; relaxant
depot: injection; reaction; therapy
depressed: fracture
depressed skull: fracture
depressive: neurosis; psychosis; reaction; stupor; syndrome
depressor: fibers; muscle of epiglottis; muscle of eyebrow; muscle of lower lip; muscle of septum; nerve of Ludwig; reflex
depressor anguli oris: muscle
depressor labii inferioris: muscle
depressor septi nasi: muscle
depressor supercilii: muscle
deprivation: amblyopia; dwarfism
depth: compensation; dose; perception; psychology; recording
de Quervain: disease; fracture; tenosynovitis; thyroiditis
derby hat: fracture
Dercum: disease
derivative: chromosome
derived: protein
dermal: bone; graft; leishmanoid; papillae; ridges; sinus; system; tuberculosis
dermal duct: tumor
dermal-fat: graft
dermatan: sulfate
dermatitis-arthritis-tenosynovitis: syndrome
dermatitis-causing: caterpillar
dermatogenic: torticollis
dermatologic: paste
dermatomal: distribution
dermatomic: area
dermatopathic: lymphadenitis; lymphadenopathy
dermoepidermal: interface
dermoid: cyst; cyst of ovary; tumor
dermolytic bullous: dermatosis
dermotuberculin: reaction
De Sanctis-Cacchione: syndrome
Desault: bandage
Descartes: law
Descemet: membrane
descending: aorta; artery of knee; branch; branch of anterior segmental artery of left and right lungs; branch of hypoglossal nerve; branch of lateral circumflex femoral artery; branch of medial

circumflex femoral artery; branch of occipital artery; branch of posterior segmental artery of left and right lungs; branch of superficial cervical artery; colon; current; degeneration; neuritis; nucleus of the trigeminus; part of aorta; part of duodenum; part of facial canal; part of iliofemoral ligament; part of trapezius (muscle); tract of trigeminal nerve
descending anterior: branch
descending genicular: artery
descending palatine: artery
descending posterior: branch
descending scapular: artery
Deschamps: needle
descriptive: anatomy; myology; psychiatry; statistics
DES (diethylstilbestrol): daughter
desensitizing: paste
desert: fever; sore
desiccated: liver; pituitary
design: denture
Desmarres: dacryoliths; retractor
desmoid: tumor
desmoplastic: fibroma; medulloblastoma; trichoepithelioma
desmoplastic cerebral: astrocytoma
desmoplastic malignant: melanoma
desmoplastic small cell: tumor
desmoteric: medicine
desoxy: sugar
despeciated: antitoxin
D'Éspine: sign
desquamative: pneumonia
desquamative inflammatory: vaginitis
desquamative interstitial: pneumonia
destructive: distillation
detachable: balloon
detached: craniotomy; retina
detached cranial: section
detector: coil
determinant: group
determinate: cleavage
detrusor: areflexia; compliance; hyperreflexia; instability; muscle; pressure; stability
detrusor sphincter: dyssynergia
Deutschländer: disease

developmental: age; anatomy; anomaly; disability; grooves; lines; psychology
developmental hip: dysplasia
Deventer: pelvis
deviational: nystagmus
Devic: disease
devil: grip
Devine: exclusion
devitalized: tooth
Devonshire: colic
dew: itch; point
Dewar: flask
de Wecker: scissors
dexamethasone suppression: test
df caries: index
Dharmendra: antigen
d'Herelle: phenomenon
dhobie mark: dermatitis
D.I.: particle
Di: antigen
diabetic: acidosis; amyotrophy; arthropathy; cataract; coma; dermopathy; diet; fetopathy; gangrene; gingivitis; glomerulosclerosis; lipemia; myelopathy; nephropathy; neuropathy; polyneuropathy; polyradiculopathy; puncture; retinitis; retinopathy
diabetic neuropathic: cachexia
diabetic thoracic: radiculopathy
diabetogenic: factor
diachronic: study
diagnosis-related: group
diagnostic: anesthesia; audiometry; cast; radiology; sensitivity; specificity; ultrasound
diagnostic diphtheria: toxin
diagonal: band; conjugate; section
diagonal conjugate: diameter
diagonalis: stria
dial: manometer
dialysis: dementia; shunt
dialysis disequilibrium: syndrome
dialysis encephalopathy: syndrome
diamond: disk; fuchsin; skin
Diamond-Blackfan: anemia; syndrome
diamond cutting: instruments
diamond-shaped: murmur
Diamond TYM: medium
Diana: complex
diaper: dermatitis; rash
diaphragm: pessary
diaphragmatic: constriction of esophagus; flutter; hernia; ligament of the mesonephros; pacemaker; part of parietal pleura; peritonitis; pleura; pleurisy; surface
diaphragmatic myocardial: infarction
diaphysial: center; dysplasia
diarthrodial: cartilage; joint
diastasis: cordis
diastatic skull: fracture
diastolic: afterpotential; murmur; pressure; shock; thrill
diastrophic: dwarfism; dysplasia
diathermic: therapy
diatomaceous: earth
diazo: reaction; reagent; stain for argentaffin granules
diazonium: salts
dibasic: acid; amino acid; ammonium phosphate; calcium phosphate; potassium phosphate; sodium phosphate
dicarboxylic acid: cycle
dicentric: chromosome
dichorial: twins
dichorionic diamnionic: placenta
Dick: method; test
Dickens: shunt
Dick test: toxin
dicrotic: notch; pulse; wave
dicumarol: resistance
didactic: analysis
dideoxy: procedure; sequencing
Diels: hydrocarbon
diencephalic: epilepsy; syndrome of infancy
dientamoeba: diarrhea
dietary: amenorrhea; fiber
Dieterle: stain
dietetic: albuminuria; treatment
diethenoid: fatty acid
O-diethylaminoethyl: cellulose
Dietl: crisis
diet quality: index
Dieuaide: diagram
Dieulafoy: erosion; lesion; theory
Di Ferrante: syndrome
difference: limen
differential: diagnosis; display; growth; manometer; stain; stethoscope; thermometer; threshold
differential blood: pressure
differential gene: expression
differential renal function: test
differential spinal: anesthesia

differential ureteral catheterization: test
differential white: blood count
diffuse: abscess; aneurysm; angiokeratoma; choroiditis; ganglion; glomerulonephritis; goiter; hyperkeratosis of palms and soles; leishmaniasis; mastocytosis; panbronchiolitis; peritonitis; phlegmon
diffuse alveolar: damage
diffuse arterial: ectasia
diffuse cutaneous: leishmaniasis; mastocytosis
diffused: reflex
diffuse deep: keratitis
diffuse esophageal: spasm
diffuse idiopathic skeletal: hyperostosis
diffuse infantile familial: sclerosis
diffuse Lewy body: disease
diffuse mesangial: proliferation
diffuse obstructive: emphysema
diffuse small cleaved cell: lymphoma
diffuse unilateral subacute: neuroretinitis
diffuse waxy: spleen
diffusible: stimulant
diffusing: capacity; factor
diffusion: anoxia; coefficient; constant; hypoxia; method; respiration; shell
digastric: branch of facial nerve; fossa; groove; muscle; notch; triangle
DiGeorge: syndrome
digestive: apparatus; enzymes; fever; glycosuria; leukocytosis; system; tract; tube; vacuole
digital: crease; dilatation; fossa; furrow; hearing aid; joints; plethysmograph; pulp; pulp of hand; radiography; reflex; veins; whorl
digital collateral: artery
digital flexion: crease
digital gray: scale
digitalis: tincture; unit
digital subtraction: angiography
digitate: dermatosis; impressions; wart
digitonin: reaction
Di Guglielmo: disease; syndrome
dihydric: alcohol
dihydrogen: phosphate

2,8-dihydroxyadenine: lithiasis
dilantin: gingivitis
dilated: cardiomyopathy; pore
dilation: thrombosis
dilator: muscle; muscle of ileocecal sphincter; muscle of pylorus
dilator pupillae: muscle
dileptic: seizure
dilute: alcohol; phosphoric acid
diluted: acetic acid; hydrochloric acid
dilution: anemia
dimensional: stability
dimidiate: hermaphroditism
Dimmer: keratitis
dimorphic: anemia
dimorphous: leprosy
dimple: sign
dinitrophenylhydrazine: test
dinner: pad
dinoflagellate: toxin
dinucleotide: domain; fold
Diogenes: cup
dioptric: aberration
diovular: twins
DIP: joints
dip: phenomenon
diphasic: complex
diphasic milk: fever
diphenylhydantoin: gingivitis
diphenylmethane: dyes; laxatives
diphtheria: antitoxin; toxin
diphtheria antitoxin: unit
diphtheria toxoid, tetanus toxoid, and pertussis: vaccine
diphtheritic: conjunctivitis; enteritis; membrane; neuropathy; paralysis; ulcer
diphyllobothrium: anemia
diploic: canals; vein
diploid: nucleus
dipolar: buffer; ions
dipole: moment; theory
direct: calorimetry; current; diuretic; embolism; flap; fracture; illumination; image; immunofluorescence; laryngoscopy; lead; method for making inlays; ophthalmoscope; ophthalmoscopy; oxidase; percussion; rays; retainer; retention; technique; transfusion; vision; zoonosis
direct acrylic: restoration
direct bone: impression
direct composite resin: restoration
direct Coombs: test
direct filling: resin

direct fluorescent antibody: test
direct inguinal: hernia
directional: atherectomy; preponderance; weakness
directive: psychotherapy
direct lateral: veins
directly observed: therapy
direct lytic: factor of cobra venom
direct nuclear: division
direct pulp: capping
direct pyramidal: tract
direct reacting: bilirubin
direct resin: restoration
direct vision: spectroscope
direct wet mount: examination
disability-adjusted life: years
disappearing bone: disease
discharging: tubule
Dische: reaction; reagent
Dische-Schwarz: reagent
disciform: degeneration; keratitis
disciform macular: degeneration
disclosing: solution
discoid: lupus erythematosus
discoidal: cleavage
disconjugate: movement of eyes
disconnection: syndrome
discontinuation: test
discontinuous: culture; phase; sterilization
discordant: alternans; alternation
discordant atrioventricular: connections
discordant changes: electrocardiogram
discrete: analyzer; character; smallpox; variable
discrete random: variable
discriminant: analysis; function; stimulus
discrimination: score
disease: determinants
disease modifying antirheumatic: drugs
dish: face
dishpan: fracture
disintegration: constant
disjoined: pyeloplasty
disjunctive: absorption
disk: electrophoresis; herniation; kidney; space; syndrome
disk sensitivity: method
disk-shaped: cataract
dislocation of: lens
dislocation: fracture
disodium: phosphate
disorganized: schizophrenia
disparity: angle

dispensing: tablet
disperse: placenta
dispersed: phase
dispersing: electrode
dispersion: colloid; medium; phase
displacement: analysis; loop; threshold
disproportionate: dwarfism
disproportionating: enzyme
disputed neurogenic thoracic outlet: syndrome
Disse: space
dissecting: aneurysm; cellulitis
dissection: tubercle
disseminated: aspergillosis; choroiditis; coccidioidomycosis; histoplasmosis; lipogranulomatosis; lupus erythematosus; sclerosis; tuberculosis
disseminated cutaneous: gangrene; leishmaniasis
disseminated gonococcal: infection
disseminated intravascular: coagulation
disseminated recurrent: infundibulofolliculitis
dissociated: anesthesia; nystagmus
dissociated horizontal: deviation
dissociated vertical: deviation
dissociation: constant; constant of an acid; constant of a base; constant of water; sensibility
dissociative: anesthesia; disorders; hysteria; reaction
dissociative identity: disorder
distal: caries; centriole; end; ileitis; myopathy; occlusion; part of prostate; part of prostatic urethra; part [TA] of anterior lobe of hypophysis; phalanx of foot; phalanx of hand; surface of tooth; tingling on percussion
distal interphalangeal: joints
distal intestinal obstructive: syndrome
distal medial striate: artery
distal radioulnar: articulation; joint
distal spiral: septum
distal splenorenal: shunt
distal tibiofibular: joint
distance: ceptor
distant: flap
distemper: virus
distention: cyst; ulcer
distilled: water
distortion: aberration

distortion-product otoacoustic: emission
distraction: conus; osteogenesis
distributed: effort
distributing: artery
distribution: coefficient; curve; leukocytosis; volume
distributive: analysis
disulfide: bond; bridge
disuse: atrophy
Dittrich: plugs; stenosis
diurnal: enuresis; periodicity; rhythm
divergence: insufficiency; paresis
divergence excess: exotropia
divergence insufficiency: exotropia
divergent: evolution; squint; strabismus
diverging: meniscus
divers': spectacles
diver's: palsy; paralysis
diverticular: disease
divided: dose; spectacles
diving: goiter; reflex
divisional: block
Dix-Hallpike: maneuver
dizygotic: twins
djenkol: poisoning
dmfs caries: index
DNA: gap; helix; homology; hybridization; polymorphism; virus
DNA-RNA: hybrid
d'Ocagne: nomogram
docking: protein
Döderlein: bacillus
Doerfler-Stewart: test
dog: disease; ear; nose; unit
dog distemper: virus
Dogiel: cells; corpuscle
dogmatic: school
Döhle: bodies; inclusions
dolichoectatic: artery
dolichopellic: pelvis
doll's eye: sign
dolorogenic: zone
dome: cell
dominance: hierarchy
dominant: character; eye; frequency; gene; hemisphere; idea; inheritance; trait
dominant lethal: trait
dominantly inherited Lévi: disease
dominant optic: atrophy
Donath-Landsteiner: phenomenon
Donath-Landsteiner cold: autoantibody
Donders: glaucoma; law; pressure; rings
Donnan: equilibrium

Donné: corpuscle
Donohue: disease; syndrome
donor: insemination
Donovan: bodies
Doose: syndrome
dopa: reaction
Doppler: echocardiography; effect; phenomenon; shift; ultrasonography
Doppler color: flow
Dor: fundoplication; procedure
Dorello: canal
Dorendorf: sign
Dorfman-Chanarin: syndrome
dorsal: artery of clitoris; artery of foot; artery of nose; artery of penis; branch; branches of first and second posterior intercostal artery; branches of the superior intercostal artery; branch of the lumbar artery; branch of the posterior intercostal arteries 3–11; branch of the posterior intercostal veins 4–11; branch of the subcostal artery; branch of the ulnar nerve; column of spinal cord; fascia of foot; fascia of hand; flexure; funiculus; hood; mesocardium; mesogastrium; muscles; nerve of clitoris; nerve of penis; nerve of scapula; nerves of toes; nucleus; nucleus of thalamus; nucleus of trapezoid body; nucleus of vagus; pallidum; pancreas; part of intertransversarii laterales lumborum (muscles); part of pons; plate of neural tube; position; reflex; root of spinal nerve; spine; striatum; surface; surface of digit (of hand or foot); surface of sacrum; surface of scapula; thalamus; tubercle of radius; vein of corpus callosum; veins of clitoris; veins of penis; vertebrae
dorsal accessory olivary: nucleus
dorsal calcaneocuboid: ligament
dorsal callosal: vein
dorsal carpal: branch of radial artery; branch of ulnar artery; ligament; network
dorsal carpal arterial: arch
dorsal carpal tendinous: sheaths
dorsal carpometacarpal: ligaments
dorsal column: stimulation
dorsal cuboideonavicular: ligament
dorsal cuneocuboid: ligament
dorsal cuneonavicular: ligaments
dorsal digital: artery; nerves; nerves of deep fibular nerve; nerves of foot; nerves of hand; nerves of superficial fibular nerve; nerves of ulnar nerve; veins of foot; veins of toes
dorsal hypothalamic: area; region
dorsal intercuneiform: ligaments
dorsal intermediate: sulcus
dorsal interossei (interosseous): muscles of foot; muscles of hand
dorsal interosseous: artery; nerve
dorsalis pedis: artery
dorsal lateral cutaneous: nerve
dorsal lateral geniculate: nucleus
dorsal lingual: branches of lingual artery; vein
dorsal longitudinal: fasciculus
dorsal medial cutaneous: nerve
dorsal median: sulcus
dorsal metacarpal: artery; ligaments; veins
dorsal metatarsal: artery; ligaments; veins
dorsal midbrain: syndrome
dorsal motor: nucleus of vagus
dorsal nasal: artery
dorsal pancreatic: artery
dorsal premammillary: nucleus
dorsal primary: ramus of spinal nerve
dorsal radiocarpal: ligament
dorsal root: ganglion
dorsal sacrococcygeal: muscle
dorsal sacrococcygeus: muscle
dorsal sacroiliac: ligaments
dorsal scapular: artery; nerve; vein
dorsal septal: nucleus
dorsal spinocerebellar: tract
dorsal supraoptic: commissure
dorsal talonavicular: bone
dorsal tarsal: ligaments
dorsal tarsometatarsal: ligaments
dorsal tegmental: decussation
dorsal thoracic: artery; nucleus
dorsal trigeminothalamic: tract
dorsal vagal: nucleus
dorsal venous: arch of foot; network of foot; network of hand
Dorset culture egg: medium
dorsiflexor: compartment of leg
dorsispinal: veins
dorsolateral: fasciculus; nucleus; plate of neural tube; sulcus; tract
dorsomedial: nucleus; nucleus of hypothalamus
dorsomedial hypothalamic: nucleus
dorsosacral: position
dorsum of: hand
dorsum pedis: reflex
dose-response: curve; relationship
dotted: tongue
double: athetosis; bind; bond; chin; consciousness; enterostomy; fracture; helix; hemiplegia; immunodiffusion; intussusception; lip; membrane; pleurisy; pneumonia; product; protrusion; quartan; refraction; salt; stain; tachycardia; tertian; vision
double antibody: immunoassay; method; precipitation
double antibody sandwich: assay
double aortic: arch; stenosis
double back: cross
double blind: experiment; study
double bubble: sign
double-channel: catheter
double compartment: hydrocephalus
double concave: lens
double congenital: athetosis
double contrast: enema
double convex: lens
double displacement: mechanism
double elevator: palsy
double flap: amputation
double (gel) diffusion precipitin: test in one dimension; test in two dimensions
double inlet atrioventricular: connections
double loop: hernia
double-masked: experiment
double minute: chromosomes
double-mouthed: uterus
double outlet right: ventricle
double pedicle: flap
double-point: threshold
double quotidian: fever
double-reciprocal: plot
double ring: sign
double-shock: sound
double-strand: break
double tertian: malaria
double track: sign
doubling: time
doubly: heterozygous
doubly armed: suture
douche: bath
doughnut: pessary
Douglas: abscess; bag; cul-de-sac; fold; line; mechanism; pouch
Douglas spontaneous: evolution
dousing: bath
dovetail stress-broken: abutment
dowager: hump
dowel: graft
Down: syndrome
downbeat: nystagmus
Downey: cell
Downs: analysis
downward: drainage
downy: hair
Doyère: eminence
Doyle: operation
Doyne honeycomb: choroidopathy
Drabkin: reagent
Dragendorff: reagent; test
Dräger: respirometer
drainage: tube
drain-trap: stomach
Draper: law
drawer: sign; test
dream: associations
dreamy: state
drepanocytic: anemia
dressing: forceps
Dressler: beat; syndrome
Dreyer: formula
dried: alum; ferrous sulfate; yeast
dried human: albumin; serum
dried human plasma protein: fraction
drift: movements
Drinker: respirator
drip: phleboclysis; transfusion
drip-suck: irrigation
drooping lily: sign
drop: attack; finger; foot; hand; heart
droplet: infection; nuclei
dropped: beat
drug: abuse; allergy; eruption; fever; pathogenesis;

psychosis; rash; resistance; tetanus
drug-induced: disease; hepatitis; lupus
drug utilization: review
drum: membrane
Drummond: sign
drumstick: appendage
dry: abscess; amputation; beriberi; bronchiectasis; cup; distillation; dressing; drowning; gangrene; hernia; labor; leprosy; nurse; pack; pericarditis; pleurisy; rale; socket; synovitis; tetter; vomiting; weight
dry cutaneous: leishmaniasis
dry eye: syndrome
D-S: test
dual: personality; relationships
dual-cure: resin
Duane: syndrome
Dubin-Johnson: syndrome
DuBois: formula
Dubois: abscesses; disease
Du Bois-Reymond: law
Duboscq: colorimeter
Dubowitz: score
Dubreuil-Chambardel: syndrome
Duchenne: disease; dystrophy; sign
Duchenne-Aran: disease
Duchenne-Erb: paralysis
duckbill: speculum
duck embryo origin: vaccine
duck hepatitis: virus
duck influenza: virus
duck plague: virus
Duckworth: phenomenon
Ducrey: bacillus; test
duct: carcinoma; papilloma
ductal: aneurysm; hyperplasia
ductless: glands
Duddell: membrane
Duffy: antigens
Duhring: disease
Dührssen: incisions
Duke bleeding time: test
Dukes: classification; disease
Dulong-Petit: law
dumb: rabies
dumbbell: ganglioneuroma
Dumdum: fever
dummy: consultand
Dumontpallier: pessary
dumping: syndrome
Duncan: disease; folds; mechanism; placenta; syndrome; ventricle
duodenal: ampulla; branches of anterior superior pancreaticoduodenal artery; branches of posterior superior pancreaticoduodenal artery;
bulb; cap; digestion; diverticulum; fistula; fossae; glands; impression on liver; smear; sphincter
duodenojejunal: angle; flexure; fold; fossa; hernia; junction; recess; sphincter
duodenomesocolic: fold
duodenorenal: ligament
Duplay: disease
duplex: kidney; transmission; ultrasonography; uterus
duplex Doppler: scan
duplication: cyst
duplicity: theory of vision
Dupré: muscle
Dupuytren: amputation; canal; contracture; disease of the foot; fascia; fracture; hydrocele; sign; suture; tourniquet
dural: part of filum terminale; sheath; sheath of optic nerve
dural cavernous sinus: fistula
dural venous: sinuses
Duran-Reynals permeability: factor
Dürck: nodes
Duret: hemorrhage; lesion
Durham: rule; tube
Duroziez: disease; murmur; sign
dust: asthma; cell; corpuscles
Dutton: disease
Dutton relapsing: fever
Duvenhage: virus
Duverney: fissures; gland; muscle
dwarf: pelvis
dwarfed: enamel
Dwyer: osteotomy
dyadic: psychotherapy; symbiosis
dye-dilution: curve
dye disappearance: test
dye exclusion: test
Dyggve-Melchior-Clausen: syndrome
dynamic: aorta; compliance of lung; CT; demography; equilibrium; force; friction; ileus; murmur; posturography; psychiatry; psychology; psychotherapy; refraction; relations; school; splint; viscosity
dynamic computed: tomography
dynein: arm
dysarthria–clumsy hand: syndrome
dysconjugate: gaze
dysembryoplastic neuroepithelial: tumor
dysenteric: diarrhea
dysenteric algid: malaria
dysentery: antitoxin; bacillus
dysfunctional uterine: bleeding
dysgranular: cortex
dysharmonious retinal: correspondence
dyshemopoietic: anemia
dyshidrotic: eczema
dysjunctive: nystagmus
dyskinesia: syndrome
dysmenorrheal: membrane
dysmnesic: syndrome
dysplastic: nevus
dysplastic nevus: syndrome
dysproteinemic: retinopathy
dysspermatogenic: sterility
dysthymic: disorder
dysthyroid: myopathy; orbitopathy
dysthyroidal: infantilism
dystonic: reaction; torticollis
dystrophic: calcification; calcinosis

E

E: rosette; selectin
EAC: rosette
EAC rosette: assay
Eadie-Hofstee: plot
Eagle-Barrett: syndrome
Eagle basal: medium
Eagle minimum essential: medium
EAHF: complex
Eales: disease
ear: bones; canal; crystals; lobe; wax
Earle: solution
Earle L: fibrosarcoma
ear lobe: crease
early: deceleration; discharge; reaction; seizure; syphilis
early diastolic: murmur
early dumping: syndrome
early infantile: autism
early latent: syphilis
early-phase: response
early posttraumatic: epilepsy
early receptor: potential
earth: wax
earthy: water
East African: trypanosomiasis
East African sleeping: sickness
eastern equine: encephalomyelitis
eastern equine encephalomyelitis: virus
eating: disorders; epilepsy
Eaton: agent
Eaton-Lambert: syndrome
EB: virus
Ebbinghaus: test
Eberth: bacillus; lines; perithelium
Ebner: glands; reticulum
Ebola: virus; virus Côte-d'Ivoire; virus Reston; virus Sudan; virus Zaire
Ebola hemorrhagic: fever
Ebstein: anomaly; disease; sign
eccentric: amputation; fixation; hypertrophy; implantation; occlusion; position; relation
ecchymotic: mask
eccrine: acrospiroma; gland; poroma; spiradenoma
ecdysial: glands
ECG: trigger
ecgonine: benzoate
echinococcus: cyst; disease
ECHO: virus
echo: beat; reaction; speech
echocardiographic: differentiation
Eck: fistula
Ecker: fissure
eclamptic: retinopathy
eclipse: blindness; period; phase
ECMO: virus
ecologic: chemistry; study
ecological: ectocrine; system
economic: coefficient
ecotropic: virus
ECSO: virus
ectatic: aneurysm; emphysema
ectatic marginal: degeneration of cornea
ectocervical: smear
ectodermal: cloaca; dysplasia
ectogenic: teratosis
ectopic: beat; decidua; eyelash; hormone; impulse; pacemaker; pinealoma; pregnancy; rhythm; schistosomiasis; tachycardia; teratosis; testis; ureter; ureterocele
ectopic ACTH: syndrome
ectoplacental: cavity
ectotrophoblastic: cavity
ectrodactyly–ectodermal dysplasia–clefting: syndrome
ectromelia: virus
eczematoid: seborrhea
eddy: sounds
Eder-Pustow: bougie
edge: enhancement
edge-to-edge: bite; occlusion
edgewise: appliance
Edinger-Westphal: nucleus
Edlefsen: reagent
Edman: method; reagent
Edridge-Green: lamp
educational: psychology
Edwards: syndrome
EEE: virus

EEG: activation
effective: conjugate; dose; half-life; stroke; temperature
effective osmotic: pressure
effective refractory: period
effective renal blood: flow
effective renal plasma: flow
effective temperature: index
effector: cell
efferent: duct; ductules of testis; fibers; lymphatic; nerve; vessel
efferent glomerular: arteriole
effervescent: lithium citrate; magnesium citrate; magnesium sulfate; potassium citrate; salts; sodium phosphate
effort-induced: thrombosis
egg: albumin; cell; membrane
Egger: line
Eggleston: method
eggshell: calcification
egg shell: nail
egg-white: injury; syndrome
Eglis: glands
ego: analysis; ideal; identity; instincts
ego-dystonic: homosexuality
Egyptian: hematuria; ophthalmia; splenomegaly
Ehlers-Danlos: syndrome
Ehrenritter: ganglion
Ehret: phenomenon
Ehrlich: anemia; phenomenon; postulate; reaction; theory
Ehrlich acid hematoxylin: stain
Ehrlich aniline crystal violet: stain
Ehrlich benzaldehyde: reaction
Ehrlich diazo: reaction; reagent
Ehrlich inner: body
Ehrlich triacid: stain
Ehrlich triple: stain
Ehrlich-Türk: line
Eichhorst: corpuscles; neuritis
Eicken: method
eidetic: image
eighth: nerve
eighth cranial: nerve [CN VIII]
eighth nerve: tumor
Einarson gallocyanin-chrome alum: stain
Einthoven: equation; law; triangle
Einthoven string: galvanometer
Eisenmenger: complex; defect; disease; syndrome; tetralogy
ejaculatory: duct

ejection: click; fraction; murmur; period; sounds
Ejrup: maneuver
Ekbom: syndrome
EKG: trigger
elastic: artery; bandage; bougie; cartilage; cone; fibers; lamella; laminae of arteries; layers of arteries; layers of cornea; ligature; limit; membrane; skin; tissue
elastic band: fixation
elastoid: degeneration
elastotic: degeneration
Elaut: triangle
elbow: bone; jerk; joint; reflex
elbowed: bougie; catheter
elder: abuse
elderly: primigravida
elective: abortion; culture; mutism
Electra: complex
electric: anesthesia; bath; cataract; cautery; chorea; irritability; retinopathy; shock; sleep
electrical: alternans; alternation of heart; axis; diastole; failure; formula; systole
electrical heart: position
electric cardiac: pacemaker
electrocardiographic: complex; wave
electrochemical: gradient
electroconvulsive: therapy
electrode: knife
electrode catheter: ablation
electrodiagnostic: medicine
electroencephalographic: dysrhythmia
electrographic: seizure
electrohydraulic shock wave: lithotripsy
electrolyte: metabolism
electromagnetic: flowmeter; induction; radiation; unit
electromechanical: dissociation; systole
electromotive: force
electromuscular: sensibility
electron: beam; capture; interferometer; interferometry; magneton; micrograph; microscope; microscopy; radiography
electron beam: tomography
electronegative: element
electronic: number; pacemaker
electronic cell: counter
electronic fetal: monitor
electronic pacemaker: load
electron paramagnetic: resonance

electron resonance: absorption
electron spin: resonance
electron transfer: flavin
electron-transport: chain; system
electron transport: particles
electrophonic: effect
electrophrenic: respiration
electropositive: element
electroshock: therapy
electrostatic: bond; unit
electrotherapeutic: sleep
electrotherapeutic sleep: therapy
electrotonic: current; junction; synapse
elementary: bodies; granule; particle
elephant: leg
elephant man's: disease
elephantoid: fever
elevator: disease; muscle of anus; muscle of prostate; muscle of rib; muscle of scapula; muscle of soft palate; muscle of thyroid gland; muscle of upper eyelid; muscle of upper lip; muscle of upper lip and wing of nose
eleventh cranial: nerve [CN XI]
elfin: facies
elfin facies: syndrome
elimination: diet
Ellik: evacuator
Elliot: operation; position
Elliott: law
ellipsoidal: joint
elliptical: amputation; anastomosis; recess of bony labyrinth
elliptocytary: anemia
elliptocytic: anemia
elliptocytotic: anemia
Ellis type 1: glomerulonephritis
Ellis type 2: glomerulonephritis
Ellis-van Creveld: syndrome
Ellsworth-Howard: test
Eloesser: flap; procedure
elongation: factor
Elschnig: pearls; spots
El Tor: vibrio
elusive: ulcer
E-M: syndrome
EMB: agar
Embden: ester
Embden-Meyerhof: pathway
Embden-Meyerhof-Parnas: pathway
embedding: agents
embolic: abscess; gangrene; infarct; pneumonia

emboliform: nucleus
embryo: transfer
embryonal: adenoma; area; carcinoma; inducer; leukemia; medulloepithelioma; rhabdomyosarcoma; tumor; tumor of ciliary body
embryonic: anideus; axis; blastoderm; cataract; cell; circulation; diapause; disk; hemoglobin; membrane; shield
embryopathic: cataract
EMC: virus
emergency: theory
emergency hormonal: contraception
emergent: evolution
emerging: viruses
emery: disks
Emery-Dreifuss muscular: dystrophy
emesis: basin
EMG: biofeedback; examination; syndrome
EMI: scan
emissary: vein
emission: electron
Emmet: needle; operation
emotional: age; amenorrhea; amnesia; attitudes; deprivation; disease; disorder; disturbance; leukocytosis; overlay
empathic: index
emphysematous: cholecystitis; cystitis; gangrene; phlegmon
empiric: risk; treatment
empirical: formula; horopter
empty: sella
empyema: tube
empyemic: scoliosis
emulsifying: wax
emulsion: colloid
enamel: cap; cell; cleavage; cleaver; crypt; cuticle; drop; dysplasia; epithelium; fibers; fissure; germ; hypocalcification; hypoplasia; lamella; layer; ledge; membrane; niche; nodule; organ; pearl; prisms; projection; pulp; rods; tuft; wall
enamel rod: inclination; sheath
enarthrodial: joint
encapsulated: delusion
encephalic: vesicle
encephalithogenic: protein
encephalitis: virus
encephaloclastic: microcephaly

encephalocraniocutaneous: lipomatosis
encephalomyelonic: axis
encephalomyocarditis: virus
encephalotrigeminal: angiomatosis
encephalotrigeminal vascular: syndrome
encounter: group
encu: method
encysted: calculus; pleurisy
end: artery; bud; bulb; cell; organ; oxidation; piece; plate; point; product; stage
endaural: incision
end-cutting: bur
end-diastolic: volume
endemic: disease; funiculitis; goiter; hematuria; hemoptysis; hypertrophy; index; influenza; neuritis; stability; syphilis; typhus
endemic nonbacterial infantile: gastroenteritis
endemic paralytic: vertigo
Endo: agar; medium
endoabdominal: fascia
endobronchial: tube
endocardial: cushions; fibroelastosis; fibrosis; murmur; sclerosis
endocardial cushion: defect
endocervical: smear
endocervical sinus: tumor
endochondral: bone; ossification
endocochlear: potential
endocrine: exophthalmos; glands; hormones; ophthalmopathy; part of pancreas; system
endodermal: canal; cell; cloaca; cyst; pouches
endodermal sinus: tumor
endodontic: stabilizer; treatment
end-of-life: care
endogenic: toxicosis
endogenous: cycle; depression; fibers; hyperglyceridemia; infection; pyrogen
endogenous creatinine: clearance
endolemniscal: nucleus
endolymphatic: duct; hydrops; sac; space
endolymphatic sac: surgery
endolymphatic shunt: operation
endomembrane: system
endometrial: ablation; canal; cyst; hyperplasia; implants; smear
endometrial stromal: sarcoma

endometrioid: carcinoma; tumor
endomyocardial: fibrosis
end-on mattress: suture
endo-osseous: implant
endopeduncular: nucleus
endopelvic: fascia
endoplasmic: reticulum
endorectal pull-through: procedure
endoscopic: biopsy
endoscopic retrograde: cholangiopancreatography
endosseous: implant
endosteal: implant
endoteric: bacterium
endothelial: cell; cyst; leukocyte; myeloma
endothelial-leukocyte adhesion: molecule
endothelial relaxing: factor
endotheliochorial: placenta
endothelio-endothelial: placenta
endothelium-derived relaxing: factor
endothoracic: fascia
endotoxin: shock
endotracheal: anesthesia; intubation; stylet; tube
endovaginal: ultrasonography
endovenous: septum
end-point: measurement; nystagmus
end product: inhibition; repression
endstage: lung
end-systolic: volume
end-tidal: sample
end-to-end: anastomosis; bite; occlusion
energy: metabolism; subtraction
energy-rich: bond; phosphates
Engelmann: disease
Engelmann basal: knobs
engine: reamer
Englisch: sinus
English: lock; position
English sweating: disease
enrichment: culture
ensheathing: callus
ensiform: cartilage; process
ensu: method
enteral: hyperalimentation
enteric: fever; tuberculosis; viruses
enteric coated: tablet
enteric cytopathogenic human orphan: virus
enteric cytopathogenic monkey orphan: virus
enteric cytopathogenic swine orphan: virus
enteric (nervous): plexus
entericoid: fever

enteric orphan: viruses
Enterobius: granuloma
enterochromaffin: cells
enterocutaneous: fistula
enterocyte cobalamin: malabsorption
enteroendocrine: cells
enterogastric: reflex
enterogenous: cyanosis; cyst; methemoglobinemia
enterohemorrhagic: *Escherichia coli*
enterohepatic: circulation
enteroinvasive: *Escherichia coli*
enterokinetic: agent
enteropathic: arthritis
enteropathogenic: *Escherichia coli*
enterotoxigenic: *Escherichia coli*
enterovaginal: fistula
enterovesical: fistula
Entner-Douderoff: pathway
entodermal: cell
entoptic: pulse
entorhinal: area
entrance: block
entrapment: neuropathy
entry: zone
envelope: conformation; flap
environmental: illness; psychology
enzootic: stability
enzootic encephalomyelitis: virus
enzygotic: twins
enzymatic: synthesis
enzyme: analog; antagonist; immunoassay; interconversion; isomerization; kinetics; parameters; regulation; repression
enzyme-catalyzed: ligation
enzyme inhibition: theory of narcosis
enzyme-linked immunosorbent: assay
enzyme-multiplied immunoassay: technique
enzyme-substrate: complex
eosin-methylene blue: agar
eosinopenic: reaction
eosinophil: adenoma; granule
eosinophil cationic: protein
eosinophil chemotactic: factor of anaphylaxis
eosinophilia-myalgia: syndrome
eosinophilic: cellulitis; cystitis; fasciitis; gastritis; gastroenteritis; granuloma; leukemia; leukocyte; leukocytosis; leukopenia; meningitis;

meningoencephalitis; pneumonia; pneumonopathy
eosinophilic endomyocardial: disease
eosinophilic pustular: folliculitis
epactal: bones; ossicles
epamniotic: cavity
eparterial: bronchus
ependymal: cell; cyst; layer; zone
ephemeral: fever
ephemeral fever: virus
epibranchial: placodes
epicanthal: fold
epicranial: aponeurosis; muscle
epicranius: muscle
epicritic: sensibility
epidemic: curve; disease; dropsy; encephalitis; exanthema; hemoglobinuria; hepatitis; hiccup; hysteria; keratoconjunctivitis; myalgia; myositis; nausea; neuromyasthenia; parotiditis; pleurodynia; polyarthritis; roseola; stomatitis; typhus; vertigo; vomiting
epidemic benign dry: pleurisy
epidemic cerebrospinal: meningitis
epidemic diaphragmatic: pleurisy
epidemic gangrenous: proctitis
epidemic gastroenteritis: virus
epidemic hemorrhagic: fever
epidemic keratoconjunctivitis: virus
epidemic myalgia: virus
epidemic myalgic: encephalomyelitis; encephalomyelopathy
epidemic nonbacterial: gastroenteritis
epidemic parotitis: virus
epidemic pleurodynia: virus
epidemic transient diaphragmatic: spasm
epidemiologic: genetics
epidemiological: distribution
epidermal: cyst; ridges
epidermal growth: factor
epidermal growth factor: receptor
epidermal-melanin: unit
epidermal ridge: count
epidermic: cell
epidermic-dermic: nevus
epidermoid: cancer; carcinoma; cyst
epidermolytic: hyperkeratosis

epidural: anesthesia; block; cavity; hematoma; meningitis; space
epifascicular: epineurium
epigastric: angle; fold; fossa; hernia; reflex; region; veins; voice
epiglottic: cartilage; folds; tubercle; vallecula
epihyal: bone; ligament
epikeratophakic: keratoplasty
epilation: dose
epilemmal: ending
epileptic: dementia; seizure; spasm
epileptiform: neuralgia
epileptogenic: zone
epiluminescence: microscopy
epimastical: fever
epimerase deficiency: galactosemia
epimyoepithelial: islands
epinephrine: reversal
epiotic: center
epipapillary: membrane
epipericardial: ridge
epiphrenic: diverticulum
epiphysial: arrest; cartilage; eye; fracture; line; plate
epiphysial aseptic: necrosis
epiploic: appendage; appendix; branches; foramen; tags
epipteric: bone
epiretinal: membrane
episcleral: artery; lamina; layer of fibrous layer of eyeball; space; veins
episodic: hypertension
episodic dyscontrol: syndrome
epistenocardiac: pericarditis
episternal: bone
epithelial: attachment; attachment of Gottlieb; body; cancer; cast; cell; cyst; downgrowth; dysplasia; ectoderm; inlay; lamina; layers; migration; nest; pearl; plug; tissue
epithelial choroid: layer
epithelial membrane: antigen
epithelial myoepithelial: carcinoma
epithelial reticular: cell
epitheliochorial: placenta
epithelioid: cell
epithelioid cell: nevus
epithermal: chemistry; neutron
epitrichial: layer
epituberculous: infiltration
epitympanic: recess; space
epizoic: commensalism
epoxy: resin
epsilon: alcoholism; wave

Epsom: salts
Epstein: disease; pearls; sign; symptom
Epstein-Barr: virus
equal: cleavage
equatorial: cleavage; division; plane; plate; staphyloma
equianalgesic: dose
equilibrium: constant; dialysis
equine: encephalitis; encephalomyelitis; gait; Morbillivirus; rhinoviruses
equine gonadotropin: unit
equiphasic: complex
equivalence: point; zone
equivalent: dose; extract; power; temperature; weight
equivalent form: reliability
equivocal: symptom
Eranko fluorescence: stain
Erb: disease; palsy; paralysis
Erb-Charcot: disease
Erb-Westphal: sign
Erdheim: disease; tumor
Erdmann: reagent
erect: illumination
erectile: tissue
erector: muscle of hair; muscle of spine
erector spinae: muscles
erector-spinal: reflex
ergot: alkaloids; poisoning
ergot alkaloid-associated heart: disease
Erlenmeyer: flask
Erlenmeyer flask: deformity
erogenous: zone
E-rosette: test
erosive: adenomatosis of nipple
erotic: zoophilism
erotomanic: disorder
erroneous: projection
error-prone: repair
error-prone polymerase chain: reaction
eruption: cyst
eruptive: fever; phase; stage; xanthoma
Erwinia **L-:** asparaginase
erythema: dose; threshold
erythematous: syphilid
erythremic: myelosis
erythroblastic: anemia
erythrocyte: indices
erythrocyte adherence: phenomenon; test
erythrocyte fragility: test
erythrocyte maturation: factor
erythrocyte sedimentation: rate
erythrocytic: cycle; series
erythrodysesthesia: syndrome
erythrogenic: toxin
erythroid: cell

erythronormoblastic: anemia
erythropoietic: hormone; porphyria; protoporphyria
Esbach: reagent
escape: beat; conditioning; contraction; impulse; interval; phenomenon; rhythm; training
escape-capture: bigeminy
escape ventricular: contraction
Escherich: sign
Escherichia coli: enterotoxin; RNase I
Esmarch: bandage; tourniquet
esodic: nerve
esophageal: achalasia; arteries; atresia; branches; branches of the inferior thyroid artery; branches of the left gastric artery; branches of the recurrent laryngeal nerve; branches of the thoracic aorta; branches of thoracic ganglia; branches of the vagus nerve; cardiogram; constrictions; dysrhythmia; glands; hiatus; impression on liver; lead; manometry; mucosa; opening; reflux; smear; spasm; speech; varices; veins; web
esophageal (nervous): plexus
esophagogastric: junction; orifice; vestibule
esophagosalivary: reflex
essential: albuminuria; amino acids; anemia; anisocoria; bradycardia; dysmenorrhea; fatty acid; fever; fructosuria; hypertension; nutrients; oils; pentosuria; pruritus; tachycardia; telangiectasia; thrombocytopenia; tremor
essential food: factors
essential progressive: atrophy of iris
Essick cell: bands
Essig: splint
established cell: line
esterified: estrogens
Estes: operation
esthesiodic: system
esthetic: dentistry; surgery
Estlander: flap
estradiol benzoate: unit
estrogen: receptor
estrogenic: hormone
estrogen replacement: therapy
estrone: unit
estrous: cycle
ether: test
ethereal: oil; solution; tincture
ethinyl: estradiol

ethmoid: angle; bone; cells; infundibulum
ethmoid air: cells
ethmoidal: bulla; cells; crest; crest of maxilla; crest of palatine bone; foramen; groove; infundibulum; labyrinth; notch; process of inferior nasal concha; sinuses; veins
ethmoidal-lacrimal: fistula
ethmoidolacrimal: suture
ethmoidomaxillary: suture
ethmovomerine: plate
ethynyl: estradiol
"e"-type: cholinesterase
eucalyptus: gum
euglobulin clot lysis: time
eugnathic: anomaly
Eulenburg: disease
eunuchoid: gigantism; state; voice
eupeptide: bond
euplastic: lymph
European: snakeroot; tarantula; typhus
European bat: Lyssavirus
euroxenous: parasite
eustachian: catheter; cushion; tonsil; tube; tuber; valve
eutectic: alloy; temperature
euthyroid: hypometabolism
euthyroid sick: syndrome
Evans: forceps; syndrome
evidence-based: medicine
evoked: electromyography; potential; response
evoked otoacoustic: emission
evolutionary: fitness
Ewart: procedure; sign
Ewing: sarcoma; sign; tumor
examining: table
exanthematous: disease; fever; typhus
excentric: amputation
excess: lactate
exchange: transfusion
excimer: laser
excision: biopsy; repair
excitable: area; gap
excitation: spectrum; wave
excitatory junction: potential
excitatory postsynaptic: potential
excited: atom; catatonia; state
exciting: cause; electrode; eye
excitor: nerve
excitoreflex: nerve
exclamation point: hair
excretory: duct; duct of seminal gland; duct of seminal vesicle; ducts of lacrimal gland; ductules of lacrimal gland; gland
exercise: bone; imaging; test
exercise-induced: amenorrhea

exercise radionuclide: angiocardiography
exertional: dyspnea; rhabdomyolysis
exfoliation: syndrome
exfoliative: cytology; dermatitis; gastritis; psoriasis
existential: psychiatry; psychology; psychotherapy
exit: block; dose
Exner: plexus
exoccipital: bone
exocelomic: membrane
exocrine: gland; part of pancreas
exocrine pancreatic: insufficiency
exodic: nerve
exoerythrocytic: cycle; stage
exogenic: toxicosis
exogenous: cycle; depression; fibers; hemochromatosis; hyperglyceridemia; ochronosis; pigmentation; pyrogens
exogenous creatinine: clearance
exophthalmic: goiter; ophthalmoplegia
exophthalmos-producing: substance
exoteric: bacterium
expandable: stent
expanded disability status: scale
expansion: arch
expansive: delusion
expectation: neurosis
experiential: aura
experimental: error; group; medicine; method; neurosis; psychology
experimental allergic: encephalitis; encephalomyelitis
experimenter: effects
expiratory: center; dyspnea; resistance; stridor
expiratory reserve: volume
expired: gas
exploratory: drive
exploring: electrode; needle
explosive: decompression; speech
exponential: distribution; growth
exposed: pulp
exposure: dose; keratitis
expressed: mustard oil
expressed skull: fracture
expression: vector
expressive: aphasia
expulsive: pains
exsanguination: transfusion

exsiccated: alum; sodium sulfite
exsiccation: fever
extemporaneous: mixture
extended: clasp; family; mediastinoscopy; pyelotomy; thymectomy
extended family: therapy
extended insulin zinc: suspension
extended radical: mastectomy
extension: bridge; form
extensor: aponeurosis; compartment of arm; compartment of forearm; compartment of leg; compartment of thigh; expansion; muscle; muscle of fingers; muscle of little finger; retinaculum
extensor carpi radialis brevis: muscle
extensor carpi radialis longus: muscle
extensor carpi ulnaris: muscle
extensor digital: expansion
extensor digiti minimi: muscle
extensor digitorum: muscle
extensor digitorum brevis: muscle; muscle of hand
extensor digitorum longus: muscle
extensor hallucis brevis: muscle
extensor hallucis longus: muscle
extensor indicis: muscle
extensor pollicis brevis: muscle
extensor pollicis longus: muscle
external: absorption; aperture of cochlear canaliculus; aperture of vestibular aqueduct; artery of nose; axis of eye; base of skull; branch of superior laryngeal nerve; branch of trunk of accessory nerve; canthus; capsule; conjugate; defibrillator; ear; fistula; fixation; genitalia; hemorrhoids; hydrocephalus; lip of iliac crest; malleolus; matrix; medium; meningitis; naris; nose; opening; opening of cochlear canaliculus; opening of urethra; ophthalmopathy; ophthalmoplegia; os of uterus; pacemaker; phase; pyocephalus; respiration; secretion; sheath of optic nerve; sphincter muscle of

anus; sphincterotomy; squint; strabismus; surface; surface of cochlear duct; surface of cranial base; surface of frontal bone; surface of parietal bone; table of calvaria; traction; urethrotomy; wall of cochlear duct
external acoustic: aperture; foramen; meatus; pore
external anal: sphincter
external arcuate: fibers
external auditory: foramen; meatus
external cardiac: massage
external carotid: artery; nerves
external carotid (nervous): plexus
external cephalic: version
external collateral: ligament of wrist
external conjugate: diameter
external cuneate: nucleus
external dental: epithelium
external exudative: retinopathy
external female genital: organs
external iliac: artery; lymph nodes; vein
external iliac lymphatic: plexus
external inguinal: ring
external intercostal: membrane; muscle
external jugular: vein
external male genital: organs
external malleolar: sign
external mammary: artery
external maxillary: artery; plexus
external medullary: lamina
external nasal: artery; branches of infraorbital nerve; veins
external nuclear: layer of retina
external oblique: muscle; reflex; ridge
external obturator: muscle
external occipital: crest; protuberance
external palatine: vein
external pillar: cells
external pin: fixation; fixation, biphase
external pterygoid: muscle
external pudendal: veins
external respiratory: nerve of Bell
external root: sheath
external salivary: gland
external saphenous: nerve

external semilunar: fibrocartilage
external spermatic: artery; fascia; nerve
external spiral: sulcus
external urethral: orifice; sphincter; sphincter of female; sphincter of male
external urinary: meatus
exterofective: system
extinction: coefficient
Exton: reagent
extra-: systole
extra-abdominal: desmoid
extraamniotic: pregnancy
extra-anatomic: bypass
extracapsular: ankylosis; fracture; ligaments
extracardiac: murmur
extracellular: cholesterolosis; enzyme; fluid; toxin
extracellular fluid: volume
extrachorial: pregnancy
extrachromosomal: DNA; element; gene; inheritance
extracoronal: retainer
extracorporeal: circulation; dialysis; photophoresis
extracorporeal shock wave: lithotripsy
extracranial: arteritis; ganglia; pneumatocele; pneumocele
extracranial-intracranial: bypass
extracting: forceps
extraction: coefficient; ratio
extradural: anesthesia; hematorrhachis; hemorrhage; space
extraembryonic: blastoderm; celom; ectoderm; membrane; mesoderm
extraglomerular: mesangium
extramammary Paget: disease
extramembranous: pregnancy
extramural: practice
extranodal marginal zone: lymphoma
extranuclear: inheritance
extraocular: muscles; part of central retinal artery and vein
extraoral: anchorage
extraoral fracture: appliance
extraperitoneal: fascia; space
extrapineal: pinealoma
extrapleural: pneumothorax
extrapyramidal: disease; dyskinesias; syndrome
extrapyramidal cerebral: palsy
extrapyramidal motor: system
extrapyramidal motor system: disease

extrasaccular: hernia
extrasensory: perception
extrasensory thought: transference
extraskeletal: chondroma
extrathyroidal: hypermetabolism
extrauterine: pregnancy
extravaginal: torsion
extravasation: cyst
extravascular: fluid
extravesical: reimplantation
extravital: ultraviolet
extremal: quotient
extreme: capsule
extrinsic: asthma; color; factor; motivation; muscles; muscles of eyeball; proteins; sphincter
extrinsic allergic: alveolitis
extrinsic incubation: period
extruded: teeth
exudation: cell; corpuscle; cyst
exudative: bronchiolitis; choroiditis; drusen; glomerulonephritis; inflammation; retinitis; tuberculosis; vitreoretinopathy
exudative discoid and lichenoid: dermatitis
exudative retinal: detachment
eye: capsule; cup; drops; lens; ointment; reflex; socket; speculum; tooth
eyeball compression: reflex
eyeball-heart: reflex
eye-closure: reflex
eye-closure pupil: reaction
eye-ear: plane
eyelash: sign
eyelid: imbrication

F

F: agent; pili; pilus; plasmid; thalassemia; waves
F-: actin
f: distribution; wave
FA: virus
FAB: classification
Fab: fragment; piece
Faber: anemia; syndrome
Fabricius: ship
Fabry: disease
face: form; peel; presentation; region; validity
face-bow: fork; record
facet: joints; rhizotomy
facial: angle; artery; aspect; axis; bones; canal; cleft; colliculus; diplegia; eminence; height; hemiatrophy; hemiatrophy of Romberg; hemiplegia; hillock; index; lymph nodes; muscles; myokymia; nerve [CN VII]; neuralgia; nucleus; palsy; paralysis; plane; plexus; profile; reflex; root; skeleton; spasm; surface of tooth; tic; triangle; trophoneurosis; vein; vision
facialis: phenomenon
facial motor: nucleus
facial nerve: area
facial recess: approach
facilitated: diffusion; transport
faciodigitogenital: dysplasia
facioscapulohumeral: atrophy
facioscapulohumeral muscular: dystrophy
factitial: dermatitis
factitious: disorder; illness by proxy; purpura; urticaria
factorial: experiments
facultative: anaerobe; heterochromatin; hyperopia; parasite; saprophyte
Faden: suture
fading: time
Faget: sign
Fahr: disease
Fahraeus-Lindqvist: effect
Fahrenheit: scale
faith: healing
falciform: cartilage; crest; ligament; ligament of liver; lobe; margin of saphenous opening; process of sacrotuberous ligament
falciform retinal: fold
falciparum: fever; malaria
fallen: arches
falling: palate; sickness
falling of the: womb
fallopian: aqueduct; arch; canal; hiatus; ligament; neuritis; pregnancy; tube
Fallot: tetrad; triad
false: agglutination; albuminuria; anemia; aneurysm; angina; ankylosis; blepharoptosis; branching; cast; chordae tendineae; conjugate; coxa vara; cyanosis; cyst; dextrocardia; diphtheria; diverticulum; dominance; glottis; hellebore; hematuria; hermaphroditism; hypertrophy; image; joint; knots; labor; lumen; macula; membrane; mole; neuroma; nucleolus; pains; paracusis; pelvis; pregnancy; projection; ribs; suture; thirst; vertebrae; waters
false memory: syndrome
false-negative: reaction
false-positive: reaction
false tendinous: cords
false vocal: cord
familial: aggregation; amyloidosis; cancer; dysautonomia; emphysema; glycinuria; goiter; hyperbetalipoproteinemia; hyperbetalipoproteinemia and hyperprebetalipoproteinemia; hypercholesterolemia; hypercholesterolemia with hyperlipemia; hyperchylomicronemia; hyperchylomicronemia with hyperprebetalipoproteinemia; hyperlipoproteinemia; hyperprebetalipoproteinemia; hypertriglyceridemia; hypobetalipoproteinemia; hypoparathyroidism; nephrosis; polyposis coli; screening; tremor
familial adenomatous: polyposis
familial aminoglycoside: ototoxicity
familial amyloid: neuropathy
familial aortic: ectasia
familial aortic ectasia: syndrome
familial bipolar mood: disorder
familial chylomicronemia: syndrome
familial combined: hyperlipemia
familial erythrophagocytic: lymphohistiocytosis
familial fat-induced: hyperlipemia
familial hemophagocytic: lymphohistiocytosis
familial high density lipoprotein: deficiency
familial hypercholesteremic: xanthomatosis
familial hypertrophic: cardiomyopathy
familial hypogonadotropic: hypogonadism
familial hypophosphatemic: rickets
familial hypoplastic: anemia
familial juvenile: nephrophthisis
familial lipoprotein lipase: inhibitor
familial Mediterranean: fever
familial microcytic: anemia
familial multiple endocrine: adenomatosis
familial nonhemolytic: jaundice
familial paroxysmal: polyserositis; rhabdomyolysis
familial partial: lipodystrophy
familial periodic: paralysis
familial pseudoinflammatory: maculopathy
familial pseudoinflammatory macular: degeneration
familial pyridoxine-responsive: anemia
familial recurrent: polyserositis
familial spinal muscular: atrophy
familial white folded: dysplasia
family: medicine; physician; practice; therapy
famine: dropsy
fan: sign
Fañanás: cell
Fanconi: anemia; pancytopenia; syndrome
FAPA: syndrome
far: point; sight
Farabeuf: amputation; triangle
Faraday: constant; laws
far-and-near: suture
Farber: disease; syndrome
Far East hemorrhagic: fever
Far East Russian: encephalitis
farmer's: lung; skin
Farnsworth-Munsell color: test
far point of: convergence
Farr: laws
Farrant mounting: fluid
Farre: line
Fas: ligand; receptor
fascia: graft
fascial: hernia; sheath of eyeball; sheaths of extraocular muscles
fascicular: block; degeneration; graft; keratitis; ophthalmoplegia; sarcoma; ulcer
fasciculata: cell
fasciolar: gyrus
fast: smear
fast component of: nystagmus
fastidious: organism
fastigial: nucleus
fastigiobulbar: fibers; tract
fastigiospinal: fibers; tract
fasting: hypoglycemia
fast-neutron radiation: therapy
fat: body; body of cheek; body of ischioanal fossa; body of ischiorectal fossa; body of orbit; cell; embolism; graft; hernia; indigestion;

metabolism; necrosis; pad; pad of ischioanal fossa; solvents; tide
fatality: rate
fate: map
father: complex
fatigue: fever; fracture; strength
fat-soluble: vitamins
fat-storing: cell
fatty: acid; alcohol; appendices of colon; ascites; atrophy; cast; change; cirrhosis; degeneration; diarrhea; folds of pleura; heart; hernia; infiltration; kidney; layer of subcutaneous tissue; layer of subcutaneous tissue of abdomen; layer of superficial fascia; liver; metamorphosis; oil; phanerosis; series; stool; tissue
fatty acid–binding: protein
fatty acid oxidation: cycle
fatty renal: capsule
faucial: branches of lingual nerve; diphtheria; paralysis; reflex; tonsil
faulty: union
faun tail: nevus
Favre: dystrophy
Favre-Durand-Nicholas: disease
Favre-Racouchot: disease; syndrome
Fazio-Londe: disease
Fc: fragment; piece; receptor
febrile: albuminuria; convulsion; crisis; psychosis; seizure; urine; urticaria
fecal: abscess; concentration; examination; fistula; impaction; incontinence; tumor; vomiting
Fechner-Weber: law
feedback: activation; inhibition; system
feed-forward: activation
feeding: center; tube
fee-for-service: insurance
feeling: tone
Feer: disease
Fehling: reagent; solution
feigned: eruption
Feiss: line
Felty: syndrome
female: catheter; circumcision; gonad; hermaphroditism; homosexuality; prostate; pseudohermaphroditism; sterility; urethra
female external: genitalia
female internal: genitalia

female pattern: alopecia
female urethral: syndrome
femininity: complex
femoral: arch; artery; branch of genitofemoral nerve; canal; fossa; hernia; muscle; nerve; opening; reflex; region; ring; septum; sheath; triangle; vein
femoral (nervous): plexus
femoral nutrient: artery
femoroabdominal: reflex
femoropatellar: joint
femoropopliteal: bypass
femoropopliteal occlusive: disease
fenestrated: capillary; membrane; sheath
fenestration: operation
Fenn: effect
Fenton: reaction
Fenwick-Hunner: ulcer
Ferguson: reflex
Fergusson: incision
fermentation *Lactobacillus casei*: factor
fermentative: dyspepsia
fern: test
Fernandez: reaction
Fernbach: flask
Ferrata: cell
Ferrein: canal; cords; foramen; ligament; pyramid; tube; vasa aberrantia
ferric: alum
ferric and ammonium acetate: solution
ferric chloride: reaction of epinephrine; test
ferruginous: bodies
Ferry: line
Ferry-Porter: law
fertile: period
fertility: agent; factor; ratio; vitamin
fertilization: membrane
fertilized: ovum
festinating: gait
fetal: attitude; bradycardia; circulation; cotyledon; death; distress; dystocia; electrocardiography; erythroblastosis; fracture; gigantism; habitus; hemoglobin; hydrops; inclusion; membrane; movement; ovoid; placenta; souffle; tachycardia; zone
fetal adrenal: cortex
fetal alcohol: syndrome
fetal aspiration: syndrome
fetal death: rate
fetal face: syndrome
fetal growth: restriction
fetal heart: rate
fetal hydantoin: syndrome

fetal scalp: stimulation
fetal trimethadione: syndrome
fetal warfarin: syndrome
fetomaternal: transfusion
fetoplacental: anasarca
Feulgen: cytometry; reaction; stain
fever: blister; therapy
feverish: urine
fiberoptic: gastroscope
fibrillar: baskets
fibrillary: astrocyte; astrocytoma; chorea; contractions; myoclonia; neuroma; waves
fibrillation: threshold
fibrillatory: waves
fibrin: calculus; thrombus
fibrin/fibrinogen degradation: products
fibrinogen-fibrin conversion: syndrome
fibrinoid: degeneration; necrosis
fibrinolytic: purpura
fibrinopurulent: inflammation
fibrinous: adhesion; bronchitis; cast; inflammation; iritis; lymph; pericarditis; pleurisy; polyp
fibrin-stabilizing: factor
fibroblast: interferon
fibrocartilaginous: ring of tympanic membrane
fibrocaseous: peritonitis
fibrocystic: condition of the breast; disease of the pancreas
fibroelastic: membrane of larynx
fibroepithelial: polyp
fibrohyaline: tissue
fibroid: cataract; inflammation; lung; tumor
fibrolamellar liver cell: carcinoma
fibromuscular: dysplasia; hyperplasia
fibromusculocartilagenous: layer of bronchi
fibromyalgia: syndrome
fibrosing: adenomatosis; adenosis; alveolitis; colonopathy; mediastinitis
fibrositic: headache
fibrotic: ophthalmoplegia
fibrous: adhesion; ankylosis; appendix of liver; capsule; capsule of kidney; capsule of liver; capsule of parotid gland; capsule of spleen; capsule of thyroid gland; cavernitis; degeneration; dysplasia of bone; dysplasia of jaws; goiter; hamartoma

of infancy; histiocytoma; joint; layer; layer of eyeball; layer of joint capsule; layer in or on deep aspect of fatty layer of subcutaneous tissue; mediastinitis; membrane of joint capsule; pericarditis; pericardium; pneumonia; polyp; protein; ring; ring of intervertebral disk; sheaths; sheaths of digits of hand; skeleton of heart; tissue; trigones of heart; tubercle; tunic of corpus spongiosum; tunic of eye; union; xanthoma
fibrous articular: capsule
fibrous bacterial: viruses
fibrous cortical: defect
fibrous digital: sheaths of foot; sheaths of hand; sheaths of toes
fibrous tendon: sheath
fibular: artery; compartment of leg; lymph node; margin of foot; node; notch; trochlea of calcaneus; veins
fibular articular: facet of tibia; surface of tibia
fibular collateral: ligament; ligament of ankle
fibularis brevis: muscle
fibularis longus: muscle
fibularis tertius: muscle
fibular nutrient: artery
fibular (peroneal): border of foot
fibular tarsal tendinous: sheaths
Fick: laws of diffusion; method; principle
Ficoll-Hypaque: technique
fictitious: feeding
Fiedler: myocarditis
field: block; carcinogenesis; fever; gradient; lens; survey
field of: consciousness
field block: anesthesia
field emission: tube
Fielding: membrane
Field rapid: stain
Fiessinger-Leroy-Reiter: syndrome
fifth: disease; finger; ventricle
fifth cranial: nerve [CN V]
fifth digit: syndrome
fig: wart
fight or flight: reaction
Figueira: syndrome
figure-of-8: abnormality; bandage; suture
filamentary: keratitis; keratopathy
filament-nonfilament: count
filamentous: bacteriophage; colony

filamentous bacterial: viruses
filament polymorphonuclear: leukocyte
filar: mass; micrometer; substance
filarial: arthritis; funiculitis; hydrocele; periodicity; synovitis
filariform: larva
Filatov: disease; flap; operation; spots
Filatov-Dukes: disease
Filatov-Gillies: flap
filial: generation
filiform: bougie; nucleus; papillae; pulse; wart
fillet: layer
filling: defect
filling internal urethral: orifice
filmless: radiography
filter: paper
filtering: bleb; cicatrix; operation
filtrable: virus
filtrate: factor; nitrogen
filtration: angle; coefficient; fraction; slits; space
fimbriated: fold of inferior surface of tongue
fimbriodentate: sulcus
final: host; impression
Finckh: test
fine: structure; tremor
fine needle: biopsy
finger: agnosia; percussion; phenomenon
finger-nose: test
fingerprint: dystrophy
finger-thumb: reflex
finger-to-finger: test
finishing: bur
Finkelstein: test
Fink-Heimer: stain
Finney: operation; pyloroplasty
fire: ant
first: dentition; finger; messenger; molar; part of duodenum; rib [I]
first arch: syndrome
first cervical: vertebra
first cranial: nerve [CN I]
first cuneiform: bone
first-degree: burn
first degree AV: block
first duodenal: sphincter
first heart: sound
first-order: reaction
first parallel pelvic: plane
first-pass: effect; metabolism
first rank: symptoms
first and second posterior intercostal: arteries
first-set: rejection
first temporal: convolution

first visceral: cleft
Fischer: projection; sign; symptom
Fischer projection: formulas
Fischer projection formulas of: sugars
fish: poison; skin
Fishberg concentration: test
Fisher: syndrome
Fisher exact: test
fish eye: disease
Fishman-Lerner: unit
fish-mouth: meatus
fish-mouth mitral: stenosis
fish-tank: granuloma
fish tapeworm: anemia
fission: fungi; product
fissural: cyst
fissure: bur; caries; sealant; sign
fissured: fracture; tongue
fistula: knife; test
FIT: test
Fitzgerald: factor
Fitz-Hugh and Curtis: syndrome
five-day: fever
five-year survival: rate
fixation: disparity; nystagmus; reaction; suppression
fixational ocular: movement
fixator: muscle
fixed: alkali; alkaloid; bridge; contracture; coupling; dressing; end; idea; macrophage; oil; pupil; torticollis; virus
fixed drug: eruption
fixed partial: denture
fixed-rate: pacemaker
fixed rate pulse: generator
fixing: eye
flaccid: ectropion; membrane; paralysis; part of tympanic membrane
Flack: node
flag: sign
flagellar: agglutinin; antigen
flagellate: diarrhea
flail: chest; joint
flame: arc; cell; figure; photometer; spots
flame emission: spectrophotometry
flammable: anesthetic
flange: contour
flank: bone; incision; position
flap: amputation; operation
flapless: amputation
flapping: tremor
flash: blindness; burn; dispersal; keratoconjunctivitis; method; point
flashing pain: syndrome
flash-lag: effect

flask: closure
flat: affect; bone; chest; condyloma; electroencephalogram; muscle; pelvis; plate; wart
Flatau: law
Flatau-Schilder: disease
flat top: waves
flatulent: dyspepsia
flatus: enema
Flaujeac: factor
flavin: nucleotide
flax-dresser's: disease
flea-bitten: kidney
flea-borne: typhus
Flechsig: areas; fasciculi; tract
Flechsig ground: bundles
fleck: dystrophy of cornea; retina of Kandori
flecked: retina
flecked retina: syndrome
Flegel: disease
Fleisch: pneumotachograph
Fleischer: ring; vortex
Fleischer-Strümpell: ring
Fleischmann: bursa
Fleischner: lines
Fleitmann: test
Flemming: fixative
Flemming triple: stain
Flesch: formula
flesh: fly
fleshy: mole; polyp
Fletcher: factor
flexible: collodion; endoscope; hysteroscope
flexion: crease
flexion-extension: injury
Flexner: bacillus
flexor: compartment of arm; compartment of forearm; compartment of leg; compartment of thigh; muscle; reflex; retinaculum; retinaculum of forearm; retinaculum of lower limb
flexor accessorius: muscle
flexor carpi radialis: muscle
flexor carpi ulnaris: muscle
flexor digiti minimi brevis: muscle of foot; muscle of hand
flexor digitorum brevis: muscle
flexor digitorum longus: muscle
flexor digitorum profundus: muscle
flexor digitorum superficialis: muscle
flexor hallucis brevis: muscle
flexor hallucis longus: muscle
flexor pollicis brevis: muscle
flexor pollicis longus: muscle
flexural: eczema; psoriasis
flick: movements

flicker: fusion; perimetry; photometer
flicker fusion frequency: technique
Flieringa: ring
flight: blindness; nurse
flight of: ideas
flight or fight: response
Flinders Island spotted: fever
Flint: arcade; murmur
flint: disease; glass
flip: angle
flittering: scotoma
floating: cartilage; kidney; organ; patella; ribs [XI–XII]; spleen; villus
floccular: fossa
flocculation: reaction; test
flocculonodular: lobe
Flood: ligament
flood: fever
floor: cell; plate
floppy valve: syndrome
Florence: crystals; flask
Florey: unit
florid oral: papillomatosis
florid osseous: dysplasia
floriform: cataract
Florschütz: formula
floss: silk
flotation: constant; method
Flourens: theory
floury: cornea
flow: cytometry; cytophotometry; diagram; void
Flower: bone
Flower dental: index
flower-spray: ending; organ of Ruffini
flowing: hyperostosis
flow-over: vaporizer
flow-volume: curve
flow-volume loop: studies
fluent: aphasia
fluid: extract; retinopexy; wave
fluid mosaic: model
fluorescein: angiography
fluorescein instillation: test
fluorescein string: test
fluorescence: microscope; microscopy; quenching; spectrum
fluorescence plus Giemsa: stain
fluorescence in situ: hybridization
fluorescent: antibody; screen; stain
fluorescent antibody: technique
fluorescent antinuclear antibody: test
fluorescent in situ: hybridization

fluorescent treponemal antibody-absorption: test
fluoridated: tooth
Flury strain: vaccine
Flury strain rabies: virus
flush: technique
flutter-fibrillation: waves
flux: density; ratio
fluxionary: hyperemia
fly: agaric; blister
flying: blister
flying spot: microscope
Flynn: phenomenon
Flynn-Aird: syndrome
FMD: virus
foam: cells
foam stability: test
foamy: agents; viruses
focal: acrohyperkeratosis; amyloidosis; appendicitis; depth; distance; epilepsy; glomerulonephritis; illumination; infection; interval; necrosis; nephritis; point; reaction; spot
focal condensing: osteitis
focal dermal: hypoplasia
focal embolic: glomerulonephritis
focal epithelial: hyperplasia
focal lymphocytic: thyroiditis
focal metastatic: disease
focal motor: seizure
focal sclerosing: glomerulopathy
focal segmental: glomerulosclerosis
focused: grid
Fogarty: clamp
Fogarty embolectomy: catheter
fogging: retinoscopy
Foix-Alajouanine: myelitis; syndrome
Foix-Cavany-Marie: syndrome
foldable intraocular: lens
fold-back: elements
folded-lung: syndrome
folding: fracture
Foley: catheter
Foley Y-plasty: pyeloplasty
foliate: papillae; papillitis
folic acid: antagonists; conjugate
folic acid deficiency: anemia
Folin: reaction; reagent; test
Folin-Looney: test
folk: medicine
Folli: process
follian: process
follicle-stimulating: hormone; principle
follicular: abscess; adenoma; antrum; carcinoma; conjunctivitis; cyst; cystitis; gland; goiter; hormone; impetigo; iritis; lymphoma; mange; mucinosis; papule; stigma; syphilid; trachoma; urethritis; vulvitis
follicular epithelial: cell
follicular ovarian: cells
follicular predominantly large cell: lymphoma
follicular predominantly small cleaved cell: lymphoma
Folling: disease
following: bougie
follow-up: study
Foltz: valvule
Fonio: solution
Fontan: operation; procedure
Fontana: canal; spaces; stain
Fontana-Masson silver: stain
food: asthma; ball; fever; impaction; poisoning
foot: bones; plate; plugger; process; yaws
foot-and-mouth: disease
foot-and-mouth disease: virus
foot-and-mouth disease virus: vaccines
football: calf
footling: presentation
foot-pound-second: system; unit
Foot reticulin impregnation: stain
foramen of Bochdalek: hernia
foraminal: herniation; lymph node; node
Forbes: disease
Forbes-Albright: syndrome
forced: alimentation; beat; cycle; duction; feeding; respiration; spirometry
forced expiratory: flow; time; volume
forced grasping: reflex
forced vital: capacity
forceps: delivery
force-velocity: curve
Forchheimer: sign
Fordyce: angiokeratoma; disease; granules; spots
forebrain: eminence; prominence; vesicle
foreign: body; protein; serum
foreign-body: appendicitis
foreign body: granuloma; salpingitis; tumorigenesis
foreign body giant: cell
foreign protein: therapy
Forel: decussation
forensic: dentistry; medicine; odontology; psychiatry; psychology
forequarter: amputation
forest: yaws
Forestier: disease
Formad: kidney
formal: operations
formaldehyde: fixative
formalin: pigment
formalin-ether sedimentation: concentration
formalin-ethyl acetate sedimentation: concentration
formative: cell
formed visual: hallucination
formol: titration
formol-calcium: fixative
formol-gel: test
formol-Müller: fixative
formol-saline: fixative
formol-Zenker: fixative
formyl-methionyl-: tRNA
fornicate: gyrus
Forsius-Eriksson: albinism
Forssman: antibody; antigen; hapten; reaction
Forssman antigen-antibody: reaction
Förster: uveitis
Fort Bragg: fever
fortification: figures; spectrum
fortified: milk
fortified vitamin D: milk
forward: conduction
forward heart: failure
Fosdick-Hansen-Epple: test
Foshay: test
Foster: frame
Foster Kennedy: syndrome
Fothergill: disease; neuralgia; operation; sign
Fouchet: reagent; stain
founder: effect; principle
foundryman's: fever
fountain: decussation; syringe
Four Corners: virus
four-headed: muscle
Fourier: analysis; transfer; transform
Fournier: disease; gangrene
four-tailed: bandage
fourth: disease; finger; toe [IV]; ventricle
fourth cranial: nerve [CN IV]
fourth heart: sound
fourth lumbar: nerve [L4]
fourth parallel pelvic: plane
fourth turbinated: bone
foveated: chest
foveolar: cells of stomach
Foville: fasciculus; syndrome
fowl: typhoid
Fowler: position
Fox-Fordyce: disease
fractional: distillation; dose; sterilization
fractional epidural: anesthesia
fractional spinal: anesthesia
fracture: bed; blister; box; dislocation
Fraenkel: pneumococcus
fragile: site
fragile X: chromosome; syndrome
fragility: test
fragment: reaction
Fraley: syndrome
frame-shift: mutagen; mutation
framework: region
Framingham Heart: Study
Franceschetti: syndrome
Franceschetti-Jadassohn: syndrome
Francke: needle
frank breech: presentation
Frankenhäuser: ganglion
Frankfort: plane
Frankfort horizontal: plane
Frankfort-mandibular incisor: angle
Franklin: disease; spectacles
franklinic: taste
Frank-Starling: curve
Fräntzel: murmur
Fraser: syndrome
Fraser-Lendrum: stain for fibrin
fraternal: twins
Fraunhofer: lines
Frazier: needle
Frazier-Spiller: operation
Fredet-Ramstedt: operation
free: association; border; border of nail; border of ovary; electrophoresis; energy; field; flap; gingiva; graft; macrophage; margin; margin of eyelids; part of lower limb; part of upper limb; radical; tenia; villus; water
free bone: flap
free-floating: anxiety
free-hand: knife
free induction: decay
free mandibular: movements
Freeman-Sheldon: syndrome
free nerve: endings
free thyroxine: index
free water: clearance
freeway: space
freeze: fracture
freezing: point
Frei: test
Freiberg: disease; infarction
Frei-Hoffmann: reaction
Frejka pillow: splint
French: chalk; scale
French-American-British: classification
Frenkel: symptom

Frenkel anterior ocular traumatic: syndrome
frequency: curve; distribution; spectrum
Frerichs: theory
fresh frozen: plasma
Fresnel: lens; prism
Freud: theory
freudian: fixation; psychoanalysis
Freund: adjuvant; anomaly; operation
Freund complete: adjuvant
Freund incomplete: adjuvant
Frey: hairs; syndrome
friction: murmur; rub; sound
frictional: attachment
Fridenberg stigometric card: test
Friderichsen-Waterhouse: syndrome
Friedländer: bacillus; pneumonia; stain for capsules
Friedländer bacillus: pneumonia
Friedman: curve
Friedreich: ataxia; phenomenon; sign
Friend: disease; virus
Friend leukemia: virus
fright: reaction
Froehde: reagent
frog: face
frog leg: position
frog-leg lateral: projection
Fröhlich: dwarfism; syndrome
Frohn: reagent
Froin: syndrome
Froment: sign
frontal: angle of parietal bone; area; artery; aspect; belly of occipitofrontalis muscle; bone; border; border of parietal bone; border of sphenoid bone; branch of middle meningeal artery; branch of superficial temporal artery; cortex; crest; eminence; fontanelle; foramen; forceps; grooves; horn; lobe; lobe of cerebrum; margin; margin of sphenoid; nerve; notch; part of corpus callosum; plane; plate; pole; pole [TA] of cerebrum; process of maxilla; process of zygomatic bone; region of head; section; sinus; squama; suture; triangle; tuber; veins
frontalis: muscle
frontal lobe: epilepsy
frontal sinus: aperture
frontoanterior: position

frontoethmoidal: suture
frontolacrimal: suture
frontomaxillary: suture
frontonasal: duct; process; prominence; suture
fronto-occipital: fasciculus
fronto-orbital: area
frontopolar: artery
frontopontine: fibers; tract
frontoposterior: position
frontosphenoidal: process
frontotemporal: tract
frontotransverse: position
frontozygomatic: suture
front-tap: contraction; reflex
Froriep: ganglion
Frost: suture
frost: itch
frosted: heart
frosted branch: angiitis
frozen: pelvis; section; shoulder
fructokinase: deficiency
fructose: malabsorption
fruit: sugar
fruiting: body
frustration: tolerance
frustration-aggression: hypothesis
FTA-ABS: test
Fuchs: adenoma; coloboma; spur; stomas; syndrome; uveitis
Fuchs black: spot
Fuchs endothelial: dystrophy
Fuchs heterochromic: cyclitis
fuchsin: bodies
fuchsinophil: cell; granule; reaction
fugitive: swelling; wart
fugu: poison
fulcrum: line
fulgurating: migraine
full: denture
fuller's: earth
full liquid: diet
full-thickness: burn; flap; graft
fulminant: hepatitis; hyperpyrexia
fulminating: dysentery; smallpox
fuming: nitric acid; sulfuric acid
functional: albuminuria; anatomy; aphasia; apoplexy; asplenia; autonomy; blindness; castration; congestion; contracture; disease; disorder; dysmenorrhea; dyspepsia; dyspnea; genomics; group; hearing impairment; hypertrophy; illness; murmur; neurosurgery; occlusion; pathology;

pleiotropy; psychosis; sphincter; splint; stricture; visual loss
functional cardiovascular: disease
functional chew-in: record
functional endoscopic sinus: surgery
functional jaw: orthopedics
functional mandibular: movements
functional neck: dissection
functional occlusal: harmony
functional orthodontic: therapy
functional prepubertal castration: syndrome
functional refractory: period
functional residual: air; capacity
functional terminal innervation: ratio
functional vocal: fatigue
fundamental: frequency; tone
fundic: glands
fundiform: ligament of clitoris; ligament of foot; ligament of penis
fundus: reflex
fungating: sore
fungiform: papillae
fungous: foot
fungus: ball
funic: souffle
funicular: graft; hydrocele; myelitis; myelosis; part of ductus deferens; process
funnel: breast; plot
funnel-shaped: pelvis
funny: bone
furcal: nerve
furfurol: reaction
furious: rabies
furnacemen's: cataract
furred: tongue
fused: kidney; silver nitrate; teeth
fusel: oil
fusible: metal
fusiform: aneurysm; cataract; cells of cerebral cortex; gyrus; layer; muscle
fusing: point
fusion: area; beat; energy; temperature (wire method)
fusional: movement
fusion-inferred threshold: test
fusospirochetal: disease; gingivitis; stomatitis
Futcher: line
futile: cycle
Fy: antigens

G

γ: hemolysis
G: antigen; cells; factor; force; proteins; syndrome; unit of streptomycin
G$_{M1}$: gangliosidosis
G$_{M2}$: gangliosidosis
G-: actin; protein
GABA: pathway
Gaboon: ulcer
Gaddum and Schild: test
Gaenslen: sign
Gaffky: scale; table
gag: reflex
Gairdner: disease
Gaisböck: syndrome
gait: apraxia
GAL: virus
galactokinase: deficiency
galactokinase deficiency: galactosemia
galactophorous: canals; ducts
galactopoietic: hormone
galactose: cataract; diabetes
galactose tolerance: test
galactosylceramide: lipoidosis
Galant: reflex
Galassi pupillary: phenomenon
Galeati: glands
Galeazzi: fracture
Galen: anastomosis; nerve
Gall: craniology
gall: bladder; duct
Gallaudet: fascia
Gallavardin: phenomenon
gallbladder: fossa
Gallego differentiating: solution
Gallie: transplant
gallop: rhythm; sound
gallstone: colic; ileus
gallus adenolike: virus
Galton: delta; law; whistle
galtonian: genetics; inheritance; trait
Galtonian-Fisher: genetics
Galton system of classification of: fingerprints
galvanic: cautery; current; nystagmus; threshold
galvanic skin: reaction; reflex; response
galvanocaustic: snare
Gambian: fever; trypanosomiasis
game: theory
gamekeeper's: thumb
gamete intrafallopian: transfer
gametic: nucleus
gametokinetic: hormone
Gamgee: tissue
gamma: alcoholism; angle; camera; cell of pancreas; crystallin; efferent;

encephalography; fibers; knife; loop; radiation; rays
gamma motor: neurons; system
Gamna: disease
Gamna-Favre: bodies
Gamna-Gandy: bodies; nodules
Gandy-Gamna: bodies
Gandy-Nanta: disease
gangliated: cord; nerve
ganglion: cell; cells of dorsal spinal root; cells of retina; ridge
ganglionic: blockade; branches of lingual nerve; branches of lingual nerve to sublingual ganglion; branches of lingual nerve to submandibular ganglion; branches of maxillary nerve; branches of maxillary nerve to pterygopalatine ganglion; branch of internal carotid artery; chain; crest; layer; layer of cerebellar cortex; layer of cerebral cortex; layer of optic nerve; saliva
ganglionic blocking: agent
ganglionic cell: layer of retina
ganglionic motor: neuron
ganglioside: lipidosis
gangrenous: appendicitis; cellulitis; emphysema; pharyngitis; pneumonia; rhinitis; stomatitis
Ganser: commissure; syndrome
Gant: clamp
Gantzer: muscle
Gantzer accessory: bundle
Ganzfeld: stimulation
gap: arthroplasty; junction; phenomenon
gap$_1$: period; phase
gap$_0$: period; phase
gap$_2$: period; phase
garapata: disease
Gardner: syndrome
Gardner-Diamond: syndrome
Gardnerella: vaginitis
gargantuan: mastitis
Gariel: pessary
Garland: triangle
Garré: disease; osteomyelitis
Gartner: canal; cyst; duct
Gärtner: method; tonometer
Gärtner vein: phenomenon
gas: abscess; bacillus; cautery; chromatography; constant; cyst; embolism; gangrene; peritonitis; phlegmon; retinopexy; thermometer
gaseous: mediastinography; pulse
gas gangrene: antitoxin

Gaskell: bridge; clamp
gas-liquid: chromatography
gasserian: ganglion
gastral: mesoderm
gastrea: theory
gastric: analysis; area; arteries; branches of anterior vagal trunk; branches of posterior vagal trunk; bypass; calculus; canal; colic; crisis; diastole; digestion; feeding; fistula; folds; follicles; freezing; glands; hemorrhage; hypersecretion; impression on liver; impression on spleen; indigestion; juice; mucin; mucosa; neurasthenia; pit; plexuses of autonomic system; rugae; smear; stapling; surface of spleen; tetany; ulcer; veins; volvulus
gastric algid: malaria
gastric inhibitory: peptide; polypeptide
gastric lymphoid: nodules
gastric nervous: plexuses
gastrocardiac: syndrome
gastrocnemius: muscle
gastrocolic: fistula; ligament; omentum; reflex
gastrocutaneous: fistula
gastrodiaphragmatic: ligament
gastroduodenal: artery; fistula; lymph nodes; orifice
gastroenteritis: virus type A; virus type B
gastroepiploic: arteries; veins
gastroesophageal: hernia; vestibule
gastroesophageal reflux: disease
gastrogenous: diarrhea
Gastrografin: swallow
gastrohepatic: omentum
gastroileac: reflex
gastrointestinal: fistula; hormone; tract
gastrointestinal autonomic nerve: tumor
gastrointestinal stromal: tumor
gastrojejunal loop obstruction: syndrome
gastrolienal: ligament
gastroomental: arteries
gastropancreatic: folds
gastrophrenic: ligament
gastrosplenic: ligament; omentum
Gatch: bed
gate-control: hypothesis; theory

gated radionuclide: angiocardiography
gating: mechanism
Gaucher: cells; disease
gauge: pressure
gauntlet: bandage
Gauss: sign
gaussian: curve; distribution
gauze: bandage
Gavard: muscle
Gay: glands
gay bowel: syndrome
Gay-Lussac: equation; law
gaze paretic: nystagmus
GB: viruses
G-banding: stain
GC: content
Ge: antigen
Geigel: reflex
Geiger-Müller: counter; tube
gel: diffusion; electrophoresis; filtration; structure
gelastic: seizure
gelatin: sugar
gelatinous: ascites; infiltration; nucleus; polyp; scleritis; substance; tissue; varix
gelatinous bone: marrow
gelatinous droplike corneal: dystrophy
gel diffusion: reactions
gel diffusion precipitin: tests; tests in one dimension; tests in two dimensions
gel filtration: chromatography
Gélineau: syndrome
Gell and Coombs: Classification; reactions
Gellé: test
Gély: suture
geminated: teeth
gemistocytic: astrocyte; astrocytoma; cell; reaction
genal: glands
gender: identity; role
gender dysphoria: syndrome
gender identity: disorders
gene: activation; deletion; duplication; expression; family; flow; frequency; mapping; mosaicism; pool; regulation; therapy
gene dosage: compensation; effect
general: anatomy; anesthesia; anesthetics; bloodletting; hospital; immunity; paresis; peritonitis; physiology; practice; sensation; stimulant; transduction
general adaptation: reaction; syndrome
general duty: nurse
general fertility: rate

generalized: anaphylaxis; chondromalacia; elastolysis; emphysema; epilepsy; gangliosidosis; glycogenosis; lentiginosis; myokymia; paralysis; seizures; tetanus; tuberculosis; vaccinia; xanthelasma
generalized anxiety: disorder
generalized cortical: hyperostosis
generalized epidermolytic: hyperkeratosis
generalized eruptive: histiocytoma
generalized plane: xanthomatosis
generalized pustular: psoriasis of Zambusch
generalized Shwartzman: phenomenon
generalized tonic-clonic: epilepsy; seizure
general somatic afferent: column
general somatic efferent: column
general visceral afferent: column
general visceral efferent: column
generated occlusal: path
generation: effect
generative: empathy
generator: potential
generic: substitution
genesial: cycle
genetic: amplification; association; burden; carrier; code; colonization; compound; counseling; death; determinant; disequilibrium; dominance; drift; engineering; epidemiology; equilibrium; female; fingerprint; fitness; fixation; heterogeneity; homeostasis; isolate; lethal; linkage; load; locus; map; marker; material; model; penetrance; polymorphism; psychology; recombination; testing
genetic human: male
Geneva lens: measure
Gengou: phenomenon
genial: tubercle
genicular: anastomosis; arteries; veins
geniculate: body; ganglion; neuralgia; otalgia; zoster
geniculatus lateralis: nucleus
geniculocalcarine: radiation; tract
genioglossal: muscle
genioglossus: muscle

geniohyoid: muscle
genital: ambiguity; branch of genitofemoral nerve; branch of iliohypogastric nerve; cord; corpuscles; duct; eminence; fold; furrow; gland; ligament; organs; phase; primacy; primordium; ridge; stage; swellings; system; tract; tubercle; wart
genitocrural: nerve
genitofemoral: nerve
genitoinguinal: ligament
genitourinary: apparatus; fistula; surgeon; system
Gennari: band; stria
genomic: clone; DNA; imprinting; library
gentian aniline: water
genucubital: position
genupectoral: position
geographic: choroidopathy; keratitis; stippling of nails; tongue
geographic information: system
geographic retinal: atrophy
geometric: isomer; isomerism; mean; sense
Gerbich: antigen
Gerbode: defect
Gerdy: fibers; fontanelle; ligament; tubercle
Gerdy hyoid: fossa
Gerdy interatrial: loop
Gerhardt: disease; reaction; test for acetoacetic acid; test for urobilin in the urine
Gerhardt-Mitchell: disease
geriatric: medicine; therapy
Gerlach: tonsil; valve; valvula
Gerlach annular: tendon
Gerlier: disease
germ: cell; layer; line; membrane; nucleus; theory; tube
German: measles
German measles: virus
germinal: aplasia; area; cell; center of Flemming; cords; disk; epithelium; localization; mosaicism; pole; rod; streak; vesicle
germinative: layer; layer of nail
Germiston: virus
germ layer: theory
germ tube: test
Gerota: capsule; fascia; method
Gerstmann: syndrome
Gerstmann-Sträussler-Scheinker: syndrome
gestalt: phenomenon; psychology; theory; therapy

gestational: age; diabetes; edema; hypertension; proteinuria; ring; sac
gestational trophoblastic: disease
Gey: solution
ghatti: gum
Gheel: colony
Ghon: complex; focus; tubercle
Ghon primary: lesion
ghost: cell; corpuscle; tooth
ghost cell: glaucoma
ghoul: hand
Giannuzzi: crescents; demilunes
Gianotti-Crosti: syndrome
giant: cell; chromosome; colon; condyloma; drusen; fibroadenoma; hives; hypertrophy of gastric mucosa; melanosome; urticaria
giant axonal: neuropathy
giant cell: aortitis; arteritis; carcinoma; carcinoma of thyroid gland; epulis; fibroma; glioblastoma multiforme; granuloma; hepatitis; myeloma; myocarditis; pneumonia; sarcoma; thyroiditis; tumor of bone; tumor of tendon sheath
giant cell hyaline: angiopathy
giant cell monstrocellular: sarcoma of Zülch
giant follicular: lymphoblastoma; thyroiditis
giant gastric: folds
giant osteoid: osteoma
giant papillary: conjunctivitis
giant pigmented: nevus
Gibb phase: rule
Gibbs: energy of activation; theorem
Gibbs-Donnan: equilibrium
Gibbs free: energy
Gibbs-Helmholtz: equation
Gibney: boot
Gibney fixation: bandage
Gibson: bandage; murmur
Giemsa: stain
Giemsa chromosome banding: stain
Gierke: cells; disease
Gierke respiratory: bundle
Gifford: reflex
gigantiform: cementoma
gigantocellular: glioma; nucleus of medulla oblongata
Gigli: operation; saw
Gilbert: disease; syndrome
Gilchrist: disease
gill: clefts

gill arch: skeleton
Gilles de la Tourette: disease; syndrome
Gillespie: syndrome
Gillette suspensory: ligament
Gilliam: operation
Gillies: operation
Gillmore: needle
Gilmer: wiring
Gil-Vernet: operation
Gimbernat: ligament
ginger: paralysis
gingival: abrasion; abscess; atrophy; clamp; cleft; contour; crest; crevice; curvature; cyst; elephantiasis; embrasure; enlargement; epithelium; festoon; fibromatosis; fistula; flap; fluid; groove; hyperplasia; margin; massage; mucosa; papilla; pocket; proliferation; recession; repositioning; resorption; retraction; septum; space; sulcus; tissues; trough; zone
gingivobuccal: groove; sulcus
gingivodental: ligament
gingivolabial: groove; sulcus
gingivolingual: groove; sulcus
ginglymoid: joint
Giordano-Giovannetti: diet
Giovannetti: diet
Girard: reagent
girdle: anesthesia; pain; sensation
Girdlestone: procedure
Gitelman: syndrome
gitter: cell
glabrous: skin
glacial: acetic acid; phosphoric acid
glairy: mucus
glancing: wound
glandular: branches; branches of facial artery; branches of inferior thyroid artery; branches of submandibular ganglion; cancer; carcinoma; epithelium; fever; lobe of hypophysis; mastitis; plague; substance of prostate; system; tularemia
glandulopreputial: lamella
glanular: hypospadias
Glanzmann: disease; thrombasthenia
glaserian: artery; fissure
Glasgow: sign
glass: body; electrode; factor; rays
glass bead: sterilizer
glass ionomer: cement
glassworker's: cataract
glassy: membrane

Glauber: salt
glaucomatocyclitic: crisis
glaucomatous: cataract; cup; excavation; halo; ring
glaucomatous nerve-fiber bundle: scotoma
Gleason: score
Gleason tumor: grade
Glenn: operation; shunt
Glenner-Lillie: stain for pituitary
glenohumeral: articulation; joint; ligaments
glenoid: cavity; cavity of scapula; fossa; labrum of scapula; ligament; surface
glenoidal: lip
Gley: glands
glia: cells
glial fibrillary acidic: protein
glial limiting: membrane
gliding: joint; occlusion
Glisson: capsule; cirrhosis; sphincter
glitter: cells
global: aphasia; burden of disease; paralysis
globin: insulin
globin zinc: insulin
globoid: cell
globoid cell: leukodystrophy
globosus: nucleus
globular: heart; leukocyte; process; protein; sputum; thrombus
globulomaxillary: cyst
glomerular: capsule; crescent; cyst; layer of olfactory bulb; nephritis; sclerosis
glomerular filtration: rate
glomerulosa: cell
glomiform: glands
glomus: body; tumor
glomus jugulare: tumor
glomus tympanicum: tumor
glossoepiglottic: ligament
glossolabiolaryngeal: paralysis
glossopalatine: arch; fold
glossopalatolabial: paralysis
glossopharyngeal: breathing; nerve [CN IX]; neuralgia; part of superior pharyngeal constrictor; tic
glossopharyngeolabial: paralysis
glossy: skin
glove: anesthesia
gloved-finger: sign
Glover: phenomenon
glover: suture
glucagonlike: peptide
glucagonlike insulinotropic: peptide
glucagonoma: syndrome

glucose-dependent insulinotropic: polypeptide
glucose oxidase: method
glucose oxidase paper strip: test
glucose-6-phosphatase hepatorenal: glycogenosis
glucose-6-phosphate dehydrogenase: deficiency
glucosephosphate isomerase: deficiency
glucose tolerance: factor; test
glucose transport: maximum
glucosidase: inhibitors
α-glucosidase: inhibitor
β-d-glucuronidase: deficiency
glue: ear
Gluge: corpuscles
γ-glutamyl: cycle
glutaraldehyde: fixative
glutathione synthetase: deficiency
gluteal: cleft; crest; fold; furrow; hernia; lines; lymph nodes; reflex; region; ridge; surface of ilium; tuberosity; veins
gluten: ataxia; enteropathy
gluten-free: diet
gluteofemoral: bursa
gluteus maximus: gait; muscle
gluteus medius: bursae; gait; muscle
gluteus minimus: bursa; muscle
glycemic: index
glycerin: suppository
glycerinated: gelatin; tincture
glycerol dehydration: test
glycerophosphate: shuttle
glycine-succinate: cycle
glycogen: cardiomegaly; granule
glycogenic: acanthosis; cardiomegaly
glycogen-storage: disease
glycol: ethers
glycolipid: lipidosis
glycosyl: compound
glycosylated: hemoglobin
glyoxylic acid: cycle
Gm: allotypes; antigens
Gmelin: test
gnathic: index
gnome's: calf
goatpox: virus
goat's milk: anemia
goblet: cell
Godélier: law
Godman: fascia
Godwin: tumor
Goeckerman: treatment
Goethe: bone
Gofman: test
Goggia: sign

gold: alloy; casting; equivalent; inlay; number
Goldblatt: hypertension; kidney; phenomenon
Goldenhar: syndrome
Goldflam: disease
Goldie-Coldman: hypothesis
Goldman: equation
Goldman-Fox: knives
Goldman-Hodgkin-Katz: equation
Goldmann: perimeter
Goldmann applanation: tonometer
Goldmann-Favre: syndrome
gold-myokymia: syndrome
Goldscheider: test
gold sol: test
Goldstein toe: sign
golfer's: skin
golf-hole ureteral: orifice
Golgi: apparatus; body; cells; complex; corpuscle; stain; zone
Golgi epithelial: cell
Golgi internal: reticulum
Golgi-Mazzoni: corpuscle
Golgi osmiobichromate: fixative
Golgi tendon: organ
Golgi type I: neuron
Golgi type II: neuron
Goll: column
Goltz: syndrome
Gombault: triangle
Gomori aldehyde fuchsin: stain
Gomori chrome alum hematoxylin-phloxine: stain
Gomori-Jones periodic acid-methenamine-silver: stain
Gomori methenamine-silver: stain
Gomori nonspecific acid phosphatase: stain
Gomori nonspecific alkaline phosphatase: stain
Gomori one-step trichrome: stain
Gomori silver impregnation: stain
Gompertz: hypothesis; law
gompholic: joint
gonad: dose; nucleus
gonadal: agenesis; aplasia; cords; dose; dysgenesis; hormones; ridge; streak
gonadal steroid-binding: globulin
gonadotrophic: cycle
gonadotropic: hormone
gonadotropin-producing: adenoma
gonadotropin-releasing: factor; hormone

gonococcal: arthritis; conjunctivitis; stomatitis
gonorrheal: conjunctivitis; ophthalmia; rheumatism; salpingitis; urethritis
Good: antigen
good: object
Goodell: dilator; sign
Goodenough draw-a-man: test
goodness of fit: test
Goodpasture: stain; syndrome
Goormaghtigh: cells
goose: flesh
Gopalan: syndrome
Gordon: reflex; sign; symptom
Gordon and Sweet: stain
Gorham: disease; syndrome
Goriaew: rule
Gorlin: cyst; formula; sign; syndrome
Gorlin-Chaudhry-Moss: syndrome
Gorman: syndrome
Gosselin: fracture
Gothic: arch; palate
Gothic arch: tracing
Göthlin: test
Gougerot and Blum: disease
Gougerot-Carteaud: syndrome
Gougerot-Sjögren: disease
Gould: suture
Gouley: catheter
gout: diet
gouty: arthritis; diathesis; pearl; tophus; urine
government: hospital
Gower: sign
Gowers: column; contraction; disease; syndrome; tract
Gr: antigen
graafian: follicle
gracile: fasciculus; habitus; lobule; nucleus; tubercle
gracilespinal: fibers
gracilis: muscle; syndrome
grade I: astrocytoma
grade II: astrocytoma
grade III: astrocytoma
grade IV: astrocytoma
Gradenigo: syndrome
gradient: elution
gradient-recalled: acquisition in the steady state
graduate: nurse
graduated: compress; pipette; tenotomy
Graefe: forceps; knife; operation; sign; spots
Graefenberg: ring
Graffi: virus
graft versus host: disease; reaction
Graham: law

Graham-Cole: test
Graham Little: syndrome
Graham Steell: murmur
grain: alcohol; itch
Gram: iodine; stain
gram: calorie; equivalent
gram-: ion
gram-atomic: weight
Gram-chromotrope: stain
gram-molecular: weight
grand: climacteric; mal; multipara
granddaughter: cyst
grandiose: delusion
grandiose type of paranoid: disorder
grand mal: epilepsy; seizure
Granger: line; projection
Granit: loop
granny: knot
granular: cast; conjunctivitis; cortex; degeneration; foveolae; kidney; layer; layer of cerebellar cortex; layer of cerebellum; layer of epidermis; layers of cerebral cortex; layer of a vesicular ovarian follicle; leukoblast; leukocyte; lids; ophthalmia; pits; pneumonocytes; trachoma; urethritis
granular cell: myoblastoma; tumor
granular corneal: dystrophy
granular endoplasmic: reticulum
granulated: opium
granulation: tissue
granule: cell of connective tissue; cells
granulocyte colony-stimulating: factor
granulocyte-macrophage colony-stimulating: factor
granulocytic: leukemia; sarcoma; series
granulomatous: arteritis; colitis; disease; encephalomyelitis; endophthalmitis; enteritis; inflammation; mastitis; nocardiosis; rosacea
granulosa: cell
granulosa cell: tumor
granulosa lutein: cells
granulovacuolar: degeneration
grape: endings; mole; sugar
graphic: aphasia; formula
graphomotor: aphasia
grasp: reflex
grasping: reflex
grass: bacillus
Grasset: law; phenomenon; sign

Grasset-Gaussel: phenomenon
Gratiolet: fibers; radiation
gratuitous: inducer
Gräupner: method
grave: wax
Graves: disease; ophthalmopathy; orbitopathy
Graves optic: neuropathy
gravid: uterus
gravidic: retinitis; retinopathy
gravitation: abscess
gravitational: ulcer; units
gravity: concentration
Grawitz: basophilia; tumor
gray: cataract; columns; commissure; degeneration; fibers; hepatization; induration; infiltration; layers of superior colliculus; literature; matter; rami communicantes; scale; substance; syndrome; tuber; tubercle; wing
gray-scale: ultrasonography
greaseless: cream
great: foramen; toe I; vein of Galen
great adductor: muscle
great alveolar: cells
great anastomotic: artery
great auricular: nerve
great cardiac: vein
great cerebral: vein; vein of Galen
greater: circulation; cul-de-sac; curvature of stomach; horn of hyoid bone; omentum; pelvis; ring of iris; trochanter; tubercle (of humerus); tuberosity of humerus; wing of sphenoid (bone)
greater alar: cartilage
greater arterial: circle of iris
greater multangular: bone
greater occipital: nerve
greater palatine: artery; canal; foramen; groove; nerve
greater pancreatic: artery
greater pectoral: muscle
greater peritoneal: cavity
greater petrosal: nerve
greater posterior rectus: muscle of head
greater psoas: muscle
greater rhomboid: muscle
greater sciatic: notch
greater splanchnic: nerve
greater superficial petrosal: nerve
greater supraclavicular: fossa
greater tympanic: spine
greater vestibular: gland
greater zygomatic: muscle
greatest: length
great horizontal: fissure
great longitudinal: fissure
great radicular: artery
great saphenous: vein
great sciatic: nerve
great segmental medullary: artery
great superior pancreatic: artery
great-toe: reflex
green: hemoglobin; pus; sickness; soap; sputum; stain; tooth; vision
Greenfield: filter
Greenhow: disease
green monkey: virus
green soap: tincture
greenstick: fracture
green tobacco: sickness
Greig: syndrome
Greig cephalopolysyndactyly: syndrome
grenz: ray; zone
Greville: bath
Grey Turner: sign
grid: ratio
Gridley: stain; stain for fungi
Griesinger: disease; sign
grinding: surface
Grisolle: sign
Gritti: operation
Gritti-Stokes: amputation
Grocco: sign; triangle
grocer: itch
Grocott-Gomori methenamine-silver: stain
Groenouw corneal: dystrophy
Grönblad-Strandberg: syndrome
groove: sign
grooved: tongue
Gross: virus
gross: anatomy; hematuria; lesion
Gross leukemia: virus
gross reproduction: rate
ground: bundles; itch; lamella; state; substance
ground-glass: cytoplasm; pattern
ground itch: anemia
group: agglutination; agglutinin; antigens; dynamics; hospital; immunity; practice; psychotherapy; reaction; test; transfer; translocation
group A: streptococci
group A streptococcal necrotizing: fasciitis
group B: streptococci
Grover: disease
growing: fracture; pains
growing ovarian: follicle
growth: curve; factors; hormone; hormone-inhibiting hormone; hormone-releasing hormone; medium; phase; plate; rate; rate of population; regulators
growth arrest: lines
growth hormone–producing: adenoma
growth hormone-releasing: factor
growth-onset: diabetes
Gruber: cul-de-sac; method; reaction
Gruber-Landzert: fossa
Gruber-Widal: reaction
Grunert: spur
Grunstein-Hogness: assay
Grynfeltt: triangle
gryposis: penis
GTP binding: proteins
guaiac: gum; test
Guama: virus
Guanarito: virus
guanine: cell
guar: gum
Guarnieri: bodies
Guaroa: virus
gubernacular: canal; cord
Gubler: line; paralysis; syndrome; tumor
Gudden: commissure; ganglion
Gudden tegmental: nuclei
Guedel: airway
Guéneau de Mussy: point
Guérin: fold; fracture; glands; sinus; valve
guide: plane; wire
guided tissue: regeneration
Guillain-Barré: reflex; syndrome
guillotine: amputation
guinea corn: yaws
Guldberg-Waage: law
Gulf War: syndrome
Gullstrand: slitlamp
gum: contour; lancet; line; resection; resin
gummatous: abscess; syphilid; ulcer
Gumprecht: shadows
Gunn: dots; phenomenon; pupil; sign; syndrome
Gunn crossing: sign
Gunning: splint
Günning: reaction
gunshot: wound
gunstock: deformity
Günz: ligament
Günzberg: reagent; test
gurgling: rale
Gussenbauer: suture
gustatory: agnosia; anesthesia; aura; bud; cells; hallucination; hyperesthesia; hyperhidrosis; lemniscus; nucleus; organ; pore; rhinorrhea
gustatory-sudorific: reflex
gustatory sweating: syndrome
gut: glucagon
gut-associated lymphoid: tissue
Guthrie: muscle; test
gutta-percha: cone; points; spreader
guttate: choroidopathy
gutter: dystrophy of cornea; fracture; wound
Guttman: scale
guttural: duct; pulse; rale
Gutzeit: test
Guyon: amputation; canal; isthmus; sign
Guyon tunnel: syndrome
GVH: disease
gym: -diol
gynecoid: obesity; pelvis
gynecophoric: canal
gyrate: atrophy of choroid and retina
gyrochrome: cell
gyromagnetic: ratio

H

H: agglutinin; antigen; band; colony; disk; fields; gene; graft; rays; reflex; shunt; substance
H-2: antigens; complex
H-: meromyosin
HA1: virus
HA2: virus
haarscheibe: tumor
Haase: rule
habenular: commissure; nuclei; sulcus; trigone
habenulointerpeduncular: tract
Haber: syndrome
Haber-Weiss: reaction
habit: chorea; cough; scoliosis; spasm; tic
habitual: abortion
HACEK: group
Haeckel: law
Haeckel gastrea: theory
Haemophilus influenzae **type B:** vaccine
Haenel: symptom
Haff: disease
Haffkine: vaccine
hafussi: bath
Hagedorn: needle
Hageman: factor
Haglund: deformity; disease
Hahn oxine: reagent
Haidinger: brushes
Hailey-Hailey: disease

hair: bulb; cast; cells; crosses; cycle; disk; follicle; papilla; root; shaft; streams; transplant; whorls
HAIR-AN: syndrome
hairline: fracture
hairpin: loops; vessels
hairy: cells; heart; leukoplakia; mole; tongue
hairy cell: leukemia
Halberstaedter-Prowazek: bodies
Haldane: apparatus; effect; relationship; transformation; tube
Haldane-Priestley: sample
Hale colloidal iron: stain
Hales: piesimeter
half: cystine; hapten
half-: life; time
half amplitude pulse: duration
half axial: view
half-axial: projection
half-chair: form
half-glass: spectacles
half and half: nail
half-value: layer
Hallé: point
Haller: ansa; anulus; arches; cell; circle; cones; habenula; insula; line; plexus; rete; tripod; tunica vasculosa; unguis; vas aberrans
Hallermann-Streiff: syndrome
Hallermann-Streiff-François: syndrome
Haller vascular: tissue
Hallervorden: syndrome
Hallervorden-Spatz: disease; syndrome
Hallgren: syndrome
Hallopeau: disease
hallucinatory: neuralgia
halo: cast; effect; melanoma; nevus; sign; sign of hydrops; traction; vision
halogen: acne
halothane: hepatitis
halothane-ether: azeotrope
Halstead-Reitan: battery
Halsted: law; operation; suture
Ham: test
hamate: bone
Hamburger: phenomenon
Hamilton: pseudophlegmon
Hamilton anxiety rating: scale
Hamilton depression rating: scale
Hamilton-Stewart: formula; method
Hamman: disease; murmur; sign; syndrome
Hamman-Rich: syndrome

Hammarsten: reagent
hammer: finger; nose; toe
Hammerschlag: method
hammock: bandage; ligament
Hammond: disease
Hampton: hump; line; maneuver; technique
hamstring: muscles; tendon
hamular: notch; process of lacrimal bone; process of sphenoid bone
Hancock: amputation
hand: eczema; ratio
hand-and-foot: syndrome
hand-foot: syndrome
hand-foot-and-mouth: disease
hand-foot-and-mouth disease: virus
Hand-Schüller-Christian: disease
Hanes: plot
hanging: drop; septum
hanging-block: culture
hangman's: fracture
Hanhart: syndrome
Hanks: dilators; solution
Hannover: canal
Hanot: cirrhosis
Hansemann: macrophage
Hansen: bacillus; disease
Hantaan: virus
hantavirus pulmonary: syndrome
haphazard: sampling
haploid: set
haploscopic: vision
happy puppet: syndrome
Hapsburg: jaw; lip
hapten: inhibition of precipitation
haptic: hallucination
Harada: disease; syndrome
Harada-Ito: procedure
Harada-Mori filter paper strip: culture
hard: cataract; chancre; corn; drusen; palate; papilloma; paraffin; pulse; rays; soap; sore; tissue; tubercle; ulcer; water
hardened: pelvis
Harden-Young: ester
Harding-Passey: melanoma
hardness: scale
Hardy-Rand-Ritter: test
Hardy-Weinberg: equilibrium; law
hare's: eye
harlequin: fetus; ichthyosis; reaction
harmonic: mean; suture
harmonious retinal: correspondence
Harrington-Flocks: test

Harris: hematoxylin; lines; migraine; syndrome; test
Harrison: groove
Harris and Ray: test
Hartel: technique
Hartman: solution
Hartmann: curette; operation; pouch; solution
Hartnup: disease; syndrome
harvester: ant
Häser: formula
Hashimoto: disease; struma; thyroiditis
Hasner: fold
Hassall: bodies
Hassall concentric: corpuscle
Hassall-Henle: bodies
Hasson: cannula; trocar
hatchet: excavator
hatching: flask
Haudek: niche
Haverhill: fever
haversian: canals; lamella; spaces; system
Hawkins impingement: sign
Hawley: appliance; retainer
Haworth: projection
Haworth conformational formulas of cyclic: sugars
Haworth perspective and conformational: formulas
Haworth perspective formulas of cyclic: sugars
Hawthorne: effect
hay: asthma; bacillus; fever
Hayem: hematoblast; solution
Hayem-Widal: syndrome
Hayflick: limit
Haygarth: nodes
hazard: rate
H and D: curve
He: antigens
Head: areas; lines; zones
head: botflies; cap; cavity; cold; fold; kidney
head: mirror; nurse; presentation; process; tremors
head-bobbing doll: syndrome
head-dropping: test
healed: tuberculosis; ulcer
health: behavior; care; indicator; promotion; psychology
health information: system
health maintenance: organization
health risk: assessment
health status: index
healthy worker: effect
Heaney: operation
hearing: instrument; level; protectors
heart: antigen; arrest; attack; beat; block; failure; hormone; massage; position; rate; sac; sounds; stroke; tamponade; tones; transplantation
heart chamber: remodeling
heart failure: cell
heart-lung: machine; preparation; transplantation
heart rate: turbulance
heart-shaped: pelvis; uterus
heart valve: prosthesis
heat: apoplexy; capacity; cramps; edema; exhaustion; hyperpyrexia; lamp; prostration; rash; rigor; stroke; treatment; urticaria
heat coagulation: test
heat-curing: resin
Heath-Edwards: grades
heat instability: test
heat-rigor: point
heat shock: proteins
heat-stable: enzyme
heavy: chain; hydrogen; metal; nitrogen; oxygen; water
heavy chain: disease
μ-heavy-chain: disease
γ-heavy-chain: disease
α-heavy-chain: disease
heavy liquid: petrolatum
heavy metal: neuropathy
hebephrenic: dementia; schizophrenia
Heberden: angina; nodes
Hebra: disease; prurigo
Hecht: pneumonia
Heck: disease
hectic: flush
hederiform: ending
Hedström: file
heel: bone; fly; jar; pad; region; spur; tap; tendon
heel-tap: reaction; test
heel-to-knee-to-toe: test
heel-to-shin: test
Heerfordt: disease
Hegar: dilators; sign
Hegglin: anomaly; syndrome
Hehner: number; value
Heidelberger: curve
Heidenhain: crescents; demilunes; law; pouch
Heidenhain azan: stain
Heidenhain iron hematoxylin: stain
height: vertigo
height of: contour
height-length: index
Heilbronner: thigh
Heim-Kreysig: sign
Heimlich: maneuver
Heineke-Mikulicz: pyloroplasty
Heinz: bodies
Heinz body: anemia; test
Heinz-Ehrlich: body
Heister: diverticulum; valve

HeLa: cells
Held: bundle; decussation
helical: CT
helical computed: tomography
helicine: arteries of penis; arteries of the uterus
helicis major: muscle
helicis minor: muscle
helicoid: choroidopathy; ginglymus
helicopod: gait
Helie: bundle
helium: speech
Heller: myotomy; operation; plexus
Hellin: law
HELLP: syndrome
Helly: fixative
helmet: cell
Helmholtz: energy; theory of accommodation; theory of color vision; theory of hearing
Helmholtz axis: ligament
Helmholtz-Gibbs: theory
helminthic: dysentery
helper: cells; virus
Helweg: bundle
Helweg-Larssen: syndrome
Helwig: bundle
hemadsorption: virus type 1; virus type 2
hemadsorption virus: test
hemagglutinating cold: autoantibody
hemagglutination: inhibition; test
hemal: arches; gland; node; spine
hemangiectatic: hypertrophy
hematinic: principle
hematogenetic: calculus
hematogenous: abscess; embolism; jaundice; metastasis; osteitis; pigment
hematoidin: crystals
hematopoietic: gland; system
hematoxylin: bodies
hematoxylin and eosin: stain
hematoxylin-malachite green-basic fuchsin: stain
hematoxylin-phloxine B: stain
hematuric bilious: fever
hemianopic: scotoma; spectacles
hemiazygos: vein
hemibody: radiation
hemic: calculus; distomiasis; murmur
hemifacial: spasm
hemilateral: chorea
hemiplegic: amyotrophy; gait; migraine
hemisulfur: mustard

hemithoracic: duct
hemizona: assay
Hemoccult: test
hemochorial: placenta
hemoclastic: reaction
hemoendothelial: placenta
hemoglobin C: disease
hemoglobin H: disease
hemoglobinuric: fever; nephrosis
hemolymph: gland; node
hemolysin: unit
hemolytic: anemia; anemia of newborn; crisis; disease of newborn; gas; jaundice; splenomegaly; streptococci
α-hemolytic: streptococci
β-hemolytic: streptococci
hemolytic plaque: assay
hemolytic uremic: syndrome
hemophilic: arthritis; joint
hemopoietic: tissue
hemorrhagic: anemia; ascites; bronchitis; colitis; cyst; cystitis; dengue; disease of the newborn; endovasculitis; fever; fever with renal syndrome; gangrene; glaucoma; infarct; iritis; measles; nephritis; pachymeningitis; pericarditis; pian; plague; pleurisy; rickets; scurvy; shock; smallpox
hemorrhagic exudative: erythema
hemorrhoidal: cushions; nerves; plexus; veins; zone
hemostatic: collodion; forceps
HEMPAS: cells
hen-cluck: stertor
Henderson-Hasselbalch: equation
Hendra: virus
Henke: space
Henle: ampulla; ansa; fissures; glands; layer; loop; membrane; reaction; sheath; spine; tubules; warts
Henle fenestrated elastic: membrane
Henle fiber: layer
Henle nervous: layer
Hennebert: sign
Henoch: chorea; purpura
Henoch-Schönlein: purpura; syndrome
Henri-Michaelis-Menten: equation
Henry: law
Henry-Gauer: response
Hensen: canal; cell; disk; duct; knot; line; node; stripe
Hensing: ligament
heparin: complement; unit

hepatic: adenoma; amebiasis; arteries; artery proper; branches of anterior vagal trunk; branches of vagus nerve; capsulitis; colic; coma; cords; cyst; duct; encephalopathy; fistula; flexure; infantilism; insufficiency; laminae; lobule; lymph nodes; porphyria; prominence; segments; steatosis; triad; veins
hepatic intermittent: fever
hepatic (nervous): plexus
hepatic portal: system; vein
hepatitis A: virus
hepatitis-associated: antigen
hepatitis B: vaccine; virus
hepatitis B core: antigen
hepatitis B e: antigen
hepatitis B surface: antigen
hepatitis C: virus
hepatitis D: virus
hepatitis delta: virus
hepatitis E: virus
hepatitis G: virus
hepatocellular: adenoma; carcinoma; jaundice
hepatocolic: ligament
hepatocystic: duct
hepatoduodenal: ligament
hepatoenteric: recess
hepatoerythropoietic: porphyria
hepatoesophageal: ligament
hepatogastric: ligament
hepatogenous: jaundice; pigment
hepatojugular: reflex; reflux
hepatolenticular: degeneration
hepatopancreatic: ampulla; sphincter
hepatophosphorylase deficiency: glycogenosis
hepatopleural: fistula
hepatorenal: ligament; pouch; recess of subhepatic space; syndrome
herald: patch
herd: immunity; instinct
hereditary: amyloidosis; angioedema; chorea; clubbing; coproporphyria; deafness; hearing impairment; hypersegmentation of neutrophils; hyperthyroidism; lymphedema; methemoglobinemia; myokymia; nephritis; photomyoclonus; pyropoikilocytosis; spherocytosis; syphilis

hereditary angioneurotic: edema
hereditary benign: telangiectasia
hereditary cerebellar: ataxia
hereditary deforming: chondrodystrophy
hereditary epithelial: dystrophy
hereditary folate: malabsorption
hereditary fructose: intolerance
hereditary hemorrhagic: telangiectasia; thrombasthenia
hereditary hypertrophic: neuropathy
hereditary hypophosphatemic: rickets
hereditary methemoglobinemic: cyanosis
hereditary multiple: exostoses; trichoepithelioma
hereditary nonpolyposis colorectal: cancer
hereditary opalescent: dentin
hereditary progressive: arthroophthalmopathy
hereditary renal: hypouricuria
hereditary sensory radicular: neuropathy
hereditary spinal: ataxia
heredofamilial: tremor
Hering: test; theory of color vision
Hering-Breuer: reflex
Hering sinus: nerve
Herlitz: syndrome
Hermann: fixative
Hermansky-Pudlak: syndrome
hernia: knife
hernial: aneurysm; sac
herniated: disk
heroin overdose: syndrome
herpes: encephalitis; virus
herpes B: encephalomyelitis
herpes simplex: encephalitis; virus
herpes zoster: virus
herpetic: fever; keratitis; keratoconjunctivitis; meningoencephalitis; ulcer; whitlow
herpetiform: aphthae
Herring: bodies; law
herring-worm: disease
Herrmann: syndrome
Hers: disease
Hershberg: test
Hertwig: sheath
hertzian: experiments
Herxheimer: reaction

herz: hormone
Heschl: gyri
Hess: law; screen; test
Hesselbach: fascia; hernia; ligament; triangle
heterochromic: cyclitis; uveitis
heterocyclic: compound
heterocytotropic: antibody
heterodetic: peptide
heterogametic: embryo
heterogeneic: antigen
heterogeneous: nucleation; radiation; system
heterogeneous nuclear: RNA
heterogenetic: antibody; antigen; parasite
heterogenous: keratoplasty; vaccine
heterogonic life: cycle
heterologous: antiserum; desensitization; graft; insemination; protein; serotype; stimulus; tumor; twins
heteromeric: cell; peptide
heterometabolous: metamorphosis
heterometric: autoregulation
heteronomous: psychotherapy
heteronymous: diplopia; hemianopia; image; parallax
heterophil: antibody; antigen; hemolysin
heterophile: antibody; antigen
heteroplastic: graft
heteropolar: bond
heteropyknotic: chromatin
heterotopic: bones; graft; pregnancy; stimulus
heterotrophic oral gastrointestinal: cyst
heterotropic: pregnancies
heterotype: mitosis
heterotypic: cortex
heterotypical: chromosome
heterovaccine: therapy
heteroxenous: parasite
Heubner: arteritis; artery
Heuser: membrane
hexacanth: embryo
hexaxial reference: system
hexazonium: salts
hexokinase: method
hexon: antigen
hexone: bases
hexose monophosphate: pathway; shunt
Hey: amputation; hernia
Heyer-Pudenz: valve
Hey internal: derangement
Heyns abdominal decompression: apparatus
HFR: strain
HG: factor
hiatal: hernia

Hib: vaccine
hibernating: gland; myocardium
Hickman: catheter
hidden: border of nail; part; part of duodenum
hidden nail: skin
hidebound: disease
hidrotic ectodermal: dysplasia
high: convex; enema; lithotomy; wine
high altitude: chamber
high-calorie: diet
high dose: tolerance
high-dose-rate: brachytherapy
high-egg-passage: vaccine
high endothelial postcapillary: venules
high-energy: compounds; phosphates
high energy phosphate: bond
higher order: conditioning; pregnancy
highest: concha
highest intercostal: artery; vein
highest nuchal: line
highest thoracic: artery
highest turbinated: bone
high-fat: diet
high-fiber: diet
high forceps: delivery
high-frequency: current; hearing impairment; ventilation
high frequency: transduction
high-grade squamous intraepithelial: lesion
high-kV: technique
high lip: line
high molecular weight: kininogen
Highmore: body
high osmolar contrast: agent; medium
high output: failure
high-pass: filter
high-performance liquid: chromatography
high-quality filter: paper
high-resolution: banding
high-resolution computed: tomography
high spinal: anesthesia
high-steppage: gait
Higoumenakia: sign
hilar: dance; lymph nodes; shadow
hilar cell: tumor of ovary
Hill: coefficient; constant; equation; operation; phenomenon; plot; reaction; sign
Hillis-Müller: maneuver
Hill's: criteria of evidence

Hill-Sachs: lesion
Hilton: law; method; sac
Hilton white: line
hilus: cells
hind: kidney
hindbrain: vesicle
hindquarter: amputation
Hines-Brown: test
hinge: axis; joint; movement; position; region
hinged: flap
Hinman: syndrome
Hinton: test
hip: bone; joint; phenomenon
hip-flexion: phenomenon
Hippel: disease
hippocampal: commissure; convolution; fissure; gyrus; sclerosis; sulcus
Hippocratic: nails
hippocratic: school; succussion
hippocratic: face; facies; fingers
hippocratic succussion: sound
Hirschberg: method; test
Hirschfeld: canals
Hirschowitz: syndrome
Hirsch-Peiffer: stain
Hirschsprung: disease
His: band; bundle; copula; line; rule; spindle
His bundle: electrogram
His perivascular: space
Hiss: stain
Histalog: test
histamine: flush; liberators; shock; test
histamine-releasing: factor
histaminic: cephalalgia; headache
His-Tawara: system
histiocytic: lymphoma
histocompatibility: antigen; complex; gene; testing
histoid: leprosy; neoplasm; tumor
histologic: accommodation
histological internal: os of uterus
histoplasmin-latex: test
histotoxic: anoxia
histrionic personality: disorder
hitchhiker: thumb
Hitzig: girdle
HIV: encephalopathy
HIV wasting: syndrome
HL-A: antigens
HLA: complex; typing
HMG CoA-reductase: inhibitors
Ho: antigen
Hoagland: sign
hobnail: cell; liver; tongue

Hoboken: gemmules; nodules; valves
Hoche: bundle; tract
Hodge: pessary
Hodgen: splint
Hodgkin: disease; lymphoma
Hodgkin-Key: murmur
Hodgson: disease
hoe: excavator; scaler
Hofbauer: cell
Hoffa: operation
Hoffman: violet
Hoffmann: duct; phenomenon; reflex; sign
Hoffmann muscular: atrophy
Hofmann: bacillus
Hofmeister: gastrectomy; operation; series
Hofmeister-Pólya: anastomosis
Hogben: number
hog cholera: vaccines; virus
Hogness: box
holandric: gene; inheritance
Holden: line
holiday: syndrome
holiday heart: syndrome
holistic: medicine; psychology
Holl: ligament
Hollander: test
Hollenhorst: plaques
Holliday: junction; structure
hollow: back; bone
Holmes: heart; stain
Holmes-Adie: pupil; syndrome
Holmes-Rahe: questionnaire
Holmgrén-Golgi: canals
Holmgren wool: test
holoblastic: cleavage
holocrine: gland
holoendemic: disease
hologynic: inheritance
holometabolous: metamorphosis
holosystolic: murmur
Holter: monitor
Holthouse: hernia
Holt-Oram: syndrome
Holzknecht: unit
Homans: sign
Home: lobe
home: monitor
home health: nurse
homeometric: autoregulation
homeostatic: equilibrium; lag
homeotic: genes
Homer-Wright: rosettes
homigrade: scale
hominal: physiology
homing: value
homocyclic: compound
homocytotropic: antibody
homodetic: peptide
homogametic: embryo

homogeneous: immersion; nucleation; radiation; system
homogenous: keratoplasty
homogonic life: cycle
homograft: reaction
homolecithal: egg
homologous: antigen; antiserum; chromosomes; desensitization; graft; insemination; proteins; recombination; series; serotype; stimulus; tumor
homologous serum: jaundice
homomeric: peptide
homonymous: diplopia; hemianopia; images; parallax
homoplastic: graft
homosexual: panic
homotypic: cortex
homovanillic acid: test
homozygous: achondroplasia
honey: urine
honeycomb: lung; macula; pattern; ringworm
Hong Kong: foot; influenza; toe
hooded: prepuce
hoof-and-mouth: disease
Hooke: law
hookean: behavior
hooked: bone; bundle of Russell; fasciculus
hook-shaped: cataract
hookworm: anemia; disease
Hoover: signs
Hopkins rod-lens: telescope
Hopmann: papilloma; polyp
horizontal: atrophy; cell of Cajal; cells of retina; fissure of right lung; fissure [TA] of cerebellum; fracture; heart; laryngectomy; osteotomy; overlap; part of duodenum; part of facial canal; planes; plate of palatine bone; resorption; transmission; vertigo
horizontal beam: film
horizontal growth: phase
hormonal: gingivitis
hormone replacement: therapy
Horner: muscle; pupil; syndrome; teeth
Horner-Trantas: dots
horny: cell; layer of epidermis; layer of nail
horsepox: virus
horseradish: peroxidases
horseshoe: fistula; kidney; placenta
Horsley bone: wax
Hortega: cells
Hortega neuroglia: stain

Horton: arteritis; cephalalgia; headache
hospital: fever; formulary; gangrene; nurse; record
hospital-acquired: pneumonia
hospital-based: physician
host: cell
hostile: behavior
hot: abscess; flash; flush; gangrene; nodule; pack; spot
hot salt: sterilizer
Hottentot: tea
hound-dog: facies
Hounsfield: number; unit
hourglass: contraction; head; murmur; pattern; stomach; vertebrae
house: staff; surgeon
housekeeping: genes
housemaid's: knee
Houssay: animal; phenomenon; syndrome
Houston: folds; muscle
Houston-Harris: syndrome
Howard: test
Howell: unit
Howell-Jolly: bodies
Howship: lacunae
Hoyer: anastomoses; canals
HR conduction: time
Hruby: lens
H-shape: vertebrae
H-type: fistula
H-type tracheoesophageal: fistula
Hu: antigens
Hubbard: tank
Hubrecht protochordal: knot
Hückel: rule
Hucker-Conn: stain
Hudson-Stähli: line
Hueck: ligament
Hueter: maneuver
Hüfner: equation
Huggins: operation
Hughes-Stovin: syndrome
Huguier: canal; circle; sinus
Huhner: test
Hull: triad
human: babesiosis; botfly; communication; ecology; ehrlichiosis; fibrinogen; genetics; herpesvirus 1; herpesvirus 2; herpesvirus 3; herpesvirus 4; herpesvirus 5; herpesvirus 6; herpesvirus 7; herpesvirus 8; insulin; serum; thrombin
human antihemophilic: factor; fraction
human antimouse: antibody
human botfly: myiasis
β-human chorionic: gonadotropin

human chorionic: gonadotropin; somatomammotropin
human chorionic somatomammotropic: hormone
human diploid cell: vaccine
human diploid cell rabies: vaccine
human eosinophilic: enteritis
human fibrin: foam
human gamma: globulin
human glandular: kallikrein 3
human granulocytic: ehrlichiosis
human immunodeficiency: virus; virus-2
humanistic: psychology
human leukocyte: antigens
human measles immune: serum
human menopausal: gonadotropin
human monocytic: ehrlichiosis
human normal: immunoglobulin
human pertussis immune: serum
human placental: lactogen
human plasma protein: fraction
human α_1-protease: inhibitor
human scarlet fever immune: serum
human serum: jaundice
human T-cell lymphoma/leukemia: virus
human T-cell lymphotropic: virus
human T lymphotrophic: virus
humeral: artery; articulation; head
humeral axillary: lymph nodes
humeral nutrient: arteries
humeroradial: articulation; joint
humeroulnar: head of flexor digitorum superficialis muscle; joint
Hummelsheim: operation; procedure
humoral: doctrine; hypercalcemia of benignancy; immunity; pathology; regulator; theory
Humphry: ligament
hunger: contractions; pain; swelling
Hunner: ulcer
Hunt: neuralgia; syndrome
Hunter: canal; glossitis; gubernaculum; ligament; line; membrane; operation; syndrome
Hunter and Driffield: curve
Hunter-Schreger: bands; lines
Hunter-Thompson: dwarfism
hunting: phenomenon; reaction
Huntington: chorea; disease
Hunt paradoxic: phenomenon
Hurler: disease; syndrome
Hurler-Scheie: syndrome
Hurst: bougies; disease
Hürthle: cell
Hürthle cell: adenoma; carcinoma
Huschke: cartilages; foramen; valve
Huschke auditory: teeth
Hutchinson: facies; freckle; incisors; mask; patch; pupil; teeth; triad
Hutchinson crescentic: notch
Hutchinson-Gilford: disease; syndrome
Hutchison: syndrome
Huxley: layer; membrane; sheath
Huygens: ocular; principle
HV: interval
HVA: test
HV conduction: time
H-Y: antigen
hyaline: bodies; bodies of pituitary; cartilage; cast; degeneration; leukocyte; membrane; thrombus; tubercle
hyaline membrane: disease of the newborn; syndrome
hyalocapsular: ligament
hyaloid: artery; body; canal; fossa; membrane
hyaloideoretinal: degeneration
hybrid: prosthesis
hydatid: cyst; disease; fremitus; polyp; pregnancy; rash; resonance; sand; thrill
hydatidiform: mole
Hyde: disease
hydralazine: syndrome
hydrate: crystal
hydrated: alumina
hydrate microcrystal: theory of anesthesia
hydraulic: conductivity
hydremic: edema
hydride: ion
hydroalcoholic: extract; tincture
hydroelectric: bath
hydrogen: acceptor; bond; carrier; donor; electrode; ion; number; pump; transport
hydrolytic: cleavage

hydrolyzing: enzymes
hydronium: ion
hydrophil: colloid
hydrophilic: ointment; petrolatum
hydrophobic: bond; colloid; interaction
hydropic: degeneration
hydrostatic: dilator; pressure
hydrous: wool fat
17-hydroxycorticosteroid: test
11-hydroxylase: deficiency
21-hydroxylase: deficiency
17-hydroxylase deficiency: syndrome
5-hydroxy tryptamine: antagonists
hygienic laboratory: coefficient
hygroscopic: expansion
hymenal: caruncula
hyobranchial: cleft
hyoepiglottic: ligament
hyoglossal: membrane; muscle
hyoglossus: muscle
hyoid: apparatus; arch; bone
hyomandibular: cleft
Hypaque: enema
hypaque: swallow
hyparterial: bronchi
hyperabduction: syndrome
hyperactive child: syndrome
hyperacute: rejection
hyperacute purulent: conjunctivitis
hyperbaric: anesthesia; chamber; medicine; oxygen; oxygenation
hyperbaric oxygen: therapy
hyperbaric spinal: anesthesia
hypercalcemic: sarcoidosis; uremia
hypercapnic: acidosis
hyperchloremic: acidosis
hyperchromatic: macrocythemia
hyperchromic: effect
hypercyanotic: angina
hyperendemic: disease
hypereosinophilic: syndrome
hyperergic: encephalitis
hyperextension-hyperflexion: injury
hyperfractionated: radiation
hyperfunctional: occlusion
hypergenic: teratosis
hyperglobulinemic: purpura
hyperglycemic-glycogenolytic: factor
hypergonadotropic: eunuchoidism; hypogonadism
hyper-IgM: syndrome
hyperimmune: serum

hyperimmunoglobulin E: syndrome
hyperkalemic periodic: paralysis
hyperkinetic: dysarthria; syndrome
hyperkinetic heart: syndrome
hyperlucent: lung
hypermature: cataract
hypermotor: seizure
hypernatremic: encephalopathy
hyperopic: astigmatism
hyperornithinemia-hyperammonemia-hypercitrullinuria: syndrome
hyperosmolar (hyperglycemic) nonketotic: coma
hyperostotic: spondylosis
hyperplastic: arteriosclerosis; gingivitis; inflammation; osteoarthritis; polyp; pulpitis
hyperprolactinemic: amenorrhea
hyperreactive malarious: splenomegaly
hyperreflexic: bladder
hypersecretion: glaucoma
hypersegmented: neutrophil
hypersensitive: dentin
hypersensitive xiphoid: syndrome
hypersensitivity: angiitis; pneumonitis; reaction; vasculitis
hypertensive: arteriopathy; arteriosclerosis; encephalopathy; retinopathy
hypertensive upper esophageal: sphincter
hyperthyroid: heart
hypertonic: bladder
hypertrophic: arthritis; cardiomyopathy; dystrophy; gastritis; pulpitis; rhinitis; rosacea; scar
hypertrophic cervical: pachymeningitis
hypertrophic hypersecretory: gastropathy
hypertrophic interstitial: neuropathy
hypertrophic pulmonary: osteoarthropathy
hypertrophic pyloric: stenosis
hypervariable: regions
hyperventilation: syndrome; test; tetany
hyperviscosity: syndrome
hypnagogic: hallucination; image
hypnogenic: spot
hypnoid: state

hypnopompic: hallucination; image
hypnotic: psychotherapy; relationship; sleep; state; suggestion
hypobaric spinal: anesthesia
hypobranchial: eminence
hypocalcemic: cataract
hypochondriac: region
hypochondriacal: melancholia; neurosis
hypochondrial: reflex
hypochromic: anemia; effect
hypochromic microcytic: anemia
hypocomplementemic: glomerulonephritis; vasculitis
hypocycloidal: tomography
hypodermic: injection; needle; syringe; tablet
hypoferric: anemia
hypofractionated: radiation
hypogastric: artery; ganglia; nerve; reflex; vein
hypoglossal: canal; eminence; nerve [CN XII]; nucleus; trigone
hypoglycemic: coma
hypogonadotropic: eunuchoidism; hypogonadism
hypohidrotic ectodermal: dysplasia
hypokalemic: nephropathy
hypokalemic periodic: paralysis
hypokinetic: dysarthria
hypometabolic: state; syndrome
hypomotor: seizure
hypoparathyroid: tetany
hypoparathyroidism: syndrome
hypopharyngeal: diverticulum
hypophyseal: cachexia; pouch
hypophyseoportal: system
hypophysial: amenorrhea; cachexia; duct; dwarf; fossa; infantilism; syndrome
hypophysial portal: circulation; system
hypophysioportal: system
hypophysiosphenoidal: syndrome
hypophysiotropic: hormone
hypoplastic: anemia; heart
hypoplastic fetal: chondrodystrophy
hypoplastic left heart: syndrome
hypopyon: ulcer
hyporeninemic: hypoaldosteronism

hypostatic: abscess; congestion; ectasia; pneumonia
hypotensive: anesthesia
hypothalamic: amenorrhea; infundibulum; obesity; obesity with hypogonadism; sulcus
hypothalamocerebellar: fibers
hypothalamohypophysial: tract
hypothalamohypophysial portal: circulation; system
hypothalamospinal: fibers
hypothenar: eminence; fascia; prominence
hypothermic: anesthesia
hypothetical mean: organism; strain
hypothyroid: dwarf; dwarfism; infantilism
hypoventilation: coma
hypovolemic: shock
hypoxanthine guanine phosphoribosyltransferase: deficiency
hypoxemia: test
hypoxia warning: system
hypoxic: hypoxia; nephrosis
hypoxic-hypercarbic: encephalopathy
hypoxic ischemic: encephalopathy
hypsiloid: angle; cartilage; ligament
Hyrtl: anastomosis; foramen; loop; sphincter
Hyrtl epitympanic: recess
hysterical: amblyopia; anesthesia; aphonia; ataxia; blindness; chorea; convulsion; gait; hearing impairment; joint; neurosis; paralysis; personality; polydipsia; pregnancy; psychosis; syncope; torticollis; tremor; vertigo
hysterical personality: disorder

I

I: antigens; band; cell; disk; pili; region
iatrogenic: pneumothorax; transmission
iatromathematical: school
ICAO standard: atmosphere
Iceland: disease; moss
I-cell: disease
ice pick: headache
ichorous: pus
ichthyosiform: erythroderma
icing: heart
iconic: signs

icterohemorrhagic: fever
ICU: psychosis
id: reaction
ideal alveolar: gas
identical: twins
identity: crisis; disorder; matrix
ideokinetic: apraxia
idiodynamic: control
idiographic: approach
idiojunctional: rhythm
idiomuscular: contraction
idionodal: rhythm
idiopathic: aldosteronism; bradycardia; cardiomyopathy; disease; epilepsy; gout; hirsutism; hypercalcemia of infants; hyperlipemia; hypertension; infantilism; megacolon; myocarditis; neuralgia; proctitis; roseola
idiopathic bilateral: vestibulopathy
idiopathic bone: cavity
idiopathic fibrous: mediastinitis; retroperitonitis
idiopathic hypercalcemic: sclerosis of infants
idiopathic hypertrophic: osteoarthropathy
idiopathic hypertrophic subaortic: stenosis
idiopathic interstitial: fibrosis
idiopathic orthostatic: hypotension
idiopathic paroxysmal: rhabdomyolysis
idiopathic pulmonary: fibrosis; hemosiderosis
idiopathic stabbing: headache
idiopathic subglottic: stenosis
idiopathic thrombocytopenic: purpura
idiosyncratic: sensitivity
idiotype: autoantibody
idiotypic: antibody
idiotypic antigenic: determinant
idioventricular: kick; rhythm
IgA: nephropathy
IgM: nephropathy
ileal: arteries; bladder; conduit; intussusception; orifice; papilla; sphincter; ureter; veins
ileoanal: pouch
ileocecal: eminence; fold; intussusception; junction; opening; orifice; valve
ileocecocolic: sphincter
ileocolic: artery; intussusception; lymph nodes; valve; vein
Ilhéus: encephalitis; fever; virus

iliac: arteries; bone; branch of iliolumbar artery; bursa; colon; crest; fascia; fossa; horn; muscle; region; roll; spine; steal; tubercle; tuberosity; veins
iliac (nervous): plexus
iliacosubfascial: fossa; hernia
iliacus: branch of iliolumbar artery
iliacus: muscle
iliacus minor: muscle
iliococcygeal: muscle; raphe
iliococcygeus: muscle
iliocostal: muscle
iliocostalis: muscle
iliocostalis cervicis: muscle
iliocostalis lumborum: muscle
iliocostalis thoracis: muscle
iliofemoral: ligament
iliohypogastric: nerve
ilioinguinal: nerve
iliolumbar: artery; ligament; vein
iliopectineal: arch; bursa; eminence; fascia; fossa; ligament; line
iliopelvic: sphincter
iliopsoas: muscle
iliopubic: eminence; tract
iliosciatic: notch
iliotibial: band; tract
iliotibial band: syndrome
iliotibial band friction: syndrome
iliotrochanteric: ligament
Ilizarov: technique
illegal: abortion
Ilosvay: reagent
image: amplifier; cytometer
imbrication: lines of von Ebner
Imerslünd-Grasbeck: syndrome
Imlach: fat-pad; ring
immature: cataract; granulocyte; neutrophil
immediate: allergy; amputation; auscultation; denture; hypersensitivity; percussion; reaction
immediate hypersensitivity: reaction
immediate insertion: denture
immediate posttraumatic: automatism; convulsion
immersion: bath; foot; lens; microscopy; objective
immobilized: enzyme
immobilizing: antibody
immotile cilia: syndrome
immovable: bandage; joint
immune: adherence; adsorption; agglutination; agglutinin; complex; deficiency; deviation; hemolysin; hemolysis; inflammation; interferon; opsonin; paralysis; precipitation; protein; reaction; response; serum; suppression; surveillance; system; thrombocytopenia
immune adherence: phenomenon
immune adhesion: test
immune complex: disease; disorder; glomerulonephritis; nephritis
immune electron: microscopy
immune fetal: hydrops
immune response: genes
immune serum: globulin
immune thrombocytopenic: purpura
immunity: deficiency
immunoblastic: lymphadenopathy; lymphoma; sarcoma
immunochemical: assay
immunodeficiency: syndrome
immunofluorescence: method; microscopy
immunofluorescent: stain
immunologic: competence; deficiency; enhancement; mechanism; paralysis; tolerance
immunological: surveillance
immunologically activated: cell
immunologically competent: cell
immunologically privileged: sites
immunologic high dose: tolerance
immunologic pregnancy: test
immunoperoxidase: technique
immunoproliferative: disorders
immunoproliferative small intestinal: disease
immunoradiometric: assay
immunoreactive: insulin
impact: factor; resistance
impacted: fetus; fracture; tooth
impaired glucose: tolerance
impedance: angle; matching; method; plethysmography
imperative: conception
imperfect: fungus; stage; state
imperforate: anus; hymen
impermeable: junction
impetiginous: cheilitis
impingement: sign; syndrome; test
implant: denture

implantation: cone; cyst; theory of the production of endometriosis
implant denture: substructure; superstructure
implanted: suture
implosive: therapy
impression: area; compound; material; tray
impressive: aphasia
impulse control: disorder
impulsive: obsession
impure: flutter
inactivated: serum
inactivated poliovirus: vaccine
inactive: mutant; repressor; tuberculosis
inadequate: personality; stimulus
inanition: fever
inapparent: infection
inappropriate: affect; hormone
inborn: errors of metabolism; reflex
inborn error of: metabolism
inborn lysosomal: disease
incarcerated: hernia; placenta
incarceration: symptom
incarial: bone
incasement: theory
inception: rate
incest: barrier
incidence: density; rate
incident: angle; point; ray
incidental: color; learning; parasite
incipient: abortion; caries
incisal: edge; embrasure; guidance; guide; margin; path; point; rest; surface
incisal guide: angle
incised: wound
incision: biopsy
incisional: hernia
incisive: bone; canals; duct; foramen; fossa; papilla; suture
incisive canal: cyst
incisor: canals; crest; foramen; tooth
inclusion: blennorrhea; bodies; cell; compound; conjunctivitis; cyst; dermoid
inclusion body: disease; encephalitis
inclusion cell: disease
inclusion conjunctivitis: viruses
incomitant: strabismus
incompatible blood transfusion: reaction
incompetent cervical: os
incomplete: abortion; achromatopsia; agglutinin;

alexia; antibody; antigen; ascertainment; cleavage; disinfectant; fistula; fracture; hemianopia; metamorphosis; neurofibromatosis; tetanus
incomplete atrioventricular: block; dissociation
incomplete conjoined: twins
incomplete foot: presentation
incongruent: nystagmus
incongruous: hemianopia
increased markings: emphysema
incremental: lines; lines of von Ebner
incrusted: cystitis
incubation: period
incubative: stage
incubatory: carrier
incudal: fold; fossa
incudiform: uterus
incudomalleolar: articulation; joint
incudostapedial: articulation; joint
indentation: hardness
independent: assortment; variable
independent practice: association
indeterminate: cleavage; leprosy
index: ametropia; case; finger; hypermetropia; myopia
index extensor: muscle
indexical: signs
India ink capsule: stain
Indian: flap; ginger; gum; podophyllum; sickness
Indian podophyllum: resin
Indian tick: typhus
indicator: system; yellow
indicator dilution: method
indicator-dilution: curve
indifference to pain: syndrome
indifferent: cell; electrode; genitalia; gonad; oxide; tissue; water
indirect: agglutination; assay; calorimetry; diuretic; fracture; immunofluorescence; laryngoscopy; lead; method for making inlays; ophthalmoscope; ophthalmoscopy; oxidase; placentography; rays; retainer; retention; technique; test; transfusion; vision
indirect Coombs: test
indirect fluorescent antibody: test
indirect hemagglutination: test

indirect inguinal: hernia
indirect nuclear: division
indirect pulp: capping
indirect pupillary: reaction
indirect reacting: bilirubin
individual: differences; psychology; therapy; tolerance
individuation: field
indocyanine green: angiography
indole: test
indolent: bubo; ulcer
indophenol: method
induced: abortion; apnea; enzyme; fever; fit; hypotension; malaria; mutation; phagocytosis; radioactivity; sensitivity; symptom; trance
induced fit: model
induced psychotic: disorder
inducer: cell
induction: chemotherapy; period
inductive: resistance
indurative: myocarditis
industrial: disease; hygiene; psychiatry; psychology
industrial methylated: spirit
indwelling: catheter
inert: gases
inertia: time
inevitable: abortion
infant: death
infantile: acropustulosis; autism; beriberi; cataract; colic; convulsion; diplegia; dwarfism; eczema; fibrosarcoma; gastroenteritis; hemiplegia; hernia; hypothyroidism; leishmaniasis; myofibromatosis; myxedema; osteomalacia; pellagra; scurvy; sexuality; spasm; tetany
infantile acute hemorrhagic: edema of the skin
infantile celiac: disease
infantile cortical: hyperostosis
infantile digital: fibromatosis
infantile G_{M2}: gangliosidosis
infantile gastroenteritis: virus
infantile, generalized G_{M1}: gangliosidosis
infantile muscular: atrophy
infantile neuroaxonal: dystrophy
infantile neuronal: degeneration
infantile progressive spinal muscular: atrophy
infantile purulent: conjunctivitis
infantile spastic: paraplegia

infant mortality: rate
infected: abortion
infection: calculus; immunity
infection-associated hemophagocytic: syndrome
infection control: nurse
infection-exhaustion: psychosis
infection transmission: parameter
infectious: anemia; disease; endocarditis; granuloma; hepatitis; icterus; jaundice; mononucleosis; myositis; nucleic acid; plasmid; polyneuritis; wart
infectious bronchitis: virus
infectious crystalline: keratopathy
infectious ectromelia: virus
infectious eczematoid: dermatitis
infectious hepatitis: virus
infectious papilloma: virus
infectious porcine encephalomyelitis: virus
infective: embolism; jaundice; thrombus
inferential: statistics
inferior: angle of scapula; belly of omohyoid muscle; border; border of body of pancreas; border of liver; border of lung; border of pancreas; border of spleen; branch; branches of transverse cervical nerve; branch of oculomotor nerve; branch of pubic bone; branch of superior gluteal artery; colliculus; extremity; extremity of kidney; eyelid; fascia of pelvic diaphragm; fascia of urogenital diaphragm; fovea; ganglion of glossopharyngeal nerve; ganglion of vagus nerve; horn; horn of falciform margin of saphenous opening; horn of lateral ventricle; horn of thyroid cartilage; laryngotomy; ligament of epididymis; limb; limb of ansa cervicalis; lobe of (left/right) lung; margin; mediastinum; member; olive; part; part of duodenum; part of lingular vein (of left superior pulmonary vein); part of trapezius (muscle); part of vestibular ganglion; part of vestibulocochlear nerve; pole; pole of kidney; pole of testis; polioencephalitis; recess of omental bursa;

retinaculum of extensor muscles; root of ansa cervicalis; segment; surface of cerebellar hemisphere; surface of petrous part of temporal bone; surface of tongue; tarsus; trunk of brachial plexus; veins of cerebellar hemisphere; vein of vermis; vena cava; wall of orbit; wall of tympanic cavity
inferior aberrant: ductule
inferior accessory: fissure
inferior alveolar: artery; nerve
inferior anal: nerves
inferior anastomotic: vein
inferior articular: facet of atlas; pit of atlas; process; surface of atlas; surface of tibia
inferior basal: vein
inferior calcaneonavicular: ligament
inferior cardiac: vein
inferior carotid: triangle
inferior cerebellar: peduncle
inferior cerebral: surface; veins
inferior cervical: ganglion
inferior cervical cardiac: branches of vagus nerve; nerve
inferior choroid: vein
inferior clunial: nerves
inferior constrictor: muscle of pharynx
inferior costal: facet; pit
inferior dental: arch; artery; branches of inferior dental plexus; canal; foramen; nerve; rami
inferior dental (nervous): plexus
inferior duodenal: flexure; fold; fossa; recess
inferior epigastric: artery; lymph nodes; vein
inferior esophageal: constriction; sphincter
inferior extensor: retinaculum
inferior fibular: retinaculum
inferior frontal: convolution; gyrus; sulcus
inferior gemellus: muscle
inferior gingival: branches of inferior dental plexus
inferior gluteal: artery; nerve; veins
inferior hemiazygos: vein
inferior hemorrhoidal: artery; nerves; plexuses; veins
inferior hypogastric (nervous): plexus
inferior hypophysial: artery

inferior ileocecal: recess
inferior internal parietal: artery
inferiority: complex
inferior labial: artery; branches of mental nerve; branch of facial artery; vein
inferior laryngeal: artery; cavity; nerve; vein
inferior lateral brachial cutaneous: nerve
inferior lateral cutaneous: nerve of arm
inferior lateral genicular: artery
inferior lingual: muscle
inferior lingular: artery; branch of lingular branch of left pulmonary artery
inferior lingular (bronchopulmonary): segment [S V]
inferior lobar: arteries
inferior longitudinal: fasciculus; muscle of tongue; sinus
inferior lumbar: triangle
inferior macular: arteriole; venule
inferior maxillary: nerve
inferior medial genicular: artery
inferior medullary: velum
inferior mesenteric: artery; ganglion; lymph nodes; vein
inferior mesenteric (nervous): plexus
inferior myocardial: infarction
inferior nasal: arteriole of retina; colliculus; concha; venule of retina
inferior nasal retinal: venule
inferior nuchal: line
inferior oblique: muscle of head
inferior oblique: muscle
inferior occipital: gyrus; triangle
inferior occipitofrontal: fasciculus
inferior olivary: complex; nucleus
inferior omental: recess
inferior ophthalmic: vein
inferior orbital: fissure
inferior palpebral: veins
inferior palpebral (arterial): arch
inferior pancreatic: artery
inferior pancreaticoduodenal: artery
inferior parietal: gyrus; lobule
inferior pelvic: aperture

inferior peroneal: retinaculum
inferior petrosal: groove; sinus; sulcus
inferior phrenic: artery; lymph nodes; vein
inferior posterior serratus: muscle
inferior pubic: ligament; ramus
inferior quadrigeminal: brachium
inferior radioulnar: joint
inferior rectal: artery; nerves; veins
inferior rectal (nervous): plexus
inferior rectus: muscle
inferior renal: segment
inferior sagittal: sinus
inferior salivary: nucleus
inferior salivatory: nucleus
inferior segmental: artery of kidney
inferior semilunar: lobule
inferior subtendinous: bursa of biceps femoris
inferior and superior lobar: arteries
inferior suprarenal: artery
inferior tarsal: muscle
inferior temporal: convolution; gyrus; line of parietal bone; sulcus; venule of retina
inferior temporal retinal: arteriole; venule
inferior thalamic: peduncle; radiation
inferior thalamostriate: veins
inferior thoracic: aperture
inferior thyroid: artery; notch; plexus; tubercle; vein
inferior tibiofibular: joint
inferior tracheobronchial: lymph nodes
inferior transverse scapular: ligament
inferior triangle: sign
inferior turbinated: bone
inferior tympanic: artery
inferior ulnar collateral: artery
inferior ventricular: vein
inferior vesical: artery
inferior vesical venous: plexus
inferior vestibular: area; nucleus
inferolateral: margin; margin of cerebral hemisphere; surface of prostate
inferolateral myocardial: infarction
inferomedial: margin of cerebral hemisphere
infertile male: syndrome

infiltration: anesthesia
infinite: distance
inflamed: ulcer
inflammatory: carcinoma; corpuscle; edema; lymph; macrophage; polyp; pseudotumor; rheumatism
inflammatory fibrous: hyperplasia
inflammatory linear verrucous epidermal: nevus
inflammatory papillary: hyperplasia
inflatable: implant; splint
influenza: bacillus; pneumonia; viruses
influenzal virus: pneumonia
influenza virus: vaccines
information: system; theory
informational: RNA
infraauricular deep parotid: lymph nodes
infraauricular subfascial parotid: lymph nodes
infrabony: pocket
infracardiac: bursa
infraclavicular: fossa; infiltrate; part of brachial plexus; triangle
infraclinoid: aneurysm
infracostal: line
infraduodenal: fossa
infraglenoid: tubercle (of scapula); tuberosity
infraglottic: cavity; space
infragranular: layer
infrahyoid: branch of superior thyroid artery; bursa; muscles
infralobar: part of posterior vein (of right superior pulmonary vein)
inframammary: region
infranatant: fluid
infraorbital: artery; canal; foramen; groove; margin; nerve; region; suture
infraorbitomeatal: plane
infrapalpebral: sulcus
infrapatellar: branch of saphenous nerve; fat-pad
infrapatellar fat: body
infrapatellar synovial: fold
infrared: cataract; light; microscope; ray; spectroscopy; spectrum; thermography
infrascapular: artery; region
infrasegmental: part; veins
infraspinatus: bursa; fascia
infraspinatus: muscle
infraspinous: fascia; fossa
infrasternal: angle
infratemporal: approach; crest of greater wing of sphenoid; fossa; surface of (body of) maxilla; surface of greater wing of sphenoid
infratrochlear: nerve
infundibular: part; recess; stalk; stem; stenosis
infundibuliform: fascia; hymen; sheath
infundibulo-ovarian: ligament
infundibulopelvic: ligament
infusion-aspiration: drainage
Ingelfinger: rule
Ingrassia: process
ingrowing: toenail
ingrown: hairs; nail
inguinal: branches of deep external pudendal arteries; canal; crest; falx; fold; fossa; hernia; ligament; ligament of the kidney; part of ductus deferens; region; triangle; trigone
inguinal aponeurotic: fold
inguinal lymphatic: plexus
inguinocrural: hernia
inguinolabial: hernia
inguinoscrotal: hernia
inguinosuperficial: hernia
inhalation: analgesia; anesthesia; anesthetic; therapy
inherited: character
inherited albumin: variants
inhibiting: antibody
inhibition: factor
inhibitory: fibers; nerve; obsession
inhibitory junction: potential
inhibitory postsynaptic: potential
initial: contact; dose; heat; hematuria; rate; velocity
initiating: agent; codon
initiation: codon; factor; tRNA
injection: flask; mass; molding
injury: potential
inkblot: test
inlay: graft; wax
innate: heat; immunity; reflex
inner: border of iris; layer of eyeball; lip of iliac crest; malleolus; membrane; sheath of optic nerve; stripes of renal medulla; table of skull; zone of renal medulla
inner cell: mass
inner dental: epithelium
innermost intercostal: muscle
inner nuclear: layer
inner plexiform: layer
inner spiral: sulcus
innervation: apraxia
innocent: murmur; tumor

innocent bystander: cell
innominate: artery; bone; fossa; substance; veins
innominate cardiac: veins
inorganic: acid; catalyst; chemistry; compound; diphosphatase; murmur; orthophosphate; phosphate; pyrophosphatase
inorganic dental: cement
inotropic: agents
inquiline: parasite
insect: viruses
insensible: perspiration; thirst
insertion: sequence
insertional: inactivation; mutagenesis
insight: learning
insoluble: soap
inspiratory: capacity; center; stridor
inspiratory reserve: volume
inspired: gas
inspissated bile: syndrome
instantaneous: vector
instantaneous electrical: axis
institutional review: board
instructive: theory
instrumental: amusia; conditioning
insufflation: anesthesia
insular: area; arteries; cortex; gyri; hypothesis; lobe; part; part of middle cerebral artery; sclerosis; veins
insulin: antagonist; injection; lipoatrophy; lipodystrophy; resistance; shock; unit
insulin coma: therapy; treatment
insulin-dependent: diabetes mellitus
insulin hypoglycemia: test
insulinlike: activity
insulinlike growth: factor
insulinopenic: diabetes
insulin receptor: substrate-1
insulin shock: treatment
insulin zinc: suspension
integral: dose; proteins
integrated rate: expression
integumentary: system
intellectual: aura
intelligence: quotient; test
intensification: chemotherapy
intensifying: screen
intensive: care; psychotherapy
intensive care: unit
intention: spasm; tremor
intentional: replantation
intention-to-treat: analysis
interaction process: analysis
interalveolar: pores; septum; space
interannular: segment
interarch: distance

interarticular: fibrocartilage; joints
interarytenoid: fold; notch
interatrial: block; foramen primum; foramen secundum; septum
interatrial conduction: time
interaural: attenuation
interauricular: arc
intercalary: neuron; staphyloma
intercalated: disk; ducts; nucleus
intercapillary: cell; glomerulosclerosis
intercapitular: veins
intercarotid: body; nerve
intercarpal: joints; ligaments
intercartilaginous: part of glottic opening; part of rima glottidis
intercavernous: sinuses
intercellular: bridges; canaliculus; cement; digestion; junctions; lymph
intercellular adhesion: molecule-1
interceptive occlusal: contact
interchondral: articulations; joints
interclavicular: ligament; notch
interclinoid: ligament
intercolumnar: fasciae; fibers; tubercle
intercondylar: eminence; fossa; line of femur; tubercle
intercondyloid: eminence; fossa; notch
intercornual: ligament
intercostal: anesthesia; arteries; ligaments; lymph nodes; membranes; nerves; neuralgia; space; veins
intercostobrachial: nerves
intercostohumeral: nerves
intercrural: fibers of superficial ring; ganglion
intercuneiform: joints; ligaments
intercurrent: disease
intercuspal: position
interdental: canals; caries; papilla; septum; splint
interdigital: folds
interdigitating reticulum: cell
interectopic: interval
interfacial: canals
interfacial surface: tension
interfascial: space
interfascicular: fasciculus
interference: beat; dissociation; microscope
interfoveolar: ligament
interganglionic: branches of sympathetic trunk

intergenic: complementation; suppression
interglobular: dentin; space; space of Owen
intergluteal: cleft
interiliac: lymph nodes
interim: denture
interjudge: reliability
interlaminar: jelly
interlobar: arteries of kidney; artery; duct; surfaces of lung; veins of kidney
interlobular: arteries; arteries of kidney; arteries of liver; duct; ductules; emphysema; pleurisy; septum; veins of kidney; veins of liver
interlocal: additivity
interlocking: gyri
intermaxillary: anchorage; bone; elastic; fixation; relation; segment; suture; traction
intermediary: metabolism; movements; nerve; system
intermediate: abutment; amputation; body of Flemming; branch of hepatic artery proper; bronchus; column; disk; filaments; ganglia; heart; hemorrhage; host; junction; lamella; layer; line of iliac crest; mass; mesoderm; nerve; part; part of adenohypophysis; part of male urethra; part of vestibular bulb; rays; region; trait; uveitis; variable; vein of forearm; zone; zone of iliac crest
intermediate acoustic: stria
intermediate antebrachial: vein
intermediate atrial: branch of left coronary artery; branch of right coronary artery
intermediate basilic: vein
intermediate cephalic: vein
intermediate cervical: septum
intermediate cubital: vein
intermediate cuneiform: bone
intermediate density: lipoprotein
intermediate dorsal cutaneous: nerve
intermediate great: muscle
intermediate hepatic: veins
intermediate hypothalamic: area; region
intermediate lacunar: lymph node; node
intermediate laryngeal: cavity
intermediate lumbar: lymph nodes

intermediate sacral: crest
intermediate supraclavicular: nerve
intermediate temporal: artery; branches of lateral occipital artery
intermediate vastus: muscle
intermediate white: layer [TA] of superior colliculus
intermediolateral: nucleus
intermediolateral cell: column of spinal cord
intermediomedial: nucleus
intermediomedial frontal: branch of callosomarginal artery
intermembrane: space
intermembranous: part of glottic opening; part of rima glottidis
intermenstrual: pain
intermesenteric arterial: anastomoses
intermesenteric (nervous): plexus
intermetacarpal: joints
intermetatarsal: articulations; joints
intermittent: albuminuria; arthralgia; claudication; cramp; hemoglobinuria; hydrarthrosis; hydrosalpinx; malaria; pulse; sterilization
intermittent acute: porphyria
intermittent explosive: disorder
intermittent malarial: fever
intermittent mandatory: ventilation
intermittent positive pressure: breathing; ventilation
intermittent self-: obturation
intermuscular: septum
intermuscular gluteal: bursa
internal: attachment; axis of eye; base of skull; branch of superior laryngeal nerve; branch of trunk of accessory nerve; canthus; capsule; conjugate; decompression; ear; energy; fistula; fixation; hemorrhage; hemorrhoids; hernia; hydrocephalus; lip of iliac crest; malleolus; medicine; meningitis; naris; nostril; ophthalmopathy; ophthalmoplegia; phase; pyocephalus; ramus of accessory nerve; representation; resorption; respiration; sheath of optic nerve; sphincter muscle of anus; squint; strabismus; surface; surface of cranial base; surface of frontal

bone; surface of parietal bone; table of calvaria; traction; urethrotomy
internal acoustic: foramen; meatus; opening; pore
internal adhesive: pericarditis
internal anal: sphincter
internal arcuate: fibers
internal auditory: artery; foramen; meatus; veins
internal capsule: syndrome
internal carotid: artery; nerve
internal carotid (nervous): plexus
internal carotid venous: plexus
internal cephalic: version
internal cerebral: veins
internal collateral: ligament of the wrist
internal conversion: electron
internal female genital: organs
internal iliac: artery; lymph nodes; vein
internal inguinal: ring
internal intercostal: membrane; muscle
internalized: homophobia
internal jugular: vein
internal lacrimal: fistula
internal male genital: organs
internal mammary: artery; plexus
internal maxillary: artery; plexus
internal medullary: lamina
internal nasal: branches
internal oblique: muscle
internal obturator: muscle
internal occipital: crest; protuberance
internal pillar: cells
internal podalic: version
internal pterygoid: muscle
internal pudendal: artery; vein
internal root: sheath
internal salivary: gland
internal saphenous: nerve
internal semilunar: fibrocartilage of knee joint
internal spermatic: artery; fascia
internal spiral: sulcus
internal thoracic: artery; plexus; vein
internal thoracic lymphatic: plexus
internal urethral: opening; orifice; sphincter
internasal: suture
international: unit
International Labour Organization: Classification

international normalized: ratio
international sensitivity: index
internet addiction: disorder
interneuromeric: clefts
internodal: segment
internuclear: ophthalmoplegia
internuncial: neuron
interobserver: error
interocclusal: clearance; distance; gap; record
interocclusal rest: space
interofective: system
interosseous: border; border of fibula; border of radius; border of tibia; border of ulna; bursa of elbow; cartilage; crest; fascia; groove; groove of calcaneus; groove of talus; margin; membrane of forearm; membrane of leg; muscles; nerve of leg
interosseous cubital: bursa
interosseous cuneocuboid: ligament
interosseous cuneometatarsal: ligaments
interosseous metacarpal: ligaments; spaces
interosseous metatarsal: ligaments; spaces
interosseous sacroiliac: ligaments
interosseous talocalcaneal: ligament
interosseous tibiofibular: ligament
interpalpebral: zone
interpapillary: ridges
interparietal: bone; sulcus; suture
interpectoral: lymph nodes
interpeduncular: cistern; fossa; ganglion; nucleus
interpersonal: conflict
interphalangeal: articulations; joints of foot; joints of hand
interpleural: space
interpolated: extrasystole; flap
interposition: arthroplasty
interpositospinal: tract
interpositus: nucleus
interproximal: papilla; space; surface of tooth
interpubic: disk; fibrocartilage
interpulmonary: septum
interradicular: alveoloplasty; septa of maxilla and mandible; space
interrater: reliability
interridge: distance
interrod: enamel

interrupted: respiration; suture
interscalene: triangle
interscapular: gland; hibernoma; reflex
interscapulothoracic: amputation
intersegmental: fasciculi; part of pulmonary vein; veins
intersemilunar: fissure
interseptovalvular: space
intersheath: spaces of optic nerve
intersigmoid: hernia; recess
interspinal: line; muscles; plane
interspinales: muscles
interspinales cervicis: muscles
interspinales lumborum: muscles
interspinales thoracis: muscles
interspinous: ligament; plane
interspongioplastic: substance
intersternebral: joints
interstitial: absorption; brachytherapy; cells; cystitis; deletion; disease; emphysema; fluid; gastritis; gland; growth; hernia; implantation; inflammation; keratitis; lamella; mastitis; myositis; nephritis; neuritis; nuclei of anterior hypothalamus; nucleus; nucleus of Cajal; nucleus of medial longitudinal fasciculus; pattern; pneumonia; pregnancy; therapy; tissue
interstitial amygdaloid: nucleus
interstitial cell: tumor of testis
interstitial cell-stimulating: hormone
interstitial plasma cell: pneumonia
interstitial pulmonary: fibrosis
interstitiospinal: tract
intertarsal: articulations; joints
intertendinous: connections of extensor digitorum
interthalamic: adhesion
intertragic: notch
intertransversarii: muscles
intertransverse: ligament; muscles
intertrochanteric: crest; fracture; line
intertropical: hyphemia
intertubercular: groove; line; plane; sulcus

intertubercular tendon: sheath
intertubular: zone
interureteric: crest; fold
intervaginal subarachnoid: space of optic nerve
interval: gout; operation; scale
intervening: sequence; variable
intervenous: tubercle (of right atrium)
interventional: angiography; radiology
interventricular: foramen; grooves; septum
interventricular septal: branches of left/right coronary artery
intervertebral: cartilage; disk; foramen; ganglion; notch; symphysis; vein
intervillous: lacuna; spaces
interzonal: mesenchyme
intestinal: anastomosis; angina; anthrax; arteries; atresia; calculus; capillariasis; cecum; digestion; emphysema; fistula; follicles; glands; intoxication; juice; lipodystrophy; lymphangiectasis; metaplasia; myiasis; rotation; sand; schistosomiasis; sepsis; stasis; steatorrhea; surface of uterus; villi
intestinal arterial: arcades
intestinal (lymphatic): trunks
in-the-canal: hearing aid
in-the-ear: hearing aid
intra-alveolar: septa
intraaortic: balloon
intra-aortic balloon: counterpulsation
intraaortic balloon: pump
intraarticular: cartilage; fracture; ligament of costal head; ligament of head of rib
intraarticular sternocostal: ligament
intraatrial: block; conduction
intraatrial conduction: time
intrabulbar: fossa
intracanalicular: fibroadenoma
intracapsular: ankylosis; fracture; ligaments
intracapsular temporomandibular joint: arthroplasty
intracardiac: catheter; lead
intracardiac pressure: curve
intracavernous: aneurysm; plexus

intracellular: canaliculus; digestion; enzyme; fluid; toxin; water
intracerebral: hemorrhage
intracorneal: implants
intracoronal: retainer
intracranial: aneurysm; cavity; ganglion; hematoma; hemorrhage; hypotension; part of optic nerve; part of vertebral artery; pneumatocele; pneumocele; pressure
intracranial granulomatous: arteritis
intractable: epilepsy; pain
intraculminate: fissure
intracutaneous: reaction
intracystic: papilloma
intracytoplasmic sperm: injection
intradermal: nevus; test
intraductal: carcinoma; papilloma
intraembryonic: mesoderm
intraepidermal: carcinoma
intraepiploic: hernia
intraepithelial: carcinoma; dyskeratosis; glands
intrafusal: fibers
intragenic: complementation; suppression
intraglandular deep parotid: lymph nodes
intraglandular parotid: lymph nodes
intragracile: sulcus
intrahepatic: cholestasis of pregnancy
intrailiac: hernia
intrajugular: process
intralaminar: nuclei of thalamus; part of intralocular part of optic nerve
intralesional: therapy
intraligamentary: pregnancy
intralobar: part of the posterior vein (of the right superior pulmonary vein)
intralobular: duct
intralocal: additivity
intramaxillary: anchorage
intramedullary: anesthesia; reamer; tractotomy; transfusion
intramembranous: ossification
intramural: hematoma; part of male urethra; practice; pregnancy
intranasal: anesthesia
in-transit: metastasis
intraobserver: error
intraocular: fluid; implant; neuritis; part of optic nerve; pressure

intraoral: anchorage; anesthesia; antrostomy
intraoral fracture: appliance
intraosseous: anesthesia; fixation
intrapapillary: drusen
intraparietal: sulcus; sulcus of Turner
intraparotid: plexus of facial nerve
intrapartum: hemorrhage; period
intrapelvic: hernia
intraperitoneal: pregnancy
intrapersonal: conflict
intrapulmonary: blood vessels; lymph nodes
intrarenal: arteries; reflux
intraretinal: space
intrasegmental: bronchi; part of pulmonary veins; veins
intraspinal: anesthesia
intratendinous: bursa of elbow
intratendinous olecranon: bursa
intrathalamic: fibers
intrathecal: injection
intrathyroid: cartilage
intratracheal: anesthesia; intubation; tube
intrauterine: amputation; contraceptive device; devices; fracture; insemination; pneumonia; transfusion
intrauterine contraceptive: devices
intrauterine growth: retardation
intravagal: glomus
intravaginal: torsion
intravascular: ligature; lymph
intravascular papillary endothelial: hyperplasia
intravenous: anesthesia; anesthetic; bolus; cholangiography; drip; narcosis; pyelography; urography
intravenous regional: anesthesia
intraventricular: block; conduction; hemorrhage; injection
intravital: stain; ultraviolet
intrinsic: asthma; color; deflection; dysmenorrhea; factor; fibers; motivation; muscles; muscles of foot; proteins; reflex; sphincter
intrinsicoid: deflection
intrinsic sympathomimetic: activity
intromittent: organ
introspective: method

intuitive: stage
intumescent: cataract
intussusceptive: growth
inulin: clearance
inundation: fever
InV: allotypes
invaginate: planula
invasive: carcinoma; mole
invasive pituitary: adenoma
inverse: anaphylaxis; symmetry; syntropy
inversed jaw-winking: syndrome
inverse ocular: bobbing
inverse-ratio: ventilation
inverse square: law
inversion: recovery
invert: sugar
inverted: image; papilloma; pelvis; reflex
inverted cone: bur
inverted follicular: keratosis
inverted radial: reflex
investigatory: reflex
investing: cartilage; fascia; layer; layer of cervical fascia; tissues
investment: cast
InV group: antigen
invisible: differentiation; light; spectrum
involuntary: guarding; muscles
involuntary nervous: system
involution: cyst; form
involutional: depression; melancholia
involved: field
iodate: reaction of epinephrine
iodide: acne
iodide transport: defect
iodinated: glycerol
iodinated ^{131}I human serum: albumin
iodinated ^{125}I serum: albumin
iodine: eruption; number; reaction of epinephrine; stain; test; value
iodine-induced: hyperthyroidism
iodized: collodion
iodophil: granule
iodotyrosine deiodinase: defect
ion: channel; pump
ion channel: disorders
ion exchange: chromatography
ion-exchange: resin
ionic: medication; strength
ionization: chamber
ionized: atom
ionizing: radiation
ion-selective: electrodes
ipecac: syrup
ipomea: resin

ipsilateral: reflex
iridescent: virus
iridial: part of retina
iridocorneal: angle
iridocorneal endothelial: syndrome
iridocorneal mesenchymal: dysgenesis
iridopupillary: lamina
IRI/G: ratio
iris: dehiscence; freckles; pits; spatula
Irish: moss
Irish moss: gelatin
iris-nevus: syndrome
iron: hematoxylin; index; line; lung; sulfate
iron-binding: capacity
iron deficiency: anemia
iron-dextran: complex
iron-storage: disease
iron-sulfur: proteins
irradiated vitamin D: milk
irreducible: hernia
irregular: astigmatism; bone; dentin; emphysema; nystagmus; pulse
irresistible: impulse
irreversible: colloid; hydrocolloid; pulpitis; reaction; shock
irritable: breast; colon
irritant contact: dermatitis
irritation: cell; fibroma
Irvine-Gass: syndrome
Isaac: syndrome
Isaac-Merton: syndrome
ischemia-modifying: factors
ischemic: contracture of the left ventricle; hypoxia; lumbago; necrosis; neuropathy
ischemic mitral: regurgitation
ischemic muscular: atrophy
ischemic optic: neuropathy
ischiadic: plexus; spine
ischial: bone; bursa; bursitis; ramus; spine; tuberosity
ischiatic: hernia; notch
ischioanal: fossa
ischiocapsular: ligament
ischiocavernous: muscle
ischiofemoral: ligament
ischiopubic: ramus
ischiorectal: abscess; fat-pad; fossa
Ishihara: test
island: disease; fever; flap
islet: cell; tissue
islet cell: tumor
isoallotypic: determinants
isobaric spinal: anesthesia
isochromic: anemia
isocyclic: compound
isodemographic: map
isodiphasic: complex

isodynamic: law
isoelectric: electroencephalogram; line; period; point; zone
isoenzyme: electrophoresis
isogeneic: graft
isogenic: strain
isogenous: chondrocytes; nest
isoimmune neonatal: thrombocytopenia
isoionic: point
isolated: abutment; dextrocardia; dyskeratosis follicularis; hypoaldosteronism; proteinuria
isolated explosive: disorder
isolated parietal: endocarditis
isolecithal: egg; ovum
isologous: graft
isomeric: function; transition
isometric: chart; contraction; exercise; period of cardiac cycle; relaxation; ruler; traction
isometric contraction: period
isometric relaxation: period
isomorphic: response
isomorphous: gliosis
isoniazid: neuropathy; polyneuropathy
isopeptide: bond
isoperistaltic: anastomosis
isophane: insulin
isoplastic: graft
isoprene: rule
isopropanol precipitation: test
isopycnic: zone
isorhythmic: dissociation
isosbestic: point
isoserum: treatment
isotonic: coefficient; contraction; exercise; traction
isotope: clearance
isotropic: disk; lipid
isovolume pressure-flow: curve
isovolumetric: relaxation
isovolumic: interval; period; relaxation
Itai-Itai: disease
Italian: flap
ITO: method
Ito: cells; nevus
Ito-Reenstierna: test
^{131}I uptake: test
Ivemark: syndrome
Ivor Lewis: esophagectomy
ivory: exostosis; membrane; vertebra
Ivy bleeding time: test
Ivy loop: wiring

J

J: chain; point
Jaboulay: amputation; pyloroplasty
Jaccoud: arthritis; arthropathy
jacket: crown
Jackson: law; membrane; rule; sign; veil
jacksonian: epilepsy; seizure
Jacobaeus: operation
Jacobson: anastomosis; canal; cartilage; nerve; organ; plexus; reflex
Jacquart facial: angle
Jacquemet: recess
Jacquemin: test
Jacques: plexus
Jacquet: erythema
Jadassohn: nevus
Jadassohn-Lewandowski: syndrome
Jadassohn-Pellizzari: anetoderma
Jadassohn-Tièche: nevus
Jaeger: test types
Jaffe: reaction; test
Jaffe-Lichtenstein: disease
Jahnke: syndrome
jail: fever
jake: paralysis
jalap: resin
Jamaican vomiting: sickness
James: fibers; tracts
Jamestown Canyon: virus
Janet: test
Janeway: lesion
Jansen: operation
Jansky: classification
Jansky-Bielschowsky: disease
Japan: wax
Japanese B: encephalitis
Japanese B encephalitis: virus
Japanese river: fever
Japanese spotted: fever
jargon: aphasia
Jarisch-Herxheimer: reaction
Jarman: score
Jarvik artificial: heart
Jatene: procedure
jaw: bone; jerk; joint; reflex; repositioning; separation; skeleton
Jaworski: bodies
jaw-winking: phenomenon; syndrome
jaw-working: reflex
JC: virus
jealous type of paranoid: disorder
Jeanselme: nodules
Jeghers-Peutz: syndrome
jejunal: arteries
jejunal and ileal: veins
jejunogastric: intussusception
jejunoileal: bypass; shunt
Jellinek: formula
Jendrassik: maneuver
Jenner: stain
Jenner-Kay: unit
Jensen: disease; sarcoma
jerk: finger
jerky: nystagmus; respiration
Jerne: technique
Jerne plaque: assay
Jervell and Lange-Nielsen: syndrome
Jesuit: tea
jet: injection; injector; nebulizer
jet ejector: pump
Jeune: syndrome
jeweller: forceps
Jewett: sound
Jewett and Strong: staging
j-g: complex
Jk: antigens
Job: syndrome
Jobbins: antigen
Jobert de Lamballe: fossa; suture
Jocasta: complex
Jod-Basedow: phenomenon
Joffroy: reflex; sign
Johanson-Blizzard: syndrome
Johnson: method
joint: branches; capsule; effusion; gamete; mice; oil; probability; sense
jojoba: oil
Jolles: test
Jolly: bodies; reaction
Jones: criteria; test; transfer
Jones I: test
Jones II: test
Jonnesco: fossa
Jonston: alopecia
Joubert: syndrome
Joule: equivalent
Js: antigen
J-sella: deformity
Judet: view
Judkins: technique
jugal: bone; ligament; point
jugular: bulb; duct; foramen; fossa; ganglion; gland; glomus; nerve; notch of occipital bone; notch of petrous part of temporal bone; notch of sternum; process of occipital bone; pulse; sinus; tubercle of occipital bone; veins; wall of middle ear
jugular foramen: syndrome
jugular lymphatic: plexus; trunk
jugular venous: arch
jugulodigastric: lymph node; node
juguloomohyoid: lymph node; node
jump: flap
jumping: disease; gene
jumping the: bite
jumping Frenchmen of Maine: disease
junction: nevus
junctional: complex; cyst; epithelium; escape; extrasystole; rhythm; tachycardia
Jung: muscle
jungian: psychoanalysis
jungle: fever
jungle yellow: fever
Jüngling: disease
Junin: virus
junk: DNA
Junod: boot
Jurkat: cells
juvenile: angiofibroma; arrhythmia; arthritis; carcinoma; cataract; cell; chorea; cirrhosis; diabetes; elastoma; hemangiofibroma; kyphosis; neutrophil; osteoporosis; papillomatosis; pattern; pelvis; periodontitis; polyp; retinoschisis; xanthogranuloma
juvenile absence: epilepsy
juvenile cerebellar: astrocytoma
juvenile chronic: arthritis
juvenile hyalin: fibromatosis
juvenile muscular: atrophy
juvenile myoclonic: epilepsy
juvenile-onset: diabetes
juvenile palmo-plantar: fibromatosis
juvenile plantar: dermatosis
juvenile spinal muscular: atrophy
juxta-articular: nodules
juxtacolic: artery
juxtacortical: chondroma
juxtacortical osteogenic: sarcoma
juxtaesophageal: lymph nodes
juxtaglomerular: apparatus; body; cells; complex; granules
juxtaglomerular cell: tumor
juxta-intestinal mesenteric: lymph nodes
juxtamedullary: glomerulus
juxtaphrenic: peak
juxtapupillary: choroiditis
juxtarestiform: body

K

K: antigens; capture; cells; complex; region; shell; virus
K-: radiation

K:A: ratio
kabure: itch
Kaffir: pox
kainate: receptor
Kaiserling: fixative
kallikrein: system
Kallmann: syndrome
kang: cancer
kangri burn: carcinoma
Kanner: syndrome
Kaplan-Meier: analysis; estimate
Kaposi: sarcoma
Kaposi varicelliform: eruption
kappa: angle; granule; particles
karaya: gum
Karman: cannula
Karmen: unit
Karnofsky: scale
Kartagener: syndrome; triad
karyochrome: cell
karyopyknotic: index
Kasabach-Merritt: syndrome
Kasai: operation
Kashin-Bek: disease
Kasokero: virus
Kast: syndrome
Kasten fluorescent Feulgen: stain
Kasten fluorescent PAS: stain
Kasten fluorescent Schiff: reagents
Katayama: disease; fever; syndrome; test
Kawasaki: disease; syndrome
Kayser-Fleischer: ring
Kazanjian: operation
Kearns-Sayre: syndrome
Keating-Hart: method
kedani: fever
keeled: chest
Keen: operation
Kegel: exercises
Kehr: sign
Keith: bundle; node
Keith and Flack: node
Kelev strain rabies: virus
Keller: bunionectomy
Keller-Madlener: operation
Kelly: clamp; operation
Kelly rectal: speculum
Kelvin: scale
Kempner: diet
Kendall: compounds; substance
Kennedy: classification; disease; syndrome
Kenny: treatment
Kenny-Caffey: syndrome
Kent: bundle
Kent-His: bundle
Kenya: fever
Kerandel: sign
keratic: precipitates

keratin: filaments; pearl
keratinized: cell
keratinous: cyst
keratogenous: membrane
keratohyalin: granules
keratoid: exanthema
keratophakic: keratoplasty
keratorefractive: surgery
keratosic: cones
Kerckring: center; folds; ossicle; valves
Kerley A: lines
Kerley B: lines
Kerley C: lines
Kernig: sign
Kernohan: notch
kern-plasma relation: theory
Kestenbaum: number; procedure; sign
α-keto acid: dehydrogenase
α-keto acid dehydrogenase: complex
ketogenic: diet
ketogenic-antiketogenic: ratio
ketogenic corticoids: test
17-ketogenic steroid assay: test
α-ketoglutarate dehydrogenase: complex
ketone: body
ketonimine: dyes
ketosis-prone: diabetes
ketosis-resistant: diabetes
ketotic: hyperglycemia; hyperglycinemia; hypoglycemia
Kety-Schmidt: method
Kew Gardens: fever
key: attachment; ridge; vein
keyhole: deformity; pupil
key-in-lock: maneuver
keyway: attachment
Ki-1+: lymphoma
kidney: carbuncle; lobes
Kiel: classification
Kienböck: atrophy; disease; dislocation; unit
Kiernan: space
Kiesselbach: area
Kikuchi: disease
Kilham rat: virus
Kilian: line
Kiliani-Fischer: reaction; synthesis
killer: cells
Killian: bundle; operation; triangle
kilogram: calorie
Kimmelstiel-Wilson: disease; syndrome
Kimura: disease
kinematic: face-bow; viscosity
kineplastic: amputation
kinesthesia: hallucination
kinesthetic: aura; sense

kinetic: analyzer; ataxia; energy; measurement; perimetry; strabismus; system; tremor
kinetochore: fibers
King: unit
King-Armstrong: unit
Kingsley: splint
kinked: aorta
Kinkiang: fever
kinky: hair
kinky-hair: disease
Kinyoun: stain
Kirk: amputation
Kirkland: knife
Kirschner: apparatus; wire
Kisch: reflex
kissing: puncta
Kitasato: bacillus
Kjeldahl: apparatus; method
Kjelland: forceps
Kjer optic: atrophy
Klatskin: tumor
Klebs-Loeffler: bacillus
Kleihauer: stain
Kleine-Levin: syndrome
Klein-Gumprecht shadow: nuclei
Klenow: fragment
Klestadt: cyst
Klinefelter: syndrome
Klinger-Ludwig acid-thionin: stain for sex chromatin
Klippel-Feil: syndrome
Klippel-Trenaunay-Weber: syndrome
Klumpke: palsy; paralysis
Klüver-Barrera Luxol fast blue: stain
Klüver-Bucy: syndrome
Km: allotypes; antigen
Knapp: streaks; striae
knee: jerk; joint; presentation; reflex
knee-ankle-foot: orthosis
knee-chest: position
knee disarticulation: amputation
knee-elbow: position
knee-jerk: reflex
Kniest: syndrome
knife: needle
knife-rest: crystal
knockout: mouse
knock-out: drops
Knoll: glands
Knoop: theory
Knoop hardness: number; test
Knott: technique
knuckle: pads; sign
Knudsen: hypothesis
Kobberling-Dunnigan: syndrome
Kobelt: tubules
Kober: test
Köbner: phenomenon

Koch: bacillus; law; node; phenomenon; postulates; triangle
Kocher: clamp; incision; sign
Kocher-Debré-Sémélaigne: syndrome
Koch old: tuberculin
Koch-Weeks: bacillus
Kock: ileostomy; pouch
Koenen: tumor
Koenig: syndrome
Koerber-Salus-Elschnig: syndrome
Koerte-Ballance: operation
Koettstorfer: number
Köhler: disease; illumination
Kohlmeier-Degos: syndrome
Kohlrausch: folds; muscle
Kohn: pores
Kohnstamm: phenomenon
Kojewnikoff: epilepsy
kok: disease
kokoi: venom
Kokoskin: stain
Kölliker: layer; reticulum
Kollmann: dilator
Kolmer: test
Kommerell: diverticulum
Kondoleon: operation
Konno: procedure
Konno-Rastan: procedure
Koongol: viruses
Koplik: spots
Korean hemorrhagic: fever
Korean hemorrhagic fever: virus
Korff: fibers
Kornberg: enzyme
Korotkoff: sounds; test
Korsakoff: psychosis; syndrome
Koshland-Némethy-Filmer: model
Kossa: stain
Kostmann: syndrome
Krabbe: disease
Kraske: operation
Krause: bone; glands; graft; ligament; valve
Krause end: bulbs
Krause respiratory: bundle
Krause-Wolfe: graft
Krebs: cycle
Krebs-Henseleit: cycle
Krebs-Kornberg: cycle
Krebs-Ringer: solution
Kretschmann: space
Kreysig: sign
Krimsky: test
Krogh: spirometer
Kromayer: lamp
Kronecker: stain
Krönig: isthmus; steps
Krönlein: hernia; operation
Krueger: instrument stop

Krukenberg: amputation; spindle; tumor; veins
Kruse: brush
krypton: laser
KTP: laser
Kufs: disease
Kugel anastomotic: artery
Kugelberg-Welander: disease
Kühne: fiber; methylene blue; phenomenon; plate; spindle
Kuhnt: spaces
Kuhnt-Junius: degeneration
Kulchitsky: cells
Külz: cylinder
Kümmell: spondylitis
Küntscher: nail
Kupffer: cells
Kürsteiner: canals
Kurtzke multiple sclerosis disability: scale
Kurzrok-Ratner: test
Kuskokwim: syndrome
Kussmaul: coma; disease; respiration; sign
Kussmaul-Kien: respiration
Kveim: antigen; test
Kveim-Siltzbach: antigen; test
Kyasanur Forest: disease
Kyasanur Forest disease: virus
kyphoscoliotic: pelvis
kyphotic: pelvis
Kyrle: disease

L

L: chain; doses; form; selectin; shell; unit of streptomycin
L⁺: dose
L-: meromyosin; radiation
ʟ-: serine dehydratase
Laband: syndrome
Labbé: triangle; vein
labeled: atom; thyroxine
labial: arch; bar; branches of mental nerve; commissure; embrasure; flange; gingiva; glands; hernia; occlusion; part of orbicularis oris (muscle); splint; sulcus; swelling; tubercle; veins; vestibule
labile: affect; current; elements; factor; hypertension; pulse
labiodental: sulcus
labiogingival: lamina
labiolingual: appliance; plane
labioscrotal: folds; swellings
labor: curve; pains
laboratory: diagnosis
labored: respiration
Labrador: keratopathy
labyrinthine: apoplexy; artery; fistula; nystagmus; placenta; reflexes; torticollis; veins; wall of middle ear; wall of tympanic cavity
labyrinthine righting: reflexes
Lac: operon
lacerated: foramen
Lachman: test
laciniate: ligament
lacis: cell
lacquer: cracks
lacrimal: apparatus; artery; bay; bone; border of maxilla; calculus; canaliculus; caruncle; conjunctivitis; fascia; fistula; fold; fossa; gland; groove; hamulus; lake; margin of maxilla; nerve; notch; opening; papilla; part of orbicularis oculi muscle; pathway; process of inferior nasal concha; punctum; reflex; sac; vein
lacrimoconchal: suture
lacrimogustatory: reflex
lacrimomaxillary: suture
La Crosse: virus
lactacid oxygen: debt
β-lactamase: inhibitors
lactase: persistence; restriction
lactate dehydrogenase: virus
lactated Ringer: injection; solution
lactating: adenoma
lactation: amenorrhea; hormone
lactational: mastitis
lacteal: cyst; fistula; vessel
lactic: acidosis
lactic acid: bacillus; fermentation
lactiferous: ampulla; ducts; gland; sinus
lactobacillary: milk
***Lactobacillus bulgaricus*:** factor
***Lactobacillus casei*:** factor
lactogenic: hormone
lacto-ovo-: vegetarian
lactophenol cotton blue: stain
lactose: intolerance
lacunar: abscess; amnesia; ligament; state; tonsillitis
lacunar-molecular: layer
Ladd: band; operation
ladder: splint
Ladd-Franklin: theory
Laënnec: cirrhosis; pearls
Lafora: body; disease
Lafora body: disease
lag: phase
lagophthalmic: keratitis
Lahey: forceps
Lahore: sore
Laimer-Haeckerman: area

Laki-Lorand: factor
laky: blood
Lallemand: bodies
Lallouette: pyramid
lamarckian: theory
Lamaze: method
LAMB: syndrome
Lambda: phage
lambdoid: border of occipital bone; margin of occipital bone; suture
Lambert: law; syndrome
Lambert-Eaton: syndrome
Lambl: excrescences
Lambrinudi: operation
lamellar: bone; cataract; granule; ichthyosis; keratoplasty
lamellated: corpuscles
laminar: flow
laminar cortical: necrosis; sclerosis
laminated: clot; cortex; epithelium; thrombus
laminated epithelial: plug
laminin: receptor
lampbrush: chromosome
Lan: antigen
Lancaster red green: test
Lancefield: classification
Lancisi: sign
land: scurvy
Landau-Kleffner: syndrome
Landolfi: sign
Landouzy-Dejerine: dystrophy
Landouzy-Grasset: law
Landry: paralysis; syndrome
Landry-Guillain-Barré: syndrome
landscape: ecology
Landschutz: tumor
Landsteiner-Donath: test
Landström: muscle
Landzert: fossa
Lane: band; disease; kink
Lange: solution; test
Langenbeck: triangle
Langendorff: method
Langer: arch; lines; muscle
Langerhans: cells; granule; islands
Langerhans cell: histiocytosis
Langer-Saldino: syndrome
Langhans: cells; layer; stria
Langhans-type giant: cells
Langley: granules
Langmuir: trough
language: game; zone
Lannelongue: foramina; ligaments
Lanterman: incisures; segments
lanugo: hair
Lanz: line

L-AP₄: receptor
laparoscopic: cannula; cholecystotomy; knot; nephrectomy; surgery
laparoscopically assisted: surgery
laparoscopic-assisted vaginal: hysterectomy; hysteroscopy
laparoscopic uterosacral nerve: ablation
laparotomy: pad
Lapicque: law
Laplace: forceps; law
Laquer: stain for alcoholic hyalin
larch: turpentine
lardaceous: liver; spleen
large: bowel; calorie; intestine; muscle of helix; pelvis; vein
large cell: carcinoma; lymphoma
large interarch: distance
large pudendal: lip
large saphenous: vein
Larmor: frequency
Laron type: dwarfism
Laroyenne: operation
Larrey: cleft
Larsen: syndrome
larval: conjunctivitis; plague
laryngeal: aditus; aperture; atresia; bursa; cavity; chorea; crisis; diphtheria; epilepsy; glands; granuloma; inlet; mask; mucosa; papillomatosis; part of pharynx; pharynx; polyp; pouch; prominence; reflex; saccule; sinus; stenosis; stridor; syncope; tonsils; veins; ventricle; vertigo; web
laryngeal lymphoid: nodules
laryngopharyngeal: branches of superior cervical ganglion
laryngospastic: reflex
laryngotracheal: diphtheria; diverticulum; groove
laryngotracheoesophageal: cleft
Lasègue: sign; syndrome
laser: corepraxy; iridotomy; microscope; photocoagulator; trabeculoplasty
laser-assisted in situ: keratomileusis
Lash: operation
Lash casein hydrolysate-serum: medium
Lassa: fever; virus
Lassa hemorrhagic: fever
Latarget: nerve; vein

late: cyanosis; deceleration; diastole; reaction; rickets; seizure; syphilis; systole
late apical systolic: murmur
late auditory-evoked: response
late benign: syphilis
late diastolic: murmur
late dumping: syndrome
late latent: syphilis
late luteal phase: dysphoria
late luteal phase dysphoric: disorder
latency: period; phase
latent: allergy; carcinoma; carrier; content; diabetes; empyema; energy; gout; heat; homosexuality; hyperopia; infection; learning; microbism; nystagmus; period; reflex; schizophrenia; stage; syphilis; typhoid; zone
latent adrenocortical: insufficiency
latent membrane: protein
latent rat: virus
late-phase: response
lateral: aberration; angle of eye; angle of scapula; angle of uterus; aperture of fourth ventricle; aspect; border; border of foot; border of forearm; border of humerus; border of kidney; border of nail; border of scapula; branches; branches of artery of tuber cinereum; branches of pontine arteries; branch of posterior rami of spinal nerves; canal; canthus; cartilage of nose; column; column of spinal cord; compartment of leg; condyle; condyle of femur; condyle of tibia; cord of brachial plexus; crus; crus of facial canal; crus of horizontal part of the facial canal; crus of the major alar cartilage of the nose; crus of the superficial inguinal ring; curvature; division of left liver; epicondyle of femur; epicondyle of humerus; excursion; fasciculus proprius; fillet; folds; fossa of brain; funiculus; funiculus of spinal cord; ginglymus; head; hermaphroditism; horn; illumination; incisor; lacunae; lacunae of superior sagittal sinus; lakes; lamina of cartilage of pharyngotympanic (auditory) tube; lemniscus; ligament of ankle; ligament of bladder; ligament of elbow; ligament of knee; ligament of malleus; ligament of temporomandibular joint; ligament of wrist; limb; lip of linea aspera; lithotomy; malleolus; margin; mass of atlas; mass of ethmoid bone; meniscus; mesoderm; movement; nucleus; nucleus of mammillary body; nucleus of medulla oblongata; nucleus of thalamus; nucleus of trapezoid body; occlusion; part of longitudinal arch of foot; part of middle lobe vein (of right superior pulmonary vein); part of occipital bone; part of posterior cervical intertransversarii (muscles); part of posterior (extensor) compartment of forearm; part of sacrum; part of vaginal fornix; plate; plate of cartilaginous auditory tube; plate of pterygoid process; pole; process of calcaneal tuberosity; process of malleus; process of septal nasal cartilage; process of talus; projection; recess of fourth ventricle; region of abdominal region; region of neck; root of median nerve; root of optic tract; segment; sinus; sulcus; surface; surface of arm; surface of fibula; surface of finger; surface of leg; surface of lower limb; surface of ovary; surface of testis; surface of tibia; surface of toe; surface of zygomatic bone; tubercle (of posterior process) of talus; vein of lateral ventricle; ventricle; vertigo; wall of middle ear; wall of orbit; wall of tympanic cavity; zone
lateral abdominal: region
lateral abdominal/pectoral cutaneous: branches of intercostal nerves
lateral aberrant thyroid: carcinoma
lateral alveolar: abscess
lateral ampullar: nerve
lateral amygdaloid: nucleus
lateral antebrachial cutaneous: nerve
lateral anterior thoracic: nerve
lateral arcuate: ligament
lateral atlantoaxial: joint
lateral atlantoepistrophic: joint
lateral atrial: branch of left coronary artery; branch of right coronary artery; vein
lateral axillary: lymph nodes
lateral basal: branch
lateral basal (bronchopulmonary): segment [S IX]
lateral basal segmental: artery
lateral bicipital: groove
lateral bronchopulmonary: segment S IV
lateral calcaneal: branches of sural nerve
lateral cartilaginous: plate
lateral central palmar: space
lateral cerebellomedullary: cistern
lateral cerebral: fissure; fossa
lateral cervical: nucleus; region
lateral circumflex: artery of thigh
lateral circumflex femoral: artery; veins
lateral collateral: ligament of ankle
lateral condylar: inclination
lateral corticospinal: tract
lateral costal: branch of internal thoracic artery
lateral costotransverse: ligament
lateral cricoarytenoid: muscle
lateral cuneate: nucleus
lateral cuneiform: bone
lateral cutaneous: branch; branches of intercostal nerves; branches of ventral primary ramus of thoracic spinal nerves; nerve of calf; nerve of forearm; nerve of thigh
lateral decubitus: radiograph
lateral direct: veins
lateral dorsal: nucleus
lateral dorsal cutaneous: nerve
lateral epicondylar: crest; ridge
lateral femoral: tuberosity
lateral femoral circumflex: artery
lateral femoral cutaneous: nerve
lateral frontobasal: artery
lateral geniculate: body; nucleus
lateral glossoepiglottic: fold
lateral great: muscle
lateral ground: bundle
lateral habenular: nucleus
lateral humeral: epicondylitis
lateral hypothalamic: area; region
lateral inferior genicular: artery
lateral inferior hepatic: area
lateral inguinal: fossa
lateral jugular: lymph nodes
lateral lacunar: lymph node; node
lateral lingual: swellings
lateral longitudinal: arch of foot; stria
lateral lumbar intertransversarii: muscles
lateral lumbar intertransverse: muscles
lateral lumbocostal: arch
lateral malleolar: arteries; branch (of fibular peroneal artery); facet of talus; ligament; network; surface of talus
lateral malleolar subcutaneous: bursa
lateral malleolus: bursa
lateral mammary: branches; branches of lateral cutaneous branches of intercostal nerves; branches of lateral cutaneous branches of thoracic spinal nerves; branches of lateral thoracic artery
(lateral and medial) palpebral: arteries
(lateral and medial) parietal: arteries
lateral and medial posterior choroidal: branches of posterior cerebral artery
lateral medullary: branches of (intracranial part of) vertebral artery; lamina [TA] of lentiform nucleus; syndrome
lateral midpalmar: space
lateral myocardial: infarction
lateral nasal: artery; branches of anterior ethmoidal nerve; branch of facial artery; fold; process; prominence
lateral oblique: radiograph
lateral occipital: artery; sulcus
lateral occipitotemporal: gyrus
lateral olfactory: gyrus
lateral orbitofrontal: artery
lateral palpebral: commissure; ligament; raphe
lateral parabrachial: nucleus
lateral patellar: retinaculum
lateral pectoral: nerve
lateral pelvic wall: triangle

lateral pericardial: lymph nodes
lateral pericuneate: nucleus
lateral periodontal: abscess; cyst
lateral pharyngeal: space
lateral plantar: artery; nerve
lateral plate: mesoderm
lateral posterior: nucleus
lateral posterior cervical intertransversarii: muscles
lateral preoptic: nucleus
lateral proprius: bundle
lateral pterygoid: muscle; plate
lateral puboprostatic: ligament
lateral pyramidal: fasciculus; tract
lateral ramus: radiograph
lateral raphespinal: tract
lateral rectus: muscle of the head
lateral rectus: muscle
lateral recumbent: position
lateral reticular: nucleus
lateral reticulospinal: tract
lateral sacral: arteries; branches of median sacral artery; crest; veins
lateral sacrococcygeal: ligament
lateral segmental: artery
lateral semicircular: canals
lateral septal: nucleus
lateral skull: radiograph
lateral spinal: sclerosis
lateral spinothalamic: tract
lateral splanchnic: arteries
lateral striate: arteries
lateral superior genicular: artery
lateral superior hepatic: area
lateral superior olivary: nucleus
lateral supraclavicular: nerve
lateral supracondylar: crest; ridge
lateral supraepicondylar: ridge
lateral sural cutaneous: nerve
lateral talocalcaneal: ligament
lateral tarsal: artery
lateral tarsal strip: procedure
lateral temporomandibular: ligament
lateral thalamic: peduncle
lateral thoracic: artery; vein
lateral thyrohyoid: ligament
lateral tuberal: nuclei
lateral umbilical: fold; ligament
lateral vaginal wall: smear
lateral vastus: muscle
lateral venous: lacunae

lateral ventral: hernia
lateral vestibular: nucleus
lateral vestibulospinal: tract
late replicating: chromosome
latex agglutination: test
latex fixation: test
latissimus dorsi: muscle
latitude: film
lattice corneal: dystrophy
latticed: layer
Latzko cesarean: section
laudable: pus
laughing: gas
laughter: reflex
Laugier: hernia
Laumonier: ganglion
Launois-Bensaude: syndrome
Launois-Cléret: syndrome
laurel: fever
Laurence-Moon: syndrome
Laurer: canal
Lauth: canal; ligament
Lavdovsky: nucleoid
Lawrence-Seip: syndrome
lazarine: leprosy
LCAT: deficiency
L-chain: disease; myeloma
LCM: virus
L-D: body
LDH: agent
LDL receptor: disorder
LE: body; cell; factors; phenomenon
Le: antigens
lead: anemia; colic; encephalitis; encephalopathy; gout; line; neuropathy; palsy; paralysis; poisoning; stomatitis
leader: sequences
lead hydroxide: stain
leading: ancestor; edge
lead-pipe: colon; rigidity
leak point: pressure
leapfrog: position
Lear: complex
learned: drive
learning: disability; set; theory
least confusion: circle
least splanchnic: nerve
least squares: estimator
leather-bottle: stomach
Le Bel-van't Hoff: rule
Leber: plexus
Leber hereditary optic: atrophy
Leber idiopathic stellate: neuroretinitis; retinopathy
LE cell: test
Le Chatelier: law; principle
lecithin/sphingomyelin: ratio
LeCompte: maneuver; operation
lectin pathway: molecule
Lederer: anemia
Ledermann: formula

Lee: ganglion
Leede-Rumpel: phenomenon
Leeuwenhoek: canals
leeway: space
Lee-White: method
Le Fort: amputation; osteotomy; sound
Le Fort I: fracture
Le Fort II: fracture
Le Fort III: fracture
Le Fort III craniofacial: dysjunction
left: atrium of heart; auricle; branch; branch of hepatic artery proper; bundle of atrioventricular bundle; crus of atrioventricular bundle; crus of diaphragm; duct of caudate lobe of liver; heart; liver; lobe; lobe of liver; part of liver; ventricle
left anterior descending: artery
(left anterior) lateral hepatic: segment [III]
left atrioventricular: orifice; valve
left auricular: appendage
left axis: deviation
left colic: artery; flexure; lymph nodes; vein
left coronary: artery; vein
left fibrous: trigone (of heart)
left gastric: artery; lymph nodes; vein
left gastroepiploic: artery; lymph nodes; vein
left gastroomental: artery; lymph nodes; vein
left heart: bypass
left hepatic: artery; duct; vein
left inferior pulmonary: vein
left lateral: division of liver
left lumbar: lymph nodes
left main: bronchus
left marginal: artery
left medial: division of liver
(left) medial hepatic: segment [IV]
left ovarian: vein
(left posterior) lateral hepatic: segment III
left pulmonary: artery
(left and right) brachiocephalic: veins
left sagittal: fissure
left-sided: appendicitis
left-sided heart: failure
left superior intercostal: vein
left superior pulmonary: vein
left suprarenal: vein
left testicular: vein
left-to-right: shunt
left triangular: ligament of liver
left umbilical: vein

left ventricular: failure; myomectomy
left-ventricular assist: device
left ventricular ejection: time
left ventricular volume reduction: surgery
leg: phenomenon
Legal: test
legal: blindness; dentistry; medicine
Legendre: sign
Legg-Calvé-Perthes: disease
Legionnaires: disease
Leichtenstern: sign
Leigh: disease
Leiner: disease
Leishman: stain
Leishman chrome: cells
Leishman-Donovan: body
leishmanin: test
Leiter International Performance: Scale
Lejeune: syndrome
Lembert: suture
lemniscal: trigone
lemon: sign
Lendrum phloxine-tartrazine: stain
Lenègre: disease; syndrome
length-breadth: index
lengthening: reaction
length-height: index
Lenhossék: processes
Lennert: classification; lymphoma
Lennox: syndrome
Lennox-Gastaut: syndrome
Lenoir: facet
lens: capsule; pits; placodes; stars; sutures; vesicle
lens-induced: uveitis
lente: insulin
lenticular: ansa; apophysis; astigmatism; bone; capsule; colony; fasciculus; fossa; ganglion; knife; loop; nucleus; papillae; process of incus; syphilid; vesicle
lenticular progressive: disease
lenticulostriate: arteries
lentiform: bone
leonine: facies
LEOPARD: syndrome
leopard: fundus; retina
Leopold: maneuvers
Lepehne-Pickworth: stain
Lepore: thalassemia
lepra: cells
lepromatous: leprosy
lepromin: reaction; test
leprosy: bacillus
leprous: neuropathy
leptomeningeal: carcinoma; carcinomatosis; cyst; fibrosis; space

leptospiral: jaundice
Leri: pleonosteosis; sign
Leriche: operation; syndrome
Leri-Weill: disease; syndrome
Lermoyez: syndrome
Lerner: homeostasis
Lesch-Nyhan: syndrome
Leser-Trélat: sign
Lesser: triangle
lesser: circulation; cul-de-sac; curvature of stomach; horn of hyoid; omentum; pancreas; pelvis; ring of iris
lesser: trochanter; tubercle (of humerus); tuberosity of humerus; wing of sphenoid (bone)
lesser alar: cartilages
lesser arterial: circle of iris
lesser internal cutaneous: nerve
lesser multangular: bone
lesser occipital: nerve
lesser palatine: artery; canals; foramina; nerves
lesser peritoneal: cavity; sac
lesser petrosal: nerve
lesser rhomboid: muscle
lesser sciatic: notch
lesser splanchnic: nerve
lesser superficial petrosal: nerve
lesser supraclavicular: fossa
lesser tympanic: spine
lesser vestibular: glands
lesser zygomatic: muscle
Lesshaft: triangle
let-down: reflex
lethal: coefficient; dose; dwarfism; equivalent; factor; gene; mutation
lethality: rate
lethal midline: granuloma
lethargic: hypnosis
letter: blindness
Letterer-Siwe: disease
leucine: hypoglycemia
leucine-induced: hypoglycemia
leucine-sensitive: hypoglycemia
Leudet: tinnitus
leukemia inhibitory: factor
leukemic: leukemia; myelosis; reticuloendotheliosis; reticulosis; retinitis; retinopathy
leukemic hyperplastic: gingivitis
leukemoid: reaction
leukocyte: cream; inclusions; interferon
leukocyte adherence assay: test
leukocyte adhesion: deficiency

leukocyte bactericidal assay: test
leukocyte common: antigen
leukocytic: pyrogens; sarcoma
leukocytoclastic: vasculitis
leukocytosis-promoting: factor
leukoerythroblastic: anemia
leukopenic: factor; index; leukemia; myelosis
leukotriene receptor: antagonist
Lev: disease; syndrome
Levaditi: stain
levator: cushion; hernia; muscle of thyroid gland; swelling
levator anguli oris: muscle
levator ani: muscle
levatores costarum: muscles
levatores costarum breves: muscles
levatores costarum longi: muscles
levator labii superioris: muscle
levator labii superioris alaeque nasi: muscle
levator palati: muscle
levator palpebrae superioris: muscle
levator prostatae: muscle
levator scapulae: muscle
levator veli palatini: muscle
Levay: antigen
LeVeen: shunt
level-dependent frequency: response
Levey-Jennings: chart
Levin: tube
levoatrio-cardinal: vein
Levret: forceps
Lewis: acid; base
Lewy: bodies
Lewy body: dementia
Leyden: ataxia; crystals; neuritis
Leyden-Möbius muscular: dystrophy
Leydig: cells
Leydig cell: tumor
Lf: dose
Lhermitte: sign
libido: theory
Libman-Sacks: endocarditis; syndrome
Liborius: method
licensed practical: nurse
licensed vocational: nurse
lichen: amyloidosis
lichenoid: amyloidosis; dermatosis; eczema; keratosis
lichen planus-like: keratosis
Lichtheim: sign
lid: reflex

lid-closure: reaction
lid crutch: spectacles
Liddell-Sherrington: reflex
Lieberkühn: follicles; glands
Liebermann-Burchard: reaction; test
Liebermeister: rule
Liebig: theory
lienal: artery
lienophrenic: ligament
lienorenal: ligament
lienteric: diarrhea
Liesegang: rings
Lieutaud: body; triangle; trigone; uvula
life: cycle; instinct; stress; table
life-belt: cataract
life-span: development
Li-Fraumeni cancer: syndrome
ligand-binding: site
ligand-gated: channel
ligase chain: reaction
ligature: wire
light: adaptation; bath; cells of thyroid; chain; difference; metal; micrograph; microscope; reflex; sense; sleep; treatment
light-activated: resin
light-adapted: eye
light chain-related: amyloidosis
light-cured: resin
light differential: threshold
lighthouse: lens
light liquid: petrolatum
light-near: dissociation
lightning: strip
light-touch: palpation
light wire: appliance
ligneous: conjunctivitis; struma; thyroiditis
Likert: scale
Lillie allochrome connective tissue: stain
Lillie azure-eosin: stain
Lillie ferrous iron: stain
Lillie sulfuric acid Nile blue: stain
lilliputian: hallucination
limb: bud; lead; myokymia
limb-girdle muscular: dystrophy
limbic: lobe; system
limb-kinetic: apraxia
lime: water
liminal: stimulus; trait
limit: dextrin; dextrinase
limited neck: dissection
limiting: angle; decision; layers of cornea; membrane of retina; sulcus; sulcus of fourth ventricle; sulcus of Reil

limulus lysate: test
Lindau: disease; tumor
Lindner: bodies
line: angle; pairs; test
linear: acceleration; accelerator; amplification; amputation; atrophy; craniectomy; fracture; phonocardiograph; scleroderma
linear absorption: coefficient
linear energy: transfer
linear epidermal: nevus
linear IgA bullous: disease in children
linear skull: fracture
lined: flap
line spread: function
Lineweaver-Burk: equation; plot
Ling: method
lingual: aponeurosis; arch; artery; bar; bone; branches; branch of facial nerve; crypt; embrasure; flange; follicles; frenulum; gingiva; goiter; gyrus; hemiatrophy; lobe; lymph nodes; mucosa; muscles; nerve; occlusion; papillae; plate; plexus; quinsy; rest; septum; splint; surface of tooth; tonsil; trophoneurosis; vein
lingual-facial-buccal: dyskinesia
lingual gingival: papilla
lingual interdental: papilla
lingual salivary gland: depression
lingular: artery; vein
linguocervical: ridge
linguofacial (arterial): trunk
linguogingival: fissure; groove; ridge
linin: network
lining: cell
linkage: analysis; disequilibrium; group; map; marker
linker: DNA
linking: number
linnaean: system of nomenclature
lion-jaw bone-holding: forceps
lip: pits; reading; reflex; sulcus
lipase: test
lipedematous: alopecia
lipemic: retinopathy
lipid: granulomatosis; histiocytosis; keratopathy; pneumonia
lipid-mobilizing: hormone
lipoatrophic: diabetes
lipogenous: diabetes

lipoid: dermatoarthritis; granuloma; nephrosis; proteinosis; theory of narcosis
lipomatous: hypertrophy; infiltration; polyp
lipomelanic: reticulosis
lipophagic: granuloma
lipophagic intestinal: granulomatosis
lipoprotein: electrophoresis; polymorphism
lipoprotein(a): hyperlipoproteinemia
lipoprotein-associated coagulation: inhibitor
lipotropic: factor; hormone
Lipschütz: cell; ulcer
liquefaction: degeneration
liquefactive: necrosis
liquefied: phenol
liquid: air; extract; glucose; paraffin; petroleum; pitch; scintillator; ventilation
liquid crystal: thermography
liquid human: serum
liquid-liquid: chromatography
Lisch: nodule
Lisfranc: amputation; joints; ligaments; operation; tubercle
Lison-Dunn: stain
lispro: insulin
Lissauer: bundle; column; fasciculus; tract
Lissauer marginal: zone
Lister: dressing; method; tubercle
listeria: meningitis
Listing: law
Listing reduced: eye
Liston: knives; shears
literal: agraphia
lithium: carmine
lithotomy: position
litigious: paranoia
Little: area; disease
little: finger; fossa of the cochlear window; fossa of the oval (vestibular) window; head of humerus; toe [V]
little: ACTH
little league: elbow
Little Leaguer's: elbow
littoral: cell
Littré: glands; hernia
Litzmann: obliquity
live: vaccine
liveborn: infant
livedo: vasculitis
livedoid: dermatitis
live oral poliovirus: vaccine
liver: acinus; breath; bud; flap; palm; spot; starch
liver of: sulfur

liver cell: carcinoma
liver filtrate: factor
liver kidney: syndrome
liver *Lactobacillus casei*: factor
liver-shod: clamp
living: anatomy
L-L: factor
Lloyd: reagent
Lo: dose
load-and-shift: maneuver
loading: dose
lobar: bronchi; pneumonia; sclerosis
Lobo: disease
Lobry de Bruyn-van Ekenstein: transformation
Lobstein: ganglion
lobster-claw: deformity
lobular: carcinoma; carcinoma in situ; glomerulonephritis; neoplasia
lobular capillary: hemangioma
local: anaphylaxis; anemia; anesthesia; anesthetics; asphyxia; bloodletting; death; epilepsy; flap; glomerulonephritis; hormone; immunity; reaction; sign; stimulant; symptom; syncope; tetanus; tic
local anesthetic: reaction
local excitatory: state
localization: agnosia
localization-related: epilepsy
localized: osteitis fibrosa; pemphigoid of Brunsting-Perry; peritonitis; scleroderma
localized nodular: tenosynovitis
localizing: electrode; symptom
lock: finger; stitch
lock-: jaw
lock-and-key: model
Locke: solutions
locked: bite; facets; knee; twins
locked-in: syndrome
Locke-Ringer: solution
locking: suture
Lockwood: ligament
locomotor: ataxia
loculated: empyema
loculated pleural: effusion
loculation: syndrome
locust: gum
lod: method
Loeb: deciduoma
Loeffler: bacillus; methylene blue; stain; syndrome I; syndrome II
Loeffler blood culture: medium

Loeffler caustic: stain
Loevit: cell
Loewenthal: bundle; reaction; tract
Löffler: disease; endocarditis; syndrome
Löffler parietal fibroplastic: endocarditis
Logan: bow
logarithmic: phase; phonocardiograph
logistic: curve; model
Logistic Organ Dysfunction: Score
logit: transformation
lognormal: distribution
Lohlein-Baehr: lesion
Lohmann: reaction
Lombard voice-reflex: test
Lon: protease
Long: coefficient; formula
long: axis; axis of body; bone; chain; crus of incus; gyrus of insula; head; limb of incus; muscle of head; muscle of neck; process of malleus; pulse; root of ciliary ganglion; sight; vinculum
long abductor: muscle of thumb
long-acting thyroid: stimulator
long adductor: muscle
long association: fibers
long axis: view
long buccal: nerve
long central: artery
long-chain 3-hydroxyacyl-CoA dehydrogenase: deficiency
long-chain/very long-chain acyl-CoA dehydrogenase: deficiency
long ciliary: nerve
long cone: technique
long extensor: muscle of great toe; muscle of thumb; muscle of toes
long fibular: muscle
long flexor: muscle of great toe; muscle of thumb; muscle of toes
long incubation: hepatitis
long interspersed: elements
longissimus: muscle
longissimus capitis: muscle
longissimus cervicis: muscle
longissimus thoracis: muscle
longitudinal: aberration; arch of foot; arc of skull; bands of cruciform ligament of atlas; canals of modiolus; dissociation; duct of epoöphoron; fold of duodenum; fracture; layer of

muscle coat of small intestine; layer of muscular coat; layers of muscular tunics; lie; ligaments; method; relaxation; section; sinus; study; sulcus of heart
longitudinal cerebral: fissure
longitudinal oval: pelvis
longitudinal pontine: bundles; fasciculi; fibers
longitudinal vertebral venous: sinus
long-leg: arthropathy
long levatores costarum: muscles
Longmire: operation
long palmar: muscle
long peroneal: muscle
long pitch helicoidal: layer
long plantar: ligament
long posterior ciliary: arteries
long QT: syndromes
long radial extensor: muscle of wrist
long saphenous: nerve; vein
long subscapular: nerve
long-term: memory
long terminal repeat: sequences
long thoracic: artery; nerve; vein
longus capitis: muscle
longus colli: muscle
loop: diuretic; excision; resection; stoma
loop electrocautery excision: procedure
loop electrosurgical excision: procedure
loose: associations; body; cartilage; skin
Looser: lines; zones
lop: ear
Lorain: disease
Lorain-Lévi: dwarfism; infantilism; syndrome
lordotic: albuminuria; pelvis
Lorenz: sign
Lorenzo: oil
Loschmidt: number
loudness discomfort: level
Lou Gehrig: disease
Louis: angle; law
Louis-Bar: syndrome
louping-ill: virus
louse: flies
louse-borne: typhus
Lovén: reflex
Lovibond: angle
Lovibond profile: sign
low: convex; wine
low-calorie: diet
low-density lipoprotein: receptors
Lowe: syndrome
low-egg-passage: vaccine

Löwenberg: canal; forceps; scala
Lowenstein-Jensen: medium
Lowenstein-Jensen culture: medium
Lower: ring; tubercle
lower: airway; extremity; eyelid; jaw; lid; limb; lip; lobe of lung; pole; pole of testis
lower abdominal periosteal: reflex
lower alveolar: point
lower dental: arcade
lower esophageal: sphincter
lower motor: neuron
lower motor neuron: dysarthria; lesion
lower nephron: nephrosis
lower respiratory tract: smear
lower ridge: slope
lower uterine: segment
lower uterine segment cesarean: section
lowest lumbar: arteries
lowest splanchnic: nerve
lowest thyroid: artery
Lowe-Terrey-MacLachlan: syndrome
low-fat: diet
low forceps: delivery
low frequency: transduction
low grade: astrocytoma
low-grade squamous intraepithelial: lesion
low lip: line
low malignant potential: tumor
low molecular weight: kininogen; proteins
Lown-Ganong-Levine: syndrome
low osmolar contrast: agent; medium
low output: failure
low-pass: filter
low purine: diet
low residue: diet
Lowry-Folin: assay
Lowry protein: assay
low salt: diet; syndrome
Lowsley: tractor
low spinal: anesthesia
low-tension: glaucoma
L-phase: variants
Lr: dose
L/S: ratio
Lu: antigens
Lubarsch: crystals
Lublows: diverticulum
lubricating: cream
Luc: operation
Lucas: groove
lucid: interval
Lucio: leprosy

Lucio leprosy: phenomenon
Lucké: virus
Lücke: test
Ludwig: angina; angle; ganglion; labyrinth; nerve; stromuhr
Luer: syringe
Luer-Lok: syringe
luetic: mask
Luft: disease
Luft potassium permanganate: fixative
Lugol iodine: solution
Lukes-Collins: classification
lumbar: appendicitis; arteries; branch of iliolumbar artery; cistern; flexure; ganglia; hernia; lordosis; lymph nodes; myelogram; nephrectomy; nerves [L1–L5]; part of diaphragm; part of spinal cord; puncture; region; rib; segments L1–L5 of spinal cord; segments of spinal cord L1–5; triangle; veins; vertebrae [L1–L5]
lumbar iliocostal: muscle
lumbar interspinal: muscle
lumbar lymphatic: plexus
lumbar (lymphatic): trunks
lumbar (nervous): plexus
lumbar puncture: needle
lumbar quadrate: muscle
lumbar rotator: muscles
lumbar splanchnic: nerves
lumberman's: itch
lumbocostal: ligament; triangle of diaphragm
lumbocostoabdominal: triangle
lumbodorsal: fascia
lumboinguinal: nerve
lumbosacral: angle; enlargement; enlargement of spinal cord; joint
lumbosacral (nerve): trunk
lumbosacral (nervous): plexus
lumbotomy: incision
lumbricals lumbrical: muscles of foot; muscles of hand
luminous: flux; intensity; retinoscope
lumpy: jaw
Luna-Ishak: stain
lunar: periodicity
lunate: bone; fissure; sulcus; surface of acetabulum
Lundh: meal
lung: bud; unit; window
lung fluke: disease
lung volume reduction: surgery
Lunyo: virus

lupoid: hepatitis; leishmaniasis; sycosis; ulcer
lupus: anticoagulant; nephritis
lupus band: test
lupus erythematosus: cell; panniculitis
lupus erythematosus cell: test
lupus-like: syndrome
Luschka: bursa; cartilage; ducts; gland; joints; ligaments; sinus; tonsil
Luschka cystic: glands
Luse: bodies
luteal: cell; phase
luteal phase: defect; deficiency
luteinized unruptured: follicle
luteinizing: hormone; principle
luteinizing hormone/follicle-stimulating hormone-releasing: factor
luteinizing hormone-releasing: factor; hormone
Lutembacher: syndrome
luteoplacental: shift
luting: agent
Lutz-Splendore-Almeida: disease
Luys: body
Lyell: disease; syndrome
Lyme: arthritis; borreliosis; disease
lymph: capillary; cell; circulation; cords; corpuscle; embolism; gland; node; nodule; sacs; scrotum; sinus; space; varix; vessels
lymphadenoid: goiter
lymphadenopathy-associated: virus
lymphangitic: carcinomatosis
lymphatic: angina; duct; edema; fistula; follicles of larynx; follicles of rectum; leukemia; nodule; plexus; ring of cardiac part of stomach; sarcoma; sinus; stroma; system; tissue; valvule; vessels
lymphatic filariasis: granuloma
lymphedematous: keratoderma
lymph node permeability: factor
lymphoblastic: leukemia; lymphoma
lymphocyte: transformation
lymphocyte function associated: antigen
lymphocyte-mediated: cytotoxicity
lymphocytic: adenohypophysitis;

choriomeningitis; hypophysitis; leukemia; leukemoid reaction; leukocytosis; leukopenia; series; thyroiditis
lymphocytic choriomeningitis: virus
lymphocytic interstitial: pneumonia; pneumonitis
lymphocytotoxic: antibodies
lymphoepithelial: cyst
lymphogenous: metastasis
lymphogranuloma venereum: antigen; virus
lymphoid: cell; hemoblast of Pappenheim; hypophysitis; leukemia; nodule; polyp; system
lymphoid interstitial: pneumonia
lymphomatoid: granulomatosis; papulosis; polyposis
lymphoplasmacellular: disorders
lymphoproliferative: syndrome
lymphostatic: verrucosis
Lynch: syndrome
Lyon: hypothesis
lyophilic: colloid
lyophobic: colloid
lyotropic: series
lysinuric protein: intolerance
lysogenic: bacterium; induction; strain
lysosomal: disease
Lyt: antigens

M

M: antigen; band; cell; concentration; line; phase; protein; shell
M2: segment of middle cerebral artery
M$_1$: antigen
MAC: complex
Macchiavello: stain
MacConkey: agar
Macewen: sign; symptom; triangle
Mach: band; effect; line; number
Machado-Guerreiro: test
Machado-Joseph: disease
machinery: murmur
Machupo: virus
Mackay-Marg: tonometer
Mackenrodt: ligament
Mackenzie: amputation; polygraph
Maclagan: test
Maclagan thymol turbidity: test

Macleod: rheumatism; syndrome
MacNeal tetrachrome blood: stain
macroaggregated: albumin
macrobiotic: diet
macrocytic: anemia; anemia of pregnancy; anemia tropical; hyperchromia
macrocytic achylic: anemia
macrofollicular: adenoma
macroglia: cell
macro-Kjeldahl: method
macromolecular: chemistry
macrophage-activating: factor
macrophage colony-stimulating: factor
macrophage inflammatory: protein
macrophage migration inhibition: test
macroscopic: anatomy; sphincter
macular: amyloidosis; area; arteries; atrophy; coloboma; degeneration; drusen; erythema; evasion; fasciculus; leprosy; retinopathy; syphilid
macular corneal: dystrophy
macular retinal: dystrophy
mad cow: disease
Maddox: rod
Madelung: deformity; disease; neck
Mad Hatter: syndrome
Madlener: operation
Madura: boil; foot
Maffucci: syndrome
Magendie: law; spaces
Magendie-Hertwig: sign; syndrome
magenta: tongue
magic: forceps
magical: thinking
Magill: forceps
Magnan: sign
Magnan trombone: movement
magnesia and alumina oral: suspension
magnet: reaction; reflex
magnetic: attraction; field; implant; inertia
magnetic field: gradient
magnetic resonance: angiography; imaging; spectroscopy
magnetogyric: ratio
magnification: angiography; radiography
magnitude: image
Magnus: sign
Mahaim: fibers
Maier: sinus

maintenance: dose
maintenance drug: therapy
Maissiat: band
maize: factor
Majocchi: disease; granulomas
major: agglutinin; amblyoscope; amputation; calices; circulus arteriosus of iris; connector; depression; epilepsy; fissure; forceps; groove; hippocampus; hypnosis; hysteria; operation; surgery; tranquilizer
major alar: cartilage
major arterial: circle of iris
major depressive: disorder
major duodenal: papilla
major histocompatibility: complex
major mood: disorder
major motor: seizure
major salivary: glands
major sublingual: duct
Makeham: hypothesis
Malabar: itch; leprosy
malabsorption: syndrome
Malacarne: pyramid; space
malar: arch; bone; flush; fold; foramen; lymph node; node; point; process
malariae: malaria
malarial: cachexia; crescent; fever; hemoglobinuria; knobs; periodicity; pigment
malarial pigment: stain
Malassez epithelial: rests
malate-aspartate: shuttle
malate-condensing: enzyme
Maldonado-San Jose: stain
male: breast; gonad; hermaphroditism; homosexuality; hypogonadism; pseudohermaphroditism; sterility; urethra
Malecot: catheter
male external: genitalia
male internal: genitalia
male pattern: alopecia; baldness
Malgaigne: amputation; fossa; hernia; luxation; triangle
Malherbe calcifying: epithelioma
malic: enzyme
malignant: anemia; bubo; dysentery; dyskeratosis; endocarditis; exophthalmos; glaucoma; granuloma; hepatoma; histiocytosis; hyperphenylalaninemia; hyperpyrexia; hypertension; hyperthermia; jaundice; lymphadenosis; lymphoma;

malnutrition; melanoma; melanoma in situ; meningioma; myopia; nephrosclerosis; pustule; scleritis; smallpox; stupor; tumor
malignant atrophic: papulosis
malignant carcinoid: syndrome
malignant catarrhal fever: virus
malignant ciliary: epithelioma
malignant external: otitis
malignant fibrous: histiocytoma
malignant lentigo: melanoma
malignant midline: reticulosis
malignant mixed müllerian: tumor
malignant mole: syndrome
malignant tertian: fever; malaria
malignant tertian malarial: parasite
Mall: formula; ridges
mallear: folds; prominence; stripe
malleolar: groove; stria; sulcus
malleolar articular: surface of fibula; surface of tibia
mallet: finger
Mallory: bodies; stain for actinomyces; stain for hemofuchsin
Mallory aniline blue: stain
Mallory collagen: stain
Mallory iodine: stain
Mallory phloxine: stain
Mallory phosphotungstic acid hematoxylin: stain
Mallory trichrome: stain
Mallory triple: stain
Mallory-Weiss: lesion; syndrome; tear
malondialdehyde-modified low-density: lipoprotein
Maloney: bougies
malpighian: bodies; capsule; cell; corpuscles; glands; glomerulus; layer; nodules; pyramid; rete; stigmas; stratum; tubules; tuft; vesicles
malt: liquor; sugar
Malta: fever
maltese: cross
malt-worker's: lung
mamillary: ducts
mamillothalamic: tract
mammary: branches; calculus; ducts; fistula; fold; gland; line; neuralgia; plexus; region; ridge; souffle
mammary cancer: virus of mice

mammary duct: ectasia
mammary tumor: virus of mice
mammillary: arteries; body; line; process of lumbar vertebra; tubercle; tubercle of hypothalamus
mammillotegmental: fasciculus
mammillothalamic: fasciculus
mammosomatotroph cell: adenoma
mammotropic: factor; hormone
managed: care
Manchester: operation; ovoid
Manchurian: fever; typhus
Manchurian hemorrhagic: fever
mandatory minute: ventilation
Mandelin: reagent
mandibular: arch; axis; canal; cartilage; condyle; dentition; disk; foramen; fossa; glide; joint; lymph node; movement; nerve [CN V3]; nodes; notch; process; protraction; reflex; retraction; symphysis; tongue; torus
mandibular dental: arcade
mandibular guide: prosthesis
mandibular hinge: position
mandibuloacral: dysostosis
mandibulofacial: dysostosis; dysplasia
mandibulofacial dysotosis: syndrome
mandibulomaxillary: fixation
mandibulo-oculofacial: syndrome
mango: dermatitis
mangrove: fly
manic: episode; excitement; psychosis
manic-depressive: disorder; illness; psychosis
manifest: content; hyperopia; strabismus; tetany; vector
manifesting: carrier; heterozygote
manna: sugar
Mann-Bollman: fistula
Mannkopf: sign
Mann methyl blue-eosin: stain
mannose-binding: protein
mannose-6-phosphate: receptors
Mann-Williamson: operation; ulcer
Manson: disease; schistosomiasis
Manson eye: worm
Mantel-Haenszel: test

mantle: layer; radiotherapy; sclerosis; zone
mantle cell: lymphoma
Mantoux: pit; test
manual: pelvimetry; ventilation
manual visual: method
manubriosternal: joint; junction; symphysis
map-dot-fingerprint: dystrophy
maple: sugar
maple bark: disease
maple syrup: urine
maple syrup urine: disease
maplike: skull
Marañón: sign; syndrome
marantic: atrophy; edema; endocarditis; thrombosis; thrombus
marasmic: kwashiorkor
marathon group: psychotherapy
marble: bones
marble bone: disease
Marburg: disease; virus
Marburg virus: disease
Marcacci: muscle
march: fracture; hemoglobinuria
Marchand: adrenals; rest
Marchand wandering: cell
Marchant: zone
Marchi: fixative; reaction; stain; tract
Marchiafava-Bignami: disease
Marchiafava-Micheli: anemia; syndrome
Marcille: triangle
Marcus Gunn: phenomenon; pupil; sign; syndrome
Marek disease: virus
Marey: law
Marfan: disease; law; syndrome
margarine: disease
marginal: arcade; artery of colon; blepharitis; branch of cingulate sulcus; branch of parietooccipital sulcus; branch [TA] of cingulate sulcus; crest of tooth; fasciculus; gingivitis; gyrus; integrity of amalgam; keratitis; layer; part of orbicularis oris (muscle); rays; ridge; sinuses of placenta; sphincter; sulcus; tubercle; tubercle (of zygomatic bone); zone
marginal atrial: branch of right coronary artery
marginal mandibular: branch of facial nerve
marginal ring: ulcer of cornea

marginal tentorial: branch of internal carotid artery
marginal zone: lymphoma
marian: lithotomy
Marie: ataxia
Marie-Robinson: syndrome
Marie-Strümpell: disease
marine: pharmacology; soap
Marine-Lenhart: syndrome
Marinesco-Garland: syndrome
Marinesco-Sjögren: syndrome
Marinesco succulent: hand
Marion: disease
Mariotte: bottle; experiment; law
Mariotte blind: spot
marital: counseling; therapy
Marjolin: ulcer
marked fetal: bradycardia
marker: chromosome; enzyme; locus; trait
marker X: syndrome
Markov: process
Marme: reagent
marmoset: virus
Maroteaux-Lamy: syndrome
Marquis: reagent
marriage: therapy
marrow: canal; cell
marrow-lymph: gland
marrow-mesenchyme: connections
Marseilles: fever
marsh: fever; gas
Marshall: method; syndrome; test
Marshall-Marchetti: test
Marshall-Marchetti-Krantz: operation
Marshall oblique: vein
Marshall vestigial: fold
marsupial: notch
Martegiani: area; funnel
Martin: bandage; disease; tube
Martin-Bell: syndrome
Martin-Gruber: anastomosis
Martinotti: cell
Martorell: syndrome
masculine: pelvis; uterus
masculinity-femininity: scale
Masini: sign
masked: epilepsy; gout; hyperthyroidism; virus
masking: dilemma
masking level: difference
masklike: face
Maslow: hierarchy
masochistic: personality
Mason-Pfizer: virus
mason's: lung
MASS: syndrome
mass: hysteria; infection; law; movement; number;
peristalsis; reflex; screening; spectrograph
mass action: principle; theory
mass-action: ratio
Masselon: spectacles
masseter: muscle; reflex
masseteric: artery; fascia; nerve; tuberosity; veins
massive: collapse
massive bowel resection: syndrome
Masson argentaffin: stain
Masson-Fontana ammoniac silver: stain
Masson trichrome: stain
mass sociogenic: illness
mast: cell; leukocyte
mast cell: leukemia
Master: test
master: cast; eye; gland
Master two-step exercise: test
mastery: motive
masticating: cycles; surface
masticator: nerve; space
masticatory: apparatus; diplegia; force; muscles; nucleus; spasm; surface; system
masticatory silent: period
mastoid: abscess; angle of parietal bone; antrum; artery; bone; border of occipital bone; branches of posterior auricular artery; branches of posterior tympanic artery; branch of occipital artery; canaliculus; cells; cortex; empyema; fontanelle; foramen; fossa; groove; lymph nodes; margin of occipital bone; notch; part of the temporal bone; process; process of petrous part of temporal bone; sinuses; wall of middle ear; wall of tympanic cavity
mastoid air: cells
mastoid emissary: vein
mat: burn; gold
matched: groups
maternal: cotyledon; death; dystocia; immunity; inheritance; morbidity; placenta
maternal death: rate
maternal deprivation: syndrome
maternal-fetal: medicine
maternal mortality: ratio
maternity: hospital
mathematical: chaos; determinant; genetics; model
mating: isolate

matrix: band; calculus; metalloproteinase; retainer; vesicles
matrix Gla: protein
mattress: suture
maturation: arrest; factor; index; value
mature: bacteriophage; cataract; neutrophil
mature cell: leukemia
mature ovarian: follicle
maturity-onset: diabetes
maturity onset: diabetes of youth
matutinal: epilepsy
Mauchart: ligaments
Maurer: clefts; dots
Mauriac: syndrome
Mauriceau: maneuver
Mauriceau-Levret: maneuver
Mauthner: sheath; test
maxillary: angle; antrum; artery; dentition; eminence; gland; hiatus; nerve [CN V2]; plexus; process of embryo; process of inferior nasal concha; protraction; sinus; surface of greater wing of sphenoid bone; surface of palatine bone; tuberosity; vein
maxillary dental: arcade
maxillary sinus: radiograph
maxillofacial: prosthetics
maxillomandibular: fixation; record; registration; relation; traction
maximal: dose; stimulus; thymectomy
maximal Histalog: test
maximal permissible: dose
Maxim-Gilbert: sequencing
Maximow: stain for bone marrow
maximum: temperature; velocity
maximum breathing: capacity
maximum intensity: projection
maximum likelihood: estimator
maximum occipital: point
maximum permissible: dose
maximum power: output
maximum tolerated: dose
maximum urea: clearance
maximum voluntary: ventilation
May apple: root
Mayaro: virus
Mayer: pessary; reflex
Mayer hemalum: stain
Mayer mucicarmine: stain
Mayer muchihematein: stain

Mayer-Rokitansky-Küster-Hauser: syndrome
May-Grünwald: stain
May-Hegglin: anomaly
Mayo: bunionectomy; operation; vein
Mayo-Robson: point; position
May-White: syndrome
Mazzoni: corpuscle
Mazzotti: reaction; test
McArdle: disease; syndrome
McArdle-Schmid-Pearson: disease
McBurney: incision; point; sign
McCall culdoplasty: procedure
McCarey-Kaufmann: media
McCarthy: reflexes
McCrea: sound
McCune-Albright: syndrome
McDonald: maneuver
McGoon: technique
McIndoe: operation
McKee: line
McKusick metaphyseal: dysplasia
McMurray: test
McNemar: test
McPhail: test
McRoberts: maneuver
McVay: operation
M:E: ratio
meadow: dermatitis
Meadows: syndrome
meal: worm
mean: calorie; temperature; vector
mean corpuscular: hemoglobin; volume
mean corpuscular hemoglobin: concentration
mean electrical: axis
mean foundation: plane
mean manifest: vector
measles: immunoglobulin; virus
measles convalescent: serum
measles immune: globulin (human)
measles, mumps, and rubella: vaccine
measles virus: vaccine
measured: intelligence
meatal: cartilage; spine
Mecca: balsam
mechanical: abrasion; alternation of the heart; antidote; corepraxy; dysmenorrhea; heart; ileus; intelligence; jaundice; strabismus; vector; ventilation; vertigo
mechanically balanced: occlusion
mechanism-based: inhibitor

mechanistic: school
mechanobullous: disease
mechanoelectric: transduction
Mecke: reagent
Meckel: band; cartilage; cavity; diverticulum; ganglion; ligament; plane; scan; space; syndrome
Meckel-Gruber: syndrome
meconial: colic
meconium: aspiration; ileus; peritonitis; plug
meconium aspiration: syndrome
meconium blockage: syndrome
medial: angle of eye; arteriole of retina; arteriosclerosis; border; border of foot; border of forearm; border of humerus; border of kidney; border of scapula; border of suprarenal gland; border of tibia; branches; branches of artery of tuber cinereum; branches of pontine arteries; branch of posterior branch of spinal nerves; branch of posterior rami of spinal nerves; canthus; compartment of thigh; condyle; condyle of femur; condyle of tibia; cord of brachial plexus; crest of fibula; crus; crus of facial canal; crus of the horizontal part of the facial canal; crus of major alar cartilage of nose; crus of the superficial inguinal ring; eminence; epicondyle of femur; epicondyle of humerus; fillet; head; lamina of cartilage of pharyngotympanic (auditory) tube; lemniscus; ligament of ankle joint; ligament of knee; ligament of talocrural joint; ligament of temporomandibular joint; ligament of wrist; limb; lip of linea aspera; malleolus; margin; meniscus; nuclei of thalamus; nucleus; nucleus of trapezoid body; part of longitudinal arch of foot; part of middle lobe vein (of right superior pulmonary vein); plate of cartilaginous auditory tube; plate of pterygoid process; pole of ovary; process of calcaneal tuberosity; root of median nerve; root of optic tract; rotator; segment; sulcus of crus cerebri; surface; surface of arytenoid cartilage; surface of cerebral hemisphere; surface of fibula; surface of lung; surface of ovary; surface of testis; surface of tibia; surface of toes; surface of ulna; tubercle (of posterior process) of talus; vein of lateral ventricle; venule of retina; wall of middle ear; wall of orbit; wall of tympanic cavity; zone
medial accessory olivary: nucleus
medial amygdaloid: nucleus
medial antebrachial cutaneous: nerve
medial anterior thoracic: nerve
medial arcuate: ligament
medial atrial: vein
medial basal: branch of pulmonary artery
medial basal bronchopulmonary: segment S VII
medial basal segmental: artery
medial bicipital: groove
medial brachial cutaneous: nerve
medial bronchopulmonary: segment S V
medial calcaneal: branches of tibial nerve
medial canthal: ligament
medial canthic: fold
medial cartilaginous: plate
medial central: nucleus of thalamus
medial cerebral: surface
medial circumflex: artery of thigh
medial circumflex femoral: artery; veins
medial clunial: nerves
medial collateral: artery; ligament of elbow
medial commisural: artery
medial crural cutaneous: branches of saphenous nerve; nerve
medial cuneiform: bone
medial cutaneous: branch of dorsal branch of posterior intercostal arteries; nerve of arm; nerve of forearm; nerve of leg
medial dorsal: nucleus [TA] of thalamus
medial dorsal cutaneous: nerve
medial epicondylar: crest; ridge
medial femoral: tuberosity

medial femoral circumflex: artery
medial forebrain: bundle
medial frontal: gyrus
medial frontobasal: artery
medial geniculate: body; nuclei; nuclei
medial great: muscle
medial habenular: nucleus
medial inferior genicular: artery
medial inguinal: fossa
medial lacunar: lymph node; node
medial longitudinal: arch of foot; bundle; fasciculus; stria
medial lumbar intertransversarii: muscles
medial lumbar intertransverse: muscles
medial lumbocostal: arch
medial magnocellular: nucleus
medial malleolar: arteries; branches (of posterior tibial artery); facet of talus; network
medial malleolar subcutaneous: bursa
medial mammary: branches
medial medullary: branches of vertebral artery; lamina [TA] of lentiform nucleus
medial midpalmar: space
medial nasal: branches of anterior ethmoidal nerve; fold; process; prominence
medial occipital: artery
medial occipitotemporal: gyrus
medial olfactory: gyrus
medial orbitofrontal: artery
medial palpebral: commissure; ligament
medial parabrachial: nucleus
medial patellar: retinaculum
medial pectoral: nerve
medial pericuneate: nucleus
medial plantar: artery; nerve
medial popliteal: nerve
medial posterior cervical intertransversarii: muscles
medial preoptic: nucleus
medial pterygoid: muscle; plate
medial puboprostatic: ligament
medial rectus: muscle
medial reticulospinal: tract
medial segmental: artery
medial septal: nucleus
medial striate: artery
medial superior genicular: artery
medial superior olivary: nucleus

medial supraclavicular: nerve
medial supracondylar: crest; ridge
medial supraepicondylar: ridge
medial sural cutaneous: nerve
medial talocalcaneal: ligament
medial tarsal: arteries
medial umbilical: fold; ligament
medial vastus: muscle
medial ventral: nucleus
medial vestibular: nucleus
medial vestibulospinal: tract
median: aperture of fourth ventricle; artery; bar of Mercier; conjugate; eminence; groove of tongue; laryngotomy; line; lithotomy; nerve; plane; rhinoscopy; section; sternotomy; strumectomy; sulcus of fourth ventricle; sulcus of tongue; vein of forearm; vein of neck
median antebrachial: vein
median anterior maxillary: cyst
median arcuate: ligament
median atlantoaxial: joint
median basilic: vein
median callosal: artery
median cephalic: vein
median commissural: artery
median cricothyroid: ligament
median cubital: vein
median glossoepiglottic: fold
median longitudinal: raphe of tongue
median mandibular: point
median maxillary anterior alveolar: cleft
median palatal: cyst
median palatine: suture
median preoptic: nucleus
median raphe: cyst of the penis
median retruded: relation
median rhomboid: glossitis
median sacral: artery; crest; vein
median thyrohyoid: ligament
median tongue: bud
median umbilical: fold; ligament
mediastinal: arteries; branches; branches of internal thoracic artery; branches of thoracic aorta; emphysema; fibrosis; lipomatosis; part of lung; part of parietal pleura; pleura; pleurisy; space; surface of lung; veins; window
mediate: auscultation; percussion; transfusion
mediator: complex
medical: anatomy; biophysics; care; diathermy; ethics; examiner; genetics; jurisprudence; model; mycology; pathology; psychology; record; selection; treatment
medical record: linkage
medicinal: charcoal; chemistry; eruption; zinc peroxide
medicinal soft: soap
mediocolic: sphincter
mediodorsal: nucleus
mediopubic: reflex
Mediterranean: fever; lymphoma
Mediterranean erythematous: fever
Mediterranean exanthematous: fever
Mediterranean spotted: fever
medium: artery; vein
medium-chain acyl-CoA dehydrogenase: deficiency
medullary: arteries of brain; callus; carcinoma; carcinoma of breast; carcinoma of thyroid; cavity; center; chemoreceptor; cone; cords; folds; groove; laminae of thalamus; layers of thalamus; membrane; plate; pyramid; pyramidotomy; ray; sarcoma; sheath; space; striae of fourth ventricle; stria of thalamus; substance; teniae; tube
medullary reticulospinal: tract
medullary spinal: arteries
medullary sponge: kidney
medullated nerve: fiber
medullopontine: sulcus
Medusa: head
Meeh: formula
Meeh-Dubois: formula
Mees: lines; stripes
Meesman: dystrophy
megacystic: syndrome
megacystitis-megaureter: syndrome
megacystitis-microcolon-intestinal hypoperistalsis: syndrome
megakaryocyte growth and development: factor
megakaryocytic: leukemia
megaloblastic: anemia
megalocytic: anemia
meibomian: blepharitis; conjunctivitis; cyst; glands; sty
Meige: disease
Meigs: syndrome
Meinicke: test
meiotic: division; drive; phase
Meischer: syndrome
Meissner: corpuscle; plexus
melamine: resin
melanocyte-stimulating: hormone
melanophore-expanding: principle
melanotic: freckle; medulloblastoma; pigment; progonoma
melanotic neuroectodermal: tumor of infancy
melanotropin release-inhibiting: hormone
melanotropin-releasing: factor; hormone
Meleney: gangrene; ulcer
Melkersson-Rosenthal: syndrome
Melnick-Needles: osteodysplasty; syndrome
melon-seed: body
melting: point; temperature; temperature of DNA
Meltzer: law
Meltzer-Lyon: test
membrane: bone; enzyme; potential; rupture; stripping
membrane attack: complex
membrane-coating: granule
membrane expansion: theory
membranoproliferative: glomerulonephritis
membranous: ampulla; ampullae of the semicircular ducts; cataract; cochlea; conjunctivitis; dysmenorrhea; glomerulonephritis; labyrinth; lamina of cartilage of pharyngotympanic (auditory) plate; laryngitis; layer; layer of subcutaneous tissue of abdomen; layer of superficial fascia; layer of superficial fascia of perineum; lipodystrophy; neurocranium; ossification; part of interventricular septum; part of male urethra; part of nasal septum; pharyngitis; septum; urethra; viscerocranium; wall of middle ear; wall of trachea; wall of tympanic cavity
memory: loop; span
memory B: cells
memory T: cells
Menangle: virus
Mendel-Bechterew: reflex
Mendeléeff: law
Mendel first: law
mendelian: character; genetics; inheritance; ratio; trait
Mendel instep: reflex
Mendel second: law
Mendelson: syndrome
Ménétrier: disease; syndrome
Menge: pessary
Mengo: encephalitis; virus
Ménière: disease; syndrome
meningeal: branch of cavernous part of internal carotid artery; branch of cerebral part of internal carotid artery; branches; branch of internal carotid artery; branch of (intracranial part of) vertebral artery; branch of mandibular nerve; branch of maxillary nerve; branch of occipital artery; branch of ophthalmic nerve; branch of spinal nerves; branch of vagus nerve; carcinoma; carcinomatosis; hernia; layer of dura mater; leukemia; neurosyphilis; plexus; veins
meningitic: streak
meningocerebral: cicatrix
meningococcal: meningitis
meningotyphoid: fever
meningovascular: neurosyphilis; syphilis
meniscofemoral: ligaments
meniscus: lens; sign
Menkes: syndrome
menopausal: syndrome
menstrual: age; colic; cycle; edema; leukorrhea; molimina; period; sclerosis
menstrual extraction: abortion
mental: aberration; age; apparatus; artery; branches of mental nerve; branch (of inferior alveolar artery); canal; chronometry; deficiency; disease; disorder; foramen; health; hospital; hygiene; illness; image; impairment; impression; nerve; point; process; protuberance; region; retardation; scotoma; spine; symphysis; tubercle (of mandible)
mentalis: muscle
mentoanterior: position
mentolabial: furrow; sulcus
mentoposterior: position
mentotransverse: position

mercapturic acid: pathway
Mercier: bar; sound; valve
mercurial: diuretics; line; manometer; stomatitis
mercury: arc; poisoning
mercury vapor: lamp
Merendino: technique
Meretoja: syndrome
meridional: aberration; amblyopia; cleavage; fibers of ciliary muscle
Merkel: corpuscle; filtrum ventriculi; fossa; muscle
Merkel cell: tumor
Merkel tactile: cell; disk
mermaid: malformation
meroblastic: cleavage
merocrine: gland
Merrifield: knife; synthesis
Méry: gland
Merzbacher-Pelizaeus: disease
mesangial: cell; nephritis
mesangial proliferative: glomerulonephritis
mesangiocapillary: glomerulonephritis
mesatipellic: pelvis
mesencephalic: flexure; nucleus of trigeminal nerve; tegmentum; tract of trigeminal nerve; veins
mesencephalic corticonuclear: fibers
mesenchymal: cells; epithelium; tissue
mesenteric: adenitis; glands; hernia; lymphadenitis; lymph nodes; portion of small intestine; veins
mesenteric artery: occlusion
mesentericoparietal: fossa; recess
mesenteroaxial: volvulus
mesethmoid: bone
mesh: graft
mesial: angle; caries; displacement; occlusion; surface of tooth
meso: compounds
mesoblastic: nephroma; segment
mesocaval: shunt
mesocolic: lymph nodes; tenia
mesodermal: factor
mesoglial: cells
mesomelic: dwarfism
mesometric: pregnancy
mesonephric: adenocarcinoma; duct; fold; rest; ridge; tissue; tubule
mesonephroid: tumor
mesopic: perimetry
mesothelial: cell
mesovarian: border of ovary; margin of ovary

messenger: RNA
messengerlike: RNA
metabisulfite: test
metabolic: acidosis; alkalosis; calculus; coma; craniopathy; disease; encephalopathy; equivalent; indican; pool
metabolized vitamin D: milk
metabotropic: receptor
metacarpal: bones [I–V]; index; veins
metacarpohypothenar: reflex
metacarpophalangeal: articulations; joints
metacarpothenar: reflex
metacentric: chromosome
metachromatic: bodies; granules; leukodystrophy; stain
metafacial: angle
metaherpetic: keratitis
metahypophysial: diabetes
metal: base; interface
metal fume: fever
metal insert: teeth
metallic: rale
metameric nervous: system
metanephric: blastema; bud; cap; diverticulum; duct; tubule
metanephrogenic: tissue
metaphyseal fibrous cortical: defect
metaphysial: dysostosis; dysplasia
metaplastic: anemia; carcinoma; ossification; polyp
metastasizing: septicemia
metastatic: abscess; calcification; carcinoma; choroiditis; mumps; ophthalmia; pneumonia; retinitis
metastatic carcinoid: syndrome
metatarsal: artery; bones [I–V]; reflex
metatarsal interosseous: ligaments
metatarsophalangeal: articulations; joints
metatropic: dwarfism
Metchnikoff: theory
Metenier: sign
meter: angle
metered-dose: inhaler
meter-kilogram-second: system; unit
methacholine challenge: test
methacrylate: resin
methamphetamine: base
methanol: fixative
methenamine silver: stain
methionine-activating: enzyme

methionine malabsorption: syndrome
methionyl: dipeptidase
methonium: compounds
3-methoxy-4-hydroxymandelic acid: test
methyl: alcohol; mercaptan
methylglucamine: iodipamide
methyl green-pyronin: stain
methylol: riboflavin
metopic: point; suture
metric: system
metroperitoneal: fistula
metrotrophic: test
Meulengracht: diet
Mexican: typhus
Mexican hat: cell; corpuscle
Mexican spotted: fever
Meyenburg: complex; disease
Meyenburg-Altherr-Uehlinger: syndrome
Meyer: cartilages; line; reagent; sinus
Meyer-Archambault: loop
Meyer-Betz: disease; syndrome
Meyerhof oxidation: quotient
Meyer-Overton: rule; theory of narcosis
Meynert: cells; commissure; decussation; layer
MHA-TP: test
MHC: restriction
miasma: theory
Mibelli: angiokeratomas; disease
Michaelis: complex; constant
Michaelis-Gutmann: body
Michaelis-Menten: constant; equation; hypothesis
Michel: malformation; spur
microangiopathic hemolytic: anemia
micro-Astrup: method
microbial: collagenase; genetics; persistence; RNase II; vitamin
micrococcal: endonuclease; nuclease
microcrystalline: cellulose
microcystic: disease of renal medulla
microcystic epithelial: dystrophy
microcytic: anemia
microdrepanocytic: anemia
microelectric: waves
microetching: technique
microfilarial: sheath
microfold: cell
microfollicular: adenoma; goiter
microglandular: adenosis
microglia: cells
microhemagglutination-Treponema pallidum: test

microhematocrit: concentration
microinvasive: carcinoma
micro-Kjeldahl: method
microlecithal: egg
micromelic: dwarfism
micrometastatic: disease
micromyeloblastic: leukemia
microophthalmia transcription factor: gene
microprecipitation: test
microscopic: anatomy; field; hematuria; polyangiitis; section; sphincter
microscopically controlled: surgery
microsphere: method
microsporidian: keratoconjunctivitis
microtubule-associated: proteins
microtubule-organizing: center
microvascular: anastomosis
microvillus inclusion: disease
microwave: therapy
micturating: cystourethrogram
micturition: reflex; syncope
midaxillary: line
midbrain: tegmentum; vesicle
midcarpal: joint
midclavicular: line
middiastolic: murmur
middle: cells; ear; finger; kidney; lobe of prostate; lobe of right lung; mediastinum; pain; phalanges of foot and hand; piece; trunk of brachial plexus
middle atlantoepistrophic: joint
middle axillary: line
middle cardiac: vein
middle carpal: joint
middle cerebellar: peduncle
middle cerebral: artery
middle cervical: fascia; ganglion
middle cervical cardiac: nerve
middle clinoid: process
middle cluneal: nerves
middle colic: artery; lymph nodes; vein
middle collateral: artery
middle constrictor: muscle of pharynx
middle costotransverse: ligament
middle cranial: fossa
middle cuneiform: bone
middle-ear: effusion
middle esophageal: constriction

middle ethmoidal: cells; sinuses
middle ethmoidal air: cells
middle fossa: approach
middle frontal: convolution; gyrus; sulcus
middle genicular: artery
middle glossoepiglottic: fold
middle gray: layer of superior colliculus
middle group of mesenteric: lymph nodes
middle hemorrhoidal: artery; plexuses; veins
middle hepatic: veins
middle latency: response
middle lobar: artery; artery of right lung
middle lobe: branch of right superior pulmonary vein; syndrome; vein
middle macular: arteriole
middle meningeal: artery; branch of maxillary nerve; nerve; veins
middle meningeal artery: groove
middle nasal: concha
middle palmar: space
middle radioulnar: joint
middle rectal: artery; lymph node; node; veins
middle rectal (nervous): plexus
middle sacral: artery
middle sacral lymphatic: plexus
middle scalene: muscle
middle superior alveolar: branch of infraorbital nerve
middle supraclavicular: nerve
middle suprarenal: artery
middle talar articular: surface of calcaneus
middle temporal: artery; branches of lateral occipital artery; branch of insular part of middle cerebral artery; convolution; gyrus; sulcus; vein
middle thyroid: vein
middle transverse rectal: fold
middle turbinated: bone
middle umbilical: fold; ligament
midforceps: delivery
midgastric transverse: sphincter
midget bipolar: cells
midlife: crisis
midline: incision; myelotomy
midline malignant reticulosis: granuloma
midpalmar: space
midsagittal: plane; section

midsigmoid: sphincter
midtarsal: joint
Miescher: elastoma; granuloma; tubes
mignon: lamp
migraine: headache
migraine-related: vestibulopathy
migrating: abscess; teeth
migration: theory
migration inhibition: test
migration-inhibitory: factor
migration inhibitory factor: test
migratory: cell; pneumonia
mika: operation
Mikulicz: aphthae; cells; clamp; disease; drain; operation; syndrome
Mikulicz-Vladimiroff: amputation
mild: silver protein
mild fetal: bradycardia
Miles: operation
miliary: abscess; aneurysm; embolism; fever; pattern; tuberculosis
milieu: therapy
military: medicine
milk of: calcium
milk: anemia; corpuscle; crust; cyst; ducts; factor; fever; gland; line; ridge; scall; sickness; spots; sugar; tetter; tooth
milk-alkali: syndrome
milk-ejection: reflex
milkers': nodes; nodules
milker's nodule: virus
milk let-down: reflex
Milkman: syndrome
milk-ring: test
milky: ascites; urine
mill: fever
Millard-Gubler: syndrome
milled-in: curves; paths
miller: asthma
Miller-Abbott: tube
Miller chemicoparasitic: theory
Millner: needle
Millon: reaction; reagent
Millon clinical multiaxial: inventory
Millon Clinical Multiaxial Inventory: test
Millon-Nasse: test
mill wheel: murmur
Milroy: disease
Milton: disease
MIM: number
mimetic: muscles; paralysis
mimic: genes
Minamata: disease
mind: blindness
mineral: water; wax

miner's: asthma; cramps; disease; elbow; lung; nystagmus
Minerva: jacket
miniature: stomach
miniature scarlet: fever
minicore-multicore: myopathy
minimal: air; dose
minimal alveolar: concentration
minimal amplitude: nystagmus
minimal anesthetic: concentration
minimal brain: dysfunction
minimal-change: disease
minimal-change nephrotic: syndrome
minimal deviation: melanoma
minimal infecting: dose
minimal inhibitory: concentration
minimal lethal: dose
minimally invasive: surgery
minimal reacting: dose
minimum: light; temperature
minimum light: threshold
minimum protein: requirement
mink enteritis: virus
Minnesota Multiphasic Personality: Inventory
Minnesota Multiphasic Personality Inventory: test
minor: agglutinin; amputation; calices; circulus arteriosus of iris; connector; fissure; forceps; groove; hippocampus; hypnosis; hysteria; operation; surgery; tranquilizer
minor alar: cartilage
minor arterial: circle of iris
minor duodenal: papilla
minor histocompatibility: complex
minor motor: seizure
minor salivary: glands
minor sublingual: ducts
Minot-Murphy: diet
minus: lens; strand
minute: output; volume
miostagmin: reaction
Mirchamp: sign
Mirizzi: syndrome
mirror: haploscope; image; speech
mirror image: dextrocardia
mirror-image: cell
misdirection: phenomenon
mismatch: repair
missed: abortion; labor; period
missense: mutation
Mitchell: disease; procedure; treatment

mite: typhus
mite-born: typhus
mitochondrial: biogenesis; chromosome; disorders; gene; matrix; membrane; myopathy; sheath
mitogenic: lectin
mitotic: cycle; division; figure; index; period; rate; spindle
mitral: area; cells; click; commissurotomy; facies; gradient; incompetence; insufficiency; murmur; orifice; regurgitation; stenosis; tap; valve; valvotomy
mitral valve: prolapse
mitral valve prolapse: syndrome
Mitrofanoff: principle
Mitsuda: antigen; reaction
Mitsuo: phenomenon
Mittendorf: dot
mixed: aphasia; astigmatism; beat; chancre; disulfide; esotropia; gland; glioma; glycerides; hearing loss; hyperlipemia; hyperlipidemia; hypoglycemia; infection; leukemia; nerve; paralysis; thrombus; tocopherols concentrate; tumor; tumor of salivary gland; tumor of skin
mixed agglutination: reaction; test
mixed connective-tissue: disease
mixed discrete-continuous random: variable
mixed expired: gas
mixed function: oxygenase
mixed hyperlipoproteinemia familial, type 5: hyperlipidemia
mixed lymphocyte: culture
mixed lymphocyte culture: reaction; test
mixed mesodermal: tumor
Mixter: clamp
Miyagawa: bodies
MLC: test
MM: virus
M-mode: echocardiography
M'Naghten: rule
mnemic: hypothesis; theory
MNSs: antigens
mobile: end; part of nasal septum; spasm
Mobitz: block
Mobitz types of atrioventricular: block
Möbius: sign; syndrome
modal: alteration
model: game

modeling: composition; compound; plastic
moderate: hypothermia
moderator: band; variable
modern: genetics
modified: milk; smallpox
modified acid-fast: stain
modified radical: hysterectomy; mastectomy; mastoidectomy
modified trichrome: stain
modified zinc oxide-eugenol: cement
modifier: gene
modulation transfer: function
Moeller: glossitis
Moeller grass: bacillus
Mogen: clamp
Mohr: pipette; syndrome
Mohrenheim: fossa; space
Mohs: chemosurgery; scale; surgery
Mohs fresh tissue chemosurgery: technique
Mohs micrographic: surgery
moist: gangrene; papule; rale; wart
Mokola: virus
molar: absorptivity; behavior; concentration; glands; mass; pregnancy; tooth; tubercle
molar absorbancy: index
molar absorption: coefficient
molar extinction: coefficient
mold: guide
mole: fraction
molecular: behavior; biology; biophysics; disease; dispersion; distillation; epidemiology; formula; genetics; heat; layer; layer of cerebellar cortex; layer of cerebellum; layer of cerebral cortex; layer of retina; layers of olfactory bulb; mass; movement; pathology; rotation; sieve; weight
molecular dispersed: solution
molecular dissociation: theory
molecular weight: ratio
Molisch: test
Moll: glands
Mollaret: meningitis
molluscum: body; conjunctivitis; corpuscle
molluscum contagiosum: virus
Moloney: test; virus
molybdenum: cofactor
molybdenum target: tube
Monakow: bundle; nucleus; syndrome; tract
Mönckeberg: arteriosclerosis; calcification; degeneration; sclerosis

Mönckeberg medial: calcification
Mondini: dysplasia; hearing impairment
Mondonesi: reflex
Mondor: disease
Monge: disease
mongolian: fold; macula; spot
moniliform: hair
monkey: hand; malaria
monkey B: virus
monkeypox: virus
monoamine: hypothesis
monoamine oxidase: inhibitor
monoamniotic: twins
monobasic: acid; ammonium phosphate; potassium phosphate
monobromated: camphor
monochorial: twins
monochorionic diamnionic: placenta
monochorionic monoamnionic: placenta
monochromatic: aberration; radiation
monoclonal: antibody; gammopathy; gammopathy of undetermined significance; gammopathy of unknown significance; immunoglobulin; peak; protein
monocrotic: pulse
monocular: diplopia; heterochromia; strabismus
monocyte chemoattractant: protein; protein-1
monocyte-derived neutrophil chemotactic: factor
monocytic: angina; leukemia; leukemoid reaction; leukocytosis; leukopenia
monocytoid: cell
Monod-Wyman-Changeux: model
monofixation: syndrome
monohydric: alcohol
monoleptic: fever
monomolecular: reaction
monomorphic: adenoma
mononuclear phagocyte: system
monophasic: complex
monophyletic: theory
monopolar: cautery
monopotassium: phosphate
monorecidive: chancre
monosodium: phosphate
monostotic fibrous: dysplasia
monotonic: sequence
monovalent: antiserum
monovular: twins
monoxenic: culture
monozygotic: twins

Monro: doctrine; foramen; line; sulcus
Monro-Kellie: doctrine
Monro-Richter: line
Monsel: solution
Monson: curve
montan: wax
Monteggia: fracture
Montenegro: test
Montevideo: units
Montgomery: follicles; glands; tubercles
mood: disorders
mood-congruent: hallucination
mood-incongruent: hallucination
mood stabilizing: agent
Moon: molars
moon: face; facies
moon shaped: face
Moore: method
Moore lightning: streaks
Mooren: ulcer
Mooser: bodies
moral: ataxia; treatment
Morand: foot; spur
Moraxella: conjunctivitis
morbid: impulse; obesity; thirst
morbidity: rate
morcellated: nephrectomy
morcellation: operation
Morel: ear
Morgagni: appendix; cartilage; caruncle; cataract; columns; concha; crypts; disease; foramen; fossa; fovea; frenum; globules; humor; hydatid; lacuna; liquor; nodule; prolapse; retinaculum; sinus; spheres; syndrome; tubercle; valves; ventricle
Morgagni-Adams-Stokes: syncope; syndrome
morgagnian: cyst
Morgagni foramen: hernia
Morgan: bacillus; fold
Morison: pouch
Mörner: test
morning: diarrhea; sickness; vomiting
morning after: pill
morning glory: anomaly; syndrome
Moro: reflex
morphine injector's: septicemia
morphogenetic: movement
morphologic: element
Morquio: disease; syndrome
Morquio-Ullrich: disease
mortality: rate
mortar: kidney
mortise: joint

Morton: metatarsalgia; neuralgia; neuroma; plane; syndrome; toe
Morvan: chorea; disease
mosaic: fundus; inheritance; pattern; wart
Moschcowitz: disease; test
Mosenthal: test
Mosler: diabetes; sign
mosquito: clamp; forceps
Moss: tube
moss: starch
Mossman: fever
Mosso: ergograph; sphygmomanometer
mossy: cell; fibers; foot
most comfortable: level
Motais: operation
moth: patch
moth-eaten: alopecia
mother: cell; colony; cyst; liquor; star; surrogate; yaw
mother of: vinegar
motile: leukocyte
motility: test
motility test: medium
motion: sickness
motor: abreaction; agraphia; amusia; aphasia; apraxia; area; ataxia; cell; cortex; decussation; endplate; fibers; image; impersistence; nerve; nerve of face; neuron; nuclei; nucleus of facial nerve; nucleus of trigeminal nerve; nucleus of trigeminus; paralysis; plate; point; root of ciliary ganglion; root of spinal nerve; root of trigeminal nerve; unit; urgency; zone
motor dapsone: neuropathy
motor neuron: disease
motor speech: center
motor system: disease
mottled: enamel; tooth
Motulsky dye reduction: test
Mounier-Kuhn: syndrome
mountain: anemia; balm; disease; sickness
mounting: medium
mouse: cancer; encephalomyelitis; unit
mouse antialopecia: factor
mouse encephalomyelitis: virus
mouse hepatitis: virus
mouse leukemia: viruses
mouse mammary tumor: virus
mouse parotid tumor: virus
mouse poliomyelitis: virus
mousepox: virus
mousetail: pulse
mouse thymic: virus
mouse-tooth: forceps

mouth: breathing; mirror; rehabilitation
mouth-to-mouth: respiration; resuscitation
movable: heart; joint; kidney; pulse; spleen; testis
Mowry colloidal iron: stain
moyamoya: disease
Mozart: ear
MP: joints
MR: angiography
MS-1: hepatitis
MSB trichrome: stain
Mu: antigen
Much: bacillus
Mucha-Habermann: disease; syndrome
mucilaginous: gland
mucin clot: test
mucinogen: granules
mucinoid: degeneration
mucinous: carcinoma
muciparous: gland
Muckle-Wells: syndrome
mucoalbuminous: cells
mucobuccal: fold
mucociliary: clearance
mucociliary clearance: rate
mucocutaneous: junction; leishmaniasis
mucocutaneous lymph node: syndrome
mucoepidermoid: carcinoma; tumor
mucoepithelial: dysplasia
mucoid: adenocarcinoma; colony; degeneration
mucoid impaction of: bronchus
mucoid medial: degeneration
mucomembranous: enteritis
mucoperichondrial: flap
mucoperiosteal: flap
mucopolysaccharide keratin: dystrophy
mucosa-associated lymphoid: tissue
mucosal: folds of gallbladder; graft; tunics; wave
mucosal disease: virus
mucosal relief: radiography
mucoserous: cells
mucous: cast; cell; colitis; cyst; diarrhea; gland; glands of auditory tube; membrane of bronchus; membrane of ductus deferens; membrane of esophagus; membrane of female urethra; membrane of gallbladder; membrane of large intestine; membrane of larynx; membrane of male urethra; membrane of nose; membrane of pharyngotympanic auditory tube; membrane of pharynx; membranes; membrane of small intestine; membrane of stomach; membrane of tongue; membrane of trachea; membrane of tympanic cavity; membrane of ureter; membrane of urinary bladder; membrane of uterine tube; membrane of vagina; patch; plaque; plug; polyp; rale; sheath of tendon
mucous connective: tissue
mucous neck: cell
mucus: blanket; impaction
mud: bed; fever
Muehrcke: bands; lines; sign
Mueller electronic: tonometer
Mueller-Hinton: agar; medium
muffle: furnace
Muir-Torre: syndrome
mulberry: calculus; molar; ovary; spots
Mulder: test
Mules: operation
mule-spinner's: cancer
mulibrey: nanism
Müller: capsule; duct; fibers; fixative; law; maneuver; muscle; sign; trigone; tubercle
müllerian: adenosarcoma; agenesis
müllerian inhibiting: factor; substance
müllerian regression: factor
Müller radial: cells
multangular: bone
multiaxial: classification; joint
multicentric: reticulohistiocytosis
multicolony-stimulating: factor
multicore: disease
multicuspid: tooth
multidrug: resistance
multienzyme: complex
multifactorial: inheritance
multifidus: muscle
multifocal: choroiditis; lens; osteitis fibrosa
multifocal atrial: tachycardia
multiform: layer; layer [TA] of cerebral cortex
multiformat: camera
multi-infarct: dementia
multilamellar: body
multilaminar primary: follicle
multilocal: genetics
multilocular: cyst; fat
multilocular adipose: tissue
multilocular hydatid: cyst
multimammate: mouse
multinodular: goiter
multinomial: distribution
multinuclear: leukocyte
multipennate: muscle
multiphasic: screening
multiple: alcohol; amputation; anchorage; embolism; exostosis; fission; fracture; myeloma; myelomatosis; myositis; neuritis; parasitism; personality; pregnancy; sclerosis; serositis; stain; sulfatase deficiency; vision
multiple chemical: sensitivity
multiple ego: states
multiple endocrine: adenomatosis; neoplasia; neoplasia 1; neoplasia 2; neoplasia 3; neoplasia 2B; neoplasia, type 1; neoplasia, type 2A
multiple endocrine deficiency: syndrome
multiple endocrine neoplasia: syndrome, type 1; syndrome, type 2A; syndrome, type 2B
multiple epiphyseal: dysplasia
multiple-gated acquisition: scan
multiple glandular deficiency: syndrome
multiple hamartoma: syndrome
multiple idiopathic hemorrhagic: sarcoma
multiple intestinal: polyposis
multiple lentigines: syndrome
multiple marker: screen
multiple mucosal neuroma: syndrome
multiple personality: disorder
multiple puncture tuberculin: test
multiple self-healing squamous: epithelioma
multiple sleep latency: test
multiple symmetric: lipomatosis
multiple system: atrophy
multiplicative: division; growth; model
multipolar: cell; mitosis; neuron
multistage: model
multivalent: vaccine
multivariate: studies
multivesicular: bodies
mummification: necrosis
mummified: pulp
mumps: meningoencephalitis; virus
mumps sensitivity: test
mumps skin test: antigen
mumps virus: vaccine
mumu: fever
Munchausen: syndrome; syndrome by proxy
Münchhausen: syndrome
mung bean: nuclease
municipal: hospital
Munro: abscess; microabscess; point
Munson: sign
mural: cell; endocarditis; pregnancy; thrombosis; thrombus
murine: leukemia; typhus
murine sarcoma: virus
Murphy: button; drip; percussion; sign
Murray Valley: encephalitis; rash
Murray Valley encephalitis: virus
Murutucu: virus
muscarinic: antagonist; receptors
muscle: bundle; curve; epithelium; fascicle; hemoglobin; layer in fatty layer of subcutaneous tissue; plasma; plate; proteins; relaxant; repositioning; resection; serum; sound; spasm; spindle
muscle contraction: headache
muscle phosphorylase: deficiency
muscle-sparing: thoracotomy
muscle-tendon: attachment; junction
muscular: arteries (of ophthalmic artery); artery; asthenopia; atrophy; branches; coat; coat of bronchi; coat of colon; coat of ductus deferens; coat of esophagus; coat of female urethra; coat of gallbladder; coat of intermediate part of male urethra; coat of large intestine; coat of male urethra; coat of pharynx; coat of prostatic urethra; coat of rectum; coat of small intestine; coat of spongy part of male urethra; coat of stomach; coat of trachea; coat of ureter; coat of urinary bladder; coat of uterine tube; coat of uterus; coat of vagina; dystrophy; fascia; fascia of extraocular muscle; fibril; hyperesthesia; incompetence; insufficiency; lacuna; layer; layer of bronchi; layer of colon; layer of ductus deferens; layer of esophagus; layer of female urethra; layer of gallbladder; layer of

intermediate part of (male) urethra; layer of large intestine; layer of male urethra; layer of mucosa; layer of pharynx; layer of prostatic urethra; layer of rectum; layer of renal pelvis; layer of seminal gland; layer of small intestine; layer of spongy (male) urethra; layer of stomach; layer of trachea; layer of ureter; layer of urinary bladder; layer of uterine tube; layer of vagina; movement; part of interventricular septum (of heart); process of arytenoid cartilage; pulley; reflex; rheumatism; sense; space of retroinguinal compartment; sphincter supracollicularis; substance of prostate; system; tissue; torticollis; triangle (of neck); trochlea; trophoneurosis; tunic of gallbladder; tunics
muscular subaortic: stenosis
musculocutaneous: flap; nerve; nerve of leg
musculophrenic: artery; veins
musculospiral: groove; nerve; paralysis
musculotendinous: cuff
musculotubal: canal
mushroom: poisoning
mushroom-worker's: lung
music: blindness
musical: agraphia; alexia; murmur
musician's: cramp
muskeag: moss
Musset: sign
Mustard: operation; procedure
mustard: gas
mutant: gene
mutation: rate
mutational: frequency
mutilating: keratoderma; leprosy
mutton-fat keratic: precipitates
mutual: resistance
mutualistic: symbiosis
MVE: virus
MWC: model
myasthenic: crisis; facies; reaction; syndrome
mycotic: aneurysm; endocarditis; keratitis
myelin: body; figure; protein A1; sheath
myelinated: nerve
myelinated nerve: fiber
myelinic: degeneration
myeloblastic: leukemia

myelocytic: crisis; leukemia; leukemoid reaction
myelodysplastic: syndrome
myelogenic: sarcoma
myeloid: cell; metaplasia; sarcoma; series; tissue
myelomonocytic: leukemia
myelophthisic: anemia
myeloproliferative: syndromes
myenteric: reflex
myenteric (nervous): plexus
mylohyoid: artery; branch (of inferior alveolar artery); fossa; groove; line; muscle; nerve; ridge
mylopharyngeal: part of superior constrictor muscle of pharynx; part of superior pharyngeal constrictor (muscle) of pharynx
myocardial: bridge; infarction; insufficiency; ischemia; rigor mortis
myocardial depressant: factor
myoclonic: seizure
myoclonic astatic: epilepsy
myoclonus: epilepsy
myocutaneous: flap
myodermal: flap
myoelastic: theory
myoepicardial: mantle
myoepithelial: cell
myofascial: syndrome
myofascial pain-dysfunction: syndrome
myofunctional: therapy
myogenic: potential; tonus
myoid: cells
myomatous: polyp
myometrial arcuate: arteries
myometrial radial: arteries
myoneural: blockade; junction
myopathic: atrophy; facies; scoliosis
myophosphorylase deficiency: glycogenosis
myopic: astigmatism; choroidopathy; conus; crescent; degeneration
myosin: filament
myotatic: contraction; irritability; reflex
myotonic: cataract; chondrodystrophy; dystrophy; response
myotubular: myopathy
myovascular: sphincter
myovenous: sphincter
myxedema: heart; voice
myxedematous: infantilism
myxoid: cyst; degeneration
myxomatosis: virus
myxomembranous: colitis
myxopapillary: ependymoma

N

N: terminus
nabothian: cyst; follicle
nacreous: ichthyosis
Nadi: reaction
Naegeli: syndrome
Naegeli type of monocytic: leukemia
Naffziger: operation; syndrome
Nagel: test
Nägele: obliquity; pelvis; rule
Nageotte: cells
nail: bed; extension; fold; horn; matrix; pits; plate; pulse; wall
nail-patella: syndrome
Nair buffered methylene blue: stain
Nakanishi: stain
naked: virus
NAME: syndrome
NANB: hepatitis
NANBNC: hepatitis
NANC: neuron
Nance-Insley: syndrome
Nance-Sweeney: chondrodysplasia
nanoid: enamel
nanukayami: fever
nape: nevus
napkin: rash
narcissistic personality: disorder
narcoleptic: tetrad
narcotic: blockade; hunger; reversal
narrow-angle: glaucoma
nasal: arch; atrium; bone; border of frontal bone; calculus; capsule; catarrh; cavity; crest; crest of horizontal plate of palatine bone; crest of palatine process of maxilla; duct; feeding; foramen; ganglion; glands; glioma; height; hemorrhage; index; margin of frontal bone; meatus; mucosa; muscle; myiasis; nerve; notch; part of frontal bone; part of pharynx; pharynx; pits; placodes; point; polyp; process; reflex; region; ridge; sacs; septum; spine of frontal bone; surface of maxilla; surface of palatine bone; valve; venules of retina; vestibule
nasalis: muscle
nasal septal: branch of superior labial branch of facial artery; cartilage
nasal venous: arch

Nasik: vibrio
nasion-pogonion: measurement
nasion-postcondylar: plane
nasion soft: tissue
Nasmyth: cuticle; membrane
nasoalveolar: cyst
nasobasilar: line
nasobregmatic: arc
nasociliary: nerve; root of ciliary ganglion
nasofrontal: vein
nasogastric: tube
nasojugal: fold
nasolabial: cyst; groove; lymph node; node; sulcus
nasolacrimal: canal; duct
nasomandibular: fixation
nasomaxillary: suture
nasomental: reflex
naso-occipital: arc
nasopalatine: groove; nerve
nasopalatine duct: cyst
nasopharyngeal: carcinoma; groove; leishmaniasis; meatus; passage
nasotracheal: intubation; tube
Nasse: law
Natal: sore
natal: cleft; tooth
natiform: skull
native: albumin; protein
natural: antibody; dentition; dyes; focus of infection; hemolysin; immunity; mutation; pigment; products; selection
natural killer: cells
natural killer cell: leukemia
natural killer cell stimulating: factor
nature-nurture: issue
Nauheim: bath; treatment
Nauta: stain
navicular: abdomen; bone of hand; fossa of urethra
navicular: bone
navicular articular: surface of talus
navigator: echo
NBT: test
ND: virus
Nd:YAG: laser
near: drowning; point; reaction; reflex; sight
nearest neighbor: frequency
near point of: convergence
near-total: thyroidectomy
nebulous: urine
necessary: cause
neck: reflexes; sign
neck-shaft: angle
necrobiotic: xanthogranuloma
necrogenic: wart
necrolytic migratory: erythema

necrosis: bacillus
necrotic: angina; arachnidism; cirrhosis; cyst; inflammation; pulp
necrotic infectious: conjunctivitis
necrotizing: angiitis; arteriolitis; cellulitis; encephalitis; encephalomyelopathy; encephalopathy; enterocolitis; fasciitis; keratitis; papillitis; scleritis; sialometaplasia
necrotizing hemorrhage: leukomyelitis
necrotizing ulcerative: gingivitis
needle: bath; biopsy; culture; forceps
needle point: tracing
Needles split cast: method
Neer impingement: sign
negative: accommodation; afterimage; anergy; catalyst; chronotropism; control; convergence; cooperativity; electrode; electrotaxis; feedback; image; meniscus; phase; politzerization; pressure; scotoma; stain; symptom; taxis; thermotaxis; transference; valence
negative base: excess
negative end-expiratory: pressure
negatively: inotropic
negative myoclonic: seizure
negative pressure: ventilation
negative strand: virus
Negishi: virus
Negri: bodies; corpuscles
Negro: phenomenon
Neisser: coccus; stain; syringe
Nélaton: catheter; dislocation; fibers; fold; line; sphincter
Nelson: syndrome; tumor
nemaline: myopathy
neonatal: anemia; apoplexy; conjunctivitis; death; diagnosis; hepatitis; herpes; hyperbilirubinemia; hypoglycemia; isoerythrolysis; jaundice; line; lupus; medicine; ring; screening; tetanus; tetany; tooth
neonatal calf diarrhea: virus
neonatal mortality: rate
neoplastic: arachnoiditis; meningitis
neotype: culture; strain
neovascular: glaucoma
nephric: blastema; duct
nephritic: factor; syndrome

nephrogenic: adenoma; cord; diabetes insipidus; tissue
nephronic: loop
nephrostomy: tube
nephrotic: edema; syndrome
nephrotomic: cavity
Neptune: girdle
Néri: sign
Nernst: equation
nerve: avulsion; block; cell; conduction; deafness; decompression; ending; fascicle; fiber; field; force; ganglion; graft; implantation; papilla; plexus; root; stroma; suture; tract; trunk
nerve block: anesthesia
nerve cell: body
nerve conduction: velocity
nerve growth: cone; factor
nerve growth factor: antiserum
nervous: asthenopia; asthma; dyspepsia; indigestion; lobe; part of retina; system; tissue; tunic of eyeball
Nessler: reagent
nested polymerase chain: reaction
net: flux; knot
Netherton: syndrome
nettle: rash
Nettleshop-Falls: albinism
nettling: hairs
Neubauer: artery
Neuberg: ester
Neufeld: reaction
Neufeld capsular: swelling
Neumann: cells; disease; law; sheath
neural: arch of vertebra; axis; canal; crest; cyst; factor; folds; groove; hearing loss; layer of optic part of retina; layer of retina; lobe of hypophysis; part of hypophysis; plate; segment; spine; tube
neural crest: syndrome
neuralgic: amyotrophy
neurasthenic: personality
neurenteric: canal; cysts
neurilemma: cells
neuritic: plaque
neuroaxonal: dystrophy
neurobiotactic: movement
neurocentral: joint; suture; synchondrosis
neurochronaxic: theory
neurocirculatory: asthenia
neurocranial granulomatous: arteritis
neurocutaneous: melanosis; syndrome
neuroectodermal: junction

neuroendocrine: cell
neuroendocrine transducer: cell
neuroepithelial: body; cells; layer of retina
neurofibrillar: network
neurofibrillary: degeneration; tangle
neurogenic: airway; atrophy; bladder; claudication; fracture; tonus
neuroglia: cells
neurohemal: organs
neurohumoral: secretion; transmission
neurohypophysial: hormones
neurolemma: cells
neuroleptic: agent
neuroleptic malignant: syndrome
neurolinguistic: programming
neuromuscular: junction; relaxant; spindle; system
neuromuscular blocking: agents
neuronal: hyperplasia
neuronal ceroid: lipofuscinosis
neuronal intestinal: dysplasia
neuronal migration: abnormality
neuron-specific: enolase
neuroparalytic: keratitis; keratopathy
neuropathic: albuminuria; arthritis; arthropathy; bladder; joint
neuropsychologic: disorder
neurosecretory: cells; substance
neurosomatic: junction
neurotendinous: organ; spindle
neurotic: disorder; excoriation; manifestation
neurotonic: reaction
neurotrophic: atrophy; keratitis
neurotropic: attraction; virus
neurovascular: bundle of Walsh; flap; sheath
Neusser: granules
neutral: axis of straight beam; element; fat; mutation; occlusion; oxide; point; reaction; spirits; stain; zone
neutral buffered formalin: fixative
neutralization: plate; test
neutralizing: antibody
neutral lipid storage: disease
neutron: radiation
neutropenic: angina
neutrophil: granule
neutrophil-activating: factor; protein

neutrophil chemotactant: factor
neutrophilic: leukemia; leukocyte; leukocytosis; leukopenia
neutrophilic eccrine: hidradenitis
nevoid: amentia; elephantiasis; hypertrichosis
nevus: cell; cell, A-type; cell, B-type; cell, C-type
new: combination; growth; methylene blue; mutation
Newcastle: disease
Newcastle disease: virus
Newcomer: fixative
New Hampshire: rule
Newton: disk; law
Newtonian: constant of gravitation
newtonian: aberration; flow; fluid; viscosity
New World: leishmaniasis
new yellow: enzyme
New York: virus
New York Heart Association: classification
Neyman-Pearson statistical: hypothesis
Nezelof: syndrome
Nezelof type of thymic: alymphoplasia
NGF: antiserum
niacin: test
Nick: procedure
nick: translation
nickel: dermatitis
Nickerson-Kveim: test
Nicol: prism
Nicolas-Favre: disease
Nicolle: stain for capsules
Nicolle white: mycetoma
nicotine: stomatitis
nicotinic: receptors
nicotinic acid: maculopathy
nicotinic cholinergic: receptor
nictitating: membrane; spasm
Nieden: syndrome
Niemann: disease; splenomegaly
Niemann-Pick: cell; disease
Niemann-Pick C1: disease
Niewenglowski: rays
night: blindness; hospital; myopia; pain; sight; soil; sweats; vision
nihilistic: delusion
Nikiforoff: method
Nikolsky: sign
nil: disease
nine mile: fever
ninhydrin: reaction
ninhydrin-Schiff: stain for proteins
ninth cranial: nerve [CN IX]
ninth-day: erythema

Nipah: virus
nipple: line; shield
nirvana: principle
Nissen: fundoplication; operation
Nissl: bodies; degeneration; granules; stain; substance
Nitabuch: layer; membrane; stria
niter: paper
nitinol: filter
nitrate: respiration
nitritoid: reaction
nitro: dyes
nitroblue: tetrazolium
nitroblue tetrazolium: test
nitrofurantoin: polyneuropathy
nitrogen: autotrophy; balance; cycle; equivalent; fixation; mustards; narcosis
nitrogenous: equilibrium
nitroid: shock
nitroprusside: test
NK: cells
NMDA: receptor
NNN: medium
Noack: syndrome
Noble: position; stain
noble: element; gases; metal
Noble-Collip: procedure
Nocardia: dacryoliths
nociceptive: reflex
nocifensor: reflex
nocturnal: amblyopia; diarrhea; dyspnea; emission; enuresis; epilepsy; myoclonus; periodicity; vertigo
nodal: bigeminy; bradycardia; fever; plane; point; rhythm; tachycardia; tissue
nodding: spasm
nodose: ganglion; rheumatism
nodoventricular: fibers
nodular: amyloidosis; arteriosclerosis; body; disease; episcleritis; fasciitis; headache; hidradenoma; hyperplasia of prostate; iritis; leprosy; lymphoma; melanoma; mesoneuritis; opacity; panencephalitis; scleritis; sclerosis; syphilid; transformation of the liver; tuberculid; vasculitis
nodular histiocytic: lymphoma
nodular nonsuppurative: panniculitis
nodular non-X: histiocytosis
nodular regenerative: hyperplasia
nodular subepidermal: fibrosis
nodus sinuatrialis: echo

noetic: anxiety
noise: pollution
noise-induced: hearing loss
Nomarski: optics
Nomarski interference: microscopy
nomenclatural: type
nominal: aphasia
nomothetic: approach
nonabsorbable: ligature
nonabsorbable surgical: suture
nonaccommodative: esotropia
nonadrenergic, noncholinergic: neuron
non–A-E: hepatitis
nonan: malaria
nonanatomic: teeth
non-A, non-B: hepatitis
non-A, non-B hepatitis: virus
non-A, non-B, non-C: hepatitis
non-arcon: articulator
nonbacterial thrombotic: endocarditis
nonbacterial verrucous: endocarditis
nonbullous congenital ichthyosiform: erythroderma
nonchromaffin: paraganglioma
nonclassical: phenylketonuria
nonclonogenic: cell
noncohesive: gold
noncommunicating: hydrocele; hydrocephalus
noncompetitive: inhibition
noncomplementary: role
nonconjugative: plasmid
noncontained disk: herniation
nonconvulsive: seizure
noncovalent: bond
non–cycle-specific: agent
nondeciduous: placenta
nondepolarizing: block; relaxant
nondepolarizing neuromuscular blocking: agent
nondiabetic: glycosuria
nondirective: psychotherapy
nonepileptic: seizure
nonessential: amino acids
nonfenestrated: forceps
nonfilament polymorphonuclear: leukocyte
nonfluent: aphasia
nongonococcal: urethritis
nongranular: leukocyte
non-heme iron: protein
non-Hodgkin: lymphoma
nonhomologous: chromosomes
nonhyperglycemic: glycosuria

nonimmune: agglutination; serum
nonimmune fetal: hydrops
noninfiltrating lobular: carcinoma
noninflammatory: edema
non-insulin-dependent: diabetes mellitus
noninvasive positive pressure: ventilation
nonionic: surfactant
nonionic contrast: agent
nonisolated: proteinuria
nonketotic: hyperglycemia; hyperglycinemia
nonlamellar: bone
nonlipid: histiocytosis
nonmedullated: fibers
nonmotile: leukocyte
nonneurogenic neurogenic: bladder
non-newtonian: fluid
nonobstructive: atelectasis; jaundice
nonoccluded: virus
nonorganic: aphonia
nonossifying: fibroma
nonosteogenic: fibroma
nonovulational: menstruation
nonparticipant: observer
nonpedunculated: hydatid
nonpenetrant: trait
nonpenetrating: keratoplasty; wound
nonphasic sinus: arrhythmia
nonpitting: edema
non-PKU: hyperphenylalaninemia
nonplasmatic: compartment
nonpolar: amino acid; compound; solvents
nonprecipitable: antibody
nonprecipitating: antibody
nonprotein: nitrogen
nonrandom: mating
non-rapid eye: movement
nonreactive: depression
nonreassuring fetal: status
nonrebreathing: anesthesia; mask; valve
nonrefractive accommodative: esotropia
nonrenal: azotemia
nonresponder: tolerance
nonrigid: connector
nonsecretory: myeloma
nonsense: codon; mutation; syndrome; triplet
nonseptate: mycelium
nonsexual: generation
nonshivering: thermogenesis
nonspecific: anergy; cholinesterase; protein; system; therapy; urethritis; vaginitis

nonspecific building-related: illnesses
nonsteroidal anti-inflammatory: drugs
nonstress: test
nonsuppressible insulinlike: activity
nonthrombocytopenic: purpura
nontoxic: goiter
nontransmural myocardial: infarction
nontropical: sprue
nontypeable: *Haemophilus influenzae*
nonvenereal: syphilis
nonvital: pulp; tooth
noogenic: neurosis
Noonan: syndrome
NOR-: banding
Nordhausen: sulfuric acid
no reflow: phenomenon
normal: animal; antibody; antithrombin; antitoxin; bite; concentration; distribution; hearing; occlusion; opsonin; ovariotomy; phosphate; serum; solution; tartrate; toxin; values
normal cholesteremic: xanthomatosis
normal electrical: axis
normal horse: serum
normal human: plasma; serum
normal human serum: albumin
normally posed: tooth
normal pressure: hydrocephalus
normal-tension: glaucoma
normochromic: anemia
normocytic: anemia
normoglycemic: glycosuria
normokalemic periodic: paralysis
normospermatogenic: sterility
normotriglyceridemic: abetalipoproteinemia
Norrie: disease
Norris: corpuscles
North American: blastomycosis
Northern blot: analysis
North Queensland tick: fever; typhus
Norton: operation
Norton-Simon: hypothesis
Norwalk: agent; virus
Norway: itch
Norwegian: scabies
Norwood: operation; procedure
nose: drops
nose-bridge-lid: reflex

nose-eye: reflex
nosocomial: gangrene; pneumonia
notched: teeth
note: blindness
Nothnagel: syndrome
no-threshold: concept
notifiable: disease
notochordal: canal; plate; process; sheath
Novy and MacNeal blood: agar
NPH: insulin
nu: body
nuchal: arm; cord; fascia; ligament; plane; rigidity; tubercle
Nuck: diverticulum; hydrocele
nuclear: atom; bag; cataract; chemistry; energy; envelope; factor-κB; family; fusion; hyaloplasm; jaundice; lamina; layers of retina; magneton; matrix; medicine; membrane; ophthalmoplegia; pacemaker; pore; reaction; RNA; sap; sclerosis; spindle; stain
nuclear bag: fiber
nuclear chain: fiber
nuclear-cytoplasmic: ratio
nuclear inclusion: bodies
nuclear magnetic: resonance
nuclear magnetic resonance: imaging; tomography
nuclear Overhauser: effect
nucleate: endonuclease
nucleic acid: base; hybridization; probe
nucleocortical: fibers
nucleolar: chromosome; organizer; zone
nucleolar-nuclear: ratio
nucleolus: organizer
nucleolus organizer: region
nucleoplasmic: index
nucleoside: pair; phosphorylases
nucleotide: deletion; sequence
nude: mouse
Nuel: space
Nuhn: gland
null: cells; hypothesis
null-cell: adenoma
numb chin: syndrome
numerical: aperture; hypertrophy; taxonomy
nummular: dermatitis; eczema; sputum; syphilid
nun's: murmur
nurse: cells
nursemaid's: elbow
nursing bottle: caries
Nussbaum: bracelet
nutmeg: liver

nutrient: agar; arteries of humerus; artery; artery of femur; artery of fibula; artery of radius; artery of the tibia; artery of ulna; canal; enema; foramen; medium; vessel
nutritional: amblyopia; anemia; cirrhosis; dropsy; edema; energy; hemosiderosis; marasmus; polyneuropathy
nutritional macrocytic: anemia
nutritional type cerebellar: atrophy
nutritive: equilibrium
nymphocaruncular: sulcus
nymphohymenal: sulcus
nystagmus: test
nystagmus blockage: syndrome
Nysten: law

O

O: agglutinin; antigen; colony; shell
ω-3: fatty acids
oasthouse urine: disease
oat: cell
oat cell: carcinoma
oatmeal-tomato paste: agar
OAV: syndrome
O'Beirne: sphincter; valve
Ober: test
Obermayer: test
Obermeier: spirillum
Obersteiner-Redlich: line; zone
obesity: index
object: blindness; constancy; glass; libido; relationship
objective: optometer; perimetry; probability; psychology; sign; symptom; synonyms
obligate: aerobe; anaerobe; parasite
oblique: amputation; bandage; bundle of pons; cord of interosseous membrane of forearm; diameter; fibers of muscular layer of stomach; fissure; fissure of lung; fracture; head; illumination; lie; ligament of elbow joint; line; line of mandible; line of thyroid cartilage; muscle of auricle; part of cricothyroid (muscle); projection; ridge; ridge of trapezium; section; sinus of pericardium; vein of left atrium
oblique arytenoid: muscle

oblique auricular: muscle
oblique facial: cleft
oblique pericardial: sinus
oblique pontine: fasciculus
oblique popliteal: ligament
obliquus capitis inferior: muscle
obliquus capitis superior: muscle
obliterative: arachnoiditis; bronchitis; pericarditis
oblong: fovea of arytenoid cartilage; pit of arytenoid cartilage
obsessional: neurosis
obsessive: behavior; personality
obsessive-compulsive: disorder; neurosis; personality
obsessive-compulsive personality: disorder
obstacle: sense
obstetric: conjugate; conjugate of pelvic outlet; hand; palsy; paralysis; position; ultrasound
obstetrical: binder; forceps
obstetric conjugate: diameter
obstructive: appendicitis; dysmenorrhea; hydrocephalus; jaundice; murmur; pneumonia; thrombus; uropathy
obstructive sleep: apnea
obturating: embolism
obturator: appliance; artery; branch of pubic branch of inferior epigastric vein; canal; crest; fascia; foramen; groove; hernia; lymph nodes; membrane; nerve; tubercle; veins
obturator externus: muscle
obturator internus: muscle
occipital: anchorage; angle of parietal bone; artery; aspect; belly of occipitofrontalis muscle; bone; border; border of parietal bone; border of temporal bone; branch; condyle; fontanelle; forceps; groove; gyri; horn; line; lobe; lobe of cerebrum; lymph nodes; margin; margin of temporal bone; neuralgia; neurectomy; neuritis; operculum; part of corpus callosum; plane; plexus; point; pole; pole [TA] of cerebrum; region of head; sinus; somite; stripe; triangle; vein
occipital cerebral: veins
occipital emissary: vein
occipital horn: syndrome

occipitalis: muscle
occipital lobe: epilepsy
occipitoanterior: position
occipitoaxial: ligaments
occipitocollicular: tract
occipitofrontal: diameter; fasciculus; muscle
occipitofrontalis: muscle
occipitomastoid: suture
occipitomental: diameter; projection
occipitopontine: fibers; tract
occipitoposterior: position
occipitotectal: fibers; tract
occipitotemporal: sulcus
occipitothalamic: radiation
occipitotransverse: position
occluded: virus
occluding: frame; ligature; paper; relation
occluding centric relation: record
occlusal: adjustment; analysis; balance; caries; clearance; correction; curvature; disharmony; embrasure; force; form; harmony; imbalance; path; pattern; pivot; plane; position; pressure; radiograph; rest; rim; scheme; surface of tooth; system; table; trauma; wear
occlusal rest: bar
occlusal vertical: dimension
occlusion: rim
occlusive: dressing; ileus; meningitis
occult: bleeding; blood; border of nail; carcinoma; fracture; hydrocephalus
occult choroidal: neovascularization
occult posterior laryngeal: cleft
occupational: disease; therapy
Ochoa: law
ochre: codon; mutation
ochronotic: arthritis
Ochsner: clamp; method
ocular: albinism; albinism 1; albinism 2; albinism 3; albinism with late-onset sensorineural deafness; albinism with sensorineural deafness; bobbing; cone; crisis; cup; dysmetria; flutter; humor; hypertelorism; larva migrans; lens; micrometer; migraine; muscles; myiasis; myopathy; nystagmus; onchocerciasis; paralysis; pemphigoid; prosthesis; rigidity; scoliosis;

sparganosis; tension;
torticollis; vertigo; vesicle
ocular cicatricial: pemphigoid
ocular larva migrans:
granuloma
ocular motor: apraxia
ocular-mucous membrane:
syndrome
oculoauriculovertebral:
dysplasia
oculobuccogenital: syndrome
oculocardiac: reflex
oculocephalic: reflex
oculocephalogyric: reflex
oculocerebrorenal: syndrome
oculocutaneous: albinism;
syndrome
oculodentodigital: dysplasia
oculodermal: melanosis
oculoencephalic: angiomatosis
oculogravic: illusion
oculogyral: illusion
oculogyric: crises
oculomandibulofacial:
syndrome
oculomotor: nerve [CN III];
nucleus; response; root of
ciliary ganglion; sulcus of
mesencephalon; system
oculopharyngeal: dystrophy;
syndrome
oculovagal: reflex
oculovertebral: dysplasia;
syndrome
oculovestibulo-auditory:
syndrome
odd: chromosome
Oddi: sphincter
Odland: body
odontoblastic: layer; process
odontogenic: cyst; dysplasia;
fibroma; keratocyst;
myxoma
odontoid: process; process of
epistropheus; vertebra
odorant binding: protein
odoriferous: gland
O'Dwyer: tube
oedipal: neurosis; period;
phase
Oedipus: complex
Oehl: muscles
Oehler: symptom
OFD: syndrome
official: formula
off label: indication
off-vertical: rotation
Ofuji: disease
Ogilvie: syndrome
Ogino-Knaus: rule
Ogston: line
Ogston-Luc: operation
Oguchi: disease
Ogura: operation
O'Hara: forceps
17-OH-corticoids: test

Ohm: law
Ohngren: line
oil: bath; cyst; embolism;
glands; immersion;
pneumonia; sugar; tumor;
vaccine
oil retention: enema
oily: granuloma
ointment: base
Okazaki: fragment
OKT: cells
Oldfield: syndrome
Old World: leishmaniasis
old yellow: enzyme
olecranon: bursitis; fossa;
process; reflex
olfactory: agnosia; angle;
area; aura; bulb; bundle;
cells; cortex; epithelium;
esthesioneuroblastoma; fila;
foramen; glands;
glomerulus; groove; groove
of nasal cavity;
hallucination; hyperesthesia;
hypesthesia; membrane;
mucosa; nerves [CN I];
neuroblastoma; organ;
peduncle; pits; placodes;
pyramid; region of mucosa
of nose; region of nasal
mucosa; region of nose;
region of tunica mucosa of
nose; roots; striae; sulcus;
sulcus of nasal cavity; tract;
trigone; tubercle
olfactory receptor: cells
oligemic: shock
oligoclonal: band
oligodendroglia: cells
olivary: body; eminence
olive: oil
olive-tipped: catheter
olivocerebellar: tract
olivocochlear: bundle; fibers;
tract; tract
olivopontocerebellar:
atrophy; degeneration
olivospinal: fibers; tract
Ollier: disease; graft; theory
Ollier-Thiersch: graft
Olmsted: syndrome
olympian: forehead
Ombrédanne: operation
omega-3: fatty acids
omega-: oxidation
omega-oxidation: theory
Omenn: syndrome
omental: appendices;
branches; bursa; eminence
of pancreas; enterocleisis;
flap; foramen; sac; tenia;
tuber; tuberosity of liver
Ommaya: reservoir
omnifocal: lens
omoclavicular: triangle
omohyoid: muscle

omotracheal: triangle
omphaloangiopagous: twins
omphalomesenteric: artery;
cord; cyst; duct
omphalomesenteric duct:
cyst
Omsk hemorrhagic: fever
Omsk hemorrhagic fever:
virus
oncocytic: adenoma;
carcinoma
oncocytic hepatocellular:
tumor
oncofetal: antigens; marker
oncogenic: virus
oncosphere: embryo
oncotic: pressure
Ondine: curse
one-carbon: fragment
one-horned: uterus
onion: bodies
onion bulb: neuropathy
onlay: graft
Onodi: cell
on-off: phenomenon
ontogenic: homeostasis
Onuf: nucleus
o'nyong-nyong: fever; virus
oophoritic: cyst
opacifying: gallstones
opal: codon; mutation
opalescent: dentin
opaline: patch
Opalski: cell
opaque: microscope
open: biopsy; bite; comedo;
cordotomy; dislocation;
drainage; fracture; hospital;
laparoscopy; pneumothorax;
reading frame; reduction of
fractures; system;
tuberculosis; wound
open-angle: glaucoma
open chain: compound
open chest: massage
open circuit: method
open drop: anesthesia
open head: injury
open heart: surgery
opening: axis; contraction;
movement; snap
open skull: fracture
opera-glass: hand
operant: behavior;
conditioning
operating: microscope; table
operative: dentistry;
myxedema
operator: gene
opercular: fold; part
ophryospinal: angle
ophthalmic: artery;
hyperthyroidism; nerve [CN
V1]; ointment; solutions;
veins; vesicle

ophthalmomandibulomelic:
dysplasia
ophthalmoplegic: migraine
opiate: receptors
opiate intoxication: syndrome
opioid: antagonists
Opitz BBB: syndrome
Opitz G: syndrome
Oppenheim: disease; reflex;
syndrome
opponens: muscle
opponens digiti minimi:
muscle
opponens pollicis: muscle
opponent: color
opportunistic: pathogen
opposer: muscle of little
finger; muscle of thumb
oppositional: disorder
oppositional defiant: disorder
opsonic: index
optic: activity; agnosia;
antipode; ataxia; axis; canal;
capsule; chiasm; cup;
decussation; density; disk;
fissure; foramen; groove;
isomerism; layer; nerve [CN
II]; neuritis; papilla; part of
retina; pit; placodes;
radiation; recess; rotation;
stalk; tract; vesicle
optical: aberration; illusion;
image; iridectomy;
keratoplasty; pachymeter
optical righting: reflexes
optic nerve: glioma; head;
hypoplasia
optic nerve sheath:
decompression; fenestration
opticokinetic: nystagmus
optic rotatory: dispersion
optimum: dose; pH;
temperature
optokinetic: nystagmus
O-R: system
oral: biology; cavity; cavity
proper; contraceptive;
fissure; hygiene; membrane;
mucosa; opening; part of
pharynx; pathology;
pharynx; phase;
physiotherapy; plate;
primacy; region; shields;
smear; stereotypy; surgeon;
surgery; teeth; vestibule
oral auditory: method
oral epithelial: nevus
oral (erosive): lichen planus
oral focal: mucinosis
oral lactose tolerance: test
oral poliovirus: vaccine
oral pontine reticular:
nucleus
oral submucous: fibrosis
Orbeli: effect

orbicular: bone; ligament; ligament of radius; muscle; muscle of eye; muscle of mouth; process; zone of hip joint
orbicularis: muscle; phenomenon
orbicularis oculi: muscle; reflex
orbicularis oris: muscle
orbicularis pupillary: reflex
orbital: abscess; artery; axis; branches of maxillary nerve; branch of middle meningeal artery; branch of pterygopalatine ganglion; cavity; cellulitis; decompression; eminence of zygomatic bone; exenteration; fasciae; fat-pad; gyri; height; hernia; implant; index; lamina of ethmoid bone; layer of ethmoid bone; margin; margin of eyelids; muscle; nerve; opening; ophthalmoplegia; part of frontal bone; part of lacrimal gland; part of optic nerve; part of orbicularis oculi (muscle); part [TA] of inferior frontal gyrus; plane; plate; plate of ethmoid bone; process of palatine bone; region; rim; septum; sulci; surface; syndrome; tubercle (of zygomatic bone); width
orbital fat: body
orbitalis: muscle
orbitofrontal: artery; cortex
orbitomeatal: line; plane
orbitonasal: index
orcinol: test
ordered: mechanism
ordered on-random off: mechanism
ordinal: scale
orf: virus
organ: culture
organic: acid; catalyst; chemistry; compound; contracture; delusions; disease; evolution; hallucinosis; headache; hearing impairment; murmur; pain; phosphate; principle; stricture; vertigo
organic brain: syndrome
organic dental: cement
organic mental: disorder
organic mood: syndrome
organification: defect
organoid: nevus; tumor
organ-specific: antigen
Oriboca: virus
oriens: layer

Oriental: boil; button; ringworm; schistosomiasis; sore; ulcer
orienting: reflex; response
Ormond: disease
Ornish prevention: diets
Ornish reversal: diet
ornithine: cycle
ornithosis: virus
oroantral: fistula
orodigitofacial: dysostosis
orofacial: fistula
orofaciodigital: syndrome
oronasal: fistula; membrane
oropharyngeal: isthmus; membrane; passage
Oropouche: fever
orotracheal: intubation; tube
Oroya: fever
orphan: disease; drugs; products; receptor; viruses
Orsi-Grocco: method
Orth: fixative; stain
orthodontic: appliance; band; therapy
orthoglycemic: glycosuria
orthognathic: surgery
orthograde: conduction
orthomolecular: psychiatry; therapy
orthopedic: surgery
orthopnea: position
orthopneic: position
orthoscopic: lens; spectacles
orthostatic: albuminuria; hypopiesis; hypotension; proteinuria; tachycardia
orthotopic: graft; ureterocele
Ortolani: maneuver; test
oscillating: vision
oscillatory: potential
Osgood-Schlatter: disease
Osler: disease; node; sign
Osler-Vaquez: disease
osmic acid: fixative
osmolal: clearance
osmotic: diuresis; diuretics; fragility; nephrosis; pressure; shock
osseous: ampulla; cell; labyrinth; lacuna; part of skeletal system; polyp; tissue
osseous hydatid: cyst
osseous spiral: lamina
ossicular: chain; reconstruction
ossific: center
ossification: center
ossifying: cartilage
osteochondrogenic: cell
osteoclast activating: factor
osteocollagenous: fibers
osteogenetic: fibers; layer
osteogenic: cell; sarcoma; tissue

osteoid: osteoma; tissue
osteomalacic: pelvis
osteomyelofibrotic: syndrome
osteopathic: medicine; physician; scoliosis
osteoperiosteal: graft
osteoplastic: amputation; craniotomy; necrotomy; obliteration of the frontal sinus
osteoplastic bone: flap
osteoporotic marrow: defect
osteoprogenitor: cell
osteosclerotic: anemia
ostial: sphincter
ostiomeatal: complex; unit
Ostrum-Furst: syndrome
Ostwald solubility: coefficient
Ot: antigen
Ota: nevus
Othello: syndrome
otic: barotrauma; capsule; ganglion; pits; placodes; vesicle
otitic: abscess; hydrocephalus; meningitis
otoacoustic: emission
otolithic: crisis; membrane; organs
otomandibular: dysostosis; syndrome
otopalatodigital: syndrome
otopharyngeal: tube
otospondylomegaepiphyseal: dysplasia
Otto: disease; pelvis
Ottoson: potential
Ouchterlony: technique; test
outer: border of iris; lip of iliac crest; malleolus; membrane; sheath of optic nerve; stripes of renal medulla; table of skull; zone of renal medulla
outer limiting: layer
outer nuclear: layer
outer plexiform: layer
outer spiral: sulcus
outlet forceps: delivery
outline: form
outpatient: anesthesia
outstanding: ear
oval: area of Flechsig; corpuscle; fasciculus; foramen; foramen of heart; fossa; window
ovale: malaria
ova and parasite: examination
ovarian: amenorrhea; artery; branches of uterine artery; bursa; colic; cortex; cycle; cyst; dysmenorrhea; fimbria; fossa; ligament; pregnancy; varicocele; veins
ovarian (nervous): plexus
ovarian tubular: adenoma

ovarian vein: syndrome
ovarioabdominal: pregnancy
overanxious: disorder
overflow: incontinence; wave
overhanging: restoration
overlap: hybridization
overlay: denture
overproduction: theory
overriding: aorta
overripe: cataract
overt: homosexuality
overvalued: idea
ovo-: vegetarian
ovular: membrane; transmigration
ovulation: inhibitor
ovulational: sclerosis
ovulocyclic: porphyria
Owen: lines
own: controls
Owren: disease
ox: bots; heart
oxalate: calculus
oxazin: dyes
Oxford: unit
oxidase: reaction; test
oxidation-reduction: electrode; indicator; potential; reaction; system
oxidative: deamination; decarboxylation; metabolism; phosphorylation
oxidized: cellulose; glutathione
oxonium: ion
oxygen: capacity; consumption; debt; deficit; effect; electrode; poisoning; tent; therapy; toxicity
oxygen affinity: anoxia; hypoxia
oxygenated: hemoglobin
oxygen deprivation: theory of narcosis
oxygen-derived free: radicals
oxygen utilization: coefficient
oxyntic: cell; gland
oxyphil: adenoma; cell; chromatin; granule
oxyphilic: carcinoma; leukocyte
oxytocin challenge: test

P

π: helix
ψ: factor
P: antigens; cell; elements; enzyme; factor; selectin; substance of Lewis; wave
P1: segment of posterior cerebral artery
P2: segment of posterior cerebral artery
P3: segment of posterior cerebral artery

P4: segment of posterior cerebral artery
PA: interval; projection
Paas: disease
pacchionian: bodies; corpuscles; depressions; glands; granulations
pacemaker: failure; output; potential; sensitivity; syndrome
Pacheco parrot disease: virus
Pachon: method; test
pachydermoperiostosis: syndrome
pacing: catheter
pacinian: corpuscles
packed cell: volume
packed human blood: cells
packing: process
PA conduction: time
Padykula-Herman: stain for myosin ATPase
Pagenstecher: circle
Paget: cells; disease
Paget-Eccleston: stain
pagetoid: cells; reticulosis
Paget-von Schrötter: syndrome
Pahvant Valley: fever; plague
pain: reaction; threshold; tolerance
painful: anesthesia; heel; hematuria; paraplegia; point; toe
painful arc: sign; syndrome
painful-bruising: syndrome
painless: hematuria; jaundice
pain-pleasure: principle
painter's: colic
paired: allosome; associates; beats; organelles
Pajot: maneuver
Palade: granule
palatal: abscess; bar; index; myoclonus; nystagmus; papillomatosis; plate; reflex; seal; shelf; triangle
palate: hook; myograph
palatine: aponeurosis; bone; crest of horizontal process of palatine bone; glands; grooves; papilla; process of maxilla; raphe; ridge; spines; surface of horizontal plate of palatine bone; tonsil; torus; uvula
palatoethmoidal: suture
palatoglossal: arch
palatoglossus: muscle
palatomaxillary: index; suture
palatopharyngeal: arch; muscle; sphincter
palatopharyngeus: muscle
palatouvularis: muscle
palatovaginal: canal; groove

pale: globe; hypertension; infarct; thrombus
paleostriatal: syndrome
Palfyn: sinus
palindromic: DNA; encephalopathy; sequence
palisade: layer
pallesthetic: sensibility
palliative: treatment
pallidal: syndrome
palm: grasp; oil; wax
palmar: aponeurosis; branch of anterior interosseous nerve; branch of median nerve; branch of ulnar nerve; crease; fascia; fibromatosis; flexion; ligaments; ligaments of interphalangeal joints of hand; ligaments of metacarpophalangeal joints; monticuli; plates; psoriasis; reflex; surfaces of fingers; syphilid
palmar carpal: branch of radial artery; branch of ulnar artery; ligament
palmar carpal tendinous: sheaths
palmar carpometacarpal: ligaments
palmar digital: veins
palmar interossei interosseous: muscles
palmar interosseous: artery
palmaris brevis: muscle
palmaris longus: muscle
palmar metacarpal: artery; ligaments; veins
palmar radiocarpal: ligament
palmar ulnocarpal: ligament
palmate: folds of cervical canal
palm-chin: reflex
Palmer acid: test for peptic ulcer
palmin: test
palmomental: reflex
palmoplantar: keratoderma
palpable: rale
palpatory: percussion
palpebral: branches of infratrochlear nerve; conjunctiva; fissure; glands; margins; part of lacrimal gland; part of orbicularis oculi (muscle); raphe; veins
palpebronasal: fold
paludal: fever
pampiniform: body
pampiniform venous: plexus
panacinar: emphysema
pancake: kidney
pancervical: smear
Pancoast: syndrome; tumor

pancreatic: abscess; branches; calculus; cholera; colic; cystoduodenostomy; deoxyribonuclease; diabetes; diarrhea; digestion; diverticula; dornase; duct; encephalopathy; infantilism; islands; islets; juice; lithiasis; lymph nodes; notch; polypeptide; RNase; sphincter; steatorrhea; veins
pancreatic hyperglycemic: hormone
pancreatic (nervous): plexus
pancreaticoduodenal: lymph nodes; transplantation; veins
pancreaticoduodenal arterial: arcades
pancreaticoenteric: recess
pancreaticosplenic: lymph nodes
pancreatogenous: diarrhea
pancreatorenal: syndrome
pancreozymin-secretin: test
Pandy: reaction; test
Paneth granular: cells
panhypopituitary: dwarfism
panic: attack; disorder
panlobular: emphysema
Panner: disease
pannicular: hernia
panniculus carnosus: muscle
panoptic: stain
panoramic: radiograph
panoramic rotating: machine
panoramic x-ray: film
Pansch: fissure
pansystolic: murmur
pantaloon: embolism; hernia
pantoate-activating: enzyme
pantoscopic: spectacles; tilt
pantropic: virus
Panum: area
PAP: technique
Pap: smear; test
Papanicolaou: examination; smear; stain
Papanicolaou smear: test
paper: autoradiography; chromatography; plate
paper mill worker's: disease
Papez: circuit
papillary: adenocarcinoma; adenoma of large intestine; carcinoma; cystadenoma lymphomatosum; ducts; foramina of kidney; hidradenoma; layer; muscle; process of caudate lobe of liver; ridges; stasis; tumor
papillary cystic: adenoma
papillary muscle: dysfunction; syndrome
papilloma: virus
Papillon-Léage and Psaume: syndrome

Papillon-Lefèvre: syndrome
pappataci: fever
pappataci fever: viruses
Pappenheim: stain
Pappenheimer: bodies
papular: acrodermatitis of childhood; dermatitis of pregnancy; fever; mucinosis; scrofuloderma; tuberculid; urticaria
papulonecrotic: tuberculid
papulosquamous: syphilid
papyraceous: scars
paraaortic: bodies
parabasal: body; filament
parabigeminal: nucleus
paraboloid: condenser
parabrachial: nuclei
paracarcinomatous: encephalomyelopathy; myelopathy
paracarmine: stain
paracellular: transport
paracelsian: method
paracentral: artery; branches of callosomarginal artery; branches (of pericallosal artery); fissure; lobule; nucleus of thalamus; scotoma; sulcus
paracentric: inversion
paracervical block: anesthesia
parachordal: cartilage; plate
parachute: deformity; reflex
parachute mitral: valve
paracicatricial: emphysema
paracoccidioidal: granuloma
paracolic: gutters; recesses
paracolon: bacillus
paracyclic: ovulation
paracystic: pouch
paradoxic: pulse
paradoxical: contraction; embolism; incontinence; movement of eyelids; pupil; reflex; respiration; sleep
paradoxical diaphragm: phenomenon
paradoxical extensor: reflex
paradoxical flexor: reflex
paradoxical patellar: reflex
paradoxical pupillary: phenomenon; reflex
paradoxical triceps: reflex
paradoxical vocal cord: movement
paraduodenal: fold; fossa; hernia; recess
paradysentery: bacillus
paraesophageal: hernia
paraffin: cancer; tumor; wax
parafollicular: cells
parafrenal: abscess
paraganglionic: cells
paragenital: tubules
paraglenoid: groove; sulcus

paraglottic: space
Paragonimus: granuloma
Paraguay: tea
parahiatal: hernia
parahippocampal: gyrus
parainfluenza: viruses
parajejunal: fossa
paralemniscal: nucleus
parallax: method; test
parallel: attachment; rays
paraluteal: cell
paralutein: cell
paralytic: dementia; ectropion; ileus; miosis; mydriasis; rabies; scoliosis; strabismus
paralyzing: vertigo
paramammary: lymph nodes
paramastoid: process
paramedial reticular: nucleus
paramedian: arteries; incision; lobule
paramedian pontine: branches of pontine arteries
paramesonephric: duct
parametric: abscess; test
paranasal: sinuses
paraneoplastic: acrokeratosis; encephalomyelopathy; pemphigus; syndrome
paranephric: abscess; body; fat
paraneural: infiltration
paranigral: nucleus
paranoid: disorder; personality; schizophrenia
paranoid personality: disorder
paranuclear: body
parapeduncular: nucleus
paraperitoneal: hernia
parapharyngeal: abscess; space
paraphysial: body; cysts
parapneumonic: effusion
pararectal: fossa; lymph nodes; pouch
parasaccular: hernia
parasagittal: plane; section
paraseptal: cartilage; emphysema
parasinoidal: sinuses
parasite-host: ecosystem
parasitic: chylocele; cyst; disease; granuloma; hemoptysis; leiomyoma; melanoderma; thyroiditis; twin
parasitophorous: vacuole
parasol: insertion
paraspinal: line
parasternal: hernia; line; lymph nodes
parastriate: area; cortex
parasympathetic: ganglia; nerve; part of autonomic division of peripheral nervous system; root of ciliary ganglion; root of otic ganglion; root of pelvic ganglia; root of pterygopalatine ganglion; root of submandibular ganglion
parasympathetic nervous: system
parasystolic: beat
parataxic: distortion
paratenic: host
paraterminal: body; gyrus
parathyroid: gland; hormone; insufficiency; osteosis; tetany
parathyroid hormonelike: protein
parathyroid hormone-related: peptide; protein
parathyroprival: tetany
paratracheal: lymph node
paratuberculous: lymphadenitis
paratyphoid: bacillus; fever
paraumbilical: veins
paraurethral: ducts; glands
parauterine: lymph nodes
paravaccinia: virus
paravaginal: hysterectomy; lymph nodes
paraventricular: nucleus; nucleus [TA] of hypothalamus
paravertebral: anesthesia; ganglia; gutter; line; triangle
paravesical: fossa; lymph nodes; pouch
paraxial: mesoderm; rays
parchment: heart; skin
parchment right: ventricle
Paré: suture
parenchymal: atelectasis; cell
parenchymatous: cartilage; cell of corpus pineale; degeneration; goiter; hemorrhage; mastitis; neuritis
parent: artery; cell; cyst
parental: generation; rejection
parenteral: absorption; alimentation; hyperalimentation; therapy
parenteric: fever
Parenti-Fraccaro: syndrome
paretic: neurosyphilis
parietal: angle; bone; border; border of frontal bone; border of sphenoid bone; border of squamous part of temporal bone; border of temporal bone; branch; branch of medial occipital artery; branch of middle meningeal artery; branch of superficial temporal artery; cell; eminence; eye; fistula; foramen; hernia; layer; layer of leptomeninges; layer of serous pericardium; layer of tunica vaginalis of testis; lobe; lobe of cerebrum; lymph nodes; margin; margin of frontal bone; margin of greater wing of sphenoid; nodes; notch; peritoneum; plate; pleura; region; thrombus; tuber; veins; wall
parietal abdominal: fascia
parietal emissary: vein
parietal lobe: epilepsy
parietal pelvic: fascia
parietomastoid: suture
parieto-occipital: branches (of anterior cerebral artery); branch (of posterior cerebral artery)
parietooccipital: artery; fissure; sulcus
parietopontine: fibers; tract
Parinaud: conjunctivitis; ophthalmoplegia; syndrome
Parinaud oculoglandular: syndrome
Paris: line
Park: aneurysm
Parker-Kerr: suture
Parkes Weber: syndrome
Parkinson: disease; facies
Park-Williams: fixative
paroccipital: process
parolfactory: area; sulci
Parona: space
paroophoritic: cyst
parosteal: fasciitis; osteosarcoma
parotid: abscess; bed; branches; bubo; duct; fascia; gland; notch; papilla; plexus of facial nerve; recess; sheath; space; veins
parotideomasseteric: fascia
paroxysmal: hypertension; sleep; tachycardia
paroxysmal cerebral: dysrhythmia
paroxysmal cold: hemoglobinuria
paroxysmal nocturnal: dyspnea; hemoglobinemia; hemoglobinuria
Parrot: disease
parrot: fever; jaw; virus
parrot-beak: nail
Parry: disease
parry: fracture
Parsonage-Turner: syndrome
partial: agglutinin; anencephaly; aneuploidy; anodontia; antigen; cystectomy; denture; denture, distal extension; enterocele; epilepsy; laryngectomy; lipoatrophy; pressure; sclerectasia; seizure; volume
partial adrenocortical: insufficiency
partial anomalous pulmonary venous: connections
partial breech: extraction
partial cricoid: cleft
partial denture: impression; retention
partial face-sparing: lipodystrophy
partial heart: block
partial ileal: bypass
partial left: ventriculectomy
partial posterior laryngeal: cleft
partial-thickness: burn; graft
partial thromboplastin: time
participant: observer
particulate wear: debris
partition: chromatography; coefficient
parturient: canal
parvilocular: cyst
PAS: stain
Pascal: law
Pascheff: conjunctivitis
Paschen: bodies
Passavant: bar; cushion; pad; ridge
passional: attitudes
passive: agglutination; anaphylaxis; atelectasis; clot; congestion; diffusion; duction; eruption; hemagglutination; hyperemia; immunity; immunization; incontinence; learning; medium; movement; prophylaxis; transference; transport; tremor; vasoconstriction; vasodilation
passive-aggressive: behavior; personality
passive cutaneous: anaphylaxis
passive cutaneous anaphylactic: reaction
passive cutaneous anaphylaxis: test
passive length-tension: curve
Pasteur: effect; pipette; vaccine
Pastia: sign
pastoral: counseling
Patau: syndrome
patch: clamp; test
patchy: atelectasis
Patein: albumin

patellar: anastomosis; fossa of vitreous; ligament; network; reflex; retinaculum; surface of femur
patellar apprehension: sign
patellar tendon: reflex
patelloadductor: reflex
patellofemoral: syndrome
patellofemoral stress: syndrome
patent: ductus arteriosus; medicine; part of umbilical artery
Paterson-Brown-Kelly: syndrome
Paterson-Kelly: syndrome
path: analysis
pathematic: aphasia
pathetic: nerve
pathogenic: occlusion
pathognomonic: symptom
pathologic: absorption; amenorrhea; amputation; calcification; diagnosis; fracture; glycosuria; histology; model; myopia; physiology; proteins; rigidity; sphincter
pathological: anatomy
pathologic retraction: ring
pathologic startle: syndromes
patient-controlled: analgesia; anesthesia
Patois: virus
Paton: lines
Patrick: test
pattern distortion: amblyopia
patterned: alopecia
pattern retinal: dystrophy
pattern-sensitive: epilepsy
Paul: reaction; test
Paul-Bunnell: test
Pauli exclusion: principle
Pauling: theory
Pauling-Corey: helix
pause: signal
Pautrier: abscess; microabscess
pavement: epithelium
Pavlov: method; pouch; reflex; stomach
pavlovian: conditioning
Pavy: disease
Paxton: disease
Payne: operation
Payr: clamp; membrane; sign
PBI: test
PCA: pump
peak: magnitude
peak expiratory: flow
peak flow: rate
Pearl: index
pearl: cyst; moss
pearl-worker's: disease
pear-shaped: area
peat: moss

peccant: humors
pecking: order
Pecquet: cistern; duct; reservoir
pecten: band
pectin: sugar
pectinate: fibers; ligaments of iridocorneal angle; ligaments of iris; line; muscles; zone
pectineal: ligament; line of femur; line of pubis; muscle
pectineus: muscle
pectiniform: septum
pectoral: branch of thoracoacromial artery; fascia; girdle; glands; reflex; region; ridge; veins
pectoral and abdominal anterior cutaneous: branch of intercostal nerves
pectoral axillary: lymph nodes
pectoralis major: muscle
pectoralis minor: muscle
pectorodorsal: muscle
pectorodorsalis: muscle
pedal: system
Pedersen: speculum
pediatric: dentistry; radiology
pedicle: flap; graft
pediculous: blepharitis
pedigree: analysis
peduncular: ansa; loop; veins
pedunculated: hydatid; polyp
pedunculomammillary: fasciculus
pedunculopontine tegmental: nucleus
peeping: testis
peg-and-socket: articulation; joint
pegged: tooth
Pel-Ebstein: disease; fever
Pelger-Huët nuclear: anomaly
peliosis: hepatitis
Pelizaeus-Merzbacher: disease
pellagra-preventing: factor
Pellegrini: disease
Pellegrini-Stieda: disease
pellet: implantation
Pellizzi: syndrome
pellucid: zone
pellucid marginal corneal: degeneration
pelvic: abscess; axis; bone; brim; canal; cavity; cellulitis; diaphragm; exenteration; fascia; ganglia; girdle; hematocele; inclination; index; inlet; kidney; limb; lymph nodes; outlet; part; part of ductus deferens; part of peripheral autonomic plexuses and

ganglia; part of ureter; part of the urogenital sinus; peritonitis; plane of greatest dimensions; plane of inlet; plane of least dimensions; plane of outlet; pole; presentation; promontory; surface of sacrum; version
pelvic inflammatory: disease
pelvic (nervous): plexus
pelvic splanchnic: nerves
pelvirectal: sphincter
pelvivertebral: angle
pelvofemoral muscular: dystrophy
pen: grasp
pencil: tenderness
Pendred: syndrome
pendular: movement; nystagmus
pendulous: abdomen; heart; palate
pendulum: rhythm
penetrant: trait
penetrating: keratoplasty; ulcer; wound
penicillin G: potassium
penile: epispadias; fibromatosis; hypospadias; implant; prosthesis; raphe; urethra
penis: envy
pennate: muscle
penopubic: epispadias
penoscrotal: hypospadias; transposition
Penrose: drain
pension: neurosis
pentagastrin: test
pentavalent gas gangrene: antitoxin
penton: antigen
pentose monophosphate: shunt
pentose phosphate: cycle; pathway
pep: pills
Pepper: syndrome
pepper and salt: fundus
peptic: cell; digestion; gland; ulcer
peptide: antibiotic; bond
peptidyl: leukotrienes
perambulating: ulcer
percept: analysis
perceptive: hearing impairment
perceptual: expansion
percussion: sound; wave
percutaneous: absorption; cholangiography; nephrostomy; stimulation
percutaneous endoscopic: gastrostomy

percutaneous radiofrequency: gangliolysis
percutaneous transhepatic: cholangiography
percutaneous transluminal: angioplasty
percutaneous transluminal coronary: angioplasty
Perez: reflex; sign
perfect: fungus; stage; state
perfectionistic: personality
perforated: layer of sclera; space; ulcer
perforating: abscess; appendicitis; arteries of hand; arteries (of deep femoral artery); arteries (of foot); arteries (of internal thoracic artery); arteries of penis; branch of anterior interosseous artery; branches; branches of internal thoracic artery; branches (of palmar metacarpal arteries); branches (of plantar metatarsal arteries); branch of fibular artery; branch of peroneal artery; fibers; folliculitis; keratoplasty; ulcer of foot; veins; wound
perforating radiate: arteries (of kidney)
performance: intensity; status; test
performic acid: reaction
perfusion: cannula
perhydrase: milk
perialveolar: wiring
periapical: abscess; curettage; cyst; granuloma; osteofibrosis; radiograph; tissue
periapical cemental: dysplasia
periappendiceal: abscess
periaqueductal gray: substance
periarterial: pad; plexus; plexus of anterior cerebral artery; plexus of ascending pharyngeal artery; plexus of choroid artery; plexuses of coronary arteries; plexus of facial artery; plexus of inferior phrenic artery; plexus of inferior thyroid artery; plexus of internal thoracic artery; plexus of lingual artery; plexus of maxillary artery; plexus of middle cerebral artery; plexus of occipital artery; plexus of ophthalmic artery; plexus of popliteal artery;

plexus of posterior auricular artery; plexus of subclavian artery; plexus of superficial temporal artery; plexus of superior thyroid artery; plexus of testicular artery; plexus of thyroid artery; plexus of vertebral artery; sympathectomy
periarterial lymphatic: sheath
periarticular: abscess
pericallosal: artery; cistern
pericanalicular: fibroadenoma
pericapillary: cell
pericardiacophrenic: artery; veins
pericardial: branch of phrenic nerve; branch of thoracic aorta; cavity; decompression; effusion; fremitus; knock; murmur; reflex; rub; symphysis; tap; veins; villi
pericardial friction: sound
pericardioperitoneal: canal
pericardiopleural: membrane
pericardium: fibrosa
pericemental: abscess; attachment
pericentral: fibrosis; scotoma
pericentric: inversion
perichondral: bone
perichoroid: space
perichoroidal: space
periclaustral: lamina
pericolic membrane: syndrome
periconchal: sulcus
pericoronal: abscess; flap
pericorpuscular: synapse
pericytic: venules
peridental: ligament; membrane
peridural: anesthesia
perifornical: nucleus
perihypoglossal: nuclei
periinfarction: block
perilimbal suction: cup
perilunar: dislocation
perilymphatic: duct; fistula; gusher; space
perimortem: delivery
perimuscular: fibrosis
perinatal: death; medicine; mortality; torsion
perinatal mortality: rate
perineal: artery; body; branches of posterior cutaneous nerve of thigh; branches of posterior femoral cutaneous nerve; fascia; flexure of anal canal; flexure of rectum; hernia; hypospadias; lithotomy; membrane; muscles; nerves; raphe; region; section; spaces; urethrostomy; urethrotomy
perineovaginal: fistula
perinephric: abscess
perineural: infiltration
perineuronal: satellite
perinuclear: cataract; space
periodic: arthralgia; biopolymer; catatonia; disease; edema; fever; filariasis; law; neutropenia; paralysis; peritonitis; polyserositis; system
periodic acid-Schiff: stain
periodic bone: pain
periodic migrainous: neuralgia
periodontal: abscess; anesthesia; atrophy; fiber; file; ligament; membrane; pocket; probe
periodontal ligament: fibers
periolivary: nuclei
periorbital: cellulitis; membrane
periosteal: bone; bud; chondroma; elevator; ganglion; graft; implantation; layer of dura mater; osteosarcoma; reaction; reflex; sarcoma
periotic: bone; cartilage
peripartum: cardiomyopathy
peripeduncular: nucleus
peripharyngeal: space
peripheral: aneurysm; arteriosclerosis; cataract; chemoreceptor; dysostosis; glare; iridectomy; part of nervous system; proteins; resistance; scotoma; seal; tabes; vision
peripheral anterior: synechia
peripheral facial: paralysis
peripheral nervous: system
peripheral ossifying: fibroma
peripheral T-cell: lymphoma, unspecified
peripolar: cell
periportal: cirrhosis; space of Mall
perirectal: abscess
perirenal: fascia; insufflation
perirenal fat: capsule
periscopic: lens; meniscus
perisinusoidal: space
peristatic: hyperemia
peristernal: perichondritis
peristriate: area; cortex
peritarsal: network
perithelial: cell
peritoneal: button; cavity; dialysis; fossae; insufflation; villi
peritoneovenous: shunt
peritonsillar: abscess
peritracheal: glands
peritrigeminal: nucleus
peritubular: dentin; zone
peritubular contractile: cells
perityphlitis: actinomycotica
periungual: fibroma
periureteral: abscess
periurethral: abscess
perivascular: cuffs
perivascular fibrous: capsule
periventricular: fibers; zone
periventricular preoptic: nucleus
perivisceral: cavity
perivitelline: space
Perlia: nucleus
Perls: test
Perls Prussian blue: stain
permanent: callus; cartilage; restoration; stricture; tooth
permanent stained smear: examination
permanent threshold: shift
permeability: coefficient; constant; theory of narcosis; vitamin
permissible exposure: limit
permissive: cell
permissive hypercapnic: ventilation
perna: disease
pernicious: anemia; malaria; vomiting
pernicious anemia type: metarubricyte; prorubricyte; rubriblast
peroneal: artery; bone; border of foot; compartment of leg; lymph node; phenomenon; pulley; retinaculum; trochlea of calcaneus; veins
peroneal anastomotic: ramus
peroneal communicating: branch; nerve
peroneal muscular: atrophy
peroneus brevis: muscle
peroneus longus: muscle
peroneus tertius: muscle
peroral: endoscopy
peroxidase: reaction; stain
perpendicular: fasciculus; plate; plate of ethmoid bone; plate of palatine bone
perpetually growing: tooth
Perrault: syndrome
persecution: complex
persecutory type of paranoid: disorder
Persian Gulf: syndrome
Persian relapsing: fever
persistent: cloaca; tremor; truncus arteriosus
persistent anterior hyperplastic primary: vitreous
persistent atrioventricular: canal
persistent ectopic: pregnancy
persistent frontal: suture
persistent generalized: lymphadenopathy
persistently growing: tooth
persistent müllerian duct: syndrome
persistent posterior hyperplastic primary: vitreous
persistent vegetative: state
personal: equation; motivation; probability; space
personal growth: laboratory
personality: disorder; formation; integration; inventory; profile; test
perspiratory: glands
Perthes: disease; test
Pertik: diverticulum
pertrochanteric: fracture
pertussis: immunoglobulin; syndrome; vaccine
pertussis immune: globulin
pertussis-like: syndrome
Peruvian: tarantula; wart
pervasive developmental: disorder
pervenous: pacemaker
pessary: cell; corpuscle
petechial: angiomas; hemorrhage
Peters: anomaly; ovum
Petit: aponeurosis; canals; hernia; herniotomy; sinus
petit: mal
petite: mutant
Petit lumbar: triangle
petit mal: epilepsy; seizure
Petri: dish
Petri dish: culture
petrooccipital: fissure; joint; synchondrosis
petrosal: bone; branch of middle meningeal artery; foramen; fossa; fossula; ganglion; impression of the pallium; sinus; vein
petrosphenoidal: fissure; syndrome
petrosquamous: fissure; suture
petrotympanic: fissure
petrous: bone; part of internal carotid artery; part of temporal bone; pyramid
Pette-Döring: disease
Petzval: surface
Peutz: syndrome
Peutz-Jeghers: syndrome
Peyer: glands; patches
Peyronie: disease
Peyrot: thorax

Pezzer: catheter
Pfannenstiel: incision
Pfaundler-Hurler: syndrome
Pfeiffer: phenomenon; syndrome
Pflüger: law
Pfuhl: sign
pH: scale; value
phacoanaphylactic: uveitis
phacogenic: glaucoma; uveitis
phacolytic: glaucoma
phacomorphic: glaucoma
phaeomycotic: cyst
phagedenic: ulcer
phagocyte: dysfunction
phagocytic: index; pneumonocyte
phagocytic dysfunction: immunodeficiency
phagocytic dysfunction disorders: immunodeficiency
phakic: eye
phalangeal: cell; joints
Phalen: maneuver
phallic: phase; tubercle
phantom: aneurysm; corpuscle; limb; pregnancy; tumor
phantom limb: pain
pharmaceutical: biology; chemistry
pharmacologic: mediators of anaphylaxis
pharmacologic stress: imaging
pharmacopeial: gel
pharmacoresistent: epilepsy
pharyngeal: arches; branch of the artery of pterygoid canal; branch of the ascending pharyngeal artery; branch of descending palatine artery; branches; branches of recurrent laryngeal nerve; branch of glossopharyngeal nerve; branch of inferior thyroid artery; branch of pterygopalatine ganglion; branch of vagus nerve; bursa; calculus; canal; cartilages; flap; fornix; glands; grooves; hypophysis; isthmus; lacuna; membranes; mucosa; nerve; opening of eustachian tube; opening of pharyngotympanic (auditory) tube; pituitary; pouches; raphe; recess; reflex; ridge; space; tonsil; tubercle (of basilar part of occipital bone); veins
pharyngeal lymphatic: ring
pharyngeal (nervous): plexus
pharyngeal pouch: syndrome

pharyngobasilar: fascia
pharyngobranchial: ducts
pharyngoconjunctival: fever
pharyngoconjunctival fever: virus
pharyngoepiglottic: fold
pharyngoesophageal: constriction; cushions; diverticulum; pads
pharyngomaxillary: space
pharyngonasal: cavity
pharyngopalatine: arch
pharyngotympanic: groove
pharyngotympanic (auditory): tube
phase: image; microscope; rule; shift
phase I: block
phase II: block
phasic: reflex
phasic sinus: arrhythmia
PH conduction: time
phenanthrene: nucleus
phenobarbital: elixir
phenol: coefficient
phenolsulfonphthalein: test
phenotypic: mixing; threshold; value
phentolamine: test
phenylhydrazine: hemolysis
phenylpyruvate: oligophrenia
phenylpyruvic: amentia
phenylthiocarbamoyl: peptide; protein
phi: phenomenon
Phialophore-type: conidiophore
Philadelphia: chromosome; cocktail
philanthropic: hospital
Philip: glands
Philippe: triangle
Philippine hemorrhagic: fever
Phillips: catheter
Phillipson: reflex
philosopher's: stone
phlebotomus: fever
phlebotomus fever: viruses
phlegmonous: abscess; cellulitis; enteritis; erysipelas; gastritis; mastitis; ulcer
phlogiston: theory
phlorizin: diabetes; glycosuria
phlyctenular: conjunctivitis; keratitis; ophthalmia; pannus
PhNCS: protein
phocomelic: dwarfism
phonemic: regression
phonetic: balance
phosphatase: unit
phosphate: diabetes; tetany
phosphogluconate: pathway
phosphohexose isomerase: deficiency

phospholipid: syndrome
phosphor: plate
phosphoroclastic: cleavage; reaction
phosphorylase-rupturing: enzyme
phosphotungstic acid: hematoxylin; stain
phosphureted: hydrogen
photechic: effect
photic: driving; stimulation
photic-sneeze: reflex
photo: cell
photoallergic: sensitivity
photochromic: lens; spectacles
photodynamic: sensitization; therapy
photoelectric: absorption; effect
photogenic: epilepsy
photomultiplier: tube
photon: density
photo-patch: test
photopic: adaptation; eye; vision
photoradiation: therapy
photoreactivating: enzyme
photoreceptor: cells
photorefractive: keratectomy
photosensor: oculography
photostimulable: phosphor
photostress: test
phototherapeutic: keratectomy
phototoxic: sensitivity
phrenic: ampulla; ganglia; nerve; nucleus; pleura; plexus; veins
phrenicoabdominal: branches of phrenic nerve
phrenicoceliac: part of suspensory muscle (ligament) of duodenum
phrenicocolic: ligament
phrenicocostal: sinus
phrenicolienal: ligament
phrenicomediastinal: recess
phrenicopleural: fascia
phrenicosplenic: ligament
phrenic pressure: test
phrenogastric: ligament
phrenopericardial: angle
phrenosplenic: ligament
phrygian: cap
phthinoid: chest
phyllodes: tumor
physaliphorous: cell
physical: age; allergy; anthropology; diagnosis; elasticity of muscle; examination; fitness; half-life; map; medicine; sign; therapy
physician-assisted: suicide
Physick: pouches

physiologic: age; albuminuria; amenorrhea; anatomy; anemia; anisocoria; antidote; chemistry; congestion; cup; dwarfism; elasticity of muscle; equilibrium; excavation; homeostasis; hypertrophy; icterus; incompatibility; jaundice; leukocytosis; occlusion; saline; sclerosis; scotoma; sphincter; tremor; unit; vertigo
physiological: drives
physiologically balanced: occlusion
physiologic dead: space
physiologic rest: position
physiologic retraction: ring
pia: mater encephali; mater spinalis
pial: filament; funnel; part of filum terminale
pial-glial: membrane
pianist's: cramp
piano: percussion
PICC: line
Picchini: syndrome
Pick: atrophy; bodies; bundle; cell; disease; syndrome
picker's: nodules
Pickles: chart
pickwickian: syndrome
pi cone: monochromatism
picrocarmine: stain
picroformol: fixative
picro-Mallory trichrome: stain
picronigrosin: stain
picture: element
picture frame: vertebra
piebald: eyelash; skin
Pierre Robin: syndrome
piezoelectric: effect; transducer
piezogenic pedal: papule
pig: skin
pigeon: breast; chest
pigment: cell; cells of iris; cell of skin; cells of retina; cirrhosis; epithelium; epithelium of optic retina; induration of the lung
pigmentary: cirrhosis; glaucoma; retinopathy; syphilid
pigment dispersion: syndrome
pigmented: ameloblastoma; dermatofibrosarcoma protuberans; epulis; layer of ciliary body; layer of iris; layer of retina; liver; part of retina
pigmented hair epidermal: nevus

pigmented keratic: precipitates
pigmented purpuric lichenoid: dermatosis
pigmented villonodular: synovitis; tenosynovitis
Pignet: formula
pigtail: catheter
pilar: cyst; tumor of scalp
pileous: gland
piliferous: cyst
pillar: cells; cells of Corti
pill-rolling: tremor
pilocytic: astrocytoma
piloid: gliosis
pilomotor: fibers; reflex
pilon: fracture
pilonidal: cyst; fistula; sinus
Piltz: sign
pilular: mass
pin: amalgam; implant
Pinard: maneuver
pincer: nail
pinch: graft
pincushion: distortion
Pindborg: tumor
pineal: body; cells; cyst; eye; gland; habenula; recess; stalk
Pinel: system
ping-pong: bone; fracture; mechanism
pinhole: pupil
pink: disease
pink bread: mold
Pinkus: tumor
pinocytotic: vesicle
Pins: sign; syndrome
pinta: fever
pinworm: vaginitis
PIP: joints
pipe: bone
Piper: forceps
pipe-smoker's: cancer
pipe stem: cirrhosis
pipestem: arteries; fibrosis
piqûre: diabetes
Pirie: bone
piriform: aperture; area; cortex; fossa; muscle; opening; recess; sinus
piriformis: muscle
piriform neuron: layer
Pirogoff: amputation; angle; triangle
Pirquet: index; reaction; test
pisciform: cataract
pisiform: joint
pisiform: bone
pisohamate: ligament
pisometacarpal: ligament
pisotriquetral: joint
pisounciform: ligament
pisouncinate: ligament
pistol-shot: sound
pistol-shot femoral: sound

piston: pulse
pit: caries
pitch: wart
pitch-worker's: cancer
pit and fissure: caries
pithecoid: theory
Pitot: tube
Pitres: area; sign
pitted: keratolysis
pitting: edema
Pittsburgh: pneumonia
Pittsburgh pneumonia: agent
pituitary: adamantinoma; adenoma; ameloblastoma; apoplexy; cachexia; diverticulum; dwarf; dwarfism; dystopia; fossa; gigantism; gland; infantilism; membrane; myxedema; stalk
pituitary gonadotropic: hormone
pituitary growth: hormone
pituitary stalk: section
pivot: joint
pivot shift: test
PJ: interval
P-K: antibodies; test
place: coding; theory
placenta: gonadotropin; protein
placental: barrier; circulation; dysfunction; dystocia; lobes; membrane; plasmodium; polyp; presentation; septa; sign; souffle; thrombosis; transfusion
placental dysfunction: syndrome
placental growth: hormone
placental parasitic: twin
placental site trophoblastic: tumor
placental sulfatase: deficiency
placental transfusion: syndrome
Placido da Costa: disk
plague: bacillus; pneumonia; septicemia; vaccine
plain: film
Planck: constant; theory
plane: joint; suture; wart
planoconcave: lens
planoconvex: lens
plant: agglutinin; antitoxin; casein; indican; RNase; toxin; viruses
plantar: aponeurosis; arch; fascia; fasciitis; fibromatosis; flexion; ligaments; ligaments of interphalangeal joints of foot; ligaments of metatarsophalangeal joints; muscle; reflex; region;

space; surface of foot; surface of toe; syphilid; wart
plantar arterial: arch
plantar calcaneocuboid: ligament
plantar calcaneonavicular: ligament
plantar cuboideonavicular: ligaments
plantar cuneocuboid: ligament
plantar cuneonavicular: ligaments
plantar digital: veins
plantarflexor: compartment of leg
plantar interossei interosseous: muscles
plantaris: muscle
plantar metatarsal: artery; ligaments; veins
plantar muscle: reflex
plantar quadrate: muscle
plantar tarsal: ligaments
plantar tarsometatarsal: ligaments
plantar tendon: sheath of fibularis longus muscle; sheath of peroneus longus muscle
plantar venous: arch; network
plasma: albumin; cell; factor X; fibronectin; layer; membrane; proteins; scalpel; stain; substitute; therapy
plasma accelerator: globulin
plasma cell: balanitis; gingivitis; hepatitis; leukemia; mastitis; myeloma
plasmacrit: test
plasma iodoprotein: disorder
plasmal: reaction
plasma labile: factor
plasma renin: activity
plasma thromboplastin: antecedent; component; factor; factor B
plasmatic: compartment
plasminogen: activator
plasmin prothrombins conversion: factor
plasmocytic: leukemoid reaction
plasmodial: trophoblast
plaster: bandage; splint
plastic: anatomy; bronchitis; corpuscle; cyclitis; induration; iritis; lymph; motor; pleurisy; surgery; teeth
plastic envelope: culture
plastic restoration: material
plastic section: stain
plate: thrombosis
plateau: iris; pulse
Plateau-Talbot: law

platelet: actomyosin; cofactor I; cofactor II; factor 3
platelet-activating: factor
platelet-aggregating: factor
platelet aggregation: test
platelet-derived growth: factor
platelet tissue: factor
platelike: atelectasis
platypellic: pelvis
platypelloid: pelvis
platysma: muscle
play: therapy
Pleasure: curve
pleasure: principle
pledgetted: suture
pleiotropic: gene
pleomorphic: adenoma; lipoma; oligodendroglioma; xanthoastrocytoma
plethysmographic: goggle
pleural: calculus; canal; cavity; cupula; effusion; fluid; fremitus; isthmus; lines; plaque; poudrage; pressure; rale; reaction; recesses; rub; sinuses; space; stripe; tap; villi
pleural friction: rub
pleuritic: pneumonia; rub
pleuroesophageal: line; muscle
pleuroesophageus: muscle
pleuropericardial: canals; fold; hiatus; membrane; murmur
pleuroperitoneal: canal; cavity; fold; hiatus; membrane; shunt
pleuropneumonia-like: organisms
pleurovenous: shunt
plexiform: layer; layer of cerebral cortex; layers of retina; neurofibroma; neuroma
plexogenic pulmonary: arteriopathy
Plimmer: bodies
plugging: instrument
Plummer: disease
Plummer-Vinson: syndrome
plural: pregnancy
pluripotent: cells
plus: lens; strand
PMA: index
pneocardiac: reflex
pneopneic: reflex
pneumatic: bone; dilator; otoscopy; retinopexy; space; tonometer
pneumatic tire: injury
pneumatized: bone
pneumatoenteric: recess
pneumococcal: empyema; polysaccharide; vaccine

pneumococcal/suppurative: keratitis
Pneumocystis carinii: pneumonia
pneumogastric: nerve
pneumogenic: osteoarthropathy
pneumonia: virus of mice
pneumonic: plague
P/O: quotient; ratio
pocketed: calculus
podalic: extraction; version
podiatric: medicine
podophyllum: resin
POEMS: syndrome
point: angle; deletion; epidemic; mutation
pointed: wart
point system: test types
Poirier: gland; line
Poiseuille: law; space
Poiseuille viscosity: coefficient
Poisson: distribution
Poisson-Pearson: formula
Poitou: colic
poker: back; spine
pokeweed: mitogen
Poland: syndrome
polar: amino acid; anemia; body; cataract; cell; compound; fibers; globule; hypogenesis; plates; presentation; ring; solvents; star; zone
polar frontal: artery
polarized: light
polarizing: microscope
polar temporal: artery
pole: ligation
Polenské: number
poliomyelitis: immunoglobulin; vaccines; virus
poliomyelitis immune: globulin (human)
poliovirus: vaccines
polishing: brush
Politzer: bag; method
Politzer luminous: cone
polka: fever
pollen: antigen; extract
Pólya: gastrectomy; operation
polyacrylamide gel: electrophoresis
polyalveolar: lobe
polyamine-methylene: resin
polyaxial: joint
polybasic: acid
polycarboxylate: cement
polychlorinated: biphenyl
polychromatic: cell; radiation
polychromatophil: cell
polychrome: methylene blue
polyclonal: activator; antibody; gammopathy

polycystic: disease of kidneys; kidney; liver; ovary
polycystic liver: disease
polycystic ovary: syndrome
polyendocrine deficiency: syndrome
polyester: resin
polygenic: inheritance
polyhedral: body
polyleptic: fever
polymerase chain: reaction
polymer fume: fever
polymorphic: neuron; reticulosis
polymorphic genetic: marker
polymorphic superficial: keratitis
polymorphocytic: leukemia
polymorphonuclear: leukocyte
polymorphous: layer; perversion
polymorphous light: eruption
polymorphous low-grade: carcinoma of salivary glands
polyol: pathway
polyoma: virus
polyostotic fibrous: dysplasia
polyovular ovarian: follicle
polyoxyethylene: alcohols
polyphenic: gene
polyphyletic: theory
polypoid: adenoma
polypous: endocarditis; gastritis
polysaccharide: sulfate esters
polysaccharide conjugated: vaccine
polysplenia: syndrome
polytene: chromosome
polyuria: test
polyvalent: allergy; antiserum; serum; vaccine
polyzygotic: twins
pomade: acne
Pomeroy: operation
Pompe: disease
pond: fracture
ponderal: index
Ponfick: shadow
pontine: angle; arteries; cistern; flexure; hemorrhage; nuclei; veins
pontine angle: tumor
pontine corticonuclear: fibers
pontine gray: matter
pontobulbar: body; nucleus
pontocerebellar: cistern; fibers; recess
ponto-geniculo-occipital: spike
pontomedullary: groove
pontomesencephalic: vein
pontoreticulospinal: tract
Pool: phenomenon
pooled: serum

Pool-Schlesinger: sign
poorly compliant: bladder
poorly crystalline: hydroxyapatite
poorly differentiated lymphocytic: lymphoma
popliteal: arch; artery; fascia; fossa; groove; line; lymph nodes; muscle; notch; plane of femur; plexus; region; space; surface of femur; vein
popliteal communicating: nerve
popliteal entrapment: syndrome
popliteus: muscle
population: genetics; pyramid
porcelain: gallbladder; inlay
porcine: graft; valve
porcine hemagglutinating encephalomyelitis: virus
porcupine: skin
Porges: method
Porges-Meier: test
porphobilinogen synthase: porphyria
Porro: hysterectomy; operation
portable: radiography
portacaval: anastomoses; shunt
portal: canals; circulation; cirrhosis; fissure; hypertension; lobule of liver; pyemia; system; triad; vein
portal hypophysial: circulation
portal-systemic: anastomoses; encephalopathy
portasystemic: shunt
Porter: fascia
Porter-Silber: chromogens; reaction
Porter-Silber chromogens: test
Portuguese: man-of-war
Portuguese-Azorean: disease
port-wine: mark; stain
Posadas: disease
position: agnosia; effect; sense
positional: cloning; nystagmus; vertigo; vertigo of Bárány
positive: accommodation; afterimage; afterpotential; anergy; chronotropism; control; convergence; cooperativity; electrode; electron; electrotaxis; feedback; meniscus; phase; rays; scotoma; stain; symptom; taxis; thermotaxis; transference; valence
positive contrast: orbitography

positive end-expiratory: pressure
positively: inotropic
positive-negative pressure: breathing
positron emission: tomography
post: dam; implant
postadrenalectomy: syndrome
postanal: dimple; gut
postarsphenamine: jaundice
postauricular: incision
postaxillary: line
postbasic: stare
postcapillary: venules
postcardiotomy: syndrome
postcaval: ureter
postcentral: area; artery; fissure; gyrus; sulcus
postcentral sulcal: artery
postcholecystectomy: syndrome
postcloacal: gut
postcoital: contraception; test
postcommissural: fibers
postcommissurotomy: syndrome
postcommunicating: part of anterior cerebral artery; part of posterior cerebral artery
postconcussion: syndrome
postcostal: anastomosis
post dam: area
postdate: pregnancy
postdiphtheritic: paralysis
postdrive: depression
posterior: aphasia; arch of atlas; asynclitism; belly of digastric muscle; blepharitis; border of eyelids; border of fibula; border of petrous part of temporal bone; border of radius; border of testis; border of ulna; branches; branch of great auricular nerve; branch of inferior pancreaticoduodenal artery; branch of lateral cerebral sulcus; branch of medial antebrachial cutaneous nerve; branch of medial cutaneous nerve of forearm; branch of obturator artery; branch of obturator nerve; branch of recurrent ulnar artery; branch of renal artery; branch of right branch of portal vein; branch of right hepatic duct; branch of right superior pulmonary vein; branch of spinal nerves; branch of superior thyroid artery; branch of ulnar recurrent artery; canaliculus of chorda tympani; cells; centriole;

chamber of eyeball; choroiditis; column; column of spinal cord; commissure; commissure of the larynx; compartment of arm; compartment of forearm; compartment of leg; compartment of thigh; cord of brachial plexus; crus of stapes; curvature; cusp of left atrioventricular valve; cusp of mitral valve; cusp of right atrioventricular valve; cusp of tricuspid valve; divisions of (trunks of) brachial plexus; embryotoxon; extremity of spleen; fascicle of palatopharyngeus muscle; fasciculus proprius; fontanelle; funiculus; horn; layer of rectus sheath; ligament of fibular head; ligament of head of fibula; ligament of incus; ligament of knee; limb of internal capsule; limb of stapes; lip of external os of uterus; liver; lobe of hypophysis; mediastinum; nares; nephrectomy; neuropore; notch of cerebellum; nucleus; nucleus of hypothalamus; nucleus of vagus nerve; occlusion; part; part of anterior commissure of brain; part of the diaphragmatic surface of the liver; part of liver; part of tongue; part of vaginal fornix; pillar of fauces; pillar of fornix; pituitary; pole of eyeball; pole of lens; probability; process of septal cartilage; process of talus; pyramid of the medulla; ramus of lateral cerebral sulcus; ramus of lateral sulcus of cerebrum; ramus of spinal nerve; recess; recess of tympanic membrane; region of arm; region of elbow; region of forearm; region of knee; region of leg; region of neck; region of thigh; region of wrist; rhinoscopy; rhizotomy; root of spinal nerve; scleritis; sclerosis; sclerotomy; segment; sinus of tympanic cavity; staphyloma; surface; surface of arm; surface of arytenoid cartilage; surface of cornea; surface of elbow; surface of eyelids; surface of fibula; surface of forearm; surface of iris; surface of kidney; surface of leg; surface of lens; surface of lower limb; surface of pancreas; surface of petrous part of temporal bone; surface of prostate; surface of radius; surface of scapula; surface of shaft of humerus; surface of suprarenal gland; surface of thigh; surface of tibia; surface of ulna; symblepharon; synechia; tooth; triangle of neck; tubercle of atlas; tubercle of cervical vertebrae; urethra; urethritis; uveitis; vaginismus; vein of corpus callosum; vein of septum pellucidum; vein(s) of left ventricle; vitrectomy; wall of middle ear; wall of stomach; wall of tympanic cavity; wall of vagina
posterior accessory olivary: nucleus
posterior acoustic: stria
posterior alveolar: artery
posterior ampullar: nerve
posterior antebrachial: nerve; region
posterior antebrachial cutaneous: nerve
posterior anterior jugular: vein
posterior articular: facet of dens; surface of dens
posterior atlanto-occipital: membrane
posterior auricular: artery; groove; nerve; plexus; vein
posterior auricular: muscle
posterior axillary: fold; line; lymph nodes
posterior basal: branch
posterior basal bronchopulmonary: segment S X
posterior basal segmental: artery of left/right lung
posterior brachial: region
posterior brachial cutaneous: nerve
posterior bronchopulmonary: segment S II
posterior cardinal: veins
posterior carpal: region
posterior cecal: artery
posterior central: convolution; gyrus
posterior cerebellar: notch
posterior cerebellomedullary: cistern
posterior cerebral: artery
posterior cervical: region
posterior cervical intertransversarii: muscles
posterior cervical intertransverse: muscles
posterior cervical (nervous): plexus
posterior choroidal: artery
posterior circumflex humeral: artery; vein
posterior clinoid: process
posterior column: cordotomy
posterior communicating: artery
posterior condyloid: foramen
posterior conjunctival: artery
posterior corneal: dystrophy
posterior coronary: plexus
posterior costotransverse: ligament
posterior cranial: fossa
posterior cricoarytenoid: ligament; muscle
posterior cruciate: ligament
posterior crural: region
posterior cubital: region
posterior cutaneous: nerve of arm; nerve of forearm; nerve of thigh
posterior dental: artery
posterior descending coronary: artery
posterior elastic: layer
posterior ethmoidal: artery; cells; nerve
posterior ethmoidal air: cells
posterior external arcuate: fibers
posterior facial: vein
posterior femoral cutaneous: nerve
posterior focal: point
posterior fossa: approach
posterior gastric: artery; branches of posterior vagal trunk
posterior glandular: branch of superior thyroid artery
posterior gray: commissure
posterior hepatic: segment I
posterior humeral circumflex: artery
posterior hypothalamic: area; nucleus; region
posterior inferior cerebellar: artery
posterior inferior cerebellar artery: syndrome
posterior inferior iliac: spine
posterior inferior nasal: branches of greater palatine nerve; nerves
posterior intercondylar: area of tibia
posterior intercostal: arteries 1–2; arteries 3–11; veins
posterior intermediate: groove; sulcus
posterior interosseous: artery; nerve
posterior interpositus: nucleus
posterior interventricular: artery; groove; sulcus
posterior interventricular branch of right coronary: artery
posterior intestinal: portal
posterior intraoccipital: joint; synchondrosis
posterior junction: line
posterior knee: region
posterior labial: arteries; branches of perineal artery; commissure; nerves; veins
posterior labial branches of internal perineal: artery
posterior lacrimal: crest
posterior laryngeal: cleft
posterior lateral nasal: arteries
posterior leukoencephalopathy: syndrome
posterior limiting: lamina of cornea; layer of cornea
posterior longitudinal: bundle; ligament
posterior lunate: lobule
posterior marginal: vein
posterior median: fissure of the medulla oblongata; fissure of spinal cord; line; sulcus of medulla oblongata; sulcus of spinal cord
posterior mediastinal: arteries; lymph nodes
posterior medullary: velum
posterior meningeal: artery
posterior meniscofemoral: ligament
posterior myocardial: infarction
posterior nasal: apertures; spine of horizontal plate of palatine bone
posterior neck: region
posterior occipitoaxial: ligament
posterior palatal: seal
posterior palatal seal: area
posterior palatine: arch; foramina; spine
posterior palpebral: margin
posterior pancreaticoduodenal: artery
posterior paracentral: gyrus
posterior parietal: artery
posterior parolfactory: sulcus
posterior parotid: veins
posterior pelvic: exenteration

posterior perforated: substance
posterior pericallosal: vein
posterior periventricular: nucleus
posterior peroneal: arteries
posterior polymorphous corneal: dystrophy
posterior primary: division
posterior quadrigeminal: body
posterior renal: segment
posterior sacroiliac: ligaments
posterior sacrosciatic: ligament
posterior sagittal: diameter
posterior scalene: muscle
posterior scapular: nerve
posterior scrotal: branches of perineal artery; branch of internal pudendal artery; nerves; veins
posterior segmental: artery; artery (of kidney)
posterior semicircular: canals
posterior septal: artery of nose; branches of sphenopalatine artery; branch of nose
posterior spinal: artery; sclerosis
posterior spinocerebellar: tract
posterior sternoclavicular: ligament
posterior subcapsular: cataract
posterior superior: fissure
posterior superior alveolar: artery; branches of maxillary nerve
posterior superior iliac: spine
posterior superior lateral nasal: branches of maxillary nerve; branches of pterygopalatine ganglion
posterior superior medial nasal: branches of maxillary nerve; branches of pterygopalatine ganglion
posterior supraclavicular: nerve
posterior talar articular: surface (of calcaneus)
posterior talocalcaneal: ligament
posterior talofibular: ligament
posterior talotibial: ligament
posterior tegmental: decussation
posterior temporal: artery; branch of middle cerebral artery
posterior thalamic: radiation

posterior thoracic: nerve; nucleus
posterior tibial: artery; lymph node; muscle; node; veins
posterior tibial recurrent: artery
posterior tibiofibular: ligament
posterior tibiotalar: ligament; part of deltoid ligament; part of medial ligament of ankle joint
posterior tooth: form
posterior transverse temporal: gyrus
posterior trigeminothalamic: tract
posterior tympanic: artery
posterior urethral: valves
posterior vaginal: hernia
posterior vestibular: branch of vestibulocochlear artery
posteroanterior: projection
posterolateral: fissure; fontanelle; groove; nucleus; sulcus; thoracotomy; tract
posterolateral central: arteries
posteromedial: nucleus
posteromedial central: arteries
posteromedial frontal: branch of callosomarginal artery
posteruption: cuticle
postextrasystolic: pause
postextrasystolic T: wave
postganglionic: fibers
postganglionic motor: neuron
postganglionic nerve: fiber
postgastrectomy: syndrome
postglenoid: foramen
posthemiplegic: athetosis; chorea
posthemorrhagic: anemia
posthepatitic: cirrhosis
posthippocampal: fissure
posthypnotic: amnesia; psychosis; suggestion
posthypoglycemic: hyperglycemia
posticus: palsy; paralysis
postinfarction ventricular septal: defect
postinfectious: bradycardia; myelitis; polyneuritis; psychosis
post-kala azar dermal: leishmanoid
postlaminar: part of intraocular part of optic nerve
postlingual: deafness; fissure
post–lumbar puncture: syndrome
postlunate: fissure

postmalaria neurologic: syndrome
post-marketing: surveillance
postmature: infant
postmaturity: syndrome
postmeiotic: phase
postmeningitic: hydrocephalus
postmenopausal: atrophy
postmitotic: phase
postmortem: clot; delivery; examination; hypostasis; livedo; lividity; pustule; rigidity; suggillation; thrombus; tubercle; wart
postmyocardial infarction: pericarditis; syndrome
postnasal: drip
postnatal: life
postnecrotic: cirrhosis
postnormal: occlusion
postobstructive: pneumonia
postoperative: bronchopneumonia; parotiditis; tetany
postoperative pressure: alopecia
postoral: arches
postpalatal: seal
postpalatal seal: area
postpartum: alopecia; amenorrhea; atony; blues; cardiomyopathy; estrus; hemorrhage; hypertension; psychosis; tetanus
postpartum pituitary necrosis: syndrome
postparturient: hemoglobinuria
postperfusion: lung
postpericardiotomy: pericarditis; syndrome
postpharyngeal: space
postphlebitic: syndrome
postprandial: lipemia; pain
postprimary: tuberculosis
postpyloric: sphincter
postpyramidal: fissure
postreduction: phase
postremal: chamber of eyeball
postrenal: albuminuria
postrhinal: fissure
postrubella: syndrome
postsphenoid: bone
poststationary: phase
post–steady: state
post-stenotic: dilation
poststeroid: panniculitis
postsulcal: part of tongue
postsynaptic: membrane
postterm: infant
postthrombotic: syndrome
posttransplant lymphoproliferative: disease

posttraumatic: delirium; dementia; epilepsy; headache; hydrocephalus; neurosis; osteoporosis; pericarditis; psychosis; syndrome
posttraumatic arterial: thrombosis
posttraumatic leptomeningeal: cyst
posttraumatic neck: syndrome
posttraumatic stress: disorder; syndrome
posttussis suction: sound
posttussive: suction
postural: albuminuria; contraction; drainage; hypotension; ischemia; position; reflex; set; syncope; tremor; version; vertigo
postural sway: response
posture: sense
postvaccinal: encephalitis; encephalomyelitis; myelitis
pot: curare
potable: water
Potain: sign
potassium: inhibition
potassium nitrate: paper
potassium sparing: diuretics
potato: nose; tumor of neck
potato dextrose: agar
potential: energy
potential acuity: meter
potentiometric: titration
Pott: abscess; aneurysm; curvature; disease; fracture; gangrene; paralysis; paraplegia
Potter: disease; facies; syndrome; version
Potter-Bucky: diaphragm
Pott puffy: tumor
Potts: anastomosis; clamp; operation
pouch: culture
poultry handler's: disease
poultryman's: itch
Poupart: ligament; line
povidone: iodine
Powassan: encephalitis; virus
powdered: gold; ipecac; opium; stomach
power: failure; injector; point
Pozzi: muscle
P-P: interval
p-p: factor
PQ: interval
PR: enzyme; interval; segment
practical: anatomy; nurse; units
practice: guidelines; parameters
Prader-Willi: syndrome

Prague: maneuver; pelvis
prairie: conjunctivitis; itch
Pratt: dilators; symptom
Prausnitz-Küstner: antibody; reaction
pravastatin: sodium
preanesthetic: medication
preauricular: groove; pit; point; sinus; sulcus
preauricular deep parotid: lymph nodes
preautomatic: pause
preaxillary: line
pre-B: lymphocyte
precancerous: lesion; melanosis of Dubreuilh
precapillary: anastomosis
prececal: lymph nodes
prececocolic: fascia
precentral: area; artery; fissure; gyrus; sulcus
precentral cerebellar: vein
precentral sulcal: artery
precervical: sinus
prechiasmatic: sulcus
prechordal: plate
precipitate: labor
precipitated: calcium carbonate; sulfur
precipitating: antibody; cause
precipitation: curve; test
precipitin: reaction; test
precision: attachment; rest
precocious: pseudopuberty; puberty
precollagenous: fibers
precommissural: bundle; fibers; septum
precommissural septal: area; nucleus
precommunical: segment of anterior cerebral artery; segment of posterior cerebral artery
precommunicating: part of anterior cerebral artery; part of posterior cerebral artery
preconceptual: stage
precordial: electrocardiography; leads
precordial catch: syndrome
precorneal: film
precostal: anastomosis
preculminate: fissure
precuneal: artery; branches (of anterior cerebral artery)
precursory: cartilage
pre-Descemet corneal: dystrophy
predictive: validity; value
predisposing: cause; factors
predorsal: bundle
preejection: period
preepiglottic: space
preexcitation: syndrome
preextraction: record

preferred provider: organization
preformation: theory
prefrontal: area; cortex; leukotomy; lobotomy; veins
preganglionic: fibers
preganglionic motor: neuron
preganglionic nerve: fibers
pregeniculate: nucleus
pregenital: organization; phase
pregnancy: cells; diabetes; gingivitis; hormone; luteoma; tumor
pregnancy-induced: hypertension
pregranulosa: cells
prehyoid: gland
preinfarction: angina; syndrome
preinterparietal: bone
prelaminar: branch of spinal branch of dorsal branch of posterior intercostal artery; part of intraocular part of optic nerve
prelaryngeal: lymph nodes
preliminary: impression
prelingual: deafness
prelogical: mind; thinking
premammary: abscess
premature: alopecia; beat; birth; contact; contraction; delivery; ejaculation; labor; menopause; systole
premature membrane: rupture
premature ovarian: failure
premature senility: syndrome
prematurity: myopia
premaxillary: bone; suture
premeiotic: phase
premenstrual: edema; syndrome; tension
premenstrual dysphoric: disorder
premenstrual salivary: syndrome
premenstrual tension: syndrome
premitotic: phase
premolar: tooth
premotor: area; cortex; syndrome
prenatal: diagnosis; life; screening
prenodular: fissure
Prentice: rule
preoccipital: notch
pre-oedipal: phase
preoperative: record
preoptic: area; region
preoral: gut
prepancreatic: artery
prepapillary: sphincter

prepared: chalk; ipecacuanha; suet
prepared mutton: tallow
prepatellar: bursa; bursitis
prepatent: period
prepericardial: lymph nodes
prepiriform: gyrus
prepontine: cistern
preprostate urethral: sphincter
preprostatic: part of male urethra; sphincter
preputial: calculus; glands; sac
prepyloric: sphincter; vein
prepyramidal: fissure; tract
prerectal: lithotomy
prereduction: phase
prerenal: albuminuria
pre-Rolandic: artery
prerubral: field; nucleus
presacral: anesthesia; fascia; nerve; neurectomy; sympathectomy
presenile: dementia
presenile spontaneous: gangrene
presenting: symptom
preseptal: cellulitis
presomite: embryo
presphenoid: bone
presplenic: fold
pressor: amine; base; fibers; nerve; substance
pressoreceptive: mechanism
pressoreceptor: nerve; reflex; system
pressure: alopecia; amaurosis; anesthesia; atrophy; collapse; dressing; epiphysis; gangrene; palsy; paralysis; plethysmograph; pneumothorax; point; reversal; sense; sore; stasis; ulcer; urticaria; waveform
pressure-controlled: respirator; ventilation
pressure pulse: differentiation
pressure-support: ventilation
pressure-volume: index
pre–steady: state
presternal: notch; region
prestriate: area
presulcal: part of tongue
presumed ocular: histoplasmosis
presumptive: region
presynaptic: membrane
presystolic: gallop; murmur; thrill
pretectal: area; nuclei; region
pretectoolivary: fibers
preterm: infant
preterm membrane: rupture
pretibial: fever; myxedema

pretracheal: fascia; layer of cervical fascia; lymph nodes
preventive: dentistry; dose; medicine; treatment
prevertebral: fascia; ganglia; layer of cervical fascia; lymph nodes; part of vertebral artery
previllous: chorion; embryo
Pribnow: box
Price-Jones: curve
prickle: cell
prickle cell: layer
prickly: heat
primal: repression; scene
primaquine: sensitivity
primary: adhesion; aerodontalgia; alcohol; aldosteronism; amenorrhea; amputation; amyloidosis; anesthetic; atelectasis; bronchus; bubo; carcinoma; cardiomyopathy; caries; cementum; center of ossification; choana; coccidioidomycosis; color; complex; constriction; curvature of vertebral column; dementia; dentin; dentition; deviation; digestion; digit of foot; disease; drives; dysmenorrhea; fissure of cerebellum; gain; gout; hair; hemochromatosis; hemorrhage; hydrocephalus; hyperoxaluria and oxalosis; hyperparathyroidism; hypertension; hyperthyroidism; hypogammaglobulinemia; hypogonadism; impression; irritant; lymphedema; lysosomes; megaureter; mesoderm; metabolism; metabolite; methemoglobinemia; narcissism; neurasthenia; nodule; nondisjunction; oocyte; organizer; palate; pentosuria; point of ossification; process; proteose; pyoderma; radiation; rays; reaction; reinforcement; rejection; screw-worm; sensation; sequestrum; shock; sodium phosphate; spermatocyte; structure; syphilis; telangiectasia; tooth; tuberculosis; union; villus; vitreous
primary adrenocortical: insufficiency
primary amebic: meningoencephalitis

primary atypical: pneumonia
primary biliary: cirrhosis
primary brain: vesicle
primary carnitine: deficiency
primary dental: lamina
primary dried: yeast
primary dye: test
primary egg: membrane
primary embryonic: cell
primary erythroblastic: anemia
primary extrapulmonary: coccidioidomycosis
primary generalized: epilepsy
primary herpetic: gingivostomatitis; stomatitis
primary idiopathic macular: atrophy
primary immune: response
primary interatrial: foramen
primary irritant: dermatitis
primary labial: groove
primary lateral: sclerosis
primary macular: atrophy of skin
primary medical: care
primary myeloid: metaplasia
primary neuroendocrine: carcinoma of the skin
primary neuronal: degeneration
primary ossification: center
primary ovarian: follicle
primary pigmentary: degeneration of retina
primary progressive cerebellar: degeneration
primary pulmonary: lobule
primary refractory: anemia
primary renal: calculus
primary renal tubular: acidosis
primary sclerosing: cholangitis
primary senile: dementia
primary sex: characters
primary skin: graft
primary visual: area; cortex
primer: extension
primitive: aorta; chorion; furrow; groove; gut; knot; meninx; node; palate; pit; ridge; streak
primitive costal: arches
primitive neuroectodermal: tumor
primitive perivisceral: cavity
primitive reticular: cell
primordial: cartilage; cell; cyst; dwarfism; gigantism; kidney
primordial germ: cell
primordial ovarian: follicle
princeps cervicis: artery
princeps pollicis: artery
Princeteau: tubercle

principal: artery of thumb; focus; piece; plane; point
principal olivary: nucleus
principal optic: axis
principal sensory: nucleus of trigeminal nerve; nucleus of the trigeminus
Pringle: disease
Prinzmetal: angina
prion: protein
prior: probability
prism: diopter
prism cover: test
prism vergence: test
prison fever: typhus
private: antigens; blood group; hospital; nurse
private duty: nurse
privet: cough
privileged: site
proacrosomal: granules
proactive: inhibition
probability: curve; sample
probe: gorget; patency; syringe
problem-oriented: record
procentriole: organizer
procerus: muscle
process: schizophrenia
prochordal: plate
procursive: chorea; epilepsy
prodromal: period; stage
prodromic: sign
product: inhibition
productive: inflammation; peritonitis; pleurisy
product-moment: correlation
Profeta: law
proficiency: samples; testing
profile: record
profound: hypothermia
profunda brachii: artery
profunda femoris: artery; vein
progestational: hormone
progesterone: receptor; unit
progesterone challenge: test
programmable: hearing aid
programmed cell: death
progress: curve
progressive: cataract; cleavage; lipodystrophy; processes; staining; vaccinia
progressive bacterial synergistic: gangrene
progressive bulbar: palsy; paralysis
progressive cerebellar: tremor
progressive cerebral: poliodystrophy
progressive choroidal: atrophy
progressive circumscribed cerebral: atrophy

progressive emphysematous: necrosis
progressive familial: scleroderma
progressive hypertrophic: polyneuropathy
progressive infantile spinal muscular: atrophy
progressive multifocal: leukoencephalopathy
progressive muscular: atrophy
progressive outer retinal: necrosis
progressive pigmentary: dermatosis
progressive spinal: amyotrophy
progressive spinal muscular: atrophy
progressive subcortical: encephalopathy
progressive supranuclear: palsy
progressive tapetochoroidal: dystrophy
projectile: vomiting
projection: angiogram; fibers; perimeter; system
projective: identification; test
prolactin: cell; unit
prolactin-inhibiting: factor
prolactin-producing: adenoma
proliferating: pleurisy
proliferating cell nuclear: antigen
proliferating systematized: angioendotheliomatosis
proliferating tricholemmal: cyst
proliferation: cyst; therapy
proliferative: arthritis; bronchiolitis; choroiditis; dermatitis; fasciitis; gingivitis; glomerulonephritis; inflammation; intimitis; myositis; retinopathy
proligerous: disk; membrane
prolonged: pregnancy
prolonged action: tablet
prometaphase: banding
prominent: heel
promontorial common iliac: nodes
promoting: agent
prompt insulin zinc: suspension
pronator: reflex; ridge; tuberosity
pronator: muscle
pronator quadratus: muscle
pronator teres: muscle; syndrome
prone: position

pronephric: duct; tubule
proof: spirit
propagated: thrombus
proparathyroid: hormone
proper: fasciculi; ligament of ovary; membrane of semicircular duct; substance
proper cochlear: artery
properdin: factor B; factor D; system
properitoneal inguinal: hernia
proper palmar digital: arteries; nerves
proper plantar digital: artery; nerves
property: emergence
prophylactic: membrane; odontotomy; treatment
proportional: counter; limit
proportional assist: ventilation
proportionate: dwarfism; infantilism
proprietary: hospital; medicine
proprioceptive: mechanism; reflexes; sensibility
proprioceptive-oculocephalic: reflex
prosecretion: granules
prosector's: tubercle; wart
proserum prothrombin conversion: accelerator
prospective: fate
prostate: gland
prostate-specific: antigen
prostatic: adenoma; branches of inferior vesical artery; branches of middle rectal artery; calculus; catheter; ducts; ductules; fluid; massage; sheath; sinus; urethra; utricle
prostatic intraepithelial: neoplasia
prostatic (nervous): plexus
prostaticovesical venous: plexus
prostatic venous: plexus
prosthetic: dentistry; group; valves
prostomial: mesoderm
protamine zinc: insulin
protease: inhibitor
protection: test
protective: block; colloid; protein; spectacles; zone
protective laryngeal: reflex
protein: factor; fever; malnutrition; metabolism; quotient; shock; synthesis
protein-bound: iodine
protein-bound iodine: test
protein-losing: enteropathy
protein shock: therapy

proteoglycan: aggregate
Proteus: syndrome
prothoracic: glands
prothrombin: accelerator; test; time
prothrombin and proconvertin: test
protochordal: knot
protodiastolic: gallop
proton: pump
proton pump: inhibitor
protopathic: sensibility
protoplasmic: astrocyte; astrocytoma; movement
prototrophic: strains
protozoan: cyst
protruded: disk
protruding: ear; teeth
protrusive: excursion; occlusion; position; record; relation
protrusive jaw: relation
protuberant: abdomen
proud: flesh
Proust: law; space
provisional: callus; cortex; denture; ligature; prosthesis; restoration
provocation: typhoid
provocative: test
provocative Wassermann: test
Prowazek: bodies
Prowazek-Greeff: bodies
proximal: border of nail; caries; centriole; contact; part of prostate; part of prostatic urethra; phalanx of foot; phalanx of hand
proximal deep inguinal: lymph node
proximal femoral focal: deficiency
proximal interphalangeal: joints
proximal medial striate: arteries
proximal myotonic: myopathy
proximal radioulnar: articulation; joint
proximal spiral: septum
proximal splenorenal: shunt
proximal tibiofibular: joint
proximal urethral: sphincter
proximate: cause; principle
prozone: reaction
prune: belly
prune-belly: syndrome
prune-juice: expectorant; sputum
pruritic urticarial: papules and plaques of pregnancy
Prussak: fibers; pouch; space
Prussian blue: stain
PSA: velocity

psalterial: cord
psammoma: bodies
psammomatous: meningioma
pseudo: psychosis
pseudo-: hemianopia
pseudoachondroplastic spondyloepiphysial: dysplasia
pseudoanaphylactic: shock
pseudobulbar: paralysis
pseudocholinesterase: deficiency
pseudochylous: ascites
pseudocoarctation of the: aorta
pseudocowpox: virus
pseudoepitheliomatous: hyperplasia
pseudoexfoliation: syndrome
pseudoexfoliative: glaucoma
pseudofusion: beat
pseudo-Gaucher: cell
pseudo-Graefe: phenomenon; sign
pseudo-Hurler: disease; polydystrophy
pseudohypertrophic muscular: dystrophy
pseudolepromatous: leishmaniasis
pseudolymphocytic choriomeningitis: virus
pseudolysogenic: strain
pseudomembranous: bronchitis; colitis; conjunctivitis; enteritis; enterocolitis; gastritis; inflammation
Pseudomonas: osteomyelitis
pseudomucinous: cyst
pseudoneurogenic: bladder
pseudoneurotic: schizophrenia
pseudoosteomalacic: pelvis
pseudoplastic: fluid
pseudorabies: virus
pseudorheumatoid: nodules
pseudosarcomatous: fasciitis
pseudostratified: epithelium
pseudotubercular: yersiniosis
pseudotubular: degeneration
pseudounipolar: cell; neuron
pseudoxanthoma: cell
psi: factor; phenomenon
psittacosis: virus
psittacosis inclusion: bodies
psoas: abscess; margin
psoas major: muscle
psoas minor: muscle
psoatic: part of iliopsoas fascia
psoriatic: arthritis
psoroptic: acariasis
psychedelic: drug; therapy
psychiatric: nosology

psychic: blindness; contagion; determinism; energy; force; impotence; inertia; overtone; seizure; tic; trauma
psychoanalytic: psychiatry; psychotherapy; situation; therapy
psychocardiac: reflex
psychodysleptic: drug
psychogalvanic: reaction; reflex; response
psychogenic: hearing impairment; pain; polydipsia; purpura; seizure; torticollis; tremor; vomiting
psychogenic nocturnal: polydipsia
psychogenic nocturnal polydipsia: syndrome
psychogenic pain: disorder
psychological: tests
psycholytic: drug
psychomotor: epilepsy; retardation; seizure; tests
psychopathic: personality
psychophysiologic: manifestation
psychosensory: aphasia
psychosexual: development; dysfunction
psychosocial: dwarfism
psychosomatic: disorder; medicine
psychotic: disorder; manifestation
psychotomimetic: drug
psychotropic: agent; drug
PTA: stain
PTC: protein
pterygium: syndrome
pterygoid: branch of maxillary artery; branch of posterior deep temporal artery; canal; chest; depression; fissure; fossa; fovea; hamulus; laminae; nerve; notch; pit; plates; process of sphenoid bone; ridge of sphenoid bone; tubercle; tuberosity (of mandible)
pterygoid venous: plexus
pterygomandibular: ligament; raphe; space
pterygomaxillary: fissure; fossa; notch
pterygomeningeal: artery
pterygopalatine: canal; fossa; ganglion; groove; nerves
pterygopharyngeal: part of superior constrictor muscle of pharynx
pterygospinal: ligament
pterygospinous: ligament; process
ptotic: organ

pubic: angle; arch; arteries; body; bone; branch of inferior epigastric artery; branch of inferior epigastric vein; branch of obturator artery; crest; hair; rami; region; spine; symphysis; tubercle
public: antigens; health; hospital
public health: dentistry; nurse
puboanalis: muscle
pubocapsular: ligament
pubococcygeal: muscle
pubococcygeus: muscle
pubofemoral: ligament
puboperinealis: muscle
puboprostatic: ligament; muscle
puboprostaticus: muscle
puborectal: muscle
puborectalis: muscle
pubourethral: triangle
pubovaginal: muscle; operation
pubovaginalis: muscle
pubovesical: ligament (of female); ligament (of male); muscle
pubovesicalis: muscle
Puchtler-Sweat: stain for basement membranes; stain for hemoglobin and hemosiderin
pudding: opium
puddle: sign
pudendal: anesthesia; canal; cleavage; cleft; hematocele; hernia; nerve; sac; slit; ulcer; veins
pudic: nerve
puerile: respiration
puerperal: eclampsia; fever; hemoglobinemia; mastitis; morbidity; period; psychosis; sepsis; septicemia; tetanus
Puestow: procedure
Pulfrich: phenomenon
pulmonary: acinus; adenomatosis; alveolus; amebiasis; anthrax; arc; area; artery; atresia; bleb; branch of autonomic nervous system; branches of pulmonary nerve plexus; bulla; cavity; circulation; cirrhosis; collapse; cone; conus; distomiasis; edema; embolism; emphysema; encephalopathy; fistula; glomangiosis; glomus; groove; hamartoma; heart; hypertension; hypostasis; incompetence; insufficiency; ligament; lymph nodes;

murmur; orifice;
osteoarthropathy; pleura;
pleurisy; pressure; ridges;
schistosomiasis; siderosis;
sinuses; stenosis; sulcus;
talcosis; toilet; transpiration;
trunk; tuberculosis;
tularemia; valve; veins;
ventilation
pulmonary alveolar:
microlithiasis; proteinosis
pulmonary artery:
anastomosis; aneurysm;
atresia; banding; catheter
pulmonary capillary wedge:
pressure
pulmonary dysmaturity:
syndrome
pulmonary (nervous): plexus
pulmonic: plague;
regurgitation; tularemia;
valve
pulmonocoronary: reflex
pulp: abscess; amputation;
atrophy; calcification;
calculus; canal; cavity;
cavity of crown; chamber;
horn; nodule; polyp;
pressure; stone; test
pulpal: wall
pulpar: cell
pulpit: spectacles
pulpless: tooth
pulsatile: hematoma
pulsatility: index
pulsating: empyema;
metastases; neurasthenia
pulse: curve; deficit;
generator; granuloma;
oximetry; period; pressure;
rate; sequence; therapy;
wave
pulse-chase: experiment
pulsed: laser
pulsed dye: laser
pulsed-field gel:
electrophoresis
pulse-field gel: electrophoresis
pulse height: analyzer
pulseless: disease
pulseless electrical: activity
pulse wave: duration
pulsion: diverticulum
pulvinar: nuclei
pump: failure; lung
pumped: laser
punch: biopsy; grafts
punchdrunk: syndrome
punctate: basophilia; cataract;
hemorrhage; hyalosis;
keratitis; keratoderma;
parotiditis; retinitis
punctuation: codon
puncture: diabetes; wound
pupillary: axis; block; border
of iris; distance; margin of

iris; membrane; reflex; ruff;
zone
pupillary block: glaucoma
pupillary light-near:
dissociation
pupillary-skin: reflex
pupillotonic: pseudotabes
pure: absence; aphasias; color;
culture
pure autonomic: failure
pure random: drift
pure red cell: anemia; aplasia
pure tone: audiogram
pure-tone: audiometer;
average
purified: cotton; ozokerite;
water
purified placental: protein
**purified protein derivative
of:** tuberculin
purine: base; bodies
purine-free: diet
purine-restricted: diet
Purkinje: cells; conduction;
corpuscles; effect; fibers;
figures; images; network;
phenomenon; shift; system
Purkinje cell: layer
Purkinje-Sanson: images
Purmann: method
pursed lips: breathing
purse-string: corepexy;
instrument; suture
Purtscher: disease;
retinopathy
purulent: conjunctivitis;
cyclitis; encephalitis;
inflammation; ophthalmia;
pericarditis; pleurisy;
pneumonia; retinitis;
synovitis
pus: basin; cell; corpuscle;
tube
push-back: procedure
pustular: blepharitis;
melanosis; miliaria;
psoriasis; syphilid
Putnam-Dana: syndrome
putrescent: pulp
putrid: bronchitis
Putti-Platt: operation;
procedure
putty: kidney
Puumala: virus
PVA: fixative
PVM: virus
pyelonephritic: kidney
pyelotubular: reflux
pyelovenous: backflow
pyemic: abscess; embolism
pyloric: antrum; artery; branch
of anterior vagal trunk;
canal; cap; constriction;
glands; incompetence;
insufficiency; lymph nodes;

orifice; part of stomach;
sphincter; stenosis; vein
pylorus-preserving:
pancreaticoduodenectomy
Pym: fever
pyogenic: arthritis; bacterium;
fever; granuloma; infection;
membrane; pachymeningitis;
salpingitis
pyramid: sign
pyramidal: bone; cataract;
cells; eminence; fibers;
fracture; layer; lobe of
thyroid gland; muscle;
muscle of auricle; process of
palatine bone; radiation;
tract; tractotomy
pyramidal auricular: muscle
pyramidal cell: layer
pyramidalis: muscle
pyridoxine: dependency with
seizure
pyriform: apparatus
pyriform aperture: wiring
pyrimidine: base; dimer
pyroligneous: alcohol; spirit;
vinegar
pyrrol: cell
pyrrole: nucleus
pyruvate dehydrogenase:
complex
pyruvate kinase: deficiency
pyruvate oxidation: factor

Q

Q: angle; bands; disks;
enzyme; fever; wave
Q-banding: stain
QR: interval
QRB: interval
QRS: complex; interval
QS$_2$: interval
Q-switched: laser
QT: interval
Q tip: test
quack: medicine
quadrangular: cartilage;
lobule; membrane; space;
therapy
quadrantic: hemianopia;
scotoma
quadrate: ligament; lobe;
lobule; muscle; muscle of
loins; muscle of sole;
muscle of thigh; muscle of
upper lip; part of liver
quadrate pronator: muscle
quadratus: muscle
quadratus femoris: muscle
quadratus lumborum: muscle
quadratus plantae: muscle
quadriceps: muscle of thigh;
reflex
quadriceps femoris: muscle

quadrigeminal: artery; bodies;
cistern; cistern; lamina;
plate; pulse; rhythm
quadrilateral: space
quadripedal extensor: reflex
quadruple: amputation;
rhythm
quail bronchitis: virus
qualitative: alteration;
analysis; trait
quality of: life
quality: control; factor
quality control: chart
Quant: sign
quantal: effect
quantitative: alteration;
analysis; genetics;
hypertrophy; perimetry
quantum: efficiency; limit;
mottle; requirement; theory;
yield
Quaranfil: virus
quarantine: period
quartan: fever; malaria;
parasite
quartz: glass
quasi-continuous wave: laser
quaternary: structure; syphilis
quaternary carbon: atom
Quatrefages: angle
Queckenstedt-Stookey: test
Queensland tick: typhus
quellung: phenomenon;
reaction; test
Quénu hemorrhoidal: plexus
Quénu-Muret: sign
Quick: method; test
quick cure: resin
quick-stop: mutant
quiet: iritis; lung
quiet hip: disease
quilted: suture
**quinacrine chromosome
banding:** stain
Quincke: disease; edema;
pulse; puncture; sign
quinhydrone: electrode
quinine carbacrylic: resin
quinine carbacrylic resin:
test
Quinlan: test
quintan: fever
quisqualate: receptor
quorum: sensing
quotidian: fever; malaria

R

ρ: factor
R: antigen; enzyme; factors;
pili; plasmids; wave
R$_f$: value
rabbit: fever; fibroma
rabbit fibroma: virus
rabbit myxoma: virus
rabbitpox: virus

rabies: immunoglobulin; vaccine; vaccine, Flury strain egg-passage; virus; virus, Flury strain; virus, Kelev strain
rabies immune: globulin (human)
raccoon: eyes
racemic: calcium pantothenate
racemose: aneurysm; gland; hemangioma
rachitic: diet; pelvis; rosary; scoliosis
racial: melanoderma
racket: amputation; nail
racquet: hypha
Radford: nomogram
radial: acceleration; artery; border of forearm; bursa; clubhand; eminence of wrist; fossa of humerus; groove; immunodiffusion; keratotomy; nerve; notch; part of posterior compartment of forearm; phenomenon; pulse; reflex; scar; tuberosity; veins
radial aplasia-thrombocytopenia: syndrome
radial collateral: artery; ligament; ligament of elbow joint; ligament of wrist joint
radial flexor: muscle of wrist
radial growth: phase
radial index: artery
radialis indicis: artery
radial recurrent: artery
radial sclerosing: lesion
radial styloid: tendovaginitis
radial tunnel: syndrome
radiant: energy; heat; intensity; layer
radiate: crown; layer of tympanic membrane; ligament; ligament of head of rib; ligament of wrist
radiate carpal: ligament
radiate sternocostal: ligaments
radiation: anemia; biology; biophysics; burn; caries; cataract; chimera; dermatosis; myelitis; myelopathy; oncologist; oncology; physics; pneumonitis; poisoning; risks; sickness; therapy
radiation weighting: factor
radical: cystectomy; hysterectomy; mastectomy; mastoidectomy; operation for hernia; pericardiectomy
radical neck: dissection
radicular: abscess; cyst; fila; pulp; syndrome

radioactive: atom; constant; cyanocobalamin; equilibrium; iodine; isotope; probe; thyroxine
radioactive iodide uptake: test
radioallergosorbent: test
radiobicipital: reflex
radiocarpal: articulation; joint
radiochemical: purity
radiofrequency: pulse
radiographic: pelvimetry
radiographic parallel line: shadow
radioimmunosorbent: test
radioiodinated serum: albumin
radioisotopic: purity
radiolabeled: thyroxine
radiologic: anatomy; enteroclysis; sphincter
radionuclide: angiocardiography; angiography; cisternography; generator; ventriculography
radionuclide ejection: fraction
radionuclidic: purity
radioperiosteal: reflex
radiopharmaceutical: chemistry; purity; synovectomy
radioreceptor: assay
radiotelemetering: capsule
radiotherapy: localization
radioulnar: disk; syndesmosis
radium: emanation
radium beam: therapy
Raeder paratrigeminal: syndrome
ragpicker's: disease
ragsorter's: disease
Rahe-Holmes social readjustment rating: scale
Rahn-Otis: sample
RAI: test
railroad: nystagmus
rainbow: symptom
Rainey: corpuscles
Raji: cell
Raji cell radioimmune: assay
Ramachandran: plot
Raman: effect; spectrum
Rambourg chromic acid-phosphotungstic acid: stain
Rambourg periodic acid-chromic methenamine-silver: stain
Ramsay Hunt: syndrome
Ramsden: ocular
Ramstedt: operation
Randall: plaques
Randall stone: forceps
random: coil; mating; mechanism; sample; sampling; variable; waves

randomized controlled: trial
random mating: equilibrium
random pattern: flap
Raney: alloy; catalyst; nickel
range of: accommodation; convergence
Ranikhet: disease
ranine: anastomosis; artery; tumor
rank-difference: correlation
Ranke: angle; complex; formula
Rankin: clamp
Rankine: scale
Ransohoff: sign
Ranvier: crosses; disks; plexus; segment
Raoult: law
raphe: nuclei
raphespinal: fibers
rapid: canities; decompression; film changer
rapid eye: movements
rapid eye movement: sleep
rapidly progressive: glomerulonephritis
rapid plasma reagin: test
Rapoport: test
Rapoport-Luebering: shunt
Rappaport: acinus; classification
rare: earths
rare-earth: screen
rare earth: elements; metal
ras: oncogene
Rasmussen: aneurysm; syndrome
raspberry: tongue
Rastelli: operation
rat-bite: disease; fever
rate: constants; equation; meter
Rathke: bundles; diverticulum; pocket; pouch
Rathke cleft: cyst
Rathke pouch: tumor
ratio: scale
rational: formula; therapy
rat mite: dermatitis
Rau: process
Rauber: layer
Rauscher: virus
Rauscher leukemia: virus
Ravius: process
raw: score
ray: fungus; therapeutics
Rayer: disease
Rayleigh: equation; test
Raynaud: disease; phenomenon; sign; syndrome
R-banding: stain
reaction: center; formation; time
reactivation: tuberculosis

reactive: arthritis; astrocyte; cell; changes; depression; hyperemia; schizophrenia
reactive airway: disease
reactive attachment: disorder
reactive perforating: collagenosis
reading-frame-shift: mutation
reaginic: antibody
REAL: classification
real: focus; image
reality: adaptation; principle; testing
real-time: echocardiography; ultrasonography
Réaumur: scale
rebound: phenomenon; tenderness
rebreathing: anesthesia; technique
Rebuck skin window: technique
recall: bias
Récamier: operation
recapitulation: theory
receiver operating: characteristic
receiver operating characteristic: curve
receptive: aphasia
receptor: protein; site
recessive: character; inheritance; trait
reciprocal: anchorage; arm; beat; bigeminy; forces; inhibition; innervation; rhythm; transfusion; translocation
reciprocating: rhythm
reciprocity: law
Recklinghausen: disease of bone
reclotting: phenomenon
recognition: time
recoil: atom; wave
recombinant: DNA; strain; vector
recombinant human: interleukin 11
recombination: fraction
recombinatorial: repair
recommended daily: allowance
reconstructive: mammaplasty; psychotherapy; surgery
record: base; linkage; rim
recovery: score; stroke
recreational: drug
recrudescent: typhus
recrudescent typhus: fever
recruiting: response
rectal: alimentation; ampulla; anesthesia; columns; folds; plexuses; reflex; shelf; sinuses; valves; valvotomy
rectal venous: plexus

rectangular: amputation
rectified: spirit; tar oil; turpentine oil
rectifier: tube
rectocardiac: reflex
rectococcygeal: muscle
rectococcygeus: muscle
rectolabial: fistula
rectolaryngeal: reflex
rectosacral: fascia
rectosigmoid: junction; sphincter
rectourethral: fistula; muscles
rectouterine: fold; muscle; pouch
rectouterinus: muscle
rectovaginal: fistula; septum
rectovaginouterine: pouch
rectovesical: fascia; fistula; fold; muscle; pouch; septum
rectovesicalis: muscle
rectovestibular: fistula
rectovulvar: fistula
rectus: muscle of abdomen; muscle of thigh; sheath
rectus abdominis: muscle
rectus capitis anterior: muscle
rectus capitis lateralis: muscle
rectus capitis posterior major: muscle
rectus capitis posterior minor: muscle
rectus femoris: muscle
recurrence: rate; risk
recurrent: abortion; albuminuria; appendicitis; artery; artery of Heubner; branch of spinal nerves; caries; encephalopathy; fever; hypopyon; jaundice of pregnancy; nerve; polyserositis; stricture
recurrent aphthous: stomatitis; ulcers
recurrent central: retinitis
recurrent corneal: erosion
recurrent herpetic: stomatitis
recurrent interosseous: artery
recurrent laryngeal: nerve
recurrent meningeal: branch of spinal nerves; nerve
recurrent pyogenic: cholangitis
recurrent radial: artery
recurrent respiratory: papillomatosis
recurrent scarring: aphthae
recurrent ulcerative: stomatitis
recurrent ulnar: artery
recurring digital: fibroma of childhood
red: atrophy; corpuscle; degeneration; fever; fibers; gum; half-moon; hepatization; induration; infarct; lead; muscle; neuralgia; nucleus; oil; precipitate; pulp; pulp of spleen; reflex; sweat; thrombus; tide; vision; wine
red blood: cell
red blood cell: cast
red bone: marrow
red cell: cast
red cell adherence: phenomenon; test
red imported fire: ant
redox: electrode; indicator; potential; system
red oxide of: lead
red pulp: cords
red strawberry: tongue
reduced: eye; glutathione; hematin; hemoglobin
reduced enamel: epithelium
reduced interarch: distance
reducible: hernia
reducing: diet; enzyme; sugar; valve
5α-reductase: inhibitors
reduction: deformity; division; mammaplasty; nucleus; phase
reduction left: ventriculoplasty
reduplicated: cataract
red, white, and blue: sign
Reed: cell
Reed-Frost: model; theory of epidemics
reed instrument: theory
Reed-Sternberg: cell
reedy: nail
re-entrant: mechanism
reentry: phenomenon; theory
Rees-Ecker: fluid
refeeding: gynecomastia
reference: electrode; method; values
referred: pain; sensation
Refetoff: syndrome
reflected: colors; light; ray
reflected inguinal: ligament
reflecting: retinoscope
reflection: coefficient
reflex: angina; arc; asthma; control; cough; dyspepsia; epilepsy; headache; incontinence; inhibition; iridoplegia; ligament; movement; otalgia; symptom; tachycardia; therapy
reflex detrusor: contraction
reflex neurogenic: bladder
reflexogenic: pressosensitivity; zone
reflex sympathetic: dystrophy
reflux: esophagitis; nephropathy; otitis media
refracted: light
refracting: angle of a prism
refractive: amblyopia; ametropia; index; keratoplasty; keratotomy
refractive accommodative: esotropia
refractory: anemia; cast; flask; investment; period; period of electronic pacemaker; rickets; state
refrigeration: anesthesia
Refsum: disease; syndrome
Regaud: fixative
regenerative: polyp
regional: anatomy; anesthesia; enteritis; enterocolitis; hypothermia; lymphadenitis; perfusion
regional granulomatous: lymphadenitis
registered: nurse
regressing atypical: histiocytosis
regression: analysis
regression of the: mean
regressive: staining
regressive-reconstructive: approach
regular: astigmatism; insulin
regular insulin: injection
regulator: gene
regulatory: albuminuria; sequence
regurgitant: fraction; murmur
regurgitation: jaundice
Rehfuss: method
Rehfuss stomach: tube
Reichel-Pólya stomach: procedure
Reichert: cartilage
Reichert cochlear: recess
Reichert-Meissl: number
Reichstein: compound; substance
Reid base: line
Reifenstein: syndrome
Reil: ansa; band; ribbon; triangle
Reinecke: salt
reinfection: tuberculosis
reinforced: anchorage
Reinke: crystalloids; space
Reinsch: test
Reis-Bücklers corneal: dystrophy
Reisseisen: muscles
Reissner: fiber; membrane
Reiter: disease; syndrome; test
relapsing: appendicitis; fever; malaria; perichondritis; polychondritis
relapsing febrile nodular nonsuppurative: panniculitis
relational: threshold
relative: accommodation; dehydration; humidity; immunity; incompetence; leukocytosis; polycythemia; risk; scotoma; sensitivity; specificity; viscosity
relative afferent pupillary: defect
relative biologic: effectiveness
relative molecular: mass
relative refractory: period
relaxation: atelectasis; response; suture; time
release: phenomenon
released: substance
releasing: factors; hormone
reliability: coefficient
relief: area; chamber
relocation: test
REM: syndrome
Remak: fibers; ganglia; plexus; reflex; sign
Remak nuclear: division
REM behavior: disorder
reminiscent: aura
remittent: fever; malaria
remittent malarial: fever
remote: memory
remote afterloading: brachytherapy
removable: bridge
removable partial: denture
renal: adenocarcinoma; agenesis; amyloidosis; artery; ballottement; branch of lesser splanchnic nerve; branch of vagus nerve; calculus; capsulotomy; carcinosarcoma; cast; colic; collar; columns; corpuscle; cortex; diabetes; epistaxis; failure; fascia; ganglia; glycosuria; hematuria; hemorrhage; hypertension; hypoplasia; impression on liver; impression of spleen; infantilism; insufficiency; labyrinth; lobe; medulla; nanism; osteitis fibrosa; osteodystrophy; papilla; pelvis; pyramids; reflex; retinopathy; rickets; segments; sinus; surface of spleen; surface of suprarenal gland; threshold; transplantation; veins
renal cell: carcinoma
renal cortical: adenoma; lobule; scan
renal fibrocystic: osteosis
renal (nervous): plexus
renal papillary: necrosis

renal portal: system
renal-splanchnic: steal
renal-splenic venous: shunt
renal tubular: acidosis
Renaut: body
Rendu-Osler-Weber: syndrome
reniform: pelvis
renin-angiotensin: system
renin-angiotensin-aldosterone: system
renovascular: hypertension
Renpenning: syndrome
Renshaw: cells
REO: virus
reovirus-like: agent
repair: enzyme
reparative: dentin; granuloma
reparative giant cell: granuloma
reperfusion: injury
repetition: rate; time
repetition-compulsion: principle
repetitive: DNA
repetitive strain: disorders
repetitive stress: disorders
replacement: bone; fibrosis; therapy
replica: plating
replication: site
replicative: form; intermediate
reportable: disease
reporting: bias
repressible: enzyme
repressor: gene
reproductive: assimilation; cycle; nucleus; system
required arch: length
resectoscope: electrode; sheath
reserve: air; force
reserve tooth: germ
reservoir: bag; host
resident: physician
residual: abscess; affinity; air; body; body of Regaud; capacity; cleft; cyst; error; inhibition; inhibitor; lumen; ridge; schizophrenia; urine; volume
residual ovary: syndrome
resin: cement
resistance: factors; form; plasmids; pyrometer; thermometer
resistance-inducing: factor
resistance-transfer: factor
resistance-transferring: episomes
resistant ovary: syndrome
resistive: movement
resolution: acuity
resolving: power
resonance: theory of hearing
resonant: frequency

resorcinol: test
resorption: atelectasis; lacunae
respirable: aerosols
respiratory: acidosis; airway; alkalosis; apparatus; arrhythmia; ataxia; bronchioles; burst; capacity; center; chain; coefficient; enzyme; epithelium; failure; frequency; gating; hippus; inhibitor; insufficiency; lobule; metabolism; metal; mucosa; murmur; pause; pigments; poison; pulse; quotient; rate; region of mucosa of nasal cavity; region of tunica mucosa of nose; scleroma; sounds; system; therapy; tract
respiratory dead: space
respiratory distress: syndrome of the newborn; syndrome type II
respiratory enteric orphan: virus
respiratory exchange: ratio
respiratory minute: volume
respiratory syncytial: virus
respirophasic: pain
respondent: behavior; conditioning
response: bias; hierarchy
response-produced: cues
rest: area; bite; body; nitrogen; pain; position; relation; seat
restiform: body; eminence
resting: cell; length; saliva; stage; tremor
resting tidal: volume
resting wandering: cell
rest jaw: relation
restless: legs
restless legs: syndrome
Reston: virus
restorative: dentistry
restorative dental: materials
restored: cycle
restrained: beam
restriction: endonuclease; enzyme; map; methylation; site
restriction fragment length: polymorphism
restriction length: polymorphism
restriction-site: polymorphism
restrictive: cardiomyopathy
restructured: cell
rest vertical: dimension
retained: menstruation; placenta
retained products of: conception
retarded: dentition

rete: cords; cyst of ovary; pegs; ridge
retention: area; cyst; form; groove; jaundice; point; polyp; suture; vomiting
retentive: arm
retentive circumferential clasp: arm
retentive fulcrum: line
reticular: cartilage; cell; degeneration; fibers; formation; lamina; layer of corium; membrane of spinal organ; nuclei of the brainstem; nuclei of medulla oblongata; nuclei of mesencephalon; nuclei of pons; nucleus of thalamus; substance; tissue
reticular activating: system
reticular erythematous: mucinosis
reticularis: cell
reticulated: bone; corpuscle
reticuloendothelial: cell; system
reticulohistiocytic: granuloma
reticulonodular: pattern
reticulospinal: tract
reticulum cell: sarcoma
retinal: adaptation; blood vessels; camera; cones; detachment; disparity; dysplasia; embolism; fold; image; migraine
retinal anlage: tumor
retinoic acid: receptor
retinoid X: receptor
retinol-binding: protein
retractile: testis
retraction: pockets; syndrome
retroactive: inhibition
retroadductor: space
retroauricular: fold; lymph nodes
retrobulbar: abscess; anesthesia; fat; neuritis
retrocalcaneal: bursa
retrocaval: ureter
retrocecal: abscess; lymph nodes; recess
retrocedent: gout
retrochiasmatic: area
retrocochlear: hearing loss
retrocuspid: papilla
retroduodenal: artery; fossa; recess
retroflex: bundle of Meynert; fasciculus
retrogasserian: neurectomy; neurotomy
retrograde: amnesia; aortography; beat; block; cardioplegia; chromatolysis; cystourethrogram; degeneration; ejaculation;

embolism; hernia; intussusception; memory; menstruation; metamorphosis; pyelography; urography
retrograde P: wave
retrograde VA: conduction
retrohyoid: bursa
retroiliac: ureter
retroinguinal: space
retrolental: fibroplasia
retrolenticular: limb of internal capsule; part of internal capsule
retrolentiform: limb of internal capsule
retromammary: mastitis
retromandibular: fossa; process of parotid gland; vein
retromolar: fossa; pad; triangle
retromylohyoid: space
retroperitoneal: fibrosis; hernia; space; veins
retropharyngeal: abscess; lymph nodes; space
retroposterior lateral: nucleus
retropubic: hernia; space
retropyloric: lymph nodes; nodes
retrorectal: lamina of endopelvic fascia; lamina of hypogastric sheath
retrosigmoid: approach
retrospective: falsification
retrosternal: hernia; space
retrotarsal: fold
retroviral: vector
retrozonular: space
retrusive: excursion; occlusion
Rett: syndrome
return: extrasystole
returning: cycle
Retzius: cavity; fibers; gyrus; ligament; space; striae; veins
Reuss: formula; test
Reuss color: tables
reverberating: circuit
Reverdin: graft
reverse: banding; bevel; curve; genetics; mutation; osmosis; transcriptase; transcription
reversed: anaphylaxis; coarctation; peristalsis; shunt
reversed paradoxical: pulse
reversed passive: anaphylaxis
reversed phase: chromatography
reversed Prausnitz-Küstner: reaction
reversed reciprocal: rhythm
reversed-three: sign

reverse Eck: fistula
reverse Kingsley: splint
reverse passive: hemagglutination
reverse pupillary: block
reverse transcriptase polymerase chain: reaction
reverse Trendelenburg: position
reversible: calcinosis; colloid; decortication; hydrocolloid; pulpitis; reaction; shock
Revilliod: sign
Reye: syndrome
Reynolds: number; pentad
Rh: antigens; factor
rhabditiform: larva
rhagiocrine: cell
Rh antigen: incompatibility
Rh blocking: test
Rh$_o$(D): immunoglobulin
RH$_o$(D) immune: globulin
rhegmatogenous retinal: detachment
Rheinberg: microscope
Rhese: projection
Rhesus: factor
rhesus: disease
rheumatic: arteritis; carditis; chorea; disease; endocarditis; fever; pericarditis; pneumonia; valvulitis
rheumatic heart: disease
rheumatoid: arteritis; arthritis; disease; factors; nodules; pocket; spondylitis
rhinal: fissure; sulcus
rhizomelic: chondrodysplasia punctata; dwarfism
Rh null: syndrome
rho: factor
Rhodesian: trypanosomiasis
rhombencephalic: isthmus; tegmentum
rhombencephalic gustatory: nucleus
rhombic: grooves; lip
rhomboid: fossa; impression; ligament
rhomboidal: sinus
rhomboid major: muscle
rhomboid minor: muscle
rhonchal: fremitus
rhus: dermatitis
Rhus toxicodendron: antigen
Rhus venenata: antigen
rhythm: method
rhythmic: chorea
rib: spreader
Ribas-Torres: disease
ribbon: arch
ribbon arch: appliance
Ribes: ganglion
riboflavin: deficiency; unit

ribosomal: RNA
ribosome-lamella: complex
Ribot: law of memory
Ricco: law
rice: body; diet; disease; itch; starch
rice-field: fever
rice-Tween: agar
rice-water: stool
Richards-Rundle: syndrome
Richter: hernia; syndrome
Richter-Monro: line
ricin-blocked: antibody
rickettsia: vaccine, attenuated
Rickles: test
Rida: virus
Riddoch: phenomenon
Rideal-Walker: coefficient; method
Ridell: operation
rider's: bone; bursa; leg; muscles
ridge: extension; relation; resorption
riding: embolism
Ridley: circle; sinus
Riedel: disease; lobe; struma; thyroiditis
Rieder: cells; lymphocyte
Rieder cell: leukemia
Riegel: pulse
Rieger: anomaly; syndrome
Riehl: melanosis
Rift Valley: fever
Rift Valley fever: virus
Riga-Fede: disease
right: atrium of heart; auricle; border of heart; branch; branch of hepatic artery proper; branch of portal vein; bundle of atrioventricular bundle; crus of atrioventricular bundle; crus of diaphragm; duct of caudate lobe of liver; heart; liver; lobe; lobe of liver; margin of heart; part of diaphragmatic surface of liver; part of liver; ventricle
right angle: clamp
right anterior lateral hepatic: segment [VI]
right atrial: branch of right coronary artery
right atrioventricular: orifice; valve
right auricular: appendage
right axis: deviation
right colic: artery; flexure; lymph nodes; vein
right coronary: artery
right descending pulmonary: artery
right fibrous: trigone (of heart)

right flexural: artery
right gastric: artery; lymph nodes; vein
right gastroepiploic: artery; lymph nodes; vein
right gastroomental: artery; lymph nodes; vein
right heart: bypass
right hepatic: artery; duct; veins
right inferior pulmonary: vein
righting: reflexes
right lateral: division of liver
(right/left): ventricles of heart
(right and left) fibrous: rings of heart
right or left lateral decubitus: film
right/left pulmonary: surfaces of heart
right lumbar: lymph nodes
right lymphatic: duct
right main: bronchus
right marginal: branch (of right coronary artery)
right medial: division of liver
right ovarian: vein
right parasternal: impulses
(right) posterior lateral hepatic: segment [VII]
(right) posterior medial hepatic: segment [VIII]
right pulmonary: artery
right sagittal: fissure
right splicing: junction
right superior intercostal: vein
right superior pulmonary: vein
right suprarenal: vein
right testicular: vein
right-to-left: shunt
right triangular: ligament of liver
right ventricular: failure; hypoplasia
rigid: connector; dysarthria
Riley-Day: syndrome
Rimini: test
Rindfleisch: cells; folds
ring: abscess; chromosome; compound; enhancement; finger; ligament; pessary; scotoma; syringe; test; ulcer of cornea
ringed: hair
Ringer: injection; lactate; solution
ringlike corneal: dystrophy
ring precipitin: test
ring-shaped: placenta
ring-wall: lesion
ringworm: yaws
Rinne: test

Riolan: anastomosis; arc; arcades; bones; bouquet; muscle
Ripault: sign
ripe: cataract
Ripstein: operation
rise: time
risk: factor
Risley rotary: prism
risorius: muscle
Ritgen: maneuver
Rittenhouse-Manogian: procedure
Ritter opening: tetanus
Ritter-Rollet: phenomenon
ritualistic: behavior
Riva-Rocci: sphygmomanometer
river: blindness
Rivero-Carvallo: effect
Rivers: cocktail
Rivière: salt
Rivinus: canals; ducts; gland; incisure; membrane; notch
RNA: enzyme; virus
RNA tumor: viruses
Ro: spatula
Roach: clasp
Roaf: syndrome
Robert: pelvis
Roberts: syndrome
Robertshaw: tube
Robertson: pupil
robertsonian: translocation
Robin: syndrome
Robinow: dwarfism; syndrome
Robinson: catheter; disease; index
Robison: ester
Robison-Embden: ester
Robison ester: dehydrogenase
ROC: curve
Rochelle: salt
rock: oil
rocket: immunoelectrophoresis
Rocky Mountain spotted: fever
Rocky Mountain spotted fever: vaccine
rod: cell of retina; disks; fiber; granule; monochromatism; myopathy; vision
rodent: ulcer
rod nuclear: cell
roentgen: ray; unit
Roesler-Dressler: infarct
Roger: bruit; disease; murmur; reflex
Roger Anderson pin fixation: appliance
Rogers: sphygmomanometer
Rohr: stria
Röhrer: index

Rokitansky: disease; hernia; pelvis
Rokitansky-Aschoff: sinuses
Rokitansky-Küster-Hauser: syndrome
rolandic: epilepsy
Rolandic sulcal: artery
Rolando: angle; area; cells; column; tubercle
Rolando gelatinous: substance
role: conflict
roll: sulfur; tube
Roller: nucleus
roller: bandage
rollerball: electrode
Rolleston: rule
Rollet: stroma
rolling: circle
roll-tube: culture
Roman: fever
Romaña: sign
Romano-Ward: syndrome
Romanowsky blood: stain
Romberg: disease; sign; syndrome; test; trophoneurosis
Römer: test
Rónne nasal: step
R-on-T: phenomenon
roof: nucleus; plate
room: temperature
root: abscess; amputation; apex; avulsion; canal of tooth; caries; dehiscence; filaments; foramen; pulp; resection; resorption; sheath; tip
root canal: file; orifice; plugger; restoration; spreader; therapy; treatment
root caries: index
root end: cyst; granuloma
root-form: implant
rooting: reflex
rope: burn
Ropes: test
Rorschach: test
rosacea-like: tuberculid
Rosai-Dorfman: disease
rosanilin: dyes
Roscoe-Bunsen: law
Rose: position
rose: cold; spots
rose bengal radioactive (^{131}I): test
Rose-Bradford: kidney
Rose cephalic: tetanus
Rosenbach: law; sign; test
Rosenbach-Gmelin: test
Rosenmüller: fossa; gland; node; recess; valve
Rosenthal: canal; fiber; vein
Rosenthaler-Turk: reagent
Roser-Nélaton: line
rosette: test

rosette-forming: cells
Rose-Waaler: test
Ross: cycle; procedure
Ross-Jones: test
Rossolimo: reflex; sign
Ross River: fever; virus
rostral: lamina; layer; neuropore
rostral transtentorial: herniation
rostrate: pelvis
rotary: joint
rotating: anode
rotating anode: tube
rotation: flap; therapy
rotational: axis; nystagmus
rotator: cuff of shoulder; muscle
rotatores: muscles
rotatores cervicis: muscles
rotatores lumborum: muscles
rotatores thoracis: muscles
rotatory: nystagmus; tic
Rotch: sign
rote: learning
Roth: spots
Rothera nitroprusside: test
Rothmund: syndrome
Rothmund-Thomson: syndrome
Rotor: syndrome
Rouget: bulb; muscle
Rouget-Neumann: sheath
rough: colony; line
rough-surfaced endoplasmic: reticulum
Roughton-Scholander: apparatus; syringe
Rougnon-Heberden: disease
rouleaux: formation
round: bur; eminence; fasciculus; foramen; heart; ligament of elbow joint; ligament of femur; ligament of liver; ligament of uterus; pelvis; window
round cell: sarcoma
rounded: atelectasis
round pronator: muscle
round window: membrane
Rous: sarcoma; tumor
Rous-associated: virus
Rous sarcoma: virus
Roussy-Lévy: disease; syndrome
Roux: method; stain
Roux-en-Y: anastomosis; operation
Rovsing: sign
royal: touch
RPR: test
R-R: interval
Rs: virus
RST: segment
Rubarth disease: virus
rubber: dam; pelvis; tissue

rubber-bulb: syringe
rubber dam: clamp
rubber dam clamp: forceps
rubber-shod: clamp
rubbing: alcohol
rubella: cataract; retinopathy; virus
rubella HI: test
rubella virus: vaccine, live
rubeola: virus
Rubin: test
Rubinstein-Taybi: syndrome
Rubner: laws of growth; test
rubrobulbar: tract
rubroolivary: fibers
rubropontine: tract
rubroreticular: fasciculi; tract
rubrospinal: decussation; tract
ruby: spots
Rud: syndrome
Ruffini: corpuscles
rufous: albinism
rugal: columns of vagina
rugger jersey: vertebra
rum: nose
rumination: disorder
Rummel: tourniquet
Rumpel-Leede: phenomenon; sign; test
runaway: pacemaker
Runeberg: formula
runner's: knee
running: time
runt: disease
runting: syndrome
Runyon: classification
Runyon group I: mycobacteria
Runyon group II: mycobacteria
Runyon group III: mycobacteria
Runyon group IV: mycobacteria
rupial: syphilid
ruptured: aneurysm; disk
rural cutaneous: leishmaniasis
Rushton: bodies
Russell: bodies; effect; sign; syndrome; traction
Russell's: viper
Russell's viper: venom
Russell's viper venom clotting: time
Russian: fly; influenza
Russian autumn: encephalitis
Russian autumn encephalitis: virus
Russian spring-summer: encephalitis (Eastern subtype); encephalitis (Western subtype)
Russian spring-summer encephalitis: virus

Russian tick-borne: encephalitis
Rust: disease; phenomenon
rusty: sputum
Ruysch: membrane; muscle; tube; veins
Ryan: stain
ryanodine: receptor
Rye: classification
Ryle: tube

S

σ: factor
S: antigen; factor; peptide; phase; potential; protein; sign of Golden; unit of streptomycin; wave
S$_7$: gallop
S-A: node
saber: shin; tibia
saber-sheath: trachea
Sabia: virus
Sabin: vaccine
Sabin-Feldman dye: test
sabot: heart
Sabouraud: agar; pastils
Sabouraud dextrose: agar
Sabouraud-Noiré: instrument
saccadic: movement
sacciform: recess of distal radioulnar joint; recess of elbow joint
saccular: aneurysm; bronchiectasis; duct; gland; nerve; recess of bony labyrinth; spot
sacculated: pleurisy
Sachs-Georgi: test
sacral: anesthesia; canal; cornu; crest; flexure; flexure of rectum; foramina; ganglia; hiatus; horn; index; kyphosis; lymph nodes; nerves [S1–S5]; part of spinal cord; plexus; promontory; region; triangle; tuberosity; veins; vertebrae [S1–S5]
sacral splanchnic: nerves
sacral venous: plexus
sacred: bone
sacroanterior: position
sacrococcygeal: disk; joint; junction; teratoma
sacrocolpopexy: procedure
sacrodural: ligament
sacrogenital: folds
sacroiliac: articulation; joint
sacropelvic: surface of ilium
sacroposterior: position
sacrosciatic: notch
sacrospinous: ligament
sacrospinous vaginal vault suspension: procedure
sacrotransverse: position

sacrotuberous: ligament
sacrouterine: fold
sacrovaginal: fold
sacrovesical: fold
saddle: back; embolism; head; joint; nose
saddleback: caterpillar
saddle block: anesthesia
sadomasochistic: relationship
Saemisch: section; ulcer
Saenger: macula; operation; sign
Saethre-Chotzen: syndrome
SAF: fixative
safe: sex
safety: lens; spectacles
sagittal: axis; border of parietal bone; crest; fontanelle; groove; line; plane; section; sulcus; suture; synostosis
sagittal split mandibular: osteotomy
sago: spleen
sagulum: nucleus
Saigon: cinnamon
sail: sound
sailor's: skin
Saint: triad
Saint Anthony: dance
Saint Ignatius: itch
Sakaguchi: reaction
Sakurai-Lisch: nodule
sakushu: fever
salaam: attack; convulsions; spasm
Salah sternal puncture: needle
salicylic acid: collodion
saline: agglutinin; purgative; solution; water
Salinem: fever; infection
Salisbury common cold: viruses
saliva: ejector; pump
salivary: calculus; colic; corpuscle; digestion; duct; fistula; gland; virus
salivary gland: disease; hormone; virus
salivary gland virus: disease
Salk: vaccine
Salla: disease
salmon: patch
Salmonella **food:** poisoning
salpingopalatine: fold
salpingopharyngeal: fold; muscle
salpingopharyngeus: muscle
salt: action; bridge; depletion; dye; edema; fever; loading; sensitivity; solution; wasting
saltatory: chorea; conduction; evolution; spasm
salt depletion: syndrome
salt-depletion: crisis

salted: plasma; serum
Salter-Harris: classification of epiphysial plate injuries
Salter incremental: lines
salt-losing: defect; nephritis; syndrome
saltpeter: paper
salt water: boils; soap
salvage: chemotherapy; cystectomy; pathway; therapy
Salzmann nodular corneal: degeneration
sampling: bias
Samter: syndrome
Sanarelli: phenomenon
Sanarelli-Shwartzman: phenomenon
Sanchez Salorio: syndrome
sand: bath; bodies; tumor
sandal: foot
sandal strap: dermatitis
sandfly: fever
sandfly fever: viruses
Sandhoff: disease
Sandifer: syndrome
Sandison-Clark: chamber
sandpaper: disks; gallbladder
Sandström: bodies
sandworm: disease
Sanfilippo: syndrome
Sanger: method; reagent
sanguineous: cyst
sanious: pus
San Joaquin: fever
San Joaquin Valley: disease; fever
San Miguel sea lion: virus
Sansom: sign
Sanson: images
Santini booming: sound
Santorini: canal; cartilage; concha; duct; fissures; incisures; labyrinth; muscle; plexus; tubercle; vein
Santorini major: caruncle
Santorini minor: caruncle
Sao Paulo: typhus
São Paulo: fever
saphenous: branch of descending genicular artery; hiatus; nerve; opening; veins
saponification: number
Sappey: fibers; plexus; veins
sarcogenic: cell
sarcoidal: granuloma
sarcomatoid: carcinoma
sarcoplasmic: reticulum
sarcoptic: acariasis; mange
sartorius: bursae; muscle
Sartwell incubation: model
satellite: abscess; cells; cell of skeletal muscle; DNA; metastasis
satellite-rich: heterochromatin
satiety: center

Sattler: veil
Sattler elastic: layer
saturated: color; fat; fatty acid; hydrocarbon; solution
saturation: analysis; index
saturation sound pressure: level
saturnine: colic; encephalopathy; gout
saucer-shaped: cataract
Saundby: test
sausage: fingers
Savage: syndrome
Savage perineal: body
Savary: bougies
Sayre: jacket
Sayre suspension: apparatus; traction
S-BP: line
scabbard: trachea
scabby: mouth
scaffold-associated: regions
scalar: electrocardiogram
scalded mouth: syndrome
scalded skin: syndrome
scalene: hiatus; tubercle; tubercle of Lisfranc
scalenus anterior: muscle; syndrome
scalenus medius: muscle
scalenus minimus: muscle
scalenus posterior: muscle
scalp: contusion; hair; infection; laceration; muscle
scaly: ringworm; tetter
scamping: speech
scanning: speech
scanning electron: microscope
scanning equalization: radiography
Scanzoni: maneuver
Scanzoni second: os
scaphoid: abdomen; bone; fossa; fossa of sphenoid bone; tuberosity
scapular: line; notch; reflex; region
scapulocostal: syndrome
scapulohumeral: atrophy; muscles; reflex
scapulohumeral muscular: dystrophy
scapuloperiosteal: reflex
scar: cancer; cancer of the lungs; carcinoma; emphysema
Scardino vertical flap: pyeloplasty
scarf: bandage; sign
scarification: test
scarlatinal: nephritis
scarlatiniform: erythema
scarlet: fever
scarlet fever: antitoxin

scarlet fever erythrogenic: toxin
Scarpa: fascia; fluid; foramina; ganglion; habenula; hiatus; liquor; membrane; method; sheath; staphyloma; triangle
scarring: alopecia
Scatchard: plot
scattered: radiation
scavenger: cell; receptor
Schacher: ganglion
Schaeffer-Fulton: stain
Schaer: reagent
Schäfer: method
Schaffer: test
Schäffer: reflex
Schamberg: dermatitis; fever
Schapiro: sign
Schardinger: dextrins; enzyme; reaction
Schatzki: ring
Schaudinn: fixative
Schaumann: bodies; lymphogranuloma; syndrome
Schauta vaginal: operation
Schede: method
scheduled: drug
Scheele: green
Scheibe: hearing impairment
Scheibler: reagent
Scheie: syndrome
Scheiner: experiment
Schellong: test
Schellong-Strisower: phenomenon
schematic: eye
Schenck: disease
Scheuermann: disease
Schick: method; test
Schick test: toxin
Schiff: base; reagent
Schiff-Sherrington: phenomenon
Schilder: disease
Schiller: test
Schilling: blood count; index; test
Schilling band: cell
Schilling type of monocytic: leukemia
Schindler: disease
schindyletic: joint
Schiötz: tonometer
Schirmer: test
schistosomal: dermatitis
schistosome: granuloma
schizencephalic: microcephaly
schizo-affective: psychosis
schizoid: personality
schizoid personality: disorder
schizophreniform: disorder
schizotypal: personality
schizotypal personality: disorder

Schlatter: disease
Schlemm: canal
Schlesinger: sign
schlieren: optics
Schmidel: anastomoses
Schmid-Fraccaro: syndrome
Schmidt: diet; syndrome
Schmidt-Lanterman: clefts; incisures
Schmidt-Strassburger: diet
Schmidt-Thannhauser: method
Schmorl: jaundice; nodule
Schmorl ferric-ferricyanide reduction: stain
Schmorl picrothionin: stain
Schneider: carmine
Schneider first rank: symptoms
schneiderian: membrane
schneiderian first rank: symptoms
Schnitzler: syndrome
Schober: test
Scholander: apparatus
Scholz: disease
Schönbein: test
Schönlein: disease; purpura
Schönlein-Henoch: syndrome
school: nurse; phobia
Schott: treatment
Schreger: lines
Schridde cancer: hairs
Schroeder: operation
Schuchardt: operation
Schüffner: dots; granules
Schüller: disease; ducts; phenomenon; syndrome
Schultz: reaction; stain
Schultz-Charlton: phenomenon; reaction
Schultz-Dale: reaction
Schultze: cells; fold; mechanism; membrane; phantom; placenta; sign
Schütz: bundle; law; rule
Schwabach: test
Schwalbe: corpuscle; nucleus; ring; spaces
Schwann: cells
Schwann cell: unit
Schwann white: substance
Schwartz: syndrome; tractotomy
Schwartz-Jampel: disease
Schweninger: method
Schweninger-Buzzi: anetoderma
sciatic: bursa of gluteus maximus; foramen; hernia; nerve; neuralgia; neuritis; plexus; scoliosis; spine
scientific: theory
scimitar: sign
scintigraphic: angiography
scintillating: scotoma

scintillation: camera; counter
scirrhous: carcinoma
scissor: gait
scleral: ectasia; resection; rigidity; ring; roll; spur; staphyloma; sulcus; veins
scleral buckling: operation
scleral venous: sinus
sclerocorneal: junction
sclerocystic: disease of the ovary
sclerosing: adenosis; agent; hemangioma; inflammation; keratitis; leukoencephalitis; mastoiditis; osteitis; therapy
sclerotic: bodies; coat; dentin; gastritis; kidney; stomach; teeth
sclerotic cemental: mass
scoliotic: pelvis
scombroid: poisoning
scorbutic: anemia
scotopic: adaptation; eye; perimetry; vision
Scott: operation
Scott-Wilson: reagent
scout: film; radiograph
scratch: test
screen: defense; memory
screening: audiometry; test
screw: arteries; elevator; joint
screwdriver: teeth
Scribner: shunt
scrivener's: palsy
scrofulous: keratitis; rhinitis
scroll: bones; ear
scrotal: arteries; hernia; hypospadias; part of ductus deferens; raphe; septum; swelling; tongue; veins
scrub: nurse; typhus
Scultetus: bandage; position
scurvy: rickets
sea: louse; scurvy; sickness
seabather's: eruption
sea-blue: histiocyte
sea-blue histiocyte: disease
sea gull: murmur
seal: fingers
sealed jar: technique
seamstress's: cramp
Seashore: test
seasonal affective: disorder
sea urchin: granuloma
sebaceous: adenoma; cyst; epithelioma; follicles; glands; horn; tubercle
Sebileau: hollow; muscle
seborrheic: blepharitis; dermatitis; dermatosis; eczema; keratosis; verruca; wart
Seckel: dwarfism; syndrome
seclusion of: pupil
second: finger; incisor; law of thermodynamics; messenger;

molar; part of duodenum; sight; sound; toe [II]; tooth
secondarily generalized tonic-clonic: seizure
secondary: adhesion; aerodontalgia; agammaglobulinemia; alcohol; aldosteronism; amenorrhea; amputation; amyloidosis; anesthetic; atelectasis; axis; calcium phosphate; carcinoma; cardiomyopathy; caries; cataract; cementum; center of ossification; choana; coccidioidomycosis; constriction; curvatures of vertebral column; dementia; dentin; dentition; deviation; dextrocardia; digestion; disease; drives; drowning; dysmenorrhea; elaboration; encephalitis; failure; fissure [TA] of cerebellum; gain; glaucoma; gout; hemochromatosis; hemorrhage; host; hydrocephalus; hyperparathyroidism; hypertension; hyperthyroidism; hypogammaglobulinemia; hypogonadism; hypothyroidism; immunodeficiency; infection; lysosomes; megaureter; mesoderm; metabolism; metabolite; methemoglobinemia; narcissism; nodule; nondisjunction; oocyte; palate; pellagra; point of ossification; process; proteose; pyoderma; radiation; rays; reinforcement; retinitis; saturation; screw-worm; spermatocyte; structure; suture; syphilid; syphilis; telangiectasia; thrombus; tuberculosis; union; villus; vitreous
secondary abdominal: pregnancy
secondary adrenocortical: insufficiency
secondary antibody: deficiency
secondary aortic: area
secondary cartilaginous: joint
secondary dye: test
secondary egg: membrane
secondary generalized: epilepsy
secondary immune: response

secondary interatrial: foramen
secondary medical: care
secondary myeloid: metaplasia
secondary ossification: center
secondary ovarian: follicle
secondary pulmonary: lobule
secondary refractory: anemia
secondary renal: calculus
secondary renal tubular: acidosis
secondary sensory: cortex; nuclei
secondary sex: characters
secondary spiral: lamina; plate
secondary tympanic: membrane
secondary visual: area; cortex
secondary X: zone
second cervical: vertebra
second cranial: nerve [CN II]
second cuneiform: bone
second-degree: burn
second degree AV: block
second gas: effect
second heart: sound
second-look: operation
second-order: conditioning
second parallel pelvic: plane
second set: rejection
second signaling: system
second temporal: convolution
second tibial: muscle
Secrétan: syndrome
secretin: test
secretomotor: nerve
secretor: factor
secretory: canaliculus; carcinoma; component; cyst; duct; granule; immunoglobulin; immunoglobulin A; nerve; otitis media
sectional: impression; radiography
sector: echocardiography; iridectomy; scan
secular: equilibrium
sedimentary: cataract
sedimentation: coefficient; constant; rate; velocity
seed: corn
Seeligmüller: sign
seesaw: murmur; nystagmus
Seessel: pocket; pouch
segmental: anesthesia; arteries of kidney; arteries of liver; atelectasis; bronchus; fracture; glomerulonephritis; neuritis; plate; sphincter; tubule; zone
segmental alveolar: osteotomy

segmental demyelinating: polyneuropathy
segmental medullary: arteries
segmentation: cavity; nucleus
segmented: cell; leukocyte; neutrophil
segmenting: body
segregation: analysis; ratio
Seidel: scotoma; sign
Seidlitz: mixture
Seignette: salt
Seiler: cartilage
Seip: syndrome
Seldinger: technique
selection: coefficient; pressure
selective: angiography; grinding; hypoaldosteronism; immunoglobulin A deficiency; inattention; inhibition; injection; medium; memory; reduction; stain; termination
selective estrogen receptor: modulator
selective norepinephrine reuptake: inhibitor
selective serotonin reuptake: inhibitor
selenium: plate
self-: concept
self-curing: resin
self-limited: disease
self-registering: thermometer
self-retaining: catheter
Selivanoff: test
sellar: diaphragm
Sellick: maneuver
Selters: water
semantic: aphasia
semi-: vegetarian
Semichon acid carmine: stain
semicircular: canals; canals of bony labyrinth; ducts; line; line of Douglas
semi-closed: circle
semiconservative: replication
semidirect: leads
semi-Fowler: position
semihorizontal: heart
semilente: insulin
semilunar: bone; cartilage; cusp; fascia; fasciculus; fibrocartilage; fold; folds of colon; ganglion; hiatus; line; notch; nucleus of Flechsig; valve
semilunar conjunctival: fold
semimembranosus: muscle; reflex
semimembranous: bursa
seminal: capsule; colliculus; duct; fluid; gland; granule; hillock; lake; vesicle
seminal vesical: cyst

seminiferous: epithelium; tubules
seminiferous tubule: dysgenesis
semioval: center
semipennate: muscle
semipermeable: membrane
semipolar: bond
semiprone: position
semispinal: muscle; muscle of head; muscle of neck; muscle of thorax
semispinalis: muscle
semispinalis capitis: muscle
semispinalis cervicis: muscle
semispinalis thoracis: muscle
semisulfur: mustard
semitendinosus: muscle
semivertical: heart
Semliki Forest: virus
Semon-Hering: theory
Semple: vaccine
Sendai: virus
Senear-Usher: disease; syndrome
Seneca: snakeroot
senegal: gum
Sengstaken-Blakemore: tube
senile: amyloidosis; arteriosclerosis; atrophoderma; atrophy; cataract; chorea; degeneration; delirium; dementia; deterioration; dwarfism; emphysema; fibroma; gangrene; halo; hemangioma; involution; keratoderma; keratoma; keratosis; lentigo; melanoderma; memory; nephrosclerosis; osteomalacia; plaque; psychosis; retinoschisis; tremor; vaginitis; wart
senile dental: caries
senile lenticular: myopia
senile sebaceous: hyperplasia
senior: synonym
Sennetsu: fever
Senning: operation
sensation: level; time
sense of: identity
sense: organs; strand
sensible: heat; perspiration; temperature
sensitivity training: group
sensitized: antigen; cell; culture
sensitizing: dose; injection
sensorial: areas
sensorimotor: area; theory
sensorineural: hearing loss
sensory: amblyopia; amusia; aphasia; ataxia; cell; cortex; crossway; decussation of medulla oblongata;

deprivation; epilepsy; ganglion; hearing impairment; image; inattention; nerve; neuron; neuronopathy; nuclei; paralysis; phantom; receptors; root of ciliary ganglion; root of pterygopalatine ganglion; root of spinal nerve; root of sublingual ganglion; root of submandibular ganglion; root of trigeminal nerve; tract; urgency
sensory acuity: level
sensory precipitated: epilepsy
sensory speech: center
sentinal node: biopsy
sentinel: animal; event; gland; lymph node; node; pile; tag
sentinel loop: sign
Seoul: virus
separating: medium; wire
separation: anxiety
separation anxiety: disorder
sepsis: syndrome
septal: area; artery; bone; branches; cartilage; cell; cusp of right atrioventricular valve; cusp of tricuspid valve; gingiva; lines
septal nasal: cartilage
septate: hymen; mycelium; uterus; vagina
septic: abortion; arthritis; endocarditis; fever; infarct; intoxication; phlebitis; pneumonia; retinitis; shock; wound
septicemic: abscess; plague
septofimbrial: nucleus
septomarginal: fasciculus; trabecula; tract
septooptic: dysplasia
sequence: hypothesis; pulse
sequence-tagged: sites
sequence-tagged site (STS): map
sequential: analysis; anastomosis
sequential multichannel: autoanalyzer
sequestration: cyst; dermoid
Sergent white: line
serial: extraction; film changer; interval; passage; radiography; section
serine: carboxypeptidase; hydrolases
serine protease: inhibitors
serofibrinous: inflammation; pleurisy
serologic: pipette
seromucous: cells; gland
serotonin norepinephrine reuptake: inhibitor

serous: cell; coat; coat of peritoneum; cyst; demilunes; diarrhea; gland; hemorrhage; inflammation; iritis; layer of peritoneum; ligament; membrane; meningitis; otitis media; pericardium; pleurisy; retinitis; synovitis; tunic
serpent: ulcer of cornea
serpentine: aneurysm
serpiginous: choroidopathy; keratitis; ulcer
serpiginous corneal: ulcer
serrate: suture
serratus anterior: muscle
serratus posterior inferior: muscle
serratus posterior superior: muscle
Serres: angle; glands
Sertoli: cells; columns
Sertoli-cell-only: syndrome
Sertoli-Leydig cell: tumor
Sertoli-stromal cell: tumor
serum: accelerator; accident; agar; agglutinin; albumin; disease; eruption; hepatitis; nephritis; proteins; rash; reaction; shock; sickness; therapy
serum accelerator: globulin
serumal: calculus
serum hepatitis: virus
serum prothrombin conversion: accelerator
Servetus: circulation
sesamoid: bone; cartilage of cricopharyngeal ligament; cartilage of larynx; cartilages of nose
sessile: hydatid; polyp
set of: idiotopes
seton: operation; wound
setting: expansion
setting sun: sign
seven-day: fever
seventh: sense
seventh cranial: nerve [CN VII]
Sever: disease
severe combined: immunodeficiency
severe postanoxic: encephalopathy
Severinghaus: electrode
severity of: illness
sewer: gas
sex: cell; chromatin; chromosomes; cords; determination; factor; hormones; linkage; object; ratio; reassignment; reversal; role
sex chromosome: imbalance

sex hormone-binding: globulin
sex-influenced: inheritance
sex-limited: inheritance
sex-linked: character; inheritance; locus
sex steroid-binding: globulin
sexual: abuse; deviation; dimorphism; disorders; dwarfism; generation; gland; infantilism; instinct; intercourse; life; neurasthenia; orientation; perversion; potency; reproduction; selection
sexually transmitted: disease
Sézary: cell; erythroderma; syndrome
shadow: cells; corpuscle; nucleus; test
Shaffer-Hartmann: method
shaggy: aorta; chorion; pericardium
shagreen: patch; skin
shake: culture; test
shaken baby: syndrome
shaking: palsy
shallow: breathing
sham: feeding; rage
sham-movement: vertigo
shared: epitope
shared psychotic: disorder
sharp: spoon
Sharpey: fibers
shave: biopsy
Shaver: disease
shaving: cramp
shawl: muscle
shear: flow; rate; stress; thinning
shearing: edge
sheath: ligaments; process of sphenoid bone
sheathed: artery
Sheehan: syndrome
sheep: bots
sheep-pox: virus
shelf: procedure
shell: nail; shock
shellac: base
Shemin: cycle
Shenton: line
Shepherd: fracture
Sherman: unit
Sherman-Bourquin: unit of vitamin B_2
Sherman-Munsell: unit
Sherrington: law; phenomenon
sherry: wine
Shibley: sign
shifting: dullness; pacemaker
Shiga: bacillus; toxin
Shiga-Kruse: bacillus
Shigalike: toxin
shilling: scars

shimamushi: disease
shin: bone
shin bone: fever
Shine-Dalgarno: sequence
ship: beriberi; fever
Shipley-Hartford: scale
shipping fever: virus
shipyard: eye
Shirodkar: operation
shivering: thermogenesis
shock: antigen; index; lung; therapy; treatment
shocking: dose
shock wave: lithotripsy
shoddy: fever
Shone: anomaly; complex; syndrome
shop: typhus
Shope: fibroma; papilloma
Shope fibroma: virus
Shope papilloma: virus
short: bone; chain; crus of incus; gyri of insula; head; head of biceps brachii; head of biceps femoris; limb of incus; process of malleus; root of ciliary ganglion; sight; vinculum
short abductor: muscle of thumb
short adductor: muscle
short association: fibers
short-bowel: syndrome
short central: artery
short-chain acyl-CoA dehydrogenase: deficiency
short ciliary: nerve
short circumferential: arteries
shortening: reaction
short extensor: muscle of great toe; muscle of thumb; muscle of toes
short fibular: muscle
short flexor: muscle of great toe; muscle of little finger; muscle of little toe; muscle of thumb; muscle of toes
short gastric: arteries; veins
short increment sensitivity: index
short incubation: hepatitis
short interspersed: elements
short levatores costarum: muscles
short palmar: muscle
short peroneal: muscle
short pitch helicoidal: layer
short posterior ciliary: artery
short radial extensor: muscle of wrist
short saphenous: nerve; vein
short-term: memory
short-term exposure: limit
short TI inversion: recovery
short wave: diathermy
shotgun: prescription

shot-silk: phenomenon; reflex; retina
shotted: suture
shoulder: dystocia; girdle; joint; presentation
shoulder apprehension: sign
shoulder-girdle: syndrome
shoulder-hand: syndrome
Shprintzen: syndrome
Shrapnell: membrane
Shulman: syndrome
shunt: cyanosis; muscle
shut-in: personality
shuttle: vector
Shwachman: syndrome
Shwachman-Diamond: syndrome
Shwartzman: phenomenon; reaction
Shy-Drager: syndrome
SI: units
Siamese: twins
Siberian tick: typhus
sibilant: rale
sibling: rivalry
Sibson: aponeurosis; fascia; groove; muscle
Sibson aortic: vestibule
sicca: complex; syndrome
sick: headache; role
sick building: syndrome
sick euthyroid: syndrome
sickle: cell; form; scotoma
sickle cell: anemia; crisis; dactylitis; disease; hemoglobin; retinopathy; test; trait
sickle cell C: disease
sickle cell-thalassemia: disease
sick sinus: syndrome
side: chain
side-chain: theory
sideroblastic: anemia
sideropenic: dysphagia
siderotic: cataract; nodules
Siegert: sign
Siegle: otoscope
sieve: bone; plate
Siggaard-Andersen: nomogram
sight: blindness
sigma: effect; factor; peptide
sigmoid: arteries; colon; flexure; fossa; groove; kidney; lymph nodes; notch; sinus; sulcus; veins; volvulus
sigmoidovesical: fistula
sign: blindness
signal: lymph node; node; void
signal-processing: circuits
signal recognition: particle
signal-to-noise: ratio
signet: ring

signet ring: cells
signet-ring cell: carcinoma
Signorelli: sign
silastic: band
silent: allele; area; electrode; gallstones; gap; ischemia; mutant; mutation; period
silent myocardial: infarction
silhouette: sign of Felson
silica: granuloma
silicate: cement; restoration
silicone: implant
silicotic: granuloma
silo-filler's: disease; lung
silver: cell; cone; point; poisoning; stain
silver-ammoniac silver: stain
silver-fork: deformity; fracture
silverized: catgut
Silverman-Lilly: pneumotachograph
silver protein: stain
Silver-Russell: dwarfism; syndrome
Silverskiöld: syndrome
silver-tin: alloy
Simbu: virus
simian: crease; fissure; hand; malaria; virus; virus 40
simian hemorrhagic: fever
simian vacuolating: virus No. 40
Simmonds: disease
Simmons citrate: medium
Simon: position; sign
Simonart: bands; ligaments; threads
Simons: disease
simple: absence; anchorage; anisocoria; beam; color; conjunctivitis; crus of semicircular duct; diplopia; dislocation; epithelium; fission; fracture; glaucoma; goiter; heterochromia; hypertrophy; joint; lipids; lobule; lymphangiectasis; mastectomy; mastoidectomy; microscope; myopia; necrosis; obesity; phobia; protein; retinitis; schizophrenia; ulcer; urethritis
simple bone: cyst
simple-central: anisocoria
simple endometrial: hyperplasia
simple hyperopic: astigmatism
simple membranous: limb of semicircular duct
simple myopic: astigmatism
simple partial: seizure
simple pulmonary: eosinophilia

simple skull: fracture
simple squamous: epithelium
Simpson: forceps
Simpson uterine: sound
Sims: position
Sims uterine: sound
simulated: hypertrophy
simultaneous: communication; contrast; perception
sincipital: presentation
Sindbis: fever; virus
Sinding-Larsen-Johansson: syndrome
singer's: nodes; nodules
single: ascertainment; bond; immunodiffusion; ventricle
single (gel) diffusion precipitin: test in one dimension; test in two dimensions
single photon emission computed: tomography
single-strand: break
single-stranded nucleate: endonuclease
singlet: oxygen; state
single vial: fixatives
singular: foramen
Sin Nombre: virus
sinoatrial: block; node
sinoatrial conduction: time
sinoatrial recovery: time
sinoauricular: block
sinoventricular: conduction
sinuatrial: chamber; node
sinuatrial nodal: artery; branch of right coronary artery
sinuatrial node: artery
sinuatrial (S-A) nodal: branch of right coronary artery
sinus: arrest; arrhythmia; barotrauma; bradycardia; histiocytosis with massive lymphadenopathy; nerve of Hering; node; pause; reflex; rhythm; septum; standstill; tachycardia; tubercle
sinus node: artery
sinusoidal: capillary
sinus venosus: syndrome
sinuvertebral: nerves
Sipple: syndrome
Sippy: diet
SISI: test
sister chromatid: exchange
Sistrunk: operation
site-directed: mutagenesis
site specific: mutation
site-specific: recombination
in situ: hybridization
situation: anxiety
situational: psychosis; test
in situ nucleic acid: hybridization

sitz: bath
sixth: disease; ventricle
sixth cranial: nerve [CN VI]
sixth venereal: disease
sixth-year: molar
Sjögren: disease; syndrome
Sjögren-Larsson: syndrome
Sjöqvist: tractotomy
skein: cell
skeletal: dysplasias; extension; muscle; survey; system; traction
skeletal muscle: fibers; tissue
skeleton: hand
Skene: glands; tubules
skew: deviation; distribution; form
Skillern: fracture
skim: milk
skin: botflies; dose; flap; furrows; graft; grooves; ligaments; pore; reaction; reflexes; ridges; stones; sulci; tag; test; traction
skinbound: disease
skin-muscle: reflexes
Skinner: box
skinnerian: conditioning
skin-puncture: test
skin-pupillary: reflex
skip: areas
skipped: generation
Sklowsky: symptom
Skoda: rale; sign; tympany
skodaic: resonance
skull: fracture
skull base: surgery
slab-off: lens
slaked: lime
slant: culture
slaty: anemia
sleep: apnea; deficit; dissociation; drunkenness; epilepsy; paralysis; spindle
sleep apnea: syndrome
sleep-induced: apnea
sleeping: sickness
sleep phase delay: syndrome
sleep terror: disorder
sleeve: graft
SLE-like: syndrome
slender: fasciculus; lobule; process of malleus
slew: rate
slide: micrometer; tracheoplasty
sliding: hernia; hook; lock
sliding esophageal hiatal: hernia
sliding filament: hypothesis
sliding hiatal: hernia
sliding oblique: osteotomy
slime: fever
sling: psychrometer
slipped: hernia
slipping: patella; rib

slipping rib: cartilage
slit: lamp; pores
slit ventricle: syndrome
slope: culture
slotted: attachment
sloughing: phagedena; ulcer
slow: combustion; fever; virus
slow channel-blocking: agent
slow component of: nystagmus
slow-reacting: factor of anaphylaxis; substance
slow virus: disease
SLR: factor
Sluder: neuralgia
sludged: blood
sluggish: layer
slurring: speech
Sly: syndrome
Sm: antigen
small: arteries; bowel; calorie; canal of chorda tympani; cell; intestine; pancreas; pelvis; trochanter; vein
small bowel: enema; series
small cardiac: vein
small cell: carcinoma
small cleaved: cell
small deep petrosal: nerve
smaller: muscle of helix
smaller pectoral: muscle
smaller posterior rectus: muscle of head
smaller psoas: muscle
smallest cardiac: veins
smallest scalene: muscle
smallest splanchnic: nerve
small increment sensitivity: index
small increment sensitivity index: test
small interarch: distance
small lymphocytic: lymphoma
small nuclear: RNA
small plaque: parapsoriasis
smallpox: vaccine; virus
small pudendal: lip
small saphenous: vein
small sciatic: nerve
smear: culture
Smellie: scissors
smelling: salts
smelter's: chills; fever; shakes
Smith: fracture; operation
Smith-Boyce: operation
Smith-Indian: operation
Smith-Lemli-Opitz: syndrome
Smith-Petersen: nail
Smith-Riley: syndrome
Smith-Robinson: operation
smoker's: patches; tongue
smooth: broach; chorion; colony; diet; leprosy; muscle
smooth muscle: relaxant; tissue
smooth muscular: sphincter

smooth surface: caries
smooth-surfaced endoplasmic: reticulum
smudge: cells
S-N: line
S-N-A: angle
snail: fever
snail track: degeneration
snap: finger
snapping: hip; reflex
S-N-B: angle
Sneddon: syndrome
Sneddon-Wilkinson: disease
sneezing: gas
Snell: law
Snellen: sign; test types
sniff: test
snout: reflex
snow: blindness; conjunctivitis
snowball: opacity; sampling
snowman: abnormality
snowshoe hare: virus
snub-nose: dwarfism
S1 nuclease: mapping
Snyder: test
soapsuds: enema
Soave: operation
social: adaptation; control; diseases; instinct; intelligence; maladjustment; medicine; phobia; psychiatry; therapy
socialized: medicine
social network: therapy
sociometric: distance
socket: joint
soda: loading
sodium: chromate Cr 51; iodide iodine-131; methylprednisolone succinate; pump
sodium-potassium: pump
sodium-responsive periodic: paralysis
Soemmerring: ganglion; ligament; muscle; spot
soft: cataract; chancre; corn; diet; drusen; palate; papilloma; parts; pulse; rays; soap; sore; sulfur; tubercle; ulcer; wart; water
soft tissue: window
Sohval-Soffer: syndrome
solar: blindness; cheilitis; comedo; dermatitis; elastosis; energy; fever; ganglia; keratosis; lentigo; maculopathy; plexus; retinopathy; therapy; treatment; urticaria
soldier's: patches
sole: nuclei; reflex
soleal: line; part of posterior (plantar flexor) compartment of leg
sole-plate: ending

sole tap: reflex
soleus: muscle
solid: edema
solid phase: immunoassay
solid-state: detector
solitariospinal: tract
solitary: bundle; fasciculus; follicles; glands; nodules of intestine; tract
solitary bone: cyst
solitary fibrous: tumor
solitary lymphatic: follicles; nodules
solitary osteocartilaginous: exostosis
solubility: test
soluble: antigen; ferric phosphate; glass; ligature; RNA; soap; starch; tartar
soluble gun: cotton
soluble specific: substance
solution: pressure
solvent: drag; ether; inhalation
somatic: agglutinin; antigen; arteries; cells; crossing-over; death; delusion; layer; mesoderm; mitosis; mutation; nerve; nucleus; reproduction; swallow; teniasis
somatic cell: genetics; hybridization
somatic motor: neuron; nuclei
somatic mutation: theory of cancer
somatic nerve: fibers
somatic sensory: cortex
somatization: disorder
somatoform: disorder; pain
somatosensory: aura
somatosensory evoked: potential
somatotropic: hormone
somatotropin release-inhibiting: factor; hormone
somatotropin-releasing: factor; hormone
somesthetic: area; system
somite: cavity
somitic: mesoderm
somnambulic: epilepsy
somnambulistic: trance
Somogyi: effect; method; phenomenon; unit
Sondermann: canal
Songo: fever
sonic: waves
sonomotor: response
sonorous: rale
soot: wart
sorbitol: pathway
sore: mouth; throat
soremouth: virus
Sörensen: scale
Soret: band; phenomenon
Sorsby: syndrome

Sorsby macular: degeneration
SOS: genes; repair
Sotos: syndrome
sound: abatement; field
soundex: code
sound pressure: level
South African tick-bite: fever
South African type: porphyria
South American: blastomycosis; trypanosomiasis
Southern blot: analysis
Southey: tubes
space: maintainer; medicine; myopia; retainer; sense; sickness
space adaptation: syndrome
spaced: teeth
spade: fingers; hand
Spallanzani: law
spallation: product
Spanish: influenza
sparing: action; phenomenon
spasmodic: asthma; dysmenorrhea; dysphonia; laryngitis; stricture; tic; torticollis
spasmophilic: diathesis
spastic: anemia; aphonia; colon; diplegia; dysarthria; dysphonia; ectropion; entropion; gait; hemiplegia; ileus; miosis; mydriasis; paraplegia; speech
spastic flat: foot
spastic spinal: paralysis
spatial: acuity; formula; localization; vector; vectorcardiography
spatula: needle
speaking: tube
special: anatomy; hospital; nurse; sense
specialized: transduction
special somatic afferent: column
special visceral efferent: column; nuclei
special visceral motor: nuclei
species: tolerance
species-specific: antigen
specific: absorbance; action; activity; anergy; antigens; antiserum; bactericide; cause; cholinesterase; compliance; disease; epithet; extinction; granules; gravity; heat; hemolysin; immunity; opsonin; parasite; phobia; reaction; serum; therapy; transduction; urethritis
specific absorption: coefficient
specific active: immunity
specific building-related: illnesses

specific capsular: substance
specific dynamic: action
specific immune: globulin (human)
specificity: constant
specific optic: rotation
specific passive: immunity
specific soluble: polysaccharide; sugar
speck: finger
spectacle: plane
spectral: phonocardiograph; sensitivity
specular: glare; image
speculum: forceps
speech: audiogram; audiometer; bulb; centers; pathology; processor; reading
speech awareness: threshold
speech detection: threshold
speech-language: pathologist; pathology
speech reception: threshold
Spens: syndrome
sperm: aster; cell; crystal; nucleus
spermacytic: seminoma
spermatic: cord; duct; filament; fistula; plexus; vein
sphagnum: moss
sphenoethmoidal: recess; suture; synchondrosis
sphenofrontal: suture
sphenoid: angle; part of middle cerebral artery; process; process of septal nasal cartilage
sphenoid: bone
sphenoidal: angle of parietal bone; border of temporal bone; conchae; crest; fissure; fontanelle; herniation; lingula; margin of temporal bone; process of palatine bone; ridges; rostrum; sinus; spine; yoke
sphenoidal emissary: foramen
sphenoidal sinus: aperture
sphenoidal turbinated: bones
sphenomandibular: ligament
sphenomaxillary: fissure; fossa; suture
sphenooccipital: joint; suture; synchondrosis
spheno-orbital: suture
sphenopalatine: artery; foramen; ganglion; neuralgia; notch
sphenoparietal: sinus; suture
sphenopetrosal: fissure; synchondrosis
sphenosquamous: suture
sphenotic: center; foramen
sphenovomerine: suture

sphenozygomatic: suture
spherical: aberration; amalgam; lens; nucleus; recess of bony labyrinth
spherical form of: occlusion
spherocylindrical: lens
spherocytic: anemia; jaundice
spheroid: articulation; colony
spheroidal: degeneration; joint
sphincter: muscle; muscle of pancreatic duct; muscle of pupil; muscle of pylorus; muscle of urethra; muscle of urinary bladder
sphincter of Oddi: dysfunction
sphincteroid: tract of ileum
sphingomyelin: lipidosis
sphygmic: interval
spica: bandage; cast
spider: angioma; cancer; cell; finger; hemangioma; mole; nevus; pelvis; telangiectasia
Spiegelberg: criteria
Spiegler-Fendt: sarcoid
Spielmeyer acute: swelling
Spielmeyer-Sjögren: disease
Spielmeyer-Stock: disease
Spielmeyer-Vogt: disease
spigelian: hernia
Spigelius: line; lobe
spike: potential
spike and wave: complex
spin: density; echo
spinach: stools
spinal: analgesia; anesthesia; anesthetic; apoplexy; arachnoid mater; arteries; ataxia; block; branches; canal; column; concussion; cord; curvature; decompression; dura mater; dysraphism; fusion; ganglion; headache; induction; instability; lamina II; lemniscus; length; marrow; muscle; muscle of head; muscle of neck; muscle of thorax; nerves; nucleus of trigeminal nerve; nucleus of the trigeminus; paralysis; part of accessory nerve; part of arachnoid; part of deltoid (muscle); part of filum terminale; point; puncture; pyramidotomy; quotient; reflex; root of accessory nerve; shock; sign; stroke; tap; tract; tractotomy; tract of trigeminal nerve; veins
spinal accessory: nerve
spinal arachnoid: mater
spinal cord: concussion
spinalis: muscle
spinalis capitis: muscle

spinalis cervicis: muscle
spinalis thoracis: muscle
spinal muscular: atrophy; atrophy, type I; atrophy, type II; atrophy, type III
spinal nerve: plexus
spinal pia: mater
spinal trigeminal: nucleus
spindle: cataract; cell; fiber
spindle cell: carcinoma; lipoma; nevus; sarcoma
spindle-celled: layer
spindle-shaped: muscle
spine: cell; sign
Spinelli: operation
spin-lattice: relaxation
spinning disk: nebulizer
spinoadductor: reflex
spinocerebellar: ataxia; tracts
spinocervical: tract
spinocervicothalamic: tract
spinocuneate: fibers
spinoglenoid: ligament
spinogracile: fibers
spinohypothalamic: fibers
spinomesencephalic: fibers
spinoolivary: fibers; tract; tract
spinoperiaqueductal: fibers
spinoreticular: fibers; tract
spinotectal: fibers; tract
spinothalamic: cordotomy; tract; tractotomy
spinous: layer; process of sphenoid; process of tibia; process of vertebra
spinovestibular: tract
spin-spin: relaxation
spiral: artery; bandage; canal of cochlea; canal of modiolus; crest; crest of cochlear duct; CT; fold of cystic duct; fracture; ganglion of cochlea; groove; hyphae; joint; ligament of cochlea; ligament of cochlear duct; line; membrane; organ; plate; prominence of cochlear duct; septum; suture; tubule; valve of cystic duct; vein of modiolus
spiral bulbar: septum
spiral cochlear: ganglion
spiral computed: tomography
spiral foraminous: tract
spiral modiolar: artery
spiral tip: catheter
spirillum: fever
spirit: lamp; thermometer
spirituous: liquor
spiro-: index
spirochetal: jaundice
spironolactone: test
spiruroid: larva migrans
Spitz: nevus

Spitzer: theory
Spitzka: nucleus
Spitzka marginal: tract; zone
Spix: spine
splanchnesthetic: sensibility
splanchnic: anesthesia; cavity; layer; mesoderm; nerve; wall
spleen: deoxyribonuclease; endonuclease; phosphodiesterases
Splendore-Hoeppli: phenomenon
splenial: gyrus
splenic: anemia; artery; branches of splenic artery; cells; cords; corpuscles; flexure; hilum; index; leukemia; lymph nodes; pulp; recess; sinus; trabeculae; vein
splenic flexure: syndrome
splenic lymph: follicles; nodules
splenic (nervous): plexus
splenic portal: venography
splenius: muscle of head; muscle of neck; muscles
splenius capitis: muscle
splenius cervicis: muscle
splenogonadal: fusion
splenorenal: ligament
splinted: abutment
splinter: hemorrhages
splintered: fracture
split: brain; fat; genes; hand; papules; pelvis; tolerance
split cast: method; mounting
split renal function: test
split-skin: graft
split-thickness: graft
splitting: enzymes
splitting of heart: sounds
split-virus: vaccine
Spondweni: virus
spondyloepiphyseal: dysplasia; dysplasia congenita; dysplasia tarda
spondylolisthetic: pelvis
sponge: biopsy; tent
spongiform: encephalopathy; pustule of Kogoj
spongy: body of penis; bone; degeneration of infancy; layer of female urethra; layer of vagina; part of the male urethra; spot; substance; urethra
spontaneous: abortion; agglutination; amputation; combustion; correction of placenta previa; evolution; fracture; gangrene of newborn; generation; mutation; phagocytosis;

pneumothorax; recovery; remission; version
spontaneous breech: extraction
spontaneous cephalic: delivery
spontaneous membrane: rupture
spoon: nail
sporotrichositic: chancre
sports: medicine
spot: film; map; test for infectious mononucleosis
spot-film: radiography
spotted: fever; sickness
spouse: abuse
sprain: fracture
spreading: depression; factor
Sprengel: deformity
spring: conjunctivitis; finger; lancet; ligament; ophthalmia
spun glass: hair
spur: cell
spur cell: anemia
spurious: ankylosis; cast; meningocele; parasite; pregnancy; torticollis
Spurling: test
sputum: smear
squamocolumnar: junction
squamomastoid: suture
squamoparietal: suture
squamosal: border; border of parietal bone; margin; margin of greater wing of sphenoid
squamotympanic: fissure
squamous: border; border of parietal bone; border of sphenoid bone; cell; margin; metaplasia; metaplasia of amnion; part of frontal bone; part of occipital bone; part of temporal bone; pearl; suture
squamous alveolar: cells
squamous cell: carcinoma; hyperplasia
squamous odontogenic: tumor
square: knot; matrix
square wave: stimuli
squint: hook
squinting: eye
squirrel plague: conjunctivitis
ST: junction; segment
stab: cell; culture; drain; neutrophil; wound
stabilized: baseplate
stabilizing circumferential clasp: arm
stabilizing fulcrum: line
stable: colloid; disease; equilibrium; factor; fracture; isotope
staccato: speech

Stader: splint
Staderini: nucleus
staff: cell
Stafne bone: cyst
staggered spondaic word: test
staghorn: calculus
stagnant: anoxia; hypoxia
stagnation: mastitis
Stahl: ear
staircase: phenomenon
stalked: hydatid
standard: atmosphere; bicarbonate; cell; deviation; pressure; score; solution; substance; temperature; volume
standard error of the: mean
standard error of: difference
standardized mortality: ratio
standard limb: lead
standard serologic: tests for syphilis
standard urea: clearance
standby pulse: generator
standing: test
standing plasma: test
Stanford-Binet intelligence: scale
Stanley cervical: ligaments
Stanley Way: procedure
Stannius: ligature
stapedial: artery; branch of posterior tympanic artery; branch of stylomastoid artery; fold; membrane; reflex
stapedius: muscle
stapes: mobilization
stapes mobilization: operation
staphylococcal: blepharitis; enterotoxin; pneumonia
staphylococcal scalded skin: syndrome
staphylococcus: antitoxin; vaccine
Staphylococcus **food:** poisoning
staphyloopsonic: index
starch: equivalent; glycerite; gum; sugar
starch-iodine: test
Stargardt: disease
Starling: curve; hypothesis; law; reflex
Starr-Edwards: valve
start: codon
starter: tRNA
starting: friction
startle: disease; epilepsy; reaction; reflex
starvation: acidosis; diabetes
stasis: cirrhosis; dermatitis; eczema; ulcer
Stas-Otto: method
state: hospital
state-dependent: learning

static: arthropathy; ataxia; compliance; friction; gangrene; hysteresis; infantilism; perimetry; reflexes; refraction; relation; scoliosis; sense; system; tremor
static bone: cyst
station: test
stationary: anchorage; cataract; phase
statistical: genetics; model; power
statoacoustic: nerve
statoconial: membrane
statokinetic: reflex
statotonic: reflexes
Staub-Traugott: effect; phenomenon
Stauffer: syndrome
steady: state
steady-state: rate; velocity
steady state: approximation
steal: phenomenon
steam-fitter's: asthma
Steele-Richardson-Olszewski: disease; syndrome
Steell: murmur
Steenbock: unit
steeple: skull
steering wheel: injury
Stein: test
Steinberg thumb: sign
Steinert: disease
Stein-Leventhal: syndrome
Steinmann: pin
stellate: abscess; block; cataract; cells of cerebral cortex; cells of liver; fracture; ganglion; hair; ligament; neuroretinitis; reticulum; veins; venules
stellate skull: fracture
Stellwag: sign
stem: bronchus; cell
stem cell: factor; leukemia
Stender: dish
Stenger: test
stenopeic: disk; iridectomy; spectacles
stenosal: murmur
stenosing: tenosynovitis
stenoxous: parasite
Stensen: duct; foramen; plexus; veins
Stent: graft
Stenvers: projection; view
steppage: gait
stercoraceous: vomiting
stercoral: abscess; appendicitis; ulcer
sterculia: gum
stereochemical: formula; isomerism
stereoscopic: acuity; microscope; parallax; vision

stereotactic: brachytherapy; cordotomy; instrument; surgery
stereotaxic: localization; surgery
sterile: abscess; cyst
sterile insect: technique
Stern: posture
sternal: angle; arteries; bar; branches of internal thoracic artery; cartilage; end of clavicle; extremity of clavicle; facet of clavicle; joints; line; line of pleural reflection; membrane; muscle; notch; part of diaphragm; plane; puncture; synchondroses
sternal articular: surface of clavicle
sternalis: muscle
Sternberg: cell; sign
Sternberg-Reed: cell
sternobrachial: reflex
sternochondral: separation
sternochondroscapular: muscle
sternoclavicular: angle; disk; joint; ligaments; muscle
sternocleidomastoid: branches of occipital artery; branch of superior thyroid artery; muscle; region; vein
sternocostal: articulations; head of pectoralis major (muscle); joints; part of pectoralis major muscle; surface of heart; triangle; triangle (of diaphragm)
sternocostalis: muscle
sternohyoid: muscle
sternomanubrial: junction
sternomastoid: artery; muscle
sternopericardial: ligaments
sternothyroid: muscle
steroid: acne; diabetes; fever; hormones; nucleus; ulcer
steroid cell: tumor
steroid metabolic clearance: rate
steroidogenic: diabetes
steroid production: rate
steroid secretory: rate
steroid withdrawal: syndrome
stertorous: breathing; respiration
stethoscopic: phonocardiograph
Stevens-Johnson: syndrome
Stewart: test
Stewart-Hamilton: method
Stewart-Holmes: sign
Stewart-Morel: syndrome
Stewart-Treves: syndrome
stichochrome: cell
Sticker: disease

Stickler: syndrome
sticky-ended: DNA
Stieda: process
Stierlin: sign
stiff: neck; toe
stiff heart: syndrome
stiff man: syndrome
stigmal: plates
Stiles-Crawford: effect
Still: disease; murmur
still: layer
stillbirth: rate
stillborn: infant
Still-Chauffard: syndrome
Stilling: canal; column; nucleus; raphe
Stilling gelatinous: substance
stimulatory: protein 1
stimulus: control; generalization; substitution; threshold
stimulus sensitive: myoclonus
stinging: caterpillar
stippled: epiphysis; tongue
Stirling modification of Gram: stain
stitch: abscess
St. John's: wort
St. Louis encephalitis: virus
Stobo: antigen
stochastic: independence; process
stock: culture; strain; vaccine
Stocker: line
Stockholm: syndrome
stocking: anesthesia
Stoffel: operation
stoichiometric: number
stoker's: cramps
Stokes: amputation; basket; law
Stokes-Adams: disease; syndrome
stomach: ache; drops; pump; reefing; tooth; tube
stomal: ulcer
stomatognathic: system
stone: basket; heart
stone-mason's: disease
Stookey-Scarff: operation
stop: codon
stop-: needle; speculum
stopping: rules
storage: disease; oscilloscope
storiform: neurofibroma
Stout: wiring
stove-pipe: colon
strabismic: amblyopia
straddling: embolism
straight: arteries; conjugate; gyrus; muscle; part of cricothyroid muscle; sinus; tubule; tubule of testis; venules of kidney
straight back: syndrome
straight seminiferous: tubule

strain: fracture; gauge
strangulated: hernia
strap: cell; muscles
Strassburg: test
Strassman: phenomenon
stratified: epithelium; sample; thrombus
stratified ciliated columnar: epithelium
stratified squamous: epithelium
stratiform: fibrocartilage
Straus: reaction; sign
straw: itch
strawberry: birthmark; cervix; gallbladder; hemangioma; mark; nevus; tongue
streak: culture; gonad; hyperostosis
streaming: movement
street: drug; virus
Streeter: bands
strength-duration: curve
streptococcal: empyema; fibrinolysin; pneumonia
streptococcal toxic shock: syndrome
streptococcus erythrogenic: toxin
Streptococcus M: antigen
streptomycin: units
stress: echocardiography; fibers; fracture; immunity; inoculation; reaction; test; ulcer
stress-bearing: area
stress-broken: connector; joint
stress-strain: curve
stress urinary: incontinence
stretch: marks; receptors; reflex
striate: area; atrophy of skin; body; cortex; keratopathy; veins
striated: border; duct; membrane; muscle
striated muscular: sphincter
striatonigral: fibers
string: sign; test
stringed instrument: theory
stringent: factor; response
strionigral: fibers
stripped: atom
stripper's: asthma
stroboscopic: disk; microscope
Stroganoff: method
stroke: output; volume
stroke work: index
stroma: plexus
stromal: hyperthecosis
stromal corneal: dystrophy
strong: silver protein
Strong vocational interest: test

structural: color; formula; gene; interface; isomerism; pleiotropy
structure: proteins
structured: abstract; noise
Strümpell: disease; phenomenon; reflex
Strümpell-Marie: disease
struvite: calculus
Stryker: frame; saw
Stryker-Halbeisen: syndrome
Stuart: factor
stuck: finger
student: nurse
Student's *t*: test
stump: cancer; hallucination; neuralgia
stunned: myocardium
stuporous: catatonia
Sturge-Kalischer-Weber: syndrome
Sturge-Weber: disease; syndrome
Sturm: conoid; interval
Sturmdorf: operation
stuttering: urination
styloauricular: muscle
styloglossus: muscle
stylohyoid: branch of facial nerve; ligament; muscle
styloid: cornu; process of fibula; process of radius; process of temporal bone; process of third metacarpal bone; process of ulna; prominence
stylomandibular: ligament
stylomastoid: artery; foramen; vein
stylomaxillary: ligament
stylopharyngeal: branch of glossopharyngeal nerve; muscle
stylopharyngeus: muscle
styloradial: reflex
stylus: tracing
"s"-type: cholinesterase
styptic: collodion; colloid; cotton
Stypven time: test
subacromial: bursa; bursitis
subacute: glomerulonephritis; hepatitis; inflammation; nephritis; rheumatism
subacute bacterial: endocarditis
subacute combined: degeneration of the spinal cord
subacute granulomatous: thyroiditis
subacute inclusion body: encephalitis
subacute lymphocyte: thyroiditis

subacute migratory: panniculitis
subacute necrotizing: encephalomyelopathy; myelitis
subacute sclerosing: leukoencephalitis; panencephalitis
subacute spongiform: encephalopathy
subadventitial: fibrosis
subanconeus: muscle
subaortic: lymph nodes; stenosis
subapical: segment
subarachnoid: anesthesia; cavity; cisterns; hemorrhage; space
subarcuate: fossa
subareolar duct: papillomatosis
subastragalar: amputation
subcaeruleus: nucleus
subcallosal: area; fasciculus; gyrus
subcapital: fracture
subcapsular: cataract
subcecal: fossa
subchorial: lake; space
subclavian: artery; duct; groove; loop; muscle; nerve; plexus; steal; sulcus; triangle; vein
subclavian lymphatic: trunk
subclavian steal: syndrome
subclavius: muscle
subclinical: coccidioidomycosis; diabetes; seizure
subcommissural: organ
subconscious: memory; mind
subcoracoid: bursa
subcoracoid-pectoralis minor tendon: syndrome
subcorneal pustular: dermatitis; dermatosis
subcoronal: hypospadias
subcortical arteriosclerotic: encephalopathy
subcostal: angle; arch; artery; groove; line; muscle; nerve; plane
subcrepitant: rale
subcrestal: pocket
subcrural: muscle
subcuneiform: nucleus
subcutaneous: bursa of the laryngeal prominence; bursa of lateral malleolus; bursa of medial malleolus; bursa of teres major; bursa of tibial tuberosity; bursa of tuberosity of tibia; emphysema; flap; implantation; mastectomy; myiasis; operation; part of

external anal sphincter; phycomycosis; portion of external anal sphincter; ring; tenotomy; tissue; tissue of penis; tissue of perineum; transfusion; veins of abdomen; wound
subcutaneous acromial: bursa
subcutaneous calcaneal: bursa
subcutaneous fat: necrosis of newborn
subcutaneous infrapatellar: bursa
subcutaneous olecranon: bursa
subcutaneous prepatellar: bursa
subcuticular: suture
subdeltoid: bursa; bursitis
subdiaphragmatic: abscess; pyopneumothorax
subdigastric: node
subdural: cavity; cleavage; cleft; hematoma; hematorrhachis; hemorrhage; hygroma; space
subendocardial: branches of atrioventricular bundles; layer
subendocardial conducting: system of heart
subendocardial myocardial: infarction
subendothelial: layer
subependymal giant cell: astrocytoma
subepidermal: abscess
subfalcial: herniation
subfascial prepatellar: bursa
subfornical: organ
subgaleal: emphysema; hemorrhage
subgerminal: cavity
subgingival: calculus; curettage; space
subhepatic: abscess; recess; space
subhyoid: bursa
subhypoglossal: nucleus
subinguinal: fossa; triangle
subjective: fremitus; insomnia; probability; psychology; sign; symptom; synonyms; vision
sublenticular: limb of internal capsule; part of internal capsule
sublentiform: limb of internal capsule
subleukemic: leukemia
sublimed: sulfur
subliminal: self; stimulus; thirst
sublingual: artery; bursa; caruncula; crescent; cyst;

fold; fossa; ganglion; gland; medication; nerve; pit; tablet; vein
submammary: mastitis
submandibular: duct; fossa; ganglion; gland; lymph nodes; triangle
submaxillary: duct; fossa; ganglion; gland; triangle
submental: artery; lymph nodes; triangle; vein
submental vertex: projection; radiograph
submentovertex: radiograph
submentovertical: projection
submerged: tonsil
submetacentric: chromosome
submitochondrial: particles
submucosal: implant
submucosal (nervous): plexus
submucous laryngeal: cleft
subnasal: point
subneural: apparatus
suboccipital: decompression; muscles; nerve; neuralgia; neuritis; part of vertebral artery; region; triangle
suboccipital venous: plexus
suboccipitobregmatic: diameter
suboccluding: ligature
subocclusal: surface
subpapillary: layer; network
subparabrachial: nucleus [TA]
subparietal: sulcus
subpellicular: fibril; microtubule
subperiodic: periodicity
subperiosteal: abscess; amputation; fracture; implant
subperitoneal: appendicitis; fascia
subphrenic: abscess; recesses; space
subplasmalemmal dense: zone
subpopliteal: recess
subpubic: angle
subpulmonic: effusion
subpyloric: lymph nodes; node
subquadricipital: muscle
subsartorial: canal; fascia
subscapular: artery; branches of axillary artery; bursa; fossa; muscle; nerves
subscapular axillary: lymph nodes
subscapularis: muscle
subsegmental: atelectasis
subseptate: uterus
subserous: layer
subserous (nervous): plexus
subsidiary atrial: pacemaker

subsistence: diet
substance: abuse; dependence
substance abuse: disorders
substance dependence: disorder
substance-induced organic mental: disorders
substernal: angle; goiter
substituted: amide
substitution: product; therapy; transfusion
substitutive: therapy
substrate: cycle; inhibition; specificity
substrate-level: phosphorylation
subsuperior: segment
subsurface: cisterna
subtalar: joint
subtemporal: decompression
subtendinous: bursae of gastrocnemius (muscle); bursa of iliacus; bursa of infraspinatus; bursa of latissimus dorsi; bursa of sartorius; bursa of subscapularis; bursa of tibialis anterior; bursa of trapezius; bursa of triceps brachii
subtendinous iliac: bursa
subtendinous prepatellar: bursa
subthalamic: fasciculus; nucleus
subthreshold: stimulus
subtotal: hysterectomy; thyroidectomy
subungual: abscess; exostosis; melanoma
subunit: vaccine
subvalvar: stenosis
subvalvular aortic: stenosis
subvocal: speech
succedaneous: dentition; tooth
succenturiate: placenta
successional: lamina
successive: contrast
succinic acid: cycle
succussion: sound
sucking: blister; cushion; louse; pad
sucking chest: wound
suckling: reflex
Sucquet: anastomoses; canals
Sucquet-Hoyer: anastomoses; canals
sucrose hemolysis: test
suction: cup; curettage; drainage; ophthalmodynamometer; plate
Sudan: virus
sudanophobic: zone
sudden: deafness; death

sudden infant death: syndrome
Sudeck: atrophy; syndrome
Sudeck critical: point
sudomotor: fibers; nerves
sudoriferous: abscess; cyst; duct; glands
sufficient: cause
suffocating: gas
suffocative: goiter
sugar: alcohol; cataract; ester; tumor
sugar-coated: spleen
suggestive: psychotherapy; therapeutics
Sugiura: procedure
suicide: gesture; inhibitor; substrate
suid: herpesvirus
sulcal: artery
sulcomarginal: tract
sulcular: epithelium; fluid
sulcus: test
sulfate: respiration; water
sulfatide: lipidosis
sulfhydryl: reagent
sulfonium: ion
sulfosalicylic acid turbidity: test
sulfur: autotrophy; mustard; water
sulfurated: lime; potash
sulfureted: hydrogen
Sulkowitch: reagent
Sulzberger-Garbe: disease; syndrome
summating: potentials
summation: beat; gallop
summer: asthma; diarrhea; itch; prurigo; rash
Sumner: sign
sump: drain; syndrome
sun: stroke
sunflower: cataract
sun protection: factor
superciliary: arch; ridge
superconducting: magnet
superfatted: soap
superficial: angioma; branch; branch of the lateral plantar nerve; branch of medial circumflex femoral artery; branch of the medial plantar artery; branch of the radial nerve; branch of the superior gluteal artery; branch of the transverse cervical artery; branch of the ulnar nerve; burn; cleavage; ectoderm; fascia; fascia of penis; fascia of perineum; fascia of scrotum; head of flexor pollicis brevis; implantation; lamina; layer; layer of deep cervical fascia; layer of the levator palpebrae superioris;

layer of temporal fascia; part of anterior (flexor) compartment of forearm; part of external anal sphincter; part of masseter muscle; part of parotid gland; part of posterior (plantar flexor) compartment of leg; reflex; vein
superficial back: muscles
superficial brachial: artery
superficial cardiac (nervous): plexus
superficial cerebral: veins
superficial cervical: artery; nerve
superficial circumflex iliac: artery; vein
(superficial and deep) external pudendal: arteries
superficial dorsal: veins of clitoris; veins of penis
superficial dorsal sacrococcygeal: ligament
superficial epigastric: artery; vein
superficial fibular: nerve
superficial flexor: muscle of fingers
superficial gray: layer [TA] of superior colliculus
superficial inguinal: lymph nodes; pouch; ring
superficial investing: fascia of perineum
superficial lateral cervical: lymph nodes
superficial linear: keratitis
superficial lingual: muscle
superficial lymph: vessel
superficial middle cerebral: vein
superficial palmar: artery; branch of radial artery
superficial palmar (arterial): arch
superficial palmar venous: arch
superficial parotid: lymph nodes
superficial perineal: pouch; space
superficial peroneal: nerve
superficial posterior sacrococcygeal: ligament
superficial punctate: keratitis
superficial pustular: perifolliculitis
superficial spreading: melanoma
superficial temporal: artery; branch of auriculotemporal nerve; plexus; veins
superficial transverse: muscle of perineum

superficial transverse metacarpal: ligament
superficial transverse metatarsal: ligament
superficial transverse perineal: muscle
superficial volar: artery
superimposed: eclampsia; preeclampsia
superior: angle of scapula; aspect; belly of omohyoid muscle; border; border of body of pancreas; border of pancreas; border of petrous part of temporal bone; border of scapula; border of spleen; border of suprarenal gland; branch; branch of the oculomotor nerve; branch of the pubic bone; branch of the right and left inferior pulmonary veins; branch of the superior gluteal artery; branch of the transverse cervical nerve; bursa of biceps femoris; cistern; colliculus; extremity; extremity of kidney; eyelid; facet of trochlear of talus; fascia of pelvic diaphragm; fovea; ganglion of glossopharyngeal nerve; ganglion of vagus nerve; horn of falciform margin of saphenous opening; horn of thyroid cartilage; laryngotomy; ligament of epididymis; ligament of incus; ligament of malleus; limb; limb of ansa cervicalis; lobe of (right/left) lung; margin of cerebral hemisphere; mediastinum; member; olive; paraplegia; part of diaphragmatic surface of liver; part of duodenum; part of lingular vein (of left superior pulmonary vein); part of vestibular ganglion; part of vestibulocochlear nerve; pole; pole of kidney; pole of testis; polioencephalitis; recess of lesser peritoneal sac; recess of omental bursa; recess of tympanic membrane; retinaculum of extensor muscles; root of ansa cervicalis; segment; surface of cerebellar hemisphere; surface of talus; tarsus; trunk of brachial plexus; veins of cerebellar hemisphere; vein of vermis; vena cava; wall of orbit
superior aberrant: ductule

superior alveolar: nerves
superior anastomotic: vein
superior articular: facet of atlas; pit of atlas; process; process of sacrum; surface of atlas; surface of tibia
superior auricular: muscle
superior azygoesophageal: recess
superior basal: vein
superior carotid: triangle
superior central tegmental: nucleus
superior cerebellar: artery; peduncle
superior cerebellar artery: syndrome
superior cerebral: veins
superior cervical: ganglion
superior cervical cardiac: branches of vagus nerve; nerve
superior choroid: vein
superior clunial: nerves
superior costal: facet; pit
superior costotransverse: ligament
superior dental: arch; branches of superior dental plexus; nerves; rami
superior dental (nervous): plexus
superior duodenal: flexure; fold; fossa; recess
superior epigastric: artery; veins
superior esophageal: sphincter
superior extensor: retinaculum
superior fibular: retinaculum
superior frontal: convolution; gyrus; sulcus
superior gastric: lymph nodes
superior gemellus: muscle
superior gingival: branches of superior dental plexus
superior gluteal: artery; nerve; vein
superior hemorrhagic: polioencephalitis
superior hemorrhoidal: artery; plexus; vein
superior hypogastric (nervous): plexus
superior hypophysial: artery
superior ileocecal: recess
superior intercostal: artery; vein
superior internal parietal: artery
superiority: complex
superior labial: artery; branches of infraorbital nerve; branch of facial artery; vein

superior laryngeal: artery; cavity; nerve; vein
superior lateral brachial cutaneous: nerve
superior lateral genicular: artery
superior limbic: keratoconjunctivitis
superior lingular: artery; branch of lingular branch of superior lobar left pulmonary artery
superior lingular bronchopulmonary: segment S IV
superior lobar: arteries
superior longitudinal: fasciculus; muscle of tongue; sinus; sulcus
superior macular: arteriole; venule
superior maxillary: nerve
superior medial genicular: artery
superior medullary: velum
superior mesenteric: artery; ganglion; lymph nodes; vein
superior mesenteric artery: syndrome
superior mesenteric (nervous): plexus
superior nasal: concha; venule of retina
superior nasal retinal: arteriole; venule
superior nuchal: line
superior oblique: muscle; muscle of head
superior occipital: gyrus; sulcus
superior occipitofrontal: fasciculus
superior olivary: complex; nucleus
superior omental: recess
superior ophthalmic: vein
superior orbital: fissure
superior palpebral: veins
superior palpebral (arterial): arch
superior parietal: gyrus; lobule
superior pelvic: aperture
superior peroneal: retinaculum
superior petrosal: sinus; sulcus
superior pharyngeal constrictor: muscle
superior phrenic: artery; lymph nodes; veins
superior posterior serratus: muscle
superior pubic: ligament; ramus

superior pulmonary sulcus: tumor
superior quadrigeminal: brachium
superior radioulnar: joint
superior rectal: artery; lymph nodes; vein
superior rectal (nervous): plexus
superior rectus: muscle
superior renal: segment
superior sagittal: sinus
superior salivary: nucleus
superior salivatory: nucleus
superior segmental: artery; artery of kidney
superior semilunar: lobule
superior suprarenal: arteries
superior tarsal: muscle
superior temporal: convolution; fissure; gyrus; line of parietal bone; sulcus; venule of retina
superior temporal retinal: arteriole; venule
superior thalamostriate: vein
superior thoracic: aperture; artery
superior thyroid: artery; notch; plexus; tubercle; vein
superior tibial: articulation
superior tibiofibular: joint
superior tracheobronchial: lymph nodes
superior transverse scapular: ligament
superior triangle: sign
superior turbinated: bone
superior tympanic: artery
superior ulnar collateral: artery
superior vena cava: syndrome
superior vermian: branch (of superior cerebellar artery)
superior vesical: artery
superior vestibular: area; nucleus
supernatant: fluid
supernormal: conduction
supernormal recovery: phase
supernumerary: breast; kidney; mamma; organs; placenta
superolateral: face of cerebral hemisphere; surface of cerebrum
superolateral cerebral: surface
superomedial: margin
supersaturated: solution
supersonic: rays; waves
supertraction: conus
supination: reflex
supinator: crest (of ulna); jerk; muscle; reflex
supine: position

supine hypotensive: syndrome
supplemental: air; groove; lobe; ridge
supplementary: menstruation
supplementary motor: cortex
supplementary motor area: epilepsy
support: medium
supporting: area; cell; reactions; reflexes
supportive: psychotherapy
suppressed: menstruation
suppression: amblyopia
suppressor: cells; mutation; tRNA
suppressor-sensitive: mutant
suppurative: appendicitis; arthritis; cerebritis; choroiditis; encephalitis; gingivitis; hepatitis; hyalitis; inflammation; mastitis; necrosis; nephritis; periodontitis; pleurisy; pneumonia; pulpitis; synovitis
supra-acetabular: groove
supraacetabular: sulcus
supra-arytenoid: cartilage
supra-auricular: point
supracallosal: gyrus
supracervical: hysterectomy
suprachiasmatic: artery; nucleus
suprachoroid: lamina of sclera; layer
supraclavicular: lymph nodes; muscle; part of brachial plexus; triangle
supraclinoid: aneurysm
supracollicular: sphincter
supracondylar: fracture; process of humerus
supracrestal: line; plane
supracristal: plane
supraduodenal: artery
supraepicondylar: process
supragingival: calculus
supraglenoid: tubercle (of scapula)
supraglottic: laryngectomy
suprahepatic: spaces
suprahisian: block
suprahyoid: branch of lingual artery; gland; muscles
suprainterparietal: bone
supralemniscal: nucleus
supramammillary: nucleus
supramarginal: convolution; gyrus
supramastoid: crest; fossa
supramaximal: stimulus
suprameatal: pit; spine; triangle
supranasal: point
supranormal: conduction; excitability

supranuclear: lesion; paralysis
supraoptic: artery; nucleus; nucleus [TA] of hypothalamus; recess
supraopticohypophysial: tract
supraorbital: arch; artery; foramen; margin; nerve; neuralgia; notch; point; reflex; ridge; vein
supraorbitomeatal: plane
suprapatellar: bursa; reflex
supraperiosteal: implant
suprapineal: recess
suprapleural: membrane
suprapubic: cystotomy; lithotomy
suprapyloric: lymph node; node
suprarenal: body; capsule; cortex; gland; impression on liver; medulla; veins
suprarenal (nervous): plexus
suprascapular: artery; ligament; nerve; notch; vein
suprasellar: cyst
supraspinalis: muscle
supraspinatus: muscle; syndrome
supraspinous: fossa; ligament; muscle
suprasternal: bones; notch; plane; pulsation; space
suprastyloid: crest of radius
supratonsillar: fossa; recess
supratragic: tubercle
supratrochlear: artery; nerve; veins
supraumbilical: reflex
supravaginal: part of cervix
supravalvar: stenosis
supravalvar aortic stenosis: syndrome
supravalvar aortic stenosis-infantile hypercalcemia: syndrome
supravalvular: stenosis
supraventricular: crest; extrasystole; tachycardia
supravesical: fossa
supravital: stain
supreme: concha
supreme intercostal: artery; vein
supreme nasal: concha
supreme turbinated: bone
sural: arteries; nerve; region
sural communicating: branch of common fibular nerve; branch of common peroneal nerve
surdocardiac: syndrome
surface: anatomy; catalysis; coil; epithelium; microscopy; tension; thermometer
surface mucous: cells of stomach
surface tension: theory of narcosis
surface thalamic: veins
surfactant-specific: proteins
surgeon's: knot
surgical: abdomen; anatomy; anesthesia; appliance; diathermy; emphysema; eruption; erysipelas; ligation; maggot; microscope; neck of humerus; orthodontics; pathology; prosthesis; rod; silk; splint; template
surgical ciliated: cyst
surging: faradism
surrogate: mother
survey: line
survival: analysis; time
susceptibility: cassette; testing
suspended: animation
suspension: colloid; laryngoscopy; stability
suspensory: bandage; ligament of axilla; ligament of clitoris; ligament of duodenum; ligament of esophagus; ligament of eyeball; ligament of gonad; ligament of lens; ligament of ovary; ligament of penis; ligaments of breast; ligaments of Cooper; ligament of testis; ligament of thyroid gland; muscle of duodenum; retinaculum of breast
sustained: pulse
sustained action: tablet
sustentacular: cell; fibers of retina
Sutton: disease; nevus; ulcer
sutural: bones; cataract; ligament
suture: abscess; joint; ligature
Suzanne: gland
SV40-adenovirus: hybrid
Svedberg: equation; unit
Sw^a: antigen
swallow: syncope
swallowing: reflex; threshold
swamp: itch
Swan-Ganz: catheter
Swann: antigens
swan-neck: deformity
sweat: duct; glands; pore; test
sweat gland: carcinoma
sweating: test
sweaty feet: syndrome
Swedish: gymnastics; movements
Sweet: disease
sweet: balm; precipitate
sweet birch: oil
Swift: disease
swim: bladder
swimmer's: ear; itch
swimming pool: conjunctivitis; granuloma
swine: erysipelas; influenza
swine encephalitis: virus
swine fever: virus
swineherd's: disease
swine influenza: viruses
swinepox: virus
swine vesicular: disease
swinging light: test
Swiss cheese: endometrium
Swiss mouse leukemia: virus
Swiss type: agammaglobulinemia
switching: site
swollen belly: disease; syndrome
Swyer: syndrome
Swyer-James: syndrome
Swyer-James-MacLeod: syndrome
Sydenham: chorea; disease
Sydney: crease; line
syllabic: speech
sylvatic: plague
Sylvest: disease
Sylvian: cistern
sylvian: angle; aqueduct; fissure; line; point; valve; ventricle
symbiotic fermentation: phenomenon
Syme: amputation; operation
Symington anococcygeal: body
Symmers clay pipestem: fibrosis
symmetric: adenolipomatosis; asphyxia; disulfide
symmetrical: gangrene
symmetric distal: neuropathy
symmetric fetal growth: restriction
sympathetic: agent; amine; blockade; branch to submandibular ganglion; ganglia; heterochromia; hormone; hypertonia; imbalance; iridoplegia; iritis; nerve; ophthalmia; part of autonomic division of peripheral nervous system; plexuses; root of ciliary ganglion; root of otic ganglion; root of pterygopalatine ganglion; root of sublingual ganglion; root of submandibular ganglion; saliva; segment; symptom; trunk; uveitis
sympathetic formative: cell
sympathetic nervous: system
sympathetic reflex: dystrophy
sympathicotropic: cells
sympathizing: eye
sympathochromaffin: cell
sympathomimetic: amine
symphysial: surface of pubis
symphysic: teratosis
symptom: complex; formation; group; score; substitution
symptomatic: epilepsy; erythema; fever; headache; nanism; neuralgia; porphyria; pruritus; reaction; tetany; torticollis; treatment; varicocele
symptomatic myeloid: metaplasia
Syms: tractor
synaptic: boutons; cleft; conduction; endings; phase; resistance; terminals; trough; vesicles
synaptinemal: complex
synaptonemal: complex
synarthrodial: joint
synchondrodial: joint
synchronic: study
synchronized intermittent mandatory: ventilation
synchronous: reflex
syncytial: bud; knot; sprout; trophoblast
syndesmodial: joint
synergic: control
synergistic: effect; muscles
syngeneic: graft
synovial: bursa; cell; chondromatosis; crypt; cyst; fluid; fold; frena; frenula; fringe; hernia; joint; joints of free lower limb; joints of free upper limb; joints of thorax; ligament; membrane; mesenchyme; osteochondromatosis; sarcoma; sheath; sheaths of digits of foot; sheaths of digits of hand; sheaths of toes; tufts; villi
synovial tendon: sheath
synovial trochlear: bursa
syntactical: aphasia
synthesis: period
synthetic: chemistry; dyes
synthetic sentence: identification
syntonic: personality
syphilitic: aneurysm; aortitis; cirrhosis; fever; leukoderma; meningoencephalitis; nephritis; osteochondritis; roseola; teeth; ulcer
Syriac: ulcer
syringomyelic: dissociation; hemorrhage

systematic: anatomy; bacteriology; desensitization
systematized: delusion; nevus
systemic: anaphylaxis; anatomy; blastomycosis; chondromalacia; circulation; heart; hyalinosis; lupus erythematosus; mastocytosis; myelitis; poisoning; scleroderma; sclerosis
systemic autoimmune: diseases
systemic capillary leak: syndrome
systemic febrile: diseases
systemic vascular: resistance
systemic venous: hypertension
systolic: bruit; click; gallop; gradient; honk; murmur; pressure; shock; thrill; whoop
systolic/diastolic: ratio
systolic gallop: rhythm
systolic time: intervals

T

T: agglutinogen; antigens; cell; enzyme; fiber; group; lymphocyte; myelotomy; system; tube; tubule; wave
Tγ: cells
Tμ: cells
T-: bandage; binder
t: distribution; test
T.A.B.: vaccine
tabby cat: striation
tabetic: arthropathy; crisis; cuirass; dissociation; neurosyphilis
table: salt
Tac: antigen
Tacaribe: complex of viruses; virus
tachybradycardia: syndrome
tachycardia: window
tachycardia-bradycardia: syndrome
tactile: agnosia; anesthesia; cell; corpuscle; disk; elevations; fremitus; hallucination; hyperesthesia; image; meniscus; organ; papilla; sense
Tactual Performance: Test
tadpole-shaped: pupil
Taenzer: stain
tagged: atom
Tahyna: virus
tail: bone; bud; fold; sheath; vertebrae
tailor's: cramp; muscle
Tait: law
Taiwan Dobrava-Belgrade: virus
Takahara: disease

Takayama: stain
Takayasu: arteritis; disease; syndrome
talar: sulcus
talar articular: surfaces of calcaneus
talc: operation
Tallerman: treatment
tallow: soap
talocalcaneal: joint; ligament
talocalcaneal interosseous: ligament
talocalcaneonavicular: joint
talocrural: articulation; joint
talon: cusp
talonavicular: joint; ligament
tambour: sound
tamed: iodine
Tamm-Horsfall: mucoprotein; protein
tangent: screen
tangential: wound
tangible body: macrophage
Tangier: disease
tank: respirator
tanned red: cells
Tanner: stage
Tanner growth: chart
tanner's: ulcer
tannic acid: glycerite
tantalum: bronchography
tapered: bougie
tapetoretinal: degeneration
Tapia: syndrome
tapir: mouth
Taq: polymerase
tar: acne; camphor; keratosis
Tardieu: ecchymoses; petechiae; spots
tardive: cyanosis; dyskinesia
target: behavior; cell; gland; organ; patient; response
target cell: anemia
Tarin: space; tenia; valve
Tarlov: cyst
Tarnier: forceps
tarry: cyst
tarsal: arch; bones; canal; cartilage; cyst; fold; glands; joints; ligaments; plates; sinus
tarsal interosseous: ligaments
tarsal tunnel: syndrome
tarsoepiphyseal: aclasis
tarsometatarsal: joints; ligaments
tarsophalangeal: reflex
tarsotibial: amputation
tart: cell
tartrated: antimony
taste: blindness; bud; bulb; cells; corpuscle; deficiency; hairs; pore; ridge
TATA: box
Taussig-Bing: disease; syndrome

tautomeric: fibers
Tawara: node
Tay cherry-red: spot
Taylor: apparatus; disease; splint
Taylor back: brace
Tay-Sachs: disease
^{99m}Tc: pyrophosphate
T cell antigen: receptors
T-cell growth: factor; factor-1; factor-2
T-cell–rich, B-cell: lymphoma
T cytotoxic: cells
T-dependent: antigen
TDTH: cells
T-E: fistula
teacher's: nodes
teaching: hospital
TEAE-: cellulose
tear: film; gas; sac; stone
technical: error
tectal: plate; stria
tectobulbar: tract
tectonic: keratoplasty
tectoolivary: fibers
tectopontine: fibers; tract
tectoreticular: fibers
tectorial: membrane of cochlear duct; membrane (of median atlantoaxial joint)
tectospinal: decussation; tract
tegmental: decussations; fields of Forel; nuclei; root of tympanic cavity; syndrome; wall of middle ear; wall of tympanic cavity
Teichmann: crystals
telangiectatic: angioma; angiomatosis; cancer; fibroma; glioma; lipoma; wart
telangiectatic osteogenic: sarcoma
telencephalic: flexure; vesicle
telephone: ear; theory
teleradium: therapy
telescopic: denture; spectacles
television: microscope
TeLinde: operation
telocentric: chromosome
telogen: effluvium
telolecithal: egg; ovum
telomeric R-banding: stain
temperate: bacteriophage; virus
temperature: coefficient; sense; spot
temperature-compensated: vaporizer
temperature-sensitive: mutant
template: RNA
temporal: aponeurosis; apophysis; arteritis; bone; branch of facial nerve; canal; cortex; crest of mandible; dispersion; fascia; fossa; horn; line; line of frontal bone; lobe; muscle; plane; pole; pole [TA] of cerebrum; process of zygomatic bone; region of head; ridge; squama; surface; veins; venules of retina
temporalis: muscle
temporal lobe: epilepsy
temporary: base; callus; cartilage; denture; memory; parasite; restoration; stricture; tooth
temporary threshold: shift
temporofrontal: tract
temporomandibular: arthrosis; articulation; joint; ligament; nerve; syndrome
temporomandibular articular: disk
temporomandibular joint: dysfunction
temporomandibular joint pain-dysfunction: syndrome
temporomaxillary: vein
temporoparietal: muscle
temporoparietalis: muscle
temporopontine: fibers; tract
temporozygomatic: suture
tenaculum: forceps
tender: lines; points; zones
tendinous: arch; arch of levator ani muscle; arch of pelvic fascia; arch of soleus muscle; chiasm of the digital tendons; cords; inscription; intersection; intersections of rectus abdominis; opening; sheath of abductor pollicis longus and extensor pollicis brevis muscles; sheath of extensor carpi radialis muscles; sheath of extensor carpi ulnaris muscle; sheath of extensor digiti minimi muscle; sheath of extensor digitorum and extensor indicis muscles; sheath of extensor digitorum longus muscle of foot; sheath of extensor hallucis longus muscle; sheath of extensor pollicis longus muscle; sheath of flexor carpi radialis muscle; sheath of flexor digitorum longus muscle (of foot); sheath of flexor hallucis longus muscle; sheath of flexor pollicis longus muscle; sheath of superior oblique muscle; sheath of tibialis anterior muscle; sheath of tibialis posterior muscle; spot; synovitis; xanthoma

tendo Achillis: reflex
tendon: advancement; bundle; cells; graft; recession; reflex; suture; transplantation
tendon sheath: syndrome
ten Horn: sign
tennis: elbow; leg; thumb
Tenon: capsule; space
tense: part of the tympanic membrane; pulse
tensile: strength; stress
tension: curve; headache; lines; pneumopericardium; pneumothorax; suture
tension-type: headache
tensor: muscle of fascia lata; muscle of soft palate; muscle) of tympanic membrane
tensor fasciae latae: muscle
tensor tarsi: muscle
tensor tympani: muscle; reflex
tensor veli palati: muscle
tenth cranial: nerve [CN X]
tentorial: angle; nerve; notch; sinus; surface
tentorial basal: branch of internal carotid artery
tentorial marginal: branch of cavernous part of internal carotid artery
teratoid: tumor
teratomatous: cyst
teres major: muscle
teres minor: muscle
term: infant
terminal: artery; bar; boutons; branches of middle cerebral artery; bronchiole; cisternae; crest; deletion; disinfection; endocarditis; filum; ganglion; hair; hematuria; ileus; infection; leukocytosis; line; nerve; notch of auricle; nucleus; oxidase; oxidation; part; plate; pneumonia; redundancy; sinus; stria; sulcus; sulcus of tongue; thread; transferases; vein; ventricle; web
terminal addition: enzyme
terminal deoxynucleotidyl: transferase
terminal duct: carcinoma
terminal hinge: position
terminal jaw relation: record
terminal nerve: corpuscles
terminal respiratory: unit
termination: codon; factor; sequence; signal
terminoterminal: anastomosis
ternary: complex
Terrien: valve

Terrien marginal: degeneration
territorial: matrix
Terry: nails; syndrome
Terson: glands; syndrome
tertian: fever; malaria; parasite
tertiary: alcohol; amyl alcohol; calcium phosphate; cortex; dentin; structure; syphilid; syphilis; villus; vitreous
tertiary egg: membrane
tertiary medical: care
Teschen disease: virus
Tesla: current
tessellated: fundus
Tessier: classification
test: cross; injection; meal; object; profile; solution; tube; type
test handle: instrument
testicular: appendage; artery; cord; duct; dysgenesis; feminization; implant; plexus; prosthesis; veins
testicular feminization: syndrome
testis: cords; ectopia
testis-determining: factor
testosterone-estrogen-binding: globulin
test-retest: reliability
test-tube: baby
tetanic: contraction; convulsion
tetanus: antitoxin; immunoglobulin; toxin; vaccine
tetanus antitoxin: unit
tetanus and gas gangrene: antitoxins
tetanus immune: globulin
tetanus-perfringens: antitoxin
tetany: cataract
Tete: viruses
tethered cord: syndrome
tetracyclic: antidepressant
tetracyclic steroid: nucleus
tetraethyl: poisoning
tetramethyl: acridine
tetrazonium: salts
Teutleben: ligament
Texas: snakeroot
text: blindness
TGE: virus
Thal: procedure
thalamic: fasciculus; syndrome; tenia
thalamic gustatory: nucleus
thalamocortical: fibers
thalamostriate: veins
thallium: poisoning
thanatophoric: dwarfism
Thane: method
Thayer-Martin: agar; medium

thebesian: circulation; foramina; valve; veins
theca: cells of stomach
theca cell: tumor
theca interna: cone
thecal: abscess; whitlow
theca lutein: cell
Theden: method
Theile: canal; glands; muscle
Theiler: virus
Theiler mouse encephalomyelitis: virus
Theiler original: virus
T helper: cells
T helper subset 1: cells
T helper subset 2: cells
thematic: paralogia; paraphasia
thematic apperception: test
thenar: eminence; prominence; space
Theobald Smith: phenomenon
therapeutic: abortion; anesthesia; angiography; community; crisis; dose; electrode; fever; group; incompatibility; index; iridectomy; malaria; nihilism; optimism; pessimism; pneumothorax; radiology; range; ratio
thermal: anesthesia; artifact; burn; capacity; sense; spectrum
thermic: fever
thermo-: stromuhr
thermodynamic: potential; theory of narcosis
thermoelectric: pile
thermogenic: action
thermolabile: opsonin
thermoluminescence: dosimetry
thermoprecipitin: reaction
thermostable: enzyme; opsonin
thermostable opsonin: test
theta: antigen; rhythm; wave
Thezac-Porsmeur: method
thiamin chloride: unit
thiamin hydrochloride: unit
thiazide: diabetes
thiazin: dyes
thick: filament; skin
Thiemann: disease; syndrome
Thiersch: canaliculi; graft
thigh: bone; joint
thin: filament; section; skin
thin-layer: chromatography; electrophoresis; immunoassay
thiochrome: method
thioclastic: cleavage
thiocyanogen: number; value
thioflavine T: stain
thiol: enzyme; ester

third: corpuscle; disease; eyelid; finger; molar; ovary; part of duodenum; sound; spacing; toe [III]; tonsil; trochanter; ventricle; ventriculostomy
third cranial: nerve [CN III]
third cuneiform: bone
third-degree: burn
third degree AV: block
third and fourth pharyngeal pouch: syndrome
third heart: sound
third occipital: nerve
third parallel pelvic: plane
third peroneal: muscle
third temporal: convolution
third-year molar: tooth
thirst: fever
Thiry: fistula
Thiry-Vella: fistula
thixotropic: fluid
Thoma: ampulla; fixative; laws
Thomas: splint
Thompson: ligament; test
Thomsen: disease
Thomson: sign
thoracic: aorta; axis; cage; cavity; compliance; constriction of esophagus; duct; fistula; ganglia; girdle; glands; goiter; index; inlet; kidney; kyphosis; limb; lymph nodes; nerves [T1–T12]; outlet; part of aorta; part of esophagus; part of iliocostalis lumborum (muscle); part of peripheral autonomic plexuses and ganglia; part of spinal cord; part of thoracic duct; part of trachea; respiration; skeleton; spine; splenosis; stomach; veins; vertebrae [T1–T12]; wall
thoracic aortic (nervous): plexus
thoracic cardiac: branches of thoracic ganglia; branches of vagus nerve; nerves
thoracic interspinal: muscle
thoracic interspinales: muscles
thoracic intertransversarii: muscles
thoracic intertransverse: muscles
thoracic longissimus: muscle
thoracic outlet: syndrome
thoracic-pelvic-phalangeal: dystrophy
thoracic pulmonary: branches of thoracic ganglia
thoracic rotator: muscles

thoracic splanchnic: ganglion; nerves
thoracoabdominal: ectopia cordis; nerves
thoracoacromial: artery; trunk; vein
thoracoappendicular: muscles
thoracodorsal: artery; nerve
thoracoepigastric: vein
thoracolumbar: aponeurosis; fascia; system
thoracolumbar nervous: system
thoracolumbosacral: orthosis
thoracoscopic: surgery
thoracostomy: tube
thorium: emanation
Thormählen: test
Thorn: syndrome; test
thorn apple: crystals
thought: disorder
thought process: disorder
threaded: implant
thready: pulse
threatened: abortion
three-chambered: heart
three-cornered: bone
three-day: fever; measles
three-dimensional: record
three-glass: test
three-headed: muscle
three-incision: esophagectomy
thresher's: lung
threshold: body; differential; pads of anal canal; percussion; shift; stimulus; substance; trait
threshold limit: value
thrombin: time
thrombocytic: series
thrombocytopenia-absent radius: syndrome
thrombocytopenic: purpura
thrombolytic: therapy
thrombopathic: syndrome
thrombopenic: purpura
thrombospondin-related adhesive: protein
thrombotic: gangrene; hydrocephalus; infarct; microangiopathy
thrombotic thrombocytopenic: purpura
through: drainage
through-and-through myocardial: infarction
through transfer: imaging
thrush: fungus
thumb: forceps; lancet; reflex
thunderclap: headache
Thygeson: disease
thyme: camphor
thymic: abscesses; agenesis; alymphoplasia; branches of internal thoracic artery; corpuscle; hypoplasia; veins
thymic lymphopoietic: factor
thymine: dimer
thymol turbidity: test
thymus: gland; treatment
thymus-dependent: zone
thymus-independent: antigen
thyroarytenoid: muscle
thyrocardiac: disease
thyrocervical (arterial): trunk
thyroepiglottic: ligament; muscle; part of thyroarytenoid (muscle)
thyroglossal: duct
thyroglossal duct: cyst
thyrohyoid: branch of ansa cervicalis; membrane; muscle
thyrohypophysial: syndrome
thyroid: axis; body; bruit; cartilage; colloid; diverticulum; eminence; foramen; gland; insufficiency; lymph nodes; storm; therapy; toxicosis; veins
thyroid articular: surface of cricoid (cartilage)
thyroid ima: artery
thyroid-stimulating: hormone; immunoglobulins
thyroid-stimulating hormone-releasing: factor
thyroid-stimulating hormone stimulation: test
thyroid suppression: test
thyrolingual: duct
thyropharyngeal: part of inferior constrictor muscle of pharynx; part of inferior pharyngeal constrictor (muscle) of pharynx
thyrotoxic: coma; crisis; encephalopathy; myopathy; serum
thyrotoxic heart: disease
thyrotropic: hormone
thyrotropin: resistance
thyrotropin-producing: adenoma
thyrotropin-releasing: factor; hormone
thyrotropin-releasing hormone stimulation: test
thyroxine-binding: globulin; prealbumin; protein
tibial: border of foot; crest; nerve; phenomenon; tuberosity
tibial collateral: ligament; ligament of ankle joint
tibial communicating: nerve
tibial intertendinous: bursa
tibialis anterior: muscle
tibialis posterior: muscle
tibial nutrient: artery
tibial tarsal tendinous: sheaths
tibiocalcaneal: ligament; part of deltoid ligament; part of medial ligament of ankle joint
tibiofemoral: index
tibiofibular: articulation; joint; ligament; syndesmosis
tibionavicular: ligament; part of deltoid ligament; part of medial ligament of ankle joint
tibiotalar: part of medial ligament of ankle joint
tick: paralysis; typhus
tick-borne: encephalitis (Central European subtype); encephalitis (Eastern subtype); virus
tick-borne encephalitis: virus
tic-tac: rhythm; sounds
tidal: air; drainage; volume; wave
Tiedemann: gland; nerve
tie-over: dressing
Tietz: syndrome
Tietze: syndrome
tiger: heart
tight: junction
tigroid: bodies; fundus; retina; striation; substance
tilt: table; test
tilting disk: valve
tilting disk valve: prosthesis
time: constant; marker; sense
time-compensated: gain
time compensation: gain
time-gain: compensation
time-lapse: microscopy
Time-Line: therapy
time-varied: gain
time-varied gain: control
tine: test
Tinel: sign
tinted: vision
tinted denture: base
tip: links
Tiselius: apparatus
Tiselius electrophoresis: cell
Tissot: spirometer
tissue: basophil; culture; displaceability; displacement; factor; fluid; hormones; lymph; molding; registration; respiration; tension; valve
tissue-bearing: area
tissue culture infectious: dose
tissue plasminogen: activator
tissue-specific: antigen
tissue thromboplastin inhibition: time
tissue weighting: factor
titratable acidity: test
Tizzoni: stain
Tj: antigen
TMJ: syndrome
TNM: staging
TO: virus
toad: skin
to-and-fro: anesthesia; murmur; sound
toasted: shins
tobacco: heart
tobacco-alcohol: amblyopia
Tobia: fever
Tobruk: splint
Tod: muscle
Todaro: tendon
Todd: paralysis; unit
toddler's: diarrhea; fracture
Todd postepileptic: paralysis
toe: clonus; itch; phenomenon
toilet: training
Toison: stain
Tokelau: ringworm
Toker: cell
tolbutamide: test
Toldt: fascia; membrane
tolerance: dose; limits
Tolosa-Hunt: syndrome
Tolu: balsam
toluidine blue: stain
Toma: sign
Tomes: fibers; processes
Tomes granular: layer
Tommaselli: disease
tone: color
tone decay: test
tongue: bone; depressor; phenomenon
tonic: contraction; control; convulsion; epilepsy; pupil; reflex; seizure
tonic-clonic: seizure
tonsillar: branches of glossopharyngeal nerve; branches of lesser palatine nerves; branch of the facial artery; calculus; crypt; fossa; fossulae; herniation; ring
tonsillolingual: sulcus
tooth: abrasion; avulsion; bud; cement; form; germ; ligation; plane; polyp; pulp; sac; socket; transplantation
tooth-and-nail: syndrome
tooth-borne: base
toothed: vertebra
toper's: nose
Töpfer: test
tophaceous: gout
topical: anesthesia; anesthetic
Topinard: line
Topinard facial: angle
Topografov: virus
topographic: anatomy
Topolanski: sign
toppling: gait
TORCH: syndrome

Torek: operation
toric: lens
Torkildsen: shunt
tornado: epilepsy
Tornwaldt: abscess; cyst; disease; syndrome
Toronto: formula for pulmonary artery banding
Torre: syndrome
torsion: disease of childhood; dystonia; fracture; neurosis
torsional: deformity
torsive: occlusion
Torsten Sjögren: syndrome
torus: fracture
total: acidity; aphasia; ascertainment; cataract; cleavage; communication; cystectomy; elasticity of muscle; energy; hematuria; hyperopia; keratoplasty; mastectomy; necrosis; placenta previa; sclerectasia; synechia; transfusion
total anomalous pulmonary venous: return
total body: hypothermia; water
total breech: extraction
total catecholamine: test
total cell: count
total cricoid: cleft
total end-diastolic: diameter
total end-systolic: diameter
total joint: arthroplasty
total lung: capacity
total parenteral: nutrition
total pelvic: exenteration
total peripheral: resistance
total push: therapy
total refractory: period
total spinal: anesthesia
totipotent: cell
totipotential: protoplasm
touch: cell; corpuscle
toughened: silver nitrate
Toupet: fundoplication
Tourette: disease; syndrome
Tournay: phenomenon; sign
tourniquet: poditis; test
Tourtual: membrane; sinus
Touton giant: cell
Tovell: tube
Towne: projection; view
Towne projection: radiograph
toxemic: jaundice; retinopathy of pregnancy
toxic: amaurosis; amblyopia; anemia; cataract; cirrhosis; cyanosis; delirium; dementia; equivalent; goiter; hemoglobinuria; hydrocephalus; megacolon; myocarditis; nephrosis; neuritis; psychosis; retinopathy; shock; tetanus; unit
toxic epidermal: necrolysis
toxicogenic: conjunctivitis
toxic shock: syndrome
toxin: unit
Toynbee: corpuscles; muscle; tube
TPHA: test
TPI: test
Tr^a: antigen
trabecular: bone; carcinoma; meshwork; network; reticulum; tissue of sclera; zone
trabeculated: bladder
trace: conditioning; elements; nutrient
trace conditioned: reflex
tracheal: bifurcation; branches; carina; cartilages; fenestration; glands; intubation; lymph nodes; mucosa; ring; triangle; tube; tug; ulceration; veins
tracheal breath: sounds
trachealis: muscle
tracheal wall: stripe
trachelobregmatic: diameter
tracheloclavicular: muscle
tracheobronchial: diverticulum; dyskinesia; groove
tracheoesophageal: fistula; puncture; shunt; speech
tracheostomy: tube
tracheotomy: hook; tube
trachoma: bodies; glands; virus
trachomatous: conjunctivitis; keratitis; pannus
traction: alopecia; atrophy; diverticulum; epiphysis
tragal: lamina
tragicus: muscle
trained: reflex
training: analysis; group
train-of-four: stimulus
trainwheel: rhythm
tram: lines
trance: coma
trans: phase
transactional: analysis; psychotherapy
transaxial: plane
transcapsular gray: bridges
transcellular: fluids; transport; water
transcendental: anatomy
transcervical: fracture; thymectomy
transcochlear: approach
transcondylar: fracture
transcortical: aphasia; apraxia
transcranial: radiograph
transcription-based chain: reaction
transducer: cell
transduodenal: sphincterotomy
transesophageal: echocardiography
transfer: coping; factor; genes; imaging; RNA
transferase deficiency: galactosemia
transference: neurosis
transferred: ophthalmia
transferring: enzymes
transfixion: suture
transformation: constant; zone
transformed: lymphocyte
transforming: agent; factor; gene
transforming growth: factor α; factor β; factors
transfusion: hepatitis; nephritis
transgenic: mice
trans-Golgi: reticulum
transhiatal: esophagectomy
transient: agammaglobulinemia; albuminuria; equilibrium; erythroblastopenia of childhood; hypogammaglobulinemia of infancy; myopia; retinopathy; tachypnea of the newborn
transient acantholytic: dermatosis
transient evoked otoacoustic: emission
transient global: amnesia
transient ischemic: attack
transition: electron; mutation
transitional: cell; convolution; denture; epithelium; gyrus; leukocyte; object; zone; zone of lips
transitional cell: carcinoma; papilloma
transjugular intrahepatic portosystemic: shunt
translabyrinthine: approach
translatory: movement
translocation: carrier; chromosome
translumbar: aortography
transmeatal: incision
transmembrane: potential
transmethylation: factor
transmissible: plasmid
transmissible gastroenteritis: virus of swine
transmitted: light
transmural: pressure
transmural myocardial: infarction
transnasal fiberoptic: laryngoscopy
transneuronal: atrophy
transnexus: channel
transorbital: leukotomy; lobotomy
transosseous: venography
transovarial: transmission
transparent: dentin; septum; ulcer of the cornea
transplantation: antigen; genetics
transplant lung: syndrome
transporionic: axis
transport: antibiotic; host; maximum; medium; number
transposable: element
transpulmonary: pressure
transpyloric: plane
transseptal: fibers; orchiopexy
transsexual: surgery
transstadial: transmission
transsynaptic: chromatolysis; degeneration
transtentorial: herniation
transthoracic: echocardiography; esophagectomy; pacemaker; pressure
transureteroureteral: anastomosis
transurethral: resection
transurethral resection: syndrome
transvaginal: scanning
transversalis: fascia
transversarial: part of vertebral artery
transverse: amputation; arch of foot; artery of neck; branch of lateral femoral circumflex artery; colon; crest; crest of internal acoustic meatus; diameter; disk; ductules of epoöphoron; fasciculi; fissure of cerebellum; fissure of the right lung; folds of rectum; foramen; fornix; fracture; head; hermaphroditism; lie; ligament of acetabulum; ligament of the atlas; ligament of elbow; ligament of knee; ligament of leg; ligament of pelvis; ligament of perineum; muscle of abdomen; muscle of auricle; muscle of chin; muscle of nape; muscle of thorax; muscle of tongue; myelitis; nerve of neck; part of iliofemoral ligament; part of left branch of portal vein; part of nasalis muscle; part of trapezius (muscle); plane;

presentation; process of vertebra; relaxation; ridge; ridges of sacrum; section; septum; sinus; sinus of pericardium; thoracosternotomy; vein of face; vein of scapula; veins of neck; velum
transverse abdominal: incision
transverse acetabular: ligament
transverse anthelicine: groove
transverse arytenoid: muscle
transverse atlantal: ligament
transverse auricular: muscle
transverse carpal: ligament
transverse cerebral: fissure
transverse cervical: artery; ligament; nerve; veins
transverse costal: facet
transverse crural: ligament
transverse facial: artery; fracture; vein
transverse genicular: ligament
transverse horizontal: axis
transverse humeral: ligament
transverse intermesocolic: fossa
transverse metacarpal: ligament
transverse metatarsal: ligament
transverse nasal: groove
transverse occipital: sulcus
transverse oval: pelvis
transverse palatine: fold; ridge; suture
transverse pancreatic: artery
transverse pericardial: sinus
transverse perineal: ligament
transverse pontine: fibers
transverse rhombencephalic: flexure
transverse scapular: artery
transverse tarsal: articulation; joint
transverse temporal: convolutions; gyri; sulcus
transverse tibiofibular: ligament
transverse vesical: fold
transversion: mutation
transversospinal: muscle
transversospinales: muscles
transversovertical: index
transversus abdominis: muscle
transversus menti: muscle
transversus nuchae: muscle
transversus thoracis: muscle
Trantas: dots
trapezium: bone
trapezius: muscle

trapezoid: body; bone; ligament; line; ridge
Trapp: formula
Trapp-Häser: formula
Traube: bruit; corpuscle; dyspnea; plugs; sign
Traube double: tone
Traube-Hering: curves; waves
Traube semilunar: space
traumatic: alopecia; amenorrhea; amnesia; amputation; anemia; anesthesia; aneurysm; asphyxia; cataract; dermatitis; encephalopathy; fever; herpes; meningocele; neurasthenia; neuritis; neuroma; neurosis; occlusion; orchitis; pneumothorax; psychosis; retinopathy; tetanus
traumatic bone: cyst
traumatic cervical: discopathy
traumatic progressive: encephalopathy
traumatogenic: occlusion
Trautmann triangular: space
traveler's: diarrhea
traveling wave: theory
Treacher Collins: syndrome
treatment: denture
treble: increase at low levels
trefoil: polypeptide; tendon
Treitz: arch; fascia; fossa; hernia; ligament; muscle
Trélat: stools
tremulous: iris
trench: fever; foot; hand; lung; mouth
Trendelenburg: gait; operation; position; radiograph; sign; symptom; test
trephine: biopsy
treponema-immobilizing: antibody
treponemal: antibody
Treponema pallidum **hemagglutination:** test
Treponema pallidum **immobilization:** reaction; test
Tresilian: sign
Treves: fold
Trevor: disease
triad: asthma
triadic: symbiosis
trial: base; case; denture; frame; lenses
trial of: labor after cesarean section
triangular: bandage; bone; cartilage; crest; disk of wrist; fascia; fold; fossa of

auricle; fovea of arytenoid cartilage; lamella; ligament; ligaments of liver; muscle; nucleus; nucleus of septum; part; pit of arytenoid cartilage; recess; ridge; uterus
triaxial reference: system
triazolopyridine: antidepressant
tribasic: calcium phosphate; magnesium phosphate
tribasilar: synostosis
TRIC: agents
tricarboxylic acid: cycle
triceps: bursa; muscle; muscle of arm; muscle of calf; muscle of hip; reflex
triceps brachii: muscle
triceps coxae: muscle
triceps surae: muscle; reflex
trichilemmal: cyst
trichinosis: granuloma
trichorhinophalangeal: syndrome
trichrome: stain
tricorn: protease
tricuspid: area; atresia; incompetence; insufficiency; murmur; orifice; stenosis; tooth; valve
tricyclic: antidepressant
trident: hand
O-**(triethylaminoethyl):** cellulose
trifacial: nerve; neuralgia
trifid: stomach
trifocal: lens
trigeminal: cave; cavity; crest; decompression; ganglion; impression; lemniscus; nerve [CN V]; neuralgia; pulse; rhizotomy; rhythm; tractotomy; tubercle
trigeminofacial: reflex
trigeminospinal: tract
trigeminothalamic: tract
trigger: area; finger; point; zone
triggered: activity
trihydric: alcohol
triiodothyronine: toxicosis
triiodothyronine uptake: test
triketohydrindene: reaction
trilaminar: blastoderm
trimalleolar: fracture
triphammer: pulse
triphenylmethane: dyes
triphyllomatous: teratoma
Tripier: amputation
triplant: implant
triple: arthrodesis; bond; helix; phosphate; point; quartan; response; rhythm; screen; vision
triple A: syndrome

triple repeat: disorders
triple symptom: complex
triplet: oxygen; state
triple X: syndrome
tripod: fracture
triquetrous: cartilage
triquetrum: bone
trisodium: phosphate
trisomy 8: syndrome
trisomy 13: syndrome
trisomy 18: syndrome
trisomy 20: syndrome
trisomy 21: syndrome
trisomy C: syndrome
trisomy D: syndrome
trispiral: tomography
tritiated: thymidine
triticeal: cartilage
triton: tumor
trochanter: reflex
trochanteric: bursa; bursae of gluteus medius; bursae of gluteus minimus; crest; fossa; syndrome
trochlear: fossa; fovea; nerve [CN IV]; notch; nucleus; pit; process; spine
trochlear synovial: bursa
trochoid: articulation; joint
Troisier: ganglion; node
Trolard: vein
Tröltsch: corpuscles; pockets; recesses
Trömner: reflex
trophic: changes; gangrene; nucleus; syndrome; ulcer
trophoblast: interferon
trophoblastic: lacuna; operculum
trophoneurotic: atrophy; leprosy
trophotropic: zone of Hess
tropic: hormones
tropical: abscess; acne; anemia; boil; bubo; diarrhea; diseases; eczema; eosinophilia; lichen; mask; measles; medicine; myositis; pyomyositis; sore; splenomegaly; sprue; typhus; ulcer
tropical splenomegaly: syndrome
trough: sign
Trousseau: point; sign; spot; syndrome
Trousseau-Lallemand: bodies
true: aneurysm; ankylosis; cementoma; cholinesterase; conjugate; diverticulum; dwarfism; glottis; hermaphroditism; hypertrophy; knot; lumen; muscles of back; pelvis; ribs [I–VII]; thirst; vertebra

true neurogenic thoracic outlet: syndrome
true precocious: puberty
true vocal: cord
truncate: ascertainment
Trunecek: sign
Trusler: rule for pulmonary artery banding
truth: serum
trypanosome: fever; stage
trypsin: inhibitor
α_1-trypsin: inhibitor
trypsin G-banding: stain
tsutsugamushi: disease; fever
tubal: abortion; branch; branch of ovarian artery; branch of the tympanic plexus; branch of the uterine artery; cartilage; colic; dysmenorrhea; extremity of ovary; glands of pharyngotympanic tube; infantilism; ligation; pregnancy; prominence; tonsil
tubal air: cells (of pharyngotympanic tube)
tube: cast; curare; tooth
tubed: flap
tubed pedicle: flap
tuberal: nuclei
tubercle: bacillus
tuberculin: test
tuberculin-type: hypersensitivity
tuberculoid: leprosy; rosacea
tuberculoopsonic: index
tuberculosis: lymphadenitis; vaccine
tuberculous: bronchopneumonia; enteritis; lymphadenitis; meningitis; nephritis; pericarditis; peritonitis; rheumatism; spondylitis; wart
tuberoinfundibular: tract
tuberomammillary: nucleus
tuberosity: reduction
tuberous: root; sclerosis
Tübinger: perimeter
tuboabdominal: pregnancy
tubo-ovarian: varicocele
tuboovarian: abscess; pregnancy
tuboreticular: structure
tubotympanic: canal; recess
tubouterine: pregnancy
tubular: adenoma; aneurysm; carcinoma; cyst; forceps; gland; maximum; respiration; vision
tubular excretory: mass
tubuloacinar: gland
tubuloalveolar: gland
tubuloglomerular: feedback
tubulointerstitial: nephritis

Tucker-McLean: forceps
tuffstone: body
tufted: cell; phalanx
tularemic: chancre; conjunctivitis; pneumonia
Tullio: phenomenon
Tulp: valve
tumbu dermal: myiasis
tumescent: liposuction
tumor: antigens; blush; embolism; marker; stage; virus
tumoral: calcinosis
tumor angiogenic: factor
tumor-associated: antigen
tumor-infiltrating: lymphocytes
tumor lysis: syndrome
tumor necrosis: factor; factor-α; factor-β
tumor-specific transplantation: antigens
tumor suppressor: gene
tungsten arc: lamp
tuning: curve; fork
tunnel: cells; disease; vision
Tuohy: needle
T$_3$ uptake: test
TUR: syndrome
turban: tumor
turbinal: varix
turbinated: body; bones; crest
Türck: bundle; column; degeneration; tract
Turcot: syndrome
Türk: cell; leukocyte
turkey gobbler: neck
Turkish: saddle
Turlock: virus
Turner: sulcus; syndrome; tooth
turnover: number
turpentine: enema; poisoning
tussive: fremitus; syncope
Tuttle: proctoscope
Tweed: triangle
Tweed edgewise: treatment
twelfth cranial: nerve [CN XII]
twelfth-year: molar
twenty-nail: dystrophy
twiddler's: syndrome
twilight: sleep; state; vision
twin: cone; crystal; helix; method; placenta; pregnancy
twin reversed arterial perfusion: sequence
twin-twin: transfusion
twist: form
twisted: hairs
two-bellied: muscle
two-carbon: fragment
two-dimensional: chromatography; echocardiography; immunoelectrophoresis

two-dimension–three-dimension: phenomenon
two-glass: test
two-headed: muscle
Twort: phenomenon
Twort-d'Herelle: phenomenon
two-step exercise: test
two-tail: test
two-way: catheter
tying: forceps
tympanic: antrum; aperture of canaliculus for chorda tympani; attic; body; bone; canal; canaliculus; cavity; cells; enlargement; ganglion; gland; groove; incisure; intumescence; labium of limbus of spiral lamina; lamella (of osseous spiral lamina); lip of limbus of spiral lamina; lip of spiral limbus; membrane; nerve; notch; opening of canaliculus for chorda tympani; opening of eustachian tube; opening of pharyngotympanic (auditory) tube; part of temporal bone; plate of temporal bone; promontory; ring; scute; sinus; sulcus; surface of cochlear duct; veins; wall of cochlear duct
tympanic air: cells
tympanic (nervous): plexus
tympanitic: resonance
tympanohyal: bone
tympanomastoid: fissure; suture
tympanosquamous: fissure
tympanostapedial: junction; syndesmosis
tympanostomy: tube
Tyndall: effect; phenomenon
type: culture; species; strain
type 1: dextrocardia; glycogenosis
type 2: dextrocardia; glycogenosis
type 3: dextrocardia; glycogenosis
type 4: dextrocardia; glycogenosis
type 5: glycogenosis
type 6: glycogenosis
type 7: glycogenosis
type A: behavior; personality
type B: behavior
Type 1 choroidal: neovascularization
Type 2 choroidal: neovascularization
Type 1 G$_{M1}$: gangliosidosis
Type I: osteogenesis imperfecta

type I: acrocephalosyndactyly; cells; collagen; diabetes; diabetes mellitus; dip; error; interferon
Type IA: achondrogenesis
Type IB: achondrogenesis
type I familial: hyperlipoproteinemia
type IH: mucopolysaccharidosis
type I H/S: mucopolysaccharidosis
Type II: achondrogenesis; osteogenesis imperfecta
type II: acrocephalosyndactyly; cells; collagen; diabetes; dip; error; interferon; mucopolysaccharidosis
type II familial: hyperlipoproteinemia
Type III: osteogenesis imperfecta
type III: acrocephalosyndactyly; collagen; mucopolysaccharidosis
type III familial: hyperlipoproteinemia
type III hypersensitivity: reaction
type III punctate palmoplantar: keratoderma
type IS: mucopolysaccharidosis
Type IV: osteogenesis imperfecta
type IV: collagen
type IVA, B: mucopolysaccharidosis
type IV familial: hyperlipoproteinemia
type V: acrocephalosyndactyly; mucopolysaccharidosis
type V familial: hyperlipoproteinemia
type VI: mucopolysaccharidosis
type VII: mucopolysaccharidosis
typhoid: bacillus; bacteriophage; cholera; fever; pleurisy; pneumonia; septicemia; vaccine
typhoid-paratyphoid A and B: vaccine
typhus: vaccine
typical: achromatopsia; drusen; pseudocholinesterase
typical antipsychotic: agent
typist's: cramp
Tyrode: solution
Tyrrell: fascia
TY1-S-33: medium
TYSGM-9: medium

Tyson: glands
Tzanck: cells; test

U

U: wave
ubiquitin-protease: pathway
Uffelmann: reagent
Uhl: anomaly
Uhthoff: sign; symptom; syndrome
ulcerating: granuloma of pudenda
ulcerative: colitis; pharyngitis; stomatitis
ulceromembranous: gingivitis; pharyngitis
Ullmann: line; syndrome
ulnar: artery; border of forearm; branch of medial antebrachial cutaneous nerve; bursa; clubhand; eminence of wrist; head; margin of forearm; nerve; notch; reflex; veins
ulnar collateral: ligament; ligament of elbow joint; ligament of wrist joint
ulnar communicating: branch of superficial radial nerve
ulnar extensor: muscle of wrist
ulnar flexor: muscle of wrist
ulnar recurrent: artery
ultimate: principle; strength
ultimobranchial: body; pouch
ultra-: microscope
ultradian: rhythm
ultrafast Pap: stain
ultrafiltration: coefficient; hemodialyzer
ultralente: insulin
ultrashortwave: diathermy
ultrasonic: cardiography; cephalometry; cleaning; lithotripsy; microscope; nebulizer; rays; scaler; therapy; waves
ultrasonic egg: recovery
ultrasound: cardiography; transducer
ultrastructural: anatomy
ultraviolet: index; keratoconjunctivitis; lamp; microscope; rays; spectrum
ultropaque: method
Ulysses: syndrome
umber: codon; mutation
umbilical: artery; cord; cyst; duct; fascia; fissure; fistula; fossa; fungus; granuloma; hernia; notch; part of left branch of portal vein; region; ring; souffle; vein; vesicle
umbilical prevesical: fascia

umbilicated: cataract
umbilicomammillary: triangle
umbilicovesical: fascia
Umbre: virus
unarmed: rostellum
unavoidable: hemorrhage
unbalanced: translocation
uncal: artery; herniation
unciform: bone; fasciculus
uncinate: attack; bundle of Russell; epilepsy; fasciculus of cerebellum; fasciculus of Russell; fit; gyrus; pancreas; process of cervical vertebra; process of ethmoid bone; process of first thoracic vertebra; process of pancreas
uncombable hair: syndrome
uncomfortable: level
uncompensated: acidosis; alkalosis
uncompetitive: inhibition; inhibitor
unconditioned: reflex; response; stimulus
unconjugated: bilirubin
unconscious: homosexuality
uncoupling: factors
uncovertebral: joints
uncrossed: diplopia
uncus: band of Giacomini
undercut: gauge
undermining: ulcer
Underwood: disease
undescended: testis
undetermined: nitrogen
undifferentiated: cell
undifferentiated cell: adenoma
undifferentiated type: fevers
undulant: fever
undulating: fever; membrane; pulse
unequal: cleavage; pulse
unequal retinal: image
unerupted: tooth
unesterified free: fatty acid
uneven: crossing-over
unformed visual: hallucination
ungual: phalanx; tuberosity
uniaxial: joint
unicameral: cyst
unicameral bone: cyst
unicanalicular: sphincter
unicellular: gland; sclerosis
unicorn: uterus
unidentified: reading frame
unidirectional: block; flux; replication
unilaminar primary: follicle
unilateral: anesthesia; hemianopia; hermaphroditism
unilateral hyperlucent: lung
unilateral lobar: emphysema

unilocular: cyst; fat; joint
unilocular hydatid: cyst
unimolecular: reaction
uninducible: mutant
uninhibited neurogenic: bladder
uninterrupted: suture
uniovular: twins
unipennate: muscle
unipolar: cell; electrocardiogram; leads; neuron
unit: character; fibrils; membrane
unit of: convergence
uniting: canal; cartilage; duct
univalent: antibody
univentricular: connections; heart
universal: antidote; appliance; donor; infantilism; solvent
unmodified zinc oxide-eugenol: cement
unmyelinated: fibers; nerve
Unna: disease; mark; nevus; stain
Unna-Pappenheim: stain
Unna-Taenzer: stain
Unna-Thost: syndrome
unpaired: allosome; chromosome
unpaired thyroid venous: plexus
unresolved: pneumonia
unroofed coronary sinus: syndrome
unsaturated: alcohols; fat; fatty acid
unsharp: masking
unstable: angina; bladder; colloid; equilibrium; fracture; hemoglobins; lie
unstable hemoglobin hemolytic: anemia
unstrained jaw: relation
unstriated: muscle
unsystematized: delusion
ununited: fracture
Unverricht: disease
unwinding: proteins
upbeat: nystagmus
upper: airway; extremity; extremity of fibula; eyelid; jaw; lid; limb; lip; lobe of lung; pole; pole of testis
upper abdominal periosteal: reflex
upper dental: arcade
upper esophageal: constriction
upper GI: series
upper jaw: bone
upper lateral cutaneous: nerve of arm
upper motor: neuron
upper motor neuron: lesion

upper subscapular: nerve
upper thoracic splanchnic: nerves
upper uterine: segment
up promoter: mutation
upregulation/downregulation: hypothesis
ur-: defenses
urachal: cyst; fistula; fold; ligament
uracil: mustard
uranium: nephritis
uranyl acetate: stain
urate crystals: stain
Urbach-Wiethe: disease
Urban: operation
urban: typhus
urban cutaneous: leishmaniasis
urea: clearance; cycle; frost; nitrogen
urea clearance: test
urease: test
urecholine supersensitivity: test
uremic: breath; colitis; coma; lung; pericarditis; pneumonia; pneumonitis; polyneuropathy
ureteral: branches; colic; ectopia; meatus; opening; reimplantation
ureteric: branches; branches of the inferior suprarenal artery; branches of the ovarian artery; branches of the patent part of umbilical artery; branches of the renal artery; branches of the testicular artery; bud; dysmenorrhea; fold; orifice; pelvis
ureteric (nervous): plexus
ureterocutaneous: fistula
ureteroileal: anastomosis
ureteropelvic: junction
ureteropelvic junction: obstruction
ureterorenal: reflux
ureterosigmoid: anastomosis
ureteroureteral: anastomosis
ureterovaginal: fistula
ureterovesical: junction; obstruction
urethral: artery; calculus; carina of vagina; caruncle; crest; crest of female; crest of male; dilation; diverticulum; fever; glands; glands of female; glands of male; groove; hematuria; lacuna; openings; papilla; plate; stricture; surface of penis; syndrome; valves
urethral pressure: profile

urethrocutaneous: fistula
urethrovaginal: fistula; sphincter
urethrovesical: angle
urge: incontinence
uric acid: infarct
uricolytic: index
urinary: apparatus; bladder; calculus; casts; cyst; fever; fistula; nitrogen; organs; reflex; sand; schistosomiasis; smear; stuttering; system; tract
urinary concentration: test
urinary exertional: incontinence
urinary tract: infection
uriniferous: tubule
urogenital: apparatus; cleft; diaphragm; fistula; membrane; mesentery; peritoneum; region; ridge; septum; sinus; system; triangle
urogenital sinus: anomaly
uropoietic: system
urorectal: fold; membrane; septum
urothelial: carcinoma; papilloma
urticarial: fever; vasculitis
u-score: method
Usher: syndrome
USP: unit
usual interstitial: pneumonia of Liebow
uterine: appendages; artery; atony; calculus; cavity; colic; contraction; dysmenorrhea; extremity of ovary; glands; horn; inertia; insufficiency; milk; opening of uterine tubes; ostium of uterine tubes; part of uterine tube; pregnancy; sinus; sinusoid; souffle; tetanus; tube; tympanites; veins
uterine venous: plexus
uteroabdominal: pregnancy
uteroepichorial: membrane
utero-ovarian: varicocele
uteroperitoneal: fistula
uteroplacental: apoplexy; sinuses
uterovaginal: canal
uterovaginal (nervous): plexus
uterovesical: fold; ligament; pouch
utilization: time
utricular: cyst; duct; nerve; recess of bony labyrinth; recess of membranous labyrinth; reflexes; spot
utriculoampullar: nerve
utriculosaccular: duct

uveal: part of trabecular reticulum; part of trabecular tissue of sclera; staphyloma; tract
uveocutaneous: syndrome
uveoencephalitic: syndrome
uveomeningitis: syndrome
uveoparotid: fever
uviol: lamp
uvular: muscle
Uzbekistan hemorrhagic: fever

V

V: antigen; gene; lead; wave
V-2: carcinoma
vaccine: bodies; lymph; virus
vaccinia: virus
vaccinoid: reaction
VACTERL: syndrome
vacuolar: degeneration; nephrosis
vacuolating: virus
vacuum: aspirator; casting; desiccator; extractor; flask; headache; investing; tube
vacuum disk: phenomenon
vacuum pack: technique
vagabond's: disease
vagal: attack; bradycardia; part of accessory nerve
vagal nerve: stimulation
vagal (nerve): trigone; trunk
vagi: eminentia
vaginal: artery; atresia; celiotomy; columns; cuff; dysmenorrhea; fornix; gland; hysterectomy; hysterotomy; introitus; laceration; lithotomy; mucosa; myomectomy; nerves; opening; orifice; part of cervix; pool; process; process of peritoneum; process of sphenoid bone; process of testis; rugae; smear
vaginal cornification: test
vaginal intraepithelial: neoplasia
vaginal mucification: test
vaginal synovial: membrane
vaginal venous: plexus
vagovagal: reflex
vagrant's: disease
vagus: area; nerve [CN X]; pulse
valence: electron
Valentin: corpuscles; ganglion; nerve
Valentine: position; test
vallate: papillae
vallecular: dysphagia
Valleix: points
valley: fever

Valsalva: antrum; ligaments; maneuver; muscle; sinus; test
valvotomy: knife
valvular: endocarditis; incompetence; insufficiency; prolapse; regurgitation; sclerosis; thrombus
vampire: bat
van Bogaert: encephalitis
van Buchem: syndrome
van Buren: disease; sound
van Deen: test
van den Bergh: test
van der Hoeve: syndrome
van der Velden: test
van der Waals: forces
van Ermengen: stain
van Gieson: stain
van Helmont: mirror
van Horne: canal
vanillylmandelic acid: test
vanished testis: syndrome
vanishing: cream; lung
vanishing lung: syndrome
Van Lohuizen: syndrome
Van Slyke: apparatus; formula
van't Hoff: equation; law; theory
vapor: density; pressure
Vaquez: disease
variable: coupling; deceleration; region
variance: ratio
variant: angina pectoris; hemoglobin
varicella: encephalitis
varicella-zoster: virus
varicose: aneurysm; bronchiectasis; eczema; ulcer; veins
variegate: porphyria
variola: virus
Varolius: sphincter
vascular: bud; cataract; circle; circle of optic nerve; cones; dementia; dentin; fold of the cecum; gland; headache; keratitis; lacuna; lamina of choroid; layer; layer of choroid coat of eye; layer of eyeball; layer of testis; leiomyoma; meninx; murmur; nerves; organ of lamina terminalis; papillae; pedicle; plexus; polyp; ring; sclerosis; sheaths; space of retroinguinal compartment; spider; spur; stripe; system; tunic of eye; zone
vasculocardiac: syndrome of hyperserotonemia
vasculogenic: impotence
vasoactive: amine
vasoactive intestinal: peptide; polypeptide

vasodepressor: substance; syncope
vasoformative: cell
vasogenic: shock
vasomotor: angina; ataxia; center; epilepsy; fibers; imbalance; nerve; paralysis; rhinitis
vasoocclusive: crisis
vasopressin-resistant: diabetes
vasopressor: reflex
vasovagal: attack; epilepsy; syncope; syndrome
vastoadductor: fascia
vastus intermedius: muscle
vastus lateralis: muscle
vastus medialis: muscle
VATER: complex
Vater: corpuscles; fold
Vater-Pacini: corpuscles
VCE: smear
VDRL: test
vector: loop
vector-borne: infection
VEE: virus
vegetable: alkali; base; calomel; charcoal; gelatin; sulfur; wax
vegetal: pole
vegetative: bacteriophage; endocarditis; life; reproduction; stage; state
vegetative nervous: system
veil: cell
veiled: cells; puff
veiling: glare
vein: stone; stripper
Vel: antigen
velamentous: insertion
veldt: sore
Vella: fistula
vellus: hair
velocardiofacial: syndrome
velocity: coefficient; constants
velopharyngeal: closure; insufficiency; seal; sphincter
Velpeau: bandage; canal; fossa; hernia
velvet: ant
Ven: antigen
vena cava: filter
vena caval: foramen
venereal: bubo; disease; lymphogranuloma; sore; ulcer; wart
Venezuelan equine: encephalomyelitis
Venezuelan equine encephalomyelitis: virus
Venezuelan hemorrhagic: fever
Venice: turpentine
Venn: diagram
venocaval: filter
venom: hemolysis

venoocclusive: disease of the liver
venorespiratory: reflex
venous: angioma; angle; artery; blood; capillary; circle of mammary gland; congestion; embolism; foramen; gangrene; grooves; heart; hum; hyperemia; insufficiency; lakes; ligament; malformation; murmur; plexus; plexus of bladder; plexus of canal of hypoglossal nerve; plexus of foramen ovale; pulse; return; segments of the kidney; sinuses; sinus of sclera; star; stasis; ulcer; valve
venous occlusion: plethysmography
venous-stasis: retinopathy
ventilation: meter
ventilation-perfusion: scan
ventilation/perfusion: ratio
ventilatory: compliance
ventral: aortas; border; branch; decubitus; funiculus; glands; hernia; horn; mesocardium; mesogastrium; nuclei of thalamus; nucleus of trapezoid body; pallidum; pancreas; part of intertransversarii laterales lumborum (muscles); part of pons; plate; plate of neural tube; rami of cervical nerves; rami of lumbar nerves; rami of sacral nerves; rami of thoracic nerves; ramus of spinal nerve; root of spinal nerve; striatum; surface of digit; thalamus
ventral acoustic: stria
ventral anterior: nucleus [TA] of thalamus
ventral apron: prepuce
ventral intermediate: nucleus [TA] of thalamus
ventral lateral: nucleus of thalamus
ventral lateral geniculate: nucleus
ventral posterior: nucleus of thalamus
ventral posterior intermediate: nucleus of thalamus
ventral posterolateral: nucleus [TA] of thalamus
ventral posteromedial: nucleus [TA] of thalamus
ventral premammillary: nucleus

ventral primary: rami of cervical spinal nerves; rami of lumbar spinal nerves; rami of sacral spinal nerves; rami of thoracic spinal nerves; ramus of spinal nerve
ventral principal: nucleus
ventral raphespinal: tract
ventral sacrococcygeal: ligament; muscle
ventral sacrococcygeus: muscle
ventral sacroiliac: ligaments
ventral spinocerebellar: tract
ventral spinothalamic: tract
ventral splanchnic: arteries
ventral tegmental: decussation
ventral thalamic: peduncle
ventral tier thalamic: nuclei
ventral trigeminothalamic: tract
ventral white: column; commissure
ventricular: aberration; afterload; aneurysm; arteries; band of larynx; bigeminy; bradycardia; capture; complex; conduction; diastole; diverticulum; escape; extrasystole; fibrillation; fluid; flutter; fold; gradient; layer; ligament; loop; plateau; preexcitation; preload; rhythm; septum; standstill; systole; tachycardia; trigone
ventricular assist: device
ventricular filling: pressure
ventricular fusion: beat
ventricular inhibited pulse: generator
ventricular late: potential
ventricular reduction: surgery
ventricular septal: defect
ventricular synchronous pulse: generator
ventricular triggered pulse: generator
ventriculoatrial: conduction
ventriculoradial: dysplasia
ventrobasal: complex; nuclei (complex)
ventrolateral: nucleus; sulcus
ventromedial: nucleus; nucleus of hypothalamus
Venturi: effect; meter; tube
verbal: agraphia; apraxia; autopsy
Veress: needle
Verga: ventricle
Verheyen: stars
Verhoeff elastic tissue: stain

vermian: fossa
vermicular: colic; movement; pulse
vermiform: appendage; appendix; process
vermilion: border; zone
verminous: abscess; appendicitis; ileus
vernal: catarrh; conjunctivitis; encephalitis; keratoconjunctivitis
Verner-Morrison: syndrome
Vernet: syndrome
Verneuil: neuroma
Vernier: acuity
vero: cytotoxin
Verocay: bodies
verrucous: carcinoma; hemangioma; hyperplasia; nevus; scrofuloderma; vegetations; xanthoma
versive: seizure
vertebral: arch; artery; body; border of scapula; canal; column; foramen; formula; fusion; ganglion; groove; line of pleural reflection; nerve; notch; part of the costal surface of the lungs; part of diaphragm; plexus; polyarthritis; pulp; region; ribs; vein; venography
vertebral-basilar: system
vertebral epidural: space
vertebral venous: plexus; system
vertebrate: hormones
vertebrated: catheter; probe
vertebroarterial: foramen
vertebrochondral: ribs
vertebrocostal: trigone
vertebromediastinal: recess
vertebropelvic: ligaments
vertebrosternal: ribs
vertex: presentation
vertical: aspect; axis; crest of internal acoustic meatus; dimension; elastic; heart; hymen; illumination; index; muscle of tongue; nystagmus; opening; osteotomy; overlap; parallax; plate; strabismus; transmission; vertigo
vertical banded: gastroplasty
vertical growth: phase
vertical retraction: syndrome
verticosubmental: view
Vesalius: bone; foramen; vein
vesical: calculus; diverticulum; fistula; gland; hematuria; lithotomy; reflex; surface of uterus; triangle; veins
vesicalis: anus
vesical (nervous): plexus
vesicating: gas

vesicle: hernia
vesicocolic: fistula
vesicocutaneous: fistula
vesicointestinal: fistula
vesicoumbilical: ligament
vesicoureteral: reflux; valve
vesicourethral: canal
vesicouterine: fistula; ligament; pouch
vesicovaginal: fistula
vesicovaginorectal: fistula
vesicular: appendages of epoophoron; appendices of uterine tube; follicle; keratitis; keratopathy; mole; murmur; rale; resonance; respiration; rickettsiosis; stomatitis; transport
vesicular breath: sounds
vesicular exanthema of swine: virus
vesicular ovarian: follicle
vesicular stomatitis: virus
vesicular venous: plexus
vesiculocavernous: respiration
vesiculotympanitic: resonance
Vesling: line
vestibular: anus; apparatus; aqueduct; area; branches of labyrinthine artery; canal; cecum of the cochlear duct; crest; fissure of cochlea; fold; fossa; ganglion; glands; labium of limbus of spiral lamina; labyrinth; lamella (of osseous spiral lamina); ligament; lip of limbus of spiral lamina; lip of spiral limbus; membrane; nerve; neurectomy; neuronitis; nuclei; nystagmus; organ; part of vestibulocochlear nerve; root; root of vestibulocochlear nerve; schwannoma; screen; surface of cochlear duct; surface of tooth; wall of cochlear duct; window
vestibular blind: sac
vestibular hair: cells
vestibulocerebellar: ataxia
vestibulocochlear: artery; nerve [CN VIII]; nuclei; organ
vestibulo-equilibratory: control
vestibuloocular: reflex
vestibulospinal: reflex; tracts
vestigial: fold; muscle; organ
Veterans Administration: hospital
veterinary: medicine
Vi: antibody; antigen
viable cell: count
vibrating: line

vibration: syndrome; tolerance
vibratory: massage; sensibility; urticaria
vicarious: hypertrophy; menstruation
vicious: cicatrix; circle; union
Vicq d'Azyr: bundle; centrum semiovale; foramen
Vidal: disease
video: fluoroscopy
video-assisted thoracic: surgery
vidian: artery; canal; nerve; vein
Vierra: sign
Vieth-Müller: circle
Vieussens: ansa; anulus; centrum; foramina; ganglia; isthmus; limbus; loop; ring; valve; veins; ventricle
view: box
villous: adenoma; atrophy; carcinoma; papilloma; placenta; tenosynovitis; tumor
Vinca: alkaloids
Vincent: angina; bacillus; disease; infection; spirillum; tonsillitis
Vincent white: mycetoma
Vineberg: procedure
vinegar: eel
vinous: liquor
violinist's: cramp
Vipond: sign
viral: cystitis; dysentery; encephalomyelitis; envelope; gastroenteritis; hemagglutination; hepatitis; hepatitis type A; hepatitis type B; hepatitis type C; hepatitis type D; hepatitis type E; load; neutralization; pericarditis; probe; strand; therapy; tropism; wart
viral hemorrhagic: fever
viral hemorrhagic fever: virus
Virchow: angle; cells; corpuscles; crystals; disease; law; node; psammoma
Virchow-Hassall: bodies
Virchow-Holder: angle
Virchow-Robin: space
virgin: generation; silk
virginal: membrane
Virginia: snakeroot
viridans: hemolysis; streptococci
virile: member
virtual: endoscopy; focus; image
virulent: bacteriophage; bubo
virulent phage: mutant

virus: blockade; hepatitis; keratoconjunctivitis
virus A: hepatitis
virus-associated hemophagocytic: syndrome
virus B: hepatitis
virus C: hepatitis
virus-transformed: cell
virus X: disease
visceral: anesthesia; arches; brain; cavity; cleft; crises; disorder; epilepsy; fascia; inversion; larva migrans; layer; layer of serous pericardium; layer of tunica vaginalis of testis; leishmaniasis; lymph nodes; lymph nodes of abdomen; mesoderm; muscle; nerve; nodes; nuclei of oculomotor nerve; pericardium; peritoneum; plate; pleura; pleurisy; sense; skeleton; surface of liver; surface of the spleen; swallow
visceral disease: virus
visceral motor: fibers; neuron; system
visceral nervous: system
visceral pelvic: fascia
visceral traction: reflex
viscerogenic: reflex
visceromotor: reflex
viscerosensory: reflex
viscerotrophic: reflex
viscoelastic: retardation
visibility: acuity
visible: spectrum
visiting: nurse
visna: virus
visual: acuity; agnosia; angle; aphasia; area; aura; axis; blackout; cortex; cycle; efficiency; extinction; field; image; inattention; inspection with acetic acid; organ; pathway; pigments; projection; purple; threshold; vertigo; violet; yellow
visual evoked: potential
visual-kinetic: dissociation
visual orbicularis: reflex
visual receptor: cells
visual-spatial: agnosia
vita: glass
vital: capacity; center; force; index; knot; node; pulp; signs; spirits; stain; statistics; tooth; tripod
vitality: test
vitamin A: unit
vitamin B$_{12}$: neuropathy
vitamin B$_2$: unit
vitamin B$_6$: unit
vitamin B$_1$ hydrochloride: unit

vitamin C: test; unit
vitamin D: milk; unit
vitamin D–binding: protein
vitamin D-resistant: rickets
vitamin E: unit
vitamin K: unit
vitelliform: degeneration
vitelliform retinal: dystrophy
vitelline: artery; cord; duct; fistula; membrane; pole; reservoir; sac; vein; vessels
vitelliruptive: degeneration
vitellointestinal: cyst
vitiated: air
vitiliginous: choroiditis
vitreoretinal choroidopathy: syndrome
vitreoretinal traction: syndrome
vitreotapetoretinal: dystrophy
vitreous: body; camera; cell; chamber; chamber of eye; detachment; hernia; humor; lamella; membrane; table
in vitro: fertilization
vivax: fever; malaria
in vivo: fertilization
Vladimiroff-Mikulicz: amputation
VMA: test
vocal: amusia; cord; fold; fremitus; ligament; muscle; process; process of arytenoid cartilage; resonance; shelf; spectrum; tract
vocal cord: nodules
vocalis: muscle
Vogel: law
Voges-Proskauer: reaction
Vogt: angle; syndrome
Vogt-Koyanagi: syndrome
Vogt-Spielmeyer: disease
Vohwinkel: syndrome
voice fatigue: syndrome
voiding: cystogram; cystourethrogram
voiding flow: rate
voiding internal urethral: orifice
volar carpal: ligament
volar interosseous: artery; nerve
volatile: anesthetic; mustard oil; oil
volatile fatty acid: number
Volhard: test
volitional: tremor
Volkmann: canals; cheilitis; contracture; spoon
Vollmer: test
Volpe-Manhold: Index
voltage-gated: channel
voltaic: taste
Voltolini: disease
volume: element; index; substitute; unit

volume-controlled: respirator
volume-displacement: plethysmograph
volume-time: curve
volumetric: analysis; flask; solution
voluntary: dehydration; guarding; hospital; muscle; mutism; nystagmus
volutin: granules
vomeral: groove; sulcus
vomerine: canal; cartilage; crest of choana; groove
vomerobasilar: canal
vomeronasal: cartilage; organ
vomerorostral: canal
vomerovaginal: canal; groove
vomiting: gas; reflex
von Economo: disease
von Gierke: disease
von Graefe: sign
von Hippel: disease
von Hippel-Lindau: syndrome
von Kossa: stain
von Recklinghausen: disease
von Spee: curve
von Willebrand: disease; factor
Voorhoeve: disease
vortex: veins
vortex corneal: dystrophy
vorticose: veins
Vossius lenticular: ring
V-pattern: esotropia; exotropia
VS: virus
V-shaped: area of esophagus
vulnerable: period; phase
vulnerable child: syndrome
Vulpian: atrophy
vulsella: forceps
vulvar: dystrophy; slit
vulvar intraepithelial: neoplasia
vulvovaginal: cystectomy; gland
Vw: antigen
V-Y: flap

W

W: chromosome; factor; rays
W-: arch
"w": hernia
Waardenburg: syndrome
Wachendorf: membrane
Wachstein-Meissel: stain for calcium-magnesium-ATPase
Wada: test
waddingtonian: homeostasis
waddling: gait
Wagner: disease; syndrome
WAGR: syndrome
waist-hip: ratio
waiter's: cramp

Walcher: position
Waldenström: macroglobulinemia; purpura; syndrome; test
Waldeyer: fossae; glands; sheath; space; tract
Waldeyer throat: ring
Waldeyer zonal: layer
Walker: chart; tractotomy
walking: typhoid
walk-through: angina
Wallenberg: syndrome
wallerian: degeneration; law
wallet: stomach
wall-eyed bilateral internuclear: ophthalmoplegia
Walsh: procedure
Walthard cell: rest
Walther: canals; dilator; ducts; ganglion; plexus
wandering: abscess; cell; erysipelas; goiter; kidney; liver; organ; pacemaker; pneumonia
Wang: test
Wangensteen: drainage; suction; tube
war: neurosis
warble: botfly; fly
Warburg: apparatus; theory
Warburg-Dickens-Horecker: shunt
Warburg-Lipmann-Dickens-Horecker: shunt
Warburg old yellow: enzyme
Warburg respiratory: enzyme
Ward: triangle
Ward-Romano: syndrome
Wardrop: disease; method
warehouseman's: itch
warm: agglutinins; autoantibody
warm-blooded: animal
warm-cold: hemolysin
warmup: phenomenon
Warren: shunt
Wartenberg: symptom
Warthin: tumor
Warthin-Finkeldey: cells
Warthin-Starry silver: stain
warty: dyskeratoma; horn
wash-: bottle
washed: sulfur
washed field: technique
washerwoman's: itch
washing: soda
washout: cannula; test
Wasmann: glands
wasserhelle: cell
Wassermann: antibody; reaction; test
wasted: ventilation
wasting: disease; syndrome
watchmaker's: cramp

water: aspirator; bath; bed; canker; depletion; diuresis; dressing; gas; glass; intoxication; itch; sore
water-clear: cell of parathyroid
water-drinking: test
water-hammer: pulse
Waterhouse-Friderichsen: syndrome
watering-can: perineum; scrotum
Waters: operation; projection; view
watershed: infarction
water-soluble: chlorophyll derivatives
Waterston: operation; shunt
Waters view: radiograph
water-trap: stomach
water wheel: murmur
waterwheel: sound
water-whistle: sound
watery: eye
Watson-Crick: helix
Watson-Schwartz: test
wave: analyzer; form; number
wax: acid; alcohol; expansion; form; pattern
wax model: denture
wax-tipped: bougie
waxy: cast; degeneration; fingers; kidney; liver; spleen
WDHA: syndrome
wear-and-tear: pigment
weaver's: cough
web: eye
Webb: antigen
webbed: fingers; neck; penis; toes
Weber: glands; law; organ; paradox; point; sign; stain; syndrome; test for hearing; triangle
Weber-Christian: disease
Weber-Cockayne: syndrome
Weber-Fechner: law
Webster: test
Wechsler-Bellevue: scale
Wechsler intelligence: scales
weddellite: calculus
Wedensky: effect; facilitation; inhibition
wedge: biopsy; bone; pressure; resection; spirometer
wedge-and-groove: joint; suture
wedge-shaped: fasciculus; tubercle
WEE: virus
weekend: hospital
Weeks: bacillus
weeping: eczema
Wegener: granulomatosis
Wegner: disease; line
Weibel-Palade: bodies

Weichselbaum: coccus
Weidel: reaction
Weigert: law; stain for actinomyces; stain for elastin; stain for fibrin; stain for myelin; stain for neuroglia
Weigert-Gram: stain
Weigert iodine: solution
Weigert iron hematoxylin: stain
weight: sense
Weil: disease
Weil basal: layer; zone
Weil-Felix: reaction; test
Weill-Marchesani: syndrome
Weinberg: reaction
Weingrow: reflex
Weir: operation
Weir Mitchell: disease; treatment
Weisbach: angle
Weiss: sign
Weitbrecht: cartilage; cord; fibers; foramen; ligament
Welch: bacillus
Welcker: angle
welder's: conjunctivitis; lung
well: counter
well-differentiated lymphocytic: lymphoma
Wells: syndrome
Wenckebach: block; period; phenomenon
Wenzel: ventricle
Wepfer: glands
Werdnig-Hoffmann: disease
Werdnig-Hoffmann muscular: atrophy
Werlhof: disease
Wermer: syndrome
Wernekinck: commissure; decussation
Werner: syndrome; test
Wernicke: aphasia; area; center; disease; encephalopathy; field; radiation; reaction; region; sign; syndrome; zone
Wernicke-Korsakoff: encephalopathy; syndrome
Wertheim: operation
Werther: disease
Wesselsbron: disease; fever
Wesselsbron disease: virus
West: syndrome
West African: fever; trypanosomiasis
West African sleeping: sickness
Westberg: space
Westergren: method
Westermark: sign
Western blot: analysis
western equine: encephalomyelitis

western equine encephalomyelitis: virus
West Indian: smallpox
West Nile: fever; virus
West Nile encephalitis: virus
Westphal-Piltz: phenomenon
Westphal pupillary: reflex
wet: beriberi; compress; cup; dream; gangrene; lung; nurse; pack; pleurisy; shock; tetter
wet cutaneous: leishmaniasis
wet and dry bulb: thermometer
wettable: sulfur
wet-technique: liposuction
wet-to-dry: dressing
Wetzel: grid
Wever-Bray: phenomenon
Weyers-Thier: syndrome
whale: fingers
Wharton: duct; jelly
wheal-and-erythema: reaction
wheal-and-flare: reaction
wheat: germ; gum
Wheatstone: bridge
Wheeler: method
Wheeler-Johnson: test
whetstone: crystals
whewellite: calculus
whey: alum; protein
whiff: test
whip: bougie
whiplash: injury; retinopathy
Whipple: disease; operation
whispered: bronchophony; pectoriloquy
whistle-tip: catheter
whistling: deformity; rale
whistling face: syndrome
Whitaker: test
white: arsenic; beeswax; bile; commissure; corpuscle; fat; fiber; fingers; forelock; gangrene; infarct; lead; line; line of anal canal; line of Toldt; matter; muscle; mustard; noise; petrolatum; piedra; pine; pitch; pulp; pulp of spleen; rami communicantes; reaction; spot; substance; thrombus; turpentine; wax; yolk
white blood: cell
white blood cell: cast
white cell: cast
whitegraft: reaction
Whitehead: deformity; operation
white limbal: girdle of Vogt
white mercuric: precipitate
white-out: syndrome
white pupillary: reflex
white soft: paraffin
white sponge: nevus
white spot: disease

Whitman: frame
Whitmore: bacillus; disease
Whitnall: tubercle
whole: blood
whole-body: counter
whole-body titration: curve
whooping: cough
whooping-cough: vaccine
whorled: enamel
WI-38: cells
Wickham: striae
Widal: reaction; syndrome
wide: plane; spectrum
wide dynamic range: compression
wide field: ocular
wide-latitude: film
Wigand: maneuver
Wilbrand: knee
wild: ginger; mandrake; tobacco; type; yeast
Wilde: cords; triangle
Wilder: diet; sign; stain for reticulum
Wildermuth: ear
Wildervanck: syndrome
wildfire: rash
wild-type: strain
Wilhelmy: balance
Wilkie: disease
Willett: forceps
Williams: factor; stain; syndrome
Williams-Beuren: syndrome
Willis: centrum nervosum; cords; pancreas; paracusis; pouch
Williston: law
Wilms: tumor
Wilson: disease; lichen; method; muscle
Wilson-Mikity: syndrome
Windigo: psychosis
window: level; width
wine: spirit
wing: cell; plate
wing-beating: tremor
winged: catheter; scapula
Winiwarter-Buerger: disease
wink: reflex
winking: spasm
Winkler: disease
Winslow: ligament; pancreas; stars
winter: eczema; itch; sleep
Winterbottom: sign
Winternitz: sound
Wintersteiner: compound F; rosettes
wire: arch; splint
wire-loop: lesion
Wirsung: canal; duct
wiry: pulse
wisdom: tooth
Wiskott-Aldrich: syndrome
Wissler: syndrome

Wistar: rats
witch's: milk
withdrawal: reflex; symptoms; syndrome
wobble: base; hypothesis
Wohlfart-Kugelberg-Welander: disease
Wolfe: graft
Wolfe-Krause: graft
Wolff: law
Wolff-Chaikoff: block; effect
wolffian: body; cyst; duct; rest; ridge; tubules
wolffian duct: carcinoma
Wolff-Parkinson-White: syndrome
Wölfler: gland
Wolf-Orton: bodies
Wolfram: syndrome
Wolfring: glands
Wollaston: doublet; theory
Wolman: disease; xanthomatosis
Wood: glass; lamp; light; units
wood: charcoal; naphtha; spirit; sugar; vinegar
woodcutter's: encephalitis
wooden: resonance
wooden-shoe: heart
wool: wax
Woolf-Lineweaver-Burk: plot
woolly: hair
woolly hair: nevus
Woolner: tip
woolsorter's: disease; pneumonia
word: deafness
Woringer-Kolopp: disease
working: bite; contacts; occlusion; side
working occlusal: surfaces
working side: condyle
worm: abscess
wormian: bones
Wormley: test
Worth: amblyoscope
Woulfe: bottle
wound: botulism; clip; dehiscence; fever; myiasis
woven: bone
Wr^a: antigen
Wright: antigens; respirometer; stain; syndrome; version
wrinkler: muscle of eyebrow
Wrisberg: cartilage; ganglia; ligament; nerve; tubercle
wrist: clonus; joint; sign
wrist clonus: reflex
wrist-hand: orthosis
writer's: cramp
writhing: number
writing: hand
wrought: wire
wry: neck
Wurster: reagent; test

Wyburn-Mason: syndrome

X

χ^2: test
X: body; disease; inactivation; zone
X-: strabismus
x: wave
x-: ray
xanthene: dyes
xanthogranulomatous: cholecystitis; pyelonephritis
xanthoprotein: reaction
xenic: culture
xenogeneic: graft
xenon-arc: photocoagulator
xenotropic: virus
xerotic: degeneration; keratitis
Xg: antigen
xiphisternal: joint
xiphisternal crunching: sound
xiphocostal: angle
xiphoid: cartilage; process
X-linked: agammaglobulinemia; gene; hypogammaglobulinemia; hypogammaglobulinemia with growth hormone deficiency; ichthyosis; inheritance; locus
X-linked lymphoproliferative: disease; syndrome
X-linked recessive bulbospinal: neuronopathy
XO: female; syndrome
X-pattern: esotropia; exotropia
x-ray: dosimetry; generator; microscope; therapy; tube
XX: male
XXX: female
XXY: male; syndrome
xylose: test
xylostyptic: ether
XYY: male; syndrome

Y

Y: body; cartilage
Y-: axis
y: wave
y-: angle
Yaba: virus
Yaba monkey: virus
Yangtze: edema
Yangtze Valley: fever
yeast: fungus; RNase
yeast artificial: chromosomes
yeast extract: agar
yellow: atrophy of the liver; body; cartilage; corallin; disease; enzyme; fever; fibers; hepatization; ligament; mercury iodide; nail; precipitate; skin; spot; vision; wax; yolk
yellow bone: marrow
yellow fever: vaccine; virus
yellow nail: syndrome
yellow soft: paraffin
yield: strength; stress
Y-linked: gene; inheritance; locus
yoke: bone
yolk: cells; cleavage; membrane; sac; stalk
yolk sac: carcinoma; tumor
Yorke autolytic: reaction
Young: modulus; rule; syndrome
Young-Helmholtz: theory of color vision
Young prostatic: tractor
Y-shaped: ligament
Yt^a: antigen
Yvon: test

Z

Z: band; disk; filament; gene; line
Z-: DNA; protein
Zaffaroni: system
Zaglas: ligament
Zahn: infarct
Zaire: virus
Zambesi: ulcer
Zappert counting: chamber
Zarit burden: interview
Zavanelli: maneuver
zebra: body
Zeeman: effect
Zeis: glands
zeisian: sty
Zellweger: syndrome
Zenker: degeneration; diverticulum; fixative; paralysis
zero: gravity
zero degree: teeth
zero end-expiratory: pressure
zero-order: reaction
zero time-binding: DNA
zeta: potential
zeta sedimentation: ratio
Ziehen-Oppenheim: disease
Ziehl: stain
Ziehl-Neelsen: stain
Ziemann: dots; stippling
Zieve: syndrome
Zika: fever; virus
Zimmerlin: atrophy
Zimmermann: corpuscle; granule; reaction; test
Zimmermann elementary: particle
zinc: colic; finger; gelatin
zinc fume: fever
zinc phosphate: cement

zinc sulfate flotation: concentration
zinc sulfate flotation centrifugation: method
Zinn: artery; corona; ligament; membrane; ring; tendon; zonule
Zinn vascular: circle
zirconium: granuloma
Zivert: syndrome
Zollinger-Ellison: syndrome; tumor
Zöllner: lines
zonal: necrosis
zonary: placenta
zone: centrifugation

zonular: band; cataract; fibers; layer; scotoma; spaces
zoo blot: analysis
Zoon: erythroplasia
zoonotic: infection; potential
zoonotic cutaneous: leishmaniasis
zooplastic: graft
zoster: encephalomyelitis
zoster immune: globulin
Zsigmondy: test
Z-tract: injection
Zubrod: scale
Zuckerkandl: bodies; convolution; fascia
zwitter: hypothesis

zwitterionic: buffer; detergent; surfactant
zygal: fissure
zygapophysial: joints
zygomatic: arch; bone; border of greater wing of sphenoid bone; branches of facial nerve; diameter; fossa; margin of greater wing of sphenoid bone; nerve; process of frontal bone; process of maxilla; process of temporal bone; region
zygomaticoauricular: index
zygomaticofacial: branch of zygomatic nerve; foramen

zygomaticomaxillary: suture
zygomatico-orbital: artery; foramen
zygomaticotemporal: branch of zygomatic nerve; foramen; suture
zygomaticus major: muscle
zygomaticus minor: muscle
zygomaxillary: point
zymogen: granule
zymogenic: cell
zymoplastic: substance
zymotic: papilloma
ZZ: genotype

A

α 1. Alfa, primeira letra do alfabeto grego; utilizada como um classificador na nomenclatura de muitas ciências. **2.** Símbolo de coeficiente (*coefficient*) de solubilidade de Bunsen. **3.** Em química, indica o primeiro em uma série, uma posição imediatamente adjacente a um grupamento carboxila, a primeira de uma série de compostos intimamente relacionados, um substituto aromático em uma cadeia alifática, ou a orientação de uma ligação química na direção oposta ao observador. **4.** Abreviatura de partícula alfa (alpha *particle*). **5.** Em química, símbolo para ângulo de rotação óptica (optic *rotation*); grau de dissociação. Para termos que começam com esse prefixo, VER o termo específico.

[α] Símbolo para rotação óptica específica (specific optic *rotation*).

α₁PI Abreviatura de human α₁-protease *inhibitor* (inibidor da α₁-protease humana).

A 1. Abreviatura de ampère; adenina; alanina. **2.** Como subscrito, refere-se a gás alveolar (alveolar *gas*). **3.** Símbolo (geralmente em letra maiúscula e em itálico) para absorbância. **4.** Símbolo para adenosina ou ácido adenílico em polinucleotídeos; alanina ou alanil em polipeptídeos; primeiro substrato em uma reação com múltiplos substratos catalisada por enzimas.

Å Símbolo para angström.

°A Símbolo para grau absoluto; substituído por K (kelvin).

A⁻ Símbolo para ânion.

A. Símbolo de absorbância; Helmholtz *energy* (energia Helmholtz).

a 1. Abreviatura de acidez total (total *acidity*); ante-; área, assimétrico; orelha (*auris*); artéria [TA]. **2.** Símbolo para atto-. **3.** Como subscrito, refere-se ao sangue arterial sistêmico.

a Símbolo de coeficiente específico de absorção (specific absorption *coefficient*); abreviatura de absortividade (absorptivity).

a-, an-. Não, sem, isento de; prefixos equivalentes ao L. in- e ao I. un-. [G. a-, privação, negação; em geral, *an-* antes de vogal]

AA, aa Abreviatura de aminoácido; aminoacil (amino acid, aminoacyl).

aa. Abreviatura de artérias [TA], arteriae [TA].

ā ā. Abreviatura do G. *ana*, de cada um; usada em prescrições após o nome de dois ou mais ingredientes.

AAA Abreviatura de aneurisma abdominal da aorta (abdominal aortic aneurysm); comumente, o procedimento para correção cirúrgica de um AAA.

Aad Abreviatura de ácido α-aminoadípico (α-aminoadipic).

AAF Abreviatura de 2-acetilaminofluoreno (2-acetylaminofluorene); 2-acetamidofluoreno (2-acetamidofluorene).

Aagenaes, O., médico norueguês. VER Aagenaes *syndrome*.

AAMC Abreviatura de *Association of American Medical Colleges* (Associação de Escolas de Medicina da América).

AAR Abreviatura de antigen-antibody *reaction* (reação antígeno-anticorpo).

Aaron, Charles D., médico norte-americano, 1866–1951. VER A. *sign*.

Aarskog, Dagfinn J., pediatra norueguês, *1928. VER A.-Scott *syndrome*.

AASH Abreviatura de adrenal androgen-stimulating *hormone* (hormônio estimulante de androgênio adrenal).

AAV Abreviatura de adeno-associated *virus* (vírus adeno-associado).

Ab Abreviatura de antibody (anticorpo).

ab-, abs-. 1. De, longe de, fora. **2.** Prefixo aplicado a unidades elétricas no sistema eletromagnético CGS (centímetro-grama-segundo) com a finalidade de distingui-las das unidades no sistema eletrostático CGS (prefixo stat-) e daquelas no sistema métrico ou SI (sem prefixo). [L. *ab*, de, geralmente *abs-* antes de c, q e t; com freqüência, *a-* antes de m, p ou v]

Abadie, Joseph Louis Irénée Jean, neurocirurgião francês, 1873–1946. VER A. *sign* de tabes dorsalis.

ab·am·pere (ā-am′pēr). Abampère; unidade eletromagnética de corrente equivalente a 10 ampères absolutos; corrente que exerce uma força de 2π dinas em um pólo magnético unitário no centro de uma espira circular de 1 cm de raio.

abap·i·cal (ā-bap′i-kăl). Abapical; oposto ao ápice.

abar·og·no·sis (ā-bar′og-nō′sis). Abarognosia; perda da capacidade de avaliar o peso dos objetos segurando-os com as mãos ou de diferenciar objetos de pesos diferentes. Quando os sentidos primários estão intactos, é causada por uma lesão do lobo parietal contralateral. [G. *a-* priv. + *baros*, peso, + *gnōsis*, conhecimento]

aba·sia (ā-bā′zē-ă). Abasia; incapacidade de andar. VER gait. [G. *a-* priv. + *basis*, passo]

atactic a., ataxic a., a. atática, a. atáxica; dificuldade de caminhar devido à ataxia das pernas.

aba·si·a-asta·si·a. Abasia-astasia VER astasia-abasia.

aba·sic (ā-bā′sik). Abásico. **1.** Afetado pela abasia ou associado a ela. **2.** Refere-se à perda dos locais de pirimidina no DNA. SIN abatic.

abate·ment (ā-bāt′ment). **1.** Diminuição ou alívio. **2.** A redução, em última análise a eliminação, de fatores prejudiciais à saúde pública, como fumaça, barulho. [abate, do I.M. *abaten*, do Fr. Ant. *abattre*, abater, do L. Tard. *batto*, bater + -ment]

sound a., termo genérico para quaisquer medidas redutoras do ruído ambiental.

abatic (ā-bat′ik). Abásico. SIN abasic.

ab·ax·i·al, ab·ax·ile (ab-ak′sē-ăl, -ak′sīl). Abaxial. **1.** Que se situa fora do eixo de qualquer parte ou corpo. **2.** Localizado na extremidade oposta do eixo de uma parte.

Abbe, Robert W., cirurgião norte-americano, 1851–1928. VER A. *flap*.

Abbé, Ernst K., físico alemão, 1840–1905. VER A. *condenser*.

Abbott, Alexander C., bacteriologista norte-americano, 1860–1935. VER A. *stain* para esporos.

Abbott, W. Osler, médico norte-americano, 1902–1943. Ver A. *tube*; Miller-A. *tube*.

Abbott ar·tery. Artéria de Abbott. VER em artery.

abciximab. Anticorpo monoclonal com propriedades antitrombóticas usado no tratamento e na prevenção de distúrbios oclusivos das artérias.

ab·cou·lomb (ab-koo-lom′). Abcoulomb; unidade de carga elétrica equivalente a 10 coulombs. A carga elétrica que passa sobre uma determinada superfície durante 1 segundo quando uma corrente de 1 abampère atravessa essa superfície. [ab + coulomb]

ab·do·men (ab-dō′men, ab′dō-men) [TA]. Abdome; a parte do tronco situada entre o tórax e a pelve. O a. não inclui a região vertebral posterior, mas alguns anatomistas consideram a pelve como parte integrante dele (cavidade abdominopélvica). Inclui a maior parte da cavidade abdominal (cavitas abdominis [TA]), sendo dividido em nove regiões por planos arbitrários. VER TAMBÉM abdominal *regions*, em *region*. SIN venter (1) [TA]. [L. *abdomen*, etimologia duvidosa]

acute a., a. agudo; qualquer condição intra-abdominal aguda grave (como apendicite), acompanhada de dor, sensibilidade à palpação e rigidez muscular, exigindo cirurgia de emergência. SIN surgical a.

carinate a., a. carinado; uma inclinação dos lados com proeminência da linha central do a.

navicular a., a. navicular. SIN scaphoid a.

a. obsti′pum, termo raramente empregado para uma deformidade do a. decorrente de músculos retos congenitamente pequenos.

pendulous a., um a. com paredes musculares muito relaxadas que se projetam sobre a região púbica.

protuberant a., a. protuberante; convexidade incomum ou saliente do a. devido a gordura subcutânea excessiva, tônus muscular insuficiente ou aumento no conteúdo intra-abdominal.

scaphoid a., a. escafóide; condição na qual a parede abdominal anterior está afundada, apresentando um contorno côncavo, ao invés de convexo. SIN navicular a.

surgical a., a. cirúrgico. SIN acute a.

ab·dom·i·nal (ab-dom′i-năl). Abdominal; relativo ao abdome.

abdomino-, abdomin-. O abdome, abdominal. [L. *abdomen, abdominis*]

ab·dom·i·no·cen·te·sis (ab-dom′i-nō-sen-tē′sis). Abdominocentese; paracentese do abdome. [abdomino- + G. *kentēsis*, punção]

ab·dom·i·no·cy·e·sis (ab-dom′i-nō-sī-ē′sis). Abdominociese. **1.** Gestação abdominal. SIN abdominal *pregnancy*. **2.** Gestação abdominal secundária. SIN secondary abdominal *pregnancy*. [abdomino- + G. *kyēsis*, gravidez]

ab·dom·i·no·cys·tic (ab-dom-i-nō-sis′tik). Abdominocístico. SIN abdominovesical. [abdomino- + G. *kystis*, bexiga]

ab·dom·i·no·gen·i·tal (ab-dom′i-nō-gen′i-tăl). Abdominogenital; relativo ao abdome e aos órgãos genitais.

ab·dom·i·no·hys·ter·ec·to·my (ab-dom′i-nō-his-ter-ek′tō-mē). Histerectomia abdominal. SIN abdominal *hysterectomy*.

ab·dom·i·no·hys·ter·ot·o·my (ab-dom′i-nō-his-ter-ot′ō-mē). Histerotomia abdominal. SIN abdominal *histerotomy*.

ab·dom·i·no·pel·vic (ab-dom′i-nō-pel′vik). Abdominopélvico; relativo ao abdome e à pelve, principalmente às cavidades abdominal e pélvica combinadas.

ab·dom·i·no·per·i·ne·al (ab-dom′i-nō-păr-i-nē′ăl). Abdominoperineal; relativo ao abdome e ao períneo, como na ressecção abdominoperineal do reto.

⌂ Formas Combinantes	☆ Termo oficial alternativo para a *Terminologia Anatomica*
🔲 Indica que o termo é ilustrado, ver Índice de Ilustrações	
SIN Sinônimo	[MIM] *Mendelian Inheritance in Man*
Cf. Comparar, confrontar	I.C. Índice de Corantes
[NA] *Nomina Anatomica*	
[TA] *Terminologia Anatomica*	**Termo de Alta Importância**

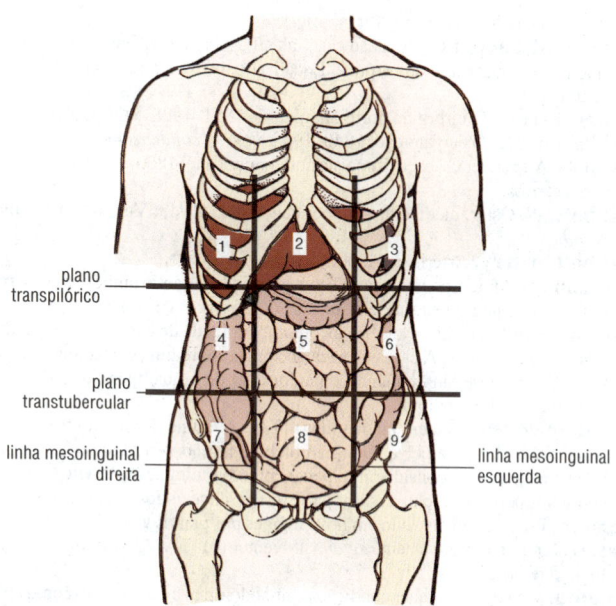

regiões abdominais: (1) hipocôndrio direito, (2) epigástrio, (3) hipocôndrio esquerdo, (4) flanco direito (lombar), (5) umbilical, (6) flanco esquerdo (lombar), (7) fossa ilíaca direita, (8) hipogástrio (suprapúbica), (9) fossa ilíaca esquerda

ab·dom·i·no·plas·ty (ab-dom′i-nō-plas-tē). Abdominoplastia; operação realizada na parede abdominal para fins estéticos. [abdomino- + G. *plastos*, formado]

ab·dom·i·nos·co·py (ab-dom-i-nos′kŏ-pē). Abdominoscopia. SIN laparoscopy. [abdomino- + G. *skopeō*, examinar]

ab·dom·i·no·scro·tal (ab-dom′i-nō-skrō′tăl). Abdominoescrotal; relativo ao abdome e ao escroto.

ab·dom·i·no·tho·rac·ic (ab-dom′i-nō-thō-ras′ik). Abdominotorácico; relativo ao abdome e ao tórax.

ab·dom·i·no·vag·i·nal (ab-dom′i-nō-vag′i-năl). Abdominovaginal; relativo ao abdome e à vagina.

ab·dom·i·no·ves·i·cal (ab-dom′i-nō-ves′i-kăl). Abdominovesical; relativo ao abdome e à bexiga, ou ao abdome e à vesícula biliar. SIN abdominocystic.

ab·duce (ab-doos′). Abduzir. SIN abduct.

ab·du·cens (ab-doo′senz). Abducente. SIN abducent. [L.]

 a. oc′uli, músculo a. dos olhos; SIN lateral rectus (*muscle*).

ab·du·cent (ab-doo′sent). Abducente. **1.** Que abduz; que se afasta, principalmente para longe do plano mediano. **2.** SIN abducent nerve [CN VI]. SIN abducens. [L. *abducens*]

ab·duct (ab-dŭkt′). Abduzir; afastar-se do plano mediano. SIN abduce.

ab·duc·tion (ab-dŭk′shŭn). Abdução. **1.** Movimento de uma parte do corpo para longe do plano mediano (do corpo, no caso dos membros; da mão ou do pé, no caso dos dedos). **2.** Rotação monoocular (dução) do olho em direção à têmpora. **3.** Uma posição resultante de tal movimento. Cf. adduction. [L. *abductio*]

ab·duc·tor (ab-dŭk′ter,-tōr). Abdutor. SIN abductor (*muscle*).

Abegg, Richard, químico dinamarquês, 1869–1910. Ver A. *rule*.

Abell-Kendall meth·od. Método de Abell-Kendall. Ver em method.

Abelson, Herbert T., pediatra norte-americano, *1941. VER A. murine leukemia *virus*.

ab·em·bry·on·ic (ab′em-brē-on′ik). Abembriônico; área do blastocisto oposta à região onde o embrião é formado. [L. *ab*, de, + embriônico]

ab·en·ter·ic (ab-en-ter′ik). Abentérico; termo raramente empregado que significa longe do intestino; diz-se de um processo mórbido que ocorre em outro local e que, normalmente, ocorreria no intestino. [L. *ab*, de, + G. *enteron*, intestino]

Abernethy, John, cirurgião e anatomista inglês, 1764–1831. VER A. *fascia*.

ab·er·rant (ab-er′ant). **1.** Aberrante; diferente do normal; em botânica ou zoologia, diz-se de certos indivíduos atípicos de uma espécie. **2.** Errante; diz-se de certos ductos, vasos ou nervos que se desviam do curso ou padrão normal. **3.** Ectópico. SIN ectopic (1). [L. *aberrans*]

ab·er·ra·tion (ab-er-ā′shŭn). Aberração. **1.** Que se desvia do curso ou padrão normal. **2.** Desenvolvimento ou crescimento divergente. VER TAMBÉM chromosome. [L. *aberratio*]

chromatic a., a. cromática; diferença no foco ou na ampliação de uma imagem devido à diferença na refração de diferentes comprimentos de onda que compõem a luz branca. SIN chromatism (2), newtonian a.

chromosome a., a. cromossômica; qualquer desvio do número ou da morfologia normais dos cromossomos; da mesma forma, as conseqüências fenotípicas desse desvio.

color a., aberração cromática SIN chromatic a.

coma a., **(1)** aberração da coma; distorção da formação de uma imagem criada quando um feixe de raios luminosos penetra em um sistema óptico não-paralelo ao eixo óptico; **(2)** em botânica, qualquer tufo, como os pêlos em uma semente ou brácteas de um rabanete ou de um abacaxi. SIN coma (3). [G. *komē*, pêlo, folhagem]

curvature a., aberração por encurvamento; falta de correspondência espacial que faz com que a imagem de um objeto reto pareça curva.

dioptric a., a. dióptrica. SIN spherical a.

distortion a., a. por distorção; formação defeituosa de uma imagem por ser a ampliação da parte periférica de um objeto diferente daquela da parte central quando observada através de uma lente. VER TAMBÉM Petzval *surface*.

lateral a., a. lateral; na a. esférica, a distância entre o foco paraxial dos raios centrais no eixo óptico.

longitudinal a., a. longitudinal; na a. esférica, a distância que separa o foco de raios paraxiais e periféricos no eixo óptico.

mental a., a. mental; pensamento ou comportamento perturbado que sugere um distúrbio psicológico ou psiquiátrico. VER delusion.

meridional a., a. meridional; a. produzida no plano de um único meridiano de uma lente.

monochromatic a., a. monocromática; defeito em uma imagem óptica devido à natureza das lentes; os principais tipos são a. esférica, da coma, por encurvamento e por distorção, além do astigmatismo de feixes luminosos oblíquos.

newtonian a., a. newtoniana. SIN chromatic a.

optical a., a. óptica; incapacidade de os raios, a partir de uma fonte puntiforme, formarem uma imagem perfeita depois de atravessarem um sistema óptico.

spherical a., a. esférica; a. monocromática que ocorre na refração em uma superfície esférica na qual os raios paraxiais e periféricos são focalizados ao longo do eixo, em diferentes pontos. SIN dioptric a.

ventricular a., a. ventricular. SIN aberrant ventricular *conduction*.

ab·er·rom·e·ter (ab-er-rom′ē-ter). Aberrômetro; instrumento para medir a aberração óptica ou qualquer erro na experimentação. [L. *aberratio*, aberração, + G. *metron*, medida]

abe·ta·lip·o·pro·tein·e·mia (ā-bā′tă-lip′ō-prō′tēn-ē′mē-ă) [MIM*200

---

aberrações cromossômicas numéricas freqüentes

	Contagem de Cromossomas
autossômicas	
trissomia G (síndrome de Down)	
1 cromossoma 21 extra	
a) cromossoma extra normal	47
com mosaicismo	46/47
b) translocação G/G do cromossoma extra, fundido com cromossoma 21 ou 22	46
c) translocação D/G do cromossoma extra, fundido com um cromossoma do grupo D	46
trissomia D (síndrome de Patau) 1 D1 extra, cromossoma (n.º 13)	47
trissomia E (síndrome de Edward) 1 cromossoma 18 extra	47
cromossomas sexuais	
monossomia X-XO (síndrome de Turner) 1 cromossoma X faltando, fenótipo feminino	45 (Ø)
trissomia XXX 1 cromossoma X extra, fenótipo feminino	47 (++)
trissomia XXY 1 cromossoma X extra, fenótipo masculino (síndrome de Klinefelter)	47 (+)
1 cromossoma Y extra, geralmente fenótipo masculino	47 (Ø)
tetrassomias (XXXY, XXYY) e pentassomias raramente são observadas	

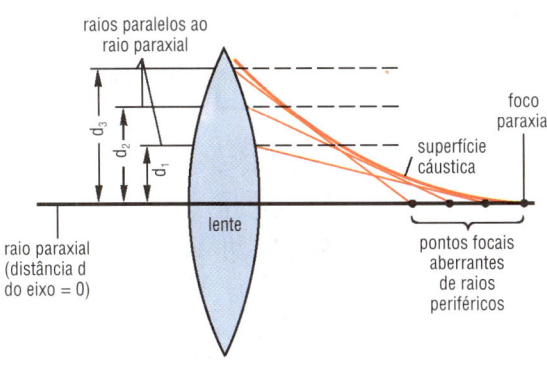

aberração (esférica)

100]. Abetalipoproteinemia; distúrbio caracterizado por ausência de lipoproteínas beta de baixa densidade, presença de acantócitos no sangue, degeneração pigmentar da retina, má absorção, ingurgitamento das células absortivas da parte superior do intestino com triglicerídeos alimentares, além de anormalidades neuromusculares; herança autossômica recessiva, causada por mutação no gene que codifica a proteína microssomial de transferência de triglicerídeos (MTP) no cromossoma 4q. SIN Bassen-Kornzweig syndrome. [G. *a-*, priv., + β + lipoproteína + *-emia*, sangue]
    normotriglyceridemic a., a. normotriglicerídêmica; a. com níveis normais de triglicerídeos. Esse distúrbio hereditário (possivelmente autossômico recessivo) deve-se, provavelmente, à ausência de apolipoproteína B-100.
abey·ance (ā-bā′ans). Latência, suspensão; estado de abolição temporária da função. [do Fr. A.]
ab·far·ad (ab-far′ad). Abfarad; unidade eletromagnética de capacidade equivalente a 10^9 farads.
ABG Abreviatura de arterial blood gas (gás sanguíneo arterial). VER blood *gases*, em *gas*.
ab·hen·ry (ab-hen′rē). Abhenry; unidade eletromagnética no sistema CGS de indutância equivalente a 10^{-9} henry.
abil·i·ty (ă-bil′i-tē). Capacidade; a competência física, mental ou legal para exercer uma função. [L. *habilitas*, aptidão]
abi·ot·ic (ā-bī-ot′ik). Abiótico. **1.** Incompatível com a vida. **2.** Sem vida.
ab·i·ot·ro·phy (ab-ē-ot′rō-fē). Abiotrofia. Manifestação, dependente da idade, de um traço geneticamente determinado. [G. *a-* priv. + *bios*, vida, + *trophē*, nutrição]
ab·ir·ri·ta·tion (ab-ir-i-tā′shŭn). Abirritação; termo obsoleto para diminuição ou abolição da irritabilidade em uma parte. [L. *ab*, de, + *irrito*, pp. *-atus*, irritar]
abl Oncogene encontrado na linhagem de Abelson do vírus da leucemia do camundongo e envolvido na translocação do cromossoma Filadélfia na leucemia granulocítica crônica.
ablas·te·mic (ā-blas-tem′ik). Ablastêmico; que não é germinativo nem blastêmico. [G. *a-* priv. + *blastēma*, broto]
ablas·tin (ă-blas′tin). Ablastina; anticorpo que parece inibir a reprodução de tripanossomas; encontrado em ratos infectados por *Trypanosoma lewisi*. [G. *a-* priv. + *blastos*, germe]
ab·late (ab-lāt′). Remover ou destruir a função de algo. [L. *au-fero*, pp. *ablatus*, remover]
ab·la·tion (ab-lā′shun). Ablação; remoção de uma parte do corpo ou destruição de sua função por meio de procedimento cirúrgico, processo mórbido ou substância nociva. [L. ver ablate]
    electrode catheter a., a. por cateter eletrodo; método de ablação do local de origem de arritmias por meio do qual uma corrente elétrica de alta energia é aplicada através de cateteres intravasculares.
    endometrial a., a. endometrial; destruição seletiva terapêutica do endométrio.
    laparoscopic uterosacral nerve a., a. laparoscópica do nervo útero-sacro; transecção laparoscópica por laser (geralmente KTP ou argônio) dos nervos úterosacros para o tratamento da dismenorréia primária.
ableph·a·ria (ā-blef-ar′ē-ă). Ablefaria; ausência congênita das pálpebras. VER TAMBÉM cryptophthalmus, microblepharon. [G. *a-* priv. + *blepharon*, pálpebra]
ab·lu·ent (ab′loo-ent). Abluente. **1.** Que limpa. **2.** Qualquer agente com propriedades de limpeza. [L. *abluens*, de *ab-luo*, lavar]
ab·lu·tion (ab-loo′shŭn). Ablução; ato de lavar ou banhar. [L. *ablutio*, lavar, limpar]
ab·ner·val (ab-ner′val). Abneural; afastado de um nervo; denota especificamente uma corrente elétrica que passa através de uma fibra muscular no sentido oposto do ponto de entrada da fibra nervosa. SIN abneural (1).

ab·neu·ral (ab-noor′āl). **1.** Abneural. SIN abnerval. **2.** Afastado do eixo neural. [L. *ab*, afastado, + G. *neuron*, nervo]
ab·nor·mal (ab-nōr′măl). Anormal; que não é normal; que difere, de algum modo, do estado, estrutura, condição ou regra habituais.
ab·nor·mal·i·ty (ab-nōr-mal′i-tē). Anormalidade. **1.** O estado ou a qualidade de ser anormal. **2.** Uma anomalia, deformidade, malformação, incapacidade ou disfunção.
    figure-of-8 a., a. em forma de oito; aspecto radiográfico associado à drenagem total anômala da circulação pulmonar venosa em uma veia cava direita aumentada e em uma veia cava superior esquerda anômala, produzindo uma densidade globular acima do coração; a silhueta sugere a forma de um 8; p. ex., RPVTA. VER TAMBÉM anomalous pulmonary venous *connections*, total or partial, em *connection*. SIN snowman a.
    neuronal migration a., a. da migração neuronal. SIN cortical *dysplasia*.
    snowman a., a. em boneco de neve. SIN figure-of-8 a.
ABO blood group. Grupo sanguíneo ABO. VER o apêndice Grupos Sanguíneos.
ab·ohm (ab′ōm). Abohm; unidade eletromagnética de resistência equivalente a 10^{-9} ohm.
ab·o·rad, ab·o·ral (ab-ō′rad,-rāl). Aboral; em sentido oposto ao da boca; o contrário de oral. [L. *ab*, de, + *os* (*or-*), boca]
abort (ă-bōrt′). Abortar. **1.** Dar à luz um embrião ou feto antes de sua viabilidade. VER TAMBÉM miscarry. **2.** Remover prematuramente os produtos da concepção a fim de destruir a prole. **3.** Interromper um processo mórbido em seus estágios iniciais. [L. *aborior*, falhar no início]
a·bor·ti·cide (ah-bōr′ti-sīd). Abortifaciente. SIN abortifacient (1). [L. *flabboriri*, abortar + *cadere*, matar]
abor·tient (ă-bōr′shent). Abortifaciente. SIN abortifacient (1).
abor·ti·fa·cient (ă-bōr-ti-fā′shent). Abortifaciente. **1.** Que induz aborto. SIN aborticide, abortient, abortigenic, abortive (3). **2.** Agente que induz um aborto. [L. *abortus*, aborto, + *facio*, fazer]
abor·ti·gen·ic (ă-bōr-ti-jen′ik). Abortifaciente. SIN abortifacient (1). [L. *abortus*, aborto, + *genesis*, produção]
abor·tion (ă-bōr′shŭn). Aborto. **1.** Expulsão de um embrião ou de um feto do útero antes do estágio de viabilidade (20.ª semana de gestação ou peso fetal < 500 g). Distinção entre a. e parto prematuro: prematuros são aqueles nascidos após o estágio de viabilidade, porém antes de 37 semanas. O a. pode ser espontâneo (que ocorre por causas naturais) ou induzido (artificial ou terapêutico). **2.** Interrupção de qualquer ação ou processo antes de sua finalização normal.
    ampullar a., a. ampular; a. resultante de gravidez na ampola da tuba de Falópio.
    complete a., a. completo; **(1)** expulsão ou extração completa de um feto ou embrião do corpo da mãe; **(2)** expulsão completa de qualquer outro produto da gestação (p. ex., ovo anembrionado).
    criminal a., a. criminoso; interrupção de uma gravidez sem respaldo. SIN illegal a.
    elective a., a. eletivo; um a. sem justificativa médica mas realizado legalmente, como nos EUA.
    habitual a., a. recorrente. SIN recurrent a.
    illegal a., a. ilegal. SIN criminal a.
    incomplete a., a. incompleto; um a. no qual parte dos produtos da concepção foi eliminada, mas outra parte (em geral a placenta) permanece no útero.
    induced a., a. induzido; a. provocado intencionalmente por medicamentos ou meios mecânicos.
    inevitable a., a. inevitável; caracterizado pela ruptura da bolsa das águas ou dilatação cervical em uma gravidez previamente viável associada a sangramento vaginal e contrações uterinas.
    infected a., a. infectado; complicação séptica de um a.
    menstrual extraction a., técnica para aspiração dos produtos iniciais da concepção do útero alguns dias após a ausência do primeiro período menstrual.
    missed a., a. oculto; a. no qual o feto falece *in utero*, mas o produto da concepção fica retido no útero durante dois meses ou mais.
    recurrent a., a. recorrente; perda de 3 ou mais gestações consecutivas antes da 20.ª semana de gravidez. SIN habitual a.
    septic a., a. séptico; a. infeccioso, complicado por febre, endometrite e parametrite.
    spontaneous a., a. espontâneo; que não foi induzido artificialmente. SIN miscarriage.
    therapeutic a., a. terapêutico; a. induzido devido a doença física ou mental da mãe, ou para evitar o nascimento de uma criança malformada ou resultante de um estupro.
    threatened a., ameaça de a.; dor em cólica e pequena perda de sangue que podem ou não ser acompanhadas pela expulsão do feto durante as primeiras 20 semanas de gestação.
    tubal a., a. tubário; ruptura de um oviduto, a sede da gravidez ectópica, ou extrusão do produto da concepção através da extremidade fimbriada do oviduto; gravidez ectópica abortada, uma gravidez originada na tuba de Falópio. SIN aborted ectopic pregnancy.

abor·tion·ist (ă-bōr′shŭn-ist). Aborteiro; aquele que interrompe uma gravidez.
abor·tive (ă-bōr′tiv). **1.** Abortado; que não alcança a finalização; p. ex., diz-se do episódio de uma doença que cede antes de inteiramente desenvolvida ou completada sua evolução. **2.** SIN rudimentary. **3.** abortifaciente. SIN abortifacient (1). [L. *abortivus*]
abor·tus (ă-bōr′tŭs). Aborto; qualquer produto (ou todos os produtos) de um aborto. [L.]
abou·lia (ă-boo′lē-ă). Abulia. SIN abulia.
ABP Abreviatura de androgen binding *protein* (proteína de ligação de androgênio).
ABPA Abreviatura de allergic bronchopulmonary aspergillosis (aspergilose broncopulmonar alérgica).
ABR Abreviatura de auditory brainstem *response* (resposta evocada do tronco cerebral). VER auditory brainstem *response*.
abra·chia (ă-brā′kē-ă). Abraquia, abraquionia; ausência congênita dos braços. VER amelia. [G. *a-* priv. + *brachion*, braço]
abra·chi·o·ceph·a·ly, abra·chi·o·ce·pha·lia (ă-brā′kē-ō-sef′ă-lē, -se-fā′lē-ă). Abraquiocefalia; ausência congênita dos braços e da cabeça. SIN acephalobrachia. [G. *a-* priv. + *brachion*, braço, + *kephale*, cabeça]
abrade (ă-brād′). **1.** Desgastar (por atrito), raspar por ação mecânica. **2.** Desbastar, parcial ou totalmente, a camada superficial de um elemento. [L. *ab-rado*, pp. *-rasus*, raspar]
Abrahams, Robert, médico norte-americano, 1861–1935. VER A. *sign*.
Abrams, Albert, médico norte-americano, 1863–1924. VER A. heart *reflex*.
abra·sion (ă-brā′zhŭn). Abrasão. **1.** Escoriação ou remoção circunscrita das camadas superficiais da pele ou da mucosa. SIN abraded wound. **2.** Raspagem de uma porção da superfície. **3.** Em odontologia, o desgaste anormal da substância do dente por métodos incorretos de escovamento, corpos estranhos, bruxismo ou causas semelhantes. SIN grinding. Cf. attrition. [ver abrade]
 brush burn a., a. por queimadura. VER brush *burn*.
 gingival a., a. gengival; lesão da gengiva resultante da remoção mecânica de parte do epitélio superficial.
 tooth a., a. dentária; perda ou desgaste da estrutura dentária causado pelas características abrasivas de substâncias que não os alimentos.
abra·sive (a-brā′siv). Abrasivo. **1.** Que causa abrasão. **2.** Qualquer material usado para produzir abrasões. **3.** Substância utilizada em odontologia para raspar, desgastar ou polir.
abra·sive·ness (ă-brā′siv-nes). Abrasividade. **1.** Propriedade de uma substância de causar desgaste em uma superfície por fricção. **2.** Qualidade de ser capaz de causar abrasão ou desgaste em outro material.
ab·re·act (ab-rē-akt′). Ab-reagir. **1.** Demonstrar forte emoção ao lembrar de uma experiência traumática anterior. **2.** Descarregar ou liberar uma emoção reprimida (catarse).
ab·re·ac·tion (ab-rē-ak′shŭn). Ab-reação. Na psicanálise freudiana, um episódio de liberação emocional ou catarse associado a recordação consciente de experiências desagradáveis previamente reprimidas.
 motor a., a. motora; liberação de um pensamento, impulso ou idéia inconsciente por meio de expressão muscular ou motora.
abrin (ab′rin). Abrina; fitotoxina obtida das sementes do jequiriti ou alcaçuz da Índia (*Abrus precatorius*); utilizada em oftalmologia.
abrup·tion (ab-rŭp′shŭn). Ruptura, rotura, separação ou descolamento.
ab·rup·tio pla·cen·tae (ab-rŭp′shē-ō pla-sen′tē). Descolamento prematuro de uma placenta normalmente situada.
Ab·rus (ā′brŭs). Gênero de plantas leguminosas. A raiz de *A. precatorius*, alcaçuz da Índia ou jequiriti, é por vezes utilizada como substituto do alcaçuz; as sementes são tóxicas e podem causar vômitos, diarréia, convulsões e morte quando mastigadas. [mais corretamente *Habrus*, do G. *habros*, gracioso]

ABSCESS

ab·scess (ab′ses). Abscesso. **1.** Coleção circunscrita de exsudato purulento freqüentemente associada a edema e outros sinais de inflamação. **2.** Cavidade formada por necrose de liquefação nos tecidos sólidos. [L. *abscessus*, partida]
 acute a., a. agudo; a. recém-formado, com pouca ou nenhuma fibrose na parede da cavidade. SIN hot a.
 alveolar a., a. alveolar; a. situado no processo alveolar das mandíbulas, mais comumente causado pela extensão da infecção de um dente adjacente sem vida. SIN dental a., dentoalveolar a., root a.
 amebic a., a. amebiano; área de necrose de liquefação do fígado ou de outro órgão contendo amebas, amiúde após disenteria amebiana. SIN tropical a.
 apical a., a. apical. SIN periapical a.
 apical periodontal a., a. periodontal. SIN periapical a.
 appendiceal a., a. apendicular; a. intraperitoneal, geralmente na fossa ilíaca

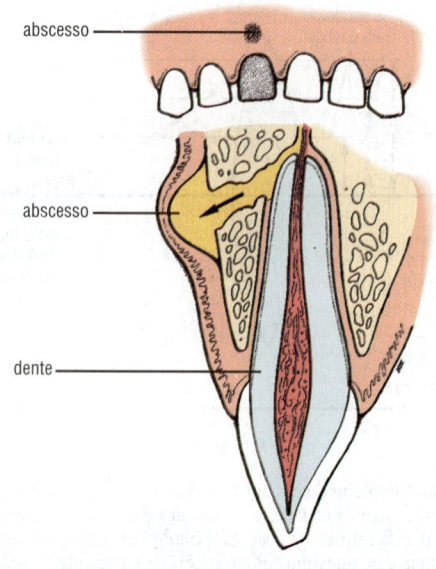

abscesso alveolar

direita, resultante da extensão de uma infecção na apendicite aguda, principalmente com perfuração do apêndice. SIN periappendiceal a.
 Bartholin a., a. de Bartholin; a. da glândula vulvovaginal.
 Bezold a., a. de Bezold; a. profundo na parte superior do músculo esternocleidomastóideo, devido à destruição supurativa das células apicais da mastóide na mastoidite.
 bicameral a., a. bicameral; a. com duas cavidades ou câmaras separadas.
 bone a., a. ósseo; supuração dentro da cavidade medular (osteomielite), no córtex ou no periósteo de um osso.
 Brodie a., a. de Brodie; a. crônico do osso, cercado por tecido fibroso denso e osso esclerótico.
 bursal a., a. da bolsa supuração dentro de uma bolsa.
 caseous a., a. caseoso; a. contendo material branco, sólido ou semi-sólido, com consistência semelhante à do queijo; geralmente tuberculoso. VER TAMBÉM cheesy a.
 cheesy a., a. caseoso; a. que contém tecido necrótico de consistência semelhante à do queijo; observado principalmente na tuberculose. VER TAMBÉM caseous a.
 cholangitic a. (kō-lan-jī′-tik), a. colangítico; área focal de formação de pus no fígado resultante de uma infecção originada no trato biliar.
 chronic a., a. crônico; coleção de pus de longa data cercada por tecido fibroso.
 cold a., a. frio; a. sem calor ou outros sinais habituais de inflamação.
 crypt a's., a. localizado nas criptas de Lieberkühn da mucosa do intestino grosso; um aspecto característico da colite ulcerativa.
 dental a., dentoalveolar a., a. dentário; a. dentoalveolar. SIN alveolar a.
 diffuse a., a. difuso; coleção de pus não circunscrita por uma cápsula bem-definida.
 Douglas a., a. de Douglas; supuração no fundo-de-saco de Douglas.
 dry a., a. seco; remanescente de um a. depois de o pus ser absorvido.
 Dubois a's, a. de Dubois; pequenos cistos do timo contendo leucócitos polimorfonucleares, mas revestidos por epitélio escamoso; relatado na sífilis congênita, mas também encontrado na ausência de sífilis. SIN Dubois disease thymic a.
 embolic a., a. embólico; a. que surge distalmente ao ponto onde um êmbolo séptico se aloja.
 fecal a., a. fecal. SIN stercoral a.
 follicular a., a. folicular; a. em um folículo piloso, tonsilar ou outro.
 gas a., a. gasoso; um a. que contém gás. Freqüentemente causado por microrganismos formadores de gás, como *Enterobacter aerogenes* ou *Escherichia coli*.
 gingival a., a. gengival; um a. confinado aos tecidos moles da gengiva. SIN gumboil, parulis.
 gravitation a., a. perfurante. SIN perforating a.
 gummatous a., a. gomoso; devido ao amolecimento e à rotura de uma goma, principalmente no osso.
 hematogenous a., a. hematogênico; a. causado por microrganismos transportados pelo sangue.
 hot a., a. quente. SIN acute a.

hypostatic a., a. hipostático. SIN perforating a.
ischiorectal a., a. isquiorretal; a. que envolve a fossa isquiorretal.
lateral alveolar a., a. alveolar lateral; a. alveolar localizado ao longo da superfície radicular lateral de um dente. SIN pericemental a.
lateral periodontal a., a. periodontal lateral; a. que se forma na porção mais profunda de uma bolsa periodontal devido à multiplicação de microrganismos piogênicos ou à presença de material estranho.
mastoid a., a. mastóideo; a. devido à coalescência das células de ar da mastóide na mastoidite.
metastatic a., a. metastático; formação de um a. secundário, distante do foco primário, como resultado do transporte de bactérias piogênicas pela circulação linfática ou pela corrente sanguínea.
migrating a., a. migratório. SIN perforating a.
miliary a., a. miliar; uma dentre numerosas e diminutas coleções de pus amplamente disseminadas por uma área ou por todo o corpo.
Munro a., a. de Munro. SIN Munro *microabscess.*
orbital a., a. orbital; coleção de pus entre o periósteo orbital e a lâmina papirácea; com freqüência, a extensão de uma infecção purulenta dos seios paranasais, geralmente os etmóides.
otitic a., a. ótico; a. cerebral, geralmente envolvendo o lobo temporal ou o hemisfério do cerebelo, secundário à supuração do ouvido médio.
palatal a., a. palatal; (1) a. periodontal lateral associado à superfície lingual de um dente maxilar; (2) a. alveolar que erodiu a placa cortical, permitindo a extensão, para os tecidos moles, do palato.
pancreatic a., a. pancreático; a. na área pancreática ou peripancreática, geralmente relacionado à pancreatite.
parafrenal a., a. parafrenal; a. que ocorre de um lado e do outro do frênulo do pênis.
parametric a., parametritic a., a. paramétrico; a. no tecido conjuntivo do ligamento largo do útero.
paranephric a., a. paranéfrico; a. na região dos rins, fora da fáscia renal.
parapharyngeal a., a. parafaríngeo; a. que ocorre lateralmente à faringe.
parotid a., a. da parótida; supuração na glândula parótida; em geral, uma complicação rapidamente progressiva da parotidite.
Pautrier a., a. de Pautrier. SIN Pautrier *microabscess.*
pelvic a., a. pélvico; a. que se desenvolve na cavidade peritoneal pélvica, como complicação da peritonite difusa ou da peritonite localizada associada a doença inflamatória abdominal ou pélvica, como a salpingite; o pus geralmente se acumula na bolsa retovesical ou retouterina.
perforating a., a. perfurante; a. que rompe as barreiras de tecido a fim de penetrar em áreas adjacentes. SIN gravitation a., hypostatic a., migrating a., wandering a.
periapical a., a. periapical; a. alveolar localizado ao redor do ápice de uma raiz dentária. SIN apical a., apical periodontal a.
periappendiceal a., a. periapendicular. SIN appendiceal a.
periarticular a., a. periarticular; a. ao redor de uma articulação, mas não necessariamente envolvendo-a.
pericemental a., a. pericemental. SIN lateral alveolar a.
pericoronal a., a. pericoronal; a. que se desenvolve no tecido folicular dentário inflamado que recobre a coroa de um dente após a sua erupção parcial.
perinephric a., a. perinéfrico; a. na fáscia de Gerota, mas fora da cápsula renal.
periodontal a., a. periodontal; a. alveolar ou a. periodontal lateral.
perirectal a., a. perirretal; a. no tecido conjuntivo adjacente ao reto ou ânus.
peritonsillar a., a. peritonsilar; extensão de infecção tonsilar além da cápsula tonsilar, com formação de abscesso entre a cápsula e a musculatura da fossa tonsilar.
periureteral a., a. periureteral; a. ao redor do ureter.

periurethral a., a. periuretral; a. que envolve os tecidos ao redor da uretra, principalmente o corpo esponjoso.
phlegmonous a., a. fleimonoso; supuração circunscrita caracterizada por intensa reação inflamatória circunjacente que produz induração e espessamento da área afetada.
Pott a., a. de Pott; a. tuberculoso da coluna vertebral.
premammary a., a. pré-mamário; a. no tecido subcutâneo que recobre a glândula mamária.
psoas a., a. do psoas; um a., geralmente tuberculoso, que se origina na espondilite tuberculosa, estendendo-se, através do músculo iliopsoas, até a região inguinal.
pulp a., a. pulpar; a. que envolve o tecido mole na câmara pulpar de um dente, em geral como seqüela de cáries ou, menos freqüentemente, de traumatismo.
pyemic a., a. piêmico; a. hematogênico resultante de piemia, septicemia ou bacteriemia. SIN septicemic a.
radicular a., a. radicular; a. alveolar, um a. ao redor da raiz de um dente.
residual a., a. residual; a. que recidiva no local de um a. anterior, como resultado da persistência de micróbios e pus.
retrobulbar a., a. retrobulbar; a. localizado posteriormente ao globo ocular.
retrocecal a., a. retrocecal; a. localizado posteriormente ao ceco, em geral resultante de perfuração de um apêndice retrocecal.
retropharyngeal a., a. retrofaríngeo; a. que surge, em geral, nos linfonodos retrofaringianos, mais comumente em lactentes.
ring a., a. anelar; inflamação purulenta aguda da periferia da córnea, na qual uma área necrótica é circundada por infiltração leucocítica.
root a., a. radicular. SIN alveolar a.
satellite a., a. satélite; a. intimamente associado a um a. primário.
septicemic a., a. septicêmico. SIN pyemic a.
stellate a., a. estrelado; área necrótica em forma de estrela, circundada por histiócitos, observada dentro de linfonodos tumefeitos no linfogranuloma venéreo e na febre da arranhadura de gato.
stercoral a., a. estercoral; uma coleção de pus e fezes. SIN fecal a.
sterile a., a. estéril; (1) a. cujo conteúdo não é causado por bactérias piogênicas; (2) um a. que, quando aspirado ou em cultura, não gera bactérias.
stitch a., a. na sutura. SIN suture a.
subdiaphragmatic a., a. subdiafragmático. SIN subphrenic a.
subepidermal a., a. subepidérmico; a. microscópico, localizado na derme, logo abaixo da epiderme.
subhepatic a., a. subepático; a. localizado imediatamente abaixo do fígado.
subperiosteal a., a. subperiósteo; a. entre o periósteo e a placa cortical do osso.
subphrenic a., a. subfrênico; a. que ocorre diretamente abaixo do diafragma. SIN subdiaphragmatic a.
subungual a., a. subungueal; supuração que se estende por baixo de uma unha, do pé ou da mão, geralmente como decorrência de paroníquia.
sudoriferous a., a. sudorífero; uma coleção de pus em uma glândula sudorípara.
suture a., a. na sutura; exsudato purulento que circunda uma sutura, principalmente uma sutura na córnea. SIN stitch a.
thymic a.'s, a. tímico. SIN Dubois a.'s.
Tornwaldt a., a. de Tornwaldt; infecção crônica da bolsa faringiana. VER TAMBÉM Tornwaldt *syndrome.*
tropical a., a. tropical. SIN amebic a.
tuboovarian a., a. tuboovariano; um grande a. que envolve a tuba uterina e um ovário aderente, resultante da extensão de uma inflamação purulenta da tuba.
verminous a., a. por vermes; a. verminado. SIN worm a.
wandering a., a. migratório. SIN perforating a.
worm a., a. verminado; a. por vermes; a. devido a vermes parasitas ou no qual são encontrados vermes. SIN verminous a.

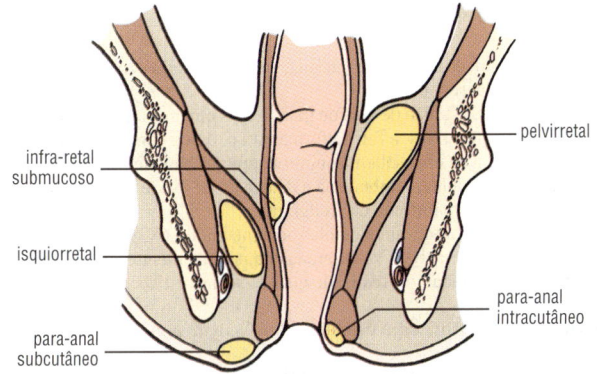

abscessos perirretais

ab·scis·sa (ab-sis′ă). Abscissa; o eixo horizontal (*x*) em um sistema plano de coordenadas cartesianas. Cf. ordinate. [L. *ab-scindo,* pp. *-scissus,* cortar de]
ab·scis·sion (ab-si′shŭn). Abscissão; corte. [L. *ab-scindo,* pp. *-scissus,* cortar de]
ab·scon·sio (ab-skon′shē-ō). Absconso; recesso, cavidade ou depressão; usado principalmente em osteologia para indicar uma cavidade óssea que acomoda a cabeça de outro osso. [L. Mod. de *abs-condo,* pp. *-conditus* ou *-consus,* esconder]
ab·sco·pal (ab-skō′păl -skop′ăl). Indica o efeito remoto que a irradiação de um tecido tem sobre outro tecido não-irradiado distante. [ab- + G. *skopos,* alvo, + -al]
ab·sence (ab′sens). Ausência; ataques paroxísmicos, decorrentes de comprometimento da consciência, acompanhados, ocasionalmente, por espasmos ou tremores dos músculos cefálicos, podendo ser, em geral, desencadeados por hiperventilação; dependendo do tipo e da gravidade da a., o ECG pode apresentar um início súbito de um padrão ponta-onda de 3 s, como na a. simples, ou, nos casos atípicos, um padrão ponta-onda de 4 s e complexos ponta mais rápidos. Os estados clínicos que acompanham essas anormalidades do ECG

podem ser classificados como: 1) a. sem manifestações francas, p. ex., a. simples; a. epiléptica; a. subclínica; 2) a. com movimentos clônicos, p. ex., a. mioclônica; 3) a. com estados atônicos, p. ex., a. atônica; 4) a. com contrações tônicas, p. ex., contração muscular hipertônica; 5) a. com automatismos, p. ex., movimentos estereotipados diversos, geralmente do rosto ou das mãos; 6) a. com manifestações atípicas, p. ex., atividade motora bizarra. [L. *absentia*]

pure a., a. pura. SIN simple a.

simple a., a. simples; um breve embotamento da consciência acompanhado pelo início súbito de complexos de ponta-onda de 3 s no ECG. SIN pure a.

abs. feb. abreviatura do L. *absente febre,* quando não há febre.

Ab·sid·ia (ab-sid′ē-ā). Absídeos; gênero de fungos (família Mucoraceae) comumente encontrado na natureza. As espécies termofílicas sobrevivem em camadas alternadas de turfa, folhas podres e esterco em temperaturas superiores a 45°C, podendo causar mucormicoses (zigomicoses) nos seres humanos.

ab·sinthe (ab′sinth). Licor que consiste em um extrato alcoólico de absinto e outras ervas amargas.

ab·sin·thin (ab′sin-thin). Absintina; um princípio amargo, $C_{30}H_{40}O_8$, obtido do absinto.

ab·sin·thi·um (ab-sin′thē-ŭm). Absinto; as folhas e os brotos secos da *Artemisia absinthium* (família Compositae). Hoje em dia a infusão raramente é usada, mas já foi utilizada como tônico; em doses elevadas ou freqüentemente repetidas provoca cefaléia, tremores e convulsões epileptiformes. SIN wormwood. [L., do G. *apsinthion*]

ab·sin·thol (ab-sin′thawl). Absintol, absintiol. SIN thujone.

ab·so·lute (ab′sō-loot). Absoluto; incondicional; ilimitado; não-combinado; não-diluído (como no caso do álcool); certo. [L. *absolutus*, completo, pp. de *ab-solvo*, liberar de]

ab·sorb (ab-sōrb′). Absorver, sorver. 1. Embeber-se de. 2. Reduzir a intensidade da luz transmitida. [L. *ab-sorbeo*, pp. *-sorptus*, sugar]

ab·sor·bance (A, A) (ab-sōr′bans). Absorvência; em espectrofotometria, o log (logaritmo) da relação entre a energia radiante da radiação incidente e a energia radiante da radiação transmitida. SIN absorbancy, absorbency, extinction (2), optic density.

specific a., a. específica; a. por unidade de concentração. VER specific absorption *coefficient.*

ab·sor·ban·cy (ab-sōr′ban-sē). Absorvência. SIN absorbance.

ab·sor·be·fa·cient (ab-sōr-bē-fā′shŭnt). Absorvente. 1. Que causa absorção. 2. Qualquer substância que possui essa qualidade. [L. *ab-sorbeo*, sugar, + *facio*, fazer]

ab·sorb·en·cy (ab-sōr′ben-sē). Absorvência. SIN absorbance.

ab·sor·bent (ab-sōr′bent). Absorvente. 1. Que tem o poder de absorver, embeber ou consumir um gás, líquido, raios luminosos ou calor. SIN absorptive, bibulous. 2. Qualquer substância que possui tal poder. 3. Material (geralmente cáustico) usado para remover dióxido de carbono de circuitos nos quais ocorre reinalação; p. ex., equipamentos de anestesia e metabolismo basal.

ab·sorb·er head (ab-sōr′ber hed) Cabeçote de absorção; parte de um circuito de reinalação de anestesia que contém um absorvente de dióxido de carbono; muitas vezes denominado recipiente químico (canister).

ab·sorp·tion (ab-sōrp′shŭn). Absorção. 1. Incorporação, tomada ou recepção de gases, líquidos, luz ou calor. Cf. adsorption. 2. Em radiologia, a captação da energia de radiação pelos tecidos ou meios através dos quais ela passa. VER half-value *layer,* photoelectric *effect,* attenuation. [L. *absorptio,* de *absorbeo,* engolir]

cutaneous a., a. cutânea. SIN percutaneous a.

disjunctive a., a. disjuntiva; a. de tecido vivo em relação imediata com uma parte necrosada, produzindo uma linha de demarcação.

electron resonance a., a. por ressonância de elétrons. VER electron spin *resonance.*

external a., a. externa; a. de substâncias pela pele, superfícies mucocutâneas ou mucosas.

interstitial a., a. intersticial; remoção de água ou substâncias, no líquido intersticial, pela circulação linfática.

parenteral a., a. parenteral; a. através de qualquer outra via que não o tubo digestivo.

pathologic a., a. anormal; a. parenteral de qualquer material anormal ou excremento. (p. ex., pus, urina, bile, etc.) para a corrente sanguínea.

percutaneous a., a. percutânea; a. de medicamentos, alérgenos e outras substâncias através de uma pele íntegra. A camada córnea da epiderme é a principal barreira. SIN cutaneous a.

photoelectric a., a. fotoelétrica; interação de um fóton gama com uma matéria na qual o fóton incidente é completamente absorvido, utilizando toda a sua energia ao deslocar e acelerar um elétron do nível mais interno. VER TAMBÉM photoelectric *effect.*

ab·sorp·tive (ab-sōrp′tiv). Absortivo. SIN absorbent (1).

ab·sorp·tiv·i·ty (a) (ab-sōrp-tiv′i-tē). 1. Coeficiente de absorção específica. SIN specific absorption *coefficient.* 2. Coeficiente de absorção molar. SIN molar absorption *coefficient.* 3. Absorvibilidade; capacidade de um material absorver radiação eletromagnética.

molar a., a. molar. SIN molar absorption *coefficient.*

ab·sti·nence (ab′sti-nens). Abstinência. O ato de evitar o uso de certos itens da alimentação, bebidas alcoólicas, substâncias ilegais, bem como relações sexuais. [L. *abs -tineo,* reter, de *teneo,* segurar]

ab·stract (ab′strakt). 1. Extrato; preparação feita a partir da evaporação de um extrato líquido para um pó e trituração com lactose. 2. Condensação ou resumo de um artigo literário ou científico ou de uma conferência. [L. *ab-straho*, pp. *-tractus*, retirar]

structured a., descrição resumida de um trabalho publicado, na qual as informações acerca do estudo relatado são colocadas de maneira estilizada e sistemática, em tópicos como objetivos, métodos, principais medidas dos desfechos, resultados e conclusões.

ab·strac·tion (ab-strak′shŭn). 1. Abstração; destilação ou separação dos constituintes voláteis de uma substância. 2. Abstração; concentração mental exclusiva. 3. Extração; obtenção de um extrato a partir da matéria-prima. 4. Má oclusão, na qual os dentes ou as estruturas associadas são mais baixas do que seu plano normal de oclusão. VER TAMBÉM odontoptosis. 5. Processo de selecionar certo aspecto de um conceito global. [L. *abs-traho*, pp. *-tractus*, retirar]

ab·stric·tion (ab-strik′shŭn). Abstrição. Nos fungos, a formação de esporos assexuais pela supressão de porções do esporóforo por meio do crescimento de partes divisórias. [L. *ab-*, de, + *strictura*, contração]

ab·ter·mi·nal (ab-ter′mi-năl). Que se afasta da extremidade em direção ao centro; indica a trajetória de uma corrente elétrica em um músculo. [L. *ab,* de, + *terminus,* fim]

γ-Abu Abreviatura de γ-aminobutyric acid (ácido γ-aminobutírico).

abu·lia (ă-boo′lē-ă). Abulia. 1. Perda ou distúrbio da capacidade de realizar ações voluntárias ou de tomar decisões. 2. Redução na fala, nos movimentos, no pensamento e nas reações emocionais; resultado comum de doença bilateral do lobo frontal. SIN aboulia. [G. *a-* priv. + *boulē*, vontade]

abu·lic (ă-boo′lik). Abúlico; relativo à abulia ou que sofre de abulia.

a·bun·dance (ă-bŭn′dans). Abundância; o número médio de tipos de macromoléculas (p. ex., mRNA) por célula.

abuse (ă-būs′). Abuso. 1. Mau uso, uso errôneo, especialmente o uso excessivo de qualquer coisa. 2. Tratamento prejudicial, lesivo ou ofensivo, como no caso de a. sexual ou a. infantil.

child a., a. infantil; o a. psicológico, emocional e sexual de uma criança, principalmente por um genitor, padrasto ou responsável. VER domestic violence.

drug a., a. de drogas; uso habitual de drogas não para fins terapêuticos, mas apenas para alterar o humor, o sentimento ou o estado de consciência, ou para afetar desnecessariamente uma função corporal (como no a. de laxantes); uso não terapêutico de drogas.

elder a., a. de idosos; o a. físico ou emocional, incluindo exploração financeira, de um idoso, por um ou mais de seus filhos, cuidadores das casas de repouso ou outros.

sexual a., a. sexual. VER domestic violence.

spouse a., spousal a., a. do cônjuge. VER domestic violence.

substance a., a. de substâncias; padrão mal adaptativo do uso de drogas, bebidas alcoólicas ou outros agentes químicos, podendo acarretar problemas sociais, profissionais, psicológicos ou físicos.

abut·ment (ă-bŭt′ment). Pivô, apoio; em odontologia, um dente natural ou um substituto implantado, usado para apoio ou ancoragem de uma prótese fixa ou removível.

auxiliary a., pivô auxiliar; um dente diferente do que apóia o retentor direto, ajudando no apoio geral de uma dentadura parcial removível.

ball and socket a., p. universal ou esférico; um p. conectado a uma dentadura parcial fixa por meio de um conector não-rígido esférico.

dovetail stress-broken a., p. conectado a uma dentadura parcial fixa por meio de um conector não-rígido transversalmente trapezóide.

intermediate a., p. intermediário; um dente natural, ou um substituto implantado, sem outros dentes naturais em contato próximo, usado juntamente com o p. mesial ou distal para apoiar uma prótese; chamado, com freqüência, de "pilar".

isolated a., p. isolado; um dente, ou raiz, solitário, usado como p. com áreas mesiais e distais desdentadas.

splinted a., p. unido; união de dois ou mais dentes em uma unidade rígida, por meio de restaurações fixas, a fim de formar um p. único com raízes múltiplas.

ABVD Abreviatura de um esquema quimioterápico à base de Adriamycin (doxorrubicina), bleomicina, vimblastina e dacarbazina; usado para o tratamento de neoplasias, como o linfoma de Hodgkin.

ab·volt (ab′vōlt). Abvolt; unidade eletromagnética do CGS de diferença de potencial equivalente a 10^{-8} V. Diferença de potencial entre dois pontos, de modo que 1 erg de trabalho é realizado quando se move 1 abcoulomb de carga de um ponto a outro.

ab·zyme (ab′zīm). Anticorpo catalítico. SIN catalytic *antibody*. [antibody + en*zyme*]

AC Abreviatura de alternating *current* (corrente alternada).

Ac Símbolo para actinium (actínio); acetyl (acetil).

aC Símbolo para arabinosylcytosine (arabinosilcitosina).

a.c. Abreviatura do L. *ante cibum*, antes de uma refeição, ou *ante cibos*, antes das refeições.

AC/A Abreviatura de accommodative convergence-accommodation *ratio* (relação convergência de acomodação/acomodação).

aca·cia (ā - kā′shē - ă). Acácia, goma arábica; exsudato gomoso desidratado da *Acacia senegal* e de outras espécies de *A*. (família Leguminosae), preparado como mucilagem e xarope; usada como emoliente, excipiente demulcente e agente suspensor em alimentos e produtos farmacêuticos; antigamente, usada como líquido de transfusão. SIN gum arabic. [G. *akakia*]

acal·cu·lia (ā′kal - kū′lē - ă). Acalculia; forma de afasia caracterizada pela incapacidade de resolver problemas matemáticos simples; encontrada em lesões de várias áreas dos hemisférios cerebrais, sendo, freqüentemente, um sinal precoce de demência. [G. *a*- priv. + L. *calculo*, calcular]

acamp·sia (ā - kamp′sē - ă). Acampsia; termo raramente empregado para o caso de endurecimento ou rigidez de uma articulação por qualquer motivo. [G. *a*- priv. + *kamptō*, dobrar]

acanth-. VER acantho-.

acan·tha (ā - kan′thă). **1.** Espinho ou processo espinhoso. **2.** O processo espinhoso de uma vértebra. [G. *akantha*, um espinho]

acan·tha·me·bi·a·sis (ā - kan′thă - mē - bī′ă - sis). Acantamebíase; infestação por amebas do gênero *Acanthamoeba* de vida livre no solo e na água, podendo resultar em invasão dérmica ou tecidual necrotizante, meningoencefalite amebiana primária fulminante e geralmente fatal, ou em encefalite amebiana granulomatosa subaguda ou crônica.

Acan·tha·moe·ba (ā - kan - thă - mē′bă). Acantameba; gênero de amebas de vida livre (família Acanthamoebidae, ordem Amoebida) caracterizado pela presença de acantópodes. A infestação humana inclui a invasão da pele ou a colonização após lesão, invasão e colonização da córnea e, possivelmente, colonização pulmonar ou genitourinária; já ocorreram alguns casos de invasão cerebral ou do SNC, mas não só pela via de entrada do epitélio olfatório, como também por infestações mais virulentas produzidas por *Naegleria fowleri*. A espécie responsável é principalmente a *A. culbertsoni*, porém já foram relatados casos envolvendo *A. castellanii, A. polyphaga* e *A. astronyxis*, embora a maioria dos casos tenha sido crônica e não fulminante e rapidamente fatal, como na infestação por *Naegleria fowleri*. [G. *akantha*, espinho, espinha, + L. Mod. *amoeba*, fr. G. *amoibē*, mudança]

ac·an·thel·la (ā - kan - thel′ă). Acantela; fase larvar intermediária dos acantocéfalos, formada dentro do hospedeiro artrópode; estágio pré-infeccioso, não-encistado, que leva à cistacanta infecciosa. [G. *akantha*, espinho, espinha]

acan·thes·the·sia (ā - kan - thes - thē′zē - ă). Acantestesia; parestesia semelhante a uma picada de alfinete. [G. *akantha*, espinho, + *aisthēsis*, sensação]

Acan·thia lec·tu·lar·ia (ā - kan′thē - ă lek - tū - lār′ē - ă). Denominação antiga de *Cimex lectularius*. [G. *akantha*, espinho; L. *lectus*, leito]

acan·thi·on (ā - kan′thē - on). Acantião; extremidade da espinha nasal anterior. SIN akanthion. [G. *akantha*, espinho]

acantho-. Processo espinhoso; espinhoso. [G. *akantha*, espinho, a coluna vertebral, de *akē*, um ponto, + *anthos*, uma flor]

Acan·tho·ceph·a·la (ā - kan - thō - sef′ă - lă). Acantocéfalos; vermes còm espinhos córneos na cabeça; um filo (considerado, antigamente, uma classe) de parasitas obrigatórios sem um canal alimentar, caracterizados por uma probóscida espinhosa anterior introvertível. Assemelham-se superficialmente aos nematódeos, mas são semelhantes aos cestódeos em outros aspectos e, por isso, agrupados como um filo distinto de helmintos. Na fase adulta, são parasitas de vertebrados, principalmente peixes e anfíbios; a fase larvar se passa nos invertebrados, principalmente crustáceos e insetos. [acantho- + G. *kephalē*, cabeça]

acan·tho·ceph·a·li·a·sis (ā - kan′thō - sef - ă - lī′ă - sis). Acantocefalíase; doença causada por infestação de uma espécie de acantocéfalos.

Acan·tho·chei·lo·ne·ma (ā - kan′thō - kī - lō - nē′mă). Gênero de filárias que parasita o homem, considerado, atualmente, parte do gênero *Mansonella*. [acantho- + G. *cheilos*, lábio, + *nēma*, fio]

acan·tho·cyte (ā - kan′thō - sīt). Acantócito; eritrócito caracterizado por múltiplas projeções citoplasmáticas espinhosas, como na acantocitose. [acantho- + G. *kytos*, célula]

acan·tho·cy·to·sis (ā - kan′thō - sī - tō′sis). Acantocitose; condição rara na qual a maioria dos eritrócitos é constituída de acantócitos; característica regular da abetalipoproteinemia; às vezes, também presente na doença hepatocelular grave. SIN acanthrocytosis.

acan·thoid (ā - kan′thoyd). Acantóide; em forma de espinha.

ac·an·thol·y·sis (ak - an - thol′i - sis). Acantólise; separação de queratinócitos epidérmicos individuais de seus vizinhos, como no pênfigo vulgar e na doença de Darier. [acantho- + G. *lysis*, afrouxamento]

ac·an·tho·ma (ak - an - thō′mă). Acantoma; tumor formado pela proliferação de células epiteliais escamosas. VER TAMBÉM keratoacanthoma. [acantho- + G. *-oma*, tumor]

   clear cell a., a. de células claras; pequeno tumor epidérmico benigno bem demarcado, de uma perna ou um braço, com acantose e acúmulo de glicogênio nos queratinócitos, que apresentam citoplasma de coloração pálida.

acan·tho·po·dia (ā - kan - thō - pō′dē - ă). Acantópodes; pseudópodos dentiformes observados em certas amebas, especialmente em membros do gênero *Acanthamoeba*. [acantho- + G. *pous, podos*, pé]

acan·thor (ā - kan′thōr). Acântor; embrião fusiforme, com acúleos rostelares e espinhos corporais, formado dentro da casca do ovo dos acantocéfalos; essa fase se esconde dentro da cavidade corporal de seu primeiro hospedeiro intermediário, geralmente um crustáceo em ciclos aquáticos ou insetos em ciclos terrestres. [G. *akantha*, espinho ou espinha]

ac·an·tho·sis (ak - an - thō′sis). Acantose; aumento da espessura do estrato espinoso da epiderme. [acantho- + G. *-osis*, condição]

   glycogenic a., a. glicogênica; placas cinza-esbranquiçado elevadas das mucosas esofágica distal ou vaginal, com epitélio espessado pela proliferação de grandes células escamosas cheias de glicogênio.

   a. ni′gricans, erupção de lesões aveludadas e verrucosas associada a hiperpigmentação que ocorre na pele das axilas, do pescoço, da área anogenital e da virilha; nos adultos, pode estar associada a processos malignos internos, distúrbios endócrinos ou obesidade; um tipo hereditário benigno ocorre em crianças. VER TAMBÉM pseudoacanthosis nigricans. [L. de *niger*, preto]

ac·an·thot·ic (ak - an - thot′ik). Acantótico; pertencente a acantose ou característico dela.

acan·thro·cyte (a - kan′thrō - sīt). Acantrócito; termo obsoleto para acantócito.

acan·thro·cy·to·sis (a - kan′thrō - sī - tō′sis). Acantrocitose; termo obsoleto para acantocitose. SIN acanthocytosis.

acap·nia (ā - kap′nē - ă). Acapnia; ausência de dióxido de carbono no sangue; termo, por vezes, usado incorretamente no lugar de hipocapnia. [G. *a*- priv. + *hapnos*, fumaça]

acarbose (ā - kar′bōs). Acarbose; oligossacarídeo inibidor da alfa-glicosidase; tratamento auxiliar no diabetes melito tipo 2, usado para neutralizar a hiperglicemia pós-prandial.

acar·dia (ā - kar′dē - ă). Acardia; ausência congênita do coração; condição que ocorre, por vezes, em um dos gêmeos monozigóticos ou em um dos gêmeos unidos quando seu companheiro monopoliza o suprimento de sangue placentário; pode ocorrer também em gestações triplas. [G. *a*- priv. + *kardia*, coração]

acar·di·ac (ā - car′dē - ak). Acardíaco; sem o coração.

acar·di·us (ā - kar′dē - ŭs). Acárdio; gêmeo sem o coração, mas que permanece viável por utilizar a circulação placentária de seu companheiro.

   a. aceph′alus, a. acéfalo; acefalocárdio; feto acardíaco, sem cabeça e órgãos torácicos; as costelas e vértebras podem estar presentes, e os membros superiores estão ausentes ou defeituosos.

   a. amor′phus, a. amorfo; concepto sem forma definida e recoberto por pele e pêlos.

   a. an′ceps, feto acardíaco com cabeça parcialmente desenvolvida e face, membros e tronco deformados.

ac·a·ri·a·sis (ak - ar - ī′ă - sis). Acaríase; qualquer doença produzida por ácaros, geralmente uma infestação cutânea. VER mange.

   psoroptic a., a. psoróptica; infestação da pele de mamíferos pelo ácaro *Psoroptes*.

   sarcoptic a., a. sarcóptica; infestação da pele por *Sarcoptes scabiei*. VER scabies (1).

acar·i·cide (ā - kar′i - sīd). Acaricida; agente que extermina ácaros; termo comumente usado para indicar produtos químicos que eliminam carrapatos. [L. Mod. *acarus*, um ácaro, do G. *akari* + L. *caedo*, cortar, matar]

ac·a·rid (ak′ă - rid). Ácaro; termo genérico para indicar um membro da família Acaridae. SIN acaridan. [G. *akari*, ácaro]

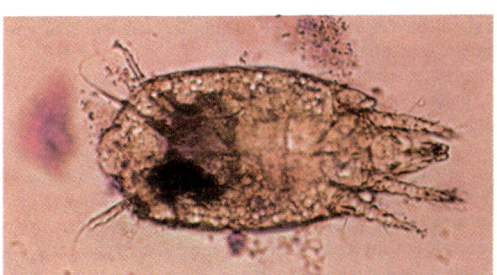

ácaro

Acar·i·dae (ă - kar′i - dē). Acarídeos; família da ordem Acarina, um grande grupo de ácaros excepcionalmente pequenos, em geral com 0,5 mm ou menos, abundantes em frutas secas e carnes, grãos e farinhas; causa comum de dermatite grave em pessoas hipersensibilizadas pelo manuseio freqüente de produtos infestados.

acar·i·dan (ă - kar′i - dan). Ácaro. SIN acarid.

Ac·a·ri·na (ak-ă-rī′nă). Ordem de aracnídeos que inclui ácaros e carrapatos. [G. *akari,* um ácaro]

ac·a·rine (ak′ă-rin). Acarino; membro da ordem Acarina.

ac·a·ro·der·ma·ti·tis (ak′ă-rō-der-mă-tī′tis). Acarodermatite; inflamação ou erupção cutânea produzida por um ácaro. [G. *akari,* ácaro, + *derma* (*dermat-*), pele]
  a. urticarioi′des, a. urticarióide; infestação pelo ácaro dos cereais *Pyemotes ventricosus.* VER grain *itch.*

ac·a·roid (ak′ă-royd). Acaróide; semelhante a um ácaro. [G. *akari,* ácaro, + *eidos,* semelhança]

ac·a·rol·o·gy (ak-ă-rol′ō-jē). Acarologia; estudo dos parasitas acarinos, carrapatos e ácaros, e das doenças que transmitem. [G. *akari,* ácaro, + *logos,* estudo]

ac·a·ro·pho·bia (ak′ă-rō-fō′bē-ă). Acarofobia; temor mórbido de pequenos parasitas, pequenas partículas ou do prurido por eles induzido. [G. *akari,* ácaro, + *phobos,* medo]

Ac·a·rus (ak′ă-rŭs). Gênero de ácaros da família Acaridae. [G. *akari,* ácaro]
  A. bala′tus, espécie tropical de ácaro que causa um tipo particularmente grave de irritação semelhante à escabiose.
  A. folliculo′rum, SIN *Demodex folliculorun.*
  A. galli′nae, SIN *Dermanyssus gallinae.*
  A. horde′i, ácaro da cevada, uma espécie que penetra por baixo da pele.
  A. rhizoglyp′ticus hyacin′thi, espécie de ácaro que se desenvolve em cebolas estragadas e pode causar dermatite.
  A. scabe′i, termo antigo para *Sarcoptes scabiei.*

acar·y·ote (ā-kar′ē-ōt). Acariócito. SIN *akaryocyte.*

acat·a·la·se·mia [MIM*115500]. Acatalassemia. SIN *acatalasie.*

acat·a·la·sia (ā-kat-ă-lā′zē-ă). [MIM*115500]. Acatalasia; ausência ou deficiência de catalase no sangue e nos tecidos, manifestada, com frequência, por infecção recorrente ou ulceração das gengivas e estruturas orais correlatas e causada por mutações no gene da catalase (CAT) em 11p. Os homozigotos podem apresentar ausência completa (variedade japonesa) ou níveis muito reduzidos (variedade suíça) de catalase; os heterozigotos apresentam níveis reduzidos de catalase (hipocatalasia), que se sobrepõem à faixa normal. SIN acatalasemia, Takahara disease.

ac·a·thec·tic (ak-ă-thek′tik). Acatético; termo raramente empregado relativo à acatexia.

ac·a·thex·ia (ak-ă-thek′sē-ă). Acatexia; termo raramente empregado para a liberação anormal de secreções. [G. *a-* priv. + *kathexis,* retenção]

ac·a·thex·is (ak-ă-thek′sis). Termo raramente empregado para um distúrbio mental no qual certos objetos ou idéias não provocam uma resposta emocional no indivíduo. [G. *a-* priv. + *kathexis,* retenção]

aca·thi·sia (ak-ă-thiz′ē-ă). Acatisia. SIN *akathisia.*

acau·dal, acau·date (ā-kaw′dăl, ă-kaw′dāt). Acaudado; que não possui cauda. [G. *a-* priv. + L. *cauda*]

ACC Abreviatura de anodal closure *contraction* (contração muscular quando do fechamento de um circuito elétrico).

ac·cel·er·ans (ak-sel′er-anz). 1. Que acelera. 2. Termo obsoleto para um nervo acelerador (simpático) do coração. [L. *accelerator*]

ac·cel·er·ant (ak-sel′er-ant). SIN *accelerator (3).*

ac·cel·er·a·tion (ak-sel-er-ā′shŭn). Aceleração. 1. Ato de acelerar. 2. O índice de aumento na velocidade por unidade de tempo; comumente expresso em unidades *g*; também expresso em centímetros ou pés por segundo ao quadrado. 3. O índice de desvio crescente a partir de uma trajetória retilínea. VER radial a. [ver accelerator]
  angular a., a. angular; o índice de mudança de uma velocidade angular; p. ex., quando a velocidade de um rotor centrífugo aumenta ou quando ocorre uma mudança simultânea na velocidade e na direção, como em uma aeronave em forte manobra de parafuso.
  linear a., a. linear; o índice de mudança de velocidade sem mudança de direção; p.ex., quando ocorre o aumento da velocidade de uma aeronave em um vôo em linha reta.
  radial a., a. radial; a. centrípeta de uma partícula ou veículo que se move ao longo de uma via curva a uma velocidade constante; p.ex., quando se faz uma curva em um automóvel, o ato de mergulhar, ou uma manobra de *loop* (em espiral) em uma aeronave. Em aviação, a. varia diretamente com o quadrado da velocidade do ar e inversamente com o raio da curva ($a = V^2/r$, na qual V é a velocidade do ar e r, o raio da curva).

ac·cel·er·a·tor (ak-sel′er-ā-ter). Acelerador. 1. Qualquer coisa que aumenta a velocidade de uma ação ou função. 2. Em fisiologia, um nervo, músculo ou substância que acelera o movimento ou a resposta. 3. Catalisador usado para acelerar uma reação química. SIN accelerant. 4. Em física nuclear, um dispositivo que acelera partículas com carga elétrica (p.ex., prótons) a uma alta velocidade, a fim de produzir reações nucleares com um alvo para o estudo da estrutura subatômica, para a produção de radionuclídeos ou para radioterapia. [L. *accelerans,* p. pres. de *ac-celero,* acelerar, apressar, de *celer,* rápido]
  linear a. (LINAC), a. linear; dispositivo que confere alta velocidade e energia a partículas atômicas e subatômicas; importante para a radioterapia.
  proserum prothrombin conversion a. (PPCA), a. da conversão da protrombina pró-sérica; termo obsoleto para o fator VIII.
  prothrombin a., a. da protrombina; termo obsoleto para o fator V.
  serum a., a. sérico; termo obsoleto para o fator VII.
  serum prothrombin conversion a. (SPCA), a. da conversão da protrombina sérica; termo obsoleto para o fator VII.

ac·cel·er·in (ak-sel′er-in). Acelerina; termo obsoleto para o que já foi considerado um produto intermediário da coagulação, mas que, hoje em dia, não se acredita que exista.

ac·cel·er·om·e·ter (ak-sel-er-om′ē-ter). Acelerômetro; instrumento que mede o índice de mudança da velocidade por unidade de tempo.

ac·cen·tu·a·tor (ak-sent′ū-ā-ter). Acentuador; substância, como a anilina, cuja presença permite a combinação entre um tecido ou elemento histológico e um corante que, de outra forma, seria impossível. [L. *accentus,* intensidade, de *cano,* cantar]

ac·cep·tor (ak-sep′ter). Aceptor. 1. Composto que recebe um grupamento químico (p.ex., um grupamento amina, um grupamento metila, um grupamento carbamoíla) de outro composto (o doador); sob a ação da alanina transaminase, o ácido L-glutâmico é um doador de aminas, enquanto o ácido pirúvico é um a. de aminas. 2. Um receptor que se liga a um hormônio. [L. *ac-cipio,* pp. *-ceptus,* aceitar]
  hydrogen a., a. de hidrogênio. SIN *hydrogen carrier.*

ac·cès per·ni·ci·eux (ak-sā′ per-ni-syu′). Uma série de ataques graves de malária falcípara, por vezes ocorrendo em casos aparentemente brandos; classificado como cerebral e álgido. [Fr., ataques ou sintomas perniciosos]

ac·cess (ak′ses). Acesso. Um meio ou maneira de abordagem ou admissão. Em odontologia: 1. O espaço necessário para se visualizar e manipular os instrumentos para a remoção das cáries e o preparo do dente para restauração. 2. Abertura na coroa de um dente necessária para permitir a admissão adequada à polpa a fim de se limpar, modelar e selar o(s) canal(is) da raiz. SIN access opening. [L. *accessus*]

ac·ces·so·ri·us (ak-ses-ō′rē-ŭs). Acessório. SIN *accessory.* [L.]
  a. willis′ii, nervo acessório de Willis. SIN *accessory nerve [CN XI].*

ac·ces·so·ry (ak-ses′ō-rē). Acessório; em anatomia, indica certos músculos, nervos, glândulas, etc. que são auxiliares ou supranumerários em relação a algo semelhante e, em geral, mais importante. SIN accessorius. [L. *accessorius,* de *ac-cedo,* pp. *-cessus,* mover em direção a]

ac·ci·dent (ak′si-dent). Acidente; um evento não-planejado ou não-intencional, mas às vezes previsível, que leva a uma lesão, como, p.ex., no trânsito, na indústria ou no lar, ou evento desse tipo que se desenvolve no curso de uma doença. [L. *ac-cido,* acontecer]
  cardiac a., a. cardíaco; catástrofe cardíaca súbita, como a que pode resultar de uma oclusão coronariana.
  cerebrovascular a. (CVA), a. vascular cerebral (AVC); termo impreciso para a lesão cerebral irreversível.
  serum a., a. sérico; choque anafilático que resulta da injeção de soro de uma espécie diferente para fins terapêuticos. VER TAMBÉM serum *sickness.*

ac·ci·dent-prone. Propenso a acidentes. 1. Que sofre um número maior de acidentes do que seria esperado para uma pessoa comum em circunstâncias semelhantes. 2. Que apresenta características de personalidade que predispõem a acidentes.

ac·cli·ma·tion (ak-li-mā′shŭn). Aclimação, aclimatação. SIN *acclimatization.*

ac·cli·ma·ti·za·tion (ă-klī′mă-ti-zā′shŭn). Aclimatização; ajuste fisiológico de um indivíduo a um clima diferente, principalmente a mudanças na temperatura ambiental ou altitude. SIN acclimation.

ac·com·mo·da·tion (ă-kom′ō-dā′shŭn). Acomodação. 1. Ato ou estado de ajuste ou adaptação. 2. Na teoria sensorimotora, a modificação de esquemas ou expectativas cognitivas para adaptação à experiência. [L. *ac-commodo,* pp. *-atus,* adaptar, de *modus,* medida]
  amplitude of a., amplitude de a.; diferença na refratariedade do olho em repouso e quando completamente acomodado.
  a. of eye, a. ocular; aumento na espessura e na convexidade da lente do olho em resposta à contração do músculo ciliar a fim de focalizar a imagem de um objeto externo na retina.
  histologic a., a. histológica; alteração no formato das células para se adaptar a condições físicas modificadas, como o achatamento de células cubóides em cistos, em consequência da pressão. SIN pseudometaplasia.
  negative a., a. negativa; redução de a. que ocorre quando se muda da visão para perto para a visão a distância.
  a. of nerve, a. do nervo; a propriedade de um nervo por meio da qual ele se ajusta a um estímulo de intensidade lentamente crescente, de modo que seu limiar de excitação é maior do que seria se a intensidade do estímulo aumentasse mais rapidamente.
  positive a., a. positiva; refratariedade ocular aumentada que ocorre quando se muda da visão de um objeto a distância para um objeto próximo.
  range of a., variação de a.; distância entre um objeto observado com refratariedade ocular mínima e outro observado com acomodação máxima.
  relative a., a. relativa; quantidade de a. necessária para uma visão binocular

accommodation

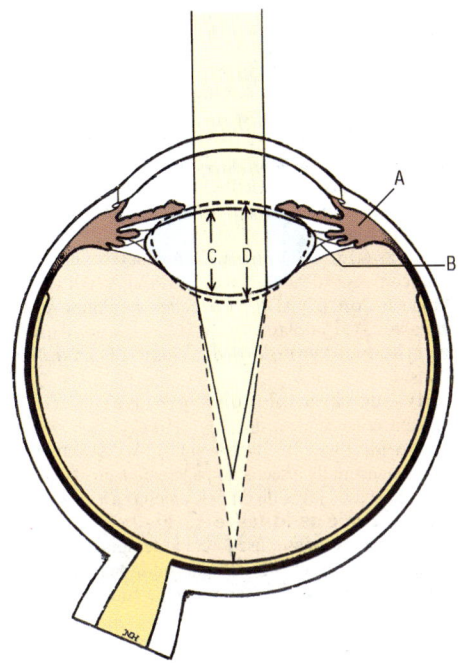

acomodação: (A) músculo ciliar, (B) ligamentos suspensores, (C) a lente do olho focaliza a imagem em frente à retina, imagem embaçada, (D) a lente se acomoda para focalizar a imagem na retina, imagem nítida

---

única para qualquer distância específica ou para qualquer grau de convergência.

ac·com·mo·da·tive (ă-kom′ŏ-dā-tiv). Acomodativo; relativo à acomodação.

ac·com·plice (ă-kom′plis). Cúmplice; uma bactéria que acompanha o agente infeccioso principal em uma infecção mista e que influencia a virulência do microrganismo principal. [I.M., do Fr. Ant., do L. *comples*, intimamente conectado]

ac·couche·ment (a-koosh-mawn′). Parto; nascimento de uma criança. VER TAMBÉM birth. [Fr. de *coucher*, deitar]

a. forcé (fōr-sā′), p. forçado; parto acelerado artificialmente por meio da utilização de fórceps, versão, etc.; originalmente aplicado à dilatação rápida do colo uterino com as mãos, com versão e extração forçada do feto.

ac·cou·cheur (a-koo-sher′). Parteiro; termo obsoleto para obstetra.

ac·cre·men·ti·tion (ak′rē-men-tish′ŭn). 1. Reprodução por brotamento ou germinação. 2. Acreção. SIN accretion (1). [L. *accresco*, pp.-*cretus*, aumentar]

ac·cre·tio cor·dis (ă-krē′shē-ō kōr′dis). Aderência do pericárdio a estruturas extracardíacas adjacentes.

ac·cre·tion (ă-krē′shŭn). Acreção. 1. Aumento pela adição à periferia de material da mesma natureza que o já existente; p.ex., o tipo de crescimento dos cristais. SIN accrementition (2). 2. Em odontologia, o material estranho (geralmente placa bacteriana ou tártaro) coletado na superfície de um dente ou em uma cavidade. 3. Um crescimento conjunto. [L. *accretio*, de *ad*, para, + *crescere*, crescer]

ac·cro·chage (ak-rō-shahj′). Sincronização intermitente de dois ritmos diferentes do coração, um influenciando o comportamento do outro, quando nenhum dos dois é dominante; observado nos casos de dissociação atrioventricular quando um batimento atrial ocorre logo após um batimento ventricular e este faz com que o batimento atrial ocorra mais cedo que o esperado. [Fr. enganchamento, atrelamento]

ac·cu·ra·cy (ak′kū-ră-sē). Acurácia; o grau de representação de uma medida, ou de uma estimativa baseada em medidas, do valor verdadeiro do atributo que está sendo medido. No laboratório, a a. de um exame é determinada, quando possível, pela comparação dos resultados do exame em questão com os resultados gerados usando-se padrões de referência ou um método de referência estabelecido.

ACD Abreviatura de acid-citrate-dextrose (ácido-citrato-dextrose).

ACE Abreviatura de angiotensin-converting *enzyme* (enzima conversora da angiotensina).

ac·e·bu·to·lol (as-ē-bū′tō-lol). Acebutolol; um agente bloqueador β-adrenérgico.

acec·li·dine (a-sek′li-dēn). Aceclidina; medicamento colinérgico usado para o tratamento tópico do glaucoma.

ac·e·dap·sone (as-ē-dap′sōn). Acedapsona; derivado da dapsona com ação mais prolongada; usada na malária para reforçar a quimioprofilaxia com quinino ou com uma combinação de cloroquina-primaquina; acredita-se que sua ação se baseia na interferência na utilização do ácido fólico.

ace·dia (ă-sē-dē′-ă). Acedia; termo obsoleto para uma síndrome mental cujas características principais são desânimo, indiferença, apatia e melancolia.

acef·yl·line pi·per·a·zine (ā-sef′i-lēn). Piperazina acefilina; um diurético e relaxante da musculatura lisa.

ACEI Abreviatura de angiotensin-converting enzyme *inhibitors*, em *inhibitor* (inibidores da enzima conversora da angiotensina).

acel·lu·lar (ā-sel′ū-lăr). Acelular. 1. Desprovido de células. SIN noncellular (2). 2. Termo aplicado a microrganismos unicelulares que não se tornam multicelulares e são completos em uma única unidade celular; freqüentemente aplicado a protozoários para enfatizar sua organização completa em uma única célula. [G. *a-* priv. + L. *cellula*, pequena câmara]

ace·lom (ă-sē′lom). Aceloma; ausência de um celoma verdadeiro ou cavidade corporal revestida de mesotélio; tipicamente encontrado em platelmintos que apresentam uma massa sincicial de células parenquimatosas em vez de uma cavidade corporal verdadeira. [G. *a-* priv. + *koilōma*, buraco (celoma)]

ace·lo·mate, ace·lo·ma·tous (ă-sē′lō-māt, ā-sē-lō′mă-tŭs). Acelomado; que não possui um celoma ou cavidade corporal.

acen·o·cou·ma·rin (ā-sē-nō-koo′mă-rin). Acenocumarina. SIN acenocoumarol.

acen·o·cou·ma·rol (ā-sē-nō-koo′mă-rol). Acenocumarol; efetivo anticoagulante sintético por via oral do tipo cumarina, com ações semelhantes. SIN acenocoumarin, nicoumalone.

acen·tric (ā-sen′trik). Acêntrico, excêntrico; sem um centro; em citogenética, indica um fragmento cromossômico sem um centrômero. [G. *a-* priv. + *kentron*, centro]

ace·pha·lia, aceph·a·lism (ā-se-fā′lē-ă, ā-sef′ă-lizm). 1. Acefalia. SIN acephaly. 2. Acéfalo SIN acephalus.

aceph·a·line (ā-sef′ă-līn). Acefalina; indica os membros da subordem de protozoários Acephalina (ordem Eugregarinida), caracterizados por corpúsculos simples não-compartimentalizados, que parasitam os invertebrados.

aceph·a·lo·bra·chia (ā-sef′ă-lō-brā′kē-ă). Acefalobraquia. SIN abrachiocephaly. [G. *a-* priv. + *kephalē*, cabeça, + *brachion*, braço]

aceph·a·lo·car·dia (ā-sef′ă-lō-kar′dē-ă). Acefalocardia; ausência da cabeça e do coração, conforme se observa no gêmeo parasita. [G. *a-* priv. + *kephalē*, cabeça, + *kardia*, coração]

aceph·a·lo·chei·ria, aceph·a·lo·chi·ria (ā-sef′ă-lō-kī′rē-ă). Acefaloquiria; ausência congênita da cabeça e das mãos. [G. *a-* priv. + *kephalē*, cabeça, + *cheir*, mão]

aceph·a·lo·cyst (ā-sef′ă-lō-sist). Acefalocisto; cisto hidático isolado; uma hidátide estéril, assim chamada porque não desenvolve escóleces (cabeças de tênias). [G. *a-* priv. + *kephalē*, cabeça, + *kystis*, bexiga]

aceph·a·lo·gas·ter·ia (ā-sef′ă-lō-gas-tēr′ē-ă). Acefalogastria; ausência congênita da cabeça, do tórax e do abdome, conforme se observa no gêmeo parasita que apresenta apenas pernas e pelve.

aceph·a·lo·po·dia (ā-sef′ă-lō-pō′dē-ă). Acefalopodia; ausência congênita da cabeça e dos pés. [G. *a-* priv. + *kephalē*, cabeça, + *pous*, pé]

aceph·a·lor·rha·chia (ā-sef′ă-lō-rak′ē-ă). Acefalorraquia; ausência congênita da cabeça e da coluna vertebral. [G. *a-* priv. + *kephalē*, cabeça, + *rhachis*, espinha]

aceph·a·lo·tho·ra·cia (ā-sef′ă-lō-thōr-asē-ă). Acefalotoracia; ausência congênita da cabeça e do tórax. [G. *a-* priv. + *kephalē*, cabeça, + *thorax*, peito]

aceph·a·lous (ā-sef′ă-lŭs). Acéfalo; sem cabeça.

aceph·a·lus (ā-sef′ă-lŭs). Acéfalo; um feto sem cabeça. SIN acephalia (2), acephalism. [G. *a-* priv. + *kephalē*, cabeça]

a. acormus (ā-kōr′mŭs), acefalia associada a acormia; condição na qual a cabeça, sem o corpo, está ligada à placenta pelo cordão umbilical.

a. dibra′chius, um feto sem cabeça mas que apresenta os dois braços reconhecidamente desenvolvidos.

a. di′pus, um feto sem cabeça mas que apresenta os dois membros inferiores reconhecidamente desenvolvidos.

a. monobra′chius, um feto sem cabeça e que apresenta apenas um braço reconhecidamente desenvolvido.

a. mon′opus, um feto sem cabeça e com fusão tão acentuada das extremidades inferiores que apenas um pé é reconhecível.

a. sym′pus, um feto sem cabeça e que apresenta fusão total dos membros inferiores.

aceph·a·ly (ā-sef′ă-lē). Acefalia; ausência congênita da cabeça. SIN acephalia (1), acephalism. [G. *a-* priv. + *kephalē*, cabeça]

ace·ro·la (ā-sē-rō-lă). Fruta de um arbusto que cresce nas Américas Central e do Sul e em Porto Rico; a fruta é a mais rica fonte conhecida de vitamina C (ácido ascórbico).

acer·vu·lus (ă-ser′vū-lŭs). Acérvulo. SIN *corpora* arenacea, em *corpus*. [L. Mod. dim. de L. *acervus*, grande quantidade]

aces·to·ma (ă-ses-tō′mă). Acestoma; granulações exuberantes que formam uma cicatriz. [G. *akestos*, curável, + *ōma*, tumor]

ace·sul·fame (ā-sē-sul-fām). Acelssulfamo; adoçante sintético, não-calórico, semelhante à sacarina.

acet-, aceto-. Formas combinantes que indicam o fragmento de dois carbonos do ácido acético.

ac·e·tab·u·la (as-ĕ-tab'ū-lă). Acetábulos; plural de acetabulum.

ac·e·tab·u·lar (as-ĕ-tab'ū-lăr). Acetabular; relativo ao acetábulo.

ac·e·tab·u·lec·to·my (as'ĕ-tab-ū-lek'tō-mē). Acetabulectomia; excisão do acetábulo. [acetábulo + G, *ektomē*, excisão]

ac·e·tab·u·lo·plas·ty (as-ĕ-tab'ū-lō-plas-tē). Acetabuloplastia; qualquer operação que visa a restauração do acetábulo a um estado mais próximo possível do normal. [acetábulo + G, *plastos*, formado]

ac·e·tab·u·lum, pl. **ac·e·tab·u·la** (as-ĕ-tab'ū-lŭm, -lă) [TA]. Acetábulo; depressão em forma de xícara, na superfície externa do osso ilíaco, na qual se encaixa a cabeça do fêmur. SIN cotyle (2), cotyloid cavity. [L. xícara rasa de vinagre]

ac·e·tal (as'e-tal). Acetal; produto da adição de 2 moles de álcool a 1 de aldeído, assim: RCHO + 2R'OH → RCH(OR')$_2$ + H$_2$O; em acetais mistos (p.ex., glicosídeos), dois alcoóis diferentes são ligados ao grupamento aldeído original. VER TAMBÉM hemiacetal, hemiketal, ketal.

a. phosphatide, a. fosfatídeo; denominação antiga para alq-1-enilglicerofosfolipídio.

ac·et·al·de·hyde (as-e-tal'dĕ-hīd). Acetaldeído; intermediário na fermentação por leveduras do carboidrato e no metabolismo do álcool. É um agente fundamental para os efeitos tóxicos do etanol. SIN acetic aldehyde, ethanal.

activated a., a. ativado; forma ativada de acetaldeído produzida durante a descarboxilação do piruvato ativo. Formada na fermentação do álcool e no metabolismo de carboidratos. SIN α-hydroxyethylthiamin pyrophosphate.

acet·a·mide (as-et-am'īd, ă-set'ă-mīd). Acetamida; CH$_3$CONH$_2$; usada em pesquisas biomédicas. SIN acetic amide.

2-ac·et·am·i·do·flu·o·rene (AAF) (as'et-am'i-dō-flōr'en). 2- acetamidofluoreno. SIN 2-acetylaminofluorene.

ac·et·a·min·o·phen (as-et-a-mē'nō-fen). Acetaminofeno; antipirético e analgésico com potência semelhante à do ácido acetilsalicílico. SIN paracetamol.

ac·et·am·in·o·sal·ol (as-ĕ-tam'in-ō-sal'ol). Acetaminosalol; usado como analgésico, antipirético e anti-séptico intestinal. SIN phenetsal.

ac·et·ar·sol (as-ĕ-tar'sol). Acetarsol. SIN acetarsone.

ac·et·ar·sone (as-ĕ-tar'son). Acetarsona; usada no tratamento da amebíase e como aplicação tópica na angina de Vincent e na vaginite por *Trichomonas*. O sal dietilamina é usado como anti-sifilítico. SIN acetarsol.

ac·e·tate (as'e-tāt). Acetato; sal ou éster do ácido acético.

active a., a. ativo. SIN acetyl-CoA.

a. kinase [EC 2.7.2.1], a. cinase; uma fosfotransferase que forma acetil fosfato e ADP a partir de ATP e acetato. Uma importante enzima na formação de fosfatos de "alta energia" em certos microrganismos. SIN acetokinase.

a. thiokinase, a. tioquinase. SIN acetyl-CoA ligase.

ac·e·tate-CoA ligase. Acetato-CoA ligase. SIN acetyl-CoA ligase.

acet·a·zol·a·mide (as'ĕ-tă-zol'ă-mīd). Acetazolamida; a sulfonamida heterocíclica, 5-acetilamido-1,3,4-tiadiazol-2-sulfonamida, que inibe a ação da anidrase carbônica nos rins aumentando a excreção urinária de sódio, potássio e bicarbonato, reduzindo a excreção de amônio, elevando o pH urinário e diminuindo o pH sanguíneo; usada na acidose respiratória para diurese e estimulação do impulso respiratório, no glaucoma para reduzir a pressão intraocular e na epilepsia. A a. sódica possui as mesmas ações e usos que a a., porém é mais solúvel e, portanto, mais adequada para administração parenteral.

acet·e·nyl (a-sē'ten-il). Acetenil. SIN ethynyl.

ace·tic (a-sē'tik, -set'ik). Acético. **1.** Denotando a presença do fragmento de dois carbonos do ácido acético. **2.** Relativo ao vinagre; acre. [L. *acetum*, vinagre]

ace·tic ac·id. Ácido acético; produto da oxidação do etanol e da destilação destrutiva da madeira; usado topicamente como um contra-irritante e, por vezes, internamente, sendo também um reagente; está contido nos vinagres. SIN ethanoic acid.

diluted a. a., a. a. diluído; contém 6% p/v (peso/volume) de a. a.

glacial a. a., a. a. glacial; contém 99% de ácido acético absoluto; um cáustico para a remoção de verrugas e calos.

ace·tic al·de·hyde. Aldeído acético. SIN acetaldehyde.

ace·tic am·ide. Amida acética. SIN acetamide.

ace·ti·co·cep·tor (a-sē'ti-kō-sep'tŏr). Aceticoceptor; cadeia lateral de moléculas com afinidade especial pelo radical ácido acético. [L. *acetum*, vinagre, + *capio*, captar]

ace·ti·fy (ă-set'i-fī). Acetificar; causar fermentação acética; fazer vinagre ou se tornar vinagre. [L. *acetum*, vinagre, + *facio*, fazer; ou *fieri*, ser feito, tornar-se]

ace·tim·e·ter (as-ĕ-tim'ĕ-ter). Acetímetro; aparelho para a determinação do conteúdo de ácido acético no vinagre ou em outro líquido. SIN acetometer. [L. *acetum*, vinagre, + G. *metron*, medida]

aceto-. VER acet-.

ac·e·to·ac·e·tate (as'e-tō-as'e-tāt). Acetoacetato; um sal ou íon do ácido acetoacético. Um corpo cetônico formado na cetogênese. SIN diacetate (1).

a. decarboxylase [EC 4.1.1.4], a. descarboxilase; uma carboxilase que cliva CO$_2$ a partir do acetoacetato para formar acetona.

ac·e·to·a·ce·tic ac·id (as'e-tō-a-sē'tik). Ácido acetoacético; um dos corpos cetônicos, formado em excesso e surgindo na urina nos casos de inanição ou diabetes.

ac·e·to·a·ce·tyl-CoA (as'e-tō-a-sē'til). Acetoacetil-CoA; intermediário na oxidação de ácidos graxos e na formação de corpos cetônicos; também formada a partir de duas moléculas de acetil-CoA; a principal função é a condensação com acetil-CoA para formar a importante β-hidróxi-β-metilglutaril-CoA. SIN acetoacetyl-coenzyme A.

a.-CoA reductase [EC 1.1.1.36], a.-CoA redutase; uma oxirredutase que catalisa a interconversão de 3-oxoacil-CoA e NADPH, e a correspondente D-3-hidroxiacil-CoA, e NADP$^+$. Uma etapa na síntese de ácidos graxos.

a.-CoA thiolase, a.-CoA tiolase. SIN acetyl-CoA acetyltransferase.

ac·e·to·a·ce·tyl-co·en·zyme A (as'e-tō-as'e-til-kō-en'zim). Acetoacetil coenzima A. SIN acetoacetyl-CoA.

ac·e·to·a·ce·tyl-suc·cin·ic thi·o·phor·ase (as'e-tō-as'e-til-sŭk-sin'ik). Tioforase acetoacetilsuccínica. SIN 3-oxoacid-CoA transferase.

ac·e·to·hex·am·ide (as-ĕ-tō-heks'ă-mid). Acetoexamida; agente hipoglicemiante oral que estimula a secreção pancreática de insulina; mais útil, terapeuticamente, nos casos leves de diabetes melito não-insulino dependente.

ac·e·to·hy·drox·a·mic ac·id (as'e-tō-hī-drok'să-mik). Ácido acetodroxâmico; inibidor da urease, usado como terapia adjuvante nas infecções urinárias crônicas causadas por microrganismos degradadores de uréia.

ac·et·o·in (as-et'-ō-in). Acetoína; produto da condensação de duas moléculas de acetaldeído.

ac·e·to·ki·nase (as'e-tō-kī'nās). Acetoquinase. SIN acetate kinase.

ac·e·tol (as'e-tol). Acetol; termo obsoleto para 1-hidroxi-2-propanona, ou hidroxiacetona; também usado como nome comercial para certos produtos.

α-ac·e·to·lac·tic ac·id (as'e-tō-lak'tik). Ácido α-acetoláctico; intermediário no catabolismo do ácido pirúvico e na biossíntese da valina.

ac·e·tol·y·sis (as-e-tol'i-sis). Acetólise; decomposição de um composto orgânico com a adição dos elementos do ácido acético no momento da decomposição; análoga à hidrólise e à fosforólise.

ac·e·to·me·naph·thone (as'e-tō-me-naf'thōn). Acetomenaftona. SIN menadiol di-acetate.

ac·e·tom·e·ter (as-ĕ-tom'ĕ-ter). Acetômetro. SIN acetimeter.

ac·e·tone (as'e-tōn). Acetona; líquido incolor, volátil e inflamável; quantidades extremamente pequenas são encontradas na urina normal, mas quantidades maiores ocorrem na urina e no sangue de diabéticos, por vezes conferindo um odor etéreo (de éter) à urina e à respiração. É um dos corpos cetônicos. A a. sintética é usada como solvente em certos preparados farmacêuticos e comerciais. SIN dimethyl ketone.

ac·e·ton·e·mia (as'e-tō-nē'mē-ă). Acetonemia; presença de acetona ou corpos cetônicos em quantidades relativamente grandes no sangue, manifestada primeiramente por cretinismo e, mais tarde, por depressão progressiva. [acetona + G. *haima*, sangue]

ac·e·to·ne·mic (as'e-tō-nē'mik). Acetonêmico; relativo à acetonemia ou causado por ela.

ac·e·to·ni·trile (as'e-tō-nī'tril). Acetonitrilo, cianeto de metila; líquido incolor de odor aromático, solúvel em água e álcool.

ac·e·to·nu·ria (as'e-tō-noor'ē-ă). Acetonúria; excreção de grandes quantidades de acetona na urina, indicando oxidação incompleta de grandes quantidades de lipídios; ocorre comumente na acidose diabética. [acetona + G. *ouron*, urina]

ac·e·to·phen·a·zine ma·le·ate (as-ĕ-tō-fē'nă-zēn mal'ē-āt). Maleato de acetofenazina; um tranqüilizante fenotiazínico.

ac·e·to·phe·net·i·din (as'ĕ-tō-fe-net'i-din). Acetofenetidina. SIN phenacetin.

ac·e·to·sul·fone so·di·um (as'ĕ-tō-sŭl'fōn). Acetossulfona sódica; um leprostático administrado por via oral.

ace·tous (as'e-tŭs). Acetoso; relativo ao vinagre; de gosto azedo.

ac·e·to·whit·en·ing (ă-sē'tō-hwīt'en-ing). Acetoclareamento; descoloração da pele ou das mucosas após a aplicação de uma solução de ácido acético a 3–5%, um sinal de aumento de proteína celular e da densidade nuclear; usado principalmente na pele e nas mucosas genitais, incluindo o colo uterino, a fim de identificar áreas de alteração da célula escamosa para biópsia e o tratamento do condiloma acuminado (condyloma acuminatum). SIN visual inspection with acetic acid. [ácido acético + branqueamento]

ac·e·tri·zo·ate so·di·um (as-ĕ-tri-zō'āt). Acetrizoato sódico; sal do ácido 3-acetamido-2,4,6-triiobenzóico, um contraste radiográfico hidrossolúvel usado antigamente.

ace·tum, pl. **ace·ta** (ă-sē'tŭm, -tă). Vinagre. SIN vinegar. [L. *vinum acetum*, vinho azedo, vinagre]

ac·e·u·rate (a-set'ū-rāt). Aceturato; contração aprovada pela USAN para o termo *N*-acetilglicinato, CH$_3$CONHCH$_2$COO$^-$.

ace·tyl (Ac) (as'e-til). Acetil, CH$_3$CO$^-$; molécula de ácido acético cujo grupamento hidroxila foi removido.

a. chloride, cloreto de acetil; líquido incolor usado como um reagente; é também um corrosivo, causando graves queimaduras devido à hidrólise a HCl.

a. phosphate, fosfato de acetil; um fosfato de "alta energia" que age como doador de acetato no metabolismo de várias bactérias.

a. transacylase, acetil transacilase. SIN ACP-acetyltransferase.

ac·e·tyl·ad·e·nyl·ate (as'e-til-ā-den'il-āt). Acetiladenilato; anidrido misto entre o grupamento carboxila do ácido acético e o resíduo fosfórico do ácido adenosina 5'-monofosfórico.

2-ace·tylami·no·flu·o·rene (AAF) (as'e-til-am'i-nō-flōr'ēn). 2-acetilaminofluoreno; um composto carcinogênico poderoso. SIN 2-acetamidofluorene.

acet·y·lase (a-set'il-ās). Acetilase; qualquer enzima que catalisa acetilação ou desacetilação, como a formação de N-acetilglutamato a partir do glutamato mais acetil-CoA, ou o contrário; em geral, as acetilases são chamadas de acetiltransferases.

N-ace·tyl·as·par·tate (as'-ē-til-as-par'tāt). N-acetilaspartato; derivado acetilado do aspartato encontrado no cérebro. Usado como marcador na ressonância magnética do cérebro e na aquisição de imagens neurais.

acet·y·la·tion (a-set-i-lā'shŭn). Acetilação; formação de um derivado acetil.

ace·tyl·car·bro·mal (ā-sē'til-kar-brō'măl). Acetilcarbromal; um sedativo que foi substituído por benzodiazepínicos e medicamentos mais modernos.

O-ace·tyl·car·ni·tine (as-e-til-kar'ni-tēn). O-acetilcarnitina; derivado acetil da carnitina formado pela carnitina acetiltransferase. Facilita o transporte de acetil para as mitocôndrias e é uma fonte energética importante para os espermatozóides.

ace·tyl·cho·line (ACH, Ach) (as-e-til-kō'lēn). Acetilcolina; o éster acético da colina, a substância neurotransmissora, nas sinapses colinérgicas, que produz inibição cardíaca, vasodilatação, peristaltismo gastrointestinal e outros efeitos parassimpáticos. É liberada pelas terminações pré- e pós-ganglionares das fibras parassimpáticas e das fibras pré-ganglionares do sistema simpático em conseqüência de lesões nervosas, agindo como transmissor no órgão efetor; é rapidamente hidrolisada em colina e ácido acético pela acetilcolinesterase, nos tecidos, e pela pseudocolinesterase, no sangue.

a. chloride, cloreto de acetilcolina; um miótico, administrado como solução oftálmica por seus efeitos parassimpaticomiméticos; usado nas cirurgias de catarata.

ace·tyl·cho·lin·es·ter·ase (as'e-til-kō-lin-es'ter-ās). Acetilcolinesterase; as colinesterases que hidrolisam a acetilcolina em acetato e colina no sistema nervoso central e nas junções neuroefetoras periféricas (p.ex., placas motoras terminais e gânglios autônomos). SIN choline esterase I, "e"-type cholinesterase, specific cholinesterase, true cholinesterase.

ace·tyl-CoA. Acetil-CoA; produto da condensação da coenzima A e do ácido acético, simbolizado por CoAS~COCH₃; intermediário na transferência do fragmento de dois carbonos, notavelmente em sua entrada no ciclo do ácido tricarboxílico e na síntese de ácidos graxos. SIN acetyl-coenzyme A, active acetate.

a.-CoA acetyltransferase, acetil-CoA acetiltransferase; uma acetiltransferase que forma acetoacetil-CoA a partir de duas moléculas de a.-CoA, liberando uma CoA. Uma etapa fundamental na cetogênese e na síntese de esterol. SIN acetoacetyl-CoA thiolase, a.-CoA thiolase, thiolase.

a.-CoA acylase, acetil-CoA acilase. SIN a.-CoA hydrolase.

a.-CoA acyltransferase, acetil-CoA aciltransferase; enzima que catalisa a clivagem tioclástica da β-cetoacil-CoA, formando uma acil-CoA com uma cadeia de carbonos dois átomos mais curta, com os dois átomos que faltam aparecendo como a.-CoA. Uma etapa na degradação de ácidos graxos. VER TAMBÉM a.-CoA acetyltransferase. SIN 3-ketoacyl-CoA thiolase, β-ketothiolase.

a.-CoA carboxylase, acetil-CoA carboxilase; uma ligase que catalisa a reação de acetil-CoA, CO_2, H_2O e ATP com um cátion divalente como catalisador e biotina ligada por covalência, para formar malonil-CoA, ADP and P_i (ou a descarboxilase inversa); a N-carboxibiotina é um intermediário. Uma enzima fundamental na síntese de ácidos graxos.

a.-CoA deacylase, acetil-CoA desacilase. SIN a.-CoA hydrolase.

a.-CoA:α-glucosaminide acetyltransferase, acetil-CoA:α-glicosaminida acetiltransferase; enzima envolvida na síntese de certas partes carboidrato em proteínas. A deficiência dessa enzima leva à mucopolissacaridose tipo III C.

a.-CoA hydrolase, acetil-CoA hidrolase; uma hidrolase que cliva acetato e coenzima A a partir de acetil-CoA. SIN a.-CoA acylase, a.-CoA deacylase.

a.-CoA ligase, acetil-CoA ligase; uma ligase que catalisa a reação de acetato e CoA e ATP para formar AMP, pirofosfato e a.-CoA. Uma etapa fundamental na ativação do acetato. SIN acetate thiokinase, acetate-CoA ligase, acetyl-activating enzyme, a.-CoA synthetase.

a.-CoA synthetase, acetil-CoA sintetase. SIN a.-CoA ligase.

a.-CoA thiolase, acetil-CoA tiolase. SIN a.-CoA acetyltransferase.

ace·tyl-co·en·zyme A (as'e-til-kō-en'zīm). Acetilcoenzima A. SIN acetyl-CoA.

ace·tyl·cys·te·ine (as'e-til-sis'tē-in). Acetilcisteína; agente mucolítico que diminui a viscosidade do muco; usada na prevenção da lesão hepática provocada por intoxicação por acetaminofeno.

ace·tyl·dig·i·tox·in (ā-sē'til-dij-i-tok'sin). Acetildigitoxina; o éster α-acetil da digitoxina, derivado do lanatosídeo A, que possui as mesmas ações e usos da digitoxina, mas com início rápido e menor tempo de ação.

ace·tyl·di·gox·in (ā-sē'til-dī-jok'sin). Acetildigoxina; glicosídeo digitálico com propriedades semelhantes às da digoxina; derivada da digilanida C.

α-N-ace·tyl·ga·lac·to·sam·in·id·ase (as'ē-til-gal-ăk-tōs-a-min-i-dās). α-N-acetilgalactosaminidase; enzima que hidrolisa 2-acetamido-2-desoxi-α-D-galactosídeos em álcool e 2-acetamido-2-desoxi-D-galactose livre. A deficiência dessa enzima resulta na doença de Schindler.

N-ace·tyl·glu·co·sam·ine (as'e-til-glu-cōs'a-mēn). N-acetilglicosamina; um amino açúcar acetilado, parte importante das glicoproteínas.

α-N-ace·tyl·glu·co·sam·in·id·ase (as'ē-til-glu-cōs-a-min-i-dās). α-N-acetilglicosaminidase; enzima que hidrolisa glicosídeos da N-acetilglicosamina produzindo álcool e N-acetilglicosamina. A deficiência dessa enzima resulta na mucopolissacaridose III B.

N-ace·tyl·glu·ta·mate (NAG) (ā-sē'til-gloo'tă-māt). N-acetilglutamato; o sal do ácido N-acetilglutâmico. Um ativador da carbamoil fosfato sintetase I durante a síntese da uréia; esse aminoácido produz uma mudança na configuração da enzima, aumentando sua atividade. A incapacidade de sintetizar acetilglutamato resulta em um defeito na biossíntese da uréia.

ace·tyl·meth·a·dol (as'ē-til-meth-ă-dol). Acetilmetadol; um analgésico opióide que existe em 4 isômeros ópticos diferentes. Os isômeros l são ativos e o l-acetilmetadol (LAM) apresenta ação prolongada, tendo sido tentado como substituto da metadona nos programas de manutenção com esse fármaco e nos programas nos quais a metadona deve ser retirada, como na dependência física de morfina.

N-ace·tyl·neu·ra·min·ic ac·id (NeuAc) (as'ē-til-nur-a-min'ik-as'id). Ácido N-acetilneuramínico; a forma mais comum de ácido siálico nos mamíferos.

ace·tyl·or·ni·thine de·a·cet·yl·ase (as'e-til-ōr'ni-thēn) [EC 3.5.1.16]. Acetilornitina desacetilase; enzima que catalisa a hidrólise de N^2-acetil-L-ornitina a L-ornitina e acetato.

3-ace·tyl·pyr·i·dine (as'e-til-pir'i-dēn). 3-acetilpiridina; um antimetabólito da nicotinamida que produz sinais e sintomas da deficiência de nicotinamida em camundongos; neurotoxina que lesiona o hipotálamo, o tronco cerebral e os gânglios basais.

ace·tyl·sal·i·cyl·ic ac·id (as'e-til-sal-i-sil'ik). Ácido acetilsalicílico (AAS). SIN aspirin.

N^4-ace·tyl·sul·fa·nil·a·mide (as'e-til-sŭl-fă-nil'ă-mīd). N^4-acetilsulfanilamida; intermediário na síntese de sulfanilamida; formada nos corpos animais por meio da acetilação da sulfanilamida. SIN p-sulfamylacetanilide.

N^1-ace·tyl·sul·fa·nil·a·mide. N^1-acetilsulfanilamida; antibacteriano à base de sulfa usado topicamente e nos olhos.

ace·tyl sul·fi·sox·a·zole. Acetil sulfisoxazol; derivado do sulfisoxazol com as mesmas ações e usos; antibacteriano à base de sulfa.

ace·tyl·tan·nic ac·id (as'e-til-tan'ik). Ácido acetiltânico; adstringente usado antigamente para o tratamento da diarréia. SIN diacetyltannic acid, tannylacetate.

ace·tyl·trans·fer·ase (as'e-til-trans'fer-ās). Aceltiltransferase; qualquer enzima que transfere grupamentos acetil de um composto a outro. VER TAMBÉM acetyl-CoA acetyltransferase, choline acetyltransferase, dihydrolipoamide S-acetyltransferase. SIN transacetylase.

AcG, ac-g Abreviatura de accelerator globulin (globulina aceleradora).

ACH, Ach Abreviatura de acetylcholine (acetilcolina).

Ach Acetilcolina. VER ACH.

acha·la·sia (ak-ā-lā'-zē-ă). Acalasia; insuficiência de relaxamento; refere-se principalmente às aberturas viscerais, como piloro, cárdia ou qualquer outra musculatura do esfíncter. [G. a- priv. + chalasis, um relaxamento]

a. of the cardia, a. do cárdia. SIN esophageal a.

cricopharyngeal a., a. cricofaríngea; obstrução funcional ao nível do esfíncter esofágico superior devido ao relaxamento insuficiente da musculatura cricofaríngea; geralmente associada a um divertículo faringoesofágico (pharyngoesophageal diverticulum). SIN a. of the upper sphincter, hypertensive upper esophageal sphincter.

esophageal a., a. esofágica; relaxamento normal insuficiente do esfíncter esofágico inferior associado a contrações não-coordenadas do esôfago torácico, resultando em obstrução funcional e dificuldade de deglutição. SIN a. of the cardia, cardiospasm.

a. of the upper sphincter, a. do esfíncter superior. SIN cricopharyngeal a.

Achard, Emile C., médico francês, 1860–1941. VER A. syndrome, A.-Thiers syndrome.

ache (āk). Dor vaga, de localização imprecisa, geralmente de intensidade média.

bone a., dor óssea; dor imprecisa em um ou mais ossos, em geral intensa; uma variedade extrema ocorre no dengue.

stomach a., dor abdominal, originando-se geralmente no estômago ou no intestino. SIN gastralgia, gastrodynia.

achei·lia (ā-kī'lē-ā). Aquilia; ausência congênita dos lábios. [G. a- priv. + cheilos, lábio]

achei·lous, achi·lous (ā-kī′lŭs). Aquiloso; caracterizado por aquilia ou relativo a ela.

achei·ria (ā-kī′rē-ă). Aquiria. **1.** Ausência congênita de uma ou ambas as mãos. **2.** Anestesia, com perda da sensação de posse, de uma ou ambas as mãos. **3.** Uma forma de disquiria na qual o paciente é incapaz de dizer em que lado do corpo foi aplicado um estímulo. [G. *a-* priv. + *cheir*, mão]

achei·rop·o·dy, achi·rop·o·dy (ā-kī-rop′ō-dē, ā-kī-rop′ō-dē) (MIM*200500). Aquiropodia; ausência congênita das mãos e dos pés; herança autossômica recessiva. [G. *a-* priv. + *cheir*, mão, + *podos*, pé]

achei·rous, achi·rous (ā-kī′rŭs). Aquiroso; caracterizado por aquiria ou relativo a ela. VER acheiria (1).

Achenbach, Walter, internista alemão do século XX. VER A. *syndrome*.

Achilles, Aquiles. Guerreiro grego mitológico, vulnerável apenas no calcanhar. VER A. *bursa, reflex, tendon*.

achil·lo·bur·si·tis (ā-kil′ō-ber-sī′tis). Bursite aquiléia, aquilobursite; inflamação de uma bolsa próxima ao tendão do calcâneo. SIN retrocalcaneobursitis.

achil·lo·ten·ot·o·my (ā-kil′ō-ten-ot′ō-mē). Tenotomia aquiléia; incisão do tendão de Aquiles. [Achilles (tendão) + G. *tenōn*, tendão, + *tomē*, incisão]

achi·ral (ā-kī′ral). Indica ausência de quiralidade. [G. *a-* priv. + *cheir*, mão]

achlor·hy·dria (ā-klōr-hī′drē-ă). Acloridria; ausência de ácido clorídrico do suco gástrico. [G. *a-* priv. + clorídrico (ácido)]

achlor·o·phyl·lous (ā-klōr-of′ĭ-lŭs). Aclorófilo; sem clorofila, como no caso dos fungos.

Acho·le·plas·ma, pl. *Acho·le·plas·ma·ta* (ā-kō-lē-plas′mă, mah-tă). Gênero de bactérias (ordem Mycoplasmatales) com características idênticas às das espécies do gênero *Mycoplasma*, exceto pelo fato de não exigirem esterol para o crescimento; ocorrem espécies saprófitas e parasitas. A espécie típica é A. *laidlawii*.

A. axan'thum, espécie encontrada originalmente em uma linhagem celular de leucemia murina; ecologia bovina, porcina, botânica.

A. laidla'wii, espécie que ocorre como saprófita no adubo, estrume, húmus e terra; a espécie típica do gênero A. SIN *Mycoplasma laidlawii*.

acho·lia (ā-kō′lē-ă). Acolia; ausência ou supressão da secreção de bile. [G. *a-* priv. + *cholē*, bile]

achol·ic (ā-kol′ik). Acólico; sem bile, como nas fezes acólicas (pálidas).

achol·u·ria (ā-kō-loo′rē-ă). Acolúria; ausência de pigmentos biliares da urina em certos casos de icterícia. [G. *a-* priv. + *cholē*, bile, + *ouron*, urina]

achol·u·ric (ā-kō-loo′rik). Acolúrico; sem bile na urina.

achon·dro·gen·e·sis (ā-kon-drō-jen′ē-sis). Acondrogênese; nanismo neonatal letal caracterizado por grave displasia óssea dos quatro membros, micromelia, crânio aumentado e tronco pequeno, com ossificação ausente ou retardada da parte inferior da coluna vertebral e dos ossos pubianos. Existem vários tipos [G. *a-* priv. + *chondros*, cartilagem, + *genesis*, origem]

Type IA a. [MIM*200600], a. tipo IA; a. com cartilagem hipervascular e osso hipercelular; padrão de herança incerto. SIN Houston-Harris syndrome.

Type IB a. (MIM*600972), a. tipo IB; a. com ossificação intracartilaginosa gravemente desorganizada; herança autossômica recessiva, causada por mutação no gene transportador de sulfato da displasia diastrófica (DTDST) no cromossoma 5q. SIN Parenti-Fraccaro syndrome.

Type II a. [MIM*200610], a. tipo II; a. com herança autossômica dominante, causada por mutação no gene do colágeno tipo II (COL2A1) no cromossoma 12q. SIN Langer-Saldino syndrome.

achon·dro·pla·sia (ā-kon-drō-plā′zē-ă) [MIM*100800 *134934]. Acondroplasia; essa condrodistrofia, caracterizada por uma anormalidade na conversão da cartilagem em osso, é a forma mais comum de nanismo de membros curtos; caracterizada por baixa estatura, com encurtamento rizomélico dos membros, cabeça grande com proeminência frontal e hipoplasia mesofacial, lordose lombar acentuada, limitação da extensão do cotovelo, joelho varo, mão em tridente, achados radiográficos do esqueleto característicos e sintomas neurológicos complicando hidrocefalia e estenose do canal espinal. Herança autossômica dominante, com a maioria dos casos sendo esporádica e causada por mutação no gene do receptor 3 do fator de crescimento de fibroblastos (FGFR3) no cromossoma 4p. [G. *a-* priv. + *chondros*, cartilagem, + *plasis*, moldagem]

homozygous a., a. homozigótica; a. grave causada pela herança de dois alelos de a., um de cada genitor; geralmente fatal no primeiro ano de vida.

achon·dro·plas·tic (ā-kon-drō-plas′tik). Acondroplásico; relativo à acondroplasia ou caracterizado por ela.

achor·da·te, achor·dal (ā-kōr′dāt, ā-kōr′dăl). Acordal; refere-se às formas animais inferiores ao filo Chordata, que não desenvolvem um notocórdio ou medula espinal.

acho·re·sis (ā-kō-rē′sis). Acorese; contração permanente de uma víscera oca, como o estômago ou a bexiga, reduzindo sua capacidade. [G. *a-* priv. + *chōreō*, dar lugar, fr. *chōros*, espaço]

Acho·ri·on (ā-kō′rē-on). Denominação antiga dos dermatófitos que hoje fazem parte do gênero *Trichophyton* ou *Microsporum*. [G. *achōr*, caspa]

achro·a·cyte (ā-krō′ā-sīt). Acroácito; uma célula incolor. [G. *a-* priv. + *chroa*, cor, + *kytos*, cavidade (célula)]

ach·ro·dex·trin (ak-rō-deks′trin). Acrodextrina. SIN achroodextrin. [G. *a-* priv. + *chroma*, cor, + dextrina]

achro·ma·cyte (ā-krō′mă-sīt). Acromócito. SIN achromocyte.

ach·ro·ma·sia (ak-rō-mā′sē-ă). Acromasia. **1.** Palidez associada a face hipocrática, emagrecimento e astenia, prenunciando com freqüência um estado moribundo. SIN cachectic pallor. 2. Acromia. SIN achromia. [G. *achrōmos*, incolor]

achro·mat (ā-krō′mat). Acromatope; pessoa que exibe acromatopsia. [G. *a-* priv. + *chroma*, cor]

ach·ro·mat·ic (ak-rō-mat′ik). Acromático. **1.** Incolor. **2.** Que não se cora prontamente. **3.** Refração da luz sem aberração cromática. [G. *a-* priv. + *chroma*, cor]

achro·ma·tin (ā-krō′mă-tin). Acromatina; componentes do núcleo que se coram fracamente, como a cariolinfa e a eucromatina.

achro·ma·tin·ic (ā-krō-mă-tin′ik). Acromatínico; que contém acromatina ou relativo a ela.

achro·ma·tism (ā-krō′mă-tizm). Acromatismo. **1.** Qualidade de ser acromático. **2.** Anulação da aberração cromática pela combinação de lentes com índices de refração e dispersão diferentes.

achro·mat·o·cyte (ā-krō-mat′ō-sīt). Acromatócito. SIN achromocyte.

achro·ma·tol·y·sis (ā-krō-mă-tol′i-sis). Acromatólise; dissolução da acromatina de uma célula ou de seu núcleo. SIN karyoplasmolysis.

achro·mat·o·phil (ā-krō-mat′ō-fil). Acromatófilo. **1.** Que não é colorido por corantes histológicos ou bacteriológicos. SIN achromophilic, achromophilous. **2.** Célula ou tecido que não pode ser corado de forma habitual. [G. *a-* priv. + *chroma*, cor, + *philos*, afinidade]

achro·mat·o·phil·ia (ā-krō′mat-ō-fil′ē-ă). Acromatofilia; condição de ser refratário aos processos de coloração.

achro·ma·top·sia, achro·ma·top·sy (ā-krō-mă-top′sē-ă, ā-krō′mă-top-sē) [MIM*216900]. Acromatopsia; esta é a forma completa de a., caracterizada por grave deficiência na percepção das cores, associada a nistagmo, fotofobia, acuidade visual reduzida e "cegueira diurna"; herança autossômica recessiva, causada por mutação no canal de cátion regulado por cGMP do fotorreceptor do cone, subunidade alfa do gene 3 (CNGA3) no cromossoma 2q. SIN achromatic vision, monochromasia, monochromasy, monochromatism (2). [G. *a-* priv. + *chroma*, cor, + *opsis*, visão]

atypical a., a. atípica; a. incompleta com acuidade visual normal sem nistagmo. Cf. dyschromatopsia.

complete a., a. completa; a. com ausência da visão em cores, nistagmo, acuidade visual reduzida e aversão à luz. SIN rod monochromatism, typical a.

incomplete a. [MIM*200930], a. incompleta; visão em cores comprometida mas não ausente, com acuidade visual menos gravemente reduzida que na a. completa, associada a fotofobia e nistagmo; herança autossômica recessiva. Existem uma forma autossômica dominante [MIM*180020] e várias formas ligadas ao X [MIM*304020, M1M*300085 e MIM*303700]

typical a., a. típica. SIN complete a.

achro·ma·to·sis (ā-krō-mă-tō′sis). Acromatose. SIN achromia. [G. *a-* priv. + *chroma*, cor]

achro·ma·tous (ā-krō′mă-tŭs). Acromatoso; incolor.

achro·ma·tu·ria (ā-krō-mă-too′rē-ă). Acromatúria; eliminação de urina incolor ou muito pálida. [G. *a-* priv. + *chroma*, cor, + *ouron*, urina]

achro·mia (ā-krō′mē-ă). Acromia. **1.** Hipopigmentação; ausência ou perda da pigmentação natural da pele e da íris; pode ser congênita ou adquirida. VER TAMBÉM depigmentation. **2.** Perda da capacidade de aceitar coloração nas células ou no tecido. SIN achromasia (2), achromatosis. [G. *a-* priv. + *chroma*, cor]

a. parasit'ica, a. parasítica; fase de diminuição ou ausência de pigmentação nas lesões cutâneas, causada pelo fungo *Malassezia furfur*. VER TAMBÉM *tinea versicolor*.

achro·mic (ā-krō′mik). Acrômico. Incolor.

Achromobacter (a′krō-mō-bak′ter). Gênero de bactérias Gram-negativas de importância clínica incerta, intimamente relacionadas com os membros da espécies de *Alcaligenes* e *Ochrobactrum*.

achro·mo·cyte (ā-krō′mō-sīt). Acromócito; eritrócito hipocrômico, em forma de crescente, que resulta provavelmente da ruptura (artefato) de uma hemácia com perda de hemoglobina. SIN achromacyte, achromatocyte, ghost corpuscle, phantom corpuscle, Ponfick shadow, shadow corpuscle, shadow (3), Traube corpuscle. [G. *a-* priv. + *chroma*, cor, + *kytos*, oco (célula)]

achro·mo·phil (ā-krō′mō-fil). Acromófilo. SIN achromatophil.

achro·mo·phil·ic, achro·moph·i·lous (ā-krō-mō-fil′ik, ā-krō-mof′ĭ-lŭs). Acromofílico, acromófilo. SIN achromatophil (1).

achro·mo·trich·ia (ā-krō-mō-trik′ē-ă). Acromotriquia; ausência ou perda do pigmento nos pêlos. VER TAMBÉM canities. [G. *a-* priv. + *chroma*, cor, + *thrix*, pêlos]

ach·ro·o·dex·trin (ak-rō′ō-deks′trin). Acroodextrina; dextrina de baixo peso molecular, formada a partir do amido em um estágio da sua digestão pela amilase; não apresenta reação colorida com o iodo. Cf. amylodextrin, erythrodextrin. SIN achrodextrin. [G. *achrōmos*, sem cor, + dextrina]

achy·lia (ā-kī′lē-ă). Aquilia. **1.** Ausência de suco gástrico ou outras secreções gástricas. **2.** Ausência de quilo. [G. *a-* priv. + *chylos*, suco]
  a. gas′trica, a. gástrica; secreção diminuída ou ausente de suco gástrico associada a atrofia da mucosa gástrica.
  a. pancreat'ica, a. pancreática; deficiência ou ausência de secreção pancreática, em geral resultando em esteatorréia, emagrecimento e desnutrição.
achy·lous (ā-kī-lŭs). **1.** Sem suco gástrico ou outras secreções digestivas. **2.** Que não possui quilo. [G. *achylos*, sem suco]
acic·u·lar (ā-sik′ū-lar). Acicular; em forma ou com ponta de agulha; aplicado principalmente a folhas e cristais. [L. *acicular*, pequeno alfinete]
ac·id (as′id). Ácido. **1.** Composto que libera um íon hidrogênio em um solvente polar (p.ex., na água); os ácidos formam sais substituindo todo o hidrogênio ionizável ou parte dele por um elemento ou radical eletropositivo. **2.** Na linguagem popular, qualquer composto químico que possui gosto acre (dado pelo íon hidrogênio). **3.** Acre; picante ao paladar. **4.** Relativo a um a.; que origina uma reação a. Para os ácidos individuais, Ver os nomes específicos. [L. *acidus*, acre]
  bile a.'s, ácidos biliares; ácidos esteróides encontrados na bile; p.ex., ácidos taurocólico e glicocólico, usados terapeuticamente quando a secreção biliar é inadequada e para os casos de cólica biliar. Suas funções fisiológicas incluem a emulsificação da gordura. Sua síntese está reduzida nos distúrbios dos peroxissomas.
  Bronsted a., a. de Bronsted; um a. que é doador de prótons.
  conjugate a., a. conjugado; o composto com prótons de dois compostos que diferem em estrutura apenas pela presença do próton lábil.
  dibasic a., a. dibásico; um a. que contém dois átomos de hidrogênio ionizáveis na molécula. VER acid (1).
  fatty a., ácido graxo; VER fatty acid.
  inorganic a., a. inorgânico; um a. constituído de moléculas que não contêm radicais orgânicos; p.ex., HCl, H_2SO_4, H_3PO_4.
  Lewis a., a. de Lewis; a. que é aceptor de um par de elétrons.
  monobasic a., a. monobásico; a. que contém um átomo ionizável de hidrogênio na molécula. VER acid (1).
  organic a., a. orgânico; a. formado por moléculas que contêm radicais orgânicos; p.ex., a. acético, a. cítrico, que contém o grupamento –COOH ionizável.
  polybasic a., a. polibásico; a. que contém mais de três átomos ionizáveis de hidrogênio na molécula. VER acid (1).
  wax a., a. monocarboxílico de cadeia longa, com número par de carbonos, em geral encontrado esterificado nas ceras (p.ex., ácido láurico).
ac·id-cit·rate-dex·trose (ACD). Ácido-citrato-dextrose; anticoagulante citrato usado para o armazenamento e a preservação do sangue total. Tem sido amplamente substituído por anticoagulantes mais modernos (CPD, Adsol) que permitem conservação mais prolongada do sangue e dos hemoderivados.
ac·i·de·mia (as-i-dē′mē-ă). Acidemia; aumento na concentração dos íons H do sangue ou uma queda no pH abaixo do normal. Tipos individuais de a. são arrolados por nomes específicos, p. ex., isovalericacidemia (isovalericacidemia), aminoacidemia, etc. [ácido + G. *haima*, sangue]
ac·id-fast (as′id-fast). Álcool-ácido-resistente; indica as bactérias que não são descoloridas por ácido-álcool após terem sido coradas por corantes como a fucsina básica; p.ex., as micobactérias e *Nocardia*.
acid·i·fy (a-sid′i-fī). Acidificar. **1.** Tornar ácido. **2.** Converter em ácido.
acid·i·ty (a-sid′i-tē). Acidez. **1.** Qualidade de ser ácido. **2.** O conteúdo ácido de um líquido.
  total a. (a), a. total; expressão obsoleta que denota o a. gástrico, a acidez sendo determinada com titulação com hidróxido de sódio, usando-se fenolftaleína como indicador.
ac·i·do·phil, ac·i·do·phile (ā-sid′ō-fil, ā-sid′ō-fīl). Acidófilo. **1.** Uma das células coradas por ácido da hipófise anterior (adeno-hipófise). **2.** Um microrganismo que cresce bem em um meio muito ácido. [ácido + G. *philos*, afinidade]
ac·i·do·phil·ic (as′i-dō-fil′ik, ā-sid′ō-fil-ik). Acidofílico; que tem afinidade por corantes ácidos; indica uma célula ou elemento tecidual que se cora por um corante ácido, como eosina. SIN oxychromatic.
ac·i·do·sis (as-i-dō′sis). Acidose; estado anormal caracterizado por aumento da concentração de íons hidrogênio no sangue arterial acima do nível normal, 40 nmol/L, ou pH 7,4; pode ser causada por acúmulo de dióxido de carbono ou produtos ácidos do metabolismo, ou por diminuição na concentração de compostos alcalinos. [ácido + G. *-osis*, condição]
  carbon dioxide a., a. respiratória. SIN respiratory a.
  compensated a., a. compensada; a. na qual o pH dos líquidos corporais é normal; a compensação é alcançada por mecanismos respiratórios ou renais.
  compensated respiratory a., a. respiratória compensada; retenção de bicarbonato pelos túbulos renais para minimizar o efeito da retenção de dióxido de carbono pelos pulmões sobre o pH do sangue, como ocorre na hiperventilação.
  diabetic a., a. diabética; tipo de a. metabólica causada pelo acúmulo de corpos cetônicos no diabetes melito.
  hypercapnic a., a. respiratória. SIN respiratory a.
  hyperchloremic a., a. hiperclorêmica. SIN renal tubular a.
  lactic a., a. láctica; tipo de a. metabólica causada pelo acúmulo de ácido láctico devido a hipóxia tecidual, efeito de medicamento ou etiologia desconhecida.
  metabolic a., a. metabólica; pH e concentração de bicarbonato diminuídos nos líquidos corporais por causa do acúmulo de ácidos ou de perdas anormais de bases fixas do corpo, como na diarréia ou na doença renal.
  primary renal tubular a., a. tubular renal primária; defeito metabólico no mecanismo de acidificação urinária que pode ser tanto do tipo transitório, com início no primeiro ano de vida, quanto do tipo persistente, com surgimento na criança ou no adulto; os dois tipos são familiares.
  renal tubular a., a. tubular renal; uma síndrome clínica caracterizada por diminuição da capacidade de acidificar a urina e por concentrações plasmáticas baixas de bicarbonato e altas de cloreto, freqüentemente com hipopotassemia; costuma ser complicada por osteomalacia, nefrocalcinose ou cálculos renais. VER TAMBÉM primary renal tubular a., secondary renal tubular a. SIN hyperchloremic a.
  respiratory a., a. respiratória; a. causada por retenção de dióxido de carbono; deve-se a ventilação pulmonar inadequada ou hipoventilação, com diminuição do pH sanguíneo, a menos que compensada por retenção renal de bicarbonato. SIN carbon dioxide a., hypercapnic a.
  secondary renal tubular a., a. renal tubular secundária; a. tubular renal que pode ocorrer como uma complicação de estados hipercalcêmicos, distúrbios hiperglobulinêmicos e em algumas outras doenças renais crônicas; um componente regular da síndrome de De Toni-Fanconi.
  starvation a., a. por inanição; cetoacidose, resultante da falta de ingestão de alimentos, o que leva ao catabolismo das gorduras a fim de fornecer energia, liberando corpos cetônicos ácidos.
  uncompensated a., a. não-compensada; a. na qual o pH dos líquidos do corpo está abaixo do normal, porque a restauração do equilíbrio ácido-básico normal não é possível ou ainda não foi atingida.
ac·i·dot·ic (as-i-dot′ik). Acidótico; pertencente à acidose ou que a indica.
ac·id red 87. Vermelho ácido 87. SIN eosin y.
ac·id red 91. SIN eosin B.
ac·i·du·ria (as-i-doo′rē-ă). Acidúria. **1.** Excreção de urina ácida. **2.** Excreção de uma quantidade anormal de qualquer ácido especificado. Os tipos individuais de a. têm como prefixo o ácido específico; p.ex., aminoacidúria, cetoacidúria. [ácido + G. *ouron*, urina]
  argininosuccinic a. [MIM*207900], a. argininossuccínica; distúrbio autossômico recessivo caracterizado por excreção urinária excessiva de ácido argininossuccínico, epilepsia, ataxia, retardo mental, doença hepática e cabelos quebradiços e em tufo; presume-se que seja conseqüência da deficiência de uma enzima responsável pela degradação do ácido argininossuccínico em arginina e ácido fumárico. SIN arginosuccinate lyase deficiency.
ac·i·du·ric (as-i-doo′rik). Acidúrico; pertencente às bactérias que toleram um ambiente ácido. [ácido + L. *duro*, resistir]
ac·i·nar (as′i-nar). Acinar; que pertence ao ácino. SIN acinic.
Ac·i·ne·to·bac·ter (as-i-nē′tō-bak′ter). Gênero de bactérias imóveis, aeróbicas (família Moraxellaceae), que contém cocóides ou bastonetes pequenos Gram-negativos ou Gram-variáveis, ou cocos, freqüentemente em pares; não produzem esporos. Essas bactérias crescem em meios comuns, sem a adição de soro. São oxidase-negativas e catalase-positivas; os carboidratos são oxidados ou não são atacados, e arginina diidrolase não é produzida. São uma causa freqüente de infecções nosocomiais; geralmente resistentes a muitos antibióticos, elas podem causar também graves infecções primárias em pessoas imunocomprometidas. A espécie típica é *A. calcoaceticus*. SIN *Lingelsheimia*.
  A. calcoacet'icus, espécie de bactérias encontradas originalmente em meio enriquecido com quinato; cepas desse microrganismo antes identificado como *Bacterium anitratum* foram encontradas no trato genitourinário; é a espécie típica do gênero *A.* SIN *Lingelsheimia anitrata*.
ac·i·ni (as′i-nī). Ácinos; plural de acinus.
acin·ic (a-sin′ik). Acinar. SIN acinar.
acin·i·form (a-sin′i-fōrm). Aciniforme, acinoso. SIN acinous. [L. *acinus*, uva, + *forma*]
ac·i·nose (as′i-nōs). Acinoso. SIN acinous.
ac·i·nous (as′i-nŭs). Acinoso; que lembra um ácino ou uma estrutura em forma de uva. SIN aciniform, acinose.
ac·i·nus. gen. e pl. **ac·i·ni** (as′i-nŭs, -nī). Ácino; uma das diminutas porções secretoras de uma glândula acinar, em forma de uva. Alguns especialistas utilizam os termos ácino e alvéolo como sinônimos enquanto outros os diferenciam pelas aberturas reduzidas do ácino no duto excretor. [L. *bago*, uva]
  liver a., a. hepático; unidade funcional do fígado, que compreende todo o parênquima hepático suprido por um ramo terminal da veia porta e artéria hepática; tipicamente envolve os segmentos de dois lóbulos que ocorrem entre duas vênulas hepáticas terminais. SIN Rappaport a.
  pulmonary a., a. pulmonar; a parte das vias respiratórias que consiste em um bronquíolo respiratório e todos os seus ramos. SIN primary pulmonary lobule, respiratory lobule.
  Rappaport a., a. de Rappaport. SIN liver a.

a·clas·ia (ă-klā′zē-ă). Áclase. SIN aclasis.

ac·la·sis (ak′lă-sis). Áclase; estado de continuidade entre o tecido normal e o anormal. SIN aclasia. [G. *a-* priv. + *klasis*, rompimento, um fragmento]

tarsoepiphyseal a. (tār′-sō-ep′ī-fiz′e-al), a. tarsoepifisária; hemimelia epifisária; afeta tornozelos e joelhos, levando à limitação do movimento. SIN Trevor, disease.

ac·me (ak′mē). Acme, clímax, apogeu; período de maior intensidade de qualquer sinal, sintoma ou processo. [G. *akmē*, o ponto mais alto]

ac·ne (ak′nē). Acne; erupção inflamatória folicular, papular e pustular que envolve o aparelho pilossebáceo. VER TAMBÉM a. vulgaris. [provavelmente uma corruptela (ou erro de reprodução) do G. *akmē*, ponto de eflorescência]

a. artificia′lis, a. artificial; a. produzida por agentes irritantes externos, como alcatrão (**clor**oacne), ou medicamentos administrados para uso interno, como **iodetos** ou brometos. SIN a. venenata.

bromide a., a. por brometo, a. brômica; erupção folicular na face, tronco e membros devido à ingestão de brometo. VER TAMBÉM bromoderma.

a. cachectico′rum, a. da caquexia; que ocorre em pessoas que sofrem de uma doença sistêmica debilitante; caracterizada por lesões grandes, purulentas, ulcerativas, císticas e fibróticas.

a. cilia′ris, a. ciliar; pápulas e pústulas foliculares presentes nas bordas livres das pálpebras.

a. congloba′ta, a. conglobada; a. cística grave, caracterizada por lesões císticas, abscessos, seios comunicantes e cicatrizes espessas e nodulares; em geral poupando a face.

a. cosmet′ica, a. cosmética; lesões acneicas discretas, não-inflamatórias, decorrentes da aplicação repetida de agentes comedogênicos presentes em cosméticos.

cystic a., a. cística; a. grave na qual as lesões predominantes são cistos foliculares que se rompem e formam cicatrizes.

a. fulminans (ak′nē ful′mi-nanz), a. fulminante; a. grave e que forma cicatriz, associada a febre, poliartralgia, lesões ulcerativas crostosas, perda de peso e anemia. [*fulmen, fulminis*, trovão, raio]

a. genera′lis, lesões acneicas que envolvem a face, o tórax e o dorso.

halogen a., a. halogênica; erupção acneiforme causada por brometos ou iodetos.

a. hypertroph′ica, a. hipertrófica; a. vulgar na qual as lesões, ao cicatrizarem, deixam cicatrizes hipertróficas.

iodide a., a. por iodeto, a. iódica; erupção folicular na face, no tronco e nos membros, devido a injeção ou ingestão de iodetos por uma pessoa hipersensível. VER TAMBÉM iododerma.

a. medicamento′sa, a. causada ou exacerbada por fármacos, como, p.ex., lítio, halógenos ou esteróides.

a. necrotica miliaris, a. necrótica miliar. SIN a. varioliformis.

a. neonato′rum, a. neonatal; condição em recém-nascidos do sexo masculino, caracterizada por pápulas, pústulas e comedões na testa e nas bochechas, que em geral desaparece em alguns meses.

pomade a., a. por pomadas; forma de a. causada pela aplicação repetida de cremes capilares contendo óleos que bloqueiam a liberação de sebo pelos folículos pilosos; observada mais comumente na testa e têmporas de jovens afro-americanos.

a. puncta′ta, a. pontilhada; a. com comedões pretos abertos.

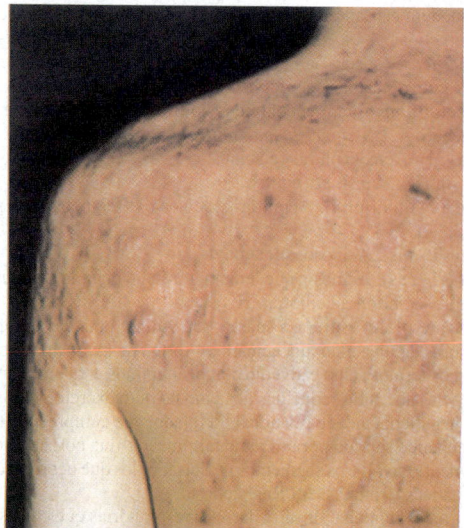

acne conglobada

a. pustulo′sa, a. vulgar na qual predominam as lesões pustulares.

a. rosa′cea, a. rosácea. SIN rosacea.

steroid a., a. por esteróides; foliculite ou hiperqueratose folicular resultante da administração tópica ou oral de esteróides.

tar a., a. por alcatrão. SIN chloracne.

tropical a., a. tropical; tipo grave de a. que acomete todo o tronco, os ombros, os braços, as nádegas e as coxas; ocorre em climas quentes e úmidos.

a. variolifor′mis, a. varioliforme; infecção piogênica envolvendo os folículos e que ocorre principalmente na testa e nas têmporas; a involução das lesões umbilicadas e crostosas é seguida pela formação de cicatrizes. SIN a. necrotica miliaris.

a. venena′ta, a. artificial SIN a. artificialis.

a. vulga′ris, a. vulgar; erupção, predominantemente da face, porção superior do dorso e tórax, composta de comedões, cistos, pápulas e pústulas de base inflamatória; a condição ocorre na maioria de pessoas durante a puberdade e a adolescência, devido ao estímulo androgênico da secreção de sebo, com entupimento dos folículos pela queratinização, associada à proliferação de *Propionibacterium acnes*. A supuração folicular pode levar à formação de cicatriz. Os tratamentos tópicos incluem tretinoína, peróxido de benzoíla e antibióticos. À luz do sol, os antibióticos sistêmicos e o ácido retinóico 13-*cis* por via oral (exceto na gravidez) são também efetivos. VER TAMBÉM acne.

ac·ne·form (ak′nē-form). Acneiforme; que lembra a acne. SIN acneiform.

ac·ne·i·form (ak-nē′i-form). Acneiforme. SIN acneform.

ac·ne·mia, ak·ne·mia (ak-nē′mē-ă). Acnemia. 1. Ausência congênita das pernas. 2. Atrofia dos músculos das panturrilhas. [G. *a-* priv. + *knēmē*, perna]

ACNM. Abreviatura de *American College of Nuclear Medicine* (*Colégio Americano de Medicina Nuclear*).

ACNP. Abreviatura de *American College of Nuclear Physicians* (*Colégio Americano de Especialistas em Medicina Nuclear*).

ac·o·kan·thera (ak′-ō-kan′ther-ă). Acocantera; suco das folhas e do caule da *Acokanthera ouabaio* (família Apocynaceae); veneno das pontas das setas sul-africanas que contêm ouabaína. [G. *akōkē*, um ponto, + *antheros*, floração]

ac·o·lous (ak′ō-lŭs). Ácolo, que não tem os membros. [G. *a-* priv. + *kōlon*, extremidade]

acon·i·tase (ă-kon′i-tās). Aconitase. SIN aconitate hydratase.

acon·i·tate hy·dra·tase (ă-kon′i-tāt). Aconitato hidratase; uma enzima contendo ferro que catalisa a desidratação do ácido cítrico em ácido *cis*-aconítico, uma reação importante no ciclo do ácido tricarboxílico. SIN aconitase.

ac·o·nite (ak′ō-nīt). Acônito; a raiz seca da *Aconitun napellus* (família Ranunculaceae); um veneno potente e de ação rápida usado outrora como antipirético, diurético, diaforético, anódino, depressor cardíaco e respiratório e, externamente, como analgésico.

***cis*-ac·o·nit·ic ac·id** (ak-ō-nit′ik). Ácido *cis*-aconítico; produto da desidratação do ácido cítrico; um intermediário ligado a enzima no ciclo do ácido tricarboxílico.

acon·i·tine (ă-kon′i-tēn). Aconitina; princípio ativo extremamente venenoso (alcalóide dipertênico) da *Aconitum* sp. e *Delphinium* sp., usado outrora como sedativo cardíaco e aplicado externamente para neuralgia.

aco·rea (ă-kō′rē-ă). Acoréia, acoria; ausência congênita da pupila dos olhos. [G. *a-* priv. + *korē*, pupila]

Acosta, Joseph (José) de, missionário jesuíta espanhol, 1539–1600. VER A. disease.

acous·tic (ă-koos′tik). Acústico; relacionado ao som, p.ex., meato acústico, nervo acústico. [Gr. *akoustikos*]

acous·ti·co·pho·bia (ă-koos′ti-kō-fō′bē-ă). Acusticofobia; medo mórbido dos sons. [G. *akoustikos*, acústico, + *phobos*, medo]

acous·tics (ă-koos′tiks). Acústica; a ciência relativa aos sons. [G. *akoustikos*, relativo aos sons]

ACP Abreviatura de acyl carrier *protein* (proteína carreadora de acil); *American College of Physicians* (*Colégio Americano de Medicina*).

ACP-ace·tyl·trans·fer·ase. ACP-acetiltransferase; enzima que transfere acetil da acetil-CoA para a ACP e libera CoA para iniciar a síntese de ácidos graxos. SIN acetyl transacylase.

ACP-mal·o·nyl·trans·fer·ase. ACP-maloniltransferase; enzima que transfere malonil da malonil-CoA para ACP e libera CoA livre; uma etapa fundamental da síntese de ácidos graxos. SIN malonyl transacylase.

ACPS abreviatura de acrocephalosyndactyly (acrocefalossindactilia).

ac·quired (ă-kwīrd′). Adquirido; indica uma doença, predisposição ou anormalidade que não é herdada. [L. *ac-quiro* (*adq-*), obter, de *quaero*, procurar]

ac·qui·si·tion (ak-wi-zish′ŭn). Aquisição; em psicologia, a demonstração empírica de aumento da força da resposta condicionada em testes sucessivos de pareamento dos estímulos condicionados e não-condicionados.

gradient-recalled a. in the steady state, um tipo de seqüência gradiente–eco com amostragem de decaimento na ressonância magnética; também chamada de "aquisição de imagens rápida com precessão em equilíbrio dinâmico". Essa família de seqüências é mais rápida do que as técnicas spin–eco, sendo usada para angiorressonância magnética e técnicas de aquisição de imagens cardíacas.

ACR abreviatura de *American College of Radiology* (*Colégio Americano de Radiologia*).

ac·ral (ak′răl). Acral; relativo às partes periféricas ou que as afeta, p.ex., membros, dedos das mãos, ouvidos, etc. [G. *akron*, extremidade]

Acra·nia (ā-krā′nē-ă). Acraniotas; grupo do filo Chordata cujos membros possuem notocórdio, brânquias e medula espinal, mas sem vértebras, costelas ou crânio; p.ex., *Amphioxus*, tunicados e cefalocordados. [G. *a-* priv. + *kranion*, crânio]

acra·nia (ā-krā′nē-ă). Acrania; ausência completa ou parcial do crânio; associada a anencefalia. [G. *a-* priv. + *kranion*, crânio]

acra·ni·al (ā-krā′nē-ăl). Acranial, acrânio; que não tem crânio; relativo à acrania ou um acrânio.

acra·ni·us. Acrânio, acrânico, acranial; feto malformado que exibe acrania.

Acrel, Olaf, cirurgião sueco, 1717–1806. VER *A. ganglion*.

Ac·re·mo·ni·um (ak-rĕ-mō′nē-ŭm). Gênero de fungos (família Moniliaceae, ordem Moniliales) que causa micetoma eumicótico; três espécies, *A. falciforme*, *A. kiliense* e *A. recifei*, produzem grãos amarelo-esbranquiçados nos tecidos. Provoca ceratomicose e, ocasionalmente, outras infecções, além de produzir o antibiótico cefalosporina.

ac·ri·bom·e·ter (ak-ri-bom′e-ter). Acribômetro; um instrumento para medir objetos muito pequenos. [G. *akribēs*, exato, + *metron*, medida]

ac·rid (ak′rid). Acre, picante, pungente ou irritante. [L. *acer* (*acr-*), pungente]

ac·ri·dine (ak′ri-dēn). Acridina; 10-Azantraceno; um corante, intermediário de um corante e precursor anti-séptico (9-aminoacridina, acriflavina, hemissulfato de proflavina) derivado do alcatrão de hulha e irritante à pele e às mucosas. SIN dibenzopyridine.

tetramethyl a., tetrametil acridina. SIN acridine orange.

ac·ri·dine or·ange [C.I. 46005]. Laranja acridina; cloridrato de 3,6-bis(dimetilamino)acridina; um corante fluorescente básico útil como marcador metacromático para ácidos nucleicos; usado também no rastreamento de esfregaços cervicais para células anormais e malignas, onde as quantidades incomuns de DNA e RNA ocorrem durante a proliferação e nos tumores (o DNA fluoresce de amarelo a verde; o RNA fluoresce de laranja a vermelho). SIN tetrametyl acridine.

ac·ri·dine yel·low. Amarelo acridina; solução amarelo-pálida com forte fluorescência violeta-azulado; usada como anti-séptico tópico e como um corante fluorescente em histologia. SIN 5-aminoacridine, hydrochloride, 9-aminoacridine hydrochloride.

ac·ri·fla·vine (ak-ri-flā′vin) [C.I. 46000]. Acriflavina; um corante acridina, uma mistura de cloreto de 3,6-diamino-10-metilacridínio e 3,6-diaminoacridina; usada outrora como anti-séptico tópico e urinário, sendo utilizada como um dos reagentes fluorescentes de Kasten Schiff para revelar polissacarídeos e DNA.

ac·ri·mo·nia (ak-ri-mō′nē-ă). Acrimonia; na patologia humoral antiga, um humor ácido, pungente, que provoca doenças. [L. pungência]

ac·ri·mo·ny (ak′ri-mo-nē). Acrimônia; a qualidade de ser intensamente irritante, mordaz ou pungente. [L. *acrimonia*, pungência]

ac·ri·nol (ak′ri-nol). Lactato de etacridina. SIN ethacridine lactate.

ac·ri·sor·cin (ak-ri-sōr′sin). Acrisorcina; um agente antifúngico tópico sintético.

acrit·i·cal (ā-krit′i-kăl, ā-). Acrítico; termo raramente empregado para: 1. Não-crítico; marcado pela ausência de crise; indica doenças que terminam por lise. 2. Prognóstico indeterminado, especialmente preocupante. [G. *a-* priv. + *kritikos*, crítico]

△ **acro-.** Forma combinante que significa: 1. Extremidade, ponta, final, pico, topo. 2. Extremo. [G. *akron*, ponto mais alto, extremidade; *akros*, posição mais ao topo, mais externa, mais interna, extrema, ponta]

ac·ro·ag·no·sis (ak′rō-ag-nō′sis). Acroagnose; perda e incapacidade de reconhecimento semi-sensorial de uma extremidade. Ausência de acrognosia.

ac·ro·an·es·the·sia (ak′rō-an-es-thē′zē-ă). Acroanestesia; anestesia de um ou mais membros. [acro- + G. *an-* priv. + *aisthēsis*, sensação]

ac·ro·ar·thri·tis (ak′rō-arth-rī′tis). Acroartrite; inflamação das articulações das mãos ou dos pés. [acro- + G. *arthron*, articulação, + *-itis*]

ac·ro·as·phyx·ia (ak′rō-as-fik′sē-ă). Acroasfixia; comprometimento da circulação digital, possivelmente uma forma leve de doença de Raynaud, marcada por uma coloração púrpura ou branco-cérea dos dedos das mãos, com temperatura local subnormal e parestesia. SIN dead fingers, waxy fingers. [acro- + G. *asphyxia*, interrupção do pulso]

ac·ro·a·tax·ia (ak′rō-ă-tak′sē-ă). Acroataxia; ataxia que afeta a porção distal dos membros, isto é, mãos e dedos das mãos, pés e artelhos. Cf. proximoataxia. [acro- + ataxia]

ac·ro·blast (ak′rō-blast). Acroblasto; componente da espermátide em desenvolvimento, composto de numerosos elementos de Golgi; contém os grânulos proacrossômicos. [acro- + G. *blastos*, germe]

ac·ro·brach·y·ceph·a·ly (ak′rō-brak-i-sef′ă-lē). Acrobraquicefalia; tipo de craniossinostose com fechamento prematuro da sutura coronal, resultando em diâmetro ântero-posterior anormalmente pequeno do crânio. [acro- + G. *brachys*, pequeno, + *kephalē*, cabeça]

ac·ro·cen·tric (ak-rō-sen′trik). Acrocêntrico; que tem o centrômero perto de uma extremidade; diz-se dos cromossomas normais 13–15 e 21–22. [acro- + G. *kentron*, centro]

ac·ro·ce·pha·lia (ak-rō-se-fā′lē-ă). Acrocefalia. SIN oxycephaly.

ac·ro·ce·phal·ic (ak-rō-se-fal′ik). Acrocefálico. SIN oxycephalic.

ac·ro·ceph·a·lo·pol·y·syn·dac·ty·ly (ak′rō-sef′ă-lō-pol′ē-sin-dak′ti-lē). Acrocefalopolissindactilia; grupo de síndromes congênitas caracterizadas por um formato anormal do crânio devido à craniossinostose, braquidactilia, sindactilia e polidactilia pré-axial das mãos e/ou pés; retardo mental é uma característica variável. Existem várias síndromes autossômicas recessivas [MIM*201000, MIM*201020 e MIM*272350] e uma forma autossômica dominante [MIM*101600]. Uma classificação antiga de a., tipos I a IV, é hoje considerada obsoleta.

ac·ro·ceph·a·lo·syn·dac·ty·ly (ACPS) (ak′rō-sef′ă-lō-sin-dak′ti-lē). Acrocefalossindactilia; grupo de síndromes congênitas caracterizadas por craniossinostoses com formato anormal do crânio e sindactilia cutânea e/ou óssea. Existem vários tipos, sendo a maioria herdada como autossômica dominante. Os fenótipos dos tipos II e IV não são bem definidos. [acrocefalia+ G. *syn*, junto, + *daktylos*, dedo da mão]

type I a., a. tipo I. SIN Apert *syndrome*.
type II a., a. tipo II. SIN Vogt cephalodactyly.
type III a., a. tipo III. SIN Saethre-Chotzen *syndrome*.
type V a., a. tipo V. SIN Pfeiffer *syndrome*.

ac·ro·ceph·a·lous (ak-rō-sef′ă-lŭs). Acrocéfalo. SIN oxycephalic.

ac·ro·ceph·a·ly (ak′rō-sef′ă-lē). Acrocefalia. SIN oxycephaly. [acro- + G. *kephalē*, cérebro]

ac·ro·chor·don (ak-rō-kōr′don). Acrocórdone. SIN skin *tag*. [acro- + G. *chordē*, corda]

ac·ro·ci·ne·sia, ac·ro·ci·ne·sis (ak′rō-si-nē′zē-ă, -ē′sis). Acrocinesia, acrocinese; movimento excessivo. SIN acrokinesia. [acro- + G. *kinēsis*, movimento]

ac·ro·con·trac·ture (ak′rō-kon-trak′choor). Acrocontratura; contratura das articulações das mãos ou pés.

ac·ro·cy·a·no·sis (ak′rō-sī-ă-nō′sis). Acrocianose; distúrbio circulatório no qual as mãos e, menos comumente, os pés ficam persistentemente frios e cianóticos; algumas formas são relacionadas ao fenômeno de Raynaud. SIN Crocq disease, Raynaud sign. [acro- + G. *kyanos*, azul, + *-osis*, condição]

ac·ro·cy·a·not·ic (ak′rō-sī-ă-not′ik). Acrocianótico; caracterizado por acrocianose.

ac·ro·der·ma·ti·tis (ak′rō-der-mă-tī′tis). Acrodermatite; inflamação da pele dos membros. [*acro-* + G. *derma*, pele, + *-itis*, inflamação]

ℹ **a. chron′ica atroph′icans,** a. atrófica crônica; manifestação cutânea tardia, gradativamente progressiva, da doença de Lyme, surgindo primeiro nos pés, mãos, cotovelos ou joelhos, e composta por placas eritematosas e induradas, que se tornam atróficas, originando uma aparência de papel de seda dos locais envolvidos.

a. contin′ua, a. contínua. SIN pustulosis palmaris et plantaris.

a. enteropath′ica [MIM*201100], a. enteropática; defeito hereditário progressivo do metabolismo do zinco em crianças pequenas (início 3 semanas a 18 meses de vida), manifestando-se, geralmente, primeiro como uma erupção bolhosa, exsudativa e crostosa em um membro ou ao redor de um dos orifícios do corpo, seguida de queda dos cabelos e diarréia ou outros distúrbios gastrointestinais; aliviada pela suplementação oral de zinco durante toda a vida; traço autossômico recessivo.

papular a. of childhood, a. papular da infância. SIN Gianotti-Crosti *syndrome*.
a. per′stans, a. persistente. SIN pustulosis palmaris et plantaris.

ac·ro·der·ma·to·sis (ak′rō-der-mă-tō′sis). Acrodermatose; qualquer afecção cutânea que envolva as porções mais distais dos membros. [acro- + G. *derma*, pele, + *-osis*, condição]

ac·ro·dont (ak-rō-dont). Acrodontia; fixação dentária em alguns vertebrados inferiores (principalmente peixes) nos quais os dentes se formam na borda do osso da mandíbula e não nos alvéolos. [acro- + G. *odous*, dente]

ac·ro·dyn·ia (ak-rō-din′ē-ă). Acrodinia. 1. Dor nas partes periféricas ou acrais do corpo. 2. Uma síndrome causada, quase exclusivamente no passado, pela intoxicação por mercúrio; em crianças, caracterizada por eritema dos membros, do tórax e do nariz, sintomas gastrointestinais e por polineurite (no Japão); nos adultos, caracterizada por anorexia, fotofobia, sudorese e taquicardia. SIN acrodynic erythema, dermatopolyneuritis, erythredema, Feer disease, pink disease. [acro- + G. *odynē*, dor]

ac·ro·dys·es·the·sia (ak′rō-dis-es-thē′zē-ă). Acrodisestesia; sensações anormais e desagradáveis nas porções periféricas dos membros. [acro- + disestesia]

ac·ro·dys·os·to·sis (ak′rō-dis-os-tō′sis) [MIM*101800]. Acrodisostose; distúrbio no qual as mãos e os pés são pequenos, com dedos curtos. O retardo do crescimento é progressivo. Retardo mental e hipoplasia nasal acentuada também ocorrem; herança autossômica dominante. [acro- + disostose]

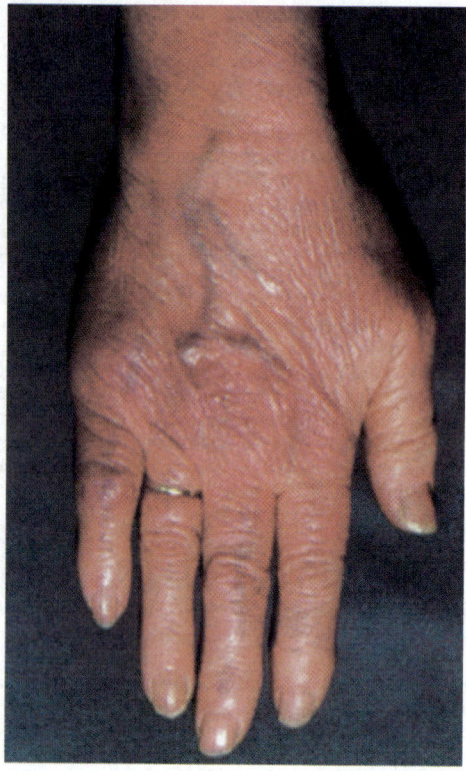

acrodermatite atrófica crônica

ac·ro·es·the·sia (ak′ro-es-the′ze-ă). Acroestesia. **1.** Grau extremo de hiperestesia. **2.** Hiperestesia de um ou mais membros. [acro- + G. *aisthēsis*, sensação]

acrog·e·nous (ak-roj′e-nŭs). Acrógeno; indica conídeos ou fungos produzidos pela célula conidiogênica na ponta de um conidióforo. [acro- + G. *genos*, nascimento]

ac·ro·ger·ia (ak-ro-jēr′e-ă) [MIM*201200]. Acrogeria; redução ou perda da gordura subcutânea e do colágeno das mãos e dos pés, dando a aparência de envelhecimento prematuro. [acro- + G. *gerōn*, velho]

ac·rog·no·sis (ak-rog-nō′sis). Acrognose; cenestesia ou percepção sensorial normal dos membros. [acro- + G. *gnōsis*, conhecimento]

ac·ro·hy·per·hi·dro·sis (ak′ro-hī′per-hi-drō′sis). Acro-hiperidrose; hiperidrose das mãos e dos pés.

acrohyperkeratosis. Acro-hiperceratose.
  focal acrohyperkeratosis, acro-hiperceratose focal. SIN acrokeratoelastoidosis.

ac·ro·ker·a·to·e·las·toi·do·sis (ak′ro-ker′a-tō-ē-las-toy-dō′sis) [MIM*101850]. Acroceratoelastoidose; ceratose papular autossômica dominante das regiões palmares e plantares, com desorganização das fibras elásticas dermais; uma condição semelhante, porém adquirida, pode resultar da lesão actínica das mãos. VER TAMBÉM keratoelastoidosis. SIN focal acrohyperkeratosis, type III punctate palmoplantar keratoderma. [acro- + G. *keras*, chifre, + *elastos*, batido, + *eidos*, semelhança, + -*ōsis*, condição]

ac·ro·ker·a·to·sis (ak′ro-ker-a-tō′sis). Acroceratose; crescimento excessivo da camada espinhosa da pele, geralmente configurações nodulares, do dorso dos dedos das mãos e dos pés, e ocasionalmente na borda da orelha e na ponta do nariz. [acro- + G. *keras*, chifre, + -*osis*, condição]
  paraneoplastic a., a. paraneoplásica; uma rara distrofia ungueal com eritema acral e descamação, associada a câncer do trato respiratório superior ou do trato alimentar alto. SIN Bazex syndrome.

ac·ro·ki·ne·sia (ak′ro-ki-ne′ze-ă). Acrocinesia. SIN acrocinesia.

ac·ro·meg·a·lia (ak-ro-mē-gā′le-ă). Acromegalia. SIN acromegaly.

ac·ro·me·gal·ic (ak-ro-mē-gal′ik). Acromegálico; relacionado à acromegalia ou caracterizado por ela.

ac·ro·meg·a·lo·gi·gan·tism (ak′ro-meg′a-lō-jī′gan-tizm). Acromegalogigantismo; gigantismo no qual as características faciais, o aumento desproporcional dos membros e outros sinais e sintomas da acromegalia são proeminentes. [acro- + G. *megas*, grande, + *gigas*, gigante]

ac·ro·meg·a·loid·ism (ak-ro-meg′a-loyd-izm). Acromegaloidismo; termo raramente empregado para uma condição na qual as proporções corporais lembram as da acromegalia.

ac·ro·meg·a·ly (ak-ro-meg′a-le). Acromegalia; distúrbio caracterizado pelo aumento progressivo das partes periféricas do corpo, principalmente a cabeça, a face, as mãos e os pés, devido à secreção excessiva de somatotropina; ocorrem organomegalia e distúrbios metabólicos; os pacientes podem apresentar diabetes melito. SIN acromegalia. [acro- + G. *megas*, grande]

ac·ro·mel·al·gia (ak-ro-mel-al′je-ă). Acromelalgia. VER erythromelalgia. [acro- + G. *melos*, membro, + *algos*, dor]

acromelia (ak-ro-mē′le-ă). Acromelia. SIN acromesomelia.

ac·ro·mel·ic (ak-ro-mel′ik). Acromélico; que afeta a parte terminal de um membro. [acro- + G. *melos*, membro]

ac·ro·mes·o·me·lia (ak-ro-mē-so-mē′le-ă). Acromesomelia. SIN acromesomelic *dwarfism*. SIN acromelia. [acro- + G. *melos*, membro, + *ia*, condição]

ac·ro·met·a·gen·e·sis (ak′ro-met-ă-jen′e-sis). Acrometagênese; crescimento anormal dos membros resultando em malformação. [acro- + G. *meta*, além, + *genesis*, origem]

acro·mi·al (ă-krō′mē-al). Acromial; relativo ao acrômio.

ac·ro·mic·ria (ak-ro-mik′re-ă, ak-ro-mī′krē-ă). Acromicria; o contrário de acromegalia; uma condição na qual os ossos da face e dos membros são pequenos e delicados; deve-se possivelmente a uma deficiência de somatotropina. [acro- + G. *mikros*, pequeno]

acro·mi·o·cla·vic·u·lar (ă-krō′mē-o-kla-vik′u-lăr). Acromioclavicular; relativo ao acrômio e à clavícula; indica a articulação e os ligamentos entre a clavícula e o acrômio da escápula. SIN scapuloclavicular (1).

acro·mi·o·cor·a·coid (ă-krō-mē-o-kōr′ă-koyd). Acromiocoracóide. SIN coracoacromial.

acro·mi·o·hu·mer·al (ă-krō-mē-o-hū′mer-ăl). Acromiumeral; relativo ao acrômio e ao úmero.

acro·mi·on (ă-krō′mē-on) [TA]. Acrômio; a extremidade lateral da espinha da escápula, que se projeta como um processo largo e achatado, sobrepondo-se à fossa glenóide; ele se articula com a clavícula e dá fixação a parte dos músculos deltóide e trapézio. Sua borda lateral é um ponto de referência palpável ("a ponta do ombro"). SIN acromial process. [G. *akrōmion*, de *akron*, ponta, + *ōmos*, ombro]

acromioplasty (ă-krō′mē-o-plas-ty). Acromioplastia; remodelagem cirúrgica do acrômio, freqüentemente realizada para remediar a compressão da porção supra-espinal do manguito rotatório da articulação do ombro entre o acrômio e o tubérculo maior do úmero.

acro·mi·o·scap·u·lar (ă-krō′mē-o-skap′u-lăr). Acromioscapular; relativo ao acrômio e ao corpo da escápula.

acro·mi·o·tho·rac·ic (ă-krō′mē-o-thō-ras′ik). Acromiotorácico. SIN thoracoacromial.

a·crom·pha·lus (ak-rom′fal-ŭs). Acrônfalo, acronfálio; projeção anormal do umbigo. [acro- + G. *omphalos*, umbigo]

ac·ro·my·o·to·nia (ak′rō-mī-o-tō′ne-ă). Acromiotonia; miotonia que afeta apenas os membros, resultando em deformidade espástica da mão ou do pé. SIN acromyotonus. [acro- + G. *mys*, músculo, + *tonos*, tensão]

ac·ro·my·ot·o·nus (ak-ro-mī-ot′o-nŭs). Acromiotônus. SIN acromyotonia.

ac·ro·os·te·ol·y·sis (ak′rō-os-tē-ol′i-sis) [MIM*102500]. Acrosteólise; condição congênita manifestada por lesões ulcerativas palmares e plantares, com osteólise envolvendo as falanges distais dos dedos das mãos e dos pés. A a. adquirida foi relatada em tabalhadores expostos ao cloreto de vinila. Existe um distúrbio autossômico, a síndrome de Cheney [MIM*102500], no qual esse achado se combina aos ossos das suturas cranianas, hipoplasia dos ramos mandibulares e osteoporose basilar. VER TAMBÉM Cheney *syndrome*. [acro- + G. *osteon*, osso, + *lysis*, afrouxamento]

ac·ro·pachy (ak′rō-pak-ē, ă-krop′ă-kē) [MIM*119900]. Acropaquia. SIN hereditary *clubbing*. [acro- + G. *pachys*, espesso]

ac·ro·pach·y·der·ma (ak′rō-pak-i-der′mă). Acropaquidermia. SIN pachydermoperiostosis. [acro- + G. *pachys*, espesso, + *derma*, pele]

ac·ro·par·es·the·sia (ak′rō-par-es-thēs′ē-a). Acroparestesia. **1.** Parestesia de um ou mais membros. **2.** Parestesia noturna envolvendo as mãos, mais freqüentemente em mulheres de meia-idade; antes atribuída a uma lesão na saída torácica, sendo hoje conhecida por ser um sintoma clássico da síndrome do túnel do carpo. [acro- + parestesia]

acrop·e·tal (ă-krop′e-tăl). Acrópeto, acropétalo. **1.** Em direção ao cimo. **2.** Produzido sucessivamente em direção ao ápice, com o conídio mais jovem formado na ponta e o mais velho, na base de uma cadeia de conídios; referente à produção de esporo assexual nos fungos por brotamento sucessivo do esporo distal em uma cadeia de esporos. [acro- + L. *peto*, procurar]

ac·ro·pho·bia (ak-ro-fō′be-ă). Acrofobia; medo mórbido de altura. [acro- + G. *phobos*, medo]

ac·ro·pig·men·ta·tion (ak′rō-pig-men-tā′shŭn). Acropigmentação; hiperpigmentação pontilhada e reticulada das superfícies dorsais dos dedos dos pés e das mãos, tendo início nos primeiros anos de vida e geralmente piorando com a idade; mais comum em asiáticos de pele mais escura.

ac·ro·pleu·rog·e·nous (ak′rō-ploo-roj′e-nŭs). Acropleurógeno. Indica esporos que se desenvolvem na ponta e ao longo das laterais das hifas fúngicas.

ac·ro·pus·tu·lo·sis (ak′rō-pŭs-tū-lō′sis). Acropustulose. Erupções pustulares das mãos e dos pés, amiúde uma forma de psoríase. [acro- + pustulose]
infantile a., a. infantil; erupção vesicopustular e crostosa, ciclicamente recorrente, geralmente em crianças negras, que surge logo após o nascimento até os 10 meses de vida; a remissão ocorre em torno dos 2 anos de idade.

ac·ro·scle·ro·der·ma (ak′rō-sklēr-ō-der′mă). Acrosclerodermia. SIN acrosclerosis. [acro- + G. *skleros*, duro, + *derma*, pele]

ac·ro·scle·ro·sis (ak′rō-sklē-rō′sis). Acroesclerose; rigidez e endurecimento da pele dos dedos das mãos, com atrofia dos tecidos moles e osteoporose das falanges distais das mãos e dos pés; forma limitada de esclerose progressiva sistêmica que ocorre com o fenômeno de Raynaud e com a esclerodermia dos antebraços. VER CREST *syndrome*. SIN acroscleroderma, sclerodactyly, sclerodactylia.

ac·ro·sin (ak′rō-sin). Acrosina; uma serina proteinase, presente nos espermatozóides, semelhante, em especificidade, à tripsina.

ac·ro·some (ak′rō-sōm). Acrossomo; uma organela ou sáculo semelhante a um capuz, derivado do aparelho de Golgi, que circunda os dois terços anteriores do núcleo de um espermatozóide. Dentro desse capuz ficam enzimas que parecem facilitar a penetração do espermatozóide pela zona pelúcida. [acro- + G. *soma*, corpo]

ac·ro·so·min (ak-rō-sō′min). Acrossomina; complexo lipoglicoproteico presente no capuz acrossômico.

ac·ro·spi·ro·ma (ak′rō-spī-rō′mă). Acrospiroma; tumor do segmento dérmico distal de uma glândula sudorípara. [acro- + G. *speira*, mola + -oma, tumor]
eccrine a., a. écrino. SIN clear cell *hidradenoma*.

ac·ro·ter·ic (ak-rō-ter′ik). Acrotérico; relativo às partes periféricas extremas ou apicais, como as pontas dos dedos das mãos e dos pés e do nariz. [G. *akrōtērion*, o ponto mais ao topo]

Ac·ro·the·ca (ak-rō-thē′kă). Denominação antiga para espécies que hoje estão colocadas no gênero *Rhinocladiella* ou *Fonsecaea*. [ver acrotheca]

ac·ro·the·ca (ak-rō-thē′kă). Nos fungos, um tipo de formação de esporos característico do gênero *Fonsecaea*, no qual conídios são formados ao longo das extremidades e laterais de conidióforos irregulares em forma de baqueta. [acro- + G. *thēkē*, caixa]

acrot·ic (ă-krot′ik). Acrótico. **1.** Marcado por pulso muito fraco ou ausente; sem pulso. [G. *a-* priv. + *krotos*, batida] **2.** Termo obsoleto que indica a superfície do corpo, principalmente as glândulas cutâneas. [G. *akrotēs*, extremidade]

ac·ro·tism (ak′rō-tizm). Acrotismo; ausência ou imperceptibilidade de pulso. [G. *a-* priv. + *krotos*, batida]

ac·ro·troph·o·dyn·ia (ak′rō-trof′ō-din′ē-a). Acrotrofodinia; dor, parestesia, perda sensorial e alterações tróficas afetando as porções distais dos membros, geralmente os pés, que podem ocorrer após exposição prolongada ao frio e à umidade. [acro- + G. *trophē*, nutrição, + *odynē*, dor]

ac·ro·troph·o·neu·ro·sis (ak′rō-trof′ō-noo-rō′sis). Acrotrofoneurose, acrotrofonevrose; trofoneurose de um ou mais membros. [acro- + G. *trophē*, nutrição, + *neuron*, nervo, + *-osis*, condição]

a·cryl·ate (ă′kril-āt). Acrilato; um sal ou éster do ácido acrílico.

acryl·ic (ă-kril′ik). Acrílico; indica certas resinas sintéticas plásticas derivadas do ácido acrílico. VER TAMBÉM acrylic *resin*.

acryl·ic ac·ids. Ácidos acrílicos; uma série de ácidos alifáticos insaturados de fórmula geral R=CH–COOH; o protótipo, ácido acrílico ($R = CH_2$) ou ácido 2-propenóico, é derivado do ácido propiônico por redução ou do glicerol por desidratação.

ACT Abreviatura de activated clotting *time* (tempo de coagulação ativado).

ACTH Abreviatura de adrenocorticotropic *hormone* (hormônio adrenocorticotrófico).
big ACTH, ACTH grande; uma forma de ACTH produzida por certos tumores; é uma molécula maior e mais ácida do que o ACTH pequeno, mas não-diferenciável imunoquimicamente dele, além de não exercer quaisquer dos efeitos biológicos característicos do ACTH; a digestão proteolítica do ACTH grande produz ACTH pequeno hormonalmente ativo.
little ACTH, ACTH pequeno; termo criado para indicar a molécula de ACTH convencional quando comparada ao ACTH grande.

ac·tin (ak′tin). Actina; um dos componentes proteicos ao qual a actomiosina pode ser dividida; pode existir sob forma fibrosa (actina F) ou globular (actina G).
F-a., actina F; associação das subunidades da a. G em uma proteína fibrosa (F) causada por um aumento na concentração de sal; a conversão de a. G para a. F é catalisada por pequenas concentrações do íon magnésio, é reversível e acompanhada pela conversão da molécula de ATP ligada em ADP e pela conversão de um grupamento -tiol em uma forma não-reativa.
G-a., a. G; subunidades globulares (G) da molécula de a., que possuem um peso molecular de 42 kd e uma molécula de ATP; é solúvel em sal diluído, polimerizando-se em a. F quando a força iônica é aumentada.

act·ing out. Representação; ato ou série de ações explícitas que possibilitam um escape emocional para a expressão de conflitos emocionais (geralmente inconscientes).

ac·tin·ic (ak-tin′ik). Actínico; relativo aos raios quimicamente ativos do espectro eletromagnético. [G. *aktis* (aktin-), um raio]

ac·tin·ides (ak′tin-īdz). Actinídios; elementos com números atômicos de 89 a 103, que correspondem aos lantanídios na Tabela Periódica. SIN actinide elements. [*actinium*, primeiro elemento de uma série]

α-ac·tin·in (ak-tin′in). α-actinina; uma proteína de ligação da F-actina nas células de vertebrados que une transversalmente filamentos de actina em arranjos paralelos regulares. É encontrada tanto na linha Z como na banda I.

ac·tin·i·um (Ac) (ak-tin′ē-ŭm). Actínio; elemento químico de número atômico 89 e peso atômico 227,05; não possui isótopos estáveis e existe na natureza apenas como um produto da desintegração do urânio e do tório. [G. *aktis*, um raio]

actino-. Forma combinante que significa um raio, como o de luz; aplicada a qualquer forma de radiação ou estrutura com partes radiantes. VER TAMBÉM radio-. [G. *aktis, aktinos*, um raio de luz, um feixe]

ac·ti·no·bac·il·lo·sis (ak′tin-ō-bas-i-lō′sis). Actinobacilose; doença de bovinos e suínos, ocasionalmente relatada em seres humanos, causada pelo *Actinobacillus lignieresii*. Ataca os tecidos moles, freqüentemente a língua e os linfonodos cervicais, onde se formam tumefações granulomatosas que, por fim, rompem-se para formar abscessos.

Ac·ti·no·ba·cil·lus (ak′tin-ō-bă-sil′lŭs). Actinobacilos; gênero de bactérias imóveis, não-formadoras de esporos, aeróbicas, anaeróbicas facultativas, contendo bastões Gram-negativos disseminados entre elementos cócicos. O metabolismo dessas bactérias é fermentativo. São patogênicas para os animais. A espécie típica é *A. lignieresii*. [actino- + L. *bacillus*, pequeno bastão]
A. actinomycetemcom'itans, uma espécie de posição taxonômica duvidosa; freqüentemente associada a doença periodontal humana, assim como a endocardite subaguda e crônica; acompanha os actinomicetos nas lesões actinomicóticas. SIN *Haemophilus actinomycetemcomitans*.
A. lignieres'ii, espécie que produz infecção no tubo digestivo superior e na boca de bovinos e suínos (actinobacilose) e lesões supurativas na pele e nos pulmões de carneiros; é a espécie típica do seu gênero.

ac·ti·no·he·ma·tin (ak′ti-nō-hē′mă-tin). Actinoematina; pigmento respiratório vermelho encontrado em certas formas de *Actinia* (anêmonas-do-mar). [actino- + G. *haima*, sangue]

Ac·ti·no·ma·du·ra (ak′ti-nō-ma-dū′-ră). Um gênero de bactérias filamentosas não-álcool-ácido-resistentes, ramificadas, Gram-positivas e aeróbicas; pode formar hifas aéreas e conter cadeias com até 15 esporos. [actino- + *Madura*, Índia]
A. africa'na, espécie bacteriana encontrada em casos de micetoma do pé na África.
A. latina, uma espécie de bactéria associada a micetoma na América do Sul.
A. madurae, actinomiceto aeróbico; uma causa de actinomicetoma.
A. pelliertieri, VER *A. latina*.

ac·ti·no·my·ce·li·al (ak′ti-nō-mī-sē′lē-ăl). Actinomicelial; relativo aos filamentos miceliformes dos Actinomicetales.

Ac·ti·no·my·ces (ak′ti-nō-mī′sēz). Um gênero de bactérias de crescimento lento, imóveis, que não formam esporos, anaeróbicas a anaeróbicas facultativas (família Actinomycetaceae) contendo filamentos Gram-positivos, corados de forma irregular; células difteróides podem ser proeminentes. Exibem ramificação verdadeira enquanto estão formando colônias do tipo micélio. O metabolismo desses quimioeterótrofos é fermentativo; os produtos da fermentação da glicose incluem os ácidos acético, fórmico, láctico e succínico, mas não o ácido propiônico. A. podem ter típicos grânulos de enxofre na secreção purulenta. Esses microrganismos são patogênicos para os seres humanos e outros animais, podendo causar infecção supurativa crônica em seres humanos. Mais de 16 espécies já foram descritas; a espécie típica é *A. bovis*. [actino- + G. *mykēs*, fungo]
A. bo'vis, uma espécie de bactéria que provoca actinomicose no gado bovino; ainda não foi comprovada infecção em seres humanos; é a espécie típica do gênero.
A. israe'lii, a espécie que mais comumente causa actinomicose em seres humanos e, às vezes, no gado bovino.
A. naeslun'dii, uma espécie cujo *habitat* natural é a cavidade oral; infecções humanas ocorrem e esses microrganismos provocam destruição periodontal em algumas espécies de animais.
A. odontoly'ticus, uma espécie cujo *habitat* normal é a cavidade oral humana; já foi isolado em cáries dentárias profundas.
A. visco'sus, uma espécie que já foi isolada na cavidade oral de seres humanos e em algumas espécies de outros animais, e já foi isolada de tártaro humano e de cáries da superfície radicular.

Ac·ti·no·my·ce·ta·ce·ae (ak′ti-nō-mī′sē-tā′sē-ē). Família de bactérias não-formadoras de esporos, imóveis, em geral anaeróbicas facultativas (algumas espécies são aeróbicas e outras são anaeróbicas), da ordem Actinomycetales, que contêm células Gram-positivas não-álcool-ácido-resistentes, predominantemente difteróides e tendendo a formar filamentos ramificados no tecido ou em alguns estágios de desenvolvimento em cultura; os filamentos se fragmentam facilmente, produzindo formas difteróides e cocóides. O metabolismo dessas bactérias quimioeterotróficas é fermentativo. Essa família contém os gêneros *Actinomyces* (gênero típico), *Arachnia, Bacterionema, Bifidobacterium* e *Rothia*.

Ac·ti·no·my·ce·ta·les (ak′ti - nō - mī′sē - tā′lēz). Actinomicetales; ordem de bactérias que consistem em formas semelhantes ao bolor, com formato de bastão, clava ou filamentosas, com tendência definida à verdadeira ramificação, sem endosporos mas, às vezes, desenvolvendo conídios; inclui as famílias Mycobacteriaceae, Actinomycetaceae e Nocardiaceae.

ac·ti·no·my·cetes (ak′ti - nō - mī - sē′tēz). Actinomicetos; termo empregado para designar os membros do gênero *Actinomyces;* por vezes, impropriamente utilizado para designar qualquer membro da família Actinomycetaceae ou da ordem Actinomycetales.

actinomycetoma (ak′tin - ō - mī - set - ō′ma). Actinomicetoma; micetoma causado por bactérias superiores. Cf. eumycetoma.

ac·ti·no·my·cin (ak′tin - ō - mī′sin). Actinomicina; grupo de agentes antibióticos peptídicos, isolados de diversas espécies de *Streptomyces* (originalmente *Actinomyces*), que são ativos contra bactérias Gram-positivas, fungos e neoplasias. As actinomicinas são cromopeptídeos. A maioria contém o cromóforo actinocina, sendo derivadas da fenoxazina, que difere nos seus aminoácidos e em sua seqüência nas cadeias peptídicas; formam complexos com DNA e, portanto, inibem a síntese de RNA, principalmente do tipo ribossômico.
   a. A, a primeira das actinomicinas isoladas em forma cristalina.
   a. C, SIN cactinomycin.
   a. D, SIN dactinomycin.
   a. F$_1$, KS4; produzida pelas cepas de *Streptomyces chrysomallus* que elaboram actinomicina C; usada como agente antineoplásico.

ac·ti·no·my·co·sis (ak′ti - nō - mī - kō′sis). Actinomicose; doença primariamente do gado bovino e dos seres humanos provocada pela bactéria *Actinomyces bovis* no gado e por *A. israelii* e *Arachnia propionica* nos seres humanos. Esses actinomicetos são parte da flora bacteriana normal da boca e da faringe, mas, quando introduzidos nos tecidos, podem produzir abscessos ou granulomas crônicos destrutivos que acabam secretando pus viscoso contendo diminutos grânulos amarelados (grânulos de enxofre). Nos seres humanos, a doença afeta comumente a área cervicofacial, o abdome ou o tórax; no gado, a lesão é comumente encontrada na mandíbula. SIN actinophytosis (1), lumpy jaw. [actino- + G. *mykēs,* fungo + *-osis,* condição]

ac·ti·no·my·cot·ic (ak′ti - nō - mī - kot′ik). Actinomicótico; relativo à actinomicose.

Ac·ti·no·myx·id·ia (ak′ti - nō - mik - sid′ē - ă). Ordem de esporozoários com duplo envoltório celular, três cápsulas polares e oito esporos; parasitas principalmente de vermes segmentados, como as minhocas comuns. [actino- + G. *myxa,* muco]

ac·tin·o·phage (ak - tin′ō - fāj). Actinófago; vírus específico dos actinomicetos. [actino(myces) + G. *phagō,* comer]

ac·ti·no·phy·to·sis (ak′ti - nō - fī - tō′sis). Actinofitose. **1.** Actinomicose. SIN actinomycosis. **2.** Botriomicose. SIN botryomycosis.

Ac·ti·no·po·da (ak - ti - nop′ō - dă). Actinópodes; subclasse da classe Sarcodina com pseudópodos delgados e possuidores de um filamento axial central. [actino- + G. *pous,* pé]

ac·tin·o·sin (ak - tin′ō - sin). Actinosina; derivado da fenoxazona, que é o cromóforo das actinomicinas.

ac·ti·no·ther·a·py (ak′ti - nō - thār′ă - pē). Actinoterapia; em dermatologia, tratamento pela luz ultravioleta ou pela luz do sol.

ac·tion (ak′shŭn). Ação. **1.** Desempenho de qualquer das funções vitais, maneira de ser de tal desempenho ou resultado do mesmo. **2.** Exercício de qualquer força ou poder, físico, químico ou mental. [L. *actio,* de *ago,* pp. *actus,* fazer]
   ball valve a., ação de válvula esférica; bloqueio intermitente de um tubo ou saída de uma cavidade por um objeto ou material que permita a passagem em uma direção, mas não na outra.
   calorigenic a., ação calorigênica; aumento da produção de calor pelo corpo, como pelo hormônio tireóideo. SIN thermogenic a.
   cumulative a., ação cumulativa. SIN cumulative *effect.*
   salt a., a. salina; qualquer efeito físico-químico produzido por concentrações hipertônicas de eletrólitos osmoticamente ativos.
   sparing a., a poupadora; a maneira pela qual um componente nutritivo não-essencial, graças à sua presença na dieta, diminui a necessidade de um componente essencial; assim, a L-cisteína não-essencial poupa a L-metionina essencial e a L-tirosina não-essencial poupa a L-fenilalanina essencial. SIN sparing phenomenon.
   specific a., a. específica; ação de um medicamento ou método de tratamento que exerce um efeito curativo direto e especial sobre uma doença, p. ex., a ação da vitamina B$_{12}$ na anemia perniciosa.
   specific dynamic a. (SDA), a. dinâmica específica; aumento da produção de calor causado pela ingestão de alimento, principalmente de proteínas.
   thermogenic a., a. termogênica. SIN calorigenic a.

ac·ti·vate (ak′ti - vāt). Ativar. **1.** Tornar ativo. **2.** Tornar radioativo.

ac·ti·va·tion (ak - ti - vā′shŭn). Ativação. **1.** Ato de tornar ativo. **2.** Aumento do conteúdo energético de um átomo ou molécula por meio da elevação da temperatura, da absorção de fótons de luz, etc., que confere maior reatividade a esse átomo ou molécula. **3.** Técnicas de estimulação do cérebro mediante luz, som, eletricidade ou substâncias químicas, visando produzir atividade anormal no eletroencefalograma. **4.** Estimulação das fibras nervosas periféricas até o ponto de serem iniciados os potenciais de ação. **5.** Estímulo da divisão celular em um óvulo mediante fertilização ou por meios artificiais. **6.** O ato de tornar radioativo. VER TAMBÉM cross-section.
   amino acid a., a. do aminoácido; formação do derivado aminoacil adenilato (p. ex., durante a biossíntese das proteínas).
   EEG a., a. do EEG; o padrão rápido e de baixa voltagem da vigília.
   feedback a., a. por retroalimentação; a. inibidora ou antiinibidora sobre uma enzima por um produto final de uma via bioquímica na qual essa enzima desempenha uma função. Por exemplo, a ativação dos fatores VIII e V pela trombina durante a coagulação do sangue.
   feed-forward a., a. ou estimulação de uma enzima por um precursor do substrato da mesma.
   gene a., a. do gene; processo de a. de um gene de modo que ele é expressado em um determinado momento. Esse processo é fundamental para o crescimento e desenvolvimento.

ac·ti·va·tor (ak′ti - vā - tor). Ativador. **1.** Substância que torna ativa outra substância, ou catalisador, ou que acelera um processo ou uma reação. **2.** Fragmento produzido pela clivagem química de um pró-ativador que induz a atividade enzimática de outra substância. **3.** Aparelho para tornar substâncias radioativas; p.ex., geradores de nêutrons, ciclotron. **4.** Tipo removível de dispositivo ortodôntico miofuncional que atua como um transmissor passivo de força, produzida pela função dos músculos ativados, para os dentes e processo alveolar que estão em contato com ele. **5.** Uma substância que se liga a uma seqüência de DNA antes da transcrição da RNA polimerase.
   catabolite gene a. (CGA), a. de catabólitos (gene). SIN catabolite (gene) activator *protein.*
   plasminogen a., a. de plasminogênio; uma proteinase que converte o plasminogênio em plasmina pela clivagem de uma única ligação (em geral Arg-Val) no primeiro. SIN urokinase.
   polyclonal a. (pol - ē - klō′năl), a. policlonal; substância que ativa células T e/ou células B independentemente de suas especificidades.

   tissue plasminogen a. (TPA, tPA), a. de plasminogênio do tecido; **(1)** serina protease trombolítica, de ocorrência natural, que catalisa a conversão de plasminogênio em plasmina; **(2)** proteína manipulada geneticamente, usada como agente trombolítico nos casos de infarto do miocárdio, AVC (acidente vascular cerebral) e trombose vascular periférica.

   Trata-se de uma glicoproteína de cadeia única, com peso molecular de cerca de 70 kD. Produzido pelas células endoteliais nos locais de lesão vascular, ele modula a trombogênese convertendo o plasminogênio ligado à fibrina em plasmina, clivando a ligação arginina-valina na posição 560–561 do plasminogênio. Como resultado, os filamentos de fibrina em um coágulo são decompostos quimicamente, e a agregação e a adesão das plaquetas ficam inibidas. O TPA exerce pouco efeito sobre o plasminogênio na ausência de fibrina, e sua liberação não reduz significativamente as concentrações sistêmicas de fibrinogênio. Alteplase, um TPA sintético produzido por tecnologia recombinante do DNA, melhora o desfecho quando administrado por via intravenosa no infarto agudo do miocárdio e em casos selecionados de AVC e isquemia periférica devido à trombose. Ele possui uma meia-vida circulante de apenas 4–6 minutos, mas permanece nos coágulos por até 7 horas. VER thrombolytic therapy.

ac·tiv·in (ak′ti - vin). Ativina; hormônio placentário que alcança níveis máximos no soro materno durante o trabalho de parto. [ativo + -in]

ac·tiv·i·ty (ak - tiv′i - tē). **1.** Em eletroencefalografia, a presença de energia elétrica neurogênica. **2.** Em físico-química, uma concentração ideal para a qual a lei da ação das massas se aplicará perfeitamente; a proporção de atividade em relação à verdadeira concentração é o coeficiente de atividade (γ), que se torna 1,00 na diluição infinita. **3.** No caso de enzimas, a quantidade de substrato consumida (ou produto formado) em um dado momento, sob determinadas circunstâncias; número de renovação (*turnover number*). **4.** O número de transformações nucleares (desintegrações) em uma determinada quantidade de um material por unidade de tempo. Unidades: curie (Ci), millicurie (mCi), becquerel (Bq), megabecquerel (MBq). VER TAMBÉM radioactivity.
   blocking a., a. bloqueadora; repressão ou eliminação de atividade elétrica no cérebro pela chegada de um estímulo sensorial.
   insulinlike a. (ILA), a. insulino-símile; medida de substâncias, geralmente no plasma, que exercem efeitos biológicos semelhantes aos da insulina em diversas análises biológicas; empregada, às vezes, como uma medida de concentrações de insulina plasmática; fornece sempre valores mais elevados do que as técnicas imunoquímicas para a dosagem de insulina.

intrinsic sympathomimetic a. (ISA), a. simpaticomimética intrínseca; propriedade de um fármaco que causa ativação dos receptores adrenérgicos de modo a produzir efeitos semelhantes à estimulação do sistema nervoso simpático.
nonsuppressible insulinlike a. (NSILA), a. não-suprimível insulino-símile. A a. plasmática insulino-símile não suprimida por anticorpos antiinsulina, presente sobretudo após pancreatectomia. Deve-se principalmente à ação dos fatores de crescimento polipeptídicos insulino-símiles IGF-I e IGF-II.
optic a., a. óptica; a capacidade de um composto em solução (um que não possua plano de simetria, em geral por causa da presença de um ou mais átomos de carbono assimétricos) para rodar o plano da luz polarizada.
plasma renin a. (PRA), atividade da renina plasmática; estimativa da renina no plasma medindo-se a velocidade de formação de angiotensina I ou II.
pulseless electrical a. (PEA), a. elétrica sem pulso. SIN electromechanical dissociation.
specific a., a. específica; (1) radioatividade por unidade de massa de um elemento ou composto; (2) para uma enzima, a quantidade de substrato consumido (ou de produto formado) em um determinado momento, sob certas condições por miligrama de proteína; (3) a. por unidade de massa do radionuclídeo determinado.
triggered a., a. deflagrada; um ou uma série de batimentos cardíacos gerados espontaneamente, originados de um potencial de ação que produz uma pós-despolarização que alcança o limiar de ativação.
ac·to·my·o·sin (ak′-tō-mī′ō-sin). Actomiosina; complexo proteico composto de actina e miosina; é a substância contrátil indispensável da fibra muscular, ativa com MgATP.
platelet a., a. da plaqueta; a proteína contrátil das plaquetas, responsável pela retração do coágulo, pela agregação plaquetária e pela liberação de ADP e outras aminas biológicas indispensáveis à função plaquetária. SIN thrombosthenin.
Ac·u·a·ria spi·ra·lis (ak-ū-a′rē-ā spi-rā′lis). Nematódeo parasita que vive no proventrículo e no esôfago e, às vezes, no intestino de galinhas, perus, faisões e outras aves. [L. *acus*. agulha; L. Mod. *spiralis*, espiral]
acu·i·ty (ā-kū′i-tē). 1. Acuidade, clareza, nitidez. 2. Gravidade. [atr. Fr., do L. *acuo*, pp. *acutus*, agudo]
absolute intensity threshold a., a. do limiar de intensidade absoluta; a luz mínima que pode ser vista.
resolution a., acuidade de resolução; detecção de um alvo que tem duas ou mais partes, freqüentemente medida utilizando-se letras ou símbolos do quadro de Snellen; indicada por dois números: o primeiro representa a distância na qual um indivíduo vê as letras do quadro (em geral, 6m ou 20 pés), e o segundo, a distância na qual as letras do quadro subtendem um ângulo de 5 minutos; p. ex., uma visão de 6/9 indica uma distância de prova de 6m e o reconhecimento de símbolos que subtendem um ângulo de 5 minutos a uma distância de 9m. SIN visual. a.
spatial a., a. espacial; detecção da forma de um objeto de prova; p.ex., a percepção de polígonos do mesmo tamanho, mas com números diferentes de lados.
stereoscopic a., a. estereoscópica; detecção de diferenças na distância pela superposição de imagens retinianas um pouco diferentes em uma única imagem para o cérebro.
Vernier a., a. de Vernier; detecção do deslocamento de parte de uma linha.
visibility a., a. de visibilidade; reconhecimento de um objeto em um fundo de caráter diferente.
visual a. (V), SIN resolution a.
acu·le·ate (a-kū′lē-āt). Aculeado; pontiagudo; coberto com espinhos afiados. [L. *aculeatus*, pontiagudo, de *acus*, agulha]
acu·men·tin (ak-ū-men′tin). Acumentina; proteína de motilidade de neutrófilos e macrófagos que se liga à molécula de actina a fim de controlar o comprimento do filamento.
acu·mi·nate (ā-kū′mi-nāt). Acuminado; pontiagudo. [L. *acumino*, pp. *-atus*, afiar]
ac·u·ol·o·gy (ak-ū-ol′ō-jē). Acuologia; estudo do uso de agulhas para fins terapêuticos, como na acupuntura. [L. *acus*, agulha, + G. *logos*, estudo]
a·cu·pres·sure. Acupressão; aplicação de pressão nos pontos usados para acupuntura com fins terapêuticos.
ac·u·punc·ture (ak-ū-punk′choor). Acupuntura; punção feita com agulhas longas e finas. 1. Sistema oriental antigo de tratamento. 2. Mais recentemente, método de anestesia (*anesthesia*) ou analgesia. [L. *acus*, agulha, + punção]
acu·sis (ā-kū′sis). Acusia; capacidade de perceber os sons normalmente. SIN normal hearing. [G. *akousis*, escutar]
acute (ā-kūt′). Agudo. 1. Que se refere a um efeito sobre a saúde, geralmente de instalação curta e nítida, não-crônica; às vezes usado popularmente para designar grave. 2. Que se refere à exposição curta, intensa, em curto prazo; em geral designa, especificamente, a exposição breve de alta intensidade. [L. *acutus*, agudo]
acy·a·not·ic (ā-sī-ā-not′ik). Acianótico; caracterizado pela ausência de cianose.
acy·clic (ā-sī′klik). Acíclico; não-cíclico; refere-se particularmente a um composto acíclico.

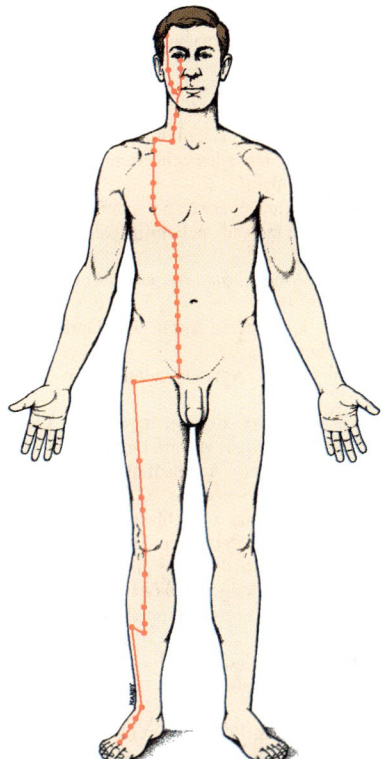

acupuntura (meridiano do estômago)

acy·clo·guan·o·sine (ā-sī-klō-gwan′ō-sēn). Acicloguanosina. SIN acyclovir.
acy·clo·vir (ā-sī′klō-vir). Aciclovir; um análogo acíclico sintético do nucleosídeo purina usado como agente antiviral no tratamento do herpes genital; o sal sódico é utilizado para terapêutica parenteral. SIN acycloguanosine.
ac·yl (as′il). Acil; radical orgânico derivado de um ácido orgânico pela remoção do grupamento hidroxila carboxílico.
ac·yl-ACP de·hy·dro·gen·ase, ac·yl-ACP re·duc·tase. Acil-ACP desidrogenase ou redutase. SIN enoyl-ACP reductase (NADPH).
ac·yl·ad·e·nyl·ate (as′il-ā-den′il-āt). Acildenilato; composto em que o grupamento acil está combinado com AMP por eliminação de H_2O entre os OH de um grupamento carboxila e do resíduo fosfato do AMP, em geral, inicialmente sob a forma de ATP e eliminando pirofosfato inorgânico na condensação.
***n*-ac·yl·a·mi·no ac·id** (as-il-am′i-nō). Ácido *n*-acilamino; aminoácido com um grupamento acil ligado ao seu *N*, como no ácido hipúrico (*N*-benzoilglicina) ou no ácido fenacetúrico.
ac·yl·a·tion (as-i-lā′shŭn). Acilação; introdução de um radical acil em um composto orgânico ou formação desse radical em um composto orgânico.
a·cyl·car·ni·tine (as′il-kar′ni-tēn). Acilcarnitina; produto da condensação de ácido carboxílico e carnitina. A forma de transporte de um ácido graxo que cruza a membrana mitocondrial interna.
ac·yl-CoA. Acil-CoA; produto de condensação de um ácido carboxílico e coenzima A; intermediário metabólico importante, notavelmente na oxidação e síntese de gorduras. SIN acyl-coenzyme A.
a.-CoA dehydrogenase (NADPH), Acil-CoA desidrogenase; enzima que catalisa a redução reversível dos derivados de enoil-CoA de cadeia com comprimento de 4–16, sendo o NADPH o doador de hidrogênio, formando a.-CoA e $NADP^+$. SIN enoyl-CoA reductase.
a.-CoA synthetase, Acil-CoA sintetase; (1) termo genérico para enzimas (EC 6.2.1.×) que formam acil-CoA, agora conhecidas como ligases; (2) especificamente, a acil-CoA ligase de ácidos graxos de cadeia longa.
ac·yl·co·en·zyme A (as′il-kō-en′zim). Acil-coenzima A. SIN acyl-CoA.
1-ac·yl·gly·ce·rol-3-phos·phate ac·yl·trans·fer·ase. 1-acilglicerol-3-fosfato aciltransferase. VER lysophosphatidic acid acyltransferase.
ac·yl-mal·o·nyl-ACP syn·thase. Acilmalonil ACP sintase. SIN 3-oxoacyl-ACP synthase.
ac·yl·mer·cap·tan (as′il-mer-kap′tan). Acilmercaptano. SIN thioester.
***N*-ac·yl·sphin·go·sine** (as-il-sfing′gō-sēn). *N*-acilesfingosina; produto de condensação de ácido orgânico com esfingosina no grupamento amino do último composto.

ac·yl·trans·fer·as·es (as-il-trans′fer-ā-sez) [EC 2.3.x.x]. Enzimas que catalisam a transferência de um grupamento acil de uma acil-CoA para vários aceptores. SIN transacylases.

acys·tia (ā-sis′tē-ā). Acistia; ausência congênita da bexiga urinária. [G. *a-* priv. + *kystis*, bexiga]

A.D. Abreviatura de *auris dexter* [L.], orelha direita.

ad-. Prefixo que indica aumento, aderência ou movimento para, em direção a; próximo; bastante. [L. *ad*, para]

-ad. Sufixo na nomenclatura anatômica com o significado do sufixo inglês *-ward*; indica em direção à parte indicada pela principal porção da palavra. [L. *ad*, para]

ADA Abreviatura de *American Dental Association* (*Associação Americana de Odontologia*).

ad·a·cr·ya (a-dak′rē-ā). Adacria; ausência de lágrimas; sem lágrimas. [G. *a-* priv. + *dakryon*, lágrima, + *-ia*]

adac·ty·lous (ā-dak′tĭ-lŭs). Adáctilo, adátilo; sem os dedos das mãos ou artelhos.

Adair-Koshland-Némethy-Filmer mod·el (AKNF). Modelo de Adair-Koshland-Némethy-Filmer. VER em model.

ad·a·man·tine (ad-ă-man′tēn). Adamantino; excessivamente duro; outrora usado em referência ao esmalte do dente. [G. *adamantinos*, muito duro]

adamantinoma. Adamantinoma, ameloblastoma; neoplasia epitelial odontogênica de tecido característico do esmalte embrionário, mas que não se diferencia a ponto de formar tecidos dentários duros.
 a. of long bones, a. dos ossos longos; tumor raro dos ossos dos membros, em geral da tíbia, que se assemelha microscopicamente a um ameloblastoma; a histogênese é incerta.
 pituitary a., a. hipofisário. SIN craniopharyngioma.

Adamkiewicz, Albert, patologista polonês, 1850–1921. VER *artery* of Adamkiewicz.

Adams, Robert, físico irlandês, 1791–1875. VER A.-Stokes *disease*; Stokes-A. *disease* ou *syndrome*; A.-Stokes *syncope, syndrome*; Morgagni-A.-Stokes *syndrome*.

Adams, Sir William, cirurgião inglês, 1760–1829.

Adam's ap·ple. Pomo-de-adão. SIN laryngeal prominence.

ad·am·site (DM) (ad′ăm-sīt). Agente emético usado no treinamento militar e no controle de protestos. [Roger *Adams*, químico norte-americano]

Adanson, Michel, naturalista francês, 1727–1806. VER adansonian *classification*.

ad·ap·ta·tion (ad-ap-tā′shŭn). Adaptação. **1.** Sobrevida preferencial de membros de uma espécie apresentando certos aspectos fenotípicos que conferem uma capacidade maior para suportar o meio ambiente, inclusive a ecologia. **2.** Mudança vantajosa na função ou constituição de um órgão ou tecido para satisfazer a novas condições. **3.** Ajustamento da sensibilidade da retina à intensidade da luz. **4.** Propriedade de certos receptores sensoriais que modifica a resposta a estímulos repetidos ou contínuos de intensidade constante. **5.** O preenchimento, a condensação ou o revestimento do material restaurador de um dente ou um gesso de modo a ficar em contato íntimo. **6.** Processo dinâmico pelo qual pensamentos, sentimentos, comportamento e mecanismos biofisiológicos do indivíduo se modificam continuamente para se adaptarem a um ambiente em transformação contínua. SIN adjustment (2) **7.** Resposta homeostática. [L. *ad-apto*, pp. *-atus*, ajustar]
 dark a., a. à escuridão; ajuste visual que ocorre sob iluminação reduzida, na qual a sensibilidade da retina à luz é aumentada. VER TAMBÉM dark-adapted *eye*, Purkinje *shift*. SIN scotopic a.
 light a., a. à luz; ajuste visual que ocorre sob iluminação aumentada, na qual a sensibilidade da retina à luz está reduzida. VER TAMBÉM light-adapted *eye*, Purkinje *shift*. SIN photopic a.
 photopic a., a. fotóptica. SIN light a.
 reality a., a. à realidade; capacidade de ajustar-se ao mundo tal qual ele existe.
 retinal a., a. retiniana; ajuste ao grau de iluminação.
 scotopic a., a. escotópica. SIN dark a.
 social a., a. social, ajuste à vida de acordo com as restrições e demandas interpessoais, bem como restrições e demandas culturais.

adapt·er, adap·tor (a-dap′ter, -tōr). Adaptador. **1.** Uma parte de união, reunindo duas peças do aparelho. **2.** Um transformador de corrente elétrica para uma forma desejada.

ad·ap·tom·e·ter (ad-ap-tom′ĕ-ter). Adaptômetro; dispositivo para determinar o curso da adaptação ocular à obscuridade e para medir o limiar luminoso mínimo.

ad·ax·i·al (ad-ak′sē-ăl). Adaxial; em direção a um eixo ou a um outro lado de um eixo.

ADC Abreviatura de AIDS dementia *complex* (complexo demencial relacionado à AIDS/SIDA).

ADCC Abreviatura de antibody-dependent cell-mediated *cytotoxicity* (citotoxicidade mediada por células e dependente de anticorpos).

add. Abreviatura do L. *adde*, adicionar; L. *addantur,* deixar ser adicionado; *addendus*, a ser adicionado; e *addendo*, por adicionamento.

ad·der. Cobra, serpente; denominação comum de muitos membros da família Viperidae (víboras), aplicado a diversos gêneros, embora as verdadeiras víboras sejam do gênero *Vipera*. [I.M. *naddre*, do I. Ant. *nǣdre*]

ad·dict (ad′ikt). Adicto; viciado; pessoa habituada a uma substância ou prática, especialmente considerada prejudicial ou ilegal.

ad·dic·tion (ă-dik′shŭn). Adicção, vício; dependência psicológica e fisiológica habitual de uma substância ou prática que esteja além do controle voluntário. [L. *ad-dico*, pp. *-dictus*, consentir, de *ad-* + *dico*, dizer]
 alcohol a., alcoolismo. SIN alcoholism.

Addis, Thomas, internista norte-americano, 1881–1949. VER A. *count*.

Addison, Christopher, anatomista inglês, 1869–1951. VER A. clinical *planes*, em *plane*.

Addison, Thomas, físico inglês, 1793–1860. VER A. *anemia, disease*; addisonian *anemia*; addisonian *crisis*; A.-Biermer *disease*.

ad·di·so·ni·an (ad-i-sō′nē-an). Adissoniano; relativo a Thomas Addison ou descrito por ele; termo empregado em relação à *anemia* perniciosa ou aos vários aspectos da doença de Addison.

ad·di·tive (ad′ĭ-tiv). Aditivo. **1.** Substância que não faz parte natural de um material (p. ex., de um alimento), mas que é deliberadamente acrescentada para um determinado propósito (p. ex., conservação). **2.** Que se tende a acrescentar ou ser acrescentado; indicando adição. **3.** Em estudos métricos (p. ex., genética, epidemiologia, fisiologia, estatística), que tem a propriedade de que o efeito total combinado de dois ou mais fatores equivale à soma de seus efeitos individuais isolados. Cf. synergism.

ad·di·tiv·i·ty (ad-i-tiv′i-tē). Qualidade ou estado de ser aditivo.
 causal a., relação entre dois ou mais componentes causais, de tal modo que seu efeito combinado seja a soma algébrica de seus efeitos individuais.
 interlocal a., relação entre efeitos quantitativos de diferentes *loci* genéticos de modo que seu efeito de união seja igual à soma de seus efeitos individuais; ausência de epistase ou interação.
 intralocal a., relação entre alelos de modo que o fenótipo quantificável do heterozigoto está no ponto médio entre aqueles para os dois homozigotos; ausência de dominância.

ad·dres·sin (ad-res′in). Adressina; molécula na superfície de uma célula que serve como um dispositivo indicador para orientar outra molécula a um local específico. [address, do Fr. Ant. *adresser*, dirigir, do L.L. *addirectiare*, do L. *ad*, para, + *directus*, direto + *-in*]

ad·du·cent (ă-doo′sent). Aducente; que traz. [L. *adducens,* pres. p. de *ad-duco,* trazer]

ad·du·cin (ă-doo′sen). Proteína que se liga a espectrina e à actina e une a "montagem" da espectrina.

ad·duct (a-dŭkt′). Aduzir. **1.** Impelir na direção do plano mediano. **2.** Um produto ou complexo de adição ou uma parte do mesmo. [L. *ad-duco*, pp. *-ductus*, trazer para]

ad·duc·tion (ă-dŭk′shŭn). Adução. **1.** Movimento de uma parte do corpo em direção ao plano mediano (do corpo, nos caso das extremidades; da mão ou do pé, no caso dos dígitos). **2.** Rotação monocular (ducção) do olho em direção ao nariz. **3.** Posição resultante desse movimento. Cf. abduction.

ad·duc·tor (ă-dŭk′ter, tōr). Adutor. SIN adductor muscle.

Ade Abreviatura de adenine (adenina).

ade·lo·mor·phous (ă-del-ō-mōr′fŭs). Adelomorfo; sem forma claramente definida. Anteriormente, esse termo era aplicado a certas células das glândulas gástricas. [G. *adēlos*, incerto, não-claro, + *morphē*, forma]

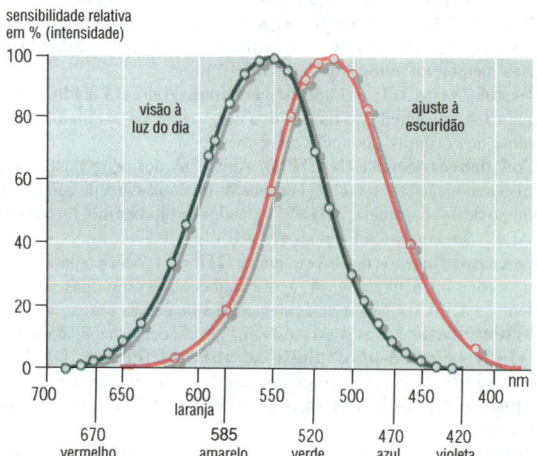

adaptação ao escuro e à luz: intensidade das cores durante o dia e à tarde

aden-. VER adeno-.

ad·e·nal·gia (ad-ē-nal′jē-ă). Adenalgia; termo raramente empregado para a dor em uma glândula. [aden- + G. *algos*, dor]

aden·dric (ā-den′drik). Adêndrico. SIN adendritic.

aden·drit·ic (ā-den-drit′ik). Adendrítico; sem dendritos. SIN adêndrico. [G. *a-* priv. + *dendron*, árvore]

ad·e·nec·to·my (ad-ē-nek′tō-mē). Adenectomia; excisão de uma glândula. [aden- + G. *ektomē*, excisão]

ad·e·nec·to·pia (ad′ē-nek-tō′pē-ă). Adenectopia; presença de uma glândula fora de sua posição anatômica normal. [aden- + G. *ek*, fora + *topos*, local]

ad·e·nem·phrax·is (ad′ē-nem-frak′sis). Adenefraxia; termo raramente empregado para uma obstrução à saída da secreção de uma glândula. [aden- + G. *emphraxis*, parada]

aden·i·form (ā-den′i-fōrm). Adeniforme. SIN adenoid (1).

Ad·e·nine (A, Ade) (ad′ē-nēn). Adenina; uma das duas purinas principais (a outra é a guanina) encontradas tanto no RNA como no DNA, como também em vários nucleotídeos livres importantes para o organismo, como o AMP (ácido adenílico), o ATP, o NAD^+, o $NADP^+$ e o FAD; em todos esses compostos menores, a adenina está condensada com a ribose no nitrogênio 9, formando adenosina. Quanto à estrutura, ver adenylic acid. SIN 6-aminopurine.

a. arabinoside, a. arabinosídeo; nome errôneo da arabinosiladenina.

a. deaminase, a. desaminase; enzima que catalisa a hidrólise de a. em amônia e hipoxantina. Parte da degradação da purina.

a. deoxyribonucleotide, a. desoxirribonucleotídeo. SIN deoxyadenylic acid.

a. nucleotide, nucleotídeo da a. SIN adenylic acid.

a. phosphoribosyltransferase, a. fosforribosiltransferase; enzima que catalisa a reação de a. com 5-fosfo-α-D-ribose 1-difosfato (PRPP) para formar AMP e pirofosfato. Uma etapa importante na recuperação da purina. A deficiência dessa enzima pode levar a cálculos de 2,8-diidroxiadenina.

a. sulfate, sulfato de a.; adenina conjugada com ácido sulfúrico; utilizada para estimular a produção de leucócitos na agranulocitose.

ad·e·ni·tis (ad-ē-nī′tis). Adenite; inflamação de um linfonodo ou de uma glândula. [aden- + G. *-itis*, inflamação]

mesenteric a., a. mesentérica; enfermidade com dor abdominal e febre devido ao aumento e à inflamação dos linfonodos mesentéricos; freqüentemente confundida com a apendicite. SIN mesenteric lymphadenitis.

ad·e·ni·za·tion (ad-ē-nī-zā′shŭn). Adenização; conversão em uma estrutura semelhante a glândula.

adeno-, aden-. Formas combinantes indicando relação com uma glândula; glandular; correspondem ao L. glandul-, glandi- [G. *adēn, adenos*, glândula]

ad·e·no·ac·an·tho·ma (ad′ē-nō-ak-an-thō′mă). Adenoacantoma; neoplasia maligna que consiste, principalmente, em epitélio glandular (adenocarcinoma), em geral bem-diferenciado, com focos de células neoplásicas escamosas (ou epidermóides).

ad·e·no·am·e·lo·blas·to·ma (ad′ē-nō-am′el-ō-blast-ō′mă). Adenoameloblastoma. SIN adenomatoid odontogenic *tumor*.

ad·e·no·blast (ad′ē-nō-blast). Adenoblasto; célula embrionária proliferativa com o potencial para formar parênquima glandular. [adeno- + G. *blastos*, germe]

ad·e·no·car·ci·no·ma (ad′ē-nō-kar-si-nō′mă). Adenocarcinoma; neoplasia maligna das células epiteliais com padrão glandular ou glanduliforme. SIN glandular cancer, glandular carcinoma.

acinic cell a., a. de célula acinar; a. originário de células secretoras de uma glândula racemosa, particularmente as glândulas salivares. SIN acinar carcinoma, acinic cell carcinoma.

alveolar a., a. alveolar; a. do pulmão no qual as células tumorais formam estruturas que lembram alvéolos.

a. in Barrett esophagus, a. no esôfago de Barrett; a. que surge no esôfago e que se tornou revestido por células colunares (mucosa de Barrett).

bronchiolar a., a. bronquiolar. SIN alveolar cell *carcinoma*.

bronchioloalveolar a., a. bronquioloalveolar. SIN alveolar cell carcinoma.

clear cell a., a. de células claras; (1) tipo histológico de a. renal; (2) tipo histológico de a. que ocorre principalmente nos tratos genitourinários masculino e feminino e que é caracterizado por crescimento celular característico (em cravo) de células neoplásicas em lâminas, papilas e glândulas coalescentes.

mesonephric a., a. mesonéfrico. SIN mesonephroma.

mucoid a., a. mucóide; às vezes aplicado ao carcinoma mucinoso, ou a. contendo células neoplásicas secretoras de mucina.

papillary a., a. papilar; a. contendo prolongamentos digitiformes de tecido conjuntivo vascular recoberto por epitélio neoplásico, projetando-se para cistos ou cavidades de glândulas ou folículos; ocorre mais freqüentemente no ovário e na glândula tireóide.

renal a., a. renal; a. originário do parênquima renal, que ocorre geralmente em pessoas de meia-idade ou mais velhas de ambos os sexos (embora mais comum no masculino). SIN clear cell carcinoma of kidney, renal cell carcinoma.

a. in si′tu, proliferação anormal não-invasiva de glândulas considerada precedente do surgimento de adenocarcinoma invasivo; relatada no endométrio, mama, intestino grosso, colo uterino e outros locais.

ad·e·no·cys·to·ma (ad′ē-nō-sis-tō′mă). Adenocistoma; adenoma em que o epitélio glandular forma cistos.

ad·e·no·cyte (ad′ē-nō-sīt). Adenócito; célula secretora de uma glândula. [adeno- + G. *kytos*, cavidade (célula)]

ad·e·no·di·as·ta·sis (ad′ē-nō-dī-as′tă-sis). Adenodiastase; separação ou ectopia de glândulas ou tecido glandular de seus locais anatômicos habituais, p.ex., glândulas pancreáticas na parede do intestino delgado, glândulas gástricas na parede do esôfago. [adeno- + *diastasis*, separação]

ad·e·no·dyn·ia (ad′ē-nō-din′ē-ă). Adenodinia; termo raramente empregado para adenalgia. [adeno- + G. *odynē*, dor]

ad·e·no·fi·bro·ma (ad′ē-nō-fī-brō′mă). Adenofibroma; neoplasia benigna composta de tecidos glandulares e fibroso, com uma proporção relativamente grande de glândulas.

ad·e·no·fi·bro·sis (ad′ē-nō-fī-brō′sis). Adenofibrose. SIN sclerosing *adenosis*.

ad·e·nog·en·ous (ad-ē-noj′en-ŭs). Adenógeno; que tem origem no tecido glandular.

ad·e·no·hy·po·phy·si·al (ad′ē-nō-hī-pō-fiz′ē-ăl). Adeno-hipofisário; relativo a adeno-hipófise.

ad·e·no·hy·poph·y·sis (ad′ē-nō-hī-pof′i-sis) [TA]. Adeno-hipófise; glândula hipofisária anterior; consiste em parte distal, parte intermédia e parte infundibular. VER TAMBÉM pituitary *gland*. SIN lobus anterior hypophyseos [TA], anterior lobe of hypophysis*, glandular lobe of hypophysis, lobus glandularis hypophyseos.

ad·e·no·hy·poph·y·si·tis (ad′ē-nō-hī-pof-ĭ-sī′tis). Adeno-hipofisite; reação inflamatória e fibriótica da adeno-hipófise, freqüentemente relacionada com a gravidez.

lymphocytic a., a. linfocitária; infiltração linfocitária difusa da adeno-hipófise, freqüentemente relacionada com a gravidez; provavelmente um distúrbio no sistema imunológico.

ad·e·noid (ad′ē-noyd). Adenóide. **1.** Glanduliforme; de aspecto glandular. SIN adeniforme. **2.** VER pharyngeal *tonsil*. [adeno- + G. *eidos*, aparência]

ad·e·noid·ec·to·my (ad′ē-noy-dek′tō-mē). Adenoidectomia; operação para a remoção de tecido adenóide na nasofaringe. [adenoid + G. *ektomē*, excisão]

ad·e·noid·i·tis (ad′ē-noy-dī′tis). Adenoidite; inflamação do tecido linfóide nasofaríngeo.

ad·e·noids (ad′ē-noydz). Adenóides. **1.** Acúmulo normal de tecido linfóide não-encapsulado na nasofaringe. Também chamado de tonsilas faríngeas. **2.** Terminologia comum para as grandes (normais) tonsilas faríngeas das crianças. [G. *adēn*, glândula, + *-eidos*, semelhança]

ad·e·no·li·po·ma (ad′ē-nō-li-pō′mă). Adenolipoma; neoplasia benigna composta de tecidos glandular e adiposo. [G. *adēn*, glândula, + *lipos*, gordura, + *-oma*, tumor]

ad·e·no·lip·o·ma·to·sis (ad′ē-nō-lip′ō-mă-tō′sis). Adenolipomatose; condição caracterizada pelo desenvolvimento de múltiplos adenolipomas.

symmetric a., a. simétrica. SIN multiple symmetric *lipomatosis*.

ad·e·no·lym·pho·cele (ad′ē-nō-lim′fō-sēl). Adenolinfocele; dilatação cística de um linfonodo após obstrução dos vasos linfáticos eferentes. [adeno- + L. *lympha*, nascente, + G. *kēlē*, tumor]

ad·e·no·lym·pho·ma (ad′ē-nō-lim-fō′mă). Adenolinfoma; termo obsoleto para tumor glandular benigno geralmente originário da glândula parótida e composto de duas fileiras de células epiteliais eosinófilas, que são freqüentemente císticas e papilares, junto com um estroma linfóide. SIN papillary cystadenoma lymphomatosum, Warthin tumor.

ad·e·no·ma (ad-ē-nō′mă). Adenoma; neoplasia benigna de tecido epitelial no qual as células tumorais formam estruturas glandulares ou glanduliformes; em geral bem-circunscrita, tendendo mais a comprimir do que infiltrar ou invadir o tecido adjacente. [adeno- + G. *-oma*, tumor]

acidophil a., a. acidófilo; tumor da adeno-hipófise no qual o citoplasma celular se cora com corantes ácidos; muitas vezes produz hormônio do crescimento. SIN eosinophil a.

ACTH-producing a., a. produtor de ACTH; tumor hipofisário composto de corticotrofos que produzem ACTH, freqüentemente um a. basófilo; pode dar origem à doença de Cushing ou à síndrome de Nelson.

adnexal a., a. dos anexos; a. que se origina ou forma estruturas semelhantes a apêndices cutâneos.

adrenocortical a., a. adrenocortical; tumor benigno das células corticais da supra-renal; os pequenos nódulos não-encapsulados do córtex da supra-renal são provavelmente áreas localizadas de hiperplasia em vez de adenomas; os verdadeiros adenomas são raros e podem apresentar-se de forma assintomática ou associados à síndrome de Cushing ou ao aldosteronismo primário.

apocrine a., a. apócrino. SIN papillary *hidradenoma*.

basal cell a., a. basocelular; tumor benigno das glândulas salivares maiores ou menores ou de outros órgãos compostos de pequenas células mostrando formação de paliçada periférica.

basophil a., a. basófilo; tumor da adeno-hipófise no qual o citoplasma celular se cora com corantes básicos; freqüentemente produz ACTH.

bronchial a., a. brônquico; termo obsoleto usado para abranger tumores carcinóides, carcinoma mucoepidermóide (mucoepidermoid *carcinoma*) e carcinoma cístico adenóide (adenoid cystic *carcinoma*). Cf. bronchial mucous gland a.
bronchial mucous gland a., a. da glândula brônquica produtora de muco; raro tumor benigno que surge das glândulas produtoras de muco da mucosa brônquica.
canalicular a. (ca-na-lik′oo-lar), a. canalicular; uma variante do a. monomórfico composta de fileiras duplas de células epiteliais em cordões longos.
chromophobe a., chromophobic a., a. cromófobo; tumor da adeno-hipófise cujas células não se coram nem com corantes ácidos, nem com básicos.
colloid a., a. colóide; a. folicular da tireóide, composto de grandes folículos contendo colóide. SIN macrofollicular a.
embryonal a., a. embrionário; neoplasia benigna na qual os elementos epiteliais glandulares não são completamente diferenciados, assemelhando-se ao tecido imaturo observado no desenvolvimento embrionário.
eosinophil a., a. eosinofílico. SIN acidophil a.
follicular a., a. folicular; a. da tireóide com padrão glandular simples.
Fuchs a., a. de Fuchs; tumor epitelial benigno do epitélio não-pigmentado do corpo ciliar raramente excedendo 1 mm de diâmetro.
gonadotropin-producing a., a. produtor de gonadotropina; tipo raro de a. hipofisário que produz FSH e LH; suas células podem ser identificadas apenas por técnicas imunoquímicas.
growth hormone-producing a., a. produtor de hormônio do crescimento; a. que produz o quadro clínico de gigantismo ou acromegalia, embora um terço das células não tenha grânulos ou então seja uma mistura de acidófilos e cromófobos; alguns tumores podem secretar tanto hormônio do crescimento como prolactina; freqüentemente um a. acidófilo ou eosinófilo.
hepatic a., a. hepático; tumor benigno do fígado, que geralmente ocorre nas mulheres durante os anos férteis em associação com o uso prolongado de contraceptivos orais. O tumor em geral é solitário, subcapsular e grande, composto de cordões de hepatócitos com tríades portas. SIN hepatocellular a.
hepatocellular a., SIN hepatic a.
Hürthle cell a., a. de células de Hürthle; tipo incomum de tumor da tireóide caracterizado por citoplasma eosinofílico abundante contendo muitas mitocôndrias. Freqüentemente maligno com metástases disseminadas; raramente capta iodo radioativo. VER TAMBÉM Hürthle cell *carcinoma*. SIN oncocystic a.
invasive pituitary a., a. pituitário invasivo; infiltrados extensos da dura-máter, dos ossos e dos seios paranasais.
lactating a., a. da lactação; adenoma incomum da mama, composto de estruturas tubuloacinares com alterações secretoras pronunciadas, como as observadas na gravidez e na lactação.
macrofollicular a., a. macrofolicular. SIN colloid a.
mammosomatotroph cell a., a da célula mamossomatotrófica; raro adenoma hipofisário, produtor de prolactina e hormônio do crescimento, composto de células ultra-estruturalmente monomórficas com diferenciação tanto somatotrófica como lactotrófica.
microfollicular a., a. microfolicular; a. fetal da tireóide, composto de folículos muito pequenos e grupos alveolares sólidos de células epiteliais da tireóide.
monomorphic a., a. monomórfico; neoplasia ductal benigna das glândulas salivares, com padrão epitelial uniforme mas sem o estroma condromixóide de um a. pleomórfico.
nephrogenic a., a. nefrogênico; tumor benigno da mucosa da bexiga urinária ou urotelial, composto de estruturas glandulares semelhantes a túbulos renais.
a. of nipple, a. do mamilo. SIN subareolar duct *papillomatosis*.
null-cell a., a. de células nulas; a. da hipófise composto de células para as quais não existe franca evidência de produção hormonal, mas que produz hipopituitarismo e distúrbios visuais pela compressão de estruturas adjacentes; aproximadamente um terço desses tumores tem células com mitocôndrias abundantes (oncócitos), um pouco maiores do que as células nulas monocíticas. SIN undifferentiated cell a.
oncocytic a., a. oncótico. SIN Hürthle cell a.
oxyphil a., a. oxifílico. SIN oncocytoma.
papillary cystic a., a. cístico papilar; a. em que a luz dos ácinos está freqüentemente distendida por líquido, e os elementos epiteliais neoplásicos tendem a formar projeções irregulares, digitiformes.
papillary a. of large intestine, a. papilar do colo. SIN villous a.
pituitary a., a. hipofisário; neoplasia benigna da hipófise que geralmente surge na adeno-hipófise.
pleomorphic a., a. pleomórfico. SIN mixed *tumor* of salivary gland.
polypoid a., a. polipóide. SIN adenomatous *polyp*.
prolactin-producing a., a. produtor de prolactina; adenoma hipofisário composto de células produtoras de prolactina; dá origem a amenorréia não-puerperal e galactorréia (síndrome de Forbes-Albright) em mulheres e impotência em homens. SIN prolactinoma.
prostatic a., a. prostático; o crescimento na hiperplasia prostática benigna.
renal cortical a., a. cortical renal; um a., geralmente pequeno, às vezes en-

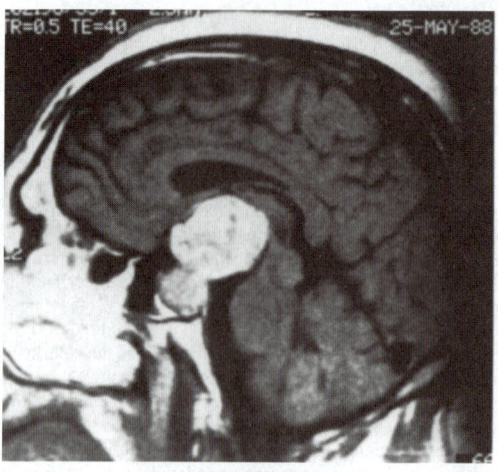

adenoma da hipófise: imagem por ressonância magnética após injeção de contraste

contrado incidentalmente no córtex renal na necropsia e derivado do tecido tubular renal.
sebaceous a., a. sebáceo; neoplasia benigna de tecido sebáceo, com predominância de células sebáceas secretoras maduras. Cf. a. sebaceum.
a. seba′ceum, a. sebáceo; denominação arcaica e errônea para um hamartoma que ocorre na face, composto de tecido fibrovascular e aparecendo como um agregado de pápulas vermelhas ou amarelas que podem estar associadas à esclerose tuberosa; glândulas sebáceas podem estar presentes, mas não estão aumentadas. Cf. sebaceous a. SIN Pringle disease.
thyrotropin-producing a., a. produtor de tireotropina; adenoma hipofisário raro, em geral associado a hipo- ou hipertireoidismo.
tubular a., a. tubular; (1) neoplasia benigna composta de tecido epitelial assemelhando-se a uma glândula tubular; (2) pólipo displásico da mucosa colônica considerado um precursor potencial do adenocarcinoma.
undifferentiated cell a., a. de células indiferenciadas. SIN null-cell a.
villous a., a. viloso; freqüentemente surge como um tumor séssil solitário, muitas vezes grande, da mucosa colônica, embora possa ocorrer em qualquer lugar do trato GI; composto de epitélio mucinoso que recobre delicadas projeções vasculares; costumam ocorrer alterações malignas com freqüência; hipersecreção ocorre raramente. Também conhecido como adenoma. SIN papillary a. of large intestine.
ad·e·no·ma·toid (ad-ē-nō′mă-toyd). Adenomatóide; semelhante a um adenoma.
ad·e·no·ma·to·sis (ad′ē-nō-mă-tō′sis). Adenomatose; condição caracterizada por proliferações glandulares múltiplas.
erosive a. of nipple, a. erosiva do mamilo. SIN subareolar duct *papillomatosis*.
familial multiple endocrine a., [MIM*131100], a. endócrino múltiplo familiar. SIN multiple endocrine *neoplasia*.
fibrosing a., a. fibrosante. SIN sclerosing *adenosis*.
multiple endocrine a., a. endócrino múltiplo. SIN multiple endocrine *neoplasia*.
pulmonary a., a. pulmonar; doença neoplásica em que os alvéolos e os brônquios distais estão cheios de muco e células epiteliais colunares secretoras de muco; caracteriza-se por escarro abundante, extremamente viscoso, calafrios, febre, tosse, dispnéia e dor pleurítica.
ad·e·nom·a·tous (ad-ē-nō′mă-tŭs). Adenomatoso; relativo a um adenoma e a alguns tipos de hiperplasia glandular.
ad·e·no·meg·a·ly (ad′ē-nō-meg′ă-lē). Adenomegalia; aumento de uma glândula. [adeno- + G. *megas*, grande]
ad·e·no·mere (ad′ē-nō-mēr). Adenômero; unidade estrutural no parênquima de uma glândula em desenvolvimento que se torna a parte funcional do órgão. [adeno- + G. *meros*, parte]
ad·e·no·my·o·ma (ad′ē-nō-mī-ō′mă). Adenomioma; neoplasia benigna do músculo (geralmente músculo liso) com elementos glandulares; ocorre mais freqüentemente no útero e nos ligamentos uterinos. [G. *adēn*, glândula, + *mys*, músculo, + *-oma*, tumor]
ad·e·no·my·o·sis (ad′ē-nō-mī-ō′sis). Adenomiose; ocorrência ectópica ou implantação difusa de tecido adenomatoso no músculo (geralmente músculo liso). [G. *adēn*, glândula, + *mys*, músculo, + *-osis*, condição]
a. u′teri, a. uterina; invasão benigna do miométrio por tecido endometrial.
ad·e·nop·a·thy (ad-ē-nop′ă-thē). Adenopatia; inflamação ou aumento mórbido dos gânglios linfáticos. [adeno- + G. *pathos*, sofrimento]
ad·e·no·phleg·mon (ad′ē-nō-fleg′mon). Adenofleimão; inflamação aguda

de uma glândula e de um tecido conjuntivo adjacente. [adeno- + G. *phlegmonē*, inflamação]

Ad·e·no·pho·ra·si·da (ad′ē-nō-fō-ras′i-dă). Adenoforasídeos; classe de nematóides sem canais laterais abrindo para o sistema excretor e sem plasmídio; com pouca ou nenhuma papila caudal, ovos não-segmentados e com tampões polares ou eclosão *in utero*. Inclui os gêneros *Trichuris*, *Capillaria* e *Trichinella* entre parasitas importantes do homem e de animais domésticos. VER TAMBÉM Secernentasida. SIN Adenophorea, Aphasmidia. [G. *adēn*, glândula, + *phōr*, ladrão]

Ad·e·no·pho·rea (ad′ē-nō-fō′rē-ă). SIN Adenophorasida.

ad·e·no·sal·pin·gi·tis (ad′ē-nō-sal-pin-jī′tis). Adenossalpingite. SIN *salpingitis isthmica nodosa*.

ad·e·no·sar·co·ma (ad′ē-nō-sar-kō′mă). Adenossarcoma; neoplasia maligna que se origina, simultânea ou consecutivamente, no tecido mesodérmico e no epitélio glandular da mesma região.

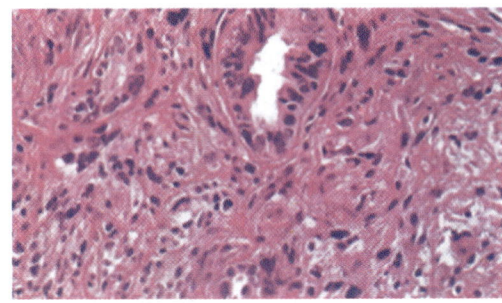

adenocarcinoma mülleriano do útero: preparado histológico mostrando componentes malignos de origem epitelial e mesenquimal

müllerian a., a. mülleriano; tumor do útero ou ovário, com baixo grau de malignidade, caracterizado por glândulas de aspecto benigno e estroma sarcomatoso.

ad·e·nose (ad′ē-nōs). Adenoso; relativo a, ou semelhante a, uma glândula.

aden·o·sine (Ado) (ă-den′ō-sēn). Adenosina. **1.** Produto da condensação da adenina e D-ribose; nucleosídeo encontrado entre os produtos da hidrólise de todos os ácidos nucleicos e dos diversos nucleotídeos da adenina. A a. se acumula na imunodeficiência combinada grave. **2.** Potente dilatador coronário usado no lugar do exercício para os estudos de perfusão miocárdica com radionuclídeos. SIN 9-β-D-ribofuranosyladenine.
a. cyclic phosphate, fosfato de adenosina cíclico. VER adenosine 3′,5′-cyclic monophosphate.
a. deaminase, a. desaminase; enzima encontrada nos tecidos de mamíferos capaz de catalisar a desaminação de adenosina, formando inosina e amônia. A deficiência de a. pode levar a uma forma de imunodeficiência combinada grave.
a. diphosphate, difosfato de adenosina. VER adenosine 5′-diphosphate.
a. kinase, a. cinase; enzima catalisadora da transferência de um grupamento fosfato do MgATP para a adenosina, formando MgADP e AMP. Uma importante etapa na recuperação de nucleosídeos.
a. monophosphate (AMP), monofosfato de adenosina; especificamente, 5′-monofosfato de adenosina. VER adenylic acid.
a. nucleosidase, enzima que hidrolisa a adenosina em adenina e D-ribose.
a. phosphate, fosfato de adenosina; especificamente, 3′- ou 5′-fosfato de adenosina. VER adenylic acid.
a. tetraphosphate, tetrafosfato de adenosina; produto da condensação de adenosina com ácido tetrafosfórico na posição 5′.
a. triphosphate, trifosfato de adenosina. SIN adenosine 5′-triphosphate.

aden·o·sine 3′,5′-cy·clic mono·phos·phate (cAMP). 3′,5′-monofosfato cíclico de adenosina (AMPc); ativador da fosforilase cinase e efetor de outras enzimas, formado no músculo a partir do ATP pela adenilato ciclase e decomposto em 5′-AMP por uma fosfodiesterase; o primeiro composto é chamado de "segundo mensageiro". É um regulador metabólico. Um composto correlato (2′,3′) também é conhecido. SIN cyclic adenylic acid, cyclic AMP, cyclic phosphate.

aden·o·sine 3′,5′-cy·clic phos·phate phos·pho·di·es·ter·ase. Fosfodiesterase de 3′,5′-fosfato cíclico de adenosina; enzima que catalisa a hidrólise de 3′,5′-fosfato cíclico de adenosina formando 5′-AMP. Etapa fundamental na regulação dos níveis celulares de 3′,5′-fosfato cíclico de adenosina. É inibida pela cafeína. SIN cAMP phosphodiesterase.

aden·o·sine 5′-di·phos·phate (ADP). 5′-difosfato de adenosina; produto da condensação de adenosina com ácido pirofosfórico, formado a partir do ATP pela hidrólise do grupamento fosfato terminal do último composto.

aden·o·sine 3′-phos·phate. 3′-fosfato de adenosina; ácido 3′-adenílico. VER adenylic acid.

aden·o·sine 5′-phos·phate. 5′-fosfato de adenosina; ácido 5′-adenílico. VER adenylic acid.

aden·o·sine 3′-phos·phate 5′-phos·pho·sul·fate (PAPS). 3′-fosfato, 5-fosfossulfato de adenosina (PAPS); intermediário na formação de sulfatos etéreos urinários, notável por conter uma ligação fosfato de "alta energia"; o 3′-OH da adenosina é substituído por –OPO$_3$H$_2$, o 5′-OH por –OP(O$_2$H) – OSO$_3$H. SIN active sulfate.

ad·e·no·sine 5′-phos·pho·sul·fate (APS). 5′-fosfossulfato de adenosina; intermediário na formação de PAPS (sulfato ativo).
adenosine 5′-phosphosulfate kinase, quinase de 5′-fosfossulfato de adenosina; enzima que catalisa a formação de sulfato ativo a partir de 5′-fosfossulfato de adenosina e ATP.

ad·e·no·sine tri·phos·pha·tase (ATPase) (a-den′ō-sēn-trī-fos′fă-tās). Adenosina trifosfatase; enzima que catalisa a liberação do grupamento fosfato terminal de 5′-trifosfato de adenosina; visualizada citoquimicamente em várias membranas celulares, mitocôndrias e na banda A de sarcômeros do músculo estriado, associada à miosina.

aden·o·sine 5′-tri·phos·phate (ATP). 5′-trifosfato de adenosina; pirofosfato de adenosina (5); adenosina com ácido trifosfórico esterificado em sua posição 5′; precursores imediatos de nucleotídeos adenina no RNA. A energia primária de troca de todas as células. SIN adenosine triphosphate.

ad·e·no·sis (ad-ĕ-nō′sis). Adenose. **1.** Termo raramente empregado para doença glandular mais ou menos generalizada. **2.** Tecido glandular em um ou mais locais nos quais ele não costuma ser encontrado.
blunt duct a., adenose da mama, em que os canais estão dilatados mas não aumentados em número.
fibrosing a., a. fibrosante. SIN sclerosing a.
microglandular a., a. microglandular; a. da mama na qual existem grupos irregulares de pequenos túbulos nos tecidos fibrosos ou adiposos, assemelhando-se ao carcinoma tubular mas sem proliferação fibroblástica do estroma.
sclerosing a., a. esclerosante; lesão nodular benigna da mama que ocorre com mais freqüência em mulheres relativamente jovens e consiste em lóbulos hiperplásicos distorcidos de tecido acinar com estroma colágeno aumentado; pode ser difícil distinguir microscopicamente as alterações de carcinoma. Além disso, uma lesão nodular microscópica benigna da próstata, que consiste em tecido acinar com estroma aumentado; a camada de células basais exibe metaplasia característica do músculo liso. SIN adenofibrosis, fibrosing adenomatosis, fibrosing a.

aden·o·syl (a-den′ō-sil). Adenosil; o radical de adenosina menos um H ou OH de um dos grupamentos OH do ribosil, em geral o 5′, p. ex., *S*-adenosil-L-metionina.

ad·e·no·sylco·bal·a·min (a-den′ō-sil-kō-bal′ă-min). Adenosilcobalamina; derivado da vitamina B$_{12}$; sua biossíntese deficiente pode levar à acidemia metilmalônica.

S-aden·o·syl-L-ho·mo·cys·te·ine (a-den′ō-sil-hō-mō-sis′te-ēn). *S*-adenosil-L-homocisteína; composto formado pela desmetilação de *S*-adenosil-L-metionina.

S-aden·o·syl-L-me·thi·o·nine (SAM, AdoMet) (a-den′ō-sil-me-thī′ō-nēn). Produto da condensação de adenosina e L-metionina, envolvendo a substituição de –OPO$_3$H$_2$ do ácido adenílico por –S$^+$(CH$_3$)CH$_2$CH$_2$CH(NH$_3^+$)CO$_2^-$ da metionina; um composto sulfônico portando um grupamento metila que é transferido nas reações de transmetilação. VER TAMBÉM *methionine* adenosyltransferase. SIN active methionine.

ad·e·not·o·my (ad-ĕ-not′ō-mē). Adenotomia; incisão de uma glândula. [adeno- + G. *tomē*, corte]

ad·e·no·ton·sil·lec·to·my (ad′ē-nō-ton-si-lek′tō-mē). Adenotonsilectomia; remoção cirúrgica de tonsilas e adenóides.

ad·e·nous (ad′ē-nŭs). Termo raramente empregado para adenose.

Ad·e·no·vi·ri·dae (ad′ē-nō-vir′i-dē). Família de vírus com DNA de duplo filamento, comumente conhecidos como adenovírus, que se desenvolvem no núcleo de células infectadas em mamíferos e aves. O vírion tem 70 a 90 nm de diâmetro, é resistente ao éter, mas não tem invólucro; os capsídeos são icosaédricos e compostos de 252 capsômeros. A família inclui dois gêneros: Mastadenovirus e Aviadenovirus.

ad·e·no·vi·rus (ad′ē-nō-vī′rŭs). Adenovírus; vírus adenóide-faríngeo-conjuntival ou A-P-C; qualquer vírus da família Adenoviridae. Mais de 40 tipos são conhecidos por infectar seres humanos causando sintomas no trato respiratório superior, doença respiratória aguda, conjuntivite, gastroenterite, cistite hemorrágica e infecções graves em neonatos. SIN A-P-C virus, adenoidal-pharyngeal-conjunctival virus. [G. *adēn*, glândula, + vírus]
canine a. 1, a. canino; vírus que causa hepatite canina infecciosa em cães. SIN Rubarth disease virus.

ad·e·nyl (ad′e-nil). Adenil; radical ou íon da adenina; utilizado freqüentemente no lugar de adenilil, como no ácido adenilsuccínico.

aden·y·late (a-den′i-lāt). Adenilato; sal ou éster do ácido adenílico.
a. cyclase, a. ciclase; enzima que age no ATP para formar AMP 3′,5′-cíclico mais pirofosfato. Uma etapa fundamental na regulação e formação de segundos mensageiros. SIN 3′,5′-cyclic AMP synthethase.

a. kinase [EC 2.7.4.3], a. cinase; cinase do ácido adenílico; uma fosfotransferase que catalisa a fosforilação reversível de uma molécula de ADP por MgADP, liberando MgATP e AMP. SIN adenylic acid kinase, myokinase.

ad·e·nyl cy·clase (ad′e-nil sī′klās). Adenil ciclase; enzima que converte monofosfato de adenosina em monofosfato cíclico de adenosina, um segundo mensageiro intracelular de ativação neural e hormonal.

ad·e·nyl·ic ac·id (ad-e-nil′ik). Ácido adenílico; produto da condensação de adenosina e ácido fosfórico; nucleotídeo encontrado entre os produtos da hidrólise de todos os ácidos nucleicos. O ácido 3′-adenílico (3′-monofosfato de adenosina) e o ácido 5′-adenílico (5′-monofosfato de adenosina [AMP]) diferem quanto ao local de fixação do ácido fosfórico na D-ribose; o ácido desoxiadenílico difere por ter um H em vez de OH na posição 2′ da D-ribose. VER TAMBÉM AMP. SIN adenine nucleotide.

cyclic a. a., a. a. cíclico. SIN adenosine 3′,5′-cyclic monophosphate.
a. a. deaminase, desaminase do a. a. SIN AMP deaminase.
a. a. kinase, cinase do a. a. SIN adenylate kinase.

ad·e·nyl·o·suc·ci·nase (ad′e-nil-ō-sŭk′sin-ās). Adenil succinase. SIN adenylosuccinate lyase.

ad·e·nyl·o·suc·ci·nate ly·ase (ad′e-nil-ō-sŭk′sin-āt). Adenililsuccinato liase; enzima catalisadora da clivagem não-hidrolítica do ácido adenilsuccínico, produzindo AMP e fumarato, e também do nucleotídeo de 4-(N-succinocarboxamido)-5-aminoimidazol para fornecer fumarato e aminoimidazol carboxamida ribosil-5-fosfato. Ambas são etapas na biossíntese do nucleotídeo da purina. SIN adenylosuccinase, adenylylosuccinate lyase.

ad·e·nyl·o·suc·ci·nate syn·thase. Adenilsuccinato sintase; ligase que catalisa a formação de adenilsuccinato, GDP e P$_i$ a partir do ácido inosínico, aspartato e GTP. Importante enzima na biossíntese do nucleotídeo da purina. SIN adenylylosuccinate synthase, IMP-aspartate ligase.

ad·e·nyl·o·suc·cin·ic ac·id (sAMP) (ad′e-nil-ō-sŭk′sin-ik). Ácido adenilsuccínico; produto da condensação de ácido aspártico e 5′-monofosfato de inosina; intermediário na biossíntese do ácido adenílico. Formalmente, trata-se do ácido adenílico com ácido succínico substituindo um H do grupamento NH$_2$, formando uma ligação C–N. SIN adenylylosuccinic acid, N-succinyladenylic acid.

aden·y·lyl (a-den′i-lil). Adenilil; o radical do ácido adenílico menos um OH do grupamento fosfórico; freqüentemente encurtado para adenil em nomes compostos, como ácido adenilsuccínico.

a. cyclase, a. ciclase; nome anterior de *adenylate* cyclase (adenilato ciclase).

aden·y·lyl·o·suc·ci·nate ly·ase (a-den′i-lil-ō-sŭk′sin-āt). Adenililsuccinato liase. SIN adenylosuccinate lyase.

aden·y·lyl·o·suc·ci·nate syn·thase, adenililsuccinato sintase. SIN adenylosuccinate synthase.

aden·y·lyl·o·suc·cin·ic ac·id (a-den′i-lil-ō-sŭk′sin-ik). Ácido adenililsuccínico. SIN adenylosuccinic acid.

aden·y·lyl·sul·fate ki·nase. Adenililsulfato cinase. VER *adenosine 5′-phosphosulfate* kinase.

a·deps, gen. **adi·pis, adi·pes** (ad′eps, ad′i-pis, -pēz). **1.** Indica gordura ou tecido adiposo. **2.** Banha de porco derretida, usada na preparação de pomadas. SIN lard. VER TAMBÉM a. lanae. [L. banha, gordura]

a. lanae, lanolina; substância gordurosa obtida da lã da ovelha *Ovis aries* (família Bovidae). Utilizada como base emoliente para cremes e pomadas. SIN hydrous wool fat, lanolin, wool wax. [L. gordura da lã]

a. re′nis, termo obsoleto para a camada de tecido adiposo ("cápsula de gordura") que envolve o rim (gordura perirrenal).

ader·mia (ā-der′mē-ā). Adermia; ausência congênita de pele. [G. *a-* priv. + *derma*, pele]

ADH Abreviatura de antidiuretic *hormone* (hormônio antidiurético); alcohol dehydrogenase (álcool desidrogenase).

ad·her·ence (ad-hēr′ens). **1.** Aderência; ato ou qualidade de aderir a alguma coisa. VER TAMBÉM adhesion. **2.** Adesão, aquiescência; o quanto um paciente continua a concordar com o modo de tratamento sem supervisão. Cf. compliance (2), maintenance. [L. *adhaereo*, aderir]

immune a., a. imune; união de células por meio de complexos antígeno-anticorpo que desencadearam a fixação do complemento; a aderência se dá com receptores do complemento apropriados.

ad·he·sins (ad-hē′zins). Adesinas; antígenos da superfície microbiana que existem freqüentemente sob a forma de projeções filamentosas (*pili* ou fímbrias) e se unem a receptores específicos nas membranas celulares epiteliais; geralmente classificadas segundo sua capacidade de induzir aglutinação de eritrócitos de diversas espécies, sua fixação diferencial a células epiteliais de diversas origens ou sua suscetibilidade à reversão dessas atividades de ligação na presença de manose. [L. *ad-haereo*, pp. *ad-haesum*, aderir + -in]

ad·he·sio, pl. **ad·he·si·o·nes** (ad-hē′zē-ō, ad-hē-zē-ō′nēz) [TA]. Adesão. SIN adhesion (1). [L]

a. interthalam′ica [TA], a. intertalâmica. SIN interthalamic adhesion.

ad·hes·i·ol·y·sis (ad-hēz-ē-ol′ō-sis). Adesiólise; separação de aderência(s) ou brida(s) feita por laparoscopia ou laparotomia. [adesão + lise]

ad·he·sion (ad-hē′zhŭn) [TA]. Adesão. **1.** Processo de aderência ou união de duas superfícies ou partes, especialmente a união de superfícies opostas de uma ferida. SIN adhesio [TA], conglutination (1). **2.** Nas cavidades pleural e peritoneal, faixas inflamatórias que unem superfícies serosas opostas. **3.** Atração física de moléculas desiguais entre si. **4.** Atração molecular existente entre superfícies de corpos em contato. [L. *adhaesio*, de *adhaereo*, aderir]

amnionic a.'s, a. amniônica. SIN amnionic band.

fibrinous a., a. fibrinosa; **(1)** uma aderência que consiste em finos filamentos de fibrina resultantes de exsudato de plasma ou linfa ou extravasamento de sangue; **(2)** múltiplos filamentos finos ou delicados de fibrina.

fibrous a., a. fibrosa; fortes filamentos fibrosos resultantes da organização de aderências fibrinosas, freqüentemente após procedimento operatório anterior, comumente observadas em pacientes com obstrução intestinal mecânica.

interthalamic a. [TA], a. intertalâmica; conexão variável entre as duas massas talâmicas através do terceiro ventrículo; ausente em cerca de 20% dos cérebros humanos. SIN adhesio interthalamica [TA], massa intermedia*, commisura cinerea, commisura grisea (1), intermediate mass.

primary a., a. primária. SIN healing by first intention.
secondary a., a. secundária. SIN healing by second intention.

ad·he·si·ot·o·my (ad-hē-sē-ot′ō-mē). Adesiotomia; secção cirúrgica ou lise de aderências.

ad·he·sive (ad-hē′siv). Adesivo. **1.** Relativo a uma aderência ou tendo suas características. **2.** Qualquer material que adere a uma superfície ou produz aderência entre superfícies.

adhib. Abreviatura de L. *adhibendus*, a ser administrado.

a·di·a·ba·tic (ā-dē-ā-bā′tik). Adiabático; que se refere a um processo termodinâmico no qual não há perda ou ganho de calor entre o sistema e seus arredores. [G. *adiabatos*, impermeável, de *a* priv. + *diabainō*, atravessar]

ad·i·ad·o·cho·ci·ne·sia, ad·i·ad·o·cho·ci·ne·sis (ā-dī′ā-dō-kō-si-nē′sē-ā,-sis). Adiadococinesia, adiadococinese. SIN adiadochokinesis. [G. *a-* priv. + *diadochos*, sucessivo, + *kinēsis*, movimento]

ad·i·ad·o·cho·ki·ne·sis (ā-dī′ā-dō-kō-kin-ē′sis). Adiadococinese; incapacidade de realizar movimentos alternativos rápidos. Uma das manifestações clínicas de disfunção cerebelar. VER TAMBÉM dysdiadochokinesia Cf. diadochokinesia. SIN adiadochocinesia, adiadochocinesis, dysdiadochokinesis. [G. *a-* priv. + *diadochos*, sucessivo, + *kinēsis*, movimento]

adi·a·pho·re·sis (ā′dī-ā-fō-rē′sis). Adiaforese. SIN anhidrosis. [G. *a-* priv. + *diaphorēsis*, transpiração]

adi·a·pho·ret·ic (ā-dī-ā-fō-ret′ik). Adiaforético. SIN anhidrotic.

adi·a·pho·ria (ā-dī-ā-fō′rē-ā). Adiaforia; incapacidade de responder a um estímulo depois de uma série de estímulos anteriormente aplicados. [G. *a-* priv. + *dia*, através, + *phoros*, condução]

adi·a·spi·ro·my·co·sis (ā′dē-ā-spī′rō-mī-kō′sis). Adiaspiromicose; rara micose pulmonar de seres humanos, de roedores e de outros animais que escavam o solo ou são aquáticos, causada pelo fungo *Emmonsia parva* var. *crescens*.

adi·a·spore (ā′dē-ā-spōr). Adiásporo; esporo fúngico que, quando cresce nos pulmões de um animal, ou é incubado *in vitro* a temperaturas elevadas, aumenta enormemente de tamanho sem reprodução ou replicação. [G. *a-* priv. + *dia*, através, + *sporos*, sementes]

adi·as·to·le (ā-dī-as′tō-lē). Adiástole; ausência ou imperceptibilidade do movimento diastólico do coração; anormalidade funcional ventricular diastólica. Uso mais freqüentemente europeu. [G. *a-* priv. + *diastolē*, dilatação]

adi·a·ther·man·cy (ā-dī-ā-ther′man-sē). Adiatermância, adicitermia. Impenetrabilidade às ondas de calor. [G. *dia-thermainō*, aquecer através de, de *a-* priv. + *dia*, através, + *thermē*, calor]

Adie, William J., médico australiano. 1886–1935. VER A. *pupil syndrome*; Holmes-Adie *pupil*; Holmes-Adie *syndrome*.

ad·i·em·or·rhy·sis (ad′i-em-ōr′i-sis). Adiemórrise; parada da circulação capilar. [G. *a-* priv. + *dia*, através, + *haima*, sangue, + *rhysis*, fluxo]

Adin·i·da (ā-din′i-dā). Subordem de dinoflagelados na qual os flagelos são livres e não permanecem em sulcos. [G. *a-* priv. + *diēn*, remoinho]

♲ **adip-, adipo-.** Adipo; gordura, gorduroso. Formas correspondentes ao G. lip-, lipo-. VER TAMBÉM lipo-. [L. *adeps, adipis*, banha mole de animais; tecido adiposo; obesidade; semelhante a G. *aleipha*, ungüento, óleo, pomada, gordura, resina; *lipos*, gordura animal, banha, sebo, óleo vegetal]

adiph·e·nine hy·dro·chlo·ride (ā-dif′ē-nen). Cloridrato de adifenina; agente espasmólico empregado para diminuir o espasmo das vias biliares, tubo digestivo, útero e ureter.

adip·ic ac·id (ā-dip′ik). Ácido adípico; ácido hexanodióico; o ácido dicarboxílico HOOC(CH$_2$)$_4$COOH.

ad·i·pi·o·done. Adipiodona. SIN iodipamide.

♲ **adipo-.** VER adip-.

ad·i·po·cel·lu·lar (ad′i-pō-sel′ū-lar). Adipocelular; relativo aos tecidos adiposo e celular ou ao tecido conjuntivo com muitas células gordurosas.

ad·i·po·cer·a·tous (ad-i-pō-ser′ā-tŭs). Adipoceratoso; relativo ao adipócero. SIN lipoceratous.

ad·i·po·cere (ad′i-pō-sēr). Adipocera; graxa de cadáveres. Substância gordurosa de consistência cérea à qual tecidos animais mortos (como os de um cadáver) são, às vezes, convertidos quando isolados do ar sob condições favoráveis de temperatura e umidade. SIN grave wax, lipocere. [adipo- + L. *cera,* cera]

ad·i·po·cyte (ad′i - pō - sit). Adipócito. SIN fat cell.
ad·i·po·gen·e·sis (ad′i - pō - jen′e - sis). Adipogênese. SIN lipogenesis.
ad·i·po·gen·ic, ad·i·pog·e·nous (ad′i - pō - jen′ik, ad - i - poj′e - nŭs). Adipogênico. SIN lipogenic.
ad·i·poid (ad′i - poyd). Adipóide. SIN lipoid. [adipo- + G. *eidos,* semelhante]
ad·i·po·ki·net·ic (ad′i - pō - ki - net′ik). Adipocinético; indica uma substância ou fator que produz mobilização dos lipídios armazenados. [adipo- + G. *kinēsis,* movimento]
ad·i·po·ki·nin (ad - i - pō - kī′nin). Adipocinina; hormônio da hipófise anterior (adeno-hipófise) que produz mobilização da gordura de tecidos adiposos. SIN adipokinetic hormone.
ad·i·pom·e·ter (ad - i - pom′e - ter). Adipômetro; instrumento para determinar a espessura da pele. [adipo- + G. *metron,* medida]
ad·i·po·ne·cro·sis (ad′i - pō - ne - krō′sis). Adiponecrose; termo raramente empregado para necrose da gordura, como na pancreatite hemorrágica.
ad·i·po·sal·gia (ad′i - pō - sal′jē - ă). Adiposalgia; condição na qual se desenvolvem áreas dolorosas de gordura subcutânea. [adipo- + G. *algos,* dor]
ad·i·pose (ad′i - pōs). Adiposo; indica gordura.
ad·i·po·sis (ad - i - pō′sis). Adipose; acúmulo local ou geral excessivo de gordura no organismo. SIN lipomatosis, liposis (1), steatosis (1). [adipo- + G. *-osis,* condição]
  a. cerebra′lis, a. cerebral; obesidade resultante de doença intracraniana, mais comumente do hipotálamo, provocando hiperfagia.
  a. doloro′sa, a. dolorosa; condição caracterizada por depósito de massas nodulares ou pendulares simétricas de gordura em várias regiões orgânicas, com desconforto ou dor. SIN Anders disease, Dercum disease, lipomatosis neurotica.
  a. or′chica, distrofia adiposogenital. SIN adiposogenital *dystrophy.*
  a. tubero′sa sim′plex, a. tuberosa simples; condição semelhante à a. dolorosa em que a gordura ocorre em pequenas massas nodulares sensíveis ao tato, podendo ser espontaneamente dolorosas no abdome ou nos membros.
  a. universa′lis, a. universal; deposição excessiva de gordura em todas as partes do organismo, incluindo as vísceras.
ad·i·pos·i·ty (ad - i - pos′i - tē). **1.** Obesidade. SIN obesity. **2.** Adiposidade; acúmulo excessivo de gordura em um local ou órgão.
ad·i·po·su·ria (ad′i - pō - soo′rē - ă). Adiposúria. SIN lipuria. [adipo- + G. *ouron,* urina]
adip·sia, adip·sy (ă - dip′sē - ă, - dip′sē). Adipsia; ausência de sede ou falta do desejo de beber. [G. *a-* priv. + *dipsa,* sede]
ad·i·tus (ad′i - tŭs) [TA]. Ádito. SIN aperture, inlet. [L. acesso, de *ad-eo,* pp. *-itus,* ir]
  a. ad an′trum [TA], a. ao antro. SIN a. to mastoid antrum.
  a. ad antrum mastoideum [TA], a. ao antro mastóideo. SIN a. to mastoid antrum.
  a. ad aqueduc′tum cer′ebri, abertura do aqueduto do mesencéfalo. SIN opening of aqueduct of mid-brain.
  a. ad infundib′ulum [TA], recesso do infundíbulo. SIN infundibular *recess.*
  a. ad sac′cum perito ne′i mino′rem, forame omental. SIN omental *foramen.*
  a. glot′tidis infe′rior, a. da glote inferior. SIN infraglottic *cavity.*
  a. glot′tidis supe′rior, a. da glote superior. SIN intermediate laryngeal *cavity.*
  laryngeal a. [TA], a. da laringe; SIN laryngeal *inlet.*
  a. laryn′gis [TA], a. da laringe. SIN laryngeal *inlet.*
  a. to mastoid antrum [TA]. a. ao antro mastóideo; orifício que vai do recesso epitimpânico ao antro mastóideo. SIN a. ad antrum mastoideum [TA], a. ad antrum [TA], aperture of mastoid antrum.
  a. or′bitae [TA], a. orbital.; SIN orbital *opening.*
  a. pel′vis, abertura da pelve. SIN pelvic *inlet.*
ad·just·ment (ă - jŭst′ment). Ajustamento. **1.** Em odontologia, qualquer modificação feita em uma prótese fixa ou removível durante ou após a sua inserção para adaptação e função perfeitas. **2.** Adaptação, acomodação. SIN adaptation (6). **3.** Procedimento de resumo para uma medida estatística no qual os efeitos das diferenças na composição de populações sendo comparadas foram minimizados por métodos estatísticos.
  occlusal a., a. oclusal; modificação das superfícies oclusivas e incisivas dos dentes para desenvolver uma relação harmoniosa entre essas superfícies.
ad·ju·vant (ad′joo - vănt). Adjuvante. **1.** Substância acrescentada a uma prescrição e que afeta a ação do ingrediente ativo de maneira previsível. **2.** Em imunologia, veículo empregado para reforçar a antigenicidade; p.ex., suspensão de minerais (alume, hidróxido ou fosfato de alumínio) em que o antígeno é absorvido; ou uma emulsão de água e óleo na qual a solução antigênica é emulsificada em óleo mineral (a. incompleto de Freund), às vezes com a inclusão de micobactérias mortas (a. completo de Freund) para aumento adicional da antigenicidade (inibe a degradação do antígeno e/ou causa influxo de macrófagos). **3.** Terapia adicional administrada para aumentar ou ampliar o efeito da terapia primária, como na adição de quimioterapia ao esquema cirúrgico. **4.** Tratamento adicionado a um tratamento curativo para prevenir a recorrência de câncer clínico a partir de doença residual microscópica. [L. *adjuvo,* pres. p. *-juvans,* ajudar]
  Freund a., a. de Freund. VER adjuvant.
  Freund complete a., a. completo de Freund; emulsão (óleo em água) de antígeno à qual se adicionam micobactérias ou bacilos da tuberculose mortos.
  Freund incomplete a., a. incompleto de Freund; emulsão de água em óleo do antígeno, sem micobactérias.
ADL. Abreviatura de activities of daily living (atividades cotidianas). VER activities of daily living *scale.*
Adler, Alfred, psiquiatra austríaco, 1870–1937. VER adlerian *psychology;* adlerian *psychoanalysis.*
Adler, Oscar, médico alemão, 1879–1932. VER A. *test.*
ad·le·ri·an (ad - ler′ē - an). Adleriano; relativo a Alfred Adler ou descrito por ele.
ad lib. Abreviatura de L. *ad libitum,* livremente, conforme o desejado, à vontade.
adm. aplicar. VER admov.
ad·me·di·al, ad·me·di·an (ad - mē′dē - ăl, - dē - an). Admediano; em direção ou próximo ao plano mediano.
ad·min·ic·u·lum, pl. **ad·min·ic·u·la** (ad - mi - nik′u - lŭm, - u - lă). Adminículo; que proporciona apoio a uma parte; em farmacologia, o que facilita a ação ou o efeito de um medicamento. [L. um repouso para a mão, prop. de *ad + manus,* mão]
  a. lin′eae al′bae, a. da linha alba; expansão fibrosa triangular, às vezes contendo algumas fibras musculares, que passa do ligamento pubiano superior para a superfície posterior da linha alba.
ad·mit·tance (ad - mit′ans). Admitância (recíproca da impedância). SIN immittance.
admov. Abreviatura de L. *admove,* aplicar.
ad·ner·val (ad - ner′val). Adneural. SIN adneural.
ad·neu·ral (ad - noor′ăl). Adneural. **1.** Localizado próximo a um nervo. **2.** Na direção de um nervo; referente a uma corrente elétrica que passa através do tecido muscular em direção ao ponto de entrada do nervo. SIN adnerval.
ad·nex·a, sing. **ad·nex·um** (ad - nek′să, - sŭm). Adnexo, anexo. SIN *accessory structures,* em *structure.* VER TAMBÉM appendage. [L. partes ligadas]
  a. o′culi, a. dos olhos. SIN accessory visual *structures,* em *structure.*
  a. u′teri, a. uterino. SIN uterine *appendages,* em *appendage.*
ad·nex·al (ad - nek′săl). Adnexo; relativo aos adnexos. SIN annexal.
ad·nex·ec·to·my (ad - nek - sek′tō - mē). Adnexectomia. **1.** Excisão de qualquer anexo. **2.** Em ginecologia, excisão da tuba de Falópio e do ovário — unilateral — ou excisão de ambas as tubas e ovários (anexos uterinos) — bilateral.
ad·nex·i·tis (ad - neks - ī′tis). Adnexite; inflamação dos adnexos uterinos. [L. *annexa,* anexos, + *-itis,* inflamação]
ad·nex·o·pexy (ad - neks′ō - pek - sē). Adnexopexia; operação para suspensão da tuba uterina e do ovário; em geral, a ooforopexia é realizada sem a suspensão da tuba. [L. *annexa,* anexos, + G. *pēxis,* fixação]
Ado Símbolo de adenosine (adenosina).
ad·o·les·cence (ad - ō - les′ens). Adolescência; período da vida que começa com a puberdade e termina com o crescimento e com a maturidade física completos. [L. *adolescentia*]
ad·o·les·cent (ad - ō - les′ent). Adolescente. **1.** Pertinente à adolescência. **2.** Indivíduo nessa fase de desenvolvimento.
AdoMet Abreviatura de *S*-adenosyl-L-methionine (*S*-adenosil-L-metionina).
adon·is (a - don′is). Planta medicinal obtida da *Adonis vernalis* (família Ranunculaceae), que cresce na Europa Ocidental e é utilizada para o tratamento de insuficiência cardíaca congestiva. Contém estrofantidina e glicosídeos cardiotônicos correlatos. SIN false hellebore. [G. *Adōnis,* figura mítica, do Fenício *adon,* lorde]
adon·i·tol (ă - don′i - tol). Adonitol. SIN ribitol.
ADP Abreviatura de adenosine 5′-diphosphate (5′-difosfato de adenosina).
ADPase. ADPase. SIN apyrase.
△ **adren-.** VER adreno-.
ad·re·nal (ă - drē′năl). **1.** Adrenal. Próximo ou sobre o rim; indicando a glândula supra-renal (glândula adrenal). **2.** Glândula supra-renal ou tecido ou produto dela separado. VER TAMBÉM suprarenal. [L. *ad,* para, + *ren,* rim]
  accessory a., a. acessória; uma ilhota de tecido cortical separada da glândula supra-renal, em geral encontrada nos tecidos retroperitoneais, rim ou órgãos genitais. SIN adrenal rest.
  Marchand a.'s, a. de Marchand; pequenas coleções de tecido a. acessório no ligamento largo do útero ou nos testículos. SIN Marchand rest.
ad·re·nal·ec·to·my (ă - drē - năl - ek′tō - mē). Adrenalectomia; remoção de uma ou de ambas as glândulas supra-renais. [adrenal + G. *ektomē,* excisão]
adren·a·line (ă - dren′ă - lin). Adrenalina, epinefrina. SIN epinephrine.
  a. oxidase, a. oxidase. SIN *amine* oxidase (flavin-containing).
ad·re·nal·ism. Adrenalismo, hiperadrenocorticalismo. SIN hypercorticoidism.
ad·re·nal·i·tis (ă - drē - năl - ī′tis). Adrenalite; inflamação da glândula supra-renal.
adren·a·lone (ă - dren′ă - lōn). Adrenalona; precursor da epinefrina em alguns processos industriais; agente adrenérgico tópico em oftalmologia.

adre·na·lop·a·thy (ă-drē-nă-lop'ă-thē). Adrenopatia; qualquer condição anormal das glândulas supra-renais. SIN adrenopathy. [adrenal + G. *pathos*, sofrimento]

ad·ren·ar·che (ad'ren-ar-kē). Adrenarca. **1.** Crescimento de pêlos axilares e púbicos durante a puberdade induzido pela hiperatividade do córtex supra-renal. **2.** Mudança fisiológica na puberdade produzida pela secreção adrenocortical de hormônios androgênicos ou seus precursores. [adren- + G. *arché*, começo]

ad·re·ner·gic (ad-rĕ-ner'jik). Adrenérgico. **1.** Relativo a células nervosas ou fibras do sistema nervoso autônomo que empregam a norepinefrina como seu neurotransmissor. Cf. cholinergic. **2.** Relativo a medicamentos que simulam as ações do sistema nervoso simpático. VER α-adrenergic *receptors*, em *receptor*, β-adrenergic *receptors*, em *receptor*. [adren- + G. *ergon*, trabalho]

adren·ic (ă-drē'nik). Adrenal; relativo à glândula supra-renal.

△ **adreno-, adrenal-, adren-.** Relativo à glândula supra-renal. [L. *ad*, para, próximo, + *ren*, rim, + -o- + -*alis*, que pertence a]

adre·no·cep·tive (ă-dren-ō-sep'tiv). Adrenoceptivo; referente a locais químicos em efetores com os quais o mediador adrenérgico se une. Cf. cholinoceptive.

adre·no·cep·tor (ă-drē'sep'tor). Adrenoceptor. SIN adrenergic *receptors*, em *receptor*.

adre·no·cor·ti·cal (ă-drē-nō-kōr'ti-kăl). Adrenocortical; que pertence ao córtex supra-renal.

adre·no·cor·ti·coid (ă-drē-nō-kor'ti-koid). Adrenocorticóide. SIN corticosteroid.

adre·no·cor·ti·co·mi·met·ic (ă-drē'nō-kōr'ti-kō-mi-met'ik). Adrenocorticomimético; que simula ou produz efeito semelhante à função adrenocortical. [adrenal + córtex + G. *mimētikos*, que imita]

adre·no·cor·ti·co·tro·pic, adre·no·cor·ti·co·tro·phic (ă-drē'nō-kōr'ti-kō-trō'pik, -trō'fik). Adrenocorticotrópico, adrenocorticotrófico; que estimula o crescimento do córtex da supra-renal ou a secreção de seus hormônios. SIN adrenotropic, adrenotrophic. [córtex da supra-renal + G. *trophé*, nutrição; *tropé*, uma volta]

adre·no·cor·ti·co·tro·pin (ă-drē'nō-kōr-ti-kō-trō'pin). Adrenocorticotropina. SIN adrenocorticotropic *hormone*.

adre·no·gen·ic, adre·nog·e·nous (ă-drē-nō-jen'ik, a-drē-noj'ē-nŭs). Adrenogênico, adrenogenoso; de origem supra-renal. [adreno- + G. -*gen*, produzindo]

adre·no·leu·ko·dys·tro·phy (ALD) (ă-drē'nō-loo-kō-dis'trō-fē). [MIM*300100]. Adrenoleucodistrofia; distúrbio recessivo ligado ao X, que acomete homens jovens, caracterizado por insuficiência adrenocortical crônica, hiperpigmentação cutânea, demência progressiva, paralisia espástica e outros distúrbios intelectuais e neurológicos; deve-se à degeneração da mielina na substância branca cerebral. O gene causador é mapeado em Xq e codifica a proteína da a. (ALDP), um transportador de ligação ao ATP localizado na membrana peroxissômica.

adre·no·lyt·ic (ă-dren-ō-lit'ik). Adrenolítico; indica antagonismo, inibição ou bloqueio da ação da epinefrina, da norepinefrina e dos simpaticomiméticos relacionados. VER TAMBÉM adrenergic blocking *agent*. [adreno- + G. *lysis*, afrouxamento, dissolução]

adre·no·meg·a·ly (ă-drē-nō-meg'ă-lē). Adrenomegalia; hipertrofia de uma ou de ambas as glândulas supra-renais. [adreno- + G. *megas*, grande]

adre·no·mi·met·ic (ă-drē'nō-mi-met'ik). Adrenomimético; que exerce ação semelhante à dos compostos epinefrina e norepinefrina liberados da medula da supra-renal e dos nervos adrenérgicos; termo proposto para substituir o termo menos exato, simpaticomimético. Cf. adrenergic, cholinomimetic. [adreno- + G. *mimētikos*, imitativo]

adre·no·my·e·lo·neu·rop·a·thy (ad-rē'nō-mī'e-lō-noo-rop'a-thē). Adrenomieloneuropatia; distúrbio que ocorre em homens adultos consistindo em insuficiência renal de longa data, hipogonadismo, mielopatia progressiva, neuropatia periférica e distúrbios esfincterianos; considerado uma variante da adrenoleucodistrofia. [adreno- + G. *myelos*, medula, + *neuron*, nervo, + *pathos*, sofrimento]

adre·nop·a·thy (ă-drē-nop'ă-thē). Adrenopatia. SIN adrenalopathy.

adrenopause. Adrenopausa; diminuição do funcionamento das glândulas supra-renais com o envelhecimento, análoga à menopausa.

adre·no·pri·val (ă-drē-nō-prī'văl). Adrenoprivo; termo raramente empregado que indica a perda de função da supra-renal em consequência de doença ou excisão cirúrgica. [adreno- + L. *privo*, privar]

adre·no·re·ac·tive (ă-drē'nō-rē-ak'tiv). Adrenorreativo; que responde às catecolaminas.

adre·no·re·cep·tors (ă-drē'nō-rē-sep'terz). Adrenorreceptores. SIN adrenergic *receptors*, em *receptor*.

adre·nos·ter·one (a-drē-nos'ter-ōn). Adrenosterona; androgênio isolado do córtex supra-renal. SIN andrenosterone.

adre·no·tox·in (ă-drē-nō-tok'sin). Adrenotoxina; substância tóxica para as glândulas supra-renais. [adreno- + toxina]

adre·no·tro·pic, adre·no·tro·phic (ă-drē-nō-trō'pik, -trō'fik). Adrenotrópico, adrenotrófico. SIN adrenocorticotropic.

adre·no·tro·pin (ă-drē-nō-trō'pin). Adrenotropina. SIN adrenocorticotropic *hormone*.

adri·a·my·cin (ā'drē-ă-mī'sin). Nome comercial da doxorrubicina. SIN doxorubicin.

ad sat Abreviatura do L. *ad saturatum*, até a saturação.

Adson, Alfred W., neurocirurgião norte-americano, 1887–1951. VER A. *test, forceps, maneuver;* Brown-A. *forceps*.

ad·sorb (ad-sōrb'). Adsorver; captar por adsorção. [L. *ad*, para, + *sorbeo*, sugar]

ad·sorb·ate (ad-sōr'bāt). Adsorbato; qualquer substância adsorvida.

ad·sorb·ent (ad-sōr'bent). Adsorvente. **1.** Substância que adsorve, isto é, uma substância sólida com a propriedade de fixar outra substância em sua superfície sem qualquer ligação covalente, p.ex., carvão ativado. **2.** Um antígeno ou anticorpo usado em adsorção imunológica.

ad·sorp·tion (ad-sōrp'shun). Adsorção; propriedade que apresenta uma substância sólida de atrair e manter em sua superfície um gás, líquido ou uma substância em solução ou em suspensão. Por exemplo, a condensação de um gás em uma superfície. Cf. adsorption. [L. *ad*, para, + *sorbeo*, sugar]

immune a., a. imunológica; **(1)** remoção de anticorpo (aglutinina ou precipitina) do anti-soro pelo uso de antígeno específico; depois de ocorrida a agregação, o complexo antígeno-anticorpo é separado por centrifugação ou filtração; **(2)** remoção de antígeno por anti-soro específico de modo semelhante.

ad·ster·nal (ad-ster'năl). Próximo ou em cima do esterno.

ad·ter·mi·nal (ad-ter'mi-năl). Em direção a terminações nervosas, inserções musculares ou extremidade de qualquer estrutura.

adult (ă-dŭlt'). **1.** Crescimento completo e maduro. **2.** Adulto; indivíduo completamente crescido e maduro. [L. *adultus*, adulto de *adolesco*, crescer]

adul·ter·ant (ă-dŭl'ter-ănt). Adulterante; uma impureza; um aditivo considerado como tendo um efeito indesejável ou que dilui o material ativo de modo a reduzir seu valor terapêutico ou monetário.

adul·ter·a·tion (ă-dŭl-ter-ā'shŭn). Adulteração; alteração de qualquer substância pela adição deliberada de um componente que não faz parte habitual dessa substância; em geral usada para significar que a substância é enfraquecida com o resultado.

adul·to·mor·phism (ă-dŭl-tō-mōr'fizm). Adultomorfismo; interpretação do comportamento de crianças em termos adultos.

adv. Abreviatura do L. *adversum*, contra.

ad·vance (ad-vans'). Avançar; mover-se para a frente. [Fr. *avancer*, mover-se para frente]

ad·vanced life sup·port. Apoio vital avançado; assistência médica de urgência definitiva, que inclui desfibrilação, desobstrução das vias respiratórias e o uso de medicamentos e tratamento clínico. Cf. basic life support.

ad·vance·ment (ad-vans'ment). Método cirúrgico no qual uma inserção tendinosa ou um retalho cutâneo é parcialmente separado ou liberado de sua inserção de modo que o tecido possa ser movido para um ponto mais distal.

capsular a., a. capsular; reinserção cirúrgica da porção anterior da cápsula de Tenon.

tendon a., a. do tendão; excisão do tendão de um músculo ocular e sua fixação em um local mais anterior no globo.

ad·ven·ti·tia (ad-ven-tish'ă). Adventícia; tecido conjuntivo mais superficial que reveste qualquer órgão, vaso ou outra estrutura que não é revestida por uma serosa; em vez disso, o revestimento é derivado apropriadamente do tecido conjuntivo circundante e não forma uma parte integrante desse órgão ou estrutura. A *Terminologia Anatomica* [TA] inclui a adventícia (*tunica adventitia*) dos seguintes órgãos: ducto deferente, esôfago, pelve renal, glândulas seminais e ureteres. SIN membrana adventitia (1), tunica adventitia. [L. *adventicius*, vindo de fora, estranho, de *ad*, para + *venio*, vir]

ad·ven·ti·tial (ad-ven-tish'ăl). Adventício; relativo ao revestimento externo de um vaso sanguíneo ou outra estrutura. SIN adventitious (3).

ad·ven·ti·tious (ad-ven-tish'ŭs). Adventício. **1.** Acessório; originário de uma fonte externa ou ocorrendo em um local ou de maneira incomuns. VER TAMBÉM extrinsic. **2.** Acidental, casual, fortuito; ocorre acidental ou espontaneamente, em oposição a causas naturais ou hereditárias. **3.** SIN adventitial.

ady·nam·ia (ă-dī-nam'ē-ă, ad-i-nā'mē-ă). Adinamia. **1.** SIN asthenia. **2.** Falta de atividade ou força motora. **3.** Termo obsoleto para íleo (*ileus*) paralítico. [G. *a-* priv. + *dynamis*, força]

a. episodica hereditaria, a.episódica hereditária; paralisia periódica hiperpotassêmica (hyperkalemic periodic *paralysis*), sem miotonia. VER entradas em paralysis.

△ **ady·nam·ic** (ă-dī-nam'ik). Adinâmico; relativo à adinamia.

△ **ae-**. No caso de palavras que começam assim e não são encontradas aqui, ver em e-.

Aeby, Christopher T., anatomista suíço, 1835–1885. VER A. *plane*.

Aedes (ā-ē'dēz). Gênero disseminado de pequenos mosquitos frequentemente encontrados em regiões tropicais e subtropicais. [G. *aēdēs*, desagradável, não-amistoso]

A. aegyp'ti, o mosquito da febre amarela, espécie que também é o vetor do patógeno do dengue; caracterizado por marcas brancas em forma de lira no tórax.

A. albopic'tus, espécie que é um vetor importante dos vírus do dengue, disseminado na bacia do Pacífico.

A. atlanticus, mosquitos da família Culicidae conhecidos por transmitirem os vírus que causam dengue, febre amarela e encefalite.

A. cabal'lus, espécie que é um vetor importante da febre do Vale Rift na África do Sul.

A. dorsalis, espécie de mosquito que é um vetor secundário ou suspeitado da encefalite eqüina do oeste.

A. leucocelae'nus, espécie que transmite a febre amarela na América do Sul.

A. melanimon, espécie de mosquito que é vetor da encefalite eqüina do oeste e do grupo Califórnia de encefalites.

A. mitchellae, espécie de mosquito que é um vetor secundário ou suspeitado da encefalite eqüina do leste.

A. nigromaculis, espécie de mosquito que é um vetor secundário ou suspeitado da encefalite eqüina do oeste e do grupo Califórnia de encefalites.

A. polynesien'sis, espécie que é um vetor importante da filaríase e do dengue na região da Polinésia.

A. sollic'itans, mosquito comum em marnotas e vetor da encefalomielite eqüina oriental do Atlântico e da Costa do Golfo nos Estados Unidos.

A. taeniorhynchus, espécie de mosquito que é um vetor da encefalite eqüina venezuelana e um vetor secundário ou suspeitado do grupo Califórnia de encefalites.

A. triseriatus, espécie de mosquito que é um vetor do grupo Califórnia de encefalites.

A. trivittatus, espécie de mosquito que é um vetor do grupo Califórnia de encefalites.

A. variegat'us, espécie vetora de parasitas filarianos nas Ilhas do Pacífico (grupo Gilbert e Ellice).

A. vexans, espécie de mosquito que é um vetor do grupo Califórnia de encefalites e um vetor secundário ou suspeitado da encefalite eqüina do leste.

Aelu·ro·stron·gy·lus (ē'loor-ō-stron'ji-lŭs). Gênero comum de verme pulmonar em gatos; caracóis e lesmas servem como hospedeiros intermediários, e os animais que ingerem lesmas podem servir como hospedeiros transportadores. [G. *ailuros,* gato, + L. Mod., do G. *strongylus,* redondo]

ae·quo·rin (ē'kwō-rin). Equorina; uma proteína bioluminescente, isolada da medusa *Aequorea,* que emite luz azul na presença de quantidades diminutas do íon cálcio; injetada por via intracelular e usada para medir íons cálcio livres transitórios dentro da célula. VER TAMBÉM fura-2, quin-2.

aer-, aero-. Formas combinantes indicando relações com o ar ou gás; aéreo, gasoso. [G. *aēr* (L. *aer*), ar]

aer·ate (ār'āte). Aerar. **1.** Suprir (o sangue) com oxigênio. **2.** Expor à circulação de ar para purificação. **3.** Suprir ou carregar (um líquido) com um gás, principalmente dióxido de carbono.

aer·en·do·car·dia (ār-en-dō-kar'dē-ă). Aerendocardia; presença de ar não-dissolvido no sangue dentro do coração. [aer- + G. *endon,* dentro, + *kardia,* coração]

aero-. VER aer-.

Aer·o·bac·ter (ār-ō-bak'ter). VER *Enterobacter.* [aero- + G. *baktērion,* um bastonete]

aer·obe (ār'ōb). Aeróbio. **1.** Organismo que consegue viver e crescer na presença de oxigênio. **2.** Organismo que consegue utilizar o oxigênio como um aceptor final de elétrons em uma cadeia respiratória. [aero- + G. *bios,* vida]

obligate a., a. obrigatório; organismo que não consegue viver nem crescer na ausência de oxigênio.

aer·o·bic (ār-ō'bik). Aeróbico, aeróbio. **1.** Aerófilo; que vive no ar. **2.** Relativo a um aeróbio. SIN aerophilic, aerophilous.

aer·o·bi·ol·o·gy (ār'ō-bī-ol'ō-jē). Aerobiologia; o estudo dos constituintes atmosféricos, vivos e não-vivos, de importância biológica, p.ex., esporos aerógenos, bactérias patogênicas, substâncias alergênicas, poluentes.

aer·o·bi·o·scope (ār-ō-bī'ō-skōp). Aerobiscópio; aparelho para determinar o teor bacteriano do ar. [aero- + G. *bios,* vida, + *skopeō,* ver]

aer·o·bi·o·sis (ār-ō-bī-ō'sis). Aerobiose; existência em uma atmosfera contendo oxigênio. [aero- + G. *biōsis,* modo de viver]

aer·o·bi·ot·ic (ār-ō-bī-ot'ik). Aerobiótico; relativo à aerobiose.

aer·o·cele (ār'ō-sēl). Aerocele; distensão de uma pequena cavidade natural com gás. [aero- + G. *kēlē,* tumor]

Aer·o·coc·cus (ār-ō-kok'ŭs). Aerococo; gênero de cocos Gram-positivos aeróbicos que ocorrem como saprófitas aerógenos; produzem α-hemólise em ágar-sangue e crescem na presença de 40% de bile. A espécie típica, *A. viridans,* é comumente isolada como parte da flora cutânea normal; apresenta baixa patogenicidade, mas tem sido relatada como uma rara causa de endocardite. [aero- + G. *kokkos,* amora]

aer·o·col·pos (ār-ō-kol'pos). Aerocolpo; termo obsoleto para distensão da vagina por gás. [aero- + G. *kolpos,* vagina, cavidade]

aer·o·der·mec·ta·sia (ar'ō-der-mek-tā'zē-ă). Aerodermectasia. SIN subcutaneous *emphysema.* [aero- + G. *derma,* pele, + *ektasis,* distensão]

aer·o·don·tal·gia (ār'ō-don-tal'jē-ă). Aerodontalgia; dor dentária produzida por pressão atmosférica aumentada ou reduzida. SIN aero-odontalgia, aero-odontodynia. [aero- + G. *odous,* dente, + *algos,* dor]

primary a., a. primária; dor dental associada à expansão de gases aprisionados dentro de um dente, como ocorre sob uma obturação ou em uma polpa infectada.

secondary a., a. secundária; dor que se irradia para a área dentária a partir de uma área de aerossinusite.

aer·o·don·tia (ār-ō-don'shē-ă). Aerodontia; a ciência dos efeitos da pressão atmosférica aumentada ou diminuída sobre os dentes. [aero- + G. *odous,* dente]

aer·o·dy·nam·ics (ār'ō-dī-nam'iks). Aerodinâmica; estudo do ar e de outros gases em movimento, das forças que os colocam em movimento e dos resultados desse movimento. [aero- + G. *dynamis,* força]

aer·o·dy·nam·ic size. Dimensão aerodinâmica; em aerossóis, o tamanho da partícula cuja densidade mais bem representa o comportamento aerodinâmico de uma partícula.

aer·o·gas·tria (ār-ō-gas'trē-ă). Aerogastria; distensão do estômago por gás.

blocked a., a. bloqueada; retenção de gases no estômago devido ao espasmo da região esfincteriana do esôfago inferior, que impede a eructação.

aer·o·gen (ār'ō-jen). Aerógeno; microrganismo formador de gás.

aer·o·gen·e·sis (ār-ō-jen'ē-sis). Aerogênese; produção de gás, como por microrganismos. [aero- + G. *genesis,* origem]

aer·o·gen·ic, aer·og·e·nous (ār-ō-jen'ik, -oj'ē-nŭs). Aerogênico, aerógeno; formador de gás.

aer·o·med·i·cine (ār-ō-med'i-sin). Aeromedicina. SIN aviation *medicine.*

aer·o·mo·nad (ār-ō-mō'nad). Aeromônada; termo vernacular usado para referir-se a qualquer membro do gênero *Aeromonas.*

Aer·o·mo·nas (ār-ō-mō'nas). Gênero de bactérias aeróbicas Gram-negativas, oxidase-positivas, anaeróbicas facultativas (família Vibrionaceae) contendo células bacilares a cocóides; as células móveis possuem um único flagelo, polar; algumas espécies não são móveis. O metabolismo desses microrganismos é tanto respiratório como fermentativo; as exigências nutricionais não são rígidas. Essas bactérias são encontradas na água e no esgoto; algumas são patogênicas para os animais de água doce e salgada e para os seres humanos. A espécie típica é a *A. hydrophila.*

A. hydroph'ila, espécie que causa celulite, infecções em feridas, diarréia aguda (veiculada por água e associada a frutos-do-mar), septicemia e infecções do trato urinário de seres humanos. Também causa a doença da perna vermelha das rãs. É a espécie típica de *Aeromonas.*

aer·o·o·don·tal·gia (ār'ō-ō-don-tal'jē-ă). Aerodontalgia. SIN aerodontalgia.

aer·o·o·don·to·dyn·ia (ār'ō-ō-don-tō-din'ē-ă). Aerodontalgia. SIN aerodontalgia

aer·o·pause (ār'ō-pawz). Aeropausa; região superior da atmosfera, entre a estratosfera e o espaço externo, na qual as partículas gasosas estão tão dispersas a ponto de quase não fornecerem suporte às exigências fisiológicas humanas ou para veículos que exigem ar para queimar combustível.

aer·o·pha·gia, aer·oph·a·gy (ār-ō-fā'jē-ă, -of'ă-jē). Aerofagia. Deglutição excessiva de ar como a observada na birra (eqüinos) e tique de ar (eqüinos) SIN pneumophagia. [aero- + G. *phagō,* comer]

aer·o·phil, aer·o·phile (ār'ō-fil, -fīl). **1.** Aerofilia; afinidade pelo ar. **2.** Aerofílico; organismo aeróbico, especialmente um aeróbio obrigatório. [aero- + G. *philos,* amigo]

aer·o·phil·ic, aer·oph·i·lous (ār-ō-fil'ik, ār-of'i-lŭs). Aerofílico, aeróbico. SIN aerobic.

aer·o·pho·bia (ār-ō-fō'bē-ă). Aerofobia; temor mórbido de ar fresco ou de ar em movimento. [aero- + G. *phobos,* temor]

aer·o·pi·e·so·ther·a·py (ār'ō-pī-e'sō-thăr'ă-pē). Aeropiesoterapia; tratamento de doença por ar comprimido (ou rarefeito). [aero- + G. *piesis,* pressão, + *therapeia,* tratamento clínico]

aer·o·plank·ton (ār-ō-plank'ton). Aeroplâncton, aeroplancto; organismo ou substância transportada pelo ar, p.ex., bactéria, grão de pólen. [aero- + G. *planktos,* ntr. *-on,* vagar]

aer·o·si·al·oph·a·gy (ār'ō-sī-al-of'ă-jē). Aerosialofagia. SIN sialoaerophagy.

aer·o·si·nus·i·tis (ār-ō-sī-nŭ-sī'tis). Aerossinusite. SIN barosinusitis.

aer·o·sis (ār-ō'sis). Aerose; formação de gás nos tecidos. [aero- + G. *-osis,* condição]

aer·o·sol (ār'ō-sol). Aerossol. **1.** Líquido ou matéria particulada dispersa no ar, no gás ou no vapor sob a forma de um fino nevoeiro com propósito terapêutico, inseticida ou outra finalidade. **2.** Produto embalado sob pressão e contendo ingredientes terapêutica ou quimicamente ativos destinados a aplicações tópicas, inalação ou introdução em orifícios corporais. [aero- + solução]

respirable a.'s, a. respirável; aerossóis com dimensões aerodinâmicas inferiores a 10 μm.

terapia com aerossol

(Relação entre o tamanho da partícula, a área-alvo e o modo de transporte)

tamanho da partícula	área-alvo	modo de transporte
< 1 µm	partículas são exaladas	permanecem no estado gasoso
1–5 µm	vias periféricas brônquicas	as partículas formam um sedimento
5–10 µm	vias respiratórias superiores e vias brônquicas centrais	rebote de partículas
> 10 µm	vias respiratórias superiores	

aer·o·sol·i·za·tion (ār-ō-sol-i-zā′shŭn). Aerossolização; dispersão no ar de um material líquido ou uma solução sob a forma de um fino nevoeiro, em geral com fins terapêuticos, especialmente para as vias respiratórias.

aer·o·ther·a·peu·tics, aer·o·ther·a·py (ār′ō-thār-ă-pū′tiks, -thār′ă-pē). Aeroterapia; tratamento de doenças por intermédio de ar fresco, de ar sob diferentes graus de pressão ou rarefação, ou pelo ar tratado de diversas maneiras.

aer·o·ti·tis me·di·a (ār-ō-tī′tis mē′dē-ă). Aerotite média. SIN barotitis media. [aero- + G. ous, ouvido, + -itis, inflamação]

aer·o·ton·om·e·ter (ār′ō-ton-om′e-ter). Aerotonômetro. 1. Instrumento para avaliar a pressão ou a tensão de um gás. 2. Tonômetro. SIN tonometer (2). [aero- + G. tonos, tensão, + metron, medida]

aes·cu·la·pi·an (es-kū-lā′pē-an). Esculapiano, medicinal; relativo a Aesculapius (Esculápio), à arte da medicina ou a um médico. SIN esculapian. [L. Aesculapius, G. Asklēpios, deus da medicina]

aes·cu·lin (es′kū-lin). SIN esculin.

aes·ti·val (es′ti-val). Estival; relativo ao verão ou à idade madura. SIN estival.

AFB 1. Abreviatura de acid-fast bacillus (bacilo álcool-ácido-resistente [BAAR]). VER acid-fast. **2.** Abreviatura de aortofemoral bypass (cirurgia de prótese vascular), do procedimento cirúrgico ou de seu resultado.

afe·brile (ā-feb′ril). Afebril; sem febre, denota apirência; que apresenta temperatura corporal normal. SIN apyretic, apyrexial.

afe·tal (ā-fē′tăl). Afetal; sem relação com o feto ou com a vida intra-uterina.

af·fect (af′fekt). Afeto; sentimentos, emoções e humor ligados a um pensamento, incluindo suas manifestações externas. [L. affectus, estado de espírito, de afficio, ter influência sobre]

blunted a., afeto embotado, transtorno do humor que ocorre em pacientes esquizofrênicos manifestado por superficialidade e grave redução na expressão dos sentimentos.

flat a., apatia, a ausência ou diminuição do tônus emocional ou das reações emocionais externas tipicamente apresentada a outras pessoas ou a si mesmo sob circunstâncias similares; uma forma mais amena é denominada afeto embotado (blunted a.)

inappropriate a., a. inadequado; tônus emocional ou reações emocionais externas em desarmonia com a idéia, objeto ou pensamento que o acompanha.

labile a., a. lábil; desvios rápidos nas expressões emocionais externas; freqüentemente associados a síndromes cerebrais orgânicas, como as intoxicações.

af·fect dis·play. Expressões de afeto; expressões faciais, posturas e gestos que indicam os estados emocionais.

af·fec·tion (ă-fek′shŭn). **1.** Afeição, simpatia, inclinação, afeto; sentimento moderado de ternura, cuidado ou amor. **2.** Doença, estado mórbido; condição anormal do corpo ou espírito. [L. affectio, de af-ficio, afetar, influence]

af·fec·tive (ă-fek′tiv). Afetivo; pertinente a emoção, sentimento, sensibilidade ou a um estado mental.

af·fec·tiv·i·ty (af-fek-tiv′i-tē). Afetividade. SIN feeling tone.

af·fec·to·mo·tor (af′fek-tō-mō′ter). Afetomotor; relativo a manifestações musculares associadas ao tônus afetivo.

af·fer·ent (af′er-ent). Aferente, influxo; que se dirige para o centro, indicando certas artérias, veias, linfáticos e nervos. Oposto de eferente. SIN centripetal (1), esodic. [L. afferens, Fr. af-fero, trazer para]

af·fin·i·ty (ā-fin′i-tē). Afinidade. **1.** Em química, a força que impele certos átomos para se unirem com outros a fim de formarem compostos; atração química. **2.** Coloração seletiva de um tecido por um corante ou captação seletiva de um corante, substância química ou outra substância por um tecido. [L. affinis, vizinhança, de ad, para, + finis, fim, limite]

residual a., a. residual; forças secundárias que capacitam átomos, íons ou moléculas aparentemente saturadas a atrair outros átomos ou grupamentos, produzindo fenômenos tais como a formação de complexos, hidratação adsorção, etc.

af·fi·nous (af′i-nŭs). Afim; parentesco que um cônjuge contrai com a família do outro cônjuge; relacionado por outros laços que não a consangüinidade. [L. affinis, relacionado por casamento, de ad, para + finis, limite]

af·fir·ma·tion (af-fer-mā′shŭn). Afirmação; fase na auto-sugestão em que se apresenta uma tendência reativa positiva. [L. affirmatio, de afirmar, enfatizar, de firmus, forte]

af·fu·sion (ă-fū′zhŭn). Afusão; aspersão de água sobre o corpo ou qualquer de suas partes com finalidade terapêutica. [L. af-fundo, aspergir]

AFH Abreviatura de anterior facial height (altura facial anterior).

afi·bril·lar (ā-fī′bri-lăr). Afibrilar; indica uma estrutura biológica que não contém fibrilas.

afi·brin·o·gen·e·mia (ā-fī′brin-ō-jĕ-nē′mē-ă). Afibrinogenemia; ausência de fibrinogênio no plasma. VER TAMBÉM hypofibrinogenemia.

congenital a. [MIM*202400], a. congênita; distúrbio raro da coagulação sanguínea no qual pouco ou nenhum fibrinogênio é encontrado no plasma devido a uma forma mutante em um dos três *loci* do fibrinogênio. Leva à agregação plaquetária defeituosa; herança autossômica recessiva.

Afipia (ă-fip′ē-ă). Gênero de bactérias Gram-negativas, oxidase-positivas, móveis, não-fermentativas, que foram colocadas na classe Proteobacteria. Morfologicamente variáveis, aparecem como bastonetes ou filamentos que se coram mal. Mais de 10 espécies já foram identificadas; originalmente relatadas como o agente causador da doença da arranhadura do gato, seu papel patogênico atual permanece incerto. A cepa típica é *A. felis*.

af·la·tox·i·co·sis (af′la-toks-ē-cō′sis). Aflatoxicose; doença causada pela ingestão de aflatoxina.

af·la·tox·in (af′lă-tok′sin). Aflatoxina; metabólicos tóxicos de algumas cepas de *Aspergillus* que incluem os fungos *Aspergillus flavus, Aspergillus parasiticus* e *Aspergillus oryzae*. Participariam na etiologia do câncer primário do fígado em seres humanos e causariam doença em animais que se alimentam com farelo de amendoim e outros alimentos contaminados por esses fungos.

AFORMED VER AFORMED Phenomenon.

AFP Abreviatura de α-*fetoproteins* (α-fetoproteína). VER fetoproteins.

af·ter·birth (af′ter-berth). Secundina, decídua; a placenta e as membranas expelidas do útero após o parto. SIN secundina, secundines.

af·ter·care (af′ter-kār). **1.** Cuidados e tratamento de um paciente depois de uma operação, um parto ou durante a convalescença de uma doença. **2.** Após uma hospitalização psiquiátrica, um programa contínuo de reabilitação destinado a reforçar os efeitos do tratamento; pode incluir hospitalização parcial, hospital-dia e ambulatorial.

af·ter·chrom·ing (af′ter-krōm′ing). Pós-cromagem; tratamento adicional de uma amostra tecidual com cromato ou mordente metálico para conferir propriedades especiais de coloração. SIN postchroming.

af·ter·con·trac·tion (af′ter-kon-trak′shŭn). Pós-contração; uma contração muscular persistente durante um tempo notável depois que cessou o estímulo.

af·ter·cur·rent (af′ter-kŭr-ent). Pós-corrente; uma corrente elétrica induzida em um músculo após a interrupção de uma corrente constante que atravessava esse músculo.

af·ter·dis·charge (af-ter-dis′charj). Pós-descarga; prolongamento da resposta de um músculo de elementos neurais depois de interrompido o estímulo. A miotonia é uma manifestação clínica de pós-descarga muscular prolongada.

af·ter·ef·fect (af′ter-ĕ-fekt′). Efeito secundário ou posterior; efeito físico, fisiológico, psicológico ou emocional que persiste após a remoção do estímulo. VER flashback.

af·ter·gild·ing (af′ter-gild′ing). Pós-douração; tratamento de uma amostra histológica fixada e endurecida de tecido nervoso com sais de ouro.

af·ter·im·age (af′ter-im′ij). Pós-imagem; persistência de uma resposta visual após interrompido o estímulo. SIN accidental image, negative image.

negative a., pós-imagem negativa; pós-imagem em que a relação luminosa é invertida; quando cromática, aparece em cores complementares.

positive a., pós-imagem positiva; pós-imagem em que a relação luminosa é igual à original; quando cromática, aparece na mesma cor.

af·ter·im·pres·sion (af′ter-im-presh′ŭn). Pós-impressão. SIN aftersensation.

af·ter·load (af′ter-lōd). Pós-carga. **1.** Disposição de um músculo de tal forma que, ao encurtar-se, desloca um peso de um suporte ajustável ou realiza um trabalho contra uma força de oposição constante à qual não está exposto em repouso. **2.** Carga ou força assim encontrada ao encurtar.

ventricular a., pós-carga ventricular; antiga e erradamente, a pressão arterial ou alguma outra medida de força que um ventrículo precisa sobrepujar enquanto se contrai durante a ejeção, recebendo as contribuições da impedância aórtica ou da artéria pulmonar, da resistência vascular periférica e da massa e da viscosidade do sangue; atualmente, é expressa de forma mais rigorosa em termos da tensão parietal, isto é, a tensão por unidade de área transversal nas fibras musculares do ventrículo (calculada por uma expansão da lei de Laplace a partir da pressão, do raio interno e da espessura da parede) necessária para produzir a pressão intracavitária necessária durante a ejeção.

af·ter·move·ment (af′ter - moov′ment). Pós-movimento; abdução involuntária do braço que se segue à contração isométrica sustentada dos músculos deltóide e supra-espinal (geralmente realizada empurrando-se o membro superior, com firmeza, contra uma superfície vertical imóvel enquanto se está ao lado e próximo desta). SIN Kohnstamm phenomenon.

af·ter·pains (af′ter - pānz). Dores pós-parto; contrações espasmódicas dolorosas do útero que ocorrem depois do parto.

af·ter·per·cep·tion (af′ter - per - sep′shŭn). Pós-percepção. SIN aftersensation.

af·ter·po·ten·tial (af′ter - pō - ten′shal). Pós-potencial; a pequena alteração no potencial elétrico em um nervo estimulado que ocorre após o potencial principal ou espícula; consiste em uma deflexão negativa inicial seguida de uma deflexão positiva no registro oscilográfico.
diastolic a., pós-potencial diastólico; no coração, a modificação de potencial transmembrana após a repolarização, que pode alcançar a magnitude limiar e produzir um distúrbio de ritmo; registrado freqüentemente na intoxicação, como na *overdose* digitálica.
positive a., pós-potencial positivo; aumento espontâneo ou induzível no potencial transmembrana de uma célula cardíaca ou nervosa após o término da repolarização. No coração, corresponde geralmente (em termos temporais) à onda U do eletrocardiograma.

af·ter·sen·sa·tion (af′ter - sen - sā′shŭn). Sensação tardia; sensação que persiste depois que cessou a causa original da ação. SIN afterimpression, afterperception.

af·ter·sound (af′ter - sownd). Som secundário; persistência subjetiva da sensação auditiva após a interrupção do estímulo.

af·ter·taste (af′ter - tāst). Gosto secundário; persistência subjetiva de uma sensação gustativa após a cessação do contato com a substância estimulante.

af·ter·touch (af′ter - tŭch). Persistência subjetiva de sensação tátil após a cessação do estímulo, uma forma de sensação tardia.

af·to·sa (af - tō′sa). Febre aftosa. SIN foot-and-mouth *disease*. [Esp. *fiebre aftosa*, febre aftosa]

Ag 1. Símbolo da prata (argentum). **2.** Abreviatura de antígeno.

ag·a·lac·tia (ā - gal - ak′shē - ā). Agalactia; ausência de leite nas mamas depois do parto. SIN agalactosis. [G. *a-* priv. + *gala (galakt-)*, leite]

aga·lac·tor·rhea (ā - ga - lak - tō - rē′ā). Agalactorréia; ausência da secreção ou do fluxo de leite da mama. [G. *a-* priv. + *gala*, leite, + *rhoia*, fluxo]

ag·a·lac·to·sis (ā - gal - ak - tō - sis). Agalactia, agalacia. SIN agalactia.

ag·a·lac·tous (ā - gal - ak′tŭs). Agaláctico; relativo à agalactia ou à diminuição ou ausência de leite da mama.

ag·a·mete (ā - gam′et, ag′a - mēt). Agameta; protozoário produzido por fissão assexual múltipla. VER TAMBÉM schizogony. [G. *a-* priv. + *gametes*, esposo]

agam·ic (ā - gam′ik). Agâmico; indica reprodução não-sexuada, como por fissão, brotamento, etc. SIN agamous.

agam·ma·glob·u·lin·e·mia (ā - gam′ă - glob′ū - li - nē′mē - ā). Agamaglobulinemia; ausência, ou níveis extremamente baixos, da fração gama da globulina sérica; usada livremente, às vezes para ausência de imunoglobulinas de modo geral. VER TAMBÉM hypogammaglobulinemia.
acquired a., a. adquirida. SIN common variable *immunodeficiency.*
Bruton a., a. de Bruton, condição ligada ao X, com hipo- ou agamaglobulinemia; a imunodeficiência se torna aparente à medida que os níveis de imunoglobulina transmitidos pela mãe diminuem nos primeiros meses de vida. SIN X-linked a.
secondary a., a. secundária. SIN secondary *immunodeficiency.*
Swiss type a., a. do tipo suíço. SIN severe combined *immunodeficiency.*
transient a., a. transitória. SIN transient *hypogammaglobulinemia* of infancy.
X-linked a., a. ligada ao X. SIN Bruton a.

agam·o·cy·tog·e·ny (ā - gam′ō - sī - tojē - nē). Agamocitogenia. SIN schizogony. [G. *agamos*, solteiro, + *kytos*, célula, + *genesis*, criação]

Agam·o·fi·lar·ia (ā - gam′ō - fī - lā′rē - ā). Nome dado a filárias imaturas, sendo o gênero das formas adultas indeterminado. [G. *agamos*, solteiro, + L. *filum*, filamento]

ag·a·mo·gen·e·sis (ag′ă - mō - jen′ē - sis, ā - gam - ō -). Agamogênese. SIN asexual *reproduction.* [G. *agamos*, solteiro, + *genesis*, criação]

ag·a·mo·ge·net·ic (ag′ă - mō - jē - net′ik, - ā - gam - ō -). Agamogenético; indica reprodução assexuada.

ag·a·mog·o·ny (ag - ā - mog′ō - nē). Agamogonia. SIN asexual *reproduction.* [G. *agamos*, solteiro, + *gonos*, descendência]

Ag·a·mo·mer·mis cu·li·cis (ag - ā - mō - mer′mis kū′li - kis). Espécie de nematódeo parasita no mosquito; foram relatados alguns casos em seres humanos, em geral formas larvárias saindo de orifícios orgânicos, presumivelmente após a ingestão de insetos infectados ou contato com terra úmida contendo estágios larvares de vida livre. [G. *agamos*, solteiro, + L. Mod., do G. *mermis*, cordão; L. *culex*, mosquito]

ag·a·mont (ag′ă - mont). Esquizonte. SIN schizont. [G. *agamos*, solteiro, + *ōn (ont-)*, ser]

ag·a·mous (ag′ā - mŭs). Agâmico. SIN agamic. [G. *agamos*, solteiro]

agan·gli·on·ic (ā - gang - glē - on′ik). Aganglônico; sem gânglios.

agan·gli·o·no·sis (ā - gang′glē - ō - nō′sis). Aganglionose; o estado de não possuir gânglios; p. ex., ausência de células ganglionares do plexo mioentérico como uma característica do megacólon congênito. [G. *ā-* priv. + gânglio + *-osis*, doença]

agap·ism (ah′gahp - izm). Agapismo; doutrina que exalta o amor não-sexual (fraterno). [G. *agape*, amor fraterno]

agar (ah′gar, ā′gar). Ágar, ágar-ágar; polissacarídeo complexo (uma galactana sulfatada) derivado da alga marinha (diversas algas vermelhas); usado como agente solidificador em meios de cultura. Apresenta a útil propriedade de derreter a 100°C, solidificando-se apenas a 49°C. [Bengalês]
bile salt a., á. de sais biliares; um meio de cultura contendo lactose, peptona, taurocolato de sódio e vermelho neutro, para o crescimento e o isolamento de bastonetes Gram-negativos.
birdseed a., meio de cultura preparado a partir das sementes de *Guizottia abyssinica*, usado na cultura e no diagnóstico presuntivo de *Cryptococcus neoformans*.
blood a., á.-sangue; mistura de sangue (geralmente de ovelha ou cavalo) e um meio de á. utilizada para cultura de muitos microrganismos clinicamente importantes.
Bordet-Gengou potato blood a., á.-sangue-batata de Bordet e Gengou; á. glicerina-batata, com 25% de sangue, usado para isolar *Bordetella pertussis*.
brain-heart infusion a., á. com infusão de cérebro e coração; meio de cultura usado para o isolamento de microrganismos exigentes, principalmente fungos.
chocolate a., á.-chocolate; á.-sangue aquecido até que o sangue se torne castanho ou achocolatado, usado especialmente para isolar *Haemophilus* ou *Neisseria* e outras espécies para as quais o sangue não-aquecido é um inibidor.
cholera a., meio de á. alcalino para cultura do *Vibrio cholerae*.
cornmeal a., meio de cultura pobre em nutrientes, muito utilizado no estudo de fungos leveduriformes e filamentosos; suprime o crescimento vegetativo ao mesmo tempo que estimula a esporulação de muitas espécies, sendo muito empregado para produzir os clamidósporos característicos de *Candida albicans*.
Czapek solution a., á. Czapek; meio de cultura usado para o cultivo de espécies de fungos e para a identificação das espécies de *Aspergillus* e *Penicillium*. SIN Czapek-Dox medium.
EMB a., á. eosina-azul-de-metileno. SIN eosin-methylene blue a.
Endo a., á. Endo; meio de cultura contendo peptona, lactose, fosfato dipotássico, ágar, sulfato de sódio, fucsina básica e água destilada; originalmente criado para o isolamento de *Salmonella typhi*, esse meio atualmente é mais útil no exame bacteriológico da água; os microrganismos coliformes fermentam a lactose, e suas colônias tornam-se vermelhas e colorem o meio vizinho; os microrganismos que não fermentam lactose produzem colônias claras, incolores, contra o fundo rosa-pálido do meio. SIN Endo medium.
eosin-methylene blue a., á. eosina-azul-de-metileno; a. composto de peptona, lactose e sacarose e contendo eosina e azul-de-metileno, usado para diferenciar bactérias Gram-negativas fermentadoras de lactose daquelas não-fermentadoras de lactose. *Escherichia* sp. apresenta um brilho característico. SIN EMB a.
MacConkey a., á. MacConkey; meio de cultura contendo peptona, lactose, sais biliares, vermelho neutro e violeta cristal, usado para identificar bacilos Gram-negativos e caracterizá-los de acordo com sua condição de fermentadores de lactose. Os fermentadores aparecem como colônias de coloração rosa, enquanto os não-fermentadores são incolores.
Mueller-Hinton a., á. Mueller-Hinton; meio de cultura contendo infusão de carne de boi ou vaca, peptona e amido, usado principalmente para o método de difusão disco-ágar nas pesquisas de suscetibilidade a antimicrobianos (antibiograma).
Novy and MacNeal blood a., á-sangue Novy e MacNeal; um a. nutriente contendo dois volumes de sangue desfibrinado de coelho; adequado para a cultura de inúmeros tripanossomas.
nutrient a., á. nutriente; meio sólido simples, contendo extrato de carne de boi ou vaca, peptona, ágar e água; usado para o crescimento de muitas bactérias heterotróficas comuns.
oatmeal-tomato paste a., á. com farinha de aveia e tomate; meio de cultura especial para a formação de ascósporos nos dermatófitos.
potato dextrose a., á. com dextrose e batata; meio de cultura muito utilizado para o cultivo de fungos; bom sobretudo para o desenvolvimento de conídios e formas esporulantes pelas quais um microrganismo é identificado microscopicamente.
rice-Tween a., á. com arroz-Tween; meio de cultura útil para o desenvolvimento de clamidósporos em *Candida albicans* e para o preparo de culturas em lâminas para outras formas de esporulação em outras espécies de fungos.
Sabouraud a., á. Sabouraud; meio de cultura para fungos contendo á. com neopeptona ou polipeptona e glicose, com pH final de 5,6; é o meio de cultura padrão, mais universalmente utilizado em micologia. **Trata-se da referência internacional.** O á. Sabouraud modificado (modificação de Emmons) com menos glicose e pH neutro é melhor para o desenvolvimento de pigmento nas colônias.
Sabouraud dextrose a., á. Sabouraud-dextrose; meio de cultura contendo peptona e dextrose que possibilita o cultivo da maioria dos fungos patogênicos.

serum a., á.-soro; meio enriquecido para a cultura de microrganismos exigentes; preparado pelo acréscimo de soro estéril ao á. dissolvido.
Thayer-Martin a., á. Thayer-Martin; á. Mueller-Hinton com 5% de sangue de carneiro hemolisado com calor e antibióticos, usado para o transporte e o isolamento primário de *Neisseria gonorrhoeae* e *Neisseria meningitidis*. SIN Thayer-Martin medium.
yeast extract a., á. com extrato de levedura; meio usado para induzir a esporulação e reduzir o crescimento vegetativo na cultura de fungos.

agar·ic (ā-gar′ik). Agárico; o fruto seco de *Polyporus officinalis* (família Polyporaceae), que ocorre sob a forma de massas leves, de coloração acastanhada ou esbranquiçada, contendo ácido agárico. SIN amadou. [G. *agarikon*, uma espécie de fungos]
deadly a. a., cogumelo-de-chapéu, cogumelo venenoso. SIN Amanita phalloides.
fly a. a., *Amanita muscaria*. SIN Amanita muscaria.

agar·ic ac·id (ā-gar′ik). Ácido agárico; obtido do agárico e responsável pela ação anidrótica do cogumelo; usado como agente anidrótico.

Agar·i·cus (ā-gar′i-kŭs). Grande gênero de cogumelos, dos quais muitos são comestíveis e outros venenosos. [L. *agaricum*, do G. *agarikon*, um fungo arbóreo]

agar·o·pec·tin (ag′ā-rō-pek′tin). Agaropectina; polissacarídeo encontrado em preparações de ágar que consiste em D-galactose ligada β1,3 glicosidicamente. Algumas das unidades galactosil são sulfatadas.

ag·a·rose (ag′ā-rōs). Agarose; a fração polissacarídica linear neutra encontrada em preparados de ágar, geralmente compostos de D-galactose e resíduos 3,6-anidrogalactose alterados; usada em cromatografia e eletroforese.

agas·tric (ā-gas′trik). Agástrico; que não possui estômago ou tubo digestivo. [G. *a*-priv. + *gastēr*, estômago]

agas·tro·neu·ria (ā-gas-tro-noor′ē-ă). Agastroneuria; redução do controle nervoso do estômago. [G. *a*- priv. + *gastēr*, estômago, + *neuron*, nervo]

AGC Abreviatura de automatic gain *control* (controle automático do ganho).

age (āj). **1.** Idade; o período decorrido desde o nascimento. **2.** Idade; um dos períodos em que é dividida a vida humana, diferenciada por evolução física, equilíbrio ou involução; p. ex. as sete idades do ser humano são: infância, meninice, adolescência, maturidade, meia-idade, senescência e senilidade. **3.** Envelhecer; as modificações estruturais desenvolvidas gradativamente e que não se devem a doenças ou traumatismos evitáveis e que estão associadas à diminuição da capacidade funcional e ao aumento da probabilidade de óbito. **4.** Produzir artificialmente o aspecto característico de alguém que viveu muito ou de alguma coisa que existiu durante muito tempo. **5.** Têmpera lenta; em odontologia, aquecer lentamente uma liga para amálgama, aumentar sua força, reduzir o fluxo e ter uma vida estável; o envelhecimento ocorre pela redução das tensões internas. [F. *âge*, L. *aetas*]
achievement a., i. de aproveitamento; relação entre a idade cronológica e a idade de aproveitamento, estabelecida por provas padronizadas.
anatomical a., i. anatômica; idade física; idade em termos de estrutura, em vez de função ou do decorrer do tempo. SIN physical a.
basal a., i. basal; o nível mais elevado da idade mental na escala de inteligência de Stanford-Binet.
Binet a., i. de Binet; idade da criança anormal (medida pela escala de Stanford-Binet) correspondente à inteligência da criança normal (o indivíduo com retardo mental grave age como uma criança de 1–2 anos; o indivíduo moderada a gravemente retardado, age como uma criança de 3 a 7 anos; o indivíduo limítrofe [*borderline*] a levemente retardado age como uma criança de 8 a 12 anos).
bone a., i. óssea; fase do desenvolvimento dos ossos (em anos) avaliada por radiografias, em contraste com a idade cronológica.
childbearing a., i. fértil; o período na vida de uma mulher entre a puberdade e a menopausa.
chronologic a. (CA), i. cronológica; idade expressa em anos e meses; utilizada como uma medida para avaliar a idade mental das crianças ao calcular seu quociente de inteligência de Stanford-Binet.
developmental a., i. do desenvolvimento; **(1)** idade fetal; idade calculada pelo desenvolvimento anatômico desde a nidação; **(2) (DA),** idade de um indivíduo calculada pelo grau de maturação anatômica, fisiológica, mental e emocional.
emotional a., i. emocional; medida da maturidade emocional por comparação com o desenvolvimento emocional médio.
gestational a., i. gestacional; **(1)** em embriologia, a i. do embrião expressa de acordo com o tempo transcorrido desde a concepção; **(2)** em obstetrícia, a i. de desenvolvimento de um feto, geralmente baseada no primeiro dia presumido do último período menstrual normal.
menstrual a., i. menstrual; i. do concepto computada a partir do início do último período menstrual da mãe.
mental a. (MA), i. mental; medida expressa em anos e meses da inteligência de uma criança, em relação às normas etárias conforme a avaliação pela escala de Stanford-Binet.
physical a., idade física. SIN anatomical a.
physiologic a., i. fisiológica; idade avaliada em termos de função.

agen·e·sis (ā-jen′ē-sis). Agenesia; ausência, formação incompleta de qualquer parte. [G. *a*- priv. + *genesis*, produção]
gonadal a., a. gonadal; ausência de uma ou de ambas as gônadas.
müllerian a., a. mülleriana. SIN Mayer-Rokitansky-Küster-Hauser *syndrome*.
renal a., a. renal; ausência de um ou dos dois rins, mais freqüentemente unilateral, com ausência do ducto paramesonéfrico ipsolateral e seus derivados; a função renal é normal enquanto o rim remanescente está íntegro; a agenesia renal bilateral ou completa está associada a fácies de Potter e óbito neonatal.
thymic a., a. tímica; ausência do timo, que pode estar associada à ausência das paratireóides na síndrome de Di George.

agen·i·tal·ism (ā-jen′i-tal-izm). Agenitalismo; ausência congênita da genitália.

agen·o·so·mia (ā-gen-ō-sō′mē-ă). Agenossomia; formação acentuadamente defeituosa ou ausência da genitália; em geral acompanhada pela protrusão das vísceras abdominais através de uma parede abdominal incompleta. [G. *a*- priv. + *genos*, sexo, + *soma*, corpo]

agent (ā′jent). Agente. **1.** Força ativa ou substância capaz de produzir um efeito. Quanto aos agentes não-apresentados, ver o nome específico. **2.** Uma doença, um fator como um microrganismo, uma substância química ou uma forma de radiação cuja presença ou ausência (como nas doenças por deficiência) resulta em enfermidade ou grau mais avançado da doença. [L. *ago*, pres. p. *agens (agent-)*, realizar]
adrenergic blocking a., a. bloqueador adrenérgico; composto que bloqueia ou inibe seletivamente as respostas à atividade de nervos adrenérgicos simpáticos (a. simpaticolítico) e à epinefrina, à norepinefrina e a outras aminas adrenérgicas (a. adrenolítico); existem duas classes diferentes: os agentes bloqueadores dos receptores alfa- e beta-adrenérgicos.
α-adrenergic blocking a., bloqueador α-adrenérgico; classe de medicamentos que competem com agonistas α-adrenérgicos pelos receptores disponíveis: alguns competem tanto por receptores α_1 como pelos α_2 (p. ex., fentolamina, dibenzilina), enquanto outros são primariamente agentes bloqueadores α_1 (p. ex., prazosina, terazosina) ou α_2 (p. ex., ioimbina). SIN α-adrenoceptor antagonist, alpha-blocker.
β-adrenergic blocking a., a. bloqueador β-adrenérgico; classe de medicamentos que competem com os agonistas β-adrenérgicos pelos receptores disponíveis; alguns competem tanto pelos receptores β_1 como pelos receptores β_2 (p. ex., propranolol), enquanto outros são primariamente bloqueadores β_1 (p. ex., metoprolol) ou β_2; usado no tratamento de várias doenças cardiovasculares quando o bloqueio β-adrenérgico é desejável. SIN β-adrenergic receptor blocking a., β-adrenoreceptor antagonist, beta-blocker.
adrenergic neuronal blocking a., a. bloqueador neuronal adrenérgico; medicamento que evita a liberação de norepinefrina pelas terminações nervosas simpáticas (p. ex., guanetidina); não inibe as respostas dos receptores adrenérgicos à epinefrina, à norepinefrina e a outras aminas adrenérgicas circulantes.
β-adrenergic receptor blocking a., a. bloqueador de receptores β-adrenérgicos. SIN β-adrenergic blocking a.
alkylating a., a. alquilante; medicamento ou substância química que, através da formação de ligações covalentes, forma um constituinte tissular derivado que contém, permanentemente, parte do medicamento ou do composto químico; embora freqüentemente carcinogênico e mutagênico, é muito usado na quimioterapia do câncer (p. ex., mostardas nitrogenadas e carmustina).
antianxiety a., a. ansiolítico; categoria funcional de medicamentos úteis no tratamento da ansiedade e capazes de reduzir a ansiedade em doses que não causam sedação excessiva. A maioria dos medicamentos comumente usados que se encaixam nessa categoria são os benzodiazepínicos, que atuam nos receptores do ácido γ-aminobutírico (GABA). Os barbitúricos eram considerados os principais agentes nessa categoria; uma nova categoria, que atua nos receptores de serotonina (5-HT$_{1A}$), é atualmente representada pela buspirona. SIN anxiolytic (1), minor tranquilizer.
antidiskinetic a., a. antidiscinético; categoria funcional de medicamentos com ação anticolinérgica, usada no tratamento da doença de Parkinson e de alguns dos distúrbios agudos do movimento causados por agentes antipsicóticos.
antifoaming a.'s, a. tensoativos; produtos químicos que baixam a tensão superficial (e, portanto, a produção de espuma), utilizados em evaporações laboratoriais e também administrados com oxigênio para aliviar a obstrução respiratória agravada pela espuma do líquido no edema pulmonar (surfactante pulmonar).
antipsychotic a., a. antipsicótico; classe funcional de medicamentos neurolépticos úteis no tratamento de psicoses e com capacidade de aliviar os transtornos do raciocínio. SIN antipsychotic (1), major tranquilizer.
atypical antipsychotic a., a. antipsicótico atípico; categoria funcional de novos medicamentos antipsicóticos. Acredita-se que sua ação se deva predominantemente ao bloqueio serotonérgico.
bacteriostatic a., a. bacteriostático. SIN bacteriostat.
Bittner a., a. Bittner. SIN mammary tumor *virus* of mice.
blister a., i. que promove a formação de bolhas ou vesículas (p. ex., calor, substâncias químicas).
blocking a., a. bloqueador; classe de medicamentos que inibem (bloqueiam) uma atividade ou um processo biológico, como condução ou transmissão por

axônios, acesso a um receptor ou movimento de íons através de uma membrana celular; freqüentemente denominados "bloqueadores" (blockers).

calcium channel-blocking a., a. bloqueadores do canal de cálcio; classe de medicamentos com capacidade para inibir o movimento dos íons cálcio através da membrana celular; valiosos sobretudo para o tratamento de distúrbios cardiovasculares por causa de efeitos farmacológicos, como a depressão da contração mecânica dos músculos cardíaco e liso, e da formação do impulso e da velocidade de condução (p. ex., verapamil, nifedipina). SIN calcium antagonist, slow channel-blocking a.

chimpanzee coryza a. (CCA), vírus sincicial respiratório. SIN respiratory syncytial virus.

cholinergic a., a. colinérgico; agente que simula a ação da acetilcolina ou do sistema nervoso parassimpático (p. ex., metacolina).

contrast a., contraste. SIN contrast medium.

cycle-specific a., a. ciclo-específico; a. que possui efeito em apenas uma parte do ciclo celular (fase S) ou apenas quando a célula se encontra em uma parte específica do ciclo celular.

delta a., a. delta. SIN hepatitis D virus.

Eaton a., a. Eaton. SIN Mycoplasma pneumoniae.

embedding a.'s, agentes de inclusão; materiais como celoidina, parafina, etc., nos quais são colocadas amostras de tecido antes de serem cortadas para exame microscópico.

enterokinetic a., a. enterocinético; agente utilizado para aliviar a atonia intestinal.

F a., a. F, termo obsoleto para F *plasmid* (plasmídeo F).

fertility a., a. de fertilidade; termo obsoleto para F *plasmid* (plasmídeo F).

foamy a.'s, retrovírus do gênero Spumavirus. SIN foamy viruses, em virus.

ganglionic blocking a., agente bloqueador ganglionar; agente que compromete (interfere) a passagem de impulsos pelos gânglios autônomos (p. ex., tetraetilamônio, trimetafano).

high osmolar contrast a., contraste de alta osmolaridade; contrastes iodados hidrossolúveis iônicos. SIN high osmolar contrast medium.

initiating a., a. iniciador. VER initiation.

inotropic a.'s, a. inotrópicos; medicamentos que aumentam a força de contração do músculo cardíaco; os exemplos incluem glicosídeos digitálicos, amrinona e epinefrina.

LDH a., a. LDH, arterivírus. SIN lactate dehydrogenase virus.

low osmolar contrast a. (LOCA), contraste de baixa osmolaridade; contraste radiográfico não-iônico hidrossolúvel. SIN low osmolar contrast medium, nonionic contrast a.

luting a., luto; massa, especialmente cimento de argila, para fixação; p. ex. gesso ou cera para fixar ataduras rígidas a um articulador ou material para fixar coroas aos dentes.

mood stabilizing a., a. estabilizador do humor; categoria funcional de medicamentos usada para normalizar o humor, reduzindo principalmente as variações de humor (p. ex., lítio e alguns anticonvulsivantes, como carbamazepina e ácido valpróico).

neuroleptic a., a. neuroléptico. SIN neuroleptic.

neuromuscular blocking a.'s, agentes bloqueadores neuromusculares; grupo de medicamentos que impedem as extremidades dos nervos motores de excitar os músculos esqueléticos. Atuam tanto por competição pelo neurotransmissor, a acetilcolina (como a D-tubocurarina, o mivacúrio e o pancurônio), quanto por estimular primeiro a membrana muscular pós-juncional e, depois, dessensibilizar as placas terminais dos músculos à acetilcolina (como a succinilcolina ou o decametônio); usados em cirurgia para produzir paralisia e facilitar a manipulação dos músculos.

non-cycle-specific a., a. não-ciclo-específico; a. cujo efeito não depende de onde esteja a célula no seu ciclo de divisão.

nondepolarizing neuromuscular blocking a., agente bloqueador neuromuscular não-despolarizante; composto que paralisa a musculatura esquelética, basicamente por inibir a transmissão de impulsos nervosos na junção neuromuscular, em vez de afetar o potencial de membrana da placa terminal motora ou as fibras neuromusculares (p. ex., curare, galamina, vecurônio).

nonionic contrast a., contraste não-iônico. SIN low osmolar contrast a.

Norwalk a., a. Norwalk; uma cepa do vírus da gastroenterite epidêmica que pertence aos calcivírus. [*Norwalk*, Ohio, primeiro local onde esse vírus foi implicado na doença]

Pittsburgh pneumonia a., a. da pneumonia de Pittsburgh. SIN Legionella micdadei.

promoting a., a. promotor. VER promotion.

psychotropic a., a. psicotrópico; composto químico que influencia a psique humana.

reovirus-like a., a. semelhante ao reovírus. SIN rotavirus.

sclerosing a., agente esclerosante; composto que age por irritação do epitélio da íntima venosa; utilizado no tratamento de veias varicosas.

slow channel-blocking a., a. bloqueador dos canais lentos. SIN calcium channel-blocking a.

sympathetic a., a. simpaticomimético. VER sympathomimetic *amine*.

transforming a., a. transformador; **(1)** SIN mitogen; **(2)** vírus que consegue transformar células.

TRIC a.'s, agentes TRIC; cepas de *Chlamydia trachomatis* que causam *tracoma* e *conjuntivite* de *inclusão*. VER Chlamydia trachomatis.

typical antipsychotic a., a. antipsicótico típico; categoria funcional de medicamentos antipsicóticos antigos. Acredita-se que exerçam sua ação predominantemente através do bloqueio dopaminérgico.

Agent Orange. Agente Laranja; herbicida e desfolhante que consiste em ácido (2,4,5-triclorofenoxi)acético, ácido (2,4-diclorofenoxi)acético e dioxina; foi muito utilizado na Guerra do Vietnã; demonstrou-se que possui propriedades carcinogênicas e teratogênicas residuais pós-exposição em seres humanos.

age·ra·sia (ā-jer-ā′zē-ă). Agerasia; aparência de juventude na velhice. [G. *agerasia,* juventude eterna, de *a-* priv. + *geras,* velhice]

ageu·sia (ā-goo′sē-ă). Ageusia, ageustia; perda ou ausência do paladar. Pode ser: 1) geral para todos os sabores (total), parcial para alguns sabores, ou específica a um ou mais sabores; 2) decorrente de distúrbios do transporte (no acesso ao interior do botão gustativo) ou transtornos sensorineurais (que afetam as células ou nervos sensoriais gustativos ou as vias neurais gustativas centrais); ou 3) hereditária ou adquirida. SIN ageustia, gustatory anesthesia. [G. *a-* priv. + *geusis,* sabor]

ageus·tia (ā-goos′tē-ă). Ageustia. SIN ageusia.

ag·ger, pl. **ag·ger·es** (aj′er, -ēz; ag′er) [TA]. Crista, eminência, saliência ou proeminência. [L. elevação]

a. na′si [TA], crista nasal; elevação na parede lateral da cavidade nasal, entre o átrio do meato médio e o sulco olfatório; é formada pela mucosa que reveste a base da crista etmoidal do maxilar. SIN nasal ridge.

a. perpendicula′ris, eminência da fossa triangular. SIN eminence of triangular fossa of auricle.

a. val′vae ve′nae, proeminência das valvas venosas. SIN prominence of venous valvular sinus.

ag·glom·er·ate, ag·glom·er·at·ed (ă-glom′er-āt). Aglomerado. SIN aggregated. [L. *ag-glomero,* soprar em uma bola, de *ad,* para, + *glomus,* uma bola]

ag·glom·er·a·tion (ă-glom-er-ā′shŭn). Aglomeração; agrupamento. SIN aggregation.

ag·glu·ti·nant (ă-gloo′ti-nant). Aglutinante; substância que aglutina ou que causa adesão das partes de um todo. [L. *ad,* para + *gluten,* cola]

ag·glu·ti·nate (ă-gloo′ti-nāt). Aglutinar; causar ou tender a causar aglutinação.

ag·glu·ti·na·tion (ă-gloo-ti-nā′shŭn). Aglutinação. **1.** O processo pelo qual bactérias, células de outras partículas suspensas são levadas a aderir e formar grumos, semelhante à precipitação, mas as partículas são maiores e estão em suspensão, e não em solução. Quanto às reações específicas de aglutinação nos diversos grupos sanguíneos, ver o Apêndice de Grupos Sanguíneos. **2.** Aderência das superfícies de uma ferida. **3.** O processo de aderir. [L. *ad,* para, + *gluten,* cola]

acid a., aglutinação ácida; o agrupamento de certos microrganismos em elevada concentração de íons hidrogênio.

bacteriogenic a., a. bacteriogênica, o agrupamento de células em conseqüência dos efeitos de bactérias ou de seus produtos.

cold a., a. fria; a. das hemácias pelo seu próprio soro (ver autoagglutination), ou por qualquer outro soro quando o sangue é resfriado abaixo da temperatura corporal, porém mais pronunciada abaixo de 25°C; o fenômeno resulta de crioaglutininas; pode ser observado ocasionalmente no sangue de pessoas aparentemente normais ou como achado anormal em pacientes com pneumonia atípica primária, mononucleose infecciosa e outras doenças virais, certas protozoonoses ou neoplasias linfoproliferativas. VER autoagglutination.

cross a., a. cruzada. SIN group a.

false a., a. falsa. SIN pseudoagglutination (1).

group a., a. cruzada; a. por anticorpos específicos para antígenos menores (de grupo) comuns a diversos microrganismos, cada qual possuindo seu próprio antígeno específico maior. SIN cross a.

immune a., a. imune; a. produzida por anticorpos (aglutininas) específicos para o microrganismo em suspensão, célula ou para um antígeno que revestiu uma partícula de tamanho adequado.

indirect a., a. indireta. SIN passive a.

nonimmune a., a. não-imune; **(1)** a. produzida por uma lectina possuidora de certa especificidade para determinado açúcar, cujo mecanismo é obscuro; **(2)** a. que resulta de fatores inespecíficos, como no caso da a. ácida ou a. espontânea.

passive a., a. passiva; a. indireta; a. de partículas que foram revestidas com antígeno solúvel, por anti-soro específico para o antígeno adsorvido. SIN indirect a.

spontaneous a., a. espontânea; agrupamento inespecífico de microrganismos em soro fisiológico, relacionado com a falta de grupamentos polares em solução eletrolítica.

ag·glu·ti·na·tive (ă-gloo′ti-nă-tiv). Aglutinativo, aglutinante; que causa ou é capaz de causar aglutinação.

ag·glu·ti·nin (ă-gloo′tĭ-nĭn). Aglutinina. **1.** Anticorpo que produz agrupamento ou aglutinação de bactérias ou outras células que estimularam a formação da aglutinina ou contêm antígeno reativo e imunologicamente semelhante. SIN agglutinating antibody, immune a. **2.** Substância, que não um anticorpo aglutinante específico, que faz com que partículas orgânicas se aglutinem, p. ex., aglutinina vegetal.
  blood group a.'s, a. dos grupos sanguíneos; ver apêndice sobre Grupos Sanguíneos.
  chief a., a principal. SIN major a.
  cold a., crioaglutinina; anticorpo que reage mais eficientemente em temperaturas abaixo de 37°C.
  cross-reacting a., a. de reação cruzada. SIN group a.
  flagellar a., a. flagelar. SIN H a. (1).
  group a., a. de reação cruzada; uma imunoaglutinina específica para um antígeno comum ou "compartilhado". SIN cross-reacting a.
  H a., a. H; **(1)** a. flagelar; uma a. formada em conseqüência da estimulação e reação, por antígeno(s) relativamente termoestável(eis) nos flagelos de cepas móveis de microrganismos. SIN flagellar a. **(2)** ver grupos sanguíneos ABO, apêndice sobre Grupos Sanguíneos.
  immune a., a. imune. SIN agglutinin (1).
  incomplete a. (ă-gloo′tĭ-nĭn), a. incompleta; anticorpo que se liga ao antígeno, mas não induz aglutinação. Esses anticorpos geralmente são da classe IgG, sendo chamados de anticorpos incompletos.
  major a., a. principal; imunoa. presente em maior quantidade em um anti-soro e evocada pelo mais dominante de um mosaico de antígenos. SIN chief a.
  minor a., a. menor; imunoa. presente em um anti-soro em menor concentração do que a a. principal. SIN partial a.
  O a., (1) a. somática; a. formada em conseqüência da estimulação por, e reação pelo(s), antígeno(s) relativamente termoestável(eis) existente(s) nas paredes celulares de certos microrganismos. SIN somatic a. **(2)** ver grupos sanguíneos ABO, apêndice sobre Grupos Sanguíneos.
  partial a., a. parcial. SIN minor a.
  plant a., a. vegetal; uma lectina.
  saline a., a. salina; anticorpo que produz aglutinação de eritrócitos quando suspensos em soro fisiológico ou em meio proteico. SIN complete antibody.
  somatic a., a. somática. SIN O a. (1).
  warm a.'s, a. quentes; a. que são mais reativas a 37°C do que a temperaturas menores.

ag·glu·tin·o·gen (ă-gloo-tĭn′ō-jen). Aglutinogênio; substância antigênica que estimula a formação de aglutinina específica, a qual pode causar aglutinação de células que contenham o antígeno ou partículas revestidas com o antígeno. SIN agglutogen. [agglutinin + G. *-gen*, produção]
  blood group a.'s, a. dos grupos sanguíneos. ver apêndice sobre Grupos Sanguíneos.
  T a., a. T., termo obsoleto para uma aglutinina formada a partir de um receptor latente nas hemácias humanas pela ação de uma enzima em culturas de certas bactérias.

ag·glu·tin·o·gen·ic (ă-gloo′tĭn-ō-jen′ĭk). Aglutinogênico; capaz de causar a produção de uma aglutinina. SIN agglutogenic.

ag·glu·tin·o·phil·ic (ă-gloo′tĭn-ō-fĭl′ĭk). Aglutinofílico; que sofre prontamente acentuada aglutinação. [agglutination + G. *phileō*, amar]

ag·glu·to·gen (ă-gloo′tō-jen). Aglutogênio. SIN agglutinogen.

ag·glu·to·gen·ic (ă-gloo-tō-jen′ĭk). Aglutogênico. SIN agglutinogenic.

ag·gre·can (ag′re-kan). Agrecano; gene candidato para a otoesclerose, localizado de 15q25 a q26.

ag·gre·gate (ag′re-gāt). **1.** Unir ou juntar em uma massa ou conjunto. **2.** O total de unidades individuais que compõem uma massa ou conjunto. [L. *aggrego*, pp. *-atus*, adicionar, de *grex* (greg-), agregar]
  proteoglycan a., a. de proteoglicanos; um grande a. de proteoglicanos ligados de maneira não-covalente a uma longa molécula de ácido hialurônico; envolvido na ligação cruzada de fibrilas de colágeno da matriz cartilaginosa.

ag·gre·gat·ed (ag′re-gā-ted). Agregado; unidos, formando assim um grupo, um conjunto ou uma massa de unidades individuais. SIN agglomerate, agglomerated, agminate, agminated.

ag·gre·ga·tion (ag-re-gā′shŭn). Aglomeração; massa agrupada de unidades independentes mas semelhantes; um grupo. SIN agglomeration.
  familial a., a. familiar; ocorrência de um traço em mais membros de uma família que pode ser prontamente atribuída ao acaso; evidência presuntiva, mas não convincente, de ação de fatores genéticos.

ag·gre·gom·e·ter (ag-re-gom′e-ter). Agregômetro; instrumento para medir a agregação de plaquetas pela monitoração, ao longo do tempo, das mudanças na densidade óptica de uma suspensão de plaquetas tratada com agentes agregadores como ADP, colágeno, epinefrina, etc.

ag·gres·sin (ă-gres′ĭn). Agressina; substância de origem microbiana tida como inibidora dos mecanismos de resistência do hospedeiro. [L. *agressor*, um assaltante, de *ad-gredio*, pp. *-gressus*, atacar]

ag·gres·sion (ă-gresh′ŭn). Agressão; atitude dominadora, violenta ou de assalto verbal ou físico contra outra pessoa como o componente motor dos sentimentos de ira, hostilidade ou raiva. [L. *aggressio*, de *aggredior*, agredir, atacar]

ag·gres·sive (ă-gres′ĭv). Agressivo. **1.** Denotando agressão. **2.** Denotando impetuosidade ou ato dissociativo como o de um padrão comportamental, um organismo patogênico ou um processo mórbido.

ag·ing (ā′jing). Envelhecimento. **1.** O processo de envelhecimento, especialmente pela incapacidade de substituir as células em número suficiente para manter a capacidade funcional plena; afeta sobretudo as células (p. ex., neurônios) incapazes de divisão mitótica. **2.** A deterioração gradativa de um organismo maduro, resultante de alterações estruturais irreversíveis e dependentes de tempo, intrínsecas a cada espécie e que acabam por levar à capacidade diminuída de enfrentar os estresses ambientais, aumentando assim a probabilidade de óbito. **3.** No sistema cardiovascular, a substituição progressiva de tipos celulares funcionais por tecido conjuntivo fibroso. **4.** Termo demográfico que significa um aumento, com o tempo, da proporção de pessoas idosas na população.
  clonal a., envelhecimento clonal; a deterioração em gerações sucessivas de um clone; assim, os paramécios e outras formas simples, quando se reproduzem assexuadamente durante algumas gerações, sofrem invariavelmente deterioração, com as características de cada grupo de descendentes afastando-se de forma progressiva das características do ancestral produzido sexuadamente.

ag·i·to·la·lia (aj′ĭ-tō-lā′lē-ă). Agitolalia. SIN agitophasia.

ag·i·to·pha·sia (aj′ĭ-tō-fā′zē-ă). Agitofasia; linguagem anormalmente rápida na qual as palavras são imperfeitamente pronunciadas ou perdidas em uma frase. SIN agitolalia. [L. *agito*, apressar, + G. *phasis*, linguagem]

aglo·mer·u·lar (ă-glō-mer′ū-lar). Aglomerular; que não possui glomérulos; refere-se especialmente a um rim cujos glomérulos foram destruídos ou aos rins de certos peixes, como, p. ex., peixe-sapo, que possui túbulos, mas não glomérulos.

aglos·sia (ă-glos′ē-ă). Aglossia; ausência congênita da língua. [G. *a-* priv. + *glōssa*, língua]

aglos·so·sto·mia (ă-glos-ō-stō′mē-ă). Aglossostomia; ausência congênita da língua, com boca anômala (geralmente fechada). [G. *a-* priv. + *glōssa*, língua, + *stoma*, boca]

aglu·con (ă-gloo′kon). Aglucona; parte de um glicosídeo diferente da glicose. [G. *a-* priv. + *glucose* + *-on*]

ag·lu·ti·tion (ă-gloo-tish′ŭn). Aglutição; incapacidade de deglutir. VER TAMBÉM dysphagia.

agly·ca, sing. **agly·con** (ă-glī′kon). Aglicones.

agly·con, a·gly·cone, pl. **agly·ca** (ă-glī′kon). Aglicona; a porção não-carboidratada de um glicosídeo (p. ex., digoxigenina). [Gr. *a-* priv. + *glykys*, doce]

a·gly·cone. Aglicona. VER aglycon.

agly·cos·u·ria (ă-glī-kō-soo′rē-ă). Aglicosúria; ausência de carboidratos na urina.

agly·cos·u·ric (ă-glī-kō-soo′rik). Aglicosúrico; relativo à aglicosúria.

ag·men, pl. **ag·mina** (ag′men, ag′min-ă) Termo obsoleto para agregação. [L. multidão]
  a. peyerian′um, nódulos linfóides agregados do intestino delgado. SIN aggregated lymphoid *nodules* of small intestine, em *nodule*.

ag·mi·nate, ag·mi·nat·ed (ag′mi-nāt, ag′mi-nā-ted). SIN aggregated. [L. *agmen*, multidão]

ag·na·thia (ăg-nā′thē-ă). Agnatia; ausência congênita da mandíbula, em geral acompanhada por aproximação das orelhas. VER TAMBÉM otocephaly, synotia. [Gr. *a-* priv. + *gnathos*, mandíbula]

ag·na·thous (ăg′nā-thŭs). Ágnato; relativo à agnatia.

ag·nea (ag-nē′ă). Agnosia. SIN agnosia. [G. *agnoia*, desejo de percepção]

ag·no·gen·ic (ag-nō-jen′nik). Agnogênico. SIN idiopathic. [G. *a-* priv. + *gnosis*, conhecimento, + *genesis*, origem]

ag·no·sia (ag-nō′zē-ă). Agnosia; comprometimento da capacidade de reconhecer, ou compreender, o significado de vários estímulos sensoriais não-atribuível a distúrbios dos receptores primários ou do intelecto geral; defeitos de recepção causados por lesões em várias porções do cérebro. SIN agnea [G. ignorância; de *a-* priv. + *gnōsis*, conhecimento]
  auditory a., a. auditiva; incapacidade de reconhecer sons, palavras ou música; causada por lesão do córtex auditivo do lobo temporal.
  color a., a. de cores; incapacidade de nomear ou identificar cores específicas através da visão; causada por lesão dos lobos occipital dominante e temporais.
  finger a., a. digital; incapacidade de nomear ou reconhecer os dedos das mãos individualmente, sejam os próprios ou os de outras pessoas; causada mais freqüentemente por lesão do giro angular (ou dos tecidos próximos) do hemisfério dominante.
  gustatory a., a. gustativo; incapacidade de classificar ou identificar um sabor, embora a capacidade de distinguir sabores diferentes ou de reconhecer sabores possa estar normal; pode ser geral, parcial ou específica.
  localization a., a. de localização; incapacidade de reconhecer a área onde a pele é tocada.
  olfactory a., a. olfatória; incapacidade de classificar ou identificar um odor,

agnosia

embora a capacidade de distinguir odores ou de reconhecê-los possa estar normal; pode ser geral, parcial ou específica.

optic a., a. óptica. SIN visual a.

position a., a. de posição; incapacidade de reconhecer a postura de uma extremidade.

tactile a., a. tátil; incapacidade de reconhecer objetos pelo tato, na presença de sensibilidade cutânea e proprioceptiva íntegra da mão; causada por uma lesão no lobo parietal contralateral. SIN astereognosis, stereoagnosis, stereoanesthesia.

visual a., incapacidade de reconhecer objetos pela visão; geralmente causada por lesões parieto-occipitais bilaterais. SIN optic a.

visual-spatial a., a. vísio-espacial; incapacidade de localizar objetos ou de avaliar distância, movimento e relações espaciais; causada por lesão no lobo occipital. Cf. simultanagnosia.

-agogue, -agog. Sufixos indicadores de promoção, estímulo ou liderança; um promotor ou estimulante. [G. *agōgos*, conduzir, de *agō*, liderar]

agom·phi·ous (a-gom′-fē-us). Agonfo. SIN anodontia.

agom·pho·sis, agom·phi·a·sis (ag-om-fō′sis, fi′a-sis). Agonfose; agonfíase. SIN anodontia. [G. *a-* priv. + *gomphos*, cavilha, tarugo]

ago·nad·al (ā-gon′a-dăl). Agonádico, indicando a ausência de gônadas.

ag·o·nal (ag′on-ăl). Agônico; relativo ao processo de morte ou ao momento da morte, assim chamado por causa da noção errônea antiga de que a morte é um processo doloroso.

ag·o·nist (ag′on-ist). Agonista. **1.** Indica um músculo em estado de contração, com referência a seu músculo oposto ou antagonista. **2.** Medicamento capaz de combinar-se com receptores para iniciar ações medicamentosas; possui afinidade e atividade intrínseca. [G. *agōn*, uma disputa]

ag·o·ny (ag′o-nē). Agonia; dor intensa ou angústia do corpo ou da mente. [G. *agōn*, luta, tentativa]

ag·o·ra·pho·bia (ag′or-ă-fō′bē-ă). Agorafobia; transtorno mental caracterizado por temor irracional de deixar o ambiente familiar e aventurar-se em espaços abertos, tão penetrante que há relutância e evitação em vivenciar um grande número de situações vitais externas, com freqüência associada a ataques de pânico. [G. *agora*, mercado + *phobos*, medo]

agor·a·pho·bic (ā-gōr-ă-fō′bik). Agorafóbico. Relativo ou característico da agorafobia.

agou·ti (ah-gu′tē). Aguti, acuti, cutia. SIN Dasyprocta. [Fr., do tupi]

-agra. Sufixo significando a instalação violenta de dor aguda. [G. *agra*, caçada, armadilha]

agraffe (ă-graf′). Agrafe, agrafo; gancho ou colchete metálico para manter juntas as bordas de uma ferida, empregado no lugar de suturas. [Fr. *agrafe*, gancho, grampo]

ag·ram·mat·i·ca (ag-ră-mat′i-kă). Agramatismo. SIN agrammatism.

agram·ma·tism (ă-gram′ă-tizm). Agramatismo; forma de afasia caracterizada pela incapacidade de construir uma sentença gramatical e pelo uso de palavras incorretas ou ininteligíveis; causada por uma lesão no lobo temporal dominante. SIN agrammatica, agrammatologia, jargon aphasia.

agram·ma·to·lo·gia (ă-gram′mă-tō-lō′jē-ă). Agramatologia. SIN agrammatism.

agran·u·lo·cyte (ă-gran′ū-lō-sīt). Agranulócito; leucócito não-granular. [G. *a-* priv. + L. *granulum*, grânulo, + G. *kytos*, célula]

agran·u·lo·cy·to·sis (ă-gran′ū-lō-sī-tō′sis). Agranulocitose; condição aguda caracterizada por leucopenia acentuada, como grande redução no número de leucócitos polimorfonucleares (freqüentemente < 500 granulócitos/mm³); é provável o aparecimento de úlceras infectadas na orofaringe, no tubo intestinal e em outras mucosas, bem como na pele. SIN agranulocytic angina, angina lymphomatosa, neutropenic angina.

agran·u·lo·plas·tic (ă-gran′ū-lō-plas′tik). Agranuloplásico; capaz de formar células não-granulares e incapaz de formar células granulosas. [G. *a-* priv. + L. *granulum*, grânulo, + G. *plastikos*, formador]

agraph·ia (ă-graf′ē-ă). Agrafia; incapacidade de escrever apropriadamente na ausência de anormalidades no membro; freqüentemente acompanha afasia e alexia; causada por lesões em várias porções do cérebro, especialmente aquelas no giro angular ou próximo a ele. SIN graphic aphasia, graphomotor aphasia. [G. *a-* priv. + *graphō*, escrever]

absolute a., a. absoluta; a. na qual o indivíduo não consegue escrever nem mesmo letras isoladas. SIN atactic a., literal a.

acoustic a., a. acústica; incapacidade de escrever palavras ditadas.

amnemonic a., a. amnemônica; a. na qual as letras e as palavras podem ser escritas, mas não reunidas em frases.

atactic a., a. absoluta. SIN absolute a.

constructional a., a. de construção; a. na qual as letras e palavras podem ser escritas corretamente, mas não arrumadas apropriadamente na superfície em que se escreve.

literal a., a. literal. SIN absolute a.

motor a., a. motora; a. devida à incoordenação muscular.

musical a., a. musical; incapacidade de escrever anotações musicais.

verbal a., a. verbal; agrafia na qual o indivíduo consegue escrever letras isoladas, mas não palavras.

agraph·ic (ā-graf′ik). Agráfico; relativo a agrafia ou acentuado por ela.

agre·tope (ag-rē′tōp). Agregatopo; parte de um antígeno processado que se liga à molécula do complexo de histocompatibilidade principal.

ague (ā′goo). **1.** Sezão; termo arcaico para a febre malárica. **2.** Calafrio. [Fr. *aigu*, agudo]

brass founder's a., febre do fundidor de bronze. SIN brass founder's *fever*.

AGUS Acrônimo para atypical glandular *cells* of undetermined significance (células glandulares atípicas de importância indeterminada), em *cell*. VER TAMBÉM Bethesda *system*.

ag·yi·o·pho·bia (aj′ē-ō-fō′bē-ă). Uma forma de agorafobia caracterizada por temor mórbido de estar na rua. [Gr. *agyia*, rua, + *phobos*, medo]

agy·ria (ā-jī′rē-ă). Agiria, falta congênita ou subdesenvolvimento do padrão de convoluções do córtex cerebral. SIN lissencephalia, lissencephaly [G. *a-* priv. + *gyros*, círculo]

ahaus·tral (ā-hos′trăl). Ausência de haustros, liso; termo que descreve a aparência do cólon intestinal em radiografias (enema baritado) na colite ulcerativa. [G. *a-* priv. + haustra]

AHF Abreviatura de antihemophilic *factor* A (fator anti-hemofílico A).

AHG Abreviatura de antihemophilic *globulin* (globulina anti-hemofílica).

aHyl Símbolo de allohydroxylysine (alo-hidroxi-lisina).

ahy·log·no·sia (ā-hī-log-nō′sē-ă). Incapacidade de reconhecer diferenças de densidade, peso e aspereza. [Gr. *a-* priv. + *hylē*, matéria, + *gnōsis*, reconhecimento]

Aicardi, J. Dennis, neurologista francês do século XX. VER A. *syndrome*.

aich·mo·pho·bia (īk-mō-fō′bē-ă). Temor mórbido de ser tocado pelo dedo da mão ou qualquer objeto delgado e pontudo. [G. *aichmē*, um ponto, + *phobos*, medo]

AID Abreviatura de donor of heterologous (artificial) insemination [doador de inseminação heteróloga (artificial)].

aid (ād). Ajuda ou assistência; por extensão, é aplicado a qualquer dispositivo graças ao qual uma função pode ser melhorada ou incrementada, como uma prótese auditiva.

programmable hearing aid, prótese auditiva de canais múltiplos que pode utilizar mais de uma estratégia de resposta de freqüência nível-dependente.

aidoi-, aidoio-. A genitália; corresponde ao L. pudend-. [G. *aidoia*, coisas indecentes, genitália]

AIDS

AIDS (ādz). AIDS/SIDA; síndrome de imunodeficiência adquirida; deficiência da imunidade celular induzida pela infecção pelo vírus da imunodeficiência humano (HIV-1) e caracterizada por doenças oportunistas, incluindo pneumonia por *Pneumocystis carinii*, sarcoma de Kaposi, leucoplaquia oral pilosa, doença por citomegalovírus, tuberculose, doença pelo complexo *Mycobacterium avium* (MAC), esofagite por *Candida*, criptosporidiose, isosporíase, criptococose, linfoma não-Hodgkin, leucoencefalopatia progressiva multifocal (LPM), herpes zoster e linfoma. O HIV é transmitido de uma pessoa para outra através da troca de líquidos orgânicos ricos em células (principalmente sêmen e sangue) por meio do contato sexual, do compartilhamento de agulhas contaminadas (como por dependentes de drogas IV) ou de outro contato com sangue contaminado (p. ex., acidentes com material biológico em profissionais de saúde). Os alvos primários do HIV são as células com a proteína de superfície CD4, incluindo principalmente linfócitos T auxiliares (*helper*). Os anticorpos anti-HIV, que surgem no soro 6 semanas a 6 meses após a infecção, servem como marcadores diagnósticos confiáveis, mas não se ligam ao HIV nem o inativam. A queda gradativa na contagem de linfócitos CD4, que tipicamente ocorre em um período de 10 a 12 anos, culmina com a perda da capacidade de resistência às infecções oportunistas; o surgimento de uma ou mais dessas infecções define o aparecimento da AIDS/SIDA. Em alguns pacientes, a linfadenopatia generalizada, a febre, a perda de peso, a demência e a diarréia crônica estão associadas aos estágios iniciais da doença. A AIDS/SIDA é uniformemente letal, com a maioria dos pacientes morrendo em decorrência de uma ou mais infecções oportunistas ou de suas complicações nos 2–5 anos seguintes ao aparecimento dos sintomas. Nos Estados Unidos, a AIDS/SIDA é a principal causa de morte de homens com 25–44 anos de idade, e a quarta causa de morte de mulheres na mesma faixa etária. Durante os últimos 5 anos, a taxa de mortalidade da doença e as taxas de transmissão perinatal diminuíram substancialmente, assim como a transmissão entre homens homossexuais e usuários de drogas intravenosas. Enquanto isso, a transmissão heterossexual e as taxas da doença em negros e hispânicos aumentaram. Estima-se que cerca de 50 milhões de pessoas estejam infectadas em todo o mundo, com a mais alta incidência em alguns países da África Central e do Leste da África, onde 1/4 da população adulta pode ser HIV-positiva. Além da profilaxia contra infecções oportunistas, o tratamento padrão da infecção pelo HIV inclui o uso de análogos nucleosídicos (didanosina, lamivudina, ribavirina, estavudina, zidovudina), inibidores da transcriptase reversa não-nucleosídicos (delavirina, efavirenz, nevirapina) e inibidores da protease (crixivan, indinavir, ritonavir, saquinavir). VER TAMBÉM human immunodeficiency *virus*. SIN acquired immunodeficiency syndrome. [acrônimo, *a*cquired *i*mmuno*d*eficiency *s*yndrome]

diagnóstico clínico de indivíduos infectados pelo HIV

contagem de células T CD4+	categorias clínicas*		
	(A)	(B)	(C)
(1) ≥ 500/µl	A1	B1	C2
(2) 200–499/µl	A2	B2	C2
(3) < 200/µl	A3	B3	C3

categoria A

assintomático: ausência de sintomas no momento da infecção pelo HIV

infecção aguda: enfermidade semelhante à mononucleose que dura algumas semanas no momento da infecção

linfadenopatia generalizada persistente: aumento dos linfonodos que persistem por 3 meses ou mais sem evidência de infecção

categoria B

angiomatose por bacilos

candidíase orofaringiana

candidíase vulvovaginal: persistente, freqüente ou que responde mal ao tratamento

displasia cervical (moderada ou grave)/carcinoma cervical *in situ*

sintomas característicos como febre ou diarréia que dura ≥ 1 mês

leucoplaquia oral (pilosa)

herpes zoster que envolve pelo menos dois episódios distintos ou mais de um dermátomo

púrpura trombocitopênica idiopática

listeriose

doença inflamatória pélvica, principalmente por abscesso tubovariano

neuropatia periférica

categoria C

candidíase dos brônquios, da traquéia ou dos pulmões

candidíase esofagiana

câncer cervical (invasivo)

coccidioidomicose disseminada ou extrapulmonar

criptococose extrapulmonar

criptosporidiose intestinal crônica (duração > 1 mês)

citomegalovirose (outra que não no fígado, no baço ou nos pulmões)

retinite por citomegalovírus (com perda da visão)

encefalopatia relacionada com o HIV

herpes simples: úlceras(s) crônica(s) (duração >1 mês) ou bronquite, pneumonite ou esofagite

histoplasmose disseminada ou extrapulmonar

isosporíase disseminada ou extrapulmonar

sarcoma de Kaposi

linfoma de Burkitt

linfoma imunoblástico

complexo de *Mycobacterium avium* ou *M. kansasii* disseminado ou extrapulmonar

outras espécies de *Mycobacterium* disseminadas ou extrapulmonares

pneumonia por *Pneumocystis carinii*

leucoencefalopatia progressiva multifocal

septicemia por *Salmonella* (recorrente)

toxoplasmose do cérebro

síndrome de emaciação decorrente do HIV

O desenvolvimento de agentes anti-retrovirais efetivos (inibidores da transcriptase reversa e inibidores da protease) e de ensaios quantitativos plasmáticos do RNA do HIV que permitem a monitoração da progressão da doença e da resposta ao tratamento mudaram o objetivo da terapia contra a AIDS/SIDA da profilaxia e tratamento das infecções oportunistas para a obtenção da remissão graças à terapia supressora. O comprometimento imunológico é monitorado por contagens seriadas de CD4; a replicação viral, pelo ensaio de RNA do HIV plasmático (carga viral). As indicações para o início da terapia anti-retroviral são o surgimento de sinais e sintomas de infecção oportunista, a queda da contagem de CD4 abaixo de 500/mm^3, ou carga viral de mais de 5.000 cópias/mL. Os inibidores da protease (IP) mostraram-se agentes anti-retrovirais bastante efetivos, e os esquemas padrões de tratamento que combinam dois inibidores da transcriptase reversa com 1 inibidor da protease ("terapia tripla") mostraram-se claramente **superiores** à monoterapia. Contudo, esses medicamentos são caros; em 1999, o custo anual da terapia e da monitoração foi superior a U$10.000. Os esquemas freqüentemente são complexos, com exigências variáveis em relação a **jejum e hora dos medicamentos**, sendo comuns efeitos colaterais e interações medicamentosas. Os inibidores da protease têm sido associados a aumento dos níveis séricos de colesterol e triglicerídeos, resistência à insulina e lipodistrofia desfigurante. Já apareceram cepas de HIV resistentes a todos os inibidores da protease disponíveis. A base racional dos esquemas de tratamento atuais contra a AIDS/SIDA é um esforço para erradicar a infecção pelo HIV através da inibição da disseminação do vírus para novas células até que todas as células infectadas tenham morrido. Entretanto, nenhuma pessoa até hoje foi curada da AIDS/SIDA. Um pequeno número de células CD4 de memória quiescentes em pacientes tratados com níveis plasmáticos indetectáveis de RNA do HIV abrigam DNA pró-viral do HIV capaz de replicação, e essas células podem sobreviver por meses ou anos. Os macrófagos e os neurônios do sistema nervoso central (SNC) atuariam como santuário anatômico para o HIV e os medicamentos anti-retrovirais não conseguem penetrar na concentração adequada. Quando se inicia precocemente a terapia anti-retroviral, as contagens de células CD4 auxiliares (*helper*) aumentam, a atividade da célula CD4 é preservada e os níveis de RNA do HIV podem permanecer indetectáveis por longos períodos. Contudo, em cerca de metade dos pacientes com doença avançada, mesmo os esquemas com múltiplos agentes não conseguem suprimir o RNA viral plasmático a níveis indetectáveis. Muitos fracassos terapêuticos resultam da desobediência aos esquemas com múltiplos agentes. Um quarto dos pacientes entrevistados admitiu "férias sem medicamentos" ocasionais. O fracasso de um esquema terapêutico freqüentemente impede o sucesso de outros esquemas devido ao alto grau de resistência cruzada entre os agentes anti-retrovirais. Após o fracasso de um esquema inicial, a pesquisa genotípica pode ser usada para identificar mutações no genoma do HIV que conferem resistência a uma ou mais classes de medicamentos anti-HIV. Em um significativo número de pacientes, as infecções oportunistas continuam, apesar do restabelecimento das contagens de CD4, provavelmente porque algumas subpopulações de células T foram aniquiladas pela infecção pelo HIV e não se recuperam mesmo após a supressão viral. Assim, a profilaxia contra as infecções oportunistas permanece um componente essencial do tratamento da doença pelo HIV. Além disso, mesmo pessoas infectadas pelo HIV que apresentam cargas virais indetectáveis ainda precisam ser consideradas infecciosas. Os padrões de tratamento da doença pelo HIV em evolução incluem terapia agressiva da fase aguda da infecção e administração profilática de terapia anti-retroviral após picadas acidentais com agulhas ou violência sexual. O desenvolvimento de uma vacina contra o HIV tem sido dificultado pelas propriedades únicas do vírus e pelo longo período de incubação da AIDS/SIDA. Uma vacina bivalente que induz a produção de anticorpos contra a proteína da camada externa do HIV está na fase III dos testes. Muitas autoridades no assunto acreditam que uma vacina efetiva também precisa estimular a imunidade mediada por células.

AIH Abreviatura de homologous (artificial) insemination [inseminação homóloga (artificial)].

AILD Abreviatura de angioimmunoblastic *lymphadenopathy* with dysproteinemia (linfadenopatia angioimunoblástica com disproteinemia).

aIle Abreviatura de alloisoleucine (aloisoleucina).

ai·lu·ro·pho·bia (ī′loo - rō - fō′bē - ă, ā′lu-). Temor mórbido de gatos ou aversão a eles. [G. *ailouros*, gato, + *phobos*, medo]

ai·nhum (ī′um). Ainhum. Dactilólise espontânea, constrição fibrosa adquirida, lentamente progressiva, dolorosa, que se desenvolve na dobra digitoplantar, em geral do quinto artelho, levando gradativamente à perda espontânea do artelho; afeta mais comumente os homens negros nos trópicos. [do. Af. (Lagos), serrar]

AIR Abreviatura de 5-aminoimidazole ribose 5′-phosphate and 5-aminoimidazole ribotide (5-aminoimidazol ribose 5′-fosfato e 5-aminoimidazol ribotídeo).

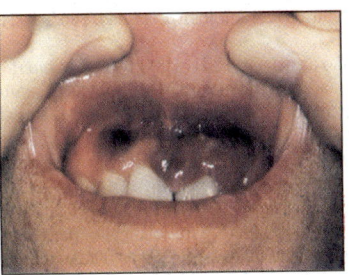 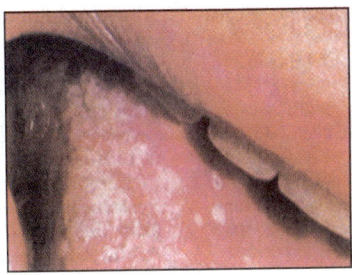 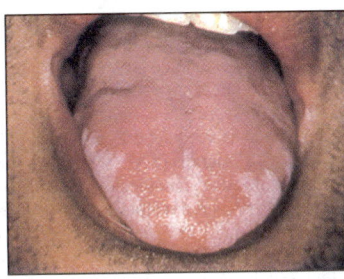

AIDS: lesões orais associadas à AIDS: (A) sarcoma de Kaposi, (B) Herpes zoster (devida a *Candida albicans*) e (C) leucoplaquia pilosa

air (ār). **1.** Ar, mistura de gases inodoros encontrados na atmosfera nas seguintes percentagens aproximadas por volume após a remoção do vapor d'água: oxigênio, 20,95; nitrogênio, 78,08; argônio 0,93; dióxido de carbono, 0,03; outros gases, 0,01. Termo outrora empregado para significar qualquer gás respiratório, independentemente de sua composição. **2.** Ventilar. SIN ventilate. [G. aēr; L. aer]
  alveolar a., gás alveolar. SIN alveolar gas.
  complemental a., volume de reserva inspiratório. SIN inspiratory reserve volume.
  complementary a., capacidade inspiratória. SIN inspiratory capacity.
  functional residual a., capacidade, residual funcional. SIN functional residual capacity.
  a. hunger, ventilação extremamente profunda como a que ocorre nos pacientes com acidose que tentam aumentar a ventilação dos alvéolos e expirar mais dióxido de carbono. VER TAMBÉM Kussmaul respiration.
  liquid a., ar líquido; ar que se tornou liquefeito devido a frio e pressão acentuados.
  minimal a., o volume de gás que permanece nos pulmões e não pode ser expelido após a retirada desses órgãos do organismo; ou depois que o tórax foi aberto.
  reserve a., volume de reserva expiratório. SIN expiratory reserve volume.
  residual a., volume residual. SIN residual volume.
  supplemental a., volume de reserva expiratório. SIN expiratory reserve volume.
  tidal a., volume corrente. SIN tidal volume.
  vitiated a., ar viciado; ar contendo uma percentagem reduzida de oxigênio.
Aird, Robert B., neurologista norte-americano, *1903. VER Flynn-A. syndrome.
air·sick·ness. Condição semelhante ao enjôo marítimo ou outras formas de cinetose, que ocorre em viagens aéreas ou espaciais em consequência da estimulação contínua e errática do ouvido interno.
air·space (ār'spās). Espaço aéreo; pertinente à porção do pulmão distal às vias aéreas condutoras ou brônquios; alveolar.
air·trap·ping (ār - trap'ing). Retenção de ar; esvaziamento lento ou incompleto de gás de todo o pulmão ou de parte dele durante a expiração; implica obstrução das vias aéreas regionais ou enfisema.
air·way (ār'wā) **1.** Qualquer parte das vias respiratórias através das quais passa o ar durante a respiração. **2.** Em anestesia ou reanimação, dispositivo para corrigir a obstrução respiratória, especialmente uma cânula orofaríngea e nasofaríngea, uma cânula endotraqueal ou um tubo de traqueotomia.
  anatomic a., espaço morto anatômico. SIN anatomic dead space.
  conducting a., vias aéreas de condução; as vias aéreas desde a cavidade nasal até um bronquíolo terminal.
  Guedel a., cânula orofaríngea usada para garantir a desobstrução das vias aéreas durante anestesia geral.
  lower a., vias aéreas inferiores; a porção das vias respiratórias que se estende da subglote até os bronquíolos terminais.
  neurogenic a., vias aéreas neurogênicas; obstrução das vias aéreas superiores devido a tônus muscular anormal; encontrada em pacientes com grave atraso do desenvolvimento ou lesão cerebral, e especialmente naqueles com tetraplegia espástica.
  respiratory a., vias respiratórias; a parte das vias aéreas onde ocorre a troca gasosa; inclui bronquíolos respiratórios, canais alveolares, sacos e alvéolos.
  upper a., vias aéreas superiores; a porção do trato respiratório que vai das narinas ou da boca até a laringe, inclusive.
Ajel·lo·my·ces cap·su·la·tum (ah - jē - lō - mī'sēz kap - soo - lā'tum). O estado ascomiceto (perfeito, sexuado, telemorfo) do *Histoplasma capsulatum*. SIN Emmonsiella capsulata.
Ajel·lo·my·ces der·ma·tit·i·dis (ah - jē - lō - mī'sēz der - mă - tit'i - dis). O estado perfeito (telemorfo) do fungo *Blastomyces dermatitidis;* os tipos masculino (+) e (−) causam doença com a mesma frequência. Esse estado sexuado é colocado na família Gymnoascaceae.
aj·ma·line (aj'mă - lēn); Ajmalina; alcalóide indol das raízes da *Rauwolfia serpentina*, relacionado com a reserpina, serpentina (serpentária) e ioimbina; usado no tratamento da hipertensão e como tranqüilizante ou sedativo.
aj·o·wan oil (aj'ō - wan). Óleo de ajovan, óleo de *ptychotis*. Óleo volátil destilado do fruto do *Carum copticum,* uma das fontes de timol; carminativo, aromático e expectorante. SIN ptychotis oil.
akan·thi·on (ă - kan'thē - on). Acantião. SIN acanthion.
akar·y·o·cyte (ă - kar'ē - ō - sīt). Acariota; célula desprovida de núcleo, como o eritrócito. SIN acaryote, akaryote. [G. *a*- priv. + *karyon*, núcleo, + *kytos*, cavidade (célula)]
akar·y·ote (ă - kar'ē - ōt). Acariota. SIN akaryocyte. [G. *a*- priv. + *karyon*, grão]
a·ka·thi·sia (ak - ă - thiz'ē - ă). Acatisia; síndrome caracterizada pela incapacidade de permanecer sentado, com inquietação motora e sensação de tremor muscular; pode surgir como efeito colateral de medicação antipsicótica e neuroléptica. SIN acathisia. [G. *a*- priv. + *kathisis*, assento]
akem·be (ă - kem'bē). Aquembe. SIN onyalai.
Åkerlund, A. Olof, radiologista sueco, 1885–1958. VER A. deformity.
aki·ne·sia (ā - ki - nē'sē - ă, ā - kī-). Acinesia, acinese. **1.** Ausência ou perda da força de movimento voluntário devido a um distúrbio extrapiramidal. **2.** Termo antigo para o intervalo pós-sistólico de repouso do coração. **3.** Neurose acompanhada por sintomas paréticos. SIN akinesis. [G. *a*- priv. + *kinēsis*, movimento]
  a. al'gera, a. álgica; condição marcada por intensa dor generalizada desencadeada por qualquer movimento; freqüentemente de origem psicogênica. [G. *algos*, dor]
  a. amnes'tica, perda de força muscular por desuso.
aki·ne·sic (ā - ki - nē'sik, ā - kī-). Acinésico, acinético. SIN akinetic.
aki·ne·sis (ā - ki - nē'sis, ā - kī-). Acinese, acinesia. SIN akinesia.
akin·es·the·sia (ā - kin'es - thē'zē - ă). Acinestesia; incapacidade de perceber o movimento ou a posição. Ausência da percepção de movimento ou da sensação muscular. [G. *a*- priv. + *kinēsis*, movimento, + *aisthēsis*, sensação]
aki·net·ic (ā - ki - net'ik, - kī - net'ik). Acinético; relativo à acinésia ou que sofre dela. SIN akinesic.
aki·ya·mi (ah - kē - yah'mē). Febre sakushu. SIN hasamiyami.
ak·lo·mide (ak'lō - mīd). Aclomida; coccidiostático usado na prática veterinária.
ak·ne·mia (ak - ne - me - a). Acnemia. VER acnemia.
AKNF Abreviatura de Adair-Koshland-Némethy-Filmer *model* (modelo de Adair-Koshland-Némethy-Filmer).
Al Símbolo de aluminum (alumínio).
ALA Abreviatura de δ-aminolevulinic acid (ácido δ-aminolevulínico).
Ala Símbolo de alanine (alanina) ou de seus mono- ou birradicais.
ala, gen. e pl. **alae** (ā'lă, ā'lē). **1.** [TA]. Asa. SIN wing. **2.** Dobras cuticulares pronunciadas, longitudinais nos nematódeos, geralmente encontradas nos estágios larvais (*Ascaris lumbricoides*), embora ocasionalmente presentes em vermes adultos (*Enterobius vermicularis*). [L. asas]
  a. au'ris, orelha externa. SIN auricle (1).
  a. cerebel'li, asa do lóbulo central. SIN wing of central lobule.
  a. cine' rea, trígono do nervo vago. SIN vagal (nerve) trigone.
  a. cris'tae gal'li [TA], asa da crista etmoidal. SIN a. of crista galli.
  a. of crista galli [TA], asa da crista etmoidal; pequena expansão lateral do osso etmóide à partir da parte frontal da crista etmoidal de cada lado e que se articula com o osso frontal, formando o forame cego. SIN a. cristae galli [TA], alar process, wing of crista galli.
  a. of ilium [TA], a. do ílio; a porção superior do ílio. SIN a. ossis ilii [TA], wing of ilium*.
  alae lin'gulae cerebel'li, língula do cerebelo. SIN lingula of cerebellum.
  a. lob'ulis centra'lis [TA], asa do lóbulo central. SIN wing of central lobule.
  a. ma'jor os'sis sphenoida'lis [TA], asa maior do esfenóide. SIN greater wing of sphenoid (bone).
  a. mi'nor os'sis sphenoida'lis [TA], asa menor do esfenóide. SIN lesser wing of sphenoid (bone).
  a. na'si [TA], asa do nariz. SIN a. of nose.

a. of nose [TA], asa do nariz; a parede externa, com maior abertura, de cada narina. SIN a. nasi [TA], pinna nasi, wing of nose.
a. orbitalis, asa menor do esfenóide. SIN lesser wing of sphenoid (bone).
a. os'sis il'ii [TA], asa do íleo. SIN a. of ilium.
a. sacra'lis [TA], asa do sacro. SIN a. of sacrum.
a. of sacrum [TA], a. do sacro; a superfície superior da parte lateral do sacro adjacente ao corpo. SIN a. sacralis [TA], wing of sacrum*.
a. tempora'lis, asa maior do esfenóide. SIN greater wing of sphenoid (bone).
a. of vomer [TA], a. do vômer; um lábio evertido de cada lado da borda superior do vômer, entre os quais se encaixa o rostro do osso esfenóide. SIN a. vomeris [TA], wing of vomer.
a. vo'meris [TA], asa do vômer. SIN a. of vomer.
alacrima (ā-lak'rē-ma). Alacrimia; ausência congênita de lágrimas. [G. a- priv.+ L. lacrima, lágrima]
Alagille, Daniel, médico francês, * 1925. VER Alagille syndrome.
Alajouanine, Théophile, neurologista francês, 1890–1980. VER Foix-Alajouanine myelitis; Foix-Alajouanine syndrome.
ala·lia (ă-la'lē-ă). Alalia; mutismo, incapacidade de falar. VER aphonia. [G. a- priv. + lalia, falar]
alal·ic (ă-lal'ik). Alálico; relacionado à alalia.
al·a·nine (A, Ala) (al'ă-nēn). Alanina; ácido 2-aminopropiônico; ácido α-aminopropiônico; o L-esteroisômero é um dos aminoácidos que ocorrem amplamente nas proteínas.
β-al·a·nine. β-alanina; ácido 3-aminopropiônico ou ácido β-aminopropiônico; produto da descarboxilação do ácido aspártico. Encontrado no cérebro, na carnosina e na coenzima A.
al·a·nine ami·no·trans·fer·ase (ALT). Alanina aminotransferase; enzima que transfere grupamentos amina da L-alanina para 2-cetoglutarato, ou o inverso (do L-glutamato para o piruvato); existe uma D-alanina transaminase que realiza a mesma reação, mas usando D-alanina e D-glutamato. A concentração sérica está aumentada na hepatite viral e no infarto do miocárdio. SIN alanine transaminase, glutamic-pyruvic transaminase, serum glutamic-pyruvic transaminase.
al·a·nine-gly·ox·y·late ami·no·trans·fer·ase. Alanina-glioxilato aminotransferase; enzima que catalisa reversivelmente a transferência de um grupamento amino da L-alanina para o glioxilato, produzindo, assim, piruvato e glicina. Um distúrbio hereditário que resulta em alteração da atividade da a.-g.a. está associado a hiperoxalúria primária do tipo I.
al·a·nine-ox·o·mal·o·nate ami·no·trans·fer·ase. Alanina-oxomalonato aminotransferase; enzima que realiza a transferência reversível de grupamentos amino da L-alanina para oxomalonato, ação semelhante à da alanina aminotransferase, produzindo piruvato e aminomalonato.
β-ala·nine-py·ru·vate ami·no·trans·fer·ase. β-alanina-piruvato aminotransferase; enzima que transfere reversivelmente o grupamento amino da β-alanina para o piruvato, produzindo, assim, L-alanina e malonato semialdeído. A deficiência dessa enzima é considerada a causa da hiper-β-alaninemia.
al·a·nine rac·e·mase. Alanina racemase; enzima que, exigindo fosfato de piridoxal como coenzima, catalisa a racemização reversível de L-alanina para D-alanina; encontrada em vários microrganismos, nos quais participaria na biossíntese dos D-aminoácidos presentes nas proteínas capsulares.
al·a·nine trans·am·i·nase. Alanina transaminase. SIN alanine aminotransferase.
alan·o·sine (ă-lan'ō-sēn). Alanosina; antibiótico produzido pelo Streptomyces alanosinicus; possui atividade antineoplásica e antiviral.
Alanson, Edward, cirurgião inglês, 1747–1823. VER A. amputation.
alan·tin (ă-lan'tin). Alantina; inulina. SIN inulin.
al·an·tol (al'an-tol). Alantol; líquido amarelado obtido por destilação da raiz de Inula helenium ou ênula; usado internamente como tônico irritante e externamente como um leve rubefaciente. SIN inulol.
al·ant starch (ă-lant'). Inulina. SIN inulin.
al·a·nyl (al'ă-nil). Alanil; radical acil da alanina.
alar (ā'lăr). **1.** Alar, relativo a asa; alado. **2.** Axilar. SIN axillary. **3.** Relativo à asa de estruturas como o nariz, o esfenóide, o sacro, etc.
ALARA. Acrônimo para a filosofia do uso da radiação com base nas dosagens tão baixas quanto razoavelmente atingíveis (as low as reasonably achievable) para alcançar o diagnóstico, o tratamento ou outro objetivo desejado.
alar·mone (ă-lar'mōn). Alarmona; substância bioquímica cuja síntese é aumentada em certas condições de estresse (p.ex., uma deficiência nutricional que afeta certas enzimas). [alarm + -mone]
alas·trim (ă-las'trim). Alastrim; forma leve de varíola causada por uma cepa menos virulenta do vírus. SIN Cuban itch, Kaffir pox, milkpox, pseudosmallpox, pseudovariola, variola minor, West Indian smallpox, whitepox. [Pg. alastrar, espalhar sobre uma superfície]
al·ba (al'bă). Substância branca. SIN white matter. [fem. de L. albus, branco]
Albarran y Dominguez, Joaquin, urologista cubano, 1860–1912. VER Albarran glands, em gland; Albarran test; A. tubules, em tubule.
al·be·do (al-bē'dō). Albedo; área branca da retina decorrente de edema ou infarto. [L. brancura]

Albers-Schönberg, Heinrich E., radiologista alemão, 1865–1921. VER Albers-Schönberg disease.
Albert, Eduard, cirurgião austríaco, 1841–1900. VER A. suture.
Albert, Henry médico norte-americano, 1878–1930. VER A. stain.
al·bi·cans, pl. **al·bi·can·tia** (al'bi-kanz, -kan'tē-ă). **1.** SIN white. **2.** Corpo albicante (ovário). SIN corpus albicans. [L.]
al·bi·du·ria (al-bi-doo'rē-ă). Albinúria; eliminação de urina pálida ou branca de baixa densidade, como na quilúria. SIN albinuria. [L. albidus, esbranquiçado, + G. ouron, urina]
al·bi·dus (al'bi-dŭs). Álbido; branco, esbranquiçado. [L.]
Albini, Giuseppe, fisiologista italiano, 1827–1911. VER A. nodules, em nodule.
al·bi·nism (al'bi-nizm). Grupo de distúrbios hereditários (geralmente autossômicos recessivos) com deficiência ou ausência de pigmento na pele, nos cabelos e nos olhos, ou apenas nos olhos, decorrentes de uma anormalidade na produção de melanina. SIN ocular a., piebaldismo. [albin + ism]

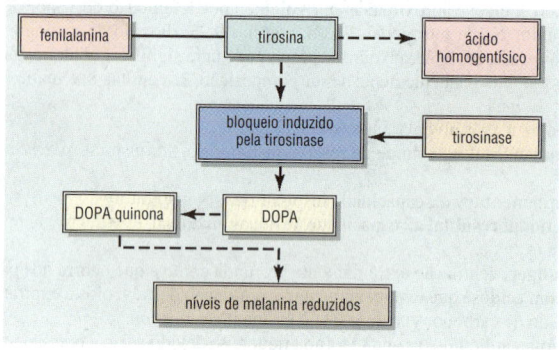

albinismo: diagrama mostrando os efeitos de tirosinase sobre a produção de melanina

Åland Island a., albinismo ocular 2. SIN ocular a. 2.
cutaneous a. [MIM* 126070], a. cutâneo. SIN piebaldism.
Forsius-Eriksson a., albinismo ocular 2. SIN ocular a. 2.
Nettleshop-Falls a., albinismo ocular 1. SIN ocular a. 1.
ocular a. [MIM*300650 & *300700], a. ocular; ausência de pigmento principalmente na íris, na coróide e no epitélio pigmentar da retina.
ocular a. 1 a. ocular. [MIM*300500], tipo de a. ocular caracterizado por despigmentação do fundo e veias coroidais proeminentes, nistagmo e titubeação; a visão geralmente é comprometida; causado por mutação no gene OA1 no cromossoma Xp; herança ligada ao X. SIN Nettleshop-Falls a.
ocular a. 2 [MIM*300600], tipo de a. ocular caracterizado por hipoplasia da fóvea, comprometimento acentuado da visão, nistagmo, miopia, astigmatismo e cegueira protanômala para cores, além de a. do fundo. SIN Åland Island a., Forsius-Eriksson a.
ocular a. 3 [MIM*203310], tipo de a. ocular caracterizado por visão comprometida, íris translucentes, nistagmo congênito, fotofobia, albinismo do fundo com hiperplasia da fóvea e estrabismo; causado por mutação no gene da conjuntivite (P) no 6q; herança autossômica recessiva.
ocular a. with late-onset sensorineural deafness [MIM* 300650], a. ocular com surdez sensorineural de início tardio. Herança ligada ao X.
ocular a. with sensorineural deafness [MIM* 103470], a. ocular com surdez sensorineural. Síndrome de Waardenburg tipo II. VER Waardenburg syndrome.
oculocutaneous a., oculocutâneo; distúrbio caracterizado por deficiência de pigmento na pele, no cabelo e nos olhos, fotofobia, acuidade visual diminuída; existem dois grupos: tirosinase-negativo [MIM*203100], no qual ocorre ausência de tirosinase, e tirosinase-positivo [MIM*203200], no qual a tirosinase normal não pode penetrar nas células pigmentares; o heterozigoto composto é normal, e, portanto, as duas formas não são alélicas. Existem várias formas de herança autossômica recessiva: a do tipo IA é caracterizada por ausência de tirosinase com ausência completa por toda a vida de melanina, fotofobia acentuada e nistagmo, causada por mutação no gene da tirosinase (TYR) no cromossoma 11q. O tipo II apresenta atividade normal da tirosinase e é o mais comum; o cabelo escurece e há o desenvolvimento de nevos e efélides; causado por mutação no gene do albinismo oculocutâneo (OCA2) em 15q. O tipo III é caracterizado por tirosinase ausente, mas com pigmentação da íris na primeira década de vida; causado por mutação no gene da proteína 1 relacionado com a tirosina (TYRP1) em 9p. O tipo IV é encontrado em africanos com tirosinase normal e o tipo V está associado a cabelos ruivos. O tipo VI é sinônimo da síndrome de Hermansky-Pudlak [MIM*203300], com tirosinase baixa a ausente e hemorragia decorrente da deficiência plaquetária, causado por mutação no gene Hermansky-Pudlak (HPS) em 10q.

rufous a., albinismo ruivo. SIN xanthism.
al·bi·no (al-bī′nō). Albino; indivíduo com albinismo. [Pg., aquele que é branco, de *albo*, branco, do L. *albus* + *-ino*, dim. sufixo]
al·bi·not·ic (al-bi-not′ik). Pertinente ao albinismo.
al·bi·nu·ria (al-bi-noo′rē-ă). Albinúria, albidúria. SIN albiduria.
Albinus (Weiss), Bernhard S., anatomista e cirurgião alemão, 1697–1770. Ver A. *muscle*.
al·bo·ci·ne·re·ous (al-bō-si-nē′rē-ŭs). Albocinério; relativo tanto à substância branca como à cinzenta do cérebro ou da medula espinal. [L. *albus*, branco, + *cinereus*, cinza, de *cinis (ciner-)*, cinzas]
Albrecht, Karl M. P., anatomista alemão, 1851–1894. VER A. *bone*.
Albright, Fuller, médico norte-americano, 1900–1969. VER A. *disease, syndrome*, hereditary *osteodystrophy*; Forbes-A. *syndrome*; McCune-A. *syndrome*.
al·bu·gin·ea (al-bū-jin′ē-ă). Albugínea; camada de tecido fibroso branca, como a túnica albugínea. VER *tunica* albuginea, *tunica* albuginea of corpus spongiosum, *tunica* albuginea of corpora cavernosa, *tunica* albuginea oculi, *tunica* albuginea of testis. [L. *albugineus*, de *albugo*, mancha branca]
al·bu·gin·e·ot·o·my (al-bū-jin-ē-ot′ō-mē). Albugineotomia. Incisão em qualquer túnica albugínea. [albuginea + G. *tomē*, cortar]
al·bu·gin·e·ous (al-bū-jin′ē-ŭs). Albugíneo. **1.** Semelhante à clara de ovo fervida. **2.** Relativo a qualquer túnica albugínea. [L. *albugineus*, de *albugo*, mancha branca]
al·bu·men (al-bū′men). Albume, albúmen. SIN ovalbumin. [ver albumin]
al·bu·min (al-bū′min). Albumina; tipo de proteína simples cujas variedades são amplamente distribuídas pelos tecidos e líquidos de vegetais e animais; a albumina é solúvel em água pura, precipitável de soluções por ácidos fortes e coagulável pelo aquecimento em solução ácida ou neutra. [L. *albumen (-min-)*, a clara de ovo]
a. A, albumina A; o tipo normal ou comum de a. do soro humano.
acetosoluble a., a. acetossolúvel. SIN Patein a.
a. B, albumina B. VER inherited albumin *variants*, em *variant*.
Bence Jones a., VER Bence Jones *proteins*, em *protein*.
blood a., a. sérica. SIN serum a.
bovine serum a. (BSA), albumina sérica bovina; fonte de albumina empregada comumente em estudos biológicos *in vitro*.
dried human a., a. humana desidratada. SIN normal human serum a.
egg a., albume. SIN ovalbumin.
a. Ghent, a. de Ghent. VER inherited albumin *variants*, em *variant*.
iodinated ^{131}I human serum a., a. sérica humana iodada (I[131]), solução estéril, tamponada e isotônica preparada para conter não menos de 10 mg de a. sérica humana normal radioiodada por mL, e ajustada para fornecer não mais do que 1 mCi de radioatividade por mL; usada como auxiliar de diagnóstico na medida do volume sanguíneo e do débito cardíaco.
iodinated ^{125}I serum a., a. sérica iodada (I[125]); a. sérica radioiodada; solução estéril, tamponada e isotônica preparada para conter não menos de 10 mg de albumina sérica humana normal radioiodada por mL, e ajustada para fornecer não mais do que 1 mCi de radioatividade por mL; usada como auxiliar de diagnóstico na determinação do volume sanguíneo e do débito cardíaco. SIN radioiodinated serum a.
macroaggregated a. (MAA), a. macroagregada (MAA); conglomerados de albumina sérica humana em suspensão; em geral, refere-se a partículas de 10 a 50 μm de tamanho; usados como agente marcador para cintilografia pulmonar.
a. Mexico, a. México. VER inherited albumin *variants*, em *variant*.
a. Naskapi, a. Naskapi. VER inherited albumin *variants*, em *variant*.
native a., a. nativa; a. existente em seu estado natural, sendo as duas formas principais a a. sérica e a. do ovo; é solúvel em água e não se precipita em ácidos diluídos.
normal human serum a., albumina sérica humana normal; preparação estéril de albumina sérica, obtida por fracionamento de proteínas plasmáticas de pessoas sadias; usada como material de transfusão e para tratar o edema devido a hipoproteinemia. SIN dried human a.
Patein a., a. de Patein; a. acetossolúvel; substância semelhante à albumina sérica, mas solúvel em ácido acético. SIN acetosoluble a.
plasma a., a. sérica. SIN serum a.
radioiodinated serum a. (RISA), a. sérica radioiodada. SIN iodinated ^{125}I serum a.
a. Reading, a. de Reading. VER inherited albumin *variants*, em *variant*.
serum a., albumina sérica; soroalbumina; a principal proteína no plasma, presente no plasma sanguíneo e em líquidos serosos. Participa no transporte de ácidos graxos e ajuda a regular a pressão osmótica do sangue. Também se liga a hormônios, bilirrubina e medicamentos. SIN blood a., plasma a., seralbumin.
a. tannate, tanato de albumina; pó adstringente obtido pela ação do ácido tânico sobre a albumina; contém cerca de 50% de ácido tânico; usado como adstringente desinfetante na diarréia e como talco.
al·bu·min·ate (al-bū′min-āt). Albuminato; produto da reação entre a albumina nativa e ácidos ou bases diluídos, resultando em albuminas ácidas ou alcalinas; os dois tipos se caracterizam pela solubilidade em álcalis ou ácidos diluídos e relativa insolubilidade em água, soluções diluídas de sais e álcool.

al·bu·mi·na·tu·ria (al-bū′mi-nă-too′rē-ă). Albuminatúria; presença de quantidade anormalmente grande de albuminatos na urina. [albuminato + G. *ouron*, urina]
al·bu·min·if·er·ous (al-bū-min-if′er-ŭs). Albuminífero; produtor de albumina. [albumina + L. *fero*, conduzir]
al·bu·min·ip·ar·ous (al-bū-min-ip′ar-ŭs). Albuminíparo; formador de albumina. [albumina + L. *pario*, produzir]
al·bu·min·og·e·nous (al-bū-min-oj′en-ŭs). Albuminógeno; produtor ou formador de albumina.
al·bu·mi·noid (al-bū′min-oyd). Albuminóide. **1.** Semelhante à albumina. **2.** Qualquer proteína. **3.** Um tipo simples de proteína, insolúvel em solventes neutros, presente em tecidos córneos e cartilaginosos e no cristalino; p.ex., ceratina, elastina, colágeno. SIN glutinoid, scleroprotein.
al·bu·mi·nol·y·sis (al-bū-min-ol′i-sis). Albuminólise; proteólise; com freqüência, especificamente a proteólise de albuminas. [albumin + G. *lysis*, dissolução]
al·bu·mi·nop·ty·sis (al-bū-mi-nop′ti-sis). Albuminoptise; expectoração albuminosa. [albumin + G. *ptysis*, escarro]
al·bu·mi·nor·rhea (al-bū-min-ō-rē′ă). Albuminorréia, albuminúria. SIN albuminuria. [albumin + G. *rhoia*, fluxo]
al·bu·min·ous (al-bū′min-ŭs). Albuminoso; relativo a, contendo ou consistindo em albumina.
al·bu·min·u·ria (al-bū-mi-noo′rē-ă). Albuminúria; presença de proteína na urina, principalmente albumina, mas também globulina; em geral, indicativa de doença, mas, às vezes, resultante de disfunção temporária ou passageira. SIN albuminorrhea, proteinuria (2). [albumin + G. *ouron*, urina]
adolescent a., a. do adolescente, a. funcional que ocorre por ocasião da puberdade; em geral é cíclica ou ortostática.
adventitious a., a. adventícia; a. falsa; a. resultante da presença de sangue escapando de algum lugar nas vias urinárias, de quilo ou de algum outro líquido albuminoso, não produzido pela filtração de albumina no sangue pelos rins. SIN false a.
a. of athletes, a. de atletas; uma forma de a. funcional após exercícios musculares excessivos.
Bamberger a., a. Bamberger; termo obsoleto para a. hematógena, às vezes observada nas últimas fases de anemia avançada.
benign a., a. benigna, a. essencial, termo coletivo para tipos que não resultam de anormalidades nos rins. SIN essential a.
cardiac a., a. cardíaca; a. provocada por insuficiência cardíaca congestiva.
colliquative a., a. coliquativa; a. que, a princípio, é discreta mas que, inesperadamente, agrava-se durante a convalescença de doença muito febril, como a febre tifóide.
cyclic a., a. cíclica; a. recidivante; a. funcional às vezes observada de forma intermitente em ciclos de 12 a 36 horas de duração, principalmente em jovens; a albuminúria costuma ser leve. SIN recurrent a.
dietetic a., a. dietética; excreção de proteínas na urina após a ingestão de certos alimentos.
essential a., a. essencial, a. benigna. SIN benign a.
false a., a. falsa. SIN adventitious a.
febrile a., a. febril; a. associada a febre.
functional a., a. funcional; termo coletivo que indica tipos de a. benigna associados a exercícios físicos ou a outras condições nas quais existem alterações fisiológicas, como a gravidez ou a adolescência. SIN physiologic a. (2).
intermittent a., a. intermitente; a. funcional que ocorre em intervalos, como a. cíclica ou a. dos atletas.
lordotic a., a. lordótica; assim chamada devido à teoria de que a albuminúria resulta da pressão devida à lordose na coluna lombar.
neuropathic a., a. neuropática; a. associada à epilepsia ou a outros distúrbios convulsivos, traumatismo cerebral e hemorragia cerebral.
orthostatic a., a. ortostática; proteinúria ortostática ou postural; aparecimento de albumina na urina quando o paciente está de pé e seu desaparecimento quando deitado. SIN orthostatic proteinuria, postural proteinuria, postural a.
physiologic a., a. fisiológica; **(1)** presença de traços de proteína em urina normal sob outros aspectos; **(2)** a. funcional. SIN a. funcional.
postrenal a., a. pós-renal; albuminúria produzida por doença distal ao rim.
postural a., a. postural. SIN orthostatic a.
prerenal a., a. pré-renal; a. produzida por doença diferente de nefropatia ou das vias geniturinárias.
recurrent a., a. recidivante. SIN cyclic a.
regulatory a., a. reguladora; a. transitória que ocorre após exercícios físicos incomuns.
transient a., a. transitória; a. de natureza temporária ou breve.
al·bu·min·u·ric (al-bū-mi-noo′rik). Albumúrico; relativo a ou caracterizado por albuminúria.
al·bu·ter·ol (al-bū′ter-ol). Albuterol; broncodilatador simpaticomimético com efeitos relativamente seletivos sobre receptores β$_2$, por inalação. SIN salbutamol.
Al·ca·lig·e·nes (al-kă-lij′en-ēz). Gênero de bactérias Gram-negativas,

baciliformes, não-fermentativas (família Achromobacteraceae), que são móveis e peritríquias ou imóveis. São estritamente aeróbicas; algumas cepas são capazes de respiração anaeróbica na presença de nitrato ou nitrito. Seu metabolismo é respiratório, nunca fermentativo. Não utilizam carboidratos. São encontradas principalmente no canal intestinal, em matérias putrefatas, em laticínios, na água e na terra; podem ser isoladas dos tratos gastrointestinal e respiratório e de feridas de seres humanos hospitalizados com sistema imunológico comprometido; ocasionalmente causam infecções oportunistas, incluindo septicemia nosocomial. A espécie típica é *A. faecalis*. [alkali + G. *-gen*, produtor]

al·cap·ton (al-kap'ton). Alcaptona. SIN homogentisic acid.

al·cap·ton·u·ria, al·kap·ton·u·ria (al-kap-tō-noo'rē-a) [MIM* 203500]. Alcaptonúria; excreção de ácido homogentísico (alcaptona) na urina decorrente de ausência congênita da enzima homogentisato 1,2-dioxigenase, que medeia uma etapa essencial no catabolismo da fenilalanina e da tirosina; a urina torna-se escura, se deixada em repouso, ou é alcalinizada (resultado da formação de produtos da polimerização do ácido homogentísico); ocorre freqüentemente através de períodos relativamente longos ou pode recidivar ou ceder em intervalos irregulares; artrite e ocronose são complicações tardias; herança autossômica recessiva; causada por mutação no gene da homogentisato 1,2-dioxigenase (HGD) no cromossoma 3q. [alkapton + G. *ouron*, urina]

al·cap·ton·ur·ic, al·kap·to·nur·ic (al-kap-tō-noo-rik; al-kap'to-nu'rik). Alcaptonúrico. 1. Relativo à alcaptonúria. 2. A pessoa com alcaptonúria.

Al·ci·an blue (al'sē-an) [C.I. 74240]. Azul alcião; complexo ftalociânico usado como corante para distinguir as sulfomucinas das sialomucinas e das mucinas do ácido urônico, para demonstrar os polissacarídeos sulfados e detectar glicoproteínas na eletroforese; empregado freqüentemente em associação com PAS ácido ou aldeído fucsina.

al·clo·fe·nac (al-klō'fē-nak). Alclofenaco; agente antiinflamatório.

al·clo·met·a·sone (al-klō-met'a-sōn). Alclometasona; corticosteróide poderoso usado como o 17,21-dipropionato no tratamento tópico da psoríase e de outras dermatoses profundas.

Alcock, Benjamin, anatomista irlandês, 1801-?. VER A. canal.

al·co·gel (al'kō-jel). Alcogel; um hidrogel com álcool em vez de água como meio de dispersão.

al·co·hol (al'kō-hol). Álcool. 1. Um de uma série de compostos orgânicos químicos nos quais um hidrogênio (H) fixado ao carbono é substituído por uma hidroxila (OH); os álcoois reagem com ácidos para formar ésteres e com álcalis metálicos para formar alcoolatos. Quanto aos álcoois individuais aqui não apresentados, ver o nome específico. 2. CH_3CH_2OH; feito de açúcar, amido e outros carboidratos por fermentação com levedo e sinteticamente a partir do etileno ou acetileno. Tem sido utilizado em bebidas e como solvente, veículo e conservante; na medicina, tem sido usado externamente como rubefaciente, refrigerante e desinfetante, e, internamente, como analgésico, tônico estomacal, sedativo e antipirético. SIN ethanol, ethyl alcohol, grain a., rectified spirit, wine spirit. 3. A mistura azeotrópica de CH_3CH_2OH e água (92,3% por peso de etanol a 15,56°C). [Ar. *al*, o, + *kohl*, pó antimonial fino; inicialmente usado para designar um pó fino e, depois, qualquer coisa impalpável (volátil)]

absolute a., álcool absoluto; (1) a. a 100% tendo-se removido a água. SIN anhydrous a. (2) a. com mínima mistura de água; no máximo a 1%. SIN dehydrated a.

acid a., álcool ácido; a. etílico (70%) contendo 1% de ácido clorídrico.

anhydrous a., a anidro, a. absoluto. SIN absolute a. (1).

bile a., a. biliar; um de um grupamento de álcoois poliidroxilados derivados do colestano.

dehydrated a., a desidratado. a. absoluto. SIN absolute a. (2).

denatured a., a. desnaturado; álcool etílico tornado impróprio para consumo como bebida pelo acréscimo de um ou mais produtos químicos para fins comerciais (p.ex., metanol, aldeol, octaacetato de sacarose). SIN industrial methylated spirit, methylated spirit.

dihydric a., a. diídrico; a. contendo dois grupamentos OH em sua molécula; p.ex. etilenoglicol.

dilute a., a. diluído; um álcool em misturas aquosas de diversas concentrações, p.ex., 90, 80, 70, 60, 50, 45, 25 e 20% volume/volume de C_2H_5OH.

fatty a., a. graxo; álcool de cadeia longa, análogo aos ácidos graxos, dos quais o álcool graxo pode ser considerado como um produto de redução, p.ex. octadecanol do ácido esteárico. É geralmente encontrado esterificado nas ceras. SIN wax a.

grain a., álcool de cereais. SIN alcohol (2).

methyl a., CH_3OH; a. metílico; líquido móvel, inflamável e tóxico, usado como solvente industrial, anticongelante e na produção de substâncias químicas; a ingestão pode causar acidose grave, comprometimento visual e outros efeitos no sistema nervoso central. SIN carbinol, methanol, pyroligneous a., pyroligneous spirit, pyroxylic spirit, wood alcohol, wood naphtha, wood spirit.

monohydric a., a. monoídrico; álcool contendo um grupamento OH.

multiple a., a. múltiplo; álcool contendo mais de um grupo OH.

polyoxyethylene a.'s, a. de polioxietileno; usado como agente emulsificante e umidificante, antiestático, solubilizante, desespumante e para outros fins industriais. O polidocanol (Laureth 9) é usado como espermaticida; auxiliar farmacêutico (surfactante).

primary a., a. primário; álcool caracterizado pelo radical univalente $-CH_2OH$.

pyroligneous a., a. metálico. SIN methyl a.

rubbing a., linimento; mistura alcoólica destinada ao uso externo; contém geralmente 70% por volume de álcool absoluto ou a. isopropílico; o restante consiste em água, desnaturantes (com e sem corantes à base de alcatrão) e óleos perfumados; usado como rubefaciente para dores musculares e articulares.

secondary a., a. secundário; a. caracterizado pelo grupamento atômico bivalente

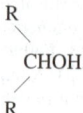

sugar a., álcool poliídrico formado pela redução do grupamento carbonila de um açúcar a um grupamento hidroxila. VER sugar alcohol.

tertiary a., a. terciário; a. caracterizado pelo grupamento atômico trivalente,

$$\begin{array}{c} R \\ | \\ R-COH. \\ | \\ R \end{array}$$

trihydric a., a. triídrico; a. contendo três grupamentos OH; p.ex., glicerol.

unsaturated a.'s, a. insaturado; os a. cujas cadeias de carbono contêm uma ou mais ligações duplas ou triplas.

wax a., álcool graxo. SIN fatty a.

al·co·hol ac·ids. Ácidos alcoólicos; um grupo de compostos que contêm tanto radicais carboxila como hidroxila; p.ex., ácido glicólico.

al·co·hol·ate (al-kō-hol'āt). Alcoolato. 1. Tintura ou outro preparado contendo álcool. 2. Composto químico no qual o íon hidrogênio no grupamento OH de um álcool é substituído por um metal alcalino (lítio, sódio, potássio, rubídio, césio e frâncio); p.ex., metilato de sódio, CH_3ONa.

al·co·hol de·hy·dro·gen·ase (ADH). Álcool desidrogenase; oxidorredutase que converte reversivelmente um álcool em aldeído (ou cetona) com NAD^+ como aceptor de H. Por exemplo, etanol + NAD^+ ↔ acetaldeído + NADH. VER TAMBÉM alcohol dehydrogenase (acceptor), alcohol dehydrogenase ($NADP^+$).

al·co·hol de·hy·dro·gen·ase (ac·cep·tor). Álcool desidrogenase (aceptor); oxidorredutase que converte reversivelmente os álcoois primários em aldeídos com um aceptor de H diferente de $NADP^+$.

al·co·hol de·hy·dro·gen·ase ($NADP^+$). Álcool desidrogenase ($NADP^+$); oxidorredutase que converte reversivelmente os álcoois em aldeídos (ou cetonas) com $NAD(P)^+$ como aceptor de H. SIN aldehyde reductase.

al·co·hol·ic (al-kō-hol'ik). Alcoólico. 1. Relativo a, contendo ou produzido por álcool. 2. Pessoa que sofre de alcoolismo. 3. Pessoa que abusa ou é dependente do álcool.

al·co·hol·ism (al'kō-hol-izm). Alcoolismo; abuso crônico, dependência ou vício do álcool; consumo crônico excessivo de bebidas alcoólicas, resultando em comprometimento da saúde e/ou do funcionamento social ou profissional, e adaptação crescente aos efeitos do álcool, o que exige doses cada vez maiores para alcançar e manter o efeito desejado; os sinais e sintomas específicos da supressão em geral se manifestam após a cessação súbita desse consumo. SIN alcohol addiction.

acute a., a. agudo; deterioração temporária da função mental, acompanhada por incoordenação e paresia musculares induzidas pela ingestão rápida de bebidas alcoólicas. SIN intoxication (2).

chronic a., a. crônico; condição patológica que afeta principalmente os sistemas nervoso e gastrentérico, produzida pelo consumo habitual de bebidas alcoólicas em quantidades tóxicas.

al·co·hol·i·za·tion (al'kō-hol-i-zā'shŭn). Alcoolização; impregnação ou saturação com álcool.

al·co·hol·o·pho·bia (al'kō-hol-ō-fō'bē-a). Alcoolofobia; temor mórbido do álcool ou de se tornar um alcoólatra. [álcool + G. *phobos*, medo]

al·co·hol·y·sis (al-kō-hol'i-sis). Alcoólise; rompimento de uma ligação química com o acréscimo de elementos do álcool no momento da divisão. [álcool + G. *lysis*, dissolução]

al·cur·o·ni·um chlo·ride (al-kūr-ō'nē-ŭm). Cloreto de acurônio; relaxante de músculos esqueléticos ativos como um agente bloqueador neuromuscular não-despolarizante, que lembra o curare.

ALD Abreviatura de adrenoleukodystrophy (adrenoleucodistrofia).

al·da·di·ene (al-da-dī'ēn). Aldadieno; metabólito da espironolactona que contém ligações duplas entre C-4 e C-5 e entre C-6 e C-7; formado pela retirada da cadeia lateral 7α-acetiltiol da espironolactona e diurético tão potente quanto o composto original.

al·dar·ic ac·id (al'dar-ik). Ácido aldárico; ácido de um grupamento de ácidos do açúcar, caracterizado pela fórmula HOOC–(CHOH)$_n$–COOH; p.ex., ácido sacárico.

al·de·hol (al'dĕ-hol). Aldeol; produto de oxidação do querosene; usado para desnaturar o álcool etílico.

al·de·hyde (al'dĕ-hīd). Aldeído; composto contendo o radical –CH=O, redutível a um álcool (CH$_2$OH), oxidável a um ácido carboxílico (COOH); p.ex., acetaldeído.

  activated glycol aldehyde, aldeído glicólico ativado; pirofosfato de 2-(1,2-diidroxietil)tiamina; intermediário no metabolismo de carboidratos e na transcetolização.

  active a., a. ativo; qualquer derivado aldeídico do pirofosfato de tiamina.

  angular a., a. angular; o grupamento a. fixado ao carbono 13 (entre o anéis C e D) do núcleo esteróide na aldosterona.

  a. reductase, aldeído redutase. SIN alcohol dehydrogenase (NADP$^+$).

al·de·hyde de·hy·dro·gen·ase (ac·yl·at·ing). Aldeído desidrogenase (acetilante); oxidorredutase que converte um aldeído e CoA em acil-CoA com NAD$^+$ como aceptor de H.

al·de·hyde de·hy·dro·gen·ase (NAD$^+$). Aldeído desidrogenase (NAD$^+$); oxidorredutase que converte, de forma reversível, aldeído em ácidos com NADP$^+$ como aceptor de H.

al·de·hyde de·hy·dro·gen·ase (NAD(P)$^+$). Aldeído desidrogenase (NAD(P)$^+$); oxidorredutase que converte, de forma reversível, aldeídos em ácidos com NAD$^+$ ou NADP$^+$ como aceptor de H.

al·de·hyde-ly·as·es [EC 4.1.2.x]. aldeído liases; enzimas que catalisam a reversão da condensação de um aldol.

Alder, Albert von. VER A. *anomaly, bodies*, em *body*.

al·dim·ine (al'dĕ-mēn). Aldimina. SIN Schiff *base*.

al·di·tol (al'di-tol). Alditol; o poliálcool derivado da redução de uma aldose; p.ex., sorbitol. VER TAMBÉM aldose reductase.

al·do·bi·u·ron·ic ac·id (al'dō-bī-ū-ron'ik). Ácido aldobiurônico; produtos de condensação de uma aldose e um ácido urônico; esses agrupamentos ocorrem entre os componentes de diversos mucopolissacarídeos, principalmente o ácido hialurônico.

al·do·cor·tin (al'dō-kōr'tin). Aldocortina. SIN aldosterone.

al·do·hex·ose (al-dō-heks'ōs). Aldo-hexose; açúcar de seis carbonos caracterizado pela presença (potencial) de um grupamento aldeído na molécula; p.ex., glicose, galactose.

al·do·ke·to·mu·tase (al'dō-kē-tō-mū'tās). Aldocetomutase. SIN lactoyl-glutathione lyase.

al·dol (al'dōl). Aldol, acetaldol. VER aldol *condensation.*

al·do·las (al'dō-lās). Aldolase. **1.** Termo genérico para aldeído liase. **2.** Nome às vezes aplicado à frutose-bifosfato aldolase.

al·don·ic ac·ids (al-don'ik). Ácidos aldônicos; derivados monossacarídeos nos quais o grupamento aldeído foi oxidado em um grupamento carboxila. Podem formar lactonas (p.ex., ácido galactônico). SIN glyconic acids.

al·do·pen·tose (al-dō-pen'tōs). Aldopentose; monossacarídeo com cinco átomos de carbono, um dos quais é um grupamento aldeído (potencial), p.ex., ribose.

al·dose (al'dōs). Aldose; monossacarídeo potencialmente contendo o grupo característico dos aldeídos, –CHO; um poliidroxialdeído.

  a. mutarotase, a. 1-epimerase. SIN aldose 1-epimerase.

  a. reductase, a. redutase, polioldesidrogenase (NADP$^+$); oxidorredutase que converte reversivelmente aldoses em alditóis (p.ex., glicose em sorbitol) com NADPH como doador de hidrogênio. Etapa importante no metabolismo do sorbitol e na formação da catarata do diabetes. VER TAMBÉM D-sorbitol-6-phosphate dehydrogenase.

al·dose 1-ep·i·mer·ase. Aldose 1-epimerase; enzima que catalisa a interconversão reversível de α- e β-aldoses (p.ex., α- e β-D-glicose); age também sobre a L-arabinose, D-xilose, D-galactose maltose e lactose. SIN aldose mutarotase; mutarotase.

al·do·side (al'dō-sīd). Aldosídeo; glicosídeo em que a porção açúcar é uma aldose.

al·dos·ter·one (al-dos'ter-ōn). Aldosterona; hormônio esteróide produzido pela zona glomerulosa do córtex supra-renal; sua principal ação é facilitar a troca de potássio por sódio no túbulo renal distal, levando à reabsorção de sódio e à perda de potássio e hidrogênio; é o principal mineralocorticóide. Existe em equilíbrio com a forma aldeído. SIN aldocortin.

al·dos·ter·on·ism (al-dos'ter-on-izm). Aldosteronismo; distúrbio causado pela secreção excessiva de aldosterona. SIN hyperaldosteronism.

  idiopathic a., a. idiopático. SIN primary a.

  primary a., a. primário; distúrbio adrenocortical causado pela secreção excessiva de aldosterona e caracterizado por cefaléia, nictúria, poliúria, fadiga, hipertensão, alcalose hipopotassêmica, depleção de potássio, hipervolemia e atividade plasmática diminuída de renina; pode estar associado a pequenos adenomas corticais benignos. SIN Conn syndrome, idiopathic a.

  secondary a., a. secundário; a. que não resulta de um defeito intrínseco ao córtex supra-renal, mas de estímulo da secreção hormonal provocado por distúrbios extra-supra-renais; associado à atividade plasmática aumentada de renina e ocorre na insuficiência cardíaca, na síndrome nefrótica, na cirrose e na hipoproteinemia.

al·do·ste·ron·o·gen·e·sis (al-dos'ter-on-ō-jen'ĕ-sis). Aldosteronogênese; formação do hormônio aldosterona. [aldosterona + G. *genesis*, produção]

al·do·tet·rose (al-dō-tet'rōs). Aldotetrose; aldose de quatro carbonos; p.ex., treose, eritrose.

al·do·tri·ose (al-dō-trī'os). Aldotriose; aldose com três carbonos; p.ex., D- ou L- gliceraldeído.

al·dox·ime (al-doks'ēm). Aldoxima; derivado composto pela reação de uma aldose com hidroxilamina, contendo assim o grupo a. –HC=NOH.

Aldrich, Robert Anderson, pediatra norte-americano, *1917. VER A. *syndrome;* Wiskott-Aldrich *syndrome.*

al·drin (al'drīn). Aldrin; hidrocarboneto clorado volátil empregado como inseticida; quando absorvido pela pele, produz sintomas tóxicos que consistem em irritabilidade acompanhada por depressão.

alec·i·thal (ā-les'i-thal). Alecítico, alécito; sem saco vitelino; indicando ovos com pouco ou nenhum deutoplasma. [G. *a-* priv. + *lekithos*, saco vitelino]

Alec·to·ro·bi·us ta·la·je (ā-lek-tōr-ō'bē-us ta-lā'jē). Um inseto, comumente encontrado no México e na América do Sul, cuja picada, da mesma forma que a dos percevejos, pode supurar.

alem·mal (ā-lem'al). Indica uma fibra nervosa que não possui neurolema. [G. *a-* priv. + *lemma*, casca]

aleu·ke·mia (ā-loo-kē'mē-ă). Aleucemia **1.** Literalmente, uma falta de leucócitos no sangue. O termo em geral é utilizado para indicar variedades de doença leucêmica nas quais o número de leucócitos no sangue circulante é normal ou abaixo do normal (isto é, sem leucocitose), mas alguns leucócitos jovens são observados; às vezes empregado de forma mais restritiva para casos incomuns de leucemia sem leucocitose e sem formas jovens no sangue. **2.** Alterações leucêmicas na medula óssea, associadas a um número subnormal de leucócitos no sangue. VER TAMBÉM subleukemic *leukemia*. [G. *a-* priv. + *leukos*, branco, + *haima*, sangue]

aleu·ke·mic (ā-loo-kē'mik). Aleucêmico; pertinente à aleucemia.

aleu·ke·moid (ā-loo-kē'moyd). Aleucemóide; semelhante, em termos sintomáticos, à aleucemia.

aleu·kia (ā-look̄'ē-ă). Aleucia. **1.** Ausência ou número extremamente diminuído de leucócitos no sangue circulante; às vezes também denominada mielose aleucêmica. **2.** Nome obsoleto para trombocitopenia. [G. *a-* priv. + *leukos*, branco]

aleu·ko·cyt·ic (ā-loo-kō-sit'ik). Aleucocítico, apresentando número extremamente reduzido (ou ausente) de leucócitos no sangue ou nas lesões.

aleu·ko·cy·to·sis (ā-loo-kō-si-tō'sis). Aleucocitose; ausência ou grande redução (relativa ou absoluta) do número de leucócitos no sangue circulante (isto é, um grau avançado de leucopenia), ou falta de leucócitos em uma lesão anatômica. [G. *a-* priv. + *leukos*, branco, + *kytos*, uma cavidade (célula)]

aleu·ri·o·con·id·i·um (ā-loo'rē-ō-kō-nid'ē-ŭm). Aleurioconídio; conídio desenvolvido a partir da extremidade em brotamento de células conidiógenas ou ramos hifais e liberado pela rotura abaixo da base de fixação. SIN aleurios-pore. [G. *aleuron*, farinha, + *conidium*]

aleu·ri·o·spore (ā-loo'rē-ō-spōr). Aleurióspore, aleurioconídio. SIN aleurioconidium.

al·eu·ron (al'oo-ron). Aleurona; grânulos de proteína no endosperma de sementes contendo supostamente as vitaminas de sementes e grãos comestíveis. [G. farinha]

aleu·ro·nate (ā-loo'rō-nāt). Aleuronato; proteína da camada de aleurona (endosperma) de grãos cereais; utilizado para fazer pão para diabético.

aleu·ro·noid (ā-loo'rō-noyd). Aleuronóide; semelhante à farinha.

Alexander, Gustav, otolaringologista austríaco, 1873–1932. VER A. *hearing impairment.*

Alexander, W. Stewart, patologista neozelandês do século XX. VER A. *disease.*

alex·ia (ā-lek'sē-ă). Alexia; incapacidade de entender o significado de palavras e sentenças escritas ou impressas, causada por lesão cerebral. Também chamada de **alexia óptica**, **sensorial** ou **visual** na diferenciação da **alexia motora** (anartria), na qual existe uma perda da capacidade de ler em voz alta, embora o significado do que está escrito ou impresso seja compreendido. SIN text blindness, word blindness, visual aphasia (1). [G. *a-* priv. + *lexis*, palavra ou frase]

  incomplete a., a. incompleta, dislexia. SIN dyslexia.

  musical a., a. musical; perda da capacidade para ler uma notação musical. SIN music blindness, note blindness.

alex·ic (ā-lek'sik). Aléxico; pertinente à alexia.

alex·in (ā-lek'sin). Alexina; termo obsoleto para as substâncias bactericidas do soro acelular, cuja atividade é destruída pelo aquecimento a 56°C; aplicado por Bordet à substância termolábil normalmente presente no soro e diferente da substância sensibilizante (anticorpo) produzida pela infecção ou imunização. Nesse sentido, é sinônimo de complemento. [G. *alexō*, precaver-se]

alex·i·thy·mia (ā-lek-si-thī'mē-ă). Alexitimia; dificuldade de reconhecer e descrever as emoções, definindo-as em termos de sensações somáticas ou reações comportamentais. [G. *a-* priv. + *lexis,* palavra, + *-thymia,* sentimentos, paixão]

al·fa·cal·ci·dol (al-fă-kal'si-dol). Alfacalcidol; derivado da vitamina D empregado no tratamento do hipoparatireoidismo, do raquitismo dependente da vitamina D e do raquitismo associado a síndromes disabsortivas.

al·fen·ta·nil hy·dro·chlo·ride (al-fen'tă-nil). Cloridrato de alfentanil; analgésico agonista de narcóticos muito potente, de ação breve, empregado como anestésico ou auxiliar na manutenção da anestesia geral.

ALG Abreviatura de antilymphocyte *globulin* (globulina antilinfócito).

al·gae (al'jē). Algas; divisão de organismos eucarióticos, fotossintéticos, que não têm florescência e inclui muitas algas marinhas. [pl. of L. *alga,* alga]
blue-green a., algas azul-esverdeadas; nome antigo para bactérias azul-esverdeadas, atualmente classificadas como cianobactérias.

al·gal (al'gal). Algal, algáceo; semelhante ou pertinente às algas.

al·ga·ro·ba (al-ga-rō'ba). Farinha de alfarroba; goma de alfarroba; fruto da *Ceratonia siliqua;* usado como adsorvente-demulcente no tratamento da diarréia. SIN carob flour, locust gum.

△ **alge-, algesi-, algio-, algo-.** Formas combinantes significando dor; corresponde ao L. dolor-. [G. *algos,* dor]

al·ge·fa·cient (al-jē-fā'shent). Agente que possui ação refrigerante. [L. *Algeo,* estar frio, + *facio,* pr. pl. *-iens,* fazer]

△ **algesi-.** VER alge-.

al·ge·sia (al-jē'zē-ă). Algesia. SIN algesthesia. [G. *algēsis,* sensação de dor]

al·ge·sic (al-jēz'ik). Algésico. **1.** Doloroso; relativo à dor ou que a causa. **2.** Relativo à hipersensibilidade à dor. SIN algetic.

al·ge·si·chron·om·e·ter (al-jē'zē-krō-nom'e-ter). Algesocronômetro; instrumento para registrar o tempo necessário para a percepção do estímulo doloroso. [G. *algēsis,* sensação de dor, + *chronos,* tempo, + *metron,* medida]

al·ge·sim·e·ter (al-jē-sim'e-ter). Algesímetro. SIN algesiometer.

al·ge·si·o·gen·ic (al-jē'zē-ō-jen'ik). Algesiogênico; que provoca dor. SIN algogenic. [G. *algēsis,* sensação de dor + *-gen,* produção]

al·ge·si·om·e·ter (al-jē-zē-om'e-ter). Algesímetro; instrumento para medir o grau de sensibilidade a um estímulo doloroso. SIN algesimeter, algometer. [G. *algēsis,* remoção de dor, + *metron,* medida]

al·ges·the·sia (al-jes-thē'zē-ă). Algesia. **1.** A apreciação da dor. **2.** Hipersensibilidade à dor. SIN algestesia. [G. *algos,* dor, + *aisthēsis,* sensação]

al·ges·the·sis (al-jes-thē'sis). Algesia. SIN algesthesia.

al·ges·tone ac·e·to·phe·nide (al-jes'ton ă-se-tō-fē'nīd). Acetofenida de algestona; um progestágeno com propriedades anticoncepcionais. SIN alphasone acetophenide.

al·get·ic (al-jet'ik). Algético, al. SIN algesic.

△ **-algia.** Sufixo que significa dor ou condição dolorosa. [G. *algos,* dor]

al·gi·cide (al'ji-sīd). Algicida; agente ativo contra algas. [algae, + L. *caedo,* matar]

al·gid (al'jid). Álgido; frio, gelado. [L. *algidus,* frio]

al·gin (al'jin). Algina; hidrato de carbono produzido pela alga marinha *Macrocystis pyrifera;* usado como gel em preparados farmacêuticos. SIN sodium alginate.

al·gi·nate (al'ji-nāt). Alginato; hidrocolóide irreversível que consiste em sais de ácido algínico, um polissacarídeo coloidal ácido obtido de algas marinhas e composto de resíduos de ácido manurônico; usado em materiais para impressão dentária.

△ **algio-.** VER alge-.

al·gi·o·mo·tor (al-jē-ō-mō'tōr). Algiomotor; que causa contrações musculares dolorosas. SIN algiomuscular. [algio- + L. *motor,* mover]

al·gi·o·mus·cu·lar (al'jē-ō-mŭs'kū-lar). Algomotor. SIN algiomotor.

al·gi·o·vas·cu·lar (al'jē-ō-vas'kū-lar). Algovascular. SIN algovascular.

△ **algo-.** VER alge-.

al·go·dys·tro·phy (al-gō-dis'trō-fē). Algodistrofia; distúrbio doloroso localizado do crescimento, em particular devido à necrose asséptica focal do osso e da cartilagem. [algo- + G. *dys-,* má, + *trophē,* nutrição]

al·go·gen·e·sis, al·go·ge·ne·sia (al-gō-jen'e-sis, -jē-nē'zē-ă). Algogenesia; produção ou origem da dor. [algo- + G. *genesis,* origem]

al·go·gen·ic (al-gō-jen'ik). Algogênico. SIN algesiogenic.

al·go·lag·nia (al-gō-lag'nē-ă). Algolagnia; termo obsoleto de algofilia (algomania). [algo- + G. *lagneia,* luxúria]

al·gol·o·gy (al-gōl'o-jē). Algologia. **1.** Estudo da dor. [G. *algos,* dor, + *-logia*] **2.** Estudo científico das algas.

al·gom·e·ter (al-gom'e-ter). Algômetro. SIN algesiometer. [algo- + G. *metron,* medida]

al·gom·e·try (al-gom'e-trē). Algometria; o processo de medir a dor.

al·go·phil·ia (al-gō-fil'ē-ă). Algofilia, algomania, algolagnia; forma de perversão sexual na qual infligir ou sentir dor aumenta o prazer do ato sexual ou causa prazer sexual independentemente do ato; inclui tanto o sadismo como o masoquismo. [algo- + G. *phileō,* amar]

al·go·pho·bia (al-gō-fō'bē-ă). Algofobia; temor anormal de dor ou sensibilidade à dor. [algo- + G. *phobos,* medo]

al·go·rithm (al'gō-rithm). Algoritmo; processo sistemático que consiste em uma seqüência ordenada de etapas, cada etapa dependendo do resultado da anterior. Na clínica médica, protocolo passo a passo para o tratamento de um problema de saúde; na tomografia computadorizada, as fórmulas usadas para o cálculo da imagem final a partir dos dados transmitidos pelos raios X. [L. Mediev. *algorismus,* em homenagem a Muhammad ibn-Musa *al-Khwarizmi,* matemático árabe, + G. *arithmos,* número]

al·gos·co·py (al-gos'kō-pē). Algoscopia. SIN cryoscopy. [L. *algor,* frio, + G. *skopeō,* ver]

al·go·spasm (al'gō-spazm). Algoespasmo; espasmo produzido pela dor. [G. *algos,* dor, + *spasmos,* convulsão]

al·go·vas·cu·lar (al-gō-vas'kū-lar). Algovascular; relativo às alterações na luz dos vasos sanguíneos que ocorrem sob a influência da dor. SIN algiovascular. [G. *algos,* dor]

al·i·ble (al'i-bl). Alíbil, nutritivo. SIN nutritive. [L. *alibilis,* nutritivo, de *alo,* nutrir]

al·i·cy·clic (al-i-sik'lik). Alicíclico; indica um composto alicíclico.

alien·a·tion (ā-lē-en-ā'shun). Alienação; condição caracterizada pela falta de relações significativas com outros, às vezes produzindo despersonalização e estranheza dos outros. [L. *alieno,* pp. *-atus,* tornar estranho]

ali·e·nia (ā-li-ē'nē-ă). Alienia; ausência congênita do baço. [G. *a-* priv. + L. *lien,* baço]

al·i·form (al'i-fōrm). Aliforme; em forma de asa, pterigóideo. [L. *ala,* + *forma,* formato]

align·ment (ā-līn'ment). Alinhamento. **1.** Posição longitudinal de um osso ou membro **2.** O ato de colocar em linha. **3.** Em odontologia, a distribuição dos dentes com relação às estruturas de apoio e dentições adjacentes e opostas. SIN alinement. [Fr. *aligner,* alinhar, do L. *linea,* linha]

al·i·ment (al'i-ment). **1.** Alimento, sustento. SIN nourishment. **2.** Na teoria sensomotora, aquilo que se encontra assimilado em um esquema; análogo a um estímulo. [L. *alo,* nutrir]

al·i·men·ta·ry (al-i-men'ter-ē). Alimentar; relativo a alimento ou nutrição. [L. *alimentarius,* de *alimentum,* nutrição]

al·i·men·ta·tion (al-i-men-tā'shŭn). Alimentação, aquilo que nutre. VER TAMBÉM feeding.
forced a., a. forçada. SIN forced *feeding.*
parenteral a., a. parenteral; nutrição por via intravenosa.
rectal a., a. retal; fornecimento de nutrição por enemas de retenção.

al·i·na·sal (al'i-nā'sal). Alinasal; relativo às asas do nariz (*alae nasi*) ou às partes móveis da narinas. [L. *ala,* + *nasus,* nariz]

aline·ment (ā-līn'ment). Alinhamento. SIN alignment.

al·in·jec·tion (al'in-jek'shŭn). Injeção de álcool para o endurecimento e a conservação de amostras anatomopatológicas e histológicas.

al·i·phat·ic (al-i-fat'ik). Alifático; indica os compostos acíclicos de carbono, cuja maioria pertence à serie de ácidos graxos. [G. *aleiphar* (*aleiphat-*), gordura, óleo]
a. acids, ácidos alifáticos; os ácidos de hidrocarbonatos não-aromáticos (p.ex., ácidos acético, propiônico, butírico); os assim chamados ácidos graxos da fórmula R–COOH, na qual R é um hidrocarbonato não-aromático (alifático).

ali·poid (ā-lip'oyd). Alipóide; caracterizado pela ausência de lipóides. [G. *a-* priv. + *lipoidēs,* semelhante a gordura]

alip·o·tro·pic (ā'lip-ō-trōp'ik). Alipotrópico; que não exerce qualquer influência sobre o metabolismo das gorduras ou sobre o movimento das gorduras para o fígado. [G. *a-* priv. + *lipos,* gordura, + *tropos,* volta]

al·i·quot (al'i-kwot). Alíquota; em química e imunologia, pertinente a uma porção do todo; livremente, qualquer uma de duas ou mais amostras de algo do mesmo volume e peso. [L. alguns, vários]

al·i·sphe·noid (al-i-sfē'noyd). Alisfenóide, alisfenoidal; relativo à asa maior do osso esfenóide. [L. *ala,* + *sphēn,* cunha]

aliz·a·rin (ă-liz'ă-rin). [C.I. 58000]. Alizarina. 1,2-diidroxiantraquinona; corante vermelho que ocorre na raiz da garança ou ruiva-dos-tintureiros (*Rubia tinctorum* e outras *Rubiaceae*) em combinação com a glicose (ácido ruberítrico) como agulhas cor de laranja, discretamente hidrossolúveis; usado pelos antigos como corante. Atualmente, produzida de forma sintética a partir do antraceno e usada na fabricação de corantes, p.ex. a. azul, a. laranja, "vermelho-alaranjado". Como indicador, muda de amarelo em pH < 5,5 para vermelho em pH > 6,8; outras alizarinas modificadas têm outras cores e mudam de cor em outros valores de pH.
a. cyanin [C.I. 58610], alizarina cianina; dissulfonato de hexaidroxiantraquinona; corante ácido empregado como corante nuclear depois do mordente e como fluorocromo na microscopia ultravioleta.
a. purpurin, purpurina. SIN purpurin (2).
a. red S [C.I. 58005], a. vermelha S; sulfonato sódico de alizarina; usado como corante para o cálcio nos ossos (o cálcio aparece vermelho-laranja, e o magnésio, o alumínio e o bário aparecem em matizes variáveis de vermelho), na determinação do flúor; como indicador, passa do amarelo para o púrpura em pH entre 3,7 e 5,2.

al·ka·di·ene (al-kă-dī'ēn). Alcadieno; hidrocarboneto acíclico (alcano) contendo duas ligações duplas.

al·ka·le·mia (al-kă-lē´mē-ă). Alcalemia; diminuição na concentração do íon H do sangue ou elevação no pH. [álcali + G. *haima*, sangue]

al·ka·li, pl. **alkalies** (al´kă-lī). **1.** Álcali; substância fortemente básica que fornece íons hidróxido (OH⁻ em solução); p.ex., hidróxido de sódio, hidróxido de potássio. **2.** Base. SIN base (3). **3.** Metal alcalino. SIN alkali metal. [Ar., *al*, o, + *qalīy*, soda calcinada]

caustic a., a. cáustico, álcali muito ionizado (em solução); p.ex., NaOH.
fixed a., a. fixo; qualquer álcali afora um fracamente ionizado, como a amônia.
vegetable a., a. vegetal; mistura de hidróxido e carbonato de potássio.

al·ka·line (al´kă-līn). Alcalino; relativo a ou tendo uma reação de álcali.

al·ka·lin·i·ty (al-kă-lin´i-tē). Alcalinidade; o estado de ser alcalino.

al·ka·lin·i·za·tion (al´kă-lin-i-zā´shŭn). Alcalinização. SIN alkalization.

al·ka·li·nu·ria (al´kă-lī-noo´rē-ă). Alcalinúria; a eliminação de urina alcalina. SIN alkaluria. [alcalino + G. *ouron*, urina]

al·ka·li·ther·a·py (al´kă-lī-thār´ă-pē). Alcaliterapia; uso terapêutico de álcalis para efeito local ou sistêmico.

al·ka·li·za·tion (al´kal-i-zā´shŭn). Alcalização, basificação; processo de tornar alcalino. SIN alkalinization.

al·ka·liz·er (al´kă-līz-er). Alcalizador; agente que neutraliza ácidos ou deixa uma solução alcalina.

al·ka·loid (al´kă-loyd). Alcalóide; originalmente, qualquer um dentre as centenas de produtos vegetais e fúngicos diferenciados pelas reações alcalinas (básicas), mas agora restritos a estruturas heterocíclicas contendo nitrogênio e, muitas vezes, complexas com atividade farmacológica; seus nomes vulgares ou populares terminam geralmente em -ina (p.ex., morfina, atropina, colchicina). Os alcalóides são sintetizados por vegetais e encontrados nas folhas, cascas, sementes e outras partes, constituindo geralmente o princípio ativo do medicamento em estado natural; representam um grupo frouxamente definido, mas que pode ser classificado segundo a estrutura química de seu núcleo principal. Para fins medicinais, devido à hidrossolubilidade aumentada, utilizam-se geralmente os sais de alcalóides (p.ex., sulfato de morfina, fosfato de codeína). Ver também individual a. ou a. class. SIN vegetable base.

ergot a.'s (er´got), a. do esporão do centeio; qualquer a. de um grande número de a. obtidos do fungo do esporão de centeio *Claviceps purpurea* ou semi-sinteticamente derivado; os exemplos incluem ergotamina, ergonovina, diidroergotamina, dietilamida do ácido lisérgico (LSD), metissergida.
fixed a., alcalóide fixo; alcalóide não-volátil.
Vinca a.'s, a. da Vinca; a. como a vincristina e a vimblastina (agentes antitumorais) extraído da mirta. SIN Catharanthus alkaloids.

al·ka·lo·sis (al-kă-lō´sis). Alcalose; estado caracterizado por diminuição na concentração do íon H no sangue arterial abaixo do nível normal, 40 nmol/L, ou pH 7,4. A condição pode ser causada por aumento da concentração de compostos alcalinos, ou por diminuição da concentração de compostos ácidos ou dióxido de carbono.

acapnial a., a. acápnica, a. respiratória. SIN respiratory a.
compensated a., a. compensada; a. em que existe modificação no bicarbonato, mas o pH dos líquidos orgânicos é quase normal; a. repiratória pode ser compensada pelo aumento da produção de ácidos metabólicos ou da excreção renal de bicarbonato; a a. metabólica raramente é compensada por hipoventilação.
compensated metabolic a., a. metabólica compensada; retenção de ácido, basicamente dióxido de carbono pelos pulmões e íons ácidos pelos túbulos renais, para reduzir o efeito sobre o pH sanguíneo do excesso de álcalis produzidos pela ingestão ou pelo metabolismo de substâncias produtoras de álcalis.
compensated respiratory a., a. respiratória compensada; excreção aumentada de íons ácidos pelos rins para minimizar o efeito sobre o pH sanguíneo da perda excessiva de dióxido de carbono pelos pulmões, como ocorre na hiperventilação.
metabolic a., a. metabólica; alcalose associada à concentração plasmática arterial aumentada de bicarbonato, possivelmente em consequência da ingestão excessiva de material alcalino ou da perda excessiva de ácido na urina ou por vômitos persistentes; o excesso de base e o bicarbonato padrão estão elevados. VER TAMBÉM compensated a.
respiratory a., a. respiratória; alcalose resultante da perda anormal de CO_2 por hiperventilação, seja ela ativa ou passiva, com redução simultânea na concentração de bicarbonato do plasma arterial. VER TAMBÉM compensated a. SIN acapnial a.
uncompensated a., a. descompensada; alcalose na qual o pH dos líquidos orgânicos está elevado devido à falta de mecanismos compensatórios da alcalose compensada.

al·ka·lot·ic (al-kă-lot´ik). Alcalótico; relativo à alcalose.

al·ka·lu·ria (al-kă-loo´rē-ă). Alcalúria. SIN alkalinuria.

al·kane (al´kān). Alcano; o termo geral para um hidrocarboneto acíclico saturado; p.ex., propano, butano.

al·kan·net (al´kă-net) [C.I. 75530, 75520]. Alcaneto; raiz de uma erva, *Alkanna*, ou *Anchusa tinctoria* (família Boraginaceae), que fornece corantes vermelhos alcanen e alcanina; usado como agente corante; também, associado ao tanino, usado como adstringente.

al·kan·nan (al´kă-nan) [C.I. 75520]. Alcanan; um componente secundário corante vermelho derivado do alcaneto.

al·kan·nin (al´kă-nin) [C.I. 75530]. Alcanina; o corante vermelho principal derivado do alcaneto; usado como adstringente e em cosméticos e alimentos; pode ser utilizado como indicador: vermelho em pH 6,8, mudando para púrpura em pH 8,8 e azul em pH 10,0; também empregado como corante de gorduras. SIN anchusin.

al·kap·ton (al-kap´ton). Alcaptona. SIN homogentisic acid. [Termo cunhado por Boedeker a partir de álcali + L + G. *kapto*, sugar vorazmente]

al·ka·tri·ene (al-kă-trī´en). Alcatrieno; hidrocarboneto acíclico contendo três ligações duplas; p.ex. 2, 4, 6 –octatrieno, CH_3–CH=CH–CH=CH–CH=CH–CH_3.

al·ka·ver·vir (al-kă-ver´vir). Alcavervir; mistura de alcalóides obtidos por extração seletiva do *Veratrum viride* com diversos solventes orgânicos; utilizado por via oral ou parenteral como agente hipotensor.

al·kene (al´kēn). Alqueno, alceno; um hidrocarboneto acíclico contendo uma ou mais ligações duplas, p.ex. eteno, propeno. SIN olefin.

al·ke·nyl (al´ken-il). Alcenil, alquenil; o radical de um alqueno.

alk-1-en·yl. Alc-1-enil; o radical de um alceno (alqueno) no qual a dupla ligação, indicada pelo "eno", está entre os carbonos 1 e 2 (o carbono 1 sendo o radical ou carbono "il"), isto é, R–CH=CH–; expresso às vezes como alc-1-en-1-il (alk-1-en-1-yl).

alk-1-en·yl·glyc·er·o·phos·pho·lip·id. Alce-1-enilglicerofosfolipídeo; um fosfatidato no qual pelo menos um dos radicais fixados ao glicerol é um alc-1-enil, em vez do habitual radical acil (isto é, derivado de um aldeído, e não de um ácido, daí os nomes habituais mais antigos de fosfatidal e acetal fosfatídeo (dato)); foi proposto o nome de "ácido plasmênico" para esses fosfatidatos.

al·kide (al´kīd). Alquila, alcoíla. SIN alkyl (2).

al·kyl (al´kil). Alquila, alcoíla. **1.** Um radical hidrocarboneto da fórmula genérica C_nH_{2n+1}. **2.** Composto, como o chumbo tetraetila, no qual um metal está associado a radicais alquila ou alcoíla. SIN alkide.
arylated a., a. arilatada. SIN aralkyl.

al·kyl·a·mine (al-kil´ă-mēn). Alquilamina; alcano contendo um grupamento –NH_2 no lugar de um átomo H; p.ex., etilamina.

al·kyl·a·tion (al´ki-lā´shŭn). Alquilação; substituição de um radical alquila por um átomo de hidrogênio; p.ex., introdução de uma cadeia lateral em um composto aromático.

ALL Abreviatura de acute lymphocytic leukemia (leucemia linfocítica aguda).

al·la·ches·the·sia (al´ă-kes-thē´zē-ă). Alaquestesia, alestesia, aloquestesia; condição em que uma sensação tátil é referida a um ponto que não aquele onde o estímulo é aplicado. VER TAMBÉM allochiria. [G. *allachē*, outro lugar, + *aisthēsis*, sensação]

allanto-, allant-. Formas combinantes de alantóide. [G. *allas, allantos*, salsicha, tripa]

al·lan·to·ate de·im·i·nase. Alantoato desiminase; enzima que catalisa a conversão de ácido alantóico em ureidoglicina, NH_3 e CO_2.

al·lan·to·cho·ri·on (ă-lan-tō-kōr´ē-on). Alantocório; membrana extraembrionária formada pela fusão da alantóide com o cório (córion).

al·lan·to·gen·e·sis (ă-lan-tō-jen´ē-sis). Alantogênese; formação e desenvolvimento de alantóide. [allanto- + G. *genesis*, origem]

al·lan·to·ic (ă-lan-tō´ik). Alantóico, alantoidiano; relativo à alantóide (membrana embrionária).

al·lan·to·ic ac·id (ă-lan-tō´ik as´id). Ácido alantóico; ácido diureidoacético; produto da degradação da alantoína. Uma importante fonte de nitrogênio nas plantas.

al·lan·toid (ă-lan´toyd). Alantóide. **1.** Botuliforme, cilindriforme; em forma de lingüiça. **2.** Relativo a ou semelhante a alantóide. [allanto- + G. *eidos*, aparência]

al·lan·toid·o·an·gi·op·a·gus (ă-lan-toyd´ō-an-jē-op´ă-gŭs). Alantoidoangiópago. SIN omphaloangiopagus. VER allantoidoangiopagous twins, em twin. [allantoid + G. *angeion*, vaso, + *pagos*, ligados]

al·lan·to·in (ă-lan´tō-in). Alantoína; substância presente no líquido alantóico, na urina fetal e em outros locais; também um produto da oxidação do ácido úrico e o produto final da administração de purina em outros animais afora o homem e demais primatas. SIN 3-ureidohydantoin, cordianine, glyoxyldiureide.

al·lan·to·in·ase (ă-lan-tō´i-nās). Alantoinase; enzima (uma amidoidrolase) que catalisa a hidrólise da alantoína a ácido alantóico.

al·lan·to·in·u·ria (ă-lan´tō-in-u´rē-ă). Alantoinúria; a excreção urinária de alantoína, normal na maioria dos mamíferos, anormal na espécie humana. [alantoína + G. *ouron*, urina]

al·lan·to·is (ă-lan´tō-is). Alantóide; membrana fetal que se desenvolve no intestino superior (ou saco vitelino nos seres humanos). Nos seres humanos é vestigial; externamente, nos mamíferos, contribui para a formação do cordão umbilical e da placenta; em aves e répteis, permanece logo abaixo da casca porosa do ovo e serve como órgão respiratório. SIN allantoid membrane. [allanto- + G. *eidos*, aparência]

al·lax·is (ă-laks´is). Metamorfose. SIN metamorphosis. [G. *allattein*, alterar]

al·lele (ă-lēl´). Alelo; qualquer de uma série de dois ou mais genes diferentes

que ocupariam a mesma posição ou *locus* em um cromossoma específico. Como os cromossomas autossômicos são pareados, cada gene autossômico é representado duas vezes nas células somáticas normais. Caso o mesmo alelo ocupe as duas unidades de *locus*, o indivíduo ou a célula é homozigoto no que se refere a esse alelo. Caso os alelos sejam diferentes, o indivíduo ou a célula é heterozigoto para os dois alelos. VER DNA makers. VER TAMBÉM *dominance* of traits. SIN allelomorph. [o. *allelon,* reciprocamente]
codominant a., a. codominante. VER codominant.
silent a., a. silencioso, a. amorfo. SIN amorph.
al·le·lic (ă-lē'lik). Relativo a um alelo. SIN allelomorphic.
al·lel·ism (al'ē-lizm). Alelismo; o estado mantido em comum por alelos. SIN allelomorphism.
al·le·lo·ca·tal·y·sis (ă-lē'lō-kă-tal'i-sis). Alelocatálise; auto-estimulação de crescimento em uma cultura bacteriana pelo acréscimo de células semelhantes. [G. *allelon,* mutuamente, reciprocamente, + *catalytikos,* capaz de dissolver]
al·le·lo·cat·a·lyt·ic (ă-lē'lō-kat-ă-lit'ik). Alelocatalítico; mutuamente catalítico; indica duas substâncias, cada uma das quais é decomposta na presença da outra.
al·le·lo·chem·i·cals (ă-lē'lō-kem'i-kălz). Aleloquímicos; substâncias sinalizadoras entre indivíduos de diferentes espécies. Cf. pheromones. [G. *allelon,* reciprocamente, + químico]
al·le·lo·morph (ă-lē'lō-mōrf). Alelomorfo. SIN allele. [G. *allelon,* reciprocamente, + *morphe,* forma]
al·le·lo·mor·phic (ă-lē'lō-mōr'fik). Alelomórfico. SIN allelic.
al·le·lo·mor·phism (ă-lē-lō-mōr'fizm). Alelomorfismo. SIN allelism.
al·le·lo·tax·is, al·le·lo·taxy (ă-lēl-ō-taks'is, -taks'ē). Alelotaxia; desenvolvimento de um órgão a partir de várias estruturas ou tecidos embrionários. [G. *allelon,* reciprocamente, + *taxis,* distribuição]
Allen, Alfred Henry, químico norte-americano, 1846–1904. VER A. *test.*
Allen, Edgar, endocrinologista norte-americano, 1892–1943. VER A.-Doisy *test, unit.*
Allen, Edgar Van Nuys, médico norte-americano, 1900–1961. VER A. *test.*
Allen, Willard Myron, ginecologista norte-americano, *1904. VER Corner-A. *test, unit;* A.-Masters *syndrome.*
al·ler·gen (al'er-jen). Alérgeno, alergênio; termo para um antígeno que induz uma resposta alérgica ou de hipersensibilidade. [alergia + G. *-gen,* produzindo]
al·ler·gen·ic (al-er-jen'ik). Alergênico, antigênico. SIN antigenic.
al·ler·gic (ă-ler'jik). Alérgico; relativo a qualquer resposta estimulada por um alérgeno.
al·ler·gic sa·lute. Saudação alérgica; um movimento característico de esfregadura do nariz (movimento transversal ou ascendente da mão), como observado em crianças com rinite alérgica.
al·ler·gist (al'er-jist). Alergista; quem se especializa no tratamento das alergias.
al·ler·gi·za·tion (al'er-ji-zā'shŭn). Alergização; sensibilização ativa como resultado de contato natural ou artificial de antígenos com tecidos suscetíveis; o processo de ser alergizado.
al·ler·gized (al'er-jīzd). Alergizado; alterado especificamente na reatividade; tornado capaz de apresentar uma ou outra manifestação alérgica.
al·ler·gol·o·gy (al-er-gol'ō-gē). Alergologia. Ciência que estuda as condições alérgicas.
al·ler·go·sis (al'er-gō'sis). Alergose; qualquer condição anormal caracterizada por alergia. [alergia + G. *-osis,* condição]
al·ler·gy (al'er-jē). Alergia. **1.** Hipersensibilidade causada pela exposição a um antígeno (alérgeno), resultando em um aumento acentuado na reatividade a esse antígeno até a exposição subseqüente, às vezes com conseqüências imunológicas perigosas. SIN acquired sensitivity, induced sensitivity. VER TAMBÉM allergic *reaction,* anaphylaxis, immune reaction. **2.** O ramo da medicina que estuda o diagnóstico e o tratamento das manifestações alérgicas. **3.** Hipersensibilidade adquirida a certos medicamentos e preparados biológicos. [G. *allos,* outro, + *ergon,* trabalho]
atopic a., a. atópica. VER atopy.
bacterial a., a. bacteriana, **(1)** reação alérgica de hipersensibilidade do tipo I causada por alérgenos bacterianos; **(2)** o tipo tardio de prova cutânea (reação de hipersensibilidade do tipo IV), assim chamado por sua associação precoce com antígenos bacterianos (p.ex., o teste tuberculínico).
cold a., sintomas físicos produzidos por hipersensibilidade ao frio.
contact a., a. de contato. SIN allergic contact *dermatitis.*
delayed a., a. tardia; reação alérgica de hipersensibilidade do tipo IV; assim chamada porque, em um indivíduo sensibilizado, a reação torna-se evidente horas após o contato com o alérgeno (antígeno), alcança seu máximo após 24 a 48 horas e, em seguida, regride lentamente. Associada a respostas mediadas por células. VER TAMBÉM delayed *reaction;* Cf. immediate a.
drug a., a. medicamentosa; sensibilidade (hipersensibilidade) a um fármaco ou substância química.
immediate a., a. imediata; reação alérgica de hipersensibilidade do tipo 1; assim chamada porque, em um indivíduo sensibilizado, a reação torna-se evidente em geral minutos após o contato com o alérgeno (antígeno), alcança seu máximo em aproximadamente uma hora e, em seguida, regride rapidamente. VER TAMBÉM immediate *reaction,* anaphylaxis; Cf. delayed a.
latent a., a. latente; não provoca sinais nem sintomas, mas pode ser revelada por meio de certas provas imunológicas com alérgenos específicos.
physical a., a. física; resposta excessiva a fatores ambientais tais como calor ou frio.
polyvalent a., a. polivalente; resposta alérgica manifestada simultaneamente a diversos e numerosos alérgenos específicos.
Al·les·che·ria boy·dii (al-es-kē'rē-ă boy'dē-ī). Nome antigo de *Pseudallescheria boydii;* o anamorfo é *Scedosporium apiosperman.*
al·les·the·sia (al-es-thē'zē-ă). Alestesia. SIN allochiria. [G. *allos,* outro, + *aisthēsis,* sensação]
al·le·thrins (al'ē-thrinz). Aletrina; ésteres de aletrolona dos ácidos crisantemomonocarboxílicos e análogos sintéticos das piretrinas, que são ésteres piretrolona dos mesmos ácidos; líquidos viscosos, insolúveis na água, que podem ser absorvidos pelos pulmões, pele e mucosas e produzir lesão hepática e renal, com congestão pulmonar; usado como inseticida.
al·leth·ro·lone (ă-leth'rō-lōn). Aletrolona; análogo da piretrolona (2-propenil substituindo o grupamento 2,4-pentadienil) usado nas aletrinas.
al·lied health pro·fes·sion·al. Indivíduo, que não um médico ou um enfermeiro, treinado para atender os pacientes; inclui vários técnicos terapeutas (p.ex., pulmonar), técnico de radiologia, fisioterapeutas, etc.
al·li·ga·tion (al-i-gā'shŭn). Regra de misturas na qual 1) o custo de uma mistura pode ser determinado pelos preços e proporções dos vários ingredientes; ou 2) em farmácia, as quantidades relativas de soluções de diferentes percentagens que têm de ser usadas para formar uma mistura de uma concentração desejada. [L. *alligatio,* de *al-ligo* (adl-), pp. *-atus,* unir a]
Allis, Oscar Huntington, cirurgião norte-americano, 1836–1921. VER A. *forceps.*
al·lit·er·a·tion (ă-lit-er-ā'shŭn). Aliteração; em psiquiatria, um distúrbio da linguagem no qual as palavras que começam com os mesmos sons, em geral consoantes, são notavelmente freqüentes. [Fr. *allitération,* do L. *ad.,* para, + *littera,* letra do alfabeto]
al·li·um (al'ē-ŭm). Alho; *Allium sativum* (família Liliaceae), cujo bulbo contém até 0,9% de óleo irritante volátil com ação anti-séptica; tem sido utilizado como diaforético, diurético e expectorante. SIN garlic. [L]
all or none. Lei do tudo-ou-nada. VER Bowditch *law.*
allo-. 1. Prefixo significando "outro" ou diferindo do normal ou habitual. **2.** Prefixo químico antes empregado junto com um aminoácido cuja cadeia lateral contém um carbono assimétrico; p.ex., as aloisoleucinas e alotreoninas.[G. *allos,* outro]
al·lo·al·bu·mi·ne·mia (al'ō-al-bū'mi-nē'mē-ă) [MIM*103600] Aloalbuminemia; condição autossômica dominante de possuir albumina sérica de uma variante que difere em mobilidade na eletroforese do tipo A habitual; os indivíduos são homozigotos ou heterozigotos para um dos alelos para as variantes de albumina, polimorfismo genético sem importância clínica conhecida. VER TAMBÉM inherited albumin *variants,* em *variant.* [allo- + albumin + G. *haima,* sangue, + -ia]
al·lo·an·ti·body (al-ō-an'ti-bod-ē). Aloanticorpo; um anticorpo específico para um aloantígeno.
al·lo·an·ti·gen (al-ō-an'ti-jen). Aloantígeno; um antígeno que ocorre em alguns, mas não em outros membros da mesma espécie.

alergias alimentares

distribuição percentual dos alimentos responsáveis por 600 casos de alergia alimentar

alimento	%
leite de vaca	42,0
ovos de galinha	
clara	14,5
gema	9,0
ovo inteiro	9,7
peixe	11,0
frutas cítricas	4,5
leguminosas	2,5
carne vermelha	2,8
vegetais	1,0
cebolas	1,0
outros (amendoim, chocolate)	2,0

al·lo·bar·bi·tal (al-ō-bar′bi-tal). Alobarbital; hipnótico com duração de ação intermediária a longa.

al·lo·cen·tric (al-ō-sen′trik). Alocêntrico; caracterizado por ou denotando interesse centrado em outras pessoas, em vez de em si mesmo. Cf. egocentric. SIN heterocentric (2). [allo- + G. *kentron*, centro]

al·lo·chi·ria, al·lo·chei·ria (al′-ō-kī′rē-ă, al-ō-kī′rē-ă). Aloquiria; forma de alaquestesia na qual a sensação de um estímulo em um membro é referida para o membro contralateral. SIN allesthesia, alloesthesia, Bamberger sign (2). [allo- + G. *cheir*, mão]

al·lo·cho·les·ter·ol (al-ō-kō-les′ter-ol). Alocolesterol; um isômero do colesterol, diferindo na posição de uma ligação dupla. SIN coprostenol.

al·lo·chro·ic (al-ō-krō′ik). Alocróico; de cor alterada ou alterável; relativo a alocroísmo.

al·lo·chro·ism (al-ō-krō′izm). Alocroísmo; alteração ou instabilidade de cor. [allo- + G. *chrōa*, cor]

al·lo·cor·tex (al′ō-kōr′teks) [TA]. Alocórtex; termo de O. Vogt indicando diversas regiões do córtex cerebral, em particular o córtex olfatório e o hipocampo, que se caracterizam por menos camadas celulares do que o isocórtex. VER TAMBÉM cerebral *cortex*. SIN heterotypic cortex. [allo- + L. *cortex*, casca]

α-al·lo·cor·tol (al-ō-kōr′tol). α-alocortol; o enantiômero 5α do α-cortol; um metabólito da hidrocortisona encontrado na urina.

β-al·lo·cor·tol. β-alocortol; o isômero 20β do α-alocortol e enantiômero 5α do β-cortol; um metabólito da hidrocortisona encontrado na urina.

α-al·lo·cor·to·lone (al-ō-kōr′tō-lōn). α-alocortolona. O enantiômero 5α da α-cortolona; um metabólito da hidrocortisona encontrado na urina.

β-al·lo·cor·to·lone. β-alocortolona; o isômero 20β da α-alocortolona e enantiômero 5α da β-cortolona; um metabólito da hidrocortisona encontrado na urina.

al·lo·de·ox·y·cho·lic ac·id (al-ō-dē-oks′e-kō′lik). Ácido alodesoxicólico; um dos ácidos biliares.

al·lo·dip·loid (al-ō-dip′loyd). Alodiplóide. VER alloploid.

al·lo·dyn·ia (al-ō-din′ē-ă). Alodinia; condição na qual estímulos normalmente não-dolorosos provocam dor. [allo- + G. *odynē*, dor]

al·lo·er·o·tism (al-ō-ār′ō-tizm). Aloerotismo; atração sexual por outra pessoa. [allo- + G. *erōs*, amor]

al·lo·es·the·sia (al-ō-es-thē′zē-ă). Alestesia. SIN allochiria.

al·log·a·my (al-og′ă-mē). Alogamia; fertilização do óvulo de um indivíduo pelo espermatozóide de outro. Cf. autogamy. [allo- + G. *gamos*, casamento]

al·lo·gen·ic, al·lo·ge·ne·ic (al-ō-jen′ik, -jē-nē′ik). Alogênico; usado na biologia de transplantes. Concernente a constituições gênicas diferentes na mesma espécie; distinto antigenicamente.

al·lo·go·tro·phia (al′ō-gō-trō′fē-ă). Alogotrofia; crescimento ou nutrição de uma parte ou tecido a expensas de outra parte do corpo. [allo-+ G. *trophē*, nutrição]

al·lo·graft (al′ō-graft). Aloenxerto; enxerto transplantado entre indivíduos geneticamente não-idênticos da mesma espécie. SIN allogeneic graft, homograft, homologous graft, homoplastic graft.

al·lo·group (al′ō-groop). Alogrupo; termo antes utilizado para indicar um haplótipo constituído por marcadores alotípicos intimamente ligados.

al·lo·hex·a·ploid (al-ō-heks′ă-ployd). Alo-hexaplóide. VER alloploid.

al·lo·hy·drox·y·ly·sine (aHyl) (ā-lō-hī-drok-sē-lī-sēn). Alo-hidroxilisina; 5-alo-hidroxilisina; um estereoisômero da 5-hidroxilisina; D-a é o diastereoisômero da D-5-hidroxilisina.

al·lo·im·mune (al′ō-im-oon′). Aloimune; imune a um antígeno alogênico. [allo- + imune]

al·lo·i·so·leu·cine (alle) (ă-lō-ī-sō-loo′sēn). Aloisoleucina; um estereoisômero da isoleucina; D-a. é o diastereoisômero da D-isoleucina.

al·lo·i·so·mer (al-ō-ī′som-er). Aloisômero; um isômero geométrico.

al·lo·ker·a·to·plas·ty (al-ō-ker′ă-tō-plas-tē). Aloceratoplastia; substituição de tecido córneo opaco por uma prótese transparente, em geral de plástico.

al·lo·ki·ne·sis (al-ō-ki-nē′sis, -kī-nē′sis). Alocinesia; movimento passivo ou reflexo; movimento não-voluntário. [allo- + G. *kinēsis*, movimento]

al·lo·lac·tose (ă-lō-lăk′tōs). Alolactose; um açúcar, isômero à lactose, que é o indutor verdadeiro do óperon *lac*.

al·lo·la·lia (al-ō-lā′lē-ă). Alolalia; qualquer defeito de linguagem, especialmente aquele causado por distúrbio cerebral. [allo- + G. *lalia*, conversa]

al·lom·er·ism (al-lom′er-izm). Alomerismo; alteração na composição química de uma substância, mas conservando sua forma cristalina. [allo- + G. *meros*, parte]

al·lom·e·tron (al-ō-me′tron). Alometria, aloiometria; mudança evolutiva no tamanho ou na proporção de seres orgânicos. [allo- + G. *metron*, medida]

al·lo·mones (ă-lō-mōn). Alomonas; feromônio que induz uma alteração comportamental ou fisiológica em um membro de outra espécie que é benéfica para o produtor. Cf. kairomones, pheromones. [G. *allos*, outro, + -mone]

al·lo·mor·phism (al-ō-mōr′fizm). Alomorfismo. **1.** Modificação na forma das células devido a causas mecânicas, como o achatamento por compressão, ou a metaplasia progressiva, como a transformação das células dos ductos biliares em células hepáticas. **2.** O estado de semelhança na composição química mas de diferença na forma (especialmente cristalina). [allo- + G. *morphē*, forma]

al·longe·ment (al-onzh′-maw). Alongamento; termo raramente usado para alongamento de uma estrutura, durante uma operação, por meio de incisões adequadas. [Fr. elongation]

al·lo·path (al′ō-path). Alopata. **1.** Médico da escola tradicional, em contraposição aos profissionais ecléticos ou homeopatas. **2.** Aquele que pratica a alopatia. SIN allopathist.

al·lo·path·ic (al-ō-path′ik). Alopático; relativo à alopatia.

al·lop·a·thist (al-op′ă-thist). Alopata. SIN allopath.

al·lop·a·thy (al-op′ă-thē). Alopatia; medicina convencional, forma tradicional de prática médica. Cf. homeopathy. SIN heteropathy (2), substitutive therapy. [allo + G. *pathos*, sofrendo]

al·lo·pen·ta·ploid (al-ō-pent′ă-ployd). Alopentaplóide. VER alloploid.

al·lo·phan·ic ac·id (al-ō-fan′ik). Ácido alofânico; ácido carbônico da uréia; sua amida é biureto (alofanamida). SIN carbamoylcarbamic acid, N-carboxyurea.

al·loph·a·sis (al-of′ă-sis). Alofasia; linguagem incoerente, desordenada [allo- + G. *phasis*, fala]

al·lo·phe·nic (al-ō-fē′nik). Alofênico; pertinente a um animal produzido pela combinação de blastômeros de genótipos diferentes (isto é, de pares diferentes de genitores). VER TAMBÉM mosaic. [allo- + G. *phainō*, aparecer, + -ic]

al·lo·phore (al′ō-fōr). Alóforo. SIN erythrophore.

al·loph·thal·mia (al-of-thal′mē-ă). Aloftalmia. SIN heterophthalmus.

al·lo·pla·sia (al-ō-plā′zē-ă). Aloplasia. SIN heteroplasia. [allo- + G. *plasis*, modelagem]

al·lo·plast (al′ō-plast). Aloplasto; material inerte usado para construir, reconstruir ou aumentar um tecido. [allo- + G. *plastos*, formado]

al·lo·plas·ty (al′ō-plas-tē). Aloplastia; reparo de defeitos por alotransplante.

al·lo·ploid (al′ō-ployd). Aloplóide; relativo a um indivíduo ou célula híbrida com dois ou mais grupos de cromossomas derivados de duas espécies ancestrais diferentes; dependendo do número de múltiplos de grupos haplóides, os aploplóides são conhecidos como alodiplóides, alotriplóides, alotetraplóides, alopentaplóides, aloexaplóides, etc. VER TAMBÉM heterokaryon. [allo- + -ploid]

al·lo·ploi·dy (al′ō-ploy′dē). Aloploidia; condição de ser aloplóide.

al·lo·pol·y·ploid (al-ō-pol′i-ployd). Alopoliplóide; um aloplóide com três ou mais grupos haplóides de cromossomas. [allo- + poliplóide]

al·lo·pol·y·ploi·dy (al-ō-pol′i-ploy-dē). Alopoliploidia; condição de ser alopoliplóide.

al·lo·preg·nane (al-ō-preg′nān). Alopregnano; nome original do 5α-pregnano. VER pregnane.

α-al·lo·preg·nane·di·ol (al′ō-preg-nan-dī′ol). α-alopregnanediol; 5α-pregnano-3α,20α-diol; um metabólito da progesterona e dos hormônios adrenocorticais; encontrado na urina.

β-al·lo·preg·nane·di·ol β-alopregnanediol; os 5α-pregnano-3β,20α(e β)-dióis; ambos são metabólitos da progesterona e de hormônios adrenocorticais; encontrados na urina.

al·lo·psy·chic (al-ō-sī′kik). Alopsíquico; indica os processos mentais em sua relação com o mundo exterior. [allo- + G. *psychē*, mente]

al·lo·pu·ri·nol (al-ō-pū′ri-nol). Alopurinol; inibidor da xantina oxidase para a inibição da formação do ácido úrico; empregado no tratamento da gota e para retardar a rápida degradação metabólica da 6-mercaptopurina.

al·lo·rhyth·mia (al-ō-rith′mē-ă). Alorritmia; irregularidade no ritmo cardíaco que se repete de forma regular. [allo- + G. *rhythmos*, ritmo]

al·lo·rhyth·mic (al-ō-rith′mik). Alorrítmico; relativo a, ou caracterizado por, alorritmia.

al·lose (al′ōs). Alose; $C_6H_{12}O_6$; uma aldoexose. D-A. é epimérico com D-glicose.

al·lo·sen·si·ti·za·tion (al′ō-sen′si-ti-zā-shŭn). Alossensibilização; exposição a um aloantígeno que induz células de memória imunológica.

al·lo·some (al′ō-sōm). Alossoma, alossomo; termo obsoleto para um dos cromossomas que diferem em aspecto e comportamento dos autossomas e, às vezes, está distribuído desigualmente entre as células germinativas. [allo- + G. *sōma*, corpo]

 paired a., diplossoma. SIN diplosome.
 unpaired a., cromossoma acessório. SIN accessory *chromosome*.

al·lo·ste·ric (al-ō-stār′ik). Alostérico; pertinente a, ou caracterizado por, alosterismo.

al·lo·ster·ism, al·lo·ste·ry (ă-los′ter-izm, -los′ter-ē). Alosteria; a influência de uma atividade enzimática, ou a ligação de um ligando a uma proteína, através de modificação na conformação da proteína, desencadeada pela união de um substrato ou outro efetor a um local (local alostérico) diferente do ponto ativo da proteína. Cf. cooperativity, hysteresis.

al·lo·tet·ra·ploid (al-ō-tet′ră-ployd). Alotetraplóide. VER alloploid. [allo- + tetraplóide]

al·lo·therm (al′ō-therm). Peciloterme. SIN poikilotherm. [allo- + G. *thermē*, calor]

al·lo·thre·o·nines (aThr) (al-o-thrē′ō-nēnz). Alotreoninas; dois dos quatro diastereoisômeros da treonina, diferindo das L-treoninas e D-treoninas na configuração do grupamento hidroxila na cadeia lateral.

al·lo·tope (al′ō-tōp). Alótopo; o determinante antigênico na região constante ou não-variável de um alótipo. [allo- + -tope]

al·lo·to·pia (al-ō-tō′pē-ă). Alotopia. SIN dystopia. [allo- + G. *topos*, lugar]

al·lo·trans·plan·ta·tion (al′ō-tranz-plan-tā′shŭn). Alotransplante; transplante de um aloenxerto. SIN homotransplantation.

al·lot·ri·o·don·tia (al-ot′rē-ō-don′shē-ă). Alotriodontia. **1.** Crescimento de um dente em algum local anormal. **2.** Transplante de dentes. [G. *allotrios*, estranho, + *odous (odont-)*, dente]

al·lot·ri·os·mia (al-ot-rē-oz′mē-ă). Alotriosmia; reconhecimento incorreto dos odores. SIN heterosmia. [G. *allotrios*, estranho, + *osmē*, olfato]

al·lo·trip·loid (al-ō-trip′loyd). Alotriplóide. VER alloploid. [allo + triplóide]

al·lo·trope (al′ō-trōp). Alótropo; um elemento em uma das formas alotrópicas que pode assumir. [allo- + G. *tropos*, circuito]

al·lo·tro·phic (al-o-trō′fik). Alotrófico; com valor nutritivo alterado. [allo- + G. *trophē*, nutrição]

al·lo·tro·pic (al-ō-trop′ik). Alotrópico. **1.** Relativo ao alotropismo. **2.** Denotando um tipo de personalidade que se caracteriza pela preocupação com as reações de outros.

al·lot·ro·pism, al·lot·ro·py (ă-lot′rō-pizm, -lot′rō-pē). Alotropismo, alotropia; a existência de certos elementos que diferem, em diversas formas, quanto às propriedades físicas; p.ex., negro-de-fumo, grafite e diamante representam carbono puro. [allo- + G. *tropos*, circuito]

al·lo·type (al′ō-tip). Alótipo; qualquer uma das diferenças antigênicas geneticamente determinadas dentro de uma determinada classe de imunoglobulina que ocorre entre membros da mesma espécie. VER TAMBÉM antibody. SIN allotypic marker. [allo- + G. *typos*, modelo]

Gm a.'s (ăl′lō-tīps), a. Gm; refere-se às cadeias pesadas da gama-imunoglobulina humana que expressam determinantes alotípicos Gm diferentes (antígenos). Cada um dos 25 a. Gm diferentes é o produto de genes dentro das regiões constantes da cadeia pesada gama humana.

InV a.'s. (ăl′lō-tīps), a. InV, a. Km. SIN Km a.'s.

Km a.'s (ăl′lō-tīps), a. Km; refere-se às cadeias leves *kapa* de imunoglobulina humana que expressam determinantes alotípicos Km diferentes (antígenos). SIN InV a.'s.

al·lo·typ·ic (al-ō-tip′ik). Alotípico; pertencente a um alótipo.

al·low·ance (a′lau-antz). **1.** Permissão, autorização, consentimento. **2.** Cota; uma porção distribuída.

recommended daily a. (RDA), cota diária recomendada (CDR); a porção diária de nutrientes considerada adequada para a manutenção da boa nutrição de um adulto médio.

al·lox·an (ă-loks′-an). Aloxana; produto da oxidação do ácido úrico, 2,4,5,6-pirimidinotetrona; a administração a animais de experimentação causa hipoglicemia devido à liberação de insulina, seguida por hiperglicemia decorrente da destruição das ilhotas de Langerhans (diabete por aloxana).

al·lox·an·tin (ă-loks′an-tin). Aloxantina; produto da condensação de duas moléculas de aloxana, formado na presença de agentes redutores; um diabetogênico. SIN uroxin.

al·lox·u·re·mia (al-oks-ū-rē′mē-ă, al-ok-soo-rē′mē-ă). Aloxuremia; a presença de purinas no sangue. [alloxan + G. *haima*, sangue]

al·lox·u·ria (al-oks-ū′rē-ă, al-ok-soo′rē-ă). Aloxúria; presença de purinas na urina. [alloxan + G. *ouron*, urina]

al·loy (al′oy). Liga; substância composta de uma mistura de dois ou mais metais.

chrome-cobalt a.'s, ligas de cobalto-cromo; ligas de cobalto e cromo contendo molibdênio e/ou tungstênio mais oligoelementos; usadas em odontologia para bases e armações protéticas, bem como outras estruturas.

eutectic a., liga eutética; geralmente quebradiça e sujeita a manchas e corrosão, com temperatura de fusão mais baixa do que qualquer um de seus componentes; usada em odontologia principalmente em soldas.

gold a., liga de ouro, liga cujo principal ingrediente é o ouro, contendo habitualmente cobre ou platina e prata; usada em odontologia para restaurações que exigem considerável estabilidade.

Raney a., liga de Raney; uma liga de Ni (níquel) e Al (alumínio) em proporções iguais, usada na preparação Raney Nickel.

silver-tin a., liga de prata-estanho; qualquer liga de prata (Ag) e estanho (Sn), comumente três partes de Ag e uma de Sn, formando Ag_3Sn, o principal composto intermetálico no amálgama dentário.

all-*trans*-ret·i·nal. Transretinal total; o retinaldeído laranja resultante da ação da luz sobre a rodopsina da retina, que converte o componente 11-*cis*-retinal da rodopsina em *trans*-retinal total mais opsina. SIN *trans*-retinal; visual yellow.

all·spice oil (awl′spīs). Óleo de pimenta. SIN pimenta oil.

al·lyl (al′il). Alilo; o radical monovalente, $CH_2=CHCH_2-$.

a. alcohol, álcool alínico; líquido incolor de odor irritante utilizado na fabricação de resinas e plastificadores; muito irritante para as mucosas e prontamente absorvido, causando depressão e coma. SIN vinyl carbinol.

a. cyanide, cianeto de alilo; encontrado em alguns óleos de mostardas.

a. isothiocyanate, isotiocianato de alilo; obtido da *Brassica nigra* ou pela ação da água sobre a sinigrina e mirosina ou produzido sinteticamente; vesicante, utilizado em solução a 10% em álcool a 50%, como contra-irritante na neuralgia. Dá à mostarda seu sabor e aroma característicos. VER TAMBÉM mustard oil. SIN volatile mustard oil.

a. sulfide, sulfeto de alilo; um constituinte do óleo de alho usado na fabricação de aromatizantes.

al·lyl·a·mine (al-il-am′ēn). Alilamina; líquido incolor derivado do óleo cru de mostarda e utilizado na indústria farmacêutica, p.ex., na fabricação de diuréticos mercuriais.

al·lyl·es·tre·nol (al-il-es′trĕ-nol). Alilestrenol; agente progestacional.

al·lyl·mer·cap·to·meth·yl·pen·i·cil·lin (al′il-mer-kap′tō-meth′il-pen-i-sil′in). Alilomercaptometilpenicilina, penicilina O. SIN penicillin O.

***N*-al·lyl·nor·mor·phine** (al′il-nor-mor′fēn). *N*-alilonormorfina, nalorfina. SIN nalorphine.

al·ly·sines (al′i-sēnz). Alisinas; dois ou mais α-aminoácidos de seis carbonos reunidos por uma união carbono–carbono; constituintes do tecido conjuntivo e de outros elementos estruturais. VER TAMBÉM desmin.

Almeida, Floriano Paulo de, médico brasileiro, *1898. VER A. *disease*; Lutz-Splendore-A. *disease*.

Almén, August Teodor, fisiologista sueco, 1833–1903. VER A. *test* for blood.

al·mond oil (aw′mŭnd, awl′mŭnd). Óleo de amêndoa; óleo extraído da amêndoa doce, dos grãos da variedade de *Prunus amygdalus*; usado em pomadas.

bitter almond a. o., óleo de amêndoas amargas; um óleo volátil de grãos de amêndoas amargas dessecados e de outras amêndoas contendo amigdalina; contém entre 2 e 4% de ácido hidrociânico e 95% de benzaldeído.

al·oe (al′ō). Aloé. **1.** O suco dessecado das folhas de plantas do gênero *Aloe* (família Liliaceae), do qual são obtidos aloína, resina, emodina e óleos voláteis. **2.** O suco dessecado das folhas de *Aloe perryi* (a. de Socotra), de *A. barbadensis* (aloé de Barbados e Curaçao) ou de *A. capensis* (do Cabo); usado como purgativo; usado topicamente em cosméticos, nos quais não apresenta valor comprovado.

al·oe-em·o·din (al′ō-em′ō-din). Aloé-emodina; o éter trimetil da emodina; usado como laxativo. VER aloin, emodin. SIN rhabarberone.

al·o·etin (al-ō-ē′tin). Aloetina. SIN aloin.

alo·gia (ă-lō′jē-ă). **1.** Alogia, afasia. SIN aphasia. **2.** Alogia; incapacidade de falar devido a deficiência ou a um episódio de demência. [G. *a-* priv. + *logos*, fala]

al·o·in (al′ō-in). Aloína; um princípio cristalino amarelo composto de aloé-emodina e glicose, obtido de aloé; usado como laxativo. SIN aloetin, barbaloin.

al·o·pe·cia (al-ō-pē′shē-ă). Alopecia; ausência ou perda de cabelo. SIN baldness, calvities, pelade. [G. *alōpekia*, doença parecida com a sarna de raposa, de *alōpex*, raposa]

a. adnata, a. adnata; subdesenvolvimento dos cílios. VER TAMBÉM a. congenitalis, milphosis. SIN madarosis (2).

androgenic a., a. androgênica; diminuição gradativa da densidade do cabelo em adultos com a transformação dos fios de cabelo terminais em fios finos, com queda desses devido à suscetibilidade familiar aumentada dos folículos pilosos a secreção de androgênios após a puberdade. Duas áreas do couro cabeludo são comumente afetadas nos homens; quando ocorre nas mulheres, está associada a outras evidências de atividade androgênica excessiva, como hirsutismo. Herança autossômica dominante. VER female pattern a., male pattern a. SIN common baldness.

a. area'ta [MIM*104000], a. em áreas, a. circunscrita; condição comum, de etiologia indeterminada, caracterizada por áreas circunscritas, não-fibróticas, geralmente assimétricas, de calvície no couro cabeludo, nas sobrancelhas e na porção com barba da face. Qualquer parte da pele do corpo com pêlos pode ser afetada; ocasionalmente, a herança é autossômica dominante. Infiltração linfocítica peribulbar e associação a distúrbios auto-imunes sugerem uma etiologia auto-imune. É comum o aumento lento com recrescimento final em 1 ano, mas a recidiva é frequente e a progressão para a a. total pode ocorrer, especialmente quando a alopecia surgiu na infância.

a. cap'itis tota'lis, a. total. SIN a. totalis.

cicatricial a., a. cicatricial. SIN scarring a. [L. *cicatrix, cicatricis*, cicatriz + sufixo -*al*, caracterizado por]

a. congenita'lis, a. congênita; ausência de todos os pêlos ao nascimento. Pode estar associada a epilepsia psicomotora [MIM*104130]; herança autossômica dominante ou ligada ao X [MIM*300042]. SIN congenital baldness, hypotrichiasis (2).

congenital sutural a., termo obsoleto para *dyscephalia* mandibulooculofacialis (discefalia mandíbulo-óculo-facial).

female pattern a., a. de padrão feminino; perda parcial difusa de cabelo na área centroparietal do couro cabeludo, com preservação das linhas de cabelo frontal e temporais; o tipo mais freqüente de a. androgênica em mulheres.

alopecia / **alternation**

a. heredita′ria, a. hereditária, a. de padrão masculino. SIN male pattern a.
a. leproti′ca, a. leprosa, a. morfética; escassez ou perda completa do terço lateral de sobrancelhas, cílios e pêlos corporais, vista na lepra; a perda do cabelo é rara.
a. limina′ris fronta′lis, a. frontal, a. marginal. SIN a. marginalis.
lipedematous a., a. lipedematosa; a. com prurido, dor ou hipersensibilidade do couro cabeludo em mulheres negras; o couro cabeludo está espessado e amolecido, a gordura subcutânea está aumentada e os fios de cabelo são escassos e curtos.
male pattern a. [MIM* 109200], a. de padrão masculino; forma mais comum de a. androgênica, vista nos homens como o retrocesso das linhas de implantação do cabelo frontal e temporais bilaterais, e uma área de calvície no vértex do crânio, que pode progredir para a. completa; a herança é autossômica dominante em homens e recessiva nas mulheres. SIN a. hereditaria, male pattern baldness, patterned a.
a. margina′lis, a. marginal; perda na linha de implantação do cabelo, condição encontrada mais comumente em negros; comumente transitória e causada por tração crônica, embora a tração continuada possa causar a. permanente. SIN a. liminaris frontalis.
a. medicamento′sa, a. medicamentosa; perda difusa do cabelo, mais notavelmente no couro cabeludo, causada pela administração de diversos tipos de medicamentos.
moth-eaten a., a. em roído-de-traça; perda irregular de cabelo nas regiões parietal e occipital do couro cabeludo, característica de sífilis secundária.
a. mucino′sa, a. mucinosa; mucinose folicular com a. surgindo nas áreas de eritema e edema na porção barbada da face ou no couro cabeludo.
patterned a., a. de padrão masculino. SIN male pattern a.
postoperative pressure a., a. por compressão pós-operatória. SIN pressure a.
postpartum a., a. pós-parto; perda temporária difusa dos fios de cabelo telógenos no fim da gravidez.
premature a., a. prematu′ra, a. prematura; calvície de padrão masculino que aparece muito precocemente.
a. preseni′lis, a. pré-senil; calvície comum ou habitual que ocorre no adulto ou na meia-idade, sem qualquer doença evidente do couro cabeludo.
pressure a., a. por compressão; perda de cabelo em uma área circunscrita, geralmente na parte posterior do couro cabeludo, resultante da compressão contínua do occipício durante um procedimento cirúrgico demorado ou da inconsciência seguinte a *overdose* farmacológica. SIN postoperative pressure a.
scarring a., a. cicatricial; a. em que os folículos pilosos são destruídos de maneira irreversível por processos fibróticos, incluindo traumatismo, queimaduras, lúpus eritematoso, líquen planopiloso, esclerodermia, foliculite descalvada ou de etiologia indeterminada (pseudopelada). SIN cicatricial a.
a. seni′lis, a. senil; a perda normal de cabelo na velhice.
a. symptomat′ica, a. sintomática; a. que ocorre no curso de várias doenças constitucionais ou locais, ou após doença febril prolongada.
a. syphilit′ica, a. sifilítica; a. da sífilis secundária (em roído-de-traça).
a. tota′lis, a. total; perda total do cabelo do couro cabeludo, em um intervalo de tempo muito curto ou durante a progressão da a. localizada, principalmente da a. em áreas. Cf. a. universalis. SIN a. capitis totalis.
a. tox′ica, a. tóxica; perda de cabelos atribuída a doença febril.
traction a., a. por tração; perda circunscrita ou difusa do cabelo resultante da tração repetitiva dos fios de cabelo ao puxar ou torcer; também ocorre depois da aplicação excessiva de "relaxantes" de cabelo, como soluções para ondas permanentes ou ferros quentes. A. marginal é uma forma de a. por tração. SIN traumatic a.
traumatic a., a. traumática. SIN traction a.
a. triangularis (trī′ang - oo - la - ris), a. triangular; retrocesso bilateral das linhas de implantação capilar temporais na a. de padrão masculino.
a. triangula′ris congenita′lis, a. triangular congênita; uma placa triangular congênita de calvície na região frontal ou temporal do couro cabeludo.
a. universa′lis, a. universal; perda total dos pêlos de todas as regiões do corpo. Cf. a. totalis.
al·o·pe·cic (al - ō - pē′sik). Alopécico; relativo à alopecia.
Alpers, Bernard J., neurologista norte-americano, 1900–1981. VER A. *disease*.
al·pha (al′fä). Alfa; primeira letra do alfabeto grego, α.
al·pha am·y·lase. Alfa-amilase; uma enzima degradadora de amido obtida a partir de uma bactéria não-patogênica da classe do *Bacillus subtilis*, empregada no tratamento de afecções inflamatórias e edema de tecidos moles associado a lesão traumática; sua utilidade terapêutica não foi plenamente estabelecida e seu modo de ação não é conhecido.
al·pha-block·er (al′fä - blok′er). Bloqueador alfa. SIN α-adrenergic blocking agent.
al·pha·di·one (al - fä - dī′on). Alfadiona; anestésico intravenoso que contém dois esteróides, alfaxalona e acetato de alfadolona, dissolvidos em 20% de óleo de rícino polioxietilado.
Al·pha·her·pes·vir·inae (al′fa - her′pez - vir′i - nē). Uma subfamília dos Herpesviridae contendo Simplesvirus e Varicellavirus.
al·pha·pro·dine (al - fa - prō′den). Alfaprodina; um analgésico narcótico relacionado à meperidina; pode desenvolver-se dependência tanto física quanto psíquica.

al·pha·sone ac·e·to·phe·nide (al′fä - son). Acetofenida de alfasona. SIN algestone acetophenide.
Al·pha·vi·rus (al′fä - vī - rus). Um dos gêneros da família Togaviridae que já foi classificado como parte dos arbovírus do "grupo A" e que inclui os vírus que causam as encefalites eqüina oriental, eqüina ocidental e venezuelana.
al·pi·dem (al - pī′dem). Alpidem; um benzodiazepínico ansiolítico/sedativo/hipnótico.
Alport, Arthur Cecil, médico sul-africano, 1880–1959. VER A. *syndrome*.
al·praz·o·lam (al - praz′ō - lam). Alprazolam; um tranqüilizante benzodiazepínico suave utilizado para o controle de transtornos da ansiedade e de pânico; o abuso pode levar ao hábito ou vício.
al·pren·o·lol hy·dro·chlo·ride (al - pren′ō - lol). Cloridrato de alprenolol; o cloridrato do 1-(*o*-alilofenoxi)-3-(isopropilamino)propan-2-ol; um agente bloqueador de β-receptores utilizado para o tratamento de arritmias cardíacas.
al·pros·ta·dil (al - pros′tä - dil). Alprostadil; vasodilatador empregado como terapia paliativa, visando manter temporariamente a permeabilidade do canal arterial em neonatos com cardiopatias congênitas. SIN prostaglandin E_1.
ALS Abreviatura para amyotrophic lateral *sclerosis* (esclerose lateral amiotrófica); antilymphocyte *serum* (soro antilinfócito).
al·ser·ox·y·lon (al′ser - ok′si - lon). Alseroxilona; uma fração alcaloidal lipossolúvel, extraída da raiz da *Rauwolfia serpentina*, contendo reserpina e outros alcalóides amorfos não-adrenolíticos; utilizada como sedativo em psicoses, na hipertensão leve e como adjunto para medicamentos hipotensores mais potentes.
Alström, Carl-Henry, geneticista sueco, *1907. VER A. *syndrome*.
ALT Abreviatura para alanine aminotransferase (alanina aminotransferase).
Altemeier, William A., cirurgião norte-americano do século XX. VER A. *operation*.
al·ter·a·tion (awl - ter - ā′shun). Alteração. **1.** Uma mudança. **2.** Uma modificação; ato de tornar diferente.
modal a., a. modal; em irritabilidade elétrica, uma mudança no modo de resposta do músculo degenerado à estimulação elétrica, com a contração tornando-se lenta em vez de rápida.
qualitative a., a. qualitativa; em irritabilidade elétrica, uma modificação na qual o músculo se contrai tão prontamente à aplicação do anódio quanto do catódio.
quantitative a., a. quantitativa; em irritabilidade elétrica, perda gradual da contratilidade em um músculo em resposta às correntes estática, farádica e galvânica, sucessivamente.
al·ter·e·go·ism (awl - ter - ē′gō - izm). Identificação com pessoas de personalidade semelhante à sua própria.
al·ter·nans (awl-ter′nanz). Alternância; com freqüência utilizada principalmente para a alternância cardíaca, elétrica ou mecânica. Que alterna; usada como nome no sentido de *pulsus* alternans [L.]
auditory a., a. auditiva. SIN auscultatory a.
auscultatory a., a. auscultatória; alternação (alternância) na intensidade das bulhas cardíacas ou dos sopros cardíacos na vigência de ritmo cardíaco regular em conseqüência de alternação mecânica do coração. SIN auditory a.
concordant a., a. concordante; ocorrência simultânea de a. ventricular direita e da artéria pulmonar com a. ventricular esquerda e do pulso periférico.
cycle lenght a., a. da duração do ciclo; uma sucessão de intervalos diastólicos longos e curtos.
discordant a., a. discordante; presença de a. ventricular direita e da artéria pulmonar com a. do pulso periférico, porém com o batimento forte do ventrículo direito coincidindo com o batimento fraco do esquerdo, e vice-versa.
electrical a., a. elétrica; alternação elétrica do coração.
Al·ter·nar·ia (al - ter - nā′rē - ä). Um gênero de fungos facilmente isolado a partir do ar e considerado um contaminante laboratorial comum e um alérgeno; ocasionalmente patogênico em seres humanos.
al·ter·na·tion (awl - ter - nā′shun). Alternação, alternância; ocorrência de duas coisas ou fases em sucessão e de maneira recorrente; usada como sinônimo de alternância.
cardiac a., a. cardíaca; a ocorrência de qualquer fenômeno cardíaco a batimentos alternados.
concordant a., a. concordante; a. na atividade mecânica ou elétrica do coração que acontece nas circulações sistêmica e pulmonar.
discordant a., a. discordante; a. nas atividades cardíacas da circulação sistêmica ou pulmonar, mas não em ambas, ou em ambas, porém com sentidos opostos entre si.
electrical a. of heart, a. elétrica cardíaca; um distúrbio em que os complexos ventriculares e/ou atriais são regulares no tempo, porém com padrão alternante; detectada por eletrocardiografia. Segmentos P, PR, QRS, T, QRS-T ou P-QRST alternam-se de forma isolada ou em combinação.
a. of generations, a. de gerações; uma sucessão de gerações de indivíduos semelhantes e diferentes dos pais originais ou uma a. de gerações sexuadas e não-sexuadas.
mechanical a. of the heart, a. mecânica do coração; distúrbio em que as contrações do coração são regulares, porém alternadamente mais fortes e mais fracas.

al·ter·na·tor (awl'ter - nā - ter). Alternador; aparelho mecânico com prateleiras transparentes móveis, nas quais se pode prender um grande número de radiografias, de modo a possibilitar a seleção e visualização em frente a uma fonte de luz estacionária. [L. *alterno*, fazer por etapas, de *alter*, outro]

al·ter·noc·u·lar (awl - ter - nok'u - lar). Alternocular; indica o uso de cada um dos olhos separadamente, em lugar da forma binocular. [L. *alternus*, por vez, + ocular]

Al·te·ro·mo·nas. Gênero de bactérias Gram-negativas com bastonetes curvos e móveis graças a um único flagelo polar; exige uma base de água salgada para o crescimento; uma causa de deterioração da carne de aves.
A. putrefa'ciens, uma espécie marinha de bactérias implicadas como uma causa da deterioração da carne de peixes, mas raramente é um patógeno humano.

al·thea (al - thē'ă). Altéia; derivado da *Althaea officinalis*, uma planta perene que é encontrada na forma silvestre em regiões úmidas da Europa. Contém uma elevada proporção de amidos, pectina e açúcares; utilizada como flavorizante e demulcente. SIN marshmallow root. [L., fr. G. *althaia*, malvaísco]

Altherr, Franz. VER Meyenburg-A.-Uehlinger *syndrome.*

alt. hor. Abreviatura para L. *alternis horis*, em horas alternadas.

al·ti·tu·di·nal (al - ti - too'di - năl). Altitudinal, altitúdico; relativo às relações verticais; p.ex., a. hemianopsia.

Altmann, Richard, histologista alemão, 1852–1900. VER A. *fixative, granule,* anilin-acid fuchsin *stain, theory*; A.-Gersh *method.*

al·trose (al'trōs). Altrose; uma aldoexose isômera da glicose, talose, alose, etc. D-altrose é o epímero de D-manose.

al·um (al'ŭm). Alume; alúmen; um sulfato duplo de alumínio e de um elemento de terra alcalina ou amônio; quimicamente, um alúmen é qualquer um dos sais duplos acentuadamente adstringentes formados por uma combinação de um sulfato de alumínio, ferro, manganês, cromo ou gálio com um sulfato de lítio, sódio, potássio, amônio, césio ou rubídio; usado localmente como estíptico. [L. *alumen*]
 burnt a., a. queimado. SIN dried a.
 cake a., torta de alume, sulfato de alumínio octadecaidratado. SIN *aluminum sulfate octadecahydrate.*
 chrome a., a. de cromo; o sulfato de cromo e potássio; empregado como mordente em coloração histológica.
 dried a., a. dessecado; a. privado de sua água de cristalização por calor; um talco adstringente. SIN burnt a.
 exsiccated a., a. exsicado; a. aquecido até o ressecamento completo; um adstringente local.
 ferric a., a. férrico. SIN *ferric* ammonium sulfate.
 whey a., a. uma preparação adstringente e estíptica feita pela fervura do a. (31 g) em leite (310 g).

al·um-he·ma·tox·y·lin (al'ŭm - hē - mă - tok'si - lin). Alume-hematoxilina; um corante nuclear púrpura utilizado em histologia; uma mistura de uma solução aquosa de alume de amônio e uma solução alcoólica de hematoxilina, a qual é amadurecida ou oxidada a hemateína.

alu·mi·na (ă - loo'mi - nă). Alumina; óxido de alumínio. SIN *aluminum* oxide.
 hydrated a., a. hidratada. SIN *aluminum* hydroxide.

alu·mi·nat·ed (ă - loo'mi - nā - ted). Aluminado; que contém alúmen.

alu·mi·non (ă - loo'min - on). O sal de amônio do ácido aurintricarboxílico, assim chamado por causa de sua utilidade na detecção de alumínio em materiais biológicos, alimentos, etc.

alu·mi·no·sis (ă - loo - min - ō'sis). Aluminose; pneumoconiose provocada pela inalação de partículas de alumínio para dentro dos pulmões.

alu·mi·num (Al) (ă - loo'min - ŭm). Alumínio; um metal branco prateado de peso muito leve; número atômico 13, peso atômico 26,981539. Muitos sais e compostos são empregados em medicina e odontologia. [L. *alumen*, alúmen]
 a. acetate, acetato de a.; usado como desinfetante por embalsamadores; proposto como pó secante e desodorante para eczema e úlceras cutâneas crônicas.
 a. acetotartrate, acetotartarato de a.; acetato básico de alumínio (70%) e ácido tartárico (30%); anti-séptico.
 a. acetylsalicylate, acetilsalicilato de alumínio. SIN a. aspirin.
 a. ammonium sulfate, sulfato de amônio e alumínio; um adstringente.
 a. aspirin, acetilsalicilato de alumínio; um analgésico e antipirético. SIN a. acetylsalicylate.
 a. bismuth oxide, óxido de bismuto e alumínio. SIN *bismuth* aluminate.
 a. carbonate, basic, carbonato básico de alumínio; um complexo carbonato-hidróxido de alumínio que consiste em grumos brancos, insolúveis em água; as suspensões aquosas se ligam ao fósforo no intestino e diminuem o fósforo inorgânico sérico, resultando em aumento da reabsorção de fósforo pelos túbulos renais e redução da excreção urinária de fósforo; diminui a formação de cálculos urinários de fosfato e a acidez gástrica.
 a. chlorate nonahydrate, cloreto de alumínio nonaidratado; um anti-séptico. SIN mallebrin.
 a. chloride hexahydrate, cloreto de alumínio hexaidratado; empregado como adstringente ou anti-séptico em solução.
 a. diacetate, diacetato de alumínio. SIN a. subacetate.
 a. hydrate, hidrato de alumínio. SIN a. hydroxide.
 a. hydroxide, hidróxido de alumínio; um pó adstringente; também utilizado internamente como antiácido adstringente brando. SIN a. hydrate, hydrated alumina.
 a. hydroxide gel, gel de hidróxido de alumínio; uma suspensão contendo Al$_2$O$_3$, principalmente na forma de hidróxido de alumínio, empregada como antiácido; uma forma desidratada, com a mesma utilização, é obtida através da secagem do produto da interação na solução aquosa de um sal de a. com carbonato de amônio ou sódio.
 a. hydroxychloride, hidroxicloreto de alumínio; um antitranspirante.
 a. magnesium silicate, silicato de magnésio e alumínio. SIN *magnesium* aluminum silicate.
 a. monostearate, monoestearato de alumínio; um composto de alumínio com uma mistura de ácidos orgânicos sólidos obtidos a partir da gordura que consiste, principalmente, em monoestearato de alumínio e monopalmitato de alumínio; utilizado como um meio de suspensão em preparações farmacêuticas.
 a. nicotinate, nicotinato de alumínio; um agente liporredutor com ação vasodilatadora periférica.
 a. oleate, oleato de alumínio; usado como pomada em determinadas afecções cutâneas e em queimaduras.
 a. oxide, óxido de alumínio; usado como abrasivo, como refratário e em cromatografia. SIN alumina.
 a. penicillin, penicilina alumínica; o sal trivalente de alumínio da penicilina. VER aluminum *penicillin.*
 a. phenolsulfonate, fenolsulfonato de alumínio; anti-séptico e adstringente para aplicação local, geralmente em úlceras cutâneas.
 a. phosphate, fosfato de alumínio; um pó infusível, insolúvel em água, mas solúvel em hidróxidos alcalinos, utilizado para cimentos dentários com sulfato de cálcio e silicato de sódio.
 a. phosphate gel, gel de fosfato de alumínio; uma suspensão aquosa com 4 a 5% de fosfato de alumínio; empregada como antiácido.
 a. potassium sulfate, sulfato de alumínio e potássio; um adstringente e estíptico; também utilizado em medicina veterinária para a estomatite ulcerativa, leucorréia e conjuntivite. SIN potassium alum.
 a. salicylate, basic, salicilato básico de alumínio; usado no tratamento da ozena e da faringite.
 a. salicylate, basic, soluble, salicilato básico solúvel de alumínio; empregado em solução como aerossol para as doenças das vias aéreas superiores.
 a. silicate, silicato de alumínio. SIN kaolin.
 a. subacetate, subacetato de alumínio; utilizado em solução (como na solução de Burow) como adstringente, como um ingrediente em colutórios e em líquidos de embalsamamento. SIN a. diacetate.
 a. sulfate octadecahydrate, sulfato de alumínio octadecaidratado; detergente adstringente para úlceras cutâneas. SIN cake alum.

alu·mi·num group. Grupo do alumínio; alumínio, boro, gálio, índio e tálio.

al·vei (al'vē - ī). Álveos; plural de alveus.

al·ve·o·al·gia (al'vē - ō - al'jē - ă). Alveoalgia; uma complicação pós-operatória da extração dentária, na qual o coágulo de sangue no alvéolo se desintegra, resultando em osteomielite focal e dor intensa. SIN alveolalgia, alveolar osteitis, dry socket. [alveolus + G. *algos*, dor]

al·ve·o·lal·gia (al'vē - ō - lal'jē - ă). Alveolalgia. SIN alveoalgia.

al·ve·o·lar (al - vē'ō - lar). Alveolar; relativo a um alvéolo.

al·ve·o·late (al - vē'ō - lāt). Alveolado; dotado de pequenas cavidades, alvéolos. [L. *alveolus*, diminutivo de *alveus*, depressão, saco oco, cavidade]

al·ve·o·lec·to·my (al'vē - ō - lek'tō - mē). Alveolectomia; a excisão cirúrgica de uma parte do processo dentoalveolar para remodelar a crista alveolar no momento da remoção do dente, visando facilitar uma prótese dentária. [alveolus + G. *ektomē*, excisão]

al·ve·o·li (al - vē'ō - lī). Alvéolos; plural de alveolus.

al·ve·o·lin·gual (al'vē - o - ling'gwăl). Alveolingual. SIN alveololingual.

al·ve·o·li·tis (al'vē - ō - lī'tis). Alveolite. 1. Inflamação dos alvéolos pulmonares. 2. Inflamação do alvéolo dentário.
 acute pulmonary a., alveolite pulmonar aguda; inflamação aguda, envolvendo exsudato para dentro dos alvéolos pulmonares e comprometimento da troca gasosa, como acontece em um portador de doenças pulmonares intersticiais, incluindo lesão alveolar difusa, doença pulmonar induzida por substâncias e lesão imunológica aguda.
 chronic fibrosing a., alveolite crônica fibrosante. SIN *idiopathic pulmonary fibrosis.*
 cryptogenic fibrosing a., alveolite criptogênica fibrosante. SIN *idiopathic pulmonary fibrosis.*
 extrinsic allergic a., alveolite alérgica extrínseca; pneumoconiose decorrente da hipersensibilidade oriunda da inalação repetida de poeira orgânica, geralmente especificada de acordo com a exposição ocupacional; na forma aguda, as manifestações respiratórias e a febre começam várias horas após a exposição à poeira; na forma crônica, acaba ocorrendo fibrose pulmonar difusa após a exposição durante alguns anos.
 fibrosing a., a. fibrosante. SIN *idiopathic pulmonary fibrosis.*

alveolo-. Formas combinantes que indicam um alvéolo, o processo alveolar; alveolar. [L. *alveolus*, um vaso côncavo, uma tigela, uma cuba, de *alveus*, uma depressão, + *-olus*, pequeno; semelhante a *alvus*, a barriga, a cavidade]

al·ve·o·lo·cla·sia (al - vē′ō - lō - klā′zē - ă). Alveoloclasia; a destruição do alvéolo. [alveolo- + G. *klasis*, rotura]

al·ve·o·lo·den·tal (al - vē′ō - lō′ - den′tăl). Alveolodental; relativo aos alvéolos e aos dentes.

al·ve·o·lo·la·bi·al (al - vē′ō - lō - lā′bē - ăl). Alveololabial; relativo à superfície labial ou vestibular (externa) dos processos alveolares da mandíbula superior ou inferior.

al·ve·o·lo·la·bi·a·lis (al - vē′ō - lō - lā - bē - ā′lis). Alveololabial; relativo à região ou sulco alveololabial. [L.]

al·ve·o·lo·lin·gual (al - vē′ō - lō - ling′gwăl). Alveololingual; relativo à superfície lingual (interna) do processo alveolar da mandíbula. SIN alveolingual.

al·ve·o·lo·pal·a·tal (al - vē′ō - lō - pal′ă - tăl). Alveolopalatal; relativo à superfície palatina do processo alveolar da maxila.

al·ve·o·lo·plas·ty (al - vē′ō - lō - plas - tē). Alveoloplastia; preparação cirúrgica das cristas alveolares para a recepção de dentaduras; a modelagem e o alisamento das bordas dos alvéolos depois da extração dos dentes com subseqüente sutura para garantir a cicatrização ótima. SIN alveoplasty. [alveolo- + G. *plasso*, formar]

interradicular a., intraseptal a., a. inter-radicular, a. intra-septal; remoção do osso inter-radicular e colapso das placas corticais para um contorno alveolar mais aceitável.

al·ve·o·los·chi·sis (al - vē - ō - los′ki - sis). Alveolosquise; uma fenda no processo alveolar. [alveolo- + G. *schisis*, separação]

al·ve·o·lot·o·my (al - vē - ō - lot′ō - mē). Alveolotomia; abertura cirúrgica de um alvéolo dentário para possibilitar a drenagem de pus a partir de um abscesso periapical ou de outro abscesso intra-ósseo. [alveolo- + G. *tome*, incisão]

al·ve·o·lus, gen. e pl. **al·ve·o·li** (al - vē′ō - lŭs, - ō - lī) [NA]. Alvéolo; uma pequena célula, cavidade ou encaixe. **1.** Alvéolo pulmonar. SIN pulmonary a. **2.** Uma das porções secretoras terminais de uma glândula alveolar ou racemosa. **3.** Uma das depressões alveolares na parede do estômago. **4.** Alvéolo dentário. SIN tooth *socket*. [L. diminutivo de *alveus*, depressão, saco oco, cavidade]

a. dentalis, pl. **alveoli dentales** [TA], alvéolo dental. SIN tooth *socket*.

pulmonary a., alvéolo pulmonar; dilatação terminal sacular de bronquíolos respiratórios, dutos alveolares e sacos alveolares, com paredes finas, através da qual ocorre a troca gasosa entre o ar alveolar e os capilares pulmonares. SIN alveolus (1) [NA], air cells (1), air vesicles, alveoli pulmonis, bronchic cells.

alveoli pulmo'nis, alvéolos pulmonares. SIN pulmonary a.

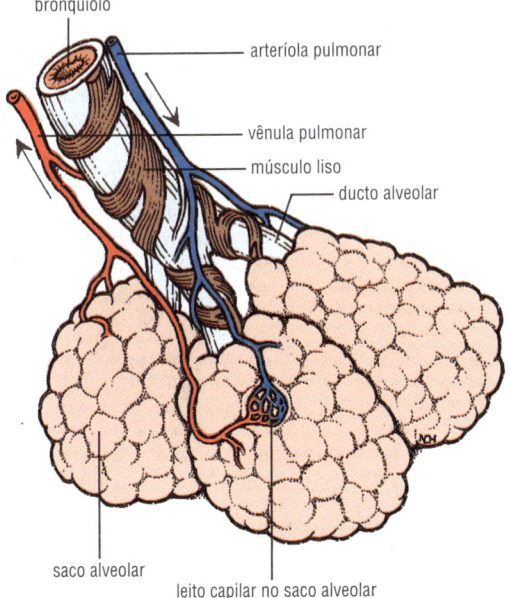

alvéolos pulmonares

al·ve·o·plas·ty (al′vē - ō - plas - tē). Alveoplastia, alveoloplastia. SIN alveoloplasty.

al·ve·us, pl. **al·vei** (al′vē - ŭs, - vē - ī). Álveo; um canal ou buraco. [L. depressão, gamela, cavidade, de *alvus*, barriga]

a. hippocam'pi [TA], álveo do hipocampo. SIN a. of hippocampus.

a. of hippocampus [TA], álveo do hipocampo; uma fina faixa branca de fibras do fórnix que reveste a superfície ventricular do hipocampo. SIN a. hippocampi [TA]

a. urogenita'lis, álveo urogenital; termo obsoleto para o prostatic *utricle* (utrículo prostático).

ALW Abreviatura para arch-loop-whorl *system* (sistema arco-alça-espiral).

alym·phia (ā - lim′fē - ă). Alinfia; ausência ou deficiência de linfa. [G. *a*- priv. + lymph + -ia]

alym·pho·cy·to·sis (ā - lim′fō - sī - tō′sis). Alinfocitose; ausência ou grande redução dos linfócitos.

alym·pho·pla·sia (ā - lim - fō - plā′zē - ă). Alinfoplasia; falta de desenvolvimento ou hipoplasia do tecido linfóide.

Nezelof type of thymic a., alinfoplasia tímica do tipo Nezelof; imunodeficiência celular com falha do desenvolvimento das células T e da função da célula T.

thymic a. alinfoplasia tímica; hipoplasia com ausência dos corpúsculos de Hassall e deficiência de linfócitos no timo e, em geral, nos linfonodos, baço e trato gastrointestinal, resultando em grave imunodeficiência combinada. VER TAMBÉM *immunodeficiency* with hipoparathyroidism.

Alzheimer, Alois, neurologista alemão, 1864–1915. VER A. *dementia, disease, sclerosis*.

al·zyme (al′zīm). Alzima; união do anticorpo e enzima para formar uma molécula catalítica híbrida.

Am Símbolo do amerício.

am Abreviatura para ammeter (amperímetro).

AMA Abreviatura para American Medical Association (Associação Americana de Medicina).

am·a·crine (am′ă - krin). Amácrina. **1.** Uma célula ou estrutura sem um processo fibroso longo. **2.** Indica essa célula ou estrutura. VER TAMBÉM amacrine *cell*. [G. *a*- priv. + *makros*, longo, + *is (in-)*, fibra]

am·a·dou (ahm′ah - doo). Agárico. SIN agaric. [Fr.]

amal·gam (ă - mal′gam). Amálgama; uma liga de um elemento ou metal com mercúrio. Em odontologia, basicamente de dois tipos: liga de prata-estanho, contendo pequenas quantidades de cobre, zinco e, talvez, outros metais, e um segundo tipo contendo mais cobre (12 a 30% por peso); são empregadas para a restauração de dentes e fabricação de corantes. [G. *malagma*, uma massa amolecida]

pin a., amálgama de pino; uma restauração com a. mantida na posição em grande parte por pequenos bastonetes metálicos que se projetam de orifícios feitos com broca na estrutura dentária.

spherical a., a. esférica; uma liga para a. dentária composta de partículas esféricas em vez de limalha.

amal·ga·mate (ă - mal′gă - māt). Amalgamar; fazer uma amálgama.

amal·ga·ma·tion (ă - mal - gă - mā′shŭn). Amalgamação; o processo de combinar mercúrio com um metal ou uma liga para formar uma nova liga.

amal·ga·ma·tor (ă - mal′gă - mā - tōr). Amalgamador; um aparelho para combinar o mercúrio com um metal ou ligar para formar uma nova liga.

Am·a·ni·ta (am - ă - nī′tă). Um gênero de fungos, do qual muitos membros são bastante venenosos. [G. *amanitai*, fungos]

A. musca'ria, uma espécie tóxica de cogumelo com um umbráculo amarelo a avermelhado e lamelas brancas; contém muscarina, um colinomimético, que provoca estados psicóides e outros sintomas. SIN fly agaric.

A. phalloi'des, uma espécie que contém princípios venenosos, inclusive faloidina e amanitina, que provocam gastrenterite, necrose hepática e necrose renal. SIN deadly agaric.

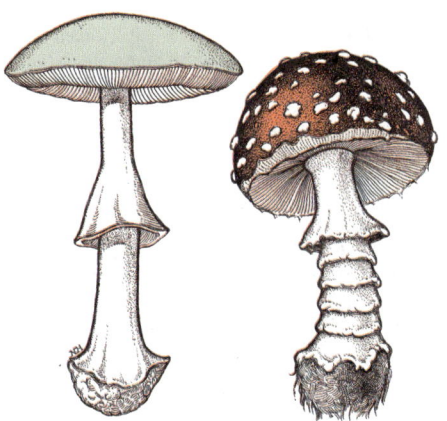

Amanita phalloides (esquerda) e ***Amanita muscaria*** (direita)

α-am·a·ni·tin (am - ă - nī′tin). α-Amanitina; um oligopeptídeo bicíclico muito tóxico, termoestável, na *Amanita phalloides*. Inibe a transcrição por certas RNA polimerases.

aman·ta·dine hy·dro·chlo·ride (ă - man′tă - dēn). Cloridrato de amantadina; um agente antiviral utilizado para a gripe; também empregado para tratar o parkinsonismo, visto que aumenta a liberação de dopamina e reduz sua recaptação nas terminações nervosas dopaminérgicas dos neurônios da substância negra.

am·a·ra (ă-mah′ră). Amargos, amaros. SIN bitters (2). [pl. neut. de L. *amarus*, amargo]

am·a·ranth, am·a·ran·thum (am′ă-ranth, am-ă-ran′thŭm). [C.I. 16185]. Amaranto; um corante azo; um pó vermelho-acastanhado solúvel, cuja coloração se modifica para vermelho-magenta em solução; usado como corante alimentar, farmacêutico e cosmético e, ocasionalmente, em histologia. [G. *amaranthon*, uma flor que nunca murcha]

am·a·rine (am′ă-rin). Amarina; um nome aplicado a vários princípios amargos derivados de plantas, especialmente a uma substância venenosa, 2,4,5-trifenilimidazolina, obtida do óleo de amêndoa amarga. [L. *amarus*, amargo]

am·a·roid (am′ă-royd). Amaróide; um extrato amargo que não pertence à classe dos glicosídeos, alcalóides ou a qualquer um dos princípios vegetais próximos conhecidos. [L. *amarus*, amargo, + G. *eidos*, semelhante]

am·a·roi·dal (am-ă-roy′dăl). Amaroidal; que se assemelha ao amargo; que possui um paladar discretamente amargo.

ama·rum (ă-mah′rŭm). Amargo; qualquer um dos componentes de uma classe de medicamentos vegetais de paladar amargo, como a genciana e a quássia, usado como aperitivos e tônicos. [neut, de L. *amarus*, amargo]

amas·tia (ă-mas′tē-ă). Amastia; ausência de mamas.[G. *a-* priv. + *mastos*, mama]

amas·ti·gote (ă-mas′ti-gōt). Amastigota. SIN Leishman-Donovan *body*. [G. *a-* priv. + *mastix*, flagelo]

am·a·tho·pho·bia (ă-math-ō-fō′bē-ă). Amatofobia; temor mórbido de poeira ou sujeira. [G. *amathos*, poeira, + *phobos*, medo]

am·a·tox·in (am-a-tok′sin). Amatoxina; um de um grupo de octapeptídeos bicíclicos dos agáricos em geral e da *Amanita phalloides*.

am·au·ro·sis (am-aw-rō′sis). Amaurose; cegueira, especialmente aquela que ocorre sem alteração aparente no próprio olho, como em decorrência de uma lesão cerebral. [G. *amauros*, escuro, obscuro, + *-osis*, condição]

a. congen′ita of Leber [MIM*204000 & MIM*204100], amaurose congênita de Leber; abiotrofia de cones e bastonetes que provoca cegueira ou visão muito reduzida ao nascer; herança autossômica recessiva em, pelo menos, 3 *loci* distintos. O tipo I é causado por mutação no gene para a guanilato ciclase retiniana (GUC2D) no cromossoma 17p, o tipo II por mutação no gene para a proteína de 65 kD específica do epitélio pigmentar retiniano (RPE65) em 1p e o tipo III por mutação no gene para o gene homeobox CRX específico do fotorreceptor em 19q.

a. fu′gax, a. fugaz; cegueira transitória que pode resultar de isquemia transitória decorrente de insuficiência da artéria carótida, embolia na artéria retiniana ou força centrífuga (blecaute visual de vôo).

pressure a., a. compressiva; perda da visão que ocorre alguns segundos depois que a pressão intra-ocular supera a pressão sistólica das artérias retinianas.

toxic a., a. tóxica; cegueira decorrente de neurite óptica provocada por álcool metílico, chumbo, arsênico, quinina ou outros venenos.

am·au·rot·ic (am-aw-rot′ik). Amaurótico; relativo a, ou que sofre de, amaurose.

amax·o·pho·bia (ă-mak-sō-fō′bē-ă). Amaxofobia; termo raramente empregado para o medo mórbido de um veículo ou de entrar nele. [G. *amaxa*, *hamaxa*, uma carruagem, + *phobos*, medo]

am·ba·geu·sia (am-bă-goo′sē-ă). Ambageusia; perda do paladar em ambos os lados da língua. [L. *ambo*, dois lados, + G. *a-* priv. + *geusis*, paladar]

am·be·no·ni·um chlo·ride (am-bē-nō′nē-ŭm). Cloreto de ambenônio; um inibidor da colinesterase semelhante à neostigmina em suas ações; empregado principalmente no controle da miastenia grave e, ocasionalmente, para a obstrução dos tratos intestinal e urinário.

AMBER (am′ber). Acrônimo para advanced multiple-beam equalization *radiography* (radiografia com equalização de múltiplos feixes).

am·ber (am′ber). Âmbar. **1.** Uma resina fossilizada endurecida, amarelo-escura a marrom-clara, derivada do pinheiro. **2.** VER amber *codon*. [Ar. *anbar*]

Amberg, Emil, otologista norte-americano, 1868–1948. VER A. lateral sinus *line*.

am·ber·gris (am′ber-gris). Âmbar-gris; uma secreção patológica acinzentada oriunda do intestino do cachalote que ocorre como uma massa cérea inflamável (ponto de fusão de aproximadamente 60°C), insolúvel em água; contém colesterol e ácido benzóico, sendo utilizado como fixador de perfumes. [L. mod. *ambra grisea*, âmbar cinza]

⚠ **ambi-.** Prefixo que significa em torno de; em todos (ambos) os lados; ambos, duplo; corresponde ao G. amphi-. VER TAMBÉM ambo-. [L. ao redor, acerca de, semelhante a *ambo*, ambos]

am·bi·dex·ter·i·ty (am-bi-deks-ter′i-tē). Ambidestrismo, ambidesteridade; a capacidade de usar ambas as mãos com igual facilidade. SIN ambidextrism.

am·bi·dex·trism (am-bi-deks′trizm). Ambidestrismo, ambidesteridade. SIN ambidexterity.

am·bi·dex·trous (am-bi-deks′trŭs). Ambidestro; ter igual facilidade (eficiência) no uso de ambas as mãos.

am·bi·ent (am′bē-ent). Ambiente; que circunda, que envolve; pertinente ao ambiente no qual um organismo ou aparelho funciona. [L. *ambiens*, o que há em torno]

am·bi·gu·i·ty (am-bi-goo′ĭ-tē). Ambigüidade; condição de ser ambíguo; incerteza.

genital a., a. genital; desenvolvimento incompleto da genitália fetal em conseqüência da ação excessiva de androgênio sobre um feto feminino ou por quantidades inadequadas de androgênio em um feto masculino. SIN ambiguous external genitalia, ambiguous genitalia.

am·big·u·ous (am-big′ū-ŭs). Ambíguo. **1.** Que possui mais de uma interpretação. **2.** Em anatomia, migratório; que possui mais de uma direção. **3.** Em neuroanatomia, aplicado a um núcleo (núcleo ambíguo) que fornece fibras eferentes viscerais especiais para os nervos vago e glossofaríngeo. [L. *ambiguus*, de *ambigo*, vaguear]

am·bi·lat·er·al (am-bi-lat′er-ăl). Ambilateral; relativo a ambos os lados. [ambi- + L. *latus*, lado]

am·bi·le·vous (am-bi-lē′vŭs). Ambílevo; inaptidão ou inabilidade no uso de ambas as mãos. SIN ambisinister, ambisinistrous. [ambi- + L. *laevus*, esquerda]

am·bi·sex·u·al (am-bi-seks′u-ăl). Ambissexual. **1.** Indica as características sexuais encontradas em ambos os sexos, p.ex., mama, pêlos pubianos. **2.** Jargão para bissexual.

am·bi·sin·is·ter (am-bi-sin′is-ter). Ambílevo. SIN ambilevous. [ambi- + L. *sinister*, esquerda]

am·bi·si·nis·trous (am′bi-sin′is-trŭs). Ambílevo. SIN ambilevous.

am·biv·a·lence (am-biv′ă-lens). Ambivalência; a coexistência de atitudes ou emoções antitéticas (antagônicas) em relação a uma determinada pessoa, coisa ou idéia, como no sentimento e expressão simultâneos de amor e ódio em relação à mesma pessoa. [ambi- + L. *valentia*, força]

am·biv·a·lent (am-biv′ă-lent). Ambivalente; relativo a, ou caracterizado por, ambivalência.

am·bi·vert (am′bi-vert). Ambivertido; aquele que se situa entre os dois extremos da introversão e extroversão, possuindo algumas das tendências de cada uma.

⚠ **ambly-.** Formas combinantes [ambli (i/o)] que indicam embotado, obscurecido, arredondado, amolecido, sem vigor. [G. *amblys*, turvo, embotado; desmaio, obscurecimento]

am·bly·geus·tia (am-bli-goos′tē-ă). Ambligeustia; diminuição do paladar. [ambly- + G. *geusis*, paladar]

amblyogenic (am′blē-ō-jen′ic). Ambliogênico; que induz a ambliopia. [amblyopia + -genic]

Am·bly·om·ma (am-blē-om′ă). Um gênero de carrapatos de couraça dura e ornada (família Ixodidae) caracterizado por ter olhos, festões e placas ventrais profundamente embebidas perto dos festões nos machos. [ambly- + G. *omma*, olho, visão]

A. america′num, o carrapato Lone Star, uma espécie que é uma praga e vetor importante da febre maculosa das Montanhas Rochosas, encontrado principalmente no sul dos Estados Unidos e norte do México; ocorre em cães e em muitos outros hospedeiros, incluindo animais domésticos, pássaros e seres humanos, aos quais pica nos estágios de larva, ninfa e adulto.

A. cajennen′se, o carrapato de Caiena, carrapato-estrela, carrapato-de-cavalo, uma espécie que é uma praga importante no sul do Texas, nas Américas Central e do Sul e nas maiores ilhas do Caribe, e um vetor da febre maculosa das Montanhas Rochosas no México e nas Américas Central e do Sul; em todos os estágios, ataca os seres humanos e muitas espécies de animais domésticos e selvagens.

A. hebrae′um, um carrapato sul-africano de antílopes, um importante vetor de uma riquetsiose fatal (*heartwater*) no sul da África.

A. macula′tum, o carrapato da costa do Golfo, uma espécie que é uma praga de animais domésticos no sudeste dos Estados Unidos.

A. variega′tum, um carrapato parasita tropical, uma praga grave de animais domésticos e um vetor importante de uma riquetsiose fatal (*heartwater*) na África e no Caribe; está intimamente associado ao desenvolvimento de dermatofilose clínica grave no gado no Caribe.

am·bly·o·pia (am-blē-ō′pē-ă). Ambliopia; a deficiência visual causada pelo desenvolvimento anormal das áreas visuais do cérebro em resposta à estimulação visual anormal durante o desenvolvimento inicial. [G. *amblyōpia*, borramento visual, fr. *amblys*, embotamento, + *ōps*, olho]

anisometropic a., a. anisometrópica; supressão da visão central decorrente de um erro de refração desigual (anisometropia) mínimo de duas dioptrias. Isto induz uma diferença tal no tamanho da imagem (aniseiconia) que as duas imagens não conseguem se fundir. Buscando evitar a confusão, a imagem mais turva é suprimida. SIN refractive a.

deprivation a., a. de privação, a. sensorial. SIN sensory a.

a. ex anop′sia, a. por supressão. SIN suppression a.

hysterical a., a. histérica; perda visual funcional.

meridional a., a. meridional; a. decorrente de um grande astigmatismo não-corrigido, durante o período ambliogênico (amblyogenic *period*) do desenvolvimento visual.

nocturnal a., a. noturna. SIN nyctalopia.

nutritional a., a. nutricional; a. resultante da falta de constituintes do complexo da vitamina B.

pattern distortion a., a. por distorção de padrão; a. decorrente de uma imagem retiniana turva durante o período ambliogênico do desenvolvimento visual.
refractive a., a. por refração. SIN anisometropic a.
sensory a., a. sensorial; supressão da visão central em um olho devido à formação deficiente da imagem; p.ex., por uma cicatriz córnea, catarata ou blefaroptose. SIN deprivation a.
strabismic a., a. estrábica; supressão da visão central decorrente de dois olhos que apontam em direções diferentes. As duas cenas não podem ser fundidas em uma imagem única, de modo que, para evitar confusão, uma das imagens é suprimida.
supression a., a. por supressão; supressão da visão central em um olho quando as imagens oriundas dos dois olhos são tão diferentes que não podem ser fundidas em uma só. Isso pode ser causado por: 1) formação defeituosa da imagem (a. sensorial); 2) uma grande diferença na refração entre os dois olhos (a. anisometrópica); ou 3) os dois olhos apontando em direções diferentes (a. estrábica). Grande parte da a. por supressão pode ser revertida quando tratada da maneira adequada antes dos 6 anos de idade. SIN a. ex anopsia.
tobacco-alcohol a., a. por tabaco e álcool; neuropatia óptica adquirida, que afeta principalmente as fibras nervosas do feixe maculopapilar, associada ao consumo excessivo de álcool e tabaco.
toxic a., a. tóxica. VER toxic *amaurosis*.
am·bly·o·pic (am-blē-ō′pik). Ambliópico; relativo a, ou que sofre de, ambliopia.
am·bly·o·scope (am′blē-ō-skōp). Amblioscópio; estereoscópio de reflexão empregado para avaliar ou simular a visão binocular. VER TAMBÉM haploscope. [amblyopia + G. *skopeō*, visualizar]
major a., a. maior; a. em que a intensidade da iluminação, bem como os alvos, pode ser variada.
Worth a., a. de Worth; o a. original; um a. manual consistindo em tubos angulados que podem ser girados para qualquer grau de convergência ou divergência.
ambo-. Prefixo que significa ao redor de; em todos (ambos) os lados; corresponde a G. ampho-. VER TAMBÉM ambi-. [L. *ambo*, ambos]
am·bo·cep·tor (am′bō-sep-tor). Ambiceptor; termo de Ehrlich para seu conceito, atualmente ultrapassado, da estrutura do anticorpo fixador de complemento; empregado hoje em dia principalmente para indicar o anticorpo antieritrócito de carneiro usado no sistema hemolítico dos testes de fixação de complemento. [ambo- + L. *capio*, tomar]
am·bo·mal·le·al (am-bō-mal′ē-āl). Ambomalear. SIN incudomalleal.
am·bro·sin (am-brō′sin). Ambrosina; um princípio existente na erva-de-santiago relacionado à absintina.
am·bu·cet·a·mide (am-bū-set′a-mīd). Ambucetamida; um antiespasmódico intestinal.
am·bu·lance (am′bū-lans). Ambulância; veículo empregado para transportar pessoas doentes ou feridas para uma instituição de tratamento. [Fr., de *(hôpital) ambulant*, hospital móvel]
am·bu·la·to·ry, am·bu·lant (am′bū-lā-tōr-ē, am′bū-lant). Ambulatorial, ambulante; que caminha ou é capaz de caminhar; indica um paciente que não está confinado ao leito ou ao hospital em conseqüência de doença ou cirurgia. [L. *ambulans*, caminhar]
am·bu·phyl·line (am-bū′fi-lin). Ambufilina; diurético e broncodilatador.
am·cin·o·nide (am-sin′ō-nīd). Ancinonida; glicocorticóide empregado por via tópica no tratamento de dermatoses.
ame·ba, pl. **ame·bae, ame·bas** (a-mē′ba, -bē, -bāz). Ameba, amebas; nome comum para *Amoeba* e protozoários sarcodíneos semelhantes, descobertos, lobosos.

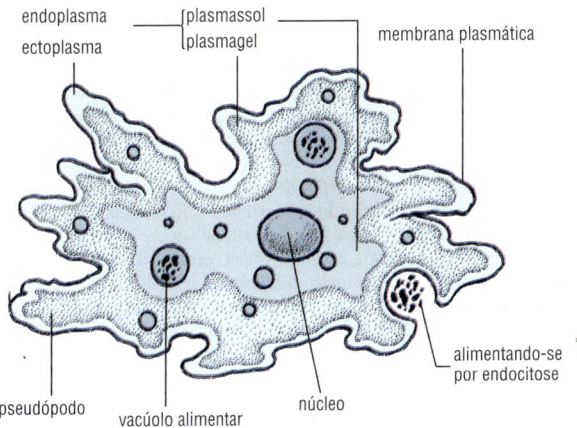

ameba

ame·ba·cide (ā-mē′ba-sīd). Amebicida. SIN amebicide.
ame·ba·ism (ā-mē′ba-izm). Ameboísmo. **1.** Movimento amebóide. SIN ameboidism (1). **2.** Ameboísmo. SIN ameboididity.
am·e·bi·a·sis (am-ē-bī′a-sis). Amebíase; infecção pelo protozoário *Entamoeba histolytica*. [ameba + G. *-iasis*, condição]
canine a., a. canina; infecção dos cães por *Entamoeba histolytica* adquirida de seres humanos; os cães raramente são eliminadores de cistos e, por conseguinte, não constituem um reservatório para a infecção humana.
a. cu′tis, a. cutânea; a. da pele que geralmente aparece como uma extensão da infecção subjacente (p.ex., perianal ou em uma colostomia ou sobre um abscesso hepático).
hepatic a., a. hepática; infecção do fígado por *Entamoeba histolytica;* pode ocorrer com ou sem disenteria amebiana antecedente.
pulmonary a., a. pulmonar; infecção do pulmão por amebas; geralmente indica a extensão da infecção por *Entamoeba histolytica* a partir de abscesso hepático, penetrando no pulmão através do diafragma.
ame·bic (ā-mē′bik). Amébico; relativo, que se assemelha a ou causado por amebas.
ame·bi·ci·dal (ā-mē-bi-sī′dal). Amebicida; destrutivo para as amebas.
ame·bi·cide (ā-mē′bi-sīd). Amebicida; qualquer agente que cause a destruição das amebas. SIN amebacide. [ameba + L. *caedo*, matar]
ame·bi·form (ā-mē′bi-fōrm). Amebiforme; com o formato ou aparência de uma ameba. [ameba + L. *forma*, forma]
am·e·bi·o·sis (am-ē-bī-ō′sis). Termo obsoleto para amebíase.
ame·bism (ā-mē′bizm). Termo obsoleto para amebíase.
ame·bo·cyte (ā-mē′bō-sīt). Amebócito. **1.** Uma célula migratória encontrada em invertebrados. **2.** Termo obsoleto para leucócito. **3.** Um leucócito em cultura de tecido *in vitro*. [ameba + *kytos*, célula]
ame·boid (ā-mē′boyd). Amebóide. **1.** Que se assemelha a uma ameba em aparência ou características. **2.** De contorno irregular com projeções periféricas; que indica o contorno de uma forma de colônia na cultura em placa. [ameba + G. *eidos*, aparência]
ame·boi·did·i·ty (ā-mē-boy-did′i-tē). Ameboidicidade; o poder de locomoção semelhante ao de uma célula amebóide. SIN amebaism (2).
ame·boid·ism (ā-mē′boyd-izm). **1.** A realização de movimentos semelhantes aos de uma ameba. SIN amebaism (1). **2.** Indica uma condição por vezes observada em determinadas células nervosas.
am·e·bo·ma (am-ē-bō′ma). Ameboma; um foco nodular, tumoriforme, de inflamação proliferativa que, por vezes, se desenvolve na amebíase crônica, em especial na parede do cólon. SIN amebic granuloma. [ameba + G. *-oma*, tumor]
ame·bu·la, pl. **ame·bu·lae** (ā-mē′bū-lā, -lē). Amébula. Termo aplicado a amebas "jovens" de espécies de *Entamoeba* que emergem dos cistos no intestino de seres humanos ou vertebrados e sua progênie imediata, geralmente totalizando oito, antes de sua localização no intestino grosso. [G. *amoibē*, alteração, mudança.]
amebule (ā-mē′būl). Amébula; uma ameba diminuta.
am·e·bu·ria (am-ē-bū′rē-ā). Amebúria; a presença de amebas na urina. [ameba + G. *ouron*, urina]
amel·a·not·ic (ā-mel-ā-not′ik). Amelanótico; que carece de melanina. [G. *a-* priv. + *melas*, negro]
ame·lia (ā-mē′lē-ā). Amelia; ausência congênita de um membro ou membros. Já foram descritas formas autossômica dominante, autossômica recessiva e ligada ao X, porém a maioria dos casos é esporádica. [G. *a-* priv. + *melos*, um membro]
ame·lio·ra·tion (ā-mēl-yō-rā′shun). Melhoria; melhora; moderação na gravidade de uma doença ou intensidade de seus sintomas. [L. *ad*, para, + *meliorо*, tornar melhor]
am·e·lo·blast (ā-mel′ō-blast, am-ē-lō′blast). Ameloblasto; uma das células epiteliais colunares da camada interna do órgão do esmalte de um dente em desenvolvimento, ligada à formação da matriz do esmalte. SIN enamel cell, enameloblast, ganoblast. [E. antigo *amel*, esmalte, + G. *blastos*, germe]
am·e·lo·blas·to·ma (am′ē-lō-blas-tō′mā). Ameloblastoma; uma neoplasia epitelial odontogênica benigna que, do ponto de vista histológico, mimetiza o órgão do esmalte embrionário, mas não se diferencia a ponto de formar os tecidos duros dentários; comporta-se como um tumor radiotransparente expansível, com crescimento lento; ocorre mais amiúde nas regiões posteriores da mandíbula e exibe uma tendência acentuada para reincidir quando é excisado de maneira inadequada. [ameloblast + G. *-oma*, tumor]
pigmented a., a. pigmentado. SIN melanotic neuroectodermal *tumor* of infancy.
pituitary a., a. hipofisário. SIN craniopharyngioma.
am·e·lo·den·tin·al (am′ē-lō-den′ti-nāl). Amelodentinário. SIN dentinoenamel.
am·e·lo·gen·e·sis (am′ē-lō-jen′ē-sis). Amelogênese; a deposição e maturação do esmalte. SIN enamelogenesis.
a. imperfec′ta, a. imperfeita; um grupo de distúrbios ectodérmicos hereditários nos quais o esmalte exibe estrutura defeituosa ou quantidade insuficiente. São reconhecidos três grupos principais: os tipos hipoplásicos, com deposição defeituosa da matriz do esmalte, mas com mineralização normal; os tipos

de hipomineralização, com matriz normal, porém mineralização defeituosa; e o tipo de hipomaturação, em que os pequenos cristais do esmalte permanecem imaturos. Os vários tipos podem ser herdados como herança autossômica dominante [MIM*104500, 104510, 104530], autossômica recessiva [MIM*204650, 204690, 204700] ou ligada ao X [MIM*301100, 301200, 301201]. SIN enamel dysplasia, enamelogenesis imperfecta.

a·mel·o·gen·ins (am'el-ō-jen'inz). Amelogeninas; uma classe de proteínas que formam grande parte da matriz orgânica durante o desenvolvimento inicial do esmalte dentário. [amelogenesis + -in]

ame·nia (ā-mē'nē-ā). Amenia; termo raramente empregado para amenorréia. [G. *a*- priv. + *mēn*, mês]

amen·or·rhea (ā-men-ō-rē'ā). Amenorréia; ausência ou cessação anormal da menstruação. [G. *a*- priv. + *mēn*, mês, + *rhoia*, fluxo]

  dietary a., a. dietética; perda da função menstrual em virtude do ganho ou da perda grave de peso.

  emotional a., a. emocional; a. causada por um forte distúrbio emocional, p.ex., temor, luto.

  exercise-induced a., a. induzida pelo exercício; cessação temporária da função menstrual decorrente de exercício extenuante diário, como na corrida, com as endorfinas aumentadas inibindo a função hipotalâmica.

  hyperprolactinemic a., a. hiperprolactinêmica; a. associada a níveis séricos extremamente elevados de prolactina; pode ser acompanhada por lactação não-fisiológica.

  hypophysial a., a. hipofisária; a. devido à secreção inadequada de gonadotrofina pelo lobo anterior da hipófise.

  hypothalamic a., a. hipotalâmica; a. secundária que se origina do estímulo hipotalâmico inadequado do lobo anterior da hipófise.

  lactation a., a. da lactação; supressão fisiológica da menstruação durante o aleitamento.

  ovarian a., a. ovariana; a. em consequência da deficiência de produção de hormônio estrogênico pelo ovário, freqüentemente referida como menopausa, quando permanente.

  pathologic a., a. patológica; a. devido à doença orgânica, uterina ou de outro tipo, p.ex., insuficiência ovariana ou hipofisária.

  physiologic a., a. fisiológica; a. da gestação ou a menopausa não associada a um distúrbio orgânico.

  postpartum a., a. pós-parto; a. permanente após o parto, em consequência da síndrome de Sheehan. VER Sheehan *syndrome*.

  primary a., a. primária; a. quando nunca ocorreu menstruação.

  secondary a., a. secundária; a. em que a menstruação apareceu na puberdade, mas cessou mais adiante.

  traumatic a., a. traumática; ausência da menstruação por causa da fibrose endometrial ou estenose cervical resultante de lesão ou doença. SIN Asherman syndrome.

amen·or·rhe·al, amen·or·rhe·ic (ā-men-ō-rē'al, -rē'ik). Amenorreico; relativo a, acompanhado por ou devido a amenorréia.

amen·tia (ā-men'shē-ā). Amência. **1.** Retardo mental. SIN mental *retardation*. **2.** Demência. SIN dementia. [L. loucura, de *ab*, de + *mens*, mente]

  nevoid a., a. nevóide. SIN Brushfield-Wyatt *disease*.

  phenylpyruvic a., a. fenilpirúvica; a. acompanhada pelo aparecimento de fenilpiruvato na urina.

amen·ti·al (ā-men'shē-al). Amencial; pertinente à amência.

***Amer·i·can Law In·sti·tute* for·mu·la·tion.** Usado em determinadas jurisdições para determinar a responsabilidade criminal em procedimentos legais. VER criminal *insanity*.

***Amer·i·can Law In·sti·tute* rule.** Ver em rule.

American National Standards Institute **(ANSI).** Organização que estabelece os padrões para as medidas físicas nos Estados Unidos.

Amer·i·can Red Cross. A sociedade nacional *Cruz Vermelha dos Estados Unidos*, estabelecida pelo Congresso para auxiliar no atendimento de doentes e feridos, servir como um elo de comunicação entre os membros das Forças Armadas norte-americanas e suas famílias, conduzir programas de alívio e prevenção de desastres e fomentar outros serviços humanitários, dos quais o maior é uma rede de bancos de sangue regionais que fornecem sangue e hemoderivados.

am·er·ci·um (Am) (am'ĕ-ris'ē-ŭm). Amerício; um elemento obtido através do bombardeio do urânio com nêutrons ou decaimento β do plutônio 241, 242 e 243; número atômico 95; peso atômico 243,06. O Am^{241} (meia-vida de 432,2 anos) tem sido empregado no diagnóstico de distúrbios ósseos. O Am^{243} possui uma meia-vida de 7.370 anos. [the Americas]

am·er·ism (am'er-izm). Amerismo; a condição ou qualidade de não se dividir em partes, segmentos ou merozoítos. [G. *a*- priv. + *meros*, parte]

am·er·is·tic (am-ĕ-ris'tik). Amerístico; dotado de amerismo; não se divide em partes ou segmentos.

Ames, Bruce N., geneticista molecular norte-americano, *1928. VER A. *assay, test*.

am·e·thop·ter·in (ā-meth-ō-ter'in, am-ĕ-thop'tĕ-rin). Ametopterina. SIN methotrexate.

ame·tria (ā-mē'trē-ā). Ametria; ausência congênita do útero; a genética é obscura. [G. *a*- priv. + *mētra*, útero]

ame·tri·o·din·ic ac·id (ā'mē-trī-ō-din'ik). Ácido ametriodínico. SIN iodamide.

am·e·tro·pia (am-ĕ-trō'pē-ā). Ametropia; a condição óptica em que existe um erro de refração, de modo que, com o olho em repouso, os raios luminosos de objetos distantes não se focalizam de forma conjugada na retina, isto é, apenas os objetos mais próximos são focalizados sobre a retina. [G. *ametros*, desproporcional, de *a*- priv. + *metron*, medida, + *ōps*, olho]

  axial a., a. axial; que resulta de um encurtamento ou alongamento do globo ocular no eixo óptico, gerando hiperopia ou miopia, respectivamente.

  index a., a. de índice; que resulta da alteração no índice de refração do cristalino do olho. SIN refractive a.

  refractive a., a. de refração. SIN index a.

am·e·tro·pic (am-ĕ-trō'pik). Ametrópico; relativo a ou que sofre de ametropia.

am·i·an·ta·ceous (am'i-an-tā'shŭs). Amiantáceo; semelhante ao asbesto; descreve as finas placas de crosta inflamatória de uma lesão cutânea. [G. *amiantus*, asbesto]

am·i·an·thoid (am-i-an'thoyd). Amiantóide; que possui uma aparência cristalina semelhante ao asbesto. SIN asbestoid. [G. *amianthus*, asbesto]

-amic. -Âmico; sufixo químico que indica a substituição de um grupamento COOH de um ácido dicarboxílico por um grupamento carboxamida (–CONH$_2$); aplicado apenas aos nomes comuns (p.ex., ácido succinâmico).

ami·cro·bic (ā-mi-krō'bik). Amicrobiano; não relacionado ou causado por microrganismos.

ami·cro·scop·ic (ā'mī-krō-skop'ik). Amicroscópico. SIN submicroscopic.

am·i·dase (am'i-dās). Amidase; uma enzima que catalisa a hidrólise das amidas monocarboxílicas em ácido livre mais NH$_3$; a ω-a. atua sobre amidas como o ácido α-cetoglutarâmico e o ácido α-cetossuccinâmico.

am·i·das·es. Amidases. SIN amidohydrolases.

am·ide (am'id, am'id). Amida; uma substância formalmente derivada da amônia através da substituição de um ou mais dos átomos de hidrogênio por grupamentos acil, R–CO–NH$_2$, ou a partir de um ácido carboxílico pela substituição de uma OH carboxílica por NH$_2$. A substituição de um átomo de hidrogênio constitui uma **a. primária**; a de dois átomos de hidrogênio, uma **a. secundária**; e a de três átomos de hidrogênio, uma **a. terciária**.

  substituted a., a. substituída; uma a. secundária ou terciária; as ligações peptídicas são amidas substituídas.

am·i·dine (am'i-din). Amidina; o radical monovalente –C(NH)–NH$_2$.

am·i·di·no·hy·dro·las·es (am'i-din-ō-hī'drō-lās-ez). [EC 3.5.3.x]. Amidinoidrolases; enzimas que clivam as amidinas lineares; p.ex. arginase, creatinase.

am·i·din·o·trans·fer·as·es (am'i-din-ō-trans'fer-ās-ez) [EC 2.1.4.x]. Amidinotransferases; enzimas que catalisam uma reação de transamidinação (p.ex., glicina-amidinotransferase). SIN transaminidases.

amido-. Prefixo que indica o radical amida, R–CO–NH– ou R–SO$_2$–NH–, etc. [am(monia) + -id(e) + -o-]

ami·do black 10B (am'i-dō) [C.I. 20470]. Negro de amida 10B; um corante ácido diazo, C$_{12}$H$_{14}$N$_6$O$_9$S$_2$Na$_2$, empregado como corante de tecido conjuntivo, para corar a proteína na cromatografia em papel e na eletroforese.

ami·do·hy·dro·las·es (am'i-dō-hī'drō-lā-sez) [EC 3.5.1.x e 3.5.2.x]. Amidoidrolases; enzimas que hidrolisam as ligações C–N das amidas e as amidas cíclicas; p.ex., asparaginase, barbiturase, urease, amidase. SIN amidases, deamidases, deamidizing enzymes.

ami·do·naph·thol red (am'i-dō-naf'thol) [C.I. 18050]. Vermelho de amidonaftol; um corante azo, C$_{18}$H$_{13}$N$_3$S$_2$Na$_2$, empregado na microscopia óptica e fluorescente como um contracorante ácido verdadeiro. SIN azophloxin.

ami·do·py·rine (am-i-dō-pī'ren). Amidopirina. SIN aminopyrine.

Am·i·dos·to·mum an·ser·is (am-i-dos'tō-mŭm an'ser-is). Uma espécie de nematódeos hematófagos, similar àqueles do gênero *Trichostrongylus*, que parasita a moela e, por vezes, também o proventrículo e o esôfago de patos e gansos domésticos e selvagens; causa substancial mortalidade nos pássaros jovens. [amido- + G. *stoma*, boca + L. *anser*, ganso]

am·i·dox·imes (am-i-doks'imz, -dok'sēmz). Amidoximas; as oximas de amidas com a fórmula geral R–C(NH$_2$)–NOH. SIN amide oximes.

am·i·dox·yl (am-i-dok'sil). Amidoxil; o radical de uma oxima de amida (amidoxima), com o H terminal (do NOH) tendo sido perdido.

am·i·ka·cin sul·fate (am-i-kā'sin). Sulfato de amicacina; um antibiótico aminoglicosídeo com atividade antimicrobiana semelhante à da canamicina; também efetivo contra *Pseudomonas aeruginosa*.

amil·o·ride hy·dro·chlo·ride (ā-mil'ō-rīd). Cloridrato de amilorida; um composto não-esteróide que exerce um efeito semelhante ao de um inibidor da aldosterona, isto é, a excreção urinária de sódio é aumentada e a excreção de potássio é reduzida; um diurético poupador de potássio.

amim·ia (ā-mim'ē-ā). Amimia. **1.** Incapacidade de expressar as idéias por comunicação não-verbal, como gestos ou sinais. **2.** Assimbolia; a incapacidade de compreender o significado dos gestos, sinais, símbolos ou imitações. [G. *a*- priv. + *minos*, uma mímica]

am·i·nac·rine hy·dro·chlo·ride (am′i-nak′rin). Cloridrato de aminacrina; agente bactericida para uso externo. VER TAMBÉM acridine yellow. SIN 5-aminoacridine hydrochloride, 9-aminoacridine hydrochloride.

am·i·nate (am′i-nāt). Aminar; combinar com amônia.

am·i·na·tion (ā-me-nā′shŭn). Aminação; a introdução de uma molécula de amina em um composto.

amine (ā-mēn′, am′in). Amina; uma substância formalmente derivada da amônia pela substituição de um ou mais átomos de hidrogênio por hidrocarboneto ou outros radicais. A substituição de um átomo de hidrogênio constitui uma **a. primária**, p.ex., NH_2CH_3; a de dois átomos, uma **a. secundária**, p.ex., $NH(CH_3)_2$; a de três átomos, uma **a. terciária**, p.ex., $N(CH_3)_3$; e a de quatro átomos, um **íon amônio quaternário**, p.ex., $^+N(CH_3)_4$, um íon com carga positiva isolado apenas em associação a um íon negativo. As aminas formam sais com os ácidos.

  adrenergic a., a. adrenérgica. SIN sympathomimetic a.
  adrenomimetic a., a. adrenomimética. SIN sympathomimetic a.
  biogenic a.'s, aminas biogênicas; uma classe de compostos, cada qual contendo um grupamento amina, produzidos por um organismo vivo. Essa classe normalmente não inclui os aminoácidos.
  a. oxidase (cooper-containing), a. oxidase (contendo cobre); uma oxirredutase que contém cobre e, talvez, piridoxal fosfato, e que realiza a mesma reação que uma a. oxidase (contendo flavina). SIN diamine oxidase, histaminase.
  a. oxidase (flavin-containing), a. oxidase (contendo flavina); uma oxirredutase que contém flavina e que oxida as aminas, com o auxílio do O_2 e água, em aldeídos ou cetonas, com liberação de NH_3 e H_2O_2. Ativada por antidepressivos. SIN adrenaline oxidase, diamine oxidase, monoamine oxidase, tyraminase, tyramine oxidase.
  pressor a., a. pressora. SIN pressor base.
  sympathetic a., a. simpática. SIN sympathomimetic a.
  sympathomimetic a., a. simpaticomimética; um agente que provoca respostas similares àquelas produzidas pela atividade nervosa adrenérgica (p.ex., epinefrina, efedrina, isoproterenol). SIN adrenergic a., adrenomimetic a., sympathetic a.
  vasoactive a., a. vasoativa; uma substância, como histamina ou serotonina, que contém grupamentos amino e que se caracteriza, do ponto de vista farmacológico, por sua ação sobre os vasos sanguíneos (alterando o diâmetro ou a permeabilidade vascular).

am·in·er·gic (ā-mēn′er-gik). Aminérgico; relativo às células ou fibras nervosas.

amino-. Prefixo que indica um composto que contém o radical $-NH_2$. [am(monia) +in(e) + -o-]

ami·no ac·id (AA, aa) (ā-mē′nō). Aminoácido; um ácido orgânico em que um dos átomos de hidrogênio em um átomo de carbono foi substituído por NH_2. Geralmente refere-se a um ácido aminocarboxílico. Entretanto, a taurina também é um aminoácido. VER TAMBÉM α-amino acid.

  acidic a.a., a. ácido; um a. com uma segunda molécula ácida, p.ex., ácido glutâmico, ácido aspártico, ácido cisteico.
  activated a.a., a. ativado. SIN aminoacyl adenylate.
  basic a.a., a. básico; um a. que contém um segundo grupamento básico (usualmente um grupamento amino); p.ex., lisina, arginina, ornitina. SIN dibasic a.a.
  a.a. dehydrogenases, a. desidrogenases; enzimas que catalisam a desaminação oxidativa de aminoácidos nos oxo(ceto)ácidos correspondentes; existem duas variedades relativamente inespecíficas, L e D, para as quais os L-aminoácidos e os D-aminoácidos são os respectivos substratos; os produtos incluem NH_3 e um aceptor de hidrogênio reduzido (NADH no caso do L); existem a. desidrogenases de maior especificidade (p.ex., glicina desidrogenase). Cf a. a. oxidases.
  dibasic a. a., a. dibásico. SIN basic a. a.
  essential a. a.'s, aminoácidos essenciais; α-aminoácidos exigidos nutricionalmente por um organismo e que têm de ser fornecidos em sua dieta (isto é, não podem ser sintetizados pelo organismo), seja como a. livre ou proteínas.
  nonessential a. a.'s, aminoácidos não-essenciais; aqueles aminoácidos que podem ser sintetizados por um organismo e que, por conseguinte, não são exigidos em sua dieta.
  nonpolar a. a., a. apolar; um α-aminoácido em que o grupamento funcional ligado ao carbono α (isto é, R em $RCH(NH_2)COOH$) possui propriedades hidrofóbicas; p.ex., valina, leucina, α-aminobutirato.
  a. a. oxidases, a. oxidases; flavoenzimas que oxidam especificamente L- ou D-aminoácidos, com O_2 e H_2O, aos 2-cetoácidos correspondentes, NH_3 e H_2O_2. Cf. a. a. dehydrogenases, yellow *enzyme*.
  polar a. a., a. polar; um α-aminoácido em que o grupamento funcional ligado ao carbono α (isto é, R em $RCH(NH_2)COOH$) possui propriedades hidrofílicas; p.ex., serina, cisteína, homocisteína.

α-ami·no ac·id. α-Aminoácido; tipicamente, um aminoácido de fórmula geral $R-CHNH_2-COOH$ (isto é, o NH_2 na posição α); as formas L desses aminoácidos são os produtos de hidrólise de proteínas. Em usos mais raros, essa classe de moléculas também inclui os ácidos α-aminofosfóricos e ácidos α-aminossulfônicos.

ami·no·ac·i·de·mia (ā-mē′nō-as-i-dē′mē-ā, am′i-nō-). Aminoacidemia; a presença de quantidades excessivas de aminoácidos específicos no sangue. [amino acid + G. *haima*, sangue]

ami·no·ac·id-tRNA li·gas·es. Aminoácido-ARNt ligases; nome recomendado para as aminoacil-ARNt sintetases, p.ex., tirosina-ARNt ligase para a tirosil-ARNt sintetase.

ami·no·ac·i·du·ria (am′i-nō-as-i-doo′rē-ā). Aminoacidúria; a excreção de aminoácidos na urina, principalmente em quantidades excessivas. SIN hyperaminoaciduria. [amino acid + G. *ouron*, urina]

  hiperbasic aminoaciduria, aminoacidúria hiperbásica; um distúrbio hereditário associado a deficiência de transporte de aminoácido dibásico. Os indivíduos tipicamente não apresentam intolerância à proteína. Cf. lysinuric protein *intolerance*.

9-ami·no·ac·ri·dine (ā-mē-nō-ak′ri-dēn). 9-Aminoacridina; um dos componentes do grupo acridina de anti-sépticos (flavinas); muito fluorescente em solução; usado topicamente como anti-séptico.

5-ami·no·ac·ri·dine hy·dro·chlo·ride, 9-ami·no·ac·ri·dine hy·dro·chlo·ride. Cloridrato de 5 ou 9-aminoacridina. SIN acridine yellow, aminacrine hydrochloride.

ami·no·ac·yl (AA, aa) (ā-mē′nō-as′il). Aminoacila; o radical formado a partir de um aminoácido pela remoção de OH de um grupamento COOH.

ami·no·ac·yl a·den·y·late (ā-mē′nō-as-il-ā-den′i-lāt). Aminoaciladenilato; o produto formado pela condensação do radical acila de um aminoácido e o 5′-monofosfato de adenosina (originariamente na forma de 5′-trifosfato de adenosina, com a eliminação de um grupamento pirofosfórico). Formado na primeira etapa da biossíntese proteica. SIN activated amino acid.

ami·no·ac·yl·ase (ā-mē′nō-as′i-lās). Aminoacilase; uma enzima que catalisa a hidrólise de uma grande variedade de N-acil-aminoácidos no aminoácido correspondente e um ânion ácido. SIN hippuricase, histozyme.

ami·no·ac·yl-tRNA. Aminoacil-ARNt; termo genérico para aqueles compostos em que os aminoácidos são esterificados através de seus grupamentos COOH a 3′-(ou 2′-)OH dos resíduos da adenosina terminal do ARN de transferência (p.ex., alanil-ARNt, glicil-ARNt); cada composto envolve um ou pequeno número de ARN de transferência de estrutura química específica. Usado na biossíntese proteica.

  a.-tRNA ligases, a.-ARNt ligases. SIN a.-tRNA syntethases.
  a.-tRNA syntethases, a.-ARNt sintetases; enzimas que catalisam a formação de um a.-ARNt específico a partir de um aminoácido e do 5′-trifosfato de adenosina com a concomitante formação de 5′-monofosfato de adenosina e pirofosfato. SIN amino acid activating enzyme, a.-tRNA ligases.

ami·no·a·dip·ic δ-sem·i·al·de·hyde syn·thase. δ-Semialdeído aminodípico sintase; uma enzima bifuncional empregada na degradação da lisina; possui atividade de lisina:α-cetoglutarato redutase, bem como atividade de sacaropina desidrogenase. A deficiência dessa enzima resulta em hiperlisinemia familial.

α-ami·no·a·dip·ic ac·id (Aad) (ā-mē′nō-ā-dip′ik). Ácido α-aminoadípico; ácido 2-amino-1,6-hexanedióico; um intermediário da biossíntese da lisina em fungos e bactérias superiores, mas não em algas e vegetais superiores. Também encontrado na degradação da lisina em mamíferos.

ami·no·ben·zene (ā-mē′nō-ben′zēn). Aminobenzeno. SIN aniline.

***o*-ami·no·ben·zo·ic ac·id** (ā-mē′nō-ben-zō′ik). Ácido *o*-aminobenzóico. SIN anthranilic acid.

***p*-ami·no·ben·zo·ic ac·id (PABA).** Ácido *p*-aminobenzóico; um fator no complexo da vitamina B, uma parte de todos os ácidos fólicos e necessária para sua formação; neutraliza os efeitos bacteriostáticos das sulfonamidas, pois fornece um fator de crescimento essencial para bactérias, cuja utilização sofre interferência das sulfonamidas; usado como um filtro para ultravioleta em loções e cremes. É produzido em um teste da função pancreática. SIN paraaminobenzoic acid, vitamin B_x.

D(-)-α-ami·no·ben·zyl·pen·i·cil·lin (ā-mē′nō-ben′zil-pen-i-sil′in). D (-)-α-aminobenzilpenicilina. SIN ampicillin.

γ-ami·no·bu·tyr·ic ac·id (GABA, γ-Abu) (ā-mē′nō-bū-tēr′ik). Ácido γ-aminobutírico; ácido 4-aminobutírico; um constituinte do sistema nervoso central; quantitativamente, o principal neurotransmissor inibitório. Usado no tratamento de inúmeros distúrbios (p.ex., epilepsia).

δ-ami·no·bu·tyr·ic ac·id amino transferase. Ácido δ-aminobutírico aminotransferase; uma enzima que catalisa a transferência reversível de um grupamento amino do ácido δ-aminobutírico em 2-oxoglutarato, formando, assim, um ácido L-glutâmico e succinato semialdeído. Uma etapa importante no catabolismo do ácido δ-aminobutírico.

ami·no·ca·pro·ic ac·id (ā-mē′nō-cā-prō′ik). Ácido aminocapróico; um agente antifibrinolítico, usado para evitar o sangramento na hemofilia, bem como depois de cirurgia cardíaca e de próstata, quando o plasminogênio ou a uroquinase podem ser ativados.

ami·no·car·bon·yl (am-i-nō-kar′bon-il). Aminocarbonil. SIN carboxamide.

ami·no·cit·ric ac·id (ā-mē′no-sit′rik). Encontrado em hidrolisados ácidos de ribonucleoproteína no baço humano.

2-ami·no-2-de·oxy-D-ga·lac·tose. 2-amino-2-desoxi-D-galactose. VER galactosamine.

ami·no·glu·teth·i·mide (ă-mē′nō-gloo-teth′i-mīd). Aminoglutetimida; um inibidor da aromatase empregado no tratamento do câncer de mama; bloqueia a síntese de estrogênio; originalmente testado como anticonvulsivante, mas não é mais utilizado para esse propósito.

am·i·no·gly·co·side (am′i-nō-glī′kō-sīd). Aminoglicosídeo; qualquer um de um grupo de antibióticos bactericidas derivados de espécies de *Streptomyces* ou *Micromonosporum* e caracterizados por dois ou mais amino açúcares unidos por uma ligação glicosídica a uma hexose central; os aminoglicosídeos agem ao provocarem a leitura errônea e a inibição da síntese proteica nos ribossomas bacterianos e são efetivos contra bacilos aeróbicos Gram-negativos e *Mycobacterium tuberculosis*. Alguns dos aminoglicosídeos comumente utilizados são a estreptomicina, neomicina e gentamicina.

p-**ami·no·hip·pu·ric ac·id (PAH)** (ă-mē′nō-hi-pūr′ik). Ácido *p*-aminohipúrico; usado nas provas de função renal para medir o fluxo plasmático renal; secretado (e filtrado) ativamente pelo rim.

  p.-a. a. synthase, sintase do ácido para-amino-hipúrico; uma enzima no fígado que catalisa a síntese de ácido *p*-amino-hipúrico a partir do ácido *p*-aminobenzóico (ou do derivado CoA) e glicina. Pode ser idêntico à glicina aciltransferase.

5-ami·no·im·id·az·ole ri·bose 5′-phos·phate (AIR) (ă-mē′nō-im-id-āz′ōl). 5-Aminoimidazol ribose 5′-fosfato; um intermediário na biossíntese das purinas. SIN 5-aminoimidazole ribotide.

5-ami·no·im·id·az·ole ri·bo·tide (AIR) (ă-mē′n′o-im-id-āz′ōl). 5-aminoimidazol ribotídeo. SIN 5-aminoimidazole ribose 5′-phosphate.

5-a·mi·no·im·id·az·ole-4-*N*-suc·ci·no·car·box·am·ide ri·bo·nu·cle·o·tide (ă-mē′nō-im-id-āz′ōl). 5-aminoimidazol-4-*N*-succinocarboxamida ribonucleotídeo; um intermediário na biossíntese da purina.

β-ami·no·iso·bu·ty·rate:py·ru·vate ami·no·trans·fer·ase. β-aminoisobutirato:piruvato aminotransferase; β-aminoisobutirato:piruvato transaminase; uma enzima que catalisa a transferência reversível de um grupamento amino do β-aminoisobutirato em piruvato, produzindo L-alanina e metilmalonato semialdeído; uma etapa na degradação da valina. A deficiência dessa enzima resulta em acidúria hiper-β-aminoisobutírica.

α-ami·no·i·so·bu·tyr·ic ac·id (ă-mē′nō-i-sō-bū-tĕr′ik). Ácido α-aminoisobutírico; ácido 2-amino-2-metilpropiônico; um aminoácido sintético útil no estudo do transporte de aminoácido através das membranas celulares e no estudo dos efeitos da citocina; não é metabolizado pela célula.

β-ami·no·i·so·bu·tyr·ic ac·id. Ácido β-aminobutírico; ácido 3-amino-2-metilpropiônico; um produto final do catabolismo da tiamina; foram observados níveis urinários elevados (200–300 mg/dia) em alguns indivíduos, devido a algum processo patológico ou seguindo um padrão genético.

α-ami·no-β-ke·to·a·dip·ic ac·id. Ácido α-amino-β-cetoadípico; um intermediário da síntese do profobilinogênio formado pela sintase do ácido-δ-aminolevulínico a partir da succinil-CoA e glicina; descarboxila rapidamente em ácido δ-aminolevulínico.

δ-ami·no·lev·u·li·nate de·hy·dra·tase (ă-mē′nō-lev-ū-lin′āt). δ-aminolevulinato desidratase. SIN *porphobilinogen* synthase.

δ-ami·no·lev·u·lin·ic ac·id (ALA) (ă-mē′nō-lev-ū-lin′ik). Ácido δ-aminolevulínico; um ácido formado pela δ-aminolevulanato sintase a partir da glicina e succinil-coenzima A; um precursor do profobilinogênio, sendo, portanto, um importante intermediário na biossíntese do heme. Os níveis de ALA mostram-se elevados nos casos de intoxicação por chumbo.

  δ-aminolevulinic acid synthase. Sintase do ácido δ-aminolevulínico; uma enzima que catalisa a reação da succinil-CoA com a glicina para formar o ácido δ-aminolevulínico, coenzima A e CO_2. A etapa obrigatória na biossíntese da porfirina.

am·i·nol·y·sis (am-i-nol′i-sis). Aminólise; a substituição de um halogênio em uma molécula de alquila ou arila por um radical amina, com eliminação do halóide de halogênio.

ami·no·met·ra·dine (ă-mē′nō-met′rā-dēn). Aminometradina. SIN aminometramide.

ami·no·met·ra·mide (ă-mē′nō-met′rā-mīd). Aminometramida; derivado sintético do uracil; um diurético efetivo por via oral que parece inibir a reabsorção de sódio pelos túbulos renais; usado no tratamento do edema decorrente da insuficiência cardíaca congestiva, doença hepática, gestação e determinados medicamentos. SIN aminometradine.

6-ami·no·pen·i·cil·lan·ic ac·id (6-APS) (ă-mē′nō-pen-i-sil-ăn′ik). Ácido 6-amino-penicilânico; um importante precursor na síntese de derivados da penicilina. Por si só, não possui atividade antibiótica. Para a estrutura, ver em penicilina, em que R = H. SIN penicin.

ami·no·pen·i·cil·lins (ă-mē′nō-pen-i-sil′inz). Aminopenicilinas; uma classe de antibióticos semelhantes à penicilina que, quimicamente, contêm um grupamento amina; essa classe compreende a ampicilina e a amoxicilina; usadas em infecções respiratórias altas, infecções do trato urinário, meningite, infecções por *Salmonella*.

ami·no·pep·ti·dase (cy·to·sol). Aminopeptidase (citosol); uma enzima de ampla especificidade, contendo zinco, e que catalisa a hidrólise do aminoácido N-terminal de um peptídeo (isto é, uma exopeptidase).

ami·no·pep·ti·dase (mi·cro·som·al). Aminopeptidase (microssomial); uma aminopeptidase de ampla especificidade, mas com preferência pela alanina e discriminação contra a prolina.

ami·no·pep·ti·das·es (ă-mē′nō-pep′ti-dās-ez) [EC 3.4.11.x]. Aminopeptidases; enzimas que catalisam a clivagem de um peptídeo, removendo o aminoácido na terminação amino da cadeia (isto é, uma exopeptidase); encontradas nas secreções intestinais.

ami·no·phen·a·zone (ă-mē′nō-fen′ā-zōn). Aminofenazona. SIN aminopyrine.

ami·no·phyl·line (ă-mē′nō-fil′in, am-i-nof′i-lin, -ēn). Aminofilina; uma forma solubilizada da teofilina; um diurético, vasodilatador e estimulante cardíaco; também usada como broncodilatador na asma e em medicina veterinária. SIN teophylline ethylenediamine.

ami·no·pro·ma·zine (ă-mē-nō-prō′mă-zēn). Aminopromazina; um antiespasmódico intestinal.

ami·no·pro·pi·on·ic ac·id (ă-mē′nō-prō-pē-on′ik). Ácido aminopropiônico. VER alanine.

p-**ami·no·pro·pi·o·phe·none (PAPP)** (ă-mē′nō-prō-pē-ō-fē′nōn). *p*-Aminopropiofenona; um antídoto para a intoxicação por cianeto.

am·i·nop·ter·in (am-i-nop′ter-in). Aminopterina; um antagonista do ácido fólico originalmente empregado no tratamento da leucemia aguda e em outras doenças neoplásicas.

6-ami·no·pu·rine (ă-mē′nō-pūr′ēn). 6-Aminopurina. SIN adenine.

4-ami·no·pyr·i·dine (am-i-nō-pir′i-dēn). 4-Aminopiridina; um antagonista do bloqueio neuromuscular não-despolarizante; desprovido de efeitos colaterais muscarínicos, mas associado à estimulação do sistema nervoso central.

ami·no·py·rine (am′i-nō-pī′rēn). Aminopirina; originalmente muito usada como antitérmico e analgésico em reumatismo, neurite e resfriado; pode provocar leucocitopenia; empregada para medir a água corporal total. SIN amidopyrine, aminophenazone, dipyrine.

amin·o·rex (ă-min′ō-reks). Aminorex; um simpaticomimético supressor do apetite.

p-**ami·no·sal·i·cyl·ic ac·id (PAS, PASA)** (am′i-nō-sal-i-sil′ik). Ácido *p*-aminossalicílico; um agente bacteriostático contra os bacilos da tuberculose, usado como um agente de segunda linha; os sais de potássio, sódio e cálcio possuem o mesmo uso.

ami·no·ter·mi·nal (ă-mē′nō-ter′min-ăl). Aminoterminal; o grupamento α-NH_2 ou o resíduo aminoacil que o contém em uma extremidade de um peptídeo ou proteína (geralmente à esquerda, como se escreve). SIN NH_2-terminal.

ami·no·trans·fer·as·es (ă-mē′nō-trans′fer-ās-ez) [EC 2.6.1.x]. Aminotransferases; enzimas que transferem os grupamentos amino entre um aminoácido para (em geral) um 2-cetoácido; p.ex., L-alanina e 2-cetoglutarato. Com freqüência, o aminoácido é um α-aminoácido. SIN transaminases.

ami·no·tri·a·zole (am′i-nō-trī′ā-zol). Aminotriazol; herbicida efetivo que também possui alguma atividade antitireóidea. SIN amitrole.

ami·no·tri·pep·tid·ase (ă-mē′nō-tri-pep′tă-dās). Aminotripeptidase; uma peptidase intestinal que age sobre os tripeptídeos, liberando um aminoácido e um dipeptídeo.

am·i·nu·ria (am-i-noo′rē-ă). Aminúria; excreção de aminas na urina. [amine + G. *ouron*, urina]

ami·o·da·rone hy·dro·chlo·ride (ă-mē′ō-dă-rōn). Cloridrato de amiodarona; agente antiarrítmico empregado no controle das arritmias ventriculares e supraventriculares. Pode provocar intoxicação pulmonar significante e distinta.

am·i·thi·o·zone (am-i-thī′ō-zōn). Amitiozona; um agente leprostático. SIN thiacetazone.

ami·to·sis (am-i-tō′sis). Amitose; divisão direta do núcleo e da célula, sem as complicadas alterações no núcleo que acontecem no processo habitual de reprodução celular. SIN direct nuclear division, Remak nuclear division. [G. *a*-priv. + mitosis]

ami·tot·ic (am-i-tot′ik). Amitótico; relativo a, ou caracterizado por, amitose.

am·i·trip·ty·line hy·dro·chlo·ride (am-i-trip′ti-lēn). Cloridrato de amitriptilina; relacionado, química e farmacologicamente, ao cloridrato de imipramina; um agente antidepressivo com propriedades tranqüilizantes brandas, usado no tratamento da depressão mental e na fase depressiva dos estados maníaco-depressivos; por vezes empregado no tratamento de distúrbios do sono e em síndromes álgicas neurogênicas.

am·i·trole (am′i-trōl). Amitrol. SIN aminotriazole.

am·lo·dip·ine (am-lō′dĭ-pēn). Amlodipina. Agente bloqueador dos canais de cálcio da série diidropiridínica; pertence à mesma classe de agentes que a nifedipina.

am·me·ter (am) (am′mē-ter). Amperômetro; um instrumento para medir a força da corrente elétrica em amperes.

Ammon, Friedrich A. von, oftalmologista e patologista alemão, 1799–1861. VER A. *fissure, prominence*.

Ammon, nome grego do deus egípcio Amun. VER A. *horn*.

am·mo·ne·mia, am·mo·ni·e·mia (am-ō-nē′mē-ă). Amonemia; a presença de amônia ou de alguns de seus compostos no sangue, creditada como sendo formada a partir da decomposição da uréia; geralmente resulta em tempe-

ammonemia, ammoniemia / **amniorrhexis**

ratura subnormal, pulso fraco, sinais e sintomas gastroentéricos e coma. SIN hyperammonemia. [ammonia + G. *haima*, sangue]

am·mo·nia (ă-mō′nē-ă). Amônia; um gás volátil e incolor, NH_3, muito solúvel em água, capaz de formar a base fraca $NH_4^+OH^-$, que se combina a ácidos para formar compostos amônio. [do L. *sal ammoniacus*, sal de Amen (G. *Ammōn*), obtido próximo a um templo de Amen na Líbia]

am·mo·ni·ac (ă-mō′nē-ak). Amoníaca; goma resina de uma planta do oeste da Ásia, *Dorema ammoniacum* (família Umbelliferae); usada internamente como estimulante e expectorante e, externamente, como um emplastro contra-irritante.

am·mo·ni·a·cal (ă-mō-nī′ă-kl). Amoniacal; relativo à amônia.

am·mo·nia-ly·as·es. Amônia liases; enzimas que removem a amônia ou um aminocomposto de forma não-hidrolítica (daí liases, classe EC 4), por ruptura de uma ligação C–N, deixando uma dupla ligação (subgrupo EC 4.3); p.ex., aspartato amônia-liase (aspartase).

am·mo·ni·at·ed (ă-mō′nē-āt-ed). Amoniacado; que contém amônia ou se combina à amônia.

ammonio-. Forma combinante indicando um grupamento amônio; p.ex., trimetilamonioetanol (colina).

am·mo·ni·um (ă-mō′nē-ŭm). Amônio; o íon NH_4^+, formado por combinação de NH_3 e H^+ (o valor de pK_a é de 9,24); comporta-se como um metal univalente na formação dos compostos de amônio.

a. benzoate, benzoato de a.; foi utilizado como estimulante, diurético, anti-séptico urinário e anti-reumático.

a. carbonate, carbonato de a.; $(NH_4)_2CO_3$; estimulante cardíaco e respiratório e expectorante carminativo.

a. chloride, cloreto de a.; NH_4Cl; estimulante expectorante e colagogo; usado para aliviar a alcalose e promover a excreção de chumbo; um acidificante urinário. SIN sal ammoniac.

dibasic a. phosphate, fosfato dibásico de a.; $(NH_4)_2HPO_4$; usado em material refratário ao fogo, no fermento em pó e como anti-reumático.

a. ferric sulfate, sulfato férrico de a. SIN *ferric* ammonium sulfate.

a. ichthosulfonate, ictossulfonato de a. SIN ichthammol.

a. iodide, iodeto de a.; NH_4I; expectorante.

a. mandelate, mandelato de a.; sal de amônio do ácido mandélico; anti-séptico urinário.

a. molybdate, molibdato de a.; usado em microscopia eletrônica como corante negativo, bem como reagente para alcalóides e outras substâncias.

monobasic a. phosphate, fosfato monobásico de a.; usado no fermento em pó.

a. nitrate, nitrato de a.; usado na produção do gás óxido nitroso, em misturas congelantes, palitos de fósforo e fertilizantes; também usado em medicina veterinária.

am·mo·ni·u·ria (ă-mō-nē-ū′rē-ă). Amoniúria; excreção de urina que contém uma quantidade excessiva de amônia. SIN ammoniacal urine. [ammonia + G. *ouron*, urina]

am·mo·nol·y·sis (ă-mō-nol′i-sis). Amoniólise; a clivagem de uma ligação química com a adição de elementos da amônia (NH_2 e H) no ponto de ruptura. [ammonia + G. *lysis*, dissolução]

am·mo·no·tel·ia (ă-mōn-ō-tēl′-e-ă). Amonotelia; o processo ou tipo de excreção de nitrogênio em que a amônia e os íons amônio constituem a forma básica de excreção de nitrogênio por um organismo. [ammonia + G. *telos*, final, resultado, + -ia]

am·mo·no·tel·ic (ă-mōn-ō-tēl′ik). Amonotélico; que possui a propriedade do amonotelismo.

am·mo·no·tel·ism (ă-mōn-ō-tēl′izm). Amonotelismo; a excreção de amônia e de íons amônio. Cf. ammonotelia.

am·ne·sia (am-nē′zē-ă). Amnésia; um distúrbio na memória de informações armazenadas na memória remota, em contraste com a memória imediata, manifestada por incapacidade total ou parcial de relembrar experiências pregressas. [G. *amnēsia*, esquecimento]

anterograde a., a. anterógrada; a. em relação aos eventos que ocorrem depois do traumatismo ou doença que causou a condição.

emotional a., a. emocional; etiologia psicológica do esquecimento ou repressão da emoção.

lacunar a., localized a., a. lacunar, a. localizada; a. em relação a eventos isolados.

posthypnotic a., a. pós-hipnótica; depois de um estado hipnótico, o esquecimento seletivo de eventos que ocorreram durante a hipnose ou das informações armazenadas na memória remota, como o próprio nome, endereço e nomes de parentes.

retrograde a., a. retrógrada; a a. em relação aos eventos que ocorreram antes do traumatismo ou doença que provocou a condição.

transient global a., a. global transitória; um distúrbio de memória, observado na meia-idade e em pessoas idosas, caracterizado por um episódio de a. e confusão que persiste por várias horas; durante o episódio, o paciente apresenta um defeito de memória para eventos presentes e pregressos recentes, mas está plenamente ativo, orientado, capaz de atividade intelectual de alto nível e apresenta um exame neurológico normal. Tipicamente, esses episódios amnésicos ocorrem de forma espontânea, e a maioria dos pacientes experimenta apenas um episódio; de etiologia incerta — provavelmente isquêmica, mas não decorrente de aterosclerose.

traumatic a., a. traumática; a perda ou o transtorno da memória após uma agressão ou lesão do cérebro do tipo que acompanha um traumatismo craniano ou pelo uso excessivo de álcool, ou após a cessação da ingestão de álcool ou de outras substâncias psicoativas; ou a perda ou transtorno da memória do tipo observado na histeria e em outras formas de transtornos dissociativos.

am·ne·si·ac (am-nē′sē-ak). Amnésico; aquele que sofre de amnésia.

am·ne·sic (am-nē′sik). Amnésico; relativo a, ou caracterizado por, amnésia. SIN amnestic (1).

am·nes·tic (am-nes′tik). **1.** Amnésico. SIN amnesic. **2.** Amnéstico; um agente que causa amnésia.

amnio-. Âmnio-. [G. *amnion*]

am·ni·o·cele (am′-nē-ō-sēl). Amniocele; onfalocele. VER omphalocele.

am·ni·o·cen·te·sis (am′nē-ō-sen-tē′sis). Amniocentese; aspiração transabdominal de líquido a partir do saco amniótico. [amnio- + G. *kentēsis*, punção]

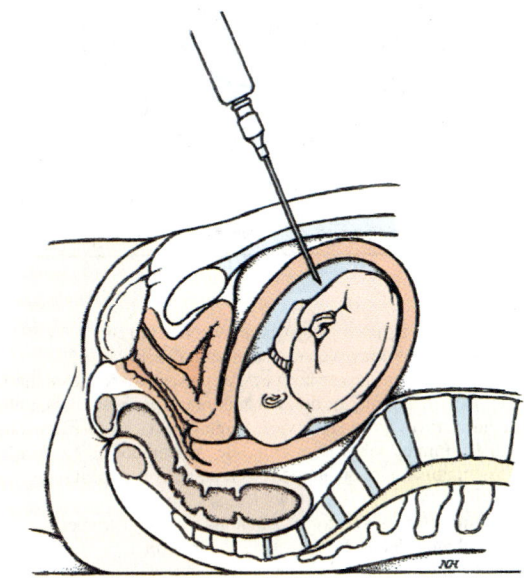

amniocentese

am·ni·o·cho·ri·al, am·ni·o·cho·ri·on·ic (am′nē-ō-kōr′e-ăl, -kōr-ē-on′ik). Amniocorial; amniocoriônico; relativo ao âmnio e ao cório.

am·ni·o·gen·e·sis (am′nē-ō-jen′e-sis). Amniogênese; formação do âmnio. [amnio- + G. *genesis*, produção]

am·ni·og·ra·phy (am-nē-og′ră-fē). Amniografia; radiografia do saco amniótico depois da injeção de solução radiopaca hidrossolúvel no saco, a qual delineia o cordão umbilical, a placenta e os tecidos moles do corpo fetal; uma técnica obsoleta. VER TAMBÉM fetography. [amnio- + G. *graphō*, escrever]

am·ni·o-hook (am′nē-ō-hook′). Instrumento destinado a fazer um orifício no saco amniótico sem lesionar o feto.

amnioinfusion (am′nē-ō-in-fyu′zhun). Amnioinfusão; a infusão de soro fisiológico aquecido através de um cateter intra-uterino durante o trabalho de parto para o comprometimento do cordão umbilical decorrente do baixo volume de líquido amniótico ou para o mecônio espesso no trabalho de parto.

am·ni·o·ma (am-nē-ō′mă). Amnioma; massa achatada e larga sobre a pele resultante da aderência pré-natal do âmnio. [amnio- + G. *-oma*, tumor]

am·ni·on (am′nē-on). Âmnio; a membrana extra-embrionária mais interna que reveste o embrião no útero e que contém o líquido amniótico; consiste em uma camada embrionária interna, com seu componente ectodérmico, e um componente mesodérmico somático externo; nos estágios mais avançados da gestação, o âmnio se expande, entrando em contato com a parede interna da vesícula coriônica e fundindo-se parcialmente a ela; derivado das células trofoblásticas. SIN amnionic sac. [G. a membrana ao redor do feto, de *amnios*, carneiro]

a. nodo'sum, a. nodoso; nódulos no a. que consistem em epitélio escamoso estratificado típico. SIN squamous metaplasia of amnion.

am·ni·on·ic (am-nē-on′ik). Amniônico; relativo ao âmnio. SIN amniotic.

am·ni·o·ni·tis (am′nē-ō-nī′tis). Amnionite; inflamação resultante de infecção do saco amniótico, que, por sua vez, resulta, em geral, da ruptura prematura das membranas (uma condição freqüentemente associada a infecção neonatal). [amnion + G. *-itis*, inflamação]

am·ni·or·rhea (am-nē-ō-rē′ă). Amnorréia; saída de líquido amniótico. [amnio- + G. *rhoia*, fluxo]

am·ni·or·rhex·is (am-nē-ō-rek′sis). Amniorrexe; ruptura da membrana amniótica. [amnio- + G. *rhēxis*, ruptura]

amnioscope   54   amphibolic

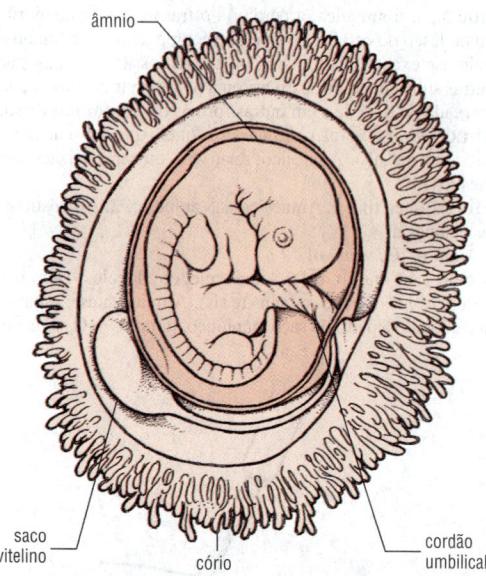

âmnio e estruturas correlatas: mostrando o embrião de 5 semanas

am·ni·o·scope (am'nē-ō-skōp). Amnioscópio; um endoscópio para estudar o líquido amniótico através do saco amniótico intacto.

am·ni·os·co·py (am-nē-os'kō-pē). Amnioscopia; exame do líquido amniótico, na parte mais inferior do saco amniótico, por meio de um endoscópio introduzido através do canal cervical. [amnio- + G. *skopeō*, visualizar]

Am·ni·o·ta (am'nē-ō'ta). Um grupo de vertebrados cujos embriões estão envoltos em um âmnio; inclui todos os répteis, aves e mamíferos.

am·ni·ot·ic (am-nē-ot'ik). Amniótico. SIN amnionic.

am·ni·o·tome (am'nē-ō-tōm). Amniotomo; um instrumento para puncionar as membranas fetais. [amnio- + G. *tomē*, cortar]

am·ni·ot·o·my (am-nē-ot'ō-mē). Amniotomia; ruptura artificial das membranas fetais como um meio de induzir ou acelerar o trabalho de parto.

am·o·bar·bi·tal (am-ō-bar'bi-tahl). Amobarbital; um depressor do sistema nervoso central com uma duração de ação intermediária; também empregado como o sal sódico.

A-mode. Na ultra-sonografia diagnóstica, uma apresentação unidimensional de uma onda sonora refletida, na qual a amplitude (A) do eco é exibida ao longo do eixo vertical e o retardo (profundidade) do eco ao longo do eixo horizontal; as informações do eco resultam das interfaces de tecido ao longo de uma única linha na direção do feixe sonoro.

am·o·di·a·quine hy·dro·chlo·ride (am-ō-dī'a-kwīn). Cloridrato de amodiaquina; medicamento antimalárico, também empregado no tratamento da hepatite amebiana; as doses grandes podem resultar em sialorréia, náuseas, vômitos, diarréia, insônia, palpitações, espasticidade e, possivelmente, convulsões.

amoeb-. Ameba, *Amoeba*.

Amoe·ba (ă-mē'bă). Um gênero de protozoários formadores de pseudópodos, lobosos e sem envoltório, da classe Sarcodina (ou Rhizopoda), que são habitantes abundantes do solo, especialmente quando rico em resíduos orgânicos, e também comumente encontrados como parasitas. Os parasitas amebianos típicos dos seres humanos são atualmente colocados nos gêneros *Entamoeba*, *Endolimax* e *Iodamoeba*. VER TAMBÉM *Naegleria*. [L. mod. de G. *amoibē*, alteração]

A. bucca'lis, denominação antiga de *Entamoeba gingivalis*.
A. co'li, nome antigo e incorreto para *Entamoeba coli*.
A. denta'lis, denominação antiga de *Entamoeba gingivalis*.
A. dysenter'iae, nome antigo e incorreto para *Entamoeba histolytica*.
A. histolyt'ica, nome antigo e incorreto para *Entamoeba histolytica*.
A. pro'teus, uma espécie não-parasitária, abundante, notável pelo número e formas variadas de seus pseudópodos.

amoebapore (ă-mē'ba-pōr). Amebaporo; um peptídeo ativo, liberado pela *Entamoeba histolytica*, que pode inserir canais iônicos nos lipossomas e que possui atividades citolíticas e bactericidas. [amoeba + G. *poros*, passagem]

Amoe·bo·tae·nia (ă-mē'bō-tē'nē-ă). Um gênero de tênias do intestino delgado de aves, que raramente possui mais de 30 segmentos. *A. cuneata* (*A. sphenoides*) é uma espécie comum nas aves domésticas; seu cisticercóide é desenvolvido em minhocas. [amoeb- + L. de G. *tainia*, faixa, fita, uma tênia]

amok (ă-mok'). Amoque, amouco. **1.** Um distúrbio mental ligado à cultura, originalmente observado na Malaia, no qual a pessoa se torna perigosamente maníaca ("amoque de corrida"). **2.** Coloquialismo que indica o comportamento maníaco, selvagem ou descontrolado que ameaça lesionar os outros. SIN amuck. [malaio, *amoq*, engajado na batalha]

amorph (ā'morf). Alelo amorfo; um alelo que não possui um produto fenotipicamente reconhecido e, portanto, sua existência só pode ser inferida a partir de evidências moleculares, dependendo da sutileza dos meios de detecção disponíveis. SIN silent allele. [G. *a-* neg + *morphē*, forma, formato]

amor·phag·no·sia (ă-mor-fag-nō'sē-ă). Amorfagnosia; incapacidade de reconhecer o tamanho e a forma dos objetos. [G. *a-* priv. + *morphē*, forma, + *gnōsis*, reconhecimento]

amor·phia, amor·phism (ă-mōr'fē-ă, -fizm). Amorfia, amorfismo; condição de ser amorfo (1). [G. *a-* priv. + *morphē*, forma]

amor·pho·syn·the·sis (ă-mōr'fō-sin'thē-sis). Amorfossíntese; transtorno de reconhecimento do lado direito do corpo nas relações espaciais, provocado por uma lesão do lobo parietal esquerdo. [G. *a-* priv. + *morphē*, forma, + synthesis]

amor·phous (ă-mōr'fŭs). Amorfo. **1.** Sem forma definida ou diferenciação visível na estrutura. **2.** Não cristalizado.

amor·phus (ă-mōr'fŭs). Amorfo; um feto malformado com cabeça, membros e coração rudimentares. [G. *ā-* priv. + *morphē*, forma, formato]

amox·a·pine (ă-mok'să-pēn). Amoxapina; um medicamento antidepressivo/antipsicótico; a *overdose* pode produzir convulsões.

amox·i·cil·lin (ă-mok-si-sil'in). Amoxicilina; uma penicilina semi-sintética com um espectro antimicrobiano semelhante ao da ampicilina.

AMP Abreviatura para *adenosine* monophosphate (monofosfato de adenosina); especificamente, o 5'-monofosfato, exceto quando modificado por um prefixo numérico. VER adenylic acid.

AMP de·am·i·nase. AMP desaminase; uma enzima que hidrolisa o ácido adenílico em ácido inosínico e NH_3. A deficiência de AMP d. nos músculos pode levar a fadiga excessiva após o exercício. SIN adenylic acid deaminase.

am·per·age (am'pēr-ij). Amperagem; intensidade de uma corrente elétrica. VER ampere.

Ampère, André-Marie, físico francês, 1775–1836. VER ampere; statampere; A. postulate.

am·pere (A) (am-pēr). Ampere; a unidade prática da corrente elétrica; o a. absoluto, prático, foi originalmente definido como tendo o valor de 1/10 da unidade eletromagnética (ver abampere e coulomb). As definições atuais são: **1.** A unidade prática da corrente elétrica; o a. absoluto, prático, foi originalmente definido como possuindo o valor de 1/10 da unidade eletromagnética (ver abampere e coulomb). **2.** Definição legal: a corrente que, fluindo durante 1 segundo, depositará 1,118 mg de prata a partir da solução de nitrato de prata. **3.** Definição científica (SI): a corrente que, quando mantida em dois condutores retos paralelos de comprimento infinito e de cortes transversais circulares desprezíveis e colocados a uma distância de 1 m entre si em um vácuo, produz entre eles a força de 2×10^{-7} N/m de comprimento. [A. *Ampère*]

am·per·om·e·try (am-pē-rom'ē-trē). Amperimetria, amperometria; a determinação da concentração de uma substância por mensuração da corrente gerada em uma reação química adequada.

amph-. VER amphi-, ampho-.

am·phe·clex·is (am-fē-klek'-sis). Anficlexe; seleção sexual recíproca, isto é, tanto masculina quanto feminina. [G. *amphi*, de dois lados, + *eklexis*, seleção]

am·phet·a·mine (am-fet'ă-mēn). Anfetamina; intimamente relacionado, em sua estrutura e ação, com a efedrina e outras aminas simpatomiméticas. Uma substância psicoestimulante que pode gerar vício.

a. (4-chlorophenoxy)acetate, (4-clorofenoxi)acetato de a.; possui as mesmas ações e usos que o sulfato de a.
a. phosphate, fosfato de a.; possui as mesmas ações e usos que o sulfato de a.
a. sulfate, sulfato de a.; exerce menor efeito vasopressor, cardíaco e brônquico que a efedrina, porém possui um maior efeito estimulador do sistema nervoso central, diminuindo a sensação de fadiga; usado no tratamento da narcolepsia e em determinados tipos de paralisia agitante, e para diminuir o apetite (temporariamente, 1–2 semanas) na obesidade.

***d*-am·phet·a·mine phos·phate.** Fosfato de *d*-anfetamina. SIN dextroamphetamine phosphate.

***d*-am·phet·a·mine sul·fate.** Sulfato de *d*-anfetamina. SIN dextroamphetamine sulfate.

amphi-. Forma combinante que significa em ambos os lados, que circunda, duplo; corresponde ao L. *ambi-*. [G. *amphi, amphi-*, em ambos os lados, a cerca de, em volta de]

am·phi·ar·thro·di·al (am'fi-ar-thrō'dē-ăl). Anfiartrodial; relativo a uma sínfise (1) (anfiartrose).

am·phi·ar·thro·sis (am'fi-ar-thrō'sis). Anfiartrose. SIN symphysis (1). [amphi- + G. *arthrōsis*, articulação]

am·phi·as·ter (am-fi-as'ter). Anfiáster; uma figura de duas estrelas formada por duas astrosferas e suas fibras fusiformes conectantes durante a mitose. SIN diaster. [amphi- + G. *astēr*, estrela]

am·phi·bol·ic (am'fi-bol'ik). Anfibólico; referente às reações ou vias biológicas que atuam tanto na biossíntese como na degradação (isto é, anabolismo e catabolismo). [amphi- + metabolic]

am·phi·ce·lous (am-fi-sē'lŭs). Anficelo, anficélico; côncavo dos dois lados, como o corpo de uma vértebra de um peixe. [amphi- + G. *koilos,* oco]

am·phi·cen·tric (am-fi-sen'trik). Anficêntrico; com um centro em ambas as extremidades, diz-se de uma rede admirável que começa por um vaso que se fragmenta em inúmeros ramos e termina quando os ramos se unem novamente para formar o mesmo vaso. [amphi- + G. *kentron,* centro]

am·phi·chro·ic (am-fi-krō'ik). Anficróico. SIN amphichromatic.

am·phi·chro·mat·ic (am'fi-krō-mat'ik). Anficromático; que possui a propriedade de exibir qualquer uma de duas cores; p.ex., tornassol, um pigmento a. que é vermelho em ácidos e azul em alcalinos. SIN amphichroic. [amphi- + G. *chrōma,* cor]

am·phi·cyte (am'fi-sīt). Anficito; uma das células localizadas ao redor dos corpos dos neurônios dos gânglios simpáticos e cerebroespinais. SIN capsule cell. [amphi- + G. *kytos,* célula]

am·phid (am'fid). Anfídio; no sistema nervoso dos nematódeos, um par de minúsculos órgãos receptores, dispostos lateralmente, na região cefálica ou cervical. [amphi- + -id]

am·phi·dip·loid (am'fi-dip'loid). Anfidiplóide; que possui um conjunto completo de cromossomas diplóides a partir de cada cepa original. [*amphi* + diploid]

am·phi·kar·y·on (am'fē-kar'ē-on). Anficário; um núcleo diplóide que contém dois conjuntos haplóides de cromossomas. [amphi- + G. *karyon,* núcleo]

am·phi·leu·ke·mic (am'fi-loo-kē'mik). Anfileucêmico; indica uma condição leucêmica que corresponde, em grau, às alterações no órgão ou tecido.

Am·phim·er·us (am-fim'er-ŭs). Um gênero de trematódeos opistorquídeos encontrados nos ductos biliares de mamíferos, aves e répteis; provavelmente transmitido pelo peixe. [amphi- + G. *meros,* segmento]

am·phi·mi·crobe (am'fi-mī'krōb). Anfimicróbio; um microrganismo que é aeróbico ou anaeróbico, de acordo com o ambiente.

am·phi·mic·tic (am'fi-mik'tik). Anfimítico; a capacidade de cruzar livremente e produzir uma prole híbrida fértil. [amphi + G. *miktos,* unido, cruzado, de *mignumi,* misturar, + -ia]

am·phi·mix·is (am'fi-mik'sis). Anfimixia. **1.** União das cromatinas paterna e materna depois da impregnação do ovo. **2.** Em psicanálise, uma combinação de erotização genital e anal. [amphi- + G. *mixis,* mistura]

am·phi·nu·cle·o·lus (am'fi-noo-klē'ō-lŭs). Anfinucléolo; um nucléolo duplo que possui tanto componentes basofílicos como oxifílicos. [amphi- + L. *nucleolus,* dim. de *nucleus,* núcleo]

am·phi·ons (am'fi-ons). Íons dipolares. SIN dipolar *ions,* em *ion.*

Am·phi·ox·us (am-fē-ok'sŭs). Anfioxo; um gênero de pequenos organismos cordados, translúcidos, semelhantes a peixes, encontrados nas águas quentes do mar. Os membros são estruturalmente similares aos vertebrados ao possuir notocórdio, guelras, trato digestivo e cordão nervoso, mas não têm barbatanas pareadas, vértebras, costelas ou crânio. [amphi- + G. *oxys,* afiado]

am·phi·path·ic (am-fē-path'ik). Anfipático; indica uma molécula, como a de detergentes ou agentes umedecedores, que contém grupamentos com propriedades caracteristicamente distintas, p.ex., propriedades hidrofílicas assim como hidrofóbicas. SIN amphiphilic, amphiphobic. [amphi- + G. *pathos,* sensação]

am·phi·phil·ic (am-fē-fil'ik). Anfifílico. SIN amphipathic. [amphi- + G. *philos,* amigo]

am·phi·pho·bic (am-fē-fōb'ik). Anfifóbico. SIN amphipathic. [amphi- + G. *phobos,* medo]

am·phis·tome (am-fis'tōm). Anfístoma; um nome comum para qualquer trematódeo do gênero *Paramphistomum.* [amphi- + G. *stoma,* boca]

am·phit·ri·chate, am·phit·ri·chous (am-fit'ri-kāt, am-fit'ri-kŭs). Anfítrico; que possui um flagelo ou flagelos nas duas extremidades de uma célula microbiana; indica determinados microrganismos. [amphi- G. *thrix,* cabelo]

am·phit·y·py (am-fit'i-pē). Anfitipia; exibição das propriedades características de dois tipos.

am·phix·en·o·sis (am-fiks-en-ō'sis). Anfixenose; uma zoonose mantida na natureza pelos seres humanos e animais inferiores, p.ex., determinadas estafilococoses. Cf. anthropozoonosis, zooanthroponosis. [amphi- + G. *xenos,* estranho, + G. *-osis,* condição]

♻ **ampho-.** Forma combinante que significa ambos os lados, que circunda, duplo. [G. *amphō,* ambos]

am·pho·chro·mat·o·phil, am·pho·chro·mat·o·phile (am'fō-krō-mat'ō-fil, -ō-fīl). Anficromatófilo. SIN amphophil (2).

am·pho·chro·mo·phil, am·pho·chro·mo·phile (am-fō-krō'mō-fil, -fīl). Anficromófilo. SIN amphophil. [ampho- + G. *chroma,* cor + *philos,* amigo]

am·pho·cyte (am'fō-sīt). Anfócito. SIN amphophil (2).

am·pho·lyte (am'fō-līt). Anfolito. SIN amphoteric *electrolyte.*

am·pho·my·cin (am-fō-mī'sin). Anfomicina; uma substância antibiótica produzida pelo *Streptomyces canus;* usada topicamente para infecções cutâneas.

am·pho·phil, am·pho·phile (am'fō-fil, -fīl). Anfófilo. **1.** Que possui afinidade por corantes ácidos e básicos. SIN amphophilic, amphophilous. **2.** Uma célula que se cora prontamente com corantes ácidos ou básicos. SIN amphochromatophil, amphochromatophile, amphocyte. SIN amphochromophil, amphochromophile. [ampho- + G. *philos,* amigo]

am·pho·phil·ic, am·phoph·i·lous (am-fō-fil'ik, am-fof'i-lŭs). Anfofílico. SIN amphophil (1).

am·phor·ic (am-fōr'ik). Anfórico; que indica o som detectado à percussão e ausculta, assemelhando-se ao ruído obtido ao soprar através da boca de uma garrafa. [G. *amphora,* uma jarra]

am·pho·ril·o·quy (am-fō-ril'ō-kwē). Anforilóquia; presença de voz anfórica. [G. *amphora,* uma jarra, + *loquor,* falar]

am·phor·oph·o·ny (am-fō-rof'ō-nē). Anforofonia. SIN amphoric *voice.* [G. *amphora,* uma jarra, + *phōnē,* voz]

am·pho·ter·ic (am-fō-tār'ik). Anfotérico, anfótero; que possui duas características opostas, principalmente que tem a capacidade de reagir como um ácido ou como uma base; p.ex. $Al(OH)_3 \equiv H_3AlO_3$ ou um aminoácido. [G. *amphoteroi* (pl.), ambos, de *amphō,* ambos]

am·pho·ter·i·cin, am·pho·ter·i·cin B (am-fō-tār'i-sin). Anfotericina, anfotericina B; $C_{46}H_{73}NO_{20}$; um antibiótico poliênico anfotérico preparado a partir do *Streptomyces nodosus* e disponível como o complexo desoxicolato sódico; também um agente antifúngico nefrotóxico empregado, com freqüência, no tratamento de micoses sistêmicas.

am·pi·cil·lin (am-pi-si'lin). Ampicilina; uma penicilina semi-sintética ácido-estável derivada do ácido 6-aminopenicilânico; possui um espectro maior de ação antimicrobiana que a penicilina G, inibe o crescimento de bactérias Gram-positivas e Gram-negativas e não é resistente a penicilinase; também disponível como a. sódica e a. triidratada. SIN D(-)-α-aminobenzylpenicillin.

ampl. Abreviatura do L. *amplus,* grande.

am·plex·us (am-plek'sŭs). Amplexo; o pareamento do macho e da fêmea no momento em que os ovos e o esperma são liberados simultaneamente nas espécies, como as rãs, em que a fertilização ocorre externamente. [L. um abraço, de *amplector,* pp. *-plexus,* enlaçar]

am·pli·fi·ca·tion (am'pli-fi-kā'shŭn). Ampliação, amplificação; o processo de tornar maior, como no aumento de um estímulo auditivo ou visual para estimular sua percepção. [L. *amplificatio,* um aumento]

genetic a., a. genética; um processo para produzir um aumento no material genético pertinente, principalmente para aumentar a proporção do DNA do plasmídio em relação ao DNA bacteriano. Inclui a produção de cópias extracromossomiais dos genes para o ARN. Esse processo é usualmente observado nas células malignas em seres humanos.

linear a., a. linear; um circuito de prótese auditiva em que todas as freqüências recebem ampliação equivalente.

am·pli·fi·er. Amplificador, ampliador. **1.** Um aparelho que aumenta a ampliação de um microscópio. **2.** Um aparelho eletrônico que aumenta a intensidade dos sinais de entrada.

image amplifier, ampliador de imagem; um aparelho que converte uma imagem fluoroscópica de baixo nível de energia em uma que possa ser observada a olho nu em um ambiente iluminado; geralmente consiste em um amplificador luminoso eletrônico ligado a um tubo de televisão. SIN image intensifier.

am·pli·tude (am'pli-tood). Amplitude; grandeza; extensão; largura ou faixa. [L. *amplitudo,* de *amplus,* grande]

a. of pulse, a. de pulso. VER average pulse *magnitude,* peak *magnitude.*

am·poule (am'pul). Ampola. VER ampule.

am·pro·tro·pine phos·phate (am'prō-trō'pēn). Fosfato de amprotropina; um antiespasmódico com ação similar à atropina.

am·pule, am·pul (am'pool). Ampola; um recipiente hermeticamente selado, geralmente feito de vidro, que contém uma solução medicinal estéril ou pó para fazer uma solução a ser utilizada para injeção subcutânea, intramuscular ou intravenosa. SIN ampoule. [L. *ampulla*]

am·pul·la, gen. e pl. **am·pul·lae** (am-pul'lă, -ē) [TA]. Ampola; uma dilatação sacular de um canal ou ducto. [L. um frasco com duas alças]

biliaropancreatic a., a. hepatopancreática *termo oficial alternativo para hepatopancreatic a.

a. biliaropancreatica, a. hepatopancreática *termo oficial alternativo para hepatopancreatic a.

bony ampullae of semicircular canals [TA], ampolas ósseas dos canais semicirculares; dilatação circunscrita de uma extremidade em cada um dos três canais semicirculares ósseos, anterior, posterior e lateral; cada uma contém uma a. semimembranosa dos canais semicirculares. SIN ampullae osseae canalium semicircularium [TA], osseae a.

a. canalic'uli lacrima'lis [TA], a. do canalículo lacrimal. SIN a. of lacrimal canaliculus.

a. chy'li, cisterna do quilo. SIN *cisterna* chyli.

a. of ductus deferens [TA], a. do ducto deferente; a dilatação do ducto deferente na base da bexiga, onde ele se aproxima de seu equivalente contralateral, exatamente antes de sua reunião com o canal da vesícula seminal para formar o canal ejaculatório. SIN a. ductus deferentis [TA], Henle a.

ampulla   56   **amputation**

a. duc'tus deferen'tis [TA], a. do ducto deferente. SIN a. of ductus deferens.
a. duc'tus lacrima'lis, termo incorreto para a a. do canalículo lacrimal.
duodenal a., (1) a. do duodeno. SIN a. of duodenum; **(2)** a. hepatopancreática. SIN hepatopancreatic a.
a. duode'ni [TA], a. do duodeno. SIN a. of duodenum.
a. of duodenum [TA], a. do duodeno; a porção dilatada da parte superior do duodeno. VER TAMBÉM duodenal *cap.* SIN a. duodeni [TA], bulbus duodeni*, duodenal a. (1).
a. of gallbladder, a. da vesícula biliar. SIN Hartmann *pouch.*
Henle a., a. de Henle, a. do ducto deferente. SIN a. of ductus deferens.
hepatopancreatic a. [TA], a. hepatopancreática; a dilatação dentro da principal papila duodenal que normalmente recebe tanto o ducto biliar (comum) como o ducto pancreático principal. SIN a. hepatopancreatica [TA], a. biliaropancreatica*, biliaropancreatic a.*, a. of Vater, duodenal a. (2).
a. hepat'opancreat'ica [TA], a. hepatopancreática. SIN hepatopancreatic a.
a. of lacrimal canaliculus [TA], a. do canalículo lacrimal; uma discreta dilatação no ângulo do canalículo lacrimal imediatamente após o ponto lacrimal. SIN a. canaliculi lacrimalis [TA].
a. lactif'era, a. lactífera. SIN lactiferous *sinus.*
lactiferous a., a. lactífera. SIN lactiferous *sinus.*
a. of lactiferous duct, a. do ducto lactífero. SIN lactiferous *sinus.*
a. membrana'cea, pl. **ampullae membrana'ceae ductuum semicircularium** [TA], a. membranácea. SIN membranous ampullae of the semicircular ducts.
membranous a., a. membranácea. SIN membranous ampullae of the semicircular ducts.
membranous ampullae of the semicircular ducts [TA], ampolas membranáceas dos canais semicirculares; uma dilatação quase esférica de uma extremidade de cada um dos três canais semicirculares, anterior, posterior e lateral, onde eles se conectam com o utrículo. Cada uma contém uma crista neuroepitelial ampular. SIN a. membranacea [TA], membranous a.
a. of milk duct, a. do ducto lactífero. SIN lactiferous *sinus.*
ampullae osseae canalium semicircularium [TA], a. ósseas dos canais semicirculares; SIN bony ampullae of semicircular canals.
osseous a., a. óssea. SIN bony ampullae of semicircular canals.
phrenic a., a. frênica; uma dilatação fisiológica localizada do esôfago distal, comumente demonstrada por esofagografia.
rectal a. [TA], a. do reto; uma porção dilatada do reto exatamente acima do diafragma pélvico e proximal ao canal anal. SIN a. recti [TA], a. of rectum.
a. rec'ti [TA], a. do reto. SIN rectal a.
a. of rectum, a. do reto. SIN rectal a.
Thoma a., a. de Thoma; uma dilatação do capilar arterial além da artéria interlobular do baço.
a. tu'bae uteri'nae [TA], a. da tuba uterina. SIN a. of uterine tube.
a. of uterine tube [TA], a. da tuba uterina; a parte larga da tuba uterina (de Falópio) próxima à extremidade fimbriada; possui uma mucosa pregueada de maneira complexa com um epitélio colunar composto, em sua maioria, por células ciliadas, entre as quais estão células secretoras. SIN a. tubae uterinae [TA].
a. of Vater, a. de Vater, a. hepatopancreática. SIN hepatopancreatic a.
am·pul·lar (am-pul´ăr). Ampular; relativo, em qualquer sentido, a uma ampola.
am·pul·li·tis (am-pul-lī´tis). Ampulite; inflamação de qualquer ampola, especialmente da extremidade dilatada do canal deferente ou da ampola de Vater. [ampulla + G. *itis,* inflamação]
am·pul·lu·la (am-pul´oo-lă). Uma dilatação circunscrita de qualquer ducto ou vaso sanguíneo ou linfático pequeno. [L. Mod. dim. de L. *ampulla*]

AMPUTATION

🛈 **am·pu·ta·tion** (am-pū-tā´shŭn). Amputação. **1.** Corte de um membro ou parte de um membro, da mama ou de outra parte que se projeta do corpo. **2.** Em odontologia, a remoção da raiz de um dente ou da polpa, ou da raiz nervosa ou gânglio; utiliza-se, portanto, um adjetivo modificador (a. da polpa; a. da raiz). [L. *amputatio,* de *am-puto,* pp. *-atus,* cortar em torno, aparar]
A-E a., abreviatura de a. acima do cotovelo.
A-K a., abreviatura de a. acima do joelho.
Alanson a., a. de Alanson; uma a. circular, sendo o coto cônico.
amnionic a., a. amniônica. SIN congenital a.
aperiosteal a., a. com a remoção do periósteo do osso no local da a.
B-E a., abreviatura para a. abaixo do cotovelo.
Bier a., a. de Bier; a. osteoplástica da tíbia e fíbula.
B-K a., abreviatura para a. abaixo do joelho.
bloodless a., a. em que, por meio de um torniquete, a saída de sangue a partir das superfícies cortadas é mínima. SIN dry a.

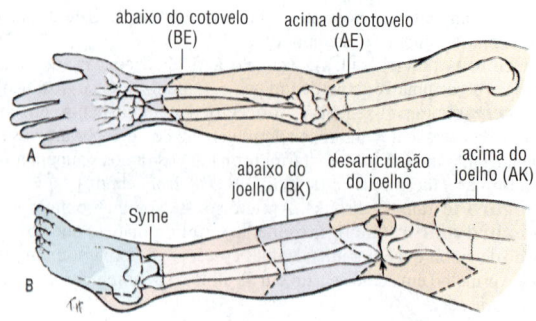

amputação: (A) níveis do membro superior, (B) níveis do membro inferior

Callander a., a. de Callander; a. tenoplástica através do fêmur no joelho. SIN knee disarticulation a.
Carden a., a. de Carden; a. transcondiliana da perna, serrando-se o fêmur através dos côndilos, logo acima da superfície articular.
central a., a. central; a. em que os retalhos são tão unidos que a cicatriz corre através da extremidade do coto.
cervical a., a. cervical; a. do colo uterino.
Chopart a., a. de Chopart; a. através da articulação mediotársica; isto é, entre as articulações tarsais navicular e calcaneocubóidea.
cinematic a., a. cinemática. SIN cineplastic a.
cineplastic a., a. cineplástica; um método de a. de um membro onde os músculos e tendões são dispostos de tal forma, no coto, que eles são capazes de executar movimentos independentes e de comunicar o movimento a uma prótese especialmente construída. SIN cinematic a., cineplastics, kineplastic a.
circular a., a. circular; a. realizada por meio de uma incisão circular através da pele, com os músculos sendo divididos de maneira semelhante em um ponto mais alto e o osso em um ponto ainda mais alto. SIN guillotine a., linear a.
congenital a. [MIM*217100], a. congênita; a. produzida *in utero;* atribuída à pressão de faixas constritivas (amnióticas). VER TAMBÉM amputation (1). SIN amnionic a., intrauterine a., spontaneous a. (1).
a. in continuity, a. em continuidade; a. através de um segmento de um membro, mas não em uma articulação.
double flap a., a. de retalho duplo; a. em que um retalho é cortado a partir das partes moles sobre um lado qualquer do membro.
dry a., a. seca. SIN bloodless a.
Dupuytren a., a. de Dupuytren; a. do braço na articulação do ombro.
eccentric a., a. excêntrica; a. com a cicatriz do coto fora do centro. SIN excentric a.
elliptical a., a. elíptica; a. circular em que a curva do bisturi não é exatamente vertical ao eixo do membro, sendo, portanto, elíptico o contorno da superfície de corte.
excentric a., a. excêntrica. SIN eccentric a.
Farabeuf a., a. de Farabeuf; **(1)** a. da perna, com o retalho sendo grande e no lado externo; **(2)** a. do pé; desarticulação do pé através da articulação subtalar e da articulação talonavicular.
flap a., a. com retalho; uma a. em que os retalhos dos tecidos muscular e cutâneo são dispostos de modo a cobrir a extremidade do osso. SIN flap operation (1).
flapless a., a. sem retalho; uma a. sem qualquer tecido para cobrir o coto.
forequarter a., a. interescapulotorácica; a. do braço com a retirada da escápula e de uma porção da clavícula. SIN interscapulothoracic a.
Gritti-Stokes a., a. de Gritti-Stokes; a. supracondiliana do fêmur, com a patela sendo preservada e aplicada na extremidade do osso, sendo removida sua cartilagem articular de modo a obter a união. SIN Gritti operation.
guillotine a., a. em guilhotina. SIN circular a.
Guyon a., a. de Guyon; acima dos maléolos, uma modificação da a. de Syme.
Hancock a., a. de Hancock; a do pé através do tálus.
Hey a., a. de Hey; a. do pé por diante da articulação tarsometatársica.
hindquarter a., hemipelvectomia. SIN hemipelvectomy.
immediate a., a. imediata; a. necessária em virtude de lesão irreparável do membro, realizada nas primeiras 12 horas após a lesão.
intermediate a., a. intermediária; uma a. realizada antigamente durante o período entre o trauma ou gangrena incipiente e a supuração. SIN primary a.
interscapulothoracic a., a. interescapulotorácica. SIN forequarter a.
intrauterine a., a. intra-uterina. SIN congenital a.
Jaboulay a., a. de Jaboulay, hemipelvectomia. SIN hemipelvectomy.
kineplastic a., a. cineplástica. SIN cineplastic a.
Kirk a., a. de Kirk; a. na extremidade inferior do fêmur, usando o tendão extensor do quadríceps para cobrir a extremidade do osso.
knee disarticulation a., a. com desarticulação do joelho. SIN Callander a.

Krukenberg a., a. de Krukenberg; uma a. cineplástica no carpo com a extremidade distal do antebraço sendo usada para criar um coto semelhante a um garfo, entre o rádio e a ulna; especialmente valiosa para os cegos porque o coto possui propriocepção.
Le Fort a., a. de Le Fort; uma modificação da a. de Pirogoff; o calcâneo é serrado no sentido horizontal, em vez de vertical, de modo que o paciente pisa sobre a mesma parte do calcanhar, como antes.
linear a., a. linear. SIN circular a.
Lisfranc a., a. de Lisfranc; a. do pé na articulação tarsometatarsal, com a região plantar sendo preservada para fazer o retalho. SIN Lisfranc operation.
Mackenzie a., a. de Mackenzie; uma modificação da a. de Syme na articulação do tornozelo, com o retalho originando-se a partir do lado interno.
major a., a. maior; a do membro inferior ou superior acima do tornozelo ou punho, respectivamente.
Malgaigne a., a. de Malgaigne. SIN subastragalar a.
Mikulicz-Vladimiroff a., a. de Mikulicz-Vladimiroff; uma ressecção osteoplástica do pé em que o tálus e o calcâneo são excisados, a fileira anterior de ossos do tarso é unida com a extremidade inferior da tíbia, as superfícies articulares de ambos são removidas. A extremidade inferior do coto consiste, portanto, na porção anterior do pé, com o paciente caminhando, daí por diante, sobre a ponta dos artelhos. SIN Vladimiroff-Mikulicz a.
minor a., a. menor; a. da mão ou do pé ou de quaisquer partes de ambos.
multiple a., a. múltipla; a. de dois ou mais membros ou de partes dos membros realizada na mesma cirurgia.
oblique a., a. oblíqua; a. em que a linha de corte através de um membro é diferente de um ângulo reto; isso confere uma aparência oval à superfície de corte (daí, por vezes, ser referida, embora raramente, como uma a. oval).
osteoplastic a., a. osteoplástica; uma, p.ex., através do tarso, em que a superfície de corte do outro osso é colocada em aposição com aquele originalmente dividido, de modo que os dois se unam, propiciando, assim, um coto melhor.
pathologic a., a. patológica; a. exigida pelo câncer ou outra doença do membro, e não por uma lesão.
Pirogoff a., a. de Pirogoff; a. do pé; as superfícies articulares inferiores são serradas e as extremidades cobertas com uma porção do calcâneo, a qual também foi serrada a partir de cima na parte posterior, para baixo e para diante.
primary a., a. primária. SIN intermediate a.
pulp a., a. da polpa. SIN pulpotomy.
quadruple a., a. quádrupla; a. de ambos os braços e de ambas as pernas.
racket a., a. em raquete; uma a. circular, ou discretamente oval, em que é feita uma longa incisão no eixo do membro.
rectangular a., a. retangular; a. em que os retalhos são modelados na forma de um retângulo.
root a., a. da raiz; remoção cirúrgica de uma ou mais raízes de um dente com múltiplas raízes, com o(s) resultante(s) canal(is) da raiz sendo tratado(s) por meios endodônticos. SIN radectomy, radiectomy, radisectomy.
secondary a., a. secundária; a. realizada algum tempo depois de uma a. prévia que não cicatrizou de maneira satisfatória.
spontaneous a., a. espontânea. (1) SIN congenital a.; (2) a. em consequência de um processo patológico, em lugar de um trauma externo.
Stokes a., a. de Stokes; uma modificação da a. de Gritti-Stokes em que a linha de corte do fêmur é um pouco mais alta.
subastragalar a., a. subtalar; a. do pé em que apenas o tálus é mantido. SIN Malgaigne a.
subperiosteal a., a. subperióstea; a. em que o periósteo é destacado do osso e recolocado depois, formando um retalho perióstico sobre a extremidade cortada.
Syme a., a. de Syme; a. do pé na articulação do tornozelo, com os maléolos sendo serrados e sendo feito um retalho com as partes moles do calcanhar. SIN Syme operation.
tarsotibial a., a. tarsotibial; a. através da articulação do tornozelo.
transverse a., a. transversa; a. em que a linha de corte através do membro é feita em ângulo reto com o eixo longitudinal.
traumatic a., a. traumática; a. decorrente de lesão acidental ou não-cirúrgica; pode ser completa ou incompleta.
Tripier a., a. de Tripier; uma modificação da a. de Chopart na qual uma parte do calcâneo também é removida.
Vladimiroff-Mikulicz a., a. de Vladimiroff-Mikulicz. SIN Mikulicz-Vladimiroff a.

am·pu·tee (am′pū-tē). Amputado; uma pessoa com um membro, ou parte do membro, amputado.
am·ri·none lac·tate (am′ri-nōn). Lactato de amrinona; um inibidor da fosfodiesterase com atividades inotrópica e vasodilatadora, usado no controle da insuficiência cardíaca congestiva.
Amsler, Marc, oftalmologista suíço, 1891–1968. VER A. *chart*; Amsler *grid*; A. *test*.
amu. Abreviatura para atomic mass *unit* (unidade de massa atômica).

amuck (ă-mŭk′). Amoque; amouco. SIN amok (2).
amu·sia (ă-mū′zē-ă). Amusia; uma forma de afasia caracterizada por incapacidade de produzir ou reconhecer a música. [G. *a-* priv. + *mousa*, música]
instrumental a., a. instrumental; perda da capacidade de tocar um instrumento musical.
motor a., a. motora; incapacidade de produzir música.
sensory a., a. sensorial; incapacidade de interpretar ou apreciar os sons musicais.
vocal a., a. vocal; a incapacidade de cantar, embora a fala permaneça intacta.
Amussat, Jean Z., cirurgião francês, 1796–1856. VER A. *valve, valvula*.
am·y·cho·pho·bia (am′ĭ-kō-fō′bē-ă). Amicofobia; medo mórbido de ser arranhado. [G. *amychē*, arranhadura, + *phobos*, medo]
Am·y·co·la·top·sis (am-ē-kō-la-top′sis). Um gênero de bactérias filamentosas Gram-positivas, definido como um gênero separado em 1986, que tende a dividir-se em fragmentos quadrados; encontrados no solo e em material vegetal; *A*. é um raro patógeno humano que foi isolado de diversas amostras clínicas, inclusive no líquido cefalorraquidiano. A espécie-protótipo é *A. orientalis*.
A. orienta'lis, subsp. *lu'rida*, uma espécie bacteriana que produz ristocetina.
amy·el·en·ce·pha·lia (ā-mī′el-en-sĕ-fā′lē-ă). Amielencefalia; ausência congênita do cérebro e da medula espinal. [G. *a-* priv. + *myelos*, medula, + *enkephalos*, cérebro]
amy·el·en·ce·phal·ic, amy·el·en·ceph·a·lous (ā-mī′el-en-se-fal′ik, -sef′ă-lŭs). Amielencefálico, amielencéfalo; denotando ou característico de amielencefalia.
amy·e·lia (ā-mī-ē′lē-ă). Amielia; ausência congênita da medula espinal, encontrada em associação à anencefalia. [G. *a-* priv. + *myelos*, medula]
amy·el·ic (ā-mī-ē′lik). Amiélico. SIN amyelous.
amy·e·li·nat·ed (ā-mī′ē-li-nā′ted). Amielinizado. SIN unmyelinated.
amy·e·li·na·tion (ā-mī′ē-li-nā′shŭn). Amielinização; falha da formação da bainha de mielina de um nervo.
amy·e·lin·ic (ā-mī′e-lin′ik). Amielínico. SIN unmyelinated.
amy·e·lo·ic, amy·e·lon·ic (ā-mī-e-lō′ik, ā-mī-e-lon′ik). Amielóico, amielônico. **1.** Amiélico. SIN amyelous. **2.** Em hematologia, por vezes usado para indicar a ausência de medula óssea ou a falta de participação funcional da medula óssea na hematopoese. [G. *a-* priv. + *myelos*, medula]
amy·e·lous (ā-mī′ē-lŭs). Amiélico; sem medula espinal. SIN amyelic, amyeloic (1), amyelonic.
amyg·da·la, gen. e pl. **amyg·da·lae** (ă-mig′dă-lă, -lē). Amígdala. **1.** Termo para as tonsilas linfáticas (faríngeas, palatinas, linguais, laríngeas e tubárias). **2.** Termo geral que descreve um núcleo no lobo temporal, o corpo amigdalóide. [L. de G. *amygdalē,* amêndoa; em L. Mediev. & Mod., tonsila]
a. cerebel′li, a. cerebelar; termo ultrapassado para cerebellar *tonsil* (tonsila cerebelar).
amyg·da·lase (ă-mig′dă-lās). Amigdalase. SIN β-D-glucosidase.
amyg·da·lin (ă-mig′dă-lin). Amigdalina; um glicosídeo cianogênico presente em amêndoas e sementes de outros vegetais da família Rosaceae; o principal componente da letrila. A emulsina cliva a a. em benzaldeído, D-glicose e ácido hidrociânico. SIN amygdaloside. [G. *amygdala,* amêndoa + *-in*]
amyg·da·line (ă-mig′dă-līn). Amigdalina. **1.** Relativo a uma amêndoa. **2.** [TA] Relativo a uma tonsila ou à estrutura cerebral chamada amígdala (tonsila) ou complexo amigdalóide [TA]. **3.** Tonsilar. SIN tonsillar.
amyg·da·loid (ă-mig′dă-loyd). Amigdalóide; que se assemelha a uma amêndoa ou a uma tonsila. [amygdala + G. *eidos,* aparência]
a·myg·dal·ose (ā-mig′dal-ōs). Amigdalose. SIN gentiobiose.
amyg·da·lo·side (ă-mig′dă-lō-sīd). Amigdalosídeo; SIN amygdalin.
am·yl (ā′mil). Amila; o radical formado a partir de um pentano, C_5H_{12}, pela retirada de um H. Existem diversas formas isoméricas, sendo as mais importantes $CH_3CH_2CH_2CH_2CH_2-$ (amila ou pentila); $(CH_3)_2CHCH_2CH_2-$ (isoamila ou isopentila); $CH_3CH_2CH_2(CH_3)-$ e $(CH_3CH_2)_2CH-$ (amila ou pentila secundária); e $CH_3CH_2C(CH_3)_3$ (amila terciária ou pentila). SIN pentyl (1).
a. alcohol, álcool amílico; usado como solvente para vernizes e óleos; extremamente tóxico, com vapores irritantes. VER TAMBÉM fusel *oil.*
a. hydrate, hidrato de amila. SIN amylene hydrate.
a. nitrite, nitrato de amila; vasodilatador utilizado na angina de peito e na intoxicação por cianeto.
tertiary a. alcohol, álcool de a. terciária. SIN amylene hydrate.
a. valerate, valerato de a.; usado como sedativo; originalmente usado no tratamento de cálculos biliares por causa de sua ação de solvente sobre o colesterol. SIN apple oil.
amyl-. Amila. **1.** VER amylo-. **2.** Pentil-. VER amyl.
am·y·la·ceous (am′i-lā′shŭs). Amiláceo; que contém amilo.
am·y·lase (am′il-ās). Amilase; membro de um grupo de enzimas amilolíticas que clivam amido, glicogênio e 1,4-α-glicanos correlatos.
α-am·y·lase. α-Amilase; uma glicanoidrolase que fornece α-glicose e maltose de modo aleatório a partir dos 1,4-α-glicanos. Uma amilase que tem sido utilizada clinicamente como adjunto digestivo. SIN glycogenase, ptyalin, Taka-diastase.

β-am·y·lase. β-Amilase; uma glicanoidrolase que fornece unidades de β-maltose a partir das terminações não-redutoras de 1,4-α-glicanos. Uma exoamilase. SIN glycogenase, saccharogen amylase.

γ-am·y·lase. γ-Amilase. SIN exo-1,4-α-D-glucosidase.

am·y·la·su·ria (am-i-lā-soo'rē-ă). Amilasúria; a excreção de amilase (por vezes denominada diastase) na urina, com quantidades principalmente aumentadas na pancreatite aguda. SIN diastasuria.

am·y·le·mia (am-i-lē'mē-ă). Amilemia; a presença hipotética de amido no sangue circulante. [amylo- + G. *haima*, sangue]

am·yl·ene (am'i-lēn). Amileno; um hidrocarboneto líquido inflamável formado pela decomposição do álcool amílico; possui propriedades anestésicas, porém ações colaterais indesejáveis. SIN trimethylethylene.
  a. chloral, a. cloral; um hipnótico.
  a. hydrate, hidrato de a.; hipnótico obsoleto utilizado como solvente para tribromoetanol. SIN amyl hydrate, tertiary amyl alcohol.

am·y·lin (am'i-lin). Amilina; a celulose de amilo; o envelope insolúvel dos grãos de amilo.

♻ **amylo-.** Amilo; da natureza ou origem do polissacarídeo. [G. *amylon,* amido, de a-, + *mylē,* um moinho]

am·y·lo·dex·trin (am-i-lō-deks'trin). Amilodextrina; o produto final da hidrólise da amilopectina pela β-amilase; a hidrólise adicional exige amilo-1,6-glicosidase, a qual ataca os pontos de ramificação. Identificada pela reação colorida com o iodo (a. fica azul). Cf. achroodextrin, erythrodextrin.

am·y·lo·gen·e·sis (am-i-lō-jen'ē-sis). Amilogênese; biossíntese do amilo. [amylo- + G. *genesis,* produção]

am·y·lo·gen·ic (am-i-lō-jen'ik). Amilogênico; relativo à amilogênese.

am·y·lo-1,4:1,6-glu·can·trans·fer·ase. Amilo-1,4:1,6-glicanotransferase. SIN 1,4-α-D-glucanbranching enzyme.

am·y·lo·glu·co·si·dase (am-i-lō-gloo'kō-si-dās). Amiloglicosidase. SIN exo-1,4-α-D-glucosidase.

am·y·lo-1,6-glu·co·si·dase. Amilo-1,6-glicosidase; uma enzima que hidrolisa as ligações α-D-1,6 (pontos de ramificação) em cadeias de resíduos de α-D-glicose com ligação 1,4, daí ser chamada fator ou enzima desramificadora; a deficiência provoca glicogenose do tipo III. SIN dextrin 6-α-D-glucosidase.

am·y·loid (am'i-loyd). Amilóide. **1.** Qualquer proteína de um grupo de proteínas quimicamente diversas que parece microscopicamente homogêneo, mas que é composto de fibrilas lineares não-ramificantes agregadas, dispostas em bainhas, quando observadas à microscopia eletrônica; essa proteína cora-se em castanho-escuro com o iodo, produz birrefringência esverdeada típica na luz polarizada depois de corada com vermelho-congo, é metacromática com a metil-violeta (rosa-avermelhado) ou violeta cristal (púrpura-avermelhado) e fluoresce em amarelo depois da coloração com tioflavina T; o a. ocorre, de maneira característica, como depósitos extracelulares patológicos (amiloidose), principalmente em associação com tecido reticuloendotelial; a natureza química das fibrilas proteináceas depende do processo patológico subjacente. **2.** Que se assemelha ao ou contém amilo. [amylo- + G *eidos,* semelhança]

am·y·loi·do·ma (am'il-oyd-ō'ma). Amiloidoma; um tumor dentro do qual é produzido amilóide. [amyloid + G *-oma,* tumor]

am·y·loi·do·sis (am'i-loy-dō'sis). Amiloidose. **1.** Uma doença caracterizada por acúmulo extracelular de amilóide em vários órgãos e tecidos do corpo; pode ser localizada ou generalizada; pode ser primária ou secundária. **2.** O processo de deposição da proteína amilóide. [amyloid + G. *-osis,* condição]
  a. of aging, a. da velhice; caracterizada por deposição de material corável por vermelho-congo, derivado de diversas proteínas, principalmente no tecido nervoso, miocárdio e pâncreas. Associada à síndrome de Alzheimer; pode resultar em insuficiência cardíaca congestiva intratável.
  chronic amyloidosis, a. crônica; a. de longa data.
  a. cu'tis, a. da pele, a. liquenóide. SIN lichenoid a.
  familial a., a. familiar. SIN familial amyloid neuropathy.
  focal a., a. focal, a. nodular. SIN nodular a.
  hereditary a., a. hereditária. SIN familial amyloid neuropathy.
  lichen a., a. do líquen. SIN lichenoid a.
  lichenoid a. (līk'en-oyd), a. liquenóide; a. cutânea localizada com pápulas castanho-avermelhadas pruriginosas, freqüentemente descamativas, mais amiúde nas pernas de pessoas de meia-idade, decorrente da infiltração amilóide da derme papilar. SIN a. cutis, lichen a. [G. *leichēn,* líquen, uma erupção semelhante ao líquen + *eidos,* semelhança]
  light chain-related a., a. de cadeia leve; a forma mais comum de a. primária, em que os depósitos de amilóide fibrilar derivam da região aminoterminal variável das cadeias leves da imunoglobulina; observada nas discrasias de linfócitos B e plasmócitos (especialmente no mieloma múltiplo) e em outras formas de gamopatias.
  macular a., a. macular; uma forma localizada de a. da pele, caracterizada por máculas reticuladas, de cor marrom, simétricas e pruriginosas, especialmente na parte superior das costas; do ponto de vista microscópico, o amilóide é depositado como pequenos glóbulos subepidérmicos.
  a. of multiple myeloma, a. do mieloma múltiplo; focos de a. nos tecidos mesenquimatosos de algumas pessoas com mieloma múltiplo; não se conhece nenhuma relação direta conclusiva entre o amilóide e a proteína de Bence-Jones.
  nodular a., a. nodular; uma forma localizada de a. em que o amilóide ocorre como massas endurecidas ou nódulos abaixo da pele ou mucosas, p.ex., na laringe, freqüentemente com infiltração local de plasmócitos; pode estar associado à discrasia plasmocitária ou à a. sistêmica. SIN amyloid tumor, focal a.
  primary a., a. primária; várias formas de a. são conhecidas, seguindo uma herança autossômica dominante [MIM*104750, *105120, *105150, *105200, *105210, *105250], recessiva [MIM 204850 e *204900] e ligada ao X [MIM 301220] e não associada a outra doença identificável. Tende a afetar de maneira difusa as paredes vasculares e tecidos mesenquimatosos na língua, pulmões, trato intestinal, pele, músculo esquelético e miocárdio, interferindo com as funções vitais; com freqüência, o amilóide não manifesta a afinidade usual pelo vermelho-congo e, por vezes, provoca uma reação inflamatória do tipo corpo estranho no tecido adjacente.
  renal a., a. renal; depósitos renais de amilóide, principalmente nas paredes dos capilares glomerulares, o que pode provocar albuminúria e a síndrome nefrótica. SIN amyloid nephrosis (1).
  secondary a., a. secundária; a. que ocorre em associação a outra doença inflamatória crônica; os órgãos principalmente atingidos são fígado, baço e rins, sendo as glândulas supra-renais afetadas com menor freqüência.
  senile a., a. senil; uma forma comum de a. nas pessoas muito idosas, geralmente branda e limitada ao coração ou vesículas seminais. VER TAMBÉM a. of aging.

am·y·lol·y·sis (am-i-lol'i-sis). Amilólise; hidrólise do amilo em produtos solúveis. [amylo- + G. *lysis,* dissolução]

am·y·lo·lyt·ic (am-i-lō-lit'ik). Amilolítico; relativo à amilólise.

am·y·lo·malt·ase (am-i-lō-mal'tās). Amilomaltase. SIN 4-α-D-glucanotransferase.

am·y·lo·pec·tin (am-i-lō-pek'tin). Amilopectina; uma poliglicose (glicano) de cadeia ramificada no amilo que contém ligações 1,4 e 1,6. Cf. amylose.

am·y·lo·pec·tin 6-glu·can·o·hy·dro·lase. Amilopectina 6-glicanoidrolase; denominação antiga da α-dextrinaendo-1,6-α-glicosidase.

am·y·lo·pec·tin 1,6-glu·co·si·dase. Amilopectina 1,6-glicosidase; denominação antiga de uma enzima atualmente conhecida como sendo, pelo menos, duas enzimas: α-dextrina endoglicanoidrolase e isoamilase.

am·y·lo·pec·tin·o·sis (am'i-lō-pek-tin-ō'sis). Amilopectinose. VER type 4 *glycogenosis*. [amylopectin + G. *-osis,* condição]

am·y·lo·pha·gia (am'i-lō-fā'jē-ă). Amilofagia; um desejo mórbido pelo amilo. SIN starch-eating. [amylo- + G. *phagō,* comer]

am·y·lo·plast (am'i-lō-plast). Amiloplasto; um grânulo no protoplasma de uma célula vegetal que é o centro de um processo de formação de amilo. SIN amylogenic body. [amylo- + G. *plastos,* formado]

am·y·lo·psin (am-il-op'sin). Amilopsina; a amilase do suco pancreático.

am·y·lor·rhea (am'i-lō-rē'ă). Amilorréia; eliminação de amilo não-digerido nas fezes, implicando deficiência de atividade de amilase no intestino. [amylo- + G. *rhoia,* fluxo]

am·y·lose (am'i-lōs). Amilose; uma poliglicose (glicano) não-ramificada no amilo, similar à celulose, contendo ligações α(1→4). Cf amylopectin.

am·y·lo·su·ria (am'i-lō-soo'rē-ă). Amilosúria; excreção de amido na urina. SIN amilúria.

am·y·lo-(1,4→1,6)-trans·glu·co·si·dase, am·y·lo-(1,4→1,6)-trans·glu·co·syl·ase. Amilo-(1,4→1,6)-transglicosidase ou transglicosilase. SIN 1,4-α-D-glucan-branching-enzyme.

am·y·lum (am'i-lŭm). Amido, amilo. SIN starch.

am·y·lu·ria (am'i-loo're-ă). Amilúria. SIN amylosuria.

amy·o·es·the·sia, amy·o·es·the·sis (ā-mī'ō-es-thē'zē-ă, -thē'sis). Amioestesia; ausência de sensibilidade no músculo. [G. *a-* priv. + *mys,* músculo, + *aisthēsis,* percepção]

amy·o·pla·sia (ā-mī-ō-plā'zē-ă). Amioplasia; formação deficiente do tecido muscular e crescimento muscular deficiente. [G. *a-,* priv. + *mys,* músculo + *plasis,* moldagem]
  a. congen'ita, a. congênita. SIN *arthrogryposis* multiplex congenita.

amy·o·sta·sia (ā-mī-ō-stā'zē-ă). Amiostasia; dificuldade em ficar de pé decorrente de tremor ou incoordenação muscular. [G. *a-* priv. + *mys,* músculo, + *stasis,* ficar em pé]

amy·o·stat·ic (ā-mī-ō-stat'ik). Amiostático; que exibe tremores musculares.

amy·os·the·nia (ā-mī'os-thē'nē-ă). Amiostenia; fraqueza muscular. [G. *a-* priv. + *mys,* músculo + *sthenos,* força]

amy·os·then·ic (ā-mī-os-then'ik). Amiostênico; relativo a ou que causa fraqueza muscular.

amy·o·taxy, amy·o·tax·ia (ā-mī'ō-tak-sē, ā-mī-ō-tak'sē-ă). Amiotaxia; ataxia muscular. [G. *a-* priv. + *mys,* músculo + *taxis,* ordem]

amy·o·to·nia (ā-mī-ō-tō'nē-ă). Amiotonia; ausência generalizada de tono muscular, usualmente associada à musculatura flácida e à amplitude aumentada de movimento passivo nas articulações. [G. *a-* priv. + *mys,* músculo, + *tonos,* tono]
  a. congen´ita, a. congênita; um termo indefinido para inúmeros transtornos

amyotonia neuromusculares congênitos que provocam a perda generalizada do tono muscular e, por vezes, fraqueza em lactentes e crianças pequenas; grande parte desses distúrbios apresenta uma evolução benigna. SIN congenital atonic pseudoparalysis, myatonia congenita, Oppenheim disease, Oppenheim syndrome.

a·my·o·tro·phia (ā-mī-ō-trō'fē-ā). Amiotrofia. SIN amyotrophy.

am·y·o·tro·phic (ā-mī-ō-trō'fik). Relativo à amiotrofia.

am·y·ot·ro·phy (ā-mī-ot'rō-fē). Amiotrofia; enfraquecimento ou atrofia muscular. SIN amyotrophia. [G. *a-* priv. + *mys*, músculo, + *trophē*, nutrição]
  diabetic a., a. diabética; um tipo de neuropatia diabética que afeta principalmente os diabéticos idosos; clinicamente caracterizada por dor unilateral ou bilateral na face anterior da coxa, fraqueza e atrofia; de instalação abrupta ou gradual e, quando bilateral, de instalação simultânea ou seqüencial, sendo, em geral, assimétrica; um tipo de polirradiculopatia diabética. Por vezes referida, de maneira errônea, como neuropatia femoral diabética.
  hemiplegic a., a. hemiplégica; atrofia muscular nos membros hemiplégicos.
  neuralgic a., a. neurálgica; um transtorno neurológico, de etiologia desconhecida, caracterizado pela súbita instalação de dor intensa, geralmente em torno do ombro e começando, com freqüência, à noite, logo seguida por fraqueza e emaciação de diversos músculos da parte anterior do ombro, em particular os músculos do cíngulo dos membros superiores; tem ocorrência esporádica e familial, sendo a primeira muito mais comum; freqüentemente precedida por algum evento antecedente, como uma infecção respiratória alta, hospitalização, vacinação ou traumatismo inespecífico; usualmente atribuída a uma lesão do plexo braquial, porque as fibras nervosas envolvidas derivam, com maior freqüência, do tronco superior, porém, na realidade, são mononeuropatias proximais múltiplas. SIN acute brachial radiculitis, brachial neuritis, brachial plexitis, brachial plexus neuropathy, Parsonage-Turner syndrome, shoulder-girdle syndrome.
  progressive spinal a., a. espinal progressiva. SIN amyotrophic lateral *sclerosis.*

am·y·ous (am'ē-ŭs). Que carece de tecido muscular ou de força muscular. [G. *a-* priv. + *mys*, músculo]

amyx·or·rhea (ā-mik-sō-rē'ā). Amixorréia; ausência de secreção normal de muco. [G. *a-* priv. + *myxa*, muco, + *rhoia*, fluxo]

⚠ **an-.** VER a-.

ANA. Abreviatura para antinuclear *antibody* (anticorpo antinuclear); *American Nurses Association (Associação Americana de Enfermagem).*

⚠ **ana-.** Prefixo que significa para cima, novamente, de novo; por vezes *an-* antes de uma vogal; corresponde ao L. *sursum-*. ADVERTÊNCIA: *an-* antes de uma vogal geralmente se distingue de *a-*, que significa não; por vezes *ana-* se torna *am-* antes de p, b ou ph. [G. *ana*, para cima]

An·a·bae·na (an-ā-bē'nā). Um gênero de cianobactérias encontrado em água potável; elas podem provocar odor nos reservatórios de água; embora não sejam patógenos invasivos, produzem potentes neurotoxinas semelhantes à saxitoxina, as quais podem envenenar animais de fazendas que ingerem água de reservatório intensamente infectada.

an·a·bi·o·sis (an'ā-bī-ō'sis). Anabiose; reanimação depois de morte aparente. [G. um reviver, de *ana*, novamente + *biōsis*, vida]

an·a·bi·ot·ic (an'ā-bī-ot'ik). Anabiótico. **1.** Que se reanima ou restaura. **2.** Um remédio restaurador; um estimulante poderoso. [ana- + G. *bios*, vida]

an·a·bol·ic (an-ā-bol'ik). Anabólico; relativo a ou que promove o anabolismo.

anab·o·lism (ā-nab'ō-lizm). Anabolismo. **1.** A construção de compostos químicos complexos, no corpo, a partir de compostos menores e mais simples (p.ex., proteínas a partir de aminoácidos), geralmente com o uso de energia. Cf. catabolism, metabolism. **2.** O somatório das reações metabólicas de síntese. [G. *anabolē*, uma construção]

anab·o·lite (ā-nab'ō-līt). Anabólito; qualquer substância formada em conseqüência de processos anabólicos.

an·a·camp·tom·e·ter (an-ā-kamp-tom'ē-ter). Anacamptômetro; instrumento para medir a intensidade dos reflexos profundos. [G. *anakampsis*, um retorno, reflexão, + G. *metron*, medir]

an·a·cat·es·the·sia (an'ā-kat'es-thē'zē-ā). Anacatestesia; sensação de flutuar no espaço. [G. *ana*, para cima, + *kata*, para baixo, + *aisthēsis*, sensação]

an·a·cid·i·ty (an-ā-sid'i-tē). Anacidez; ausência de acidez; usada especialmente para indicar a ausência de ácido clorídrico no suco gástrico.

anac·la·sis (ā-nak'lā-sis). Anáclase. **1.** Reflexão da luz ou som. **2.** Refração do meio ocular. [G. um retorno, reflexão]

an·a·clit·ic (an-ā-klit'ik). Anaclítico; dependente; em psicanálise, relativo à dependência do lactente em relação à mãe ou substituto da mãe. VER anaclitic *depression*. [G. *ana*, no sentido de + *klino*, inclinar]

an·a·crot·ic (an-ā-krot'ik). Anacrótico; que se refere a elevação (ões) na onda ascendente do traçado do pulso arterial; uma forma abreviada para anadicrótico, batimento duplo na ascensão. SIN anadicrotic.

anac·ro·tism (ā-nak'rō-tizm). Anacrotismo; peculiaridade da onda do pulso. VER anacrotic *pulse*. SIN anadicrotism. [G. *ana*, para cima, + *krotos*, um batimento]

an·a·cu·sis (an'ā-koo'sis). Anacusia; perda ou ausência total da capacidade de perceber o som como tal. SIN anakusis. [G. *an-* priv. + *akousis*, audição]

an·a·de·nia (an-ā-dē'nē-ā). Anadenia; termo obsoleto para a ausência de glândulas ou suspensão da função glandular. [G. *an-* priv. + *adēn*, glândula]
  a. ventric′uli, a. ventricular; ausência de glândulas no estômago.

an·a·di·crot·ic (an-ā-dī-krot'ik). Anadicrótico. SIN anacrotic.

an·a·di·cro·tism (an-ā-dik'rō-tizm). Anadicrotismo. SIN anacrotism. [G. *ana*, para cima + *di-krotos*, batimento duplo]

an·a·did·y·mus (an-ā-did'i-mŭs). Anadídimo. SIN *duplicitas* posterior. [G. *ana*, para cima, + *didymos*, gêmeo]

an·a·dip·sia (an-ā-dip'sē-ā). Anadipsia; termo raramente utilizado para a sede intensa. VER TAMBÉM polydipsia. [G. *ana*, intenso + *dipsa*, sede]

an·ad·re·nal·ism (an-ā-drē'nal-izm). Anadrenalismo; ausência completa da função das supra-renais.

an·ad·ro·mous (an-a-drō'mŭs). Anádromo; que migra da água do mar para a água doce para desovar; alguns desses peixes alojam patógenos humanos. VER TAMBÉM catadromous.

an·aer·obe (an'ār-ōb, an-ār'ōb). Anaeróbio; um microrganismo que consegue viver e crescer na ausência de oxigênio. [G. *an-* priv. + *aēr*, ar, + *bios*, vida]
  facultative a., a. facultativo; um a. que cresce na presença de ar ou sob condições de pressão de oxigênio reduzida.
  obligate a., a. obrigatório; um a. que somente crescerá na ausência de oxigênio livre.

an·aer·o·bic (an-ār-ō'bik). Anaeróbico; relativo a um anaeróbio; que vive sem oxigênio.

an·aer·o·bi·o·sis (an-ār-ō-bī-ō'sis). Anaerobiose; a existência em uma atmosfera isenta de oxigênio. [G. *an-* priv. + *aēr*, ar, + *biōsis*, modo de viver]

An·aer·o·bo·plasma (an-ār-ō'bō-plaz'ma). Uma ordem na classe Molicutes que é sensível ao oxigênio. Não foi definida uma função na doença humana.

an·aer·o·gen·ic (an-ār-ō-jen'ik). Anaerogênico; que não produz gás. [G. *an-* priv. + *aēr*, ar, + *-gen*, que produz]

an·aer·o·phyte (an-ār'ō-fīt). Anaerófito. **1.** Um vegetal que cresce sem ar. **2.** Uma bactéria anaeróbica. [G. *an-* priv. + *aēr*, ar + *phyton*, planta]

an·aer·o·plas·ty (an-ār'ō-plas-tē). Anaeroplastia; tratamento de feridas pela exclusão do ar. [G. *an-* não + *aēr*, ar, + *plastos*, formado]

an·a·gen (an'ā-jen). Anágeno; fase de crescimento do ciclo do cabelo, que dura cerca de 3–6 anos no cabelo humano. [G. *ana*, para cima, + *-gen*, que produz]

an·a·gen·e·sis (an-ā-jen'ē-sis). Anagênese. **1.** Reparação do tecido. **2.** Regeração das partes perdidas. [G. *ana*, para cima, + *genesis*, produção]

an·a·ge·net·ic (an'ā-jē-net'ik). Anagenético; pertinente à anagênese.

an·a·ges·tone ac·e·tate (an-ā-jes'ton). Acetato de anagestona; um agente progestágeno.

Anagnostakis, Andreas, oftalmologista cretense, 1826–1897.

an·a·go·gy (an-ā-gō'jē). Anagogia, anagoge; termo raramente utilizado para o conteúdo psíquico de natureza idealista ou espiritual. [G. *anagōgē*, de *an-ago*, levantar]

an·a·kat·a·did·y·mus, an·a·cat·a·did·y·mus (an'ā-kat-ā-did'i-mŭs). Anacatadídimo; gêmeos unidos pelo meio, porém separados por cima e por baixo. SIN dichepalus dipygus. [G. *ana*, para cima + *kata*, para baixo + *didymos*, gêmeos]

an·á·khré (an-ah-krā'). Anacré. SIN goundou. [Fr. de Af. termo nativo que significa "nariz grande"]

an·ak·me·sis (an-ak'mē-sis). Anacmese; parada da maturação dos leucócitos em seus centros de produção, resultando, assim, em maior número de formas jovens e proporções progressivamente menores de células granulares maduras na medula óssea, conforme observado na agranulocitose. [G. *an-* priv. + *akmēnos*, crescimento pleno, de *akmē*, ponto mais elevado]

an·a·ku·sis (an-ā-koo'sis). Anacusia. SIN anacusis.

anal (ā'nal). Anal; relativo ao ânus.

an·al·bu·mi·ne·mia (an'al-boo-mi-nē'mē-ā). Analbuminemia; ausência de albumina no soro. [G. *an-* priv. + albumin + G. *haima*, sangue]

an·a·lep·tic (an-ā-lep'tik). Analéptico. **1.** Que fortalece, estimula ou revigora. **2.** Um remédio restaurador. **3.** Um estimulante do sistema nervoso central, particularmente empregado para indicar os agentes que revertem a função deprimida do sistema nervoso central. [G. *analēptikos*, restaurador]

an·al·ge·sia (an-āl-jē'zē-ā). Analgesia; um estado neurológico ou farmacológico em que os estímulos dolorosos são tão moderados que, embora ainda percebidos, não são mais dolorosos. Cf. anesthesia. [G. insensibilidade, de *an-* priv. + *algēsis*, sensação de dor]
  conduction a., a. de condução. SIN regional *anesthesia.*
  inhalation a., a. por inalação; a. produzida pela inalação de um gás ou vapor depressor do sistema nervoso central (principalmente óxido nitroso).
  patient-controlled a. (PCA), a. controlada pelo paciente; um método para controle da dor baseado em uma bomba para a infusão intravenosa constante

ou, menos amiúde, epidural de uma solução de narcótico diluída, que inclui um mecanismo para a auto-administração em intervalos predeterminados de uma dose predeterminada de solução narcótica, caso a infusão não alivie a dor. SIN outpatient anesthesia, patient-controlled anesthesia.
spinal a., a. espinal; eufemismo para spinal *anesthesia* (anestesia espinal).
an·al·ge·sic (an-ăl-jē′zik). **1.** Analgésico, analgético; um composto capaz de produzir analgesia, isto é, aquele que alivia a dor por modificar a percepção dos estímulos nociceptivos sem produzir anestesia ou perda da consciência. SIN analgetic (1). **2.** Antálgico; caracterizado por resposta reduzida aos estímulos dolorosos. SIN antalgic.
an·al·ge·sim·e·ter (an′ăl-jē-zim′i-ter). Analgesímetro; um aparelho para produzir estímulos dolorosos a fim de medir a dor sob condições experimentais. [analgesia + G. *metron*, medir]
an·al·get·ic (an-ăl-jet′ik). Analgético. **1.** SIN analgesic (1). **2.** Associado à percepção diminuída da dor.
anal·i·ty (ā-nal′i-tē). Analidade; relativo à organização psíquica derivada e característica do período anal de Freud do desenvolvimento psicossexual.
an·al·ler·gic (an-ă-ler′jik). Analérgico; não-alérgico.
an·a·log (an′ă-log). Análogo. **1.** Um de dois órgãos ou partes em espécies diferentes de animais ou vegetais que diferem na estrutura ou desenvolvimento, mas que são similares na função. **2.** Um composto que se assemelha a outro em estrutura, mas que não é necessariamente um isômero (p.ex., o 5-fluorouracil é um análogo da timina); os análogos são freqüentemente empregados para bloquear as reações enzimáticas ao se combinarem com as enzimas (p.ex., isopropil tiogalactosídeo *vs.* lactose). SIN analogue. [G. *analogos*, proporcional]
enzyme a., a. enzimático. SIN synzyme.
anal·o·gous (ă-nal′ō-gŭs). Análogo; que possui uma semelhança funcional, porém apresenta uma origem ou estrutura diferente.
an·a·logue (an′ă-log). Análogo. SIN analog.
an·al·pha·lip·o·pro·tein·e·mia (an-al′fă-lip′ō-prō′tēn-ē′mē-ă) [MIM*205400]. Analfalipoproteinemia; deficiência de lipoproteína de alta densidade; um transtorno hereditário do metabolismo lipídico caracterizado por ausência quase completa de lipoproteínas de alta densidade no plasma, e pelo armazenamento de ésteres do colesterol nas células espumosas, aumento de tonsilas, coloração alaranjada ou amarelo-acinzentada das mucosas da faringe e reto, hepatoesplenomegalia, linfadenopatia, opacificação da córnea e neuropatia periférica; herança autossômica recessiva. SIN familial high density lipoprotein deficiency, Tangier disease. [G. *an-* priv. + *alpha*, α, + lipoprotein + *-emia*, sangue]
anal·y·sand (ă-nal′i-sand). Analisando; em psicanálise, a pessoa que está sendo analisada. [analysis + L. *-andus*, terminação do gerúndio]
anal·y·sis, pl. **anal·y·ses** (ă-nal′i-sis, -sēz). Análise. **1.** A decomposição de um composto ou mistura química nos elementos mais simples; um processo pelo qual se determina a composição de uma substância. **2.** O exame e estudo de um todo em relação às partes que o compõem. **3.** VER psychoanalysis. [G. uma decomposição, de *ana*, para cima, + *lysis*, uma liberação]
accumulation a., a. por acúmulo; uma técnica em que um intermediário de uma via metabólica se acumula devido à inibição seletiva de determinada etapa nessa via ou em um mutante que está deficiente de certa etapa. Então, o intermediário é isolado, analisado e identificado.
activation a., a. por ativação; a identificação e quantificação de elementos desconhecidos a partir de suas emissões características e constantes de decaimento depois que eles se tornaram radioativos através da exposição à radiação com nêutron ou partícula carregada.
amino acid a., a. de aminoácido; **(1)** determinação e identificação do conteúdo de aminoácidos de uma macromolécula; **(2)** identificação de um aminoácido específico em macromoléculas, freqüentemente uma proteína que sofreu mutação; **(3)** identificação e quantificação do conteúdo de aminoácidos no plasma sanguíneo ou urina; um auxiliar diagnóstico importante.
bite a., a. de mordida. SIN occlusal a.
blood gas a., a. de gases sanguíneos; a medição direta por eletrodo da pressão parcial de oxigênio e de gás carbônico no sangue.
bradykinetic a., a. bradicinética; a a. do movimento por meio de cinematografia lenta.
breath a., a. respiratória. SIN breath *test.*
cephalometric a., a. cefalométrica; um estudo das relações do esqueleto e dentárias utilizado na a. de caso ortodôntica.
character a., a. de caráter; a. das defesas e traços de personalidade que caracterizam o indivíduo.
cluster a., a. de conjunto; um grupo de métodos estatísticos empregado para agrupar variáveis ou observações em subgrupos fortemente inter-relacionados.
content a., a. de conteúdo; qualquer uma das diversas técnicas para a classificação e estudo dos produtos verbais de indivíduos normais e psicologicamente incapacitados.
decision a., a. de decisão; um derivado de pesquisa de operações e teoria de jogos que envolve a identificação de todas as opções disponíveis e os resultados potenciais de cada uma delas, em uma série de decisões que têm de ser tomadas sobre o cuidado do paciente — procedimentos diagnósticos, esquemas terapêuticos, expectativas de prognóstico; a faixa de opções pode ser plotada em um fluxograma de decisão.
didactic a., a. didática. SIN training a.
discriminant a., a. discriminativa; uma técnica analítica estatística utilizada com variáveis dependentes discretas, preocupadas com a separação de grupos dos valores observados e na alocação de novos valores; uma alternativa para a análise de regressão.
displacement a., a. de deslocamento. SIN competitive binding *assay.*
distributive a., a. distributiva; a a. das informações obtidas sobre o paciente e sua distribuição pelo médico, como indicado pela queixa e sintomas do paciente.
Downs a., a. de Down; uma série de critérios cefalométricos empregados como auxílio no diagnóstico ortodôntico.
ego a., a. do ego; estudo psicoanalítico dos modos pelos quais o ego lida com os conflitos intrapsíquicos.
Fourier a., a. de Fourier; uma aproximação matemática de uma função como o somatório das funções periódicas (ondas de seno e/ou cosseno) de diferentes freqüências; um método para converter uma função do tempo ou espaço em uma função de freqüência; usada na reconstrução de imagens na tomografia computadorizada e no imageamento por ressonância magnética em radiologia e na análise de qualquer tipo de sinal quanto ao seu conteúdo de freqüência. SIN Fourier transfer, Fourier transform.
gastric a., a. gástrica; medição do pH e do débito ácido do conteúdo gástrico; o débito ácido basal pode ser determinado ao se coletar a secreção gástrica durante toda a noite ou por meio de uma coleta por 1 hora; o débito ácido máximo é determinado após a injeção de histamina; o débito é medido pela titulação com uma base forte.
intention-to-treat a., a. da intenção de tratar; método para analisar os resultados de um estudo controlado randomizado que inclui na a. todos os casos que deviam ter recebido um esquema terapêutico, mas que, por qualquer motivo, não o receberam. Todos os casos alocados em cada ramo do estudo são analisados em conjunto, como representativos desse braço de tratamento, quer tenham ou não recebido ou completado o regime prescrito.
interaction process a., a. do processo de interação; em psicologia, a a. do comportamento de um pequeno grupo em relação a 12 categorias específicas, p.ex., solidariedade, liberação de tensão, concordância.
Kaplan-Meier a., a. de Kaplan-Meier; um método para calcular a sobrevida de uma população de pacientes em que os aumentos constituem os tempos de sobrevida reais dos pacientes.
linkage a., a. de vinculação; a avaliação das relações de vinculação entre dois *loci* pelo exame dos dados nos heredogramas. A preocupação clássica refere-se à estimativa das frações de recombinação e (por causa de sua elasticidade, eficiência e outras propriedades ótimas) o método preferido é a estimativa de probabilidade máxima. Entretanto, existem outras preocupações mais recentes, notadamente a determinação da ordem dos *loci*, testes para as propriedades aditivas e interativas na função de mapeamento e a reconciliação dos dados do heredograma com as evidências de outros métodos (p.ex., citogenética, exames de hibridização *in situ*, etc.)
Northern blot a., a. da mancha do Norte; um procedimento similar à Southern blot a., usado para separar e identificar fragmentos de RNA; tipicamente, por meio da transferência de fragmentos de RNA de um gel de agarose para um filtro de nitrocelulose, seguido pela detecção com uma sonda adequada. [cunhado para diferenciá-lo do epônimo Southern blot a.]
occlusal a., a. oclusal; um estudo das relações das superfícies oclusais de dentes opostos e seus efeitos sobre as estruturas correlatas. SIN bite a.
path a., a. de trajetória; uma modalidade de a. que envolve as suposições a respeito da direção das relações causais entre seqüências ligadas e as configurações das variáveis.
pedigree a., a. de heredograma; o estudo formal do padrão de um traço em um heredograma para determinar certas propriedades, como seu modo de herança, idade no estabelecimento e variabilidade no fenótipo.
percept a., a. de percepção; análise psicológica da personalidade de um indivíduo empregando a série de manchas de Rorschach.
qualitative a., a. qualitativa; a determinação da natureza, em oposição à quantidade, de cada um dos elementos que compõem uma substância.
quantitative a., a. quantitativa; a determinação da quantidade, bem como da natureza, de cada um dos elementos que compõem uma substância.
regression a., a. de regressão; o método estatístico para encontrar o "melhor" modelo matemático para descrever uma variável como função de outra.
saturation a., a. de saturação. SIN competitive binding *assay.*
segregation a., a de segregação; em genética, a enumeração da progênie de acordo com fenótipos distintos e mutuamente exclusivos; usada como um teste de um suposto padrão de herança, p.ex., mendeliana, autossômica dominante, epistática, idade-dependente.
sequential a., a seqüencial; um método estatístico que permite que uma experiência seja terminada logo que se obtenha um resultado com a precisão desejada.
Southern blot a., a. de Southern blot; um procedimento para separar e identi-

ficar seqüências de DNA; os fragmentos de DNA são separados por eletroforese em um gel de agarose, transferidos (*blotted*) para uma membrana de nitrocelulose ou náilon, e hibridizados com sondas de ácido nucleico complementar (marcado).

survival a., a. de sobrevida; uma classe de procedimentos estatísticos para estimar as taxas de sobrevida e tirar as conclusões sobre os efeitos do tratamento, fatores prognósticos, etc.

training a., a. de treinamento; tratamento psicanalítico com o objetivo de treinar um candidato a analista, realizado sob os auspícios oficiais de uma instituição de treinamento psicanalítico. SIN didactic a.

transactional a., a. transacional; um sistema de psicoterapia, usado no tratamento individual ou em grupo, envolvendo uma compreensão sistemática das qualidades das interações interpessoais nas sessões de tratamento; inclui quatro componentes: 1) análise estrutural dos fenômenos intrapsíquicos; 2) a própria a. transacional, que consiste na determinação do ego atualmente dominante (pai, filho ou adulto) de cada participante; 3) análise de jogos, que consiste na identificação dos jogos efetuados em suas interações e das gratificações recebidas; 4) análise do *script*, que é a revelação das causas dos problemas emocionais do paciente.

a. of variance (ANOVA), a. de variância; uma técnica estatística que isola e avalia a contribuição de variáveis de categoria independentes para a variação na média de uma variável dependente contínua.

volumetric a., a. volumétrica; a. quantitativa pela adição de quantidades graduadas de uma solução de teste padronizada a uma solução de uma quantidade conhecida da substância analisada, até que a reação esteja exatamente no fim; depende da natureza estoiquiométrica da reação entre a solução de teste e a desconhecida.

Western blot a., a. de Western blot; um procedimento em que as proteínas, separadas por eletroforese em gel de poliacrilamida, são transferidas (*blotted*) para membranas de nitrocelulose ou náilon e são identificadas por formarem complexos específicos com anticorpos que são pré- ou pós-marcados com uma proteína secundária marcada. VER TAMBÉM immunoblot. SIN Western blot, Western blotting. [cunhado para diferenciá-lo do epônimo Southern blot a.]

zoo blot a., a. de zoo blot; um procedimento que emprega a a. de Southern blot para testar a capacidade de uma amostra de ácido nucleico de uma espécie de sofrer hibridização com o fragmento de DNA de outra espécie.

an·a·lyst (an′ă-list). Analista. 1. Aquele que faz determinações analíticas. 2. Termo abreviado para psicanalista.

an·a·lyte (an′ă-līt). Analisado; qualquer substância química ou material sujeito a análise.

an·a·lyt·ic, an·a·lyt·i·cal (an-ă-lit′-ik, -i-kăl). Analítico. 1. Relativo à análise. 2. Relativo à psicanálise.

an·a·lyz·er, an·a·lyz·or (an′ă-līz-er, -ŏr). Analisador. 1. Qualquer instrumento que realize uma análise. 2. O prisma, em um polariscópio, através do qual se examina a luz polarizada. 3. A base neural do reflexo condicionado; inclui a totalidade do lado sensorial do arco reflexo e suas conexões centrais. 4. Um aparelho que determina eletronicamente a freqüência e a amplitude de um determinado canal de um eletroencefalograma.

batch a., a. de lote; um pequeno a. químico automático em que o sistema do instrumento realiza, de maneira seqüencial, um único teste em cada um dos componentes de um grupo de amostras.

centrifugal fast a., a. de centrifugação; um espectrofotômetro automático que emprega a força centrífuga para misturar amostras e reagentes, e impulsiona os reagentes em alta velocidade diante de um detector que faz múltiplas leituras de absorção.

continuous flow a., a. de fluxo contínuo; um a. químico automático em que as amostras e reagentes são continuamente bombeados através de um sistema de módulos interligados por tubos.

discrete a., a. descontínuo; um a. químico automático em que o instrumento realiza os testes em amostras que são mantidas em recipientes separados, em contraste com um analisador de fluxo contínuo.

kinetic a., a. cinética; um instrumento que mede a taxa de alteração em uma substância química; usada principalmente para a medição enzimática.

pulse height a., a. da altura de pulso; circuito eletrônico que determina a energia das cintilações registradas por um detector, possibilitando o uso de um discriminador para selecionar os fótons de um tipo específico.

wave a., a. de ondas; um aparelho que avalia uma mistura complexa de formas de onda através da separação de suas freqüências componentes e da demonstração de sua distribuição.

an·am·ne·sis (an-am-nē′sis). 1. Anamnese, anamnesia; o ato de relembrar. 2. Anamnese; a história médica ou de desenvolvimento de um paciente. [G. *anamnēsis*, lembrança]

an·am·nes·tic (an-am-nes′tik). Anamnéstico, anamnésico. 1. Auxiliar a memória. SIN mnemonic. 2. Relativo à história médica de um paciente.

an·am·ni·on·ic, an·am·ni·ot·ic (an-am-nē-on′ik, -ot′ik). Anamniônico, anamniótico; sem um âmnio.

An·am·ni·o·ta (an-am-nē-ō′tă). Um grupo de vertebrados cujos embriões não ficam envoltos em um âmnio; inclui os ciclóstomos, peixes e anfíbios.

an·a·morph. Anamorfo; uma estrutura somática ou reprodutora que se origina sem recombinação nuclear (reprodução assexuada); a parte imperfeita do ciclo de vida dos fungos. [G. *ana*, para cima, + *morphē*, forma]

an·a·mor·pho·sis (an′ă-mōr-fō′sis). Anamorfose. 1. Em filogenia, uma série progressiva de alterações na evolução de um grupo de animais ou vegetais. 2. Em óptica, o processo de correção de uma imagem distorcida com um espelho curvo. [G. *ana*, para cima + *morphē*, forma]

an·an·a·sta·sia (an′an-ă-stā′zē-ă). Ananastasia; incapacidade de se levantar. [G. *a*-, priv. + *anastasis*, levantar]

an·an·casm (an′an-kazm). Anancasma; qualquer forma de comportamento estereotipado repetitivo que, quando evitado, resulta em ansiedade. [G. *anankasma*, compulsão]

an·an·cas·tia (an-an-kas′tē-ă). Anancastia; obsessão em que uma pessoa se sente forçada a agir ou pensar contra sua vontade. [G. *anankastos*, compelido]

an·an·cas·tic (an-an-kas′tik). Anancástico; pertinente ao anancasma ou anancastia.

an·an·dria (an-an′drē-ă). Anandria; ausência de masculinidade. [G. falta de virilidade, de *an*- priv. + *anēr*- (*andr*-), homem]

an·an·gi·o·pla·sia (an-an′jē-ō-plā′zē-ă). Anangioplasia; vascularização imperfeita de uma região devido a não-formação de vasos ou de vasos com diâmetro inadequado. [G. *an*- priv. + *ageion*, vaso + *plastos*, formado]

an·an·gi·o·plas·tic (an-an′jē-ō-plas′tik). Anangioplásico; relativo a, caracterizado por ou decorrente de anangioplasia.

ANAP Abreviatura de anionic neutrophil-activating *peptide* (peptídeo ativador de neutrófilos aniônico).

an·a·phase (an′ă-fāz). Anáfase; o estágio da mitose ou meiose em que os cromossomas se movem da placa equatorial para os pólos da célula. Na mitose, um conjunto completo de cromossomas (46 nos seres humanos) desloca-se no sentido de cada pólo. Na primeira divisão da meiose, cada membro de cada par homólogo (23 nos seres humanos), consistindo em duas cromátides unidas no centrômero, desloca-se no sentido de cada pólo. Na segunda divisão da meiose, o centrômero sofre divisão e as duas cromátides separam-se, cada uma se deslocando para cada pólo. [G. *ana*, para cima + *phasis*, aparência]

an·a·phia (an-ā′fē-ă, an-af′ē-ă). Anafia; ausência da sensação do tato. SIN anhaphia. [G. *an*- priv. + *haphē*, tato]

an·a·pho·re·sis (an′ă-fō-rē′sis). Anaforese; movimento de partículas com cargas elétricas negativas (ânions) em uma solução ou suspensão no sentido do anodo na eletroforese. Cf. cataphoresis. [G. *ana*-, para cima + *phorēsis*, transportado]

an·aph·o·ret·ic (an′ă-fō-ret′ik). Anaforético; relativo à anaforese (1).

an·aph·ro·di·si·ac (an′af-rō-diz′ē-ak). Anafrodisíaco. 1. Relativo à anafrodisia. 2. Que reprime ou destrói o desejo sexual. 3. Um agente que diminui ou abole o desejo sexual. SIN antaphrodisiac, anthaphroditic (1). [G. *an*- priv + *aphrodisia*, prazer sexual]

an·a·phy·lac·tic (an′ă-fi-lak′tik). Anafilático; relativo à anafilaxia; que manifesta sensibilidade muito grande à proteína não-própria ou a outro material.

an·a·phy·lac·to·gen (an′ă-fi-lak′tō-jen). Anafilactógeno; uma substância (antígeno) capaz de tornar um indivíduo suscetível à anafilaxia; uma substância (antígeno) que provocará uma reação anafilática em um indivíduo sensível a ela.

an·a·phy·lac·to·gen·e·sis (an′ă-fi-lak-tō-jen′ĕ-sis). Anafilactogênese; a produção de anafilaxia.

an·a·phy·lac·to·gen·ic (an′ă-fi-lak-tō-jen′ik). Anafilactogênico; que produz anafilaxia; pertinente às substâncias (antígenos) que fazem com que um indivíduo se torne suscetível à anafilaxia.

an·a·phy·lac·toid (an′ă-fi-lak′toyd). Anafilactóide; que se assemelha à anafilaxia. SIN pseudoanaphylactic. [anaphylaxis + G. *eidos*, semelhança]

an·a·phyl·a·tox·in (an′ă-fil-ă-tok′sin). Anafilatoxina; substâncias de baixo peso molecular produzidas pela ativação do complemento; os componentes biologicamente ativos do complemento derivam de C3, C4 e C5 e levam a aumento da permeabilidade vascular em conseqüência da desgranulação principalmente dos mastócitos; a liberação de mediadores de hipersensibilidade imediata (Tipo I), isto é, histamina, ocorre após a desgranulação dos mastócitos. SIN anaphylotoxin. [anaphylaxis + toxin]

an·a·phyl·a·tox·in in·ac·ti·va·tor. Inativador da anafilatoxina; uma α-globulina (PM 300.000) que destrói a atividade de fragmentos anafilatóxicos do complemento. VER anaphylatoxin.

an·a·phy·lax·is (an′ă-fi-lak′sis). Anafilaxia; sensibilidade sistêmica ou generalizada induzida; por vezes, o termo a. é empregado para o choque anafilático. O termo é comumente utilizado para indicar o tipo imediato e transitório de reação imunológica (alérgica), caracterizada por contração dos músculos lisos e dilatação dos capilares em decorrência da liberação de substâncias farmacologicamente ativas (histamina, bradicinina, serotonina e substância de reação lenta), classicamente iniciada pela combinação do antígeno (alérgeno) com o anticorpo citofílico (principalmente IgE) fixado ao mastócito; a reação pode ser iniciada, também, por quantidades relativamente grandes de agrega-

anaphylaxis

dos séricos (complexos antígeno-anticorpo e outros) que, aparentemente, ativam o complemento, levando à produção de anafilatoxinas. SIN anaphylactic reaction. [G. *ana*, caminho de, de volta para + *phylaxis*, proteção]

active a., a. ativa; reação que ocorre após a inoculação do antígeno em uma pessoa previamente sensibilizada para o antígeno específico, em contraste com a passive a.

aggregate a., a. agregada; uma reação anafilática iniciada pela formação de complexos antígeno-anticorpo que ativam o complemento.

antiserum a., a. passiva. SIN passive a.

chronic a., a. crônica. SIN *enteritis* anaphylactica.

generalized a., a. generalizada; a resposta imediata, envolvendo os músculos lisos e capilares por todo o organismo de uma pessoa sensibilizada, que sucede à injeção intravenosa (e, ocasionalmente, intracutânea) do antígeno (alérgeno). VER TAMBÉM anaphylactic *shock*. SIN systemic a.

inverse a., a. inversa; choque anafilático em um animal (p.ex., cobaia), cujos tecidos contêm o antígeno de Forssman, resultante de uma injeção intravenosa do soro que contém o anticorpo de Forssman.

local a., a. local; o tipo imediato e transitório de resposta que sucede à injeção de antígeno (alérgeno) na pele de uma pessoa sensibilizada e que se limita à área circunvizinha do sítio de inoculação. VER TAMBÉM skin *test*.

passive a., a. passiva; uma reação resultante da inoculação do antígeno em um animal previamente inoculado por via intravenosa com o anti-soro específico obtido de outro animal, havendo necessidade de um período latente entre as duas inoculações. SIN antiserum a.

passive cutaneous a. (PCA), a. cutânea passiva; uma reação que acontece em cobaias, quando o anti-soro é injetado na pele e, 6 a 24 horas depois, o antígeno específico e um corante, como o azul de Pontamina ou o azul de Evans, são inoculados por via intravenosa; o tamanho das áreas azuladas nos locais das injeções de anticorpo constitui uma medida do grau de alteração de permeabilidade para a albumina ligada ao corante.

reversed a., a. passiva reversa. SIN reversed passive a.

reversed passive a., a. passiva reversa; uma reação anafilática induzida em um animal injetado com um antígeno específico, o qual se ligará ao tecido reativo e, em seguida, depois de um período de latência, com o soro de outro animal previamente sensibilizado para o mesmo antígeno. SIN reversed a.

systemic a., a. sistêmica. SIN generalized a.

an·a·phyl·o·tox·in (an′ă-fil-ō-tok′sin). Anafilotoxina. SIN anaphylatoxin.

an·a·pla·sia (an-ă-plā′sē-ă). Anaplasia; perda da diferenciação estrutural, observada principalmente na maioria das neoplasias malignas, porém não em todas. SIN dedifferentiation (2). [G. *ana*, novamente + *plasis*, uma modelagem]

an·a·plas·tic (an-ă-plas′tik). Anaplástico. **1.** Relativo à anaplasia. **2.** Caracterizado por ou pertinente à anaplasia. **3.** Que cresce sem forma ou estrutura.

an·a·plas·to·lo·gy (an′ă-plas-tol′ō-jē). Anaplastologia; aplicação de materiais protéticos para a construção e/ou reconstrução de uma parte ausente do corpo. [G. *ana*, novamente + *plastos*, formado]

an·a·ple·ro·sis (an′ă-pler-ō′sis). Anaplerose; o processo de reposição de intermediários depletados do ciclo ou via metabólica; refere-se, mais amiúde, ao ciclo do ácido tricarboxílico. [G. enchimento, de *ana-*, para cima + *plerosis*, enchimento, de *pleroō*, encher]

an·a·ple·rot·ic (an′ă-pler-ō′tik). Anaplerótico; que se refere às reações ou vias que contribuem para a anaplerose.

an·a·poph·y·sis (an-ă-pof′i-sis). Anapófise; um processo espinal acessório de uma vértebra, encontrado principalmente nas vértebras torácicas ou lombares. [G. *ana*, atrás + *apophysis*, broto]

anap·tic (ă-nap′tik). Anáptico; relativo à anafia.

an·a·rith·mia (an-ă-rith′mē-ă). Anarritmia; afasia caracterizada por incapacidade de contar ou usar números. [G. *an-* priv. + *arithmos*, número]

an·ar·thria (an-ar′thrē-a). Anartria; perda do poder da fala articulada. VER TAMBÉM aphasia, alexia, dysarthria. [G. de *an-anthos*, sem articulações; (de som) inarticulado]

an·a·sar·ca (an-ă-sar′kă). Anasarca; infiltração generalizada de líquido de edema no tecido conjuntivo subcutâneo. SIN hydrosarca. [G. *ana*, através de, + *sarx (sark-)*, carne]

fetoplacental a., a. fetoplacentária; edema do feto e da placenta, como aquele encontrado na hidropisia fetal.

an·a·sar·cous (an-ă-sar′kŭs). Anasarco, anasárcico; caracterizado por anasarca.

an·a·stig·mat·ic (an′as-tig-mat′ik). Anastigmático; não-astigmata.

an·as·tig·mats. Anastigmata. **1.** Lente com a qual o astigmatismo é corrigido. **2.** Lente com a qual o astigmatismo e a curvatura do campo são corrigidos.

an·as·to·le (an-as′tō-lē). Anástole; termo obsoleto para a abertura de uma ferida. [G. *anastole*, as bordas expostas de uma ferida]

anas·to·mose (ă-nas′tō-mōs). Anastomosar. **1.** Abrir uma estrutura diretamente dentro da outra ou conectando canais, com referência a vasos sanguíneos, linfáticos e vísceras ocas; também incorretamente aplicado a nervos. **2.** Unir, por meio de uma anastomose ou conexão, estruturas originalmente separadas.

anas·to·mo·sis, pl. **anas·to·mo·ses** (ă-nas′tō-mō′sis, -sez). Anastomose, anastomoses. **1.** Uma comunicação natural, direta ou indireta, entre dois vasos sanguíneos ou outras estruturas tubulares. VER communication. **2.** Uma união cirúrgica de duas estruturas (p.ex., vasos, ureteres, nervos). **3.** Uma abertura, criada por cirurgia, traumatismo ou doença, entre dois ou mais órgãos ou espaços normalmente separados. [G. *anastomōsis*, de *anastomoō*, prover com uma abertura]

acromial a. of the thoracoacromial artery [TA], a. acromial da artéria toracoacromial; uma rede vascular entre o acrômio e a pele do ombro, formada por anastomoses do ramo acromial da artéria supra-escapular com o ramo acromial da artéria toracoacromial. SIN rete acromiale arteriae thoracoacromialis [TA], acromial arterial network, acromial plexus.

arteriolovenular a. [TA], a. arteriolovenular; vasos através dos quais o sangue é desviado das arteríolas para as vênulas, sem passar pelos capilares. O termo "a. arteriovenosa" é amplamente utilizado, mas não é a forma preferida, pois a conexão se faz entre as arteríolas e vênulas, em vez de artérias e veias. SIN a. arteriolovenularis*, a. arteriovenosa, arteriovenous a.

a. arteriolovenularis, a. arteriolovenular; *termo alternativo oficial para arteriolovenular a.

a. arteriovenoʼsa, a. arteriovenosa. SIN arteriolovenular a.

arteriovenous a. (ava), a. arteriovenosa. SIN arteriolovenular a.

Béclard a., a. de Béclard. SIN ranine a.

bevelled a., a. em bisel; a. realizada após cortar cada uma das estruturas a ser unida de maneira oblíqua.

Billroth I a., a. à Billroth I; restabelecimento da continuidade intestinal por uma gastroduodenostomia. VER TAMBÉM Billroth *operation* I.

Billroth II a., a. à Billroth II; restabelecimento da continuidade intestinal por meio de uma gastrojejunostomia em alça. VER TAMBÉM Billroth *operation* II.

Braun a., a. de Braun; depois de uma gastrenterostomia, a a. entre as alças aferente e eferente do jejuno.

calcaneal a. [TA], a. do calcâneo; uma rede superficial sobre o calcâneo, formada por ramos das artérias fibular e tibial posterior e ramificações da rede maleolar. SIN rete calcaneum [TA], calcaneal arterial network.

cavopulmonary a., a. cavopulmonar; um meio de aliviar a cardiopatia cianótica através da anastomose da artéria pulmonar direita com a veia cava superior. SIN cavopulmonary shunt, Glenn shunt.

Clado a., a. de Clado; a. no ligamento levantador direito do ovário, entre as artérias apendicular e ovariana.

conjoined a., a. conjugada; reunião de dois pequenos vasos sanguíneos por meio de a. elíptica látero-lateral para criar um único estoma maior para posterior anastomose término-terminal.

cruciate a., crucial a., a. crucial; uma a. de quatro componentes entre os ramos do primeiro ramo perfurante da artéria femoral profunda, artérias glútea inferior e femorais circunflexas medial e lateral, localizada atrás da parte superior do fêmur. Outrora descrita como habitual, as pesquisas mostram que ela raramente ocorre no padrão "cruzado" com quatro vias.

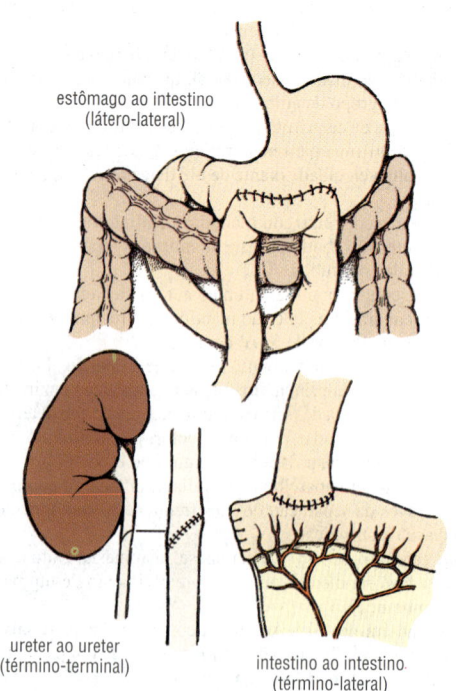

anastomoses cirúrgicas

cubital a. [TA], a. cubital; redes vasculares na região do cotovelo, compostas por anastomoses entre ramos das artérias radial e colateral média, colaterais ulnares superior e inferior, recorrente radial, recorrente interóssea e recorrente ulnar. SIN rete articulare cubiti [TA], articular vascular network of elbow.

Damus-Stancel-Kaye a., a. de Damus-Stancel-Kaye. SIN Damus-Kaye-Stancel *procedure*.

elliptical a., a. elíptica; uma modificação da a. direta pela qual uma ou ambas as estruturas tubulares são previamente espatuladas, criando, dessa maneira, uma elipse de maior corte transversal e de maior diâmetro do que a que seria possível com uma a. em bisel ou circular.

end-to-end a., a. término-terminal; a. realizada depois de cortar cada estrutura a ser unida em um plano perpendicular para ultimar o fluxo através das estruturas.

Galen a., a. de Galen. SIN communicating *branch* of internal laryngeal nerve with recurrent laryngeal nerve.

genicular a. [TA], a. genicular; uma rede arterial sobre as partes anterior e laterais do joelho, formada por ramos da artéria genicular descendente, das cinco artérias geniculares originárias da artéria poplítea, da artéria tibial anterior recorrente e de ramos circunflexos fibulares da tibial posterior. SIN rete articulare genus [TA], articular vascular network of knee.

Hofmeister-Pólya a., a. de Hofmeister-Pólya. VER Hofmeister *operation*, Pólya *operation*.

Hoyer anastomoses, anastomoses de Hoyer. SIN Sucquet-Hoyer *canals*, em *canal*.

Hyrtl a., a. de Hyrtl. VER Hyrtl *loop*.

intermesenteric arterial anastomoses, anastomoses arteriais intermesentéricas. SIN intestinal arterial *arcades*, em *arcade*.

intestinal a., a. intestinal. SIN enteroenterostomy.

isoperistaltic a., a. isoperistáltica; uma a. que permite o fluxo do conteúdo na mesma direção normal.

Jacobson a., a. de Jacobson; uma parte do plexo timpânico.

Martin-Gruber a., a. de Martin-Gruber; uma anomalia de nervos no antebraço, consistindo em uma comunicação entre os nervos mediano e ulnar; também referida como um cruzamento mediano-ulnar.

microvascular a., a. microvascular; a. de vasos sanguíneos muito pequenos realizada sob um microscópio cirúrgico.

patellar a. [TA], a. patelar; a porção superficial da rede vascular articular do joelho. SIN rete pattelare [TA], patellar network.

portacaval anastomoses, anastomoses portocavas. SIN portal-systemic anastomoses.

portal-systemic anastomoses, anastomoses portossistêmicas; **(1)** comunicações venosas naturais entre as tributárias do sistema venoso porta e as tributárias do sistema venoso sistêmico. As principais anastomoses portossistêmicas incluem: 1) ramos esofágicos da veia gástrica esquerda com as veias esofágicas; 2) veia retal superior com as veias retais média e inferior; 3) veias paraumbilicais com as veias subcutâneas da parede abdominal anterior; 4) veias retroperitoneais com os ramos venosos das veias do cólon e da área desnuda do fígado, e 5) um canal venoso permeável que une o ramo esquerdo da veia porta à veia cava inferior (raro). Essas anastomoses são clinicamente importantes, fornecendo a circulação colateral durante a obstrução ou hipertensão porta, embora elas possam tornar-se varicosas. VER *caput* medusae, esophageal *varices*, em *varix*, hemorrhoids; **(2)** comunicações criadas cirurgicamente, entre a veia porta e a veia cava inferior ou suas tributárias, para aliviar a hipertensão porta. SIN portacaval anastomoses.

postcostal a., a. pós-costal; a. longitudinal das artérias intersegmentares que origina a artéria vertebral.

Potts a., a. de Potts. SIN Potts *operation*.

precapillary a., a. pré-capilar; uma a. entre arteríolas exatamente antes que elas se transformem em capilares.

precostal a. (prē-kos′-tal). a. pré-costal; a. longitudinal das artérias intersegmentares no embrião que dá origem aos troncos tireocervical e costocervical.

pulmonary artery a., a. da artéria pulmonar; 40–50% estão associadas a defeitos cardíacos congênitos.

ranine a., a. da rânula; uma a. entre os ramos terminais direito e esquerdo da artéria lingual profunda. SIN arcus raninus, Béclard a.

Riolan a., a. de Riolan; a porção específica da artéria marginal do cólon que se une às artérias cólicas média e esquerda. SIN Ryolan arc (3).

Roux-en-Y a., a. em Y de Roux; a. da extremidade distal do jejuno dividido ao estômago, ducto biliar ou outra estrutura, com o implante da extremidade proximal na parte lateral do jejuno a uma distância adequada (geralmente > 40 cm) abaixo da primeira a., com o intestino formando, então, um padrão em Y.

Schmidel anastomoses, anastomoses de Schmidel; canais anormais de comunicação entre os sistemas venosos porta e cava.

sequential a., a. seqüencial; duas ou mais anastomoses criadas a partir de um único conduto, p.ex., duas ou mais artérias coronárias a partir de um único enxerto venoso ou da artéria mamária.

Sucquet anastomoses, anastomoses de Sucquet. SIN Sucquet-Hoyer *canals*, em *canal*.

Sucquet-Hoyer anastomoses, anastomoses de Sucquet-Hoyer. SIN Sucquet-Hoyer *canals*, em *canal*.

terminoterminal a., a. término-terminal; uma cirurgia em que a extremidade central de uma artéria é conectada à extremidade periférica da veia correspondente, e a extremidade periférica da artéria à extremidade central da veia.

transureteroureteral a., a. transureteroureteral. SIN transureteroureterostomy.

ureteroileal a., a. ureteroileal: a. entre o ureter e um segmento isolado do íleo. VER TAMBÉM Bricker *operation*.

ureterosigmoid a., a. ureterossigmóide; a. entre o ureter e um segmento ou todo o cólon sigmóide. VER TAMBÉM ureterosigmoidostomy.

ureteroureteral a., a. ureteroureteral; a. a partir de uma parte de um ureter com outra parte do mesmo ureter.

anas·to·mo·tic (a-nas-tō-mot′ik). Anastomótico; pertinente a uma anastomose.

an·as·tral (an-as′trăl). Anastral; que não tem uma astrosfera.

an·a·tom·i·cal (an′ă-tom′i-kăl). Anatômico. **1.** Relativo à anatomia. **2.** Estrutural. SIN structural. **3.** Indica um aspecto estritamente morfológico independentemente de suas considerações fisiológicas ou cirúrgicas, p.ex., colo anatômico do útero, espaço morto anatômico, lobulação anatômica do fígado.

an·a·tom·i·co·med·i·cal (an-ă-tom′i-kō-med′i-kăl). Anatomomédico; que se refere à medicina e à anatomia.

an·a·tom·i·co·path·o·log·ic (an-ă-tom′i-kō-path-ō-loj′i-kăl). Anatomopatológico; relativo à anatomia patológica.

an·a·tom·i·co·sur·gi·cal (an-ă-tom′i-kō-ser′ji-kăl). Anatomocirúrgico; relativo à anatomia cirúrgica.

an·a·tom·ic snuff·box (snŭf′boks). Tabaqueira anatômica; um oco observado na face radial do punho quando o polegar está totalmente estendido; é limitada, posteriormente, pelas proeminências do tendão do extensor longo do polegar e, anteriormente, dos tendões do extensor curto do polegar e abdutor longo do polegar. A artéria radial cruza o assoalho, que é formado pelos ossos escafóide e trapézio. SIN tabatière anatomique.

anat·o·mist (ă-nat′ō-mist). Anatomista; um especialista na ciência da anatomia.

anat·o·my (ă-nat′ō-mē) [TA]. Anatomia. **1.** A estrutura morfológica de um organismo. **2.** A ciência da morfologia ou estrutura dos organismos. **3.** SIN dissection. **4.** Um trabalho que descreve a forma e a estrutura de um organismo e suas várias partes. [G. *anatomē*, dissecção, de *ana*, separado + *tomē*, corte]

applied a., a. aplicada. SIN clinical a.

artificial a., a. artificial; a fabricação de modelos de estruturas anatômicas ou o estudo da a. a partir desses modelos.

artistic a., a. artística; o estudo da a. para fins artísticos, conforme aplicado na pintura, desenho ou escultura.

clastic a., a. clástica; a construção ou estudo de modelos em camadas, podendo estas ser removidas uma após outra para mostrar a estrutura do organismo e/ou órgão. SIN plastic a.

clinical a., a. clínica; a aplicação prática do conhecimento anatômico ao diagnóstico e tratamento. SIN applied a.

comparative a., a. comparada; o estudo comparativo da estrutura animal com relação a partes ou órgãos homólogos.

dental a., a. dentária; o ramo da a. macroscópica relacionado à morfologia dos dentes, suas localizações, posição e relações.

descriptive a., a. descritiva; uma descrição, em especial um tratado descritivo, da estrutura física, mais particularmente a do homem. SIN systematic a.

developmental a., a. do desenvolvimento; a. das alterações estruturais de um indivíduo, desde a fertilização até a vida adulta; inclui embriologia, fetologia e desenvolvimento pós-natal.

functional a., a. funcional; a. estudada em sua relação com a função. SIN morphophysiology, physiologic a.

general a., a. geral; o estudo das estruturas macroscópicas e microscópicas, bem como da composição do organismo, seus tecidos e líquidos.

gross a., a. macroscópica; a. geral, até onde ela possa ser estudada sem o emprego de um microscópio; comumente utilizada para indicar o estudo da a. através da dissecção de um cadáver. VER practical a. SIN macroscopic a.

living a., a. viva; o estudo da a. no ser vivo por meio da inspeção.

macroscopic a., a. macroscópica. SIN gross a.

medical a., a. clínica; a. em suas relações com o diagnóstico e tratamento das doenças.

microscopic a., a. microscópica; o ramo da a. em que a estrutura das células, tecidos e órgãos é estudada à microscopia óptica. VER histology.

pathological a., a. anatomopatológica. SIN anatomic *pathology*.

physiologic a., a. fisiológica. SIN functional a.

plastic a., a. plástica. SIN clastic a.

practical a., a. prática; a. estudada por meio de dissecção. VER gross a.

radiologic a., a. radiológica; o estudo da estrutura corpórea pelo uso de radiografias e outros métodos de imageamento.

regional a., a. regional; uma abordagem para o estudo anatômico com base

nas regiões, partes ou divisões do corpo (p.ex., o pé ou a região inguinal), enfatizando as relações entre as diversas estruturas sistêmicas (p.ex., músculos, nervos e artérias) dentro de uma área; distinto da a. sistêmica. SIN topographyc a., topology (1).
special a., a. especial; a a. de determinados órgãos ou grupos de órgãos definidos envolvidos na realização de funções especiais; a. descritiva que lida com os sistemas em separado.
surface a., a. de superfície; o estudo da configuração da superfície do corpo, especialmente em sua relação com as partes mais profundas.
surgical a., a. cirúrgica; a. aplicada em relação ao diagnóstico cirúrgico, dissecção ou tratamento.
systematic a., a. sistemática. SIN descriptive a.
systemic a., a. sistêmica; a. dos sistemas do corpo; uma conduta para o estudo anatômico organizado pelos sistemas corporais, p.ex., o sistema cardiovascular, enfatizando uma revisão do sistema por todo o corpo; diferenciada da a. regional.
topographic a., a. topográfica. SIN regional a.
transcendental a., a. transcendental; as teorias e deduções baseadas na morfologia dos órgãos e partes individuais do corpo.
ultrastructural a., a. ultra-estrutural; o estudo ultramicroscópico das estruturas muito pequenas para serem observadas à microscopia óptica.
anat·o·pism (ă-nat'ō-pizm). Anatopismo; falha em moldar-se ao padrão cultural. [G. *ana*, para trás + *topos*, local]
an·a·tox·ic (an-ă-tok'sik). Anatóxico; pertinente às propriedades características da anatoxina (toxóide).
an·a·tox·in (an-ă-tok'sin). Anatoxina; toxóide. SIN toxoid.
an·a·tri·crot·ic (an'ă-tri-krot'ik). Anatricrótico; caracterizado por anatricrotismo; indica um traçado esfigmográfico com três ondas no ramo ascendente.
an·a·tric·ro·tism (an'ă-trik'rō-tizm). Anatricrotismo; uma condição do pulso manifestada por um batimento triplo no ramo ascendente do traçado esfigmográfico. [G. *ana*, para cima + *tri*-, três, *krotos*, batimento]
an·a·trip·sis (an-ă-trip'sis). Anatripsia; uso terapêutico de atrito ou fricção, com ou sem aplicação simultânea de um medicamento. [G. um atrito, de *anatribō*, de *ana*, intenso + *tribō*, atritar]
an·a·trip·tic (an-ă-trip'tik). Anatríptico. 1. Pertinente à anatripsia. 2. Um remédio a ser aplicado por meio de atrito ou fricção.
an·ax·on, an·ax·one (an-aks'on, -aks'ōn). Anaxônio; que não possui axônio; indica determinadas células nervosas, primeiramente descritas por S. Ramón y Cajal como células amácrinas na retina, sendo posteriormente descobertas em várias regiões cerebrais. [G. *an*- priv. + *axōn*, eixo]
an·a·zo·tu·ria (an'az-ō-too'rē-ă). Anazotúria; deficiência ou carência de produtos metabólicos nitrogenados excretados na urina; relaciona-se especialmente a quantidades muito pequenas de uréia na urina. [G. *an*- priv. + azoturia]
ANCA Abreviatura para antineutrophil cytoplasmic *antibodies* (anticorpos contra o citoplasma de neutrófilos), em *antibody*.
AnCC Abreviatura para anodal closure *contraction* (contração de fechamento anódico).
an·ces·tor. Ancestral; uma pessoa na linha direta de ascendência da qual provém o paciente avaliado (pais, avós, etc.; mas não colaterais ou descendentes).
leading ancestor, ancestral principal; em genética, o aconselhamento fornecido a um consultado não-afetado, mas possivelmente portador da doença ou com a doença latente; o ancestral mais recente na linha direta de descendência conhecido como tendo tido o gene afetado em questão.
an·chor·age (ang'kŏr-ij). Ancoragem. 1. Fixação cirúrgica de órgãos abdominais ou pélvicos frouxos ou prolapsados. 2. A parte em que algo é preso. Em odontologia, um dente ou substituto dentário implantado no qual se prende uma dentadura parcial fixa ou removível, coroa ou restauração. 3. A natureza e o grau de resistência oferecidos ao deslocamento por uma unidade anatômica, quando usada com a finalidade de efetuar o movimento dentário. [L. *ancora*, de G. *ankyra*, âncora]
cervical a., a. cervical; a. em que a parte posterior do pescoço é usada para a resistência por meio de uma faixa cervical.
extraoral a., a. extra-oral; a. em que a unidade de resistência está fora da cavidade oral; p.ex., a. craniana, occipital ou cervical.
intermaxillary a., a. intermaxilar; a. em que as unidades em um maxilar são usadas para efetuar o movimento dentário no outro maxilar.
intramaxillary a., a. intramaxilar; a. em que as unidades de resistência situam-se, sem exceção, no mesmo maxilar.
intraoral a., a. intra-oral; a. em que as unidades de resistência localizam-se, sem exceção, dentro da cavidade oral.
multiple a., a. múltipla; a. em que mais de um tipo de unidade de resistência é utilizada. SIN reinforced a.
occipital a., a. occipital; a. em que o ápice e a parte posterior da cabeça são usados para a resistência por meio de um boné.
reciprocal a., a. recíproca; a. em que o movimento de um ou mais dentes é balanceado contra o movimento de um ou mais dentes opostos.
reinforced a., a. reforçada. SIN multiple a.
simple a., a. simples; a. em que a resistência ao movimento de um ou mais dentes origina-se unicamente da resistência ao movimento executado da unidade de a.
stationary a., a. estacionária; a. em que a resistência ao movimento de um ou mais dentes advém da resistência ao movimento corporal da unidade de a.; um conceito questionável, pois os dentes selecionados permanecem apenas relativamente estáveis.
an·chor·in (ang'kŏr-in). Ancorina. SIN ankyrin [anchor + -in]
an·chu·sin (an'koo-sin). Ancusina. SIN alkannin.
an·cil·lary (an'si-lār-ē). Servente, auxiliar, acessório ou secundário. [L. *ancillaris*, relacionado a um serviçal]
an·cip·i·tal, an·cip·i·tate, an·cip·i·tous (an-sip'i-tăl, -i-tāt, -i-tŭs). Ancipital; que tem duas cabeças; dois ramos. [L. *anceps*, duas cabeças]
an·con (ang'kŏn). Cotovelo. SIN elbow (2). [L. *ankon*, cotovelo]
an·co·nad (ang'kō-nad). Ancôneo; no sentido do cotovelo. [G. *ankōn*, cotovelo + L. *ad*, para]
an·co·nal, an·co·ne·al (ang'kō-năl, ang-kō'nē-ăl). Ancôneo. 1. Relativo ao cotovelo (ancon). 2. Relativo ao músculo ancôneo.
an·co·ne·us (ang-kō'nē-ŭs). Ancôneo. SIN anconeus *muscle*. [L.]
an·co·noid (ang'kō-noyd). Anconóide; que se assemelha ao cotovelo.
an·crod (an'krod). Uma fração obtida do veneno da serpente *Angkistrodon rhodostoma*, que contém uma enzima de clivagem do fibrinogênio; produz hipofibrinogenemia e diminuição da viscosidade do sangue total e do plasma para a melhoria das propriedades reológicas do sangue, sendo utilizada no tratamento da doença vascular periférica crônica.
△**ancylo-.** Ancilo-; VER ankylo-.
An·cy·los·to·ma (an-si-los'tō-mă, an-ki-). Ancilóstomo; um gênero de nematódeos, o ancilóstomo do Velho Mundo, cujos membros são parasitas no duodeno. Eles se fixam às vilosidades na mucosa, sugam o sangue e podem provocar um estado de anemia, principalmente nos casos de desnutrição. Os ovos são eliminados com as fezes e as larvas se desenvolvem no solo úmido para se transformarem em larvas de terceiro estágio (filariformes) infecciosas que penetram no corpo humano através da pele e, possivelmente, da água potável; elas migram pela corrente sanguínea até os alvéolos pulmonares, são transportadas até os brônquios e traquéia, engolidas e passam para o intestino, onde amadurecem. VER TAMBÉM ancylostomiasis, *Necator*. SIN *Ankylostoma* (1). [G. *ankylos*, curvado, com gancho + *stoma*, boca]
A. brazilien'se, uma espécie caracterizada por um par de dentes bucais ventrais, normalmente um parasita intestinal de cães e gatos, mas também encontrado em seres humanos como uma causa de larva migrans cutânea.
A. cani'num, uma espécie que possui três pares de dentes ventrais na cavidade oral; comum em cães, mas que também ocorre na pele humana como uma causa de larva migrans cutânea.
A. ceylan'icum, uma espécie encontrada no almiscareiro do Ceilão; raramente relatado a partir de seres humanos como um parasita intestinal no sudeste da Ásia.
A. duodena'le, o ancilóstomo de seres humanos do Velho Mundo, uma espécie disseminada nas áreas temperadas, em contraste com a distribuição mais tropical do ancilóstomo do Novo Mundo, *Necator americanus*, que é o único ancilóstomo encontrado nos Estados Unidos.
A. tubaeforme, uma espécie de nematódeo encontrada no gato; a larva migrans cutânea é observada nos seres humanos.
an·cy·lo·sto·mat·ic (an'si-lō-stō-mat'ik, an'ki-). Ancilostomático; que se refere aos ancilóstomos do gênero *Ancylostoma*.
an·cy·lo·sto·mi·a·sis (an'si-lō-stō-mī'ă-sis, an'ki-). Ancilostomíase; doença causada pelo nematódeo *Ancylostoma duodenale* e caracterizada por eosinofilia, anemia, emagrecimento, dispepsia e, em crianças com infestações crônicas graves, distensão do abdome com desenvolvimento físico e mental deficiente. SIN ankylostomiasis, intertropical hyphemia, tropical hyphemia, miner's disease (1), tunnel disease, uncinariasis.
cutaneous a., a. cutânea; larva migrans cutânea. SIN cutaneous *larva migrans*.
an·cy·roid (an'si-royd). Anciróide; com forma semelhante à de uma âncora ou gancho; indica o corno dos ventrículos laterais do cérebro e o processo coracóide da escápula. SIN ankyroid. [G. *ankyra*, âncora, + *eidos*, semelhança]
Andernach, Johann W. (Guenther von Andernach), médico alemão, 1505–1574. VER A. *ossicles*, em *ossicle*.
Anders, James Meschter, médico norte-americano, 1854–1936. VER A. *disease*.
Andersch, Carolus Samuel, anatomista alemão, 1732–1777. VER A. *ganglion, nerve*.
Andersen, Dorothy Hansine, pediatra norte-americana, 1901–1963. VER A. *disease*.
Anderson, Evelyn, médica norte-americana, *1899. VER A.-Collip *test*.
Anderson, James C., urologista britânico, *1899.
Anderson, Roger, cirurgião norte-americano, 1891–1971. VER A. *splint*; Roger A. pin fixation *appliance*.
an·di·ra (an-dī'ră). Andira; a casca de *Andira inermis*, uma árvore da família das leguminosas da América tropical, usada como emético, purgativo e anti-helmíntico. SIN cabbage tree, worm bark. [nome nativo da Índia Ocidental]

Andral, Gabriel, médico francês, 1797–1876. VER A. *decubitus*.
an·dre·nos·ter·one (an - drē - nos′ter - ōn). Andrenosterona; adrenosterona. SIN adrenosterone.
an·dri·at·rics, an·dri·a·try (an - dri - at′riks, - drī′ā - trē). Andriatria; ciência médica relacionada às doenças dos órgãos genitais masculinos e dos homens em geral. [G. *anēr*, um homem, + *iatreia*, tratamento médico]
andro-. Andro-; masculino. [G. *anēr, andros*, um ser humano do sexo masculino]
an·dro·gen (an′drō - jen). Androgênio; termo genérico para um agente, usualmente um hormônio (p.ex., androsterona, testosterona), que estimula a atividade dos órgãos sexuais masculinos acessórios, encoraja o desenvolvimento das características sexuais masculinas ou evita alterações nestas que sucedem à castração; os andrógenios naturais são esteróides, derivados do androstano. SIN testoid (2).
  adrenal a., a. supra-renal; qualquer hormônio androgênico com origem no córtex da supra-renal; p.ex., desidroepiandrosterona (e seu sulfato), androstenediona, 11β-hidroxiandrostenediona.
an·dro·gen·e·sis (an - drō - jen′e - sis). Androgênese; desenvolvimento na presença apenas dos cromossomas paternos. [andro + G. *genesis*, produção]
an·dro·gen·ic (an - drō - jen′ik). Androgênico; relativo a um androgênio; que possui efeito masculinizante. SIN testoid (1).
an·drog·e·nous (an - droj′e - nŭs). Andrógeno; que faz nascer predominantemente machos ou elementos masculinos.
an·drog·y·nism (an - droj′i - nizm). Androginismo. SIN female *pseudohermaphroditism*.
an·drog·y·noid (an - droj′i - noyd). Androginóide; um homem que se assemelha a uma mulher ou que possui caracteres femininos. [andro- + G. *gynē*, mulher, + *eidos*, semelhança]
an·drog·y·nous (an - droj′i - nŭs). Andrógino; pertinente à androginia.
an·drog·y·ny (an - droj′i - nē). Androginia. **1.** SIN female *pseudohermaphroditism.* **2.** Que possui características masculinas e femininas, como nas atitudes e comportamentos que contêm aspectos de papéis sexuais estereotipados, culturalmente sancionados, tanto no homem como na mulher. [andro- + G. *gynē*, mulher]
an·droid (an′droyd). Andróide. SIN andromorphous. [andro- + G. *eidos*, semelhança]
an·drol·o·gy (an - drol′ō - jē). Andrologia; o ramo da medicina ligado às doenças próprias do sexo masculino, principalmente infertilidade e disfunção sexual. SIN andro- + G. *logos*, tratar]
an·drom·e·do·tox·in (an - drom′e - dō - tok′sin). Andromedotoxina; um princípio ativo fortemente emético obtido de várias espécies de *Andromeda* e *Rhododendron* (família Ericaceae); é um veneno cardíaco que, primeiro, estimula e, em seguida, paralisa o vago; também paralisa as terminações nervosas motoras na musculatura estriada.
an·dro·mor·phus (an - drō - mōr′fŭs). Andróide; que possui a forma ou o biotipo masculino. SIN android. [andro- + G *morphē*, forma]
an·drop·a·thy (an - drop′ā - thē). Andropatia; qualquer doença, como a prostatite, peculiar ao sexo masculino. [andro- + G. *pathos*, sofrimento]
andropause. Andropausa; uma suposta diminuição na função das gônadas masculinas com o envelhecimento, análoga à menopausa.
an·dro·pho·bia (an - drō - fō′bē - ā). Androfobia; medo mórbido de homens ou do sexo masculino. [andro- + G. *phobos*, medo]
an·dro·stane (an′drō - stān). Androstano; o hidrocarboneto original dos esteróides androgênicos. Para a estrutura, veja steroids.
an·dro·stane·di·ol (an - drō - stān′dī - ol). Androstanediol; 5α-androstano-3β,17β-diol; um metabólito esteróide, do qual também são conhecidos isômeros 5β.
an·dro·stane·di·one (an - drō - stān′dī - ōn). Androstanediona; 5α-androstano-3,17-diona; um metabólito esteróide do qual também se conhece o isômero 5β. É um precursor da testosterona e da estrona. É secretado pelas suprarenais.
an·dro·stene (an′drō - stēn). Androsteno; androstano com uma ligação insaturada (isto é, –CH=CH–) na molécula.
an·dro·stene·di·ol (an - drō - stēn′dī - ol). Androstenediol; 5-androsteno-3β,17β-diol; um metabólito esteróide que difere do androstanediol por possuir uma dupla ligação entre C-5 e C-6.
an·dro·stene·di·one (an - drō - stēn′dī - ōn). Androstenediona; 4-androsteno-3,17-diona; androstanediona com uma dupla ligação entre C-4 e C-5; um esteróide androgênico cuja potência biológica é mais fraca do que a da testosterona; secretado pelos testículos, pelos ovários e pelo córtex da supra-renal.
androstenol. Androstenol; uma substância que é um suposto feromônio; é encontrada no suor do homem, onde é oxidada a androstenona. Nos testes, as mulheres gostam do odor almiscarado seco do androstenol, mas acham que a androstenona possui um odor químico desagradável, semelhante ao da urina; entretanto, as mulheres em fase de ovulação reagem de forma neutra.
an·dro·sten·o·lone (an - drō - stēn - ō - lōn). Androstenolona. SIN dehydro-3-epiandrosterone.
an·dros·ter·one (an - dros′ter - ōn). Androsterona; *cis*-androsterona; 3α-hidroxi-5α-androstan-17-ona; um metabólito esteróide, encontrado na urina masculina, que possui potência androgênica fraca. Formado no testículo a partir da progesterona.
an·ec·dot·al (ă - nek′dō - tal). Relato de experiências clínicas baseadas em casos individuais, em vez de uma pesquisa organizada com controles apropriados, etc. [G. *anekdota*, itens não-publicados, de *an*- priv. + *ekidomi*, publicar]
an·e·cho·ic (an - ē - kō′ik). Anecóico; a propriedade de ser isento de eco ou de aparecer sem ecos em uma imagem ultra-sonográfica; um cisto cheio de líquido claro mostra-se anecóico. VER transonic. SIN echo-free. [G. *an-*, priv. + echo + ic]
Anel, Dominique, cirurgião francês, 1679–1725. VER A. *method.*
an·e·lec·tro·ton·ic (an - ē - lek - trō - ton′ik). Aneletrotônico; relativo ao aneletrotônus.
an·e·lec·trot·o·nus (an′ē - lek - trot′ō - nŭs). Aneletrotônus; as alterações na excitabilidade e condutividade em uma célula nervosa ou muscular nas proximidades do anódio durante a passagem de uma corrente elétrica constante. [anelectrode + G. *tônus*, tensão]

ANEMIA

ane·mia (ă - nē′mē - ă). Anemia; qualquer condição na qual o número de eritrócitos por mm^3, a quantidade de hemoglobina em 100 ml de sangue e/ou o volume de eritrócitos concentrados por 100 ml de sangue estejam abaixo do normal; clinicamente, diz respeito, em geral, à concentração de material de transporte de oxigênio em um volume designado de sangue, em contraste com as quantidades totais, como na oligocitemia, oligocromemia e oligoemia (hipovolemia). A a. manifesta-se, com freqüência, por palidez da pele e das mucosas, dispnéia, palpitações cardíacas, sopros sistólicos suaves, letargia e fadiga. [G. *anaimia*, de *an*- priv. + *haima*, sangue]
  achlorhydric a., a. aclorídrica; uma forma de a. microcítica hipocrômica crônica associada à acloridria ou aquilia gástrica; observada com maior freqüência em mulheres da terceira à quinta década de vida. SIN Faber a., Faber syndrome.
  achrestic a., a. acrescente; uma forma de a. macrocítica progressiva crônica que pode ser fatal, na qual as alterações na medula óssea e no sangue circulante se assemelham muito àquelas da a. perniciosa, mas na qual existe apenas uma resposta transitória ou ausente à terapia com vitamina B$_{12}$; não se observam glossite, distúrbios gastrointestinais, doença do sistema nervoso central e pirexia, e há apenas discreto sangramento ou hemólise. [G. *a-*, priv. + *chrēsis*, uma utilização]
  acquired hemolytic a., a. hemolítica adquirida; a. aguda ou crônica, não-hereditária, associada a ou causada por fatores extracorpusculares, p.ex., determinados agentes infecciosos, substâncias químicas (inclusive auto-anticorpos ou agentes terapêuticos), queimaduras, materiais tóxicos provenientes de formas de vegetais superiores e animais.
  Addison a., a. de Addison; a. perniciosa. SIN pernicious a.
  addisonian a., a. addisoniana; a. perniciosa. SIN pernicious a.
  angiopathic hemolytic a., a. hemolítica angiopática; uma rara a. pós-parto de etiologia desconhecida associada a uremia e nefrosclerose; pode ser uma complicação rara após o uso de esteróides contraceptivos.
  aplastic a., a. aplásica; a. caracterizada por formação muito diminuída de eritrócitos e hemoglobina, usualmente associada a granulocitopenia e trombocitopenia pronunciadas, em conseqüência de medula óssea hipoplásica ou aplásica. SIN a. gravis, Ehrlich a.
  asiderotic a., a. asiderótica; clorose. SIN chlorosis.
  autoimmune hemolytic a., a. hemolítica auto-imune; **(1)** tipo crioanticorpo, causada por anticorpo hemaglutinante (usualmente da classe IgM) com atividade máxima a 4°C; e resultante de hemólise grave na doença da crioemaglutinina; **(2)** tipo anticorpo quente (que é o mais comum), a. hemolítica adquirida decorrente de auto-anticorpos séricos (usualmente da classe IgG), com atividade máxima a 37°C, que reagem com os eritrócitos do paciente; varia em gravidade, ocorre em todos os grupos etários de ambos os sexos e pode ser idiopática ou secundária a doença neoplásica, auto-imune ou a outra doença.
  Bartonella a., a. por *Bartonella*; a. que ocorre na infecção por *Bartonella bacilliformis* e caracterizada por uma a. febril aguda, com início rápido e elevada taxa de mortalidade. Ocorre na região central dos Andes, ao norte da América do Sul; o vetor é o mosquito flebótomo, *Lutzomyia*.
  Belgian Congo a., a. do Congo Belga. SIN kasai.
  Biermer a., a. de Biermer; a. perniciosa. SIN pernicious a.
  brickmaker's a., a. do oleiro; a. associada à ancilostomíase.
  chlorotic a., clorose. SIN chlorosis.
  congenital a., a. congênita; eritroblastose fetal. SIN *erythroblastosis fetalis.*
  congenital aplastic a., a. aplásica congênita; a. de Fanconi. SIN Fanconi a.
  congenital dyserythropoietic a., a. diseritropoética congênita; um grupo de

anemias caracterizado por eritropoese não-efetiva, multinuclearidade eritroblástica da medula óssea e hemocromatose secundária. Três tipos são descritos: **tipo I** [MIM224120], a. macrocítica megaloblástica com pontes de cromatina internucleares eritroblásticas; **tipo II,** [MIM*224100], a. normoblástica com eritroblastos multinucleados; **tipo III**, a. macrocítica com multinuclearidade eritroblástica e gigantoblastos [MIM*105600]. Tanto o tipo I como o tipo II são herdados de maneira autossômica recessiva, enquanto o tipo III tem herança autossômica dominante.

congenital hemolytic a., a. hemolítica congênita; destruição acelerada dos eritrócitos devido a um defeito hereditário, como na membrana na esferocitose hereditária.

congenital hypoplastic a. [MIM*205900], a. hipoplásica congênita; a. macrocítica que resulta de hipoplasia congênita da medula óssea, que é flagrantemente deficiente em precursores eritróides, enquanto outros elementos estão normais; a a. é progressiva e grave, mas as contagens de leucócitos e plaquetas se mostram normais ou pouco reduzidas; a sobrevida dos eritrócitos transfundidos é normal; anomalias congênitas menores são encontradas em alguns pacientes. Já foram descritas formas autossômicas dominante e recessiva, causadas por mutação no gene codificador da proteína ribossomial S19 (RBS19) no cromossoma 19q. SIN congenital nonregenerative a., Diamond-Blackfan a., Diamond-Blackfan syndrome, erythrogenesis imperfecta, familial hypoplastic a., pure red cell a.

congenital nonregenerative a., a. não-regenerativa congênita. SIN *congenital hypoplastic a.*

Cooley a., a. de Cooley. SIN *thalassemia major.*

cow milk a., a. do leite de vaca; a. que ocorre em lactentes alimentados com leite de vaca sem suplementação de ferro, atribuída à reação alérgica no trato intestinal que leva à perda de sangue e, daí, à deficiência de ferro.

deficiency a., a. por deficiência. SIN *nutritional a.*

Diamond-Blackfan a., a. de Diamond-Blackfan. SIN *congenital hipoplastic a.*

dilution a., a. por diluição. SIN *hydremia.*

dimorphic a., a. dimórfica; a. em que duas formas distintas de eritrócitos estão circulando.

diphyllobothrium a., uma rara forma de a. macrocítica associada à infestação por *Diphyllobothrium latum*, principalmente na Finlândia. SIN *fish tapeworm a.*

drepanocytic a., a. drepanocítica; a. falciforme. SIN *sickle cell a.*

dyshemopoietic a., a. disemopoética; qualquer a. que resulte da função defeituosa da medula óssea.

Ehrlich a., a. de Ehrlich. SIN *aplastic a.*

elliptocytary a. (ē-lip′tō-sī′tar-ē), a. eliptocitária; a. com eliptocitose; um grupo heterogêneo de anemias hereditárias que possuem em comum eritrócitos elípticos no esfregaço sanguíneo. O defeito pode consistir em disfunção ou deficiência de proteínas no esqueleto da membrana eritrocitária. SIN elliptocytotic a.

elliptocytotic a. (ē-lip′tō-sī-tot′ik), a. eliptocitótica. SIN *elliptocytary a.*

erythroblastic a., a. eritroblástica; a. caracterizada pela presença de numerosos eritrócitos nucleados (normoblastos e eritroblastos) no sangue periférico. Observada em neonatos com a. hemolítica, devido à iso-imunização, como aquela provocada por incompatibilidade Rh ou ABO. VER TAMBÉM *erythroblastosis* fetalis. SIN erythronormoblastica a.

erythronormoblastic a. (ē-rith′rō-nōr′mō-blast-ik), a. eritronormoblástica. SIN *erythroblastic a.*

essential a., a. essencial; termo obsoleto para a. perniciosa; também usado outrora para qualquer tipo de a. por mecanismo desconhecido.

Faber a., a. de Faber. SIN *achlorhydric a.*

false a., a. falsa. SIN *pseudoanemia.*

familial hypoplastic a., a. hipoplásica familial. SIN *congenital hypoplastic a.*

familial microcytic a. [MIM*206200], a. microcítica familial; um raro tipo de a. microcítica hipocrômica, autossômica recessiva, associada a um defeito no metabolismo do ferro caracterizado por ferro sérico alto, depósitos hepáticos de ferro e ausência de reservas de ferro coráveis na medula óssea.

familial pyridoxine-responsive a. [MIM*206000], a. familial responsiva à piridoxina; uma rara a. hipocrômica, autossômica recessiva; responsiva à piridoxina.

Fanconi a., a. de Fanconi; um tipo de a. refratária hereditária, caracterizado por pancitopenia, hipoplasia da medula óssea e anomalias congênitas, que ocorre em membros da mesma família (um traço autossômico recessivo em, pelo menos, cinco tipos não-alélicos [MIM*227650, 227660, 227645, 227646, 600901]); a a. é normocítica ou ligeiramente macrocítica, os macrócitos e as células-alvo podem ser encontrados no sangue circulante e a leucopenia geralmente se deve à neutropenia. As anomalias congênitas incluem baixa estatura; microcefalia; hipogenitalismo; estrabismo; anomalias dos polegares, rádios, rins e trato urinário; retardo mental; e microftalmia. SIN congenital aplastic a., congenital pancytopenia, Fanconi pancytopenia, Fanconi syndrome (1).

fish tapeworm a., a. associada a Diphyllobothrium latum. SIN *diphyllobothrium a.*

folic acid deficiency a., a. por deficiência de ácido fólico; a. devido à deficiência de ácido fólico, caracterizada por eritrócitos grandes (macrocitose) e presença de grandes núcleos nas células precursoras eritróides (megaloblastos) na medula óssea.

goat's milk a., a. do leite de cabra; a. nutricional em lactentes mantidos principalmente com leite de cabra, o qual é relativamente pobre em conteúdo de ferro.

a. gra'vis, a. grave. SIN *aplastic a.*

ground itch a., a. associada à ancilostomíase.

Heinz body a., a. do corpúsculo de Heinz. VER unstable hemoglobin hemolytic a.

ℹ️ **hemolytic a.,** a. hemolítica; qualquer a. decorrente de uma taxa aumentada de destruição eritrocitária.

hemolytic a. of newborn, a. hemolítica do recém-nascido. SIN *erythroblastosis fetalis.*

hemorrhagic a., a. hemorrágica; a. que resulta diretamente da perda de sangue.

hookworm a., a. ancilostomiásica; a. associada à infestação maciça por *Ancylostoma duodenale* ou *Necator americanus.*

hypochromic a., a. hipocrômica; a. caracterizada por diminuição na relação entre o peso da hemoglobina e o volume do eritrócito, isto é, a concentração de hemoglobina corpuscular média (CHCM) é menor que a normal; cada hemácia contém menos hemoglobina do que em condições ótimas e coram-se com menor intensidade.

hypochromic microcytic a., a. microcítica hipocrômica; a. causada por deficiência de ferro ou talassemia, caracterizando-se por volume corpuscular médio (VCM), hemoglobina corpuscular média (HCM) e concentração de hemoglobina corpuscular média (CHCM) menores que o normal.

hypoferric a., a. ferropriva. SIN *iron deficiency a.*

hypoplastic a., a. hipoplásica; a. não-regenerativa progressiva que resulta da medula óssea muito deprimida e funcionando de maneira inadequada; à medida que o processo persiste, pode ocorrer a a. aplásica.

infectious a., a. infecciosa; a. que se desenvolve como uma complicação da infecção; resulta provavelmente da formação deprimida e da curta sobrevida dos eritrócitos (hemácias) e do metabolismo anormal do ferro.

iron deficiency a., a. por deficiência de ferro; a. ferropriva; a. microcítica hipocrômica caracterizada por ferro sérico baixo, aumento da capacidade de fixação de ferro, ferritina sérica diminuída e diminuição das reservas medulares de ferro. SIN hypoferric a.

isochromic a., a. isocrômica. SIN *normochromic a.*

lead a., a. por chumbo; a. associada à intoxicação por chumbo; atribuída a um defeito na síntese da hemoglobina com base na falha do ferro de se combinar no anel porfirínico.

leukoerythroblastic a., a. leucoeritroblástica. SIN *leukoerythroblastosis.*

local a., a. localizada; a. decorrente de suprimento sanguíneo diminuído para uma região, como na oclusão de um vaso.

macrocytic a., a. macrocítica; qualquer a. em que o tamanho médio dos eritrócitos circulantes seja maior que o normal, isto é, o volume corpuscular médio (VCM) é ≥ 94 μm^3 (faixa normal, 82–92 μm^3), incluindo determinadas síndromes, como a a. perniciosa, espru, doença celíaca, a. macrocítica da gestação, a. da difilobotríase e outras. SIN megalocytic a.

macrocytic achylic a., a. aquílica macrocítica. SIN *pernicious a.*

macrocytic a. of pregnancy, a. macrocítica da gestação; a. que ocorre na gestação, relacionada à deficiência de folato e caracterizada por nível baixo de hemoglobina e número reduzido de eritrócitos, os quais são maiores que o normal (macrócitos).

macrocytic a. tropical, a. macrocítica tropical; a a. macrocítica megaloblástica do espru tropical.

malignant a., a. maligna. SIN *pernicious a.*

Marchiafava-Micheli a., a. de Marchiafava-Micheli. SIN *paroxysmal nocturnal hemoglobinuria.*

megaloblastic a., a. megaloblástica; qualquer a. em que exista um número predominante de eritroblastos megaloblásticos e relativamente poucos normoblastos entre as células eritróides hiperplásicas na medula óssea (como na a. perniciosa).

megalocytic a., a. megalocítica. SIN *macrocytic a.*

metaplastic a., a. metaplásica; a. perniciosa na qual os vários elementos formados no sangue estão alterados, p.ex., neutrófilos multissegmentados, incomumente grandes (macropolicitos), células mielóides imaturas, plaquetas bizarras.

microangiopathic hemolytic a., a. hemolítica microangiopática; hemólise decorrente da fragmentação intravascular de eritrócitos; pode ser causada por lesões microcirculatórias ou pela inserção de próteses cardíacas ou intravasculares.

ℹ️ **microcytic a.,** a. microcítica; qualquer a. em que o tamanho médio dos eritrócitos circulantes é menor que o normal, isto é, o volume corpuscular médio (VCM) é ≤ 80 μm^3 (faixa normal, 82–92 μm^3).

microdrepanocytic a., a. microdrepanocítica. SIN *sickle cell-thalassemia disease.*

milk a., a. do leite; um tipo de a. microcítica hipocrômica que resulta da deficiência de ferro, ocorrendo em lactentes que se alimentam de leite por um período muito longo.
mountain a., a. da montanha; termo por vezes utilizado para o mal das montanhas (transtorno relacionado às grandes altitudes).
myelophthisic a., myelopathic a., a. mieloftísica, a. mielopática, leucoeritroblastose. SIN leucoerythroblastosis.
neonatal a., a. neonatal; eritroblastose fetal. SIN *erythroblastosis* fetalis.
a. neonato'rum, a. neonatal; eritroblastose fetal. SIN *erythroblastosis* fetalis.
normochromic a., a. normocrômica; qualquer a. em que a concentração de hemoglobina nos eritrócitos está dentro da faixa de normalidade, isto é, a concentração de hemoglobina corpuscular média está entre 32 e 36%. SIN isochromic a.
normocytic a., a. normocítica; qualquer a. em que os eritrócitos têm tamanho normal, isto é, o volume corpuscular médio (VCM) varia de 82 a 92 μm^3.
nutritional a., a. nutricional; qualquer a. que resulte da deficiência dietética de materiais essenciais para a formação eritrocitária, p.ex., ferro, vitaminas (especialmente ácido fólico), proteína. SIN deficiency a.
nutritional macrocytic a., a. macrocítica nutricional; anemia macrocítica megaloblástica decorrente da deficiência de folato ou vitamina B_{12}.
osteosclerotic a., a. osteosclerótica; a. decorrente do comprometimento da eritropoese causado por osteosclerose.
ℹ **pernicious a.** [MIM*361000], uma a. progressiva crônica dos idosos (que ocorre mais amiúde durante a quinta década de vida e depois, raramente, antes de 30 anos de idade); devido à falha da absorção de vitamina B_{12}, resultante usualmente de um defeito no estômago acompanhado por atrofia de mucosa e associado à falta de secreção de fator "intrínseco"; caracterizada por dormência e formigamento, fraqueza e uma língua lisa e dolorosa, bem como por dispnéia após os esforços leves, desmaio, palidez da pele e das mucosas, anorexia, diarréia, perda de peso e febre; os exames laboratoriais comumente revelam contagens de eritrócitos muito diminuídas, níveis baixos de hemoglobina, numerosos eritrócitos macrocíticos com formato oval característico (índice de coloração maior que o normal, mas não verdadeiramente hipercrômico) e hipo- ou acloridria, em associação a um número predominante de megaloblastos e um número relativamente pequeno de normoblastos na medula óssea; a contagem de leucócitos no sangue periférico pode revelar valor menor que o normal, com linfocitose relativa e neutrófilos hipersegmentados; nível baixo de vitamina B_{12} é encontrado nos eritrócitos periféricos; a administração de vitamina B_{12} resulta em uma característica resposta de reticulócitos, alívio dos sintomas e aumento nos eritrócitos, desde que a a. perniciosa não esteja complicada por outra doença; a condição não é realmente "perniciosa" como ocorria antes da disponibilidade da terapia com vitamina B_{12}. Pelo menos duas formas autossômicas recessivas são conhecidas. Em uma, existe um defeito do fator intrínseco [MIM*26100] e, em outra, existe absorção defeituosa de vitamina B_{12} a partir do intestino [MIM*261100]. SIN Addison a., Addison-Biermer disease, addisonian a., Biermer a., Biermer disease, macrocytic achylic a., malignant a.
physiologic a., a. fisiológica; um termo obsoleto para a a. aparente causada por volume aumentado de líquido no sangue (hidratação excessiva).
polar a., a. polar; uma forma de a. por vezes observada nos nativos de climas temperados quando migram para regiões árticas ou antárticas.
posthemorrhagic a., a. pós-hemorrágica; a. aguda causada por perda de sangue bastante rápida e súbita, como por laceração traumática de um vaso relativamente grande, erosão de artéria em úlcera duodenal ou hemorragia em gravidez ectópica. SIN traumatic a.
primary erythroblastic a., a. eritroblástica primária. Talassemia major. SIN *thalassemia* major.
primary refractory a., a. refratária primária; qualquer uma de um grupo de condições anêmicas em que existe a. persistente, freqüentemente avançada, que não é tratada com sucesso por qualquer meio, exceto por transfusões de sangue, e que não está associada a outra doença primária.
pure red cell a., a. eritrocitária pura. SIN congenital hypoplastic a.
radiation a., a. por radiação; a. hipoplásica que, por vezes, ocorre depois de exposição aguda a radiação ionizante de alto nível ou exposição crônica a radiação ionizante de baixo nível.
refractory a., a. refratária; a. progressiva que não responde a outras formas de terapia diferente de transfusão. VER primary refractory a., secondary refractory a.
scorbutic a., a. do escorbuto; a. que ocorre em pacientes com escorbuto, geralmente causada por deficiência nutricional coincidente; p.ex., a "a. megaloblástica do escorbuto" é causada por deficiência concomitante de ácido fólico.
secondary refractory a., a. refratária secundária, qualquer a. persistente que só é tratada com sucesso por transfusões de sangue e que está associada a outra patologia.
ℹ **sickle cell a.** [MIM*141900], a. falciforme; a. autossômica recessiva caracterizada por eritrócitos com formato em crescente ou afoiçados e hemólise acelerada, decorrente da substituição de um único aminoácido (valina por ácido glutâmico) na sexta posição da cadeia β da hemoglobina, cujo gene está no cromossoma 11; os homozigotos afetados possuem 85 a 95% de Hb S e anemia grave, enquanto os heterozigotos (ditos como portadores do traço falciforme) possuem 40 a 45% de Hb S, com o restante sendo formado por hemoglobina A normal; a baixa pressão de oxigênio causa polimerização das cadeias β anormais, distorcendo, assim, a forma dos eritrócitos para a forma afoiçada. Os homozigotos desenvolvem episódios de "crise" de dor intensa decorrente de oclusões microvasculares, infartos ósseos, úlceras de perna e atrofia do baço associada a suscetibilidade aumentada às infecções bacterianas, em especial à pneumonia estreptocócica. Ocorre mais amiúde nos indivíduos de ascendência africana. SIN drepanocytic a., sickle cell disease, vasoocclusive crisis.
sideroblastic a., sideroachrestic a., a. sideroblástica; a. refratária caracterizada pela presença de sideroblastos na medula óssea.
slaty a., a. cinzenta; uma palidez acinzentada na intoxicação por acetanilida ou prata (argiria).
spastic a., a. espástica; a. local resultante da contração intrínseca não-transitória dos vasos arteriais que irrigam a região afetada.
spherocytic a., a. esferocítica. SIN hereditary *spherocytosis*.
splenic a., a. esplênica. SIN Banti *syndrome*.
spur cell a., a. acantocítica; a. em que os eritrócitos apresentam um aspecto espiculado (acantócitos) e são destruídos prematuramente, sobretudo no baço; pode ser observada em pacientes com doença hepática grave, em conseqüência de anormalidade no conteúdo de colesterol da membrana eritrocitária.
target cell a., a. da célula em alvo; qualquer a. com um número conspícuo de células em alvo no sangue periférico; característico das talassemias e também encontrada em diversas hemoglobinopatias.
toxic a., a. tóxica; qualquer a. que resulte dos efeitos destrutivos de uma substância química, veneno metabólico, toxina bacteriana, veneno e materiais similares.
traumatic a., a. traumática. SIN posthemorrhagic a.
tropical a., a. tropical; várias síndromes freqüentemente observadas em pessoas nos climas tropicais, geralmente resultando de deficiências nutricionais ou de ancilostomíase ou de outras doenças parasitárias.
unstable hemoglobin hemolytic a., a. hemolítica da hemoglobina instável; uma a. hemolítica congênita decorrente da herança autossômica de uma das muitas hemoglobinas instáveis. A a. exibe gravidade variável e caracteriza-se pela presença *in vivo* ou *in vitro* de corpúsculos de Heinz.

ane·mic (ā - nē′mik). Anêmico; pertinente à anemia ou que manifesta os vários aspectos desta.
an·e·mom·e·ter (an - ē - mom′ē - ter). Anemômetro; um instrumento para medir a velocidade do fluxo aéreo. [G. *anemos*, vento + *metron*, medida]
a·nem·o·nol (ă - nem′ō - nol). Anemonol; um óleo volátil que possui propriedades acentuadamente tóxicas, obtido a partir de plantas do gênero *Anemone*.
an·e·mo·pho·bia (an′e - mō - fō′bē - ă). Anemofobia; medo mórbido do vento. [G. *anemos*, vento + *phobos*, medo]
an·e·mot·ro·phy (an - ē - mot′rō - fē). Anemotrofia; falta de substâncias essenciais para a formação do sangue, resultando, assim, em anemia hipoplásica. [G. *an-* priv. + *haima*, sangue + *trophē*, nutrição]
an·en·ce·pha·lia (an′en - se - fā′lē - ă). Anencefalia. SIN anencephaly.
an·en·ce·phal·ic (an - en - se - fal′ik). Anencefálico; relativo à anencefalia. SIN anencephalous.
an·en·ceph·a·lous (an - en - sef′ă - lŭs). Anencéfalo. SIN anencephalic.
an·en·ceph·a·ly (an′en - sef′ă - lē). Anencefalia; desenvolvimento defeituoso congênito do cérebro, com ausência dos ossos da calota craniana e hemisférios cerebrais e cerebelares, tronco cerebral e gânglios da base ausentes ou rudimentares. SIN anencephalia. [G. *an-* priv. + *enkephalos*, cérebro]
  partial a., a. parcial. SIN hemicephalia.
an·en·ter·ous (an - en′ter - ŭs). Anêntero; que não possui intestino; indica determinados parasitas, como os cestódeos. [G. *an-* priv. + *entera*, intestinos]
an·en·zy·mia (an - en - zī′mē - ă). Anenzimia; ausência congênita de uma enzima.
aneph·ric (ā - nef′rik). Anéfrico; que carece de rins. [*a-* priv. + G. *nephros*, rim]
an·ep·i·plo·ic (an - ep - i - plō′ik). Anepiplóico; que carece de um epíploo.
an·er·gia (an - er′jē - ă). Anergia. SIN anergy (2).
an·er·gic (an - er′jik). Anérgico; relativo a, ou marcado por, anergia.
an·er·gy (an′er - jē). Anergia. **1.** Ausência da capacidade de gerar uma reação de sensibilidade às substâncias esperadas como sendo antigênicas (imunogênicas, alergênicas) em determinado indivíduo. **2.** Falta de energia. SIN anergia. [G. *an-* priv. + *energeia*, energia, de *ergon*, trabalho]
negative a., a. negativa; redução das respostas imunológicas normais ou usuais por causa de doença interveniente não-correlata. SIN nonspecific a.
nonspecific a., a. inespecífica. SIN negative a.
positive a., a. positiva; redução da resposta imunológica normal ou usual decorrente de uma reação a um alérgeno específico. SIN specific a.
  specific a., a. específica. SIN positive a.
an·er·oid (an′er-oyd). Aneróide; sem líquido; indica uma forma de barômetro

sem mercúrio, no qual a pressão variável do ar é indicada por um ponteiro governado pelo movimento da parede elástica de uma câmara esvaziada. Também utilizado para indicar um calibrador de pressão sem mercúrio utilizado em alguns esfigmomanômetros. [G. *a-* priv. + *nēros,* umidade + *eidos,* forma]

an·e·ryth·ro·pla·sia (an´ē - rith - rō - plā´zē - ă). Aneritroplasia; uma condição em que não há formação de eritrócitos. [G. *an-,* priv. + erythro- (cyte) + G. *plasis,* um molde]

an·e·ryth·ro·plas·tic (an´ē - rith - rō - plas´tik). Aneritroplástico; pertinente a, ou caracterizado por, aneritroplasia.

an·e·ryth·ro·re·gen·er·a·tive (an - ē - rith´thrō - rē - jen´er - ă - tiv). Aneritrorregenerativo; pertinente a, ou caracterizado por, falta de regeneração dos eritrócitos.

an·es·the·ci·ne·sia (an - es´thē - si - nē´zē - ă). Anestecinesia. SIN anesthekinesia.

an·es·the·ki·ne·sia (an - es´thē - ki - nē´zē - ă). Anestecinesia; paralisia motora e sensorial combinada. SIN anesthecinesia. [G. *an-,* priv. + *aisthēsis,* sensação, + *kinēsis,* movimento]

ANESTHESIA

an·es·the·sia (an´es - thē´zē - ă). Anestesia. 1. Perda da sensibilidade resultante de depressão farmacológica da função nervosa ou de disfunção neurológica. 2. Termo genérico para anestesiologia como uma especialidade clínica. [G. *anaisthēsia,* do *an-* priv. + *aisthēsis,* sensação]

acupuncture a., a. por acupuntura; a inserção percutânea de, e estímulo por, agulhas posicionadas em áreas críticas do organismo para produzir a perda da sensibilidade em outra área.

ambulatory a., a. ambulatorial; a. fornecida fora do ambiente hospitalar.

axillary a., a. axilar; a perda da sensibilidade nos dois terços distais do membro superior após a injeção de uma solução anestésica local em torno dos troncos nervosos na axila.

balanced a., a. equilibrada; uma técnica de a. geral baseada no conceito de que a administração de uma mistura de pequenas doses de vários depressores neuronais reúne as vantagens, mas não as desvantagens, dos componentes individuais da mistura.

basal a., a. basal; administração parenteral de um ou mais sedativos para produzir um estado de consciência deprimida antes de uma a. geral.

block a., bloqueio anestésico. SIN conduction a.

brachial a., a. braquial; anestesia do membro superior por injeção de solução de anestésico local em torno do plexo braquial.

caudal a., a. caudal; a. regional por injeção da solução anestésica local no espaço epidural através do hiato sacral.

cervical a., a. cervical; a. regional do pescoço através da injeção de uma solução de anestésico local em torno dos nervos cervicais ou no espaço epidural cervical.

circle absorption a., a. de absorção circular; a. inalatória em que um circuito com absorvente de dióxido de carbono é empregado para a reinalação completa (fechada) ou parcial (semiaberta) dos gases exalados.

closed a., a. fechada; a. inalatória em que existe reinalação total de todos os gases exalados, exceto o dióxido de carbono, que é absorvido; o fluxo de gás para dentro do circuito anestésico consiste apenas em oxigênio, em quantidades iguais ao consumo metabólico do paciente, mais pequenas quantidades de outros gases (p.ex., óxido nitroso) que sofrem captação e distribuição contínuas no paciente.

compression a., a. de compressão. SIN pressure a.

conduction a., a. de condução; a. regional em que uma solução anestésica local é injetada em torno dos nervos para inibir a transmissão nervosa; inclui a. espinal, a. epidural, bloqueio de nervos e bloqueio de campo, mas não a a. local ou tópica. SIN block a.

continuous epidural a., a. epidural contínua; inserção de um cateter no espaço epidural lombar ou caudal para a injeção repetida de soluções anestésicas locais como um meio de prolongar a duração da anestesia. SIN fractional epidural a.

continuous spinal a., a. espinal contínua; inserção de um cateter no espaço subaracnóide e deixado no local para permitir a injeção intermitente seriada da solução anestésica local para a a. espinal prolongada. SIN fractional spinal a.

crossed a., a. cruzada; de um lado da cabeça e do outro lado do corpo devido a uma lesão do tronco cerebral.

dental a., a. dentária; a. geral, de condução, local ou tópica para cirurgias nos dentes, gengivas ou estruturas associadas.

diagnostic a., a. diagnóstica; a. induzida para avaliação do mecanismo responsável por uma condição dolorosa.

differential spinal a., a. espinal diferenciada; uma forma de a. espinal diagnóstica que produz bloqueio de diferentes tipos de nervos no espaço subaracnóide, baseada em suas diferenças na sensibilidade ao anestésico local; também observada durante a a. espinal cirúrgica.

dissociated a., a. dissociada; perda de alguns tipos de sensibilidade com a persistência de outros; usada mais amiúde no contexto dos bloqueios de nervos, nos quais ocorre perda da sensibilidade álgica e térmica, sem perda da sensibilidade tátil.

dissociative a., a. dissociativa; uma forma de a. geral, mas não necessariamente de inconsciência completa, caracterizada por catalepsia, catatonia e amnésia, em especial aquela produzida por compostos da fenilcicloexilamina, inclusive a cetamina.

a. doloro'sa, a. dolorosa; dor espontânea grave que ocorre em uma área anestésica. SIN painful a.

electric a., a. elétrica; a., comumente a. geral, produzida por aplicação de uma corrente elétrica.

endotracheal a., a. endotraqueal; técnica de a. inalatória em que o anestésico e os gases respiratórios passam por um tubo colocado na traquéia através da boca ou nariz. SIN intratracheal a.

epidural a., a. epidural; a. regional produzida por injeção da solução anestésica local no espaço peridural. SIN peridural a.

extradural a., a. extradural; anestesia, por anestésico local, dos nervos próximos ao canal espinal, externos à dura-máter; refere-se, com freqüência, à a. epidural, mas pode incluir a a. paravertebral.

field block a., a. de bloqueio de campo; a. de condução em que os pequenos nervos não são anestesiados individualmente, como no bloqueio anestésico de nervo, mas, em vez disso, são bloqueados *em masse* (em bloco) por solução de anestésico local injetada para formar uma barreira proximal ao local cirúrgico.

fractional epidural a., a. epidural fracionada. SIN continuous epidural a.

fractional spinal a., a. espinal fracionada. SIN continuous spinal a.

general a., a. geral; perda da capacidade de perceber a dor associada à perda da consciência produzida por agentes anestésicos intravenosos ou inalatórios.

girdle a., a. em cinta; a. distribuída como uma faixa que envolve o tronco.

glove a., a. em luva; perda da sensibilidade na parte distal do membro superior, isto é, a mão e os dedos.

gustatory a., a. gustativa. SIN ageusia.

high spinal a., a. espinal alta; a. espinal em que o nível de denervação sensorial estende-se até o segundo ou terceiro dermátomo torácico.

hyperbaric a., a. hiperbárica; inalação de gases ou vapores depressores em pressões maiores que 1 atmosfera, em especial como um meio de produzir a. geral com agentes muito fracos para produzir a. a 1 atmosfera.

hyperbaric spinal a., a. espinal hiperbárica; a. espinal em que a disseminação da solução de anestésico local no espaço subaracnóide é controlada ao se ajustar a posição do paciente quando a densidade do anestésico local torna-se maior que a densidade do líquido cefalorraquidiano (isto é, hiperbárica) pela adição de glicose.

hypobaric spinal a., a. espinal hipobárica; a. espinal em que a disseminação da solução de anestésico local no espaço subaracnóide é controlada por meio do ajuste da posição do paciente, quando a densidade da solução anestésica local torna-se menor que a densidade do líquido cefalorraquidiano (isto é, hipobárica) pela adição de água destilada.

hipotensive a., a. hipotensora; a. em que a hipotensão arterial é deliberadamente induzida como um meio de diminuir a perda sanguínea operatória.

hypothermic a., a. hipotérmica; a. geral administrada em conjunto com a diminuição artificial da temperatura corpórea.

hysterical a., a. histérica; a. como uma manifestação da histeria, envolvendo geralmente as áreas de superfície do corpo que não são compatíveis com a distribuição neuroanatômica.

infiltration a., a. por infiltração; a. produzida pela injeção de solução de anestésico local diretamente em uma área que é dolorosa ou prestes a ser operada.

inhalation a., a. inalatória; a. geral que resulta da respiração de gases ou vapores anestésicos.

insufflation a., a. por insuflação; manutenção da a. por inalação por liberação de gases ou vapores anestésicos diretamente na via aérea de um paciente com respiração espontânea.

intercostal a., a. intercostal; a. regional produzida por injeção de anestésico local em torno dos nervos intercostais.

intramedullary a., a. intramedular; método de a. geral, raramente empregado, por injeção do(s) agente(s) anestésico(s) intravenoso(s) no canal medular dos ossos longos. SIN intraosseous a.

intranasal a., a. intranasal; (1) a. por insuflação, em que um anestésico inalatório é acrescentado ao ar inalado que passa através do nariz ou da nasofaringe; (2) a. das vias nasais por infiltração e aplicação tópica de solução anestésica local na mucosa nasal.

intraoral a., a. intra-oral; (1) a. por insuflação em que um anestésico inalatório é acrescentado ao ar que passa através da boca; (2) a. regional da boca e estruturas associadas quando as soluções anestésicas orais são utilizadas por aplicação tópica na mucosa oral, por infiltração local ou como bloqueios nervosos.

intraosseous a., a. intra-óssea. SIN intramedullary a.

intraspinal a., a. intra-espinal; sinônimo inexato para a a. espinal; as soluções anestésicas locais não são injetadas dentro da medula espinal.
intratracheal a., a. intratraqueal. SIN endotracheal a.
intravenous a., a. intravenosa; a. geral produzida por injeção de depressores do sistema nervoso central na circulação venosa.
intravenous regional a., a. regional intravenosa; a. regional por injeção intravenosa da solução de anestésico local distal a um torniquete oclusivo em um membro previamente exsanguinado por pressão ou gravidade. SIN Bier method (1).
isobaric spinal a., a. espinal isobárica; a. espinal de mesma densidade que o líquido cefalorraquidiano, de tal forma que o nível da a. não seja influenciado por uma modificação na posição do paciente.
local a., a. local; termo genérico que se refere à a. por aplicação tópica, infiltração, bloqueio de campo ou bloqueio de nervo, mas, geralmente, não à a. epidural ou espinal. VER TAMBÉM local *anesthetics*, em *anesthetic*.
low spinal a., a. espinal baixa; a. espinal em que o nível da denervação sensorial se estende até o décimo ou décimo primeiro dermátomo.
nerve block a., a. por bloqueio de nervo; a de condução em que a solução anestésica local é injetada em torno de nervos, troncos nervosos ou plexos nervosos.
nonrebreathing a., a. sem reinalação; uma técnica de a. inalatória em que as válvulas fazem a exaustão de todo o ar expirado do circuito.
open drop a., a. de gotejamento aberto; a. inalatória por vaporização de um anestésico líquido colocado gota a gota sobre uma máscara de gaze que cobre a boca e o nariz.
outpatient a., a. ambulatorial. SIN patient-controlled *analgesia.*
painful a., a. dolorosa. SIN a. dolorosa.
paracervical block a., a. de bloqueio paracervical; a. regional do colo uterino por injeção de solução de anestésico local nos tecidos adjacentes ao colo uterino.
paravertebral a., a. paravertebral; **(1)** a. por injeção da solução anestésica local em torno dos nervos, à medida que eles saem do canal vertebral; **(2)** bloqueio pré-sináptico, pós-sináptico e ganglionar combinado por injeção de solução de anestésico local em torno das cadeias simpáticas paravertebrais.
patient-controlled a. (PCA), analgesia controlada pelo paciente. SIN patient-controlled *analgesia.*
peridural a., a. peridural. SIN epidural a.
periodontal a., a. periodontal; a do ligamento periodontal, produzida por injeção de um anestésico local.
presacral a., a. pré-sacral; injeção de solução de anestésico local anterior ao sacro, para bloquear os nervos à medida que eles saem dos forames sacrais.
pressure a., a. por compressão; perda da sensibilidade produzida por compressão de um nervo. SIN compression a.
pudendal a., a. pudenda; a. local produzida por bloqueio dos nervos pudendos próximo aos processos espinais do ísquio; usado em obstetrícia.
rebreathing a., a. com reinalação; uma técnica de a. inalatória em que uma parte ou a totalidade dos gases expirados é subseqüentemente inalada depois que o dióxido de carbono foi absorvido.
rectal a., a. retal; a. geral produzida por instilação de uma solução contendo um depressor do sistema nervoso central dentro do reto.
refrigeration a., a. por refrigeração. SIN cryoanesthesia.
regional a., a. regional; uso de soluções de anestésicos locais para produzir áreas circunscritas de perda da sensibilidade; um termo genérico que inclui a. de condução, bloqueio de nervo, a. regional, epidural, bloqueio de campo, infiltração e a. tópica. SIN conduction analgesia.
retrobulbar a., a. retrobulbar; injeção de um anestésico local atrás do olho para produzir a desnervação sensorial do olho.
sacral a., a. sacral; a. regional limitada às áreas inervadas pelos nervos sensoriais sacrais.
saddle block a., bloqueio anestésico em sela; uma forma de a. espinal limitada na área das nádegas, períneo e superfícies internas das coxas.
segmental a., a. segmental; perda da sensibilidade limitada a uma área suprida por uma ou mais raízes nervosas espinais.
spinal a., a. espinal; **(1)** perda da sensibilidade produzida pela injeção de soluções de anestésicos locais no espaço subaracnóide espinal. SIN subarachnoid a.; **(2)** perda da sensibilidade produzida por doença da medula espinal.
splanchnic a., a. esplâncnica; perda da sensibilidade nas áreas do peritônio visceral inervadas pelos nervos esplâncnicos. SIN visceral a.
stocking a., a. em meia; perda da sensibilidade na parte distal do membro inferior, isto é, o pé e os artelhos.
subarachnoid a., a. subaracnóide. SIN spinal a. (1).
surgical a., a. cirúrgica; **(1)** qualquer a. administrada com a finalidade de permitir a realização de um procedimento cirúrgico, conforme diferenciada da a. obstétrica, diagnóstica e terapêutica; **(2)** perda da sensibilidade com relaxamento muscular adequado para um procedimento cirúrgico.
tactile a., a. tátil; perda ou comprometimento da sensação do tato.
therapeutic a., a. terapêutica; administração de um anestésico como um meio de tratamento.

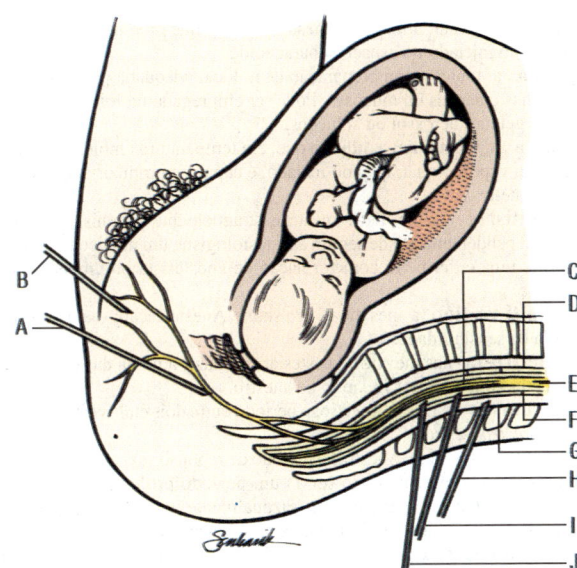

anestesia regional para o delivramento: sítios de injeção; (A) bloqueio pudendo, (B) infiltração local do períneo, (C) pia-máter, (D) dura-máter; (E) medula espinal, (F) espaço subaracnóide, (G) espaço epidural, (H) bloqueio epidural lombar, (I) bloqueio espinal lombar, (J) bloqueio em sela

thermal a., thermic a., a. térmica; perda da apreciação da temperatura.
to-and-fro a., a. de vaivém; a. que utiliza um circuito de a. fechada sem válvula, no qual os gases respirados se movem através de um absorvente de dióxido de carbono interposto entre o paciente e a bolsa-reservatório de respiração.
topical a., a. tópica; perda superficial da sensibilidade na conjuntiva, mucosas ou pele, produzida pela aplicação direta de soluções, pomadas ou geléias anestésicas locais.
total spinal a., a. espinal total; a. espinal suficientemente extensa para produzir a perda da sensibilidade em todas as raízes extracranianas.
traumatic a., a. traumática; perda da sensibilidade decorrente de lesão de nervo.
unilateral a., a. unilateral. SIN hemianesthesia.
visceral a., a. visceral. SIN splanchnic a.

an·es·the·si·ol·o·gist (an′es - thē - zē - ol′ō - jist). Anestesiologista. **1.** Médico que se especializa unicamente em anestesiologia e nas áreas correlatas. **2.** Indivíduo com grau de doutorado que é certificado e legalmente qualificado para administrar anestesia e as técnicas correlatas. Cf. anesthetist.
an·es·the·si·ol·o·gy (an′es - thē - zē - ol′ō - jē). Anestesiologia; a especialidade médica relacionada às bases farmacológica, fisiológica e clínica da anestesia e dos campos correlatos, incluindo reanimação, cuidados respiratórios intensivos e dor aguda e crônica. [anesthesia + G. *logos*, tratar]
an·es·thet·ic (an-es-thet′ik). Anestésico. **1.** Composto que deprime de forma reversível a função neuronal, produzindo perda da capacidade de perceber a dor e/ou outras sensações. **2.** Designação coletiva para os agentes anestesiantes administrados a um indivíduo em determinado momento. **3.** Caracterizado pela perda da sensação ou capaz de produzir a perda da sensibilidade. **4.** Associado com ou decorrente do estado de anestesia.
fammable a., a. inflamável; a. inalatório que suporta a combustão e forma misturas explosivas com os gases oxidantes.
general a.'s, anestésicos gerais; substâncias empregadas por via intravenosa ou inalatória que tornam a pessoa inconsciente e incapaz de perceber a dor, como poderia acontecer, de outra forma, na cirurgia.
inhalation a., a. inalatório; gás ou líquido com pressão de vapor suficiente para produzir anestesia geral, quando inspirado.
intravenous a., a. intravenoso; composto que produz anestesia quando injetado por via intravenosa.
local a.'s, anestésicos locais; substâncias usadas para a interrupção da transmissão nervosa das sensações dolorosas. Elas agem no local da aplicação para impedir a percepção da dor; os exemplos compreendem a procaína e a lidocaína.
primary a., a. primário; o composto que contribui com a maior parte da perda da sensibilidade quando se administra uma mistura de anestésicos.
secondary a., a. secundário; um composto que contribui para a perda da sensibilidade, mas não é o principal responsável por essa perda, quando dois ou mais anestésicos são administrados de maneira simultânea.

spinal a., a. espinal; um agente anestésico local que produz a perda da sensação quando injetado no espaço subaracnóide.
topical a., a. tópico; uma preparação de a. local adequada para anestesiar as superfícies cutâneas ou mucosas. Pode ser empregado na forma de pomadas, cremes, geléias, aerossol ou soluções.
volatile a., a. volátil; um a. líquido que, em temperatura ambiente, volatiliza-se em um vapor, o qual, quando inalado, é capaz de produzir anestesia geral. SIN anesthetic *vapor*.
anes·the·tist (ă - nes′thĕ - tist). Anestesista; aquele que administra um anestésico, independentemente de ser um anestesiologista, um médico não-anestesiologista, uma enfermeira com formação de anestesista ou um assistente de anestesia.
anes·the·ti·za·tion (ă - nes′thĕ - ti - zā′shun). Anestesiação; o ato de produzir a perda da sensibilidade.
anes·the·tize (ă - nes′thĕ - tīz). Anestesiar; produzir a perda da sensibilidade.
an·es·trous (an - es′trŭs). Relativo ao anestro.
a·nes·trum (an - es′trŭm). Anestro; o período entre dois ciclos éstricos. [G. *an*- priv. + *oistros*, estro]
an·es·trus (an - es′trŭs). Anestro; o período de repouso sexual entre dois ciclos éstricos dos mamíferos; pode ser 1) um período prolongado nos animais monoéstricos (cães) ou em animais sazonalmente poliéstricos (carneiro), ou 2) um período prolongado de falha da menstruação em animais poliéstricos maduros, não-grávidos. [G. *a*- priv. + *oistros*, um moscardo, um desejo ruim (estro)]
ane·tho·path (ă - nē′thō - path). Anetopata; uma pessoa moralmente desinibida. [G. *an*- priv. + *ethos*, hábito, + *pathos*, doença]
an·e·to·der·ma (an - ĕ - tō - der′mă). Anetodermia; atrofodermia em que a pele se torna semelhante a um saco e enrugada ou deprimida, com perda da elasticidade dérmica. SIN atrophia maculosa varioliformis cutis, atrophoderma maculatum, macular atrophy, primary idiopathic macular atrophy, primary macular atrophy of skin. [G. *anetos*, relaxado, + *derma*, pele]
Jadassohn-Pellizzari a., a. de Jadassohn-Pellizzari; atrofia cutânea precedida por lesões eritematosas ou urticariformes inflamatórias do tronco e regiões superiores dos membros, e que aumentam até 2 a 3 cm antes de entrarem em involução.
Schweninger-Buzzi a., a. de Schweninger-Buzzi; aparecimento súbito de lesões permanentes, semelhantes a um balão, branco-azuladas e não-inflamatórias, moles e facilmente depressíveis, principalmente no tronco das mulheres.
an·eu·ploid (an′ū - ployd). Aneuplóide; que possui um número anormal de cromossomas que não é um múltiplo exato do número haplóide, em contraste com os números anormais de haplóides completos da série de cromossomas, como diplóides, triplóides, etc. [G. *an*- priv. + *euploid*]
an·eu·ploi·dy (an′ū - ploy - dē). Aneuploidia; estado de ser aneuplóide.
partial a., a. parcial; um tipo de mosaicismo em que algumas células possuem um número normal de cromossomas e outras apresentam um número anormal.
an·eu·rine (an′ū - rēn). Aneurina. SIN thiamin.
a. hydrochloride, cloridrato de a. SIN *thiamin* hydrochloride.
a. pyrophosphate, pirofosfato de a. SIN *thiamin* pyrophosphate.
aneu·ro·lem·mic (ă - noo - rō - lem′ik). Aneurolêmico; sem um neurolema.
an·eu·rysm (an′ū - rizm). Aneurisma. 1. Dilatação circunscrita de uma artéria ou compartimento cardíaco, uma comunicação direta com a luz, geralmente devido a debilidade adquirida ou congênita da parede da artéria ou compartimento. 2. Dilatação circunscrita de uma câmara cardíaca comumente provocada por debilidade adquirida ou congênita da parede do coração. [G. *aneurysma* (*-mat-*), uma dilatação, de *eurys*, amplo]
ampullary a., a. ampular. SIN saccular a.
a. by anastomosis, a. por anastomose; uma massa de vasos anastomosantes dilatados que produz um tumor pulsátil, geralmente em uma posição superficial.
aortic a., a. aórtico; dilatação difusa ou circunscrita de uma parte da aorta (p.ex., a. de aorta abdominal, a. do arco aórtico). VER TAMBÉM dissecting a.
aortic sinus a., a. do seio aórtico; dilatação anormal de um ou mais dos três seios aórticos situados atrás das três cúspides da valva aórtica.
arteriosclerotic a., a. arterioesclerótico. SIN atherosclerotic a.
arteriovenous a., a. arteriovenoso; **(1)** derivação (*shunt*) arteriovenosa dilatada; **(2)** comunicação entre uma artéria e uma veia, geralmente congênita ou associada às alterações ateroscleróticas; denominada de maneira mais adequada como fístula arteriovenosa ou malformação arteriovenosa.
atherosclerotic a., a. aterosclerótico; o tipo mais comum de a., que ocorre na aorta abdominal e em outras artérias calibrosas, principalmente no idoso. Freqüentemente associado a alterações ateroscleróticas nos vasos sanguíneos em outras regiões do corpo. SIN arteriosclerotic. a.
axial a., a. axial; um a. que envolve toda a circunferência de um vaso sanguíneo.
benign bone a., a. ósseo benigno; termo obsoleto para aneurysmal bone *cyst* (cisto ósseo aneurismático).
Bérard a., a. de Bérard; um a. arteriovenoso nos tecidos adjacentes à veia lesionada.

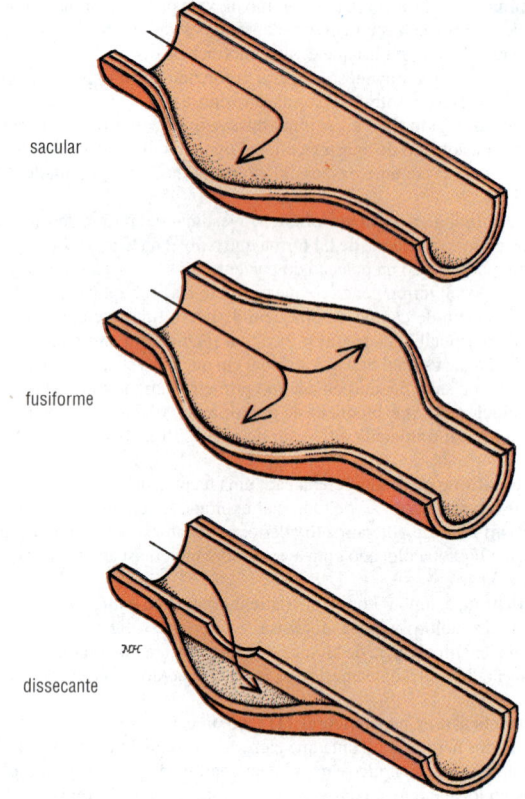

aneurisma

berry a., a. saculado; a. sacular de uma artéria cerebral que se assemelha a uma baga. Esses aneurismas podem romper-se, gerando hemorragia subaracnóide.
cardiac a., a. cardíaco, a. ventricular. SIN ventricular a.
Charcot-Bouchard a., a. de Charcot-Bouchard. SIN miliary a.
cirsoid a., a. cirsóide; dilatação de um grupo de vasos sanguíneos devido à malformação congênita com derivação arteriovenosa. SIN cirsoid varix, racemose a., racemose hemangioma.
compound a., a. composto; um a. em que algumas das camadas da artéria estão rompidas, outras intactas.
congenital cerebral a., a. cerebral congênito; dilatação localizada de um vaso cerebral; comumente um a. saculado.
consecutive a., a. consecutivo; dois ou mais aneurismas ao longo do trajeto do fluxo sanguíneo.
coronary artery a., a. de artéria coronária; a. da artéria coronária, raramente congênito, geralmente causado por aterosclerose, processos inflamatórios ou por uma fístula coronária.
cylindroid a., a. cilindróide. SIN tubular a.
diffuse a., a. difuso; um a. que aumentou e espalhou-se para os tecidos circunvizinhos em conseqüência da ruptura de suas paredes.
dissecting a., a. dissecante; condição que resulta quando sangue passa da luz verdadeira de uma artéria para uma luz falsa dentro da parede arterial; as camadas da parede estão efetivamente separadas; deve-se mais amiúde à necrose da camada média, como na *síndrome* de Marfan, e com a laceração originando-se na aorta torácica ascendente (tipo A) ou descendente (tipo B), ou, ocasionalmente, em artérias menores, como as carótidas; a *luz* falsa pode sofrer trombose, romper-se, reentrar na luz (*lúmen*) verdadeira a jusante e/ou romper por cisalhamento os ramos arteriais vitais; denominada com maior propriedade de dissecção aórtica em vez de aneurisma, pois o processo não é transmural. VER TAMBÉM aortic *dissection*.
ductal a., a. do canal arterial persistente, ocorre em lactantes ou adultos. SIN ductus diverticulum.
ectatic a., a. ectásico; um a. em que todas as camadas da artéria, embora distendidas, não estão rompidas.
false a., a. falso. SIN pseudoaneurysm.
fusiform a., a. fusiforme; uma dilatação alongada, em formato de fuso, de uma artéria.
hernial a., a. herniário; a protrusão das camadas internas distendidas de uma artéria através de um defeito na adventícia.

infraclinoid a., a. infraclinóide; um a. intracraniano que ocorre abaixo do nível do processo clinóide anterior do osso esfenóide.

intracavernous a., a. intracavernoso; um a. da artéria carótida dentro do seio cavernoso.

intracranial a., a. intracraniano; qualquer a. localizado dentro do crânio.

miliary a., a. miliar; dilatação no diâmetro das pequenas artérias e arteríolas secundária à lipo-hialinose por hipertensão de longa duração; associado a hematomas intracerebrais. SIN Charcot-Bouchard a.

mural aneurysm, a. mural. SIN ventricular a.

mycotic a., a. micótico; um a. causado pelo crescimento de fungos ou bactérias dentro da parede vascular, geralmente após a impactação de um êmbolo séptico.

Park a., a. de Park; um a. arteriovenoso em que a artéria braquial se comunica com as veias braquial e basílica mediana.

peripheral a., a. periférico; **(1)** um a. sacular que se origina de um lado de uma artéria; **(2)** um a. de um dos ramos menores de uma artéria.

phantom a., a. fantasma; uma aorta pulsátil palpável, confundida com um a. por examinadores inexperientes.

Pott a., a. de Pott. SIN aneurysmal varix.

pulmonary artery a., a. de artéria pulmonar; pode ser secundário a estenose infundibular ou valvar congênita; alguns são aneurismas micóticos (q.v.)

racemose a., a. racemoso. SIN cirsoid a.

Rasmussen a., a. de Rasmussen; dilatação aneurismática de um ramo da artéria pulmonar, em uma cavidade tuberculosa, cuja ruptura pode provocar hemoptise grave.

a. of right ventricle or right ventricular outflow patch, a. do ventrículo direito ou do trato de saída do ventrículo direito; a. que ocorre após ventriculotomia direita; o a. pode ser falso ou verdadeiro.

ruptured a., a. roto; um a. que está sangrando para dentro de sua parede ou para os tecidos circunvizinhos.

saccular a., sacculated a., a. sacular; a. saculado; abaulamento sacular em um lado de uma artéria. SIN ampullary a.

serpentine a., a. em serpentinado; dilatação e tortuosidade de uma artéria, afetando por vezes as artérias temporal, esplênica ou ilíaca no idoso.

a. of sinus of Valsalva, a. do seio de Valsalva; uma evaginação congênita de paredes finas com um trajeto totalmente intracardíaco, geralmente no seio direito ou não-coronário, que pode romper-se para dentro das câmaras cardíacas direitas ou, raramente, esquerdas, formando uma fístula aortocardíaca.

supraclinoid a., a. supraclinóide; um a. intracraniano localizado imediatamente acima do processo clinóide anterior do osso esfenóide.

syphilitic a., a. sifilítico; um a., comumente envolvendo a aorta torácica, que resulta da aortite da sífilis terciária.

traumatic a., a. traumático; um a. resultante da lesão física da parede de uma artéria; geralmente falso ou arteriovenoso.

true a., a. verdadeiro; dilatação localizada de uma artéria com uma luz expandida revestida pelos resíduos distendidos da parede arterial.

tubular a., a. tubular; a dilatação uniforme de um segmento grande de uma artéria. SIN cylindroid a.

varicose a., a. varicoso; um saco contendo sangue, que se comunica com uma artéria e uma veia.

ventricular a., a. ventricular; adelgaçamento, estiramento e abaulamento de uma parede ventricular enfraquecida, geralmente em conseqüência de infarto do miocárdio; raramente pós-inflamatório ou congênito. SIN cardiac a., mural aneurysm.

a. of the ventricular portion of the membranous septum, a. da porção ventricular do septo membranoso; um a. que se abaúla para a direita na sístole, consistindo, com freqüência, no folheto anterior da valva tricúspide.

an·eu·rys·mal, an·eu·rys·mat·ic (an - ū - riz′mǎl, - riz - mat′ik). Aneurismático; relativo a um aneurisma.

an·eu·rys·mec·to·my (an - ŭ - riz - mek′tō - mē). Aneurismectomia; excisão de um aneurisma. [aneurysm + G. *ektomē*, excisão]

an·eu·rys·mo·plas·ty (an - ŭ - riz′mō - plas - tē). Aneurismoplastia; reparação de um aneurisma através da abertura do saco e sutura de suas paredes para restaurar a dimensão normal da luz da artéria. VER TAMBÉM aneurysmorrhaphy. SIN endoaneurysmoplasty, endoaneurysmorrhaphy. [aneurysm + G. *plastos*, formado]

an·eu·rys·mor·rha·phy (an′ū - riz - mōr′a - fē). Aneurismorrafia; fechamento por sutura do saco de um aneurisma para restaurar as dimensões normais da luz. [aneurysm + G. *rhaphē*, sutura]

an·eu·rys·mot·o·my (an′ū - riz - mot′ō - mē). Aneurismotomia; incisão dentro do saco de um aneurisma. [aneurysm + G. *tomē*, incisão]

ANF Abreviatura para antinuclear *factor* (fator antinuclear), atrial natriuretic *factor* (fator natriurético atrial).

angei-. VER angio-.

an·gel·i·ca root (an - jel′i - kǎ). Raiz de angélica; a raiz da *Angelica archangelica* (família Umbelliferae); um tônico e estimulante que pode causar náuseas; usado como carminativo, diurético e, externamente, como contra-irritante.

Angelucci, Arnaldo, oftalmologista italiano, 1854–1934. VER A. *syndrome*.

Anger, Hal, engenheiro elétrico norte-americano, *1920. VER A. *camera*.

angi-. VER angio-.

an·gi·ec·ta·sia, an·gi·ec·ta·sis (an - jē - ek - tā′zē - ǎ, - ek′tǎ - sis). Angiectasia; dilatação de um vaso linfático ou sanguíneo. [angio- + G. *ektasis*, um estiramento]

congenital dysplastic a., a. displásica congênita. SIN Klippel-Trenaunay-Weber syndrome.

an·gi·ec·tat·ic (an - jē - ek - tat′ik). Angiectático; caracterizado pela presença de vasos sanguíneos dilatados. [angio- + G. *ektatos*, capaz de extensão]

an·gi·ec·to·pia (an - jē - ek - tō′pē - ǎ). Angiectopia; localização anormal de um vaso sanguíneo. SIN angioplany. [angio- + G. *ektopos*, fora do lugar]

an·gi·i·tis, an·gi·tis (an - jē - ī′tis, an - jī′tis). Angiíte; inflamação de um vaso sanguíneo (arterite, flebite) ou vaso linfático (linfangite). SIN vasculitis. [angio- + G. *-itis*, inflamação]

allergic granulomatous a., a. alérgica granulomatosa. SIN Churg-Strauss syndrome.

consecutive a., a. consecutiva; a. causada por extensão do processo inflamatório a partir dos tecidos circunvizinhos.

frosted branch a., a. de galho congelado; a. caracterizada pela inflamação dos vasos sanguíneos com o embainhamento gerando o aspecto dos galhos em uma árvore.

hypersensitivity a., a. por hipersensibilidade; reação inflamatória em um vaso sanguíneo, o resultado de uma reação específica a uma substância antigênica (alérgica) ou a outros agentes aos quais o indivíduo expressa sensibilização vascular incomum.

necrotizing a., a. necrotizante; reação inflamatória dos vasos sanguíneos resultando em necrose fibrinóide do tecido, em especial da parede dos vasos sanguíneos.

an·gi·na (an′ji - nǎ, an - jī′nǎ). Angina. **1.** Dor intensa, freqüentemente constritiva, geralmente referente à de peito. **2.** Termo antigo para uma faringite por qualquer etiologia. [L. amigdalite]

abdominal a., a. abdom′inis, a. abdominal; dor abdominal intermitente, que ocorre freqüentemente em um horário fixo depois da alimentação, causada pela inadequação da circulação mesentérica devido a arterioesclerose ou a outra doença arterial. SIN intestinal a.

agranulocytic a., a. agranulocítica. SIN agranulocytosis.

crescendo a., a. em crescendo; a. de peito que ocorre com freqüência crescente.

a. cru′ris, a. da perna; claudicação intermitente da perna.

a. decu′bitus, a. de decúbito; a. de peito relacionada à posição corporal horizontal, geralmente em decúbito dorsal.

a. of effort, a. de esforço; a. de peito precipitada pelo esforço físico.

false a., a. falsa; sensação semelhante a a. na ausência de isquemia miocárdica.

Heberden a., a. de Heberden. SIN a. pectoris.

hypercyanotic a., a. hipercianótica; dor anginosa em pacientes cianóticos com cardiopatia congênita ou doença pulmonar crônica, com a dor se desenvolvendo com a intensificação da cianose durante a atividade.

intestinal a., a. intestinal. SIN abdominal a.

a. inver′sa, a. inversa. SIN Prinzmetal a.

Ludwig a., a. de Ludwig; celulite, usualmente de origem odontogênica, que afeta bilateralmente os espaços submaxilar, sublingual e submentoniano, resultando em tumefação dolorosa do assoalho da boca, elevação da língua, disfasia, disfonia e, por vezes, comprometimento das vias aéreas. [W. F. Ludwig]

lymphatic a., a. linfática; afecção semelhante à doença de Vincent, caracterizada pelo aumento do número de linfócitos no sangue.

a. lymphomato′sa, a. linfomatosa. SIN agranulocytosis.

neutropenic a., a. neutropênica. SIN agranulocytosis.

a. pec′toris, a. de peito; dor constritiva intensa no tórax, freqüentemente irradiando-se do precórdio para um ombro (geralmente o esquerdo) e para baixo pelo braço, devido à isquemia do músculo cardíaco, comumente causada por doença coronária. SIN breast pang, coronarism (2), Heberden a., Rougnon-Heberden disease, stenocardia.

a. pec′toris decu′bitus, a. de peito de decúbito; dor anginosa que se desenvolve enquanto a pessoa está deitada.

a. pec′toris si′ne dolor′e, a. de peito indolor; SIN Gairdner disease.

a. pec′toris vasomoto′ria, a. de peito vasomotora; a. de peito em que a dor torácica é comparativamente discreta, mas a palidez, seguida por cianose, e o resfriamento e dormência dos membros são acentuados. SIN a. spuria, a. vasomotoria, pseudangina, pseudoangina, reflex a., vasomotor a.

preinfarction a., a. pré-infarto; termo obsoleto para a. instável, incluindo a a. em crescendo.

Prinzmetal a., a. de Prinzmetal; uma forma de a. de peito caracterizada por dor que não é precipitada por trabalho cardíaco, tem duração mais longa, é geralmente mais intensa e está associada a manifestações eletrocardiográficas incomuns, incluindo segmentos ST elevados nas derivações que estão habitualmente deprimidas na a. típica e, em geral, sem alterações ST recíprocas; ocorre à noite, no leito. SIN a. inversa, variant a. pectoris.

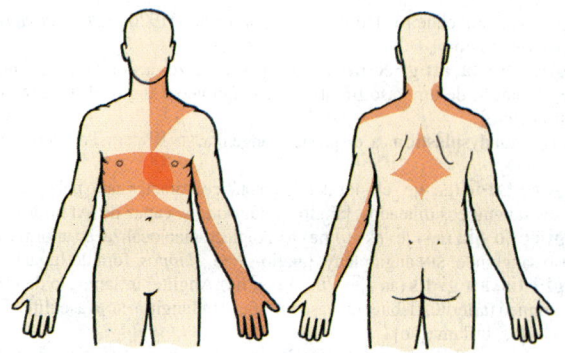

angina de peito: zonas de dor

reflex a., a. reflexa. SIN a. pectoris vasomotoria.
a. si'ne do'lore, a. indolor; os sintomas de insuficiência coronariana ocorrem sem dor.
a. spu'ria, a. espúria. SIN a. pectoris vasomotoria.
unstable a., a. instável; (1) a. de peito caracterizada por dor no tórax de origem coronariana, que ocorre em resposta a esforços cada vez menores ou a outros estímulos menores que os comumente exigidos para produzir a a.; leva, com freqüência, ao infarto do miocárdio, quando não tratada; (2) a. que não atingiu um padrão constante ou reprodutível em 30 ou 60 dias.
variant a. pectoris, a. de peito variante. SIN Prinzmetal a.
vasomotor a., a. vasomotora. SIN a. pectoris vasomotoria.
a. vasomotor'ia, a. vasomotora. SIN a. pectoris vasomotoria.
Vincent a., a. de Vincent; infecção ulcerativa dos tecidos moles orais, incluindo as tonsilas e a faringe, causada por microrganismos fusiformes e espiroquetas; está comumente associada à gengivite ulcerativa necrotizante e pode progredir para a noma. Pode ocorrer morte por sufocação ou sépsis.
walk-through a., uma circunstância em que, apesar da atividade continuada, como a caminhada, a dor da a. de peito diminui ou desaparece.
an·gi·nal (an'ji-nǎl, an-jī'). Anginoso; relativo à angina em qualquer sentido.
an·gi·ni·form (an-jin'i-form). Anginiforme; que se assemelha à angina.
an·gi·noid (an'jin-oid). Anginóide; termo raramente empregado para algo que se assemelhe a uma angina, especialmente à angina de peito.
an·gin·o·pho·bia (an'ji-nō-fō'bē-ǎ). Anginofobia; medo extremo de uma crise de angina de peito. [angina + G. *phobos*, medo]
an·gi·nose, an·gi·nous (an'ji-nōs, -ji-nŭs). Anginoso; termo raramente empregado para relacionar-se a qualquer angina.
angio-, angi-. Formas combinantes relativas a vasos sanguíneos ou linfáticos; revestimento, envoltório; corresponde ao L. vas-, vaso-, vasculo-. [G. *angeion*, um vaso ou cavidade do corpo, de *angos*, um vaso, tanque, balde, + *-eion*, pouco, pequeno]
an·gi·o·ar·chi·tec·ture (an'jē-ō-ar'ki-tek-choor). Angioarquitetura. 1. A disposição e distribuição dos vasos sanguíneos de qualquer órgão. 2. A estrutura vascular de um órgão ou tecido.
an·gi·o·blast (an'jē-ō-blast). Angioblasto. 1. Uma célula que toma parte na formação do vaso sanguíneo. SIN vasoformative cell. 2. Tecido mesenquimal primordial a partir do qual são diferenciadas as células sanguíneas embrionárias e o endotélio vascular. SIN angioderm. [angio- + G. *blastos*, germe]
an·gi·o·blas·to·ma (an'jē-ō-blas-tō'mǎ). Angioblastoma, hemangioblastoma. SIN hemangioblastoma.
a. of Nakagawa, a. de Nakagawa. SIN acquired tufted *angioma*.
an·gi·o·car·di·og·ra·phy (an'jē-ō-kar-dē-og'ra-fē). Angiocardiografia; imageamento do coração e dos grandes vasos por raios X que se tornam visíveis graças à injeção de uma solução radiopaca. SIN coronary *angiography*. SIN cardioangiography. [angio- + G. *kardia*, coração, + *graphō*, escrever]
exercise radionuclide a., a. de esforço com radionuclídeo; uma a. com radionuclídeo enquanto o paciente está realizando exercício físico, como em uma esteira rolante ou bicicleta ergométrica.
gated radionuclide a., a. com radionuclídeo com colimador; a. com radionuclídeo que emprega um colimador cardíaco para combinar as imagens a partir de vários ciclos cardíacos, visando melhorar a qualidade das imagens de fases separadas (p.ex., sístole e diástole).
radionuclide a., a. com radionuclídeo; a demonstração, por meio de uma câmera de cintilação estacionária, da passagem pelo coração de uma dose de substância farmacológica radioativa rapidamente injetada. SIN radionuclide ventriculography.
an·gi·o·car·di·o·ki·net·ic, an·gi·o·car·di·o·ci·net·ic (an'jē-ō-kar'dē-ō-ki-net'ik, -dē-ō-si-net'ik). Angiocardiocinético; que causa dilatação ou contração do coração e dos vasos sanguíneos. [angio- + G. *kardia*, coração, + *kinēsis*, movimento]

an·gi·o·car·di·op·a·thy (an'jē-ō-kar-dē-op'ǎ-thē). Angiocardiopatia; doença que afeta o coração e os vasos sanguíneos. [angio- + G. *kardia*, coração + *pathos*, doença]
an·gi·o·cho·li·tis (an'jē-ō-kō-lī'tis). Angiocolite; colangite. SIN cholangitis.
an·gi·o·cyst (an'jē-ō-sist). Angiocisto; uma pequena agregação vesicular de células mesodérmicas embrionárias que originaria o endotélio vascular e as células sanguíneas.
an·gi·o·derm (an'jē-ō-derm). Angioderma; angioblasto (2). SIN angioblast (2).
an·gi·o·dys·pla·sia (an'jē-ō-dis-plā'zē-ǎ). Angiodisplasia; anormalidade estrutural congênita ou degenerativa da vasculatura normalmente distribuída.
an·gi·o·dys·tro·phy, an·gi·o·dys·tro·phia (an'jē-ō-dis'trō-fē, -dis-trō'fē-ǎ). Angiodistrofia; formação ou crescimento defeituoso associado a alterações vasculares acentuadas. [angio- + G. *dys-*, ruim, + *trophē*, nutrição]
an·gi·o·e·de·ma (an'jē-ō-ē-dē'mǎ). Angioedema; grandes áreas circunscritas e recorrentes de edema de tecido subcutâneo ou mucosa de estabelecimento súbito, que geralmente desaparecem em 24 horas; acomete principalmente mulheres jovens, freqüentemente como uma reação alérgica a alimentos ou medicamentos. SIN angioneurotic edema, giant hives, giant urticaria, periodic edema.
hereditary a., a. hereditário; uma doença hereditária, autossômica dominante, caracterizada pelo aparecimento episódico de edema não-depressível, que afeta mais amiúde os membros, mas que pode envolver qualquer parte do corpo, inclusive as superfícies de mucosa, como as do intestino (gerando dor abdominal) ou do trato respiratório (causando asfixia, que pode exigir intubação para evitar a morte). Associado à deficiência de inibidor do primeiro componente da via do complemento (C1). O tratamento de emergência com epinefrina e em longo prazo, com vários agentes, é efetivo.
an·gi·o·el·e·phan·ti·a·sis (an'jē-ō-el'ē-fan-tī'ǎ-sis). Angioelefantíase; aumento significativo da vasculatura do tecido subcutâneo, produzindo espessamento importante simulando a formação de um grande angioma difuso.
an·gi·o·en·do·the·li·o·ma·to·sis (an'jē-ō-en-dō-thē'lē-ō-mǎ-tō'sis). Angioendoteliomatose; proliferação das células endoteliais dentro dos vasos sanguíneos.
proliferating systematized a., a. proliferativa sistemática; rara proliferação intracapilar generalizada das células endoteliais viscerais e cutâneas, com obstrução e trombose vascular. A condição foi dividida em um tipo reativo benigno e um tipo neoplásico rapidamente fatal; entretanto, a maioria dos últimos casos mostrou ser de linfomas intravasculares de células grandes.
an·gi·o·fi·bro·li·po·ma (an'jē-ō-fī'brō-li-pō'mǎ). Angiofibrolipoma; uma neoplasia composta de fibroblastos, capilares e tecido adiposo. SIN angiolipofibroma.
an·gi·o·fi·bro·ma (an'jē-ō-fī-brō'mǎ). Angiofibroma. SIN telangiectatic *fibroma*.
juvenile a., a. juvenil; tumor fibroso acentuadamente vascular que ocorre na nasofaringe dos homens, usualmente na segunda década de vida; epistaxe e invasão local podem acontecer, mas regressão espontânea pode ocorrer depois da maturidade sexual. SIN juvenile hemangiofibroma.
an·gi·o·fi·bro·sis (an'jē-ō-fī-brō'sis). Angiofibrose; fibrose das paredes dos vasos sanguíneos.
an·gi·o·gen·e·sis (an'jē-ō-jen'ě-sis). Angiogênese; desenvolvimento de novos vasos sanguíneos. [angio- + G. *genesis*, produção]
an·gi·o·gen·ic (an'jē-ō-jen'ik). Angiogênico. 1. Relativo à angiogênese. 2. De origem vascular.
an·gi·o·gli·o·ma (an'jē-ō-glī-ō'mǎ). Angioglioma; um glioma e angioma misto.
an·gi·o·gli·o·ma·to·sis (an'jē-ō-glī'ō-mǎ-tō'sis). Angiogliomatose; a ocorrência de múltiplas áreas de capilares e neuróglia em proliferação ou de múltiplos angiogliomas.
an·gi·o·gli·o·sis (an'jē-ō-glī-ō'sis). Angiogliose; fibrose glial em torno de um vaso sanguíneo. Uma forma de arteriosclerose dos vasos cerebrais, caracterizada por aumento da neuróglia.
an·gi·o·gram (an'jē-ō-gram). Angiograma; radiografia obtida na angiografia. [angio- + G. *gramma*, uma escrita]
projection a., a. de projeção; uma a. digital, como no imageamento por tomografia computadorizada ou ressonância magnética, reconstruída por computador para aparecer como uma a. radiográfica.
an·gi·o·graph·ic (an'jē-ō-graf'ik). Angiográfico; relativo ou que usa angiografia.
an·gi·og·ra·phy (an'jē-og'rǎ-fē). Angiografia; radiografia dos vasos depois da injeção de um contraste radiopaco; geralmente exige a inserção percutânea de um cateter radiopaco e o posicionamento sob controle fluoroscópico. VER TAMBÉM arteriography, venography. [angio- + G. *graphō*, escrever]
biplane a., a. biplana; a. sincrônica em dois planos em ângulos retos entre si ou em dois planos ortogonais.
cerebral a., a. cerebral; visualização radiográfica dos vasos sanguíneos que irrigam o cérebro, incluindo as porções extracranianas; a injeção de contraste pode ser feita por via percutânea, por exposição aberta e punção da artéria carótida ou por cateterismo após a introdução do cateter em um local distante. SIN cerebral arteriography.

angiography

coronary a., a. coronária; imageamento da circulação do miocárdio através de injeção de contraste, usualmente por cateterismo seletivo de cada artéria coronária, originalmente por injeção não-seletiva na raiz da aorta.
digital subtraction a. (ASD), angiografia por subtração digital; a. radiográfica assistida por computador que permite a visualização das estruturas vasculares sem as densidades de ossos e tecidos moles superpostos; a subtração das imagens feita antes e depois da injeção de contraste remove as estruturas não realçadas pelo contraste. Outros processamentos de imagem podem ser realizados. O contraste pode ser injetado por via intravenosa ou intra-arterial em uma dose menor que a usual.

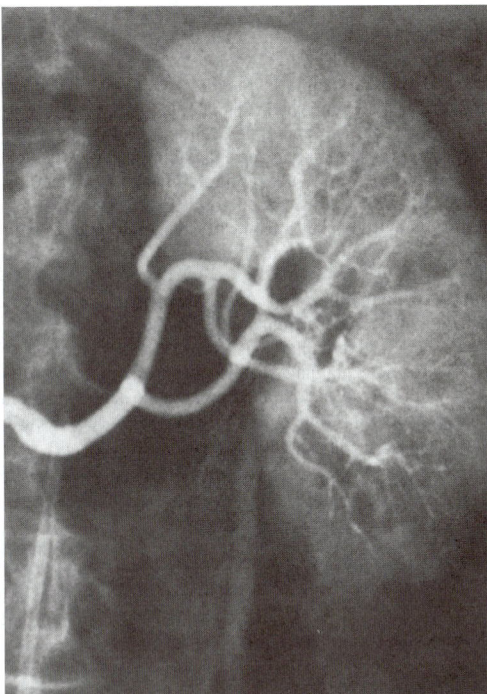

angiografia renal

fluorescein a., a. por fluoresceína; visualização fotográfica da passagem de fluoresceína através dos vasos intra-oculares depois de injeção intravenosa.
indocyanine green a., a. com verde de indocianina; um exame para estudar a vascularização coroidal pela qual o corante verde de indocianina, que absorve a luz infravermelha em 805 nm e emite a 835 nm, é injetado por via intravenosa e fotografado quando ele flui através dos vasos retinianos e coroidais.
interventional a., a. intervencionista. SIN angioplasty.

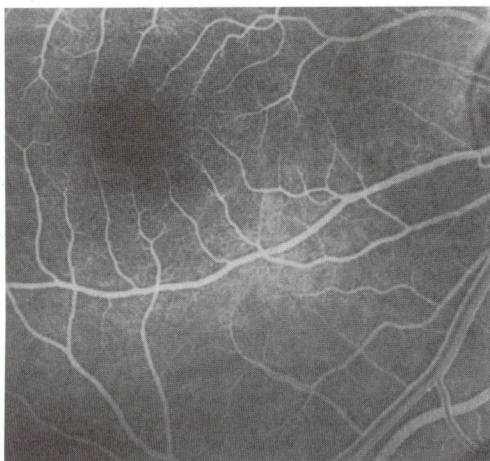

angiografia com fluoresceína: a angiografia com fluoresceína (fase venosa inicial; o enchimento do sistema capilar retiniano fica nítido)

angioma

magnetic resonance a., angiorressonância magnética. SIN MR a.
magnification a., a. com ampliação; imageamento aumentado dos pequenos vasos sanguíneos empregando uma distância aumentada entre o indivíduo e o filme, como na radiografia de ampliação.
MR a. (MRA), angiorressonância magnética (ARM); imageamento dos vasos sanguíneos empregando seqüências especiais de ressonância magnética (RM) que estimulam o sinal do fluxo de sangue e suprimem aquele de outros tecidos. SIN magnetic resonance a.
radionuclide a., a. com radionuclídeo; imageamento da perfusão tecidual com câmera de cintilação através da injeção intravascular de uma substância radioativa. VER TAMBÉM radionuclide *angiocardiography*. SIN scintigraphic a.
scintigraphic a., a. cintigráfica. SIN radionuclide a.
selective a., a. seletiva; a. em que a visualização é melhorada pela concentração do contraste na região a ser estudada através da injeção por meio de um cateter posicionado em uma artéria regional, p.ex., a. coronária.
therapeutic a., a. terapêutica; uso dos cateteres angiográficos que foram modificados para reduzir ou aumentar o fluxo sanguíneo regional, ou para administrar agentes medicinais; a. intervencionista. VER angioplasty, balloon *catheter*, interventional a.

an·gi·o·hy·a·li·no·sis (an′jē-ō-hī′ă-li-nō′sis). Angioialinose; degeneração hialina das paredes dos vasos sanguíneos. [angio- + G. *hyalos*, vidro, + *-osis*, condição]
an·gi·o·hy·per·to·nia (an′jē-ō-hī-per-tō′nē-ă). Angioipertonia; vasospasmo. SIN vasospasm. [angio- + G. *hyper*, acima, + *tonos*, tensão]
an·gi·o·hy·po·to·nia (an′jē-ō-hī-pō-tō′nē-ă). Angioipotonia; vasoparalisia. SIN vasoparalysis. [angio- + G. *hypo*, embaixo + *tonos*, tensão]
an·gi·oid (an-jē-oyd). Angióide; que se assemelha a vasos sanguíneos; um padrão arborizante. [angio- + G. *eidos*, semelhança]
an·gi·o·in·va·sive (an′jē-ō-in-vā′siv). Angioinvasivo; indica uma neoplasia ou outra condição patológica capaz de penetrar no leito vascular.
an·gi·o·ker·a·to·ma (an′jē-ō-ker-ă-tō′mă). Angioceratoma; telangiectasia capilar intradérmica superficial adquirida, sobre a qual existe hiperceratose verruciforme e acantose. SIN keratoangioma, telangiectasia verrucosa, verruga telangiectásica. [angio- + G. *keras*, corno, + *-ōma*, tumor]
diffuse a., a. difusa. SIN Fabry *disease.*
Fordyce a., a. de Fordyce; pápulas vasculares assintomáticas do escroto que aparecem nos adultos.
Mibelli a.'s, a. de Mibelli; pequenas pápulas telangiectásicas dos membros, comuns em meninas adolescentes.
an·gi·o·ker·a·to·sis (an′jē-ō-ker-ă-tō′sis). Angioceratose; a ocorrência de múltiplos angioceratomas.
an·gi·o·lei·o·my·o·ma (an′jē-ō-lī′ō-mī-ō′mă). Angioleiomioma. SIN vascular *leiomyoma.*
an·gi·o·lip·o·fi·bro·ma (an′jē-ō-lip′ō-fi-brō′mă). Angiolipofibroma. SIN angiofibrolipoma.
an·gi·o·li·po·ma (an′jē-ō-li-pō′mă). Angiolipoma; um lipoma que contém um número incomumente grande, ou focos, de canais vasculares freqüentemente dilatados, proliferados, semelhantes à neoplasia. SIN lipoma cavernosum, telangiectatic lipoma.
an·gi·o·lith (an′jē-ō-lith). Angiolito; um arteriólito ou flebólito. [angio- + G. *lithos*, pedra]
an·gi·o·lith·ic (an′jē-ō-lith′ik). Angiolítico; relativo a um angiólito.
an·gi·o·lo·gia (an′jē-ō-lō′jē-ă). Angiologia. SIN angiology. [angio- + G. *logos*, tratado, discurso]
an·gi·ol·o·gy (an-jē-ol′ō-jē). Angiologia; a ciência relacionada com os vasos sanguíneos e linfáticos em todas as suas relações. SIN angiologia. [angio- + G. *logos*, tratado, discurso]
an·gi·ol·y·sis (an-jē-ol′i-sis). Angiólise; obliteração de um vaso sanguíneo, como a que acontece no neonato após a laqueadura do cordão umbilical. [angio- + G. *lysis*, destruição]
an·gi·o·ma (an-jē-ō′mă). Angioma; tumefação ou tumor decorrente da proliferação, com ou sem dilatação, dos vasos sanguíneos (hemangioma) ou linfáticos (linfangioma). [angio- + G. *-ōma*, tumor]
acquired tufted a., angioblastoma de Nakagawa; placas e máculas eritematosas expansivas, em crianças e adultos, compostas, ao nível microscópico, de lóbulos ou capilares e células fusiformes que se projetam para dentro das fendas dérmicas venulares de paredes finas. SIN angioblastoma of Nakagawa.
capillary a., a. capilar; hemangioma capilar. SIN capillary *hemangioma.*
cavernous a., a. cavernoso; malformação vascular composta de vasos sinusoidais sem uma grande artéria nutrícia; pode ser múltiplo, em especial quando herdado como um traço autossômico dominante. SIN nevus cavernosus.
cherry a., hemangioma senil. SIN senile *hemangioma.*
petechial a.'s, a. petequial; múltiplas lesões que se assemelham a petéquias, mas decorrentes da dilatação das paredes dos capilares; elas são obliteradas por pressão.

a. serpigino'sum, a. serpiginoso; a presença de anéis de manchas avermelhadas na pele, especialmente em crianças do sexo feminino, as quais tendem a alargar-se perifericamente, devido à dilatação dos capilares superficiais. SIN essential telangiectasia (2), primary telangiectasia.
spider a., a. aracneiforme; uma arteríola telangiectásica na pele com ramos capilares que se irradiam, simulando as pernas de uma aranha; característico, mas não patognomônico, da doença hepática parenquimatosa; também observado na gestação, desaparecendo, com freqüência, após o parto e, por vezes, em pessoas normais. SIN arterial spider, nevus araneus, spider hemangioma, spider nevus, spider telangiectasia, vascular spider.
superficial a., a. superficial; hemangioma capilar. SIN capillary *hemangioma*.
telangiectatic a., a. telangiectásica; a. composto de vasos dilatados.
a. veno'sum racemo'sum, a. venoso racemoso; inchação tortuosa causada por varicosidades das veias superficiais.
venous a., a. venoso; anomalia vascular composta de veias anômalas. SIN venous malformation.

an·gi·o·ma·toid (an - jē - ō'mă - toyd). Angiomatóide; que se assemelha a um tumor de origem vascular.

an·gi·o·ma·to·sis (an'jē - ō - mă - tō'sis). Angiomatose; uma condição caracterizada por múltiplos angiomas.
bacillary a., a. bacilar; (**1**) uma infecção de pacientes imunocomprometidos por uma espécie de Rickettsia recentemente reconhecida, *Rochalimaea henselae*, caracterizada por febre e nódulos cutâneos granulomatosos e por peliose hepática em alguns casos. A biopsia cutânea mostra proliferação vascular e infiltração das paredes vasculares por neutrófilos e massas de microrganismos observadas à coloração por prata de Warthin-Starry. (**2**) Doença infecciosa caracterizada por febre e lesões granulomatosas cutâneas. Existem duas formas. Em uma, associada à *Bartonella henselae*, as mordeduras e arranhaduras por cães são predisponentes; os linfonodos e vísceras podem ser afetados, podendo acontecer a peliose bacilar do fígado e do baço. Uma forma separada, associada à *B. quintana*, está ligada a condições de má higiene (infestação por piolhos, rendimentos baixos, alojamento deficiente ou inexistente); as lesões subcutâneas e ósseas são mais predominantes.
cephalotrigeminal a., a. cefalotrigêmea; a. encefalotrigêmea. SIN Sturge-Weber *syndrome*.
cerebroretinal a., a. retinocerebral. SIN von Hippel-Lindau *syndrome*.
congenital dysplastic a. [MIM*185300 & MIM149000], a. displásica congênita; a. autossômica dominante em que existe displasia dos tecidos subjacentes, por vezes com crescimento excessivo do osso (síndrome de Klippel-Trenaunay-Weber), ou a. encefalotrigêmea (síndrome de Sturge-Weber), na qual existe um angioma na distribuição de um ou mais ramos do nervo trigêmeo, com anomalias vasculares e calcificação do córtex cerebral.
cutaneomeningospinal a., a. cutaneomeningoespinal. SIN Cobb *syndrome*.
encephalotrigeminal a., a. encefalotrigêmea. SIN Sturge-Weber *syndrome*.
oculoencephalic a. [MIM*185300], a. óculo-encefálica; uma forma frustra da síndrome de Sturge-Weber, consistindo em angiomas apenas da coróide e meninges; provável herança autossômica dominante.
telangiectatic a., a. telangiectásica; malformações vasculares venosas e capilares disseminadas, dos hemisférios cerebrais e leptomeninges, que ocorrem na síndrome de Sturge-Weber.

an·gi·o·ma·tous (an'jē - ō'mă - tŭs). Angiomatoso; relativo a ou que se assemelha a um angioma.

an·gi·o·meg·a·ly (an'jē - ō - meg'ă - lē). Angiomegalia; aumento dos vasos sanguíneos ou linfáticos. [angio- + G. *megas*, grande]

an·gi·o·my·o·car·di·ac (an'jē - ō - mī'ō - kar'dē - ak). Angiomiocárdico; relativo aos vasos sanguíneos e ao músculo cardíaco. [angio- + G. *mys*, músculo, + *kardia*, coração]

an·gi·o·my·o·fi·bro·ma (an'jē - ō - mī'ō - fi - brō'mă). Angiomiofibroma; leiomioma vascular. SIN vascular *leiomyoma*.

an·gi·o·my·o·li·po·ma (an'jē - ō - mī'ō - li - pō'mă). Angiomiolipoma; neoplasia benigna do tecido adiposo (lipoma) em que as células musculares e as estruturas vasculares são razoavelmente evidentes; mais amiúde um tumor renal que contém músculo liso; freqüentemente associada à esclerose tuberosa. [angio- + G. *mys*, músculo, + *lipos*, gordura, + *-oma*, tumor]

an·gi·o·my·o·ma (an'jē - ō - mī - ō'mă). Angiomioma; leiomioma vascular. SIN vascular *leiomyoma*. [angio- + G. *mys*, músculo, + *-ōma*, tumor]

an·gi·o·my·op·a·thy (an'jē - ō - mī - op'ă - thē). Angiomiopatia; qualquer doença dos vasos sanguíneos que envolva a camada muscular. [angio- + G. *mys*, músculo, + *pathos*, sofrimento]

an·gi·o·my·o·sar·co·ma (an'jē - ō - mī'ō - sar - kō'mă). Angiomiossarcoma; um miossarcoma que apresenta um número incomumente grande de canais vasculares proliferados, freqüentemente dilatados.

an·gi·o·myx·o·ma (an'jē - ō - miks - ō'mă). Angiomixoma; um mixoma em que existe um número incomumente grande de estruturas vasculares.
aggressive a., a. agressivo; um tumor localmente invasivo, porém não-gerador de metástases, dos órgãos genitais em mulheres jovens.

an·gi·o·neu·rec·to·my (an'jē - ō - noo - rek'tō - mē). Angioneurectomia; a excisão de vasos e nervos de uma região. [angio- + G. *neuron*, nervo, + *ektomē*, um corte]

an·gi·o·neu·rop·a·thy (an'jē - ō - noo - rop'ă - thē). Angioneuropatia; transtorno vascular atribuído a anormalidade das fibras do sistema nervoso autônomo que inervam os vasos sanguíneos (isto é, o sistema vasomotor).

an·gi·o·neu·rot·ic (an'jē - ō - noo - rot'ik). Angioneurótico, angioneuropático; relativo à angioneurose (angioneuropático). VER angioneuropathy.

an·gi·o·neu·rot·o·my (an'jē - ō - noo - rot'ō - mē). Angioneurotomia; divisão de nervos e vasos de uma região. [angio- + G. *neuron*, nervo, + *tomē*, um corte]

an·gi·o·pa·ral·y·sis (an'jē - ō - pă - ral'i - sis). Angioparalisia. SIN vasoparalysis.

an·gi·o·pa·re·sis (an'jē - ō - pă - rē'sis, - par'ē - sis). Angioparesia; vasoparesia. SIN vasoparesis.

an·gi·o·path·ic (an'jē - ō - path'ik). Angiopático; relativo à angiopatia.

an·gi·op·a·thy (an - jē - op'ă - thē). Angiopatia; qualquer doença dos vasos sanguíneos ou linfáticos. SIN angiosis. [angio- + G. *pathos*, sofrimento]
amyloid a., a. amilóide; deposição de material hialino acelular nas pequenas artérias e arteríolas das leptomeninges e córtex cerebral no idoso, com resultante predileção para hematomas intraparenquimatosos lobares recorrentes.
cerebral amyloid a., a. amilóide cerebral; uma condição patológica dos pequenos vasos cerebrais caracterizada por depósitos de amilóide nas paredes vasculares, os quais podem levar a infartos ou hemorragia; também pode ocorrer na doença de Alzheimer ou na síndrome de Down. VER TAMBÉM congophilic a.
congophilic a., a. congofílica; uma condição dos vasos sanguíneos caracterizada por depósitos, nas paredes vasculares, de uma substância, usualmente amilóide, que capta o corante vermelho-congo. VER TAMBÉM cerebral amyloid a.
giant cell hyaline a., a. hialina de células gigantes; um infiltrado inflamatório que contém células gigantes do tipo corpo estranho e material eosinofílico. Os fragmentos do material estranho, assemelhando-se à substância vegetal, podem estar inclusos. SIN pulse granuloma.

an·gi·o·phac·o·ma·to·sis, an·gi·o·phak·o·ma·to·sis (an'jē - ō - fak'ō - mă - tō'sis). Angiofacomatose; as facomatoses angiomatosas, p.ex., doença de von Hippel-Lindau e a síndrome de Sturge-Weber.

an·gi·o·pla·ny (an'jē - ō - plā - nē). Angioplania; angiectopia. SIN angiectopia. [angio- + G. *planē*, uma viagem]

an·gi·o·plas·ty (an'jē - ō - plas - tē). Angioplastia; reconstituição ou recanalização de um vaso sanguíneo; pode envolver a dilatação por balão, desnudamento mecânico da camada íntima, injeção forçada de fibrinolíticos ou colocação de um *stent*. SIN interventional angiography. [angio- + G. *plastos*, formado, moldado]
percutaneous transluminal a. (PTA), a. transluminal percutânea; cirurgia para alargar uma luz vascular estreitada por insuflar e retirar, através de uma região estenótica, um balão na extremidade de um cateter angiográfico; pode incluir a colocação de um *stent* endoluminal intravascular.

percutaneous transluminal coronary a. (PTCA), a. coronária transluminal percutânea (PTCA); cirurgia para dilatar uma luz vascular estreitada por insuflar e retirar um balão na extremidade de um cateter angiográfico através de uma região estenótica.

A PTCA é um procedimento cirúrgico pouco invasivo para o tratamento da aterosclerose coronária. Um cateter com balão na extremidade é inserido, por via percutânea, na circulação arterial, sendo avançado até a raiz da aorta e direcionado, com um guia flexível, até a estenose coronária. Uma vez posicionado dentro do segmento arterial estreitado, o balão é insuflado de modo a distender a luz e/ou fraturar a placa obstrutiva. A angioplastia por balão é considerada bem-sucedida quando existe um aumento superior a 20% no calibre da artéria estenótica, com a restauração de, pelo menos, 50% da permeabilidade normal, sem complicações agudas. O procedimento apresenta uma taxa de sucesso imediato de, aproximadamente, 90%. Ele oferece vantagens na melhoria dos sintomas e tolerância aos esforços, quando comparado à terapia clínica, principalmente em curto prazo, e é menos perigoso e apresenta um menor tempo de recuperação em relação ao enxerto em artéria(s) coronária(s). A taxa de mortalidade cirúrgica situa-se em 2%. Existe um risco de 1 a 3% de infarto agudo do miocárdio não-fatal durante o procedimento, bem como um risco de 1 a 3% de que haverá necessidade de um enxerto em artéria coronária de emergência. Portanto, o procedimento está contra-indicado, a menos que uma equipe cirúrgica esteja imediatamente disponível. Ele também está contra-indicado para os pacientes sem obstrução vascular significativa demonstrada, bem como para aqueles com doença grave em múltiplos vasos ou estenose superior a 50% da artéria coronária esquerda. Apesar das vantagens da PTCA, há necessidade de repetir a angioplastia por balão ou de enxerto em artéria coronária para reestenose em 6 meses em 30 a 50% dos pacientes. A inserção de um *stent* de aço inoxidável no momento da angioplastia por balão, visando manter a

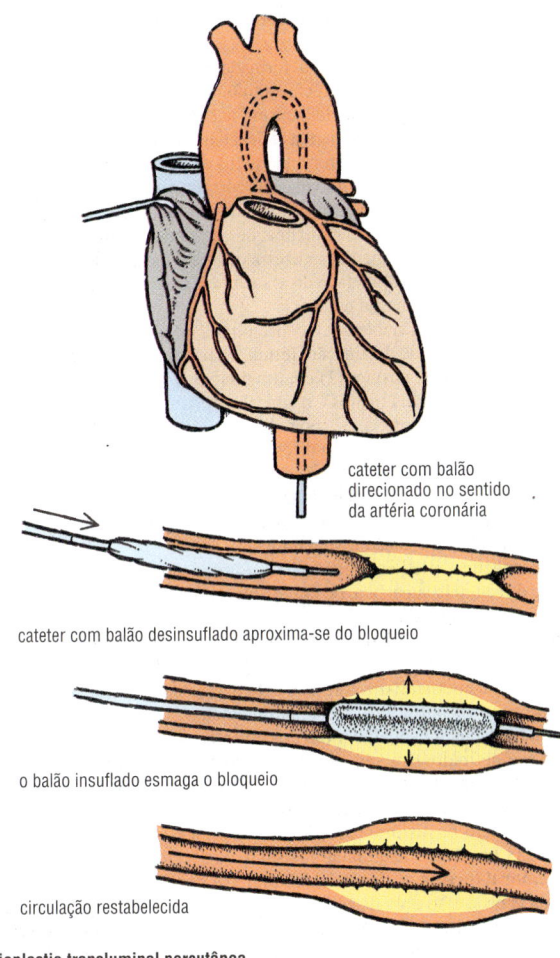

cateter com balão direcionado no sentido da artéria coronária

cateter com balão desinsuflado aproxima-se do bloqueio

o balão insuflado esmaga o bloqueio

circulação restabelecida

angioplastia transluminal percutânea

permeabilidade arterial, melhorou o sucesso inicial e reduziu a taxa de reestenose com 6 meses. O verapamil em dose alta também foi associado a taxas menores de reestenose.

an·gi·o·poi·e·sis (an'jē-ō-poy-ē'sis). Angiopoese; formação de vasos sanguíneos ou linfáticos. SIN vasifaction, vasoformation. [angio- + G. *poiesis*, formação]

an·gi·o·poi·et·ic (an'jē-ō-poy-et'ik). Angiopoético; relativo à angiopoese. SIN vasifactive, vasofactive, vasoformative.

an·gi·or·rha·phy (an-jē-ōr'ă-fē). Angiorrafia; reparação por sutura de qualquer vaso, especialmente de um vaso sanguíneo. [angio- + G. *rhaphē*, uma costura]

an·gi·o·sar·co·ma (an'jē-ō-sar-kō'mă). Angiossarcoma; uma rara neoplasia maligna que ocorre mais amiúde nos tecidos moles; acredita-se que se origina das células endoteliais dos vasos sanguíneos; composta microscopicamente por células fusiformes, algumas das quais revestem pequenos espaços que se assemelham a fendas vasculares.

an·gi·o·scope (an'jē-ō-skōp). Angioscópio; um microscópio modificado para estudar os vasos capilares e um instrumento utilizado para visualizar vasos mais calibrosos. [angio- + G. *skopeō*, ver]

an·gi·os·co·py (an-jē-os'kō-pē). Angioscopia. **1.** Visualização, com um microscópio, da passagem de substâncias (p. ex., contrastes, agentes radiopacos) pelos capilares após a injeção intravenosa. **2.** Visualização do interior dos vasos sanguíneos, sobretudo das artérias pulmonares, usando um cateter de fibra óptica inserido através de uma artéria periférica. [angio- + G. *skopeō*, ver]

an·gi·o·sco·to·ma (an'jē-ō-skō-tō'mă). Angioscotoma; defeito dos campos visuais, em forma de faixa, provocado pelos vasos retinianos que se sobrepõem aos fotorreceptores. [angio- + G. *skotoma*, tonteira, vertigem]

an·gi·o·sco·tom·e·try (an'jē-ō-skō-tom'e-trē). Angioscotometria; a mensuração ou projeção do padrão do angioscotoma.

an·gi·o·sis (an-jē-ō'sis). Angiose; angiopatia. SIN angiopathy.

angiosome. Angiossoma; territórios vasculares anatômicos compostos de pele e músculos, tendões, nervos e ossos subjacentes, baseados na segmentação ou distribuição das artérias.

an·gi·o·spasm (an'jē-ō-spazm). Angiospasmo; vasospasmo. SIN vasospasm.

an·gi·o·spas·tic (an'jē-ō-spas'tik). Angiospástico; vasospástico. SIN vasospastic.

an·gi·o·ste·no·sis (an'jē-ō-stē-nō'sis). Angiostenose; estreitamento de um ou mais vasos sanguíneos. [angio- + G. *stenōsis*, um estreitamento]

an·gi·o·stron·gy·lo·sis (an'jē-ō-stron-ji-lō'sis). Angiostrongilose; infestação de animais e seres humanos por nematódeos do gênero *Angiostrongylus*. SIN eosinophilic meningitis.

An·gi·o·stron·gy·lus (an'jē-ō-stron'ji-lŭs). Um gênero de nematódeos metastrôngilos parasitas no sistema respiratório ou circulatório de roedores, carnívoros e marsupiais. SIN *Parastrongylus*. [G. *angeion*, vaso, + *strongylos*, redondo]

A. cantonen'sis, parasita do pulmão de roedores, uma espécie transmitida por moluscos infestados ingeridos pelos roedores; as larvas desenvolvem-se no cérebro e migram para os pulmões, onde são encontrados os vermes adultos; acredita-se que provoquem a encefalomeningite eosinofílica em seres humanos na bacia do Pacífico; larvas já foram removidas do líquido cefalorraquidiano e da câmara anterior do olho em pessoas na Tailândia que ingeriram lesmas cruas.

A. costaricen'sis, um nematódeo parasita de ratos e outros roedores na América Central, recentemente encontrado em seres humanos infestados, nos quais se localizam nas artérias mesentéricas; larvas infecciosas de terceiro estágio já foram encontradas na lesma *Vaginulus plebeius*. SIN *Morerastrongylus costaricensis*.

A. malaysien'sis, espécie de *A.* encontrada na Malásia, um parasita comum de roedores semelhante a *A. cantonensis* e um agente causal real ou potencial de meningite eosinofílica naquela região.

an·gi·o·te·lec·ta·sis, an·gi·o·tel·ec·ta·sia (an'jē-ō-tē-lek'tă-sis, -tel'ek-tā'sē-ă). Angiotelectasia; telangectasia. SIN telangiectasia. [angio- + G. *telos*, término, + *ektasis*, uma dilatação]

an·gi·o·ten·sin (an'jē-ō-ten'sin). Angiotensina; uma família de peptídeos de seqüência conhecida e similar, com atividade vasoconstritora, produzida pela ação enzimática da renina sobre a angiotensina. VER angiotensin I, angiotensin II, angiotensin III.

an·gi·o·ten·sin I. Angiotensina I; um decapeptídeo de seqüência discretamente variável, dependendo da origem animal, formado a partir do tetradecapeptídeo angiotensinogênio pela retirada de quatro resíduos aminoácido, uma reação catalisada pela renina; uma peptidase cliva um dipeptídeo (histidil-leucina) para gerar a angiotensina II, a forma fisiologicamente ativa.

an·gi·o·ten·sin II. Angiotensina II; um octapeptídeo vasoativo produzido pela ação da enzima conversora de angiotensina sobre a angiotensina I; produz estimulação da musculatura lisa vascular, promove a produção de aldosterona e estimula o sistema nervoso simpático.

an·gi·o·ten·sin III. Angiotensina III; um heptapeptídeo vasoativo menos potente que a angiotensina II sobre a musculatura lisa vascular, mas quase igualmente ativo na promoção da secreção de aldosterona.

an·gi·o·ten·sin am·ide. Amida da angiotensina; uma substância sintética intimamente relacionada à angiotensina II de ocorrência natural; um potente agente vasopressor útil no controle de determinados tipos de choque e colapso circulatório.

an·gi·o·ten·sin·ase (an'jē-ō-ten'sin-ās). Angiotensinase; nome original para a enzima responsável pela conversão da angiotensina I em II; atualmente aplicado à enzima que degrada a angiotensina II. Hidrolisa uma ligação peptídica entre um resíduo tirosil e um isoleucil.

an·gi·o·ten·sin·o·gen (an'jē-ō-ten-sin'ō-jen). Angiotensinogênio; o substrato para a renina. Graças à ação enzimática sobre o a., a angiotensina I é liberada; uma α_2-globulina abundante que circula no plasma sanguíneo. SIN angiotensin precursor.

an·gi·o·ten·sin·o·gen·ase (an'jē-ō-ten-sin'ō-jen-ās). Angiotensinogenase. SIN renin.

an·gi·o·ten·sin pre·cur·sor. Precursor da angiotensina; SIN angiotensinogen.

an·gi·ot·o·my (an'jē-ot'ō-mē). Angiotomia; o seccionamento de um vaso sanguíneo ou a criação de uma abertura em um vaso antes de sua reparação. [angio- + G. *tomē*, corte]

Angle, Edward Hartley, ortodontista norte-americano, 1855–1930. VER A. *classification* of malocclusion.

ANGLE

an·gle (θ) (ang'gl) [TA]. Ângulo; o ponto de encontro de duas linhas ou planos; a figura formada pela junção de duas linhas ou planos; o espaço limitado em dois lados por linhas ou planos que se encontram. Para os ângulos não arrolados adiante, ver o termo descritivo; p.ex., axioincisal, distobuccal, labiogingival, linguogingival (2), mesiogingival, proximobuccal, etc. SIN angulus [TA]. [L. *angulus*]

acromial a. [TA], a. acromial; o ângulo proeminente na junção das bordas posterior e lateral do acrômio. SIN angulus acromii [TA].

acute a., a. agudo; qualquer a. menor que 90°.

adjacent a., a. adjacente; um a. com uma linha em comum com outro a.

alpha a., a. alfa; (1) o a. entre os eixos visual e óptico quando eles se cruzam no ponto nodal do olho; (2) o a. entre a linha visual e o eixo principal da elipse córnea.

alveolar a., a, alveolar; o a. entre o plano horizontal e uma linha que une a base da espinha nasal e o ponto médio da projeção do alvéolo da maxila.

anorectal a., a. anorretal; flexura anorretal. SIN anorectal *flexure.*

a. of antetorsion, a. de antetorção. SIN a. of anteversion.

a. of anteversion, a. de anteversão; o a. formado por uma linha traçada através do centro do eixo longitudinal do colo do fêmur encontrando uma linha traçada no eixo transversal dos côndilos, quando o osso é visto por cima diretamente para baixo, através da cabeça do fêmur; usado para ilustrar o grau normal de anteversão de aproximadamente 12° do colo do fêmur, que pode estar aumentado ou diminuído em algumas doenças. SIN a. of antetorsion.

a. of aperture, a. de abertura; o a. formado por linhas traçadas a partir das extremidades do diâmetro de uma lente até seu ponto focal. VER TAMBÉM angular *aperture.*

apical a., a. apical; o a. entre duas superfícies planas de um prisma. SIN refracting a. of a prism.

axial a., a. axial; a. formado por duas superfícies de um corpo, cuja linha de união é paralela ao seu eixo; os ângulos axiais de um dente são distobucal, distolabial, distolinguais, mesiobucal, mesiolabial e mesiolingual.

basilar a., a. basilar; a. formado pela intersecção no básio das linhas que vêm da espinha nasal e do ponto nasal.

Bennett a., a. de Bennett; o a. formado pelo plano sagital e pelo trajeto do côndilo em progressão durante o movimento mandibular lateral, quando visto no plano horizontal.

beta a., a. beta; o a. formado por uma linha que une o bregma e o hórmio, encontrando o *radius fixus* (linha reta do hórmio até o ínio).

biorbital a., a. biorbitário; um a. formado pelo encontro dos eixos das órbitas.

Broca a.'s, a. de Broca; (1) SIN Broca basilar a.; (2) SIN Broca facial a.; (3) SIN occipital a. of parietal bone (1).

Broca basilar a., a. basilar de Broca; o a. formado no básio das linhas traçadas a partir do násio e do ponto alveolar. SIN Broca a.'s (1).

Broca facial a., a. facial de Broca; o a. formado pela intersecção no eixo biauricular das linhas traçadas desde o ponto supra-orbitário e o ponto alveolar. SIN Broca a.'s (2).

buccal a.'s, a. bucal; os ângulos formados pela superfície bucal de um dente com as outras superfícies.

bucco-occlusal a., a. bucooclusal; a linha de junção das superfícies bucal e oclusal de um dente.

cardiodiaphragmatic a., a. cardiodiafragmático. SIN cardiophrenic a.

cardiohepatic a., a. cardioepático; o a. formado pela borda superior do fígado e borda direita do coração, principalmente quando definido pela percussão. SIN cardiohepatic triangle.

cardiophrenic a., a. cardiofrênico; o a. entre o coração e o diafragma na extremidade lateral da projeção cardíaca nos exames de imagem (geralmente na radiografia de tórax). O a. cardiofrênico direito normalmente não se distingue do a. cardioepático por meios radiográficos. SIN cardiodiaphragmatic a., phrenopericardial a.

carrying a., a. de transporte; o a. feito pelos eixos do braço e antebraço quando o cotovelo se encontra em extensão plena.

cavity line a., a. de linha da cavidade; em odontologia, o a. formado por duas paredes de uma cavidade, p.ex., uma cavidade dentária, que se reúnem ao longo de uma linha.

cavosurface a., a. cavossuperficial; o a. formado pela junção de uma parede de cavidade com a superfície do dente.

cephalic a., a. cefálico; um de vários ângulos formados pela intersecção de duas linhas que passam através de determinados pontos da face ou do crânio.

cephalomedullary a., a. cefalomedular; o a. formado pela junção do cérebro com o tronco cerebral.

cerebellopontile a., a. cerebelopontino. SIN cerebellopontine a.

cerebellopontine a., a. cerebelopontino; o a. formado na junção do cerebelo, da ponte e da medula oblonga; o tumor mais comum encontrado nessa localização é o neuroma do acústico. SIN angulus pontocerebellaris [TA], cerebellopontile a., pontine a., pontocerebellar recess.

costal a., a. costal. SIN a. of rib.

costophrenic a., a. costofrênico; o a. entre as pleuras parietais costal e diafragmática quando elas se encontram na linha costodiafragmática da reflexão pleural. Usado como sinônimo em radiologia para identificar o recesso costodiafragmático. VER TAMBÉM costodiaphragmatic *recess.*

costovertebral a., a. costovertebral; o a. agudo formado entre a décima segunda costela e a coluna vertebral.

costoxiphoid a., a. costoxifóide; o a. formado entre o arco costal direito ou esquerdo e o eixo longitudinal do processo xifóide (usualmente idêntico à linha média); é metade do a. infra-esternal. VER TAMBÉM infrasternal a. SIN xiphocostal a.

craniofacial a., a. craniofacial; o a. formado pelos eixos basifacial e basicraniano no ponto médio da sutura esfenoetmoidal.

critical a., a. crítico; o a. de incidência em que um raio de luz, ao passar entre dois meios, muda da refração para a reflexão total. SIN limiting a.

cusp a., a. cúspide; (1) o a. formado pelos declives de uma cúspide com o plano que passa através da extremidade da cúspide e que é perpendicular a uma linha que corta duas vezes a cúspide, medida no sentido mesiodistal ou bucolingual; (2) o a. formado pelas inclinações de uma cúspide com uma linha perpendicular que secciona duas vezes a cúspide, medida no sentido mesiodistal ou bucolingual; (3) metade do a. incluído entre as inclinações da cúspide bucal e lingual ou mesial e distal.

Daubenton a., a. de Daubenton. SIN occipital a. of parietal bone (2).

a. of declination, a. de declinação; termo arcaico para o a. de anteversão.

a. of deviation, a. de desvio; (1) em um prisma, o somatório dos ângulos de incidência e emergência menos o a. apical do prisma; (2) em óptica, a. de refração; (3) no estrabismo, a. de anomalia.

disparity a., a. de disparidade; a diferença na posição das imagens na retina, mas ainda permitindo a fusão.

duodenojejunal a., a. duodenojejunal. SIN duodenojejunal *flexure.*

a. of eccentricity, a. de excentricidade; no estrabismo, o a. entre a linha de fixação e a linha de fixação foveal normal.

a. of emergence, a. de emergência; o a. formado por um raio luminoso que emerge da segunda superfície de um prisma e uma linha paralela ao raio incidente. Cf. a. of deviation.

epigastric a., a. epigástrico; o a. formado pelo processo xifóide com o corpo do esterno.

ethmoid a., a. etmoidal; o a. formado pelo plano da placa cribriforme do osso etmóide ao se encontrar com o eixo basicraniano.

facial a., a. facial; (1) qualquer um dos diversos ângulos variadamente denominados e definidos que têm sido empregados para quantificar a protrusão facial; (2) em odontologia, o a. formado pela intersecção do plano orbitomeatal (Frankfort) com a linha násio-pogônio (a. inferior interno), que estabelece a relação ântero-posterior da mandíbula com a face superior no plano orbitomeatal. SIN Frankfort-mandibular incisor a.

a. of femoral torsion, a. de torção femoral; o a. formado entre o eixo longitudinal da cabeça e do colo do fêmur, proximalmente, e o eixo transversal dos côndilos femorais, distalmente, quando o fêmur é visto ao longo do eixo de sua diáfise; normalmente, esse a. tem aproximadamente 15° nos adultos, mas é consideravelmente maior no lactente.

filtration a., a. de filtração. SIN iridocorneal a.

flip a., a. de inversão; em uma seqüência de pulso de ressonância magnética, o desvio no sentido do plano transversal do eixo médio dos prótons induzido pelos sinais de radiofreqüência; ângulos baixos são empregados nas seqüências de imagens do sangue rápidas ou brilhantes.

Frankfort-mandibular incisor a., a. incisivo mandibular de Frankfort. SIN facial a. (2).

frontal a. of parietal bone [TA], a. frontal do osso parietal; o a. ântero-superior do osso parietal. SIN angulus frontalis ossis parietalis [TA].

a. of Fuchs, a. de Fuchs; fenda entre as zonas ciliar e pupilar da íris formada por atrofia das camadas superficiais da íris na zona pupilar.

gamma a., a. gama; o a. formado entre uma linha que une o ponto de fixação ao centro do olho e o eixo óptico.

hypsiloid a., a. hipsilóide. SIN y-a.

impedance a., a. de impedância; um termo que expressa a relação entre a resistência elétrica e a capacitância elétrica (ohms/microfarads) nos tecidos do corpo ou em qualquer outra substância.

a. of incidence, a. de incidência; (1) o a. que um raio, penetrando em um meio refratário, faz com uma linha desenhada perpendicular à superfície desse meio; (2) o a. que um raio que colide com uma superfície refletora faz com uma linha perpendicular a essa superfície. SIN incident a.

incident a., a. de incidência. SIN a. of incidence.

incisal guide a., a. de guia incisal; o a. formado com o plano horizontal ao desenhar uma linha no plano sagital entre as bordas incisais dos incisivos centrais maxilares e mandibulares quando os dentes estão em oclusão central.

a. of inclination, a. de inclinação; o a. formado pela reunião de uma linha traçada através da diáfise de um osso longo com aquela que passa através do eixo longitudinal de seu colo femoral; normalmente se refere ao fêmur e ao úmero. SIN neck-shaft a.

inferior a. of scapula [TA], a. inferior da escápula; o a. agudo formado pela junção das bordas lateral e medial da escápula. SIN angulus inferior scapulae [TA].

infrasternal a. [TA], a. infra-esternal; o a. entre as bordas inferiores das cartilagens costais dos dois lados, quando elas se aproximam do esterno. SIN angulus infrasternalis [TA], subcostal a.*, subcostal arch*, substernal a.

iridocorneal a. [TA], a. iridocorneal; o a. agudo entre a íris e a córnea na periferia da câmara anterior do olho. SIN angulus iridocornealis [TA], a. of íris, angulus iridis, filtration a.

a. of iris, a. da íris. SIN iridocorneal a.
Jacquart facial a., a. facial de Jacquart; um a. facial com a intersecção sempre no ponto da espinha nasal; a variação adicional utiliza o ponto supra-orbitário, em vez de a glabela, sendo esta última versão também conhecida como a. facial ofrioespinhal ou a. facial de Topinard.
a. of jaw, a. da mandíbula. SIN a. of mandible.
kappa a., a. kapa; o a. entre o eixo pupilar e o eixo visual; é positivo quando o eixo pupilar é nasal em relação ao eixo visual, e negativo quando o eixo pupilar é temporal em relação ao eixo visual.
lateral a. of eye [TA], a. lateral do olho; o a. formado pela junção das partes laterais das pálpebras superior e inferior. SIN angulus oculi lateralis [TA], angulus oculi temporalis, external canthus, lateral canthus.
lateral a. of scapula [TA], a. lateral da escápula; a cabeça côncava e obtusa da escápula formando a cavidade glenóide na junção das bordas superior e lateral do osso. SIN angulus lateralis scapulae [TA].
lateral a. of uterus, a. lateral do útero; a parte superior do lado do útero no ponto de sua junção com a tuba uterina.
limiting a., a. crítico. SIN critical a.
line a., a. da linha; em odontologia, a junção de duas superfícies da coroa de um dente ou de uma cavidade dentária (a. da linha da cavidade).
Louis a., a. de Louis. SIN sternal a.
Lovibond a., a. de Lovibond; o a. feito na reunião da prega ungueal proximal com a placa ungueal quando visto a partir da face radial; normalmente, inferior a 180°, mas supera esse limite no baqueteamento dos dedos das mãos. SIN Lovibond profile sign.
Ludwig a., a. de Ludwig. SIN sternal a.
lumbosacral a., a. lombossacro; o a. entre o eixo longitudinal da parte lombar da coluna vertebral e o do sacro.
a. of mandible [TA], a. da mandíbula; o a. formado pela margem inferior do corpo e margem posterior do ramo da mandíbula. SIN angulus mandibulae [TA], a. of jaw.
mastoid a. of parietal bone [TA], a. mastóide do parietal; o ponto póstero-inferior do osso parietal. SIN angulus mastoideus ossis parietalis [TA].
maxillary a., a. maxilar; o a. formado por uma linha traçada desde o ófrio e outra desde o ponto da mandíbula e que se encontram entre os dentes incisivos superior e inferior.
medial a. of eye [TA], a. medial do olho; o a. formado pela união das pálpebras superior e inferior medialmente. SIN angulus oculi medialis [TA], angulus oculi nasalis, internal canthus, medial canthus.
mesial a., a. mesial; o a. formado pela reunião da superfície mesial com a labial (ou bucal) ou lingual de um dente.
metafacial a., a. metafacial; o a. entre os processos pterigóide e a base do crânio. SIN Serres a.
meter a., a. medidor; a convergência necessária para ver binocularmente um objeto a 1 m de distância e exercendo 1 dioptria de acomodação. SIN unit of ocular convergence.
a. of mouth [TA], a. da boca; o limite lateral da fissura oral. VER TAMBÉM labial *commissure*. SIN angulus oris [TA].
neck-shaft a., a. colo-diáfise; a. de inclinação. SIN a. of inclination.
occipital a. of parietal bone [TA], a. occipital do parietal; (1) o ângulo póstero-superior do osso parietal. SIN Broca a.'s (3); (2) a. formado pela junção, no opístio, de linhas que provêm do básio e da projeção, no plano mediano, da borda inferior das órbitas. SIN angulus occipitalis ossis parietalis [TA], Daubenton a. VER TAMBÉM Daubenton line, Daubenton plane.
olfactory a., a. olfatório; o a. formado pelo plano da lâmina cribriforme com o eixo basicraniano.
ophryospinal a., a. ofrioespinal. VER Jacquart facial a.
parietal a., a. parietal; um a. formado pela reunião do prolongamento de duas linhas tangenciais à parte mais proeminente do arco zigomático e à sutura parietofrontal em cada lado; quando as linhas permanecem paralelas, o a. é zero; quando elas divergem, ele é negativo. SIN Quatrefages a.
pelvivertebral a., a. pelvivertebral; o a. formado pela pelve, conforme definido pelo plano da abertura pélvica superior com o eixo geral do tronco ou da coluna vertebral. VER TAMBÉM pelvic *inclination*.
phrenopericardial a., a. frenopericárdico. SIN cardiophrenic a.
Pirogoff a., a. de Pirogoff. SIN venous a. (1).
point a., a. do ponto; a junção de três superfícies da coroa de um dente ou das paredes de uma cavidade.
a. of polarization, a. de polarização; o a. de incidência em que a luz refletida é totalmente polarizada.
pontine a., a. pontino. SIN cerebellopontine a.
pubic a., a. púbico. SIN subpubic a.
Q a., a. Q; o a. formado por linhas que representam a tração do músculo quadríceps e o eixo do tendão patelar.
Quatrefages a., a. de Quatrefages. SIN parietal a.
Ranke a., a. de Ranke; o a. formado pelo plano horizontal da cabeça e uma linha que passa desde o centro da margem do arco alveolar da maxila, abaixo da espinha nasal até o centro da sutura frontonasal. [J. Ranke]

a. of reflection, a. de reflexão; o a. que um raio refletido a partir de uma superfície forma com uma linha traçada perpendicularmente a essa superfície; é igual ao a. de incidência (2).
refracting a. of prism, a. de refração do prisma. SIN apical a.
a. of refraction, a. de refração; o a. que um raio que deixa um meio de refração faz com uma linha traçada perpendicularmente à superfície desse meio.
a. of retroversion, a. de retroversão; o a. formado por uma linha traçada através do centro do eixo longitudinal do colo e da cabeça do úmero que se encontra com uma linha traçada ao longo do eixo transversal dos côndilos, quando a base é visualizada por cima, olhando diretamente para baixo, a partir de um ponto acima da cabeça do úmero; o a. normal de retroversão do úmero situa-se entre 20° e 40°.
a. of rib [TA], a. costal; a mudança algo abrupta na curvatura do corpo de uma costela posteriormente, de tal modo que o colo e a cabeça da costela fiquem direcionados para cima. SIN angulus costae [TA], costal a.
Rolando a., a. de Rolando; o a. que a fissura de Rolando (sulco central) faz com o plano médio.
Serres a., a. de Serres. SIN metafacial a.
S-N-A a., a. S-N-A; em cefalometria, um a. que mede a relação ântero-posterior do arco basal maxilar na base craniana anterior; mostra o grau de prognatismo do maxilar. VER TAMBÉM subspinale. [sella-nasion-subspinale (ou point A)]
S-N-B a., a. S-N-B; um a. que mostra o limite anterior do arco basal mandibular em relação à base craniana anterior. VER TAMBÉM supramentale. [sella-nasion-supramentale (ou point B)]
sphenoid a., sphenoidal a., a. do esfenóide; (1) a. formado pela intersecção, no ápice da sela turca (dorso da sela), das linhas que se originam do ponto nasal e da extremidade do rostro do esfenóide; (2) SIN sphenoidal a. of parietal bone.
sphenoidal a. of parietal bone [TA], a. esfenoidal do parietal; o a. ântero-inferior do osso parietal. SIN angulus sphenoidalis ossis parietalis [TA], sphenoid a. (2), sphenoidal a., Welcker a.
sternal a. [TA], a. esternal; o a. entre o manúbrio e o corpo do esterno na junção manubrioesternal. Marca o nível da segunda cartilagem costal (costela) para a contagem de costelas ou espaços intercostais. Indica o nível do arco aórtico, da bifurcação da traquéia e do disco intervertebral T4/T5. SIN angulus sterni [TA], Louis a., Ludwig a., manubriosternal junction.
sternoclavicular a., a. esternoclavicular; o a. formado pela junção da clavícula com o esterno.
subcostal a., a. subcostal; *termo oficial alternativo para infrasternal a.
subpubic a. [TA], a. subpúbico; o a. formado entre os ramos inferiores dos ossos púbicos. Na mulher, o a. é quase igual ao a. entre os dedos polegar e indicador bem esticados (90°); no homem, aproxima-se do a. formado entre os dedos indicador e médio bastante abduzidos (60°). VER TAMBÉM pubic *arch*. SIN angulus subpubicus [TA], pubic a.
subesternal a., a. subesternal. SIN infrasternal a.
superior a. of scapula [TA], a. superior da escápula; originalmente denominado de ângulo medial, localiza-se na junção das bordas superior e medial do osso. SIN angulus superior scapulae [TA].
sylvian a., a. de Sylvius; o a. formado pela linha de Sylvius e uma linha perpendicular ao plano horizontal, tangencial ao ponto mais elevado do hemisfério.
tentorial a., a. tentorial; o a. formado pelo plano do tentório com o eixo basicraniano.
Topinard facial a., a. facial de Topinard. VER Jacquart facial a.
a. of torsion, a. de torção; a rotação de um osso longo ao longo de seu eixo ou entre dois eixos, medida em graus; quando esse a. está orientado anteriormente, é referido como o a. de anteversão e descreve, mais amiúde, o fêmur; quando esse a. está orientado posteriormente, é o a. de retroversão e descreve mais comumente o úmero.
urethrovesical a., a. uretrovesical; o a. entre a uretra feminina e a parede vesical posterior (normalmente ~ 90°); o estreitamento desse ângulo na cistocele predispõe à incontinência por estresse.
venous a., a. venoso; (1) a junção das veias jugular interna e subclávia, para a qual convergem as veias jugulares externa e anterior e as veias vertebrais, o ducto torácico no a. esquerdo e o ducto linfático direito no a. direito. SIN Pirogoff a.; (2) em neurorradiologia, o a. de união da veia talamoestriada superior (*vena terminalis*) com a veia cerebral interna, usualmente muito próximo à parte posterior do forame interventricular (de Monro).
Virchow a., a. de Virchow; a. formado pela reunião de uma linha traçada a partir do meio da sutura nasofrontal até a base da espinha nasal anterior com uma linha traçada a partir deste último ponto até o centro do meato auditivo externo. SIN Virchow-Holder a.
Virchow-Holder a., a. de Virchow-Holder. SIN Virchow a.
visual a., a. visual; o a. formado na retina pela reunião de linhas traçadas a partir da periferia do objeto observado.
Vogt a., a. de Vogt; um a. craniométrico formado pelas linhas nasobasilar e alveolonasal. [K. Vogt]
Weisbach a., a. de Weisbach; um a. craniométrico formado pela junção, no ponto alveolar, de linhas que passam desde o básio e desde o meio da sutura frontonasal.

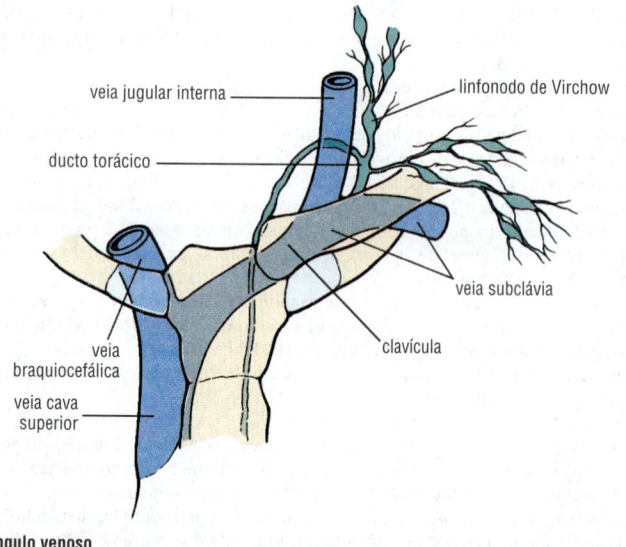

ângulo venoso

Welcker a., a. de Welcker. SIN sphenoidal a. of parietal bone.
xiphocostal a., a. xifocostal. SIN costoxiphoid a.
y-a., a. y; em craniometria, o a. na união formada por linhas traçadas a partir do hórmio e lambda. SIN hypsiloid a.

an·gor (ang′or). Termo raramente empregado para a perturbação extrema ou angústia mental. [L. angústia, angina]
  a. an′imi, a sensação de estar morrendo, diferindo do medo da morte ou do desejo de morrer; um sintoma que pode ocorrer com a angina de peito e, ocasionalmente, nas doenças da medula oblonga. SIN a. pectoris (2).
  a. pec′toris, a. de peito; (1) SIN Gairdner *disease*; (2) SIN a. animi.
Ångström, Anders J., físico sueco, 1814–1874. VER angström; A. *law, unit, scale.*
ang·ström (Å) (ang′strŏm). Uma unidade de comprimento de onda, 10^{-10} m, aproximadamente o diâmetro de um átomo; equivalente a 0,1 nm. [AJ Ångström]
An·guil·lu·la (ang - gwil′loo - la). Nome antigo para um gênero de nematódeos de vida livre. VER *Turbatrix*. [L. mod. dim. de L. *anguilla*, enguia]
an·gu·la·tion (ang′goo - lā′shŭn). Angulação. 1. Formação de um ângulo; um ângulo anormal ou curvado em um órgão. 2. Em ortopedia, um método de descrição do alinhamento dos ossos longos que foram afetados por lesão ou doença; pode ser descrito nos planos ântero-posterior e lateral.
  apex anterior a., a. apical anterior; a a. no plano lateral em que o ápice do ângulo está dirigido anteriormente.
  apex posterior a., a. apical posterior; a a. no plano lateral em que o ápice do ângulo está dirigido posteriormente.
an·gu·lus, gen. e pl. **an·gu·li** (ang′gŭ - lŭs, - lī) [TA], Ângulo. SIN angle. [L.]
  a. acromii [TA], a. acromial. SIN acromial *angle*.
  a. cos′tae [TA], a. costal. SIN *angle* of rib.
  a. fronta′lis os′sis parieta′lis [TA], a. frontal do osso parietal. SIN frontal *angle* of parietal bone.
  a. infe′rior scap′ulae [TA], a. inferior da escápula. SIN inferior *angle* of scapula.
  a. infrasterna′lis [TA], a. infra-esternal. SIN infrasternal *angle*.
  a. ir′idis [TA], a. da íris. SIN iridocorneal *angle*.
  a. iridocornea′lis [TA], a. iridocorneano. SIN iridocorneal *angle*.
  a. latera′lis scap′ulae [TA], a. lateral da escápula. SIN lateral *angle* of scapula.
  a. mandib′ulae [TA], a. da mandíbula. SIN *angle* of mandible.
  a. mastoid′eus os′sis parieta′lis [TA], a. mastóideo do osso parietal. SIN mastoyd *angle* of parietal bone.
  a. occipita′lis os′sis parieta′lis [TA], a. occipital do osso parietal. SIN occipital *angle* of parietal bone (2).
  a. oc′uli latera′lis [TA], a. lateral do olho. SIN lateral *angle* of eye.
  a. oc′uli media′lis [TA], a. medial do olho. SIN medial *angle* of eye.
  a. oc′uli nasa′lis [TA], a. nasal do olho. SIN medial *angle* of eye.
  a. oc′uli temporalis, a. temporal do olho. SIN lateral *angle* of eye.
  a. o′ris [TA], a. da boca. SIN *angle* of mouth.
  a. pontocerebellaris [TA], a. pontocerebelar. SIN cerebellopontine *angle*.
  a. sphenoida′lis os′sis parieta′lis [TA], a. esfenoidal do osso parietal. SIN sphenoidal *angle* of parietal bone.
  a. ster′ni [TA], a. esternal. SIN sternal *angle*.

  a. subpu′bicus [TA], a. subpúbico. SIN subpubic *angle*.
  a. supe′rior scap′ulae [TA], a. superior da escápula. SIN superior *angle* of scapula.
an·haph·ia (an - haf′e - a). Anafia. SIN anaphia.
an·he·do·nia (an - hē - dō′nē - a). Anedonia; ausência de prazer a partir da realização de atos que comumente seriam agradáveis. [G. *an-* priv. + *hedonē*, prazer]
an·hi·dro·sis (an - hī - drō′sis). Anidrose; ausência de glândulas sudoríparas ou ausência de suor, p.ex., devido a medicamentos anticolinérgicos. SIN adiaphoresis. [G. *an-* priv. + *hidrōs*, suor]
an·hi·drot·ic (an - hī - drot′ik). Anidrótico. 1. Relativo a, ou caracterizado por, anidrose. 2. SIN antiperspirant (2). 3. Indica redução ou ausência de glândulas sudoríparas, característica de defeito ectodérmico congênito e displasia ectodérmica anidrótica. SIN adiaphoretic.
an·his·tic, an·his·tous (an - his′tik, - tŭs). Anístico; sem estrutura aparente. [G. *an-*, priv. + *histos*, rede]
an·hy·drase (an - hī′drās). Anidrase; uma enzima que catalisa a retirada de água de um composto; muitas dessas enzimas são atualmente conhecidas como hidrases, hidroliases ou desidratases.
  carbonic a., a. carbônica; uma enzima que contém zinco que catalisa a interconversão do CO_2 com HCO_3^- e H^+. Existem pelo menos sete isoenzimas humanas que aparecem predominantemente nos eritrócitos, tecidos secretores, músculo, etc. A deficiência da a. carbônica II pode resultar em osteopetrose e acidose metabólica. A inibição da a. carbônica IV e, possivelmente, da a. carbônica II por sulfonamidas é a atual terapia do glaucoma. SIN carbonate dehydratase, carbonate hydro-lyase.
an·hy·dra·tion (an - hī - drā′shŭn). Anidratação. SIN dehydration (1).
an·hy·dride (an - hī′drīd). Anidrido; um óxido que pode combinar-se com água para formar um ácido ou que é derivado de um ácido pela retirada de água.
♻ **anhydro-**. Anidro-; prefixo químico que indica a retirada de água. Cf. pyro- (2). [G. *an-* priv. + *hydōr*, água]
3,6-an·hy·dro·ga·lac·tose (an - hī′drō - ga - lak′tōs). 3,6-Anidrogalactose; um derivado da galactose encontrado em inúmeros polissacarídeos (p.ex., agarose).
an·hy·dro·gi·tal·in (an - hī′drō - jit′a - lin). Anidrogitalina. SIN gitoxin.
an·hy·dro·leu·cov·o·rin (an - hī′drō - loo - kō - vor′in). Anidroleucovorina; um intermediário formado na interconversão glicina-serina catalisada por ácido fólico. SIN N^5, N^{10}-methenyltetrahydrofolic acid.
an·hy·dro·sug·ars (an - hī′drō - shug - ărz). Anidroaçúcares; açúcares dos quais uma ou mais moléculas de água foram eliminadas, diferente da água de cristalização. SIN dehydrosugars.
an·hy·drous (an - hī′drŭs). Anidroso; que não contém água, em especial água de cristalização.
a·ni·a·cin·am·i·do·sis (ā - nī′a′ - sin - am - i - dō′sis). Aniacinamidose; termo raramente empregado para a deficiência de niacinamida que pode estar associada à pelagra. [G. *a-* priv. + niacinamide + *-osis*, condição]
a·ni·a·cin·o·sis (ā - nī′a - sin - ō′sis). Aniacinose; termo raramente utilizado para a aniacinamidose. [G. *a-* priv. + niacin + *-osis*, condição]
an·ic·ter·ic (an - ik - ter′ik). Anictérico; não-ictérico.
an·id·e·an (an - id′e - an). Anídeo; sem forma; indica uma massa disforme de tecido. SIN anidous. [ver anideus]
an·id·e·us (an - id′e - ŭs). Anídeo; um feto parasita que consiste em uma massa mal diferenciada de tecido com indicações discretas das partes. VER TAMBÉM *holoacardius amorphus*. [G. *an-*. priv. + *eidos*, forma]
  embryonic a., a. embrionário; um blastoderma sem organização axial.
an·i·dous (an - ī′dŭs). Anídeo. SIN anidean.
an·i·ler·i·dine (an - i - ler′i - dēn). Anileridina; agente analgésico relacionado, química e farmacologicamente, ao cloridrato de meperidina; usado para alívio da dor moderada a grave; também discretamente anti-histamínico e espasmolítico; a capacidade de viciar é equivalente à da morfina.
an·i·lide (an′i-lid). Anilida; uma *N*-acil anilina; p.ex., acetanilida.
ani·linc·tion, ani·linc·tus (ā - ni - lingk′shŭn, - lingk′tŭs). Anilíngua. SIN anilingus.
an·i·line (an′i - lin, - lēn). Anilina, $C_6H_5(NH_2)$; um líquido oleoso, incolor ou acastanhado, de odor aromático e paladar acre, que é a substância de origem de muitos corantes sintéticos; derivado do benzeno por substituição do grupamento $-NH_2$ por um dos átomos de hidrogênio. A a. é muito tóxica, pode causar intoxicação industrial e ser carcinogênica. SIN aminobenzene, benzeneamine, phenylamine. [Ar. *an-nil*, índigo]
an·i·line blue [C.I. 42755]. A. azul; uma mistura de corantes trifenilmetano sulfonatados amplamente utilizados como corante de tecido conjuntivo e contracorante.
ani·lin·gus (ā - ni - ling′gŭs). Anilíngua; estimulação sexual por lamber ou beijar o ânus; um tipo de atividade sexual orogenital. SIN anilinction, anilinctus. [L. *anus*, + *lingo*, lamber]
an·i·lin·ism (an′i - lin - izm). Anilismo. SIN anilism.
an·i·li·no·phil, an·i·li·no·phile (an - i - lin′ō - fil, - fīl). Anilinófilo; que indica uma célula ou estrutura histológica que se cora prontamente com um corante de anilina. SIN anilinophilous. [aniline + G. *philos*, ligação]

an·i·li·noph·i·lous (an - i - li - nof′ĭ - lŭs). Anilinófilo. SIN anilinophil.
an·il·ism (an′i-lizm). Anilismo; intoxicação crônica por anilina caracterizada por debilidade gástrica e cardíaca, vertigem, depressão muscular, pulso intermitente e cianose. SIN anilinism.
an·i·ma (an′i - mă). Alma. **1.** O espírito ou alma. VER animus (4). **2.** Em psicologia jungiana, o ser interno, em contraste com a persona; um arquétipo feminino em um homem. Cf animus (5). [L. respiração, alma]
an·i·mal (an′i - măl). Animal. **1.** Um organismo vivo, sensível, que apresenta paredes celulares membranosas, precisa de oxigênio e alimentos orgânicos, e é capaz de se movimentar voluntariamente, diferente de um vegetal ou mineral. **2.** Um dos organismos animais inferiores que se diferenciam dos seres humanos. [L.]
  cold-blooded a., a. de sangue frio; pecilotérmico. SIN poikilotherm.
  control a., a. de controle; em pesquisa, um a. submetido às mesmas condições que os outros usados para a experiência, mas sem ser submetido ao fator crucial (como a injeção de antídoto, a administração de um medicamento, etc.). VER TAMBÉM control, control *experiment*.
  conventional a., a. convencional; um a. colonizado pela massa de microrganismos residentes, normalmente associada à sua espécie particular.
  Houssay a., a. de Houssay; um a. que foi pancreatectomizado e hipofisectomizado. Homenagem ao descobridor do princípio que os animais são mais sensíveis à insulina depois da retirada da hipófise e que, depois dessa cirurgia, a intensidade do diabetes, em animais despancreatectomizados, diminui.
  normal a., a. normal; em pesquisa, um a. experimental que não sofreu um ataque de determinada doença, nem recebeu uma injeção de um microrganismo específico ou de sua toxina.
  sentinel a., a. sentinela; um a. deliberadamente colocado em determinado ambiente para detectar a presença de um agente infeccioso, como um vírus.
  warm-blooded a., a. de sangue quente; a. homeotérmico. SIN homeotherm.
an·i·mal black. Carvão animal. SIN animal *charcoal*.
an·i·mal·cule (an - i - mal′kŭl). Animálculo; termo utilizado pelos adeptos da teoria de pré-formação para designar a suposta miniatura corporal contida em um gameta. VER homunculus. [L. mod. *animalculum*, dim. de L. *animal*, um ser vivo]
an·i·ma·tion (an - i - mā′shŭn). Animação. **1.** O estar vivo. **2.** Vivacidade; espírito elevado. [L. *animo*, pp. *-atus*, tornar vivo; *anima*, respiração, alma]
  suspended a., a. suspensa; um estado temporário que se assemelha à morte, com cessação da respiração; também pode referir-se a determinadas formas de hibernação em animais ou à formação de endosporos por algumas bactérias.
an·i·ma·tism (an′i - mă - tizm). Animatismo; atribuição de qualidades mentais ou espirituais aos seres vivos e a coisas inanimadas. VER TAMBÉM animism.
an·i·mism (an′i-mizm). Animismo; a visão de que todas as coisas na natureza, tanto animadas quanto inanimadas, contêm um espírito ou alma; crença mantida pelos povos primitivos e crianças pequenas. VER TAMBÉM animatism. [L. *anima*, alma]
an·i·mus (an′i - mŭs). **1.** Um espírito animador ou energizante. **2.** Ânimo; intenção de fazer algo; disposição. **3.** Em psiquiatria, sentimento de hostilidade ativa ou de rancor. **4.** A imagem ideal almejada por uma pessoa. **5.** Na psicologia jungiana, um arquétipo masculino em uma mulher. Cf. anima (2). [L. *animus*, respiração, alma racional no homem, desejo]
an·i·on (A^-) (an′ĭ - on). Ânion; um íon cuja carga elétrica é negativa, indo, portanto, para o anódio com carga elétrica positiva; nos sais, os radicais ácidos são ânions.
an·i·on ex·change. Troca de ânion; processo pelo qual um ânion em uma fase móvel (líquida) troca com outro ânion previamente ligado a uma fase sólida, positivamente carregada, sendo a última um permutador de ânions. Ocorre quando um Cl^- é trocado por OH^- na dessalinização. A reação é Cl^- (na solução) + (OH^- no permutador de ânion⁺) → (Cl^- no permutador de ânion) + OH^- (na solução); combinado a uma troca de cátion, o NaCl é removido da solução. A troca de ânion também pode ser utilizada por meio cromatográfico, para separar ânions, e para fins medicinais, para remover um ânion (p.ex., Cl^-) do conteúdo gástrico ou dos ácidos biliares no intestino.
an·i·on ex·chang·er. Permutador de ânion; um sólido insolúvel, usualmente polistireno ou um polissacarídeo, com grupamentos de cátions (p.ex., $-NR_3^+$ ou $-NR_2H^+$), que pode atrair e manter os ânions que passam em uma solução móvel em troca dos ânions previamente ligados.
an·i·on·ic (an - ī - on′ik). Aniônico; que se refere a um íon com carga elétrica negativa.
an·i·on·ot·ro·py (an′ - ī - on - ot′rō - pē). Anionotropia; a migração de um íon negativo em alterações tautoméricas.
an·i·rid·ia (an - i - rid′ē - ă) [MIM*106200]. Aniridia; ausência da íris; quando congênita, geralmente existe uma raiz rudimentar de íris. Cerca de 60% dos casos têm herança autossômica dominante, embora manifestada de forma algo irregular. Cf. irideremia. [G. *an-* priv. + *irid-* + *-ia*]
an·i·sa·ki·a·sis (an′i - să - kī′a - sis). Anisaquíase; a infestação da parede intestinal por larvas de *Anisakis marina* e outros gêneros de nematódeos anisaquídeos (*Contracaecum, Phocanema*), caracterizada por granuloma intestinal eosinofílico e sintomas semelhantes àqueles da úlcera péptica ou tumor. SIN herring-worm disease. [G. *anisos*, desigual, + *akis*, um ponto, + *-iasis*, condição]
an·i·sa·kid (an - i - să′kid). Nome comum dos nematódeos da família Anisakidae.
An·i·sa·ki·dae (an - i - să′ki - dē). Família de grandes nematódeos (superfamília Heterocheilidae) encontrados no estômago e intestinos de aves comedoras de peixes e mamíferos marinhos, sendo a infestação adquirida a partir do peixe marinho; casos humanos de anisaquíase já foram relatados no Japão. VER TAMBÉM *Anisakis*.
An·i·sa·kis (an - i - să′kis). Gênero de nematódeos (família Anisakidae) que inclui muitos parasitas comuns de aves que comem peixes marinhos e mamíferos marinhos. [G. *anisos*, desigual, + *akis*, um ponto]
an·is·ate (an′ī - sāt). Anisado; um sal do ácido anísico, que geralmente possui propriedades anti-sépticas.
an·ise (an′is). Anis; o fruto da *Pimpinella anisum* (família Umbelliferae); um aromático e carminativo que se assemelha ao funcho.
an·is·ei·ko·nia (an′ī - sī - kō′nē - ă). Anisoconia; uma condição ocular em que a imagem de um objeto em um olho difere no tamanho ou formato da imagem do mesmo objeto no outro olho. SIN unequal retinal image. [G. *anisos*, desigual, + *eikōn*, uma imagem]
anis·ic (an-is′ik). Anísico; relativo ao anis.
anis·ic ac·id (an-is′ik). Ácido anísico; um ácido volátil cristalino obtido a partir do anis; seus compostos são os anisados anti-sépticos. SIN 4-methoxy-benzoic acid.
an·i·sin·di·one (an′i - sin - dī′ōn). Anisindiona; um anticoagulante com ações farmacológicas similares às da fenindiona e diidroxicumarina.
aniso-. Forma combinante que indica desigual, dessemelhante, diferente. [G. *anisos*, desigual, de *an-*, não, + *isos*, igual]
an·i·so·ac·com·mo·da·tion (an - ī′sō - ă - kom - ō - dā′shŭn). Anisoacomodação; variação entre os dois olhos na capacidade de acomodação. [aniso- + L. *accommodo*, adaptar]
an·i·so·chro·ma·sia (an - ī′sō - krō - mā′zē - ă). Anisocromasia; a distribuição desigual da hemoglobina nos eritrócitos, de tal modo que a periferia fica pigmentada e a região central é quase incolor, conforme observado nos esfregaços de sangue de pessoas com determinadas formas de anemia causadas por deficiência de ferro; os eritrócitos normais mostram a. branda por causa de seu formato bicôncavo. [aniso- + G. *chrōma*, cor]
an·i·so·chro·mat·ic (an - ī′sō - krō - mat′ik). Anisocromático; a falta de uniformidade de uma cor.
an·i·so·co·ria (an - ī - sō - kō′rē - ă). Anisocoria; uma condição em que as duas pupilas não possuem o mesmo tamanho. [aniso- G. *korē*, pupila]
  essential a., a. essencial. SIN simple a.
  physiologic a., a. fisiológica. SIN simple a.
  simple a., a. simples; desigualdade benigna comum (20% dos indivíduos normais) das pupilas que pode mudar de uma hora para outra. SIN essential a., physiologic a., simple-central a.
  simple-central a., a. central simples. SIN simple a.
an·i·so·cy·to·sis (an - ī′sō - sī - tō′sis). Anisocitose; variação considerável no tamanho das células que são normalmente uniformes, especialmente em relação aos eritrócitos. [aniso- + G. *kytos*, célula, + *-osis*, condição]
an·i·so·dac·ty·lous (an - ī′sō - dak′ti - lŭs). Anisodáctilo; relativo à anisodactilia.
an·i·so·dac·ty·ly (an - ī′sō - dak′ti - lē). Anisodactilia; comprimento desigual nos dedos das mãos correspondentes. [aniso- + G. *daktylon*, dedo da mão]
an·i·sog·a·my (an′ - i - sog′ă - mē). Anisogamia; fusão de dois gametas desiguais em tamanho ou forma; fertilização quando diferenciada da isogamia ou conjugação. [aniso- + G. *gamos*, casamento]
an·i·sog·na·thous (an - i - sog′nă - thŭs). Anisognato; que possui maxilares desiguais em tamanho, sendo o superior mais largo que o inferior. [aniso- + G. *gnathos*, mandíbula]
an·i·so·kar·y·o·sis (an - ī′sō - kar - ē - ō′sis). Anisocariose; variação no tamanho dos núcleos, maior que a faixa normal para um tecido. [aniso- + G. *karyon*, núcleo, + *-osis*, condição]
an·is·ole (an′i - sōl). Anisol; obtido a partir do ácido anísico; usado em perfumaria.
an·i·so·mas·tia (an - i - sō - mas′tē - ă). Anisomastia; mamas desiguais em tamanho. [aniso- + G. *mastos*, mama]
an·i·so·me·lia (an - i - sō - mē′lē - ă). Anisomelia; desigualdade entre dois membros pareados. [aniso- + G. *melos*, membro]
an·i·so·me·tro·pia (an - ī′sō - me - trō′pē - ă). Anisometropia; uma diferença no poder de refração dos dois olhos. [aniso- + G. *metron*, medida, + *ōps*, visão]
an·i·so·me·tro·pic (an - ī′sō - me - trop′ik). Anisometrópico. **1.** Relativo à anisometropia. **2.** Que possui olhos com poder de refração diferente.
an·i·so·pi·e·sis (an - ī - sō - pi - ē′sis). Anisopiese; pressão arterial desigual nos dois lados do corpo. [aniso- + G. *piesis*, pressão]
an·i·sor·rhyth·mia (an - ī - sō - ridth′mē - ă). Anisorritmia; ação irregular do coração ou ausência de sincronismo na freqüência dos átrios e ventrículos. [aniso- + G. *rhythmos*, ritmo]

an·i·so·sphyg·mia (an-ī-sō-sifg'mē-ă). Anisosfigmia; diferença no volume, força ou tempo do pulso nas artérias correspondentes nos dois lados do corpo, p.ex., as duas radiais ou femorais. [aniso- + G. *sphygmos*, pulso]

an·i·sos·then·ic (an-ī-sos-then'ik). Anisostênico; com força desigual; indica dois músculos ou grupos de músculos que são pareados ou antagonistas. [aniso- + G. *sthenos*, força]

an·i·so·ton·ic (an-ī-sō-ton'ik). Anisotônico; que não tem tensão igual; que possui pressão osmótica desigual. [aniso- + G. *tonus*, tensão]

an·i·so·tro·pic (an-ī-sō-trop'ik). Anisotrópico; que não possui propriedades que sejam idênticas em todas as direções. [aniso- + G. *tropos*, uma volta]

an·i·so·tro·pine meth·yl·bro·mide (an'i-sō-trō'pēn). Metilbrometo de anisotropina; anticolinérgico e antiespasmódico intestinal.

Anitschkow, Nikolai, patologista russo, 1885–1964. VER A. *cell, myocyte*.

an·kle (ang'kl). Tornozelo. **1.** SIN ankle *joint*. **2.** A região de uma articulação do tornozelo. **3.** Tálus. SIN talus.

ankylo-. Anquilo-, ancilo-; forma combinante que indica dobrado, curvo, rígido, fixo, fechado. VER TAMBÉM ancylo-. [G. *ankylos*, curvo, dobrado; *ankylōsis*, enrijecimento das articulações, de *ankos*, uma dobra, uma cavidade]

an·ky·lo·bleph·a·ron (ang'ki-lō-blef'ă-ron). Anciloblefáro, anquiloblefáro; aderência congênita ou adquirida das pálpebras superior e inferior por faixas de tecido. SIN blepharocoloboma, filiform adnatum. [ankylo- + G. *blepharon*, pálpebra]

an·ky·lo·dac·ty·ly, an·ky·lo·dac·tyl·ia (ang'ki-lō-dak'ti-lē, -dak-til'ē-ă). Ancilodactilia, anquilodactilia; aderência entre dois ou mais dedos das mãos ou artelhos. VER TAMBÉM syndactyly. [ankylo- + G. *daktylos*, dedo]

an·ky·lo·glos·sia (ang'ki-lō-glos'ē-ă) [MIM 106280]. Anciloglossia, anquiloglossia; fusão parcial ou completa da língua com o assoalho da boca; encurtamento anormal do frênulo lingual. SIN tongue-tie. [ankylo- + G. *glōssa*, língua]

an·ky·lo·me·le (ang'ki-lō-mē'lē). Ancilômelo; sonda curva ou dobrada. [ankylo- + G. *mēlē*, sonda]

an·ky·losed (ang'ki-lōst). Ancilosado, anquilosado; preso por aderências; indica uma articulação em estado de ancilose.

an·ky·lo·sis (ang'ki-lō'sis). Ancilose, anquilose; enrijecimento ou fixação de uma articulação em consequência de um processo patológico, com união fibrosa ou óssea através da articulação. [G. *ankylōsis*, enrijecimento de uma articulação]

  artificial a., a. artificial; artrodese. SIN arthrodesis.
  bony a., a. óssea; sinostose. SIN synostosis.
  dental a., a. dentária; união óssea da superfície radicular de um dente ao osso alveolar circunvizinho em uma área de reabsorção prévia parcial da raiz.
  extracapsular a., a. extracapsular; enrijecimento de uma articulação devido à induração ou ossificação heterotópica dos tecidos circunvizinhos. SIN spurious a.
  false a., a. falsa. SIN fibrous a.
  fibrous a., a. fibrosa; enrijecimento de uma articulação devido à presença de faixas fibrosas entre e ao redor dos ossos formadores da articulação. SIN false a., pseudoankylosis.
  intracapsular a., a. intracapsular; enrijecimento de uma articulação devido à presença de aderências ósseas ou fibrosas entre as superfícies articulares da articulação.
  spurious a., a. espúria. SIN extracapsular a.
  true a., a. verdadeira. SIN synostosis.

An·ky·los·to·ma (ang'ki-los'tō-mă). **1.** VER *Ancylostoma*. **2.** SIN trismus. [ankylo- + G. *stoma*, boca]

an·ky·lo·sto·mi·a·sis (ang'ki-lō-stō-mī'ă-sis). Ancilostomíase. SIN ancylostomiasis.

an·ky·lot·ic (ang-ki-lot'ik). Ancilótico, anquilótico; caracterizado por ou pertinente à ancilose.

an·ky·rin (ang'ki-rin). Ancirina; uma proteína da membrana eritrocitária que se liga à espectrina. A deficiência na ancirina pode levar a um tipo de esferocitose hereditária. SIN anchorin, syndein. [G. *ankyra*, âncora, + -in]

an·ky·roid (an'ki-royd). Anciróide. SIN ancyroid.

an·la·ge, pl. **an·la·gen** (ahn'lah-ge, -gen). **1.** Primórdio. SIN primordium. **2.** Em psicanálise, a predisposição genética para um determinado traço ou característica de personalidade. [Al. plano, esboço]

an·neal (an-nēl'). Temperar. **1.** Amolecer ou temperar um metal através do aquecimento controlado e resfriamento. O processo torna um metal mais facilmente adaptado, dobrado ou maleável, e menos quebradiço. **2.** Em odontologia, aquecer a folha de ouro na preparação para sua inserção em uma cavidade, de modo a remover os gases adsorvidos e outros contaminantes. **3.** O pareamento de faixas únicas complementares de DNA ou do DNA-RNA. **4.** A fixação das extremidades de duas macromoléculas; p.ex., dois microtúbulos que se fundem para formar um microtúbulo maior. **5.** Em biologia molecular, a remodelagem é um processo em que seções curtas de um DNA de filamento único a partir de uma fonte são ligadas a um filtro e incubadas com o DNA de filamento único, conjugado por meios radioativos, a partir de uma segunda fonte. Nos locais onde os dois grupos de DNA possuem sequências complementares de nucleotídeos, acontece a ligação. O grau de correlação (homologia) de dois grupos de DNA é, então, estimado de acordo com o nível de radioatividade do filtro. Essa técnica é fundamental para a classificação de bactérias e vírus. SIN nucleic acid hydribization. [A. S., *anaelan*, queimar]

an·nec·tent (a-nek'tent). Ligado com; unido. [L. *an-necto*, pres. p. *-nectere*, pp. *-nexus*, unir a]

An·nel·i·da (an'nĕ-li'dă). Um ramo que inclui os vermes segmentados ou verdadeiros, como a minhoca.

an·ne·lids (an'nĕ-lids). Anelídios; nome comum para os membros do ramo Annelida.

an·nel·lide (an'ĕ-līd). Anelídeo; uma célula conidiogenosa que produz conídios em sucessão, cada um deixando um colar anular na parede da célula quando liberado. [Fr. *annelide*, do L. *anellus*, um anel]

an·nel·lo·co·nid·i·um (an'ĕ-lō-kō-nid'ē-um). Aneloconídio; um conídio produzido por um anelídeo.

an·nexa (a-nek'să). Anexos, adnexos. SIN accessory *structures,* em *structure*.

an·nex·al (a-neks-ăl). Anexal, adnexal. SIN adnexal.

an·nex·ins (a-nek'sinz). Anexinas; uma família com pelo menos 13 proteínas de ligação de fosfolipídio dependentes de Ca^{2+} que podem atuar como mediadores dos sinais de cálcio intracelular.

an·not·to (ă-not'ō). Anoto; material de coloração extraído das sementes da *Bixa orellana*; contém bixina e vários outros pigmentos amarelados a vermelho-alaranjados; usado para colorir manteiga, margarina, queijo e óleos.

an·nu·lar (an'ū-lăr). Anular. SIN anular. [L. *anulus*, anel]

an·nu·lo·plasty (an'ū-lō-plas-tē). Anuloplastia; reconstrução do anel (ou ânulo) de uma valva cardíaca. [L. *anulus*, anel, + G. *plastos*, formado]

an·nu·lor·rha·phy (an-ū-lōr'ă-fē). Anulorrafia; fechamento de um anel herniário por sutura. [L. *anulus*, anel, + G. *rhaphē*, costura]

an·nu·lus (an'ū-lŭs). Ânulo, anel. SIN ring.

AnOC. Abreviatura para anodal opening *contraction* (contração de abertura anódica).

an·o·chro·ma·sia (an'ō-krō-mā'zē'ă). Anocromasia. **1.** Falha das células ou de outros elementos de se corar da maneira usual quando tratados com um corante (ou corantes). **2.** Acúmulo de hemoglobina na zona periférica dos eritrócitos, resultando, dessa maneira, em uma porção central pálida, quase incolor. [G. *anō*, para cima, + *chrōma*, cor]

ano·ci·as·so·ci·a·tion (ă-nō'sē-ă-sō-sē-ā'shŭn). Anociassociação; teoria de que os estímulos aferentes, especialmente a dor, contribuem para o desenvolvimento do choque cirúrgico e, como corolário, que a anestesia de condução no campo cirúrgico e a sedação pré-cirúrgica protegem contra o choque. [G. *a-* priv. + L. *noceo*, lesionar, + associação]

ano·coc·cyg·e·al (a-nō-kok-sij'ē-ăl). Anococcígeo; relativo ao ânus e ao cóccix.

anod·al (an-ōd'ăl). Anódico; de, pertinente ou que emana de um anódio. SIN anodic.

an·ode (an'ōd). Anódio. **1.** O pólo positivo de uma bateria galvânica ou o eletrodo a ele conectado; um eletrodo no sentido do qual migram os íons com carga elétrica negativa (ânions). **2.** A porção, geralmente feita de tungstênio, de um tubo de raios X, de onde são liberados os raios X pelo bombardeamento por raios catódicos (elétrons). SIN positive electrode. [G. *anodos*, um caminho para cima, de *ana*, para cima, + *hodos*, um caminho]

  rotating a., a. rotatório; em radiografia diagnóstica, um anódio em forma de cogumelo nos modernos equipamentos de raios X que gira rapidamente para evitar o acúmulo local de calor decorrente do impacto de elétrons durante a geração dos raios X.

an·o·derm (ā'nō-derm). Anoderma; revestimento do canal anal imediatamente inferior à linha dentada e que se estende por cerca de 1,5 cm até a borda anal; é desprovido de pêlos e glândulas sebáceas e sudoríparas, portanto, não é pele verdadeira, embora seja epitélio escamoso; é pálido, liso, fino e delicado, e brilhoso quando distendido; é particularmente vulnerável à abrasão (como a decorrente do uso de papel higiênico áspero), irritantes químicos (sabões) e é bem provido com terminações táteis e nociceptivas (dor, prurido) supridas pelo nervo retal inferior (pudendo).

an·od·ic (an-ōd'ik). Anódico. SIN anodal.

an·o·don·tia (an-ō-don'shē-ă). Anodontia; ausência congênita dos dentes; por desenvolvimento, não por extração ou impacto. SIN agomphious, agomphosis, agomphiasis. [G. *an-*, priv. + *odous*, dente]

  partial a., a. parcial; hipodontia. SIN hypodontia.

an·o·dont·ism (an-ō-dont'izm). Anodontia; ausência congênita do desenvolvimento do germe dentário.

an·o·dyne (an'ō-dīn). Anódico; um composto menos potente que um anestésico ou um narcótico, porém capaz de aliviar a dor. [G. *an-* priv. + *odynē*, dor]

an·o·et·ic (an-ō-et'ik). Anoético; que carece da força da compreensão, como nos níveis grave e profundo de retardo mental. [G. *anoēsia*, de *a-*, priv. + *noos*, percepção]

ano·gen·i·tal (ā'nō-jen'ī-tăl). Anogenital; relativo, em qualquer maneira, às regiões anal e genital.

anom·a·lad (ā - nom´a - lad). Anomalia; uma malformação juntamente com suas alterações estruturais subseqüentemente derivadas. [ver anomaly]

anom·a·lo·scope (a - nom´a - lō - skōp). Anomaloscópio; instrumento utilizado para diagnosticar anormalidades da percepção das cores, no qual metade de um campo da cor é emparelhado pela mistura de duas outras cores. [G. *anōmalos,* irregular, + *skopeō,* examinar]

anom·a·ly (ā - nom´a - lē). Anomalia; desvio da média ou da norma; qualquer coisa que seja estruturalmente incomum ou irregular ou contrária a uma regra geral. Os defeitos congênitos constituem um exemplo da definição de anomalia. [G. *anōmalia,* irregularidade]

Alder a., a. de Alder; granulação azurofílica grosseira dos leucócitos, principalmente granulócitos, que pode estar associada a gargolismo e síndrome (*syndrome*) de Morquio.

Aristotle a., a. de Aristóteles; quando um objeto pequeno é mantido entre o primeiro e o segundo dedos da mão, cruzados de tal modo que esse objeto toque ou pressione as superfícies cutâneas que comumente não são pressionadas simultaneamente por um único objeto, ele é percebido falsamente como dois objetos.

Chédiak-Steinbrinck-Higashi a., a. de Chédiak-Steinbrinck-Higashi. SIN Chédiak-Higashi *syndrome.*

developmental a., a. de desenvolvimento; uma a. estabelecida durante a vida intra-uterina; uma a. congênita.

Ebstein a., a. de Ebstein; deslocamento para baixo (congênito) da valva tricúspide, para dentro do ventrículo direito. SIN Ebstein disease.

eugnathic a., a. eugnática. SIN eugnathia.

Freund a., a. de Freund; estreitamento da abertura superior do tórax pelo encurtamento da primeira costela e sua cartilagem; acreditava-se, originalmente, que predispunha à tuberculose por causa da expansão defeituosa do ápice pulmonar.

Hegglin a., a. de Hegglin; um distúrbio em que os neutrófilos e eosinófilos contêm estruturas basofílicas conhecidas como corpúsculos de Döhle ou de Amato e no qual existe maturação defeituosa das plaquetas, com trombocitopenia; herança autossômica dominante. SIN May-Hegglin a.

May-Hegglin a., a. de May-Hegglin. SIN Hegglin a.

morning glory a., a. em ipoméia; a. congênita do disco óptico em que a cabeça do nervo é afunilada, com uma mancha de tecido esbranquiçada no fundo da escavação, e é circundada por um ânulo pigmentado elevado; os vasos retinianos observados são múltiplas faixas estreitas na borda do disco.

Pelger-Huët nuclear a. [MIM*169400], a. nuclear de Pelger-Huët; inibição congênita da lobulação nos núcleos dos leucócitos neutrofílicos; a maioria das células é bilobulada ou assemelha-se a bastões (leucócitos prematuros), e apenas uma célula ocasional mostra-se trilobulada; não está associada a doença, mas pode ser confundida com o "desvio para a esquerda" dos leucócitos; herança autossômica dominante.

Peters a., a. de Peters. SIN anterior chamber cleavage *syndrome.*

Rieger a., a. de Rieger; disgenesia mesodérmica iridocorneal.

Shone a., a. de Shone; coartação da aorta, estenose subaórtica e anel estenosante do átrio esquerdo encontrados em associação a uma valva mitral em pára-quedas.

Uhl a., a. de Uhl; aplasia miocárdica ventricular direita, provocando um ventrículo direito dilatado, com paredes finas, sem sopros; a morte ocorre nos primeiros anos de vida. SIN parchment right ventricle.

urogenital sinus a., a. do seio urogenital. SIN hypospadias.

an·o·mer (an´ō - mer). Anômero; uma de duas moléculas de açúcar que são epímeras no átomo de carbono hemiacetal (carbono 1 nas aldoses, carbono 2 na maioria das cetoses); p.ex., α-D-glicose e β-D-glicose. VER TAMBÉM sugars. Cf. epimer.

ano·mia (a - nō´mē - ā). Anomia. SIN nominal *aphasia.* [G. *a-* priv. + *ōnoma,* nome]

an·o·mie (an´ō - mē). Anomia. **1.** Ilegalidade; ausência ou enfraquecimento das normas ou valores sociais, com correspondente erosão da coesão social. **2.** Em psiquiatria, a ausência ou enfraquecimento das normas ou valores individuais; caracterizada por ansiedade, isolamento e desorientação pessoal. [Fr. do G. *anomia,* ilegalidade]

an·o·nych·ia, an·o·ny·cho·sis (an - ō - nik´ē - ā, an - ō - nī - kō´sis). Anoníquia; ausência das unhas. [G. *an-* priv. + *onyx* (*onych-*), unha]

anon·y·ma (a - non´i - mā). Inominado. SIN innominate. [G. *an-* priv. + *onyma,* nome]

Anoph·e·les (ā - nof´ē - lēz). Um gênero de mosquitos (família Culicidae; subfamília Anophelinae). O ciclo esporogenoso do parasita da malária passa-se na cavidade corporal das fêmeas dos mosquitos de determinadas espécies desse gênero; alguns vetores selecionados (dentre mais de 90 espécies) são arrolados adiante. [G. *anōpheles,* sem uso, perigoso, de *an-* priv. + *ōpheleō,* ser de valor]

A. aconitus, espécie de mosquito que é um vetor da malária na Indonésia, Tailândia e Camboja.

A. albima'nus, uma espécie que possui patas traseiras brancas, um portador comum do parasita da malária nas Índias Ocidentais e América Central.

A. albitar'sus, uma espécie da América do Sul que transmite a malária.

A. annularis, espécie de mosquito que é um vetor acidental da malária na Índia.

A. annulipes, espécie de mosquito que é um vetor da malária na Austrália.

A. aquasalis, espécie de mosquito que é um vetor da malária nas Antilhas menores, Trinidad e Brasil.

A. arabiensis, espécie de mosquito que é um vetor importante da malária nas áreas áridas ou montanhosas desde a África subsaariana até o Quênia e o Sudão.

A. aztecus, espécie de mosquito que é um vetor da malária nas regiões mais elevadas do México.

A. balabacen'sis, uma espécie vetora no Sudeste Asiático, Birmânia e Índia.

A. barbirostris, espécie de mosquito que é um vetor da malária na Indonésia e Península da Malásia.

A. bellator, espécie de mosquito que é um vetor da malária em Trinidad e no Brasil.

A. brunnipes, espécie de mosquito que é um vetor acidental da malária em toda a África tropical.

A. campestris, espécie de mosquito que é um vetor da malária na Malásia.

A. crucians, espécie de mosquito que é um vetor secundário ou suspeito da malária, encefalite eqüina venezuelana e encefalite eqüina ocidental no território dos Estados Unidos.

A. cruzi, espécie de mosquito que é um vetor da malária no Brasil.

A. culicifa´cies, espécie de mosquito que é um vetor comum da malária na Índia e Sri Lanka, China e em outros pontos no Oriente.

A. darling'i, uma espécie sul-americana, um importante carreador do parasita da malária.

A. flavirostris, espécie de mosquito que é um importante vetor da malária nas Filipinas, Java e norte das Célebes.

A. fluviatil'is, uma espécie que é um vetor importante na Índia e Paquistão.

A. freebor'ni, espécie de mosquito que é um vetor no oeste dos Estados Unidos (embora não haja mais casos endêmicos).

A. funes'tus, uma importante espécie de mosquito africano que transmite malária.

A. gam'biae, uma espécie de mosquito africano que é um vetor muito importante da malária.

A. jeyporien'sis, espécie de mosquito que é um vetor da malária no sul da China.

A. karwa'ri, espécie de mosquito que é um vetor da malária na Nova Guiné.

A. kwei'yangen'sis, espécie de mosquito que é um importante vetor de malária na província de Szechuan, na China.

A. labranch'iae, espécie de mosquito que é um importante vetor de malária onde quer que seja encontrado na região Paleártica.

A. les'teri, espécie de mosquito que é um importante vetor da malária na parte baixa do Vale do Yangtze, na China.

A. leucosphy'rus, espécie de mosquito que é um importante vetor da malária em Bornéu.

A. macula'tus, espécie de mosquito que é um vetor na Malásia e Indonésia.

A. maculipen'nis, a espécie típica desse gênero; suas asas são marcadas por manchas formadas de coleções de escamas; uma das espécies mais amplamente distribuídas, ativa na disseminação da malária (outrora um importante vetor na Europa continental).

A. mes'seae, espécie de mosquito que é um vetor da malária em regiões da Hungria e no leste da Romênia.

A. min'imus, espécie de mosquito que é um importante vetor da malária onde quer que seja encontrado por todo o Oriente.

A. pseudopunctipen'nis, uma espécie de mosquito-vetor na América do Sul.

A. quadricula'tus, espécie de mosquito que já foi um importante vetor da malária no sul dos Estados Unidos.

A. stephen'si, uma espécie de mosquito disseminada que é um importante vetor da malária na Ásia.

A. sundai'cus, espécie de mosquito que é um importante vetor no Oriente e no Sudeste Asiático.

A. superpic'tus, espécie de mosquito que é um importante vetor na região do Mediterrâneo, Oriente Médio e sul da Ásia.

anoph·e·li·cide (ā - nof´ē - li - sīd). Anofelicida; um agente que destrói o mosquito *Anopheles.*

anoph·e·li·fuge (ā - nof´ē - li - fooj). Anofelífugo; um agente que afasta ou evita a picada pelos mosquitos *Anopheles.*

Anoph·e·li·nae (an - of - ē - li´nē). Uma subfamília dos mosquitos (Culicidae) que consiste em vários gêneros, inclusive *Anopheles.*

anoph·e·line (ā - nof´ē - līn). Anofelino; relativo ao mosquito *Anopheles.*

Anophe·li·ni (ā - nof - ē - li´nī). Anofelinos; a tribo de mosquitos (família Culicidae) que inclui o gênero *Anopheles.* [G. *anōphelēs,* inútil, problemático]

anoph·e·lism (ā - nof´ē - lizm). Anofelismo; a presença habitual de mosquitos *Anopheles* em qualquer região.

an·oph·thal·mia (an - of - thal´mē - ā). Anoftalmia; ausência congênita de todos os tecidos dos olhos. SIN anophthalmos. [G. *an-* priv. + *ophthalmos,* olho]

anophthalmos. Anoftalmia. SIN anophthalmia.

ano·plas·ty (a̅'no̅ - plas - te̅). Anoplastia; reconstrução do ânus, freqüentemente empregando retalhos de avanço. [L. *anus* + G. *plastos*, formado]

An·o·plo·ceph·a·la (an - op'lo̅'sef'a̅ - la̅). Um gênero de grandes tênias (família Anoplocephalidae) com forte segmentação linear, numerosos testículos disseminados e ovos com aparelho piriforme; eles são parasitas em herbívoros, com ácaros terrestres servindo como hospedeiros intermediários. [G. *anoplos*, sem braços, + *kephale̅*, cabeça]

A. perfolia'ta, uma espécie cosmopolita do cavalo, mula, burro e zebra; as larvas cisticercóides são encontradas em artrópodes. SIN *Taenia equina*, *Taenia quadrilobata*.

An·o·plu·ra (an - o̅ - ploo'ra̅). A ordem de insetos que inclui o piolho hematófago dos mamíferos, com cerca de 450 espécies dispostas em 6 famílias, das quais 4 contêm espécies de importância médica ou veterinária: *Haematopinus*, *Linognathus* e *Solenopotes*, de mamíferos domésticos, e o piolho hematófago humano *Pediculus humanus*. [G. *anoplos*, sem braços + *oura*, cauda]

an·or·chia (an - o̅r'ke̅ - a̅). Anorquia; anorquidia. SIN anorchism.

an·or·chism (an - o̅r'kizm). Anorquia, anorquidia; ausência de testículos; pode ser congênita ou adquirida. SIN anorchia. [G. *an-*, priv. + *orchis*, testículo]

ano·rec·tal (a̅'no̅ - rek'tal). Anorretal; relativo ao ânus e reto.

an·o·rec·tic, an·o·ret·ic (an - o̅ - rek'tic, - ret'ik). Anorético. **1.** Relativo a, caracterizado por ou que sofre de anorexia, em especial anorexia nervosa. **2.** Um agente que provoca anorexia. SIN anorexic.

an·o·rex·ia (an - o̅ - rek'se̅ - a̅). Anorexia; apetite diminuído; aversão ao alimento. [G. de *an-* priv. + *orexis*, apetite]

a. nervo'sa, a. nervosa; um distúrbio mental manifestado por medo extremo de ficar obeso e aversão a comida, que ocorre comumente em mulheres jovens e resultando, com freqüência, em perda de peso com risco de vida, acompanhado por distúrbio na imagem corporal, hiperatividade e amenorréia.

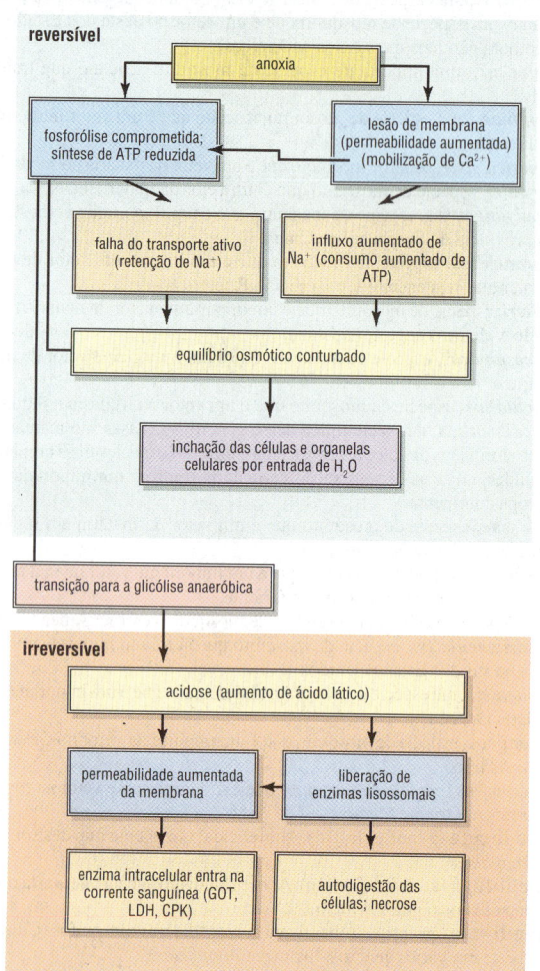

anoxia: patogenia da destruição celular anóxica; ATP, adenosina 5´-trifosfato; TGO, transaminase glutâmico-oxalacética; LDH, desidrogenase láctica; CPK, creatinofosfoquinase

an·o·rex·i·ant (an - o̅ - rek'se̅ - ant). Anorexiante; um medicamento ("pílulas de emagrecimento"), processo ou evento que leva à anorexia.

an·o·rex·ic (an - o̅ - rek'sik). Anorético. SIN anorectic.

an·o·rex·i·gen·ic (an'o̅ - rek - si - jen'ik). Anorexigênico; que promove a anorexia ou leva a esta.

an·or·gas·my, an·or·gas·mia (an - o̅r - gaz'me̅, - gaz'me̅ - a̅). Anorgasmia; incapacidade de experimentar um orgasmo; pode ser biogênica (secundária a um distúrbio físico ou medicamento), psicogênica (secundária a fatores psicológicos ou situacionais) ou uma combinação dos dois. [G. *an-*, priv. + orgasmo + -ia]

ano·scope (a̅'no̅ - sko̅p). Anoscópio; um pequeno espéculo para examinar o canal anal e a parte inferior do reto.

Bacon a., a. de Bacon; um instrumento que se assemelha a um espéculo retal, com uma longa fenda em um lado e uma forte luminosa no lado oposto.

ano·sig·moid·os·co·py (a̅'no̅ - sig - moy - dos' - ko̅ - pe̅). Anossigmoidoscopia; endoscopia do ânus, reto e cólon sigmóide.

an·os·mia (an - oz'me̅ - a̅). Anosmia; perda ou ausência da sensação do olfato. Pode ser: 1, geral para todos os odores (total), parcial para alguns odores ou específica para um ou mais odores; 2, decorrente de distúrbios de transporte (na obstrução nasal) ou distúrbios sensorioneurais (afetando o neuroepitélio olfativo ou as vias neurais olfativas centrais); ou 3, hereditária ou adquirida. [G. *an-* priv. + *osme̅*, sensação do olfato]

an·os·mic (an - oz'mik). Anósmico; relativo à anosmia.

ano·so·di·a·pho·ria (a̅ - no̅'so̅ - di̅ - a̅ - fo̅r'e̅ - a̅). Anosodiaforia; indiferença, real ou presumida, em relação à presença de doença, especificamente de paralisia. [G. *a-*, priv. + *nosos*, doença, + *diaphora*, diferença]

ano·sog·no·sia (a̅ - no̅'sog - no̅'se̅ - a̅). Anosognosia; ignorância da presença da doença, especificamente da paralisia. Observada mais amiúde em pacientes com lesões do lobo parietal não-dominante, que negam suas hemiparesias. [G. *a-* priv. + *nosos*, doença + *gno̅sis*, conhecimento]

ano·sog·no·sic (a̅ - no̅ - sog - no̅'sik). Anosognósico; relativo à anosognosia.

ano·spi·nal (a̅'no̅ - spi̅'nal). Anoespinal; relativo ao ânus e à medula espinal.

an·os·te·o·pla·sia (an - os'te̅ - o̅ - pla̅'ze̅ - a̅). Anosteoplasia; incapacidade de formação óssea. [G. *an-* priv. + *osteon*, osso, + *plasso̅*, formar]

an·os·to·sis (an - os - to̅'sis). Anostose; insuficiência de ossificação. [G. *an-*, priv. + *osteon*, osso]

an·o·tia (an - o̅'she̅ - a̅). Anotia; ausência congênita de uma ou de ambas as orelhas. [G. *an-* priv. + *ous*, ouvido]

ANOVA Acrônimo para *analysis of variance* (análise de variância).

ano·ves·i·cal (a̅'no̅ - ves'i - kal). Anovesical; relativo, de alguma maneira, ao ânus e à bexiga.

an·ov·u·lar (an - ov'u̅ - lar). Anovulatório. SIN anovulatory.

an·ov·u·la·tion (an - ov - u̅ - la̅'shun). Anovulação; suspensão ou cessação da ovulação.

an·ov·u·la·to·ry (an - ov'u̅ - lă - to̅r - e̅). Anovulatório; ausência do desenvolvimento de um folículo de Graaf maduro e/ou liberação do óvulo durante um ciclo menstrual. SIN anovular.

an·ox·e·mia (an - ok - se̅'me̅ - a̅). Anoxemia; ausência de oxigênio no sangue arterial; termo que já foi muito utilizado para incluir a diminuição moderada no oxigênio, atualmente adequadamente diferenciado como hipoxemia. [G. *an-* priv. + oxigênio + G. *haima*, sangue]

an·ox·ia (an - ok'se̅ - a̅). Anoxia, anóxia; ausência completa ou quase completa de oxigênio a partir dos gases inspirados, sangue arterial ou tecidos; a ser diferenciada da hipoxia. [G. *an-* priv. + oxigênio]

anemic a., a. anêmica; um termo que já foi considerado sinônimo de hipoxia anêmica, porém atualmente reservado para casos extremamente graves em que o oxigênio e o volume eritrocitário funcional estão ausentes quase por completo.

anoxic a., a. anóxica; um termo que já foi considerado sinônimo de hipoxia hipóxica, mas atualmente reservado para casos extremamente graves em que o oxigênio está quase completamente ausente.

diffusion a., a. de difusão; hipoxia de difusão suficientemente grave para resultar na ausência de oxigênio no gás alveolar.

histotoxic a., a. histotóxica; intoxicação dos sistemas de enzimas respiratórias dos tecidos, como na inibição da citocromo oxidase por cianetos; devido à incapacidade das células teciduais de utilizar o oxigênio, sua pressão no sangue arterial e capilar é geralmente maior que a normal.

a. neonator'um, a. neonatal; qualquer a. observada em neonatos.

oxigen affinity a., a. por afinidade de oxigênio; a. decorrente da incapacidade da hemoglobina de liberar oxigênio.

stagnant a., a. estagnante; hipoxia estagnante suficientemente grave para resultar na ausência de oxigênio nos tecidos.

an·ox·ic (an-ok'sik). Anóxico; denotador ou característico de anoxia.

ANP Abreviatura para atrial natriuretic *peptide* (peptídeo natriurético atrial).

Anrep, G. V., fisiologista libanês do século XX na Grã-Bretanha. VER *A. phenomenon*.

ANS Abreviatura para anterior nasal *spine* (espinha nasal anterior); autonomic nervous *system* (sistema nervoso autônomo).

an·sa, gen e pl. **an·sae** (an'sa̅, - se̅) [TA]. Alça; qualquer estrutura anatômica na forma de uma alça ou de um arco. VER TAMBÉM loop. [L. alça, cabo]

a. cervica′lis [TA], a. cervical; uma alça no plexo cervical que consiste em fibras originárias dos três primeiros nervos cervicais. As fibras de uma alça entre os nervos espinais C1 e C2 acompanham o nervo hipoglosso por uma curta distância, deixando-o como a raiz superior da a. cervical. As fibras oriundas de uma alça entre os nervos espinais C2 e C3 formam a raiz inferior da a. cervical. Mais amiúde, as raízes se misturam, formando a a. cervical, a qual origina os ramos que inervam os músculos infra-hióideos. SIN cervical loop, loop of hypoglossal nerve.
Haller a., a. de Haller. SIN communicating branch of facial nerve with glossopharyngeal nerve.
Henle a., a. de Henle. SIN nephronic loop.
a. hypoglos′si, a. do hipoglosso; termo obsoleto para a a. cervicalis.
lenticular a., a. lenticular. SIN lenticular loop.
a. lenticula′ris [TA], a. lenticular. SIN lenticular loop.
ansae nervo′rum spina′lium, a. dos nervos espinais. SIN loops of spinal nerves, em loop.
peduncular a., a. peduncular. SIN a. peduncularis.
a. peduncula′ris [TA], a. peduncular; um complexo feixe de fibras que se curva ao redor da borda medial da cápsula interna e que une a parte anterior do lobo temporal (córtex temporal), amígdala e córtex olfativo com o núcleo mediodorsal do tálamo; entra no tálamo como um componente do pedúnculo talâmico inferior, o qual também contém uma parte importante das fibras que conectam o núcleo mediodorsal ao córtex orbitofrontal. SIN peduncular a., peduncular loop, Reil a.
Reil a., a. de Reil. SIN a. peduncularis.
a. sacra′lis, a. sacral; um cordão nervoso que une um ou ambos os troncos nervosos simpáticos ao gânglio ímpar.
a. subcla′via [TA], a. da subclávia; um cordão nervoso que une os gânglios cervical médio e cervical inferior ou simpático estrelado, formando uma alça ao redor da artéria subclávia. SIN subclavian loop, Vieussens a., Vieussens loop.
Vieussens a., a. de Vieussens, a. da subclávia. SIN a. subclavia.
an·sate (an′sāt). Alçado. SIN ansiform.
an·ser·ine. Anserino. **1** (an′ser-in).Que se assemelha ou tem características de um ganso. VER *cutis* anserina, *pes* anserinus. **2** (an′ser-ēn). $N^α$-(β-Alanil)-π-metil-L-histidina; presente no músculo e cérebro. SIN *N*-methylcarnosine. [L. *anserinus*, de *anser*, ganso]
ANSI Abreviatura de *American National Standards Institute* (*Instituto de Normas Nacionais Norte-Americanas*).
an·si·form (an′si-fōrm). Ansiforme; em formato de alça ou arco. SIN ansate. [L. *ansa*, cabo + *forma*, forma]
an·sot·o·my (an-sot′ō-mē).Ansotomia. **1**. Divisão cirúrgica de uma alça, usualmente uma alça que faz constrição. **2**. Secção da alça lenticular para tratamento de síndromes estriadas. [L. *ansa*, alça, + G. *tomē*, corte]
♲ **ant-**. VER anti-.
ant. Formiga; um dos insetos mais numerosos (ordem Hymenoptera), caracterizado por um extraordinário desenvolvimento de vida colonial e especialização de castas.
black imported fire a., f. do fogo negra importada. SIN *Solenopsis richteri*.
fire a., formiga-de-fogo; qualquer uma das várias espécies no gênero *Solenopsis* cuja picada provoca uma sensação causticante, de queimação e, por vezes, reações alérgicas graves. VER TAMBÉM solenopsin A.
harvester a., formiga-cortadeira. SIN *Pogonomyrmex*.
red imported fire a., f. -de-fogo vermelha importada. SIN *Solenopsis invicta*.
velvet a., formiga-feiticeira, formiga-vespa; uma vespa sem asa e provida de muitos opérculos (família Mutilidae, ordem Hymenoptera) conhecida por sua picada venenosa.
ant·ac·id (ant-as′id). Antiácido. **1**. Que neutraliza um ácido. **2**. Qualquer agente que reduz ou neutraliza a acidez, como a do suco gástrico ou qualquer outra secreção (p.ex., carbonato de cálcio, hidróxido de magnésio). SIN antiacid.
an·tag·o·nism (an-tag′on-izm). Antagonismo. **1**. Indica a oposição mútua na ação entre estruturas, agentes, doenças ou processos fisiológicos. Cf. sinergism. **2**. A situação em que o efeito combinado de dois ou mais fatores é menor que o efeito isolado de qualquer um dos fatores. SIN mutual resistance. [G. *antagōnisma*, de *anti*, contra, + *agōnizomai*, lutar, de *agōn*, uma luta]
bacterial a., a. bacteriano; a inibição de uma bactéria por outra.
an·tag·o·nist (an-tag′ō-nist). Antagonista; algo que se opõe ou resiste à ação de outro; certas estruturas, agentes, doenças ou processos fisiológicos que tendem a neutralizar ou impedir a ação ou efeito de outros. Cf. synergist.
α-adrenoceptor a., a. do α-adrenorreceptor. SIN α-adrenergic blocking *agent*.
β-adrenoceptor a., a. do β-adrenorreceptor. SIN β-adrenergic blocking *agent*.
aldosterone a., a. da aldosterona; um agente que se opõe à ação do hormônio supra-renal aldosterona sobre a retenção tubular renal de mineralocorticóide; esses agentes, p.ex., espironolactona, são úteis no tratamento da hipertensão do hiperaldosteronismo primário ou da retenção de sódio do hiperaldosteronismo secundário.
associated a., a. associado; um de dois músculos ou grupos musculares que tracionam em direções quase opostas, mas que, quando atuam em conjunto, movimentam uma região em uma trajetória entre suas linhas divergentes de ação.
calcium a., a. do cálcio. SIN calcium channel-blocking *agent*.
competitive a., a. competitivo; um antimetabólito.
enzyme a., a. enzimático; um antimetabólito ou inibidor da ação da enzima.
folic acid a.'s, antagonistas do ácido fólico; pterinas modificadas, como a aminopterina e o metotrexato, que interferem com a ação do ácido fólico e, dessa maneira, provocam sintomas de deficiência de ácido fólico; têm sido empregados na quimioterapia contra o câncer e em distúrbios inflamatórios.
5-hydroxy tryptamine a.'s, antagonistas da 5-hidroxitriptamina; agentes que bloqueiam os receptores de serotonina e, portanto, interferem com as ações biológicas da serotonina (5-HT).
insulin a., a. da insulina; substâncias nas frações β- e γ-globulina ou $β_1$-lipoproteína do soro que podem induzir uma deficiência funcional de insulina; podem incluir anticorpos não-precipitantes contra a insulina não-humana.
leukotriene receptor a., a. do receptor de leucotrieno; uma classe de agentes dos quais os mais conhecidos são zileuton, montelukast e zafirlukast, usados no tratamento profilático e crônico da asma em crianças maiores e em adultos; esses medicamentos não são, *per se*, broncodilatadores, mas interferem com o processo inflamatório mediado por leucotrieno presente na asma.
muscarinic a., a. muscarínico; substâncias que se ligam aos receptores colinérgicos muscarínicos, mas não os ativam, evitando, assim, o acesso a acetilcolina; os exemplos incluem atropina, escopolamina, propantelina e pirenzepina.
opioid a.'s, antagonistas de opióide; agentes, como a naloxona e a naltrexona, que possuem afinidade significativa por receptores de opiáceos, mas que não os ativam. Esses medicamentos bloqueiam os efeitos dos opióides administrados por via exógena, como morfina, heroína, meperidina e metadona, ou das endorfinas e encefalinas liberadas endogenamente.
ant·al·ge·sia (ant-al-jē′zē-ă). Antalgesia; termo raramente utilizado para a diminuição de uma elevação prévia no limiar de dor. [anti- +G. *algēsis*, sensação de dor]
ant·al·gic (ant-al′jik). Antálgico. SIN analgesic (2).
ant·al·ka·line (ant-al′kă-līn). Antialcalino; que reduz ou neutraliza a alcalinidade.
ant·aph·ro·di·si·ac (ant′af-rō-diz′ē-ak). Antiafrodisíaco. SIN anaphrodisiac.
ant·aph·ro·dit·ic (ant′af-rō-dit′ik). **1**. Antiafrodisíaco. SIN anaphrodisiac. **2**. Antivenéreo. SIN antivenereal.
ant·ar·thrit·ic (ant′ar-thrit′ik). Antiartrítico; termo raramente empregado para antiartrítico. SIN antiarthritic.
ant·as·then·ic (ant-as-then′ik). Antiastênico. **1**. Que fortalece ou revigora. **2**. Um agente que possui essas qualidades. [anti- + G. *astheneia*, fraqueza]
ant·asth·mat·ic (ant-az-mat′ik). Antiasmático. SIN antiasthmatic.
ant·a·tro·phic (ant-ă-trof′ik). Antiatrófico. **1**. Que impede ou cura a atrofia. **2**. Um agente que promove a restauração das estruturas atrofiadas.
an·taz·o·line hy·dro·chlo·ride (an-taz′ō-lēn). Cloridrato de antazolina; um agente antagonista da histamina empregado no tratamento da alergia; também disponível como fosfato de antazolina. SIN phenazoline hydrochloride.
♲ **ante-**. Prefixo que indica antes, na frente de (no tempo, espaço ou ordem). VER TAMBÉM pre-, pro- (1). [L. *ante*, antes, na frente de]
an·te·brach·i·al (an′te-brā′kē-ăl). Antebraquial; relativo ao antebraço.
an·te·bra·chi·um (an-te-brā′kē-ŭm) [TA]. Antebraço. SIN forearm. [ante- + L. *brachium*, braço]
an·te·car·di·um (an-te-kar′dē-ŭm). Precórdio. SIN precordia.
an·te·ced·ent (an-te-sē′dent). Antecedente; um precursor. [L. *antecedo*, ir antes]
plasma thromboplastin a. (PTA), a. da tromboplastina plasmática (PTA). SIN *factor* XI.
an·te ci·bum (an′tē-sī′bŭm). Antes de uma refeição; o plural é ante cibos, antes das refeições. [L.]
an·te·cu·bi·tal (an-te-kū′bi-tăl). Antecubital; por diante do cotovelo. [ante- + L. *cubitum*, cotovelo]
an·te·fe·brile (an-te-feb′ril). Antifebril; termo raramente utilizado para antipirético. [ante- + L. *febris*, febre]
an·te·flex (an′te-fleks). Antefletir; curvar anteriormente (para diante) ou provocar a curvatura para a frente. [ante- + L. *flecto*, pp. *flexus*, curvar]
an·te·flex·ion (an-te-flek′shŭn). Anteflexão; inclinação (flexão) para diante; uma curva ou angulação aguda para diante; indica especialmente a curvatura anterógrada normal no útero na junção do corpo com o colo uterino.
a. of iris, a. da íris; termo raramente empregado para uma íris que está, em parte, curvada para diante depois de uma iridodiálise grave, de modo que a camada pigmentada fique voltada para diante.
an·te·grade (an′te-grād). Anterógrado; na direção do movimento normal, como no fluxo sanguíneo ou na peristalse. [ante- + L. *gradior*, caminhar]
an·te·mor·tem (an′te-mōr-tem). Antes da morte. Cf. postmortem. [ante- + L. *mors* (*mort*-), morte]
an·te·na·tal (an-te-nā′tăl). Pré-natal. SIN prenatal. [ante- + L. *natus*, nascimento]

an·te·par·tum (an′te-par-tŭm). Anteparto; antes do trabalho de parto ou do parto. Cf. intrapartum, postpartum. [ante- + L. *pario*, pp. *partus*, dar à luz]

an·te·po·si·tion (an′te-pō-si′shŭn). Anteposição; posição anterior ou para a frente.

an·te·py·ret·ic (an′te-pī-ret′ik). Antipirético; antes da ocorrência da febre; antes do período de reação após o choque. [ante- + G. *pyretos*, febre]

an·te·ri·or (an-tēr′ē-or). Anterior. **1** [NA]. Na anatomia humana, que indica a superfície ventral do corpo; freqüentemente empregado para indicar a posição de uma estrutura em relação a outra, isto é, situado mais próximo da parte frontal do corpo. SIN ventral (2) [TA], ventralis [TA]. **2.** Próximo da cabeça ou da extremidade rostral de determinados embriões. **3.** Substituto indesejável e confuso para *cranial* em quadrúpedes. Em anatomia veterinária, a. restringe-se às partes do olho e do ouvido interno. **4.** Antes, em relação ao tempo ou espaço. [L.]

antero-. Prefixo que indica anterior. [L. *anterior*, mais à frente, mais cedo, de *ante*, antes + -r- -*ior*, mais]

an·ter·o·ex·ter·nal (an′ter-ō-eks-ter′nal). Ântero-externo; na frente e do lado externo.

an·ter·o·grade (an′ter-ō-grād). Anterógrado. **1.** Que se move para diante. Cf. antegrade. **2.** Que se estende para diante a partir de um determinado ponto no tempo; usado em referência à amnésia. [L. *gradior*, pp. *gressus*, andar, ir]

an·ter·o·in·fe·ri·or (an′ter-ō-in-fēr′ē-or). Ântero-inferior; por diante e abaixo.

an·ter·o·in·ter·nal (an′ter-ō-in-ter′nal). Ântero-interno; por diante e voltado para o lado interno.

an·ter·o·lat·er·al (an′ter-ō-lat′er-al). Ântero-lateral; por diante e afastado da linha média.

an·ter·o·me·di·al (an′ter-ō-mē′dē-al). Anteromedial; por diante e no sentido da linha média.

an·ter·o·me·di·an (an′ter-ō-mē′dē-an). Anteromediano; por diante e na linha central.

an·ter·o·pos·te·ri·or (an′ter-ō-pos-tēr-ē-er). Ântero-posterior. **1.** Relativo tanto à frente quanto às costas. **2.** Nas técnicas de imagem por raios X, descreve a direção do feixe através do paciente (incidência), da parte anterior para a posterior, p.ex., uma incidência A-P do abdome; ou a direção do exame (exame A-P) quando uma radiografia é vista como se você estivesse de frente para o paciente (anterior para posterior), independentemente da incidência.

an·ter·o·su·pe·ri·or (an′ter-ō-soo-pē′rē-er). Ântero-superior; em frente e acima.

ant·e·rot·ic (ant-er-ot′ik). Antierótico; relativo a um esforço para evitar os sentimentos eróticos. [anti- + G. *erōtikos*, relativo ao amor]

an·te·sys·to·le (an-te-sis′tō-lē). Ante-sístole; ativação prematura do ventrículo responsável pela síndrome de pré-excitação dos tipos Wolff-Parkinson-White ou Lown-Ganong-Levine.

an·te·ver·sion (an-te-ver′shŭn). Anteversão; virar para frente, inclinar para diante como um todo sem se curvar. [ante- + L. Mediev. *versio*, uma volta]

an·te·vert·ed (an-te-vert′ed). Antevertido; inclinado para frente; em uma posição de anteversão.

ant·hel·ix (ant′hē-liks, an′thē-liks). Antélice. SIN antihelix. [anti- + G. *helix*, mola]

ant·hel·min·thic (ant-hel-min′thik). Anti-helmíntico. SIN anthelmintic (1).

ant·hel·min·tic (ant-hel-min′tik, an-thel-). Anti-helmíntico. **1.** Um agente que destrói ou expulsa os vermes intestinais. SIN anthelminthic, anti-helminthic, helminthagogue, helminthic (2), helmintic (2), vermifuge. **2.** Que possui o poder de destruir ou expelir os vermes intestinais. SIN vermifugal. [anti- + G. *helmins*, verme]

an·the·lone (an′thē-lōn). Antelona. SIN urogastrone.

a. E, a. E; enterogastrona. SIN enterogastrone.

a. U, a. U; urogastrona. SIN urogastrone.

an·ther·id·i·um (an′ther-id′ē-um). Anterídio; o gametângio masculino produzido na parte teleomorfa do ciclo de vida dos fungos. [L. mod. *anthera*, flor, do G. *antēros*, em flor, de *anthēo*, florescer, + sufixo dim. -*idium*, de G. -*idion*]

an·thi·o·li·mine (an-thī-ō′li-mēn). Antiolimina; usada no tratamento da filaríase e esquistossomíase.

an·tho·cy·a·nins (an-thō-sī′a-ninz). Antocianinas; um grupo de pigmentos florais, que existem como glicosídeos em combinação com moléculas de glicose ou celobiose, variando desde o vermelho até o azul e, com freqüência, pH-dependentes; solúveis em água e álcool, mas não em éter. As antocianinas são divididas nos derivados da pelargonidina, cianidinas e delfinidinas. Algumas foram utilizadas como substitutos da hematoxilina. [G. *anthos*, flor + *kyanos*, uma substância azul]

An·tho·my·ia (an-thō-mī′ya). Um gênero de moscas muscóides semelhantes em aparência à mosca comum. [G. *anthos*, flor, + *myia*, mosca]

A. canicula′ris, uma pequena mosca preta, cujas larvas foram relatadas como parasitas acidentais no intestino de seres humanos, onde eclodem a partir de ovos ingeridos; os sintomas de irritação gastrentérica podem ser causados por ela; os adultos podem transportar ovos da mosca tropical humana para os seres humanos, *Dermatobia hominis*, uma causa de miíase.

an·thra·ce·mia (an-thră-sē′mē-ă). Antracemia; a presença do *Bacillus anthracis* no sangue circulante, resultando geralmente de antraz previamente desenvolvido na pele ou nos pulmões. SIN anthrax septicemia.

an·thra·cene (an′thră-sēn). Antraceno. **1.** Um hidrocarboneto obtido do alcatrão; ele oxida para antraquinona, que é convertida em corantes alizarinas. **2.** Um composto contendo a. (1) como parte de sua estrutura. [G. *anthrax*, carvão]

an·thrac·ic (an-thras′ik). Antrácico; relativo ao antraz.

an·thra·cin (an′thră-sin). Antracina, antraceno. SIN anthracene (1).

anthraco- (an′thră-kō-). Antraco-; forma combinante relacionada ao carvão, carbono; carbúnculo; corresponde ao L. carb-, carbo-. [G. *anthrax, anthrakos*, carvão, um carvão vivo; um carbúnculo, uma pústula]

an·thra·co·sil·i·co·sis (an′thră-kō-sil′i-kō′sis). Antracossilicose; pneumoconiose decorrente do acúmulo de carbono e sílica (da poeira de carvão inalada) nos pulmões; o teor de sílica produz nódulos fibrosos. SIN coal worker's pneumoconiosis. [antraco- + silicose]

an·thra·co·sis (an-thră-kō′sis). Antracose; pneumoconiose resultante do acúmulo de carbono oriundo da fumaça ou poeira de carvão inalada nos pulmões. VER TAMBÉM pneumomelanosis. SIN collier lung, miner's lung (1). [antraco- + G. -*osis*, condição]

an·thra·cot·ic (an-thră-kot′ik). Antracótico; caracterizado por antracose.

anthracycline (an-thra-sīk′lin, -lēn). Antraciclina; agente anticâncer que consiste em 3 moléculas: uma aglicona pigmentada, um amino-açúcar e uma cadeia lateral. Os exemplos são doxorrubicina, daunorrubicina e daunomicina.

an·thra·lin (an′thră-lin). Antralina; usada como substituto para a crisarobina em pomada para tratamento da psoríase e infestação por tinha. SIN dithranol.

an·thra·mu·cin (an-thră-mū′sin). Antramucina; material oriundo da cápsula do *Bacillus anthracis* que neutraliza a ação antimicrobiana do soro e tecido.

an·thra·nil·ic ac·id (an-thră-nil′ik). Ácido antranílico; um dos produtos do catabolismo do triptofano. SIN *o*-aminobenzoic acid.

an·thra·nil·o·yl (an-thră-nil′ō-il). Antraniloíla; o radical acil do ácido antranílico.

an·thra·pur·pu·rin (an′thră-poor′poo-rin). Antrapurpurina; $C_{14}H_8O_5$; 1,2,7-triidroxiantraquinona; um corante púrpura usado em histologia como reagente para o cálcio, embora sua especificidade tenha sido questionada.

9,10-an·thra·qui·none (an′thră-kwi′nōn). 9,10-Antraquinona. **1.** A base dos princípios catárticos naturais em vegetais; usado como reagente. **2.** Um composto contendo 9,10-antraquinona (1) como parte de sua estrutura; essa classe de compostos compreende o maior grupo de quinonas de ocorrência natural.

an·thrax (an′thraks). Antraz. **1.** Uma doença em seres humanos causada pela infecção por antraz cutâneo (q. v.), seguida por septicemia pela bactéria *Bacillus anthracis* a partir de animais infectados através da pele; caracterizada por hemorragia e derrames serosos em diversos órgãos e cavidades corporais e por sintomas de prostração extrema. Em raros casos, a infecção é transmitida pelo ar, causando pneumonia rapidamente fatal. Essa é a forma mais grave. **2.** Uma doença infecciosa de animais, em especial de herbívoros, devido à presença, no sangue, do *Bacillus anthracis*. SIN charbon. [G. *anthrax (anthrak-)*, carvão, carbono, um carbúnculo]

cerebral a., a. cerebral; uma forma de a. associada ao a. pulmonar ou intestinal, na qual os bacilos específicos invadem os capilares do cérebro, provocando delírio violento; freqüentemente associado à meningite hemorrágica.

cutaneous a., a. cutâneo; a lesão característica da infecção da pele pelo *B. anthracis*, que começa como uma pápula e logo se transforma em uma vesícula e se rompe, liberando um soro sanguinolento; a base dessa vesícula, em cerca de 36 horas, torna-se uma massa necrótica preto-azulada; os sinais e sintomas constitucionais da septicemia são graves: febre alta, vômitos, sudorese profusa e prostração extrema; a infecção é freqüentemente fatal. SIN malignant pustule.

intestinal a., a. intestinal; uma forma usualmente fatal de a. caracterizada por calafrio, febre alta, dor na cabeça, nas costas e nos membros, vômitos, diarréia sanguinolenta, colapso cardiovascular e, com freqüência, hemorragias a partir das mucosas e na pele (petéquias). VER TAMBÉM *mycosis* intestinalis.

pulmonary a., a. pulmonar; uma forma de a. adquirida por inalação de poeira contendo o *Bacillus anthracis*; existe calafrio inicial seguido por dor nas costas e nas pernas, respiração rápida, dispnéia, tosse, febre, pulso rápido e colapso cardiovascular extremo. SIN ragpicker's disease, ragsorter's disease, woolsorter's disease, woolsorter's pneumonia.

an·throne (an′thrōn). Antrona; 9,10-diidro-9-oxoantraceno; um reagente usado na detecção de carboidratos.

anthropo-. Antropo-; forma combinante que significa humano; homem. [G. *anthrōpos*, um ser humano (de ambos os sexos)]

an·thro·po·bi·ol·o·gy (an′thrō-pō-bī-ol′ō-jē). Antropobiologia; o estudo das relações biológicas do ser humano como uma espécie.

an·thro·po·cen·tric (an′thrō-pō-sen′trik). Antropocêntrico; com uma tendenciosidade humana; sob a suposição de que os seres humanos são o fato central do universo. [antropo- + G. *kentron*, centro]

an·thro·po·gen·e·sis (an′thrō-pō-jen′ē-sis). Antropogênese. SIN antropogeny.

an·thro·po·gen·ic, an·thro·po·ge·net·ic (an′thrō-pō-jen′ik, -jĕ-net′ik). Antropogênico; relativo à antropogenia.

an·thro·pog·e·ny (an-thrō-poj′ē-nē). Antropogenia; origem e desenvolvimento do homem, tanto em termos individuais como raciais. SIN anthropogenesis, anthropogony. [antropo- + G. *genesis*, origem]

an·thro·pog·o·ny (an-thrō-poj′ō-nē). Antropogonia; antropogenia. SIN antropogeny.

an·thro·pog·ra·phy (an-thrō-pog′ră-fē). Antropografia; a distribuição geográfica das variedades de seres humanos. [antropo- + G. *graphō*, escrever]

an·thro·poid (an′thrō-poyd). Antropóide. **1.** Que se assemelha aos seres humanos em estrutura e forma. **2.** Um dos macacos semelhantes aos seres humanos; um símio. [G. *anthrōpos-eidēs*, semelhante ao homem]

An·thro·poi·dea (an′thrō-pō-id′ē-ă). Uma subordem de mamíferos da ordem dos Primatas, que engloba as famílias Cebidae (macacos do Novo Mundo), Callithricidae (sagüis), Cercopithecidae (macacos do Velho Mundo), Pongidae (gibão, gorila, chimpanzé e orangotango) e Hominidae (seres humanos).

an·thro·pol·o·gy (an-thrō-pol′ō-jē). Antropologia; o ramo da ciência relacionado à origem e ao desenvolvimento dos seres humanos em todas as suas relações físicas, sociais e culturais. [antropo- + G. *logos*, tratado]
  applied a., a. aplicada; uma fusão da moderna a. cultural e alguns aspectos da sociologia no estudo de povos literatos em suas culturas e aplicações derivantes.
  criminal a., a. criminal; a. em relação às características físicas e mentais, hereditariedade e relações sociais do criminoso. VER TAMBÉM criminology.
  cultural a., a. cultural; o estudo de todos os aspectos da cultura resultantes do comportamento humano, inclusive, entre outros, da fala e linguagem, sistemas de raciocínio, sistemas sociais e os artefatos produzidos por uma cultura.
  physical a., a. física; o estudo dos atributos físicos dos seres humanos.

an·thro·pom·e·ter (an-thrō-pom′ē-ter). Antropômetro; um instrumento para medir as diversas dimensões do corpo humano.

an·thro·po·met·ric (an-thrō-pō-met′rik). Antropométrico; relativo à antropometria.

an·thro·pom·e·try (an-thrō-pom′ē-trē). Antropometria; o ramo da antropologia relacionado às mensurações comparativas do corpo humano. [antropo- + G. *metron*, medida]

an·thro·po·mor·phism (an′thrō-pō-mōr′fizm). Antropomorfismo; atribuição da forma ou das qualidades humanas a criaturas não-humanas ou objetos inanimados. Cf. theriomorphism. [antropo- + G. *morphē*, forma]

an·thro·pon·o·my (an-thrō-pon′ō-mē). Antroponomia; o estudo das leis que governam o desenvolvimento da espécie humana e a relação com o ambiente. [antropo- + G. *nomos*, lei]

an·thro·pop·a·thy (an-thrō-pop′ă-thē). Antropatia; atribuição de sentimentos humanos a seres não-humanos, p.ex., a deuses ou animais inferiores. [antropo- + G. *pathos*, sofrimento]

an·thro·po·phil·ic (an′thrō-pō-fil′ik). Antropofílico; que busca ou prefere o ser humano, especialmente com relação a: 1) artrópodos hematófagos, indicando a preferência de um parasita pelo hospedeiro humano como uma fonte de sangue ou tecidos em relação a um hospedeiro animal; e 2) fungos dermatofíticos que crescem preferencialmente nos seres humanos em vez de outros animais. [antropo- + G. *phileō*, amar]

an·thro·po·pho·bia (an′thrō-pō-fō′bē-ă). Antropofobia; aversão mórbida pela ou medo da companhia humana. [antropo- + G. *phobos*, medo]

an·thro·pos·co·py (an′thrō-pos′kō-pē). Antroposcopia; o julgamento do tipo e da constituição corporal por inspeção. [antropo- + G. *skopeō*, visualizar]

an·thro·po·so·ma·tol·o·gy (an′thrō-pō′sō-mă-tol′ō-jē). Antropossomatologia; a parte da antropologia relacionada com o corpo humano, p.ex., anatomia, fisiologia ou patologia. [antropo- + G. *sōma*, corpo, + *logos*, estudo]

an·thro·po·zo·o·no·sis (an′thrō-pō-zō′ō-nō′sis). Antropozoonose; uma zoonose mantida na natureza por animais e transmissível para os seres humanos; p.ex., raiva, brucelose. Cf. zooanthroponosis, amphixenosis. [antropo- + G. *zōon*, animal, + *nosos*, doença]

△ **anti-**. Anti-. **1.** Contra, em oposição a, em relação a sintomas e doenças, curativo. **2.** Prefixo que indica um anticorpo (imunoglobulina) específico para a substância indicada; p.ex., antitoxina (anticorpo específico para uma toxina). [G. *anti*, contra, oposto a, em vez de]

an·ti·ac·id (an-tē-as′id). Antiácido. SIN antacid.

an·ti·ad·ren·er·gic (an′tē-ad-rē-ner′jik). Antiadrenérgico; antagonista à ação das fibras simpáticas ou de outras fibras adrenérgicas. VER TAMBÉM sympatholytic.

an·ti·ag·glu·ti·nin (an′tē-ă-gloo′ti-nin). Antiaglutinina; um anticorpo específico que inibe ou destrói a ação de uma aglutinina.

an·ti·a·lex·in (an′tē-ă-lek′sin). Antialexina; anticomplemento. SIN anticomplement.

an·ti·al·ler·gic (an′tē-ă-ler′jik). Antialérgico; relativo a qualquer agente ou medida que previna, iniba ou alivie uma reação alérgica.

an·ti·an·a·phy·lax·is (an′tē-an′ă-fi-lak′sis). Antianafilaxia, dessensibilização. SIN desensitization (1).

an·ti·an·dro·gen (an-tē-an′drō-jen). Antiandrogênio; qualquer substância capaz de evitar a expressão plena dos efeitos biológicos dos hormônios andro-

grupos de antibióticos
aminoglicosídeos   (p.ex., estreptomicina, gentamicina, sisomicina, tobramicina, amicacina)
ansamicinas   (p.ex., rifamicina)
antimicóticos   *polienos*   (p.ex., nistatina, pimaricina, anfotericina B, pecilocina)   *derivados benzofuranos*   (griseofulvina)
antibióticos β-lactâmicos   *penicilinas*   (penicilina G e seus derivados, penicilinas orais, penicilinas fixadas por penicilinase, penicilinas de amplo espectro, penicilinas ativas contra Proteus e *Pseudomonas*)   *cefalosporinas*   (p.ex., cefalotina, cefaloridina, cefalexina, cefazolina, cefotaxima)
grupo do cloranfenicol   (cloranfenicol, tianfenicol, azidanfenicol)
Imidazol   fluconazol, itraconazol
linosamidas   (lincomicina, clindamicina)
macrolídeos   (p.ex., azitromicina, eritromicina, oleandomicina, espiramicina, claritromicina)
peptídeos, peptolídeos, polipeptídeos   (p.ex., polimixina B e E, bacitracina, tirotricina, capreomicina, vancomicina)
quinolonas   (ácido nalidíxico, ofloxacina, ciprofloxacina, norfloxina)
tetraciclinas   (p.ex., tetraciclina, oxitetraciclina, minociclina, doxiciclina)
outros antibióticos   (fosfomicina, ácido fusídico)

gênicos ou de tecidos responsivos, seja pela produção de efeitos antagonistas no tecido-alvo, como fazem os estrogênios, seja pela simples inibição dos efeitos androgênicos, como por competir pelos locais de fixação na superfície celular.

an·ti·a·ne·mic (an′tē-ă-nē′mik). Antianêmico; relativo aos fatores ou substâncias que impedem ou corrigem as condições anêmicas.

an·ti·an·ti·body (an′tē-an′tē-bod-ē). Antianticorpo; anticorpo específico para outro anticorpo.

an·ti·an·ti·tox·in (an′tē-an-tē-tok′sin). Antiantitoxina; um antianticorpo que inibe uma antitoxina ou se opõe aos efeitos desta.

an·ti·a·rach·nol·y·sin (an-tē-ar-ak-nol′i-sin). Antiaracnolisina; um antiveneno que se contrapõe ao veneno (lisina) de uma aranha. [anti- + G. *arachnē*, aranha, + lisina]

an·ti·ar·rhyth·mic (an′tē-ă-rith′mik). Antiarrítmico; que combate uma arritmia. SIN antidysrhythmic.

an·ti·ar·thrit·ic (an′tē-ar-thrit′ik). Antiartrítico. **1.** Que alivia a artrite. **2.** Um remédio para a artrite. SIN antarthritic.

an·ti·asth·mat·ic (an′tē-az-mat′ik). Antiasmático. **1.** Que tende a aliviar ou evitar a asma. **2.** Um agente que evita ou aborta uma crise asmática. SIN antasthmatic.

an·ti·au·tol·y·sin (an′tē-aw-tol′i-sin). Antiautolisina; um anticorpo que inibe ou neutraliza a atividade de uma autolisina.

an·ti·bac·te·ri·al (an′tē-bak-tēr′ē-ăl). Antibacteriano; destrutivo para as bactérias ou que evita seu crescimento.

an·ti·bech·ic (an-tē-bek′ik). Antitussígeno. SIN antitussive. [anti- + G. *bēx* (*bēch*-), tosse]

an·ti·bi·ont (an-tē-bī′ont). Antibionte; um microrganismo que produz substância antimicrobiana.

an·ti·bi·o·sis (an′tē-bī-ō′sis). Antibiose. **1.** Uma associação de dois organismos que é deletéria para um deles, em contraste com a probiose. **2.** A produção de um antibiótico por bactérias ou outros organismos inibitórios para outros seres vivos, especialmente entre os micróbios do solo. [anti- + G. *biōsis*, vida]

an·ti·bi·ot·ic (an′tē - bī - ot′ik). Antibiótico. **1.** Relativo à antibiose. **2.** Prejudicial à vida. **3.** Uma substância solúvel derivada de um mofo ou bactéria que inibe o crescimento de outros microrganismos. **4.** Relativo a uma ação desse tipo.
broad-spectrum a., a. de largo espectro; um a. que possui uma ampla faixa de atividade contra microrganismos Gram-positivos e Gram-negativos.
peptide a., a. peptídico; a. composto de peptídeos; a ação antibacteriana baseia-se na ruptura física das membranas celulares.
transport a., a. de transporte; uma substância que torna permeáveis as biomembranas a determinados íons.
an·ti·bi·ot·ic-re·sis·tant. Antibiótico-resistente; indica microrganismos que continuam a multiplicar-se, embora expostos a agentes antibióticos.
an·ti·bi·o·tin (an - tē - bī′ō - tin). Antibiotina, avidina. SIN avidin.
an·ti·blen·nor·rhag·ic (an′tē - blen - ō - raj′ik). Antiblenorrágico; termo raramente utilizado para: **1.** Preventivo ou curativo de corrimento mucoso (blenorragia). **2.** Um remédio que possui essas propriedades.

ANTIBODY

an·ti·body (Ab) (an′tē - bod - ē). Anticorpo (Ac); uma molécula de imunoglobulina produzida por células linfóides B com uma seqüência específica de aminoácidos incitada, nos seres humanos ou em outros animais, por um antígeno (imunógeno). Essas moléculas caracterizam-se por reagir especificamente com o antígeno de alguma forma demonstrável, sendo antígeno (Ag) e anticorpo (Ac) definidos em termos um do outro. Os Ac também podem existir naturalmente, ou seja, sem correlação com estímulo fornecido pela introdução de um antígeno; os Ac são encontrados no sangue e nos líquidos corporais; embora a estrutura básica da molécula consista em duas cadeias leves e duas pesadas, os Ac também podem ser encontrados como dímeros, trímeros ou pentâmeros. VER TAMBÉM immunoglobulin. SIN immune protein, protective protein, sensitizer (2).
affinity a., afinidade por a.; a força de ligação entre um anticorpo e um antígeno. Essa interação é reversível.
agglutinating a., a. aglutinante; aglutinina. SIN agglutinin (1).
anaphylactic a., a. anafilático; a. citotrópico. SIN cytotropic a.
anti-basement membrane a., a. antimembrana basal; auto-anticorpos contra antígenos da membrana basal glomerular renal.
anticardiolipin a.'s, a. anticardiolipina; anticorpos contra a cardiolipina, um éster polissacarídico fosforilado de ácidos graxos encontrado nas membranas celulares. Associado a doenças imunomediadas, sífilis e acidentes vasculares cerebrais; acredita-se que resultem de um estado hipercoagulável.
antiidiotype a., a. antiidiótipo; um antianticorpo cuja atividade é dirigida especificamente contra os determinantes antigênicos (idiótipo) de determinada molécula de imunoglobulina (anticorpo). SIN idiotypic a.
anti-MAG a., a. anti-MAG; um a. específico contra a glicoproteína associada à mielina; o mais importante dos anticorpos específicos contra a mielina identificados até o momento, presente na maioria dos pacientes com polineuropatias associadas à IgM.

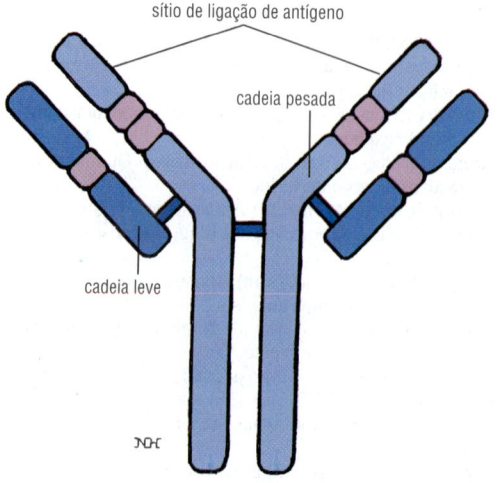

anticorpo

antineutrophil cytoplasmic a.'s (ANCA), a. anticitoplasma de neutrófilo; auto-anticorpos encontrados em algumas doenças auto-imunes, reconhecidos por suas reatividades com antígenos citoplasmáticos nos neutrófilos; dois grupos são reconhecidos: c-ANCA, que reage com a proteinase 3, é encontrado na poliangiite e na síndrome de Churg-Strauss; p-ANCA, que reage com a mieloperoxidase, é encontrado na granulomatose de Wegener.
antinuclear a. (ANA), a. antinuclear; um a. que mostra afinidade para antígenos nucleares, incluindo DNA, e encontrado no soro de um elevado percentual de pacientes com lúpus eritematoso sistêmico, artrite reumatóide e certas doenças de colágeno, em alguns de seus parentes saudáveis; também é encontrado em cerca de 1% dos indivíduos normais.
antiphospholipid a.'s, anticorpos antifosfolipídio; anticorpos contra ésteres polissacarídicos fosforilados de ácidos graxos; incluem anticoagulante lúpico, VDRL e anticardiolipina. Associados às doenças imunomediadas, sífilis e acidente vascular cerebral; acredita-se que se originem de um distúrbio hipercoagulável.
antithyroglobulin a., a. antitireoglobulina; a. contra a tireoglobulina.
avidity a., avidez do a.; o somatório total da força de ligação funcional entre um a. polivalente e seu antígeno. A força de ligação total representa o somatório da força de todas as ligações de afinidade.
bivalent a., a. bivalente; a. que provoca uma reação visível com o antígeno específico como na aglutinação, precipitação e assim por diante; assim chamado porque, de acordo com a "teoria da rede", a agregação acontece quando a molécula de anticorpo possui dois ou mais locais de ligação que podem fazer uma ligação cruzada entre uma partícula de antígeno e outra; provavelmente uma característica da classe de imunoglobulina.
blocking a., a. bloqueador; **(1)** a. que, em determinadas concentrações, não provoca precipitação após se combinar ao antígeno específico e que, nesse estado combinado, "bloqueia" a atividade do a. adicionado para aumentar a concentração até um nível em que a precipitação comumente aconteceria; **(2)** a classe IgG das imunoglobulinas que se combina especificamente com um alérgeno atópico, mas que não provoca uma reação alérgica do tipo I, o a. IgG combinado "bloqueando" a atividade do a. da classe IgE (reagínico) disponível.
blood group a.'s, a. de grupo sanguíneo. VER apêndice sobre Grupos Sanguíneos.
catalytic a., a. catalítico; um a. que foi alterado para dar a ele uma atividade catalítica. SIN abzyme.
cell-bound a., a. ligado à célula; um termo empregado para o a. nas superfícies celulares que pode estar ligado através de locais de combinação de antígeno ou de outros sítios, como a região Fc.
CF a., a. FC; a. fixador de complemento. SIN complement-fixing a.
chimeric a., a. quimérico; a. que teria o fragmento FAB de uma espécie fundido ao fragmento FC da cadeia pesada de outra espécie.
cold a., crioaglutinina. VER cold *agglutinin*.
cold-reactive a., crioaglutinina. VER cold *agglutinin*.
complement-fixing a., a. fixador de complemento (FC); a. que se combina ao antígeno que conduz à ligação e ativação do complemento, o que pode resultar em lise da célula. SIN CF a.
complete a., a. completo. SIN saline *agglutinin*.
cross-reacting a., a. de reação cruzada; **(1)** a. específico para um epítopo compartilhado por membros de um grupo, isto é, aqueles com epítopos funcionais idênticos; **(2)** a. contra antígenos que possuem grupamentos funcionais de estrutura química similar, porém não idêntica.
cytophilic a., a. citofílico; a. citotrópico. SIN cytotropic a.
cytotropic a., a. citotrópico; a. com afinidade por determinados tipos de células, além de (e não relacionada a) sua afinidade específica para o antígeno que o induziu, por causa das propriedades da porção Fc da cadeia pesada. VER TAMBÉM heterocytotropic a., homocytotropic a., cytotropic antibody *test*. SIN anaphylactic a., cytophilic a.
fluorescent a., a. fluorescente; uma imunoglobulina (anticorpo) ao qual foi preso um corante fluorescente.
Forssman a., a. de Forssman; um a. heterogenético específico para o grupo Forssman de antígenos heterogenéticos. SIN heterophil a., heterophile a.
heterocytotropic a., a. heterocitotrópico; um a. citotrópico (principalmente da classe IgG) semelhante em atividade ao a. homocitotrópico, mas possuindo uma afinidade por células de uma espécie diferente, em vez de células da mesma espécie ou de espécies intimamente correlatas.
heterogenetic a., a. heterogenético; um a. que reage com um antígeno heterogenético.
heterophil a., a. heterófilo. SIN Forssman a.
heterophile a., a. heterófilo. SIN Forssman a.
homocytotropic a., a. homocitotrópico; a. geralmente da classe IgE que possui uma afinidade por tecidos (notadamente mastócitos) da mesma espécie ou de espécies intimamente correlatas e que, ao se combinar com o antígeno específico, deflagra a liberação de mediadores farmacológicos da anafilaxia pelas células ao qual se ligou; o tropismo parece ser dependente da porção Fc da molécula do anticorpo; na anafilaxia em cobaias, o a. homocitotrópico envolvido é da classe γG. SIN reagin (4), reaginic a.

human antimouse a. (HAMA), a. humano anticamundongo; a. produzido após a exposição às proteínas do camundongo.
idiotypic a., a. idiotípico; um a. que se liga a um idiótipo de outro a. SIN antiidiotype a.
immobilizing a., a. imobilizante. SIN treponema-immobilizing a.
incomplete a., a. incompleto; **(1)** SIN univalent a.; **(2)** não-aglutinante.
inhibiting a., a. inibidor. SIN univalent a.
lymphocytotoxic a.'s, anticorpos linfocitotóxicos; anticorpos específicos contra antígenos de linfócitos e que, ao se combinarem com os antígenos, induzem lesão celular ou morte.

monoclonal a. (MAB, MoAb), a. monoclonal; um a. produzido por um clone ou população de células híbridas fundidas, geneticamente homogêneas, isto é, hibridoma; as células híbridas são clonadas para estabelecer linhagens celulares, produzindo um a. específico, que é química e imunologicamente homogêneo.

A técnica para a produção de anticorpos monoclonais, inventada em 1975 pelos biologistas moleculares Cesar Milstein e Georges Kohler, tornou-se um alicerce da pesquisa imunológica e do diagnóstico médico. Os MoAb servem como sondas experimentais em biologia celular, bioquímica e parasitologia, e são empregados na purificação de substâncias biológicas e determinados medicamentos (p.ex., interferons). Por causa de suas elevadas especificidades na ligação a antígenos-alvo, eles fornecem ensaios muito mais acurados que o anti-soro convencional. Marcados com radionuclídeos, eles têm sido empregados para liberar doses de radiação diretamente nos tecidos cancerosos.

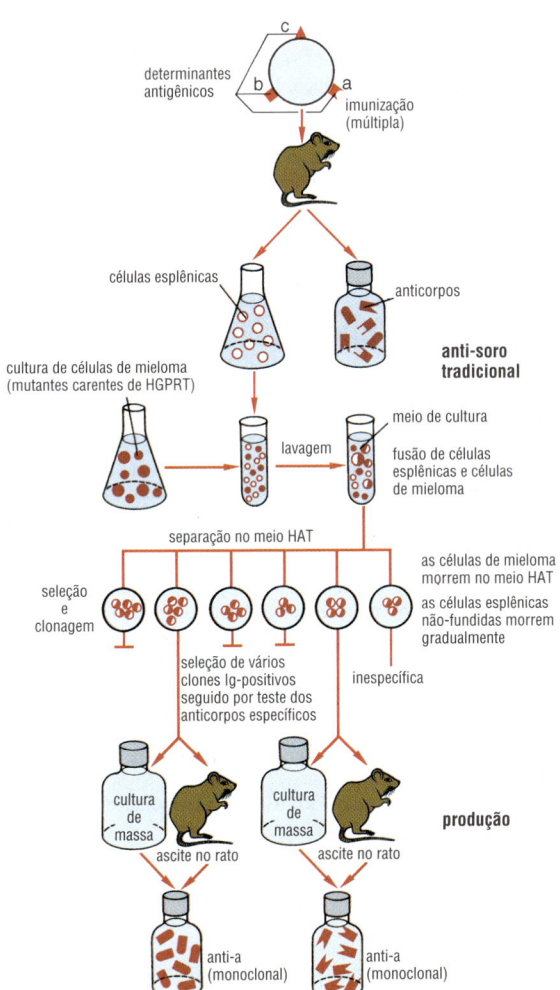

anticorpos monoclonais: preparação

natural a., a. natural. SIN normal a.
neutralizing a., a. neutralizante; uma forma de a. que reage com um agente infeccioso (geralmente um vírus) e destrói ou inibe sua infectividade e virulência; pode ser detectado ao se misturar o soro com a suspensão de agente infeccioso e, em seguida, injetando a mistura em animais ou culturas de células que sejam suscetíveis ao agente em questão.
nonprecipitable a., a. não-precipitável; a. não-precipitante. SIN nonprecipitating a.
nonprecipitating a., a. não-precipitante; a. que, sob as condições normalmente empregadas nos testes de precipitação, é refratário à precipitação por a. específico, demonstrável quando o antígeno é adicionado de forma seriada em pequenas quantidades; o a. não-precipitável precipitará em condições especiais, como quando da adição de complemento. SIN nonprecipitable a.
normal a., a. normal; a. demonstrável no soro ou plasma de várias pessoas ou animais que, sabidamente, não foram estimulados por antígeno específico, por meios artificiais ou por contato de ocorrência natural. SIN natural a.
P-K a.'s, a. P-K; anticorpos IgE envolvidos na reação de Prausnitz-Küstner.
polyclonal a. (pol - ē - klō′nal), a. policlonal; a. que deriva de diferentes clones de plasmócitos, mas que reage com diferentes epítopos de determinado antígeno.
Prausnitz-Küstner a., a. de Prausnitz-Küstner; um anticorpo da classe IgE demonstrado pela primeira vez por Prausnitz e Küstner por transferência passiva para a pele. VER homocytotropic a. SIN atopic reagin.
precipitating a., a. precipitante; precipitina. VER precipitin.
reaginic a., a. reagínico; a. homocitotrópico. SIN homocytotropic a.
ricin-blocked a., a. bloqueado por ricina; a. ao qual foi acoplada ricina.
treponema-immobilizing a., a. imobilizador de treponema; a. evocado durante as infecções sifilíticas, que possui afinidade específica por *Treponema pallidum* e que, na presença de complemento, imobiliza esse microrganismo. SIN immobilizing a., treponemal a.
treponemal a., a. imobilizador de treponema. SIN treponemal-immobilizing a.
univalent a., a. univalente; uma forma "incompleta" de a. que possui um único local de ligação; no caso dos eritrócitos Rh+, anticorpo anti-Rh desse tipo pode recobrir as células, mas não faz com que elas se aglutinem em soro fisiológico; entretanto, a aglutinação realmente acontece quando essas células revestidas são suspensas em soro ou em outros meios proteicos, como albumina, sendo portanto chamados de aglutinina sérica. SIN incomplete a. (1), inhibiting a.
Vi a., a. Vi; uma forma de a. que aglutina cepas muito virulentas de *Salmonella typhi*, isto é, células com antígeno Vi; essas bactérias não são aglutináveis com o anti-soro O, até que o antígeno Vi seja destruído. VER Vi antigen.
Wassermann a., a. de Wassermann; um a. inespecífico, evocado durante as infecções sifilíticas, que se combina à cardiolipina na presença de lecitina e colesterol; é diferente do a. imobilizador de treponema.

an·ti·bra·chi·al (an - tē - brā′kē - ăl). Antebraquial; soletração incorreta de antebrachial (antebraquial).
an·ti·bra·chi·um (an - tē - brā′kē - ŭm). Antebraço; soletração incorreta de antebrachium (antebraço).
an·ti·bro·mic (an - tē - brō′mik). Antibrômico. **1.** Desodorizante. **2.** Um desodorizador. [anti- + G. *brōmos,* odor]
an·ti·cal·cu·lous (an - tē - kal′kū - lŭs). Anticalculoso. SIN antilithic.
an·ti·car·i·ous (an′tē - kăr′ē - ŭs). Anticarioso; que evita ou inibe cárie.
an·ti·ca·thex·is (an′tē - kă - thek′sis). Anticatexia; em psicanálise, o deslocamento de uma carga emocional para um impulso ou ação de caráter oposto; p.ex., aversão inconsciente expressa como amor intencional. SIN counterinvestment.
an·ti·ceph·a·lal·gic (an′tē - sef - ă - lal′jik). Anticefalálgico; que impede ou evita a cefaléia.
an·ti·chol·a·gogue (an - tē - kol′ă - gog). Anticolagogo; termo raramente empregado para um agente ou processo que reduz ou suspende o fluxo da bile.
an·ti·cho·lin·er·gic (an′tē - kol - i - ner′jik). Anticolinérgico; antagonista para a ação das fibras nervosas parassimpáticas ou outras fibras nervosas colinérgicas (p.ex., atropina).
an·ti·cho·lin·es·ter·ase (an′tē - kō - lin - es′ter - ās). Anticolinesterase; um dos medicamentos que inibem ou inativam a acetilcolinesterase, seja reversivelmente (p.ex., fisostigmina), seja irreversivelmente (p.ex., pirofosfato de tetraetila).
α_1-**an·ti·chy·mo·tryp·sin** (an′ti - kī′mō - trip - sin). α_1-Antiquimotripsina; uma proteína inibidora da protease digestiva, quimotripsina.
an·tic·i·pate (an - tis′i - pāt). Antecipar; chegar antes da hora marcada; diz-se de um sintoma ou doença periódica, como o paroxismo da malária, quando ele reincide a intervalos cada vez mais curtos. [L. *anticipo,* pp. *-cipatus,* antecipar, de *anti* (forma antiga de *ante*), antes, + *capio,* tomar]
an·tic·i·pa·tion (an - tis - i - pā′shŭn). Antecipação. **1.** Aparecimento antes do período previsto de um sintoma ou sinal periódico. **2.** Idade cada vez mais precoce de manifestação de uma doença hereditária em gerações sucessivas; pode

ser artificial (por causa da consciência aumentada para os sinais iniciais da doença ou porque eles são mais evidentes no jovem) ou autêntica (por causa da perda progressiva de genes epistáticos e modificadores por recombinação e segregação, ou por causa da expansão de alelos instáveis em gerações sucessivas). **3.** Agravamento de um fenótipo em gerações sucessivas de uma família, freqüentemente associado a aumento do número de repetições de trinucleotídeos em um gene causal (p.ex., síndrome do X frágil, distrofia miotônica, doença de Huntington).

an·ti·cli·nal (an - tē - klī′nal). Anticlinal; inclinado em direções opostas, como dois lados de uma pirâmide. [anti- + G. *klinō*, inclinar]

an·tic·ne·mi·on (an - tik - nē′mē - on). Borda anterior da tíbia. SIN anterior border of tibia. [G. *antiknēmion*]

an·ti·co·ag·u·lant (an′tē - kō - ag′ū - lant). Anticoagulante. **1.** Que impede a coagulação. **2.** Um agente que possui essa ação (p.ex., warfarin).

  lupus a., a. lúpico; anticorpo antifosfolipídio que provoca o prolongamento do tempo de tromboplastina parcial; associado à trombose venosa e arterial.

an·ti·co·don (an - tē - kō′don). Anticódon; a seqüência trinucleotídica complementar a um códon encontrada em uma alça da molécula de ARNt; p.ex., se um códon é A–G–C, seu anticódon é U (ou T)–C–G. O princípio da complementaridade origina-se do pareamento de bases de Watson-Crick, no qual A é complementar a U (ou T) e G é complementar a C. Por vezes denominado de "nodoc".

an·ti·com·ple·ment (an - tē - kom′plē - ment). Anticomplemento; uma substância que se combina a um componente do complemento e neutraliza sua ação por evitar sua união com um anticorpo. SIN antialexin.

an·ti·com·ple·men·ta·ry (an′tē - kom - plē - men′ta - rē). Anticomplementar; que indica uma substância que consegue diminuir ou abolir a ação de um complemento.

an·ti·con·ta·gious (an′tē - kon - tā′jŭs). Anticontagioso; que impede o contágio.

an·ti·con·vul·sant (an′tē - kon - vŭl′sant). Anticonvulsivante. **1.** Que impede ou interrompe uma convulsão. **2.** Um agente que exerça essa ação. SIN anticonvulsive, antiepileptic.

an·ti·con·vul·sive (an′tē - kon - vŭl′siv). Anticonvulsivo; anticonvulsivante. SIN anticonvulsant.

an·ti·cu·ra·re (an - tē - koo - ra′rē). Anticurare; uma propriedade medicamentosa que se refere à capacidade de reverter a paralisia muscular produzida pela *d*-tubocurarina e outros medicamentos bloqueadores neuromusculares semelhantes ao curare. Os exemplos incluem neostigmina, piridostigmina e edrofônio.

an·ti·cus (an - tī′kŭs). Termo na nomenclatura anatômica para designar um músculo ou outra estrutura que, dentre todas as estruturas semelhantes, é a mais próxima da superfície anterior ou ventral. A *Nomina Anatomica* utiliza "anterior" em lugar desse termo. [L. o mais a frente, de *ante*, antes]

an·ti·cy·to·tox·in (an′tē - sī - tō - tok′sin). Anticitotoxina; um anticorpo específico que inibe ou destrói a atividade de uma citotoxina.

an·ti·de·pres·sant (an′tē - dē - pres′ant). Antidepressivo. **1.** Que se contrapõe à depressão. **2.** Um agente utilizado no tratamento da depressão.

  tetracyclic a., a. tetracíclico; uma classe de a. semelhante aos a. tricíclicos e também relacionada aos antipsicóticos fenotiazínicos; p.ex., maprotilina.

  triazolopyridine a., a. triazolpiridínico; uma classe de a. estrutural e farmacologicamente distintos dos outros a.; a efetividade clínica parece ser equivalente à dos a. tricíclicos, porém com menos efeitos colaterais anticolinérgicos; p.ex., trazodona.

  trycyclic a., a. tricíclico; um grupo químico de substâncias antidepressivas que compartilham um núcleo com 3 anéis; p.ex., amitriptilina, imipramina, desipramina e nortriptilina.

an·ti·di·a·bet·ic (an′tē - dī - ă - bet′ik). Antidiabético; que se contrapõe ao diabetes; indica um agente que reduz a glicemia (p.ex., tolbutamida, insulina).

an·ti·di·ar·rhe·al, an·ti·di·ar·rhet·ic (an′tē - dī - ă - rē′al, - dī - ă - ret′ik). Antidiarreico. **1.** Que possui a propriedade de se opor ou corrigir a diarréia. **2.** Um agente que exerça essa ação (p.ex., loperamida).

an·ti·di·u·re·sis (an′tē - dī - ū - rē′sis). Antidiurese; redução do volume urinário.

an·ti·di·u·ret·ic (an′tē - dī - ū - ret′ik). Antidiurético; um agente que reduz o débito urinário.

an·ti·dot·al (an -tē - dō′tăl). Antidotal; que se relaciona a ou atua como um antídoto.

an·ti·dote (an′tē - dōt). Antídoto; um agente que neutraliza um veneno ou contrapõe-se a seus efeitos. [G. *antidotos*, de *anti*, contra, + *dotos*, o que é dado, de *didōmi*, dar]

  chemical a., a. químico; uma substância que se une a um veneno para formar um composto químico inócuo.

  mechanical a., a. mecânico; uma substância que impede a absorção de um veneno.

  physiologic a., a. fisiológico; um agente que produz efeitos sistêmicos contrários àqueles de determinado veneno.

  universal a., a. universal; uma mistura obsoleta de 2 partes de carvão ativado,

1 parte de ácido tânico e 1 parte de óxido de magnésio destinada a ser administrada a pacientes que consumiram veneno. A mistura não é efetiva e não é mais utilizada; o carvão ativado é útil.

an·ti·drom·ic (an - tē - drom′ik). Antidrômico; que indica a propagação de um impulso ao longo de um sistema de condução (p.ex., fibra nervosa) na direção oposta à que ele normalmente percorre.

an·ti·dys·en·ter·ic (an′tē - dis - en - ter′ik). Antidisentérico; que alivia ou evita a disenteria.

an·ti·dys·rhyth·mic (an′tē - dis - rith′mik). Antiarrítmico. SIN antiarrhythmic.

an·ti·dys·u·ric (an′tē - dis - ū′rik). Antidisúrico; que evita ou alivia a estrangúria ou desconforto à micção.

an·ti·e·met·ic (an′tē - ē - met′ik). Antiemético. **1.** Que evita ou interrompe o vômito. **2.** Um remédio que tende a controlar a náusea e o vômito. [anti- + G. *emetikos*, emético]

an·ti·e·ner·gic (an′tē - en - er′jik). Antienérgico; que atua contra ou se opõe. [anti- + G. *energos*, ativo]

an·ti·en·zyme (an - tē - en′zim). Antienzima; um agente ou princípio que retarda, inibe ou destrói a atividade de uma enzima; pode ser uma enzima inibitória ou um anticorpo contra uma enzima (p.ex., antitripsina sérica).

an·ti·ep·i·lep·tic (an′tē - ep - i - lep′tik). Antiepiléptico. SIN anticonvulsant.

an·ti·es·tro·gen (an′tē - es′trō - jen). Antiestrogênio; qualquer substância capaz de evitar a expressão plena dos efeitos biológicos dos hormônios estrogênicos sobre os tecidos responsivos, seja promovendo efeitos antagonistas sobre o tecido-alvo, como os androgênios e progestogênios o fazem, seja competindo com os estrogênios pelos receptores destes ao nível celular (p.ex., tamoxifeno).

an·ti·fe·brile (an - tē - fē′brīl, - feb′ril). Antifebril; antipirético. SIN antipyretic (1). [anti- + L. *febris*, febre]

an·ti·fi·bril·la·tory (an′tē - fi′bri - lă - tōr - ē). Antifibrilatório; qualquer medida ou medicamento que tenda a suprimir as arritmias fibrilares (fibrilação atrial, fibrilação ventricular).

an·ti·fi·bri·nol·y·sin (an′tē - fī - bri - nol′i - sin). Antifibrinolisina. SIN antiplasmin.

an·ti·fi·bri·no·lyt·ic (an′tē - fī - brin - ō - lit′ik). Antifibrinolítico; indica uma substância que diminui a degradação da fibrina; p.ex. ácido aminocapróico.

an·ti·fo·lic (an - tē - fō′lik). Antifólico. **1.** Antagonista para a ação do ácido fólico. **2.** Qualquer agente com esse efeito. VER TAMBÉM folic acid *antagonists*, em *antagonist*.

an·ti·fun·gal (an - tē - fŭng′al). Antifúngico, antimicótico. SIN antimycotic.

an·ti-G. No sentido estrito, um termo que significa "antigravidade", mas, da maneira comumente utilizada, um adjetivo que implica proteção contra os efeitos da gravidade (p.ex., *roupa* anti-G).

ANTIGEN

an·ti·gen (Ag) (an′ti-jen). Antígeno (Ag); qualquer substância que, em conseqüência de entrar em contato com células apropriadas, induz um estado de sensibilidade e/ou responsividade imune após um período latente (dias a semanas) e que reage, de uma maneira demonstrável, com os anticorpos e/ou células imunes do indivíduo sensibilizado *in vivo* ou *in vitro*. O uso moderno tende a reter o amplo significado de um a., empregando os termos "determinante antigênico" ou "grupo determinante" para o grupamento químico em questão de uma molécula que confere a especificidade antigênica. VER TAMBÉM hapten. SIN immunogen. [anti (body) + G. *-gen*, que produz]

  ABO a.'s, a. ABO. ver grupo sanguíneo ABO, apêndice de Grupos Sanguíneos.

  acetone-insoluble a., cardiolipina. SIN cardiolipin.

  allogeneic a. (al′ō - je - ne′ik), a. alogênico; variações genéticas dos mesmos antígenos em uma determinada espécie.

  Am a.'s, a. Am; determinantes alotípicos (antígenos) na cadeia pesada das moléculas de IgA humanas.

  Au a., a. Au; **(1)** VER grupo sanguíneo Auberger no apêndice de Grupos Sanguíneos; **(2)** SIN Australia a.

  Aus a., a. Aus. SIN Australia a.

  Australia a., a. Austrália; assim chamado porque foi reconhecido pela primeira vez em um aborígene da Austrália, mas, hoje em dia, sabe-se que nada mais é que subunidades do antígeno de superfície do vírus da hepatite B. SIN Au a. (2), Aus a.

  Beᵃ a.'s, a. Beᵃ; VER grupos sanguíneos de baixa freqüência, no apêndice de Grupos Sanguíneos. SIN Becker a.

  Becker a., a. de Becker. SIN Beᵃ a.'s.

  Bi a., a. Bi. VER grupos sanguíneos de baixa freqüência no apêndice de Grupos Sanguíneos. SIN Bile a.

  Bile a., a. Bile. SIN Bi a.

blood group a., a. de grupo sanguíneo; termo genérico para designar qualquer antígeno herdado encontrado na superfície dos eritrócitos que determine uma reação de tipagem sanguínea com anti-soro específico; os Ag dos grupos sanguíneos ABO e Lewis também podem ser encontrados na saliva e em outros líquidos corporais; os genes que controlam o desenvolvimento dos antígenos de grupo sanguíneo variam em freqüência nos diferentes grupos étnicos e populacionais. VER TAMBÉM apêndice de Grupos Sanguíneos. SIN blood group substance.
By a., a. By. VER grupos sanguíneos de baixa freqüência, no apêndice de Grupos Sanguíneos.
CA-125 a., a. CA-125; marcador tumoral elevado em 85% das mulheres com câncer de ovário avançado. VER TAMBÉM cancer antigen 125 *test.*
CA-15-3 a., a. CA-15-3; a. presente em algumas pacientes com câncer de mama.
CA-19-9 a., a. CA-19-9; a. tumoral presente em colangiossarcomas e carcinomas pancreáticos.
capsular a., a. capsular; aquele encontrado apenas nas cápsulas de determinados microrganismos; p.ex., os polissacarídeos específicos dos vários tipos de pneumococos.
carcinoembryonic a. (CEA), a. carcinoembrionário; uma glicoproteína constituinte do glicocálice do epitélio endodérmico embrionário, que pode estar elevada no soro de alguns pacientes com câncer de cólon e outros tipos específicos de câncer e no soro dos tabagistas.
Casoni a., a. de Casoni; a. de teste cutâneo composto de líquido hidático estéril; usado no teste para a doença hidática.
C carbohydrate a., a. do carboidrato C; um antígeno encontrado na parede celular de espécies de *Streptococcus* e que indica diferentes cepas. VER β-hemolytic *streptococci,* em *streptococcus.*
CDE a.'s, a. CDE. VER grupo sanguíneo Rh no apêndice de Grupos Sanguíneos.
cholesterinized a., cardiolipina à qual foi acrescentado o colesterol.
Chr^a a.'s, a. Chr^a. VER grupos sanguíneos de baixa freqüência no apêndice de Grupos Sanguíneos.
class I a.'s, antígenos de classe I; glicoproteínas ligadas à membrana celular encontradas na maioria das células nucleadas que são codificadas por genes do principal complexo de histocompatibilidade (MHC).
class II a.'s, antígenos de classe II; uma glicoproteína da membrana celular codificada por genes do principal complexo de histocompatibilidade (MHC). Esses antígenos estão distribuídos nas células apresentadoras de a., como macrófagos, células B e células dendríticas.
class III a.'s, antígenos de classe III; moléculas não-pertencentes à membrana celular que são codificadas pela região S do principal complexo de histocompatibilidade (MHC). Esses antígenos não estão envolvidos na determinação da histocompatibilidade e incluem as proteínas do complemento, bem como determinados genes de citocinas, isto é, fatores α e β de necrose tumoral.
cluster of differentiation (CD) a., a. de grupo de diferenciação (CD); um antígeno (marcador) na superfície de uma célula, geralmente um linfócito.
common a., a. comum; a. de reação cruzada (epítopo); um a. comum que ocorre em duas ou mais moléculas ou organismos diferentes.
complete a., a. completo; qualquer a. capaz de estimular a formação de anticorpo com o qual reage *in vivo* e *in vitro,* conforme diferenciado do a. incompleto (hapteno).
conjugated a., a. conjugado. SIN conjugated *hapten.*
D a., a. D; um dos 6 antígenos que compõem o *locus* Rh. O anticorpo induzido pelo antígeno D é a causa mais freqüente de doença hemolítica do recém-nascido.
delta a., a. delta. SIN hepatitis D *virus.*
Dharmendra a., a. de Dharmendra; uma suspensão de *Mycobacterium leprae* extraída pelo clorofórmio-éter usada para produzir a reação de Fernandez em um teste de lepromina.
Di a., a. Di. VER grupo sanguíneo Diego, no apêndice de Grupos Sanguíneos.
Duffy a., a. Duffy. VER grupo sanguíneo Duffy no apêndice de Grupos Sanguíneos.
epithelial membrane a. (EMA), a. da membrana epitelial; uma proteína complexa de 70 kd, maciçamente glicosilada, isolada pela primeira vez na globulina da gordura do leite humano. Esse a. está presente em diversos epitélios glandulares, principalmente nas células do carcinoma de mama, mas também pode ser observado em fibroblastos cultivados, células linfóides e em algumas células do estroma. A coloração imuno-histoquímica pode ser empregada no diagnóstico desses tecidos.
flagellar a., a. flagelar; os antígenos termolábeis associados aos flagelos de bactérias, em contraste com o a. somático. VER TAMBÉM H a.
Forssman a., a. de Forssman; um tipo de a. heterogenético encontrado em cães, cavalos, gatos, carneiros, tartarugas, ovos de alguns peixes, em certas bactérias (p.ex., algumas cepas de microrganismos entéricos e pneumococos) e variedades de milho; geralmente encontrado em tecidos e órgãos (não no sangue), mas existe nos eritrócitos de carneiro, mas não nos tecidos desse animal; com a exceção de cobaias e *hamsters,* o a. de Forssman não é encontrado em roedores ou em rãs, porcos e na maioria dos primatas; o anticorpo que se desenvolve na mononucleose infecciosa dos seres humanos reage especificamente com o a. de Forssman.
Fy a.'s, a. Fy. VER grupo sanguíneo Duffy no apêndice de Grupos Sanguíneos.
G a., a. G; uma glicoproteína antigênica freqüentemente associada às superfícies virais. [Al. *gebundenes,* ligado]
Ge a., a. Ge. VER grupos sanguíneos de alta freqüência no apêndice de Grupos Sanguíneos.
Gerbich a., a. de Gerbich; glicoforina C. VER glucophorins.
Gm a.'s, antígenos Gm; determinantes alotípicos (antígenos) que existem na cadeia pesada da imunoglobulina G. Existem 25 determinantes distintos presentes por toda a população humana.
Good a., a. de Good. VER grupos sanguíneos de baixa freqüência no apêndice de Grupos Sanguíneos.
Gr a., a. Gr. SIN Vw a. VER Vw a. em grupo sanguíneo MNSs no apêndice de Grupos Sanguíneos.
group a.'s, antígenos de grupo; antígenos que existem em diferentes organismos.
H a., a. H; **(1)** o a. nos flagelos de bactérias móveis; importante na classificação sorológica das bactérias entéricas. VER TAMBÉM o a. (1); **(2)** o precursor químico dos antígenos do *locus* do grupo sanguíneo ABO.
H-2 a.'s, antígenos H-2; antígenos que são codificados pelo complexo H-2 dos genes no camundongo e que estão envolvidos no reconhecimento do próprio/não-próprio (*self/nonself*).
He a.'s, a. He. VER grupo sanguíneo MNSs no apêndice de Grupos Sanguíneos. SIN Hu a.'s
heart a., cardiolipina. SIN cardiolipin.
hepatitis-associated a. (HAA), a. associado à hepatite; um termo empregado para o a. de superfície do vírus da hepatite B antes que sua natureza fosse estabelecida. VER hepatitis B surface a.
hepatitis B core a. (HB$_c$Ab, HB$_c$Ag), a. do cerne da hepatite B; o a. encontrado no cerne da partícula Dane (que é o vírus completo) e também nos núcleos de hepatócitos nas infecções por hepatite B.
hepatitis B e a. (HB$_e$Ab, HBe, HB$_e$Ag), a. e da hepatite B; um a., ou grupo de a., associado à hepatite B e diferente do a. de superfície (HB$_s$Ag) e do a. do cerne (HB$_c$Ag); está associado ao nucleocapsídio viral. Sua presença indica que o vírus está se replicando e que o indivíduo é potencialmente infeccioso.
hepatitis B surface a. (HB$_s$Ab, HB$_s$Ag), a. de superfície da hepatite B; a. das pequenas (20 nm) formas esféricas e filamentosas do a. da hepatite B e um a. de superfície da grande partícula Dane (42 nm) (vírus infeccioso completo da hepatite B). VER TAMBÉM hepatitis B core a., hepatitis B e a.
heterogeneic a., a. heterogênico. VER heterophile a.
heterogenetic a., a. heterogênico. SIN heterophile a.
heterophil a., a. heterófilo. SIN heterophile a.
heterophile a., a. heterófilo; **(1)** um a. ou determinante antigênico que é encontrado em diferentes tecidos em mais de uma espécie; **(2)** um a. que é possuído por várias espécies não-correlatas e filogeneticamente diferentes; p.ex., os vários antígenos específicos para órgãos e tecidos, a proteína cristalina α e β da lente do olho e o a. de Forssman. SIN heterogenetic a., heterophil a.
hexon a., a. hexon, subunidade viral. VER hexon.
histocompatibility a., a., de histocompatibilidade; um a. na superfície das células nucleadas, principalmente de leucócitos e trombócitos. VER TAMBÉM H-2 a.'s. SIN transplantation a.
HL-A a.'s, antígenos HL-A; atualmente obsoleto, esta era a designação original para *human leukocyte histocompatibility a.* O sistema de histocompatibilidade HLA em seres humanos é composto pelas classes I, II e III do MHC. VER major histocompatibility *complex.*
Ho a., a. Ho. VER grupos sanguíneos de baixa freqüência no apêndice de Grupos Sanguíneos.
homologous a., a. homólogo; o a. específico que gera a formação de um anticorpo, que, por sua vez, pode reagir com esse antígeno.
Hu a.'s, a. Hu. SIN He a.'s.
human leukocyte a.'s (HLA) [MIM*142560], antígenos dos leucócitos humanos; sistema de designação para os produtos genéticos de, pelo menos, quatro *loci* ligados (A, B, C e D) e de um número de *subloci* no sexto cromossoma humano que mostraram ter uma forte influência sobre o alotransplante humano, transfusões em pacientes refratários e determinadas associações de doenças; mais de 50 alelos são reconhecidos, muitos dos quais estão nos *loci* HLA-A e HLA-B; herança autossômica dominante.
H-Y a., a. H-Y; um fator antigênico, dependente do cromossoma Y, responsável pela diferenciação do embrião humano em um fenótipo masculino por induzir a gônada embrionária inicialmente bipotencial para se desenvolver em um testículo; na ausência desse a., a gônada indiferenciada desenvolve-se em um ovário. Existem pelo menos dois *loci* envolvidos, um gene autossômico que gera o a. [MIM*143170] e um que produz o receptor [MIM*143150].
I a.'s, a. I. VER grupo sanguíneo I no apêndice de Grupos Sanguíneos.
incomplete a., a. incompleto. SIN hapten.
InV group a., a. do grupo InV. SIN Km a.
Jk a.'s, a. JK. VER grupo sanguíneo Kidd no apêndice de Grupos Sanguíneos.

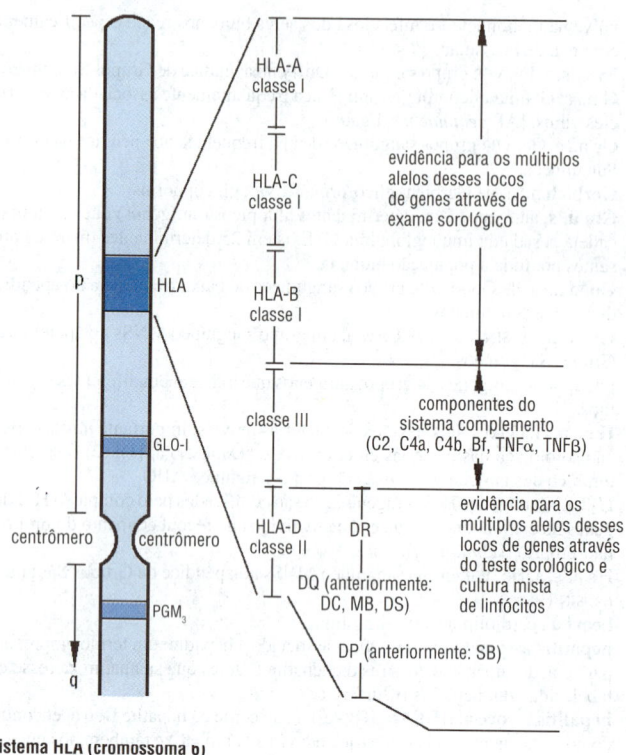

sistema HLA (cromossoma 6)

Jobbins a., a. de Jobbins. VER grupos sanguíneos de baixa freqüência no apêndice de Grupos Sanguíneos.
Js a., a. Js. VER grupo sanguíneo Sutter no apêndice de Grupos Sanguíneos.
K a.'s, a. K. VER grupo sanguíneo Kell no apêndice de Grupos Sanguíneos.
Km a., a. Km; antígenos alotípicos que são encontrados na cadeia leve kapa da imunoglobulina humana. SIN InV group a.
Kveim a., a. de Kveim; uma suspensão salina de tecido sarcóide humano preparada a partir do baço de um indivíduo com sarcoidose ativa; usado no teste de Kveim. SIN Kveim-Siltzbach a.
Kveim-Siltzbach a., a. de Kveim-Siltzbach. SIN Kveim a.
Lan a., a. de Lan. VER grupos sanguíneos de alta freqüência no apêndice de Grupos Sanguíneos.
Le a.'s, a. de Le. VER grupo sanguíneo Lewis no apêndice de Grupos Sanguíneos.
leukocyte common a. (loo'kō-sit), a. leucocitário comum; uma família de glicoproteínas encontradas na maioria dos leucócitos e ausente em células de outros tipos. Esses antígenos de superfície celular podem compreender até 10% das proteínas de membrana.
Levay a., a. de Levay. VER grupos sanguíneos de baixa freqüência no apêndice de Grupos Sanguíneos.
Lu a.'s, a. de Lu. VER grupo sanguíneo Lutheran no apêndice de Grupos Sanguíneos.
lymphocyte function associated a. (LFA) (lim f'ō-sit), a. associado à função do linfócito; um membro da família das integrinas que é expresso em todos os leucócitos e que se liga ao ICAM-1 e ICAM-2 em diversas células.
lymphogranuloma venereum a., a. do linfogranuloma venéreo; uma preparação estéril de clamídias inativadas e cultivadas no saco vitelino de aves domésticas e usado como a. no teste de Frei.
Lyt a.'s, a. de Lyt; um grupo de aloantígenos que são encontrados nos linfócitos T ou B murinos, p.ex., Lyt 2,3 é equivalente ao CD8 humano.
M a., a. M; um antígeno encontrado na célula do *Streptococcus pyogenes*; associado à virulência. VER β-hemolytic *streptococci*, em *streptococcus*.
M_1 a., M^g a., M^c a., M_2 a., VER grupo sanguíneo MNSs, no apêndice de Grupos Sanguíneos.
Mitsuda a., a. de Mitsuda; uma suspensão autoclavada de tecido humano naturalmente infectado por *Mycobacterium leprae*; usada para produzir a reação de Mitsuda em um teste de lepromina.
MNSs a.'s, antígenos MNSs. VER grupo sanguíneo MNSs no apêndice de Grupos Sanguíneos.
Mu a., a. Mu. VER grupo sanguíneo MNSs no apêndice de Grupos Sanguíneos.
mumps skin test a., a. do teste cutâneo de caxumba; uma suspensão estéril de vírus da caxumba mortos em solução de cloreto de sódio isotônica, usada para determinar a suscetibilidade à caxumba ou para confirmar a exposição prévia.
O a., a. O; **(1)** a. somático de bactérias entéricas Gram-negativas. A parte externa do lipopolissacarídeo da parede celular. VER TAMBÉM H a. (1); **(2)** VER grupo sanguíneo ABO no apêndice de Grupos Sanguíneos.
oncofetal a.'s, antígenos oncofetais; antígenos associados a tumor presentes no tecido fetal e em alguns tumores malignos, mas não no tecido adulto normal, incluindo a α-fetoproteína.
organ-specific a., a. órgão-específico; um antígeno heterogenético com especificidade por determinado órgão; p.ex., além do a. específico para a espécie, o rim de uma espécie contém antígenos que são idênticos àqueles no rim de outras espécies. SIN tissue-specific a.
Ot a., a. Ot. VER grupos sanguíneos de baixa freqüência no apêndice de Grupos Sanguíneos.
P a.'s, antígenos P. VER grupo sanguíneo P no apêndice de Grupos Sanguíneos.
partial a., a. parcial. SIN hapten.
penton a., penton. VER penton.
pollen a., a. de pólen; um extrato da proteína antigênica oriunda do pólen das plantas; isto é, alérgeno do pólen, usado no diagnóstico e na prevenção da febre do feno.
private a.'s, a. particular. VER grupos sanguíneos de baixa freqüência no apêndice de Grupos Sanguíneos.
proliferating cell nuclear a., a. nuclear de proliferação celular; uma proteína nuclear não-histona com um peso molecular de 36 kd que participa na iniciação da proliferação celular através do aumento da DNA polimerase; a coloração para o a. nuclear de proliferação celular em tumores correlaciona-se com o grau e com a atividade mitótica.

prostate-specific a. (PSA), a. específico da próstata; uma glicoproteína de cadeia única, com 31 kDa, com 240 resíduos aminoácidos e 4 cadeias laterais de carboidratos; uma protease calicreína produzida pelas células epiteliais da próstata e normalmente encontrada no líquido seminal e no sangue circulante. As elevações do PSA sérico são muito órgão-específicas, mas ocorrem no câncer (adenocarcinoma) e na doença benigna (hiperplasia prostática benigna, prostatite). Um número significativo de pacientes com câncer confinado à próstata tem valores normais de PSA. SIN human glandular kallikrein 3.

Os níveis de PSA abaixo de 4 ng/dl são considerados normais, enquanto os níveis acima de 10 ng/dl são fortemente indicativos de carcinoma da próstata. Aproximadamente 30% dos pacientes com níveis de PSA entre esses limites apresentarão câncer de próstata detectável por biopsia no decorrer de 1 ano. A mensuração do PSA livre e do PSA em complexo com o inibidor de protease α-1 antiquimotripsina (PSA-ACT) aumenta a sensibilidade do teste para o carcinoma nos homens com níveis totais de PSA entre 4 e 10 ng/dl. O percentual de PSA livre é menor no soro dos homens com câncer de próstata do que nos pacientes com próstatas normais ou doença benigna. Um nível de PSA livre que é de 25% ou mais do PSA total em um paciente com uma próstata benigna palpável descarta efetivamente a necessidade de biopsia da próstata, quando o PSA total está abaixo de 10 ng/dl. Um PSA livre de 15% ou menos sugere fortemente um carcinoma. Um nível de 20% ou mais pode ser observado no adenocarcinoma, quando a próstata está aumentada. Durante a década de 80, o uso aumentado do rastreamento por PSA levou a um aparente deslocamento na incidência de carcinoma de próstata, com um número proporcionalmente maior de diagnósticos em homens com menos de 70 anos de idade e menor em homens acima de 70 anos, bem como a uma maior incidência de doença inicial ou restrita ao órgão. Esse deslocamento atingiu o máximo em 1992; atualmente, a estatística de incidência quase retornou aos níveis pré-rastreamento com PSA. A taxa de mortalidade por câncer de próstata diminuiu substancialmente desde 1990. Muitos observadores atribuem esse declínio à capacidade do rastreamento com PSA de detectar o câncer em um estágio curável. Entretanto, o uso do teste de PSA, bem como de outras manobras diagnósticas para avaliar os homens idosos assintomáticos para o câncer de próstata, é controverso, pois muitos homens com câncer de próstata não morrem em conseqüência dessa neoplasia, e, para muitos observadores, as conseqüências do tratamento agressivo, que podem incluir a incontinência urinária e a impotência, parecem piores que a doença.

public a.'s, a. público. VER grupos sanguíneos de alta freqüência no apêndice de Grupos Sanguíneos.
R a., a. R. VER β-hemolytic *streptococci*, em *streptococcus*.
Rh a.'s, antígenos Rh. VER grupo sanguíneo Rh no apêndice de Grupos Sanguíneos.
Rhus toxicodendron a., a. do *Rhus toxicodendron*; um extrato de folhas fres-

cas de erva venenosa, com 0,4% de cloridrato de procaína; usado por injeção intradérmica para determinar a sensibilidade ao veneno do *Rhus toxicodendron*.
Rhus venenata a., a. da *Rhus venenata*; um extrato de folhas frescas do sumagre venenoso; usado para determinar a sensibilidade à planta ou para aliviar a dermatite causada pelo contato com suas folhas.
S a., a. S. SIN soluble a.
sensitized a., a. sensibilizado; o complexo formado quando o a. se combina ao anticorpo específico; assim chamado porque o a., através da mediação do anticorpo, torna-se sensível à ação do complemento.
shock a., a. de choque; um a. capaz de produzir choque anafilático em um animal que foi sensibilizado a ele.
Sm a., a. Sm. VER grupos sanguíneos de alta freqüência no apêndice de Grupos Sanguíneos.
soluble a., a. solúvel; um a. viral que permanece em solução depois que as partículas do vírus foram removidas por meio de centrifugação; no caso dos vírus influenza, é a estrutura helicoidal interna, livre do envelope externo. SIN S a.
somatic a., a. somático; um a. localizado na parede celular de uma bactéria em contraste com um antígeno no flagelo (a. flagelar) ou na cápsula (a. capsular).
species-specific a., a. espécie-específico; componentes antigênicos nos tecidos e líquidos de membros de uma espécie de animal, por meio dos quais as várias espécies podem ser imunologicamente diferenciadas; p.ex., a albumina sérica dos cavalos é imunologicamente diferente daquela do homem, cães, carneiro e assim por diante.
specific a.'s, a. específico; antígenos que caracterizam um único gênero de microrganismos.
Stobo a., a. de Stobo. VER grupos sanguíneos de baixa freqüência no apêndice de Grupos Sanguíneos.
Streptococcus M a., a. M do estreptococo; o a. somático associado à virulência e especificidade de tipo dos estreptococos do grupo A. É antifagocítico e existem mais de 80 tipos diferentes. SIN M protein (1).
Sw^a a., a. Sw^a. VER grupos sanguíneos de baixa freqüência no apêndice de Grupos Sanguíneos.
Swann a,'s, a. de Swann. VER grupos sanguíneos de baixa freqüência no apêndice de Grupos Sanguíneos.
T a.'s, antígenos T; antígenos tumorais associados à replicação e transformação por determinados DNA vírus tumorais, incluindo adenovírus e papovavírus. VER TAMBÉM β-hemolytic *streptococci*, em *streptococcus*, tumor a.'s
Tac a., a. Tac; um determinante antigênico do receptor da interleucina 2 humana que se identifica por um anticorpo monoclonal murino, anti-Tac. A ligação desse antígeno com os anticorpos anti-Tac evita a proliferação das células T, as quais são normalmente estimuladas pela ligação com a interleucina-2.
T-dependent a., a. T-dependente; um a. que necessita das células T auxiliares, além das células B apropriadas. A maioria dos antígenos é T-dependente.
theta a. (thā'tä), a. teta; uma glicoproteína de superfície encontrada nos timócitos e nas células T maduras de camundongos e ratos.
thymus-independent a., a. timo-independente; um a. que não necessita da ativação da célula T auxiliar a fim de que as células B do hospedeiro sejam estimuladas. Os polímeros repetidos, como os polissacarídeos, são exemplos de a. T-independente.
tissue-specific a., a. tecido-específico. SIN organ-specific a.
Tj a., a. Tj. VER grupo sanguíneo P, no apêndice de Grupos Sanguíneos.
Tr^a a., a. Tr^a. VER grupos sanguíneos de baixa freqüência no apêndice de Grupos Sanguíneos.
transplantation a., a. do transplante. SIN histocompatibility a.
tumor a.'s, antígenos tumorais; (1) antígenos que podem estar freqüentemente associados a tumores ou que podem ser especificamente encontrados em células tumorais de mesma origem (tumor-específico); (2) os antígenos tumorais também podem estar associados à replicação e transformação por determinados vírus DNA tumorais, incluindo adenovírus e papovavírus. SIN neoantigens. VER TAMBÉM T a.'s.
tumor-associated a., a. associado ao tumor; antígenos que guardam uma elevada correlação com determinadas células tumorais. Eles não são usualmente encontrados ou são encontrados em menor extensão nas células normais.
tumor-specific transplantation a.'s (TSTA), a. de transplante tumor-específico; antígenos de superfície das células tumorais transformadas por DNA vírus, os quais provocam uma rejeição imune das células sem vírus quando transplantadas para um animal que foi imunizado contra o vírus específico transformador de células.
V a., a. V; a. viral que está intimamente associado à partícula do vírus, é de natureza protéica, possui múltiplas antigenicidades e é cepa-específico; o anticorpo contra esse a. é demonstrável como anticorpo protetor ou neutralizante, como as projeções de hemaglutinina na superfície do vírus influenza.
Vel a., a. Vel. VER grupos sanguíneos de alta freqüência no apêndice de Grupos Sanguíneos.
Ven a., a. Ven. VER grupos sanguíneos de baixa freqüência no apêndice de Grupos Sanguíneos.
Vi a., a. VI; "a. de virulência"; um a. capsular externo das enterobactérias que já se acreditou estar ligado à virulência aumentada.
Vw a., a. Vw. VER grupo sanguíneo MNSs no apêndice de Grupos Sanguíneos. SIN Gr a.
Webb a., a. Webb. VER grupos sanguíneos de baixa freqüência no apêndice de Grupos Sanguíneos.
Wr^a a., a. Wr^a. VER grupos sanguíneos de baixa freqüência no apêndice de Grupos Sanguíneos.
Wright a.'s (Wr^a), a. de Wright. VER grupos sanguíneos de baixa freqüência no apêndice de Grupos Sanguíneos.
Xg a., a. Xg. VER grupo sanguíneo Xg no apêndice de Grupos Sanguíneos.
Yt^a a., a. Yt^a. VER grupos sanguíneos de alta freqüência no apêndice de Grupos Sanguíneos

an·ti·ge·ne·mia (an'ti-jĕ-nē'mē-ă). Antigenemia; persistência do antígeno no sangue circulante; p.ex., antigenemia HB$_s$ (presença do antígeno de superfície da hepatite B no soro sanguíneo). [antígeno + G. *haima*, sangue]
an·ti·gen·ic (an-ti-jen'ik). Antigênico; que possui as propriedades de um antígeno (alérgeno). SIN allergenic, immunogenic.
an·ti·ge·nic·i·ty (an'ti-jĕ-nis'i-tē). Antigenicidade; o estado ou propriedade de ser antigênico. SIN immunogenicity.
anti·gen·ome. Antigenoma; o filamento de RNA positivo complementar sobre o qual é feito o genoma de filamento negativo dos vírus.
an·ti·gon·or·rhe·ic (an'tē-gon-ō-rē'ik). Antigonorreico; que cura a gonorréia.
an·ti·grav·i·ty (an-tē-grav'i-tē). Antigravidade. VER anti-G.
an·ti·HB$_e$. Anti-HB$_e$; anticorpo para o antígeno e (e *antigen*) da hepatite B (HB$_e$Ag).
an·ti·HB$_c$. Anti-HB$_c$; anticorpo contra o antígeno do cerne (core *antigen*) da hepatite B (HB$_c$Ag).
an·ti·HB$_s$. Anti-HB$_s$; anticorpo contra o antígeno de superfície (surface *antigen*) da hepatite B (HB$_s$Ag).
an·ti·he·lix (an-tē-hē'liks)[TA]. Antélice; uma crista elevada da cartilagem anterior e aproximadamente paralela à porção posterior da hélice do ouvido externo. SIN anthelix.
an·ti·hel·min·thic (an'tē-hel-min-th'ik). Anti-helmíntico. SIN anthelmintic (1).
an·ti·hem·ag·glu·ti·nin (an'tē-hē-mă-gloo'ti-nin, an'tē-hem-ă-). Anti-hemaglutinina; uma substância (inclusive anticorpo) que inibe ou evita a hemaglutinação.
an·ti·he·mo·ly·sin (an'tē-hē-mol'i-sin, an'tē-hem-ol'-). Anti-hemolisina; uma substância (inclusive anticorpo) que inibe ou evita os efeitos da hemolisina.
an·ti·he·mo·lyt·ic (an'tē-hē-mō-lit'ik, an'tē-hem-ō-). Anti-hemolítico; que impede a hemólise.
an·ti·hem·or·rhag·ic (an'tē-hem-ō-rāj'ik). Anti-hemorrágico; que interrompe a hemorragia. SIN hemostatic (2).
an·ti·his·ta·mines (an-tē-his'tă-mēnz). Anti-histaminas; medicamentos que possuem ação antagônica àquela da histamina sobre receptores H$_1$ ou H$_2$; a. do tipo H$_1$ são usados no tratamento de sintomas de alergia, enquanto os a. do tipo H$_2$ reduzem a acidez gástrica na doença ulcerosa e no refluxo gastroesofágico.
an·ti·his·ta·min·ic (an'tē-his-tă-min'ik). Anti-histamínico. **1.** Que tende a neutralizar ou antagonizar a ação da histamina ou inibir sua produção no corpo. **2.** Um agente que possui esse efeito pode ser utilizado para aliviar os sintomas de alergia ou hipersensibilidade.
an·ti·hor·mones (an-tē-hōr'mōnz). Anti-hormônios; substâncias demonstráveis no soro que inibem ou evitam os efeitos usuais de determinados hormônios, p.ex., anticorpos específicos.
an·ti·hy·drop·ic (an'tē-hī-drop'ik). Anti-hidrópico. **1.** Que alivia o edema. **2.** Um agente que mobiliza líquidos acumulados.
an·ti·hy·per·ten·sive (an'tē-hī-per-ten'siv). Anti-hipertensivo; indicando um medicamento ou modo de tratamento que reduz a pressão arterial de indivíduos hipertensos.
an·ti·hyp·not·ic (an'te-hip-not'ik). Anti-hipnótico. **1.** Que evita ou tende a evitar o sono. **2.** Um agente despertador, ou um antagonista do sono.
an·ti·hy·po·ten·sive (an'tē-hī'pō-ten'siv). Anti-hipotensivo; qualquer medida ou medicamento que tende a elevar a pressão arterial reduzida.
an·ti·ic·ter·ic (an'tē-ik-ter'ik). Antiictérico; termo raramente utilizado para a prevenção ou cura da icterícia.
an·ti·in·flam·ma·to·ry (an'tē-in-flam'ă-tō-rē). Antiinflamatório; que reduz a inflamação por agir sobre as respostas corporais, sem antagonizar diretamente o agente causal; indica agentes como glicocorticóides e ácido acetilsalicílico (AAS).
an·ti·in·su·lin. Antiinsulina; um fator, geralmente um anticorpo, que antagoniza a ação da insulina.
an·ti·ke·to·gen·e·sis (an'tē-kē-tō-jen'ē-sis). Anticetogênese; prevenção ou redução de cetose por produção diminuída ou por utilização aumentada dos corpos cetônicos.

an·ti·ke·to·gen·ic (an′tē - kē - tō - jen′ik). Anticetogênico; que inibe a formação de corpos cetônicos ou acelera sua utilização.

an·ti·leu·koc·i·din (an′tē - loo - kos′i - din, loo - kō - sī′din). Antileucocidina. **1.** Uma substância que inibe ou evita os efeitos da leucocidina. **2.** Um anticorpo específico contra a leucocidina.

an·ti·leu·ko·tox·in (an′tē - loo - kō - tok′sin). Antileucotoxina; uma substância (inclusive anticorpos) que inibe ou evita os efeitos da leucocitoxina; freqüentemente considerado sinônimo de antileucocidina.

an·ti·leu·ko·tri·ene (an - tē - loo - ko - trī - ēn). Antileucotrieno; um medicamento que evita ou alivia a broncoconstrição na asma por bloquear a produção ou ação dos leucotrienos de ocorrência natural; também pode ser útil na psoríase.

Em 1940, um mediador de ocorrência natural da broncoconstrição asmática, diferente da histamina e com ação mais prolongada, foi isolado e nomeado substância de reação lenta da anafilaxia (SRS-A). A análise mostrou que esse agente consistia em três leucotrienos cisteinil, chamados C4, D4 e E4. Este último leucotrieno, do qual os outros são precursores, é o mais potente. Os leucotrienos são eicosanóides derivados do ácido araquidônico, que é encontrado nas membranas celulares. Constatou que os leucotrienos cisteinil, que são produzidos pelos mastócitos broncopulmonares, eosinófilos e, provavelmente, macrófagos alveolares, medeiam a broncoconstrição induzida por exercício, hiperventilação em ar frio, ácido acetilsalicílico e alérgenos inalados; eles agem através da estimulação de um receptor específico, conhecido como receptor de leucotrieno cisteinil do tipo 1 (CysLT1). Os antileucotrienos com utilidade clínica na asma compreendem o zileuton, que inibe a 5-lipoxigenase, uma enzima crítica na biossíntese dos leucotrienos, e os antagonistas dos receptores de leucotrieno (cinalukast, montelukast, zafirlukast e outros). Os antileucotrienos revertem menos a broncoconstrição na asma que os agonistas β_2-adrenérgicos, mas seus efeitos são aditivos aos destes últimos agentes. Na asma crônica, os antileucotrienos melhoram o fluxo máximo e a VEF_1 e reduzem a freqüência e a gravidade das crises asmáticas agudas, a necessidade de β_2-agonistas e a necessidade de corticosteróides. Eles são particularmente efetivos na profilaxia da asma induzida por exercício e ácido acetilsalicílico; em contrapartida, muitas pessoas com asma alérgica mostram pouca ou nenhuma resposta. Os antileucotrienos não estão indicados no tratamento de uma crise asmática aguda nem na asma branda e intermitente controlada de modo adequado com o uso ocasional de β_2-agonistas inalados. Eles não foram recomendados como substituto para o corticosteróide inalado na profilaxia da asma. Um antagonista do receptor de leucotrieno LTB4 nas células cutâneas mostrou-se promissor no tratamento da psoríase. Os antileucotrienos são administrados por via oral ou por inalação. Tanto o início como o desaparecimento dos efeitos clínicos são graduais. Os efeitos colaterais são mínimos, mas as interações medicamentosas podem ocorrer por causa da interferência com as enzimas citocromo P-450. Raras elevações transitórias da aminotransferase hepática foram relatadas com alguns agentes.

an·ti·lew·is·ite (an - tē - loo′i - sīt). Dimercaprol. SIN dimercaprol.
an·ti·lip·o·tro·pic (an - tē - lip - ō - trop′ik). Antilipotrópico; pertinente às substâncias que deprimem a síntese de colina (p.ex., por competir pelos grupamentos metil) e, assim, estimulam a esteatose hepática de origem dietética.
an·ti·lith·ic (an - tē - lith′ik). Antilítico. **1.** Que evita a formação de cálculos ou promove sua dissolução. **2.** Um agente com essa ação. SIN anticalculous. [anti- + G. *lithos*, pedra]
an·ti·lo·bi·um (an - tē - lō′bē - ŭm). Trago. SIN tragus (1). [L. de G. *antilobion*.]
an·ti·lu·te·o·gen·ic (an′tē - loo - tē - ō - jen′ik). Antiluteogênico; que inibe o crescimento ou acelera a involução do corpo lúteo.
an·ti·ly·sin (an - tē - lī′sin). Antilisina; um anticorpo que inibe ou evita os efeitos da lisina.
an·ti·ma·lar·i·al (an′tē - ma - lā′rē - ăl). Antimalárico. **1.** Que evita ou cura a malária. **2.** Um agente farmacológico que inibe ou destrói os parasitas da malária.
an·ti·mere (an′ti - mēr). Antímero. **1.** Um segmento do corpo de um animal formado por planos que cortam o eixo do corpo em ângulos retos. **2.** Uma das partes simétricas de um organismo bilateral. **3.** A metade direita ou esquerda do corpo. [anti- + G. *meros*, uma parte]
an·ti·mes·en·ter·ic (an′tē - mez′en - ter′ik). Antimesentérico; pertinente à parte do intestino que se situa em ponto oposto à fixação do mesentério.
an·ti·me·tab·o·lite (an′tē - me - tab′ō - līt). Antimetabólito; uma substância que compete com, substitui ou antagoniza um determinado metabólito; p.ex., a etionina é um a. da metionina.
an·ti·me·tro·pia (an′tē - me - trō′pē - ă). Antimetropia; uma forma de anisometropia em que um olho é míope e o outro hipermétrope. [anti- + G. *metron*, medida, + *ōps*, olho]

an·ti·mi·cro·bi·al (an′tē - mī - krō′bē - ăl). Antimicrobiano; que tende a destruir os micróbios, evitar sua multiplicação ou crescimento, ou evitar sua ação patogênica.
an·ti·mi·tot·ic (an′tē - mī - tot′ik). Antimitótico. **1.** Que tem uma ação de parada da mitose. **2.** Um medicamento com esse efeito; p.ex., um antagonista do ácido fólico que é utilizado na leucemia para inibir a multiplicação dos leucócitos.
an·ti·mon·gol·oid (an - tē - mon′gō - loyd). Antimongolóide; a condição em que a porção lateral da fissura palpebral é mais baixa que a porção medial.
an·ti·mo·nid (an - tē - mō′nid). Antimonídeo; um composto químico que contém antimônio em união com um elemento mais positivo; p.ex., a. sódico, Na_3Sb.
an·ti·mo·nous ox·ide (an - ti - mō′nŭs). Óxido de antimônio. SIN antimony trioxide.
an·ti·mo·ny (Sb) (an′ - ti - mō - nē). Antimônio (Sb); um elemento metálico, número atômico 51, peso atômico 121,757, valências 0, -3, $+3$, $+5$; usado em ligas; tóxico e irritante para a pele e mucosas. SIN stibium. [G. *anti* + *monos*, não encontrado sozinho]
a. chloride, cloreto de a. SIN a. trichloride.
a. dimercaptosuccinate, dimercaptosuccinato de a.; um antiparasitário efetivo contra *Schistosoma mansoni* e *S. haematobium*. SIN stibocaptate.
a. oxide, óxido de a.; SIN a. trioxide.
a. potassium tartrate, tartarato potássico de a.; um composto usado como expectorante e no tratamento da esquistossomíase japonesa, embora seja extremamente tóxico e precise ser administrado muito lentamente por via intravenosa; as manifestações tóxicas comuns são flebite, taquicardia e hipotensão. Mortes súbitas já foram descritas, principalmente por colapso circulatório. SIN potassium antimonyltartrate, tartar emetic, tartrated a.
a. sodium gluconate, gluconato sódico de a. SIN stibogluconate *sodium* (1).
a. sodium tartrate, tartarato sódico de a. usado no tratamento da esquistossomíase e como emético. SIN sodium antimonyl tartrate.
a. sodium thioglycollate, tioglicolato sódico de a.; um composto de trióxido de a. e ácido tioglicólico usado para parasitas tropicais.
tartrated a., tartarato de a. SIN a. potassium tartrate.
a. thioglycollamide, tioglicolamida de a.; a triamida do ácido tioglicólico de a.; usado no tratamento da tripanossomíase, calazar e filaríase.
a. trichloride, tricloreto de a.; combina-se com a vitamina A para formar um composto azulado e com β-caroteno para formar um esverdeado, como um método de pesquisa dessas substâncias; também usado externamente como cáustico. SIN a. chloride.
a. trioxide, trióxido de a.; usado tecnicamente em tintas e materiais à prova de fogo; também usado originalmente como expectorante e emético. SIN antimonous oxide, a. oxide, flowers of antimony.
an·ti·mo·nyl (an - tim′ō - nil). Antimonil; o radical univalente, SbO–, do antimônio.
an·ti·mus·ca·rin·ic (an′tē - mŭs′kă - rin′ik). Antimuscarínico; que inibe ou evita as ações de agentes muscarínicos e de agentes muscarina-símiles, ou os efeitos da estimulação parassimpática na junção neuroefetora (p.ex., atropina).
an·ti·mu·ta·gen (an - tē - mū′tă - jen). Antimutágeno; um fator que reduz, ou interfere com, as ações mutagênicas ou os efeitos de uma substância.
an·ti·mu·ta·gen·ic (an′tē - mū - tă - jen′ik). Antimutagênico; pertinente a ou característico de um antimutágeno.
an·ti·my·as·then·ic (an′tē - mī′as - then′ik). Antimiastênico; que tende no sentido da correção dos sintomas da miastenia grave, p.ex., como na ação da neostigmina.
an·ti·my·cot·ic (an′ - tē - mī - kot′ik). Antimicótico; antagonista dos fungos. SIN antifungal. [anti- + G. *mykēs*, fungo]
an·ti·nau·se·ant (an - tē - naw′sē - ant). Antinauseante; que evita a náusea.
an·ti·ne·o·plas·tic (an′tē - nē - ō - plas′tik). Antineoplásico; que impede o desenvolvimento, a maturação ou a disseminação de células neoplásicas.
an·ti·neo·plas·tons (an′tē - nē - ō - plas′ - tonz). Misturas de várias substâncias químicas, como aminoácidos e peptídeos, com suporte teórico como auxílios da defesa natural contra o câncer e várias outras doenças.
an·ti·neu·ro·tox·in (an - tē - noo - rō - tok′sin). Antineurotoxina; um anticorpo para uma neurotoxina.
an·tin·i·ad (an - tin′ē - ad). Antinial; no sentido do antínio.
an·tin·i·al (an - tin′ē - ăl). Antinial; relativo ao antínio.
an·tin·i·on (an - tin′ē - on). Antínio; o espaço entre as sobrancelhas; o ponto do crânio oposto ao ínio. VER TAMBÉM glabella. [anti- + G. *inion*, nuca]
an·tin·o·my (an - tin′ō - mē). Antinomia; uma contradição entre dois princípios, cada qual sendo considerado verdadeiro. [anti- + G. *nomos*, lei]
an·ti·nu·cle·ar (an - tē - noo′klē - er). Antinuclear; que possui afinidade ou que reage com o núcleo da célula.
an·ti·o·don·tal·gic (an′tē - ō - don - tăl - jik). Antiodontálgico. **1.** Que alivia a dor de dentes. **2.** Um remédio para dor de dentes. [anti- + G. *odous*, dente, + *algos*, dor]
antioncogene. Antioncogene. SIN tumor supressor *gene*.

an·ti·ox·i·dant (an - tē - oks′ĭ - dant). Antioxidante; um agente que inibe a oxidação; uma de numerosas substâncias químicas, incluindo determinados produtos corporais naturais e nutrientes, que conseguem neutralizar o efeito oxidante de radicais livres e de outras substâncias.

Os radicais livres, formados no curso do metabolismo e da respiração celular normais, e de forma mais abundante sob a influência de determinadas substâncias químicas ambientais e luz solar, foram implicados na geração de vários tipos de lesão tecidual, principalmente aquelas envolvidas na aterosclerose, no processo do envelhecimento e no desenvolvimento do câncer. Um radical livre é qualquer átomo ou molécula que possua 1 ou mais elétrons não-pareados e, portanto, é muito reativo, procurando adquirir elétrons de outras substâncias. Os radicais livres são normalmente depurados dos tecidos pelas enzimas antioxidantes superóxido dismutase e glutationa peroxidase. Acredita-se também que a ubidecarenona (coenzima Q10) atue como um antioxidante em reações da respiração mitocondrial. Além disso, inúmeras substâncias nutrientes, vitaminas e minerais comprovadamente contribuem para as funções antioxidantes, geralmente por servir como co-fatores ou coenzimas. Estas incluem selênio, β-caroteno e as vitaminas C e E. Postulou-se que um desequilíbrio entre a produção de radicais livres e os processos antioxidantes naturais seria um importante fator causal no envelhecimento e em muitos distúrbios crônicos e degenerativos, tendo alguns especulado que os nutrientes antioxidantes participariam na prevenção da doença. A oxidação do LDL-colesterol realmente parece ser responsável pela formação da célula espumosa na gênese das placas ateroscleróticas. Além disso, já foi constatado que os radicais livres lesionam o DNA de várias formas, podendo culminar em alteração maligna. Todavia, a oxidação também ocorre em muitos processos benéficos, incluindo a quimiotaxia das células com funções imunológicas, fagocitose, mecanismos de coagulação e apoptose. Ademais, os antioxidantes não exercem seus efeitos apenas de uma maneira, mas podem agir durante o início ou a propagação das reações em vários pontos intracelulares e extracelulares e, em algumas circunstâncias, podem ser pró-oxidantes. As alegações de que as vitaminas e outros nutrientes, quando tomados em doses maciças, conseguem evitar o infarto do miocárdio ou o câncer ou retardar o envelhecimento, não se baseiam em evidências científicas. Embora um consumo alto de nutrientes antioxidantes (fontes alimentares) pareça oferecer algumas vantagens para a saúde, não há, no momento, evidências inequívocas de que algum nutriente antioxidante, quando ingerido além das cotas dietéticas normais, tenha valor na prevenção ou no tratamento da doença cardiovascular, câncer ou qualquer outro processo anormal, exceto aquele que possa estar associado a deficiência nutricional ou vitamínica franca. Na verdade, embora os nutrientes antioxidantes de ocorrência natural sejam componentes vitais da dieta, eles podem provocar efeitos adversos quando grandes quantidades são ingeridas por períodos prolongados. Um estudo controlado de β-caroteno e retinol não apenas falhou em mostrar qualquer benefício, como foi interrompido quando as estatísticas mostraram grandes aumentos no risco de morte por câncer de pulmão e doença cardiovascular.

an·ti·pain (an′tē - pā - in). Um peptídeo que inibe as enzimas proteolíticas papaína, tripsina e plasmina. [anti- + pa*pain*]

an·ti·par·al·lel (an - tē - par′ă - lel). Antiparalelo; que indica moléculas que estão em paralelo, mas que possuem polaridade direcional oposta; p.ex., os dois filamentos de uma dupla hélice de ADN.

an·ti·par·a·sit·ic (an′tē - par - ă - sit′ik). Antiparasitário; destrutivo para os parasitas.

an·ti·pe·dic·u·lar (an′tē - pe - dik - ū - lăr). Pediculicida; destrutivo para o piolho.

an·ti·pe·dic·u·lot·ic (an′tē - pe - dik - ū - lot′ik). Antipediculótico; efetivo no tratamento da pediculose, indicando especialmente um agente desse tipo.

an·ti·pe·ri·od·ic (an′tē - pēr - ē - od′ik). Antiperiódico; que evita a recorrência regular de uma doença (p.ex., malária) ou de um sintoma.

an·ti·per·i·stal·sis (an′tē - per - i - stal′sis). Antiperistalse. SIN reversed *peristalsis*.

an·ti·per·i·stal·tic (an′tē - per - i - stal′tik). Antiperistáltico. **1.** Relativo à antiperistalse. **2.** Que compromete ou interrompe a peristalse.

an·ti·per·spi·rant (an′tē - per′spi - rant). Antiperspirante. **1.** Que tem ação inibitória sobre a secreção do suor. **2.** Um agente que possui essa ação (p.ex., cloreto de alumínio). SIN anhydrotic (2).

an·ti·phag·o·cyt·ic (an′tē - fag - ō - sit′ik). Antifagocítico; que compromete ou evita a ação dos fagócitos.

an·ti·phlo·gis·tic (an′tē - flō - jis′tik). Antiflogístico. **1.** Termo antigo que indica a prevenção ou o alívio da inflamação. **2.** Um agente que reduz a inflamação. SIN antipyrotic (1). [anti- + G. *phogistos*, inflamado]

an·ti·pho·bic (an - tē - fō′bik). Antifóbico; um mecanismo ou medicamento destinado a controlar as fobias.

an·ti·plas·min (an - tē - plaz′min). Antiplasmina; uma substância que inibe ou evita os efeitos da plasmina; encontrada no plasma e em alguns tecidos, especialmente no baço e fígado. SIN antifibrinolysin.

an·ti·plate·let (an - tē - plāt′let). Antiplaquetário; uma substância que manifesta ação lítica ou aglutinante sobre as plaquetas sanguíneas, inibindo ou destruindo, assim, os efeitos destas.

an·ti·pneu·mo·coc·cic (an′tē - noo - mō - kok′sik). Antipneumocócico; destrutivo para, ou que reprime o crescimento de, pneumococos (p.ex., penicilina).

an·tip·o·dal (an - tip′ō - dăl). Antípoda; que indica posições opostas; posicionado em lados opostos de uma célula ou de outro corpo.

an·ti·pode (an′ti - pōd). Antípoda; que é diametralmente oposto. [G. *antipous*, com os pés opostos]

  optic a., a. óptico. SIN enantiomer.

an·ti·port (an′tē - pōrt). Contratransporte; transporte acoplado de duas moléculas ou íons diferentes através de uma membrana em direções opostas por um mecanismo transportador comum (contratransportador). Cf. symport, uniport. [anti- + L. *porto*, carregar]

an·ti·por·ter (an′tē - pōr - ter). Contratransportador; uma proteína responsável por mediar o transporte de duas moléculas ou íons diferentes ao mesmo tempo, em direções opostas, através de uma membrana.

an·ti·pre·cip·i·tin (an′tē - prē - sip′ĭ - tin). Antiprecipitina; um anticorpo específico que inibe ou evita os efeitos de uma precipitina.

an·ti·pro·ges·tin (an′tē - prō - jes′tin). Antiprogestina; uma substância que inibe a formação de progesterona, que interfere com seu transporte ou estabilidade no sangue, ou que reduz sua captação pelos órgãos-alvo ou seus efeitos sobre ele (p.ex., RU-486).

an·ti·pro·throm·bin (an′tē - prō - throm′bin). Antiprotrombina; um anticoagulante que inibe ou evita a conversão da protrombina em trombina; os exemplos são a heparina, que existe em diversos tecidos (especialmente no fígado), e a dicumarina, que é isolada a partir do meliloto (trevo-cheiroso) parcialmente decomposto.

an·ti·pru·rit·ic (an′tē - proo - rit′ik). Antiprurítico, antipruriginoso. **1.** Que evita ou alivia o prurido. **2.** Um agente que alivia o prurido.

an·ti·psy·chot·ic (an′tē - sī - kot′ik). Antipsicótico. **1.** SIN antipsychotic *agent*. **2.** Que indica as ações de um agente desse tipo (p.ex., clorpromazina).

an·ti·pu·rine (an′tē - pūr′ēn). Antipurina; um análogo das purinas e nucleotídeos da purina que atua como antimetabólito.

an·ti·py·o·gen·ic (an′tē - pī - ō - jen′ik). Antipiogênico; que evita a supuração. [anti- + G. *pyos*, pus, + *-gen*, produção]

an·ti·py·re·sis (an′tē - pī - rē′sis). Antipirese; tratamento sintomático da febre em vez da doença subjacente.

an·ti·py·ret·ic (an′tē - pī - ret′ik). Antipirético. **1.** Que reduz a febre. SIN antifebrile, febrifugal. **2.** Um agente que diminui a febre (p.ex., acetaminofeno, ácido acetilsalicílico). SIN febrifuge. [anti- + G. *pyretos*, febre]

an·ti·py·rim·i·dine (an′tē - pir - im′ĭ - dēn). Antipirimidina; um análogo das pirimidinas e dos nucleotídeos da pirimidina que atua como antimetabólito.

an·ti·py·rine (an - tē - pī′rin, - pī′ren). Antipirina; analgésico e antipirético obsoleto.

  a. acetylsalicylate, acetilsalicilato de antipirina; um composto de a. e ácido acetilsalicílico; um anti-reumático e analgésico.

  a. salicylacetate, salicilacetato de a.; analgésico, anti-reumático e antipirético.

  a. salicylate, salicilato de a.; analgésico e antipirético; empregado originalmente na dismenorréia, gripe (*influenza*) e rinite aguda nos estágios iniciais.

an·ti·py·rot·ic (an′tē - pī - rot′ik). Antipirótico. **1.** Antiflogístico. SIN antiphlogistic. **2.** Que alivia a dor e promove a cura das queimaduras superficiais. **3.** Uma aplicação tópica para queimaduras. [anti- + G. *pyrotikos*, queimadura, inflamação]

an·ti·ra·chit·ic (an′tē - ră - kit′ik). Anti-raquítico; que promove a cura do raquitismo ou evita seu desenvolvimento (p.ex., preparações de vitamina D).

an·ti·rheu·mat·ic (an′tē - roo - mat′ik). Anti-reumático. **1.** Indica um agente que suprime as manifestações da doença reumática; usualmente aplicado aos agentes antiinflamatórios ou agentes que são capazes de retardar a progressão do processo patológico básico na artrite inflamatória. **2.** Um agente que possui essas propriedades (p.ex., compostos de ouro).

an·ti·ri·cin (an - tē - rī′sin). Anti-ricina; um anticorpo ou antitoxina que inibe ou evita os efeitos da ricina.

an·ti·ru·mi·nant (an - tē - roo′mi - nănt). Anti-ruminante; indica um método para 1) controlar a regurgitação do alimento ou 2) interromper uma tendência compulsiva do pensamento. [anti- + L. *rumino*, ruminar, de *rumen*, garganta]

an·ti-S. Anti-S. VER grupo sanguíneo MNS no apêndice de Grupos Sanguíneos.

an·ti·scor·bu·tic (an′tē - skōr - bū′tik). Antiescorbútico. **1.** Que evita ou cura o escorbuto. **2.** Um tratamento para o escorbuto (p.ex., vitamina C).

an·ti·seb·or·rhe·ic (an′tē - seb - ō - rē′ik). Anti-seborreico. **1.** Que evita ou alivia a secreção excessiva de sebo; que evita ou alivia a dermatite seborreica. **2.** Um agente com essas ações.

an·ti·se·cre·to·ry (an'tē - sē - krē'tō - rī). Anti-secretório; inibidor da secreção; diz-se de determinados medicamentos que reduzem ou suprimem a secreção gástrica (p.ex., ranitidina, omeprazol).

an·ti·sense (an'tē - sens). Anti-sentido. VER antisense DNA, antisense RNA.

an·ti·sep·sis (an - tē - sep'sis). Anti-sepsia; prevenção da infecção por inibir o crescimento dos agentes infecciosos. VER TAMBÉM disinfection. [anti- + G. *sēpsis*, putrefação]

an·ti·sep·tic (an - tē - sep'tik). Anti-séptico. **1.** Relativo à anti-sepsia. **2.** Um agente ou substância capaz de efetuar a anti-sepsia.

an·ti·se·rum (an - tē - sē'rŭm). Anti-soro; soro que contém anticorpo demonstrável ou anticorpos específicos contra um (a. monovalente ou específico) ou mais (a. polivalente) antígenos; pode ser preparado a partir do sangue de animais inoculados com um material antigênico ou a partir do sangue de animais e pessoas que foram estimulados por contato natural com um antígeno (como naqueles que se recuperam de uma crise de doença). SIN immune serum.
blood group a.'s, a. de grupo sanguíneo. VER apêndice de Grupos Sanguíneos.
heterologous a., a. heterólogo; um a. que reage com (p.ex., aglutina) determinados microrganismos ou outros complexos de antígenos, ainda que o a. tenha sido produzido por meio de estimulação com um microrganismo ou material antigênico diferente. VER TAMBÉM homologous a.
homologous a., a. homólogo; um a. em que existe correspondência completa entre o teor de anticorpos e o material antigênico utilizado para produzir o a.
monovalent a., a. monovalente. VER antiserum.
nerve growth factor a., a. contra o fator de crescimento nervoso; um a. contendo anticorpos contra o fator de crescimento nervoso; quando injetado em animais recém-nascidos, a maioria das células ganglionares simpáticas são destruídas para sempre, resultando em hipoinervação dos tecidos periféricos. SIN NGF a.
NGF a., a. NGF. SIN nerve growth factor a.
polyvalent a., a. polivalente. VER antiserum.
specific a., a. específico. VER antiserum.

an·ti·shock gar·ment. Roupa antichoque. VER military antishock trousers, pneumatic antishock *garment.*

an·ti·si·al·a·gogue (an - tē - sī - al'ă - gog). Anti-sialagogo; um agente que diminui ou interrompe o fluxo da saliva (p.ex., atropina). [anti- + G. *sialon*, saliva, + *agōgos*, que conduz]

an·ti·si·der·ic (an - tē - sid'er - ik). Anti-siderótico; que se contrapõe à ação fisiológica do ferro, provavelmente por quelação ou precipitação. [anti- + G. *sideros*, ferro]

an·ti·so·cial (an - tē - sō'shŭl). Anti-social; oposto aos direitos dos indivíduos ou às normas legais da sociedade; p.ex., a personalidade anti-social, o psicopata. Cf. asocial.

an·ti·spas·mod·ic (an'tē - spaz - mod'ik). Antiespasmódico. **1.** Que evita ou alivia os espasmos musculares (cãibras). **2.** Um agente que termina o espasmo.

an·ti·staph·y·lo·coc·cic (an'tē - staf'i - lō - kok'sik). Antiestafilocócico; antagonista dos estafilococos ou de suas toxinas.

an·ti·staph·y·lol·y·sin (an'tē - staf - i - lol'i - sin). Antiestafilolisina; uma substância que antagoniza ou neutraliza a ação da estafilolisina.

an·ti·ste·ap·sin (an - tē - ap'sin). Antiesteapsina; anticorpo que se contrapõe à ação da triacilglicerol lipase (esteapsina).

an·ti·strep·to·coc·cic (an'tē - strep - tō - kok'sik). Antiestreptocócico; destrutivo para os estreptococos ou antagonista de suas toxinas.

an·ti·strep·to·ki·nase (an'tē - strep - tō - kī'nāz). Antiestreptocinase; um anticorpo que inibe ou evita a dissolução de fibrina pela estreptocinase.

an·ti·strep·tol·y·sin (an'tē - strep - tol'i - sin). Antiestreptolisina; um anticorpo que inibe ou evita os efeitos da estreptolisina O elaborada por estreptococos do grupo A; a concentração de a. no soro está freqüentemente aumentada durante e após a doença estreptocócica, podendo os títulos comparativos ser valiosos para fins diagnósticos e prognósticos.

an·ti·tac (an' - tē - tak). Anticorpo monoclonal que reconhece a cadeia alfa do receptor de IL-2.

anti·ter·min·a·tion. Antiterminal; um estado da RNA polimerase bacteriana onde ela é resistente a sinais de pausa, parada ou término. VER TAMBÉM hesitant, overdrive.

an·ti·te·tan·ic (an'tē - te - tan'ik). Antitetânico; que evita ou alivia a contração muscular.

an·ti·the·nar (an - tē - thē'nar). Antitenar. SIN hypothenar *eminence.*

an·ti·throm·bin (an - tē - throm'bin). Antitrombina; qualquer substância que iniba ou evite os efeitos da trombina, de tal modo que o sangue não coagula. A deficiência de a. resulta em comprometimento da inibição dos fatores da coagulação IIa, IXa e Xa no plasma, provocando trombose recorrente.
a. III, a. III; um processo da α_2-globulina plasmática que inibe a trombina e que possui atividades anticoagulantes. A deficiência [MIM*107300] é comumente herdada como um traço autossômico dominante, causado por mutação no gene da antitrombina III (AT_3) ou no cromossoma 1q; esse é um dos poucos distúrbios mendelianos conhecidos, a partir do qual ocorre doença trombótica.
normal a., a. normal; uma a. de ocorrência natural no sangue e em determinados tecidos sob condições normais em contraste com os estados anormais ou da a. originária de outras fontes.

an·ti·thy·roid (an - tē - thī'royd). Antitireóideo; relativo a um agente que suprime a função tireoidiana (p.ex., propiltiouracil).

an·ti·ton·ic (an - tē - ton'ik). Antitônico; que diminui o tônus muscular ou vascular.

an·ti·tox·ic (an - tē - tok'sik). Antitóxico; que neutraliza a ação de um veneno; especificamente, relativo a uma antitoxina. VER TAMBÉM antidotal.

an·ti·tox·i·gen (an - tē - toks'i - jen). Antitoxígeno. SIN antitoxinogen.

an·ti·tox·in (an - tē - tok'sin). Antitoxina; anticorpo formado em resposta a substâncias venenosas antigênicas de origem biológica, como as exotoxinas bacterianas (p.ex., aquelas elaboradas por *Clostridium tetani* ou *Corynebacterium diphtheriae*), fitotoxinas e zootoxinas; em uso geral, a. refere-se ao soro total ou à fração globulina do soro, de pessoas ou animais (geralmente cavalos) imunizados por injeções do toxóide específico. A a. neutraliza os efeitos farmacológicos de sua toxina específica *in vitro* e também *in vivo*, quando a toxina ainda não está fixada às células teciduais. [anti- + G. *toxikon*, veneno]
bivalent gas gangrene a., a. bivalente da gangrena gasosa; a. específica para as toxinas do *Clostridium perfringens* e *C. septicum.*
bothropic a., a. botrópica; a. específica para o veneno de víboras do gênero *Bothrops* (*Bothrophora*) da família Crotalidae. SIN Bothrops a.
Bothrops a., a. botrópica. SIN bothropic a.
botulinum a., a. botulínica. SIN botulism a.
botulism a., a. botulínica; a. específica para uma toxina de uma ou outra cepa de *Clostridium botulinum.* SIN botulinum a.
bovine a., a. bovina; a. preparada a partir do gado, em vez de cavalos, usada no tratamento de pessoas que são sensíveis ao soro eqüino; o gado bovino é imunizado contra a toxina para a qual se deseja a a. específica.
Crotalus a., a. crotálica; a. específica para o veneno de cascavéis (espécies de *Crotalus*).
despeciated a., um soro antitóxico tratado de uma maneira apropriada para alterar a proteína espécie-específica, de modo que não seja provável que uma pessoa sensibilizada à proteína animal tenha uma reação grave quando a a. for administrada.
diphtheria a., a. diftérica; a. específica para a toxina de *Corynebacterium diphtheriae.*
dysentery a., a. disentérica; a. específica para a neurotoxina de *Shigella dysenteriae.*
gas gangrene a., a. da gangrena gasosa; a. específica para a toxina de uma ou mais espécies de *Clostridium* que provocam a gangrena gasosa e a toxemia associada, especialmente *C. perfringens, C. novyi, C. histolyticum*, sendo as preparações comercialmente disponíveis em geral polivalentes, isto é, contém a. para duas ou mais espécies. SIN pentavalent gas gangrene a.
normal a., a. normal; soro que é capaz de neutralizar uma quantidade equivalente de uma solução normal de toxina.
pentavalent gas gangrene a., a. pentavalente da gangrena gasosa. SIN gas gangrene a.
plant a., a. vegetal; a. específica para uma fitotoxina.
scarlet fever a., a. da escarlatina; a. específica para a toxina eritrogênica de determinadas cepas de estreptococos β-hemolíticos do grupo A.
staphylococcus a., a. estafilocócica; um soro contendo globulinas antitóxicas ou seus derivados que neutraliza especificamente as propriedades hemolíticas, necrotizantes cutâneas e letais da α-toxina do *Staphylococcus aureus.*
tetanus a., a. tetânica; a. específica para a toxina de *Clostridium tetani.*
tetanus and gas gangrene a.'s, a. da gangrena gasosa e tetânica; uma mistura de anticorpos obtida de animais imunizados contra as toxinas de *Clostridium tetani, C. perfringens* e *C. septicum.*
tetanus-perfringens a., a. do tétano e *C. perfringens*; uma a. preparada a partir de animais imunizados contra as toxinas do *Clostridium tetani* e *C. perfringens (C. welchii).*

an·ti·tox·in·o·gen (an'tē - tok'sin'ō - jen). Antitoxinogênio; qualquer antígeno que estimule a formação de antitoxina em um animal ou pessoa, isto é, uma toxina ou toxóide. SIN antitoxigen. [antitoxina + G. *-gen*, que produz]

an·ti·trag·i·cus (an'tē - traj'i - kŭs). Músculo antitrágico. VER antitragicus (*muscle*).

an·ti·tra·go·hel·i·cine (an'tē - trā'gō - hel'i - sēn). Fissura antitrago-helicina. VER antitragohelicine *fissure.*

an·ti·tra·gus (an - tē - trā'gŭs) [TA]. Antitrago; uma projeção da cartilagem da aurícula, por diante da cauda da hélice, exatamente acima do lóbulo e posterior ao trago, do qual é separada pela incisura intertrágica. [G. *anti-tragos*, a eminência do ouvido externo, de *anti*, oposto, + *tragos*, cabra, trago]

an·ti·trep·o·ne·mal (an'tē - trep - ō - nē'măl). Antitreponêmico. SIN treponemicidal.

an·ti·tris·mus (an - tē - triz'mŭs). Antitrismo; uma condição de espasmo muscular tônico que impede o fechamento.

an·ti·trope (an′ti - trōp). Antítropo; um órgão ou apêndice que forma um par simetricamente invertido com outro do mesmo tipo, p.ex., as pernas direita e esquerda de um vertebrado. [anti- + G. *tropē*, uma volta]

an·ti·tro·pic (an - tē - trō′pik). Antitrópico; similar, bilateralmente simétrico, mas em uma localização oposta (como em uma imagem especular), p.ex., o polegar direito em relação ao polegar esquerdo.

an·ti·tryp·sic (an - tē - trip′sik). Antitríptico. SIN antityptric.

an·ti·tryp·sin (an - tē - trip′sin). Antitripsina; uma substância que inibe ou evita a ação da tripsina.

α₁-a., α₁-antitripsina; uma glicoproteína que é o principal inibidor de protease do soro humano, é sintetizada no fígado e é geneticamente polimórfica devido à presença de 25 alelos; os indivíduos adequadamente homozigotos são deficientes em α₁-tripsina e estão predispostos ao enfisema pulmonar e cirrose hepática juvenil por causa de alterações nos componentes de aminoácido e ácido siálico da glicoproteína. A a. também inibe a trombina e a elastase. SIN α₁-trypsin inhibitor, human α₁-protease inhibitor.

an·ti·tryp·tic (an - tē - trip′tik). Antitríptico; que possui propriedades de antitripsina. SIN antitrypsic.

an·ti·tu·mor·i·gen·e·sis (an′tē - too - mōr - i - jen′e - sis). Antitumorigênese; inibição do desenvolvimento de uma neoplasia.

an·ti·tus·sive (an - tē - tŭs′iv). Antitussivo, antitussígeno. **1.** Que alivia a tosse. **2.** Um remédio para a tosse (p.ex., codeína). SIN antibechic. [anti- + L. *tussis*, tosse]

an·ti·ty·phoid (an - tē - tī′foyd). Antitifóide; que previne ou cura a febre tifóide.

an·ti·ve·nene (an - tē - vĕ - nēn′). Antiveneno. SIN antivenin.

an·ti·ve·ne·re·al (an′tē - ve - nē′rē - al). Antivenéreo; termo raramente empregado para aquilo que previne ou cura as doenças venéreas. SIN antaphroditic (2).

an·ti·ven·in (an - tē - ven′in). Antivenina; antitoxina específica para um veneno de animal ou inseto. SIN antivenene. [anti- + L. *venenum*, veneno]

an·ti·vi·ral (an - tē - vī′ral). Antiviral; que se opõe a um vírus; que interfere com sua replicação; que enfraquece ou abole sua ação (p.ex., zidovudina, aciclovir).

an·ti·vi·ta·min (an - tē - vī′tă - min). Antivitamina; uma substância que evita que uma vitamina exerça seus efeitos biológicos típicos. Muitas antivitaminas apresentam estruturas químicas semelhantes às das vitaminas (p.ex., piridoxina e sua a., desoxipiridoxina) e parecem funcionar como antagonistas competitivos; algumas antivitaminas têm efeitos adicionais, que não estão relacionados ao antagonismo da vitamina.

an·ti·viv·i·sec·tion (an′tē - viv - i - sek′shŭn). Antivivissecção; oposição ao uso de animais vivos em experiências. VER vivisection.

an·ti·xe·roph·thal·mic (an′tē - zē - rof - thal′mik). Antixeroftálmico; indica agentes (vitamina A e ácido retinóico) que inibem o ressecamento patológico da conjuntiva (xeroftalmia). [anti- G. *xēros*, seco, + *ophthalmos*, olho]

an·ti·xe·rot·ic (an′tē - zē - rot′ik). Antixerótico; que previne a xerose.

Anton, Gabriel, neuropsiquiatra alemão, 1858–1933. VER A. *syndrome*.

Antoni, Nils R., neurologista sueco, 1887–1968. VER A. type *neurilemoma*, type B *neurilemoma*.

an·tra (an′tră). Antros; plural de antrum.

an·tral (an′tral). Antral; relativo a um antro.

an·trec·to·my (an - trek′tō - mē). Antrectomia; remoção de parte das paredes do antro maxilar. Remoção do antro (metade distal) do estômago; freqüentemente combinada à excisão bilateral de porções dos troncos do nervo vago (vagotomia) no tratamento da úlcera péptica. A restauração da continuidade do trato alimentar pode ser feita por uma gastroduodenostomia (Billroth I) ou por uma gastrojejunostomia em alça (Billroth II). [antro + G. *ektomē*, incisão]

♻ **antro-.** Forma combinante que indica relação com qualquer antro; um antro. [L. *antrum*, de G. *antron*, uma caverna]

an·tro·na·sal (an - trō - nā′sal). Antronasal; relativo a um seio maxilar e à cavidade nasal correspondente.

an·tro·phose (an′trō - fōz). Antrofosia; sensação subjetiva de luz ou cor que se origina nos centros visuais do cérebro. VER TAMBÉM phosphene. [antro- + G. *phos*, luz]

an·tro·py·lo·ric (an′trō - pī - lōr′ik). Antropilórico; relacionado ao ou que afeta o antro pilórico.

an·tro·scope (an′trō - skōp). Antroscópio; um instrumento para auxiliar no exame visual de qualquer cavidade, principalmente do antro de Highmore (seio maxilar). [antro- + G. *skopeō*, visualizar]

an·tros·co·py (an - tros′cō - pē). Antroscopia; exame de qualquer cavidade, especialmente do antro de Highmore (seio maxilar), por meio de um antroscópio.

an·tros·to·my (an - tros′tō - mē). Antrostomia; formação de uma abertura permanente em qualquer antro (seio maxilar). [antro- + G. *stoma*, boca]

  intraoral a., a. intra-oral. SIN Caldwell-Luc *operation*.

an·trot·o·my (an - trot′ō - mē). Antrotomia; incisão através da parede de qualquer antro. [antro- + G. *tomē*, incisão]

an·tro·to·nia (an - trō - tō′nē - ă). Antrotonia; tônus das paredes musculares de um antro, como o do estômago.

an·tro·tym·pan·ic (an′trō - tim - pan′ik). Antrotimpânico; relativo ao antro da mastóide e à cavidade timpânica.

an·trum, gen. **an·tri,** pl. **an·tra** (an′trŭm, - trī, - tră) [TA]. **1.** Antro; qualquer cavidade quase fechada, principalmente aquela com paredes ósseas. **2.** Antro pilórico. SIN pyloric a. [L. do G. *antron*, uma caverna]

  a. au′ris, a. acústico externo. SIN external acoustic *meatus*.

  cardiac a., a. cárdico; uma dilatação que, ocasionalmente, ocorre na parte abdominal do esôfago. VER TAMBÉM abdominal *part* of esophagus. SIN . a. cardiacum, forestomach.

  a. cardi′acum, a. cárdico. SIN cardiac a.

  antra ethmoida′lia, células etmoidais. SIN ethmoid *cells,* em *cell*.

  follicular a., a. folicular; a cavidade de um folículo ovariano preenchida com líquido folicular.

  a. of Highmore, a. de Highmore, seio maxilar. SIN maxillary *sinus*.

  mastoid a. [TA], a. mastóideo; uma cavidade, na porção petrosa do osso temporal, que se comunica, posteriormente, com as células mastóideas e, anteriormente, com o recesso epitimpânico da orelha média por meio da abertura do a. mastóideo. SIN a. mastoideum [TA], tympanic a., Valsalva a.

  a. mastoid′eum [TA], a. mastóideo. SIN mastoid a.

  maxillary a., seio maxilar. SIN maxillary *sinus*.

  pyloric a. [TA], a. pilórico; a porção inicial da parte pilórica do estômago, que pode, temporariamente, ficar separada, de forma total ou parcial, do restante do estômago durante a digestão por contração peristáltica do "esfíncter" pré-pilórico; é, por vezes, demarcada da segunda parte da parte pilórica do estômago (canal pilórico) por um discreto sulco. SIN a. pyloricum [TA], antrum (2) [TA], lesser cul-de-sac.

  a. pylor′icum [TA], a. pilórico. SIN pyloric a.

  tympanic a., a. mastóideo. SIN mastoid a.

  Valsalva a., a. mastóideo. SIN mastoid a.

ANTU Abreviatura para α-naphthylthiourea (α-naftiltiouréia).

Antyllus, médico grego, *ca.* 150 d.C. VER A. *method*.

ANUG Abreviatura para acute necrotizing ulcerative *gingivitis* (gengivite ulcerativa necrotizante aguda).

an·u·lar (an′ū - lar). Anular; em forma de anel. SIN annular.

an·u·lus, pl. **an·u·li** (an′ū - lŭs, - lī) [TA]. Anel. SIN ring (1). [L.]

  a. abdomina′lis, a. inguinal profundo. SIN deep inguinal *ring*.

  a. cilia′ris, corpo ciliar. SIN ciliary *body*.

  a. conjuncti′vae [TA], a. da conjuntiva. SIN conjunctival *ring*.

  a. femora′lis [TA], a. femoral. SIN femoral *ring*.

  a. fibrocartilagin′eus membra′nae tympa′ni [TA], a. fibrocartilagíneo da membrana timpânica. SIN fibrocartilaginous *ring* of tympanic membrane.

  a. fibro′sus [TA], a. fibroso; **(1)** SIN (right and left) fibrous *rings* of heart, em *ring*; **(2)** SIN a. fibrosus of intervertebral disk.

  a. fibro′sus dexter/sinister cordis, a. fibroso direito/esquerdo do coração. SIN (right and left) fibrous *rings* of heart, em *ring*.

  a. fibro′sus dis′ci intervertebra′lis [TA], a. fibroso do disco intervertebral. SIN a. fibrosus of intervertebral disk.

  a. fibrosus of intervertebral disk [TA], a. fibroso do disco intervertebral; o anel de tecido fibrocartilagíneo e fibroso que forma a circunferência do disco intervertebral; circunda o núcleo pulposo, que está propenso a herniação quando o a. fibroso está comprometido. SIN a. fibrosus disci intervertebralis [TA], a. fibrosus (2) [TA], fibrous ring of intervertebral disk, fibrous ring (2).

  a. of fibrosus sheath, parte anular da bainha fibrosa dos dedos das mãos e dos pés. SIN anular *part* of fibrous digital sheath of digits of hand and foot.

  Haller a., a. de Haller, ínsula de Haller. SIN Haller *insula*.

  a. hemorrhoida′lis, a. hemorroidal. SIN hemorrhoidal *zone*.

  a. inguina′lis profun′dus [TA], a. inguinal profundo. SIN deep inguinal *ring*.

  a. inguina′lis superficia′lis, a. inguinal superficial. SIN superficial inguinal *ring*.

  a. ir′idis [TA], a. da íris. SIN *border* of iris.

  a. iridis major [TA], a. maior da íris. SIN outer *border* of iris.

  a. iridis minor [TA], a. menor da íris. SIN inner *border* of iris.

  a. lymphat′icus car′diae [TA], a. linfático cárdico. SIN lymph nodes around cardia of stomach, em *lymph node*.

  a. lymphoideus pharyngis [TA], a. linfático da faringe. SIN pharyngeal lymphatic *ring*.

  a. ova′lis, limbo da fossa oval. SIN *limbus* fossae ovalis.

  a. tendin′eus commu′nis, a. tendíneo comum do bulbo do olho. SIN common tendinous *ring* of extraocular muscles.

  a. tympan′icus, a. timpânico. SIN tympanic *ring*.

  a. umbilica′lis, a. umbilical. SIN umbilical *ring*.

  a. urethra′lis, esfíncter interno da uretra. SIN internal urethral *sphincter*.

  Vieussens a., a. de Vieussens, limbo da fossa oval. SIN *limbus* fossae ovalis.

  a. of Zinn, a. de Zinn, anel tendíneo comum do olho. SIN common tendinous *ring* of extraocular muscles.

an·u·ria (an - ū′rē - ă). Anúria; ausência de formação da urina.

an·u·ric (an - ūr′ik). Anúrico; relativo à anúria.

anus, gen. e pl. **ani** (ā′nŭs, - nī) [TA]. Ânus; a abertura inferior do trato digestivo, que se situa na fenda entre as nádegas, através da qual é expelido o material fecal. SIN anal orifice. [L.]

Bartholin a., abertura do aqueduto do mesencéfalo. SIN opening of aqueduct of midbrain.

a. cer'ebri, a. cerebral; termo obsoleto para a abertura do aqueduto do mesencéfalo (opening of aqueduct of midbrain).

imperforate a., a. imperfurado, atresia anal. SIN anal atresia.

a. vesica'lis, a. vesical; esvaziamento retal na bexiga.

vesicalis a. (ve-sī′kal-is).a. vesical; a. imperfurado com abertura do a. na bexiga.

vestibular a., vulvovaginal a., a. vestibular, a. vulvóvaginal; uma malformação congênita em que o a. é imperfurado, porém o reto se abre na vagina, exatamente acima da vulva.

an·vil. Bigorna. SIN incus.

anx·i·e·ty (ang-zī′e-tē).Ansiedade. 1. Medo, apreensão ou temor de perigo iminente e acompanhado por inquietação, tensão, taquicardia e dispnéia, não ligados a um estímulo claramente identificável. 2. Em psicologia experimental, um impulso ou estado motivacional aprendido e, depois disso, associado a indícios previamente neutros. [L. *anxietas*, de *anxius*, perturbado, de *ango*, comprimir, atormentar]

a. attack, crise de a.; um episódio agudo de ansiedade.

castration a., a. de castração. SIN castration complex.

free-floating a., a. de livre flutuação; em psicanálise, uma expectativa não-realista e infiltrante que não está ligada a um conceito claramente formulado ou a um objeto de medo; observada principalmente na neurose da a. e pode ser percebida em alguns casos de esquizofrenia latente.

noetic a., a. noética; em psicoterapia experimental, a. causada por confusão ou perda do significado na vida.

separation a., a. da separação; a apreensão ou medo de uma criança associado ao afastamento ou perda de um dos pais ou de outra pessoa significativa.

situation a., a. de situação; a. relacionada a problemas atuais da vida.

anx·i·o·lyt·ic (ang′zē-ō-lit′ik).Ansiolítico. 1. SIN antianxiety agent. 2. Indica as ações de um agente desse tipo (p.ex., diazepam). [ansiedade + G. *lysis*, uma dissolução ou afrouxamento]

AOC Abreviatura para anodal opening *contraction* (contração de abertura anódica).

Aon·cho·the·ca (ā-on-kō-the′ka).Um dos três gêneros de nematódeos trichuríedos, comumente referidos como *Capillaria*.

aor·ta, gen. e pl. **aor·tae** (ā-or′tă, ā-or′tē)[TA]. Aorta; uma grande artéria do tipo elástica, que é o principal tronco do sistema arterial sistêmico, originando-se da base do ventrículo esquerdo e terminando no lado esquerdo do corpo da quarta vértebra lombar ao se dividir para formar as artérias ilíacas comuns direita e esquerda. A a. é subdividida em: a. ascendente; arco aórtico; e a. descendente, a qual, por sua vez, é dividida em a. torácica e a. abdominal. SIN artéria aorta. [L. Mod. de G. *aortē*, de *aeirō*, levantar]

abdominal a. [TA], a. abdominal; a parte da a. descendente que supre as estruturas abaixo do diafragma. SIN pars abdominalis aortae [TA], a. abdominalis*, abdominal part of aorta.

a. abdomina'lis, a. abdominal; *termo oficial alternativo para abdominal a.

a. angus'ta, a. estreita; estreitamento congênito da a.

a. ascen'dens, a. ascendente; *termo oficial alternativo para ascending a.

ascending a. [TA], a. ascendente; a parte da a. antes do arco aórtico, de onde se originam as artérias coronárias. SIN pars ascendens aortae [TA], a. ascendens*, ascending part of aorta.

buckled a., pseudocoartação. SIN pseudocoarctation.

a. descen'dens, a. descendente; *termo oficial alternativo para descending a.

descending a. [TA], a. descendente; uma parte da a., subdividida em a. torácica e a. abdominal. SIN pars descendens aortae [TA], a. descendens*, descending part of aorta.

dynamic a., a. dinâmica; pulsações anormalmente acentuadas da a.

kinked a., pseudocoartação. SIN pseudocoarctation.

overriding a., a. acavalgada; a. congenitamente malposicionada, cuja origem se sobrepõe ao septo ventricular e, assim, recebe o sangue ejetado do ventrículo direito, bem como do esquerdo; é encontrada especialmente na tetralogia de Fallot.

primitive a., a. primitiva; os primórdios aórticos pareados nos embriões jovens.

pseudocoarctation of the a., pseudocoartação da aorta; uma rara anormalidade constritiva do arco da a. mas que não é uma coartação verdadeira, visto que não há invasão significativa da luz.

shaggy a., uma descrição coloquial, porém adequada, para a degeneração grave da aorta, cuja superfície é extremamente friável e provável causa de ateroembolia.

thoracic a. [TA], a. torácica; a parte da a. descendente que supre as estruturas até o diafragma. SIN pars thoracica aortae [TA], a. thoracica*, thoracic part of aorta.

a. thorac'ica, a. torácica; *termo oficial alternativo para thoracic a.

ventral aortas, aortas ventrais; os vasos pareados, ventrais à faringe, que originam os arcos aórticos.

aor·tal (ā-or′tăl).Aórtico. SIN aortic.

aor·tal·gia (ā-or-tal′jē-ă).Aortalgia; dor atribuída a aneurisma ou outras condições patológicas da aorta. [aorta + G. *algos*, dor]

aor·tarc·tia (ā-or-tark′shē-ă).Estenose da aorta. SIN aortostenosis. [aorta + L. *arcto*, corretamente *arto*, estreitar]

aor·tar·tia (ā-or-tar′shē-ă).Estenose da aorta. SIN aortostenosis.

aor·tec·ta·sis, aor·tec·ta·sia (ā-or-tek′tă-sis, -tek-tā′zē-ă).Aortectasia; dilatação da aorta. [aorta + G. *ektasis*, distensão]

aor·tec·to·my (ā-or-tek′tō-mē).Aortectomia; excisão de uma porção da aorta. [aorta + G *ektomē*, excisão]

aor·tic (ā-or′tik).Aórtico; relativo à aorta ou ao orifício aórtico do ventrículo esquerdo do coração. SIN aortal.

aor·tic cur·tain. Cortina aórtica; uma lâmina intertrigonal de tecido fibroso entre o ânulo aórtico e o folheto anterior da valva mitral.

aor·ti·co·re·nal (ā-or-ti-kō-rē′năl).Aortorrenal; relativo à aorta e ao rim, especificamente ao gânglio aortorrenal.

aor·ti·tis (ā-or-tī′tis).Aortite; inflamação da aorta.

giant cell a., a. de células gigantes; arterite de células gigantes envolvendo a aorta.

syphilitic a., a. sifilítica; uma manifestação comum da sífilis terciária, envolvendo a aorta torácica, onde a destruição do tecido elástico na camada média resulta em dilatação e formação de aneurisma.

aor·to·cor·o·nary (ā-or′tō-kōr′ō-nar-ē).Aortocoronário; relativo à aorta e às artérias coronárias.

aor·to·gram (ā-or′tō-gram).Aortograma; a imagem ou conjunto de imagens resultantes da aortografia.

aor·tog·ra·phy (ā-or-tog′ra-fē).Aortografia. 1. Imagens radiográficas da aorta e seus ramos, ou de uma parte da aorta, através da injeção de contraste. 2. Obtenção de imagens da aorta por ultra-som ou ressonância magnética. [aorta + G. *grapho*, escrever]

retrograde a., a. retrógrada; a. por injeção de contraste na aorta através de um de seus ramos, p.ex., artéria braquial, em uma direção contrária ao fluxo de sangue arterial normal.

translumbar a., a. translombar; método antigo de a. através da injeção na aorta abdominal por meio de uma agulha exatamente abaixo da décima segunda costela e a quatro dedos transversos à esquerda do processo espinhoso da vértebra.

aor·top·a·thy (ā-or-top′ă-thē).Aortopatia; doença que afeta a aorta. [aorta + G. *pathos*, doença]

aor·to·pex·y. Aortopexia; um procedimento cirúrgico usado para tratar a traqueomalacia ou a compressão traqueal.

aor·to·plas·ty (ā-or′tō-plas′tē).Aortoplastia; um procedimento para o reparo cirúrgico da aorta.

aor·top·to·sia, aor·top·to·sis (ā-or-top-tō′zē-ă, -top-tō′sis).Aortoptose; deslocamento da aorta abdominal para baixo na esplancnoptose. [aorta + G. *ptōsis*, uma queda]

aor·tor·rha·phy (ā-or-tōr′ă-fē). Aortorrafia; a sutura da aorta. [aorta + G. *rhaphē*, costura]

aor·to·scle·ro·sis (ā-or′tō-skler-ō′sis).Aortoesclerose; arteriosclerose da aorta.

aor·to·ste·no·sis (ā-or-tō-stē-nō′sis).Aortoestenose; estreitamento da aorta. SIN aortactia, aortartia. [aorta + G. *stenōsis*, estreitamento]

aor·tot·o·my (ā-or-tot′ō-mē).Aortotomia; incisão da aorta. [aorta + G. *tomē*, corte]

AP Abreviatura para *area* postrema (área postrema).

APA Abreviatura para antipernicious anemia *factor* (fator contra a anemia perniciosa).

apall·es·the·sia (ā-pal-es-thē′zē-ă).Apalestesia. SIN pallanesthesia. [G. *a*- priv. + *pallo*, tremor, sacudir + *aithēsis*, sensação]

apal·lic (ă-pal′ik). Apálico. SIN apallic state. [G. *a*- priv. + L. *pallium*, manto cerebral (córtex cerebral)]

apan·cre·at·ic (ā-pan-krē-at′ik).Apancreático; sem um pâncreas.

apar·a·lyt·ic (ā-par′ă-lit′ik). Aparalítico; sem paralisia; que não causa paralisia.

apar·a·thy·re·o·sis (ā-par-ă-thī′rē-ō-sis). Aparatireose; hipoparatireoidismo, principalmente aquele causado pela remoção das glândulas paratireóides. [G. *a*- priv. + paratireóide + *-osis*, condição]

apar·a·thy·roid·ism (ā-par-ă-thī′royd-izm). Aparatireoidismo; ausência congênita, deficiência ou remoção cirúrgica das glândulas paratireóides.

apa·reu·nia (ā-par-ū′nē-ă). Apareunia; ausência ou impossibilidade do coito. [G. *a*- priv. + *para*, junto de, + *eunē*, cama]

ap·a·thet·ic (ap-ă-thet′ik). Apático; que exibe apatia; indiferente.

ap·a·thism (ap′ă-thizm).Apatismo, apatia; lentidão da reação.

ap·a·thy (ap′ă-thē).Apatia; indiferença; ausência de interesse no ambiente. Freqüentemente um dos sinais mais precoces de doença cerebral. [G. *apatheia*, de *a*- priv. + *pathos*, sofrimento]

ap·a·tite (ap′ă-tīt). Apatita. 1. Nome genérico para uma classe de minerais com composições que são variantes da fórmula D_5T_3M, onde D é um cátion divalente, T é um íon composto tetraédrico trivalente e M é um ânion monovalente; as apatitas de fosfato de cálcio são importantes constituintes minerais de ossos e dentes. VER hydroxyapatite. **2.** $Ca_5(PO_4)_3(OH,F,Cl)$.

APC Acrônimo para *a*cetylsalicylic acid (ácido acetilsalicílico), *p*henacetin (fenacetina) e *c*affeine (cafeína) combinados como um antipirético e analgésico muito utilizado antigamente; antigen-presenting *cells* (células apresentadoras de antígeno), em *cell*.

A-P-C 1. Abreviatura para adenoidal-pharyngeal-conjunctival (adenóidea-faríngea-conjuntival). **2.** Célula apresentadora de antígeno.

apel·lous (a-pel′us). **1.** Sem pele. **2.** Sem prepúcio; circuncidado. [G. *a-* priv. + L. *pellis*, pele]

ap·en·ter·ic (ap-en-ter′ik). Termo antigo para abenteric. [G. *apo*, de + *enteron*, intestino]

apep·sin·ia (a-pep-sin′e-a). Apepsinia; termo raramente empregado para a falta de pepsina no suco gástrico.

ape·ri·od·ic (a-pēr-e-od′ik). Aperiódico; que não ocorre periodicamente.

aper·i·stal·sis (a′per-i-stal′sis). Aperistalse; ausência de peristalse.

aper·i·tive (a-per′i-tiv). Aperitivo; que estimula o apetite. [Fr. *apéritif*, de L. *aperio*, abrir]

Apert, Eugène, pediatra francês, 1868–1940. VER A. *syndrome*.

aper·to·gnath·ia (a-per-to-nath′e-a). Apertognatia; uma deformidade da mordida aberta, um tipo de má oclusão caracterizado por oclusão posterior prematura e ausência de oclusão anterior. SIN open bite (2). [L. *apertus*, aberto, + G. *gnathos*, mandíbula]

ap·er·tom·e·ter (ap-er-tom′e-ter). Apertômetro; instrumento para medir a abertura angular da objetiva de um microscópio.

ap·er·tu·ra, pl. **ap·er·tu·rae** (ap-er-too′ra, -re) [TA]. Abertura; SIN aperture. [L. de *aperio*, pp. *apertus*, abrir]

a. aqueductus cerebri, a. do aqueduto do mesencéfalo; *termo oficial alternativo para opening of aqueduct of midbrain.

a. aqueductus mesencephali [TA]. a. do aqueduto do mesencéfalo. SIN opening of aqueduct of midbrain.

a. canal′uli coch′leae, a. externa do canalículo da cóclea. SIN external opening of cochlear canaliculus.

a. canaliculi vestib′uli, a. do canalículo do vestíbulo. SIN opening of vestibular canaliculus.

a. latera′lis ventric′uli quar′ti [TA]. a. lateral do quarto ventrículo. SIN lateral aperture of fourth ventricle.

a. media′na ventric′uli quar′ti [TA]. a. medial do quarto ventrículo. SIN median aperture of fourth ventricle.

a. pel′vis infe′rior [TA]. a. inferior da pelve. SIN pelvic outlet.

a. pel′vis mino′ris, a. inferior da pelve. SIN pelvic outlet.

a. pel′vis supe′rior [TA]. a. superior da pelve. SIN pelvic inlet.

a. pirifor′mis [TA]. a. piriforme. SIN piriform aperture.

a. si′nus fronta′lis [TA]. a. do seio frontal. SIN opening of frontal sinus.

a. si′nus sphenoidal′is [TA]. a. do seio esfenoidal. SIN opening of the sphenoidal sinus.

a. thora′cis infe′rior [TA]. a. inferior do tórax. SIN inferior thoracic aperture.

a. thora′cis supe′rior [TA]. a. superior do tórax. SIN superior thoracic aperture.

a. tympan′ica canalic′uli chor′dae tym′pani [TA]. a. timpânica do canalículo da corda do tímpano. SIN tympanic aperture of canaliculus for chorda tympani.

ap·er·ture (ap′er-choor) [TA]. Abertura. **1.** Uma entrada para uma cavidade ou canal; em anatomia, um espaço aberto ou orifício. VER TAMBÉM fossa, ostium, orifice, pore. **2.** O diâmetro da objetiva de um microscópio. SIN aditus [TA], apertura [TA]. [L. *apertura*, uma abertura]

angular a., a. angular; o ângulo, no ar, da luz que emana de um objeto até as bordas do diâmetro da lente frontal da objetiva do microscópio.

external acoustic a., poro acústico externo, *termo oficial alternativo para external acoustic pore.

external a. of cochlear canaliculus, a. externa do canalículo da cóclea. SIN external opening of cochlear canaliculus.

external a. of vestibular aqueduct, a. do canalículo do vestíbulo. SIN opening of vestibular canaliculus.

frontal sinus a., a. do seio frontal. SIN opening of frontal sinus.

inferior pelvic a., a. inferior da pelve. SIN pelvic outlet.

inferior thoracic a. [TA]. a. inferior do tórax; o limite inferior do tórax ósseo composto pela décima segunda vértebra e pelas margens inferiores do gradil costal e esterno. SIN apertura thoracis inferior [TA], thoracic outlet (1).

laryngeal a., a. laríngea. SIN laryngeal inlet.

lateral a. of fourth ventricle [TA]. a. lateral do quarto ventrículo; uma das duas aberturas laterais do quarto ventrículo para o espaço subaracnóide (a cisterna cerebelobulbar lateral) no ângulo pontinocerebelar. SIN apertura lateralis ventriculi quarti [TA], foramen lateralis ventriculi quarti, foramen of Key-Retzius, foramen de Luschka, foramen de Retzius.

a. of mastoid antrum, ádito do antro mastóideo. SIN aditus to mastoid antrum.

median a. of fourth ventricle [TA]. a. mediana do quarto ventrículo; a grande abertura na linha média, na parte ínfero-posterior do teto do quarto ventrículo, que une o ventrículo à cisterna cerebelobulbar posterior. SIN apertura mediana ventriculi quarti [TA], arachnoid foramen, foramen of Magendie.

numerical a. (N.A.), a. numérica; definida pela fórmula *n* seno de *a*, onde *n* é o índice de refração do meio entre o objeto e a objetiva e *a* é o ângulo entre o raio central e o raio marginal que penetram na objetiva.

a. of orbit, a. da órbita. SIN orbital opening.

piriform a. [TA]. a. piriforme; a abertura nasal anterior no crânio. SIN apertura piriformis [TA], piriform opening.

posterior nasal a.'s, cóanos; *termo oficial alternativo para choanae.

sphenoidal sinus a., a. do seio esfenoidal. SIN opening of sphenoidal sinus.

superior pelvic a., a. superior da pelve. SIN pelvic inlet.

superior thoracic a. [TA]. a. superior do tórax; o limite superior do tórax ósseo composto da primeira vértebra torácica e margens superiores das primeiras costelas e do manúbrio do esterno. Nota: os médicos referem-se à abertura torácica superior como a "saída torácica", como na "síndrome da saída torácica". SIN apertura thoracis superior [TA], thoracic inlet, thoracic outlet (2).

tympanic a. of canaliculus for chorda tympani [TA]. a. timpânica do canalículo da corda do tímpano; a pequena abertura do canal encontrada lateral à eminência piramidal na parede posterior da cavidade da orelha média, da qual emerge o nervo da corda do tímpano para se dirigir anteriormente entre os ossículos, acompanhado por um ramo da artéria estilomastóidea. SIN apertura tympanica canaliculi chordae tympani [TA], tympanic opening of canaliculus for chorda tympani.

apex, gen **ap·i·cis,** pl. **ap·i·ces** (a′peks, ap′i-sis, ap′i-ses) [TA]. Ápice, ápex; a extremidade de uma estrutura cônica ou piramidal, como o coração ou pulmão. [L. cume ou ponta]

a. of arytenoid cartilage [TA], ápice da cartilagem aritenóidea; a extremidade superior afilada da cartilagem que suporta a cartilagem corniculada e a prega ariepiglótica. SIN a. cartilaginis arytenoideae [TA].

a. of auricle [TA], ápice da orelha; uma ponta que se projeta para cima e para trás a partir da margem curva livre da hélice, um pouco posterior à sua extremidade superior. SIN a. auriculae [TA], tip of ear*, a. satyri, tip of auricle, Woolner tip.

a. auric′ulae [TA], ápice da orelha. SIN a. of auricle.

a. cap′itis fib′ulae [TA], ápice da cabeça da fíbula. SIN a. of head of fibula.

a. cartila′ginis arytenoi′deae [TA], ápice da cartilagem aritenóidea. SIN a. of arytenoid cartilage.

a. cor′dis [TA], ápice do coração. SIN a. of heart.

a. cor′nus posterio′ris [TA], ápice do corno posterior. SIN a. of posterior horn.

a. cus′pidis den′tis [TA], ápice da cúspide dentária. SIN a. of cusp of tooth.

a. of cusp of tooth [TA], ápice da cúspide dentária; a extremidade de projeções semelhantes a picos a partir da coroa de um dente. SIN a. cuspidis dentis [TA].

a. of dens [TA], ápice do dente; a extremidade do dente do eixo à qual está preso o ligamento apical do dente. SIN a. dentis [TA].

a. den′tis [TA], ápice do dente. SIN a. of dens.

a. of head of fibula [TA], ápice da cabeça da fíbula; a extremidade superior afilada da cabeça da fíbula, na qual se inserem o ligamento poplíteo arqueado e parte do tendão do bíceps femoral. SIN a. capitis fibulae [TA], styloid process of fibula.

a. of heart [TA], ápice do coração; a extremidade romba do coração formada pelo ventrículo esquerdo. VER apex *beat*. SIN a. cordis [TA], vertex cordis.

a. lin′guae [TA], ápice da língua. SIN a. of tongue.

a. of lung [TA], ápice do pulmão; a extremidade superior arredondada de cada pulmão que se estende para a cúpula da pleura. SIN a. pulmonis [TA].

a. na′si [TA], ápice do nariz. SIN a. of nose.

a. of nose [TA], ápice do nariz; extremidade afilada mais anterior da porção externa do nariz. SIN a. nasi [TA], tip of nose*.

a. of orbit, ápice da órbita; a parte posterior da órbita na qual se abre o canal óptico; forma a ponta do espaço piramidal.

a. os′sis sa′cri [TA], ápice do sacro. SIN a. of sacrum.

a. par′tis petro′sae ossis temporalis [TA], ápice da parte petrosa do osso temporal. SIN a. of petrous part of temporal bone.

a. of patella [TA], ápice da patela; a extremidade inferior afilada da patela por onde passa o ligamento patelar para se inserir na tuberosidade tibial. SIN a. patellae [TA].

a. patel′lae [TA], ápice da patela. SIN a. of patella.

a. of petrous part of temporal bone [TA], ápice da parte petrosa do osso temporal; a extremidade anteromedial irregular da porção petrosa sobre a qual se abre a extremidade anterior do canal carótico. SIN a. partis petrosae ossis temporalis [TA].

a. of posterior horn [TA], ápice do corno posterior; a extremidade afilada de cada coluna cinzenta posterior ou corno da medula espinal. SIN a. cornus posterioris [TA], tip of posterior horn.

a. pro′statae [TA], ápice da próstata. SIN a. of prostate.

a. of prostate [TA], ápice da próstata; a parte mais inferior da próstata, situada sobre o diafragma urogenital. SIN a. prostatae [TA].

a. pulmo′nis [TA], ápice do pulmão. SIN a. of lung.

a. rad′icis den′tis [TA], ápice da raiz do dente. SIN root a.

root a. [TA], ápice da raiz do dente; a extremidade da raiz dentária, a parte mais distante do lado incisal ou oclusal. SIN a. radicis dentis [TA], root tip, tip of tooth root.

a. of sacrum [TA], ápice do sacro; a extremidade inferior afunilada do sacro que se articula com o cóccix. SIN a. ossis sacri [TA].

a. sat'yri, ápice da orelha. SIN a. of auricle.

a. of tongue [TA], a da língua; o extremo anterior da língua que pode ser afilado para sentir ou sondar e que repousa contra a face lingual dos dentes incisivos. SIN a. linguae [TA], tip of tongue*.

a. of (urinary) bladder [TA], a. da bexiga; a junção das superfícies superior e ântero-inferior da bexiga, contínua, acima, com o ligamento umbilical mediano. SIN a. vesicae.

a. vesi'cae, a. da bexiga. SIN a. of (urinary) bladder.

apex·car·di·o·gram (a - peks - kar'de - o - gram). Apexcardiograma; registro gráfico dos movimentos da parede torácica produzidos pelo batimento apical do coração.

apex·car·di·og·ra·phy (a'peks - kar'de - og - ra - fe). Apexcardiografia; registro gráfico não-invasivo das pulsações cardíacas da região do ápice, geralmente do ventrículo esquerdo, e que se assemelha à curva de pressão ventricular.

apex·i·fi·ca·tion (a - pek'si - fi - ka'shun). Apicificação; desenvolvimento induzido da raiz dentária ou fechamento do ápice da raiz por deposição de tecido duro.

apex·i·graph (a - pek'si - graf). Apexígrafo; um dispositivo para determinar o tamanho e a posição do ápice de uma raiz dentária. [ápice + G. *grapho*, escrever]

APF Abreviatura para animal protein *factor* (fator proteico animal).

Apgar, Virginia, neonatologista norte-americana, 1909–1974. VER A. score.

apha·gia (a - fa'je - a). Afagia; incapacidade de comer. [G. *a*- priv. + *phago*, comer]

apha·kia (a - fa'ke - a). Afaquia, afacia; ausência da lente do olho. [G. *a*- priv. + *phakos*, lentilha, qualquer coisa com forma semelhante a uma lentilha]

apha·lan·gia (a - fa - lan'je - a). Afalangia; ausência congênita de um dedo ou, mais especificamente, ausência de um ou mais dos ossos longos (falanges) de um dedo ou artelho. [G. *a*- priv. + falange]

apha·sia (a - fa'ze - a). Afasia; comprometimento ou ausência da compreensão ou da produção de, ou comunicação por, fala, escrita ou sinais, decorrente de uma lesão adquirida do hemisfério cerebral dominante. SIN alogia (1). [G. sem fala, de *a*- priv. + *phasis*, fala]

acoustic a., a. acústica, a. auditiva. SIN auditory a.
acquired epileptic a., a. epiléptica adquirida. SIN Landau-Kleffner *syndrome*.
amnestic a., amnesic a., a. amnésica. SIN nominal a.
anomic a., a. anômica. SIN nominal a.
anterior a., a. anterior, a. motora. SIN motor a.
associative a., a. associativa. SIN conduction a.
ataxic a., a. atáxica, a. motora. SIN motor a.
auditory a., a. auditiva; comprometimento da compreensão das formas auditivas da linguagem e comunicação, incluindo a capacidade para escrever a partir de ditado na presença de audição normal. A fala espontânea, a leitura e a escrita não são afetadas. SIN acoustic a., word deafness.
Broca a., a. de Broca, a. motora. SIN motor a.
conduction a., a. de condução; uma forma de a. em que o paciente compreende as palavras escritas e faladas, está consciente de seu déficit e consegue falar e escrever, porém omite ou repete palavras, ou substitui uma palavra por outra (parafasia); a repetição de palavras está gravemente comprometida. A lesão responsável ocorre nos tratos de associação que unem os vários centros da linguagem. SIN associative a.
crossed a., a. cruzada; a. na pessoa destra devido a uma lesão cerebral somente no lado direito.
expressive a., a. motora. SIN motor a.
fluent a., a. sensorial. SIN sensory a.
functional a., a. funcional; a. não-orgânica relacionada a histeria de conversão.
global a., a. global; na qual todos os aspectos da fala e comunicação estão gravemente comprometidos. No máximo, os pacientes conseguem compreender ou falar apenas algumas palavras ou frases; eles não conseguem ler nem escrever. SIN mixed a., total a.
graphic a., agrafia. SIN agraphia.
graphomotor a., agrafia. SIN agraphia.
impressive a., a. sensorial. SIN sensory a.
jargon a., agramatismo, jargonofasia. SIN agrammatism.
mixed a., a. global. SIN global a.
motor a., a. motora; um tipo de a. em que existe deficiência na produção da fala ou débito da linguagem, freqüentemente acompanhada por um déficit na comunicação por escrita, sinais, etc. O paciente está ciente do comprometimento. SIN anterior a., ataxic a., Broca a., expressive a., nonfluent a.
nominal a., a. nominal; uma a. em que o principal déficit é a dificuldade em nomear as pessoas e objetos observados, ouvidos ou sentidos; devido a lesões em várias partes da área da linguagem. SIN amnestic a., amnesic a., anomia, anomic a.
nonfluent a., a. motora. SIN motor a.
pathematic a., mutismo ligado à raiva ou fortes emoções.
posterior a., a. sensorial. SIN sensory a.
psychosensory a., a. sensorial. SIN sensory a.
pure a,'s, afasias puras; raras afasias que afetam apenas um tipo de comunicação, p.ex., leitura, enquanto formas de comunicação correlatas, como escrita, compreensão auditiva, etc., permanecem intactas.
receptive a., a. sensorial. SIN sensory a.
semantic a., a. semântica; a. em que os objetos são nomeados corretamente; há pouco distúrbio na articulação das palavras; as palavras individuais são compreendidas, mas a pessoa não consegue apreender o significado mais amplo do que é ouvido.
sensory a., a. sensorial; a. em que existe comprometimento na compreensão das palavras faladas e escritas, associada à fala e escrita sem esforço, articulada, porém parafrásica; palavras malformadas, palavras substituídas e neologismos são característicos. Quando grave e a fala é incompreensível, é chamada jargonofasia (agramatismo). Com freqüência, o paciente parece não estar ciente do déficit. SIN fluent a., impressive a., posterior a., psychosensory a., receptive a., Wernicke a.
syntactical a., a. sintática; a. em que as palavras são razoavelmente bem pronunciadas, porém são faladas em frases curtas ou frases mal construídas sem artigos, preposições ou conjunções.
total a., a. global. SIN global a.
transcortical a., a. transcortical; uma a. em que as áreas de linguagem sensoriais e motoras não-afetadas estão isoladas do restante do córtex hemisférico. Subdividida em a. transcortical sensorial e a. transcortical motora.
visual a., a. visual; (1) SIN alexia; (2) impropriamente utilizado como um sinônimo para anomia.
Wernicke a., a. de Wernicke, a. sensorial. SIN sensory a.

apha·si·ac, apha·sic (a - fa'ze - ak, a - fa'sik). Afásico; relativo a ou que sofre de afasia.

apha·si·ol·o·gist (a - fa'ze - ol'o - gist). Afasiologista; um especialista que lida com os distúrbios da fala causados por disfunção das áreas da linguagem no cérebro.

apha·si·ol·o·gy (a - fa'ze - ol'o - ge). Afasiologia; a ciência dos distúrbios da fala causados por disfunção das áreas de linguagem cerebrais.

aphas·mid (a - faz'mid). Afasmídio. 1. Que carece de fasmídios, conforme observado nos nematódeos da classe Adenophorasida (Aphasmidia). 2. Nome comum para um membro da classe Aphasmidia, atualmente Adenophorasida.

Aphas·mid·ia (a - faz - mid'e - a). Afasmídios. SIN Adenophorasida.

aph·e·li·ot·ro·pism (ap - he - le - ot'ro - pizm). Afeliotropismo; heliotaxia negativa. [G. *apo*, longe + *helios*, sol + *tropein*, virar]

apher·e·sis (a - fer - e'sis). Aférese; infusão do sangue do próprio paciente do qual foram retirados determinados elementos celulares ou líquidos (plasma, leucócitos, plaquetas, etc.). [G. *aphairesis*, retirada]

aphil·op·o·ny (a - fil - op'o - ne). Afilofonia; termo obsoleto para a aversão, ou falta de desejo, de trabalhar. [G. *a*- priv. + *philo*, gostar, + *ponos*, trabalho]

apho·nia (a - fo'ne - a). Afonia; perda da voz em consequência de doença ou lesão da laringe. [G. *a*- priv. + *phone*, voz]

hysterical a., a. histérica; perda da voz por motivos psicogênicos, como em algumas variedades de histeria. SIN nonorganic a.
nonorganic a., a. não-orgânica, a. histérica. SIN hysterical a.
a. paralyt'ica, a. paralítica; a. devido à paralisia das cordas vocais.
spastic a., a. espástica; a. causada por contração espasmódica dos músculos adutores da laringe provocada por tentativa de fonação.

aphon·ic (a - fon'ik). Afônico; relativo à afonia. SIN aphonous.

aph·o·nous (af'o - nus). Afônico. SIN aphonic.

apho·tes·the·sia (a - fo - tes - the'ze - a). Afotestesia; sensibilidade diminuída da retina à luz causada por exposição excessiva à luz solar. [G. *a*- priv. + *phos*, luz, + *aisthesis*, percepção]

aphra·sia (a - fra'ze - a). Afrasia; incapacidade de falar, de qualquer causa. [G. *a*- priv. + *phrasis*, fala]

aph·ro·di·sia (af - ro - diz'e - a). Afrodisia; desejo sexual, especialmente quando excessivo. [G. *aphrodisios*, relativo à Afrodite]

aph·ro·di·si·ac (af - ro - diz'e - ak). Afrodisíaco. 1. Que aumenta o desejo sexual. 2. Qualquer coisa que desperte ou aumente o desejo sexual.

aph·ro·di·si·o·ma·nia (af - ro - diz'e - o - ma'ne - a). Afrodisiomania; interesse erótico anormal e excessivo. [G. *aphrodisia*, prazeres sexuais, + *mania*, insanidade]

aph·tha, pl. **aph·thae** (af'tha, af'the). Afta. 1. No singular, uma pequena úlcera em uma mucosa. 2. No plural, estomatite caracterizada por episódios intermitentes de úlceras orais dolorosas, de etiologia desconhecida, que estão cobertas por exsudato acinzentado, são circundadas por um halo eritematoso e variam desde alguns milímetros a 2 cm de diâmetro; elas se limitam às mucosas orais que não estão ligadas ao periósteo, ocorrem como lesões solitárias ou múltiplas e curam espontaneamente em 1–2 semanas. SIN aphthae minor, aphthous stomatitis, canker sores, recurrent aphthous stomatitis, recurrent aphthous ulcers, recurrent ulcerative stomatitis, ulcerative stomatitis. [G. ulceração]

Bednar aphthae, aftas de Bednar; úlceras traumáticas localizadas bilateralmente em ambos os lados da rafe do palato em lactentes.

herpetiform aphthae, aftas herpetiformes; uma variante das aftas orais, de etiologia desconhecida, caracterizada por até várias dúzias de úlceras, com 2–3 mm de diâmetro, organizadas em uma distribuição herpetiforme agrupada.

aphthae ma'jor, aftas maiores; uma forma grave de aftas caracterizada por úlceras freqüentes, profundas, grandes e muito numerosas; a cura pode levar até 6 semanas e resultar em fibrose. SIN Mikulicz aphthae, periadenitis mucosa necrotica recurrens, recurrent scarring aphthae, Sutton disease.

Mikulicz aphthae, aftas de Mikulicz, aftas maiores. SIN aphthae major.

aphthae mi'nor, aftas menores. SIN aphtha (2).

recurrent scarring aphthae, aftas fibróticas recorrentes. SIN aphthae major.

aph·thoid (af′thoyd). Aftóide; que se assemelha a aftas.

aph·tho·sis (af - thō′sis). Aftose; qualquer condição caracterizada pela presença de aftas.

aph·thous (af′thŭs). Aftoso; caracterizado por ou relativo a aftas ou à aftose.

Aph·tho·vi·rus (af′thō - vī′rus). Um gênero na família Picornaviridae associado a febre aftosa no gado.

aphy·lac·tic (ā - fī - lak′tik). Afilático; termo obsoleto para pertinente a, ou caracterizado por, afilaxia.

aphy·lax·is (ā - fī - lak′sis). Afilaxia; termo antigo para a falta de proteção contra a doença. SIN nonimmunity. [G *a*- priv. + *phylaxis*, uma defesa]

ap·i·cal (ap′i - kăl) [TA]. Apical. **1.** Relativo ao ápice ou extremidade de uma estrutura piramidal ou puntiforme. **2.** Situado mais próximo ao ápice de uma estrutura em relação a um ponto de referência específico; oposto a basal. SIN apicalis [TA].

ap·i·ca·lis (ap - i - kā′lis)[TA]. Apical. SIN apical, apical. [L.]

ap·i·cec·to·my (ap - i - sek′tō - mē). Apicectomia. **1.** Abertura e exenteração das células aéreas no ápice da porção petrosa do osso temporal. **2.** Em cirurgia dentária, um sinônimo obsoleto para apicoectomy. [L. *apex*, extremidade ou cume + G. *ektomē*, excisão]

apic·e·ot·o·my (ā - pis - ē - ot′ō - mē). Apicotomia. SIN apicotomy.

ap·i·ces (ap′i - sēs). Ápices; plural de apex.

apico-. Forma combinante relativa a um ápice. [L. *apex*, *apicis*, um cume ou extremidade + -o-]

ap·i·co·ec·to·my (ap′i - kō - ek′tō - mē). Apicectomia; remoção cirúrgica do ápice de uma raiz dentária. SIN root resection. [apico- + G. *ektomē*, excisão dentária]

ap·i·co·lo·ca·tor (ap′i - kō - lō′kā - tor). Apicolocalizador; um dispositivo para localizar o ápice da raiz de um dente.

ap·i·col·y·sis (ap - i - kol′i - sis). Apicólise; o colapso cirúrgico da porção superior do pulmão por descolamento cirúrgico da pleura parietal, permitindo o deslocamento inferomedial do ápice pulmonar. [apico- + G. *lysis*, destruição]

Api·com·plexa (ap - i - kom - plek′sa). Um filo do sub-reino Protozoa, que inclui a classe Sporozoea e as subclasses Coccidia e Piroplasmia, e caracteriza-se pela presença de um complexo apical. [L. *apex*, pl. *apicis*, extremidade, cume, + *complexus*, tecido junto]

ap·i·co·stome (ap′i - kō - stōm). Apicóstomo; o trocarte e a cânula usados em apicostomia.

ap·i·cos·to·my (ap - i - kos′tō - mē). Apicostomia; uma cirurgia em que a placa alveolar labial ou bucal é perfurada com um trocarte e cânula; feita para atingir o ápice da raiz e obter culturas bacterianas a partir dessa área. [apico- + G. *stoma*, boca]

ap·i·cot·o·my (ap - i - kot′ō - mē). Apicotomia; incisão em uma estrutura apical. SIN apiceotomy. [apico + G. *tomē*, um corte]

apic·u·late (ā - pik′ū - lāt). Apiculado; que termina abruptamente com uma pequena ponta. [L. *apiculus*, uma extremidade ou ponta]

apic·u·lus (ā - pik′ū - lŭs). Apículo; uma projeção pequena e aguda em uma extremidade de um esporo fúngico no ponto de fixação ou na parede de uma hifa ou conidióforo. [L.]

ap·i·cu·ret·tage (ap - i - kū′rĕ - tahzh). Apicuretagem; curetagem apical depois da remoção de um dente infectado.

apin·e·al·ism (ā - pin′ē - al - izm). Apinealismo; ausência adquirida da glândula pineal.

api·pho·bia (ā - pi - fō′bē - ā). Apifobia; medo mórbido de abelhas. SIN melissophobia. [L. *apis*, abelha, + G. *phobos*, medo]

api·tu·i·tar·ism (ā - pi - tooʹi - tăr - izm). Apituitarismo; carência total de tecido hipofisário funcional; pode ser iatrogênico (p.ex., como conseqüência de hipofisectomia) ou como resultado de um processo patológico espontâneo.

apla·cen·tal (ā - pla - sen′tăl). Aplacentário; sem uma placenta; indica os monotremados (que depositam ovos e não possuem placenta) e os marsupiais (que apresentam um saco vitelino placentário transitório).

ap·la·nat·ic (ap-la-nat′ik). Aplanático; pertinente ao aplanatismo ou a uma lente aplanática.

aplan·a·tism (ā - plan′ă - tizm). Aplanatismo; livre da aberração esférica; diz-se de uma lente. [G. *a*- priv. + *planētos*, errante]

apla·sia (ā - plā′zē - ā). Aplasia. **1.** Desenvolvimento defeituoso ou ausência congênita de um órgão ou tecido. **2.** Em hematologia, desenvolvimento incompleto, retardado ou defeituoso, ou cessação do processo regenerativo usual. [G. *a*- priv. + *plastis*, um molde]

congenital a. of thymus, a. congênita do timo. SIN DiGeorge *syndrome*.

a. cu'tis congen'ita [MIM*107600, *207700, *207730], a. congênita da pele; ausência ou deficiência congênita de uma área localizada da pele, com a base do defeito coberta por uma fina membrana translúcida; mais amiúde, uma única área próxima ao vértice do couro cabeludo, mas podendo ocorrer em outras áreas; as estruturas subjacentes também podem ser afetadas; herança autossômica, quer dominante, quer recessiva.

germinal a., a. germinal. SIN seminiferous tubule *dysgenesis*.

gonadal a., a. gonadal; ausência congênita de quase todos os tecidos gonadais; a genitália externa e os canais genitais são femininos, mas, quando há células intersticiais de Leydig, a genitália externa é comumente ambígua e os canais genitais são femininos. VER TAMBÉM gonadal *dysgenesis*, gonadal *agenesis*; Cf. Klinefelter *syndrome*, Turner *syndrome*.

pure red cell a., a. eritrocitária pura; uma parada transitória da produção de eritrócitos que pode acontecer durante uma anemia hemolítica, freqüentemente precedida por infecção, ou como uma complicação de determinados medicamentos; quando a parada persiste, pode sobrevir anemia grave. VER TAMBÉM congenital hipoplastic *anemia*.

aplas·tic (ā - plas′tik, ă-). Aplásico; pertinente à aplasia ou a condições caracterizadas por regeneração defeituosa, como na anemia a.

apleu·ria (ā - ploor′ē - ā). Apleuria; ausência congênita de uma ou mais costelas; em geral associada à ausência de processos transversos. [*a*- priv. + G. *pleura*, costela]

ap·nea (ap′nē - ā). Apnéia; ausência de respiração. [G. *apnoia*, desejo de respirar]

central a., a. central; a. em conseqüência de depressão bulbar, que inibe o movimento respiratório.

deglutition a., a. da deglutição; inibição da respiração durante a deglutição.

induced a., a. induzida; parada respiratória intencional durante a anestesia geral produzida por hipocapnia, pelo uso de relaxante muscular, por depressão do centro respiratório ou pela súbita cessação da respiração controlada.

obstructive sleep a., a. obstrutiva do sono; um distúrbio, descrito pela primeira vez em 1965, caracterizado por interrupções recorrentes da respiração durante o sono devido à obstrução temporária das vias aéreas por tecidos faríngeos frouxos, excessivamente volumosos ou malformados (palato mole, úvula e, por vezes, tonsilas), com resultante hipoxemia e letargia crônica.

> As manifestações da apnéia obstrutiva do sono são ronco alto, episódios apneicos recorrentes, durante o sono, seguidos por inspiração ofegante, com despertar parcial ou completo, inquietação noturna e sonolência diurna. Os episódios de apnéia duram 10 a 120 segundos e podem ser acompanhados por bradicardia sinusal ou bloqueio atrioventricular. O efeito cumulativo dos episódios recorrentes de apnéia é a hipoxemia e o sono superficial, não-reparador, o que pode levar a sonolência excessiva, alteração da personalidade, comprometimento da função intelectual e tendência exacerbada a acidentes durante o período de vigília. Contudo, são frágeis as evidências estabelecendo a apnéia obstrutiva do sono como um fator de risco independente para os acidentes com veículos a motor, infarto do miocárdio, acidente vascular cerebral e morte súbita. Cerca de 15% das pessoas com esse distúrbio desenvolvem hipertensão pulmonar persistente. A apnéia obstrutiva do sono afeta cerca de 4% dos homens e 2% das mulheres entre 30 e 60 anos. Obesidade, hipotireoidismo, fumo, álcool e alguns hipnóticos (principalmente benzodiazepínicos) predispõem a esse distúrbio, e sua incidência aumenta com o avançar da idade. O diagnóstico é confirmado por polissonografia (mensuração contínua do fluxo aéreo, atividade respiratória, eletromiografia do queixo, ECG, EEG, eletrooculograma e saturação de oxigênio arterial durante o sono) e por avaliação do formato e tamanho do trato respiratório superior. A perda de peso, cessação do fumo e prevenção contra os hipnóticos benzodiazepínicos são aconselhados para todos os pacientes. Um dispositivo de avanço mandibular, usado dentro da boca à noite, reduz os sintomas em alguns pacientes. Um tratamento efetivo, porém algo incômodo, consiste no uso noturno de pressão positiva contínua nas vias aéreas, o que fornece um fluxo constante de ar ambiente em baixa pressão através do nariz, visando superar a obstrução respiratória alta intermitente. Alguns pacientes beneficiam-se de procedimentos cirúrgicos, como a uvulopalatofaringoplastia (remodelagem e redução da úvula e do palato mole), que pode ser realizada por ablação com laser ou radiofreqüência sob anestesia local, e a osteotomia mandibular com avanço do músculo genioglosso.

sleep a., a. do sono; a. central e/ou periférica durante o sono, associada ao despertar freqüente e, com freqüência, à sonolência diurna. Cf. sleep-induced a.

sleep-induced a., a. induzida pelo sono; a. resultante da incapacidade do centro respiratório de estimular a respiração adequada durante o sono; dividida em pausa respiratória (cessação do fluxo de ar por menos de 10 segundos) e pausa apneica (cessação do fluxo de ar superior a 10 segundos).

ap·ne·ic (ap'nē'ik). Apneico; relativo à ou que sofre de apnéia.

a·pneu·mia (a - pnoo'mē - ă). Apneumia; ausência congênita dos pulmões. [G. *a-* priv. + *pneumōn*, pulmão]

ap·neu·sis (ap - noo'sis). Apneuse; um padrão respiratório anormal que consiste em uma pausa na inspiração plena; uma parada inspiratória prolongada causada por uma lesão ao nível pontino médio ou caudal do tronco cerebral. [G. *a-* priv. + *pneusis*, respiração, de *pneō*, respirar]

apo. Abreviatura de *apoenzyme* (apoenzima); *apolipoprotein* (apolipoproteína).

△ **apo-.** Forma combinante que, geralmente, significa separado de ou derivado de. [G. *apo*, separado, afastado; *apo-* torna-se *ap-*, especialmente antes de uma vogal ou h]

ap·o·bi·o·sis (ap - ō - bī - ō'sis). Apobiose; morte, especialmente morte local de uma parte do organismo. [G. morte, de *apo*, de + *biōsis*, vida]

ap·o·crine (ap'ō - krin). Apócrino; denotando um mecanismo de secreção glandular em que a porção apical das células secretoras é desprendida e incorporada na secreção. VER TAMBÉM apocrine *gland*. [G. *apo - krinō*, separar]

ap·o·crus·tic (ap - ō - krus - tik). Apocrústico. 1. Adstringente e repelente. 2. Um agente com essa ação. [G. *apokroustikos*, capaz de repelir, de *apo*, fora, + *krouō*, bater]

a·po·dal (ā - pō'dal). Ápode; relativo à apodia. SIN apodous. [G. *a-* priv. + *pous*, pé]

apo·dia (ā - pō'dē - ă). Apodia; ausência congênita dos pés. SIN apody. [G. *a-* priv. + *pous*, pé]

ap·o·dous (ap'ō - dŭs). Ápode. SIN apodal.

ap·o·dy (ap'ō - dē). Apodia. SIN apodia.

ap·o·en·zyme (apo) (ap'ō - en - zīm). Apoenzima; a porção proteica de uma enzima, contrastada com a porção não-proteica, coenzima, ou porção prostética (quando presente na proteína intacta).

ap·o·fer·ri·tin (ap - ō - fer'i - tin). Apoferritina, uma proteína, na parede intestinal, que se combina com um composto de hidróxido férrico-fosfato para formar a ferritina, o primeiro estágio na absorção do ferro.

ap·o·gam·ia, apog·a·my (ap - ō - gam'ē - ă, ă - pog'ă - mē). Apogamia. SIN parthenogenesis. [G. *apo*, longe, + *gameō*, casar]

apo·gee. Apogeu; o pico de gravidade das manifestações clínicas de uma doença. [Fr. do L. Mod. *apogaeum*, de G. *apogaios*, longe da terra. de *apo* + gaia, terra]

ap·o·in·duc·er (ā'pō - in - doos'er). Apoindutor; uma proteína que se liga ao DNA para ativar a transcrição.

apo-2L. apo-2L. SIN TRAIL.

apo·lar (ā - pō'lar). Apolar. 1. Sem pólos; indica especificamente as células nervosas embrionárias (neuroblastos) que ainda não começaram os processos de brotamento. 2. Hidrofóbico. SIN hydrophobic (2).

ap·o·lip·o·pro·tein (apo) (ap'ō - lip - ō - prō'tēn). Apolipoproteína; o componente proteico de qualquer complexo lipoproteico que é um constituinte normal dos quilomícrons plasmáticos, HDL, LDL e VLDL em seres humanos.

a. A-I, a. A-I; uma a. encontrada no HDL e nos quilomícrons. É um ativador de LCAT e um ligante para o receptor de HDL. A deficiência dessa a. foi associada a baixos níveis de HDL e à doença de Tangier.

a. A-II, a. A-II; uma a. encontrada na HDL (lipoproteína de alta densidade) e em quilomícrons; estabiliza a HDL.

a. A-IV, a. A-IV; uma a. secretada com quilomícrons e também encontrada na HDL. Participa no catabolismo de quilomícrons e VLDL. Também é necessária para a ativação da lipase lipoproteica.

a. B, a. B; apolipoproteínas encontradas nos quilomícrons, LDL, VLDL e IDL. Elevadas no plasma de pessoas com hiperlipoproteinemia familial.

a. B-100, a. B-100; uma a. encontrada em LDL, VLDL e IDL. O ligante para o receptor; ausente em determinados tipos de abetalipoproteinemia.

a. B-48, a. B-48; uma a. encontrada em quilomícrons e resquícios de quilomícrons. Retida no intestino de indivíduos com a doença de retenção de quilomícrons.

a. C-I, a. C-I; uma a. encontrada em VLDL e quilomícrons. Modula a interação de a. E com VLDL.

a. C-II, uma a. encontrada em VLDL, HDL e quilomícrons; um ativador da lipase lipoproteica; a deficiência resultará em acúmulo de quilomícrons e triacilgliceróis.

a. C-III, a. C-III; uma a. encontrada em VLDL e quilomícrons. Inibe inúmeras lipases.

a. D, a. D; uma a. encontrada em HDL. Forma um complexo com LCAT e parece estar envolvida no transporte da bilina.

a. E, a. E; uma a. encontrada em VLDL, HDL, quilomícrons e resquícios de quilomícrons. Elevada nos indivíduos com hiperlipoproteinemia do tipo III. Possui uma função importante no transporte do colesterol.

ap·o·mix·ia (ap - ō - mik'sē - ă). Apomixia. SIN parthenogenesis. [G. *apo*, de, + *mixis*, uma mistura]

ap·o·mor·phine hy·dro·chlo·ride (ap - ō - mōr'fēn). Cloridrato de apomorfina; um derivado da morfina usado como emético por via parenteral.

ap·o·neu·rec·to·my (ap'ō - noo - rek'tō - mē). Aponeurectomia; excisão de uma aponeurose. [aponeurose + G. *ektomē*, excisão]

ap·o·neu·ror·rha·phy (ap'ō - noo - rōr'ă - fē). Aponeurorrafia. SIN fasciorraphy. [aponeurosis + G. *rhaphē*, sutura]

ap·o·neu·ro·sis, pl. **ap·o·neu·ro·ses** (ap'ō - noo - rō'sis, - sēz). [TA]. Aponeurose; uma lâmina fibrosa ou um tendão expandido achatado, que fornece inserção para fibras musculares e serve como um meio de origem ou inserção de um músculo plano; por vezes, também age como fáscia para outros músculos. [G. no final do músculo onde ele se torna tendão, de *apo*, de + *neuron*, tendão]

bicipital a., a. bicipita'lis [TA], a. bicipital; fibras que se irradiam do tendão de inserção do bíceps, formando uma faixa triangular que passa obliquamente através do orifício do cotovelo até o lado ulnar e misturam-se na fáscia profunda do antebraço, fornecendo, dessa maneira, uma inserção indireta para a borda subcutânea da ulna. Originalmente chamada de fáscia "da graça de Deus", serve para proteger a artéria braquial e o nervo mediano durante a flebotomia da veia cubital mediana. SIN a. musculi bicipitis brachii [TA], lacertus fibrosus*, bicipital fascia, semilunar fascia.

Denonvilliers a., a. de Denonvilliers, septo retovesical. SIN rectovesical *septum*.

epicranial a. [TA], a. epicrânica; a aponeurose ou tendão intermediário que une o ventre frontal e o ventre occipital do músculo occipitofrontal para formar — com o temporoparietal — o epicrânio. SIN galea aponeurotica [TA], a. epicranialis*, galea (2).

a. epicrania'lis, a. epicrânica; *termo oficial alternativo para epicranial a.

extensor a., expansão digital extensora. SIN extensor digital *expansion*.

a. of external oblique muscle, a. do músculo oblíquo externo do abdome; a porção tendinosa, plana e larga, do músculo oblíquo externo do abdome. As fibras carnosas da extremidade muscular na a. ao longo de uma linha que desce verticalmente, desde a articulação costocondral da nona costela, virando em seguida lateralmente, logo abaixo do nível do umbigo, em direção à espinha ilíaca ântero-superior. As fibras da aponeurose correm medial e inferiormente, contribuindo para a parede anterior da bainha do músculo reto do abdome e decussando com aquelas da a. contralateral na linha alba mediana. Ínfero-medialmente, a a. está inserida na borda superior da sínfise do púbis, na crista púbica e no tubérculo púbico. Entre a espinha ilíaca ântero-superior e o tubérculo púbico, torna-se espessada e virada para baixo, formando os ligamentos inguinais. A porção da a. presa ao osso púbico forma o anel inguinal superficial por desdobrar-se nas cruzes medial e lateral. VER TAMBÉM external spermatic *fascia*, inguinal *ligament*, lacunar *ligament*, pectineal *ligament*, reflected inguinal *ligament*, superficial inguinal *ring*, rectus *sheath*.

a. of insertion, a. de inserção; uma lâmina tendinosa que serve para a inserção de um músculo largo.

a. of internal oblique muscle, a. do músculo oblíquo interno; a porção tendinosa plana e larga do músculo oblíquo interno do abdome. As fibras carnosas do músculo terminam na a. lateralmente à linha semilunar. A porção mais superior da a. está inserida nas superfícies externas e nas bordas inferiores da sétima à nona cartilagem costal. Da porção que se estende entre a margem costoxifóide e o púbis, os dois terços superiores dividem-se nas lâminas anterior e posterior, na borda lateral do músculo reto do abdome, para contribuir para as paredes anterior e posterior da bainha do músculo reto do abdome, quando elas se estendem até a linha alba média. O terço inferior da a. não se divide, mas une-se às aponeuroses dos músculos oblíquo externo e transverso do abdome para formar a parede anterior da bainha do músculo reto do abdome. As fibras da porção da a. que contribuem para a bainha dos retos decussam com aquelas da a. contralateral na linha alba. A porção mais inferior da a. mistura-se com a a. do músculo transverso do abdome para formar o tendão conjunto, inserindo-se na crista púbica e, com freqüência, pécten do púbis, formando, assim, a parede posterior do canal inguinal no anel inguinal superficial. VER TAMBÉM cremasteric *fascia*, inguinal *falx*, rectus *sheath*.

a. of investment, a. de revestimento; uma membrana fibrosa que recobre e mantém em posição um músculo ou grupo de músculos.

a. lin'guae [TA], a. da língua. SIN lingual a.

lingual a. [TA], a. da língua; a lâmina própria espessada da língua na qual se inserem os músculos linguais. SIN a. linguae [TA].

a. mus'culi bicip'itis bra'chii [TA], a. do músculo bíceps braquial. SIN bicipital a.

a. of origin, a. de origem; uma expansão tendinosa que serve como inserção de origem de um músculo largo.

a. palati'na [TA], a. palatina. SIN palatine a.

palatine a. [TA], a. palatina; os tendões expandidos dos músculos tensores do véu palatino nos dois terços anteriores do palato mole, nos quais os outros músculos palatinos se inserem. SIN a. palatina [TA].

palmar a. [TA], a. palmar; a porção central expandida da fáscia que embainha a mão; irradia-se no sentido das bases dos dedos a partir do tendão do músculo palmar longo. VER TAMBÉM palmar *fascia*. SIN a. palmaris [TA], Dupuytren fascia.

a. palma'ris [TA], a. palmar. SIN palmar a.

Petit a., a. de Petit; a camada posterior do ligamento largo do útero. [P. Petit]
a. pharyn'gea, fáscia faringobasilar. SIN pharyngobasilar *fascia*.
plantar a. [TA], a. plantar; a porção central, muito fina, da fáscia que reveste os músculos plantares; irradia-se no sentido dos artelhos, a partir do processo medial da tuberosidade do calcâneo, e fornece inserção para o músculo flexor curto dos dedos. VER TAMBÉM plantar *fascia*. SIN a. plantaris [TA].
a. planta'ris [TA], a. plantar. SIN plantar a.
Sibson a., a. de Sibson, membrana suprapleural. SIN suprapleural *membrane*.
temporal a., fáscia temporal. SIN temporal *fascia*.
thoracolumbar a., fáscia toracolombar. SIN thoracolumbar *fascia*.
a. of vastus muscles, a. dos músculos vastos. VER patellar *retinaculum*, medial patellar *retinaculum*, lateral patellar *retinaculum*.

ap·o·neu·ro·si·tis (ap'ō - noo - rō - sī'tis). Aponeurosite; inflamação de uma aponeurose.

ap·o·neu·rot·ic (ap'ō - noo - rot'ik). Aponeurótico; relativo a uma aponeurose.

ap·o·neu·ro·tome (ap - ō - noo'rō - tōm). Aponeurótomo; obsoleto. Instrumento para dividir uma aponeurose. [aponeurose + G. *tome*, um corte]

ap·o·neu·rot·o·my (ap'ō - noo - rot'ō - mē). Aponeurotomia; incisão de uma aponeurose.

ap·o·phy·lax·is (ap'ō - fī - lak'sis). Apofilaxia; termo obsoleto para designar a diminuição da proteção conferida pelos líquidos orgânicos, como por vezes observada na fase negativa da terapia com agentes imunizantes.

apoph·y·sary (ā - pof'i - sā - rē). Apofisário. SIN apophysial.

ap·o·phys·i·al, apoph·y·se·al (ā - pō - fiz'ē - ăl). Apofisário; relativo ou que se assemelha a uma apófise. SIN apophysary.

apoph·y·sis, pl. **apoph·y·ses** (ă - pof'i - sis, - sēz) [TA]. Apófise; uma proliferação ou projeção, especialmente a partir de um osso. Um processo ou proliferação óssea que carece de um centro independente de ossificação. [G. um broto]

basilar a., parte basilar do osso occipital. SIN basilar *part* of occipital bone.
a. con'chae, eminência da concha. SIN eminence of concha.
a. hel'icis, espinha da hélice. SIN spine of helix.
lenticular a., processo lenticular da bigorna. SIN lenticular *process* of incus.
temporal a., processo mastóide. SIN mastoid *process*.

apoph·y·si·tis (ă - pof - i - sī'tis). Apofisite; inflamação de qualquer apófise.
calcaneal a., a. do calcâneo. SIN Sever *disease*.
a. tibia'lis adolescen'tium, a. tibial do adolescente. SIN Osgood-Schlatter *disease*.

Apophysomyces (ap - ō - fiz - ō - mī'sēz). Um gênero de fungos da família Mucoraceae; uma causa de mucormicose.

ap·o·plas·mia (ap - ō - plaz'mē - ă). Apoplasmia; termo obsoleto para a diminuição do volume de plasma sanguíneo.

ap·o·plec·tic (ap - ō - plek'tik). Apoplético; relativo a, que sofre de ou predisposto a apoplexia (acidente vascular cerebral).

ap·o·plec·ti·form (ap - ō - plek'ti - fōrm). Apoplectiforme; que se assemelha à apoplexia (acidente vascular cerebral).

ap·o·plexy (ap'ō - plek - sē). Apoplexia, acidente vascular cerebral (AVC). SIN stroke (1). [G. *apoplexia*]
abdominal a., a. abdominal; hemorragia, trombose ou embolia mesentérica envolvendo os vasos sanguíneos abdominais ou mesentéricos.
adrenal a., a. adrenal; hemorragia para as glândulas supra-renais ou trombose das veias supra-renais, seguida por insuficiência aguda das supra-renais, que ocorre na síndrome de Waterhouse-Friderichsen.
bulbar a., a. bulbar; a. devido a lesão vascular no tronco cerebral.
functional a., a. funcional; uma condição que simula a. sem qualquer lesão cerebral; uma forma de histeria de conversão.
heat a., (1) hiperpirexia maligna. SIN heatstroke; **(2)** hiperpirexia da malária intermitente. SIN ardent *fever*.
labyrinthine a., a. labiríntica; uma síndrome clínica manifestada como uma crise única e repentina de vertigem grave, náuseas e vômitos, com perda permanente da função do labirinto em um lado, mas sem perda associada da audição ou zumbido. Atribuída à oclusão do ramo labiríntico da artéria auditiva interna.
neonatal a., a. neonatal; hemorragia intracraniana em recém-nascidos.
pituitary a., a. hipofisário; o estabelecimento súbito de perda visual, oftalmoplegia e dor meníngea decorrente do infarto de um adenoma apoplético, levando à compressão do quiasma e do seio cavernoso e a alguma hemorragia subaracnóide.
spinal a., a. espinal; acidente vascular cerebral envolvendo a medula espinal.
uteroplacental a., a. uteroplacentária, útero de Couvelaire. SIN Couvelaire *uterus*.

ap·o·pro·tein (ap - ō - prō'tēn). Apoproteína; uma cadeia polipeptídica (proteína) que ainda não formou um complexo com o grupo prostético necessário para formar a holoproteína ativa.

ap·o·pto·sis (ap'op - tō'sis, ap'ō - tō'sis). Apoptose; morte celular programada; deleção de células individuais por fragmentação em partículas ligadas à membrana, as quais são fagocitadas por outras células. SIN programmed cell death. [G. queda ou gotejamento, de *apo*, fora + *ptosis*, uma queda]

Enquanto algumas células (p. ex., fibras musculares cardíacas e esqueléticas, neurônios do SNC) duram toda a vida, outras (p.ex., células epiteliais e glandulares, eritrócitos) possuem períodos de vida limitados, ao final dos quais elas são geneticamente programadas para se autodestruírem, geralmente para serem substituídas por outras formadas por mitose a partir das células sobreviventes. As células nas culturas de tecido sofrem espontaneamente apoptose após cerca de 50 divisões celulares. Ao contrário da morte celular causada por lesão, infecção ou comprometimento circulatório, a apoptose não provoca resposta inflamatória nas células e tecidos adjacentes. Os aspectos da apoptose detectáveis por métodos histológicos e histoquímicos incluem o encolhimento celular, decorrente principalmente de desidratação; permeabilidade aumentada da membrana, com aumento do cálcio intracelular e queda do pH; endonucleólise (fragmentação do DNA nuclear); e, por fim, formação de corpúsculos apoptóticos, que são absorvidos e removidos pelos macrófagos. Além de ser decorrente de programação genética, a apoptose pode ser induzida por lesão do DNA celular, como por irradiação e alguns agentes citotóxicos usados para tratar o câncer. Ela pode ser suprimida por fatores de ocorrência natural (p.ex., citocinas) e por alguns medicamentos (p.ex., inibidores da protease).Tipicamente, a apoptose não acontece em células malignas. Portanto, essas células escapam do destino de suas precursoras não-malignas e diz-se que são imortais. A imortalização pode ocorrer de diversas maneiras. O gene bcl-2, presente em muitos cânceres, dirige a produção de uma enzima que bloqueia a apoptose e imortaliza as células afetadas. A lesão do DNA normalmente deflagra a apoptose por ativar o gene supressor tumoral p53, que está ausente ou mutado em cerca de metade de todos os cânceres humanos. As células sem gene conseguem sobreviver à quimioterapia e à radiação destinadas a destruir as células cancerosas. O fato de não ocorrer apoptose também está envolvido em algumas doenças degenerativas, incluindo o lúpus eritematoso sistêmico, e seria responsável pela lesão celular causada por determinados vírus, incluindo o HIV.

ap·o·re·pres·sor (ap - ō - rē - pres'er). Aporrepressor; uma proteína reguladora que, quando combinada a outro co-repressor, sofre transformação alostérica, podendo assim combinar-se com um *locus* operador e inibir a transcrição de determinados genes.

ap·o·some (ap'ō - sōm). Apossoma; uma inclusão citoplasmática produzida pela própria célula. [G. *apo*, de, + *sōma*, corpo]

ap·o·stax·is (ap - ō - staks'is). Apostaxia; hemorragia discreta ou sangramento por gotas. [G. destilação]

apos·thia (ă - pos'thē - ă). Apostia; ausência congênita de prepúcio. [G *a*- priv. + *posthē*, prepúcio]

ap·o·stilb (ap'ō - stilb). Apostilb (candela por cm²); uma unidade de brilho igual a 0,1 mililambert. [G. *apo*, de, + *stilbē*, lâmpada]

ap·o·tha·na·sia (ap'ō - thă - nā'zē - ă). Apotanásia; adiamento da morte; prolongamento da vida, em oposição a eutanásia. [G. *apo*, fora + *thanatos*, morte]

apoth·e·cary (ă - poth'ē - kăr - ē). Boticário; termo obsoleto para farmacêutico ou droguista. [G. *apothēkē*, depósito, armazém, de *apo*, de, + *thēkē*, uma caixa]

ap·o·them, ap·o·theme (ap'ō - them, ap'ō - thēm). Apótemo; um precipitado provocado pela fervura prolongada de uma infusão vegetal ou por sua exposição ao ar. [G. *apo*, de, + *thema*, algo depositado, de *tithēmi*, colocar]

ap·ox·e·sis (ap - ok - sē'sis). Curetagem subgengival. SIN subgingival *curettage*. [G. *apo*, fora, + *xeein*, raspar]

ap·o·zem, apoz·e·ma (ap'ō - zem, ap - oz'ē - mă). Apózema, decocção. SIN decoction. [apo- + G. *zema*, algo fervido]

ap·pa·ra·tus (ap - ă - ra'tus). Aparelho. **1.** Uma coleção de instrumentos adaptados para uma finalidade especial. **2.** Um instrumento feito de várias partes. **3** [TA]. Um grupo ou sistema de glândulas, canais, vasos sanguíneos, músculos ou outras estruturas anatômicas envolvido na realização de alguma função. VER TAMBÉM system. [L. equipamento, de *ap-paro*, pp. -*atus*, preparar]
accessory visual a., a. visual acessório. SIN accessory visual *structures,* em structure.
achromatic a., a. acromático; ásteres não-coráveis e fibras fusiformes em uma célula em divisão.
alimentary a., a. alimentar. SIN alimentary *system*.
attachment a., a. de fixação; os tecidos que fixam o dente no processo alveolar: cemento, membrana periodontal e osso alveolar.
Barcroft-Warburg a., a. de Bancroft-Warburg. SIN Warburg a.
Beckmann a., a. de Beckmann; a. para a medição exata dos pontos de fusão e pontos de ebulição em conexão com as determinações do peso molecular.
Benedict-Roth a., a. de Benedict-Roth; um aparelho empregado para medir o volume de oxigênio utilizado na respiração tranqüila, no estado basal, para a estimativa da taxa metabólica basal; a pessoa reinala o oxigênio através da soda

cáustica de um espirômetro de registro.
branchial a., a. branquial; o agregado de arcos, bolsas, fendas e membranas faríngeos, observado no embrião de vertebrados em desenvolvimento.
central a., a. central; o centrossoma e a centrosfera.
chromatic a., a. cromático; a massa intensamente corada de cromossomas em uma célula em divisão.
chromidial a., a. cromidial; o agregado da rede extranuclear, filamentos irregulares e massas de material basofílico que permeia o protoplasma da célula. VER TAMBÉM ribosome, endoplasmic *reticulum*.
dental a., a. dentário. SIN masticatory *system*.
digestive a., a. digestivo. SIN alimentary *system*.
digesto'rius, a. digestivo. SIN alimentary *system*.
genitourinary a., a. genitourinário. SIN urogenital *system*.
Golgi a., a. de Golgi; um sistema membranáceo de cisternas e vesículas localizado entre o núcleo e o pólo secretor ou superfície de uma célula; relacionado com o revestimento e transporte intracelular de proteínas secretoras ligadas à membrana, e à síntese de polissacarídeos e glicoproteínas. SIN dictyosome, Golgi body, Golgi complex, Golgi internal reticulum, Holmgrén-Golgi canals.
Haldane a., a. de Haldane; um dispositivo empregado para a análise dos gases respiratórios.
hyoid a., a. hióide; um termo de anatomia veterinária para os ossos hióides, uma porção modificada do antigo esqueleto branquial consistindo em uma cadeia articulada de ossos que se estende desde a região mastóidea do crânio, em ambos os lados, até a base da língua; nos seres humanos, é reduzido a um único osso, o hióide; em um mamífero típico (o cão), consiste em uma cartilagem tímpano-hióidea, presa ao crânio, seguida pelos ossos estilo-hióideo, epihióideo, cerato-hióideo, basi-hióideo e tireo-hióideo. SIN a. hyoideus.
a. hyoi'deus, a. hióideo. SIN hyoid a.
juxtaglomerular a., a. justaglomerular. SIN juxtaglomerular *complex*.
Kirschner a., fio de Kirschner. SIN Kirschner *wire*.
Kjeldahl a., a de Kjeldahl; um a. para destilar amônia que se origina da decomposição ácida de um composto orgânico. Usado em análise de nitrogênio.
lacrimal a. [TA], a. lacrimal; consistindo na glândula lacrimal, lago lacrimal, canais lacrimais, saco lacrimal e ducto nasolacrimal. SIN a. lacrimalis [TA].
a. lacrima'lis [TA], a. lacrimal. SIN lacrimal a.
a. ligamento'sus col'li, ligamento nucal. SIN *ligamentum nuchae*.
a. ligamento'sus weitbrecht'i, a. ligamentoso de Weitbrecht, membrana tectória (da articulação atlantoaxial mediana) SIN tectorial *membrane* (of median atlantoaxial joint).
masticatory a., a. mastigador; (**1**) SIN masticatory *system*; (**2**) SIN stomatognathic *system*.
mental a., a. mental; estrutura mental que consiste em pensamentos, sentimentos, cognições e memórias; em psicanálise, a estrutura topográfica da mente.
pyriform a., a. piriforme; uma estrutura em forma de pêra na casca de ovo de determinadas tênias (família Anoplocephalidae), de função indeterminada.
a. respirato'rius, a. respiratório. SIN respiratory *system*.
respiratory a., a. respiratório. SIN respiratory *system*.
Roughton-Scholander a., a. de Roughton-Scholander; um dispositivo semelhante a uma seringa para analisar os gases respiratórios em uma pequena amostra de sangue. SIN Roughton-Scholander syringe.
Scholander a., a. de Scholander; um dispositivo empregado para determinar o percentual de oxigênio e dióxido de carbono em 0,5 ml de um gás respiratório.
subneural a., a. subneural; sarcoplasma modificado em uma placa terminal motora.
a. suspenso'rius len'tis, zônula ciliar. SIN cilliary *zonule*.
Taylor a., a. de Taylor. SIN Taylor back *brace*.
Tiselius a., a. de Tiselius; um a. para separar proteínas em solução por eletroforese e, dessa maneira, para determinar o ponto isoelétrico, peso molecular e propriedades físicas correlatas; a direção e a taxa de migração da proteína e as características da fase limitante entre a solução de proteína e a solução de sal sobrenadante são registrados por fotografia das alterações no índice de refração na fase limitante.
urinary a., a. urinário. SIN urinary *system*.
urogenital a., a. urogenital. SIN urogenital *system*.
a. urogenita'lis, a. urogenital. SIN urogenital *system*.
Van Slyke a., a. de Van Slyke; um a. para determinar as quantidades de gases respiratórios no sangue.
vestibular a., a. vestibular; o órgão receptor da porção vestibular do 8.º nervo craniano, consistindo em três canais semicirculares e no otólito, localizado dentro da porção petrosa do osso temporal do crânio.
Warburg a., a. de Warburg; um a. para medir o consumo de oxigênio de fatias de tecido incubado por mensuração manométrica das alterações na pressão de gás produzidas pela absorção de oxigênio em um frasco fechado. SIN Barcroft-Warburg a.
ap·par·ent (ă - păr'ent). Aparente. **1.** Manifesto; óbvio; evidente; p.ex., uma infecção clinicamente a. **2.** Freqüentemente usado (de forma errada) para significar "parecendo com", ostensível, pseudo-. [L. *apparens*, visível, de *appareo*, vir à luz]

ap·pend·age (ă - pen'dij). Apêndice; qualquer parte, subordinada em função ou tamanho, presa a uma estrutura principal. VER TAMBÉM accessory *structures*, em *structure*. SIN appendix (1). [L. *appendix*]
atrial a., a. atrial. SIN auricles (of atria), em *auricle*.
auricular a., a. auricular; (**1**) SIN right *auricle*; (**2**) um pequeno apêndice cutâneo congênito geralmente localizado anterior ao trago do ouvido, freqüentemente chamado de um apêndice cutâneo; mais amiúde unilateral que bilateral.
drumstick a., a. em baqueta de tambor; um a. do núcleo que representa o cromossoma X heterocromático inativo observado em 3% dos leucócitos neutrófilos do sexo feminino humano. VER sex *chromatin*, lyonization.
epiploic a., a. epiplóico. SIN omental *appendices*, em *appendix*.
a.'s of eye, apêndices dos olhos. SIN accessory visual *structures*, em *structure*.
a.'s of fetus, a. do feto; âmnio, saco vitelino e a parte fetal (coriônica) da placenta, juntamente com o cordão umbilical.
left auricular a., a. do átrio esquerdo. SIN left *auricle*.
right auricular a., a. do átrio direito. SIN right *auricle*.
a.'s of skin. apêndices da pele; os pêlos, unhas e glândulas sudoríparas, sebáceas e mamárias.
testicular a., a. testicular. SIN *appendix* of testis.
uterine a.'s, apêndices uterinos; os ovários, trompas uterinas (de Falópio) e os ligamentos associados. SIN adnexa uteri.
vermiform a., a. vermiforme. SIN appendix (2).
vesicular a.'s of epoophoron [TA], apêndices vesiculares do epoóforo; um pequeno cisto cheio de líquido ligado a um pedículo fino na extremidade fimbriada da trompa uterina; um resquício vestigial do ducto mesonéfrico embrionário. SIN appendix vesiculosa [TA], Morgagni hydatid, morgagnian cyst, stalked hydatid, vesicular appendices of uterine tube.
ap·pen·dal·gia (ap - pen - dal'jē - ă). Apendalgia; termo obsoleto para a dor no quadrante inferior direito do abdome, na região do apêndice vermiforme. [apêndice + G. *algos*, dor]
ap·pen·dec·to·my (ap - pen - dek'tō - mē). Apendectomia; remoção cirúrgica do apêndice vermiforme. SIN appendicectomy. [apêndice + G. *ektome*, excisão]
auricular a., a. auricular; excisão do apêndice auricular de um átrio, usualmente o esquerdo.
ap·pen·di·cal (ă - pen'di - kăl) Apendicular. SIN appendiceal.
ap·pen·dic·e·al (ă - pen - dis'ē - ăl). Apendicular; relativo a um apêndice. SIN appendical.
ap·pen·di·cec·ta·sis (ap - pen - di - sek'tă - sis). Apendicectasia; ectasia do apêndice.
ap·pen·di·cec·to·my (ap - pen - di - sek'tō - mē). Apendicectomia. SIN appendectomy.
ap·pen·di·cism (ă - pen'di - sizm). Apendicismo; termo raramente utilizado para qualquer doença crônica do apêndice vermiforme ou um mal-estar sintomático nessa área.
ap·pen·di·ci·tis (ă - pen - di - sī'tis). Apendicite; inflamação do apêndice vermiforme. [apêndice + G. *-itis*, inflamação]
actinomycotic a., a. actinomicótica; a. supurativa crônica devido à infecção por *Actinomyces israelii*.
acute a., a. aguda; inflamação aguda do apêndice, geralmente causada por infecção bacteriana, a qual pode ser precipitada pela obstrução da luz por um fecalito; os sintomas variáveis, freqüentemente consistindo em dor periumbilical em cólica e vômitos, podem ser seguidos por febre, leucocitose, dor persistente e sinais de irritação peritoneal no quadrante inferior direito do abdome; a perfuração ou formação de abscesso são complicações freqüentes da intervenção cirúrgica tardia.
bilharzial a., a. esquistossomótica; a. causada pela deposição de ovos de *Schistosoma mansoni* no apêndice vermiforme.
chronic a., a. crônica; aderências fibrosas, fibrose ou deformidade do apêndice depois da diminuição da a. aguda; a obliteração fibrosa da luz distal não é anormal em pessoas idosas; termo freqüentemente utilizado em referência às repetidas crises brandas de a. aguda.
focal a., a. focal; a. aguda envolvendo apenas parte do apêndice, por vezes no local de uma obstrução da luz ou distalmente a esta.
foreign-body a., a. por corpo estranho; a. causada por obstrução da luz do apêndice por uma substância estranha, como um corpo estranho particulado.
gangrenous a., a. gangrenosa; a. aguda com necrose da parede do apêndice, desenvolvendo-se mais amiúde na a. obstrutiva e causando, com freqüência, perfuração e peritonite aguda.
left-sided a., a. do lado esquerdo; a. que ocorre no lado esquerdo do abdome, geralmente no quadrante inferior esquerdo, devido à rotação anormal do intestino (como no *situs inversus*).
lumbar a., a. lombar; a. aguda em um apêndice retrodisposto na região lombar.
obstructive a., a. obstrutiva; a. aguda decorrente da infecção da secreção retida por trás de uma obstrução da luz por um fecalito ou alguma outra causa, incluindo o carcinoma do ceco.
perforating a., a. perfurante; inflamação do apêndice levando à perfuração da parede do apêndice para a cavidade peritoneal, resultando em peritonite.

recurrent a., a. recorrente; episódios recorrentes de dor abdominal no quadrante inferior direito atribuídos à recorrência da inflamação do apêndice em um indivíduo que não sofreu uma apendicectomia para os episódios anteriores. SIN relapsing a.

relapsing a., a. recidivante. SIN recurrent a.

stercoral a., a. estercoral; a. após o alojamento de material fecal no apêndice.

subperitoneal a., a. subperitoneal; a. de um apêndice com localização subperitoneal.

suppurative a., a. supurativa; a. aguda com exsudato purulento na luz e parede do apêndice.

verminous a., a. verminosa; a. causada por obstrução ou resposta a vermes parasitas, como *Ascaris lumbricoides*, *Strongyloides stercoralis* ou o oxiúro *Enterobius vermicularis*.

appendico-. Apendico-; um apêndice, geralmente o apêndice vermiforme. [L. *appendix*, *appendicis* um apêndice, de *appendo*, pendurar algo em alguma coisa, de *ad-*, *ap-*, para, em, + *pendo*, pendurar, + -o-]

ap·pen·di·co·cele (ă-pen'di-kō-sēl). Apendicocele; o apêndice vermiforme em um saco herniário. [appendico- + G. *kēlē*, hérnia]

ap·pen·di·co·lith (ă-pen'di-kō-lith). Apendicolito; uma concreção calcificada no apêndice visível em uma radiografia abdominal; considerado diagnóstico de apendicite no abdome agudo. [appendico- + G. *lithos*, pedra]

ap·pen·di·co·li·thi·a·sis (ă-pen'di-kō-li-thī'ă-sis). Apendicolitíase; a presença de concreções no apêndice vermiforme. [appendico- + G. *lithos*, pedra]

ap·pen·di·col·y·sis (ă-pen-di-kol'i-sis). Apendicólise; operação para liberar o apêndice de suas aderências. [appendico- + G. *lysis*, um afrouxamento]

ap·pen·di·cos·to·my (ă-pen-di-kos'tō-mē). Apendicostomia; cirurgia para abrir o intestino através da extremidade do apêndice vermiforme, previamente preso à parede abdominal anterior. [appendico- + G. *stoma*, boca]

ap·pen·di·co·ves·i·cos·to·my (ă-pen-di-kō'ves'ĭ-kos-tō-mē). Apendicovesicostomia; uso de um apêndice isolado em um pedículo vascularizado como uma via de acesso cateterizável para a bexiga a partir da pele. VER TAMBÉM Mitrofanoff *principle*. [appendico- + L. *vesica*, bexiga, + G. *stoma*, boca]

ap·pen·dic·u·lar (ap'en-dik'ŭ-lăr). Apendicular. **1.** Relativo a um apêndice ou anexo. **2.** Relativo aos membros, em oposição a axial, que se refere ao tronco e cabeça.

ap·pen·dix, gen. **ap·pen·di·cis**, pl. **ap·pen·di·ces** (ă-pen'diks, -di-sis, -di-sēs). Apêndice. **1.** SIN appendage. **2** [TA]. Um divertículo intestinal vermiforme que se estende a partir da extremidade cega do ceco; ele varia em comprimento e termina em uma extremidade cega. SIN a. vermiformis [TA], a. ceci, processus vermiformis, vermiform appendage, vermiform a., vermiform process, vermix. [L. apêndice, de *ap-pendo*, pendurar algo em]

appendices adiposae coli, apêndices adiposos do cólon; *termo oficial alternativo para omental appendices.

auricular a., a. auricular. SIN *auricles* (of atria), em *auricle*.

a. ce'ci, a. cecal. SIN appendix (2).

a. epididym'idis [TA], a. do epidídimo. SIN a. of epydidimis.

a. of epididymidis, a do epidídimo; um pequeno corpo pedunculado, freqüentemente preso à cabeça do epidídimo, constituindo um vestígio do duto mesonéfrico embrionário. SIN a. epididymidis [TA], pedunculated hydatid.

epiploic a., a. adiposo do cólon. SIN omental appendices.

a. epiplo'ica, pl. **appen'dices epiplo'icae,** a. adiposo do cólon. SIN omental appendices.

fatty appendices of cólon, apêndices adiposos do cólon; *termo oficial alternativo para omental appendices.

a. fibro'sa hep'atis [TA], a. hepático fibroso. SIN fibrous a. of liver.

fibrous a. of liver [TA], a. hepático fibroso; um processo fibroso, no qual a extremidade do lobo esquerdo do fígado pode afilar-se, que passa com o ligamento triangular esquerdo para se inserir no diafragma. SIN a. fibrosa hepatis [TA].

Morgagni a., a. de Morgagni, lobo piramidal da glândula tireóide. SIN pyramidal *lobe* of thyroid gland.

omental appendices [TA], a. adiposos do cólon; inúmeros processos ou sacos pequenos do peritônio cheios de tecido adiposo e que se projetam a partir do revestimento seroso do intestino grosso, exceto no reto; são mais evidentes sobre o cólon transverso e sigmóide, sendo mais numerosos ao longo da borda livre. SIN appendices omentales [TA], appendices adiposae coli*, fatty appendices of colon*, a. epiploica, epiploic appendage, epiploic a., epiploic tags.

appendices omentales [TA], a. adiposo do cólon. SIN omental appendices.

a. tes'tis [TA], a. do testículo. SIN a. of testis.

a. of the testis, a. do testículo. SIN a. of testis.

a. of testis, a. do testículo; uma estrutura vesicular apedunculada fixada ao pólo cefálico do testículo; um vestígio da extremidade cefálica do duto paramesonéfrico (mülleriano) SIN a. testis [TA], a. of the testis, nonpedunculated hydatid, ovarium masculinum, sessile hydatid, testicular appendage.

a. ventric'uli laryn'gis, sáculo da laringe. SIN laryngeal *saccule*.

vermiform a., a. vermiforme. SIN appendix (2).

a. vermifor'mis [TA], a. vermiforme. SIN appendix (2).

vesicular appendices of uterine tube, apêndices vesiculosos do epoóforo. SIN vesicular *appendages* of epoophoron, em *appendage*.

a. vesiculo'sa, pl. **appen'dices vesiculo'sae** [TA], apêndices vesiculosos do epoóforo. SIN vesicular *appendages* of epoophoron, em *appendage*.

ap·per·cep·tion (ap-er-sep'shŭn). Apercepção. **1.** O estágio final da percepção consciente em que algo é claramente aprendido e, dessa maneira, é relativamente proeminente na consciência; a apreensão plena de qualquer conteúdo psíquico. **2.** O processo de referir a percepção de idéias para a personalidade da própria pessoa. [L. *ad*, para, + *per- cipio*, pp. *-ceptus*, tomar completamente, preencher]

ap·per·cep·tive (ap-er-sep'tiv). Aperceptivo; relativo a, envolvido em, ou capaz da apercepção.

ap·per·son·a·tion, ap·per·son·i·fi·ca·tion (ă-per'sō-nā'shŭn, ap-er-son'i-fi-kā'shŭn). Apersonação, apersonificação; uma ilusão em que alguém assume o caráter de outra pessoa.

ap·pe·stat (ap'e-stat). O mecanismo no cérebro (possivelmente no hipotálamo) relacionado com o apetite e controle da ingestão de alimento. [apetite + G. *statos*, de pé]

ap·pe·tite (ap'ĕ-tīt). Apetite; um desejo ou motivo derivado de uma necessidade biológica ou psicológica para alimento, água, sexo ou afeição; desejo ou ânsia de satisfazer qualquer necessidade física ou mental consciente. SIN orexia (2). [L. *ad-peto*, pp. *-petitus*, tentar alcançar, desejar]

ap·pla·na·tion (ap'lan-ā'shŭn). Aplanação; em tonometria, o achatamento da córnea por pressão. A pressão intra-ocular é diretamente proporcional à pressão externa e inversamente proporcional à área achatada. VER TAMBÉM applanation *tonometer*. [L. *ad*, no sentido de, + *planum*, plano]

ap·pla·nom·e·try (ap-lan-om'ĕ-trē). Aplanometria; o uso de um tonômetro de aplanação.

ap·ple oil. Amil valerato. SIN amyl valerate.

ap·pli·ance (ă-plī'ans). Dispositivo; um dispositivo empregado para melhorar a função de uma parte ou para fins terapêuticos. [do, Fr. Ant. *aplier*, aplicar, do L. *applico*, dobrar junto]

craniofacial a., d. craniofacial; um dispositivo empregado para imobilizar e/ou reduzir fraturas de mandíbula ou mediofaciais. VER TAMBÉM fixation.

edgewise a., um d. ortodôntico fixo, com múltiplas faixas, usando um braço de fixação cuja ranhura recebe um fio dentário retangular horizontalmente, permitindo o controle preciso do movimento dentário em todos os três planos espaciais.

extraoral fracture a., d. extra-oral de fraturas; um d. empregado para a redução e fixação extra-orais de fraturas da maxila ou mandíbula, no qual pinos, grampos ou parafusos, interligados por conectores metálicos ou de acrílico, são utilizados para alinhar os segmentos fraturados. VER TAMBÉM external pin *fixation*.

Hawley a., d. de Hawley. SIN Hawley *retainer*.

intraoral fracture a., d. intra-oral de fraturas; um dispositivo metálico ou de acrílico fixado aos dentes por guia ou cimento; usado para imobilizar fraturas da maxila e mandíbula.

labiolingual a., d. labiolingual; um d. que consiste em um fio em arco labial maxilar e um fio em arco lingual mandibular.

light wire a., um d. ortodôntico que utiliza pequenos fios labiais chanfrados, com alças de expansão e contração integradas, presos por ligaduras adaptadas a cada dente; por vezes chamado de técnica de força diferencial de fio fino de Begg.

obturator a., d. obturador; um d. utilizado para obliterar defeitos congênitos ou adquiridos do palato e estruturas circunvizinhas, geralmente feito de acrílico ou borracha.

orthodontic a., d. ortodôntico; um mecanismo para a aplicação da força aos dentes e seus tecidos de sustentação para produzir alterações na relação dos dentes e/ou estruturas ósseas correlatas.

ribbon arch a., um d. que consiste em um fio retangular inserido em um suporte especialmente idealizado preso às superfícies labial e bucal dos dentes.

Roger Anderson pin fixation a., d. de fixação com pino de Roger Anderson; um d. empregado na fixação extra-oral de fraturas mandibulares e correções de prognatismo, no qual os pinos colocados nos segmentos ósseos são unidos por bastonetes de conexão metálicos. VER TAMBÉM external pin *fixation*.

surgical a., d. cirúrgico; um d. metálico ou de plástico construído antes de uma cirurgia e usado para imobilizar ou suportar o tecido durante a fase pós-operatória.

universal a., d. universal; uma combinação das técnicas de perfil e de arco de borracha, conferindo o controle exato de cada dente em todos os planos espaciais.

applicand. Abreviatura para *applicandus*, a ser aplicado. [L.]

ap·pli·ca·tor (ap'li-kā-tōr). Aplicador; um bastonete fino de madeira, metal flexível ou material sintético, no qual, em uma extremidade, está preso um chumaço de algodão ou outra substância para fazer aplicações locais a qualquer superfície acessível. [L. *ap-plico*, acoplar]

ap·po·si·tion (ap-ō-zish'ŭn). Aposição. **1.** A colocação em contato de duas substâncias. **2.** A condição de ser colocado ou ajustado. **3.** A relação dos fragmentos de uma fratura entre si. **4.** O processo de espessamento da parede celular. [L. *ap-pono*, pp. *-positus*, colocar em ou justapor]

bayonet a., a. em baioneta; a relação de dois fragmentos de fratura que se situam próximos entre si, em vez de estarem em contato término-terminal.

ap·proach (ă-prōch′). Abordagem. **1.** Em psiquiatria, um termo empregado para descrever como são negociadas as relações interpessoais. **2.** O trajeto ou método empregado para expor o campo cirúrgico durante uma cirurgia. [I.M., do Fr. Ant., de L.L. *appropio*, ficar mais próximo, de *ad*, para + *propius*, mais próximo]

facial recess a., a. do recesso facial; uma a. cirúrgica para o ouvido médio, a partir da mastóide, através do recesso lateral ao canal do nervo facial.

idiographic a., a. idiográfica; o estudo abrangente de um indivíduo como uma base para a compreensão do comportamento humano em geral.

infratemporal a., a. infratemporal; a. cirúrgica da base do crânio e seu conteúdo a partir da parte inferior do osso temporal.

middle fossa a. a. da fossa média; a. cirúrgica para o ângulo pontocerebelar através da porção do assoalho da fossa média do crânio correspondente à superfície anterior da pirâmide petrosa do osso temporal.

nomothetic a., a. nomotética; uma estrutura de referência psicológica que tenta fornecer normas e princípios gerais de comportamento pelo estudo de grupos.

posterior fossa a., a. da fossa posterior; a. cirúrgica para o ângulo pontocerebelar através do processo mastóideo do osso temporal.

regressive-reconstructive a., a. regressivo-reconstrutiva; uma forma de psicoterapia em que a regressão, a fim de fazer ressurgir algum trauma psíquico original, é uma parte integrante do tratamento.

retrosigmoid a., a. retrossigmóide; uma a. cirúrgica do ângulo pontocerebelar através do osso occipital, posterior ao seio sigmóide.

transcochlear a., a. transcoclear; uma a. cirúrgica para o canal auditivo interno através da cóclea.

translabyrinthine a., a. translabiríntica; a. cirúrgica do ângulo pontocerebelar através do ouvido interno.

ap·prox·i·mate (ă-prok′si-māt). Aproximar; colocar junto. Em odontologia: **1.** Aproximar, indicando as superfícies de contato, quer mesiais, quer distais, de dois dentes adjacentes. **2.** Colocar junto; indicando o dente na mandíbula humana, conforme diferenciado dos dentes separados em determinados animais inferiores. [L. *ad*, para + *proximus*, mais perto]

ap·prox·i·ma·tion (ă-prok-si-mā′shŭn). Aproximação; em cirurgia, colocar as bordas dos tecidos juntas na aposição desejada para a sutura.

steady state a., a. em equilíbrio dinâmico; uma suposição na derivação da expressão de uma taxa enzimática em que a velocidade de alteração da concentração de qualquer espécie de enzima é zero ou muito menor que d[P]/d*t*.

APR Abreviatura para abdominoperineal *resection* (ressecção abdominoperineal).

aprac·tag·no·sia (ā-prak-tag-nō′sē-ă). Apractagnosia. SIN constructional apraxia. [G. *a-* priv. + *praktea*, coisas a serem feitas, + *gnōsis*, reconhecimento]

aprac·tic (ă-prak′tik). Apráxico. SIN apraxic.

aprag·ma·tism (ă-prag′mă-tizm). Apragmatismo; um interesse na teoria ou dogmatismo em vez de nos resultados práticos. [G. *a-* priv. + pragmatismo]

aprax·ia (ă-prak′sē-ă). Apraxia. **1.** Um distúrbio do movimento voluntário, consistindo no comprometimento no desempenho de movimentos intencionais, não obstante a preservação da compreensão, força muscular, sensibilidade e coordenação em geral; decorrente da doença cerebral adquirida. **2.** Um defeito psicomotor em que o uso correto de um objeto não pode ser efetuado, embora o objeto possa ser nomeado e seus usos descritos. [G. *a-*, priv. + *prattō*, fazer]

constructional a., a. de construção; a. manifestada como um comprometimento na atividade, como construir, reunir e desenhar; causada por lesões do lobo parietal. SIN apractagnosia.

cortical a., a. cortical, a. motora. SIN motor a.

gait a., a. da marcha; a. para caminhar, acompanhada por incapacidade de fazer os movimentos de deambulação com as pernas.

ideokinetic a., ideomotor a., a. ideocinética, a. ideomotora; uma forma de a. em que atos simples são incapazes de serem realizados, provavelmente porque as conexões entre os centros corticais que controlam a volição e o córtex motor estão interrompidas. SIN transcortical a.

innervation a., a. motora. SIN motor a.

limb-kinetic a., a. motora. SIN motor a.

motor a., a. motora; incapacidade de fazer os movimentos ou de usar objetos para a finalidade pretendida. SIN cortical a., innervation a., limb-kinetic a.

ocular motor a., a. oculomotora; incapacidade congênita de iniciar os movimentos sacádicos horizontais. As crianças com essa condição freqüentemente movem bruscamente a cabeça para olhar para a esquerda ou direita.

transcortical a., a. transcortical, a. ideocinética. SIN ideokinetic a.

verbal a., a. verbal; distúrbio da fala em que as substituições de fonema são constantemente utilizadas para a sílaba ou palavra desejada.

aprax·ic (ă-prak′sik). Apráxico; marcado por ou pertinente à apraxia. SIN apractic.

ap·ri·cot ker·nel oil (ā′pri-kot). Óleo de semente de damasco. VER persic oil.

aproc·tia (ā-prok′shē-ă). Aproctia; ausência congênita ou imperfuração do ânus. [G. *a-* priv. + *prōktos*, ânus]

ap·ro·fen, ap·ro·fene, ap·ro·phen (ap′rō-fen, ap′rō-fēn, ap′rō-fen). Aprofeno; analgésico e antiespasmódico.

apros·o·dy (ă-pros′ō-dē). Aprosodia; ausência, na fala, do timbre, do ritmo e das variações de ênfase normais. [G. *a-* priv. + *prosōdia*, modulação da voz]

ap·ro·so·pia (ap-rō-sō′pē-ă). Aprosopia; ausência congênita da porção maior ou totalidade da face, usualmente associada a outras malformações. [G. *a-* priv. + *prosōpon*, face]

apro·ti·nin (ă-prō′ti-nin). Aprotinina; um inibidor da protease e calicreína obtido a partir de órgãos de animais; um polipeptídeo com um peso molecular de aproximadamente 6.000. Pode ser útil no tratamento da pancreatite e na prevenção do sangramento após a cirurgia envolvendo derivação (*bypass*) cardiopulmonar.

APS Abreviatura para adenosine 5′-phosphosulfate (5′-fosfossulfato de adenosina).

6-APS Abreviatura para 6-aminopenicillanic acid (ácido 6-aminopenicilânico).

aPTT Abreviatura para activated partial thromboplastin *time* (tempo de tromboplastina parcial ativada).

APUD Designação proposta para um grupo de células em diferentes órgãos, as quais secretam hormônios polipeptídicos ou neurotransmissores. As células nesse grupo possuem determinadas características bioquímicas em comum, cujas primeiras letras formam o nome: elas contêm *a*minas, como catecolamina e 5-hidroxitriptamina; captam precursores dessas aminas *in vivo* e contêm descarboxilase de aminoácidos. [*a*mine precursor *u*ptake, *d*ecarboxilase]

apu·rin·ic ac·id (ă-pū-rin′ik). Ácido apurínico; DNA do qual as bases de purina foram removidas por tratamento com ácido brando.

apyk·no·mor·phous (ă-pik-nō-mōr′fŭs). Apicnomorfo; indica uma célula ou outra estrutura que não se cora profundamente porque o material corável ou cromófilo não está bem agregado. [G. *a-* priv. + *pyknos*, espesso, + *morphē*, forma]

ap·y·rase (ă-pī′rās). Apirase; uma enzima que catalisa a remoção hidrolítica de dois resíduos ortofosfato da 5′-trifosfato de adenosina para fornecer 5′-monofosfato de adenosina; isto é, $ATP + 2 H_2O \rightarrow AMP + 2 P_i$. SIN ADPase, ATP-diphosphatase.

apy·ret·ic (ā-pī-ret′ik). Apirético. SIN afebrile.

apy·rex·ia (ā-pī-rek′sē-ă). Apirexia; ausência de febre. [G. *a-* priv. + *pirexis*, febre]

apy·rex·i·al (ā-pī-rek′sē-ăl). Apirético. SIN afebrile.

apy·rim·i·din·ic ac·id (ă-pī′rim-i-din′ik). Ácido apirimidínico; DNA do qual as bases pirimidínicas foram retiradas por tratamento químico (p.ex., exposição à hidrazina).

aq. Abreviatura para L. *acqua*, água.

aq. bull. Abreviatura para L. *aqua bulliens*, água fervente.

aq. dest. Abreviatura para L. *aqua destillata*, água destilada.

aq. ferv. Abreviatura para L. *aqua fervens*, água fervendo.

aq. frig. Abreviatura para L. *aqua frigida*, água fria.

aq·ua, gen. e pl. **aq·uae** (ak′wă, ah′kwah). Água; H_2O. As águas farmacêuticas, aquae, são soluções aquosas de substâncias voláteis (p.ex., água-de-rosas). As soluções farmacêuticas são soluções aquosas de substâncias não-voláteis. VER water (3), solution (3). [L.]

a. re′gia, a. rega′lis, a. - régia. SIN nitrohydrochloric acid. [L. água real, assim chamada por sua capacidade de dissolver o ouro]

aq·ua·co·bal·a·min (ak′wă-kō-bal′ă-min). Aquacobalamina; vitamina B_{12a} (tautomérica com a B_{12b}); um derivado da cobalamina em que a sexta ligação coordenada do íon cobáltico está ligada a uma molécula de água. VER TAMBÉM *vitamin* B_{12}. SIN aquocobalamin.

aq·ua·pho·bia (ak-wă-fō′bē-ă). Aquafobia; temor mórbido da água. [L. *aqua*, água, + G. *phobos*, medo]

aq·ua·punc·ture (ak-wă-pŭnk′chŭr). Aquapuntura; termo raramente utilizado para uma injeção hipodérmica de água. [L. *aqua*, água, + *punctura*, punção]

Aq·ua·spi·ril·lum (ah-kwah-spī-ril′ŭm). Um gênero de bactérias aeróbicas, móveis, não-formadoras de esporos (família Spirillaceae), Gram-negativas, com curvatura helicoidal ou helicoidais, rígidas, com 0,2 a 1,5 μm de diâmetro. As células móveis contêm fascículos de flagelos em um ou ambos os pólos. Algumas espécies conseguem crescer em anaerobiose com nitrato, em lugar do oxigênio, como o aceptor de elétron terminal. Esses microrganismos são químio-organotrópicos, possuindo um metabolismo estritamente respiratório. Elas não fermentam carboidratos; algumas espécies conseguem oxidar uma gama limitada de carboidratos. O *habitat* desses microrganismos é a água doce. A espécie protótipo é *A. serpens*. [L. *aqua*, água, + *spirillum*, mola]

aquat·ic (ă-kwat′ik). Aquático. **1.** De ou pertinente à água. **2.** Indica um organismo que vive na água.

aq·ue·duct (ak′we-dŭkt). Aqueduto; um conduto ou canal. SIN aqueductus. [L. *aquaeductus*]

cerebral a., a. do mesencéfalo; um canal revestido de epêndima no mesencé-

falo com cerca de 20 mm de comprimento, ligando entre si o terceiro e quarto ventrículos. SIN aqueductus mesencephali [TA], aqueductus cerebri*, a. of cerebrum, aqueductus sylvii, iter a tertio ad quartum ventriculum, sylvian a.
a. of cerebrum, a. do mesencéfalo. SIN cerebral a.
cochlear a. [TA], a. da cóclea; um canal delicado, no osso temporal, que se abre acima para o canal timpânico, unindo o espaço perilinfático da cóclea com o espaço subaracnóide. SIN aqueductus cochleae [TA], ductus perilymphaticus, perilymphatic duct.
Cotunnius a., a. do vestíbulo. SIN vestibular a.
fallopian a., canal do nervo facial. SIN facial canal.
sylvian a., a. do mesencéfalo. SIN cerebral a.
vestibular a. [TA], a. do vestíbulo; um canal ósseo que sai do vestíbulo e desemboca na superfície posterior da porção petrosa do osso temporal, dando passagem ao ducto endolinfático e a uma pequena veia. SIN aqueductus vestibuli [TA], aqueductus cotunnii, Cotunnius a., Cotunnius canal.

aq·ue·duc·tus (ak-we-dŭk′tŭs). Aqueduto. SIN aqueduct. [L. de *aqua*, água, + *ductus*, um canal, de *duco*, pp. *ductus*, levar]
a. cer′ebri [alt. ofic.], a. do mesencéfalo; *termo oficial alternativo para cerebral *aqueduct.*
a. coch′leae [TA], a. da cóclea. SIN cochlear *aqueduct.*
a. cotun′nii [TA], a. do vestíbulo. SIN vestibular *aqueduct.*
a. fallo′pii, canal do nervo facial. SIN facial *canal.*
a. mesencephali, a. mesencefálico. SIN cerebral *aqueduct.*
a. syl′vii, a. do mesencéfalo. SIN cerebral *aqueduct.*
a. vestib′uli [TA], [NA] a. do vestíbulo. SIN vestibular *aqueduct.*

aque·ous (ak-we-ŭs, ā′kwē-ŭs). Aquoso; de, semelhante a ou que contém água.
aquip·ar·ous (ā-kwip′er-ŭs). Que secreta ou excreta um líquido aquoso. [L. *aqua*, água, + *pario*, parir]
aq·uo·co·bal·a·min (ak′wō-kō-bal′ă-min). Aquocobalamina. SIN aquacobalamin.
aq·uo·i·on (ak′wō-ī′on). Um íon hidratado; um íon que contém uma ou mais moléculas de água; p.ex., $Cu(H_2O)_4^{2+}$.
aquos·i·ty (ă-kwos′i-tē). Aquosidade. 1. O estado de ser aquoso. 2. Umidade.
Ar Símbolo do argônio.
Ara Símbolo para arabinose, ou seu mono- ou dirradical.
ara-. Prefixo para arabinose ou arabinosil.
arab-. Forma combinante para goma arábica; substâncias viscosas semelhantes. [G. *Araps, Arabos*, um árabe]
ar·a·ban (a′ră-ban). Arabana; um polissacarídeo que fornece arabinose na hidrólise; um constituinte de algumas pectinas.
ar·a·bic (a′ră-bik). Arábico; relativo a ou derivado de várias espécies de *Acacia* que possuem um exsudato viscoso ou resinoso.
ar·a·bic ac·id. Ácido arábico. SIN arabin.
ar·a·bin (a′ră-bin). Arabina; uma goma de carboidrato que hidrolisa a D-arabinose e hexoses, encontrada naturalmente em união com íons de cálcio, potássio e magnésio, sendo então chamada de goma arábica. SIN arabic acid.
ar·a·bi·no·a·den·o·sine (a′ră-bin-ō-ah-den′ō-sēn). Arabinoadenosina. SIN arabinosyladenine.
ar·a·bi·no·cy·ti·dine (a′ră-bin-ō-sī′ti-dēn). Arabinocitidina. SIN arabinosylcytosine.
ara·bin·o·fur·a·no·syl·ad·e·nine (a′ră-bin-ō-foor′ă-nō-sil-ad′ĕ-nēn) Arabinofuranosiladenina; um arabinosídeo que possui atividade antiviral.
ar·a·bi·no·fu·ra·no·syl·cy·to·sine (a′ră-bin-ō-foor′ă-nō-sil-sī′tō-sēn). Arabinofuranosilcitosina. SIN arabinosylcytosine.
arab·i·nose (Ara) (ă-rab′i-nōs, a′ră-bin-ōs). Arabinose; uma pentose; seus dois enantiômeros estão amplamente distribuídos em vegetais, geralmente em polissacarídeos complexos; usada em meios de cultura. O D-A é um epímero da D-ribose. [arabina + -ose (1)]
a. 5-phosphate, 5-fosfato de a.; uma a. fosforilada que é um intermediário na via da pentose fosfato.
a. 5-phosphate, 2-epimerase, 2-epimerase de 5-fosfato de a.; uma enzima na via da pentose fosfato que interconverte, de forma reversível, a a. e 5-fosfato de a.
ar·a·bi·no·side (ă-rab′i-nō-sīd). Arabinosídeo; um ribonucleotídeo em que a molécula de açúcar é a arabinose. Freqüentemente possui atividade antibiótica.
arab·i·no·sis (ă-rab-i-nō′sis). Arabinose; transtorno do metabolismo da arabinose.
ar·a·bi·no·su·ria (ă-rab′i-nō-soo′rē-ă). Arabinosúria; excreção de arabinose na urina.
ar·a·bi·no·syl·ad·e·nine (a′ră-bin-ō-sil-ă′den-ēn). Arabinosiladenina; usada para o herpes simples da córnea e na ceratite da vacínia. SIN arabinoadenosine.
ar·a·bi·no·syl·cy·to·sine (aC, araC) (a′ră-bin-ō-sil-sī′tō-sēn). Arabinosilcitosina; um composto de arabinose e citosina, análogo à ribosilcitosina (citidina), que inibe a biossíntese do DNA; usado como agente quimioterápico por causa das propriedades antiviral e de inibição do crescimento tumoral. SIN arabinocytidine, arabinofuranosylcitosine, cytarabine.

arab·i·tol (ă-rab′i-tol). Arabitol; um álcool de açúcar obtido da redução da arabinose.
AraC. Abreviatura para *cytosine* arabinoside (citosina arabinosídeo).
araC Símbolo de arabinosylcytosine (arabinosilcitosina).
arach·ic ac·id (ă-rak′ik). Ácido aráquico. SIN arachidic acid.
ar·a·chid·ic ac·id (a-ră-kid-ik). Ácido araquídico; um ácido graxo contido no óleo de amendoim, manteiga e outras gorduras. SIN arachic acid, *n*-eicosanoic acid, *n*-icosanoic acid. [*Arachis*, de G. *arakis*, planta leguminosa]
ar·a·chi·don·ic ac·id (ă-rak-i-don′ik). Ácido araquidônico; ácido 5,8,11,14-eicosatetraenóico (icosatetraenóico); um ácido graxo insaturado, geralmente essencial na nutrição; o precursor biológico das prostaglandinas, tromboxanos e leucotrienos (coletivamente conhecidos como eicosanóides).
ar·a·chi·don·ic ac·id cas·cade. Cascata do ácido araquidônico; via de síntese de eicosanóides.
ar·a·chis oil (ar′ă-kis). Óleo de amendoim. SIN peanut oil.
arach·ne·pho·bia (ă-rak-nē-fō′bē-ă). Aracnofobia; temor mórbido de aranhas. SIN arachnophobia. [G. *arachne*, aranha, + *phobos*, medo]
Arach·nia (ă-rak′nē-ă). Um gênero de bactérias imóveis, não-formadoras de esporos, anaeróbicas facultativas (família Actinomycetaceae) e que contêm bastonetes difteróides ramificados, Gram-positivos, não-álcool-ácido-resistentes (0,2–0,3 por 3,0–5,0 μm ou mais). Esses microrganismos produzem microcolônias filamentosas. Seu metabolismo é fermentativo. São produzidos basicamente ácidos propiônico e acético a partir da glicose. A catalase não é produzida. A parede celular contém ácido diaminopimélico, mas não arabinose. Esses microrganismos são patogênicos para os seres humanos, causando canaliculite lacrimal e actinomicose típica. A espécie protótipo é *A. propionica*.
A. propio′nica, uma espécie que causa canaliculite lacrimal e actinomicose típica; é a espécie protótipo do gênero *A.* SIN *Propionibacterium propionicus*.
Arach·ni·da (ă-rak′ni-dă). Aracnídeos; uma classe de artrópodos no subfilo Chelicerata, consistindo em aranhas, escorpiões, pernilongos, ácaros, carrapatos e correlatos. [G. *arachnē*, aranha]
arach·nid·ism (ă-rak′ni-dizm). Aracnidismo; intoxicação sistêmica após a picada de uma aranha (especialmente da viúva-negra).
necrotic a., a. necrótico; a. causado por aranhas que pertencem ao gênero *Loxosceles*; a necrose cutânea desenvolve-se no local da picada, com cura lenta e possível desfiguração.
arach·no·dac·ty·ly (ă-rak-nō-dak′ti-lē). Aracnodactilia; condição em que as mãos e os dedos das mãos, e, com freqüência, os pés e artelhos, são anormalmente longos e finos; uma característica da síndrome de Marfan [MIM*154700], da síndrome de Achard [MIM*100700], da síndrome MASS [MIM*157700] e de distúrbios hereditários correlatos do tecido conjuntivo. SIN spider finger. [G. *arachnē*, aranha, + *daktylos*, dedo]
arach·noid (ă-rak′noyd). Aracnóide-máter. SIN a. mater. [G. *arachnē*, aranha, + *eidos*, semelhança]
a. of brain, aracnóide-máter. SIN cranial a. mater.
cranial a. mater [TA], aracnóide-máter; a porção da a. que se localiza dentro da cavidade craniana e circunda o cérebro e a porção craniana do espaço subaracnóide. Em vários locais está relativamente muito afastada da pia-máter, criando as cisternas cranianas subaracnóides. VER TAMBÉM a. mater. SIN arachnoidea mater cranialis [TA], arachnoidea mater encephali*, a. mater cranialis, a. mater encephali, a. of brain, cerebral part of arachnoid.
a. mater [TA], uma membrana fibrosa, delicada, que forma a porção média dos três revestimentos do sistema nervoso central. Na vida, a a. (especificamente a camada de células de barreira aracnóide) está tenuemente ligada à dura-máter externamente adjacente (especificamente as células da borda dural) e não existe espaço natural na interface dura-aracnóide. Dessa maneira, em uma punção espinal, a dura-máter e a a. são penetradas simultaneamente, como uma camada única. A separação da a. da dura-máter (geralmente através da camada de células da borda dural) pode resultar de processos traumáticos ou patológicos que criam o que é comumente, porém de forma incorreta, denominado um hematoma subdural. A a. é assim chamada por causa de seus filamentos delicados em forma de teia de aranha, que se estendem desde sua superfície profunda, através do líquor do espaço subaracnóide, até a pia-máter. VER TAMBÉM leptomeninx. SIN arachnoidea mater, arachnoides [TA], arachnoid membrane, arachnoid, parietal layer of leptomeninges.
a. mater cranialis, a. -máter. SIN cranial a. mater.
a. mater encephali, a. -máter. SIN cranial a. mater.
a. mater and pia mater, leptomeninge, pia-aracnóide; a pia-máter e a aracnóide juntas (unidade funcional). SIN pia-arachnoid, leptomeninx.
a. of spinal cord, a. da medula espinal. SIN spinal a. mater.
spinal a. mater [TA], a. espinal; a porção da a. que se situa dentro do canal vertebral e que circunda a medula espinal e a porção vertebral do espaço subaracnóide. Estende-se desde o forame magno, acima, até o nível vertebral S2. Como a medula espinal termina no nível vertebral L2, ocorre uma ampla separação entre a a. e a pia-máter, a cisterna lombar, cheia de líquido cefalorraquidiano, na qual está suspensa a cauda eqüina. SIN arachnoidea mater spinalis [TA], a. of spinal cord, a. spinalis, spinal part of arachnoid.
a. spina′lis, a. espinal. SIN spinal a. mater.

ar·ach·noi·dal (ă-rak'noy'dăl). Aracnoidal; relativo à aracnóide ou membrana aracnóidea.
ar·ach·noi·dea mater, ar·ach·noi·des (ă-rak-noyd'ē-ă, -dēz) [TA]. Aracnóide-máter. SIN *arachnoid mater*. [L. Mod. *arachnoideus* do G. *arachnē*, aranha, + *eidos*, semelhança]
  a.'s spinalis [TA], a. espinal. SIN spinal *arachnoid* mater.
arach·noid·i·tis (ă-rak-noy-dī'tis). Aracnoidite; inflamação da aracnóide, freqüentemente com envolvimento do espaço subaracnóide adjacente. VER TAMBÉM leptomeninges. [aracnóide + *-itis*, inflamação]
  adhesive a., a. adesiva; espessamento das leptomeninges, por vezes com obliteração do espaço subaracnóide; comumente relacionada à leptomeningite aguda ou crônica de origem bacteriana ou química. VER TAMBÉM leptomeningeal *fibrosis*. SIN obliterative a.
  neoplastic a., a. neoplásica. SIN neoplastic *meningitis*.
  obliterative a., a. obliterativa. SIN adhesive a.
arach·no·ly·sin (ă-rak-nol'ĭ-sin). Aracnolisina; uma substância hemolítica no veneno de determinadas aranhas.
arach·no·pho·bia (ă-rak-nō-fō'bē-ă). Aracnofobia. SIN arachnephobia.
ar·al·kyl (ă-ral'kil). Aralquila; um radical em que um grupamento arila é substituído por um átomo de hidrogênio de um grupamento alquila; p.ex., $C_6H_5CH_2-$. SIN arylated alkyl.
Aran, François A., médico francês, 1817–1861. VER A.-Duchenne *disease*; Duchenne-A. *disease*.
arane·ism (ă-rān'ism). Termo raramente utilizado para aracnidismo.
Arantius, (Aranzio), Giulio C., anatomista e médico italiano, 1530–1589. VER A. *ligament, nodule, ventricle*; *corpus* arantii; *ductus* venosus arantii.
ara·phia (ă-rā'fē-ă). Raquisquise total. SIN holorachischisis. [G. *a-* priv. + *rhaphē*, uma costura]
ar·bor, pl. **ar·bo·res** (ăr'bŏr, ar-bō'rēz). Árvore; em anatomia, uma estrutura arboriforme com ramificações. [L. árvore]
  a. vitae [TA], árvore-da-vida; o aspecto arborescente das substâncias cinzenta e branca nos cortes sagitais do cerebelo.
  a. vi'tae u'teri, a.-da-vida do útero, pregas palmadas. SIN palmate *folds of cervical canal*, em *fold*.
ar·bo·res·cent (ar-bō-res'ent). Arborescente. SIN dendriform.
ar·bo·ri·za·tion (ar'bŏr-i-zā'shŭn). Arborização. **1.** A ramificação terminal das fibras nervosas ou dos vasos sanguíneos em um padrão arboriforme ramificado. **2.** O padrão ramificado formado sob determinadas condições por um esfregaço seco de muco cervical.
ar·bo·rize (ăr'bŏr-īz). Arborizar; espalhar-se em um padrão ramificado arboriforme.
ar·bo·roid (ăr'bŏr-oyd). Arboróide; que indica uma colônia de protozoários, cada um dos quais permanece preso a outra célula ou a um tronco principal em um ponto, formando uma figura de ramificação ou dendrítica. [L. *arbor*, árvore, + G. *eidos*, semelhança]
ar·bor·vi·rus (ăr'bŏr-vī'rŭs). Termo obsoleto para arbovírus.
ar·bo·vi·rus (ăr'bō-vī'rŭs). Arbovírus; um nome antigo para um grande e heterogêneo grupo de RNA vírus. Existem cerca de 500 espécies, as quais são distribuídas entre diversas famílias (Togaviridae, Flaviviridae, Bunyaviridae, Arenaviridae, Rhabdoviridae, Reoviridae) e que foram isoladas de artrópodos, morcegos e roedores; a maioria, mas nem todos, são transmitidos por artrópodos. Esses vírus de animais taxonomicamente distintos são unificados por um conceito epidemiológico, isto é, a transmissão entre hospedeiros vertebrados por vetores artrópodos hematófagos (que se alimentam de sangue), como mosquitos, carrapatos, mosquitos-pólvora e mosquitos-borrachudos. Embora cerca de 100 espécies possam infectar os seres humanos, na maioria dos casos as doenças produzidas por esses vírus são de natureza muito branda e difícil de distinguir das doenças causadas por vírus de outros grupos taxonômicos. As infecções aparentes podem ser separadas em várias síndromes clínicas: febres do tipo indiferenciado (doença febril sistêmica), hepatite, febres hemorrágicas e encefalites. [*ar*, artrópodo, + *bo*, transportado, + vírus]
ARC Abreviatura para AIDS-related *complex* (complexo relacionado à AIDS/SIDA).
arc (ark). Arco. **1.** Uma linha curva ou segmento de um círculo. **2.** A passagem luminosa contínua de uma corrente elétrica em um gás ou vácuo entre dois ou mais carvões separados ou outros eletrodos. [L. *arcus*, um arqueamento]
  auricular a., binauricular a., a. auricular, a. binauricular; uma linha que passa sobre o crânio desde o centro de um meato auditivo externo até o do outro. SIN interauricular a.
  bregmatolambdoid a., a. bregmatolambdóide; uma linha que corre ao longo da sutura sagital, desde o bregma até o ápice da sutura lambdóide.
  crater a., a. da cratera; um a. de corrente direta que forma uma escavação semelhante a uma fóvea no pólo positivo.
  flame a., a. de chama; um a. entre dois eletrodos impregnados que causa a volatilização do núcleo com a chama resultante.
  interauricular a., a. interauricular. SIN auricular a.
  longitudinal a. of skull, a. longitudinal do crânio; uma linha que passa sobre o crânio na linha média, desde o násio até o opístio.
  mercury a., a. de mercúrio; uma descarga elétrica através do vapor de mercúrio entre os eletrodos, um dos quais é usualmente de mercúrio; fornece uma rica fonte de raios ultravioleta terapêuticos; o tubo contendo o mercúrio geralmente é de quartzo; também pode ser de vidro com uma janela de fluoreto.
  nasobregmatic a., a. nasobregmático; uma linha que corre através da linha média da frente, desde o násio até o bregma.
  naso-occipital a., a. naso-occipital; o a. na linha média desde a raiz do nariz até o limite inferior da protuberância occipital externa.
  pulmonary a., a. pulmonar; o contorno radiograficamente demonstrado da artéria pulmonar principal na radiografia frontal do tórax.
  reflex a., a. reflexo; a via percorrida pelos impulsos nervosos na produção de um ato reflexo, desde o órgão receptor periférico através do nervo aferente até a sinapse do sistema nervoso central e, em seguida, através do nervo eferente até o órgão efetor.
  Riolan a., a. de Riolan; **(1)** Arcos arteriais intestinais. SIN intestinal arterial *arcades*, em *arcade*; **(2)** Artéria marginal do colo. SIN marginal *artery* of colon; VER TAMBÉM Riolan *anastomosis*; **(3)** Anastomose de Riolan, arcada de Riolan, arco justacólico. SIN Riolan *anastomosis*.
ar·cade (ar-kād'). Arcada; uma estrutura anatômica ou estruturas (principalmente um vaso sanguíneo) que toma a forma de uma série de arcos. [L. *arcus*, arco, arqueamento]
  anomalous mitral a., a. mitral anômalo; cordas tendíneas curtas que se estendem desde os músculos papilares até a porção central do folheto anterior da valva mitral e resultam na estenose ou incompetência da valva.
  arterial a.'s, arcadas arteriais; uma série de arcos arteriais anastomosantes, como as arcadas arteriais intestinais entre os ramos das artérias jejunal e ileal no mesentério e as artérias pancreatoduodenais na cabeça do pâncreas.
  Flint a., a. de Flint; uma série de arcos vasculares nas bases das pirâmides do rim.
  intestinal arterial a.'s, arcadas arteriais intestinais; a série de arcos arteriais formada no mesentério pelas anastomoses entre as artérias jejunal e ileal adjacentes e a partir das quais surgem os vasos retos. As arcadas arteriais do íleo são mais curtas e mais complexas que aquelas do jejuno. VER TAMBÉM arterial *arches of ileum*, em *arch*; arterial *arches of jejunum*, em *arch*; marginal *artery* of colon. SIN intermesenteric arterial anastomoses, Riolan arc (1), Riolan a.'s.
  lower dental a., a. dental inferior; *termo oficial alternativo para mandibular dental a.
  mandibular dental a. [TA], a. dental mandibular; os dentes suportados pela parte alveolar da mandíbula, quer os 10 dentes decíduos, quer os 16 dentes permanentes. SIN arcus dentalis inferior*, lower dental a.*, inferior dental arch, mandibular dentition.
  marginal a., a. marginal; *termo oficial alternativo para marginal *artery* of colon.
  maxillary dental a. [TA], a. dental maxilar; os dentes suportados pelos processos alveolares das duas maxilas, quer os 10 dentes decíduos, quer os 16 dentes permanentes. SIN arcus dentalis maxillaris [TA], arcus dentalis superior*, upper dental a.*, maxillary dentition, superior dental arch.
  pancreaticoduodenal arterial a.'s, arcadas arteriais pancreatoduodenais; as anastomoses entre as artérias pancreatoduodenais anterior e posterior (a partir da artéria gastroduodenal) e as artérias pancreatoduodenais anterior e posterior (a partir da artéria mesentérica superior) nas faces anterior e posterior da cabeça do pâncreas e no duodeno, irrigando as duas estruturas.
  Riolan a.'s, arcada de Riolan, arco justacólico. SIN intestinal arterial a.'s. VER TAMBÉM Riolan *anastomosis*.
  upper dental a., a. dental maxilar; *termo oficial alternativo para maxillary dental a.
Ar·can·o·bac·te·ri·um (ar-kā'nō-bac-tēr'ē-um). Um gênero de bactérias imóveis, facultativamente anaeróbicas, contendo bastonetes finos, irregulares e Gram-positivos, por vezes mostrando extremidades claiformes que podem estar em formação de V sem filamentos. Esses microrganismos são parasitas obrigatórios da faringe em animais de criação e seres humanos, causando, ocasionalmente, lesões na faringe ou na pele. A espécie protótipo é *A. haemolyticum.*
  A. haemolyticum, uma espécie que provoca faringite e úlceras cutâneas crônicas em seres humanos, assim como em animais de criação.
ar·cate (ar'kāt). Arqueado. SIN arcuate.

ARCH

arch [TA]. Arco; aquilo que é curvado ou arqueado; segmento de uma curva. Em anatomia, qualquer estrutura curva ou arqueada. VER arcus. SIN arcus [TA]. [do Fr. Ant. do L. *arcus*, arqueamento]
  abdominothoracic a., a. abdominotorácico; uma linha campanular definida pela extremidade inferior do esterno e pelos arcos costais de cada lado, cons-

tituindo uma linha limítrofe entre as porções ântero-laterais das paredes torácica e abdominal.

alveolar a. of mandible [TA], a. alveolar da mandíbula; a borda livre do processo alveolar da mandíbula. SIN arcus alveolaris mandibulae [TA], limbus alveolaris (1).

alveolar a. of maxilla [TA], a. alveolar da maxila; a borda livre do processo alveolar. SIN arcus alveolaris maxillae [TA], limbus alveolaris (2).

anterior a. of atlas [TA], a. anterior do atlas; um arco que une as massas laterais do atlas anteriormente e articula-se com a faceta articular anterior do dente da segunda vértebra cervical. SIN arcus anterior atlantis [TA].

anterior palatine a., a. palatino anterior. SIN palatoglossal a.

a. of aorta, a. da aorta. SIN aortic a. (1).

aortic a., a. aórtico; **(1)** a porção curva entre as partes ascendente e descendente da aorta; começa como uma continuação da aorta ascendente posterior ao ângulo do esterno, corre posteriormente e um pouco para a esquerda, quando passa sobre a raiz do pulmão esquerdo, e transforma-se na aorta descendente quando atinge e começa o trajeto ao longo da coluna vertebral; origina o tronco braquiocefálico, as artérias carótida comum esquerda e subclávia esquerda. SIN a. of the aorta; **(2)** qualquer membro dos vários pares de canais arteriais que envolvem a faringe embrionária no mesênquima dos arcos branquiais; existem potencialmente seis pares, mas, nos mamíferos, o quinto par está mal desenvolvido ou ausente. O primeiro e segundo pares somente são funcionais nos embriões muito jovens; o terceiro par está envolvido na formação das carótidas; o quarto arco à esquerda é incorporado ao a. da aorta; o sexto par forma a parte proximal das artérias pulmonares. SIN arcus aortae.

aortic a.'s, arcos aórticos; uma série de canais arteriais que circundam a faringe embrionária no mesênquima dos arcos branquiais. Existem potencialmente seis pares, mas, nos mamíferos, o quinto par apresenta-se mal desenvolvido ou ausente. O primeiro e segundo pares somente são funcionais nos embriões muito jovens; o terceiro par está envolvido na formação das carótidas; o quarto arco à esquerda é incorporado ao a. da aorta; o sexto par forma a parte proximal das artérias pulmonares.

arterial a.'s of colon, arcos arteriais do cólon; anastomoses entre ramos adjacentes das artérias cólicas que formam arcos no mesocólon, a partir dos quais são irrigadas as paredes do cólon. Quando esses arcos formam uma artéria paracólica contínua, isso é referido como a artéria marginal do cólon. VER marginal *artery* of colon.

arterial a.'s of ileum, arcos arteriais do íleo; arcos formados no mesentério por ramos da artéria mesentérica superior, a partir dos quais se originam vasos (*vasa* recta, em *vas*) que irrigam a parede do íleo. VER TAMBÉM intestinal arterial *arcades*, em *arcade*.

arterial a.'s of jejunum, arcos arteriais do jejuno; arcos formados no mesentério por ramos da artéria mesentérica superior, a partir dos quais se originam vasos (*vasa* recta, em *vas*) que irrigam as paredes do jejuno. VER TAMBÉM intestinal arterial *arcades*, em *arcade*.

arterial a. of lower eyelid, a. arterial da pálpebra inferior. SIN inferior palpebral (arterial) a.

arterial a. of upper eyelid, a. arterial da pálpebra superior. SIN superior palpebral (arterial) a.

axillary a., a. axilar. SIN pectorodorsalis *muscle*.

branchial a.'s, arcos branquiais; tipicamente, 6 arcos nos vertebrados; nos vertebrados inferiores, eles dão origem às guelras; nos vertebrados superiores, aparecem de forma transitória e originam estruturas especializadas na cabeça e no pescoço. SIN pharyngeal a.'s, visceral a.'s.

carpal a.'s, arcos carpais; dois ramos arteriais anastomóticos que correm no sentido transverso através do pulso; o *palmar* ou *anterior* situa-se na frente do carpo, sendo formado pelos ramos carpianos palmares das artérias radial e ulnar; o *dorsal* ou *posterior* situa-se na superfície dorsal do carpo, sendo formado pelos ramos carpianos dorsais das artérias radial e ulnar.

coracoacromial a., a. coracoacromial; um a. protetor formado pela face inferior lisa do acrômio e processo coracóide da escápula, com o ligamento coracoacromial formando uma ponte sobre eles. Essa estrutura osseoligamentosa superpõe-se à cabeça do úmero, evitando seu deslocamento para cima a partir da fossa glenóide.

Corti a., a. de Corti; o a. formado pela junção das "cabeças" das células dos pilares interno e externo de Corti.

cortical a.'s of kidney, arcos corticais do rim; as porções da substância renal (córtex) que se interpõem entre as bases das pirâmides e a cápsula do rim.

costal a., a. costal; *termo oficial alternativo para costal *margin*.

a. of cricoid cartilage [TA], a. da cartilagem cricóide; a parte estreita da cartilagem que envolve a passagem de ar anterior à lâmina. SIN arcus cartilaginis cricoideae [TA].

crural a., ligamento inguinal. SIN inguinal *ligament*.

deep crural a., trato iliopúbico. SIN iliopubic *tract*.

deep palmar (arterial) a. [TA], a. palmar profundo (arterial); o arco arterial localizado profundamente aos tendões do flexor longo na mão. É formado pela parte terminal da artéria radial em conjunto com o ramo palmar profundo da artéria ulnar. O a. origina as artérias metacarpiana palmar e principal do polegar. SIN arcus palmaris profundus, arcus volaris profundus.

deep palmar venous a. [TA], a. venoso palmar profundo; o arco venoso que acompanha o arco arterial palmar profundo; geralmente consiste nas veias acompanhantes pareadas. SIN arcus venosus palmaris profundus [TA].

dental a., a. dentário; a estrutura composta curva da dentição natural e as cristas residuais ou resquícios destas depois da perda de alguns ou de todos os dentes naturais.

dorsal carpal arterial a. [TA], a. arterial carpal dorsal; uma rede vascular sobre a superfície dorsal das articulações carpianas, formada por anastomoses dos ramos dos interósseos anteriores e posteriores e ramos carpianos dorsais das artérias radial e ulnar. SIN rete carpale dorsale [TA], dorsal carpal network, rete carpi posterius.

dorsal venous a. of foot [TA], a. venoso dorsal do pé; o arco no tecido subcutâneo do dorso do pé formado pelas veias dorsal e digital; une-se medialmente com a veia dorsal do polegar para formar a veia safena maior e, lateralmente, com a veia dorsal do dedo mínimo para formar a safena menor. SIN arcus venosus dorsalis pedis [TA].

double aortic a., a. aórtico duplo; malformação congênita da aorta que se divide e apresenta um a. direito e um a. esquerdo, em lugar de um a. único.

expansion a., a. de expansão; um dispositivo ortodôntico que move as estruturas dentárias distal, bucal ou labialmente, criando largura de um molar ao outro e o comprimento do arco.

fallen a.'s, arcos diminuídos; uma diminuição dos arcos do pé, quer no sentido longitudinal, quer no transversal ou em ambos; a deformidade resultante é o pé plano (longitudinal) e/ou chato (transversal).

fallopian a., ligamento inguinal. SIN inguinal *ligament*.

femoral a., ligamento inguinal. SIN inguinal *ligament*.

a.'s of the foot, arcos do pé. VER longitudinal a. of foot, plantar a.

glossopalatine a., a. palatoglosso. SIN palatoglossal a.

Gothic a., a. gótico. SIN needle point *tracing*.

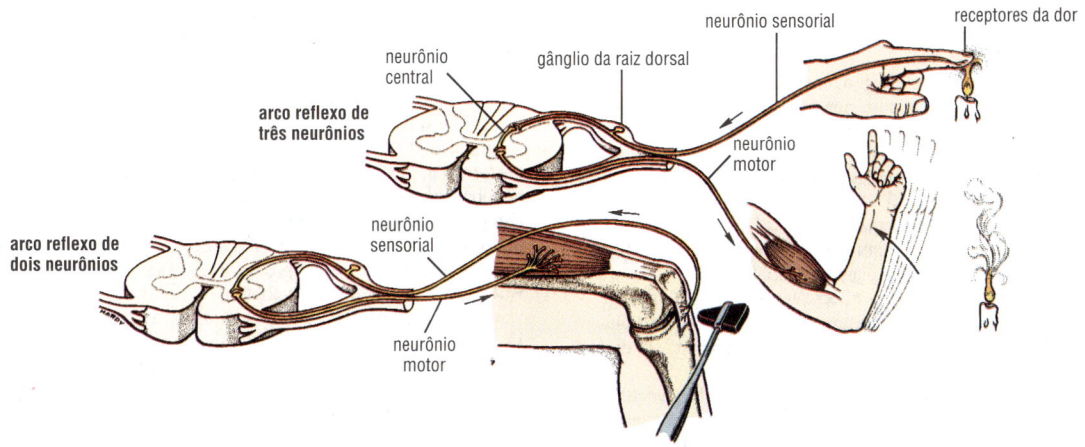

arcos reflexos: (acima) reflexo flexor, (abaixo) reflexo extensor

Haller a.'s, arcos de Haller. VER lateral arcuate *ligament*, medial arcuate *ligament*.

hemal a.'s, arcos hemáticos; **(1)** os arcos que, coletivamente, compreendem o arcabouço torácico, cada qual consistindo em uma vértebra (corpo, pedículo e processos transversos), o par correspondente de costelas e suas cartilagens articulares, e a porção do esterno na qual eles se inserem; **(2)** três ou quatro ossos em forma de V localizados ventralmente aos corpos da terceira à sexta vértebra coccígea; eles representam intercentros e, em geral, envolvem a artéria e veia caudais ventrais.

hyoid a., a. hióide; o segundo a. branquial ou visceral; o segundo a. pós-oral na série de arcos branquiais.

iliopectineal a. [TA], a. iliopectíneo; uma faixa espessada das fáscias ilíaca e do psoas fundidas que passa da face posterior do ligamento inguinal, anteriormente, através da frente do nervo femoral para se inserir na eminência iliopectínea do osso do quadril, posteriormente. O a. iliopectíneo forma, assim, um septo que subdivide o espaço profundo ao ligamento inguinal em uma lacuna muscular lateral e uma lacuna vascular medial. Quando um músculo psoas menor está presente, seu tendão de inserção mistura-se com o a. iliopectíneo. SIN arcus iliopectineus [TA], iliopectineal ligament, ligamentum iliopectineale.

inferior dental a., a. dental mandibular. SIN mandibular dental *arcade*. SIN arcus dentalis mandibularis [TA].

inferior palpebral (arterial) a. [TA], a. palpebral inferior (arterial); formado pela artéria palpebral medial, que se comunica com um ramo da artéria lacrimal ao longo da margem tarsal. SIN arcus palpebralis inferior [TA], arterial a. of lower eyelid.

jugular venous a. [TA], a. venoso jugular; uma veia que faz conexão entre as duas veias jugulares anteriores no espaço supra-esternal. SIN arcus venosus juguli [TA].

labial a., a. labial; um a. ortodôntico de arame que aproxima as superfícies labiais dos dentes.

Langer a., a. de Langer, alça tendínea anômala. SIN pectorodorsalis *muscle*.

lateral longitudinal a. of foot, a. longitudinal lateral do pé; formado pelo calcâneo, cubóide e dois metatarsos laterais; o a. combinado é suportado normalmente por ligamentos, músculos intrínsecos e tendões dos músculos extrínsecos do pé. SIN arcus pedis longitudinalis pars lateralis.

lateral lumbocostal a., ligamento arqueado lateral. SIN lateral arcuate *ligament*.

lingual a., a. lingual; um a. ortodôntico de arame que aproxima as superfícies linguais dos dentes.

longitudinal a. of foot, a. longitudinal do pé. VER medial longitudinal a. of foot, lateral longitudinal a. of foot. SIN arcus pedis longitudinalis.

malar a., a. zigomático. SIN zygomatic a.

mandibular a., a. mandibular; o primeiro a. pós-oral na série de arcos branquiais. SIN mandibular process.

medial longitudinal a. of foot, a. longitudinal medial do pé; formado pelo calcâneo, talo, navicular, três cuneiformes e três metatársicos mediais. SIN arcus pedis longitudinalis pars medialis.

medial lumbocostal a., ligamento arqueado medial. SIN medial arcuate *ligament*.

nasal a., a. nasal; crista do nariz, o teto arqueado para cima da abertura piriforme formado pelos processos nasais da maxila de cada lado e pelos ossos nasais entre si. Os óculos repousam centralmente sobre várias partes desse arco.

nasal venous a., a. venoso nasal; um a. formado na raiz do nariz pelas duas veias supratrocleares ligadas por uma veia transversa.

neural a. of vertebra, a. vertebral. SIN vertebral a.

a. of the palate, a. do palato; o teto abobadado da boca.

palatoglossal a. [TA], a. palatoglosso; uma de duas cristas ou pregas da mucosa que passam do palato mole até o lado da língua; envolve o músculo palatoglosso e forma a margem posterior da fossa tonsilar. Também separa a cavidade oral do istmo da face. SIN arcus palatoglossus [TA], anterior pillar of fauces*, plica anterior faucium*, anterior palatine a., arcus glossopalatinus, glossopalatine a., glossopalatine fold.

palatopharyngeal a. [TA], a. palatofaríngeo; uma de duas cristas ou pregas da mucosa que se dirigem da margem posterior do palato mole para a parede lateral da faringe. Envolve o músculo palatofaríngeo e forma a margem posterior da fossa tonsilar. Também separa o istmo da fauce da orofaringe. SIN arcus palatopharingeus [TA], plica posterior faucium*, posterior pillar of fauces*, pharyngopalatine a., posterior palatine a.

pharyngeal a.'s, arcos faríngeos. SIN branchial a.'s

pharyngopalatine a., a. palatofaríngeo. SIN palatopharyngeal a.

plantar a., a. plantar profundo. SIN deep plantar (arterial) *arch*.

plantar arterial a., a. plantar profundo. SIN deep plantar (arterial) *arch*.

plantar venous a. [TA], a. venoso plantar; o arco formado pelas veias digitais plantares desde os artelhos, acompanhando o arco arterial plantar. SIN arcus venosus plantaris [TA].

popliteal a., ligamento poplíteo arqueado. SIN arcuate popliteal *ligament*.

posterior a. of atlas [TA], a. posterior do atlas; o arco posterior do atlas que se liga às massas laterais do atlas posteriormente, formando a parede posterior do canal vertebral nesse nível. SIN arcus posterior atlantis [TA].

posterior palatine a., a. palatofaríngeo. SIN palatopharyngeal a.

postoral a.'s, arcos pós-orais; a série de arcos branquiais caudais à boca; o primeiro é o mandibular, o segundo é o hióide; caudal ao hióide, os arcos não possuem nome, sendo designados apenas por seu número pós-oral.

primitive costal a.'s, arcos costais primitivos; os arcos formados na região torácica da coluna vertebral, no embrião, a partir dos processos costais ou elementos costais, os quais originam as costelas.

pubic a. [TA], a. púbico; o arco formado pela sínfise, corpos e ramos inferiores dos ossos do púbis. VER TAMBÉM subpubic *angle*. SIN arcus pubis [TA].

ribbon a., a. de fita; um a. ortodôntico de arame, retangular, fino, com formato de fita, aplicado aos arcos dentários, de modo que a sua maior dimensão fique paralela às superfícies labial ou bucal dos dentes.

subcostal a., a. infra-esternal; *termo oficial alternativo para infrasternal *angle*.

superciliary a. [TA], a. superciliar; uma massa que se estende lateralmente, a partir da glabela, em ambos os lados, acima da margem orbital do osso frontal. SIN arcus superciliaris [TA], superciliary ridge.

superficial palmar (arterial) a. [TA], a. palmar superficial (arterial); o arco arterial na mão localizado superficialmente aos tendões do flexor longo, aproximadamente ao nível de uma linha traçada através da palma desde o lado distal do polegar esticado. É formado principalmente pelo término da artéria ulnar superficial e comumente completado por uma comunicação com o ramo palmar superficial da artéria radial. O a. origina as artérias digitais palmares comuns. SIN arcus palmaris superficialis [TA], arcus volaris superficialis.

superficial palmar venous a., a. venoso palmar superficial; o arco venoso que acompanha o arco arterial palmar superficial; consiste usualmente nas veias acompanhantes pareadas e é drenado pelas veias ulnar superficial e radial. SIN arcus venosus palmaris superficialis [TA].

superior dental a., a. dental maxilar. SIN maxillary dental *arcade*.

superior palpebral (arterial) a., [TA], a. palpebral superior (arterial); formada por ramos comunicantes das artérias palpebral medial e lateral. Freqüentemente existem dois arcos, um próximo à borda livre da placa tarsal e outro ao longo da borda superior do tarso. SIN arcus palpebralis superior [TA], arterial a. of upper eyelid.

supraorbital a., margem supra-orbital. SIN supraorbital *margin*.

tarsal a., a. tarsal. VER inferior palpebral (arterial) a., superior palpebral (arterial) a.

tendinous a. [TA], a. tendíneo; **(1)** uma faixa branca e fibrosa, presa ao osso e/ou músculo, que forma um arco superiormente e, dessa maneira, protege os elementos neurovasculares que passam abaixo dela contra a compressão lesiva; **(2)** um espessamento linear da fáscia profunda de um músculo que fornece inserção para ligamentos e/ou fibras musculares. SIN arcus tendineus [TA].

tendinous a. of levator ani muscle [TA], a. tendinoso do músculo levantador do ânus; uma porção espessada da fáscia obturadora que se estende em uma linha arqueada desde o púbis, posteriormente, até a espinha isquiática, dando origem a parte do músculo levantador do ânus. SIN arcus tendineus musculi levatoris ani [TA], arcus tendineus of obturador fascia, arcus tendineus of pelvic diaphragm.

tendinous a. of pelvic fascia [TA], a. tendíneo da fáscia pélvica; espessamento linear da fáscia superior do diafragma pélvico que se estende posteriormente a partir do corpo do púbis ao longo da lateral da bexiga (e vagina na mulher) e que fornece inserção para os ligamentos de sustentação das vísceras pélvicas. SIN arcus tendineus fasciae pelvis [TA].

tendinous a. of soleus muscle [TA], a. tendíneo do músculo sóleo; um arco tendinoso sobre os vasos poplíteos — e que define o término desses vasos — entre a tíbia e a fíbula e dá origem à porção central do músculo solear. SIN arcus tendineus musculi solei [TA].

a. of thoracic duct [TA], a. do ducto torácico; porção terminal do ducto torácico que se vira abruptamente para a esquerda, comumente ao nível de C7, para entrar na face súpero-lateral da junção das veias subclávia esquerda e jugular interna. VER TAMBÉM thoracic *duct*. SIN arcus ductus thoracici [TA].

transverse a. of foot, a. transverso do pé; o arco formado pelas partes proximais dos metatarsos, pelos três ossos cuneiformes e pelo cubóide. SIN arcus pedis transversalis.

Treitz a., a. de Treitz. SIN paraduodenal *fold*.

vertebral a. [TA], a. vertebral; a projeção posterior a partir do corpo de uma vértebra que envolve o forame vertebral; consiste em pedículos pareados e lâminas; os processos espinhosos, transversos e articulares originam-se a partir do arco. Em conjunto, os arcos venosos — e os ligamentos amarelos que os unem — formam a parede posterior do canal vertebral (espinal). SIN arcus vertebrae [TA], neural a. of vértebra.

visceral a.'s, arcos viscerais, a. branquiais. SIN branchial a.'s.

W-a., a. W; um dispositivo de expansão maxilar fixo preso à parte lingual dos molares, com braços de extensão bilaterais ou unilaterais.

wire a., a. de arame; arame conformado ao a. dental; usado para restaurar a curvatura normal da dentadura.

zygomatic a. [TA], a. zigomático; o arco formado pelo processo temporal do osso zigomático que une o processo zigomático do osso temporal. SIN arcus zygomaticus [TA], cheek bone (2), malar a., zygoma (2).

arch-, arche-, archi-. Formas combinantes que significam primitivo ou ancestral; originalmente, também indicavam primeiro, principal, extremo. [G. *archē*, origem, início, + -o-]

ar·chae·o·cer·e·bel·lum (ar'kē-ō-ser'ē-bel'ŭm). Arquicerebelo. SIN archicerebellum. [G. *archaios*, antigo, + cerebelo]

ar·chae·us (ar-kē'ŭs). Arqueísmo; termo primeiramente utilizado por Valentine e, mais adiante, por Paracelsus e van Helmont para indicar um espírito que presidia e governava os processos corporais. SIN archeus. [L. do G. *archaios*, principal, líder]

ar·cha·ic (ar-kā'ik). Arcaico; antigo; ancestral; na psicologia junguiana, indica o passado ancestral dos processos mentais. [G. *archaikos*, ancestral]

Archambault, LaSalle, neurologista norte-americano, 1879–1940. VER Meyer-A. *loop*.

arche-. VER arch-.

arch·en·ter·on (ark-en'ter-on). Arquêntero, arquênteron. SIN primitive *gut*. [G. *archē*, início, + *enteron*, intestino]

ar·che·o·cer·e·bel·lum (ar-kē-ō-ser'-ē-bel'ŭm). Vestibulocerebelo, arquicerebelo. SIN vestibulocerebellum.

ar·che·o·ki·net·ic (ar-kē-ō-ki-net'ik). Arqueocinético; indica um tipo baixo e primitivo de mecanismo nervoso motor, como aquele encontrado no sistema nervoso periférico e ganglionar. Cf. neokinetic, paleokinetic. [G. *archaios*, antigo, + *kinētikos*, relativo a movimento]

ar·che·type (ar'kē-tip). Arqueótipo. **1.** Um plano estrutural primitivo a partir do qual evoluíram várias modificações. **2.** Em psicologia junguiana, a manifestação estrutural do inconsciente coletivo. SIN imago (2). [G. *archetypos*, padrão, modelo, de *archē*, início, + *typō*, estampar]

ar·che·us (ar-kē'ŭs). Arqueísmo. SIN archaeus.

archi-. Arqui-. VER arch-.

ar·chi·cer·e·bel·lum (ar'ki-ser-ē-bel'ŭm) [TA]. Arquicerebelo; a pequena porção filogeneticamente mais antiga do cerebelo, por vezes chamada de vestibulocerebelo, porque seus aferentes originam-se principalmente do gânglio e núcleos vestibulares; nos mamíferos, é representado por quatro subdivisões do cerebelo: nódulo, verme da úvula, flóculo e língula do cerebelo. SIN archaeocerebellum. [arqui- + L. *cerebellum*.

ar·chi·cor·tex (ar'ki-kōr'teks) [TA]. Arquicórtex. **1.** Tipicamente, as partes filogeneticamente mais antigas do córtex cerebral. **2.** Mais especificamente, o córtex que forma o hipocampo. VER TAMBÉM allocortex, cerebral *cortex*. SIN archipallium. [arqui- + L. *cortex*]

ar·chil (ar'kil) [I.C. antigo 1242). Rocela; corante violeta a partir dos liquens *Rocella tinctoria* e *R. fuciformis*. SIN orchella, orchil, roccellin.

ar·chin (ar'kin). Emodina. SIN emodin.

ar·chi·pal·li·um (ar-ki-pal'ē-ŭm). Arquicórtex. SIN archicortex. [arqui- + L. *pallium*]

ar·chi·tec·ton·ics (ar-ki-tek-ton'iks). Arquitetônico. SIN cytoarchitecture.

arch·wire (arch'wīr). Freio dentário; um dispositivo que consiste em um arame moldado para o arco alveolar ou dental, usado como uma fixação na correção de irregularidades na posição dos dentes. SIN arch wire.

ar·ci·form (ar'si-fōrm). Arciforme. SIN arcuate.

Ar·co·bac·ter (ar-kō-bak'ter). Um gênero de bactérias da família Campylobacteraceae que são Gram-negativas, aerotolerantes e capazes de crescer a 15° C. A cepa protótipo é *Arcobacter butzleri*.

***A. butzleri*,** uma espécie de bactéria do gênero *Arcobacter* encontrada em aves e na carne de vaca; foi associada a doenças diarreicas e sistêmicas em seres humanos.

arc·ta·tion (ark-tā'shŭn). Arctação; um estreitamento, contração, estenose ou coartação. [L. *arto* (improp. *arcto*), pp. *-atus*, apertar]

ar·cu·al (ar'kū-ăl). Arcual, arciforme; relativo a um arco.

ar·cu·a·te (ar'kū-āt). Arqueado; indica uma forma que é arqueada ou que apresenta a forma de um arco. SIN arcate, arciform. [L. *arcuatus*, arqueado]

ar·cu·a·tion (ar-kū-ā'shŭn). Arqueamento; uma curvatura.

ARCUS

ar·cus (ar'kus) [TA]. Arco. SIN arch. [L. um arco]

a. adipo'sus, a. adiposo, a. senil. SIN a. senilis.
a. alveola'ris mandib'ulae [TA], a. alveolar da mandíbula. SIN alveolar *arch* of mandible.
a. alveola'ris maxil'lae [TA], a. alveolar da maxila. SIN alveolar *arch* of maxilla.
a. ante'rior atlan'tis [TA], a. anterior do atlas. SIN anterior *arch* of atlas.
a. aor'tae, a. da aorta. SIN aortic *arch* (2).
a. cartila'ginis crico'ideae [TA], a. da cartilagem cricóidea. SIN *arch* of cricoid cartilage.
a. cornea'lis, a. senil. SIN a. senilis.
a. costa'lis [TA], a. costal. SIN costal *margin*.
a. costa'rum, a. costal. SIN costal *margin*.
a. denta'lis infe'rior, a. dental mandibular; *termo oficial alternativo para mandibular dental *arcade*.
a. dentalis mandibularis [TA], a. dental mandibular. SIN inferior dental *arch*.
a. dentalis maxillaris [TA], a. dental maxilar. SIN maxillary dental *arcade*.
a. denta'lis supe'rior, a. dental maxilar; *termo oficial alternativo para maxillary dental *arcade*.
a. ductus thoracici [TA], a. do ducto torácico. SIN *arch* of thoracic duct.
a. glossopalati'nus, a. palatoglosso. SIN palatoglossal *arch*.
a. iliopectin'eus [TA], a. iliopectíneo. SIN iliopectineal *arch*.
a. inguina'lis, ligamento inguinal; *termo oficial alternativo para inguinal *ligament*.
a. juveni'lis, a. juvenil; a. da córnea, a. senil. SIN a. senilis.
a. lipoi'des, a. lipóide, a. senil. SIN a. senilis.
a. lumbocosta'lis latera'lis, ligamento arqueado lateral. SIN lateral arcuate *ligament*.
a. lumbocosta'lis media'lis, ligamento arqueado medial. SIN medial arcuate *ligament*.
a. marginalis coli, a. marginal do cólon; *termo oficial alternativo para marginal *artery* of colon.
a. palati'ni, a. palatino. VER palatoglossal *arch*, palatopharyngeal *arch*.
a. palatoglos'sus [TA], a. palatoglosso. SIN palatoglossal *arch*.
a. palatopharyn'geus [TA], a. palatofaríngeo. SIN palatopharyngeal *arch*.
a. palma'ris profun'dus, a. palmar profundo. SIN deep palmar (arterial) *arch*.
a. palma'ris superficia'lis [TA], a. palmar superficial. SIN superficial palmar (arterial) *arch*.
a. palpebra'lis infe'rior [TA], a. palpebral inferior. SIN inferior palpebral (arterial) *arch*.
a. palpebra'lis supe'rior [TA], a. palpebral superior. SIN superior palpebral (arterial) *arch*.
a. pe'dis longitudina'lis, a. longitudinal do pé. SIN longitudinal *arch* of foot.
a. pe'dis longitudina'lis pars lateralis, a. longitudinal lateral do pé. SIN lateral longitudinal *arch* of foot.
a. pe'dis longitudina'lis pars medialis, a. longitudinal medial do pé. SIN medial longitudinal *arch* of foot.
a. pe'dis transversa'lis, a. transverso do pé. SIN transverse *arch* of foot.
a. plantaris profundus [TA], a. plantar profundo. SIN deep plantar (arterial) *arch*.
a. poste'rior atlan'tis, a. posterior do atlas. SIN posterior *arch* of atlas.
a. pu'bis [TA], a. púbico. SIN pubic *arch*.
a. rani'nus, a. da rânula. SIN ranine *anastomosis*.
a. seni'lis, a. senil; um anel opaco e acinzentado na periferia da córnea, exatamente na junção esclerocorneal, de ocorrência freqüente no idoso; resulta do depósito de grânulos gordurosos na lamela e células da córnea, ou da degeneração hialina de ambas. SIN anterior embryotoxon, a. adiposus, a. cornealis, a. juvenilis, a. lipoides, gerontoxon, linea corneae senilis, lipoidosis corneae.
a. supercilia'ris [TA], a. superciliar. SIN superciliary *arch*.
a. tar'seus, a. tarsal. VER inferior palpebral (arterial) *arch*, superior palpebral (arterial) *arch*.
a. tendin'eus [TA], a. tendíneo. SIN tendinous *arch*.
a. tendin'eus fas'ciae pel'vis [TA], a. tendíneo da fáscia da pelve. SIN tendinous *arch* of pelvic fascia.
a. tendin'eus mus'culi levato'ris ani [TA], a. tendíneo do músculo levantador do ânus. SIN tendinous *arch* of levator ani muscle.
a. tendin'eus mus'culi so'lei [TA], a. tendíneo do músculo sóleo. SIN tendinous *arch* of soleus muscle.
a. tendineus of obturator fascia, a. tendíneo do músculo levantador do ânus. SIN tendinous *arch* of levator ani muscle.
a. tendineus of pelvic diaphragm, a. tendíneo do músculo levantador do ânus. SIN tendinous *arch* of levator ani muscle.
a. un'guium, lúnula da unha. SIN lunule of nail.
a. veno'sus dorsa'lis pe'dis [TA], a. venoso dorsal do pé. SIN dorsal venous *arch* of foot.
a. veno'sus jug'uli [TA], a. venoso jugular. SIN jugular venous *arch*.
a. veno'sus palma'ris profun'dus [TA], a. venoso palmar profundo. SIN deep palmar venous *arch*.
a. veno'sus palma'ris superficia'lis [TA], a. venoso palmar superficial. SIN superficial palmar venous *arch*.
a. veno'sus planta'ris [TA], a. venoso plantar. SIN plantar venous *arch*.
a. ver'tebrae [TA], a. vertebral. SIN vertebral *arch*. VER TAMBÉM hemal *arches*, em *arch*.
a. vola'ris profun'dus, a. palmar profundo. SIN deep palmar (arterial) *arch*.
a. vola'ris superficia'lis, a. palmar superficial. SIN superficial palmar (arterial) *arch*.
a. zygomat'icus [TA], a. zigomático. SIN zygomatic *arch*.

ar·dor (ar'dōr). Ardor; termo antigo para uma sensação de calor ou queimação. [L. fogo, calor]

ARDS Abreviatura para adult respiratory distress *syndrome* (síndrome de angústia respiratória do adulto [SARA]).

AREA

ar·ea (a), pl. **ar·e·ae** (ār'ē-ă, -ē). Área. **1.** [TA]. Qualquer superfície ou espaço circunscrito. **2.** A totalidade da região suprida por uma determinada artéria ou nervo. **3.** Uma região de um órgão que possui uma função especial, como a a. motora do cérebro. VER TAMBÉM regio, region, space, spatium, zone. [L. um pátio]

acoustic a., a. vestibular; o assoalho do recesso lateral do quarto ventrículo, que se estende medialmente até o sulco limitante e sobrejacente aos núcleos coclear e vestibular do rombencéfalo. SIN a. vestibularis [TA], a. acústica.

a. acu'stica, a. vestibular. SIN acoustic a.

amygdaloclaustral a. [TA], a. amigdaloclaustral; a região no lobo temporal onde as porções laterais do núcleo amigdalóide estão em íntima aposição às faces ventrais do claustro ou se fundem com elas. SIN a. amygdaloclaustralis [TA].

a. amygdaloclaustralis [TA], a. amigdaloclaustral. SIN amygdaloclaustral a.

a. amygdaloidea anterior [TA], a. amigdalóidea anterior. SIN anterior amygdaloid a.

amygdalopiriform transition a. [TA], a. de transição amigdalopiriforme; a área onde os grupos de células que formam o núcleo amigdalóide estão intimamente adjacentes ao córtex piriforme. SIN a. transitionis amygdalopiriformis [TA].

anterior amygdaloid a. [TA], a. amigdalóidea anterior; a porção mais rostral do complexo amigdalóide composta de células espalhadas que representam uma transição para as divisões mais nitidamente organizadas da amígdala. SIN a. amygdaloidea anterior [TA].

anterior hypothalamic a., a. hipotalâmica rostral; a porção rostral (anterior) do hipotálamo geralmente interna à região do quiasma óptico; contém os seguintes núcleos: núcleo hipotalâmico anterior [TA] (nucleus anterior hypothalami [TA]), núcleo periventricular anterior [TA] (nucleus periventricular ventralis [TA]), núcleos intersticiais do hipotálamo anterior [TA] (nuclei interstitiales hypothalami anteriores [TA]), núcleo pré-óptico lateral [TA] (nucleus preopticus lateralis [TA]), núcleo pré-óptico medial [TA] (nucleus preopticus medialis [TA]), núcleo pré-óptico mediano [TA] (nucleus preopticus medianus [TA]), nucleus paraventricularis [TA] (nucleus paraventricularis hypothalami [TA]), núcleo periventricular pré-óptico [TA] (nucleus preopticus periventricularis [TA]) núcleo supraquiasmático [TA] (nucleus suprachiasmaticus [TA]) e o núcleo supra-óptico [TA] (nucleus supraopticus [TA]). O último grupo de células consiste nas partes dorsomedial, ventromedial e dorsolateral. VER TAMBÉM hypothalamus. SIN a. hypothalamica rostralis [TA], anterior hypothalamic region*.

anterior intercondylar a. of tibia [TA], a. intercondilar anterior da tíbia; a ampla a. deprimida entre os côndilos da tíbia anteriormente, na qual se inserem as extremidades anteriores dos meniscos e o ligamento cruzado anterior. SIN a. intercondylaris anterior tibiae [TA].

aortic a. (of auscultation), foco aórtico (de ausculta); a região da parede torácica sobre a segunda cartilagem costal direita, onde os sons produzidos pelo orifício aórtico são, com freqüência, mais bem auscultados.

apical a., a. apical; a a. sobre a extremidade da raiz de um dente.

association areas, áreas de associação. SIN association *cortex*.

auditory a., córtex auditivo. SIN auditory *cortex*.

bare a. of liver [TA], a. nua do fígado; a a. na superfície póstero-superior (diafragmática) do fígado, limitada pelo ligamento coronário, mas ela mesma desprovida de peritônio, de modo que o diafragma e o fígado ficam em contato direto e são aderentes entre si, não revestidos por peritônio. SIN a. nuda hepatis [TA].

bare a. of stomach [TA], a. nua do estômago; a parte da superfície posterior do fundo do estômago, entre as duas camadas divergentes do ligamento gastrofrênico, que não é revestida pelo peritônio.

basal seat a., a. da sede basal; a porção das estruturas orais que está disponível para suportar uma dentadura.

Broca a., a. de Broca. SIN Broca *center*.

Broca parolfactory a., a. paraolfatória de Broca. SIN parolfactory a.

Brodmann areas, áreas de Brodmann; áreas do córtex cerebral mapeadas com base nos padrões da citoarquitetura cortical. VER cerebral *cortex*.

a. of cardiac dullness, a. de macicez cardíaca; uma área triangular determinada por percussão da face anterior do tórax; corresponde à parte do coração que não é coberta pelo tecido pulmonar.

catchment a., a. de atuação; um termo relativo ao centro comunitário de saúde mental que delimita a área geográfica que circunda cada centro, e, assim, a população de indivíduos que se qualifica para os serviços de saúde mental em cada centro.

a. centra'lis, a. central. SIN *macula* of retina.

a. coch'leae [TA], a. coclear. SIN cochlear a.

cochlear a. [TA], a. coclear; a a. inferior à crista transversa do fundo do meato auditivo interno através da qual os filamentos do nervo coclear passam para entrar na cóclea; forma a base do modíolo cônico sobre o qual o canal coclear forma a espiral. VER *base* of modiolus of cochlea. SIN a. cochleae [TA].

Cohnheim a., a. de Cohnheim; uma figura poligonal, semelhante a um mosaico, no corte transversal de uma fibra muscular esquelética ao microscópio; um artefato de enrugamento de fixação. SIN Cohnheim field.

contact a., a. de contato; a parte da superfície proximal de um dente que toca o dente adjacente mesial ou distalmente. SIN contact point, point of proximal contact.

cribriform a. of the renal papilla [TA], a. cribriforme da papila renal; o ápice de uma papila renal perfurado por 10 a 22 aberturas dos ductos papilares, os forames papilares. SIN a. cribosa papillae renalis [TA].

a. cribro'sa papillae renalis [TA], a. cribriforme da papila renal. SIN cribriform a. of the renal papilla.

denture-bearing a., a. de sustentação da prótese dentária. SIN denture foundation a.

denture foundation a., a. de sustentação; a porção dos tecidos orais que suporta a base de uma prótese parcial ou total sob a carga oclusal. SIN basal seat, denture-bearing a., denture-supporting a., stress-bearing a. (1), supporting a. (2), tissue-bearing a.

denture-supporting a., a. de sustentação da prótese dentária. SIN denture foundation a.

dermatomic a., a. do dermátomo. SIN dermatome (3).

dorsal hypothalamic a. [TA], a. hipotalâmica dorsal; uma região relativamente pequena do hipotálamo localizada ventralmente ao sulco hipotalâmico; contém os seguintes núcleos: porções do núcleo dorsomedial [TA] (nucleus dorsomedialis [TA]), núcleo endopeduncular [TA] (nucleus endopeduncularis [TA]), e partes do núcleo da alça lenticular [TA] (nucleus ansae lenticularis [TA]). VER TAMBÉM hypothalamus. SIN a. hypothalamica dorsalis [TA], dorsal hypothalamic region*.

embryonal a., embryonic a., a. embrionária; a a. do blastoderma em ambos os lados e imediatamente cefálica ao traço primitivo onde as camadas celulares componentes tornam-se espessadas.

entorhinal a., a. entonasal; a. de Brodmann 28, uma a. citoarquiteturalmente bem definida de córtex cerebral multilaminado na face medial do giro parahipocampal, imediatamente caudal ao córtex olfatório do uncus; a a. constitui a origem do principal sistema de fibras aferentes para o hipocampo, a chamada via perfurante.

excitable a., a. excitável. SIN motor *cortex*.

facial nerve a. [TA], a. do nervo facial; a a. do fundo do meato acústico interno superior à crista transversa através da qual passa o nervo facial para entrar no canal facial. SIN a. nervi facialis [TA].

Flechsig areas, áreas de Flechsig; três divisões (anterior, lateral, posterior) de cada metade lateral da medula, conforme observado no corte transversal, marcadas por fibras das raízes dos nervos hipoglosso e vago.

frontal a., a. frontal. SIN frontal *cortex*.

fronto-orbital a., a. fronto-orbital. SIN orbitofrontal *cortex*.

fusion a., a. de fusão. SIN Panum a.

gastric a. [TA], a. gástrica; uma das inúmeras pequenas áreas poligonais, com 1 a 6 mm de diâmetro, separadas por depressões lineares na superfície da mucosa do estômago; elas contêm as pequenas depressões gástricas, onde várias glândulas gástricas se abrem em cada depressão. SIN a. gastrica [TA].

a. gas'trica [TA], a. gástrica. SIN gastric a.

germinal a., a. germinati'va, a. germinativa; o local no blastoderma onde o embrião começa a ser formado. SIN germinal *disk*.

Head areas, áreas de Head; áreas da pele que exibem hiperestesia reflexa e hiperalgesia devido à doença visceral.

a. hypothalamica dorsalis [TA], a. hipotalâmica dorsal. SIN dorsal hypothalamic a.

a. hypothalamica intermedia [TA], a. hipotalâmica intermédia. SIN intermediate hypothalamic a.

a. hypothalamica lateralis [TA], a. hipotalâmica lateral. SIN lateral hypothalamic a.

a. hypothalamica posterior [TA], a. hipotalâmica posterior. SIN posterior hypothalamic a.

a. hypothalamica rostralis [TA], a. hipotalâmica rostral. SIN anterior hypothalamic a.

impression a., a. de impressão; em odontologia, a superfície que é registrada em uma impressão.

inferior vestibular a. [TA], a. vestibular inferior; a a. do fundo do meato acústico interno inferior à crista transversal através da qual passa a porção inferior do nervo vestibular (sacular). SIN a. vestibularis inferior [TA].

insular a., ínsula. SIN insula (1).

a. intercondyla'ris ante'rior tibiae [TA], a. intercondilar anterior da tíbia. SIN anterior intercondylar a. of tibia.

a. intercondyla'ris poste'rior tibiae [TA], a. intercondilar posterior da tíbia. SIN posterior intercondylar a. of tibia.
intermediate hypothalamic a. [TA], a. hipotalâmica intermédia; a porção do hipotálamo geralmente interna à região do infundíbulo; contém os seguintes núcleos: núcleo dorsal [TA], (nucleus dorsalis hypothalami [TA]), partes do núcleo dorsomedial [TA] (nucleus dorsomedialis [TA]), núcleo arqueado [TA] (nucleus arcuatus [TA]), núcleo periventricular posterior [TA] (nucleus periventricularis posterior [TA]), área retroquiasmática [TA], (area retrochiasmatica [TA]), núcleos tuberosos laterais [TA] (nuclei tuberales laterales [TA]) e o núcleo ventromedial [TA] (nucleus ventromedialis hypothalami [TA]). VER TAMBÉM hypothalamus. SIN intermediate hypothalamic region*, a. hypothalamica intermedia.
Kiesselbach a., a. de Kiesselbach; uma a., na porção anterior do septo nasal, rica em capilares (plexo de Kiesselbach) e, com freqüência, a origem da epistaxe. SIN Little a.
a. of Laimer, a. de Laimer; uma a. triangular (ou em forma de V) na face posterior do esôfago proximal, com seu ápice voltado para baixo na linha média e o músculo cricofaríngeo formando sua base, que é uma a. de fraqueza devido à ausência quase total de músculo longitudinal; local potencial de herniação da mucosa faríngea ou esofágica. SIN Laimer-Haeckerman a., V-shaped a. of esophagus.
Laimer-Haeckerman a., a. de Laimer-Haeckerman. SIN a. of Laimer.
lateral hypothalamic a. [TA], a. hipotalâmica lateral; a porção do hipotálamo localizada geralmente lateral a uma linha rostrocaudal traçada através da coluna do fórnice e do trato mamilotalâmico; contém as fibras que, coletivamente, compreendem o feixe medial do prosencéfalo [TA] e os seguintes núcleos: porções da área pré-óptica [TA] (area preoptica [TA]), porções dos núcleos tuberosos laterais [TA] (nuclei tuberales laterales [TA]), o núcleo perifornicial [TA] (nucleus perifornicalis [TA]) e o núcleo tuberomamilar [TA] (nucleus tuberomammillaris [TA]). VER TAMBÉM hypothalamus. SIN a. hypothalamica lateralis [TA].
lateral inferior hepatic a., segmento lateral anterior do fígado. SIN (left anterior) lateral hepatic segment [III].
lateral superior hepatic a. [TA], segmento lateral posterior do fígado. SIN (left posterior) lateral hepatic segment [III].
Little a., a. de Little. SIN Kiesselbach a.
macular a., a. macular. SIN macula of retina.
Martegiani a., a. de Martegiani. SIN Martegiani funnel.
mitral a., a. mitral; a região do tórax sobre o ápice do coração, onde os sons, normais ou patológicos, produzidos na valva mitral, são usualmente auscultados de forma mais nítida.
motor a., córtex motor. SIN motor cortex.
a. ner'vi facia'lis [TA], a. do nervo facial. SIN facial nerve a.
a. nu'da hep'atis [TA], a. nua do fígado. SIN bare a. of liver.
olfactory a., substância perfurada anterior. SIN anterior perforated substance.
oval a. of Flechsig, a. oval de Flechsig, fascículo interfascicular. VER semilunar fasciculus.
Panum a., a. de Panum; a. no espaço que circunda o horóptero empírico, onde a visão binocular única é observada, apesar da estimulação de pontos retinianos não-correspondentes. SIN fusion a.
parastriate a., córtex visual. VER visual cortex.
a. parolfacto'ria [TA], a. paraolfatória. SIN parolfactory a.
parolfactory a. [TA], a. paraolfatória; uma pequena região do córtex cerebral, na superfície medial do lobo frontal, formada pela junção do giro reto com o giro cingulado, demarcada do giro paraterminal pelo sulco paraolfatório posterior. SIN a. parolfactoria [TA], Broca parolfactory a.
pear-shaped a., coxim retromolar. SIN retromolar pad.
peristriate a., córtex visual. VER visual cortex.
piriform a., a. piriforme. SIN piriform cortex.
Pitres a., a. de Pitres; córtex pré-frontal do hemisfério cerebral. VER frontal cortex.
postcentral a., a. pós-central; o córtex do giro pós-central.
post dam a., a. de vedação palatal posterior. SIN posterior palatal seal a.
posterior hypothalamic a. [TA], a. hipotalâmica posterior; a porção do hipotálamo localizada geralmente na região dos corpos mamilares; contém os seguintes núcleos: núcleo pré-mamilar dorsal [TA] (nucleus premammillaris dorsalis [TA]), núcleo lateral do corpo mamilar [TA] (nucleus mammillaris medialis [TA]), núcleo supramamilar [TA] (nucleus supramammillaris [TA]) e núcleo pré-mamilar ventral [TA] (nucleus premammillaris ventralis [TA]). O núcleo posterior do hipotálamo [TA] está localizado na interface das áreas hipotalâmicas intermediária e posterior e, por vezes, é considerada como parte da última. VER TAMBÉM hypothalamus, posterior hypothalamic region. SIN a. hypothalamica posterior [TA].
posterior intercondylar a. of tibia [TA], a. intercondilar posterior da tíbia; uma profunda incisura entre os côndilos tibiais, posteriormente, na qual se insere o ligamento cruzado posterior. SIN a. intercondylaris posterior tibiae [TA].
posterior palatal seal a., a. de vedação palatal posterior; os tecidos moles ao longo da junção dos palatos duro e mole sobre os quais a pressão dentro dos limites fisiológicos dos tecidos pode ser aplicada por uma prótese para auxiliar na retenção da mesma. SIN post dam a., postpalatal seal a.
postpalatal seal a., a. de vedação palatal posterior. SIN posterior palatal seal a.
a. postre'ma (AP) [TA], a. postrema; uma pequena área elevada na parede lateral do recesso inferior do quarto ventrículo; um dos poucos locais no cérebro onde não há barreira hematoencefálica; uma área quimiorreceptora associada ao vômito.
precentral a., a. pré-central; o córtex do giro pré-central.
precommissural septal a., giro paraterminal. SIN subcallosal gyrus.
prefrontal a., a. pré-frontal. VER frontal cortex.
premotor a., a. pré-motora. SIN premotor cortex.
preoptic a. [TA], a. pré-óptica. SIN preoptic region.
a. preoptica [TA], a. pré-óptica. SIN preoptic region.
prestriate a., córtex visual. VER visual cortex.
pretectal a. [TA], a. pré-tectal; uma zona rostral estreita do teto mesencefálico, orientada transversalmente, limitada caudalmente pelo colículo superior, rostralmente pelo trígono habenular e lateralmente pelo pulvinar do tálamo; a área pré-tectal contém vários núcleos que recebem fibras do trato óptico; apresenta conexões eferentes bilaterais com o núcleo de Edinger-Westphal do complexo nuclear oculomotor por meio do qual ela media o reflexo pupilar luminoso. SIN pretectal region, pretectum.
primary visual a., a. visual primária. VER visual cortex.
pulmonary a., a. pulmonar; a região do tórax no segundo espaço intercostal esquerdo, onde os sons produzidos na valva pulmonar do ventrículo direito são auscultados de maneira mais nítida.
relief a., a. de alívio; em odontologia, a porção da a. de sustentação da prótese dentária sobre a qual a base da dentadura é alterada para diminuir a pressão funcional.
rest a., a. de repouso; a porção de uma estrutura dentária ou de uma restauração em um dente que é preparada para receber a base positiva do apoio oclusal, incisal, lingual ou cíngulo metálico de uma prótese removível. SIN rest seat.
retention a., a. de retenção; uma a. de um dente criada durante sua preparação para a restauração, a qual auxiliará na manutenção da posição da restauração. VER TAMBÉM retention groove, retention point.
retrochiasmatic a. [TA], a. retroquiasmática; VER intermediate hypothalamic a. SIN a. retrochiasmatica [TA].
a. retrochiasmatica [TA], a. retroquiasmática. SIN retrochiasmatic a. VER intermediate hypothalamic a.
Rolando a., a. de Rolando. SIN motor cortex.
secondary aortic a., foco aórtico secundário; a região do tórax na base mesoesternal esquerda, onde os sopros diastólicos são, com freqüência, mais bem auscultados.
secondary visual a., a. visual secundária. VER visual cortex.
sensorial areas, sensory areas, áreas sensoriais. VER cerebral cortex.
sensorimotor a., a. sensoriomotora; o giro pré-central [TA] e o giro pós-central [TA] do córtex cerebral.
septal a. [TA], a. septal; a região do hemisfério cerebral que se estende como uma fina lâmina de tecido cerebral entre o feixe fornicial e a superfície ventral do corpo caloso, formando a parede medial do corno frontal do ventrículo lateral; estende-se ventralmente, através do estreito intervalo entre a comissura anterior e o rostro do corpo caloso, como o septo pré-comissural ou giro paraterminal, que é contínuo caudalmente com a a. pré-óptica e com o hipotálamo, bem como, mais lateralmente, com a substância inominada; suas principais conexões funcionais são com o hipocampo e com o hipotálamo. É composta de um núcleo septal dorsal [TA], núcleo septal lateral [TA], núcleo septal medial [TA], núcleo septofimbrial [TA] e núcleo triangular do septo [TA]. O órgão subfornicial [TA] também é encontrado nessa área.
silent a., a. silenciosa; qualquer a. do cérebro ou cerebelo em que as lesões não causem sintomas sensoriais ou motores definitivos.
skip areas, áreas salteadas; segmentos subsidiários de intestino ou cólon doentio na enterite regional ou colite de Crohn, separados da região de envolvimento principal.
somesthetic a., a. somestésica. SIN somatic sensory cortex.
stress-bearing a., a. de sustentação de pressão; (**1**) área de sustentação da prótese dentária. SIN denture foundation a.; (**2**) superfícies das estruturas orais que resistem às forças, tensões ou pressões impostas a elas durante a função.
striate a., córtex visual. VER visual cortex.
a. subcallo'sa [TA], giro paraterminal. SIN subcallosal gyrus.
subcallosal a. [TA], giro paraterminal. SIN subcallosal gyrus.
superior vestibular a. [TA], a. vestibular superior; a a. no fundo do meato acústico interno superior à crista transversal, através da qual passa a parte superior do nervo vestibular (utriculoampular) para atingir a mácula do utrículo e a ampola dos canais semicirculares anterior e lateral. SIN a. vestibularis superior [TA].
supporting a., (**1**) as áreas das cristas maxilar e mandibular desdentadas que são consideradas mais adequadas para suportar as forças de mastigação quando as dentaduras estão em funcionamento; (**2**) área de sustentação da prótese dentária. SIN denture foundation a.

tissue-bearing a., a. de sustentação da prótese dentária. SIN denture foundation a.
a. transitionis amygdalopiriformis [TA], a. de transição amigdalopiriforme. SIN amygdalopiriform transition a.
tricuspid a., foco tricúspide; a região da parede torácica sobre a parte inferior do corpo do esterno onde os sons produzidos na valva tricúspide são auscultados de maneira mais nítida.
trigger a., ponto-gatilho. SIN trigger point.
vagus a., a. do vago; a porção do assoalho do quarto ventrículo que se sobrepõe aos núcleos vagoglossofaríngeos.
vestibular a. [TA], a. vestibular; a área no assoalho do quarto ventrículo lateral ao sulco limitante [TA] e medial ao corpo restiforme [TA] que se sobrepõe aos núcleos vestibulares e às porções dos núcleos cocleares. VER TAMBÉM inferior vestibular a., superior vestibular a.
a. vestibularis [TA], a. vestibular. SIN acoustic a.
a. vestibula'ris infe'rior [TA], a. vestibular inferior. SIN inferior vestibular a.
a. vestibula'ris supe'rior [TA], a. vestibular superior. SIN superior vestibular a.
visual a., córtex visual. SIN visual cortex.
V-shaped a. of esophagus, a. de Laimer. SIN a. of Laimer.
Wernicke a., a. de Wernicke. SIN Wernicke center.

ar·e·a·tus, ar·e·a·ta (ā-rē-ā′tŭs, -tā). Que ocorre em placas ou áreas circunscritas. [L.]
Are·ca (ar′ē-kă). Um gênero de palmeiras da Índia e do Arquipélago Malaio. Uma espécie, *A. catechu*, (arequeira), fornece nozes-de-areca ou avelã-da-índia, que contêm arecolina e 15% de tanino vermelho; nas Índias Orientais, esses frutos costumam ser mastigados (bétele), com ação anti-helmíntica e estimulante. VER TAMBÉM betel nut. [Malaio]
arec·ai·dine (ă-rek′ā-dēn). Arecaidina; um alcalóide cristalino que se assemelha à betaína, derivado da noz-de-areca. SIN arecaine.
are·caine (ar′ē-kān). Arecaína, arecaidina. SIN arecaidine.
arec·o·line (ă-rek′ō-lēn). Arecolina; um alcalóide oleoso incolor a partir da noz-de-areca.
are·flex·ia (ā-rē-flek′sē-ă). Arreflexia; ausência de reflexos.
detrusor a., a. do detrusor; incapacidade do músculo detrusor de contrair reflexamente, ainda que a bexiga tenha alcançado ou excedido sua capacidade.
ar·e·na·ceous (ar-ĕ-nā′shŭs). Arenáceo; arenoso; com consistência semelhante à da areia. [L. *arena*, areia]
Are·na·vi·ri·dae (ā-rē-nă-vir′i-dē). Uma família de cerca de 15 vírus RNA, muitos dos quais parasitas naturais de roedores, entre eles o vírus da coriomeningite linfocítica, o vírus Lassa e o complexo de vírus Tacaribe. Os vírions têm 50 a 300 nm (média de 100 nm) de diâmetro, têm envoltório, são éter-sensíveis e contêm 2 moléculas de ARN monofilamentar (peso molecular de 3 a 5 × 10⁶); eles também apresentam grânulos elétron-densos, contendo RNA (20 a 30 nm de diâmetro) que se assemelham a ribossomas, com um aspecto arenoso à microscopia eletrônica. [L *arena* (*harena*), areia]
Are·na·vi·rus (ā-rē′nă-vī′rŭs). Gênero da família Arenaviridae que está associado à coriomeningite linfocítica e a numerosas febres hemorrágicas.
are·o·la, pl. **are·o·lae** (ă-rē′ō-lă, -lē). Aréola. **1** [NA]. Uma pequena área. **2.** Um dos espaços ou interstícios no tecido areolar. **3.** Aréola da mama. SIN a. of breast. **4.** Uma zona pigmentada, despigmentada ou eritematosa que circunda uma pápula, pústula, urticária ou neoplasia cutânea. SIN halo (3). [L. dim de *area*]
a. of breast [TA], a. da mama; uma área pigmentada circular em torno do mamilo (papila mamária); sua superfície é pontilhada com pequenas projeções de glândulas areolares subjacentes. SIN a. mammae [TA], a. of nipple, a. papillaris, areola (3).
a. mam'mae [TA], a. da mama. SIN a. of breast.
a. of nipple, a. da mama. SIN a. of breast.
a. papilla'ris, a. da mama. SIN a. of breast.
a. umbilicus, a. do umbigo; um anel pigmentado ao redor do umbigo nas gestantes.
are·o·lar (ă-rē′ō-lăr). Areolar; relativo a uma aréola.
ar·e·om·e·ter (ar-ē-om′ĕ-ter). Areômetro. SIN hydrometer. [G. *araios*, fino, + G. *metron*, medir]
Arg Símbolo da arginine (arginina) ou de seus mono- ou dirradicais.
Argas. Um gênero de carrapatos de carapaça mole da família Argasidae, algumas espécies infestam pássaros (ectoparasitas), mas podem atacar os seres humanos.
A. reflex'us, o carrapato do pombo, uma espécie que pode provocar lesão inflamatória cutânea nos seres humanos.
ar·ga·sid (ar-gas′id). Argasídeo; nome comum para os membros da família Argasidae.
Argas·i·dae (ar-gas′i-dē). Família de carrapatos (superfamília Ixodoidea, ordem Acarina), os carrapatos de carapaça mole, assim chamados por causa de sua aparência enrugada, coriácea, tuberculada, que aumenta de volume e torna-se lisa quando o carrapato está ingurgitado de sangue. A. contém 4 gêneros: *Argas, Ornithodoros, Otobius* e *Antricola*; carrapatos argasídeos, principalmente espécies de *Ornithodoros*, alojam-se e transmitem espiroquetas do gênero *Borrelia* que provocam febre recidivante em pássaros e mamíferos.
ar·gen·taf·fin, ar·gen·taf·fine (ar-jen′tă-fin, -fēn). Argentafim; pertinente a elementos celulares ou teciduais que reduzem os íons de prata em solução, tornando-se, assim, tintos de castanho ou preto. [L. *argentum*, prata, + *affinitas*, afinidade]
ar·gen·ta·tion (ar-fen-tā′shŭn). Argentação; impregnação por um sal de prata. VER TAMBÉM argyria. [L. *argentum*, prata]
ar·gen·tic (ar-jen′tik). Argêntico. **1.** Relativo à prata. SIN argyric (1). **2.** Indica um composto químico que contém prata como o dicátion raro (Ag^{2+}).
ar·gen·tine (ar′jen-tēn). Argentino; relativo ou semelhante a ou que contém prata.
ar·gen·to·phil, ar·gen·to·phile (ar-jen′tō-fil, -fīl). Argentófilo. SIN argyrophil.
ar·gen·tous (ar-jen′tŭs). Argentoso; que indica um composto químico que contém prata como um íon de carga elétrica única (Ag^+). A grande maioria dos compostos de prata contém o íon a.; quando o estado iônico da prata não é especificamente afirmado, como no nitrato de prata, presume-se o estado a.
ar·gen·tum, gen. **ar·gen·ti** (ar-jen′tŭm, -jen′tī). Prata. SIN silver. [L.]
ar·gi·nase (ar′ji-nās). Arginase; uma enzima do fígado que catalisa a hidrólise da L-arginina em L-ornitina e uréia; a enzima principal do ciclo da uréia. A deficiência de a. leva à argininemia. SIN canavanase.
ar·gi·nine (Arg) (ar′ji-nēn). Arginina; ácido 2-amino-5-guanidinopentanóico; um dos aminoácidos que ocorrem entre os produtos de hidrólise das proteínas, abundante sobretudo nas proteínas básicas, como histonas e protaminas. Um aminoácido dibásico.
a. deiminase, a. desiminase; uma enzima que catalisa a desaminação hidrolítica da L-a. em L-citrulina e amônia. Cf. *nitric oxide* synthase.
a. glutamate, glutamato de a.; um composto formado de arginina e ácido glutâmico, administrado por via intravenosa para desintoxicar a amônia; usado no tratamento da amoniemia decorrente de disfunção hepática.
a. hydrochloride, cloridrato de a.; uma forma de a. usada para administração intravenosa como um auxiliar no tratamento das encefalopatias associadas às doenças hepáticas e azotemia amoniacal.
a. phosphate, fosfato de a. SIN phosphoarginine.
ar·gi·ni·no·suc·ci·nase (ar′ji-ni-nō-sŭk′si-nās). Argininossuccinase. SIN argininosuccinate lyase.
ar·gi·ni·no·suc·ci·nate ly·ase (ar′ji-ni-nō-sŭk′si-nāt). Argininossuccinato liase; uma enzima que cliva o L-argininossuccinato de maneira não-hidrolítica em L-arginina e fumarato; a deficiência dessa enzima leva à argininossuccinúria; uma etapa primordial no ciclo da uréia. SIN argininosuccinase.
ar·gi·ni·no·suc·cin·ic ac·id (ar′ji-ni-nō-sŭk-sin′ik). Ácido argininossuccínico; formado como um intermediário na conversão da L-citrulina em L-arginina no ciclo da uréia.
ar·gi·ni·no·suc·cin·ic·ac·i·du·ria (ar-ji-nin′ō-sŭk-sin′ik-as-i-doo′rē-ă) [MIM*207900]. Argininossuccinicacidúria; um distúrbio do ciclo da uréia devido à deficiência de argininossuccinatoliase; caracterizada por retardo físico e mental, epilepsia, ataxia, doença hepática, cabelos quebradiços e em tufos e por excreção urinária excessiva de ácido argininossuccínico. Herança autossômica recessiva, causada por mutação no gene da argininossuccinato liase (ASL) no cromossomo 7q.
ar·gin·yl (ar′jin-il). Arginil; o radical aminoacil da arginina.
ar·gi·pres·sin (ar-ji-pres′in). Argipressina. SIN arginine vasopressin.
ar·gon (Ar) (ar′gon). Argônio (Ar); um elemento gasoso, número atômico 18, peso atômico 39,948, presente no ar seco na proporção de aproximadamente 0,94%; um dos gases nobres. [G. neut. de *argos*, preguiçoso, inativo, de *a-* priv. + *ergon*, trabalho]
Argyll Robertson, Douglas, oftalmologista escocês, 1837–1909. VER A. R. - *pupil*.
ar·gyr·ia (ar-jir′ē-ă, -jī′rē-ă). Argiria; uma coloração ligeiramente acinzentada ou azulada da pele e dos tecidos profundos, devido à deposição de albuminato insolúvel de prata, que ocorre depois da administração medicinal de um sal solúvel de prata por um longo período; originalmente bastante comum devido ao uso, no nariz e nos seios paranasais, de preparações comerciais de materiais contendo prata. SIN argyrism, silver poisoning. [G. *argyros*, prata]
ar·gyr·ic (ar-jir′ik). Argírico. **1.** Argêntico. SIN argentic (1). **2.** Relativo à argiria.
ar·gy·rism (ar′ji-rizm). Argirismo. SIN argyria.
ar·gy·rol. Argirol. SIN mild silver protein.
ar·gyr·o·phil, ar·gyr·o·phile (ar-ji′rō-fil, -fīl). Argirófilo; pertinente a elementos teciduais que são capazes de impregnação com íons de prata e de se tornarem visíveis depois que é empregado um agente redutor externo. SIN argentophil, argentophile. [G. *argyros*, prata, + *philos*, ligação]
arhin·ia (ă-rin′ē-ă). Arrinia; ausência congênita do nariz. SIN arrhinia.
Arias-Stella, Javier, patologista peruano, *1924. VER Arias-Stella *effect*; Arias-Stella *phenomenon*; Arias-Stella *reaction*.

a·ri·bo·fla·vin·o·sis (ā-rī'bō-flā-vi-nō'sis). Arriboflavinose; mais adequadamente, hiporriboflavinose; condição nutricional produzida por deficiência de riboflavina na dieta, caracterizada por queilose e língua magenta, usualmente associada a outras manifestações de deficiência de vitamina B.

ar·is·to·loch·ic ac·id (ă-ris-tō-lō'kik). Ácido aristolóquico; um aromático amargo derivado de vegetais do gênero *Aristolochia*.

ar·is·to·te·lian (ar'is-tō-tē'lē-an, ar'i-stō-tēl'yan). Aristotélico; atribuído ou descrito por Aristóteles.

Aristotle. Aristóteles de Estagira; filósofo e cientista grego, de origem macedônica, 384–322 a.C. VER Aristotle *anomaly*, aristotelian *method*.

arith·mo·ma·nia (ă-rith-mō-mā'nē-ă). Aritmomania; um impulso mórbido para contar. [G. *arithmeō*, contar, de *arithmos*, número, + *mania*, loucura]

A·ri·zo·na (ar'i-zō-nă). Nome antigo de *Salmonella enterica*, subespécie *arizonae*.

A. hinshawii, nome antigo de *Salmonella enterica*, subespécie *arizonae*.

Arlt, Carl Ferdinand von, oftalmologista austríaco, 1812–1887. VER A. *operation, sinus*.

arm [TA]. Braço, ramo. **1.** Braço, especificamente o segmento do membro superior entre o ombro e o cotovelo; comumente usado para significar a totalidade do membro superior. SIN brachium (1) [TA], brachio-. **2.** Uma extensão anatômica que se assemelha a um b. **3.** Uma extensão especificamente moldada e posicionada de uma estrutura de prótese dentária parcial removível. **4.** Um grupo de casos ou pessoas em um estudo epidemiológico, especialmente um estudo controlado randomizado, em que as comparações ou contrastes estão sendo feitos entre os grupos. [L. *armus*, quarto dianteiro de um animal; G. *harmos*, uma articulação do ombro]

bar clasp. a., braço de gancho de barra; braço de gancho que tem sua origem na base da dentadura ou no conector principal; consiste em um braço que atravessa as estruturas gengivais sem entrar em contato com elas, e numa extremidade terminal que aproxima seu contato com o dente em uma oclusão gengivoclusal.

brawny a., um braço aumentado de volume por causa de linfedema, pode ser observado após mastectomia radical ipsolateral.

circumferential clasp a., braço de gancho circunferencial; um braço de gancho que tem sua origem em um conector menor e que segue o contorno do dente em um plano aproximadamente perpendicular à via de inserção da dentadura parcial.

clasp a., braço de gancho; uma parte de um gancho de uma prótese dentária parcial removível que se projeta a partir do corpo do gancho e ajuda a reter a prótese dentária parcial em posição na boca. VER clasp (2).

dynein a., b. de dineína; uma estrutura que se estende no sentido horário, a partir de um túbulo de cada um dos 9 microtúbulos duplos para o par oposto, observada no axonema dos cílios ou flagelos (incluindo as caudas dos espermatozóides humanos); a ausência congênita de dineína, refletida estruturalmente por ausência dos braços de dineína, pode resultar nos sintomas observados na síndrome de Kartagener, uma síndrome de cílios imóveis.

nuchal a., situação no parto vaginal com o feto de nádegas, na qual um ou ambos os braços são encontrados ao redor da nuca, interferindo com o parto.

reciprocal a., b. recíproco; um braço de garra ou outra extensão usada em uma dentadura parcial removível para se opor à ação de alguma outra parte ou partes do dispositivo.

retentive a., retention a., braço de retenção; um segmento flexível de uma prótese dentária parcial removível que se encaixa em um corte feito por baixo de um ponto de apoio e que se destina a reter a dentadura.

retentive circumferential clasp a., braço de retenção circunferencial; um braço que é flexível e que se encaixa na protuberância inferior na extremidade terminal do braço.

stabilizing circumferential clasp a., braço de estabilização circunferencial; um braço que é relativamente rígido e que envolve todo o contorno do dente.

ar·ma·men·tar·i·um (ar'mă-men-tar'ē-ŭm). Arsenal; todos os meios terapêuticos disponíveis para os profissionais de saúde exercerem seu ofício. [L. um arsenal, de *armamenta*, implementos, de *arma*, armas]

Armanni, Luciano, patologista italiano, 1839–1903. VER A.-Ebstein *kidney, change*.

ar·mar·i·um (ar-mar'ē-ŭm). Termo raramente utilizado para a biblioteca do médico, como parte de seu armamento. [L. um armário, tórax, de *arma*, arma]

Ar·mil·li·fer (ar-mil'i-fer). Um gênero de Pentastomida (ordem Porocephalida, família Porocephalidae); os adultos são encontrados nos pulmões dos répteis, e os jovens em muitos mamíferos, incluindo os seres humanos. [Fr. Ant. *armille*, de L. *armilla*, um bracelete]

A. armilla'tus, espécie que infesta as serpentes pitonídeas, com a larva ou a ninfa sendo encontrada, ocasionalmente, em seres humanos. SIN *Porocephalus armillatus*.

Armitage, Peter, estatístico inglês (1924-). VER A.-Doll *model*.

arm·pit. Axila. SIN axilla.

Armstrong, Arthur Riley, médico canadense, *1904. VER King-A. *unit*.

Armstrong, Henry E., médico britânico.

ARN Acrônimo para acute retinal *necrosis* (necrose retiniana aguda).

Arndt, Rudolph G., psiquiatra alemão, 1835–1900. VER A. *law*.

Arneth, Joseph, médico alemão, 1873–1956. VER A. *classification, count, formula, index, stages,* em *stage*.

ar·ni·ca (ar'ni-kă). Arnica; a ponta da flor seca da *Arnica montana* (família Compositae); sedativo cardíaco obsoleto raramente administrado por via interna; usado externamente para entorses e equimoses; outrora amplamente empregado como linimento contra-irritante. SIN leopard's bane. [L. Mod]

Arnold, Friedrich, anatomista alemão, 1803–1890. VER A. *bundle, canal, ganglion, nerve, tract; foramen* of A.

Arnold, Julius, patologista alemão, 1835–1915. VER A. *bodies,* em *body*; A.-Chiari *deformity, malformation, syndrome*.

ar·o·mat·ic (ar-ō-mat'ik). Aromático. **1.** Que tem um odor agradável, algo pungente, picante. **2.** Um de um grupo de fitoterápicos com odor fragrante e propriedades discretamente estimulantes. **3.** VER aromatic *compound*. [G. *arōmatikos*, de *arōma*, condimento, erva aromática]

ar·o·mat·ic D-amino ac·id de·car·box·yl·ase. L-aminoácido aromático descarboxilase; uma enzima que catalisa a descarboxilação da L-dopa em dopamina, do L-triptofano em triptamina e do L-hidroxitriptofano em serotonina; importante na via biossintética das catecolaminas e melanina. SIN dopa decarboxylase, hydroxytryptophan decarboxylase, tryptophan decarboxylase.

arotinoid (ă-rot'in-oyd). Arotinóide; um derivado retinóide poliaromático semi-sintético da vitamina A. VER TAMBÉM retinoid, retinoic acid. [*aromatic* + *retinoid*]

ar·o·yl (a'rō-il). Aroil; o radical de um ácido aromático (p.ex., benzoil); análogo ao acil, o termo mais geral.

ar·rack (a-rak'). Arraque; um líquor alcoólico forte, destilado a partir de tâmaras, arroz, seiva do coqueiro e outras substâncias. [Ar. doce suco]

ar·rec·tor, pl. **ar·rec·to·res** (ă-rek'tor, ă-rek-tō'rēz). Eretor, levantador. SIN erector. [L. aquilo que levanta, de *ar-rigo*, pp. *-rectus*, levantar]

ar·rest (ă-rest'). Parar. **1.** Parar, reter, restringir. **2.** Uma parada; interferência com, ou retenção do, curso regular de uma doença, sintoma ou desempenho de uma função. **3.** Inibição de um processo de desenvolvimento, usualmente no estágio final do desenvolvimento; a parada prematura pode levar a uma anormalidade congênita. [Fr. Ant. *arester*, de LL. *adresto,* parar por trás]

cardiac a. (CA), parada cardíaca; cessação completa da atividade cardíaca, elétrica e/ou mecânica; pode ser propositalmente induzida por motivos terapêuticos. SIN heart a.

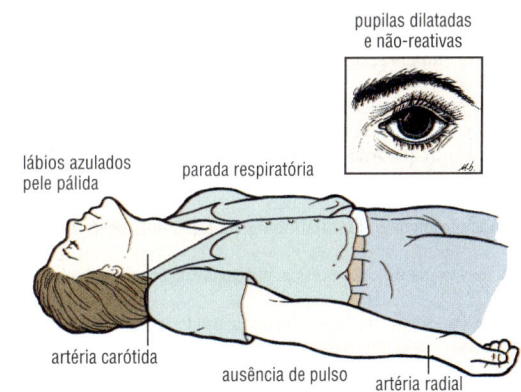

parada cardíaca (sintomas)

cardioplegic a., parada cardioplégica; a cessação intencional temporária da atividade cardíaca elétrica e mecânica, geralmente por soluções contendo potássio, usada para proteger o músculo cardíaco por diminuir sua demanda metabólica durante a cirurgia à coração aberto com *bypass* (derivação) cardiopulmonar.

cardiopulmonary a., parada cardiopulmonar; parada resultando na ausência de atividade cardíaca e pulmonar.

circulatory a., parada circulatória; **(1)** cessação da circulação do sangue em conseqüência de parada ou fibrilação ventricular; **(2)** cessação intencional da circulação por interromper temporariamente o fluxo acessório cardiopulmonar durante determinadas cirurgias da aorta torácica; associada a hipotermia corporal total profunda intencional para proteger os órgãos vitais.

deep hypothermic a., parada hipotérmica profunda; interrupção da atividade cardíaca elétrica e mecânica que ocorre quando o coração é resfriado.

epiphysial a., parada epifisária; fusão precoce e prematura entre a epífise e a diáfise.

heart a., parada cardíaca. SIN cardiac a.
a. of labor, parada do trabalho de parto; ausência de progressão do trabalho de parto ativo (conforme definido por dilatação cervical e descida da parte apresentada) por 2 horas ou mais.
maturation a., parada da maturação; cessação da diferenciação completa das células em um estágio imaturo; na parada da maturação espermatogênica, os túbulos seminíferos contêm espermatócitos, mas não espermatozóides desenvolvidos.
sinus a., parada sinusal; cessação da atividade sinusal; os ventrículos podem continuar a bater sob controle atrial ectópico, juncional A-V ou idioventricular. VER TAMBÉM sinus *standstill*, atrial *standstill*.
ar·rhaph·i·a Arrafia. SIN *status dysraphicus.*
ar·rhen·ic (ă-ren′ik). Arrênico; relativo ao arsênico. [G. *arrhenikon* (var.), arsênico]
Arrhenius, Svante, químico sueco e laureado com o prêmio Nobel, 1859–1927. VER A. *doctrine, equation, law*; A-Madsen *theory*.
ar·rhe·no·blas·to·ma (ă-rē′nō-blas-tō-mă). Arrenoblastoma. SIN Sertoli-Leydig cell *tumor*. [G. *arrhēn*, masculino, + *blastos*, germe, + *-oma*, tumor]
ar·rhin·en·ceph·a·ly, ar·rhin·en·ce·pha·lia, a·rhin·en·ceph·aly (ă-rin-en-sef′ă-lē, -se-fā′lē-ă). Arrinencefalia; ausência congênita ou estado rudimentar do rinencéfalo ou lobo olfatório do cérebro, em um ou em ambos os lados, com a carência correspondente do desenvolvimento dos órgãos olfatórios externos. [G. *a-* priv. + *rhis* (*rhin-*), nariz, + *enkephalos*, cérebro]
ar·rhin·ia (ă-rin′ē-ă). Arrinia. SIN arhinia [G. *a-* priv. + *rhis* (*rhin-*), nariz]
ar·rhyth·mia (ă-rith′mē-ă). Arritmia; perda ou anormalidade do ritmo; indica especialmente uma irregularidade do batimento cardíaco. Ver também as entradas em rhythm. Cf. dysrhythmia. [G. *a-*. priv. + *rhythmos*, ritmo]
cardiac a., a. cardíaca. VER cardiac *dysrhythmia*.
continuous a., a. contínua; termo obsoleto para atrial *fibrillation* (fibrilação atrial).
juvenile a., a. sinusal. SIN sinus a.
nonphasic sinus a., a. sinusal não-fásica; a. sinusal em que as variações no ritmo não estão relacionadas às fases da respiração.
phasic sinus a., a. sinusal fásica; a. sinusal em que a irregularidade está relacionada às fases da respiração, sendo a freqüência mais rápida na inspiração e mais lenta na expiração.
respiratory a., a. respiratória; a. sinusal fásica ou qualquer outra flutuação do ritmo induzida por flutuação respiratória.
sinus a., a. sinusal; irregularidade rítmica repetitiva do batimento cardíaco, estando o coração sob o controle de seu marcapasso normal, o nódulo sinoatrial. SIN juvenile a.
ar·rhyth·mic (ă-ridh′mik, ā-). Arrítmico; marcado pela perda do ritmo; pertinente à arritmia.
ar·rhyth·mo·gen·ic (ă-ridh-mō-jen′ik). Arritmogênico; capaz de induzir arritmias cardíacas. [G. *a-* priv. + *rhythmos*, ritmo, + *-gen*, produção]
ar·row·root (ar′ō-root). Araruta, maranta; o rizoma da *Maranta arundinacea*, uma planta da América tropical, que é a fonte de uma forma de amido empregado outrora como suplemento dietético.
Arruga, Conde Hermenegildo, oftalmologista espanhol, 1886–1972. VER A. *forceps*.
ar·sa·ce·tin (ar-să-sē′tin). Arsacetina; usada outrora como um agente antisifilítico.
ar·sen·a·mide (ar-sen′ă-mīd). Arsenamida; usada no tratamento da filaríase.
ar·se·nate (ar-sē-nāt). Arseniato; um sal do ácido arsênico.
ar·sen·i·a·sis (ar-sen-ī′ă-sis). Arseníase; intoxicação arsenical crônica. SIN arsenicalism.
ar·se·nic (ar-sen′ik). Arsênico; indica o elemento arsênico ou um de seus compostos, especialmente o ácido arsênico.
ar·se·nic (As) (ar′sĕ-nik). Arsênico (As); um elemento metálico, número atômico 33, peso atômico 74,92159; forma inúmeros compostos venenosos, alguns empregados em medicina. SIN arsenium, ratsbane. [L. *arsenicum*, G. *arsenikon*, do Pers. *zarnik*]
a. acid, o hidrato do óxido de arsênico ou pentóxido de arsênico que forma arseniatos com determinadas bases.
a. trihydride, triidreto de a., arsenamina. SIN arsine.
a. trioxide, trióxido de arsênico; As_2O_3; dissolve em água para gerar ácido arsenoso, H_3AsO_3; usado no tratamento de doenças cutâneas e malária, e como tônico; também empregado externamente como cáustico. SIN arsenous oxide, white a.
white a., trióxido de arsênico. SIN a. trioxide.
ar·sen·i·cal (ar-sen′i-kăl). Arsenical. **1.** Um medicamento ou agente cujo efeito depende de seu conteúdo de arsênico. **2.** Indica ou contém arsênico.
ar·sen·i·cal·ism (ar-sen′i-kăl-izm). Arsenicalismo, arseníase. SIN arseniasis.
ar·se·nic-fast. Arsênico-resistente; resistente à ação venenosa do arsênico; indica especialmente os espiroquetas e outros protozoários que adquirem resistência após a administração repetida do medicamento.
ar·se·nide (ar-sē-nīd). Arsenieto; um composto do arsênico com um metal ou outros átomos ou grupamentos com carga elétrica positiva em que o arsênico não está ligado a quaisquer átomos de carbono. SIN arseniuret.
ar·se·ni·ous (ar-sēn′ē-ŭs). Arsenioso; arsênico (adj.).
ar·se·ni·um (ar-sē′nē-ŭm). Arsênico, arsênio. SIN arsenic.
ar·sen·iu·ret (ar-sē′nū-ret). Arsenieto. SIN arsenide.
ar·se·no·ther·a·py (ar′sen-ō-thār′ă-pē). Arsenoterapia; tratamento com arsênico.
ar·se·nous (ar′-sen-ŭs). Arsenioso. **1.** Indica um composto de arsênico com uma valência de +3. **2.** Arsênico (adj.).
ar·se·nous ac·id. Ácido arsenioso. VER *arsenic* trioxide.
ar·se·nous hy·dride. Hidreto de arsênico. VER arsine.
ar·se·nous ox·ide. Óxido de arsênico, trióxido de arsênico. SIN arsenic trioxide.
ar·se·nox·i·des (ar-sē-nok′i-dēs). Arsenóxidos; produtos de oxidação das arsfenaminas no corpo; acredita-se que sejam agentes ativos contra espiroquetas.
ar·sine (ar′sēn). Arsenamina, arseniato de hidrogênio; um veneno celular e sangüíneo; muitos de seus derivados orgânicos têm sido utilizados na guerra química. SIN arsenic trihydride, arseniureted hydrogen, arsenous hydride.
ar·son·ic ac·id (ar-son′ik). Ácido arsônico; um derivado do ácido arsênico pela substituição de um grupamento hidroxila por um radical orgânico.
ar·so·ni·um (ar-son′ē-ŭm). Arsônio; o íon com carga elétrica positiva, AsH_4^+; análogo ao íon amônio, NH_4^+.
ars·phen·a·mine (ars-fen′ă-min). Arsfenamina; utilizada outrora no tratamento da sífilis, bouba e em algumas outras doenças de origem protozoária, após neutralização com NaOH. A síntese da a. em 1907 e a demonstração de sua utilidade como um agente terapêutico por Paul Ehrlich e colaboradores (1909) marcou o início da quimioterapia. SIN phenarsenamine.
ars·thi·nol (ars′thī-nol). Arstinol; um amebicida.
ar·te·fact (ar′tĕ-fakt). Artefato. VER artifact.
artemether (ar-tem′ĕ-ther). Artemetro; derivado semi-sintético da artemisinina utilizado no tratamento da malária cerebral.
Artemisia annua. Um vegetal da família Compositae a partir do qual é produzido um medicamento antimalárico e antiesquistossomótico.
artemisinin (ar-te-mis′in-in). Artemisinina; um medicamento sesquiterpênico antimalárico e antiesquistossomótico derivado da *Artemisia annua*; a a. é um potente esquizontocida sanguíneo, de ação rápida, relatado como sendo muito útil no tratamento da malária cerebral; ativo contra *P. falciparum* cloroquina-resistente e *P. falciparum* e *P. vivax* cloroquina-sensíveis.
ar·te·re·nol (ar′ter-ē-nol). Arterenol; o sal cloridrato da norepinefrina. VER norepinephrine.
⟳ **arteri-.** VER arterio-

ARTERIA

ar·te·ria (a), gen. e pl. **ar·te·ri·ae (aa)** (ar-tēr′ē-ă, ar-tēr′ī-e). [TA]. Artéria. SIN artery. VER TAMBÉM branch. [L. de G. *artēria*, a traquéia, depois uma artéria em diferenciação a uma veia].
a. acetab′uli, ramo acetabular. SIN acetabular *branch.*
arteriae alveola′res superio′res anterio′res [TA], artérias alveolares superiores anteriores. SIN anterior superior alveolar *arteries*, em *artery.*
a. alveola′ris infe′rior [TA], a. alveolar inferior. SIN inferior alveolar *artery.*
a. alveola′ris supe′rior poste′rior [TA], a. alveolar superior posterior. SIN posterior superior alveolar *artery.*
a. anastomot′ica auricula′ris mag′na, ramo anastomótico atrial do ramo circunflexo da artéria coronária esquerda. SIN atrial anastomotic *branch* of circumflex branch of left coronary artery.
a. anastomot′ica mag′na, (1) a. colateral ulnar inferior. SIN inferior ulnar collateral *artery;* **(2)** a. descendente do joelho. SIN descending genicular *artery.*
a. angula′ris [TA], ramo para o giro angular. SIN *branch* to angular gyrus.
a. aorta, aorta. SIN aorta.
a. appendicula′ris [TA], a. apendicular. SIN appendicular *artery.*
arte′riae arcua′tae renis [TA], artérias arqueadas do rim. SIN arcuate *arteries* of kidney, em *artery.*
a. arcua′ta (pedis) [TA], a. arqueada (do pé). SIN arcuate *artery* (of foot) (inconstante).
a. articula′ris az′ygos, a. média do joelho. SIN middle genicular *artery.*
a. ascen′dens [TA], **(1)** ramo cólico da a. ileocólica. SIN colic *branch* of ileocolic artery; **(2)** a. ascendente. SIN ascending *artery* (2).
arteriae atria′les, artérias atriais. SIN atrial *arteries*, em *artery.*
a. auditi′va inter′na, a. do labirinto. SIN labyrinthine *artery.*
a. auricula′ris poste′rior [TA], a. auricular posterior. SIN posterior auricular *artery.*

a. auricula'ris profun'da [TA], a. auricular profunda. SIN deep auricular artery.
a. axilla'ris [TA], a. axilar. SIN axillary artery.
a. basila'ris [TA]. a. basilar (a. do labirinto). SIN basilar artery.
a. brachia'lis [TA], a. braquial. SIN brachial artery.
a. brachia'lis superficia'lis [TA], a. braquial superficial. SIN superficial brachial artery.
a. bucca'lis [TA], a. bucal. SIN buccal artery.
a. bul'bi pe'nis [TA], a. do bulbo do pênis. SIN artery of bulb of penis.
a. bul'bi ure'thrae, a. do bulbo do pênis. SIN artery of bulb of penis.
a. bulbi vaginae, a. do bulbo do vestíbulo. SIN artery of bulb of vestibule.
a. bul'bi vestib'uli [TA], a. do bulbo do vestíbulo. SIN artery of bulb of vestibule.
a. calcari'na, Ramo calcarino da a. occipital medial. SIN calcarine branch of medial occipital artery.
a. callosa mediana [TA], a. calosa mediana. SIN median callosal artery.
a. callo'somargina'lis [TA], a. calosomarginal. SIN callosomarginal artery.
a. cana'lis pterygoid'ei [TA], a. do canal pterigóide. SIN artery of pterygoid canal.
arte'riae carot'icotympan'icae (arteriae carotidis internae) [TA], artérias caroticotimpânicas (das artérias carótidas internas). SIN caroticotympanic arteries (of internal carotid artery), em artery.
a. carot'is commu'nis [TA], a. carótida comum. SIN common carotid artery.
a. carot'is exter'na [TA], a. carótida externa. SIN external carotid artery.
a. carot'is inter'na [TA], a. carótida interna. SIN internal carotid artery.
a. cau'dae pancrea'tis [TA], a. da cauda do pâncreas. SIN artery to tail of pancreas.
a. ceca'lis ante'rior [TA], a. cecal anterior. SIN anterior cecal artery.
a. ceca'lis poste'rior [TA], a. cecal posterior. SIN posterior cecal artery.
a. celi'aca, tronco celíaco. SIN celiac (arterial) trunk.
arte'riae centra'les anterolatera'les [TA], artérias centrais ântero-laterais. SIN anterolateral central arteries, em artery.
arte'riae centra'les anteromedia'les [TA], artérias centrais anteromediais. SIN anteromedial central arteries, em artery.
arte'riae centra'les posterolatera'les [TA], artérias centrais póstero-laterais. SIN posterolateral central arteries, em artery.
arte'riae centra'les posteromedia'les [TA], artérias centrais póstero-mediais. SIN posteromedial central arteries, em artery.
a. centra'lis brev'is, artérias estriadas mediais proximais. SIN proximal medial striate arteries, em artery.
a. centra'lis ret'inae [TA], a. central da retina. SIN central retinal artery.
a. cer'ebri ante'rior [TA], a. cerebral anterior. SIN anterior cerebral artery.
a. cer'ebri me'dia [TA], a. cerebral média. SIN middle cerebral artery.
a. cer'ebri poste'rior [TA], a. cerebral posterior. SIN posterior cerebral artery.
a. cervica'lis ascen'dens [TA], a. cervical ascendente. SIN ascending cervical artery.
a. cervica'lis profun'da [TA], a. cervical profunda. SIN deep cervical artery.
a. cervica'lis superficia'lis [TA], ramo superficial da a. cervical transversa. SIN superficial cervical artery. VER TAMBÉM superficial branch of the transverse cervical artery.
a. cervicovagina'lis, a. cervicovaginal. SIN cervicovaginal artery.
a. choroi'dea ante'rior [TA], a. corióidea anterior. SIN anterior choroidal artery.
a. choroi'dea poste'rior [TA], a. corióidea posterior. SIN posterior choroidal artery.
arteriae cilia'res anterio'res, artérias ciliares anteriores. SIN anterior ciliary arteries, em artery.
arteriae cilia'res posterio'res lon'gae, artérias ciliares posteriores longas. SIN long posterior ciliary arteries, em artery.
a. cilia'ris poste'rior bre'vis [TA], artéria ciliar posterior curta. SIN short posterior ciliary artery.
arteriae circumferentiales brevis [TA], artérias circunferenciais curtas. SIN short circumferential arteries, em artery.
a. circumflex'a fem'oris latera'lis [TA], a. circunflexa femoral lateral. SIN lateral circumflex femoral artery.
a. circumflex'a fem'oris media'lis [TA], a. circunflexa femoral medial. SIN medial circumflex femoral artery.
a. circumflex'a hu'meri ante'rior [TA], a. circunflexa anterior do úmero. SIN anterior circumflex humeral artery.
a. circumflex'a hu'meri poste'rior [TA], a. circunflexa posterior do úmero. SIN posterior circumflex humeral artery.
a. circumflex'a ili'aca profun'da [TA], a. ilíaca circunflexa profunda. SIN deep circumflex iliac artery.
a. circumflex'a ili'aca superficia'lis [TA], a. ilíaca circunflexa superficial. SIN superficial circumflex iliac artery.
a. circumflex'a scap'ulae [TA], a. circunflexa da escápula. SIN circumflex scapular artery.
a. cochlearis communis [TA], a. coclear comum. SIN common cochlear artery.
a. cochlearis propria [TA], a. coclear própria. SIN proper cochlear artery.

a. col'ica dex'tra [TA], a. cólica direita. SIN right colic artery.
a. col'ica me'dia [TA], a. cólica média. SIN middle colic artery.
a. col'ica sinis'tra [TA], a. cólica esquerda. SIN left colic artery.
a. collatera'lis me'dia [TA], a. colateral média. SIN middle collateral artery.
a. collatera'lis radia'lis [TA], a. colateral radial. SIN radial collateral artery.
a. collatera'lis ulna'ris infe'rior [TA], a. colateral ulnar inferior. SIN inferior ulnar collateral artery.
a. collatera'lis ulna'ris supe'rior [TA], a. colateral ulnar superior. SIN superior ulnar collateral artery.
a. collicularis [TA], a. colicular. SIN collicular artery.
a. co'mes ner'vi phren'ici, a. pericardicofrênica. SIN pericardiacophrenic artery.
a. com'itans ner'vi ischiad'ici [TA], a. acompanhante do nervo isquiático. SIN artery to sciatic nerve.
a. co'mitans ner'vi media'ni [TA], a. acompanhante do nervo mediano. SIN median artery.
a. commissuralis mediana [TA], a. da comissura mediana. SIN median commissural artery.
a. commu'nicans ante'rior [TA], a. comunicante anterior. SIN anterior communicating artery.
a. commu'nicans poste'rior [TA], a. comunicante posterior. SIN posterior communicating artery.
a. conjunctiva'lis ante'rior [TA], a. conjuntival anterior. SIN anterior conjunctival artery.
a. conjunctiva'lis poste'rior [TA], a. conjuntival posterior. SIN posterior conjunctival artery.
a. corona'ria dex'tra [TA], a. coronária direita. SIN right coronary artery.
a. corona'ria sinis'tra [TA], a. coronária esquerda. SIN left coronary artery.
arteriae corticales radiatae [TA], artérias corticais radiais. SIN cortical radiate arteries, em artery.
a. cremaster'ica [TA], a. cremastérica. SIN cremasteric artery.
a. cys'tica [TA], a. cística. SIN cistic artery.
a. deferentia'lis, a. do ducto deferente. SIN artery to ductus deferens.
a. descen'dens ge'nus [TA], a. descendente do joelho. SIN descending genicular artery.
arteriae digitales palmares propriae [TA], artérias digitais palmares próprias. SIN proper palmar digital arteries, em artery.
arteriae digita'les planta'res pro'priae, artéria digital plantar própria. SIN proper plantar digital artery.
a. digita'lis dorsa'lis [TA], a. digital dorsal. SIN dorsal digital artery.
a. digita'lis palma'ris commu'nis [TA], a. digital palmar comum. SIN common palmar digital artery.
a. digita'lis palma'ris pro'pria, a. digital palmar própria. SIN proper palmar digital arteries, em artery.
a. digita'lis planta'ris commu'nis [TA], a. digital plantar comum. SIN common plantar digital artery.
a. digitalis plantaris propria [TA], a. digital plantar própria. SIN proper plantar digital artery.
a. dorsa'lis clitor'idis [TA], a. dorsal do clitóris. SIN dorsal artery of clitoris.
a. dorsa'lis na'si [TA], a. dorsal do nariz. SIN dorsal nasal artery.
a. dorsa'lis pe'dis [TA], a. dorsal do pé. SIN dorsalis pedis artery.
a. dorsa'lis pe'nis [TA], a. dorsal do pênis. SIN dorsal artery of penis.
a. dorsa'lis scap'ulae [TA], a. dorsal da escápula. SIN dorsal scapular artery.
a. duc'tus deferen'tis, a. do ducto deferente. SIN artery to ductus deferens.
arteriae encephali [TA], artérias do encéfalo. SIN arteries to brain, em artery.
a. epigas'trica infe'rior [TA], a. epigástrica inferior. SIN inferior epigastric artery.
a. epigas'trica superficia'lis [TA], a. epigástrica superficial. SIN superficial epigastric artery.
a. epigas'trica supe'rior [TA], a. epigástrica superior. SIN superior epigastric artery.
a. episclera'lis [TA], a. episcleral. SIN episcleral artery.
a. ethmoida'lis ante'rior [TA], a. etmoidal anterior. SIN anterior ethmoidal artery.
a. ethmoida'lis poste'rior [TA], a. etmoidal posterior. SIN posterior ethmoidal artery.
a. facia'lis [TA], a. facial. SIN facial artery.
a. femora'lis [TA], a. femoral. SIN femoral artery.
a. fibula'ris [TA], a. fibular. SIN fibular artery.
a. flexurae dextrae [TA], a. da flexura direita. SIN right flexural artery.
a. fronta'lis, a. supratroclear. SIN supratrochlear artery.
a. frontobasa'lis latera'lis [TA], a. frontobasilar lateral. SIN lateral frontobasal artery.
a. frontobasa'lis media'lis [TA], a. frontobasilar medial. SIN medial frontobasal artery.
a. gas'trica dex'tra [TA], a. gástrica direita. SIN right gastric artery.
arte'riae gas'tricae bre'ves [TA], artérias gástricas curtas. SIN short gastric arteries, em artery.

a. gastrica posterior [TA], a. gástrica posterior. SIN posterior gastric *artery*.
a. gas'trica sinis'tra [TA], a. gástrica esquerda. SIN left gastric *artery*.
a. gastroduodena'lis [TA], a. gastroduodenal. SIN gastroduodenal *artery*.
a. gastroepiplo'ica dex'tra, a. gastromental direita. SIN right gastroomental *artery*.
arteriae gastroepiploicae, artérias gastromentais; *termo oficial alternativo para gastroomental *arteries*, em *artery*.
a. gastroepiplo'ica sinis'tra, a. gastromental esquerda. SIN left gastroomental *artery*.
arteriae gastro-omentales [TA], artérias gastromentais. SIN gastroomental *arteries*, em *artery*.
a. gastromenta'lis dex'tra [TA], a. gastromental direita. SIN right gastroomental *artery*.
a. gastromenta'lis sinis'tra [TA], a. gastromental esquerda. SIN left gastromental *artery*.
a. ge'nus infe'rior latera'lis, a. inferior lateral do joelho. SIN inferior lateral genicular *artery*.
a. ge'nus infe'rior media'lis, a. inferior medial do joelho. SIN inferior medial genicular *artery*.
a. ge'nus me'dia, a. média do joelho. SIN middle genicular *artery*.
a. glu'tea infe'rior [TA], a. glútea inferior. SIN inferior gluteal *artery*.
a. glu'tea supe'rior [TA], a. glútea superior. SIN superior gluteal *artery*.
a. gy'ri angula'ris [TA], ramo do giro angular. SIN branch to angular gyrus.
arteriae helicinae penis [TA], artérias helicinas do pênis. SIN helicine *arteries* of penis, em *artery*.
arteriae helicinae uteri [TA], artérias helicinas do útero. SIN helicine *arteries* of the uterus, em *artery*.
a. hepat'ica commu'nis [TA], a. hepática comum. SIN common hepatic *artery*.
a. hepat'ica pro'pria, a. hepática própria. SIN hepatic *artery* proper.
a. hyaloi'dea [TA], hialóide. SIN hyaloid *artery*.
a. hypogas'trica, a. ilíaca interna. SIN internal iliac *artery*.
a. hypophysia'lis infe'rior [TA], a. hipofisária inferior. SIN inferior hypophysial *artery*.
a. hypophysia'lis supe'rior [TA], a. hipofisária superior. SIN superior hypophysial *artery*.
arte'riae ilea'les [TA], artérias ileais. SIN ileal arteries, em *artery*.
a. ileocol'ica [TA], a. ileocólica. SIN ileocolic *artery*.
a. ili'aca commu'nis [TA], a. ilíaca comum. SIN common iliac *artery*.
a. ili'aca exter'na [TA], a. ilíaca externa. SIN external iliac *artery*.
a. ili'aca inter'na [TA], a. ilíaca interna. SIN internal iliac *artery*.
a. iliolumba'lis [TA], a. iliolombar. SIN iliolumbar *artery*.
a. infe'rior ante'rior cerebel'li [TA], a. cerebelar anterior inferior. SIN anterior inferior cerebellar *artery*.
a. inferior lateralis genus [TA], a. inferior lateral do joelho. SIN inferior lateral genicular *artery*.
a. inferior medialis genus [TA], a. inferior medial do joelho. SIN inferior medial genicular *artery*.
a. infe'rior poste'rior cerebel'li [TA], a. cerebelar inferior posterior. SIN posterior inferior cerebellar *artery*.
a. infraorbita'lis [TA], a. infra-orbital. SIN infraorbital *artery*.
arte'riae insula'res [TA], artérias insulares. SIN insular *arteries*, em *artery*.
arte'riae intercosta'les posterio'res I et II, primeira e segunda artérias intercostais posteriores. SIN first and second posterior intercostal *arteries*, em *artery*.
arteriae intercosta'les poste'riores III-XI [TA], artérias intercostais posteriores 3–11. SIN posterior intercostal *arteries* 3–11, em *artery*.
arteriae intercostales posteriores prima et secunda [TA], primeira e segunda artérias intercostais posteriores. SIN first and second posterior intercostal *arteries*, em *artery*.
a. intercosta'lis supre'ma [TA], a. intercostal suprema. SIN supreme intercostal *artery*.
arte'riae interloba'res re'nis [TA], artérias interlobares do rim. SIN interlobar *arteries* of kidney, em *artery*.
arteriae interlobula'res [TA], artérias interlobulares. SIN interlobular *arteries*, em *artery*.
a. interlobula'res (hepatis), artérias interlobulares (do fígado). SIN interlobular *arteries* of liver, em *artery*.
a. interlobula'res (renis), artérias interlobulares (do rim). SIN cortical radiate *arteries*, em *artery*.
a. intermesenter'ica, a. mesentérica inferior (a. ascendente). SIN ascending *artery* (2).
a. interos'sea ante'rior [TA], a. interóssea anterior. SIN anterior interosseous *artery*.
a. interos'sea commu'nis [TA], a. interóssea comum. SIN common interosseous *artery*.
a. interos'sea poste'rior [TA], a. interóssea posterior. SIN posterior interosseous *artery*.

a. interos'sea recur'rens [TA], a. interóssea recorrente. SIN recurrent interosseous *artery*.
a. interos'sea vola'ris, a. interóssea anterior. SIN anterior interosseous *artery*.
arte'riae intestina'les, artérias intestinais. VER ileal *arteries*, em *artery*, jejunal *arteries*, em *artery*.
arteriae intrarenales [TA], artérias intra-renais. SIN intrarenal *arteries*, em *artery*.
a. ischiad'ica, a. ischiat'ica, a. glútea inferior. SIN inferior gluteal *artery*.
arteriae jejuna'les [TA], artérias jejunais. SIN jejunal *arteries*, em *artery*.
a. juxtacolica, a. justacólica; *termo oficial alternativo para marginal *artery* of colon.
arte'riae labia'les anterio'res, ramos labiais anteriores da a. pudenda externa profunda. SIN anterior labial *branches* of deep external pudendal artery, em *branch*.
a. labia'lis infe'rior, ramo inferior da a. facial. SIN inferior *branch* of facial *artery*.
a. labia'lis supe'rior [TA], ramo labial superior da a. facial. SIN superior labial *branch* of facial artery.
a. labyrin'thi [TA], a. do labirinto (a. basilar). SIN labyrinthine *artery*.
a. lacrima'lis [TA], a. lacrimal. SIN lacrimal *artery*.
a. laryn'gea infe'rior [TA], a. laríngea inferior. SIN inferior laryngeal *artery*.
a. laryn'gea supe'rior [TA], a. laríngea superior. SIN superior laryngeal *artery*.
a. liena'lis, a. esplênica; *termo oficial alternativo para splenic *artery*.
a. ligamen'ti tere'tis u'teri, a. do ligamento redondo do útero. SIN *artery* of round ligament of uterus.
a. lingua'lis [TA], a. lingual. SIN lingual *artery*.
a. lingularis [TA], a. lingular. VER left pulmonary *artery*.
a. lingularis inferior [TA], a. lingular inferior. SIN inferior lingular *artery*. VER left pulmonar *artery*.
a. lingularis superior [TA], a. lingular superior. SIN superior lingular *artery*. VER left pulmonary *artery*.
arteriae lobares inferiores [TA], artérias lobares inferiores. VER left pulmonary *artery*, right pulmonary *artery*.
arteriae lobares inferior et superior [TA], artérias lobares inferior e superior. VER left pulmonary *artery*, right pulmonary *artery*.
arteriae lobares superiores [TA], artérias lobares superiores. VER left pulmonary *artery*, right pulmonary *artery*.
a. lobaris media [TA], a. lobar média. VER left pulmonary *artery*, right pulmonary *artery*.
a. lobaris media pulmonis dextri [TA], a. lobar média. VER right pulmonary *artery*.
a. lo'bi cauda'ti [TA], a. do lobo caudado. SIN *artery* of caudate lobe.
arteriae lumba'les [TA], artérias lombares. SIN lumbar *arteries*, em *artery*.
arteriae lumba'les i'mae [TA], artérias lombares imas. SIN lowest lumbar *arteries*, em *artery*.
a. luso'ria, uma a. subclávia direita aberrante que se origina da aorta descendente; passa posteriormente ao esôfago, muitas vezes provocando disfagia.
arte'riae malleola'res posterio'res latera'les, ramo maleolar lateral da a. fibular. SIN lateral malleolar *branch* (of fibular peroneal artery).
arte'riae malleola'res posterio'res media'les, ramos maleolares mediais da a. tibial posterior. SIN medial malleolar *branches* (of posterior tibial artery), em *branch*.
a. malleola'ris ante'rior latera'lis [TA], a. maleolar anterior lateral. SIN anterior lateral malleolar *artery*.
a. malleola'ris ante'rior media'lis [TA], a. maleolar anterior medial. SIN anterior medial malleolar *artery*.
a. mamma'ria inter'na, a. torácica interna. SIN internal thoracic *artery*.
arteriae mammillares [TA], artérias mamilares. SIN mammillary *arteries*, em *artery*.
a. marginalis coli [TA], a. marginal do cólon. SIN marginal *artery* of colon.
a. masseter'ica [TA], a. massetérica. SIN masseteric *artery*.
a. maxilla'ris [TA], a. maxilar. SIN maxillary *artery*.
a. maxilla'ris exter'na, a. facial. SIN facial *artery*.
a. media genus [TA], artéria média do joelho. SIN middle genicular *artery*.
a. media'na, a. mediana. SIN median *artery*.
arteriae medullares segmentales [TA], artérias medulares segmentares. SIN segmental medullary *arteries*, em *artery*.
arteriae membri inferioris [TA], artérias do membro inferior. SIN *arteries* of lower limb, em *artery*.
arteriae membri superioris [TA], artérias do membro superior. SIN *arteries* of upper limb, em *artery*.
a. menin'gea ante'rior [TA], ramo meníngeo anterior da a. etmoidal anterior. SIN anterior meningeal *branch* (of anterior ethmoidal artery).
a. menin'gea me'dia [TA], a. meníngea média. SIN middle meningeal *artery*.
a. menin'gea posterior [TA], a. meníngea posterior. SIN posterior meningeal *artery*.
a. menta'lis, ramo mentual da a. alveolar inferior. SIN mental *branch* (of inferior alveolar artery).

arteria

a. mesenter'ica infe'rior [TA], a. mesentérica inferior. SIN inferior mesenteric artery.
a. mesenter'ica supe'rior [TA], a. mesentérica superior. SIN superior mesenteric artery.
a. metacarpa'lis dorsa'lis [TA], a. metacarpal dorsal. SIN dorsal metacarpal artery.
a. metacarpa'lis palma'ris [TA], a. metacarpal palmar. SIN palmar metacarpal artery.
a. metatarsa'lis [TA], a. metatarsal. SIN metatarsal artery.
a. metatarsa'lis dorsa'lis [TA], a. metatarsal dorsal. SIN dorsal metatarsal artery.
a. metatarsa'lis planta'ris [TA], a. metatarsal plantar. SIN plantar metatarsal artery.
arteriae musculares (arteriae ophthalmicae) [TA], artérias musculares (artérias oftálmicas). SIN muscular arteries (of ophthalmic artery), em artery.
a. musculophren'ica [TA], a. musculofrênica. SIN musculophrenic artery.
arte'riae nasa'les posterio'res latera'les [TA], artérias nasais posteriores laterais. SIN posterior lateral nasal arteries, em artery.
a. nasa'lis poste'rior sep'ti, ramo septal posterior do nariz. SIN posterior septal branch of nose.
a. na'si exter'na, a. nasal dorsal. SIN dorsal nasal artery.
arteriae nervo'rum, artérias dos nervos; artérias para os nervos.
a. nutri'cia [TA], a. nutrícia. SIN nutrient artery.
a. nutriciae femoris [TA], a. nutrícia do fêmur. SIN nutrient artery of femur.
arte'riae nutri'ciae hu'meri [TA], artérias nutrícias do úmero. SIN humeral nutrient arteries, em artery.
a. nutricia tibiae [TA], a. nutrícia da tíbia. SIN tibial nutrient artery.
a. nutricia ulnae [TA], a. nutrícia da ulna. SIN nutrient artery of ulna.
a. nutriens femoris, a. nutrícia do fêmur; *termo oficial alternativo para nutrient artery of femur.
a. nu'triens fib'ulae, a. nutrícia da fíbula; *termo oficial alternativo para fibular nutrient artery.
a. nutriens humeri, artérias nutrícias do úmero; *termo oficial alternativo para nutrient arteries of humerus, em artery.
a. nutriens radii, a. nutrícia do rádio; *termo oficial alternativo para nutrient artery of radius.
a. nutriens tibiae, a. nutrícia da tíbia; *termo oficial alternativo para tibial nutrient artery.
a. nu'triens tibia'lis, a. nutrícia da tíbia. SIN tibial nutrient artery.
a. nutriens ulnae, a. nutrícia da ulna; *termo oficial alternativo para nutrient artery of ulna.
a. obturato'ria [TA], a. obturatória. SIN obturator artery.
a. obturato'ria accesso'ria [TA], a. obturatória acessória. SIN acessory obturator artery.
a. occipita'lis [TA], a. occipital. SIN occipital artery.
a. occipita'lis latera'lis [TA], a. occipital lateral. SIN lateral occipital artery.
a. occipita'lis media'lis [TA], a. occipital medial. SIN medial occipital artery.
a. ophthal'mica [TA], a. oftálmica. SIN ophthalmic artery.
a. orbitofronta'lis, latera'lis, a. frontobasilar lateral; *termo oficial alternativo para lateral frontobasal artery.
a. orbitofronta'lis media'lis, a. frontobasilar medial; *termo oficial alternativo para medial frontobasal artery.
a. ova'rica [TA], a. ovárica. SIN ovarian artery.
a. palati'na ascen'dens [TA], a. palatina ascendente. SIN ascending palatine artery.
a. palati'na descen'dens [TA], a. palatina descendente. SIN descending palatine artery.
a. palati'na major, a. palatina maior. SIN greater palatine artery.
a. palati'na mi'nor, a. palatina menor. SIN lesser palatine artery.
arte'riae palpebra'les (laterales et mediales) [TA], artérias palpebrais (lateral e medial). SIN (lateral and medial) palpebral arteries, em artery.
a. pancreat'ica dorsa'lis [TA], a. pancreática dorsal. SIN dorsal pancreatic artery.
a. pancreat'ica infe'rior [TA], a. pancreática inferior. SIN inferior pancreatic artery.
a. pancreat'ica mag'na, a. pancreática magna. SIN greater pancreatic artery.
a. pancreat'icoduodena'lis infe'rior [TA], a. pancreaticoduodenal inferior. SIN inferior pancreaticoduodenal artery.
a. pancreat'icoduodena'lis supe'rior (anterior et posterior), a. pancreaticoduodenal superior (anterior e posterior). SIN (anterior and posterior) superior pancreaticoduodenal artery.
a. paracentra'lis, ramos paracentrais da a. pericalosa. SIN paracentral branches (of pericallosal artery), em artery.
a. parieta'lis anterior [TA], a. parietal anterior. SIN anterior parietal artery.
arte'riae parieta'les (laterales et mediales) [TA], artérias parietais (lateral e medial). SIN (lateral and medial) parietal arteries, em artery.
a. parieta'lis posterior [TA], a. parietal posterior. SIN posterior parietal artery.

arteriae pari'eto-occipita'les, ramos parieto-occipitais da a. cerebral anterior. SIN parieto-occipital branches (of anterior cerebral artery), em branch.
arteriae perforantes anteriores [TA], artérias perfurantes anteriores. SIN anterior perforating arteries, em artery.
arte'riae perforan'tes arteriae profundae femoris [TA], artérias perfurantes da a. femoral profunda. SIN perforating arteries (of deep femoral artery), em artery.
arteriae perforantes penis [TA], artérias perfurantes do pênis. SIN perforating arteries of penis, em artery.
arteriae perforantes radiatae (renis) [TA], artérias perfurantes radiadas (intra-renais). SIN perforating radiate arteries (of kidney), em artery.
a. pericallo'sa [TA], a. pericalosa. SIN pericallosal artery.
a. pericardiacophreni'ca [TA], a. pericardifrênica. SIN pericardiacophrenic artery.
a. perinea'lis [TA], a. perineal. SIN perineal artery.
a. perone'a, a. fibular; *termo oficial alternativo para fibular artery.
a. pharyn'gea ascen'dens [TA], a. faríngea ascendente. SIN ascending pharyngeal artery.
a. phren'ica infe'rior [TA], a. frênica inferior. SIN inferior phrenic artery.
a. phren'ica supe'rior [TA], a. frênica superior. SIN superior phrenic artery.
a. planta'ris latera'lis [TA], a. plantar lateral. SIN lateral plantar artery.
a. planta'ris media'lis [TA], a. plantar medial. SIN medial plantar artery.
a. plantaris profunda arteriae dorsalis pedis [TA], a. plantar profunda. SIN deep plantar artery.
a. plantaris profundus [TA], ramo plantar profundo da a. pediosa dorsal. SIN deep plantar branch of dorsalis pedis artery.
a. polaris frontalis [TA], a. polar frontal. SIN polar frontal artery.
a. polaris temporalis [TA], a. polar temporal. SIN polar temporal artery.
arte'riae pont'is [TA], artérias pontinas. SIN pontine arteries, em artery.
a. poplit'ea [TA], a. poplítea. SIN popliteal artery.
a. precunea'lis, ramos precuneais. SIN precuneal branches (of anterior cerebral artery), em branch.
a. prepancreatica [TA], a. pré-pancreática. SIN prepancreatic artery.
a. prin'ceps pol'licis [TA], a. principal do polegar. SIN princeps pollicis artery.
a. profun'da bra'chii [TA], a. braquial profunda. SIN profunda brachii artery.
a. profun'da clitor'idis [TA], a. profunda do clitóris. SIN deep artery of clitoris.
a. profun'da fem'oris, a. profunda do fêmur. SIN deep artery of thigh.
a. profun'da lin'guae [TA], a. profunda da língua. SIN deep lingual artery.
a. profun'da pe'nis [TA], a. profunda do pênis. SIN deep artery of penis.
a. pterygomeningealis [TA], a. pterigomeníngea. SIN pterygomeningeal artery.
arte'riae puden'dae exter'nae [TA], artérias pudendas externas (superficial e profunda). SIN (superficial and deep) external pudendal arteries, em artery.
a. puden'da inter'na [TA], a. pudenda interna. SIN internal pudendal artery.
a. pulmona'lis, a. pulmonar. SIN pulmonary trunk.
a. pulmona'lis dex'tra [TA], a. pulmonar direita. SIN right pulmonary artery.
a. pulmona'lis sinis'tra [TA], a. pulmonar esquerda. SIN left pulmonary artery.
a. quadrigeminalis, a. colicular; *termo oficial alternativo para collicular artery.
a. radia'lis [TA], a. radial. SIN radial artery.
a. radia'lis in'dicis [TA], a. radial do indicador. SIN radialis indicis artery.
arteriae radiculares (anterior et posterior), artérias radiculares (anterior e posterior). SIN (anterior and posterior) radicular arteries, em artery.
a. radicula'ris mag'na, a. medular segmentar maior. SIN great segmental medullary artery.
a. radii nutricia [TA], a. nutricial do rádio. SIN nutrient artery of radius.
a. rani'na, a. profunda da língua; SIN deep lingual artery.
a. recta'lis infe'rior [TA], a. retal inferior. SIN inferior rectal artery.
a. recta'lis me'dia [TA], a. retal média. SIN middle rectal artery.
a. recta'lis supe'rior [TA], a. retal superior. SIN superior rectal artery.
a. recur'rens, a. recorrente. SIN medial striate artery.
a. recur'rens radia'lis [TA], a. recorrente radial. SIN radial recurrent artery.
a. recur'rens tibia'lis ante'rior [TA], a. recorrente tibial anterior. SIN anterior tibial recurrent artery.
a. recur'rens tibia'lis poste'rior [TA], a. recorrente tibial posterior. SIN posterior tibial recurrent artery.
a. recur'rens ulna'ris [TA], a. recorrente ulnar. SIN ulnar recurrent artery.
a. rena'lis [TA], a. renal. SIN renal artery.
arte'riae re'nis [TA], artérias segmentares do rim. SIN segmental arteries of kidney, em artery.
a. ret'inae centra'lis, a. central da retina. SIN central retinal artery.
a. retroduodena'lis [TA], a. retroduodenal. SIN retroduodenal artery.
arteriae sacra'les latera'les, artérias sacrais laterais. SIN lateral sacral arteries, em artery.
a. sacra'lis media'na [TA], a. sacral mediana. SIN median sacral artery.
a. scapula'ris descen'dens, a. dorsal da escápula. SIN dorsal scapular artery.

a. scapula'ris dorsa'lis, a. dorsal da escápula. SIN dorsal scapular *artery*.
a. segmentalis anterior [TA], a. segmentar anterior (a. pulmonar). VER left pulmonary *artery*, right pulmonary *artery*.
a. segmentalis apicalis [TA], a. segmentar apical (a, pulmonar). VER left pulmonary *artery*, right pulmonary *artery*.
a. segmentalis basalis anterior [TA], a. segmentar basilar anterior. SIN anterior basal segmental *artery*.
a. segmentalis basalis lateralis [TA], a. segmentar basilar lateral. SIN lateral basal segmental *artery*.
a. segmentalis basalis medialis [TA], a. segmentar basilar medial. SIN medial basal segmental *artery*.
a. segmentalis lateralis [TA], a. segmentar lateral. SIN lateral basal segmental *artery*. VER left pulmonary *artery*, right pulmonary *artery*.
a. segmentalis medialis [TA], a. segmentar medial. SIN medial basal segmental *artery*; VER left pulmonary *artery*, right pulmonary *artery*.
a. segmentalis posterior [TA], a. segmentar posterior. VER left pulmonary *artery*, right pulmonary *artery*.
a. segmentalis superior [TA], a. segmentar superior. VER left pulmonary *artery*, right pulmonary *artery*.
a. segmen'ti anterio'ris inferio'ris re'nis [TA], a. do segmento anterior inferior do rim (a. renal). VER segmental *arteries* of kidney, em *artery*.
a. segmen'ti anterio'ris superio'ris re'nis [TA], a. do segmento anterior superior do rim. VER segmental *arteries* of kidney, em *artery*.
arteriae segmenti hepaticae, artérias dos segmentos hepáticos. SIN segmental *arteries* of liver, em *artery*.
a. segmen'ti inferio'ris re'nis [TA], a. do segmento inferior do rim. VER segmental *arteries* of kidney, em *artery*.
a. segmen'ti posterio'ris re'nis [TA], a. do segmento posterior do rim. VER segmental *arteries* of kidney, em *artery*.
a. segmen'ti superio'ris re'nis [TA], a. do segmento superior do rim. VER segmental *arteries* of kidney, em *artery*.
arte'riae sigmoi'deae [TA], artérias sigmóides. SIN sigmoid *arteries*, em *artery*.
a. spermat'ica inter'na [TA], a. espermática interna. SIN testicular *artery*.
a. sphe'nopalati'na [TA], a. esfenopalatina. SIN sphenopalatine *artery*.
a. spina'lis ante'rior [TA], a. espinal anterior. SIN anterior spinal *artery*.
a. spina'lis poste'rior [TA], a. espinal posterior. SIN posterior spinal *artery*.
a. sple'nica [TA], a. esplênica. SIN splenic *artery*.
a. striata medialis distalis [TA], a. estriada medial distal. SIN medial striate *artery*.
a. stylomastoi'dea [TA], a. estilomastóidea. SIN stylomastoid *artery*.
a. subcla'via [TA], a. subclávia. SIN subclavian *artery*.
a. subcosta'lis [TA], a. subcostal. SIN subcostal *artery*.
a. sublingua'lis [TA], a. sublingual. SIN sublingual *artery*.
a. submenta'lis [TA], a. submentual. SIN submental *artery*.
a. subscapula'ris [TA], a. subescapular. SIN subscapular *artery*.
a. sul'ci centra'lis [TA], a. do sulco central. SIN *artery* of central sulcus.
a. sul'ci postcentra'lis [TA], a. do sulco pós-central. SIN *artery* of postcentral sulcus.
a. sul'ci precentra'lis [TA], a. do sulco pré-central. SIN *artery* of precentral sulcus.
a. supe'rior cerebel'li [TA], a. cerebelar superior. SIN superior cerebellar *artery*.
a. supe'rior latera'lis ge'nus [TA], a. superior lateral do joelho. SIN superior lateral genicular *artery*.
a. supe'rior media'lis ge'nus [TA], a. superior medial do joelho. SIN superior medial genicular *artery*.
a. suprachiasmatica [TA], a. supraquiasmática. SIN suprachiasmatic *artery*.
a. supraduodena'lis [TA], a. supraduodenal. SIN supraduodenal *artery*.
a. supraoptica [TA], a. supra-óptica. SIN supraoptic *artery*.
a. supraorbita'lis [TA], a. supra-orbital. SIN supraorbital *artery*.
arteriae suprarena'les supe'riores [TA], artérias supra-renais superiores. SIN superior suprarenal *arteries*, em *artery*.
a. suprarena'lis infe'rior [TA], a. supra-renal inferior. SIN inferior suprarenal *artery*.
a. suprarena'lis me'dia [TA], a. supra-renal média. SIN middle suprarenal *artery*.
a. suprascapula'ris [TA], a. supra-escapular. SIN suprascapular *artery*.
a. supratrochlea'ris [TA], a. supratroclear. SIN supratrochlear *artery*.
arteriae sura'les [TA], artérias surais. SIN sural *arteries*, em *artery*.
a. tar'sea latera'lis [TA], a. tarsal lateral. SIN lateral tarsal *artery*.
a. tar'sea media'lis [TA], a. tarsal medial. SIN medial tarsal *arteries*, em *artery*.
a. tempora'lis ante'rior [TA], a. temporal anterior. SIN anterior temporal *branch*.
a. tempora'lis interme'dia, ramo temporal médio da parte insular da a. cerebral média. SIN middle temporal *branch* of insular part of middle cerebral *artery*.
a. tempora'lis media [TA], a. temporal média. SIN middle temporal *artery*.
a. tempora'lis poste'rior, ramo temporal posterior da a. cerebral média. SIN posterior temporal *branch* of middle cerebral *artery*.
a. tempora'lis profun'da [TA], a. temporal profunda. SIN deep temporal *artery*.
a. tempora'lis superficia'lis [TA], a. temporal superficial. SIN superficial temporal *artery*.
a. testicula'ris [TA], a. testicular. SIN testicular *artery*.
arte'riae thalamostria'tae anterolatera'les, artérias centrais ântero-laterais. SIN ântero-lateral central *arteries*, em *artery*.
arte'riae thalamostria'tae anteromedia'les, artérias centrais anteromediais. SIN anteromedial central *arteries*, em *artery*.
a. thora'cica inter'na [TA], a. torácica interna. SIN internal thoracic *artery*.
a. thora'cica latera'lis [TA], a. torácica lateral. SIN lateral thoracic *artery*.
a. thora'cica supe'rior [TA], a. torácica superior. SIN superior thoracic *artery*.
a. thoracoacromia'lis [TA], a. tóraco-acromial. SIN thoracoacromial *artery*.
a. thoracodorsa'lis [TA], a. toracodorsal. SIN thoracodorsal *artery*.
a. thyroi'dea i'ma [TA], a. tireóidea ima. SIN thyroid ima *artery*.
a. thyroi'dea infe'rior [TA], a. tireóidea inferior. SIN inferior thyroid *artery*.
a. thyroi'dea supe'rior [TA], a. tireóidea superior. SIN superior thyroid *artery*.
a. tibia'lis ante'rior [TA], a. tibial anterior. SIN anterior tibial *artery*.
a. tibia'lis poste'rior [TA], a. tibial posterior. SIN posterior tibial *artery*.
a. transver'sa cer'vicis, a. cervical transversa; *termo oficial alternativo para transverse cervical *artery*.
a. transver'sa col'li [TA], a. cervical transversa. SIN transverse cervical *artery*.
a. transver'sa facie'i [TA], a. facial transversa. SIN transverse facial *artery*.
a. tuberis cinerei [TA], a. do túber cinéreo. SIN *artery* of tuber cinereum.
a. tympan'ica ante'rior [TA], a. timpânica anterior. SIN anterior tympanic *artery*.
a. tympan'ica infe'rior [TA], a. timpânica inferior. SIN inferior tympanic *artery*.
a. tympan'ica poste'rior [TA], a. timpânica posterior. SIN posterior tympanic *artery*.
a. tympan'ica supe'rior [TA], a. timpânica superior. SIN superior tympanic *artery*.
a. ulna'ris [TA], a. ulnar. SIN ulnar *artery*.
a. umbilica'lis [TA], a. umbilical. SIN umbilical *artery*.
a. uncalis [TA], a. do unco (a. carótida interna). SIN uncal *artery*.
a. urethra'lis [TA], a. urethral. SIN urethral *artery*.
a. uteri'na [TA], a. uterina. SIN uterine *artery*.
a. vagina'lis [TA], a. vaginal. SIN vaginal *artery*.
arte'riae ventricula'res [TA], artérias. ventriculares. SIN ventricular *arteries*, em *artery*.
a. vertebra'lis [TA], a. vertebral. SIN vertebral *artery*.
a. vesica'lis infe'rior, a. vesical inferior. SIN inferior vesical *artery*.
a. vesica'lis supe'rior [TA], a. vesical superior. SIN superior vesical *artery*.
a. vestibularis anterior [TA], a. vestibular anterior. SIN anterior vestibular *artery*.
a. vestibuli, a. vestibular anterior; *termo oficial alternativo para anterior vestibular *artery*.
a. vestibulocochlearis [TA], a. vestibulococlear. SIN vestibulocochlear *artery*.
a. vitelli'na, a. vitelina. SIN vitelline *artery*.
a. vola'ris ind'icis radia'lis, a. radial do indicador. SIN radialis indicis *artery*.
a. zigomat'ico-orbitalis [TA], a. zigomático-orbital. SIN zygomatico-orbital *artery*.

ar·te·ri·al (ar-tē'rē-ăl). Arterial; relativo a uma ou mais artérias ou a todo o sistema de artérias.
ar·te·ri·al·i·za·tion (ar-tē'rē-ăl-ī-zā'shŭn). Arterialização. **1.** Que faz ou torna arterial. **2.** Aeração ou oxigenação do sangue, por meio da qual ele troca de caráter de venoso para arterial. **3.** Vascularização. SIN vascularization. **4.** Conversão de uma estrutura venosa para funcionar como uma artéria.
ar·te·ri·ec·ta·sis, ar·te·ri·ec·ta·sia (ar-tēr-ē-ek'tă-sis, -ek-tā'zē-ă). Arteriectasia; termo obsoleto para a vasodilatação das artérias. [L. *arteria*, artéria, + G. *ektasis*, distensão]
ar·te·ri·ec·to·my (ar-tēr-ē-ek'tō-mē). Arteriectomia; a excisão de parte de uma artéria. [L. *arteria*, artéria, + G. *ektomē*, excisão]
△ **arterio-, arteri-.** Formas combinantes que significam artéria. [L. *arteria*, de G. *artēria*, uma traquéia, uma artéria]
ar·te·ri·o·at·o·ny (ar-tēr'ē-ō-at'ō-nē). Arterioatonia; um estado anormalmente relaxado das paredes arteriais. [arterio- + G. *atonia*, atonia]
ar·te·ri·o·cap·il·lary (ar-tēr'ē-ō-cap'i-lār-ē). Arteriocapilar; relativo a artérias e capilares.
ar·te·ri·o·gram (ar-tēr'ē-ō-gram). Arteriograma; demonstração radiográ-

arteriogram

fica de uma artéria após a injeção de contraste na mesma. [arterio- + G. *gramma*, algo escrito]

ar·te·ri·o·graph·ic (ar-tēr′ē-ō-graf′ik). Arteriográfico; relativo a ou que se utiliza da arteriografia.

ar·te·ri·og·ra·phy (ar-tēr-ē-og′ră-fē). Arteriografia; demonstração de uma artéria ou artérias por imagem radiográfica após a injeção de um contraste radiopaco. [arterio- + G. *graphō*, escrever]

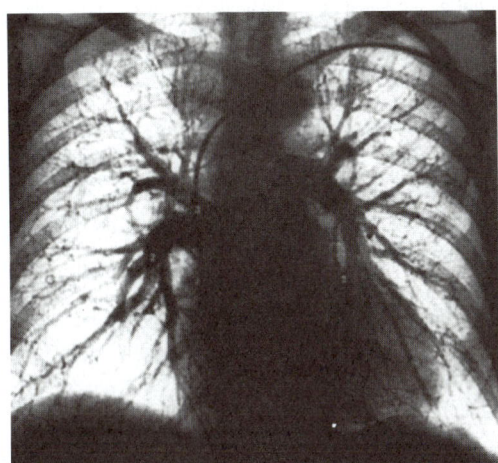

arteriografia: estudo normal das artérias pulmonares

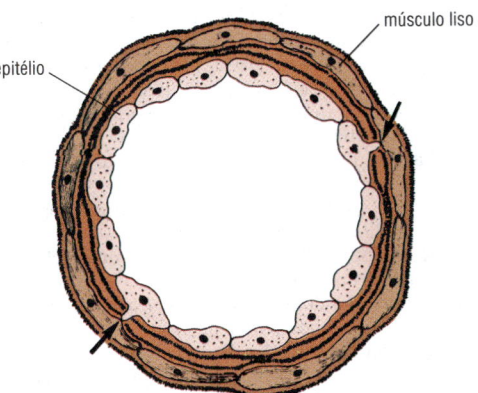

arteríola: as setas mostram os pontos de contato entre o epitélio e o músculo liso

    bronchial a., a. brônquica; radiografia das artérias brônquicas por injeção seletiva das artérias intercostais das quais se originam.
    cerebral a., a. cerebral. SIN cerebral *angiography.*

ar·te·ri·o·la, pl. **ar·te·ri·o·lae** (ar-tēr-ē-ō′la, -ō′lē) [TA]. Arteríola. SIN arteriole. [L. Mod. dim. de *arteria*, artéria]
    a. glomerula'ris af'ferens [TA], a. glomerular aferente. SIN afferent glomerular *arteriole.*
    a. glomerula'ris ef'ferens [TA], a. glomerular eferente. SIN efferent glomerular *arteriole.*
    a. maculae medius [TA], a. macular média. SIN middle macular *arteriole.*
    a. macula'ris infe'rior [TA], a. macular inferior. SIN inferior macular *arteriole.*
    a. macula'ris supe'rior [TA], a. macular superior. SIN superior macular *arteriole.*
    a. media'lis ret'inae [TA], a. macular média. SIN middle macular *arteriole.*
    a. nasa'lis ret'inae infe'rior [TA], a. nasal inferior da retina. SIN inferior nasal *arteriole* of retina.
    a. nasa'lis ret'inae supe'rior [TA], a. nasal superior da retina. SIN superior nasal retinal *arteriole.*
    arteriolae rectae [TA], arteríolas retas. SIN *vasa recta renis*, em *vas.*
    a. tempora'lis ret'inae infe'rior [TA], a. temporal inferior da retina. SIN inferior temporal retinal *arteriole.*
    a. tempora'lis ret'inae supe'rior [TA], a. temporal superior da retina. SIN superior temporal retinal *arteriole.*

ar·te·ri·o·lar (ar-ter-ē-ō′lăr). Arteriolar; de ou pertinente a uma arteríola ou às arteríolas coletivamente.

ar·te·ri·ole (ar-tēr′ē-ōl) [TA]. Arteríola; uma artéria pequena com uma túnica média que compreende apenas uma ou duas camadas de células musculares lisas; uma artéria terminal contínua com a rede capilar. SIN arteriola [TA].
    afferent glomerular a. [TA], a. glomerular aferente; um ramo de uma artéria interlobular do rim que conduz o sangue para o glomérulo. SIN arteriola glomerularis afferens [TA], afferent vessel (2), vas afferens.
    capillary a., a. capilar; uma artéria diminuta que termina em um capilar.
    efferent glomerular a. [TA], a. glomerular eferente; o vaso que leva o sangue da rede capilar glomerular para o leito capilar do túbulo contornado proximal; coletivamente, esses vasos constituem o sistema porta renal. SIN arteriola glomerularis efferens [TA], efferent vessel, vas efferens (2).
    inferior macular a. [TA], a. macular inferior; *origem*, artéria central da retina; *distribuição*, parte inferior da mácula. SIN arteriola macularis inferior [TA].
    inferior nasal a. of retina [TA], a. nasal inferior da retina; o ramo da artéria central da retina que irriga a porção medial inferior, ou nasal, da retina. SIN arteriola nasalis retinae inferior [TA].
    inferior temporal retinal a. [TA], a. temporal inferior da retina; o ramo da artéria central da retina que passa inferior, sob a mácula, para irrigar a parte lateral inferior ou temporal da retina. SIN arteriola temporalis retinae inferior [TA].
    medial a. of retina, a. macular média. SIN middle macular a.
    middle macular a. [TA], a. macular média; uma arteríola que irriga a parte da retina entre o disco óptico e a mácula. SIN arteriola medialis retinae [TA], medial a. of retina.
    superior macular a. [TA], a. macular superior; *origem*, artéria central da retina; *distribuição*, parte superior da mácula. SIN arteriola macularis superior [TA].
    superior nasal retinal a. [TA], a. nasal superior da retina; o ramo da artéria central da retina que passa para a parte medial superior, ou nasal, da retina. SIN arteriola nasalis retinae superior [TA].
    superior temporal retinal a. [TA], a. temporal superior da retina; o ramo da artéria central da retina que passa lateralmente acima da mácula para irrigar a parte lateral superior ou temporal da retina. SIN arteriola temporalis retinae superior [TA].

ar·te·ri·o·lith (ar-tēr′ē-ō-lith). Arteriólito; um depósito calcário em uma parede ou trombo arterial. [L. *arteria*, artéria, + G. *lithos*, uma pedra]

ar·te·ri·o·li·tis (ar-tēr′ē-ō-lī′tis). Arteriolite; inflamação da parede das arteríolas. [L. *arteriola*, arteríola, + G. *-itis*, inflamação]
    necrotizing a., a. necrotizante; necrose na camada média das arteríolas, característica da hipertensão maligna. SIN arteriolonecrosis.

arteriolo-. Forma combinante que significa arteríola; as arteríolas. [L. Mod. *arteriola*, arteríola]

ar·te·ri·ol·o·gy (ar-tēr′ē-ol′ō-jē). Arteriologia; a anatomia das artérias; usualmente associada ao estudo de outros vasos sob o nome angiologia. [L. *arteria*, artéria. + G. *logos*, estudo]

ar·te·ri·o·lo·ne·cro·sis (ar-tēr-ē-ō′lō-nĕ-krō′sis). Arteriolonecrose. SIN necrotizing *arteriolitis.* [L. *arteriola*, arteríola, + G. *nekrōsis*, uma morte]

ar·te·ri·o·lo·neph·ro·scle·ro·sis (ar-tēr-ē-ō′lō-nef′rō-skler-ō′sis). Arteriolonefroscrose. SIN arteriolar *nephrosclerosis.*

ar·te·ri·o·lo·scle·ro·sis (ar-tēr-ē-ō′lō-skler-ō′sis). Arteriolosclerose; a arteriosclerose que afeta principalmente as arteríolas, observada principalmente na hipertensão crônica. SIN arteriolar sclerosis.

ar·te·ri·o·lo·ve·nous (ar-tēr-ē-ō′lō-vē′nŭs). Arteriolovenoso; que envolve arteríolas e veias. SIN arteriolovenular.

ar·te·ri·o·lo·ven·u·lar (ar-tēr-ē-ō′lō-vē′nū-lăr). Arteriolovenular. SIN arteriolovenous.

ar·te·ri·o·ma·la·cia (ar-tēr′ē-ō-mă-lā′shē-ă). Arteriomalacia; amolecimento das artérias. [arterio- + G. *malakia*, maciez]

ar·te·ri·om·e·ter (ar-tēr-ē-om′ĕ-ter). Arteriômetro; um instrumento para medir o diâmetro de uma artéria, ou sua alteração em tamanho durante a pulsação. [arterio- + G. *metron*, medida]

ar·te·ri·o·mo·tor (ar-tēr′ē-ō-mō′ter). Arteriomotor; que provoca alterações no calibre de uma artéria; vasomotor, com referência especial às artérias.

ar·te·ri·o·my·o·ma·to·sis (ar-tēr′ē-ō-mī′ō-mă-tō′sis). Arteriomiomatose; espessamento das paredes de uma artéria por crescimento excessivo de fibras musculares dispostas irregularmente, fazendo interseção entre si, sem qualquer relação definida com o eixo do vaso. [arterio- + G. *mys*, músculo, + *-oma*, tumor, + *-osis*, condição]

ar·te·ri·o·neph·ro·scle·ro·sis (ar-tēr′ē-ō-nef′rō-skler-ō′sis). Arterionefroscrose. SIN arterial *nephrosclerosis.*

ar·te·ri·o·pal·mus (ar-tēr′ē-ō-pal′mŭs). Sensação subjetiva de batida da artéria. [arterio- + G. *palmos*, batimento]

ar·te·ri·op·a·thy (ar-tēr′ē-op′ă-thē). Arteriopatia; qualquer doença das artérias. [arterio- + G. *pathos*, sofrimento]
    hypertensive a., a. hipertensiva; degeneração arterial resultante da hipertensão.
    plexogenic pulmonary a., a. pulmonar plexogênica. SIN Ayerza *syndrome.*

ar·te·ri·o·pla·nia (ar-tēr′ē-ō-plā′nē-ă). Arterioplania; presença de uma anomalia no trajeto de uma artéria. [arterio- + G. *planē*, um erro]

ar·te·ri·o·plas·ty (ar-tēr′ē-ō-plas-tē). Arterioplastia; qualquer cirurgia para a reconstrução da parede de uma artéria. [arterio- + G. *plastos*, formado]

ar·te·ri·o·pres·sor (ar-tēr′ē-ō-pres′ser). Arteriopressor; que aumenta a pressão sanguínea arterial.

ar·te·ri·or·rha·phy (ar-tēr-ē-ōr′ă-fē). Arteriorrafia; sutura de uma artéria. [arterio- + G. *rhaphē*, costura]

ar·te·ri·or·rhex·is (ar-tēr′ē-ō-rek′sis). Arteriorrexia; ruptura de uma artéria. [arterio- + G. *rhēxis*, ruptura]

ar·te·ri·o·scle·ro·sis (ar-tēr′ē-ō-skler-ō′sis). Arteriosclerose; endurecimento das artérias; os tipos geralmente reconhecidos são: aterosclerose, a. de Mönckeberg e arteriolosclerose. SIN arterial sclerosis, vascular sclerosis. [arterio- + G. *sklērōsis*, endurecimento]
  coronary a., a. coronária; alterações degenerativas e metabólicas das paredes das artérias coronárias, começando geralmente com ateroma da camada íntima e prosseguindo até envolver a média; também, lesões calcificadas conhecidas como a. de Mönckeberg.
  hyperplastic a., a. hiperplásica; hiperplasia da camada íntima e da camada elástica interna e hipertrofia da média, independentemente de lesões ateromatosas.
  hypertensive a., a. hipertensiva; aumento progressivo nos tecidos muscular e elástico das paredes arteriais, resultante da hipertensão; na hipertensão de longa data, o tecido elástico forma numerosas camadas concêntricas na camada íntima, observando-se também substituição do músculo por fibras colágenas e espessamento hialino da camada íntima das arteríolas; essas alterações podem desenvolver-se com o aumento da idade na ausência de hipertensão e, então, são denominadas a. senil.
  medial a., a. da média. SIN Mönckeberg a.
  Mönckeberg a., a. de Mönckeberg; esclerose que envolve as artérias periféricas, especialmente das pernas das pessoas idosas, com deposição de cálcio na camada medial (artérias em tubo de cachimbo), mas com pouca ou nenhuma invasão da luz. SIN medial a., Mönckeberg calcification, Mönckeberg degeneration, Mönckeberg medial calcification, Mönckeberg sclerosis.
  nodular a., a. nodular; ateromas que ocorrem na camada íntima arterial como tumores bem definidos.
  a. oblit'erans, a. obliterante; a. que produz estreitamento e oclusão da luz arterial.
  peripheral a., a. periférica; a. em qualquer um dos vasos além da aorta; refere-se mais comumente aos membros inferiores.
  senile a., a. senil; a. similar à a. hipertensiva, mas em conseqüência da idade avançada em lugar da hipertensão.

ar·te·ri·o·scle·rot·ic (ar-tēr′ē-ō-skler-ot′ik). Arteriosclerótico; relativo a, ou afetado por, arteriosclerose.

ar·te·ri·o·spasm (ar-tēr′ē-ō-spazm). Arteriospasmo; espasmo de uma artéria ou artérias.

ar·te·ri·o·ste·no·sis (ar-tēr′ē-ō-stē-nō′sis). Arterioestenose; estreitamento do calibre de uma artéria, quer temporário, através de vasoconstrição, quer permanente, através da arteriosclerose. [arterio- + G. *stenōsis*, um estreitamento]

ar·te·ri·ot·o·my (ar-tēr-ē-ot′ō-mē). Arteriotomia; qualquer incisão cirúrgica na luz de uma artéria, p.ex., para remover um êmbolo. [arterio- + G. *tomē*, incisão]

ar·te·ri·o·ve·nous (AV) (ar-tēr′ē-ō-vē′nŭs). Arteriovenoso (AV); relativo a uma artéria e uma veia ou às artérias e veias em geral; tanto arterial quanto venoso, como em uma "anastomose AV".

ar·te·ri·tis (ar-ter-ī′tis). Arterite; inflamação ou infecção que envolve uma artéria ou artérias. [L. *arteria*, artéria, + G. *-itis*, inflamação]
  brachiocephalic a., a. braquiocefálica; a. de célula gigante observada nos idosos; caracterizada por lesões inflamatórias nas artérias de médio calibre, mais comumente na área da cabeça, pescoço e/ou cintura escapular; as lesões incluem elastina fragmentada, macrófagos e células gigantes. A velocidade de hemossedimentação está, em geral, bastante aumentada. A perda visual pode acontecer.
  coronary a., a. coronária; inflamação de uma ou de todas as camadas das paredes da artéria coronária.
  cranial a., a. temporal. SIN temporal a.
  extracranial a., a. temporal. SIN temporal a.
  giant cell a., a. temporal. SIN temporal a.
  granulomatous a., a. temporal. SIN temporal a.
  Heubner a., a. de Heubner; inflamação das artérias do polígono de Willis secundária à meningite basal crônica causada pelo bacilo da tuberculose ou por determinados fungos, como *Cryptococcus*, *Histoplasma* ou *Coccidioides*.
  Horton a., a. temporal. SIN temporal a.
  intracranial granulomatous a., a. granulomatosa intracraniana; uma a. de células gigantes, de pequenos vasos, que afeta apenas os vasos sanguíneos intracranianos, de etiologia desconhecida e com manifestações clínicas diversas, inclusive aquelas observadas com um tumor cerebral involuindo, e com meningite discreta, levando a infarto de uma porção do cérebro ou cerebelo. SIN neurocranial granulomatous a.
  neurocranial granulomatous a., a. granulomatosa neurocraniana. SIN intracranial granulomatous a.
  a. nodo'sa, poliarterite nodosa. SIN polyarteritis nodosa.
  a. oblit'erans, obliterating a., a. obliterante. SIN endarteritis obliterans.
  rheumatic a., a. reumática; a. devido à febre reumática; os corpúsculos de Aschoff são freqüentemente encontrados na adventícia de pequenas artérias, especialmente no miocárdio, e podem levar à fibrose e constrição das luzes.
  rheumatoid a., a. reumatóide; a. associada à artrite reumatóide; pode estar relacionada à aortite, com incompetência da valva aórtica que acompanha a espondilite anquilosante.
  Takayasu a., a. de Takayasu; arterite obliterativa progressiva, de etiologia desconhecida, que envolve a inflamação crônica do arco aórtico com fibrose e acentuado estreitamento luminal, afetando a aorta e seus ramos, freqüentemente com oclusão completa ou quase total dos segmentos da aorta; mais comum em mulheres. VER TAMBÉM aortic arch *syndrome*. SIN pulseless disease, Takayasu disease, Takayasu syndrome.
  temporal a., a. temporal; a. granulomatosa subaguda que afeta as artérias carótidas externas, principalmente a artéria temporal; ocorre em idosos e pode ser manifestada por sintomas constitucionais, principalmente cefaléia grave e, por vezes, cegueira unilateral súbita. Compartilha muitos dos sintomas da polimialgia reumática (polymyalgia rheumatica). SIN crànial a., extracranial a., giant cell a., granulomatous a., Horton a.

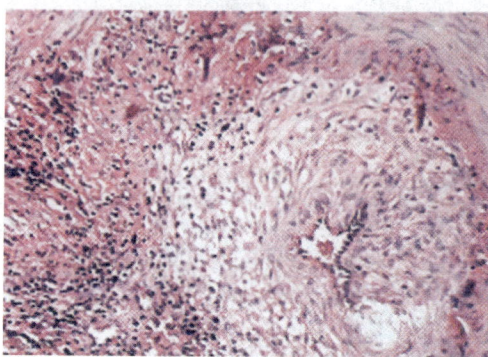

arterite temporal (arterite de células gigantes): corte transversal mostrando a infiltração da túnica média por um processo granulomatoso, com formação de células gigantes e acentuado estreitamento da luz

ARTERY

ar·tery (a) (ar′ter-ē) [TA]. Artéria; um vaso sanguíneo pulsátil, muscular, com paredes relativamente espessas, que conduz o sangue para longe do coração. Com exceção das artérias pulmonar e umbilical, as artérias contêm sangue oxigenado ou vermelho. Nas principais artérias, os ramos arteriais são arrolados em separado, seguindo a designação *branches* (ramos). SIN arteria [TA]. [L. *arteria*, do G. *artēria*]
  Abbott a., a. de Abbott; uma a. anômala que se origina da aorta descendente proximal posteromedial, importante durante a reparação da coartação.
  aberrant a., a. aberrante; uma a. que possui uma origem ou trajeto incomum.
  aberrant obturator a. [TA], a. obturatória aberrante. VER pubic *branch* of inferior epigastric artery.
  accessory meningeal a., a. pterigomeníngea. SIN pterygomeningeal a.
  accessory obturator a. [TA], a. obturatória acessória; termo aplicado à anastomose do ramo púbico da a. epigástrica inferior com o ramo púbico da a. obturadora, quando ela contribui com um aporte significante através do canal obturador. SIN arteria obturatoria accessoria [TA], ramus obturatorius arteriae epigastricae inferioris.
  acetabular a., ramo acetabular. SIN acetabular *branch*.
  acromial a., ramo acromial da a. tóraco-acromial. SIN acromial *branch* of thoracoacromial artery.
  acromiothoracic a., a. tóraco-acromial. SIN thoracoacromial a.
  a. of Adamkiewicz, a. de Adamkiewicz, a. medular segmentar. SIN great segmental medullary a.
  alar a. of nose, a. aliforme do nariz; um ramo da a. angular que irriga a asa do nariz.

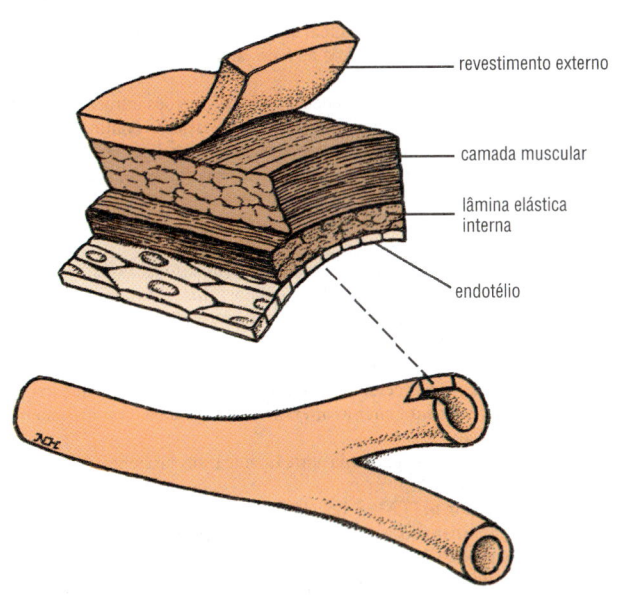

artéria: mostrando as camadas da parede

angular a. [TA], a. angular; **(1)** o ramo terminal da a. facial; *distribuição*, músculos e pele do lado do nariz; *anastomoses*, artérias nasal lateral, dorsal do nariz e palpebrais a partir da a. oftálmica, fornecendo, assim, uma anastomose arterial carotídea externa-interna; **(2)** ramo para o giro angular. SIN branch to angular gyrus.
a. of angular gyrus, ramo para o giro angular. SIN branch to angular gyrus.
anterior basal segmental a. [TA], ramo basilar anterior das artérias basilares superiores dos lobos inferiores direito e esquerdo dos pulmões direito e esquerdo. SIN arteria segmentalis basalis anterior [TA], ramus basalis anterior.
anterior cecal a. [TA], a. cecal anterior; *origem*, artéria ileocólica; *distribuição*, região anterior do ceco. SIN arteria cecalis anterior [TA].
anterior cerebral a. [TA], a. cerebral anterior; um dos dois ramos terminais (com a a. cerebral média) da a. carótida interna; passa anteriormente, contorna o joelho do corpo caloso e, depois, a fissura inter-hemisférica, juntamente com seu par do lado oposto, sendo as duas unidas pela a. comunicante anterior [TA]; para fins descritivos, é dividida em duas partes: a parte pré-comunicante [TA] (segmento A_1 da terminologia clínica), que origina as artérias central anteromedial [TA], que consiste nas artérias estriadas mediais proximais [TA], a a. supra-óptica [TA], artérias perfurantes centrais [TA] e artérias pré-ópticas [TA], e uma parte pós-comunicante [TA] (segmento A_2), que origina uma a. estriada medial distal [TA], a. frontobasal medial [TA], a. frontal polar [TA] e dois grandes ramos terminais: a artéria pericalosa [TA] e a a. calosomarginal [TA]. As duas últimas apresentam ramos que servem a regiões específicas do córtex. SIN arteria cerebri anterior [TA].
anterior choroidal a. [TA], a. corióidea anterior; *origem*, artéria carótida interna ou (raramente) cerebral média; *distribuição*, ramos nomeados [TA] para o plexo coróide do ventrículo lateral e do terceiro ventrículo, quiasma e trato ópticos, cápsula interna (joelho, ramo posterior, ramo retrolentiforme), corpo geniculado lateral, globo pálido, cauda do núcleo caudado, hipocampo, corpo amigdalóide, túber cinéreo, núcleos hipotalâmicos, núcleos talâmicos, substância negra, núcleo vermelho e cruz do cérebro. SIN arteria choroidea anterior [TA].
anterior ciliary a.'s, artérias ciliares anteriores; uma das várias artérias derivadas dos ramos musculares da oftálmica que perfuram a parte anterior da esclera e anastomosam-se com as artérias ciliares posteriores. SIN arteriae ciliares anteriores.
anterior circumflex humeral a. [TA], a. circunflexa anterior do úmero; *origem*, axilar; *distribuição*, articulação do ombro e músculo bíceps; *anastomoses*, a. umeral circunflexa posterior. SIN arteria circumflexa humeri anterior [TA], anterior humeral circumflex a.
anterior communicating a. [TA], a. comunicante anterior; um pequeno vaso que une as duas artérias cerebrais anteriores e que completa o círculo arterial cerebral (polígono de Willis) anteriormente. SIN arteria communicans anterior [TA].
anterior conjunctival a. [TA], a. conjuntival anterior; um dos inúmeros ramos pequenos das artérias ciliares anteriores que nutrem a conjuntiva. SIN arteria conjunctivalis anterior [TA], conjunctival a.'s
anterior ethmoidal a. [TA], a. etmoidal anterior; *origem*, oftálmica; *distribuição*, membranas cerebrais na fossa craniana anterior, células etmoidais anteriores, seio frontal, parte superior anterior da mucosa nasal, pele do dorso do nariz. SIN arteria ethmoidalis anterior [TA].
anterior humeral circumflex a., a. circunflexa anterior do úmero. SIN anterior circumflex humeral a.
anterior inferior cerebellar a. [TA], a. cerebelar inferior anterior; *origem*, basilar; *distribuição*, superfície inferior dos lobos laterais do cerebelo, plexo coróide no ângulo cerebelopontino; *anastomoses*, a. cerebelar póstero-inferior; origem usual da a. do labirinto. SIN arteria inferior anterior cerebelli [TA].
anterior inferior segmental a. of kidney [TA], a. do segmento anterior inferior do rim; *origem*, ramo anterior da a. renal. VER segmental a.'s of kidney. SIN a. of anterior inferior segment of kidney.
a. of anterior inferior segment of kidney, a. do segmento anterior inferior do rim. SIN anterior inferior segmental a. of kidney.
anterior intercostal a.'s, ramos intercostais anteriores da a. torácica interna. SIN anterior intercostal branches of internal thoracic artery, em branch.
anterior interosseous a. [TA], a. interóssea anterior; *origem*, a. interóssea comum; *distribuição*, partes profundas do antebraço anteriormente; *anastomoses*, a. interóssea posterior. SIN arteria interossea anterior [TA], arteria interossea volaris, volar interosseous a.
anterior interventricular a., ramo interventricular anterior da a. coronária esquerda. SIN anterior interventricular branch of left coronary artery.
anterior labial a.'s, ramos labiais anteriores da a. pudenda externa. SIN anterior labial branches of deep external pudendal artery, em branch.
anterior lateral malleolar a. [TA], a. maleolar anterior lateral; *origem*, tibial anterior; *distribuição*, articulação do tornozelo; *anastomoses*, fibular, tarsal lateral. SIN arteria malleolaris anterior lateralis [TA].
anterior medial malleolar a. [TA], a. maleolar anterior medial; *origem*, tibial anterior; *distribuição*, articulação do tornozelo e tegumento circunvizinho; *anastomoses*, ramos da tibial posterior. SIN arteria malleolaris anterior medialis [TA].
anterior mediastinal a.'s, ramos mediastinais anteriores da a. torácica interna. SIN mediastinal branches of internal thoracic artery, em branch.
anterior meningeal a., ramo meníngeo anterior da a. etmoidal anterior. SIN anterior meningeal branch (of anterior ethmoidal artery).
anterior parietal a. [TA], a. parietal anterior; um dos ramos terminais da parte insular da a. cerebral média, distribuído para a parte anterior do lobo parietal. SIN arteria parietalis anterior [TA].
anterior perforating a.'s [TA], artérias perfurantes anteriores; *origem*, como parte das artérias centrais anteromediais que se originam da parte pré-comunicante (segmento A_1) da a. cerebral anterior; penetra na substância perfurada anterior da base do crânio. SIN arteriae perforantes anteriores [TA].
anterior peroneal a., a. fibular anterior. VER perforating branches, em branch.
(anterior and posterior) radicular a.'s, artérias radiculares (anterior e posterior); ramos das artérias espinais distribuídos para as raízes dorsal e ventral dos nervos espinais e seus revestimentos. VER spinal a.'s, segmental medullary a.'s. SIN arteriae radiculares (anterior et posterior).
(anterior and posterior) superior pancreaticoduodenal a., a. pancreaticoduodenal superior (anterior e posterior); *origem*, a. gastroduodenal; uma das duas artérias, anterior e superior; *distribuição*, cabeça do pâncreas, duodeno, ducto biliar comum; *anastomoses*, pancreaticoduodenal inferior, esplênica. SIN arteria pancreaticoduodenalis superior (anterior et posterior).
anterior segmental a., a. segmentar anterior (a. pulmonar). VER left pulmonary a., right pulmonary a.
anterior spinal a., a. espinal anterior [TA]; *origem*, parte intracraniana da a. vertebral; *distribuição*, porção anteromedial da medula espinal e pia-máter adjacente; *anastomoses*, espinal das artérias intercostal e lombar. SIN arteria spinalis anterior [TA].
anterior superior alveolar a.'s, artérias alveolares superiores anteriores; *origem*, artéria infra-orbital no canal infra-orbital; *distribuição*, através dos canais alveolares anteriores até os incisivos superiores e dentes caninos, mucosa do seio maxilar. SIN arteriae alveolares superiores anteriores [TA], anterior superior dental a.'s.
anterior superior dental a.'s, artérias alveolares superiores anteriores. SIN anterior superior alveolar a.'s.
anterior superior segmental a. of kidney [TA], a. do segmento anterior superior do rim; *origem*, ramo anterior da a. renal. VER segmental a.'s of kidney. SIN a. of anterior superior segment of kidney.
a. of anterior superior segment of kidney, a. do segmento anterior superior do rim. SIN anterior superior segmental a. of kidney.
anterior temporal a., ramo temporal anterior. SIN anterior temporal branch.
anterior tibial a., a. tibial anterior; *origem*, poplítea; *distribuição*, artérias tibiais recorrentes posterior e anterior, maleolares anteriores lateral e medial, dorsal do pé, tarsal lateral, tarsal medial, arqueada, metatarsal dorsal e digital dorsal. SIN arteria tibialis anterior [TA].
anterior tibial recurrent a [TA], a. tibial recorrente anterior; um ramo da a. tibial anterior que ascende para nutrir as partes anterior e laterais da articulação do joelho, contribuindo, assim, para a rede articular do joelho. SIN arteria recurrens tibialis anterior [TA].

anterior tympanic a. [TA], a. timpânica anterior; *origem*, primeira parte (retromandibular) da a. maxilar; *distribuição*, orelha média; *anastomoses*, ramos timpânicos das a. carótida interna e faríngea ascendente e estilomastóidea. SIN arteria tympanica anterior [TA], glaserian a.

anterior vestibular a., a. vestibular anterior; *origem*, como um ramo terminal, com a a. coclear comum, da a. do labirinto; *ramo*: a. vestibulococlear; *distribuição*: para o gânglio vestibular, utrículo e (especialmente a ampola) ductos semicirculares lateral e posterior. SIN arteria vestibularis anterior [TA], arteria vestibuli*.

anterolateral central a.'s [TA], artérias centrais ântero-laterais; numerosos pequenos ramos a partir da parte esfenoidal das artérias cerebrais médias que nutrem as partes lateral e anterior do corpo estriado. SIN arteriae centrales anterolaterales [TA], lenticulostriate a.'s (1)*, anterolateral striate a.'s, anterolateral thalamostriate a.'s, arteriae thalamostriatae anterolaterales, a.'s of cerebral hemorrhage, lateral striate a.'s

anterolateral striate a.'s, artérias estriadas ântero-laterais. SIN anterolateral central a.'s.

anterolateral thalamostriate a.'s, artérias centrais ântero-laterais. SIN anterolateral central a.'s.

anteromedial central a.'s [TA], artérias centrais anteromediais; vários pequenos ramos da parte pré-comunicante (segmento A1) da a. cerebral anterior ou da a. comunicante anterior; elas se distribuem para a parte anteromedial da parte do corpo estriado do tálamo. SIN arteriae centrales anteromediales [TA], anteromedial thalamostriate a.'s, arteriae thalamostriatae anteromediales.

anteromedial thalamostriate a.'s, artérias centrais anteromediais. SIN anteromedial central a.'s.

apical segmental a. [TA], a. segmentar apical (a. pulmonar). VER left pulmonary a., right pulmonary a.

apical segmental a. of superior lobar artery of right lung [TA], a. segmentar apical da artéria lobar superior do pulmão direito; ramo (do ramo lobar inferior) da a. pulmonar direita que serve ao segmento apical do lobo inferior do pulmão direito. SIN apical branch of inferior lobar branch of right pulmonary artery*, ramus apicalis lobi inferioris arteriae pulmonalis dextrae*.

apicoposterior a., a. apicoposterior; um ramo da a. pulmonar para o segmento apicoposterior esquerdo do lobo superior.

appendicular a. [TA], a. apendicular; o ramo da a. ileocólica que desce posterior ao íleo terminal no mesoapêndice para nutrir o apêndice vermiforme. SIN arteria appendicularis [TA].

arciform a.'s, artérias arqueadas. SIN arcuate a.'s of kidney.

arcuate a.'s of kidney, artérias arqueadas do rim; artérias curvas, na borda corticomedular, que se originam das artérias interlobares e dão origem às artérias interlobulares. SIN arteriae arcuatae renis [TA], arciform a.'s.

arcuate a. (of foot) (inconstant) [TA], a. arqueada (do pé) (inconstante); *origem*, dorsal do pé; *ramos*, passa lateralmente, dorsal às bases dos metatarsos, originando a segunda, a terceira e a quarta artérias metatarsais ao nível do osso cuneiforme medial. SIN arteria arcuata (pedis) [TA].

ascending a. [TA], a. ascendente; **(1)** ramo cólico da a. ileocólica. SIN colic branch of ileocolic artery; **(2)** ramo da a. cólica esquerda (a partir da a. mesentérica inferior) que passa anteriormente ao rim esquerdo para o mesocólon transverso, onde se anastomosa com a a. cólica média. Dessa maneira, forma uma anastomose entre as a. mesentéricas superior e inferior, sendo um componente da a. marginal (Drummond) do cólon. SIN arteria ascendens (2) [TA], arteria intermesenterica, ascending branch of inferior mesenteric artery.

ascending cervical a. [TA], a. cervical ascendente; *origem*, usualmente um ramo terminal do tronco tireocervical (juntamente com a a. tireóidea inferior); *distribuição*, músculos do pescoço e da medula espinal; *anastomoses*, ramos das a. vertebral, occipital, faríngea ascendente e cervical profunda. SIN arteria cervicalis ascendens [TA], cervicalis ascendens (2).

ascending palatine a. [TA], a. palatina ascendente; *origem*, facial; *distribuição*, paredes laterais da faringe, tonsilas, canais auditivos e palato mole; *anastomoses*, ramo tonsilar da facial, lingual dorsal e palatina descendente. SIN arteria palatina ascendens [TA].

ascending pharyngeal a. [TA], a. faríngea ascendente; *origem*, carótida externa; *distribuição*, parede da faringe e palato mole, fossa craniana posterior. SIN arteria pharyngea ascendens [TA].

atrial a.'s, artérias atriais; ramos das artérias coronárias direita e esquerda distribuídos para o músculo dos átrios. SIN arteriae atriales.

a. to atrioventricular node, a. para o nódulo atrioventricular. SIN atrioventricular nodal branch.

axillary a. [TA], a. axilar; a continuação da a. subclávia depois de cruzar a primeira costela para entrar na axila; transforma-se na a. braquial ao passar a borda inferior do músculo redondo maior. É acompanhada pelos cordões do plexo braquial e está envolta com eles e com a veia axilar na bainha axilar, quando atravessa a axila. São descritas partes da a. axilar: proximal, posterior e distal ao músculo peitoral menor. Ramos: primeira parte — a. torácica superior; segunda parte — tronco toracoacromial, a. torácica lateral; terceira parte — a. subescapular, artérias umerais circunflexas anterior e posterior. SIN arteria axillaris [TA].

azygos a. of vagina, a. ázigo da vagina; uma das duas artérias que correm longitudinalmente na linha média sobre as faces anterior e posterior da vagina; elas se originam da a. uterina.

basilar a. [TA], a. basilar; formada pela união das porções intracranianas das duas artérias vertebrais; corre ao longo do sulco na cisterna pontina do espaço subaracnóide, desde a borda inferior até a superior da ponte, onde se bifurca nas duas artérias cerebrais posteriores; *ramos*, artéria cerebelar anterior inferior [TA], artérias pontinas [TA], artéria cerebelar anterior inferior [TA], artéria cerebelar superior [TA] e artéria cerebral posterior [TA]. SIN arteria basilaris [TA].

brachial a. [TA], a. braquial; *origem*, é uma continuação da axilar, que começa na borda inferior do músculo redondo maior; *ramos*, braquial profundo, colateral ulnar superior, colateral ulnar inferior, muscular e nutriente; termina na fossa cubital (nível do cotovelo) ao bifurcar-se nas artérias radial e ulnar. SIN arteria brachialis [TA], humeral a.

a.'s of brain [TA], artérias cerebrais; as artérias e ramos arteriais que irrigam o cérebro; são derivadas do círculo arterial cerebral e da a. coróide anterior. SIN arteriae encephali [TA].

bronchial a.'s, ramos brônquicos da aorta torácica. SIN bronchial branches of thoracic aorta, em branch.

buccal a., buccinator a. [TA], a. bucal; *origem*, maxilar; *distribuição*, músculo bucinador, pele e mucosa da bochecha; *anastomoses*, ramo bucal do facial. SIN arteria buccalis [TA].

buckled innominate a., a. inominada curva; prolongamento da a. inominada que se manifesta como uma massa pulsátil no espaço supraclavicular direito e com um aspecto radiográfico que mimetiza um aneurisma ou tumor do ápice do pulmão direito ou do mediastino superior.

a. of bulb of penis [TA], a. do bulbo do pênis; um ramo da a. pudenda interna que irriga o bulbo do pênis, incluindo a uretra bulbar. SIN arteria bulbi penis [TA], arteria bulbi urethrae.

a. of bulb of vestibule [TA], a. do bulbo do vestíbulo; o ramo da a. pudenda interna, na mulher, que irriga o bulbo do vestíbulo. SIN arteria bulbi vestibuli [TA], arteria bulbi vaginae.

calcaneal a.'s, ramos calcâneos. SIN calcaneal branches, em branch.

calcarine a., ramo calcarino da a. occipital medial. SIN calcarine branch of medial occipital artery.

a. of calf, a. sural. SIN sural a.'s.

callosomarginal a. [TA], a. calosomarginal; o segundo ramo da artéria pericalosa que corre no sulco cingulado e emite ramos para irrigar parte das superfícies medial e súpero-lateral do hemisfério cerebral. SIN arteria callosomarginalis [TA].

caroticotympanic a.'s (of internal carotid artery) [TA], artérias caroticotimpânicas (da artéria carótida interna); pequenos ramos da porção petrosa da artéria carótida interna que irrigam a cavidade timpânica; anastomosam-se com as artérias timpânica e maxilar. SIN arteriae caroticotympanicae (arteriae carotidis internae) [TA], rami caroticotympanici.

carotid a.'s, artérias carótidas. VER common carotid a., external carotid a., internal carotid a.

carpal a., artérias relacionadas à articulação do punho e que a irrigam. VER dorsal carpal branch of radial artery, dorsal carpal branch of ulnar artery, palmar carpal branch of radial artery, palmar carpal branch of ulnar artery.

caudal pancreatic a., a. da cauda do pâncreas. SIN a. to tail of pancreas.

a. of caudate lobe [TA], a. do lobo caudado; *origem*, ramo esquerdo da a. hepática própria; *distribuição*, lobo caudado do fígado. SIN arteria lobi caudati [TA].

cavernous a.'s, ramo cavernoso da parte cavernosa da a. carótida interna. SIN cavernous branch of cavernous part of internal carotid artery.

cecal a.'s, artérias cecais. VER anterior cecal a., posterior cecal a.

celiac a., tronco celíaco. SIN celiac (arterial) trunk.

central a., a. do sulco central. SIN a. of central sulcus.

central a. of retina, a. central da retina. SIN central retinal a.

central retinal a. [TA], a. central da retina; um ramo da a. oftálmica que penetra no nervo óptico 1 cm atrás do olho (parte extra-ocular) para penetrar no olho (parte intra-ocular) na papila óptica, na retina; divide-se nos ramos temporais e nasais superiores e inferiores. SIN arteria centralis retinae [TA], arteria retinae centralis, central a. of retina, Zinn a.

central sulcal a., a. do sulco central. SIN a. of central sulcus.

a. of central sulcus [TA], a. do sulco central; um ramo da parte terminal da a. cerebral média distribuído para o córtex dos dois lados do sulco central. SIN arteria sulci centralis [TA], central a., central sulcal a., Rolandic sulcal a.

cerebellar a.'s, artérias cerebelares; artérias relacionadas ao cerebelo e que o irrigam. VER anterior inferior cerebellar a., posterior inferior cerebellar a., superior cerebellar a.

cerebral a.'s, artérias do encéfalo; artérias relacionadas ao córtex cerebral e que o irrigam. VER anterior cerebral a. middle cerebral a., posterior cerebral a.

a.'s of cerebral hemorrhage, artérias centrais ântero-laterais. SIN anterolateral central a.'s.

cervicovaginal a., a. cervicovaginal; uma comunicação anastomótica entre a

a. uterina e a a. vaginal; faz trajeto ao longo da face lateral do colo e da vagina. SIN arteria cervicovaginalis.

Charcot a., a. de Charcot. SIN lenticulostriate a.'s (2).
chief a. of thumb, a. principal do polegar. SIN princeps pollicis a.
circumflex femoral a.'s, artérias circunflexas femorais. VER lateral circumflex femoral a., medial circumflex femoral a.
circumflex fibular a., ramo fibular circunflexo da a. tibial posterior. SIN circumflex fibular branch (of posterior tibial artery).
circumflex humeral a.'s, artérias circunflexas do úmero. VER anterior circumflex humeral a., posterior circumflex humeral a.
circumflex iliac a.'s, artérias ilíacas circunflexas. VER deep circumflex iliac a., superficial circumflex iliac a.
circumflex scapular a. [TA], artéria circunflexa da escápula; *origem*, ramo terminal (com a a. toracodorsal) da subescapular; *distribuição*, músculos da região do ombro e da escápula; *anastomoses*, ramos da supra-escapular e cervical transversa. SIN arteria circumflexa scapulae [TA].
coiled a. of the uterus, a. espiral do útero. SIN spiral a.
colic a.'s, artérias cólicas; artérias que nutrem o cólon. VER left colic a., middle colic a., right colic a.
collateral a., a. colateral; **(1)** aquela que corre em paralelo a um nervo ou outra estrutura; **(2)** aquela através da qual se estabelece uma circulação colateral. VER articular vascular *network*.
collateral digital a., a. digital palmar própria. SIN proper palmar digital a.'s.
collicular a. [TA], a. colicular; *origem*, parte pré-comunicante (segmento P1) da a. cerebral posterior; *distribuição*, para os colículos superior e inferior (corpos quadrigêmeos) do teto do mesencéfalo. SIN arteria collicularis [TA], arteria quadrigeminalis*, quadrigeminal a. *.
comitant a. of median nerve, a. acompanhante do nervo mediano. SIN median a.
common carotid a. [TA], a. carótida comum; *origem*, à direita, a partir da braquiocefálica; à esquerda, a partir do arco da aorta; faz trajeto para cima, no pescoço, e divide-se na borda superior oposta da cartilagem tireóidea (nível vertebral C-4) nos *ramos terminais*, carótidas externa e interna. SIN arteria carotis communis [TA].
common cochlear a. [TA], a. coclear comum; *origem*, como um ramo terminal, com a a. vestibular anterior, da a. do labirinto; *distribuição*, corre no eixo coclear do modíolo, irrigando os gânglios espirais; envia a a. coclear própria para o canal coclear e supre as duas voltas apicais da a. espiral do modíolo. SIN arteria cochlearis communis [TA].
common hepatic a. [TA], a. hepática comum; *origem*, celíaca; *ramos*, gástrica direita, gastroduodenal e hepática própria. SIN arteria hepatica communis [TA].
common iliac a. [TA], a. ilíaca comum; um dos dois ramos terminais da aorta abdominal; anterior à articulação sacroilíaca no nível do promontório sacral, ela se bifurca para formar a ilíaca interna e a ilíaca externa. SIN arteria iliaca communis [TA].
common interosseous a. [TA], a. interóssea comum; *origem*, ulnar; *ramos*, interósseas posterior e anterior. SIN arteria interossea communis [TA].
common palmar digital a. [TA], a. digital palmar comum; uma das três artérias que se originam do arco palmar superficial e que fazem trajeto para as fendas interdigitais, onde cada uma se divide em duas artérias digitais palmares próprias. SIN arteria digitalis palmaris communis [TA].
common plantar digital a. [TA], a. digital plantar comum; uma das quatro artérias que se originam de um arco plantar superficial, quando presente como uma variação. Elas se unem com os arcos metatársicos plantares, distalmente aos ramos perfurantes. SIN arteria digitalis plantaris communis [TA].
communicating a., a. comunicante; uma a. que une duas artérias maiores. VER anterior communicating a., posterior communicating a.
companion a. to sciatic nerve, a. acompanhante do nervo isquiático. SIN a. to sciatic nerve.
conjunctival a.'s, artérias conjuntivais. SIN anterior conjunctival a., posterior conjunctival a.
coronary a., a. coronária; **(1)** VER right coronary a., left coronary a.; **(2)** SIN left gastric a.
cortical a.'s, artérias corticais; ramos das artérias cerebrais anterior, média e posterior que nutrem o córtex cerebral.
cortical radiate a.'s [TA], artérias corticais radiais; os ramos das artérias arqueadas do rim que se irradiam para fora, através das colunas renais e do córtex, e nutrem os glomérulos. SIN arteriae corticales radiatae [TA], arteria interlobulares (renis), interlobular a.'s of kidney.
costocervical a., tronco costocervical. SIN costocervical (arterial) *trunk*.
cremasteric a. [TA], a. cremastérica; *origem*, epigástrica inferior; *distribuição*, revestimentos do cordão espermático; *anastomoses*, a. pudenda externa, espermática e perineal. SIN arteria cremasterica [TA], external spermatic a.
cricothyroid a., a. cricotireóidea; SIN cricothyroid branch of superior thyroid artery.
cystic a. [TA], a. cística; *origem*, ramo direito da hepática; *distribuição*, vesícula biliar e superfície visceral do fígado. SIN arteria cystica [TA].

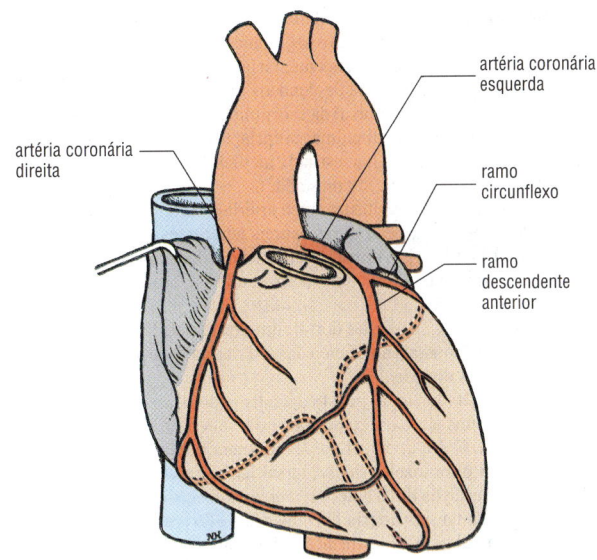

artérias coronárias

deep a. of arm, a. braquial profunda; *termo oficial alternativo para profunda brachii a.
deep auricular a. [TA], a. auricular profunda; *origem*, primeira parte da maxilar; *distribuição*: articulação da mandíbula, glândula parótida, meato auditivo externo e membrana timpânica externa; *anastomoses*, ramos auriculares da temporal superficial e auricular posterior. SIN arteria auricularis profunda [TA].
deep brachial a., a. braquial profunda. SIN profunda brachii a.
deep cervical a. [TA], a. cervical profunda; *origem*, ramo terminal do tronco costocervical (juntamente com a artéria intercostal superior); *distribuição*, músculos posteriores profundos do pescoço; *anastomoses*, ramos da occipital, cervical ascendente e vertebral. SIN arteria cervicalis profunda [TA].
deep circumflex iliac a. [TA], a. ilíaca circunflexa profunda; *origem*, ilíaca externa; *distribuição,* músculos e pele da parte inferior do abdome, sartório e tensor da fáscia lata; *anastomoses*, lombar, epigástrica inferior, glútea superior, iliolombar e ilíaca circunflexa superficial. SIN arteria circumflexa iliaca profunda [TA].
deep a. of clitoris [TA], a. profunda do clitóris; o ramo terminal profundo da artéria pudenda interna na mulher; nutre o ramo do clitóris. SIN arteria profunda clitoridis [TA].
deep epigastric a., a. epigástrica inferior. SIN inferior epigastric a.
deep lingual a. [TA], a. profunda da língua; término da artéria lingual; *distribuição*, músculos e mucosa sob a superfície inferior da língua. SIN arteria profunda linguae [TA], arteria ranina, deep a. of tongue, ranine a.
deep a. of penis [TA], a. profunda do pênis; *origem*, ramo terminal (com a. dorsal do pênis) da artéria pudenda interna; *distribuição*, corpo cavernoso do pênis, através dos leitos capilares e das artérias helicinas e de anastomoses arteriovenosas para produzir a ereção. SIN arteria profunda penis [TA].
deep plantar a. [TA], a. plantar profunda; ramo plantar profundo da a. arqueada ou ramo de sua primeira a. metatársica que penetra no pé, entre o primeiro e o segundo metatársicos, para se anastomosar com o término do arco arterial plantar. SIN arteria plantaris profunda, arteriae dorsalis pedis [TA], deep plantar branch of dorsalis pedis artery, ramus plantaris profundus arteriae dorsalis pedis.
deep temporal a., a. temporal profunda, em número de duas, anterior e posterior; *origem*, maxilar; *distribuição*, músculo e periósteo temporais, osso e osso díploe da fossa temporal; *anastomoses*, ramos da temporal superficial, lacrimal e meníngea média. SIN arteria temporalis profunda [TA].
deep a. of thigh [TA], a. profunda do fêmur; *origem*, femoral; *ramos*, femoral circunflexo lateral, femoral circunflexo medial, terminando em três ou quatro artérias perfurantes. SIN arteria profunda femoris, profunda femoris a.
deep a. of tongue, a. profunda da língua. SIN deep lingual a.
deferential a., a. do ducto deferente. SIN a. to ductus deferens.
descending genicular a. [TA], a. descendente do joelho; *origem*, femoral, no canal adutor; *distribuição*, penetra na fáscia do vastoadutor para nutrir a articulação do joelho e partes adjacentes; *anastomoses*, artérias genicular superior medial, genicular inferior medial, genicular superior lateral, genicular inferior lateral e tibial anterior recorrente, isto é, a rede articular do joelho. SIN arteria descendens genus [TA], arteria anastomotica magna (2), a. descending of knee, great anastomotic a. (2).
descending a. of knee, a. descendente do joelho. SIN descending genicular a.

descending palatine a. [TA], a. palatina descendente; *origem*, maxilar; *distribuição*, palato mole, gengivas, ossos e mucosa do palato duro; *anastomoses*, esfenopalatina, palatina ascendente, faríngea ascendente e ramos tonsilares da facial. SIN arteria palatina descendens [TA].
descending scapular a., a. dorsal da escápula. SIN dorsal scapular a.
digital collateral a., a. digital palmar própria. SIN proper palmar digital a.'s
distal medial striate a. [TA], a. estriada medial. SIN medial striate a.
distributing a., a. muscular. SIN muscular a.
dolichoectatic a., a. dolicoectásica; uma artéria distorcida, dilatada e alongada que pode comprimir as estruturas neurais adjacentes.
dorsal a. of clitoris [TA], a. dorsal do clitóris; um dos dois ramos terminais da a. pudenda interna na mulher, com o outro sendo a a. profunda da clitóris. SIN arteria dorsalis clitoridis [TA].
dorsal digital a. [TA], a. digital dorsal; um dos ramos digitais colaterais das artérias metatarsais dorsais no pé e/ou das artérias metacarpais dorsais na mão. SIN arteria digitalis dorsalis [TA].
dorsal a. of foot, a. dorsal do pé. SIN dorsalis pedis a.
dorsal interosseous a., a. interóssea posterior. SIN posterior interosseous a.
dorsalis pedis a. [TA], a. dorsal do pé; continuação da artéria tibial anterior depois de cruzar o tornozelo; *ramos*, tarsal lateral, arqueada, metatarsal dorsal; uma continuação da tibial anterior; *anastomoses*, com a plantar lateral para formar o arco plantar. SIN arteria dorsalis pedis [TA], dorsal a. of foot.
dorsal metacarpal a. [TA], a. metacarpal dorsal; uma das quatro artérias que se originam do arco carpal dorsal e que correm sobre a face posterior dos músculos interósseos da mão. SIN arteria metacarpalis dorsalis [TA].
dorsal metatarsal a. [TA], a. metatarsal dorsal; uma das quatro artérias que se originam da dorsal do pé (I) e arqueada (II–IV) e que correm sobre o dorso dos músculos interósseos do pé. SIN arteria metatarsalis dorsalis [TA].
dorsal nasal a. [TA], a. dorsal do nariz; *origem*, artéria externa do nariz; *distribuição*, pele da parte lateral da raiz do nariz; *anastomoses*, a. angular. SIN arteria dorsalis nasi [TA], external nasal a.*, arteria nasi externa, dorsal a. of nose, external a. of nose.
dorsal a. of nose, a. dorsal do nariz. SIN dorsal nasal a.
dorsal pancreatic a. [TA], a. pancreática dorsal; *origem*, esplênica; *distribuição*, cabeça e corpo do pâncreas; *anastomoses*, pancreaticoduodenal superior. SIN arteria pancreatica dorsalis [TA], great superior pancreatic a.
dorsal a. of penis [TA], a. dorsal do pênis; o ramo terminal dorsal da artéria pudenda interna no homem. SIN arteria dorsalis penis [TA].
dorsal scapular a. [TA], a. dorsal da escápula; *origem*, inconstante; subclávia (quando esse termo é preferido) ou como ramo profundo da cervical transversa; *distribuição*, passa profundamente aos músculos rombóides, nutrindo-os e a outros músculos e a pele ao longo da borda vertebral da escápula; *anastomoses*, supra-escapular e circunflexa escapular. SIN arteria dorsalis scapulae [TA], rami profundi arteriae transversae cervicis [TA], ramus profundus arteriae transversae colli [TA], arteria scapularis descendens, arteria scapularis dorsalis, deep branch of the transversae cervical artery, descending scapular a., ramus profundus arteriae scapularis descendentis.
dorsal thoracic a., a. toracodorsal. SIN thoracodorsal a.
a. of Drummond, A. de Drummond. SIN marginal a. of colon.
a. to ductus deferens [TA], a. do ducto deferente; *origem*, divisão anterior da ilíaca interna ou, por vezes, vesical superior; *distribuição*, canal deferente, vesículas seminais, testículo, ureter; *anastomoses*, testicular, artérias cremastéricas. SIN a. to vas deferens*, arteria deferentialis, arteria ductus deferentis, deferential a.
elastic a., a. elástica; uma grande a., como a aorta ou a a. pulmonar, que possui muitas lamelas elásticas em sua túnica média.
end a., a. terminal; uma a. com anastomoses insuficientes para manter a viabilidade do tecido nutrido se ocorrer oclusão da a. SIN terminal a.
episcleral a. [TA], a. episcleral; um dos muitos ramos pequenos das artérias ciliares anteriores que se originam quando estas perfuram a esclerótica próximo à junção córneo-esclerótica e avançam na esclerótica. SIN arteria episcleralis [TA].
esophageal a.'s, ramos esofágicos das seguintes: 1) a. tireóidea inferior; 2) a. gástrica esquerda; 3) aorta torácica.
external carotid a. [TA], a. carótida externa; *origem*, a. carótida comum ao nível vertebral C–4; *ramos*, tireóidea superior, lingual, facial, occipital, auricular posterior, faríngea ascendente e *ramos terminais*, maxilar e temporal superficial ao nível do colo da mandíbula. SIN arteria carotis externa [TA].
external iliac a. [TA], a. ilíaca externa; *origem*, a. ilíaca comum; *ramos*, epigástrico inferior, ilíaco circunflexo profundo; transforma-se na a. femoral no ligamento inguinal. SIN arteria iliaca externa [TA].
external mammary a., a. torácica lateral. SIN lateral thoracic a.
external maxillary a., a. facial. SIN facial a.
external nasal a., a. dorsal do nariz; *termo oficial alternativo para dorsal nasal a.
external a. of nose, a. dorsal do nariz. SIN dorsal nasal a.
external spermatic a., a. cremastérica. SIN cremasteric a.
facial a. [TA], a. facial; *origem*, carótida externa; *ramos*, palatina ascendente, ramos tonsilar e glandular, submentual, labial inferior, labial superior, massetérica, bucal, ramos nasais laterais e angular. SIN arteria facialis [TA], arteria maxillaris externa, external maxillary a.
femoral a. [TA], a. femoral; *origem*, continuação da ilíaca externa, começando no ligamento inguinal; *ramos*, pudenda externa, epigástrica superficial, ilíaca circunflexa superficial, femoral profunda, descendente do joelho, terminando como a a. poplítea quando atravessa o hiato adutor para penetrar no espaço poplíteo. SIN arteria femoralis [TA].
femoral nutrient a. [TA], a. nutrícia do fêmur; uma das duas artérias, superior e inferior, que se originam da primeira e na terceira artérias perfurantes, respectivamente (por vezes segunda e quarta). SIN nutrient a. of femur.
fibular a. [TA], a. fibular; *origem*, tibial posterior; *distribuição*, músculos solear, tibial posterior, flexor longo dos dedos, fibulares, articulação tibiofibular inferior e articulação do tornozelo; *anastomoses*, maleolar lateral anterior, tarsal lateral, plantar lateral, dorsal do pé. SIN arteria fibularis [TA], arteria peronea*, peroneal a. *.
fibular nutrient a. [TA], a. nutrícia da fíbula; *origem*, fibular (peroneira); *distribuição*, fíbula. SIN arteria nutriens fibulae*, nutrient a. of fibula.
first and second posterior intercostal a.'s [TA], primeira e segunda artérias intercostais posteriores; ramos terminais da a. intercostal superior (a partir do tronco costocervical) que nutrem os dois espaços intercostais superiores. SIN arteriae intercostales posteriores I et II, posterior intercostal a.'s 1–2.
frontal a., a. supratroclear. SIN supratrochlear a.
frontopolar a. [TA], a. polar frontal. SIN polar frontal a.
gastric a.'s, artérias gástricas; artérias que nutrem o estômago ao longo da curvatura menor. SIN left gastric a., right gastric a.
gastroduodenal a. [TA], a. gastroduodenal; *origem*, hepática; *ramos*, terminais, gastroepiplóica direita, pancreaticoduodenal superior. SIN arteria gastroduodenalis [TA].
gastroepiploic a.'s, artérias gastromentais; *termo oficial alternativo para gastroomental a.'s; VER left gastroomental a., right gastroomental a.
gastroomental a.'s [TA], artérias gastromentais; artérias que nutrem o estômago e o omento maior, à medida que avançam ao longo da curvatura maior do estômago. SIN arteriae gastro-omentales [TA], arteriae gastroepiploicae*, gastroepiploic a.'s*.
genicular a.'s, artérias do joelho; artérias que contribuem para a rede arterial do joelho. VER descending genicular a, inferior lateral genicular a., inferior medial genicular a., middle genicular a., superior lateral genicular a., superior medial genicular a.
glaserian a., a. timpânica anterior. SIN anterior tympanic a.
great anastomotic a., (1) SIN inferior ulnar collateral a. **(2)** SIN descending genicular a. **(3)** SIN great segmental medullary a.
greater palatine a. [TA], a. palatina maior; ramo anterior da artéria palatina descendente, que nutre as gengivas e a mucosa do palato duro. SIN arteria palatina major [TA].
greater pancreatic a. [TA], a. pancreática magna; *origem*, esplênica; *distribuição*, cauda do pâncreas; *anastomoses*, a. pancreática inferior e artérias da cauda do pâncreas. SIN arteria pancreatica magna.
great radicular a., a. medular segmentar maior. SIN great segmental medullary a.
great segmental medullary a., a. medular segmentar magna; a maior das artérias medulares que irrigam a medula espinal ao se anastomosarem com a a. espinal anterior (longitudinal); origina-se a partir de uma a. intercostal inferior ou lombar superior (no lado esquerdo em cerca de 65% das vezes), fornecendo a maior parte do sangue para os dois terços inferiores da a. espinal ant. VER medullary a.'s of brain. SIN arteria radicularis magna, a. of Adamkiewicz, great anastomotic a. (3), great radicular a.
great superior pancreatic a., a. pancreática dorsal. SIN dorsal pancreatic a.
helicine a.'s of penis [TA], artérias helicinas do pênis; os ramos terminais espiralados das artérias profunda e dorsal do pênis. A estimulação parassimpática faz com que se retifiquem, possibilitando que o sangue na pressão arterial encha o tecido cavernoso, gerando a ereção. SIN arteriae helicinae penis [TA].
helicine a.'s of uterus [TA], artérias helicinas do útero; os ramos terminais espiralados da a. uterina na musculatura uterina (miométrio). SIN arteriae helicinae uteri [TA].
hepatic a.'s, artérias hepáticas; as artérias envolvidas no fornecimento de sangue para o fígado. VER common hepatic a., hepatic a. proper, left *branch* of hepatic artery proper, right *branch* of hepatic artery proper.
hepatic a. proper [TA], a. hepática própria; *origem*, hepática comum; *ramos*, hepáticas direita e esquerda. SIN arteria hepatica propria.
Heubner., a. de Heubner. SIN medial striate a.
a. of Heubner, a. de Heubner. SIN medial striate a.
highest intercostal a., a. intercostal suprema. SIN supreme intercostal a.
highest thoracic a., a. torácica superior. SIN superior thoracic a.
humeral a., a. braquial. SIN brachial a.
humeral nutrient a.'s [TA], artérias nutrícias do úmero; *origem*, braquial profunda; *distribuição*, a cavidade medular do úmero. SIN arteriae nutriciae humeri [TA], nutrient a.'s of humerus.

hyaloid a., a. hialóide; o ramo terminal da artéria oftálmica primitiva, que forma, no embrião, uma extensa ramificação no vítreo primário e uma túnica vascular ao redor do cristalino; em torno de 8,5 meses, esses vasos atrofiam-se quase por completo, mas alguns resquícios persistentes são evidentes dentro do olho como moscas volantes. SIN arteria hyaloidea [TA].

hypogastric a., a. ilíaca interna. SIN internal iliac a.

ileal a.'s [TA], artérias ileais; *origem*, mesentérica superior; *distribuição*, íleo; *anastomoses*, outros ramos da mesentérica superior. SIN arteriae ileales [TA].

ileocolic a., a. ileocólica; *origem*, mesentérica superior, freqüentemente por um tronco comum com a cólica direita; *distribuição*, parte terminal do íleo, ceco, apêndice vermiforme e cólon ascendente; *anastomoses*, cólica direita e ileal. SIN arteria ileocolica [TA].

iliac a.'s, artérias ilíacas; artérias relacionadas ao ílio. VER common iliac a., deep circumflex iliac a., external iliac a., internal iliac a., superficial circumflex iliac a.

iliolumbar a. [TA], a. iliolombar; *origem*, ilíaca interna; *distribuição*, músculos e ossos pélvicos; *anastomoses*, ilíaca circunflexa profunda, lombar. SIN arteria iliolumbalis [TA].

inferior alveolar a. [TA], a. alveolar inferior; *origem*, 1.ª parte da a. maxilar; *distribuição*, através do forame/canal mandibular para os dentes inferiores e queixo; *ramos*, a. para o milo-hióide, a. mentoniana, a. dental. SIN arteria alveolaris inferior [TA], inferior dental a.

inferior dental a., a. alveolar inferior. SIN inferior alveolar a.

inferior epigastric a. [TA], a. epigástrica inferior; *origem*, ilíaca externa; *ramos*, cremastérica, muscular e púbica; *anastomoses*, epigástrica superior, obturadora. Com o peritônio suprajacente, forma o ligamento umbilical lateral e forma uma base para distinguir os tipos de hérnia inguinal: as hérnias diretas passam medialmente à a.; as hérnias indiretas passam lateralmente. SIN arteria epigastrica inferior [TA], deep epigastric a.

inferior gluteal a. [TA], a. glútea inferior; *origem*, ilíaca externa; *distribuição*, articulação do quadril e região glútea; *anastomoses*, ramos da pudenda interna, sacral lateral, glútea superior, obturadora, femoral circunflexa medial e lateral. SIN arteria glutea inferior [TA], arteria ischiadica, arteria ischiatica.

inferior hemorrhoidal a., a. retal inferior. SIN inferior rectal a.

inferior hypophysial a. [TA], a. hipofisária inferior; um pequeno ramo da parte cavernosa da carótida interna para a hipófise. SIN arteria hypophysialis inferior [TA].

inferior internal parietal a., ramos precuneais da a. cerebral anterior. SIN precuneal *branches* (of anterior cerebral artery), em *branch*.

inferior labial a., ramo labial inferior da a. labial. SIN inferior labial branch of facial artery.

inferior laryngeal a. [TA], a. laríngea inferior; *origem*, tireóidea inferior; *distribuição*, músculos e mucosa da laringe; *anastomoses*, laríngea superior. SIN arteria laryngea inferior [TA].

inferior lateral genicular a. [TA], a. inferior lateral do joelho; *origem*, poplítea; *distribuição*, articulação do joelho; *anastomoses*, genicular superior e tibial recurrente anterior (e posterior); isto é, a *rede* vascular articular do joelho. SIN arteria inferior lateralis genus [TA], arteria genus inferior lateralis, lateral inferior genicular a.

inferior lingular a. [TA], a. lingular inferior; ramo (do ramo lingular) da a. pulmonar esquerda que serve o segmento lingular inferior do lobo superior do pulmão esquerdo. VER left pulmonary a. SIN arteria lingularis inferior [TA], inferior lingular branch of lingular branch of left pulmonary artery, ramus lingularis inferior.

inferior lobar a.'s [TA], artérias lobares inferiores. VER left pulmonary a., right pulmonary a.

inferior medial genicular a. [TA], a. inferior medial do joelho; *origem*, poplítea; *distribuição*, articulação do joelho; *anastomoses*, tibial recurrente anterior e posterior e genicular superior medial, isto é, a *rede* vascular articular do joelho. SIN arteria inferior medialis genus [TA], arteria genus inferior medialis, medial inferior genicular a.

inferior mesenteric a. [TA], a. mesentérica inferior; *origem*, aorta abdominal; *ramos*, cólica esquerda, sigmóide, retal superior; *anastomoses*, cólica média e retal média. SIN arteria mesenterica inferior [TA].

inferior pancreatic a. [TA], a. pancreática inferior; *origem*, pancreática dorsal; *distribuição*, corpo e cauda do pâncreas; *anastomoses*, a. pancreática magna. SIN arteria pancreatica inferior [TA], transverse pancreatic a.

inferior pancreaticoduodenal a. [TA], a. pancreaticoduodenal inferior; *origem*, mesentérica superior; uma das duas artérias, anterior e posterior; *distribuição*, cabeça do pâncreas, duodeno; *anastomoses*, pancreaticoduodenal superior. SIN arteria pancreaticoduodenalis inferior [TA].

inferior phrenic a. [TA], a. frênica inferior; *origem*, o primeiro ramo pareado a partir da aorta abdominal, inferior ao diafragma; *distribuição*, diafragma; *anastomoses*, frênica superior, torácica interna e musculofrênica. SIN arteria phrenica inferior [TA].

inferior rectal a. [TA], a. retal inferior; *origem*, pudenda interna; *distribuição*, canal anal, músculos e pele da região anal, e pele das nádegas; *anastomoses*, retal média, perineal e glútea. SIN arteria rectalis inferior [TA], inferior hemorrhoidal a.

inferior segmental a. of kidney [TA], a. do segmento inferior do rim; *origem*, ramo anterior da renal. VER segmental a.'s of kidney. SIN a. of inferior segment of kidney.

a. of inferior segment of kidney, a. do segmento inferior do rim. SIN inferior segmental a. of kidney

inferior and superior lobar a.'s [TA], artérias lobares inferior e superior. VER left pulmonary a., right pulmonary a.

inferior suprarenal a. [TA], a. supra-renal inferior; *origem*, renal; *distribuição*, glândula supra-renal. SIN arteria suprarenalis inferior [TA].

inferior thyroid a. [TA], a. tireóidea inferior; *origem*, ramo terminal do tronco tireocervical (com artéria cervical ascendente); *ramos*, laríngea inferior e muscular, esofágico e traqueal. SIN arteria thyroidea inferior [TA].

inferior tympanic a. [TA], a. timpânica inferior; *origem*, faríngea ascendente; *distribuição*, ouvido médio; *anastomoses*, ramos timpânicos de outras artérias. SIN arteria tympanica inferior [TA].

inferior ulnar collateral a., a. colateral ulnar inferior; *origem*, braquial; *distribuição*, músculos do braço na parte posterior do cotovelo; *anastomoses*, ulnar recurrente anterior e posterior; colateral ulnar superior, braquial profunda e interóssea recurrente, como parte da rede articular do cotovelo. SIN arteria collateralis ulnaris inferior [TA], arteria anastomotica magna (1), great anastomotic a. (1).

inferior vesical a. [TA], a. vesical inferior; *origem*, ilíaca interna; *distribuição*, base da bexiga, ureter e (no homem) vesículas seminais, canal deferente e próstata; *anastomoses*, retal média e outros ramos vesicais. SIN arteria vesicalis inferior [TA].

infraorbital a. [TA], a. infra-orbital; *origem*, terceira parte da maxilar; *distribuição*, dentes caninos e incisivos superiores, músculos reto inferior e oblíquo inferior, pálpebra inferior, saco lacrimal, seio maxilar e lábio superior; *anastomoses*, ramos da oftálmica, facial, labial superior, facial transversa e bucal. SIN arteria infraorbitalis [TA].

infrascapular a., a. infra-escapular; um pequeno ramo da a. escapular circunflexa.

innominate a., a. inominada; termo obsoleto para brachiocephalic (arterial) *trunk* [tronco braquiocefálico (arterial)].

insular a.'s [TA], artérias insulares; ramos da parte insular (segmento M2) da artéria cerebral média distribuídos para o córtex da ínsula. SIN arteriae insulares [TA].

intercostal a.'s, artérias intercostais; artérias que fazem trajeto na parede torácica entre as costelas. VER anterior intercostal *branches* of internal thoracic artery, em *branch*, first and second posterior intercostal a.'s, posterior intercostal a.'s 3–11, supreme intercostal a.

interlobar a., a. interlobar; a a. pulmonar descendente direita, que é contígua com os lobos médio e inferior direito e os perfunde.

interlobar a.'s of kidney [TA], artérias interlobares do rim; os ramos das artérias segmentares do rim; elas fazem trajeto entre os lobos renais e originam as artérias arqueadas. SIN arteriae interlobares renis [TA].

interlobular a.'s [TA], artérias interlobulares; artérias que passam entre os lóbulos de um órgão. VER interlobular a.'s of liver, cortical radiate a.'s. SIN arteriae interlobulares [TA].

interlobular a.'s of kidney, artérias interlobulares do rim. SIN cortical radiate a.'s.

interlobular a.'s of liver, artérias interlobulares do fígado; os muitos ramos terminais da a. hepática que passam entre os lóbulos hepáticos. SIN arteriae interlobulares (hepatis).

intermediate temporal a., ramo temporal médio da parte insular da a. cerebral média. SIN middle temporal *branch* of insular part of middle cerebral artery.

internal auditory a., a. do labirinto. SIN labyrinthine a.

internal carotid a. [TA], a. carótida interna; origina-se da carótida comum, oposta à borda superior da cartilagem tireóidea (nível vertebral C–4) e termina na fossa craniana média, ao se dividir nas artérias cerebrais anterior e média; para fins descritivos, divide-se em quatro partes: cervical, petrosa, cavernosa e cerebral. SIN arteria carotis interna [TA].

internal iliac a. [TA], a. ilíaca interna; *origem*, ilíaca; *ramos*, iliolombar, sacral lateral, obturadora, glútea superior, glútea inferior, umbilical, vesical superior, vesical inferior, retal média e pudenda interna. SIN arteria iliaca interna [TA], arteria hypogastrica, hypogastric a.

internal mammary a., a. torácica interna. SIN internal thoracic a.

internal maxillary a., a. maxilar. SIN maxillary a.

internal pudendal a. [TA], a. pudenda interna; *origem*, ilíaca interna; *ramos*, retal inferior, perineal, escrotal (ou labial) posterior, uretral, a. do bulbo do pênis (ou do vestíbulo), a. profunda do pênis (ou clitóris), a. dorsal do pênis (ou clitóris). SIN arteria pudenda interna [TA].

internal spermatic a., a. testicular. SIN testicular a.

internal thoracic a., a. torácica interna; *origem*, subclávia; *ramos*, ramos pericardiacofrênico, intercostal anterior, esternal, mediastinal, tímico, brônquico, musculares e perfurantes, e bifurca-se na musculofrênica e epigástrica superior. SIN arteria thoracica interna [TA], arteria mammaria interna, internal mammary a.

intestinal a.'s, artérias intestinais. VER ileal a.'s, jejunal a.'s.
intrarenal a.'s [TA], artérias intra-renais; artérias e ramos arteriais distribuídos dentro do rim; originam-se como ramos e derivados das artérias dos segmentos renais. SIN arteriae intrarenales [TA].
jejunal a.'s [TA], artérias jejunais; *origem*, mesentérica superior; *distribuição*, jejuno; *anastomoses*, por uma série de arcos entre elas e com as artérias ileais. SIN arteriae jejunales [TA].
juxtacolic a., a. justacólica; *termo oficial alternativo para marginal a. of colon.
a.'s of kidney, artérias dos segmentos do rim. SIN segmental a.'s of kidney.
Kugel anastomotic a., a. anastomótica de Kugel. SIN atrial anastomotic *branch of circumflex branch of left coronary artery.*
a. of labyrinth, a. do labirinto. SIN labyrinthine a.
labyrinthine a. [TA], a. do labirinto; ramo do meato auditivo interno; um ramo da artéria basilar que penetra no labirinto através do meato auditivo interno. SIN arteria labyrinthi [TA], arteria auditiva interna, a. of labyrinth, internal auditory a., ramus meatus acustici interni.
lacrimal a. [TA], a. lacrimal; *origem*, oftálmica; *distribuição*, glândula lacrimal, músculos retos lateral e superior, pálpebra superior, fronte e fossa temporal. SIN arteria lacrimalis [TA].
lateral basal segmental a. [TA], a. segmentar basilar lateral; ramo basilar lateral dos seguintes: 1) parte basilar do ramo lobar inferior da a. pulmonar direita; 2) parte basilar do ramo lobar inferior da a. pulmonar esquerda. SIN arteria segmentalis basalis lateralis [TA], arteria segmentalis lateralis [TA], lateral basal branch, ramus basalis lateralis.
lateral circumflex femoral a. [TA], a. circunflexa femoral lateral; *origem*, femoral profunda; *distribuição*, articulação do quadril, músculos da coxa; *anastomoses*, femoral circunflexa medial, glútea inferior, glútea superior. SIN arteria circumflexa femoris lateralis [TA], lateral circumflex a. of thigh, lateral femoral circumflex a.
lateral circumflex a. of thigh, a. circunflexa femoral lateral. SIN lateral circumflex femoral a.
lateral femoral circumflex a., a. circunflexa femoral lateral. SIN lateral circumflex femoral a.
lateral frontobasal a. [TA], a. frontobasilar lateral; um ramo da parte insular da a. cerebral média distribuído para o córtex da parte inferior lateral do lobo frontal. SIN arteria frontobasalis lateralis [TA], arteria orbitofrontalis lateralis*, lateral orbitofrontal a. *.
lateral inferior genicular a., a. inferior lateral do joelho. SIN inferior lateral genicular a.
lateral malleolar a.'s, artérias maleolares laterais. SIN lateral malleolar *branch (of fibular peroneal artery).*
(lateral and medial) palpebral a.'s [TA], artérias palpebrais (lateral e medial); ramos da oftálmica que suprem as pálpebras superior e inferior, consistindo em dois grupos: lateral e medial. SIN arteriae palpebrales (laterales et mediales) [TA].
(lateral and medial) parietal a.'s [TA], artérias parietais (laterais e mediais); ramos da parte terminal da a. cerebral média, dividida em dois ramos: a. parietal anterior e a. parietal posterior. SIN arteriae parietales (laterales et mediales) [TA].
lateral nasal a., ramo nasal lateral da a. facial. SIN lateral nasal *branch* of facial artery.
lateral occipital a. [TA], a. occipital lateral; um dos ramos terminais da artéria cerebral posterior; supre as porções medial e ventral do lobo temporal por meio dos ramos temporais anterior, intermediário, medial e posterior; pode ser chamada de segmento P3 da a. cerebral posterior. SIN arteria occipitalis lateralis [TA], P3 segment of posterior cerebral artery [TA], segmentum P3 arteriae cerebri posterioris [TA].
lateral orbitofrontal a., a. frontobasilar lateral; *termo alternativo oficial para lateral frontobasal a.
lateral plantar a. [TA], a. plantar lateral; o maior dos dois ramos terminais da a. tibial posterior; *distribuição*, forma o arco plantar e, através dele, nutre a planta do pé e as superfícies plantares dos artelhos; *anastomoses*, plantar medial, dorsal do pé. SIN arteria plantaris lateralis [TA].
lateral sacral a.'s [TA], artérias sacrais laterais; geralmente uma das duas artérias que se originam da a. ilíaca interna ou de seus ramos; elas suprem os músculos e a pele nas vizinhanças e enviam ramos para o canal sacral, nutrindo as artérias radicular e espinal e continuando até a pele e tecidos subcutâneos que se sobrepõem ao sacro. SIN arteriae sacrales laterales.
lateral segmental a. [TA], a. segmentar lateral. VER left pulmonary a., right pulmonary a.
lateral splanchnic a.'s, artérias esplâncnicas laterais; artérias que se originam no embrião, a partir da aorta dorsal, e suprem o mesonéfron, testículos ou ovários e a glândula supra-renal.
lateral striate a.'s, artérias centrais ântero-laterais. SIN anterolateral central a.'s.
lateral superior genicular a., a. superior lateral do joelho. SIN superior lateral genicular a.

lateral tarsal a. [TA], a. tarsal lateral; *origem*, a. dorsal do pé; *distribuição*, articulações társicas e músculo extensor curto dos dedos; *anastomoses*, arqueada, fibular, plantar lateral, maleolar lateral anterior. SIN arteria tarsea lateralis [TA].
lateral thoracic a. [TA], a. torácica lateral; *origem*, terceira parte da axilar; *distribuição*, passa ao redor da borda lateral dos músculos peitorais, suprindo-os e a outros músculos do tórax e a glândula mamária. SIN arteria thoracica lateralis [TA], external mammary a., long thoracic a.
left anterior descending a., ramo interventricular anterior da a. coronária esquerda. SIN anterior interventricular *branch* of left coronary artery.
left colic a. [TA], a. cólica esquerda; *origem*, mesentérica inferior; *distribuição*, cólon descendente e flexura esplênica; *anastomoses*, cólica média, sigmóide. SIN arteria colica sinistra [TA].
left coronary a. [TA], a. coronária esquerda; *origem*, seio aórtico esquerdo; *distribuição*, divide-se em dois ramos principais: um interventricular anterior, que desce no sulco interventricular anterior, e um ramo circunflexo, que passa até à superfície diafragmática do ventrículo esquerdo; fornece ramos atriais, ventriculares e atrioventriculares. SIN arteria coronaria sinistra [TA].
left gastric a. [TA], a. gástrica esquerda; *origem*, celíaca; *distribuição*, cárdia do estômago na curvatura menor, parte abdominal do esôfago e, com freqüência, uma porção do lobo esquerdo do fígado através de um ramo hepático esquerdo aberrante; *anastomoses*, esofágica, gástrica direita. SIN arteria gastrica sinistra [TA], coronary a. (2).
left gastroepiploic a., a. gastromental esquerda. SIN left gastroomental a.
left gastroomental a. [TA], a. gastromental esquerda; *origem*, esplênica; *distribuição*, curvatura maior do estômago e omento maior; *anastomoses*, artérias gastroepiplóica direita e gástrica curta. SIN arteria gastroomentalis sinistra [TA], arteria gastroepiploica sinistra, left gastroepiploic a.
left hepatic a., ramo esquerdo da a. hepática própria. SIN left *branch* of hepatic artery proper.
left marginal a. [TA] ramo marginal esquerdo da a. coronária esquerda; um grande ramo ventricular do ramo circunflexo da a. coronária esquerda que faz trajeto ao longo do centro da superfície pulmonar esquerda (margem obtusa) do coração, usualmente até o ápice. SIN ramus marginalis sinister arteriae coronariae sinistrae [TA].
left pulmonar a. [TA], a. pulmonar esquerda; o mais curto dos dois ramos terminais do tronco pulmonar; perfura o pericárdio para penetrar no hilo do pulmão esquerdo. São emitidos ramos que se distribuem com os brônquios segmentares e subsegmentares; ocorrem variações freqüentes. *Ramos típicos*: das artérias lobares superiores [TA] (*arteriae* lobares superiores, em *arteria* [TA]) são a a. do segmento apical [TA] (*arteria* segmentalis apicalis [TA]), a. do segmento anterior [TA] (*arteria* segmentalis anterior [TA]) e a. do segmento posterior [TA] (*arteria* segmentalis posterior [TA]), com as duas últimas apresentando ramos ascendente e descendente [TA] (rami ascendens et descendens [TA]); da artéria lingular [TA] (*arteria* lingularis [TA]) são a a. lingular superior [TA] (*arteria* lingularis superior [TA]) e a. lingular inferior [TA] (*arteria* lingularis inferior [TA]); e das artérias lobares inferiores [TA] (*arteriae* lobares inferiores, em *arteria* [TA]) são a artéria do segmento superior [TA] (*arteria* segmentalis superior [TA]) e uma parte basal [TA] (pars basalis [TA]) que dá origem às artérias dos segmentos basais anterior, posterior, lateral e medial [TA] (arteriae segmentales basales anterior, posterior, lateralis et medialis [TA]). SIN arteria pulmonalis sinistra [TA].
lenticulostriate a.'s, artérias lenticuloestriadas; **(1)** *termo oficial alternativo para anterolateral central a.'s; **(2)** qualquer uma das várias pequenas artérias que entram na base do cérebro através da substância perfurada anterior e que nutrem o estriado, globo pálido e cápsula interna; a maioria dessas artérias perfurantes são ramos do segmento M_1 (terminologia clínica) da a. cerebral média e (raramente) da coróide anterior. SIN Charcot a.
lesser palatine a. [TA], a. palatina menor; um dos vários ramos posteriores da palatina descendente no canal palatino maior, distribuída para o palato mole e tonsila. SIN arteria palatina minor [TA].
lienal a., a. esplênica. SIN splenic a.
lingual a. [TA], a. lingual; *origem*, carótida externa; *distribuição*, corre ao longo da superfície da língua, termina como a a. lingual profunda; *ramos*, ramos suprahióideo e do dorso da língua e artéria sublingual. SIN arteria lingualis [TA].
lingular a. [TA], a. pulmonar esquerda. VER left pulmonary a.
long central a., a. estriada medial. SIN medial striate a.
long posterior ciliary a.'s [TA], artérias ciliares posteriores longas; um dos dois ramos da oftálmica que correm para diante, entre os revestimentos esclerótico e coróide da íris, em cujas margens interna e externa formam dois círculos por meio de anastomoses. SIN arteriae ciliares posteriores longae.
long thoracic a., a. torácica lateral. SIN lateral thoracic a.
a.'s of lower limb [TA], artérias do membro inferior; artérias que nutrem o membro inferior, as quais derivam, sem exceção, da a. ilíaca externa. SIN arteriae membri inferioris.
lowest lumbar a.'s [TA], artérias lombares imas; *origem*, sacral média; *distribuição*, sacro e músculo ilíaco; *anastomoses*, a. ilíaca circunflexa profunda. SIN arteriae lumbales imae [TA].

lowest thyroid a., a. tireóidea ima. SIN thyroid ima a.
lumbar a.'s [TA], artérias lombares; *origem*, aorta abdominal; um dos quatro ou cinco pares; *distribuição*, vértebras lombares, músculos das costas, parede abdominal; *anastomoses*, intercostal, subcostal, epigástricas superior e inferior, ilíaca circunflexa profunda e iliolombar. SIN arteriae lumbales [TA].
macular a.'s, arteríolas maculares. VER macular *arteriole*, superior macular *arteriole*.
mammillary a.'s [TA], artérias mamilares; *origem*, artéria comunicante posterior; *distribuição*, para os corpos mamilares do hipotálamo. SIN arteriae mammillares [TA].
marginal a. of colon [TA], a. justacólica, arco justacólico; a. formada por anastomoses entre as artérias cólicas direita e esquerda; passa para baixo, a partir da flexura cólica esquerda até a extremidade aboral do cólon pélvico. SIN arteria marginalis coli [TA], arcus marginalis coli*, arteria juxtacolica*, juxtacolic a.*, marginal arcade*, a. of Drummond, Riolan arc (2).
masseteric a. [TA], a. massetérica; *origem*, segunda parte (infratemporal) da maxilar; *distribuição*, músculo masseter através da incisura mandibular, articulação temporomandibular; *anastomoses*, ramos da facial transversa e ramos massetéricos da facial. SIN arteria masseterica [TA].
mastoid a., ramo mastóideo da a. occipital. SIN mastoid branch of occipital artery.
maxillary a. [TA], a. maxilar; *origem*, carótida externa; *ramos*, primeira parte (retromandibular): auricular profunda, timpânica profunda; segunda parte (infratemporal): meníngea média, alveolar inferior, massetérica, temporal profunda, bucal; terceira parte (pterigopalatina): alveolar superior posterior, infraorbitária, palatina descendente, arteria do canal pterigóide, esfenopalatina. SIN arteria maxillaris [TA], internal maxillary a.
medial basal segmental a. [TA], a. segmentar basilar medial; origina-se da parte basal das artérias lobares inferiores dos pulmões esquerdo e direito. SIN arteria segmentalis basalis medialis [TA], arteria segmentalis medialis [TA], medial basal branch of pulmonary artery, ramus basalis medialis.
medial circumflex femoral a. [TA], a. circunflexa femoral medial; *origem*, femoral profunda; *distribuição*, articulação do quadril, músculos da coxa; *anastomoses*, glútea inferior, glútea superior, circunflexa lateral do fêmur. SIN arteria circumflexa femoris medialis [TA], medial circumflex a. of thigh, medial femoral circumflex a.
medial circumflex a. of thigh, a. circunflexa femoral medial. SIN medial circumflex femoral a.
medial collateral a. [TA], a. colateral medial. SIN middle collateral a.
medial commisural a. [TA], a. comissural medial; *origem*, a. comunicante anterior; *distribuição*, para a comissura supra-óptica, quiasma óptico.
medial femoral circumflex a., a. circunflexa femoral medial. SIN medial circumflex femoral a.
medial frontobasal a. [TA], a. frontobasilar medial; o primeiro ramo da parte pós-comunicante (segmento A2) da a. cerebral anterior (a. pericalosa); nutre a metade medial da superfície inferior do córtex frontal. SIN arteria frontobasalis medialis [TA], arteria orbitofrontalis medialis*, medial orbitofrontal a.*, orbital a.
medial inferior genicular a., a. inferior medial do joelho. SIN inferior medial genicular a.
medial malleolar a.'s, ramos maleolares mediais da a. tibial posterior. SIN medial malleolar branches (of posterior tibial artery), em branch.
medial occipital a. [TA], a. occipital medial; um dos ramos terminais da a. cerebral posterior; distribui-se para o corpo caloso, faces mediais da face caudal do lobo parietal e lobo occipital médio, incluindo o córtex visual pelos ramos próprios, que compreendem o ramo dorsal do corpo caloso, ramo parietal, ramo parieto-occipital, ramo occipito-temporal e ramo calcarino; pode ser chamado de segmento P4 da artéria cerebral posterior. SIN arteria occipitalis medialis [TA], P4 segment of posterior cerebral artery*, segmentum P1 arteriae cerebri posterioris*, segmentum P4 arteriae cerebri posterioris.
medial orbitofrontal a., frontobasilar medial; *termo oficial alternativo para medial frontobasal a.
medial plantar a. [TA], a. plantar medial; um dos ramos terminais da tibial posterior; *distribuição*, lado medial da planta do pé; *anastomoses*, dorsal do pé, plantar lateral. SIN arteria plantaris medialis [TA].
medial segmental a. [TA], a. segmentar medial. VER left pulmonary a., right pulmonary a.
medial striate a., a. estriada medial; origina-se na a. comunicante anterior [TA] ou exatamente distal a ela; *distribuição*, caudado anterior e putâmen e ramo anterior da cápsula interna. VER distal medial striate a., proximal medial striate a.'s. SIN arteria striata medialis distalis [TA], distal medial striate a. [TA], arteria recurrens, a. of Heubner, Heubner a., long central a., recurrent a. of Heubner, recurrent a. (2).
medial superior genicular a., a. superior medial do joelho. SIN superior medial genicular a.
medial tarsal a.'s [TA], artérias tarsais mediais; dois pequenos ramos da a. dorsal do pé; *distribuição*, para a margem interna do pé. SIN arteriae tarsae medialis [TA].

median a. [TA], a. acompanhante do nervo mediano; *origem*, interóssea anterior; *distribuição*, acompanha o nervo mediano até a região palmar; *anastomoses*, ramos do arco palmar superficial. SIN arteria comitans nervi mediani [TA], arteria mediana, comitant a. of median nerve.
median callosal a. [TA], a. calosa mediana; *origem*: a. comunicante anterior; *distribuição*, lâmina terminal e rostro do corpo caloso. SIN arteria callosa mediana [TA].
median commissural a. [TA], a. comissural mediana; *origem*, a. comunicante anterior; *distribuição*: para a comissura supra-óptica e quiasma óptico. SIN arteria commissuralis mediana [TA].
median sacral a. [TA], a. sacral mediana; *origem*, face posterior da aorta abdominal, exatamente acima da bifurcação; *distribuição*, vértebras lombares inferiores, sacro e cóccix; *anastomoses*, sacral lateral, retais superior e média. SIN arteria sacralis mediana [TA], middle sacral a.
mediastinal a.'s, ramos mediastinais. SIN mediastinal branches, em branch.
medium a., a. muscular. SIN muscular a.
medullary a.'s of brain, artérias medulares do cérebro; ramos das artérias corticais que penetram e nutrem a substância branca do cérebro.
medullary spinal a.'s, artérias da medula espinal. SIN segmental medullary a.'s.
mental a., ramo mentual da a. alveolar inferior. SIN mental branch (of inferior alveolar artery).
metatarsal a. [TA], a. metatarsal; uma das quatro artérias dorsais ou quatro plantares que fazem trajeto em relação aos ossos metatársicos, cada uma se dividindo distalmente em uma a. digital medial e lateral que supre a face dorsal ou plantar dos lados adjacentes dos dois artelhos. VER dorsal metatarsal a., plantar metatarsal a. SIN arteria metatarsalis [TA].
middle cerebral a. [TA], a. cerebral média; um dos dois grandes ramos terminais (com a a. cerebral anterior) da artéria carótida interna; passa lateralmente ao redor do pólo do lobo temporal, em seguida posteriormente, na profundidade da fissura cerebral lateral; para fins descritivos, divide-se em três partes: 1) a parte esfenoidal (segmento M_1 da terminologia clínica), que fornece ramos perfurantes para a cápsula interna, tálamo e corpo estriado; 2) a parte insular, que fornece ramos para a ínsula e áreas corticais adjacentes; e 3) a parte terminal ou parte cortical, que nutre uma grande parte da convexidade cortical central (as duas últimas formando, em conjunto, o segmento M_2). SIN arteria cerebri media [TA].
middle colic a. [TA], a. cólica média; *origem*, mesentérica superior; *distribuição*, cólon transverso; *anastomoses*, cólicas direita e esquerda. SIN arteria colica media [TA].
middle collateral a., a. colateral média; o ramo terminal posterior da braquial profunda, anastomosando-se com as artérias que formam a rede articular do cotovelo. SIN arteria collateralis media [TA], medial collateral a.
middle genicular a. [TA], a. média do joelho; *origem*, poplítea; *distribuição*, membrana sinovial e ligamentos cruzados da articulação do joelho. SIN arteria media genus [TA], arteria articularis azygos, arteria genus media.
middle hemorrhoidal a., a. retal média. SIN middle rectal a.
middle lobar a. [TA], a. lobar média. VER left pulmonary a., right pulmonary a.
middle lobar a. of right lung [TA], a. lobar média do pulmão direito. VER right pulmonary a.
middle meningeal a. [TA], a. meníngea média; *origem*, maxilar; *ramos*, petrosa, timpânica superior, frontal e parietal; *distribuição*, para as partes mencionadas e através dos ramos terminais para as fossas cranianas anterior e média; *anastomoses*, ramos meníngeos da occipital, faríngea ascendente, oftálmica e lacrimal, estilomastóidea, ramo meníngeo acessório da maxilar e temporal profunda. SIN arteria meningea media [TA].
middle rectal a. [TA], a. retal média; *origem*, ilíaca interna; *distribuição*, porção média do reto; *anastomoses*, retal inferior e retal superior. Como a última é uma tributária do sistema porta, esta é uma anastomose portossistêmica ou portocava. SIN arteria rectalis media [TA], middle hemorrhoidal a.
middle sacral a., a. sacral mediana. SIN median sacral a.
middle suprarenal a. [TA], a. supra-renal média; *origem*, aorta; *distribuição*, glândula supra-renal. SIN arteria suprarenalis media [TA].
middle temporal a. [TA], a. temporal média; *origem*, temporal superficial; *distribuição*, fáscia e músculo temporal; *anastomoses*, ramos da maxilar. VER TAMBÉM middle temporal branch of insular part of middle cerebral artery, posterior temporal branch of middle cerebral artery. SIN arteria temporalis media [TA].
muscular a., a. muscular; uma a. com uma túnica média composta principalmente de músculo liso com arranjo circular. SIN distributing a., medium a.
muscular a.'s (of ophthalmic artery) [TA], artérias musculares (da artéria oftálmica); ramos diretos ou indiretos da a. oftálmica que nutrem os músculos extra-oculares. SIN arteriae musculares (arteriae ophthalmicae) [TA].
musculophrenic a. [TA], a. musculofrênica; *origem*, o ramo terminal lateral da torácica interna; *distribuição*, diafragma e músculos intercostais; *anastomoses*, ramos das artérias pericardiacofrênica, frênica inferior e intercostal posterior. SIN arteria musculophrenica [TA].
mylohyoid a., ramo milo-hióideo da a. alveolar inferior. SIN mylohyoid branch (of inferior alveolar artery).

myometrial arcuate a.'s, artérias arqueadas do miométrio; ramos das artérias uterina e ovariana.
myometrial radial a.'s, artérias radiais do miométrio; continuações das artérias arqueadas do miométrio.
Neubauer a., a. de Neubauer. SIN thyroid ima a.
nutrient a. [TA], a. nutrícia; uma artéria de origem variável que nutre a cavidade medular de um osso longo. SIN arteria nutricia [TA], nutrient vessel.
nutrient a. of femur, a. nutrícia do fêmur. SIN femoral nutrient a. SIN arteria nutriciae femoris [TA], arteria nutriens femoris*.
nutrient a. of fibula, a. nutrícia da fíbula. SIN fibular nutrient a.
nutrient a.'s of humerus, artérias nutrícias do úmero. SIN humeral nutrient a.'s. SIN arteria nutriens humeri*.
nutrient a. of radius [TA], a. nutrícia do rádio; *origem*, radial a.; *distribuição:* cavidade medular do rádio. SIN arteria radii nutricia [TA], arteria nutriens radii*.
nutrient a. of the tibia, a. nutrícia da tíbia. SIN tibial nutrient a.
nutrient a. of ulna [TA], a. nutrícia da ulna; *origem*, a. ulnar; *distribuição*, cavidade medular da ulna. SIN arteria nutricia ulnae [TA], arteria nutriens ulnae*.
obturator a. [TA], a. obturatória; *anastomoses,* iliolombar, epigástrica inferior, circunflexa femoral medial; *origem*, divisão anterior da ilíaca interna; *distribuição*, ílio, púbis, músculos obturatório e adutor; *ramos*, púbico, acetabular, anterior e posterior. SIN arteria obturatoria [TA].
occipital a. [TA], a. occipital; *origem*, carótida externa; *ramos*, esternocleidomastóidea, meníngea, auricular, occipital, mastóidea e descendente. SIN arteria occipitalis [TA].
omphalomesenteric a., a. onfalomesentérica; termo antigo para a a. vitelina.
ophthalmic a. [TA], a. oftálmica; *origem*, carótida interna; *ramos*, ciliar, artéria central da retina, meníngea anterior, lacrimal, conjuntival, episcleral, supra-orbital, etmoidal, palpebral, dorsal nasal e supratroclear. SIN arteria ophthalmica [TA].
orbital a., a. frontobasilar medial. SIN medial frontobasal a.
orbitofrontal a., a. frontobasilar. VER lateral frontobasal a., medial frontobasal a.
ovarian a. [TA], a. ovárica; *origem*, aorta; *distribuição*, ureter, ovário, ligamento ovariano e trompa uterina; *anastomoses*, uterina. SIN arteria ovarica [TA].
palmar interosseous a., a. metacarpal palmar. SIN palmar metacarpal a.
palmar metacarpal a. [TA], a. metacarpal palmar; uma das três artérias que se originam a partir do arco palmar profundo que correm nos três espaços metacárpicos interósseos mediais; anastomosam-se com a palmar comum e, através de ramos perfurantes, com as artérias metacarpais dorsais. SIN arteria metacarpalis palmaris [TA], palmar interosseous a.
paracentral a., ramos paracentrais da a. pericalosa. SIN paracentral branches (of pericallosal artery), em branch.
paramedian a.'s, artérias centrais póstero-mediais; *termo oficial alternativo para posteromedial central a.'s.
parent a., a.-mãe; a a. que dá origem a uma determinada a.; a. da qual uma determinada a. é um ramo.
parietooccipital a., ramos parieto-occipitais da a. cerebral anterior. SIN parieto-occipital branches (of anterior cerebral artery), em branch.
a.'s of penis, artérias do pênis. VER dorsal a. of penis, deep a. of penis.
perforating a.'s of hand, ramos perfurantes do arco palmar profundo. SIN perforating branches of deep palmar arch.
perforating a.'s (of deep femoral artery) [TA], artérias perfurantes (da artéria femoral profunda); *origem*, a. profunda femoris; *distribuição*, como três ou quatro vasos que passam através da aponeurose do adutor magno para os compartimentos posterior e anterior da coxa. SIN arteriae perforantes arteriae profundae femoris [TA].
perforating a.'s (of foot), ramos perfurantes das artérias metatarsais plantares. SIN perforating branches (of plantar metatarsal arteries), em branch.
perforating a.'s (of internal thoracic artery), ramos perfurantes (da artéria torácica interna). SIN perforating branches of internal thoracic artery, em branch.
perforating a.'s of penis [TA], artérias perfurantes do pênis; ramos da a. dorsal do pênis que perfuram a túnica albugínea ao longo do dorso do pênis, especialmente próximo à glande, para nutrir a glande e suplementar a a. profunda do pênis na irrigação dos espaços cavernosos do corpo cavernoso. SIN arteriae perforantes penis [TA].
perforating radiate a.'s (of kidney) [TA], artérias radiais perfurantes (do rim); continuações das artérias radiais corticais que perfuram a cápsula do rim e contribuem para o plexo vascular capsular. VER TAMBÉM cortical radiate a.'s. SIN arteriae perforantes radiatae (renis) [TA].
pericallosal a. [TA], a. pericalosa; a continuação da a. cerebral anterior depois da a. comunicante anterior; fornece ramos para o córtex cerebral, à medida que passa ao longo do corpo caloso. SIN arteria pericallosa [TA].
pericardiacophrenic a. [TA], a. pericardiofrênica; *origem,* torácica interna; *distribuição,* pericárdio, diafragma e pleura; *anastomoses,* musculofrênica, frênica inferior, ramos mediastinal e pericárdico da torácica interna. SIN arteria pericardiacophrenica [TA], arteria comes nervi phrenici.

perineal a. [TA], a. perineal; *origem*, pudenda interna; *distribuição*, estruturas superficiais do períneo; *anastomoses*, external pudendal arteries. SIN arteria perinealis [TA].
peroneal a., a. fibular; *termo oficial alternativo para fibular a.
pipestem a.'s, artérias em tubo de cachimbo; artérias endurecidas por calcificação, conforme observado na arteriosclerose de Mönckeberg; descritivo da sensação característica para o dedo do examinador.
plantar metatarsal a. [TA], a. metatarsal plantar; um dos quatro ramos do arco arterial plantar que se dividem em artérias digitais plantares para suprirem os artelhos. SIN arteria metatarsalis plantaris [TA].
polar frontal a. [TA], artéria polar frontal; *origem,* como o segundo ramo principal da parte pós-comunicante (segmento A2) da a. cerebral anterior (a. pericalosa); *distribuição*, face medial do lobo frontal, envolvendo o lobo frontal do cérebro. SIN arteria polaris frontalis [TA], frontopolar a. [TA].
polar temporal a. [TA], a. polar temporal; *origem*, ramo temporal anterior da a. cerebral média; *distribuição*, face súpero-medial do lobo temporal, estendendo-se até o pólo temporal, do cérebro. SIN arteria polaris temporalis [TA].
pontine a.'s, a.'s of pons [TA], artérias da ponte; ramos da a. basilar que nutrem a ponte; divididas em ramos medial [TA] (rami mediales [TA] ou ramos pontinos paramedianos [TA alternativa]) e ramos laterais [TA] (rami laterales [TA] ou ramos pontinos circunferenciais [TA alternativa]); as artérias pontinas circunferenciais são, por vezes, designadas como ramos circunferencial curto e circunferencial longo. SIN arteriae pontis [TA], rami ad pontem.
popliteal a. [TA], a. poplítea; continuação da a. femoral no espaço poplíteo, bifurcando-se (na borda inferior do músculo poplíteo, quando passa profundamente ao arco tendíneo do músculo solear) nas artérias tibiais anterior e posterior; *ramos*, artérias superior lateral e medial do joelho, média do joelho, inferior lateral e medial do joelho e sural. SIN arteria poplitea [TA].
postcentral a., a. do sulco pós-central. SIN a. of postcentral sulcus.
postcentral sulcal a., a. do sulco pós-central. SIN a. of postcentral sulcus.
a. of postcentral sulcus [TA], a. do sulco pós-central; um ramo da parte terminal da a. cerebral média que se distribui para o córtex em ambos os lados do sulco pós-central. SIN arteria sulci postcentralis [TA], postcentral a., postcentral sulcal a.
posterior alveolar a., a. alveolar superior posterior. SIN posterior superior alveolar a.
posterior auricular a. [TA], a. auricular posterior; *origem*, face posterior da carótida externa, exatamente acima do músculo digástrico; *trajeto*, ascende primeiramente entre a glândula parótida e o processo estilóide e, em seguida, entre a cartilagem da aurícula e o processo mastóideo; *ramos*, musculares (digástrico, estilo-hióideo e esternocleidomastóideo), glandular (parótida), a. estilomastóidea, occipital e auricular; *anastomoses*, a. timpânica anterior (através da a. estilomastóidea) e a. occipital. SIN arteria auricularis posterior [TA].
posterior basal segmental a. of left/right lung, a. segmentar basilar posterior do pulmão esquerdo/direito. SIN posterior basal branch, ramus basalis posterior.
posterior cecal a. [TA], a. cecal posterior; *origem*, artéria ileocólica; *distribuição*, região posterior do ceco. SIN arteria cecalis posterior [TA].
posterior cerebral a. [TA], a. cerebral posterior; formada pela bifurcação da a. basilar; passa ao redor do pedúnculo cerebral até atingir a face medial do hemisfério; para fins descritivos, divide-se em três partes: 1) parte pré-comunicante (segmento P_1 da terminologia clínica), que origina as artérias centrais póstero-mediais [TA], artérias comunicantes curtas [TA], a a. perfurante do tálamo [TA] e a a. colicular [TA]; 2) a parte pós-comunicante (P_2), que origina as artérias centrais póstero-laterais [TA], ramos coróides posteriores mediais [TA], ramos coróides posteriores laterais [TA], ramos pedunculares [TA], a a. talamogeniculada [TA]; e 3) a parte terminal ou cortical, que consiste na a. occipital lateral [TA] (P_3), cujos ramos nutrem a face medial do lobo temporal, e a a. occipital medial [TA] (P_4), cujos ramos nutrem a superfície medial do lobo occipital; os últimos incluem os ramos calcarino e parieto-occipital. SIN arteria cerebri posterior [TA].
posterior choroidal a., a. corióidea posterior; usualmente observada como dois ramos do segmento P_2 da a. cerebral posterior [TA] que nutrem o plexo corióide do terceiro ventrículo (a. corióidea posterior medial [TA]) e partes do plexo corióide do ventrículo lateral (a. corióidea posterior lateral [TA]). SIN arteria choroidea posterior.
posterior circumflex humeral a. [TA], a. circumflexa posterior do úmero; *origem*, axilar; *distribuição*, músculos e estruturas da articulação do ombro; *anastomoses*, circunflexa anterior do úmero, supra-escapular, tóraco-acromial e braquial profunda. SIN arteria circumflexa humeri posterior [TA], posterior humeral circumflex a.
posterior communicating a. [TA], a. comunicante posterior; *origem*, carótida interna; *distribuição*, trato óptico, pilares do cérebro, região interpeduncular e giro do hipocampo; *anastomoses*, com a cerebral posterior para formar o círculo arterial cerebral (polígono de Willis). SIN arteria communicans posterior [TA].
posterior conjunctival a. [TA], a. conjuntival posterior; um de uma série de ramos a partir dos arcos arteriais das pálpebras superior e inferior que nutrem a conjuntiva. SIN arteria conjunctivalis posterior [TA], conjunctival a.'s

posterior dental a., a. alveolar posterior superior. SIN posterior superior alveolar a.

posterior descending coronary a., ramo interventricular posterior da a. coronária direita. SIN posterior interventricular branch of right coronary a.

posterior ethmoidal a. [TA], a. etmoidal posterior; *origem*, oftálmica; *distribuição*, células etmoidais posteriores e parte posterior superior da parede lateral da cavidade nasal. SIN arteria ethmoidalis posterior [TA].

posterior gastric a. [TA], a. gástrica posterior; *origem*, a. esplênica; *distribuição*, ascende por via retroperitoneal na parede posterior da bolsa omental no sentido do fundo do estômago para atingir (e nutrir) a parede gástrica por meio da dobra gastrofrênica. Omitida de muitos relatos do aporte sanguíneo do estômago, sua presença inesperada pode complicar a cirurgia na cárdia do estômago. SIN arteria gastrica posterior [TA].

posterior humeral circumflex a., a. circunflexa posterior do úmero. SIN posterior circumflex humeral a.

posterior inferior cerebellar a. [TA], a. cerebelar inferior posterior; *origem*, parte intracraniana da vertebral; *distribuição*, medula lateral, plexo coróide do quarto ventrículo e cerebelo; *anastomoses*, cerebelar superior e cerebelar anterior inferior; origina a artéria espinal posterior [TA], ramo cerebelar tonsilar [TA] e ramo corióideo para o quarto ventrículo [TA]. SIN arteria inferior posterior cerebelli [TA].

posterior intercostal a.'s 1-2, primeira e segunda artérias intercostais posteriores. SIN first and second posterior intercostal a.'s.

posterior intercostal a.'s 3-11 [TA], terceira à décima primeira artéria intercostal posterior; um dos nove pares de artérias que se originam da aorta torácica e se distribuem para os nove espaços intercostais inferiores, coluna vertebral e músculos e tegumento das costas; anastomosam-se com os ramos da musculofrênica, torácica interna, epigástrica superior, subcostal e lombar. SIN arteriae intercostales posteriores III–XI [TA].

posterior interosseous a. [TA], a. intercostal posterior; *origem*, artéria interóssea comum; *distribuição*, compartimento posterior do antebraço. SIN arteria interossea posterior [TA], dorsal interosseous a.

posterior interventricular a., ramo interventricular posterior da a. coronária direita. SIN posterior interventricular branch of right coronary a.

posterior interventricular branch of right coronary a. [TA], ramo interventricular posterior da a. coronária direita; continuação da a. coronária direita no sulco interventricular posterior; desce até o ápice para se anastomosar com a a. interventricular anterior; nutre a maior parte da face diafragmática dos ventrículos e o terço posterior do septo interventricular. SIN ramus interventricularis posterior arteriae coronariae dextrae [TA], posterior descending coronary a., posterior interventricular a.

posterior labial a.'s, ramos labiais posteriores da a. perineal interna. SIN posterior labial branches of internal perineal *artery*.

posterior lateral nasal a.'s [TA], artérias nasais posteriores laterais; ramos da a. esfenopalatina que nutrem as partes posteriores das conchas nasais e a parede lateral do nariz. SIN arteriae nasales posteriores laterales [TA].

posterior mediastinal a.'s, ramos mediastinais posteriores da aorta torácica. SIN mediastinal *branches* of thoracic aorta, em *branch*.

posterior meningeal a. [TA], a. meníngea posterior; *origem*, faríngea ascendente; *distribuição*, dura-máter da fossa craniana posterior; *anastomoses*, ramos da meníngea média e vertebral. SIN arteria meningea posterior [TA].

posterior pancreaticoduodenal a., a. pancreaticoduodenal posterior. SIN retroduodenal a.

posterior parietal a. [TA], a. parietal posterior; o ramo do segmento M2 da a. cerebral média distribuído para a parte posterior do lobo parietal. SIN arteria parietalis posterior [TA].

posterior peroneal a.'s, ramo maleolar lateral da a. fibular. SIN lateral malleolar branch (of fibular peroneal artery).

posterior segmental a. [TA], a. do segmento posterior ou a. segmentar posterior. VER left pulmonary a., right pulmonary a., segmental a.'s of kidney.

posterior segmental a. (of kidney) [TA], a. do segmento posterior (do rim); *origem*, continuação do ramo posterior da renal. VER TAMBÉM segmental a.'s of kidney. SIN a. of posterior segment of kidney.

a. of posterior segment of kidney, a. do segmento posterior do rim. SIN posterior segmental a. (of kidney).

posterior septal a. of nose, ramo septal posterior do nariz. SIN posterior septal branch of nose.

posterior spinal a. [TA], a. espinal posterior; *origem*, parte intracraniana da vertebral; *distribuição*, bulbo, medula espinal e pia-máter; *anastomoses*, ramos espinais das artérias intercostais. SIN arteria spinalis posterior [TA].

posterior superior alveolar a. [TA], a. alveolar superior posterior; *origem*, terceira parte da a. maxilar dentro da fossa pterigopalatina; *distribuição*, dentes molares e pré-molares, gengiva, mucosa do seio maxilar. SIN arteria alveolaris superior posterior [TA], posterior alveolar a., posterior dental a.

posterior temporal a., ramo temporal posterior da a. cerebral média. SIN posterior temporal *branch* of middle cerebral artery.

posterior tibial a. [TA], a. tibial posterior; o maior e a continuação mais direta dos dois ramos terminais da poplítea; *ramos*, fibular, nutrícia da fíbula, maleolares posteriores lateral e medial, a. nutrícia da tíbia, plantares medial e lateral. SIN arteria tibialis posterior [TA].

posterior tibial recurrent a. [TA], a. recorrente tibial posterior; um ramo inconstante da a. tibial posterior (ou, ocasionalmente, da a. tibial anterior), que ascende anteriormente ao músculo poplíteo, faz anastomose com os ramos da a. poplítea e envia um ramo para a articulação tibiofibular. SIN arteria recurrens tibialis posterior [TA].

posterior tympanic a. [TA], a. timpânica posterior; *origem*, estilomastóidea; *distribuição*, ouvido médio; *anastomoses*, outras artérias timpânicas. SIN arteria tympanica posterior [TA].

posterolateral central a.'s [TA], artérias centrais póstero-laterais; os ramos mesencefálicos circunflexos, vários pequenos ramos da parte pós-comunicante (segmento P2) da a. cerebral posterior que se distribuem para a parte posterior lateral do mesencéfalo. SIN arteriae centrales posterolaterales [TA].

posteromedial central a.'s [TA], artérias centrais póstero-mediais; os ramos perfurantes interpedunculares, vários pequenos ramos da parte pré-comunicante (segmento P1) da a. cerebral posterior e da a. comunicante posterior que suprem a parte medial posterior do mesencéfalo. SIN arteriae centrales posteromediales [TA], paramedian a.'s.

precentral a., a. do sulco pré-central. SIN a. of precentral sulcus.

precentral sulcal a., a. do sulco pré-central. SIN a. of precentral sulcus.

a. of precentral sulcus [TA], a. do sulco pré-central; um ramo da parte terminal da a. cerebral média que se distribui para o córtex dos dois lados do sulco pré-central. SIN arteria sulci precentralis [TA], pre-Rolandic a., precentral a., precentral sulcal a.

precuneal a., ramos precuneais da a. cerebral anterior. SIN precuneal *branches (of anterior cerebral artery),* em *branch.*

prepancreatic a. [TA], a. pré-pancreática; *origem*, origina-se da a. pancreática dorsal como seu ramo terminal esquerdo; *distribuição*, freqüentemente dupla, ela corre entre o colo e o processo uncinado do pâncreas para formar um arco (arcada) arterial com a a. pancreaticoduodenal superior anterior. SIN arteria prepancreatica [TA].

pre-Rolandic a., a. do sulco pré-central. SIN a. of precentral sulcus.

princeps cervicis a., ramo descendente da a. occipital. SIN descending *branch of occipital artery.*

princeps pol'licis a. [TA], a. principal do polegar; *origem*, radial (arco palmar (arterial) profundo); *distribuição*, superfície palmar e lados do polegar; *anastomoses*, artérias no dorso do polegar. SIN arteria princeps pollicis [TA], chief a. of thumb, princeps pollicis, principal a. of thumb.

principal a. of thumb, a. principal do polegar. SIN princeps pollicis a.

profunda brachii a. [TA], a. braquial profunda; *origem*, braquial; *distribuição*, úmero e músculos e tegumento do braço; *anastomoses*, a. circunflexa posterior do úmero, a. recorrente radial, a. interóssea recorrente, a. ulnar colateral, isto é, a rede vascular articular do cotovelo (articular vascular *network* of elbow). SIN arteria profunda brachii [TA], ramus deltoideus arteriae profundae brachii [TA], deep a. of arm*, deep brachial a.

profunda fem'oris a., a. femoral profunda. SIN deep a. of thigh.

proper cochlear a. [TA], a. coclear própria; *origem*, a. coclear comum no modíolo; *distribuição*, para o canal coclear. SIN arteria cochlearis propria [TA].

proper palmar digital a.'s [TA], a. digital palmar própria; ramos terminais da a. digital palmar comum que passam para o lado de cada dedo. SIN arteriae digitales palmares propriae [TA], arteria digitalis palmaris propria, collateral digital a., digital collateral a.

proper plantar digital a. [TA], a. digital plantar própria; um dos ramos digitais das artérias metatarsais plantares. SIN arteria digitalis plantaris propria [TA], arteriae digitales plantares propriae.

proximal medial striate a.'s [TA], artérias estriadas mediais proximais; *origem*, parte pré-comunicante (segmento A1) da a. cerebral anterior; *distribuição*, superfície inferior do lobo frontal do cérebro, estendendo-se para o tálamo e o corpo estriado. SIN arteria centralis brevis, short central a.

a. of pterygoid canal [TA], a. do canal pterigóide; *origem*, geralmente origina-se da terceira parte da a. maxilar, mas, com freqüência, surge da a. palatina maior na fossa pterigopalatina. Dirige-se posteriormente para fazer trajeto, através do canal pterigóide, com o nervo correspondente, irrigando o conteúdo e a parede do canal, a mucosa da porção superior da faringe, o canal auditivo e a cavidade timpânica. SIN arteria canalis pterygoidei [TA], vidian a.

pterygomeningeal a. [TA], a. pterigomeníngea; *origem*, a. maxilar ou meníngea média; *distribuição*, atravessa o forame oval para penetrar na cavidade craniana, onde nutre o gânglio trigêmeo, a dura-máter e o osso do assoalho da fossa craniana média; entretanto, sua principal distribuição é extracraniana para os músculos pterigóide e tensor do tímpano, osso esfenóide e nervos mandibulares e seu gânglio ótico. SIN arteria pterygomeningealis [TA], accessory meningeal a., accessory meningeal branch, ramus meningeus accessorius.

pubic a.'s, ramos púbicos. VER pubic *branch* of inferior epigastric artery, pubic *branch* of obturator artery.

pulmonary a., a. pulmonar. SIN pulmonary *trunk*; VER TAMBÉM right pulmonary a., left pulmonary a.

a. of pulp, a. da polpa; a primeira parte de um penicilo do baço.

pyloric a., a. gástrica direita. SIN right gastric a.
quadrigeminal a., a. colicular; *termo oficial alternativo para collicular a.
radial a. [TA], a. radial; *origem*, braquial; *ramos*, recorrente radial, carpais e metacarpais dorsais e palmares, digital dorsal, principal do polegar, radial do indicador, palmar e muscular, e perfurante; geralmente termina como o arco palmar profundo. SIN arteria radialis [TA].

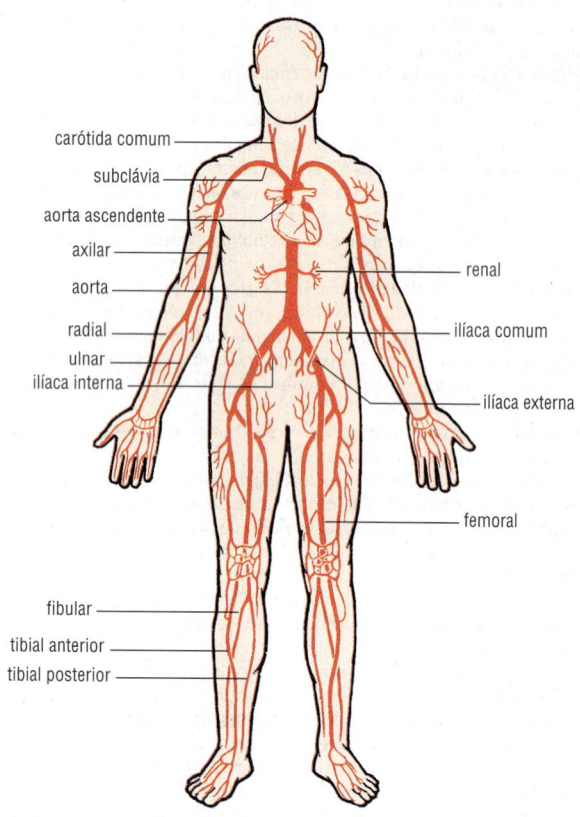

principais artérias do corpo

radial collateral a. [TA], a. colateral radial; um ramo terminal anterior da a. braquial profunda, que se anastomosa com a a. recorrente radial, formando parte do plexo vascular articular do cotovelo. SIN arteria collateralis radialis [TA].
radial index a., a. radial do indicador. SIN radialis indicis a.
radialis indicis a. [TA], a. radial do indicador; *origem*, radial; *distribuição*, lado radial do dedo indicador. SIN arteria radialis indicis [TA], arteria volaris indicis radialis, radial index a.
radial recurrent a. [TA], a. recorrente radial; *origem*, radial; *distribuição*, ascende ao redor da face lateral da articulação do cotovelo; *anastomoses*, a. colateral radial, a. interóssea recorrente. SIN arteria recurrens radialis [TA], recurrent radial a.
ranine a., a. profunda da língua. SIN deep lingual a.
recurrent a., a. recorrente; **(1)** uma a. que, no seu local de origem, ou logo depois, reflete-se ou vira agudamente e segue um trajeto oposto ao de sua a.-mãe; **(2)** a. estriada medial. SIN medial striate a.
recurrent a. of Heubner, a. recorrente de Heubner. SIN medial striate a.
recurrent interosseous a. [TA], a. interóssea recorrente; *origem*, a. interóssea posterior; *distribuição*, articulação do cotovelo; *anastomoses*, ramos da a. braquial profunda e da a. colateral ulnar inferior, isto é, a rede vascular articular do cotovelo; articular vascular *network* of elbow. SIN arteria interossea recurrens [TA].
recurrent radial a., a. recorrente radial. SIN radial recurrent a.
recurrent ulnar a., a. recorrente ulnar. SIN ulnar recurrent a.
renal a. [TA], a. renal; *origem*, aorta; *ramos*, segmentar, ureteral e supra-renal inferior; *distribuição*, rim. SIN arteria renalis [TA].
retroduodenal a. [TA], a. pancreaticoduodenal posterior; *origem*, um dos vários pequenos ramos da a. gastroduodenal posterior para o duodeno; *distribuição*, primeira parte do duodeno. SIN arteria retroduodenalis [TA], posterior pancreaticoduodenal a.
right colic a. [TA], a. cólica direita; *origem*, mesentérica superior, por vezes por um tronco comum com a. ileocólica; *distribuição*, colo ascendente; *anastomoses*, a. cólica média, a. ileocólica. SIN arteria colica dextra [TA].

right coronary a. [TA], a. coronária direita; *origem*, seio aórtico direito; *distribuição*, passa ao redor do lado direito do coração no sulco coronário, fornecendo ramos para o átrio e ventrículo direitos, inclusive os ramos atrioventriculares e o ramo interventricular posterior. SIN arteria coronaria dextra [TA].
right descending pulmonary a. (RDPA), a. pulmonar descendente direita; a. que irriga os lobos médio e inferior direito e que compõe a maior parte do hilo direito na radiografia frontal do tórax.
right flexural a. [TA], a. da flexura direita; *origem*, a. mesentérica superior; ramo variante que se origina entre as artérias cólicas direita e média ou no lugar de uma delas, passando diretamente para a flexura cólica direita. SIN arteria flexurae dextrae [TA].
right gastric a. [TA], a. gástrica direita; *origem*, hepática; *distribuição*, porção pilórica na curvatura menor do estômago; *anastomoses*, a. gástrica esquerda. SIN arteria gastrica dextra [TA], pyloric a.
right gastroepiploic a., a. gastromental direita; *termo oficial alternativo para right gastroomental a.
right gastroomental a. [TA], a. gastromental direita; *origem*, gastroduodenal; *distribuição*, curvatura maior e paredes do estômago e omento maior; *anastomoses*, freqüentemente une-se com a gastromental esquerda, e ramos, a partir desse arco, anastomosam-se com os ramos das artérias gástricas direita e esquerda. SIN arteria gastroomentalis dextra [TA], right gastroepiploic a.*, arteria gastroepiploica dextra.
right hepatic a., ramo direito da a. hepática própria. SIN right branch of hepatic artery proper.
right pulmonary a. [TA], a. pulmonar direita; o mais longo dos dois ramos terminais do tronco (artéria) pulmonar, atravessa transversalmente a linha média no mediastino superior, passando inferiormente ao arco aórtico até penetrar no hilo do pulmão direito como parte de sua raiz. Os ramos dividem-se e são distribuídos com os brônquios segmentares e subsegmentares; ocorrem variações freqüentes. *Ramos típicos*: das artérias lobares superiores [TA], (arteriae lobares superiores [TA]) são a a. segmentar apical [TA] (arteria segmentalis apicalis [TA]), a. segmentar anterior (arteria segmentalis anterior [TA]) e a. segmentar posterior [TA] (arteria segmentalis posterior [TA]), com as duas últimas apresentando ramos ascendente e descendente [TA] (rami ascendens et descendens [TA]); da a. lobar média [TA] (arteria lobaris media [TA]) são a a. segmentar medial [TA] (arteria lobaris media [TA]) e a a. segmentar lateral [TA] (arteria segmentalis laterales [TA]); e das artérias lobares inferiores [TA] (arteriae lobares inferiores [TA]) são a a. segmentar superior [TA] (arteria segmentalis superior [TA]) e uma parte basilar [TA] (pars basalis [TA]) que origina as artérias segmentares basilares anterior, posterior, lateral e medial [TA] (arteriae segmentales basales anterior, posterior, lateralis et medialis [TA]). SIN arteria pulmonalis dextra [TA].
Rolandic sulcal a., a. do sulco central. SIN a. of central sulcus.
a. of round ligament of uterus, a. do ligamento redondo do útero; *origem*, a. epigástrica inferior; *distribuição*, ligamento redondo do útero. SIN arteria ligamenti teretis uteri.
a. to sciatic nerve [TA], a. acompanhante do nervo isquiático; *origem*, a. glútea inferior; *distribuição*, nervo isquiático; *anastomoses*, ramos da. femoral profunda. SIN arteria comitans nervi ischiadici [TA], companion a. to sciatic nerve.
screw a.'s, artérias espiraladas na mucosa uterina ou na região macular da retina.
scrotal a.'s, ramo escrotal anterior da a. pudenda externa profunda. VER anterior scrotal *branch* of deep external pudendal artery, posterior scrotal *branch* of internal pudendal artery, em *branch*.
segmental a.'s of kidney [TA], artérias dos segmentos renais; os ramos da. renal que irrigam os segmentos anatômicos do rim. Geralmente em número de cinco, elas constituem artérias terminais e emitem as artérias interlobares, arqueadas e interlobulares em seqüência. Estas últimas emitem as arteríolas aferentes para os glomérulos, bem como ramos para a cápsula renal. As artérias dos segmentos renais são identificadas como: (1) a. do segmento anterior inferior (arteriae segmenti anterioris inferioris renis [NA]); (2) a. do segmento anterior superior (arteriae segmenti anterioris superioris renis [NA]); (3) a. do segmento inferior (arteriae segmenti inferioris renis [NA]); (4) a. do segmento posterior (arteriae segmenti posterioris renis [NA]); e (5) a. do segmento superior (arteriae segmenti superioris renis [NA]). SIN arteriae renis [TA], a.'s of kidney.
segmental a.'s of liver [TA], artérias dos segmentos hepáticos; as artérias dos segmentos anterior e posterior que se originam do ramo direito da a. hepática, e as artérias dos segmentos medial e lateral, que se originam do ramo esquerdo da a. hepática; as artérias dos segmentos irrigam quatro das cinco principais divisões do fígado e, em seguida, ramificam-se, de modo que cada segmento hepático receba um aporte sanguíneo independente. SIN arteriae segmenti hepaticae.
segmental medullary a.'s [TA], artérias medulares segmentares; uma a. espinal ou radicular calibrosa cujo trajeto é central ao longo de uma raiz dorsal ou ventral, talvez nutrindo-a e às meninges circunvizinhas, da mesma forma que qualquer a. espinal/radicular, mas que prossegue até alcançar a a. espinal anterior ou posterior (longitudinal), anastomosando-se com ela. Apenas 4–9 das

artery (a)

artérias espinais são artérias espinais medulares; encontradas principalmente nos níveis cervical inferior, torácico inferior e lombar superior, das quais a maior é a a. medular segmentar. VER TAMBÉM great segmental medullary a., spinal a.'s (anterior and posterior), radicular a.'s. SIN arteriae medullares segmentales [TA], medullary spinal a.'s

septal a., a. septal; um ramo da a. labial superior que nutre a parte inferior do septo nasal.

sheated a., a. embainhada; uma subdivisão do penicilo do baço circundada por macrófagos e por um estroma reticular.

short central a., a. estriada proximal medial. SIN proximal medial striate a.'s.

short circumferential a.'s [TA], artérias circunferenciais curtas; ramos curtos da parte pré-comunicante (segmento P1) da a. cerebral posterior. SIN arteriae circumferentiales brevis [TA].

short gastric a.'s [TA], artérias gástricas curtas; quatro ou cinco pequenas artérias originadas da a. esplênica, que avançam através do ligamento gastro-esplênico até o fundo do estômago, ao longo da curvatura maior, anastomosando-se com as outras artérias nessa região. SIN arteriae gastricae breves [TA], vasa brevia.

short posterior ciliary a. [TA], a. ciliar posterior curta; um de aproximadamente sete ramos da a. oftálmica que contornam o nervo óptico para irrigar o globo ocular. Dividindo-se em cerca de 15–20 ramos, penetram na esclerótica, adjacentes ao nervo óptico, nutrindo a coróide e os processos ciliares. *Anastomoses:* com a a. central da retina e com as artérias ciliares longa e anterior (na ora serrata). SIN arteria ciliaris posterior brevis [TA].

sigmoid a.'s [TA], artérias sigmóideas; *origem,* a. mesentérica inferior; *distribuição,* cólon descendente e flexura sigmóide; *anastomoses,* a. cólica esquerda, a. retal superior. SIN arteriae sigmoideae [TA].

sinuatrial nodal a., ramo do nó sinoatrial da a. coronária direita. SIN sinuatrial (S-A) nodal *branch* of right coronary artery.

a. to the sinoatrial (S-A) node, ramo do nó sinoatrial (S-A) da a. coronária direita. SIN sinuatrial (S-A) nodal *branch* of right coronary artery.

sinuatrial node a., ramo do nó sinoatrial da a. coronária direita. SIN sinuatrial (S-A) nodal *branch* of right coronary artery.

sinus node a., ramo do nó sinoatrial da a. coronária direita. SIN sinuatrial (S-A) nodal *branch* of right coronary artery.

small a.'s, artérias pequenas; artérias musculares sem nome, usualmente com menos de seis ou sete camadas de músculo.

somatic a.'s, artérias somáticas; artérias que se originam no embrião a partir da aorta dorsal e que nutrem a parede corporal; elas persistem quase inalteradas como as artérias intercostal posterior, subcostal e lombar.

sphenopalatine a. [TA], a. esfenopalatina; *origem,* terceira parte da a. maxilar; *distribuição,* porção posterior do septo e da parede lateral do nariz; *anastomoses,* ramos das artérias palatina descendente, labial superior e infra-orbital. SIN arteria sphenopalatina [TA].

spinal a.'s, ramos espinais. SIN rami radiculares. SIN spinal *branches,* em *branch.*

spiral a., a. espiralada do útero; uma das artérias semelhantes a saca-rolhas no endométrio pré-menstrual ou progestacional. SIN coiled a. of uterus.

spiral modiolar a. [TA], a. espiral do modíolo; é paralela ao gânglio espiral da cóclea na raiz da lâmina espiral do modíolo, que nutre o gânglio e os canais cocleares e seu conteúdo; é formada por contribuições da a. coclear comum (que nutre as duas voltas apicais da cóclea) e do ramo coclear da a. vestibulococlear (que nutre a volta basilar).

splenic a. [TA], a. esplênica; *origem,* tronco celíaco; *ramos,* pancreático, gastromental esquerdo, gástrico curto e esplênico (próprio). VER great segmental medullary a. SIN arteria splenica [TA], arteria lienalis*, lienal a.

stapedial a., a. estapédica; uma pequena a. no embrião que atravessa o anel do estribo e que, mais adiante, é obliterada; na maioria das pessoas, é uma derivação do segundo arco aórtico.

sternal a.'s, ramos esternais da a. torácica interna. SIN sternal *branches* of internal thoracic artery, em *branch.*

sternomastoid a., ramo esternocleidomastóideo. VER sternoclidomastoid *branch* of superior thyroid artery, sternoclidomastoid *branches* of occipital artery, em *branch.*

straight a.'s, artérias retas; *termo oficial alternativo para vasa recta renis, em vas.

stylomastoid a. [TA], a. estilomastóidea; *origem,* auricular posterior; *distribuição,* meato acústico externo, células da mastóide, canais semicirculares, músculo estapédio e vestíbulo; *anastomoses,* ramos timpânicos das artérias carótida interna e faríngea ascendente e a. do labirinto. SIN arteria stylomastoidea [TA].

subclavian a. [TA], a. subclávia; *origem,* à direita da a. braquiocefálica, à esquerda do arco da aorta; *ramos,* vertebral, tronco tireocervical, torácico interno; tronco costocervical, descendente da escápula; continua como a. axilar depois de cruzar a primeira costela. SIN arteria subclavia [TA].

subcostal a. [TA], a. subcostal; *origem,* aorta torácica; *distribuição,* inferior até a décima segunda costela, de forma semelhante às artérias intercostais posteriores. SIN arteria subcostalis [TA].

sublingual a. [TA], a. sublingual; *origem,* a. lingual; *distribuição,* músculos extrínsecos da língua, glândula sublingual, mucosa da região; *anastomoses,* a. artéria do lado oposto e submental. SIN arteria sublingualis [TA].

submental a. [TA], a. submentual; *origem,* a. facial; *distribuição,* músculo milo-hióide, glândulas submandibulares e sublinguais e estruturas do lábio inferior; *anastomoses,* a. labial inferior, ramo mentual das artérias alveolar inferior e sublingual. SIN arteria submentalis [TA].

subscapular a. [TA], a. subescapular; *origem,* a. axilar; *ramos,* circunflexo da escápula, toracodorsal; *distribuição,* músculos do ombro e região escapular; *anastomoses,* ramos das artérias cervical transversa, supra-escapular, torácica lateral e intercostais. SIN arteria subscapularis [TA].

sulcal a., a. do sulco; um pequeno ramo da a. espinal anterior que avança na fissura mediana anterior da medula espinal.

superficial brachial a. [TA], a. braquial superficial; uma variação ocasional em que a a. braquial é superficial ao nervo mediano no braço. SIN arteria brachialis superficialis [TA].

superficial cervical a. [TA], a. cervical superficial; *origem,* ramo do tronco tireocervical que avança junto com o nervo espinal acessório, profundamente ao músculo trapézio. VER TAMBÉM superficial *branch* of the transverse cervical artery. SIN ramus superficialis arteriae transversae cervicis [TA], arteria cervicalis superficialis.

superficial circumflex iliac a., a. circunflexa superficial; *origem,* a. femoral; *distribuição,* linfonodos inguinais e tegumento daquela região; músculos sartório e tensor da fáscia lata; *anastomoses,* a. ilíaca circunflexa profunda. SIN arteria circumflexa iliaca superficialis [TA].

(superficial and deep) external pudendal a.'s [TA], artérias pudendas externas (superficial e profunda); *origem,* na a. femoral como duas artérias que passam superficial e profundamente à veia femoral; *distribuição,* pele sobre o púbis, pele sobre o pênis e pele da bolsa escrotal ou lábios maiores do pudendo, através dos ramos escrotais (labiais) anteriores; *anastomoses,* a. dorsal do pênis ou do clitóris, ramos escrotais ou labiais posteriores. SIN arteriae pudendae externae [TA].

superficial epigastric a. [TA], a. epigástrica superficial; *origem,* femoral; *distribuição,* linfonodos inguinais e tegumento do abdome inferior; *anastomoses,* artérias epigástrica inferior, ilíaca circunflexa superficial e pudenda externa. SIN arteria epigastrica superficialis [TA].

superficial palmar a., ramo palmar superficial da a. radial. SIN superficial palmar *branch* of radial artery.

superficial temporal a. [TA], a. temporal superficial; *origem,* um ramo terminal da a. carótida externa (com a a. maxilar); *ramos,* facial transverso, temporal médio, orbitário, parotídeo, auricular anterior, frontal e parietal. SIN arteria temporalis superficialis [TA].

superficial volar a., ramo palmar superficial da a. radial. SIN superficial palmar *branch* of radial artery.

superior cerebellar a. [TA], a. cerebelar superior; *origem,* a. basilar; *distribuição,* superfície superior do cerebelo, colículos e maioria dos núcleos cerebelares; *anastomoses,* a. cerebelar inferior posterior; origina os ramos mediais [TA] e os ramos laterais [TA]. SIN arteria superior cerebelli [TA].

superior epigastric a. [TA], a. epigástrica superior; *origem,* o ramo terminal medial da a. torácica interna; *distribuição,* músculos e tegumento abdominais; ligamento falciforme; *anastomoses,* a. epigástrica inferior. SIN arteria epigastrica superior [TA].

superior gluteal a. [TA], a. glútea superior; *origem,* a. ilíaca interna; *distribuição,* região glútea; *anastomoses,* a. sacral lateral, a. glútea inferior, a. pudenda interna, a. ilíaca circunflexa profunda a. circunflexa femoral lateral. SIN arteria glutea superior [TA].

superior hemorrhoidal a., a. retal superior. SIN superior rectal a.

superior hypophysial a. [TA], a. hipofisária superior; um pequeno ramo da parte cerebral da a. carótida interna que nutre a hipófise. SIN arteria hypophysalis superior [TA].

superior intercostal a., a. intercostal suprema. SIN supreme intercostal a.

superior internal parietal a., ramos parieto-occipitais da a. cerebral anterior. SIN parieto-occipital *branches* (of anterior cerebral artery), em *branch.*

superior labial a., ramo labial superior da a. facial. SIN superior labial *branch* of facial artery.

superior laryngeal a. [TA], a. laríngea superior; *origem,* a. tireóidea superior; *distribuição,* músculos e mucosa da laringe; *anastomoses,* ramo cricotireóideo da a. tireóidea superior e ramos terminais da a. laríngea inferior. SIN arteria laryngea superior [TA].

superior lateral genicular a. [TA], a. superior lateral do joelho; *origem,* poplítea; *distribuição,* articulação do joelho; *anastomoses,* a. circunflexa femoral lateral, terceiro ramo perfurante, recorrente anterior da tíbia, lateral inferior do joelho, isto é, a rede vascular articular do joelho. SIN arteria superior lateralis genus [TA], lateral superior genicular a.

superior lingual a. [TA], a. lingual superior; ramificação (do ramo lingular) da a. pulmonar esquerda que irriga o segmento lingular superior do lobo superior do pulmão esquerdo. VER left pulmonary a. SIN arteria lingularis superior [TA], ramus lingularis superior, superior lingular *branch* of lingular *branch* of superior lobar left pulmonary artery.

superior lobar a.'s [TA], artérias lobares superiores. VER left pulmonary a., right pulmonary a.

superior medial genicular a. [TA], a. superior medial do joelho; *origem*, a. poplítea; *distribuição*, articulação do joelho; *anastomoses*, a. descendente do joelho, a. lateral superior do joelho, isto é, a rede vascular articular do joelho. SIN arteria superior medialis genus [TA], medial superior genicular a.

superior mesenteric a. [TA], a. mesentérica superior; *origem*, aorta abdominal; *ramos*, artérias pancreaticoduodenal inferior, jejunal, ileal, ileocólica, apendicular, cólica direita, cólica média; *anastomoses*, a. pancreaticoduodenal superior e a. cólica esquerda. SIN arteria mesenterica superior [TA].

superior phrenic a. [TA], a. frênica superior; uma de um par de pequenas artérias emitidas da aorta torácica exatamente acima do diafragma; *distribuição*, diafragma; *anastomoses*, a. musculofrênica, a. pericardicofrênica e a. frênica inferior. SIN arteria phrenica superior [TA].

superior rectal a. [TA], a. retal superior; *origem*, a. mesentérica inferior; *distribuição*, parte superior do reto; *anastomoses*, a. retais média e inferior. Como uma tributária da veia porta, sua anastomose com essas artérias forma uma anastomose portossistêmica ou portocava. SIN arteria rectalis superior [TA], superior hemorrhoidal a.

superior segmental a. [TA], a. segmentar superior ou a. do segmento superior. VER left pulmonary a., right pulmonary a., segmental a.'s of kidney.

superior segmental a. of kidney [TA], a. do segmento superior do rim; *origem*, ramo anterior da a. renal. VER segmental a.'s of kidney. SIN a. of superior segment of kidney.

a. of superior segment of kidney, a. do segmento superior do rim. SIN superior segmental a. of kidney.

superior suprarenal a.'s [TA], artérias supra-renais superiores; *origem*, a. frênica inferior; *distribuição*, glândula supra-renal. SIN arteriae suprarenales superiores [TA].

superior thoracic a. [TA], a. torácica superior; *origem*, axilar; *distribuição*, músculos da parte superior do tórax; *anastomoses*, ramos da a. supra-escapular, a. torácica interna e a. tóraco-acromial. SIN arteria thoracica superior [TA], highest thoracic a.

superior thyroid a. [TA], a. tireóidea superior; *origem*, a. carótida externa; *ramos*, infra-hióideo, laríngeo superior, esternocleidomastóideo, cricotireóideo e dois ramos terminais. SIN arteria thyroidea superior [TA].

superior tympanic a. [TA], a. timpânica superior; *origem*, a. meníngea média; *distribuição*, ouvido médio; *anastomoses*, outras artérias timpânicas. SIN arteria tympanica superior [TA].

superior ulnar collateral a. [TA], a. colateral ulnar superior; *origem*, a. braquial; *distribuição*, articulação do cotovelo; *anastomoses*, a. recorrente ulnar posterior e a. colateral ulnar inferior, como parte da rede vascular articular do cotovelo. SIN arteria collateralis ulnaris superior [TA].

superior vesical a. [TA], a. vesical superior; *origem*, a. umbilical; *distribuição*, bexiga, úraco, ureter; *anastomoses*, outros ramos vesicais. SIN arteria vesicalis superior [TA].

suprachiasmatic a. [TA], a. supraquiasmática; *origem*, a. comunicante anterior; passa acima do quiasma óptico para nutrir a região do recesso óptico, área hipotalâmica. SIN arteria suprachiasmatica [TA].

supraduodenal a. [TA], a. supraduodenal; *origem*, gastroduodenal; *distribuição*, primeira parte do duodeno. SIN arteria supraduodenalis [TA].

supraoptic a. [TA], a. supra-óptica; *origem*, parte pré-comunicante (segmento A1) da a. cerebral anterior; *distribuição*, passa superiormente ao nervo óptico para a superfície orbital do lobo frontal do cérebro. SIN arteria supraoptica [TA].

supraorbital a. [TA], a. supra-orbital; *origem*, a. oftálmica; *distribuição*, músculo frontal e couro cabeludo; *anastomoses*, ramos das artérias temporal superficial e supratroclear. SIN arteria supraorbitalis [TA].

suprascapular a. [TA], a. supra-escapular; *origem*, tronco tireocervical; *distribuição*, clavícula, escápula, músculos do ombro e articulação do ombro; *anastomoses*, a. cervical transversa, a. circunflexa da escápula. SIN arteria suprascapularis [TA], transverse scapular a.

supratrochlear a. [TA], a. supratroclear; *origem*, a. oftálmica; *distribuição*, porção anterior do couro cabeludo; *anastomoses*, ramos da a. supra-orbital. SIN arteria supratrochlearis [TA], arteria frontalis, frontal a.

supreme intercostal a. [TA], a. intercostal suprema; *origem*, tronco costocervical; *distribuição*, estruturas do primeiro e do segundo espaços intercostais através de seus ramos terminais, primeira e segunda artérias intercostais posteriores; *anastomoses*, ramos intercostais anteriores da a. torácica interna. SIN arteria intercostalis suprema [TA], highest intercostal a., superior intercostal a.

sural a.'s [TA], artérias surais; uma das quatro ou cinco artérias que se originam (por vezes por um tronco comum) da a. poplítea; *distribuição*, músculos e tegumento da panturrilha; *anastomoses*, a. tibial posterior, artérias inferiores medial e lateral do joelho. SIN arteriae surales [TA], a. of calf.

a. to tail of pancreas [TA], a. da cauda do pâncreas; *origem*, a. esplênica próximo à a. gastromental esquerda; *distribuição*, a cauda do pâncreas; *anastomoses*, com outras artérias pancreáticas. SIN arteria caudae pancreatis [TA], caudal pancreatic a.

terminal a., a. terminal. SIN end a.

testicular a. [TA], a. testicular; *origem*, aorta; *ramos*, ureteral, cremastérico, epididimário; *distribuição*, testículo e partes designadas pelos nomes dos ramos; *anastomoses*, ramos das artérias renal, epigástrica inferior e do canal deferente. SIN arteria testicularis [TA], arteria spermatica interna, internal spermatic a.

thoracoacromial a. [TA], a. tóraco-acromial; *origem*, axilar; *distribuição*, músculos e pele do ombro e parte superior do tórax; *anastomoses*, ramos das artérias torácica superior, torácica interna, torácica lateral, circunflexas posterior e anterior do úmero e supra-escapular. SIN arteria thoracoacromialis [TA], ramus deltoideus arteriae thoracoacromialis [TA], acromiothoracic a., thoracic aixs (1), thoracoacromial trunk.

thoracodorsal a. [TA], a. toracodorsal; *origem*, a. subescapular; *distribuição*, músculos da parte superior das costas; *anastomoses*, ramos da a. torácica lateral. SIN arteria thoracodorsalis [TA], dorsal thoracic a.

thyroid ima a. [TA], a. tireóidea ima; *origem*, arco da aorta ou a. braquiocefálica; *distribuição*, glândula tireóide. SIN arteria thyroidea ima [TA], lowest thyroid a., Neubauer a.

tibial nutrient a. [TA], a. nutrícia da tíbia; a. derivada da parte superior da a. tibial posterior; penetra através do forame nutrício na superfície posterior da tíbia. SIN arteria nutricia tibiae [TA], arteria nutriens tibiae*, arteria nutriens tibialis, nutrient a. of the tibia.

transverse cervical a. [TA], a. cervical transversa; *origem*, tronco tireocervical; *ramos*, superficial (cervical superficial) e profundo (descendente da escápula). SIN arteria transversa colli [TA], arteria transversa cervicis*, transverse a. of neck.

transverse facial a. [TA], a. facial transversa; *origem*, a. temporal superficial; *distribuição*, glândula parótida, canal parotídeo, músculo masseter e pele suprajacente; *anastomoses*, ramos infra-orbital e bucal da a. maxilar e ramos bucal e massetérico da a. facial. SIN arteria transversa faciei [TA].

transverse a. of neck, a. cervical transversa. SIN transverse cervical a.

transverse pancreatic a., a. pancreática inferior. SIN inferior pancreatic a.

transverse scapular a., a. supra-escapular. SIN suprascapular a.

a. of tuber cinereum [TA], a. do túber cinéreo; pequena a. originada da a. comunicante posterior, que dá origem aos ramos lateral e medial que irrigam o túber cinéreo. SIN arteria tuberis cinerei [TA].

ulnar a. [TA], a. ulnar; *origem*, a. braquial; *ramos*, a. recorrente ulnar, a. interóssea comum, ramos carpais dorsal e palmar, ramo palmar profundo e arco palmar superficial, com seus ramos digitais. SIN arteria ulnaris [TA].

ulnar recurrent a. [TA], a. recorrente ulnar; *origem*, a. ulnar; *distribuição*, dois ramos, anterior e posterior, que passam medialmente por diante e por trás da articulação do cotovelo; *anastomoses*, artérias colaterais ulnares superior e inferior, isto é, com o plexo vascular articular do cotovelo. SIN arteria recurrens ulnaris [TA], recurrent ulnar a.

umbilical a. [TA], a. umbilical; antes do nascimento, essa a. é uma continuação da a. ilíaca interna; depois do nascimento, é obliterada entre a bexiga e o umbigo, formando o ligamento umbilical medial, com a porção restante, entre a a. ilíaca interna e a bexiga, sendo reduzida em tamanho e originando as artérias vesicais superiores. SIN arteria umbilicalis [TA].

uncal a. [TA], a. do unco; *origem*, parte cerebral da a. carótida interna ou, ocasionalmente, a partir da parte esfenoidal (segmento M1) da a. cerebral média; *distribuição*, para o unco. SIN arteria uncalis [TA].

a.'s of upper limb [TA], artérias do membro superior; artérias que suprem o membro superior; todas são derivadas da a. axilar. SIN arteriae membri superioris [TA].

urethral a. [TA], a. uretral; *origem*, a. perineal; *distribuição*, uretra membranosa. SIN arteria urethralis [TA].

uterine a. [TA], a. uterina; *origem*, a. ilíaca interna; *distribuição*, útero, parte superior da vagina, ligamento redondo e parte medial da tuba uterina; *anastomoses*, a. ovárica, a. vaginal, a. epigástrica inferior. Supre a circulação materna para a placenta durante a gestação. SIN arteria uterina [TA].

vaginal a. [TA], a. vaginal; *origem*, a. ilíaca interna; *distribuição*, vagina, base da bexiga, reto; *anastomoses*, a. uterina, a. pudenda interna. SIN arteria vaginalis [TA].

a. to vas deferens, a. do ducto deferente; *termo oficial alternativo para a. to ductus deferens.

venous a., tronco pulmonar. SIN pulmonary *trunk*.

ventral splanchnic a.'s, artérias esplâncnicas ventrais; artérias que se originam no embrião a partir da aorta dorsal e são distribuídas para o tubo digestivo.

ventricular a.'s, artérias ventriculares; ramos das artérias coronárias direita e esquerda distribuídos para o músculo dos ventrículos. SIN arteriae ventriculares [TA].

vertebral a. [TA], a. vertebral; o primeiro ramo da a. subclávia; para fins descritivos, dividida em quatro partes: 1) pré-vertebral, a porção anterior à sua penetração no forame do processo transverso da sexta vértebra cervical; 2) cervical, a porção nos forames transversos das seis primeiras vértebras cervicais; 3) suboccipital, a porção que corre ao longo do arco posterior do atlas, e 4) intracraniana, a porção dentro da cavidade craniana até sua união com a artéria contralateral para formar a artéria basilar. SIN arteria vertebralis [TA].

vestibulocochlear a. [TA], a. vestibulococlear; *origem*, a. vestibular anterior; *ramos*, sacular, coclear e vestibular posterior. SIN arteria vestibulocochlearis [TA].
vidian a., a. do canal pterigóide. SIN a. of pterygoid canal.
vitelline a., a. vitelina; uma a. que conduz o sangue até o saco vitelino a partir do embrião. SIN arteria vitellina.
volar interosseous a., a. interóssea anterior. SIN anterior interosseous a.
Zinn a., a de Zinn, a. central da retina. SIN central retinal a.
zygomatico-orbital a. [TA], a. zigomático-orbital; *origem*, a. temporal superior, por vezes a. temporal média; *distribuição*, músculo orbicular do olho e porções da órbita; *anastomoses*, ramos lacrimal e palpebral da a. oftálmica. SIN arteria zygomatico-orbitalis [TA].

♻ **arthr-.** VER arthro-.
ar·thral (ar′thrăl). Articular. SIN articular.
ar·thral·gia (ar-thral′jē-ă). Artralgia; dor em uma articulação, especialmente aquela que não tem caráter inflamatório. SIN arthrodynia. [G. *arthron*, articulação, + *algos*, dor]
intermittent a., a. intermitente, a. periódica. SIN periodic a.
periodic a. [MIM*112270], a. periódica; uma condição na qual há dor e tumefação; atribuída originalmente às articulações, mas hoje se sabe que envolve as diáfises dos ossos longos; ocorre a intervalos regulares; por vezes, há dor abdominal, púrpura ou edema associados. SIN intermittent a., periodic bone pain.
a. saturni′na, a. saturnina; dor intensa, principalmente na flexão das articulações dos membros inferiores, na intoxicação plúmbica (saturnismo).
ar·thral·gic (ar-thral′jik). Artrálgico; relativo a, ou afetado por, artralgia.
ar·threc·to·my (ar-threk′tō-mē). Artrectomia; excisão de uma articulação. [G. *arthron*, articulação, + *ektomē*, excisão]
ar·thres·the·sia (ar-thres-thē′ze-ă). Artrestesia. SIN articular *sensibility*. [G. *arthron*, articulação, + *aisthesis*, sensação]
ar·thrit·ic (ar-thrit′ik). Artrítico; relativo à artrite.
ar·thrit·i·des (ar-thrit′i-dēz). Artrítide; plural de artrite.
ar·thri·tis, pl. **ar·thrit·i·des** (ar-thrī′tis, ar-thrit′i-dēz). Artrite; inflamação de uma articulação ou um estado caracterizado por inflamação das articulações. SIN articular rheumatism. [G. de *arthron*, articulação, + *-itis*, inflamação]
acute rheumatic a., a. reumática aguda; a. decorrente da febre reumática.
chronic absorptive a., a. absortiva crônica, a. mutilante. SIN a. mutilans.
chylous a., a. quilosa; a. com elevado teor de linfa no líquido sinovial, geralmente decorrente de filaríase.
a. defor′mans, a. deformante, a. reumatóide. SIN rheumatoid a.
degenerative a., a. degenerativa, osteoartrite. SIN osteoarthritis.
enteropathic a., a. enteropática; uma forma de a. que, por vezes, assemelha-se à a. reumatóide e pode complicar a evolução da colite ulcerativa, doença de Crohn ou outra doença intestinal.
filarial a., a. por filárias; a. que ocorre na filaríase, provavelmente causada por extravasamento de linfa rica em lipídios (semelhante ao quilo) para o espaço articular.
gonococcal a., a. gonocócica; infecção do espaço articular em seres humanos causada por disseminação da *Neisseria gonorrhoeae;* caracteristicamente monoarticular, mas pode ser poliarticular. SIN gonorrheal arthritis.
gonorrheal arthritis, a. gonocócica. SIN gonococcal a.
gouty a., a. gotosa; inflamação das articulações na gota.
hemophilic a., a. hemofílica; doença articular resultante do sangramento hemofílico para dentro de uma articulação.
hypertrophic a., a. hipertrófica; variante da osteoartrite caracterizada por formação de osteófitos periarticulares aferentes.
Jaccoud a., a. de Jaccoud; uma forma rara de a. crônica, relatada como ocorrendo após crises de febre reumática aguda, caracterizada por uma forma incomum de erosão óssea das cabeças dos metacarpos e por desvio ulnar dos dedos das mãos; assemelha-se à a. reumatóide, porém com inflamação mais suave e ausência do fator reumatóide. SIN Jaccoud arthropathy.
juvenile a., juvenile rheumatoid a., a. juvenil, a. reumatóide juvenil (ARJ); a. crônica que começa na infância, com a maioria dos casos sendo pauciarticulares, isto é, afetando poucas articulações. Já foram identificados diversos padrões da doença: em um subgrupo, que afeta principalmente meninas, a irite é comum, assim como o achado de anticorpo antinuclear; outro subgrupo, que afeta principalmente os meninos, inclui, com freqüência, a. espinal, assemelhando-se à espondilite anquilosante; alguns casos são de a. reumatóide verdadeira, começando na infância e caracterizando-se por fator reumatóide e alterações articulares deformantes destrutivas, que freqüentemente sofrem remissão na puberdade. VER TAMBÉM Still *disease*. SIN juvenile chronic a.
juvenile chronic a., a. juvenil crônica. SIN juvenile a.
Lyme a., a. de Lyme; a manifestação artrítica da doença de Lyme.
a. mu′tilans, a. mutilante; uma forma de a. reumatóide crônica na qual ocorre osteólise com extensa destruição das cartilagens e superfícies ósseas com deformidades pronunciadas, principalmente das mãos e pés; alterações semelhantes ocorrem em alguns casos de a. psoriática. SIN chronic absorptive a.
neuropathic a., a. neuropática; a. associada a um distúrbio neurológico subjacente, p.ex., siringomielia, tabes dorsal, diabetes melito.
a. nodo′sa, a. nodosa; termo obsoleto para a a. reumatóide.
ochronotic a., a. ocronótica; osteoartrite que ocorre como complicação da ocronose.
proliferative a., a. proliferativa; termo para descrever a a. reumatóide baseado na característica proliferação da membrana sinovial percebida nas articulações afetadas pela doença.
psoriatic a., a. psoriática; a concorrência da psoríase e poliartrite, assemelhando-se à a. reumatóide, mas considerada uma entidade patológica específica, soronegativa para o fator reumatóide e envolvendo, com freqüência, os dedos. VER TAMBÉM a. mutilans. SIN arthropathia psoriatica.
pyogenic a., a. piogênica. SIN suppurative a.
reactive a., a. reativa; poliartropatia estéril, geralmente transitória, após várias doenças infecciosas.
rheumatoid a., a. reumatóide; uma doença generalizada, que ocorre com maior freqüência nas mulheres, afetando principalmente o tecido conjuntivo; a a. é a manifestação clínica dominante, envolvendo muitas articulações, principalmente as das mãos e pés, acompanhada por espessamento do tecido mole articular, com extensão do tecido sinovial sobre as cartilagens articulares, que sofrem erosão; a evolução é variável, mas, com freqüência, é crônica e progressiva, levando a deformidades e incapacidade. SIN a. deformans, nodose rheumatism (1).
septic a., a. séptica. SIN suppurative a.
suppurative a., a. supurativa; inflamação aguda das membranas sinoviais, com derrame purulento para dentro de uma articulação, devido à infecção bacteriana; a via usual de infecção é a hematológica para o tecido sinovial, gerando destruição da cartilagem articular, podendo tornar-se crônica, com formação de seio, osteomielite, deformidade e incapacidade. SIN purulent synovitis, pyarthrosis, pyogenic a., septic a., suppurative synovitis.

♻ **arthro-, arthr-.** Artro-; uma articulação; corresponde ao L. articul-. [G. *arthron*, uma articulação, de *arariskō*, unir, formar um conjunto]
Arth·ro·bac·ter (ar-thrō-bak′ter). Um gênero de bactérias Gram-positivas, estritamente aeróbicas (família Corynebacteriaceae), cujas células passam de uma forma cocóide para uma forma de bastonete após transferência para um meio de crescimento complexo fresco. Embora encontrada basicamente no solo, espécies identificadas como pertencentes a esse gênero já foram encontradas na frente em expansão de lesões de cárie dentária. A espécie protótipo é A. *globiformis*. [G. *arthron*, articulação, + *baktron*, bastão ou mastro]
ar·thro·cen·te·sis (ar′thrō-sen-tē′sis). Artrocentese; aspiração de líquido de uma articulação realizada por punção com agulha. [arthro- + G. *kentēsis*, punção]
ar·thro·chon·dri·tis (ar′thrō-kon-drī′tis). Artrocondrite; inflamação de uma cartilagem articular. [arthro- + G. *chondros*, cartilagem, + *-itis*, inflamação]
ar·thro·cla·sia (ar-thrō-klā′ze-ă). Artroclasia; a ruptura forçada de aderências na anquilose. [arthro- + G. *klasis*, uma ruptura]
ar·thro·co·nid·i·um (ar′thrō-kō-nid′ē-um). Artroconídio; um conídio liberado pela fragmentação ou separação no septo das células da hifa. SIN arthrospore. [G. *arthron*, articulação, + conídio]
Arth·ro·der·ma (ar′thrō-der′ma). Um gênero de fungos ascomicetosos composto de espécies anamorfas dos gêneros *Microsporium* e *Trychophyton*.
ar·throd·e·sis (ar-thrōd′ē-sis, ar-thrō-dē′sis). Artrodese; a fixação de uma articulação por meios cirúrgicos. SIN artificial ankylosis. [arthro- + G. *desis*, uma ligação em conjunto]
triple a., a. tríplice; fusão cirúrgica das articulações talonavicular, talocalcânea e calcâneo-cubóide.
ar·thro·dia (ar-thrō′dē-ă). Artródia, articulação plana. SIN plane *joint*. [G. *arthrōdia*, uma articulação deslizante, de *arthron*, articulação, + *eidos*, forma]
ar·thro·di·al (ar-thrō′dē-al). Artrodial; relativo à artródia.
ar·thro·dyn·ia (ar-thrō-din′ē-ă). Artrodinia. SIN arthralgia. [arthro- + G. *odynē*, dor]
ar·thro·dyn·ic (ar-thrō-din′ik). Artrodínico. SIN arthralgic.
ar·thro·dys·pla·sia (ar′thrō-dis-plā′ze-ă). Artrodisplasia; defeito congênito hereditário do desenvolvimento articular. [arthro- G. *dys*, ruim, + *plasis*, uma modelagem]
ar·thro·en·dos·co·py (ar′thrō-en-dos′kō-pē). Artroendoscopia, artroscopia. SIN arthroscopy.
ar·thro·e·rei·sis (ar′thrō-ĕ-rī′sis). Artrorise. SIN arthrorisis.
ar·throg·e·nous (ar-throj′ē-nŭs). Artrógeno. **1.** De origem articular; que começa a partir de uma articulação. **2.** Que forma uma articulação.
ar·thro·gram (ar′thrō-gram). Artrograma; obtenção de imagens de uma articulação após a introdução de um contraste na cápsula articular para melhorar a visualização das estruturas intra-articulares. [arthro- + G. *gramma*, uma escrita]
ar·throg·ra·phy (ar-throg′ră-fē). Artrografia; o ato de fazer um artrograma. [arthro- + G. *graphō*, descrever]

ar·thro·gry·po·sis (ar′thrō - gri - pō′sis). Artrogripose; defeito congênito dos membros caracterizado por contraturas graves de múltiplas articulações. [arthro- + G. *gryphōsis*, curvo]
  a. mul′tiplex congen′ita, a. congênita múltipla; limitação da amplitude do movimento articular e contraturas ao nascimento, geralmente envolvendo múltiplas articulações; uma síndrome provavelmente de etiologia diversa que pode resultar de alterações na medula espinal, músculo ou tecido conjuntivo. Existem várias formas, autossômica dominante [MIM*108110, 108120, 108130, 108140, 108145, 108200], recessiva [MIM*208080, 208081, 208085, 208100, 208150, 208155, 208200] e ligada ao X [MIM*301830]. SIN amyoplasia congenita.
ar·thro·ka·tad·y·sis (ar′thrō - kă - tad′i - sis). Artrocatadise; uma condição de uma articulação com erosão significativa da superfície côncava, resultando em migração medial da superfície convexa. VER TAMBÉM Otto *disease*. [arthro- + G. *katadysis*, uma queda, uma colocação, de *dyō*, escoar]
ar·thro·lith (ar′thrō - lith). Artrólito; um corpo frouxo em uma articulação. [arthro- + G. *lithos*, pedra]
ar·thro·li·thi·a·sis (ar′thrō - li - thī′a - sis). Artrolitíase; termo raramente utilizado para a gota articular (articular *gout*).
ar·thro·lo·gia (ar - thrō - lō′jē - ā). Artrologia. SIN arthrology.
ar·throl·o·gy (ar - throl′ō - jē). Artrologia; o ramo da anatomia relacionado com as articulações. SIN arthrologia, syndesmologia, syndesmology, synosteology. [arthro- + G. *logos*, estudo]
ar·throl·y·sis (ar - throl′i - sis). Artrólise; restauração da mobilidade em articulações rígidas e anquilosadas através do processo de ruptura de aderências intra-articulares e extra-articulares. [arthro- + G. *lysis*, um amolecimento]
ar·throm·e·ter (ar - throm′ĕ - ter). Artrômetro, goniômetro. SIN goniometer (3).
ar·throm·e·try (ar′throm′ĕ - trē). Artrometria; medição da amplitude de movimento em uma articulação. [arthro- + G. *metron*, medida]
ar·thro·oph·thal·mop·a·thy (ar′thrō - of′thal - mop′ă - thē). Artroftalmopatia; doença que afeta articulações e olhos. [arthro- + ophthalmo- + G. *pathos*, doença]
  hereditary progressive a.-o [MIM*108300], a. progressiva hereditária; displasia esquelética associada à displasia múltipla das epífises, tubulação excessiva dos ossos longos com alargamento metafisário, corpos vertebrais achatados, anormalidades ósseas pélvicas, hipermobilidade das articulações, fenda palatina, miopia progressiva, descolamento de retina e surdez. Herança autossômica dominante causada por mutação no gene COL2A1 no 12q, gene COL11A1 em 1p ou gene COL11A2 em 6p. SIN Stickler syndrome.
arthropatia psoriatica. Artropatia psoriática. SIN psoriatic *arthritis.*
ar·thro·pa·thol·o·gy (ar′thrō - pa - thol′ō - jē). Artropatologia; o estudo das doenças das articulações.
ar·throp·a·thy (ar - throp′ă - thē). Artropatia; qualquer doença que afete uma articulação. [arthro- + G. *pathos*, doença]
  diabetic a., a. diabética; a. neuropática que ocorre no diabetes.
  Jaccoud a., a. de Jaccoud. SIN Jaccoud *arthritis.*
  long-leg a., a. da perna comprida; uma doença articular degenerativa que se desenvolve, depois de muitos anos, no quadril e/ou joelho da perna mais longa de uma pessoa cujas pernas têm comprimento desigual.
  neuropathic a., a. neuropática. SIN neuropathic *joint.*
  static a., a. estática; envolvimento secundário de uma articulação depois de doença em uma articulação do mesmo membro; p.ex., envolvimento do joelho ou tornozelo na doença do quadril.
  tabetic a., a. tabética; a. neuropática que ocorre com o tabes dorsal (neurossífilis tabética). VER TAMBÉM neuropathic *joint*.
ar·thro·plas·ty (ar′thrō - plas - tē). Artroplastia. **1.** Criação de uma articulação artificial para corrigir artrite degenerativa avançada. **2.** Uma cirurgia para restaurar o máximo possível a integridade e a força funcional de uma articulação. [arthro- + G. *plastos*, formado]
  Charnley hip a., a. de quadril de Charnley; uma forma de artroplastia coxofemoral total, consistindo na colocação de um cálice acetabular e de uma prótese de cabeça de fêmur; o termo é uma homenagem a John Charnley, considerado o pioneiro no desenvolvimento desse procedimento.
  gap a., a. correção cirúrgica de anquilose ao criar um espaço entre a parte anquilosada de uma articulação e a porção para a qual se deseja o movimento.
  interposition a., a. de interposição; a correção cirúrgica da anquilose através da separação da parte imóvel de uma articulação da parte mobilizada e interposição de uma substância (p.ex., fáscia, cartilagem, metal ou plástico) entre elas.
  intracapsular temporomandibular joint a., a. intracapsular da articulação temporomandibular; a remodelagem cirúrgica da superfície articular do côndilo mandibular sem a retirada do disco articular.
  total joint a., a. articular total; a. em que as duas superfícies articulares são substituídas por materiais artificiais, usualmente composta de metal e plástico de alta densidade; sendo atualmente realizada para quadril, joelho, ombro e cotovelo.
ar·thro·pneu·mo·ra·di·og·ra·phy (ar′thrō - noo′mō - rā - dē - og′ră - fē).

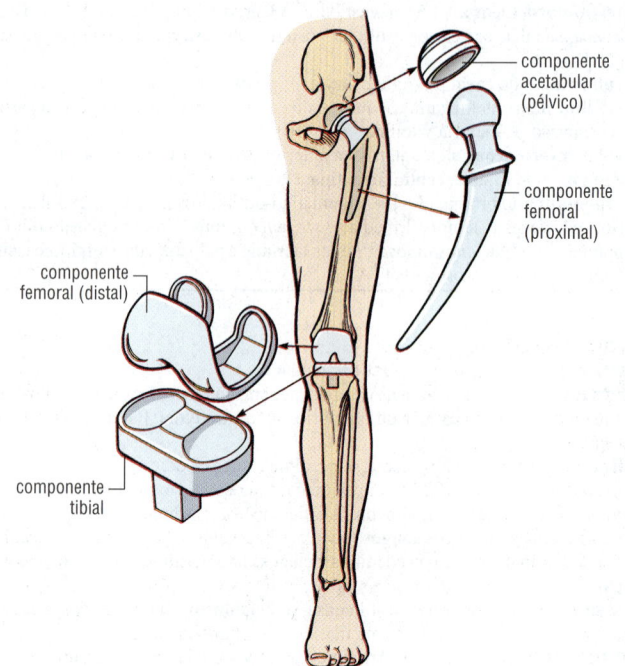

artroplastia: mostrando a substituição de quadril e joelho

Artropneumorradiografia; exame radiográfico de uma articulação depois que foi injetado ar nela. [arthro- + pneumo- + radiography]
ar·thro·pod (ar - thrō - pod). Artrópodo; um membro do filo dos artrópodes. [arthro- + G. *pous*, pé]
Ar·throp·o·da (ar - throp′ō - dă). Filo dos Metazoa que inclui as classes Crustacea (caranguejos, camarões, lagostas, siris), Insecta, Arachnida (aranhas, escorpiões, ácaros, carrapatos), Chilopoda (centopéias), Diplopoda (milipedes), Merostomata (*Limulus polyphemus*) e vários outros grupos extintos ou menos conhecidos. Os artrópodes formam o maior conjunto de microrganismos vivos, 75% dos insetos, dos quais se conhece cerca de um milhão de espécies. [arthro- + G. *pous*, pé]
ar·thro·po·di·a·sis (ar′thrō - pō - dī′ă - sis). Artropodíase; efeitos diretos dos artrópodes sobre os vertebrados, incluindo acaríase, alergia, dermatose, entomofobia e ações de toxinas de contato.
ar·thro·pod·ic, ar·throp·o·dous (ar - thrō - pō′dik, ar - throp′ō - dŭs). Artropódico; pertinente aos artrópodes.
ar·thro·py·o·sis (ar′thrō - pī - ō′sis). Artropiose; supuração em uma articulação. [arthro- + G. *pyōsis*, supuração]
ar·thro·ri·sis (ar′thrō - rī′sis). Artrórise; cirurgia para limitar o movimento de uma articulação nos casos de mobilidade indevida devido a paralisia, geralmente por meio de bloqueio ósseo. SIN arthroereisis. [arthro- + G. *ereisis*, um levantamento]
ar·thro·scle·ro·sis (ar′thrō - skler - ō′sis). Artrosclerose; rigidez das articulações, especialmente no idoso. [arthro- + G. *sklērōsis*, endurecimento]
ar·thro·scope (ar′thrō - skōp). Artroscópio; um endoscópio para examinar a anatomia interna de uma articulação.
ar·thros·co·py (ar - thros′kō - pē). Artroscopia; exame endoscópico do interior de uma articulação. SIN arthroendoscopy. [arthro- + G. *skopeō*, visualizar]
ar·thro·sis (ar - thrō′sis). **1.** Articulação. SIN joint. [G. *arthrōsis*, uma articulação] **2.** Osteoartrite. SIN osteoarthritis. [arthro- + G. *-osis*, condição]
  temporomandibular a., a. temporomandibular (ATM); disfunção degenerativa não-infecciosa da articulação ATM caracterizada por dor, estalido e abertura mandibular limitada. VER TAMBÉM myofascial pain-dysfunction *syndrome*.
ar·thro·spore (ar′thrō - spōr). Artrósporo. SIN arthroconidium. [arthro- + G. *sporos*, semente]
ar·thros·to·my (ar - thros′tō - mē). Artrostomia; estabelecimento de uma abertura temporária dentro de uma cavidade articular. [arthro- + G. *stoma*, boca]
ar·thro·sy·no·vi·tis (ar′thrō - sin - ō - vī′tis). Artrossinovite; inflamação da membrana sinovial de uma articulação.
ar·thro·tome (ar′thrō - tōm). Artrótomo; um bisturi grande e forte usado no corte de cartilagens e outras estruturas articulares.
ar·throt·o·my (ar - throt′ō - mē). Artrotomia; corte de uma articulação para expor seu interior. [arthro- + G. *tomē*, um corte]
ar·thro·tro·pic (ar - thrō - trop′ik). Artrotrópico; que tende a afetar as articulações. [arthro- + G. *tropos*, uma volta]

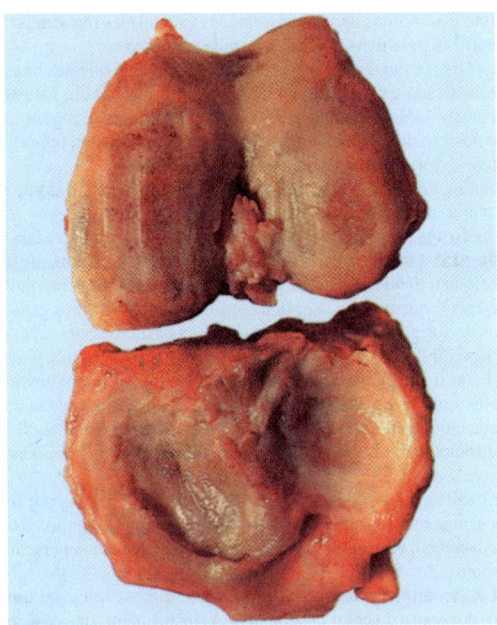
artrose: a cartilagem do joelho está quase destruída

ar·thro·ty·phoid (ar-thrō-tī′foyd). Artrotifóide; termo obsoleto para febre tifóide com o envolvimento articular sendo decorrente da infecção metastática.

Arthus, Maurice, bacteriologista francês, 1862–1945. VER A. *phenomenon, reaction.*

ar·tic·u·lar (ar-tik′ū-lar). Articular; relativo a uma articulação. SIN arthral.

ar·tic·u·la·re (ar-tik-ū-lā′rē). Articular; em cefalometria, o ponto de intersecção do contorno dorsal externo do côndilo mandibular e osso temporal; o ponto médio é utilizado quando uma radiografia de perfil mostra as projeções duplas dos ramos.

ar·tic·u·late (ar-tik′ū-lit). **1.** Articulado. SIN articulated. **2.** Capaz de fala significante nítida e conectada. (ar-tik′yū-lāt). **3.** Articular; unir ou conectar-se frouxamente para permitir o movimento entre as partes. **4.** Articular; pronunciar, falar de maneira clara e coerente. [L. *articulo,* pp. *-atus,* articular]

ar·tic·u·lat·ed (ar-tik′ū-lā-ted). Articulado; unido. SIN articulate (1).

ARTICULATIO

ar·tic·u·la·tio, pl. **ar·tic·u·la·ti·o·nes** (ar-tik-ū-lā′shē-ō, -lā-shē-ō′nēz). Articulação, a. sinovial; *termo oficial alternativo para sinovial joint. [L. um fila de peças]
- **a. acromioclavicula′ris** [TA], a. acromioclavicular. SIN acromioclavular *joint.*
- **a. atlantoaxia′lis latera′lis** [TA], a. atlantoaxial lateral. SIN lateral atlantoaxial *joint.*
- **a. atlantoaxia′lis media′na** [TA], a. atlantoaxial mediana. SIN median atlantoaxial *joint.*
- **a. atlan′to-occipita′lis** [TA], a. atlantoccipital. SIN atlanto-occipital *joint.*
- **a. bicondyla′ris** [TA], a. bicondilar. SIN bicondylar *joint.*
- **a. calca′neocuboi′dea** [TA], a. calcaneocubóidea. SIN calcaneocuboid *joint.*
- **a. capi′tis cos′tae** [TA], a. da cabeça da costela. SIN *joint* of head of rib.
- **articulationes carpi** [TA], articulações do carpo. SIN carpal *joints,* em *joint.*
- **a. carpi** [TA], articulações do carpo. SIN carpal *joints,* em *joint.*
- **articulatio′nes carpometacarpa′les** [TA], articulações carpometacarpais. SIN carpometacarpal *joints,* em *joint.*
- **a. carpometacar′palis pol′licis,** a. carpometacarpal do polegar. SIN carpometacarpal *joint* of thumb.
- **a. cartilag′inis,** a. cartilagínea. SIN cartilaginous *joint.*
- **articulatio′nes cin′guli mem′bri inferio′ris,** articulações do cíngulo do membro inferior. SIN *joints* of pelvic girdle, em *joint.*
- **articulationes cinguli pectoralis,** articulações do cíngulo do membro superior; *termo oficial alternativo para *joints* of pectoral girdle, em *joint.*
- **articulationes cinguli pelvici** [TA], articulações do cíngulo do membro inferior. SIN *joints* of pelvic girdle, em *joint.*
- **articulatio′nes cin′guli mem′bri superio′ris,** articulações do cíngulo do membro superior. SIN *joints* of pectoral girdle, em *joint.*
- **a. complex′a,** a. composta. SIN complex *joint.*
- **a. compos′ita** [TA], a. composta. SIN complex *joint.*
- **a. condyla′ris,** a. elipsóidea. SIN condylar *joint.*
- **articulationes costochondra′les** [TA], articulações costocondrais. SIN costochondral *joints,* em *joint.*
- **a. cos′totransversa′ria,** a. costotransversária. SIN costotransverse *joint.*
- **articulatio′nes costovertebra′les** [TA], articulações costovertebrais. SIN costovertebral *joints,* em *joint.*
- **a. cotyl′ica,** a. cotilóidea. SIN ball and socket *joint.*
- **a. cox′ae** [TA], a. coxofemoral. SIN hip *joint.*
- **a. coxofemoralis,** a. coxofemoral; *termo oficial alternativo para hip *joint.*
- **articulationes cranii** [TA], articulações sinoviais do crânio. SIN cranial synovial *joints,* em *joint.*
- **a. cricoarytenoid′ea** [TA], a. cricoaritenóidea. SIN cricoarytenoid *joint.*
- **a. cricothyroid′ea** [TA], a. cricotireóidea. SIN cricothyroid *joint.*
- **a. cu′biti** [TA], a. do cotovelo. SIN elbow *joint.*
- **a. cuneonavicula′ris** [TA], a. cuneonavicular. SIN cuneonavicular *joint.*
- **a. cylindrica** [TA], a. cilíndrica. SIN cylindrical *joint.*
- **a. dentoalveola′ris,** gonfose. SIN gomphosis.
- **a. ellipsoi′dea** [TA], a. elipsóidea. SIN condylar *joint.*
- **a. fibro′sa,** a. fibrosa. SIN fibrous *joint.*
- **a. ge′nus** [TA], a. do joelho. SIN knee *joint.*
- **a. glenohumeralis,** a. do úmero; *termo oficial alternativo para glenohumeral *joint.*
- **a. hu′meri** [TA], a. do úmero. SIN glenohumeral *joint.*
- **a. humeroradia′lis** [TA], a. umerorradial. SIN humeroradial *joint.*
- **a. humeroulna′ris** [TA], a. umeroulnar. SIN humeroulnar *joint.*
- **a. incudomallea′ris** [TA], a. incudomalear. SIN incudomalleolar *joint.*
- **a. incudostape′dia** [TA], a. incudoestapedial. SIN incudostapedial *joint.*
- **articulatio′nes intercarpa′les,** articulações intercarpais; *termo oficial alternativo para carpal *joints,* em *joint.*
- **articulatio′nes interchondra′les** [TA], articulações intercondrais. SIN interchondral *joints,* em *joint.*
- **articulationes intercuneiformes** [TA], articulações intercuneiformes. SIN intercuneiform *joints,* em *joint.*
- **articulatio′nes intermetacarpa′les** [TA], articulações intermetacarpais. SIN intermetacarpal *joints,* em *joint.*
- **articulatio′nes intermetatarsa′les** [TA], articulações intermetatarsais. SIN intermetatarsal *joints,* em *joint.*
- **articulatio′nes interphalan′geae ma′nus** [TA], articulações interfalângicas da mão. SIN interphalangeal *joints* of hand, em *joint.*
- **articulatio′nes interphalan′geae pe′dis** [TA], articulações interfalângicas do pé. SIN interphalangeal *joints* of foot, em *joint.*
- **articulatio′nes intertar′seae,** articulações intertarsais. SIN intertarsal *joints,* em *joint.*
- **a. lumbosacra′lis** [TA], a. lombossacral. SIN lumbosacral *joint.*
- **a. mandibula′ris,** a. temporomandibular. SIN temporomandibular *joint.*
- **articulatio′nes ma′nus** [TA], articulações da mão. SIN *joints* of hand, em *joint.*
- **a. mediocarpa′lis** [TA], a. mediocarpal. SIN midcarpal *joint.*
- **articulatio′nes mem′bri inferio′ris li′beri** [TA], articulações da parte livre do membro inferior. SIN synovial *joints* of free lower limb, em *joint.*
- **articulatio′nes mem′bri superio′ris li′beri** [TA], articulações da parte livre do membro superior. SIN synovial *joints* of free upper limb, em *joint.*
- **articulatio′nes metacarpophalan′geae** [TA], articulações metacarpofalângicas. SIN metacarpophalangeal *joints,* em *joint.*
- **articulatio′nes metatarsophalan′geae** [TA], articulações metatarsofalângicas. SIN metatarsophalangeal *joints,* em *joint.*
- **articulationes ossiculorum auditoriorum,** articulações dos ossículos da audição; *termo oficial alternativo para *joints* of auditory ossicles, em *joint.*
- **articulatio′nes ossiculo′rum audi′tus** [TA], articulações dos ossículos da audição. SIN *joints* of auditory ossicles, em *joint.*
- **a. os′sis pisifor′mis** [TA], a. do pisiforme. SIN pisiform *joint.*
- **a. ovoida′lis,** a. selar. SIN saddle *joint.*
- **articulatio′nes pe′dis** [TA], articulações do pé. SIN *joints* of foot, em *joint.*
- **a. pla′na** [TA], a. plana. SIN plane *joint.*
- **a. radiocar′palis** [TA], a. radiocarpal. SIN wrist *joint.*
- **a. radioulna′ris dista′lis** [TA], a. radioulnar distal. SIN distal radioulnar *joint.*
- **a. radioulna′ris proxima′lis** [TA], a. radioulnar proximal. SIN proximal radioulnar *joint.*
- **a. sacrococcy′gea** [TA], a. sacrococcígea. SIN sacrococcygeal *joint.*
- **a. sacroili′aca** [TA], a. sacroilíaca. SIN sacroiliac *joint.*
- **a. sellar′is** [TA], a. selar. SIN saddle *joint.*
- **a. sim′plex** [TA], a. simples. SIN simple *joint.*
- **a. spheroi′dea** [TA], a. esferóidea. SIN ball and socket *joint.*
- **a. sternoclavicula′ris** [TA], a. esternoclavicular. SIN sternoclavicular *joint.*

articulatio'nes sternocosta'les [TA], articulações esternocostais. SIN sternocostal *joints*, em *joint*.
a. subtala'ris [TA], a. talocalcânea. SIN subtalar *joint*.
a. synovia'lis, a. sinovial. SIN synovial *joint*.
a. talocalcanea, a. talocalcânea; *termo oficial alternativo para subtalar *joint*.
a. tal'ocalca'neonavicula'ris [TA], a. talocalcaneonavicular. SIN talocalcaneonavicular *joint*.
a. talocrura'lis [TA], a. talocrural. SIN ankle *joint*.
a. tar'si transver'sa [TA], a. transversa do tarso. SIN transverse tarsal *joint*.
articulatio'nes tarsometatarsa'les [TA], articulações tarsometatarsais. SIN tarsometatarsal *joints*, em *joint*.
a. temporomandibula'ris [TA], a. temporomandibular. SIN temporomandibular *joint*.
articulationes thoracis [TA], articulações do tórax. SIN synovial *joints* of thorax, em *joint*.
a. tibiofibula'ris [TA], a. tibiofibular. SIN tibiofibular *joint*.
a. trochoid'ea [TA], a. trocóidea. SIN pivot *joint*.
articulatio'nes zygapophysia'les [TA], articulações zigapofisárias. SIN zygapophysial *joints*, em *joint*.

ar·tic·u·la·tion (ar-tik-ū-lā'shŭn). Articulação. **1.** SIN joint. **2.** Uma articulação ou união frouxa de modo a permitir a movimentação entre as partes. **3.** Fala ou enunciação clara e distinta. **4.** Em odontologia, a relação de contato das superfícies de oclusão dos dentes durante a movimentação da mandíbula. [ver articulatio]
arthrodial a., a. plana. SIN plane *joint*.
atlanto-occipital a., a. atlantoccipital. SIN atlanto-occipital *joint*.
balanced a., mordida equilibrada. SIN balanced *occlusion*.
bicondylar a., a. bicondilar. SIN bicondylar *joint*.
cartilaginous a., a. cartilagínea. SIN cartilaginous *joint*.
compound a., a. composta. SIN complex *joint*.
condylar a., a. condilar. SIN condylar *joint*.
confluent a., a. confluente; tendência para misturar de forma confusa as sílabas na fala.
cricoarytenoid a., a. cricoaritenóidea. SIN cricoarytenoid *joint*.
cricothyroid a., a. cricotireóidea. SIN cricothyroid *joint*.
cuneonavicular a., a. cuneonavicular. SIN cuneonavicular *joint*.
dental a., a. dentária; a relação de contato das superfícies de oclusão dos dentes superiores e inferiores quando estes se movimentam para dentro e para fora da oclusão cêntrica. SIN gliding occlusion.
distal radioulnar a., a. radioulnar distal. SIN distal radioulnar *joint*.
a.'s of foot, articulações do pé. SIN joints of foot, em *joint*.
glenohumeral a., a. gleno-umeral. SIN glenohumeral *joint*.
a.'s of hand, articulações da mão. SIN joints of hand, em *joint*.
humeral a., a. do úmero. SIN glenohumeral *joint*.
humeroradial a., a. umerorradial. SIN humeroradial *joint*.
incudomalleolar a., a. incudomalear. SIN incudomalleolar *joint*.
incudostapedial a., a. incudoestapedial. SIN incudostapedial *joint*.
interchondral a.'s, articulações intercondrais. SIN interchondral *joints*, em *joint*.
intermetatarsal a.'s, articulações intermetatarsais. SIN intermetatarsal *joints*, em *joint*.
interphalangeal a.'s, articulações interfalângicas. SIN interphalangeal *joints* of hand, em *joint*.
intertarsal a.'s, articulações intertarsais. SIN intertarsal *joints*, em *joint*.
metacarpophalangeal a.'s, articulações metacarpofalângicas. SIN metacarpophalangeal *joints*, em *joint*.
metatarsophalangeal a.'s, articulações metatarsofalângicas. SIN metatarsophalangeal *joints*, em *joint*.
peg-and-socket a., gonfose. SIN gomphosis.
a. of pisiform bone, a. do pisiforme. SIN pisiform *joint*.
proximal radioulnar a., a. radioulnar proximal. SIN proximal radioulnar *joint*.
radiocarpal a., a. radiocarpal. SIN wrist *joint*.
sacroiliac a., a. sacroilíaca. SIN sacroiliac *joint*.
spheroid a., a. esferóidea. SIN ball and socket *joint*.
sternocostal a.'s, articulações esternocostais. SIN sternocostal *joints*, em *joint*.
superior tibial a., a. tibiofibular. SIN tibiofibular *joint*.
talocrural a., a. talocrural. SIN ankle *joint*.
temporomandibular a., a. temporomandibular. SIN temporomandibular *joint*.
tibiofibular a., **(1)** a. tibiofibular. SIN tibiofibular *joint*; **(2)** sindesmose tibiofibular. SIN tibiofibular *syndesmosis*.
transverse tarsal a., a. transversa do tarso. SIN transverse tarsal *joint*.
trochoid a., a. trocóidea. SIN pivot *joint*.

ar·tic·u·la·tor (ar-tik'ū-lā-tōr). Articulador dentário; um dispositivo mecânico que representa as articulações temporomandibulares e os componentes da mandíbula aos quais podem ser fixados os modelos maxilares e mandibulares. SIN occluding frame.
adjustable a., a. ajustável; **(1)** um a. que pode ser ajustado para permitir o movimento dos moldes dentro das relações excêntricas registradas; **(2)** um a. capaz de ajuste para mais de uma posição excêntrica.
arcon a., **(1)** um a. dentário com as guias condilares equivalentes fixas na porção superior da arcada e o eixo da dobradiça na inferior; **(2)** um instrumento que mantém uma relação constante entre o plano de oclusão e as guias do arco em qualquer posição do membro superior, possibilitando, assim, reproduções mais exatas de movimentos mandibulares.
non-arcon a., um a. com as guias condilares equivalentes fixas na porção inferior e o eixo da dobradiça na superior.

ar·tic·u·la·to·ry (ar-tik'ū-la-tō-rē). Articulatório; relativo à fala articulada.
ar·tic·u·lo·stat (ar-tik'ū-lō-stat). Articulostato; um instrumento de pesquisa que posiciona a dentição de uma pessoa e a cabeça de uma máquina de raios X, de tal modo que os filmes obtidos em momentos distintos possam ser superpostos de forma acurada. [articulo- + G. *stasis*, uma parada]
ar·tic·u·lus (ar-tik'ū-lŭs). Articulação. SIN joint. [L. articulação]
ar·ti·fact (ar'ti-fakt). Artefato. **1.** Qualquer coisa, principalmente em uma amostra histológica ou em um registro gráfico, que é provocada pela técnica empregada e que não reflete a amostra ou experimento original. **2.** Uma lesão cutânea produzida ou perpetuada pela ação auto-infligida, como na dermatite factícia. [L. *ars*, arte, + *facio*, pp. *factus*, fazer]
chemical shift a., a. por deslocamento químico; nas imagens por ressonância magnética, uma faixa escura causada por uma diferença bioquímica na freqüência de ressonância das regiões adjacentes, em vez de uma separação anatômica verdadeira.
thermal a., a. térmico; distorção da estrutura microscópica em uma amostra de tecido, por causa do calor produzido pelo instrumento (p.ex., eletrocautério de alça) usado para obter a amostra.

ar·ti·fac·ti·tious (ar'ti-fak-tish'ŭs). Artificial. SIN artifactual.
ar·ti·fac·tu·al (ar-ti-fak'chū-ăl). Artificial; produzido ou causado por um artefato. SIN artifactitious.
Ar·ti·o·dac·ty·la (ar'ti-ō-dak'ti-lă). Uma ordem de ungulados que têm dois ou quatro dedos, com o eixo entre o terceiro e o quarto; p.ex., porco e hipopótamo, com quatro; camelo, cervo, girafa, antílope e vaca, com dois. [G. *artios*, igual em número, + *daktylos*, dedo]
ar·y·ep·i·glot·tic (ar'ē-ep-i-glot'ik). Ariepiglótico; relativo à cartilagem aritenóidea e à epiglote; indica uma prega da mucosa (prega ariepiglótica) e um músculo nela contido (músculo ariepiglótico). SIN arytenoepiglottidean.
ar·yl (ar'il). Aril, arila; um radical orgânico derivado de um composto aromático por remoção de um átomo de hidrogênio.
a. acylamidase, aril acilamidase; uma amidoidrolase que cliva o grupamento acila de uma anilida por hidrólise, produzindo anilina e um ânion ácido. SIN arylamidase.
ar·yl·am·i·dase (ar-il-am'i-dās). Arilamidase. SIN aryl acylamidase.
ar·yl·ar·son·ic ac·id (ar'il-ar-son'ik). Ácido arilarsônico; um ácido arsônico que contém um radical arila; p.ex., ácido arsenílico.
ar·yl·sul·fa·tase (ar-il-sŭl'fă-tās). Arilsulfatase; uma enzima que cliva os fenóis sulfatados, incluindo os cerebrosídios sulfatados (isto é, um fenol sulfatado + H_2O → um fenol + ânion sulfato). Algumas arilsulfatases são inibidas pelo sulfato (tipo II) e algumas não o são (tipo I). SIN sulfatase (2).
ar·y·te·no·ep·i·glot·tid·e·an (a-rit'ē-nō-ep'i-glo-tid'ē-an). Aritenoepiglótico. SIN aryepiglottic.
ar·y·te·noid (ar-i-tē'noyd) [TA]. Aritenóide; indica uma cartilagem (cartilagem aritenóide) e os músculos (músculos aritenóides oblíquo e transverso) da laringe. [ver arytenoideus]
ar·y·te·noi·dec·to·my (ar'ī-tē-noy-dek'tō-mē). Aritenoidectomia; excisão de uma cartilagem aritenóide, usualmente na paralisia bilateral de cordas vocais, para melhorar a respiração. [arytenoid + G. *ektomē*, excisão]
ar·y·te·noi·de·us (ar-ī-tē-noy'dē-ŭs). Aritenóideo. SIN oblique arytenoid *muscle*, transverse arytenoid (muscle). [G. *arytainoeides*, em forma de concha, aplicado à cartilagem da laringe, de *arytaina*, uma concha, + *eidos*, semelhança]
ar·yt·e·noi·di·tis (ā-rit'ē-noy-dī'tis). Aritenoidite; inflamação de uma articulação cricoaritenóidea, cartilagem aritenóidea ou seu revestimento mucoso.
ar·y·te·noi·do·pexy (ar'ī-tē-noy'dō-pek'sē). Aritenoidopexia; fixação por cirurgia de uma cartilagem aritenóidea. [arytenoid + G. *pēxis*, fixação]
A.S. Abreviatura para *auris sinistra* [L.], ouvido esquerdo.
As Símbolo do arsenic (arsênico).
as·a·fet·i·da (as-ă-fet'ī-dă). Assa-fétida; goma resinosa, o exsudato espesso da raiz da *Ferula foetida* (família Umbelliferae); material com odor fétido usado como repelente de cães, gatos e coelhos e outrora empregado como antiespasmódico; na Ásia, usado como condimento e agente flavorizante. [Pers. *aza*, goma, + L. *fetidus*, fétido]
As·a·rum (as'ar-ŭm). Um gênero de plantas da família Aristolochiaceae. [L., de G. *asarom*, gengibre]
A. canaden'se, estimulante aromático e diaforético. SIN Canada snakeroot, Indian ginger, wild ginger.
A. europae'um, emético e catártico. SIN European snakeroot, hazelwort.

as·bes·toid (as-bes′toyd). Asbestóide. SIN amianthoid.
as·bes·tos (as-bes′tos). Asbesto; o produto comercial, depois de minerado e processado, de uma família de silicatos hidratados fibrosos divididos mineralogicamente em anfibólios (amosita, antrofilita e crocidolita) e serpentinas (crisotila); é virtualmente insolúvel e é empregado para proporcionar força e capacidade de modelagem, isolamento térmico e resistência ao fogo, calor e corrosão; a inalação de partículas de a. pode provocar asbestose, placas pleurais, fibrose pleural, derrame pleural, mesotelioma e câncer do pulmão. [G. inextinguível; chamado assim pela crença errônea de que, quando aquecido, não poderia ser extinto]
as·bes·to·sis (as-bes-tō′sis). Asbestose; pneumoconiose devido à inalação de fibras de asbesto suspensas no ar ambiente; por vezes complicada por mesotelioma pleural ou carcinoma broncogênico; os corpúsculos ferruginosos são a característica histológica da exposição ao asbesto.
as·ca·ri·a·sis (as-kă-rī′ă-sis). Ascaríase; doença causada por infestação por *Ascaris* ou nematódeos ascarídeos correlatos. [G. *askaris*, um verme intestinal, + *-iasis*, condição]
as·ca·ri·cide (as-kar′i-sīd). Ascaricida. **1.** Que causa a morte de nematódeos ascarídeos. **2.** Um agente que possui essas propriedades. [ascarid + L. *caedo*, matar]
as·ca·rid (as′kă-rid). Ascarídeo. **1.** Um nome geral para qualquer nematódeo da família Ascarididae. **2.** Pertinente a esses nematódeos.
As·car·i·dae (as-kar′i-dē). Grafia antiga de Ascarididae.
As·car·i·da·ta (as-kă-rid′ă-tă). Ascaridida. SIN Ascaridida.
As·car·i·di·a (as-kă-rid′i-dă). Uma ordem de vermes nematódeos que inclui muitos parasitas importantes de seres humanos, animais domésticos e aves, como *Ascaris*, *Ascaridia*, *Subuluris*, *Heterakis* e *Anisakis*. SIN Ascaridata, Ascarididea, Ascaridorida.
As·car·i·di·dae (as-kă-rid′i-dē). Uma família de grandes nematódeos intestinais que inclui o importante nematódeo dos seres humanos, *Ascaris lumbricoides*, o nematódeo abundante do suíno, *Ascaris suum*, e os ascarídeos comuns de cães e gatos, espécies *Toxocara* e *Toxascaris*. [G. *askaris*, um verme intestinal]
As·car·i·did·ea (as-kar-i-did′e-ă). Ascaridida. SIN Ascaridida.
As·car·i·doi·dea (as-kă-ri-doy′dē-ă). Superfamília de nematódeos intestinais trilabiados que inclui a família Ascarididae.
as·car·i·dole (as-kar′i-dōl). Ascaridol; um importante constituinte do óleo de quenopódio; um anti-helmíntico.
As·car·i·dor·i·da (as-kări-dōr′i-dă). Ascaridida. SIN Ascaridida.
As·ca·ris (as′kă-ris). Um gênero de grandes parasitas nematódeos corpulentos no intestino delgado; abundante em seres humanos e em muitos outros vertebrados. [G. *askaris*, um verme intestinal]
 A. equo′rum, SIN *Parascaris equorum.*
 A. lumbricoi′des, a. lombricóide; um grande nematódeo de seres humanos, um dos parasitas humanos mais comuns (22 a 33 cm de comprimento); vários sintomas, como inquietação, febre e, por vezes, diarréia, são atribuídos à sua presença, mas, em geral, ele não provoca sintomas definidos; a espécie similar *A. suum* (ou *A. lumbricoides suum*) é muito comum no suíno, mas não é prontamente transmitida para seres humanos, e vice-versa; os tipos são semelhantes do ponto de vista morfológico e imunológico, mas aparentemente são tipos que se adaptam ao hospedeiro, considerados como espécies ou raças distintas.
As·ca·roi·dea (as-kă-roy′dē-ă). Grafia antiga para Ascaridoidea.
as·car·on (as-kă-ron). Ascaron; uma peptona tóxica presente em helmintos, especialmente os ascarídeos; os sinais e sintomas da intoxicação por a. são semelhantes aos do choque anafilático. [G. *askaris*, um verme intestinal, + *hormōn*, part. pres. de *hormaō*, excitar]
As·ca·rops stron·gy·li·na (as′kă-rops stron-ji-lī′nă). Um pequeno verme hematófago encontrado no estômago de porcos e porcos selvagens em muitas partes do mundo. As larvas dessa espécie desenvolvem-se em besouros coprófagos; os vermes aderem à mucosa gástrica do porco e podem provocar inflamação e ulceração nas infestações maciças. [G. *askaris*, um verme intestinal; *strongylos*, redondo]
as·cen·dens (as-sen′denz). Ascendente; que ascende. Ir para cima, subir, no sentido de uma posição mais elevada. [L.]
as·cen·sus (ă-sen′sus). Ascensão; movimento para cima; que possui uma posição anormalmente elevada. [L. ascensão]
as·cer·tain·ment (as-ser-tān′ment). Determinação, averiguação; em pesquisa epidemiológica e genética, o método pelo qual uma pessoa, heredograma ou agrupamento recebe a atenção de um pesquisador; influencia a interpretação de relações de segregação, taxas de concordância, análise de ligação e outros aspectos de probabilidade.
 complete a., d. completa; método pelo qual todas as famílias com pelo menos um indivíduo afetado em uma população são destacadas ou possuem uma probabilidade igual de serem identificadas por levantamento epidemiológico ou por uma técnica de amostragem randomizada apropriada.
 incomplete a., d. incompleta; método de localizar os indivíduos afetados em que a probabilidade de localizar qualquer paciente específico possui um valor conhecido entre 0 e 1. SIN truncate a.
 single a., d. isolada; método de d. de localizar os indivíduos afetados por internação hospitalar ou outro meio em que a probabilidade de encontrar a mesma família duas vezes se aproxima de zero; dessa maneira, a probabilidade de que uma família será descoberta é proporcional ao número de membros afetados.
 total a., d. total; método pelo qual todos os membros de uma população em risco de um traço são destacados ou é igualmente provável que estejam contidos em uma amostra.
 truncate a., d. truncada, d. incompleta. SIN incomplete a.
Asc·hel·min·thes (ask-hel-min′thēz). Um antigo filo dos Metazoa (metazoários) que incluía a classe Nematoda e um agrupamento dessemelhante variado de outros pseudocelomados. Agora, cada um está em filos distintos; eles são não-assegmentados, bilateralmente simétricos e cilíndricos ou filiformes, com uma cavidade corporal (pseudocele) e extremidades arredondadas ou afiladas; variam consideravelmente em tamanho e o macho é usualmente menor que a fêmea.
Ascher, Karl W., oftalmologista norte-americano, 1887–1971. VER A. aqueous influx *phenomenon*, *syndrome*.
Aschner, Bernhard, ginecologista austríaco, 1883–1960. VER A.′*phenomenon*, *reflex*; A.-Dagnini *reflex*.
Aschoff, Karl Ludwig, patologista alemão, 1866–1942. VER A. *bodies*, em *body*; *nodules*, em *nodule*; *node* of A. and Tawara; Rokitansky-A. *sinuses*, em *sinus*; A. *cell*.
as·ci·tes (ă-sī′tēz). Ascite; acúmulo de líquido seroso na cavidade peritoneal. SIN abdominal dropsy, hidroperitoneum, hidroperitonia. [L. de G. *askos*, uma bolsa, + *-ites*]
 a. adipo′sus, a. quilosa. SIN chylous a.
 chyliform a., a. quilosa. SIN chylous a.
 chylous a., a. chylo′sus, a. quilosa; presença, na cavidade peritoneal, de um líquido leitoso que contém gordura suspensa, comumente causada por obstrução ou lesão do ducto ou do cisterna torácica. SIN a. adiposus, chyliform a., chyloperitoneum, fatty a., milky a.
 fatty a., a. quilosa. SIN chylous a.
 gelatinous a., pseudomixoma peritoneal. SIN *pseudomyxoma* peritonei.
 hemorrhagic a., a. hemorrágica; líquido sanguinolento, ou seroso tinto de sangue, que, freqüentemente, resulta de carcinoma metastático na cavidade peritoneal.
 milky a., a. quilosa. SIN chylous a.
 pseudochylous a., a. pseudoquilosa; presença no peritônio de um líquido opalescente ou turvo que não contém gordura.
as·cit·ic (ă-sit′ik). Ascítico; de ou relativo à ascite.
as·ci·tog·e·nous (as-i-toj′e-nŭs). Ascitógeno; que produz ascite.
as·co·carp (as′kō-karp). Ascocarpo; estrutura de fungo, de complexidade variável, que contém ascos e ascósporos. [G. *askos*, bolsa, + *karpos*, fruta]
as·cog·e·nous (as-koj′e-nŭs). Ascógeno; indica hifas ou células portadoras de ascos.
as·co·go·ni·um (as-kō-gō′ne-ŭm). Ascogônio; a célula feminina em um ascomiceto que é fertilizada pela célula masculina.
Ascoli, Alberto, sorologista italiano, 1877–1957. VER Ascoli *reaction*; Ascoli *test*.
As·co·my·ce·tes (as′kō-mi-sē′tēz). Classe de fungos caracterizada pela presença de ascos e ascósporos. Esses fungos possuem, em geral, duas fases reprodutivas distintas: o estágio sexual ou perfeito e o estágio assexuado ou imperfeito. *Ajellomyces capsulatum* e *Ajellomyces dermatitidis* são membros patogênicos dessa classe. [G. *askos*, uma bolsa, + *mykēs*, cogumelo]
as·co·my·ce·tous (as′kō-mī′se-tus). Ascomicetoso; fungos relacionados aos Ascomycota.
As·co·my·co·ta (as′kō-mī-kō-tă). Um filo de fungos caracterizados pela presença de ascos e ascósporos. Alguns micologistas mudaram a classe Ascomycetes para o nível de filo ou divisão.
as·cor·base (as-kōr′bās). Ascorbase, ascorbato oxidase. SIN *ascorbate* oxidase.
as·cor·bate (as′kōr′bāt). Ascorbato; um sal ou éster do ácido ascórbico.
 a. oxidase, a. oxidase; uma enzima portadora de cobre que catalisa a oxidação do ácido L-ascórbico com O_2 em ácido L-desidroascórbico. Algumas formas de a. também utilizam $NADP^+$. Usado como enzima antitumoral. SIN ascorbase.
ascor·bic ac·id (as-kōr′bik). Ácido ascórbico; usado na prevenção do escorbuto como um forte agente redutor e como antioxidante. SIN antiscorbutic vitamin, cevitamic acid, vitamin C. [G. *a-* priv. + L. Mod. *scorbutus*, escorbuto, do alemão]
ascor·byl pal·mi·tate (as-kōr′bil pal′mi-tāt). Palmitato de ascorbila; usado como conservante em preparações farmacêuticas.
as·co·spore (as′kō-spōr). Ascósporo; um esporo formado dentro de um asco; o esporo sexual dos Ascomicetos. [G. *askos*, bolsa, + *sporos*, semente]
ASCUS No sistema Bethesda, acrônimo para atypical squamous *cells* of undetermined significance (células escamosas atípicas de importância indeterminada), em *cell*. VER TAMBÉM Bethesda *system*.
as·cus, pl. **as·ci** (as′kŭs, as′ī). Asco; a célula saculiforme dos Ascomycetes

em que os ascósporos se desenvolvem após a fusão nuclear e a meiose. [G. *askos*, bolsa]

♻ **-ase.** Sufixo que indica uma enzima; é sufixo do nome da substância (substrato) sobre o qual a enzima atua; p.ex., fosfatase, lipase, proteinase. Também pode indicar a reação catalisada, p.ex., decarboxilase, oxidase. As enzimas que receberam nomes antes do estabelecimento da convenção geralmente possuem uma terminação -ina; p.ex., pepsina, ptialina, tripsina. [De *(diast)ase*, uma amilase que converte o amido em maltose, de G. *diastasis*, separação, de *dia-*, através, separado, + *stasis*, uma parada]

ase·cre·to·ry (ā-sē-krē′tō-rē). Não-secretório; sem secreção.

Aselli (Asellius, Asellio), Gasparo, anatomista italiano em Cremona, 1581–1626. VER A. *pancreas*.

asep·sis (ă-sep′sis, ā-). Assepsia; uma condição na qual não há organismos patogênicos vivos; um estado de esterilidade (2). [G. *a-*, priv. + *sēpsis*, putrefação]

asep·tate (ā-sep′tāt, ā-). Asseptado; nos fungos, um termo que descreve a ausência das paredes cruzadas em um filamento de hifa ou em um esporo. [G. *a-* priv. + L. *saeptum*, uma partição]

asep·tic (ā-sep′tik, ā-). Asséptico; caracterizado por ou relativo à assepsia.

asep·ti·cism (ā-sep′ti-sizm, ā-). Assepticismo; a prática da cirurgia asséptica.

ase·quence (ā-sē′kwens). Falta da seqüência normal, especificamente entre as contrações atrial e ventricular.

asex·u·al (ā-seks′ū-ăl). Assexual. **1.** Referente à reprodução sem fusão nuclear em um organismo. **2.** Que não possui desejo ou interesse sexual. [G. *a-* priv. + sexual]

Ashby, Winifred, hematologista no século XX. VER Ashby *method*.

Asherman, Joseph G., ginecologista tcheco-eslovaco, *1889. VER A. *syndrome*.

Ashman, R., fisiologista norte-americano no século XX. VER A. *phenomenon*.

asialism (ā′syal-izm). Assialismo; ausência de saliva. [G. *a-* priv. + *sialon*, saliva + *-ism*]

asi·a·lo·gly·co·pro·tein (ā-sī-al′ō-glī-kō-prō-tēn). Assialoglicoproteína; uma glicoproteína sem uma porção de ácido siálico; essas proteínas são reconhecidas por receptores de a. e são direcionadas para a degradação.

asit·ia (ā-sish′ē-ă). Assitia; aversão perante a visão ou pensamento sobre alimentos. [G. *a-* priv. + *sitos*, alimento]

Askanazy, Max, patologista alemão, 1865–1940. VER A. *cell*.

Ask-Upmark, Erik, patologista sueco do século XX. VER Ask-Upmark *kidney*.

ASL Abreviatura de American Sign *Language* (linguagem americana de sinais).

Asn (Asx). Símbolo para asparagine (asparagina) ou seu mono- ou diradical.

aso·cial (ā-sō′shŭl). Associal; não-social; isolado da sociedade; indiferente às regras ou costumes sociais; p.ex., um recluso, uma pessoa esquizofrênica regredida, uma personalidade esquizóide. Cf. antisocial.

aso·ma, pl. **aso·ma·ta** (ā-sō′mă, -sō′mă-tă). Assoma; um feto com apenas um corpo rudimentar. [G. *a-* priv. + *sōma*, corpo]

Asp (Asx) Símbolo de aspartic acid (ácido aspártico) ou suas formas radicais.

as·pal·a·so·ma (as-pal-ă-sō′mă). Aspalassoma; termo obsoleto para um feto malformado com eventração na parte inferior do abdome, apresentando aberturas separadas para intestino, bexiga e órgãos sexuais. [G. *aspalax*, uma mola + *sōma*, corpo]

as·par·a·gi·nase (as-par′ă-ji-nās). Asparaginase. **1.** Uma enzima que catalisa a hidrólise da L-asparagina em ácido L-aspártico e amônia. **2.** A enzima da *Escherichia coli*, usada no tratamento da leucemia aguda e outras doenças neoplásicas.

Erwinia **L-a.,** L-a. das bactérias *Erwinia*, usada em pacientes que são alérgicos à L-a. da *Escherichia coli*. VER TAMBÉM asparginase.

as·par·a·gine (N, Asn) (as-par′ă-jin). Asparaginase; $NH_2COCH_2CH(NH_3^+COO^-)$; a β-amida do ácido aspártico, o L-isômero é um aminoácido nutricionalmente não-essencial que ocorre em proteínas; um diurético.

a. ligase, a. ligase; uma ácido:amônia ligase (amida sintetase) formando a L-asparagina e L-glutamato a partir do L-aspartato e L-glutamina, com a clivagem concomitante do ATP em AMP e pirofosfato. Em condições não-fisiológicas, a enzima dos mamíferos pode usar amônia como o doador de nitrogênio. A a. também exibe atividade semelhante à glutaminase. SIN a. synthetase.

a. synthetase, a. sintetase. SIN a. ligase.

as·pa·rag·i·nyl (as-par′ă-jin-il). Asparaginil; o radical aminoacil da asparagina.

As·par·a·gus (as-par′ă-gŭs). Aspargo; um gênero de plantas da família Liliaceae. *A. officinalis* é um vegetal comestível, cujo rizoma e as raízes, juntamente com os brotos novos comestíveis, foram empregados como diurético. [L. de G. *asparagos*]

as·par·tame (as′pŭr-tām). Aspartame; um agente adoçante com baixa caloria, cerca de 200 vezes mais doce que a sacarose, utilizado por pessoas que precisam restringir a ingesta de açúcar e calorias.

as·par·tase (as-par′tās). Aspartase, aspartato amônia-liase. SIN aspartate ammonia-lyase.

as·par·tate (as-par′tāt). Aspartato; um sal ou éster do ácido aspártico.

a. aminotransferase (AST), a. aminotransferase; uma enzima que catalisa a transferência reversível de um grupamento amino do ácido L-glutâmico para o ácido oxalacético, formando o ácido α-cetoglutárico e o ácido L-aspártico; um exame diagnóstico na hepatite viral e no infarto do miocárdio. SIN a. transaminase, glutamic-aspartic transaminase, glutamic-oxaloacetic transaminase, serum glutamic-oxaloacetic transaminase.

a. ammonia-lyase, a. amônia-liase; uma enzima não existente em mamíferos que catalisa a conversão do ácido L-aspártico em ácido fumárico, liberando amônia. SIN aspartase, fumaric aminase.

a. carbamoyltransferase, a. carbamoiltransferase; uma enzima que catalisa a formação do ureidossuccinato (N-carbamoil-L-aspartato) e ortofosfato pela transferência de uma porção carbamoil do carbamoilfosfato para o grupamento amino do L-aspartato; participa na biossíntese da pirimidina.

a. kinase, a. cinase; uma enzima que catalisa a fosforilação pelo ATP do L-aspartato para formar 4-fosfo-L-aspartato (β-aspartil fosfato) e ADP.

a. transaminase, a. transaminase. SIN a. aminotransferase.

as·par·tate 1-de·car·box·yl·ase. Aspartato 1-descarboxilase. SIN *glutamate decarxylase*.

as·par·tate 4-de·car·box·yl·ase. Aspartato 4-descarboxilase; aspartato β-descarboxilase; uma carboxi-liase que converte L-aspartato em L-alanina (liberando CO_2); descarboxila aminomalonato e (nas bactérias) remove SO_2 da cisteinossulfinato. VER TAMBÉM desulfinase.

as·par·tic ac·id (Asp) (as-par′tik). Ácido aspártico; $HOOC-CH_2-CH-NH_2)-COOH$; o L-isômero é um dos aminoácidos que ocorrem naturalmente em proteínas. O D-isômero é encontrado nas paredes celulares de muitas bactérias.

as·par·tyl (as-par′til). Aspartil; o radical aminoacil do ácido aspártico.

β-as·par·tyl (ace·tyl·glu·cos·a·mine) (as-par′til-as′e-til-gloo′kō-să-mēn). β-Aspartil (acetilglicosamina); nome errôneo para 1-(β-asparagino)-N-acetilglicosamina ou 1-(β-aspartamido)-N-acetilglicosamina, ou, originalmente, 1-(β-L-aspartamido)-N-2-acetamido-1,2-didesoxi-β-D-glicose. Um composto da N-acetilglicosamina e asparagina, ligado através do nitrogênio da amida do último e do carbono-1 do primeiro. Uma importante ligação estrutural em muitas glicoproteínas. Níveis elevados são encontrados em certos casos de retardo mental progressivo.

as·par·tyl·gly·co·sa·mine (as-par′til-glī′kō-să-mēn). Aspartilglicosamina; termo genérico para compostos da asparagina e um açúcar 2-amino; p.ex., β-aspartil(acetilglicosamina).

as·par·tyl·gly·cos·a·mi·nid·ase (as-par′til-glī′kō-să-mi-ni-dās). Aspartilglicosaminidase; uma enzima hidrolítica que cliva o L-aspartato de aspartilglicosaminas. A deficiência de a. pode resultar em aspartilglicosaminúria.

as·par·tyl·gly·cos·a·mi·nu·ria (as-par′til-glī′kō-să-mi-noor′ē-ă) [MIM*208400]. Aspartilglicosaminúria; um distúrbio lipossomial devido à deficiência da aspartoglicosaminidase, resultando em acúmulo de aspartilglicosamina na urina e no líquido espinal; caracterizado por sintomas usualmente nos primeiros meses de vida, com infecções recorrentes e diarréia; retardo mental, convulsões, aspectos faciais rudes e anormalidades esqueléticas são evidenciados pela adolescência. Herança autossômica recessiva, causada por mutação no gene da aspartoglicosaminidase (AGA) em 4q.

as·pect (as′pekt). Aspecto, face, norma. **1.** A maneira do aparecimento; aparência. **2.** O lado de um objeto que é dirigido em qualquer direção designada. SIN norma (1). [L. *aspectus*, de *a-spicio*, pp. *-spectus*, olhar em]

facial a. [TA], a. facial; o contorno do crânio visto por diante. SIN norma facialis [TA], frontal a. *, norma frontalis*, norma anterior.

frontal a., a. frontal; *termo oficial alternativo para *facial a.*

lateral a. [TA], a. lateral; o perfil do crânio; o contorno do crânio visto a partir de um lado. SIN norma lateralis [TA], norma temporalis.

occipital a. [TA], a. occipital; o contorno do crânio visto por trás. SIN norma occipitalis [TA], norma posterior.

superior a., [TA], a. superior; o contorno da superfície do crânio visto por cima. SIN norma superior [TA], norma verticalis*, vertical a.*

vertical a., a. vertical; *termo oficial alternativo para *superior a.*

Asperger, Hans, psiquiatra austríaco do século XX. VER A. *disorder*.

as·per·gil·lic ac·id (as-per-jil′ik). Ácido aspergílico; produzido por *Aspergillus flavus*; um agente antibiótico moderadamente ativo contra bactérias Gram-positivas e Gram-negativas, mas tóxico para os tecidos animais.

as·per·gil·lin (as-per-jil′in). Aspergilina; um pigmento preto obtido a partir da várias espécies de *Aspergillus*; termo inadequadamente utilizado para designar vários antibióticos obtidos a partir do *Aspergillus*.

ℹ **as·per·gil·lo·ma** (as′per-ji-lō′mă). Aspergiloma; uma massa de hifas de *Aspergillus* semelhante a uma bola que coloniza uma cavidade existente no pulmão. [aspergillus + *-oma*, tumor]

as·per·gil·lo·sis (as′per-ji-lō′sis). Aspergilose; a presença do fungo *Aspergillus* nos tecidos ou invadindo tecidos (a. invasivo) ou colonizando cavidades corporais contendo ar. VER TAMBÉM aspergillio.

acute invasive a., a. invasiva aguda; uma infecção agressiva, principalmente em pessoas gravemente imunocomprometidas, que consiste na invasão dos vasos sanguíneos e infarto tecidual por *Aspergillus fumigatus*. Com freqüência, a doença mimetiza os sinais e sintomas de pneumonia bacteriana aguda.

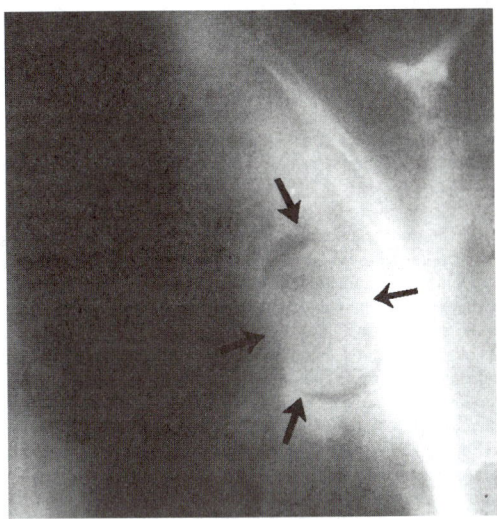

aspergiloma: tomografia mostrando a massa fúngica em uma cavidade pulmonar preexistente resultante de tuberculose

allergic bronchopulmonary a., a. broncopulmonar alérgica; uma doença em que o fungo cresce no muco (provocado por inflamação), que pode ser expectorado como cilindros brônquicos amarelos e provoca obstrução brônquica intermitente, com infiltrados transitórios observados em radiografias; é freqüente a ocorrência de asma e a destruição da parede brônquica acaba resultando em uma forma proximal de bronquiectasia.
chronic necrotizing a., a. necrotizante crônica; uma infecção indolente, porém lentamente progressiva, dos pulmões em pacientes com doença pulmonar subjacente, causada por *Aspergillus*. A maioria dos pacientes afetados apresenta discreta depressão do sistema imune, causada por doenças como o diabetes.
disseminated a., a. disseminada; uma variedade da a. broncopulmonar caracterizada por infecção generalizada do pulmão por *Aspergillus*, que geralmente acontece em pessoas com resposta imune defeituosa.
As·per·gil·lus (as-per-jil'ŭs). Um gênero de fungos (classe Ascomycetes) que contém muitas espécies, das quais várias apresentam esporos pretos, acastanhados ou esverdeados. Algumas espécies são patogênicas para os seres humanos, aves e outros animais. Existem cerca de 300 espécies nesse gênero. [L. Med. um aspersório, de L. *aspergo*, aspergir]
A. clava'tus, uma espécie de fungo isolada do solo e das fezes; produz uma micotoxina carcinogênica conhecida como patulina.
A. fla'vus, uma espécie de fungo com conídios amarelo-esverdeados que é encontrado crescendo em grãos; pode produzir aflatoxina, que é a causa da aflatoxicose em aves e no gado, e é carcinogênico para ratos e, possivelmente, para seres humanos; causa aspergilose invasiva em seres humanos e animais.
A. fumiga'tus, uma espécie de fungo que fornece os antibióticos fumigacina e fumigatina, sendo a causa comum da aspergilose em seres humanos e pássaros.
A. nid'ulans, uma espécie que causa uma forma de micetoma e, ocasionalmente, causa aspergilose em seres humanos e em outros animais.
A. ni'ger, uma espécie com esporos pretos, freqüentemente presente no meato acústico externo, mas raramente patogênica; usada na fabricação comercial dos ácidos cítrico e glucônico.
A. ter'reus, uma espécie que produz o antibiótico citrinina; foi isolado a partir de otomicose, principalmente no Japão e Formosa, e, ocasionalmente, causa aspergilose em seres humanos e animais.
asper·mat·o·gen·ic (ā-sper'mă-tō-jen'ik' ā-sper'). Aspermatogênico; que não consegue produzir espermatozóide. [G *a-* priv. + *sperma*, semente, + *-gen*, produção]
asper·mia (ā-sper'mē-ă, ā-sper'). Aspermia; falta da secreção ou da expulsão de sêmen após a ejaculação.
as·per·sion (as-per'zhŭn). Aspersão; uma forma de hidroterapia na qual a água, em determinada temperatura, é aspergida sobre o corpo. [L. *aspersio*, um aspersório]
aspher·ic (ā-sfer'ik). Asférico, anesférico; indica uma superfície parabolóide, especialmente uma lente ou espelho, que elimina a aberração esférica. [G. *a-* priv. + *sphaira*, esfera]
as·phyg·mia (as-fig'mē-ă). Asfigmia; ausência temporária do pulso. [G. *a-* priv. + *phygmos*, pulso]
as·phyx·ia (as-fik'sē-ă). Asfixia; troca comprometida ou ausente de oxigênio e dióxido de carbono (conceito ventilatório); hipercapnia e hipoxia (ou anoxia) combinadas. [G. *a.* priv. + *sphyzō*, pulsar]

cyanotic a., a. cianótica; a. até o ponto de destruição suficiente da hemoglobina para produzir cianose.
local a., a. local; estagnação da circulação, por vezes resultando em gangrena local, especialmente dos dedos das mãos; um dos sintomas geralmente associados à doença de Raynaud.
symmetric a., a. simétrica. SIN Raynaud *syndrome.*
traumatic a., a. traumática; a. cianótica devido a traumatismo; o extravasamento de sangue para a pele e as conjuntivas, produzido por aumento mecânico súbito na pressão venosa, análogo ao teste de Rumpel-Leede; é comum em pessoas que foram enforcadas e é observado ocasionalmente em lesões por esmagamento. SIN pressure stasis.
as·phyx·i·al (as-fik'sē-ăl). Asfíxico, asfixioso; relativo à asfixia.
as·phyx·i·ant (as-fik'sē-ănt). Asfixiante. **1.** Que produz asfixia. SIN asphyxiating. **2.** Qualquer coisa, especialmente um gás, que produza asfixia.
as·phyx·i·ate (as'fik'sē-āt). Asfixiar; induzir asfixia.
as·phyx·i·at·ing (as-fik'sē-āt-ing). Asfixiante. SIN asphyxiant (1).
as·phyx·i·a·tion (as-fik-sē-ā'shŭn). Asfixia; a produção ou o estado de asfixia.
As·pic·u·lu·ris tet·rap·tera (as-pik-ū-loo'ris tet-rap'ter-ă). O oxiúro do camundongo, um nematódeo oxiurídio abundante no ceco ou no intestino grosso do camundongo, juntamente com outro oxiurídeo do camundongo, *Syphacia obvelata*; também é encontrado em outros roedores, incluindo *Rattus*. [Pers. *espic*, do L. *spica*, ouvido, espiga; *tetra-* + *pteron*, asa]
as·pid·in (as-pid'in). Aspidina; um princípio tóxico ativo, $C_{25}H_{32}O_8$, contido no aspídio (*Dryopteris*).
as·pid·i·nol (as-pid'i-nol). Aspidinol; um álcool, $C_{12}H_{16}O_4$, ocorrendo no aspídio (*Dryopteris*).
as·pid·i·um (as-pid'ē-ŭm). Aspídio; rizomas e extremidades do *Dryopteris filix-mas* (dentebrura ou feto-macho) ou do *Dryopteris marginalis* (a. -americano ou feto-marginal, família Polypodiaceae); usado no tratamento da infestação por tênias, usualmente na forma da oleorresina ou extrato, mas, por causa de sua toxicidade potencial, seu uso é restrito aos pacientes que não respondem ao tratamento com medicamentos mais seguros, como diclorofeno, niclosamida ou quinacrina. [G. *aspidion*, um pequeno escudo, dim. de *aspis*, escudo]
as·pi·do·sam·ine (as'pi-dō-sam'ēn). Aspidosamina; uma base forte, $C_{22}H_{28}N_2O_2$, derivada de quebracho; um irritante tóxico.
as·pi·do·sper·mine (as'pi-dō-sper'mēn). Aspidospermina; um alcalóide, $C_{22}H_{30}N_2O_2$, obtido a partir do quebracho, um irritante.
as·pi·rate. 1. Aspirar; remover por sucção. **2.** (as'pi-rāt'). Aspirar; inalar para as vias aéreas material particulado estranho, como vômito. **3.** (as'pi-rit). Aspirado; corpo estranho, alimento, conteúdo gástrico ou líquido, incluindo saliva, que é inalado. [L. *a-spiro*, pp. *-atus*, para respirar, fazer o som de H]
as·pi·ra·tion (as-pi-rā'shŭn). Aspiração. **1.** Remoção, por sucção, de um gás, líquido ou tecido a partir de uma cavidade corporal ou órgão pelo acúmulo incomum ou a partir de um recipiente. **2.** Sucção respiratória de líquido ou qualquer material estranho, principalmente de conteúdo gástrico ou alimento, nas vias aéreas. **3.** Uma técnica cirúrgica para catarata, exigindo uma pequena incisão na córnea, rotura da cápsula da lente do olho, fragmentação do material da lente do olho e retirada com uma agulha. [L. *aspiratio*, de *aspira*, respirar]
meconium a., a. mecânica; a. intra-uterina pelo feto de líquido amniótico contaminado por mecônio resultando de angústia hipóxica fetal.
as·pi·ra·tor (as'pi-rā'-ter, -tōr). Aspirador; um aparelho para remover o líquido, ar ou tecido por sucção de qualquer uma das cavidades corporais; consiste geralmente em uma agulha oca (trocarte) e cânula, conectados por um equipo a um recipiente com vácuo por uma seringa ou bomba de ar (aspiração) de sentido inverso.
vacuum a., a. a vácuo; um instrumento para remover os produtos de concepção por aspiração depois da dilatação cervical.
water a., a. de água; uma bomba ejetora operada à água e comumente usada como uma bomba de sucção laboratorial.
as·pi·rin (as'pi-rin). Nome comercial do ácido acetilsalicílico; um agente analgésico, antipirético e antiinflamatório amplamente utilizado; também usado como agente antiplaquetário. SIN acetylsalicylic acid.
asple·nia (ā-splē'nē-ă). Asplenia; ausência congênita ou adquirida do baço (p.ex., depois da remoção cirúrgica).
functional a., a. funcional; ausência da função esplênica devido ao infarto espontâneo do baço, como acontece na anemia falciforme.
a. with cardiovascular anomalies, a. com anomalias cardiovasculares. SIN polisplenia.
asplen·ic (ā-splen'ik). Asplênico; que não possui baço.
aspo·rog·e·nous (as-pō-roj'e-nŭs). Asporogenoso; que não produz esporos. [G *a-* priv. + *sporos*, semente, + *-gen*, produção]
aspo·rous (as-pōr'ŭs). Ásporo; incapaz de produzir esporos. [G *a-* priv. + *sporos*, semente]
aspor·u·late (as-pōr'ū-lāt). Asporulado; que não forma esporo.
as·say (as'sā, ā-sā'). **1.** Análise, ensaio; a avaliação quantitativa ou qualitativa de uma substância à procura de impurezas, toxidez, etc.; os resultados des-

sa avaliação. **2.** Examinar; sujeitar a análise. **3.** Teste de pureza; estudo. [I. M., do Fr. Ant. *essaier*, do L. Tard. *exagium*, uma ponderação]
  Ames a., a. de Ames. SIN Ames *test*.
  biologic a., a. biológica. SIN biotest.
  clonogenic a., a. clonogênica; cultura *in vitro* de células neoplásicas para testar suas radiossensibilidades ou quimiossensibilidades, e provável eficácia clínica de um agente terapêutico.
  competitive binding a., a. de união competitiva; termo geral para uma a. em que uma substância compete pelo ligante marcado *versus* o não-marcado; após a separação do ligante livre e ligado, a concentração do ligante livre é inversamente proporcional à quantidade do ligante ligado marcado. Os valores são comparados a padrões conhecidos. VER TAMBÉM enzyme-linked immunosorbent a., radioreceptor a., immunoassay, enzyme-multiplied *immunoassay* technique, radioimmunoassay. SIN displacement analysis, saturation analysis.
  complement binding a., a. de união de complemento. SIN complement *fixation*.
  double antibody sandwich a., a. dupla com anticorpo; para detectar antígenos; uma aplicação do método ELISA, no qual o material a ser testado quanto à presença de antígeno é acrescentado a reservatórios revestidos com anticorpo conhecido; a presença de antígeno fixado à camada de anticorpo pode ser determinada por meios diretos, através do acréscimo de anticorpo ligado à enzima do sistema indicador, ou por meios indiretos, através do acréscimo, primeiramente, de anticorpo conhecido não-marcado, cuja fixação ao antígeno pode ser demonstrada pela adição de anticorpo imunoglobulina-específico ligada à enzima.
  EAC rosette a. (ro-zet′as′sā), análise da roseta EAC. VER EAC *rosette*.
  enzyme-linked immunosorbent a. (ELISA), a. imunossorvente ligado a enzima; uma a. de união *in vitro* na qual uma enzima e seu substrato (em lugar de uma substância radioativa) servem como o sistema indicador; nos testes positivos, os dois produzem uma substância colorida ou facilmente reconhecida de outra forma; os testes são realizados em reservatórios de poliestireno ou outro material aos quais as imunoglobulinas ou preparações antigênicas são prontamente adsorvidas; a enzima é ligada à imunoglobulina (ou antígeno) conhecida e, em testes positivos, permanece no reservatório como parte do complexo antígeno-anticorpo (Ag-Ac) disponível para reagir com seu substrato, quando adicionado.
  Grunstein-Hogness a., a. de Grunstein-Hogness; um procedimento para identificar clones de plasmídios pela hibridização de colônias.
  hemizona a. (hem′ē-zō-nä), a. da hemizona; teste diagnóstico que avalia a capacidade de ligação do espermatozóide à zona pelúcida.
  hemolytic plaque a., a. da placa hemolítica. SIN Jerne plaque a.
  immunochemical a., imunoensaio. SIN immunoassay.
  immunoradiometric a., a. imunorradiométrica; uma a. que difere do radioimunoensaio convencional pelo fato de que o composto a ser medido combina-se diretamente com os anticorpos com marcação radioativa.
  indirect a., a. indireta; para anticorpo; uma aplicação do método ELISA no qual o soro a ser examinado (à procura do anticorpo) é colocado em poços revestidos com o antígeno conhecido; a presença do anticorpo ligado à camada de antígeno pode ser determinada pela adição de anticorpo imunoglobulina-específico que está ligado à enzima do sistema indicador, seguida pela adição de substrato ao agregado lavado.
  Jerne plaque a., a. de placa de Jerne; uma a. que enumera as células formadoras de anticorpos individuais. SIN hemolytic plaque a.
  Lowry-Folin a., a. de Lowry-Folin. SIN Lowry protein a.
  Lowry protein a., a. da proteína de Lowry; um método para determinar as concentrações de proteína usando o reagente de Folin-Ciocalteu. SIN Lowry-Folin a.
  radioreceptor a., a. de rádio-receptor; uma a. de união competitiva em que o fixador é uma membrana ou tecido receptor, em lugar de um anticorpo.
  Raji cell radioimmune a., a. radioimune da célula Raji, para imunocomplexos; um procedimento pelo qual imunocomplexos adsorvidos de um soro-teste por uma preparação padronizada de células linfoblastóides (Raji) são analisados quanto à sua capacidade de fixar anticorpo marcado com I^{125} a imunoglobulina.
assessment. Avaliação; estimativa.
  health risk a. (h.r.a.), a. de risco de saúde; método para descrever a possibilidade de uma pessoa adoecer ou morrer de uma afecção especificada, com base nos cálculos atuariais que comparam a chance de contrair a afecção com a chance da população geral, expressa como a idade esperada em que a doença ou morte ocorrerá, e idealizada como um meio de chamar a atenção da pessoa para as prováveis consequências do comportamento de risco para a saúde.
Asségzat, Jules, antropólogo francês, 1832–1876. VER A. *triangle*.
as·sim·i·la·ble (ă-sim′i-lă-bl). Assimilável; capaz de sofrer assimilação. VER assimilation.
as·sim·i·la·tion (ă-sim-i-lā′shŭn). Assimilação. **1.** Incorporação nos tecidos de materiais digeridos a partir de alimentos. **2.** Amalgamação e modificação das informações e experiências recentemente percebidas na estrutura cognitiva existente. [L. *as-similo*, pp. *-atus*, tornar semelhante]
  ammonia a., a. da amônia; a utilização da amônia (ou de íons amônio) na síntese final de moléculas contendo nitrogênio, p.ex., glutamina sintetase. SIN ammonia fixation.
  reproductive a., a. reprodutiva; na teoria sensoriomotora é um processo cognitivo ativo pelo qual a experiência passada é aplicada a situações novas.
Assmann, Herbert, clínico alemão, 1882–1950. VER A. tuberculous *infiltrate*.
as·so·ci·ate (ă-sō′shi-āt) **1.** Associado; qualquer item ou indivíduo agrupado com outros por algum fator comum. **2** (ă-sō′shē-āt). Associar; realizar uma associação.
  paired a.'s, associações pareadas; palavras, sílabas ou outros itens aprendidos aos pares, de modo que, quando um é apresentado, sua a. deva ser lembrada.
as·so·ci·a·tion (ă-sō-sē-ā′shŭn). Associação. **1.** Uma conexão de pessoas, coisas ou idéias por algum fator comum. **2.** Uma conexão funcional de duas idéias, eventos ou fenômenos fisiológicos estabelecida através do aprendizado ou da experiência. VER TAMBÉM conditioning. **3.** Dependência estatística entre dois ou mais eventos, características ou outras variáveis. **4.** Em genética médica, um agrupamento de anomalias congênitas encontrado em conjunto com maior freqüência que seria a esperada; o uso desse termo implica que a causa é desconhecida. [L. *as-socio*, pp. *-sociatus*, unir; *ad + socius*, companhia]
  CHARGE a., a. CHARGE; um agrupamento particular de anomalias congênitas encontradas em conjunto com uma freqüência maior que a esperada. As pessoas afetadas apresentam *c*oloboma ocular, defeitos cardíacos (*h*earts) (tipicamente tetralogia de Fallot, persistência do canal arterial ou defeito do septo interventricular ou interatrial), *a*tresia de cóanos, anomalias *r*enais e retardo do crescimento e/ou desenvolvimento, anomalias *g*enitais nos homens, como pênis pequeno ou criptorquidismo, e anormalidades dos ouvidos (*e*ars) ou surdez. SIN CHARGE *syndrome*.
  clang a., a. do tinido; associações psíquicas resultantes de sons; freqüentemente encontradas na fase maníaca da psicose maníaco-depressiva.
  dream a.'s, associações de sonhos; as memórias e emoções mencionadas por um paciente que tenta compreender um sonho diante da solicitação de um psicanalista.
  free a., a. livre; uma técnica psicanalítica investigativa em que o paciente verbaliza, sem reservas ou censura, o conteúdo que lhe passa na mente; os conflitos verbalizados que emergem constituem resistências que constituem a base das interpretações do psicanalista.
  genetic a., a. genética; a ocorrência em conjunto, em uma população, com freqüência maior que a que pode ser explicada pela probabilidade, de dois ou mais traços, dos quais pelo menos um é conhecido como sendo de origem genética.
  independent practice a. (IPA), a. de prática independente; uma a. de médicos independentes ou de pequenos grupos de médicos formada com a finalidade de fazer contrato com uma ou mais organizações de cuidados gerenciados da saúde. Os médicos afiliados fornecem os serviços médicos para os pacientes da organização em seus próprios consultórios e podem realizar serviços particulares. VER TAMBÉM managed *care*, health maintenance *organization*.
  loose a.'s, associações fracas; manifestação de um distúrbio do pensamento pelo qual as respostas do paciente não se relacionam com as perguntas do entrevistador ou um parágrafo, uma sentença ou frase não se liga de maneira lógica àquela que ocorre antes ou depois.
as·so·ci·a·tion·ism (ă-sō-sē-ā′shŭn-izm). Associacionismo; em psicologia, a teoria de que a compreensão do mundo pelo homem ocorre através de idéias associadas à experiência sensorial e não através de idéias inatas.
as·sort·ment (ă-sōrt′ment). Agrupamento; em genética, a relação entre traços genéticos não-alélicos que são transmitidos de pai para filho de forma mais ou menos independente, de acordo com o grau de ligação entre os respectivos *loci*.
  independent a., a. independente; o padrão de transmissão de *loci* não-ligados.
as·sump·tion. Suposição, pressuposição; crença adquirida no final de um argumento como uma base para dedução e inferência. Comumente confundida com uma hipótese, uma conclusão no final do argumento ou uma inferência baseada em dados empíricos.
AST Abreviatura para *aspartate* aminotransferase (aspartato aminotransferase).
as·ta·sia (ă-stā′zē-ă). Astasia; incapacidade, decorrente de incoordenação muscular, de ficar em pé. [G. oscilação, de *a-* priv. + *stasis*, ficar em pé]
as·ta·sia-aba·sia (ă-stā′zē-ă-ă-bā′zē-ă). Astasia-abasia; a incapacidade de ficar em pé ou caminhar de uma maneira normal; a marcha é bizarra e não é sugestiva de uma lesão orgânica específica; freqüentemente o paciente oscila muito e quase cai, mas se recupera no último momento; um sintoma de reação de histeria de conversão. SIN Blocq disease.
astat·ic (ă-stat′ik). Astático; pertinente à astasia.
as·ta·tine (At) (as′tă-tēn). Astatínio; um elemento radioativo artificial da série halogenada; número atômico 85, peso atômico 211. [G. *astatos*, instável]
aste·a·to·sis (ă-stē-ă-tō′sis). Asteatose; secreção diminuída ou interrompida das glândulas sebáceas. [G. *a-* priv. + *stear* (*steat-*), gordura]
  a. cu′tis, a. cutânea; pele seca e descamativa com diminuição da secreção sebácea.
astem·i·zole. Astemizol; uma substância bloqueadora da histamina, do tipo H-1, com baixa tendência sedativa.
as·ter (as′ter). Áster. SIN astrosphere. [L. Mod. de G. *astēr*, uma estrela]

sperm a., a. espermático. SIN sperm-aster.
as·ter·e·og·no·sis (ă-stēr-og-nō′sis). Estereognose, estereognosia. SIN tactile agnosia. [G. *a-* priv. + *stereos*, sólido, + *gnōsis*, conhecimento]
as·te·ri·on (ăs-tē′rē-on) [TA]. Astério; um ponto craniométrico na região da fontanela póstero-lateral, ou mastóide, na junção das suturas lambdóide, occipitomastóidea e parietomastóidea. [G. *asterios*, estrelar]
as·ter·i·o·sap·on·ins (ă-stēr′ē-ō-sap′ō-ninz). Asteriossaponinas. SIN asteriotoxins.
as·ter·i·o·tox·ins (ă-stēr′ē-ō-tok′sinz). Asteriotoxinas; esteróides tóxicos produzidos pela estrela-do-mar (Asteroidea). SIN asteriosaponins.
aster·ix·is (as-ter-ik′sis). Asterixe; movimentos de contratura involuntária, especialmente nas mãos, mais bem percebidos ao se pedir que o paciente estenda os braços, faça a dorsiflexão dos punhos e abra os dedos das mãos; decorrente de lapsos arrítmicos da postura sustentada; observado basicamente com várias encefalopatias metabólicas e tóxicas, sobretudo encefalopatia hepática. SIN flapping tremor. [G. *a-* priv. + *stērixis*, posição fixa]
aster·nal (ā-ster′năl). **1.** Asternal; que não se articula com o esterno, p.ex., uma costela. **2.** Sem um esterno. [G. *a-* priv. + *sternon*, tórax]
aster·nia (ā-ster′nē-ă). Asternia; ausência congênita do esterno.
As·ter·o·coc·cus. *Mycoplasma.* SIN *Mycoplasma.* [L Mod. de G. *astēr*, uma estrela, + *kokkos*, uma baga]
as·ter·oid (as′tē-royd). Asteróide; semelhante a uma estrela. [G. *astēr*, estrela, + *eidos*, semelhança]
as·the·nia (as-thē′nē-ă). Astenia; fraqueza ou debilidade. SIN adynamia (1). [G. *astheneia*, fraqueza, de *a-* priv. + *sthenos*, força]
neurocirculatory a., a. neurocirculatória; um termo obsoleto para um tipo de neurose de ansiedade originalmente encontrada, com freqüência, entre militares durante os tempos de guerra, na qual os sintomas cardiorrespiratórios, como palpitação, pulso rápido e dor precordial, eram proeminentes.
as·the·nic (as-then′ik). Astênico. **1.** Relativo à astenia. **2.** Indica um tipo corporal magro, delicado.
as·the·no·pia (as-thē-nō′pē-ă). Astenopia; sintomas subjetivos de fadiga ocular, desconforto, lacrimejamento e cefaléias que se originam do uso dos olhos. SIN eyestrain. [G. *astheneia*, fraqueza, + *ōps*, olho]
accommodative a., a. acomodativa; a. decorrente de erros de refração e contração excessiva do músculo ciliar.
muscular a., a. decorrente do desequilíbrio dos músculos oculares extrínsecos.
nervous a., a. nervosa; a. devido a doença nervosa funcional ou orgânica.
as·the·nop·ic (as-thē-nop′ik). Astenópico; relativo a ou que sofre de astenopia.
as·the·no·sper·mia (as-thē-nō-sper′mē-ă). Astenospermia. SIN asthenozoospermia. [G. *astheneia*, fraqueza, + *sperma*, semente, sêmen]
asthenozoospermia (as′thē-nō-zō-ō-sperm′ē-ă). Astenozoospermia; perda ou redução da mobilidade dos espermatozóides, freqüentemente associada a infertilidade. SIN asthenospermia. [G. *astheneia*, fraqueza, + *zōos*, vivo, + *sperma*, semente, sêmen, + -ia]
asth·ma (az′mă). Asma; uma doença inflamatória dos pulmões caracterizada por obstrução reversível das vias aéreas (na maioria dos casos). Originalmente, um termo empregado para "dificuldade de respirar"; hoje utilizado para indicar a. brônquica. SIN reactive airway disease. [G.]
atopic a., a. atópica; a. brônquica decorrente da atopia.

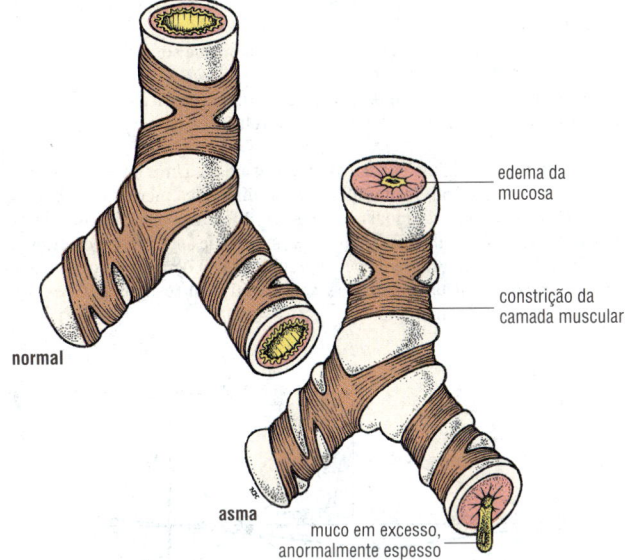

asma: mostrando as alterações no bronquíolo durante a crise de asma

bronchial a., a. brônquica; um distúrbio agudo ou crônico caracterizado por redução ampla e, em grande parte, reversível no calibre dos brônquios e bronquíolos, devido a graus variados de espasmos da musculatura lisa, edema de mucosa e muco excessivo na luz das vias aéreas; os sintomas cardeais são dispnéia, sibilos e tosse; as crises ou exacerbações podem ser induzidas por alérgenos transportados pelo ar (p.ex., mofos, pólen, pêlos de animais, poeira de ácaros e antígenos de barata), irritantes inalados (p.ex., ar frio, fumaça de cigarro, ozônio), exercício físico, infecção respiratória, estresse psicológico ou outros fatores; os sinais e sintomas da a. brônquica são causados pela liberação local de espasmógenos e mediadores inflamatórios (histaminas, leucotrienos, prostaglandinas) e outras substâncias a partir dos mastócitos, eosinófilos, linfócitos, neutrófilos e células epiteliais; o calibre das vias aéreas pode ser reduzido de forma abrupta e drástica durante um paroxismo ou depois de um teste diagnóstico com metacolina ou histamina, e pode retornar rapidamente à normalidade depois da administração de um broncodilatador (agonista β-adrenérgico inalado ou epinefrina subcutânea).

A asma é uma doença comum, com uma incidência de cerca de 5% nos Estados Unidos, e é uma causa importante de doença e incapacidade em pessoas entre 2 e 17 anos de idade. É responsável por 14,5 milhões de consultas ambulatoriais e 5.000 mortes por ano nesse país. De 1980 a 1994, a prevalência da asma aumentou em 75%; a incidência máxima (160%) ocorreu em crianças com menos de 5 anos de idade. É mais provável que a asma que se manifesta pela primeira vez na infância seja de origem alérgica e mostre variação sazonal. A sinusite crônica e a doença do refluxo gastroesofágico estão estatisticamente correlacionadas à asma. Um subgrupo de pessoas com asma alérgica também apresenta pólipos nasais e sensibilidade ao ácido acetilsalicílico e muitos outros agentes antiinflamatórios não-esteróides. A exposição ocupacional a irritantes ou alérgenos transportados pelo ar é cada vez mais reconhecida como uma causa de asma crônica em adultos. Os conceitos atuais da fisiopatologia da asma enfatizam seu componente inflamatório e o risco de remodelação gradual e irreversível das vias aéreas devido à fibrose subepitelial na asma mal controlada. As recomendações atuais para o tratamento da asma crônica ou grave exigem o uso de agentes antiinflamatórios (principalmente corticosteróides inalados). Os outros tratamentos compreendem broncodilatadores β_2-adrenérgicos (albuterol, terbutalina, salmeterol), xantinas (teofilina, oxitrifilina, difilina), estabilizadores dos mastócitos (cromolin, nedocromil) e antileucotrienos (montelukast, zafirlukast, zileuton). A automonitoração da taxa de fluxo respiratório máximo com um dispositivo portátil simples ajuda os pacientes a ajustar as doses do medicamento para o efeito ótimo. A prevenção dos alérgenos, irritantes e outros deflagradores conhecidos é essencial para o bom controle.

bonchitic a., a. bronquítica; a. precipitada pela bronquite. SIN catarrhal a.
cardiac a., a. cardíaca; uma crise asmática, sendo a broncoconstrição secundária à congestão pulmonar e edema da insuficiência ventricular esquerda.
catarrhal a., a. catarral. SIN bronchitic a.
cotton-dust a., bissinose. SIN byssinosis.
dust a., a. da poeira; a. agravada pela inalação de poeira, observada principalmente como doença ocupacional decorrente da poeira de algodão.
extrinsic a., a. extrínseca; a. brônquica resultante de uma reação alérgica a substâncias estranhas, como partículas inaladas, vapores ou gases, ou alimentos ingeridos, bebidas ou medicamentos.
food a., a. alimentar; a. causada por reação alérgica a um item da dieta.
hay a., a. do feno; um estágio asmático da febre do feno.
intrinsic a., a. intrínseca; a. brônquica em que nenhuma causa extrínseca pode ser identificada, e presumivelmente causada por processo endógeno, possivelmente alérgico.
miller a., a. do moleiro; a. causada por alérgenos da farinha de trigo ou outro cereal.
miner's a., a. do mineiro; a dispnéia da antracose ou de outras pneumoconioses em mineiros.
nervous a., a. nervosa; a. precipitada por estresse psíquico.
reflex a., a. reflexa; a. que ocorre como um reflexo na doença das vísceras, do nariz ou de outras partes.
spasmodic a., a. espasmódica; a. decorrente do espasmo dos bronquíolos.
steam-filter's a., a. do operário que instala e conserta caldeiras a vapor; a. associada a asbestose adquirida por exposição aos componentes de encanamento e aquecimento forrados com asbesto.
stripper's a., a. do debulhador; a. associada à bissinose.
summer a., a. de verão; a. associada à febre do feno ou alergia à vegetação do verão.

triad a., síndrome que compreende pólipos nasais, asma e intolerância ao ácido acetilsalicílico.

asth·mat·ic (az-mat′ik). Asmático; relativo a ou que sofre de asma.

asth·ma-weed. 1. SIN lobelia. 2. SIN *Euphorbia pilulifera*.

asth·mo·gen·ic (az-mō-jen′ik). Asmogênico; que causa asma.

as·tig·mat·ic (as′tig-mat′ik). Astigmático; relativo a ou que sofre de astigmatismo.

astig·ma·tism (ă-stig′mă-tizm). Astigmatismo. 1. Uma lente ou sistema óptico que possui refratividade diferente em diferentes meridianos. 2. Uma condição de curvaturas desiguais ao longo de diferentes meridianos em uma ou mais das superfícies de refração (córnea, superfície anterior ou posterior do cristalino) do olho, em conseqüência do que os raios de um ponto luminoso não são focalizados em um único ponto sobre a retina. SIN astigmia. [G. *a-* priv. + *stigma (stigmat-)*, um ponto]

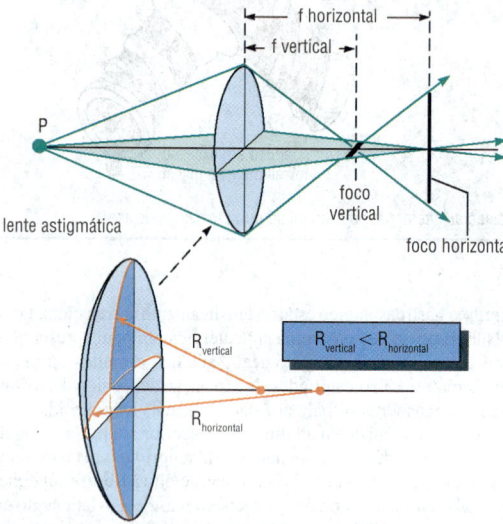

astigmatismo: em um cristalino astigmático, as curvaturas (R) nos dois meridianos são desiguais; dessa maneira, o cristalino possui duas distâncias focais diferentes e um ponto P aparece como uma linha (foco horizontal e vertical); na região entre os dois pontos focais, P aparece como uma elipse

a. against the rule, a. inverso; a. quando a curvatura ou força de refração maior está no meridiano horizontal.

compound hyperopic a., a. hiperópico composto; a. em que todos os meridianos são hiperópicos, mas em graus diferentes.

compound myopic a., a. miópico composto; a. em que todos os meridianos são miópicos, mas em graus diferentes.

corneal a., a. córneo; a. devido a um defeito na curvatura da superfície da córnea.

hyperopic a., a. hiperópico; forma de a. em que um meridiano é hiperópico e aquele em ângulo reto com ele não possui um erro de refração. SIN simple hyperopic a.

irregular a., a. irregular; a. em que diferentes partes do mesmo meridiano apresentam diferentes graus de curvatura.

lenticular a., a. lenticular; a. devido a defeito na curvatura, posição ou índice de refração da lente do olho.

mixed a., a. misto; a. em que um meridiano é hiperópico, enquanto aquele em ângulo reto com ele é miópico.

myopic a., a. miópico; forma de a. na qual um meridiano é miópico e aquele em ângulo reto com ele não exibe erro de refração. SIN simple myopic a.

a. of oblique pencils, uma aberração que ocorre quando um feixe de raios luminosos colide com um meio de refração em alguma direção diferente daquela paralela ao eixo do cristalino.

regular a., a. regular; a. em que a curvatura de cada meridiano é igual durante todo o seu trajeto e os meridianos de curvatura máxima e mínima estão em ângulos retos entre si.

simple hyperopic a., a. hiperópico simples. SIN hyperopic a.

simple myopic a., a. miópico simples. SIN myopic a.

a. with the rule, a. direto; a. quando a curvatura ou força de refração maior está no meridiano vertical.

astig·ma·tom·e·try, as·tig·mom·e·try (ă-stig-mă-tom′e-trē, as-tig-mom′e-trē). Astigmatometria, astigmometria; determinação da forma e medição do grau de astigmatismo.

astig·mia (ă-stig′mē-ă). Astigmatismo. SIN astigmatism.

asto·ma·tous (ă-stō′mă-tŭs). Astomatoso; sem uma boca. SIN astomous.

asto·mia (ă-stō′mē-ă). Astomia; ausência congênita da boca. [G. *a-* priv. + *stoma*, boca]

asto·mous (ă-stō′mŭs). Astomoso. SIN astomatous.

as·trag·a·lar (as-trag′ă-lar). Talar; relativo ao tálus.

as·trag·a·lec·to·my (as-trag-ă-lek′tō-mē). Remoção do tálus. [astragalus, + G. *ektomē*, excisão]

as·trag·a·lo·cal·ca·ne·an (as-trag′ă-lō-kal-kā′nē-an). Talocalcâneo; relativo ao tálus e ao calcâneo.

as·trag·a·lo·fib·u·lar (as-trag′ă-lō-fib′ū-lar). Talofibular; relativo ao tálus e à fíbula.

as·trag·a·lo·scaph·oid (as-trag′ă-lō-scaf′oyd). Talonavicular. SIN talonavicular.

as·trag·a·lo·tib·i·al (as-trag′ă-lō-tib′ē-ăl). Talotibial; relativo ao tálus e à tíbia.

As·trag·a·lus (as-trag′ă-lŭs). Gênero de plantas (família Leguminosae), notadamente *A. mollissimus* (astrágalo) nas pastagens do oeste norte-americano, capaz de captar o selênio do solo e provocar intoxicação em carneiros, gado e cavalos. *A. gummifer* é uma fonte de tragacanto.

as·tral (as′tral). Astral; relativo a uma astrosfera.

as·tra·po·pho·bia (as′tră-pō-fō′bē-ă). Astrapofobia; medo mórbido de relâmpagos e trovões. [G. *astrapē*, iluminação, + *phobos*, medo]

as·tric·tion (as-trik′shŭn). 1. Ação adstringente. 2. Compressão para estancar a hemorragia.

as·trin·gent (as-trin′jent). Adstringente. 1. Que causa contração ou enrugamento dos tecidos, parada da secreção ou controla a hemorragia. 2. Um agente que possui esses efeitos. [L. *astringens*]

as·tro·blast (as′trō-blast). Astroblasto; uma célula primitiva que se desenvolve em um astrócito. [G. *astron*, estrela, + *blastos*, germe]

as·tro·blas·to·ma (as′trō-blas-tō′mă). Astroblastoma; um glioma relativamente mal diferenciado de células neoplásicas jovens e imaturas da série dos astrócitos, freqüentemente disposto de forma radial com as fibrilas curtas, terminando em pequenos vasos sanguíneos. [astro- + G. *blastos*, germe, + *-oma*, tumor]

as·tro·ce·le (as′trō-sēl). Astrocele. SIN centrosphere. [G. *astron*, estrela, + *koilia*, cavidade]

as·tro·cyte (as′trō-sīt). Astrócito; uma das grandes células da neuróglia do tecido nervoso. VER TAMBÉM neuroglia. SIN astroglia cell, astroglia, Cajal cell (2), Deiters cells (2), macroglia cell, macroglia, spider cell (1). [G. *astron*, estrela, + *kytos*, cavidade (célula)]

Alzheimer tipe I a., a. do tipo I de Alzheimer; astrócitos multinucleados freqüentemente aumentados, observados na leucoencefalopatia multifocal progressiva.

Alzheimer tipe II a., a. do tipo II de Alzheimer; astrócitos aumentados com núcleos vesiculares e um ou mais nucléolos basofílicos pequenos, observados na doença hepatocerebral e doença de Wilson.

fibrillary a., fibrous a., a. fibrilar, a. fibroso; célula astrocítica estrelada com processos longos encontrada na substância branca do cérebro e da medula espinal, caracterizada por apresentar feixes de filamentos gliais em seu citoplasma; origem da maioria dos astrocitomas.

gemistocytic a., a. gemistocítica; célula astrocítica arredondada a oval com citoplasma abundante e um núcleo excêntrico; pode conter dois núcleos na célula; hipertrofia dos astrócitos. SIN gemistocyte, gemistocytic cell, reactive a., reactive cell.

protoplasmic a., a. protoplasmática; uma forma de a., encontrada principalmente na substância cinzenta, que possui poucas fibrilas e numerosos processos de ramificação.

reactive a., a. reativo. SIN gemistocytic a.

as·tro·cy·to·ma (as′trō-si-tō′mă). Astrocitoma; um glioma derivado de astrócitos. [G. *astron*, estrela, + *kytos*, célula, + *-oma*, tumor]

anaplastic a., a. anaplásico; um a. de grau intermediário caracterizado por celularidade aumentada, pleomorfismo celular, mitoses e proliferação endotelial vascular variável.

cerebellar a., a. cerebelar; uma variante do a. localizado no cerebelo que ocorre na maioria das crianças; consiste em dois padrões de arquitetura na microscopia, incluindo um padrão reticular frouxo e um padrão celular mais compacto, freqüentemente fusiforme. SIN juvenile cerebellar a.

desmoplastic cerebral a., a. cerebral desmoplásico; uma rara variante do a. que ocorre com maior freqüência na infância, tendo o tumor um aspecto de célula fusiforme.

fibrillary a., a. fibrilar; a. derivado de astrócitos fibrilares.

gemistocytic a., a. gemistocítico; um astrocitoma composto principalmente de astrócitos do tipo gemistocítico. SIN gemistocytoma.

grade I a., a. de grau I; a. sólido ou cístico de baixo grau; a designação da *Organização Mundial de Saúde (OMS)* que inclui o a. pilocítico e outras variantes de a. de baixo grau.

grade II a., a. de grau II; a. de baixo grau; designação da *Organização Mundial de Saúde (OMS)* que inclui o a. fibrilar bem diferenciado.

astrocytoma | **ataxia**

grade III a., a. de grau III; a. de grau intermediário; designação da *Organização Mundial de Saúde (OMS).* VER TAMBÉM anaplastic a.
grade IV a., a. de grau IV; a. de alto grau; designação da *Organização Mundial de Saúde (OMS).* VER TAMBÉM glioblastoma multiforme.
juvenile cerebellar a., a. cerebelar juvenil. SIN cerebellar a.
low grade a., a. de baixo grau; a. caracterizado por celularidade aumentada de distribuição desigual e pleomorfismo nuclear brando.
pilocytic a., a. pilocítico; um a. de crescimento lento composto histologicamente de astrócitos alongados; freqüentemente localizado na região do quiasma óptico do terceiro ventrículo, hipotálamo ou cerebelo, predominantemente em indivíduos mais jovens. SIN piloid astrocytoma.
piloid astrocytoma, a. pilóide. SIN pilocytic a.
protoplasmic a., a. protoplasmático; uma neoplasia composta principalmente de astrócitos do tipo protoplasmático.
subependymal giant cell a., a. de célula gigante subependimária; um raro a., freqüentemente localizado na parede do ventrículo lateral, formado por grandes células gliais com citoplasma eosinofílico abundante e astrócitos alongados entremeados, associados à esclerose tuberosa.
as·tro·cy·to·sis (as′trō-sī-tō′sis). Astrocitose; aumento no número de astrócitos, freqüentemente observado em uma zona irregular, mal ou moderadamente bem-definida, adjacente às lesões degenerativas (p.ex., encefalomalacia), inflamações focais (p.ex., abscessos) ou determinadas neoplasias no cérebro; em alguns casos, o a. pode ser difuso em uma região relativamente grande; o a. representa um mecanismo de reparação.
a. cer′e·bri, gliomatose a. cerebral. SIN gliomatosis cerebri.
as·tro·ep·en·dy·mo·ma (as′trō-ē-pen′di-mō′mă). Astroependimoma; neoplasia glial composta de uma população mista de células astrocíticas e ependimárias.
as·trog·lia (as-trog′lē-ă). Astróglia. SIN astrocyte. [G. *astron*, estrela, + neuroglia]
as·troid (as′troyd). Astróide; em formato de estrela. [G. *astroeidēs*, de *astron*, estrela, + *eidos*, semelhança]
as·tro·ki·net·ic (as-trō-ki-net′ik). Astrocinético; relativo ao movimento do centrossoma e da astrosfera de uma célula em divisão. [G. *astron*, estrela, + *kinēsis*, movimento]
as·tro·sphere (as′trō-sfēr). Astrosfera; um grupo de microtúbulos que se irradiam, estendendo-se para fora do citocentro e da centrosfera de uma célula em divisão. SIN aster, attraction sphere, Lavdovsky nucleoid, paranuclear body. [G. *astron*, estrela, + *sphaira*, bola]
As·tro·vi·rus (as-′trō-vī′rus). Um pequeno RNA vírus e o único gênero na família Astroviridae; está associado à diarréia e é detectado nas fezes de inúmeros animais.
Astrup, Poul, químico clínico dinamarquês, *1915. VER micro-A. *method*.
Astwood, Edwin B., endocrinologista norte-americano, 1909–1976. VER A. *test*.
as·ver·in (as′ver-in). Asverina; um antitussígeno.
Asx Símbolo que significa Asp (ácido aspártico) ou Asn (asparagina).
asyl·la·bia (ā-si-lā′bē-ă). Assilabia; forma de alexia em que uma pessoa reconhece as letras individuais, mas não consegue compreendê-las quando dispostas coletivamente em sílabas ou palavras. [G. *a-* priv. + *syllablē*, sílaba]
asy·lum (ā-sī′lŭm). Asilo; termo antigo para uma instituição para alojar e cuidar daqueles que, por motivo de idade ou enfermidades mentais ou corporais, eram incapazes de cuidar de si próprios. [L. do G. *asylon*, um santuário, de *a-* priv. + *sylē*, direito de violar]
asym·bo·lia (ā-sim-bō′lē-ă). Assimbolia; uma forma de afasia em que o significado dos sinais e símbolos não é apreciado. SIN sight blindness. [G. *a-* priv. + *symbolon*, um símbolo]
asym·met·ric (a) (ā-sim-et′rik). Assimétrico; não-simétrico; indica falta de simetria entre duas ou mais partes iguais.
asym·me·try (ā-sim′e-trē). Assimetria. **1.** Falta de simetria; desproporção entre duas partes normalmente iguais. **2.** Diferença de significado na amplitude ou freqüência da atividade do EEG registrada simultaneamente a partir de dois lados do cérebro em condições idênticas. SIN dissymmetry.
asymp·tom·at·ic (ā′simp-to-mat′ik). Assintomático; sem sintomas ou que não produz sintomas.
asymp·tot·ic (ā′simp-tot′ik). Assimptótico, assintótico; pertinente a um valor limitado, por exemplo de uma variável dependente, quando a variável independente se aproxima de zero ou do infinito (assimptota).
asyn·cli·tism (ā-sin′kli-tizm). Assinclitismo; ausência de sinclitismo ou paralelismo; pode ser usado, p.ex., em referência ao eixo da parte apresentada da criança e aos planos pélvicos no nascimento, aos arcos dentários ou aos planos do crânio. SIN obliquity. [G. *a-* priv. + *syn-klinō*, inclinar em conjunto]
anterior a., a. anterior. SIN Nägele *obliquity*.
posterior a., a. posterior. SIN Litzmann *obliquity*.
a. of the skull, a. do crânio, plagocefalia. SIN plagiocephaly.
asyn·ech·ia (ā-si-nek′ē-ă). Assinéquia; descontinuidade da estrutura. [G. *a-* priv. + *synecheia*, continuidade]
asy·ner·gia (ā-sin-er′jē-ă). Assinergia. SIN asynergy. [G. *a-* priv. + *syn*, com, + *ergon*, trabalho]

asyn·er·gic (ā′sin-er′jik). Assinérgico; caracterizado por assinergia.
asyn·er·gy (ā-sin′er-jē). Assinergia; falta de coordenação entre vários grupamentos musculares durante a realização de movimentos complexos, resultando na perda da habilidade e da velocidade. Quando grave, resulta em decomposição do movimento, onde os atos mais complexos são realizados em uma série de movimentos isolados; causada por distúrbios cerebelares. SIN asynergia.
asy·ne·sia, asyn·e·sis (ā-si-nē′zē-ă, -nē′sis). Assinesia; falta de compreensão fácil e de inteligência prática. [G. *a-* priv. + *synesis*, união, compreensão]
asys·tem·at·ic (ā′sis-tē-mat′ik). Assistemático; não-sistemático; não relacionado a um sistema ou conjunto de órgãos.
asys·to·le (ā-sis′tō-lē). Assistolia; ausência de contrações do coração. SIN asystolia, cardiac standstill. [G. *a-* priv. + *systolē*, uma contração]
asys·to·lia (ā-sis-tō′lē-ă). Assistolia. SIN asystole.
asys·tol·ic (ā-sis-tol′ik). Assistólico. **1.** Relativo à assistolia. **2.** Não-sistólico.
AT Abreviatura para o par de bases ligadas por hidrogênio adenina-tiamina nos polinucleotídeos de filamento duplo; adenina: tiamina.
At Símbolo para astatine (astatina).
ata Abreviatura para *atmosphere* absolute (atmosfera absoluta).
at·a·brine hy·dro·chlo·ride (a′tē-brin). Cloridrato de atabrina. SIN quinacrine hydrochloride.
atac·til·ia (ā-tak-til′ē-ă). Atactilia; perda da sensação do tato. [G. *a-* priv. + L. *tactilis*, relativo ao tato, de *tango*, pp. *tactus*, tocar]
at·a·rac·tic (at-ă-rak′tik). Atarático. **1.** Que possui efeito calmante ou tranqüilizante. **2.** Um tranqüilizante. SIN ataraxic. [G. *ataraktos*, calma]
at·a·rax·ia (at-ă-rak′sē-ă). Ataraxia; calma e paz da mente; tranqüilidade. [G *a-* priv. + *taraktos*, conturbado, + -ia]
at·a·rax·ic (at-ă-rak′sik). Ataráxico. SIN ataractic.
at·a·vism (at′ă-vizm). Atavismo; o aparecimento em uma pessoa de características que, supostamente, estiveram presentes em algum ancestral remoto; a reversão para um tipo biológico inferior, um retrocesso. [L. *atavus*, um ancestral remoto]
at·a·vis·tic (at-ă-vis′tik). Atávico; relativo ao atavismo.
atax·ia (ā-tak′sē-ă). Ataxia; incapacidade de coordenar a atividade muscular durante o movimento voluntário; causada com maior freqüência por distúrbios do cerebelo ou das colunas posteriores da medula espinal; pode envolver os membros, a cabeça ou o tronco. SIN ataxy, incoordenation. [G. *a-* priv. + *taxis*, ordem]
acute a., a. aguda; a. generalizada de estabelecimento repentino, causada mais amiúde por intoxicações medicamentosas, envenenamentos ou neuronite vestibular.
Briquet a., a. de Briquet; enfraquecimento da sensibilidade muscular e sensibilidade aumentada da pele na histeria. SIN hysterical a.
Bruns a., a. de Bruns; dificuldade na iniciação do movimento dos pés quando eles estão em contato com o solo, uma condição ligada à lesão do lobo frontal.
cerebellar a., a. cerebelar; perda da coordenação muscular causada por distúrbios do cerebelo.
chronic a., a. crônica; a. persistente, causada mais amiúde por distúrbios cerebelares hereditários ou metabólicos.
a. cor′dis, fibrilação atrial. SIN atrial *fibrillation*.
Friedreich a. [MIM*229300], a. de Friedreich; distúrbio neurológico caracterizado por a., disartria, escoliose, pé com arco alto ou pés cavos e paralisia dos músculos, principalmente dos membros inferiores; o início ocorre geralmente na infância ou juventude, com esclerose das colunas posterior e lateral da medula espinal; herança autossômica recessiva, causada por mutação envolvendo a expansão de repetição de trinucleotídeo no gene da ataxia de Friedreich (FRDA) no cromossoma 9q. SIN hereditary spinal a., heredotaxia.
gluten a., a. por glúten; a. resultante da lesão imunológica do cerebelo, colunas espinais posteriores e nervos periféricos nas pessoas sensíveis ao glúten.
hereditary cerebellar a., a. cerebelar hereditária; **(1)** uma doença de fase final da infância e início da vida adulta, marcada por marcha atáxica, fala hesitante e explosiva, nistagmo e, por vezes, neurite óptica. Provavelmente, compreende várias condições distintas, com padrões diversos de herança; **(2)** termo coletivo para inúmeros distúrbios hereditários em que os sinais cerebelares constituem o achado mais proeminente.
hereditary spinal a. [MIM*229300], a. espinal hereditária. SIN Friedreich a.
hysterical a., a. histérica. SIN Briquet a.
kinetic a., a. cinética. SIN motor a.
Leyden a., a. de Leyden. SIN pseudotabes.
locomotor a., a. locomotora; a ataxia grave da marcha observada na neurossífilis tabética. Os pacientes caminham com os pés bem afastados, batendo-os desajeitadamente no chão a cada passo, e dependem de indícios visuais para manter o equilíbrio. VER TAMBÉM tabetic *neurosyphilis*.
Marie a., a. de Marie; termo obsoleto para várias ataxias hereditárias não-Friedreich.
motor a., a. motora; a. que se desenvolve na tentativa de realizar os movimentos musculares coordenados. SIN kinetic a.

optic a., a. óptica; incapacidade de guiar a mão em direção a um objeto usando informações visuais; observada na síndrome de Balint (Balint *syndrome*).
respiratory a., a. respiratória. SIN Biot *respiration*.
sensory a., a. sensorial; a. decorrente do comprometimento da propriocepção causada por lesões localizadas em algum ponto ao longo das vias sensoriais centrais ou periféricas.
spinal a., a. espinal; a. devido a doença da medula espinal, como tabes dorsal.
spinocerebellar a., a. espinocerebelar; a a. hereditária mais comum, com início da metade para o final da infância, manifestada como a. de membro, nistagmo, cifoescoliose e pés cavos; as principais alterações histopatológicas são encontradas nas colunas posteriores da medula espinal; mais amiúde, herança autossômica recessiva.
static a., a. estática; incapacidade de preservar o equilíbrio enquanto fica em pé, devido à perda da mioestesia; presente durante o estado de repouso.
a. telangiectasia, ataxia-telangiectasia, a.-telangiectasia; distúrbio multissistêmico lentamente progressivo com as seguintes manifestações: a. que surge com o início da deambulação; telangiectasias nas conjuntivas e na pele da face, do pescoço e dos ouvidos; atetose e nistagmo; e infecções recorrentes do sistema respiratório provocadas por deficiências de imunoglobulinas. Devido a um traço autossômico recessivo, com importantes alterações histopatológicas que afetam o córtex cerebelar, as colunas posteriores, as vias espinocerebelares, as células do corno anterior, as raízes dorsais e os nervos periféricos. Um elevado percentual de pacientes apresenta deficiência concomitante de IgA, com função diminuída da célula T-auxiliadora. Existem inúmeras rupturas cromossomiais e os níveis séricos de α-fetoproteína estão usualmente elevados; gerada por várias mutações no gene da PI3´cinase. SIN ataxia telangiectasia syndrome, Louis-Bar syndrome.
vasomotor a., a. vasomotora; uma forma de a. autônoma que provoca irregularidade na circulação periférica, caracterizada por alternâncias de palidez e transpiração, devido ao espasmo dos vasos sanguíneos de menor calibre.
vestibulocerebellar a., a. vestibulocerebelar; a. decorrente de doença do sistema vestibular central ou de seus componentes cerebelares, manifestada clinicamente por marcha desequilibrada, nistagmo e incoordenação dos movimento de braço e perna.
atax·i·a·dy·nam·ia (ă-tak′sē-ă-dī-nam′ē-ă). Ataxiadinamia; fraqueza muscular combinada à incoordenação.
atax·i·a·gram (ă-tak′sē-ă-gram). Ataxiograma; o registro feito por um ataxiógrafo.
atax·i·a·graph (ă-tak′sē-ă-graf). Ataxiógrafo; um instrumento para medir o grau e a direção da oscilação do corpo e da cabeça na ataxia estática, com os olhos da pessoa fechados. SIN ataxiameter.
atax·i·a·me·ter (ă-tak′sē-ă-mē′ter). Ataxômetro. SIN ataxiagraph.
atax·i·a·pha·sia (ă-tak′sē-ă-fā′zē-ă). Ataxiafasia; incapacidade de formar frases conectadas, embora as palavras isoladas possam, talvez, ser utilizadas de forma inteligível. [G. *a-* priv. + *taxis*, ordem, + *phasis*, uma afirmação, fala]
atax·ia-tel·an·gi·ec·ta·sia. Ataxia-telangiectasia. VER *ataxia* telangiectasia.
atax·ic (ă-tak′sik). Atáxico; relativo a, marcado por ou que sofre de ataxia.
atax·i·o·pho·bia (ă-tak′sē-ō-fō′bē-ă). Ataxiofobia; temor mórbido de distúrbio ou negligência. [G. *a-* priv. + *taxis*, ordem, + *phobos*, medo]
ataxy (ă-tak′sē). Ataxia. SIN ataxia.
♻ **-ate.** -ato; terminação empregada como um substituto para "ácido -ico", quando o ácido é neutralizado. (p.ex., acetato de sódio) ou esterificado (p.ex., acetato de etila).
at·el·ec·ta·sis (at-ĕ-lek′tă-sis). Atelectasia; ar diminuído ou ausente em todo o pulmão ou em parte dele, com a resultante perda de volume pulmonar. A perda do próprio volume pulmonar. VER TAMBÉM pulmonary *collapse*. [G. *atelēs*, incompleto, + *ektasis*, extensão]
adhesive a., a. adesiva; colapso alveolar na vigência de vias aéreas permeáveis, principalmente quando o surfactante é inativado ou está ausente, em especial na síndrome de angústia respiratória do recém-nascido, pneumotórax por radiação aguda ou pneumonia viral. SIN microatelectasis, nonobstructive a.
cicatrization a., a. por fibrose; (1) a diminuição do ar por unidade de volume pulmonar decorrente de fibrose, causando diminuição da complacência pulmonar e aumento dos tecidos; (2) a. devido a cicatrização ou fibrose pulmonar.
a. of the middle ear, a. da orelha média; a redução no volume do orelha média por causa da obstrução da tuba auditiva seguida por absorção do oxigênio da orelha média e subseqüente retração medial da membrana timpânica.
nonobstructive a., a. não-obstrutiva. SIN adhesive a.
passive a., a. passiva; o colapso pulmonar que ocorre devido a um processo intratorácico que ocupa espaço, como pneumotórax ou hidrotórax. SIN relaxation a.
patchy a., a. difusa; aeração diminuída e colapso de múltiplas pequenas áreas do pulmão.
platelike a., a. laminar. SIN subsegmental a.
primary a., a. primária; não-expansão dos pulmões depois do nascimento, encontrada em todos os natimortos e em neonatos vivos que morrem antes que se estabeleça a respiração.

relaxation a., a. passiva. SIN passive a.
resorption a., a. de reabsorção; o lento colapso parcial de um lobo que ocorre quando a comunicação entre os alvéolos e a traquéia é obstruída.
rounded a., a. redonda; uma área de pulmão atelectásico causada por pregueamento parenquimatoso devido a fibrose pleural, mais amiúde a partir da exposição ao asbesto; aparece como uma lesão hipotransparente semelhante a uma massa, podendo ser confundida com câncer de pulmão; pode estar associada a um sinal da cauda do cometa (comet tail *sign*); o maior realce pelo contraste na tomografia computadorizada dinâmica (dynamic computed *tomography*) auxilia o diagnóstico. SIN folded-lung syndrome.
secondary a., a. secundária; colapso pulmonar em qualquer idade, mas principalmente nos lactentes, devido a doença da membrana hialina ou encolhimento elástico dos pulmões enquanto morrem por outras causas.
segmental a., a. segmentar; colapso parcial de um ou mais segmentos pulmonares individuais.
subsegmental a., a. subsegmentar; colapso da porção do pulmão distal a um brônquio subsegmentar obstruído, manifestado como uma opacificação linear na radiografia de tórax. VER Fleischner *lines*, em *line*. SIN platelike a.
at·e·lec·tat·ic (at-ĕ-lek-tat′ik). Atelectásico; relativo à atelectasia.
ate·lia (ă-tē′lē-ă). Ateliose. SIN ateliosis.
atel·i·o·sis (ă-tē′lē-ō′sis). Ateliose; desenvolvimento incompleto do corpo ou de qualquer de suas partes, como no infantilismo e nanismo. SIN atelia. [G. *atelēs*, incompleto, + *-osis*, condição]
atel·i·ot·ic (ă-tē-lē-ot′ik). Ateliótico; marcado por ateliose.
atel·op·id·tox·in (ă-tel-op′id-tok′sin). Atelopitoxina; um veneno potente da pele do sapo *Atelopus zeteki* das Américas Central e do Sul.
aten·o·lol (ă-ten′ō-lol). Atenolol; um agente bloqueador β-adrenérgico relativamente cárdio-seletivo empregado principalmente no tratamento da angina de peito e hipertensão arterial; é menos lipossolúvel que outros membros dessa classe e, portanto, causa aparentemente menos efeitos colaterais sobre o sistema nervoso central.
athe·lia (ă-thē-lē-ă). Atelia; ausência congênita de mamilos. [G. *a-* priv. + *thēlē*, mamilo]
ath·er·ec·to·my (ath-e-rek′tō-mē). Aterectomia; qualquer remoção por cirurgia ou cateterismo especializado de um ateroma na artéria coronária ou em qualquer outra artéria.
coronary a., a. coronária; remoção instrumental, por meio de cateter, de ateromas nas artérias coronárias.
directional a., a. direcional; remoção do aterômetro coronariano com o cateter instrumentado.
ather·man·cy (ă-ther′man-sē). Atermancia, adiatermia; impermeabilidade ao calor. [G. *athermantos*, não-aquecido, de *a-* priv. + *thermaino*, aquecer, de *thermē*, calor]
ather·ma·nous (ă-ther′mă-nŭs). Atérmano, adiatérmico; que absorve calor radiante; não-permeável aos raios de calor.
ather·mo·sys·tal·tic (ă-ther′mō-sis-tal′tik). Atermossistáltico; não-contraído ou constringido por variações comuns da temperatura; diz-se de determinados tecidos. [G. *a-* priv. + *thermos*, calor, + *systaltikos*, constringente]
♻ **athero-.** Atero-; material pastoso, mole, semelhante a mingau; ateroma, ateromatoso. [G. *athērē*, mingau, papa]
ath·er·o·em·bo·lism (ath′er-ō-em′bō-lizm). Ateroembolismo; embolia por colesterol, com ou sem matéria calcificada, que se origina a partir de ateroma da aorta ou outra artéria enferma.
ath·er·o·gen·e·sis (ath′er-ō-jen′ĕ-sis). Aterogênese; formação do ateroma, importante na patogenia da arteriosclerose.
ath·er·o·gen·ic (ath-er-ō-jen′ik). Aterogênico; que possui a capacidade de iniciar, aumentar ou acelerar o processo da aterogênese.
ath·er·o·ma (ath-er-ō′mă). Ateroma; os depósitos de lipídios na íntima das artérias produz uma tumefação amarelada na superfície endotelial; uma característica da aterosclerose. SIN atherosis. [G. *athērē*, mingau, + *-ōma*, tumor]
ath·er·om·a·tous (ath-er-ō′mă-tŭs). Ateromatoso; relativo a ou afetado por ateroma.

🛈 **ath·er·o·scle·ro·sis** (ath′er-ō-skler-ō′sis). Aterosclerose; arteriosclerose caracterizada por depósitos lipídicos irregularmente distribuídos na camada íntima de artérias de grosso e médio calibres, provocando o estreitamento das luzes arteriais e evoluindo, por fim, para fibrose e calcificação; as lesões geralmente são focais e progridem de forma lenta e intermitente. A limitação do fluxo sanguíneo é responsável pela maioria das manifestações clínicas, as quais variam com a distribuição e gravidade das lesões. Nos animais inferiores, a. dos suínos e aves assemelham-se muito à a. dos seres humanos. SIN nodular sclerosis. [G. *athērē*, mingau, + sclerosis]

> A aterosclerose, a forma mais comum de arteriosclerose, é um processo complexo que começa com o aparecimento de macrófagos preenchidos por colesterol (células espumosas) na íntima de uma artéria. As células musculares lisas proliferam em resposta à presença de lipídios, sob in-

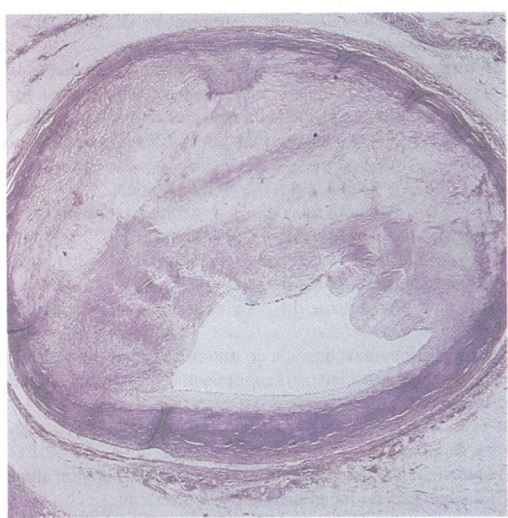

aterosclerose: corte transversal da artéria renal mostrando estreitamento luminal significativo por aterosclerose; hematoxilina e eosina, × 10

fluência de fatores plaquetários. Uma placa forma-se no local, consistindo em células musculares lisas, leucócitos e deposição adicional de lipídio; com o tempo, a placa torna-se fibrótica e pode calcificar-se. A expansão de uma placa aterosclerótica leva a obstrução gradualmente crescente da artéria e isquemia dos tecidos por ela irrigados. Ulceração, trombose ou embolização de uma placa, ou hemorragia e dissecção da camada íntima, podem causar o comprometimento mais agudo e grave do fluxo sanguíneo, com o risco de infarto. Estes são os principais mecanismos da doença da artéria coronária (cardiopatia arteriosclerótica com ou sem insuficiência cardíaca, angina de peito, infarto do miocárdio), doença vascular periférica (principalmente a doença oclusiva do membro inferior causando claudicação intermitente ou gangrena) e acidente vascular cerebral (infarto cerebral devido à oclusão da artéria carótida ou intracraniana). Os fatores de risco independentes para a aterosclerose são sexo masculino, envelhecimento, pós-menopausa, história familiar de aterosclerose, tabagismo, hipertensão, diabetes melito, LDL-colesterol plasmático elevado, homocisteína plasmática elevada, peso acima do ideal e estilo de vida sedentário. As evidências crescentes sugerem que a elevação dos níveis plasmáticos de triglicerídeos, insulina em jejum, fibrinogênio, apolipoproteínas A e B e lipoproteína (a) também constituem fatores de risco independentes. O diagnóstico de aterosclerose baseia-se, usualmente, na história e exame físico e é confirmado por angiografia, ultra-sonografia com Doppler e outras técnicas de imagem. O tratamento é, em grande parte, mecânico: estiramento por balão, ablação a laser ou remoção cirúrgica das placas, e vários procedimentos de *bypass* (derivação) e enxerto. A prevenção da aterosclerose é um objetivo importante da medicina moderna. As medidas preventivas incluem a prática regular de exercícios vigorosos, dieta pobre em lipídios e colesterol, manutenção de um peso saudável, abstinência do fumo e uso de agentes farmacológicos conforme indicado (p.ex., controle rigoroso da hipertensão e diabetes melito, redução do colesterol elevado, terapia de reposição de estrogênio depois da menopausa). VER free radical; low-fat diet.

ath·er·o·scle·rot·ic (ath′er-ō-skler-ot′ik). Aterosclerótico; relativo a, ou caracterizado por, aterosclerose.
ath·er·o·sis (ath-er-ō′sis). Ateroma. SIN atheroma.
ath·er·o·throm·bo·sis (ath′er-ō-throm-bō′sis). Aterotrombose; formação de trombo em um vaso ateromatoso.
ath·er·o·throm·bot·ic (ath′er-ō-throm-bot′ik). Aterotrombótico; que indica, característico de ou causado por aterotrombose.
ath·e·toid (ath′e-toyd). Atetóide; que se assemelha à atetose.
ath·e·to·sic, ath·e·tot·ic (ath-ē-tō′sik, -tot′ik). Atetósico, atetótico; pertinente a, ou marcado por, atetose.
ath·e·to·sis (ath-ē-tō′sis). Atetose; condição na qual existe uma sucessão constante de movimentos convulsivos lentos e involuntários de flexão, extensão, pronação e supinação dos dedos das mãos e das mãos, e, por vezes, dos artelhos e dos pés. Geralmente causado por uma lesão extrapiramidal. SIN extrapiramidal cerebral palsy, Hammond disease. [G. *athetos*, sem posição ou local]
double a., a. dupla; um tipo de paralisia cerebral manifestada predominantemente como movimentos involuntários bilaterais, começando com cerca de 3 anos de idade, e continuado por hipotonia generalizada e desenvolvimento motor retardado. Existem várias causas, incluindo *kernicterus* e hipoxia neonatal. SIN congenital choreoathetosis, double congenital a., Vogt syndrome.
double congenital a., a. dupla congênita. SIN double a.
posthemiplegic a., a. pós-hemiplégica; atetose unilateral que envolve os membros hemiplégicos, geralmente observada em crianças. SIN posthemiplegic chorea.
aThr Abreviatura para allothreonines (alotreoninas). VER allothreonines.
athrep·sia, ath·rep·sy (ā-threp′sē-ā, ath′rep-sē). Atrepsia. **1.** Termo obsoleto para marasmo. **2.** Conforme utilizado por Ehrlich, a imunidade para as células neoplásicas transplantadas devido à ausência de nutrição no sentido de deficiência das supostas substâncias necessárias para o desenvolvimento dessas células. [G. *a*- priv. + *threpsis*, nutrição]
ath·ro·cy·to·sis (ath′rō-sī-tō′sis). Atrocitose; a capacidade das células de absorver e reter os colóides eletronegativos, conforme demonstrado por macrófagos e na superfície apical das células do túbulo contornado proximal do rim. [G. *athrō*, reunido, + *kytos*, célula, + *-osis*, condição]
athrom·bia (ā-throm′bē-ā) [MIM*209050]. Atrombia; um distúrbio hemorrágico hereditário caracterizado por tempo de sangramento prolongado, aderência e agregação plaquetárias diminuídas, mas tempo de coagulação e retração do coágulo normais, contagem de plaquetas normal com disponibilidade do fator 3 plaquetário; provavelmente herança autossômica recessiva. [G. *a*- priv. + thrombin]
athy·mia (ā-thī′mē-ā). Atimia. **1.** Ausência de afeto ou emotividade; impassividade mórbida. **2.** Ausência congênita da glândula timo, freqüentemente com a imunodeficiência associada. SIN athymism. [G. *a*- priv. + *thymos*, mente, também timo]
athy·mism (ā-thī′mizm). Atimia. SIN athymia (2).
athy·rea (ā-thī′rē-ā). **1.** Hipotireoidismo. SIN hypothyroïdism. **2.** Atireoidismo. SIN athyroidism.
athy·roid·ism (ā-thī′royd-izm). Atireoidismo; ausência congênita da glândula tireóide ou supressão ou ausência de sua secreção hormonal. VER hypothyroidism. SIN athyrea (2), athyrosis.
athy·ro·sis (ā-thī-rō′sis). Atireoidismo. SIN athyroidism.
athy·rot·ic (ā-thī-rot′ik). Atireóideo; relativo ao atireoidismo.
ATL Abreviatura para adult T-cell *leukemia* (leucemia de células T do adulto) ou adult T-cell *lymphoma* (linfoma de células T do adulto).
at·lan·tad (at-lan′tad). Na direção do atlas.
at·lan·tal (at-lan′tăl). Atlóide; relativo ao atlas. SIN atloid.
♻ **atlanto-, atlo-.** O atlas (a vértebra que suporta o crânio). [G. *Atlas, Atlantos*, Atlas, o mítico Titã que apoiava a cúpula do céu sobre seus ombros]
at·lan·to·ax·i·al (at-lan′tō-ak′sē-ăl). Atlantoaxial; pertinente ao atlas e ao áxis, indica a articulação entre as duas primeiras vértebras cervicais. SIN atlantoepistrophic, atlantoxoid.
at·lan·to·did·y·mus (at-lan′tō-did′ē-mŭs). Atlantodídimo; gêmeos unidos por duas cabeças em um pescoço e um único corpo. SIN atlodidymus. [atlanto- + G. *didymos*, gêmeo]
at·lan·to·ep·i·stroph·ic (at-lan′tō-ep′i-strof′ik). Atlantoaxial. SIN atlantoaxial.
at·lan·to·oc·cip·i·tal (at-lan′tō-ok-sip′i-tăl). Atlantoccipital; relativo ao atlas e ao osso occipital. SIN atlo-occipital.
at·lan·to·odon·toid (at-lan′tō-ō-don′toyd). Atlanto-odontóide; relativo ao atlas e ao dente do áxis.
at·las (at′las) [TA]. Atlas; primeira vértebra cervical, que se articula com o osso occipital e que roda ao redor do dente do áxis. SIN vertebra C1*, first cervical vertebra. [G. *Atlas*, na mitologia grega, um Titã que sustentava os céus sobre seus ombros]
♻ **atlo-.** VER atlanto-.
at·lo·ax·oid (at-lō-ak′soyd). Atlantoaxial. SIN atlantoaxial.
at·lo·did·y·mus (at-lō-did′ē-mŭs). Atlantodídimo. SIN atlantodidymus.
at·loid (at′loyd). Atlóide. SIN atlantal.
at·lo·oc·cip·i·tal (at′lō-ok-sip′i-tăl). Atlantoccipital. SIN atlanto-occipital.
atm. Símbolo de standard *atmosphere* (atmosfera padrão).
♻ **atmo-.** Prefixo que indica vapor ou fumaça; ou derivado por ação de fumaça ou vapor. [G. *atmos*, fumaça, vapor]
at·mol·y·sis (at-mol′i-sis). Atmólise; separação de gases misturados ao passá-los através de um diafragma poroso, com os gases mais leves difundindo-se mais rapidamente. [atmo- + G. *lysis*, dissolução]
at·mom·e·ter (at-mom′ĕ-ter). Atmômetro, atmidômetro; um instrumento para medir a velocidade de evaporação. [atmo- + G. *metron*, medida]
at·mos. Abreviatura obsoleta para uma unidade de pressão; substituído por atm. [abreviatura de atmosphere]
at·mos·phere (at′mos-fēr). Atmosfera. **1.** Qualquer gás que circunda determinado corpo; um meio gasoso. **2.** Uma unidade da pressão de ar igual a 101,325 kPa. VER TAMBÉM standard a., torr. [atmo- + G. *sphaira*, esfera]
a. absolute (ata), a. absoluta; uma unidade de pressão absoluta (também conhecida como pressão barométrica) expressa em atm.

ICAO standard a., a. padrão ICAO; a a. padrão adotada pela *International Civil Aviation Organization*, usada para calibrar altímetros e para expressar as pressões de câmaras hiperbáricas em relação à altitude equivalente; ela ignora muitos desvios encontrados na natureza.

standard a. (atm), a. padrão; (1) a pressão da a. ao nível do mar médio em 273,15 K, equivalente a 1.013.250 dinas/cm² ou 101,325 Pa (N/m² no sistema SI); (2) uma expressão padronizada da relação da pressão barométrica, temperatura e outras variáveis atmosféricas como uma função da altitude acima do nível do mar.

at·mo·spher·i·za·tion (at′mŏ-sfēr-i-zā′shŭn). Atmosferização; conversão do sangue venoso em arterial.

At·mungs·fer·ment (aht′mungz-fer-ment). **1.** Um sistema de citocromos e suas oxidases que participam nos processos respiratórios. **2.** Com freqüência, de maneira específica, citocromo-oxidase. SIN Warburg respiratory enzyme. [Alemão]

at·om (at′ŏm). Átomo; outrora considerada a última partícula de um elemento, considerada indivisível, como indica seu nome. A descoberta da radioatividade mostrou que existem partículas subatômicas, notadamente prótons, nêutrons e elétrons, com os dois primeiros compreendendo a maior parte da massa do núcleo atômico. Atualmente, sabemos que as partículas subatômicas são subdivididas em hadrons, leptons e quarks. [G. *atomos*, indivisível, não-seccionável]

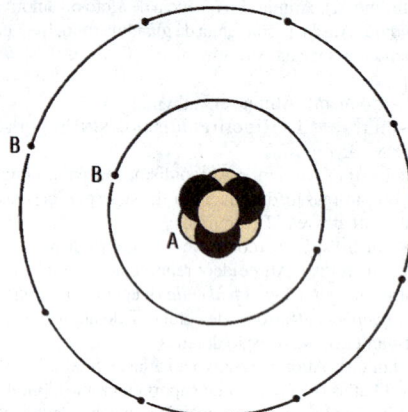

estrutura de um átomo: (A) núcleo, contendo prótons (laranja) e nêutrons (escuros); (B) elétrons, percorrendo as órbitas em torno do núcleo

activated a., a. excitado; um a. que possui energia maior que a normal, em consequência de ganho de energia. VER TAMBÉM excited *state*. SIN excited a.

Bohr a., a. de Bohr; um conceito ou modelo de a. em que os elétrons com carga elétrica negativa se movem em órbitas circulares ou elípticas ao redor do núcleo com carga elétrica positiva, sendo a energia emitida ou absorvida quando os elétrons mudam de uma órbita para outra.

excited a., a. excitado. SIN activated a.

ionized a., a. ionizado; um a. que possui uma carga eletrostática em consequência da perda ou ganho de elétrons; p.ex., H^+, Ca^{2+}, Cl^-, O^{2-}.

labeled a., a. marcado; um a. radioativo ou um a. estável, porém raro, que, por sua presença em uma molécula, ajuda a localização ou medição da mesma. SIN tagged a.

nuclear a., a. nuclear; um conceito ou modelo do a. caracterizado pela presença de um pequeno núcleo maciço em seu centro.

quaternary carbon a., a. de carbono quaternário; um a. de carbono ao qual estão ligados quatro outros átomos de carbono.

radioactive a., a. radioativo; um a. com um núcleo instável, que emite radiação particulada ou eletromagnética (emissão radioativa) para atingir maior estabilidade. VER radionuclide, half-life, Becquerel.

recoil a., a. de rechaço; o restante de um a. do qual uma partícula nuclear foi emitida ou ejetada em alta velocidade; o restante recolhe-se com uma velocidade inversamente proporcional à sua massa.

stripped a., a. desnudado; um a. menos todos os seus elétrons; um núcleo.

tagged a., a. marcado. SIN labeled a.

atom·ic (ă-tom′ik). Atômico; relativo a um átomo.

at·om·ism (at′ŏm-izm). Atomismo; a abordagem para o estudo de um fenômeno psicológico através da análise de partes elementares, das quais se presume que ele seja composto. Cf. holism.

at·om·is·tic (at-ŏm-is′tik). Atomístico, atomista; pertinente ao atomismo ou à psicologia atomística.

at·om·i·za·tion (at-ŏm-i-zā′shŭn). Atomização; produção de um aerossol; redução de um líquido em pequenas gotículas.

at·om·iz·er (at′ŏm-ī-zer). Atomizador, nebulizador; um dispositivo utilizado para fragmentar o medicamento líquido a partículas finas na forma de um aerossol ou *spray*; útil na aplicação de medicamento nos pulmões, no nariz e na garganta. VER TAMBÉM nebulizer, vaporizer. [G. *atomos*, partícula indivisível]

ato·nia (ă-tō′nē-ă). Atonia. SIN atony. [G. languidez]

aton·ic (ă-ton′ik). Atônico; relaxado; sem o tono ou tensão normal.

at·o·nic·i·ty (at-ō-nis′i-tē). Atonia. SIN atony.

at·o·ny (at′ō-nē). Atonia; relaxamento, flacidez ou falta de tônus ou tensão. SIN atonia, atonicity. [G. *atonia*, languidez]

postpartum a., a. pós-parto; a. das paredes uterinas após dar à luz. SIN metratonia.

uterine a., a. uterina; incapacidade do miométrio de se contrair depois da liberação da placenta; associada ao sangramento excessivo oriundo do local de implantação placentário.

at·o·pen (at′ō-pen). Atópeno; um termo antigo para indicar a causa de qualquer forma de atopia.

atop·ic (ă-top′ik). Atópico. **1.** Relativo a, ou caracterizado por, atopia. **2.** Alérgico. [G. *atopos*, fora do lugar; estranho]

Ato·po·bium (at-ō-pō′bē-um). Um gênero de bactérias Gram-positivas, obrigatoriamente anaeróbicas, não-formadoras de esporos, que aparecem como cocos e cocobacilos, por vezes em cadeias curtas. A espécie protótipo é *Atopobium parvulus*, um microrganismo de crescimento lento que forma diminutas colônias em meios de cultura padronizados, originalmente chamado de *Peptostreptococcus parvulus* e *Streptococcus parvulus*.

atop·og·no·sia, atop·og·no·sis (ă-top-og-nō′zē-ă, -og-nō′sis). Atopognosia; desatenção sensorial; incapacidade de localizar adequadamente uma sensação. Geralmente causada por lesão do lobo parietal contralateral. [G. *a*- priv. + *topos*, local, + *gnōsis*, conhecimento]

at·o·py (at′ō-pē). Atopia; um estado geneticamente determinado de hipersensibilidade a alérgenos ambientais. A reação alérgica do tipo I está associada ao anticorpo IgE e a um grupo de doenças, principalmente asma, febre do feno e dermatite atópica. [G. *atopia*, singularidade, de *a*- priv. + *topos*, um local]

atox·ic (ă-tok′sik). Atóxico; não-tóxico.

ATP Abreviatura para adenosine 5′-triphosphate (5′trifosfatase da adenosina).

ATPase. Abreviatura para adenosine triphosphatase (adenosina trifosfatase).

ATP cit·rate ly·ase. ATP-citrato liase. VER ATP *citrate (pro-3S)*-lyase.

ATPD Abreviatura de ambient temperature and pressure, dry; símbolo que indica que um volume de gás foi expresso como se ele tivesse sido secado em temperatura e pressão ambientes.

ATP-di·phos·pha·tase. ATP-difosfatase. SIN apyrase.

ATPS. Abreviatura de Ambient **t**emperature and **p**ressure, **s**aturated with water vapor; símbolo que indica que um volume de gás foi expresso como se ele estivesse saturado com vapor d'água em pressão barométrica e temperatura ambientes; a condição de um gás expirado em um espirômetro.

ATP sul·fur·y·lase. ATP-sulfurilase. SIN sulfate adenylyltransferase.

atrac·to·syl·id·ic ac·id (ă-trak′tō-sil-id′ik). Ácido atractossilídico. SIN atractyligenin.

atrac·tyl·ic ac·id (ă-trak′til-ik). Ácido atractílico; um glicosídeo esteróide muito venenoso da *Atractylis gummifera L. (Compositae)*, que possui uma ação semelhante à estricnina e provoca convulsões de natureza hipoglicêmica; a aglícona, a atractiligenina, combina-se à glicose e ao ácido isovalérico, sendo o princípio tóxico. O a. interfere com as reações oxidativas, ciclo do ácido cítrico e condução nervosa.

atrac·tyl·i·gen·in (ă-trak′til-i-jen′in). Atractiligenina; a aglícona aglicônio esteróide e princípio tóxico do ácido atractílico. SIN atractosylidic acid, atractylin.

atrac·tyl·in (ă-trak′til-in). Atractilina. SIN atractyligenin.

atra·cu·ri·um be·syl·ate (a-tră-kūr′ē-ŭm). Besilato de atracúrio; relaxante neuromuscular não-despolarizante com duração de ação intermediária; usado como adjunto para a anestesia geral; um agente semelhante ao curare.

atrep·sy (ă-trep′sē). Atrepsia. SIN athrepsia (2). [G. *a*- priv. + *trephō*, nutrir]

atre·sia (ă-trē′zē-ă). Atresia; ausência congênita de uma abertura normal ou luz normalmente pérvia. SIN clausura. [G. *a*- priv. + *trēsis*, um orifício]

anal a., a. a'ni, a. anal; ausência congênita de uma abertura anal devido à presença de um septo membranoso (persistência da membrana da cloaca) ou à ausência completa do canal anal. SIN imperforate anus, proctatresia.

aortic a., a. aórtica; a ausência congênita do orifício valvar na aorta.

biliary a., a. biliar; a. dos principais canais biliares, provocando colestase e icterícia, que não se torna aparente até vários dias depois do nascimento; a fibrose periporta desenvolve-se e leva à cirrose, com proliferação dos pequenos canais biliares, que quando estes também sejam atrésicos; também ocorre transformação das células hepáticas em células gigantes. Cf. neonatal *hepatitis*.

bronchial a., a. brônquica; estreitamento focal grave ou obliteração de um brônquio segmentar, subsegmentar ou lobar, geralmente associado ao aprisionamento de ar distal e impacção mucóide brônquica distal à obstrução.

choanal a., a. de cóano; a. decorrente da falha congênita de um ou ambos os cóanos em se abrir devido à ausência de involução da membrana buconasal. Resulta em obstrução nasal e cria uma emergência nos recém-nascidos, pois eles são respiradores nasais obrigatórios.

esophageal a., a. esofágica; a ausência congênita de desenvolvimento da luz da totalidade do esôfago; freqüentemente associada a fístula tráqueo-esofágica.

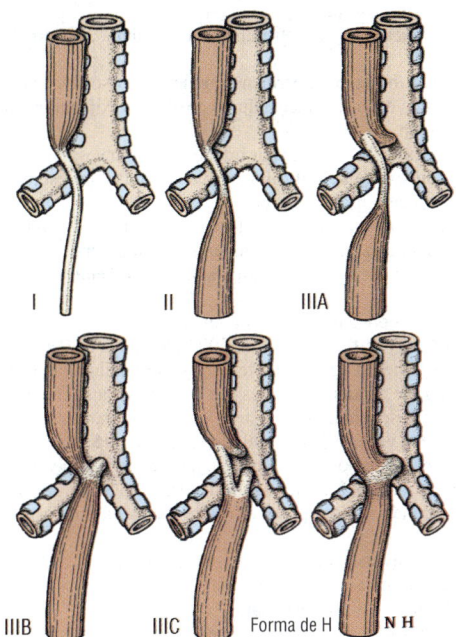

classificação de Vogt da atresia de esôfago: I-IIIC e o chamado tipo em forma de H

a. follic'uli, a. folicular; um processo normal que afeta os folículos ovarianos primordiais, no qual a morte do óvulo resulta em degeneração cística seguida por fechamento cicatricial.
intestinal a., a. intestinal; obliteração da luz do intestino delgado, com o íleo envolvido em 50% dos casos e o jejuno e duodeno em seguida na freqüência; causa mais freqüente de obstrução intestinal no neonato; a etiologia estaria relacionada à ausência de recanalização durante o desenvolvimento inicial ou a algum comprometimento do aporte sanguíneo durante a vida intra-uterina.
a. i'ridis, a. da íris; ausência congênita da abertura pupilar. SIN atretopsia.
laryngeal a., a. laríngea; ausência congênita do desenvolvimento da abertura laríngea, resultando em obstrução parcial ou total na glote ou logo acima ou abaixo dela.
pulmonary a., a. pulmonar; ausência congênita do orifício da valva pulmonar.
pulmonary artery a., a. da artéria pulmonar; ausência de uma artéria pulmonar, geralmente da a. direita.
tricuspid a., a. tricúspide; ausência congênita do orifício tricúspide.
vaginal a., a. vaginal; imperfuração ou oclusão, congênita ou adquirida, da vagina ou adesão das paredes da vagina. SIN colpatresia.
atre·sic (ā-trē′zik). Atrético. SIN atretic.
atret·ic (ā-tret′ik). Atrético; relativo à atresia. SIN atresic, imperforate.
atreto-. Prefixo que indica ausência de abertura. [G. atrētos, imperfurado, de a-, não + trētos, perfurado, de tetrainō, titrēmi, perfurar, atravessar]
atre·to·ble·pha·ria (ā-trē′tō-ble-far′ē-ă). Atretoblefaria. SIN symblepharon. [atreto- + G. blepharon, pálpebra]
atre·to·cys·tia (ā-trē′tō-sis′tē-ă). Atretocistia; termo obsoleto para ausência congênita ou adquirida de abertura da bexiga. [atreto- + G. kystis, bexiga]
atre·to·gas·tria (ā-trē′tō-gas′trē-ă). Atretogastria; ausência congênita de uma abertura do estômago. [atreto- + G. gaster, estômago]
atre·top·sia (ā-trē-top′sē-ă). Atretopsia, atresia da íris. SIN atresia iridis. [atreto- + G. ōps, olho]
atria (ā′trē-ă) [TA]. Átrios; plural de atrium.
atri·al (ā′trē-ăl). Atrial; relativo ao átrio.
atrich·ia (ā-trik′ē-ă). Atriquia; ausência de cabelos, congênita ou adquirida. SIN atrichosis. [G. a- priv. + thrix (trich-), cabelo]
atri·cho·sis (at-ri-kō′sis). Atricose. SIN atrichia.
atrio-. O átrio; atrial. [L. atrium, um hall de entrada]

atri·o·meg·a·ly (ā′trē-ō-meg′ă-lē). Atriomegalia; dilatação do átrio. [átrio- + G. megas, grande]
atri·o·nec·tor (ā-trē-ō-nek′ter, -tōr). Nó sinoatrial. SIN sinuatrial node. [átrio- + L. necto, unir]
atri·o·pep·tin (ā′trē-ō-pep′tin). Atriopeptina. SIN atrial natriuretic peptide. [atrio- + peptide + sufixo -in, material]
atri·o·sep·to·plas·ty (ā′trē-ō-sep′tō-plas-tē). Atriosseptoplastia; reparação cirúrgica de um defeito do septo interatrial. [atrio- + L. septum, partição, + G. plastos, formado]
atri·o·sep·tos·to·my (ā′trē-ō-sep-tos′tō-mē). Atriosseptostomia. SIN atrial septostomy. [atrio- + L. septum, partição, + G. stoma, boca]
balloon a., a. por balão; laceração ou aumento do forame oval por tração de um cateter com balão através do septo interatrial com a finalidade de aumentar a mistura interatrial do sangue no tratamento da cardiopatia congênita cianótica.
atri·ot·o·my (ā-trē-ot′ō-mē). Atriotomia; abertura cirúrgica de um átrio. [atrio- + G. tomē, incisão]
atri·o·ven·tric·u·lar (AV) (ā′trē-ō-ven-trik′u-lar). Atrioventricular; relativo aos átrios e ventrículos do coração, especialmente no tocante à transmissão comum, ortógrada, da condução ou do fluxo sanguíneo.
atrip·li·cism (ă-trip′li-sizm). Atriplicismo; uma intoxicação causada pela ingestão de determinadas espécies de Atriplex, ingerido como verduras na China; caracteriza-se por dor e edema dos dedos das mãos, propagando-se para o antebraço; formam-se bolhas e úlceras, e os dedos das mãos podem tornar-se gangrenosos. [L. atriplex (-plic-), armole, um vegetal]
atri·um, pl. **atria** (ā′trē-ŭm, ā′trē-ă). Átrio, átrios. 1 [TA]. Um compartimento ou uma cavidade à qual estão conectados vários compartimentos ou vias de passagem. 2. Átrios do coração. SIN a. of heart. 3. A parte da cavidade timpânica que se situa imediatamente profunda à membrana timpânica. 4. Átrio do meato médio. SIN a. of middle nasal meatus. 5. No pulmão, uma subdivisão do ducto alveolar a partir da qual se abre o saco alveolar. [L. um hall de entrada]
accessory a., a. acessório. SIN cor triatriatum.
a. cor'dis [TA], a. do coração. SIN a. of heart.
a. cordis dextrum [TA], a. direito do coração. SIN right a. of heart.
a. cordia sinistrum [TA], a. esquerdo do coração. SIN left a. of heart.
a. dex'trum cordis, a. direito do coração. SIN right a. of heart.
a. glot'tidis, vestíbulo da laringe. SIN vestibule of larynx.
a. of heart [TA], a. do coração; o compartimento superior de cada metade do coração. SIN a. cordis [TA], atrium (2).
a. of lateral ventricle [TA], a. do ventrículo lateral; porção do ventrículo lateral do cérebro comum aos cornos frontal, occipital e temporal. SIN a. ventriculi lateralis [TA], a. ventriculus lateralis [TA].
a. of lateral ventricle [TA], a. do ventrículo lateral; a porção do ventrículo lateral onde o corpo (ou parte central), corno posterior e corno temporal convergem; contém a dilatação coróide.
left a. of heart [TA], a. esquerdo do coração; a. do lado esquerdo do coração que recebe o sangue das veias pulmonares. SIN a. cordis sinistrum [TA], a. pulmonale, a. sinistrum cordis.
a. mea'tus me'dii, a. do meato médio. SIN a. of middle nasal meatus.
a. meatus medii nasalis [TA], a. do meato médio. SIN a. of middle nasal meatus.
a. of middle nasal meatus [TA], a. do meato médio; a porção anterior expandida do meato médio do nariz, exatamente acima do vestíbulo. SIN a. meatus medii nasalis [TA], a. meatus medii, atrium (4), nasal a.
nasal a., a. do meato. SIN a. of middle nasal meatus.
a. pulmona'le, a. esquerdo do coração. SIN left a. of heart.
right a. of heart [TA], a. direito do coração; a. do lado direito do coração que recebe o sangue das veias cava e do seio coronário. SIN a. cordis dextrum [TA], a. dextrum cordis.
a. sinis'trum cordis, a. esquerdo do coração. SIN left a. of heart.
a. ventriculi lateralis [TA], a. do ventrículo lateral. SIN a. of lateral ventricle.
a. ventriculus lateralis [TA], a. do ventrículo lateral. SIN a. of lateral ventricle.
At·ro·pa (at′rō-pă). Um gênero de plantas (família Solanaceae) da qual a A. belladonna é típica. VER belladonna. [G. Atropos, uma das Parcas que cortava o fio da vida, por causa dos efeitos letais da planta]
atro·phia (ă-trō′fē-ă). Atrofia. SIN atrophy. [G. de a- priv. + trophē, nutrição]
a. cu'tis, a. da pele, atrofodermia. SIN atrophoderma.
a. maculo'sa variolifor'mis cu'tis, a. maculosa varioliforme da pele, anetodermia. SIN anetoderma.
a. pilo'rum pro'pria, a. própria do pêlo; termo geral que inclui a tricoptilose, tricorrexe nodosa, monilietriquia e atrofia capilar.
atroph·ic (ă-trof′ik). Atrófico; que indica atrofia.
atro·phie blanche (ā′trō-fi blahnsh′). Atrofia branca; pequenas áreas branco-ebúrneas lisas, com bordas hiperpigmentadas e telangiectasia, que se desenvolvem em cicatrizes estrelares atróficas; observadas principalmente nas pernas e nos tornozelos de mulheres de meia-idade e associadas ao livedo reticular e à vasculite hialinizante dérmica. [Fr.]
at·ro·phied (at′rō-fēd). Atrofiado; caracterizado por atrofia.
at·ro·pho·der·ma (at′rō-fō-der′mă). Atrofodermia; atrofia da pele que pode

acontecer em áreas bem localizadas ou em áreas espalhadas. VER TAMBÉM anetoderma. SIN atrophia cutis.
a. al'bidum, a. álbida; tipo de atrofia em meia que afeta os membros, provavelmente congênita; observada pela primeira vez nos primeiros anos de vida nos membros inferiores como um adelgaçamento simétrico que torna as regiões sensíveis.
a. diffu'sum, a. difusa; atrofia cutânea idiopática difusa.
a. macula'tum, a. maculosa, anetodermia. SIN anetoderma.
a. neurit'icum, a. neurítica. SIN glossy skin.
a. of Pasini e Pierini, a. de Pasini e Pierini; uma forma de atrofia cutânea com coloração de ardósia que ocorre em lesões bem definidas, com 2 cm ou mais, isoladas ou múltiplas; ocasionalmente é confluente, aumentando em número e tamanho durante um período de anos e, em seguida, permanecendo constante; alguns acreditam que existem dois tipos: um que é precedido por morféia e o outro que aparece sem nenhuma patologia precedente identificável.
senile a., a. seni'lis, a. senil; a perda do colágeno, com adelgaçamento e elasticidade diminuída da pele associada ao envelhecimento.
a. stria'tum, a. estriada. SIN striae cutis distansae, em stria.
at·ro·pho·der·ma·to·sis (at'rō-fō-der-mă-tō'sis). Atrofodermatose; qualquer afecção cutânea na qual um sintoma proeminente é a atrofia da pele.
at·ro·phy (at'rō-fē). Atrofia; desgaste dos tecidos, órgãos ou de todo o corpo, como o causado pela morte, e reabsorção das células, proliferação celular diminuída, volume celular diminuído, pressão, isquemia, desnutrição, função diminuída ou alterações hormonais. SIN atrophia. [G. *atrophia*, de *a-* priv. + *trophē*, nutrição]
acute reflex bone a., a. óssea reflexa aguda. SIN Sudeck a.
acute yellow a. of the liver, necrose maciça aguda do fígado. SIN acute massive liver necrosis.
alveolar a., a. alveolar; diminuição no tamanho dos tecidos de sustentação dos dentes decorrente da falta de função, aporte sanguíneo reduzido ou causas desconhecidas.
arthritic a., a. artrítica; a. dos músculos tornados inativos por uma articulação cronicamente inflamada ou fixa.
blue a., a. azul; cicatrizes atróficas azuladas, deprimidas, devido a injeções na pele de substâncias impuras, conforme observado em viciados em narcóticos.
brown a., a. parda; a. da parede do coração, especialmente no idoso, na qual o músculo fica castanho-avermelhado escuro e reduzido em volume; as fibras musculares tornam-se pigmentadas, principalmente em torno dos núcleos, por grânulos lipocrômicos.
Buchwald a., a. de Buchwald; uma forma progressiva de a. cutânea.
central areolar choroidal a., a. areolar central da coróide. SIN areolar choroidopathy.
cerebellar a., a. cerebelar; degeneração do cerebelo, principalmente das células de Purkinje, como resultado da abiotrofia ou dos agentes tóxicos, como no alcoolismo.
choroidal vascular a., a. vascular da coróide; uma a. que afeta todos os vasos da coróide ou apenas os capilares corióideos, ocorrendo de forma difusa ou confinada ao pólo posterior do olho.
congenital cerebellar a., a. cerebelar congênita; distúrbio familiar que causa degeneração de várias células no cerebelo. São reconhecidos dois tipos, em um dos quais as células da camada granular degeneram e, no outro, as células de Purkinje degeneram.
congenital microvillus a., a. congênita das microvilosidades. SIN microvillus inclusion disease.
cyanotic a., a. cianótica; a. causada por destruição das células parenquimatosas de um órgão em consequência de congestão venosa crônica. SIN red a.
cyanotic a. of the liver, a. cianótica do fígado; seqüela da congestão hepática duradoura devido à alta pressão no átrio direito, como na pericardite constritiva crônica e na insuficiência ventricular direita grave e protraída.
dentatorubral cerebellar a. with polymyoclonus, a. cerebelar dentatorubral com polimioclonia. SIN dyssynergia cerebellaris myoclonica.
disuse a., a. por desuso; enfraquecimento muscular causado por imobilização, como no aparelho gessado.
dominant optic a., a. óptica dominante; neuropatia óptica autossômica dominante bilateral, caracterizada por perda insidiosa da visão no período pré-escolar. SIN Kjer optic a.
essential progressive a. of iris, a. essencial progressiva da íris; a. progressiva da íris sem sinais inflamatórios, caracterizada por perda difusa de todas as camadas da íris com a formação de uma cavidade, migração da pupila, degeneração do endotélio da córnea, sinéquias anteriores periféricas e glaucoma secundário; geralmente unilateral, afetando predominantemente as mulheres de meia-idade. VER TAMBÉM iridocorneal syndrome.
facioscapulohumeral a., a. facioescapuloumeral. SIN facioscapulohumeral muscular dystrophy.
familial spinal muscular a., a. muscular facial familial. SIN spinal muscular a., type I.
fatty a., a. gordurosa; infiltração gordurosa secundária à a. dos elementos essenciais de um órgão ou tecido.

geographic retinal a., a. retiniana geográfica; um padrão de a. bem demarcada do epitélio pigmentado retiniano associada à camada coriocapilar e à a. dos fotorreceptores, levando à perda da visão.
gingival a., a. gengival. SIN gingival recession.
gyrate a. of choroid and retina [MIM*258870], a. convoluta da coróide e retina; a. lentamente progressiva dos coriocapilares, do epitélio pigmentar e da retina sensorial, com áreas atróficas confluentes irregulares e ornitinúria associada; herança autossômica recessiva; devido a deficiência de ornitina δ-aminotransferase, causada por mutação no gene da ornitina δ-aminotransferase (OAT) no cromossoma 10q.
Hoffmann muscular a., a. muscular de Hoffmann. SIN spinal muscular a., type I.
horizontal a., a. horizontal; perda progressiva de osso alveolar e de sustentação ao redor dos dentes, começando no nível mais coronal do osso. SIN horizontal resorption.
infantile muscular a., a. muscular infantil. SIN spinal muscular a. type I.
infantile progressive spinal muscular a., a. muscular espinal progressiva infantil. SIN spinal muscular a., type I.
ischemic muscular a., a. muscular isquêmica. VER Volkmann contracture.
juvenile muscular a., a. muscular juvenil. SIN spinal muscular a., type III.
juvenile spinal muscular a., a. muscular espinal juvenil. SIN spinal muscular a., type III.
Kjer optic a., a. óptica de Kjer. SIN dominant optic a.
Leber hereditary optic a. [MIM*535000], a. óptica degenerativa de Leber; degeneração do nervo óptico e do feixe maculopapular com resultante perda da visão central e cegueira, progressiva durante várias semanas, geralmente tornando-se, em seguida, estacionária, com escotoma central permanente; a idade do início é variável, mais amiúde na terceira década de vida; é afetado um número maior de homens do que de mulheres. Herança mitocondrial ou citoplasmática, através da linhagem materna, causada por mutação no(s) gene(s) mitocondrial(ais), que atua(m) de forma autônoma ou em associação entre si.
linear a., a. linear. SIN striae cutis distansae, em stria.
macular a., a. macular. SIN anetoderma.
marantic a., marasmo. SIN marasmus.
multiple system a., a. de múltiplos sistemas; doença neurodegenerativa não-hereditária de etiologia desconhecida, caracterizada clinicamente pelo desenvolvimento de parkinsonismo, ataxia, insuficiência autônoma ou sinais do trato piramidal, em diversas combinações. Ao nível histopatológico, há perda das células nervosas, gliose e acúmulo de estruturas tubulares anormais no citoplasma e núcleo dos oligodendrócitos e neurônios nos gânglios da base, cerebelo e colunas intermediolaterais da medula espinal; pode apresentar-se como parkinsonismo predominante, como ataxia predominante ou como uma combinação de parkinsonismo, ataxia e insuficiência autônoma; é um distúrbio com progressão relativamente rápida e fatal.
muscular a., a. muscular; atrofia do tecido muscular. Cf. myopathic a. SIN myatrophy, myoatrophy.
myopathic a., a. miopática; a. muscular provocada por um distúrbio primário do músculo.
neurogenic a., a. neurogênica. SIN neurotrophic a.
neurotrophic a., anormalidades da pele, dos cabelos, das unhas, dos tecidos subcutâneos e do osso causadas por lesões de nervos periféricos. SIN neurogenic a., trophoneurotic a.
nutritional type cerebellar a., a. cerebelar do tipo nutricional; um tipo restrito de degeneração cortical cerebelar, afetando principalmente as células de Purkinje das porções anterior e superior do verme; provavelmente causada por deficiência de tiamina; observada com mais freqüência nos alcoólicos crônicos e, em seguida, chamada de degeneração cerebelar alcoólica.
olivopontocerebellar a., a. olivopontocerebelar; um grupo de doenças neurológicas geneticamente distintas, em sua maioria autossômicas dominantes, caracterizadas por perda de neurônios no córtex cerebelar, parte basilar da ponte e núcleos olivares inferiores; resulta em ataxia, tremor, movimento involuntário e disartria; cinco tipos clínicos (quatro com herança dominante, um com recessiva) já foram descritos, com cada tipo caracterizado por achados adicionais, como perda sensorial, degeneração da retina, oftalmoplegia e sinais extrapiramidais. Estão envolvidos vários *loci*, autossômicos dominantes [MIM*164400 a *164600] e recessivos [MIM*258300]. VER TAMBÉM spinocerebellar *ataxia*. SIN olivopontocerebellar degeneration.
periodontal a., a. periodontal; diminuição no tamanho e/ou elementos celulares peridentários, depois que eles alcançaram a maturidade normal.
peroneal muscular a., a. muscular fibular; um grupo de distúrbios neuromusculares periféricos que compartilha o aspecto comum do desgaste acentuado das partes distais dos membros, principalmente dos grupos musculares fibulares, resultando em pernas longas e finas; geralmente afeta as pernas antes dos braços, com o pé cavo sendo, com freqüência, o primeiro sinal. Existem duas formas de polineuropatias sensorimotoras hereditárias, isto é, um tipo desmielinizante e um tipo com perda axônica. Existem formas autossômica dominante [MIM*118200 e MIM*118220], autossômica recessiva [MIM*214400]

atrophy

e recessiva ligada ao X [MIM*302800, MIM*302801 e MIM*302802]. SIN Charcot-Marie-Tooth disease.

Pick a., a. de Pick; a. circunscrita do córtex cerebral. SIN lobar sclerosis, progressive circumscribed cerebral a.

postmenopausal a., a. pós-menopausa; a. após a menopausa, como dos órgãos genitais.

pressure a., a. por compressão; a atrofia de tecidos moles e duros decorrente da pressão excessiva aplicada aos tecidos pela base de uma prótese dentária.

primary idiopathic macular a., a. macular idiopática primária. SIN anetoderma.

primary macular a. of skin, a. macular primária da pele. SIN anetoderma.

progressive choroidal a., a. progressiva da coróide. SIN choroideremia.

progressive circumscribed cerebral a., a. cerebral circunscrita progressiva. SIN Pick a.

progressive infantile spinal muscular a., a. infantil progressiva da musculatura paravertebral. SIN spinal muscular a., type I.

progressive muscular a., a. muscular progressiva. SIN amyotrophic lateral sclerosis.

progressive spinal muscular a., a. progressiva da musculatura paravertebral; um dos subgrupos da doença do neurônio motor; distúrbio degenerativo progressivo dos neurônios motores da medula espinal, manifestado como desgaste e fraqueza progressivos, freqüentemente simétricos, que começam tipicamente nas porções distais dos membros, principalmente nos membros superiores, e que se disseminam no sentido proximal; potenciais de fasciculação são comuns, mas sem evidências de doença do trato corticoespinal (p.ex., reflexos tendinosos profundos exacerbados, sinal de Babinski).

pulp a., a. pulpar; diminuição do tamanho e/ou dos elementos celulares da polpa dentária devido à interferência com o aporte sanguíneo.

red a., a. ciano. SIN cyanotic a.

scapulohumeral a., a. escapuloumeral. SIN Vulpian a.

senile a., a. senil; desgaste dos tecidos e órgãos com o envelhecimento por causa de processos catabólicos ou anabólicos diminuídos, por vezes devido às alterações endócrinas, uso diminuído ou isquemia. SIN geromarasmus.

spinal muscular a. (SMA), a. da musculatura paravertebral; um grupo heterogêneo de doenças degenerativas das células do corno anterior na medula espinal e nos núcleos motores do tronco cerebral; todas caracterizam-se por fraqueza. Os neurônios motores superiores permanecem normais. Essas doenças incluem a doença de Werdnig-Hoffmann (SMA do tipo 1), SMA do tipo 2 e doença de Kugelberg-Welander (SMA do tipo 3). VER TAMBÉM Fazio-Londe *disease*.

spinal muscular a., type I [MIM*253300], a. da musculatura espinal do tipo 1; a forma infantil inicial, caracterizada por desgaste substancial da musculatura e atrofia que surge por ocasião do nascimento ou logo após; a morte geralmente acontece antes de 2 anos de idade. Herança autossômica recessiva, causada por mutação no gene de sobrevida do neurônio motor (SMN1) em 5q. Cerca de metade dos pacientes também não têm homólogos em um gene vizinho que codifica a proteína inibitória da apoptose neuronal (NAIP), cuja perda se acredita influencie a gravidade da doença. SIN familial spinal muscular a., Hoffmann muscular a., infantile muscular a., infantile progressive spinal muscular a., progressive infantile spinal muscular a., Werdnig-Hoffmann disease, Werdnig-Hoffmann muscular a.

spinal muscular a., type II [MIM*253550], a. da musculatura paravertebral do tipo II; uma forma intermediária em termos de gravidade entre a forma infantil (SMA do tipo I) e a forma juvenil (SMA do tipo III); caracterizada por fraqueza muscular proximal com o início geralmente entre 3 e 15 meses e sobrevida até a adolescência; herança autossômica recessiva, causada por mutação no gene SMN1 em 5q.

spinal muscular a., type III [MIM*253400], a. da musculatura paravertebral do tipo III; a forma juvenil com início na infância ou adolescência, caracterizada por fraqueza e desgaste progressivos da musculatura proximal, principalmente nas pernas, seguindo-se envolvimento da musculatura distal, causada por degeneração dos neurônios motores nos cornos anteriores da medula espinal; herança autossômica recessiva, causada por mutação no gene SMN1 em 5q. SIN juvenile muscular a., juvenile spinal muscular a., Kugelberg-Welander disease, Wohlfart-Kugelberg-Welander disease.

striate a. of skin, a. estriada da pele. SIN *striae* cutis distansae, em *stria*.

Sudeck a., a. de Sudeck; a. dos ossos, comumente dos ossos do carpo ou tarso, após uma lesão leve, como uma distensão. VER TAMBÉM causalgia, reflex sympathetic *dystrophy*. SIN acute reflex bone a., posttraumatic osteoporosis, Sudeck syndrome.

traction a., a. de tração. SIN *striae* cutis distansae, em *stria*.

transneuronal a., a. transneuronal. SIN transsynaptic degeneration.

trophoneurotic a., a. trofoneurótica. SIN neurotrophic a.

villous a., a. vilosa; anormalidade da mucosa do intestino delgado com hiperplasia das criptas, resultando em achatamento da mucosa e aparecimento da a. das vilosidades; clinicamente observada nas síndromes de má absorção, como o espru.

Vulpian a., a. de Vulpian; a. progressiva da musculatura paravertebral que começa no ombro. SIN scapulohumeral a.

attack

Werdnig-Hoffmann muscular a., a. muscular de Werdnig-Hoffmann; SIN spinal muscular a., type I.

yellow a. of the liver, necrose maciça aguda do fígado. VER acute yellow a. of the liver.

Zimmerlin a., a. de Zimmerlin; uma variedade de a. muscular progressiva hereditária em que a a. começa na metade superior do corpo.

at·ro·pine (at′rō‐pēn). Atropina; uma mistura racêmica de d- e l-hiosciamina, alcalóides obtidos das folhas e raízes da *Atropa belladonna*; um anticolinérgico com efeitos diversos (taquicardia, midríase, cicloplegia, constipação, retenção urinária, anti-sudoral) atribuíveis ao bloqueio competitivo reversível da acetilcolina nos receptores colinérgicos do tipo muscarínico; usada no tratamento do envenenamento por inseticidas organofosforados ou gases dos nervos. A forma (−) é, sem dúvida, a forma mais ativa. SIN *dl*-hyoscyamine, tropine tropate.

a. methonitrate, metonitrato de a.; o metilnitrato de a., com as mesmas ações e usos de a., porém menos lipossolúvel (devido à presença de um átomo de amônio quaternário que limita a penetração da barreira hematoencefálica) e, portanto, com menos efeitos sobre o sistema nervoso central; um composto quaternário.

a. methylbromide, metilbrometo de a. SIN methylatropine bromide.

a. sulfate, sulfato de a.; anticolinérgico, um sal solúvel de atropina amplamente utilizado.

atrop·in·ic (at′rō‐pin‐ik). Atropínico; termo utilizado para indicar a partilha das propriedades farmacológicas com a atropina. Isso significa o bloqueio das junções neuroefetoras assimpáticas que levam a inúmeros efeitos, incluindo taquicardia, retenção urinária, ressecamento da boca, constipação, midríase, cicloplegia e outros efeitos anticolinérgicos.

at·ro·pin·ism (at′rō‐pin‐izm). Atropinismo; sintomas de intoxicação por atropina ou beladona.

at·ro·pin·i·za·tion (at‐rō′pin‐i‐zā′shŭn). Atropinização; administração de atropina ou beladona até o ponto de conseguir o efeito farmacológico.

atros·cine. Atroscina; *dl*-escopolamina. VER scopamine. [atropine + hyoscine]

at·ro·tox·in (at‐rō‐toks′in). Atrotoxina; um componente do veneno da cascavel *Crotalus atrox*, que aumenta de forma específica e reversível as correntes de íon cálcio voltagem-dependentes em miócitos isolados.

at·tach·ment (ă‐tach′ment). Conexão, fixação. **1.** Uma conexão de uma parte com outra. **2.** Em odontologia, um dispositivo mecânico para a fixação e estabilização de uma prótese dentária.

bar clip a.'s, articulações de barra. SIN bar-sleeve a.'s

bar-sleeve a.'s, articulações de barra fixa ou unidades de barra rígida usadas para dar suporte a contrafortes com grampos ou bainhas removíveis dentro da dentadura parcial para o suporte e/ou retenção da prótese. SIN bar clip a.'s.

epithelial a., epitélio juncional. SIN junctional *epithelium*.

epithelial a. of Gottlieb, epitélio juncional. SIN junctional *epithelium*.

frictional a., conexão friccional. SIN precision a.

internal a., conexão interna. SIN precision a.

key a., conexão de precisão. SIN precision a.

keyway a., conexão de precisão. SIN precision a.

muscle-tendon a., conexão musculotendínea; a união de um músculo e fibra tendinosa em que o sarcolema intervém entre os dois; a extremidade da fibra muscular pode ser arredondada, cônica ou afilada. SIN muscle-tendon junction.

parallel a., conexão de precisão. SIN precision a.

pericemental a., i. pericimental; os tecidos que circundam o cimento do dente, isto é, o ligamento periodontal e o osso alveolar.

precision a., conexão de precisão; **(1)** uma unidade friccional ou mecanicamente retida utilizada em prótese odontológica removível ou fixa, consistindo em partes macho e fêmea bem ajustadas; **(2)** uma conexão que pode ser rígida na função ou pode incorporar uma unidade de controle de estresse móvel para diminuir o torque sobre o ponto de apoio. SIN frictional a., internal a., key a., keyway a., parallel a., slotted a.

slotted a., conexão de precisão. SIN precision a.

at·tack (ă‐tak′). Ataque, crise, episódio; uma doença súbita ou um episódio ou exacerbação da doença crônica ou recorrente.

brain a., acidente vascular cerebral. SIN stroke (1).

drop a., episódios de queda; um episódio de queda súbita que acontece ao ficar em pé ou caminhar, sem aviso prévio e sem perda da consciência, vertigem ou comportamento pós-ictal. Os pacientes geralmente são idosos e apresentam eletroencefalogramas normais, de etiologia desconhecida.

heart a., infarto do miocárdio. SIN myocardial *infarction*.

panic a., a. de pânico; início súbito de apreensão intensa, medo, terror ou morte iminente acompanhado por atividade aumentada do sistema nervoso autônomo e por vários distúrbios constitucionais, despersonalização e perda do sentido da realidade.

salaam a., espasmos de aquiescência, crises de salamaleque. SIN nodding *spasm*.

transient ischemic a. (TIA), a. isquêmico transitório (AIT); súbita perda focal da função neurológica com recuperação completa, geralmente em 24 ho-

ras; causado por um breve período de perfusão inadequada em uma porção do território das artérias carótida ou basilar vertebral.
uncinate a., epilepsia uncinada. SIN uncinate *epilepsy.*
vagal a., a. vagal. SIN Gowers *syndrome.*
vasovagal a., a vasovagal. SIN Gowers *syndrome.*
at·tar of rose (at'ăr). Óleo de rosa. SIN rose oil, oil of rose. [Pers. *attara,* odor doce]
at·tend·ing (ă-tend'ing). Dedicação; em psicologia, uma disposição exacerbada para observar (compreender), por meio da audição ou visão; a focalização dos órgãos do sentido está, por vezes, envolvida. [L. *attendo,* atender, noticiar]
at·ten·u·ant (ă-ten'ū-ănt). Atenuante, atenuador. **1.** Denotando aquilo que atenua. **2.** Um agente, meio ou método que atenua.
at·ten·u·ate (ă-ten'ū-āt). Atenuar; diluir, tornar menos espesso, amolecer, adelgaçar, enfraquecer, abrandar. [L. *at-tenuo,* pp. *-tenuatus,* tornar mais fino ou fraco; de *tenuis,* fino]
at·ten·u·a·tion (ă-ten-ū-ā'shŭn). Atenuação. **1.** O ato de atenuar. **2.** Diminuição da virulência em uma cepa de um organismo, obtido através da seleção de variantes que ocorrem naturalmente ou através de meios experimentais. **3.** Perda da energia de um feixe de energia radiante devido à absorção, dispersão, divergência do feixe e outras causas, enquanto o feixe se propaga através de um meio. **4.** Regulação do término da transcrição; envolvido no controle da expressão do gene em tecidos específicos.
interaural a., a. interaural; a redução feita pela cabeça na intensidade do som apresentado a um canal auditivo antes que ele chegue ao outro ouvido; para a condução pelo ar, a redução aproxima-se de 35 dB, mas, para a condução óssea, ela é de apenas cerca de 10 dB.
at·ten·u·a·tor (ă-ten'ū-ā-tŏr, -tōr). Atenuador. **1.** Um sistema elétrico de resistências e capacitores usado para diminuir a força dos sinais elétricos em uma ultra-sonografia. **2.** A seqüência terminal no DNA em que ocorre atenuação.
at·tic (at'ik). Ático, recesso.
tympanic a., Recesso epitimpânico. SIN epitympanic *recess.*
at·ti·co·mas·toid (at'i-kō-mas'toyd). Relativo ao recesso epitimpânico e às células ou ao antro mastóideo.
at·ti·cot·o·my (at-i-kot'ō-mē). Abertura cirúrgica para o recesso epitimpânico. [attic + G. *tomē,* incisão]
at·ti·tude (at'i-tood). Atitude. **1.** Posição do corpo e dos membros. **2.** Maneira de agir. **3.** Em psicologia social ou clínica, uma predisposição ou disposição relativamente estável e resistente para se comportar ou reagir de determinada maneira em relação a pessoas, objetos, instituições ou questões. [L. Mediev. *aptitudo,* do L. *aptus,* apto].
emotional a.'s, atitudes emocionais. SIN passional a.'s.
fetal a., posição fetal. SIN fetal *habitus.*
passional a.'s, atitudes passionais; atitudes expressivas de qualquer uma das grandes paixões; p.ex., raiva, luxúria. SIN emotional a.'s.
at·ti·tu·di·nal (at-i-too'di-năl). Atitudinal; relativo a uma postura do corpo; p.ex., reflexo a. (estatônico).
atto- (a). Ato; prefixo utilizado no SI e sistema métrico para significar um quintilionésimo (10^{-18}). [Dinamarquês *atten,* dezoito]
at·tol·lens (ă-tol'ens). Elevado; em anatomia, a ação muscular que eleva. [L. *at-tollo,* pp. *-tollens,* levantar]
a. au'rem, a. auric'ulam, músculo auricular superior. SIN auricularis superior (*muscle*).
a. oc'uli, músculo superior do bulbo do olho. SIN superior rectus (*muscle*).
at·trac·tin (a-trak'tin). Atractina; uma glicoproteína oriunda da célula T envolvida no agrupamento da célula T e do movimento do monócito.
at·trac·tion (ă-trak'shŭn). Atração; a tendência de dois corpos para se aproximarem um do outro. [L. *at-traho,* pp. *-tractus,* tender para]
capillary a., a. capilar; a força que faz com que os líquidos se elevem em tubos muito finos ou atravessem os poros de um material frouxo.
chemical a., a. química; a força que impele os átomos de diferentes elementos ou moléculas a se unirem para formar novas substâncias ou compostos.
magnetic a., a. magnética; a força que dirige o ferro ou o magnésio no sentido de um magneto.
neurotropic a., a. neurotrópica; a atração de um axônio em regeneração em direção à placa motora terminal.
at·tra·hens (at'ră-henz). Atraente; que se inclina no sentido de, indicando um músculo (auricular superior) rudimentar no homem, que tende a mover o pavilhão auricular para diante. VER auricularis anterior (*muscle*). [ver attraction]
at·tri·tion (ă-trish'ŭn). Atrito. **1.** Desgaste por fricção ou raspagem. **2.** Em odontologia, a perda fisiológica da estrutura dentária causada pelo caráter abrasivo do alimento ou a partir do bruxismo. Cf. abrasion. [L. *at-tero,* pp. *-tritus,* esfregar contra, atritar]
at. wt. Abreviatura para atomic *weight* (peso atômico).
atyp·ia (ă-tip'ē-ă). Atipia; o estado de não ser típico. SIN atypism.
atyp·i·cal (ă-tip'i-kal). Atípico; não-típico; que não corresponde à forma ou tipo normal. [G. *a-* priv. + *typikos,* conformado a um tipo]

atyp·ism (ă-tip'izm). Atipia. SIN atypia.
A. U. Abreviatura para *auris uterque* [L.], cada orelha ou as duas orelhas.
Au Símbolo do ouro (aurum).
Aub, Joseph C., médico norte-americano, 1890–1973. VER A.-DuBois *table.*
Auberger blood group, Au blood group, grupo sanguíneo Auberger ou Au. Ver apêndice de Grupos Sanguíneos.
Aubert, Hermann, fisiologista alemão, 1826–1892. VER A. *phenomenon.*
AUC Área sob a curva de concentração plasmática de medicamento *versus* tempo; uma medida da exposição do medicamento. [abrev. de *area under the curve*]
Auch·mer·o·my·ia (awk'mer-ō-mī'yă). Um gênero de moscas-varejeiras hematófagas (família Calliphoridae, ordem Diptera). [G. *auchmeros,* sem chuva, daí não lavado, esquálido, + *myia,* uma mosca]
A. lute'ola, a larva hematófaga dessa espécie de mosca é encontrada na África, ao sul do Saara, geralmente em habitações de seres humanos ou próximo a elas; as larvas resistentes rastejam para os seres humanos durante o sono, sugando-lhes o sangue por 15 a 20 minutos; a seguir, desprendem-se e escondem-se, repetindo esses ataques noturnos durante seu período de desenvolvimento; não se conhece nenhuma doença transmitida por esse inseto.
[198]Au col·loid. Colóide de ouro radiológico. SIN radiogold colloid.
au·dile (aw'dil). **1.** Auditivo; relativo à audição. **2.** Pessoa do tipo auditivo; denotando o tipo que lembra mais prontamente aquilo que foi ouvido do que o que foi visto ou lido (isto é, que possui um sistema de representação auditiva). Cf. motile. **3.** SIN auditive.
audio-. Forma combinante relativa à audição. [L. *audio,* ouvir]
au·di·o·an·al·ge·sia (aw'dē-ō-an-ăl-jē'zē-ă). Audioanalgesia; uso de música ou som (por meio de fones de ouvido) para mascarar a dor durante procedimentos dentários ou cirúrgicos.
au·di·o·gen·ic (awdē-ō-jen'ik). Audiogênico; causado por som, especialmente um ruído alto. [audio- + G. *genesis,* produção]
au·di·o·gram (aw'dē-ō-gram). Audiograma; o registro gráfico feito a partir dos resultados dos testes de audição com um audiômetro, o qual traça o limiar da audição em várias freqüências em relação à intensidade do som em decibéis. [audio- + G. *gramma,* um desenho]

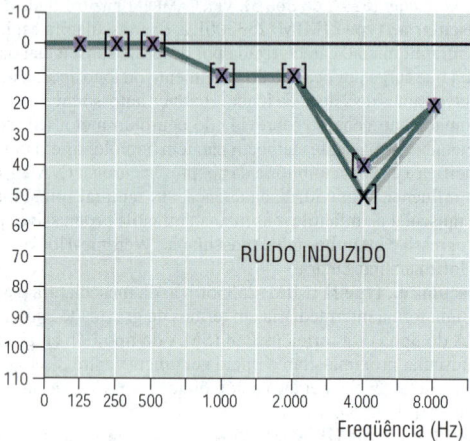

audiograma: padrão anormal típico da perda auditiva induzida por ruído

pure tone a., a. de tom puro, a. tonal; um gráfico do limiar para a audição em várias freqüências usualmente expressos em decibéis em relação ao limiar normal e, em geral, cobrindo as freqüências de 250–8.000 Hz.
speech a., a. da fala, a. vocal; o registro dos limiares para listas de palavras esporádicas e escores para listas de palavras foneticamente balanceadas.
au·di·ol·o·gist (aw-dē-ol'ōjist). Audiólogo, audiologista; um especialista na avaliação e reabilitação daqueles cujos distúrbios de comunicação se originam, em parte ou totalmente, do comprometimento da audição.
au·di·ol·o·gy (aw-dē-ol'ō-jē). Audiologia; o estudo dos distúrbios da audição através da identificação e medição do comprometimento da audição, bem como da reabilitação das pessoas com comprometimentos da audição.
au·di·om·e·ter (aw-dē-om'ĕ-ter). Audiômetro; um aparelho eletrônico usado na medição do limiar da audição para tons puros de freqüências, que geralmente variam entre 125 e 8.000 Hz e a fala (registrada nos termos de decibéis). [audio- + G. *metron,* medida]
automatic a., a. automático. SIN Békésy a.

audiometer / auricula

Békésy a., a. de Békésy; um a. automático em que o tom oscila na escala audiométrica, enquanto o paciente controla a intensidade ao pressionar um botão quando o tom é ouvido e libera-o quando o tom não pode ser ouvido; pode ser operado em uma freqüência fixa ou em freqüências mutáveis.
pure-tone a., a. de tom puro; um a. que gera tons puros de freqüências selecionadas com intensidade variável. Os estímulos são transmitidos por condução aérea e condução óssea para diferenciar a perda auditiva por condução, sensorioneural ou mista.
speech a., a. da fala; um a. que fornece o material falado em níveis de pressão sonora controlada para obter os limiares de recepção da fala, tolerância para a fala alta e capacidade de discriminação, quer usando uma voz viva por um microfone, quer uma voz gravada. Fornece uma medição do desempenho global na audição, compreensão e resposta à fala e uma estimativa do grau de incapacidade auditiva.
au·di·o·met·ric (aw-dē-ō-met′rik). Audiométrico; relacionado à medição dos níveis de audição ou a um audiômetro.
au·di·om·e·trist (aw-dē-om′ē-trist). Audiometrista; uma pessoa treinada no uso de um audiômetro no teste da audição.
au·di·om·e·try (aw-dē-om′ē-trē). Audiometria. **1.** A medição da audição. **2.** O uso de um audiômetro. **3.** A medição rápida da audição de uma pessoa ou de um grupo contra um limite predeterminado da normalidade; são testadas as respostas auditivas a diferentes freqüências apresentadas em um nível de intensidade constante. SIN screening a.
automatic a., a. automática; a. em que a pessoa controla os aumentos e diminuições na intensidade em uma freqüência fixa ou, mais amiúde, à medida que a freqüência do estímulo é gradualmente alterada, de modo que o indivíduo é avaliado ao longo do limiar de audição. SIN Békésy a.
behavioral observation a., a. por observação comportamental; um método de observar as respostas motoras de crianças pequenas para testar as intensidades sonoras para determinar o limiar de audição.
Békésy a., a. de Békésy. SIN automatic a.
cortical a., a. cortical; medição dos potenciais que se originam no sistema auditivo acima do nível do tronco cerebral.
diagnostic a., a. diagnóstica; medição dos níveis de limiar de audição para determinar a natureza e o grau de comprometimento da audição (isto é, por condução, sensorioneural ou misto).
screening a., a. de triagem. SIN audiometry (3).
au·di·o·vi·su·al (aw′dē-ō-vizh′ū-ăl). Audiovisual; pertinente a uma técnica de comunicação ou ensino que combina símbolos audíveis e visíveis.
au·dit. Auditoria; um exame ou revisão que estabelece a extensão em que uma condição, processo ou desempenho se conforma aos padrões ou critérios predeterminados. [L. *auditus*, uma audição, de *audio*, ouvir]
au·di·tion (aw-dish′ŭn). Audição. SIN hearing. [L. *auditio*, uma audição, de *audio*, ouvir]
chromatic a., a. cromática. SIN color hearing.
au·di·tive (aw′di-tiv). Pessoa do tipo auditivo, ou seja, que se lembra mais facilmente daquilo que foi ouvido. SIN audile (3).
au·di·to·ry (aw′di-tōr-ē). **1.** Auditivo; pertinente ao sentido da audição ou ao sistema que serve à audição. **2.** Pessoa do tipo auditivo; termo usado para descrever uma pessoa que utiliza preferencialmente imagens mentais verbais. VER TAMBÉM internal *representation*. [L. *audio*, pp. *auditus*, ouvir]
Auenbrugger, Leopold, médico austríaco, 1722–1809. VER A. *sign*.
Auer, John, médico norte-americano, 1875–1948. VER A. *bodies*, em *body*, *rods*, em *rod*.
Auerbach, Leopold, anatomista alemão, 1828–1897. VER A. *ganglia*, em *ganglion*, *plexus*.
Aufrecht, Emanuel, médico alemão, 1844–1933. VER A. *sign*.
Auger (aw′gĕr). Pierre-Victor, físico francês, 1899–1993. VER Auger *electron*.
aug·na·thus (awg-nā′thŭs). Augnato. SIN dignathus. [G. *au*, novamente, + *gnathos*, mandíbula]
Aujeszky, Aládar, patologista húngaro, 1869–1933. VER A. disease *virus*.
aur Abreviatura para auris (orelha).
au·ra, pl. **au·rae** (aw′ră, -rē). Aura. **1.** Fenômeno/fenômenos ictais epilépticos percebidos apenas pelo paciente. **2.** Sintomas subjetivos no início de uma enxaqueca. [L. brisa, odor, raio de luz]
abdominal a., a. abdominal; a. epiléptica caracterizada por desconforto abdominal, incluindo náuseas, indisposição, dor e fome; alguns fenômenos refletem disfunção autônoma ictal. VER TAMBÉM aura (1).
auditory a., a. auditiva; a. epiléptica caracterizada por ilusões ou alucinações sonoras. VER TAMBÉM aura (1).
experiential a., a. de experiência; a. epiléptica caracterizada por percepção alterada do ambiente interno e/ou externo da pessoa; pode envolver percepções auditiva, visual, olfativa, gustativa, somatossensorial ou emocional alteradas. Quando uma das percepções alteradas é nitidamente predominante, deve ser utilizada a classificação da a. específica. VER TAMBÉM aura (1).
gustatory a., a. gustativa; a. epiléptica caracterizada por ilusões ou alucinações do paladar. VER TAMBÉM aura (1).
intellectual a., a. intelectual; uma a. reminiscente, desprendida ou onírica. SIN reminiscent a.
kinesthetic a., a. cinestésica; a. que consiste em sensação subjetiva de movimento de uma parte do corpo.
olfactory a., a. olfativa; a. epiléptica caracterizada por ilusões ou alucinações do olfato. VER TAMBÉM aura (1).
reminiscent a., a. reminiscente. SIN intellectual a.
somatosensory a., a. somatossensorial; a. epiléptica caracterizada por parestesias ou somatognosia abdominal com uma distribuição regional bem definida. VER TAMBÉM aura (1).
visual a., a. visual; a. epiléptica caracterizada por ilusões ou alucinações visuais, formadas ou disformes, incluindo cintilações, teicopsia. VER TAMBÉM aura (1).
au·ral (aw′răl). Aural. **1.** Relativo à orelha (auris). **2.** Relativo a uma aura.
au·ra·mine O (aw′ră-mēn). [C.I. 41000]. Auramina; um corante fluorescente amarelo, usado como corante para o bacilo da tuberculose e como corante para DNA na coloração de Feulgen fluorescente de Kasten.
au·ran·o·fin (aw-ran′ō-fin). Auranofina; uma forma oral de complexo de ouro usada no tratamento da artrite reumatóide.
au·re·o·lic ac·id (aw-rē-ō′lik). Ácido aureólico. SIN mithramycin.
auri-. Forma combinante que indica a orelha. VER TAMBÉM ot-, oto-. [L. *auris*, um ouvido]
au·ri·a·sis (aw-rī′ă-sis). Auríase, aurocromodermia. SIN chrysiasis.
au·ric (aw′rik). Áurico, áureo; relativo ao ouro (aurum).
au·ri·cle (aw′ri-kl). [TA]. **1.** A estrutura em forma de concha que se projeta no lado da cabeça, constituindo, com o meato acústico externo, a orelha externa. SIN auricula (1) [TA], ala auris, pinna (1). **2.** Aurículas dos átrios. SIN a.'s (of atria).
accessory a.'s, aurículas acessórias; pregas ou nódulos carnosos pequenos, por vezes com a cartilagem de sustentação, ocasionalmente encontrados ao longo das margens das fendas branquiais embrionárias.
atrial a., a. do átrio. SIN a.'s (of atria). VER TAMBÉM left *atrium* of heart, right *atrium* of heart.
cervical a., a. cervical; a. acessória no pescoço.
left a. [TA], a. do átrio esquerdo; a pequena projeção cônica a partir do átrio esquerdo do coração. SIN auricula atrii sinistra [TA], a. of left atrium, left auricular appendage.
a. of left atrium, a. do átrio esquerdo. SIN left a.
a.'s (of atria) [TA], aurículas (dos átrios); uma pequena projeção sacular cônica ("em forma de concha") a partir da porção ântero-superior de cada átrio do coração, aumentando um pouco o volume atrial. VER left a., right a. SIN auricle (2) [TA], auricula (2) [TA], auriculae atrii [TA], atrial appendage, atrial a., atrial auricula, auricular appendix.
right a. [TA], a. do átrio direito; a pequena projeção cônica do átrio direito do coração. SIN auricula atrii dextra [TA], a. of right atrium, auricular appendage (1), right auricular appendage.
a. of right atrium, a. do átrio direito. SIN right a.
au·ric·u·la, pl. **au·ric·u·lae** (aw-rik′ū-lă, -lē) [TA]. Aurícula. **1.** SIN auricle (1). **2.** Aurículas dos átrios. SIN *auricles* (of atria), em *auricle*. [L. a orelha externa, dim. de *auris*, orelha]

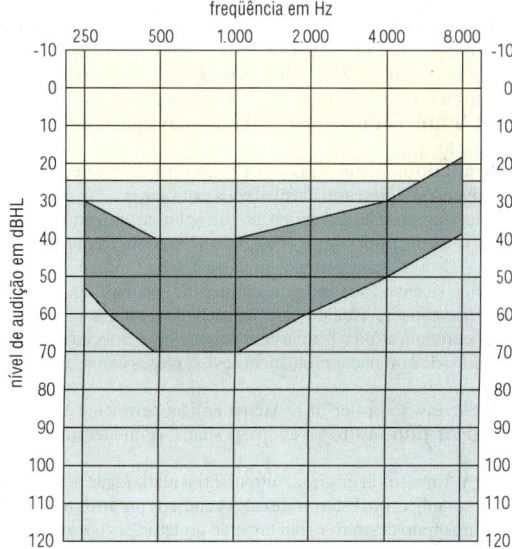

audiograma de tom puro: a área amarela indica os limites da audição normal; a área verde-escura ilustra a freqüência e a intensidade dos fonemas em inglês; dBHL = decibéis (de) perda auditiva

atrial a., a. do átrio. SIN *auricles (of atria)*, em *auricle*. VER TAMBÉM left *atrium* of heart, right *atrium* of heart.
  auriculae atrii [TA], aurículas dos átrios. SIN *auricles (of atria)*, em *auricle*. VER left *atrium* of heart, right *atrium* of heart.
   a. atrii dex'tra [TA], a. do átrio direito. SIN right *auricle*.
   a. atrii sinis'tra [TA], a. do átrio esquerdo. SIN left *auricle*.
au·ric·u·lar (aw-rik′u-lăr). Auricular; relativo à orelha ou a uma aurícula em qualquer sentido.
au·ric·u·la·re, pl. **au·ric·u·lar·ia** (aw-rik-u-lā′rē, -rē-ă). Ponto auricular; um ponto craniométrico no centro da abertura do meato acústico externo; ou, em certos casos, no meio da borda superior dessa abertura. SIN auricular point. [L. *auricularis*, pertinente à orelha]
au·ric·u·lo·cra·ni·al (aw-rik′u-lō-krā′nē-ăl). Auriculocranial; relativo à orelha externa e ao crânio.
au·ric·u·lo·tem·po·ral (aw-rik′u-lō-tem′pō-răl). Auriculotemporal; relativo à orelha externa e à região temporal.
au·ric·u·lo·ven·tric·u·lar (aw-rik′u-lō-ven-trik′u-lăr). Auriculoventricular; sinônimo obsoleto para atrioventricular.
au·rid, pl. **au·ri·des** (aw′rid, aw′ri-dēz). Áuride; uma lesão cutânea decorrente da injeção de sais de ouro. [L. *aurum*, ouro, + *-id* (1)]
au·ri·form (aw′ri-form). Auriforme; em formato de orelha.
au·rin (aw′rin) [C.I. 43800]. Aurina; um derivado trifenilmetano usado como indicador (muda de amarelo para vermelho quando o pH 6,8 passa para 8,2) e como corante intermediário; também usado para ajudar a diferenciar o bacilo da tuberculose de outros microrganismos álcool-ácido-resistentes. SIN corallin, *p*-rosolic acid.
au·rin·tri·car·box·yl·ic ac·id (aw′rin-trī′kar-boks-il′ik). Ácido aurintricarboxílico; agente quelante que possui uma afinidade especial pelo berílio e alguns outros materiais, podendo, portanto, ser usado no combate à intoxicação por berílio; o sal de amônio é conhecido como aluminon.
au·ris (a, a, aur), pl. **au·res** (aw′ris, aw′rēz) [TA]. Orelha. SIN ear. [L.]
   a. exte'rna, o. externa. SIN external *ear*.
   a. inter'na, o. interna. SIN internal *ear*.
   a. me'dia, o. média. SIN middle *ear*.
au·ro·chro·mo·der·ma (aw′rō-krō-mō-der′mă). Aurocromodermia. SIN chrysiasis. [L. *aurum*, ouro, + *chrōma*, cor, + *derma*, pele]
au·ro·mer·cap·to·ac·et·an·i·lid (aw′rō-mer-kap′tō-as-ĕ-tan′i-lid). Auromercaptoacetanilida; um composto orgânico de ouro, insolúvel em água; usado no tratamento da artrite reumatóide e administrado por injeção intramuscular; absorvido mais lentamente que os sais hidrossolúveis de ouro. SIN aurothioglycanide.
au·rone (aw′ron). Aurona. **1.** O composto original de uma série de pigmentos vegetais; estes são cumarononas substituídas e podem ser formados a partir de calconas. Com freqüência, são encontrados como glicosídeos. **2.** Uma classe de compostos baseados na a. (1). SIN benzalcoumaran-3-one.
au·ro·ther·a·py (aw-rō-thār′ă-pē). Auroterapia. SIN chrysotherapy. [L. *aurum*, ouro]
au·ro·thi·o·glu·cose (aw′rō-thī-ō-gloo′kōs). Aurotioglicose; preparação de ouro orgânico com o grupamento –SAu em lugar do grupamento 1-OH da glicose; usado no tratamento da artrite reumatóide e lúpus eritematoso discóide. Possivelmente detém progressão da doença. SIN gold thioglucose.
au·ro·thi·o·gly·ca·nide (aw′-rō-thī-ō-glī′kă-nīd). Aurotioglicanida. SIN auromercaptoacetanilid.
au·rum (aw′rŭm). Ouro. SIN gold. [L.]
aus·cul·tate, aus·cult (aws′kŭl-tāt, aws-kŭlt′). Auscultar; realizar a ausculta.
aus·cul·ta·tion (aws-kŭl-tā′shŭn). Ausculta; ouvir os sons feitos pelas várias estruturas corporais como um método diagnóstico. [L. *ausculto*, pp. *-atus*, ouvir]
   immediate a., direct a., a. imediata, a. direta; a. pela aplicação da orelha à superfície do corpo.
   mediate a., a. mediata; a. realizada com o uso de um estetoscópio.
aus·cul·ta·to·ry (aws-kŭl′tă-tō-rē). Auscultatório; relativo à ausculta.
Auspitz, Heinrich, médico austríaco, 1835–1886. VER Auspitz sign.
Austin Flint, Austin Flint. VER Flint.
aut-. VER auto-.
au·ta·coid (aw-tā′-koyd). Autacóide. SIN autocoid. [aut- + G. *akos*, alívio, recurso]
au·te·cic, au·te·cious (aw-tē′sik, aw-tē′shŭs). Autécico; indica um parasita que infecta, durante toda a sua existência, o mesmo hospedeiro. [G. *autos*, idêntico, + *oikion*, casa]
au·te·me·sia (aw-tĕ-mē′zē-ă). Autemésia. Termo raramente utilizado para: **1.** Vômito idiopático ou funcional. **2.** Vômito decorrente da indução do reflexo do vômito. [G. *autos*, próprio, + *emesis*, vômito]
au·then·tic·i·ty (aw-then-tis′i-tē). Autenticidade. **1.** A qualidade de ser autêntico, genuíno e válido. **2.** Em funcionamento psicológico e personalidade, aplicado aos sentimentos conscientes, percepções e pensamentos que alguém expressa e comunica de forma honesta e genuína. [G. *authentikos*, original, primário]

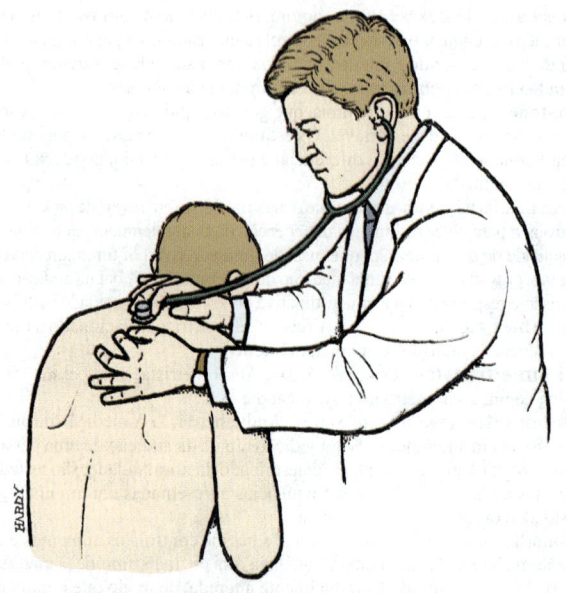

ausculta: mediada

au·tism (aw′tizm). Autismo; distúrbio mental caracterizado por desenvolvimento bastante anormal da interação social e das habilidades de comunicação verbal e não-verbal. Os indivíduos afetados (autistas) podem aderir a rituais ou rotinas inflexíveis e não-funcionais. Eles podem ficar aborrecidos mesmo com alterações triviais no ambiente. Com freqüência, a faixa de interesses é limitada, mas podem ficar preocupados com uma faixa estreita de indivíduos ou atividades. Os autistas parecem incapazes de compreender os sentimentos dos outros e, amiúde, não mantêm contato ocular com outras pessoas. Podem ocorrer oscilações imprevisíveis do humor. Muitos apresentam maneirismos motores estereotipados, como agitar as mãos ou os dedos das mãos, balançar o corpo ou inclinar o corpo como para mergulhar. O distúrbio é causado, provavelmente, por disfunção orgânica do sistema nervoso central, principalmente na capacidade de processar as informações sociais ou emocionais ou a linguagem. [G. *autos*, próprio]
   early infantile a., a. infantil precoce. SIN infantile a.
   infantile a., a. infantil; grave distúrbio emocional da infância caracterizado por comprometimento qualitativo da interação social recíproca e da comunicação, linguagem e desenvolvimento social. SIN childhood schizophrenia, early infantile a., Kanner syndrome.
au·tis·tic (aw-tis′tik). Autista; pertinente a, ou caracterizado por, autismo.
auto-, aut-. Prefixos que significam próprio, idêntico. [G. *autos*, próprio]
au·to·ac·ti·va·tion (aw′tō-ak-ti-vā′shŭn). Auto-ativação. SIN autocatalysis.
au·to·ag·glu·ti·na·tion (aw′tō-ă-gloo-ti-nā′shŭn). Auto-aglutinação. **1.** Aglutinação inespecífica de células (p.ex., bactérias, eritrócitos) devido a fatores físicos e/ou químicos. **2.** A aglutinação dos eritrócitos por auto-anticorpos específicos presentes no próprio soro da pessoa.
au·to·ag·glu·ti·nin (aw′tō-ă-gloo′ti-nin). Auto-aglutinina; um auto-anticorpo aglutinante.
   anti-Pr cold a., crioauto-aglutinina anti-Pr; uma crioauto-aglutinina específica para o antígeno Pr (protease-sensível) dos eritrócitos.
   cold a., crioauto-aglutinina; um anticorpo que aglutina antígenos particulados (isto é, bactérias) em temperaturas abaixo de 37°C, com freqüência de forma mais ativa a 4°C; a maioria pertence à classe IgM de imunoglobulinas com afinidade para o sistema Ii de antígenos eritrocitários, mas algumas são auto-aglutininas a frio anti-Pr; crioauto-aglutininas podem estar associadas a infecção (p.ex., pneumonia atípica primária, mononucleose infecciosa e outras infecções por vírus, determinadas protozoonoses), e, nesses casos, elas geralmente não são ativas *in vivo*.
au·to·al·ler·gic (aw′tō-ă-ler′jik). Auto-alérgico; pertinente à auto-alergia.
au·to·al·ler·gi·za·tion (aw′tō-al′er-ji-zā′shŭn). Auto-alergização; indução da auto-alergia.
au·to·al·ler·gy (aw-tō-al′er-jē). Auto-alergia; reatividade alterada em que anticorpos (auto-anticorpos) são produzidos contra os próprios tecidos da pessoa, gerando um efeito destrutivo, em lugar de protetor. SIN autoimmunity (1).
au·to·a·nal·y·sis (aw′tō-ă-nal′i-sis). Auto-análise; tentativa de análise ou psicanálise de si próprio. SIN self-analysis.
au·to·an·a·lyz·er (aw-tō-an′ă-līz-er). Auto-analisador; um instrumento capaz de conduzir automaticamente as análises; comumente utilizado em análises químicas.

sequential multichannel a. (SMA), a. seqüencial multicanal; um instrumento automatizado capaz de realizar múltiplas análises (geralmente químicas) de maneira simultânea ao impulsionar as amostras e reagentes em um fluxo contínuo ao longo de tubos até os mecanismos detectores.

au·to·an·a·phy·lax·is (aw′tō-an′ă-fĭ-lak′sis). Auto-anafilaxia; termo obsoleto para determinados tipos de auto-imunidade.

au·to·an·ti·body (aw-tō-an′ti-bod-ē). Auto-anticorpo; anticorpo que ocorre em resposta aos constituintes antigênicos do tecido hospedeiro contra o antígeno próprio (*self*) e que reage com o componente tecidual incitante.
antiidiotype a., a. antiidiotípico. SIN idiotype a. VER antiidiotype *antibody*.
cold a., crioauto-anticorpo um a. que reage em temperaturas abaixo de 37°C.
Donath-Landsteiner cold a., crioauto-anticorpo de Donath-Landsteiner; um a. da classe IgG responsável pela crioemoglobinúria paroxística; é adsorvido aos eritrócitos apenas em temperaturas ≤ 20°C, fazendo com que os eritrócitos sofram lise na presença de complemento em temperaturas mais elevadas; ele possui uma especificidade dentro do grupo sanguíneo P; também é ocasionalmente encontrado durante curtos períodos de tempo após sarampo e outras infecções, e outrora foi freqüentemente associado à sífilis. SIN cold hemolysin.
hemagglutinating cold a., crioauto-anticorpo. hemaglutinante; uma crioautoaglutinina.
idiotype a., a. idiotípico. SIN antiidiotype a.
warm a., a. quente; um a. que reage de forma ótima a 37°C.

au·to·an·ti·com·ple·ment (aw′tō-an-ti-com′plĕ-ment). Auto-anticomplemento; um anticomplemento que é formado no corpo de um animal e inibe ou destrói o complemento do mesmo animal.

au·to·an·ti·gen (aw-to-an′ti-jen). Auto-antígeno; um antígeno "próprio"; qualquer constituinte tecidual que provoque uma resposta imune pelo hospedeiro.

au·to·as·say (aw′tō-as-ā). Auto-ensaio; detecção ou estimativa da quantidade de uma substância produzida em um organismo por meio de um objeto de teste nesse organismo, como, p. ex., o uso do coração desnervado *in situ* de um gato para pesquisar epinefrina ou simpatina liberada para a sua corrente sanguínea.

au·to·aug·men·ta·tion (aw′-tō-awg′men-tā-shŭn). Autocistoplastia; aumento da bexiga através da incisão e excisão do músculo detrusor, deixando apenas o epitélio da bexiga. SIN autocystoplasty.

au·to·blast (aw′tō-blast). Autoblasto. **1.** Uma célula independente. **2.** Um micróbio simples e independente, protozoário ou organismo monocelular (acelular). [auto- + G. *blastos*, germe]

au·to·ca·tal·y·sis (aw′tō-kă-tal′ĭ-sis). Autocatálise; uma reação na qual um ou mais dos produtos formados agem catalisando a reação; começando de forma lenta, a velocidade dessa reação aumenta rapidamente. Cf. chain *reaction*. SIN autoactivation.

au·to·cat·a·lyt·ic (aw′tō-kat-ă-lit′ik). Autocatalítico; relativo à autocatálise.

au·to·cath·e·ter·i·za·tion, au·to·cath·e·ter·ism (aw′tō-kath-ĕ-ter-i-zā′shŭn, -kath′ĕ-ter-izm). Autocateterismo; passagem de um cateter pelo paciente.

au·toch·thon·ous (aw-tok′thon-ŭs). Autóctone. **1.** Nativo do local; aborígene. **2.** Que se origina no local onde foi encontrado; diz-se de uma doença que se origina na parte do corpo onde foi encontrada ou de uma doença contraída no local onde o paciente está. [auto- + G. *chthon*, terra, solo, país]

au·toc·la·sis, au·to·cla·sia (aw-tok′lă-sis, aw-tō-klā′zē-ă). Autoclasia. **1.** Fragmentação ou ruptura por causas intrínsecas ou internas. **2.** Destruição tecidual progressiva imunologicamente induzida. [auto- + G. *klasis*, quebra]

au·to·clave (aw′tō-klāv). **1.** Autoclave; um aparelho para esterilização por vapor sob pressão; consiste em uma caldeira fechada e potente que contém um pequeno volume de água e uma cesta de arame, na qual são colocados os artigos a serem esterilizados. **2.** Esterilizar em uma autoclave. [auto- + L. *clavis*, uma chave, no sentido de autofechamento]

au·to·coid (aw′tō-koyd). Autocóide; uma substância química produzida por um tipo de célula que afeta a função de diferentes tipos de células na mesma região, funcionando, dessa maneira, como um hormônio local ou mensageiro. SIN autacoid substance, autacoid. [G. *autos*, próprio, + *eidos*, forma]

au·to·crine (aw′tō-krin). Autócrino; denotando auto-estimulação através da produção celular de um fator e de um receptor específico para ele. [auto- + G. *krino*, separar]

au·to·cys·to·plas·ty (aw-tō-sis′tō-plas-tē). Autocistoplastia. SIN autoaugmentation. [auto- + G. *kystis*, bexiga, + *plastos*, formado]

au·to·cy·to·ly·sin (aw′tō-sī-tol′ĭ-sin). Autocitolisina. SIN autolysin.

au·to·cy·tol·y·sis (aw′tō-sī-tol′ĭ-sis). Autocitólise. SIN autolysis.

au·to·cy·to·tox·in (aw′tō-sī-tō-toks′in). Autocitotoxina; um auto-anticorpo citotóxico.

au·to·der·mic (aw-tō-der′mik). Autodérmico; relativo à própria pele da pessoa; indica especialmente um enxerto autodérmico ou dermatoautoplastia. [auto- + G. *derma*, pele]

au·to·di·ges·tion (aw′tō-dī-jes′chŭn). Autodigestão, autólise. SIN autolysis.

au·to·dip·loid (aw-tō-dip′loyd). Autodiplóide. VER autoploid.

au·to·drain·age (aw-tō-drān′ij). Autodrenagem; drenagem para os tecidos contíguos.

au·to·ech·o·la·lia (aw′tō-ek-ō-lā′lē-ă). Auto-ecolalia; uma repetição mórbida das palavras de uma outra pessoa ou da própria pessoa. [auto- + echolalia]

au·to·e·rot·ic (aw′tō-ĕ-rot′ik). Auto-erótico; pertinente ao auto-erotismo.

au·to·e·rot·i·cism (aw′tō-ĕ-rot′ĭ-sizm). Auto-eroticismo; estímulo ou gratificação sexual usando o próprio corpo, como na masturbação. SIN autoerotism. [auto- + G. *erōtikos*, relativo ao amor]

au·to·er·o·tism (aw-tō-ăr′ō-tizm). Auto-erotismo. SIN autoeroticism. [auto- + G. *erōtikos*, relativo ao amor]

au·to·flu·o·ro·scope (aw-tō-flōr′ō-skōp). Autofluoroscópio; um tipo de câmara de cintilação de uma matriz de cristais isolados de iodeto de sódio, cada um com seu cachimbo de luz separado e tubo fotomultiplicador; usado para procedimentos de imagens com radioisótopos.

au·tog·a·mous (aw-tog′ă-mŭs). Autógamo; relativo a, ou caracterizado por, autogamia.

au·tog·a·my (aw-tog′ă-mē). Autogamia; uma forma de auto-fertilização em que a fissão do núcleo da célula ocorre sem divisão da célula, com os dois pronúcleos assim formados se reunindo para formar o sincárion; em outros casos, o corpo da célula também se divide, mas as duas células-filhas se conjugam imediatamente. SIN automixis. [auto- + G. *gamos*, casamento]

au·to·gen·e·sis (aw-tō-jen′ĕ-sis). Autogênese. **1.** A origem de matéria viva dentro do próprio organismo. **2.** Em bacteriologia, o processo pelo qual a vacina é feita a partir de bactérias obtidas do próprio corpo do paciente. [auto- + G. *genesis*, produção]

au·to·ge·net·ic, au·to·gen·ic (aw′tō-jĕ-net′ik, jen′ik). Autogenético, autogênico. SIN autogenous (1).

au·tog·e·nous (aw-toj′ĕ-nŭs). Autógeno. **1.** SIN autogenetic, autologous. **2.** Que se origina dentro do corpo, aplicado às vacinas preparadas a partir de bactérias ou outras células obtidas da pessoa afetada. Cf. endogenous. [G. *autogenēs*, autoproduzido]

au·tog·no·sis (aw-tog-nō′sis). Autognose; reconhecimento das características, tendências e peculiaridades próprias. SIN self-knowledge. [auto- + G. *gnōsis*, conhecimento]

au·to·graft (aw′tō-graft). Auto-enxerto; tecido ou órgão transferido para uma nova posição no corpo do mesmo indivíduo. SIN autogeneic graft, autologous graft, autoplastic graft, autotransplant. [auto- + A.S. *graef*]

au·to·graft·ing (aw-tō-graft′ing). Auto-enxerto. SIN autotransplantation.

au·to·gram (aw′tō-gram). Autograma; uma lesão semelhante a um vergão na pele após compressão por um instrumento não-pontiagudo ou por coçadura. [auto- + G. *gramma*, algo escrito]

au·tog·ra·phism (aw-tog′ră-fizm). Autografismo, dermatografismo. SIN dermatographism.

au·to·hem·ag·glu·ti·na·tion (aw′tō-hē′mă-gloo-ti-nā′shŭn). Auto-hemaglutinação; auto-aglutinação de eritrócitos autólogos.

au·to·he·mo·ly·sin (aw′tō-hē-mol′i-sin). Auto-hemolisina; um auto-anticorpo que causa lise dos eritrócitos na presença do complemento.

au·to·he·mol·y·sis (aw′tō-hē-mol′ĭ-sis). Auto-hemólise; hemólise que ocorre em determinadas doenças em conseqüência de uma auto-hemolisina.

au·to·hex·a·ploid (aw-tō-heks′ă-ployd). Auto-hexaplóide. VER autoploid.

au·to·hyp·no·sis (aw′tō-hip-nō′sis). Auto-hipnose; hipnose auto-induzida, realizada ao se concentrar no pensamento auto-absorvente ou na idéia de ser hipnotizado. SIN autohypnotism, idiohypnotism.

au·to·hyp·not·ic (aw′tō-hip-not′ik). Auto-hipnótico; relativo à auto-hipnose.

au·to·hyp·no·tism (aw-tō-hip′nō-tizm). Auto-hipnose. SIN autohypnosis.

au·to·im·mune (aw-tō-i-mūn′). Auto-imune; células e/ou anticorpos que surgem e são direcionados contra os tecidos da própria pessoa, como na doença auto-imune.

au·to·im·mu·ni·ty (aw′tō-i-mū′ni-tē). Auto-imunidade. **1.** Em imunologia, a condição em que os próprios tecidos da pessoa estão sujeitos aos efeitos deletérios do sistema imune, como na auto-alergia e na doença auto-imune; a resposta imune humoral ou celular específica contra os tecidos do próprio corpo. SIN autoallergy. **2.** Literalmente, a condição em que o "próprio" não é reconhecido.

au·to·im·mu·ni·za·tion (aw′tō-im′ū-ni-zā′shŭn). Auto-imunização; indução da auto-imunidade.

au·to·im·mu·no·cy·to·pe·nia (aw-tō-im′oo-nō-sī-tō-pē′nē-ă). Auto-imunocitopenia; anemia, trombocitopenia e leucopenia resultantes de reações citotóxicas auto-imunes.

au·to·in·fec·tion (aw′tō-in-fek′shŭn). Auto-infecção ou auto-infestação. **1.** Reinfecção por micróbios ou organismos parasitas que já passaram por um ciclo infeccioso. **2.** Auto-infestação por contágio direto, como ocorre com os ovos de oxiúros (*Enterobius vermicularis*) eliminados no estado infeccioso e transmitidos pelas unhas (via oroanal). SIN autoreinfection, self-infection.

au·to·in·fu·sion (aw′tō-in-fū′shŭn). Auto-infusão; forçar o sangue dos membros ou de outras áreas, como o baço, através da aplicação de uma ataduꟷ

algumas doenças auto-imunes em seres humanos

doen	auto-antígeno	resposta imune
doenças auto-imunes específicas por órgãos		
doença de Addison	células da supra-renal	auto-anticorpos
anemia hemolítica auto-imune	proteínas da membrana eritrocitária	auto-anticorpos
síndrome de Goodpasture	membranas basais renais e pulmonares	auto-anticorpos
doença de Graves	receptor do hormônio tireoestimulante	auto-anticorpos (estimulando)
tireoidite de Hashimoto	células e proteínas tireóideas	células T$_{DTH}$, auto-anticorpos
púrpura trombocitopênica idiopática	proteínas da membrana plaquetária	auto-anticorpos
diabetes melito do tipo 1	células beta-pancreáticas	células T$_{DTH}$, auto-anticorpos
miastenia grave	receptores de acetilcolina	auto-anticorpo (bloqueando)
anemia perniciosa	células parietais gástricas, fator intrínseco	auto-anticorpo
glomerulonefrite pós-estreptocócica	rim	complexos antígeno-anticorpo
infertilidade espontânea	esperma	auto-anticorpos
doenças auto-imunes sistêmicas		
espondilite anquilosante	vértebras	complexos imunes
esclerose múltipla	substância branca do cérebro e medula espinal	células T$_{DTH}$ e células T$_C$, auto-anticorpos
artrite reumatóide	tecido conjuntivo, IgG	auto-anticorpos, complexos imunes
esclerodermia	núcleos, coração, pulmões, trato gastrointestinal, rim	auto-anticorpos
síndrome de Sjögren	glândula salivar, fígado, rim, tireóide	auto-anticorpos
lúpus eritematoso sistêmico (SLE)	DNA, proteína nuclear, membranas eritrocitárias e plaquetárias	auto-anticorpos, complexos imunes

ra ou dispositivo compressivo, visando aumentar a pressão arterial e encher os vasos sanguíneos nos centros vitais; utilizada depois da perda excessiva de sangue ou de outros líquidos corporais. Cf. autotransfusion.

au·to·in·oc·u·la·ble (aw′tō-in-ok′ū-lă-bl). Auto-inoculável; suscetível de auto-inoculação.

au·to·in·oc·u·la·tion (aw′tō-in-ok-ū-lā′shŭn). Auto-inoculação; uma infecção secundária que se origina de um foco de infecção já existente no corpo.

au·to·in·tox·i·cant (aw′tō-in-toks′i-kant). Auto-intoxicante; um agente tóxico endógeno que causa auto-intoxicação. SIN autotoxin.

au·to·in·tox·i·ca·tion (aw′tō-in-toks-i-kā′shŭn). Auto-intoxicação; um distúrbio resultante da absorção de produtos residuais do metabolismo, da matéria decomposta a partir do intestino ou dos produtos do tecido morto e infectado como na gangrena. SIN autotoxicosis, endogenic toxicosis, enterotoxication, enterotoxism, intestinal intoxication, self-poisoning.

au·to·i·sol·y·sin (aw′tō-i-sol′i-sin). Auto-isolisina; um anticorpo que, na presença de complemento, causa lise de células na pessoa em cujo corpo a lisina é formada, bem como em outros da mesma espécie.

au·to·ker·a·to·plas·ty (aw-tō-ker′ă-tō-plas-tē). Autoceratoplastia; enxerto de tecido da córnea de um olho de um paciente no outro olho. [auto- G. *keras*, chifre, + *plastos*, formado]

au·to·ki·ne·sia, au·to·ki·ne·sis (aw-tō-ki-ne′sē-ă, aw-tō-ki-nē′sis). Autocinesia; movimento voluntário. [auto- + G. *kinēsis*, movimento]

au·to·ki·net·ic (aw-tō-ki-net′ik). Autocinético; relativo à autocinesia.

au·to·le·sion (aw-tō-lē′zhŭn). Autolesão; uma lesão auto-infligida.

au·tol·o·gous (aw-tol′ŏ-gŭs). Autólogo. **1.** Que ocorre natural e normalmente em determinado tipo de tecido ou em uma estrutura específica do corpo. **2.** No transplante, refere-se a um enxerto em que as áreas doadora e receptora pertencem ao mesmo indivíduo, ou ao sangue que o doador doou previamente e, em seguida, recebe de volta, geralmente durante a cirurgia. **3.** Por vezes usado para indicar uma neoplasia derivada das células que ocorrem normalmente naquele lugar, p.ex., um carcinoma de células escamosas na parte superior do esôfago. SIN autogenous (1). [auto- + G. *logos*, relação]

au·tol·y·sate (aw-tol′i-sāt). Autolisado; a mistura de substâncias que resultam de autólise.

au·to·lyse (aw′tō-līs). Autolisar. SIN autolyze.

au·tol·y·sin (aw-tol′i-sin). Autolisina; um anticorpo que, na presença de complemento, provoca a lise das células e tecidos no corpo do indivíduo em que a lisina é formada. SIN autocytolysin.

au·tol·y·sis (aw-tol′i-sis). Autólise. **1.** Digestão enzimática de células (especialmente mortas ou degeneradas) por enzimas presentes dentro delas (autógenas). **2.** Destruição de células em conseqüência de uma lisina formada nessas células ou em outras do mesmo organismo. SIN autocytolysis, autodigestion, isophagy. [auto- + G. *lysis*, dissolução]

au·to·lyt·ic (aw-tō-lit′ik). Autolítico; pertinente a ou que causa autólise.

au·to·ly·ze (aw-tō-līz). Autolisar; que sofre autólise. SIN autolyse.

au·to·mal·let (aw′tō-mal-et). Termo obsoleto para obturador automático (automatic *plugger*) ou condensador.

au·tom·a·tism (aw-tom′ă-tizm). Automatismo. **1.** O estado de ser independente da volição (arbítrio) ou inervação central; aplicável, p. ex., à ação do coração. **2.** Uma crise epiléptica que consiste em fenômenos psíquicos, sensoriais ou motores estereotipados realizados em um estado de comprometimento da consciência e do qual o indivíduo geralmente não tem conhecimento. **3.** Uma condição em que um indivíduo é compelido de maneira consciente ou inconsciente, mas involuntária, ao desempenho de determinados atos motores ou verbais, freqüentemente sem propósito e, por vezes, tolos ou perigosos. SIN telergy. [G. *automatos*, auto-movimentação, + -in]

ambulatory a., o desempenho automático de uma ação ou série de ações por uma pessoa sem estar consciente dos processos envolvidos no desempenho.

immediate posttraumatic a., a. pós-traumático imediato; estado pós-traumático em que o paciente age automaticamente sem memória imediata ou posterior de seu comportamento.

au·to·mat·o·graph (aw-tō-mat′ō-graf). Automatógrafo; um instrumento para registrar os movimentos automáticos.

au·to·mix·is (aw-tō-miks′is). Automixia, autogamia. SIN autogamy. [auto- + G. *mixis*, intercurso]

au·tom·ne·sia (aw-tom-nē′zē-ă). Automnésia; lembrança espontânea das memórias de uma condição mais precoce da vida. [auto- + G. *mnēsis*, uma lembrança]

au·to·my·so·pho·bia (aw′tō-mis-ō-fō′bē-ă). Automisofobia; medo mórbido da falta de higiene pessoal. [auto- + G. *mysos*, sujeira, + *phobos*, medo]

au·to·nom·ic (aw-tō-nom′ik). Autônomo; relativo ao sistema nervoso autônomo.

au·to·nom·o·tro·pic (aw-tō-nom-ō-trop′ik). Autonomotrópico; que atua sobre o sistema nervoso autônomo. [autonomic + G. *trepo*, virar]

au·ton·o·mous (aw-ton′ō-mŭs). Autônomo; que possui independência ou liberdade do controle por forças externas ou, em um sentido estrito, pelos centros nervosos cerebroespinais.

au·ton·o·my (aw-ton′ō-mē). Autonomia; a condição ou estado de ser autônomo, capaz de tomar decisões sem o auxílio dos outros. [auto- + G. *nomos*, lei]

functional a., a. funcional; em psicologia social, a tendência de um sistema motivacional desenvolvido (p. ex., motivo da aquisição) para se tornar independente do estímulo primário ou inato a partir do qual ele se originou (p. ex., necessidade de alimento).

au·to-ox·i·da·tion (aw′tō-oks-i-dā′shŭn). Auto-oxidação; a combinação direta de uma substância com oxigênio molecular em temperaturas comuns. SIN autoxidation.

au·to-ox·i·diz·a·ble (aw′tō-oks-i-dīz′ă-bl). Auto-oxidável; indica a substância que reage diretamente com o oxigênio (p.ex., hemocromógeno b em citocromo) e não exige a ação de desidrogenases.

au·to·path·ic (aw-tō-path′ik). Autopático; sinônimo raramente utilizado para idiopathic (idiopático).

au·to·pen·ta·ploid (aw-tō-pen′tă-ployd). Autopentaplóide. VER autoploid.

au·to·pep·sia (aw-tō-pep′sē-ă). Autopepsia; termo raramente utilizado para a autodigestão, refere-se à ulceração da mucosa gástrica por sua própria secreção, ou digestão da pele ao redor de uma abertura de gastrostomia ou colostomia. [auto- + G. *pepsis*, digestão]

au·to·pha·gia (aw-tō-fā′jē-ă). Autofagia. **1.** Que morde a própria carne;

p.ex., como um sintoma da síndrome de Lesch-Nyhan. **2.** Manutenção da nutrição de todo o corpo por consumo metabólico de parte dos tecidos corporais. **3.** SIN autophagy. [auto- + G. *phagō*, comer]

au·to·pha·gic (aw-tō-fā′jik). Autofágico; relativo a, ou caracterizado por, autofagia.

au·to·pha·go·ly·so·some (aw-tō-fā-gō-lī′sō-sōm). Autofagolisossoma; o vacúolo digestivo da autofagia que resulta da fusão de um lisossoma primário com um vacúolo autofágico.

au·toph·a·gy (aw-tof′ă-jē). Autofagia; segregação e remoção das organelas lesionadas dentro de uma célula. SIN autophagia (3). [auto- + G. *phagō*, comer]

au·to·pho·bia (aw-tō-fō′bē-ă). Autofobia; medo mórbido da solidão ou de si próprio. [auto- + G. *phobos*, medo]

au·toph·o·ny (aw-tof′ō-nē). Autofonia; audição aumentada da própria voz, sons respiratórios, sopros arteriais, etc., notada especialmente na doença da orelha média ou das fossas nasais. SIN tympanophonia, tympanophony. [auto- G. *phōne*, som]

au·to·ploid (aw′tō-ployd). Autoplóide; relativo a um indivíduo ou célula com duas ou mais cópias de um único conjunto haplóide; dependendo do número de múltiplos da série haplóide, os autoplóides são referidos como autodiplóides, autotriplóides, autotetraplóides, autopentaplóides, auto-hexaplóides, etc. [auto- + -ploid]

au·to·ploi·dy (aw′tō-ploy-dē). Autoploidia; a condição de ser autoplóide.

au·to·plug·ger (aw′tō-plŭg-er). Termo obsoleto para automatic *plugger*, obturador automático.

au·to·pod (aw′tō-pod). Autópode. SIN autopodium.

au·to·po·di·um, pl. **au·to·po·dia** (aw′tō-pō′dē-ŭm, dē-ă). Autópode; a principal subdivisão distal de um membro (mão ou pé). SIN autopod. [auto- + G. *pous* (*pod*-), pé]

au·to·poi·son·ous (aw-tō-poy′zŭn-ŭs). Autovenenoso. SIN autotoxic.

au·to·pol·y·mer (aw-tō-pol′i-mer). Autopolímero. VER autopolymer *resin*.

au·to·pol·y·mer·i·za·tion (aw-tō-pol′i-mer-i-zā′shŭn). Autopolimerização; polimerização sem o uso do calor externo, em conseqüência da adição de um ativador e de um catalisador.

au·to·pol·y·ploid (aw-tō-pol′i-ployd). Autopoliplóide; um autoplóide que possui dois ou mais múltiplos de conjuntos haplóides de cromossomas.

au·to·pol·y·ploi·dy (aw-tō-pol′i-ploy-dē). Autopoliploidia; a condição de ser autopoliplóide.

au·top·sy (aw′top-sē). **1.** Necropsia; exame dos órgãos de um corpo morto para determinar a causa da morte ou para estudar as alterações patológicas presentes. SIN necropsy. **2.** Na terminologia da antiga escola grega de empíricos, a reprodução intencional de um efeito, evento ou circunstância que ocorreu no curso de uma doença e observação de sua influência na melhoria ou no agravamento dos sintomas do paciente. SIN postmortem examination. [G. *autopsia*, observar com os próprios olhos]

verbal a., método de obter o máximo possível de informações sobre uma pessoa falecida através de perguntas à família e a outras pessoas que possam descrever o modo da morte e das circunstâncias que precederam à morte; usado sobretudo nos países em desenvolvimento e nos ambientes e situações em que o exame histopatológico *post-mortem* não é possível.

au·to·ra·di·o·gram (aw-tō-rā′dē-ō-gram). Auto-radiograma. SIN autoradiograph. [auto- + radiogram]

au·to·ra·di·o·graph (aw-tō-rā′dē-ō-graf). Auto-radiografia; imagem da distribuição e concentração da radioatividade em um tecido ou outra substância feita ao colocar uma emulsão fotográfica sobre a superfície da substância ou em íntima proximidade com esta. SIN autoradiogram.

au·to·ra·di·og·ra·phy (aw′tō-rā-dē-og′ră-fē). Auto-radiografia; o processo de produzir um auto-radiograma. SIN radioautography.

paper a., a. de papel; a. em que os compostos são separados por cromatografia em papel.

autoreceptor (au′tō-rē-sep-tor, tōr). Auto-receptor; um local em um neurônio que se liga ao neurotransmissor liberado por esse neurônio, que, em seguida, regula a atividade do neurônio. [auto- + receptor]

au·to·reg·u·la·tion (aw′tō-reg-ū-lā′shŭn). Auto-regulação. **1.** A tendência do fluxo sanguíneo para um órgão ou região permanecer ou retornar ao mesmo nível, apesar das alterações pressóricas na artéria que conduz o sangue para esse órgão ou região. **2.** Em geral, qualquer sistema biológico equipado com sistemas de retroalimentação inibitória, de tal modo que determinada alteração tende a ser contraposta em grande parte ou por completo; p.ex., os reflexos de barorreceptor formam uma base para a auto-regulação da pressão arterial sistêmica.

heterometric a., a. heterométrica; regulação intrínseca da força de contração cardíaca em função do comprimento (volume) diastólico da fibra, independentemente da pós-carga, nervos autônomos e outras influências extrínsecas. A a. heterométrica também é conhecida como relação comprimento–tensão, relação entre o volume diastólico final e a pressão diastólica final, lei de Starling do coração e curva de Frank-Starling.

homeometric a., a. homeométrica; a regulação intrínseca da força da contração cardíaca em resposta às influências que não dependem da alteração no comprimento da fibra, isto é, a curva de Frank-Starling (p.ex., o efeito Anrep em que a força aumenta em resposta à pós-carga aumentada, e o efeito Bowditch em que a força aumenta em resposta à freqüência cardíaca aumentada) e não depende de regulação extrínseca (p.ex., em que a força aumenta em resposta a estimulação nervosa simpática ou à norepinefrina).

au·to·re·in·fec·tion (aw′tō-rē-in-fek′shŭn). Auto-reinfecção. SIN autoinfection.

au·to·re·pro·duc·tion (aw′tō-rē-prō-duk′shŭn). Auto-reprodução; a capacidade de um gene ou vírus, ou geralmente a molécula de nucleoproteína, iniciar a síntese de outra molécula idêntica a ela mesma a partir de moléculas menores dentro da célula.

au·tor·rha·phy (aw-tōr′ă-fē). Auto-rafia; o fechamento da ferida usando filamentos da fáscia a partir das bordas da ferida. [auto- + G. *rhaphē*, costura]

au·to·sen·si·tize (aw-tō-sen′si-tīz). Auto-sensibilizar; sensibilizar contra as células do próprio corpo. SIN isosensitize.

au·to·sep·ti·ce·mia (aw′tō-sep-ti-sē′mē-ă). Auto-septicemia; septicemia que se origina aparentemente a partir de microrganismos existentes dentro do indivíduo, ou seja, não-exógenos. [auto- + G. *sēpsis*, decaimento, + *haima*, sangue]

au·to·se·ro·ther·a·py (aw′tō-sē-rō-thār′ă-pē). Auto-soroterapia; o tratamento de determinadas condições, como dermatoses, através da injeção do soro do próprio paciente.

au·to·se·rum (aw-tō-sē′rŭm). Auto-soro; soro obtido a partir do sangue do próprio paciente e utilizado na auto-soroterapia.

au·to·site (aw′tō-sīt). Autosito; aquele membro de gêmeos conjugados anormais e desiguais que é capaz de viver de forma independente e de nutrir o outro membro (parasita) do par. [auto- + G. *sitos*, alimento]

au·tos·mia (aw-toz′mē-ă). Autosmia; a sensação de olfato do odor do próprio corpo. [auto- + G. *osmē*, olfato]

au·to·so·mal (aw-tō-sō′mal). Autossômico; pertinente a um autossoma.

au·to·so·ma·tog·no·sis (aw-tō-sō′mă-tog-nō′sis). Auto-somatognose; a sensação de que uma parte amputada do corpo ainda existe. VER phantom *limb*. [auto- + G. *sōma*, corpo, + *gnōsis*, reconhecimento]

au·to·so·ma·tog·nos·tic (aw-to-sō′mă-tog-nos′tik). Auto-somatognóstico; pertinente à auto-somatognose.

au·to·some (aw′tō-sōm). Autossoma; qualquer cromossoma diferente de um cromossoma sexual; os autossomas ocorrem normalmente aos pares em células somáticas e isoladamente nos gametas. SIN euchromosome. [auto- + G. *sōma*, corpo]

au·to·sug·gest·i·bil·i·ty (aw′tō-sŭg-jes-tī-bil′i-tē). Auto-sugestibilidade; um estado mental em que a auto-sugestão (1) ocorre de imediato.

au·to·sug·ges·tion (aw′tō-sŭg-jes′chŭn). Auto-sugestão. **1.** Convivência constante com uma idéia ou conceito, induzindo, portanto, alguma alteração nas funções mentais ou corporais. VER TAMBÉM autohypnosis. **2.** Reprodução no cérebro de impressões previamente recebidas, as quais, então, tornam-se o ponto de partida de novos atos ou idéias.

au·to·syn·noia (aw′tō-sin-noy′ă). Auto-sinóia; um distúrbio mental em que a pessoa jamais tem um pensamento desligado de si próprio. SIN self-centeredness. [auto- + G. *synnoia*, pensamento profundo, de *syn*, com + *noeō*, pensar]

au·to·syn·the·sis (aw-tō-sin′thē-sis). Auto-síntese; auto-reprodução ou auto-replicação.

au·to·te·lic (aw-tō-tel′ik). Autotélico; indica aqueles traços intimamente associados aos propósitos centrais de um indivíduo. [auto- + G. *telos*, fim, término, finalidade]

au·to·tem·nous (aw-tō-tem′nŭs). Autóteno; indica uma célula que se propaga por fissão sem conjugação prévia. [auto- + G. *temnō*, cortar]

au·to·tet·ra·ploid (aw-tō-tet′ră-ployd). Autotetraplóide. VER autoploid.

au·to·ther·a·py (aw-tō-thār′ă-pē). Autoterapia. **1.** Autotratamento. **2.** Cura espontânea.

au·tot·o·my (aw-tot′ō-mē). Autotomia; o ato de desprender uma parte do corpo como um meio de escape; p.ex., o membro de um caranguejo ou a cauda de um lagarto. [auto- + G. *tomē*, um corte]

au·to·top·ag·no·sia (aw′tō-top′ag-nō′zē-ă). Autotopagnosia; incapacidade de reconhecer ou orientar qualquer parte do próprio corpo; causada por lesão do lobo parietal. Cf. somatotopagnosis. [auto- + G. *topos*, local, + G. *a-* priv. + *gnōsis*]

au·to·tox·e·mia (aw′tō-tok-sē′mē-ă). Autotoxemia; auto-intoxicantes presentes no sangue, resultando comumente em auto-intoxicação.

au·to·tox·ic (aw-tō-toks′ik). Autotóxico; relativo à auto-intoxicação. SIN autopoisonous.

au·to·tox·i·co·sis (aw′tō-tok-si-kō′sis). Autotoxicose. SIN autointoxication.

au·to·tox·in (aw-tō-tok′sin). Autotoxina. SIN autointoxicant.

au·to·trans·fu·sion (aw′tō-tranz-fū′zhŭn). Autotransfusão; retirada e reinjeção/transfusão do sangue do próprio paciente; comumente, o sangue do próprio paciente é coletado em várias ocasiões para ser reinfundido durante um procedimento cirúrgico, quando se prevê perda sanguínea substancial. Cf. autoinfusion.

au·to·trans·plant (aw-tō-tranz′plant). Autotransplante. SIN autograft.

au·to·trans·plan·ta·tion (aw′tō-tranz-plan-tā′shŭn). Autotransplante; a realização de um auto-enxerto. SIN autografting.

au·to·trip·loid (aw-tō-trip′loyd). Autotriplóide. VER autoploid.

au·to·troph (aw′tō-trōf). Autótrofo; um microrganismo que utiliza apenas materiais inorgânicos como sua fonte de nutrientes; o dióxido de carbono serve como a única fonte de carbono. [auto- + G. *trophē*, nutrição]

au·to·tro·phic (aw-tō-trof′ik). Autotrófico. **1.** Autonutriente. A capacidade de um organismo de produzir o alimento a partir de compostos inorgânicos. **2.** Pertinente a um autótrofo.

au·to·tro·phy (aw′tō-trof-ē). Autotrofia; o estado de ser auto-sustentável e capaz de produzir o alimento a partir de compostos inorgânicos, com o dióxido de carbono servindo como a única fonte de carbono.

  carbon a., a. de carbono; capacidade de assimilar CO_2 do ar.

  nitrogen a., a. de nitrogênio; capacidade de assimilar nitrato ou de empreender a fixação de nitrogênio.

  sulfur a., a. de enxofre; capacidade de assimilar sulfato.

au·to·vac·ci·na·tion (aw′tō-vak-si-nā′shŭn). Autovacinação; uma segunda vacinação com vírus oriundo de uma ferida vacinal ou liberação de produtos antigênicos derivados de microrganismos invasores no mesmo indivíduo.

au·tox·i·da·tion (aw-tok-si-dā′shŭn). Auto-oxidação. SIN auto-oxidation.

au·to·zy·gous (aw-tō-zī′gŭs). Indica os genes, em um homozigoto, que são cópias do gene original idêntico em consequência de um cruzamento consanguíneo. [auto- + G. *zygōtos*, emparelhar]

△ **auxano-, auxo-, aux-.** Prefixos que indicam aumento, p.ex., no tamanho, intensidade, velocidade. [G. *auxanō*, aumentar]

aux·an·o·gram (awk-san′ō-gram). Auxanograma; uma placa de cultura de bactérias à qual são fornecidas condições variáveis, a fim de determinar o efeito dessas condições sobre o crescimento das bactérias. [auxano- + G. *gramma*, algo escrito]

aux·an·o·graph·ic (awk′san-ō-graf′ik). Auxanográfico; pertinente ao auxanograma ou à auxanografia.

aux·a·nog·ra·phy (awk-sa-nog′ra-fē). Auxanografia; o estudo, usando auxanogramas, dos efeitos de condições diferentes sobre o crescimento de bactérias.

aux·an·ol·o·gy (awk-sa-nol′ō-jē). Auxanologia; o estudo do crescimento. [auxano + G. *logos*, estudo]

aux·e·sis (awk-sē′sis). Auxese; aumento no tamanho, especialmente como na hipertrofia. [G. aumento]

aux·il·ia·ry (og-zil′yă-rē). Auxiliar. **1.** Que funciona em capacidade crescente; suplementar. **2.** Que funciona como um subordinado; secundário.

aux·il·i·o·mo·tor (awg-zil′ē-ō-mō-tor). Auxiliomotor; que ajuda o movimento.

aux·i·lyt·ic (awk′si-lit′ik). Auxilítico; que aumenta o poder de destruição de uma lisina ou que favorece a lise. [G. *auxō*, aumentar, + *lysis*, dissolução]

△ **auxo-.** VER auxano-.

aux·o·car·dia (awk-sō-kar′dē-ă). **1.** Aumento do coração, por hipertrofia ou por dilatação. **2.** Diástole do coração. [auxo- + G. *kardia*, coração]

aux·o·chrome (awk′sō-krōm). Auxocromo; o grupamento químico em uma molécula de corante graças ao qual o corante é ligado a grupamentos terminais reativos nos tecidos. O a. aumenta a intensidade da absorção. [auxo- + G. *chrōma*, coloração]

aux·o·drome (awk′sō-drōm). Auxódromo; uma trajetória de crescimento como a plotada na placa de Wetzel. [auxo- + G. *dromos*, trajetória]

aux·o·flore (awk′sō-flōr). Auxofloro; um átomo ou grupamento de átomos que, por sua presença em uma molécula, desloca a radiação fluorescente da última na direção do comprimento de onda mais curto, ou aumenta a fluorescência. Cf. bathoflore.

aux·o·gluc (awk′sō-gluk). Auxoglico; um grupamento atômico que, quando presente em uma molécula, intensifica sua doçura. [G. *auxanō*, aumentar, + *glykys*, doce]

aux·o·ton·ic (awk-sō-ton′ik). Auxotônico; indica a condição em que um músculo em contração se encurta contra uma carga crescente. Cf. isometric (2), isotonic (3).

aux·o·tox (awk′sō-toks). Auxotóxico; um grupamento atômico que, quando presente em uma molécula, intensifica suas características venenosas. [G. *auxanō*, aumentar, + *toxikon*, veneno]

aux·o·troph (awk′sō-trōf). Auxotrofo; um microrganismo mutante que precisa de algum nutriente que não é necessário pelo organismo (prototrofo) do qual derivou o mutante. Cf. polyauxotroph, monoauxotroph. [auxo- + G. *trophē*, nutrição]

aux·o·tro·phic (awk-sō-trof′ik, -trō′fik). Auxotrófico; pertinente a um auxótrofo.

AV Abreviatura para arteriovenous (arteriovenoso); atrioventricular (atrioventricular).

ava Abreviatura para arteriovenous *anastomosis* (anastomose arteriovenosa).

aval·vu·lar (ā-val′vū-lăr). Avalvar; não-valvar; sem valvas.

avas·cu·lar (ā-vas′kū-ler, -ă). Avascular; sem vasos linfáticos ou sanguíneos; pode ser um estado normal, como em certas formas de cartilagem, ou o resultado da doença. SIN nonvascular.

avas·cu·lar·i·za·tion (ā-vas′kū-lar-ī-zā′shŭn, ā-). Avascularização. **1.** Expulsão do sangue de uma parte, como por meio de um torniquete ou outros meios de compressão arterial. **2.** Perda da vascularização, como por cicatrização (fibrose).

AVC Abreviatura para atrioventricular *conduction* (condução atrioventricular).

AVD Abreviatura para atrioventricular *dissociation* (dissociação atrioventricular).

Avellis, Georg, laringologista alemão, 1864–1916. VER A. *syndrome*.

ave·nin (ā-vē′nin). Avenina; uma prolamina, contendo cerca de 25% de resíduos glutamil, encontrados na aveia (*Avena*) e em vários legumes; considerada muito nutritiva. SIN legumin, plant casein.

av·er·age. Média; um valor que representa ou sumariza os aspectos relevantes de um conjunto de valores; geralmente é computado por uma manipulação matemática dos valores individuais em um grupo. [I.M, *averays*, perda a partir da lesão para embarcar ou carregar, do It. *avaris*, do Ar. *awariya*, bens prejudicados, + *damage*]

  pure-tone average, média de tom puro; média em decibéis dos limiares para tons puros em 500, 1.000 e 2.000 Hz.

avermectins. Avermectinas; um grupo de medicamentos endectocidas que inclui a ivermectina.

aVF, aVL, aVR Abreviaturas para as derivações eletrocardiográficas aumentadas a partir do pé (esquerdo), braço esquerdo e braço direito, respectivamente.

Avi ad·e·no·vi·rus (ā′vē-ad′ē-nō-vī′rŭs). Um gênero de vírus (família Adenoviridae) que inclui tipos de vírus encontrados nos pássaros. [L. *avis*, pássaro, + G. *adēn*, glândula, + virus]

avi·an (ā′vē-ăn). Aviário; pertinente aos pássaros. [L. *avis*, pássaro]

av·i·din (av′i-din). Avidina; uma glicoproteína, obtida das claras dos ovos, que possui uma elevada afinidade pela biotina. Permite-se que a a. marcada se ligue a anticorpos marcados com biotina, a fim de ampliar as reações antígeno-anticorpo que podem ser de difícil visualização. A ingestão de a. pode causar deficiência de biotina. SIN antibiotin. [L. *avidus*, ávido, de *aveo*, ansiar, + -in]

avid·i·ty (ă-vid′ĭ-tē). Avidez; a força de ligação de um anticorpo com um antígeno. [L. *avidus*, ansioso, ávido, de *aveo*, ansiar]

A vi pox vi rus (ā′vē-poks-vī′rŭs). O gênero de vírus (família Poxviridae) que inclui os poxvírus de pássaros, inclusive os dos canários e galinhas. [L. *avis*, pássaro, + pox + virus]

avir·u·lent (ā-vir′ū-lent). Avirulento; não-virulento.

avi·ta·min·o·sis (ā-vī′tă-min-ō′sis). Avitaminose; mais corretamente, hipovitaminose.

  conditioned a., a. condicionada; a. causada por qualquer um dos inúmeros estados patológicos ou disfunções em que o aporte de uma vitamina absorvido pelo corpo é inadequado para as necessidades em determinadas circunstâncias; p.ex., a síntese bacteriana reduzida das vitaminas no canal alimentar produzido por agentes antibióticos.

avive·ment (ah-vēv-maw′). Avivamento; termo obsoleto para a excisão das bordas de uma ferida para auxiliar o processo de cicatrização. [Fr. *aviver*, avivar, reviver]

AV node. Nó AV; abreviatura para atrioventricular *node* (nó atrioventricular).

Avogadro, Amadeo, físico italiano, 1776–1856. VER A. *constant, hypothesis, law, number, postulate*.

av·oir·du·pois (av′er-du-poyz′). Um sistema de pesos em que 16 onças perfazem uma libra, equivalente a 453,59237 g. Ver apêndice de Pesos e Medidas. [Fr. ter peso, corruptela do Fr. Ant. *avoir*, propriedade, + *de*, de, + *pois*, peso]

AVP Abreviatura de antiviral *protein* (proteína antiviral); arginine *vasopressin* (arginina vasopressina).

A-V shunt Desvio A-V; abreviatura de arteriovenous *shunt* (derivação ou desvio arteriovenoso).

avul·sion (ă-vŭl′shŭn). Avulsão; laceração ou separação forçada. Cf. evulsion. [L. *a-vello*, pp. -*vulsus*, rasgar]

  nerve a., a. do nervo; a laceração de um nervo periférico em seu ponto de origem a partir de seu nervo original devido a tração.

  root a., a. da raiz; a laceração das raízes nervosas primárias anteriores e posteriores a partir da medula espinal, devido a tração espinal; mais frequentemente, as raízes de C5 a T1 são afetadas.

  tooth a., a. do dente; a separação traumática de um dente de seu alvéolo.

AW Abreviatura para atomic *weight* (peso atômico).

ax Abreviatura para axis (eixo).

axen·ic (ā-zen′ik). Axênico; estéril, que indica especialmente uma cultura pura. Também utilizado para indicar animais "livres de germes" e criados em um ambiente estéril. VER TAMBÉM gnotobiote. [G. *a-* priv. + *xenos*, estranho]

ax·er·oph·thol (ak′ser-of′thol). Vitamina A. SIN vitamin A. [antixerophthalmic + -ol]

ax·es (ak′sēz). Eixos; plural de axis.
ax·i·al (ak′sē-al). Axial. **1** [TA]. Relativo a um eixo. SIN axialis [TA], axile. **2.** Relativo a ou situado na parte central do corpo, na cabeça e tronco, conforme distinguido a partir dos membros, p.ex., esqueleto axial. **3.** Em odontologia, relativo a ou em paralelo com o eixo longitudinal de um dente. **4.** Em radiologia, uma imagem axial é aquela obtida por rodar em torno do eixo do corpo, produzindo uma imagem planar transversa, isto é, um corte transversal ao eixo.
axialis [TA]. Axial. SIN axial (1).
ax·if·u·gal (ak-sif′ū-găl). Axífugo; que se estende além de um eixo ou axônio. SIN axofugal. [L. *axis* + *fugio*, fugir de]
ax·il (ak′sil). Axila. SIN axilla.
ax·ile (ak′sīl). Axial. SIN axial (1).
ax·il·la, gen. e pl. **ax·il·lae** (ak′sil′ă, ak-sil′ē). [TA]. Axila; o espaço sob a articulação do ombro limitado pelo músculo peitoral maior, anteriormente, pelo músculo latíssimo do dorso, posteriormente, pelo músculo serrátil anterior, medialmente, e pelo úmero, lateralmente; apresenta uma abertura superior entre a clavícula, a escápula e a primeira costela (canal cervicoaxilar) e uma abertura inferior ou assoalho coberto pela fáscia axilar e pele; contém a artéria e a veia axilares, a parte infraclavicular do plexo braquial, linfonodos e vasos linfáticos axilares, e tecido areolar. SIN armpit, axil, axillary cavity, axillary fossa, axillary space, fossa axillaris, maschale. [L.]
ax·il·lary (ak′sil-ār-ē). Axilar; relativo à axila. SIN alar (2).
△ **axio-.** Um eixo. VER TAMBÉM axo-. [L. *axis*]
ax·i·o·buc·cal (ak′sē-ō-bŭk′ăl). Axiobucal; que se refere à junção dos planos axial e bucal de um dente, usualmente uma linha.
ax·i·o·buc·co·gin·gi·val (ak′sē-ō-bŭk-ō-jin′ji-val). Axiobucogengival; refere-se à junção dos planos axial, bucal e gengival dos dentes; usualmente um ponto.
ax·i·o·in·ci·sal (ak′sē-ō-in-sī′săl). Axioincisal; refere-se ao ângulo da linha formada pela junção da borda incisal e pelas paredes axiais de um dente.
ax·i·o·la·bi·al (ak′sē-ō-lā′bē-ăl). Axiolabial; refere-se ao ângulo da linha de uma cavidade formada pela junção das paredes axial e labial de um dente.
ax·i·o·la·bi·o·lin·gual (ak′sē-ō-lā′bē-ō-ling′gwăl). Axiolabiolingual; refere-se a uma secção em sentido labiolingual ao longo do eixo longitudinal de um dente.
ax·i·o·lin·gual (ak′sē-ō-ling′gwăl). Axiolingual; refere-se ao ângulo da linha de uma cavidade formada pela junção de uma parede axial e uma lingual de um dente.
ax·i·o·lin·guo·cer·vi·cal (ak′sē-ō-ling′gwō-ser′vi-kăl). Axiolinguocervical; refere-se ao ângulo triédrico formado pela junção de uma parede axial, lingual e cervical (gengival) de uma cavidade dentária.
ax·i·o·lin·guo·clu·sal (ak′sē-ō-ling′gwō-kloo′săl). Axiolinguoclusal; refere-se ao ângulo triédrico formado pela junção das paredes axial, lingual e oclusal da cavidade de um dente.
ax·i·o·lin·guo·gin·gi·val (ak′sē-ō-ling′gwō-jin′ji-văl). Axiolinguogengival; refere-se ao ângulo formado pela junção das paredes axial, lingual e gengival (cervical) de uma cavidade dentária.
ax·i·o·me·si·al (ak′sē-ō-mē′zē-ăl). Axiomesial; refere-se ao ângulo da linha de uma cavidade dentária pela junção das paredes axial e mesial.
ax·i·o·me·si·o·cer·vi·cal (ak′sē-ō-mē′zē-ō-ser′vi-kăl). Axiomesiocervical; refere-se ao ângulo triédrico formado pela junção das paredes axial, mesial e cervical (gengival) de uma cavidade dentária.
ax·i·o·me·si·o·dis·tal. Axiomesiodistal. VER axiomesiodistal *plane*.
ax·i·o·me·si·o·gin·gi·val (ak′sē-ō-mē′zē-ō-jin′ji-văl). Axiomesiogengival; refere-se ao ângulo triédrico formado pelas paredes axial, mesial e gengival (cervical) de uma cavidade dentária.
ax·i·o·me·si·o·in·ci·sal (ak′sē-ō-mē′zē-ō-in-sī′săl). Axiomesioincisal; refere-se ao ângulo triédrico formado pela junção das paredes axial, mesial e incisal de uma cavidade dentária.
ax·i·on (ak′sē-on). O cérebro e a medula espinal (eixo cerebroespinal).
ax·io-oc·clu·sal (ak′sē-ō-ō-kloo′săl). Axioclusal; pertinente ao ângulo de linha formado pela junção das paredes axial e oclusal de um dente.
ax·i·o·plasm (ak′sē-ō-plazm). Axioplasma. SIN axoplasm.
ax·i·o·po·di·um, pl. **ax·i·o·po·dia** (ak′sē-ō-pō′dē-ŭm, -dē-ă). Axiopódio. SIN axopodium.
ax·i·o·pul·pal (ak′sē-ō-pŭl′păl). Axiopulpar; refere-se ao ângulo de linha formado pela junção das paredes axial e pulpar de uma cavidade dentária.
ax·i·o·ver·sion (ak′sē-ō-ver′zhŭn). Axioversão; inclinação anormal do eixo longitudinal de um dente.
ax·ip·e·tal (ak-sip′e-tăl). Axípeto. SIN centripetal (2). [L. *axis* + *peto*, procurar]
ax·i·ram·if·i·cate (ak′sē-ram-if′i-kāt). Axirramificar; indica uma célula nervosa cujo axônio, geralmente curto, divide-se em muitos ramos, p.ex, células de Golgi do tipo II. [G. *axōn*, eixo, + *grapho*, escrever]
ax·is (ax), pl. **ax·es** (ak′sis, ak′sēz). **1** [TA]. Eixo; uma linha reta que une dois pólos opostos de um corpo esférico, em torno do qual o corpo pode virar. **2** [TA]. A linha central do corpo ou qualquer uma de suas partes. **3.** A coluna vertebral. **4.** O sistema nervoso central. **5** [TA]. Áxis; a segunda vértebra cervical. SIN vertebra C2*, epistropheus, odontoid vertebra, second cervical vertebrae, toothed vertebra, vertebra dentata. **6.** Tronco; uma artéria que se divide, imediatamente após sua origem, em inúmeros ramos, p.ex., tronco celíaco. VER trunk. [L. axle, eixo]
basibregmatic a., eixo basibregmático; uma linha que se estende do básio ao bregma.
basicranial a., eixo basicraniano; uma linha traçada do básio até o ponto médio da sutura esfenoetmoidal.
basifacial a., e. basifacial; uma linha traçada do ponto subnasal até o ponto médio da sutura esfenoetmoidal. SIN facial a.
biauricular a., e. biauricular; uma linha reta que une as duas aurículas. Cf. auriculare.
celiac a., tronco celíaco. SIN celiac (arterial) *trunk*.
cephalocaudal a., eixo cefalocaudal. SIN long a. of body.
cerebrospinal a., e. cefaloespinal; o sistema nervoso central; o cérebro e a medula espinal. SIN encephalomyelonic a., neural a.
condylar a., eixo condilar; uma linha através dos dois côndilos mandibulares, em torno dos quais a mandíbula pode rodar durante uma parte do movimento de abertura. SIN condyle cord.
conjugate a., eixo conjugado. SIN median *conjugate*.
craniofacial a., eixo craniofacial; uma linha reta que passa através do osso mesetmóide, do osso pré-esfenóide, do corpo do esfenóide e da parte basilar do osso occipital.
electrical a., eixo elétrico; a direção geral das forças eletromotivas desenvolvidas no coração durante sua ativação, usualmente representada no plano frontal. VER triaxial reference *system*.
embryonic a., eixo embrionário; o eixo cefalocaudal estabelecido no embrião pela linha primitiva.
encephalomyelonic a., e. cefaloespinal. VER cerebrospinal a.
external a. of eye [TA], eixo externo do bulbo do olho; a parte do eixo óptico a partir do ponto médio, da superfície anterior da córnea até a superfície posterior do pólo posterior da superfície externa da esclerótica. SIN a. externus bulbi oculi [TA].
a. exter′nus bul′bi oculi [TA], e. externo do bulbo do olho. SIN external a. of eye.
facial a., eixo facial. SIN basifacial a.
axes of Fick, eixos de Fick; três eixos que passam através do centro do bulbo do olho vertical (Z) e horizontalmente, no plano coronal (X), e horizontalmente, no plano sagital (Y). Todas as rotações oculares podem ser descritas por rotação ao longo desses eixos.
hinge a., eixo horizontal transverso, eixo mandibular. SIN transverse horizontal a.
instantaneous electrical a., eixo elétrico instantâneo; o eixo resultante das forças eletromotoras que se desenvolvem no coração em dado momento.
internal a. of eye [TA], eixo interno do bulbo do olho; a parte do e. óptico a partir do ponto médio da superfície posterior da córnea até a superfície anterior da retina, oposta ao pólo posterior. SIN a. internus bulbi oculi [TA].
a. inter′nus bul′bi oculi [TA], eixo interno do bulbo do olho. SIN internal a. of eye.
a. of lens, eixo da lente do olho; uma linha que une os pólos anterior e posterior da lente do olho. SIN a. lentis.
a. len′tis, eixo da lente do olho. SIN a. of lens.
long a., eixo longitudinal; uma linha que se estende no sentido longitudinal através do centro de um objeto; em odontologia, a linha que se estende no sentido inciso (ocluso)-cervical em paralelo com as superfícies axiais de um dente.
long a. of body, eixo longitudinal do corpo; a linha reta imaginária, no plano mediano, que quase faz intersecção com o centro de todos os planos transversos através do corpo, correndo desde o ápice do crânio através do centro do períneo e continuando entre os membros inferiores, paralelo e eqüidistante dos eixos longitudinais dos membros; na teoria, essa é a linha sobre a qual a massa do corpo se distribui uniformemente. VER TAMBÉM embryonic a. SIN cephalocaudal a.
mandibular a., eixo horizontal transverso, eixo mandibular. SIN transverse horizontal a.
mean electrical a., eixo elétrico médio; a magnitude e a direção médias de todas as forças eletromotoras desenvolvidas durante o evento cardíaco em consideração; p.ex., despolarização atrial ou ventricular, ou repolarização ventricular. VER TAMBÉM axis *deviation*.
neural a., eixo cefaloespinal. SIN cerebrospinal a.
neutral a. of straight beam, eixo neutro do feixe reto; o e. perpendicular ao plano de carga de um feixe sob esforço dentro do limite proporcional; situa-se no eixo de gravidade do corte transversal do feixe.
normal electrical a., eixo elétrico normal; eixo elétrico médio do coração situado entre −30° e +90°. VER hexaxial reference *system*.
opening a., eixo de abertura; uma linha imaginária em torno da qual os côndilos mandibulares podem girar durante os movimentos de abertura e fechamento. Cf. fulcrum *line*.

optic a. [TA], eixo óptico; o eixo do bulbo do olho que conecta os pólos anterior e posterior; geralmente diverge do e. visual em cinco graus ou mais. SIN a. opticus [TA].
a. op'ticus [TA], eixo óptico. SIN optic a.
orbital a., eixo orbital; a linha originária no centro do forame óptico (ápice da órbita) que se estende anterior, lateral e inferiormente até o meio da abertura orbital.
pelvic a., eixo da pelve. SIN a. of pelvis.
a. pel'vis [TA], eixo da pelve. SIN a. of pelvis.
a. of pelvis [TA], eixo da pelve; uma linha curva hipotética que une o ponto central de cada um dos quatro planos da pelve, marcando o centro da cavidade pélvica em todos os níveis. SIN a. pelvis [TA], pelvic a., plane of pelvic canal.
principal optic a., eixo óptico principal; uma linha que passa através do centro da lente de um sistema de refração em ângulos retos com sua superfície.
pupillary a., eixo pupilar; uma linha perpendicular à superfície da córnea, passando através do centro da pupila; a "direção do olhar".
rotational a., eixo de rotação. SIN fulcrum line.
sagittal a., eixo sagital; em odontologia, a linha no plano frontal ao redor do qual o côndilo do lado funcional gira durante o movimento mandibular.
secondary a., eixo secundário; qualquer raio que passa através do centro óptico de uma lente.
a. of symmetry, eixo de simetria; um eixo através de uma partícula (p.ex., um vírus) em um plano tal que, quando a partícula é girada no eixo, existem duas ou mais posições em que a partícula parece idêntica.
thoracic a., (1) Artéria tóraco-acromial. SIN thoracoacromial artery; (2) Veia tóraco-acromial. SIN thoracocromial vein.
thyroid a., tronco (arterial) tireocervical. SIN thyrocervical (arterial) trunk.
transporionic a., eixo transporiônico; uma linha imaginária que une os pontos centrais superiores dos meatos acústicos externos; usada na cefalometria radiográfica. VER porion.
transverse horizontal a., eixo horizontal transverso, eixo mandibular; uma linha imaginária em torno da qual a mandíbula pode rodar através do plano horizontal. SIN hinge a., mandibular a.
vertical a., eixo vertical; em odontologia, a linha em torno da qual o côndilo do lado funcional gira no plano horizontal durante o movimento mandibular.
visual a., eixo visual; a linha reta que se estende desde o objeto observado, através do centro da pupila, até a mácula lútea da retina. SIN line of vision.
Y-a., eixo Y; um indicador cefalométrico das coordenadas vertical e horizontal do crescimento mandibular expresso em graus do ângulo facial inferior, formado pela intersecção do plano sela-gnátio com o plano horizontal de Frankfort.

axo-. Forma combinante que significa eixo e geralmente relacionada a um axônio. [G. axōn, eixo]

ax·o·ax·on·ic (ak'sō-ak-son'ik). Axoaxônico; relativo ao contato sináptico entre o axônio de uma célula nervosa e o de outra. VER synapse.

ax·o·den·drit·ic (ak'sō-den-drit'ik). Axodendrítica; pertinente à relação sináptica de um axônio com um dendrito de outro neurônio. VER synapse.

ax·of·u·gal (ak-sof'ū-gǎl). Axofugo. SIN axifugal. [axo- + L. fugio, fugir]

ax·o·graph (ak'sō-graf). Axógrafo; um aparelho para registrar as escalas ou eixos de magnitude predeterminada nos registros cimográficos. [axo- + G. graphō, escrever]

ax·o·lem·ma (ak'sō-lem'ǎ). Axolema; a membrana plasmática do axônio. SIN Mauthner sheath. [axo- + G. lemma, casca]

ax·ol·y·sis (ak-sol'i-sis). Axólise; destruição ou dissolução de um axônio nervoso. [axo- + G. lysis, dissolução]

ax·on (ak'son). Axônio; o processo único de uma célula nervosa que, em condições normais, conduz os impulsos nervosos para longe do corpo celular e seus processos remanescentes (dendritos). É um processo filamentoso relativamente uniforme, que varia em espessura de cerca de 0,25 μm a mais de 10 μm. Em contraste com os dendritos, que raramente excedem 1,5 mm de comprimento, os axônios podem estender-se por grandes distâncias a partir do corpo celular original (alguns axônios do trato piramidal têm 40 a 50 cm de comprimento). Os axônios com 0,5 μm de espessura ou mais são geralmente envolvidos por uma bainha de mielina segmentada, formada por células da oligodendróglia (no cérebro e na medula espinal) ou por células de Schwann (nos nervos periféricos). Como os dendritos e corpos da célula nervosa, os axônios contêm um grande número de neurofibrilas. Com algumas exceções, as células nervosas transmitem sinapticamente impulsos para outras células nervosas ou para as células efetoras (células musculares, células glandulares) exclusivamente por meio das terminações sinápticas de seus axônios. [G. axōn, eixo]

ax·o·nal (ak'sō-nǎl). Axonal; pertinente a um axônio.

ax·o·neme (ak'sō-nēm). **1.** Axonema; o filamento central que corre no eixo do cromossoma. **2.** Filamento axial. SIN axial filament. **3.** O arranjo peculiar dos microtúbulos no núcleo dos cílios eucarióticos e flagelos que compreendem um par central circundado por um feixe de nove microtúbulos duplos. [axo- + G. nēma, um filamento]

ax·on·og·ra·phy (ak-sō-nog'rǎ-fē). Axonografia; o registro das alterações elétricas nos axônios. SIN electroaxonography.

ax·o·nop·a·thy (aks'on-op'ǎ-thē). Axonopatia; um distúrbio que afeta principalmente os axônios das fibras nervosas periféricas (embora ocorra desmielinização secundária), em contraste com aquele que afeta apenas a mielina (mielinopatia).

ax·on·ot·me·sis (ak'son-ot-mē'sis). Axonotmese; a interrupção dos axônios de um nervo seguida por degeneração completa do segmento periférico, sem ruptura das estruturas de sustentação do nervo; essa lesão pode resultar de pinçamento, esmagamento ou compressão prolongada. VER TAMBÉM neurapraxia, neurotmesis. [axon + G. tmēsis, um corte]

ax·op·e·tal (ak-sop'ě-tǎl). Axópeto; que se estende para um axônio. [axo- + L. peto, procurar]

ax·o·plasm (ak'sō-plazm). Axoplasma; neuroplasma do axônio. SIN axioplasm.

ax·o·po·di·um, pl. **ax·o·po·dia** (ak-sō-pō'dē-ŭm, -ǎ). Axópodo; um pseudópodo permanente que contém um filamento axial rígido de protoplasma diferenciado. SIN axiopodium. [L. Mod. de L. axis + G. podion, dim. de pous (pod-), pé]

ax·o·so·mat·ic (ak-sō-sō-mat'ik). Axossomático; relativo à relação sináptica de um axônio com um corpo celular nervoso. VER synapse. [axo- + G. sōma, corpo]

ax·o·style (ak'sō-stīl). Axóstilo; um bastão ou túbulo de sustentação alongado que percorre o comprimento de determinados protozoários flagelados, projetando-se, com frequência, para fora da extremidade posterior. Isolados ou múltiplos, filamentosos ou rígidos, eles variam com a espécie, mas servem como uma estrutura de endoesqueleto e também podem funcionar na locomoção. [axo- + G. stylos, pilar]

ax·ot·o·my (ak'sot'ō-mē). Axotomia; incisão ou transecção de um axônio. [axo- + G. tomē, cortar]

ay·a·hua·sca (ī'ǎ-wa-skǎ). Ayahuasca, caapi. SIN caapi.

Ayala, G., neurologista italiano, 1878–1943. VER A. index, quotient.

Ayerza, L., médico argentino, 1861–1918. VER A. disease, syndrome.

Ayre, James Ernest, ginecologista norte-americano, *1910. VER A. brush.

aza·crine (ā'zǎ-krēn). Azacrina; um antimalárico; um esquizonticida efetivo na infecção aguda por Plasmodium falciparum.

aza·cy·clo·nol hy·dro·chlo·ride (ā'zǎ-sī'klō-nol). Cloridrato de azaciclonol; um isômero estrutural do cloridrato de pipradol, parcialmente antagonista às suas ações, usado com resultados variáveis no tratamento de alucinações e confusões.

9-aza·flu·o·rene (ā'zǎ-flōr'ēn). 9-azafluoreno. SIN carbazole.

8-aza·gua·nine (ā-zǎ-gwah'nēn). 8-azaguanina; guanina com N em lugar do C na posição 8; um antagonista da guanina que tem sido empregado no tratamento da leucemia aguda. SIN guanazolo, triazologuanine.

aza·me·tho·ni·um bro·mide (ā-zǎ-me-thō'nē-ŭm). Brometo de azametônio; um agente bloqueador ganglionar.

aza·per·one (ā'zǎ-per-ōn). Azaperona; um tranquilizante.

azap·e·tine phos·phate (ā-zap'ě-tēn). Fosfato de azapetina; um potente agente bloqueador adrenérgico (α-receptor), com ação e usos semelhantes aos da tolazolina; usado no tratamento das doenças vasculares periféricas.

aza·pir·ones (ā-zǎ-pī'rōnz). Azapironas; ansiolíticos que agem através de ação agonista nos receptores 1-A da serotonina.

azar·i·bine (ā-zar'i-bēn). Azaribina; agente antipsoriático que não é mais utilizado por causa de uma alta incidência de reações adversas graves.

aza·ser·ine (ā-zǎ-ser'ēn). Azasserina; O-diazoacetil-L-serina; um antibiótico inibidor da síntese da purina; análogo da glutamina; mutagênico e antimorigênico. Retarda o crescimento de neoplasias animais transplantáveis.

aza·spi·ro·dec·ane·di·one (ā-zǎ-spī'rō-dek-ān-dī'ōn). Azaspirodecanodiona; uma classe de agentes ansiolíticos não relacionados química ou farmacologicamente a outras classes de medicamentos sedativos e ansiolíticos; p.ex., cloridrato de buspirona.

azat·a·dine ma·le·ate (ā-zat'ǎ-dēn). Maleato de azatadina; um anti-histamínico com propriedades anticolinérgicas e anti-serotonina.

aza·thi·o·prine (ā-zǎ-thī'ō-prēn). Azatioprina; um derivado da 6-mercaptopurina, empregado como agente citotóxico e imunossupressor em transplante de órgãos e no tratamento de doenças auto-imunes, como anemias hemolíticas, lúpus eritematoso sistêmico, artrite reumatóide e leucemias.

6-aza·thy·mine (ā-zǎ-thī'mēn). 6-azatimina; timina com N em lugar de C na posição 6; um antimetabólito da timina.

6-az·au·ri·dine (AZUR) (az-aw'ri-dēn). 6-azauridina; uridina com N em lugar de C na posição 6; um análogo triazínico da uridina e um antimetabólito com seletividade para os leucócitos neoplásicos humanos; produz remissões parciais em determinadas leucemias agudas de adultos.

aze·o·trope (ā-zē'ō-trōp). Azeótropo; uma mistura de dois ou mais líquidos que ferve sem alteração na proporção das substâncias, seja na fase líquida seja na de vapor; p.ex., etanol a 95% (na realidade 94,9% por volume, o restante sendo água). [G. a- priv. + zeō, ferver, + tropos, volta]

halothane-ether a., a. éter-halotano; uma mistura azeotrópica nas proporções de 68 para o halotano e 32 para o éter, por volume, que combina as vantagens de cada anestésico, embora não seja inflamável.

aze·o·tro·pic (āʹzē-ō-tropʹik). Azeotrópico; que indica ou caracteriza um azeótropo.

az·ide (azʹīd). Azida; um composto que contém o grupamento –N₃ monovalente.

az·i·do·thy·mi·dine (AZT) (azʹi-dō-thīʹmi-dēn). Azidotimidina (AZT). SIN zidovudine.

az·lo·cil·lin so·di·um (az-lōʹ-silʹin). Azlocilina sódica; uma penicilina de amplo espectro usada no tratamento de infecções causadas por *Pseudomonas aeruginosa*, *Escherichia coli* e *Haemophilus influenzae*.

♻ **azo-.** Prefixo que indica a presença de uma molécula do grupamento ≡C–N=N–C≡. Cf. diazo-. [Fr. *azote*, nome para o nitrogênio proposto por AL Lavoisier 1743–1794).]

az·o·bi·li·ru·bin (azʹō-bil-i-rooʹbin). Azobilirrubina; o pigmento vermelho-violáceo formado pela condensação do ácido sulfanílico diazotado com a bilirrubina na reação de van den Bergh.

az·o·car·mine (āʹzō-karʹmin). Azocarmim; uma série de corantes azo utilizados na preparação de colorações histológicas.

az·o·car·mine B, az·o·car·mine G (az-ō-karʹmin) [C.I. 50090, C.I. 50085]. Azocarmim B, azocarmim G; corantes ácidos vermelhos, sendo o primeiro mais hidrossolúvel e útil na coloração de Heidenhain.

azo·ic (ā-zōʹik, āʹ-). Azóico; que não contém seres vivos; sem vida orgânica. [G. *a-* priv. + *zōikos*, relativo a um animal]

az·ole (azʹōl). Azol. SIN pyrrole.

az·o·lit·min (az-ō-litʹmin) [antiga C.I. 1242]. Azolitimina; uma matéria de coloração vermelho-púrpura obtida do litmo natural ou sintetizada por oxidação do orcinol na presença de amônia, lima e potassa; usada como um indicador amplo de pH (vermelho em 4,5, azul em 8,3).

a·zo·o·sper·mia (ā-zō-ō-sperʹmē-ā). Azospermia; ausência de espermatozóides vivos no sêmen; falha da espermatogênese. VER TAMBÉM aspermia. [G. *a-* priv. + *zōon*, animal, + *sperma*, semente]

az·o·phlox·in (az-ō-flokʹsin). Azofloxina. SIN amidonaphthol red.

az·o·pro·tein (az-ō-prōʹtēn). Azoproteína; qualquer uma das proteínas modificadas produzidas por tratamento com derivados diazônio de diversas aminas aromáticas; usada para provocar a formação de anticorpos e demonstrar a especificidade do anticorpo.

az·o·sul·fa·mide (az-ō-sŭlʹfa-mīd). Azossulfamida; um derivado avermelhado, hidrossolúvel, menos tóxico, porém menos efetivo que a sulfanilamida; deve sua atividade antibacteriana à sulfanilamida liberada.

az·o·te·mia (az-ō-tēʹmē-ā). Azotemia; aumento anormal na concentração da uréia e outras substâncias nitrogenadas no plasma sanguíneo. VER TAMBÉM uremia. [azo- (azote) + G. *haima*, sangue]
 nonrenal a., prerenal a., a. não-renal, a. pré-renal; retenção de nitrogênio resultante de algo diferente de uma doença renal primária.

az·o·tem·ic (az-ō-tēmʹik). Azotêmico; relativo à azotemia.

az·o·ther·mia (az-ō-therʹmē-ā). Azotermia; termo raramente utilizado para a febre decorrente da uremia. [azote + G. *therme*, calor]

azo·tu·ria (az-ō-toorʹē-ā). Azotúria; eliminação aumentada de uréia na urina. [azo- (azote) + G. *ouron*, urina]

az·o·van blue (azʹō-van). Azul de Evans. SIN Evans blue.

AZT Abreviatura para azidothymidine (azidotimidina).

az·tre·o·nam (az-trēʹō-nam). Aztreonam; antibiótico monolactâmico bactericida sintético com um amplo espectro de atividade contra patógenos aeróbicos Gram-negativos.

az·ul (azhʹŭl). Pinta. SIN pinta. [Sp. blue]

AZUR Abreviatura para 6-azauridine (6-azauridina).

az·ure (azhʹūr). Azur; um termo para um grupo de corantes básicos metacromáticos, metiltioninícios ou fenotiazínicos, usados como corantes biológicos, principalmente nas colorações de sangue e nucleares.
 a. A [C.I. 52005¶, aʹ. A; cloreto de dimetiltionina assimétrica; um corante azul empregado como componente do corante sanguíneo tetracromo de MacNeal e nos corantes sanguíneos do tipo Romanowsky; também utilizado como um corante para mucinas, ácidos nucleicos e grânulos de mastócitos; fornece uma coloração metacromática do violeta ao vermelho para substâncias muito ácidas nos tecidos.
 a. B [C.I. 52010], a. B; cloreto de trimetiltionina; um corante azul usado de forma semelhante ao a. A; também como o brometo de a. B para fornecer coloração metacromática do RNA e DNA.
 a. C [C.I. 52002], a. C; cloreto de monometiltionina; um corante tiazínico azul-violeta empregado na coloração metacromática de mucinas e cartilagem.
 a. I, a. I; uma mistura de a. A e B. SIN methylene azure.
 a. II, a. II; uma mistura de a. I e azul de metileno; o eosinato, a. II-eosina, é o principal ingrediente da coloração de Giemsa.

az·u·res·in (azhʹū-resʹin). Azurresina; um complexo de azur A e resina carbacrílica; usado como indicador para a detecção da acloridria gástrica sem intubação. SIN quinine carbacrylic resin.

az·u·ro·phil, az·u·ro·phile (azhʹū-rō-fil, -fīl). Azurófilo; que se cora prontamente com um corante do tipo azur, indicando principalmente a hipercromatina e os grânulos vermelho-purpúreos de determinadas células sanguíneas. [azure + G. *philos*, ligação]

az·u·ro·phil·ia (azʹū-rō-filʹē-ā). Azurofilia; uma condição em que o sangue contém células com granulações azurófilas.

azy·go·gram (azʹi-gō-gram). Azigograma; demonstração radiográfica do sistema venoso ázigos depois da injeção de contraste. [azygos + G. *gramma*, uma escrita]

azy·gog·ra·phy (azʹi-gogʹra-fē). Azigografia; radiografia do sistema venoso ázigos depois de injeção de contraste.

az·y·gos (azʹi-gos). **1.** Ázigo; uma estrutura anatômica ímpar. **2.** Veia ázigo. SIN azygos vein. [G. *a-* priv. + *zygon*, parelha]
 a. continuation (of the inferior vena cava), continuação ázigo (da veia cava inferior), uma anomalia congênita em que a porção infra-hepática da veia cava não se forma e a drenagem venosa da metade inferior do corpo é mantida através de uma veia supracardinal direita persistente, a qual se transforma em uma grande veia ázigo.

az·y·gous (azʹi-gŭs, ā-zīʹgŭs). Ázigo; ímpar. [G. *azygos*]

B

β 1. Segunda letra do alfabeto grego, beta. **2.** Em química, indica o segundo em uma série, o segundo carbono a partir de um grupamento funcional (p.ex., carboxílico), ou a direção de uma ligação química no sentido do observador. Para os termos que possuem esse prefixo, veja o termo específico.
β-. Símbolo para electron (elétron).
β+. Símbolo para positron (pósitron).
B 1. Símbolo do boron (boro); símbolo do aspartic acid (ácido aspártico) ou asparagine (asparagina) quando não se sabe qual dos dois aminoácidos está presente; símbolo de bromouridine (bromouridina); segundo substrato em uma reação catalisada por enzima com múltiplos substratos. **2.** Como subscrito, refere-se a barometric *pressure* (pressão barométrica).
b 1. Como subscrito, refere-se a blood (sangue). **2.** Abreviatura de bis [L.].
Ba Símbolo de barium (bário).
Babbitt, Isaac, inventor norte-americano, 1799–1862. VER B. *metal*.
Babcock, Stephen M., químico norte-americano, 1843–1931. VER B. *tube*.
Babès, Victor, bacteriologista romeno, 1854–1926. VER *Babesia*; B. *nodes*, em *node*.
Ba·be·sia (bă-bē′zē-ă). O gênero economicamente mais importante dos protozoários da família Babesiidae; caracterizado por multiplicação nos eritrócitos do hospedeiro para formar pares e tétrades; causa a babesiose (piroplasmose) na maioria dos tipos de animais domésticos, e duas espécies provocam a doença em pessoas esplenectomizadas ou normais; os vetores são os carrapatos ixodídeos ou argasídeos. [V. *Babès*]
B. diver′gens, a causa da babesiose bovina nas regiões oeste e central da Europa; o carrapato vetor é o *Ixodes ricinus*; causou babesiose humana em indivíduos esplenectomizados na Europa; também encontrada na rena.
B. micro′ti, um protozoário semelhante ao da malária que parasita naturalmente determinados roedores (espécies de *Peromyscus* e *Microtus*) na América do Norte; inúmeros casos humanos foram reportados nos Estados Unidos. O carrapato vetor local é o *Ixodes scapularis*. O número e os níveis de infecção desse carrapato aumentaram muito nos últimos anos com o aumento da população de cervos, que lhe servem como uma fonte abundante de sangue. VER TAMBÉM *Borrelia burgdorferi*.
Ba·be·si·el·la (ba-bē-zē-el′ă). VER *Babesia*.
Ba·be·si·i·dae (ba′bē-zī′i-dē, -zē′i-dē). Uma família de protozoários parasitas (classe Sporozoea, ordem Piroplasmida) que ocorrem nos eritrócitos de vários mamíferos. Os microrganismos são piriformes, arredondados ou ovais e se reproduzem por esquizogonia para formar tétrades ou por fissão binária para formar pares nos eritrócitos; a transmissão é feita por carrapatos. A família inclui os gêneros *Babesia*, *Echinozoon* e *Entopolypoides*; atualmente, acredita-se que *Aegyptianella*, originalmente incluída, é uma riquétsia. VER TAMBÉM Theileriidae.
ba·be·si·o·sis (bă-bē′zē-ō′sis). Babesiose; uma doença causada por infecção por uma espécie do protozoário *Babesia*, transmitido por carrapatos. Em animais, a doença caracteriza-se por febre, indisposição, inquietação, anemia grave e hemoglobinúria; a taxa de mortalidade freqüentemente é mais elevada nos animais adultos que nos mais jovens. SIN piroplasmosis.
human b., b. humana; uma rara doença humana causada por infecção por espécies de *Babesia* (mais freqüentemente *B. divergens* na Europa e *B. microti* nos Estados Unidos) que tem sido fatal em alguns indivíduos esplenectomizados.
Babinski, Joseph F., neurologista francês, 1857–1932. VER B. *phenomenon, sign, reflex, syndrome*.
ba·by (ba′bē) Bebê; um lactente; um recém-nascido.
blue b., b. azul; uma criança que nasce cianótica por causa de um defeito cardíaco ou pulmonar congênito que causa oxigenação incompleta do sangue.
blueberry muffin b., um neonato com lesões cutâneas purpúreas, cujo aspecto foi comparado ao de um *muffin* (bolinho semelhante a um sonho). As lesões são causadas por eritropoese dérmica e são observadas nas infecções congênitas, como a infecção por citomegalovírus, toxoplasmose ou rubéola. A infecção interfere com a produção normal de eritrócitos na medula óssea.
collodion b. [MIM*146600], bebê-colódio; neonato com ictiose lamelar; ao nascimento, a pele é vermelho-viva, brilhante, translúcida e repuxada, gerando um aspecto distorcido (como se tivesse sido pintada com colódio) de imobilização da face; a contração da pele provoca ectrópio, um aspecto nasal achatado e abertura exagerada da boca e dos lábios; herança autossômica recessiva.
test-tube b., b. de proveta; termo popular para um b. nascido depois de implante uterino de um ovo materno fertilizado *in vitro*.
bac·am·pi·cil·lin hy·dro·chlo·ride (bak′am-pi-sil′in). Cloridrato de bacampicilina; penicilina semi-sintética com as mesmas atividades e usos da ampicilina, porém mais bem absorvida na administração oral.
bac·cate (bak′āt). Baciforme; semelhante a uma baga. [L. *bacca*, baga]
Baccelli, Guido, médico italiano, 1832–1916. VER B. *sign*.
bac·ci·form (bak′sĭ-fōrm). Baciforme; em formato de baga. [L. *bacca*, baga]
Bachman, George W., parasitologista norte-americano, *1890. VER B.-Pettit *test*.
Bachmann, Jean George, fisiologista norte-americano, 1877–1959. VER B. *bundle*.

Bachmann, VER Rivinus.
Ba·cil·la·ce·ae (ba-si-lā′sē-ē). Família de bactérias aeróbicas ou anaeróbicas facultativas, formadoras de esporos, comumente móveis (ordem Eubacteriales), que contêm bastonetes Gram-positivos. Esses microrganismos são químio-heterotróficos. Algumas espécies são patogênicas. Geralmente dois gêneros, *Bacillus* e *Clostridium*, são incluídos. O gênero típico é *Bacillus*.
ba·cil·lar, bac·il·la·ry (bas′i-lar, bas′i-lā-rē). Bacilar; com formato de um bastão; consiste em bastonetes ou elementos semelhantes a bastonetes.
ba·cil·le Calmette-Guérin (BCG) (bah′sel′). Bacilo de Calmette-Guérin; cepa atenuada de *Mycobacterium bovis* utilizada na preparação da vacina BCG, que é empregada para a imunização contra a tuberculose e na quimioterapia para o câncer. SIN Calmette-Guérin bacillus. [Fr.]
bac·il·le·mia (bas-i-lē′mē-ă). Bacilemia; a presença de bacilos no sangue circulante. [bacillus + G. *haima*, sangue]
ba·cil·li (bă-sil′ī). Bacilos; plural de bacillus.
ba·cil·li·form (ba-sil′i-fōrm). Baciliforme; em formato de bastão. [L. *bacillus*, um bastão, + *forma*, forma]
ba·cil·lin (ba-sil′in). Bacilina; uma substância antibiótica produzida pelo *Bacillus subtilis*.
ba·cil·lo·myx·in (ba-sil-ō-mik′sin). Bacilomixina; um antibiótico ativo contra determinados fungos patogênicos obtido a partir de culturas de *Bacillus subtilis*. [*Bacillus* + G. *mykēs*, fungo, + -in]
ba·cil·lo·sis (bas-i-lō′sis). Bacilose; infecção generalizada por bacilos.
bac·il·lu·ria (bas-i-loo′rē-ă). Bacilúria; a presença de bacilos na urina. [bacillus + G. *ouron*, urina]
Ba·cil·lus (ba-sil′ŭs). Gênero de bactérias aeróbicas ou anaeróbicas facultativas, formadoras de esporos, comumente móveis (família Bacillaceae), que contêm bastonetes Gram-positivos. As células móveis são peritríquias; os esporos têm paredes espessas e se coram mal pelo método de Gram; esses microrganismos são químio-heterotróficos e são encontrados principalmente no solo. Algumas espécies são patógenos de animais; algumas espécies provocam produção de anticorpo. A espécie típica é *B. subtilis*. [L. dim. de *baculus*, bastão, bastonete]
B. an′thracis, espécie bacteriana que provoca antraz em seres humanos, gado, suínos, carneiros, coelhos, cobaias e camundongos; contém plasmídeos de virulência associados à cápsula e à produção de toxina.
B. bre′vis, espécie bacteriana encontrada no solo, ar, poeira, leite e queijo; algumas cepas produzem o antibiótico gramicidina ou tirocidina.
B. ce′reus, espécie bacteriana que causa um tipo emético e um tipo diarréico de intoxicação alimentar em seres humanos, podendo provocar infecções em seres humanos e em outros mamíferos. Pode causar uma infecção altamente destrutiva no olho traumatizado.
B. circulans, espécie bacteriana encontrada no solo, que foi incriminada em infecções de seres humanos, inclusive na septicemia, infecções por abscessos mistos e infecções de feridas.
B. hemoly′ticus, nome original do *Clostridium haemolyticum*.
B. histoly′ticus, nome original do *Clostridium histolyticum*.
B. megate′rium, espécie bacteriana saprofítica de interesse experimental; as cepas produzem bacteriocinas (megacinas).
B. polymyx′a, espécie bacteriana encontrada no solo, água, leite, fezes e vegetais em decomposição; algumas cepas produzem o antibiótico polimixina.
B. pumilis, espécie usualmente saprofítica de bactérias que foi associada à intoxicação alimentar e, raramente, à formação de abscesso ou de fístula intestinal.
B. sphae′ricus, espécie bacteriana que é um patógeno de insetos e que foi associada a infecções ocasionais em seres humanos e em outros mamíferos, principalmente em hospedeiros imunocomprometidos; as infecções em seres humanos incluíram meningite, endocardite e intoxicação alimentar.
B. subti′lis, espécie bacteriana encontrada no solo e na matéria orgânica em decomposição; algumas cepas produzem o antibiótico subtilina, subtenolina ou bacilomicina; foi associada a infecções em seres humanos, principalmente em pacientes imunocomprometidos, e a intoxicação alimentar. É a espécie típica do gênero *B.* SIN grass bacillus, hay bacillus.

⌂ Formas Combinantes	☆ Termo oficial alternativo para a *Terminologia Anatomica*
🛈 Indica que o termo é ilustrado, ver Índice de Ilustrações	
SIN Sinônimo	[MIM] Mendelian Inheritance in Man
Cf. Comparar, confrontar	I.C. Índice de Corantes
[NA] *Nomina Anatomica*	
[TA] *Terminologia Anatomica*	Termo de Alta Importância

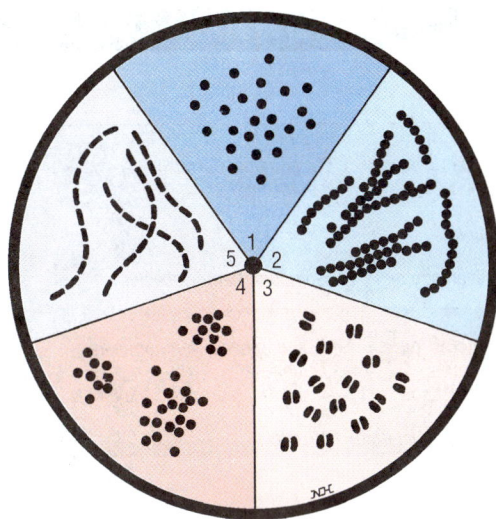

bactérias: (1) cocos, (2) estreptococos, (3) diplococos, (4) estafilococos, (5) bacilos

B. thuringien'sis, espécie bacteriana que é um patógeno de insetos, usada para controle de vetor, que foi implicada em infecções em seres humanos e em mamíferos. No laboratório, pode ser erroneamente diagnosticada como uma cepa do *B. cereus.*

ba·cil·lus, pl. **ba·cil·li** (ba-sil′ŭs, -ī). Bacilo. 1. Um termo vernacular utilizado para se referir a qualquer membro do gênero de bactérias *Bacillus.* 2. Termo empregado para referir-se a qualquer bactéria em formato de bastonete. [L. dim. de *baculus,* um bastão, bastonete]
  abortus b., *Brucella abortus.* SIN *Brucella abortus.*
  Battey b., b. de Battey. SIN *Mycobacterium intracellulare.* [Hospital Battey em Roma, GA]
  blue pus b., *Pseudomonas aeruginosa.* SIN *Pseudomonas aeruginosa.*
  Bordet-Gengou b., b. de Bordet-Gengou. SIN *Bordetella pertussis.*
  Calmette-Guérin b., b. de Calmette-Guérin. SIN bacille Calmette-Guérin.
  cholera b., *Vibrio cholerae.* SIN *Vibrio cholerae.*
  coliform bacilli (kō′li-fōrm, kol′i-fōrm), bacilos coliformes; nome comum para *Escherichia coli,* que é utilizado como um indicador de contaminação fecal da água, medida em relação à contagem de coliformes; ocasionalmente empregado para referir-se a todas as bactérias entéricas fermentadoras da lactose.
  colon b., *Escherichia coli.* SIN *Escherichia coli.*
  comma b., *Vibrio cholerae.* SIN *Vibrio cholerae.*
  Döderlein b., b. de Döderlein; grande bactéria Gram-positiva que ocorre em secreções vaginais normais; embora creditado por alguns como sendo idêntico ao *Lactobacillus acidophilus,* a identidade do b. de Döderlein ainda é duvidosa.
  Ducrey b., b. de Ducrey. SIN *Haemophilus ducreyi.*
  dysentery b., b. da disenteria; um microrganismo do gênero *Shigella* que provoca a disenteria.
  Eberth b., b. de Eberth. SIN *Salmonella typhi.*
  Flexner b., b. de Flexner. SIN *Shigella flexneri.*
  Friedländer b., b. de Friedländer. SIN *Klebsiella pneumoniae.*
  gas b., b. da gangrena gasosa. SIN *Clostridium perfringens.*
  grass b., *Bacillus subtilis.* SIN *Bacillus subtilis.*
  Hansen b., b. de Hansen. SIN *Mycobacterium leprae.*
  hay b., *Bacillus subtilis.* SIN *Bacillus subtilis.*
  Hofmann b., b. de Hofmann. SIN *Corynebacterium pseudodiphtheriticum.*
  influenza b., *Haemophilus influenzae.* SIN *Haemophilus influenzae.*
  Kitasato b., b. de Kitasato. SIN *Yersinia pestis.*
  Klebs-Loeffler b., b. de Klebs-Loeffler. SIN *Corynebacterium diphtheriae.*
  Koch b., b. de Koch. SIN *Mycobacterium tuberculosis.*
  Koch-Weeks b., b. de Koch-Weeks. SIN *Haemophilus aegyptius.*
  lactic acid b., um membro do gênero *Lactobacillus.*
  leprosy b., b. da lepra. SIN *Mycobacterium leprae.*
  Loeffler b., b. de Loeffler. SIN *Corynebacterium diphtheriae.*
  Moeller grass b., *Mycobacterium phlei.* SIN *Mycobacterium phlei.*
  Morgan b., b. de Morgan. SIN *Morganella morganii.*
  Much b., b. de Much; uma suposta forma granular não-álcool-ácido-resistente do b. da tuberculose; não é demonstrável pelo corante de Ziehl, mas capta um corante de Gram modificado; diz-se que é a forma presente na lesão cutânea da tuberculose.
  necrosis b., *Fusobacterium necrophorum.* SIN *Fusobacterium necrophorum.*
  paracolon b., qualquer uma das inúmeras bactérias entéricas que não fermentam rapidamente a lactose.
  paradysentery b., *Shigella flexneri.* SIN *Shigella flexneri.*
  paratyphoid b., b. paratifóide; qualquer um dos três microrganismos que causam as três formas (A, B, C) da febre paratifóide. VER TAMBÉM paratyphoid *fever.*
  plague b., *Yersinia pestis.* SIN *Yersinia pestis.*
  Shiga b., b. Shiga. SIN *Shigella dysenteriae.*
  Shiga-Kruse b., b. Shiga-Kruse. SIN *Shigella dysenteriae.*
  tubercle b., (1) SIN *Mycobacterium tuberculosis;* **(2)** SIN *Mycobacterium bovis.*
  typhoid b., *Salmonella typhi.* SIN *Salmonella typhi.*
  Vincent b., b. de Vincent; provavelmente *Fusobacterium nucleatum.*
  Weeks b., b. de Weeks. SIN *Haemophilus influenzae.*
  Welch b., b. de Welch. SIN *Clostridium perfringens.*
  Whitmore b., b. de Whitmore. SIN *Pseudomonas pseudomallei.*

bac·i·tra·cin (bas-i-trā′sin). Bacitracina; polipeptídeo antibiótico (antibacteriano) de estrutura química conhecida, isolado a partir de culturas de um bacilo aeróbico, Gram-positivo, formador de esporos (membro do grupo do *Bacillus subtilis*); ativo contra estreptococos hemolíticos, estafilococos e vários tipos de microrganismos Gram-positivos, aeróbico, em formato de bastão; usualmente aplicado localmente. Também existe b. zíncica. [*Bacillus* + Margaret *Tracy,* fonte da cultura original]

back (bak). **1.** Dorso; face posterior do tronco, abaixo do pescoço e acima das nádegas; **2.** Coluna vertebral com os músculos associados (eretor da espinha e espinotransversais) e o tegumento suprajacente. VER dorsum.
  adolescent round d., doença de Scheuermann. SIN Scheuermann *disease.*
  hollow b., lordose. SIN lordosis.
  poker b., espondilite deformante. SIN spondylitis deformans.
  saddle b., lordose. SIN lordosis.

back·ache (bak′āk). Dorsalgia; termo inespecífico utilizado para descrever a dor nas costas; geralmente refere-se à dor abaixo do nível cervical.

back·bone (bak′bōn). Coluna vertebral. SIN vertebral *column.*

back·cross (bak′kros). **1.** Cruzamento de um indivíduo heterozigoto em um ou mais *loci* com um indivíduo homozigoto nos mesmos *loci.* **2.** SIN testcross.

back·flow. Fluxo invertido; a inversão do fluxo normal de um líquido ou corrente. VER TAMBÉM regurgitation.
  pyelovenous backflow, fluxo pielovenoso retrógrado; o movimento retrógrado de líquido (urina ou contraste injetado) da pelve renal para o sistema venoso renal. Isso acontece sob condições de obstrução distal ou injeção de soluções no sistema coletor renal.

background (bak′grownd). Base, antecedente, fundamento; instrumento de resposta na ausência de uma amostra.

back·ing (bak′ing). Apoio; em odontologia, um suporte metálico que serve para fixar um revestimento à prótese.

back-knee (bak′nē′). Joelho recurvado. SIN *genu* recurvatum.

back·pro·jec·tion (bak′prō-jek′shŭn). Projeção por trás (da tela); em tomografia computadorizada ou outras técnicas de imagem que exigem a reconstrução de múltiplas incidências, um algoritmo para calcular a contribuição de cada voxel da estrutura para os raios medidos, a fim de gerar uma imagem; o método mais antigo e mais simples de reconstrução de imagem. Cf. Fourier *analysis.* SIN apical lordotic projection. Cf. Fourier *analysis.*

back·scat·ter (bak′skat-er). Retrodifusão, difusão de retorno; radiação secundária defletida mais que 90° a partir do feixe primário. VER scattered *radiation.*

back·track·ing. Retrocesso; o movimento retrógrado da RNA-polimerase ao longo do molde de DNA até um estado mais estável que aquele encontrado quando alguns pares de bases rompem a ligação da extremidade 3′ a partir do sítio de transcrição ativa.

bac·lo·fen (bak′lō-fen). Baclofeno; relaxante muscular utilizado no tratamento sintomático de lesões raquimedulares e esclerose múltipla; um agonista nos receptores $GABA_b$.

Bacon, Harry E., proctologista norte-americano, *1900. VER B. *anoscope.*

bac·te·re·mia (bak-tēr-ē′mē-ă). Bacteriemia; a presença de bactérias viáveis no sangue circulante; pode ser transitória após traumatismo, como manipulação dentária ou outra manipulação iatrogênica, ou pode ser persistente ou recorrente em conseqüência da infecção. SIN bacteremia. [bacteria + G. *haima,* sangue]

bacteri-. VER bacterio-.

bac·te·ria (bak-tēr′ē-ă). Bactérias; plural de bacterium.
  blue-green b., b. verde-azuladas. VER Cyanobacteria.
  cell wall-defective b., b. com parede celular defeituosa; as b. com paredes celulares ausentes ou lesionadas; morfologicamente, podem tornar-se esferoplastos, estruturas arredondadas com pouca ou nenhuma parede celular, ou podem desenvolver formas filamentosas, com ou sem porções bulbosas, extrudadas.
  coryneform b., b. corineformes; nome comum para as corinebactérias não-diftéricas, um componente não-patogênico da flora cutânea e orofaríngea em seres humanos e animais pode causar infecções oportunistas no hospedeiro imunocomprometido.

bac·te·ri·al (bak-tēr′ē-ăl). Bacteriano; relativo às bactérias.

classificação de bactérias

reino: procariontes ou procariotas ou procariotos (Prokaryotae)
divisão I: gracilicutes (maioria das bactérias Gram-negativas)

Espiroquetas
ordem I Spirochaetales

| | família I | Spirochaetaceae | gêneros: p.ex., | Treponema, Borrelia |
| | família II | Leptospiraceae | gênero: | Leptospira |

bactérias Gram-negativas aeróbicas ou microaerofílicas, móveis, espiraladas ou curva

gêneros: p.ex., Spirillum, Campylobacter

cocos e bacilos aeróbicos Gram-negativos

	família I	Pseudomonadaceae	gêneros: p.ex.,	Pseudomonas, Xanthomonas
	família VII	Legionellaceae	gêneros:	Legionella
	família VIII	Neisseriaceae	gêneros: p.ex.,	Neisseria, Moraxella, Acinetobacter, Kingella

outros gêneros: p.ex., Alcaligenes, Brucella, Bordetella, Flavobacterium, Francisella

bacilos anaeróbicos facultativos Gram-negativos

	família I	Enterobacteriaceae	gêneros:	Escherichia, Shigella, Salmonella, Citrobacter, Klebsiella, Enterobacter, Erwinia, Serratia, Hafnia, Edwardsiella, Proteus, Providencia, Morganella, Yersinia
	família II	Vibrionaceae	gêneros: p.ex.,	Vibrio, Aeromonas, Plesiomonas
	família III	Pasteurellaceae	gêneros:	Pasteurella, Haemophilus, Actinobacillus

outros gêneros: Zymomonas, Chromobacterium, Cardiobacterium, Calymmatobacterium, Gardnerella, Eikenella, Streptobacillus

bacilos anaeróbicos Gram-negativos, retos, curvos e espiralados

| | família | Bacteroidaceae | gêneros: p.ex., | Bacteroides, Fusobacterium, Leptotrichia |

cocos anaeróbicos Gram-negativos

| | família | Veillonellaceae | gêneros: p.ex., | Veillonella, outros |

Riquétsias
ordem I Rickettsiales

	família I	Rickettsiaceae	gêneros: p.ex.,	Rickettsia, Coxiella
		Ehrlichiaceae	gêneros: p.ex.,	Ehrlichia
	família II	Bartonellaceae	gênero: p.ex.,	Bartonella
ordem II Chlamydiales	família I	Chlamydiaceae	gênero:	Chlamydia

divisão II: firmicutes (Gram-positivos)

cocos Gram-positivos

| | família | Micrococcaceae | gêneros: | Micrococcus, Stomatococcus, Planococcus, Staphylococcus |
| | família | Deinococcaceae | gênero: | Deinococcus |

outros microrganismos: p.ex., estreptococos, pediococos, peptococos, peptostreptococos

bacilos e cocos Gram-positivos formadores de endosporos

gêneros: p.ex., Bacillus, Clostridium

bacilos Gram-positivos asporogenos, regularmente formados

gêneros: p.ex., Lactobacillus, Listeria, Erysipelothrix

bacilos Gram-positivos asporogenos, irregularmente formados

gêneros: p.ex., Corynebacterium, Gardnerella, Brevibacterium, Propionibacterium, Eubacterium, Actinomyces, Bifidobacterium

| Micobactérias | Família | Mycobacteriaceae | gênero: | Mycobacterium |

Nocardioformes

gênero: p.ex., Nocardia

divisão III: Tenericutes (sem parede celular)
ordem I Mycoplasmatales

| | classe I: | Mollicutes | | |
| | família I: | Mycoplasmataceae | gênero: | Mycoplasma, Ureaplasma |

divisão IV: Mendosicutes;
classe I: Archaeobacteria (parede celular sem ácido murâmico)

bactérias metanógenas,
b. extremamente halofílicas,
b. extremamente termofílicas

bac·te·ri·cho·lia (bak′tēr-i-kō′lē-ă). Bactericólia; bactérias na bile.
bac·te·ri·cid·al (bak-tēr′i-sī′dăl). Bactericida; que causa a morte das bactérias. Cf. bacteriostatic. SIN bactericidal.
bac·te·ri·cide (bak-tēr′i-sīd). Bactericida; agente que destrói bactérias. Cf. bacteriostat. SIN bacteriocide. [bacteria + L. *caedo*, matar]
 specific b., b. específico; substância bacteriolítica, i.e., soro imune destrutivo para um único gênero ou espécie bacteriana.
bac·ter·id (bak′ter-id). Bactéride. **1.** Erupção recorrente ou persistente de pústulas estéreis bem-definidas das regiões palmares e plantares, considerada uma resposta alérgica para a infecção bacteriana em um sítio remoto. **2.** Disseminação de uma infecção cutânea bacteriana previamente localizada. [bacteria + -id (1)]
bac·te·ri·e·mia (bak-tēr-ē-ē′mē-ă). Bacteriemia. SIN bacteremia.
bacterio-, bacteri-. Formas combinantes relativas a bactérias. [ver bacterium]
bac·te·ri·o·ag·glu·ti·nin (bak′tēr′ē-ō-ă-gloo′ti-nin). Bacterioaglutinina; anticorpo que aglutina bactérias.
bac·te·ri·o·chlo·rin (bak-tēr′-ē-ō-klōr′in). Bacterioclorina; 7,8,17,18-tetraidroporfirina; a estrutura básica das bacterioclorofilas.
bac·te·ri·o·chlo·ro·phyll (bak-tēr-ē-ō-klōr′ō-fil). Bacterioclorofila; qualquer forma de clorofila em bactérias fotossintéticas: 1) b. *a*, $-CH=CH_2$ substituído por $-CO-CH_3$ na estrutura da clorofila α, dois hidrogênios também sendo acrescentados; os pigmentos fotossintéticos das bactérias púrpuras; 2) b. *b*, $-CH=CH_2$ substituído por $-CO-CH_3$ e $-CH_2-CH_3$ substituído por $-C≡CH$ na estrutura da clorofila β, com dois hidrogênios também sendo acrescentados.
bac·te·ri·o·cid·al (bak-tēr′ē-ō-sī′dăl). Bactericida. SIN bactericidal.
bac·te·ri·o·cide (bak-tēr′ē-ō-sīd). Bactericida. SIN bactericide.
bac·te·ri·o·cid·in (bak-tēr′ē-ō-sī′din). Bacteriocidina; anticorpo que possui atividade bactericida.
bac·te·ri·o·cin·o·gens (bak-tēr′ē-ō-sin′ō-jenz). Bacteriocinógenos. SIN bacteriocinogenic *plasmids*, em *plasmid*.
bac·te·ri·o·cins (bak-tēr′ē-ō-sinz). Bacteriocinas; proteínas produzidas por determinadas bactérias que possuem plasmídeos bacteriocinogênicos e que exercem efeito letal sobre as bactérias intimamente correlatas; em geral, as b. têm uma faixa mais estreita de atividade que os antibióticos e são mais potentes.
bac·te·ri·o·flu·o·res·cin (bak-tēr′ē-ō-flōr-es′in). Bacteriosfluoresceína; material fluorescente produzido por bactérias.
bac·te·ri·o·gen·ic (bak-tēr′ē-ō-jen′ik). Bacteriogênico; causado por bactérias.
bac·te·ri·og·e·nous (bak′tēr-ē-oj′e-nŭs). Bacteriógeno. **1.** Que produz bactérias. **2.** De origem ou causa bacteriana.
bac·te·ri·oid (bak-tēr′ē-oyd). Bacterióide. **1.** Semelhante a bactéria. **2.** Formas intracelulares de *Rhizobium* spp. nos nódulos das raízes de vegetais leguminosos. [bacterio- + G. *eidos*, semelhança]
bac·te·ri·o·log·ic, bac·te·ri·o·log·i·cal (bak′tēr-ē-ō-loj′ik, -i-kăl). Bacteriológico; relativo às bactérias ou à bacteriologia.
bac·te·ri·ol·o·gist (bak′ter-ē-ol′ō-jist). Bacteriologista; aquele que estuda ou trabalha principalmente com bactérias.
bac·te·ri·ol·o·gy (bak-tēr-ē-ol′ō-jē). Bacteriologia; o ramo da ciência relacionado com o estudo de bactérias. [bacterio- + G. *logos*, estudo]
 systematic b., b. sistemática; o ramo da b. relacionado com a nomenclatura e com a classificação (taxonomia).
bac·te·ri·o·ly·sin (bak-tēr-ē-ol′i-sin). Bacteriolisina; anticorpo específico que se combina com as células bacterianas (i.e., antígeno) e, na presença do complemento, causa lise ou dissolução das células.
bac·te·ri·ol·y·sis (bak-tēr-ē-ol′i-sis). Bacteriólise; a dissolução de bactérias, p. ex., por meio das enzimas, soluções hipotônicas ou anticorpo e complemento específicos. [bacterio- + G. *lysis*, dissolução]
bac·te·ri·o·lyt·ic (bak-tēr-ē-ō-lit′ik). Bacteriolítico; pertinente à destruição lítica de bactérias; que manifesta a capacidade de causar a dissolução das células bacterianas.
bac·te·ri·o·lyze (bak-tēr′ē-ō-līz). Bacteriolisar; causar a digestão ou a dissolução das células bacterianas.
bac·te·ri·o·pexy (bak-tēr′ē-ō-pek-sē). Bacteriopexia; imobilização das bactérias por células fagocíticas. [bacterio- + G. *pexis*, fixação]
bac·te·ri·o·phage (bak-tēr′ē-ō-fāj). Bacteriófago; vírus com afinidade específica por bactérias. Os bacteriófagos foram encontrados em associação com quase todos os grupos de bactérias, incluindo Cyanobacteria; como outros vírus, eles contêm RNA ou DNA (mas nunca ambos) e variam em estrutura desde vírus bacterianos filamentosos aparentemente simples a formas relativamente complexas com "caudas" contráteis; suas relações com as bactérias do hospedeiro são altamente específicas e, como no caso do b. temperado, podem ser geneticamente íntimas. Os bacteriófagos são denominados de acordo com as espécies, os grupos ou as cepas de bactérias para os quais são específicos, p. ex., corinebacteriófago, colifago; inúmeras famílias são reconhecidas, e foram atribuídos nomes provisórios: Corticoviridae, Cystoviridae, Fuselloviridae, Inoviridae, Leviviridae, Lipothrixviridae, Microviridae, Myoviridae, Plasmaviridae, Podoviridae, Styloviridae e Tectiviridae. VER TAMBÉM coliphage. SIN phage. [bacterio- + G. *phago*, comer]

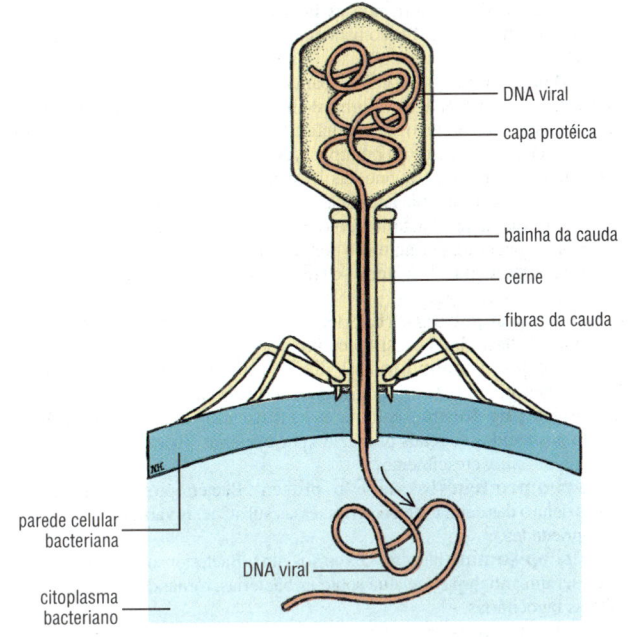

bacteriófago

 defective b., b. defeituoso; b. temperado mutante cujo genoma não contém todos os componentes normais e não consegue se transformar em um vírus completamente infeccioso, embora possa replicar-se indefinidamente no genoma bacteriano como um pró-bacteriófago defeituoso; muitos b. defeituosos são mediadores da transdução. SIN defective phage.
 filamentous b., b. filamentoso; b. que tem formato de bastonete e alongado, não tendo a estrutura de cabeça e cauda que é característica de muitos bacteriófagos.
 mature b., b. maduro; a forma completa e infecciosa de b.
 temperate b., b. temperado; o b. cujo genoma incorpora-se e se replica no da bactéria hospedeira; a dissociação (e o resultante desenvolvimento do b. vegetativo) ocorre mais lentamente e resulta, às vezes, na lise de uma bactéria e na

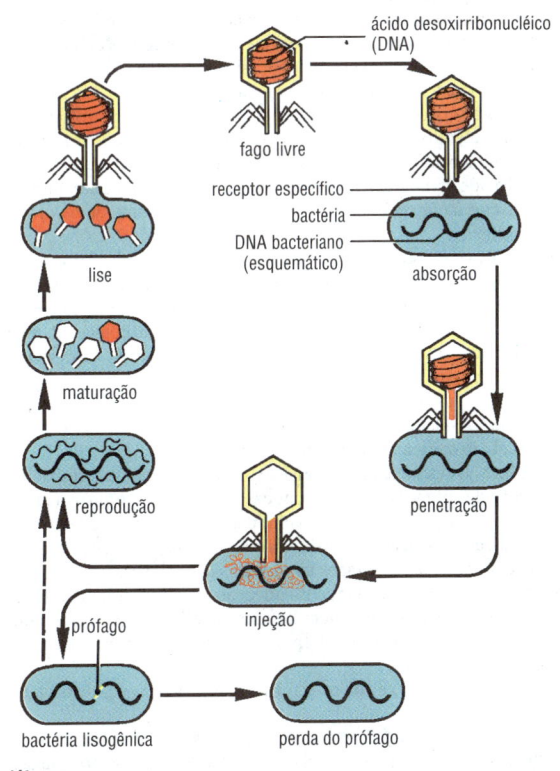

bacteriófagos

liberação do b. maduro, tornando, assim, a cultura bacteriana capaz de induzir a lise geral, quando transferido para uma cultura de uma cepa bacteriana suscetível.
typhoid b., b. tifóide; b. específico para a *Salmonella typhi*.
vegetative b., b. vegetativo; a forma do b. em que o ácido nucléico do b. (que carece de seu revestimento) se multiplica livremente dentro da bactéria hospedeira, independentemente da multiplicação bacteriana.
virulent b., b. virulento; b. que regularmente causa lise das bactérias que ele infecta; pode existir em uma das duas formas, vegetativa ou madura; não possui uma forma de pró-bacteriófago (i.e., seu genoma não se incorpora ao da bactéria hospedeira), portanto não efetua a lisogenização.
bac·te·ri·o·pha·gia (bak-tēr'ē-ō-fā'jē-ā). Bacteriofagia; lise de bactérias por um bacteriófago.
bac·te·ri·o·pha·gol·o·gy (bak-tēr'ē-ō-fa-gol'ō-jē). Bacteriofagologia; o estudo dos bacteriófagos. SIN protobiology.
bac·te·ri·o·phe·o·phor·bin (bak-tēr'ē-ō-fē-ō-fōr'bin). Bacteriofeoforbina; bacteriofeoforbida desesterificada, derivada da bacterioclorina.
bac·te·ri·o·phy·to·ma (bak-tēr'ē-ō-fi-tō'mā). Bacteriofitoma; crescimento nos tecidos vegetais produzido por bactérias. [bacterio- + G. *phytos*, vegetal, + *-oma*, crescimento]
bac·te·ri·o·pro·tein (bak-tēr'ē-ō-prō'tēn). Bacterioproteína; uma das proteínas dentro das células de bactérias; essas substâncias variam em seu caráter e propriedades.
bac·te·ri·op·so·nin (bak-tēr-ē-op'sō-nin). Bacteriopsonina; opsonina que pode ser um anticorpo que atua sobre as bactérias, tornando-as suscetíveis às células fagocitárias.
bac·te·ri·o·sis (bak-tēr-ē-ō'sis). Bacteriose; uma infecção bacteriana localizada ou generalizada.
bac·te·ri·o·sper·mia (bak'ter-ē-ō-sper-mē-ā). Bacteriospermia; bactérias no sêmen ou ejaculadas.
bac·te·ri·o·sta·sis (bak-tēr-ē-os'tā-sis). Bacterioestase; parada ou retardo do crescimento das bactérias. [bacterio- + G. *stasis*, uma parada]
bac·te·ri·o·stat (bak-tēr'ē-ō-stat). Bacteriostato; qualquer agente que inibe ou retarda o crescimento bacteriano. SIN bacteriostatic agent.
bac·te·ri·o·stat·ic (bak-tēr'ē-ō-stat'ik). Bacteriostático; que inibe ou retarda a multiplicação de bactérias.
bac·te·ri·o·tox·ic (bak-tēr'ē-ō-tok'sik). Bacteriotóxico; venenoso ou tóxico para as bactérias.
bac·te·ri·o·tro·pic (bak-tēr'ē-ō-trop'ik). Bacteriotrópico; que se volta ou se movimenta em direção às bactérias; que possui afinidade por bactérias. [bacterio- + G. *tropē*, uma volta]
bac·te·ri·ot·ro·pin (bak-tēr-ē-ot'rō-pin). Bacteriotropina; constituinte do sangue, usualmente um anticorpo específico, i.e., opsonina, que combina com as células bacterianas e as torna mais suscetíveis para os fagócitos.
bac·te·ri·o·tryp·sin (bak-tēr'ē-ō-trip'sin). Bacteriotripsina; enzima semelhante à tripsina produzida por bactérias, principalmente pelo *Vibrio cholerae*.
Bac·te·ri·um (bak-tēr'ē-ŭm). Nome genérico de bactérias colocadas na lista de nomes rejeitados pela Judicial Commission e pelo International Committee on Systematic Bacteriology da International Association of Microbiological Societies. Como consequência, *B.* não é mais usado em bacteriologia. Os microrganismos identificáveis originalmente colocados no gênero *B.* foram todos transferidos para outros gêneros. Especificamente, *B. anitratum* é atualmente conhecido como *Acinetobacter calcoaceticus*; *B. coli* é atualmente chamado de *Escherichia coli*. [L. mod. do G. *baktērion*, dim. de *baktron*, uma equipe ou clube]
bac·te·ri·um (bak-tēr'ē-ŭm). Bactéria; um microrganismo procariótico unicelular que comumente se multiplica por divisão celular e tem uma parede celular que fornece uma constância de forma; podem ser aeróbicas ou anaeróbicas, móveis ou não-móveis, e de vida livre, saprofítica, comensal, parasitária ou patogênica. VER TAMBÉM Cyanobacteria. [L. mod. do G. *baktērion*, dim. de *baktron*, uma equipe]
blue-green b., b. azul-esverdeada. VER Cyanobacteria.
endoteric b., b. endotérica; b. que forma endotoxina.
exoteric b., b. exotérica; b. que secreta exotoxina.
lysogenic b., b. lisogênica; um genoma de b. inclui o genoma (pró-bacteriófago) de um bacteriófago temperado; em casos ocasionais, o pró-bacteriófago dissocia-se do genoma bacteriano, evolui para bacteriófago vegetativo e, em seguida, amadurece, causando lise da respectiva b. hospedeira e liberação para o meio de cultura de bacteriófagos temperados infecciosos.
pyogenic b., b. piogênica; b. que causa infecção piogênica usualmente associada a exsudato purulento que contém leucócitos polimorfonucleares, como os cocos piogênicos (estafilococos, estreptococos, pneumococos, meningococos) e *Haemophilus influenzae*.
bac·te·ri·u·ria (bak-tēr-ē-oo'rē-ā). Bacteriúria; a presença de bactérias na urina.
bac·te·roid (bak'ter-oyd). Bacteróide; que se assemelha às bactérias.
Bac·te·roi·da·ce·ae (bak'ter-oy-dā'sē-ē). Família de bactérias anaeróbicas obrigatórias (podem ocorrer espécies microaerofílicas), não-formadoras de esporos (ordem Eubacteriales), contendo bastonetes Gram-negativos, cujo tamanho varia desde formas pequenas filtráveis até formas longas, filamentosas e ramificadoras; pode ocorrer pleomorfismo pronunciado. Existem espécies móveis e não-móveis; as células móveis são peritríquias. Líquidos corporais são freqüentemente necessários para o crescimento. A maioria das espécies fermenta carboidratos, freqüentemente com produção de ácido; gás pode ser produzido em meios com glicose ou peptona. Esses microrganismos ocorrem principalmente nos tratos intestinais inferiores e nas mucosas dos animais de sangue quente. Eles podem ser patogênicos. O gênero típico é *Bacteroides*.
Bac·te·roi·des (bak-ter-oy'dēz). Gênero que inclui muitas espécies de bactérias anaeróbicas obrigatórias, não-formadoras de esporos (família Bacteroidaceae), contendo bastonetes Gram-negativos. Existem espécies móveis e não-imóveis; as células móveis são peritríquias. Algumas espécies fermentam carboidratos e produzem combinações de ácidos succínico, lático, acético, fórmico ou propiônico, por vezes com alcoóis de cadeia curta; o ácido butírico não é um produto importante. As espécies que não fermentam carboidratos produzem, a partir da peptona, quantidades mínimas a moderadas dos ácidos succínico, fórmico, acético e lático ou quantidades importantes de ácidos acético e butírico, com quantidades moderadas de alcoóis e ácidos isovalérico, propiônico e isobutírico. Eles fazem parte da flora normal do trato intestinal e, em menor grau, das cavidades respiratória e urogenital de seres humanos e animais; muitas espécies originalmente classificadas como *B.* foram reclassificadas como pertencentes ao gênero *Prevotella*. Muitas espécies podem ser patogênicas. A espécie típica é *B. fragilis*. [G. *bacterion* + *eidos*, forma]
B. bivius, espécie usualmente isolada a partir de infecções urogenitais e abdominais e ligada à doença inflamatória pélvica.
B. cappilo'sus, espécie bacteriana isolada a partir de cistos e feridas, boca e fezes de seres humanos e a partir do trato intestinal de alguns animais. Suas propriedades diferem daquelas da maioria das espécies de *B.*; é provável a futura reclassificação.
B. corro'dens, nome original para *Eikenella corrodens*.
B. di'siens, SIN *Prevotella disiens*.
B. distasonis, espécie bacteriana que faz parte da flora fecal humana normal; causa ocasional de infecções intra-abdominais.
B. frag'ilis, espécie bacteriana encontrada nos tratos intestinais de seres humanos e animais. Embora represente apenas cerca de 10-20% das espécies de *B.* encontradas no colo, é a espécie primária associada a abscessos intra-abdominais e outras infecções subdiafragmáticas em seres humanos, incluindo peritonite, abscessos retal, feridas cirúrgicas abdominais e infecção do trato urogenital. Sua cápsula é capaz de induzir, de maneira independente, a formação de abscesso; caracteristicamente, essa espécie produz uma β-lactamase que inativa os antibióticos β-lactâmicos, como as penicilinas e as cefalosporinas; é a espécie típica do gênero *B*.
B. furco'sus, nome original do *Anaerohabdus furcosis*.
B. melaninogenicus, SIN *Prevotella melaninogenica*.
B. nodo'sus, espécie bacteriana que provoca a deterioração das patas em carneiros e cabras; pode ser encontrada no trato intestinal humano e foi associada a infecções em seres humanos; esse microrganismo tem muitas propriedades diferentes de outras espécies de *B.*, e sua classificação final é incerta. SIN *Dichelobacter nodosus*.
B. ora'lis, nome original da *Prevotella oralis*.
B. o'ris, nome original da *Prevotella oris*.
B. pneumosin'tes, nome original do *Dialister pneumosintes*.
B. praeacu'tus, espécie isolada dos tratos intestinais de crianças e adultos, lesões gangrenosas, abscessos pulmonares e sangue. SIN *Tissierella praeacuta*.
B. putredi'nis, espécie isolada das fezes, de casos de apendicite aguda e de abscessos abdominais e retais; também encontrada em patas deterioradas de carneiros e do solo de fazendas. Suas propriedades divergem daquelas da maioria das espécies de *B*.
B. splanchnicus, espécie de grupo indol-positivo, encontrada na flora colônica humana normal e, ocasionalmente, em amostras humanas com propriedades metabólicas singulares, as quais incluem a produção de grandes quantidades de ácido N-butírico; parece estar intimamente relacionado com o gênero *Porphyromonas*.
B. thetaiotamicron, espécie de bactéria encontrada no trato intestinal; em seu gênero, fica atrás apenas do *B. fragilis* como causa de infecções subdiafragmáticas humanas.
B. ureolyt'icus, espécie isolada de infecções dos tratos respiratório e intestinal, e da cavidade bucal, do trato intestinal, do trato urogenital e do sangue após uma extração dentária. Está intimamente relacionado às espécies de *Campylobacter*.
bac·te·roi·do·sis (bak'ter-oy-dō'sis). Bacteroidose; termo raramente utilizado para uma infecção por *Bacteroides*.
bac·u·li·form (bā-kū'li-fōrm). Baculiforme; em formato de bastonete. [L. *baculum*, um bastonete, + *forma*, forma]
Bac·u·lo·vi·ri·dae (bak-ū-lō-vir'i-dē). Família de vírus que se multiplicam apenas em artrópodes; os víreons são em formato de bastonete e medem 30-35 nm por 250-400 nm; os genomas são de DNA com dois filamentos,

superespiralados (90-160 kb). Os vetores derivados do baculovírus são freqüentemente utilizados para expressar genes estranhos nas células de insetos. [L. *baculum*, bastonete]

bac·u·lo·vi·rus (bak'oo-lō-vī-rŭs). Baculovírus; vírus que infecta as células de insetos; usado extensamente em sistemas de expressão para proteínas recombinantes que necessitam de sistemas de processamento eucariótico. [L. *baculum*, um bastonete, + vírus]

Baehr, George, médico norte-americano, 1887–1978. VER B.-Lohlein *lesion*; Lohlein-B. *lesion*.

Baelz, Erwin O., médico alemão em Tóquio, 1849–1913. VER B. *disease*.

BAER. Abreviatura de brainstem auditory evoked response (resposta auditiva evocada do tronco cerebral). VER evoked *response*.

Baer, Karl E. von, embriologista russo-germânico. 1792–1876. VER B. *law*.

Baeyer, Johann F. W. A. von, químico alemão laureado com o Prêmio Nobel, 1835–1917. VER B. *theory*.

bag. Bolsa; um saco, divertículo ou receptáculo. [A.S. *baelg*]
  Ambu b., b. de Ambu; marca registrada de uma b. auto-insuflante com válvulas unidirecionais para fornecer ventilação com pressão positiva durante a reanimação com oxigênio ou ar.
  breathing b., b. de respiração; reservatório colabável a partir do qual os gases são inalados e para dentro do qual os gases podem ser expirados durante a anestesia geral ou ventilação artificial. SIN reservoir b.
  colostomy b., b. de colostomia; b. usada sobre uma conexão cirurgicamente produzida entre o colo e a pele para coletar as fezes.
  Douglas b., b. de Douglas; uma grande bolsa em que o gás expirado é coletado por vários minutos para determinar o consumo de oxigênio em seres humanos sob condições de trabalho real. [C. G. Douglas]
  nuclear b., b. nuclear; a agregação de núcleos que ocorre no centro não-estriado de uma fibra muscular intrafuso de um feixe neuromuscular.
  Politzer b., b. de Politzer; b. de borracha piriforme usada para forçar o ar através da tuba auditiva pelo método de Politzer.
  reservoir b., b. reservatório. SIN breathing b.
  b. of waters, b. das águas; coloquialismo para o saco amniótico e o líquido amniótico contido.

bag·as·so·sis (bag-ă-sō'sis). Bagaçose; a alveolite alérgica extrínseca após exposição à poeira da fibra da cana-de-açúcar (bagaço); foi atribuída à inalação de esporos de fungos do solo e, particularmente, aos actinomicetos termofílicos.

Baggenstoss, Archie H., patologista norte-americano, *1908. VER B. *change*.
Bagolini, oftalmologista italiano do século 20. VER B. *test*.
Baillarger, Jules G. F., neurologista francês, 1809–1891. VER B. *bands,* em *band, lines,* em *line*.
Bailliart, Paul, oftalmologista francês, 1877–1969. VER B. *ophthalmodynamometer*.
Bainbridge, Francis A., fisiologista inglês, 1874–1921. VER B. *reflex*.
Baker, James Porter, médico norte-americano, *1902. VER Charcot-Weiss-B. *syndrome*.
Baker, John Randal, zoólogo inglês, *1900. VER B. pyridine *extraction,* acid *hematein*.
Baker, William M., cirurgião inglês, 1839–1896. VER B. *cyst*.
BAL Abreviatura de British anti-Lewisite (dimercaprol).
BAL Abreviatura de bronchoalveolar *lavage* (lavado broncoalveolar).
Balamuthia (bal-ă-moo'thē-ă). Gênero de amebas de vida livre que provoca a encefalite amebiana granulomatosa.
balan-. VER balano-.
bal·ance (bal'ans). **1.** Balança; um aparelho para pesar. **2.** Equilíbrio; o estado normal de ação e reação entre duas ou mais partes ou órgãos do corpo. **3.** Quantidades, concentrações e quantidades proporcionais dos constituintes orgânicos. **4.** Balanço; a diferença entre o aporte e a utilização, o armazenamento ou a excreção de uma substância pelo corpo. VER TAMBÉM equilibrium. [L. *bi-*, duas vezes, + *lanx*, prato, escala]
  acid-base b., equilíbrio ácido-básico; o equilíbrio normal entre ácidos e bases no plasma sangüíneo, expresso na concentração de íon hidrogênio ou pH, resultando das quantidades relativas de materiais ácidos e básicos ingeridos e produzidos pelo metabolismo corporal, comparado com as quantidades relativas de materiais ácidos e básicos excretadas do corpo e consumidas pelo metabolismo corporal; o estado normal do equilíbrio ácido-básico não é de neutralidade, com concentrações iguais de íons hidrogênio e hidroxila, mas um estado mais alcalino com um certo excesso de íons hidroxila. SIN acid-base equilibrium.
  nitrogen b., balanço nitrogenado; a diferença entre o aporte total de nitrogênio por um organismo e sua perda total de nitrogênio. Um balanço nitrogenado zero é observado em adultos normais saudáveis; $N_{aporte} > N_{perda}$ é um balanço nitrogenado positivo e $N_{aporte} < N_{perda}$ é um balanço nitrogenado negativo.
  occlusal b., b. oclusal; condição em que existem contatos simultâneos das unidades oclusoras dos arcos dentários opostos nas posições cêntrica e excêntrica dentro da faixa funcional.
  phonetic b., b. fonético; propriedade pela qual um grupo de palavras usadas na mensuração da audição apresenta os vários fonemas que ocorrem em uma freqüência aproximadamente igual àquela em que eles ocorrem na conversação comum naquela língua; listas de palavras foneticamente balanceadas são utilizadas na determinação da pontuação de discriminação.
  Wilhelmy b., b. de Wilhelmy; dispositivo para medir a tensão superficial em relação à tração exercida sobre uma placa fina de platina ou de outro material suspenso verticalmente através da superfície; usado em uma tina de Langmuir para estudar o surfactante pulmonar.

ba·lan·ic (ba-lan'ik). Balânico; relativo à glande do pênis ou do clitóris. [G. *balanos*, bolota, glande]

Ba·la·ni·tes ae·gyp·ti·a·ca (bal-ă-nī'tēz ē-jip-tī'ă-kă). Gênero de árvores que cresce no Oriente Próximo cujas bagas contêm um princípio ativo que é mortal para moluscos, miracídios, cercárias, girinos e peixes e que é utilizado como profilático contra a esquistossomíase ao ser adicionado à água potável. [L. *balanos*, bolota]

bal·a·ni·tis (bal-ă-nī'tis). Balanite; inflamação da glande do pênis ou do clitóris. [G. *balanos*, bolota, glande, + *-itis*, inflamação]
  b. circumscripta plasmacellularis, b. circunscrita plasmocitária. SIN plasma cell b.
  b. diabet'ica, b. diabética; inflamação da glande em diabéticos relacionada com infecção urinária ou postite concomitante.
  plasma cell b., b. plasmocitária; b. circunscrita benigna caracterizada microscopicamente por infiltração subepitelial de plasmócitos e clinicamente por pequenas lesões papulares eritematosas. SIN b. circumscripta plasmacellularis.
  b. xerot'ica oblit'erans, b. xerótica obliterante; líquen escleroso e atrófico da glande do pênis, o qual pode resultar em estenose do meato.

balano-, balan-. Formas combinantes que indicam a glande do pênis. [G. *balanos*, bolota, glande]

bal·a·no·plas·ty (bal'an-ō-plas-tē). Balanoplastia; reconstrução cirúrgica da glande do pênis. [balano- + G. *plastos*, formado]

bal·a·no·pos·thi·tis (bal'an-ō-pos-thī'tis). Balanopostite; inflamação da glande do pênis e do prepúcio suprajacente. [balano- + G. *posthē*, prepúcio, + *-itis*, inflamação]

bal·an·ti·di·a·sis (bal'an-ti-dī'ă-sis). Balantidíase; doença causada pela presença do *Balantidium coli* no intestino grosso; caracterizada por diarréia, disenteria e, ocasionalmente, ulceração. SIN balantidosis.

Ba·lan·ti·di·um (bal-an-tid'ē-ŭm). Gênero de ciliados (família Balantidiidae) encontrados no trato digestivo de vertebrados e invertebrados. [G. *balantidion*, dim. de *ballantion*, uma bolsa]
  ***B. co'li*,** espécie de ciliados parasitas muito grandes, usualmente com 50-80 μm de comprimento, alcançando até 200 μm em porcos, encontrados no ceco ou intestino grosso, nadando ativamente em sua luz; geralmente inócuo nos seres humanos, porém pode invadir e ulcerar a parede intestinal, provocando colite que se assemelha à disenteria amebiana.
  ***B. su'is*,** espécie originalmente considerada separada do parasita ciliado do homem, *B. coli*, mas que atualmente é considerada sinônimo dele; não-patogênica nos suínos.

bal·an·ti·do·sis (bal'an-ti-dō'sis). Balantidose. SIN balantidiasis.

bal·a·nus (bal'ă-nŭs). Bálano. SIN *glans* penis. [G. *balanos*, bolota, glande do pênis]

bald (bawld). Calvo; que não possui cabelo ou que apresenta redução do número de fios de cabelo no couro cabeludo. [M. E. *balled*]

bald·ness (bawld'nes). Calvície, alopecia. SIN alopecia.
  common b., c. comum. SIN androgenic *alopecia*.
  congenital b., c. congênita. SIN *alopecia* congenitalis.
  male pattern b., c. de padrão masculino. SIN male pattern *alopecia*.

Balint, Rudolph, neurologista e psiquiatra húngaro, 1874–1930. VER B. *syndrome*.
Ball, Sir Charles B., cirurgião irlandês, 1851–1916. VER B. *operation*.
ball. 1. Bola; uma massa arredondada. VER bezoar. **2.** Em medicina veterinária, um bolo ou pílula grande.
  chondrin b., b. de condrina; uma das massas globulares formada por um grupo de células envolvidas em uma cápsula, na cartilagem hialina.
  food b., fitobezoar. SIN phytobezoar.
  b. of the foot, b. do pé; a porção acolchoada da sola, na extremidade anterior das cabeças metatarsais, sobre a qual repousa o peso quando o calcanhar é levantado.
  fungus b., b. de fungos; massa compacta de micélios fúngicos e resíduos celulares, com 1 a 5 cm de diâmetro, localizada dentro de uma cavidade pulmonar, seio paranasal ou trato urinário; o aspergiloma é um tipo de b. de fungo do pulmão.

Ballance, Sir Charles A., cirurgião inglês, 1856–1936. VER B. *sign*; Koerte-B. *operation*.

bal·ism (bal'izm). Balismo. SIN ballismus.

bal·lis·mus (bal-iz'mŭs). Balismo; um tipo de movimento involuntário que afeta a musculatura proximal do membro, manifestado por movimentos de contração súbita e violenta do membro; causado por lesão do núcleo subtalâmico contralateral ou próximo a ele. Geralmente apenas um lado do corpo é afetado, resultando em hemibalismo. SIN ballism. [G. *ballismos*, um salto]

bal·lis·to·car·di·o·gram (bal - is - tō - kar′dē - ō - gram). Balistocardiograma; um registro do recuo do corpo provocado por contração cardíaca, ejeção do sangue para a aorta e forças de enchimento ventricular; tem sido empregado como base para calcular o débito cardíaco no homem, mas sua falta de acurácia e reprodutibilidade fez com que deixasse de ser usado. [G. *ballō*, arremessar, + *kardia*, coração, + *gramma*, algo escrito]

bal·lis·to·car·di·o·graph (BCG) (bal - is - tō - kar′dē - ō - graf). Balistocardiógrafo; instrumento para obter um balistocardiograma, consistindo em uma mesa móvel suspensa no teto ou em um aparelho que repousa sobre o corpo do paciente, usualmente sobre a face anterior das pernas, juntamente com um sistema de registro gráfico.

bal·lis·to·car·di·og·ra·phy (bal - is - tō - kar - dē - og′ra - fē). Balistocardiografia. **1.** O registro gráfico dos movimentos do corpo impostos pelas forças balísticas (contração cardíaca e ejeção do sangue, enchimento ventricular, aceleração e desaceleração do fluxo sangüíneo através dos grandes vasos); esses pequenos movimentos são amplificados e registrados em um papel de gráfico em movimento após serem traduzidos em um potencial elétrico por um aparelho de captação. **2.** O estudo e a interpretação dos balistocardiogramas.

bal·lis·to·pho·bia (bal - is - tō - fō′bē - ă). Balistofobia; temor mórbido de um projétil ou míssil. [G. *ballista*, catapulta, do G. *ballistēs*, de *ballō*, + *phobos*, medo]

bal·loon (bă - loon). **1.** Balão; dispositivo ovóide ou esférico insuflável usado para reter tubos ou cateteres dentro de várias estruturas corporais, ou para fornecer apoio para elas. **2.** Balão; dispositivo distensível empregado para estirar ou ocluir uma víscera ou vaso sangüíneo. **3.** Distender uma cavidade corporal com um gás ou líquido para facilitar seu exame, dilatar uma estrutura ou ocluir sua luz. [Fr. *ballon*, do It. *ballone*, de *balla*, bola, do Alemão]
  angioplasty b., b. de angioplastia; b. próximo à extremidade de um cateter angiográfico, destinado a distender vasos estreitados. VER balloon-tip *catheter*.
  detachable b., b. destacável; um pequeno balão preso à extremidade de um cateter, que pode ser liberado para ocluir um vaso.
  intraaortic b., b. intra-aórtico. VER intraaortic balloon *pump*.

bal·lot·ta·ble (bal - ot′ă - bl). Rechaçável; capaz de exibir o fenômeno do rechaço.

bal·lotte·ment (bal - ot - maw′). Rechaço. **1.** Manobra utilizada no exame físico para estimar o tamanho de um órgão afastado da superfície, principalmente quando existe ascite, por meio de um piparote (com a mão ou os dedos) similar àquele envolvido no drible com uma bola de basquete. **2.** Um método obsoleto de diagnóstico da gravidez: com a extremidade do dedo indicador na vagina, uma pequena pancada é feita contra o segmento inferior do útero; o feto, quando presente, é empurrado para cima, e (quando o dedo é mantido na posição) será percebida uma colisão contra as paredes do útero à medida que ele cai. [Fr. *balloter*, sacudir]
  abdominal b., r. abdominal; o exame do abdome através da palpação para detectar o excesso de líquido (ascite) ao fazer com que os órgãos se movimentem para cima e para baixo no meio líquido.
  renal b., r. renal; manobra em que o rim é movido pela pressão por trás, permitindo que ele seja palpado entre as mãos e que sejam determinados seu tamanho, formato e mobilidade.

balm (bawlm). **1.** Bálsamo. SIN balsam. **2.** Pomada, ungüento, especialmente com uma fragrância. **3.** Uma aplicação suavizante. [L. *balsamum*, do G. *balsamon*, árvore balsâmica]
  b. of Gilead, b. de Meca, opobálsamo; oleorresina obtida da *Commiphora opobalsamum* (família Burseraceae), provavelmente a mirra da Bíblia; usada em perfumaria. SIN Mecca balsam, opobalsamum.
  mountain b., b.-da-montanha. SIN eriodictyon.
  sweet b., melissa. SIN melissa.

bal·ne·o·ther·a·peu·tics, bal·ne·o·ther·a·py (bal′nē - ō - thăr - ă - pū′tiks, - thăr′ă - pē). Balneoterapia; a imersão de parte ou de todo o corpo em um banho de água mineral como uma forma de terapia. [L. *balneum*, banho]

Baló, Jozsef, médico húngaro, *1896. VER B. *disease*.

bal·sam (bawl′sam). Bálsamo; exsudato oleoso, perfumado, resinoso ou espesso, obtido de várias árvores e vegetais. SIN balm (1), oleoresin (3). [G. *balsamon*; L. *balsamum*]
  Canada b., b.-do-canadá; resina líquida amarelada obtida do pinheiro balsâmico, *Abies balsamea* (família Pinaceae); contém os acetatos cinêmico e bornílico; usada para montar peças histológicas e como um cimento para lentes. SIN Canada turpentine.
  b. of copaiba, b. de copaíba, copaíba. SIN copaiba.
  Mecca b., b. de Meca. SIN balm of Gilead.
  b. of Peru, b.-do-peru; um líquido espesso, castanho-escuro, obtido da *Toluifera pereirae* (família Leguminosae), contendo 60% de cinameína; usado como aplicação cicatrizante em feridas.
  Tolu b., b.-de-tolu; massa macia amarelo-acastanhada obtida da *Toluifera balsamum* (família Leguminosae), contendo ácidos e ésteres cinêmico e benzóico; usado como expectorante estimulante.

bal·sam·ic (bawl - sam′ik). Balsâmico. **1.** Relativo ao bálsamo. **2.** Aromático.

BALT Abreviatura de bronchus-associated lymphoid *tissue* (tecido linfóide associado ao brônquio).

Bamberger, Eugen, médico austríaco, 1858–1921. VER B.-Marie *disease*, *syndrome*.

Bamberger, Heinrich von, médico austríaco, 1822–1888. VER B. *albuminuria*, *disease*, *sign*.

ba·mif·yl·line hy·dro·chlo·ride (bă - mif′i - lin). Cloridrato de bamifilina; vasodilatador e relaxante da musculatura lisa.

bam·i·pine (bam - i - pēn). Bamipina; anti-histamínico.

ban·crof·ti·a·sis, ban·crof·to·sis (ban - krof - ti′ă - sis, - tō′sis). Bancroftíase, bancroftose; infecção por *Wuchereria bancrofti*.

band. Faixa. **1.** Qualquer aplicação ou parte de um aparelho que envolva ou se ligue a uma parte do corpo. VER TAMBÉM zone. **2.** Qualquer estrutura anatômica semelhante a uma corda ou em formato de cinta que circunda ou liga outra estrutura e que junta duas ou mais partes. VER fascia, line, linea, stripe, stria, tenia. **3.** Uma faixa estreita que contém uma ou mais macromoléculas (ocasionalmente, pequenas moléculas) detectadas na eletroforese ou em determinados tipos de cromatografia.
  A b.'s, faixas A; discos A; as estriações cruzadas anisotrópicas coradas em escuro nas miofibrilas das fibras musculares, compreendendo as regiões de superposição dos filamentos espesso (miosina) e fino (actina). SIN A disks, anisotropic disks, Q b.'s (1), Q disks.
  absorption b., f. de absorção; a faixa de comprimentos de onda ou freqüências no espectro eletromagnético na qual a energia radiante é absorvida pela passagem através de uma substância gasosa, líquida ou dissolvida; é explorada para fins analíticos em colorimetria ou espectofotometria e, em geral, é descrita em relação ao comprimento de onda em que acontece a absorbância máxima (i.e., λ_{max}).
  amnionic b. [MIM*217100], f. amniótica; as faixas do âmnio após sua ruptura, que podem se enrolar ao redor dos membros, dedos, face e órgãos internos, provocando constrição e amputação; a genética disso é incerta. VER TAMBÉM congenital *amputation*. SIN amnionic adhesions, amnionic band syndrome, anular b., constriction ring (2), Simonart b.'s (1), Simonart ligaments.
  anogenital b., f. anogenital; a primeira indicação do períneo no embrião.
  anular b., f. anular. SIN amnionic b.
  atrioventricular b., feixe atrioventricular. SIN atrioventricular *bundle*.
  Baillarger b.'s, linhas de Baillarger. SIN Baillarger lines, em *line*.
  Bechterew b., estria de Bechterew. SIN b. of Kaes-Bechterew.
  Broca diagonal b., estria diagonal de Broca; estria diagonal da parte basilar do telencéfalo; feixe de fibras brancas que desce no septo pré-comissural no sentido da base do prosencéfalo, imediatamente rostral à lâmina terminal; esse feixe consiste em um ramo horizontal [TA] (cruz horizontal [TA]), um ramo vertical [TA] (crus vertical [TA]) e as células associadas ao f. formam o núcleo da estria diagonal [TA] (núcleo estriado diagonal [TA]); na base, o feixe vira-se na direção caudolateral; atravessa um estrato ventral da substância inominada, ao longo do trato óptico, desaparecendo antes de alcançar a amígdala. SIN diagonal b. [TA], stria diagonalis [TA].
  chromosome b., banda cromossômica; uma região mais escura ou que se cora de forma contrastante através da largura de um cromossoma; o padrão das faixas é característico para a maioria dos cromossomas. VER banding.
  Clado b., f. de Clado. SIN suspensory *ligament* of ovary.
  b.'s of colon, tênias do colo. SIN teniae coli, em *tenia*.
  contraction b., f. de contração; alteração microscópica nas células miocárdicas em que a contração excessiva, associada ao cálcio intracelular e à norepinefrina sérica elevados, provoca a formação da f. transversa amorfa nas fibras, que ficam, então, incapacitadas de se contrair novamente. SIN contraction bands necrosis.
  diagonal b. [TA], estria diagonal. SIN Broca diagonal b.
  Essick cell b.'s, faixas de células de Essick; grupos de células no rombencéfalo em desenvolvimento que migram em duas faixas, uma das quais forma, mais adiante, o núcleo olivar inferior e o núcleo arqueado, e a outra, os núcleos pontinos.
  Gennari b., f. de Gennari. SIN line of Gennari.
  b. of Giacomini, f. de Giacomini. SIN uncus b. of Giacomini.
  H b., faixa H; a área mais pálida no centro da faixa A de uma fibra muscular estriada, compreendendo a porção central dos filamentos espessos (miosina) que não estão superpostos pelos filamentos finos (actina). SIN H disk, Hensen disk, Hensen line.
  His b., feixe de His. SIN atrioventricular *bundle*.
  Hunter-Schreger b.'s, faixas de Hunter-Schreger; linhas claras e escuras alternantes observadas no esmalte dentário que começam na junção do dente com o esmalte e terminam antes que alcancem a superfície do esmalte; representam áreas de colunas de esmalte cortadas transversalmente, dispersas entre áreas de colunas cortadas longitudinalmente. SIN Hunter-Schreger lines, Schreger lines.
  I b., faixa I; uma faixa clara em cada lado da linha Z das fibras musculares estriadas, compreendendo uma região do sarcômero onde os filamentos finos (actina) não estão sobrepostos aos filamentos espessos (miosina). SIN I disk, isotropic disk.

iliotibial b., trato iliotibial. SIN *iliotibial tract.*
b. of Kaes-Bechterew, estria de Kaes-Bechterew, estria da lâmina molecular; a f. de fibras mielinizadas horizontais na parte mais superficial da terceira camada do isocórtex. SIN stria laminae molecularis [TA], stria of molecular layer [TA], Bechterew b., layer of Bechterew, line of Bechterew, line of Kaes.
Ladd b., f. de Ladd; inserção peritoneal de um ceco rodado de maneira incompleta, encontrada na má-rotação do intestino; pode causar obstrução do duodeno.
Lane b., f. de Lane; uma f. congênita no íleo distal que pode se estender para dentro da fossa ilíaca direita, provocando estase. SIN Lane kink.
longitudinal b.'s of cruciform ligament of atlas [TA], fascículos longitudinais do ligamento cruciforme do atlas [TA]; faixas ligamentosas que formam o feixe "ereto" ou vertical do ligamento cruciforme do atlas. SIN fasciculi longitudinales ligamenti cruciformis atlantis [TA].
M b., f. M. SIN *M line.*
Mach b., f. de Mach; faixa relativamente brilhosa ou escura percebida em uma zona onde o brilho aumenta ou diminui rapidamente.
Maissiat b., f. de Maissiat. SIN *iliotibial tract.*
matrix b., faixa matricial; faixa metálica ou plástica fixada ao redor da coroa de um dente para confinar o material de restauração a ser adaptado dentro de uma cavidade preparada.
Meckel b., f. de Meckel; a porção do ligamento anterior do martelo que se estende a partir da base do processo anterior através da fissura petrotimpânica, para se inserir na espinha do esfenóide. VER anterior *ligament* of malleus. SIN Meckel ligament.
moderator b., trabécula septomarginal. SIN *septomarginal trabecula.*
Muehrcke b.'s, faixas de Muehrcke; leuconíquia aparente com faixas brancas em paralelo com a lânula das unhas, observada na hipoalbuminemia. SIN Muehrcke sign.
oligoclonal b., f. oligoclonal; pequenas faixas discretas na região da gamaglobulina da eletroforese do líquido cefalorraquidiano, indicando a produção local de IgG no sistema nervoso central; as faixas são freqüentemente observadas nos pacientes com esclerose múltipla, mas também podem ser encontradas em outras patologias do sistema nervoso central, inclusive sífilis, sarcoidose e inflamação ou infecção crônica.
orthodontic b., f. ortodôntica; uma fina faixa de metal intimamente adaptada à coroa de um dente, na qual os fios podem ser presos para o movimento do dente.

pecten b., faixa pectínea; induração fibrosa do pécten anal resultante de congestão passiva ou de uma forma crônica de inflamação nessa região.
Q b.'s, feixes Q. (1) SIN *A. b's;* (2) VER Q-banding *stain.*
Reil b., f. de Reil. (1) SIN *septomarginal trabecula;* (2) SIN *medial lemniscus.*
silastic b. (si'lăs-tik), f. de Silastic; um pequeno anel de Silastic (borracha siliconizada) colocado ao redor de cada trompa de Falópio para alcançar a esterilização permanente.
Simonart b.'s, faixas de Simonart; (1) SIN *amnionic b.;* (2) faixa ou tecido em forma de rede que preenche parcialmente o hiato entre as porções medial e lateral de um lábio leporino.
Soret b., f. de Soret; a faixa de absorção de todas as porfirinas em cerca de 400 nm.
uncus b. of Giacomini, feixe unciforme de Giacomini; um feixe esbranquiçado e delgado, a continuação anterior atenuada do giro denteado (fáscia denteada), que cruza transversalmente a superfície da parte recurvada do giro para-hipocampal. SIN b. of Giacomini, cauda fasciae dentatae, frenulum of Giacomini, tail of dentate gyrus.
ventricular b. of larynx, prega ventricular. SIN *vestibular fold.*
Z b., faixa Z. SIN *Z line.*
zonular b., zona orbicular. SIN *zona orbicularis (articulationis coxae).*

ban·dage (ban'dij). **1.** Bandagem, atadura; um pedaço de tecido ou outro material, de tamanho e formato variados, aplicado a uma parte do corpo para comprimir, proteger de contaminação, evitar ressecamento, absorver drenagem, evitar o movimento e reter curativos cirúrgicos. **2.** Bandar; cobrir uma parte do corpo através da aplicação de uma b.
adhesive b., b. adesiva; curativo de gaze absorvente simples, afixada a plástico ou a tecido coberto com um adesivo sensível à pressão.
Barton b., b. de Barton; b. em figura de 8 que sustenta a mandíbula, abaixo e anteriormente; utilizada na fratura de mandíbula.
capeline b., b. em gorro; b. que cobre a cabeça ou um coto de amputação semelhante a um gorro. [L. *capella,* um gorro]
circular b., b. circular; aquela que circunda um membro ou parte dele ou o tronco.
cravat b., b. em gravata; b. feita ao se trazer a ponta de uma b. triangular para o meio da base e, em seguida, dobrando longitudinalmente na largura desejada.
crucial b., b. crucial; uma b. na forma de cruz; p.ex., uma b. em T.
demigauntlet b., b. em meia-luva; b. em luva que cobre apenas a mão, deixando os dedos expostos.

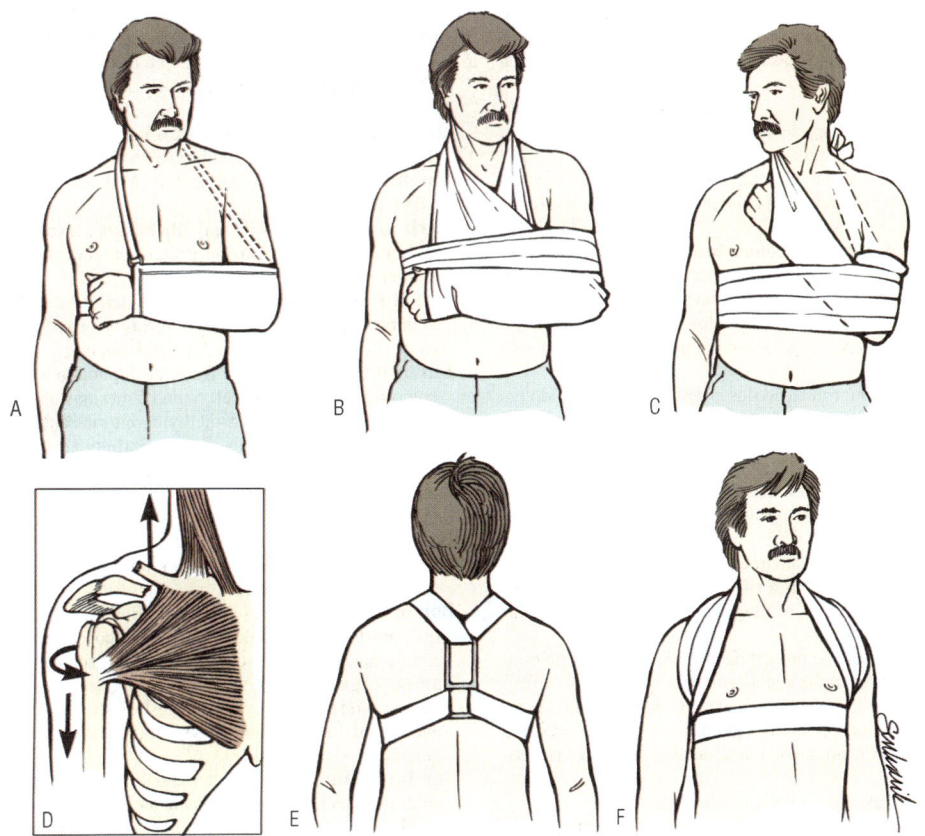

bandagens de imobilização: utilizadas para fraturas da porção proximal do úmero, (A) tipóia e atadura comerciais, (B) tipóia e atadura convencionais, (C) Velpeau (atadura e luva); (D) usada para fraturas de clavícula: (E) suporte clavicular, vista posterior, (F) suporte clavicular, vista anterior

Desault b., b. de Desault; b. para fratura da clavícula; o cotovelo é fixado ao lado, com acolchoamento colocado na axila.

elastic b., b. elástica; b. que contém material distensível; usada para proporcionar compressão local.

Esmarch b., b. de Esmarch. SIN Esmarch *tourniquet.*

figure-of-8 b., b. em forma de 8; b. aplicada alternadamente a duas partes, usualmente dois segmentos de um membro acima e abaixo da articulação, de tal modo que as voltas descrevem a figura de 8; bandagem específica utilizada para o tratamento de fraturas da clavícula.

four-tailed b., b. de quatro pontas; uma faixa de tecido dividida em dois, exceto para a parte central colocada sob o queixo, com quatro pontas atadas sobre a cabeça; usada para limitar a movimentação da mandíbula.

gauntlet b., b. em manopla; b. em forma de 8 que cobre a mão e os dedos.

gauze b., b. de gaze. VER gauze.

Gibney fixation b., b. de fixação de Gibney; enfaixamento do pé e da perna em forma de espinha de arenque para o entorse do tornozelo.

Gibson b., b. de Gibson; b. que se assemelha à b. de Barton para estabilizar uma fratura da mandíbula.

hammock b., b. em rede; b. para reter curativos sobre a cabeça; os curativos são cobertos por uma ampla faixa de gaze, cujas extremidades são trazidas para baixo sobre as orelhas e mantidas, enquanto uma b. circular estreita é passada ao redor da cabeça; as extremidades da faixa de gaze são, então, viradas sobre a b. circular e outras voltas são feitas fixando-as de modo firme.

immovable b., b. imóvel; b. de tecido impregnada com gesso, vidro líquido ou material semelhante, que endurece logo depois de sua aplicação.

Martin b., b. de Martin; b. cilíndrica de borracha macia usada para comprimir um membro no tratamento de veias varicosas ou úlceras.

oblique b., b. oblíqua; b. em que as voltas sucessivas prosseguem de maneira oblíqua para cima ou para baixo no membro.

plaster b., b. gessada; b. roliça impregnada com gesso e aplicada úmida; usada para fazer um curativo rígido para uma fratura ou articulação lesionada.

roller b., b. uma atadura, de largura variável, que é enrolada em um cilindro compacto para facilitar sua aplicação.

scarf b., b. em cachecol. SIN triangular *b.*

Scultetus b., b. de Scultetus; um grande tecido oblongo, cujas extremidades são cortadas em faixas estreitas, que é aplicado ao tórax ou abdome, com as faixas sendo apertadas ou sobrepostas e presas com alfinete.

spica b., b. em espiga; faixas sucessivas de material aplicadas ao corpo e à primeira parte de um membro, ou à mão e a um dedo, que se sobrepõem discretamente em V, assemelhando-se a uma espiga de milho. [L. *spica,* espiga]

spiral b., b. em espiral; b. oblíqua que envolve um membro, com as voltas sucessivas se sobrepondo àquelas anteriores.

suspensory b., b. em suspensório; uma bolsa de tecido distensível para apoiar a bolsa escrotal e seu conteúdo.

T-b., b. em T. SIN *T-binder.*

triangular b., b. triangular; um pedaço de tecido cortado na forma de um triângulo de ângulo reto, usada como tipóia. SIN scarf b.

Velpeau b., b. de Velpeau; uma b. que serve para imobilizar o braço contra a parede torácica, com o antebraço posicionado obliquamente através e para cima por diante do tórax.

band·ing. Padrão de bandas; o processo de coloração diferencial de (usualmente) cromossomas das células em metáfase para revelar os padrões característicos das faixas que permitem a identificação de cromossomas individuais e o reconhecimento de segmentos ausentes; cada um dos 22 pares de cromossomas humanos e os cromossomas X e Y possuem um padrão identificador de bandas.

BrDu-b., padrão de bandas BrDu; rotulação dos cromossomas no tecido em proliferação por acrescentar um excesso de bromodesoxiuridina, que substitui a uridina incorporada ao RNA e fluoresce na luz ultravioleta; as bandas resultam de trocas de cromátides irmãs.

high-resolution b., padrão de bandas em alta resolução; a b., especialmente na prófase, que aumenta a clareza e o número de faixas cromossomiais discerníveis.

NOR-b., padrão de bandas NOR; um procedimento que utiliza um corante de prata que se acumula preferencialmente nas regiões organizadoras de nucléolos (*nucleoli-organizing regions*), i.e., as regiões satélites de cromossomas acrocêntricos.

prometaphase b., padrão de bandas da prometáfase; o processo feito no estágio da mitose intermediária entre a prófase e a metáfase.

pulmonary artery b., ligadura da artéria pulmonar; método cirúrgico de redução do fluxo sanguíneo pulmonar e, por conseguinte, redução da sobrecarga de volume do ventrículo esquerdo, aliviando a ICC em determinados defeitos cardíacos congênitos.

reverse b., padrão de bandas invertido. VER R-banding *stain.*

band·width. Largura de banda; a gama de freqüência ou de comprimentos de onda sobre a qual um aparelho pretende operar.

ban·dy-leg (ban′dē-leg). Joelho varo. SIN *genu varum.*

bane (bān). Veneno; um veneno ou ferrugem. [Ing. Ant. *bana*]

Bang, Bernhard L. F., veterinário e médico dinamarquês, 1848–1932. VER B. *disease.*

ba·nis·te·rine (ba-nis′tĕ-rēn). Banisterina. SIN harmine.

Banti, Guido, médico italiano, 1852–1925. VER B, *disease, syndrome.*

Banting, Sir Frederick G., médico canadense, 1891–1941, um dos ganhadores do Prêmio Nobel de 1923 por isolar a insulina a partir do pâncreas.

bap·ti·tox·ine. Baptitoxina. SIN cytisine.

bar. 1. Bar; uma unidade de pressão atmosférica igual a 1 megadina (10^6 dinas) por cm² no sistema CGS, 0,9869233 atmosfera, ou 10^5 Pa (N/m²) no sistema SI. **2.** Conector; um segmento metálico cujo comprimento é maior que a largura; conecta duas ou mais partes de uma dentadura parcial removível. VER TAMBÉM major *connector.* **3.** Um segmento de tecido ou osso que une duas ou mais estruturas semelhantes.

arch b., conector em arco; qualquer um dos vários tipos de arames, barras ou talas que se adequa ao arco dos dentes, estendendo-se de um lado do arco até o outro e localizado labialmente ou lingualmente; usado para o tratamento de fraturas de mandíbula e/ou estabilização de dentes lesionados.

b. of bladder, prega interuretérica. SIN interureteric *crest.*

clasp b., fecho, colchete. VER clasp.

connector b., conector. VER major *connector,* minor *connector.*

labial b., conector labial; importante conector localizado labialmente ao arco dentário que une duas ou mais partes bilaterais de uma dentadura parcial mandibular removível.

lingual b., conector lingual; importante conector localizado lingualmente ao arco dentário que une duas ou mais partes bilaterais de uma dentadura parcial mandibular removível.

median b. of Mercier, barra de Mercier; faixa proeminente de tecido fibromuscular que envolve a prega interuretérica ou o colo da bexiga urinária, resultando ocasionalmente em obstrução urinária.

Mercier b., barra de Mercier. SIN interureteric *crest.*

occlusal rest b., barra oclusal de repouso; conector menor usado para fixar um repouso oclusal a uma parte maior de uma dentadura parcial removível.

palatal b., barra palatina; um conector importante que cruza o palato e une duas ou mais partes de uma dentadura maxilar parcial removível.

Passavant b., saliência de Passavant. SIN Passavant *ridge.*

sternal b., barra esternal; uma das unidades transversas do esterno em desenvolvimento formadas pela união de primórdios pareados.

terminal b., barra terminal; barras ou máculas negras (dependendo do plano de corte) no limite lateral entre as extremidades apicais das células colunares epiteliais; essa região corresponde à área do complexo juncional e dos filamentos finos que ancoram a zônula aderente.

bar·ag·no·sis (bar-ag-nō′sis). Baragnose; perda da capacidade de apreciar o peso dos objetos seguros na mão ou de diferenciar objetos de pesos diferentes. Quando os sentidos primários estão intactos, causada por uma lesão do lobo parietal contralateral. [G. *baros,* peso, + *a-* priv., + *gnōsis,* um conhecimento]

Bárány, Robert, otologista austro-húngaro e laureado com o Prêmio Nobel, 1876–1936. VER B. *sign,* caloric *test;* positional *vertigo* de B.

bar·ba (bar′bă). [TA]. Barba. **1.** [NA] A barba. **2.** O pêlo da barba. SIN beard [TA]. [L.]

barb·al·o·in (bar-bal′ō-in). Barbaloína. SIN aloin.

Barber, Glenn, cirurgião ortopédico norte-americano do século 20. VER Blount-Barber *disease.*

bar·bi·e·ro (bar-bē-ā′rō). Barbeiro; termo brasileiro para o inseto triatomídeo hemíptero, hematófago, *Panstrongylus megistus,* um importante vetor da doença de Chagas, causada pelo *Trypanosoma cruzi.* [Port. o barbeiro]

bar·bi·tal (bar′bi-tawl). Barbital; hipnótico e sedativo antigo; disponível como b. sódico (b. solúvel), com os mesmos usos; freqüentemente utilizado como um tampão. SIN 5,5-diethylbarbituric acid, Veronal.

bar·bi·tu·rate (bar-bich′ūr-āt). Barbitúrico; derivado do ácido barbitúrico, inclusive fenobarbital e outros, que atua como depressor do SNC, sendo prescrito por causa de seus efeitos tranqüilizantes, hipnóticos e anticonvulsivantes; a maioria dos barbitúricos possui o potencial para o vício.

bar·bi·tu·ric ac·id (bar-bi-chūr′ik). Ácido barbitúrico; um ácido dibásico cristalino do qual derivam o barbital e outros barbitúricos; não possui ação sedativa. SIN malonylurea.

bar·bi·tu·rism (bar′bi-chūr-izm). Barbiturismo; intoxicação crônica por qualquer um dos derivados do ácido barbitúrico; os sintomas, que não são muito distintos, incluem erupção cutânea acompanhada por calafrios, febre e cefaléia.

bar·bo·tage (bar-bō-tahzh′). Barbotagem; um método de anestesia espinal em que uma porção da solução anestésica é injetada no líquido cefalorraquidiano, o qual é, então, aspirado de volta para a seringa e reinjetado. [Fr. *barboter,* borrifar]

bar·bu·la hir·ci (bar′bū-lă hir′sī). Os pêlos que crescem a partir do trago, antitrago e incisura intertrágica da orelha de homens depois de 27 anos de idade. [L. dim. of *barba,* barba, + gen. sing. de *hircus,* cabra]

Barclay, Alfred E., médico inglês, 1877–1949. VER B.-Baron *disease.*

Barcroft, Sir Joseph F., fisiologista inglês, 1872–1947. VER B.-Warburg *apparatus, technique.*

Bard, Philip, fisiologista norte-americano, 1898–1945. VER Cannon-B. *theory*.
Bardet, Georges, médico francês, *1885. VER B.-Biedl *syndrome*.
Bardinet, Barthélemy A., médico francês, 1809–1874. VER B. *ligament*.
bar·es·the·sia (bar-es-thē′zē-ā). Barestesia. SIN pressure sense. [G. *baros*, peso, + *aisthēsis*, sensação]
bar·es·the·si·om·e·ter (bar′es-thē′zē-om′e-ter). Barestesiômetro; instrumento para medir a sensação de pressão. [G. *baros*, peso, + *aisthēsis*, sensação, + *metron*, medida]
bar·i·at·ric (bar-ē-at′rik). Bariátrico; relativo à bariatria.
bar·i·at·rics (bar-ē-at′riks). Bariatria; ramo da medicina relacionado com o controle (prevenção ou controle) da obesidade e doenças aliadas. [G. *baros*, peso, + *iatreia*, tratamento médico]
ba·ric (ba′rik). Bárico; relativo à pressão barométrica (como em isobar) ou ao peso no geral.
ba·ric·i·ty (ba-ris′i-tē). Baricidade; o peso de uma substância comparado ao peso de um volume igual de outra substância na mesma temperatura. [G. *baros*, peso]
ba·ril·la (ba-ril′ā). Barrilha; sulfato e carbonato de sódio comercial, usualmente impuro.
bar·i·to·sis (bar-i-tō′sis). Baritose; uma forma de pneumoconiose causada pela barita ou pó de bário.
bar·i·um (Ba) (ba′rē-ŭm, bā′rē-ŭm). Bário; elemento metálico, alcalino, terroso, divalente; no. atômico 56, peso atômico 137,327. Os sais insolúveis são freqüentemente utilizados em radiologia como contraste. [G. *barys*, pesado]
b. chloride, cloreto de b.; utilizado outrora como tônico cardíaco e para veias varicosas; extremamente tóxico.
b. hydroxide, hidróxido de b.; composto cáustico combinado com o hidróxido de cálcio em um absorvente de dióxido de carbono; usado nos circuitos anestésicos. VER TAMBÉM absorbent (3).
b. meal, a administração oral de suspensão de sulfato de b. para o estudo radiográfico do trato gastrintestinal superior (termo usado no Reino Unido).
b. oxide, b. monoxide, óxido de b., monóxido de b.; é cáustico, formando uma base forte, $Ba(OH)_2$ em água; usado como agente desidratante. SIN baryta.
b. sulfate, s. de bário; fornecido como suspensão por via oral, retal ou através de um tubo, para demonstração radiográfica de uma parte do trato gastrintestinal. VER enteroclysis, barium *enema*.
b. sulfide, sulfeto de b.; pó venenoso amarelo-acinzentado, usado como depilatório.
b. swallow, suspensão de b.; a administração oral de suspensão de sulfato de b. para a investigação radiográfica da hipofaringe e esôfago.
bark. 1. Casca; o envoltório ou revestimento das raízes, tronco e ramos das plantas. As cascas importantes em termos farmacológicos não listadas adiante são colocadas sob os nomes específicos na ordem alfabética. **2.** Cinchona. SIN cinchona.
cinchona b., cinchona. SIN cinchona.
cotton-root b., c. da raiz do algodão; a casca da raiz seca do *Gossypium herbaceum* e outras espécies de *Gossypium* (família Malvaceae). Tem sido utilizada como abortifaciente e ocitócico.
Barkan, Otto, oftalmologista norte-americano, 1887–1958. VER Barkan *membrane*; B. *operation*.
Barkman, Åke, clínico sueco do século 20. VER B. *reflex*.
Barkow, Hans K. L., anatomista alemão, 1798–1873. VER B. *ligaments*, em *ligament*.
Barlow, John B., cardiologista sul-africano, *1924. VER B. *syndrome*.
Barlow, Sir Thomas, médico britânico, 1845–1945. VER B. *disease*.
barn (b). *Barn*; unidade de área para o corte transversal efetivo dos núcleos atômicos com relação aos mísseis atômicos; igual a 10^{-24} cm². [de "grande como o lado de um celeiro" pela comparação humorística com áreas muito menores]
Barnard, Christiaan, cirurgião sul-africano, 1922–2002, realizou o primeiro transplante cardíaco bem-sucedido em 1967.
Barnes, Robert, obstetra britânico, 1817–1907. VER B. *curve*, *zone*.
Barnes, Stanley, médico britânico, 1875–1955.
baro-. Forma combinante relativa a peso, pressão. [G. *baros*, peso]
bar·o·cep·tor (bar′ō-sep-ter, -tōr). Baroceptor. SIN baroreceptor.
bar·og·no·sis (bar′og-nō′sis). Barognose; capacidade de apreciar o peso dos objetos ou de diferenciar os objetos de pesos diferentes. [G. *baros*, peso, + *gnōsis*, conhecimento]
bar·o·graph (bar′ō-graf). Barógrafo; aparelho que fornece um registro contínuo da pressão barométrica. SIN barometrograph.
bar·o·met·ro·graph (bar-ō-met′rō-graf). Barometrógrafo. SIN barograph.
Baron. VER Barclay-Baron *disease*.
bar·o·phil·ic (bar′ō-fil′ik). Barofílico; que se desenvolve melhor sob alta pressão ambiental; aplicado a microrganismos. [G. *baros*, peso, + *phileō*, amar]
bar·o·re·cep·tor (bar′ō-rē-sep′ter, -tor). Barorreceptor. **1.** Em geral, qualquer sensor das alterações de pressão. **2.** A terminação nervosa sensorial na parede dos átrios do coração, veia cava, arco aórtico e seio carotídeo, sensível ao estiramento da parede resultante da pressão interna aumentada e funcionando como o receptor dos mecanismos reflexos centrais que tendem a reduzir essa pressão. SIN baroceptor, pressoreceptor. [G. *baros*, peso, + receptor]

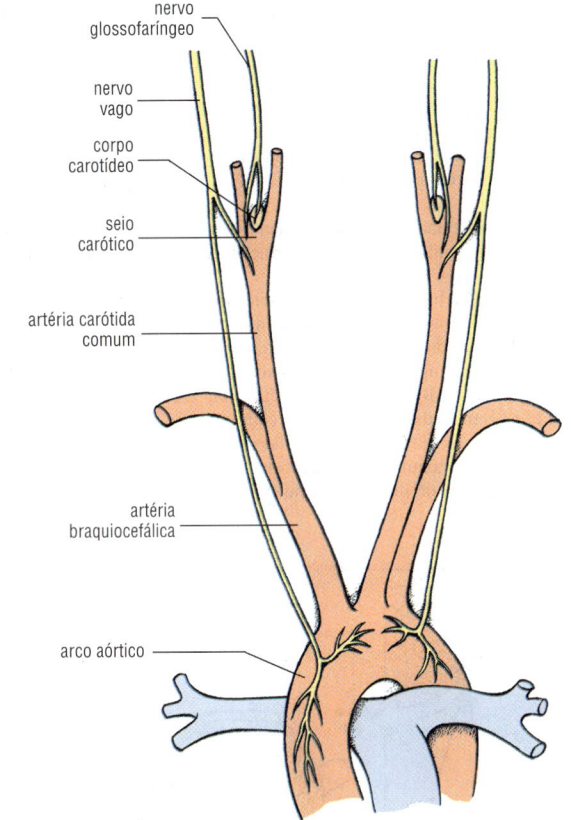

barorreceptores: na área dos seios carotídeos e no arco aórtico

bar·o·re·flex (bar-ō-rē′fleks). Barorreflexo; reflexo deflagrado por estimulação de um barorreceptor.
bar·o·scope (bar′ō-skōp). Baroscópio; instrumento que mede as alterações na pressão atmosférica.
bar·o·si·nus·i·tis (bar′ō-sī-nus-ī′tis). Barossinusite; inflamação da mucosa dos seios paranasais causada pela diferença de pressão no seio paranasal em relação à pressão ambiental, secundária à obstrução do óstio sinusal e que ocorre durante a descida de altitude. SIN aerosinusitis. [G. *baros*, peso, pressão, + sinusitis]
bar·o·stat (bar′ō-stat). Barostato; aparelho ou estrutura que regula a pressão, como os barorreceptores do seio carotídeo e arco aórtico, quando conectado aos efetores que fornecem a retroalimentação negativa. [G., *baros*, peso, pressão, + *statos*, feito para ficar em pé]
bar·o·tax·is (bar-ō-tak′sis). Barotaxia; a reação do tecido vivo às alterações na pressão. SIN barotropism. [G. *baros*, peso, + *taxis*, ordem]
bar·o·ti·tis me·di·a (bar-ō-tī′tis mē′dē-ā). Barotite média; inflamação da mucosa da orelha média causada por diferença de pressão na orelha média relativa à pressão ambiental, secundária à obstrução da tuba auditiva ou sua falha em abrir; com freqüência ocorre na descida de locais altos. SIN aerotitis media.
bar·o·trau·ma (bar′ō-traw′mă). Barotrauma; termo previamente utilizado para descrever a lesão do ouvido médio e dos seios paranasais, resultando do desequilíbrio entre a pressão ambiental e aquela dentro da cavidade afetada. Atualmente, é utilizado com maior freqüência para indicar a lesão do pulmão decorrente da pressão, como a que acontece quando um paciente está sendo ventilado mecanicamente e está sujeito à pressão alta nas vias aéreas (barotrauma pulmonar). [G. *baros*, peso, + trauma]
otic b., b. auditivo; a lesão causada ao ouvido pelo desequilíbrio na pressão entre o ar ambiente e o ar na orelha média. VER TAMBÉM barotitis media.
sinus b., b. sinusal; lesão dos seios paranasais, resultante do desequilíbrio na pressão entre o ar ambiente e o ar nos seios paranasais. VER TAMBÉM barosinusitis.
bar·ot·ro·pism (bar-ot′rō-pizm). Barotropismo. SIN barotaxis. [G. *baros*, peso, + *tropē*, uma volta]
Barr, Murray L., microanatomista canadense, *1908. VER B. chromatin *body*.
Barr, Yvonne M., virologista inglesa, *1932. VER Epstein-B. *virus*.
Barraquer, Ignacio, oftalmologista espanhol, 1884–1965. VER B. *method*.
Barraquer Roviralta, Luis, médico espanhol, 1855–1928. VER Barraquer *disease*.

Barré, Jean A., neurologista francês, *1880. VER B. *sign;* Guillain-B. *reflex, syndrome;* Landry-Guillain-B. *syndrome.*

bar·ren (bar'en). Estéril; incapaz de engravidar. [I. M. *bareyne*]

Barrett, Norman R., médico britânico, *1903. VER *adenocarcinoma* em B. esophagus; B. *esophagus, epitelium, syndrome;* Barrett *metaplasia.*

bar·ri·er (bar'ē-er). Barreira. **1.** Um obstáculo ou impedimento. **2.** Em psiquiatria, um agente de conflito que bloqueia o comportamento que poderia ajudar a resolver um conflito pessoal. [I. M., do Fr. Ant. *barriere*, do L. L. *barraria*]

blood-air b., b. hematoaérea; o material entre o ar alveolar e o sangue; consiste em uma película não-estrutural ou surfactante, epitélio alveolar, lâmina basal e endotélio.

blood-aqueous b., b. hematoaquosa; b. seletivamente permeável entre o leito capilar nos prolongamentos do corpo ciliar e o humor aquoso na câmara anterior do olho; consiste em duas camadas de epitélio cubóide simples unidas em suas superfícies apicais com complexos juncionais.

blood-brain b. (BBB), b. hematoencefálica; um mecanismo seletivo que se opõe à passagem da maioria dos íons e compostos de grande peso molecular do sangue para o tecido cerebral localizado em uma camada contínua de células endoteliais por zônulas aderentes; os pequenos capilares são encontrados na retina, na íris, na orelha interna e no endonêurio dos nervos periféricos.

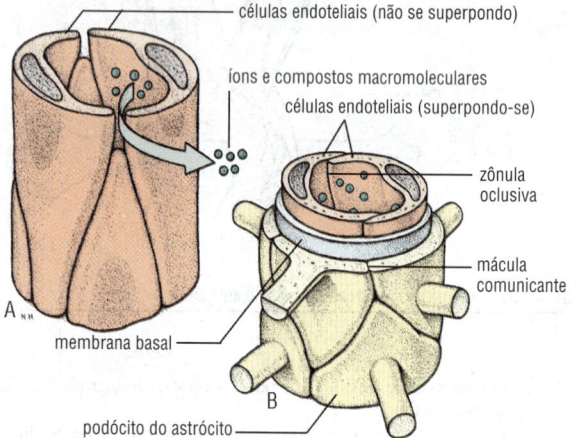

barreira hematoencefálica: (A) nos capilares não-neuronais, determinados íons e moléculas atravessam as lacunas entre as células endoteliais; (B) em um capilar neural, a barreira criada por zônulas de oclusão entre as células endoteliais, a membrana basal e os podócitos dos astrócitos opõem-se à passagem dessas substâncias

blood-cerebrospinal fluid b., blood-CSF b., b. hematoliquórica; uma b. localizada nas zônulas aderentes que circundam e conectam as células epiteliais cubóides na superfície do plexo coróide; os capilares e o estroma de tecido conjuntivo da coróide não representam uma b. para os marcadores proteicos ou corantes.

blood-testis b., b. hematotesticular; b. oclusora formada pelas células de Sertoli nos ductos seminíferos do testículo, que separa as células mais maduras da espermatogênese no compartimento adluminal do ducto dos produtos derivados do sangue no compartimento basal.

blood-thymus b., b. hematotímica; bainha de pericitos e células reticulares epiteliais ao redor dos capilares tímicos que impede os linfócitos T do timo em desenvolvimento de serem expostos aos antígenos circulantes.

incest b., b. incestuosa; em psicanálise, o aprendizado ou a internalização das proibições parentais e sociais contra o incesto.

placental b., membrana placentária. SIN placental *membrane.*

Bart, Bruce J., dermatologista norte-americano, *1936. VER B. *syndrome.*

Bartels, Peter H., cientista alemão nos Estados Unidos que se especializou em ótica e ciência da computação, *1929.

Barth, Jean B. P., médico de Estrasburgo, 1806–1877. VER B. *hernia.*

Bartholin, Casper, anatomista dinamarquês, 1655–1738. VER B. *abscess, cyst, cystectomy, duct, gland.*

Bartholin, Thomas, anatomista dinamarquês, 1616–1680. VER B. *anus.*

bar·tho·lin·i·tis (bar-tō-lin-ī'tis). Bartolinite; inflamação de uma glândula vulvovaginal (Bartholin).

Bartley, Samuel H., psicólogo norte-americano, *1901. VER Brücke-B. *phenomenon.*

Barton, John Rhea, cirurgião norte-americano, 1794–1871. VER B. *bandage, forceps, fracture.*

Bar·ton·el·la (bar-tō-nel'ā). Gênero de bactérias encontrado em seres humanos e em vetores artrópodes; cresce lentamente em meios artificiais e pode ser isolada de hemoculturas de pacientes infectados; pode ser observada no nível intracelular nos tecidos e eritrócitos. B. é um microrganismo cocobacilar, Gram-negativo e pequeno, que pode parecer curvo; pode provocar uma doença progressiva, maldefinida e indolente nos pacientes imunocomprometidos, inclusive aqueles com infecções por HIV. [A. L. *Barton*]

B. bacillifor'mis, espécie encontrada no sangue e em células epiteliais dos linfonodos, baço e fígado na febre de Oroya (é a causa da febre de Oroya) e no sangue e elementos eruptivos na verruga peruana; provavelmente também é encontrado em mosquitos-pólvora (*Phlebotomus verrucarum*); conhecido por estar estabelecido apenas no continente sul-americano e, talvez, na América Central; é a espécie típica do gênero *B.*

B. henselae, espécie bacteriana que provoca a *doença* da arranhadura do gato nas pessoas com imunidade normal e angiomatose bacilar nas pessoas com AIDS/SIDA. VER TAMBÉM catscratch *disease.*

B. quintana, outrora a espécie típica do gênero *Rochalimaea,* esse microrganismo causa a febre da trincheira (*trench fever*) e, nos pacientes com AIDS/SIDA, está associada a septicemia e endocardite; o artrópode vetor é *Pediculus humanus,* o piolho do corpo.

Bar·ton·el·la·ceae (bar-ton-el-ā'sē-ē). Família de bactérias que atualmente inclui o gênero *Bartonella.* Com base nos estudos do RNAr S16, os gêneros anteriores de *Rochalimaea* e *Grahamella* misturaram-se com o gênero *Bartonella,* retendo seus nomes de espécie.

bar·ton·el·lo·sis (bar-tō-nel-ō'sis). Bartonelose; doença causada pela infecção por uma espécie de bactérias que pertencem ao gênero *Bartonella.*

Bart's. Apelido do St. Bartholomew's Hospital em Londres, onde a hemoglobina de Bart foi isolada pela primeira vez de um paciente.

Bartter, Frederic C., médico norte-americano, 1914–1983. VER B. *syndrome.*

Baruch, Simon, médico norte-americano, 1840–1921. VER B. *law.*

bar·u·ria (bar-ū'rē-ā). Barúria; termo raramente utilizado para a excreção da urina que apresenta densidade incomumente elevada, p. ex., maior que 1,025 a 1,030. [G. *barys,* pesado, + *ouron,* urina]

bary-. Forma combinante que indica pesado. [G. *barys*]

bar·ye (ba'rē). A unidade de pressão CGS, igual a 1 dina/cm² ou 10^{-6} bar. VER bar (1). [G. *barys,* pesado]

ba·ry·ta (ba-rī'tā). Barita. SIN barium oxide. [G. *barytēs,* peso]

baryto-. Barito-; prefixo que indica a presença de bário em um mineral.

ba·sad (bā'sad). Basal; em direção à base de qualquer objeto ou estrutura.

ba·sal (bā'sal) [TA]. Basal. **1.** Situado mais próximo à base de um órgão em formato de pirâmide em relação a um ponto de referência específico; oposto de apical. SIN basalis [TA]. **2.** Em odontologia, que indica o assoalho de uma cavidade na superfície molar de um dente. **3.** Indica um estado padrão ou de referência de uma função, como uma base para a comparação. Mais especificamente, indica as condições exatas para a mensuração da taxa metabólica basal (basal metabolic *rate*) (*q.v.*); as condições basais nem sempre indicam um valor mínimo, p.ex., a taxa metabólica no sono é usualmente menor que a taxa b., mas é inconveniente para a mensuração de padrão.

ba·sa·lis (bā-sā'lis) [TA]. Basal. SIN basal (1). [L.]

ba·sa·loid (bā'sā-loyd). Basalóide; que se assemelha ao que é basal, mas não é necessariamente basal em sua origem ou posição.

ba·sal ra·tion. Cota basal; dieta mínima que contém apenas os componentes essenciais.

base (bās) [TA]. Base. **1.** A parte inferior ou fundo; a parte de uma pirâmide ou estrutura cônica oposta ao ápice; a base. SIN basis [TA], basement (1). **2.** Em farmácia, o ingrediente principal de uma mistura. **3.** Em química, um elemento eletropositivo (cátion) que se une a um ânion para formar um sal; um composto ionizante para formar o íon hidroxila. SIN alkali (2). VER TAMBÉM Brønsted b., Lewis b. **4.** Compostos orgânicos portadores de nitrogênio (p.ex., purinas, pirimidinas, aminas, alcalóides, ptomaínas) que agem como bases de Brønsted. **5.** Cátions ou substâncias formadoras de cátions. [L. e G. *basis*]

acrylic resin b., base de resina acrílica; uma fôrma feita de resina acrílica moldada para adaptar-se aos tecidos do processo alveolar e usada para apoiar os dentes de uma prótese.

anterior cranial b., fossa craniana anterior. SIN anterior cranial *fossa.*

b. of arytenoid cartilage [TA], b. da cartilagem aritenóidea; a parte da cartilagem aritenóidea que se articula com a cartilagem cricóide e a partir da qual o processo muscular se estende lateralmente e o processo vocal se projeta anteriormente. SIN basis cartilaginis arytenoideae [TA].

b. of bladder, b. da bexiga. SIN *fundus of bladder.*

b. of brain, b. do cérebro; a superfície inferior do cérebro, principalmente do tronco cerebral, quando observado por baixo; comumente estendido para incluir a superfície inferior das partes adjacentes do hemisfério cerebral. SIN basis cerebri, inferior cerebral surface.

Brønsted b., b. de Brønsted; qualquer molécula ou íon que se combina a um próton; p.ex., OH^-, CN^-, NH_3; essa definição substitui os conceitos antigos e mais limitados de base (3).

cavity preparation b., b. de preparação da cavidade. SIN cement b.

cement b., b. de cimento; em odontologia, uma camada de cimento dentário, por vezes medicamentosa, que é colocada na porção profunda na preparação de uma cavidade para proteger a polpa, reduzir a massa de uma restauração metálica ou eliminar rebaixamentos. SIN cavity preparation b.

b. of cochlea [TA], b. da cóclea; a parte dilatada da cóclea que está dirigida posterior e medialmente e se situa próximo ao meato acústico interno. SIN basis cochleae [TA].

cranial b. [TA], b. do crânio; o assoalho inclinado da cavidade craniana. Compreende a b. externa do crânio (vista externa) e a b. interna do crânio (vista interna). SIN basis cranii [TA], basicranium*, b. of skull.

denture b., b. da dentadura; **(1)** a parte de uma dentadura que repousa sobre a mucosa oral e na qual são presos os dentes; **(2)** a parte de uma dentadura completa ou parcial que repousa sobre o assento basal e à qual os dentes estão presos. SIN saddle (2).

external b. of skull, b. externa do crânio. SIN external *surface* of cranial base.

b. of heart [TA], b. do coração; a parte do coração que se situa em oposição ao ápice, formada principalmente pelo átrio esquerdo, mas, em uma pequena extensão, pela parte posterior do átrio direito; é dirigida para trás e para a direita, sendo separada da coluna vertebral pelo esôfago e pela aorta. SIN basis cordis [TA].

hexone b.'s, histone b.'s, bases hexônicas, bases histônicas; os α-aminoácidos arginina, histidina e lisina, que são básicos em virtude da presença nas cadeias de um grupamento guanidina, imidazol e amina, respectivamente; o termo "hexona" é um nome errôneo, pois a histidina não possui seis carbonos.

b. of hyoid bone, corpo do osso hióide. SIN *body* of hyoid bone.

internal b. of skull, face interna do crânio. SIN internal *surface* of cranial base. VER TAMBÉM cranial b.

Lewis b., b. de Lewis; uma b. que é um doador de par de elétron.

b. of lung [TA], b. do pulmão; a parte côncava inferior do pulmão que repousa sobre a convexidade do diafragma. SIN basis pulmonis [TA].

b. of mandible, b. da mandíbula; a borda inferior arredondada do corpo da mandíbula. SIN basis mandibulae [TA].

b. of metacarpal [TA], b. metacarpal; a extremidade proximal estendida de cada metacárpico que se articula com um ou mais ossos da fileira distal do carpo. SIN basis ossis metacarpalis [TA].

metal b., b. metálica; uma porção metálica de uma b. de dentadura que forma uma parte da parede da superfície basal da dentadura; ela serve como uma b. para a inserção da parte plástica (resina) da dentadura e dos dentes.

b. of metatarsal [TA], b. metatarsal; a extremidade proximal expandida de cada osso metatársico; articula-se com um ou mais dos ossos da fileira distal do tarso. SIN basis ossis metatarsalis [TA].

methamphetamine b., b. de metanfetamina; uma forma de metanfetamina que pode ser prontamente volatilizada.

b. of modiolus of cochlea [TA], b. do modíolo da cóclea; a parte do modíolo envolvida pela volta basal da cóclea; volta-se para a extremidade lateral do meato acústico interno. VER cochlear *area*. SIN basis modioli cochleae [TA].

nucleic acid b., b. de ácido nucléico; uma purina ou pirimidina; encontrada em ácidos nucléicos de ocorrência natural, como o DNA.

ointment b., b. de pomada; o veículo no qual os ingredientes ativos podem ser incorporados. O petrolato ou vaselina (que pode ser enrijecido com cera) é a base graxa mais utilizada e é adequada para a incorporação de materiais oleaginosos. As bases que contêm lanolina absorverão água (e os materiais dissolvidos) e formam emulsões do tipo água-em-óleo. As bases hidrossolúveis (laváveis) são frequentemente derivadas de polímeros do etileno glicol (PEGS); essas absorverão água e ingredientes dissolvidos na água. As bases de pomada são, em geral, farmacologicamente inertes, porém podem reter a água e servir para impedir que a pele resseque ou para fornecer uma película protetora emoliente.

b. of patella [TA], b. da patela; a borda superior da patela na qual o tendão do reto femoral se insere. SIN basis patellae [TA].

b. of phalanx, b. da falange; a extremidade proximal expandida de cada falange na mão e no pé que se articula com a cabeça do osso proximal a seguir no dedo. SIN basis phalangis.

b. of phalanx of foot [TA], b. da falange do pé; a extremidade proximal, côncava e de articulação dos ossos dos artelhos. SIN basis phalangis pedis [TA].

b. of phalanx of hand [TA], b. da falange da mão; a extremidade proximal, côncava e de articulação dos ossos dos dedos. SIN basis phalangis manus [TA].

pressor b., b. pressora; **(1)** um dos vários produtos da putrefação intestinal que se acredita causar a hipertensão funcional, quando absorvido; **(2)** qualquer substância alcalina que aumenta a pressão arterial. SIN pressor amine, pressor substance.

b. of prostate [TA], b. da próstata; a superfície superior mais ampla da próstata contígua à parede vesical. SIN basis prostatae [TA].

purine b., b. purínica; uma purina.

pyrimidine b., b. pirimidínica; uma pirimidina.

record b., b. de registro. SIN baseplate.

b. of renal pyramid, b. da pirâmide renal; a porção externa larga de uma pirâmide renal que se situa próximo ao córtex. SIN basis pyramidis renis.

b. of sacrum [TA], b. do sacro; a extremidade superior do sacro que se articula com o corpo da quinta vértebra lombar na linha média e as asas em ambos os lados. SIN basis ossis sacri [TA].

Schiff b., b. de Schiff; os produtos de condensação de aldeídos e cetonas com as aminas primárias; os compostos são estáveis quando existe pelo menos um grupamento arila no nitrogênio ou carbono. Cf. ketimine. SIN aldimine.

shellac b., goma-laca; material resinoso adaptado a moldes maxilares ou mandibulares para formar as placas basais.

b. of skull, b. do crânio. SIN cranial b. VER TAMBÉM internal *surface* of cranial base.

b. of stapes [TA], b. do estribo; a porção plana do estribo que se adapta na janela oval. SIN basis stapedis [TA], footplate (1), foot-plate*.

temporary b., b. temporária. SIN baseplate.

tinted denture b., b. dentária colorida; b. dentária que simula a coloração e o sombreado dos tecidos orais naturais.

b. of tongue, b. da língua. SIN *root* of tongue.

tooth-borne b., b. de sustentação de dente; a b. da dentadura que restaura uma área edentulosa que possui pinos de fixação de dente em cada extremidade para o apoio; o tecido que ela cobre não é usado para apoio.

trial b., b. experimental. SIN baseplate.

vegetable b., b. vegetal. SIN alkaloid.

wobble b., a base do códon 3´ que está especificada de forma menos rígida no código genético. VER TAMBÉM wobble, wobble *hypothesis*.

bas·e·doid (bahz'e-doyd). Basedóide; termo raramente utilizado que indica uma condição semelhante à doença de Graves (doença de Basedow), mas sem manifestações tóxicas.

Basedow, Karl A. von, médico alemão, 1799–1854. VER B. *disease, pseudoparaplegia;* Jod-B. *phenomenon;* B. *goiter*.

ba·se·dow·i·an (bahz-e-dō'e-an). Basedoviano; raramente usado para denotar termos descritos por ou atribuídos a K. Basedow.

base·ment (bās'ment). **1.** Fundamento; base. SIN base (1). **2.** Uma cavidade ou espaço parcial ou completamente separado de um espaço maior acima dele.

base·plate (bās'plāt). Placa básica; uma forma temporária que representa a base de uma dentadura; usada para fazer os registros da relação maxilo-mandibular e para a disposição dos dentes. SIN record base, temporary base, trial base.

stabilized b., placa basal estabilizada; uma placa basal revestida com material plástico para melhorar sua adaptação e estabilidade.

base-stack·ing. Um arranjo de bases de DNA ou RNA em que as bases ficam umas sobre as outras.

bas-fond (bah-fawn') Fundo. SIN *fundus* of bladder.

Basham mix·ture. Mistura de Basham. SIN ferric and ammonium acetate *solution*.

basi-, basio-, baso-. Formas combinantes que indicam base. [G. e L. *basis*]

ba·si·a·lis (bā-sē-ā'lis). Basal; relativo a uma base ou ao básio.

ba·si·al·ve·o·lar (bā'sē-al-vē'ō'lar). Base alveolar; relativo ao básio e aos pontos alveolares; indica especialmente o comprimento da b., ou a distância mais curta entre esses dois pontos.

ba·sic (bā'sik). Básico; relativo a uma base.

ba·sic·i·ty (bā-sis'i-tē). Basicidade. **1.** A valência ou força de combinação de um ácido, ou o número de átomos substituíveis de hidrogênio em sua molécula. **2.** A característica de ser uma base química.

ba·sic life sup·port. Suporte básico de vida; reanimação cardiopulmonar de emergência, controle de hemorragia, tratamento de choque, acidose e intoxicação, estabilização de lesões e feridas e primeiros socorros básicos.

ba·si·cra·ni·al (bā'si-krā'nē-ăl). Basecranial; relativo à base do crânio.

ba·si·cra·ni·um. Base do crânio; termo oficial alternativo* para cranial *base*.

Ba·sid·i·ob·o·lus (bā-sid'ē-ob'ō-lŭs). Basidíobolos; um gênero de fungos que pertence à classe dos Zigomicetos. *B. haptosporus* foi isolado a partir de casos de zigomicose (entomoftoramicose por basidiobolos) em seres humanos, especialmente na Indonésia, África tropical e Sudeste da Ásia. [L. Mod. *basidium*, dim. do G. *basis*, base, + L. *bolus*, do G. *bolos*, protuberância ou torrão]

Ba·sid·i·o·my·ce·tes (ba-sid'ē-ō-mī-sēt'ez). Basidiomicetos; uma das quatro classes principais de fungos, caracterizada por um órgão formador de esporos (basídio), usualmente uma célula claviforme única, que comporta os basidiósporos depois da cariogamia e meiose. A classe compreende as ferrugens, mofos, cogumelos e bufa de lobo. Excluindo-se as micotoxinas, existe apenas um patógeno humano, o estágio basidiomicetoso do *Cryptococcus neoformans*. [L. Mod. *basidium*, dim. do G. *basis*, base, + *mikēs (mikēt)*, fungo]

Ba·sid·i·o·my·co·ta (ba-sid'ē-ō-mī-kō'ta). Um filo de fungos caracterizado por um órgão formador de esporos, o basídio, que, em geral, é uma célula claviforme que comporta os basidiósporos depois da cariogamia e meiose. Alguns micologistas elevaram a classe dos Basidiomicetos a um nível de filo ou divisão.

ba·sid·i·o·spore (ba-sid'ē-ō-spōr). Basidiosporo; um esporo fúngico originado em um basídio, característico da classe dos Basidiomicetos. [G. *basidon*, pequena base, + *sporos*, semente]

ba·sid·i·um, pl. **ba·sid·ia** (ba-sid'ē-ŭm, ā). Basídio; uma célula ou órgão formador de esporos, geralmente no formato de uma clava, que é característico dos Basidiomicetos. Transporta os basiodiosporos externamente depois da cariogamia e meiose. É composta de uma célula terminal edemaciada situada em um pedículo fino, e origina filamentos finos (esterigmas), geralmente em número de quatro, a partir das extremidades das quais se desenvolvem os basidiosporos. [L., do G. *basis*, base]

ba·si·fa·cial (ba'si-fa'shăl). Basifacial; relativo à porção inferior da face.

ba·si·hy·al (ba'si-hi'ăl). Base ou corpo do osso hióide. SIN *body* of hyoid bone.

ba·si·hy·oid (ba-ze-hi'oyd). Base ou corpo do osso hióide. SIN *body* of hyoid bone.

bas·i·lar, bas·i·la·ris (bas'i-lăr, bas-i-la'ris) [TA]. Basilar; relativo à base de uma estrutura piramidal ou larga.

ba·si·lat·er·al (ba'si-lat'er-ăl). Basilateral; relativo à base e a um ou mais lados de qualquer parte.

ba·si·lem·ma (ba-si-lem'ă). Basilema. SIN basement *membrane*. [basi- + G. *lemma*, casca]

ba·sil·i·cus (ba-sil'i-kŭs). Basílico; indica uma parte ou estrutura proeminente ou importante. [L. do G. *basilikos*, real]

ba·sin (ba'sin). Bacia, cuba; um receptáculo para líquidos.
  emesis b., kidney b., cuba em rim; uma b. rasa de design curvo, em forma de rim, usada para coletar os líquidos corporais ou como um recipiente para vários outros líquidos.
  pus b., um receptáculo curvo de modo a se adaptar intimamente à superfície à qual ele é aplicado, usado para receber o pus de uma ferida durante drenagem, limpeza e/ou troca de curativo.

ba·si·na·sal (ba'si-na'săl). Basinasal; relativo ao básio e ao násio; indica principalmente o comprimento b. ou a distância mais curta entre os dois pontos.

△ **basio-.** VER basi-.

ba·si·oc·cip·i·tal (ba'se-ok-sip'i-tăl). Basioccipital; relativo ao processo basilar do osso occipital.

ba·si·oc·ci·put (ba-ze-ok'se-put). Basioccipital. SIN basilar *part* of occipital bone.

ba·si·o·glos·sus (ba-se-o-glos'ŭs). Basioglosso; a porção do músculo hioglosso que se origina do corpo do osso hióide.

ba·si·on (ba'se-on) [TA]. Básio; o ponto médio da margem anterior do forame magno, oposto ao opístion. [G. *basis*, uma base]

ba·sip·e·tal (ba-sip'e-tăl). Basípeto. **1.** Em uma direção no sentido da base. **2.** Pertinente à produção assexuada de conídios nos fungos, na qual o brotamento bem-sucedido dos conídios basais forma uma cadeia não-ramificada com os mais jovens na base. [basi- + L. *peto*, procurar]

bas·i·pho·bia (bas-i-fo'be-ă). Basifobia; medo mórbido de caminhar. [G. *basis*, uma passada, + *phobos*, medo]

ba·sis (ba'sis) [TA]. Base. SIN base (1). [L. e G.]
  b. cartilag'inis arytenoi'deae [TA], base da cartilagem aritenóide. SIN *base* of arytenoid cartilage.
  b. cer'ebri, b. do cérebro. SIN *base* of brain.
  b. coch'leae [TA], b. da cóclea. SIN *base* of cochlea.
  b. cor'dis [TA], b. do coração. SIN *base* of heart.
  b. cra'nii [TA], b. do crânio. SIN cranial *base*.
  b. cra'nii exter'na [TA], b. externa do crânio. SIN external *surface* of cranial base.
  b. cra'nii inter'na [TA], b. interna do crânio. SIN internal *surface* of cranial base.
  b. mandib'ulae [TA], b. da mandíbula. SIN *base* of mandible.
  b. modi'oli coch'leae [TA], b. do modíolo da cóclea. SIN *base* of modiolus of cochlea.
  b. os'sis metacarpa'lis [TA], b. do osso metacárpico. SIN *basis* of metacarpal.
  b. os'sis metatarsa'lis [TA], b. do osso metatársico. SIN *base* of metatarsal.
  b. os'sis sa'cri [TA], b. do osso sacro. SIN *base* of sacrum.
  b. patel'lae [TA], b. da patela. SIN *base* of patella.
  b. pedun'culi [TA], b. do pedúnculo; a base do mesencéfalo que consiste na cruz do cérebro e substância negra. VER TAMBÉM cerebral *peduncle*.
  b. phalan'gis, b. da falange. SIN *base* of phalanx.
  b. phalangis manus [TA], b. da falange da mão. SIN *base* of phalanx of hand.
  b. phalangis pedis [TA], b. da falange do pé. SIN *base* of phalanx of foot.
  b. pontis, b. da ponte. SIN basilar *part* of pons.
  b. pro'statae [TA], b. da próstata. SIN *base* of prostate.
  b. pulmo'nis [TA], b. do pulmão. SIN *base* of lung.
  b. pyram'idis re'nis, b. da pirâmide renal. SIN *base* of renal pyramid.
  b. stape'dis [TA], b. do estribo. SIN *base* of stapes.

ba·si·sphe·noid (ba'si-sfe'noyd). Basiesfenóide; relativo à base ou corpo do osso esfenóide; indica o centro independente de ossificação no embrião que forma a porção posterior do corpo do osso esfenóide.

ba·si·tem·po·ral (ba'si-tem'po-răl). Basitemporal; relativo à parte inferior da região temporal.

ba·si·ver·te·bral (ba'si-ver'te-brăl). Basivertebral; relativo ao corpo de uma vértebra.

bas·ket. 1. Uma arborização em forma de cesta do axônio das células no córtex cerebelar que circunda o corpo celular das células de Purkinje. **2.** Qualquer dispositivo ou estrutura em forma de cesta. [I. M. do Celta]
  fibrillar b.'s, cestas fibrilares; a terminação escleral das fibras de Müller da neuróglia que, como fibrilas finas, e com largura decrescente e semelhantes a

agulha, ascendem nas partes proximais dos cones e bastonetes, conferindo a elas um aspecto fibrilar.
  Stokes b., c. de Stokes; maca de salvamento trançada em metal.
  stone b., c. de cálculo; um instrumento introduzido em um endoscópio para capturar e extrair cálculos urinários.

Basle Nom·i·na An·a·tom·i·ca (BNA). Nomenclatura Anatômica da Basiléia; o nome adotado em 1895 na Basiléia, Suíça (pronúncia francesa, Basle) por membros da Sociedade Anatômica Alemã que se reuniram para compilar uma nomenclatura latina dos termos anatômicos. As revisões da nomenclatura resultante foram publicadas em intervalos até que, em 1955 em Paris, França, o colegiado internacional do Congress of Anatomists adotou uma modificação da terminologia da Nomenclatura Anatômica da Basiléia. Essa modificação omitiu a referência ao local do encontro original. VER Nomina Anatomica, *Terminologia Anatomica*.

△ **baso-.** VER basi-.

ba·so·cyte (ba'so-sit). Basócito. SIN basophilic *leukocyte*. [G. *basis*, base, + *kytos*, célula]

ba·so·cy·to·pe·nia (ba'so-si-to-pe'ne'ă). Basocitopenia. SIN basophilic *leukopenia*.

ba·so·cy·to·sis (ba'so-si-to'sis). Basocitose. SIN basophilic *leucocytosis*.

ba·so·e·ryth·ro·cyte (ba'so-e-rith'ro-sit). Basoeritrócito; eritrócito que manifesta alterações de degeneração basofílica, como a granulação basófila, basofilia puntiforme ou grânulos basófilos.

ba·so·e·ryth·ro·cy·to·sis (ba'so-ĕ-rith'ro-si-to'sis). Basoeritrocitose; aumento de eritrócitos com alterações degenerativas basófilas, freqüentemente observado em doenças caracterizadas por anemia hipocrômica prolongada.

ba·so·lat·er·al (ba'so-lat'er-ăl). Basolateral; basal e lateral; especificamente utilizado para se referir a uma das duas principais divisões citológicas do complexo amigdalóide. VER amigdaloid *body*.

ba·so·met·a·chro·mo·phil, ba·so·met·a·chro·mo·phile (ba'so-met-ă-kro'mo-fil, -fil). Basometacromófilo; que se cora metacromaticamente com um corante básico. VER metachromasia.

ba·so·pe·nia (ba-so-pe'ne-ă). Basopenia. SIN basophilic *leukopenia*. [baso- + G. *penia*, pobreza]

ⓘ **ba·so·phil, ba·so·phile** (ba'so-fil, -fil). Basófilo. **1.** Uma célula com grânulos que se coram especificamente com corantes básicos. **2.** SIN basophilic. **3.** Um leucócito fagocítico do sangue caracterizado por inúmeros grânulos basofílicos contendo heparina e histamina e leucotrienos; exceto por seu núcleo segmentado, é morfologicamente e fisiologicamente similar ao mastócito, embora elas se originem de diferentes células primordiais na medula óssea. [baso- + G. *phileo*, amar]
  tissue b., b. tecidual. SIN mast *cell*.

ba·so·phil·ia (ba-so-fil'e-ă). Basofilia. **1.** Uma condição em que existe um número maior que o usual de leucócitos basófilos no sangue circulante (leucocitose basofílica) ou um aumento na proporção de células basofílicas parenquimatosas em um órgão (na medula óssea, hiperplasia basofílica). **2.** Uma condição em que os eritrócitos basófilos são encontrados no sangue circulante, como em determinados casos de leucemia, anemia avançada, malária e plumbismo. SIN Grawitz b. **3.** A reação de eritrócitos imaturos aos corantes básicos, por meio da qual as células aparecem azuis ou contêm grânulos azulados. SIN basophilism.
  Grawitz b., b. de Grawitz. SIN basophilia (2).
  punctate b., b. puntiforme. SIN stippling (1).

ba·so·phil·ic (ba'so-fil'ik). Basofílico; indica os componentes do tecido que possuem uma afinidade por corantes básicos. SIN basophil (2), basophile.

ba·soph·i·lism (ba-sof'i-lizm). Basofilia. SIN basophilia.
  Cushing b., síndrome de Cushing. SIN Cushing *syndrome*.
  Cushing pituitary b., doença de Cushing. SIN Cushing *disease*.

ba·so·phil·o·cyte (ba'so-fil'o-sit). Basofilócito. SIN basophilic *leukocyte*.

ba·so·plasm (ba'so-plazm). Basoplasma; a parte do citoplasma que se cora prontamente com os corantes básicos.

Bassen, Frank A., médico norte-americano, *1903. VER B.-Kornzweig *syndrome*.

Bassini, Edoardo, cirurgião italiano, 1844–1924. VER B. *operation*; Bassini *herniorrhaphy*.

Bassler, Anthony, médico norte-americano, 1874–1959. VER B. *sign*.

bas·sor·in (bas'or-in). Bassorina; a porção insolúvel (60 a 70%) de tragacanto que se incha e forma um gel; ela contém ácidos metoxilados complexos, particularmente o ácido bassórico.

Bastedo, Walter A., médico norte-americano, 1873–1952. VER B. *sign*.

bastokinin. Bastocinina. SIN uteroglobin.

bat. Morcego; um membro dos mamíferos da ordem Chiroptera. [I. M. *bakke*]
  vampire b., m. vampiro; um membro do gênero *Desmodus*; um hospedeiro reservatório importante do vírus da raiva nas Américas Central e do Sul.

bath. 1. Banho; imersão do corpo ou de qualquer de suas partes em água ou qualquer outro meio líquido ou produtivo, ou aplicação desse meio em qualquer forma ao corpo ou a qualquer uma de suas partes. **2.** Aparelho usado para dar um b. de qualquer forma, qualificado de acordo com o meio utilizado, temperatura do meio, forma na qual o meio é aplicado, o medicamento adicionado ao meio, ou de acordo com a parte banhada. **3.** Líquido utilizado para a manutenção das atividades metabólicas ou do crescimento dos organismos vivos, p. ex., células derivadas do tecido corporal. [A.S. *baeth*]

colloid b., b. de colóide; um b. preparado ao se adicionar agentes suavizantes, como bicarbonato de sódio ou aveia, à água do banho, de modo a aliviar a irritação e o prurido.

contrast b., b. de contraste; um b. em que uma parte é imersa em água quente por um período de alguns minutos e, em seguida, na água fria, com períodos quentes e frios alternados regularmente em intervalos, usualmente de meia hora; usado para aumentar o fluxo sangüíneo para a região.

douche b., b. de ducha; a aplicação local de água na forma de uma corrente ou jato grande.

dousing b., um b. de ar quente elétrico e luminoso administrado em uma temperatura muito quente.

electric b., electrotherapeutic b., b. elétrico, b. eletroterapêutico; **(1)** um b. em que o meio é carregado com eletricidade. SIN hydroelectric b. **(2)** aplicação terapêutica de eletricidade estática, com o paciente posicionado sobre uma plataforma isolada.

Greville b., b. de Greville; tratamento obsoleto com ar quente elétrico não-luminoso fornecido em uma temperatura muito alta.

hafussi b., uma modificação do tratamento de Nauheim, apenas com as mãos e os pés do paciente sendo imersos em água quente, através da qual o gás de dióxido de carbono é passado. [Alemão, *hand*, mão, + *fuss*, pé]

hydroelectric b., b. hidroelétrico. SIN electric b. (1).

immersion b., b. de imersão; um b. terapêutico em que a pessoa como um todo ou uma parte do corpo é totalmente imersa em substância terapêutica.

light b., b. de luz; exposição terapêutica da pele à luz radiante.

Nauheim b., b. de Nauheim. SIN Nauheim *treatment*.

needle b., b. de agulha; um b. em que a água é projetada forçadamente contra o corpo em muitos jatos bastante finos.

oil b., b. de óleo; em química, um vaso que contém óleo, em que um recipiente contendo uma substância a ser aquecida ou evaporada pode ser imersa.

sand b., b. de areia; em química, um arranjo pelo qual uma substância a ser tratada está em um vaso protegido da ação direta do fogo por uma camada de areia.

sitz b., b. de assento; a imersão apenas do períneo e das nádegas, com as pernas ficando para fora da banheira. [Alemão *sitzen*, sentar]

water b., b. de água; em química, um vaso que contém água, no qual pode ser imerso um recipiente que retém uma substância a ser aquecida ou evaporada.

batho-. Forma combinante relativa a profundidade. VER TAMBÉM bathy-. [G. *bathos*, profundidade]

bath·o·chro·mic (bath-ō-krō′mik). Batocrômico; indicando o deslocamento de um espectro de absorção máximo para um comprimento de onda maior. Oposto de hipsocrômico. [batho- + G. *chrōma*, coloração]

bath·o·flore (bath′ō-flōr). Batofloro; um átomo ou grupo de átomos que, por sua presença em uma molécula, desloca a radiação fluorescente da última na direção do comprimento de onda mais longo, ou reduz a fluorescência. Cf. auxoflore.

bath·o·pho·bia (bath-ō-fō′bē-ă). Batofobia; medo mórbido de locais profundos ou de olhar para eles. [G. *bathos*, profundidade, + *phobos*, medo]

bathy-. Forma combinante que indica profundidade. VER TAMBÉM batho-. [G. *bathys*, profundo]

bath·y·an·es·the·sia (bath′ē-an-es-thē′zē-ă). Batianestesia; perda da sensibilidade profunda, i.e., dos músculos, ligamentos, tendões, ossos e articulações. [G. *bathys*, profundo, + *an-*, priv., + *aisthēsis*, sensação]

bath·y·car·dia (bath-ē-kar′dē-ă). Baticardia; condição em que o coração ocupa uma posição inferior que o normal, mas é fixa aqui, conforme distinguido da cardioptosia. [G. *bathys*, profundo, + *kardia*, coração]

bath·y·es·the·sia (bath′ē-es-thē′zē-ă). Batiestesia; termo genérico para toda sensação a partir dos tecidos abaixo da pele, i.e., músculos, ligamentos, tendões, ossos e articulações. VER TAMBÉM myesthesia. SIN deep sensibility. [G. *bathys*, profundo, + *aisthēsis*, sensação]

bath·y·gas·try (bath-ē-gas′trē). Batigastria. SIN gastroptosis. [G. *bathys*, profundo, + *gastēr*, estômago]

bath·y·hy·per·es·the·sia (bath-ē-hī′per-es-thē′zē-ă). Bati-hiperestesia; sensibilidade exagerada das estruturas profundas, p.ex., tecido muscular. [G. *bathys*, profundo, + *hyper*, acima, + *aisthēsis*, sensação]

bath·y·hyp·es·the·sia (bath-ē-hip′es-thē′zē-ă). Bati-hipestesia; comprometimento da sensação das estruturas abaixo da pele, p.ex., tecido muscular. [G. *bathys*, profundo, + *hypo*, sob, + *aisthēsis*, sensação]

Batista, Randas, cirurgião cardíaco brasileiro do século 20. VER B. *procedure*.

ba·trach·o·tox·in (ba-tra-kō-tok′sin). Batracotoxina; uma neurotoxina a partir de rãs venenosas colombianas (*Phyllobates* spp.). É atóxica quando ingerida. Quando é injetada ou quando existe a presença de úlceras, isso provocará um aumento irreversível na permeabilidade de íons sódio na membrana nervosa, produzindo paralisia; usada em estudos farmacológicos experimentais da transmissão neuromuscular. [G. *batrachos*, rã, + toxin]

Batson, Oscar V., otorrinolaringologista norte-americano, 1894–1979. VER B. *plexus*; Carmody-B. *operation*.

Batten, Frederick E., oftalmologista britânico, 1865–1918. VER B.-Mayou *disease*; B. *disease*.

bat·tery (bat′er-ē). Bateria; um grupo ou série de testes administrados para fins analíticos ou diagnósticos. [I. M. *batri*, metal batido, do Fr. Ant. *batre*, bater]

Halstead-Reitan b., b. de Halstead-Reitan; uma b. de exames neuropsicológicos (teste de categoria, teste de desempenho do tato, teste de Seashore, teste de percepção de sons da fala, teste de oscilação de dedos, teste de elaboração de trajeto, dinamômetro para medir a força de preensão) usada para estudar as funções de comportamento humano, incluindo a determinação dos efeitos da lesão cerebral no comportamento. SIN Tactual Performance Test.

Battle, William H., cirurgião inglês, 1855–1936. VER B. *sign*.

Bauer, Hans, anatomista alemão do século 20. VER B. chromic acid leucofuchsin *stain*.

Bauer, Walter, clínico norte-americano, *1898. VER B. *syndrome*.

Bauhin, Gaspard, anatomista suíço, 1560–1624. VER B. *gland*, *valve*.

Baumé, Antoine, químico e farmacêutico francês, 1728–1804. VER B. *scale*.

Baumès symp·tom. Sintoma de Baumès. Ver em symptom.

Baumgarten, Paul Clemens von, patologista alemão, 1848–1928. VER B. *veins*, em *vein*; Cruveilhier-B. *disease*, *murmur*, *sign*, *syndrome*.

bay (bā). Recesso, baía. **1.** Em anatomia, um recesso que contém líquido. **2.** Especialmente, o r. lacrimal.

celomic b., r. celômico; **(1)** os recessos medial e lateral em ambos os lados do mesentério urogenital do embrião; **(2)** recesso superior do vestíbulo do espaço peritoneal menor; com a formação do diafragma, uma porção do recesso direito é cortada e se torna a bolsa infracardíaca; a porção abaixo do diafragma se torna o recesso superior do saco peritoneal menor; o recesso esquerdo é perdido. SIN pneumatoenteric.

lacrimal b., r. lacrimal. SIN lacrimal *lake*.

bay·ber·ry bark (bā′ber-ē). Casca de cereira. SIN myrica.

Bayes, Thomas, matemático britânico, 1702–1761. VER B. *theorem*.

Bayle, Antoine L. J., médico francês, 1799–1858.

Bayley, Nancy, psicóloga norte-americana, *1899. VER B. *Scales of Infant Development*, em *scale*.

bay·lis·as·car·i·a·sis (bā-lē-sas′kar-ī-a-sis). Bailisascaríase; a doença provocada pelos parasitas nematódeos do gênero *Baylisascaris*; as larvas migratórias do parasita do guaxinim *B. procyonis* podem causar uma doença grave do sistema nervoso central em várias espécies de animais selvagens e domésticas e, raramente, em seres humanos; a doença humana foi manifestada como uma meningoencefalite eosinofílica fatal ou uma neurorretinite subaguda unilateral difusa.

Bay·lis·as·ca·ris (bāy-lis-as′kā-ris). Gênero de nematódeos ascarídeos encontrado no intestino de mamíferos.

B. procyonis, um grande verme comumente encontrado em guaxinins; é a causa da larva migrans visceral humana e da larva migrans ocular, após a ingestão acidental dos ovos *B. procyonis* embrionado nas fezes de guaxinins infectados. VER TAMBÉM visceral *larva migrans*.

bay·o·net (bā-ō-net′). Baioneta; instrumento que tem uma lâmina ou extremidade pontiaguda que se salienta e fica em paralelo com a diáfise. [Fr. *bayonette*, de *Bayonne*, França, onde foi fabricado pela primeira vez]

Bazett, Henry C., cardiologista inglês, *1885. VER Bazett *formula*.

Bazex, A., médico francês do século 20. VER Bazex *syndrome*.

Bazin, Antoine P. E., dermatologista francês, 1807–1878. VER B. *disease*.

BBB Abreviatura de blood-brain *barrier* (barreira hematoencefálica).

BBC Abreviatura de bromobenzylcyanide (bromobenzilcianeto).

BBOT Abreviatura de 2,5-bis(5-*t*-butilbenzoxazol-2-il)tiofeno, um cintilador líquido.

BCG Abreviatura de bacille Calmette-Guérin (bacilo de Calmette-Guérin); de ballistocardiograph (balistocardiógrafo).

BCL-2. Um oncogene que inibe apoptose.

BCNU Carmustina. + carmustine.

bdel·lin (del′in). Bdelina; um de um grupo de inibidores da protease a partir da sanguessuga. [G. *bdella*, sanguessuga, + -in]

Bdellovibrio.

B.D.S. Abreviatura de Bachelor of Dental Surgery (Bacharel em Cirurgia Dentária).

B.D.Sc. Abreviatura de Bachelor of Dental Science (Bacharel em Ciência Dentária).

Be Símbolo de berilium (berílio).

bead·ed (bēd′ed). **1.** Caracterizado por pequenas e numerosas projeções arredondadas, freqüentemente dispostas em fileira semelhante às contas de um rosário. **2.** Aplicado a uma série de colônias bacterianas não-contínuas ao longo da linha da inoculação em uma cultura repicada. **3.** Indicando as bactérias coradas em que os grânulos mais intensamente corados estão em intervalos regulares.

bead·ing (bē′ding). **1.** Numerosas projeções arredondadas e pequenas, freqüentemente em fileira semelhantes às contas de um rosário. **2.** A elevação arredondada ao longo da borda da superfície tecidual dos principais conectores de

uma prótese dentária maxilar. **3.** A proteção das bordas formadas das impressões finais para uma prótese dentária feita pela colocação de bastões de cera ou uma combinação de gesso e pedra-pome adjacente às bordas antes de formar o molde-mestre.
b. of the ribs, rosário raquítico. SIN rachitic *rosary.*
beak (bēk). Bico. **1.** O bico de alicate usado em odontologia para contornar e ajustar dispositivos dentários metálicos ou fundidos. **2.** Por vezes usado para descrever uma estrutura anatômica em formato de bico. VER rostrum. [L. *beccus*]
beak·er (bē′ker). Copázio; um vaso de vidro fino, com um lábio (bico) para despejar, usado como recipiente para líquidos.
Beale, Lionel S., médico britânico, 1828–1906. VER B. *cell.*
beam (bēm). Viga. **1.** Qualquer barra cujas curvaturas se modificam sob a carga; em odontologia, freqüentemente utilizado em lugar de "barra". **2.** Uma emissão colimada de radiação luminosa ou de outra radiação, como uma v. de raio X. [O. H. G. *Boum*]
Balkan b., b. de Balkan. SIN Balkan *frame.*
cantilever b., b. em cantiléver; em odontologia, um b. que é apoiado apenas por um suporte fixo em apenas uma de suas extremidades.
continuous b., b. contínuo; em odontologia, um b. que continua sobre três ou mais suportes, com aqueles que suportam não nas extremidades da b. sendo suportes igualmente livres.
electron b., b. de elétron; uma forma de radiação usada principalmente na radioterapia superficial. VER betatron.
restrained b., b. reprimida; em odontologia, uma b. que tem dois ou mais suportes, pelo menos um dos quais permite alguma liberdade de rotação até o ponto de sustentação, mas não tanto como se o suporte fosse um suporte livre.
simple b., b. simples; em odontologia, uma b. reta que apresenta apenas dois suportes, um em cada extremidade.
bean (bēn). Feijão; a semente achatada, contida em uma vagem, de várias plantas leguminosas. Os feijões de significado farmacológico são colocados em ordem alfabética pelo nome específico. [I. Ant. *bean*]
beard [TA]. Barba. SIN barba.
bear·ing (bār′ing). Conexão; um ponto ou superfície de sustentação.
central b., c. central; em odontologia, a aplicação de forças entre o maxilar e a mandíbula em um único ponto localizado como o mais próximo possível do centro de áreas de apoio das mandíbulas superior e inferior; usado para a finalidade de distribuir as forças de oclusão de maneira uniforme por todas as áreas das estruturas de sustentação durante o registro das relações maxilo-mandibulares e durante a correção de erros de oclusão.
bear·ing down. O esforço expulsivo de uma parturiente no segundo estágio do trabalho de parto.
beat (bēt). Batida, batimento. **1.** Bater; vibrar ou pulsar. **2.** Um batimento, impulso ou pulsação, como a do coração ou pulso. **3.** A atividade de um compartimento cardíaco produzida por capturar um estímulo produzido em outro ponto no coração. **4.** A percepção de um terceiro tom quando dois tons de freqüências ligeiramente diferentes são apresentados. **5.** Um de uma série de tons regularmente pulsantes criados pelo reforço mútuo periódico de dois tons que soam ao mesmo tempo, os quais diferem discretamente na freqüência. [A. S. *beatan*]
apex b., b. apical; a pulsação visível e/ou palpável feita pelo ápice do ventrículo esquerdo quando ele colide com a parede torácica na sístole; normalmente no quinto espaço intercostal, cerca de 10 cm à esquerda da linha média.
atrial capture b., b. de captura atrial; o ciclo cardíaco que resulta quando, depois de um período de dissociação A-V, os átrios recuperam o controle dos ventrículos; a despolarização atrial devido à transmissão retrógrada a partir de um batimento ectópico ventricular ou um impulso ventricular eletronicamente estimulado.
atrial fusion b., b. de fusão atrial; um b. que acontece quando os átrios são ativados em parte pelo impulso sinusal e, em parte, por um impulso ectópico ou retrógrado a partir da junção A-V ou ventrículo.
automatic b., b. automático; em contraste com o b. forçado, um b. ectópico que surge *de novo* e não é precipitado pelo b. precedente; dessa maneira, os batimentos escapados e parassistólicos são automáticos. SIN automatic contraction.
combination b., b. de combinação. SIN fusion b.
coupled b.'s, batimentos acoplados; os batimentos (geralmente prematuros) que reincidem em um intervalo fixo a partir de um batimento precedente (usualmente normal).
dependent b., b. dependente. SIN forced b.
Dressler b., b. de Dressler; o b. de fusão que interrompe uma taquicardia ventricular e que produz um complexo QRS normalmente estreito como uma conseqüência da fusão dos dois impulsos, um impulso a partir da taquicardia ventricular e outro de um foco supraventricular; os batimentos de Dressler suportam fortemente o diagnóstico de taquicardia ventricular por sua interrupção.
dropped b., b. solto; b. cardíaco que falha em aparecer.
echo b., b. repetido; a extra-sístole produzida pelo retorno de um impulso no coração retrógrado a um foco próximo à sua origem, que, então, retorna de forma anterógrada para produzir uma segunda despolarização.

ectopic b., b. ectópico; um b. cardíaco que se origina em algum ponto no nódulo sinoatrial.
escape b., b. de escape; um b. automático, originando-se usualmente na junção AV ou no ventrículo, que ocorre depois que falhou o próximo b. normal esperado; portanto, ele sempre é um b. tardio terminando em um ciclo mais longo que o normal. SIN escape contraction.
forced b., b. forçado; **(1)** uma extra-sístole supostamente precipitada por algum modo pelo b. normal precedente ao qual está acoplado; **(2)** uma extra-sístole causada por estimulação artificial do coração. SIN dependent b.
fusion b., b. de fusão; um b. deflagrado por mais de um impulso elétrico, quando as frentes de onda coincidem em agir juntas sobre uma única via final de atividade; no eletrocardiograma, o complexo atrial ou ventricular quando os átrios ou os ventrículos são ativados em conjunto por dois impulsos invasores simultâneos ou quase simultâneos. SIN combination b., mixed b., summation b.
heart b., b. cardíaco; um ciclo cardíaco completo, incluindo a disseminação do impulso elétrico e a conseqüente contração mecânica. SIN ictus cordis.
interference b., b. de interferência; captura ventricular na forma de dissociação AV decorrente da interferência.
mixed b., b. misto. SIN fusion b.
paired b.'s, batimentos pareados. VER bigeminy.
parasystolic b., b. parassistólico. SIN parasystole.
premature b., b. prematuro. SIN extrasystole.
pseudofusion b., b. de pseudofusão; uma representação eletrocardiográfica de uma despolarização cardíaca produzida por superposição de um estímulo de marca-passo eletrônico ineficaz após um complexo QRS que se origina de um foco espontâneo dentro do coração; o estímulo do marca-passo é ineficaz porque a descarga eletrônica, que ele representa graficamente, ocorreu dentro do período refratário absoluto do batimento espontâneo e, portanto, não é indicativo do mau funcionamento do marca-passo.
reciprocal b., b. recíproco. VER reciprocal *rhythm.*
retrograde b., b. retrógrado; um b. que ocorre como uma ativação elétrica de uma porção de um compartimento cardíaco para o compartimento de origem, p.ex., um b. atrial deflagrado por um impulso que se origina no ventrículo.
summation b., b. de somação. SIN fusion b.
ventricular fusion b., b. de fusão ventricular; um b. de fusão que ocorre quando os ventrículos são ativados parcialmente pelo seio descendente ou impulso juncional AV e parcialmente por um impulso ventricular ectópico.
Beau, Joseph H. S., médico francês, 1806–1865. VER B. *lines,* em *line.*
Beau·var·ia (bō - vā′rē - ā). Um gênero de fungos (classe Hyphomycetes). O *B. bassiana* é patogênico para insetos, é promissor no controle biológico dos insetos e produz infecção em seres humanos.
be·can·thone hy·dro·chlo·ride (be - can′thōn). Cloridrato de becantona; um esquistossomicida.
Bechterew, Vladimir M. von, neurologista russo, 1857–1927. VER B. *band; disease; layer* of B.; B. *nucleus, sign; line* of B.; *band* of Kaes-B.; B.-Mendel *reflex;* Mendel-B. *reflex.*
Beck, Claude S., cirurgião norte-americano, 1894–1971. VER B. *triad.*
Beck, Emil G., cirurgião norte-americano, 1866–1932. VER B. *method.*
Beck, E. V. V., médico russo. VER Bek.
Becker, J. P. VER B. *disease.*
Becker, Peter Emil, geneticista alemão, *1908. VER B.-type tardive muscular *dystrophy,* B. muscular *dystrophy.*
Becker, Samuel W., dermatologista norte-americano, 1894–1964. VER B. *nevus.*
Becker stain for spi·ro·chetes. Corante de Becker para espiroquetas; ver em *stain.*
Beckmann, Ernst O., químico alemão, 1853–1923. VER B. *apparatus.*
Beckwith, John Bruce, patologista norte-americano, *1933. VER B.-Wiedemann *syndrome.*
Béclard, Pierre A., anatomista francês, 1785–1825. VER ranine *anastomosis;* B. *hernia, triangle.*
be·clo·meth·a·sone di·pro·pi·o·nate (be - klō - meth′a - sōn). Dipropionato de beclometasona; um agente antiinflamatório tópico; freqüentemente utilizado por inalação na asma.
Becquerel, Antoine H., físico francês e laureado com o Prêmio Nobel, 1852–1908. VER becquerel; B. *rays,* em *ray.*
bec·que·rel (Bq) (bek - ā - rel′). Bequerel; a unidade SI de mensuração da radioatividade, igual a 1 desintegração por segundo; 1 Bq = $0{,}027 \times 10^{-9}$ Ci. [AH *Becquerel*]
bed. Leito. **1.** Em anatomia, uma base ou estrutura que suporta outra estrutura. **2.** Um pedaço de mobília utilizado para o repouso, recuperação ou tratamento.
b. of breast, l. da mama; as estruturas contra as quais a superfície posterior da mama se posiciona; inclui principalmente o músculo peitoral maior, mas também parte do músculo serrátil anterior e oblíquo externo do abdome; estende-se da segunda à sexta costela e da linha para-esternal até a axilar anterior.
capillary b., l. capilar; os capilares considerados coletivamente e suas capacidades de volume para o sangue.
fracture b., l. de fratura; um l. estreito, extrafirme, para o tratamento de fraturas; geralmente incorpora uma estrutura por sobre a cabeça para o aparelho de tração.

Gatch b., l. de Gatch; um l. com partes divididas para a elevação independente da cabeça e joelhos de um paciente.

mud b., l. de barros; um l. em que o colchão consiste em barro semilíquido de argila especial, coberto com uma lâmina de material de plástico; usado para distribuir amplamente a pressão do peso do corpo sobre a superfície dependente, para pacientes com queimaduras ou grandes áreas anestesiadas.

nail b., l. ungueal. SIN nail matrix.

parotid b., l. parotídeo; as estruturas que circundam e fazem contato com a parótida, formando os limites do espaço parotídeo: anteriormente, o ramo da mandíbula flanqueado pelo massêter e músculos pterigóides mediais; medialmente, a parede faríngea, a bainha carotídea e as estruturas que se originam do processo estilóide; posteriormente, o processo mastóide, o músculo esternocleidomastóideo e a porção carnosa posterior do músculo digástrico; superiormente, a articulação temporomandibular e o osso timpânico e a porção cartilaginosa do meato acústico externo.

b. of parotid gland, l. da glândula parótida. SIN parotid space.

b. of stomach, l. do estômago; as estruturas contra as quais a superfície pósteroinferior do estômago se posiciona, e a partir da qual é separada, em sua maior parte, pela bolsa omental; inclui o diafragma, a glândula supra-renal esquerda, a parte superior do rim esquerdo, a artéria esplênica, a face anterior do corpo e da cauda do pâncreas, a flexura cólica esquerda e o mesocólon transverso.

water b., colchão d'água; um colchão na forma de uma bolsa de borracha fechada cheia com a água; usado para evitar ou tratar as úlceras de decúbito por equalizar a distribuição do peso do paciente contra o apoio.

bed·bug. Percevejo; veja as entradas em *Cimex.*

bed·lam (bed'lăm). **1.** Coloquialismo pejorativo para uma instituição ou hospital mental. **2.** Um local ou cena de comportamento selvagem ou revoltoso. **3.** Um tumulto conturbador. [corruptela ou contração do St. Mary of *Bethlehem Hospital* em Londres]

Bednar, Alois, médico austríaco, 1816–1888. VER B. *aphthae,* em *aphtha.*

Bednar, Blahoslav, patologista checo do século 20. VER B. *tumor.*

bed·sore (bed'sōr). Úlcera de decúbito. SIN decubitus ulcer.

bed-wet·ting. Enurese. SIN nocturnal enuresis.

bee. Abelha; um inseto do gênero *Apis;* a abelha do mel, *A. mellifica,* é a fonte do mel e da cera. [A. S. *beó, bī*]

beech oil. Óleo de faia. SIN beechwood tar.

beech·wood tar (bēch'wud). Alcatrão de faia; um líquido espesso, oleoso, castanho-escuro, com o odor de creosoto; usado em grande parte como uma fonte de creosoto. SIN beech oil.

Beer, August, físico alemão, 1825–1863. VER B.-Lambert *law;* B. *law.*

Beer, Georg J., oftalmologista austríaco, 1763–1821. VER B. *knife.*

bees·wax (bēz'waks) Cera de abelha. SIN wax (1).

white b., cera branca de abelha. SIN white wax.

bee·tu·ria (bē-too'rē-ă). Betacianinúria; excreção urinária da betacianina depois da ingestão de beterrabas, encontrada na maioria dos indivíduos com deficiência de ferro e em algumas pessoas normais. SIN betacyaninuria.

Beevor, Charles E., neurologista inglês, 1854–1908. VER B. *sign.*

Begbie, James, médico escocês, 1798–1869.

Begg, P. Raymond, ortodontista australiano, *1898. VER B. light wire differential force *technique.*

Béguez César, Antonio, pediatra cubano. VER B. C. *disease.*

be·hav·ior (bē-hāv'yer). Comportamento. **1.** Qualquer resposta emitida ou provocada a partir de um organismo. **2.** Qualquer ato ou atividade mental ou motora. **3.** Especificamente, as partes de um padrão de resposta total. [I. M., do Fr. Ant. *avoir,* ter]

adaptive b., c. adaptativo; qualquer c. que possibilite que um organismo se ajuste a uma determinada situação ou movimento.

appetitive b., c. apetitivo; o movimento de um organismo no sentido de um determinado tipo de estímulo, como o alimento. Cf. aversive b.

aversive b., c. relutante; movimento de um organismo para longe de um determinado tipo de estímulo, como o choque elétrico. Cf. appetitive b.

coronary-prone b., c. propenso à doença coronária; o c. hostil que aumenta o risco de doença cardíaca.

health b., c. de saúde; a combinação de conhecimento, práticas e atitudes que, em conjunto, contribuem para motivar as ações que empreendemos no sentido da saúde.

hookean b., c. huquiano; o c. de um corpo perfeitamente elástico; i.e., o esforço é diretamente proporcional ao estresse. VER TAMBÉM Hooke *law.*

hostile b., c. hostil; o c. que aumenta o risco de doença cardíaca.

molar b., c. molar; em psicologia, o c. descrito em grandes unidades de resposta em vez das menores. Cf. molecular b.

molecular b., c. molecular; em psicologia, o c. descrito em pequenas unidades de resposta em lugar das maiores; uma resposta específica. Cf. molar b.

obsessive b., c. obsessivo; o c. estilizado repetitivo observado na neurose obsessivo-compulsiva.

operant b., c. operante; o c. cuja continuação e freqüência são determinadas por suas conseqüências sobre o autor; o elemento central de teoria de condicionamento comportamental. VER conditioning.

passive-aggressive b., c. passivo-agressivo; o c. aparentemente complacente, com as qualidades obstrutivas ou inflexíveis intrínsecas, para cobrir os sentimentos agressivos profundamente percebidos que não podem ser expressos de forma mais direta.

respondent b., c. respondente; o c. em resposta a um estímulo específico; usualmente associado ao condicionamento clássico. VER conditioning.

ritualistic b., c. ritualista; o c. automático de origem psicogênica ou cultural.

target b., c.-alvo; **(1)** SIN operant; **(2)** na terapia de modificação do c., o c. prescrito.

type A b., c. do tipo A; padrão de c. caracterizado por agressividade, ambição, inquietação e forte sensação de urgência de tempo. Novas pesquisas revelam que é a hostilidade, que pode ser entremeada com outros traços do tipo A, que está associada ao risco aumentado de cardiopatia coronária.

type B b., c. do tipo B; padrão de c. caracterizado pela ausência ou o reverso das características do c. de tipo A.

be·hav·ior·al (bē-hāv'yer-ăl). Comportamental; pertinente ao comportamento.

be·hav·ior·al sci·enc·es. Ciências comportamentais; termo coletivo para as disciplinas ou ramos da ciência, como a psicologia, a sociologia e a antropologia, e que derivam suas teorias, conceitos e condutas a partir da observação e do estudo do comportamento dos organismos vivos.

be·hav·ior·ism (bē-hāv'yer-izm). Behaviorismo; ramo da psicologia que formula, através da observação e experimentação sistemáticas, as leis e os princípios que fundamentam o comportamento de seres humanos e animais; suas principais contribuições foram feitas nas áreas de condicionamento e aprendizado. SIN behavioral psychology.

be·hav·ior·ist (bē-hāv'yer-ist). Behaviorista; partidário do behaviorismo.

Behçet, Hulusi, dermatologista turco, 1889–1948. VER B. *disease, syndrome.*

be·hen·ic ac·id (bē-hen'ik). Ácido behênico; $CH_3(CH_2)_{20}COOH$; um constituinte da maioria das gorduras e óleos de peixe; grandes quantidades são encontradas na semente de mostarda, óleo de semente de colza e cerebrosídeos. SIN *n-*docosanoic acid.

Behr, Carl J. P., oftalmologista alemão, 1874–1943. VER B. *disease, syndrome.*

Behring, Emil A. von, bacteriologista alemão e laureado com o Prêmio Nobel, 1854–1917. VER B. *law.*

BEI. Abreviatura para butanol-extractable *iodine* (iodo extraído do butanol).

bej·el. Bejel; sífilis endêmica não-venérea agora encontrada principalmente em crianças árabes; aparentemente causada pelo *Treponema pallidum.* VER TAMBÉM nonvenereal *syphilis.* [Ár. *bajlah*]

Bek (ou Beck), E. V., médico russo. VER Kashin-B. *disease.*

Békésy, Georg von, biofísico húngaro nos Estados Unidos e laureado com o Prêmio Nobel, 1899–1972. VER B. *audiometer, audiometry.*

bel. Bel; unidade que expressa a intensidade relativa de um som. A intensidade em bels é o logaritmo (de base 10) da proporção da potência do som para aquela de um som de referência. Comumente, supõe-se que o som de referência seja aquele com uma potência de 10^{-16} watts por cm^2, aproximadamente o limiar de um ouvido humano normal a 1000 Hz. [A. G. *Bell,* cientista escocês-norteamericano, 1847–1922]

belch·ing. Eructação. SIN eructation. [A. S. *baelcian*]

bel·em·noid (be-lem'noyd). Belemnóide; em forma de flecha. [G. *belemnon,* uma flecha, + *eidos,* semelhança]

Bell, John, cirurgião e anatomista escocês, 1763–1820. VER B. *muscle.*

Bell, Sir Charles, cirurgião, anatomista e fisiologista escocês, 1774–1842. VER B. *law,* B.-Magendie *law;* B. respiratory *nerve, palsy, spasm;* external respiratory *nerve* of B.

bel·la·don·na (bel-ă-don'ă). Beladona; *Atropa belladonna* (família Solanaceae); uma erva perene com flores púrpuras escuras e sementes pretas purpúreas e brilhantes; as folhas (0,3% de alcalóides da beladona) e a raiz (0,5% dos alcalóides da beladona) eram originalmente a fonte da atropina e dos alcalóides correlatos, que são anticolinérgicos; a B. é usada como um pó (0,3% dos alcalóides da beladona, calculados como hiosciamina) e tintura na diarréia, asma, cólica e hiperacidez. SIN deadly nightshade. [It. *bella,* bonita, + *donna,* dama]

bel·la·don·nine (bel-ă-don'ēn). Beladonina; um alcalóide artificial derivado da atropina por aquecimento com o ácido clorídrico.

bell-crowned (bel'krownd). Coroa em forma de sino; indica um dente cuja coroa apresenta um diâmetro transverso muito maior que o colo.

belle in·dif·fér·ence. Bela indiferença; VER la belle indifférence.

Bellini, Lorenzo, médico e anatomista italiano, 1643-1704. VER B. *ducts,* em *duct, ligament.*

bel·ly (bel'ē). Ventre. **1.** O abdome. **2.** A parte ampla e tumefata de um músculo. SIN venter (2) [TA]. **3.** Popularmente, o estômago ou a barriga. [I. A. *belig,* saco]

anterior b. of digastric muscle [TA], v. anterior do músculo digástrico; a porção do músculo digástrico que se estende anteriormente a partir do tendão intermediário e se insere na face posterior da mandíbula. SIN venter anterior musculi digastrici [TA].

b.'s of digastric muscle, ventres do músculo digástrico. VER anterior b. of digastric muscle, posterior b. of digastric muscle.

frontal b. of occipitofrontalis muscle [TA], v. frontal do músculo occipitofrontal; o v. anterior do músculo occipitofrontal. VER occipitofrontalis (*muscle*). SIN venter frontalis musculi occipitofrontalis [TA], frontalis muscle.
inferior b. of omohyoid b. [TA], v. inferior do músculo omoióide; o v. inferior do músculo omoióide, inserido na borda superior da escápula. SIN venter inferior musculi omohyoidei [TA].
occipital b. of occipitofrontalis muscle [TA], v. occipital do músculo occipitofrontal; o v. posterior do músculo occipitofrontal. VER occipitofrontalis (*muscle*). SIN venter occipitalis musculi occipitofrontalis [TA], occipitalis muscle.
b.'s of omohyoid muscle, ventres do músculo omoióide. VER inferior b. of omohyoid b., superior b. of omohyoid muscle.
posterior b. of digastric muscle [TA], v. posterior do músculo digástrico; porção do músculo digástrico posterior ao tendão intermediário, que se insere no sulco digástrico do osso temporal. SIN venter posterior musculi digastrici [TA].
prune b., v. de ameixa seca. SIN abdominal muscle deficiency *syndrome*.
superior b. of omohyoid muscle [TA], v. superior do músculo omoióide; o v. superior do músculo omoióide, inserido no osso hióide. SIN venter superior musculi omohyoidei [TA].
bel·ly·ache (bel′ē - āk). Dor de barriga; coloquialismo para a dor abdominal, usualmente em cólica.
bel·ly but·ton (bel′ē - but′ŏn). Umbigo. SIN umbilicus.
bel·o·ne·pho·bia (bel′ō - nē - fō′bē - ă). Belonefobia; medo mórbido de agulhas, alfinetes e outros objetos pontiagudos. [G. *belonē*, agulha, + *phobos*, medo]
Belsey, Ronald, cirurgião britânico do século 20. VER Belsey *fundoplication*; B. Mark *operation*, *procedure*; Collis-Belsey *fundoplication*; Collis-B. *procedure*.
bem·e·gride (bem′ē - grīd). Bemegrida; um estimulante do sistema nervoso central originalmente utilizado como um analéptico em intoxicações decorrentes de barbitúricos e outros medicamentos depressores do sistema nervoso central.
ben. Abreviatura para L. *bene*, bem.
ben·ac·ty·zine hy·dro·chlo·ride (ben - ak′ti - zēn). Cloridrato de benactizina; um medicamento anticolinérgico com as mesmas ações, mas com aproximadamente um quinto da atividade da atropina; acredita-se que eleve o limiar da reação emocional aos estímulos externos; agora raramente utilizado como um agente psicoterápico e tranqüilizante.
Bence Jones, Henry, médico britânico, 1814–1873. VER B. J. *albumin*, *cylinders*, em *cylinder*, *myeloma*, *proteins*, em *protein*, *reaction*.
ben·da·zac (ben′dă - zak). Bendazac; um agente antiinflamatório tópico.
Bender, Lauretta, psiquiatra norte-americana, 1897–1987. VER B. gestalt *test*. Visual Motor Gestalt *test*.
ben·dro·flu·a·zide (ben - drō - flooā - zīd). Bendrofluazida. SIN bendroflumethiazide.
ben·dro·flu·me·thi·a·zide (ben′drō - floo′mĕ - thīā - zīd). Bendroflumetiazida; um diurético tiazídico e agente anti-hipertensivo. SIN bendrofluazide.
bends (bendz). Mal dos mergulhadores; coloquialismo para a doença do caixão; doença da descompressão. [da postura convulsiva daqueles afetados]
ben·e·cep·tor (ben′ē - sep′ter, tōr). Beneceptor; um mecanismo ou órgão nervoso (ceptor) para a apreciação e transmissão dos estímulos de um caráter benéfico. Cf. nociceptor. [L. *bene*, bem, + *capio*, captar]
Benedek, Ladislaus (László), neurologista austríaco, 1887–1945. VER B. *reflex*.
Benedict, Francis G., metabolista norte-americano, 1870–1957. VER B.-Roth *apparatus*, *calorimeter*.
Benedict, Stanley R., químico norte-americano, 1884–1936. VER B. *solution*, *test* for glucose; B.-Hopkins-Cole *reagent*.
Benedikt, Moritz, médico austríaco, 1835–1920. VER B. *syndrome*.
ben·e·fi·cence (be - nef′ĭ - sens). Beneficência; o princípio ético de fazer o bem. [L. *beneficentia*, de *bene*, bem, + *facio*, fazer]
be·nign (bē - nīn′). Benigno; indica o caráter brando de uma doença ou o caráter não-maligno de uma neoplasia. [através do Fr. Ant., do L. *benignus*, benévolo]
ben·ne oil. (ben′nĕ). Óleo de gergelim. SIN sesame oil.
Bennett, Edward H., cirurgião irlandês, 1837–1907. VER B. *fracture*.
Bennett, Norman G., dentista britânico, 1870–1947. VER B. *angle*, *movement*.
Bennhold, H., médico alemão, *1893. VER B. Congo red *stain*.
ben·ox·a·pro·fen (ben - oks - ă - prō′fen). Benoxaprofeno; agente antiinflamatório não-esteróide e analgésico, não mais utilizado clinicamente.
ben·per·i·dol (ben - per′ĭ - dol). Benperidol; tranqüilizante. SIN benzperidol.
ben·ser·a·zide (ben - ser′ă - zīd). Benserazida; um inibidor da descarboxilase do aminoácido *l*-aromático (dopa-descarboxilase) que se assemelha à carbidopa em ação; administrada em combinação com a levodopa como um esquema antiparkinsoniano. A benserazida evita a destruição periférica da levodopa e, dessa maneira, reduz os efeitos colaterais cardiovasculares do tratamento.
Bensley, Robert R., anatomista canadense-norte-americano, 1867–1956. VER B. specific *granules*, em *granule*.

ben·tir·o·mide (ben - tir′ō - mīd). Bentiromida; um peptídeo utilizado em um teste de rastreamento para a insuficiência pancreática exócrina e para monitorar a adequação da terapia pancreática suplementar.
ben·ton·ite (ben′ton - īt). Bentonita; silicato de alumínio hidratado coloidal natural; uma argila absorvente encontrada no oeste dos Estados Unidos; é por vezes utilizada no tratamento de diarréia e de distúrbios cutâneos, tendo sido usada como um agente de suspensão em loções. [Fort *Benton*, Montana, + -ite)
△ **benz-.** Forma combinante que indica a associação com o benzeno.
ben·zal·ac·e·to·phe·none (ben′zal - as - e - tō - fē′nōn). Benzalacetofenona. SIN chalcone.
ben·zal·cou·mar·an-3-one (ben - zal - kooˊmar - an - thrē′ōn). Benzalcumaran-3-ona. SIN aurone.
benz·al·de·hyde (ben - zal′dĕ - hīd). Benzaldeído; um aldeído produzido artificialmente ou obtido do óleo de amêndoa amarga, contendo não menos que 80% de b.; um agente flavorizante utilizado em medicamentos administrados por via oral. SIN benzoic aldehyde.
ben·zal·ko·ni·um chlo·ride (ben - zal - kō′nē - ŭm). Cloreto de benzalcônio. Uma mistura de cloretos de alquilbenzildimetilamônio em que as alquilas são compostos de cadeia longa (C_8 a C_{18}); um germicida superficial ativo para muitas bactérias patogênicas não-formadoras de esporos e fungos. As soluções aquosas desse agente apresentam uma baixa tensão superficial, e possuem propriedades detergentes, ceratolíticas e emulsificantes que auxiliam na penetração e no umedecimento das superfícies dos tecidos.
benz[*a*]an·thra·cene (ben - zan′thră - sēn). Benzantraceno; 1,2-benzantraceno; um hidrocarboneto carcinogênico. SIN benzanthrene.
ben·zan·threne (ben - zan′thren). Benzantreno. SIN benz[*a*]anthracene.
ben·zene (ben′zēn). Benzeno; a estrutura básica na maioria dos compostos aromáticos; um hidrocarboneto altamente tóxico a partir do óleo do alcatrão leve; usado como um solvente. SIN benzol, coal tar naphtha. [*benzoin* + -ene]
b. bromide, brometo de b.; gás lacrimejante.
ben·zene·a·mine (ben - zēn′ă - mēn). Benzenoamina. SIN aniline.
(γ)-ben·zene hex·a·chlo·ride. Cloreto de (γ)-benzeno. VER lindane.
ben·zes·trol (ben - zes′trol). Benzestrol; uma substância estrogênica sintética.
benz·e·tho·ni·um chlo·ride (benz - ĕ - thō′nē - ŭm). Cloreto de benzetônio; um composto de amônio quaternário sintético, um da classe catiônica dos detergentes; germicida e bacteriostático.
ben·zi·dine (ben′zi - dēn). Benzidina; um composto incolor e cristalino utilizado para detectar sulfatos na análise da água, para a identificação de sangue, e como um reagente em corantes especiais; como foi identificado como um carcinógeno, tem uso atual é limitado.
benz·im·id·az·ole (benz - im - id - ā′z - ōl). Benzimidazol. **1.** Um sistema de anel compreendido por um anel benzênico fundido com um anel imidazólico; ocorre na natureza como parte da molécula da vitamina B_{12}. **2.** Uma classe de anti-helmínticos, freqüentemente utilizados para tratar nematódeos e cestódeos.
ben·zin, ben·zine (ben′zin, ben - zēn). Benzina. SIN petroleum benzin.
ben·zin·da·mine hy·dro·chlo·ride (ben - zin′dă - mēn). Cloridrato de benzidamina. SIN benzydamine hydrochloride.
ben·zi·o·da·rone (ben - zē′ō - dă - rōn). Benziodarona; um vasodilatador coronariano.
ben·zo·ate (ben′zō - āt). Benzoato; um sal ou éster do ácido benzóico. Os sais são freqüentemente utilizados como conservantes farmacêuticos ou alimentares.
ben·zo·at·ed (ben′zō - āt - ed). Benzoatado; que contém ácido benzóico ou um benzoato, usualmente benzoato de sódio.
ben·zo·caine (ben′zō - kān). Benzocaína; o éster etílico do ácido *p*-aminobenzóico; um agente anestésico tópico. SIN ethyl aminobenzoate.
ben·zo·di·az·e·pine (ben′zō - dī - az′ĕ - pēn). Benzodiazepina. **1.** O composto original para a síntese de inúmeros compostos psicoativos (p.ex., diazepam, clordiazepóxido). **2.** Benzodiazepínicos; uma classe de compostos com propriedades ansiolíticas, hipnóticas, anticonvulsivantes e relaxantes da musculatura esquelética.
ben·zo·ic (ben - zō′ik). Benzóico; relativo ou derivado da benzoína.
ben·zo·ic ac·id. Ácido benzóico; ocorre naturalmente na benzoína; é utilizado como um conservante alimentar, localmente como um fungistático e oralmente como um anti-séptico. É rapidamente excretado como ácido hipúrico. SIN benzoyl hydrate, flowers of benzoin.
ben·zo·ic al·de·hyde. Aldeído benzóico. SIN benzaldehyde.
ben·zo·in (ben′zō - in, ben′zoyn). Benzoína; uma resina balsâmica obtida a partir do *Styrax benzoin* (família Styracaceae), usado como um expectorante estimulante, mas, em geral, por inalação na laringite e bronquite; retarda a rancidificação de gorduras e é utilizado, com essa finalidade, no toucinho benzoinatado oficial. [It. *benzoino*, do Ár. *lubān jāwī*, incenso de Java]
ben·zol (ben′zol). Benzol. SIN benzene.
ben·zo·mor·phan (ben - zō - mōr′fan). Benzomorfan; o composto original de uma série de analgésicos, incluindo a pentazocina e a fenazocina; não possui propriedades analgésicas próprias.
ben·zo·na·tate (ben - zō′nă - tāt). Benzonatato; um agente antitussígeno relacionado quimicamente à tetracaína; acredita-se que atue por deprimir os mecanorreceptores nos pulmões.

ben·zo·pur·pu·rin 4B (ben - zō - per′pū - rin) [C. I. 23500]. Benzopurpurina 4B; um corante ácido vermelho, originalmente usado como um corante e como um indicador (alterações do violeta para o vermelho na faixa de pH de 1,2 a 4,0).

1,4-ben·zo·qui·none (ben - zō - kwin′ōn). 1,4-benzoquinona. **1.** Uma parte essencial da coenzima Q e da vitamina E, redutível em hidroquinona. SIN quinone (2). **2.** Um de uma classe de derivados da benzoquinona.

ben·zo·qui·no·ni·um chlo·ride (ben′zō - kwi - nō′ne - ŭm). Cloreto de benzoquinônio; um relaxante muscular esquelético.

ben·zo·res·in·ol (ben - zō - res′i - nol). Benzorresinol; um constituinte resinoso da benzoína.

ben·zo·sul·fi·mide (ben - zō - sŭl′fi - mīd). Benzossulfimida. SIN saccharin.

ben·zo·thi·a·di·a·zides (ben′zō - thī - a - dī′a - zīdz). Benzotiadiazidas; uma classe de diuréticos que aumentam a excreção de sódio e cloreto e um volume acompanhante de água, independentemente das alterações no equilíbrio ácido-básico; a maioria dos compostos nesse grupo é formada por análogos do 1,2,4-benzotiadiazina-1,1-dióxido. VER TAMBÉM benzthiazide.

ben·zox·i·quine (ben - zoks′i - kwin). Benzoxiquina; um desinfetante. SIN benzoxyline.

ben·zox·y·line (ben - zoks′i - lēn). Benzoxilina. SIN benzoxiquine.

ben·zo·yl (ben - zō - il). Benzoil; o radical do ácido benzóico, C_6H_5CO-, que forma benzoil compostos.
  b. chloride, cloreto de benzoíla; um líquido incolor de odor pungente; um reagente para reações de acilação.
  b. hydrate, hidrato de benzoíla. SIN benzoic acid.
  b. peroxide, peróxido de benzoíla; feito pela interação do peróxido de sódio e cloreto de benzoíla; usado em óleos como uma aplicação em úlceras e queimaduras e escaldaduras, na promoção da polimerização das resinas dentárias, e como um ceratolítico no tratamento da acne.

benz·oy·lec·gon·ine (ben′zō - il - ek′gō - nēn). Benzoilecgonina; um metabólito da cocaína produzido por hidrólise; pode ser encontrada na urina. SIN ecgonine benzoate.

ben·zo·yl·pas cal·ci·um (ben - zō′il - pas). Benzoil-PAS-cálcio; um agente antituberculoso.

benz·per·i·dol (benz - per′i - dol). Benzoperidol. SIN benperidol.

benz·phet·a·mine hy·dro·chlo·ride (benz - fet′a - mēn). Cloridrato de benzofetamina; um agente simpaticomimético usado como um anoréxico.

benz·py·rene (benz - pī′rēn). Benzopireno; um carcinógeno ambiental encontrado na exaustão de combustível de jatos, fumaça de cigarro e metais muito aquecidos em carvão; um poderoso indutor enzimático.

benz·pyr·in·i·um bro·mide (benz - pī - rin′ē - ŭm). Brometo de benzopirínio; um medicamento colinérgico com ação e usos similares àqueles da neostigmina. SIN benzstigminum bromidum.

benz·quin·a·mide (benz - kwin′a - mīd). Benzoquinamida; uma amida da benzoquinolina usada como um agente antiemético.

benz·stig·mi·num bro·mi·dum (benz - stig′mi - nŭm). Brometo de benzoestigmina. SIN benzpyrinium bromide.

benz·thi·a·zide (benz - thī′a - zīd). Benzotiazida; um diurético e agente anti-hipertensivo.

benz·tro·pine mes·y·late (benz - trō′pēn). Mesilato de benzotropina; agente parassimpaticolítico com ações semelhantes às da atropina e anti-histamínicas.

ben·zyd·a·mine hy·dro·chlo·ride (ben - zid′a - mēn). Cloridrato de benzidamina; analgésico e antipirético. SIN benzindamine hydrochloride.

ben·zyl (ben′zil). Benzila; o radical de hidrocarboneto, $C_6H_5CH_2-$.
  b. alcohol, álcool benzílico; $C_6H_5CH_2OH$; possui propriedades anestésicas locais e bacteriostáticas. SIN phenmethylol, phenylcarbinol.
  b. benzoate, benzoato de benzila; um agente que reduz a contratilidade do tecido muscular liso, possuindo acentuadas propriedades antiespasmódicas; usado atualmente com um pediculicida e escabicida.
  b. benzoate-chlorophenothane-ethyl aminobenzoate, benzoato de benzila-clorofenotano-etil aminobenzoato; uma mistura de três componentes utilizados em emulsões ou pomadas.
  b. carbinol, carbinol benzílico. SIN phenylethyl alcohol.
  b. cinnamate, cinamato benzílico; um constituinte de bálsamo-do-peru, bálsamo-de-tolu e estoraque. SIN cinnamein.
  b. fumarate, fumarato de benzila; usado para os mesmos propósitos do benzoato de b.
  b. mandelate, mandelato de benzila; o éster de benzila do ácido mandélico, que possui ação antiespasmódica similar à do benzoato de benzila.
  b. succinate, succinato de b.; a ação e dosagem são idênticas às do benzoato de benzila.

ben·zyl·ic (ben - zil′ik). Benzílico; relativo a ou que contém benzila.

ben·zyl·i·dene (ben - zil′i - dēn). Benzilideno; o radical de hidrocarboneto, $C_6H_5CH=$.

ben·zyl·iso·quin·o·lines (ben′zil - ī - sō - kwin - ō - linz). Benzilisoquinolinas; um grupo de alcalóides encontrados principalmente nos vegetais da papoula (Papaveraceae). Os alcalóides do curare são bisbenzilisoquinolinas.

ben·zyl·ox·y·car·bon·yl (Z, Cbz) (ben′zil - ok - sē - kar′bon - il). Benziloxicarbonila; radical amino-protetor usado (como o cloreto) na síntese peptídica, fornecendo $PhCH_2OCO-NHR$. SIN carbobenzoxy-.

ben·zyl·pen·i·cil·lin (ben′zil - pen - i - sil′in). Benzilpenicilina. SIN penicillin G.

be·phen·i·um hy·drox·y·naph·tho·ate (be - fen′ē - ŭm hī - droks′ē - naf′thō - āt). Hidroxinaftoato de befênio; um medicamento utilizado contra *Ancylostoma duodenale* e *Necator americanus* (nematódeos do homem); atualmente substituído em grande parte pelo mebendazol.

BER Abreviatura para basic electrical *rhythm* (ritmo elétrico básico).

Beradinelli, Waldemar, médico argentino, 1903–1956. VER B. *syndrome.*

Bérard, Auguste, cirurgião francês, 1802–1846. VER B. *aneurysm.*

Béraud, Bruno J., cirurgião francês, 1825–1865. VER B. *valve.*

ber·ber·ine (ber′ber - ēn). Berberina; um alcalóide do *Hydrastis canadensis* (família Berberidaceae); tem sido utilizado como um antimalárico, antipirético e carminativo, e externamente para úlceras indolentes.

be·reave·ment (bē - rēv - ment). Perda; um estado agudo de tristeza psicológica intensa e de sofrimento experimentados depois da perda trágica de uma pessoa amada ou de alguma posse inestimável. [I. M., *bireven,* privar, + -ment]

Berger, Emil, oftalmologista austríaco, 1855–1926. VER B. *space.*

Berger, Hans, neurologista alemão, 1873–1941. VER B. *rhythm.*

Berger, Jean, nefrologista francês do século 20. VER B. *disease,* focal *glomerulonephritis.*

Berger cells. Células de Berger, Ver em cell.

Bergman, Harry, urologista norte-americano, 1912–1998. VER B. *sign.*

Bergmann, Gottlieb H., neurologista e anatomista alemão, 1781–1861. VER B. *cords,* em *cord, fibers,* em *fiber.*

Bergmeister, O; oftalmologista austríaco, 1845–1918. VER B. *papilla.*

Berg stain. Corante de Berg. Ver em stain.

ber·i·beri, beri beri (ber′ē - ber′ē). Beribéri; síndrome de deficiência nutricional específica que ocorre na forma endêmica no Leste e Sudeste da Ásia, esporadicamente em outras partes do mundo sem referência ao clima e, por vezes, em alcoólatras, resultando principalmente de deficiência de tiamina na dieta; a forma "seca" é caracterizada por polineurite dolorosa; é mais provável que os nervos sensoriais sejam mais afetados que os nervos motores, com os sintomas começando nos pés e ascendendo; as mãos são afetadas numa fase avançada da doença; a forma "úmida" caracteriza-se por edema que resulta de uma forma de alto débito de insuficiência cardíaca. VER TAMBÉM nutritional *polyneuropathy.* SIN endemic neuritis. [Senegalês, fraqueza extrema]
  dry b., b. seca; b. paraplégica, afetando principalmente os nervos periféricos; seu padrão clínico é predominantemente o de uma polineuropatia sem insuficiência cardíaca associada.
  infantile b., b. infantil; b. que aparece em lactentes aleitados, cujas mães possuem b. decorrente de deficiência de tiamina. É principalmente a forma "úmida" de b., caracterizada por insuficiência cardíaca com edema periférico acentuado (algo incomum na insuficiência cardíaca no lactente). Uma doença frequentemente fatal, com estabelecimento agudo, que era originalmente comum nos países do Extremo Oriente, onde o arroz é consumido; reversível com tiamina.
  ship b., b. do navio; forma de deficiência de tiamina observada em marinheiros.
  wet b., b. úmida; b. edemaciada, na qual insuficiência cardíaca congestiva acompanha a polineuropatia.

berke·li·um (Bk) (berk′lē - um). Berquélio, berkélio; elemento radioativo transurânico artificial; número atômico 97, peso atômico 247,07. [*Berkeley,* CA, cidade onde foi preparado pela primeira vez]

Berlin, Rudolf, oftalmologista alemão, 1833–1897. VER B. *edema.*

Ber·lin blue [C.I. 77510]. Azul da Prússia; ferrocianeto férrico; um corante usado para os estudos de injeção dos vasos sangüíneos e vasos linfáticos, e na coloração de siderócitos. SIN Prussian blue.

Bernard, Claude, fisiologista francês, 1813–1878. VER B. *canal, duct, puncture;* B.-Cannon *homeostasis;* B.-Horner *syndrome;* B.-Sergent *syndrome.*

Bernard, Jean, médico francês, *1907. VER B.-Soulier *disease, syndrome.*

Bernays, Augustus C., cirurgião norte-americano, 1854–1907. VER B. *sponge.*

Bernhardt, Martin, neurologista alemão, 1844–1915. VER B. *disease;* B.-Roth *syndrome.*

Bernhardt for·mu·la. Fórmula de Bernhardt. Ver em formula.

Bernheim, P., médico francês do início do século 20. VER Bernheim *syndrome.*

Bernoulli, Daniel, matemático suíço, 1700–1782. VER B. *effect, law, principle, theorem.*

Bernoulli tri·al. Ensaio de Bernoulli; um evento ao acaso único para o qual existem dois e apenas dois resultados possíveis que são mutuamente excludentes e têm *a priori* probabilidades fixas (e complementares) de resultado. O ensaio é a realização desse processo. De maneira convencional, um resultado é denominado um sucesso e é atribuída a pontuação 1, o outro é um fracasso e tem pontuação zero. Dessa maneira, o resultado poderia ser 0 (nenhuma cabeça, uma cauda) ou 1 (1 cabeça, nenhuma cauda).

Bernstein, Lionel M., clínico norte-americano, *1923. VER B. *test.*

Berry, Sir James, cirurgião canadense, 1860–1946. VER B. *ligaments,* em *ligament.*

Berson, Solomon A., clínico norte-americano, 1918–1972. VER B. *test.*

Berthelot, Pierre Eugene Marcellin, químico francês, 1827–1907. VER B. *reaction*.
Berthollet, Claude L., químico francês, 1748–1822. VER B. *law*.
Bertiella studeri (ber-tē-el′ă stood-er′ē). Cestódeo comum encontrado em primatas; foram reportadas infecções zoonóticas acidentais em seres humanos nos trópicos.
ber·ti·el·lo·sis (ber′tē-ĕ-lō′sis). Bertielose; infecção de primatas, inclusive seres humanos, com cestódeos do gênero *Bertiella*.
Bertin, Exupère Joseph, anatomista francês, 1712–1781. VER B. *bones*, em *bone*, *columns*, em *column*, *ligament*, *ossicles*, em *ossicle*.
Bertrand, Ivan Georges, neurologista francês do século 20. VER Canavan-van Bogaert-Bertrand *disease*.
be·ryl·li·o·sis (be-ril-ē-ō′sis). Beriliose; intoxicação por berílio caracterizada por pneumonia aguda ou fibrose granulomatosa intersticial crônica, especialmente dos pulmões, decorrente da inalação do berílio.
be·ryl·li·um (Be) (be-ril′ē-ŭm). Berílio; elemento metálico branco que pertence aos alcalinos terrosos; número atômico 4, peso atômico 9,012 182. [G. *beryllos*, berílio]
Berzelius, J. J., químico sueco, 1779–1848.
Besnier, Ernest H., dermatologista francês, 1831–1909. VER B. *prurigo*, B.-Boeck-Schaumann *syndrome*.
Bes·noi·ti·i·dae (bes-noy′tē-i-dē). Família de protozoários parasitas similares aos da família Toxoplasmatidae, à qual o gênero *Besnoitia* pertence.
Best, Franz, patologista alemão, 1878–1920. VER B. *disease*, carmine *stain*.
bes·ti·al·i·ty (bes-tē-al′i-tē). Bestialidade. SIN zoophilia. [L. *bestia*, fera]
be·syl·ate (bes′il-āt). Besilato; contração aprovada pela USAN para benzenossulfonato.
be·ta (β) (bā′tă). Beta; segunda letra do alfabeto grego, β (ver entrada no início da letra B.) [G.]
be·ta-block·er (bā′tă-blok′er). Betabloqueador. SIN β-adrenergic blocking agent.
be·ta·cism (bā′tă-sizm). Betacismo; defeito na fala em que o som do *b* é conferido a outras consoantes. [G. *bēta*, a segunda letra do alfabeto]
be·ta·cy·a·nin (bā′tă-sī-ă-nin). Betacianina; um dos vários pigmentos vegetais vermelhos; uma betalaína. Um exemplo é a betanina. Elevado na urina dos indivíduos com betacianinúria. [L. *beta*, beterraba, + G. *kyanos*, substância azul-escura, + -in]
be·ta·cy·a·ni·nu·ria (bā-tă-sī′ă-ni-noo′rē-ă). Betacianinúria. SIN beeturia. [betacyanin + G. *ouron*, urina]
Be·ta·her·pes·vir·i·nae (bā′tă-her′pez-vir′i-nē). Uma subfamília de Herpesviridae que contém Cytomegalovirus e Roseolovirus.
be·ta·his·tine hy·dro·chlo·ride (bā-tă-his′tēn). Cloridrato de beta-histamina; inibidor da diamina oxidase utilizado como agente semelhante à histamina para o tratamento da doença de Ménière.
be·ta·i·ne (bē′tă-ēn). Betaína. **1.** Um produto de oxidação da colina e um intermediário transmetilante no metabolismo. **2.** Uma classe de compostos relacionados com a b. (1) (i.e., R$_3$N$^+$–CHR′–COO$^-$), p.ex., betaína glicina. SIN glycine betaine.
b. aldehyde, aldeído betaínico; intermediário na interconversão da betaína e colina.
b. hydrochloride, cloridrato de betaína; agente acidificante usado no tratamento de acloridria e hipocloridria.
be·ta·ine-al·de·hyde de·hy·dro·gen·ase. Aldeído betaínico desidrogenase; enzima oxidante que catalisa a oxidação do aldeído betaínico com NAD$^+$ e água em betaína e NADH; parte do sistema colina oxidase e do metabolismo da colina.
bet·a·lains (bā′tă-lāns). Betalaínas; um grupo de pigmentos vegetais encontrado quase exclusivamente na família Centrospermae, p.ex., betanina. Existem dois grupos: betacianinas (em vegetais de coloração vermelho-violeta) e betaxantinas (em vegetais de coloração amarelada).
be·ta·meth·a·sone (bā-tă-meth′ă-sōn). Betametasona; um glicocorticóide semi-sintético com efeitos antiinflamatórios e toxicidade similares aos do cortisol; inútil no tratamento da insuficiência da supra-renal, porque provoca pouca retenção de sódio. Para a terapia sistêmica e tópica, suas ações são similares às da prednisona, porém mais potentes. Também disponível como fosfato sódico de b., acetato de b. e valerato de b.
be·tan·i·dine sul·fate (be-tan′i-dēn). Sulfato de betanidina. SIN bethanidine sulfate.
be·tan·in (bā′tă-nin). Betanina; o pigmento vermelho nas beterrabas (*Beta vulgaris*); elevada na urina dos indivíduos com betacianinúria. [de *betacyanin*]
be·ta sheets. Lâminas beta; estrutura de proteínas em que o peptídeo é estendido e estabilizado pela ligação de hidrogênio entre os grupamentos NH e CO de diferentes estruturas de cadeias de polipeptídeos ou regiões separadas da mesma cadeia.
be·ta·tron (bā′tă-tron). Betatron; acelerador eletrônico circular que é uma fonte de elétrons de alta energia ou de raios X.

be·tax·o·lol hy·dro·chlo·ride (be-taks′ō-lol). Cloridrato de betaxolol; agente bloqueador β-adrenérgico utilizado principalmente no tratamento da hipertensão ocular e do glaucoma crônico de ângulo aberto.
be·ta·zole hy·dro·chlo·ride (bā′tă-zōl). Cloridrato de batazol; análogo da histamina que estimula a secreção gástrica por uma ação sobre os receptores H$_2$ com menor tendência para produzir os efeitos colaterais observados com a histamina; utilizado, em lugar da histamina, para medir a resposta secretora gástrica.
be·tel (bē′tl). Betel; as folhas secas da *Piper betle* (família Piperaceae), uma planta trepadeira da Índia Oriental; usado como estimulante e narcótico. [Pg. *betel*, *betle*, do Malaio ou Tamil *vetilla*]
be·tel nut. Noz de areca; a noz da palmeira areca, *Areca catechu* (família Palmae), das Índias Orientais, mastigada pelos nativos; contém arecolina; produz estimulação do sistema nervoso central; tinge os dentes e a gengiva de vermelho.
be·tha·ne·chol chlo·ride (be-than′ē-kol). Cloreto de betanecol; agente parassimpaticomimético, usado para aliviar a constipação, o íleo paralítico e a retenção urinária.
be·than·i·dine sul·fate (be-than′i-dēn). Sulfato de betanidina; agente bloqueador adrenérgico usado para o tratamento paliativo da hipertensão. SIN betanidine sulfate.
Bethesda-Ballerup Group. Grupo Bethesda-Ballerup; grupo de bactérias que fermentam lentamente a lactose e utilizam o citrato (família Enterobacteriaceae) e que compartilham uma série de antígenos similares com as citrobactérias fermentadoras da lactose; esses organismos estão atualmente incluídos no gênero *Citrobacter* sem uma diferenciação entre a fermentação imediata e lenta da lactose.
Betke-Kleihauer test. Teste de Betke-Kleihauer. Ver em test.
Bettendorff, Anton J., químico alemão, 1839–1902. VER B. *test*.
bet·u·la (bet′ū-lă). Bétula; madeira branca européia, casca e folhas da *Betula alba* (família Betulaceae); nativa da Europa, norte da Ásia e América do Norte, norte da Pennsylvania. Contém betulina (cânfora de bétula), ácido betulorresínico, óleo volátil, saponinas, betulol (álcool sesquiterpina), apigenina, éter dimetílico, betulosida, gaulterina, salicilato de metila e ácido ascórbico; apresenta odor de gaultéria e é utilizada como um adjunto farmacêutico (flavorizante/aromático).
Betz, Vladimir A., anatomista russo, 1834–1894. VER B. *cells*, em *cell*.
Beuren, Alois J., cardiologista alemão do século 20. VER Beuren *syndrome*.
Bevan-Lewis, William, médico e fisiologista inglês, 1847–1929. VER Bevan-Lewis *cells*, em *cell*.
bev·el (bev′el). Bisel. **1.** Uma superfície que possui uma borda enviesada ou oblíqua. **2.** A inclinação que uma superfície ou linha faz com outra quando não em ângulos retos. **3.** A borda de um instrumento cortante. **4.** Criar uma borda oblíqua sobre uma estrutura corporal.
cavosurface b., b. cavo-superficial; a inclinação do ângulo cavo-superficial de uma parede cavitária preparada em relação ao plano da parede do esmalte.
reverse b., b. invertido; a borda inclinada de um instrumento cortante.
be·vo·ni·um meth·yl sul·fate (be-vō′nē-ŭm). Metil sulfato de bevônio; agente anticolinérgico. SIN pyribenzyl methyl sulfate.
be·zoar (bē′zōr). Bezoar; concreção formada no canal alimentar dos animais e, ocasionalmente, dos seres humanos; originalmente considerado um remédio útil com propriedades mágicas e aparentemente ainda utilizado para essa finalidade em alguns países; de acordo com a substância formadora, pode ser denominado tricobezoar (de pêlos), tricofitobezoar (pêlos e fibras vegetais misturados) ou fitobezoar (bola de alimento). [Pers. *padzahr*, antídoto]
Bezold, Albert von, fisiologista alemão, 1836–1868. VER B. *ganglion*; B.-Jarisch *reflex*.
Bezold, Friedrich, otologista alemão, 1842–1908. VER B. *abscess*.
BGP Abreviatura de bone G1a *protein* (proteína G1a óssea).
BHA Abreviatura para butylated hydroxyanisole (hidroxianisol butilado).
bhang (bang). Nome dado no Oriente à preparação em pó da *Cannabis sativa* que é mastigada ou fumada pelos habitantes locais. VER TAMBÉM cannabis. [Hind.]
BHN Abreviatura de Brinell hardness *number* (número da dureza de Brinell).
BHT Abreviatura de butylated hydroxytoluene (hidroxitolueno butilado).
Bi Símbolo do bismuth (bismuto).
bi-. 1. Prefixo que significa duas vezes ou duplo, referindo-se a estruturas duplas ou ações duplicadas. **2.** Em química, usado para indicar um ácido parcialmente neutralizado (um sal ácido); p.ex., bissulfato. Cf. bis-, di-. [L.]
Bial, Manfred, médico alemão, 1869–1908. VER B. *test*.
Bianchi, Giovanni B., anatomista italiano, 1681–1761. VER B. *nodule*.
bi·ar·tic·u·lar (bī′ar-tik′ū-lăr). Biarticular. SIN diarthric.

bi·as (bī′-as). Tendenciosidade, viés, distorção, *bias*. **1.** A discrepância sistemática entre uma medida e o valor real; pode ser constante ou proporcional e pode afetar de maneira adversa os resultados do teste. **2.** Qualquer tendência na coleta, análise, interpretação, publicação ou revisão de dados que possa levar a conclusões que diferem de maneira sistemática da verdade; o desvio sistemático de resultados ou inferências da verdade, ou os processos que levam ao desvio. [Fr. *biais*, obliqüidade, talvez do L. *bifax*, duas faces]

Não existem preconceito, sectarismo ou outro fator subjetivo ou emocional que se comparem ao desejo do investigador de alcançar um determinado resultado. Mais de 100 variedades de tendenciosidades já foram descritas, porém todas caem em uma de um número bastante restrito de categorias distintas: 1. Variação unilateral sistemática das mensurações a partir do valor verdadeiro (SIN systematic error, instrumental error ou bias). 2. Variação das medidas de resumo estatístico (médias, taxas, medidas de associação etc.) a partir de seus valores verdadeiros como uma conseqüência da variação sistemática de instrumentos, outras falhas na coleta de dados ou falhas no projeto ou na análise do estudo. 3. Desvio de deduções da verdade como resultado de falhas no projeto, na coleta ou na análise dos dados ou na interpretação dos resultados do estudo. 4. Tendência dos procedimentos no projeto, na coleta de dados, na análise dos dados, na interpretação dos dados ou na revisão dos dados ou na publicação do estudo, visando a fornecer resultados ou conclusões que se afastam da verdade. 5. Preconceito levando à seleção consciente ou inconsciente de procedimentos de estudo que se afastam da verdade em um determinado sentido, ou à unilateralidade na interpretação dos resultados. Essa forma de tendenciosidade pode originar-se ou ser decorrente de métodos científicos de má qualidade ou, de maneira deliberada, quando os pesquisadores se comportam de forma fraudulenta para representar erroneamente a verdade.

ascertainment b., t. de verificação; falha sistemática para representar igualmente todas as classes de casos ou pessoas que deveriam estar em uma amostra.
cross-level b., t. cruzada; tendenciosidade decorrente da agregação no nível populacional das causas e/ou efeitos que são distintos no nível individual; pode ocorrer em estudos ecológicos.
recall b., t. de lembrança; erro sistemático decorrente de diferenças na acurácia ou totalidade da lembrança da memória de eventos ou experiências pregressas.
reporting b., t. de relato; revelação ou supressão seletiva de informações sobre a história patológica pregressa, p.ex., detalhes de exposição a doenças sexualmente transmitidas.
response b., t. de resposta; erro sistemático devido a diferenças nas características entre aqueles que escolhem ou são voluntários para tomar parte em um estudo e aqueles que não o são.
sampling b., t. de amostragem; erro sistemático devido ao estudo de uma amostra não-randomizada de uma população.
bi·as·te·ri·on·ic (bī-as-ter-ē-on'ik). Biasteriônico; relativo aos astérios, principalmente o diâmetro b. ou largura biasteriônica, com a distância mais curta entre um astério e outro.
bi·au·ric·u·lar (bī-aw-rik'ū-lār). Biauricular; relativo às duas aurículas, em qualquer sentido.
bib. Abreviatura do L. *bibe*, beber.
bib·li·o·ma·ni·a (bib'lē-ō-mā'nē-ā). Bibliomania; desejo morbidamente intenso de coletar e possuir livros, especialmente livros raros. [G. *biblion*, livro, + *mania*, mania]
bib·u·lous (bib'ū-lŭs). Bíbulo. SIN absorbent (1). [L. *bibulus*, beber livremente, absorver]
bi·cam·er·al (bī-kam'er-āl). Bicameral; que possui duas câmaras; indica especialmente um abscesso dividido por um septo mais ou menos completo. [bi- + L. *camera*, câmara]
bi·cap·su·lar (bī-kap'soo-lăr). Bicapsular; que possui uma cápsula dupla.
bi·car·bon·ate (bī-kar'bon-āt). Bicarbonato; HCO_3^-; o íon que resta depois da primeira dissociação do ácido carbônico; um agente de tamponamento central no sangue.
standard b., b.-padrão; a concentração plasmática de b. de uma amostra de sangue total que foi equilibrada a 37°C com uma pressão de dióxido de carbono de 40 mm Hg e uma pressão de oxigênio superior a 100 mm Hg; os valores anormalmente altos ou baixos indicam alcalose ou acidose metabólica, respectivamente.
bi·car·di·o·gram (bī-kar'dē-ō-gram). Bicardiograma; a curva composta de um eletrocardiograma que representa os efeitos combinados dos ventrículos direito e esquerdo.
bi·cel·lu·lar (bī-sel'ū-lăr). Bicelular; que possui duas células ou subdivisões.
bi·ceph·a·lus (bī-sef'ā-lŭs). Bicéfalo. SIN dicephalus.
bi·ceps (bī'seps). Bíceps; um músculo com duas origens ou cabeças. Comumente utilizado para referir-se ao bíceps braquial (*muscle*). [bi- + L. *caput*, cabeça]
Bichat, Marie F. X., anatomista, médica e bióloga francesa, 1771–1802. VER B. *canal, fat-pad, fissure, fossa, ligament, membrane, protuberance, tunic*.
bi·cho (bē'cho). Bicho. SIN epidemic gangrenous *proctitis*.
bi·cil·i·ate (bī-sil'ē-āt). Biciliado; que possui dois cílios.
bi·cip·i·tal (bī-sip'i-tăl). Bicipital. **1.** Que possui duas cabeças. **2.** Relativo a um músculo bíceps. [bi- + L. *caput*, cabeça]
Bickel, Gustav, médico alemão do século 19. VER B. *ring*.

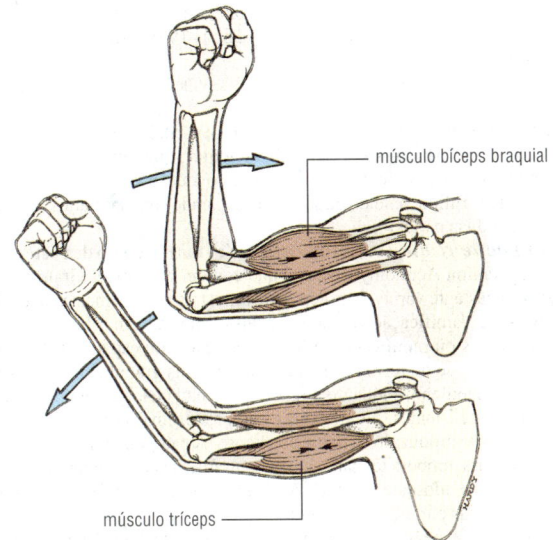

músculos bíceps e tríceps: durante a flexão (acima) e a extensão (abaixo)

bi·clo·nal (bī-klō'năl). Biclonal; pertinente a ou caracterizado pela biclonalidade.
bi·clon·al·i·ty (bī-klōn-al'i-tē). Biclonalidade; uma condição em que algumas células possuem marcadores de uma linhagem celular e outras células têm marcadores de outra linhagem celular, como nas leucemias biclonais.
bi·con·cave (bī-kon'kāv). Bicôncavo; côncavo em dois lados; indica especialmente uma forma de lente. SIN concavoconcave.
bi·con·vex (bī-kon'veks). Biconvexo; convexo em dois lados; indica especialmente uma forma de lente. SIN convexoconvex.
bi·cor·nous, bi·cor·nu·ate, bi·cor·nate (bī-kōr'nŭs, -noo-āt, -nāt). Bicorne, bicornado, bicórneo; com dois cornos; que possui dois processos ou projeções. [bi- + L. *cornu*, corno]
bicro-. SIN pico- (2).
bi·cron (bī'kron). Milimícron. SIN picometer.
bi·cu·cul·line (bī'coo-cu-lēn). Bicuculina; um alcalóide de ocorrência natural na forma *d*; encontrada na *Dicentra cucullaria* e na *Adlumia fungosa* (família Fumariaceae) e em várias espécies de *Corydalis*; um poderoso convulsivante que atua por antagonizar o ácido γ-aminobutírico, um neurotransmissor inibitório.
bi·cus·pid (bī-kŭs'pid). Bicúspide. **1.** Que possui dois pontos, bicos ou cúspides. **2.** Os dentes que têm duas cúspides. Os seres humanos têm oito dentes bicúspides ou pré-molares: dois na frente de cada grupo de molares. VER bicuspid *tooth*. [bi- + L. *cuspis*, ponto]
b. aortic valve, valva aórtica bicúspide. VER familial aortic ectasia *syndrome*.
bi·cus·pi·di·za·tion (bī-kŭs'pi-di-zā'shŭn). Bicuspidização; alteração cirúrgica de uma valva tricúspide normal em uma válvula bicúspide funcionante; realizado na correção da doença valvar tricúspide.
b.i.d. Abreviatura do L. *bis in die*, duas vezes ao dia.
bi·dac·ty·ly (bī-dak'ti-lē). Bidactilia; anormalidade em que os dedos mediais estão ausentes, com apenas o primeiro e o quinto representados. VER TAMBÉM lobster-claw *deformity*, ectrodactyly. [bi- + G. *daktylos*, dedo]
bi·det (bē-dā'). Bidé; bacia oblonga para um banho de assento, que também possui um dispositivo para aplicar infusões vaginais ou retais. [Fr. um pequeno cavalo]
bi·dis·coi·dal (bī'dis-koy'dăl). Bidiscoidal; que se assemelha ou consiste em dois discos.
BIDS [MIM*234050]. Acrônimo de *b*rittle hair, *i*mpaired intelligence, *d*ecreased fertility e *s*hort stature (cabelos quebradiços, distúrbio da inteligência, diminuição da fertilidade e baixa estatura); os cabelos quebradiços podem ser decorrentes de uma deficiência herdada de uma proteína rica em enxofre; herança autossômica recessiva.
bid·u·ous (bid'ū-ŭs). Bíduo; termo raramente utilizado que indica a duração de dois dias. [L. *biduus*, que dura dois dias, de *bi-*, + *dies*, dia]
Biebl, M. VER B. *loop*.
Biebrich scar·let red (C.I. 26905). Vermelho-escarlate de Biebrich. SIN scarlet red. [*Biebrich*, Alemanha]
Biederman, Joseph, médico norte-americano, *1907. VER B. *sign*.
Biedl, Artur, médico austríaco, 1869–1933. VER Bardet-B. *syndrome*.
Bielschowsky, Alfred, oftalmologista alemão, 1871–1940. VER B. *sign*.
Bielschowsky, Max, neuropatologista alemão, 1869–1940. VER B. *disease, stain*; Jansky-B. *disease*.

Biemond, Avic, neurologista francês, *1902. VER B. *syndrome*.
Bier, August K. G., cirurgião alemão, 1861–1949. VER B. *amputation, hyperemia, method*.
Biermer, Anton, médico alemão, 1827–1892. VER B. *anemia, disease;* Addison-B. *disease*.
Biesiadecki, Alfred von, médico polonês, 1839–1888. VER B. *fossa*.
bi·fas·cic·u·lar (bī-fă-sik′ū-lar). Bifascicular; que envolve dois dos três principais supostos fascículos do sistema de condução ventricular do coração.
bi·fid (bī′fid). Bífido; fendido ou separado; separado em duas partes. [L. *bifidus*, fendido em duas partes]
Bi·fi·do·bac·te·ri·um (bī-fi-dō-bak-tēr′ē-ŭm). Gênero de bactérias anaeróbicas (família Actinomycetaceae) que contém bastonetes Gram-positivos de aspecto bastante variável; as cepas em amostras frescas mostram, de forma característica, ramificação verdadeira e falsa, com as formas bifurcadas em V e Y, uniformes ou ramificadas, e formas em clava ou espatuladas. Com freqüência, coram-se de forma irregular; dois ou mais grânulos podem corar-se com azul de metileno, enquanto o restante da célula não se cora. Elas não são álcool-ácido-resistentes, são imóveis e não produzem esporos; os ácidos acético e lático são produzidos a partir da glicose. A patogenicidade para os seres humanos é rara, embora tenham sido encontradas nas fezes e no trato alimentar de lactentes, idosos e animais. A espécie típica é *B. bifidum.* [L. *bifidus*, fendido em duas partes, + bacterium]
B. bi′fidum, a espécie típica do gênero *Bifidobacterium*; é encontrado nas fezes e no trato alimentar de lactentes amamentados ou que recebem leite em pó e de pessoas idosas, ratos, perus e galinhas; também encontrado no rúmen do gado; a patogenicidade para seres humanos e outros animais é rara. Associado a um fator de crescimento pertencente a um grupo de polissacarídeos portadores de *N* com um elevado conteúdo de hexosamina e conhecido como fator bífido.
B. dentium, espécie bacteriana isolada em associação com a cárie dentária e a doença periodontal. Também é um patógeno oportunista, recuperado em infecções mistas associadas à formação de abscesso.
bi·fo·cal (bī-fō′kăl). Bifocal; que possui dois focos.
bi·fo·rate (bī-fō′rāt) Bifurado; que possui duas aberturas. [bi- + L. *foro*, pp. -*atus*, furar, perfurar]
bi·func·tion·al (bī-fŭnc′shŭn-ăl). Bifuncional; que se refere a uma molécula que contém dois grupamentos funcionais reativos; os reagentes cruzados são compostos bifuncionais.
bi·fur·cate, bi·fur·cat·ed (bī-fer′kăt, -kā-ted). Bifurcar, bifurcado; em forma de garfo; com dois ramos. [bi- + L. *furca*, garfo]
bi·fur·ca·tio (bī′fer-kā′shē-ō) [TA]. Bifurcação. SIN bifurcation.
  b. aor′tae [TA], b. da aorta. SIN aortic *bifurcation*.
  b. tra′cheae [TA], b. da traquéia. SIN tracheal *bifurcation*.
  b. trun′ci pulmona′lis [TA], b. do tronco pulmonar. SIN *bifurcation* of pulmonary trunk.
bi·fur·ca·tion (bī-fer-kā′shŭn) [TA]. Bifurcação; separação; uma divisão em dois ramos. SIN bifurcatio [TA].
  b. of aorta, b. da aorta. SIN aortic b.
  aortic b. [TA], b. da aorta; a divisão da aorta nas artérias ilíacas comuns direita e esquerda; ocorre no nível da quarta e quinta vértebras lombares. SIN bifurcatio aortae [TA], b. of aorta.
  b. of pulmonary trunk [TA], b. do tronco pulmonar; a divisão do tronco pulmonar nas artérias pulmonares direita e esquerda. SIN bifurcatio trunci pulmonalis [TA].
  b. of trachea, b. da traquéia. SIN tracheal b.
  tracheal b. [TA], b. da traquéia; a divisão da traquéia nos brônquios principais direito e esquerdo; ocorre no nível do quinto ou sexto corpo vertebral torácico e é marcada internamente por uma carina ou crista em forma de quilha entre os brônquios divergentes. SIN bifurcatio tracheae [TA], b. of trachea.
Bigelow, Henry J., cirurgião norte-americano, 1818–1890. VER B. *ligament, septum*.
bi·gem·i·na (bī-jem′i-nă). Bigêmeo. SIN bigeminal *pulse*.
bi·gem·i·nal (bī-jem′i-năl). Bigeminal; pareado; duplo; gêmeo.
bi·gem·i·ni (bī-jem′i-nī). Bigeminismo. SIN bigeminy.
bi·gem·i·num (bī-jem′i-nŭm). Bigêmeo; um dos corpos bigêmeos. [L. neut. de *bigeminus*, duplicado]
bi·gem·i·ny (bī-jem′i-nē) Bigeminismo; pareamento; especialmente, a ocorrência de batimentos cardíacos aos pares. SIN bigemini. [bi- + L. *geminus*, gêmeo]
  atrial b., b. atrial; o emparelhamento dos batimentos atriais, como quando uma extra-sístole atrial é acoplada a cada batimento sinusal.
  atrioventricular junctional b., b. atrioventricular juncional; batimentos emparelhados, com cada par consistindo em uma extra-sístole nodal AV acoplada a um batimento do ritmo dominante, usualmente sinusal. SIN nodal b.
  escape-capture b., b. de escape-captura; batimentos emparelhados, com cada dupla consistindo em um batimento de escape seguido por um batimento sinusal conduzido ou um batimento de escape seguido por um batimento ectópico conduzido (usualmente atrial com onda P retrógrada).
  nodal b., b. nodal. SIN atrioventricular junctional b.
  reciprocal b., b. recíproco; batimentos emparelhados, com cada par consistindo em um batimento nodal AV seguido por um batimento recíproco.
  ventricular b., b. ventricular; batimentos ventriculares emparelhados, com a forma comum consistindo em extra-sístoles ventriculares acopladas a batimentos sinusais.
bi·ger·min·al (bī-jer′min-ăl). Bigerminal; relativo a dois ovos ou germes.
bi·git·a·lin (bī-jit′ă-lin). Bigitalina. SIN gitoxin.
bi·gly·can (bī′glī-kan). Biglicano; um pequeno proteoglicano intersticial que contém duas cadeias de glicosaminoglicanos. SIN proteoglycan I.
Bignami, Amico, médico italiano, 1862–1929. VER Marchiafava-B. *disease*.
bi·kun·in (bik′oo-nin). Bicunina; glicoproteína plasmática que é encontrada em estado livre e sob ligação covalente com as cadeias pesadas de determinados inibidores da protease. Pode participar no crescimento celular, na expansão do cúmulo do oócito e na estabilização.
bi·labe (bī′lāb). Litolábio; pinça para capturar e remover pequenos cálculos vesicais ou uretrais. [bi- + L. *labium*, lábio]
bi·lat·er·al (bī-lat′er-ăl). Bilateral; relativo a, ou que possui dois lados. [bi- + L. *latus*, lado]
bi·lat·er·al·ism (bī-lat′er-ăl-izm) Bilateralismo; condição em que os dois lados são simétricos.
bile (bīl). Bile; o líquido esverdeado ou amarelo-acastanhado secretado pelo fígado e liberado para o duodeno, onde auxilia na emulsificação de gorduras, aumenta a peristalse e retarda a putrefação; contém glicocolato de sódio e taurocolato de sódio, colesterol, biliverdina e bilirrubina, muco, gorduras, lecitina, células e resíduos celulares. SIN gall (1). [L. *bilis*]
  A b., b. A; a b. do ducto comum.
  B b., b. B; b. da vesícula biliar.
  C. b., b. C; b. do ducto hepático.
  white b., b. branca; que designa o líquido relativamente claro, quase incolor, víscido, que ocorre na vesícula biliar e/ou nos intestinos como conseqüência da obstrução dos ductos biliares em vários sítios; na realidade, a secreção da mucosa, sem a coloração usual decorrente dos pigmentos biliares. SIN leukobilin.
Bilharz, Theodor M., especialista alemão em doenças tropicais, 1829–1862. VER *Bilharzia*; bilharzial *appendicitis*; bilharzial *dysentery*; bilharzial *granuloma*.
Bil·har·zia (bil-har′zē-ă). Um nome antigo para o *Schistosoma*. [T. *Bilharz*]
bil·har·zi·a·sis (bil-har-zī′ă-sis). Bilharzíase. SIN schistosomiasis.
bil·har·zi·o·ma (bil-har-zē-ō′mă). Bilharzioma; tumefação inflamatória e fibrosa, semelhante a um tumor, da serosa intestinal, do mesentério ou da pele, causada por esquistossomíase.
bil·har·zi·o·sis (bil-har-zē-ō′sis). Bilharziose. SIN schistosomiasis.
bili-. Forma combinante que indica bile. [L. *bilis*, bile]
bil·i·ary (bil′ē-ār-ē). Biliar; relativo à bile ou ao trato biliar. SIN bilious (1).
bil·i·fac·tion, bil·i·fi·ca·tion (bil-i-fak′shŭn, -fi-kā′shŭn). Bilificação; termos raramente utilizados para a formação da bile. [bili- + L. *facio*, pp. *factus*, fazer]
bil·if·er·ous (bil-if′er-ŭs). Bilífero; termo raramente utilizado para significar contendo ou transportando bile.
bil·i·gen·e·sis (bil-i-jen′ē-sis). Biligênese; produção de bile. [bili- + G. *genesis*, produção]
bil·i·gen·ic (bil-i-jen′ik). Biligênico; que produz bile.
bi·lin, bi·line (bī′lin). Bilina; a cadeia de quatro resíduos pirrólicos que resulta da clivagem em uma ligação de um dos quatro resíduos metilideno da porção porfina de uma porfirina; especificamente, o tetrapirrol não-substituído; a bilirrubina e a biliverdina são bilinas.
bil·ious (bil′yŭs). Bilioso. 1. SIN biliary. 2. Relativo a ou característico da biliosidade. 3. Originalmente, indica um temperamento caracterizado por um temperamento irritável, rápido. SIN choleric.
bil·ious·ness (bil′yŭs-nes). Biliosidade; distúrbio congestivo delineado de forma imprecisa com anorexia, língua saburrosa, constipação, cefaléia, tonteira, palidez cutânea e, raramente, icterícia discreta; presumido como decorrente de disfunção hepática.
bil·i·ra·chia (bil-i-rā′kē-ă). Bilirraquia; ocorrência de pigmentos biliares no líquido espinhal. [bili- + G. *rhachis*, coluna vertebral]
bil·i·ru·bin (bil-i-roo′bin). Bilirrubina; pigmento biliar amarelo encontrado como bilirrubinato de sódio (solúvel) ou como um sal de cálcio insolúvel nos cálculos biliares; formada a partir da hemoglobina durante a destruição normal e anormal dos eritrócitos pelo sistema reticuloendotelial; uma bilina com substitutos nos átomos de carbono 2, 3, 7, 8, 12, 13, 17 e 18 e com oxigênio nos carbonos 1 e 19. A b. em excesso está associada à icterícia. [bili- + L. *ruber*, vermelho]
  conjugated b., b. conjugada. SIN direct reacting b.
  delta b., b. delta; a fração da b. que se liga de forma covalente à albumina; nos métodos convencionais, é medida como parte da b. conjugada. Por causa de sua ligação covalente durante a fase de recuperação da icterícia hepatocelular, ela pode persistir no sangue durante uma semana ou mais depois que a urina volta ao normal.

direct reacting b., b. de reação direta; a fração da b. sérica que foi conjugada com o ácido glicurônico na célula hepática para formar o diglicuronídeo da bilirrubina; assim chamada porque reage diretamente com o reagente diazo de Ehrlich; os níveis aumentados são encontrados nas doenças hepatobiliares, especialmente da variedade obstrutiva. SIN conjugated b.

indirect reacting b., b. de reação indireta; a fração da b. sérica que não foi conjugada com o ácido glicurônico na célula hepática; assim chamada porque reage com o reagente diazo de Ehrlich apenas quando o álcool é adicionado; os níveis aumentados são encontrados na doença hepática e nas condições hemolíticas. SIN unconjugated b.

b. UDPglucuronyltransferase (gloo - koo'ron - il - trans'fer - ās), UDPglicuroniltransferase da bilirrubina; enzima que catalisa a reação do UDPglicuronato e a bilirrubina, formando UDP e bilirrubina-glicuronosídeo; a deficiência dessa enzima está associada à síndrome de Crigler-Najjar.

unconjugated b., b. não-conjugada. SIN indirect reacting b.

bi·li·ru·bi·ne·mia (bil'i - roo - bin - ē'mē - ā). Bilirrubinemia; a presença de bilirrubina no sangue, onde está normalmente presente em quantidades relativamente pequenas; o termo é comumente utilizado em relação às concentrações aumentadas observadas em diversas condições patológicas, em que existe destruição excessiva dos eritrócitos ou interferência com o mecanismo de excreção na bile. A determinação da quantidade da bilirrubina no soro sangüíneo revela duas frações, a saber, a bilirrubina de reação direta (conjugada) e a de reação indireta (não-conjugada); a determinação da bilirrubina conjugada e total no soro é um exame laboratorial clínico freqüentemente solicitado. [bilirubin + G. *haima*, sangue]

bi·li·ru·bi·glob·u·lin (bil - i - roo'bin - glob'ū - lin). Complexo bilirrubinaglobulina; uma forma de transporte da bilirrubina até o fígado, onde a bilirrubina é convertida em um derivado do ácido diglicurônico e passa para dentro da bile.

bi·li·ru·bin-glu·cu·ron·o·side glu·cu·ron·o·syl trans·fer·ase. Bilirrubina glicuronídeo glicuronosiltransferase; bilirrubina monoglicuronídeo transglicuronidase; transferase que transfere um glicuronosídeo de uma molécula de bilirrubina glicuronosídeo para outra, formando a bilirrubina biglicuronosídeo e a bilirrubina não-conjugada (uma etapa no catabolismo do heme).

bi·li·ru·bin·oids (bil - i - roo'bin - oydz). Bilirrubinóides; termo genérico que indica os intermediários na conversão da bilirrubina em estercobilina pelas enzimas redutoras nas bactérias intestinais. Estão incluídos a mesobilirrubina, o mesobilano, o mesobileno-b, o urobilinogênio, a urobilina, os produtos de redução do mesobilano (estercobilinogênio) e o mesobileno (estercobilina) e a mesobiliviolina; a maioria é encontrada na urina e nas fezes normais. Os produtos relacionados com esses intermediários e encontrados nas condições patológicas (p.ex., icterícia, doença hepática) são as probilifuscinas e propendiopentes encontrados na vesícula biliar.

bi·li·ru·bi·nu·ria (bil'i - roo - bi - noo'rē - ā). Bilirrubinúria; a presença de bilirrubina na urina. [bilirubin + G. *ouron*, urina]

bil·i·ther·a·py (bil - i - thār'ā - pē). Biliterapia; o tratamento com bile ou sais biliares.

bil·i·u·ria (bil - ē - ū'rē - ā). Biliúria; a presença de vários sais biliares ou bile na urina. SIN choleuria, choluria. [bili- + G. *ouron*, urina]

bil·i·ver·din, bil·i·ver·dine (bil - i - ver'din). Biliverdina; pigmento biliar esverdeado formado a partir da oxidação do heme; uma bilina com uma estrutura quase idêntica à da bilirrubina. SIN dehydrobilirubin, verdine.

Bill, Arthur H., obstetra norte-americano, 1877–1961. VER B. *maneuver*.

Billings, J. J., ginecologista australiano do século 20. VER B. *method*.

Billroth, Christian A. T., cirurgião austríaco, 1829–1894. VER B. *cords*, em *cord, operation* I, *operation* II, *venae* cavernosae, em *vena*, I *anastomosis*, II *anastomosis*.

bi·lo·bate, bi·lobed (bī - lō'bāt, bī'lōbd). Bilobado; que possui dois lobos.

bi·lo·bec·to·my (bī'lōb - ek'tō - mē). Bilobectomia; excisão cirúrgica de dois lobos do pulmão direito, quer o superior direito e o médio, quer o inferior direito e o médio.

bi·lob·u·lar (bī - lob'ū - lār). Bilobular; que possui dois lóbulos.

bi·loc·u·lar, bi·loc·u·late (bī - lok'ū - lār, - ū - lāt). Biloculado; que possui dois compartimentos ou espaços. [bi- + L. *loculus*, dim. de *locus*, um lugar]

bi·man·u·al (bī - man'ū - āl). Bimanual; relativo a, ou realizado pelas duas mãos. [bi- + L. *manus*, mão]

bi·mas·toid (bī - mas'toyd). Bimastóide; relativo a ambos os processos mastóides.

bi·max·il·lary (bī - mak'si - lār - e). Bimaxilar; relativo às partes direita e esquerda da maxila; por vezes utilizado quando se descreve algo que afeta as duas partes da maxila.

bi·mod·al (bī - mō'dāl). Bimodal; indicando uma curva de freqüência caracterizada por dois picos.

bi·mo·lec·u·lar (bī - mō - lek'ū - lār). Bimolecular; que envolve duas moléculas, como em uma reação b.

bin·an·gle (bin - ang'ŭl). Biângulo. **1.** O segundo ângulo dado à haste de um instrumento angulado para fazer com que sua extremidade funcional fique em relação direta com o eixo do cabo, a fim de evitar que esse gire em torno do eixo. **2.** Instrumento dentário que possui as características acima. [L. *bini*, par, + *angulus*, ângulo]

bi·na·ry (bī'nar - ē). Binário. **1.** Que compreende dois componentes, elementos, moléculas etc. **2.** Indica uma escolha de dois resultados mutuamente excludentes para um evento (p.ex., homem ou mulher, cabeças ou caudas, afetados ou não-afetados). [L. *binarius*, que consiste em dois, de *bini*, dois por vez]

bin·au·ral (bin - aw'rāl). Binauricular; relativo às duas orelhas. SIN binotic. [L. *bini*, um par, + *auris*, orelha]

bind (bīnd). **1.** Ligar; confinar ou envolver com uma faixa ou bandagem. **2.** Ligar; unir com uma faixa ou ligadura. **3.** Ligar; combinar ou unir as moléculas por meio de grupos reativos, quer em moléculas por si, quer em uma substância química acrescentada para essa finalidade; freqüentemente utilizado em relação às ligações químicas que podem ser rompidas com muita facilidade (i.e., não-covalente), como na ligação de uma toxina com uma antitoxina, ou de um metal pesado com um agente quelante etc. **4.** Ligação; relacionamento íntimo em que uma pessoa se sente compelida a agir de uma certa maneira para obter a aprovação de outra pessoa. [A.S. *bindan*]

double b., ligação dupla; um tipo de interação pessoal em que uma pessoa recebe duas instruções ou ordens mutuamente conflitantes, verbais ou não-verbais, a partir da mesma pessoa ou de indivíduos diferentes, resultando em uma situação em que a transigência ou intransigência com uma das alternativas ameaça uma relação necessária.

bind·er (bīnd'er). **1.** Uma bandagem larga, especialmente aquela que envolve o abdome. **2.** Qualquer coisa que liga. VER bind (3).

obstetrical b., bandagem obstétrica; bandagem que recobre o abdome desde as costelas até os trocanteres, firmemente presa no dorso, conferindo suporte após o parto ou, raramente, durante o parto.

T-b., bandagem em T; duas faixas de tecido em ângulos retos; usada para reter um curativo, como sobre o períneo. SIN T-bandage.

Binet, Alfred, psicólogo francês, 1857–1911. VER B. *age, scale, test;* B.-Simon *scale*; Stanford-B. *intelligence scale*.

Bing, Paul Robert, neurologista alemão, 1878–1956. VER B. *reflex*.

Bing, Richard J., médico norte-americano, *1909. VER Taussig-B., *disease, syndrome*.

Bingham, Eugene C., químico norte-americano, 1878–1945. VER B. *flow, model, plastic*.

bin·oc·u·lar (bin - ok'ū - lār). Binocular; adaptado para o uso de ambos os olhos; diz-se de um instrumento óptico. [L. *bini*, pareado, + *oculus*, olho]

bi·no·mi·al (bī - nō'mē - āl). Binomial; um grupo de dois termos ou nomes; no sentido probabilístico ou estatístico, corresponde a uma experiência de Bernoulli. VER TAMBÉM binary *combination*. [bi- + G. *nomos*, nome]

bin·ot·ic (bin - ot'ik). Binótico. SIN binaural. [L. *bini*, um par, + G. *ous* (ōt-), ouvido]

Binswanger, Otto Ludwig, neurologista alemão, 1852–1929. VER B. *disease, encephalopathy*.

bi·nu·cle·ar, bi·nu·cle·ate (bī - noo'klē - ar, - klē - āt). Binuclear, binucleado; que possui dois núcleos.

bi·nu·cle·o·late (bī - noo'klē - ō - lāt). Binucleolado; que possui dois nucléolos.

bio-. Forma combinante que indica vida. [G. *bios*, vida]

bi·o·a·cous·tics (bī'ō - ā - koos'tiks). Bioacústica; a ciência que lida com os efeitos do campo sonoro ou as vibrações mecânicas dos organismos vivos.

bi·o·ac·tive (bī'ō - āk'tiv). Bioativo; refere-se a uma substância que pode ser afetada por um organismo vivo ou por um extrato de um organismo vivo.

bi·o·as·say (bī - ō - as'ā). Bioensaio; a determinação da potência ou concentração de um composto por seu efeito sobre os animais, tecidos isolados ou microrganismos, quando comparado a uma análise de suas propriedades químicas ou físicas.

bi·o·as·tro·nau·tics (bī'ō - as - tro - naw'tiks). Bioastronáutica; o estudo dos efeitos de viajar pelo espaço e habitar o espaço sobre os organismos vivos.

bi·o·a·vail·a·bil·i·ty (bī'ō - ā - vāl'ā - bil'i - tē). Biodisponibilidade; a disponibilidade fisiológica de uma determinada quantidade de um medicamento, conforme diferenciado de sua potência química; a proporção da dose administrada que é absorvida para a corrente sangüínea.

bi·o·bur·den (bī'ō - ber'den). Biocarga; o grau de contaminação microbiana ou carga microbiana; o número de microrganismos que contamina um objeto.

bi·o·cat·a·lyst (bī'ō - kat - ā - list). Biocatalisador; substância de origem biológica que pode catalisar uma reação; p.ex., uma enzima.

bi·o·ce·no·sis (bī - ō - se - nō'sis). Biocenose; um agrupamento de espécies vivendo em um biótopo particular. SIN biotic community. [bio- + G. *koinos*, comum]

bi·o·chem·i·cal (bī - ō - kem'i - kāl). Bioquímico; relativo à bioquímica.

bi·o·chem·is·try (bī - ō - kem'is - trē). Bioquímica; a química de organismos vivos e das alterações químicas, moleculares e físicas que ocorrem neles. SIN biologic chemistry, physiologic chemistry.

bi·o·chem·or·phic (bī'ō - kem - or'fik). Bioquimórfico; indica a relação entre a ação biológica e a estrutura química, como no alimento e em medicamentos.

bi·o·chrome (bī′ō - krōm). Biocromo, pigmento natural. SIN natural *pigment*. [bio- + G. *chrōma*, coloração]

bi·o·cid·al (bī - ō - sī′dăl). Biocida; destruidor da vida; pertinente em particular aos microrganismos. [bio- + L. *caedo*, matar]

bi·o·cli·ma·tol·o·gy (bī - ō - klī - mă - tol′ō - jē). Bioclimatologia; a ciência da relação dos fatores climáticos com a distribuição, os números e os tipos de organismos vivos; um aspecto da ecologia.

biocompatibility (bī′ō - kom - pat - i - bil′i - tē). Biocompatibilidade; a capacidade relativa de um material de interagir favoravelmente com um sistema biológico. [bio- + compatibility]

bi·o·cy·ber·net·ics (bī′ō - sī - ber - net′iks). Biocibernética; a ciência da comunicação e controle dentro de um organismo vivo, principalmente em uma base molecular.

bi·o·cy·tin (bī - ō - sī′tin). Biocitina; ε-*N*-Biotinil-L-lisina; a biotina condensada através de seu grupamento carboxila com o grupamento ε-amino de um resíduo lisil nas apoenzimas para as quais a biotina é a coenzima; a ligação predominante em que a biotina é encontrada. SIN biotinyllysine.

bi·o·cy·tin·ase (bī - ō - sī′tin - ās). Biocitinase; enzima no sangue que catalisa a hidrólise da biocitina em biotina e lisina (ou, resíduo de lisina quando a lisina está em uma proteína).

bi·o·de·grad·a·ble (bī - ō - dē - grăd′ă - bl). Biodegradável; indica uma substância que pode ser quimicamente degradada ou decomposta por efetores naturais (p.ex., tempo, bactérias do solo, vegetais, animais).

bi·o·de·gra·da·tion. Biodegradação. SIN biotransformation.

bi·o·dy·nam·ic (bī′ō - dī - nam′ik). Biodinâmica; relativo à biodinâmica.

bi·o·dy·nam·ics (bī′ō - dī - nam′iks). Biodinâmica; a ciência que lida com a força ou energia da matéria viva. [bio- + G. *dynamis*, força]

bi·o·e·col·o·gy (bī - ō - ē - kol′ō - jē). Bioecologia. SIN ecology.

bi·o·el·e·ment (bī′ō - el′ĕ - ment). Bioelemento; elemento necessário a um organismo vivo.

bi·o·en·er·get·ics (bī′ō - en - er - jet′iks). Bioenergética. **1.** O estudo das alterações de energia envolvidas nas reações químicas dentro do tecido vivo. **2.** O estudo das trocas de energia entre os organismos vivos e seus ambientes.

bi·o·en·gi·neer·ing (bī′ō - en - jin - ēr′ing). Bioengenharia. VER biomedical *engineering*.

bi·o·feed·back (bī - ō - fēd′bak). *Biofeedback*; técnica de treinamento que possibilita a um indivíduo ganhar algum elemento do controle voluntário sobre as funções autônomas do corpo; baseado no princípio de aprendizagem de que uma resposta desejada é aprendida quando as informações recebidas, como um aumento registrado na temperatura cutânea (retroalimentação), indicam que um complexo ou ação específico do pensamento produziu a resposta fisiológica desejada.
EMG b., b. da EMG; uma forma de b. que utiliza uma medida eletromiográfica da tensão muscular como um sintoma físico a ser descondicionado, de tal modo que a tensão no músculo frontal na cabeça pode causar cefaléias.

bi·o·fla·vo·noids (bī - ō - flăv′on - oydz). Bioflavonóides; os derivados da flavona ou da cumarina de ocorrência natural, comumente encontrados nas frutas cítricas, que possuem a atividade da chamada vitamina P, notadamente a rutina e a esculina.

bi·o·gen·e·sis (bī - ō - jen′ĕ - sis). Biogênese. **1.** Termo dado por Huxley ao princípio de que a vida se origina apenas da vida preexistente e nunca do material não-vivo. VER spontaneous *generation*, recapitulation *theory*. **2.** SIN biosynthesis. [bio- + G. *genesis*, origem]
mitochondrial b., b. mitocondrial; o processo pelo qual a mitocôndria aumenta sua capacidade de produzir trifosfato de adenosina por sintetizar complexos enzimáticos respiratórios adicionais.

bi·o·ge·net·ic (bī′ō - jĕ - net′ik). Biogenética; relativo à biogênese.

bi·o·gen·ic (bī′ō - jen - ik). Biogênico; produzido por um organismo vivo.

bi·o·geo·chem·is·try (bī′ō - jē - ō - kem′is - trē). Biogeoquímica; o estudo da influência dos organismos vivos e dos processos vitais sobre a estrutura química e a história da terra.

bi·o·grav·ics (bī - ō - grav′iks). Biogravimetria; esse campo de estudo lida com o efeito sobre os organismos vivos (principalmente os seres humanos) dos efeitos gravitacionais anormais produzidos, p.ex., por aceleração ou por queda livre; no primeiro caso, no peso maior que o normal é induzido, e, no último, a imponderabilidade. [bio- + L. *gravis*, peso]

bioinformatics. Bioinformática; uma disciplina científica que engloba todos os aspectos da aquisição, do processamento, do armazenamento, da distribuição, da análise e da interpretação das informações biológicas que combina os instrumentos e as técnicas da matemática, da ciência da computação e da biologia com o objetivo de compreender o significado biológico de vários dados.

bi·o·in·stru·ment (bī′ō - in′stroo - ment). Bioinstrumento; um sensor ou dispositivo usualmente preso ou implantado no corpo humano ou em outro animal vivo para registrar e transmitir os dados fisiológicos a uma central receptora e de monitoramento.

bi·o·ki·net·ics (bī′ō - ki - net′iks). Biocinética; o estudo das alterações do crescimento e dos movimentos que sofrem os organismos em desenvolvimento. [bio- + G. *kinēsis*, movimento]

bi·o·log·ic, bi·o·log·i·cal (bī′ō - loj′ik, - loj′i - kăl). Biológico; relativo à biologia.

bi·ol·o·gist (bī - ol′ō - jist). Biólogo; especialista ou experiente em biologia.

bi·ol·o·gy (bī - ol′ō - jē). Biologia; a ciência que trata dos fenômenos da vida e dos organismos vivos. [bio- + G. *logos*, estudo]
cellular b., b. celular. SIN cytology.
molecular b., b. molecular; o estudo dos fenômenos biológicos em termos das interações moleculares (ou químicas); tradicionalmente, o foco da b. molecular é mais específico que o da bioquímica pelo fato de que ela apresenta uma ênfase sobre as interações químicas envolvidas na replicação do DNA, sua "transcrição" em RNA e sua "tradução" ou expressão em proteína, i.e., nas reações químicas que conectam o genótipo e o fenótipo.
oral b., b. oral; o aspecto da b. devotado ao estudo dos fenômenos biológicos associados à cavidade oral na saúde e na doença (p.ex., cárie dentária, mastigação, doença periodontal).
pharmaceutical b., b. farmacêutica. SIN pharmacognosy.
radiation b., b. da radiação; campo da ciência que estuda os efeitos biológicos da radiação ionizante.

bi·o·lu·mi·nes·cence (bī′ō - loo - min - es′ens). Bioluminescência. **1.** Luz produzida por determinados organismos a partir da oxidação das luciferinas através da ação das luciferases e com produção desprezível de calor, sendo a energia química convertida diretamente em energia luminosa. SIN cold light (1). **2.** Qualquer luz produzida por um organismo vivo. [bio- + L. *lumen* (-*inis*), luz]

bi·ol·y·sis (bī - ol′i - sis). Biólise; desintegração da matéria orgânica através da ação química de organismos vivos. [bio- + G. *lysis*, dissolução]

bi·o·lyt·ic (bī - ō - lit′ik). Biolítico. **1.** Relativo à biólise. **2.** Capaz de destruir a vida.

bi·o·mac·ro·mol·e·cule (bī′ō - măk - rō - mol′ĕ - kūl). Biomacromolécula; uma substância de grande peso molecular de ocorrência natural (p.ex., proteína, DNA).

bi·o·mass (bī′ō - mas). Biomassa; o peso total de todas as coisas vivas em uma determinada área, comunidade biótica, população de espécies ou hábitat; uma medida da produtividade biótica total.

biomaterial (bī′ō - ma - tē′rē - al). Biomaterial; um material sintético ou semi-sintético utilizado em um sistema biológico para construir uma prótese implantável e escolhido por sua biocompatibilidade. [bio- + material]

bi·ome (bī′ōm). Bioma; o complexo total das comunidades bióticas que ocupam e caracterizam uma determinada zona ou área geográfica. [bio- + -ome]

bi·o·me·chan·ics (bī - ō - mĕ - kan′iks). Biomecânica; a ciência relacionada com a ação das forças, internas ou externas, sobre o corpo vivo.
dental b., b. dentária. SIN dental *biophysics*.

bi·o·med·i·cal (bī - ō - med′i - kăl). Biomédico. **1.** Pertinente àqueles aspectos das ciências naturais, principalmente as ciências biológicas e fisiológicas, que se relacionam com ou fundamentam a medicina. **2.** Biológico e médico, i.e., que engloba a ciência e a arte da medicina.

bi·o·mem·brane (bī - ō - mem′brăn). Biomembrana; estrutura que liga uma célula ou organela celular; contém lipídios, proteínas, glicolipídios, esteróides etc. SIN membrane (2).

bi·om·e·ter (bī - om′ĕ - ter). Biômetro; um dispositivo para medir o dióxido de carbono eliminado por organismos e, daí, para determinar a quantidade de matéria viva presente. [bio- + G. *metron*, medida]

bi·o·me·tri·cian (bī - ō - me - trish′an). Biômetro; aquele que se especializa na ciência da biometria.

bi·om·e·try (bī - om′ĕ - trē). Biometria; a aplicação de métodos estatísticos ao estudo dos dados numéricos baseados nas observações e fenômenos biológicos. [bio- + G. *metron*, medida]
b. fetal, b. fetal; a mensuração ultra-sônica das dimensões fetais para avaliar a idade gestacional do tamanho fetal.

bi·o·mi·cro·scope (bī - ō - mī′krō - skōp). Biomicroscópio. SIN slitlamp.

bi·o·mi·cros·co·py (bī - ō - mī - kros′kō - pē). Biomicroscopia. **1.** O exame microscópico de tecido vivo no corpo. **2.** Exame da córnea, humor aquoso, lente, humor vítreo e retina pelo uso de uma lâmpada de fenda combinada a um microscópio binocular.

Bi·om·pha·la·ria (bī - om - fă - lā′rē - ă). Gênero importante de lesmas de água doce (família Planorbidae, subfamília Planorbinae), da qual várias espécies servem como hospedeiros intermediários do *Schistosoma mansoni* na África, Arábia Saudita e Iêmen, América do Sul e no Caribe. As lesmas hospedeiras foram originalmente colocadas nos gêneros *Australorbis*, *Tropicorbis* e *Taphius*, mas não são mais consideradas genericamente distintas.

bi·on (bī′on). Um ser vivo. [G. pas. pres. neut. de *bioō*, viver]

Biondi, Aldolpho, patologista italiano, 1846–1917. VER B.-Heidenhain *stain*.

bi·o·ne·cro·sis (bī - ō - ne - krō′sis). Bionecrose.

bi·on·ic (bī - on′ik). Biônico; relativo a ou desenvolvido a partir da biônica.

bi·on·ics (bī - on′iks). Biônica. **1.** A ciência das funções e mecanismos biológicos conforme aplicados à química eletrônica; como computadores empregando vários aspectos da física, da matemática e da química; p.ex., melhorando a engenharia cibernética por referência à organização do sistema nervoso dos vertebrados. **2.** A ciência de aplicar o conhecimento obtido através do estudo das características dos organismos vivos à formulação de aparelhos e técnicas não-orgânicos. [bio- + electronics]

bi·o·nom·ics (bī′ō-nom′iks). Bionomia. **1.** SIN bionomy. **2.** SIN ecology.

bi·on·o·my (bī-on′ō-mē). Bionomia; as leis da vida; a ciência relacionada com as leis que regulam as funções vitais. SIN bionomics (1). [bio- + G. *nomos*, lei]

bi·o·phage (bī′ō-fāj). Biófago; organismo que se nutre de outro organismo vivo.

bi·oph·a·gism (bī-of′ă-jizm). Biofagismo; o ato de se nutrir de organismos vivos. SIN biophagy. [bio- + G. *phagō*, comer]

bi·oph·a·gous (bī-of′ă-gŭs). Biófago; que se alimenta nos organismos vivos; indicando determinados parasitas.

bi·oph·a·gy (bī-of′ă-jē). Biofagia. SIN biophagism.

bi·o·phar·ma·ceu·tics (bī′ō-far-mă-soo′tiks). Biofarmacêutica; o estudo das propriedades físicas e químicas de um medicamento, e sua forma de dosagem, conforme relacionado ao início, à duração e à intensidade de ação da substância, incluindo os co-constituintes e a modalidade de fabricação.

bi·o·phy·lac·tic (bī′ō-fī-lak′tik). Biofilático; relativo à biofilaxia.

bi·o·phy·lax·is (bī′ō-fī-lak′sis). Biofilaxia; as reações de defesa inespecíficas do corpo, p.ex., fagocitose, reações vasculares e outras reações dos processos inflamatórios. [bio- + G. *phylaxis*, proteção]

bi·o·phys·ics (bī-ō-phyz′iks). Biofísica. **1.** O estudo dos processos e materiais biológicos por meio das teorias e instrumentos da física; a aplicação de métodos físicos para analisar os problemas e processos biológicos. **2.** O estudo dos processos físicos (p.ex., eletricidade, luminescência) que ocorrem nos organismos.

cellular b., b. celular; a b. relacionada com os processos celulares.

dental b., b. dentária; a relação entre o comportamento biológico das estruturas orais e a influência física de uma restauração dentária. SIN dental biomechanics.

medical b., b. médica; a b. relacionada com o diagnóstico e a terapia.

molecular b., b. molecular; a b. relacionada com os processos da membrana, as propriedades conformacionais e configuracionais das macromoléculas, os fenômenos bioelétricos etc.

radiation b., b. da radiação; o estudo dos efeitos da radiação sobre as células, os tecidos, as biomoléculas e os organismos vivos.

bi·o·plasm (bī′ō-plazm). Bioplasma; protoplasma, especialmente em sua relação aos processos vivos e ao desenvolvimento. [bio- + G. *plasma*, coisa formada]

bi·o·plas·mic (bī-ō-plas′mik). Bioplásmico; relativo ao bioplasma.

bi·o·pol·y·mer (bī′ō-pol′ē-mer). Biopolímero; composto de ocorrência natural que é um polímero que contém subunidades idênticas ou similares.

aperiodic b., b. aperiódico; b. que consiste em subunidades não-idênticas existentes em uma seqüência não-periódica.

periodic b., b. periódico; b. em que existem subunidades idênticas e repetitivas.

bi·op·sy (bī′op-sē). Biopsia. **1.** Processo de remoção de tecido a partir de pacientes para o exame diagnóstico. **2.** Uma amostra obtida por b. [bio- + G. *opsis*, visão]

aspiration b., b. por aspiração. SIN needle b.

brush b., b. por escova; obtida através da abrasão da superfície de uma lesão com uma escova para obter as células e tecidos para o exame microscópico.

chorionic villus b., b. de vilosidade coriônica; a amostragem transcervical ou transabdominal das vilosidades coriônicas para análise genética.

endoscopic b., b. endoscópica; b. obtida por instrumentos inseridos através de um endoscópio ou obtida por uma agulha introduzida sob orientação endoscópica.

excision b., b. excisional; a excisão de tecido para os exames macroscópico e microscópico, de tal maneira que toda a lesão seja removida.

fine needle b., b. com agulha fina; a aspiração e remoção de tecido ou suspensões das células através de uma pequena agulha.

incision b., b. incisional; a remoção apenas de uma parte de uma lesão ao fazer uma incisão nela.

needle b., b. por agulha; qualquer método em que a amostra para a b. é removida por aspiração dela através de uma agulha ou trocarte apropriado que perfura a pele, ou a superfície externa de um órgão, e dentro do tecido subjacente a ser examinado. SIN aspiration b.

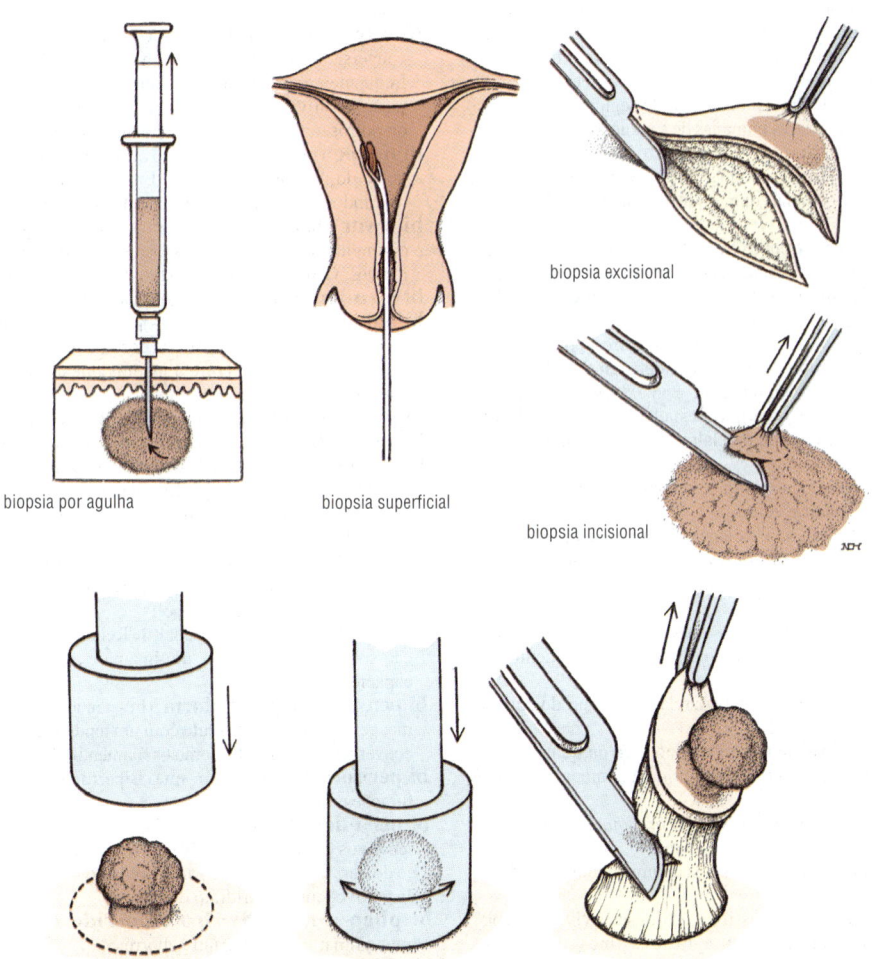

biopsia por agulha
biopsia superficial
biopsia excisional
biopsia incisional
biopsia em saca-bocado (*punch*)

biopsia

open b., b. aberta; a incisão ou excisão cirúrgica da região a partir da qual a b. é obtida.

punch b., b. por punção; qualquer método que remove uma pequena amostra cilíndrica para b. por meio de um instrumento especial que perfura diretamente o órgão ou através da pele ou de uma pequena incisão na pele. SIN trephine b.

sentinal node b., b. de gânglio sentinela; a b. precedida por injeção de um corante ou radioisótopo proximal a um tumor para a identificação, visando à excisão do linfonodo primário que drena a área; usada para determinar a extensão da disseminação de uma malignidade.

shave b., b. por raspagem; técnica de b. realizada com uma lâmina cirúrgica ou uma lâmina de barbeador; usada para lesões que são elevadas acima do nível da pele ou confinadas à epiderme e à derme superior, ou para protrusões das lesões a partir de sítios internos.

sponge b., b. por esponja; abrasão de uma lesão com uma esponja adequada.

trephine b., b. por trépano. SIN punch b.

wedge b., b. em cunha; a excisão de uma amostra cuneiforme.

bi·op·sy·chol·o·gy (bī′ō-sī-kol′ō-jē). Biopsicologia; uma área interdisciplinar de estudo envolvendo psicologia, biologia, fisiologia, bioquímica, as ciências neurais e os campos relacionados.

bi·op·sy·cho·so·cial (bī-ō-sī′kō-sō-shăl). Biopsicossocial; que envolve a inter-relação das influências biológica, psicológica e social.

bi·op·ter·in (bī-op′ter-in). Biopterina; pterina encontrada no fermento, na mosca das frutas e na urina humana normal. A forma reduzida da b. serve como uma coenzima para inúmeras reações catalisadas por enzima.

bi·op·tome (bī-op′tōm). Biótomo; instrumento de biopsia introduzido através de um cateter dentro do coração para se obter pedaços de tecido para o diagnóstico. [biopsy + G. tomē, um corte]

bi·or·bit·al (bī-ōr-bī-tăl). Biorbital; relativo a ambas as órbitas. [bi- + G. orbita, órbita]

bi·o·rhe·ol·o·gy (bī′ō-rē-ol′ō-jē). Biorreologia; a ciência que trata da deformação e do fluxo nos sistemas biológicos. [bio- + G. rheō, fluir, + logos, estudo]

bi·o·rhythm (bī′ō-rith-m). Biorritmo; variação cíclica biologicamente inerente ou recidiva de um evento ou estado, como o ciclo do sono, ritmos circadianos ou doenças periódicas. [bio- + G. rhythmos, ritmo]

bi·o·safe·ty (b-ī′ō-saf′tē). Biossegurança; as medidas de segurança aplicadas ao manuseio dos materiais ou organismos biológicos com um potencial conhecido para provocar doença em seres humanos. As atuais recomendações do Centers for Disease Control and Prevention são as de seguir as precauções universais, que é tratar todas as amostras humanas de sangue e líquidos corporais como se elas fossem infecciosas.

bi·o·sis (bī-ō′sis). Biose; a vida, em um sentido geral. [G. biōsis meio de vida]

bi·o·so·cial (bī-ō-sō′shŭl). Biossocial; que envolve a inter-relação das influências biológicas e sociais.

bi·o·spec·trom·e·try (bī′ō-spek-trom′e-trē). Bioespectrometria; a determinação espectroscópica dos tipos e quantidades de várias substâncias no tecido vivo ou líquido a partir de um corpo vivo. SIN clinical spectrometry. [bio- + L. spectrum, uma imagem, + G. metron, medida]

bi·o·spec·tros·co·py (bī′ō-spek-tros′kō-pē). Bioespectroscopia; o exame espectroscópico do tecido vivo, incluindo os líquidos dele removidos. SIN clinical spectroscopy. [bio- + L. spectrum, imagem, + G. skopeō, examinar]

bi·o·spe·le·ol·o·gy (bī′ō-spē′lē-ol′ō-jē). Bioespeleologia; o estudo dos organismos cujo hábitat natural é total ou parcialmente subterrâneo. [bio- + G. spēliaion, caverna]

bi·o·sphere (bī′ō-sfēr). Biosfera; todas as regiões no mundo onde são encontrados seres vivos. [bio- + G. sphaira, esfera]

bi·o·stat·ics (bī-ō-stat′iks). Bioestático; a ciência da relação entre a estrutura e a função nos organismos. [bio- + G. statikos, que faz ficar de pé]

bi·o·sta·tis·tics (bī′ō-stă-tis′tiks). Bioestatística; a ciência da estatística aplicada a dados biológicos ou médicos.

bi·o·syn·the·sis (bī-ō-sin′thĕ-sis). Biossíntese; a formação de um composto químico por enzimas, quer no organismo (in vivo), quer por fragmentos ou extratos de células (in vitro). SIN biogenesis (2).

bi·o·syn·thet·ic (bī′ō-sin-thet′ik). Biossintético; relativo a ou produzido por biossíntese.

bi·o·sys·tem (bī′ō-sis-tem). Biossistema; organismo vivo ou qualquer sistema completo de coisas vivas que podem, direta ou indiretamente, interagir com outros.

Biot, Camille, médica francesa do século 19. VER B. *breathing, respiration, breathing sign, sign.*

bi·o·ta (bī-ō′tă). Biota; o conjunto da flora e fauna de uma região. [L. Mod., do G. bios, vida]

bi·o·tax·is (bī-ō-tak′sis). Biotaxia. **1.** A classificação dos seres vivos de acordo com suas características anatômicas. **2.** SIN cytoclesis. [bio- + G. taxis, arranjo]

bi·o·tech·nol·ogy (bī′ō-tek-nol′ō-jē). Biotecnologia. **1.** O campo devotado a aplicar as técnicas da bioquímica, da biologia celular, da biofísica e da biologia molecular para abordar as questões práticas relacionadas aos seres humanos, à agricultura e ao ambiente. **2.** O uso das tecnologias do DNA recombinante ou do hibridoma para a produção de moléculas úteis, ou para a alteração dos processos biológicos para estimular alguma propriedade desejada.

bi·o·te·lem·e·try (bī-ō-tel-em′e-trē). Biotelemetria; a técnica de monitorar os processos vitais e transmitir os dados sem fios até um ponto distante da pessoa.

bi·o·test (bī′ō-test). Bioteste; um método para avaliar o efeito de um composto, técnica ou procedimento sobre um organismo. SIN biologic assay.

bi·ot·ic (bī-ot′ik). Biótico; pertinente à vida.

bi·ot·ics (bī-ot′iks). Biótica; a ciência relacionada com as funções da vida ou atividade e força vitais. [G. biōtikos, relativo à vida]

bi·o·tin (bī′ō-tin). Biotina; o componente D-isômero do complexo da vitamina B_2 que ocorre ou é necessário pela maioria dos organismos e inativado pela avidina; participa nas carboxilações biológicas. É uma pequena molécula com alta afinidade pela avidina que pode ser prontamente acoplada a um anticorpo previamente marcado, a fim de permitir a visualização por meios enzimáticos ou histoquímicos. VER TAMBÉM avidin. SIN coenzyme R, vitamina H, W factor.
b. carboxylase, biotina carboxilase; uma subunidade de inúmeras enzimas (p.ex., acetil-CoA carboxilase). Catalisa a formação da carboxibiotina (em uma proteína transportadora de biotina), ADP e P_i a partir de ATP, CO_2 e biotina.
b. oxidase, b. oxidase; uma enzima (provavelmente inespecífica) que catalisa a beta-oxidação da cadeia lateral da biotina.

bi·o·tin·i·dase (bī-ō-tin′i-dās). Biotinidase; enzima que catalisa a hidrólise da biotinamida (formando biotina e amônia), biocitina (formando biotina e lisina) e outras biotinidas. A deficiência da b. pode levar à acidemia orgânica.

bi·ot·i·nides (bī-ot′i-nīdz). Biotinidas; compostos da biotina; p.ex., biocitina.

bi·o·tin·yl·ly·sine (bī′ō-tin-il-lī′sin). Biotinilisina. SIN biocytin.

bi·o·tope (bī′ō-tōp). Biótopo; a menor área geográfica que fornece condições uniformes para a vida; a parte física de um ecossistema. [G. bios, vida, + topos, local]

bi·o·tox·i·col·o·gy (bī-ō-tok-si-kol′ō-jē). Biotoxicologia; o estudo dos venenos produzidos pelos organismos vivos.

bi·o·tox·in (bī-ō-tok′sin). Biotoxina; qualquer substância tóxica formada em um corpo animal, e demonstrável em seus tecidos ou líquidos corporais, ou ambos.

bi·o·trans·for·ma·tion (bī′ō-trans-fōr-mā′shŭn). Biotransformação; a conversão das moléculas de uma forma para outra dentro de um organismo, freqüentemente associada a alteração (aumento, diminuição ou pequena alteração) na atividade farmacológica; refere-se especialmente aos medicamentos ou outros xenobióticos. SIN biodegradation.

bi·o·type (bī′ō-tīp). Biótipo. **1.** Uma população ou grupo de indivíduos composto do mesmo genótipo. **2.** Em bacteriologia, o nome antigo para biovar, referindo-se a uma cepa variante de bactéria. [bio- + G. typos, modelo]

bi·o·var (bī′ō-var). Um grupo (infra-subespecífico) de cepas bacterianas distinguíveis de outras cepas da mesma espécie com base nos caracteres fisiológicos. Originalmente chamado de biótipo. [bio- + variant]

bi·o·vu·lar (bī′ov-ū-lar). Biovular. SIN diovular.

bi·pal·a·ti·noid (bī-pal′ă-ti-noyd). Bipalatinóide; uma cápsula com dois compartimentos, usada para fazer remédios na forma nascente; a reação entre as duas substâncias ocorre à medida que a cápsula se dissolve no estômago, ativando dessa maneira o remédio.

bi·par·a·sit·ism (bī-par′ă-sit-izm). SIN hyperparasitism.

bi·pa·ren·tal (bī-pa-ren′tăl). Que tem dois genitores, macho e fêmea.

bi·pa·ri·e·tal (bī-pa-rī′e-tăl). Biparietal; relativo a ambos os ossos parietais do crânio. [bi- + L. paries, parede]

bip·a·rous (bip′ă-rŭs). Bíparo; que produz descendência dupla. [bi- + L. pario, dar à luz]

bi·par·tite (bī-par′tīt). Bipartite; que consiste em duas partes ou divisões.

bi·ped (bī′ped). Bípede. **1.** Que possui dois pés. **2.** Qualquer animal com apenas dois pés. [bi- + L. pes, pé]

bi·ped·al (bī′ped-ăl). Bipedal. **1.** Relativo a um bípede. **2.** Capaz de locomoção sobre dois pés; p.ex., um iguana e alguns outros lagartos possuem essa capacidade.

bi·pen·nate, bi·pen·ni·form (bī-pen′āt, pen′i-fōrm). Bipenado, bipeniforme; pertinente a um músculo com um tendão central no sentido em que as fibras convergem de cada lado como os filamentos de uma pena. [bi- + L. penna, pena]

bi·per·fo·rate (bī-per′fō-rāt). Biperfurado; que possui dois forames ou perfurações.

bi·per·i·den (bī-per′i-den). Biperideno; agente anticolinérgico com efeitos sedativos e centrais sobre os núcleos da base; usado no tratamento sintomático do parkinsonismo e do parkinsonismo induzido por medicamento. Também disponível como cloridrato de b.

bi·phen·a·mine hy·dro·chlo·ride (bī-fen′ă-mēn). Cloridrato de bifenamina; um agente anti-seborréico.

bi·phe·no·ty·pic (bī′fē-nō-tip′ik). Bifenotípico; pertinente a ou caracterizado por bifenotipia.

bi·phe·no·ty·py (bī-fē′nō-tī′pē) Bifenotipia; a expressão dos marcadores de mais de um tipo de célula pela mesma célula, como em determinadas leucemias.

bi·phen·yl (bī-fen′il). Bifenil, difenil. SIN diphenyl.
  polychlorinated b. (PCB), b. policloretado; o b. em que alguns ou todos os átomos de hidrogênio ligados aos carbonos do anel são substituídos por átomos de cloro; um provável carcinógeno e teratógeno humano.
bi·po·lar (bī-pō′ler). Bipolar; que possui dois pólos, extremidades ou extremos.
Bipolaris (bī-pō-la′ris). Gênero de fungos dematiáceos que estão entre as causas de feoifomicose; algumas espécies de *Drechslera* e *Helminthosporium* são atualmente classificadas como espécies de *B*.
  B. australiensis, espécie de fungos dematiáceos que está entre as causas de feoifomicose.
  B. hawaiiensis, espécie de fungos dematiáceos que está entre as causas de feoifomicose.
  B. spicifera, espécie de fungos dematiáceos que está entre as causas de feoifomicose.
bi·po·ten·ti·al·i·ty (bī′pō-ten-shē-al′i-tē). Bipotencialidade; a capacidade de diferenciar ao longo de dois trajetos de desenvolvimento. Um exemplo é a capacidade da gônada de evoluir para ovário ou testículo.
bi·ra·mous (bī-rā′mŭs). Birramoso; que possui dois ramos. [bi- + L. *ramus*, ramo]
Birbeck, Michael S., pesquisador britânico contemporâneo sobre o câncer. VER B. *granule*.
Birch-Hirschfeld, Felix V., patologista alemão, 1842–1899. VER Birch-Hirschfeld *stain*.
birch tar (berch). Alcatrão da bétula. SIN birch tar oil.
birch tar oil. Óleo de alcatrão de bétula; óleo pirolenhoso obtido pela destilação seca da madeira de *Betula alba* e retificado pela destilação a vapor; usado externamente no tratamento de doenças cutâneas. SIN birch tar.
Bird, Samuel D., médico australiano, 1833–1904. VER B. *sign*.
bi·re·frin·gence (bī-rē-frin′jens). Birrefringência. SIN double *refraction*.
bi·re·frin·gent (bī-rē-frin-jent). Birrefringente; que refrata duas vezes, dividindo um raio luminoso em dois.
Bir·na·vi·ri·dae (bir′nă-vī′rā-dā). Uma família de vírus icosaédricos não-envelopados, com 60 nm de diâmetro, cujo genoma consiste em dois segmentos de RNA linear com filamento duplo.
Bir·navi·rus (bir′nă-vī-rŭs). Um vírus na família Birnaviridae que inclui o vírus da doença infecciosa da bursa de galinhas, patos e perus, e o vírus da necrose pancreática infecciosa do peixe. [bi- + RNA + virus]
bi·ro·ta·tion (bī-rō-tā′shŭn). Birrotação. SIN mutarotation.
birth (berth). Parto, nascimento. **1.** Passagem da prole do útero para o mundo exterior; o ato de nascimento. **2.** Especificamente, no ser humano, a expulsão completa ou extração de um feto a partir de sua mãe, independentemente da idade gestacional, e independentemente de se o cordão umbilical foi cortado ou não e se a placenta está presa ou não.
  b. certificate, certidão de nascimento; documento legal oficial que registra os detalhes de um nascido vivo, geralmente compreendendo o nome, a data, o local, a identidade dos pais e, por vezes, informações adicionais, como o peso de n.
  premature b., nascimento prematuro; o nascimento de um feto que alcançou uma gestação mínima de 20 semanas ou o peso de nascimento mínimo de 500 g, mas antes de 37 semanas.
birth·ing (bir′thing). Parto; o ato de dar à luz.
birth·mark (berth′mark). Marca de nascimento; uma lesão visível permanente, usualmente na pele, identificada no nascimento ou próximo a ele; comumente um nevo ou hemangioma. VER nevus (1).
  strawberry b., nevo em morango. SIN strawberry *nevus.*
bis-. 1. Prefixo que significa dois ou duplo. **2.** Em química, usado para indicar a presença de dois grupos complexos idênticos, porém separados, em uma molécula. Cf. bi-, di-. [L.]

medidas médias ao nascimento	
comprimento	49–52 cm
diâmetro suboccipitobregmático	9,5 cm
diâmetro occipitofrontal	12,0 cm
diâmetro occipitomentual	13,5 cm
perímetro suboccipitobregmático	32,0 cm
perímetro occipitofrontal	34,0 cm
perímetro occipitomentual	35,0 cm
largura interescapular	12,0 cm
perímetro escapular	35,0 cm
largura do quadril	10–11 cm
perímetro do quadril	27,0 cm

bis·ac·o·dyl (bis-ak′ō-dil). Bisacodil; um laxativo utilizado por via oral ou retal para a constipação. A mesma classe da fenolftaleína.
bis·a·cro·mi·al (bis′a-krō′mē-āl). Bisacromial; relativo aos dois processos acromiais.
bis·al·bu·mi·ne·mia (bis′al-bū′mi-nē′mē-ă). Bisalbuminemia; a presença simultânea de dois tipos de albumina sérica que diferem na mobilidade na eletroforese: albumina normal (albumina A) e qualquer um dos diversos tipos variantes que migram em outras velocidades; os indivíduos são heterozigotos para o gene para a albumina A e o gene para a variante do tipo albumina. VER TAMBÉM inherited albumin *variants*, em *variant*.
bis·ax·il·lary (bis-ak′si-lār-ē). Biaxilar; relativo às duas axilas.
bis·ben·zy·liso·quinoline al·ka·loids (bis-benz′il-ī-sō-kwin′ō-lin al-ka-loids). Alcalóides da dibenzilisoquinolina; um grupo de alcalóides cuja estrutura básica é formada por dois anéis de isoquinolina fundidos; p.ex., alcalóides do curare.
2,5-bis(5-*t*-bu·tyl·ben·zox·a·zol-2·yl)thi·o·phene (BBOT). 2,5-bis(5-*t*-butilbenzoxazol-2-il)tiofeno (BBOT); cintilador utilizado nas mensurações da radioatividade pela contagem de cintilação.
Bischof, W., neurocirurgião alemão do século 20. VER B. *myelotomy*.
bis·cuit (bis′kit). Biscoito; termo associado à queima da porcelana e aplicado ao artigo queimado antes de ser vidrado. Pode ser em qualquer estágio depois que os fluxos fluíram o suficiente para fornecer a rigidez à estrutura até o estágio em que o encolhimento é completo. Referido como b. baixo, médio ou alto, dependendo da totalidade da vitrificação, também como b. duro ou mole.
bis·cuit-bake. Queima de biscoito; a queima inicial feita para fundir a porcelana em temperaturas inferiores às de vitrificação para controlar o encolhimento durante o processo de fabricação da restauração dentária. SIN biscuit-firing.
biscuit-fir·ing. Queima de biscoito. SIN biscuit-bake.
bis·de·qua·lin·i·um chlo·ride (bis′de-kwă-lin′ē-ŭm). Cloreto de bisdequalínio; um anti-séptico.
bis in die (b.i.d.) (bis in dē′ă). Duas vezes ao dia [L.].
bi·sex·u·al (bī-seks′ū-ăl). Bissexual. **1.** Que possui as gônadas de ambos os sexos. VER TAMBÉM hermaphroditism. **2.** Indica um indivíduo que mantém relacionamentos heterossexuais e homossexuais.
bis·fer·i·ent (bis-fer′ē-ent). SIN bisferious.
bis·fer·i·ous (bis-fer′ē-ŭs). Bisfério; que bate duas vezes; diz-se do pulso. SIN bisferient. [L. *bis*, duas vezes, + *ferio*, colidir]
Bishop, Louis F., médico norte-americano, 1864–1941. VER B. *sphygmoscope*.
bis·hy·drox·y·cou·ma·rin (bis-hī-droks′ē-koo′mă-rin). Bisidroxicumarina. SIN dicumarol.
bis·il·i·ac (bis-il′ē-ak). Bisilíaco; relativo a quaisquer duas partes ou estruturas ilíacas correspondentes, como os ossos ilíacos ou as fossas ilíacas.
Bismarck brown R [C. I. 21010]. Castanho de Bismarck; um corante diazo similar ao castanho de Bismarck Y.
Bismarck brown Y [C.I. 21000]. Castanho de Bismarck Y; corante diazo utilizado para colorir a mucina e a cartilagem em cortes histológicos, na técnica de Papanicolaou para os esfregaços vaginais, e como um dos reagentes do tipo Kasten Schiff nas colorações PAS e Feulgen. SIN vesuvin. [Alemão *bismarckbraun*, em homenagem a Otto von *Bismarck*, chanceler alemão]
bis·muth (Bi) (biz′mŭth). Bismuto; um elemento metálico trivalente; número atômico 83, peso atômico 20,98037. Vários de seus sais são utilizados em medicina; alguns contêm BiO^+, em lugar de Bi^{3+}, e são chamados de subsais. [Alemão *Wismut*, *weisse Masse*, massa branca]
  b. aluminate, aluminato de b.; um antiácido gástrico. SIN aluminum bismuth oxide.
  b. ammonium citrate, amoniocitrato de b.; um adstringente intestinal.
  b. carbonate, carbonato de b. SIN b. subcarbonate.
  b. chloride oxide, oxicloreto de b. SIN b. oxychloride.
  b. citrate, citrato de b.; usado na fabricação de citrato de amônio e b.
  b. hydroxide. hidróxido de b.; usado na detecção de açúcares redutores.
  b. iodide, iodeto de b.; BiI_3; usado na microscopia eletrônica para revelar sinapses. SIN b. triiodide.
  b. oxide, óxido de b.; usado para as mesmas finalidades que o subnitrato.
  b. oxycarbonate, oxicarbonato de b. SIN b. subcarbonate.
  b. oxychloride, oxicloreto de b.; cloreto básico de b., utilizado para as mesmas finalidades que o subnitrato. SIN b. chloride oxide, bismuthyl chloride.
  b. oxynitrate, oxinitrato de b. SIN b. subnitrate.
  b. salicylate, salicilato de b. VER b. subsalicylate.
  b. sodium tartrate, tartarato sódico de b.; um tartarato sódico básico de b.; um agente anti-sifilítico.
  b. sodium triglycollamate, triglicolamato sódico de b.; um complexo sódico de b. do ácido nitrilotriacético.
  b. subcarbonate, subcarbonato de b.; usado para os mesmos propósitos que o subnitrato de b., porém apresenta menor toxicidade. SIN b. carbonate, b. oxycarbonate, bismuthyl carbonate.
  b. subgallate, subgalato de b.; usado internamente na diarréia e externamente como adstringente e polvilho protetor.

b. subnitrate, subnitrato de b.; um sal básico, cuja composição varia com as condições de preparação; usado internamente como adstringente intestinal e externamente como adstringente brando e anti-séptico; o metal é utilizado como um corante de microscopia eletrônica para os ácidos nucléicos. SIN b. oxynitrate.
b. subsalicylate, subsalicilato de bismuto; usado como anti-séptico intestinal.
b. tribromophenate, b. tribromophenol, tribromofenato de b., tribromofenol de b.; usado externamente como anti-séptico.
b. trichloride, tricloreto de b.; $BiCl_3$; a adição de água resulta na formação de oxicloreto de bismuto. SIN butter of bismuth.
b. triiodide, triiodeto de b. SIN b. iodide.

bis·mu·tho·sis (bis-mū-thō′sis). Bismutose; intoxicação crônica por bismuto.

bis·muth·yl (biz′mŭ-thil). Bismutila; o grupamento, BiO^+, que se comporta quimicamente como o íon de um metal univalente; seus sais são subsais de bismuto.
b. carbonate, carbonato de bismutila. SIN bismuth subcarbonate.
b. chloride, cloreto de bismutila. SIN bismuth oxychloride.

bis·ox·a·tin ac·e·tate (bis-ok′sa-tin). Acetato de bizoxatina; um laxativo.

1,4-bis(5-phen·yl·ox·a·zol-2-yl)ben·zene. 1,4-bis(5-feniloxazol-2-il)benzeno; um agente de cintilação líquido utilizado na mensuração de radioisótopo.

1,3-bis·phos·pho·glyc·er·ate (1,3-P_2Gri) (dī-fos′fō-glis′er-āt). 1,3-bifosfoglicerato (1,3-P_2Gri); um intermediário na glicólise que reage enzimaticamente com o ADP para produzir ATP e 3-fosfoglicerato.

2,3-bis·phos·pho·glyc·er·ate (2,3-P_2Gri). 2,3-bifosfoglicerato (2,3-P_2Gri); um intermediário na via metabólica de Rapoport-Luebering, formado entre 1,3-bifosfoglicerato e 3-fosfoglicerato; um importante regulador da afinidade da hemoglobina pelo oxigênio; um intermediário da fosfoglicerato mutase.
2,3-b. mutase, 2,3-b. mutase; uma enzima da via metabólica de Rapoport-Luebering; catalisa a interconversão reversível do 1,3-bifosfoglicerato em 2,3-b.; também apresenta atividade de fosfatase, que converte o 2,3-b. em ortofosfato e 3-fosfoglicerato; a deficiência de 2,3-b. mutase pode resultar em eritrocitose branda.

bis·phos·pho·nates (bis-fos′fō-nāts). Bifosfonatos; os análogos sintéticos do pirofosfato que inibem a reabsorção osteoclástica do osso.

bi·ste·phan·ic (bī′stē-fan′ik). Biestefânico; relativo aos dois estefânios; indica principalmente a largura b. do crânio ou o diâmetro b., a distância mais curta de um estefânio a outro.

bi·ste·roid (bī-stēr′oyd). Biesteróide; uma molécula composta de duas moléculas de um determinado esteróide unidas por uma ligação de carbono a carbono.

bis·tou·ry (bis′too-rē). Bisturi; uma faca com lâmina estreita e longa, com uma borda reta ou curva e uma ponta afiada ou cega (ponto de sondagem); usado para a abertura ou incisão de cavidades ou estruturas ocas. [Fr. *bistouri*, do dialeto Ital. *bistori*, talvez de *Pistoia*, Itália]

bi·stra·tal (bī-strā′tal). Biestratificado; que possui dois estratos ou camadas.

bi·sul·fate (bī-sŭl′fāt). Bissulfato; um sal que contém HSO_4^-. SIN acid sulfate.

bi·sul·fide (bī-sŭl′fīd). Bissulfeto; um composto do ânion HS^-; um sulfeto ácido.

bi·sul·fite (bī-sŭl′fīt). Bissulfeto; um sal ou íon de HSO_3^-.

bit. *Bit.* 1. A menor unidade de informação digital expressa no sistema de notação binária (quer 0, quer 1). 2. O sinal elétrico utilizado em computadores eletrônicos. SIN binary digit.

bi·tar·trate (bī-tar′trāt). Bitartarato; um sal ou ânion que resulta da neutralização de um dos dois grupamentos ácidos do ácido tartárico.

bitch. Cadela; um cão do sexo feminino em idade de procriação. [O. E. *bicche*]

bite (bīt). 1. Morder; incisar ou prender com os dentes. 2. Mordida; o ato da incisão ou preensão com os dentes. 3. Um pedaço de alimento mantido entre os dentes. 4. Mordida; termo utilizado para indicar a quantidade de pressão desenvolvida no fechamento dos maxilares. 5. Jargão indesejável para termos como o registro interoclusal, o registro maxilomandibular, o espaço dentário e a distância entre arcadas. 6. Mordida, picada; uma ferida ou punção da pele feita por animal ou inseto. [A. S. *bītan*]
balanced b., mordida equilibrada. SIN balanced occlusion.
biscuit b., registro maxilomandibular. SIN maxillomandibular record.
close b., mordida próxima. SIN small interarch distance.
closed b., mordida fechada; a distância vertical reduzida entre arcadas com sobreposição vertical excessiva dos dentes anteriores.
deep b., mordida profunda; uma sobreposição vertical anormalmente grande dos dentes anteriores na oclusão cêntrica.
edge-to-edge b., oclusão término-terminal. SIN edge-to-edge occlusion.
end-to-end b., oclusão término-terminal. SIN edge-to-edge occlusion.
jumping the b., uma técnica ortodôntica para corrigir uma mordida cruzada, usualmente anterior.
locked b., mordida bloqueada; oclusão em que a disposição da cúspide restringe as excursões laterais.
normal b., mordida normal. SIN normal occlusion (1).
open b., mordida aberta. (1) SIN large interarch distance; (2) SIN apertognathia.

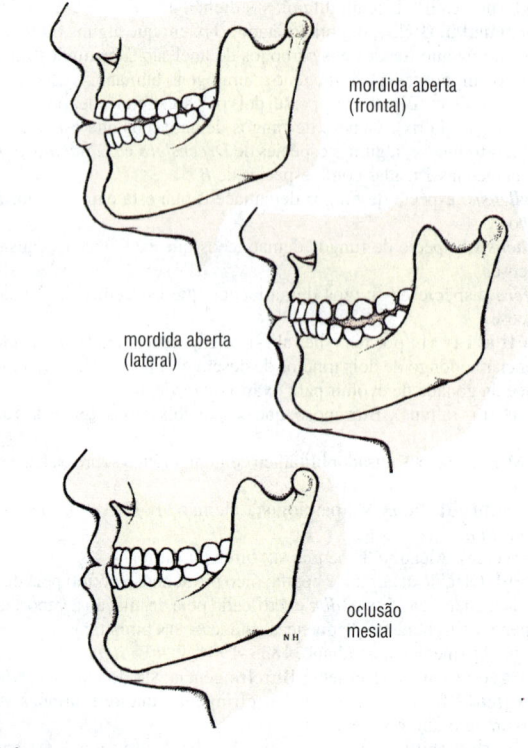

mordedura

rest b., mordida em repouso; um nome errôneo para physiologic rest *position of the mandible* (posição de repouso fisiológico da mandíbula).
working b., contatos funcionais. SIN working contacts, em contact.

bi·tem·po·ral (bī-tem′pō-ral). Bitemporal; relativo a ambas as têmporas ou ossos temporais.

bite·plate, bite·plane (bīt′plāt, bīt′plān). Placa de mordida, plano de mordida; um dispositivo removível que incorpora um plano de acrílico projetado para ocluir com os dentes opostos.

bite·wing (bīt′wing). "Asa mordida". VER bitewing *radiograph*.

bi·thi·o·nol (bī-thī′ō-nol). Bitinol; um agente antiparasitário utilizado para o tratamento do *Paragonimus westermani* e da fascíola hepática oriental, *Clonorchis sinensis*; também usado como bacteriostático em sabões e detergentes; o bitionato sódico é usado como bactericida tópico e fungicida.

bi·tol·ter·ol mes·y·late (bī-tol′ter-ol). Mesilato de bitolterol; um broncodilatador simpaticomimético utilizado na profilaxia e no tratamento da asma brônquica e do broncoespasmo reversível.

Bitot, Pierre A., médico francês, 1822–1888. VER B. *spots*, em *spot*.

bi·tro·chan·ter·ic (bī-trō-kan-ter′ik). Bitrocantérico; relativo a dois trocanteres, quer aos dois trocanteres de um fêmur, quer aos trocanteres maiores.

bi·tro·pic (bī-trop′ik). Bitrópico; que tem uma afinidade dupla, como nos tecidos ou organismos. [bi- + G. *tropē*, uma volta]

bit·ter ap·ple. Colocinto, coloquíntida. SIN colocynth.

bit·ters. 1. *Bitter*; aperitivo alcoólico no qual substâncias vegetais amargas (p.ex., quinina, genciana) foram mergulhadas. **2.** Medicamentos vegetais amargos (p.ex., quássia, genciana, cinchona), comumente utilizados como tônicos. SIN amara.
aromatic b., amargos aromáticos; amargo com sabor aromático agradável.

Bittner, John J., oncologista norte-americano, 1904–1961. VER B. *agent*, milk *factor*.

Bittorf, Alexander, médico alemão, 1876–1949. VER B. *reaction*.

bi·u·ret (bī-oo-ret′). Biureto; derivado da uréia obtido por aquecimento, eliminando um NH_3 entre as duas uréias. Usado nas determinações de proteínas. SIN carbamoylurea.

bi·va·lence, bi·va·len·cy (bī-vā′lens, bī-vā′len-sē). Bivalência; uma força de combinação (valência) de 2. SIN divalence, divalency.

bi·va·lent (bī-vā′lent, biv′a-lent). Bivalente. **1.** Que possui uma força de combinação (valência) de 2. SIN divalent. **2.** Em citologia, uma estrutura que consiste em dois cromossomas homólogos pareados, cada um dividindo-se em duas cromátides irmãs, conforme observado durante o estágio paquíteno da prófase na meiose. VER TAMBÉM tetrad.

bi·ven·ter (bī-ven′ter). Biventre; dois ventres; indica os músculos com dois ventres. [bi- + L. *venter*, ventre]

b. cer'vicis, músculo espinal da cabeça. SIN spinalis capitis (*muscle*).
b. mandib'ulae, músculo digástrico. SIN digastric (*muscle*) (1).
bi·ven·tral (bī-ven'tral). Biventral. SIN digastric (1).
bi·ven·tric·u·lar (bī-ven-trik'oo-lar). Biventricular; pertinente aos ventrículos direito e esquerdo.
bix·in (bik'sin). Bixina; éster monometílico de um ácido dicarboxílico insaturado ramificado com 24 carbonos; um carotenóide (um ácido carotenodióico); a substância com coloração amarelo-avermelhada obtida das sementes da *Bixa orellana*; o éster etílico é empregado como corante alimentar e medicamentoso. VER TAMBÉM annotto.
bi·zy·go·mat·ic (bī'zī-gō-mat'ik). Bizigomático; pertinente aos arcos ou ossos zigomáticos.
Bizzozero, Giulio, médico italiano, 1846–1901. VER B. *corpuscle*.
Bjerrum, Jannik P., oftalmologista dinamarquês, 1851–1920. VER B. *scotoma, screen, sign*.
Björk, V. O., cirurgião cardiotorácico sueco do século 20. VER B.-Shiley *valve*.
Björnstad, R. dermatologista escandinavo do século 20. VER B. *syndrome*.
Bk Símbolo do berkelium (berquélio, berkélio).
Black, Douglas A. K., médico escocês, *1909. VER B. *formula*.
Black, Greene V., dentista norte-americano, 1836–1915. VER B. *classification*.
Blackfan, Kenneth D., médico norte-americano, 1883–1941. VER Diamond-B. *anemia, syndrome*.
black·out (blak'owt). *Blackout*, blecaute. **1.** Perda temporária da consciência devido ao fluxo sangüíneo diminuído para o cérebro. **2.** Perda momentânea da consciência, como na crise de ausência. **3.** Perda temporária da visão, sem alteração da consciência, decorrente de forças g (gravidade) positivas; causada por fluxo sangüíneo diminuído temporário na artéria central da retina e observada mais amiúde em aviadores. **4.** Um episódio transitório que acontece durante um estado de intoxicação intensa (*blackout* alcoólico) do qual a pessoa não tem lembrança, embora não fique inconsciente (conforme observado pelos outros).
 visual b., *blackout* visual. VER amaurosis fugax.
black root. SIN leptandra.
blad·der (blad'er) [TA]. Bexiga. **1.** Um órgão músculo-membranoso distensível que serve como um receptáculo para o líquido, como a bexiga urinária ou a vesícula biliar. VER detrusor. **2.** SIN urinary b. [A.S. *blaedre*]
 air b., b. natatória; um saco de dois compartimentos cheios de gás que existe na maioria dos peixes e funciona como um órgão hidrostático; está localizada abaixo da coluna vertebral e está ligada ao esôfago em alguns peixes. SIN swim b.
 allantoic b., b. alantóica; um tipo de b. formado como um crescimento da cloaca.
 atonic b., b. atônica; b. urinária grande, dilatada e que não se esvazia; geralmente decorrente de distúrbio da inervação ou de obstrução crônica.
 autonomic neurogenic b., b. neurogênica autônoma; mau funcionamento da b. urinária, secundário a lesões baixas na medula espinal.
 gall b., vesícula biliar. SIN gallbladder.
 hyperreflexic b., b. hiper-reflexa; b. que exibe instabilidade do detrusor.
 hypertonic b., b. hipertônica; b. com complacência deficiente.
 ileal b., conduto ileal. SIN ileal *conduit*.
 neurogenic b., b. neurogênica. SIN neuropathic b.
 neuropathic b., b. neuropática; qualquer funcionamento defeituoso da bexiga decorrente de comprometimento da inervação, p.ex., b. medular, b. neuropática. SIN neurogenic b.
 nonneurogenic neurogenic b., b. neurogênica não-neurogênica; a incoordenação do esfíncter-detrusor com incontinência urinária, constipação, infecção do trato urinário, alterações do trato superior. SIN Hinman syndrome, pseudoneurogenic b.
 poorly compliant b., b. com complacência deficiente; b. que apresenta pressão alta em volumes baixos na ausência de atividade do detrusor.
 pseudoneurogenic b., b. pseudoneurogênica. SIN nonneurogenic neurogenic b.
 reflex neurogenic b., b. neurogênica reflexa; uma condição anormal da função da b. urinária por meio da qual a b. é separada do controle do neurônio motor superior, mas o arco do neurônio motor inferior ainda permanece intacto.
 swim b., b. natatória. SIN air b.
 trabeculated b., b. trabeculada; caracterizada por parede espessa e feixes musculares hipertrofiados. Tipicamente observada nos casos de obstrução crônica.
 uninhibited neurogenic b., b. neurogênica desinibida; disfunção, quer congênita, quer adquirida, da b. urinária na qual o controle inibitório normal pelo sistema nervoso central da função do detrusor é comprometido ou está mal desenvolvido, resultando em urgência ou enurese.
 unstable b., b. instável; caracterizada por contrações não-inibidas do detrusor.
 urinary b. [TA], b. urinária; uma bolsa elástica músculo-membranosa que serve como um local de armazenamento para a urina. SIN bladder (2) [TA], vesica urinaria [TA], vesica (1) [TA], cystis urinaria, urocyst, urocystis.
blad·der·worm (blad'er-werm). *Cysticercus*. SIN *Cysticercus*.

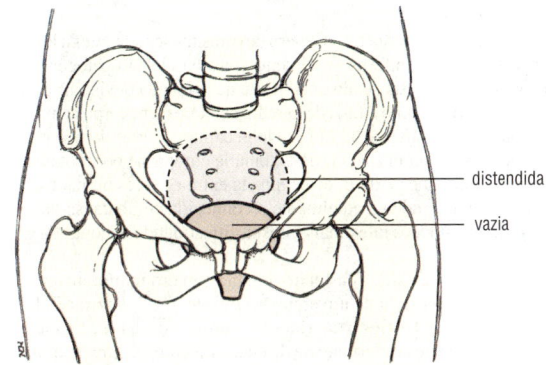

bexiga urinária: mostrada nos estados vazio e distendido

blade·vent (blād'vent). Um fino implante metálico endósteo em forma de cunha que é inserido em um sulco cirurgicamente preparado na maxila ou mandíbula.
Blagden, Sir Charles, médico britânico, 1748–1820. VER B. *law*.
Blainville, Henri Marie Ducrotay de, zoólogo e antropólogo francês, 1777–1850. VER B. *ears*, em *ear*.
Blair, Vilray P., cirurgião norte-americano, 1871–1955.
Blakemore, Arthur H., cirurgião norte-americano, 1897–1970. VER Sengstaken-B. *tube*.
Blalock, Alfred, cirurgião norte-americano, 1899–1964. VER B. *shunt*; B.-Hanlon *operation*; B.-Taussig *operation, shunt*.
Blandin, Phillippe Frédéric, anatomista e cirurgião francês, 1798–1849. VER B. *gland*.
blank. Uma solução que consiste em todos os componentes analíticos exceto o composto a ser medido; é utilizada para estabelecer a intensidade de mensuração padrão com a qual o composto de interesse é comparado. [Ing. Mod. branco, do Fr. Ant. *blanc*, do alemão]
blanket. Cobertor; um revestimento.
 mucus b., c. de muco; o muco que reveste o epitélio respiratório.
blas. Termo inventado por van Helmont para indicar um destilado místico ou força vital que presidiu e governou os vários processos do corpo. Supunha-se que cada função corporal tinha seu próprio b. especial; o b. parece ser a contraparte do archaeus de Paracelsus. [uma variante da I. M. *blast*]
Blaschko, Alfred, dermatologista austríaco, 1858–1922. VER *lines* of B., em *line*.
Blasius, Gerhard (Blaes), anatomista holandês, 1626(?)–1692. VER B. *duct*.
blast (blāst). Blasto; termo genérico para a célula imatura ou precursora. [G. *blastos*, germe]
-blast. Sufixo que indica uma célula precursora imatura do tipo indicado pela palavra precedente. [G. *blastos*, germe]
blas·te·ma (blas-tē'mă). Blastema. **1.** A massa celular primordial (precursora) a partir da qual se forma um órgão ou parte. **2.** Um grumo de células competentes para iniciar a regeneração de uma estrutura comprometida ou extirpada. [G. um brotamento]
 metanephric b., b. metanéfrico. SIN metanephric *cap*.
 nephric b., b. néfrico; a extensão do tecido do cordão nefrogênico, caudal ao mesonefro, em direção ao qual os brotos uretéricos crescem para iniciar o desenvolvimento do rim definitivo do mamífero. SIN nephroblastema.
blas·tem·ic (blas-tem'ik). Blastêmico; relativo ao blastema.
blas·tic (blas'tik) Blástico. **1.** Descreve a formação de um conídio pelo processo de brotamento de uma hifa fértil antes de ser limitado por um septo. **2.** Termo coloquial para osteoblástico. [G. *blastos*, germe, + -ic]
blasto-. Forma combinante que indica o processo de brotamento (e a formação dos brotos) por células ou tecidos. [G. *blastos*, germe]
blas·to·cele (blas'tō-sēl). Blastocele; a cavidade na blástula de um embrião em desenvolvimento. SIN blastocoele, cleavage cavity, segmentation cavity. [blasto- + G. *koilos*, oco]
blas·to·cel·ic (blas-tō-sē'lik). Blastocélico; relativo à blastocele. SIN blastocoelic.
blas·to·coele (blas'tō-sēl). Blastocele. SIN blastocele.
blas·to·coel·ic (blas'tō-sē'lik). Blastocélico. SIN blastocelic.
blas·to·co·nid·i·um (blas'tō-cō-nid'ē-ŭm). Blastoconídio; um conídio holoblástico que é produzido isoladamente ou em cadeias e desprendido na maturidade, deixando uma cicatriz de brotamento, como no brotamento de uma célula de levedura. SIN blastospore. [blasto- + conidium]
blas·to·cyst (blas'tō-sist). Blastocisto; o estágio de blástula modificado dos embriões de mamíferos, consistindo na massa de células interna e em uma fina

camada trofoblástica envolvendo a blastocele. SIN blastodermic vesicle. [blasto- + G. *kystis*, bexiga]

Blas·to·cys·tis (blas′tō-sis′tis). Gênero de parasitas semelhantes a leveduras no trato digestivo dos mamíferos; geralmente considerado não-patogênico. Sua relação com os fungos está sendo atualmente questionada devido às características de protozoários, como a falta de paredes celulares, um corpo central ligado à membrana, pseudópodos, aparelho de Golgi e mitocôndrias do tipo protozoário e reprodução por esporulação ou fissão binária em vez de por brotamento.
  B. hominis, uma espécie de *B.* disseminada entre os seres humanos, originalmente considerada inócua, atualmente reconhecida como causa de diarréia e de outras manifestações intestinais e eosinofilia, quando encontrada em infecções maciças.

blas·to·cyte (blas′tō-sīt). Blastócito; um blastômero indiferenciado do estágio de mórula ou blástula de um embrião. [blasto- + G. *kytos*, célula]

blas·to·derm, blas·to·der·ma (blas′tō-derm, -tō-der′ma). Blastoderma; a massa celular fina e em formato de disco de um embrião jovem e suas extensões extra-embrionárias sobre a superfície do vitelo; quando completamente formado, todas as três camadas germinativas primárias (ectoderma, endoderma e mesoderma) estão presentes. SIN germ membrane, germinal membrane, membrana germinativa. [blasto- + G. *derma*, pele]

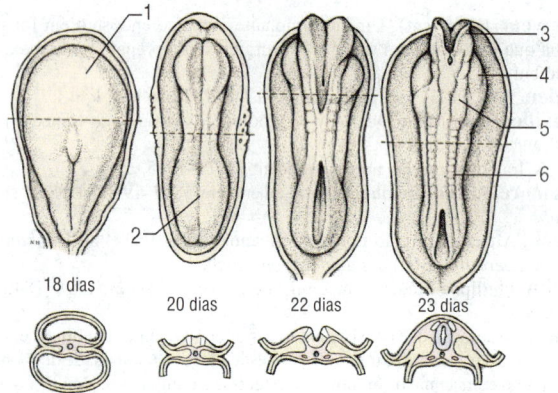

blastoderma: (acima) vistas dorsais, (abaixo) vistas transversais; (1) placa neural, (2) estria primitiva, (3) prega neural, (4) coração, (5) placódio auditivo, (6) somito

bilaminar b., b. bilaminar; o b. de um embrião jovem quando consiste em apenas duas das três camadas germinativas primárias que ele finalmente terá.
embryonic b., b. embrionário; a parte do b. que entra na formação do corpo embrionário.
extraembryonic b., b. extra-embrionário; a parte do b. que não é incorporada ao embrião, mas que forma as membranas relacionadas com sua nutrição e proteção.
trilaminar b., b. trilaminar; o b. depois que todas as três camadas germinativas primárias foram estabelecidas.

blas·to·der·mal, blas·to·der·mic (blas-tō-der′mal, -der′mik). Blastodérmico; relativo ao blastoderma.

blas·to·disk (blas′tō-disk). Blastodisco. **1.** O disco de citoplasma ativo no pólo animal de um ovo telolécito. **2.** O blastoderma, principalmente nos estágios muito jovens, quando sua extensão é pequena.

blas·to·gen·e·sis (blas-tō-jen′e-sis). Blastogênese. **1.** Reprodução de microrganismos unicelulares por brotamento. **2.** Desenvolvimento de um embrião durante a clivagem e a formação da camada germinativa. **3.** Transformação de pequenos linfócitos do sangue periférico humano na cultura de tecido em células grandes, semelhantes ao blasto, morfologicamente primitivas, capazes de sofrer mitose; pode ser induzida por vários agentes, incluindo a fito-hemaglutinina, a concanavalina A, determinados antígenos para os quais a célula doadora foi previamente imunizada e leucócitos de um indivíduo sem parentesco. [blasto- + G. *genesis*, origem]

blas·to·ge·net·ic, blas·to·gen·ic (blas′tō-je-net′ik, -tō-jen′ik). Blastogenético, blastogênico; relativo à blastogênese.

blas·tol·y·sis (blas-tol′i-sis). Blastólise; dissolução ou destruição do blastocisto ou das células blásticas e a morte subseqüente. [blasto- + G. *lysis*, desintegração]

blas·to·lyt·ic (blas-tō-lit′ik). Blastolítico; relativo à blastólise.

blas·to·ma (blas-tō′ma). Blastoma; uma neoplasia composta principalmente ou totalmente de células indiferenciadas imaturas que se assemelham àquelas que formam o blastema ou o primórdio do órgão em que o tumor surgiu. [blasto- + G. *-oma*, tumor]

blas·to·mere (blas′tō-mer). Blastômero; uma das células em que o ovo se divide depois de sua fertilização. SIN cleavage cell, embryonic cell. [blasto- + G. *meros*, parte]

blas·to·mer·ot·o·my (blas′tō-mer-ot′ō-me). Blastomerotomia. SIN blastotomy. [blastomere + G. *tomē*, incisão]

blas·to·mo·gen·ic (blas′tō-mō-jen′ik). Blastomogênico; que causa ou produz um blastoma.

Blas·to·my·ces der·ma·tit·i·dis (blas-tō-mī′sēz der-ma-tit′i-dis). Fungo dimórfico do solo que causa blastomicose, cresce nos tecidos dos mamíferos como células em brotamento e na cultura como um fungo filamentoso branco a amarelo que porta conídios esféricos ou ovóides nos conidiosporos finos e curtos terminais ou laterais. Em seu estado perfeito (teleomorfo), é conhecido como *Ajellomyces dermatitidis*. [blasto- + G. *mykēs*, fungo]

blas·to·my·cin (blas-tō-mī′sin). Blastomicina; um antígeno para teste intradérmico preparado a partir de filtrados estéreis de culturas da forma filamentosa de *Blastomyces dermatitidis*.

blas·to·my·co·sis (blas′tō-mī-kō′sis). Blastomicose; uma doença granulomatosa crônica e supurativa causada pelo *Blastomyces dermatitidis*; origina-se como uma infecção respiratória e se dissemina, usualmente com envolvimento pulmonar, ósseo e/ou cutâneo predominante. Originalmente chamada de b. norte-americana, a doença tem sido atualmente encontrada em países africanos, bem como no Canadá e nos Estados Unidos. SIN Gilchrist disease.
  Brazilian b., b. brasileira; termo obsoleto para a paracoccidioidomicose.
  cutaneous b., b. cutânea; as lesões cutâneas verrucosas ou ulcerativas observadas na infecção por *Blastomyces dermatitidis*.
  North American b., b. norte-americana. VER blastomycosis.
  South American b., b. sul-americana. SIN paracoccidioidomycosis.
  systemic b., b. sistêmica; a infecção por *Blastomyces dermatitidis* que se estende além da pele ou do pulmão, as portas de entrada usuais; o envolvimento dos ossos e do trato genitourinário (sobretudo da próstata e do epidídimo) é mais freqüente.

blas·to·neu·ro·pore (blas′tō-noo′rō-pōr). Blastoneuroporo; uma abertura temporária formada em alguns embriões pela união do blastoporo e neuroporo. [blasto- + neuropore]

blas·to·phore (blas-tō-fōr). Blastóforo; um estágio inicial da divisão de um esquizonte coccidiano em que as estruturas esferoidais ou elipsóides são formadas com uma única camada periférica de núcleos; os merozoítos formam-se na superfície do n. sobre cada núcleo, crescem no sentido radial e separam-se do corpo residual (resquício do b.); em um esquizonte de primeira geração, como *Eimeria bovis*, são produzidos cerca de 120.000 merozoítos. [blasto- + G. *phorōs*, produtivo]

blas·to·pore (blas′tō-pōr). Blastóporo; a abertura para o arquêntero, formada pela invaginação da blástula para formar uma gástrula. SIN protostoma, protostome. [blasto- + G. *poros*, abertura]

Blas·to·schiz·o·my·ces (blas′tō-skiz-ō-mī′sēz). Um gênero de fungos semelhantes a leveduras.
  B. capitatus, espécie de fungo que causa infecção disseminada grave em pacientes imunossuprimidos; originalmente classificado como uma espécie de *Geotrichum*.

blas·to·spore (blas′tō-spōr). Blastosporo. SIN Blastoconidium. [blasto- + G. *sporos*, semente]

blas·tot·o·my (blas-tot′ō-me). Blastotomia; a destruição experimental de um ou mais blastômeros. SIN blastomerotomy; [blasto- + G. *tomē*, incisão]

blas·tu·la (blas′tū-la). Blástula; estágio inicial de um embrião formado pelo rearranjo dos blastômeros da mórula para formar uma esfera oca. [G. *blastos*, germe]

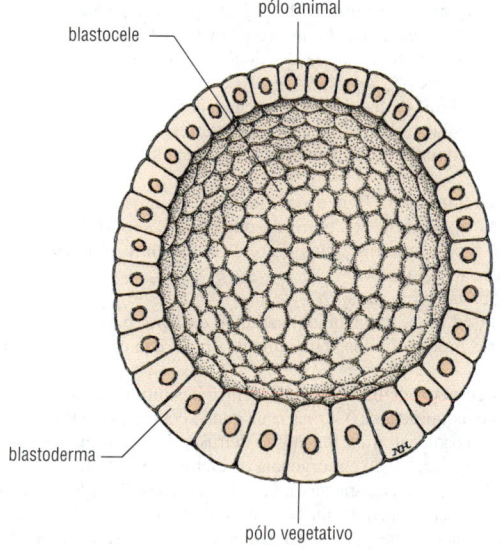

blástula: hemisseccionada

blas·tu·lar (blas′tū-lar) Blastular; pertinente à blástula.

blas·tu·la·tion (blas-tū-lā′shŭn). Blastulação; formação da blástula ou blastocisto a partir da mórula.

Blatin, Marc, médico francês, *1878. VER B. *syndrome*.

Blat·ta (blat′ā). Gênero de insetos (família Blattidae) que inclui a abundante barata-oriental, *B. orientalis*. O inseto seco fornece a anti-hidropina, um princípio diurético. [L. barata]

Blat·tel·la (bla-tel′ā). Gênero de baratas (família Blattidae) que inclui a *B. germanica*, a barata-alemã, provavelmente a mais familiar e disseminada das baratas. [L. *blatta*, barata]

Blat·ti·dae (blat′i-dē). Família de insetos (ordem Blattaria) que consiste em cerca de 4.000 espécies de baratas, em grande parte tropicais, mas com distribuição mundial, incluindo inúmeros insetos abundantes em domicílios, cozinhas e instituições, onde quer que exista alimento; nocivo sempre que encontrado, embora não tenha sido positivamente incriminado até agora na transmissão natural de microrganismos patogênicos para o homem. Os insetos domiciliares comuns englobam a barata-alemã, *Blattella germanica*, a barata-americana, *Periplaneta americana*, e a barata-oriental, *Blatta orientalis*. [L. *blatta*, barata]

bleb (blĕb). **1.** Flictena; uma grande vesícula, flácida. **2.** Vesícula; um cisto pulmonar adquirido, usualmente com menos de 1 cm de diâmetro, similar a uma bolha, porém menor, que se acredita que seja a causa mais comum de pneumotórax espontâneo. As vesículas ocorrem principalmente no ápice do pulmão.

filtering b., vesícula de filtração; uma vesícula da conjuntiva que resulta da cirurgia do glaucoma, através da qual um retalho da esclerótica é criado na parede ocular, permitindo que o *humor* aquoso seja filtrado para fora do olho, para baixo da conjuntiva, diminuindo, dessa maneira, a pressão intra-ocular. SIN filtering cicatrix.

pulmonary b., vesícula pulmonar; a dilatação alveolar cheia de ar com menos de 1 cm de diâmetro na borda do pulmão no ápice do lobo superior ou do segmento superior do lobo inferior; geralmente ocorre nas pessoas jovens e pode romper-se, produzindo pneumotórax primário. Cf. pulmonary *bulla*.

bleed (blēd). Sangrar; perder sangue em conseqüência de ruptura ou corte dos vasos sangüíneos.

bleed·er (blēd′er). **1.** Coloquialismo para uma pessoa que sofre de hemofilia, doença de Christmas, doença de Osler ou outro distúrbio da coagulação. **2.** Sangrante; um vaso sangüíneo cortado durante um procedimento cirúrgico.

bleed·ing (blēd′ing). Sangramento. **1.** A perda de sangue em conseqüência de ruptura ou corte dos vasos sangüíneos. **2.** Flebotomia; a saída de sangue.

dysfunctional uterine b., s. uterino disfuncional; o s. uterino decorrente de anormalidade endócrina benigna em vez de alguma doença orgânica.

occult b., s. oculto. VER occult *blood*.

blem·ish. 1. Defeito, mancha, imperfeição; uma pequena alteração circunscrita da pele considerada inestética, porém insignificante. **2.** Alterar a pele, gerando um aspecto inestético.

blen·nad·e·ni·tis (blen-ad-ē-nī′tis). Blenadenite; a inflamação das glândulas mucosas. [G. *blennos*, muco, + *adēn*, glândula, + *-itis*, inflamação]

blen·ne·me·sis (blen-em′ē-sis). Blenêmese; termo raramente utilizado para o vômito de muco. [G. *blennos*, muco, + *emesis*, vômito]

blenno-, blenn-. Formas combinantes que indicam muco. [G. *blenna, blennos*]

blen·no·gen·ic (blen-ō-jen′ik). Blenogênico. SIN muciparous. [blenno- + G. *-gen*, produzir]

blen·nog·e·nous (ble-noj′ē-nŭs). Blenógeno. SIN muciparous.

blen·noid (blen′oyd). Blenóide. SIN muciform. [blenno- + G. *eidos*, semelhança]

blen·noph·thal·mia (blen-of-thal′mē-ā). Blenoftalmia. **1.** SIN conjunctivitis. **2.** SIN gonorrheal *ophthalmia*.

blen·nor·rhag·ic (blen-ō-raj′ik). Blenorrágico. SIN blennorheal.

blen·nor·rhea (blen-ō-rē′ā). Blenorréia. **1.** Termo raramente utilizado para qualquer secreção mucosa, especialmente da uretra ou da vagina. **2.** No uso oftálmico, era sinônimo de conjuntivite, mas, hoje em dia, é obsoleto. [blenno- + G. *rhoia*, um fluxo]

b. conjunctiva′lis, b. conjuntival. SIN gonorrheal *ophthalmia*.

inclusion b., b. de inclusão; uma conjuntivite neonatal causada pela *Chlamydia trachomatis*.

b. neonato′rum, b. neonatal. SIN ophthalmia neonatorum.

blen·nor·rhe·al (blen-ō-rē′al). Blenorrágico; termo raramente utilizado relativo à blenorréia. SIN blennorrhagic.

blen·nos·ta·sis (blen-os′tā-sis). Blenostase; termo raramente utilizado para a diminuição ou supressão da secreção das mucosas. [blenno- + G. *stasis*, estase]

blen·no·stat·ic (blen-ō-stat′ik). Blenostático; termo raramente utilizado para a diminuição da secreção mucosa.

blen·nu·ria (ble-noo′rē-ā). Blenúria; excreção de excesso de muco na urina. [blenno- + G. *ouron*, urina]

ble·o·my·cin sul·fate (blē-ō-mī′sin). Sulfato de bleomicina; antibiótico antineoplásico obtido do *Streptomyces verticillus*. Freqüentemente produz fibrose pulmonar.

blephar-. VER blepharo-.

bleph·ar·ad·e·ni·tis (blef′ar-ad-ē-nī′tis). Blefaroadenite; a inflamação das glândulas meibomianas ou das glândulas marginais de Moll ou Zeis. SIN blepharoadenitis. [blephar- + G. *adēn*, glândula, + *-itis*, inflamação]

bleph·a·ral (blef′ā-ral). Blefário; referente às pálpebras.

bleph·a·rec·to·my (blef′a-rek′tō-mē). Blefarectomia; excisão da totalidade ou de parte de uma pálpebra. [blepharo- + G. *ektomē*, excisão]

bleph·ar·e·de·ma (blef′ar-ē-dē′mā). Blefaredema; edema das pálpebras, causando tumefação e, com freqüência, uma aparência empapuçada.

bleph·a·ri·tis (blef′ā-rī′tis). Blefarite; inflamação das pálpebras. [blepharo- + G. *-itis*, inflamação]

b. acar′ica, b. acárica. SIN demodectic b.

b. angula′ris, b. angular; inflamação das margens palpebrais nos ângulos da comissura.

ciliary b., b. ciliar. SIN b. marginalis.

demodectic b., b. acárica; inflamação da pálpebra associada ao *Demodex folliculorum*. SIN b. acarica.

b. follicula′ris, b. folicular; inflamação supurativa de localização profunda dos folículos ciliares e das glândulas de Zeis e Moll da pálpebra. SIN pustular b.

marginal b., b. marginal. SIN b. marginalis.

b. margina′lis, inflamação das margens das pálpebras. SIN ciliary b., marginal b.

meibomian b., b. meibomiana; inflamação da margem palpebral e das glândulas meibomianas.

b. parasit′ica, b. parasitária; b. marginal devido à presença de piolho. SIN b. phthiriatica, pediculous b.

pediculous b., b. pediculosa. SIN b. parasitica.

b. phthiriat′ica, b. parasitária. SIN b. parasitica.

posterior b., b. posterior; inflamação das margens palpebrais caracterizada por inspissação e oclusão dos orifícios das glândulas tarsais.

pustular b., b. pustular. SIN b. follicularis.

b. rosa′cea, b. rosácea; inflamação das margens das pálpebras em associação a acne rosácea.

seborrheic b., b. seborréica; um tipo comum de inflamação crônica das margens das pálpebras com eritema e escamas brancas; freqüentemente acompanha-se de dermatite seborréica do couro cabeludo e da face.

b. sic′ca, b. seca; inflamação das margens das pálpebras em que os cílios estão polvilhados por escamas esbranquiçadas.

staphylococcal b., b. estafilocócica; inflamação das pálpebras caracterizada por escamas endurecidas e brilhosas ao longo da base dos cílios.

b. ulcero′sa, b. ulcerosa; b. marginal com ulceração.

blepharo-, blephar-. Formas combinantes que indicam a pálpebra. [G. *blepharon*, uma pálpebra]

bleph·a·ro·ad·e·ni·tis (blef′ā-rō-ad-ē-nī′tis). Blefaroadenite. SIN blepharadenitis.

bleph·a·ro·ad·e·no·ma (blef′ā-rō-ad-ē-nō′mā). Blefaroadenoma; um tumor ou adenoma de uma glândula da pálpebra. [blepharo- + G. *adēn*, glândula, + *-oma*, tumor]

bleph·a·ro·chal·a·sis (blef′ā-rō-kal′ā-sis). Blefarocalasia; condição em que existe redundância da pele das pálpebras superiores, de modo que uma prega da pele pende, freqüentemente escondendo a margem tarsal quando o olho é aberto. SIN ptosis adiposa. [blepharo- + G. *chalasis*, relaxamento]

bleph·a·roc·lo·nus (blef-ar-ō-ok′lō-nŭs). Blefaroclono; espasmo clônico das pálpebras. [blepharo- + G. *klonos*, um tumulto]

bleph·a·ro·col·o·bo·ma (blef′ā-rō-kol-ō-bō′mā). Blefarocoloboma. SIN ankyloblepharon. [blepharo- + coloboma]

bleph·a·ro·con·junc·ti·vi·tis (blef′ā-rō-kon-jŭnk-ti-vī′tis). Blefaroconjuntivite; inflamação da conjuntiva palpebral.

bleph·a·ro·di·as·ta·sis (blef′ā-rō-di-as′tā-sis). Blefarodiastase; a separação anormal ou incapacidade de fechar por completo as pálpebras. [blepharo- + G. *diastasis*, separação]

bleph·a·ro·ker·a·to·con·junc·ti·vi·tis (blef′ā-rō-ker′ā-tō-kon-jŭnk′ti-vī′tis). Blefaroconjuntivite; inflamação que afeta pálpebras, córnea e conjuntivas.

bleph·a·ron (blef′ā-ron). Pálpebra. SIN eyelid. [G. *blepharon*, pálpebra]

bleph·a·ro·phi·mo·sis (blef′ā-rō-fi-mō′sis). Blefarofimose; diminuição na largura da abertura palpebral sem fusão das margens palpebrais. SIN blepharostenosis. [blepharo- + G. *phimōsis*, uma obstrução]

bleph·a·ro·plast (blef′ā-rō-plast). Blefaroplasto. SIN basal *body*. [blepharo- + G. *plastos*, formado]

bleph·a·ro·plas·tic (blef′ā-rō-plas′tik). Blefaroplástico; relativo à blefaroplastia.

bleph·a·ro·plas·ty (blef′ā-rō-plas-tē). Blefaroplastia; qualquer operação para a correção de um defeito nas pálpebras. [blepharo- + G. *plassō*, formar]

bleph·a·ro·ple·gia (blef′ā-rō-plē′jē-ā). Blefaroplegia; paralisia de uma pálpebra. [blepharo- + G. *plēgē*, golpe]

bleph·a·rop·to·sis, bleph·ar·op·to·sia (blef′ā-rop′tō-sis, -rop-tō′sē-ā). Blefaroptose; queda da pálpebra superior. SIN ptosis (2). [blepharo- + G. *ptōsis*, uma queda]

b. adipo'sa, b. adiposa; b. com acúmulo de tecido adiposo subcutâneo fazendo com que a pele penda sobre a borda livre da pálpebra.
false b., b. falsa, pseudoptose. SIN pseudoptosis.
bleph·a·ro·spasm, bleph·a·ro·spas·mus (blef′a-ro-spazm, -spaz′mŭs). Blefaroespasmo; contração espasmódica involuntária do músculo orbicular da órbita; pode ocorrer isoladamente ou estar associado a outras contrações distônicas dos músculos faciais, mandibulares ou cervicais; usualmente iniciado ou agravado por emoção, fadiga ou medicamentos.
bleph·a·ro·stat (blef′a-ro-stat). Blefarostato. SIN eye *speculum*. [blepharo- + G. *statos*, fixo]
bleph·a·ro·ste·no·sis (blef′a-ro-ste-no′sis). Blefaroestenose. SIN blepharophimosis. [blepharo- + G. *stenosis*, estreitamento]
bleph·a·ro·syn·ech·ia (blef′a-ro-sin-ek′e-a). Blefarossinéquia; a aderência das pálpebras entre si ou ao globo ocular. [blepharo- + G. *synecheia*, continuidade, de *syn- echo*, manter junto]
bleph·a·rot·o·my (blef-a-rot′o-me). Blefarotomia; cirurgia de incisão em uma pálpebra. [blepharo- + G. *tome*, incisão]
blind (blīnd). Cego; incapaz de enxergar; sem visão útil. VER blindness.
blind·ness (blīnd′nes). Cegueira. **1.** Perda da visão; a c. absoluta indica a não-percepção da luz. VER TAMBÉM amblyopia, amaurosis. **2.** Perda da apreciação visual de objetos, embora a acuidade visual esteja normal. **3.** Ausência de sensibilidade, p.ex., c. do paladar. SIN typhlosis.
change b., c. de alteração; a falha em perceber grandes alterações no campo visual que ocorrem simultaneamente com distúrbios breves.
color b., c. para cores; termo errôneo para a visão em cores anômala ou deficiente; a c. completa para as cores é a ausência de um dos pigmentos primários do cone da retina. VER protanopia, deuteranopia, tritanopia.
cortical b., c. cortical; a perda da visão decorrente de lesão orgânica no córtex visual.
day b., c. diurna, hemeralopia. SIN hemeralopia.
eclipse b., maculopatia solar. SIN solar *maculopathy*.
flash b., c. por clarão; perda temporária da visão produzida quando os pigmentos retinianos sensíveis à luz são descorados pela luz mais intensa que aquela a que a retina está fisiologicamente adaptada naquele momento.
flight b., c. fugaz; a cegueira visual em aviadores. VER TAMBÉM *amaurosis* fugax.
functional b., c. funcional; a perda aparente da visão relacionada à sugestibilidade.
hysterical b., c. histérica; perda da visão ou borramento visual após um evento psicologicamente traumático, como ver uma criança ser morta em um acidente.
legal b., c. legal; geralmente, a acuidade visual inferior a 6/60 ou 20/200 usando os tipos do teste de Snellen, ou a restrição do campo visual a 20° ou menos no melhor olho; os critérios empregados para definir a cegueira legal variam entre diferentes grupos.
letter b., c. literal; a agnosia visual para letras, na qual as letras são vistas, mas não são identificadas; causada por uma lesão no córtex occipital.
mind b., c. mental; a agnosia visual para objetos, em que os objetos são vistos mas não são identificados; causada por uma lesão na área 18 do córtex occipital. SIN object b., psychanopsia, psychic b.
music b., c. musical. SIN musical *alexia*.
night b., c. noturna. SIN nyctalopia.
note b., c. musical. SIN musical *alexia*.
object b., c. para objetos. SIN mind b.
psychic b., c. psíquica. SIN mind b.
river b., c. de rio. SIN ocular *onchocerciasis*.
sight b., assimbolia. SIN asymbolia.
sign b., c. de sinal; agnosia visual para sinais.
snow b., c. da neve; fotofobia grave secundária à ceratoconjuntivite por luz ultravioleta.
solar b., c. solar. SIN solar *maculopathy*.
taste b., c. de paladar; incapacidade de apreciar os estímulos gustativos.
text b., word b., c. verbal. SIN alexia.
blink (blink). Piscar; fechar e abrir rapidamente os olhos; um ato involuntário através do qual as lágrimas são espalhadas sobre a conjuntiva, mantendo-a umedecida. VER wink.
blis·ter. 1. Vesícula; uma estrutura de paredes finas, cheia de líquido, sob a epiderme ou dentro dela (subepidérmica ou intradérmica). **2.** Formar uma v. com calor ou algum outro agente vesicante.
blood b., v. sanguinolenta; v. que contém sangue; resultante de uma lesão por pinçamento ou esmagamento.
fever b., v. febril; coloquialismo para o herpes simples labial.
fly b., v. causada pela secreção de um líquido corporal vesicante por determinados besouros, principalmente os membros da família Meloidae, que produzem a cantaridina, p.ex., *Lytta (Cantharis) vesicatoria*, a notória "mosca-espanhola"; o líquido vesicante sem cantaridina é produzido por outros besouros, como os potós (família Staphylinidae), especialmente o gênero *Paederus*, cujo líquido, em contato com a pele, produz uma v. muito dolorosa.

fracture b., v. da fratura; epidermólise superficial que acontece em associação, mais comumente, com as fraturas da perna e do tornozelo e do antebraço e punho; a etiologia representa uma combinação de tumefação excessiva e lesão por torção dos tecidos moles suprajacentes.
sucking b., v. da sucção; lesão cutânea bolhosa superficial no braço do neonato provavelmente resultante de sucção pré-natal vigorosa.
blis·ter·ing. Vesiculação. SIN vesiculation (1).
bloat, bloat·ing (blot, blot′ing). **1.** Distensão abdominal a partir do ar deglutido ou do gás intestinal originário da fermentação. **2.** Distensão do rúmen do gado, causada pelo acúmulo de gases da fermentação, particularmente provável de ocorrer quando os animais pastam em locais ricos em leguminosas; quando não-aliviada, a condição pode levar rapidamente à morte.
Bloch, Bruno, dermatologista suíço, 1878–1933. VER B.-Sulzberger *disease, syndrome*.
Bloch, Marcel, médico francês, 1885–1925. VER B. *reaction*.
block (block). **1.** Bloquear; obstruir; interromper a passagem. **2.** Bloqueio; uma condição em que a passagem de um impulso elétrico é interrompida, total ou parcialmente, de maneira temporária ou permanente. **3.** Bloqueio atrioventricular. SIN atrioventricular b. [Fr. *bloquer*]
alveolocapillary b., bloqueio alveolocapilar; a presença de material que compromete a difusão dos gases entre o ar nos espaços alveolares e o sangue nos capilares alveolares; o b. pode ser causado por edema, infiltrado celular, fibrose ou tumor, e resulta na hipossaturação com oxigênio do sangue arterial periférico.
antegrade b., b. anterógrado. SIN anterograde b.
anterograde b., b. anterógrado; o b. de condução de um impulso que parte de um ponto qualquer em sua direção habitual, por exemplo, a partir do nó sinoatrial para o miocárdio ventricular. SIN antegrade b.
arborization b., b. de arborização; o b. intraventricular supostamente provocado pelo bloqueio disseminado nas ramificações de Purkinje e manifestado no eletrocardiograma por um padrão semelhante ao bloqueio de ramo, mas com complexos de baixa amplitude.
atrioventricular b., AV b., bloqueio atrioventricular, BAV; b. parcial ou completo dos impulsos elétricos que se originam no átrio ou no nó sinusal, impedindo que eles alcancem o nó atrioventricular e os ventrículos. No BAV de primeiro grau, existe o prolongamento do tempo de condução AV (intervalo PR); no BAV de segundo grau, alguns, mas não todos, impulsos atriais não alcançam os ventrículos, portanto alguns dos batimentos ventriculares não ocorrem; no BAV completo (terceiro grau), ocorre dissociação atrioventricular completa (2); nenhum impulso consegue atingir os ventrículos, apesar de uma freqüência ventricular baixa (< 45/min); os átrios e os ventrículos contraem-se de forma independente. SIN block (3), heart b.
bone b., b. ósseo; procedimento cirúrgico em que um enxerto ósseo é posicionado adjacente a uma articulação para limitar mecanicamente o movimento da articulação ou para melhorar a estabilidade da articulação, p.ex., na articulação do tornozelo para corrigir o pé em gota, ao impedir que a flexão plantar ultrapasse 0°, mas permitindo a dorsiflexão além de 0°, p.ex., na articulação gleno-umeral para evitar a instabilidade posterior.
bundle-branch b., b. de ramo; o b. intraventricular decorrente da interrupção da condução em um dos dois principais ramos do fascículo (feixe) de His e manifestado no eletrocardiograma pelo prolongamento acentuado do complexo QRS; o b. de cada ramo apresenta morfologia distinta do QRS.
complete AV b., b. AV completo; **(1)** VER atrioventricular b.; (2) SIN complete atrioventricular *dissociation*. VER atrioventricular b.
conduction b., b. de condução; a falha da transmissão do impulso em algum ponto ao longo de um nervo, embora a condução ao longo dos segmentos proximal e distal a ele não seja afetada; clinicamente, o resultado mais freqüente de uma área de desmielinização focal; quando causado por trauma focal, é denominado neurapraxia.
congenital heart b., b. atrioventricular congênito; o BAV presente *in utero* ou no nascimento e usualmente de grau avançado ou completo.
depolarizing b., b. despolarizante; paralisia da musculatura esquelética associada à perda de polaridade da placa motora terminal, como acontece após a administração de succinilcolina.
divisional b., b. divisional; parada do impulso em uma das duas supostas divisões do ramo esquerdo do feixe de His; i.e., na divisão anterior (superior) ou na divisão posterior (inferior). SIN hemiblock.
entrance b., b. de entrada. SIN protective b.
epidural b., b. epidural; obstrução no espaço epidural; usado de forma não-acurada para referir-se à anestesia epidural.
exit b., b. de saída; a incapacidade de um impulso para sair de seu ponto de origem, para o qual o mecanismo é concebido como uma zona envolvente de tecido refratário que negue a passagem ao impulso emergente.
fascicular b., b. fascicular; condição baseada no contestado conceito de que o ramo esquerdo do fascículo (feixe) de His fornece dois dos três principais fascículos de um sistema de condução, do qual o ramo do feixe direito constitui o terceiro, para a transmissão do impulso cardíaco a partir do átrio, acima, até os ventrículos abaixo do nó AV; o bloqueio pode ocorrer em qualquer um ou em

todos os fascículos, com todos os três em conjunto produzindo o bloqueio AV completo. VER TAMBÉM hemiblock.

field b., b. de campo; a anestesia regional produzida por infiltração com solução anestésica local nos tecidos que circundam um campo cirúrgico.

first degree AV b., BAV de primeiro grau. VER atrioventricular b.

heart b., BAV. SIN atrioventricular b.

incomplete atrioventricular b., b. atrioventricular incompleto. SIN partial heart b.

interatrial b., b. intra-atrial. SIN intraatrial b.

intraatrial b., b. intra-atrial; condução comprometida através dos átrios, manifestada por ondas P alargadas e, com freqüência, com chanfradura no eletrocardiograma. SIN interatrial b.

intraventricular b. (IVB), IV b., b. intraventricular (BIV), b. IV; condução retardada no sistema de condução ventricular ou miocárdio, incluindo os bloqueios de ramo, bloqueios peri-infarto, bloqueio fascicular, BIV inespecífico e síndrome de Wolff-Parkinson-White (pré-excitação).

Mobitz b., b. de Mobitz; b. atrioventricular de segundo grau em que existe uma proporção de duas ou mais deflexões (ondas P) para as respostas ventriculares.

Mobitz types of atrioventricular b., tipos Mobitz do b. atrioventricular; tipo I, o batimento falho do fenômeno de Wenckebach; tipo II, um ciclo cardíaco falho que ocorre sem alteração na condução dos intervalos precedentes.

nerve b., b. nervoso; interrupção da condução dos impulsos nos nervos periféricos ou troncos nervosos por injeção de solução anestésica local.

nondepolarizing b., b. não-despolarizante; a paralisia da musculatura esquelética que não se acompanha de alterações na polaridade da placa motora terminal, como acontece depois da administração de tubocurarina.

partial heart b., b. atrioventricular parcial; os impulsos penetram na junção atrioventricular em alguma relação com a freqüência ventricular. SIN incomplete atrioventricular b.

periinfarction b., b. peri-infarto; anormalidade eletrocardiográfica associada a infarto do miocárdio e causada por ativação retardada do miocárdio na região do infarto; caracterizado por um vetor inicial dirigido para longe da região infartada com o vetor terminal direcionado para ele.

phase I b., b. de fase I; inibição da transmissão do impulso nervoso através da junção mioneural associada à despolarização da placa motora terminal, como na paralisia muscular produzida por succinilcolina.

phase II b., b. de fase II; inibição da transmissão do impulso nervoso através da junção mioneural não-acompanhada por despolarização da placa motora terminal, como na paralisia muscular produzida pela tubocurarina.

protective b., b. protetor; um mecanismo compreendido de forma incompleta por meio do qual um marca-passo é protegido de ser descarregado pelo impulso oriundo de outro centro; o mecanismo, usualmente concebido como uma zona envolvente de tecido refratário em sentido unidirecional que permite a saída do impulso a partir do centro, mas evitando o acesso ao centro, é observado na parassistolia ventricular, em que o centro parassistólico é protegido contra a descarga pelo marca-passo sinusal e, assim, é capaz de manter inalterado seu ritmo intrínseco. SIN entrance b., protection.

pupillary b., b. pupilar; resistência aumentada ao fluxo do *humor* aquoso através da pupila, a partir do compartimento posterior para o anterior, levando ao arqueamento anterior da íris periférica sobre a rede trabecular (trabecular *meshwork*) e ao glaucoma de ângulo fechado (angle-closure *glaucoma*).

retrograde b., b. retrógrado; o comprometimento da condução para trás a partir dos ventrículos ou do nó AV para os átrios.

reverse pupillary b., b. pupilar invertido; a resistência aumentada ao fluxo do humor aquoso (através da pupila) da câmara anterior para a posterior, levando ao arqueamento posterior da íris periférica contra as zônulas; um possível mecanismo do glaucoma pigmentar.

second degree AV b., BAV de segundo grau. VER atrioventricular b.

sinoatrial b., S-A b., sinus b., b. sinoatrial, b. S-A, sinusal; o bloqueio do impulso que deixa o nó sinoatrial antes que possa ativar o músculo atrial. SIN sinoauricular b.

sinoauricular b., b. sinoatrial. SIN sinoatrial b.

spinal b., b. espinal; obstrução do fluxo do líquido cefalorraquidiano no espaço subaracnóide espinal; usado de maneira incorreta para se referir à anestesia espinal.

stellate b., b. estrelado; a injeção de solução anestésica local nas vizinhanças do gânglio estrelado.

suprahisian b., b. supra-his; retardo da condução atrioventricular que ocorre acima ou cefálico ao feixe de His.

third degree AV b., BAV de terceiro grau. SIN complete atrioventricular *dissociation.* VER atrioventricular b.

unidirectional b., b. unidirecional; o b. que impede a passagem de um impulso quando ele se aproxima de uma direção, mas não de outra, como quando o nó AV evita a condução anterógrada para os ventrículos, enquanto a condução retrógrada para os átrios permanece intacta.

Wenckebach b., b. de Wenckebach; uma forma de b. em qualquer tecido cardíaco (mais amiúde a junção atrioventricular) em que existe prolongamento progressivo da condução (condução decrescente) até que o batimento não ocorra.

Wolff-Chaikoff b., b. de Wolff-Chaikoff; o bloqueio da ligação orgânica do iodo e sua incorporação no hormônio provocado por grandes doses de iodo; usualmente um efeito transitório, mas, em grandes doses nos indivíduos suscetíveis, pode ser prolongado e causar mixedema por iodo. SIN Wolff-Chaikoff effect.

block·ade (blok′ād). Bloqueio. **1.** A injeção intravenosa de grandes quantidades de corantes coloidais ou de outras substâncias a fim de bloquear as células reticuloendoteliais (p.ex., a fagocitose é temporariamente evitada). **2.** O bloqueio do receptor, bloqueando o efeito de um hormônio na superfície da célula. **3.** Parada da condução ou transmissão do nervo periférico nas junções sinápticas autônomas, receptores autônomos ou junções mioneurais por um medicamento. **4.** A ocupação dos receptores por um antagonista, de modo que os agonistas usuais são relativamente não-efetivos.

adrenergic b., b. adrenérgico; a inibição seletiva por um medicamento das respostas das células efetoras aos impulsos adrenérgicos dos nervos simpáticos (simpaticolíticos) e à epinefrina e às aminas correlatas (adrenolíticas).

cholinergic b., b. colinérgico; **(1)** inibição da transmissão do impulso nervoso por um medicamento nas sinapses ganglionares autonômicas (b. ganglionar), nas células efetoras parassimpáticas pós-ganglionares (p.ex., por atropina) e na junção mioneural (b. mioneural); **(2)** a inibição de um agente colinérgico.

ganglionic b., b. ganglionar; inibição da transmissão do impulso nervoso nas sinapses ganglionares autonômicas por substâncias como a nicotina ou o hexametônio.

myoneural b., b. mioneural; a inibição da transmissão do impulso nervoso nas junções mioneurais por uma substância como o curare.

narcotic b., b. narcótico; o uso de substâncias para inibir os efeitos de narcóticos, como a naloxona.

sympathetic b., b. simpático; a interrupção da transmissão nos gânglios simpáticos ou da condução dos impulsos nas fibras nervosas simpáticas pré- ou pós-ganglionares.

virus b., b. viral; a interferência de um vírus por outro, quer atenuado, quer sem relação.

block·er (blok′er) Bloqueador. **1.** Um instrumento usado para obstruir uma passagem. **2.** VER blocking *agent.*

angiotensin receptor b.'s, bloqueadores do receptor de angiotensina; agentes, como o losartan, que se ligam aos receptores de angiotensina, evitando, assim, o acesso da angiotensina II ao receptor e, por conseguinte, reduzindo a vasoconstrição provocada por esse agonista; usado no tratamento da hipertensão.

calcium channel b., b. do canal de cálcio; uma classe de medicamentos com a capacidade de evitar que os íons de cálcio atravessem as membranas biológicas. Esses agentes são usados para tratar a hipertensão, a angina de peito e arritmias cardíacas; os exemplos incluem nifedipina, diltiazem, verapamil, amlodipina.

block·ing (blok′ing). Bloqueio. **1.** Que obstrui; parada da passagem, condução ou transmissão. **2.** Em psicanálise, uma ruptura súbita na livre associação que ocorre quando se toca em um assunto doloroso ou emocionalmente reprimido. **3.** A súbita interrupção dos pensamentos e da fala, que pode indicar a presença de um grave distúrbio do pensamento ou uma psicose.

alpha b., b. alfa; a atenuação do ritmo alfa occipital (ondas cerebrais de 8-14 Hz conforme observado em um eletroencefalograma), produzida pela abertura dos olhos ou por intensa concentração mental.

block·out (blok′owt). Embocar; a eliminação das escavações através do enchimento dessas áreas por um meio, como cera ou pedra-pome úmida.

Blocq, Paul O., médico francês, 1860–1896. VER B. *disease.*

Blom, Eric D., patologista da fala-linguagem norte-americano do século 20. VER B.-Singer *valve.*

blood (blŭd). Sangue; o "tecido circulante" do corpo; o líquido e seus elementos formados suspensos que são circulados através do coração, artérias, capilares e veias; o s. é o meio pelo qual 1) o oxigênio e os nutrientes são transportados até os tecidos, e 2) o dióxido de carbono e vários produtos metabólicos são removidos para a excreção. O s. consiste em um líquido amarelo pálido ou amarelo-acinzentado, o plasma, no qual estão suspensos os eritrócitos (hemácias), leucócitos e plaquetas. VER TAMBÉM arterial b., venous b. [A. S blōd]

arterial b., s. arterial; o s. que é oxigenado nos pulmões, encontrado nos compartimentos cardíacos à esquerda e nas artérias, e relativamente vermelho vivo.

cord b., s. de cordão; o s. presente nos vasos umbilicais no momento do parto. É de origem fetal.

laky b., s. hemolisado; o s. que está sofrendo ou que sofreu hemólise. VER lake (2), laky.

occult b., s. oculto; o s. nas fezes em quantidades muito pequenas para serem observadas, porém detectáveis por exames químicos.

sludged b., s. aglutinado; o s. em que os corpúsculos, em consequência de algum estado geral anormal, p.ex., queimaduras, choque traumático e estresses similares, foram aglomerados nos capilares e, dessa maneira, bloqueiam os vasos ou se movem de forma mais lenta através deles.

venous b., s. venoso; o s. que atravessou os capilares de vários tecidos, exceto os pulmões, e é encontrado nas veias, nos compartimentos cardíacos à direita

blood

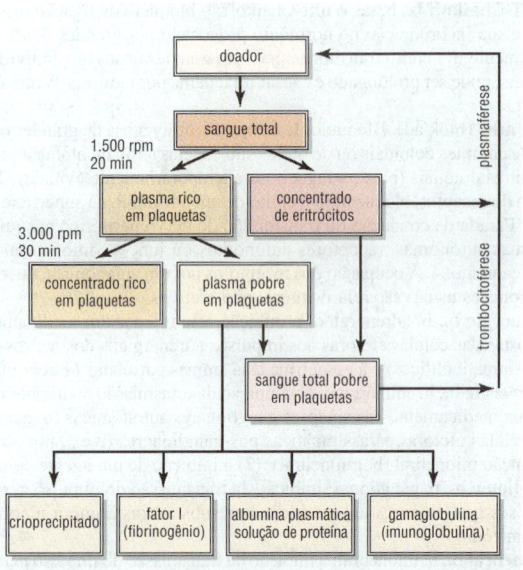

separação dos componentes sangüíneos

e nas artérias pulmonares; em geral, é vermelho-escuro em conseqüência do menor conteúdo de oxigênio.
   whole b., s. total; o s. coletado de um doador selecionado sob rígidas precauções assépticas; contém o íon citrato ou heparina como anticoagulante; utilizado como repositor de s.
blood bank. Banco de sangue; um local, comumente uma parte separada ou divisão de um laboratório hospitalar ou de uma instituição livre, em que o sangue é coletado dos doadores, classificado, separado em vários componentes e/ou preparado para a transfusão para receptores.
blood count. Contagem sangüínea; o cálculo do número de eritrócitos (RBC) ou leucócitos (WBC) em um milímetro cúbico de sangue, por meio da contagem das células em um volume exato de sangue diluído.
   complete b. c. (CBC), hematimetria completa, hemograma completo; uma combinação das seguintes determinações: contagem de eritrócitos, contagem de leucócitos, índices eritrocitários, hematócrito, contagem diferencial e, por vezes, contagem de plaquetas.
   differential white b. c., contagem diferencial de leucócitos; uma estimativa do percentual de cada tipo de leucócito que compõe a contagem de leucócitos totais.
   Schilling b. c., contagem sangüínea de Schilling; um método de contagem sangüínea em que os neutrófilos polimorfonucleares são separados em quatro grupos de acordo com o número e a disposição das massas nucleares nessas células. SIN Schilling index.
blood dust. Hemoconia. SIN hemoconia.
blood group. Grupo sangüíneo. **1.** Um sistema de antígenos sob o controle de locos alelos intimamente ligados na superfície do eritrócito. Por causa das diferenças antigênicas existentes entre os indivíduos, os grupos sangüíneos são importantes nas transfusões sangüíneas, incompatibilidades materno-fetais (doença hemolítica do recém-nascido), transplante de tecidos e órgãos, casos de paternidade e nos estudos genéticos e antropológicos; determinados grupos sangüíneos podem estar relacionados à suscetibilidade ou resistência a determinadas doenças. Freqüentemente utilizado como sinônimo de tipo sangüíneo. Veja o apêndice de Grupos Sangüíneos para os grupos individuais: ABO, Auberger, Diego, Duffy, I, Kell, Kidd, Lewis, Lutheran, MNSs, P, Rh, Sutter, Xg e os grupos sangüíneos de baixa freqüência e alta freqüência. **2.** A classificação das amostras sangüíneas por meio de exames laboratoriais de suas reações de aglutinação em relação a um ou mais grupos sangüíneos. Em geral, uma suspensão de eritrócitos a ser testada é exposta a um anti-soro específico conhecido; a aglutinação dos eritrócitos indica que eles possuem o antígeno para o qual o anti-soro é específico. Determinados anti-soros exigem condições de teste especiais.
   private b. g., grupo sangüíneo particular; um grupo sangüíneo que é conhecido por ter ocorrido em apenas uma família e é rastreável para uma única pessoa.
blood·less (blŭd′les). Exsangue; sem sangue.
blood·let·ting (blŭd′let - ing). Sangria; remover o sangue, usualmente de uma veia; originalmente empregado como uma medida terapêutica geral, porém utilizada, hoje em dia, na insuficiência cardíaca congestiva e na policitemia. VER phlebotomy.
   general b., sangria geral; remoção do sangue por arteriotomia ou flebotomia.
   local b., sangria local; a retirada do sangue de vasos menores, originalmente por uma ventosa ou sanguessuga.
blood rel·a·tive. Parente de sangue; um termo popular que descreve um parente de uma pessoa que compartilha um ancestral comum. Nenhuma importância especial se liga ao sangue como um veículo de herança. Os cônjuges não são comumente parentes de sangue e, quando o são, o casamento é consangüíneo e comporta um risco mais elevado que a média de progenia homozigótica por descender de ancestrais comuns. Esses casamentos são desencorajados e, dentro de determinados graus de parentesco, podem ser ilegais.
blood·shot (blŭd′shot). Congestão sangüínea; indica os pequenos vasos sangüíneos localmente congestos em uma região (p.ex., as conjuntivas) que estão dilatados e visíveis.
blood·stream (blŭd′strēm). Corrente sangüínea; o sangue que flui como ele é encontrado no sistema circulatório, diferente do sangue que foi removido do sistema circulatório ou seqüestrado em uma região; dessa maneira, pode-se esperar que algo acrescentado ao sangue se torne distribuído para todas as partes do corpo através das quais o sangue está fluindo.
blood type. Tipo sangüíneo; o padrão de aglutinação específico dos eritrócitos de uma pessoa para o anti-soro de um grupo sangüíneo; p.ex., o grupo sangüíneo ABO consiste em quatro tipos sangüíneos principais: O, A, B e AB. Essa classificação depende da presença ou ausência de dois antígenos principais: A ou B. O tipo O acontece quando nenhum dos dois está presente, e o tipo AB, quando ambos estão presentes. O tipo sangüíneo é o fenótipo genético do indivíduo para um sistema de grupo sangüíneo e pode ser determinado com o uso de anti-soros diferentes disponíveis para o teste. Veja o apêndice de Grupos Sangüíneos.
blood ves·sel [TA]. Vaso sangüíneo; qualquer vaso que conduza o sangue: artérias, arteríolas, vênulas, veias transportam o sangue. SIN vas sanguineum [TA].
   choroid b. v.'s, vasos sangüíneos corióides; as artérias e veias que, com o tecido conjuntivo frouxo e as células pigmentadas que formam suas matrizes, compreendem a lâmina vascular da corióide. SIN vasa sanguinea choroideae [TA].
   intrapulmonary b. v.'s [TA], vasos sangüíneos intrapulmonares; os ramos intra-segmentares da artéria e da veia pulmonares que atravessam o parênquima dos pulmões. SIN vasa sanguinea intrapulmonalia [TA].
   retinal b. v.'s [TA], vasos sangüíneos retinianos; a vasculatura sangüínea da retina, incluindo os ramos e tributárias da artéria e da veia centrais da retina, respectivamente, e o círculo vascular do nervo óptico. SIN vasa sanguinea retinae [TA].
blood·worm (blŭd′werm). **1.** A filária do carneiro, *Elaeophora schneideri*. **2.** As larvas aquáticas vermelhas de determinados mosquitos dípteros. **3.** Anelídeos marinhos da família Terebellidae com corpos flexíveis e sangue vermelho. **4.** Vermes que habitam o sangue, como os trematódeos do sangue humano no gênero *Schistosoma*.
Bloom, David, dermatologista norte-americano. *1892. VER B. *syndrome*.
blot. Mancha. VER Northern blot *analysis*, Southern blot *analysis*. Western bot *analysis*, zoo blot *analysis*.
blotch. Erupção cutânea; termo comumente utilizado para indicar uma lesão pigmentada ou eritematosa.
Blount, Walter P., cirurgião ortopédico norte-americano, *1900. VER B. *disease*, B.-Barber *disease*.
blow·fly. Varejeira. VER *Calliphora, Lucilia, Phormia regina*.
blue (bloo). Azul; a cor entre o verde e o violeta no espectro. Para os corantes azuis individuais, veja o nome específico. SIN ceruleán.
blues (blooz). Depressão; estado de depressão ou tristeza. [gíria, de *blue devils*]
   postpartum b., depressão pós-parto; o transtorno do humor (incluindo insônia, choro, depressão, ansiedade e irritabilidade) experimentado por até 50% das mulheres na primeira semana pós-parto; aparentemente precipitada pela queda abrupta dos níveis de progesterona.
Blum, Paul, médico francês, 1878–1933. VER Gougerot and B. *disease*.
Blumberg, Jacob M., cirurgião e ginecologista alemão, 1873–1955. VER B. *sign*.
Blumenau, Leonid W., neurologista russo, 1862–1932. VER B. *nucleus*.
Blumenbach, Johann F., fisiologista alemão, 1752–1840. VER B. *clivus*.
Blumer, George A., médico norte-americano, 1858–1940. VER B. *shelf*.
blunt-end (blunt-end). Extremidade cega; refere-se ao DNA com dois filamentos em que não existem bases pareadas na extremidade do polinucleotídeo.

grupo sangüíneo ABO

grupo sangüíneo	genótipo	freqüência nos Estados Unidos (%)	antígenos dos eritrócitos	anticorpos no soro
A	AA ou AO	39	A	anti-B (β)
B	BB ou BO	11	B	anti-A (α)
AB	AB	4	A e B	nenhum
O	OO	46	nem A, nem B	α e β

blush (blŭsh).. Rubor. **1.** Vermelhidão súbita e breve da face e do pescoço devido à emoção. **2.** Em angiografia, usado de maneira metafórica para descrever a neovascularização ou, em alguns casos, o extravasamento. [I. M., do I. Ant. *blyscan*]
  tumor b., r. tumoral; estimulação do tumor nos exames radiológicos através da administração de contrastes.
BLV Abreviatura para bovine leukemia *virus* (vírus da leucemia bovina).
B-mode. Modo B; uma apresentação ultra-sonográfica diagnóstica bidimensional das interfaces produtoras de eco; a intensidade do eco é representada pela modulação do brilho da mancha, e a posição do eco é determinada a partir da posição angular do transdutor e do tempo de trânsito do pulso acústico e de seu eco.
BMR Abreviatura para basal metabolic *rate* (taxa metabólica basal).
BNA Abreviatura para Basle Nomina Anatomica (Nomina Anatômica da Basiléia).
board. Comitê.
  institutional review b. (IRB), comitê de revisão institucional; o comitê permanente em um hospital ou outra instituição que é responsável pela segurança e pelo bem-estar dos seres humanos envolvidos em pesquisa.
bob·bing (bob´ing). Oscilação; um movimento para cima e para baixo.
  inverse ocular b., o. ocular inversa; o movimento ocular lento para baixo seguido pelo retorno para cima rápido e retardado.
  ocular b., oscilação ocular; o desvio dos olhos súbito, conjugado e para baixo, com um lento retorno para a posição normal; observado em alguns pacientes comatosos com lesões hemisféricas bilaterais.
bob·i·er·rite (bŏb´-ē-er-īt). Bobierita; o octaidrato do fosfato de magnésio; por vezes encontrada nos cálculos renais. Cf. newberyite, struvite. [Pierre A. Bobierre, químico francês, + - ite]
BOC, *t*-**BOC.** Abreviaturas utilizadas outrora para *t*-butoxycarbonyl (*t*-butoxicarbonila); o uso atual é Boc.
Boc Abreviatura de *t*-butoxycarbonyl (*t*-butoxicarbonila).
Bochdalek, Vincent A., anatomista checoslovaco, 1801–1883. VER B. *foramen, ganglion, gap;* foramen de B. *hernia;* B. *muscle, valve;* flower basket of B.
Bock, August C., anatomista alemão, 1782–1833. VER B. *ganglion*.
Bockhart, Max, médico alemão, 1883–1921. VER B. *impetigo*.
BOD Abreviatura para biochemical oxygen *demand* (demanda bioquímica de oxigênio).
Bodansky, Aaron, bioquímico norte-americano, 1887–1961. VER B. *unit*.
Bödecker, Charles F., histologista oral, embriologista e patologista norte-americano, *1880. VER B. *index*.
Bodian, David, anatomista norte-americano, *1910. VER B. copper-PROTARGOL *stain*.
Bo·do (bō´dō). Um gênero de protozoários de vida livre, ovóides ou discretamente piriformes, com dois flagelos, um projetando-se anteriormente e outro posteriormente; podem ser ingeridos como formas encistadas no alimento ou na bebida, ou possivelmente depositados nas fezes ou urina depois da excreção; em ambos os casos, os cistos freqüentemente evoluem para trofozoítos quando se permite que a amostra permaneça na temperatura ambiente por algumas horas antes do exame; esses microrganismos não são patogênicos para os seres humanos.
  B. cauda´tus, uma espécie que é encontrada em amostras de fezes humanas (principalmente nas regiões tropicais); os microrganismos são freqüentemente denominados flagelados coprozóicos.
  B. sal´tans, uma espécie do trato intestinal por vezes observada em úlceras.
  B. urina´rius, uma espécie encontrada ocasionalmente na urina.

BODY

body (bod´ē) Corpo; corpúsculo. **1.** A cabeça, pescoço, tronco e membros. O corpo humano, consistindo em cabeça (caput), pescoço (collum), tronco (truncus) e membros (membra). **2.** A parte material de um ser humano, conforme diferenciado da mente e da alma. **3.** A principal massa de qualquer estrutura. **4.** Uma coisa; uma substância. VER TAMBÉM corpus, soma. SIN corpus (1) [TA]. [A.S. *bodig*]
  acetone b., corpo cetônico. SIN ketone b.
  adrenal b., glândula supra-renal. SIN suprarenal *gland*.
  alcoholic hyaline b.'s, corpúsculos hialinos alcoólicos. SIN Mallory b.´s.
  Alder b.'s, corpúsculos de Alder; inclusões granulares nos leucócitos polimorfonucleares; tornam-se escuros com o corante de Giemsa-Wright e reagem de forma metacromática com o azul de toluidina. VER TAMBÉM Alder *anomaly*.
  alveolar b., processo alveolar da maxila. SIN alveolar *process* of maxilla.
  amygdaloid b. [TA], c. amigdalóide; uma massa arredondada de substância cinzenta no lobo temporal, interna ao córtex do giro cingulado e imediatamente anterior ao corno inferior do ventrículo lateral; seus principais aferentes são o olfatório e suas conexões eferentes são com o hipotálamo e o núcleo mediodorsal do tálamo, também se associando de maneira recíproca com o córtex do lobo temporal; é subdividido em dois grupos nucleares principais: basolateral e corticomedial. Os núcleos individuais do corpo amigdalóide (ou complexo) são o núcleo da amígdala basilar lateral [TA], o núcleo da amígdala basilar medial [TA], o núcleo central da amígdala [TA], o núcleo cortical da amígdala [TA] o núcleo intersticial da amígdala [TA], o núcleo lateral da amígdala [TA], o núcleo medial da amígdala [TA] e o núcleo lateral do trato olfatório [TA]. SIN amygdaloid complex [TA], corpus amygdaloideum [TA], amygdaloid nucleus, nucleus amygdalae.
  amylogenic b., amiloplasto SIN amyloplast.
  anococcygeal b., c. anococcígeo. SIN anococcygeal *ligament*.
  anterior quadrigeminal b., colículo superior. SIN superior *colliculus*.
  aortic b.'s, glomos para-aórticos. SIN paraaortic b.´s
  Arnold b.'s, corpúsculos de Arnold; pequenas porções ou fragmentos diminutos de eritrócitos (por vezes confundidos com as plaquetas sangüíneas) ou pequenos "fantasmas" de eritrócitos.
  asbestos b.'s, corpúsculos de asbesto; corpúsculos ferruginosos com fibras de asbesto como um núcleo; uma característica histológica da exposição ao asbesto.
  Aschoff b.'s, corpúsculos de Aschoff; nódulos de Aschoff; uma forma de inflamação granulomatosa observada caracteristicamente na cardite reumática aguda; os corpúsculos de Aschoff plenamente desenvolvidos consistem na alteração fibrinóide no tecido conjuntivo, linfócitos, plasmócitos ocasionais e histiócitos com características anormais. SIN Aschoff nodules.
  asteroid b., c. asteróide; **(1)** uma inclusão eosinofílica que se assemelha a uma estrela com linhas radiadas delicadas, que ocorre em uma área vacuolada do citoplasma de uma célula gigante multinucleada; particularmente freqüente na sarcoidose, mas também observado em outros granulomas; **(2)** uma estrutura que é característica da esporotricose, quando encontrada na pele ou em lesões secundárias dessa micose; circunda os 3 a 5 μm de diâmetro da levedura ovóide do *Sporothrix schenckii*.
  Auer b.'s, corpúsculos de Auer; estruturas em forma de bastonete de natureza incerta no citoplasma das células mielóides imaturas, especialmente os mieloblastos, na leucemia mielocítica aguda; podem ser uma forma anormal de lisossomas; contêm peroxidase e fosfatase, e se coram em vermelho pelos corantes azur-eosina. SIN Auer rods.
  Barr chromatin b., corpúsculo cromatínico de Barr. SIN sex *chromatin*.
  basal b., corpúsculo basal; estrutura centriolar alongada situada na base de cada cílio na margem apical de uma célula. SIN basal corpuscle, basal granule, blepharoplast, kinetosome.
  bigeminal b.'s, corpos bigêmeos; tumefação bilateral única da placa do teto do mesencéfalo embrionário que, mais adiante no desenvolvimento, subdivide-se em um colículo superior e um inferior. VER quadrigeminal b.'s. SIN corpora bigemina.
  b. of bladder [TA], c. da bexiga; a porção da bexiga entre o ápice e o fundo. SIN corpus vesicae [TA].
  brassy b., corpúsculo bronzeado; eritrócito de cor escura, geralmente enrugado, no qual existe um plasmódio.
  b. of breast [TA], c. da mama; a parte principal da mama, consistindo em tecido glandular e seu tecido fibroso de sustentação. Forma uma massa cônica que converge no sentido do mamilo e é circundada por tecido adiposo. SIN corpus mammae [TA], b. of mammary gland.
  Cabot ring b.'s, corpúsculos anulares de Cabot; as estruturas em forma de anel ou em figura de oito que se coram em vermelho pelo corante de Wright, encontradas nos eritrócitos nas anemias graves, possivelmente um resquício da membrana nuclear; uma forma de processo degenerativo basofílico.
  Call-Exner b.'s, corpos de Call-Exner; pequenos espaços cheios de líquido entre as células granulosas nos folículos ovarianos e nos tumores de célula granulosa ovariana; podem formar uma estrutura semelhante a uma roseta.
  carotid b. [TA], glomo carótico; pequena estrutura epitelióide localizada logo acima da bifurcação da artéria carótida comum em cada lado. Consiste em células principais granulares e células de sustentação não-granulares, um leito vascular sinusóide e uma rica rede de fibras sensoriais do nervo glossofaríngeo. Serve como órgão quimiorreceptor responsivo à carência de oxigênio, ao excesso de dióxido de carbono e à concentração aumentada de íon hidrogênio. SIN glomus caroticum [TA], intercarotid b., nodulus caroticus.
  b. of caudate nucleus [TA], c. do núcleo caudado; a parte supratalâmica do núcleo caudado que se situa no assoalho da parte central (o corpo) do ventrículo lateral. SIN corpus nuclei caudati [TA].
  cavernous b.'s of anal canal, dilatações do plexo venoso retal superior. SIN anal *cushions*, em *cushion*.
  cavernous b. of clitoris, c. cavernoso do clítoris. SIN *corpus* cavernosum of clitoris.
  cavernous b. of penis, c. cavernoso do pênis. SIN *corpus* cavernosum penis.
  cell b., c. celular; a parte da célula que contém o núcleo.
  central b., c. central. SIN cytocentrum.

central fibrous b., c. fibroso central; a área fibrosa onde os folhetos das valvas aórtica, mitral e tricúspide se encontram no coração.
chromaffin b., c. cromafínico. SIN paraganglion.
chromatin b., c. cromatínico; o aparelho genético das bactérias. VER nucleus (2).
ciliary b. [TA], c. ciliar; a porção espessada da túnica vascular do olho entre a corióide e a íris; consiste em três partes ou zonas: ciliar orbicular, ciliar da coroa e músculo ciliar. SIN corpus ciliare [TA], anulus ciliaris.
Civatte b.'s, corpos de Civatte; corpos esféricos hialinos eosinofílicos observados na epiderme, no líquen plano e em outros distúrbios cutâneos; formados por apoptose de células basais individuais. SIN colloid b.'s.
b. of clavicle, c. da clavícula; termo oficial alternativo* para *shaft* of clavicle.
b. of clitoris, c. do clitóris; a diáfise ou porção pendulosa do clitóris, composta de dois corpos cavernosos fundidos do clitóris, cuja extremidade distal é a glande do clitóris. SIN corpus clitoridis [TA].
coccygeal b. [TA], glomo coccígeo; anastomose arteriovenosa (arteriolovenular) suprida pela artéria sacral média e localizada na superfície pélvica do cóccix. Foi originalmente chamada de glândula (de Luschka) ou glomo e incluída com os paragânglios. SIN corpus coccygeum [TA], arteriococcygeal gland, coccygeal gland, glomus coccygeum.
colloid b.'s, c. de Civatte. SIN Civatte b.'s.
compressible cavernous b.'s, corpos cavernosos compressíveis; plexos venosos submucosos encontrados no nível da junção faringoesofágica e do canal anal que auxiliam na redução ou obliteração da luz.
conchoidal b.'s, corpúsculos de Schaumann. SIN Schaumann b.'s.
b. of corpus callosum, tronco do corpo caloso; termo oficial alternativo* para *trunk* of corpus callosum.
Councilman b., Councilman hyaline b., c. (hialinos) de Councilman; glóbulo eosinofílico observado no fígado na febre amarela, derivado da apoptose de uma única célula hepática.
Cowdry type A inclusion b.'s, corpúsculos de inclusão do tipo A de Cowdry; massas semelhantes a gotículas de material acidófilo circundadas por halos claros dentro dos núcleos, com a marginação da cromatina na membrana nuclear, conforme observado nas células infectadas pelo herpesvírus humano.
Cowdry type B inclusion b.'s, corpúsculos de inclusão do tipo B de Cowdry; termo obsoleto para massas semelhantes a gotículas de material acidófilo circundadas por halos claros dentro dos núcleos, sem outras alterações nucleares durante os estágios iniciais do desenvolvimento da inclusão conforme observado na poliomielite.
creola b.'s, grandes aglomerados compactos de células colunares ciliadas encontrados no escarro de alguns pacientes asmáticos.
cyanobacteriumlike b.'s, cyclospora. SIN *Cyclospora*.
cytoid b.'s, corpos citóides; fibras nervosas retinianas edemaciadas que, à microscopia óptica, assemelham-se a células quando cortadas no plano transverso; a correlação histopatológica de placas retinianas algodoadas.
cytoplasmic inclusion b.'s, corpúsculos de inclusão citoplasmática. VER inclusion b.'s.
Deetjen b.'s, corpúsculos de Deetjen; termo obsoleto para plaqueta.
demilune b., c. semilunar; um c. circular de transparência extrema exceto por uma substância pontilhada em forma de crescente em uma extremidade, que contém hemoglobina. O c. é muito maior que um eritrócito, mas se acredita que, possivelmente, seja um eritrócito degenerado e edemaciado por embebição; foi encontrado na malária e na convalescença da febre tifóide; a porção transparente é chamada de c. vítreo.
dense b.'s, corpúsculos densos; grânulos no granulômero central das plaquetas sangüíneas que captam e armazenam serotonina do plasma. Acredita-se que os corpúsculos elétron-densos que contêm α-actinina no citoplasma das células musculares lisas associadas à membrana celular são homólogos às linhas Z do músculo estriado.
Döhle b.'s, corpúsculos de Döhle; corpúsculos arredondados ou ovais, bem-definidos, que variam de diâmetro desde apenas visíveis até 2 μm, que se coram em azul-celeste a azul-acinzentado com os corantes de Romanowsky, encontrados nos neutrófilos de pacientes com infecções, queimaduras, trauma, gravidez ou câncer. SIN Döhle inclusions, leukocyte inclusions.
Donovan b.'s, corpúsculos de Donovan; grumos de condensações cromatínicas bipolares que se coram em azul ou negro nas grandes células mononucleares no tecido de granulação infectado por *Calymmatobacterium granulomatis*.
Ehrlich inner b., c. interno de Ehrlich; um c. oxifílico arredondado encontrado no eritrócito no caso da hemocitólise por tóxico sangüíneo específico. SIN Heinz-Ehrlich b.
elementary b.'s, corpos elementares; **(1) (E.B., EB),** termos obsoletos para vírions, principalmente as partículas virais maiores, visíveis à microscopia óptica quando coradas; como nas lesões da varíola, vacínia; **(2)** SIN platelet.
b. of epididymis [TA], c. do epidídimo; a parte média que se estende para baixo, da cabeça para a cauda do epidídimo, na superfície posterior do testículo. SIN corpus epididymidis [TA].
epithelial b., glândula paratireóide. SIN parathyroid *gland*.
fat b., c. adiposo; termo alternativo oficial* para fat-pad.
fat b. of cheek, corpo adiposo da bochecha. SIN buccal *fat-pad*.

fat b. of ischioanal fossa [TA], c. adiposo da fossa isquioanal; o tecido adiposo na fossa isquiorretal. SIN corpus adiposum fossae ischiorectalis, fat b. of ischiorectal fossa, ischiorectal fat-pad.
fat b. of ischiorectal fossa, corpo adiposo da fossa isquiorretal. SIN fat b. of ischioanal fossa.
fat b. of orbit, corpo adiposo da órbita. SIN retrobulbar *fat*.
b. of femur, c. do fêmur; termo alternativo oficial* para *shaft* of femur (diáfise do fêmur).
ferruginous b.'s, corpos ferruginosos; nos pulmões, fibras inorgânicas ou orgânicas estranhas revestidas por complexos de hemossiderina e glicoproteínas, que se acredita que sejam formadas por macrófagos que fagocitaram as fibras. VER TAMBÉM asbestos b.'s.
b. of fibula, c. da fíbula; termo oficial alternativo* para *shaft* of tibia (diáfise da tíbia).
foreign b., c. estranho; qualquer material nos tecidos ou cavidades do c. que tenha sido introduzido lá e que não seja rapidamente absorvido.

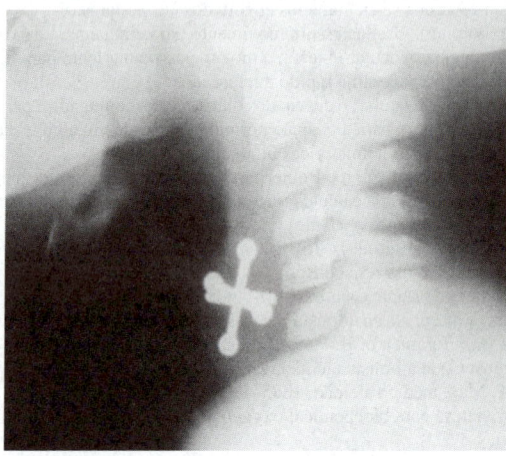

corpo estranho: radiografia de uma criança com 4 anos de idade com uma peça de um jogo infantil na porção cervical do esôfago; a incidência lateral do pescoço mostra a posição das projeções afiladas e a resultante compressão traqueal

b. of fornix [TA], c. do fórnice; a parte média do fórnice situada ventralmente ao corpo caloso. SIN corpus fornicis [TA].
fruiting b., c. frugal; qualquer estrutura fúngica que produza esporos.
fuchsin b.'s, corpos fucsínicos; **(1)** SIN Russell b.'s; **(2)** SIN hyaline b.'s.
b. of gallbladder [TA], c. da vesícula biliar; a parte principal da vesícula biliar que termina no fundo arredondado abaixo e que continua para dentro do colo da vesícula biliar acima. SIN corpus vesicae biliaris [TA], corpus vesicae felleae*.
Gamna-Favre b.'s, corpúsculos de Gamna-Favre; corpúsculos de inclusão basofílicos intracitoplasmáticos característicos, relativamente grandes, observados nas células endoteliais no linfogranuloma venéreo; provavelmente compostos de material nuclear degenerado. VER TAMBÉM Miyagawa b.'s.
Gamna-Gandy b.'s, corpúsculos de Gamna-Gandy; pequenos focos firmes, esferoidais ou irregulares, que são amarelo-acastanhados, acastanhados ou cor de ferrugem e ocorrem principalmente no baço em determinadas condições como a esplenomegalia congestiva e a doença falciforme e consistem em tecido fibroso relativamente denso ou fibras colagenosas impregnadas com pigmento de ferro e sais de cálcio; provavelmente resultam de organização e fibrose dos locais onde ocorreram pequenas hemorragias perivasculares. SIN Gamna-Gandy nodules, Gandy-Gamna b.'s, siderotic nodules.
Gandy-Gamna b.'s, corpúsculos de Gandy-Gamna. SIN Gamna-Gandy b.'s.
geniculate b., c. geniculado. VER lateral geniculate b., medial geniculate b.
glass b., c. vítreo. VER demilune b.
glomus b., c. glomoso. SIN glomus (2).
Golgi b., c. de Golgi. SIN Golgi *apparatus*.
Guarnieri b.'s, corpúsculos de Guarnieri; corpúsculos de inclusão intracitoplasmáticos acidófilos observados nas células epiteliais na varíola e na vacínia, e que incluem agregados dos corpúsculos de Paschen ou partículas virais.
Halberstaedter-Prowazek b.'s, corpúsculos de Halberstaedter-Prowazek. SIN trachoma b.'s
Hassall b.'s, corpúsculos de Hassall. SIN thymic *corpuscle*.
Hassall-Henle b.'s, corpúsculos de Hassall-Henle; os corpúsculos hialinos na superfície posterior da membrana de Descemet na periferia da córnea. SIN Henle warts.

Heinz b.'s, corpúsculos de Heinz; as inclusões intracelulares usualmente ligadas à membrana do eritrócito, compostas de hemoglobina desnaturada; ocorrem na talassemia, nas enzimopatias, nas hemoglobinopatias e após esplenectomia. A visualização desses geralmente exige o exame dos eritrócitos, usando corantes supravitais ou por microscopia de fase.
Heinz-Ehrlich b., c. de Heinz-Ehrlich. SIN Ehrlich inner b.
hematoxylin b.'s, hematoxyphil b.'s, corpúsculos hematoxilínicos, corpúsculos hematoxifílicos; remanescentes basofílicos homogêneos, maldefinidos, de núcleos integrais, um achado ocasional nos tecidos fixos dos pacientes com lúpus eritematoso sistêmico, mas observados com maior freqüência nos glomérulos renais e nas paredes dos vasos sangüíneos, e provavelmente relacionados com o fenômeno LE; assim denominados por causa de suas afinidades pelo corante hematoxilina.
Herring b.'s, corpúsculos de Herring; acúmulos de grânulos neurossecretores nas terminações finais dilatadas dos axônios na neuro-hipófise.
Highmore b., c. de Highmore. SIN *mediastinum* of testis.
Howell-Jolly b.'s, corpúsculos de Howell-Jolly; grânulos esféricos ou ovóides, excentricamente localizados, com aproximadamente 1 μm de diâmetro, por vezes observados no estroma dos eritrócitos circulantes, em especial nas preparações coradas (conforme comparado com esfregaços a fresco não-corados); provavelmente representam resquícios nucleares, visto que podem ser corados com os corantes que são bastante específicos para a cromatina; a importância desses corpúsculos não é exatamente conhecida; eles ocorrem mais amiúde depois da esplenectomia ou na anemia megaloblástica ou hemolítica grave. SIN Jolly b.'s.
b. of humerus, corpo do úmero, termo oficial alternativo* para *shaft* of humerus (diáfise do úmero).
hyaline b.'s, corpúsculos hialinos; inclusões eosinofílicas homogêneas no citoplasma das células epiteliais; nos túbulos renais, os corpúsculos hialinos representam gotículas de proteína reabsorvidas a partir da luz. VER TAMBÉM Mallory b.'s, drusen. SIN fuchsin b.'s (2).
hyaline b.'s of pituitary, corpúsculos hialinos da hipófise; acúmulos de uma substância neurossecretora gelatinosa nos axônios do trato hipotálamo-hipofisário no lobo posterior da hipófise.
hyaloid b., c. vítreo. SIN vitreous b.
b. of hyoid bone [TA], c. do osso hióide; o corpo do osso hióide, a partir do qual se estendem os cornos maior e menor. SIN corpus ossis hyoidei [TA], base of hyoid bone, basihyal, basihyoid.
b. of ilium [TA], c. do ílio; forma os dois quintos superiores do acetábulo e une o púbis e o ísquio no acetábulo. Continua acima para dentro da asa do ílio. SIN corpus ossis ilii [TA].
inclusion b.'s, corpúsculos de inclusão; estruturas distintas freqüentemente formadas no núcleo ou citoplasma (ocasionalmente em ambas as localizações) nas células infectadas por determinados vírus filtráveis; podem ser demonstrados por meio de diversos corantes, especialmente pelas técnicas de azul de metileno-eosina de Mann ou de Giemsa e visíveis à microscopia óptica. Os corpúsculos de inclusão nuclear são usualmente acidófilos e são de dois tipos morfológicos: 1) corpúsculos granulares, hialinos ou amorfos de vários tamanhos, i.e., os corpúsculos de inclusão do tipo A de Cowdry, que ocorrem em certas doenças como a infecção por vírus herpes simples ou febre amarela; 2) corpúsculos mais circunscritos, freqüentemente com vários no mesmo núcleo (e nenhuma reação no tecido adjacente), i.e., os corpúsculos do tipo B, que acontecem em determinadas doenças como a febre do vale Rift e a poliomielite. Os corpúsculos de inclusão citoplasmáticos podem ser: 1) acidófilos, relativamente grandes, esféricos ou ovóides e algo granulares, como na varíola ou vacínia, raiva e molusco contagioso; 2) combinações complexas basofílicas, relativamente grandes, de material viral e celular, como no tracoma, na psitacose e no linfogranuloma venéreo. Em alguns casos, os corpúsculos de inclusão são sabidamente infecciosos e provavelmente representam agregados de partículas virais em combinação com o material celular, enquanto em outros são aparentemente inócuos e representariam apenas produtos anormais formados pela célula em resposta à lesão.
b. of incus [TA], corpo da bigorna; a parte principal da bigorna que se articula com o martelo e a partir do qual se originam os ramos curto e longo. SIN corpus incudis [TA].
infrapatellar fat b., c. adiposo infrapatelar. SIN infrapatellar *fat-pad*.
intercarotid b., glomo carótico. SIN carotid b.
intermediate b. of Flemming, c. intermediário de Flemming. SIN midbody.
b. of ischium [TA], c. do ísquio; o ísquio inteiro, com a exceção do ramo. SIN corpus ossis ischii [TA].
Jaworski b.'s, corpúsculos de Jaworski; filamentos de muco no conteúdo gástrico na hipercloridria.
Jolly b.'s, corpúsculos de Jolly. SIN Howell-Jolly b.'s
juxtaglomerular b., c. justaglomerular; coleção de células musculares lisas modificadas ao redor das arteríolas glomerulares renais que contêm grânulos citoplasmáticos, provavelmente compostos de renina. SIN periarterial pad.
juxtarestiform b. [TA], c. justa-restiforme; subdivisão medial (menor) do pedúnculo cerebelar inferior composta de fibras que conectam de forma recíproca os núcleos vestibulares e o cerebelo, em particular o nódulo do último, flóculo e úvula do verme. Ele também carrega as fibras sensoriais primárias a partir dos gânglios vestibulares para o cerebelo, bem como as projeções cerebelares para a formação reticular rombencefálica e núcleos vestibulares. SIN corpus juxtarestiforme.
ketone b., c. cetônico; uma de um grupo de cetonas que inclui o ácido acetoacético, seu produto de redução, ácido β-hidroxibutírico e seu produto de descarboxilação, a acetona; níveis elevados são encontrados nos tecidos e nos líquidos corporais na cetose. SIN acetone b., acetone compound.
Lafora b. [MIM*254780], c. de Lafora; distúrbio autossômico recessivo caracterizado por corpúsculos de inclusão intracitoplasmáticos intraneurais compostos de mucopolissacarídeos ácidos, observado na epilepsia mioclônica familial.
Lallemand b.'s, corpúsculos de Lallemand; (1) termo obsoleto para pequenas concreções gelatinóides por vezes observadas no líquido seminal; (2) termo obsoleto para Bence Jones *cylinders* (cilindros de Bence Jones), em *cylinder*. SIN Trousseau-Lallemand b.'s.
lateral geniculate b., c. geniculado lateral; a massa lateral de um par de pequenas massas ovais que se projetam discretamente da face póstero-inferior do tálamo; comumente considerado parte do metatálamo. SIN corpus geniculatum laterale [TA], corpus geniculatum externum.
b. of lateral ventricle, parte central do ventrículo lateral. SIN *pars* centralis ventriculi lateralis.
L-D b., c. L-D. SIN Leishman-Donovan b.
LE b., corpúsculos LE; corpúsculo arredondado e amorfo no citoplasma de uma célula LE.
Leishman-Donovan b., c. de Leishman-Donovan; a forma intracitoplasmática, não-flagelada, de determinados parasitas intracelulares, como espécies de *Leishmania* ou a forma intracelular do *Trypanosoma cruzi*; originalmente utilizado para *Leishmania donovani* parasitas nas células esplênicas ou hepáticas infectadas no calazar. SIN amastigote, L-D b.
Lewy b.'s, corpúsculos de Lewy; inclusão neuronal intracitoplasmática; corpúsculos especialmente percebidos nos neurônios pigmentados do tronco cerebral e observados na doença de Parkinson.

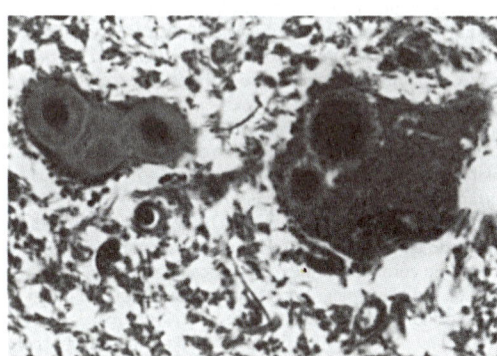

Corpúsculos de Lewy: observados em dois neurônios com cerne central proeminente e halo; hematoxilina e eosina, ampliação original 1.000×

Lieutaud b., c. de Lieutaud. SIN *trigone* of bladder.
Lindner b.'s, corpúsculos de Lindner; os corpúsculos iniciais que se assemelham aos corpúsculos de inclusão encontrados em raspados de células epiteliais infectadas pelo tracoma.
loose b., c. livre; um fragmento de tecido sólido que fica livre em uma cavidade corporal, principalmente em uma articulação ou na cavidade peritoneal; p. ex., *joint mice, melon-seed b., rice b.*
Luse b.'s, corpúsculos de Luse; fibras de colágeno com espaçamento anormalmente longo (superando 1.000 Å) entre faixas elétron-densas.
Luys b., c. de Luys. SIN subthalamic *nucleus*.
Mallory b.'s, corpúsculos de Mallory; acúmulos grandes e maldefinidos de material eosinofílico no citoplasma das células hepáticas lesionadas em determinadas formas de cirrose, principalmente aquela provocada pelo alcoolismo. SIN alcoholic hyalin, alcoholic hyaline b.'s.
malpighian b.'s, corpúsculos de Malpighi. SIN splenic limph *follicles*, em *follicle*.
b. of mammary gland, c. da mama. SIN b. of breast.
mammillary b. [TA], c. mamilar; um grupo de células pequenas, arredondadas e pareadas que se projeta para a fossa interpeduncular a partir da face inferior do hipotálamo. Recebe as fibras do hipocampo através do fórnice e projeta fibras para os núcleos talâmicos anteriores e para dentro do tegmento do tronco cerebral. SIN corpus mammillare [TA], mammillary tubercle of hypothalamus.

b. of mandible [TA], c. da mandíbula; a porção horizontal pesada da mandíbula, em formato de U, que se estende posteriormente até o ângulo onde continua com o ramo; dá suporte para os dentes inferiores. SIN corpus mandibulae [TA].
b. of maxilla, c. da maxila; a porção central da maxila, escavada pelo seio maxilar; apresenta as superfícies orbitária, nasal, anterior e infratemporal e sustenta quatro processos: frontal, zigomático, palatino e alveolar. SIN corpus maxillae [TA].
medial geniculate b., c. geniculado medial; a massa medial de um par de pequenas massas que se projetam da parte póstero-inferior do tálamo; comumente considerado parte do metatálamo. SIN corpus geniculatum mediale [TA], corpus geniculatum internum.
melon-seed b., c. em semente de melão; um pequeno corpo fibroso frouxo em uma articulação ou bainha tendinosa.
b. of metacarpal, c. do metacarpal; termo oficial alternativo* para shaft of metacarpal (diáfise do metacarpal).
metachromatic b.'s, corpúsculos metacromáticos; depósitos concentrados que consistem principalmente no polimetafosfato e que ocorrem em muitas bactérias, bem como nas algas, fungos e protozoários; os corpos metacromáticos diferem nas propriedades de coloração do protoplasma circunvizinho. VER metachromasia.
b. of metatarsal, diáfise do metatarsal; termo oficial alternativo* para shaft of metatarsal.
Michaelis-Gutmann b., c. de Michaelis-Gutmann; um c. arredondado, homogêneo ou concentricamente laminado, com 1 a 10 μ de diâmetro, contendo cálcio e ferro; encontrado dentro dos macrófagos na malacoplaquia.
Miyagawa b.'s, corpúsculos de Miyagawa; termo obsoleto para Chlamydia trachomatis (Miyagawanella lymphogranulomatosis), os corpos elementares que se desenvolvem nas microcolônias intracitoplasmáticas do linfogranuloma venéreo.
molluscum b., c. de molusco; c. esférico citoplasmático nítido nas lesões do molusco contagioso provocadas por um membro da família Poxviridae; consiste em citoplasma degenerado e no vírus. SIN molluscum corpuscle.
Mooser b.'s, corpúsculos de Mooser; um termo utilizado para referir-se às riquétsias encontradas no exsudato (e no tecido) da túnica vaginal no tifo endêmico (causado pela Rickettsia typhi).
multilamellar b., c. multilamellar. SIN cytosome (2).
multivesicular b.'s, corpúsculos multivesiculares; corpos ligados à membrana, com 0,5 a 1,0 μm de largura, que ocorrem no citoplasma das células e contêm inúmeras vesículas pequenas; as hidrolases (especialmente a fosfatase ácida) ocorrem na matriz.
myelin b., c. mielínico. SIN myelin figure.
b. of nail [TA], c. da unha; a porção exposta da unha distal à sua raiz. SIN corpus unguis [TA].
Negri b.'s, corpúsculos de Negri; corpúsculos de inclusão eosinofílicos, nitidamente delineados, patognomônicos (2 a 10 μm de diâmetro), encontrados no citoplasma de determinadas células nervosas, contendo o vírus da raiva, principalmente no corno de Ammon do hipocampo.
nerve cell b., c. da célula nervosa; a parte do neurônio que inclui o núcleo, mas exclui os prolongamentos.
neuroepithelial b., c. neuroepitelial; um agregado corpuscular de células não-ciliadas bastante inervadas, que contém a substância neurossecretora encontrada no epitélio intrapulmonar normal, principalmente nas bifurcações dos brônquios.
Nissl b.'s, corpúsculos de Nissl. SIN Nissl substance.
nodular b., c. nodular; nos fungos, uma estrutura compacta, grosseiramente esférica ou quadrada, formada por espiralamento e torção da extremidade de uma hifa; considerado como sendo crescimentos abortados no sentido da reprodução sexual.
nu b., c. nu. SIN nucleosome.
nuclear inclusion b.'s, corpúsculos de inclusão nuclear. VER inclusion b.'s.
Odland b., c. de Odland. SIN keratinosome.
olivary b., oliva. SIN oliva.
orbital fat b., c. adiposo da órbita; termo oficial alternativo* para retrobulbar fat.
pacchionian b.'s, corpúsculos de Pacchioni. SIN arachnoid granulations, em granulation.
pampiniform b., epoóforo. SIN epoophoron.
b. of pancreas [TA], c. do pâncreas; a parte do pâncreas desde o ponto em que ele cruza a veia porta até o ponto em que ele entra no ligamento lienorrenal. SIN corpus pancreatis [TA].
Pappenheimer b.'s, corpúsculos de Pappenheimer; fagossomas, contendo grânulos ferruginosos, encontrados nos eritrócitos em doenças como anemia sideroblástica, anemia hemolítica e doença falciforme; pode contribuir para as contagens espúrias de plaquetas por contadores eletro-ópticos.
paraaortic b.'s [TA], corpúsculos paraaórticos; pequenas massas de tecido cromafim encontradas próximo aos gânglios simpáticos ao longo da aorta; são mais proeminentes durante a vida fetal. As células cromafins secretam norepinefrina; as terminações quimiorreceptoras monitoram os níveis gasométricos. SIN corpora para-aortica [TA], glomus aorticum [TA], aortic glomera*, glomera aortica*, aortic b.'s, corpus aorticum, organs of Zuckerkandl, Zuckerkandl b.'s.
parabasal b., c. parabasal; um termo originalmente equivalente ao cinetoplasto do DNA, parte da mitocôndria gigante de determinados parasitas flagelados. Originalmente, acreditava-se que o c. parabasal mais o c. basal formavam um cinetoplasto, ou aparelho locomotor, mas, atualmente, o cinetoplasto é restrito a parte da mitocôndria gigante do DNA e o c. parabasal é uma estrutura distinta próximo ao núcleo, provavelmente equivalente ao aparelho de Golgi dos metazoários.
paranephric b., c. paranéfrico; uma massa de tecido adiposo que se situa atrás da fáscia renal.
paranuclear b., astrosfera. SIN astrosphere.
paraphysial b., c. parafisário. SIN paraphysis.
paraterminal b., c. paraterminal. SIN subcallosal gyrus.
Paschen b.'s, corpúsculos de Paschen; partículas de vírus observadas em número relativamente grande em células escamosas da pele (ou a córnea de cobaias) na varíola ou vacínia.
b. of penis [TA], c. do pênis; a porção pendulosa livre do pênis, consistindo no corpo e na glande do pênis. SIN corpus penis [TA], scapus penis.
perineal b., c. do períneo. SIN central tendon of perineum.
b. of phalanx, c. da falange; termo oficial alternativo* para shaft of phalanx.
Pick b.'s, corpúsculos de Pick; corpúsculos de inclusão neuronal intracitoplasmáticos argentofílicos observados na doença de Pick.
pineal b. [TA], glândula pineal; um corpo pequeno, não-pareado, achatado, com formato algo semelhante a uma pinha, preso em seu pólo anterior à região das comissuras posterior e habenular, e dispondo-se na depressão entre os dois colículos superiores abaixo do esplênio do corpo caloso; é uma estrutura glandular, composta de folículos com células epitelióides e concreções calcáreas, denominadas areia cerebral; apesar de sua inserção no cérebro, parece receber fibras nervosas exclusivamente do sistema nervoso autônomo periférico. Produz melatonina. SIN corpus pineale [TA], glandula pinealis [TA], pineal gland [TA], conarium, epiphysis cerebri, pinus.
polar b., c. polar; uma das duas pequenas células formadas pela primeira e segunda divisões meióticas dos oócitos; a primeira é usualmente liberada pouco antes da ovulação, a segunda não é liberada até a liberação do ovo a partir do ovário; nos mamíferos, o s. corpo polar pode não se formar, a menos que o ovo tenha sido penetrado por um espermatozóide. SIN polar cell, polar globule, polocyte.
polyhedral b., c. poliédrico; um corpúsculo de inclusão associado à replicação de determinados vírus de insetos.
pontobulbar b., c. pontobulbar; uma coleção de células nervosas na parte inferior da medula oblonga, formando uma crista que atravessa obliquamente o corpo restiforme. SIN corpus pontobulbare.
posterior quadrigeminal b., c. quadrigêmeo posterior. SIN inferior colliculus.
Prowazek b.'s, corpúsculos de Prowazek; termo histórico para os dois tipos de corpúsculos de inclusão associados a determinadas doenças: 1) corpúsculos do tracoma; 2) formas diminutas, ovóides, granulares, freqüentemente aos pares, observadas no citoplasma e nos corpos de Guarnieri nas células escamosas cutâneas de seres humanos e animais infectados pelo vírus da varíola ou da vacínia; provavelmente idênticos aos corpúsculos de Paschen.
Prowazek-Greeff b.'s, corpúsculos de Prowazek-Greeff. SIN trachoma b.'s.
psammoma b.'s, corpúsculos de psammoma; **(1)** corpúsculos mineralizados que ocorrem nas meninges, no plexo coróide e em determinados meningiomas; compostos usualmente de um capilar central circundado por espirais concêntricas de meningócitos em vários estágios de alteração hialina e mineralização; também podem acontecer nos tumores epiteliais benignos e malignos (como o carcinoma papilar ovariano ou tireóideo). SIN sand b.'s. **(2)** SIN corpora arenacea, em corpus; **(3)** SIN calcospherite.
psittacosis inclusion b.'s, corpúsculos de inclusão da psitacose; microcolônias intracitoplasmáticas de clamídias observadas nas células epiteliais brônquicas infectadas por Chlamydia psittaci.
pubic b., b. of pubic bone, c. do púbis. SIN b. of pubis.
b. of pubis [TA], c. do púbis; a porção medial achatada do púbis que participa na sínfise pubiana. A partir dele se estendem os ramos superior e inferior. SIN corpus ossis pubis [TA], pubic b., p. of pubic bone.
purine b.'s, corpos purínicos; qualquer purina.
quadrigeminal b.'s, colículo. VER inferior colliculus, superior colliculus. SIN corpora quadrigemina.
b. of radius, c. do rádio; termo oficial alternativo* para shaft of radius.
Renaut b., c. de Renaut; estrutura subperineurial composta de fibras de colágeno frouxamente dispostas e orientadas ao acaso em um material fibrilar fino, observado no nervo normal, bem como em determinados estados patológicos.
residual b., c. residual; vacúolo citoplasmático (lisossoma) que contém produtos particulados acumulados do metabolismo, p.ex., lipofuscina.
residual b. of Regaud, c. residual de Regaud; o citoplasma em excesso que se separa do espermatozóide durante a espermiogênese.

rest b., c. de repouso; uma pequena massa de citoplasma que permanece depois que o núcleo e o citoplasma do esquizonte de determinados esporozoários se dividiram em esporos assexuados ou merozoítos.

restiform b. [TA], c. restiforme; subdivisão lateral (maior) do pedúnculo cerebelar inferior localizada na face dorsolateral da medula oblonga e composta de uma gama de fibras, incluindo, mas não se limitando a, olivocerebelares, reticulocerebelares, cuneocerebelares, trigeminocerebelares e espinocerebelares dorsais. VER TAMBÉM inferior cerebellar *peduncle*. SIN corpus restiforme [TA], eminentia restiformis, restiform eminence.

b. of rib [TA], c. da costela; a diáfise de uma costela; a porção que se estende lateral, anterior e, em seguida, medialmente a partir do tubérculo. SIN corpus costae [TA].

rice b., c. riciforme; um dos corpúsculos pequenos e frouxos encontrado em higromas, bainhas tendinosas e articulações; usualmente um dos muitos corpos pequenos e frouxos.

Rushton b., c. de Rushton; corpúsculos hialinos lineares ou curvos, presumivelmente de origem hematogênica, encontrados no revestimento epitelial dos cistos odontogênicos.

Russell b.'s, corpúsculos de Russell; corpúsculos hialinos, acidófilos, intracitoplasmáticos, esféricos, com tamanho variado, bem-definidos e pequenos, que se coram intensamente com a fucsina; ocorrem nos plasmócitos na inflamação crônica e nos distúrbios malignos, e consistem em imunoglobulina. SIN fuchsin b.'s (1).

sand b.'s, corpúsculos arenáceos. SIN psammoma b.'s (1).
Sandström b.'s, corpúsculos de Sandström. VER parathyroid *gland*.
Savage perineal b., c. perineal de Savage. SIN central *tendon* of perineum.
Schaumann b.'s, corpúsculos de Schaumann; corpúsculos calcificados concentricamente laminados encontrados nos granulomas, principalmente na sarcoidose. SIN conchoidal b.'s.
sclerotic b.'s, corpúsculos escleróticos; células muriformes vegetativas, arredondadas, de fungos dematiáceos, característicos dos agentes causais da cromoblastomicose no tecido. SIN copper pennies.
segmenting b., esquizonte. SIN schizont.
b. of sphenoid [TA], c. do esfenóide; a porção central do osso esfenóide a partir da qual se originam as asas maior e menor e os processos pterigóides. Os seios esfenoidais se localizam dentro dele. SIN corpus ossis sphenoidalis.
spongy b. of penis, c. esponjoso do pênis. SIN *corpus* spongiosum penis.
b. of sternum [TA], c. do esterno; a porção média e maior do esterno, que se localiza entre o manúbrio, superiormente, e o processo xifóide, inferiormente. SIN corpus sterni [TA], gladiolus, mesosternum, midsternum.
b. of stomach [TA], c. gástrico; a parte do estômago que se situa entre o fundo, acima, e o antro pilórico, abaixo; seus limites são mal delimitados. SIN corpus gastricum [TA].
striate b., c. estriado; os núcleos caudado e lentiforme (lenticular); o aspecto estriado no corte é causado pelos fascículos finos de fibras mielinizadas. Histologicamente, o c. estriado pode ser subdividido em células geralmente pequenas, consistindo no núcleo caudado e no segmento externo do núcleo lentiforme (o putâmen), e no globo pálido de células grandes, composto de dois segmentos. SIN corpus striatum [TA].
suprarenal b., glândula supra-renal. SIN suprarenal *gland*.
b. of sweat gland, c. da glândula sudorípara; a porção secretora tubular espiralada de uma glândula sudorípara localizada no tecido subcutâneo ou profundamente no cório e conectado à superfície da pele por um longo duto. SIN corpus glandulae sudoriferae.
Symington anococcygeal b., c. anococcígeo de Symington. SIN anococcygeal *ligament*.
b. of talus [TA], c. do tálus; a grande parte posterior do tálus que forma a tróclea, acima, para a articulação com a tíbia e a fíbula e articulando abaixo com o calcâneo. SIN corpus tali [TA].
b. of thigh bone, c. do fêmur. SIN *shaft* of femur.
threshold b., substância limiar. SIN threshold *substance*.
thyroid b., glândula tireóide. SIN thyroid *gland*.
b. of tibia [TA], c. da tíbia; termo oficial alternativo* para *shaft* of tibia.
tigroid b.'s, corpos tigróides. SIN Nissl *substance*.
b. of tongue [TA], c. da língua; a parte oral da língua anterior ao sulco terminal. SIN corpus linguae [TA].
trachoma b.'s, corpúsculos de tracoma; formas intracitoplasmáticas complexas e distintas encontradas nas células epiteliais da conjuntiva das pessoas em fase aguda de tracoma, menos freqüentes nos estágios mais avançados, variando desde 1) grânulos acidófilos bem-definidos (aproximadamente 250 nm de diâmetro), a 2) grumos irregulares desse material embebido em uma matriz basofílica, 3) corpúsculos basofílicos relativamente grandes (aproximadamente 700–1000 nm de diâmetro), até 4) grandes corpúsculos basofílicos que incluem grânulos acidófilos diminutos e bem-definidos. SIN Halberstaedter-Prowazek b.'s, Prowazek-Greef b.'s.
trapezoid b. [TA], c. trapezóide; uma placa de fibras transversas que correm sobre a borda dorsal (profunda) dos núcleos da ponta; é formado por fibras auditivas ascendentes que cruzam para o lado oposto do tronco cerebral. SIN corpus trapezoideum [TA], trapezoid (4) [TA].

Trousseau-Lallemand b.'s, corpúsculos de Trousseau-Lallemand. SIN Lallemand b.'s.
tuffstone b., c. de lava; grânulos elétron-densos ligados à membrana, medindo cerca de 0,5 μm de diâmetro, encontrados principalmente nas células de Schwann dos pacientes que sofrem de leucodistrofia metacromática; o nome alude à sua semelhança ao calcáreo vulcânico.
turbinated b., (1) uma concha com seu revestimento da mucosa e outras partes moles. SIN turbinal; **(2)** concha. SIN inferior nasal *concha*, middle nasal *concha*, superior nasal *concha*, supreme nasal *concha*.
tympanic b., glândula timpânica. SIN tympanic *gland*.
b. of ulna, c. da ulna; termo oficial alternativo* para *shaft* of ulna.
ultimobranchial b., c. ultimobranquial; um divertículo a partir da quarta bolsa faríngea de um embrião, considerado, por alguns, uma quinta bolsa faríngea rudimentar e, por outros, um primórdio tireóideo lateral; os corpos ultimobranquiais dos vertebrados inferiores contêm grandes quantidades de calcitonina; nos mamíferos, os corpos ultimobranquiais fundem-se com a glândula tireóide e se acredita que se desenvolvam nas células parafoliculares. VER TAMBÉM ultimobranchial *pouch*.
b. of uterus [TA], c. do útero; a parte do útero acima do istmo, compreendendo cerca de dois terços do órgão não-grávido. SIN corpus uteri [TA].
vaccine b.'s, corpos de vacina; termo obsoleto pertinente aos corpúsculos intracelulares que se acreditava, erroneamente, serem formas no ciclo de vida de um protozoário, *Cytorhyctes vaccinae*, postulado como sendo o agente etiológico da vacínia.
Verocay b.'s, corpúsculos de Verocay; áreas acelulares hialinizadas compostas de membrana basal reduplicada, delineada por fileiras opostas de núcleos paralelos; observados microscopicamente nos neurilemomas.
b. of vertebra, corpo vertebral. SIN vertebral b.
vertebral b. [TA], c. vertebral; a porção principal de uma vértebra anterior ao canal vertebral, conforme distinto dos arcos. SIN corpus vertebrae [TA], b. of vertebra.
Virchow-Hassall b.'s, corpúsculos de Virchow-Hassall. SIN thymic *corpuscle*.
vitreous b. [TA], c. vítreo; a substância transparente, semelhante à gelatina, que preenche o interior do globo ocular atrás da lente; é composto de uma delicada rede (estroma vítreo) que envolve, em sua trama, um líquido aquoso (humor vítreo). SIN corpus vitreum [TA], hyaloid b., vitreous (2), vitreum.
Weibel-Palade b.'s, corpúsculos de Weibel-Palade; os feixes de microtúbulos em formato de bastonete observados à microscopia eletrônica nas células endoteliais vasculares.
wolffian b., c. de Wolff. SIN mesonephros.
Wolf-Orton b.'s, corpúsculos de Wolf-Orton; os corpúsculos de inclusão intranuclear observados nas células de neoplasias malignas, especialmente aquelas de origem nas células gliais.
Y b., c. Y; uma única mancha fluorescente que se origina no braço longo do cromossoma Y e visível nos núcleos somáticos de esfregaços bucais.
yellow b., corpo lúteo. SIN *corpus* luteum.
zebra b., c. zebróide; grânulos ligados à membrana que se coram de maneira metacromática, com 0,5-1 μm de diâmetro e contendo lamelas com um espaçamento de 5,8 nm, reportados nas células de Schwann e macrófagos de pacientes que sofrem de leucodistrofia metacromática.
Zuckerkandl b.'s, corpúsculos de Zuckerkandl. SIN paraaortic b.'s.

body bur·den. Carga de corpo; a atividade de um radiofármaco retido pelo corpo em um intervalo de tempo específico após a administração.

Boeck, Caesar P. M., dermatologista norueguês, 1845–1917. VER B. *disease*, *sarcoid*; Besnier-B.-Schaumann *disease*, *syndrome*.

Boeck, Carl W., médico norueguês, 1808–1875. VER Danielssen-B. *disease*.

Boehmer, F. VER B. *hematoxylin*.

Boerhaave, Hermann, médico holandês, 1668–1738. VER B. *syndrome*.

bog·bean (bog′bēn) Trevo aquático. SIN buckbean.

Bogros, Antoine, anatomista francês do século 19. VER B. serous *membrane*.

Bogros, Jean-Annet, anatomista francês, 1786–1823. VER B. *space*.

Bohn, Heinrich, médico alemão, 1832–1888. VER B. *nodules*, em nodule.

Bohr, Christian, fisiologista dinamarquês, 1855–1911. VER B. *effect*, *equation*.

Bohr, Niels H. D., físico dinamarquês e laureado com o Prêmio Nobel, 1885–1962. VER B. *atom*, *magneton*, *theory*.

boil (boyl). Furúnculo. SIN furuncle. [A. S. *byl*, uma inchação]
 Aleppo b., Bagdad b., f. de Aleppo, f. de Bagdá; a lesão que ocorre na leishmaniose cutânea. VER cutaneous *leishmaniasis*. SIN Biskra b.
 Biskra b., f. de Biskra. SIN Aleppo b.
 blind b., f. cego; um furúnculo que não apresenta um ponto central flutuante; aparece como uma pápula dolorosa avermelhada e inerte.
 date b., Delhi b., Jericho b., f. de Delhi, f. de Jericó; a lesão que ocorre na leishmaniose cutânea.
 Madura b., f. de Madura. SIN mycetoma.
 Oriental b., f. oriental; a lesão que ocorre na leishmaniose cutânea.

salt water b.'s, furúnculos da água salgada; furúnculos nas mãos e antebraços de pescadores.
tropical b., f. tropical; a lesão que acontece na leishmaniose cutânea.
bol. Abreviatura de bolus.
bol·din (bol′din). Boldina; um glicosídeo a partir do boldo; um colagogo e diurético. SIN boldoglucin.
bol·dine (bol′dēn). Bondina; alcalóide amargo obtido do boldo.
boldine dimethyl ether. Éter dimetílico de bondina. SIN glaucine.
bol·do (bol′dō). Boldo. SIN boldus.
bol·do·glu·cin (bol-dō-gloo′sin). Boldoglucina. SIN boldin.
bol·dus (bol′dŭs). Boldo; as folhas do *Boldu boldus* ou *Peumus boldus* (família Monimiaceae), arbusto conífero do Chile; usado em vários distúrbios da função hepática. SIN boldo. [Chileno]
Boley gauge. Medidor de Boley. Ver em gauge.
Boll, Franz C., histologista e fisiologista alemão, 1849–1879. VER B. *cells*, em *cell*.
Bollinger, Otto, patologista alemão, 1843–1909. VER B. *granules*, em *granule*.
Bollman, Jesse L., fisiologista norte-americano, *1896. VER Mann-B. *fistula*.
Bolognini symp·tom. Sintoma de Bolognini. Ver em symptom.
bo·lom·e·ter (bō-lom′ĕ-ter). Bolômetro. **1.** Um instrumento para determinar graus diminutos de calor radiante. **2.** Um instrumento obsoleto para medir a força do batimento cardíaco conforme diferenciada da pressão arterial. [G. *bolē*, um arremesso, um raio solar, + *metron*, medir]
bo·lus (bol) (bō′lŭs). Bolo. **1.** Uma quantidade única, relativamente grande, de uma substância, geralmente aquela destinada para uso terapêutico, como uma dose maciça de um medicamento injetado por via intravenosa. **2.** Um pedaço mastigado de alimento ou de outra substância pronta para ser deglutida, como um bolo de bário para exames radiográficos. **3.** Na radioterapia de alta energia, uma quantidade de material tecido-equivalente colocada no feixe de radiação, sobre a superfície da região irradiada, para aumentar a dose absorvida pelos tecidos superficiais. [L. do G. *bōlos*, nodosidade, argila]
intravenous b., b. intravenoso; volume de líquido relativamente grande ou dose de uma substância ou substância de teste administrado por via intravenosa e de forma rápida para acelerar ou ampliar uma resposta; em radiologia, a injeção rápida de uma grande dose de contraste para aumentar a opacificação dos vasos sangüíneos.
bom·bard. Bombardeio; expor uma substância a radiações particuladas ou eletromagnéticas com a finalidade de torná-la radioativa. [L. Mediev, *bombarda*, agressão por artilharia, de *bombus*, um som de estrondo]
bom·be·sin (bomb′ĕ-sin) Bombesina; tetradecapeptídeo farmacologicamente ativo encontrado na pele de anfíbios europeus da família Discoglossidae, principalmente *Bombina bombina* e *Bombina variegata variegata*. Um potente estimulador das secreções gástrica e pancreática; um peptídeo imunorreativo, semelhante à bombesina, é encontrado no cérebro e no intestino. As outras ações compreendem as atividades hipertensiva, antidiurética e hiperglicêmica. Possui um forte efeito sobre a diminuição da temperatura central em ratos. Também foram encontrados altos níveis intracelulares de bombesina no carcinoma pulmonar do tipo pequenas células humano.
bond (bond). Ligação, união; em química, a força que mantém dois átomos vizinhos em posição e que impede sua separação; uma l. é eletrovalente quando consiste na atração entre grupamentos com cargas elétricas opostas, ou é covalente quando resulta do compartilhamento de um, dois ou três pares de elétrons pelos átomos ligados.
acylmercaptan b., ligação acilmercaptânica; –CO–S–; uma ligação de "alta energia" formada pela condensação de um grupamento carboxila (–COOH) e um grupamento mercaptana (ou tiol) (–SH); amplamente formada durante o metabolismo intermediário, notadamente na oxidação das gorduras, onde o –SH faz parte da coenzima A e o –COOH faz parte do ácido graxo a ser oxidado.
apolar b., l. apolar. VER hydrophobic *interaction*.
conjugated double b.'s, ligações duplas conjugadas; duas ou mais duplas ligações separadas por uma ligação simples.
coordinate covalent b., l. covalente coordenada. SIN semipolar b.
disulfide b., l. dissulfeto; ligação simples entre dois átomos de enxofre; especificamente, a ligação –S–S– que une duas cadeias peptídicas (ou partes diferentes de uma cadeia peptídica); também ocorre como parte da molécula do aminoácido, cistina, e é importante como um determinante estrutural em muitas moléculas peptídicas e protéicas, p.ex., queratina, insulina e ocitocina. Um dissulfeto simétrico é R–S–S–R; R′–S–S–R é um dissulfeto misto ou assimétrico.
double b., l. dupla; l. covalente que resulta do compartilhamento de dois pares de elétrons, p.ex., $H_2C=CH_2$ (etileno).
electrostatic b., l. eletrostática; a l. entre átomos ou grupamentos com cargas elétricas opostas (ou, em alguns casos, as alterações parciais). SIN heteropolar b., salt bridge.
energy-rich b., l. rica em energia. VER high-energy *compounds*, em *compound*.
eupeptide b., l. eupeptídica; l. peptídica entre o grupamento α-carboxila de um aminoácido e o grupamento α-amino de outro aminoácido. Cf. peptide b., isopeptide b.
heteropolar b., l. heteropolar. SIN electrostatic b.

high energy phosphate b., l. fosfato de alta energia. VER high-energy *phosphates*, em *phosphate*.
hydrogen b., ligação de hidrogênio; l. que se origina do compartilhamento de um átomo de hidrogênio, ligado de forma covalente a um elemento fortemente eletronegativo (p.ex., N ou O), com outro elemento fortemente eletronegativo (p.ex., N, O ou um halogênio). Nas substâncias da importância biológica, as ligações de hidrogênio mais comuns são aquelas em que as ligações de H unem o N ao O ou ao N; essas ligações unem purinas em um filamento às pirimidinas no outro filamento dos ácidos nucléicos, mantendo assim as estruturas de filamento duplo como na hélice de Watson-Crick.
hydrophobic b., l. hidrofóbica. VER hydrophobic *interaction*.
isopeptide b., l. isopeptídica; l. amida entre um grupamento carboxila de um aminoácido e um grupamento amino de outro aminoácido em que pelo menos um desses grupos não é o carbono α de um dos aminoácidos; p.ex., a ligação entre o resíduo glutamil e o resíduo cisteinil do glutatião. Cf. peptide b., eupeptide b.
noncovalent b., l. não-covalente; a l. em que os elétrons não são compartilhados entre os átomos; p.ex., l. eletrostática, l. de hidrogênio.
peptide b., l. peptídica; a l. comum (–CO–NH–) entre aminoácidos nas proteínas, na verdade uma amida substituída, formada através da eliminação do H_2O entre o –COOH de um aminoácido e o H_2N– de outro. Cf. eupeptide b., isopeptide b.
semipolar b., l. semipolar; l. em que os dois elétrons compartilhados por um par de átomos pertenciam originalmente a apenas um dos átomos; com freqüência, representada por uma pequena seta apontando no sentido do elétron-receptor; p.ex., ácido nítrico, $O(OH)N{\rightarrow}O$; ácido fosfórico, $(OH)_3P{\rightarrow}O$. SIN coordinate covalent b.
single b., l. simples; l. covalente resultante do compartilhamento de um par de elétrons; p.ex., $H_3C–CH_3$ (etano).
triple b., ligação tripla; l. covalente que resulta do compartilhamento de três pares de elétrons; p.ex., $HC{\equiv}CH$ (acetileno).
bonding (bon′ding). Ligação, vínculo, elo; formação de uma ligação emocional íntima e resistente, como entre pai e filho, amantes ou marido e mulher.

BONE

bone (bōn) [TA]. Osso; tecido conjuntivo duro que consiste em células embebidas em uma matriz de substância fundamental mineralizada e fibras colágenas. As fibras são impregnadas com uma forma de fosfato de cálcio similar à hidroxiapatita, bem como com quantidades substanciais do carbonato, citrato de sódio e magnésio; através do peso, o osso é composto de 75% de material

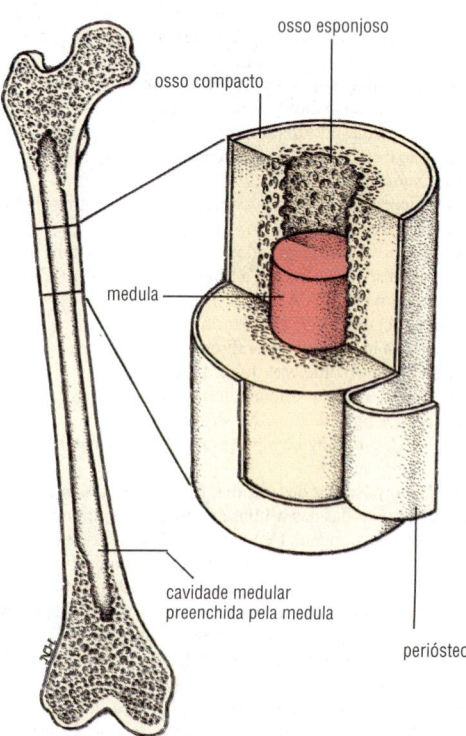

OSSO

inorgânico e 25% de material orgânico; parte do tecido ósseo de tamanho e formato definido, formando uma parte do esqueleto animal; em seres humanos, existem 200 ossos distintos no esqueleto, não incluindo os ossículos auditivos da cavidade timpânica ou os ossos sesamóides diferentes das duas patelas. O osso consiste em uma camada externa densa de substância compacta ou substância cortical coberta pelo periósteo e uma substância esponjosa frouxa interna; a porção central de um osso longo é preenchida com a medula. SIN os [TA]. [A.S. bān]

Albrecht b., osso de Albrecht; um pequeno o. entre o basioccipital e o basiesfenóide.
alveolar b., (1) Processo alveolar da maxila. SIN alveolar process of maxilla; (2) alvéolo dental; em odontologia, a estrutura óssea especializada que dá suporte aos dentes; consiste no o. cortical que compreende o alvéolo dentário, no qual as raízes do dente se adaptam, e é suportado pelo o. trabecular. SIN alveolar supporting b.
alveolar supporting b., alvéolo alveolar. SIN alveolar b. (2).
ankle b., tálus. SIN talus.
arm b., úmero. SIN humerus.
basal b., o. basal; o tecido ósseo da mandíbula e da maxila, excetuando-se os processos alveolares.
basilar b., o. basilar; o processo basilar em desenvolvimento do o. occipital que se une com as porções condilares em torno do quarto ou quinto ano, transformando-se na parte basilar do osso occipital. VER TAMBÉM basilar part of occipital bone. SIN basioccipital b., os basilare.
basioccipital b., o. basioccipital. SIN basilar b.
basisphenoid b., o. basiesfenóide; em anatomia comparada, o o. no assoalho da caixa craniana na região da hipófise. VER body of sphenoid.
Bertin b.'s, ossos de Bertin. SIN sphenoidal conchae, em concha.
blade b., escápula. SIN scapula.
breast b., esterno. SIN sternum.
Breschet b.'s, ossos de Breschet. SIN suprasternal b.'s.
brittle b.'s, osteogênese imperfeita. SIN osteogenesis imperfecta.
bundle b., o. fusiforme; o o. imaturo que contém feixes espessos de fibras de colágeno dispostos quase em paralelo entre si, com osteócitos de um tipo similar de o. é encontrado nas regiões penetradas pelas fibras de Sharpey, como nas inserções ligamentares e tendíneas.
calcaneal b., calcâneo. SIN calcaneus (1).
calf b., fíbula. SIN fíbula. [N. Antigo kalfi, fibula]
cancellous b., o. esponjoso. SIN substantia spongiosa.
capitate b., capitato. SIN capitate (1).
carpal b.'s [TA], ossos carpais; os oito ossos dispostos em duas fileiras que se articulam proximalmente com o rádio e indiretamente com a ulna e distalmente com os cinco ossos metacarpais; nos mamíferos domésticos, os ossos da fileira proximal são chamados radial, intermediário, ulnar e acessório, enquanto aqueles da fileira distal são denominados primeiro, segundo, terceiro e quarto ossos carpais. SIN carpus (2) [TA], ossa carpi [TA].
cartilage b., o. endocondral. SIN endochondral b.
central b., o. central. SIN os centrale.
central b. of ankle, navicular. SIN navicular.
cheek b., (1) osso zigomático. SIN zygomatic b.; (2) arco zigomático. SIN zygomatic arch.
coccygeal b., cóccix. SIN coccyx.
collar b., clavícula. SIN clavicle.
compact b. [TA], o. compacto; a porção compacta, não-esponjosa do o. que consiste, em grande parte, em osteons lamelares concêntricos e lamelas intersticiais. SIN substantia compacta [TA], compact substance, substantia compacta ossium.
convoluted b., concha. VER inferior nasal concha, middle nasal concha, superior nasal concha, supreme nasal concha.
cortical b. [TA], o. cortical; a camada fina superficial do osso compacto. SIN substantia corticalis [TA], cortical substance.
coxal b., osso do quadril; termo oficial alternativo* para hip b.
cranial b.'s, ossos do crânio. SIN b.'s of cranium.
b.'s of cranium [TA], ossos do crânio; os ossos pareados conchas nasais inferiores, lacrimais, maxilas, nasais, palatinos, parietais, temporais e zigomáticos; e os ossos não-pareados etmóide, frontal, occipital, esfenóide e vômer. SIN ossa cranii [TA], b.'s of skull, cranial b.'s.
cubital b., o. piramidal. SIN triquetrum.
cuboid (b.), o. cubóide; o o. lateral da fileira distal do tarso, que se articula com o calcâneo, cuneiforme lateral, navicular (ocasionalmente) e o quarto e quinto ossos metatarsais. SIN cuboideum.
cuneiform b., o. cuneiforme. VER triquetrum, intermediate cuneiform (b.), lateral cuneiform (b.), medial cuneiform (b.).
dermal b., o. dérmico; um o. formado pela ossificação da pele.
b.'s of digits, ossos dos dedos; as falanges e ossos sesamóides dos dedos das mãos e dos pés. SIN ossa digitorum*.
dorsal talonavicular b., o. talonavicular dorsal; o. anômalo do pé localizado próximo à cabeça do tálus. SIN Pirie b.

ear b.'s, ossículos da audição. SIN auditory ossicles, em ossicle.
elbow b., olécrano. SIN olecranon.
endochondral b., o. endocondral; o. que se desenvolve em ambiente cartilaginoso depois que o último é parcial ou totalmente destruído por calcificação e subseqüente reabsorção. SIN cartilage b., replacement b.
epactal b.'s, ossos suturais. SIN sutural b.'s.
epihyal b., o. epiial; um ligamento estilomastóideo ossificado.
epipteric c., o. epiptérico; um o. sutural ocasionalmente presente no ptérion ou junção dos ossos parietal, frontal, asa maior do esfenóide e porção escamosa do temporal. SIN Flower b.
episternal b., o. episternal. SIN suprasternal b.'s.
ethmoid b. [TA], o. etmóide; o. em formato irregular que se situa entre as placas orbitárias do frontal e anterior ao o. esfenóide; consiste em duas massas laterais de finas placas que englobam as células aéreas, fixadas acima até uma lâmina horizontal perfurada, a placa cribriforme, a partir da qual desce uma placa vertical mediana ou perpendicular no intervalo entre as duas massas laterais; o o. articula-se com os ossos esfenóide, frontal, maxila, lacrimal e palatino, concha nasal inferior e o vômer; entra na formação da fossa craniana anterior, das órbitas e da cavidade nasal.
exoccipital b. (eks-ok-sip'i-tăl), parte lateral do o. occipital. SIN lateral part of occipital bone.
facial b.'s, ossos da face; os ossos que circundam a boca e o nariz e contribuem para as órbitas; eles são os ossos pareados maxilas, zigomáticos, nasais, lacrimais, palatinos e conchas nasais inferiores e os ossos não-pareados etmóide, vômer, mandíbula e hióide. SIN b.'s of visceral cranium, ossa faciei.
first cuneiform b., o. cuneiforme medial. SIN medial cuneiform (b.)
flank b., SIN ilium.
flat b. [TA], o. plano; tipo de o. caracterizado por sua forma plana e achatada, como a escápula ou determinados ossos do crânio. SIN os planum [TA].
Flower b., o. de Flower. SIN epipteric b.
b.'s of foot [TA], ossos do pé; os ossos que coletivamente compreendem o esqueleto do pé; incluem os ossos tarsais, os ossos metatarsais [I-V], as falanges e os ossos sesamóides. SIN ossa pedis [TA], foot b.'s.
foot b.'s, ossos do pé. SIN b.'s of foot.
fourth turbinated b., concha nasal suprema. SIN supreme nasal concha.
frontal b. [TA], o. frontal; o grande osso único que forma a fronte e a margem superior e o teto da órbita em ambos os lados; articula-se com os ossos parietais, nasais, etmóide, maxilares e zigomáticos e com as asas menores do esfenóide. SIN os frontale [TA], coronale (1).
funny b., nome coloquial para a extremidade do olécrano.
Goethe b., o. de Goethe. SIN preinterparietal b.
greater multangular b., trapézio. SIN trapezium b.
hamate (b.) [TA], o. hamato; o o. no lado medial (ulnar) da fileira distal do carpo; articula-se com o quarto e o quinto metacarpais, piramidal, lunar e capitato. SIN hamatum, hooked b., os hamatum, unciform b., unciforme, uncinatum.
heel b., calcâneo. SIN calcaneus (1).
heterotopic b.'s, ossos heterotópicos; os ossos que não pertencem ao esqueleto principal, mas que regularmente se desenvolvem em determinados órgãos, p.ex., o coração, pênis, clítoris e a tromba de alguns animais.
highest turbinated b., concha nasal suprema. SIN supreme nasal concha.
hip b. [TA], osso do quadril; um grande osso plano formado pela fusão do ílio, ísquio e púbis (no adulto), constituindo a metade lateral da pelve; articula-se com seu companheiro anteriormente e com o fêmur lateralmente. SIN os coxae [TA], coxal b.*, pelvic b.*, innominate b., os innominatum.
hollow b., o. oco. SIN pneumatized b.
hooked b., hamato. SIN hamate (b.).
hyoid b., o. hióide; (1) um osso em forma de U que se situa entre a mandíbula e a laringe, suspenso dos processos estilóides pelos delicados ligamentos estilo-hióideos; (2) VER hyoid apparatus. SIN lingual b., os hyoideum, tongue b.
iliac b., SIN ilium.
incarial b., o. interparietal. SIN interparietal b.
incisive b. [TA], o. incisivo; a porção anterior e interna da maxila, que, no feto e por vezes no adulto, é um o. separado; a sutura incisiva corre desde o canal incisivo, entre o incisivo central e o canino; de acordo com K. Albrecht, o o. incisivo é dividido por uma sutura entre os dois dentes incisivos em cada lado em dois ossos, o endognático e o mesognático. SIN os incisivum [TA], premaxilla (1)*, intermaxilla, intermaxillary b., os intermaxillare, os premaxillare, premaxillary b.
b.'s of inferior limb, ossos do membro inferior. SIN b.'s of lower limb.
inferior turbinated b., concha nasal inferior. SIN inferior nasal concha.
innominate b., o. do quadril. SIN hip b.
intermaxillary b., o. intermaxilar. SIN incisive b.
intermediate cuneiform (b.) [TA], o. cuneiforme intermédio; um o. da fileira distal do tarso; articula-se com os cuneiformes medial e lateral, navicular e o segundo metatarsal. SIN mesocuneiform, middle cuneiform b., os cuneiforme intermedium, second cuneiform b., wedge b.

interparietal b. [TA], o. interparietal; a parte superior da escama do osso occipital, desenvolvida na membrana em vez de na cartilagem como acontece com o restante do occipital e, ocasionalmente (principalmente nos antigos crânios do Peru), existindo como um osso separado, destacado do restante do occipital pela sutura occipital transversa. SIN os interparietale [TA], incarial b., os incae.

irregular b. [TA], o. irregular; um de um grupo de ossos que possuem formas complexas ou peculiares, p.ex., vértebras, muitos dos ossos cranianos. SIN os irregulare [TA].

ischial b., ísquio. SIN ischium.

jaw b., mandíbula. SIN mandible.

jugal b., zigomático. SIN zygomatic b.

Krause b., o. de Krause; pequeno o. (centro de ossificação secundária) na cartilagem trirradiada entre o ílio, o ísquio e o púbis no acetábulo em crescimento.

lacrimal b. [TA], o. lacrimal; uma placa fina, irregularmente retangular, que forma parte da parede medial da órbita atrás do processo frontal da maxila; articula-se com a concha nasal inferior, etmóide, frontal e maxilar. SIN os lacrimale [TA], os unguis.

lamellar b., o. lamelar; o tipo normal de osso do mamífero adulto, quer esponjoso, quer compacto, composto de lamelas paralelas no primeiro e lamelas concêntricas no último; a organização lamelar reflete um padrão repetido de fibroarquitetura do colágeno.

lateral cuneiform (b.) [TA], o. cuneiforme lateral; um o. da fileira distal do tarso; articula-se com o cuneiforme intermédio, cuboide, navicular e o segundo, terceiro e quarto metatarsais. SIN os cuneiforme laterale [TA], third cuneiform b., wedge b.

lenticular b., processo lenticular da bigorna. SIN lenticular process of incus.

lentiform b., pisiforme. SIN pisiform (b.).

lesser multangular b., o. trapezóide. SIN trapezoid (b.).

lingual b., o. hióide. SIN hyoid b.

long b. [TA], osso longo; um dos ossos alongados dos membros, consistindo em uma haste tubular (diáfise) e duas extremidades (epífises), usualmente mais largas que a diáfise; a diáfise é composta de osso compacto que circunda uma cavidade medular central. Cf. short b. SIN os longum [TA], pipe b.

b.'s of lower limb [TA], ossos do membro inferior; esses incluem o cíngulo do membro inferior (o. do quadril) e o esqueleto do membro inferior livre (fêmur, tíbia, fíbula, patela, tarso, metatarso e ossos dos dedos dos pés). SIN ossa membri inferioris [TA], b.'s of inferior limb.

lunate (b.), osso semilunar; um da fileira proximal no carpo entre o escafóide e o piramidal; articula-se com o rádio, o escafóide, o piramidal, o hamato e o capitato. SIN os lunatum [TA], lunare, os intermedium.

malar b., o. zigomático. SIN zygomatic b.

marble b.'s, osteopetrose. SIN osteopetrosis.

mastoid b., processo mastóide. SIN mastoid process.

medial cuneiform (b.), o. cuneiforme medial; o maior dos três ossos cuneiformes, o o. medial da fileira distal do tarso, articulando-se com o cuneiforme intermediário, o navicular e o primeiro e segundo metatarsais. SIN os cuneiforme mediale [TA], first cuneiform b., wedge b.

membrane b., o. membranáceo; o. que se desenvolve embriologicamente dentro de uma membrana de tecido mesenquimatoso primitivo vascularizado sem a formação prévia de cartilagem.

mesethmoid b., o. mesetmóide; em anatomia comparada, o o. presente em algumas espécies como o o. mais anterior do assoalho da caixa craniana.

metacarpal (b.'s) [I-V] [TA], ossos metacarpais [I-V]; os cinco ossos longos (numerados de I a V, começando no o. no lado radial ou polegar), formando o esqueleto do metacarpo ou na região palmar; articulam-se com os ossos da fileira distal do carpo e com as cinco falanges proximais. SIN ossa metacarpi [TA], ossa metacarpalia I-V.

metatarsal (b.'s) [I-V], ossos metatarsais, os cinco ossos longos (numerados de I a V, começando com o osso no lado medial) que formam o esqueleto da porção anterior do pé, articulando-se posteriormente com os três ossos cuneiformes e o osso cuboide e anteriormente com as cinco falanges proximais. SIN ossa metatarsi [TA], ossa metatarsalia I-V.

middle cuneiform b., o. cuneiforme intermédio. SIN intermediate cuneiform (b.).

middle turbinated b., concha nasal média. SIN middle nasal concha.

multangular b., trapézio. VER trapezium, trapezoid (b.).

nasal b. [TA], o. nasal; um o. retangular alongado que, com seu companheiro, forma a ponte do nariz; articula-se com o osso frontal superiormente, o etmóide e o processo frontal da maxila posteriormente e seu companheiro medialmente. SIN os nasale [TA].

navicular (b.), o. navicular. SIN navicular.

navicular b. of hand, o. escafóide. SIN scaphoid (b.).

nonlamellar b., o. não-lamelar. SIN woven b.

occipital b. [TA], o. occipital; um osso na parte inferior e posterior do crânio, consistindo em três partes (basilar, condilar e escamosa), englobando um grande orifício oval, o forame magno; articula-se com os ossos parietal e temporal em ambos os lados, com o esfenóide anteriormente e com o atlas abaixo. SIN os occipitale [TA].

orbicular b., processo lenticular da bigorna. SIN lenticular process of incus.

palatine b. [TA], o. palatino; osso de formato irregular posterior à maxila, que entra na formação da cavidade nasal, da órbita e do palato duro; articula-se com os ossos maxilares, a concha nasal inferior, o esfenóide e o etmóide, o vômer e seu companheiro do lado oposto. SIN os palatinum [TA].

parietal b. [TA], o. parietal; osso plano, curvado, de formato quadrangular irregular, em ambos os lados da calota do crânio; articula-se com seu companheiro medialmente, com o frontal anteriormente, com o occipital posteriormente e com o temporal e o esfenóide inferiormente. SIN os parietale [TA].

pelvic b., o. do quadril; termo oficial alternativo* do hip b.

perichondral b., o. pericondral; no desenvolvimento de um o. longo, um colar ou manguito de tecido ósseo se forma no pericôndrio do modelo cartilaginoso; a membrana de tecido conjuntivo desse o. pericondral, que, em seguida, se transforma no periósteo. SIN periosteal b.

periosteal b., o. pericondral. SIN perichondral b.

periotic b., parte petrosa do osso temporal. SIN petrous part of temporal bone.

peroneal b., fíbula. SIN fibula.

petrosal b., parte petrosa do osso temporal. SIN petrous part of temporal bone.

petrous b., parte petrosa da artéria carótida interna. SIN petrous part of internal carotid artery.

ping-pong b., o. pingue-pongue; a fina concha de tecido ósseo na periferia de um tumor de células gigantes em um o.

pipe b., o. longo. SIN long b.

Pirie b., o. de Pirie. SIN dorsal talonavicular b.

pisiform (b.), o. pisiforme; um pequeno osso que se assemelha a uma ervilha em tamanho e formato, na fileira proximal do carpo, situando-se sobre a superfície anterior do piramidal, com o qual se articula; fornece a inserção para o tendão do músculo flexor ulnar do carpo. SIN os pisiforme [TA], lentiform b.

pneumatic b., o. pneumático. SIN pneumatized b.

pneumatized b. [TA], o. pneumático; um o. que é oco ou que contém muitas células aéreas, como o processo mastóideo do osso temporal. SIN os pneumaticum [TA], hollow b., pneumatic b.

postsphenoid b., o. pós-esfenóide; a porção posterior do corpo do o. esfenóide.

preinterparietal b., o. pré-interparietal; grande o. sutural ocasionalmente encontrado destacado da porção anterior do osso interparietal. SIN Goethe b.

premaxillary b., o. incisivo. SIN incisive b.

presphenoid b., o. pré-esfenóide; na anatomia comparada, o o. no assoalho da caixa craniana anterior ao o. basiesfenóide.

pubic b., monte do púbis. SIN mons pubis.

pyramidal b., o. piramidal. SIN triquetrum.

replacement b., o. endocondral. SIN endochondral b.

reticulated b., o. reticulado. SIN woven b.

rider's b., o. dos cavaleiros ou de exercício; ossificação heterotópica do tendão do músculo adutor longo a partir da pressão ao montar a cavalo.

Riolan b.'s, ossos de Riolan; vários pequenos ossos suturais por vezes existentes na sutura petro-occipital.

sacred b., o. sacro. SIN sacrum. [assim chamado a partir da crença na indestrutibilidade do osso como a base para a ressurreição]

scaphoid (b.), o. escafóide; o maior o. da fileira proximal do carpo no lado lateral (radial), articulando-se com o rádio, o semilunar, o capitato, o trapézio e o trapezóide. SIN os scaphoideum [TA], navicular b. of hand, os naviculare manus.

scroll b.'s, concha. VER inferior nasal concha, middle nasal concha, superior nasal concha, supreme nasal concha.

second cuneiform b., cuneiforme intermédio. SIN intermediate cuneiform (b.).

semilunar b., o. semilunar; termo obsoleto para lunate (b.)

septal b., septo interalveolar. SIN interalveolar septum.

sesamoid b. [TA], o. sesamóide; um osso formado depois do nascimento em um tendão onde ele passa por cima de uma articulação, p.ex., a patela. SIN os sesamoideum [TA].

shin b., tíbia. SIN tibia.

short b. [TA], o. curto; aquele cujas dimensões são aproximadamente iguais; consiste em uma camada de substância cortical englobando a substância esponjosa e a medula. Cf. long b. SIN os breve [TA].

b. sialoprotein 1, sialoproteína 1 óssea. SIN osteopontin.

sieve b., lâmina cribriforme do osso etmóide. SIN cribriform plate of ethmoid bone.

b.'s of skull, ossos do crânio. SIN b.'s of cranium.

sphenoid (b.), o. esfenóide; um o. de formato mais irregular que ocupa a base do crânio; é descrito como consistindo em uma porção central, ou corpo, e seis processos: duas asas maiores, duas asas menores e dois processos pterigóides; articula-se com o occipital, o frontal, o etmóide e o vômer, e com os ossos pareados temporais, parietais, zigomáticos, palatinos e conchas esfenoidais. SIN os sphenoidale [TA], sphenoid (2) [TA].

sphenoidal turbinated b.'s, conchas esfenoidais. SIN sphenoidal conchae, em concha.

spongy b. [TA], o. esponjoso. **(1)** SIN substantia spongiosa; **(2)** um osso turbinado.

b.'s of superior limb, ossos do membro superior. SIN b.'s of upper limb.
superior turbinated b., concha nasal superior. SIN superior nasal *concha*.
suprainterparietal b., o. supra-interparietal; um o. sutural na porção posterior da sutura sagital.
suprasternal b.'s [TA], o. supra-esternal; um dos pequenos ossículos ocasionalmente encontrados nos ligamentos da articulação esternoclavicular. SIN ossa suprasternalia [TA], Breschet b.'s, episternal b.
supreme turbinated b., concha nasal suprema. SIN supreme nasal *concha*.
sutural b.'s [TA], ossos suturais; pequenos ossos irregulares encontrados ao longo das suturas do crânio, principalmente relacionados ao o. parietal. SIN os suturarum [TA], Andernach ossicles, epactal b.'s, epactal ossicles, wormian b.'s.
tail b., cóccix. SIN coccyx.
tarsal b.'s [TA], ossos tarsais; os sete ossos do pé: os ossos tálus, calcâneo, navicular, três cuneiformes e cubóide. SIN ossa tarsi [TA], tarsale [TA], ossa tarsalia*.
temporal b. [TA], o. temporal; um grande o. irregular situado na base e no lado do crânio; consiste em três partes, escamosa, timpânica e petrosa, que estão distintas ao nascimento; a parte petrosa contém o órgão vestibulococlear; o o. articula-se com os ossos esfenóide, parietal, occipital e zigomático, e, através de uma articulação sinovial, com a mandíbula. SIN os temporale [TA].
thigh b., fêmur; termo oficial alternativo* para thigh.
third cuneiform b., cuneiforme lateral. SIN lateral cuneiform (b.).
three-cornered b., o. piramidal. SIN triquetrum.
tongue b., o. hióide. SIN hyoid b.
trabecular b., o. trabecular; termo oficial alternativo* para a *substantia spongiosa*.
trapezium b., o. trapézio; o o. lateral (radial) na fileira distal do carpo; articula-se com o primeiro e segundo metacarpais e os ossos escafóide e trapezóide. SIN greater multangular b., os multangulum majus, os trapezium, trapezium (2).
trapezoid (b.), o. trapezóide; um o. na fileira distal do carpo; articula-se com o segundo metacarpal, o trapézio, o capitato e o escafóide. SIN os trapezoideum [TA], trapezoid (3) [TA], lesser multangular b., os multangulum minus.
triangular b., o. trígono. SIN *os trigonum*.
triquetrum b., o. piramidal. SIN triquetrum.
turbinated b.'s, concha. VER inferior nasal *concha*, middle nasal *concha*, superior nasal *concha*, supreme nasal *concha*.
tympanic b., anel timpânico. SIN tympanic *ring*.
tympanohyal b., o. timpano-hióide; um pequeno nódulo de o. que forma a base do processo estilóide cartilaginoso do o. temporal ao nascimento.
unciform b., hamato. SIN hamate (b.).
upper jaw b., maxila. SIN maxilla.
b.'s of upper limb [TA], ossos do membro superior; esses incluem o cíngulo do membro superior (escápula e clavícula) e o esqueleto do membro superior livre (úmero, rádio, ulna, ossos do punho, metacarpo e ossos dos dedos). SIN ossa membri superioris [TA], b.'s of superior limb.
Vesalius b., o. de Vesalius. SIN *os vesalianum*.
b.'s of visceral cranium, ossos do crânio visceral. SIN facial b.'s.
wedge b., o. cuneiforme. SIN intermediate cuneiform (b.), lateral cuneiform (b.), medial cuneiform (b.).
wormian b.'s, ossos suturais. SIN sutural b.'s.
woven b., o. reticulado; o tecido ósseo característico do esqueleto embrionário, em que as fibras de colágeno da matriz estão dispostas irregularmente na forma de redes entrelaçadas. SIN nonlamellar b., reticulated b.
yoke b., o. zigomático. SIN zygomatic b.
zygomatic b. [TA], o. zigomático; um o. em forma de quadrilátero que modela a proeminência da bochecha; articula-se com os ossos frontal, esfenóide, temporal e maxilar. SIN os zygomaticum [TA], cheek b. (1), jugal b., mala (2), malar b., os malare, yoke b., zygoma (1).

bone ar·chi·tec·ture. Arquitetura óssea; o padrão de trabéculas e estruturas associadas. VER TAMBÉM Wolff *law*.
bone ash. Fosfato tribásico de cálcio. SIN tribasic calcium phosphate.
bone black. Carvão animal. SIN animal *charcoal*.
bone·let (bŏn'let). Ossículo. SIN ossicle.
bone-salt. Sal ósseo; o principal composto químico no osso, depositado como pequenos cristais amorfos em uma matriz de fibras colagenosas, reticuladas, contendo colágeno; assemelha-se muito à fluoroapatita de ocorrência natural $3Ca_3(PO_4)_2 \cdot CaF_2$, mas é provavelmente uma hidroxiapatita, na qual o F é substituído por OH.
Bonhoeffer, Karl, psiquiatra alemão, 1868–1948. VER B. *sign*.
Bonnet, Amédée, cirurgião francês, 1802–1858. VER B. *capsule*.
Bonnevie, Kristine, médica alemã, 1872–1950.
Bonnier, Pierre, médico francês, 1861–1918. VER B. *syndrome*.
Bonwill, William G. A., odontólogo norte-americano, 1833–1899. VER B. *triangle*.
Böök, Jan A., geneticista sueco, *1915. VER B. *syndrome*.

BOOP Abreviatura de *bronchiolitis* obliterans with organizing pneumonia (bronquiolite obliterante com pneumonia em organização), uma forma idiopática de bronquiolite obliterante.
boost·er. Reforço. VER booster *dose*.
boot (boot). Bota; um dispositivo em formato de bota. [Ing. M. *bote*, do Fr. Ant.] **Gibney b.,** b. de Gibney; tratamento com fita adesiva de um entorse de tornozelo ou condição similar, aplicado da forma de trança de cesta sob a região plantar do pé e ao redor da parte posterior da perna.
bo·rac·ic ac·id (bō-ras'ik). Ácido bórico. SIN boric acid.
bo·rate (bōr'āt). Borato; um sal do ácido bórico.
bo·rat·ed (bōr'āt - ed). Boratado; misturado ou impregnado com bórax ou ácido bórico.
bo·rax (bō'raks). Bórax. SIN *sodium borate*. [Pers. *būraq*]
bor·bo·ryg·mus, pl. **bor·bo·ryg·mi** ((bōr - bō - rig'mus, - rig'mī). Borborigmo; ruído de gargarejo ou ruflar produzido pelo movimento de gás, líquido ou de ambos no canal alimentar, e audível a uma distância. [G. *borborygmos*, ruídos nos intestinos]
Bordeau (Bordeu), Théophile de, médico francês, 1722–1776.
bor·der (bōr'der) [TA]. Margem; a parte de uma superfície que forma seu limite externo. VER TAMBÉM edge, margin, border. SIN margo [TA].
alveolar b., (1) a borda mais oclusal do osso alveolar; **(2)** SIN alveolar *process* of maxilla.
anterior b. [TA], m. anterior; a margem ventral ou mais anterior de uma estrutura. SIN margo anterior [TA], anterior margin, ventral b.
anterior b. of body of pancreas [TA], m. anterior do corpo do pâncreas; a borda afilada entre as superfícies anterior e inferior do pâncreas. SIN margo anterior corporis pancreatis [TA], anterior b. of pancreas, margo anterior pancreatis.
anterior b. of eyelids, m. anterior das pálpebras. SIN anterior palpebral *margin*.
anterior b. of fibula [TA], m. anterior da fíbula; crista na diáfise da fíbula na qual se insere o septo intermuscular anterior da perna. SIN margo anterior fibulae [TA].
anterior b. of lung [TA], m. anterior do pulmão; uma borda ântero-medial ou esternal fina do pulmão que se sobrepõe ao saco pericárdico anteriormente e forma o limite entre as superfícies mediastinal e costal. SIN margo anterior pulmonis [TA].
anterior b. of pancreas, m. anterior do pâncreas. SIN anterior b. of body of pancreas.
anterior b. of radius [TA], m. anterior do rádio; a crista na diáfise do rádio estendendo-se desde a tuberosidade radial até a parte anterior do processo estilóide. SIN margo anterior radii [TA].
anterior b. of testis [TA], m. anterior do testículo; linha convexa imaginária que demarca as superfícies lateral e medial. SIN margo anterior testis [TA].
anterior b. of tibia [TA], m. anterior da tíbia; a crista subcutânea afiada da tíbia que se estende desde a tuberosidade até a parte anterior do maléolo medial. SIN margo anterior tibiae [TA], anticnemion, shin, tibial crest.
anterior b. of ulna [TA], m. anterior da ulna; a crista no corpo da ulna que se estende desde a tuberosidade até a parte anterior do processo estilóide. SIN margo anterior ulnae [TA].
brush b., b. em escova; a superfície epitelial apical que apresenta microvilosidades intimamente acondicionadas com cerca de 2 μm de comprimento, como a que ocorre nas células do túbulo proximal do néfron. SIN limbus penicillatus.
ciliary b. of iris, m. ciliar da íris. SIN ciliary *margin* of iris.
denture b., (1) o limite ou margem circunferencial de uma base dentária; **(2)** a margem da base dentária na junção da superfície polida com a superfície de impressão (tecidual); **(3)** as bordas extremas de uma base dentária nos limites bucolabial, lingual e posterior. SIN denture edge, periphery (2).
b.'s of eyelids, margens das pálpebras. SIN palpebral *margins*, em *margin*.
fibular (peroneal) b. of foot, m. fibular do pé; termo oficial alternativo* para lateral b. of foot.
free b. [TA], m. livre; a borda sem inserção de uma estrutura, freqüentemente oposta à borda inserida. VER free b. of nail, free b. of ovary. SIN margo liber [TA], free margin.
free b. of nail [TA], m. livre da unha; a m. distal da unha que se projeta na extremidade do dedo. SIN margo liber unguis [TA].
free b. of ovary [TA], m. livre do ovário; a margem posterior livre do ovário. SIN margo liber ovarii [TA].
frontal b. [TA], m. frontal; a borda de um osso que se articula com o osso frontal. VER frontal b. of parietal bone, frontal *margin* of sphenoid. SIN margo frontalis [TA], frontal margin.
frontal b. of parietal bone [TA], m. frontal do osso parietal; a margem do osso parietal que se articula com o osso frontal. SIN margo frontalis ossis parietalis [TA].
frontal b. of sphenoid bone, m. frontal do osso esfenóide. SIN frontal *margin* of sphenoid.
hidden b. of nail [TA], m. oculta da unha; a m. proximal da unha totalmente encoberta pela parede da unha. SIN margo occultus unguis [TA], occult b. of nail, proximal b. of nail.

inferior b. [TA], m. inferior; a margem caudal ou mais inferior de uma estrutura. SIN margo inferior [TA], inferior margin.
inferior b. of body of pancreas [TA], m. inferior do corpo do pâncreas; a b. do pâncreas que separa as superfícies inferior e posterior. SIN margo inferior corporis pancreatis [TA], inferior b. of pancreas, margo inferior corporis splenis, margo inferior pancreatis.
inferior b. of liver [TA], m. inferior do fígado; a borda afilada do fígado que separa as superfícies diafragmática e visceral. SIN margo inferior hepatis [TA].
inferior b. of lung [TA], m. inferior do pulmão; a m. afilada do pulmão que separa a superfície diafragmática das superfícies costal e mediastinal. SIN margo inferior pulmonis [TA].
inferior b. of pancreas, m. inferior do pâncreas. SIN inferior b. of body of pancreas.
inferior b. of spleen [TA], m. inferior do baço; a m. mais inferior do baço, que separa a superfície visceral inferior (área da impressão renal) a partir da superfície diafragmática inferior. SIN margo inferior splenis [TA].
inner b. of iris [TA], m. interna da íris; a zona interna estreita da íris. SIN anulus iridis minor [TA], lesser ring of iris.
interosseous b. [TA], m. interóssea; a borda de um osso na qual se insere uma membrana fibrosa (interóssea), na qual o osso se insere em outro osso. VER interosseous b. of fibula, interosseous b. of radius, interosseous b. of tibia, interosseous b. of ulna. SIN margo interosseus [TA], interosseous crest, interosseous margin.
interosseous b. of fibula [TA], m. interóssea da fíbula; a crista ao longo da m. medial da fíbula na qual se insere a membrana interóssea. SIN margo interosseus fibulae [TA].
interosseous b. of radius [TA], m. interóssea do rádio; a crista ao longo do lado medial do rádio na qual se insere a membrana interóssea. SIN margo interosseus radii [TA].
interosseous b. of tibia [TA], m. interóssea da tíbia ao longo da m. lateral da tíbia à qual se insere a membrana interóssea. SIN margo interosseus tibiae [TA].
interosseous b. of ulna [TA], m. interóssea da ulna; a crista ao longo do lado lateral do corpo da ulna na qual se insere a membrana interóssea. SIN margo interosseus ulnae [TA].
b. of iris [TA], m. da íris; qualquer uma das duas zonas na superfície anterior da íris, separada por uma linha circular concêntrica com a m. pupilar. SIN anulus iridis [TA], ring of iris.
lacrimal b. of maxilla, m. lacrimal da maxila. SIN lacrimal margin of maxilla.
lambdoid b. of occipital bone [TA], m. lambdóidea do osso occipital; a margem da escama do occipital que se articula com os ossos parietais na sutura lambdóidea. SIN margo lambdoideus ossis occipitalis [TA], lambdoid margin of occipital bone, margo lambdoideus squamae occipitalis.
lateral b. [TA], m. lateral; a m. ou borda de uma estrutura que está mais afastada da linha média. SIN margo lateralis [TA], lateral margin.
lateral b. of foot [TA], m. lateral do pé; a m. do pé entre o pequeno artelho e o calcanhar. SIN margo lateralis pedis [TA], fibular (peroneal) b. of foot*, margo fibularis pedis*, peroneal b. of foot*, fibular margin of foot.
lateral b. of forearm, m. lateral do antebraço; termo oficial alternativo* para radial b. of forearm.
lateral b. of humerus [TA], m. lateral do úmero; a crista no úmero que se estende desde o tubérculo maior até o epicôndilo lateral. SIN margo lateralis humeri [TA].
lateral b. of kidney [TA], m. lateral do rim; a borda estreita convexa que separa as superfícies anterior e posterior. SIN margo lateralis renis [TA].
lateral b. of nail [TA], m. lateral da unha; os lados da unha que se estendem desde a borda proximal até as bordas livres. SIN margo lateralis unguis [TA].
lateral b. of scapula [TA], m. lateral da escápula; a borda da escápula que se estende desde a fossa glenóide até o ângulo inferior. SIN margo lateralis scapulae [TA].
mastoid b. of occipital bone [TA], m. mastóide do osso occipital; a margem da escama occipital que se articula com o osso temporal. SIN margo mastoideus ossis occipitalis [TA], margo mastoideus squamae occipitalis, mastoid margin of occipital bone.
medial b. [TA], m. medial; a m. de uma estrutura mais próxima ao plano medial. SIN margo medialis [TA], medial margin.
medial b. of foot [TA], m. medial do pé; a m. interna do pé que se estende desde o calcanhar até o hálux. SIN margo medialis pedis [TA], margo tibialis pedis*, tibial b. of foot*.
medial b. of forearm, m. medial do antebraço; termo oficial alternativo* para ulnar b. of forearm.
medial b. of humerus [TA], m. medial do úmero; a crista no úmero que se estende desde a crista do tubérculo menor até o epicôndilo medial. SIN margo medialis humeri [TA].
medial b. of kidney [TA], m. medial do rim; a m. côncava do rim. SIN margo medialis renis [TA].
medial b. of scapula [TA], m. medial da escápula; a borda da escápula mais próxima à coluna vertebral, estendendo-se desde o ângulo superior até o ângulo inferior. SIN margo medialis scapulae [TA], vertebral b. of scapula.

medial b. of suprarenal gland [TA], m. medial da glândula supra-renal; a borda paravertebral da glândula supra-renal. SIN margo medialis glandulae suprarenalis [TA].
medial b. of tibia [TA], m. medial da tíbia; a m. arredondada da tíbia que separa as superfícies posterior e medial. SIN margo medialis tibiae [TA].
mesovarian b. of ovary [TA], m. mesovárica do ovário; a m. do ovário na qual se insere o mesovário. SIN margo mesovaricus ovarii, mesovarian margin of ovary.
nasal b. of frontal bone, m. nasal do osso frontal. SIN nasal margin of frontal bone.
occipital b. [TA], m. occipital; a borda de um osso que se articula com o osso occipital. VER occipital b. of parietal bone, occipital margin of temporal bone. SIN margo occipitalis [TA], occipital margin.
occipital b. of parietal bone [TA], m. occipital do osso parietal; a m. posterior do osso parietal que se articula com a escama occipital. SIN margo occipitalis ossis parietalis [TA].
occipital b. of temporal bone, m. occipital do osso temporal. SIN occipital margin of temporal bone.
occult b. of nail, m. oculta da unha. SIN hidden b. of nail.
outer b. of iris [TA], m. externa da íris; a mais externa e mais larga das duas zonas da íris. SIN anulus iridis major [TA], greater ring of iris.
parietal b. [TA], m. parietal; a borda de um osso que se articula com o osso parietal. VER parietal margin of frontal bone, parietal margin of greater wing of sphenoid, parietal b. of squamous part of temporal bone. SIN margo parietalis [TA], parietal margin.
parietal b. of frontal bone, m. parietal do osso frontal. SIN parietal margin of frontal bone.
parietal b. of sphenoid bone, m. parietal do osso esfenóide. SIN parietal margin of greater wing of sphenoid.
parietal b. of squamous part of temporal bone [TA], m. parietal da parte escamosa do osso temporal; a m. da parte escamosa do osso temporal que se articula com o osso parietal. SIN margo parietalis partis squamosae ossis temporalis [TA], margo parietalis ossis temporalis, parietal b. of temporal bone.
parietal b. of temporal bone, m. parietal do osso temporal. SIN parietal b. of squamous part of temporal bone.
peroneal b. of foot, m. lateral do pé; termo oficial alternativo* para lateral b. of foot.
posterior b. of eyelids, m. posterior das pálpebras. SIN posterior palpebral margin.
posterior b. of fibula [TA], m. posterior da fíbula; a crista na face posterior da fíbula que se estende da cabeça da face medial do sulco fibular. SIN margo posterior fibulae [TA].
posterior b. of petrous part of temporal bone [TA], m. posterior da porção petrosa do osso temporal; a margem da porção petrosa do osso temporal que se estende desde o ápice até a incisura jugular; articula-se com as porções basal e jugular do osso occipital. SIN margo posterior partis petrosae ossis temporalis [TA].
posterior b. of radius [TA], m. posterior do rádio; a crista no rádio que se estende desde a tuberosidade até o tubérculo na face posterior da extremidade distal. SIN margo posterior radii [TA].
posterior b. of testis [TA], m. posterior do testículo; a porção posterior arredondada do testículo na qual penetram os vasos. SIN margo posterior testis [TA].
posterior b. of ulna [TA], m. posterior da ulna; a crista subcutânea sinuosa palpável na face posterior da ulna que se estende desde próximo ao olecrânio até o processo estilóide, demarcando os compartimentos "anterior" (flexor) do "posterior" (extensor) do antebraço. SIN margo posterior ulnae [TA].
proximal b. of nail, m. proximal da unha. SIN hidden b. of nail.
pupillary b. of iris, m. pupilar da íris. SIN pupillary margin of iris.
radial b. of forearm [TA], m. radial do antebraço; uma linha imaginária que corre ao longo da extensão mais externa do antebraço, separando as superfícies anterior e posterior lateralmente. SIN margo radialis antebrachii [TA], lateral b. of forearm*, margo lateralis antebrachii*.
right b. of heart [TA], m. direita do coração; a m. entre as superfícies esternocostal e diafragmática do coração; é muito bem definida em corações fixados, porém é arredondada e indefinida no coração vivo. SIN margo dexter cordis [TA], right margin of heart.
sagittal b. of parietal bone [TA], m. sagital do osso parietal; a borda medial do osso parietal que entra na sutura sagital. SIN margo sagittalis ossis parietalis [TA].
sphenoidal b. of temporal bone, m. esfenoidal do osso temporal. SIN sphenoidal margin of temporal bone.
squamosal b. [TA], m. escamosa; borda de um osso que se articula com a parte escamosa do osso temporal. SIN margo squamosus [TA], squamous b., squamous margin.
squamosal b. of parietal bone [TA], m. escamosa do osso parietal; a m. lateral do osso parietal que se articula com a parte escamosa do osso temporal. SIN margo squamosus ossis parietalis [TA], squamous b. of parietal bone.
squamous b., m. escamosa. SIN squamosal b. VER squamosal b. of parietal bone, squamosal margin of greater wing of sphenoid.
squamous b. of parietal bone, m. escamosa do osso parietal. SIN squamosal b. of parietal bone.

squamous b. of sphenoid bone, m. escamosa do osso esfenóide. SIN squamosal margin of greater wing of sphenoid.
striated b., m. estriada; a superfície livre das células colunares absortivas do intestino formadas por microvilosidades intimamente acondicionadas, com cerca de 1 μm de comprimento, dando o aspecto de estriações paralelas. SIN limbus striatus.
superior b., m. superior; a margem craniana ou mais superior de uma estrutura.
superior b. of body of pancreas [TA], m. superior do corpo do pâncreas; a m. mais superior do corpo do pâncreas que separa as superfícies anterior e posterior. SIN margo superior corporis pancreatis [TA], margo superior pancreatis, superior b. of pancreas.
superior b. of pancreas, m. superior do pâncreas. SIN superior b. of body of pancreas.
superior b. of petrous part of temporal bone [TA], m. superior da porção petrosa do osso temporal; a m. que separa as superfícies anterior e posterior da porção petrosa do osso temporal e a parte lateral da fossa craniana média a partir da fossa craniana posterior. SIN margo superior partis petrosae ossis temporalis [TA], crest of petrous part of temporal bone, crest of petrous temporal bone.
superior b. of scapula [TA], m. superior da escápula; a m. da escápula que se estende desde a fossa glenóide até o ângulo superior. SIN margo superior scapulae [TA].
superior b. of spleen [TA], m. superior do baço; a m. esplênica com incisura que separa as superfícies visceral (gástrica) e diafragmática. SIN margo superior splenis [TA].
superior b. of suprarenal gland [TA], m. superior da glândula supra-renal; a m. da glândula supra-renal na junção superior das superfícies anterior e posterior. SIN margo superior glandulae suprarenalis [TA].
tibial b. of foot, m. medial do pé; termo oficial alternativo* para medial b. of foot.
ulnar b. of forearm [TA], m. ulnar do antebraço; uma linha imaginária extrapolada desde o epicôndilo medial do úmero até o processo estilóide da ulna, formando uma m. entre as superfícies anterior e posterior. SIN margo ulnaris antebrachii [TA], margo medialis antebrachii*, medial b. of forearm*, ulnar margin of forearm.
b. of uterus [TA], m. do útero; a margem direita ou esquerda do útero ao longo da qual se insere o ligamento largo. A tuba uterina e o ligamento redondo se inserem no útero na parte superior da borda. SIN margo uteri [TA].
ventral b., m. ventral. SIN anterior b.
vermilion b., m. vermelha; a margem vermelha do lábio superior e inferior que começa na borda exterior da mucosa labial intra-oral ("linha úmida") e se estende para fora, terminando na junção cutânea labial extra-oral; tipo finamente queratinizado do epitélio escamoso estratificado perfurado profundamente por papilas dérmicas, as quais conferem, através da epiderme translúcida, o típico aspecto avermelhado dos lábios. SIN vermilion zone, vermilion transitional zone.
vertebral b. of scapula, m. medial da escápula. SIN medial b. of scapula.
zygomatic b. of greater wing of sphenoid bone, m. zigomática da asa maior do osso esfenóide. SIN zygomatic margin of greater wing of sphenoid bone.
Bordet, Jules, bacteriologista belga e laureado com o Prêmio Nobel, 1870–1961. VER *Bordetella*; B.-Gengou potato blood *agar, bacillus, phenomenon*; B. and Gengou *reaction*.
Bor·de·tel·la (bōr-dĕ-tel′ă). Gênero de bactérias estritamente aeróbicas (família Brucellaceae) contendo pequenos cocobacilos Gram-negativos, não-formadores de esporos. Existem espécies móveis e imóveis; as células móveis são peritríquias. O metabolismo desses microrganismos é respiratório. Eles exigem ácido nicotínico, cisteína e metionina; hemina (fator X) e coenzima I (fator V) não são necessárias. Eles são parasitas e patógenos do trato respiratório dos mamíferos; a espécie típica é *B. pertussis*. [J. *Bordet*]
B. bronchiseptica, espécie bacteriana encontrada em uma ampla faixa de espécies animais, causando rinite atrófica de suínos, broncopneumonia em roedores e broncopneumonia altamente contagiosa em cães. É uma causa rara de infecção oportunista do trato respiratório em pacientes imunocomprometidos.
B. hinzii, espécie bacteriana recentemente descrita, isolada de algumas hemoculturas e secreções respiratórias de seres humanos, bem como de secreções respiratórias de aves.
B. holmesii, espécie bacteriana recentemente descrita isolada de hemoculturas de humanos, principalmente de pacientes imunocomprometidos.
B. parapertus'sis, espécie bacteriana que causa uma doença semelhante à coqueluche, geralmente mais branda que aquela observada com a *B. pertussis*.
B. pertus'sis, a espécie bacteriana que é o agente causal da coqueluche, uma infecção do trato respiratório que, em lactentes e crianças pequenas, é potencialmente fatal; a tosse intensa, progredindo para uma forma paroxística depois de 7-10 dias, está associada à produção da toxina da coqueluche, uma proteína que consiste em 5 subunidades B que ligam a molécula às células epiteliais respiratórias, e uma subunidade A, uma ADP-ribosil-transferase que interfere com as proteínas associadas com a transdução do sinal normal; a patologia também está associada a secreção mucosa intensa e a hipóxia decorrente da tosse paroxística e do bloqueio das passagens aéreas com muco. SIN Bordet-Gengou bacillus.

bo·ric ac·id (bō′rik). Ácido bórico; ácido muito fraco, usado como talco anti-séptico, em solução saturada como um colírio, e com glicerina nas aftas e na estomatite. SIN boracic acid.
bor·ism (bōr′izm). Borismo; sinais e sintomas causados pela ingestão de bórax ou de qualquer composto de boro.
Börjeson, Mats, médico sueco, *1922. VER B.-Forssman-Lehmann *syndrome*.
Born, Gustav Jacob, embriologista alemão, 1851–1900. VER B. *method* of wax plate reconstruction.
bor·nane (bōr′năn). Bornano; o monoterpeno de origem dos borneóis, canfeno e óleos essenciais similares (terpenos).
bo·ro·glyc·er·in (bō-rō-glis′er-in). Boroglicerina; massa macia obtida por aquecimento de glicerina e ácido bórico; um anti-séptico, comumente usado misturado em partes iguais de glicerina, constituindo a glicerita. SIN boroglycerol, glyceryl borate.
bo·ro·glyc·er·ol (bō-rō-glis′er-ol). Boroglicerol. SIN boroglycerin.
bo·ron (B) (bōr′on). Boro; elemento não-metálico trivalente, número atômico 5, peso atômico 10,811; ocorre como uma massa cristalina dura ou como um pó acastanhado, e forma boratos e ácido bórico. Uma necessidade nutricional foi reportada para as gestantes. [Pers. *Burah*].
Borrel, Amédée, bacteriologista francês, 1867–1936. VER B. blue *stain*.
Bor·rel·ia (bō-rē′lē-ă, bo-rel′ē-ă). Gênero de bactérias (família Treponemataceae) contendo células de 8 a 16 μm de comprimento, com espirais grosseiras, superficiais e irregulares e extremidades finas que se afilam progressivamente. Esses microrganismos são parasitas em muitas formas da vida animal, geralmente são hematofíticos, ou são encontrados nas mucosas; a maioria é transmitida para os animais ou seres humanos por picadas de artrópodes. A espécie típica é *B. anserina*. [A. *Borrell*]
B. afzelii, genoespécie bacteriana da *Borrelia burgdorferi sensu lato* que causa a doença de Lyme na Europa e na Ásia; transmitida pelo carrapato *Ixodes ricinus* na Europa central e ocidental e pelo carrapato *Ixodes persulcatus* na Eurásia a partir do Mar Báltico até o Oceano Pacífico. VER TAMBÉM *B. burgdorferi sensu stricto*.
B. anseri'na, espécie bacteriana que causa a espiroquetose em aves domésticas; encontrada no sangue de gansos, patos, outras aves e nos carrapatos vetores; é a espécie típica do gênero *B*.
B. burgdor'feri, espécie bacteriana que causa a doença de Lyme em seres humanos e a borreliose em cães, gado e, possivelmente, cavalos. O vetor transmissor desse espiroqueta para seres humanos é o carrapato ixodídeo, *Ixodes dammini*.
B. burgdorferi sensu lato, um complexo bacteriano causando a doença de Lyme, que é composta de várias genoespécies, incluindo *Borrelia burgdorferi sensu stricto*, *Borrelia garinii* e *Borrelia afzelii*.
B. burgdorferi sensu stricto, genoespécie bacteriana da *Borrelia burgdorferi sensu lato* que causa a doença de Lyme na América do Norte e na Europa; transmitida pelo carrapato *Ixodes scapularis* nas regiões leste e central dos Estados Unidos, pelo carrapato *Ixodes pacificus* no oeste dos Estados Unidos, e pelo carrapato *Ixodes ricinus* na Europa. VER TAMBÉM *B. garinii*.
B. cauca'sica, espécie bacteriana encontrada como uma causa de febre recidivante no Cáucaso; transmitido por *Ornithodoros verrucosus*.
B. crocidu'rae, espécie bacteriana que causa febre recidivante na África do Norte, no Oriente Próximo e na Ásia central e é transmitido pela variedade pequena do carrapato *Ornithodoros erraticus*.
B. dutto'nii, espécie bacteriana que causa a febre recidivante da África Central e do Sul; transmitido por um carrapato, *Ornithodoros moubata*.
B. garinii, genoespécie bacteriana da *Borrelia burgdorferi sensu lato* que causa a doença de Lyme na Europa e na Ásia; transmitido pelo carrapato *Ixodes ricinus* nas regiões central e ocidental da Europa e pelo carrapato *Ixodes persulcatus* na Eurásia, desde o Mar Báltico até o Oceano Pacífico. VER TAMBÉM *B. burgdorferi sensu stricto*.
B. herm'sii, espécie bacteriana encontrada como uma causa de febre recidivante na Colúmbia Britânica, Califórnia, Colorado, Idaho, Nevada, Oregon e Washington; transmitida por um carrapato, *Ornithodoros hermsi*.
B. hispan'ica, espécie bacteriana que causa febre recidivante na Espanha, Portugal e noroeste da África, transmitida pela variedade grande do carrapato *Ornithodoros erratica*.
B. latysche'wii, espécie bacteriana que causa a febre recidivante no Irã e na Ásia central; transmitido pelo carrapato *Ornithodoros tartakovskyi* de roedores e répteis.
B. mazzot'tii, espécie bacteriana que causa a febre recidivante no México e nas Américas Central e do Sul; transmitido pelo carrapato *Ornithodoros talajé*.
B. par'keri, espécie bacteriana encontrada como uma causa de febre recidivante no oeste dos Estados Unidos; transmitido por um carrapato, *Ornithodoros parkeri*.
B. per'sica, espécie bacteriana que causa febre recidivante no Oriente Médio e Ásia central; o vetor é o carrapato *Ornithodoros tholozani*.
B. recurren'tis, espécie bacteriana que causa febre recidivante na América do Sul, Europa, África e Ásia; transmitido pelo percevejo, *Cimex lectularius*, e pelo piolho, *Pediculus humanus* subesp. *humanus*. SIN Obermeier spirillum, *Spirochaeta obermeieri*.

B. turica'tae, espécie bacteriana encontrada como uma causa de febre recidivante no México, Novo México, Texas, Oklahoma e Kansas; transmitido por *Ornithodoro turicata.*
B. venezuelen'sis, espécie bacteriana que causa a febre recidivante espiroquética nas Américas Central e do Sul; transmitido por *Ornithodoros rudis* e *O. venezuelensis.*
bor·re·li·o·sis (bō - rē - lē - ō'sis). Borreliose; a doença causada por bactérias do gênero *Borrelia.*
  Lyme b., b. de Lyme. SIN Lyme *disease.*
Borst, Maximilian, patologista alemão, 1869–1946. VER B.-Jadassohn type intraepidermal *epithelioma.*
Bosin dis·ease. Doença de Bosin. Ver em disease.
boss (baws). Bossa. **1.** Protuberância; tumefação arredondada circunscrita. **2.** A proeminência de uma cifose. [I. M. *boce,* do Fr. Ant.]
bos·se·lat·ed (baws'e - lā - ted). Bosselado; marcado por numerosas bossas ou protuberâncias arredondadas. [Fr. *bosseler,* realçar]
bos·se·la·tion (baws - ē - lā'shun). Bosselação. **1.** Uma bossa. **2.** Condição na qual existem uma ou mais bossas, ou protuberâncias arredondadas.
Boston, Leonard N., médico norte-americano, 1871–1931.
Botallo (Botallus), Leonardo, médico italiano em Paris, 1530–ca.1587. VER B. *duct, foramen, ligament.*
bot·fly (bot'flī). Mosca de berne; mosca robusta, pilosa, da ordem Diptera, com freqüência nitidamente marcada em negro e amarelo ou cinza, cujas larvas produzem vários tipos de miíase em seres humanos e em vários animais domésticos, principalmente em herbívoros.
  head b.'s, moscas da carne de famílias de dípteros Oestridae e Cuterebridae; moscas robustas, pilosas, negras, amarelas ou cinzas que, enquanto voam, depositam as larvas recém-nascidas ou, em alguns casos, ovos, nas narinas, ou próximo a elas, de carneiros, cabras, cervos, cavalos, camelos e, raramente, seres humanos.
  human b., SIN *Dermatobia hominis.*
  skin b.'s, SIN *Dermatobia hominis.* VER TAMBÉM *Cuterebra.*
  warble b., mosca do berne. SIN *Dermatobia hominis.* VER TAMBÉM *Hypoderma.*
both·ria (both'rē - ā). Bótrios; plural de bothrium.
both·ri·o·ceph·a·li·a·sis (both'rē - ō - sef - ā - lī'ā - sis). Difilobotríase. SIN diphyllobothriasis.
Both·ri·o·ceph·a·lus (both'rē - ō - sef'ā - lŭs). Gênero de tênias pseudofilídeas com estágios plerocercóides e adulto nos peixes; por vezes, historicamente confundidos com *Diphyllobothrium.* [G. *bothrion,* dim. de *bothros,* cova ou trincheira, + *kephalē,* cabeça]
  B. corda'tus, espécie de tênia comum em cães e seres humanos na Groenlândia.
  B. la'tus, nome original do *Diphyllobothrium latum.*
  B. manso'ni, nome original de *Spirometra mansoni.*
  B. mansonoi'des, nome original de *Spirometra mansonoides.*
both·ri·um, pl. **both·ria** (both'rē - um, - rē - ā). Um dos sulcos sugadores em forma de fenda encontrados no escólex de tênias pseudofilídeas, como a tênia do homem, *Diphyllobothrium latum.* [G. *bothros,* cova ou trincheira]
bot·ry·oid (bot'rē - oyd). Que possui numerosas protuberâncias arredondadas semelhantes a um cacho de uvas. SIN staphyline, uviform. [G. *botryoeidēs,* como um cacho de uvas (*botrys*)]
Bot·ry·o·my·ces (bot'rē - ō - mī'sēz). Nome genérico aplicado a um suposto fungo que causa a botriomicose. Como essa doença é atualmente conhecida como sendo causada por vários tipos de bactérias, mais amiúde por estafilococos, o nome é inválido e raramente utilizado. O nome da doença foi retido, contudo, para indicar um tipo peculiar de reação tecidual. [G. *botrys,* um cacho de uvas, + *mykēs,* fungo]
bot·ry·o·my·co·sis (bot'rē - ō - mī - kō'sis). Botriomicose; condição granulomatosa crônica de cavalos, gado, suínos e seres humanos que usualmente envolve a pele e, ocasionalmente, as vísceras, e caracterizada por grânulos no pus, consistindo em massas de bactérias, geralmente estafilococos, mas, por vezes, em outros tipos, circundadas por uma cápsula hialina que, por vezes, exibe corpúsculos claviformes ao redor de sua periferia; a estrutura anatômica da lesão assemelha-se à da actinomicose e do micetoma. SIN actinophytosis (2). [de *Botryomyces*]
bot·ry·o·my·cot·ic (bot'rē - ō - mī - kot'ik). Botriomicótico; relativo a ou afetado por botriomicose.
bots. Bernes; as larvas de várias espécies de moscas. [Gael. *boiteag,* vareja]
  ox b., larva de bovinos; larva da mosca do berne, *Hypoderma bovis* e *H. lineatum.*
  sheep b., berne dos ovinos; larvas de *Oestrus ovis.*
Böttcher, Arthur, anatomista estoniano, 1831–1889. VER B. *canal, cells,* em *cell, crystals,* em *crystal, ganglion, space;* Charcot-B. *crystalloids,* em *crystalloid.*
bot·tle (bot'tl). Frasco, garrafa; um recipiente para líquidos.
  Mariotte b., frasco de Mariotte; frasco arrolhado com saída pelo fundo, usado como reservatório para infusões constantes; o ar entra apenas por borbulhamento através de um tubo que se estende através da rolha quase até o fundo; um vácuo parcial, dessa maneira, suporta a altura variável do líquido acima da entrada do ar, proporcionando uma gravidade constante para o fluxo.
  wash-b., frasco de lavagem; **(1)** um frasco com um tubo que passa até o fundo, através do qual os gases são forçados para dentro da água para purificá-los; **(2)** um frasco arrolhado com dois tubos, um terminando acima e outro abaixo de um líquido, de modo que o borbulhamento de ar através do tubo mais curto força o líquido em uma pequena corrente a partir da extremidade longa livre; usado para a lavagem de aparelhos químicos.
  Woulfe b., frasco de Woulfe; um frasco com dois ou três colos, usado em uma série, conectado com tubos, para trabalhar com gases (lavagem, secagem, absorção etc.).
bot·u·lin (bot'ū - lin). Botulina. SIN botulinus *toxin.*
bot·u·lin·o·gen·ic (bot'ū - lin - ō - jen'ik). Botulinogênico. SIN botulogenic.
bot·u·lism (bot'ū - lizm). Botulismo; intoxicação alimentar usualmente causada pela ingestão da neurotoxina produzida pela bactéria *Clostridium botulinum* a partir do alimento inadequadamente enlatado ou preservado; afeta principalmente os seres humanos, galinhas, aves aquáticas, bovinos, carneiros e cavalos, e é caracterizado por paralisia em todas as espécies; pode ser fatal; suínos, cães e gatos são um pouco mais resistentes. Em alguns casos (p.ex., em lactentes), o b. pode ser formado no trato gastrintestinal por organismos ingeridos. VER TAMBÉM *Clostridium botulinum.* [L. *botulus,* salsicha]
  wound b., b. da ferida; b. que resulta da infecção de uma ferida.
bot·u·lis·mo·tox·in (bot'ū - liz - mō - tok'sin). Botulismotoxina. SIN botulinus *toxin.*
bot·u·lo·gen·ic (bot'ū - lō - jen'ik). Botulogênico; que produz botulismo. SIN botulinogenic.
bou·bas (boo'bahs). Bouba. SIN yaws. [termo nativo brasileiro]
Bouchard, Charles Jacques, médico francês, 1837–1915. VER B. *disease.*
bouche de ta·pir (boosh - dē - tā'pir). Boca de tapir. SIN tapir *mouth.* [Fr.]
Bouchut, Jean A. E., médico francês, 1818–1891. VER B. *tube.*
bou·gie (boo - zhē'). Vela; um instrumento cilíndrico, usualmente algo flexível e maleável, usado para calibrar ou dilatar áreas constringidas em órgãos tubulares, como a uretra ou o esôfago; por vezes, contendo um medicamento para aplicação local. [Fr. vela]
  b. à boule (boo - zhē'ā - bool'), vela bulbar; v. com a extremidade bulbosa.
  bulbous b., vela bulbosa; v. com uma extremidade em formato de bulbo, algumas das quais são modeladas como uma bolota ou uma oliva.
  Eder-Pustow b., v. de Eder-Pustow; v. metálica, em formato de oliva, com um sistema de dilatação metálico flexível (para a estenose esofágica).
  elastic b., v. elástica; v. feita de borracha, látex ou outro material igualmente flexível.
  elbowed b., v. acotovelada; v. com uma curvatura agudamente angulada próximo à sua extremidade.
  filiform b., v. filiforme; v. muito fina usada para a exploração delicada de estenoses nos tratos fistulosos de pequeno diâmetro, onde passagens falsas podem ser encontradas ou criadas; a extremidade de entrada pode consistir em uma extremidade reta ou espiralada, e a extremidade de saída usualmente consiste em um cilindro afilado em que pode ser inserida a ponta aparafusada de uma v. acompanhante.
  following b., v. acompanhante; v. flexível afunilada com uma ponta em parafuso onde é inserida na extremidade de saída de uma v. filiforme, a fim de possibilitar a dilatação progressiva sem o risco de criar passagens falsas.
  Hurst b., v. de Hurst; uma série de tubos com extremidade arredondada, cheios de mercúrio, com diâmetro graduado, para dilatar a região cardioesofágica.
  Maloney b., v. de Maloney; uma série de velas similares às velas de Hurst, mas apresentando extremidades em forma de cone.
  Savary b.'s, velas de Savary; as velas de Silastic (borracha siliconizada) com extremidade afunilada utilizadas sobre um fio-guia na dilatação esofágica.
  tapered b., v. afunilada; uma v. com calibre gradualmente crescente, usada para dilatar as estenoses.
  wax-tipped b., v. com ponta de cera; uma longa v. flexível e fina, com uma extremidade de cera, empregada para a passagem endoscópica para dentro do ureter, visando a confirmar a presença de um cálculo pelos arranhões na superfície da extremidade com as bordas agudas do cálculo.
  whip b., v. móvel; uma v. afunilada até uma ponta filiforme na extremidade.
bou·gie·nage (boo - zhē - nahzh'). O exame ou tratamento do interior de qualquer canal através da passagem de uma vela ou cânula.
bouil·lon (boo - yawn'). Caldo; um caldo de carne ralo. [Fr. caldo de cultura, de *bouillir,* ferver]
Bouin, Paul, histologista francês, 1870–1962. VER B. *fixative.*
bou·lim·i·a (boo - lim'ē - ā). Bulimia. SIN bulimia *nervosa.*
bound (bownd). **1.** Limitado, circunscrito; envolvido. **2.** Indica uma substância, como iodo, fósforo, cálcio, morfina ou outro medicamento, que não está na forma prontamente difusível, mas existe na combinação com uma substância de alto peso molecular, especialmente a proteína. **3.** Fixado a um receptor, como em uma parede celular.
bou·quet (boo - ka'). Buquê; um cacho ou feixe de estruturas, especialmente dos vasos sangüíneos, sugerindo um b. [Fr.]

Riolan b., b. de Riolan; os músculos e os ligamentos, as flores vermelhas e brancas, que se originam do processo estilóide.

Bourgery, Marc-Jean, anatomista e cirurgião francês, 1797–1849. VER B. *ligament*.

Bourneville, Désiré-Magloire, médico francês, 1840–1909. VER B. *disease*; B.-Pringle *disease*.

Bourquin, Anne, química norte-americana, *1897. VER Sherman-B. *unit* of vitamin B_2.

bou·ton (boo-ton′). Um botão, pústula ou inchação do tipo calosidade. [Fr. botão]

  axonal terminal b.'s, terminações axônicas. SIN axon *terminals*, em *terminal*.
  b. de Baghdad, b. de Bagdá, a lesão que ocorre na leishmaniose cutânea. SIN bouton de Biskra.
  b. en chemise, b. de camisa; pequeno abscesso da mucosa intestinal que acontece na disenteria amebiana.
  b.'s en passage, botões em trajeto; as sinapses consecutivas ao longo do trajeto de um axônio.
  synaptic b.'s, terminações sinápticas. SIN axon *terminals*, em *terminal*.
  terminal b.'s, b. terminaux, botões terminais. SIN axon *terminals*, em *terminal*.

bou·ton de Bis·kra. Botão de Biskra. SIN bouton de Baghdad.

bou·ton·niè·re (boo-ton-nir′, -nar′). Botoeira; uma fenda ou abertura semelhante a uma botoeira produzidas de forma traumática. [Fr. botoeira]

Bo·vic·o·la (bō-vik′o-la). Gênero de piolhos mordedores que é considerado por alguns como sendo um subgênero de *Damalinia*; inclui as espécies *B. bovis* (*Trichodectes scalaris*), o piolho vermelho comum ou piolho mordedor de bovinos; *B. caprae* (*Trichodectes climax*), encontrado em carneiros e cabras; *B. equi* (*Trichodectes parumpilosus*), o piolho mordedor comum de eqüinos; *B. ovis* (*Trichodectes sphaerocephalus*), o piolho mordedor comum dos carneiros. VER TAMBÉM *Trichodectes*.

Bovie. Um instrumento utilizado para a dissecção eletrocirúrgica e hemostasia. Freqüentemente utilizado como verbo, i.e., *to Bovie*, algo é dissecar ou cauterizar com o instrumento Bovie.

bo·vine (bō′vin, -vin). Bovino; relativo ao gado. [L. *bos* (*bov*-), boi]

bow (bō). Arco; qualquer dispositivo curvado em uma curva simples ou semicírculo e que possui flexibilidade. [A.S. *boga*]

  Cupid's b., a. do cupido; o contorno da margem superior do lábio superior.
  Logan b., a. de Logan; arame de aço inoxidável firme curvado em arco e ligado a ambas as bochechas para proteger um lábio leporino recentemente reparado.

Bowditch, Henry P., fisiologista norte-americano, 1840–1911. VER B. *law*, *effect*.

bow·el. Intestino. SIN intestine. VER small bowel *series*. [através do Fr. do L. *botulus*, salsicha]

  large b., intestino grosso; o colo.
  small b., intestino delgado; a porção proximal do intestino distal ao estômago, compreendendo o duodeno, o jejuno e o íleo.

Bowen, John T., dermatologista norte-americano, 1857–1941. VER B. *disease*, precancerous *dermatosis*; bowenoid *papulosis*; Bowenoid *cells*, em *cell*.

Bowie, Donald James, médico canadense, *1887. VER Bowie *stain*.

bow·leg, bow-b. (bō′leg). Joelho varo. SIN genu varum.

Bowles type steth·o·scope. Estetoscópio do tipo Bowles. Ver em stethoscope.

Bowman, Sir William, oftalmologista, anatomista e fisiologista inglês, 1816–1892. VER B. *capsule, disks,* em *disk, gland, membrane, muscle, probe, space*.

box (boks). Caixa; recipiente; receptáculo. [L.L. *buxis*, do G. *puxis*, caixa]

  black b., caixa preta; **(1)** (Jargão) descritivo de um método de raciocínio ou estudo de um problema em que os métodos e procedimentos não são descritos, explicados ou, talvez, até mesmo, compreendidos: as conclusões relacionam-se exclusivamente às relações empíricas observadas; **(2)** em alguns contextos, o termo pode significar um pedaço de aparelho ou uma cobaia em que a via farmacológica ou toxicológica ainda não foi elaborada.
  brain b., caixa cerebral; termo oficial alternativo* para neurocranium.
  CAAT b., caixa CAAT; uma seqüência de nucleotídeos encontrada em uma região conservada do DNA localizada "a montante" (direção 5′) dos pontos de partida das unidades de transcrição eucarióticas; os fatores de transcrição específicos parecem se associar a ela; encontrada em muitos promotores em −75 bp com a seqüência de consenso: GG(T/C)CAATCT. Acredita-se que determine a eficiência da transcrição.
  Hogness b., c. de Hogness. VER homeobox.
  Pribnow b., c. de Pribnow. VER homeobox.
  Skinner b., c. de Skinner; um aparelho experimental em que um animal pressiona uma alavanca para obter uma recompensa ou receber uma punição.
  TATA b., c. TATA, uma seqüência de DNA bacteriano altamente conservada encontrada a cerca de 25 bp acima do ponto de partida de transcrição dos genes, usualmente flanqueada por seqüências ricas em GC; sítio de ligação de fatores de transcrição, mas não da RNA-polimerase.
  view b., negatoscópio; uma caixa luminosa para demonstrar as radiografias ou outras transparências fotográficas.

box·ing (boks′ing). Encaixotamento; em odontologia, a construção de paredes verticais, geralmente em cera, ao redor de uma impressão dentária depois de emoldurar, a fim de produzir o tamanho e a forma desejados do modelo dentário, bem como para preservar determinadas marcas da impressão.

Boyce, William H., urologista norte-americano, *1918. VER Smith-B. *operation*.

Boyden, Edward A., anatomista norte-americano, 1886–1976. VER B. *meal, sphincter*.

Boyer, Baron Alexis, cirurgião francês, 1757–1833. VER B. *bursa, cyst*.

Boyle, Hon. Robert, químico e físico britânico, 1627–1691. VER B. *law*.

Bozeman, Nathan G., cirurgião norte-americano, 1825–1905. VER B. *operation, position*; B.-Fritsch *catheter*.

Bozzolo, Camillo, médico italiano, 1845–1920. VER B. *sign*.

BP Abreviatura de blood *pressure* (pressão arterial); British Pharmacopoeia (Farmacopéia Britânica)

b.p. Abreviatura de boiling *point* (ponto de ebulição); base *pair* (par de bases).

Bq Abreviatura de becquerel.

Br Símbolo de bromine (bromo).

Braasch, William F., urologista norte-americano, 1878–1975. VER B. *bulb, catheter*.

brace (brās). Suporte; uma órtose ou dispositivo ortopédico que suporta ou mantém na posição correta uma parte do corpo e pode possibilitar a movimentação nas articulações adjacentes, em contraste com uma tala, que impede a movimentação da parte. [I. M., do Fr. Ant., do L. *bracchium*, braço, do G. *brachion*]

  Taylor back b., suporte dorsal de Taylor; um suporte espinhal de aço. SIN Taylor apparatus, Taylor splint.

brac·es (brā′sez). Suportes, coletes; coloquialismo para aparelhos ortodônticos.

bra·chia (brā′kē-a). Plural de brachium (braço).

brach·i·al (brā′kē-al). Braquial; relativo ao braço.

bra·chi·al·gia (brā-kē-al′jē-a). Braquialgia; dor no braço. [L. *brachium*, braço, + *algos*, dor]

  b. stat′ica paresthet′ica, b. estática parestésica; dor no braço e parestesia transitória que ocorre somente à noite.

△ **brachio-.** Braquio-. SIN arm (1). [L. *brachium*]

bra·chi·o·ce·phal·ic (brā′kē-ō-se-fal′ik). Braquiocefálico; relativo ao braço e à cabeça.

bra·chi·o·cru·ral (brā′kē-ō-kroo′ral). Braquiocrural; relativo ao braço e à coxa.

bra·chi·o·cu·bi·tal (brā′kē-ō-kū′bi-tal). Braquicubital; relativo ao braço e ao cotovelo ou ao braço e ao antebraço.

bra·chi·o·gram (brā′kē-ō-gram). Braquiograma; o traçado do pulso da artéria braquial.

bra·chi·um, pl. **bra·chia** (brā′kē-um, brak′; -ā) [TA]. Braço. **1.** SIN arm (1). **2.** Uma estrutura anatômica que se assemelha a um braço. [L. braço, provavelmente semelhante ao G. *brachiōn*]

  b. collic′uli inferio′ris [TA], b. do colículo inferior. SIN b. of inferior colliculus.
  b. collic′uli superio′ris [TA], b. do colículo superior. SIN comissure of superior colliculus.
  b. conjuncti′vum cerebel′li, pedúnculo cerebelar superior. SIN superior cerebellar *peduncle*.
  b. of inferior colliculus [TA], b. do colículo inferior; um feixe de fibras que passa do colículo inferior, em ambos os lados do tronco cerebral, ao longo da borda lateral do colículo superior, até a parte posterior do tálamo, onde penetra no corpo geniculado medial. Forma parte da principal via auditiva ascendente. SIN b. colliculi inferioris [TA], b. quadrigeminum inferius, inferior quadrigeminal b.
  inferior quadrigeminal b., b. do colículo inferior. SIN b. of inferior colliculus.
  b. pon′tis, pedúnculo cerebelar médio. SIN middle cerebellar *peduncle*.
  b. quadrigem′inum infe′rius, b. do colículo inferior. SIN b. of inferior colliculus.
  b. quadrigem′inum supe′rius, b. do colículo superior. SIN b. of superior colliculus.
  b. of superior colliculus [TA], b. do colículo superior; uma faixa de fibras do trato óptico que se desvia do corpo geniculado lateral para terminar no colículo superior e na região pré-tectal. SIN b. quadrigeminum superius, superior quadrigeminal b.
  superior quadrigeminal b., b. do colículo superior. SIN b. of superior colliculus.

Bracht, Erich Franz, ginecologista e obstetra alemão, *1882. VER B. *maneuver*.

Bracht, E., patologista alemão do século 20. VER B.-Wächter *lesion*.

△ **brachy-.** Braqui-; forma combinante que indica curto. [G. *brachys*, curto]

brach·y·ba·sia (brak-e-bā′sē-a). Braquibasia; a marcha desajeitada característica da doença do trato piramidal. [brachy- + G. *basis*, uma passada]

brach·y·ba·so·camp·to·dac·ty·ly (brak-e-bā′sō-kamp-tō-dak′ti-lē). Braquibasocamptodactilia; o encurtamento e encurvação desproporcionais combinados dos dedos. [brachy- + G. *basis*, base, + *campylos*, curvado, + *daktylos*, dedo]

brach·y·ba·so·pha·lan·gia (brak-ē-bā′sō-fā-lan′jē-a). Braquibasofalangia; o encurtamento anormal das falanges proximais. [brachy- + G. *basis*, base, + falange]

brach·y·car·dia (brak - ē - kar'dē - ă). Braquicardia. SIN bradycardia.
brach·y·ce·pha·lia (brak - ē - se - fā'lē - ă). Braquicefalia. SIN brachycephaly.
brach·y·ce·phal·ic (brak - ē - se - fal'ik). Braquicefálico; relativo a ou caracterizado por braquicefalia. SIN brachycephalous.
brach·y·ceph·a·lism (brak - ē - sef'ă - lizm). Braquicefalismo. SIN brachycephaly. [brachy- + G. *kephalē*, cabeça]
brach·y·ceph·a·lous (brak - ē - sef'ă - lŭs). Braquicefálico. SIN brachycephalic.
brach·y·ceph·a·ly (brak - ē - sef'ă - lē). Braquicefalia; encurtamento desproporcional da cabeça, com o crânio apresentando um índice cefálico superior a 80; entre as raças braquicefálicas estão os indígenas norte-americanos, os malaios e os birmaneses. SIN brachycephalia, brachycephalism. [brachy- + G. *kephalē*, cabeça]
brach·y·chei·lia, brach·y·chi·lia (brak'ē - kī'lē - ă). Braquiqueilia; encurtamento anormal dos lábios. [brachy- + G. *cheilos*, lábio]
brach·y·cne·mic (brak - ē - nē'mik). Braquicnêmico; que possui pernas curtas; especificamente, relativo a um índice tibiofemoral inferior a 82, com a perna desproporcionalmente mais curta que a coxa. [brachy- + G. *knēmē*, perna]
brach·y·cra·nic (brak - ē - krā'nik). Braquicrânico; braquicefálico com um índice cefálico de 80,0 a 84,9. [brachy- + G. *kranion*, crânio]
brach·y·dac·tyl·ia (brak - ē - dak - til'ē - ă). Braquidactilia. SIN brachydactyly. [brachy- + G. *daktylos*, dedo]
brach·y·dac·tyl·ic (brak - ē - dak - til'ik). Braquidactílico; indica a braquidactilia.
brach·y·dac·ty·ly (brak - ē - dak'ti - lē). Braquidactilia; encurtamento anormal dos dedos. SIN brachydactylia. [brachy- + G. *daktylos*, dedo]
brach·y·e·soph·a·gus (brak'ē - e - sof'ă - gŭs). Braquiesôfago; um esôfago anormalmente curto. [brachy- + esôfago]
brach·y·fa·cial (brak - ē - fā'shăl). Braquifacial. SIN brachyprosopic.
brach·y·glos·sal (brak - ē - glos'ăl). Braquiglosso; indica uma língua anormalmente curta. [brachy- + G. *glōssa*, língua]
bra·chyg·na·thia (brak - ig - nā'thē - ă). Braquignatia; encurtamento ou recessão anormal da mandíbula. VER TAMBÉM micrognathia. SIN bird face. [brachy- + G. *gnathos*, mandíbula]
bra·chyg·na·thous (brak - ig'nā - thŭs). Braquignato; que possui uma mandíbula recuada.
brach·y·ker·kic (brak - ē - ker'kik). Braquiquérquico; relativo a um índice rádio-umeral inferior a 75, com um antebraço relativamente mais curto que o braço superior. [brachy- + G. *kerkis*, rádio]
brach·y·me·lia (brak - ē - mē'lē - ă). Braquimelia; encurtamento desproporcional dos membros. [brachy- + G. *melos*, membro]
brach·y·me·so·pha·lan·gia (brak - ē - mes'ō - fă - lan'jē - ă). Braquimesofalangia; encurtamento anormal das falanges médias. [brachy- + G. *mesos*, meio, + phalanx]
brach·y·met·a·car·pa·lia, brach·y·met·a·car·pa·lism (brak'ē - met - ă - kar - pā'lē - ă, - met - ă - kar'pă - lizm). Braquimetacarpalia. SIN brachymetacarpia.
brach·y·met·a·car·pia (brak - ē - met - ă - car'pē - ă). Braquimetacarpia; encurtamento anormal dos metacarpais, especialmente do quarto e quinto. SIN brachymetacarpalia, brachymetacarpalism.
brach·y·me·tap·o·dy (brak'ē - me - tap'ō - dē). Braquimetapodia; encurtamento aparente dos artelhos e dedos decorrente do encurtamento ou hipoplasia dos metacarpais ou metatarsais. [brachy- + G. *meta-* (tarsal) + *pous* (*pod-*), pé]
brach·y·met·a·tar·sia (brak'ē - met - ă - tar'sē - ă). Braquimetatarsia; encurtamento anormal dos metatarsais.
brach·y·mor·phic (brak'ē - mōr'fik). Braquimórfico; que possui, ou indica, uma forma mais curta que aquela usualmente aceita. [brachy- + G. *morphē*, forma]
brach·y·o·dont (brak'ē - ō - dont). Braquiodôntico; que possui dentes anormalmente curtos. [brachy- + G. *odous*, dente]
brach·y·o·nych·ia (brak'ē - ō - nik'ē - ă). Braquioníquia; unhas curtas, em que a largura da placa da unha e do leito ungueal é maior que o comprimento; pode ser congênita ou resulta de roer unhas, de reabsorção da unha no hiperparatireoidismo ou de artropatia psoriática. [G. *brachys*, curto, + *onyx*, *onychos*, unha, + sufixo *-ia*, condição]
brach·y·pel·lic (brak - ē - pel'ik). Braquipélico; indica uma pelve oval transversa. VER brachypellic *pelvis*. SIN brachypelvic. [brachy- + pelvis]
brach·y·pel·vic (brak - ē - pel'vik). Braquipélvico. SIN brachypellic.
brach·y·pha·lan·gia (brak'ē - fă - lan'jē - ă). Braquifalangia; encurtamento anormal das falanges. [brachy- + falange]
bra·chyp·o·dous (bra - kip'ō - dŭs). Braquípode; que possui pés anormalmente curtos. [brachy- + G. *pous*, pé]
brach·y·pro·sop·ic (brak - ē - prō - sop'ik). Braquiprosópico; que possui uma face desproporcionalmente curta. SIN brachyfacial. [brachy- + G. *prosōpikos*, facial]
brach·y·rhi·nia (brak - ē - rī'nē - ă). Braquirrinia; encurtamento anormal do nariz. [brachy- + G. *rhis*, nariz]

brach·y·rhyn·chus (brak - ē - ring'kŭs). Braquirrinco; encurtamento anormal do nariz e do maxilar, freqüentemente associado à ciclopia. [brachy- + G. *rhynchos*, focinho]
brach·y·skel·ic (brak - ē - skel'ik). Braquisquélico; relativo a pernas anormalmente curtas. [brachy- + G. *skelos*, perna]
brach·y·staph·y·line (brak - ē - staf'i - lin). Braquistafilino; que possui um palato curto; que possui um índice palatomaxilar acima de 85. [brachy- + G. *staphylē*, úvula]
brach·y·syn·dac·ty·ly (brak'ē - sin - dak'ti - lē). Braquissindactilia; encurtamento anormal dos dedos ou artelhos combinado a uma rede entre os dedos adjacentes. [brachy- + syndactyly]
brach·y·te·le·pha·lan·gia (brak - ē - tel'ē - fă - lan'jē - ă). Braquitelefalangia; encurtamento anormal das falanges distais. [brachy- + G. *telos*, fim, + phalanx]
brach·y·ther·a·py (brak - ē - ther'ă - pē). Braquiterapia; a radioterapia em que a fonte de irradiação é posicionada próximo à superfície do corpo ou dentro de uma cavidade corporal; p.ex., aplicação de rádio ao colo.
   high-dose-rate b., b. em dose alta; a b. em dose alta com o passar do tempo.
   interstitial b., b. intersticial; a radioterapia por implante de agulhas radioativas ou outras fontes diretamente dentro e ao redor do tecido a ser irradiado.
   remote afterloading b., b. em pós-carga remota; radioterapia aplicada localmente, que é carregada a distância, em receptáculos previamente implantados.
   stereotactic b., b. estereotáxica; a radioterapia liberada com a ajuda de localização tecidual orientada por TC.
brach·y·type (brak'ē - tīp). SIN endomorph.
brac·ing (brās'ing). Reforço; em odontologia, a resistência aos componentes horizontais da força mastigatória. VER *component* of force.
brack·et (brak'et). Suporte angulado; em odontologia, uma pequena inserção metálica que é soldada ou fundida a uma faixa ortodôntica ou ligada diretamente aos dentes, servindo para apertar o arco à faixa ou ao dente.
Bradbury, Samuel, médico norte-amerciano. VER B.-Eggleston *syndrome*.
Bradford, Edward H., ortopedista norte-americano, 1848–1926. VER B. *frame*.
△ **brady-.** Bradi-; forma combinante que indica lento. [G. *bradys*, lento]
bra·dy·ar·rhyth·mia (brad'ē - ă - rith'mē - ă). Bradiarritmia; qualquer distúrbio do ritmo cardíaco que resulta (por convenção) em uma freqüência inferior a 50 batimentos por min. [bradi-] [G. *a-* priv. + *rhythmos*, ritmo]
bra·dy·arth·ria (brad - ē - arth'rē - ă). Bradiartria; uma forma de disartria caracterizada por lentidão anormal ou deliberação na fala. SIN bradyglossia (2), bradylalia, bradylogia. [brady- + G. *arthroō*, pronunciar distintamente, de *arthron*, uma articulação]
bra·dy·car·dia (brad - ē - kar'dē - ă). Bradicardia; lentidão da freqüência cardíaca, usualmente definida (por convenção) como uma freqüência inferior a 50 batimentos/min. SIN brachycardia, bradyrhythmia. [brady- + G. *kardia*, coração]
   central b., b. central; a b. devido à doença do sistema nervoso central, usualmente com pressão intracraniana aumentada.
   essential b., b. essencial; pulso lento para o qual nenhuma causa pode ser descoberta. SIN idiopathic b.
   fetal b., b. fetal; freqüência cardíaca fetal inferior a 120 batimentos/min.
   idiopathic b., b. idiopática. SIN essential b.
   marked fetal b., b. fetal acentuado; freqüência cardíaca fetal inferior a 100 batimentos por minuto.
   mild fetal b., b. fetal leve; freqüência cardíaca fetal entre 100 e 120 batimentos por minuto.
   nodal b., b. nodal. SIN atrioventricular junctional *rhythm*.
   postinfectious b., b. pós-infeccioso; b. tóxico que ocorre durante a convalescença de várias doenças infecciosas, como a influenza.
   sinus b., b. sinusal; b. que se origina no marca-passo sinoatrial normal.
   vagal b., b. vagal; qualquer lentificação cardíaca excessiva decorrente da estimulação dos nervos vagais.
   ventricular b., b. ventricular; lentificação da freqüência ventricular, geralmente implicando a presença de bloqueio atrioventricular.
brad·y·car·di·ac (brad - ē - kar'dē - ăk). Bradicardíaco; relativo a ou caracterizado por bradicardia. SIN bradycardic.
bra·dy·car·dic (brad - ē - kar'dik). Bradicárdico. SIN bradycardiac.
bra·dy·ci·ne·sia (brad - ē - si - nē'sē - ă). Bradicinesia. SIN bradykinesia.
bra·dy·crot·ic (brad - ē - krot'ik). Bradicrótico; relativo a ou caracterizado por um pulso lento. [brady- + G. *krotos*, uma pulsação]
bra·dy·di·as·to·le (brad - ē - dī - as'tō - lē). Bradidiástole; prolongamento da diástole do coração.
bra·dy·es·the·sia (brad - ē - es - thē'zē - ă). Bradiestesia; percepção sensorial lenta. [brady- + G. *aisthēsis*, sensação]
bra·dy·glos·sia (brad - ē - glos'ē - ă). Bradiglossia. **1.** Movimento lento ou difícil da língua. **2.** SIN bradyarthria. [brady- + G. *glōssa*, língua]
bra·dy·ki·ne·sia (brad - ē - kin - ē'zē - ă). Bradicinesia; diminuição na espontaneidade e no movimento. Um dos aspectos dos distúrbios extrapiramidais, como a doença de Parkinson. SIN bradycinesia. [brady- + G. *kinēsis*, movimento]
bra·dy·ki·net·ic (brad - ē - ki - net'ik). Bradicinético; caracterizado ou pertinente ao movimento lento.

bra·dy·ki·nin (brad-ē-kī'nin). Bradicina; o nonapeptídeo Arg-Pro-Pro-Gli-Fen-Ser-Pro-Fen-Arg, produzido a partir do decapeptídeo calidina (bradicininogênio), que é produzido a partir da α_2-globulina por calicreína, normalmente presente no sangue em uma forma inativa e similar à tripsina na ação; a b. é uma das inúmeras cininas plasmáticas, é um vasodilatador potente e é um dos mediadores fisiológicos da anafilaxia liberados a partir de mastócitos cobertos por anticorpos citotrópicos após a reação com o antígeno (alérgeno) específico para o anticorpo. SIN kallidin 9, kallidin 1, kinin 9. [brady- + G. *kineō*, mover]

bra·dy·ki·nin·o·gen (brad'ē-ki-nin'ō-jen). Bradicininogênio. SIN kallidin.

bra·dy·ki·nin po·ten·ti·a·tor B. Potencializador B da bradicinina; Glp-Gli-Leu-Pro-Pro-Arg-Pro-Lis-Ile-Pro-Pro; o precursor undecapeptídeo da bradicinina e das angiotensinas.

bra·dy·la·lia (brad-ē-lā'lē-ă). Bradilalia. SIN bradyarthria. [brady- + G. *lalia*, fala]

bra·dy·lex·ia (brad-ē-lek'sē-ă). Bradilexia; lentidão anormal na leitura. [brady- + G. *lexis*, palavra]

bra·dy·lo·gia (brad-ē-lō'jē-ă). Bradilogia. SIN bradyarthria. [brady- + G. *logos*, palavra]

bra·dy·pep·sia (brad-ē-pep'sē-ă). Bradipepsia; lentidão da digestão. [brady- + G. *pepsis*, digestão]

bra·dy·pha·gia (brad-ē-fā'jē-ă). Bradifagia; lentidão na alimentação. [brady- + G. *phagō*, comer]

bra·dy·pha·sia (brad-ē-fā'zē-ă). Bradifasia; uma forma de afasia caracterizada por lentidão anormal da fala. SIN bradyphemia. [brady- + G. *phasis*, falar]

bra·dy·phe·mia (brad-ē-fē'mē-ă). Bradifemia. SIN bradyphasia. [brady- + G. *phēmē*, fala]

bra·dyp·nea (brad-ip-nē-ă). Bradipnéia; lentidão anormal da respiração, especificamente uma baixa freqüência respiratória. [brady- + G. *pnoē*, respiração]

bra·dy·psy·chia (brad-ē-sī'kē-ă). Bradipsiquia; lentidão das reações mentais. [brady- + G. *psichē*, alma]

bra·dy·rhyth·mia (brad-ē-rith'mē-ă). Bradirritmia. SIN bradycardia.

bra·dy·sper·ma·tism (brad-ē-sper'mă-tizm). Bradispermatismo; ausência de força ejaculatória, de modo que o sêmen é eliminado lentamente. [brady, + G. *sperma* (spermat-), semente, + ism]

bra·dy·sphyg·mia (brad-ē-sfing'mē-ă). Bradisfigmia; lentidão do pulso; pode ocorrer sem bradicardia, como no bigeminismo ventricular, quando cada batimento alternado pode falhar em produzir um pulso periférico. [brady- + G. *sphygmos*, pulso]

bra·dy·stal·sis (brad-ē-stahl'sis). Bradistalsia; movimento intestinal lento. [G. *bradys*, lento, + *(peri)stalsis*, que se contrai em torno]

bra·dy·tel·e·o·ci·ne·sia (brad'ē-tel-ē-ō-sin-ē'sē-ă). Bradileocinesia; parada súbita de um movimento exatamente antes de seu término desejado, em seguida, depois de uma pausa, ele é completado lentamente ou por contração; um sintoma de doença cerebelar. SIN bradyteleokinesis. [brady- + G. *teleos*, completo, + *kenēsis*, movimento]

bra·dy·tel·e·o·ki·ne·sis (brad'ē-tel-ē-ō-ki-nē'sis). Bradileocinese. SIN bradyteleocinesia.

bra·dy·u·ria (brad-ē-ū'rē-ă). Bradiúria; micção lenta. [brady- + G. *ouron*, urina]

bra·dy·zo·ite (brad-ē-zō'īt). Bradizoíto; uma forma encistada, de multiplicação lenta, de parasitas esporozoários típicos da infecção crônica por *Toxoplasma gondii*. Também é chamada de um merozoíto ou zoíto; os complexos de bradizoítos dentro de uma membrana envolvente também são chamados de um pseudocisto, embora, atualmente, ele seja considerado um cisto verdadeiro. [brady- + G. *zōē*, vida]

braille (brāl). Braile; um sistema de escrita e impressão por meio de pontos elevados que correspondem a letras, números e pontuação, a fim de possibilitar que o cego leia através do tato. [Louis *Braille*, professor francês de pessoas cegas, 1809–1852]

Brailsford, James Frederick, radiologista inglês, 1888–1961. VER B.-Morquio *disease*.

Brain, Walter Russell, Lord, médico inglês, 1895–1966. VER B. *reflex*.

brain (brān) [TA]. Cérebro; a parte do sistema nervoso central contida dentro do crânio. Cf. cerebrum, cerebellum. [A.S. *braegen*]
split b., um c. em que o corpo caloso e, em geral, as comissuras anterior e posterior foram seccionados; usualmente para tratar determinadas epilepsias refratárias.
visceral b., sistema límbico. SIN limbic *system*.

brain·case (brān'kās). Neurocrânio. SIN neurocranium.

brai·stem, brain stem (brān'stem) [TA]. Tronco encefálico; originalmente, toda a subdivisão não-pareada do cérebro, composta de (em seqüência anterior) rombencéfalo, mesencéfalo e diencéfalo, conforme diferenciado da única subdivisão pareada, o telencéfalo. Mais recentemente, a conotação do termo sofreu várias modificações arbitrárias; alguns utilizam-na para indicar não mais que o rombencéfalo mais o mesencéfalo, diferenciando aquele complexo do prosencéfalo (diencéfalo mais telencéfalo); outros restringem-no ainda mais para se referir exclusivamente ao rombencéfalo. Dos pontos de vista de desenvolvimento e de arquitetura, a interpretação original parece ser preferível. SIN truncus encephali [TA].

brain·wash·ing (brān'wash'ing). Lavagem cerebral; induzir uma pessoa a modificar as atitudes e o comportamento em determinadas direções através de várias formas de pressão psicológica ou tortura.

bran. Farelo; um subproduto da moagem do milho, contendo aproximadamente 20% de celulose não-digerível; catártico de massa, geralmente tomado na forma de cereal ou produtos de farelo especial.

branch [TA]. Ramo; uma ramificação; em anatomia, uma das divisões primárias de um nervo ou vaso sangüíneo. Um ramo. VER ramus, artery, nerve, vein. SIN ramus (1) [TA].
accessory meningeal b., artéria pterigomeníngea. SIN pterygomeningeal *artery*.
accessory meningeal b. of middle meningeal artery, r. acessório da artéria meníngea média. SIN accessory b. of middle meningeal artery.
acessory b. of middle meningeal artery [TA], r. acessório da artéria meníngea média; r. da artéria meníngea média ou maxilar na fossa infratemporal e que passa superiormente através do forame oval para irrigar o gânglio trigeminal, a dura-máter e a tábua interna do osso. SIN ramus accessorius arteriae meningeae mediae [TA], accessory meningeal b. of middle meningeal artery, ramus meningeus accessorius arteriae meningeae mediae.
acetabular b. [TA], r. acetabular; r. arterial que supre o acetábulo; duas artérias, a obturatória e a circunflexa femoral medial, possuem esses ramos. SIN ramus acetabularis [TA], acetabular artery, arteria acetabuli.
acromial b. of suprascapular artery [TA], r. acromial da artéria supra-escapular; r. da artéria supra-escapular que perfura a origem do músculo trapézio durante seu trajeto até o acrômio; *anastomoses*, r. acromial da artéria toracoacromial. SIN ramus acromialis arteriae suprascapularis [TA].
acromial b. of thoracoacromial artery [TA], r. acromial da artéria toracoacromial; r. da artéria toracoacromial que corre sobre o processo coracóide e sob o músculo deltóide. SIN ramus acromialis arteriae thoracoacromialis [TA], acromial artery.
anastomotic b. [TA], r. anastomótico; um vaso sangüíneo que interliga dois vasos vizinhos. O termo não deve ser utilizado para descrever a comunicação entre nervos no sistema nervoso, porque não existe analogia entre um ramo vascular anastomosante e uma conexão entre nervos ou suas subdivisões. SIN ramus anastomoticus [TA].
anastomotic b. of middle meningeal artery with lacrimal artery [TA], r. anastomótico da artéria meníngea média com a artéria lacrimal; um r. da artéria meníngea média que se origina na cavidade craniana que corre anteriormente através da fissura orbital superior para se anastomosar com a artéria lacrimal. VER orbital b. of middle meningeal artery. SIN ramus anastomoticus arteriae meningeae mediae cum arteriae lacrimali [TA].
b. to angular gyrus [TA], r. do giro angular; o último r. da porção terminal da artéria cerebral média distribuído para as regiões dos lobos temporal, parietal

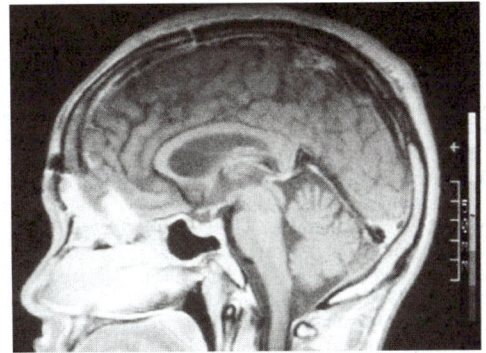
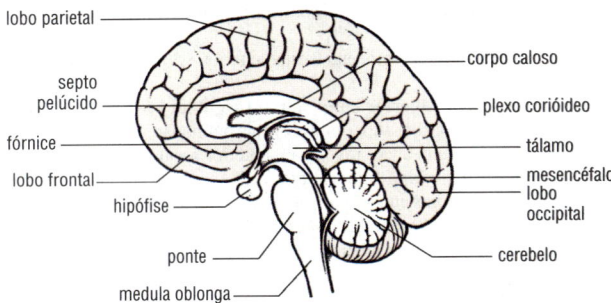

cérebro: (acima) ressonância magnética (RM) de um cérebro normal, (abaixo) ilustração da mesma incidência mediossagital

e occipital. SIN angular artery (2) [TA], artéria angularis [TA], arteria gyri angularis [TA], artery of angular gyrus.

anterior b. [TA], r. anterior; o ramo anterior dos seguintes: 1) nervo auricular magno; 2) veias pulmonares superiores esquerda e direita; 3) nervo cutâneo dorsal medial do antebraço; 4) artéria obturatória; 5) nervo obturatório; 6) artéria renal; 7) ramo direito da veia porta; 8) ducto hepático direito; 9) artéria recorrente ulnar. SIN ramus anterior [TA].

anterior abdominal cutaneous b. of intercostal nerve [TA], r. cutâneo abdominal anterior do nervo intercostal; continuação dos ramos ventrais dos nervos espinais (nervos intercostais) T7-T11 distais à origem dos nervos cutâneos laterais; distribuídos para a parede abdominal anterior. VER TAMBÉM thoracoabdominal *nerves*, em *nerve*. SIN ramus cutaneous anterior abdominalis nervi intercostalis [TA].

anterior auricular b.'s of superficial temporal artery [TA], ramos auriculares anteriores da artéria temporal superficial; *distribuição*, orelha, lóbulo da orelha e meato acústico externo. SIN rami auriculares anteriores arteriae temporalis superficialis [TA].

anterior basal b., artéria segmentar basilar anterior. SIN anterior basal segmental *artery*.

anterior basal b. of superior basal vein (of right and left inferior pulmonary veins), r. veia basilar superior (das veias pulmonares inferiores direita e esquerda); termo oficial alternativo* para anterior basal *vein*.

anterior cutaneous b.'s of femoral nerve [TA], ramos cutâneos anteriores do nervo femoral; ramos cutâneos do nervo femoral distribuídos para as faces anterior e medial da coxa; conduz a sensibilidade geral. SIN rami cutanei anteriores nervi femoralis [TA], anterior femoral cutaneous nerves.

anterior cutaneous b. of iliohypogastric nerve [TA], r. cutâneo anterior do nervo ilio-hipogástrico; *distribuição*, pele sobre o púbis. SIN ramus cutaneus anterior nervi iliohypogastrici [TA], genital b. of iliohypogastric nerve.

anterior cutaneous b.'s of intercostal nerves, ramos cutâneos anteriores dos nervos intercostais; ramos mamários mediais dos ramos cutâneos anteriores dos ramos ventrais primários dos nervos espinais torácicos. VER medial mammary b.'s.

anterior gastric b.'s of anterior vagal trunk [TA], ramos gástricos anteriores do tronco vagal anterior; os ramos gástricos anteriores do vago; ramos do tronco vagal anterior para a superfície anterior do estômago. SIN rami gastrici anteriores trunci vagalis anterioris [TA], gastric b.'s of anterior vagal trunk, rami gastrici anteriores nervi vagi.

anterior glandular b. of superior thyroid artery [TA], r. glandular anterior da artéria tireóidea superior; ramos que passam profundamente ao músculo esternotireóideo, descem ao longo do lado medial do pólo superior do lobo lateral e, em seguida, da margem superior do istmo, anastomosando-se com a artéria contralateral; eles irrigam principalmente a face anterior da tireóide. SIN ramus glandularis anterior arteriae thyroideae superioris [TA].

anterior intercostal b.'s of internal thoracic artery [TA], ramos intercostais anteriores da artéria torácica interna; uma das artérias que irrigam as porções anteriores dos espaços intercostais da parede torácica. As artérias intercostais anteriores 1 a 6 originam-se como ramos da artéria torácica interna; as artérias intercostais anteriores 7 a 11 são ramos da artéria musculofrênica. SIN rami intercostales anteriores arteriae thoracicae internae [TA], anterior intercostal arteries, rami intercostales anteriores.

anterior interventricular b. of left coronary artery [TA], r. interventricular anterior da artéria coronária esquerda; r. terminal (com o ramo circunflexo da artéria coronária esquerda; desce no sulco interventricular anterior até o ápice, anastomosando-se com o ramo interventricular posterior. Supre a maior parte da face esternal dos ventrículos e os dois terços anteriores do septo interventricular, incluindo o fascículo atrioventricular do tecido de condução. SIN ramus interventricularis anterior arteriae coronariae sinistrae [TA], anterior interventricular artery, left anterior descending artery.

anterior labial b.'s of deep external pudendal artery [TA], ramos labiais anteriores da artéria pudenda externa profunda; ramos para os lábios maiores do pudendo. SIN rami labiales anteriores arteriae pudendae externae profundae [TA], anterior labial arteries, arteriae labiales anteriores.

anterior/lateral/posterior glandular b.'s of superior thyroid artery, ramos glandulares anterior/lateral/posterior da artéria tireóidea superior; ramos dos ramos da artéria tireóidea superior para a glândula tireóide. SIN ramus glandulares anterior/lateralis/posterior arteriae thyroideae superioris.

anterior lateral nasal b.'s of anterior ethmoidal artery [TA], ramos nasais anteriores laterais da artéria etmoidal anterior; ramos da parte intracraniana da artéria etmoidal anterior que atravessam as lâminas cribriformes do osso etmóide, descem para a cavidade nasal com os nervos etmoidais anteriores, para correrem em um sulco na superfície profunda do osso nasal, e suprem a face ântero-superior da parede lateral da cavidade. SIN rami nasales anteriores laterales arteriae ethmoidalis anterioris [TA].

anterior meningeal b. (of anterior ethmoidal artery) [TA], r. meníngeo anterior (da artéria etmoidal anterior); *origem*, artéria etmoidal anterior; *distribuição*, meninges na fossa anterior do crânio; *anastomoses*, ramos da artéria meníngea média e ramos meníngeos das artérias carótida interna e lacrimal. SIN arteria meningea anterior [TA], ramus meningeus anterior arteriae ethmoidalis anterioris [TA], anterior meningeal artery.

anterior pectoral cutaneous b. of intercostal nerves [TA], r. cutâneo anterior do tórax dos nervos intercostais; a continuação dos ramos ventrais dos nervos espinais (nervos intercostais) T1-T6 distais à origem dos ramos cutâneos laterais; tornam-se cutâneos na linha para-esternal e se dividem nos ramos medial (esternal) e lateral (mamário); distribuem-se para a parede anterior do tórax. SIN ramus cutaneus anterior pectoralis nervi intercostalis [TA].

anterior b. of the renal artery [TA], r. anterior da artéria renal. VER segmental *arteries* of kidney, em *artery*.

anterior scrotal b. of deep external pudendal artery [TA], r. escrotal anterior da artéria pudenda externa profunda; *distribuição*, pele da porção anterior da bolsa escrotal; *anastomoses*, ramos escrotais posteriores da artéria pudenda interna. SIN rami scrotales anteriores arteriae pudendae externae profundae [TA].

anterior septal b.'s of anterior ethmoidal artery [TA], ramos septais anteriores da artéria etmoidal anterior; os ramos da parte intracraniana da artéria etmoidal anterior que passam através das lâminas cribriformes do osso etmóide, descem para a cavidade nasal com os nervos etmoidais anteriores e irrigam a face ântero-superior do septo nasal. SIN rami septales anteriores arteriae ethmoidalis anterioris [TA].

anterior superior alveolar b.'s of infraorbital nerve, ramos alveolares superiores anteriores do nervo infra-orbital. SIN anterior superior alveolar *nerves*, em *nerve*.

anterior temporal b. [TA], r. temporal anterior; um r. da parte insular da artéria cerebral média distribuído para o córtex da parte anterior do lobo temporal. SIN ramus temporalis anterior [TA], anterior temporal artery, arteria temporalis anterior.

anteromedial central b.'s, ramos centrais ântero-mediais; ramos da artéria comunicante anterior que irrigam parte do hipotálamo (artéria supraquiasmática [TA], artéria comissural mediana [TA]) e uma área medial do corpo caloso (artéria calosa mediana [TA]). SIN rami centrales anteromediales [TA].

anteromedial frontal b. of callosomarginal artery [TA], r. frontal ântero-medial da artéria calosomarginal; r. da porção inicial da artéria calosomarginal para a porção ântero-inferior da face medial do lobo frontal do cérebro. SIN ramus frontalis anteromedialis arteriae callosomarginalis [TA].

apical b. of inferior lobar branch of right pulmonary artery, artéria segmentar apical da artéria lobar superior do pulmão direito; termo oficial alternativo* para apical segmental *artery* of superior lobar artery of right lung.

apical b. of right superior pulmonary vein, veia apical; termo oficial alternativo* para apical *vein*.

apicoposterior b. of left superior pulmonary vein, r. apicoposterior; termo oficial alternativo* para apicoposterior *vein*.

articular b.'s [TA], ramos articulares; os ramos distribuídos para as articulações. Quase todo vaso ligado a uma articulação emitirá ramos articulares. Muitas articulações recebem ramos articulares dos ramos intramusculares dos nervos motores que inervam os músculos que cruzam a articulação (veja Hilton *law*). A Terminologia Anatômica, no entanto, reconhece especificamente apenas: (1) os ramos articulares da artéria descendente do joelho (ramos articulares da artéria descendente do joelho) [TA]: irrigam a articulação do joelho; (2) os ramos articulares de vários nervos espinais (ramos cutâneos de vários nervos) e (3) o ramo articular do ramo posterior dos nervos obturatórios que inervam a articulação do quadril. SIN rami articulares [TA], joint b.'s.

ascending b. [TA], r. ascendente; um r. com orientação superior. A Terminologia Anatômica reconhece um ramo ascendente do seguinte: 1) artérias segmentares anteriores dos pulmões esquerdo e direito (ramo ascendente das artérias segmentares anteriores das artérias pulmonares esquerda e direita), 2) artéria circunflexa ilíaca profunda (ramo ascendente da artéria circunflexa ilíaca profunda), 3) artéria epigástrica inferior (ramo ascendente das artérias epigástricas inferiores), 4) artérias circunflexas femorais lateral e medial (ramos ascendentes das artérias circunflexas femorais lateral e medial), 5) artérias segmentares posteriores dos pulmões esquerdo e direito (ramo ascendente das artérias segmentares pulmonares esquerda e direita) e 6) artéria cervical superficial (ramo ascendente dos ramos superficiais das artérias transversais do pescoço). SIN ramus ascendens [TA].

ascending b. of the inferior mesenteric artery, artéria ascendente da artéria mesentérica inferior. SIN ascending *artery* (2).

ascending b. of superficial cervical artery [TA], r. ascendente da artéria cervical transversa; o ramo ascendente da artéria cervical transversa que passa superiormente e profundamente à parte superior (cervical) do trapézio, irrigando-o, aos músculos adjacentes e aos linfonodos cervicais; anastomosa-se com o ramo descendente da artéria occipital. VER TAMBÉM superficial b. of transverse cervical artery. SIN ramus ascendens arteriae superficialis cervicalis [TA].

atrial b.'s [TA], ramos atriais; os ramos da artéria coronária direita e r. circunflexo da artéria coronária esquerda distribuídos para os átrios direito e esquerdo, respectivamente. SIN rami atriales [TA].

atrial anastomotic b. of circumflex branch of left coronary artery [TA], r. anastomótico atrial do ramo circunflexo da artéria coronária esquerda; um vaso de origem variável, mais amiúde um r. da artéria circunflexa, que avança por trás da base do septo interatrial no sentido da cruz do coração, anastomosando-se com os ramos da artéria coronária que irrigam o nó atrioventricular, o fascículo atrioventricular (feixe de His) e as paredes posteriores superiores do ventrículo esquerdo. SIN ramus atrialis anastomoticus ramus circumflexus arteriae coronariae sinistrae [TA], arteria anastomotica auricularis magna, Kugel anastomotic artery.

atrioventricular nodal b. [TA], r. do nó atrioventricular; os ramos atrioventriculares, as pequenas artérias que irrigam o nó atrioventricular; em geral, originam-se da artéria coronária direita, onde começam a descer o sulco interventricular. SIN ramus nodi atrioventricularis [TA], artery to atrioventricular node, b. to atrioventricular node.

b. to atrioventricular node, r. do nó atrioventricular. SIN atrioventricular nodal b.

auricular b. of occipital artery [TA], r. auricular da artéria occipital; *distribuição*, parte posterior da orelha; *anastomose*: artéria auricular posterior. SIN ramus auricularis arteriae occipitalis [TA].

auricular b. of posterior auricular artery [TA], r. auricular da artéria auricular posterior; origina-se no sulco entre a cartilagem auricular e o processo mastóide, ascende profundamente aos músculos auriculares posteriores e se ramifica na face craniana da orelha. SIN ramus auricularis arteriae auricularis posterioris [TA].

auricular b. of vagus nerve [TA], r. auricular do nervo vago, r. do gânglio superior do nervo vago que inerva a parte posterior da orelha externa e o meato acústico externo. SIN Arnold nerve, ramus auricularis nervi vagi.

b.'s of auriculotemporal nerve to tympanic membrane [TA], ramos para a membrana timpânica do nervo auriculotemporal; r. sensorial do nervo auriculotemporal que inerva a superfície externa da membrana timpânica. SIN rami membranae tympani nervi auriculotemporalis [TA], nerve of tympanic membrane.

basal tentorial b. of internal carotid artery, r. basilar do tentório da parte cavernosa da artéria carótida interna. SIN tentorial basal b. of internal carotid artery.

bronchial b.'s of thoracic aorta [TA], ramos bronquiais da parte torácica da aorta; os ramos ou artérias, vasos ou nervos distribuídos para os brônquios; os seguintes elementos apresentam ramos assim nomeados: 1) aorta torácica; 2) artéria torácica interna; 3) nervos vago. SIN bronchial arteries, rami bronchiales.

buccal b.'s of facial nerve, ramos bucais do nervo facial; ramos motores do nervo facial distribuídos para o músculo bucinador e outros músculos da expressão facial abaixo da órbita e acima do queixo. SIN rami buccales nervi facialis [TA].

calcaneal b.'s [TA], ramos calcâneos; os ramos ou artérias do calcâneo, ramos para as estruturas na região do calcanhar que provêm 1) da artéria tibial posterior e 2) da artéria fibular. SIN rami calcanei [TA], calcaneal arteries.

calcarine b. of medial occipital artery [TA], r. calcarino da artéria occipital medial; r. da artéria occipital medial que corre em relação ao sulco calcarino. SIN ramus calcarinus arteriae occipitalis medialis [TA], arteria calcarina, calcarine artery.

capsular b.'s of intrarenal arteries [TA], ramos capsulares das artérias intra-renais; os ramos das artérias que percorrem o córtex renal (artérias corticais e perfurantes radiadas) que suprem a cápsula fibrosa do rim. SIN rami capsulares arteriorum interenalium [TA].

capsular b.'s of renal artery [TA], ramos capsulares da artéria renal; ramos que se originam da artéria renal fora do rim que são distribuídos para a cápsula renal. SIN rami capsulares arteriae renalis [TA].

carotid b. of glossopharyngeal nerve (CN IX), r. para o seio carótico do nervo glossofaríngeo (NC IX); um ramo do nervo glossofaríngeo que inerva os barorreceptores na parede do seio carotídeo e os quimiorreceptores no glomo carótico. SIN ramus sinus carotici nervi glossopharyngei CN IX [TA], ramus sinus carotici [TA], carotid sinus b., carotid sinus nerve, Hering sinus nerve, intercarotid nerve, nerve to carotid sinus, sinus nerve of Hering.

carotid sinus b., r. para o seio carótico do nervo glossofaríngeo. SIN carotid b. of glossopharyngeal nerve (CN IX).

caudate b.'s of left branch of portal vein [TA], ramos do lobo caudado do ramo esquerdo da veia porta do fígado; ramos da parte transversa do ramo esquerdo da veia porta distribuídos para o lobo caudado antes que a veia entre no fígado. SIN rami lobi caudati rami sinistri venae portae hepatis [TA].

cavernous b. of cavernous part of internal carotid artery [TA], r. do seio cavernoso da parte cavernosa da artéria carótida interna; inúmeros ramos pequenos da parte cavernosa da artéria carótida interna. VER b.'s of internal carotid artery to trigeminal ganglion, tentorial basal b. of internal carotid artery, marginal tentorial b. of internal carotid artery. SIN ramus sinus cavernosi partis cavernosae arteriae carotidis internae [TA], cavernous arteries, cavernous sinus b. of internal carotid artery, ramus sinus cavernosi arteriae carotidis arteriae, nus sinus cavernosi arteriae carotidis internae.

cavernous sinus b. of internal carotid artery, r. do seio cavernoso da parte cavernosa da artéria carótida interna. SIN cavernous b. of cavernous part of internal carotid artery.

celiac b.'s of posterior vagal trunk [TA], ramos celíacos do tronco vagal posterior; ramos terminais do tronco vagal posterior que conduzem as fibras parassimpáticas pré-sinápticas para — e fibras aferentes viscerais de — o plexo celíaco. SIN rami celiaci trunci vagi posterioris [TA], celiac b.'s of vagus nerve, rami celiaci nervi vagi.

celiac b.'s of vagus nerve, ramos celíacos do tronco vagal posterior. SIN celiac b.'s of posterior vagal trunk.

cervical b. of facial nerve [TA], r. cervical do nervo facial; o r. mais inferior do plexo intraparotídeo do nervo facial, desce para inervar o músculo platisma. SIN ramus colli nervi facialis [TA], ramus cervicalis nervi facialis*.

choroid b.'s, ramos corióideos: ramos corióideos posteriores laterais [TA], os ramos posteriores laterais da artéria cerebral posterior distribuídos para o plexo corióideo do ventrículo lateral; ramos corióideos posteriores mediais [TA], os ramos corióideos posteriores mediais da artéria cerebral posterior distribuídos para o plexo corióideo do terceiro ventrículo; ramos corióideos do ventrículo lateral [TA], os ramos corióideos do ventrículo lateral da artéria corióidea anterior para o plexo do ventrículo lateral; ramos corióideos do terceiro ventrículo [TA], ramos corióideos da artéria corióidea anterior para o terceiro ventrículo; ramo corióideo do quarto ventrículo [TA], o ramo corióideo do quarto ventrículo da artéria cerebelar inferior posterior. SIN rami choroidei.

cingular b. of callosomarginal artery [TA], r. do cíngulo da artéria calosomarginal; r. terminal (com o r. frontal póstero-medial) da artéria calosomarginal que corre no sulco do cíngulo da face medial do cérebro. SIN ramus cingularis arteriae callosomarginalis [TA].

circumferential pontine b.'s of pontine arteries, ramos laterais das artérias da ponte; termo oficial alternativo* para lateral b.'s of pontine arteries.

circumflex fibular b. (of posterior tibial artery) [TA], r. circunflexo fibular da artéria tibial posterior; um r. da parte inicial (superior) da artéria tibial posterior que serpenteia ao redor do colo da fíbula e liga as anastomoses ao redor da articulação do joelho. SIN ramus circumflexus fibularis arteriae tibialis posterioris [TA], circumflex b. of posterior tibial artery*, circumflex peroneal b. of posterior tibial artery*, ramus circumflexus peronealis arteriae tibialis posterioris*, circumflex fibular artery.

circumflex b. of left coronary artery [TA], r. circunflexo da artéria coronária esquerda; o r. terminal (com o ramo interventricular anterior) da artéria coronária esquerda que corre para a esquerda e, em seguida, posteriormente no sulco coronário que irriga os ramos atrial e ventricular. SIN ramus circumflexus arteriae coronariae sinistrae [TA].

circumflex peroneal b. of posterior tibial artery, r. circunflexo fibular da artéria tibial posterior; termo oficial alternativo* para circumflex fibular b. (of posterior tibial artery) (r. circunflexo fibular (da artéria tibial posterior)).

circumflex b. of posterior tibial artery, r. circunflexo da artéria tibial posterior; termo oficial alternativo* para circumflex fibular b. (of posterior tibial artery).

clavicular b. of thoracoacromial artery [TA], r. clavicular da artéria toracoacromial; *distribuição*, músculo subclávio e articulação esternoclavicular. SIN ramus clavicularis arteriae thoracoacromialis [TA].

clivus b.'s of cerebral part of internal carotid artery [TA], ramos do clivo da parte cerebral da artéria carótida interna; pequenos ramos que se originam próximo à artéria oftálmica que passam medial e inferiormente à porção esfenoidal do clivo. SIN rami clivales partis cerebralis arteriae carotidis internae [TA].

cochlear b. of labyrinthine artery, r. coclear da artéria vestibulococlear. SIN cochlear b. of vestibulocochlear artery.

cochlear b. of vestibulocochlear artery [TA], r. coclear da artéria vestibulococlear; r. terminal (com o ramo vestibular posterior) da artéria vestibulococlear; faz anastomose com um r. da artéria coclear comum, formando a artéria espiral do modíolo; o ramo coclear supre especificamente o gânglio espiral e o ducto coclear da base da cóclea. SIN ramus cochlearis arteriae vestibulocochlearis [TA], cochlear b. of labyrinthine artery, ramus cochlearis arteriae labyrinthi.

colic b. of ileocolic artery [TA], r. cólico da artéria ileocólica; o r. do r. inferior da artéria ileocólica que passa superiormente até o colo ascendente para se comunicar com um r. da artéria cólica direita e irrigar o colo ascendente. SIN arteria ascendens (1) [TA], ascending artery (1) [TA], ramus colicus arteriae ileocolicae [TA].

collateral b. of intercostal nerves [TA], r. colateral dos nervos intercostais; r. inferior de um nervo intercostal que se origina medialmente (proximal) aos ângulos das costelas e corre no espaço intercostal ao longo da borda superior da costela abaixo, acompanhando o trajeto do nervo intercostal (ao longo da borda inferior da costela acima). SIN ramus collateralis nervorum intercostalium [TA].

collateral b.'s of posterior intercostal arteries 3-11 [TA], ramos colaterais das artérias intercostais posteriores 3-11; os ramos que se originam próximo ao ângulo da costela e descem ao longo da borda superior da costela abaixo; *distribuição*, metade inferior dos espaços intercostais 3-11; *anastomoses*, ramos colaterais das artérias intercostais anteriores. SIN ramus collateralis arteriarum intercostalium posteriorum III-XI [TA].

communicating b. [TA], r. comunicante; um feixe de fibras nervosas que passam de um nervo para se unir a outro. O termo "ramo comunicante" é utilizado no sistema nervoso para substituir o "ramo anastomosante" inadequado para os sistemas vasculares. SIN ramus communicans [TA].

communicating b. of anterior interosseous nerve with ulnar nerve [TA], r. comunicante do nervo interósseo anterior com o nervo ulnar; a conexão que ocorre ocasionalmente entre os nervos interósseo anterior e ulnar no antebraço proximal. SIN ramus communicans nervi interossei antebrachii anterioris cum nervi ulnari [TA].

communicating b.'s of auriculotemporal nerve with facial nerve [TA], ramos comunicantes do nervo auriculotemporal com o nervo facial; os ramos que conduzem fibras do nervo auriculotemporal para o nervo facial. SIN rami communicantes nervi auriculotemporalis cum nervo faciali [TA].

communicating b. of chorda tympani to lingual nerve, ramos comunicantes do nervo lingual com a corda do tímpano. SIN communicating b. of chorda tympani with lingual nerve.

communicating b. of chorda tympani with lingual nerve [TA], r. comunicante do nervo lingual com a corda do tímpano, ramo terminal da corda do tímpano que se une ao nervo lingual na fossa infratemporal; conduz as fibras sensoriais para o paladar dos dois terços anteriores da língua e as fibras parassimpáticas pré-sinápticas destinadas ao gânglio submandibular para a inervação das glândulas salivares submandibular e sublingual. SIN ramus communicans cum chorda tympani (1) [TA], communicating b. of chorda tympani to lingual nerve, ramus communicans nervi lingualis cum chorda tympani.

communicating b. of facial nerve with glossopharyngeal nerve [TA], r. comunicante do nervo facial com o nervo glossofaríngeo; um pequeno ramo do ramo digástrico do nervo facial para o nervo glossofaríngeo. SIN ramus communicans nervi facialis cum nervo glossopharyngeo [TA], Haller ansa, ramus communicans cum nervo glossopharyngeo (1).

communicating b. of facial nerve with tympanic plexus, r. comunicante do nervo intermédio com o plexo timpânico. SIN communicating b. of intermediate nerve with tympanic plexus.

communicating b. of fibular artery [TA], r. comunicante da artéria fibular; o r. comunicante da artéria fibular. SIN ramus communicans arteriae fibularis [TA], communicating b. of peroneal artery*, ramus communicans arteriae peroneae*.

communicating b. of glossopharyngeal nerve with auricular branch of vagus nerve, r. comunicante do nervo glossofaríngeo com o ramo auricular do nervo vago. SIN communicating b. of tympanic plexus with auricular branch of vagus nerve.

communicating b. of intermediate nerve with tympanic plexus [TA], r. comunicante do nervo intermédio com o plexo timpânico; um fino r. do nervo facial que se une ao ramo timpânico do nervo glossofaríngeo. SIN ramus communicans nervi intermedii cum plexu tympanico [TA], communicating b. of facial nerve with tympanic plexus, ramus communicans nervi facialis cum plexu tympanico.

communicating b. of internal laryngeal nerve with recurrent laryngeal nerve [TA], r. comunicante do ramo interno do nervo laríngeo superior com o nervo laríngeo recorrente; r. do ramo interno do nervo laríngeo superior que se comunica com o nervo laríngeo recorrente na parede da laringofaringe, fornecendo as fibras sensoriais para esta. SIN ramus communicans nervi laryngei interni cum nervo laryngeo recurrent [TA], communicating b. of superior laryngeal nerve with recurrent laryngeal nerve, Galen anastomosis, Galen nerve, ramus communicans nervi laryngei recurrentis cum ramo laryngeo interno, ramus communicans nervi laryngei superioris cum nervo laryngeo recurrenti.

communicating b. of lacrimal nerve with zygomatic nerve [TA], r. comunicante do nervo lacrimal com o nervo zigomático; o r. nervoso pelo qual as fibras parassimpáticas pós-sinápticas (secretomotoras) do gânglio pterigopalatino são transferidas do nervo zigomático para o nervo lacrimal (daí por diante, puramente sensorial) para distribuição para a glândula lacrimal. SIN ramus communicans nervi lacrimalis cum nervo zygomatico [TA].

communicating b.'s of lingual nerve with hypoglossal nerve [TA], ramos comunicantes do nervo lingual com o nervo hipoglosso; os ramos comunicantes entre o nervo lingual (do nervo mandibular) e do nervo hipoglosso que formam um plexo no músculo hipoglosso. SIN rami communicantes nervi lingualis cum nervo hypoglosso [TA].

communicating b. of median nerve with ulnar nerve [TA], r. comunicante do nervo mediano com o nervo ulnar; o r. do nervo mediano que se une ao nervo ulnar na mão; o r. interósseo anterior do nervo mediano também pode comunicar-se com o nervo ulnar na porção proximal do antebraço. SIN ramus communicans nervi mediani cum nervo ulnari.

communicating b. of nasociliary nerve with ciliary ganglion, raiz sensitiva do gânglio ciliar. SIN sensory root of ciliary ganglion.

communicating b. of otic ganglion to auriculotemporal nerve, r. comunicante do gânglio ótico com o nervo auriculotemporal; um r. do gânglio ótico que se une às raízes do nervo auriculotemporal para conduzir as fibras parassimpáticas pós-sinápticas para a glândula parótida. SIN ramus communicans ganglii otici cum nervo auriculotemporali.

communicating b. of otic ganglion to chorda tympani, r. comunicante do gânglio ótico com a corda do tímpano. SIN communicating b. of otic ganglion with chorda tympani.

communicating b. of otic ganglion with chorda tympani, r. comunicante do gânglio ótico com a corda do tímpano; um pequeno r. do gânglio auditivo que conduz as fibras sensoriais para a corda do tímpano. SIN ramus communicans cum chorda tympani (2) [TA], communicating b. of otic ganglion to chorda tympani, ramus communicans ganglii otic cum chorda tympani.

communicating b. of otic ganglion with medial pterygoid nerve, r. comunicante do gânglio ótico com o nervo pterigóideo medial; r. do gânglio ótico que se une ao nervo para o músculo pterigóideo medial. SIN ramus communicans ganglii otici cum nervo pterygoideo mediali.

communicating b. of otic ganglion with meningeal branch of mandibular nerve, r. comunicante do gânglio ótico com o ramo meníngeo do nervo mandibular; um r. do gânglio ótico com o ramo meníngeo do nervo mandibular para conduzir as fibras parassimpáticas pós-sinápticas que correm para trás até o tronco principal do nervo mandibular para distribuição para a glândula parótida por meio do nervo auriculotemporal. SIN ramus communicans ganglii otici cum ramo meningeo nervi mandibularis.

communicating b. of peroneal artery, r. comunicante da artéria fibular; termo oficial alternativo* para communicating b. of fibular artery.

communicating b. of radial nerve with ulnar nerve [TA], r. comunicante do nervo radial com o nervo ulnar; a conexão entre o r. superficial do nervo radial e o r. dorsal do nervo ulnar no dorso da mão. SIN ramus communicans nervi radialis cum nervi ulnari [TA].

communicating b.'s of spinal nerves, ramos comunicantes brancos do tronco simpático. SIN white rami communicantes, em ramus.

communicating b. of superficial radial nerve with ulnar nerve, r. comunicante do ramo superficial do nervo radial com o nervo ulnar; o r. comunicante ulnar do r. superficial do nervo radial, unindo o ramo dorsal do nervo ulnar na mão, transportando a sensibilidade da face dorsal dos lados adjacentes dos dedos médio e anelar. SIN ramus communicans ulnaris nervi radialis, ulnar communicating b. of superficial radial nerve.

communicating b. of superior laryngeal nerve with recurrent laryngeal nerve, r. comunicante do nervo laríngeo superior com o nervo laríngeo recorrente. SIN communicating b. of internal laryngeal nerve with recurrent laryngeal nerve.

communicating b.'s of sympathetic trunk, ramos comunicantes cinzentos do tronco simpático. SIN gray rami communicantes, em ramus:

communicating b. of tympanic plexus with auricular branch of vagus nerve [TA], r. comunicante do nervo glossofaríngeo com o ramo auricular do nervo vago; pequeno r. do nervo glossofaríngeo que une o r. auricular do nervo vago, conduzindo as fibras táteis. SIN ramus communicans plexus tympanici cum ramo auriculari nervi vagi [TA], communicating b. of glossopharyngeal nerve with auricular branch of vagus nerve, ramus communicans cum nervo glossopharyngeo (2), ramus communicans nervi glossopharyngei cum auriculari nervi vagi.

cricothyroid b. of superior thyroid artery [TA], r. cricotireóideo da artéria tireóidea superior; pequeno ramo da artéria tireóidea superior que irriga o músculo cricotireóideo. SIN cricothyroid artery, ramus cricothyroideus (arteriae thyroideae superioris).

cutaneous b. of anterior branch of obturator nerve [TA], r. cutâneo do ramo anterior do nervo obturatório; r. do ramo anterior do nervo obturatório que inerva a pele da porção medial da coxa acima do joelho. SIN ramus cutaneus rami anterioris nervi obturatorii [TA], cutaneous b. of obturator nerve.

cutaneous b. of mixed nerve [TA], r. cutâneo de nervos mistos; r. de um nervo espinal misto (ou seus derivados) que inervam a pele; esses ramos conduziriam a maior parte da inervação sensorial somática, mas também fibras motoras viscerais (fibras simpáticas pós-sinápticas para a vasomovimentação e pilomovimentação). SIN ramus cutaneus nervi mixti [TA].

cutaneous b. of obturator nerve, r. cutâneo do ramo anterior do nervo obturatório. SIN cutaneous b. of anterior branch of obturator nerve.

deep b. [TA], r. profundo; o r. que passa profundamente, abaixo ou mais distante da superfície; usualmente em contraste com um r. superficial. SIN ramus profundus [TA].

deep b. of the lateral plantar nerve [TA], r. profundo do nervo plantar lateral; r. motor do nervo plantar lateral que inerva os músculos lumbricais 2–4, interósseos plantares e dorsais e adutor do hálux. SIN ramus profundus nervi plantaris lateralis [TA].

deep b. of medial circumflex femoral artery [TA], r. profundo da artéria circunflexa femoral medial; distribuído para a face posterior da cabeça e colo do fêmur. SIN ramus profundus arteriae circumflexae femoris medialis [TA].

deep b. of medial plantar artery [TA], r. profundo da artéria plantar medial; o r. que corre profundamente ao adutor do hálux, irrigando-o e ao músculo flexor curto do hálux, profundamente à artéria e à pele do lado medial da parte distal do pé. SIN ramus profundus arteriae plantaris medialis [TA].

deep palmar b. of ulnar artery [TA], r. palmar profundo da artéria ulnar; o r. da artéria ulnar que nutre os músculos hipotenares, dirigindo-se em seguida profundamente para dentro da palma até os tendões dos flexores e se anastomosando com o arco palmar profundo, oriundo da artéria radial. SIN ramus palmaris profundus arteriae ulnaris [TA].

deep plantar b. of dorsalis pedis artery, artéria plantar profunda. SIN deep plantar *artery.* SIN arteria plantaris profundus [TA].

deep b. of radial nerve [TA], r. profundo do nervo radial; origina-se na fossa cubital (com o ramo superficial) como terminação do nervo radial (comum); perfura o músculo supinador, inervando-o e a outros músculos extensores do antebraço. Sua porção terminal é o nervo interósseo posterior, que faz trajeto sobre a membrana interóssea no terço distal do antebraço. VER TAMBÉM posterior interosseous *nerve.* VER ramus profundus nervi radialis [TA].

deep b. of the superior gluteal artery [TA], r. profundo da artéria glútea superior; r. da artéria glútea superior que se estende lateralmente, entre os músculos glúteos médio e mínimo, acompanhando o nervo glúteo superior. SIN ramus profundus arteriae gluteae superioris [TA].

deep b. of transverse cervical artery, artéria dorsal da escápula. SIN dorsal scapular *artery.*

deep b. of the ulnar nerve [TA], r. profundo do nervo ulnar; acompanha o r. palmar profundo da artéria ulnar e o arco palmar profundo para inervar a articulação do punho, os músculos lumbricais 3 e 4, os interósseos palmar e dorsal, o adutor do polegar e a porção profunda do flexor curto do polegar. SIN ramus profundus nervi ulnaris [TA].

deltoid b. [TA], r. deltóideo; os ramos relacionados ao músculo deltóide. A Terminologia Anatômica lista os ramos deltóideos: 1) da artéria tóraco-acromial (ramo deltóideo da artéria tóraco-acromial [TA]); 2) da artéria braquial profunda (ramo deltóideo da artéria braquial profunda [TA]). SIN ramus deltoideus [TA].

dental b.'s [TA], ramos dentais; ramos para os dentes. A Terminologia Anatômica lista os ramos dentais: 1) artéria alveolar superior anterior (ramos dentais da artéria alveolar superior anterior [TA]); 2) da artéria alveolar inferior (ramos dentais da artéria alveolar inferior [TA]); 3) artéria alveolar superior posterior (ramos dentais da artéria alveolar superior posterior [TA]). SIN rami dentales [TA], dental rami.

descending b. [TA], r. descendente; o r. de uma artéria ou nervo que passa inferiormente. Os ramos descendentes já descritos são: (1) r. descendente do nervo hipoglosso, raiz superior da alça cervical; (2) r. descendente da artéria circunflexa femoral lateral; (3) r. descendente da artéria occipital. SIN ramus descendens [TA].

descending anterior b., r. descendente da artéria segmentar anterior dos pulmões direito e esquerdo. SIN descending b. of anterior segmental artery of left and right lungs.

descending b. of anterior segmental artery of left and right lungs [TA], r. descendente da artéria segmentar anterior dos pulmões esquerdo e direito; o r. descendente anterior das artérias lobares superiores das artérias pulmonares direita e esquerda. SIN ramus descendens arteriae segmentalis anterioris pulmonis dextri et sinistri [TA], descending anterior b., ramus anterior descendens.

descending b. of hypoglossal nerve, raiz superior da alça cervical. SIN superior *root* of ansa cervicalis.

descending b. of lateral circumflex femoral artery [TA], r. descendente da artéria circunflexa femoral lateral; um r. importante da artéria circunflexa femoral lateral que acompanha o nervo para o músculo vasto lateral ao longo da margem anterior daquele músculo e predominantemente ao músculo reto femoral, irrigando os dois músculos. *Anastomoses*: com a artéria genicular superior lateral, i.e., ela contribui para a rede articular do joelho. SIN ramus descendens arteriae circumflexae femoris lateralis [TA].

descending b. of medial circumflex femoral artery [TA], r. descendente da artéria circunflexa femoral medial; a grande artéria que passa profundamente ao músculo reto femoral, acompanhando o r. muscular do nervo femoral para o músculo vasto lateral; termina por se anastomosar com a artéria genicular superior lateral. SIN ramus descendens arteriae circumflexae femoris medialis [TA].

descending b. of occipital artery [TA], r. descendente da artéria occipital; *origem*, artéria occipital no sulco occipital; *distribuição*: músculos posteriores do pescoço e músculo trapézio do pescoço; *anastomoses*: artérias cervicais superficiais e profundas, artéria vertebral. SIN ramus descendens arteriae occipitalis [TA], princeps cervicis artery, princeps cervicis.

descending posterior b., r. descendente da artéria segmentar posterior dos pulmões direito e esquerdo. SIN descending b. of posterior segmental artery of left and right lungs.

descending b. of posterior segmental artery of left and right lungs [TA], r. descendente da artéria segmentar posterior dos pulmões esquerdo e direito; o r. descendente das artérias lobares superiores das artérias pulmonares esquerda e direita. SIN ramus descendens arteriae segmentalis posterioris pulmonis dextri et sinistri [TA], descending posterior b., ramus posterior descendens.

descending b. of superficial cervical artery [TA], r. descendente do ramo superficial da artéria cervical transversa; r. descendente do r. superficial da artéria cervical transversa que passa inferiormente com o nervo acessório, profundamente às porções média e inferior do músculo trapézio, as quais ele nutre. SIN ramus descendens rami superficialis arteriae transversae cervicis [TA].

digastric b. of facial nerve [TA], r. digástrico do nervo facial; r. do nervo facial que inerva o ventre posterior do músculo digástrico. SIN ramus digastricus nervi facialis [TA].

dorsal b., r. dorsal ou posterior. (1) SIN posterior *ramus* of spinal nerve; (2) ramo com orientação posterior.

dorsal carpal b. of radial artery [TA], r. carpal dorsal da artéria radial; r. da artéria radial que passa para a parte posterior do punho para se unir à rede carpal dorsal. SIN ramus carpalis dorsalis arteriae radialis [TA], ramus carpeus dorsalis arteriae radialis.

dorsal carpal b. of ulnar artery [TA], r. carpal dorsal da artéria ulnar; r. da artéria ulnar que passa para o lado dorsal do carpo para entrar na rede carpal dorsal. SIN ramus carpalis dorsalis arteriae ulnaris [TA], ramus carpeus dorsalis arteriae ulnaris.

dorsal b.'s of first and second posterior intercostal artery [TA], ramos dorsais da primeira e segunda artérias intercostais posteriores; os ramos da 1.ª e 2.ª artérias intercostais posteriores que se originam como ramos da artéria intercostal suprema. A distribuição é idêntica à dos ramos dorsais das outras artérias intercostais posteriores no nível vertebral T1-T2. SIN rami dorsales arteriarum intercostalium posteriorum primae et secundae [TA], dorsal b.'s of the superior intercostal artery, rami dorsales arteriae intercostalis supremae.

dorsal lingual b.'s of lingual artery [TA], ramos dorsais da língua da artéria lingual; os ramos da artéria lingual para o terço posterior ou raiz da língua. SIN rami dorsales linguae arteriae lingualis [TA].

dorsal b. of the lumbar artery [TA], r. dorsal das artérias lombares; r. terminal (com o r. ventral) das artérias lombares 4-5, distribuídos para a porção lombar do dorso, coluna vertebral posterior e medula espinal. SIN ramus dorsalis arteriae lumbalis [TA].

dorsal b. of posterior intercostal arteries 3-11 [TA], r. dorsal das artérias intercostais posteriores 3-11; r. terminal (com o r. ventral) da 3.ª a 11.ª artérias intercostais posteriores, distribuídos para a porção torácica da coluna vertebral posterior, medula espinal e vizinhanças. SIN ramus dorsalis arteriarum intercostalium posteriorum III-XI [TA].

dorsal b. of the posterior intercostal veins 4-11 [TA], r. dorsal das veias intercostais posteriores; principal tributária da 4.ª a 11.ª veias intercostais posteriores; a área drenada é idêntica àquela suprida pelo r. dorsal das artérias intercostais posteriores. SIN ramus dorsalis venarum intercostalium posteriorum IV-XI [TA].

dorsal b. of the subcostal artery, r. dorsal da artéria subcostal; r. terminal (com o r. ventral) da artéria subcostal, distribuído para a coluna vertebral posterior, a medula espinal e vizinhanças e o dorso no nível vertebral T12-L1. SIN ramus dorsales arteriae subcostalis [TA], rami dorsales arteriae subcostalis.

dorsal b. of the subcostal artery [TA], r. dorsal da artéria subcostal; r. da artéria subcostal que nutre os músculos das costas e a pele suprajacente, imediatamente abaixo do nível da 12.ª costela.

dorsal b.'s of the superior intercostal artery, ramos dorsais da primeira e segunda artérias intercostais posteriores. SIN dorsal b.'s of first and second posterior intercostal artery.

dorsal b. of the ulnar nerve [TA], r. dorsal do nervo ulnar; r. que se origina do nervo ulnar proximal ao punho para distribuição para o lado medial do dorso da mão e porção proximal do dedo mínimo e lado medial do dedo anelar. SIN rami dorsales nervi ulnaris [TA].

duodenal b.'s of anterior superior pancreaticoduodenal artery [TA], ramos duodenais da artéria pancreaticoduodenal superior anterior; os ramos que se estendem para o duodeno a partir da arcada arterial anterior à cabeça do pâncreas na concavidade do duodeno. SIN rami duodenales arteriae pancreaticoduodenalis superioris anterioris [TA].

duodenal b.'s of posterior superior pancreaticoduodenal artery [TA], ramos duodenais da artéria pancreaticoduodenal superior posterior; os ramos que se estendem para o duodeno a partir da arcada arterial que se localiza posterior à cabeça do pâncreas na concavidade do duodeno.

epiploic b.'s, ramos epiplóicos. SIN omental b.'s.

esophageal b.'s [TA], ramos esofágicos; os ramos para o esôfago. SIN rami esophagei [TA], rami esophageales*.

esophageal b.'s of inferior thyroid artery [TA], ramos esofágicos da artéria tireóidea inferior; *distribuição*: quarto superior do esôfago; *anastomoses*: ramos esofágicos da aorta torácica. SIN rami esophageales arteriae thyroideae inferioris [TA].

esophageal b.'s of left gastric artery [TA], ramos esofágicos da artéria gástrica esquerda; ascende através do hiato esofágico do diafragma para nutrir a parte mais inferior (cárdica) do esôfago; *anastomoses*: ramos esofágicos da aorta torácica. SIN rami esophageales arteriae gastricae sinistrae [TA].

esophageal b.'s of the recurrent laryngeal nerve [TA], ramos esofágicos do nervo laríngeo recorrente; fornecem as fibras motoras e sensoriais para o esôfago cervical no lado direito e para as porções cervical e torácica superior à esquerda. SIN rami esophagei nervi laryngei recurrentis [TA].

esophageal b.'s of the thoracic aorta [TA], ramos esofágicos da parte torácica da aorta; ramos que se originam diretamente da face anterior da porção torácica da aorta adjacente ao esôfago, através dos quais a maior parte do esôfago é nutrida. SIN rami esophageales partis thoracicae aortae [TA], rami esophageales aortae thoracicae*.

esophageal b.'s of thoracic ganglia [TA], ramos esofágicos dos gânglios torácicos; os nervos esplâncnicos que conduzem as fibras aferentes viscerais e simpáticas pós-sinápticas oriundas dos gânglios paravertebrais torácicos superiores dos troncos simpáticos para o plexo esofágico dos nervos. SIN rami esophageales gangliorum thoracicorum [TA].

esophageal b.'s of the vagus nerve [TA], ramos esofágicos do nervo vago; incluem ambos os ramos que passam diretamente do vago e os ramos originários dos nervos laríngeos recorrentes que formam o plexo nervoso esofágico, o qual circunda o esôfago, inervando-o e às porções adjacentes do pericárdio. VER TAMBÉM esophageal (nervous) *plexus*. SIN rami esophagei nervi vagi.

external nasal b.'s of infraorbital nerve [TA], ramos nasais externos do nervo infra-orbital; ramos para a face externa do nariz. Existem: 1) nervo infra-orbital, ramos nasais externos do nervo infra-orbital [TA], 2) nervo nasociliar, ramos nasais externos do nervo etmoidal anterior [TA]. SIN rami nasales externi nervi infraorbitalis.

external b. of superior laryngeal nerve [TA], r. externo do nervo laríngeo superior; r. terminal do nervo laríngeo superior (com o nervo laríngeo interno) que fornece a inervação motora para o músculo cricotireóideo. SIN ramus externus nervi laryngei superioris [TA].

external b. of trunk of accessory nerve [TA], r. externo do tronco do nervo acessório; porção do tronco do nervo acessório que sai independentemente do forame jugular, comportando fibras da raiz espinal do nervo acessório para os músculos esternoclidomastóideo e trapézio. SIN ramus externus trunci nervi accessorii [TA].

faucial b.'s of lingual nerve, ramos para o istmo das fauces do nervo lingual. SIN b.'s of lingual nerve to isthmus of fauces.

femoral b. of genitofemoral nerve [TA], r. femoral do nervo genitofemoral; r. do nervo genitofemoral distribuído para a pele da porção mais superior da região anterior da coxa. SIN ramus femoralis nervi genitofemoralis [TA].

frontal b. of middle meningeal artery [TA], r. frontal da artéria meníngea média; o r. anterior e terminal maior (com o r. parietal) da artéria meníngea média; corre na profundidade do sulco ósseo, freqüentemente perfurando o osso em sua porção mais lateral do crista esfenoidal, nutrindo a porção anterior da dura-máter lateral e superior e do crânio. SIN ramus frontalis arteriae meningeae mediae [TA].

frontal b. of superficial temporal artery [TA], r. frontal da artéria temporal superficial (com r. parietal) que nutre a porção ântero-lateral do couro cabeludo e a musculatura subjacente, o periósteo e a tábua externa do crânio; *anastomose*: através da linha média com o congênere contralateral; artérias supratrocleares e supra-orbital. SIN ramus frontalis arteriae temporalis superficialis [TA].

ganglionic b. of internal carotid artery, r. ganglionar da artéria carótida interna. SIN b.'s of internal carotid artery to trigeminal ganglion.

ganglionic b.'s of lingual nerve, ramos do nervo lingual para o gânglio submandibular. SIN sensory root of submandibular ganglion.

ganglionic b.'s of lingual nerve to sublingual ganglion, ramos do nervo lingual para o gânglio sublingual; termo oficial alternativo* para sensory root of sublingual ganglion.

ganglionic b.'s of lingual nerve to submandibular ganglion, ramos do nervo lingual para o gânglio submandibular; termo oficial alternativo* para sensory root of sublingual ganglion.

ganglionic b.'s of maxillary nerve, raiz sensorial do gânglio pterigopalatino. SIN sensory root of pterygopalatine ganglion.

ganglionic b.'s of maxillary nerve to pterygopalatine ganglion, raiz sensorial do gânglio pterigopalatino; termo oficial alternativo* para sensory root of pterygopalatine ganglion.

gastric b.'s of anterior vagal trunk, ramos gástricos anteriores do tronco vagal anterior. SIN anterior gastric b.'s of anterior vagal trunk.

gastric b.'s of posterior vagal b., ramos gástricos do r. vagal posterior; os ramos gástricos posteriores; os ramos do tronco vagal posterior para a superfície posterior do estômago. SIN rami gastrici posteriores nervi vagi.

genital b. of genitofemoral nerve [TA], r. genital do nervo genitofemoral; r. do nervo genitofemoral distribuído para a pele da parte anterior da bolsa escrotal (masculino) ou lábios maiores do pudendo (feminino) e para a porção adjacente da coxa, fornecendo um r. motor para o músculo cremaster. Usualmente passa através do anel e canal inguinal profundo. SIN ramus genitalis nervi genitofemoralis [TA], external spermatic nerve, nervus spermaticus externus.

genital b. of iliohypogastric nerve, r. cutâneo anterior do nervo iliohipogástrico. SIN anterior cutaneous b. of iliohypogastric nerve.

glandular b.'s [TA], ramos glandulares; os ramos distribuídos para as glândulas. SIN rami glandulares [TA].

glandular b.'s of facial artery [TA], ramos glandulares da artéria facial; ramos da artéria facial para a glândula submandibular. SIN rami glandulares arteriae facialis [TA].

glandular b.'s of inferior thyroid artery [TA], ramos glandulares da artéria tireóidea inferior; os ramos da artéria tireóidea inferior para as glândulas tireóide e paratireóides, anastomosando-se com ramos da artéria tireóide superior. SIN rami glandulares arteriae thyroideae inferioris [TA].

glandular b.'s of submandibular ganglion, raiz sensitiva do gânglio submandibular; os ramos do gânglio submandibular que conduzem as fibras parassimpáticas pós-sinápticas para as glândulas submandibular e sublingual. SIN rami ganglii submandibularis, rami glandulares ganglii submandibularis.

b. of glossopharyngeal nerve to stylopharyngeus muscle, r. do nervo glossofaríngeo para o músculo estilofaríngeo. SIN stylopharingeal b. of glossopharyngeal nerve.

hepatic b.'s of anterior vagal trunk, ramos hepáticos do tronco vagal anterior; ramos dos troncos vagais anterior e posterior distribuídos para o fígado. SIN rami hepatici trunci vagi anterior [TA], hepatic b.'s of vagus nerve, rami hepatici nervi vagi.

hepatic b.'s of vagus nerve, ramos hepáticos do nervo vago. SIN hepatic b.'s of anterior vagal trunk.

iliac b. of iliolumbar artery, r. ilíaco da artéria iliolumbar. SIN iliacus b. of iliolumbar artery.

iliacus b. of iliolumbar artery [TA], r. ilíaco da artéria iliolumbar; r. terminal da artéria iliolumbar (com o r. lombar) distribuído para a fossa ilíaca para nutrir os músculos ilíaco, ílio e porções dos músculos que se inserem na crista ilíaca. SIN ramus iliacus arteriae iliolumbalis [TA], iliac b. of iliolumbar artery.

inferior b. [TA], r. inferior; r. dirigido para baixo (caudalmente) ou posicionado muito baixo, geralmente em contraste com outro r. (r. superior) direcionado para cima (rostralmente) ou com posição alta. SIN ramus inferior [TA].

inferior cervical cardiac b.'s of vagus nerve, ramos cardíacos cervicais inferiores do nervo vago; o mais inferior dos ramos cervicais do nervo vago que conduz as fibras parassimpáticas pré-sinápticas para, e as fibras aferentes reflexas de, o plexo cardíaco; ramificações dos vagos na raiz do pescoço. SIN rami cardiaci cervicales inferiores nervi vagi. [TA].

inferior dental b.'s of inferior dental plexus [TA], ramos dentários inferiores do plexo dental inferior; os ramos que fazem trajeto do plexo dentário inferior até as raízes dos dentes da mandíbula. SIN rami dentales inferiores plexus dentalis inferioris [TA], rami dentales inferiores [TA], inferior dental rami.

inferior gingival b.'s of inferior dental plexus [TA], ramos gengivais inferiores do plexo dental inferior; os ramos do plexo dentário inferior para a gengiva da mandíbula. SIN rami gingivales inferiores plexus dentalis inferioris [TA].

inferior labial b. of facial artery [TA], r. labial inferior da artéria facial; *origem*, facial; *distribuição*: estruturas do lábio inferior; *anastomoses*, as artérias do lado oposto, mentual e sublabial. SIN arteria labialis inferior, inferior labial artery, ramus labialis inferior arteriae facialis.

inferior labial b.'s of mental nerve, ramos labiais do nervo mentual. SIN labial b.'s of mental nerve.

inferior lingular b. of lingular branch of left pulmonary artery, artéria lingular inferior. SIN inferior lingular *artery*.

inferior b. of oculomotor nerve [TA], r. inferior do nervo oculomotor; o r. do nervo oculomotor que fornece os ramos motores para os músculos retos medial e inferior e oblíquo inferior e conduz fibras parassimpáticas pré-sinápticas que passam para o gânglio ciliar através da raiz parassimpática. SIN ramus inferior nervi oculomotorii [TA].

inferior b. of pubic bone, r. inferior do púbis; termo obsoleto para inferior pubic *ramus*.

inferior b. of superior gluteal artery [TA], r. inferior da artéria glútea superior; *distribuição*: músculos glúteo médio e mínimo; *anastomose*: lateral circumflex femoral artery. SIN ramus inferior arteriae gluteae superioris [TA].

inferior b.'s of transverse cervical nerve [TA], ramos inferiores do nervo cervical transverso; r. do nervo cervical transverso que fornece a inervação cutânea na parte inferior do triângulo anterior do pescoço. SIN rami inferiores nervi transversi colli*, rami inferiores nervi transversi cervicalis [colli].

infrahyoid b. of superior thyroid artery [TA], r. infra-hióideo da artéria tireóidea superior; pequeno ramo a partir da parte inicial da artéria tireóidea superior que corre ao longo do osso hióide profundamente ao músculo tireohióideo para se anastomosar com seu congênere contralateral. SIN ramus infrahyoideus arteriae thyroideae superioris [TA].

infrapatellar b. of saphenous nerve [TA], r. infrapatelar do nervo safeno; r. do nervo safeno que inerva a pele acima e abaixo da patela. SIN ramus infrapatellaris nervi sapheni [TA].

inguinal b.'s of deep external pudendal arteries [TA], ramos inguinais das artérias pudendas externas profundas; ramos para a região inguinal que podem se originar como ramos das artérias pudendas externas ou como ramos diretos da artéria femoral. Nutrem a pele e os tecidos subcutâneos, incluindo os linfonodos inguinais. SIN rami inguinales arteriarum pudendarum externarum profundarum [TA].

interganglionic b.'s of sympathetic trunk [TA], ramos interganglionares do tronco simpático; os filamentos nervosos que interligam os gânglios do tronco simpático; consistem em fibras pré- ou pós-ganglionares que se dirigem para os níveis superiores ou inferiores do tronco. SIN rami interganglionares trunci sympathici [TA].

intermediate atrial b. of left coronary artery [TA], r. atrial intermédio da artéria coronária esquerda; r. que se origina do r. circunflexo da artéria coronária esquerda entre os ramos anteriores (distribuídos para o átrio esquerdo) e o tronco dos ramos atriais posteriores. SIN ramus atrialis intermedius arteriae coronariae sinistrae [TA], lateral atrial b. of left coronary artery.

intermediate atrial b. of right coronary artery [TA], r. atrial intermédio da artéria coronária direita [TA]; origina-se da face superior da artéria coronária direita ou logo depois que ela cruza a margem direita do coração; nutre a parede póstero-lateral (porção do sulco/crista terminal) do átrio direito. SIN ramus atrialis intermedius arteriae coronariae dextrae [TA], lateral atrial b. of right coronary artery, marginal atrial b. of right coronary artery, right atrial b. of right coronary artery.

intermediate b. of hepatic artery proper [TA], r. intermediário da artéria hepática própria; o menor e mais central dos geralmente três ramos intra-hepáticos principais da artéria hepática; serve principalmente o segmento mediano (IV) do fígado. SIN ramus intermedius arteriae hepaticae propriae [TA].

intermediate temporal b.'s of lateral occipital artery [TA], ramos temporais médios da artéria occipital lateral; o ramo médio dos três ramos temporais da artéria occipital lateral (a partir da artéria cerebral posterior) distribuído para as faces medial e inferior do lobo temporal do cérebro. SIN rami temporales intermedii arteriae occipitalis lateralis [TA], middle temporal b.'s of lateral occipital artery✫, rami temporales medii arteriae occipitalis lateralis✫.

intermediomedial frontal b. of callosomarginal artery [TA], r. frontal intermédio-medial da artéria calosomarginal; o r. da porção média da artéria calosomarginal para a porção ântero-superior da face medial do lobo frontal do cérebro. SIN ramus frontalis intermediomedialis arteriae callosomarginalis [TA].

b.'s of internal carotid artery to trigeminal ganglion [TA], ramos ganglionares trigeminais da artéria carótida interna; r. para o gânglio trigêmeo; um pequeno r. da parte cavernosa da artéria carótida interna para o gânglio trigêmeo. SIN ramus ganglionares trigeminales arteriae carotidis internae [TA], ganglionic b. of internal carotid artery, ramus ganglii trigeminalis.

internal nasal b.'s [TA], ramos nasais internos; ramos para a cavidade nasal. Ramos nasais internos de 1) nervo infra-orbital (ramos nasais internos dos nervos infra-orbitais [NA]); 2) nervo etmoidal anterior (ramos nasais internos do nervo etmoidal anterior [NA]). SIN rami nasales interni [TA].

internal b. of superior laryngeal nerve [TA], r. interno do nervo laríngeo superior; r. terminal do nervo laríngeo superior (com o r. externo) que conduz as fibras sensoriais para a laringe supraglótica. SIN ramus internus nervi laryngei superioris [TA].

b.'s to internal capsule, genu [TA], ramos do joelho da cápsula interna. SIN rami capsulae internae, em ramus.

b.'s to internal capsule, posterior limb [TA], ramos do ramo posterior da cápsula interna. SIN rami capsulae internae, em ramus.

b.'s to internal capsule, retrolentiform limb, ramos da parte retrolentiforme da cápsula interna. SIN rami capsulae internae, em ramus.

internal b. of trunk of accessory nerve [TA], r. interno do tronco do nervo acessório; r. do tronco do nervo acessório que conduz fibras desde a raiz craniana e que se unem ao nervo vago no forame jugular. VER TAMBÉM accessory nerve [CN XI]. SIN ramus internus trunei nervi acesssorii [TA], internal ramus of accessory nerve.

interventricular septal b.'s of left/right coronary artery, ramos interventriculares septais das artérias coronárias esquerda/direita; os ramos interventriculares septais; os ramos das artérias interventriculares anterior e posterior distribuídos para o músculo do septo interventricular. SIN rami interventriculares septales arteriae coronariae sinistrae/dextrae, rami interventriculares septales, septal b.'s.

joint b.'s, ramos articulares. SIN articular b.'s.

labial b.'s of mental nerve, ramos labiais do nervo mentual; ramos do nervo mentual para o lábio inferior. SIN rami labiales nervi mentalis [TA], inferior labial b.'s of mental nerve, rami labiales inferiores nervi mentalis.

laryngopharyngeal b.'s of superior cervical ganglion [TA], ramos laringofaríngeos do gânglio cervical superior; ramos que conduzem fibras simpáticas pós-ganglionares do gânglio cervical superior para o plexo faríngeo. SIN rami laryngopharyngei ganglii cervicalis superioris [TA].

lateral b.'s [TA], ramos laterais; ramos direcionados para longe da linha média, para o lado. A Terminologia Anatômica lista os ramos laterais: 1) do ramo interventricular anterior da artéria coronária esquerda (ramus lateralis interventricularis anterioris arteriae coronariae sinistrae [TA]); 2) das artérias centrais ântero-laterais (rami laterales arteriarum centralium anterolateralium [TA]); 3) dos ramos posteriores primários dos nervos espinais cervicais/torácicos/lombares/sacrais/coccígeos (rami laterales ramorum posteriorum nervorum cervicalium/thoracalium/lumbalium/sacralium/coccygeum); 4) da parte umbilical do r. esquerdo da veia porta do fígado (rami laterales partis umbilici rami sinistri venae portae hepatis [TA]); 5) do ducto hepático esquerdo (ramus lateralis ductus hepatici sinistri [TA]); 6) da artéria lobar média (do pulmão direito) (ramus lateralis arteriae lobaris mediae (pulmonis dextrum) [TA]); 7) do nervo supra-orbital (ramus lateralis nervi supraorbitalis [TA]). SIN rami laterales [TA].

lateral abdominal/pectoral cutaneous b.'s of intercostal nerves, ramos cutâneos peitorais/abdominais laterais dos nervos intercostais; ramos que se originam aproximadamente na linha axilar anterior no nível do segundo ao sexto espaços intercostais. SIN lateral cutaneous b.'s of intercostal nerves, lateral cutaneous b.'s of ventral primary ramus of thoracic spinal nerves, ramus cutaneus lateralis abdominalis/pectoralis nervorum intercostalium.

lateral b.'s of artery of tuber cinereum [TA], ramos laterais da artéria do túber cinéreo; ramos que se originam da face lateral da artéria do túber cinéreo. VER TAMBÉM artery of tuber cinereum. SIN rami laterales arteriarum tuberis cinerei [TA].

lateral atrial b. of left coronary artery, r. atrial intermédio da artéria coronária esquerda. SIN intermediate atrial b. of left coronary artery.

lateral atrial b. of right coronary artery, r. atrial intermédio da artéria coronária direita. SIN intermediate atrial b. of right coronary artery.

lateral basal b., artéria segmentar basilar lateral. SIN lateral basal segmental artery.

lateral calcaneal b.'s of sural nerve [TA], ramos calcâneos laterais do nervo sural; ramos do nervo sural responsáveis pela inervação cutânea da face posterior da parte distal da perna e face lateral da porção proximal do pé. SIN rami calcanei laterales nervi suralis [TA].

lateral costal b. of internal thoracic artery [TA], r. costal lateral da artéria torácica interna; r. variável da artéria torácica interna que corre lateralmente e em paralelo à artéria torácica interna sobre a superfície profunda do gradil costal; anastomose: artérias intercostais posteriores. SIN ramus costalis lateralis arteriae thoracicae internae [TA].

lateral cutaneous b. [TA], r. cutâneo lateral; ramos cutâneos laterais: 1) do nervo ílio-hipogástrico (ramus cutaneus lateralis nervi iliohypogastrici [TA]); 2) do ramo dorsal das artérias intercostais posteriores (ramus cutaneus lateralis ramorum posteriorum arterieae intercostalium [TA]); 3) artéria intercostal posterior (ramus cutaneus lateralis arteriae intercostales posteriores [TA]). SIN ramus cutaneus lateralis [TA].

lateral cutaneous b.'s of intercostal nerves, ramos cutâneos peitoral/abdominal laterais dos nervos intercostais. SIN lateral abdominal/pectoral cutaneous b.'s of intercostal nerves.

lateral cutaneous b.'s of ventral primary ramus of thoracic spinal nerves, ramos cutâneos peitoral/abdominal laterais dos nervos intercostais. SIN lateral abdominal/pectoral cutaneous b.'s of intercostal nerves.

lateral malleolar b. (of fibular peroneal artery) [TA], ramos maleolares laterais (da artéria fibular). SIN rami malleolares laterales arteriae fibularis (peronei) [TA], arteriae malleolares posteriores laterales, lateral malleolar arteries, posterior peroneal arteries.

lateral mammary b.'s, ramos mamários laterais; ramos principalmente distribuídos para a porção lateral da mama. SIN rami mammarii laterales.

lateral mammary b.'s of lateral cutaneous branches of intercostal nerves, ramos mamários laterais dos ramos cutâneos laterais dos nervos intercostais. SIN lateral mammary b.'s of lateral cutaneous branches of thoracic spinal nerves.

lateral mammary b.'s of lateral cutaneous branches of thoracic spinal nerves, ramos mamários laterais dos ramos cutâneos laterais dos nervos intercostais; ramos que se originam dos ramos cutâneos laterais dos ramos ventrais primários dos nervos espinais (nervos intercostais) T-3 a T-6, os quais fazem trajeto anteriormente para inervar a face lateral da mama. SIN lateral mammary b.'s of lateral cutaneous branches of intercostal nerves, rami mammarii laterales ramorum cutaneorum lateralis nervorum thoracicorum, rami mammarii laterales ramorum cutaneorum lateralium nervorum intercostalium.

lateral mammary b.'s of lateral thoracic artery [TA], ramos mamários laterais da artéria torácica lateral; ramos da artéria torácica lateral que se estendem ao redor das bordas laterais dos músculos peitorais para nutrir a face lateral da mama e a glândula mamária. SIN rami mammarii laterales arteriae thoracicae lateralis [TA].

lateral and medial posterior choroidal b.'s of posterior cerebral artery [TA], ramos corióideos posteriores laterais e mediais da artéria cerebral posterior; um dos dois ramos corióideos (posterior lateral e posterior medial) do segmento P_2 da artéria cerebral posterior que nutrem o plexo corióide do corpo do ventrículo lateral e do terceiro ventrículo. SIN rami choroidei posteriores arteriae cerebri posteriores laterales et mediales [TA].

lateral medullary b.'s of (intracranial part of) vertebral artery [TA], ramos medulares laterais da artéria vertebral (da parte intracraniana); ramos pequenos da artéria vertebral (ou seus ramos maiores) que avançam lateralmente ao longo da face ventral da medula oblonga. SIN rami medullares laterales (partis intracranialis) arteriae vertebralis [TA].

lateral nasal b.'s of anterior ethmoidal nerve [TA], ramos nasais laterais do nervo etmoidal anterior; ramos do nervo nasociliar distribuídos para as paredes da cavidade nasal. SIN rami nasales laterales nervi ethmoidalis anterioris [TA].

lateral nasal b. of facial artery [TA], r. nasal lateral da artéria facial; r. da artéria facial para o lado do nariz (asa e dorso); anastomosa-se com seu congênere contralateral, bem como com os ramos septal e alar da artéria labial superior, r. nasal dorsal da artéria oftálmica, e o r. infra-orbital da artéria maxilar. SIN ramus lateralis nasi arteriae facialis [TA], lateral nasal artery.

lateral b.'s of pontine arteries [TA], ramos laterais das artérias da ponte; os ramos mais longos da artéria basilar que se estendem através da superfície inferior da ponte para atingir as faces laterais. SIN rami laterales arteriae pontis [TA], circumferential pontine b.'s of pontine arteries*.

lateral b. of posterior rami of spinal nerves, r. lateral dos ramos posteriores dos nervos espinais; r. terminal (com o r. medial) do ramo posterior dos nervos espinais. Na região torácica, os ramos laterais dos nervos espinais torácicos superiores são apenas musculares, não atingindo a pele; os ramos laterais dos nervos espinais torácicos inferiores são musculocutâneos, inervando e continuando além dos músculos das costas para alcançar a pele suprajacente.

lateral sacral b.'s of median sacral artery [TA], ramos sacrais laterais da artéria sacral mediana; ramos da porção sacral da artéria sacral mediana que passam lateralmente para se anastomosarem com as artérias sacrais laterais e enviam ramos para dentro dos forames sacrais anteriores. SIN rami sacrales laterales arteriae sacralis medianae [TA].

left b. [TA], r. esquerdo; de um par de ramos, o r. que passa para o lado esquerdo do corpo, para o membro esquerdo de um par bilateral de estruturas, ou para a porção esquerda de uma estrutura única; o outro membro do par é o r. direito. A Terminologia Anatômica relaciona os ramos esquerdos 1) do fascículo atrioventricular (crus sinistrum fasciculus atrioventricularis [TA]); 2) da artéria hepática própria (ramus sinister arteriae hepaticae proprii [TA]); 3) da veia porta do fígado (ramus sinister venae portae hepatis [TA]). SIN ramus sinister [TA].

left b. of hepatic artery proper [TA], r. esquerdo da artéria hepática própria; ramificação terminal da artéria hepática própria que nutre o lobo esquerdo do fígado. SIN ramus sinister arteriae hepaticae propriae [TA], left hepatic artery.

lingual b.'s, ramos linguais; ramos para a língua. A Terminologia Anatômica relaciona os ramos linguais 1) do nervo acessório (rami linguales nervi accessori [TA]); 2) do nervo facial (inconstante) (ramus linguales nervi facialis); 3) do nervo lingual (rami linguales nervi lingualis [TA]); 4) do nervo glossofaríngeo (rami linguales nervi glossopharyngei [TA]). SIN rami linguales.

lingual b. of facial nerve, r. lingual do nervo facial (inconstante) do r. estilo-hióideo do nervo facial. SIN ramus lingualis nervi facialis.

b.'s of lingual nerve to isthmus of fauces [TA], ramos para o istmo das fauces do nervo lingual. SIN rami isthmi faucium nervi lingualis [TA], faucial b.'s of lingual nerve, rami fauciales nervi lingualis.

lumbar b. of iliolumbar artery [TA], r. lombar da artéria iliolumbar; r. terminal da artéria iliolumbar (com o r. ilíaco) que ascende para nutrir os músculos psoas maior e quadrado do lombo; *anastomose*: quarta artéria lombar. SIN ramus lumbalis arteriae iliolumbalis [TA].

mammary b.'s, ramos mamários. VER lateral mammary b.'s, medial mammary b.'s.

marginal atrial b. of right coronary artery, r. atrial intermédio da artéria coronária direita. SIN intermediate atrial b. of right coronary artery.

marginal b. of cingulate sulcus [TA], r. marginal do sulco do cíngulo; extremidade posterior do sulco do cíngulo do cérebro que se dirige superiormente até a margem súpero-medial do lobo parietal. SIN ramus marginalis sulci cinguli [TA].

marginal mandibular b. of facial nerve [TA], r. marginal da mandíbula do nervo facial; r. do nervo facial que corre em paralelo à margem mandibular, inervando o músculo risório e os músculos do lábio inferior e do queixo. SIN ramus marginalis mandibulae nervi facialis [TA].

marginal b. of parietooccipital sulcus [TA], r. marginal do sulco parietooccipital; ramificação do sulco menor do sulco parietooccipital quando ele cruza a margem póstero-medial do cérebro. SIN ramus marginalis sulci parietoccipitalis [TA].

marginal b. [TA] of cingulate sulcus, r. marginal do sulco do cíngulo. SIN marginal *sulcus*.

marginal tentorial b. of internal carotid artery, r. marginal do tentório (parte cavernosa) da artéria carótida interna. SIN tentorial marginal b. of cavernous part of internal carotid artery.

mastoid b. of occipital artery [TA], r. mastóideo da artéria occipital; a artéria que atravessa o forame mastóideo; *distribuição*, células aéreas da mastóide; *anastomose*, r. meníngeo médio. SIN ramus mastoideus arteriae occipitalis [TA], mastoid artery.

mastoid b.'s of posterior auricular artery, ramos mastóideos da artéria auricular posterior. SIN mastoid b.'s of posterior tympanic artery.

mastoid b.'s of posterior tympanic artery, ramos mastóideos da artéria auricular posterior; ramos do r. estilomastóideo da artéria auricular posterior que se originam no canal facial, distribuídos para as células aéreas da mastóide. SIN rami mastoidei arteriae tympanicae posterioris [TA], mastoid b.'s of posterior auricular artery, rami mastoidei arteriae auricularis posterioris.

medial b.'s [TA], ramos mediais; ramos direcionados no sentido da linha média, para o meio. A Terminologia Anatômica relaciona os ramos mediais (ramus medialis/rami mediales): 1) das artérias centrais ântero-laterais (rami mediales arteriarum centralium anterolateralium [TA]); 2) das artérias do túber cinéreo (ramus medialis arteriae tuberis cinerei [TA]); 3) do ramo primário posterior dos nervos espinais cervicais/torácicos/lombares/sacrais/coccígeos (rami medialis ramorum posteriorum nervorum cervicalium/thoracicalium/lumbalium/sacralium/coccygeum); 4) da parte umbilical do r. esquerdo da veia porta do fígado (rami mediales portis umbilici rami sinistri venae portae hepatis [TA]); 5) do ducto hepático esquerdo (ramus medialis ductus hepatici sinistri [TA]); 6) da artéria lobar média (do pulmão direito) (ramus medialis arteriae lobaris mediae (pulmonis dextrum) [TA]); 7) do nervo supra-orbital (ramus medialis nervi supraorbitalis [TA]). SIN rami mediales [TA].

medial b.'s of artery of tuber cinereum [TA], ramos mediais das artérias do túber cinéreo; ramos que se originam da face medial da artéria do túber cinéreo. SIN rami mediales arteriarum tuberis cinerei [TA].

medial basal b. of pulmonary artery, artéria segmentar basilar medial. SIN medial basal segmental *artery*.

medial calcaneal b.'s of tibial nerve [TA], ramos calcâneos mediais do nervo tibial; ramos cutâneos do nervo tibial distribuídos para as porções inferior e medial do calcanhar. SIN rami calcanei mediales nervi tibialis [TA].

medial crural cutaneous b.'s of saphenous nerve, ramos cutâneos crurais mediais do nervo safeno. SIN medial cutaneous *nerve* of leg.

medial cutaneous b. of dorsal branch of posterior intercostal arteries [TA], r. cutâneo medial do ramo dorsal das artérias intercostais posteriores; a Terminologia Anatômica relaciona os ramos cutâneos mediais: 1) do ramo dorsal dos nervos torácicos (rami cutaneus medialis ramorum dorsalium nervorum thoracicorum [NA]); 2) do ramo dorsal das artérias intercostais posteriores (ramus cutaneus medialis rami dorsalis arteriarum intercostalium posteriorum III-XI [NA]). SIN ramus cutaneus medialis rami dorsalis arteriarum intercostalium posteriorum III-XI.

medial malleolar b.'s (of posterior tibial artery) [TA], ramos maleolares mediais (da artéria tibial posterior); ramos que se originam da face medial da artéria tibial posterior no nível da porção mais estreita da perna, passando para os tecidos na região da face posterior do maléolo medial; anastomosam-se com os ramos maleolares mediais da artéria tibial anterior. SIN rami malleolares mediales arteriae tibialis posterioris [TA], arteriae malleolares posteriores mediales, medial malleolar arteries.

medial mammary b.'s, ramos mamários mediais; distribuídos principalmente para a porção medial da mama. A Terminologia Anatômica relaciona os ramos mamários mediais (rami mammarii mediales...): 1) dos ramos cutâneos anteriores dos nervos intercostais (...rami cutanei anterioris nervorum intercostalium); os nervos que acompanham os ramos perfurantes da artéria torácica interna; 2) dos ramos perfurantes da artéria torácica interna (...rami perforantes arteriae thoracicae internae [TA]). SIN rami mammarii mediales.

medial medullary b.'s of vertebral artery [TA], ramos medulares mediais da artéria vertebral; diminutos ramos da artéria vertebral que entram na fissura mediana anterior da medula oblonga. SIN rami medullares mediales arteriae vertebralis [TA].

medial nasal b.'s of anterior ethmoidal nerve [TA], ramos nasais mediais do nervo etmoidal anterior; ramos do nervo nasociliar distribuídos para o septo nasal. SIN rami nasales mediales nervi ethmoidalis anterioris [TA].

medial b.'s of pontine arteries [TA], ramos mediais das artérias da ponte; ramos mais curtos da artéria basilar que se estendem até a porção medial da superfície inferior da ponte. SIN rami mediales arteriae pontis [TA], paramedian pontine b.'s of pontine arteries*.

medial b. of posterior branch of spinal nerves, r. medial do r. posterior dos nervos espinais; termo oficial alternativo* para medial b. of posterior rami of spinal nerves.

medial b. of posterior rami of spinal nerves, r. medial dos ramos posteriores dos nervos espinais; r. terminal (com o r. lateral) dos ramos posteriores dos nervos espinais. Na região torácica, os ramos mediais dos nervos espinais torácicos superiores são musculocutâneos, inervando e continuando através dos músculos do dorso para atingir a pele suprajacente; os ramos mediais dos nervos espinais torácicos inferiores são apenas musculares, terminando antes de alcançar a pele. SIN medial b. of posterior branch of spinal nerves*, ramus medialis ramorum dorsalium nervorum spinalis.

mediastinal b.'s [TA], ramos mediastinais; ramos distribuídos para o mediastino. SIN rami mediastinales [TA], mediastinal arteries.

mediastinal b.'s of internal thoracic artery [TA], ramos mediastinais da artéria torácica interna; pequenas ramificações que nutrem as estruturas mediastinais anteriores: principalmente o timo e os linfonodos. SIN rami mediastinales arteriae thoracicae internae [TA], anterior mediastinal arteries, rami thymici.

mediastinal b.'s of thoracic aorta [TA], ramos mediastinais da parte torácica da aorta; inúmeras pequenas artérias que nutrem a pleura e os linfonodos do mediastino posterior. SIN rami mediastinales aortae thoracicae [TA], posterior mediastinal arteries.

meningeal b.'s [TA], ramos meníngeos; ramos dos vasos ou nervos distribuídos para os revestimentos do cérebro e da medula espinal. SIN rami meningei [TA].

meningeal b. of cavernous part of internal carotid artery, r. meníngeo da porção cavernosa da artéria carótida interna; r. da porção cavernosa da artéria carótida interna para as meninges da fossa anterior do crânio. SIN ramus meningeus partis cavernosae arteriae carotidis internae [TA], meningeal b. of internal carotid artery, ramus meningeus arteriae carotidis internae.

meningeal b. of cerebral part of internal carotid artery [TA], r. meníngeo da parte cerebral da artéria carótida interna, pequena artéria que cruza a asa menor do esfenóide para nutrir a dura-máter e o osso da fossa anterior do crânio e se anastomosa com o r. meníngeo da artéria etmoidal posterior. SIN ramus meningeus partis cerebralis arteriae carotidis internae [TA].

meningeal b. of internal carotid artery, r. meníngeo da parte cavernosa da artéria carótida interna. SIN meningeal b. of cavernous part of internal carotid artery.

meningeal b. of (intracranial part of) vertebral artery [TA], r. meníngeo (da parte intracraniana) da artéria vertebral; um de um ou dois ramos da parte intracraniana da artéria vertebral, originando-se próximo ao forame magno, que se ramifica entre a dura-máter e a tábua interna do osso da fossa posterior do crânio, nutrindo a dura-máter (incluindo a foice do cerebelo), a tábua óssea interna e o díploe. SIN ramus meningeus (partis intracranialis) arteriae vertebralis [TA].

meningeal b. of mandibular nerve [TA], r. meníngeo do nervo mandibular; r. recorrente do nervo mandibular que passa superiormente através do forame espinhoso para ser distribuído com a divisão posterior da artéria meníngea média para as meninges da porção posterior da fossa craniana média. SIN ramus meningeus nervi mandibularis [TA], nervus spinosus*.

meningeal b. of maxillary nerve, r. meníngeo do nervo maxilar; r. recorrente do nervo maxilar distribuído com o r. anterior da artéria meníngea média para as meninges da porção anterior da fossa média do crânio. SIN ramus meningeus nervi maxillaris [TA], middle meningeal b. of maxillary nerve, middle meningeal nerve, ramus meningeus medius nervi maxillaris.

meningeal b. of occipital artery [TA], r. meníngeo da artéria occipital; um dos ramos variáveis da artéria occipital que podem passar através dos forames jugular ou parietal ou do canal condilóide para alcançar a dura-máter e o osso da fossa posterior do crânio, bem como as porções intracranianas dos quatro nervos cranianos caudais. SIN ramus meningeus arteriae occipitalis [TA].

meningeal b. of ophthalmic nerve, r. meníngeo do nervo oftálmico. VER tentorial *nerve*.

meningeal b. of spinal nerves [TA], r. meníngeo dos nervos espinais; r. oriundo da porção inicial (misto) de cada nervo espinal que passa de forma recorrente para trás, através do forame intervertebral, para inervar as meninges espinais, o ligamento longitudinal posterior, a periferia póstero-lateral do disco intervertebral e o periósteo das vértebras. SIN ramus meningeus nervorum spinalium [TA], recurrent b. of spinal nerves*, recurrent meningeal b. of spinal nerves, sinuvertebral nerves.

meningeal b. of vagus nerve [TA], r. meníngeo do nervo vago; r. do gânglio superior do vago que inerva as meninges da fossa posterior do crânio. SIN ramus meningeus nervi vagi [TA].

mental b.'s of mental nerve [TA], ramos mentuais do nervo mentual; ramos do nervo mentual que fornecem a inervação sensorial geral para a pele do queixo. SIN rami mentales nervi mentalis [TA].

mental b. (of inferior alveolar artery) [TA], r. mentual (da artéria alveolar inferior); *distribuição*, queixo; o ramo terminal da alveolar inferior; *anastomoses*, artéria labial inferior. SIN ramus mentalis arteriae alveolaris inferioris [TA], arteria mentalis, mental artery.

middle lobe b. of right superior pulmonary vein, veia do lobo médio. SIN middle lobe *vein*.

middle meningeal b. of maxillary nerve, r. meníngeo médio do nervo maxilar. SIN meningeal b. of maxillary nerve.

middle superior alveolar b. of infraorbital nerve [TA], r. alveolar superior médio do nervo infra-orbital; o ramo alveolar superior médio, um ramo do nervo alveolar superior que contribui para o plexo dental superior. SIN ramus alveolaris superior medius nervi infraorbitalis [TA].

middle temporal b. of insular part of middle cerebral artery [TA], r. temporal médio da parte insular da artéria cerebral média; r. da parte insular (segmento M2) da artéria cerebral média que nutre o córtex do lobo temporal entre as artérias temporais anterior e posterior. SIN ramus temporalis medius partis insularis arteriae cerebrae mediae [TA], arteria temporalis intermedia, intermediate temporal artery.

middle temporal b.'s of lateral occipital artery, ramos temporais médios da artéria occipital lateral; termo oficial alternativo* para intermediate temporal b.'s of lateral occipital artery.

muscular b.'s [TA], ramo muscular; ramos dos nervos ou vasos que suprem os músculos. Muitos não possuem nome. A Terminologia Anatômica relaciona os ramos musculares: 1) do nervo acessório (rami musculares nervi accessorii); 2) do ramo anterior do nervo obturatório (rami musculares rami anterioris nervi obturatorii); 3) do nervo interósseo anterior do antebraço (rami musculares nervi interossei antebrachii anterior); 4) do nervo axilar (rami musculares nervi axillaris); 5) do nervo fibular profundo (rami musculares nervi fibulares profundi); 6) do nervo femoral (rami musculares nervi femoralis); 7) de nervos intercostais (rami musculares nervorum intercostalium); 8) do nervo mediano (rami musculares nervi mediani); 9) do nervo musculocutâneo (rami musculares nervi musculocutanei); 10) dos nervos perineais (rami musculares nervorum perinealium); 11) do ramo posterior do nervo obturatório (rami musculares rami posterioris nervi obturatorii); 13) de nervos espinais (rami musculares nervorum spinalium); 14) do nervo fibular superficial (rami musculares nervi fibularis superficialis); 15) da parte supraclavicular do plexo braquial (rami musculares partis supraclavicularis plexus brachialis); 16) do nervo tibial (rami musculares nervi tibialis); 17) do nervo ulnar (rami musculares nervi ulnaris); 18) da artéria vertebral (rami musculares arteriae vertebralis). SIN rami musculares [TA].

mylohyoid b. (of inferior alveolar artery) [TA], r. milo-hióideo da artéria alveolar inferior; ramo da artéria alveolar inferior para o músculo milo-hióideo. SIN ramus mylohyoideus arteriae alveolaris inferioris [TA], mylohyoid artery.

nasal septal b. of superior labial branch of facial artery [TA], r. do septo nasal da artéria labial superior; o r. da artéria labial superior oriunda da artéria facial que avança para cima e se ramifica na face ântero-inferior do septo nasal. SIN ramus septi nasi arteriae labialis superioris [TA].

obturator b. of pubic branch of inferior epigastric artery [TA], r. obturatório do ramo púbico da artéria epigástrica inferior; r. do ramo púbico da artéria epigástrica inferior que desce sobre a margem pélvica para se anastomosar com o r. púbico da artéria obturatória; em 20-30% das pessoas, esse r. é maior que a artéria obturatória ou a substitui. SIN ramus obturatorius pubici arteriae epigastricae inferioris [TA].

occipital b. [TA], r. occipital; a Terminologia Anatômica relaciona os ramos occipitais 1) da artéria auricular posterior, rami occipitalis arteriae auricularis posterior [TA]; 2) do nervo auricular posterior (rami occipitalis nervi auricularis posterioris [TA]); e 3) artéria occipital, rami occipitales arteriae occipitis [TA]. SIN rami occipitalis [TA].

b. of oculomotor nerve to ciliary ganglion, raiz parassimpática do gânglio ciliar. SIN parasympathetic *root* of ciliary ganglion.

omental b.'s [TA], ramos omentais das artérias gastromentais; ramos para o omento maior; ramos epiplóicos que se originam das artérias gastromentais esquerda e direita (rami omentales arteriae gastro-omentalis sinistrae et dextrae [NA]), em oposição aos ramos gástricos (rami gastrici [NA]), ao longo da curvatura maior do estômago. SIN rami omentales [TA], epiploic b.'s, rami epiploicae.

orbital b.'s of maxillary nerve, ramos orbitais do nervo maxilar; ramos do gânglio pterigopalatino que atravessam a fissura orbitária inferior, distribuído na órbita, para a periórbita e mucosa dos seios etmoidal e esfenoidal. SIN rami orbitales nervi maxillaris [TA], orbital b.'s of pterygopalatine ganglion, ramus orbitalis ganglii pterygopalatini.

orbital b. of middle meningeal artery [TA], r. orbital da artéria meníngea média; o r. da artéria meníngea média que atravessa a fissura orbitária superior e que avança para a glândula lacrimal. VER anastomotic b. of middle meningeal artery with lacrimal artery. SIN ramus orbitalis arteriae meningeae mediae [TA].

orbital b.'s of pterygopalatine ganglion, ramos orbitais do nervo maxilar. SIN orbital b'.s of maxillary nerve.

ovarian b. of uterine artery [TA], r. ovárico da artéria uterina; r. terminal da artéria uterina (com o r. tubário) que atravessa o mesovário, nutrindo o ovário desde a face medial e se anastomosando com o r. ovárico da artéria ovárica. SIN rami ovarici arteriae uterinae [TA].

palmar b. of anterior interosseous nerve, r. palmar do nervo mediano; r. do nervo mediano que se origina proximal ao retináculo flexor e que corre superficialmente a ele para suprir a pele da região palmar central proximal e a eminência tenar. Como não atravessa o túnel do carpo, ele não é afetado pela síndrome do túnel do carpo, mesmo que ele inerve a pele distal ao túnel do carpo. SIN ramus palmaris nervi interossei antebrachii anterioris [TA], palmar b. of median nerve, ramus palmaris nervi mediani.

palmar carpal b. of radial artery [TA], r. carpal palmar da artéria radial; pequeno r. da artéria radial que passa medialmente através do punho para suprir as articulações carpais; anastomosa-se com o ramo carpal dorsal da artéria ulnar. SIN ramus carpalis palmaris arteriae radialis [TA], ramus carpeus palmaris arteriae radialis.

palmar carpal b. of ulnar artery [TA], r. carpal palmar da artéria ulnar; r. da artéria ulnar que irriga as articulações carpais e se comunica com o r. carpal dorsal da artéria radial. SIN ramus carpalis palmaris arteriae ulnaris [TA], ramus carpeus palmaris arteriae ulnaris.

palmar b. of median nerve, r. palmar do nervo mediano. SIN palmar b. of anterior interosseous nerve.

palmar b. of ulnar nerve [TA], r. palmar do nervo ulnar; r. do nervo ulnar que se origina na parte distal do antebraço e que acompanha a artéria palmar para dentro da mão, onde inerva a pele do dedo mínimo e a metade medial do dedo anelar e as partes adjacentes da região palmar. SIN ramus palmaris nervi ulnaris [TA].

palpebral b.'s of infratrochlear nerve [TA], ramos palpebrais do nervo infratroclear; os ramos do nervo infratroclear que inervam a pele das faces mediais das pálpebras superior e inferior. SIN rami palpebrales nervi infratrochlearis [TA].

pancreatic b.'s [TA], ramos pancreáticos; ramos para o pâncreas. A Terminologia Anatômica relaciona os ramos pancreáticos (1) da artéria esplênica, rami pancreatici arteriae splenicae [TA]; 2) das artérias pancreaticoduodenais superiores (anterior e posterior), rami pancreatici arteriae pancreaticoduodenalis superioris (anterior et posterior) [TA]. SIN rami pancreatici [TA].

paracentral b.'s of callosomarginal artery [TA], ramos paracentrais da artéria calosomarginal; ramos terminais do r. do cíngulo da artéria calosomarginal distribuídos para o lóbulo paracentral do cérebro. SIN rami paracentrales arteriae callosomarginalis [TA].

paracentral b.'s (of pericallosal artery), ramos paracentrais (da artéria pericalosa); ramos inconstantes da artéria pericalosa que nutrem o córtex cerebral do lóbulo paracentral e ambos os lados da parte medial do sulco central. SIN ramus paracentrales [TA], arteria paracentralis, paracentral artery.

paramedian pontine b.'s of pontine arteries, ramos mediais das artérias da ponte; termo oficial alternativo para medial b.'s of pontine arteries.

parietal b. [TA], r. parietal; (1) ramos que acompanham e suprem o osso parietal ou o lobo parietal do cérebro; (2) ramos distribuídos para as paredes do corpo e membros (as "paredes") em oposição aos ramos viscerais distribuídos para as cavidades corporais. Por exemplo, os ramos comunicantes cinzentos são os ramos parietais dos troncos simpáticos (vs. os nervos esplâncnicos, que são os ramos viscerais dos troncos). SIN rami parietales [TA].

parietal b. of medial occipital artery [TA], r. parietal da artéria occipital medial; r. anterior da artéria occipital medial que nutre a porção posterior do lobo parietal do cérebro. SIN ramus parietalis arteriae occipitalis medialis [TA].

parietal b. of middle meningeal artery [TA], r. parietal da artéria meníngea média; r. terminal menor (com o r. frontal) da artéria meníngea média que nutre a porção posterior da dura-máter lateral e superior e do crânio. SIN ramus parietalis arteriae meningeae mediae [TA].

parietal b. of superficial temporal artery [TA], r. parietal da artéria temporal superficial; ramos que acompanham e/ou nutrem o lobo parietal do cérebro. SIN ramus parietalis arteriae temporalis superficialis [TA].

parieto-occipital b.'s (of anterior cerebral artery) [TA], ramos parieto-occipitais (da artéria cerebral anterior); os maiores ramos corticais da artéria pericalosa que nutrem as superfícies medial e súpero-lateral do lobo parietal posterior ao lóbulo paracentral; raramente, eles se prolongam para nutrir parte do lobo occipital. SIN arteriae parieto-occipitales, parietooccipital artery, superior internal parietal artery.

parieto-occipital b. (of posterior cerebral artery) [TA], r. parieto-occipital (da artéria cerebral posterior); um r. posterior da artéria occipital medial que nutre a superfície medial do lobo occipital, estendendo-se até a área do sulco parieto-occipital do cérebro. SIN ramus parieto-occipitalis arteriae occipitalis medialis [TA].

parotid b.'s [TA], ramos parotídeos; ramos para a glândula parótida: a Terminologia Anatômica lista 1) os ramos parotídeos do nervo auriculotemporal, rami parotidei nervi auriculotemporalis [TA]; 2) as veias parotídeas oriundas da veia facial profunda, rami parotidei venae facialis profundus [TA]; 3) os ramos parotídeos da artéria auricular posterior, ramus parotidei arteriae auricularis posterior [TA]; 4) os ramos parotídeos da artéria temporal superficial, ramus arteriae temporalis superficialis [TA]. SIN rami parotidei [TA].

pectoral and abdominal anterior cutaneous b. of intercostal nerves, ramos cutâneos anteriores peitoral e abdominal dos nervos intercostais. SIN thoracoabdominal nerves, em nerve.

pectoral b.'s of thoracoacromial artery, ramos peitorais da artéria toracoacromial; ramos da artéria tóraco-acromial que descem entre os músculos peitorais maior e menor e os nutrem, continuando, em seguida, para nutrir o músculo serrátil anterior e, na mulher adulta, a porção superior da mama. SIN rami pectorales arteriae thoracoacromialis [TA].

perforating b.'s [TA], ramos perfurantes; ramos arteriais que penetram em uma parede ou passam da face ou compartimento anterior para a face ou compartimento posterior de uma estrutura, como a mão ou o pé, a fim de se anastomosarem ou de serem distribuídos. SIN ramus perforans [TA].

perforating b. of anterior interosseous artery [TA], r. perfurante da artéria interóssea anterior; r. da artéria interóssea anterior que perfura a membrana interóssea na parte distal do antebraço para se anastomosar com (e, na realidade, substituir distalmente) a artéria interóssea posterior. SIN ramus perforans arteriae interossei anterioris [TA].

perforating b. of fibular artery, r. perfurante da artéria fibular; o r. da artéria fibular que perfura a membrana interóssea exatamente acima do ligamento tibiofibular anterior. SIN ramus perforans arteriae fibularis [TA], perforating b. of peroneal artery*.

perforating b.'s of internal thoracic artery [TA], ramos perfurantes da artéria torácica interna; pequenos ramos da artéria torácica interna que correm entre as cartilagens costais para nutrir a pele e os tecidos subcutâneos subjacentes. SIN rami perforantes arteriae thoracicae internae [TA], perforating arteries (of internal thoracic artery).

perforating b.'s (of palmar metacarpal arteries), ramos perfurantes (das artérias metacarpais palmares). VER perforating *branches* of deep palmar arch.

perforating b.'s (of plantar metatarsal arteries) [TA], ramos perfurantes (das artérias metatarsais plantares); os ramos perfurantes das artérias metatarsais plantares, três pequenas artérias que passam dorsalmente através do segundo, terceiro e quarto espaços interósseos do pé oriundas das artérias metatarsais plantares. SIN rami perforantes arteriarum metatarsearum plantarium [TA], perforating arteries (of foot).

perforating b. of peroneal artery, r. perfurante da artéria fibular; termo oficial alternativo* para perforating b. of fibular artery.

pericardial b. of phrenic nerve [TA], r. pericárdico do nervo frênico; um dos ramos do nervo frênico distribuídos para o pericárdio e para a pleura parietal mediastinal adjacente. SIN ramus pericardiacus nervi phrenici [TA].

pericardial b.'s of thoracic aorta [TA], ramos pericárdicos da parte torácica da aorta; pequenos ramos da parte torácica da aorta distribuídos para o pericárdio e para linfonodos pré-vertebrais. SIN rami pericardiaci aortae thoracicae [TA].

perineal b.'s of posterior cutaneous nerve of thigh, ramos perineais do nervo cutâneo femoral posterior, ramos do nervo cutâneo femoral posterior que conduzem fibras sensoriais para a pele da porção mais lateral do períneo e porções adjacentes da parte medial superior da coxa. SIN rami perineales nervi cutanei femoris posterioris [TA], perineal b.'s of posterior femoral cutaneous nerve*.

perineal b.'s of posterior femoral cutaneous nerve, ramos perineais do nervo cutâneo femoral posterior; termo oficial alternativo* para perineal b.'s of posterior cutaneous nerve of thigh.

peroneal communicating b., r. fibular comunicante do nervo fibular comum. SIN sural communicating b. of common fibular nerve.

petrosal b. of middle meningeal artery [TA], r. petroso da artéria meníngea média; primeiro r. intracraniano da artéria meníngea média; *anastomose*: artéria estilomastóidea através do hiato do canal facial. SIN ramus petrosus arteriae meningeae mediae [TA].

pharyngeal b.'s [TA], ramos faríngeos; ramos para a faringe. SIN rami pharyngei [TA], rami pharingeales*, pharyngei.

pharyngeal b. of the artery of pterygoid canal [TA], r. faríngeo da artéria do canal pterigóideo; distribuído para a porção mais superior da nasofaringe (recessos faríngeos). SIN ramus pharyngeus arteriae canalis pterygoidei [TA].

pharyngeal b. of the ascending pharyngeal artery [TA], r. faríngeo da artéria faríngea ascendente; *distribuição*: paredes da orofaringe e da nasofaringe. SIN rami pharyngeales arteriae pharyngeae ascendentis [TA].

pharyngeal b. of descending palatine artery [TA], r. faríngeo da artéria palatina descendente; pode originar-se como um r. separado ou como uma continuação da artéria palatina menor. SIN ramus pharyngeus arteriae palatinae descendentis [TA].

pharyngeal b. of glossopharyngeal nerve [TA], r. faríngeo do nervo glossofaríngeo; conduz as fibras sensoriais gerais para a mucosa da orofaringe através do plexo faríngeo. SIN rami pharyngei nervi glossopharyngei [TA].

pharyngeal b. of inferior thyroid artery [TA], r. faríngeo da artéria tireóidea inferior; distribuído para a laringofaringe. SIN rami pharyngeales arteriae thyroideae inferioris [TA].

pharyngeal b. of pterygopalatine ganglion, r. faríngeo do gânglio pterigopalatino. SIN pharyngeal *nerve*.

pharyngeal b.'s of recurrent laryngeal nerve [TA], ramos faríngeos do nervo laríngeo recorrente; ramos do nervo laríngeo recorrente que continuam além da laringe para a porção inferior da faringe. SIN rami pharyngei nervi laryngei recurrentis [TA].

pharyngeal b. of vagus nerve [TA], r. faríngeo do nervo vago; conduz as fibras motoras oriundas da raiz craniana do nervo acessório para os músculos constritores da faringe, os músculos intrínsecos do palato mole e o músculo levantador do véu palatino; também pode conduzir algumas fibras sensoriais gerais para o plexo faríngeo. SIN rami pharyngei nervi vagi [TA].

phrenicoabdominal b.'s of phrenic nerve, ramos frenicoabdominais do nervo frênico; os ramos terminais do nervo frênico que fornecem a inervação motora do diafragma e a inervação sensorial para o diafragma e para a pleura e o peritônio diafragmáticos. SIN rami phrenicoabdominales nervi phrenici [TA].

posterior b.'s [TA], ramos posteriores; ramos direcionados dorsalmente ou para trás. SIN rami posteriores [TA].

posterior basal b., artéria segmentar basilar posterior dos pulmões esquerdo/direito. SIN posterior basal segmental *artery* of left/right lung.

posterior gastric b.'s of posterior vagal trunk [TA], ramos gástricos posteriores do tronco vagal posterior; ramos do tronco vagal posterior que passam posteriores à artéria gástrica esquerda no ligamento hepatogástrico para se ramificar sobre a face póstero-inferior do estômago. SIN rami gastrici posteriores trunci vagalis posterioris [TA].

posterior glandular b. of superior thyroid artery, r. glandular posterior da artéria tireóidea superior; r. da artéria tireóidea superior que desce para nutrir a porção apical do lobo ipsolateral da tireóide, continuando ao longo da margem posterior da glândula até se anastomosar com a artéria tireóidea inferior. SIN ramus glandularis posterior arteriae thyroideae superioris [TA], posterior b. of superior thyroid artery, ramus posterior arteriae thyroideae superioris.

posterior b. of great auricular nerve [TA], r. posterior do nervo auricular magno; fornece as fibras sensoriais gerais para a pele da parte posterior da orelha e sobre o processo mastóide. SIN ramus posterior nervi auricularis magni [TA].

posterior inferior nasal b.'s of greater palatine nerve, ramos nasais póstero-inferiores do nervo palatino maior. SIN posterior inferior nasal *nerves,* em *nerve.*

posterior b. of inferior pancreaticoduodenal artery [TA], r. posterior da artéria pancreaticoduodenal inferior; o mais dorsal dos dois ramos em que a artéria pancreaticoduodenal inferior se bifurca; nutre o processo uncinado e a cabeça do pâncreas, bem como a terceira e quarta partes do duodeno; anastomosa-se com o ramo posterior da artéria pancreaticoduodenal superior. SIN ramus posterior arteriae pancreaticoduodenalis inferioris [TA].

posterior labial b.'s of perineal artery [TA], ramos labiais posteriores da artéria perineal; os ramos superficiais da artéria perineal que nutrem as porções posteriores dos lábios maiores e menores do pudendo.

posterior labial branches of internal pudendal artery [TA], ramos labiais posteriores da artéria pudenda interna; os ramos da artéria pudenda para a porção posterior dos lábios maiores do pudendo. SIN rami labiales posteriores arteriae perinealis [TA], posterior labial arteries, rami labiales posteriores arteriae pudendae internae.

posterior b. of lateral cerebral sulcus, r. posterior do sulco lateral do mesencéfalo. SIN posterior *ramus* of lateral cerebral sulcus.

posterior b. of medial antebrachial cutaneous nerve, r. posterior do nervo cutâneo medial do antebraço. SIN posterior b. of medial cutaneous nerve of forearm.

posterior b. of medial cutaneous nerve of forearm, r. posterior do nervo cutâneo medial do antebraço; r. do nervo cutâneo medial do antebraço que nutre a pele da porção medial dos dois terços proximais do lado dorsal do antebraço. SIN ramus posterior nervi cutanei antebrachii medialis [TA], posterior b. of medial antebrachial cutaneous nerve, ramus ulnaris nervi cutanei antebrachii medialis, ulnar b. of medial antebrachial cutaneous nerve.

posterior b. of obturator artery, r. posterior da artéria obturatória; r. da artéria obturatória originando o r. acetabular e nutrindo os músculos inseridos no ísquio. SIN ramus posterior arteriae obturatoriae [TA].

posterior b. of obturator nerve [TA], r. posterior do nervo obturatório; r. que inerva o músculo obturador externo, passando, então, posterior ao músculo adutor curto, inervando-o e à porção adutora do músculo adutor magno. SIN ramus posterior nervi obturatorii [TA].

posterior b. of recurrent ulnar artery, r. posterior da artéria recorrente ulnar. SIN posterior b. of ulnar recurrent artery.

posterior b. of renal artery [TA], r. posterior da artéria renal; r. terminal da artéria renal (com o r. anterior) tornando-se a artéria segmentar posterior do rim. VER segmental *arteries* of kidney, em *artery.* SIN ramus posterior arteriae renalis [TA].

posterior b. of right branch of portal vein [TA], r. posterior do ramo direito da veia porta do fígado; r. segmentar posterior da veia porta; r. para os segmentos posteriores do lobo direito do fígado. SIN ramus posterior rami dextri venae portae hepatis [TA].

posterior b. of right hepatic duct [TA], r. posterior do ducto hepático direito; o r. do ducto hepático que drena a bile dos segmentos posteriores do lobo direito do fígado. SIN ramus posterior ductus hepatici dextri [TA].

posterior b. of right superior pulmonary vein [TA], r. posterior da veia pulmonar direita superior; drena a porção posterior do lobo superior do pulmão direito. SIN ramus posterior venae pulmonalis dextrae superioris [TA].

posterior scrotal b.'s of internal pudendal artery, ramos escrotais posteriores da artéria pudenda interna. SIN posterior scrotal b.'s of perineal artery.

posterior scrotal b.'s of perineal artery, ramos escrotais posteriores da artéria perineal; ramos da artéria perineal que nutrem a pele da porção posterior da bolsa escrotal. SIN rami scrotales posteriores arteriae perinealis [TA], posterior scrotal b.'s of internal pudendal artery, rami scrotales posteriores arteriae pudendae internae.

posterior septal b. of nose [TA], ramos septais posteriores da artéria esfenopalatina; um dos ramos da artéria esfenopalatina que nutre o septo nasal e acompanha o nervo nasopalatino. SIN ramus septi posterioris nasalis [TA], arteria nasalis posterior septi, posterior septal artery of nose, posterior septal b.'s of sphenopalatine artery.

posterior septal b.'s of sphenopalatine artery, ramos septais posteriores da artéria esfenopalatina. SIN posterior septal b. of nose.

posterior b. of spinal nerves, r. posterior dos nervos espinais. VER dorsal primary *ramus* of spinal nerve.

posterior superior alveolar b.'s of maxillary nerve [TA], ramos alveolares superiores posteriores do nervo maxilar; os ramos dos nervos alveolares superiores que inervam o seio maxilar e os dentes molares. SIN rami alveolares superiores posteriores nervi maxillaris [TA].

posterior superior lateral nasal b.'s of maxillary nerve, ramos nasais pósteros-laterais do nervo maxilar; os ramos do gânglio pterigopalatino para a porção posterior superior da parede lateral da cavidade nasal, incluindo a concha/meato nasal superior e média, e os seios etmoidais posteriores. SIN posterior superior lateral nasal b.'s of pterygopalatine ganglion, rami nasales posteriores superiores laterales ganglii pterygopalatini, rami nasales posteriores superiores laterales nervi maxillaris.

posterior superior lateral nasal b.'s of pterygopalatine ganglion, ramos nasais posteriores súpero-laterais do nervo maxilar. SIN posterior superior lateral nasal b.'s of maxillary nerve.

posterior superior medial nasal b.'s of maxillary nerve [TA], ramos nasais posteriores súpero-mediais do nervo maxilar; geralmente ramos do nervo nasopalatino para a porção súpero-posterior do septo nasal. SIN rami nasales posteriores superiores mediales nervi maxillaris [TA], posterior superior medial nasal b.'s of pterygopalatine ganglion, rami nasales posteriores superiores mediales ganglii pterygopalatini.

posterior superior medial nasal b.'s of pterygopalatine ganglion, ramos nasais posteriores súpero-mediais do nervo maxilar. SIN posterior superior medial nasal b.'s of maxillary nerve.

posterior b. of superior thyroid artery, r. glandular posterior da artéria tireóidea superior. SIN posterior glandular b. of superior thyroid artery.

posterior temporal b. of middle cerebral artery [TA], artéria temporal posterior da artéria cerebral média; um ramo da parte insular (segmento M2) da artéria cerebral média distribuída para o córtex da parte posterior do lobo temporal. SIN ramus temporalis posterior arteriae cerebri mediae [TA], arteria temporalis posterior, posterior temporal artery.

posterior b. of ulnar recurrent artery, r. posterior da artéria recorrente ulnar; contribui para o aporte sangüíneo do flexor ulnar do carpo e para a rede articular do cotovelo. SIN ramus posterior arteriae recurrentis ulnaris [TA], posterior b. of recurrent ulnar artery.

posterior vestibular b. of vestibulocochlear artery [TA], r. vestibular posterior da artéria vestibulococlear; *origem:* r. terminal, com o r. coclear, da artéria vestibulococlear; *distribuição:* utrículo e (especialmente a ampola do) ducto semicircular posterior. SIN ramus vestibularis posterior arteriae vestibulocochlearis [TA].

posteromedial frontal b. of callosomarginal artery [TA], r. frontal pósteros-medial da artéria calosomarginal; r. terminal (com o r. do cíngulo) da artéria calosomarginal para a porção posterior da face medial do lobo frontal do cérebro. SIN rami frontalis posteromedialis arteriae callosomarginalis [TA].

precuneal b.'s (of anterior cerebral artery) [TA], ramos precuneais (da artéria cerebral anterior); o último r. cortical da artéria pericalosa; nutrem a parte inferior do pré-cúneo. SIN rami precuneales arteriae cerebri anterioris [TA], arteria precunealis, inferior internal parietal artery, precuneal artery.

prelaminar b. of spinal branch of dorsal branch of posterior intercostal artery [TA], r. pré-laminar dos ramos espinais do r. dorsal das artérias intercostais posteriores; *origem:* artéria espinal no forame intervertebral; *distribuição:* para a superfície anterior da lâmina e dos ligamentos amarelos das vértebras torácicas e as faces anteriores das articulações zigapofisárias. SIN ramus prelaminaris rami spinalis rami dorsalis arteriae intercostalis posterioris [TA].

prostatic b.'s of inferior vesical artery [TA], ramos prostáticos da artéria vesical inferior; os ramos da artéria vesical inferior que descem para a próstata, compreendendo seu principal aporte arterial. SIN rami prostatici arteriae vesicalis inferioris [TA].

prostatic b.'s of middle rectal artery [TA], ramos prostáticos da artéria retal média; ramos da artéria retal média que se anastomosam com os ramos prostáticos da artéria vesical inferior e se unem na nutrição da próstata. SIN rami prostatici arteriae rectalis mediae [TA].

pterygoid b.'s of maxillary artery, ramos pterigóideos da artéria temporal profunda posterior. SIN pterygoid b. of posterior deep temporal artery.

pterygoid b. of posterior deep temporal artery, ramos pterigóideos da artéria temporal profunda posterior; ramos pterigóideos da artéria meníngea média. SIN ramus pterygoideus arteriae temporalis profundae posterioris [TA], pterygoid b.'s of maxillary artery, rami pterygoidei arteriae maxillaris.

pubic b. of inferior epigastric artery [TA], r. púbico da artéria epigástrica inferior; r. que se origina na artéria epigástrica inferior medialmente ao anel inguinal profundo; corre medialmente ao anel femoral para a parte posterior do púbis; anastomose, r. púbico da artéria obturatória. Essa anastomose freqüentemente é grande, sendo referida como "artéria obturatória acessória". Em 20-30% dos pacientes, essa anastomose substitui a artéria obturatória, como uma artéria obturatória "aberrante" ou "substituída". SIN ramus pubicus arteriae epigastricae inferioris [TA].

pubic b. of inferior epigastric vein [TA], r. púbico da veia epigástrica inferior; r. da veia epigástrica inferior que se origina medialmente ao anel inguinal profundo e que dá origem a um r. superior, que se anastomosa através da linha média com seu congênere contralateral, e um r. inferior que desce sobre a face posterior do púbis; esse último origina uma veia obturatória. VER TAMBÉM obturator b. of pubic branch of inferior epigastric vein. SIN ramus pubicus venae epigastricae inferioris [TA].

pubic b. of obturator artery [TA], r. púbico da artéria obturatória; r. que se origina da artéria obturatória exatamente antes de sua passagem através do canal obturatório; o r. passa superiormente sobre a face posterior do púbis. *Anastomose:* com o congênere contralateral e o r. púbico da artéria epigástrica inferi-

or. VER accessory obturator *artery*, pubic b. of inferior epigastric artery. SIN ramus pubicus arteriae obturatoriae [TA].
pulmonary b.'s of autonomic nervous system, ramos pulmonares do sistema nervoso autônomo. VER pulmonary b.'s of pulmonary nerve plexus, thoracic pulmonary b.'s of thoracic ganglia. SIN rami pulmonales systematis autonomici.
pulmonary b.'s of pulmonary nerve plexus [TA], ramos pulmonares do plexo pulmonar; ramos do plexo nervoso pulmonar que se estendem ao longo da raiz dos pulmões, alcançando os pulmões esquerdo e direito. SIN rami pulmonales plexi nervosi pulmonalis [TA].
pyloric b. of anterior vagal trunk [TA], r. pilórico do tronco vagal anterior do nervo vago; r. do tronco vagal anterior que passa através do ligamento hepatogástrico com os ramos hepáticos do nervo vago para alcançar o piloro. Nos procedimentos de vagotomia seletiva, esse r. é poupado para evitar problemas com o esvaziamento gástrico. SIN ramus pyloricus trunci vagalis anterioris [TA].
recurrent meningeal b. of spinal nerves, r. meníngeo dos nervos espinais. SIN meningeal b. of spinal nerves.
recurrent b. of spinal nerves, r. meníngeo dos nervos espinais; termo oficial alternativo* para meningeal b. of spinal nerves.
renal b. of lesser splanchnic b. [TA], r. renal do nervo esplâncnico menor; r. do nervo esplâncnico menor para o plexo/gânglio aorticorrenal. SIN ramus renalis nervi splanchnici minoris [TA].
renal b.'s of vagus nerve [TA], ramos renais do nervo vago; ramos do nervo vago para o rim através do plexo celíaco. SIN rami renales nervi vagi [TA].
right b. [TA], r. direito; de um par de ramos, o r. que passa para o lado direito do corpo, para o membro direito de um par bilateral de estruturas ou para a porção direita de uma estrutura ímpar; o outro membro do par é um ramo esquerdo. SIN ramus dexter [TA].
right atrial b. of right coronary artery, r. atrial direito da artéria coronária direita. SIN intermediate atrial b. of right coronary artery.
right b. of hepatic artery proper [TA], r. direito da artéria hepática própria; r. terminal da artéria hepática própria que nutre o lobo direito do fígado; *ramo:* artéria cística. SIN ramus dexter arteriae hepaticae propriae [TA], right hepatic artery.
right marginal b. (of right coronary artery) [TA], r. marginal direito (da artéria coronária direita); geralmente o maior dos ramos ventriculares da artéria coronária direita; corre ao longo da margem direita do coração e tem calibre e comprimento suficientes para atingir o ápice. SIN ramus marginalis dexter (arteriae coronariae dextrae) [TA].
right b. of portal vein [TA], r. direito da veia porta do fígado; r. terminal da veia porta do fígado distribuído para o lobo direito da tributária hepática: veia cística. SIN ramus dexter venae portae hepatis [TA].
saphenous b. of descending genicular artery [TA], r. safeno da artéria descendente do joelho; r. da artéria descendente do joelho que nutre a pele da parte superior da face medial da perna; *anastomose:* artéria inferior medial do joelho (rede vascular articular do joelho). SIN ramus saphenus arteriae descendentis genicularis [TA].
b.'s of segmental bronchi, brônquios intra-segmentares. SIN intrasegmental *bronchi*, em *bronchus*.
septal b.'s, ramos interventriculares septais das artérias coronárias esquerda/direita. SIN interventricular septal b.'s of left/right coronary artery.
sinuatrial nodal b. of right coronary artery, r. do nó sinoatrial da artéria coronária direita. SIN sinuatrial (S-A) nodal b. of right coronary artery.
b. to sinuatrial node, r. do nó sinoatrial da artéria coronária direita. SIN sinuatrial (S-A) nodal b. of right coronary artery.
sinuatrial (S-A) nodal b. of right coronary artery [TA], r. do nó sinoatrial (S-A) da artéria coronária direita; ramo atrial ascendente, originando-se geralmente (55%) do tronco anterior da artéria coronária direita (mas 35-45% originam-se do ramo circunflexo da artéria coronária esquerda), que corre ao redor da base da veia cava superior para alcançar o nó sinoatrial. SIN ramus nodi sinuatrialis arteriae coronariae dextrae [TA], artery to the sinoatrial (S-A) node, b. to sinuatrial node, sinuatrial nodal artery, sinuatrial nodal b. of right coronary artery, sinuatrial node artery, sinus node artery.
spinal b.'s [TA], ramos espinhais; ramos das seguintes artérias que nutrem as meninges, as raízes dos nervos espinais e, em alguns casos, a medula espinal: 1) vertebral, 2) cervical ascendente, 3) r. dorsal das artérias intercostais posteriores I a XI, 4) r. dorsal da artéria subcostal, 5) r. dorsal das artérias lombares, 6) r. lombar da artéria iliolombar, 7) sacral lateral; todas as artérias espinais originam artérias que nutrem as raízes dorsal e ventral dos nervos espinais; muitas terminam no suprimento das raízes como artérias radiculares, porém algumas (4 a 9) são suficientemente grandes para alcançar e se anastomosar com as artérias espinais anteriores e posteriores e são designadas, em vez disso, artérias medulares segmentares. VER great segmental medullary *artery*, segmental medullary *arteries*, em *artery*. SIN rami spinales (1) [TA], spinal arteries.
splenic b.'s of splenic artery [TA], ramos esplênicos da artéria esplênica; os ramos das artérias esplênicas próprias; a artéria que penetra no baço na altura do hilo. SIN rami splenici arteriae splenicae [TA], rami lienales arteriae lienalis*.

stapedial b. of posterior tympanic artery, r. do estapédio da artéria timpânica posterior; r. que se origina diretamente da artéria timpânica posterior ou de sua artéria de origem, a artéria estilomastóidea; nutre o músculo estapédio. SIN ramus stapedius arteriae tympanicae posterioris [TA], ramus stapedius arteriae stylomastoideae, stapedial b. of stylomastoid artery.
stapedial b. of stylomastoid artery, r. do estapédio da artéria timpânica posterior. SIN stapedial b. of posterior tympanic artery.
sternal b.'s of internal thoracic artery [TA], ramos esternais da artéria torácica interna; ramos da artéria torácica interna que passam medialmente para nutrir o músculo transverso do tórax e a parte posterior do esterno. SIN rami sternales arteriae thoracicae internae [TA], sternal arteries.
sternocleidomastoid b.'s of occipital artery, ramos esternocleidomastóideos da artéria occipital; ramos da artéria occipital para o músculo esternocleidomastóideo. Com freqüência, um ramo forma um gancho ao redor do nervo hipoglosso. Pode originar-se como um r. independente da artéria carótida externa, quando é denominado artéria esternocleidomastóidea. SIN rami sternocleidomastoidei arteriae occipitalis.
sternocleidomastoid b. of superior thyroid artery [TA], r. esternocleidomastóideo da artéria tireóidea superior; r. da artéria tireóidea superior para o músculo esternocleidomastóideo. SIN ramus sternocleidomastoideus arteriae thyroideae superioris [TA].
stylohyoid b. of facial nerve [TA], r. estilo-hióideo do nervo facial; r. do nervo facial para o músculo estilo-hióideo. SIN ramus stylohyoideus nervi facialis [TA].
stylopharyngeal b. of glossopharyngeal nerve [TA], r. para o músculo estilofaríngeo do nervo glossofaríngeo; r. motor único do nervo glossofaríngeo para o músculo estilofaríngeo. SIN ramus musculi stylopharyngei nervi glossopharyngei [TA], b. of glossopharyngeal nerve to stylopharyngeus muscle.
subendocardial b.'s of atrioventricular bundles, ramos subendocárdicos dos fascículos atrioventriculares; fibras entrelaçadas formadas por células de músculo cardíaco modificadas com protoplasma granulado central, contendo um ou dois núcleos e uma porção periférica com estriações transversais; são as ramificações terminais do sistema de condução do coração encontrado sob o endocárdio dos ventrículos. VER TAMBÉM conducting *system* of heart. SIN rami subendocardiales fasciculi atrioventricularis [TA], Purkinje fibers.
subscapular b.'s of axillary artery [TA], ramos subescapulares da artéria axilar; ramos da artéria axilar que passam diretamente para o músculo subescapular. SIN rami subscapulares arteriae axillaris [TA].
superficial b. [TA], r. superficial; r. que passa acima ou mais próximo à superfície; usualmente em contraste com um r. profundo. SIN ramus superficialis [TA].
superficial b. of the lateral plantar nerve [TA], r. superficial do nervo plantar lateral; o r. mais cutâneo do dedo mínimo do pé e da metade lateral dos quatro dedos do pé e da face lateral da planta do pé, mas também inerva o músculo flexor curto do dedo mínimo e os músculos interósseos dorsais e plantares mais laterais. SIN ramus superficialis nervi plantaris lateralis [TA].
superficial b. of medial circumflex femoral artery [TA], r. superficial da artéria circunflexa femoral medial; pequeno r. que se origina da porção inicial da artéria circunflexa femoral medial que passa superficialmente na porção súpero-medial da coxa; depois de originar o r. superficial, a artéria circunflexa femoral medial continua como o r. profundo. SIN ramus superficialis arteriae circumflexae femoris medialis [TA].
superficial b. of the medial plantar artery [TA], r. superficial da artéria plantar medial; origina as artérias digitais superficiais dos três dedos dos pés mediais. SIN ramus superficialis arteriae plantaris medialis [TA].
superficial palmar b. of radial artery [TA], r. palmar superficial da artéria radial; o ramo palmar superficial da artéria radial que nutre os músculos tenares, em seguida penetra na região palmar para se comunicar com o arco palmar superficial oriundo da artéria ulnar. SIN ramus palmaris superficialis arteriae radialis [TA], superficial palmar artery, superficial volar artery, superficialis volae.
superficial b. of the radial nerve [TA], r. superficial do nervo radial; r. cutâneo terminal (com o r. profundo) que avança sob o revestimento do músculo braquiorradial até o punho, inervando, em seguida, a pele da porção proximal das faces dorsais dos dedos polegar, indicador, médio e metade lateral dos dedos anelares e a porção do dorso da mão localizada proximalmente. SIN ramus superficialis nervi radialis [TA].
superficial b. of the superior gluteal artery [TA], r. superficial da artéria glútea superior; para a porção superior do músculo glúteo máximo. SIN ramus superficialis arteriae gluteae superioris [TA].
superficial temporal b.'s of auriculotemporal nerve [TA], ramos temporais superficiais do nervo auriculotemporal; ramos do nervo auriculotemporal para a porção ântero-lateral do couro cabeludo. SIN rami temporales superficiales nervi auriculotemporalis [TA].
superficial b. of the transverse cervical artery [TA], r. superficial da artéria cervical transversa; r. da artéria cervical transversa que acompanha o nervo espinal acessório sobre a superfície profunda do músculo trapézio. De forma alternativa, origina-se como um ramo direto do tronco tireocervical, em cujo caso é denominado artéria cervical superficial. SIN ramus superficialis arteriae transversae colli [TA].

superficial b. of the ulnar nerve [TA], r. superficial do nervo ulnar; r. que inerva a pele da face palmar do dedo mínimo e a metade medial do dedo anelar, a porção da região palmar próxima a eles e o músculo palmar curto. SIN ramus superficialis nervi ulnaris [TA].

superior b. [TA], r. superior; o r. que é direcionado para cima ou cranialmente ou que está em uma posição elevada, usualmente em contraste com um r. inferior. SIN ramus superior [TA].

superior cervical cardiac b.'s of vagus nerve [TA], ramos cardíacos cervicais superiores do nervo vago; os mais superiores dos ramos do nervo vago que conduzem as fibras parassimpáticas pré-sinápticas para, e as fibras aferentes reflexas do, o plexo cardíaco; ramificações a partir do vago próximo à base do crânio. SIN rami cardiaci cervicales superiores nervi vagi [TA].

superior dental b.'s of superior dental plexus [TA], ramos dentais superiores do plexo dental superior; ramos que passam do plexo dental superior para as raízes dos dentes da maxila. SIN rami dentales superiores plexus dentalis superioris [TA], rami dentales superiores [TA], superior dental rami.

superior gingival b.'s of superior dental plexus [TA], ramos gengivais superiores do plexo dental superior; ramos do plexo dental superior para a gengiva da maxila. SIN rami gingivalis superiores plexus dentalis superioris [TA].

superior labial b. of facial artery [TA], artéria labial superior da artéria facial; *origem*, facial; *distribuição*, estruturas do lábio superior e, através de um ramo septal, para as porções anteriores e inferiores do septo nasal; *anastomoses*: a artéria do lado oposto e a artéria esfenopalatina. SIN arteria labialis superior [TA], ramus labialis superior arteriae facialis, superior labial artery.

superior labial b.'s of infraorbital nerve [TA], ramos labiais superiores do nervo infra-orbital; ramos do nervo infra-orbital para o lábio superior. SIN rami labiales superiores nervi infraorbitalis [TA].

superior lingular b. of lingular branch of superior lobar left pulmonary artery, artéria lingular superior. SIN superior lingular *artery.*

superior b. of the oculomotor nerve [TA], r. superior do nervo oculomotor; r. do nervo oculomotor que inerva os músculos reto superior do bulbo do olho e levantador da pálpebra superior. SIN ramus superior nervi oculomotorii [TA].

superior b. of pubic bone, r. superior do púbis. SIN superior pubic *ramus.*

superior b. of the right and left inferior pulmonary veins [TA], veia superior das veias pulmonares inferiores direita e esquerda; tributário das veias pulmonares inferiores direita e esquerda que recebe sangue oxigenado dos segmentos broncopulmonares superiores [S6] dos lobos inferiores dos pulmões direito e esquerdo. SIN ramus superior venae pulmonalis dextrae/sinistrae inferioris.

superior b. of the superior gluteal artery [TA], r. superior da artéria glútea superior; faz trajeto entre os músculos glúteos médio e mínimo, nutrindo a ambos e prosseguindo até alcançar o músculo tensor da fáscia lata. SIN ramus superior arteriae gluteae superioris [TA].

superior b. of the transverse cervical nerve [TA], r. superior do nervo cervical transverso na parte superior do triângulo anterior do pescoço. SIN ramus superior nervi transversalis cervicalis (colli) [TA].

superior vermian b. (of superior cerebellar artery) [TA], artéria superior do verme (da artéria cerebelar superior); *origem*: r. medial da artéria cerebelar superior; *distribuição:* parte superior do verme do cerebelo. SIN ramus vermis superior [TA].

suprahyoid b. of lingual artery [TA], r. supra-hióideo da artéria lingual; r. da artéria lingual que corre ao longo do osso hióide; *anastomose*: r. infra-hióideo da artéria tireóidea superior e, através da linha média, com sua congênere contralateral. SIN ramus suprahyoideus arteriae lingualis [TA].

sural communicating b. of common fibular nerve [TA], r. fibular comunicante do nervo fibular comum; origina-se do nervo fibular comum no espaço poplíteo e passa sobre a cabeça lateral do músculo gastrocnêmio para o terço médio da perna, onde se une com o nervo cutâneo dorsal medial da fíbula para formar o nervo fibular. SIN ramus communicans fibularis nervi fibularis communis [TA], ramus communicans nervi fibularis communis cum nervo cutaneo surae mediali*, ramus communicans nervi peronei communis cum nervo cutaneo surae mediali*, ramus communicans peroneus nervi peronei communis*, sural communicating b. of common peroneal nerve*, nervus communicans fibularis, nervus communicans peroneus, peroneal anastomotic ramus, peroneal communicating b., peroneal communicating nerve.

sural communicating b. of common peroneal nerve, r. fibular comunicante do nervo fibular comum; termo oficial alternativo* para sural communicating b. of common fibular nerve.

sympathetic b. to submandibular ganglion, raiz simpática do gânglio submandibular. SIN sympathetic *root* of submandibular ganglion.

temporal b.'s of facial nerve [TA], ramos temporais do nervo facial; ramos do nervo facial que inervam a porção superior do músculo orbicular do olho e outros músculos da expressão facial acima do olho. SIN rami temporales facialis [TA].

tentorial basal b. of internal carotid artery [TA], r. basilar do tentório da parte cavernosa da artéria carótida interna; um pequeno r. que vai da porção cavernosa da artéria carótida interna até a base do tentório. SIN ramus basalis tentorii arteriae carotidis internae [TA], basal tentorial b. of internal carotid artery.

tentorial marginal b. of cavernous part of internal carotid artery, r. marginal do tentório da parte cavernosa da artéria carótida interna; um pequeno r. da parte cavernosa da artéria carótida interna para a margem livre do tentório. SIN ramus marginalis tentorii partis cavernosae arteriae carotidis internae [TA], marginal tentorial b. of internal carotid artery, ramus marginalis tentorii arteriae carotidis internae.

terminal b.'s of middle cerebral artery [TA], ramos terminais da artéria cerebral média; derivados da artéria cerebral média, originando-se distalmente ao segmento M1 (tronco principal) profundamente no sulco lateral entre o lobo temporal e a ínsula; estão incluídos os ramos (corticais) terminais superior e inferior (troncos) e as artérias insulares. SIN rami terminales arteriae cerebri medii [TA], M2 segment of middle cerebral artery*.

thoracic cardiac b.'s of thoracic ganglia, ramos cardíacos torácicos dos gânglios torácicos; parte dos nervos esplâncnicos cardiopulmonares do segundo ao quinto segmentos do tronco simpático torácico que avançam medial e anteriormente para entrar no plexo cardíaco; conduzem fibras simpáticas pós-sinápticas para, e fibras aferentes viscerais (álgicas) oriundas do, coração. SIN rami cardiaci thoracici gangliorum thoracicorum [TA], nervi cardiaci thoracici, thoracic cardiac nerves, upper thoracic splanchnic nerves.

thoracic cardiac b.'s of vagus nerve [TA], ramos cardíacos torácicos do nervo vago, ramos do nervo vago para o plexo cardíaco que se ramificam a partir do vago nos níveis torácicos, conduzindo as fibras parassimpáticas pré-sinápticas para o, e as fibras aferentes reflexas a partir do, plexo cardíaco. SIN rami cardiaci thoracici nervi vagi [TA].

thoracic pulmonary b.'s of thoracic ganglia [TA], ramos pulmonares torácicos dos gânglios torácicos; nervos esplâncnicos cardiopulmonares que se originam dos gânglios torácicos paravertebrais do tronco simpático que conduzem fibras simpáticas pós-sinápticas e aferentes viscerais para os plexos pulmonares. SIN rami pulmonales thoracici gangliorum thoracicorum [TA].

thymic b.'s of internal thoracic artery [TA], ramos tímicos da artéria torácica interna; ramos mediastinais da porção proximal (superior) da artéria torácica interna que se dirigem para o timo. SIN rami thymici arteriae thoracicae internae [TA].

thyrohyoid b. of ansa cervicalis, r. tireo-hióideo da alça cervical; derivado do plexo cervical, contém fibras do primeiro e segundo nervos cervicais que acompanham o nervo hipoglosso até a região supra-hióidea, ramificando-se, em seguida, a partir dele, para alcançar o músculo tireo-hióideo. SIN ramus thyrohyoideus ansae cervicalis [TA], nerve to thyrohyoid muscle.

tonsillar b. of the facial artery [TA], r. tonsilar da artéria facial; suprimento sangüíneo primário para a tonsila palatina, com extensas anastomoses com outras artérias tonsilares. SIN ramus tonsillaris arteriae facialis [TA].

tonsillar b.'s of glossopharyngeal nerve [TA], ramos tonsilares do nervo glossofaríngeo; os ramos do nervo glossofaríngeo que conduzem as fibras sensoriais da fossa tonsilar palatina. SIN rami tonsillares nervi glossopharyngei.

tonsillar b.'s of lesser palatine nerves [TA], ramos tonsilares dos nervos palatinos inferiores; os ramos dos nervos palatinos inferiores que se estendem até a tonsila palatina e/ou seu leito. SIN rami tonsillares nervi palatini minores [TA].

tracheal b.'s [TA], ramos traqueais; ramos para a traquéia. A Terminologia Anatômica lista os ramos traqueais 1) da artéria tireóidea inferior (rami tracheales arteriae thyroideae inferioris [TA]); 2) da artéria torácica interna (rami tracheales arteria thoracicae internae [TA]); e 3) do nervo laríngeo recorrente (rami tracheales nervi laryngei recurrentis [TA]). SIN rami tracheales [TA].

transverse b. of lateral femoral circumflex artery [TA], r. transverso da artéria circunflexa femoral lateral; o r. inicial da artéria circunflexa femoral lateral que penetra na substância do músculo vasto lateral e forma inúmeras anastomoses. SIN ramus transversus arteriae circumflexae femoris lateralis [TA].

b. to trigeminal ganglion, ramos ganglionares trigeminais; ramos ganglionares da artéria carótida interna.

tubal b. [TA], r. tubário; r. para uma estrutura tubular. SIN ramus tubarius [TA].

tubal b. of ovarian artery [TA], r. tubário da artéria ovárica; r. terminal (com o r. ovárico) da artéria ovárica que passa para a parte distal da tuba uterina e avança centralmente para se anastomosar com o r. tubário da artéria uterina própria. SIN ramus tubarius arteriae ovaricae [TA].

tubal b. of the tympanic plexus [TA], r. tubário do plexo timpânico; r. sensorial do plexo timpânico (do nervo glossofaríngeo) para a tuba auditiva. SIN ramus tubarius plexus tympanici [TA].

tubal b. of uterine artery [TA], r. tubário da artéria uterina; r. terminal da artéria uterina (com o r. ovárico) que nutre a porção medial da tuba uterina, anastomosando-se com o r. tubário da artéria ovárica. SIN ramus tubarius arteriae uterinae [TA].

ulnar communicating b. of superficial radial nerve, r. comunicante com o nervo ulnar do ramo superficial do nervo radial. SIN communicating b. of superficial radial nerve with ulnar nerve.

ulnar b. of medial antebrachial cutaneous nerve, r. posterior do nervo cutâneo medial do antebraço. SIN posterior b. of medial cutaneous nerve of forearm.

ureteral b.'s, ramos uretéricos. SIN ureteric b.'s.

ureteric b.'s [TA], ramos uretéricos; ramos distribuídos para o ureter. Os ramos uretéricos também originam-se regularmente 1) da parte abdominal da aorta; 2) da artéria ilíaca comum e 3) da artéria ilíaca interna. Os ramos uretéricos da artéria vesical inferior são de ocorrência constante e nutrem a porção terminal do ureter. SIN rami ureterici [TA], ureteral b.'s.
ureteric b.'s of the inferior suprarenal artery [TA], ramos uretéricos da artéria supra-renal inferior; ramos da artéria supra-renal inferior direita ou esquerda que descem para nutrir, com os ramos uretéricos da artéria renal, a porção mais superior do ureter. SIN rami ureterici arteriae suprarenalis inferioris [TA].
ureteric b.'s of the ovarian artery [TA], ramos uretéricos da artéria ovárica; r. da artéria ovárica que se originam quando ela cruza o ureter na mulher, nutrindo a porção média do ureter. SIN rami ureterici arteriae ovaricae [TA].
ureteric b.'s of the patent part of umbilical artery [TA], ramos uretéricos da parte pérvia da artéria umbilical; nutrem a porção pélvica do ureter. SIN rami ureterici partis patentis arteriae umbilicalis [TA].
ureteric b.'s of the renal artery, ramos uretéricos da artéria renal; nutrem a pelve uretérica (renal) e a porção superior do ureter. SIN rami ureterici arteriae renalis.
ureteric b.'s of the testicular artery [TA], ramos uretéricos da artéria testicular; r. da artéria testicular que se origina quando ela cruza o ureter no homem; nutrem a porção média do ureter. SIN rami ureterici arteriae testicularis [TA].
ventral b., r. ventral. SIN ramus ventralis. VER ventral primary *rami* of cervical spinal nerves, em *ramus*; ventral primary *rami* of lumbar spinal nerves, em *ramus*, ventral primary *rami* of sacral spinal nerves, em *ramus*, anterior *ramus* of spinal nerve.
vestibular b.'s of labyrinthine artery, ramos vestibulares da artéria do labirinto. VER posterior vestibular b. of vestibulocochlear artery, anterior vestibular *artery*.
zygomatic b.'s of facial nerve, ramos zigomáticos do nervo facial; ramos do nervo facial que cruzam a parte superior da bochecha para inervar o músculo orbicular do olho. SIN rami zygomatici nervi facialis.
zygomaticofacial b. of zygomatic nerve [TA], r. zigomaticofacial do nervo zigomático; penetra o osso zigomático para nutrir a pele sobre o zigoma. SIN ramus zygomaticofacialis nervi zygomatici [TA].
zygomaticotemporal b. of zygomatic nerve [TA], r. zigomaticofacial do nervo zigomático; penetra o processo frontal do osso zigomático para nutrir a pele da face lateralmente à órbita. SIN ramus zygomaticotemporalis nervi zygomatici [TA].
bran·chia, pl. **bran·chi·ae** (brang'kē-ă, -ē). Brânquias; as brânquias ou órgãos da respiração em animais de vida aquática. [G. brânquia]
bran·chi·al (brang'kē-ăl). Branquial. **1.** Relativo às brânquias. **2.** Em embriologia, indica as diversas estruturas que constituem o aparelho branquial (ver branchial *apparatus*).
branching. Ramificação; que se divide em partes; que emite ramificações; bifurcando-se. SIN ramose, ramous. [Fr. *branche*, relativo ao L. *branchium*, braço]
false b., r. falsa; em bacteriologia, o aparecimento de r. produzida quando uma célula é retirada da linha geral do crescimento e desenvolve uma nova linha de crescimento, enquanto as células restantes continuam a se desenvolver ao longo da linha original de crescimento.
bran·chi·o·gen·ic, bran·chi·og·en·ous (brang'kē-ō-jen'ik, -kē-oj'en-ŭs) Branquiogênico; que se origina dos arcos branquiais. [G. *branchia*, brânquia, *-gen*, produzir]
bran·chi·o·mere (brang'kē-ō-mēr). Branquiômero; um segmento embrionário a partir do qual se desenvolve um arco branquial. [G. *branchia*, brânquia, + *meros*, parte]
bran·chi·om·er·ism (brang-kē-om'er-izm). Branquiomerismo; disposição em branquiômeros.
bran·chi·o·mo·tor (brang'kē-ō-mō'tor). Branquiomotor; relativo a ou que controla o movimento dos músculos associados aos arcos branquiais.
bran·dy. Conhaque; um líquido alcoólico obtido pela destilação do suco fermentado de uvas frescas e que, em geral, contém 48 a 54% de álcool etílico. [Hol. *brandewijn*, vinho queimado (destilado)]
Branham, H. H., cirurgião norte-americano do século 19. VER B. *sign*.
Branham, Sara Elizabeth, bacteriologista norte-americana, 1888–1962. VER *Branhamella*.
Bran·ha·mel·la (bran-hă-mel'ă). Subgênero de bactérias aeróbicas, imóveis, não-formadoras de esporos, que contêm cocos Gram-negativos que ocorrem aos pares, com lados adjacentes achatados; esses microrganismos são atualmente considerados intimamente relacionados ao gênero *Moraxella*. Ocorrem nas mucosas do trato respiratório superior. A espécie típica é *B. catarrhalis*. [Sara Branham]
B. catarrha'lis. SIN *Moraxella catarrhalis*.
bran·ny (bran'ē). Farelento; indica a descamação de pequenas escamas similares à palha de milho. [I. Med. *bran*, revestimento rompido do cereal em grão]
Brasdor, Pierre, cirurgião francês, 1721–1798. VER B. *method*.
Braun, Christopher Heinrich, cirurgião alemão, 1847–1911. VER B. *anastomosis*.
Braune, Christian W., anatomista alemão, 1831–1892. VER B. *muscle*, *valve*.
brawny (brahw'nē). Espessado (liquenificado) e mosqueado (com uma coloração escurecida), como de uma tumefação. [I. Med. carnoso]
Braxton Hicks, John, ginecologista britânico, 1823–1897. VER B. H. *contraction*, *sign*.
Bray, Charles William, otologista norte-americano, *1904. VER Wever-B. *phenomenon*.
Brazelton, T. Berry, pediatra norte-americano, *1918. VER Brazelton Neonatal Behavioral Assessment *Scale*, em *scale*.
bra·zil·ein (bră-zil'ē-in). Brasileína; um produto vermelho da oxidação da brasilina.
braz·i·lin (bră-zil'in). [C. I. 75280]. Brasilina; corante vermelho natural, $C_{16}H_{14}O_5$, obtido da casca de várias espécies de árvores tropicais e oxidado no corante vermelho ativo brasileína; assemelha-se à hematoxilina em sua origem, química e utilização; usado como corante nuclear e como indicador (vermelho em álcalis, amarelo em ácidos).
braz·ing (brā'zing). Soldadura; em odontologia, soldagem.
BrDu Abreviatura de bromodeoxyuridine (bromodesoxiuridina).
break (brāk). Ruptura; separação em partes.
double-strand b., r. de filamento duplo; r. no DNA de filamento duplo em que os dois filamentos foram clivados; entretanto, os dois filamentos não se separam.
single-strand b., r. de filamento único; r. no DNA de filamento duplo em que apenas um dos filamentos foi clivado; ambos os filamentos não se separam.
breakpoint (brāk'poynt). Ponto de ruptura; na epidemiologia dos helmintos, a carga média crítica de vermes em uma comunidade, abaixo da qual a freqüência de cruzamento dos helmintos é muito baixa para manter a reprodução. Abaixo desse nível, a helmintíase na comunidade diminuirá progressivamente, chegando, por fim, a zero.
break·through (brāk'throo). Penetração; manifestação súbita de novos *insights* e de atitudes mais construtivas após um período de resistência durante a psicoterapia.
breast (brest) [TA]. Peito, mama. **1.** A superfície peitoral do tórax. **2.** O órgão feminino de secreção de leite; uma das duas projeções comumente hemisféricas anteriores aos músculos peitorais, incluindo as glândulas mamárias, dentro de uma quantidade altamente variável de tecido adiposo da camada subcutânea e comportando o mamilo, superficialmente, em ambos os lados do tórax da mulher madura; é rudimentar no homem. SIN mamma [TA], teat (2). [A.S. *brēost*]
accessory b. [TA], mama acessória; uma glândula secretora de leite localizada em algum local diferente do posicionamento normal no tórax e que existe além das duas mamas usuais. SIN mamma accessoria [TA], supernumerary b., supernumerary mamma.
chicken b., peito de pombo. SIN *pectus carinatum*.
funnel b., peito afunilado. SIN *pectus excavatum*.
irritable b., mama irritável; edema e induração da mama, não decorrente de uma neoplasia, e usualmente de duração comparativamente curta.
male b. [TA], mama masculina; uma das duas glândulas mamárias, comumente rudimentares, e os mamilos suprajacentes do homem. SIN mamma masculina [TA], mamma virilis.
pigeon b., peito de pombo. SIN *pectus carinatum*.
supernumerary b., mama supranumerária. SIN accessory b.

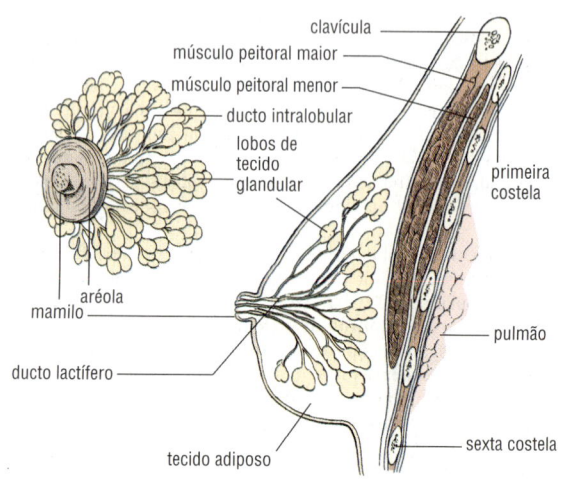

mama: tecido glandular e ductos da glândula mamária

breath (breth). Respiração. **1.** O ar inspirado. **2.** Uma inspiração. [A.S. *braeth*]
liver b., respiração hepática. SIN *fetor* hepaticus.
uremic b., respiração urêmica; odor característico da r. em pacientes com insuficiência renal crônica, descrita de forma variada como "piscosa", "amoniacal" e "fétida", o que é indicativo do acúmulo sistêmico de metabólitos voláteis, usualmente excretados na urina; a dimetilamina e a trimetilamina foram identificadas e correlacionadas com o clássico odor de peixe.
breath-holding (breth′hōld - ing). Interrupção respiratória; a cessação voluntária ou involuntária da respiração; freqüentemente observada como uma resposta à frustração.
breath·ing (brēth′ing). Respiração; inspiração e expiração do ar ou de misturas gasosas. SIN pneusis.
  apneustic b., r. apnêusica; pausas no ciclo respiratório na inspiração plena, causadas por lesão dos centros de controle respiratório na porção mais caudal da ponte.
  ataxic b., r. atáxica. SIN Biot *respiration.*
  Biot b., r. de Biot. SIN Biot *respiration.*
  bronchial b., r. brônquica; ruídos respiratórios de qualidade áspera ou soprosa, feitos pela movimentação do ar nos grandes brônquios e pouco ou nada modificados pelo pulmão interveniente; a duração do som expiratório é tão longa quanto ou mais longa que a do som inspiratório; pode ser ouvido sobre um pulmão consolidado, acima de um derrame pleural devido a um pulmão comprimido subjacente, e raramente sobre uma cavidade pulmonar; a pectorilóquia sussurrada é outra manifestação que, em geral, pode ser provocada quando a r. brônquica está presente.
  glossopharyngeal b., r. glossofaríngea; a respiração não-auxiliada pelos músculos primários usuais da respiração; o ar é forçado para dentro dos pulmões pelo uso da língua e dos músculos da faringe.
  intermittent positive pressure b. (IPPB), r. com pressão positiva intermitente; modalidade ventilatória mecânica em que o paciente deflagra uma respiração limitada por pressão. Método ultrapassado de fornecimento de terapia com aerossol para os pulmões.
  mouth b., r. bucal; respiração habitual através da boca em vez do nariz, usualmente causada por obstrução das vias nasais.
  positive-negative pressure b. (PNPB), r. com pressão positiva-negativa; a insuflação dos pulmões com pressão positiva e desinsuflação com pressão negativa por um ventilador automático.
  pursed lips b., r. com lábios franzidos; uma técnica em que o ar é inspirado lentamente através do nariz e da boca e expirado lentamente com os lábios franzidos; usada por pacientes com doença pulmonar obstrutiva crônica para melhorar a respiração por aumento da resistência ao fluxo aéreo, dilatando forçadamente os pequenos brônquios.
  shallow b., r. superficial; um tipo de r. com volume corrente anormalmente baixo.
  stertorous b., r. estertorosa. SIN stertorous *respiration.*
Breda, Achille, dermatologista italiano, 1850–1933. VER B. *disease.*
bre·douille·ment (brā - dwē - mahn′). Omissão de partes de palavras relacionada com a fala extremamente rápida. [Fr.]
breech (brēch). Nádegas. SIN buttocks. [A.S. *brēc*]
breed·ing (brēd′ing). Geração; cruzamento selecionado de indivíduos para produzir uma cepa que é desejável ou de interesse científico. VER TAMBÉM hybridization, linebreeding, inbreeding. [cruzar, do I. Med. *breden*, do I. Ant. *brēdan*, + -ing]
breg·ma (breg′mă). [TA]. Bregma; o ponto no crânio que corresponde à junção das suturas coronal e sagital. [G. a parte anterior da cabeça]
breg·mat·ic (breg - mat′ik). Bregmático; relativo ao bregma.

músculos utilizados na respiração

músculos inspiratórios	músculos auxiliares (inspiração)
diafragma	esternocleidomastóideo
intercostal externo	escalenos anterior, médio e posterior
intercostal interno, parte paraesternal (intercartilaginosa)	peitoral maior
	peitoral menor
	serrátil posterior superior
	serrátil anterior

músculos da expiração	músculos auxiliares (expiração)
intercostal interno	reto do abdome
transverso do tórax	transverso do abdome
subcostal	oblíquo externo do abdome
	oblíquo interno do abdome
	eretor da espinha
	quadrado do lombo
	serrátil posterior inferior

brei (brī). Um tecido moído ou esmagado, fino e uniforme, no qual as células permanecem, em sua maior parte, intactas. Cf. homogenate. [Alemão pasta]
brems·strah·lung (bremz′strah - lŭng). Irradiação de espectro contínuo produzida pela lentificação dos elétrons em um feixe pelos núcleos em suas vizinhanças. [Alemão *Bremsstrahlung*, radiação freada]
Brenn, Lena, pesquisadora norte-americana do século 20. VER Brown-B. *stain.*
Brenner, Fritz, patologista alemão, *1877. VER B. *tumor.*
brepho-. Brefo-; prefixo que indica um estágio primitivo de desenvolvimento. [G. *brephos*, embrião ou recém-nascido]
Breschet (Brechet), Gilbert, anatomista francês, 1784–1845. VER B. *bones*, em *bone, canals*, em *canal, hiatus, sinus, vein.*
Brescia, Michael J., nefrologista norte-americano, *1933. VER B.-Cimino *fistula.*
Breslow, Alexander, patologista norte-americano, 1928–1980. VER B. *thickness.*
bre·tyl·i·um. Bretílio. **1.** Um anti-hipertensivo que, sob a dosagem oral crônica, primeiramente libera e em seguida diminui a liberação de norepinefrina a partir das terminações nervosas não-adrenérgicas. **2.** Um antiarrítmico utilizado para tratar as arritmias ventriculares com risco de vida; bloqueia os canais de potássio.
bre·tyl·i·um tos·yl·ate (bre - til′ē - ŭm). Tosilato de bretílio; um agente simpaticolítico que evita a liberação de norepinefrina a partir da terminação nervosa; empregado no tratamento de hipertensão essencial. VER TAMBÉM bretylium.
Breuer, Josef, clínico austríaco, 1842–1925. VER Hering-B. *reflex.*
bre·ve·tox·ins (BTX) (brev′ē - tok′sins). Brevetoxinas; neurotoxinas estruturalmente ímpares produzidas pelo dinoflagelado "vermelho" *Ptychodiscus brevis Davis* (*Gymnodinium breve Davis*). Uma alga responsável por grandes mortandades de peixes e moluscos e por intoxicação alimentar humana no Golfo do México e ao longo da costa da Flórida. Diferentemente das toxinas de dinoflagelados previamente isoladas, como a saxitoxina, que são bloqueadores hidrossolúveis dos canais de cálcio, as brevetoxinas são ativadores lipossolúveis dos canais de sódio. Usadas como instrumentos na pesquisa neurobiológica.
Brev·i·bac·ter·i·um (brev - ē - bak - tēr′ē - um). Um gênero de bactérias de bastonetes Gram-positivos, imóveis e não-formadores de esporos, encontrados como flora cutânea humana normal, no leite cru e sobre a superfície de queijos; algumas espécies, recuperadas a partir de pacientes com septicemia e a partir do peritônio de pacientes que sofrem diálise peritoneal, parecem ser patógenos humanos oportunistas.
brev·i·col·lis (brev - ē - kol′is). Brevícolo; pescoço anormalmente curto. [L. *brevis*, curto, + *collum*, pescoço]
bre·vis (brev′is). Breve; curto. [L. curto]
Brewer, George E., cirurgião norte-americano, 1861–1939. VER B. *infarcts*, em *infarct.*
Bricker, Eugene M., urologista norte-americano, *1908. VER B. *operation.*
bridge (bridj). Ponte. **1.** A parte superior da crista do nariz formada pelos ossos nasais. **2.** Um dos filamentos de protoplasma que parecem passar de uma célula para outra. **3.** SIN fixed partial *denture.*
  arteriolovenular b., p. arteriolovenular; o maior capilar que une a arteríola à vênula.
  cantilever b., p. em cantiléver; uma ponte dentária parcial fixa em que o pôntico é preso em apenas um lado por um dente pivô. SIN extension b.
  caudolenticular gray b.'s [TA], pontes caudolenticulares cinzentas; filamentos de corpos neuronais que se estendem sobre a cápsula interna, principalmente seu ramo anterior, entre o núcleo caudado e o putame. SIN pontes grisei caudolenticulares [TA], transcapsular gray b.'s*.
  cell b.'s, pontes celulares. SIN intercellular b.'s.
  cystine b., p. de cistina. SIN dissulfide b.
  cytoplasmic b.'s, pontes citoplasmáticas. SIN intercellular b.'s.
  dentin b., p. de dentina; um depósito de dentina ou de outras substâncias calcificadas para reparação, o qual se forma através do tecido da polpa dentária exposta e torna a selá-lo.
  disulfide b., p. dissulfeto; **(1)** uma ligação dissulfeto entre dois resíduos cisteinil em um poli- ou oligopeptídeo ou em uma proteína; **(2)** qualquer ligação dissulfeto entre quaisquer moléculas portadoras de tióis de uma molécula maior. SIN cystine b.
  extension b., p. de extensão. SIN cantilever b.
  fixed b., p. fixa. SIN fixed partial *denture.*
  Gaskell b., p. de Gaskell. SIN atrioventricular *bundle.*
  intercellular b.'s, pontes intercelulares; filamentos citoplasmáticos delgados que conectam células adjacentes; nos cortes histológicos da epiderme e de outros epitélios escamosos estratificados, as pontes são processos presos por um desmossoma e são artefatos enrugados pela fixação; as pontes verdadeiras com a confluência citoplasmática existem entre células germinativas que sofreram divisão incompleta. SIN cell b.'s, cytoplasmic b.'s.
  myocardial b., p. miocárdica; uma p. de fibras musculares cardíacas que se estende sobre a face epicárdica de uma artéria coronária; esse achado, nos casos de morte súbita inexplicada, leva à especulação de que a contração cardíaca durante o esforço poderia fazer a constrição da artéria coronária.

removable b., p. removível. SIN removable partial *denture.*
salt b., p. salina. SIN electrostatic *bond.*
transcapsular gray b.'s, pontes transcapsulares cinzentas; termo oficial alternativo* para caudolenticular gray b.'s.
Wheatstone b., p. de Wheatstone; um aparelho para medir a resistência elétrica; quatro resistores são conectados para formar os quatro lados ou "braços" de um quadrado; uma voltagem é aplicada a um par diagonal de conexões, enquanto a voltagem entre o outro par diagonal é medida, p.ex., por um galvanômetro; a ponte é "equilibrada" quando a voltagem medida é zero; em seguida, as proporções dos dois pares de resistências unidas devem ser idênticas.
bridge-work (bridj′wŏrk). Ponte dentária. SIN partial *denture.*
bri·dle (brī′dl). Brida. **1.** SIN frenum. **2.** Um feixe de material fibroso que se estende através da superfície de uma úlcera ou outra lesão ou que forma aderências entre as superfícies serosas ou mucosas opostas. [I. Med. *bridel*]
b. of clitoris, b. do clitóris; termo obsoleto para o freio do clitóris.
Bright, Richard, patologista e clínico inglês, 1789–1858. VER B. *disease.*
Brill, Nathan E., médico norte-americano, 1860–1925. VER B. *disease*; B.-Zinsser *disease.*
bril·liant cres·yl blue. Azul cresil brilhante. VER cresyl blue.
bril·liant green [C. I. 42040]. Verde brilhante; o sulfato de di-(*p*-dietilamino)-trifenil carbinolanidrido. Um corante indicador que muda de amarelo para verde em pH 0,0 a 2,6; também utilizado como um anti-séptico tópico e como um agente bacteriostático seletivo em meios de cultura. SIN ethyl green.
bril·liant vi·tal red. Vermelho vital brilhante. SIN vital red.
bril·liant yel·low [C. I. 13085]. Amarelo brilhante; um indicador que muda do amarelo para o laranja ou vermelho em pH de 6,4 a 8,0.
brim. Margem; a borda ou orla superior de uma estrutura oca.
pelvic b., m. pélvica. SIN pelvic *inlet.*
brim·stone (brim′stōn). Enxofre. SIN sulfur. [A.S. *brinnan*, queimar]
brin·dle (brin′dl). Cor rajada; uma camada de cabelos em que existe uma mistura uniforme de cabelos com coloração acinzentada ou amarelo-acastanhada com outros de cor branca ou negra; uma coloração composta. [diminutivo do I. Ant. *brinded*]
Brinell, Johan A., metalúrgico sueco, 1849–1925. VER B. hardness *number.*
Briquet, Paul, médico francês, 1796–1881. VER B. *ataxia, syndrome.*
brise·ment (brēz-maw′) Rompimento; procedimento raramente utilizado para tratar o ombro congelado em que uma manipulação forçada é realizada para restaurar a amplitude de movimento que, em geral, resulta na laceração de aderências e da cápsula articular adjacente. [Fr. ruptura forçada]
Brissaud, Edouard, médico francês, 1852–1909. VER B. *disease, infantilism, reflex*; B.-Marie *syndrome.*
Brit·ish an·ti-Lew·is·ite (BAL) (brit′ish an-tē-loo′is-īt). SIN dimercaprol.
Brit·ish Phar·ma·co·poe·ia (BP). Farmacopéia britânica. VER Pharmacopeia.
broach (brōch). Broca; um instrumento dentário para remover a polpa de um dente ou para explorar um canal.
barbed b., b. farpada; um instrumento para o canal da raiz que contém farpas; usado para remover uma polpa dentária, resquícios de tecido da polpa ou resíduos de dentina.
smooth b., b. lisa; um instrumento de exploração usado na prática endodôntica; uma ponta de canal da raiz.
Broadbent, Sir William H., médico britânico, 1835–1907. VER B. *law, sign.*
broad-spec·trum. Amplo espectro. VER *spectrum.*
Broca, Pierre P., cirurgião, neurologista e antropólogo francês, 1824–1880. VER B. *angles*, em *angle, aphasia,* basilar *angle,* facial *angle, area,* parolfactory *area,* diagonal *band, center, field, fissure, formula,* visual *plane, pouch.*
Brock, Sir Russell C., cirurgião britânico, *1903. VER B. *syndrome, operation.*
Brockenbrough, E. C., cirurgião norte-americano, *1930. VER B. *sign.*
bro·cre·sine (brō-krē′sēn). Brocresina; um inibidor da histidina descarboxilase.
Brödel, Max, artista médico alemão nos Estados Unidos, 1870–1941. VER B. bloodless *line.*
Brodie, Sir Benjamin C., cirurgião britânico, 1783–1862. VER B. *abscess, bursa, disease, knee.*
Brodie, Charles Gordon, cirurgião e anatomista escocês, 1860–1933. VER B. *ligament.*
Brodie, Thomas Gregor, fisiologista britânico, 1866–1916. VER B. *fluid.*
Brodmann, Korbinian, neurologista alemão, 1868–1918. VER B. *areas*, em *area.*
Broesike, Gustav, anatomista alemão, *1853. VER B. *fossa.*
♻ **brom-, bromo-. 1.** Odor fétido. **2.** Prefixo que indica a presença de bromo em um composto. [G. *brōmos*, mau cheiro]
bro·mate (brō-māt). Bromato; sal ou ânion do ácido brômico.
bro·mat·ed (brō′māt-ĕd). Bromado; combinado ou saturado com bromo ou qualquer um de seus compostos. SIN brominated.
bro·ma·ze·pam (brō-ma′zĕ-pam). Bromazepam; um agente ansiolítico da classe dos benzodiazepínicos.
bro·ma·zine hy·dro·chlo·ride (brō′ma-zēn). Cloridrato de bromazina. SIN bromodiphenhydramine hydrochloride.

brom·cre·sol green (brom-krē′sol). Verde de bromocresol; um corante substituto de trifenilmetano (pK_a 4,7), pouco solúvel em água mas prontamente solúvel em álcool, éter dietílico e etil acetato; usado como um indicador de pH (amarelo em pH 3,8, verde-azulado em pH 5,4).
brom·cre·sol pur·ple. Púrpura de bromocresol; um corante substituto de trifenilmetano (pK_a 6,3), praticamente insolúvel em água, mas solúvel em álcool e álcalis diluídos; usado como um indicador de pH (amarelo em pH de 5,2, púrpura em pH de 6,8).
bro·me·lain, bro·me·lin (brō′mĕ-lān, -lin) Bromelina; uma de um grupo de hidrolases peptídicas, todas tiol-proteinases, obtidas a partir do abacaxi; utilizadas no amaciamento de carnes e na produção de hidrolisados de proteínas; administrada por via oral no tratamento da inflamação e edema de tecidos moles associados a lesão traumática.
Bromelius, C., botânico sueco, 1639–1705. VER bromelain.
brom·hex·ine hy·dro·chlo·ride (brom-hek′sēn). Cloridrato de bromexina; um expectorante com propriedades mucolíticas, antitussígeno e broncodilatador.
brom·hi·dro·sis (brom-hi-drō′sis). Bromidrose. SIN bromidrosis.
bro·mic (brō′mik). Brômico; relativo ao bromo; indica especialmente o ácido brômico, $HBrO_3$.
bro·mide (brō′mīd). Brometo; o ânion Br^-; sal do brometo de hidrogênio (HBr); vários sais originalmente utilizados como sedativos, hipnóticos e anticonvulsivantes.
bro·mi·dro·si·pho·bia (brō′mi-drō-si-fō′bē-ă). Bromidrosifobia; medo mórbido de apresentar um mau cheiro a partir do corpo, por vezes com a crença de que tal odor está presente. [bromidrosis + G. *phobos*, medo]
bro·mi·dro·sis (brōm-i-drō′sis). Bromidrose; perspiração com odor fétido ou desagradável. A b. apócrina afeta as axilas depois da puberdade, sendo que a b. ecrina é generalizada, com sudorese excessiva. SIN bromhidrosis. [G. *brōmos*, um mau cheiro, + *hidrōs*, perspiração]
bro·min·at·ed (brō′min-āt-ĕd). Bromado. SIN bromated.
bro·min·di·one (bro-min-dī′ōn). Bromindiona; um anticoagulante oral.
bro·mine (Br) (brō′mēn, -min). Bromo; um elemento líquido, volátil, avermelhado e não-metálico; número atômico 35, peso atômico 79,904; valências 1-7, inclusive; ele se liga ao hidrogênio para formar ácido bromídrico, e esse reage com muitos metais para formar brometos, alguns dos quais são utilizados em medicamentos. [Fr. *brome*, bromo, do G. *bromos*, um mau cheiro]
bro·mism, bro·min·ism (brō′mizm, -min-izm). Bromismo, brominismo; intoxicação crônica por brometo, caracterizada por cefaléia, sonolência, confusão e, ocasionalmente, delírio violento, fraqueza muscular, depressão cardíaca, erupção acniforme, hálito fétido, anorexia e desconforto gástrico.
♻ **bromo-.** VER brom-.
bro·mo·ben·zyl·cy·an·ide (BBC) (brō′mō-benz-il-sī′a-nīd). Cianeto de bromobenzila; um lacrimejante usado em gases lacrimejantes no treinamento e controle de tumultos.
bro·mo·cre·sol green (brō-mō-krē′sol). Verde de bromocresol; tetrabromo-m-cresol-sulfonftaleína; um corante indicador que muda de amarelo para azul em pH de 4,7; usado para rastrear o DNA na eletroforese em agarose e em um método de ligação de corante para análise da albumina sérica.
bro·mo·crip·tine (brō-mō-krip′tēn). Bromocriptina; um derivado semi-sintético do esporão de centeio que diminui o *turnover* da dopamina, inibe a secreção de prolactina e a liberação de prolactina pelo hormônio liberador de tireotropina e retarda o crescimento tumoral, e, por conseguinte, é empregado no tratamento da hiperprolactinemia associada a diversos tumores hipofisários; um agonista nos receptores de dopamina também utilizado na doença de Parkinson.
bro·mo·de·ox·y·ur·i·dine (BrDu) (brō′mō-dē-ok′sē-ūr′i-dēn). Bromodesoxiuridina; um composto que compete com a uridina para a incorporação no RNA e que exibe fluorescência na luz ultravioleta; utilizado na análise de bandas BrDu.
bro·mo·der·ma (brō-mō-der′mă). Bromoderma; uma erupção acneforme ou granulomatosa decorrente de hipersensibilidade ao brometo. [bromide + G. *derma*, pele]
bro·mo·di·phen·hy·dra·mine hy·dro·chlo·ride (brō′mō-dī-fen-hī′dră-mēn). Cloridrato de bromodifenidramina; um anti-histamínico que pode causar sonolência e xerostomia. SIN bromazine hydrochloride.
bro·mo·hy·per·hi·dro·sis, bro·mo·hy·per·i·dro·sis (brō′mō-hī′per-hi-drō′sis, -hī′per-i-drō′sis). Bromoiperidrose; a secreção excessiva de suor que possui um odor fétido, geralmente ecrino e generalizado ou que afeta os pés. [G. *brōmos*, um mau cheiro, + *hyper*, acima de, + *hidrōsis*, sudorese]
bro·mo·phe·nol blue (brō-mō-fē′nol). Azul de bromofenol. SIN bromphenol blue.
bro·mo·sul·fo·phtha·lein (brō′mō-sŭl′fō-thal′ē-in). Bromossulfoftaleína. SIN sulfobromophthalein sodium.
5-bro·mo·u·ra·cil (brō-mō-ū′ră-sil). 5-bromouracil; análogo sintético (antimetabólito) da timina, em que um átomo de bromo substitui o grupamento metila na timina; um mutageno.

brom·phen·ir·a·mine ma·le·ate (brōm-fen-ir′ă-mēn). Maleato de bromofeniramina; um potente agente anti-histamínico.

brom·phe·nol blue (brom-fē-nol). Azul de bromofenol; um corante substituído de trifenilmetano (PM 670, pK 4,0) usado principalmente como indicador ácido-base (amarelo em pH < 3,1 e azul em pH > 4,7); também é utilizado para demonstração histoquímica e eletroforética de proteínas. SIN bromophenol blue.

brom·sul·fo·phtha·lein (brom-sŭl′fō-thal′ē-in). Bromossulfotaleína; SIN sulfobromophthalein sodium.

brom·thy·mol blue (brom-thī′mol). Azul de bromotimol; um corante com trifenilmetano substituído (PM 624, pK 7,0), usado principalmente como indicador de íon hidrogênio (amarelo em pH 6,0, azul em pH 7,6); também um corante vital fraco, mas tóxico.

bron·ca·tar (bron′kă-tar). Broncatar; composto do ácido canfórico (neutralizado) com 2-amino-2-tiazolina (1:2); um antitussígeno e estimulante respiratório.

bronch-. Bronc-, bronqui-. VER broncho-.

bron·chi (brong′kī). Brônquios; plural de bronchus (brônquio).

bronchi-. Bronqui-; VER broncho-.

bron·chia (brong′kē-ă). Tubos brônquicos; as menores divisões dos brônquios. VER TAMBÉM bronchus, bronchiole. SIN bronchial tubes. [G. pl. de *bronchion*, dim. de *bronchos*, traquéia]

bron·chi·al (brong′kē-al). Brônquico; relativo aos brônquios.

bron·chi·ec·ta·sia (brong′kē-ek-tā′zē-ă). Bronquiectasia. SIN bronchiectasis.
b. sicca, b. seca. SIN dry bronchiectasis.

bron·chi·ec·ta·sis (brong-kē-ek′tă-sis). Bronquiectasia; dilatação crônica dos brônquios ou bronquíolos como uma seqüela de doença inflamatória ou obstrução freqüentemente associada à produção intensa de escarro. SIN bronchiectasia. [bronchi- + G. *ektasis*, uma dilatação]

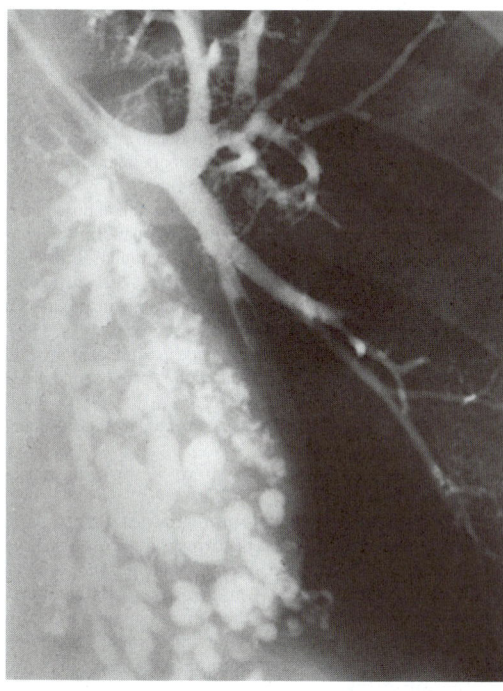

bronquiectasia: broncografia póstero-anterior esquerda de uma criança com 10 anos de idade com bronquiectasia e atelectasia do lobo inferior esquerdo secundária a pneumonia grave

congenital b., b. congênita; uma forma rara de b. decorrente da parada do desenvolvimento na árvore traqueobrônquica; pode ser unilateral ou bilateral.
cylindrical b., b. cilíndrica; b. que resulta em brônquios dilatados de formato cilíndrico; i.e., de calibre uniforme.
cystic b., b. cística; b. em que os brônquios terminam em sacos cegos maiores no diâmetro que os brônquios de drenagem. VER TAMBÉM saccular b.
dry b., b. seca; b. caracterizada por ausência de tosse produtiva e por hemoptise ocasional. SIN bronchiectasia sicca.
saccular b., b. sacular; b. que resulta em brônquios dilatados de formato sacular ou irregular. VER TAMBÉM cystic b.
varicose b., b. varicosa; b. cilíndrica com constrições irregulares que se assemelham às veias varicosas em formato.

bron·chi·ec·tat·ic (brong-kē-ek-tat′ik). Bronquiectásico; relativo à bronquiectasia.

bron·chil·o·quy (brong′kil′ō-kwē). Bronquiloquia; termo raramente utilizado para a broncofonia. [bronchi- + L. *loquor*, falar]

bron·chi·o·gen·ic (brong-kē-ō-jen′ik). Broncogênico. SIN bronchogenic.

bron·chi·ole (brong′kē-ōl) [TA]. Bronquíolo; uma das aproximadamente seis gerações de subdivisões cada vez mais finas dos brônquios, todas com menos de 1 mm de diâmetro, e não apresentando cartilagem em suas paredes, mas com fibras elásticas e musculatura lisa relativamente abundantes. SIN bronchiolus [TA].
respiratory b.'s, bronquíolos respiratórios; os menores bronquíolos (0,5 mm de diâmetro) que unem os bronquíolos terminais aos ductos alveolares; os alvéolos originam-se de parte da parede. SIN bronchioli respiratorii.
terminal b., b. terminal; a extremidade da via aérea de condução não-respiratória; o revestimento é de epitélio colunar simples ou cubóide, sem células caliciformes mucosas; muitas das células são ciliadas, porém ocorrem algumas células secretoras serosas não-ciliadas. SIN bronchiolus terminalis.

bron·chi·o·lec·ta·sia (brong′kē-ō-lek′tā′zē-ă). Bronquiolectasia. SIN bronchiolectasis.

bron·chi·o·lec·ta·sis (brong′kē-ō-lek′tă′sis). Bronquiolectasia; bronquiectasia que envolve os bronquíolos. SIN bronchiolectasia. [bronchiole + G. *ektasis*, uma dilatação]

bron·chi·o·li (brong-kē′ō-lī). Bronquíolos; plural de bronchiolus (bronquíolo).

bron·chi·ol·i·tis (brong-kē-ō-lī′tis). Bronquiolite; inflamação dos bronquíolos, freqüentemente associada à broncopneumonia. [bronchiole + *-itis*, inflamação]
constrictive b., b. constritiva; obliteração dos bronquíolos por cicatrização após a b. obliterante. Cf. proliferative b.
exudative b., b. exsudativa; inflamação dos bronquíolos, com exsudação fibrinosa.
b. fibro′sa oblit′erans, b. fibrosa obliterante; obstrução dos bronquíolos e dos ductos alveolares por tecido de granulação fibrosa induzido por ulceração da mucosa; a condição pode seguir à inalação de gases irritantes (ver silofiller's *lung*) ou pode complicar a pneumonia (ver BOOP); associada a achados obstrutivos (ver unilateral hyperlucent *lung*, Swyer-James *syndrome*). SIN b. obliterans.
b. oblit′erans, b. obliterante. SIN b. fibrosa obliterans.
b. obliterans with organizing pneumonia (BOOP), b. obliterante com pneumonia em organização; b. fibrosa obliterante complicada por pneumonia com organização.
proliferative b., b. proliferativa; b. com obliteração da luz bronquiolar e dos alvéolos por proliferação epitelial, que pode suceder à influenza e à pneumonia de células gigantes.

bronchiolo-. Bronquíolo; forma combinante que indica bronquíolo. [L. *bronchiolus*]

bron·chi·o·lo·pul·mo·nary (brong′kē-ō-lō-pul′mō-nār-ē). Bronquiolopulmonar; relativo aos bronquíolos e aos pulmões.

bron·chi·o·lus, pl. **bron·chi·o·li** (brong-kē′ō-lŭs, -ō-lī) [TA]. Bronquíolo, bronquíolos. SIN bronchiole. [L. Mod. dim. de *bronchus*]
bronchi′oli respirato′rii, bronquíolos respiratórios. SIN respiratory bronchioles, em bronchiole.
b. termina′lis, b. terminal. SIN terminal bronchiole.

bron·chi·o·ste·no·sis (brong′kē-ō-sten-ō′sis). Bronquiostenose. SIN bronchial stenosis.

bron·chit·ic (brong-kit′ik). Bronquítico; relativo à bronquite.

bron·chi·tis (brong-kī′tis). Bronquite; inflamação da mucosa dos tubos brônquicos.
asthmatic b., b. asmática; b. que causa ou agrava o broncoespasmo.
Castellani b., b. de Castellani. SIN hemorrhagic b.
chronic b., b. crônica; uma condição da árvore brônquica caracterizada por tosse, hipersecreção de muco e expectoração de escarro durante um longo período de tempo, associado a freqüentes infecções brônquicas; geralmente decorrente da inspiração, durante um intervalo prolongado, de ar contaminado por poeira ou gases nocivos de combustão.
croupous b., termo obsoleto para fibrinous b. (b. fibrinosa).
fibrinous b., b. fibrinosa; inflamação da mucosa brônquica, acompanhada por uma exsudação fibrinosa, que, com freqüência, forma um molde da árvore brônquica com grave obstrução do fluxo de ar. SIN plastic b., pseudomembranous b.
hemorrhagic b., b. hemorrágica; a b. crônica decorrente da infecção por espiroquetas (embora outras bactérias estejam usualmente presentes e contribuam para a infecção) e caracterizada por tosse e escarro sanguinolento. SIN bronchopulmonary spirochetosis, bronchospirochetosis, Castellani b.
obliterative b., b. oblit′erans, b. obliterante; b. fibrinosa em que o exsudato se torna organizado, obliterando a porção afetada dos tubos brônquicos com conseqüente colapso permanente das porções afetadas do pulmão.
plastic b., b. plástica. SIN fibrinous b.
pseudomembranous b., b. pseudomembranosa. SIN fibrinous b.
putrid b., b. pútrida; b. acompanhada por uma expectoração de escarro com odor fétido.

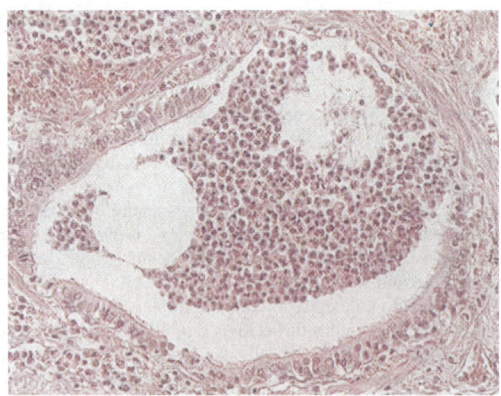
bronquiolite: massa espessa de granulócitos em uma luz bronquiolar

bron·chi·um (brong′kē-ŭm). Brônquio. SIN **bronchus.** [L. Mod. do G. *bronchion*]

△ **broncho-, bronch-, bronchi-.** Formas combinantes que indicam o brônquio e, em um uso mais anterior, a traquéia. [G. *bronchos*, traquéia]

bron·cho·al·ve·o·lar (brong′kō-al-vē′ō-lăr). Broncoalveolar. SIN **bronchovesicular.**

bron·cho·cav·ern·ous (brong-kō-kav′er-nŭs). Broncocavernoso; relativo a um brônquio ou tubo brônquico e uma cavidade pulmonar patológica.

bron·cho·cele (brong′kō-sēl). Broncocele; uma dilatação circunscrita de um brônquio. [broncho- + G. *kēlē*, hérnia]

bron·cho·con·stric·tion (brong-kō-kon-strik′shŭn). Broncoconstrição; redução no calibre de um brônquio ou brônquios, usualmente referindo-se a um processo dinâmico como na asma ou enfisema, em vez de uma constrição fixa (a última constitui uma estenose brônquica). Cf. bronchospasm.

bron·cho·con·stric·tor (brong-kō-kon-strik′ter, -tōr). Broncoconstritor. **1.** Que causa uma redução no calibre de um brônquio ou tubo brônquico. **2.** Um agente que possui essa ação (p.ex., histamina, acetilcolina).

bron·cho·di·la·ta·tion (brong′kō-dil-ă-tā′shŭn). Broncodilatação. SIN **bronchodilation.**

bron·cho·di·la·tion (brong′kō-dī-lā′shŭn). Broncodilatação. **1.** Aumento no calibre dos brônquios e bronquíolos em resposta a substâncias farmacologicamente ativas ou à atividade nervosa autonômica. **2.** Termo raramente utilizado para bronquiectasia. SIN **bronchodilatation.**

bron·cho·di·la·tor (brong-kō-dī-lā′ter, -tōr). Broncodilatador. **1.** Que causa um aumento no calibre de um brônquio ou tubo brônquico. **2.** Um agente que possui essa capacidade (p.ex., epinefrina, albuterol).

bron·cho·e·de·ma (brong′kō-ĕ-dē′mă). Broncoedema; edema da mucosa dos brônquios.

bron·cho·e·soph·a·gol·o·gy (brong′kō-ē-sof-ă-gol′ō-jē). Broncoesofagologia; a especialidade relacionada com o diagnóstico e o tratamento das doenças da árvore traqueobrônquica e do esôfago por endoscopia e outros meios. [broncho- + G. *oisophagos*, esôfago, + *logos*, estudo]

bron·cho·e·soph·a·gos·co·py (brong′kō-ē-sof-ă-gos′kŏ-pē). Broncoesofagoscopia; exame da árvore traqueobrônquica e do esôfago através dos endoscópios apropriados.

bron·cho·fi·ber·scope (brong-kō-fī′ber-skōp). Broncofibroscópio. SIN **bronchoscope.**

bron·cho·gen·ic (brong-kō-jen′ik). Broncogênico; de origem brônquica; que emana a partir dos brônquios. SIN **bronchiogenic.**

bron·cho·gram (brong′kō-gram). Broncograma; uma radiografia obtida por broncografia; visualização radiográfica de um brônquio. [broncho- + G. *gramma*, uma escrita]

air b., b. aéreo; aparecimento radiográfico de um brônquio cheio de ar circundado por espaços aéreos cheios de líquido.

bron·chog·ra·phy (brong-kog′ră-fē). Broncografia; exame radiográfico da árvore traqueobrônquica após a introdução de um material radiopaco, usualmente um composto iodado em uma suspensão viscosa; raramente realizada neste momento, tendo sido superada pela tomografia computadorizada de alta resolução. [broncho- + G. *graphē*, um desenho]

tantalum b., b. com tântalo; historicamente, a b. que emprega o pó de tântalo metálico insuflado.

bron·cho·lith (brong′kō-lith). Broncolito; uma concreção endurecida em um brônquio, geralmente resultando da erosão de um linfonodo tuberculoso ou de outro linfonodo granulomatoso através da parede brônquica para dentro da luz. SIN **bronchial calculus.** [broncho- + G. *lithos*, pedra]

bron·cho·li·thi·a·sis (brong′kō-li-thī′ă-sis). Broncolitíase; inflamação ou obstrução brônquica causada por broncolitos.

bron·cho·ma·la·cia (brong′kō-mă-lā′shē-ă). Broncomalacia; degeneração dos tecidos elásticos e conjuntivos dos brônquios e da traquéia. [broncho- + G. *malakia*, um amolecimento]

bron·cho·mo·tor (brong-kō-mō′ter). Broncomotor. **1.** Relativo a uma alteração no calibre, dilatação ou contração de um brônquio ou bronquíolo. **2.** Um agente que possui essa ação. [broncho- + L. *motor*, mover]

bron·cho·my·co·sis (brong′kō-mī-kō′sis). Broncomicose; qualquer doença fúngica dos tubos brônquicos ou dos brônquios. [broncho- + G. *mykēs*, fungo]

bron·choph·o·ny (brong-kof′ō-nē). Broncofonia; intensidade e clareza aumentadas dos sons vocais ouvidos sobre um brônquio circundado por tecido pulmonar consolidado. VER TAMBÉM tracheophony. SIN **bronchial voice.** [broncho- + G. *phōnē*, voz]

whispered b., b. sussurrada. SIN **whispered *pectoriloquy*.**

bron·cho·plas·ty (brong′kō-plas-tē). Broncoplastia; a alteração cirúrgica da configuração de um brônquio. [broncho- + G. *plastos*, formado]

bron·cho·pneu·mo·nia (brong′ko-nu-mō′nī-ă). Broncopneumonia; inflamação aguda das paredes dos tubos brônquicos de menor calibre, com quantidades variadas de consolidação pulmonar devido à disseminação da inflamação para dentro dos alvéolos peribronquiolares e dos ductos alveolares; pode tornar-se confluente ou pode ser hemorrágica. SIN **bronchial pneumonia.**

postoperative b., b. pós-operatória; a pneumonia em placas que se desenvolve em um paciente pós-operatório, geralmente sucedendo a cirurgia da parte superior do abdome, com movimentação diafragmática restrita em virtude da dor na inspiração, resultando em hipoventilação das porções mais inferiores dos pulmões, com correspondente movimentação inadequada das secreções, possibilitando o desenvolvimento de infecção; a probabilidade é minimizada pela mobilização pós-operatória precoce e por exercícios de respiração profunda.

tuberculous b., b. tuberculosa; uma forma aguda de tuberculose pulmonar caracterizada por consolidações em placa disseminadas.

bron·cho·pul·mo·nary (brong-kō-pul′mō-nār-ē). Broncopulmonar; relativo aos brônquios e aos pulmões.

bron·chor·rha·phy (brong-kōr′ă-fē). Broncorrafia; a sutura de uma ferida do brônquio. [broncho- + G. *rhaphē*, uma costura]

bron·chor·rhea (brong′kō-rē′ă). Broncorréia; as secreções excessivas a partir da mucosa brônquica, resultando em produção copiosa de escarro fino e provocadas, mais amiúde, por carcinoma broncoalveolar difuso ou proteinose alveolar pulmonar. [broncho- + G. *rhoia*, um fluxo]

bron·cho·scope (brong′kō-skōp). Broncoscópio; um endoscópio para a inspeção do interior da árvore traqueobrônquica, quer para fins diagnósticos (inclusive a biopsia), quer para a remoção de corpos estranhos. Existem dois tipos: flexível e rígido. SIN **brochofiberscope.** [broncho- + G. *skopeō*, visualizar]

bron·chos·co·py (brong-kos′kŏ-pē). Broncoscopia; inspeção do interior da árvore traqueobrônquica através de um broncoscópio.

bron·cho·spasm (brong′kō-spazm). Broncoespasmo; contração dos músculos lisos nas paredes dos brônquios e bronquíolos, provocando o estreitamento da luz. Cf. bronchoconstriction.

bron·cho·spas·mo·lyt·ic (brong′kō-spazm-mō-li-tik). Broncoespasmolítico; que alivia um broncoespasmo.

bron·cho·spi·ro·che·to·sis (brong′kō-spī′rō-kē-tō′sis). Broncospiroquetose. SIN **hemorrhagic *bronchitis*.**

bron·cho·spi·rog·ra·phy (brong′kō-spī-rog′ră-fē). Broncospirografia; uso de um tubo endobrônquico de luz única para a mensuração da função ventilatória de um pulmão. [broncho- + L. *spiro*, respirar, + G. *graphō*, escrever]

bron·cho·spi·rom·e·ter (brong′kō-spī-rom′e-ter). Broncospirômetro; um dispositivo raro para a mensuração de freqüências e volumes do fluxo aéreo para dentro de cada pulmão em separado, usando um tubo endobrônquico de luz dupla. [broncho- + L. *spiro*, respirar, + G. *metron*, medir]

bron·cho·spi·rom·e·try (brong′kō-spī-rom′e-trē). Broncospirometria; uso de um broncospirômetro para medir a função ventilatória de cada pulmão em separado.

bron·cho·stax·is (brong′kō-stak′sis). Broncostaxia. SIN **hemoptysis.** [broncho- + G. *stasis*, um gotejamento]

bron·cho·ste·no·sis (brong-kō-sten-ō′sis). Broncostenose; estreitamento crônico de um brônquio.

bron·chos·to·my (brong-kos′tō-mē). Broncostomia; formação cirúrgica de uma nova abertura em um brônquio. [broncho- + G. *stoma*, boca]

bron·chot·o·my (brong-kot′ō-mē). Broncotomia; incisão de um brônquio.

bron·cho·tra·che·al (brong-kō-trā′kē-ăl). Broncotraqueal; relativo à traquéia e aos brônquios.

bron·cho·ve·sic·u·lar (brong′kō-vĕ-sik′ū-lăr). Broncovesicular; relativo aos brônquios e alvéolos nos pulmões, especialmente quando considera o som pulmonar ouvido através da ausculta. SIN **bronchoalveolar.**

bron·chus, pl. **bron·chi** (brong′kŭs, brong′kī) [TA]. Brônquio, brônquios; uma das duas subdivisões da traquéia que servem para conduzir o ar para e a partir dos pulmões. A traquéia divide-se nos brônquios principais direito e esquerdo, os quais, por sua vez, formam os brônquios lobares, segmentares e intra-segmentares. Na estrutura, os brônquios intra-segmentares possuem um revestimento de epitélio colunar ciliado pseudo-estratificado e uma lâmina própria com abundantes redes longitudinais de fibras elásticas; existem feixes de músculos lisos dispostos em espiral, inúmeras glândulas mucosserosas, e, na parte externa da parede, placas irregulares de cartilagem hialina. SIN bronchium. [L. Mod., do G. *bronchos*, traquéia]

eparterial b., b. epiarterial; b. lobar superior direito que passa acima da artéria pulmonar direita.

hyparterial bronchi, brônquios hipoarteriais; aqueles brônquios que fazem trajeto abaixo das artérias pulmonares, i.e., brônquios lobares inferior e médio direitos e os brônquios lobares superior e inferior esquerdos.

intermediate b., b. intermediário; a porção do b. principal direito entre o b. lobar superior e a origem dos brônquios lobares médio e inferior. SIN b. intermedius.

b. intermedius, b. intermédio. SIN intermediate b.

intrasegmental bronchi [TA], brônquios intra-segmentares; ramos dos brônquios segmentares para os segmentos broncopulmonares dos pulmões. SIN bronchi intrasegmentales [TA], branches of segmental bronchi, rami bronchiales segmentorum.

bronchi intrasegmentales [TA], brônquios intra-segmentares. SIN intrasegmental bronchi.

left main b. [TA], b. principal esquerdo; origina-se na bifurcação da traquéia, passa por diante do esôfago e penetra no hilo do pulmão esquerdo, onde se divide em um b. do lobo superior e um b. do lobo inferior. É mais longo, de calibre mais estreito e mais horizontalizado que o b. principal direito, portanto, os objetos aspirados entram nele com menor freqüência. SIN b. principalis sinister [TA].

lobar bronchi [TA], brônquios lobares; as divisões dos brônquios principais que suprem os lobos dos pulmões; b. lobar superior (b. lobaris superior [TA]); b. lobar médio (b. lobaris medius [TA]); e b. lobar inferior (b. lobaris inferior [TA]) são os três brônquios lobares à direita; b. lobar superior (b. lobaris superior [TA]) e b. lobar inferior (b. lobaris inferior [TA]) são os dois à esquerda. Os brônquios lobares dividem-se em brônquios segmentares. SIN bronchi lobares [TA].

bronchi loba'res [TA], brônquios lobares. SIN lobar bronchi.

mucoid impaction of b., impacção mucóide do b.; o tamponamento da luz dos brônquios devido ao muco espessado, interferindo com a ventilação dos segmentos pulmonares correspondentes e levando às características densidades radiológicas agrupadas lineares e semelhantes a cachos, e, ocasionalmente, a atelectasia e pneumonia; observada de modo característico na fibrose cística, mas pode ocorrer em diversos estados patológicos.

primary b., b. primário; o b. principal na bifurcação traqueal e que se estende para dentro do pulmão em desenvolvimento do embrião.

b. principa'lis dex'ter [TA], b. principal direito. SIN right main b.

b. principa'lis sinis'ter [TA], b. principal esquerdo. SIN left main b.

right main b. [TA], b. principal direito; origina-se na bifurcação da traquéia e entra no hilo do pulmão direito, emitindo o b. lobar superior e continuando para baixo para gerar os brônquios lobares médio e inferior. É mais curto, de maior calibre e mais verticalizado que o b. principal esquerdo, sendo que, dessa maneira, os objetos aspirados alojam-se com maior freqüência no lado direito. SIN b. principalis dexter [TA].

segmental b. [TA], b. segmentar; uma das divisões do b. lobar que supre um segmento broncopulmonar. No pulmão direito, existem comumente dez: *no lobo superior*, o b. segmentar apical (B_1), b. segmentalis apicalis (BI) [TA]; b. segmentar posterior (B_2), b. segmentalis posterior (BII) [TA]; e o b. segmentar anterior (B_3), b. segmentalis anterior (BIII) [TA]; *no lobo médio*, b. segmentar lateral (B_4), b. segmentalis lateralis (BIV) [TA]; e b. segmentar medial (B_5), b. segmentalis medialis (BV) [TA]; *no lobo inferior*, b. segmental superior (B_6), b. segmentalis superior (BVI) [TA]; b. segmental basal medial (B_7), b. segmentalis basalis medialis (BVII) [TA]; b. segmentar basal anterior (B_8), b. segmentalis basalis anterior (BVIII) [TA]; b. segmentar basal lateral (B_9), b. segmentalis basalis lateralis (BIX) [TA]; e b. segmentar basal posterior (B_{10}), b. segmentalis basalis posterior (BX) [TA]. No pulmão esquerdo, existem, em geral, nove: *no lobo superior*, b. segmentar apicoposterior (B_{1+2}), b. segmentalis apicoposterior (BI + II) [TA]; b. segmentar anterior (B_3), b. segmentalis anterior superior (BIII) [TA]; b. segmentar lingular superior (B_4), b. lingularis superior (BIV) [TA]; e b. segmentar lingular inferior (B_5), b. lingularis inferior (BV) [TA]; *no lobo inferior*, b. segmentar superior (B_6), b. segmentalis superior (BVI) [TA]; b. segmentar basal medial (B_7), b. segmentalis basalis medialis (cardiacus) (BVII) [TA]; b. segmentar basal anterior (B_8), b. segmentalis basalis anterior (BVIII) [TA]; b. segmentar basal lateral (B_9), b. segmentalis basalis lateralis (BIX) [TA]; e b. segmentar basal posterior (B_{10}), b. segmentalis basalis posterior (BX) [TA].

b. segmenta'lis [TA], b. segmentar. SIN segmental b.

stem b., b. principal; o b. principal a partir do qual se originam os ramos da árvore brônquica.

Brønsted, Johannes N., físico-químico dinamarquês, 1879–1947. VER B. *acid, base, theory*.

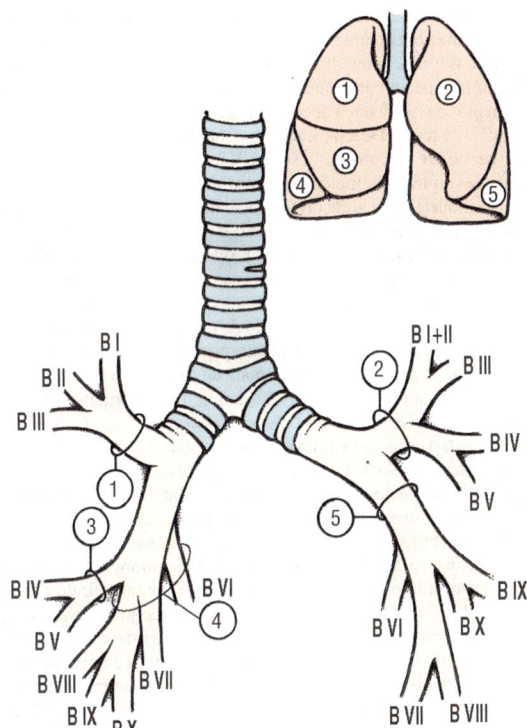

brônquios, segmentos: pulmão direito: (B I) apical, (B II) posterior, (B III) anterior, (B IV) lateral, (B V) medial, (B VI) apical, (B VII) basal medial, (B VIII) basal anterior, (B IX) basal lateral, (B X) basal posterior; pulmão esquerdo: (B I+ II), apicoposterior, (B III) anterior (B IV) lingular superior, (B V) lingular inferior, (B VI) apical, (B VII) basal medial, (B VIII) basal anterior, (B IX) basal lateral, (B X) basal posterior; lobos dos pulmões supridos: (1) superior direito, (2) superior esquerdo, (3) médio direito, (4) inferior direito, (5) inferior esquerdo

bron·to·pho·bia (bront-ō-fō′bē-a). Brontofobia; medo mórbido de trovão. SIN tonitrophobia. [G. *brontē*, trovão, + *phobos*, medo]

brood (brood). Ninhada. **1.** SIN litter (2). **2.** Refletir ansiosamente; meditar de forma mórbida.

Brooke, Bryan N., cirurgião britânico, *1915. VER B. *ileostomy*.

Brooke, Henry A. G., dermatologista inglês, 1854–1919. VER B. *tumor*.

bro·tiz·o·lam (brō′tiz-ō-lam). Brotizolam; um derivado triazol-benzodiazepínico com um átomo de enxofre e de bromo na molécula. Usado como um sedativo e hipnótico.

Broviac, J. W., cirurgião norte-americano do século 20. VER B. *catheter*.

brow. Testa. **1.** A sobrancelha. VER eyebrow. **2.** SIN forehead. [A.S. brū]

Brown, Harold W., oftalmologista norte-americano, *1898. VER B. *syndrome*.

Brown, James, cirurgião plástico norte-americano, 1899–1971. VER B.-Adson *forceps*.

Brown, James H., microbiologista norte-americano, *1884. VER B.-Brenn *stain*.

Brown, Robert, botânico inglês, 1773–1858. VER brownian *motion*; brownian *movement*; brownian-Zsigmondy *movement*.

Browne, Sir Denis John, cirurgião britânico, *1892. VER Denis B. *pouch*; Denis B. *splint*.

brown·i·an (brown′ē-an). Browniano; relativo ou descrito por Robert Brown.

Browning, William, anatomista e neurologista norte-americano, 1855–1941. VER B. *vein*.

Brown-Séquard, Charles E., fisiologista e neurologista francês, 1817–1894. VER Brown-Séquard *paralysis*; Brown-Séquard *syndrome*.

Bruce, Robert A., cardiologista norte-americano. VER B. *protocol*.

Bruce, Sir David, cirurgião britânico, 1855–1931. VER *Brucella*; brucellosis.

Bru·cel·la (broo-sel′la). Um gênero de bactérias encapsuladas, imóveis (família Brucellaceae), contendo células Gram-negativas, curtas, em formato de bastonetes a cocóides. Esses organismos não produzem gás a partir de carboidratos, são parasitas, invadem todos os tecidos animais e provocam infecção dos órgãos genitais, glândula mamária e tratos respiratório e intestinal, e são patogênicos para os seres humanos e várias espécies de animais domésticos. A espécie típica é a *B. melitensis*.

B. abor'tus, uma espécie bacteriana que causa aborto em vacas (brucelose bovina), éguas e ovelhas, febre ondulante em seres humanos e uma doença degenerativa em galinhas. SIN abortus bacillus.

B. ca'nis, uma espécie bacteriana que provoca epididimite, brucelose e aborto em cães; ocasionalmente provoca doença humana.

B. meliten'sis, uma espécie bacteriana que causa brucelose em seres humanos, aborto em cabras e uma doença degenerativa em galinhas; pode infectar vacas e porcos e ser excretada em seu leite; é a espécie típica do gênero *B.*
B. su'is, uma espécie bacteriana que causa aborto nos suínos, brucelose em seres humanos e uma doença degenerativa em galinhas; também pode infectar cavalos, cães, vacas, macacos, cabras e cobaias.

Bru·cel·la·ce·ae (broo-sel-ā'sē-ē). Uma família de bactérias (ordem Eubacteriales) que contêm células Gram-negativas pequenas, com formato cocóide a bastonete, as quais ocorrem isoladamente, aos pares, em cadeias curtas ou em grupos. As células podem mostrar, ou não, coloração bipolar. Ocorrem espécies móveis e imóveis; as células móveis são peritríquias. Os fatores V (nucleotídio fosfopiridina) e/ou X (hemina) são, por vezes, necessários para o crescimento. O soro sangüíneo pode ser necessário ou pode estimular o crescimento. A pressão aumentada de dióxido de carbono também pode favorecer o crescimento, em especial sob isolamento primário. Esses organismos são parasitas e patógenos que afetam os animais de sangue quente, incluindo os seres humanos, raramente os animais de sangue frio; originalmente denominados Parvobacteriaceae; o gênero típico é a *Brucella.*

bru·cel·ler·gin (broo-sel'er-jin). Brucelergina. VER brucellin.

bru·cel·lin (broo-sel'in). Brucelina; uma preparação de material antigênico a partir de várias espécies de *Brucella*; usada no diagnóstico da brucelose como um teste cutâneo similar àquele empregado para a tuberculose.

bru·cel·lo·sis (broo-sel-ō'sis). Brucelose; uma doença infecciosa causada pela bactéria *Brucella*, caracterizada por febre, sudorese, fraqueza, dores e astenia, transmitida para os seres humanos por contato direto com animais doentes ou através da ingestão de carne, leite ou queijo infectados, e particularmente perigosa para os veterinários, fazendeiros e trabalhadores em abatedouros; embora possa ocorrer algum cruzamento entre espécies, *Brucella melitensis, B. abortus, B. canis* e *B. suis* afetam caracteristicamente cabras, gado, cães e suínos, respectivamente. SIN febris undulans, Malta fever, Mediterranean fever (1), undulant fever, undulating fever.
bovine b., b. bovina; uma doença no gado causada por *Brucella abortus*; nas vacas grávidas, caracterizada por aborto no final da gestação, seguido por placenta retida e metrite; nos touros, podem ocorrer a orqueíte e a epididimite; o organismo pode localizar-se no úbere e, dessa maneira, aparecer no leite a partir das vacas infectadas. SIN Bang disease.

Bruch, Carl W. L., anatomista alemão, 1819–1884. VER B. *glands*, em *gland, membrane.*

bru·cine (broo-sēn, -in). Brucina; um alcalóide a partir de *Strychnos nux-vomica* e *S. ignatii* (família Loganiaceae), que produz paralisia dos nervos sensoriais e dos nervos motores periféricos; a ação convulsiva, que é característica da estricnina, está quase completamente ausente; originalmente utilizada como um anódino local e tônico. [de *Brucea* sp., um arbusto, em homenagem a James Bruce, explorador escocês, † 1794]

Bruck, Alfred, médico alemão, *1865. VER B. *disease.*
Brücke, Ernst W. von, fisiologista austríaco, 1819–1892. VER B. *muscle, tunic;* B.-Bartley *phenomenon.*
Brudzinski, Josef von, médico polonês, 1874–1917. VER B. *sign.*

Bru·gi·a (broo'jē-ā). Um gênero de filárias transmitidas por mosquitos para seres humanos, primatas, felinos carnívoros e vários outros mamíferos.
ℹ️ **B. mala'yi,** a espécie de filária da Malásia; um importante agente de filaríase e elefantíase humanas no Sudeste da Ásia e Indonésia, transmitida para os seres humanos por espécies de mosquitos *Mansonia* e *Anopheles*; os parasitas adultos causam linfangite e linfadenite, mas há menor envolvimento da região genital e dos membros inferiores e uma incidência relativamente maior de doença nos membros superiores que com a infecção por *Wuchereria bancrofti*. Originalmente chamado de *Wuchereria malayi.*

bruise (brooz). Contusão; lesão que provoca hematoma ou extravasamento difuso do sangue sem ruptura da pele. [I. Med. *bruisen*, do Fr. Ant., do Alemão]
bruisse·ment (brwēs-mawhn') Vibração; um som de ausculta semelhante ao ronronar do gato. [Fr.]

bru·it (broo-ē'). Ruído; um som de ausculta intermitente, áspero ou musical, especialmente quando anormal. [Fr.]
aneurysmal b., r. aneurysmático; r. soproso auscultado sobre um aneurisma.
carotid b., r. carotídeo; um sopro sistólico ouvido no pescoço, mas não na área aórtica; qualquer r. produzido pelo fluxo sangüíneo turbulento em uma artéria carótida.
b. de canon, r. de canhão, a primeira bulha cardíaca hiperfonética auscultada de forma intermitente no bloqueio atrioventricular completo e na interferência-dissociação, quando os ventrículos contraem logo depois dos átrios. SIN cannon sound.
b. de claquement (broo-ē dĕ klak-maw'), o som dos cliques cardíacos. VER click.
b. de cuir neuf (broo-ē dĕ kwēr nuf), o som de couro novo (também *bruit de craquement*); atrito pericárdico em rangido auscultado principalmente na pericardite crônica.
b. de diable, sopro venoso. SIN venous hum. [Fr. pião]
b. de frolement (broo-ē dĕ frōl-maw), som áspero, sussurrado, feito por um atrito pleural ou pericárdico. [Fr. sussurrar]
b. de galop, r. de galope. SIN gallop. [Fr.]
b. de la roue de moulin, r. de roda de moinho; sons de gargarejo ou de roda de moinho quando há líquido e ar no saco pericárdico. [Fr. moinho]
b. de lime, r. de lima; introduzido por R. Laënnec para descrever um sopro áspero. [Fr. lima]
b. de rappel, rufar; aplicado por J. B. Bouillaud para descrever a cadência de uma segunda bulha cardíaca desdobrada, ou seguido por um estalido de abertura ou uma terceira bulha cardíaca. SIN double-shock sound. [Fr. batida de tambor]
b. de Roger, sopro de Roger. SIN Roger *murmur.*
b. de scie (broo-ē'dĕ sē), r. de serra; um sopro cardíaco áspero ouvido na sístole e diástole cujo som se assemelha ao de uma serra. [Fr. serra]
b. de scie ou de rape, r. de serra; introduzido por R. Laënnec para descrever sopros ásperos ou rangidos. [Fr. serra]
b. de soufflet, r. de sopro; introduzido por R. Laënnec para descrever um sopro sussurrado. [Fr. fole]
b. de tabourka, r. de tambor; uma segunda bulha cardíaca hiperfonética, semelhante a um tambor ou sino, ouvido no foco aórtico na aortite sifilítica. [Fr. tambor]
b. de tambour (broo-ē'dĕ tăm-bur'), rufar; tom musical reverberante ouvido como o segundo batimento cardíaco sobre a área aórtica, associado à doença sifilítica pregressa da válvula aórtica. SIN tambour sound. [Fr. som de rufar]
b. de triolet, b. de triolé; introduzido por L. Gallavardin para descrever a cadência tripla produzida por um estalido sistólico acrescido às primeira e segunda bulhas cardíacas. [Fr. um pequeno trio]
Roger b. (broo-ē'), r. de Roger. SIN Roger *murmur.*
systolic b., r. sistólico; qualquer som anormal ou qualquer sopro ouvido durante a sístole.
thyroid b., r. tireóideo; sopro vascular auscultado sobre a glândula tireóide hiperativa, devido ao fluxo sangüíneo aumentado.
Traube b., r. de Traube. SIN gallop.

Brunn, Albert von, anatomista alemão, 1849–1895. VER B. *membrane, nest.*
Brunn, Fritz, médico tchecoslovaco do século 20. VER B. *reaction.*
Brunner, Johann C., anatomista suíço, 1653–1727. VER B. *glands*, em *gland.*
Bruns, Ludwig von, neurologista alemão, 1858–1916. VER B. *ataxia, nystagmus.*
Brunschwig, Alexander, cirurgião norte-americano, 1901–1969. VER B. *operation.*

brush (brŭsh). Escova; um instrumento feito de algum material flexível, como cerdas, preso a um manúbrio ou à extremidade de um cateter. [A.S. *byrst*, cerda]
Ayre b., e. de Ayre; um aparelho que consiste em um longo tubo flexível com uma e. na extremidade distal para coletar células da mucosa gástrica em exames de detecção de câncer; depois do posicionamento no estômago, a e. é rodada e "varre" as células da mucosa.
bronchoscopic b., e. broncoscópica; uma pequena escova para a inserção através de um broncoscópio para raspar as células para identificação microscópica na suspeita de carcinoma brônquico e na obtenção de material microbiológico para coloração e cultura.
denture b., e. dentária; uma e. utilizada para limpar dentaduras removíveis.
Haidinger b.'s, pincéis de Haidinger; a percepção de dois pincéis ou tufos amarelo-escuros que se irradia cerca de 5 graus do ponto de fixação, quando uma superfície com iluminação uniforme, como o céu azul, é visualizada através de uma lente polarizada.
Kruse b., e. de Kruse; um feixe de finos fios de platina presos a um cabo; usada em trabalhos bacteriológicos para espalhar o material sobre a superfície de um meio de cultura.
polishing b., e. de polimento; uma e. geralmente montada em um instrumento rotatório, usada para polir os dentes ou substitutos artificiais.

ℹ️ **Brushfield,** Thomas, médico britânico, 1858–1937. VER B. *spots*, em *spot*; B.-Wyatt *disease.*

brush·ite (brŭsh'īt). Bruchita; um fosfato de cálcio ácido de ocorrência natural, ocasionalmente encontrado no cálculo dentário e nos cálculos renais.

Bruton, Ogden C., pediatra norte-americana, *1908. VER Bruton *agammaglobulinemia.*

brux·ism (brŭk'sizm). Bruxismo; apertar dos dentes, associado a movimentos laterais ou protrusivos vigorosos da mandíbula, resultando em atrito ou rangido com os dentes, geralmente durante o sono; por vezes uma condição patológica. [G. *bruchō*, ranger os dentes]

Bryant, Sir Thomas, cirurgião inglês, 1828–1914. VER B. *traction.*

BSA Abreviatura de bovine serum *albumin* (albumina sérica bovina).
BSE Abreviatura de bovine spongiform *encephalopathy* (encefalopatia espongiforme bovina).
BSER Abreviatura de brainstem evoked *response* (resposta evocada do tronco cerebral). VER auditory brainstem *response.*

Bt$_2$cAMP Monofosfato de $N^6,O^{2'}$-dibutiriladenosina 3':5'-cíclico, um derivado dibutiril do cAMP.

BTPS Indica que um volume gasoso foi expresso como se estivesse saturado com vapor d'água na temperatura corporal (37°C) e na pressão barométrica ambiente; usado para mensurações dos volumes pulmonares.

BTU Abreviatura de British thermal *unit* (unidade térmica britânica).
BTX Abreviatura de brevetoxins (brevetoxinas).
bu·a·ki (boo - a′kē). Buaque; uma doença nutricional (deficiência de proteína) observada em nativos do Congo e caracterizada por edema, lesões cutâneas e anemia; possivelmente relacionado ao *kwashiorkor*.
bu·ba mad·re (boo′ba mah′dre) Buba-mãe. SIN mother *yaw*.
bu·bas (boo′bahs). Buba. SIN mucocutaneous *leishmaniasis*.
  b. brazilia'na, b. brasileira. SIN espundia.
bu·bo (boo′bō). Bubão; tumefação inflamatória de um ou mais linfonodos, usualmente na virilha; a massa confluente de linfonodos usualmente supura e drena pus. [G. *boubōn*, a virilha, uma tumefação na virilha]
  bullet b., edema duro e indolor de linfonodo na virilha, que acompanha um cancro.
  chancroidal b., b. cancróide; b. em ulceração, causado por *Haemophilus ducreyi*. SIN virulent b.
  indolent b., b. indolente; hipertrofia endurecida de um linfonodo inguinal.
  malignant b., b. maligno; linfonodo hipertrofiado associado à peste bubônica.
  parotid b., b. parotídeo; edema da glândula parótida devido a infecção séptica secundária.
  primary b., b. primário; b. que ocorre como o primeiro sinal de infecção venérea.
  tropical b., linfogranuloma venéreo. SIN venereal *lymphogranuloma*.
  venereal b., b. venéreo; linfonodo aumentado na virilha associado a qualquer doença sexualmente transmitida, especialmente cancróide.
  virulent b., b. virulento. SIN chancroidal b.
bu·bon·al·gia (boo′bon - al′jē - ā). Bubonalgia; termo raramente utilizado para dor na virilha. [G. *boubōn*, virilha, + *algos*, dor]
bu·bon·ic (boo - bon′ik). Bubônico; relativo, de qualquer modo, a um bubão.
bu·bon·u·lus (boo - bon′ū - lŭs). Bubônulo. 1. Um abscesso que acontece ao longo do trajeto de um vaso linfático. 2. Um dentre inúmeros nódulos endurecidos que, com freqüência, se abrem em úlceras, as quais se formam ao longo do trajeto de vasos linfáticos agudamente inflamados do dorso do pênis. [L. Mod. dim de *bubo*]
bu·car·dia (bū - kar′dē - ā). Bucardia. SIN ox *heart*. [G. *bous*, boi, + *kardia*, coração]
buc·ca, gen. e pl. **buc·cae** (bŭk′ā, bŭk′sē). Bochecha. SIN cheek. [L.]
buc·cal (bŭk′al). Bucal; pertinente a, adjacente a ou na direção da bochecha.
buc·ci·na·tor. Bucinador. VER buccinator (*muscle*).
△ **bucco-**. Buco-; bochecha. [L. *bucca*]
buc·co·ax·i·al (bŭk - ō - ak′sē - al). Bucoaxial; refere-se ao ângulo formado pelas paredes bucal e axial de uma cavidade.
buc·co·ax·i·o·cer·vi·cal (bŭk′ō - ak′sē - ō - ser′vi - kal). Bucoaxiocervical; refere-se ao ângulo puntiforme formado pela junção das paredes bucal, axial e cervical (gengival) de uma cavidade.
buc·co·ax·i·o·gin·gi·val (bŭk′ō - ak′sē - ō - jin′ji - val) Bucoaxiogengival; refere-se ao ângulo puntiforme formado pela junção de uma parede bucal, axial e gengival (cervical).
buc·co·cer·vi·cal (bŭk - ō - ser′vi - kal). Bucocervical. 1. Refere-se à bochecha e ao pescoço. 2. Em anatomia dentária, refere-se àquela porção da superfície bucal de um dente bicúspide ou molar adjacente à sua junção cemento-esmalte.
buc·co·clu·sal (bŭk - ō - kloo′sal). Bucoclusal; termo incorreto que se refere ao ângulo linear formado pela junção de uma parede bucal e uma pulpar. VER buccopulpal.
buc·co·dis·tal (buk - ō - dis′tal). Bucodistal; refere-se ao ângulo linear formado pela junção de uma parede bucal e uma distal de uma cavidade.
buc·co·gin·gi·val (bŭk - ō - jin′ji - val). Bucogengival; relativo à bochecha e à gengiva.
buc·co·la·bi·al (bŭk - ō - lā′bē - al). Bucolabial. 1. Relativo à bochecha e ao lábio. 2. Em odontologia, refere-se àquela face do arco dentário ou àquelas superfícies dos dentes em contato com a mucosa do lábio e da bochecha.
buc·co·lin·gual (bŭk - ō - ling′wal). Bucolingual. 1. Pertinente à bochecha e à língua. 2. Em odontologia, refere-se àquela face do arco dentário ou àquelas superfícies dos dentes em contato com a mucosa do lábio ou da bochecha e com a língua.
buc·co·me·si·al (bŭk - ō - mē′zē - al). Bucomesial; refere-se ao ângulo linear formado pela junção de uma parede bucal e uma parede mesial de uma cavidade.
buc·co·pha·ryn·ge·al (bŭk′ō - fā - rin′jē - al). Bucofaríngeo; relativo à bochecha ou boca e à faringe.
buc·co·pul·pal (buk - ō - pŭl′pal). Bucopulpar; relativo ao ângulo linear formado pela junção de uma parede bucal e uma parede pulpar de uma cavidade.
buc·co·ver·sion (bŭk′ō - ver - zhŭn). Bucoversão; posição errônea de um dente posterior a partir da linha normal de oclusão no sentido da bochecha.
buc·cu·la (bŭk - ū - la). Búcula; uma intumescência gordurosa sob o queixo. SIN double chin. [L. dim. de *bucca*, bochecha]
Büchner, Eduard, químico alemão e laureado com o Prêmio Nobel, 1860–1917. VER B. *extract, funnel*.

Büchner, Hans E. A., bacteriologista alemão, 1850–1902. VER B. *extract*.
bu·chu (boo′koo). Bucho; as folhas secas de *Barosma betulina, B. crenulata* ou *B. serratifolia* (família Rutaceae), um arbusto que cresce na África do Sul; usado como carminativo, diurético e anti-séptico urinário. SIN Hottentot tea. [nativo]
Buchwald, Hermann Edmund, médico alemão, *1903. VER B. *atrophy*.
Buck, Gordon, cirurgião norte-americano, 1807–1877. VER B. *extension, fascia, traction*.
buck·bean. Fava dos pântanos; as folhas da *Menyanthes trifoliata* (família Gentianaceae); considerado com propriedades emenagogas, antiescorbúticas e amargo simples. SIN bogbean, menyanthes.
Bücklers, Max, oftalmologista alemão, 1895–1969. VER Reis-Bücklers corneal *dystrophy*.
buck·thorn (bŭk′thorn). Espinheiro. SIN Rhamnus.
Bucky, Gustav, radiologista norte-americano, 1880–1963. VER B. *diaphragm*.
bu·cli·zine hy·dro·chlo·ride (bu′kli - zēn). Cloridrato de buclizina; sedativo brando utilizado para a cinetose, a vertigem e a ansiedade que acompanham os distúrbios psicossomáticos.
buc·lo·sa·mide (buk - lō′sa - mid). Buclosamida; agente antifúngico tópico.
bu·cry·late (bū - kri - lāt). Bucrilato; tecido aderente utilizado em cirurgia.
Bucy, Paul C., neurocirurgião norte-americano, 1904–1992. VER Klüver-B. *syndrome*.
bud (bŭd). Botão. 1. Uma protuberância que se assemelha ao b. de uma planta, usualmente pluripotencial, e capaz de se diferenciar e se desenvolver em uma estrutura definitiva. 2. Produzir tal protuberância. VER TAMBÉM gemmation. 3. Uma pequena protuberância a partir de uma célula-mãe; uma forma de reprodução assexuada.
  bronchial b., b. brônquico; uma das proliferações do tubo laringotraqueal endodérmico primordial que origina os brônquios principais. VER laryngotracheal *diverticulum*.
  end b., b. terminal. SIN tail b.
  gustatory b., b. gustativo. SIN taste b.
  limb b., b. de membro; proliferação mesenquimatosa revestida por ectoderma no flanco embrionário que origina o membro anterior ou posterior.
  liver b., b. hepático; o divertículo celular primordial do endoderma do intestino anterior que dá origem ao parênquima do fígado.
  lung b., divertículo traqueobrônquico. SIN tracheobronchial *diverticulum*.
  median tongue b., b. mediano da língua. SIN *tuberculum* impar.
  metanephric b., b. metanéfrico; a proliferação celular primordial a partir do ducto mesonéfrico que origina o revestimento epitelial do ureter, da pelve e dos cálices renais, e dos túbulos coletores retos. SIN ureteric b.
  periosteal b., b. periósteo; um b. de tecido conjuntivo vascular a partir do pericôndrio que invade o centro de ossificação do modelo cartilaginoso de um osso longo em desenvolvimento.
  syncytial b., b. sincicial. SIN syncytial *knot*.
  tail b., b. caudal; uma massa de células com proliferação rápida na extremidade caudal do embrião; resquício do nódulo primitivo. SIN end b.
  taste b., b. gustativo; um dos inúmeros nichos de células em formato de frasco localizados no epitélio das papilas circunvaladas, fungiformes e foliadas da língua e também no palato mole, epiglote e parede posterior da faringe; consiste em células de sustentação, gustativas e basais entre as quais terminam as fibras nervosas sensoriais intragemais. SIN caliculus gustatorius, gustatory b., Schwalbe corpuscle, taste bulb, taste corpuscle.
  tooth b., b. dentário; as estruturas primordiais a partir das quais se forma um dente; o órgão do esmalte, a papila dentária e o saco dentário envolvendo-os.
  ureteric b., b. ureteral. SIN metanephric b.
  vascular b., b. vascular; um brotamento endotelial que se origina de um vaso sangüíneo.
Budd, George, médico inglês, 1808–1882. VER B. *syndrome*; B.-Chiari *syndrome*.
Budde, E., engenheiro sanitarista dinamarquês, *1871. VER B. *process*.
bud·ding (bŭd′ing). Brotamento. SIN gemmation.
Budge, Julius L., fisiologista alemão, 1811–1888. VER B. *center*.
Budin, Pierre C., ginecologista francês, 1846–1907. VER B. obstetrical *joint*.
Buerger, Leo, médico austríaco-americano, 1879–1943. VER Winiwarter-B. *disease*; B. *disease*.
△ **bufa-, bufo-**. Formas combinantes que indicam a origem a partir de sapos; usado em nomes sistemáticos e comuns de substâncias tóxicas (geninas) isoladas a partir de vegetais e animais que contêm a estrutura da bufanolídea; prefixos que indicam a espécie de origem estão freqüentemente associados. [L. *bufo*, sapo]
bu·fa·di·en·o·lide (boo - fā - dī - en′ō - līd). Bufadienolídeo. VER bufanolide.
bu·fa·gen·ins (boo′fā - jen - inz). Bufageninas. SIN bufagins.
bu·fa·gins (boo′fā - jinz). Bufaginas; um grupo de esteróides (bufanolídeos) no veneno de uma família de sapos (Bufonidae) que possui uma ação semelhante ao digitálico sobre o coração; os glicosídeos cardíacos que possuem uma lactona com seis membros. VER TAMBÉM bufotoxins. SIN bufagenins, bufogenins.
bu·fan·o·lide (boo - fan′ō - līd). Bufanolídeo; a lactona esteróide fundamental de diversos venenos ou toxinas vegetais (p.ex., cila) e animais (p.ex., sapo);

também encontrado na forma de glicosídeos nos vegetais (p.ex., digitálico). O esteróide é, essencialmente, um 5β-androstano, com um 14β H. A lactona em C-17 está estruturalmente relacionada ao radical –CH(CH$_3$)–CH$_2$CH$_2$CH$_3$ preso ao C-17 nos colanos, e tem a mesma configuração do colesterol (i.e., 20R); em algumas espécies, o b. é formado a partir do colesterol. Vários derivados do b., portadores de insaturação no anel lactônico (20, 22) ou em outro ponto (4), são conhecidos como **bufenolídeos** (uma dupla ligação), **bufadienolídeos** (duas duplas ligações), **bufatrienolídeos** (três duplas ligações) etc.; eles possuem quantidades variadas de grupamentos hidroxila nas posições 3, 5, 14 e 16, e esses podem ser substituídos mais adiante. Para a estrutura, ver steroids.

bu·fa·tri·en·o·lide (boo-fă-trī-en′ō-līd). Bufatrienolídeo. VER bufanolide.
bu·fen·o·lide (boo-fen′ō-līd). Bufenolídeo. VER bufanolide.
buff′er (bŭf′er). **1.** Tampão; uma mistura de um ácido e sua base conjugada (sal), como H$_2$CO$_3$/HCO$_3^-$; H$_2$PO$_4^-$/HPO$_4^{2-}$, que, quando presente em uma solução, reduz quaisquer alterações no pH que, de outra forma, ocorreriam na solução quando o ácido ou o álcali é adicionado a ela; dessa maneira, o pH do sangue e dos líquidos corporais é mantido relativamente constante (pH 7,45), embora os metabólitos ácidos estejam sendo continuamente formados nos tecidos e o CO$_2$ seja perdido nos pulmões. VER TAMBÉM conjugate acid-base *pair*.
2. Tamponar; acrescentar um t. a uma solução e, dessa maneira, conferir-lhe a propriedade de resistir a uma alteração no pH quando se acrescenta uma quantidade limitada de ácido ou álcali.
 dipolar b., t. bipolar. SIN zwitterionic b.
 zwitterionic b., t. bipolar; t. cuja estrutura pode incluir cargas elétricas opostas. SIN dipolar b.
△ **bufo-**. VER bufa-.
bu·fo·gen·ins (boo-fō-jen-inz). Bufogeninas. SIN bufagins.
Bu·fon·i·dae (boo-fon′ĭ-dē). Família de sapos cujas glândulas dérmicas secretam vários tipos de substâncias farmacologicamente ativas portadoras de uma ação cardíaca similar à dos digitálicos. [L. *bufo*, sapo]
bu·for·min (boo-fōr′min). Buformina; agente hipoglicemiante oral semelhante à metformina.
bu·fo·ten·ine (boo-fō-ten′ēn). Bufotenina; um agente psicotomimético isolado a partir do veneno de determinados sapos (família Bufonidae) e também presente em diversas plantas e um dos princípios ativos da cooba; aumenta a pressão arterial através de uma ação vasoconstritora e produz efeitos psíquicos, inclusive alucinações. SIN mappine.
bu·fo·tox·ins (boo-fō-toks′inz). Bufotoxinas. **1.** Um grupo de lactonas esteróides (conjugados de bufaginas e suberilarginina em C-3) do digitálico presente nos venenos de sapos (família Bufonidae); seus efeitos são similares, porém mais fracos, que aqueles das bufaginas. **2.** Especificamente, a principal toxina do sapo europeu (*Bufo vulgaris*).
bug. Percevejo; inseto pertencente à subordem Heteroptera. Para os organismos assim chamados, veja o termo específico.
 assassin b., p. assassino; inseto da família Reduviidae (ordem Hemiptera) que inflige picadas irritativas e dolorosas em animais e seres humanos; relacionado aos percevejos com nariz em cone (triatomíneos), um vetor da tripanossomíase americana. [Fr., do It. *assassino*, do Ár. *hashshāshin*, aqueles viciados em haxixe]
bug·gery (bŭg′ger-ē). Bestialidade. SIN sodomy. [Fr. Ant. *bougre*, herético, do L. Med. *Bulgarus*, um búlgaro (portanto, um herético)]
bulb (bŭlb) [TA]. Bulbo. **1.** Qualquer estrutura globular ou fusiforme. SIN bulbus [TA]. **2.** Um caule curto, vertical e subterrâneo de vegetais, como a cebola e o alho. [L. *bulbus*, uma raiz bulbosa]
 aortic b., b. da aorta; a primeira parte dilatada da aorta contendo as valvas aórticas semilunares e os seios da aorta. SIN arterial b., bulbus aortae.
 arterial b., b. da aorta. SIN aortic b.
 Braasch b., cateter de Braasch. SIN Braasch *catheter*.
 carotid b., b. carótico. SIN carotid *sinus*.
 b. of corpus spongiosum, b. do pênis. SIN b. of penis.
 dental b., b. dentário; a papila, derivada do mesoderma, que forma a parte do primórdio de um dente que está situado dentro do órgão do esmalte em forma de cálice.
 duodenal b., ampola duodenal. SIN duodenal *cap*.
 end b., b. terminal; um dos corpúsculos ovalados ou arredondados em que terminam as fibras nervosas sensoriais na mucosa.
 b. of eye, b. do olho. SIN eyeball.
 hair b., b. piloso. SIN b. of hair.
 b. of hair, b. piloso; o bulbo do cabelo, a extremidade inferior expandida do folículo piloso que se adapta como uma capa sobre a papila pilosa. SIN bulbus pili, hair b.
 jugular b., b. da veia jugular. SIN b. of jugular vein.
 b. of jugular vein [TA], b. da veia jugular; uma das duas partes dilatadas da veia jugular interna: (1) o bulbo superior (divertículo de Heister) é uma dilatação no início da veia jugular interna na fossa jugular do osso temporal (bulbus superior venae jugularis [TA]); (2) o bulbo inferior é uma porção dilatada da veia exatamente antes que ela alcance a veia braquiocefálica (bulbus inferior venae jugularis [TA]). SIN jugular b. SIN bulbus venae jugularis [TA].
 Krause end b.'s, bulbos terminais de Krause; terminações nervosas na pele, na boca, na conjuntiva e em outras regiões, consistindo em uma cápsula laminada do tecido conjuntivo que envolve a extremidade terminal, ramificada e contornada de uma fibra nervosa aferente; em geral, acredita-se que sejam sensíveis ao frio. SIN bulboid corpuscles, corpuscula bulboidea.
 b. of occipital horn [TA], b. do corno posterior; uma elevação arredondada na parte dorsal da parede medial do corno posterior do ventrículo lateral, produzida pelo fórceps maior. SIN bulbus cornus posterioris [TA].
 olfactory b. [TA], b. olfatório; a extremidade rostral acinzentada e expandida do trato olfatório, situando-se na lâmina cribriforme do etmóide e recebendo os filamentos olfatórios. SIN bulbus olfactorius [TA].
 b. of penis [TA], b. do pênis; a parte proximal (posterior) expandida do corpo esponjoso do pênis, situando-se no intervalo entre a cruz do pênis e contendo a porção algo dilatada e angulada da uretra esponjosa. SIN bulbus penis [TA], b. of corpus spongiosum, b. of urethra, bulbus urethrae.
 b. of posterior horn of lateral ventricle of brain, b. do corno posterior. SIN bulbus cornus posterioris.
 Rouget b., b. de Rouget; plexo venoso na superfície do ovário.
 speech b., b. da fala; prótese de fala usada para fechar uma fenda ou outra abertura no palato duro ou mole, ou para substituir o tecido ausente necessário para a produção da boa fala.
 taste b., botão gustativo. SIN taste *bud*.
 b. of urethra, b. do pênis. SIN b. of penis.
 b. of vestibule [TA], b. do vestíbulo; massa de tecido erétil em ambos os lados da vagina unida anteriormente à uretra pela comissura bulbar. SIN bulbus vestibuli vaginae [TA].
bul·bar (bŭl′bar). Bulbar. **1.** Relativo a um bulbo. **2.** Relativo ao rombencéfalo (cérebro posterior). **3.** Em formato de bulbo; que se assemelha a um bulbo.
bul·bi (bŭl′bī). Bulbos; plural de bulbus.
bul·bi·tis (bŭl-bī′tis). Bulbite; inflamação da porção bulbosa da uretra.
△ **bulbo-**. Forma combinante relativa a um bulbo ou bulbos. [L. *bulbus*]
bul·bo·cap·nine (bŭl′bō-kap′nin). Bulbocapnina; droga derivada das raízes da *Corydalis cava* e *C. tuberosa* (família Fumariaceae) e *Dicendra canadensis* (família Papaveraceae); bloqueia os efeitos da dopamina sobre os receptores periféricos.
bul·bo·cav·er·no·sus (bŭl′bō-kav-er-nō′sus). Bulbocavernoso; VER *musculus* bulbocavernosus.
bul·boid (bŭl′boyd). Bulbóide; em formato de bulbo. [bulbo- + G. *eidos*, semelhança]
bul·bo·nu·cle·ar (bŭl-bō-noo′klē-ar). Bulbonuclear; relativo aos núcleos na medula oblonga.
bul·bo·pon·tine (bŭl-bō-pon′tēn). Bulbopontino; relativo à porção rostral do rombencéfalo composta da ponte e tegmento suprajacente.
bul·bo·sa·cral (bŭl′bō-sā′kral). Bulbossacral. VER bulbosacral *system*.
bul·bo·spi·nal (bŭl-bō-spī′nal). Bulbospinal; relativo à medula oblonga e à medula espinal, principalmente às fibras nervosas que interligam as duas. SIN spinobulbar.
bul·bo·u·re·thral (bŭl′bō-ū-rē′thral). Bulbouretral; relativo ao bulbo do pênis e à uretra. SIN urethrobulbar.
bul·bus, gen. e pl. **bul·bi** (bŭl′bus, -bī) [TA]. Bulbo, bulbos. SIN bulb (1). [L. um bulbo vegetal]
 b. aor′tae, b. da aorta. SIN aortic *bulb*.
 b. cor′dis, b. cardíaco; uma dilatação transitória no coração embrionário onde o tronco arterial se une às raízes ventrais dos arcos aórticos.
 b. cor′nus posterior′is [TA], b. do corno posterior. SIN bulb of occipital horn. SIN bulb of posterior horn of lateral ventricle of brain.
 b. duodeni, b. duodenal; termo oficial alternativo* para *ampulla* of duodenum.
 b. oc′uli [TA], b. do olho. SIN eyeball.
 b. olfacto′rius [TA], b. olfatório. SIN olfactory *bulb*.
 b. pe′nis [TA], b. do pênis. SIN *bulb* of penis.
 b. pi′li, b. piloso. SIN *bulb* of hair.
 b. ure′thrae, b. do pênis. SIN *bulb* of penis.
 b. ve′nae jugula′ris [TA], b. da veia jugular. SIN *bulb* of jugular vein.
 b. vestib′uli vaginae [TA], b. do vestíbulo. SIN *bulb* of vestibule.
bu·le·sis (boo-lē′sis). Desejo; vontade. [G. *boulēsis*, um desejo]
bu·lim·ia (boo-lim′ē-ă). Bulimia. SIN b. nervosa. [G. *bous*, boi, + *limos*, fome]
 b. nervo′sa, bulimia; distúrbio mórbido crônico que envolve episódios secretos repetidos de ingerir alimentos, caracterizados pela ingestão rápida e descontrolada de grandes quantidades de alimento durante um curto intervalo de tempo, seguida pelo vômito auto-induzido, uso de laxativos ou diuréticos, jejum ou exercício vigoroso, a fim de evitar o ganho de peso; freqüentemente acompanhada por sentimentos de culpa, depressão ou autodesaprovação. SIN boulimia, bulimia, hiperorexia.
bu·lim·ic (boo-lim′ik). Bulímico; relativo a ou que sofre de bulimia.
Bu·li·nus (bū-lī′nŭs). Gênero e subgênero de caracóis de água doce na família Planorbidae (subfamília Bulininae), que inclui muitas espécies que se cons-

tituem em hospedeiros intermediários do trematódeo sangüíneo humano, *Schistosoma haematobium*, na África e no Oriente Médio; dividido em dois subgêneros, *Physopsis* e *Bulinus*, sendo o primeiro responsável pela transmissão de *S. haematobium* ao sul do Saara e o último responsável pela transmissão desse trematódeo sangüíneo no norte da África e no Oriente Médio. As espécies importantes englobam o *B. truncatus* e o *B. forskalii*, hospedeiros para os esquistossomas humano e de animais e para vários trematódeos anfístomas de animais domésticos.

bulk·age (bŭlk′ij). Massa; qualquer coisa, como o ágar, que aumente o volume do material no intestino, estimulando, assim, a peristalse.

bull. Abreviatura de L. *bulliens, bulliat* ou *bulliant*, ferver, deixar ferver.

bul·la, gen. e pl. **bul·lae** (bul′ă, -ē). Bolha. **1.** Uma grande vesícula cheia de líquido, com mais de 10 mm de diâmetro, que aparece como uma área circunscrita de separação da epiderme a partir da estrutura subepidérmica (**b. subepidérmica**) ou como uma área circunscrita de separação de células epidérmicas (**b. intra-epidérmica**) causada pela presença de soro ou, ocasionalmente, por uma substância injetada. **2** [NA]. Uma estrutura semelhante a uma bolha. [L. bolha]
   ethmoidal b. [TA], b. etmoidal; abaulamento da parede interna do labirinto etmoidal no meato médio do nariz, exatamente abaixo da concha nasal média; é considerada uma concha rudimentar. SIN b. ethmoidalis [TA].
   b. ethmoida′lis [TA], b. etmoidal. SIN ethmoidal b.
   pulmonary b., b. pulmonar; espaço enfisematoso cheio de ar maior que um centímetro, usualmente localizado na periferia pulmonar; pode alcançar um grande diâmetro e causar sintomas por compressão do tecido pulmonar normal. Cf. pulmonary *bleb*.

bul·lec·to·my (bul - ek′tō - mē). Bulectomia; ressecção de uma bolha; valiosa no tratamento de algumas formas de enfisema bolhoso, nas quais bolhas gigantes comprimem o tecido pulmonar funcional.

bul·lous (bul′ŭs). Bolhoso; relativo a, da natureza de ou marcado por bolhas.

bu·met·a·nide (bū - met′a - nīd). Bumetanida; diurético empregado no tratamento do edema associado a insuficiência cardíaca congestiva, cirrose hepática e doença renal, semelhante à furosemida.

Bumke, Oswald C. E., neurologista alemão, 1877–1950. VER B. *pupil*.

BUN Abreviatura de blood urea *nitrogen* (uréia).

bun·am·i·dine hy·dro·chlo·ride (bŭn - am′i - dēn). Cloridrato de bunamidina; anti-helmíntico.

bun·dle (bŭn′dl) [TA]. Fascículo, feixe; estrutura composta de um grupo de fibras, musculares ou nervosas; um fascículo. SIN fasciculus (3) [TA].
   aberrant b.'s, feixes aberrantes; um grupo, ou grupos, de fibras oriundas do trato corticobulbar ou corticonuclear, direcionado para cada um dos núcleos motores dos nervos cranianos.
   anterior ground b., f. próprio. SIN *fasciculus* proprius anterior. VER *fasciculi* proprii, em *fasciculus*.
   Arnold b., f. de Arnold. SIN temporopontine *tract*.
   atrioventricular b. [TA], f. atrioventricular; o feixe de fibras musculares cardíacas modificadas que começa no nó atrioventricular como o tronco do feixe atrioventricular e atravessa o anel fibroso atrioventricular direito para a porção membranácea do septo interventricular, onde o tronco se divide em dois ramos, o f. direito do f. atrioventricular e o f. esquerdo do f. atrioventricular; os dois ramos ramificam-se no subendocárdio de seus respectivos ventrículos. SIN fasciculus atrioventricularis [TA], atrioventricular band, Gaskell bridge, His band, His b., Keith b., Kent b. (1), Kent-His b., truncus fascicularis atrioventricularis, trunk of atrioventricular bundle, ventriculonector.
   Bachmann b., f. de Bachmann; divisão do teórico trato internodal anterior que continua para dentro do átrio esquerdo, proporcionando um trajeto especializado para a condução interatrial. A realidade anatômica dessa estrutura tem sido contestada.
   comma b. of Schultze, f. em vírgula de Schultze. SIN semilunar *fasciculus*.
   Flechsig ground b.'s [TA], fascículos próprios de Flechsig; fascículo próprio anterior e fascículo próprio lateral. VER *fasciculi* proprii, em *fasciculus*.
   Gantzer accessory b., f. acessório de Gantzer. VER Gantzer *muscle*.
   Gierke respiratory b., f. respiratório de Gierke. SIN solitary *tract*.
   ground b.'s, fascículos próprios. SIN *fasciculi* proprii, em *fasciculus*.
   Held b., f. de Held. SIN tectospinal *tract*.
   Helie b., f. de Helie; f. verticalmente arqueado de fibras na camada superficial do miométrio.
   Helweg b., f. de Helweg. SIN olivospinal *tract*.
   Helwig b., f. de Helwig. SIN olivospinal *fibers*, em *fiber*.
   His b., f. de His. SIN atrioventricular b.
   Hoche b., f. de Hoche. VER semilunar *fasciculus*.
   hooked b. of Russell, f. uncinado de Russell. SIN uncinate *fasciculus* of cerebellum.
   Keith b., f. de Keith. SIN atrioventricular b.
   Kent b., f. de Kent; **(1)** SIN atrioventricular b.; **(2)** f. de fibras musculares no coração dos mamíferos abaixo do nó atrioventricular; também pode ocorrer em seres humanos.
   Kent-His b., f. de Kent-His. SIN atrioventricular b.
   Killian b., f. de Killian. VER inferior constrictor (*muscle*) of pharynx.
   Krause respiratory b., f. respiratório de Krause. SIN solitary *tract*.
   lateral ground b., f. próprio. VER *fasciculi* proprii, em *fasciculus*.
   lateral proprius b., f. próprio lateral. SIN *fasciculi* proprii, em *fasciculus*.
   left b. of atrioventricular bundle [TA], f. esquerdo do f. atrioventricular; o ramo esquerdo do f. atrioventricular que se separa do f. atrioventricular logo abaixo da porção membranácea do septo interventricular para descer a parede septal do ventrículo esquerdo e começa a se ramificar no nível subendocárdico. SIN crus sinistrum fasciculi atrioventricularis, left crus of atrioventricular bundle.
   Lissauer b., f. de Lissauer. SIN dorsolateral *fasciculus*.
   Loewenthal b., f. de Loewenthal. SIN tectospinal *tract*.
   longitudinal pontine b.'s, fascículos longitudinais da ponte. SIN longitudinal pontine *fasciculi*, em *fasciculus*.
   medial forebrain b. [TA], f. medial do telencéfalo; um sistema de fibras que avança longitudinalmente através da zona (área) lateral do hipotálamo, unindo-o, de forma recíproca, com o tegmento mesencefálico e com vários componentes do sistema límbico; também carrega fibras oriundas de grupos de células com norepinefrina e serotonina no tronco cerebral para o hipotálamo e para o córtex cerebral, bem como fibras com dopamina oriundas da substância negra para o núcleo caudado e o putame. SIN fasciculus medialis telencephali [TA].
   medial longitudinal b., f. longitudinal medial. SIN medial longitudinal *fasciculus*.
   Monakow b., f. de Monakow. SIN rubrospinal *tract*.
   muscle b., f. muscular; um grupo de fibras musculares envolto por tecido conjuntivo (perimísio).
   neurovascular b. of Walsh, f. neurovascular de Walsh; a estrutura anatômica composta de artérias e veias capsulares para a próstata e nervos cavernosos que fornecem o marco macroscópico utilizado durante a cirurgia pélvica radical com poupança nervosa.
   oblique b. of pons, f. oblíquo da ponte. SIN oblique pontine *fasciculus*.
   olfactory b., f. olfatório; um sistema de fibras, descrito por E. Zuckerkandl como "Reichbündel", que desce do septo pelúcido por diante da comissura anterior no sentido da base do cérebro anterior; contém as fibras pré-comissurais do fórnice, fibras do septo para o hipotálamo e substância inominada, bem como fibras que ascendem para o septo e hipocampo oriundas do hipotálamo e mesencéfalo; não comporta relação especial com o sentido do olfato.
   olivocochlear b., trato olivococlear. VER olivocochlear *tract*.
   Pick b., f. de Pick; um f. de fibras nervosas que se curva no sentido rostral a partir do trato piramidal na medula oblonga e que se acredita que consista em fibras corticonucleares.
   posterior longitudinal b., f. longitudinal posterior. SIN medial longitudinal *fasciculus*.
   precommissural b., f. pré-comissural. VER olfactory b.
   predorsal b., trato tetospinal. SIN tectospinal *tract*.
   b. of Rasmussen, f. de Rasmussen. SIN olivocochlear *tract*.
   Rathke b.'s, feixes de Rathke. SIN *trabeculae* carneae (of right and left ventricles), em *trabecula*.
   retroflex b. of Meynert, f. retroflexo de Meynert. SIN retroflex *fasciculus*.
   right b. of atrioventricular bundle [TA], f. direito do f. atrioventricular; o ramo direito do f. atrioventricular que se desvia do ramo esquerdo logo abaixo da porção membranácea do septo interventricular para descer a parede septal do ventrículo direito e se ramificar abaixo do endocárdio. SIN crus dextrum fasciculi atrioventricularis [TA], right crus of atrioventricular bundle.
   Schütz b., f. de Schütz. SIN dorsal longitudinal *fasciculus*.
   solitary b., trato solitário. SIN solitary *tract*.
   tendon b., fascículo tendinoso; um grupo de fibras tendinosas circundado por uma bainha de tecido conjuntivo irregular (peritendíneo).
   Türck b., f. de Türck. SIN anterior corticospinal *tract*.
   uncinate b. of Russell, f. uncinado de Russell. SIN uncinate *fasciculus* of cerebellum.
   Vicq d´Azyr b., f. de Vicq d´Azyr. SIN mammillothalamic *fasciculus*.

bun·gar·o·tox·ins (bung′gă - rō - tok′sinz). Bungarotoxinas; proteínas constituintes do veneno de uma cobra do sul da Ásia *Bungarus multicinctus*, da família Elapidae. Usadas como instrumentos farmacológicos no estudo da função neuromuscular.

bung·pag·ga (bŭng - păg′ă). Piomiosite tropical. SIN tropical *pyomyositis*.

bun·ion (bŭn′yŭn). Joanete; tumefação localizada na face medial ou dorsal da primeira articulação metatarsofalângica, causada por uma bolsa inflamatória; j. medial está usualmente associado ao hálux valgo. [Fr. Ant. *buigne*, inchaço na cabeça]

bun·ion·ec·to·my (bŭn - yŭn - ek′tō - mē). Excisão de um joanete.
   Keller b., excisão da porção proximal da falange proximal do primeiro artelho.
   Mayo b., excisão da cabeça do primeiro metatarsal.

Bunnell, Sterling, cirurgião norte-americano, 1882–1957. VER B. *suture*; Paul-B. *test*.

bu·no·dont (boo′nō-dont). Bunodonte; que possui dentes molares com cúspides arredondadas ou cônicas baixas, em contraste com o lofodonte. [G. *bounos*, pontículos, + *odous* (*odont-*), dente]

bu·no·lol hy·dro·chlo·ride (bū′nō-lol). Cloridrato de bunolol; agente bloqueador β-adrenérgico para o tratamento de arritmias cardíacas.

bu·no·loph·o·dont (boo-nō-lof′ō-dont). Bunolofodonte; que tem dentes molares com cristas transversais e cúspides arredondadas na superfície oclusal. [G. bunos, pontículos, + *lophos*, crista, + *odous*, dente]

bu·no·se·le·no·dont (boo′nō-sē-len′ō-dont). Bunosselenodonte; que possui dentes molares com cristas em crescente e cúspides arredondadas na superfície oclusal. [*bunos*, + *selēnē*, lua, + *odous*, dente]

Bu·nos·to·mum (bū-nos′to′mum). Gênero de nematódeos (família Ancylostomatidae, subfamília Necatorinae) encontrados no gado e em outros herbívoros; similar ao *Necator*. [G. *bounos*, colina, montículo, + *stoma*, boca]

B. phlebot'omum, espécie que ocorre no gado, carneiro e alguns ruminantes selvagens em muitas partes do mundo.

B. trigonoceph'alum, espécie de nematódeo cosmopolita no intestino delgado de carneiros e cabras.

Bunsen, Robert W., químico e físico alemão, 1811–1899. VER B. burner, solubility *coefficient*; B.-Roscoe *law*.

Bunsen burn·er. Bico de Bunsen; uma lâmpada de gás dotada de aberturas laterais que permitem a admissão de ar suficiente, de modo que o carbono é completamente queimado, fornecendo, assim, uma chama muito quente, porém apenas discretamente luminosa. [RW Bunsen, 1811–1899]

Bun·ya·vir·i·dae (bŭn-yă-vir′i-dē). Família de arbovírus composta de mais de 200 sorotipos de vírus e contendo, pelo menos, cinco gêneros: Bunyavirus, Hantavirus, Phlebovirus, Nairovirus e Tospovirus. Os víríons em todos os gêneros, exceto no Hantavirus, replicam-se em artrópodes. Os víríons têm 80-120 nm de diâmetro, são sensíveis aos solventes lipídicos e enveloped com projeções superficiais de glicopeptídeos; o nucleocapsídeo é de simetria helicoidal, contendo 3 moléculas de RNA de filamento simples (PM 5-8 × 10^6). [*Bunyamwere*, Uganda]

Bun·ya·vi·rus (bun′ya-vī-rus). Vírus do gênero da família Bunyaviridae que inclui pelo menos 160 tipos, i.e., vírus da encefalite da Califórnia e vírus da encefalite LaCrosse.

buph·thal·mia, buph·thal·mus, buph·thal·mos (boof-thal′mē-ă, -thal′mŭs, -thal′mos). Buftalmo, buftalmia; afecção do primeiro ano de vida, caracterizada por aumento da pressão intra-ocular com aumento do bulbo do olho. SIN congenital glaucoma, hydrophthalmia, hydrophthalmos, hydrophthalmus. [G. *bous*, boi, + *ophthalmos*, olho]

bu·piv·a·caine (bū-piv′ă-kān). Bupivacaína; anestésico local potente, com ação prolongada, usado na anestesia regional, infiltração articular e infiltração em pontos de deflagração.

bu·pre·nor·phine hy·dro·chlo·ride (boo-pre-nōr′fēn). Cloridrato de buprenorfina; analgésico opióide semi-sintético empregado para o alívio da dor moderada a grave.

bu·pro·pi·on hy·dro·chlo·ride (boo-prō′pē-on). Cloridrato de bupropiona; antidepressivo. Hoje em dia amplamente utilizado como auxiliar na abstinência do fumo.

bur (bŭr). Broca. **1.** Um instrumento cortante giratório. **2.** Em oftalmologia, um aparelho usado para remover anéis ferruginosos embebidos na córnea. SIN burr.

cross-cut b., b. de corte cruzado; b. com lâminas localizadas em ângulos retos com seu eixo longitudinal.

end-cutting b., b. de corte terminal; b. com lâminas apenas em sua extremidade.

finishing b., b. de acabamento; b. com numerosas lâminas de corte finas dispostas próximas entre si; usada para modelar restaurações metálicas.

fissure b., b. de fissura; instrumento cortante giratório cilíndrico ou que afila progressivamente destinado a estender ou alargar fissuras em um dente, ou reduzir a superfície geral da substância dentária.

inverted cone b., b. em cone invertido; instrumento cortante giratório na forma de um cone truncado, com a extremidade menor presa à haste; geralmente utilizada para penetrar em orifícios cariados ou criar cortes por baixo nas preparações cavitárias.

round b., b. redonda; b. dentária com lâminas de corte dispostas esfericamente.

Burchard, H., químico alemão do século 19. VER B.-Liebermann *reaction*; Liebermann-B. *test*.

Burdach, Karl F., anatomista e fisiologista alemão, 1776–1847. VER B. *column, fasciculus, nucleus, tract*.

bur·den (ber′den). Carga. VER body burden.

clinical b., c. clínica; uma c. que difere da c. genética principalmente no acréscimo do componente morbidade; um traço que não é clínica nem geneticamente letal, pode ser bastante incapacitante.

genetic b., c. genética; o débito genético decorrente da mutação perigosa, mas ainda não evidenciado. (Em uma grande população de tamanho fixo, toda mutação com aptidão genética diminuída acabará extinta e, dependendo dos detalhes da herança e do fenótipo, tem de ser "paga" por um número fixo de mortes genéticas por mutação, o débito genético.)

global b. of disease, c. global da doença; medida matemática da perda de anos de vida saudável devido a doenças incapacitantes na população de um país. VER TAMBÉM disability-adjusted life *years*, em *year*.

bu·ret, bu·rette (boo-ret′). Bureta; um tubo de vidro graduado com uma torneira em sua extremidade inferior; usado para medir líquidos em análise química volumétrica. [Fr.]

Bürger, Max T. F., médico alemão, *1885. VER B.-Grütz *syndrome, disease*.

Burger tri·an·gle. Triângulo de Burger. Ver em triangle.

Burk, Dean, cientista norte-americano, *1904. VER Lineweaver-B. *equation, plot*.

Burk·hol·deria (burk-hol-der′ē-ă). Gênero de bastonetes Gram-negativos, móveis, não-formadores de esporos, contendo espécies significativas de patógenos humanos originalmente classificados como membros do gênero *Pseudomonas*.

B. cepacia, espécie bacteriana encontrada em cebolas podres e em amostras clínicas; comumente encontrada em secreções respiratórias nos pacientes com fibrose cística, é freqüentemente resistente a muitos antibióticos. SIN *Pseudomonas cepacia*.

B. mallei, espécie bacteriana infecciosa para cavalos e asnos, provocando mormo e farcinose. SIN *Pseudomonas mallei*.

B. pseudomallei, espécie encontrada nos casos de melioidose em seres humanos e em outros animais e no solo e na água nas regiões tropicais.

Burkitt, Denis P., médico britânico em Uganda, 1911–1993. VER B. *lymphoma*.

Burlew disk. Disco de Burlew. VER em disk.

Burlew wheel. Roda de Burlew. VER em wheel.

Burn, Joshua Harold, 1892–1981. VER B. and Rand *theory*.

burn (bern). **1.** Queimar; causar uma lesão por calor ou uma lesão semelhante por algum outro agente. **2.** Uma sensação de dor causada por calor excessivo ou dor similar por qualquer outra causa. **3.** Queimadura; lesão causada por calor ou qualquer agente cauterizante, incluindo atrito, agentes cáusticos, eletricidade ou energia eletromagnética; os tipos de queimaduras resultantes de diferentes agentes são relativamente específicos e diagnósticos. A divisão das queimaduras em três graus (primeiro grau, segundo grau e terceiro grau) reflete a gravidade da lesão cutânea (eritema, bolhas, carbonização, respectivamente). [A.S. *baernan*]

brush b., q. por escovamento; q. causada por atrito de um objeto em movimentação rápida contra a pele ou chão contra a pele.

chemical b., q. química; q. decorrente de uma substância química cáustica.

first-degree b., q. de primeiro grau; q. que envolve apenas a epiderme e que provoca eritema e edema sem vesiculação. SIN superficial b.

flash b., q. por clarão; q. devido a exposição muito curta ao calor radiante intenso; a típica q. produzida por explosão atômica.

full-thickness b., q. de espessura total. SIN third-degree b.

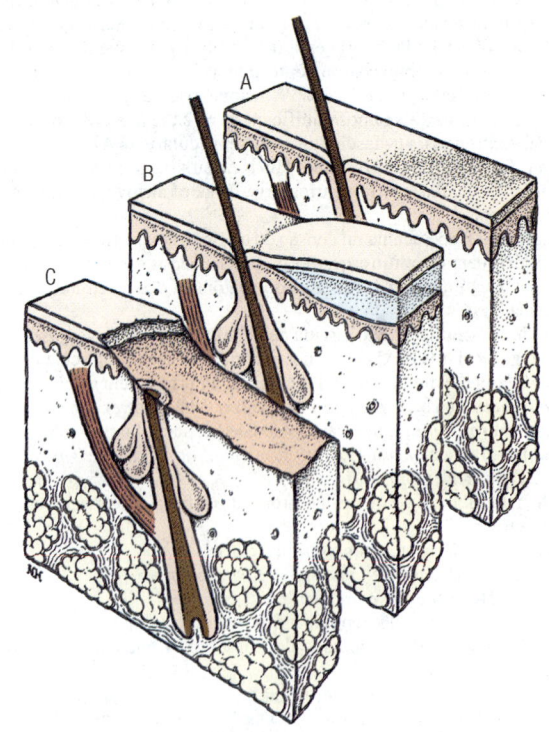

queimaduras: (A) primeiro grau, (B) segundo grau, (C) terceiro grau

mat b., q. por escovamento. SIN brush b.
partial-thickness b., q. de espessura parcial. SIN second-degree b.
radiation b., q. por radiação; q. causada por exposição a rádio, raios X, energia atômica de qualquer forma, raios ultravioleta etc.
rope b., q. por escovamento. VER brush b.
second-degree b., q. de segundo grau; q. que envolve a epiderme e a derme, em geral formando bolhas que podem ser superficiais, ou por necrose dérmica profunda, seguida por regeneração epitelial, estendendo-se a partir dos apêndices cutâneos. SIN partial-thickness b.

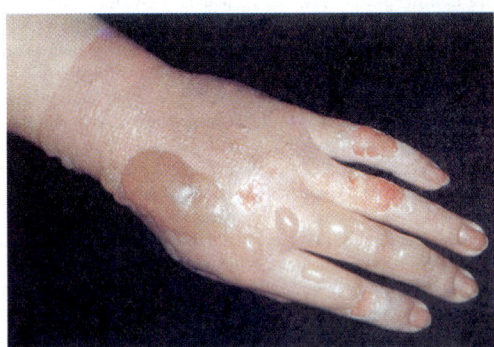

queimadura de 2.º grau: formação de bolhas

superficial b., q. superficial. SIN first-degree b.
thermal b., q. térmica; q. causada por calor.
third-degree b., q. de terceiro grau; q. com destruição de toda a pele; as queimaduras profundas e de terceiro grau estendem-se para o tecido adiposo subcutâneo, o músculo ou o osso e, com freqüência, provocam muito mais fibrose. SIN full-thickness b.
burn·ers (bern′erz). Episódios de dor em caráter de queimação no membro superior. VER TAMBÉM burner *syndrome*. SIN stingers.
Burnett, Charles H., médico norte-americano, 1901–1967. VER B. *syndrome*.
bur·nish·er (bŭr′nish-er). Polidor; um instrumento para alisar e polir a superfície ou borda de uma restauração dentária. [Fr. Ant. *burnir*, polir]
burn·out (bern′owt). **1.** Em odontologia, a eliminação, por calor, de um padrão de revestimento de um aparelho a fim de preparar o molde para receber o metal fundido. **2.** Um estado psicológico de exaustão física e emocional atribuído a uma reação de estresse à capacidade reduzida de satisfazer às demandas profissionais de uma pessoa; os sintomas incluem fadiga, insônia, comprometimento do desempenho no trabalho e uma suscetibilidade aumentada à doença física e dependência química.
Burns, Allan, anatomista escocês, 1781–1813. VER B. *ligament*, falciform *process, space.*
Burow, Karl A. von, cirurgião alemão, 1809–1874. VER B. *solution, triangle, vein.*
burr (bŭr). Trépano. SIN bur.
bur·row (ber′ō). Escavação. **1.** Um túnel ou trato subcutâneo feito por um parasita, como o ácaro da escabiose. **2.** Um seio ou fístula. **3.** Escavar ou criar um túnel ou trato através ou abaixo de vários planos teciduais.

BURSA

bur·sa, pl. **bur·sae** (ber′să, ber′sē) [TA]. Bolsa; um saco fechado ou envelope revestido com a membrana sinovial e contendo líquido, usualmente encontrado ou formado nas áreas sujeitas a atrito; p. ex., sobre uma parte do corpo exposta ou proeminente ou onde um tendão passa sobre um osso. [L. Mediev., uma bolsa]
Achil'les b., b. de Aquiles. SIN b. of tendo calcaneus.
b. achil'lis, b. de Aquiles. SIN b. of tendo calcaneus.
b. of acromion, b. subcutânea acromial. SIN subcutaneous acromial b.
adventitious b., b. adventícia; cisto semelhante a uma bolsa formada entre duas partes como conseqüência de atrito.
b. anseri'na [TA], b. anserina. SIN anserine b.
anserine b. [TA], b. anserina; a b. entre o ligamento colateral tibial da articulação do joelho e os tendões dos músculos sartório, grácil e semitendinoso. SIN b. anserina [TA], tibial intertendinous b.
anterior tibial b., b. subtendínea b. do músculo tibial anterior. SIN subtendinous b. of tibialis anterior.
bicipitoradial b. [TA], b. bicipitorradial; a b. entre o tendão do músculo bíceps braquial e a parte anterior da tuberosidade do rádio. SIN b. bicipitoradialis [TA].
b. bicip'itoradia'lis [TA], b. bicipitorradial. SIN bicipitoradial b.
Boyer b., b. de Boyer. SIN retrohyoid b.
Brodie b., b. de Brodie; **(1)** b. subtendínea medial do músculo gastrocnêmio; **(2)** SIN semimembranous b.
b. of calcaneal tendon, b. tendínea calcânea; termo oficial alternativo* para b. of tendo calcaneus.
Calori b., b. de Calori; uma b. entre o arco da aorta e a traquéia.
coracobrachial b. [TA], b. do músculo coracobraquial; uma b. freqüentemente presente entre o tendão do músculo coracobraquial e o músculo subescapular. SIN b. musculi coracobrachialis [TA], subcoracoid b.
b. cubita'lis interos'sea [TA], b. interóssea do cotovelo. SIN interosseous cubital b.
deep infrapatellar b. [TA], b. infrapatelar profunda; a b. entre a parte superior da tíbia e o ligamento patelar. SIN b. infrapatellaris profunda [TA].
b. of extensor carpi radialis brevis muscle, bainha dos tendões do músculo extensor radial curto do carpo; a b. entre o tendão do músculo extensor radial curto do carpo e a base do terceiro metacarpal. SIN b. musculi extensoris carpi radialis brevis.
b. fabric'ii, bursa de Fabricius; a b. de Fabricius nas aves, uma estrutura sacular cega localizada na parede póstero-dorsal da cloaca; realiza uma função semelhante ao timo. SIN b. of Fabricius.
b. of Fabricius, bursa de Fabricius. SIN b. fabricii.
Fleischmann b., b. de Fleischmann. SIN sublingual b.
b. of gastrocnemius, b. subtendíneas do músculo gastrocnêmio. SIN subtendinous bursae of gastrocnemius (muscle).
bursae of gastrocnemius, b. subtendíneas do músculo gastrocnêmio. SIN subtendinous bursae of gastrocnemius (muscle).
gluteofemoral b., b. intermuscular do glúteo. SIN intermuscular gluteal b.
gluteus medius bursae, bolsas trocantéricas do músculo glúteo médio. SIN trochanteric bursae of gluteus medius.
gluteus minimus b., b. trocantéricas do músculo glúteo mínimo. SIN trochanteric bursae of gluteus minimus.
b. of great toe, bainha do tendão do primeiro dedo do pé; a b. entre o lado lateral da base do primeiro osso metatarsal e o lado medial da diáfise do segundo metatarsal.
b. of hyoid, b. infra-hióidea. SIN retrohyoid b.
iliac b., b. subtendínea do músculo ilíaco. SIN subtendinous b. of iliacus.
b. iliopecti'nea [TA], b. iliopectínea. SIN iliopectineal b.
iliopectineal b., [TA], b. iliopectínea; uma grande b. entre o músculo iliopsoas e a eminência iliopúbica. SIN b. iliopectinea [TA].
inferior subtendinous b. of biceps femo'ris [TA], b. subtendínea inferior do músculo bíceps femoral; a b. entre o tendão do músculo bíceps femoral e o ligamento colateral da fíbula da articulação do joelho. SIN b. subtendinea musculi bicipitis femoris inferior [TA].
infracardiac b., um pequeno saco seroso por vezes presente no lado medial da base do pulmão direito no embrião. VER TAMBÉM pneumatoenteric *recess*, celomic *bay*.
infrahyoid b. [TA], b. infra-hióidea; uma b. por vezes encontrada abaixo da margem inferior do corpo do osso hióide entre o músculo esterno-hióideo e a membrana tireo-hióidea mediana. SIN b. infrahyoidea [TA].
b. infrahyoi'dea [TA], b. infra-hióidea. SIN infrahyoid b.
b. infrapatella'ris profun'da [TA], b. infrapatelar profunda. SIN deep infrapatellar b.
infraspinatus b., b. subcutânea do músculo infra-espinal. SIN subtendinous b. of infraspinatus.
intermuscular gluteal b. [TA], b. intermuscular dos músculos glúteos; duas ou três pequenas bolsas entre o tendão do músculo glúteo máximo e a linha áspera. SIN b. intermuscularis musculorum gluteorum [TA], gluteofemoral b.
b. intermuscula'ris musculo'rum gluteor'um [TA], b. intermuscular dos músculos glúteos. SIN intermuscular gluteal b.
interosseous cubital b. [TA], b. interóssea do cotovelo; uma b. inconstante localizada entre o tendão do músculo bíceps braquial e a ulna ou o tendão oblíquo. SIN b. cubitalis interossea [TA], interosseous b. of elbow.
interosseous b. of elbow, b. interóssea do cotovelo. SIN interosseous cubital b.
b. intratendin'ea olecra'ni [TA], b. intratendínea do olécrano. SIN intratendinous olecranon b.
intratendinous b. of elbow, b. intratendínea do olécrano. SIN intratendinous olecranon b.
intratendinous olecranon b. [TA], b. intratendínea do olécrano; uma b. por vezes presente no tendão de inserção do músculo tríceps braquial. SIN b. intratendinea olecrani [TA], b. of Monro, intratendinous b. of elbow.
b. ischiad'ica mus'culi glu'tei max'imi [TA], b. isquiática do músculo glúteo máximo. SIN sciatic b. of gluteus maximus.
b. ischiad'ica mus'culi obturato'ris inter'ni, b. isquiática do músculo obturador interno. SIN bursae of obturator internus (1).
ischial b., b. isquiática do músculo glúteo máximo. SIN sciatic b. of gluteus maximus.

laryngeal b., b. subcutânea da proeminência laríngea. SIN subcutaneous b. of laryngeal prominence.
lateral malleolar subcutaneous b., b. subcutânea do maléolo lateral. SIN subcutaneous b. of lateral malleolus.
lateral malleolus b., b. subcutânea do maléolo lateral. SIN subcutaneous b. of lateral malleolus.
b. of latiss'imus dor'si, b. subtendínea do músculo latíssimo do dorso. SIN subtendinous b. of latissimus dorsi.
Luschka b., b. de Luschka. SIN pharyngeal b.
medial malleolar subcutaneous b., b. subcutânea do maléolo medial. SIN subcutaneous b. of medial malleolus.
b. of Monro, b. de Monro. SIN intratendinous olecranon b.
b. muco'sa, b. mucosa. SIN synovial b.
b. mus'culi bicip'itis femo'ris supe'rior [TA], b. superior do músculo bíceps femoral. SIN superior b. of biceps femoris.
b. mus'culi coracobrachia'lis [TA], b. do músculo coracobraquial. SIN coracobrachial b.
b. mus'culi extenso'ris car'pi radia'lis bre'vis, bainha do músculo extensor radial curto do carpo. SIN b. of extensor carpi radialis brevis muscle.
b. mus'culi pirifor'mis, b. do músculo piriforme. SIN b. of piriformis.
b. mus'culi semimembrano'si, b. do músculo semimembranáceo. SIN semimembranous b.
b. mus'culi tenso'ris ve'li palati'ni [TA], b. do músculo tensor do véu palatino. SIN b. of tensor veli palatine.
bursae of ob'turator inter'nus, b. subtendínea do músculo obturador interno; (1) a bolsa isquiática grande e constante do músculo obturador interno entre o tendão do obturador interno e a incisura isquiática menor; SIN b. ischiadica musculi obturatoris interni. (2) a b. subtendínea entre o tendão do músculo obturador interno e a cápsula da articulação do quadril. SIN b. subtendinea musculi obturatoris interni.
b. of olecranon, b. do olécrano. SIN subcutaneous olecranon b.
omental b. [TA], b. omental; uma porção isolada da cavidade peritoneal que se localiza dorsalmente ao estômago e se estende cranialmente, posterior ao fígado e ao diafragma, e caudalmente para o omento maior; abre-se na cavidade peritoneal geral no forame omental. SIN b. omentalis [TA], lesser peritoneal cavity, lesser peritoneal sac, omental sac.
b. omenta'lis [TA], b. omental. SIN omental b.
ovarian b., fossa ovárica; o recesso peritoneal entre a face medial do ovário e a mesossalpinge. SIN b. ovarica.
b. ovar'ica, fossa ovárica. SIN ovarian b.
b. pharyn'gea, b. faríngea. SIN pharyngeal b.
pharyngeal b., b. faríngea; um resquício notocórdico cístico encontrado de forma inconstante na parede posterior da nasofaringe na extremidade inferior da tonsila faríngea. SIN b. pharyngea, Luschka b.
b. of piriformis [TA], b. do músculo piriforme; uma pequena b. localizada entre os tendões do músculo piriforme e o gêmeo superior e o fêmur. SIN b. musculi piriformis.
b. of popliteus, recesso poplíteo. SIN subpopliteal recess.
prepatellar b., b. subcutânea pré-patelar. SIN subcutaneous prepatellar b.
b. quadra'ti fem'oris, b. do quadrado femoral; entre a face anterior do músculo quadrado femoral e o trocanter menor do fêmur.
radial b., bainha do tendão do músculo flexor longo do polegar. SIN tendinous sheath of flexor pollicis longus muscle.
retrocalcaneal b. [TA], b. tendínea calcânea; termo oficial alternativo* para b. of tendo calcaneus.
retrohyoid b. [TA], b. infra-hióidea; uma b. entre a superfície posterior do corpo do osso hióide e a membrana tireóidea. SIN b. retrohyoidea [TA], Boyer b., b. of hyoid, subhyoid b.
b. retrohyoi'dea [TA], b. infra-hióidea. SIN retrohyoid b.
rider's b., b. do cavaleiro; uma b. adventícia no lado interno do joelho causada por cavalgar.
sartorius bursae, bolsas subtendíneas do músculo sartório. SIN subtendinous b. of sartorius.
sciatic b. of gluteus maximus [TA], b. isquiática do músculo glúteo máximo; a b. entre o músculo glúteo máximo e a tuberosidade do ísquio. SIN b. ischiadica musculi glutei maximi [TA], ischial b.
b. of semimembranous muscle, b. do músculo semimembranáceo. SIN semimembranous b.
semimembranous b. [TA], b. do músculo semimembranáceo; situa-se entre o músculo semimembranáceo, a cabeça do gastrocnêmio e a articulação do joelho. SIN Brodie b. (2), b. musculi semimembranosi, b. of semembranosus muscle.
subacromial b. [TA], b. subacromial; entre o acrômio e a cápsula da articulação do ombro. SIN b. subacromialis [TA].
b. subacromia'lis [TA], b. subacromial. SIN subacromial b.
subcoracoid b., bolsa do músculo coracobraquial. SIN coracobrachial b.
b. subcuta'nea acromia'lis [TA], b. subcutânea acromial. SIN subcutaneous acromial b.
b. subcuta'nea calca'nea [TA], b. subcutânea calcânea. SIN subcutaneous calcaneal b.
b. subcuta'nea infrapatella'ris [TA], b. subcutânea infrapatelar. SIN subcutaneous infrapatellar b.
b. subcuta'nea malle'oli latera'lis [TA], b. subcutânea do maléolo lateral. SIN subcutaneous b. of lateral malleolus.
b. subcuta'nea malle'oli media'lis [TA], b. subcutânea do maléolo medial. SIN subcutaneous b. of medial malleolus.
b. subcuta'nea ole'crani [TA], b. subcutânea do olécrano. SIN subcutaneous olecranon b.
b. subcuta'nea prepatella'ris, b. subcutânea pré-patelar. SIN subcutaneous prepatellar b.
b. subcuta'nea prominen'tiae laryn'geae [TA], b. subcutânea da proeminência laríngea. SIN subcutaneous b. of the laryngeal prominence.
b. subcuta'nea trochanter'ica, b. subcutânea trocantérica. SIN trochanteric b. (1).
b. subcuta'nea tuberosita'tis tib'iae, b. subcutânea da tuberosidade da tíbia. SIN subcutaneous b. of tuberosity of tibia.
subcutaneous acromial b. [TA], b. subcutânea acromial; a b. de ocorrência freqüente entre o acrômio e a pele. SIN b. subcutanea acromialis [TA], b. of acromion.
subcutaneous calcaneal b. [TA], b. subcutânea calcânea; uma b. entre a pele e a superfície posterior do calcâneo. SIN b. subcutanea calcanea [TA].
subcutaneous infrapatellar b. [TA], b. subcutânea infrapatelar; b. entre o ligamento patelar e a pele. SIN b. subcutanea infrapatellaris [TA].
subcutaneous b. of the laryngeal prominence [TA], b. subcutânea da proeminência laríngea; a b. localizada entre a junção da lâmina da cartilagem tireóidea e a pele. SIN b. subcutanea prominentiae laryngeae [TA], laryngeal b.
subcutaneous b. of lateral malleolus [TA], b. subcutânea do maléolo lateral; a b. entre o maléolo lateral e a pele. SIN b. subcutanea malleoli lateralis [TA], lateral malleolar subcutaneous b., lateral malleolus b.
subcutaneous b. of medial malleolus [TA], b. subcutânea do maléolo medial; a b. entre o maléolo medial e a pele. SIN b. subcutanea malleoli medialis [TA], medial malleolar subcutaneous b.
subcutaneous olecranon b. [TA], b. subcutânea do olécrano; a b. entre o olécrano da ulna e a pele. SIN b. subcutanea olecrani [TA], b. of olecranon.
subcutaneous prepatellar b. [TA], b. subcutânea pré-patelar; b. entre a pele e a parte inferior da patela. SIN b. subcutanea prepatellaris, prepatellar b.
subcutaneous b. of teres major [TA], b. subtendínea do músculo redondo maior; a b. sob o tendão do músculo redondo maior próximo à sua inserção. SIN b. subtendinea musculi teretis majoris [TA], b. of teres major.
subcutaneous b. of tibial tuberosity, b. subcutânea da tuberosidade da tíbia. SIN subcutaneous b. of tuberosity of tibia.
subcutaneous b. of tuberosity of tibia [TA], b. subcutânea da tuberosidade da tíbia; a b. localizada superficialmente à tuberosidade tibial, quer subcutânea, quer subfascial. SIN b. subcutanea tuberositatis tibiae, subcutaneous b. of tibial tuberosity.
subdeltoid b. [TA], b. subdeltóidea; a b. entre o músculo deltóide e a cápsula da articulação do ombro. Pode estar combinada à b. subacromial. SIN b. subdeltoidea [TA].
b. subdeltoi'dea [TA], b. subdeltóidea. SIN subdeltoid b.
b. subfascia'lis prepatella'ris [TA], b. subfascial pré-patelar. SIN subfascial prepatellar b.
subfascial prepatellar b. [TA], b. subfascial pré-patelar; uma b. de ocorrência habitual entre a fáscia lata e o tendão do quadríceps anterior à patela. SIN b. subfascialis prepatellaris [TA].
subhyoid b., b. infra-hióidea. SIN retrohyoid b.
sublingual b., b. sublingual; b. serosa inconstante no nível do freio da língua entre a superfície do músculo genioglosso e a mucosa do assoalho da boca. SIN b. sublingualis, Fleischmann b.
b. sublingua'lis, b. sublingual. SIN sublingual b.
subscapular b., b. subtendínea do músculo subescapular. SIN subtendinous b. subscapularis.
b. subtendin'eae mus'culi gastrocne'mii, bolsas subtendíneas do músculo gastrocnêmio. SIN subtendinous bursae of gastrocnemius (muscle).
bursae subtendin'eae mus'culi sarto'rii [TA], bolsas subtendíneas do músculo sartório. SIN subtendinous b. of sartorius.
b. subtendin'ea ili'aca [TA], b. subtendínea do músculo ilíaco. SIN subtendinous b. of iliacus.
b. subtendin'ea mus'culi bicip'itis fem'oris infe'rior [TA], b. subtendínea inferior do músculo bíceps femoral. SIN inferior subtendinous b. of biceps femoris.
b. subtendin'ea mus'culi infraspina'ti [TA], b. subtendínea do músculo infraespinal. SIN subtendinous b. of infraspinatus.
b. subtendin'ea mus'culi latis'simus dor'si [TA], b. subtendínea do músculo latíssimo do dorso. SIN subtendinous b. of latissimus dorsi.
b. subtendin'ea mus'culi obturatoris inter'ni, b. subtendínea do músculo obturador interno. SIN bursae of obturator internus (2).
b. subtendin'ea mus'culi subscapula'ris [TA], b. subtendínea do músculo subescapular. SIN subtendinous b. of subscapularis.

b. subtendin'ea mus'culi tere'tis majo'ris [TA], b. subtendínea do músculo redondo maior. SIN subtendinous b. of teres major.
b. subtendin'ea mus'culi tibia'lis anterio'ris [TA], b. subtendínea do músculo tibial anterior. SIN subtendinous b. of tibialis anterior.
b. subtendin'ea mus'culi trape'zii [TA], b. subtendínea do músculo trapézio. SIN subtendinous b. of trapezius.
b. subtendin'ea mus'culi trici'pitis bra'chii [TA], b. subtendínea do músculo tríceps braquial. SIN subtendinous b. of triceps brachii.
b. subtendin'ea prepatella'ris [TA], b. subtendínea pré-patelar. SIN subtendinous prepatellar b.
bursae subtendineae musculi gastrocnemii [TA], bolsas subtendíneas do músculo gastrocnêmio. SIN subtendinous bursae of gastrocnemius (muscle).
subtendinous bursae of gastrocnemius (muscle), bolsas subtendíneas do músculo gastrocnêmio; consistem em uma b. lateral e uma medial [b. de Brodie (1)] entre as cabeças do músculo gastrocnêmio e a cápsula da articulação do joelho. SIN bursae subtendineae musculi gastrocnemii [TA], b. of gastrocnemius, b. subtendineae musculi gastrocnemii, bursae of gastrocnemius.
subtendinous iliac b., b. subtendínea do músculo ilíaco. SIN subtendinous b. of iliacus.
subtendinous b. of iliacus [TA], b. subtendínea do músculo ilíaco; a b. na inserção do músculo iliopsoas no trocanter menor. SIN b. subtendinea iliaca [TA], iliac b., subtendinous iliac b.
subtendinous b. of infraspinatus [TA], b. subtendínea do músculo infra-espinal; a b. localizada entre o tendão do músculo infra-espinal e a cápsula da articulação do ombro. SIN b. subtendinea musculi infraspinati [TA], infraspinatus b.
subtendinous b. of latissimus dorsi [TA], b. subtendínea do músculo latíssimo do dorso; b. constante entre os tendões dos músculos redondo maior e latíssimo do dorso, próximo às suas interseções. SIN subtendinea musculi latissimus dorsi [TA], b. of latissimus dorsi.
subtendinous prepatellar b. [TA], b. subtendínea pré-patelar; uma b. inconstante entre o tendão do músculo quadríceps e a patela. SIN b. subtendinea prepatellaris [TA].
subtendinous b. of sartorius [TA], b. subtendínea do músculo sartório; bolsas, por vezes separadas da b. anserina, localizadas entre os tendões dos músculos sartório, semitendíneo e grácil. SIN bursae subtendineae musculi sartorii [TA], sartorius bursae.
subtendinous b. of subscapularis [TA], b. subtendínea do músculo subescapular; a b. entre o tendão do músculo subescapular e o colo da escápula; comunica-se com a articulação do ombro. SIN b. subtendinea musculi subscapularis [TA], subscapular b.
subtendinous b. of tibialis anterior, b. subtendínea do músculo tibial anterior; a pequena b. entre a superfície medial do osso cuneiforme medial e o tendão do tibial anterior. SIN b. subtendinea musculi tibialis anterioris [TA], anterior tibial b.
subtendinous b. of trapezius [TA], b. subtendínea do músculo trapézio; uma b. entre o tendão do músculo trapézio e a extremidade medial da espinha da escápula. SIN b. subtendinea musculi trapezii [TA], b. of trapezius.
subtendinous b. of triceps brachii [TA], b. subtendínea do músculo tríceps braquial; a b. localizada profundamente ao tendão do tríceps braquial próximo à sua inserção no olécrano. SIN b. subtendinea musculi tricipitis brachii [TA], triceps b.
superior b. of biceps femoris [TA], b. superior do músculo bíceps femoral; b. freqüentemente encontrada entre o tendão da cabeça longa do músculo bíceps femoral e a tuberosidade isquiática e o tendão do músculo semimembranáceo. SIN b. musculi bicipitis femoris superior [TA].
suprapatellar b. [TA], b. suprapatelar; uma grande b. entre a parte inferior do fêmur e o tendão do músculo quadríceps femoral. Em geral, comunica-se com a cavidade da articulação do joelho e está patologicamente distendida por sangue ou líquido sinovial na bursite suprapatelar ("água no joelho"). SIN b. suprapatellaris [TA].
b. suprapatella'ris [TA], b. suprapatelar. SIN suprapatellar b.
synovial b. [TA], b. sinovial; um saco contendo líquido sinovial que ocorre nos locais de atrito, como entre um tendão e um osso, sobre o qual ele se move, ou, no nível subcutâneo, sobre uma proeminência óssea. A Terminologia Anatômica lista os seguintes tipos: b. subcutânea, [TA]; b. submuscular [TA]; b. subfascial [TA]; e b. subtendínea [TA]. SIN b. synovialis [TA], b. mucosa.
b. synovia'lis [TA], b. sinovial. SIN synovial b.
synovial trochlear b., bainha tendínea do músculo oblíquo superior. SIN tendinous *sheath* of superior oblique muscle.
b. ten'dinis calca'nei, b. tendínea calcânea. SIN b. of tendo calcaneus.
b. of tendo calca'neus [TA], b. tendínea calcânea; a b. entre o tendão do calcâneo e a parte superior da superfície posterior do calcâneo. SIN b. of calcaneal tendon*, retrocalcaneal b*, Achilles b., b. achillis, b. tendinis calcanei.
b. of tensor veli palatine [TA], b. do músculo tensor do véu palatino; uma pequena b. localizada onde o tendão do tensor passa ao redor do hâmulo pterigóideo. SIN b. musculi tensoris veli palatini [TA].

b. of teres major, b. subtendínea do músculo redondo maior. SIN subcutaneous b. of teres major.
tibial intertendinous b., b. anserina. SIN anserine b.
b. of trapezius, b. subtendínea do músculo trapézio. SIN subtendinous b. of trapezius.
triceps b., b. subcutânea do músculo tríceps braquial. SIN subtendinous b. of triceps brachii.
trochanteric b. [TA], b. trocantérica; (1) b. subcutânea trocantérica entre o trocanter maior do fêmur e a pele. SIN b. subcutanea trochanterica. (2) b. trocantérica multilocular do músculo glúteo máximo entre os músculos glúteo máximo e trocanter maior do fêmur. SIN b. trochanterica musculi glutei maximi. (3) b. trocantérica do glúteo médio entre o glúteo médio e o trocanter maior. SIN bursae trochantericae musculi glutei medii [TA]. (4) b. trocantérica do glúteo mínimo. SIN b. trochanterica musculi glutei minimi [TA]. SIN b. trochanterica [TA].
b. trochanterica [TA], b. trocantérica. SIN trochanteric b.
bur'sae trochanter'icae mus'culi glu'tei me'dii [TA], bolsas trocantéricas do músculo glúteo médio. SIN trochanteric b. (3).
b. trochanter'ica mus'culi glu'tei max'imi, b. trocantérica do músculo glúteo máximo. SIN trochanteric b. (2)
b. trochanter'ica mus'culi glu'tei min'imi [TA], b. trocantérica do músculo glúteo mínimo. SIN trochanteric b. (4)
trochanteric bursae of gluteus medius [TA], bolsas trocantéricas do glúteo médio; a b. entre o tendão do glúteo médio e o trocanter maior e a b. entre os músculos piriforme e glúteo médio. SIN gluteus medius bursae.
trochanteric bursae of gluteus minimus [TA], bolsas trocantéricas do glúteo mínimo; uma b. bastante grande geralmente localizada entre o glúteo mínimo e o trocanter maior. SIN gluteus minimus b.
trochlear synovial b., bainha tendínea do músculo oblíquo superior. SIN tendinous *sheath* of superior oblique muscle.
ulnar b., bainha comum dos tendões dos músculos flexores (da mão). SIN common flexor *sheath* (of hand).

bur·sal (ber'săl). Relativo a uma bolsa.
bur·sec·to·my (ber-sek'tō-mē). Bursectomia; A remoção cirúrgica de uma bolsa. [bursa + G. *ektomē*, excisão]
bur·si·tis (ber-sī'tis). Bursite; inflamação de uma bolsa. SIN bursal synovitis.
anserine b., b. anserina; a inflamação da bolsa anserina que se situa entre o *pes anserinus* e a superfície medial superior da tíbia.
calcific b., b. calcificada; a inflamação de uma bolsa que resulta na deposição de sais de cálcio; associada mais amiúde à bursite subdeltóidea.
ischial b., b. isquiática; inflamação da bolsa suprajacente à tuberosidade isquiática da pelve.
olecranon b., b. do olécrano; inflamação da bolsa subcutânea do olécrano, suprajacente à proeminência do cotovelo.
prepatellar b., b. pré-patelar. SIN housemaid's *knee*.
subacromial b., b. subacromial; a inflamação da bolsa subacromial que se situa entre o acrômio, acima, e o manguito rotatório, abaixo; pode ser contínua com a bolsa subdeltóidea (subdeltoid *bursa*).
subdeltoid b., b. subdeltóidea; a inflamação da bolsa subdeltóidea que se localiza entre o músculo deltóide e a porção proximal do úmero e o manguito rotatório subjacentes; pode ser contínua com a bolsa subacromial.
bur·so·lith (ber'sō-lith). Cálculo formado em uma bolsa. [bursa + G. *lithos*, pedra]
bur·sop·a·thy (ber-sop'ă-thē). Qualquer doença de uma bolsa.
bur·sot·o·my (ber-sot'ō-mē). A incisão através da parede de uma bolsa. [bursa + G. *tomē*, um corte]
burst (berst). Explosão; um aumento súbito na atividade.
respiratory b., e. respiratória; o aumento acentuado na atividade metabólica que ocorre nos fagócitos e em outras células através da ligação de partículas, resultando em aumento do consumo de oxigênio, formação de ânion superóxido, formação de peróxido de hidrogênio e ativação da via metabólica da hexose monofosfato.
b. size, e. de tamanho; o número de fagos produzidos por uma célula infectada.
bur·su·la (ber'soo-lă). Pequena bolsa ou saco. [L. Mod. dim. do L. Mediev. *bursa*, bolsa]
b. tes'tium, termo arcaico para scrotum.
Burton, Henry, médico inglês, 1799–1849. VER B. *line*.
Busacca, Archimede, médico italiano, 1893. VER Busacca *nodules*, em *nodule*.
Buschke, Abraham, dermatologista alemão, 1868–1943. VER B. *disease*: B.-Ollendorf *syndrome*.
bu·spi·rone hy·dro·chlo·ride (bū-spī'rŏn). Cloridrato de buspirona; agente ansiolítico não-benzodiazepínico utilizado no controle dos transtornos da ansiedade de ou para o alívio a curto prazo dos sintomas de ansiedade.
Busquet, G. Paul, médico francês, 1865–1930. VER B. *disease*.
Busse, Otto, médico alemão, 1867–1922.

bu·sul·fan, bu·sul·phan (bū-sŭl'fan). Bussulfam; agente alquilante antineoplásico empregado no tratamento da leucemia mielocítica crônica; sabidamente teratogênico em seres humanos.

bu·ta·bar·bi·tal (bū-tă-bar'bĭ-tawl). Butabarbital; antigo sedativo e hipnótico com duração de ação intermediária; disponível como b. sódico, com os mesmos usos.

bu·ta·caine sul·fate (bū'tă-kān). Sulfato de butacaína; um anestésico local.

bu·tam·ben (bū-tam'ben). Butil aminobenzoato. SIN *butyl aminobenzoate.*

bu·tane (bū'tān). Butano; C_4H_{10}; hidrocarboneto gasoso presente no gás natural; dois isômeros são conhecidos, os quais são ativos do ponto de vista anestésico: o n-butano é $CH_3(CH_2)_2CH_3$, e o isobutano é $CH_3CH(CH_3)$–CH_3 (ou 2-metilpropano).

bu·ta·no·ic ac·id (bū-tă-nō'ik). Ácido butanóico; nome sistemático para o ácido n-butírico normal.

bu·ta·nol (bū-tă-nol). Butanol; nome químico preferido para o álcool n-butílico.

bu·tan·o·yl (bū'tan-ō-il). Butanoil; o radical do ácido butanóico. SIN butyryl.

bu·ta·per·a·zine (bū-tă-per'ă-zēn). Butaperazina; antipsicótico.

bu·tav·er·ine (bū-tav'er-ēn). Butaverina; antiespasmódico (na forma cloridrato).

bu·teth·a·mate (bū-teth'ă-māt). Butetamato; agente antiespasmódico intestinal.

bu·thet·a·mine hy·dro·chlo·ride (bū-teth'ă-mēn). Cloridrato de butetamina; anestésico local.

bu·thi·a·zide (bū-thī'ă-zīd). Butiazida; possui ações diurética e anti-hipertensiva. SIN thiabutazide.

buthionine sulfoximine (boo-thī-ō-nēn sul-fox'ĭ-mēn). Butionina sulfoximina; composto que diminui a glutationa intracelular por inibição de sua síntese.

bu·to·con·a·zole ni·trate (bū-tō-kō'nă-zōl). Nitrato de butoconazol; agente antifúngico prescrito principalmente para a candidíase vulvovaginal; similar ao cetoconazol e ao itraconazol.

bu·to·py·ro·nox·yl (bū'tō-pī-rō-nok'sil). Butopironoxil; um repelente de insetos, efetivo contra a mosca dos estábulos (*Stomoxys calcitrans*).

bu·tor·pha·nol tar·trate (bū-tōr'fă-nōl). Tartarato de butorfanol; potente agente analgésico narcótico agonista/antagonista misto, utilizado por injeção e na forma de *spray* nasal.

bu·tox·a·mine hy·dro·chlo·ride (bū-tok'să-mēn). Cloridrato de butoxamina; agente antilipêmico.

***t*-bu·tox·y·car·bon·yl (BOC, *t*-BOC, Boc)** (bū-toks-ē-kar'bŏn-il). *t*-Butoxicarbonila; grupamento amino-protegido usado na síntese de peptídeos. SIN *tert*-butyloxycarbonyl.

bu·trip·ty·line hy·dro·chlo·ride (bū-trip'tĭ-lēn). Cloridrato de butriptilina; antidepressivo.

butt (bŭt). **1.** Unir duas extremidades quadradas quaisquer a fim de formar uma articulação. **2.** Em odontologia, colocar uma restauração diretamente contra os tecidos que revestem a crista alveolar.

but·ter (bŭt'er). Manteiga. **1.** Uma massa aderente de gordura do leite, obtida a partir do creme batido até que os glóbulos de gordura separados se unam, deixando um resíduo líquido, ou soro. **2.** Um sólido macio cuja consistência é semelhante à da m. [L. *butyrum*, G. *boutyros*, prov. de *bous*, vaca, + *tyros*, queijo]
 b. of antimony, m. de antimônio; uma solução ácida concentrada de tricloreto de antimônio.
 b. of bismuth, m. de bismuto. SIN *bismuth* trichloride.
 cacao b., cocoa b., m. de cacau. SIN *theobroma* oil. VER TAMBÉM cacao.
 b. of tin, m. de estanho; cloreto estânico pentaidratado, $SnCl_4·5H_2O$.
 b. of zinc, m. de zinco. SIN *zinc* chloride.

but·ter·fly (bŭt'er-flī). Borboleta. **1.** Qualquer estrutura ou aparelho com formato semelhante a uma borboleta com as asas abertas. **2.** Uma lesão eritematosa descamativa em cada bochecha, unida por uma estreita faixa através do nariz; observada no lúpus eritematoso e na dermatite seborréica. SIN butterfly eruption, butterfly patch, butterfly rash.

but·ter·milk. Soro de leite; o líquido que contém caseína e ácido lático, que fica depois do processo de fabricação da manteiga.

but·ter yel·low [C. I. 11160]. Amarelo de metila; corante amarelo lipossolúvel (PM 225) que possui ação carcinogênica hepática em cobaias; usado como indicador do pH (vermelho em pH 2,9; amarelo em pH 4,0). SIN dimethylaminoazobenzene, methyl yellow.

but·tocks (bŭt'oks). [TA]. Nádegas; a proeminência formada pelos músculos glúteos em ambos os lados. SIN nates [TA], clunes*, breech.

but·ton (bŭt'on). Botão; estrutura, lesão ou dispositivo em forma de botão. [Ing. Med. do Fr. Ant. *bouton*, de *bouter*, golpear, do Alemão]
 Biskra b., b. de Biskra. SIN *Oriental b.*
 Murphy b., b. de Murphy; dispositivo utilizado para anastomose intestinal; consiste em dois cilindros ocos e redondos que são inseridos em cada uma das extremidades do intestino transeccionado; o intestino é fixado em cada um dos componentes com uma sutura e as terminações são aproximadas e os dois cilindros unidos com um mecanismo de trava; o aparelho é degradável e em cerca de 10 dias dissolve e é desprendido para a luz do intestino. Uma modificação de um antigo aparelho metálico com o mesmo nome.
 Oriental b., b. oriental; a lesão que ocorre na leishmaniose cutânea. SIN Biskra b.
 peritoneal b., b. peritoneal; um dispositivo empregado para drenar o líquido ascítico para o espaço subcutâneo.

but·ton·hole (bŭt'on-hōl). Botoeira. **1.** Um corte reto e curto feito através da parede de uma cavidade ou canal. **2.** A contração de um orifício até atingir uma fenda estreita; i.e., a chamada b. mitral na estenose mitral extrema. VER buttonhole *stenosis*.

bu·tyl (bū'til). Butila; $CH_3(CH_2)_3$–; um radical do n-butano.
 b. alcohol, álcool butílico; várias formas isoméricas são conhecidas: **álcool butílico primário**, 1-butanol, propilcarbinol, o álcool butílico da fermentação; **álcool isobutílico**, isopropilcarbinol, 2-metil-1-propanol, que é narcótico em concentrações elevadas; **álcool butílico secundário**, etilmetilcarbinol, 2-butanol; e **álcool butílico terciário**, trimetilcarbinol, 2-metil-2-propanol, um desnaturante para o etanol.
 b. aminobenzoate, aminobenzoato de butila, anestésico local, muito insolúvel e apenas discretamente absorvido. SIN butamben.

bu·tyl·at·ed hy·drox·y·an·is·ole (BHA) (boo-tĭ-lăt'ed hī'drok-sē-an'ĭ-sol). Hidroxianisol butilado; exibe propriedades antioxidantes; freqüentemente utilizado com o hidroxitolueno de propil galato butilado, hidroquinona, metionina, lecitina, ácido tiodipropiônico etc. Usado como antioxidante, especialmente nos alimentos.

bu·tyl·at·ed hy·drox·y·tol·u·ene (BHT). Hidroxitolueno butilado; antioxidante para alimento, ração animal, derivados de petróleo, borrachas sintéticas, plásticos, óleos animais e vegetais, sabão; também é agente antiaglutinante em tintas.

***tert*-bu·tyl·ox·y·car·bon·yl (tBoc)** (bū'til-oks'ē-kar'bŏn-il). *terc*-Butiloxicarbonila. SIN *t-butoxycarbonyl.*

bu·tyl·par·a·ben (bū-til-par'ă-ben). Butilparabeno; conservante antifúngico.

bu·ty·ra·ce·ous (bū-ti-rā'shĭ-us). Butiráceo; de consistência amanteigada.

bu·ty·rate (bū'ti-rāt). Butirato; um sal ou éster do ácido butírico.

bu·ty·rate-CoA li·gase. Butirato-CoA ligase; tiocinase de ácido graxo (cadeia média), uma ligase que forma acil-CoA a partir de ácidos graxos de cadeia média e CoA com a conversão do ATP em AMP e pirofosfato. Uma etapa importante na ativação de ácidos graxos. SIN acyl-activating enzyme (2), butyryl-CoA synthetase, octanoyl-CoA synthetase.

bu·tyr·ic (bū-tir'ik). Butírico; relativo à manteiga.

bu·tyr·ic ac·id (bū-tir'ik). Ácido butírico; ácido de odor desagradável que ocorre na manteiga, no óleo de fígado de bacalhau, no suor e em muitas outras substâncias. Existe em duas formas: **a. butírico normal** (também escrito como ácido n-butírico), ácido butanóico, que ocorre em combinação com o glicerol na manteiga de vaca; e **ácido isobutírico**, ácido 2-metilpropanóico, um dos intermediários no catabolismo da valina, encontrado na combinação com o glicerol no óleo de cróton e em outros locais.

γ-bu·tyr·o·be·taine (bū-tir'ō-be-tān). γ-butirobetaína; uma betaína do ácido γ-aminobutírico; precursor da carnitina por hidroxilação do carbono β.

bu·tyr·o·cho·lin·es·ter·ase (bū'tir-ō-kō-lin-es'ter-ās). Butirocolinesterase; pseudocolinesterase ou colinesterase plasmática. Precisa ser diferenciada da colinesterase verdadeira ou tecidual. VER TAMBÉM cholinesterase. SIN butyrylcholine esterase, pseudocholinesterase.

bu·ty·roid (bū'ti-royd). **1.** Amanteigado. **2.** Que se assemelha à manteiga.

bu·tyr·om·e·ter (bū-ti-rom'ĕ-ter). Butirômetro; um instrumento para determinar a quantidade de manteiga no leite. [G. *boutyron*, manteiga, + *metron*, medida]

bu·ty·ro·phe·none (bū'tir-ō-fē'nōn). Butirofenona; de um de um grupo de derivados da 4-fenilbutilamina que possuem atividade neuroléptica; p.ex., haloperidol.

bu·tyr·ous (bū'ti-rŭs). Butiroso, butiriáceo; indica um crescimento tecidual ou bacteriano de consistência amanteigada.

bu·tyr·yl (bū'ti-ril). Butiril. SIN *butanoyl.*

bu·tyr·yl·cho·line es·ter·ase (bū'ti-ril-kō'len es'ter-ās). Butirilcolinesterase. SIN *butyrocholinesterase.*

bu·tyr·yl-CoA. Butiril-CoA; produto de condensação de coenzima A e ácido n-butanóico; intermediário na degradação do ácido graxo e na biossíntese.
 b.-C. synthetase, b.-C. sintetase. SIN *butyrate-CoA ligase.*

Buzzard, Thomas, médico inglês, 1831–1919. VER B. *maneuver.*

Buzzi, Fausto, colaborador de Ernst Schweninger. VER Schweninger-B. *anetoderma.*

Byars, Louis T., cirurgião norte-americano do século 20, (1906-). VER B. *flap.*

Byler, família Amish nos Estados Unidos. VER Byler *disease.*

by·pass (bī'pas). **1.** Desvio, derivação; fluxo auxiliar. **2.** Desviar; criar o novo fluxo de uma estrutura para outra através de um canal de desvio. VER TAMBÉM shunt.
 aortocoronary b., d. aortocoronário. SIN *coronary artery b.*
 aortoiliac b., d. aortoilíaco; cirurgia em que uma prótese vascular é unida com a aorta e a artéria ilíaca para aliviar a obstrução da aorta abdominal inferior, sua bifurcação e os ramos ilíacos proximais.

aortorenal b., b. aortorrenal; prótese vascular de material sintético, tecido autólogo ou tecido heterólogo que evita a obstrução da artéria renal.
bowel b., d. intestinal. SIN jejunoileal b.
cardiopulmonary b., d. cardiopulmonar; desvio do fluxo sangüíneo que retorna para o coração através de uma bomba oxigenadora (máquina coração-pulmão) que, em seguida, o devolve para o lado arterial da circulação; usado em cirurgias no coração para manter a circulação extracorpórea.

coronary artery b., d. da artéria coronária; conduto, usualmente um enxerto venoso ou da artéria torácica (mamária) interna, cirurgicamente interposto entre a aorta e um ramo da artéria coronária para desviar o sangue da coronária para além de uma obstrução. SIN aortocoronary b.
extra-anatomic b., d. extra-anatômico; um d. vascular que não se adapta à anatomia preexistente.
extracranial-intracranial b., d. extracraniano-intracraniano; um desvio vascular criado pela anastomose de um vaso extracraniano a um vaso intracraniano, usualmente a artéria temporal superficial com um ramo cortical da artéria cerebral média.
femoropopliteal b., d. femoropoplíteo; prótese vascular de material sintético, tecido autólogo ou tecido heterólogo que cria um desvio em torno de uma obstrução na artéria femoral.
gastric b., d. gástrico; divisão alta do estômago, anastomose da pequena bolsa superior do estômago com o jejuno e fechamento da porção distal do estômago que fica retida; usado para o tratamento da obesidade grave.
jejunoileal b., d. jejunoileal; anastomose da porção superior do jejuno com o íleo terminal para o tratamento da obesidade grave. SIN bowel b., jejunoileal shunt.
left heart b., d. do coração esquerdo; qualquer procedimento que desvie o sangue que retorna da circulação pulmonar para a circulação sistêmica sem passar através do coração esquerdo. Isso é utilizado durante algumas cirurgias cardíacas e, experimentalmente, durante a insuficiência cardíaca esquerda grave ou choque cardiogênico.
partial ileal b., d. ileal parcial; divisão do intestino delgado cerca de 100 cm proximalmente à válvula ileocecal, fechamento da extremidade distal e anastomose da extremidade proximal com o ceco.
right heart b., d. do coração direito; introdução de um circuito que desvia o sangue oriundo das veias cavas em torno do átrio e ventrículo direitos e diretamente para a artéria pulmonar.

bys·si·no·sis (bis-i-nō′sis). Bissinose; doença obstrutiva das vias aéreas nas pessoas que trabalham com algodão, linho ou cânhamo cru; causada por reação ao material na poeira e que se acredita que inclua endotoxina por contaminação bacteriana. Por vezes chamada de "asma da manhã de segunda-feira", pois os pacientes melhoram quando estão longe do trabalho no fim-de-semana. SIN cotton-dust asthma, cotton-mill fever, mill fever. [G. *byssos*, linho, + *-osis*, condição]
byte. *Byte*; um grupo de bits adjacentes, comumente 4, 6 ou 8, que atuam como uma unidade para o armazenamento e a manipulação de dados em um computador.

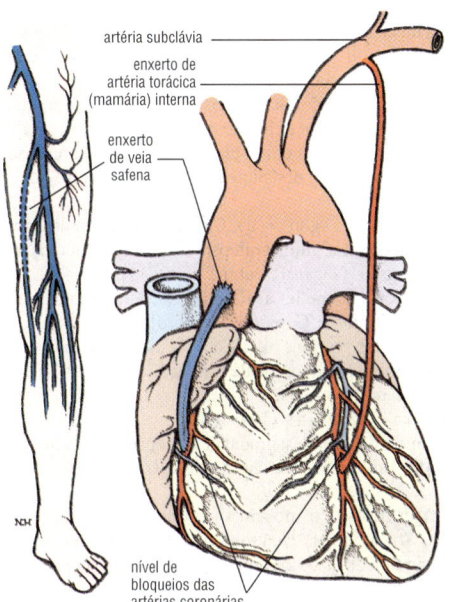

derivação (*bypass*) coronária: derivação dupla completa usando a artéria mamária interna e a veia safena

C

C 1. Abreviatura ou símbolo de grande caloria (large *calorie*); carbono; catódico; catodo; Celsius; vértebra cervical (C1–C7); fechamento (de um circuito elétrico); côngio (galão); contração; coulomb; curie; cilindro; lente cilíndrica (cylindrical *lens*); citidina; cisteína; citosina; componente do complemento (*component* of complement) (C1–C9); terceiro substrato em uma reação catalisada por enzima com múltiplos substratos. **2.** Quando seguido por letras subscritas, como, p. ex., C_{in}, indica depuração renal de uma substância (p. ex., inulina). Quando seguido por números subscritos, como, p. ex., C_{19}, indica o número de átomos de carbono em uma molécula, p. ex., 19.
c 1. Abreviatura ou símbolo de centi-; pequena caloria (small *calorie*); cento; concentração; velocidade da luz no vácuo; circunferência. Abreviatura de curie. **2.** Como subscrito, refere-se ao capilar sanguíneo (blood *capillary*).
c̄ Abreviatura do L. *cum*, com.
^{11}**C** Símbolo do carbono-11 (C^{11}).
^{12}**C** Símbolo do carbono-12 (C^{12}), a forma mais comum de carbono.
^{13}**C** Símbolo do carbono-13 (C^{13}).
^{14}**C** Símbolo do carbono-14 (C^{14}).
CA Abreviatura de câncer; a cada; parada cardíaca (cardiac *arrest*); idade cronológica (chronologic *age*); citosina arabinosídeo (*cytosine* arabinoside).
CA-125. Abreviatura de teste para antígeno do câncer 125 (cancer antigen 125 *test*).
CA125 Abreviatura de teste para antígeno do câncer 125 (cancer antigen 125 *test*).
Ca 1. Abreviatura de catodo. **2.** Símbolo do cálcio.
^{45}**Ca** Símbolo do cálcio-45 (Ca^{45}).
^{47}**Ca** Símbolo do cálcio-47 (Ca^{47}).
ca. Abreviatura do L. *circa* (cerca de, aproximadamente).
caa·pi (ka'pē). Caapi; iagê; inebriana; preparação alucinógena obtida da *Banisteria caapi* (família Malpighaceae), planta trepadeira da floresta sul-americana; contém harmina e outros princípios psicotomiméticos. SIN ayahuasca.
cab·bage tree (kab'ij trē). Angelim branco; andira-uchi; angelim-liso; cumaruana; morcegueira; pau-palmeira. SIN andira.
Cabot, Richard C., médico norte-americano, 1868–1939. VER C. ring *bodies*, em *body*; C.-Locke *murmur*.
⬯ **cac-.** VER caco-.
ca·cao (kă - ka'ō). Cacau; cacau preparado; pó preparado a partir dos grãos centrais secos e torrados da semente madura do *Theobroma cacao Linné* (família Sterculiaceae); a árvore fornece uma gordura, o óleo de teobroma. SIN theobroma. [origem mexicana nativa]
    c· oil, manteiga de cacau. SIN theobroma oil.
CaCC Abreviatura de cathodal closure *contraction* (contração de fechamento catódico).
Cacchione, Aldo, psiquiatra italiano do século XX. VER De Sanctis-C. *syndrome*.
ca·chec·tic (kă - kek'tik). Caquético; relativo a, ou que sofre de, caquexia.
ca·chec·tin (ka - kek'tin). Caquetina; uma citocina polipeptídica, produzida por macrófagos ativados por endotoxina, que tem a capacidade de modular o metabolismo dos adipócitos, lisar células tumorais *in vitro* e induzir necrose hemorrágica de alguns tumores transplantáveis *in vivo*. SIN tumor necrosis factor. [G. *kakos*, mau, + *hexis*, condição do corpo]
ca·chet (kă - shā'). Cápsula ou hóstia em forma de selo feita de farinha para revestir pós de sabor desagradável. A dosagem selada é umedecida e engolida. [Fr. um selo]
ca·chex·ia (kă - kek'sē - ă). Caquexia; perda de peso geral e desgaste muscular que ocorrem no curso de uma doença crônica ou distúrbio emocional. [G. *kakos*, mau, + *hexis*, condição do corpo]
    c. aphtho'sa, c. aftosa. SIN sprue (1).
    c. aquo'sa, c. aquosa; forma edematosa de ancilostomíase.
    diabetic neuropathic c., c. neuropática diabética; síndrome clínica observada quase exclusivamente em homens diabéticos idosos, que consiste no início algo súbito de forte dor nos membros, emagrecimento acentuado, depressão e impotência. Esses pacientes parecem ter uma combinação de polineuropatia diabética grave, polirradiculopatia diabética bilateral difusa e neuropatia autônoma diabética.
    hypophyseal c., c. hipofisária. SIN panhypopituitarism.
    c. hypophys'eopri'va, c. hipofisiopriva; condição após remoção total da hipófise, resultando em pan-hipopituitarismo caracterizado por queda da temperatura corporal, desequilíbrio eletrolítico e hipoglicemia, seguidos por coma e morte.
    hypophysial c., c. hipofisária. SIN panhypopituitarism.
    malarial c., c. malárica. SIN chronic malaria.
    pituitary c., c. hipofisária. SIN Sheehan syndrome.
    c. strumipri'va, c. tireopriva. SIN c. thyropriva.
    c. thyroid'ea, c. tireóidea. SIN c. thyropriva.
    c. thyropri'va, c. tireopriva; sinais e sintomas de hipotireoidismo (com ou sem mixedema) resultando da perda de tecido tireóideo, seja por cirurgia, radioterapia ou doença. SIN c. strumipriva, c. thyroidea.
cach·in·na·tion (kak - i - nā'shŭn). Caquinação; riso sem causa aparente, freqüentemente observado na esquizofrenia. [L. *cachinno*, rir alto e excessivamente]
⬯ **caco-, caci-, cac-.** Mau; doentio. Cf. mal-. [G. *kakos*]
cac·o·dyl (kak'ō - dil). Cacodilo; óleo resultante da destilação conjunta de ácido arsênico e acetato de potássio. SIN dicacodyl, tetramethyldiarsine. [G. *kakōdēs*, fétido]
cac·o·dyl·ate (kak'ō - dil - āt). Cacodilato; sal ou éster do ácido cacodílico. VER cacodylic acid.
cac·o·dyl·ic (kak - ō - dil'ik). Cacodílico; relativo ao cacodilo; designa principalmente o ácido cacodílico.
cac·o·dyl·ic ac·id. Ácido cacodílico; preparado pelo tratamento do cacodilo e do óxido cacodílico com óxido de mercúrio, e forma cacodilatos com várias bases que foram usadas em doenças cutâneas, tuberculose, malária e outras afecções nas quais o arsênico foi considerado útil. SIN dimethylarsinic acid.
cac·o·geu·sia (kak - ō - goo'sē - ă). Cacogeusia; gosto desagradável devido a uma substância de sabor ruim, epilepsia uncinada ou alucinação. VER TAMBÉM dysgeusia. [caco- + G. *geusis*, sabor]
cac·o·me·lia (kak - ō - mē'lē - ă). Cacomelia; deformidade congênita de um ou mais membros. [caco- + G. *melos*, membro]
cac·o·plas·tic (kak - ō - plas'tik). Cacoplástico. **1.** Relativo a, ou que causa, crescimento anormal. **2.** Incapaz de formação normal ou perfeita. [caco- + G. *plastikos*, formado]
ca·cos·mia (kă - koz'mē - ă). Cacosmia; percepção de um mau cheiro devido a uma substância de odor desagradável, epilepsia uncinada ou alucinação. VER dysosmia. [G. *kakosmia*, mau cheiro, de *kakos*, mau, + *osmē*, o sentido do olfato]
cac·ti·no·my·cin (kak'ti - nō - mī'sin). Cactinomicina; actinomicina C; produzida pelo *Streptomyces chrysomallus*. Uma mistura de actinomicinas C_1 (dactinomicina), C_2 e C_3 usada como agente imunossupressor, antineoplásico. VER TAMBÉM actinomycin. SIN actinomycin C.
cac·u·men, pl. **cac·u·mi·na** (kak - ū'men, - mi - nă). Cacume, cacúmen; o topo ou ápice de uma planta ou uma estrutura anatômica. [L. cume]
cac·u·mi·nal (kak - ū'mi - nal). Cacumial; relativo ao topo ou ápice, particularmente de uma planta ou estrutura anatômica.
ca·dav·er (kă - dav'er). Cadáver; corpo morto. SIN corpse. [L. de *cado*, cair]
ca·dav·er·ic (kă - dav'er - ik). Cadavérico; relativo a um corpo morto.
ca·dav·er·ine (kă - dav'er - in). Cadaverina; 1,5-pentanodiamina; 1,5-diaminopentano; uma diamina de odor fétido formada por descarboxilação bacteriana da lisina; venenosa e irritante para a pele; encontrada na carne e no peixe em decomposição.
ca·dav·er·ous (kă - dav'er - ŭs). Cadavérico; que possui a palidez e o aspecto semelhantes aos de um cadáver.
cade oil (kād). Óleo de cade. SIN juniper tar.
cad·her·in (kad - hēr' - in). Caderina; qualquer uma de uma classe de glicoproteínas que fazem parte integral da membrana, que participa na adesão entre células e é importante na morfogênese e diferenciação; a c. E também é conhecida como uvomorulina e é concentrada no desmossoma nas células epiteliais; a c. N é encontrada nas células nervosas, musculares e do cristalino e ajuda a manter a integridade dos agregados neuronais; a c. P é expressa nas células placentárias e epidérmicas. [cell + adhere + -in]
cad·mi·um (Cd) (kad'mē - ŭm). Cádmio; elemento metálico, n.º atômico 48, peso atômico 112,411; seus sais são venenosos e pouco usados em medicina. Vários compostos do cádmio são usados comercialmente nas áreas de metalurgia, fotografia, eletroquímica, etc.; alguns foram usados como ascaricidas, anti-sépticos e fungicidas. [L. *cadmia*, do G. *kadmeia* ou *kadmia*, minério de zinco, calamina]
ca·du·ca (kă - doo'kă). Caduca; decídua. SIN deciduous membrane. [L. fem. de *caducus*, caído, caindo]

⬯ Formas Combinantes	★ Termo oficial alternativo para a *Terminologia Anatomica*
🔳 Indica que o termo é ilustrado, ver Índice de Ilustrações	[MIM] Mendelian Inheritance in Man
SIN Sinônimo	I.C. Índice de Corantes
Cf. Comparar, confrontar	
[NA] *Nomina Anatomica*	**Termo de Alta Importância**
[TA] *Terminologia Anatomica*	

ca·du·ce·us (kă-doo′sē-ŭs). Caduceu; bastão com duas serpentes enroladas em sentido oposto e encimado por duas asas; emblema do Corpo Médico do Exército dos Estados Unidos. Na medicina veterinária, a serpente dupla foi alterada em 1972 para a sua forma atual com apenas uma serpente. VER TAMBÉM staff of Aesculapius [L. o bastão de Mercúrio; G. *kēryx* mensageiro, o bastão de Hermes]

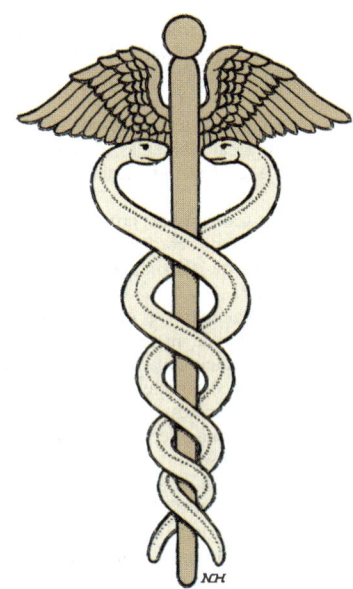

caduceu

cae-. No caso de palavras começando desse modo, ver em ce-.
caecum. Ceco. SIN cecum.
caf·fe·a·rine (kaf′e-ă-rin). Cafearina. SIN trigonelline.
caf·feine (kaf′ēn). Cafeína; alcalóide obtido das folhas secas de *Thea sinensis*, chá, ou das sementes dessecadas de *Coffea arabica*, café; usada como estimulante do sistema nervoso central, diurético, estimulante circulatório e respiratório, e como auxiliar no tratamento das cefaléias. SIN guaranine, thein.
  c. citrate, citrato de c.; c. citratada; uma mistura de partes iguais de c. e ácido cítrico; mais hidrossolúvel que a cafeína.
  c. hydrate, hidrato de c.; monoidrato de c., um estimulante do sistema nervoso central.
  c. and sodium salicylate, c. e salicilato de sódio; uma mistura de salicilato de sódio e c. usada antigamente para alívio de cefaléia e neuralgia.
caf·fein·ism (kaf′ēn-izm). Cafeinismo; intoxicação por cafeína caracterizada por agitação, tremor, nervosismo, excitação, insônia, rubor facial, diurese e queixas gastrointestinais, produzida pela ingestão de excesso de substâncias contendo cafeína.
Caffey, John Patrick, médico radiologista e pediatra norte-americano, "o pai da radiologia pediátrica", 1895–1978. VER C. *disease*, *syndrome*; C.-Kempe *syndrome*; C.-Silverman *syndrome*.
cage (kāj). Gaiola, caixa **1.** Recinto fechado composto, parcial ou completamente, de aberturas e comumente usado para abrigar animais. **2.** Uma estrutura semelhante a esse recinto. [I.M., do Fr. Ant., do L. *cavea*, cavidade, estábulo]
  thoracic c. [TA], caixa torácica; o esqueleto do tórax que consiste nas vértebras torácicas, costelas, cartilagens costais e esterno. SIN cavea thoracis [TA], compages thoracis.
Cajal (Ramón y Cajal), Santiago, histologista espanhol e Prêmio Nobel em 1906, 1852–1934. VER C. *cell*; horizontal *cell* of C.; C. astrocyte *stain*; intersticial *nucleus* of C.
caj·e·put oil, caj·u·put oil (kaj′ĕ-pŭt, -ū-pŭt). Óleo de cajepute; óleo volátil destilado das folhas frescas do *Cajuputi viridiflora*, uma árvore da Ásia tropical e da Austrália; um estimulante, contra-irritante e expectorante.
caj·e·put·ol, caj·u·put·ol (kaj′ĕ-pū-tol, -ŭ-pū-tol). Cajeputol; eucaliptol. SIN cineole.
Cal Abreviatura de large *calorie* (grande caloria, quilocaloria).
cal Abreviatura de small *calorie* (pequena caloria, caloria).
Cal·a·bar bean (kal′ă-bar bēn). Fava-de-calabar. SIN physostigma.
cal·a·mine (kal′ă-mīn). Calamina; óxido de zinco com pequena quantidade de óxido férrico ou carbonato de zinco básico corado adequadamente com óxido férrico, usado em talcos, loções e pomadas, como adstringente leve e agente protetor para distúrbios cutâneos. [L. Mediev. *calamina*, do L. *cadmia*, do G. *kadmia*, Theban (terra), de *Kadmos*, fundador de Tebas]

cal·a·mus (kal′ă-mŭs). Cálamo. **1.** O rizoma seco e descascado de *Acorus calamus* (família Araceae), cultivado em Burma e no Sri Lanka (antigo Ceilão), antifisético e anti-helmíntico. **2.** Estrutura em forma de caniço. [L. caniço, caneta]
  c. scripto'rius, ventrículo de Arantius; parte inferior da fossa rombóide; a extremidade inferior estreita do quarto ventrículo entre os tubérculos grácil. SIN Arantius ventricle. [L. pena de escrever]
cal·ca·ne·al, cal·ca·ne·an (kal-kā′nē-al, kal-kā′nē-an). Calcâneo; relativo ao calcâneo, ou osso do calcanhar.
calcaneo-. O calcâneo. [L. *calcaneum*, calcanhar]
cal·ca·ne·o·a·poph·y·si·tis (kal-kā′nē-ō-ă-pof-i-sī′tis). Calcaneoapofisite; inflamação na parte posterior do calcâneo, na inserção do tendão de Aquiles.
cal·ca·ne·o·as·trag·a·loid (kal-kā′nē-ō-as-trag′ă-loyd). Talocalcâneo; relativo ao calcâneo e ao tálus.
cal·ca·ne·o·cav·us (kal-kā′nē-ō-kā′vus). Calcaneocavo; combinação de talipe calcâneo e talipe cavo.
cal·ca·ne·o·cu·boid (kal-kā′nē-ō-kū′boyd). Calcaneocubóide; relativo ao calcâneo e ao osso cubóide.
cal·can·e·o·dyn·ia (kal-kā′nē-ō-din′ē-ă). Calcaneodinia. SIN painful *heel*. [calcaneo- + G. *odynē*, dor]
cal·ca·ne·o·na·vic·u·lar (kal-kā′nē-ō-na-vik′ū-lăr). Calcaneonavicular; relativo ao calcâneo e ao osso navicular. SIN calcaneoscaphoid.
cal·ca·ne·o·scaph·oid (kal-kā′nē-ō-skaf′oyd). Calcaneoescafóide. SIN calcaneonavicular.
cal·ca·ne·o·tib·i·al (kal-kā′nē-ō-tib′ē-ăl). Calcaneotibial; relativo ao calcâneo e à tíbia.
cal·ca·ne·o·val·go·cav·us (kal-kā′nē-ō-val′-go-kā′vus). Calcaneovalgocavo; combinação de talipe calcâneo, vago e cavo.
cal·ca·ne·o·val·gus (kal-kā′nē-ō-val′gus). Calcaneovalgo. VER *talipes* calcaneovalgus.
cal·ca·ne·o·var·us (kal-kā′nē-ō-vā′rus). Calcaneovaro. VER *talipes* calcaneovarus.
cal·ca·ne·um (kal-kā′nē-ŭm). Calcâneo. SIN calcaneus (1). [L. o calcanhar]
cal·ca·ne·us, gen. e pl. **cal·ca·nei** (kal-kā′nē-ŭs, -kā′nē-ī). **1.** [TA]. Calcâneo; o maior dos ossos tarsais; forma o calcanhar e articula-se com o cubóide, anteriormente, e o tálus, acima. SIN calcaneal bone, calcaneum, heel bone, os calcis. **2.** Talipe. SIN *talipes* calcaneus. [L. o calcanhar (outra forma de *calcaneum*)]
cal·car (kal′kar) [TA]. Esporão. **1.** Uma pequena projeção de qualquer estrutura; esporões internos (septos) ao nível de divisão das artérias e confluências das veias quando as ramificações ou raízes formam um ângulo agudo. VER TAMBÉM vascular *spur*. **2.** Uma espinha obtusa ou projeção de um osso. SIN spur [TA]. [L. esporão, espora de galo]
  c. a'vis [TA], calcar avis. SIN calcarine *spur*.
  c. femora'le, esporão femoral; esporão ósseo originado na face inferior do colo do fêmur acima e anterior ao trocanter menor, aumentando a resistência desta parte do osso. SIN Bigelow septum.
  c. pedis, esporão do calcanhar. SIN calx (2).
  c. sclerae [TA], esporão da esclera. SIN scleral *spur*.
cal·car·e·ous (kal-kā′rē-ŭs). Calcário; relativo a, ou que contém, cal ou cálcio, ou material calcificado. [L. *calcarius*, relativo à cal; de *calx*, cal]
cal·ca·rine (kal′kă′-rēn). Calcarino. **1.** Relativo a um esporão. **2.** Em forma de esporão.
cal·car·i·u·ria (kal-kar-ē-ū′rē-ă). Calcariúria; excreção de sais de cálcio (cal) na urina. [L. *calcarius*, de cal, + G. *ouron*, urina]
cal·cer·gy (kal′ser-jē). Calcergia; calcificação local de tecidos moles que ocorre no local da injeção de determinadas substâncias químicas, como acetato de chumbo ou cloreto de cério; depósitos de hidroxiapatita são encontrados nas áreas calcificadas. [L. *calx*, giz, cálcio, + G. *ergon*, trabalho, produção]
cal·ces (kal′sēz). Plural de calx.
cal·cic (kal′sik). Cálcico; relativo à cal.
cal·ci·co·sis (kal-si-kō′sis). Calcicose; pneumoconiose causada pela inalação de pó de calcário.
cal·ci·di·ol (kal-sĭ-dī′ol). Calcidiol; 25-hidroxicolecalciferol (um 3,25-diol); a primeira etapa na conversão biológica de vitamina D_3 na forma mais ativa, calcitriol; é mais potente que a vitamina D_3. SIN 25-hydroxycholecalciferol, calcifediol.
  c. 1α-hydroxylase, 25-hydroxycholecalciferol 1α-hydroxylase, calcidiol 1α-hidroxilase, 25-hidroxicolecalciferol 1α-hidroxilase; a monooxigenase que forma calcitriol a partir do calcidiol utilizando O_2 e NADPH; uma deficiência dessa enzima pode resultar em características de uma deficiência de vitamina D.
cal·ci·fe·di·ol (kal-sĭ-fē-dī′ol). Calcifediol. SIN calcidiol.
cal·cif·er·ol (kal-sif′er-ol). Calciferol. SIN ergocalciferol.
cal·cif·er·ous (kal-sif′er-ŭs). Calcífero. **1.** Que contém cal. **2.** Que produz qualquer um dos sais de cálcio. SIN calcophorous.
cal·cif·ic (kal-sif′ik). Que forma ou deposita sais de cálcio.

cal·ci·fi·ca·tion (kal′si-fi-kā′shŭn). Calcificação. **1.** Deposição de cal ou de outros sais de cálcio insolúveis. **2.** Um processo no qual o tecido ou material acelular no corpo endurece em virtude de precipitados ou depósitos maiores de sais insolúveis de cálcio (e também magnésio), principalmente carbonato e fosfato de cálcio (hidroxiapatita) normalmente ocorrendo apenas na formação de ossos e dentes. SIN calcareous infiltration. [L. *calx*, cal, + *facio*, fazer]

dystrophic c., c. distrófica; c. que ocorre em tecido degenerado ou necrótico, como em cicatrizes hialinizadas, focos degenerados em leiomiomas e nódulos caseosos.

eggshell c., c. em casca de ovo; uma fina camada de c. ao redor de um linfonodo intratorácico, geralmente na silicose, observada em uma radiografia de tórax.

metastatic c., c. metastática; c. que ocorre em tecido viável, não-ósseo (isto é, tecido não-degenerado nem necrótico), como no estômago, pulmões e rins (e raramente em outros locais); as células desses órgãos secretam materiais ácidos, e, em determinadas condições, em casos de hipercalcemia, a alteração do pH causa precipitação de sais de cálcio nesses locais.

Mönckeberg c., c. de Mönckeberg. SIN Mönckeberg *arteriosclerosis.*

Mönckeberg medial c., c. medial de Mönckeberg. SIN Mönckeberg *arteriosclerosis.*

pathologic c., c. anormal; c. que ocorre em vias excretoras ou secretoras como cálculos, e em outros tecidos além dos ossos e dentes.

pulp c., c. da polpa. SIN endolith.

cal·ci·fy (kal′si-fī). Calcificar; depositar sais de cálcio, como na formação de osso.

cal·cig·er·ous (kal-sij′er-us). Calcígero; que produz ou transporta sais de cálcio. [calcium + L. *gero*, carregar]

cal·ci·na·tion (kal-si-nā′shŭn). Calcinação; o processo de calcinar.

cal·cine (kal′sēn). Calcinar; expelir água e material volátil pelo calor.

cal·ci·neu·rin (kal-sē-noor′in). Calcineurina; uma serina-treonina fosfatase cálcio-dependente envolvida na transcrição de sinais das células T; a cascata de reação na qual se situa é denominada via da calcineurina. [calcium + G. *neuron*, nervo, + -in]

cal·ci·no·sis (kal-si-nō′sis). Calcinose; distúrbio caracterizado pela deposição de sais de cálcio em focos nodulares em vários tecidos além das vísceras com parênquima; as duas formas bem conhecidas, c. circunscrita e c. universal, não estão associadas a lesão tecidual nem a doença metabólica demonstrável; outras formas resultam do metabolismo anormal de cálcio e/ou fósforo. VER metastatic *calcification*. [calcium + -*osis*, condição]

c. circumscrip′ta, c. circunscrita; depósitos localizados de sais de cálcio na pele e nos tecidos subcutâneos, geralmente circundados por uma zona de inflamação granulomatosa; clinicamente, as lesões se assemelham aos tofos da gota.

c. cu′tis, c. cutânea; um depósito de cálcio na pele; geralmente secundário a uma dermatose inflamatória, degenerativa ou neoplásica preexistente, sendo observada freqüentemente na esclerodermia. VER metastatic *calcification*. SIN dystrophic c.

dystrophic c., c. distrófica. SIN c. cutis.

c. intervertebra′lis, c. intervertebral; depósito de cálcio no disco intervertebral.

reversible c., c. reversível; uma forma de c. que pode ser revertida, como se observa em pacientes que ingerem constantemente grandes quantidades de leite e medicamentos alcalinos, como no tratamento da úlcera péptica. VER TAMBÉM milk-alkali *syndrome*.

tumoral c., c. tumoral; **(1)** calcificação de colágeno, principalmente no local de grandes articulações, em negros sul-africanos; provavelmente genética. **(2)** c. que se desenvolve associada a distúrbios neoplásicos.

c. universa′lis, c. universal; depósitos difusos de sais de cálcio na pele e nos tecidos subcutâneos, tecido conjuntivo e outros locais; pode estar associada à dermatomiosite, é mais freqüente em jovens e muitas vezes é fatal; os níveis séricos de cálcio e fósforo geralmente estão dentro dos limites normais.

cal·ci·o·ki·ne·sis (kal′sē-ō-ki-nē′sis). Calciocinesia; mobilização do cálcio armazenado. [calcium + G. *kinēsis*, movimento]

cal·ci·o·ki·net·ic (kal′sē-ō-ki-net′ik). Calciocinético; relativo a, ou que causa, calciocinesia.

cal·ci·ol (kal′sē-ol). Calciol. SIN cholecalciferol.

cal·ci·or·rha·chia (kal′sē-ō-ra′kē-ă). Calciorraquia; a presença de cálcio no líquido cefalorraquidiano. [calcium + G. *rhachis*, coluna vertebral + -ia]

cal·ci·o·stat (kal′sē-ō-stat). Calciostato; termo raramente empregado para designar um suposto mecanismo pelo qual a produção de paratormônio (PTH) está aumentada quando o cálcio sérico está baixo, e diminuída quando ele está elevado. [calcium + G. *statos*, situação]

cal·ci·o·trau·mat·ic (kal′sē-ō-traw-mat′ik). Calciotraumático; relativo à linha de calcificação alterada que aparece na dentina dos dentes incisivos de ratos jovens submetidos a uma dieta raquitogênica: rica em cálcio e pobre em fósforo, sem vitamina D.

cal·ci·pec·tic (kal-si-pek′tik). Calcipéctico; relativo à calcipexia.

cal·ci·pe·nia (kal-si-pē′nē-ă). Calcipenia; condição na qual há uma quantidade insuficiente de cálcio nos tecidos e líquidos do corpo. [calcium + G. *penia*, pobreza]

cal·ci·pe·nic (kal-si-pē′nik). Calcipênico; relativo à calcipenia.

cal·ci·pex·ic (kal-si-pek′sik). Calcipéxico; relativo ou pertinente à calcipexia.

cal·ci·pex·is, cal·ci·pexy (kal-si-pek′sis, kal′si-pek-sē). Calcipexia; fixação de cálcio nos tecidos, causa eventual de tetania em lactentes. [calcium + G. *pēxis*, fixação]

cal·ci·phil·ia (cal-si-fil′ē-ă). Calcifilia; condição na qual os tecidos apresentam uma afinidade incomum por, e fixação de, sais de cálcio circulando no sangue. [calcium + G. *phileō*, amar]

cal·ci·phy·lax·is (kal′si-fī-lak′sis). Calcifilaxia; condição de hipersensibilidade sistêmica induzida na qual os tecidos respondem a agentes incitantes apropriados com calcificação local súbita mas, algumas vezes, efêmera.

cal·ci·priv·ia (kal-si-priv′ē-ă). Calciprivia; ausência ou privação de cálcio na dieta.

cal·ci·priv·ic (kal-si-priv′ik). Calciprívico; privado de cálcio.

cal·cite (kal′sīt). Calcita; mineral de ocorrência natural encontrado em várias formas, como, p. ex., giz, espato-de-islândia, calcário, mármore. VER TAMBÉM *calcium* carbonate. SIN calcspar.

cal·ci·tet·rol (kal-si-tet′rol). Calcitetrol; o 1,24,25-triol (daí, um 1,3,24,24-tetrol) de colecalciferol; o produto da inativação do calcitriol.

cal·ci·to·nin (kal-si-tō′nin). Calcitonina; um hormônio peptídico, do qual se conhecem oito formas em cinco espécies; composto de 32 aminoácidos e produzido pelas glândulas paratireóides, tireóide e timo; sua ação é oposta à do paratormônio porque a c. aumenta a deposição de cálcio e fosfato no osso e reduz o nível sanguíneo de cálcio; seu nível sanguíneo é aumentado pelo glucagon e pelo Ca^{2+} e, assim, opõe-se à hipercalcemia pós-prandial. SIN thyrocalcitonin. [calci- + G. *tonos*, tensão, + -in]

cal·ci·tri·ol (kal-si-trī′ol). Calcitriol; 1α,25-diidroxicolecalciferol (daí, um 1,3,25-triol); a formação de c. é a segunda etapa na conversão biológica da vitamina D_3 a sua forma ativa; é mais potente que o calcidiol.

CALCIUM

cal·ci·um (Ca), gen. **cal·′cii** (kal′sē-ŭm, -sē-ī). Cálcio; elemento metálico bivalente; n.º atômico 20, peso atômico 40,078, densidade 1,55, ponto de fusão 842°C. O óxido de c. é terra alcalina, CaO, cal, que, com a adição de água, se torna hidrato de c., $Ca(OH)_2$, cal extinta. Alguns sais de c. orgânicos, não apresentados a seguir, aparecem sob o nome da parte ácida orgânica. Muitos sais de c. têm empregos fundamentais no metabolismo e na medicina. Os sais de c. são responsáveis pela radiopacidade do osso, cartilagem calcificada e placas arterioscleróticas nas artérias. [L. Mod. do L. *calx*, cal]

c. alginate, alginato de cálcio; hemostático tópico.

c. aminosalicylate, aminossalicilato de cálcio; sal cálcico do ácido *p*-aminossalicílico, com os mesmos empregos.

c. benzoylpas, benzamidossalicilato de cálcio; agente antituberculoso.

c. bromide, brometo de cálcio; usado para atender às mesmas indicações que o brometo de potássio.

c. carbide, carbonato de cálcio; argila negra cristalina que, quando em contato com a água, produz gás acetileno.

c. carbimide, carbimida de cálcio; fertilizante e exterminador de ervas daninhas que também possui atividade antitireóidea; como o dissulfiram, compromete o metabolismo do etanol; os trabalhadores de fábricas produtoras de cianamida exibem sintomas sistêmicos ("doença da manhã de segunda-feira") após a ingestão de álcool. SIN c. cyanamide.

c. carbonate, carbonato de cálcio; adstringente, antiácido e suplemento alimentar de cálcio. VER TAMBÉM calcite. SIN chalk, creta.

c. caseinate, caseinato de cálcio; forma de caseína presente no leite de vaca; usado em preparações dietéticas; tem sido usado para tratamento de diarréia em lactentes.

c. chloride, cloreto de cálcio; usado para corrigir deficiências de cálcio e no tratamento da intoxicação por magnésio e da insuficiência cardíaca.

citrated c. carbimide, carbimida de cálcio citratada; uma mistura de 2 partes de ácido cítrico e 1 parte de carbimida de cálcio; no metabolismo do etanol, torna mais lenta a conversão de acetaldeído em acetato, usada no tratamento do alcoolismo.

crude c. sulfide, sulfeto de cálcio em estado natural; usado externamente no tratamento da acne, escabiose e tinha. SIN sulfurated lime.

c. cyanamide, cianamida de cálcio. SIN c. carbimide.

dibasic c. phosphate, fosfato dibásico de cálcio; usado como suplemento dietético de cálcio e fósforo. SIN c. monohydrogen phosphate, secondary c. phosphate.

c. folinate, folinato de cálcio. SIN *leucovorin* calcium.

c. glubionate, glubionato de cálcio; reabastecedor de cálcio.
c. gluceptate, gliceptato de cálcio; usado como nutriente. SIN c. glucoheptonate.
c. glucoheptonate, glicoeptonato de cálcio. SIN c. gluceptate.
c. gluconate, gluconato de cálcio; um sal de c. com sabor mais agradável que o cloreto de c., algumas vezes usado como suplemento de cálcio.
c. glycerophosphate, glicerofosfato de cálcio; um suplemento alimentar de cálcio e fósforo.
c. hippurate, hipurato de cálcio; considerado solvente de areias e cálculos de urato.
c. hydroxide, hidróxido de cálcio; usado como absorvente de dióxido de carbono.
c. hypophosphite, hipofosfito de cálcio; tem sido usado para tratamento do raquitismo e de distúrbios da nutrição.
c. iodate, iodato de cálcio; usado como talco e, em loções e pomadas, como anti-séptico e desodorante.
c. iodobehenate, iodobeenato de cálcio; um sal de cálcio $(C_{21}H_{42}ICOO)_2Ca$, anteriormente usado para atender às indicações dos iodetos comuns.
c. ipodate, ipodato de cálcio; meio radiopaco usado em colangiografia e colecistografia.
c. lactate, lactato de cálcio; usado como reabastecedor de cálcio.
c. lactophosphate, lactofosfato de cálcio; mistura de lactato de cálcio, lactato ácido de cálcio e fosfato ácido de cálcio; usado como suplemento alimentar de cálcio e fósforo.
c. leucovorin, leucovorina cálcica. VER *leucovorin* calcium.
c. levulinate, levulinato de cálcio; um sal de cálcio hidratado do ácido levulínico; possui os efeitos habituais do cálcio administrado por via oral ou intravenosa.
c. mandelate, mandelato de cálcio; sal cálcico do ácido mandélico; agente antiinfeccioso urinário.
milk of c., leite de cálcio; líquido densamente calcificado, encontrado radiograficamente mais amiúde na vesícula biliar em associação a obstrução crônica.
c. monohydrogen phosphate, fosfato monoidrogenado de cálcio. SIN dibasic c. phosphate.
c. oxalate, oxalato de cálcio; encontrado como sedimento na urina e em cálculos urinários. Produto final tóxico do consumo de etilenoglicol.
c. oxide, óxido de cálcio. SIN lime (1).
c. pantothenate, pantotenato de cálcio; o sal cálcico do ácido pantotênico; um fator filtrado da vitamina B.
precipitated c. carbonate, carbonato de cálcio precipitado; usado como antiácido no tratamento de úlceras pépticas e outros distúrbios de hiperacidez gástrica.
c. propionate, propionato de cálcio; o sal cálcico do ácido propiônico; um agente antifúngico.
racemic c. pantothenate, pantotenato de cálcio racêmico; uma mistura dos sais de cálcio dos isômeros dextrorrotatórios e levorrotatórios do ácido pantotênico, tem os mesmos empregos que o pantotenato de cálcio.
c. saccharate, sacarato de cálcio; usado como antiácido na dispepsia e flatulência, como antídoto no envenenamento por ácido carbólico e como estabilizador na solução de gluconato de cálcio para administração parenteral.
secondary c. phosphate, fosfato secundário de cálcio. SIN dibasic c. phosphate.
c. stearate, estearato de cálcio; sabão usado no preparo de comprimidos como lubrificante para a máquina de comprimidos e para manter o fluxo das misturas de pó.
c. sulfate, sulfato de cálcio; CaO_4S; usado na forma dessecada para fazer gesso. VER TAMBÉM gypsum.
c. sulfite, sulfito de cálcio; usado como anti-séptico intestinal e, localmente, no tratamento de doenças cutâneas parasitárias.
tertiary c. phosphate, fosfato terciário de cálcio. SIN tribasic c. phosphate.
tribasic c. phosphate, fosfato tribásico de cálcio; usado como antiácido. SIN bone ash, bone phosphate, tertiary c. phosphate, tricalcium phosphate, whitlockite.
c. trisodium pentetate, pentetato trissódico de cálcio. SIN pentetate trisodium calcium.

cal·ci·um-45 (^{45}Ca). Cálcio-45 (Ca^{45}); isótopo do cálcio-45 radioativo mais facilmente disponível; beta-emissor com meia-vida de 162,7 dias; usado como marcador.
cal·ci·um-47 (^{47}Ca). Cálcio-47 (Ca^{47}); radioisótopo do cálcio com meia-vida de 4,54 dias, usado no diagnóstico de distúrbios do metabolismo do cálcio.
cal·ci·um group. Grupo do cálcio; os metais das terras alcalinas: berílio, magnésio, cálcio, estrôncio, bário e rádio.
cal·ci·u·ria (kal-sē-ū′rē-ā). Calciúria; a excreção urinária de cálcio; usada algumas vezes como sinônimo de hipercalciúria.
cal·coph·or·ous (kal-kof′er-ŭs). Calcóforo. SIN calciferous. [L. *calx*, cal, + G. *phoros*, que produz]
cal·co·sphe·rite (kal-ko-sfēr′īt). Calcosferita; um corpo pequeno, esferóide, concentricamente laminado contendo depósitos acretivos de sais de cálcio; encontrado mais freqüentemente no carcinoma papilar da tireóide e do ovário, e no meningioma, provavelmente em virtude de alterações degenerativas no estroma fibrovascular. SIN psammoma bodies (3). [L. *calx*, cal, + G. *sphaira*, esfera]

calc·spar (kalk′spar) Calcita. SIN calcite.
cal·cu·li (kal′kū-lī). Cálculos; plural de calculus.
cal·cu·lo·sis (kal-kū-lō′sis). Calculose; a tendência ou predisposição para formar cálculos. [L. *calculus*, pequena pedra, + G. *-osis*, condição]
cal·cu·lus, gen. e pl. **cal·cu·li** (kăl′kū-lŭs, -lī). Cálculo; uma concreção formada em qualquer parte do corpo, mais comumente nas vias biliares e urinárias, geralmente composta de sais de ácidos inorgânicos ou orgânicos, ou de outra substância, como o colesterol. SIN stone (1). [L. uma pedra, um cálculo]
apatite c., c. de apatita; um c. no qual o componente cristalóide consiste em fluorofosfato de cálcio.
arthritic c., c. artrítico. SIN gouty *tophus.*
biliary c., c. biliar. SIN gallstone.
bladder c., c. vesical. SIN bladder *stone,* em *stone.*
blood c., c. sanguíneo; um angiolito ou concreção de sangue coagulado. SIN hemic c.
branched c., c. coraliforme. SIN staghorn c.
bronchial c., c. brônquico. SIN broncholith.
cerebral c., c. cerebral. SIN encephalolith.
coral c., c. coraliforme. SIN staghorn c.
cystine c., c. de cistina; um c. composto de cistina, substância mole e levemente radiopaca.
dendritic c., c. dendrítico. SIN staghorn c.
dental c., (1) Odontólito; depósitos ou concreções calcificadas formadas ao redor dos dentes; pode aparecer como concreção subgengival ou supragengival; (2) tártato SIN tartar (2).
encysted c., c. encistado; um c. urinário encerrado em um saco desenvolvido a partir da parede da bexiga. SIN pocketed c.
fibrin c., c. de fibrina; c. urinário formado principalmente por fibrinogênio no sangue.
gastric c., c. gástrico. SIN gastrolith.
hematogenetic c., c. hematogênico. SIN serumal c. (1).
hemic c., c. hêmico. SIN blood c.
infection c., c. associado a infecção. SIN secondary renal c.
intestinal c., c. intestinal; concreção intestinal, seja um coprólito ou enterólito.
lacrimal c., c. lacrimal. SIN dacryolith.
mammary c., c. mamário; uma concreção em um dos ductos mamários.
matrix c., c. de matriz; um c. urinário branco-amarelado ou castanho-claro contendo sais de cálcio, com a consistência de massa de vidraceiro; composto principalmente de uma matriz orgânica que consiste em uma mucoproteína e um mucopolissacarídio sulfatado, e geralmente está associado a infecção crônica.
metabolic c., c. metabólico; um cálculo, geralmente renal, causado por uma anormalidade metabólica que resulta em aumento da excreção de uma substância de baixa solubilidade na urina, como urato ou cistina.
mulberry c., c. em amora; c. urinário nodular e duro composto de oxalato de cálcio, assim denominado devido à sua semelhança com uma amora.
nasal c., c. nasal. SIN rhinolith.
oxalate c., c. de oxalato; um c. urinário duro de oxalato de cálcio; alguns são cobertos por minúsculos espinhos afiados que conseguem causar abrasões no epitélio pélvico renal, enquanto outros são lisos.
pancreatic c., c. pancreático; concreção, geralmente múltipla, no ducto pancreático, associada à pancreatite crônica. SIN pancreatolith, pancreolith.
pharyngeal c., c. faríngeo. SIN pharyngolith.
pleural c., c. pleural. SIN pleurolith.
pocketed c., c. encistado. SIN encysted c.
preputial c., c. prepucial; c. que ocorre sob o prepúcio. SIN postholith.
primary renal c., c. renal primário; c. formado em um trato urinário aparentemente saudável, geralmente composto de oxalatos, uratos ou cistina.
prostatic c., c. prostático; concreção formada na próstata, composta principalmente de carbonato e fosfato de cálcio (corpos amiláceos). SIN prostatolith.
pulp c., c. da polpa. SIN endolith.
renal c., c. renal; c. que ocorre no sistema coletor renal. SIN nephrolith.
salivary c., c. salivar; c. em um ducto ou glândula salivar.
secondary renal c., c. renal secundário; c. associado a infecção e/ou obstrução, geralmente composto de estruvita (fosfato de amônio-magnésio). SIN infection c.
serumal c., (1) depósito calcáreo esverdeado ou castanho-escuro no dente, geralmente apical à margem gengival. SIN hematogenetic c. (2) subgengival SIN subgingival c.
staghorn c., c. coraliforme; c. observado na pelve renal, com ramos que se estendem até os infundíbulos e cálices. SIN branched c., coral c., dendritic c.
struvite c., c. de estruvita; c. no qual o componente cristalóide consiste em fosfato de amônio-magnésio; geralmente associado à infecção do trato urinário causada por bactérias produtoras de urease.

subgingival c., c. subgengival; depósito calcáreo encontrado no dente apical à margem gengival. SIN serumal c. (2).
supragingival c., c. supragengival; placas calcificadas aderentes às superfícies dentárias coronais à margem gengival livre.
tonsillar c., c. tonsilar. SIN tonsillolith.
urethral c., c. uretral; cálculo impactado na uretra. Pode ter se formado em local proximal e ficado retido na uretra, ou pode ter se formado na uretra; é incomum.
urinary c., c. urinário; c. no rim, ureter, bexiga ou uretra. SIN urolith.
uterine c., c. uterino; mioma uterino calcificado. SIN uterolith.
vesical c., c. vesical; c. urinário formado ou retido na bexiga. SIN cystolith.
weddellite c., c. de weddellita; c. no qual o componente cristalóide consiste em oxalato diidratado de cálcio.
whewellite c., c. de whewellita; c. no qual o componente cristalóide consiste em oxalato monoidratado de cálcio.
Cal·cu·lus Sur·face In·dex (CSI). Índice Superficial de Cálculo (ISC); índice que mede apenas cálculos (concreções) dentários, usado para avaliar a formação de novos cálculos em um grande grupo de indivíduos examinados.
Caldani, Leopoldo M.A., anatomista italiano, 1725–1813. VER C. *ligament.*
cal·des·mon (kal-des'mon). Caldesmona; proteína de ligação cruzada F-actina que, em níveis de cálcio baixos ou na ausência de cálcio, liga-se à tropomiosina e actina e impede a ligação à miosina. [calcium + G. *desmos*, ligação, de *deō*, ligar]
Caldwell, Eugene W., radiologista norte-americano, 1870–1918. VER C. *projection, view.*
Caldwell, George W., otolaringologista norte-americano, 1834–1918. VER C.-Luc *operation.*
Caldwell, William E., obstetra norte-americano, 1880–1943. VER C.-Moloy *classification.*
cal·e·fa·cient (kal-e-fā'shent). Calefaciente. 1. Que produz calor. 2. Agente que causa sensação de calor na parte em que é aplicado. [L. *calefacio*, de *caleo*, estar quente, + *facio*, fazer]
calf, pl. **calves** (kaf, kavz). Bezerro, macho ou fêmea. [Gael. *kalpa*]. Também pode ser a panturrilha.
calf-bone. 1. Fíbula. SIN fibula. 2. Osso de vitelo usado em reconstrução ortopédica.
cal·i·ber (kal'i-ber). Calibre; diâmetro de uma estrutura tubular oca. [Fr. *calibre*, de etimologia incerta]
cal·i·brate (kal'i-brāt). Calibrar. 1. Graduar ou padronizar qualquer instrumento de medida. 2. Medir o diâmetro de uma estrutura tubular.
cal·i·bra·tion (kal-i-brā'shŭn). Calibragem; calibração; o ato de padronizar ou calibrar um instrumento ou procedimento laboratorial.
cal·i·bra·tor (kal'ĭ-brā-ter, -tōr). Calibrador; material ou substância padrão ou de referência usada para padronizar ou calibrar um instrumento ou procedimento laboratorial.
cal·i·ce·al (kal'i-se'al). Calicial; relativo ao cálice. SIN calyceal.
cal·i·cec·ta·sis (kal-i-sek'ta-sis). Calicectasia; caliectasia. SIN caliectasis. [calix + G. *ektasis*, dilatação]
cal·i·cec·to·my (kal-i-sek'tō-me). Calicectomia; caliectomia. SIN calicotomy. [calix + G. *ektome*, excisão]
ca·li·ces (kal'i-sēz). Cálices; plural de calix.
cal·ic·i·form (kă-lis'i-fōrm). Caliciforme; com o formato de um cálice ou taça. SIN calyciform. [L. *calix* + *forma*, forma]
cal·i·cine (kal'i-sēn). Calicino; da natureza de, ou semelhante a, um cálice. SIN calycine.
Cal·i·ci·vi·ri·dae (kal'i-sē-vī'rā-dē). Família de vírus de RNA de filamento único de sentido positivo, icosaédricos, desnudos, com 30-38 nm de diâmetro, associados à gastroenterite viral epidêmica e a algumas formas de hepatite em seres humanos.
Ca·lic·i·vi·rus (kă-lis'i-vī'rŭs). Gênero da família Caliciviridae que está associado à gastroenterite. VER hepatitis E *virus*, Norwalk *agent*. [G. *kalyx*, cálice, + virus]
ca·li·co·plas·ty (kā'lĭ-so-plas-tē). Calicoplastia; calioplastia. SIN calioplasty. [calix, + G. *plastos*, formado]
cal·i·cot·o·my (kal-ĭ-sot'ō-me). Calicotomia; caliotomia; incisão em um cálice, geralmente para remover um cálculo. SIN calicectomy, caliotomy. [calix + G. *tome*, corte]
ca·lic·u·lus, pl. **ca·lic·u·li** (kă-lik'ū-lŭs, -lī). Calículo; estrutura em forma de broto ou taça, semelhante ao cálice fechado de uma flor. SIN calycle, calyculus. [L. dim. do G. *kalyx*, botão de flor]
 c. gustato'rius, c. gustatório. SIN taste bud.
 c. ophthal'micus, c. oftálmico. SIN optic cup.
ca·li·ec·ta·sis (kā-lē-ek'ta-sis). Caliectasia; dilatação dos cálices, geralmente causada por obstrução ou infecção. SIN calicectasis, pyelocaliectasis.
cal·i·for·ni·um (Cf) (kal-i-fōr'nē-ŭm). Califórnio (CF); elemento transurânico artificial, símbolo Cf, n.º atômico 98, peso atômico 251,08; a meia-vida do Cf[251] (o isótopo mais estável conhecido) é de 900 anos. [*California*, estado e universidade onde foi preparado pela primeira vez]

ca·li·o·plas·ty (kā'lē-ō-plas-tē). Calioplastia; reconstrução cirúrgica de um cálice, geralmente designada para aumentar sua luz no infundíbulo. SIN calicoplasty.
ca·li·or·rha·phy (kā'lē-ōr-a-fē). Caliorrafia. 1. Sutura de um cálice. 2. Cirurgia plástica de um cálice dilatado ou obstruído para melhorar a drenagem urinária, exigindo freqüentemente associação de dois ou mais cálices ou o movimento maciço da mucosa pélvica renal para reconstruir o sistema de drenagem caliceal. [calix, + G. *raphē*, sutura, bainha]
ca·li·ot·o·my (kā-lē-ot'ō-me). Caliotomia. SIN calicotomy.
cal·i·pers (kal'i-perz). Compasso de calibre; instrumento usado para medir diâmetros. [corruptela de *caliber*]
cal·is·then·ics (kal-is-then'iks). Calistenia; prática sistemática de vários exercícios físicos com o objetivo de preservar a saúde e aumentar a força física. [G. *kalos*, belo, + *sthenos*, força]
ca·lix, pl. **ca·li·ces** (kā-liks, kal'i-sēz). Cálice; estrutura em forma de flor ou funil; especificamente um dos ramos ou recessos da pelve renal para o qual se projetam os orifícios das pirâmides renais de Malpighi. SIN calyx. [L. do G. *kalyx*, cálice de uma flor]
 major calices, cálices renais maiores; as subdivisões primárias da pelve renal, geralmente duas ou três. SIN calices renales majores.
 minor calices, cálices renais menores; as subdivisões dos cálices maiores, variando em número de 7 a 13, que recebem as papilas renais. SIN calices renales minores.
 calices rena'les majo'res, cálices renais maiores. SIN major calices.
 calices rena'les mino'res, cálices renais menores. SIN minor calices.
Calkins, Leroy Adelbert, obstetra-ginecologista norte-americano, 1894–1960. VER C. *sign.*
Call, Friedrich von, médico austríaco, 1844–1917. VER C.-Exner *bodies*, em *body*.
Callahan, John R., endodontista norte-americano, 1853–1918. VER C. *method.*
Callander, Latimer, cirurgião de San Francisco, 1892–1947. VER C. *amputation.*
Calleja (Calleja y Sanchez), Camilo, anatomista espanhol, †1913. VER *islands* of C., em *island.*
Cal·liph·o·ra (kă-lif'ō-ra). Gênero de moscas varejeiras (família Calliphoridae, ordem Diptera), varejeira azul, cujas larvas se alimentam da carne de animais mortos. C. *vomitoria* e C. *vicina* são espécies comuns nos Estados Unidos. [G. *kalli*, belo, + *phoros*, portador]
Callison, James S., médico norte-americano, *1873. VER C. *fluid.*
Cal·li·tro·ga (kal-i-trō'ga). Nome antigo da *Cochliomyia.*
cal·lo·sal (ka-lō'sal). Caloso; relativo ao corpo caloso.
cal·lose (kal'ōs). Calose; um 1,3-β-D-glucano linear formado por algumas enzimas a partir da UDP-glicose, diferindo da celulose (um β-1,4-glucano formado a partir da GDP-glicose) e da amilose do amido (um α-1,4-glucano formado a partir da ADP-glicose). Encontrado em determinadas paredes celulares vegetais.
cal·los·i·ty (ka-los'i-tē). Calosidade; espessamento circunscrito da camada de queratina da epiderme devido a fricção repetida ou compressão intermitente. SIN callus (1), keratoma (1), poroma (1). [L. de *callosus*, de pele espessa]
cal·lo·so·mar·gin·al (ka-lō'sō-mar'jin-āl). Calosomarginal; relativo ao corpo caloso e ao giro cingulado; designa o sulco entre eles. VER TAMBÉM *sulcus* of corpus callosum.
cal·lous (kal'ŭs). Caloso; relativo a um calo ou calosidade.
cal·lus (kal'ŭs). 1. Calosidade. SIN callosity. 2. Calo; uma massa composta de tecido que se forma em um local de fratura para estabelecer continuidade entre as extremidades ósseas; é composta inicialmente de tecido fibroso não-calcificado e cartilagem e, finalmente, de osso. [L. pele dura]
 central c., c. central; o c. na cavidade medular de um osso fraturado. SIN medullary c.
 definitive c., c. definitivo; o c. que foi convertido em tecido ósseo. SIN permanent c.
 ensheathing c., c. de embainhamento; a massa de calo ao redor da parte externa do osso fraturado.
 medullary c., c. medular. SIN central c.
 permanent c., c. permanente. SIN definitive c.
 provisional c., c. provisório; o c. que se desenvolve para manter as extremidades do osso fraturado em aposição; é absorvido após a consolidação completa. SIN temporary c.
 temporary c., c. temporário. SIN provisional c.
calm·a·tive (kahl'ma-tiv). Calmante; sedativo; redutor da excitação; indica tal agente.
Calmette, Leon A., bacteriologista francês, 1863–1933. VER bacille C.-Guérin; bacillus C. *vaccine*; C. *test*; C.-Guérin *bacillus, vaccine.*
cal·mod·u·lin (kal-mod'ū-lin). Calmodulina; proteína pequena, eucariótica, onipresente, que se liga aos íons cálcio, tornando-se assim o agente de muitos efeitos celulares antes atribuídos aos íons cálcio. Esse complexo cálcio-proteína liga-se à apoenzima para formar a holoenzima de determinadas fosfodiesterases; através desses ou de outros mecanismos ainda desconhecidos, o complexo regula a adenilato e a guanilato ciclases, muitas cinases, a atividade da fosfolipase A_2 e outras funções celulares básicas. [calcium + *modul*ate]

calo: parte do processo de consolidação da fratura óssea

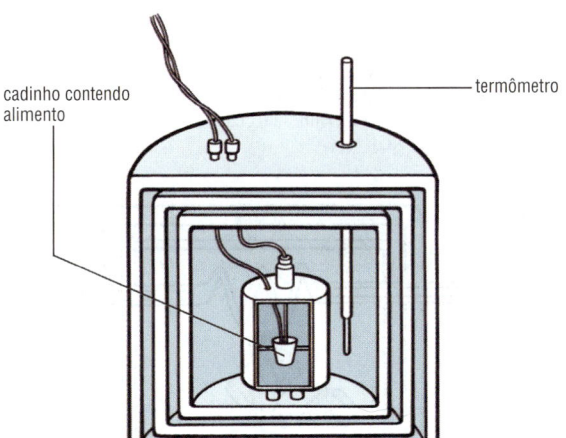

calorímetro de bomba: mede o calor produzido pela combustão completa da amostra de comida

Calodium (ka-lō′dē-oom). Um dos três gêneros de nematódeos relacionados com *Trichuris*, comumente denominado *Capillaria*.

cal·o·mel (kal′ō-mel). Calomelano; cloreto mercuroso; monocloreto, protocloreto ou subcloreto de mercúrio; tem sido usado como anti-séptico intestinal e laxativo; substituído por agentes mais seguros. SIN mercurous chloride, sweet precipitate. [L. Mediev., do G. *kalos*, belo, + *melas*, preto]
  vegetable c., c. vegetal. SIN podophyllum.

ca·lor (kā′lōr). Calor; um dos quatro sinais da inflamação (calor, rubor, tumor, dor) enunciados por Celsus. [L.]

Calori, Luigi, anatomista italiano, 1807–1896. VER C. *bursa*.

ca·lor·ic (ka-lōr′ik). Calórico. 1. Relativo a uma caloria. 2. Relativo a calor. [L. *calor*, calor]
  c. intake, ingestão calórica; o número total de calorias na alimentação diária.

cal·o·rie (kal′ō-rē). Caloria; unidade de conteúdo de calor ou energia. A quantidade de calor necessária para elevar a temperatura de 1 g de água de 14,5° para 15,5° (pequena c.). A caloria está sendo substituída pelo joule, a unidade SI igual a 0,239 caloria. VER TAMBÉM British thermal *unit*. SIN calory. [L. *calor*, calor]
  gram c., c. pequena. SIN small c.
  kilogram c. (kcal), quilocaloria. SIN large c.
  large c. (Cal, C), grande caloria; quilocaloria; a quantidade de energia necessária para elevar a temperatura de 1 kg de água em 1°C (mais precisamente de 14,5°-15,5°C); corresponde a 1.000 vezes o valor da pequena caloria; usada em medidas da produção de calor de reações químicas, incluindo aquelas envolvidas em biologia. SIN kilocalorie, kilogram c.
  mean c., c. média; um centésimo da energia necessária para elevar a temperatura de 1 g de água de 0 para 100°C.
  small c. (cal, c), caloria pequena; a quantidade de energia necessária para elevar a temperatura de 1 g de água em 1°C, ou de 14,5 para 15,5°C no caso de c. normal ou padrão. SIN gram c.

cal·o·rif·ic (cal-ō-rif′ik). Calorífico; que produz calor. [L. *calor*, calor]

ca·lor·i·gen·ic (kā-lōr-i-jen′ik). Calorífero. 1. Capaz de gerar calor. 2. Estimulante da produção metabólica de calor. SIN thermogenetic (2), thermogenic. [L. *calor*, calor, + G. *genesis*, produção]

cal·o·rim·e·ter (kal-ō-rim′ĕ-ter). Calorímetro; aparelho para medir a quantidade de calor liberada em uma reação química. [L. *calor*, calor, + G. *metron*, medida]
  Benedict-Roth c., c. de Benedict-Roth. VER Benedict-Roth *apparatus*.
  bomb c., c. de bomba; instrumento para determinar a energia potencial (valores caloríficos) de substâncias orgânicas, incluindo as contidas em alimentos. Consiste em um recipiente oco de aço, revestido com platina e cheio de oxigênio puro, dentro do qual se coloca uma quantidade pesada da substância e aceso por um dispositivo elétrico; o calor produzido é absorvido pela água que cerca a bomba, pelo aumento da temperatura, as calorias liberadas são calculadas.

cal·o·ri·met·ric (kă′lōr-i-met′rik). Calorimétrico; relativo à calorimetria.

cal·o·rim·e·try (kal-ō-rim′ĕ-trē). Calorimetria; medida da quantidade de calor produzido por uma reação ou um grupo de reações (como por um organismo).

direct c., c. direta; medida do calor produzido por uma reação, distinto dos métodos indiretos, que envolvem a medida de outra coisa que não a própria produção de calor.

indirect c., c. indireta; determinação da produção de calor de uma reação de oxidação através da medida da captação de oxigênio e/ou liberação de dióxido de carbono e excreção de nitrogênio, calculando-se depois a quantidade de calor produzido.

ca·lor·i·tro·pic (kă-lōr′i-trop′ik). Calorítropico; relativo a termotropismo.

cal·o·ry (kal′ō-rē). Caloria. SIN calorie.

Calot, Jean-François, cirurgião francês, 1861–1944. VER Calot *triangle*.

cal·pains (kal′pāns). Calpaínas; tiol proteinases cálcio-dependentes. Enzimas citoplasmáticas encontradas nos mamíferos. [calcium + sufixo *-pain*, protease, de *papain*]

cal·se·ques·trin (kal′sē-kwes′trin). Calseqüestrina; proteína ligadora de cálcio encontrada no retículo sarcoplasmático dos músculos. Libera íons cálcio nos canais de cálcio. [calcium + sequester + -in]

ca·lum·ba (kă-lŭm′bă). Columbo; calumba; a raiz seca da *Jateorrhiza palmata* (família Menispermaceae), uma planta trepadeira alta do leste da África; usada como tônico amargo.

ca·lum·bin (kal′ŭm-bin). Columbina; princípio amargo do columbo, responsável pelo sabor amargo da substância bruta.

cal·u·ster·one (kal-ū′stĕ-rōn). Calusterona; agente antineoplásico.

cal·var·ia, pl. **cal·var·i·ae** (kal-vā′rē-ă, -vā′rē-ē) [TA]. Calvária; calota craniana; a porção superior do crânio, em forma de cúpula. SIN roof of skull, skullcap. [L. um crânio]

cal·var·i·al (kal-vār′ē-ăl). Relativo à calvária.

cal·var·i·um (kal-vār′ē-ŭm). Forma incorreta para calvária.

Calvé, Jacques, cirurgião ortopédico francês, 1875–1954. VER C.-Perthes *disease*; Legg-C.-Perthes *disease*.

cal·vi·ti·es (kal-vish′e-ēz). Calvície. SIN alopecia. [L. de *calvus*, calvo]

calx, gen. **cal·cis,** pl. **cal·ces** (kalks, kal′sis, kal-sēs). 1. Cal. SIN lime (1). [L. limestone] 2. Calcanhar; a extremidade arredondada posterior do pé. SIN heel (2) [TA], calcar pedis. [L. calcanhar]

cal·y·ce·al (kal′i-sē′al). Caliceal. SIN caliceal.

ca·ly·ces (kal′i-sēz). Cálices. Plural de calyx.

ca·lyc·i·form (kă-lis′i-fōrm). Caliciforme. SIN caliciform.

ca·ly·cine (kal′i-sēn). Calicina. SIN calicine.

ca·ly·cle, ca·lyc·u·lus (kal′i-kl, kă-lik′ū-lŭs). Calículo. SIN caliculus.

Ca·lym·ma·to·bac·te·ri·um (kă-lim′mă-tō-bak-tēr′ē-ŭm). Gênero de bactérias imóveis (de classificação taxonômica incerta) contendo bacilos pleomórficos, Gram-negativos, com condensações de cromatina uni ou bipolares; as células são encontradas isoladamente ou em grupos. Fora do corpo humano, crescem apenas no saco vitelino ou no líquido amniótico de um embrião de pinto em desenvolvimento ou em meios de cultura contendo vitelo embrionário; os microrganismos são patogênicos apenas para os seres humanos. A espécie típica é *C. granulomatis*. [G. *kalymma*, capuz, véu, + *baktērion*, bacilo]

C. granulo′matis, uma espécie bacteriana que causa lesões granulomatosas (granuloma inguinal ou granuloma venéreo) (donovanose) em seres humanos, sobretudo na região inguinal; a espécie típica do gênero *C*.

ca·lyx, pl. **ca·ly·ces** (kā′liks, kal′i-sēz). Cálice. SIN calix. [G. cálice de uma flor]

CAM Abreviatura de cell adhesion *molecule* (molécula de adesão celular).

cam·ben·da·zole (kam-ben′dah-zōl). Cambendazol; anti-helmíntico.

cam·bi·um (kam′bē-ŭm). Câmbio; a camada interna do periósteo na ossificação membranosa. [L. *exchange*]

cam·era, pl. **cam·er·ae, cam·er·as** (kam′er-ă, -ē) [TA]. **1.** Câmara. SIN anterior *chamber* of eyeball. **2.** Câmera; caixa fechada; principalmente contendo uma lente, obturador e filmes ou chapas fotográficas fotossensíveis para fotografia. [L. *abóbada*]

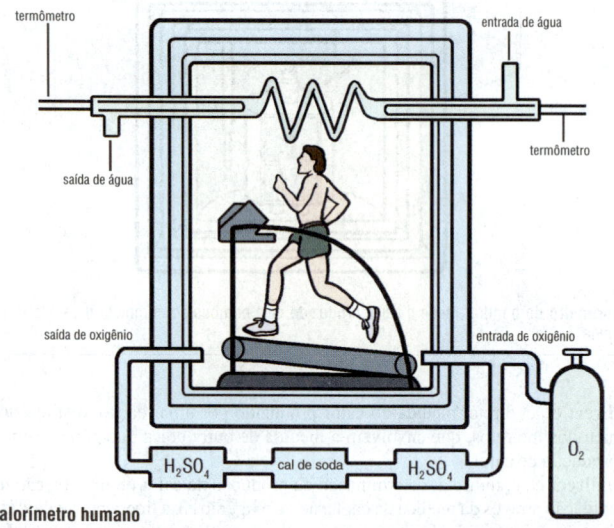

calorímetro humano

Anger c., câmera de Anger; sistema de imagem cintigráfico ou tipo de câmera gama, empregando um único cristal fino e múltiplos circuitos fotodetectores, que observa todo o campo de uma só vez e é mais efetivo na faixa energética de 100 a 511 keV.
c. ante′rior bul′bi [TA], câmara anterior do bulbo. SIN anterior *chamber* of eyeball.
camerae bulbi [TA], câmaras do bulbo. SIN *chambers* of eyeball, em *chamber*.
gamma c., câmera gama; qualquer uma dentre várias câmeras cintigráficas que registram simultaneamente contagens de todo o campo de visão. SIN scintillation c.

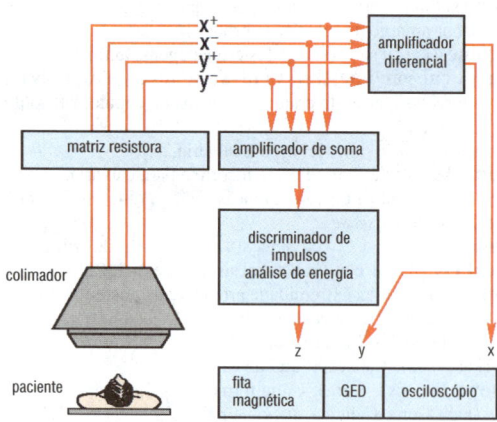

função da câmera gama (câmera de Anger): são representados sinais coordenados de apenas um fotomultiplicador (GDE, gerenciamento de dados eletrônicos)

multiformat c., câmera multiforme; impressora fotográfica ou a laser para registrar número variável de imagens digitais em uma folha de filme, como na tomografia computadorizada ou na ultra-sonografia.
c. oc′uli, ante′rior, câmara anterior do bulbo do olho. SIN anterior *chamber* of eyeball.
c. oc′uli ma′jor, câmara principal do bulbo do olho. SIN anterior *chamber* of eyeball.
c. oc′uli mi′nor, câmara menor do bulbo do olho. SIN posterior *chamber* of eyeball.
c. oc′uli poste′rior, câmara posterior do bulbo do olho. SIN posterior *chamber* of eyeball.
c. poste′rior bul′bi [TA], câmara posterior do bulbo do olho. SIN posterior *chamber* of eyeball.
c. postrema [TA], câmara postrema*. SIN postremal *chamber* of eyeball.
retinal c., câmera retiniana; instrumento para fotografar o fundo do olho.
scintillation c., câmera de cintilação. SIN gamma c.
c. vitrea, câmara vítrea; *termo oficial alternativo para postremal *chamber* of eyeball.
c. vi′trea bul′bi, c. vítrea do olho; *termo oficial alternativo para postremal *chamber* of eyeball.
vitreous c., câmara vítrea. SIN postremal *chamber* of eyeball.

cam·er·o·stome (kam′er-ō-stōm). Camerostoma; depressão ventral do cefalotórax anterior dos carrapatos (família Argasidae) onde se localizam as partes bucais (capítulo). [L. *camera*, abóbada, + G. *stoma*, boca]

cam·i·sole (kam′i-sōl). Camisa-de-força. SIN straitjacket.

cam·o·mile (kam′ō-mil). Camomila. SIN chamomile.

cAMP AMPc; abreviatura de adenosine 3′,5′-cyclic monophosphate (cyclic AMP) (monofosfato de adenosina 3′,5′-cíclico) (AMP cíclico [AMPc]).

Campbell, Meredith F., urologista pediátrico norte-americano, 1894–1969. VER C. *sound*.

Campbell, William F., cirurgião norte-americano, 1867–1926. VER C. *ligament*.

Camper, Pieter, médico e anatomista holandês, 1721–1789. VER C. *chiasm*; fatty *layer* of subcutaneous tissue of abdomen; C. *ligament, line, plane*.

cam·phene (kam′fēn). Canfano; terpenóide encontrado em muitos óleos essenciais, como, p. ex., terebintina, cânfora, citronela.

cam·phor (kam′fŏr). Cânfora; cetona destilada da casca e da madeira do *Cinnamonum camphora*, uma árvore perene de Formosa e do Sudeste Asiático e ilhas vizinhas, e também preparada sinteticamente a partir do óleo de terebintina; usada em vários produtos comerciais e como antiinfeccioso e antipruriginoso tópico. [L. mediev., do Ar. *kāfure*]
cantharis c., cantaridina. SIN cantharidin.
c. liniment, ungüento de cânfora; mistura de cânfora e óleo de semente de algodão, ou cânfora e óleo de amendoim; leve contra-irritante. SIN camphorated oil.
monobromated c., c. monobromada; designação obsoleta de um antiespasmódico, soporífero e sedativo.
tar c., naftaleno. SIN naphthalene.
thyme c., timol. SIN thymol.

cam·pho·ra·ceous (kam-fō-rā′shŭs). Canforáceo; semelhante à cânfora em aspecto, consistência ou odor.

cam·phor·at·ed (kam′fō-rā-ted). Canforado; que contém cânfora.

cam·phor·at·ed oil. Óleo canforado. SIN camphor liniment.

cam·pi fo·reli (kam′pē fōr-el′ē). Campos de Forel. SIN *fields* of Forel, em *field*. [L. pl. de *campus*, campo]

cam·pim·e·ter (kam-pim′e-ter). Campímetro; pequena tela tangencial usada para medir o campo visual central. [L. *campus*, campo, + G. *metron*, medida]

camp·lo·dac·ty·ly. Campilodactilia. SIN camptodactyly.

campothecins (kam-pō-thā′sinz). Campotecinas; agentes antitumorais que atuam como inibidores da topoisomerase; incluem irinotecan e topotecan.

cAMP phos·pho·di·es·ter·ase. AMPc fosfodiesterase. SIN adenosine 3′,5′-cyclic phosphate phosphodiesterase.

camp·to·cor·mia (kamp-tō-kōr′mē-ă). Camptocormia; flexão estática para a frente do corpo freqüentemente acentuada; em geral é uma manifestação de reação de conversão. SIN camptospasm, prosternation. [G. *kamptos*, curvo, + *kormos*, tronco de árvore]

camp·to·dac·ty·ly, camp·to·dac·tyl·ia (kamp-tō-dak′ti-lē, -dak-til′ē-ă). Camptodactilia; flexão permanente de uma ou ambas as articulações interfalângicas de um ou mais dedos das mãos, geralmente o dedo mínimo; freqüentemente de origem congênita. SIN camplodactyly, streblodactyly. [G. *kamptos*, curvo, + *daktylos*, dedo]

camp·to·me·lia (kamp-tō-mē′lē-ă). Camptomelia; displasia do esqueleto caracterizada por curvatura dos ossos longos dos membros, resultando em arqueamento ou curvatura permanente da parte afetada. [G. *kamptos*, curvo, + *melos*, membro]

camp·to·mel·ic (kamp-tō-mel′ik). Camptomélico; indicador, ou característico, de camptomelia. VER camptomelic *syndrome*.

camp·to·spasm (kamp′tō-spazm). Camptoespasmo. SIN camptocormia.

camptothecin (kamp-tō-thek′in). Camptotecina; alcalóides vegetais que consistem em uma estrutura pentacíclica com um anel lactona; inibidores da topoisomerase I, isto é, topotecan e irinotecan (CPT-11) [*Camptotheca*, gênero de fonte botânica]

Cam·py·lo·bac·ter (kam′pi-lō-bak′ter). Gênero de bactérias contendo bacilos Gram-negativos, não-formadores de esporos, em espirais ou em forma de S com um único flagelo em uma ou ambas as extremidades da célula; as células também podem tornar-se esféricas em condições adversas; são móveis, com um movimento espiral e não-sacarolíticas. A espécie típica é *C. fetus*. [G. *campylos*, curvo, + *baktron*, bastão]

---

*N.R.: Segundo a Terminologia Anatômica Internacional (2001).

C. coli, espécie bacteriana termofílica que causa primeiro diarréia aquosa e, depois, inflamatória em seres humanos e leitões.
C. concisus, espécie bacteriana catalase-negativa isolada na flora fecal humana normal, nas fendas gengivais na doença periodontal e, algumas vezes, no sangue.
C. fe'tus, espécie bacteriana que contém várias subespécies passíveis de causar infecção humana bem como abortamento em ovinos e bovinos; é a espécie típica do gênero C.
C. fetus subsp. ***jejuni,*** designação anterior do *C. jejuni*.
C. hyointestinalis, espécie bacteriana que causa enteropatia em porcos; foi isolada de amostras fecais em seres humanos com diarréia e proctite, mas seu papel patogênico não foi definido.
C. jejuni, espécie bacteriana termofílica que causa, em seres humanos, uma gastroenterite aguda de início súbito com sintomas constitucionais (mal-estar, mialgia, artralgia e cefaléia) e dor abdominal em caráter de cólica; tem sido associada a uma seqüela desmielinizante, que pode apresentar-se com paralisia ascendente. Possíveis fontes de infecção humana incluem aves domésticas, bovinos, ovinos, suínos e cães. Essa espécie também causa abortamento em ovelhas.
C. lari, espécie bacteriana encontrada basicamente em aves, mas associada à enterite transmitida pela água e, ocasionalmente, à septicemia em seres humanos.
C. pylori, SIN *Helicobacter pylori.*
C. sputo'rum, espécie facultativa, microaerofílica, catalase-negativa, encontrada no trato genital e nas fezes de ovinos e bovinos e na cavidade oral humana; uma causa de bronquite humana.
cam·py·lo·bac·te·ri·o·sis (kam'pi - lo - bak'ter - ē - ō'sis). Campilobacteriose; infecção causada por bactérias microaerofílicas do gênero *Campylobacter*.
Canada, Wilma J., radiologista norte-americana. VER Cronkhite-C. *syndrome.*
can·a·dine (kan'a - dēn). Canadina; $C_{20}H_{21}NO_4$; alcalóide presente no *Hydrastis canadensis* (família Ranunculaceae) e no *Corydalis cava* (família Fumaraceae) com propriedades sedativas e relaxantes musculares. SIN xanthopuccine.

CANAL

ca·nal (kā - nal') [TA]. Ducto ou canal; estrutura tubular. VER TAMBÉM canal, duct. SIN canalis [TA]. [L. *canalis*]
abdominal c., c. abdominal. SIN inguinal c.
accessory c., c. acessório; canal que vai da polpa radicular, lateralmente, até o tecido periodontal, passando pela dentina; pode ser encontrado em qualquer lugar na raiz do dente, porém é mais comum no terço apical da raiz. SIN lateral c.
adductor c. [TA], c. adutor; o espaço no terço médio da coxa entre os músculos vasto medial e adutor, convertido em um canal pelo músculo sartório sobrejacente. Dá passagem aos vasos femorais e ao nervo safeno, terminando no hiato adutor. SIN canalis adductorius [TA], Hunter c., subsartorial c.
Alcock c., c. de Alcock. SIN pudendal c.
alimentary c., c. alimentar. SIN digestive *tract.*
alveolar c.'s of maxilla [TA], canais alveolares do maxilar; canais no corpo do maxilar que dão passagem a nervos e vasos dos forames alveolares até os dentes maxilares. SIN canales alveolares corporis maxillae [TA], alveolodental c.'s, dental c.'s.
alveolodental c.'s, canais alveolodentários. SIN alveolar c.'s of maxilla.
anal c. [TA], c. anal; porção terminal do canal alimentar; tem cerca de 4 cm de comprimento, começa na junção anorretal, onde a ampola retal se estreita de forma bastante abrupta, quando o canal alimentar perfura o diafragma pélvico (levantador do ânus), e termina na borda anal, quando a derme anal que reveste a parte inferior do canal anal se transforma em pele perianal pilosa; circundado pelos esfíncteres anais interno e externo. SIN canalis analis [TA].
anterior condyloid c. of occipital bone, c. condilóide anterior do osso occipital. SIN hypoglossal c.
anterior semicircular c.'s, canais semicirculares anteriores. VER semicircular c.'s of bony labyrinth.
archenteric c., c. arquentérico; invaginação do blastoporo para o processo notocórdico a fim de formar uma cavidade. VER neurenteric c. SIN notochordal c.
Arnold c., c. de Arnold. SIN hiatus for lesser petrosal nerve.
arterial c., c. arterial. SIN ductus arteriosus.
atrioventricular c., c. atrioventricular; o c. no coração embrionário que vai da câmara sinoatrial comum até o ventrículo.
auditory c., c. auditivo. SIN external acoustic *meatus.*
basipharyngeal c., c. basifaríngeo. SIN vomerovaginal c.
Bernard c., c. de Bernard. SIN accessory pancreatic *duct.*
Bichat c., c. de Bichat. SIN quadrigeminal *cistern.*
birth c., c. do parto; cavidade do útero e vagina através da qual passa o feto. SIN parturient c.
blastoporic c., c. blastopórico; designação obsoleta de primitive *pit* (depressão primitiva).
bony semicircular c.'s, canais semicirculares ósseos. SIN semicircular c.'s of bony labyrinth.
Böttcher c., c. de Böttcher. SIN utriculosaccular *duct.*
Breschet c.'s, canais de Breschet. SIN diploic c.'s.
carotid c. [TA], c. carotídeo; passagem através da parte petrosa do osso temporal, de sua superfície inferior para cima, medialmente e para a frente até o ápice, onde se abre posterior e superiormente ao local do forame esfenótico. Dá passagem à artéria carótida interna e a plexos de veias e nervos autônomos. SIN canalis caroticus [TA].
carpal c., c. do carpo. (1) SIN carpal *tunnel;* (2) SIN carpal *groove.*
caudal c., c. caudal; espaço ocupado pela extensão sacral do espaço peridural.
central c. [TA], c. central. SIN canalis centralis medullae spinalis [TA], syringocele (1), tubus medullaris. SIN central c. of spinal cord.
central c.'s of cochlea, canais centrais da cóclea. SIN longitudinal c.'s of modiolus.
central c. of spinal cord [TA], canal central da medula espinhal; a luz (cavidade) do tubo neural revestida por epêndima, cuja parte cerebral permanece pérvia para formar os ventrículos cerebrais, enquanto a parte espinhal, no adulto, freqüentemente é reduzida a um filamento sólido de epêndima modificado. SIN central c. [TA]
central c. of the vitreous, c. central do vítreo. SIN hyaloid c.
cervical c. [TA], c. cervical; canal fusiforme que se estende do istmo uterino até a abertura do útero para a vagina. SIN canalis cervicis uteri [TA].
cervicoaxillary c., c. cervicoaxilar; abertura superior para a axila, limitada pela clavícula anteriormente, escápula posteriormente e primeira costela medialmente. Dá passagem aos vasos axilares e ao plexo braquial.
ciliary c.'s, canais ciliares. SIN spaces of iridocorneal angle, em *space.*
Civinini c., c. de Civinini. SIN anterior canaliculus of chorda tympani.
Cloquet c., c. de Cloquet. SIN hyaloid c.
cochlear c., c. coclear. SIN spiral c. of cochlea.
condylar c. [TA], c. condilar; c. condilóide; a abertura inconstante através do osso occipital posterior ao côndilo de cada lado, que dá passagem à veia emissária occipital. SIN canalis condylaris [TA], condyloid c., posterior condyloid foramen.
condyloid c., c. condilóide. SIN condylar c.
Corti c., c. de Corti. SIN Corti *tunnel.*
Cotunnius c., c. de Cotunnius. SIN vestibular *aqueduct.*
craniopharyngeal c., c. craniofaríngeo. SIN pituitary *diverticulum.*
deferent c., c. deferente. SIN ductus deferens.
dental c.'s, canais dentários. SIN alveolar c.'s of maxilla.
dentinal c.'s, canais dentinários. SIN canaliculi dentales, em *canaliculus.*
diploic c.'s [TA], canais diplóicos; canais na díploe que acomodam as veias diplóicas. SIN canales diploici [TA], Breschet c.'s.
Dorello c., c. de Dorello; canal ósseo algumas vezes encontrado na extremidade do osso temporal, que encerra o nervo abducente e o seio petroso inferior quando essas duas estruturas entram no seio cavernoso.
Dupuytren c., c. de Dupuytren. SIN diploic *vein.*
ear c., c. auditivo. SIN external acoustic *meatus.*
endodermal c., c. endodérmico. SIN primitive *gut.*
endometrial c. [TA], endométrio. SIN tunica mucosa uteri.
facial c. [TA], c. facial; a passagem óssea no osso temporal através da qual passa o nervo facial; o c. facial começa no meato auditivo interno com a parte horizontal que passa primeiro anteriormente (pilar medial do canal facial), depois volta-se posteriormente no genículo do c. facial, para seguir medial à cavidade timpânica (pilar lateral do canal facial); finalmente, volta-se para baixo (parte descendente do canal facial) para chegar ao forame estilomastóideo. SIN canalis nervi facialis [TA], aqueductus fallopii, fallopian aqueduct, fallopian c.
fallopian c., c. de Falópio. SIN facial c.
femoral c. [TA], c. femoral; o compartimento medial da bainha femoral freqüentemente ocupado pelo linfonodo inguinal profundo intermediário (de Cloquet), dando passagem aos linfáticos que seguem do membro inferior para o tronco e facilitando a expansão da veia femoral adjacente, como quando esta aumenta durante uma manobra de Valsalva (Valsalva *maneuver*). SIN canalis femoralis [TA].
Ferrein c., c. de Ferrein. SIN lacrimal *pathway.*
Fontana c., c. de Fontana. SIN scleral venous *sinus.*
galactophorous c.'s, canais galactóforos. SIN lactiferous *ducts,* em *duct.*
Gartner c., c. de Gartner. SIN longitudinal *duct* of epoöphoron.
gastric c. [TA], c. gástrico; sulco formado temporariamente entre as pregas longitudinais da mucosa gástrica ao longo da pequena curvatura durante a deglutição; observado radiográfica e endoscopicamente, é formado devido à fixação firme da mucosa gástrica à camada muscular, que é desprovida de uma camada oblíqua nesse local; diz-se que forma uma passagem preferida pela

saliva e por pequenas quantidades de alimento mastigado e outros líquidos quando fluem do cárdia para a junção gastroduodenal. SIN canalis gastricus [TA], magenstrasse.

greater palatine c. [TA], c. palatino maior; o c. formado entre os ossos maxilar e palatino; dá passagem à artéria palatina descendente e ao nervo palatino maior. SIN canalis palatinus major [TA], pterygopalatine c.

gubernacular c., c. gubernacular; pequeno c. localizado entre o germe dentário permanente e o ápice do dente decíduo, contendo remanescentes da lâmina dentária e tecido conjuntivo.

c. of Guyon, c. de Guyon; passagem através do ligamento transverso do carpo pela qual o nervo e a artéria ulnares entram na palma da mão; está intimamente relacionado ao osso pisiforme e ao hâmulo do osso hamato.

Guyon c., c. de Guyon; o c. superficial entre o retináculo flexor da mão e o flexor ulnar do carpo pelo qual passam o nervo ulnar e a rede vascular entre o antebraço e a mão.

gynecophoric c., c. ginecóforo; sulco ventral em todo o comprimento do esquistossoma macho, no qual se aloja a fêmea filiforme.

Hannover c., c. de Hannover; espaço virtual entre a zônula ciliar e o corpo vítreo.

haversian c.'s, canais de Havers; canais vasculares que seguem longitudinalmente no centro dos sistemas de Havers do tecido ósseo compacto. SIN Leeuwenhoek c.'s.

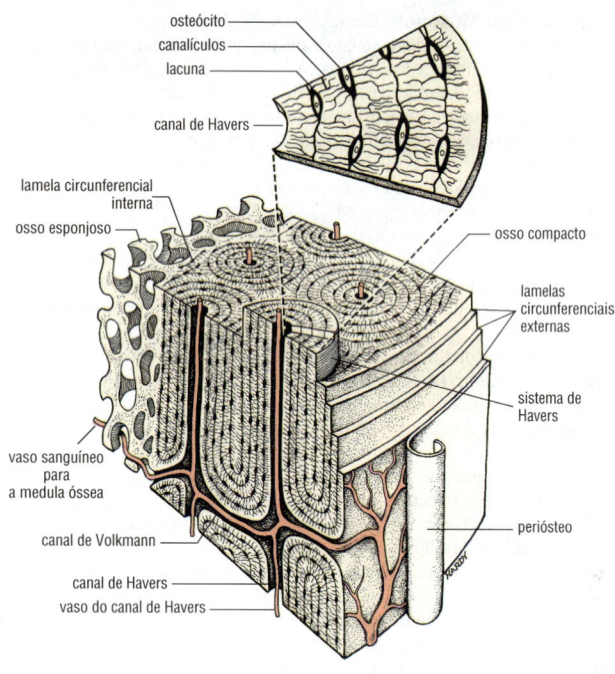

canais de Havers: observados em cunha de tecido ósseo compacto

Hensen c., c. de Hensen. SIN ductus reuniens.
c. of Hering, c. de Hering. SIN cholangiole.
Hirschfeld c.'s, canais de Hirschfeld. SIN interdental c.'s.
Holmgrén-Golgi c.'s, canais de Holmgrén-Golgi. SIN Golgi apparatus.
c. of Hovius, c. de Hovius; círculo anastomótico entre os ramos anteriores das veias vorticosas nos olhos de alguns animais, mas não em olhos humanos normais.
Hoyer c.'s, canais de Hoyer. SIN Sucquet-Hoyer c.'s.
Huguier c., c. de Huguier. SIN anterior canaliculus of chorda tympani.
Hunter c., c. de Hunter. SIN adductor c.
hyaloid c. [TA], c. hialóide; um minúsculo canal que atravessa o vítreo, do disco óptico até o cristalino, contendo, durante a vida fetal, um prolongamento da artéria central da retina, a artéria hialóide. VER vitreous, hyaloid artery. SIN canalis hyaloideus [TA], central c. of the vitreous, Cloquet c., Stilling c.
hypoglossal c. [TA], c. hipoglosso; canal através do qual o nervo hipoglosso emerge do crânio. SIN canalis hypoglossalis [TA], anterior condyloid c. of occipital bone, anterior condyloid foramen.
incisive c.'s [TA], canais incisivos; vários canais ósseos que vão do assoalho da cavidade nasal até a fossa incisiva na superfície palatina do maxilar; dão passagem aos nervos nasopalatinos e aos ramos das artérias palatinas maiores que se anastomosam com o ramo septal da artéria esfenopalatina. SIN canales incisivi [TA], incisor c.'s.

incisor c.'s, canais incisivos. SIN incisive c.'s.
inferior dental c., c. dentário inferior. SIN mandibular c.
infraorbital c. [TA], c. infra-orbitário; canal sob a borda orbitária do maxilar desde o sulco infra-orbitário, no assoalho da órbita, até o forame infra-orbitário; dá passagem à artéria e ao nervo infra-orbitários. SIN canalis infraorbitalis [TA].
inguinal c. [TA], c. inguinal; a passagem oblíqua através das camadas musculoaponeuróticas da parede abdominal inferior por onde passa o cordão espermático, no homem, e o ligamento redondo, na mulher, desde a cavidade pélvica até o escroto ou lábio maior do pudendo, respectivamente. SIN canalis inguinalis [TA], abdominal c., Velpeau c.
interdental c.'s, canais interdentários; canais que se estendem verticalmente, através do osso alveolar, entre as raízes dos incisivos mandibulares e maxilares e dentes bicúspides maxilares. SIN Hirschfeld c.'s.
interfacial c.'s, canais interfaciais; espaços intercelulares que ocorrem em relação às fixações intercelulares por desmossomas no epitélio escamoso estratificado, geralmente resultantes da retração de um artefato de fixação.
Jacobson c., c. de Jacobson. SIN tympanic canaliculus.
Kürsteiner c.'s, canais de Kürsteiner; um complexo fetal de estruturas vesiculares, canaliculares e semelhantes a glândulas, derivadas das paratireóides, do timo ou do cordão tímico; são rudimentares e não têm função, exceto se persistirem após o nascimento, quando podem ocorrer como estruturas císticas adjacentes à paratireóide III e ao timo III. Kürsteiner descreveu três tipos, sendo os canais do tipo II associados à tireoaplasia.
lateral c., c. lateral. SIN accessory c.
lateral semicircular c.'s, canais semicirculares laterais. VER semicircular c.'s of bony labyrinth.
Laurer c., c. de Laurer; tubo que se origina na superfície do ootipo dos trematódeos, orientado dorsalmente até a superfície ou próxima desta; pode ter originalmente servido como uma vagina ou, possivelmente, como reservatório do excesso de material de revestimento.
Lauth c., c. de Lauth. SIN scleral venous sinus.
Leeuwenhoek c.'s, canais de Leeuwenhoek. SIN haversian c.'s.
lesser palatine c.'s [TA], canais palatinos menores; canais localizados na parte posterior do osso palatino. SIN canales palatini minores [TA], c.'s for lesser palatine nerves.
c.'s for lesser palatine nerves, canais para os nervos palatinos menores. SIN lesser palatine c.'s.
longitudinal c.'s of modiolus [TA], canais longitudinais do modíolo; canais centrais que dão passagem aos vasos e nervos até as voltas apicais da cóclea. SIN canales longitudinales modioli [TA], central c.'s of cochlea.
Löwenberg c., c. de Löwenberg. SIN cochlear duct.
mandibular c. [TA], c. mandibular; o canal na mandíbula que dá passagem ao nervo e vasos alveolares inferiores. Sua abertura posterior é o forame mandibular. SIN canalis mandibulae [TA], inferior dental c.
marrow c., c. medular. SIN root c. of tooth.
mental c., c. mentoniano. SIN mental foramen.
musculotubal c. [TA], c. musculotubário; canal que começa na borda anterior da porção petrosa do osso temporal próximo à sua junção com a porção escamosa, seguindo até a cavidade timpânica; é dividido pelo processo cocleariforme em dois semicanais: um para a tuba faringotimpânica (auditiva) e o outro para o músculo tensor do tímpano. SIN canalis musculotubarius [TA].
nasolacrimal c. [TA], c. nasolacrimal; o canal ósseo, formado pelo maxilar, osso lacrimal e concha inferior, que dá passagem ao ducto nasolacrimal da órbita até o meato inferior do nariz. SIN canalis nasolacrimalis [TA].
neural c., c. neural; o c. situado dentro do tubo neural embrionário; o primórdio do c. central.
neurenteric c., c. neurentérico; comunicação transitória entre o tubo neural, canal notocórdico e endoderma intestinal em embriões de vertebrados.
notochordal c., c. notocórdico. SIN archenteric c.
c. of Nuck, c. de Nuck. VER processus vaginalis of peritoneum.
nutrient c. [TA], c. nutrício; canal na diáfise de um osso longo ou em outras localizações em ossos irregulares através do qual a artéria nutrícia entra no osso. SIN canalis nutricius [TA].
obturator c. [TA], c. obturador; abertura na parte superior da membrana obturadora através da qual o nervo e os vasos obturadores seguem da cavidade pélvica até a coxa. SIN canalis obturatorius [TA].
optic c. [TA], c. óptico; o canal curto, através da asa menor do osso esfenóide no ápice da órbita, que dá passagem ao nervo óptico e à artéria oftálmica. SIN canalis opticus [TA], foramen opticum, optic foramen.
palatovaginal c. [TA], c. palatovaginal; na superfície inferior do processo vaginal do osso esfenóide, um sulco que é transformado em um canal pelo processo esfenóide do osso palatino; dá passagem ao ramo faríngeo da artéria maxilar e ao nervo faríngeo do gânglio pterigopalatino. SIN canalis palatovaginalis, pharyngeal c.
parturient c., c. do parto. SIN birth c.
pelvic c. c., pélvico; a passagem da abertura superior da pelve até a abertura inferior.

pericardioperitoneal c., c. pericardioperitoneal; a porção do celoma embrionário que une a cavidade pericárdica à cavidade peritoneal, transformando-se nas cavidades pleurais. SIN pleural c.
persistent atrioventricular c., c. atrioventricular persistente; persistência do canal atrioventricular; condição causada pela falta de união dos septos interatrial e interventricular, como no desenvolvimento normal, resultando em um defeito do septo interatrial baixo e do septo interventricular alto ou um c. atrioventricular comum. SIN endocardial cushion defect.
Petit c.'s, canais de Petit. SIN zonular spaces, em space.
pharyngeal c., c. faríngeo. SIN palatovaginal c.
c. for pharyngotympanic (auditory) tube [TA], c. para a tuba faringotimpânica (auditiva); a divisão inferior do canal musculotubário que forma a parte óssea da tuba faringotimpânica (auditiva). SIN semicanalis tubae auditivae [TA], semicanal of auditory tube, semicanalis t'ubae audito'riae.
pleural c., c. pleural. SIN pericardioperitoneal c.
pleuropericardial c.'s, canais pleuropericárdicos; no embrião, espaços ou canais, um de cada lado, unindo as cavidades pericárdica e pleural.
pleuroperitoneal c., c. pleuroperitoneal; comunicação entre as cavidades pleural e peritoneal embrionárias.
portal c.'s, canais portais; espaços de tecido conjuntivo na substância do fígado que são ocupados por ramificações pré-terminais dos ductos biliares, veia porta e artéria hepática, bem como nervos e linfáticos.
posterior semicircular c.'s, canais semicirculares posteriores. VER semicircular c.'s of bony labyrinth.
pterygoid c. [TA], c. pterigóide; abertura através da base do processo pterigóide medial do osso esfenóide pela qual passam a artéria, a veia e o nervo do canal pterigóide. SIN canalis pterygoideus [TA], vidian c.
pterygopalatine c., c. pterigopalatino. SIN greater palatine c.
pudendal c. [TA], c. pudendo; o espaço na fáscia interna do obturador que reveste a parede lateral da fossa isquioanal (isquiorretal), por onde passam os vasos pudendos e os nervos pudendos internos. SIN canalis pudendalis [TA], Alcock c.
pulp c., c. da polpa. SIN root c. of tooth.
pyloric c. [TA], c. pilórico; o segmento aboral (cerca de 2–3 cm de comprimento) do estômago; este sucede o antro e termina na junção gastroduodenal. SIN canalis pyloricus [TA].
Rivinus c.'s, canais de Rivinus. VER major sublingual duct, minor sublingual ducts, em duct.
root c. of tooth [TA], c. radicular do dente; câmara da polpa dentária situada na porção radicular de um dente. SIN canalis radicis dentis [TA], marrow c., pulp c.
Rosenthal c., c. de Rosenthal. SIN spiral c. of cochlea.
sacral c. [TA], c. sacral; a continuação do canal vertebral no sacro. SIN canalis sacralis [TA].
Santorini c., c. de Santorini. SIN accessory pancreatic duct.
c.'s of Scarpa, canais de Scarpa; canais distintos para os nervos e vasos nasopalatinos. Esses canais normalmente se fundem para formar o c. incisivo.
Schlemm c., c. de Schlemm. SIN scleral venous sinus.
semicircular c., c. semicircular. VER semicircular c.'s of bony labyrinth.
semicircular c.'s of bony labyrinth [TA], canais semicirculares do labirinto ósseo; o órgão do equilíbrio; os três tubos ósseos no labirinto do ouvido nos quais estão localizados os ductos semicirculares membranosos; situam-se em planos que formam ângulos retos entre si e são conhecidos como canal semicircular anterior, canal semicircular posterior e canal semicircular lateral. SIN bony semicircular c.'s, canales semicirculares ossei.
small c. of chorda tympani, canalículo da corda do tímpano. SIN posterior canaliculus of chorda tympani.
Sondermann c., c. de Sondermann; uma evaginação de fundo cego do c. de Schlemm, que se estende em direção à câmara anterior do olho, mas não se comunica com esta.
spinal c., c. vertebral. SIN vertebral c.
spiral c. of cochlea [TA], c. espiral da cóclea; o tubo sinuoso do labirinto ósseo que dá duas voltas e meia em torno do modíolo da cóclea; é dividido incompletamente em dois compartimentos por uma prateleira óssea sinuosa, a lâmina espiral óssea. SIN canalis spiralis cochleae [TA], cochlear c., Rosenthal c.
spiral c. of modiolus [TA], c. espiral do modíolo; o espaço no modíolo em que está situado o gânglio espiral do nervo coclear. SIN canalis spiralis modioli [TA].
Stilling c., c. de Stilling. SIN hyaloid c.
subsartorial c., c. adutor. SIN adductor c.
Sucquet c.'s, canais de Sucquet. SIN Sucquet-Hoyer c.'s.
Sucquet-Hoyer c.'s, canais de Sucquet-Hoyer; anastomoses arteriovenulares que controlam o fluxo sanguíneo para as anastomoses arteriovenosas glomeriformes nos dedos. SIN Hoyer anastomoses, Hoyer c.'s, Sucquet anastomoses, Sucquet c.'s, Sucquet-Hoyer anastomoses.
tarsal c., c. do tarso. SIN tarsal sinus.
temporal c., c. temporal; canal no osso zigomático que dá passagem aos nervos e vasos zigomaticofacial e zigomaticotemporal.
c. for tensor tympani muscle [TA], c. para o músculo tensor do tímpano; semicanal do músculo tensor do tímpano; a divisão superior do canal musculotubário que contém o músculo tensor do tímpano. SIN semicanalis musculi tensoris tympani [TA], semicanal for tensor tympani muscle.
Theile c., c. de Theile. SIN transverse pericardial sinus.
tubotympanic c., c. tubotympânico. VER tubotympanic recess.
tympanic c., c. timpânico. SIN tympanic canaliculus.
uniting c., ducto de união. SIN ductus reuniens.
uterovaginal c., c. uterovaginal; estrutura tubular mediana produzida no embrião por fusão das partes caudais dos ductos paramesonéfricos.
van Horne c., c. de van Horne. SIN thoracic duct.
Velpeau c., c. de Velpeau, canal inguinal. SIN inguinal c.
vertebral c. [TA], c. vertebral; o canal que contém a medula espinhal, as meninges espinhais e estruturas relacionadas. É formado pelos forames vertebrais de vértebras sucessivas da coluna vertebral articulada. SIN canalis vertebralis [TA], spinal c., tubus vertebralis.
vesicourethral c., c. vesicouretral; a porção cranial do seio urogenital primitivo a partir da qual se desenvolve a bexiga e parte da uretra.
vestibular c., c. vestibular. SIN scala vestibuli.
vidian c., c. pterigóide. SIN pterygoid c.
Volkmann c.'s, canais de Volkmann; canais vasculares no osso compacto que, ao contrário daqueles do sistema de Havers, não são circundados por lamelas ósseas concêntricas; na maioria das vezes, seguem transversalmente, perfurando as lamelas do sistema de Havers, e comunicam-se com os canais daquele sistema.
vomerine c., c. vomerovaginal. SIN vomerovaginal c.
vomerobasilar c., c. vomerobasilar. SIN vomerorostral c.
vomerorostral c. [TA], c. vomerorrostral; pequeno canal entre a borda superior do vômero e o rostro do osso esfenóide. SIN canalis vomerorostralis [TA], vomerobasilar c.
vomerovaginal c. [TA], c. vomerovaginal; abertura entre o processo vaginal do esfenóide e a asa do vômer de cada lado. Dá passagem a um ramo da artéria esfenopalatina. SIN canalis vomerovaginalis [TA], basipharyngeal c., vomerine c.
Walther c.'s, canais de Walther. SIN minor sublingual ducts, em duct.
Wirsung c., c. de Wirsung. SIN pancreatic duct.

ca·na·les (kă-nā′lēz). Canais; plural de canalis.
can·a·lic·u·lar (kan-ă-lik′ū-lar). Canalicular; relativo a um canalículo. [L. canaliculis, canal pequeno, dim. de canalis, canal, + sufixo -ar, relativo a]
can·a·lic·u·li (kan-ă-lik′ū-lī). Canalículos; plural de canaliculus.
can·a·lic·u·li·tis (kan′ă-lik-ū-lī′tis). Canaliculite; inflamação do canalículo lacrimal. [canaliculus + G. -itis, inflamação]
can·a·lic·u·li·za·tion (kan-ă-lik′ū-lī-zā′shŭn). Canaliculização; formação de canalículos, ou pequenos canais, em qualquer tecido.
can·a·lic·u·lus, pl. **can·a·lic·u·li** (kan-ă-lik′ū-lŭs, -lī). [TA]. Canalículo; pequeno canal. VER TAMBÉM iter. [L. dim de canalis, canal]
anterior c. of chorda tympani, c. anterior da corda do tímpano; canal na fissura petrotimpânica ou de Glaser, próximo de sua borda posterior, através do qual o nervo corda do tímpano sai do crânio. SIN Civinini canal, Huguier canal, iter chordae anterius.
auricular c., c. auricular. SIN mastoid c.
biliary c., c. biliar; um dos canais intercelulares, com cerca de 1 μm de diâmetro ou menos, presentes entre os hepatócitos, que formam a primeira porção do sistema biliar. SIN bile capillary.
bone c., c. ósseo; c. que interliga as lacunas ósseas entre si ou com um canal de Havers; contém os processos citoplasmáticos conectores dos osteócitos.
caroticotympanic canaliculi [TA], canalículos caroticotimpânicos; pequenas aberturas no canal carotídeo que asseguram a passagem, até a cavidade timpânica, de ramos da artéria carótida interna e plexo simpático carotídeo. SIN canaliculi caroticotympanici [TA].
canaliculi caroticotympan'ici [TA], canalículos caroticotimpânicos. SIN caroticotympanic canaliculi.
c. chor'dae tym'pani [TA], c. da corda do tímpano. SIN posterior c. of chorda tympani.
c. of chorda tympani, c. da corda do tímpano. SIN posterior c. of chorda tympani.
c. coch'leae [TA], c. da cóclea. SIN cochlear c.
cochlear c. [TA], c. coclear; canal minúsculo, no osso temporal, que sai da cóclea inferiormente para se abrir na frente da face medial da fossa jugular. Contém o ducto perilinfático. SIN canaliculus cochleae [TA].
canalic'uli denta'les, canalículos dentários; minúsculos tubos ou canais ramificados céreos na dentina; contém os longos processos citoplasmáticos dos odontoblastos e estendem-se radialmente da polpa até a junção dentina–esmalte. SIN dental tubules, dentinal canals, dentinal tubules, tubuli dentales.
c. innomina'tus, c. inominado. SIN foramen petrosum.
intercellular c., c. intercelular; um dos finos canais entre células secretoras adjacentes, como aqueles entre as células serosas nas glândulas salivares.

intracellular c., c. intracelular; um canal fino formado pela invaginação da membrana celular para o citoplasma de uma célula, como aqueles das células parietais do estômago.
lacrimal c. [TA], canalículo lacrimal; um canal curvo que começa no orifício lacrimal na margem de cada pálpebra, próximo a comissura medial, e corre transversal e medialmente para escoar (junto com seu par) no saco lacrimal. SIN c. lacrimalis [TA].
lacrima'lis c. [TA], c. lacrimal. SIN lacrimal c.
mastoid c. [TA], c. mastóide; o canal que se estende lateralmente a partir da fossa jugular através do processo mastóide. Dá passagem ao ramo auricular do vago. SIN c. mastoideus [TA], auricular c.
c. mastoid'eus [TA], c. mastóide. SIN mastoid c.
posterior c. of chorda tympani, c. posterior da corda do tímpano; canal que vai do canal facial até a cavidade timpânica, através do qual o nervo corda do tímpano entra nessa cavidade. SIN c. chordae tympani [TA], c. of chorda tympani, iter chordae posterius, small canal of chorda tympani.
c. reu'niens, ducto de união. SIN *ductus* reuniens.
secretory c., c. secretor. VER intercellular c., intracellular c.
Thiersch canaliculi, canalículos de Thiersch; pequenos canais no tecido reparador recém-formado, permitindo a circulação de líquidos nutritivos, precursores da nova vascularização.
tympanic c. [TA], c. timpânico; pequeno canal que segue da superfície inferior da porção petrosa do osso temporal, entre a fossa jugular e o canal carotídeo, até o assoalho da cavidade timpânica. Localizado na cunha óssea que separa o canal jugular e o canal carotídeo, dá passagem ao ramo timpânico do nervo glossofaríngeo. SIN c. tympanicus [TA], Jacobson canal, tympanic canal.
c. tympan'icus [TA], c. timpânico. SIN tympanic c.
ca·na·lis, pl. **ca·na·les** (ka-nā'lis, -lēz) [TA], canal. SIN canal. [L.]
c. adductor'ius [TA], c. adutor. SIN adductor *canal*.
cana'les alveola'res corporis maxillae [TA], canais alveolares do corpo maxilar. SIN alveolar *canals* of maxilla, em *canal*.
c. ana'lis [TA], c. anal. SIN anal *canal*.
c. carot'icus [TA], c. carotídeo. SIN carotid *canal*.
c. car'pi [TA], c. do carpo. SIN carpal *tunnel*.
c. centra'lis medul'lae spina'lis [TA], c. central da medula espinhal. SIN central *canal*.
c. cerv'icis u'teri [TA], c. cervical do útero. SIN cervical *canal*.
c. condyla'ris [TA], c. condilar. SIN condylar *canal*.
cana'les diplo'ici [TA], canais diplóicos. SIN diploic *canals*, em *canal*.
c. femora'lis [TA], c. femoral. SIN femoral *canal*.
c. gastricus [TA], c. gástrico. SIN gastric *canal*.
c. hyaloid'eus [TA], c. hialóide. SIN hyaloid *canal*.
c. hypoglossa'lis [TA], c. hipoglosso. SIN hypoglossal *canal*.
canales incisi'vi [TA], canais incisivos. SIN incisive *canals*, em *canal*.
c. infraorbita'lis [TA], c. infra-orbitário. SIN infraorbital *canal*.
c. inguina'lis [TA], c. inguinal. SIN inguinal *canal*.
cana'les longitudina'les modi'oli [TA], canais longitudinais do modíolo. SIN longitudinal *canals* of modiolus, em *canal*.
c. mandib'ulae [TA], c. mandibular. SIN mandibular *canal*.
c. musculotuba'rius [TA], c. musculotubário. SIN musculotubal *canal*.
c. nasolacrima'lis [TA], c. nasolacrimal. SIN nasolacrimal *canal*.
c. ner'vi facia'lis [TA], c. do nervo facial. SIN facial *canal*.
c. ner'vi petro'si superficial'is mino'ris, c. do nervo petroso superficial menor. SIN *hiatus* for lesser petrosal nerve.
c. nutri'cius [TA], c. nutrício. SIN nutrient *canal*.
c. obturato'rius [TA], c. obturador. SIN obturator *canal*.
c. op'ticus [TA], c. óptico. SIN optic *canal*.
cana'les palati'ni mino'res [TA], canais palatinos menores. SIN lesser palatine *canals*, em *canal*.
c. palati'nus ma'jor [TA], c. palatino maior. SIN greater palatine *canal*.
c. palatovagina'lis, c. palatovaginal. SIN palatovaginal *canal*.
c. pterygoi'deus [TA], c. pterigóide. SIN pterygoid *canal*.
c. pudenda'lis [TA], c. pudendo. SIN pudendal *canal*.
c. pylor'icus [TA], c. pilórico. SIN pyloric *canal*.
c. rad'icis den'tis [TA], c. radicular do dente. SIN root *canal* of tooth.
c. reu'niens, c. de união. SIN *ductus* reuniens.
c. sacra'lis [TA], c. sacral. SIN sacral *canal*.
canales semicircularis anterior, canais semicirculares anteriores. VER semicircular *canals* of bony labyrinth, em *canal*.
canales semicircularis lateralis, canais semicirculares laterais. VER semicircular *canals* of bony labyrinth, em *canal*.
cana'les semicircula'ris os'sei, canais semicirculares ósseos. SIN semicircular *canals* of bony labyrinth, em *canal*.
canales semicircularis posterior, canais semicirculares posteriores. VER semicircular *canals* of bony labyrinth, em *canal*.
c. spira'lis coch'leae [TA], c. espiral da cóclea. SIN spiral *canal* of cochlea.
c. spira'lis modi'oli [TA], c. espiral do modíolo. SIN spiral *canal* of modiolus.
c. umbilica'lis, c. umbilical. SIN umbilical *ring*.
c. vertebra'lis [TA], c. vertebral. SIN vertebral *canal*.
c. vomerorostra'lis [TA], c. vomerorrostral. SIN vomerorostral *canal*.
c. vomerovagina'lis [TA], c. vomerovaginal. SIN vomerovaginal *canal*.
can·a·li·za·tion (kan-ăl-ī-zā'shŭn). Canalização; a formação de canais em um tecido.
Canavan, Myrtelle M., patologista norte-americano, 1879–1953. VER C. *disease, sclerosis*; C.-van Bogaert-Bertrand *disease*.
can·av·a·nase (kan-ăv'a-nās). Canavanase. SIN arginase.
can·a·van·ine (kan-ă-van'īn). Canavanina; ácido 2-amino-4-guanidinoidroxibutírico; análogo da arginina encontrado em determinados legumes; usada em estudos de sistemas arginina-dependentes; também é um potente inibidor do crescimento. [*Canavalia* + -ine]
can·cel·lat·ed (kan'sĕ-lā-ted). Esponjoso, reticulado, canceloso. SIN cancellous. [L. *cancello*, fazer um trabalho de trama]
can·cel·lous (kan'sĕ-lŭs). Esponjoso; designa o osso que tem uma estrutura reticular ou esponjosa. SIN cancellated.
can·cel·lus, pl. **can·cel·li** (kan-sel'ŭs, -lī). Uma estrutura reticular, como no osso esponjoso. [L. grade, rede]
can·cer (CA) (kan'ser). Câncer; termo geral freqüentemente usado para indicar qualquer de vários tipos de neoplasias malignas, a maioria das quais invadem os tecidos adjacentes, podendo lançar metástases para vários locais, e é provável que reapareçam após tentativa de ressecção, causando a morte do paciente se não forem adequadamente tratadas; especialmente, qualquer carcinoma ou sarcoma, mas, no uso geral, principalmente o primeiro. [L. caranguejo, câncer]
betel c., c. de bétel; carcinoma da mucosa da bochecha, observado em alguns nativos da Índia Oriental, provavelmente causado pela irritação ao mastigar uma preparação da noz de bétel e cal enrolada na folha dessa árvore. SIN buyo cheek c.
buyo cheek c., c. de betel. SIN betel c. [Filipino *buyo*, bétel]
chimney sweep's c., c. dos limpadores de chaminé; carcinoma de células escamosas da pele do escroto, que ocorre como doença ocupacional em limpadores de chaminé. A primeira forma descrita de câncer ocupacional (por Sir Percival Pott).
colloid c., c. colóide. SIN mucinous *carcinoma*.
conjugal c., c. conjugal; c. a dois que ocorre em marido e mulher.
c. à deux, c. a dois; carcinomas que ocorrem quase simultaneamente, ou em sucessão muito próxima, em duas pessoas que vivem juntas. [Fr. *deux*, dois]
c. en cuirasse (on-kwē-rahs', Fr. couraça), c. em couraça; carcinoma que envolve uma porção considerável da pele de um ou de ambos os lados do tórax. [Fr. couraça]
epidermoid c., c. epidermóide. SIN epidermoid *carcinoma*.
epithelial c., c. epitelial; qualquer neoplasia maligna originada no epitélio, isto é, um carcinoma.
familial c., c. familiar; c. que ocorre em parentes por consangüinidade; raramente a forma de herança é claramente mendeliana, seja dominante, como no retinoblastoma, síndrome do nevo basocelular, neurofibromatose e polipose intestinal, ou recessiva, como na xerodermia pigmentosa. VER TAMBÉM cancer *family*.
glandular c., c. glandular. SIN adenocarcinoma.
hereditary nonpolyposis colorectal c., c. colorretal hereditário não ligado a polipose; predisposição autossômica dominante ao câncer do cólon e do reto.
kang c., kangri c., carcinoma da pele da coxa ou do abdome observado em alguns trabalhadores indianos ou chineses; acredita-se que seja decorrente da irritação causada pelo calor de um forno para tijolos quente (*kang*) ou de um cesto contendo carvão incandescente levado junto ao corpo no inverno para se aquecer (*kangri*). SIN kangri burn carcinoma.
mouse c., c. do camundongo; qualquer um dos vários tipos de neoplasias malignas que ocorrem naturalmente em camundongos, principalmente em determinadas "cepas c." submetidas a cruzamentos consangüíneos usadas em pesquisa.
mule-spinner's c., c. dos fiadores; carcinoma do escroto ou da pele adjacente exposta ao óleo, observado em alguns indivíduos que trabalham com tecelagem de algodão.
paraffin c., c. de parafina; carcinoma de pele que ocorre como doença ocupacional em pessoas que trabalham com parafina.
pipe-smoker's c., c. do fumante de cachimbo; carcinoma de células escamosas dos lábios encontrado em fumantes de cachimbo.
pitch-worker's c., c. dos trabalhadores em asfalto; carcinoma da pele da face ou pescoço, braços e mãos ou do escroto, resultante da exposição a carcinógenos do piche, encontrado naturalmente no asfalto, ou como resíduo na destilação do alcatrão.
scar c., c. de cicatriz. SIN scar *carcinoma*.
scar c. of the lungs, c. cicatricial dos pulmões; c. pulmonar intimamente relacionado a uma área localizada de fibrose do parênquima.
stump c., c. do coto; carcinoma do estômago que se desenvolve após gastroenterostomia ou ressecção gástrica para tratamento de doença benigna.
telangiectatic c., c. telangiectástico; c. com numerosos capilares dilatados e "lagos" de sangue em canais relativamente grandes, revestidos de endotélio.

can·cer·o·pho·bia (kan′ser-ō-fō′bē-ă). Cancerofobia; medo mórbido de uma neoplasia maligna. SIN carcinophobia. [cancer + G. *phobos*, medo]

can·cer·ous (kan′ser-ŭs). Canceroso; relativo ou pertinente a uma neoplasia maligna ou a ser afetado por esse processo.

can·cra (kang′krā). Cancros; plural de cancrum.

can·cri·form (kang′kri-fōrm). Cancriforme; canceriforme; cancróide; semelhante ao câncer. SIN cancroid (1).

can·croid (kang′kroyd). Cancróide. **1.** SIN cancriform. **2.** Termo obsoleto para designar uma neoplasia maligna que apresenta um menor grau de malignidade que o freqüentemente observado no carcinoma ou sarcoma. [cancer + G. *eidos*, semelhança]

can·crum, pl. **can·cra** (kang′krŭm, -krā). Cancro; lesão gangrenosa, ulcerativa, inflamatória. [L. Mod., do L. *cancer*, caranguejo]

  c. na'si, c. nasal; rinite gangrenosa, necrotizante e ulcerativa, particularmente em crianças.

  c. o'ris, c. oral. SIN noma.

can·de·la (cd) (kan′de-lā). Candela; unidade SI de intensidade luminosa, 1 lúmen por m^2; a intensidade luminosa, em uma determinada direção, de uma fonte que emite radiação monocromática de freqüência 540×10^{12} Hz e que possui uma intensidade radiante na direção de 1/683 W por esterorradiano (unidade de medida em ângulos sólidos). SIN candle. [L.]

can·di·cans (kan′di-kanz). Um dos corpos albicantes (*corpora albicantia*). [L. *candico*, part. pres. *-ans*, esbranquiçado]

can·di·ci·din (kan-di-sī′din). Candicidina; agente antibiótico polieno fungistático e fungicida derivado de um actinomiceto encontrado no solo, semelhante ao *Streptomyces griseus*; usada no tratamento da candidíase vaginal.

Can·di·da (kan′did-ă). *Candida*; gênero de fungos leveduriformes comumente encontrados na natureza; algumas espécies são isoladas na pele, nas fezes e nos tecidos vaginal e faríngeo, mas o trato gastrointestinal é a origem da espécie mais importante, *C. albicans*. [L. *candidus*, branco ofuscante]

  C. al'bicans, espécie de fungo que comumente faz parte da flora gastrointestinal normal dos seres humanos, mas que se torna patogênico quando há perturbação do equilíbrio da flora ou comprometimento das defesas do hospedeiro por outras causas; os estados mórbidos resultantes podem variar de infecções cutâneas ou cutâneo-mucosas limitadas ou generalizadas, até doenças sistêmicas graves e fatais, incluindo endocardite, septicemia e meningite. SIN thrush fungus.

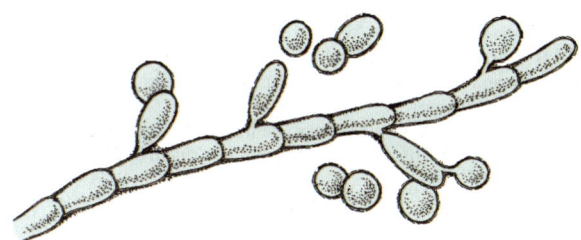

Candida albicans

  C. glabrata, espécie de fungo que causa candidíase humana; anteriormente classificado como *Torulopsis glabrata*.

  C. parapsilosis, espécie de patogenicidade limitada que pode causar endocardite, paroníquia e otite externa.

  C. tropicalis, espécie ocasionalmente associada à candidíase.

can·di·de·mia (kan-di-dē′mē-ă). Candidemia; presença de células de espécies de *Candida* no sangue periférico. [*Candida* + G. *haima*, sangue]

can·di·di·a·sis (kan-di-dī′ă-sis). Candidíase; infecção ou doença causada por *Candida*, particularmente *C. albicans*. Esta doença geralmente resulta de debilitação (como na imunossupressão e principalmente na AIDS/SIDA), alteração fisiológica, administração prolongada de antibióticos, iatrogenia e ruptura de barreira. SIN candidosis, moniliasis.

can·di·do·sis (kan-di-dō′sis). Candidíase. SIN candidiasis.

can·dle (kan′dl). Vela; candeia; candela. SIN candela.

can·dle-me·ter (kan′dl-mē′ter). Lux. SIN lux.

can·dle-pow·er (kan′dl-pow′er). Vela (unidade de intensidade luminosa); potência em velas; intensidade luminosa expressa em candelas. SIN luminous intensity.

Can·i·dae (kan′i-dē). Família da ordem Carnivora, que inclui cães, coiotes, lobos e raposas. [L. *canis*, cão]

ca·nine (kā′nīn). Canino. **1.** Relativo a um cão. **2.** Relativo aos dentes caninos. **3.** Canino. SIN canine *tooth*. **4.** Referente à cúspide do dente. [L. *caninus*]

ca·ni·ni·form (ka-nī′ni-fōrm). Caniniforme; semelhante a um dente canino.

can·is·ter (kan′is-ter). Caixa ou recipiente; canister; recipiente de cal sodada; em anestesiologia, o recipiente para o absorvente de dióxido de carbono.

ca·ni·ti·es (kă-nish′ē-ēz). Canície, poliose; embranquecimento dos cabelos. VER TAMBÉM poliosis. [L. de *canus*, grisalho, cinza]

  canities c., cílios ectópicos. SIN ectopic *eyelash.*

  c. circumscrip'ta, c. circunscrita, poliose ciliar. SIN piebald *eyelash.*

  rapid c., c. rápida; embranquecimento do cabelo durante a noite ou em alguns dias; neste último caso, pode ser observado na alopecia assimétrica, quando os cabelos pigmentados remanescentes caem primeiro que os cabelos grisalhos.

can·ker (kang′ker). Cancro. **1.** Em cães e gatos, inflamação aguda do ouvido externo e do canal auditivo. VER aphtha. **2.** No cavalo, um processo semelhante, porém mais avançado que a moniliíase; por baixo da ranilha córnea, geralmente há um exsudato esbranquiçado, semelhante a queijo, e toda a sola e até mesmo a lateral do casco podem ser corroídas. [L. *cancer*, caranguejo, crescimento maligno]

  water c., c. hídrico, noma. SIN noma.

can·na·bi·di·ol (kan-ă-bi-dī′ol). Canabidiol; um constituinte da *Cannabis*, relacionado com o canabinol.

can·nab·i·noids (ka-nab′i-noydz). Canabinóides; substâncias orgânicas presentes na *Cannabis sativa*, que possuem várias propriedades farmacológicas.

can·na·bi·nol (ka-nab′i-nol). Canabinol; um constituinte do exsudato resinoso das flores pistiladas da *Cannabis sativa*; não possui a ação psicotomimética dos derivados tetraidro isolados da maconha.

can·na·bis (kan′ă-bis). Canábis; cânhamo; maconha; haxixe; flores secas das plantas pistiladas de *Cannabis sativa* (família Moraceae) contendo tetraidrocanabinóis isoméricos, canabinol e canabidiol. As preparações de c. são fumadas ou ingeridas por membros de várias culturas e subculturas para induzir efeitos psicotomiméticos, como euforia, alucinações, sonolência e outras alterações mentais. Antigamente, a c. era empregada como sedativo e analgésico; hoje é disponível para uso restrito no tratamento da anorexia iatrogênica, principalmente aquela associada à quimioterapia e radioterapia para processos oncológicos. Conhecida nos Estados Unidos por muitos nomes coloquiais ou gírias, como marihuana; marijuana; pot; grass; bhang; charas; ganja; hashish. [L., do G. *kannabis*, cânhamo]

can·na·bism (kan′ă-bizm). Canabismo; intoxicação por preparações de canábis.

Cannizzaro, Stanislao, químico italiano, 1826–1910. VER C. *reaction*.

Cannon, Walter B., fisiologista norte-americano, 1871–1945. VER C. *ring, theory*; C.-Bard *theory*; Bernard-C. *homeostasis*.

can·nu·la (kan′ū-lā). Cânula; tubo que pode ser introduzido em uma cavidade, geralmente por meio de um trocarte que enche sua luz; após a introdução da c., o trocarte é retirado e a c. permanece como um canal para o transporte de líquido. [L. dim. de *canna*, junco, cana]

  Hasson c., c. de Hasson; instrumento laparoscópico para instituição aberta (e não insuflação às cegas por agulha) da abertura inicial. A c. de Hasson tem um obturador de ponta romba, em vez de um trocarte cortante, com um balão na porção distal da bainha para mantê-la no lugar. SIN laparoscopic c.

  Karman c., c. de Karman; uma c. de plástico flexível usada para realizar um aborto (extração menstrual) precoce.

  laparoscopic c., c. laparoscópica. SIN Hasson c.

  perfusion c., (1) c. de perfusão; c. de tubo duplo usada para irrigação de uma cavidade: o líquido de lavagem entra na cavidade por um tubo e sai pelo outro. **(2)** c. usada para perfundir um órgão, isto é, usada para irrigar um órgão doador no preparo para transplante.

  washout c., c. de irrigação; c. que pode ser irrigada sem que seja removida da artéria.

can·nu·la·tion, can·nu·li·za·tion (kan-ū-lā′shŭn, -ū-li-zā′shŭn). Canulação; inserção de uma cânula.

Cantelli sign. Sinal de Cantelli. VER em sign.

can·thal (kan′thal). Relativo a um canto (ângulo) do olho.

can·thar·i·dal (kan-thar′i-dăl). Cantarídico; relativo a, ou que contém, cantáridas.

can·thar·i·date (kan-thar′i-dāt). Cantaridato; um sal do ácido cantarídico.

can·thar·i·des (kan-thar′i-dēz). Cantáridas; plural de cantharis.

can·thar·i·dic ac·id (kan-thar′i-dik). Ácido cantarídico; um ácido, derivado da cantárida, que forma sais (cantaridatos) com álcalis.

can·thar·i·din (kan-thar′i-din). Cantaridina; cânfora da cantárida; o princípio ativo da cantárida; o anidrido do ácido cantárico. SIN cantharis camphor.

can·tha·ris, gen. **can·thar·i·dis,** pl. **can·thar·i·des** (kan′thar-is, kan-thar′i-dis, -dēz). Cantárida; besouro seco, *Lytta (Cantharis) vesicatoria*, usado como contra-irritante e vesicatório. SIN Russian fly, Spanish fly. [L., do G. *kantharis*, besouro].

can·thec·to·my (kan-thek′tō-mē). Cantectomia; excisão de um canto (ângulo) palpebral. [G. *kanthos*, canto, + *ektomē*, excisão]

can·thi (kan′thī). Cantos; plural de canthus.

can·thi·tis (kan-thī′tis). Cantite; inflamação de um canto (ângulo) do olho.

can·thol·y·sis (kan-thol′i-sis). Cantólise. SIN canthoplasty (1). [G. *kanthos*, canto, + *lysis*, afrouxamento]

can·tho·plas·ty (kan'thō-plas-tē). Cantoplastia. **1.** Operação para alongar a fissura palpebral por incisão através do ângulo (canto) lateral. SIN cantholysis. **2.** Operação para restauração do ângulo do olho. [G. *kanthos*, canto, + *plassō*, formar]

can·thor·rha·phy (kan-thōr'ă-fē). Cantorrafia; sutura das pálpebras no canto. [G. *kanthos*, canto, + *rhaphē*, sutura]

can·thot·o·my (kan-thot'ō-mē). Cantotomia; incisão do canto. [G. *kanthos*, canto, + *tomē*, incisão]

can·thus, pl. **can·'thi** (kan'thŭs, -thī). Canto; o ângulo do olho. [G. *kanthos*, ângulo do olho]
  external c., c. externo. SIN lateral *angle* of eye.
  internal c., c. interno. SIN medial *angle* of eye.
  lateral c., c. lateral. SIN lateral *angle* of eye.
  medial c., c. medial. SIN medial *angle* of eye.

Cantor, Meyer O., médico norte-americano, *1907. VER C. *tube*.

CaOC Abreviatura de cathodal opening *contraction* (contração de abertura catódica).

CAP Abreviatura de catabolite (gene) activator *protein* [proteína ativadora de catabólito (gene)].

cap (kap). **1.** Qualquer estrutura anatômica semelhante a um capuz ou cobertura. **2.** Revestimento protetor para um dente incompleto. **3.** Coroa; coloquialismo para restauração da parte coronária de um dente natural por meio de uma coroa artificial. **4.** A estrutura nucleotídica encontrada na extremidade 5′ de muitos RNA mensageiros eucarióticos, que consiste em um resíduo 7-metilguanosina unido, via seu grupamento 5′-hidroxila, por um grupamento trifosfato ao grupamento 5′-hidroxila do primeiro nucleosídeo codificado pelo DNA; geralmente representado como $m^7G^{5'}ppp^{5'}N$, onde N é o nucleosídeo número 1 no RNAm transcrito e freqüentemente ele próprio metilado; é acrescentada após a transcrição.
  acrosomal c., c. acrossômico; capuz cefálico; vesícula membranosa colapsada que cobre a parte anterior do núcleo do espermatozóide, derivada do grânulo acrossômico; a substância rica em carboidratos do capuz está associada a enzimas hidrolíticas que ajudam o espermatozóide a penetrar na zona pelúcida do óvulo. SIN head c.
  apical c., c. apical; sombra curva no ápice de um ou de ambos os hemitórax na radiografia de tórax; causado por fibrose pleural pulmonar ou, à esquerda, por sangue proveniente de uma ruptura traumática da aorta.
  cervical c., capuz cervical; diafragma contraceptivo encaixado sobre o colo uterino.
  chin c., mentoneira; aparelho extra-oral desenhado para exercer força para cima e para trás na mandíbula mediante aplicação de pressão ao queixo, assim evitando o crescimento para a frente.
  cradle c., crosta láctea; termo coloquial para dermatite seborreica do couro cabeludo do recém-nascido, uma descamação cérea, vermelha, observada na terceira e quarta semanas de vida.
  dental c.'s, dentes molares decíduos do cavalo que permanecem presos aos dentes permanentes que estão ecloindindo.
  duodenal c., bulbo duodenal; a primeira porção do duodeno, observada em radiografia ou por fluoroscopia. SIN duodenal bulb.
  enamel c., o esmalte que cobre a coroa de um dente.
  head c., capuz cefálico. SIN acrosomal c.
  metanephric c., capuz metanéfrico; a massa concentrada de células mesodérmicas ao redor do broto metanéfrico em um embrião jovem; as células do capuz formam os túbulos uriníferos do rim permanente. SIN metanephric blastema.
  phrygian c., barrete frígio; em colecistografia, um septo incompleto ou uma prega na vesícula biliar, cujo formato lembra o barrete da liberdade da Revolução Francesa.
  pyloric c., c. pilórico; termo obsoleto para bulbo duodenal.

ca·pac·i·tance (kă-pas'i-tans). Capacitância; quantidade de carga elétrica que pode ser armazenada num corpo por unidade de potencial elétrico; expressa em farads, abfarads ou statfarads.

ca·pac·i·ta·tion (kă-pas'i-tā'shŭn). Capacitação; processo pelo qual o revestimento de glicoproteína é modificado e as proteínas seminais são removidas da superfície do espermatozóide. Não há alterações morfológicas. A c. ocorre na fertilização *in vitro*; após a c., pode haver reação acrossômica. [L. *capacitas*, de *capax*, capaz de]

ca·pac·i·tor (kă-pas'i-ter, -tōr). Capacitor, condensador; dispositivo para concentrar carga elétrica. SIN condenser (4).

ca·pac·i·ty (kă-pas'i-tē). Capacidade. **1.** Volume cúbico, cubagem; o conteúdo cúbico potencial de uma cavidade ou receptáculo. **2.** Aptidão, poder de fazer. VER TAMBÉM volume. [L. *capax*, capaz de conter; de *capio*, tomar]
  buffer c., c. tampão; quantidade de íons hidrogênio (ou íons hidroxila) necessária para produzir uma alteração específica do pH em determinado volume de um tampão. VER TAMBÉM buffer *value*.
  carrying c., c. de carga, carga máxima; estimativa do número de pessoas que uma região, uma nação ou o planeta consegue sustentar.
  cranial c., c. craniana; o conteúdo cúbico do crânio obtido mediante determinação do volume de pequenas esferas, sementes ou contas necessárias para encher o crânio.
  diffusing c. (símbolo, D, seguido por subscritos indicando a localização e a espécie química), c. de difusão; quantidade de oxigênio captada pelo sangue capilar pulmonar por minuto, por unidade de gradiente de pressão média de oxigênio entre o gás alveolar e o sangue capilar pulmonar; as unidades são: ml/min/mm Hg; também aplicada a outros gases como o monóxido de carbono, que é usado na medida clínica padrão da c. de difusão.
  forced vital c. (FVC), c. vital forçada (CVF); c. vital medida com o indivíduo expirando o mais rápido possível; dados relacionados a volume, fluxo expiratório e tempo formam a base de outras provas de função pulmonar, p. ex., curva de fluxo–volume (volufluxograma), volume expiratório forçado, tempo expiratório forçado; fluxo expiratório forçado.
  functional residual c. (FRC), c. residual funcional (CRF); o volume de gás que permanece nos pulmões ao fim de uma expiração normal; é a soma do volume de reserva expiratório e do volume residual. SIN functional residual air.
  heat c., c. térmica; quantidade de calor necessária para elevar em 1°C a temperatura de um sistema. SIN thermal c.
  inspiratory c., c. inspiratória; o volume de ar que pode ser inspirado após uma expiração normal; é a soma do volume corrente e do volume de reserva inspiratório. SIN complementary air.
  iron-binding c. (IBC), capacidade de ligação ao ferro; a c. de uma proteína de ligação do ferro no soro (transferrina) de se ligar ao ferro sérico.
  maximum breathing c. (MBC), c. ventilatória máxima (CVM). SIN maximum voluntary *ventilation*.
  oxygen c., c. de oxigênio; a quantidade máxima de oxigênio que se combinará quimicamente à hemoglobina em uma unidade de volume de sangue; normalmente é de 1,34 ml de O_2 por g de Hb ou 20 ml de O_2 por 100 ml de sangue.
  residual c., c. residual. SIN residual *volume*.
  respiratory c., c. respiratória. SIN vital c.
  thermal c., c. térmica. SIN heat c.
  total lung c. (TLC), c. pulmonar total (CPT); a c. inspiratória mais a c. residual funcional; isto é, o volume de ar contido nos pulmões ao fim de uma inspiração máxima; também é igual à c. vital mais volume residual.
  vital c. (VC), c. vital (CV); o maior volume de ar que pode ser expirado dos pulmões após uma inspiração máxima. SIN respiratory c.

cap·ac·tins (kap-ak'tinz). Capactinas; classe de proteínas que cobrem as extremidades dos filamentos de actina.

CAPD Acrônimo para continuous ambulatory peritoneal *dialysis* (diálise peritoneal ambulatorial contínua).

Capgras, Jean Marie Joseph, psiquiatra francês, 1873–1950. VER C. *phenomenon*, *syndrome*.

cap·il·lar·ec·ta·sia (kap'i-lar-ek-tā'zē-ă). Capilarectasia; termo raramente empregado para indicar dilatação dos vasos sanguíneos capilares. [capillary + G. *ektasis*, extensão]

Ca·pil·la·ria (kap'i-lā'rē-ă). Gênero de nematódeos afasmídios, caracterizados pelo aspecto filiforme; relacionado ao *Trichuris*. [L. *capillaris*, de *capillus*, cabelo]
  C. hepat'ica, espécie de nematódeos que infesta o fígado em roedores; ocasionalmente descrita em seres humanos.
  C. philippinen'sis, espécie de nematódeos que foi implicada como causa da capilaríase intestinal entre pescadores do norte das Filipinas.

ca·pil·la·ri·a·sis (kap'i-lar-ī'ă-sis). Capilaríase; doença causada por infestação por nematódeos do gênero *Capillaria*.
  intestinal c., c. intestinal; doença diarreica, semelhante ao espru, causada por infestação por *Capillaria philippinensis*, que formam grandes populações por auto-infestação interna na mucosa intestinal; caracterizada por dor abdominal, edema, diarréia, caquexia, hipoproteinemia, hipotensão, insuficiência cardíaca e hiporreflexia; a infestação grave freqüentemente se manifesta como um distúrbio fulminante que pode ser fatal.

cap·il·lar·i·o·mo·tor (kap-i-lār'ē-ō-mō'tor). Capilariomotor; vasomotor, com referência especial aos capilares.

cap·il·lar·i·os·co·py (kap'i-lar-ē-os'kō-pē). Capilarioscopia; visualização dos capilares cutâneos na base da unha dos dedos da mão pelo microscópio de pequeno aumento. SIN capillaroscopy, microangioscopy.

cap·il·lar·i·tis (kap'i-lar-ī'tis). Capilarite; inflamação de um capilar ou capilares.

cap·il·lar·i·ty (kap-i-lar'i-tē). Capilaridade; a ascensão de líquidos em tubos estreitos ou através dos poros de um material frouxo, em virtude de ação capilar.

cap·il·la·ron (kap'i-lā-ron). Módulo anatômico composto de células parenquimatosas juntamente com seus capilares sanguíneos e líquido extracapilar em uma cápsula complacente; funciona como uma unidade hidráulica que fornece uma base teórica para propor que o fluxo sanguíneo é regulado no capilar.

cap·il·la·rop·a·thy (kap'i-lă-rop'ă-thē). Capilaropatia; microangiopatia; qualquer doença dos capilares, termo freqüentemente aplicado a alterações vasculares no diabetes melito. SIN microangiopathy. [capillary + G. *pathos*, doença]

cap·il·lar·os·co·py (kap'i-lar-os'kō-pē). Capilaroscopia. SIN capillarioscopy.

cap·il·lary (kap′i-lār-ē) [TA]. Capilar. **1.** Semelhante a um fio de cabelo; fino; pequeno. **2.** Um vaso capilar; p. ex., c. sanguíneo; c. linfático. SIN vas capillare [TA], capillary vessel. **3.** Relativo a um vaso c. sanguíneo ou linfático. [L. *capillaris*, relativo ao cabelo]

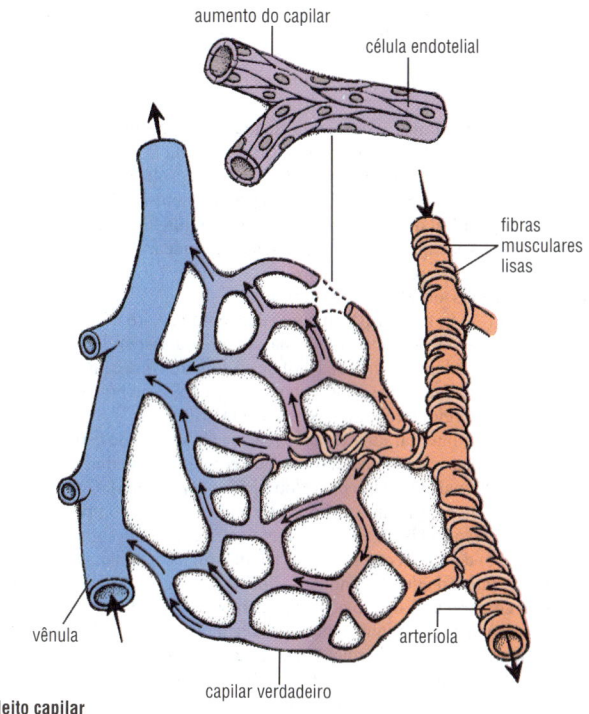

leito capilar

arterial c., c. arterial; abertura c. de uma arteríola ou metarteríola.
bile c., c. biliar. SIN biliary *canaliculus.*
blood c. (símbolo c, como subscrito), c. sanguíneo; vaso cuja parede consiste em endotélio e sua membrana basal; seu diâmetro, quando o c. está aberto, tem cerca de 8 μm; à microscopia eletrônica, podem ser distinguidos capilares fenestrados e capilares contínuos.
continuous c., c. contínuo; c. no qual há numerosas pequenas vesículas (cavéolas) e não há poros.
fenestrated c., c. fenestrado; c. encontrado nos glomérulos renais, vilosidades intestinais e glândulas endócrinas, nos quais são observados poros ultramicroscópicos de tamanhos variados; geralmente esses capilares são fechados por um delicado diafragma, por vezes ausente em alguns.
lymph c., c. linfático; o início do sistema linfático de vasos; é revestido por um endotélio altamente atenuado com membrana basal pouco desenvolvida e uma luz de calibre variável. VER lacteal (2).
sinusoidal c., c. sinusoidal. SIN sinusoid.
venous c., c. venoso; c. que se abre para uma vênula.
ca·pi·ta (kap′i-tă). Plural de caput (cabeça).
cap·i·tate (kap′i-tāt) [TA]. Capitato. **1.** O maior dos ossos carpais; localizado na fileira distal. SIN os capitatum [TA], capitate bone, magnum, os magnum. **2.** Em forma de cabeça; que possui uma extremidade arredondada. [L. *caput* (*capit-*), cabeça]
capitation (kap-i-tā′shun). Capitação; sistema de reembolso médico por meio do qual o profissional recebe um pagamento anual por paciente coberto por uma seguradora ou outra fonte financeira, cujos pagamentos somados têm por objetivo reembolsar todos os serviços prestados. [L.L. *capitatio*, de *caput*, cabeça]
cap·i·tel·lum (kap-i-tel′ŭm). Capítulo. **1.** SIN capitulum (1). **2.** *capitulum of humerus.* [L. dim. de *caput*, cabeça]
cap·i·to·ped·al (kap-i-tō-ped′ăl). Capitopodálico; relativo à cabeça e aos pés. [L. *caput*, cabeça, + *pes* (*ped-*), pé]
ca·pit·u·la (kă-pit′ū-lă). Plural de capitulum (capítulo).
ca·pit·u·lar (kă-pit′ū-lăr). Capitular; relativo a um capítulo.
ca·pit·u·lum, pl. **ca·pit·u·la** (kă-pit′ū-lŭm, -lă) [TA]. **1.** [NA]. Capítulo; pequena cabeça ou extremidade articular arredondada de um osso. SIN capitellum (1). VER TAMBÉM caput. **2.** A porção bucal sugadora de sangue, exploradora, responsável pela sensibilidade e sustentação de um carrapato, incluindo a estrutura de sustentação basal; o tamanho relativo e o formato do aparelho bucal que forma o c. são característicos dos gêneros de carrapatos rígidos. [L. dim. de *caput*, cabeça]

c. hu'meri [TA], c. do úmero. SIN c. of humerus.
c. of humerus [TA], c. do úmero; a pequena eminência arredondada na metade lateral da extremidade distal do úmero para articulação com o rádio. SIN c. humeri [TA], capitellum (2), little head of humerus.
Caplan, Anthony, médico inglês, 1907–1976. VER C. *nodules,* em nodule, syndrome.
Cap·no·cy·to·pha·ga (kap′nō-sī-tof′a-ga). Gênero de bactérias fusiformes, Gram-negativas; necessita de dióxido de carbono para crescer e move-se por deslizamento; associado à doença periodontal humana; a espécie típica é *C. ochracea* (anteriormente denominada *Bacteroides ochracea*).
C. canimor'sus, espécie de bactéria relacionada a infecções por mordidas de cachorro (incluindo bacteriemia, endocardite e meningite). Anteriormente designada DF-2 pelo CDC. Essas infecções geralmente ocorrem em pacientes com comprometimento do sistema imune.
cap·no·gram (kap′nō-gram). Capnograma; registro contínuo do teor de dióxido de carbono do ar expirado. [G. *kapnos*, fumaça, + *gramma*, algo escrito]
cap·no·graph (kap′nō-graf). Capnógrafo; instrumento pelo qual se obtém um gráfico contínuo do teor de dióxido de carbono no ar expirado.
capnometry (cap′nom-ĕ-trē). Capnometria; medida de CO_2 nas vias aéreas proximais durante a inspiração e a expiração. O CO_2 corrente final (ou CO_2 ao fim da expiração) é particularmente útil clinicamente.
cap·ping. Capeamento. **1.** Cobertura. **2.** A agregação em uma extremidade de uma célula de antígenos de superfície unidos e submetidos à ligação cruzada por anticorpos; essa cobertura é então endocitada pela célula.
direct pulp c., c. pulpar direto; procedimento para cobertura e proteção da polpa vital exposta.
indirect pulp c., c. pulpar indireto; aplicação de uma suspensão de hidróxido de cálcio a uma fina camada de dentina que recobre a polpa (quase exposta) para estimular a formação secundária de dentina e proteger a polpa.
Capps, Joseph A., médico norte-americano, 1872–1964. VER C. *reflex.*
cap·rate (kap′rāt). Caprato; um sal ou éster do ácido cáprico.
cap·re·o·my·cin sul·fate (kap′rē-ō-mī′sin). Sulfato de capreomicina; sal sulfato do antibiótico peptídio cíclico obtido do *Streptomyces capreolus*, usado no tratamento da tuberculose.
***n*-cap·ric ac·id** (kap′rik). Ácido n-cáprico; ácido graxo encontrado entre os produtos da hidrólise da gordura no leite de cabra, no leite de vaca e em outras substâncias. Cf. *n*-caproic acid, caprylic acid. SIN *n*-decanoic acid.
ca·pril·o·quism (kă-pril′ō-kwizm). Capriloquismo. SIN egophony. [L. *capter*, cabra, + *loquor*, falar]
cap·rin (kap′rin). Caprina; uma das substâncias encontradas na manteiga e da qual depende seu sabor. SIN decanoin, glyceryl tricaprate.
cap·rine (kā′prin). Caprino; relativo a cabras; semelhante a cabras. [L. *caprinus*, de cabras]
Cap·ri·pox·vi·rus (kap′ri-poks-vī′rŭs). O gênero de Poxviridae que inclui os vírus da varíola ovina e caprina. [L. *capra*, cabra, + vírus]
cap·ri·zant (kap′ri-zant). Caprizante; saltador; pulador; indica uma forma de batimento do pulso. [De, pulador, do L. *caper*, cabra]
cap·ro·ate (kap′rō-āt). Caproato. **1.** Sal ou éster do ácido n-capróico. **2.** Contração aprovada pelo USAN para hexanoato, $CH_3(CH_2)_4COO^-$.
***n*-ca·pro·ic ac·id** (kap-rō′ik). Ácido n-capróico; ácido graxo encontrado entre os produtos da hidrólise da gordura na manteiga, óleo de coco e algumas outras substâncias. SIN *n*-hexanoic acid.
cap·ro·yl (kap′rō-il). Caproíla; o radical acila do ácido capróico. SIN hexanoyl.
cap·ro·y·late (kap′rō-i-lāt). Caproilato; sal ou éster do ácido capróico. SIN hexanoate.
cap·ry·late (kap′ri-lāt). Caprilato; sal ou éster do ácido caprílico. SIN octanoate.
ca·pryl·ic ac·id (kap-ril′ik). Ácido caprílico; ácido graxo encontrado entre os produtos da hidrólise da gordura contida na manteiga, no óleo de coco e em outras substâncias. SIN octanoic acid.
cap·sa·i·cin (kap-sā′i-sin). Capsaicina; princípio alcalóide presente nos frutos de várias espécies de *Capsicum*, com os mesmos usos deste. Causa depleção da substância P das terminações nervosas sensitivas (sensoriais). Algumas vezes é usada para alívio da dor na neuralgia pós-herpética.
cap·si·cin (kap′sī-sin). Capsicina; oleorresina vermelho-amarelada que contém o princípio ativo do cápsico.
cap·si·cum (kap′si-kŭm). Cápsico; pimenta-de-caiena, africana ou vermelha, o fruto maduro seco do *Capsicum frutescens* (família Solanaceae); usado como antifisético, estimulante gastrointestinal e, externamente, como rubefaciente.
cap·sid (kap′sid). Capsídeo. VER virion.
cap·so·mer, cap·so·mere (kap′sō-mēr). Capsômero; subunidade do revestimento proteico ou capsídeo de uma partícula viral. VER TAMBÉM hexon, penton, virion.
cap·sul·a, gen. e pl. **cap·su·lae** (kap′soo-lă, -lē) [TA]. Cápsula. **1.** SIN capsule (2). [L. dim. de *capsa*, baú ou caixa]
c. adiposa perirenalis [TA], c. adiposa perirrenal. SIN paranephric *fat.*
c. adipo'sa re'nis, c. adiposa renal; gordura paranéfrica. SIN paranephric *fat.*
c. articula'ris [TA], c. articular. SIN joint *capsule.*

capsula — capsule

c. articula′ris cricoarytenoi′dea [TA], c. articular cricoaritenóidea. SIN *capsule* of cricoarytenoid joint.
c. articula′ris cricothyroi′dea [TA], c. articular cricotireóidea. SIN *capsule of cricothyroid joint.*
c. bul′bi, c. do bulbo ocular. SIN fascial *sheath* of eyeball.
c. cor′dis, pericárdio. SIN pericardium.
c. exter′na [TA], c. externa. SIN external *capsule*.
c. extre′ma [TA], c. extrema. SIN extreme *capsule*.
c. fibro′sa, c. fibrosa. SIN fibrous *capsule*.
c. fibro′sa glan′dulae thyroi′deae [TA], c. fibrosa da glândula tireóide. SIN fibrous *capsule* of thyroid gland.
c. fibro′sa per′ivascula′ris, c. fibrosa perivascular. SIN fibrous *capsule* of liver (1).
c. fibro′sa re′nis [TA], c. fibrosa do rim. SIN fibrous *capsule* of kidney.
c. glomer′uli, c. glomerular. SIN glomerular *capsule*.
c. inter′na [TA], c. interna. SIN internal *capsule*.
c. len′tis [TA], c. da lente. SIN *capsule* of lens.
c. li′enis [TA], c. do baço. SIN fibrous *capsule* of spleen.
c. vasculo′sa len′tis, c. vascular da lente; no embrião, a cápsula mesenquimal vascular que envolve a lente do olho; os vasos da parte profunda da cápsula são ramos da artéria hialóide; aqueles da parte superficial são derivados das artérias ciliares anteriores; normalmente todos os vasos estão atrofiados no final do oitavo mês de vida intra-uterina.
cap·su·lar (kap′soo-lăr). Capsular; relativo a qualquer cápsula.
cap·su·la·tion (kap-soo-lā′shŭn). Encapsulação; encerramento em uma cápsula.
cap·sule (kap′sool) [TA]. Cápsula. **1.** Estrutura membranosa, geralmente tecido conjuntivo colagenoso denso, que envolve um órgão, uma articulação ou qualquer outra parte. **2.** Estrutura anatômica semelhante a uma cápsula ou envelope. SIN capsula (1) [TA]. **3.** Camada de tecido fibroso envolvendo um órgão ou tumor, principalmente se benigno. **4.** Forma de apresentação sólida na qual o medicamento está encerrado em um recipiente solúvel, duro ou flexível, ou "revestimento" de uma forma adequada de gelatina. **5.** Revestimento hialino de polissacarídios em torno de uma célula fúngica ou bacteriana. As bactérias também podem ter uma c. polipeptídica ou uma camada viscosa ao redor da célula. [L. *capsula*, dim. de *capsa*, caixa]
adipose c., c. adiposa. SIN paranephric *fat*.
adrenal c., glândula supra-renal. SIN suprarenal *gland*.
articular c., c. articular; *termo oficial alternativo para joint c.
atrabiliary c., c. supra-renal. SIN suprarenal *gland*.
auditory c., c. auditiva. SIN otic c.
bacterial c., c. bacteriana; camada viscosa de composição variável que cobre a superfície de algumas bactérias; células encapsuladas de bactérias patogênicas geralmente são mais virulentas que células sem cápsulas porque as primeiras são mais resistentes à ação fagocítica.
Bonnet c., c. de Bonnet; a parte anterior dos bulbos vaginais.
Bowman c., c. de Bowman. SIN glomerular c.
brood c.'s, pequenas projeções ocas da membrana de revestimento de um cisto hidático de onde se originam os escólices.
cartilage c., c. cartilaginosa; a matriz mais intensamente basófila e metacromática na cartilagem hialina que circunda as lacunas de condrócitos, resultante de concentrações relativamente altas de proteínas condromuco. SIN territorial matrix.
cricoarytenoid articular c., c. articular cricoaritenóide. SIN c. of cricoarytenoid joint.
c. of cricoarytenoid joint [TA], c. da articulação cricoaritenóide; a cápsula que encerra a articulação entre as cartilagens aritenóide e cricóide. SIN capsula articularis cricoarytenoidea [TA], cricoarytenoid articular c.
cricothyroid articular c., c. articular cricotireóidea. SIN c. of cricothyroid joint.
c. of crycothyroid joint [TA], c. da articulação cricotireóidea; a cápsula que encerra a articulação cricotireóidea. SIN capsula articularis cricothyroidea [TA], cricothyroid articular c.
Crosby c., c. de Crosby; uma fixação à extremidade de um tubo flexível, usada para biópsia peroral do intestino delgado, pela qual se aspira um fragmento de mucosa através de uma abertura na cápsula, cortando-a em seguida.
crystalline c., c. do cristalino. SIN c. of lens.
external c. [TA], c. externa; uma lâmina fina de substância branca que separa o claustro do putâmen. Une-se à cápsula interna em uma das extremidades do putâmen, formando uma cápsula de substância branca externa ao núcleo lenticular. SIN capsula externa [TA], periclaustral lamina.
extreme c. [TA], c. extrema; camada de substância branca que separa o claustro do córtex da ínsula, provavelmente representando, em grande parte, as fibras corticípetas e corticífugas do córtex insular. SIN capsula extrema [TA].
eye c., c. do bulbo ocular. SIN fascial *sheath* of eyeball.
fatty renal c., c. gordurosa renal. SIN paranephric *fat*.
fibrous c. [TA], c. fibrosa; qualquer revestimento fibroso de um órgão. SIN capsula fibrosa de um órgão. SIN stratum fibrosum [TA], tunica fibrosa [TA], capsula fibrosa, stratum fibrosum capsulae articularis.
fibrous articular c., c. articular fibrosa. SIN fibrous *layer* of joint capsule.

fibrous c. of kidney [TA], c. fibrosa do rim; uma membrana fibrosa que envolve o rim. SIN capsula fibrosa renis [TA], tunica fibrosa renis.
fibrous c. of liver [TA], c. fibrosa do fígado; **(1)** uma camada de tecido conjuntivo que cobre a superfície externa do fígado e também a artéria hepática, veia porta e ductos biliares quando estes se ramificam no fígado; SIN capsula fibrosa perivascularis, perivascular fibrous c. **(2)** cápsula de tecido conjuntivo que circunda a superfície externa do fígado, mas é contínua com septos em alguns animais, como, por exemplo, o porco, que divide o parênquima em lóbulos, e com a cápsula fibrosa perivascular na porta hepática. SIN tunica fibrosa hepatis [TA], Glisson c.
fibrous c. of parotid gland, c. fibrosa da glândula parótida. SIN parotid *fascia*.
fibrous c. of spleen [TA], c. fibrosa do baço; a cápsula fibrosa do baço, que contém colágeno, fibras elásticas e músculo liso. SIN capsula lienis [TA], tunica fibrosa splenis*, tunica fibrosa lienis, tunica propria lienis.
fibrous c. of thyroid gland [TA], c. fibrosa da glândula tireóide; a bainha fibrosa da tireóide. SIN capsula fibrosa glandulae thyroideae [TA].
Gerota c., c. de Gerota. SIN renal *fascia*.
Glisson c., c. de Glisson. SIN fibrous c. of liver (2).
glomerular c. [TA], c. glomerular; o início expandido de um néfron composto de uma camada interna e uma externa; a camada visceral consiste em podócitos que circundam um tufo de capilares (glomérulo); a camada parietal consiste em epitélio escamoso simples que se torna cúbico no pólo tubular. SIN Bowman c., capsula glomeruli, malpighian c. (1), Müller c.
internal c. [TA], c. interna; uma camada maciça (8-10 mm de espessura) de substância branca separando o núcleo caudado e o tálamo (medial) do núcleo lentiforme situado mais lateralmente (globo pálido e putâmen). Consiste em: 1) fibras ascendentes do tálamo até o córtex cerebral, que compõem, entre outras, as radiações visuais, auditivas e sensitivas (sensoriais) somáticas, e 2) fibras que descem do córtex cerebral até o tálamo, região subtalâmica, mesencéfalo, metencéfalo e medula espinhal. A cápsula interna é a principal via pela qual o córtex cerebral está ligado ao tronco cerebral e à medula espinhal. Lateral e superiormente, é contínua com a coroa radiada, que forma uma grande parte da substância branca do hemisfério cerebral; caudal e medialmente, contínua, com tamanho muito reduzido, como a base do pedúnculo cerebral, que contém, entre outras, fibras corticoespinhais. Ao corte horizontal, aparece na forma de um V que se abre lateralmente; o ângulo obtuso do V é denominado joelho (*genu*); seus ramos anterior e posterior são, respectivamente, a base anterior do pedúnculo e a base posterior do pedúnculo. A cápsula interna consiste em um ramo anterior [TA], joelho da cápsula interna [TA], ramo posterior [TA], ramo retrolentiforme (ou retrolenticular) [TA] e ramo sublentiforme (ou sublenticular) [TA]. SIN capsula interna [TA].
joint c. [TA], c. articular; bolsa que envolve as extremidades articulares dos ossos que compõem uma articulação sinovial, formada por uma cápsula articular fibrosa externa e uma membrana sinovial interna. SIN capsula articularis [TA], articular c.*
lens c., c. do cristalino. SIN c. of lens.

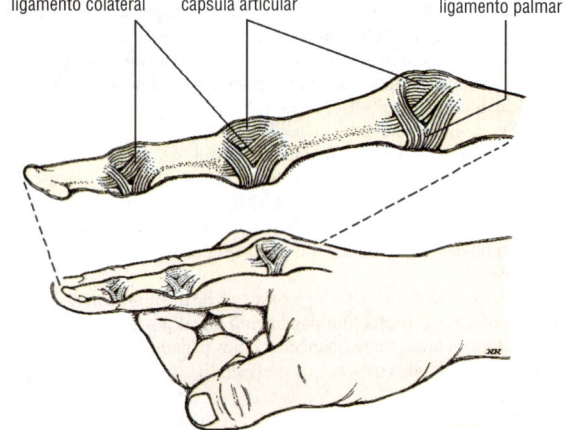

cápsulas interfalângicas: e ligamentos colaterais e palmares associados

c. of lens [TA], c. do cristalino; a cápsula que encerra o cristalino do olho. SIN capsula lentis [TA], crystalline c., lens c., lenticular c., phacocyst.
lenticular c., c. do cristalino. SIN c. of lens.
malpighian c., c. de Malpighi, **(1)** SIN glomerular c.; **(2)** membrana fibrosa fina envolvendo o baço e contínua sobre os vasos que entram no hilo.
Müller c., c. de Müller. SIN glomerular c.
nasal c., c. nasal; a cartilagem ao redor da cavidade nasal em desenvolvimento do embrião.

optic c., c. óptica; a zona concentrada de mesênquima ao redor do cálice óptico em desenvolvimento; primórdio da esclerótica do olho.
otic c., c. ótica; a cápsula cartilaginosa que circunda o mecanismo do ouvido interno; em elasmobrânquios, permanece cartilaginosa no adulto; nos embriões de vertebrados superiores, é cartilaginosa no início, mas depois torna-se óssea (com aproximadamente 23 semanas em seres humanos). SIN auditory c.
perirenal fat c., c. de gordura perirrenal. SIN paranephric fat.
perivascular fibrous c., c. fibrosa perivascular. SIN fibrous c. of liver (1).
radiotelemetering c., c. radiotelemétrica; radiopílula; instrumento que transmite medidas por impulsos de rádio do interior do corpo; p. ex., medidas de pressão do intestino delgado. SIN radiopill.
seminal c., c. seminal. SIN seminal gland.
suprarenal c., c. supra-renal. SIN suprarenal gland.
Tenon c., c. de Tenon. SIN fascial sheath of eyeball.
cap·sul·ec·to·my· Capsulectomia; remoção de uma cápsula, como a situada ao redor de um implante ou tecido fibrosado.
cap·su·li·tis (kap'soo-lī'tis). Capsulite; inflamação da cápsula de um órgão ou parte, como do fígado, do cristalino, ou que circunda uma articulação.
adhesive c., c. adesiva; condição na qual há limitação do movimento em uma articulação devido ao espessamento inflamatório da cápsula; uma causa comum de rigidez no ombro. SIN frozen shoulder.
hepatic c., c. hepática. SIN perihepatitis.
cap·su·lo·len·tic·u·lar (kap'sŏ-lō-len-tik'ū-lăr). Capsulolenticular; referente ao cristalino e à sua cápsula.
cap·su·lo·plas·ty (kap'sŏo-lō-plas-tē). Capsuloplastia; rearranjo da parede de uma cápsula; freqüentemente uma cápsula articular. [L. *capsula*, cápsula, + G. *plastos*, formado]
cap·su·lor·rha·phy (kap-soo-lōr'ă-fē). Capsulorrafia; sutura de uma laceração ou incisão cirúrgica em qualquer cápsula; especificamente, sutura de uma cápsula articular para evitar luxação recorrente da articulação. [L. *capsula*, cápsula, + *rhaphē*, sutura]
capsulorrhexis (kap-soo-lō-reks'sis). Capsulorrexe; técnica usada na cirurgia de catarata, na qual é feita uma incisão circular contínua na cápsula anterior do cristalino. [L. *capsula*, cápsula, + G. *rhēxis*, ruptura]
cap·su·lo·tome (kap'sŏo-lō-tōm). Capsulótomo. SIN cystotome (2).
cap·su·lot·o·my (kap-soo-lot'ō-mē). Capsulotomia. **1.** Divisão de uma cápsula como ao redor de um implante mamário. **2.** Criação de uma abertura através de uma cápsula; p. ex., de uma cicatriz fibrótica que poderia se formar em torno de um corpo estranho. **3.** Incisão da cápsula do cristalino na cirurgia extracapsular da catarata. [L. *capsula*, cápsula, + G. *tomē*, corte]
renal c., c. renal; incisão da cápsula renal.
cap·to·pril (kap'tō-pril). Captopril; um inibidor da enzima de conversão da angiotensina usado no tratamento da hipertensão arterial e da insuficiência cardíaca congestiva.
cap·ture (kap'choor). Captura; captura e manutenção de uma partícula ou um impulso elétrico originado em outra parte. [L. *capio*, pp. *-tus*, capturar, tomar]
atrial c., c. atrial; controle dos átrios por um ou mais batimentos após um período de batimento independente, como no bloqueio AV incompleto ou nas extra-sístoles juncionais ou ventriculares ou taquicardias por um impulso retrógrado.
electron c., c. do elétron; uma forma de desintegração radioativa, na qual um elétron orbital, geralmente na camada K, é capturado pelo núcleo, convertendo-do um próton em um nêutron com ejeção de um neutrino e emissão de um raio gama, e emissão de raios X característicos quando o elétron que falta na camada K é substituído. SIN K c.
K c., c. K. SIN electron c.
ventricular c., c. ventricular; captura do(s) ventrículo(s) por um impulso originado nos átrios ou na junção A-V.
Capuron, Joseph, médico francês, 1767–1850. VER C. points, em *point*.
ca·put, gen. **ca·pi·tis,** pl. **ca·pi·ta** (kap'ut, ka'put; kap'i-tis; kap'ī-tă). [TA]. Cabeça. [TA] SIN head. [L.]
c. angula're quadra'ti la'bii superio'ris, músculo levantador do lábio superior e da asa do nariz. SIN levator labii superioris alaeque nasi (*muscle*).
c. bre've [TA], a cabeça do músculo mais próxima da inserção, no caso de músculos com duas origens. SIN short head.
c. breve musculi bicipitis brachii [TA], c. curta do músculo bíceps braquial. SIN short head of biceps brachii.
c. breve musculi bicipitis fem'oris [TA], c. curta do músculo bíceps femoral. SIN short head of biceps femoris.
c. cos'tae [TA], c. da costela. SIN head of rib.
c. epididymid'is [TA], c. do epidídimo. SIN head of epididymis.
c. fem'oris [TA], c. do fêmur. SIN head of femur.
c. fib'ulae [TA], c. da fíbula. SIN head of fibula.
c. gallinaginis, designação obsoleta de colículo seminal (seminal *colliculus*). [L. Mod. cabeça de narceja]
c. humera'le [TA], c. do úmero. SIN humeral head.
c. humerale musculi flexoris carpi ulnaris, c. umeral do músculo flexor ulnar do carpo. VER humeral head.
c. humerale musculi pronatoris teretis, c. umeral do músculo redondo pronador. VER humeral head.
c. hu'meri [TA], c. do úmero. SIN head of humerus.
c. humeroulna're musculi flexoris digitorum superficialis [TA], c. umeroulnar do músculo flexor superficial dos dedos. SIN humeroulnar head of flexor digitorum superficialis muscle.
c. infraorbita'le quadra'ti la'bii superio'ris, c. infra-orbital do quadrado superior do lábio. SIN levator labii superioris (*muscle*).
c. latera'le [TA], c. lateral. SIN lateral head.
c. laterale musculi gastrocnemii, c. lateral do músculo gastrocnêmio. VER lateral head.
c. laterale musculi tricipitis brachii, c. lateral do músculo tríceps braquial. VER lateral head.
c. long'um [TA], c. longa. SIN long head.
c. longum musculi bicipitis brachii, c. longa do músculo bíceps braquial. VER long head.
c. longum musculi bicipitis fem'oris, c. longa do músculo bíceps femoral. VER long head.
c. longum musculi tricipitis brachii, c. longa do músculo tríceps braquial. VER long head.
c. mal'lei [TA], c. do martelo. SIN head of malleus.
c. mandib'ulae [TA], c. da mandíbula. SIN head of mandible.
c. media'le [TA], c. medial. SIN medial head.
c. mediale musculi gastrocnemii, c. medial do músculo gastrocnêmio. VER medial head.
c. mediale musculi tricipitis brachii, c. medial do músculo tríceps braquial. VER medial head.
c. medu'sae, c. de medusa; (1) veias varicosas que se irradiam do umbigo, observadas na síndrome de Cruveilhier-Baumgarten; (2) artérias ciliares dilatadas envolvendo o limbo corneoesclerótico na rubeose irídica. SIN Medusa head. [*Medusa*, G. personagem mitológico]
c. nu'clei cauda'ti [TA], c. do núcleo caudado. SIN head of caudate nucleus.
c. obli'quum [TA], c. oblíqua. SIN oblique head.
c. obliquum musculi adductoris hallucis, c. oblíqua do músculo adutor do hálux. VER oblique head.
c. obliquum musculi adductoris pollicis, c. oblíqua do músculo adutor do polegar. VER oblique head.
c. os'sis fem'oris, c. do fêmur. SIN head of femur.
c. os'sis metacarpa'lis [TA], c. do osso metacarpal. SIN head of metacarpal.
c. os'sis metatarsa'lis [TA], c. do osso metatarsal. SIN head of metatarsal.
c. pancrea'tis [TA], c. do pâncreas. SIN head of pancreas.
c. phalan'gis (manus et pedis) [TA], c. da falange (mão e pé). SIN head of phalanx (of hand or foot).
c. profun'dum musculi flexoris pollicis brevis [TA], c. profunda do músculo flexor curto do polegar. SIN deep head of flexor pollicis brevis.
c. quadra'tum, c. quadrada; c. grande e de formato quadrado, devido ao espessamento das eminências parietal e frontal, observada em crianças raquíticas.
c. ra'dii [TA], c. do rádio. SIN head of radius.
c. stape'dis [TA], c. do estribo. SIN head of stapes.
c. succeda'neum, bossa serosa; tumefação edematosa formada na porção de apresentação do couro cabeludo de um feto durante o parto; o derrame recobre o periósteo e consiste em edema; ao contrário do cefaloematoma, no qual o derrame se localiza sob o periósteo e consiste em sangue.
c. superficia'le musculi flexoris pollicis brevis [TA], c. superficial do músculo flexor curto do polegar. SIN superficial head of flexor pollicis brevis.

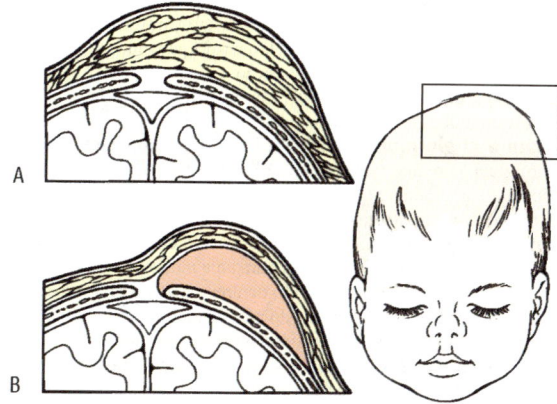

bossa serosa (A) e **cefalematoma** (B): na bossa serosa, o edema entre o crânio e o couro cabeludo atravessa a linha de sutura; no cefalematoma, a hemorragia subperiosteal pára na linha de sutura

c. ta'li [TA], c. do tálus. SIN head of talus.
c. transver'sum [TA], c. transversa. SIN transverse head.
c. transversum musculi adductoris hallucis, c. transversa do músculo adutor do hálux. VER transverse head.
c. transversum musculi adductoris pollicis, c. transversa do músculo adutor do polegar. VER transverse head.
c. ul'nae [TA], c. da ulna. SIN head of ulna.
c. ulna're [TA], c. ulnar. SIN ulnar head.
c. ulnare musculi flexoris carpi ulnaris, c. ulnar do músculo flexor ulnar do carpo. VER ulnar head.
c. ulnare musculi pronatoris teretis, c. ulnar do músculo redondo pronador. VER ulnar head.
c. zygomat'icum quadra'ti la'bii superio'ris, c. zigomática do quadrado do lábio superior. SIN zygomaticus minor (muscle).
Carabelli, Georg (Edler von Lunkaszprie), dentista austríaco, 1787–1842. VER cusp of C.; C. tubercle.
car·a·mel (kar'ă-mel). Caramelo; açúcar queimado; solução concentrada da substância obtida pelo aquecimento do açúcar com um álcali; um líquido marrom-escuro, espesso, usado como corante e aromatizante em medicamentos e alimentos. [Esp., do L.L. calamellus, do L. calamus, cana]
ca·ram·i·phen eth·ane·di·sul·fo·nate (ka-ram'i-fen eth'ān-dī-sŭl'fō-nāt). Etanodissulfonato de caramifeno; antitussígeno.
ca·ram·i·phen hy·dro·chlo·ride. Cloridrato de caramifeno; espasmolítico sintético; usado no tratamento de doenças dos gânglios da base, p. ex., doença de Parkinson e degeneração hepatolenticular.
ca·ra·te (kă-rah'tĕ). Carate, caraté, mal-da-pinta. SIN pinta.
carb-, carbo-. Prefixos que indicam carbono, principalmente a fixação de um grupamento contendo um átomo de carbono. [L. carbo, carvão]
car·ba·chol (kar'bă-kol). Carbacol; parassimpático usado localmente no olho para tratamento do glaucoma.
car·ba·dox (kar'bă-doks). Carbadox; agente antibacteriano.
car·ba·mate (kar'bă-māt). Carbamato. **1.** Sal ou éster do ácido carbâmico que constitui a base de hipnóticos uretano. **2.** Grupo de inseticidas inibidores da colinesterase semelhantes aos organofosforados; o carbamato mais freqüente é o carbaril. SIN carbamoate, carbaril.
c. kinase, c. cinase; fosfotransferase que catalisa a reação do fosfato de carbamoil e ADP para formar ATP, NH_3 e CO_2.
car·bam·az·e·pine (kar-bam-az'ē-pēn). Carbamazepina; anticonvulsivante; também usado no alívio da dor na neuralgia do trigêmeo e de outras síndromes dolorosas neurogênicas.
car·bam·ic ac·id (kar-bam'ik). Ácido carbâmico; um ácido hipotético, NH_2-COOH, que forma carbamatos; o radical acil é o carbamoil.
car·bam·ide (kar'bă-mīd). Carbamida; designação obsoleta da uréia.
carb·a·mi·no·he·mo·glo·bin (kar-bam'i-nō-hē-mō-glō'bin). Carbaminoemoglobina; dióxido de carbono ligado à hemoglobina por meio de um grupamento amino reativo da última, isto é, Hb-NHCOOH; aproximadamente 20% do conteúdo total de dióxido de carbono no sangue está associados à hemoglobina dessa forma. SIN carbhemoglobin, carbohemoglobin.
car·ba·moate (kar'bă-mōt). Carbamoato. SIN carbamate.
car·bam·o·yl (kar'bă-mō-il). Carbamoil; o radical acil, NH_2-CO-, cuja transferência desempenha um papel importante em determinadas reações bioquímicas; p. ex., no ciclo da uréia, através do fosfato de carbamoil.
car·bam·o·yl·as·par·tate de·hy·drase (kar'bă-mō-il-as-par'tāt). Carbamoilaspartato desidrase. SIN dihydro-orotase.
***N*-car·bam·o·yl·as·par·tic acid** (kar'bă-mō-il-as-par'tik). Ácido *N*-carbamoilaspártico. SIN ureidosuccinic acid.
car·bam·o·yl·a·tion (kar-bă-mō-il-ā'shŭn). Carbamoilação; transferência do carbamoil de uma molécula contendo carbamoil (p. ex., fosfato de carbamoil) para uma porção aceptora como um grupamento amino; a segunda etapa no ciclo da uréia é uma carbamoilação.
car·bam·o·yl·car·bam·ic ac·id (kar'bă-mō-il-kar-bam'ik). Ácido carbamoilcarbâmico. SIN allophanic acid.
***N*-car·bam·o·yl·glu·tam·ic ac·id** (kar'bă-mō-il-gloo-tam'ik). Ácido *N*-carbamoilglutâmico; intermediário na carbamoilação da ornitina em citrulina no ciclo da uréia; usado no tratamento de pessoas com deficiência da enzima que sintetiza *N*-acetilglutamato.
car·bam·o·yl phos·phate. Carbamoil fosfato; intermediário reativo capaz de transferir seu grupamento carbamoil para uma molécula aceptora, formando citrulina a partir da ornitina no ciclo da uréia, e ácido ureidossuccínico a partir do ácido aspártico na formação do anel pirimidina.
c. p. synthetase, carbamoil fosfato sintetase; fosfotransferase que catalisa a formação de carbamoil fosfato. Há duas isozimas significativas. A carbamoil fosfato sintetase I é uma enzima mitocondrial que catalisa a reação de 2ATP, NH_3, CO_2 e H_2O em carbamoil fosfato, 2ADP e ortofosfato. É ativada pelo *N*-acetilglutamato e participa da biossíntese da uréia. A deficiência de carbamoil fosfato sintetase I pode resultar em hiperamonemia. A carbamoil fosfato sintetase II é uma enzima do citosol que, em condições fisiológicas, usa L-glutamina como fonte de nitrogênio (produzindo L-glutamato) em vez do NH_3, não é ativada pelo *N*-acetilglutamato e participa da biossíntese da pirimidina.
car·bam·o·yl·trans·fer·as·es (kar'bă-mō-il-trans'fer-ās-ez). [EC 2.1.3.x]. Carbamoiltransferases; enzimas que transferem os grupamentos carbamoil de uma substância para outra (p. ex., aspartato carbamoiltransferase, ornitina carbamoiltransferase). SIN transcarbamoylases.
car·bam·o·yl·u·rea (kar'bă-mō-il-ū-rē'ă). Carbamoiluréia. SIN biuret.
car·ba·myl (kar'bă-mil). Carbamoil; grafia antiga de carbamoyl.
car·ba·myl·a·tion (kar'bă-mil-ā'shŭn). Carbamilação; grafia antiga de carbamoylation.
carb·an·i·on (karb-an'ī-on). Carbaníon; um ânion orgânico no qual a carga negativa se encontra num átomo de carbono; os nomes específicos são formados pelo acréscimo de -ida, -diida, etc., ao nome da substância original; p. ex., metanida, $(CH_3)^-$.
car·ba·pe·nems. Carbapenêmicos; uma classe de antibióticos β-lactâmicos bactericidas de amplo espectro que se ligam à proteína 2 de ligação à penicilina e assim interferem com a estrutura da parede celular; são muito resistentes às β-lactamases e penetram facilmente nas paredes bacterianas.
car·bar·il (car-bar-il'). Carbaril. SIN carbamate.
car·bar·sone (kar-bar'sōn). Carbarsona; um amebicida.
car·bar·yl (kar'bă-ril). Carbaril; inseticida de contato inibidor da colinesterase. Um pediculicida e ectoparasiticida. Tóxico para os seres humanos, causando náuseas, vômitos, diarréia, broncoconstrição, borramento visual, salivação excessiva, espasmos musculares, cianose, convulsões, coma, insuficiência respiratória.
car·ba·zides (kar'bă-zīdz). Carbazidas; 1,3-diaminouréias. SIN carbohydrazides.
car·baz·o·chrome sa·lic·y·late (kar-baz'ō-krōm). Salicilato de carbazocromo; produto da oxidação da epinefrina usado no controle sistêmico do sangramento capilar associado ao aumento da permeabilidade capilar.
car·ba·zole (kar'bă-zōl). Carbazol; reage com carboidratos (incluindo uronatos e desoxipentoses) produzindo cores características do tipo de açúcar; usado para ensaio e análise de carboidratos e formaldeído, e como corante intermediário; sensível à luz ultravioleta. SIN 9-azafluorene, diphenylenimine.
carb·a·zot·ic ac·id (kar-bă-zot'ik). Ácido carbazótico. SIN picric acid.
car·ben·i·cil·lin di·so·di·um (kar-ben-i-sil'in). Carbenicilina dissódica; penicilina semi-sintética de espectro ampliado ativa contra várias bactérias Gram-positivas e Gram-negativas.
car·be·ni·um (kar-ben'ē-ŭm). Carbênio. VER carbonium.
car·be·ta·pen·tane cit·rate (kar'be-tă-pen'tăn). Citrato de carbetapentano; possui ações semelhantes às da atropina e anestésica local e suprime efetivamente a tosse aguda causada por infecções comuns das vias respiratórias superiores.
carb·he·mo·glo·bin (karb'hē-mō-glō'bin). Carboemoglobina. SIN carbaminohemoglobin.
car·bide (kar'bīd). Carboneto, carbureto; composto de carbono com um elemento mais eletropositivo do que ele próprio; p. ex., CaC_2, carboneto de cálcio.
car·bi·do·pa (kar-bi-dō'pă). Carbidopa; um inibidor da dopa descarboxilase que não entra no cérebro usado em conjunto com a levodopa no tratamento da doença de Parkinson para reduzir as doses de L-dopa e os efeitos colaterais.
car·bi·ma·zole (kar-bī'mă-zōl). Carbimazol; usado no tratamento do hipertireoidismo.
car·bi·nol (kar'bi-nol). Carbinol. SIN methyl alcohol.
car·bi·nox·a·mine ma·le·ate (kar-bi-nok'să-mēn). Maleato de carbinoxamina; anti-histamínico.
car·bo. Carvão. SIN charcoal. [L. carvão].
carbo-. VER carb-.
car·bo·ben·zoxy- (Z, Cbz) (kar'bō-ben-zok'sē). Carbobenzoxi. SIN benzyloxycarbonyl.
car·bo·cat·i·on (kar-bō-kat'ī-on). Carbocátion. VER carbonium.
car·bo·gen (kar'bō-jen). Carbogênio; uma mistura de 10% de dióxido de carbono e 90% de oxigênio usada em terapia inalatória a fim de produzir vasodilatação. [carbon dioxide + oxygen]
car·bo·he·mo·glo·bin (kar'bō-hē-mō-glō'bin). Carboemoglobina. SIN carbaminohemoglobin.
car·bo·hy·drates (kar-bō-hī'drāts). Carboidratos; designação da classe dos derivados aldeídicos ou cetônicos de álcoois poliídricos; o nome deriva do fato de que os exemplos mais comuns dessas substâncias têm fórmulas que podem ser escritas da seguinte forma: $C_n(H_2O)_n$ (p. ex., glicose, $C_6(H_2O)_6$; sacarose, $C_{12}(H_2O)_{11}$), embora não sejam hidratos verdadeiros e o nome seja, dessa forma, errôneo. O grupo inclui substâncias com moléculas relativamente pequenas, como os açúcares simples (monossacarídios, dissacarídios etc.), bem como substâncias macromoleculares (poliméricas) como amido, glicogênio e celulose. Os carboidratos mais típicos da classe contêm apenas carbono, hidrogênio e oxigênio, mas intermediários metabólicos dos carboidratos nos tecidos também contêm fósforo. VER saccharides.

car·bo·hy·drat·u·ria (kar′bō - hī - drā - too′rē - ā). Carboidratúria; termo genérico que designa a excreção de um ou mais carboidratos na urina (p. ex., glicose, galactose, lactose, pentose), assim incluindo condições como glicosúria (melitúria), galactosúria, lactosúria, pentosúria etc.

car·bo·hy·dra·zides (kar - bō - hī′drā - zīdz). Carboidrazidas. SIN carbazides.

car·bo·late (kar′bō - lāt). **1.** Carbólico, fênico. SIN phenate. **2.** Carbolizar.

car·bo·lat·ed (kar′bō - lā - ted). Carbolizado. SIN phenolated.

car·bol·fuch·sin (kar′bol-fuk′sin). Carbolfucsina. **1.** VER Ziehl *stain*. **2.** VER carbol-fuchsin *paint*.

car·bol·ic ac·id (kar-bol′ik). Ácido carbólico. SIN phenol.

car·bo·lize (kar′bō - līz). Carbolizar; misturar com ou acrescentar ácido carbólico (fenol).

car·bo·lu·ria (kar - bō - loo′rē - ā). Carbolúria; a presença de fenol (ácido carbólico) na urina. [carbolic acid + G. *ouron*, urina]

car·bo·mer (kar′bō - mer). Carbômero; um polímero de ácido acrílico que faz ligação cruzada com um composto polifuncional, portanto, um poli (ácido acrílico) ou poliacrilato; um agente suspensor para medicamentos.

car·bom·e·try (kar - bom′e - trē). Carbometria. SIN carbonometry.

car·bo·my·cin (kar′bō - mī′sin). Carbomicina; antibiótico macrolídeo isolado do *Streptomyces halstedii*; semelhante à eritromicina e usado como antibacteriano e antimicrobiano.

car·bon (C) (kar′bŏn). Carbono; elemento tetravalente, não-metálico, de n.° atômico 6, peso atômico 12,011; o principal bioelemento. Possui dois isótopos naturais, C^{12} e C^{13} (o primeiro, estabelecido em 12,00000, sendo o padrão para todos os pesos moleculares), e dois isótopos artificiais, radioativos, de interesse, C^{11} e C^{14}. O elemento ocorre em três formas puras (diamante, grafite e nos fulerenos), na forma amorfa (no carvão, coque e fuligem) e na atmosfera como CO_2. Seus compostos são encontrados em todos os tecidos vivos, e o estudo de seu grande número de compostos constitui a maior parte da química orgânica. [L. *carbo*, carvão]

active c. dioxide, activated c. dioxide, dióxido de c. ativo, dióxido de c. ativado; complexo de *N*-carboxibiotina (biotina + CO_2) e uma enzima; a forma na qual o dióxido de c. é adicionado às outras moléculas nas carboxilações; p. ex., à metilcrotonil-CoA para formar β-metilglutaconil no catabolismo da leucina, e à acetil-CoA para formar malonil-CoA. VER TAMBÉM *acetyl-CoA* carboxylase.

anomeric c., c. anômero; o c. redutor de um açúcar; C-1 de uma aldose, C-2 de uma 2-cetose.

c. bisulfide, bissulfeto de c. SIN disulfide.

c. dichloride, dicloreto de c. SIN tetrachlorethylene.

c. dioxide, dióxido de c.; CO_2; o produto da combustão do c. com um excesso de ar; em concentração não inferior a 99,0% por volume de CO_2, é usado como estimulante respiratório. SIN carbonic acid gas, carbonic anhydride.

c. dioxide snow, neve carbônica; dióxido de c. sólido usado no tratamento de verrugas, lúpus, nevos e outras afecções cutâneas e como refrigerante. SIN dry ice.

c. disulfide, dissulfeto de c.; líquido tóxico, incolor, extremamente inflamável (ponto de inflamação −30°C) com odor etéreo característico (fétido quando impuro); é parasiticida. SIN c. bisulfide.

c. monoxide (CO), monóxido de c. (CO); gás incolor, praticamente inodoro e venenoso, formado pela combustão incompleta do c.; sua ação tóxica é devida à sua forte afinidade por hemoglobina, mioglobina e citocromos, reduzindo o transporte de oxigênio e bloqueando a utilização deste.

c. tetrachloride, tetracloreto de c.; líquido móvel, incolor, que possui odor etéreo característico semelhante ao do clorofórmio; é usado como líquido de limpeza e como extintor de incêndios, e tem sido usado como anti-helmíntico, principalmente contra anciióstomo. SIN tetrachloromethane.

car·bon-11 (^{11}C). Carbono-11 (C^{11}); radioisótopo do carbono produzido por ciclotron, emissor de pósitrons, com uma meia-vida de 20,3 minutos; usado na tomografia por emissão de pósitrons (PET).

car·bon-12 (^{12}C). Carbono-12 (C^{12}); o padrão de massa atômica, 98,90% do carbono natural.

car·bon-13 (^{13}C). Carbono-13 (C^{13}); isótopo natural estável, 1,1% do carbono natural.

car·bon-14 (^{14}C). Carbono-14 (C^{14}); β-emissor com uma meia-vida de 5.715 anos, amplamente usado como marcador no estudo de vários aspectos do metabolismo; o C^{14} de ocorrência natural, formado em decorrência do impacto de raios cósmicos, é usado para determinar a idade de relíquias que contêm materiais carbonáceos naturais.

car·bon·ate (kar′bŏn - āt). Carbonato. **1.** Sal do ácido carbônico. **2.** O íon CO_3^{2-}.

c. dehydratase, c. desidratase. SIN carbonic *anhydrase*.

c. hydro-lyase, c. hidroliase. SIN carbonic *anhydrase*.

car·bon·ic (kar-bon′ik). Carbônico; relativo ao carbono. Ver também em carbonate.

car·bon·ic ac·id. Ácido carbônico; H_2CO_3, formado a partir de H_2O e CO_2.

car·bon·ic an·hy·dride. Anidrido carbônico. SIN *carbon* dioxide.

car·bo·ni·um (kar - bŏn′e - ŭm). Carbônio; cátion orgânico no qual a carga positiva está localizada em um átomo de carbono; p. ex., $(CH_3)^+$. Atualmente recomenda-se o uso de carbocátion como nome da classe e de carbênio em nomes de compostos específicos.

car·bo·nom·e·ter (kar - bō - nom′ē - ter). Carbonômetro; dispositivo obsoleto usado em carbonometria. [L. *carbo* (*carbon*-), carvão, + G. *metron*, medida]

car·bo·nom·e·try (kar - bō - nom′ē - trē). Carbonometria; método obsoleto para determinar a presença e a proporção de dióxido de carbono no ar ambiente ou expirado pela precipitação de carbonato de cálcio da água de cal (hidróxido de cálcio). SIN carbometry.

car·bo·nu·ria (kar - bo - noo′rē - ā). Carbonúria; termo raramente usado, que designa a excreção de dióxido de carbono ou outros compostos de carbono na urina.

car·bon·yl (kar′bŏn - il). Carbonila; o grupamento característico, —CO—, das cetonas, aldeídos e ácidos orgânicos.

car·bo·plat·in (kar′bō - pla′tin). Carboplatina; agente de combate ao câncer que contém platina, muito semelhante à cisplatina, porém mais tóxico para os elementos mielóides da medula óssea. Causa menos náuseas e é menos tóxico para os sistemas neurológico, auditivo e renal; usada na quimioterapia de tumores sólidos.

car·bo·prost tro·meth·a·mine (kar′bō - prost trō - meth′a - mēn). Carboprost-trometamina; prostaglandina usada como abortivo e no tratamento da hemorragia pós-parto refratária.

car·box·am·ide (kar - boks′am - īd). Carboxamida; configuração molecular (—$CONH_2$) que, juntamente com as carboximidas relacionadas (iminocarbonilas) (—CONH—), é um componente de muitos hipnóticos, incluindo barbitúricos, hidantoínas e tiazinas. SIN aminocarbonyl.

car·box·im·ide (kar - boks′im - īd). Carboximida. VER carboxamide.

carboxy-. Carboxi; forma combinante que indica acréscimo de CO ou CO_2.

***N*-car·box·y·an·hy·drides** (kar - bok′sē - an - hī′drīdz). *N*-carboxianidridos; derivados heterocíclicos de aminoácidos a partir dos quais podem ser sintetizados polipeptídios.

car·box·y·ca·thep·sin (kar - bok′sē - kă - thep′sin). Carboxicatepsina. SIN peptidyl dipeptidase A.

car·box·y·dis·mu·tase (kar - bok - sē - dis′moo - tās). Carboxidismutase. SIN ribulose-1,5-bisphosphate carboxylase.

4-car·box·y·glu·tam·ic ac·id (Gla) (kar - bok′sē - gloo - tam′ik). Ácido 4-carboxiglutâmico; forma carboxilada de ácido glutâmico encontrada em determinadas proteínas (p. ex., protrombina, fatores VII, IX e X, osteocalcina). Sua síntese depende de vitamina K.

car·box·y·he·mo·glo·bin (HbCO) (kar - bok′sē - hē - mō - glō′bin). Carboxiemoglobina; união bastante estável entre monóxido de carbono e hemoglobina. A formação de carboxiemoglobina impede a transferência normal de dióxido de carbono e oxigênio durante a circulação sanguínea; assim, níveis crescentes de c. resultam em vários graus de asfixia, incluindo morte. SIN carbon monoxide hemoglobin, carbonmonoxy myoglobin.

car·box·y·he·mo·glo·bi·ne·mia (kar - bok′sē - hē′mō - glō - bi - nē′mē - ā). Carboxiemoglobinemia; presença de carboxiemoglobina no sangue, como no envenenamento por monóxido de carbono.

car·box·yl (kar-bok′sil). Carboxila; o grupo característico (—COOH) de determinados ácidos orgânicos; p. ex., HCOOH (ácido fórmico), CH_3COOH (ácido acético), $CH_3CH(NH_2)COOH$ (alanina), etc. Cf. carboxylic acid.

car·box·yl·ase (kar - bok′sil′ - ās). Carboxilase. **1.** Uma das várias carboxilases, comumente denominadas carboxilases ou descarboxilases (EC 4.1.1.x), catalisando o acréscimo de CO_2 a outra molécula inteira ou a parte dela para criar outro grupamento —COOH (p. ex., ribulose-1,5-bifosfato carboxilase). **2.** Designação obsoleta de *pyruvate* decarboxylase.

car·box·yl·a·tion (kar - bok - si - lā′shŭn). Carboxilação; acréscimo de CO_2 a um aceptor orgânico, como na formação de malonil-CoA ou na fotossíntese, para produzir um grupamento —COOH; catalisada por carboxilases.

car·box·yl·ic ac·id (kar-bok′sil-ik). Ácido carboxílico; ácido orgânico com grupo carboxila. Cf. carboxyl.

activated c. a., a. c. ativado; derivado de um grupamento carboxila que é mais suscetível ao ataque nucleofílico que um grupamento carboxila livre; p. ex., anidridos ácidos, tioésteres.

car·box·yl·trans·fer·as·es (kar - bok - sil - trans′fer - ās - ez). [EC 2.1.3.x] Carboxiltransferases; enzimas que transferem grupamentos carboxila de uma substância para outra. SIN transcarboxylases.

car·box·y·meth·yl·cel·lu·lose (kar - bok - sē - meth′il - sel′ū - lōs). Carboximetilcelulose; um derivado da celulose que forma uma dispersão coloidal na água; indigerível e inabsorvível sistemicamente; absorve água e é usado como laxante de volume. Também pode ser usado como agente suspensor.

car·box·y·pep·ti·dase (kar - bok - sē - pep′ti - dās). Carboxipeptidase; hidrolase que remove o aminoácido na extremidade carboxila livre de uma cadeia polipeptídica; uma exopeptidase.

acid c., c. ácida. SIN serine c.

serine c., c. serina; c. de ampla especificidade para resíduos aminoácidos terminais de peptídios; o pH ideal é de 4,5 a 6,0; sensível ao diisopropil fluorofosfato; contém uma serina no local ativo. SIN acid c.

car·box·y·pep·ti·dase A. Carboxipeptidase A; hidrolase que libera aminoácidos com terminação C, com a exceção dos resíduos arginil, lisil e prolil com terminação C. Uma exopeptidase que contém zinco.

car·box·y·pep·ti·dase B. Carboxipeptidase B; hidrolase que libera preferencialmente resíduos lisil ou arginil com terminação C. Uma exopeptidase que contém zinco. SIN protaminase.

car·box·y·pep·ti·dase C. Carboxipeptidase C. VER serine *carboxypeptidase*.

car·box·y·pep·ti·dase G. Carboxipeptidase G. SIN γ-glutamyl hydrolase.

***N*-car·box·y·u·rea** (kar - bok′sē - ū - rē′a). *N*-carboxiuréia. SIN allophanic acid.

car·bro·mal (kar′brō - mal). Carbromal; agente hipnótico obsoleto que é uma bromina contendo monouréida.

car·bun·cle (kar′bŭng - kl). Carbúnculo; infecção pirogênica profunda da pele e dos tecidos subcutâneos, geralmente originada em vários folículos pilosos contíguos, com formação de fístulas de união. [L. *carbunculus*, dim. de *carbo*, carvão vivo, carbúnculo]

kidney c., renal c., c. renal; designação antiga para abscessos intra-renais múltiplos e coalescentes.

car·bu·ret (kar′boo-ret). **1.** Carbureto; designação arcaica para carboneto. **2.** Combinar-se com o carbono. **3.** Enriquecer um gás com hidrocarbonetos voláteis, como em um carburador.

car·bu·ta·mide (kar - boo′tă - mĭd). Carbutamida; agente hipoglicemiante oral, p. ex., tolbutamida.

car·bu·te·rol hy·dro·chlo·ride (kar - boo′tĕ - rol). Cloridrato de carbuterol; agente simpaticomimético com atividade broncodilatadora.

car·cass (kar′kăs). Carcaça; o corpo de um animal morto; em referência a animais usados como alimento humano, o corpo após a retirada da pele, cabeça, cauda, membros e vísceras. [F. *carcasse*, do It. *carcassa*]

♢ **carcino-, carcin-.** Câncer; caranguejo. [G. *karkinos*, caranguejo, câncer]

car·ci·no·em·bry·on·ic (kar′si - nō - em - brē - on′ik). Carcinoembrionário; relativo a uma substância associada ao carcinoma presente no tecido embrionário, como um antígeno c.

car·cin·o·gen (kar - sĭn′ō - jen, kar′si - nō - jen). Carcinógeno; qualquer substância ou organismo produtor de câncer, como hidrocarbonetos aromáticos policíclicos, ou agente como em determinados tipos de irradiação. [carcino- + G. *-gen*, geração]

complete c., c. completo; um c. químico capaz de induzir câncer sem provocação por um agente promotor de câncer introduzido durante o tratamento.

car·ci·no·gen·e·sis (kar′si - nō - jen′ĕ - sis). Carcinogênese; a origem, produção ou desenvolvimento de câncer, incluindo carcinomas e outras neoplasias malignas. [carcino- + G. *genesis*, geração]

field c., c. de campo; aumento da suscetibilidade de toda uma área ao c.; o trato aerodigestivo superior e o cólon, p. ex., tendem a desenvolver cânceres sincrônicos e metacrônicos.

car·ci·no·gen·ic (kar′si - nō - jen′ik). Carcinogênico; que causa câncer.

carcinogenicity (kar′sin - ō - jen - is′ĭ - tē). Carcinogenicidade; capacidade de causar câncer.

car·ci·noid (kar′si-noyd). Carcinóide. VER carcinoid *tumor*, carcinoid *syndrome*.

car·ci·no·lyt·ic (kar′si - nō - lit′ik). Carcinolítico; destrutivo para as células do carcinoma. [carcino- + G. *lytikos*, que causa uma solução]

CARCINOMA

car·ci·no·ma (CA), pl. **car·ci·no·mas, car·ci·no·ma·ta** (kar - si - nō′mă, - măz). Carcinoma; qualquer dos vários tipos de neoplasias malignas derivadas das células epiteliais, principalmente glandulares (adenocarcinoma) ou escamosos (c. de células escamosas); o tipo de câncer mais comum. [G. *karkinōma*, de *karkinos*, câncer, + *-oma*, tumor]

Como outras neoplasias malignas, os carcinomas exibem proliferação celular descontrolada, anaplasia (regressão de células e tecidos para um estado mais primitivo ou indiferenciado) e tendência a invadir tecidos adjacentes e a se disseminar para locais distantes por metástase. Um carcinoma origina-se de uma única célula cujo genoma contém uma aberração hereditária (oncogene) ou adquiriu uma aberração em consequência de mutação espontânea ou lesão por toxinas químicas (carcinógenos), radiação, infecção viral, inflamação crônica ou outra agressão externa. Provavelmente é preciso ocorrer uma seqüência complexa de lesões bioquímicas e genéticas para o desenvolvimento de um carcinoma. Alguns carcinomas (p. ex., próstata, mama) dependem parcialmente da presença de hormônios (andrógênio, estrogênio) para sua proliferação. Os carcinomas são classificados histologicamente de acordo com as evidências de capacidade de invasão e alterações que indicam anaplasia; isto é, perda da polaridade dos núcleos, perda da maturação ordenada das células (principalmente nos tipos de células escamosas), variação no tamanho e formato das células, hipercromatismo dos núcleos com aglomeração de cromatina e aumento da razão nuclear-citoplasmática. Os carcinomas podem ser indiferenciados, ou o tecido neoplásico pode assemelhar-se em vários graus a um dos tipos de epitélio normal. Os carcinomas podem secretar vários fatores hormonais capazes de induzir efeitos sistêmicos (paraneoplásicos) (p. ex., hipercalcemia, tromboflebite). O local mais comum de origem do carcinoma em ambos os sexos é a pele; o segundo local mais comum em homens é a próstata e nas mulheres a mama. Entretanto, o carcinoma letal mais freqüente em ambos os sexos é o carcinoma broncogênico.

---

acinar c., c. acinar. SIN acinic cell *adenocarcinoma*.

acinic cell c., c. de célula acinosa. SIN acinic cell *adenocarcinoma*.

adenoid cystic c., c. adenóide cístico; tipo histológico de c. caracterizado por grandes massas epiteliais apresentando espaços ou cistos redondos, semelhantes a glândulas, que freqüentemente contêm muco ou colágeno e são limitados por algumas ou muitas camadas de células epiteliais sem estroma interposto, formando um padrão cribriforme semelhante a uma fatia de queijo suíço; invasão perineural e metástases hematogênicas são comuns; incide mais nas glândulas salivares e na pele. SIN cylindromatous c.

adenosquamous c., c. adenoescamoso; um tipo de tumor pulmonar que exibe áreas de diferenciação de células escamosas e glandulares bem definidas.

adnexal c., c. anexial; c. que se origina das glândulas sudoríparas ou sebáceas.

adrenal cortical carcinoma, c. corticossupra-renal; c. originado no córtex supra-renal que pode causar virilismo ou síndrome de Cushing.

alveolar cell c., c. de células alveolares; um subtipo de adenocarcinoma, considerado derivado do epitélio dos bronquíolos terminais, no qual o tecido neoplásico se estende ao longo das paredes alveolares e cresce em pequenas massas no interior dos alvéolos; o envolvimento pode ser uniformemente difuso e maciço, nodular ou lobular; microscopicamente, as células neoplásicas são cubóides ou colunares e formam estruturas papilares; pode-se encontrar mucina em algumas das células e no material presente nos alvéolos, que também inclui células desnudas; metástases para os linfonodos regionais, e mesmo para locais mais distantes, são conhecidas, mas são incomuns. SIN bronchiolar adenocarcinoma, bronchiolar c., bronchiolo-alveolar c., bronchioloalveolar adenocarcinoma, bronchoalveolar c.

anaplastic c., c. anaplásico; c. com ausência de diferenciação estrutural epitelial.

apocrine c., c. apócrino; **(1)** um c. composto predominantemente de células com citoplasma granular eosinofílico abundante, ocorrendo na mama ou em outros locais; **(2)** um c. das glândulas apócrinas.

basal cell c., c. basocelular; neoplasia de crescimento lento, invasiva, mas geralmente sem metástases, lembrando células basais normais da epiderme ou folículos pilosos, mais comumente originando-se na pele lesada pelo sol de pessoas idosas e de pele clara. SIN basal cell epithelioma.

basaloid c., c. basalóide. SIN cloacogenic c.

basal squamous cell c., SIN basosquamous c.

basosquamous c., basisquamous c., de células escamosas basais; c. basoescamoso; c. cutâneo cuja estrutura e comportamento são considerados de transição entre os carcinomas basocelular e de células escamosas. O termo não deve ser usado para a forma ceratótica de c. basocelular, que é muito mais comum, no qual as células tumorais são do tipo basal, mas com pequenos focos de queratinização abrupta. SIN basal squamous cell c.

bronchiolar c., c. bronquiolar. SIN alveolar cell c.

bronchiolo-alveolar c., c. bronquioloalveolar. SIN alveolar cell c.

bronchoalveolar c., c. broncoalveolar. SIN alveolar cell c.

bronchogenic c., c. broncogênico; originalmente descrito apenas como um c. originado em um brônquio, geralmente de células escamosas ou pequenas células, havendo agora, porém, consenso geral de que se refere a qualquer câncer de pulmão. Inclui o c. escamoso ou epidermóide, de pequenas células ou grandes células, e o adenocarcinoma. Observado radiologicamente como massa tumoral em crescimento; as células tumorais malignas podem ser detectadas no escarro. Esse c. dá metástases precoces para os linfonodos torácicos e para o cérebro, glândulas supra-renais e outros órgãos através da corrente sanguínea.

canine c. 1, c. canino 1; um dos poucos tumores transplantáveis de animais.

---

c. of the breast, c. de mama; tumor maligno originado nas células epiteliais da mama feminina (e, ocasionalmente, da mama masculina), geralmente adenocarcinoma originado do epitélio ductal.

O impacto do câncer de mama sobre a sociedade ocidental é enorme. O câncer de mama é a neoplasia maligna não-cutânea mais comum em mulheres. O risco de uma mulher desenvolver câncer de mama é de 8%, e anualmente são diagnosticados cerca de 182.000 novos casos nos Estados Unidos. Com 46.000 mortes por ano, figura em segundo lugar,

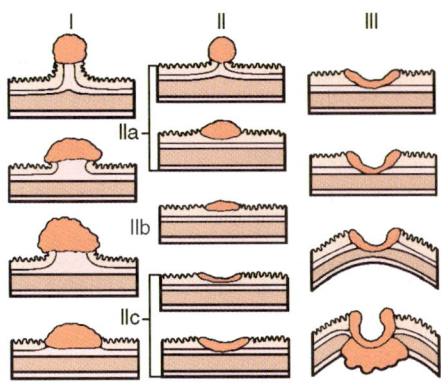

carcinoma: padrões de desenvolvimento em carcinomas do estômago; I, polipóide ou fungiforme; II, extensão superficial (a, elevada; b, semelhante a placa; c, deprimida); III, ulcerativo

perdendo apenas para o câncer de pulmão, como causa de mortes por câncer em mulheres. A maioria dos cânceres de mama é representada por adenocarcinomas estrogênio-dependentes. Muitos fatores, incluindo idade, raça, história familiar e história reprodutiva, influenciam o risco de uma mulher desenvolver câncer de mama. O risco aumenta com a idade: é menor que 0,1% aos 30 anos, de cerca de 2% aos 50 anos e de 10% aos 80 anos. As mulheres afro-americanas apresentam as maiores taxas de mortalidade e as menores taxas de sobrevida por câncer de mama. As mulheres asiáticas residentes nos Estados Unidos têm as menores taxas, mas alguns estudos sugerem que seu risco de câncer aumenta à medida que são aculturadas. O risco de câncer de mama é um pouco aumentado pela nuliparidade ou primeira gravidez após os 35 anos e pela menarca precoce ou menopausa tardia. Cerca de 10% dos cânceres de mama são induzidos por mutações genéticas hereditárias (particularmente mutações BRCA1 e BRCA2, que, juntas, são responsáveis por cerca de um terço dos cânceres de mama familiares); os outros são induzidos por mutações espontâneas, não-hereditárias. O oncogene HER-2/neu, que codifica uma oncoproteína transmembrana de 185 kDa, é amplificado e/ou excessivamente expresso em 10–30% dos cânceres de mama invasivos e em 40-60% dos carcinomas de mama intraductais. A detecção desse gene no tecido canceroso por hibridização fluorescente *in situ* está associada a prognóstico sombrio (probabilidade 30% mais alta de recidiva e de morte por câncer). As mulheres com forte história familiar de câncer de mama tendem a desenvolvê-lo mais cedo, podendo também haver risco de neoplasias malignas do ovário e de outros locais. Outros fatores de risco são tabagismo (cigarro), consumo diário de álcool, exposição ao radônio ambiental, radiação terapêutica e diagnóstica, incluindo aquela emitida por mamografias, e possivelmente terapia de reposição estrogênica (com ou sem um progestogênio associado). As opções preventivas, diagnósticas e terapêuticas continuam a ser vigorosamente exploradas. A possibilidade de identificar oncogenes hereditários causou controvérsia em relação à conveniência da mastectomia profilática para mulheres sob risco

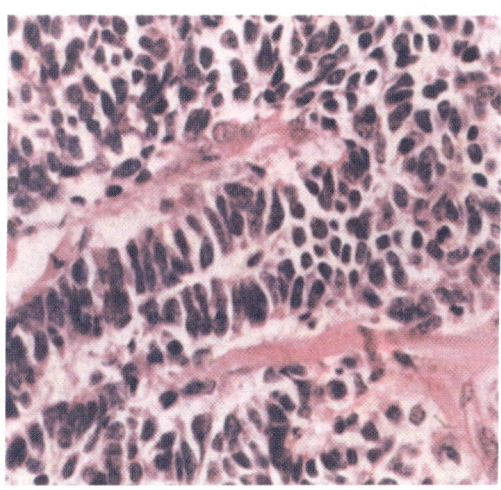

carcinoma broncogênico: pequenas células

de desenvolver carcinoma mamário precoce. Constatou-se que o tamoxifeno, um antagonista do estrogênio usado no tratamento do câncer de mama estrogênio-dependente, é efetivo na redução do risco daquelas mulheres com forte história familiar de câncer de mama. Os especialistas recomendam mamografia anual a partir dos 40 anos para todas as mulheres, e a partir dos 25 anos para as mulheres de alto risco (aquelas com forte história familiar de câncer de mama ou submetidas à radioterapia para doença de Hodgkin). Como cerca de 10% dos cânceres de mama que podem ser palpados ao exame não são diagnosticados à mamografia, também é recomendado o exame anual das mamas por um médico. Estudos recentes não mostraram vantagem em termos de sobrevida nas mulheres que realizam auto-exame da mama. Os tratamentos do câncer de mama incluem ressecção cirúrgica, limitada ou extensa, com ou sem dissecção radical e remoção dos linfonodos axilares; radioterapia; e quimioterapia, dependendo do tipo e do estágio da doença. A ressecção limitada de pequenos tumores invasivos, com preservação da mama, assegura taxas de sobrevida semelhantes àquelas observadas após mastectomia radical modificada. Os agentes quimioterápicos em uso rotineiro incluem doxorrubicina, epirrubicina, ciclofosfamida e paclitaxel. O trastuzumab, um anticorpo monoclonal contra o oncogene HER-2/neu, diminui o tamanho de tumores que contêm esse gene, mas seu uso está associado a uma alta incidência de disfunção cardíaca. Metástases conhecidas ou suspeitas de um tumor que responde ao estrogênio são tratadas com tamoxifeno ou ooforectomia. Ver Também BRCA1 gene, BRCA2 gene, mammography, tamoxifen.

c. of the prostate, c. da próstata; neoplasia maligna originada das células epiteliais glandulares da próstata.

O adenocarcinoma prostático (AP) é o câncer mais comum em homens, figurando em segundo lugar como causa de mortes por câncer em homens, perdendo apenas para o câncer de pulmão. Anualmente são diagnosticados 200.000 novos casos nos Estados Unidos, e mais de 38.000 homens morrem por causa da doença. À necrópsia são encontrados focos de AP em 40% dos homens que morrem após os 50 anos de idade. A neoplasia é androgênio-dependente e não ocorre em eunucos. É mais comum e mais agressiva em homens afro-americanos. Uma história familiar de AP e, possivelmente, a vasectomia são outros fatores de risco. É necessário fazer o diagnóstico diferencial entre AP e hiperplasia prostática benigna, que não é uma lesão pré-maligna. O AP geralmente surge na periferia da glândula e pode estender-se através da cápsula até os tecidos periprostáticos, vesículas seminais e linfonodos regionais. No momento do diagnóstico, a doença já se disseminou além da glândula em mais de 40% dos pacientes. Os ossos do esqueleto axial são os locais habituais de metástases distantes; o fígado, os pulmões e o cérebro são outros locais comuns. A doença incipiente é assintomática; freqüentemente, o diagnóstico é feito por rastreamento de homens aparentemente saudáveis através do toque retal e/ou ensaio do antígeno próstata-específico (PSA). A doença avançada pode apresentar-se como obstrução urinária ou dor óssea causada por metástase. Homens com assimetria nodular, endurecimento da próstata ao toque retal ou elevação do PSA são avaliados por ultra-sonografia transretal da próstata, com biópsia por agulha orientada pela ultra-sonografia. A pesquisa de metástases ósseas inclui dosagem da fosfatase alcalina sérica, cintigrafia óssea, tomografia computadorizada e ressonância magnética. O AP é classificado pelo método de Gleason, que reflete o grau de diferenciação histológica nos dois focos malignos mais proeminentes. O estagiamento anatômico baseia-se na extensão do tumor além da cápsula prostática, e não no tamanho do tumor. Um nível baixo ou indetectável de proteína p27 no tecido prostático é um indicador de neoplasia maligna mais agressiva. O tratamento depende do grau e do estágio da doença, bem como da idade e da condição geral do paciente. Em homens idosos e naqueles com doença concomitante que ameace a vida, a "negligência" benigna pode ser o tratamento de escolha. A prostatectomia radical (remoção de toda a glândula juntamente com as vesículas seminais) geralmente é reservada para pacientes com doença incipiente ou limitada e uma expectativa de vida mínima de 10 anos. Esse tratamento está associado a um risco significativo de incontinência urinária e impotência. A radioterapia com feixe externo ou implante transperineal de isótopos radioativos pode ser associada a cirurgia ou substituí-la. O bloqueio androgênico por orquidectomia ou por administração de estrogênio, um antagonista do androgênio ou um hormônio liberador de gonadotrofina é paliativo na doença avançada. Entre 1984 e 1992, o número de casos de AP diagnosticado quase duplicou, aparentemente devido ao extenso rastreamento por PSA. Desde 1992 o número de novos casos regrediu, quase voltando ao seu nível anterior. A taxa de mortalidade por AP diminuiu significativamente desde 1990.

Muitos observadores atribuem esse declínio à capacidade de o rastreamento de PSA detectar câncer em um estágio curável. Além disso, um grande estudo de casos-controles mostrou que a probabilidade de homens que morreram por AP terem sido submetidos ao toque retal durante os 10 anos anteriores correspondia à metade da probabilidade de controles da população. Alguns especialistas são contra o toque retal e o rastreamento por PSA de homens assintomáticos com expectativas de vida inferiores a 10 anos, com a alegação de que os riscos de resultados falso-negativos e das conseqüências adversas do tratamento agressivo superam qualquer possível benefício na sobrevida ou na qualidade de vida.

---

clear cell c., c. de células claras. SIN mesonephroma.
clear cell c. of kidney, c. de células claras renal. SIN renal adenocarcinoma.
clear cell c. of salivary glands, c. de células claras das glândulas salivares; um tumor maligno, que compreende vários subtipos, como oncocitoma de células claras, carcinoma de células claras hialinizantes, c. epitelial-mioepitelial (ducto intercalado).
cloacogenic c., c. cloacogênico; **(1)** tipo de c. de células escamosas do ânus originado em tecidos provenientes, ou em remanescentes, da cloaca. **(2)** em oncologia, câncer anal com origem proximal à linha pectinada. SIN basaloid c., cuboidal c. [cloaca + -genic]
colloid c., c. colóide. SIN mucinous c.
cuboidal c., c. cubóide. SIN cloacogenic c.
cylindromatous c., c. cilindromatoso. SIN adenoid cystic c.
cystic c., c. cístico; c. no qual se formam cistos verdadeiros revestidos de epitélio, ou alterações degenerativas podem resultar em espaços semelhantes a cistos.
duct c., ductal c., c. ductal; c. derivado do epitélio ductal, p. ex., na mama ou no pâncreas.
embryonal c., c. embrionário; neoplasia maligna do testículo ou ovário, composta de células anaplásicas com bordas celulares indistintas, citoplasma anfofílico e núcleos ovóides, redondos ou reniformes que podem ter grandes nucléolos; em alguns casos, as células neoplásicas podem formar estruturas tubulares ou papilares.
endometrioid c., c. endometrióide; adenocarcinoma do ovário ou da próstata semelhante ao adenocarcinoma endometrial.
epidermoid c., c. epidermóide; c. de células escamosas da pele ou pulmão. SIN epidermoid cancer.
epithelial myoepithelial c. (mī′yō-ep-i-thē′lē-al), c. mioepitelial epitelial; neoplasia maligna da glândula salivar composta de uma camada interna de células ductais circundada por uma camada de células mioepiteliais claras.
fibrolamellar liver cell c., c. fibrolamelar do hepatócito; c. hepático primário no qual hepatócitos malignos são cruzados por faixas laminadas fibrosas. SIN oncocytic hepatocellular tumor.
follicular carcinoma, carcinoma folicular; c. da tireóide composto de folículos epiteliais bem ou mal diferenciados sem formação papilar, difícil de distinguir do adenoma; os critérios incluem invasão dos vasos sanguíneos e o achado de metástases do tecido folicular da tireóide em outras estruturas como os linfonodos cervicais e o osso; o c. folicular pode captar iodo radioativo.
giant cell c., c. de células gigantes; neoplasia epitelial maligna caracterizada por células anaplásicas incomumente grandes.
giant cell c. of thyroid gland, c. de células gigantes da tireóide; c. indiferenciado rapidamente progressivo observado na tireóide, caracterizado por numerosas células anaplásicas, incomumente grandes, derivadas do epitélio glandular da tireóide.
glandular c., c. glandular. SIN adenocarcinoma.
hepatocellular c., c. hepatocelular; tumor maligno composto de hepatócitos neoplásicos; pode ser bem, moderadamente ou pouco diferenciado; secreta α-fetoproteína, que serve como marcador sorológico útil. SIN hepatocarcinoma, liver cell c., malignant hepatoma.
Hürthle cell c., c. de células de Hürthle; c. salivar ou tireóideo composto de células com citoplasma eosinofílico. VER TAMBÉM Hürthle cell adenoma. SIN oncocytic c., oxyphilic c.
inflammatory c., c. inflamatório; c. da mama que se apresenta com edema, hiperemia, dor à palpação e rápido aumento da mama; microscopicamente, há extensa invasão dos linfáticos dérmicos pelo c.
intraductal c., c. intraductal; uma forma de c. derivada do revestimento epitelial dos ductos; especialmente na mama, onde a maioria dos carcinomas originam-se do epitélio ductal; as células neoplásicas proliferam em projeções ou massas irregulares, ocupando as luzes, que são sólidas, cribriformes ou têm necrose central; o c. intraductal é uma forma de c. in situ, pois é contido pela membrana basal ductal; quando invade o estroma adjacente ou metastatiza, é denominado c. ductal.
intraepidermal c., c. intra-epidérmico; c. in situ da pele; p. ex., doença de Bowen.
intraepithelial c., c. intra-epitelial. SIN c. in situ.
invasive c., c. invasivo; neoplasia na qual coleções de células epiteliais infiltram ou destroem o tecido adjacente.
juvenile c., c. juvenil. SIN secretory c.
kangri burn c., c. da queimadura por kangri. SIN kang cancer.
large cell c., c. de células grandes; c. anaplásico, particularmente o c. broncogênico, composto de células muito maiores que aquelas no c. pulmonar de pequenas células.
latent c., c. latente; neoplasia epitelial com características microscópicas de malignidade que se acredita ter permanecido localizada e assintomática por um longo período; p. ex., pequeno c. da próstata em homens idosos, freqüentemente encontrado incidentalmente à necrópsia.
lateral aberrant thyroid c., c. da tireóide aberrante lateral; designação obsoleta para um nódulo cervical de c. da tireóide situado fora da tireóide, anteriormente considerado originário do tecido tireóideo ectópico, mas agora creditado como metastático de um c. oculto na glândula.
leptomeningeal c., c. leptomeníngeo. SIN meningeal c.
liver cell c., c. do hepatócito. SIN hepatocellular c.
lobular c., c. lobular; uma forma de adenocarcinoma, principalmente da mama, onde o c. lobular é menos comum que o c. ductal e geralmente é composto de pequenas células.
lobular c. in situ, c. lobular in situ. SIN noninfiltrating lobular c.
medullary c., c. medular; neoplasia maligna, de consistência comparativamente mole e cerebróide, que consiste principalmente em células epiteliais neoplásicas, com estroma fibroso escasso.
medullary c. of breast, c. medular da mama; um subtipo de c. de mama composto por lâminas de grandes células epiteliais circundadas por escasso estroma fibroso; é de consistência mole e bem circunscrito. Seu prognóstico é melhor do que o do c. ductal invasivo.
medullary c. of thyroid, c. medular da tireóide; neoplasia maligna da tireóide composta de células C produtoras de calcitonina e estroma rico em amilóide; pode ser esporádico ou familiar; a forma familiar pode ser parte da síndrome de neoplasia endócrina múltipla, tipos 2A e 2B.
meningeal c., c. meníngeo; infiltração de células carcinomatosas no espaço aracnóide e subaracnóide; pode ser primário ou secundário. SIN leptomeningeal c., leptomeningeal carcinomatosis, meningeal carcinomatosis.
metaplastic c., c. metaplásico; c. no qual algumas células tumorais são fusiformes, sugerindo um sarcoma, ou no qual o estroma mostra focos de osso ou cartilagem; esses carcinomas ocorrem nos tratos respiratório superior ou alimentar ou na mama.
metastatic c., c. metastático; c. que surgiu em uma região distante de seu local de origem, como na metástase (2). SIN secondary c.
microinvasive c., c. microinvasivo; variedade de c. mais freqüente no colo uterino, no qual o c. in situ do epitélio escamoso, na superfície ou substituindo o revestimento das glândulas, é acompanhado por pequenas coleções de células epiteliais anormais que se infiltram por uma distância muito curta no estroma; este representa o estágio inicial da invasão.
mucinous c., c. mucinoso; variedade de adenocarcinoma na qual as células neoplásicas secretam pequenas quantidades de mucina, e, conseqüentemente, a neoplasia tende a ser brilhante, viscosa e gelatinóide. SIN colloid cancer, colloid c.
mucoepidermoid c., c. mucoepidermóide; comumente um c. da glândula salivar com baixo grau de malignidade composto de células mucosas, epidermóides e intermediárias, com células mucosas abundantes apenas no c. de baixo grau; a recorrência é freqüente, e o c. de alto grau metastatiza para linfonodos cervicais. SIN mucoepidermoid tumor.
nasopharyngeal c., c. nasofaríngeo; c. de células escamosas originado do epitélio superficial da nasofaringe; são reconhecidos três tipos histológicos: c. queratinizante, não-queratinizante e indiferenciado.
noninfiltrating lobular c., c. lobular não-infiltrativo; c. da mama no qual pequenas células tumorais preenchem ácinos preexistentes nos lóbulos, sem invadir o estroma circundante. SIN lobular c. in situ, lobular neoplasia.
oat cell c., c. de pequenas células. SIN small cell c.
occult c., c. oculto; c. pequeno, assintomático ou que dá origem a metástases sem sintomas devidos ao c. primário.
oncocytic c., c. oncocítico. SIN Hürthle cell c.
oxyphilic c., c. oxifílico. SIN Hürthle cell c.
papillary c., c. papilar; neoplasia maligna caracterizada pela formação de numerosas projeções digitiformes e irregulares de estroma fibroso coberto por uma camada superficial de células epiteliais neoplásicas.
polymorphous low-grade c. of salivary glands, c. polimorfo de baixo grau das glândulas salivares; tumor maligno de baixo grau das glândulas salivares que exibe vários padrões histológicos, como crescimento cribriforme, ductal e papilar. SIN terminal duct c.
primary c., c. primário; c. no local de origem, com invasão local do órgão.
primary neuroendocrine c. of the skin, c. neuroendócrino primário da pele. SIN Merkel cell tumor.
renal cell c., c. de células renais. SIN renal adenocarcinoma.
sarcomatoid c., c. sarcomatóide. SIN spindle cell c.
scar c., c. de cicatriz; c. pulmonar, geralmente adenocarcinoma, originado de uma cicatriz pulmonar periférica ou associado à fibrose intersticial em um pulmão em favo de mel. SIN scar cancer.

scirrhous c., c. cirroso; c. de consistência dura, de natureza fibrosa, resultante de uma reação desmoplásica do estroma à presença de epitélio neoplásico.
secondary c., c. secundário. SIN metastatic c.
secretory c., c. secretor; c. da mama com células de coloração pálida que exibem atividade secretora proeminente, conforme observado na gravidez e na lactação, mas encontrado principalmente em crianças. SIN juvenile c.
signet-ring cell c., c. de células em anel de sinete; adenocarcinoma mal diferenciado composto de células com uma gotícula citoplasmática de muco que comprime o núcleo para um lado ao longo da membrana celular; origina-se freqüentemente no estômago, ocasionalmente no intestino grosso ou em outra parte.
c. in si'tu (CIS), c. *in situ*; lesão caracterizada por alterações citológicas do tipo associado ao c. invasivo, mas com o processo histopatológico limitado ao epitélio de revestimento e sem evidências histológicas de extensão para estruturas adjacentes; as alterações características geralmente são mais aparentes no núcleo, isto é, variação no tamanho e no formato, aumento da cromatina e numerosas mitoses (incluindo algumas atípicas) em todas as camadas do epitélio, com perda da maturação ordenada. Presume-se que a lesão seja o precursor histologicamente reconhecível do c. invasivo, isto é, uma fase localizada e curável de c. SIN intraepithelial c.
small cell c., c. de pequenas células; **(1)** c. anaplásico composto de pequenas células; **(2)** carcinoma anaplásico, extremamente maligno e geralmente broncogênico, composto de pequenas células ovóides com citoplasma muito escasso. SIN oat cell c.
spindle cell c., c. de células fusiformes; c. composto de células alongadas, freqüentemente um c. escamoso mal diferenciado, podendo ser difícil distingui-lo de um sarcoma. SIN sarcomatoid c.
squamous cell c., c. de células escamosas; neoplasia maligna derivada do epitélio escamoso estratificado, mas que também pode ocorrer em locais como a mucosa brônquica, onde normalmente há epitélio glandular ou colunar; são formadas quantidades variáveis de queratina, em relação ao grau de diferenciação, e, se a queratina não estiver na superfície, pode acumular-se na neoplasia como uma pérola de queratina; quando as células são bem diferenciadas, podem ser observadas pontes intercelulares entre células adjacentes.
sweat gland c., c. das glândulas sudoríparas; geralmente um tumor solitário, nodular e fixo à pele e às estruturas subjacentes, apresentando crescimento lento por longos períodos seguido por crescimento rápido e disseminação.
terminal duct c., c. dos ductos terminais. SIN polymorphous low-grade c. of salivary glands.
trabecular c., c. trabecular. SIN Merkel cell *tumor*.
transitional cell c., c. de células de transição. SIN urothelial c.
tubular c., c. tubular; forma bem diferenciada de c. de mama ductal com invasão do estroma por pequenos túbulos epiteliais.
urothelial c., c. urotelial; neoplasia maligna, derivada do epitélio de transição, que ocorre principalmente na bexiga, nos ureteres ou nas pelves renais (principalmente se bem diferenciada); freqüentemente papilar; esses carcinomas são classificados de acordo com o grau de anaplasia. O denominado c. de células de transição das vias respiratórias superiores é mais apropriadamente classificado como c. de células escamosas. O c. de células de transição também é um tumor raro do ovário. SIN trasitional cell c.
V-2 c., c. V-2; c. extremamente maligno, transplantável de animais experimentais, desenvolvido em virtude de alteração maligna em um papiloma induzido por vírus de um coelho doméstico.
verrucous c., c. verrucoso; c. de células escamosas papilares bem diferenciado da cavidade oral ou pênis, que pode invadir localmente, mas raramente dá metástases; não existem as características citológicas habituais de malignidade. O c. verrucoso genital pode estar associado a condiloma acuminado preexistente.
villous c., c. viloso; forma de c. na qual há numerosas projeções papilares, bem acondicionadas, de tecido epitelial neoplásico.
wolffian duct c., c. do ducto de Wolff. SIN mesonephroma.
yolk sac c., c. do saco vitelino. SIN endocervical sinus *tumor*.

car·ci·no·ma ex ple·o·mor·phic ad·e·no·ma. Carcinoma ex-adenoma pleomórfico; carcinoma originado em um tumor misto benigno de uma glândula salivar, caracterizado por aumento rápido e dor.
car·ci·no·ma·ta (kar-si-nō′mă-tă). Plural alternativo de carcinoma.
car·ci·no·ma·to·sis (kar′si-nō-mă-tō′sis). Carcinomatose; condição resultante da ampla disseminação do carcinoma em múltiplos locais em vários órgãos ou tecidos do corpo; algumas vezes também usado em relação ao envolvimento de uma região relativamente grande do corpo.
leptomeningeal c., c. leptomeníngea. SIN meningeal *carcinoma*.
lymphangitic c., c. linfangítica; distúrbio no qual os vasos linfáticos são preenchidos por células tumorais ou bloqueados por células tumorais.
meningeal c., c. meníngea. SIN meningeal *carcinoma*.
car·ci·nom·a·tous (kar′si-nom′ă-tŭs). Carcinomatoso; relativo a, ou que manifesta as propriedades características de, carcinoma.
car·ci·no·pho·bia (kar′sin-ō-fō′bē-ă). Carcinofobia. SIN cancerophobia.

car·ci·no·sar·co·ma (kar′si-nō-sar-kō′mă). Carcinossarcoma; neoplasia maligna que contém elementos de carcinoma e sarcoma tão misturados que indicam neoplasia do tecido epitelial e mesenquimal. VER TAMBÉM collision *tumor*.
car·ci·no·stat·ic (kar′si-nō-stat′ik). Carcinoestático. **1.** Relativo a um efeito de interrupção ou inibição do desenvolvimento ou progressão de um carcinoma. **2.** Um agente que manifesta esse efeito.
car·co·ma (kar-kō′mă). Carcoma; material granular castanho-avermelhado escuro ou cor de mogno encontrado nas fezes humanas em regiões tropicais; produz uma reação química semelhante à do urobilinogênio, e é composto por óxido de cálcio, ferro, ácidos fosfórico e carbônico, urobilinogênio, coleritrogênio e outras substâncias orgânicas em proporções variadas. [Esp. pó de madeira sob a casca de uma árvore, causado pelo cupim]
car·da·mom (kar′dă-mom). Cardamomo; grãos do paraíso; sementes maduras secas de *Elettaria cardamomum*; usado como aromatizante em assados, artigos de confeitaria, *curry* em pó e na fabricação do *óleo* de cardamomo que é usado como aromatizante de licores. Auxiliar farmacêutico (aromatizante); adjuvante e antifisético.
Carden, Henry D., cirurgião inglês, †1872. VER C. *amputation*.
car·den·o·lide (kar-den′ō-līd). Cardenolídeo; classe de glicosídeos cardíacos que contêm um anel lactona de cinco ramos (p. ex., os glicosídeos do *Digitalis*).
cardi-. VER cardio-.
car·dia (kar′dē-ă) [TA]. Cárdia; a área do estômago próxima da abertura esofágica que contém as glândulas cardíacas. SIN pars cardiaca gastricae [TA], cardiac part of stomach, cardial part of stomach, gastric cardia, pars cardiaca ventriculi. [G. *kardia*, coração]
car·di·ac (kar′dē-ak). **1.** Cardíaco; relativo ao coração. **2.** Cardíaco; relativo à abertura esofágica do estômago. **3.** (Obsoleto). Cardiotônico; um remédio para cardiopatia. [L. *cardiacus*]
car·di·ac bal·let (kar′dē-ak bal-ā′). Balé cardíaco; curtos períodos de arritmias cardíacas que consistem em seqüências uniformes de extra-sístoles multiformes repetitivas; assim denominado devido ao seu aspecto ondulante, originalmente descrito por Bellet. VER TAMBÉM torsade de pointes.
car·di·al·gia (kar-dē-al′jē-ă). Cardialgia. **1.** Termo obsoleto para pirose. **2.** SIN cardiodynia. [cardi- + G. *algos*, dor]
car·di·a·tax·ia (kar′dē-ă-tak′sē-ă). Cardiotaxia; extrema irregularidade na atividade cardíaca. [cardi- + G. *ataxia*, distúrbio]
car·di·a·te·lia (kar′dē-ă-tē′lē-ă). Cardiotelia; desenvolvimento incompleto do coração. [cardi- + G. *atelēs*, incompleto]
car·di·ec·ta·sia (kar′dē-ek-tā′zē-ă). Cardiectasia; dilatação do coração. [cardi- + G. *ektasis*, dilatação]
car·di·ec·to·my (kar-dē-ek′tō-mē). Cardiectomia; ressecção da parte cardíaca do estômago. [cardi-(2) + G. *ektomē*, excisão]
car·di·ec·to·pia (kar-dē-ek-tō′pē-ă). Cardiectopia; posicionamento anormal do coração. VER *ectopia* cordis. [cardi- + G. *ektopos*, fora de lugar]
car·di·nal (kar′di-năl). Cardinal; principal; em embriologia, relativo à drenagem venosa principal. [L. *cardinalis*, principal]
card·ing. Cardagem; procedimento para colocar séries individuais de dentes anteriores ou posteriores em bandejas revestidas com uma faixa de cera.
cardio-, cardi-. 1. O coração. **2.** A cárdia (*ostium cardiacum*). [G. *kardia*, coração]
car·di·o·ac·cel·er·a·tor (kar′dē-ō-ak-sel′er-ā-ter). Cardioacelerador; acelerador dos batimentos cardíacos.
car·di·o·ac·tive (kar′dē-ō-ak′tiv). Cardioativo; que influencia o coração.
car·di·o·an·gi·og·ra·phy (kar′dē-ō-an-jē-og′ra-fē). Cardioangiografia. SIN angiocardiography.
car·di·o·a·or·tic (kar′dē-ō-ā-ōr′tik). Cardioaórtico; relativo ao coração e à aorta.
car·di·o·ar·te·ri·al (kar′dē-ō-ar-tēr′ē-ăl). Cardioarterial; relativo ao coração e às artérias.
Car·di·o·bac·te·ri·um (kar′dē-ō-bak-tē′rē-ŭm). Gênero de bactérias baciliformes imóveis, pleomórficas, Gram-negativas, anaeróbicas facultativas, encontradas na flora nasal e associadas à endocardite em seres humanos. A espécie típica é *C. hominis*.
C. hom′inis, espécie de bactéria que causa endocardite em seres humanos. A espécie típica de *Cardiobacterium*. VER HACEK *group*.
C. violaceum, bacilo móvel, Gram-negativo, não formador de esporos, encontrado no solo em regiões tropicais e subtropicais; causa de infecções humanas incluindo septicemia, pneumonia, infecções de feridas e abscessos; pode ser rapidamente fatal, com possível recidiva após a interrupção da antibioticoterapia.
car·di·o·cele (kar′dē-ō-sēl). Cardiocele; herniação ou protrusão do coração através de uma abertura no diafragma, ou através de uma ferida. [cardio- + G. *kēlē*, hérnia]
car·di·o·cha·la·sia (kar′dē-ō-kă-lā′zē-ă). Cardiocalásia; acalásia da cárdia.

car·di·o·di·o·sis (kar′dē-ō-dē-ō′sis). Cardiodiose; termo raramente usado para designar a manobra realizada para dilatar a cárdia gástrica. [cardio- (2) + G. *diōsis*, abertura ampla]

car·di·o·dy·nam·ics (kar′dē-ō-dī-nam′iks). Cardiodinâmica; mecânica da atividade cardíaca, incluindo seu movimento e as forças assim produzidas.

car·di·o·dyn·ia (kar′dē-ō-din′ē-a). Cardiodinia; dor no coração. SIN cardialgia (2). [cardio- + G. *odynē*, dor]

car·di·o·e·soph·a·ge·al (kar′dē-ō-ē-sof-a-jē′al). Cardioesofágico; indica a área na junção entre o esôfago e a parte cardíaca do estômago.

car·di·o·gen·e·sis (kar-dē-ō-gen′e-sis). Cardiogênese; formação do coração no embrião. [cardio- + G. *genesis*, origem]

car·di·o·gen·ic (kar′dē-ō-jen′ik). Cardiogênico; de origem cardíaca.

car·di·o·gram (kar′dē-ō-gram). Cardiograma. **1.** O traçado gráfico feito pelo estilete de um cardiógrafo. **2.** Geralmente usado para qualquer registro derivado do coração, subentendendo-se prefixos como apex-, eco-, eletro-, fono- ou vetor-. [cardio- + G. *gramma*, diagrama]
esophageal c., c. esofágico; traçado das contrações atriais esquerdas feito por registro de deslocamentos da coluna de ar em um tubo ou fio transdutor esofágico equipado com sensor.

car·di·o·graph (kar′dē-ō-graf). Cardiógrafo; instrumento para registro gráfico dos movimentos do coração, construído sob o princípio do esfigmógrafo. [cardio- + G. *graphō*, escrever]

car·di·og·ra·phy (kar-dē-og′ra-fē). Cardiografia; uso do cardiógrafo. VER TAMBÉM electrocardiography.
ultrasonic c., ecocardiografia. SIN echocardiography.
ultrasound c., ecocardiografia. SIN echocardiography.

car·di·o·he·mo·throm·bus (kar′dē-ō-hē-mō-throm′bus). Cardioemotrombo. SIN cardiothrombus.

car·di·o·he·pat·ic (kar′dē-ō-hē-pat′ik). Cárdio-hepático; relativo ao coração e ao fígado.

car·di·o·he·pa·to·meg·a·ly (kar′dē-ō-hep′a-tō-meg′a-lē). Cárdio-hepatomegalia; aumento do coração e do fígado.

car·di·oid (kar′dē-oyd). Cardióide; semelhante ao coração. [cardi- + G. *eidos*, semelhança]

car·di·o·in·hib·i·to·ry (kar′dē-ō-in-hib′i-tō-rē). Cardioinibidor; que interrompe ou lentifica a ação do coração.

car·di·o·ky·mo·gram (kar′dē-ō-kī′mō-gram). Cardiocimograma; cardioquimograma; registro feito por um cardiocimógrafo.

car·di·o·ky·mo·graph (kar′dē-ō-kī′mō-graf). Cardiocimógrafo; cardioquimógrafo; aparelho não-invasivo, colocado sobre o tórax, capaz de registrar o movimento da parede segmentar anterior do ventrículo esquerdo; consiste em uma placa transdutora capacitiva de 5 cm de diâmetro como parte de um oscilador de alta freqüência e baixa potência com sonda de registro; alterações no movimento da parede afetam o campo magnético e, portanto, a freqüência oscilatória, que é então registrada em um polígrafo analógico multicanal.

car·di·o·ky·mog·ra·phy (kar′dē-ō-ki-mog′ra-fē). Cardiocimografia; cardioquimografia; uso de um cardiocimógrafo.

car·di·o·lip·in (kar′dē-ō-lip′in). Cardiolipina; 1,3-bis(fosfatidil)glicerol encontrado em muitas biomembranas com propriedades imunológicas; usado no diagnóstico sorológico da sífilis. Quando misturada à lecitina e ao colesterol, a c. se combina com o anticorpo de Wassermann, mas não com o anticorpo imobilizador do *Treponema*. SIN acetone-insoluble antigen, heart antigen.

car·di·ol·o·gist (kar-dē-ol′ō-jist). Cardiologista; médico especializado em cardiologia.

car·di·ol·o·gy (kar-dē-ol′ō-jē). Cardiologia; a especialidade médica relacionada com o diagnóstico e tratamento das doenças cardíacas. [cardio- + G. *logos*, estudo]

car·di·ol·y·sis (kar-dē-ol′i-sis). Cardiólise; operação obsoleta para romper as aderências na mediastinopericardite crônica; o acesso é feito por ressecção de uma parte do esterno e das cartilagens costais correspondentes. [cardio- + G. *lysis*, afrouxamento]

car·di·o·ma·la·cia (kar′dē-ō-mā-lā′shē-a). Cardiomalacia; amolecimento das paredes do coração. [cardio- + G. *malakia*, amolecimento]

car·di·o·meg·a·ly (kar-dē-ō-meg′a-lē). Cardiomegalia; aumento do coração. SIN macrocardia, megacardia, megalocardia. [cardio- + G. *megas*, grande]
glycogen c., c. por glicogênio; uma forma de glicogenose devida ao armazenamento anormal de glicogênio nas células musculares cardíacas.
glycogenic c., c. glicogênica; aumento do coração devido à doença por depósito de glicogênio; na maioria das vezes ocorre no tipo II (deficiência de glucosidase ácida lisossômica), principalmente na lactância e na infância.

car·di·om·e·try (kar-dē-om′e-trē). Cardiometria; medida das dimensões do coração ou da força de sua ação. [cardio- + G. *metron*, medida]

car·di·o·mo·til·i·ty (kar′dē-ō-mō-til′i-tē). Cardiomotilidade; movimentos do coração.

car·di·o·mus·cu·lar (kar′dē-ō-mŭs′kū-lar). Cardiomuscular; relativo à musculatura cardíaca.

car·di·o·my·op·a·thy (kar′dē-ō-mī-op′a-thē). Miocardiopatia; doença do miocárdio. Como classificação de doença, o termo é empregado com vários sentidos diferentes, mas é limitado pela Organização Mundial de Saúde a: "processo mórbido primário do músculo cardíaco na ausência de uma etiologia subjacente conhecida" quando se refere à miocardiopatia idiopática. SIN myocardiopathy. [cardio- + G. *mys*, músculo, + *pathos*, doença]
alcoholic c., m. alcoólica; doença do miocárdio que ocorre em alguns alcoólatras crônicos; pode resultar de intoxicação alcoólica, deficiência de tiamina ou ter patogenia desconhecida. SIN alcoholic myocardiopathy, beer heart.
congestive c., m. congestiva. SIN dilated c.
dilated c., m. dilatada; diminuição da função do ventrículo esquerdo associada à sua dilatação; a maioria dos pacientes apresenta hipocinesia global, embora possa haver anormalidades bem definidas de movimento da parede regional; geralmente se manifesta por sinais de insuficiência cardíaca geral, com achados congestivos, e também por fadiga indicativa de um estado de baixo débito. SIN congestive c.
familial hypertrophic c., m. hipertrófica familiar; ocorrência familiar de m. hipertrófica com um padrão autossômico dominante de herança. A m. familiar de vários tipos tem herança autossômica dominante [MIM*115200]. Também há uma forma assimétrica que afeta os ventrículos e o septo interventricular [MIM*192600].
hypertrophic c., m. hipertrófica; espessamento do septo interventricular e das paredes do ventrículo esquerdo com acentuado desarranjo das miofibrilas; freqüentemente está associada a maior espessamento do septo que da parede livre, resultando em estreitamento do trato de saída ventricular esquerdo e gradiente de efluxo dinâmico; a complacência diastólica está muito comprometida.
idiopathic c., m. idiopática. SIN primary c. (1).
peripartum c., m. periparto; insuficiência cardíaca devida à doença do músculo cardíaco no período anterior, simultâneo ou posterior ao parto.
postpartum c., m. pós-parto; cardiomegalia e insuficiência cardíaca congestiva que ocorrem no puerpério na ausência de causas conhecidas de doença cardíaca.
primary c., m. primária; **(1)** m. de causa desconhecida ou obscura. SIN idiopathic c. **(2)** doença que afeta principalmente o músculo cardíaco, poupando outras estruturas cardíacas e geralmente resultando em fibrose e/ou hipertrofia.

classificação etiológica das miocardiopatias

envolvimento primário do miocárdio

idiopático (D, R, H)	familiar (D, H)
doença endomiocárdica eosinofílica (R)	fibrose endomiocárdica (R)

envolvimento secundário do miocárdio

miocardite infecciosa (D)	
viral	bacteriana
fúngica	por protozoários
por metazoários	por espiroquetas
por riquétsias	
metabólicas (D)	
doença de depósito familiar (D, R)	
doença por depósito de glicogênio	mucopolissacaridoses
hemocromatose	doença de Fabry
deficiência (D)	
eletrolítica	nutricional
distúrbios do tecido conjuntivo (D)	
lúpus eritematoso sistêmico	poliarterite nodosa
artrite reumatóide	esclerose sistêmica progressiva
dermatomiosite	
infiltração e granulomas (R, D)	
amiloidose	sarcoidose
malignidade	
neuromuscular (D)	
distrofia muscular	distrofia miotônica
ataxia de Friedreich (H, D)	
reações de sensibilidade e tóxicas (D)	
álcool	radiação
drogas	
cardiopatia periparto (D)	

NOTA: A principal manifestação (ou manifestações) clínica de cada grupo etiológico é indicada por miocardiopatia D (dilatada), R (restritiva) ou H (hipertrófica).

FONTE: Adaptado do relato da força-tarefa da OMS/SFIC (Sociedade e Federação Internacional de Cardiologia) sobre a definição e a classificação das miocardiopatias, 1980.

restrictive c., m. restritiva; um grupo diverso de condições caracterizadas por restrição do enchimento diastólico; freqüentemente confundida com pericardite constritiva e com as miocardiopatias infiltrativas; o tamanho do ventrículo esquerdo e a função sistólica podem ser preservados, mas a dispnéia resulta basicamente de aumento da pressão diastólica ventricular esquerda; os sinais de insuficiência ventricular direita podem ser proeminentes.
secondary c., m. secundária; doença que afeta o miocárdio secundariamente à doença sistêmica, infecção ou doença metabólica.

car·di·o·my·o·plas·ty. Miocardioplastia; cirurgia que usa o músculo grande dorsal estimulado para auxiliar a função cardíaca. O músculo grande dorsal é mobilizado da parede torácica e deslocado para o tórax atravessando o leito da 2.ª ou 3.ª costela ressecada. O músculo então é passado ao redor dos ventrículos esquerdo e direito e estimulado a se contrair durante a sístole cardíaca por meio de um marcapasso implantado. SIN cardiac muscle wrap.

car·di·o·my·ot·o·my (kar′dē-ō-mī-ot′ō-mē). Miocardiotomia. SIN esophagomyotomy. [cardio- (2) + G. *mys*, músculo, + *tomē*, corte]

car·di·o·nat·rin. Cardionatrina, peptídeo natriurético atrial. SIN atrial natriuretic *peptide*. [cardio- + L. Mod. *natrium*, sódio, + sufixo –in, material]

car·di·o·ne·cro·sis (kar′dē-ō-ne-krō′sis). Cardionecrose; necrose do miocárdio.

car·di·o·nec·tor (kar′dē-ō-nek′tor, -tōr). Cardionector; termo arcaico algumas vezes usado para o sistema condutor do coração (conducting *system* of heart). [cardio- + L. *necto*, unir]

car·di·o·neph·ric (kar′dē-ō-nef′rik). Cardionéfrico. SIN cardiorenal.

car·di·o·neu·ral (kar′dē-ō-noor′al). Cardioneural; relativo ao controle nervoso do coração. [cardio- + G. *neuron*, nervo]

car·di·o·neu·ro·sis (kar′dē-ō-noo-rō′sis). Cardioneurose. SIN cardiac neurosis.

car·di·o·o·men·to·pexy (kar′dē-ō-ō-men′tō-pek-sē). Cardioomentopexia; cirurgia para a fixação do omento ao coração com o objetivo de melhorar seu suprimento sanguíneo. [cardio- + omentum, + G. *pēxis*, fixação]

car·di·o·pal·u·dism (kar′dē-ō-pal′oo-dizm). Cardiopaludismo; irregularidade da atividade cardíaca devido à malária. [cardio- + paludismo, malária, do L. *palus*, pântano]

car·di·o·path (kar′dē-ō-path). Cardiopata; aquele que sofre de cardiopatia.

car·di·o·path·ia ni·gra (kar-dē-ō-path′ē-a nī′gra). Cardiopatia negra. SIN Ayerza *syndrome*.

car·di·op·a·thy (kar-dē-op′a-thē). Cardiopatia; qualquer doença do coração. [cardio- + G. *pathos*, doença]

car·di·o·pho·bia (kar′dē-ō-fō′bē-a). Cardiofobia; medo mórbido de cardiopatia.

car·di·o·phone (kar′dē-ō-fōn). Cardiófono; estetoscópio especialmente modificado para ajudar a ouvir os sons do coração. [cardio- + G. *phōnē*, som]

car·di·oph·o·ny (kar′dē-of′ō-nē). Cardiofonia; termo raramente usado para fonocardiografia (1).

car·di·o·phre·nia (kar′dē-ō-frē′nē-a). Cardiofrenia. SIN phrenocardia.

car·di·o·plas·ty (kar′dē-ō-plas-tē). Cardioplastia; cirurgia na cárdia. SIN esophagogastroplasty. [cardio- (2) + G. *plastos*, formado]

car·di·o·ple·gia (kar′dē-ō-plē′jē-a). Cardioplegia. **1.** Paralisia do coração. **2.** Interrupção eletiva temporária da atividade cardíaca por injeção de substâncias químicas, hipotermia seletiva ou estímulos elétricos. [cardio- + G. *plēgē*, acesso]
antegrade c., c. anterógrada; c. produzida por administração de soluções através das artérias coronárias.
retrograde c., c. retrógrada; c. produzida pela administração de soluções através das veias coronárias.

car·di·o·ple·gic (kar-dē-ō-plē′jik). Cardioplégico; relativo à cardioplegia.

car·di·op·to·sia (kar′dē-op-tō′sē-a). Cardioptose; distúrbio no qual o coração apresenta-se indevidamente móvel e deslocado para baixo, diferentemente da baticardia. VER TAMBÉM *cor* mobile, *cor* pendulum. SIN drop heart. [cardio- + G. *ptōsis*, queda]

car·di·o·pul·mo·nary (kar′dē-ō-pŭl′mo-nār-ē). Cardiopulmonar; relativo ao coração e aos pulmões. SIN pneumocardial.

car·di·o·py·lo·ric (kar′dē-ō-pi-lōr′ik, -pi-lōr′ik). Cardiopilórico; relativo às extremidades cárdica e pilórica do estômago.

car·di·o·re·nal (kar′dē-ō-rē′nal). Cardiorrenal; relativo ao coração e ao rim. SIN cardionephric, nephrocardiac, renicardiac.

car·di·or·rha·phy (kar-dē-or′a-fē). Cardiorrafia; sutura da parede cardíaca. [cardio- + G. *rhaphē*, sutura]

car·di·or·rhex·is (kar-dē-ō-rek′sis). Cardiorrexe; ruptura da parede cardíaca. [cardio- + G. *rhēxis*, ruptura]

car·di·o·scope (kar′dē-ō-skōp). Cardioscópio; instrumento para inspecionar o interior do coração vivo. [cardio- + G. *skopeō*, ver]

car·di·o·se·lec·tive (kar′dē-ō-sē-lek′tiv). Cardiosseletivo; que designa ou possui as propriedades de cardiosseletividade.

car·di·o·se·lec·tiv·i·ty (kar′dē-ō-sē-lek′tiv′i-tē). Cardiosseletividade; o efeito farmacológico cardiovascular relativamente predominante de um agente com múltiplos efeitos farmacológicos; usado principalmente ao se descrever agentes beta-bloqueadores.

car·di·o·spasm (kar′dē-ō-spazm). Cardioespasmo. SIN esophageal *achalasia*.

car·di·o·sphyg·mo·graph (kar′dē-ō-sfig′mō-graf). Cardioesfigmógrafo; instrumento para registrar graficamente os movimentos do coração e o pulso radial. [cardio- + G. *sphygmos*, pulso, + *graphō*, escrever]

car·di·o·ta·chom·e·ter (kar′dē-ō-ta-kom′e-ter). Cardiotacômetro; instrumento para medir a freqüência cardíaca. [cardio- + G. *tachos*, velocidade, + *metron*, medida]

car·di·o·throm·bus (kar′dē-ō-throm′bŭs). Cardiotrombo; coágulo de sangue no interior de uma das câmaras cardíacas. SIN cardiohemothrombus.

car·di·o·thy·ro·tox·i·co·sis (kar′dē-ō-thī-rō-tok-si-kō′sis). Cardiotireotoxicose; hipertireoidismo com complicações cardíacas.

car·di·ot·o·my (kar-dē-ot′ō-mē). Cardiotomia. **1.** Incisão de uma parede cardíaca. **2.** Incisão na cárdia. [cardio- + G. *tomē*, incisão]

car·di·o·ton·ic (kar′dē-ō-ton′ik). Cardiotônico; que exerce um efeito favorável, denominado tônico, sobre a atividade cardíaca; geralmente com o objetivo de indicar aumento da força de contração. [cardio- + G. *tonos*, tensão]

car·di·o·tox·ic (kar′dē-ō-tok′sik). Cardiotóxico; que tem um efeito prejudicial sobre a ação do coração, devido à intoxicação do músculo cardíaco ou de seu sistema de condução. [cardio- + G. *toxikon*, veneno]

car·di·o·tox·in (kar′dē-ō-tok′sin). Cardiotoxina. **1.** Um glicosídeo tóxico com efeitos cardíacos específicos. Por exemplo, causa despolarização irreversível das membranas celulares. **2.** Especificamente, um dos princípios tóxicos do veneno de cobra. **3.** Qualquer substância que possa causar lesão cardíaca em doses tóxicas.

car·di·o·val·vu·li·tis (kar′dē-ō-val-vū-lī′tis). Cardiovalvite; inflamação das valvas cardíacas.

car·di·o·vas·cu·lar (CV) (kar′dē-ō-vas′kū-lăr) [TA]. Cardiovascular; relativo ao coração e aos vasos sanguíneos ou à circulação. SIN cardiovasculare [TA], vasculocardiac. [cardio- + L. *vasculum*, vaso]

cardiovasculare [TA], cardiovascular. SIN cardiovascular.

car·di·o·vas·cu·lo·re·nal (kar′dē-ō-vas′kū-lō-rē′nal). Cardiovasculorrenal; relativo ao coração, artérias e rins, principalmente à função ou doença.

car·di·o·ver·sion (kar′dē-ō-ver′zhŭn). Cardioversão; restauração do ritmo cardíaco normal por contrachoque elétrico ou por medicamentos (cardioversão química). [cardio- + con*version*, conversão]

car·di·o·vert (kar′dē-ō-vert). Cardioverter; o ato da cardioversão.

car·di·o·ver·ter (kar′dē-ō-ver′ter). Cardioversor; aparelho usado para cardioversão.

Car·di·o·vi·rus (kar′dē-ō-vī-rŭs). Gênero de vírus RNA da família Picornaviridae, que raramente estão associados à doença humana e são isolados freqüentemente de roedores, isto é, Columbia S.K. virus, mengo virus.

car·di·tis (kar-dī′tis). Cardite; inflamação do coração.
rheumatic c., c. reumática; pancardite que ocorre na febre reumática, caracterizada por formação de corpúsculos de Aschoff no tecido intersticial cardíaco; pode estar associada à insuficiência cardíaca aguda, endocardite com pequenas vegetações de fibrina nas margens de fechamento das cúspides valvulares (principalmente a mitral) e pericardite fibrinosa; freqüentemente é sucedida por fibrose das válvulas.

care (kār). Assistência; cuidado; atenção, atendimento; em medicina e saúde pública, um termo geral para a aplicação de conhecimentos para benefício de uma comunidade ou indivíduo.
comprehensive medical c., assistência médica global, integral ou abrangente; conceito que inclui não apenas a assistência tradicional do paciente com enfermidade aguda ou crônica, mas também a prevenção e a detecção precoce da doença e a reabilitação do paciente incapacitado.

end-of-life c., assistência terminal; assistência física, emocional e espiritual multidimensional e multidisciplinar do paciente com doença terminal, incluindo apoio à família e cuidadores.

A assistência terminal tem recebido atenção cada vez maior nos últimos anos. Os estudos pioneiros de Elisabeth Kübler-Ross sobre morte e agonia, iniciados na década de 1960, proporcionaram descobertas úteis sobre as emoções, experiências e necessidades em transformação da pessoa agonizante. Os profissionais de saúde reconheceram formalmente a importância de tornar humana e competente a assistência até o fim da vida, de forma a preservar a dignidade e a autonomia do paciente. Os médicos, particularmente oncologistas, que tratam pacientes com doença terminal concentraram-se na necessidade de distinguir claramente entre formas agressivas e paliativas de tratamento e de estabelecer parâmetros para o tratamento de pacientes que não se beneficiarão de tratamento adicional voltado para a cura. Em particular, eles reconheceram a importância de proporcionar alívio adequado da dor em pessoas com câncer avançado. Também foi dada maior atenção ao controle das náuseas e dispnéia, freqüentes na doença terminal. Estudos mostraram que o alívio da dor, em pacientes terminais, freqüentemente é inadequado porque os médicos temem induzir o vício em narcóticos ou vir a serem acusados de apressar a morte. O maior uso de analgésicos opióides e o desenvolvimento de sistemas de analgesia e anestesia controladas pelo paciente melhoraram o controle da dor no câncer terminal e na AIDS/SIDA. Os enfermeiros abraçaram a responsabilidade pelo alívio do sofrimento, conforto, companhia e, quando possível, uma morte de acordo com os desejos do paciente. O movimento das casas de apoio estabeleceu programas e instalações dentro do sistema de assistência médica organizada que se concentram nas necessidades especiais das pessoas agonizantes de conforto e cuidados, em vez de tentativas de cura. Esses programas incluem apoio aos cuidadores e parentes durante e após a doença final do paciente. A assistência terminal enfatiza a importância de discussão franca, oportuna e de apoio sobre questões como preferências por tratamento para prolongamento da vida, incluindo reanimação cardiopulmonar, antes que essas medidas sejam necessárias. A legislação procurou preservar a dignidade e a independência de pessoas que estejam próximas do fim da vida, permitindo que estabeleçam orientações antecipadas para seu tratamento no caso de uma situação de incompetência ou coma. A integridade da relação entre pacientes e profissionais de saúde foi ameaçada pela crescente tolerância social e legal ao suicídio assistido por médico. A American Medical Association e a American Nurses Association publicaram posições oficiais contrárias ao suicídio assistido. Ver Também advance directive; physician-assisted suicide.

health c., assistência de saúde; serviços prestados a pessoas ou comunidades por agentes dos serviços de saúde ou classes profissionais com o objetivo de promover, manter, monitorizar ou restabelecer a saúde.
intensive c., terapia intensiva; tratamento e assistência de pacientes em estado grave. VER TAMBÉM intensive care *unit*.

managed c., atendimento gerenciado; acordo contratual no qual o pagador (p. ex., seguradora, plano de saúde, órgão do governo ou corporação) atua como intermediário entre médicos e pacientes, negociando honorários por serviço e supervisionando os tipos de tratamento administrados. VER TAMBÉM health maintenance *organization*.

O atendimento gerenciado substituiu, em grande escala, os planos de seguro tradicionais de remuneração médica, nos quais o pagamento é automático e os procedimentos supervisionados são mínimos. No atendimento gerenciado, o pagador controla encaminhamentos a especialistas, principalmente através da indicação de médicos de atendimento primário como "controladores"; restringe o escopo de serviços cobertos (particularmente procedimentos diagnósticos, escolha de medicamentos prescritos e duração da internação hospitalar) para cada diagnóstico; e exige revisão antes da autorização para internação hospitalar e uma segunda opinião antes de cirurgia eletiva. Os padrões de assistência são controlados por parâmetros de atendimento, podendo estes ser estabelecidos por algoritmos excessivamente simplificados que apresentam opções binárias (sim/não). As alternativas de prescrição são tipicamente restritas aos medicamentos relacionados no formulário do plano. Parâmetros de atendimento, escolhas de medicação e outras políticas que afetam o tratamento do paciente incorporam padrões profissionais e de conhecimento médico atuais, mas também refletem fortemente estratégias para controle de perdas e para a distribuição uniforme dos riscos atuariais por todos os beneficiários. O plano pode barganhar com médicos, hospitais, laboratórios e farmácias por preços atacadistas, ou pode remunerar os profissionais por capitação em vez de pagamentos por serviços. As organizações de atendimento gerenciado tipicamente empregam medidas de contenção de custos, como ênfase em medicina preventiva, auditorias de prontuários, revisão intensiva de queixas e punição de prestadores de serviços que desobedecem aos ditames impostos.

medical c., assistência médica; a parte do tratamento sob orientação de um médico.
primary medical c., assistência médica primária; assistência a um paciente por um membro do sistema de saúde que tem contato inicial com o paciente.
secondary medical c., assistência médica secundária; assistência por um médico que atua como consultor (dá pareceres) ao ser solicitado pelo médico primário.
tertiary medical c., assistência médica terciária; consulta especializada, geralmente por encaminhamento de um profissional de assistência médica primária ou secundária, com especialistas que trabalham em um centro com equipe e instalações para investigação e tratamento especiais.
ca·ri·bi (kă-rē′bē). Caribe. SIN epidemic gangrenous *proctitis.*
car·i·ca (kar′i-kă). SIN papaya.

car·ies (kār′ēz). **1.** Cárie; destruição microbiana ou necrose dos dentes. **2.** Termo obsoleto para tuberculose dos ossos ou articulações. [L. raiz seca]
active c., c. ativa; lesões dos dentes induzidas por micróbios que aumentam progressivamente.
arrested dental c., c. dentária estagnada; lesões cariadas que se tornaram inativas e pararam de progredir; podem exibir alterações da cor e/ou consistência.
buccal c., c. bucal; c. que começa com decaimento da superfície bucal de um dente.
cemental c., c. do cemento; c. do cemento de um dente.
compound c., c. composta; **(1)** c. que envolve mais de uma superfície de um dente; **(2)** duas ou mais lesões cariadas unidas para formar uma cavidade.
dental c., c. dentária; doença localizada, progressivamente destrutiva dos dentes, que começa na superfície externa (geralmente o esmalte) com a aparente dissolução dos componentes inorgânicos por ácidos orgânicos produzidos na vizinhança imediata do dente pela ação enzimática de massas de microrganismos (na placa bacteriana) ou carboidratos; a desmineralização inicial é seguida por destruição enzimática da matriz proteica com subseqüente cavitação e invasão bacteriana direta; na dentina, a desmineralização das paredes dos túbulos é seguida por invasão bacteriana e destruição da matriz orgânica. SIN saprodontia.
distal c., c. distal; perda da estrutura na superfície dentária em direção oposta ao plano mediano do arco dentário.
fissure c., c. de fissura; c. que começa em uma fissura nas superfícies oclusais dos dentes posteriores.
incipient c., c. incipiente; c. inicial.
interdental c., c. interdentária; c. entre os dentes.
mesial c., c. mesial; c. na superfície dentária voltada para o plano mediano do arco dentário.
nursing bottle c., c. de mamadeira; c. e erosão do esmalte dentário observadas em lactentes e crianças que vão dormir bebendo intermitentemente uma mamadeira de leite em pó, leite integral ou suco de frutas. SIN baby bottle syndrome.
occlusal c., c. oclusal; c. que começa na superfície oclusal de um dente.
pit c., c. de fóssula; lesão cariada, geralmente pequena, que começa em uma fóssula na superfície labial, bucal, lingual ou oclusal de um dente.

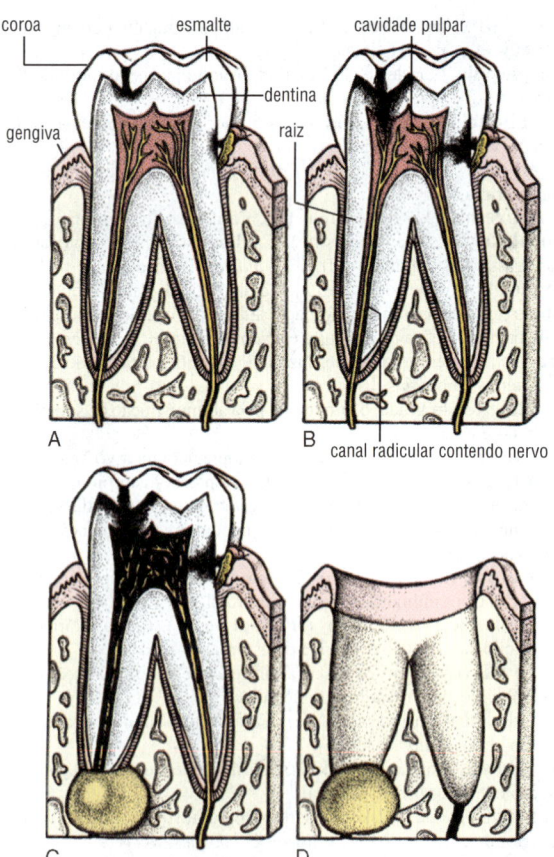

cárie: (A) ácido e/ou enzimas produzidos por bactérias orais degradam o esmalte e formam cavidades; (B) bactérias penetram na dentina para invadir a cavidade pulpar; (C) infecção destrói a polpa e se estende, através do canal radicular esquerdo, para causar doença periapical; (D) o dente foi perdido, deixando cisto periapical à esquerda

pit and fissure c., c. de fóssula e fissura; c. iniciada nas áreas onde estão localizadas fóssulas e fissuras do desenvolvimento na superfície do dente.
primary c., c. primária; lesões iniciais produzidas por extensão direta de uma superfície externa.
proximal c., c. proximal; c. que ocorre na superfície proximal, distal ou mesial, de um dente.
radiation c., c. de radiação; c. das regiões cervicais dos dentes, bordas incisivas e extremidades das cúspides secundária à xerostomia induzida pela radioterapia da cabeça e do pescoço.
recurrent c., c. recorrente; c. que recorre em uma área devido à remoção inadequada da cárie inicial, geralmente sob uma restauração ou nova cárie em um local onde já houve cáries anteriormente.
root c., c. radicular; c. da superfície radicular de um dente, que geralmente se apresenta como um defeito superficial largo na área da junção cemento–esmalte.
secondary c., c. secundária; c. de esmalte que começa na junção dente–esmalte devido à rápida disseminação lateral da cárie a partir da cárie original.
senile dental c., c. dentária senil; c. que ocorre na idade avançada, geralmente em posição interproximal e no cemento.
smooth surface c., c. da superfície lisa; c. iniciada nas superfícies lisas dos dentes.
ca·ri·na, pl. **ca·ri·nae** (kā-rī'nă, -rī'nē). Carina. **1.** Em seres humanos, termo aplicado ou aplicável a várias estruturas anatômicas que formam uma crista central projetada. **2.** Aquela parte do esterno de uma ave, morcego ou toupeira que serve como origem dos músculos peitorais; não é encontrada em aves não-voadoras nem na maioria dos mamíferos. [L. quilha de um barco]
c. for'nicis, c. do fórnice; crista que corre ao longo da superfície inferior do fórnice cerebral.
c. of trachea [TA], c. da traquéia; a crista que separa as aberturas dos brônquios-fonte direito e esquerdo em sua junção com a traquéia. SIN c. tracheae [TA], tracheal c.
c. tra'cheae [TA], c. da traquéia. SIN c. of trachea.
tracheal c., c. traqueal. SIN c. of trachea.
c. urethra'lis vagi'nae, c. uretral da vagina. SIN urethral c. of vagina.
urethral c. of vagina, c. uretral da vagina; a crista formada pela parte inferior da coluna anterior das pregas vaginais em relação à uretra, que é paralela à vagina entalhando a parede nesse lugar. SIN c. urethralis vaginae, c. vaginae.
c. vagi'nae, c. vaginal. SIN urethral c. of vagina.
car·i·nate (kar'i-nāt). Carinado; em forma de quilha; relativo, ou semelhante, a uma carina.
cario-. Cárie. [L. *caries*]
car·i·o·gen·e·sis (ka̱rē-ō-jen'ē-sis). Cariogênese; o processo de produzir cáries; o mecanismo de produção de cáries.
car·i·o·gen·ic (ka̱rē-ō-jen'ik). Cariogênico; que produz cáries; geralmente se diz de dietas.
car·i·o·ge·nic·i·ty (ka̱'rē-ō-jē-nis'i-tē). Cariogenicidade; potencial de produção de cáries.
car·i·ol·o·gy (ka-rē-ol'ō-jē). Cariologia; o estudo das cáries dentárias e da cariogênese.
car·i·o·stat·ic (kār-ē-ō-stat'ik). Cariostático; que exerce ação inibidora sobre o progresso das cáries dentárias.
car·i·ous (kār'ē-oos). Cariado; relativo a ou afetado pela cárie.
car·i·so·pro·date (kar'i-sō-prō-dāt). Carisoprodol. SIN carisoprodol.
car·i·so·pro·dol (kar'i-sō-prō'dol). Carisoprodol; um relaxante do músculo esquelético, quimicamente relacionado ao meprobamato e que pode viciar. SIN carisoprodate.
ca·ris·in (ka-ris'sin). Carissina; glicosídeo obtido da *Carissa ovata stolonifera* da Austrália; forte veneno cardíaco.
Carlen, Eric, otorrinolaringologista sueco do século XX. VER Carlen *tube*.
carm·al·um (kar-mal'ŭm). Carmalume; solução a 1% de carmim em alúmen dissolvido em água a 10%, usado como corante em histologia.
Carman, Russell D., radiologista norte-americano, 1875–1926. VER Carman *sign*.
car·mi·nate (kar'mi-nāt). Carminado; sal vermelho do ácido carmínico.
car·min·a·tive (kar-min'ă-tiv). Carminativo; antiflatulento; antifisético. **1.** Que evita a formação ou causa a expulsão de flatos. **2.** Um agente que alivia a flatulência. [L. *carmino*, pp. *–atus*, cardar lã; uso especial do L. Mod., expelir vento]
car·mine (kar'min, kar'mēn). [C.I. 75470]. Carmim; substância corante vermelha, usada como corante em histologia, produzida a partir da cochinelina, derivada da cochonilha; o tratamento da cochinelina com alúmen forma alumínio-laca de ácido carmínico, o constituinte essencial do carmim. [L. Mediev. *carminus*, contr. de *carmisinus*, do Ar. *qirmizē*, o inseto cochonilha]
lithium c., c. de lítio; corante vital para macrófagos.
Schneider c., c. de Schneider; corante que consiste em uma solução de c. a 10% em ácido acético a 45%, usado para preparações cromossômicas a fresco.
car·min·ic ac·id (kar-min'ik). Ácido carmínico; glicosídeo de um ácido carboxílico antracenoquinona; o constituinte essencial do carmim.

car·min·o·phil, car·min·o·phile, car·mi·noph·i·lous (kar-mi-n'ō-fil, -fil, kar-mi-nof'i-lŭs). Carminófilo; que se cora facilmente com corantes carmim. [G. *phileō*, amar]
Carmody, Thomas Edward, cirurgião oral norte-americano, *1875. VER C.-Batson *operation*.
car·mus·tine (kar-mŭs'tēn). Carmustina; agente antineoplásico. SIN BCNU.
car·nas·si·al (kar-nas'ē-ăl). Carniceiro; adaptado para cortar carne; indica aqueles dentes usados para cortar carne. [Fr. *carnassier*, carnívoro, do L. *caro*, carne]
car·ne·ous (kar'nē-ŭs). Carnoso; carnudo. [L. *carneus*]
car·nes (kar'nēz). Plural de caro. [L.]
Carnett, J.B., médico norte-americano do século XX. VER Carnett *sign*.
Carney, J.A., médico norte-americano contemporâneo. VER Carney *complex*.
Carney, J. Aldan, patologista norte-americano, *1934. VER C. *complex*.
car·ni·fi·ca·tion (kar'ni-fi-kā'shŭn). Carnificação; alteração nos tecidos, tornando-os carnosos, semelhantes ao tecido muscular. [L. *caro* (*carn-*), carne, + *facio*, fazer]
car·ni·tine (kar'ni-tēn). Carnitina; um derivado trimetilamônio (betaína) do ácido γ-amino-β-hidroxibutírico, formado a partir de $N^\varepsilon,N^\varepsilon,N^\varepsilon$-trimetillisina e de γ-butirobetaína; o L-isômero é um inibidor da tireóide encontrado em extratos de músculo, fígado e coração; L-c. é um transportador acil em relação à membrana mitocondrial; assim, estimula a oxidação de ácidos graxos. SIN B_T factor, vitamin B_T. [L. *caro carn-*, carne + *ine*]
c. acetyltransferase, c. acetiltransferase; enzima encontrada nas mitocôndrias que catalisa a transferência reversível de um grupo acetil da acetil-CoA para a c., formando *O*-acetilcarnitina e coenzima A. A acetilcarnitina é uma importante fonte de combustível nos espermatozóides.
c. acylcarnitine translocase, c. acilcarnitine translocase; proteína de transporte encontrada na membrana mitocondrial interna. Transporta derivados da acilcarnitina para o interior da mitocôndria e c. para fora da mitocôndria. Uma etapa importante na oxidação dos ácidos graxos.
c. palmitoyltransferase, c. palmitoiltransferase; **(1)** enzima que produz reversivelmente acilcarnitinas e coenzima A a partir da carnitina e acilcoenzima A (freqüentemente, palmitoil-CoA); importante na oxidação dos ácidos graxos. A deficiência da isozima I resulta em cetogênese e hipoglicemia; a deficiência da isozima II afeta basicamente o músculo esquelético.
Car·niv·o·ra (kar-niv'ō-ră). Ordem de mamíferos que comem principalmente carne fresca e na qual se incluem gatos, cães, ursos, civetas, visões e hienas, bem como o guaxinim e o panda; algumas espécies são onívoras ou herbívoras. [L. *carnivorous*, de *caro* (*carn-*), carne, + *voro*, devorar]
car·ni·vore (kar'ni-vōr). Carnívoro; pertencente à ordem Carnivora.
car·niv·o·rous (kar-niv'ō-rŭs). Carnívoro; que come carne; que subsiste alimentando-se de animais. SIN zoophagous.
car·nos·in·ase (kar'nō-si-nās). Carnosinase; enzima encontrada em mamíferos que catalisa a hidrólise de carnosina, produzindo histidina e β-alanina; a deficiência da enzima sérica causa elevação dos níveis de carnosina.
car·no·sine (kar'nō-sēn). Carnosina; *N*-β-alanil-L-histidina; o componente nitrogenado não-proteico dominante do tecido cerebral, encontrado pela primeira vez em quantidades relativamente grandes no músculo; quela o cobre e ativa a miosina ATPase. SIN ignotine, inhibitine. [L. *carnosus*, carnoso, de *caro*, carne, + *-ia*]
car·nos·i·ne·mia (kar'nō-si-nē'mē-ă). Carnosinemia; doença congênita autossômica recessiva, caracterizada por quantidades excessivas de carnosina no sangue e na urina, e causada por deficiência genética da enzima carnosinase. Clinicamente caracterizada por lesão neurológica progressiva, retardo mental acentuado e convulsões mioclônicas. [carnosine + G. *haima*, sangue + -ia]
car·nos·i·ty (kar-nos'i-tē). Carnosidade. **1.** Corpulência. **2.** Uma protuberância carnosa.
Carnoy, Jean Baptiste, biólogo francês, 1836–1899. VER C. *fixative*.
ca·ro, gen. **car·nis,** pl. **car·nes** (kā'ro, kar'nis, -nes). Carne; as partes carnosas do corpo; tecidos muscular e adiposo. [L.]
c. quadra'ta syl'vii, músculo quadrado plantar. SIN quadratus plantae (*muscle*).
car·ob flour (kar'ob). Farinha de alfarroba. SIN algaroba.
Caroli, J., médico francês do século XX. VER C. *disease*.
car·o·ten·ase (kar'-ō-ten-ās). Carotenase. SIN β-carotene 15,15′-dioxygenase.
car·o·tene (kar'ō-tēn). Caroteno; classe de carotenóides, pigmentos amarelo-avermelhados (lipocromos) amplamente distribuídos em vegetais e animais, notavelmente nas cenouras, e cuja estrutura está intimamente relacionada às xantofilas e licopenos e ao esqualeno de cadeia aberta; são de interesse particular porque incluem precursores das vitaminas A (carotenóides da pró-vitamina A). Quimicamente, consistem em 8 unidades isopreno em uma cadeia simétrica com os dois isoprenos em cada extremidade ciclizada, formando α-caroteno ou β-caroteno (γ-caroteno tem apenas uma extremidade ciclizada). As extremidades cíclicas do β-caroteno são estruturas tipo β-ionina idênticas; assim, na fissão oxidativa, o β-caroteno produz 2 moléculas de vitamina A. As extremidades cíclicas do α-caroteno são diferentes: uma é uma α-ionona, a

outra uma β-ionona; à fissão, o α-caroteno, como o γ-caroteno, produz 1 molécula de vitamina A (um derivado β-ionona).
c. oxidase, c. oxidase. SIN lipoxygenase.
β-ca·ro·tene 15,15'-di·ox·y·gen·ase. β-caroteno 15,15'-dioxigenase; uma enzima que catalisa a reação do β-caroteno mais O_2, produzindo retinais. SIN β-carotene-cleavage enzyme, carotenase.
car·o·ten·e·mia (kar'ō - te - nē'mē - ă). Carotenemia; caroteno no sangue, refere-se principalmente a quantidades aumentadas, que, algumas vezes, causam pigmentação amarelo-avermelhada pálida da pele, podendo assemelhar-se à icterícia. SIN carotinemia, xanthemia.
car·o·ten·o·der·ma (ka - rot'en - ō - der - mă). Carotenodermia. SIN carotenosis cutis. [carotene + G. *derma*, pele]
ca·rot·e·noid (ka - rot'e - noyd). Carotenóide. **1.** Semelhante ao caroteno; que possui cor amarela. **2.** Um dos carotenóides.
ca·rot·e·noids (ka - rot'e - noydz). Carotenóides; termo geral para uma classe de carotenos e seus derivados oxigenados (xantofilas), que consistem em 8 unidades isoprenóides (portanto, tetraterpenos) unidas de forma que sua orientação seja invertida no centro, colocando os dois grupamentos metilas centrais em uma relação 1,6 em contraste com a relação 1,5 dos outros. Todos os c. podem ser formalmente derivados da estrutura $C_{40}H_{56}$ acíclica conhecida como licopeno, com sua cadeia longa central de ligações duplas conjugadas por hidrogenação, desidrogenação, oxidação, ciclização ou combinações destes. São incluídos como carotenóides alguns compostos originados de determinados rearranjos ou degradações do esqueleto do carbono, mas não retinol e compostos C_{20} correlatos. Os grupamentos terminais de nove carbonos podem ser acíclicos, com ligações duplas 1,2 e 5,6, ou cicloexanos, com uma única ligação dupla em 5,6 ou 5,4, ou grupamentos ciclopentanos ou aril; estes agora são designados por prefixos de letras gregas precedendo o "caroteno" (α e δ, que são usados nos nomes comuns, α-caroteno e δ-caroteno, não são usados por essa razão). Os sufixos (ácido -óico, -oato, -al-, -ona, -ol) indicam determinados grupamentos contendo oxigênio (ácido, éster, aldeído, cetona, álcool); todas as outras substituições aparecem como prefixos (alcoxi-, epoxi-, hidro- etc.). A configuração em todas as ligações duplas é *trans*, a não ser que apareçam *cis* e números de localização. O prefixo *retro-* é usado para indicar um desvio de uma posição de todas as ligações simples e duplas; *apo-* indica encurtamento da molécula. Muitos carotenóides possuem atividades anticâncer.
car·o·ten·o·pro·tein (ka - rot'en - ō - prō - tēn). Carotenoproteína; uma proteína com um carotenóide com ligação covalente.
car·o·te·no·sis cu·tis (kar - ō - te - nō'sis kū'tis). Carotenose cutânea; coloração amarelada reversível e inofensiva da pele causada por aumento do conteúdo de caroteno; a esclera não é envolvida. SIN carotenoderma, carotinosis cutis.
ca·rot·ic (kă - rot'ik). Carótico, torporoso. SIN stuporous. [G. *karōtikos*, entorpecente]
ca·rot·i·co·tym·pan·ic (ka - rot'i - kō - tim - pan'ik). Caroticotimpânico; relativo ao canal carotídeo e ao tímpano.
ca·rot·id (ka - rot'id). Carotídeo; relativo a qualquer estrutura c. [G. *karōtides*, as artérias carotídeas, de *karoō*, colocar para dormir (porque a compressão da artéria carótida resulta em inconsciência)]
ca·rot·i·dyn·ia (kă - rot'i - din'ē - ă). Carotidinia. SIN carotodynia.
car·o·tin·e·mia (kar'ō - ti - nē'mē - ă). Carotinemia. SIN carotenemia.
ca·rot·i·no·sis cu·tis (ka - rot - i - nō'sis kū'tis). Carotenose cutânea. SIN carotenosis cutis.
ca·rot·o·dyn·ia (kă - rot'ō - din'ē - ă). Carotodinia; dor causada por compressão da artéria carotídea. SIN carotidynia. [G. *odynē*, dor]
car·pal (kar'păl). Carpal; relativo ao carpo.
car·pec·to·my (kar - pek'tō - mē). Carpectomia; excisão parcial ou total do carpo. [G. *karpos*, punho, + *ektomē*, excisão]
Carpenter, George Alfred, médico inglês, 1859–1910. VER C. *syndrome*.
Carpentier, Alain, cirurgião cardiotorácico francês do século XX. VER Carpentier-Edwards *valve*.
car·phen·a·zine ma·le·ate (kar - fen'ă - zēn). Maleato de carfenazina; um tranqüilizante fenotiazina do grupo da piperazina. Funcionalmente classificado como agente antipsicótico, é usado no tratamento da esquizofrenia aguda e crônica; também possui ações antiemética, adrenolítica, anticolinérgica e bloqueadora de dopamina.
car·po·car·pal (kar - pō - kar'păl). Carpocarpal. SIN midcarpal (2).
Car·po·gly·phus (kar - pō - glif'us). Gênero de ácaros, incluindo *C. passularum*, o ácaro de frutas, que causa dermatite entre os que lidam com frutas secas. [G. *karpos*, fruta, + *glyphō*, entalhar]
car·po·met·a·car·pal (kar'pō - met - ă - kar'păl). Carpometacarpal; relativo ao carpo e ao metacarpo.
car·po·ped·al (kar'pō - ped'ăl). Carpopodal; relativo ao punho e ao pé, ou às mãos e aos pés; designa principalmente o espasmo c. [G. *karpos*, punho, + L. *pes* (*ped-*), pé]
car·pop·to·sis, car·pop·to·sia (kar - pop - tō'sis, - tō'zē - ă). Carpoptose. SIN wrist-drop. [G. *karpos*, punho, + *ptōsis*, queda]

Carpue, Joseph C., cirurgião inglês, 1764–1846.
car·pus, gen. e pl. **car·pi** (kar'pus, kar'pī) [TA]. **1.** Punho; SIN wrist. **2.** Ossos carpais. SIN carpal *bones*, em *bone*. [L. Mod. do Gr. *karpos*]
c. cur'vus, carpo curvo. SIN Madelung *deformity*.
Carr, Francis H., químico inglês, *1874. VER C.-Price *reaction*.
car·ra·geen, car·ra·gheen (kar'ă - jēn, - gēn). Carragena. **1.** SIN chondrus (2). **2.** SIN carrageenan.
car·ra·gee·nan, car·ra·gee·nin (kar - ă - gē'nan, - nin). Carragenina; goma vegetal polissacarídica obtida do musgo irlandês; sulfato de galactosana com estrutura molecular semelhante à do ágar. SIN carrageen (2), carragheen. [*Carragheen*, povoado irlandês]
car·re-four sen·si·tif (kar - foor'son - sē - tēf'). Termo dado por Charcot à porção posterior do ramo caudal da cápsula interna. [Fr. cruzamentos sensoriais]
Carrel, Alexis, cirurgião franco-americano e prêmio Nobel, 1873–1944. VER C. *treatment;* C.-Lindbergh *pump*; Dakin-C. *treatment*.
car·ri·er (ka'rē - er). Portador; transportador. **1.** Pessoa ou animal que abriga um agente infeccioso específico na ausência de doença clínica evidente e serve como fonte potencial de infecção. **2.** Qualquer substância química capaz de aceitar um átomo, radical ou partícula subatômica de um composto, depois passando-a para outro; p. ex., citocromos são transportadores de elétrons; a homocisteína é um transportador de metila. **3.** Uma substância que, possuindo propriedades químicas intimamente relacionadas ou indistinguíveis de um marcador radioativo, é capaz de transportar o marcador através de uma precipitação ou procedimento químico semelhante; os melhores transportadores são os isótopos não-radioativos do marcador em questão. VER TAMBÉM label, tracer. **4.** Um grande imunógeno que, quando associado a um hapteno, facilitará uma resposta imune ao hapteno. **5.** Um componente de uma membrana que causa a transferência de uma substância de um lado da membrana para o outro. **6.** A fase móvel na cromatografia.
amalgam c., transportador de amálgama; instrumento usado para transportar amálgama triturado para uma cavidade preparada, onde é depositado.
convalescent c., portador convalescente; indivíduo clinicamente recuperado de uma doença infecciosa, mas ainda capaz de transmitir o agente infeccioso para outros.
genetic c., portador genético; pessoa heterozigota para um alelo mutante que, na forma homozigota, causa uma condição recessiva.
hydrogen c., transportador de hidrogênio; molécula que, em conjunto com um sistema enzimático tecidual, transporta hidrogênio de um metabólito (oxidante) para outro (aceptor) ou para oxigênio molecular a fim de formar H_2O. SIN hydrogen acceptor.
incubatory c., portador incubador; indivíduo capaz de transmitir um agente infeccioso para outros durante o período de incubação da doença.
latent c., portador latente; uma pessoa, que tipicamente pretende ter filhos, que possui o genótipo apropriado de um traço (homozigoto para recessivo, homozigoto ou heterozigoto para dominante, hemizigoto ou homozigoto para ligado ao X) e que só manifesta o traço em determinadas condições, p. ex., idade, uma agressão ambiental, etc.
manifesting c., portador manifesto. SIN manifesting *heterozygote*.
translocation c., portador de translocação; uma pessoa com translocação balanceada.
car·ri·er-free. Isento de carreador; diz-se de uma substância na qual se encontra um átomo radioativo ou outro átomo marcado em todas as moléculas; a maior atividade específica possível.
Carrión, Daniel A., estudante de medicina peruano, 1859–1885, que inoculou em si mesmo uma doença posteriormente designada doença de Carrión, da qual morreu. VER C. *disease*.
carry-over (kar'ē - ō'ver). Transporte; remanescente; o fenômeno pelo qual parte do analisado presente em uma amostra parece estar presente na próxima ou nas próximas amostras no mesmo processo analítico. Este é mais notável quando uma amostra de baixa concentração de analisado sucede uma amostra de concentração muito alta.
Carteaud, Alexandre, médico francês, *1897. VER Gougerot-C. *syndrome*.
car·te·sian (kar - tē'zhun). Cartesiano; relativo a Cartesius, forma latinizada de Descartes.
car·tha·mus (kar'tha - mŭs). Cártamo; flóculos secos de *Carthamus tinctorius* (família Compositae). VER TAMBÉM safflower oil. SIN safflower. [Ar. *qurtum*, de *qartama*, tinta; a planta fornece um corante]

CARTILAGE

car·ti·lage (kar'ti - lij) [TA]. Cartilagem; tecido conjuntivo caracterizado por sua ausência de vascularização e consistência firme; consiste em células (condrócitos), uma matriz intersticial de fibras (colágeno) e uma substância fundamental (proteoglicanos). Há três tipos de c.: c. hialina, c. elástica e fibrocartilagem. Tecido conjuntivo avascular, elástico, flexível, encontrado basicamente nas articulações, na parede torácica e em estruturas tubulares como a laringe, vias aéreas e ouvidos; constitui a maior parte do esqueleto no início da vida fetal, mas é lentamente substituído por osso. Para descrição anatômica macroscópica, ver cartilago e suas subentradas. SIN cartilago [TA], chondrus (1), gristle. [L. *cartilago* (*cartilagin-*), cartilagem]

accessory c., c. acessória; uma c. sesamóide.
accessory nasal c.'s [TA], cartilagens nasais acessórias; pequenas placas variáveis de cartilagem, localizadas no intervalo entre as cartilagens alar maior e nasal lateral. SIN cartilagines nasales accessoriae [TA], sesamoid c.'s of nose.
accessory quadrate c., c. alar menor. SIN minor alar c.
c. of acoustic meatus [TA], c. do meato acústico; a cartilagem que forma a parede da parte lateral do meato acústico externo. É incompleta acima e está firmemente fixada às margens da parte óssea do meato externo. SIN cartilago meatus acustici [TA], meatal c.
alisphenoid c., c. alisfenóide; a c. no embrião da qual se desenvolve a asa maior do osso esfenóide.
anular c., c. anular. SIN cricoid c.
arthrodial c., c. artrodial, c. sinovial. SIN articular c.
articular c., c. articular; a cartilagem que recobre as superfícies articulares dos ossos que participam de uma articulação sinovial. SIN arthrodial c., cartilago articularis, diarthrodial c., investing c.
arytenoid c. [TA], c. aritenóidea; uma de um par de pequenas cartilagens laríngeas piramidais triangulares que se articulam com a lâmina da cartilagem cricóidea. Fornece inserção em seu processo vocal orientado anteriormente para a parte posterior do ligamento vocal correspondente e para vários músculos em seu processo muscular orientado lateralmente. A base da cartilagem é hialina, mas o ápice é elástico. SIN cartilago arytenoidea [TA], triquetrous c. (2).
c. of auditory tube, c. da tuba auditiva. SIN c. of pharyngotympanic tube.
auricular c. [TA], cartilagem da orelha. SIN cartilago auriculae [TA], c. of ear, conchal c.
basilar c., c. basilar; a c. que ocupa o forame lacerado. SIN basilar fibrocartilage, fibrocartilago basalis.
branchial c.'s, cartilagens branquiais; cartilagens que se desenvolvem nos arcos branquiais embrionários; elas formam o viscerocrânio cartilaginoso. SIN pharyngeal c.'s.
calcified c., c. calcificada; c. na qual sais de cálcio se depositam na matriz; ocorre antes da substituição por tecido ósseo e, algumas vezes, em cartilagens envelhecidas.
cellular c., c. celular; um estágio embrionário ou imaturo de c. em que ela consiste principalmente em células com pouca matriz. SIN parenchymatous c.
ciliary c., c. ciliar; termo incorreto aplicado algumas vezes aos tarsos inferior e superior. VER tarsus (2).
circumferential c., c. circumferencial; (1) SIN acetabular *labrum*; (2) SIN glenoid *labrum* of scapula.
conchal c., c. da orelha. SIN auricular c.
connecting c., c. de união; a c. em uma articulação cartilaginosa como a sínfise púbica. SIN interosseous c., uniting c.
corniculate c. [TA], c. corniculada, c. supra-aritenóidea; um nódulo cônico de cartilagem elástica, situado sobre o ápice de cada cartilagem aritenóidea. SIN cartilago corniculata [TA], corniculum laryngis, Santorini c., supra-arytenoid c.
costal c. [TA], c. costal; a cartilagem que forma a continuação anterior de uma costela, sendo o meio pelo qual ela alcança o esterno e com ele se articula. SIN cartilago costalis [TA], costicartilage.
cricoid c. [TA], c. cricóidea; a parte mais inferior das cartilagens laríngeas; tem o formato de um anel de sinete, sendo expandida em uma lâmina quase quadrilátera posteriormente; a porção anterior é denominada arco. SIN cartilago cricoidea [TA], anular c.
cuneiform c. [TA], c. cuneiforme; um pequeno bastão não-articulado de cartilagem elástica na prega ariepiglótica ântero-lateral e um pouco superior à cartilagem corniculada. SIN cartilago cuneiformis [TA], Morgagni c., Morgagni tubercle, Wrisberg c.
diarthrodial c., c. diartrodial. SIN articular c.
c. of ear, c. da orelha. SIN auricular c.
elastic c., c. elástica; c. na qual as células são circundadas por uma matriz capsular territorial fora da qual há uma matriz interterritorial contendo redes de fibras elásticas além de fibras colágenas tipo II e substância fundamental. SIN yellow c.
ensiform c., ensisternum c., c. ensiforme; termo obsoleto para processo xifóide (xiphoid *process*).
epiglottic c. [TA], c. epiglótica; uma fina lâmina de cartilagem elástica que forma a porção central da epiglote. SIN cartilago epiglottica [TA].
epiphysial c. [TA], c. epifisial; tipo particular de c. nova produzida pela epífise de um osso longo em crescimento; localizada na face epifisária (distal) da c. da zona de crescimento; é uma zona de condrócitos relativamente quiescentes (a zona de repouso) da placa epifisial (de crescimento) que une a epífise à diáfise. VER TAMBÉM epiphysial *plate*. SIN cartilago epiphysialis [TA].

falciform c., menisco medial. SIN medial *meniscus*.
floating c., c. flutuante; um pedaço solto de c. em uma cavidade articular, que se desprendeu da c. articular ou de um menisco. SIN loose c.
greater alar c., c. da asa maior. SIN major alar c.
Huschke c.'s, cartilagens de Huschke; dois bastões cartilaginosos horizontais na borda do septo cartilaginoso do nariz.
hyaline c., c. hialina; c. que possui um aspecto de vidro fosco, com substância intersticial contendo fibras colágenas tipo II finas encobertas pela substância fundamental; na c. do adulto, as células estão presentes em grupos isógenos.
hypsiloid c., c. hipsilóide. SIN Y c.
interosseous c., c. interóssea. SIN connecting c.
intervertebral c., c. intervertebral. SIN intervertebral *disk*.
intraarticular c., (1) disco articular. SIN articular *disk*; (2) SIN meniscus *lens*.
intrathyroid c., c. intratireóidea; uma estreita faixa de c. algumas vezes encontrada unindo as lâminas da c. tireóidea da laringe na infância.
investing c., c. de revestimento. SIN articular c.
Jacobson c., c. de Jacobson. SIN vomeronasal c.
c.'s of larynx, cartilagens da laringe. VER thyroid c., cricoid c., arytenoid c., cuneiform c., triticeal c., corniculate c., sesamoid c. of cricopharyngeal ligament, epiglottic c. SIN cartilagines laryngis.
lateral c. of nose, c. lateral do nariz. SIN lateral *process* of septal nasal cartilage.
lesser alar c.'s, cartilagens alares menores. SIN minor alar c.
loose c., c. flutuante. SIN floating c.
Luschka c., c. de Luschka; pequeno nódulo cartilaginoso algumas vezes encontrado na porção anterior da corda vocal.
major alar c. [TA], c. alar maior; uma de um par de cartilagens que se formam na extremidade do nariz. Consiste em um pilar medial que se estende até o septo nasal com seu par do lado oposto, e um pilar lateral que forma a parte anterior da asa do nariz. SIN cartilago alaris major, greater alar c.
mandibular c., c. mandibular; barra cartilaginosa, no arco mandibular, que forma uma estrutura de sustentação temporária na mandíbula do embrião; os primórdios cartilaginosos do martelo e da bigorna desenvolvem-se a partir de sua extremidade proximal, dando também origem aos ligamentos esfenomandibular e maleolar anterior. SIN Meckel c.
meatal c., c. meatal. SIN c. of acoustic meatus.
Meckel c., c. de Meckel. SIN mandibular c.
Meyer c.'s, cartilagens de Meyer; as cartilagens sesamóideas anteriores nas fixações anteriores dos ligamentos vocais.
minor alar c. [TA], c. alar menor; as 2–4 lâminas cartilaginosas da asa do nariz posteriores à cartilagem da asa maior. SIN accessory quadrate c., cartilagines alares minores, lesser alar c.'s.
Morgagni c., c. de Morgagni. SIN cuneiform c.
nasal septal c., c. do septo nasal. SIN septal nasal c.
c. of nasal septum, c. do septo nasal. SIN septal nasal c.
c.'s of nose, cartilagens nasais. VER lateral *process* of septal nasal cartilage, major alar c., septal nasal c., vomeronasal c., minor alar c., accessory nasal c.'s. SIN cartilagines nasi.
ossifying c., c. ossificante. SIN temporary c.
parachordal c., c. paracórdica; c. primitiva adjacente de cada lado da porção cefálica da notocorda em embriões jovens; representa uma etapa inicial na formação do condrocrânio.
paraseptal c., c. vomeronasal. SIN vomeronasal c.
parenchymatous c., c. parenquimatosa. SIN cellular c.
periotic c., c. periótica; massa cartilaginosa de cada lado do condrocrânio circundando a vesícula auditiva em desenvolvimento no feto; a cápsula ótica em seu estágio cartilaginoso inicial.
permanent c., c. permanente; c. que não é substituída por osso.

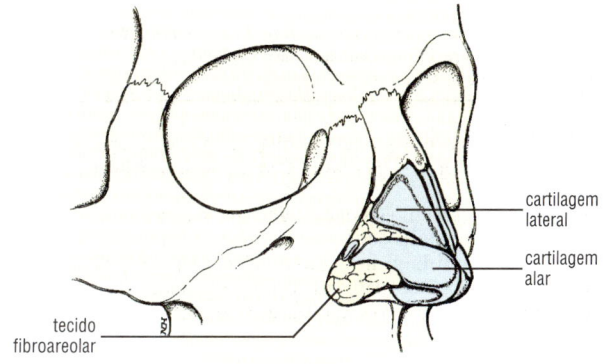

cartilagem do nariz

pharyngeal c.'s, cartilagens faríngeas. SIN branchial c.'s.
c. of pharyngotympanic tube [TA], c. da tuba auditiva; a cartilagem em forma de gamela que forma a parede medial, o teto e parte da parede lateral do tubo faringotimpânico. SIN cartilago tubae auditivae [TA], c. of auditory tube, tubal c.
precursory c., c. precursora. SIN temporary c.
primordial c., c. primordial; c. em um estágio inicial de seu desenvolvimento.
quadrangular c., c. do septo nasal. SIN septal nasal c.
Reichert c., c. de Reichert; uma c. no mesênquima do segundo arco branquial no embrião, a partir da qual se desenvolvem o estribo, os processos estilóides, os ligamentos estilóides e o corno menor do osso hióide.
reticular c., retiform c., c. reticular; termos raramente empregados para fibrocartilagem.
Santorini c., c. de Santorini. SIN corniculate c.
Seiler c., c. de Seiler; um pequeno bastão de c. fixado ao processo vocal da c. aritenóidea.
semilunar c., c. semilunar; um dos meniscos articulares da articulação do joelho. VER lateral *meniscus*, medial *meniscus*.
septal c., c. do septo nasal. SIN septal nasal c.
septal nasal c. [TA], c. do septo nasal; uma lâmina cartilaginosa fina situada entre o vômer, a lâmina perpendicular do etmóide e os ossos nasais, e que completa o septo nasal anteriormente. SIN cartilago septi nasi [TA], c. of nasal septum, cartilaginous septum, nasal septal c., pars cartilaginea septi nasi, quadrangular c., septal c.
sesamoid c. of cricopharyngeal ligament [TA], c. sesamóidea do ligamento cricofaríngeo; um pequeno nódulo de cartilagem elástica algumas vezes presente na borda lateral da cartilagem aritenóidea. SIN cartilago sesamoidea ligamentum cricopharyngeum [TA], cartilago sesamoidea laryngis, sesamoid c. of larynx.
sesamoid c. of larynx, c. sesamóidea da laringe. SIN sesamoid c. of cricopharyngeal ligament.
sesamoid c.'s of nose, cartilagens sesamóideas do nariz. SIN accessory nasal c.'s.
slipping rib c., c. costal deslizante; subluxação da c. costal, na junção costocondral, causando dor e estalido audível.
sternal c., c. esternal; c. costal de uma das costelas verdadeiras.
supra-arytenoid c., c. supra-aritenóidea. SIN corniculate c.
tarsal c., c. tarsal; termo incorreto algumas vezes aplicado aos tarsos inferior e superior. VER tarsus (2).
temporary c., c. temporária; c. que normalmente é substituída por osso, para formar uma parte do esqueleto. SIN ossifying c., precursory c.
thyroid c. [TA], c. tireóidea; a maior das cartilagens da laringe; é formada por duas lâminas aproximadamente quadriláteras unidas anteriormente em um ângulo de 90–20°, a proeminência assim formada constituindo a proeminência laríngea (pomo-de-adão). SIN cartilago thyroidea [TA].
tracheal c.'s [TA], cartilagens traqueais; os 16–20 anéis incompletos de cartilagem hialina que formam o esqueleto da traquéia; os anéis são deficientes na parte posterior em um quinto a um terço de sua circunferência. SIN cartilagines tracheales [TA], tracheal ring.
triangular c., c. triangular. SIN articular *disk* of distal radioulnar joint.
triquetrous c., (1) SIN articular *disk* of distal radioulnar joint; **(2)** SIN arytenoid c.
triticeal c. [TA], c. tritícea; um nódulo arredondado de cartilagem, do tamanho de um grão de trigo, ocasionalmente presente na margem posterior do ligamento tiroióide lateral. SIN cartilago triticea [TA], corpus triticeum, triticeum.
tubal c., c. da tuba auditiva. SIN c. of pharyngotympanic tube.
uniting c., c. de união. SIN connecting c.
vomerine c., c. vomeronasal. SIN vomeronasal c.
vomeronasal c. [TA], c. vomeronasal; uma faixa estreita de c. localizada entre a borda inferior da c. do septo nasal e o vômer. SIN cartilago vomeronasalis [TA], Jacobson c., paraseptal c., vomer cartilagineus, vomerine c.
Wietbrecht c., c. de Wietbrecht. SIN articular *disk* of acromioclavicular joint.
Wrisberg c., c. de Wrisberg. SIN cuneiform c.
xiphoid c., c. xifóide. SIN xiphoid *process*.
Y c., Y-shaped c., c. em Y; c. hipsilóide; a c. de união para o ílio, ísquio e púbis; estende-se através do acetábulo. SIN hypsiloid c.
yellow c., c. amarela. SIN elastic c.

---

car·ti·la·gi·nes (kar-ti-laj'i-nēz). Cartilagens; plural de cartilago.
car·ti·lag·i·noid (kar-ti-laj'i-noyd). Cartilaginóide; condróide. SIN chondroid (1).
car·ti·lag·i·nous (kar-ti-laj'i-nŭs). Cartilaginoso; relativo a, ou que consiste em, cartilagem. SIN chondral.
car·ti·la·go, pl. **car·ti·la·gi·nes** (kar-ti-lā'gō, -laj'i-nēs) [TA]. Cartilagem. SIN cartilage. Para descrição histológica, ver cartilage. [L. cartilagem]
cartila'gines ala'res mino'res, cartilagens alares menores. SIN minor alar *cartilage*.
c. ala'ris ma'jor, c. alar maior. SIN major alar *cartilage*.
c. articula'ris, c. articular. SIN articular *cartilage*.
c. arytenoi'dea [TA], c. aritenóidea. SIN arytenoid *cartilage*.
c. auric'ulae [TA], c. da orelha. SIN auricular *cartilage*.
c. cornicula'ta [TA], c. corniculada. SIN corniculate *cartilage*.
c. costa'lis [TA], c. costal. SIN costal *cartilage*.
c. cricoi'dea [TA], c. cricóidea. SIN cricoid *cartilage*.
c. cuneifor'mis [TA], c. cuneiforme. SIN cuneiform *cartilage*.
c. epiglot'tica [TA], c. epiglótica. SIN epiglottic *cartilage*.
c. epiphysialis [TA], c. epifisial. SIN epiphysial *cartilage*.
cartila'gines laryn'gis, cartilagens da laringe. SIN *cartilages* of larynx, em *cartilage*.
c. mea'tus acus'tici [TA], c. do meato acústico. SIN *cartilage* of acoustic meatus.
cartila'gines nasa'les accessor'iae [TA], cartilagens nasais acessórias. SIN accessory nasal *cartilages*, em *cartilage*.
cartila'gines na'si, cartilagens nasais. SIN *cartilages* of nose, em *cartilage*.
c. na'si latera'lis, c. lateral do nariz. SIN lateral *process* of septal nasal cartilage.
c. sep'ti na'si [TA], c. do septo nasal. SIN septal nasal *cartilage*.
c. sesamoi'dea laryn'gis, c. sesamóidea da laringe. SIN sesamoid *cartilage* of cricopharyngeal ligament.
c. sesamoidea ligamentum cricopharyngeum [TA], c. sesamóidea do ligamento cricofaríngeo. SIN sesamoid *cartilage* of cricopharyngeal ligament.
c. thyroid'ea [TA], c. tireóidea. SIN thyroid *cartilage*.
cartila'gines trachea'les [TA], cartilagens traqueais. SIN tracheal *cartilages*, em *cartilage*.
c. tritic'ea [TA], cartilagem tritícea. SIN triticeal *cartilage*. [L. *triticum*, trigo]
c. tu'bae auditi'vae [TA], c. da tuba auditiva. SIN *cartilage* of pharyngotympanic tube.
c. vomeronasa'lis [TA], c. vomeronasal. SIN vomeronasal *cartilage*.
ca·run·cle (kar'ŭng-kl) [TA], Carúncula; pequena protuberância carnosa ou qualquer estrutura que sugira esse formato. SIN caruncula (1). [TA].
lacrimal c. [TA], c. lacrimal; pequeno corpo avermelhado, no ângulo medial do olho, contendo glândulas sebáceas e sudoríparas modificadas. SIN caruncula lacrimalis [TA].
Morgagni c., c. de Morgagni. SIN middle *lobe* of prostate.
Santorini major c., c. maior de Santorini. SIN major duodenal *papilla*.
Santorini minor c., c. menor de Santorini. SIN minor duodenal *papilla*.
urethral c., c. uretral; pequena protrusão carnosa, algumas vezes dolorosa, da mucosa do meato uretral feminino; pode ser telangiectásica, papilomatosa ou composta de tecido de granulação.
ca·run·cu·la, pl. **ca·run·cu·lae** (kă-rŭng'kū-lă, -lē) [TA]. Carúncula. **1.** [TA]. SIN caruncle. **2.** Em ungulados, uma das quase 200 áreas específicas em forma de disco do endométrio uterino que, em conjunto com o cotilédone fetal, forma um placentoma da placenta; como um local de contato materno-fetal, a c. permanece em posição constante, mas aumenta muito durante a gravidez. [L. pequena massa carnosa, de *caro*, carne]
hymenal c. [TA], c. himenal; uma das muitas saliências ou projeções que circundam o orifício da vagina. SIN c. hymenalis [TA], c. myrtiformis.
c. hymena'lis, pl. **carun'culae hymena'les** [TA], c. himenais. SIN hymenal c.
c. lacrima'lis [TA], c. lacrimal. SIN lacrimal *caruncle*.
c. myrtifor'mis, pl. **carun'culae myrtifor'mes,** c. himenais. SIN hymenal c.
c. saliva'ris, c. salivar. SIN sublingual c.
sublingual c. [TA], c. sublingual; uma papila de cada lado do frênulo lingual marcando a abertura do ducto submandibular. SIN c. sublingualis [TA], c. salivaris.
c. sublingua'lis [TA], c. sublingual. SIN sublingual c.
Carus, Karl G., anatomista e zoólogo alemão, 1789–1869. VER C. *circle*, *curve*.
car·va·crol (kar'vă-krol). Carvacrol; isômero do timol presente em vários óleos voláteis (manjerona, orégano, segurelha e tomilho), com propriedades e atividade muito semelhantes às do timol; possui propriedades anti-sépticas, mas é usado principalmente como perfume.
Carvallo, VER Rivero-Carvallo.
car·ve·di·lol (kar'vĕ-dil-ol). Carvedilol; agente usado como anti-hipertensivo e antianginoso, e na insuficiência cardíaca congestiva.
carv·er (kar'ver). Entalhador; instrumento manual odontológico, disponível com muitos tipos de ponta, usado para esculpir cera, materiais de obturação, etc.
caryo-. Cário; núcleo. VER karyo-. [G. *karyon*, noz, núcleo]
car·y·o·phyl·lus, car·y·o·phyl·lum (kar'ē-ō-fi'lŭs, -ŭm). Cariófilo; *Dianto*; cravo-da-terra. [G. *karyophyllon*, craveiro, de *karyon*, noz, + *phyllon*, folha]
car·y·o·the·ca (kar'ē-ō-thē'kă). Carioteca. SIN nuclear *envelope*. [caryo- + G. *thēkē*, bainha, caixa]
Casal, Gasper, médico espanhol, 1691–1759. VER C. *necklace*.
cas·a·mi·no ac·ids (kăs'ă-mē'nō). Casaminoácidos; termo trivial para designar a mistura de aminoácidos obtidos por hidrólise da caseína; usados em meios de cultura bacterianos e similares.
cas·cade (kas-kād'). **1.** Cascata; série de interações seqüenciais, como as de um processo fisiológico, que, uma vez iniciada, continua até o fim; cada interação é ativada pela precedente, algumas vezes com efeito cumulativo. **2.** Derramar, principalmente com rapidez. [Fr., do It. *cascare*, cair]

cas·ca·ra (kas-kar′ă). Cáscara; cáscara sagrada. SIN c. sagrada.
  c. amara, c. amarga; c. de Honduras; a casca seca de uma espécie de *Picramnia* (família Simarubaceae); usada como laxante. SIN Honduras bark.
  c. sagrada, c. sagrada; a casca seca de *Rhamnus purshiana* (família Rhamnaceae); usada como laxante. SIN cascara.
case (kās). **1.** Caso; um caso ilustrativo de doença com suas circunstâncias associadas. Cf. *patient.* **2.** Uma caixa ou estojo. [L. *casus,* ocorrência]
  borderline c., caso limítrofe; um paciente cujos achados clínicos são sugestivos, mas não totalmente convincentes, de um diagnóstico específico.
  index c., caso índice; c. indicador. SIN proband.
  trial c., caixa de provas; em refração, uma caixa que contém lentes para provas.
ca·se·a·tion (kā′sē-ā′shŭn). Caseificação; forma de necrose de coagulação na qual o tecido necrótico se assemelha a queijo e contém uma mistura de proteína e gordura que é absorvida muito lentamente; ocorre particularmente na tuberculose. VER TAMBÉM caseous *necrosis.* SIN tyrosis (2). [L. *caseus,* queijo]
ca·sein (kā′sē-in, kā′sēn). Caseína; a principal proteína do leite de vaca e o principal constituinte do queijo. É insolúvel em água, solúvel em soluções alcalinas e salinas diluídas, forma um plástico duro insolúvel com formaldeído e é usada como constituinte de algumas colas; vários componentes são designados α-, β- e κ-caseínas. A β-caseína é convertida em γ-caseína pelas proteases do leite. Há várias isoformas de α-c. A κ-c. não é precipitada por íons cálcio.
  c. iodine, iodinated c., iodeto de c.; c. iodada; composto de c. com iodo formado por incubação da proteína com o elemento, que se fixa aos grupamentos tirosina na proteína. SIN caseo-iodine.
  plant c., c. vegetal. SIN avenin.
ca·sein·ate (kā′sē-in-āt). Caseinato; um sal de caseína.
ca·sein·o·gen (kā-sē-in′ō-jen). Caseinogênio; caseína "solúvel" ou κ-caseína que, quando sofre a ação da quimosina, é convertida em paracaseína.
ca·seo·io·dine (kā′sē-ō-i′ō-dīn). Iodeto de caseína. SIN casein iodine.
ca·se·ose (kā′sē-ōs). Caseose; termo indefinido para produto resultante da hidrólise ou digestão da caseína.
ca·se·ous (kā′sē-ŭs). Caseoso; relativo a, ou que apresenta, as características macro e microscópicas de tecido afetado por caseificação.
Casoni, Tommaro, médico italiano, 1880–1933. VER Casoni *antigen*; C. *intradermal test*, *skin test.*
cas·sa·va starch (kă-sah′vah). Fécula de mandioca; tapioca. SIN tapioca.
Casselberry, William E., laringologista norte-americano, 1858–1916. VER C. *position.*
Casser (Casserio), Giulio, anatomista italiano, 1556–1616. VER C. *fontanelle,* perforated *muscle.*
cas·se·ri·an (ka-sē′rē-an). Relativo a, ou descrito por, Casser.
cas·sette (kă-set′). **1.** Chassi; porta-placa, filme ou fita para uso em fotografia ou radiografia. Um chassi radiológico contém dois *écrans* intensificadores e uma folha de filme de raios X. **2.** Cassete; uma caixa perfurada na qual são colocados blocos de tecido para inclusão em parafina. [Fr., dim. de *casse,* caixa]
  susceptibility c., epítopo reumatóide ou compartilhado; seqüência comum de aminoácidos nos resíduos 70–74 nas cadeias HLA-DRB1, encontrada em alelos associados à artrite reumatóide. É uma dentre duas variações: glutamina[Q]-lisina[K]-arginina[R]-alanina[A]-alanina[A] ou QRRAA. Esses epítopos são encontrados em muitos alelos DRB1 diferentes. As cadeias alfa e beta que formam essas moléculas de apresentação do antígeno possuem uma configuração semelhante a uma gamela ou uma calha para recolher a água da chuva; os antígenos são ligados por seqüências de aminoácidos em uma bolsa ao longo da parte inferior e das laterais da gamela ou cavidade, e esse complexo forma um heterotrímero com o receptor de células T nas células CD4+. SIN rheumatoid pocket, shared epitope.
cas·sia bark (kash′yă). Casca de canela; canela; pau-canela. SIN cinnamon.
cas·sia fis·tu·la. Cássia imperial; chuva-de-ouro; o fruto maduro seco de *Cassia fistula,* usado como laxante. SIN purging cassia.
cas·sia oil. Óleo de cássia. SIN cinnamon oil.
cast (kast). **1.** Molde, objeto formado pela solidificação de um líquido derramado em uma fôrma. **2.** Aparelho; encerramento rígido de uma parte, como com gesso, plástico ou fibra de vidro, com o objetivo de imobilização. **3.** Cilindro; um molde alongado ou cilíndrico formado em uma estrutura tubular (p. ex., túbulo renal, bronquíolo) que pode ser observado em cortes histológicos ou em material como urina ou escarro; resulta do espessamento do material líquido secretado ou excretado nas estruturas tubulares. **4.** Contenção de um animal grande, geralmente um cavalo, com cordas e arreios, em uma posição deitada. **5.** Molde; em odontologia, uma reprodução positiva da forma dos tecidos maxilares ou mandibulares, que é feita pela solidificação de gesso, metal, etc., derramado em uma fôrma negativa, e sobre o qual podem ser produzidas bases de dentaduras ou outras restaurações dentárias. [I.M. *kasten,* de Esc. ant. *kasta*]
  bacterial c., cilindro bacteriano; um c. na urina composto de bactérias.
  blood c., cilindro hemático; c. geralmente formado nos túbulos renais, mas que pode ser encontrado nos bronquíolos; consiste em material espessado que inclui vários elementos do sangue (isto é, eritrócitos, leucócitos, fibrina, e assim por diante), resultante de hemorragia para o glomérulo ou túbulo, ou para o alvéolo ou bronquíolo.
  coma c., cilindro do coma; c. renal de grânulos fortemente refráteis, considerados indicativos de coma iminente no diabetes. SIN Külz cylinder.
  decidual c., molde decidual; um molde do interior do útero formado pela mucosa esfoliada em casos de gestação extra-uterina.
  dental c., molde dentário; reprodução positiva de uma parte ou partes da cavidade oral.
  diagnostic c., molde diagnóstico; réplica positiva da forma dos dentes e tecidos obtida a partir de uma impressão.
  epithelial c., cilindro epitelial; cilindro que contém células epiteliais e seus resquícios; é mais freqüente nos túbulos renais e na urina como um indicador de necrose tubular renal.
  false c., cilindro falso; filamento alongado, mucoso, semelhante a uma fita, com bordas mal definidas e extremidades pontiagudas ou fendidas, freqüentemente confundido com um cilindro urinário verdadeiro. SIN cylindroid, mucous c., pseudocast, spurious c.
  fatty c., cilindro gorduroso; um c. renal ou urinário que consiste, principalmente, em glóbulos de gordura; aqueles que contêm corpos duplamente refráteis (compostos de colesterol) são encontrados na síndrome nefrótica.
  fibrinous c., cilindro fibrinoso; cilindro amarelo que se assemelha um pouco a um cilindro céreo; encontrado mais provavelmente na urina de determinados pacientes com nefrite aguda.
  granular c., cilindro granular; c. urinário denso, relativamente escuro de resíduos celulares grosseiros ou finos e outro material proteináceo, freqüentemente observado na doença renal crônica, mas também na fase de recuperação da insuficiência renal aguda. VER TAMBÉM waxy c.
  hair c., cilindro piloso; cilindro composto de escamas paracerotáticas fixadas ao fio de cabelo, mas que se movem livremente para cima e para baixo no fio; encontrado na dermatite descamativa do couro cabeludo, incluindo a caspa, psoríase e dermatite seborreica. SIN pseudonit.
  halo c., halo craniano; aparelho aplicado aos ombros no qual são colocadas barras de metal que se estendem sobre a cabeça até um halo, a partir do qual se pode aplicar tração à cabeça por meio de pinças ou de uma corda.
  hyaline c., cilindro hialino; cilindro renal relativamente transparente, observado na urina, e composto de material proteináceo derivado da desintegração de células; observado em pacientes com doença renal ou, transitoriamente, durante exercício, febre, insuficiência cardíaca congestiva e tratamento com diurético.
  investment c., molde de revestimento. SIN refractory c.
  master c., molde-mestre; uma réplica das superfícies dentárias preparadas, áreas de bordas residuais e/ou outras partes da arcada dentária reproduzidas de um molde por impressão.
  mucous c., cilindro mucoso. SIN false c.
  red blood cell c., cilindro hemático ou eritrocitário; cilindro urinário composto de uma matriz contendo hemácias em vários estágios de degeneração e visibilidade, característico de doença glomerular ou hemorragia do parênquima renal. SIN red cell c.
  red cell c., cilindro hemático ou eritrocitário. SIN red blood cell c.
  refractory c., molde refratário; molde feito de material que resiste às altas temperaturas de fundição ou soldagem de metais sem se romper. SIN investment c.

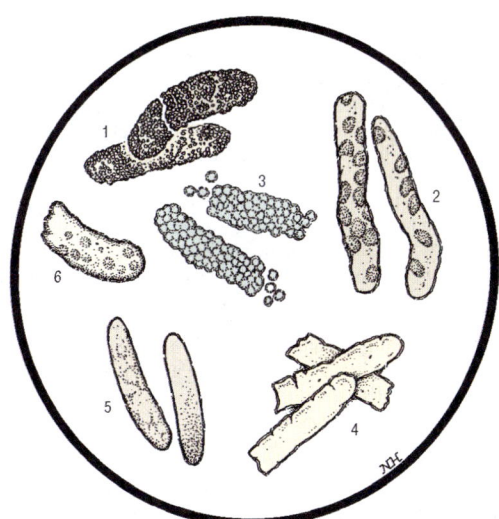

cilindros urinários: (1) cilindros granulares grosseiros; (2) cilindros de células epiteliais; (3) cilindros hemáticos; (4) cilindros céreos; (5) cilindros hialinos; (6) cilindros com piócitos

renal c., cilindro renal; qualquer tipo de cilindro formado em um túbulo renal e encontrado na urina que consiste em vários materiais, p. ex., albumina, células, sangue. SIN tube c.
spica c., gesso em oito; aparelho gessado de camadas superpostas com um padrão em V, que cobre duas partes do corpo de tamanhos muito diferentes, como o quadril e a cintura, o polegar e o punho, etc.
spurious c., cilindro espúrio. SIN false c.
tube c., cilindro tubular. SIN renal c.
urinary c.'s, cilindros urinários; cilindros eliminados na urina.
waxy c., cilindro céreo; uma forma de cilindro urinário que consiste em material proteináceo homogêneo de alto índice de refração, em contraste com o baixo índice de refração dos cilindros hialinos; os cilindros céreos provavelmente representam um estágio avançado do processo de desintegração que resulta em cilindros grosseira e finamente granulares, geralmente indicando doença renal avançada.
white blood cell c., cilindro leucocitário; cilindro urinário composto de leucócitos polimorfonucleares, característico da doença tubulointersticial, principalmente pielonefrite.
white cell c., cilindro leucocitário; um cilindro urinário composto de leucócitos.
cast brace (kast brās). Órtese; aparelho gessado ou plástico sob medida, que incorpora dobradiças e outros componentes de apoio; usado no tratamento de fraturas para imobilização e para promover atividade e movimento da articulação precoces.
Castellani, Sir Aldo, médico italiano, 1877–1971. VER C. *bronchitis, paint.*
cast·ing (kas′ting). **1.** Objeto metálico feito em uma fôrma. **2.** O ato de fazer um molde em uma fôrma.
  centrifugal c., modelagem centrífuga; modelagem de metal fundido em uma fôrma pela rotação do metal em um cadinho na extremidade de um braço de rotação.
  ceramo-metal c., molde cerâmico-metálico; molde feito de ligas contendo ou excluindo metais preciosos, às quais se pode fundir porcelana dentária.
  gold c., molde de ouro; molde feito de ouro, geralmente formado para representar e substituir uma estrutura dentária perdida.
  vacuum c., modelagem a vácuo; modelagem de um metal na presença de vácuo.
Castle, William B., médico norte-americano, 1897–1991. VER C. intrinsic *factor.*
Castleman, Benjamin, patologista norte-americano, 1906–1982. VER C. *disease.*
cas·tor bean (kas′ter bēn). Mamona, carrapateira. SIN Ricinus.
cas·tor oil. Óleo de rícino; óleo fixo obtido das sementes da *Ricinus communis* (família Euphorbiaceae); um purgante.
  aromatic c. o., óleo de rícino aromático; contém óleo de canela 3, óleo de cravo 1, vanilina 1, sacarina 0,5, álcool 30, em óleo de rícino para produzir 1.000; um catártico.
cas·trate (kas′trāt). Castrar; remover os testículos ou os ovários. [L. *castro,* pp. *-atus,* privar do poder de reprodução (masculino ou feminino)]
cas·tra·tion (kas - trā′shŭn). Castração. **1.** Remoção dos testículos ou dos ovários. **2.** VER castration *complex,* castrate.
  functional c., c. funcional; atrofia gonadal produzida por tratamento prolongado com hormônios sexuais.
ca·su·al·ty (kazh′oo - ăl - tē). Casualidade; sinistro; acidente; vítima de acidente; uma lesão ou a vítima de um acidente.
CAT Abreviatura de *chloramphenicol* acetyl transferase (cloranfenicol acetil transferase); abreviatura obsoleta de computerized axial *tomography* (CT) (tomografia computadorizada axial).
cata-. Forma combinante que significa para baixo; oposto de ana-. VER TAMBÉM kata-. Cf. de-. [G. *kata,* para baixo]
cat·a·ba·si·al (kat - ă - bā′sē - ăl). Catabasial; designa um crânio no qual o básio é mais baixo que o opístio. [cata- + L. Mod. *basion*]
cat·a·bi·ot·ic (kat′ă - bī - ot′ik). Catabiótico; usado na realização dos processos vitais além do crescimento, ou no desempenho das funções, referindo-se à energia derivada do alimento. [cata- + G. *biōtikos,* relativo à vida]
cat·a·bol·ic (kat - ă - bol′ik). Catabólico; relativo a, ou que promove, catabolismo.
ca·tab·o·lism (kă - tab′ō - lizm). Catabolismo. **1.** A decomposição no corpo de substâncias químicas complexas em formas mais simples (p. ex., glicogênio em CO_2 e H_2O), freqüentemente acompanhada por liberação de energia. **2.** A soma de todos os processos de degradação. SIN dissimilation (2). Cf. anabolism, metabolism. [G. *katabolē,* degeneração]
ca·tab·o·lite (kă - tab′ō - līt). Catabólito; qualquer produto do catabolismo.
cat·a·chron·o·bi·ol·o·gy (kat′ă - kron′ō - bī - ol′ō - jē). Catacronobiologia; estudo dos efeitos prejudiciais do tempo sobre um sistema vivo. [cata- + G. *chronos,* tempo, + biology]
cat·a·crot·ic (kat - ă - krot′ik). Catacrótico; designa um traçado de pulso no qual a linha de descida é interrompida por uma ou mais ondas ascendentes.
ca·tac·ro·tism (kă - tak′rō - tizm). Catacrotismo; uma condição do pulso na qual há uma ou mais expansões secundárias da artéria após o batimento principal, produzindo ondas ascendentes secundárias na linha de descida do traçado do pulso. [cata- + G. *krotos,* batimento]
cat·a·di·crot·ic (kat′ă - dī - krot′ik). Catadicrótico; designa um traçado de pulso no qual há duas pequenas elevações interrompendo a linha de descida.

cat·a·di·cro·tism (kat - ă - dī′krō - tizm). Catadicrotismo; distúrbio do pulso caracterizado por duas pequenas expansões da artéria após o batimento principal, produzindo duas ondas ascendentes secundárias na porção descendente do traçado do pulso. [cata + G. *di-,* dois, + *krotos,* batimento]
cat·a·did·y·mus (kat - ă - did′di - mŭs). Catadídimo. SIN duplicitas anterior. [cata- + G. *didymus,* gêmeo]
cat·a·di·op·tric (kat - ă - dī - op′trik). Catadióptrico; que emprega tanto sistemas ópticos de reflexão quanto de refração.
cat·a·dro·mous (kat - a - dro′mus). Catádromo; que migra da água doce para o oceano para desova. VER TAMBÉM anadromous.
cat·a·gen (kat′ă - jen). Catágeno; fase de regressão do ciclo de crescimento dos pêlos durante a qual a proliferação celular cessa, o folículo piloso diminui e é produzido um conglomerado piloso firme.
cat·a·gen·e·sis (kat - ă - jen′ĕ - sis). Catagênese. SIN involution. [cata- + G. *genesis,* origem]
cat·a·lase (kat′ă - lās). Catalase; hemoproteína que catalisa a decomposição do peróxido de hidrogênio em água e oxigênio ($2H_2O_2 \rightarrow O_2 + 2H_2O$); a deficiência de catalase está associada à acatalasemia.
cat·a·lep·sy (kat′ă - lep - sē). Catalepsia; condição caracterizada por rigidez cérea dos membros, que podem ser colocados em diversas posições mantidas por algum tempo, por ausência de resposta a estímulos, mutismo e inatividade; ocorre em algumas psicoses, principalmente esquizofrenia catatônica. [G. *katalēpsis,* convulsão, catalepsia, de *kata,* para baixo, + *lēpsis,* uma convulsão]
cat·a·lep·tic (kat - ă - lep′tik). Cataléptico; relativo a, ou que sofre de, catalepsia.
cat·a·lep·toid (kat - ă - lep′toyd). Cataleptóide; que simula ou se assemelha à catalepsia.
ca·tal·y·sis (kă - tal′i - sis). Catálise; o efeito que um catalisador exerce sobre uma reação química. [G. *katalysis,* dissolução]
  contact c., c. de contato; processo no qual o catalisador é um sólido e a reação catalisada é produzida após os reagentes (geralmente gases) entrarem em contato com o sólido.
  surface c., c. de superfície; catálise na superfície de uma partícula ou interface sólida, ou de uma macromolécula.
cat·a·lyst (kat′ă - list). Catalisador; substância que acelera uma reação química, mas não é consumida nem modificada permanentemente por ela. SIN catalyzer.
  inorganic c., c. inorgânico; um c. como um metal finamente dividido (Pt, Rh), carbono, etc.
  negative c., c. negativo; c. que retarda uma reação.
  organic c., c. orgânico; **(1)** SIN enzyme, ribozyme; **(2)** c. que está em uma molécula orgânica.
  Raney c., c. de Raney. SIN Raney Nickel.
cat·a·lyt·ic (kat - ă - lit′ik). Catalítico; relativo a, ou que realiza, catálise.
cat·a·lyze (kat′ă - līz). Catalisar; agir como catalisador.
cat·a·lyz·er (kat′ă - līz - er). Catalisador. SIN catalyst.
cat·am·ne·sis (kat - am - nē′sis). Catamnese; a história médica de um paciente após uma doença; a história de acompanhamento. [cata- + G. *mnēmē,* memória]
cat·am·nes·tic (kat - am - nes′tik). Catamnésico; relativo à catamnese.
cat·a·pasm (kat′ă - pazm). Catapasma; pó secante aplicado a superfícies cruentas ou úlceras. [G. *katapasma,* pó; *katapassō,* pulverizar]
cat·a·pho·re·sis (kat′ă - fō - rē′sis). Cataforese; movimento de partículas positivamente carregadas (cátions) em uma solução ou suspensão em direção ao catodo na eletroforese. Cf. anaphoresis. [cata- + G. *phorēsis,* transporte]
cat·a·pho·ret·ic (kat′ă - fō - ret′ik). Cataforético; relativo à cataforese.
cat·a·pla·sia, cat·a·pla·sis (kat - ă - plā′sē - ă, - plā′sis). Cataplasia; alteração degenerativa nas células ou tecidos que é o inverso da alteração construtiva ou evolutiva; um retorno a um estágio anterior ou embrionário. SIN retrograde metamorphosis (1), retrogression, retromorphosis. [cata- + G. *plasis,* moldagem]
cat·a·plasm (kat′ă - plazm). Cataplasma. SIN poultice. [G. *kataplasma,* cataplasma, de *kataplassō,* espalhar sobre]
cat·a·plec·tic (kat - ă - plek′tik). Catapléctico. **1.** Que se desenvolve subitamente. **2.** Relativo à cataplexia.
cat·a·plexy (kat′ă - plek - sē). Cataplexia; ataque transitório de fraqueza generalizada extrema, freqüentemente precipitada por uma resposta emocional, como surpresa, medo ou raiva, um componente da narcolepsia. [cata- + G. *plēxis,* um golpe, pancada]

CATARACT

cat·a·ract (kat′ă - rakt). Catarata; opacidade completa ou parcial do cristalino do olho. SIN cataracta. [L. *cataracta,* do G. *katarrhaktēs,* queda, catarata, de *katarrhēgnymi,* romper, correr para baixo]

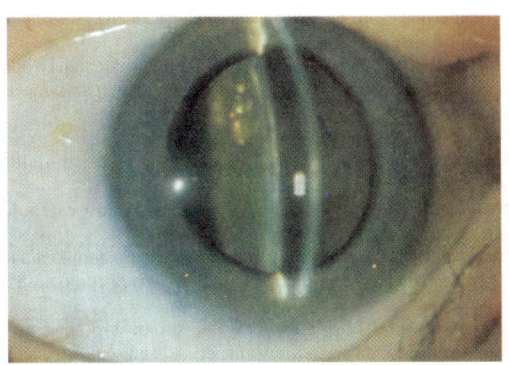
catarata

anular c., c. anular; c. congênita na qual uma membrana branca central substitui o núcleo. SIN disk-shaped c., life-belt c., umbilicated c.
atopic c., c. atópica; c. associada à dermatite atópica.
axial c., c. axial; opacidade lenticular no eixo visual do cristalino.
black c., c. negra; c. na qual o cristalino está endurecido e tem coloração marrom-escura. No século XIX, a c. negra alemã significava cegueira de etiologia desconhecida (q.v.). SIN cataracta brunescens, cataracta nigra.
blue c., c. azul; c. coronária de cor azulada. SIN cataracta cerulea.
capsular c., c. capsular; c. na qual a opacidade afeta apenas a cápsula.
capsulolenticular c., c. capsulolenticular; c. na qual há envolvimento tanto do cristalino quanto de sua cápsula. VER TAMBÉM membranous c.
central c., c. central; c. congênita limitada ao núcleo embrionário.
cerulean c. [MIM*115660], c. cerúlea; c. congênita com coloração azulada e lesões radiais; herança autossômica dominante em alguns casos.
complete c., c. completa. SIN mature c.
complicated c., c. complicada. SIN secondary c. (1).
concussion c., c. por concussão; c. traumática que ocorre com ou sem um orifício na cápsula do cristalino.
congenital c., c. congênita; c. geralmente bilateral, presente ao nascimento. Observada como um distúrbio autossômico recessivo em novilhos da raça Jersey. Em seres humanos, aproximadamente 25% das cataratas congênitas bilaterais são autossômicas dominantes [MIM*116200, *116700]; também existem formas ligadas ao X [MIM*302200, *302300]. A maioria das cataratas congênitas é esporádica; algumas são resultantes de prematuridade, infecção intra-uterina, intoxicação medicamentosa, traumatismo ou distúrbios cromossomiais ou metabólicos.
copper c., c. por cobre. SIN chalcosis lentis.
coralliform c., c. coraliforme; c. congênita com processos redondos ou alongados que se irradiam do centro do cristalino.
coronary c., c. coronária; c. de desenvolvimento cortical periférico que ocorre logo após a puberdade; transmitida como uma característica hereditária dominante.
cortical c., c. cortical; c. na qual a opacidade afeta o córtex do cristalino. SIN peripheral c.
crystalline c., c. cristalina; c. hereditária com um acúmulo coraliforme ou em forma de agulha de cristais na região axial de um cristalino transparente.
cuneiform c., c. cuneiforme; c. cortical na qual as opacidades se irradiam da periferia como raios de uma roda.
cupuliform c., c. cupuliforme; uma forma comum de c. senil freqüentemente limitada a uma região imediatamente dentro da cápsula posterior. SIN saucer-shaped c.
dendritic c., c. dendrítica; uma c. sutural congênita com ramificação complicada.
diabetic c., c. diabética; c. encontrada no diabetes melito insulino-dependente.
disk-shaped c., c. discóide. SIN anular c.
electric c., c. elétrica; c. produzida por contato com uma corrente elétrica de alta tensão ou por um raio. SIN cataracta electrica.
embryonic c. [MIM*115650], c. embrionária; c. congênita situada próxima da sutura anterior em Y do núcleo do cristalino fetal. Herança heterogênea.
embryopathic c., c. embriopática; c. congênita resultante de infecção intra-uterina, p. ex., rubéola.
fibroid c., fibrinous c., c. fibróide, c. fibrinosa; endurecimento esclerótico da cápsula do cristalino, após iridociclite exsudativa.
floriform c., c. floriforme; c. congênita com opacidades dispostas como as pétalas de uma flor.
furnacemen's c., c. do foguista. SIN infrared c.
fusiform c., c. fusiforme. SIN spindle c.
galactose c., c. por galactose; c. neonatal associada ao acúmulo de álcool de galactose (galactitol) no cristalino. VER galactosemia.
glassworker's c., c. do vidraceiro. SIN infrared c.
glaucomatous c., c. glaucomatosa; opacidade nuclear geralmente observada no glaucoma absoluto.
gray c., c. cinzenta; c. de coloração acinzentada, geralmente observada na c. senil, madura ou cortical.
hard c., c. dura. SIN nuclear c.
hook-shaped c., c. unciforme; c. congênita com figuras em forma de gancho entre os núcleos fetal e embrionário.
hypermature c., c. hipermadura; c. na qual o córtex do cristalino torna-se líquido, com o núcleo depositando-se na cápsula (c. de Morgagni). SIN overripe c.
hypocalcemic c., c. hipocalcêmica; c. que ocorre na vigência de baixo nível sérico de cálcio.
immature c., c. imatura; um estágio de opacificação parcial do cristalino.
infantile c., c. do lactente; c. que acomete uma criança muito pequena.
infrared c., c. por infravermelho; c. secundária à absorção de calor pelo cristalino, ou por transmissão a partir da íris adjacente. SIN furnacemen's c., glassworker's c.
intumescent c., c. intumescente; c. edemaciada devido à absorção de líquido.
juvenile c., c. juvenil; c. mole que acomete crianças ou adultos jovens.
lamellar c., c. lamelar; c. na qual a opacidade é limitada ao córtex. SIN zonular c.
life-belt c., c. anular. SIN anular c.
mature c., c. madura; c. na qual tanto o núcleo quanto o córtex são opacos. SIN complete c., ripe c.
membranous c., c. membranosa; c. secundária composta por remanescentes da cápsula espessada e fibras do cristalino degeneradas.
Morgagni c., c. de Morgagni; c. hipermadura na qual o núcleo deposita-se no fundo da cápsula. SIN sedimentary c.
myotonic c., c. miotônica; c. que ocorre na distrofia miotônica.
nuclear c., c. nuclear; c. que envolve o núcleo. SIN hard c.
overripe c., c. hipermadura. SIN hypermature c.
perinuclear c., c. perinuclear; c. lamelar na qual o núcleo é transparente, mas circundado por um anel de opacidade.
peripheral c., c. periférica. SIN cortical c.
pisciform c., c. pisciforme; c. hereditária com opacidades bilaterais em forma de peixe na região axial do núcleo fetal.
polar c., c. polar; c. capsular limitada a uma área do pólo anterior ou posterior do cristalino.
posterior subcapsular c. c. subcapsular posterior; c. envolvendo o córtex no pólo posterior do cristalino.
progressive c., c. progressiva; c. na qual o processo de opacificação progride para envolver todo o cristalino.
punctate c., c. pontilhada; c. incompleta na qual há pontos opacos dispersos por todo o cristalino.
pyramidal c., c. piramidal; c. polar anterior, cônica.
radiation c., c. por radiação; c. causada por exposição excessiva ou prolongada a raios ultravioleta, raios X, rádio, raios gama, calor ou isótopos radioativos.
reduplicated c., c. reduplicada; tipo de c. congênita com opacidades situadas em vários níveis no cristalino.
ripe c., c. madura. SIN mature c.
rubella c., c. da rubéola; c. embriopática secundária à infecção intra-uterina pelo vírus da rubéola.
saucer-shaped c., c. cupuliforme. SIN cupuliform c.
secondary c., c. secundária; (1) c. associada a ou que sucede alguma outra doença ocular, como uveíte. SIN complicated c., (2) c. que ocorre no cristalino ou cápsula retida após a extração de uma catarata.
sedimentary c., c. sedimentar. SIN Morgagni c.
senile c., c. senil; c. que ocorre espontaneamente em idosos; principalmente uma c. cuneiforme, c. nuclear ou c. subcapsular posterior, isolada ou associada.
siderotic c., c. siderótica; c. resultante da deposição de ferro a partir de um corpo estranho intra-ocular contendo ferro.
soft c., c. mole; c. avançada ou madura na qual o núcleo não está bem desenvolvido.
spindle c., c. fusiforme; c. na qual a opacidade é fusiforme, estendendo-se de um pólo ao outro. SIN fusiform c.
stationary c., c. estacionária; c. que não progride.
stellate c., c. estrelada; c. congênita com opacidades do cristalino que se irradiam em direção à periferia, com alterações subcapsulares e corticais.
subcapsular c., c. subcapsular; c. na qual as opacidades estão concentradas sob a cápsula.
sugar c., c. por açúcar; qualquer c. associada ao acúmulo de álcoois de pentose ou hexose no cristalino.
sunflower c., c. em girassol. SIN chalcosis lentis.
sutural c., c. sutural; tipo congênito de c. com opacidades ao longo das suturas em Y do núcleo do cristalino fetal; geralmente não afeta a visão.
tetany c., c. da tetania; c. que se desenvolve na hipocalcemia.
total c., c. total; c. que envolve todo o cristalino.
toxic c., c. tóxica; c. causada por drogas/fármacos ou substâncias químicas.
traumatic c., c. traumática; c. causada por contusão, ruptura ou por um corpo estranho.

umbilicated c., c. umbilicada. SIN anular c.
vascular c., c. vascular; c. congênita na qual o cristalino degenerado é substituído por tecido mesodérmico. SIN cataracta adiposa, cataracta fibrosa.
zonular c., c. zonular. SIN lamellar c.

cat·a·rac·ta (kat - ă - rak′tă). Catarata. SIN cataract. [L.]
  c. adipo'sa, c. adiposa. SIN vascular *cataract.*
  c. brunes'cens, c. negra. SIN black *cataract.*
  c. ceru'lea, c. cerúlea. SIN blue *cataract.*
  c. elec'trica, c. elétrica. SIN electric *cataract.*
  c. fibro'sa, c. fibrosa. SIN vascular *cataract.*
  c. ni'gra, c. negra. SIN black *cataract.*
cat·a·rac·to·gen·e·sis (kat′ă - rak - tō - jen′ĕ - sis). Cataratogênese; o processo de formação de catarata. [caratact- + G. *genesis*, produção]
cat·a·rac·to·gen·ic (kat′ă - rak - tō - jen′ik). Cataratogênico; que produz catarata.
cat·a·rac·tous (kat - ă - rak′tŭs). Catarátoso; relativo a uma catarata.
ca·tar·ia (ka - tā′rē - ă). Catária; gatária; erva-de-gato; erva-dos-gatos; os cumes floridos secos da *Nepeta cataria* (família Labiatae); emenagogo e antiespasmódico; também foi descrita a produção de efeitos psíquicos. SIN catnep, catnip. [L. *cattus*, gato macho (pós-classe)]
ca·tarrh (kă - tahr′). Inflamação de uma mucosa com aumento do fluxo de muco ou exsudato. [G. *katarrheō*, fluir para baixo]
  nasal c., rinite. SIN rhinitis.
  vernal c., conjuntivite vernal. SIN vernal *conjunctivitis.*
ca·tarrh·al (kă - tah′răl). Catarral; relativo a, ou afetado por, inflamação de mucosas.
cat·a·stal·sis (kat - ă - stal′sis). Catastalse; onda de contração semelhante à peristalse comum, mas não precedida por uma zona de inibição. [G. *katastellō*, colocar em ordem, verificar]
cat·a·stal·tic (kat - ă - stal′tik). Catastáltico; inibitório, restritivo ou contentor. [cata- + G. *staltos*, contraído, de *stellō*, contrair]
ca·tas·ta·sis (kă - tas′tă - sis). Catástase. **1.** Uma condição ou estado. **2.** Restabelecimento de uma condição normal ou um local normal. [G.]
cat·a·to·nia (kat - ă - tō′nē - ă). Catatonia; síndrome de distúrbios psicomotores caracterizada por períodos de rigidez física, negativismo ou torpor; pode ocorrer na esquizofrenia, em distúrbios do humor ou em distúrbios mentais orgânicos. [G. *katatonos*, estirado, deprimido, de *kata*, para baixo, + *tonos*, tônus]
  excited c., c. excitada; c. em que o paciente apresenta-se excitado, impulsivo, hiperativo e combativo.
  periodic c., c. periódica; fases de excitação catatônica que reaparecem regularmente.
  stuporous c., c. torporosa; c. na qual o paciente se apresenta reprimido, mudo e negativista, acompanhado por combinações variadas de olhar fixo, rigidez e cataplexia.
cat·a·ton·ic, cat·a·to·ni·ac (kat - ă - ton′ik, -tō′nē - ak). Catatônico; relativo a, ou caracterizado por, catatonia.
cat·a·tri·chy (kat′ă - tri - kē). [MIM*116850]. Catatriquia; presença de uma mecha de cabelo separada ou de aspecto diferente; pode ser herdada de forma autossômica dominante. VER Waardenburg *syndrome*. [cata- + G. *thrix*, pêlo]
cat·a·tri·crot·ic (kat′ă - trī - krot′ik). Catatricrótico; designa um traçado de pulso com três pequenas elevações interrompendo o ramo descendente.
cat·a·tri·cro·tism (kat - ă - trī′krō - tizm). Catatricrotismo; condição do pulso caracterizada por três pequenas expansões da artéria após o batimento principal, produzindo três ondas ascendentes secundárias no ramo descendente do pulso. [cata- + G. *tri*, três, + *krotos*, batimento]
cat·e·chase (kat′ē - kās). Catecase. SIN catechol 1,2-dioxygenase.
cat·e·chin (kat′ē - kin). Catequina; derivada do catechu e usada como adstringente na diarréia e como corante. SIN catechinic acid, catechuic acid, cyanidol.
cat·e·chin·ic ac·id (kat - ē - kin′ik). Ácido catequínico. SIN catechin.
cat·e·chol (kat′ē - kol). Catecol. **1.** SIN pyrocatechol. **2.** Termo amplamente empregado para catequina, que contém uma porção *o*-catecol, e como a raiz das catecolaminas, que são derivados pirocatecol.
  c.-O-methyltransferase, c.-*O*-metiltransferase; transferase que catalisa a metilação do grupamento hidroxila na posição 3 do anel aromático dos catecóis, incluindo as catecolaminas norepinefrina e epinefrina (assim convertendo em normetanefrina e metanefrina, respectivamente); o grupamento metila provém da *S*-adenosil-L-metionina. Uma etapa importante no catabolismo das catecolaminas.
  c. oxidase, c. oxidase; enzima que oxida os catecóis em 1,2-benzoquinonas, com O_2. VER TAMBÉM monophenol monooxygenase. SIN diphenol oxidase, *o*-diphenolase.
  c. oxidase (dimerizing), c. oxidase (dimerizante); enzima que oxida um c., com O_2, em uma difenilenodióxido quinona (p. ex., 4 c. + $3O_2 \rightarrow$ 2 dibenzo[1,4]-2,3-diona + $6H_2O$).
cat·e·chol·a·mines (kat - ē - kol′ă - mēnz). Catecolaminas; pirocatecóis com uma cadeia lateral alquilamina; são exemplos de interesse bioquímico: epinefrina, norepinefrina e L-dopa. As catecolaminas são elementos importantes em respostas ao estresse.
cat·e·chol 1,2-di·ox·y·gen·ase. Catecol 1,2-dioxigenase; uma oxidorredutase que catalisa a oxidação do pirocatecol, com O_2, em *cis-cis*-muconato. SIN catechase, pyrocatechase.
cat·e·chol 2,3-di·ox·y·gen·ase. Catecol 2,3-dioxigenase; uma oxidorredutase que oxida catecol, com O_2, em 2-hidroximuconato semialdeído. SIN metapyrocatechase.
cat·e·chu·ic ac·id (kat - ē - choo′ik-, - koo′ik). Ácido catéquico; ácido catecóico. SIN catechin.
cat·e·chu ni·grum. Catechu; cato; catechu negro; extrato do núcleo da madeira da *Acacia catechu* (família Leguminosae), usado como adstringente na diarréia. SIN cutch.
cat·e·lec·trot·o·nus (kat′ē - lek - trot′ō - nŭs). Cateletrotônus; as alterações na excitabilidade e condutividade em um nervo ou músculo adjacente ao catodo durante a passagem de uma corrente elétrica constante. [cathode + electrotonus]
cat·en·ate (kat′en - āt). Concatenar; encadear; unir em uma série de ligações como uma cadeia; por exemplo, dois anéis de DNA mitocondrial freqüentemente estão concatenados. [L. *catenatus*, encadeado, de *catena*, cadeia]
cat·e·nat·ing (kat′en - āt - ing). Concatenado; encadeado; que ocorre em uma cadeia ou série. [L. *catenatus*, encadeado]
cat·en·in (ka - tĕn′in). Catenina; molécula citoplasmática que serve como elo entre caderinas e o citoesqueleto das células, permitindo a formação de junções aderentes. Há dois tipos: β-c., que está ligada à própria caderina, e α-c., que está associada a microfilamentos de actina. [L. *catena*, cadeia, + -in]
cat·e·noid (kat′ē - noyd). Catenóide. **1.** Semelhante a uma cadeia, como uma cadeia de esporos fúngicos ou uma colônia de protozoários na qual os indivíduos são unidos pelas extremidades. SIN catenulate. **2.** Superfície de curvatura zero gerada pela rotação de uma catenária (curva de repouso de uma cadeia suspensa); o septo interventricular do coração na estenose subaórtica hipertrófica idiopática assemelha-se a um catenóide, o que o torna inefetivo no aumento da pressão intracavitária ou na redução de seu volume, conforme definido na lei de Laplace. [L. *catena*, cadeia, + G. *eidos*, semelhança]
ca·ten·u·late (ka - ten′ū - lāt). Catenulado. SIN catenoid (1).
cat·er·pil·lar (kat′er - pil′er). Lagarta; larva; o estágio larvar de uma borboleta ou mariposa. [I.M. *catirpeller*, do Fr. ant. *cate*, gato, + *pelose*, piloso]
  dermatitis-causing c., lagarta causadora de dermatite; uma das várias espécies cujos pêlos podem causar dermatite alérgica; a l. selada (*Sabine stimulea*) e a mariposa de cauda marrom (*Euproctis chrysorrhoea*) são exemplos comuns.
  saddleback c., *Sabine stimulea*, uma causa de dermatite por lagarta.
  stinging c., lagarta urticante; lagarta com pêlos ou espinhos urticantes que causam dermatite alérgica, p. ex., a mariposa Io (*Automeris Io*).
cat·gut (kat′gŭt). Categute; fio de sutura cirúrgica absorvível, feito com as fibras colágenas da submucosa de alguns animais (geralmente ovelha ou vacas); erroneamente denominado categute. [provavelmente de *kit*, um pequeno violino, pela confusão com *kit*, gato pequeno]
  chromic c., c. cromado; c. impregnado com sais de cromo para prolongar sua resistência à tração e retardar sua absorção.
  silverized c., c. prata; c. preparado por imersão em uma solução coloidal de prata a 2% por 1 semana e, depois, em álcool a 95% por 15 a 30 minutos.
Catha ed·u·lis (kath′ă ed′ū - lis). Khat; qat; planta da Etiópia e Arábia (família Celastraceae), cultivada para uso como estimulante; o khat (as folhas e brotos frescos) é mastigado ou usado no preparo de uma bebida; o princípio ativo é farmacologicamente relacionado às anfetaminas, provavelmente *d*-norisoefedrina. [Ar. *khat*]
Cath·ar·an·thus al·ka·loids (kath - ăr - ran′thus). Alcalóides de Catharanthus. SIN Vinca *alkaloids*, em *alkaloid.*
ca·thar·sis (kă - thar′sis). Catarse. **1.** Purgação. SIN purgation. **2.** Psicocatarse; liberação ou descarga de tensão emocional por reavivação emocional, psicanaliticamente orientada, de eventos passados, principalmente reprimidos. SIN psychocatharsis. [G. *katharsis*, purificação, de *katharos*, puro]
ca·thar·tic (kă - thar′tik). Catártico. **1.** Relativo à catarse. **2.** Um agente que tem ação purgativa.
ca·thec·tic (kă - thek′tik). Catético; relativo à catexia.
ca·them·o·glo·bin (ka - thĕm - ō - glō′bin). Catemoglobina; derivado artificial da hemoglobina no qual a globina é desnaturada e o ferro oxidado.
ca·thep·sin (kă - thep′sin). Catepsina; uma dentre várias proteinases e peptidases intracelulares (todas endopeptidases) de tecidos animais de várias especificidades.
cath·e·ther (kath′ē - ter). Cateter. **1.** Instrumento tubular para permitir a entrada ou saída de líquido de uma cavidade corporal ou vaso sanguíneo. VER TAMBÉM line (4). **2.** Particularmente um c. elaborado para ser introduzido através da uretra até a bexiga para drenar a urina retida. [G. *kathetēr*, de *kathiēmi*, mandar para baixo]
  acorn-tipped c., c. com ponta em bolota; c. usado em ureteropielografia para ocluir o orifício ureteral e evitar refluxo do ureter durante e após a injeção de um meio opaco.

angiography c., c. de angiografia; tubo de paredes finas adequado para inserção percutânea e injeção de contraste para radiografia; o diâmetro do cateter é medido na escala French. VER Seldinger *technique*.
balloon c., c. balão; c. usado em embolectomia arterial ou para flutuar na artéria pulmonar.
balloon-tip c., c. com extremidade em balão; um tubo de luz única ou dupla com um balão em sua extremidade que pode ser insuflado ou esvaziado sem remoção depois de instalado; o balão pode ser insuflado para facilitar a passagem do tubo através de um vaso sanguíneo (impelido pela corrente sanguínea) ou para ocluir o vaso quando o tubo isolado permitiria fluxo livre; esses cateteres são usados para entrar na artéria pulmonar e facilitar medidas hemodinâmicas. VER TAMBÉM Swan-Ganz c.
bicoudate c., c. bicoudé (bī-koo-dā′), cateter bicurvado; cateter angulado com duas curvas. [bi + Fr. *coudé*, curva]
Bozeman-Fritsch c., c. de Bozeman-Fritsch; c. uterino de canal duplo, ligeiramente curvo, com várias aberturas na extremidade.
Braasch c., c. de Braasch; c. com extremidade bulbosa empregado para dilatação e calibragem. SIN Braasch bulb.
Broviac c., c. de Broviac; tipo de c. venoso central para uso prolongado com uma abertura externa para administração de medicamento.
brush c., cateter com escova; cateter ureteral com uma extremidade com escova de cerdas finas que é introduzida endoscopicamente no ureter ou na pelve renal e, através de delicados movimentos de vaivém, escova as células da superfície de tumores suspeitos.
cardiac c., cateter cardíaco. SIN intracardiac c.
central venous c., c. venoso central; c. introduzido em uma veia periférica ou central, terminando na veia cava superior ou no átrio direito, para medida da pressão venosa central, ou para infusão de soluções hiperosmolares.
conical c., c. cônico; c. com extremidade cônica designado para dilatar o ureter.
c. coudé (koo-da′), cateter angulado; cateter com uma curva angular próxima à extremidade; usado para ultrapassar obstrução prostática. SIN elbowed c., prostatic c. [Fr. *coudé*, curvo]
c. à demeure (ā-dem-ër′), c. de demora; termo obsoleto para um c. mantido na uretra por um período considerável. [Fr. *demeurer*, demora]
de Pezzer c., c. de Pezzer; c. de auto-retenção com uma extremidade bulbosa.
double-channel c., cateter de canal duplo; cateter com duas luzes, permitindo irrigação e aspiração ou injeção e medida da pressão. SIN two-way c.
elbowed c., c. angulado. SIN c. coudé.
eustachian c., cateter de Eustáquio; cateter para uso no ouvido médio através da tuba de Eustáquio.
female c., c. feminino, c. curto, quase reto, para introdução na uretra feminina.
Fogarty embolectomy c., c. de Fogarty para embolectomia; c. com um balão inflável próximo de sua extremidade; usado para remover êmbolos e trombos de vasos sanguíneos ou para remover cálculos dos ductos biliares.
Foley c., cateter de Foley; cateter uretral com balão de retenção.

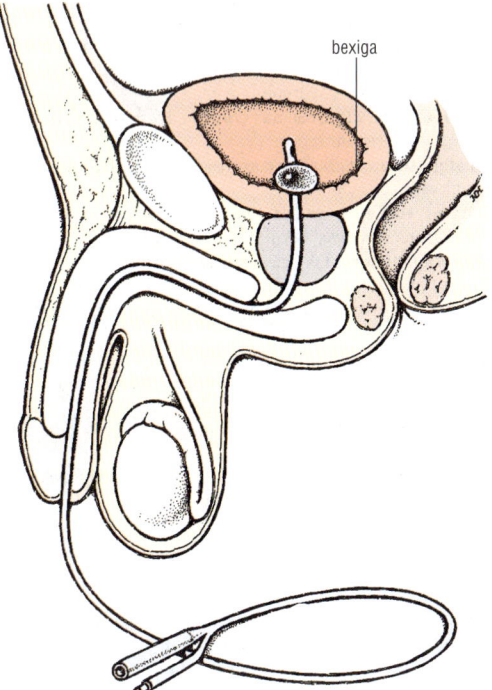

cateter de Foley

Gouley c., cateter de Gouley; instrumento sólido curvo, feito de aço, com um sulco em sua superfície inferior, de forma a poder ser passado sobre um fio-guia através de uma estenose uretral.
Hickman c., cateter de Hickman; c. venoso central de demora, para uso prolongado, com abertura(s) externa(s).
indwelling c., cateter de demora; cateter deixado na bexiga, geralmente um cateter com balão.
intracardiac c., cateter intracardíaco; c. que pode ser introduzido no coração através de uma veia ou artéria, para colher amostras de sangue, medir pressões nas câmaras cardíacas ou nos grandes vasos e injetar contraste; usado principalmente no diagnóstico e na avaliação de lesões congênitas, reumáticas e da artéria coronária para avaliar a função cardíaca sistólica e diastólica. SIN cardiac c.
Malecot c., cateter de Malecot; cateter com duas ou quatro asas.
Nélaton c., cateter de Nélaton; um cateter flexível de borracha vermelha.
olive-tipped c., cateter com extremidade em oliva; cateter ureteral com extremidade em forma de oliva, usado para dilatar um orifício ureteral contraído; os de maior calibre também são usados para dilatar ou calibrar estenoses uretrais.
pacing c., cateter marcapasso; cateter cardíaco com um ou mais eletrodos em sua extremidade que pode ser usado para estimular artificialmente o ritmo cardíaco.
Pezzer c., c. de Pezzer. VER de Pezzer c.
Phillips c., cateter de Phillips; cateter com guia filiforme para a uretra.
pigtail c., c. "rabo de porco"; c. com extremidade muito enrolada e múltiplos orifícios laterais para reduzir o impacto do líquido injetado sobre a parede do vaso, ou para permanecer em uma câmara ou espaço para drenagem.
prostatic c., cateter prostático. SIN c. coudé.
pulmonary artery c., c. arterial pulmonar. SIN Swan-Ganz c.
Robinson c., cateter de Robinson; cateter uretral reto com dois a seis orifícios para facilitar a drenagem, particularmente na presença de coágulos sanguíneos que podem ocluir uma ou mais aberturas.
self-retaining c., cateter de auto-retenção; cateter construído de forma a permanecer na uretra e na bexiga até ser removido, p. ex., cateter de demora; cateter de Foley.
spiral tip c., cateter com extremidade espiralada; cateter com extremidade filiforme helicoidal.
Swan-Ganz c., c. de Swan-Ganz; c. flexível com extremidade em balão, comumente usado no tratamento de pacientes em estado grave; introduzido através de uma grande veia periférica, geralmente jugular ou subclávia, e levado pela onda de pressão, com ou sem fluoroscopia, seqüencialmente através do átrio direito, ventrículo direito e artéria pulmonar, até finalmente se encunhar, quando o balão é insuflado, em um pequeno ramo arterial, onde a extremidade mede a pressão retrógrada transmitida do lado esquerdo do coração, que se supõe representar a pressão diastólica final ventricular esquerda; os orifícios laterais permitem medida da pressão venosa central; com o balão desinsuflado, o c. mede as pressões sistólica, diastólica e média na artéria pulmonar; também permite infusão através do cateter; alguns cateteres possuem eletrodos marcapasso. SIN pulmonary artery c.
two-way c., cateter de duas vias. SIN double-channel c.
vertebrated c., cateter vertebrado; cateter feito de vários segmentos que se movem uns sobre os outros como os elos de uma corrente.
whistle-tip c., cateter com abertura terminal e lateral.
winged c., cateter alado; cateter de borracha macia com pequenas abas de cada lado da extremidade, a fim de se manter na bexiga.
cath·e·ter·i·za·tion (kath′ĕ-ter-ī-zā′shŭn). Cateterização; cateterismo; passagem de um cateter.
  clean intermittent bladder c. (CIC), c. vesical intermitente limpa; forma comum de os pacientes com bexiga neurogênica, que não esvazia normalmente, esvaziarem a bexiga rotineiramente.
cath·e·ter·ize (kath′ĕ-ter-īz). Cateterizar; passar um cateter.
cath·e·ter·o·stat (kath′ĕ-ter-ō-stat). Cateterostato; suporte para cateteres. [catheter + G. *statos*, suporte]
ca·thex·is (kă-thek′sis). Catexia, catexe; vinculação consciente ou inconsciente de energia psíquica a uma idéia, objeto ou pessoa. [G. *kathexis*, manutenção, retenção]
cath·o·dal (C) (kath′ō-dăl). Catódico; de, relativo a, ou que emana de, um catodo. SIN cathodic.
cath·ode (Ca, C) (kath′ōd). Catodo; o pólo negativo de uma bateria galvânica ou o ligado a ela; o eletrodo para o qual íons positivamente carregados (cátions) migram e são reduzidos, e no qual elétrons são alimentados de sua fonte (anodo ou gerador). Cf. anode. SIN negative electrode. [G. *kathodos*, caminho para baixo, de *kata*, para baixo, + *hodos*, caminho]
ca·thod·ic (kă-thod′ik). Catódico. SIN cathodal.
cath·ol·y·sis (kath-ol′ĕ-sis). Católise; eletrólise com uma agulha catódica.
cat·i·on (kat′ī-on). Cátion; um íon que possui uma carga de eletricidade positiva, indo assim para o catodo negativamente carregado. [G. *katīon*, que vai para baixo]
cat·i·on ex·change. Troca de cátions; o processo pelo qual um cátion em fase líquida é trocado por outro cátion presente como o contra-íon de um polímero

sólido negativamente carregado (permutador de cátion). Uma reação de troca de cátion na remoção do Na^+ de uma solução de cloreto de sódio é $RSO_3^-H^+ + Na^+ \rightarrow RSO_3^-Na^+ + H^+$ (R é o polímero, RSO_3^- é o permutador de cátion); se isso for combinado com a reação de troca de ânions, NaCl é removido da solução (retirada do sal). A troca de cátions também pode ser usada, cromatograficamente, para separar cátions e, na medicina, para remover um cátion; p. ex., H^+ do conteúdo gástrico, ou Na^+ e K^+ no intestino. VER anion exchange.

cat·i·on ex·chang·er. Permutador catiônico; sólido insolúvel (geralmente um polistireno ou um polissacarídio) possuindo radicais negativamente carregados ligados a si (p. ex., $-COO^-$, $-SO_3^-$), que pode atrair e reter cátions que passam em uma solução em movimento, se estes forem mais atraídos para os grupamentos ácidos que o contra-íon presente.

cat·i·on·ic (kat - ī - on′ik). Catiônico; que se refere a íons positivamente carregados e suas propriedades.

cat·i·on·o·gen (kat - ī - on′ō - jen). Cationógeno; substância que dá origem a íons positivamente carregados.

cat·lin, cat·ling (kat′lin, -ling). Catlin; faca longa, pontiaguda, de duplo gume, usada em amputações.

cat·nep, cat·nip (kat′nep, kat′nip). Catária. SIN cataria.

cat·o·chus (kat′ō - kŭs). A fase da catalepsia semelhante a um transe na qual o paciente está consciente, mas não pode mover-se nem falar. [G. *katochē*, epilepsia (Galeno), de *katechō*, segurar firme]

ca·top·tric (ka - top′trik). Catóptrico; relativo à luz refletida. [G. *katoptron*, espelho]

cau·da, pl. **cau·dae** (kaw′dă, kaw′dē) [TA]. Cauda. SIN tail (1). [L. cauda]
  c. epididym′idis [TA], c. do epidídimo. SIN *tail* of epididymis.
  c. equi′na [TA], c. eqüina; o feixe de raízes nervosas espinhais originado do aumento lombossacro e do cone medular e correndo através da cisterna lombar (espaço subaracnóide) no canal vertebral abaixo da primeira vértebra lombar; compreende as raízes de todos os nervos espinhais abaixo do primeiro lombar. [L. cauda de cavalo]
  c. fas′ciae denta′tae, c. da fáscia dentada. SIN uncus *band* of Giacomini.
  c. hel′icis [TA], c. da hélice. SIN *tail* of helix.
  c. nu′clei cauda′ti [TA], c. do núcleo caudado. SIN *tail* of caudate nucleus.
  c. pancrea′tis [TA], c. do pâncreas. SIN *tail* of pancreas.
  c. stria′ti [TA], c. estriada. SIN *tail* of caudate nucleus.

cau·dad (kaw′dad). Caudal. **1.** Em direção à cauda. **2.** Situado mais próximo da cauda em relação a um ponto de referência específico; oposto a cranial. VER TAMBÉM inferior.

cau·dal (kaw′dăl) [TA]. Caudal; relativo à cauda. SIN caudalis [TA]. [L. Mod. *caudalis*]

cau·da·lis (kaw - dā′lis) [TA]. Caudal. SIN caudal.

cau·date (kaw - dāt). Caudado. **1.** Que possui cauda. **2.** SIN caudate *nucleus*.

cau·da·to·len·tic·u·lar (kaw - dā′tō - len - tik′ū - lăr). Caudatolenticular; relativo aos núcleos caudado e lenticular. SIN caudolenticular.

cau·da·tum (kaw - dā′tŭm). Caudado. SIN caudate *nucleus*.

cau·do·ceph·a·lad (kaw - dō - sef′ăl - ad). Caudocefálico; em direção da cauda para a cabeça.

cau·do·len·tic·u·lar (kaw′dō - len - tik′ū - lăr). Caudolenticular. SIN caudatolenticular.

caul, cowl (kawl). **1.** O âmnio, seja como um pedaço de membrana que cobre a cabeça do bebê ao nascer ou toda a membrana quando é eliminada com o bebê, sem se romper. SIN galea (4), veil (2), velum (2). **2.** Epíploo, omento maior. SIN greater *omentum*. [Gaélico, *call*, véu]

cau·sal·gia (kaw - zal′jē - ă). Causalgia; dor em queimação intensa e persistente, geralmente após lesão de um nervo periférico (principalmente dos nervos mediano e tibial) ou do plexo braquial, acompanhada por alterações tróficas. [G. *kausis*, queimação, + *algos*, dor]

cau·sal·i·ty (kawz′ăl - i - tē). Causalidade; a relação entre as causas e os efeitos que produzem; a patogenia da doença e a epidemiologia estão relacionadas em grande parte à causalidade.

cause (kawz). Causa; o que produz um efeito ou condição; o que causa uma alteração mórbida ou doença. [L. *causa*]
  constitutional c., c. constitucional; c. que atua a partir ou através de algum processo sistêmico ou erro congênito.
  exciting c., c. excitante; c. provocadora direta de um distúrbio. SIN procatarxis (1).
  necessary c., c. necessária; fator etiológico sem o qual não ocorrerá um resultado em questão; a ocorrência do resultado é prova de que o fator está operando.
  precipitating c., c. precipitante; fator que causa o início de manifestações de um processo mórbido.
  predisposing c., c. predisponente; qualquer coisa que produza uma suscetibilidade ou disposição a uma condição sem realmente causá-la.
  proximate c., c. próxima; c. imediata que precipita uma condição.
  specific c., c. específica; c. cuja ação definitivamente pode produzir o distúrbio em questão.
  sufficient c., c. suficiente; fator etiológico que garante que ocorrerá um resultado em questão; a não-ocorrência do resultado é uma prova de que o fator não está operando.

caus·tic (kaws′tik). Cáustico. **1.** Que exerce um efeito químico semelhante a uma queimadura. **2.** Um agente que produz esse efeito. **3.** Designa uma solução de um álcali forte; p. ex., soda cáustica, NaOH. SIN pyrotic (2). [G. *kaustikos*, de *kaiō*, queimar]

cau·ter·ant (kaw′ter - ant). Cauterizador. **1.** Que cauteriza. **2.** Um agente cauterizante.

cau·ter·i·za·tion (kaw - ter - ī - zā′shŭn). Cauterização; o ato de cauterizar. VER TAMBÉM cautery.

cau·ter·ize (kaw′ter - īz). Cauterizar; aplicar um cautério; queimar com cautério.

cau·tery (kaw′ter - ē). **1.** Cautério; um agente ou dispositivo usado para cicatrizar, queimar ou cortar a pele ou outros tecidos por meio de calor, frio, corrente elétrica, ultra-som ou substâncias químicas cáusticas. **2.** Uso de um cautério. [G. *kautērion*, ferro de marcar]
  actual c., c. real ou efetivo; um c., como um eletrocautério, que atua diretamente através do calor e não por meios químicos. SIN technocausis.
  BICAP c., c. BICAP; forma de eletrocoagulação bipolar freqüentemente usada para interromper a hemorragia gastrointestinal.
  bipolar c., c. bipolar; eletrocautério por corrente elétrica de alta freqüência passada através do tecido (de um eletrodo ativo para um eletrodo passivo); usado para hemostasia.
  chemical c., quimiocautério. SIN chemocautery.
  cold c., criocautério. SIN cryocautery.
  electric c., eletrocautério. SIN electrocautery.
  gas c., c. de gás; c. que atua por meio de um volume medido de um jato de gás em combustão.
  monopolar c., c. monopolar; eletrocautério por corrente elétrica de alta freqüência passada a partir de um único eletrodo, onde ocorre a cauterização, com o corpo do paciente servindo como terra.

ca·va (kā′vă). Cava. VER inferior *vena* cava, superior *vena* cava.

ca·va·gram (kā′vă - gram). Cavagrama. SIN cavogram.

ca·val (kā′văl). Cava; relativo à veia cava.

cave (kāv) [TA]. Caverna; cavidade; espaço oco ou fechado ou cavidade. VER cavity, cavitas, cavernous *space*. SIN cavea.
  trigeminal c., [TA], cavidade trigeminal; a fenda na camada meníngea da duramáter da fossa craniana média próxima da extremidade da parte petrosa do osso temporal; encerra as raízes do nervo trigêmeo e o gânglio do trigêmeo. SIN cavum trigeminale [TA], trigeminal cavity*, Meckel cavity, Meckel space.

cavea. Cavidade. SIN cave.
  cavea thoracis [TA], cavidade torácica. SIN thoracic *cage*.

cav·e·o·la, pl. **cav·e·o·lae** (kav - ē - ō′lă, - lē). Cavéola, pl. cavéolas; pequena bolsa, vesícula, cavidade ou recesso que se comunica com o exterior de uma célula e se estende para dentro, entalhando o citoplasma e a membrana celular. Essas cavéolas podem separar-se e formar vesículas livres no citoplasma. São consideradas locais de captação de substâncias para o interior da célula, expulsão de substâncias da célula, ou locais de acréscimo ou remoção de membrana celular (unidade) da superfície celular. [L.]

cav·ern (kav′ern). Caverna. SIN cavernous *space*.
  c.'s of corpora cavernosa, cavernas dos corpos cavernosos. SIN cavernous *spaces* of corpora cavernosa, em *space*.
  c.'s of corpus spongiosum, cavernas do corpo esponjoso. SIN cavernous *spaces* of corporus spongiosum, em *space*.

ca·ver·na, pl. **ca·ver·nae** (kă - ver′nă, - nē). Caverna, pl. cavernas. SIN cavernous *space*. [L. gruta, de *cavus*, oco]
  cavernae cor′poris spongio′si [TA], cavernas do corpo esponjoso. SIN cavernous *spaces* of corporus spongiosum, em *space*.
  cavernae cor′porum cavernoso′rum [TA], cavernas dos corpos cavernosos. SIN cavernous *spaces* of corpora cavernosa, em *space*.

cav·er·nil·o·quy (kav - er - nil′ō - kwē). Cavernilóquia; pectorilóquia ressonante de tonalidade grave ouvida sobre uma cavidade pulmonar. [L. *caverna*, caverna, + *loquor*, falar]

cav·er·ni·tis (kav - er - nī′tis). Cavernite; inflamação do corpo cavernoso do pênis. SIN cavernositis.
  fibrous c., c. fibrosa; c. ocasionalmente associada à doença de Peyronie.

cav·er·no·si·tis (kav′er - nō - sī′tis). Cavernosite. SIN cavernitis.

cav·ern·ous (kav′er - nŭs). Cavernoso; relativo a uma caverna ou cavidade; que contém muitas cavidades.

Ca·via (kā′vē - ă). Gênero da família Caviidae que inclui as cobaias. [L. Mod., do hindu nativo]
  C. porcel′lus, cobaia, porquinho-da-índia, roedor com cauda muito curta que não é visível externamente; nativo da América do Sul, onde é criado para alimentação; amplamente usado como animal de laboratório em pesquisa médica. SIN guinea pig.

cav·i·tary (kav′i - tă - rē). **1.** Cavitário; relativo a uma cavidade ou que possui uma cavidade ou cavidades. **2.** Designa qualquer parasita animal que tenha um canal entérico ou cavidade corporal e que vive dentro do corpo do hospedeiro.

cav·i·tas, pl. **cav·i·ta·tes** (kav′i-tas, -tā′tēs). Cavidade, pl. cavidades. SIN cavity. [L. Mod.]
- **c. abdomina'lis** [TA], c. abdominal. SIN abdominal cavity.
- **c. abdominis et pelvis** [TA], c. abdominopélvica. SIN abdominopelvic cavity.
- **c. articula'ris** [TA], c. articular. SIN articular cavity.
- **c. conchae** [TA], c. da concha. SIN cavity of concha.
- **c. coronae** [TA], c. da coroa. SIN crown cavity.
- **c. corona'lis,** c. pulpar da coroa. SIN pulp cavity of crown.
- **c. cranii** [TA], c. do crânio. SIN cranial cavity.
- **c. den'tis** [TA], c. pulpar. SIN pulp cavity.
- **c. glenoida'lis,** fossa mandibular. SIN mandibular fossa.
- **c. glenoidalis scapulae** [TA], c. glenoidal da escápula. SIN glenoid cavity of scapula.
- **c. infraglottica** [TA], c. infraglótica. SIN infraglottic cavity.
- **c. infraglot'ticum,** c. infraglótica. SIN infraglottic cavity.
- **c. laryn'gis** [TA], c. da laringe. SIN laryngeal cavity.
- **c. medulla'ris** [TA], c. medular. SIN medullary cavity.
- **c. na'si** [TA], c. nasal. SIN nasal cavity.
- **c. o'ris** [TA], c. oral. SIN oral cavity.
- **c. o'ris pro'pria** [TA], c. própria da boca. SIN oral cavity proper.
- **c. pelvina,** c. pélvica;* termo oficial alternativo para pelvic cavity.
- **c. pel'vis** [TA], c. pélvica. SIN pelvic cavity.
- **c. pericardiaca** [TA], c. pericárdica. SIN pericardial cavity.
- **c. peritonea'lis** [TA], c. peritoneal. SIN peritoneal cavity.
- **c. pharyn'gis** [TA], c. da faringe. SIN cavity of pharynx.
- **c. pleura'lis** [TA], c. pleural. SIN pleural cavity.
- **c. pulparis,** c. pulpar;* termo oficial alternativo para pulp cavity.
- **c. thora'cis** [TA], c. torácica. SIN thoracic cavity.
- **c. tympan'ica** [TA], c. timpânica. SIN tympanic cavity.
- **c. u'teri** [TA], c. uterina. SIN uterine cavity.

cav·i·ta·tion (kav-i-tā′shŭn). **1.** Cavitação; formação de uma cavidade, como no pulmão na tuberculose ou com desenvolvimento de um abscesso pulmonar bacteriano. **2.** A produção de pequenas bolhas ou cavidades contendo vapor em um líquido ou tecido por ultra-sonografia.

ca·vi·tis (kā-vī′tis). Cavite, celoflebite. SIN celophlebitis.

cav·i·ty (kav′i-tē). Cavidade. **1.** Um espaço oco; cavidade, vestíbulo. VER cave, cavity, cavitas, cavernous space. **2.** Termo leigo para a perda da estrutura dentária devido a cáries dentárias. SIN cavum [TA], cavitas. [L. cavus, oco]
- **abdominal c.** [TA], c. abdominal; o espaço limitado pelas paredes abdominais, diafragma e pelve; em geral é arbitrariamente separada da cavidade pélvica por um plano através da abertura superior da pelve; entretanto, pode incluir a pelve com o abdome (ver abdominopelvic c.); na cavidade estão a maior parte dos órgãos da digestão, o baço, os rins e as glândulas supra-renais. SIN cavitas abdominalis [TA], cavum abdominis, enterocele (2).
- **abdominopelvic c.** [TA], c. abdominopélvica; as cavidades abdominal e pélvica combinadas e contínuas. VER TAMBÉM abdominal c. SIN cavitas abdominis et pelvis [TA].
- **amniotic c.,** c. amniótica; a c. cheia de líquido no âmnio que contém o embrião em desenvolvimento.
- **articular c.** [TA], c. articular; uma cavidade articular, o espaço virtual limitado pela membrana sinovial e cartilagens articulares de todas as articulações sinoviais. Normalmente, a c. articular contém apenas líquido sinovial suficiente para lubrificar as superfícies internas. SIN cavitas articularis [TA], cavum articulare.
- **axillary c.,** c. axilar. SIN axilla.
- **body c.,** c. corporal; a c. visceral coletiva do tronco (c. torácica mais c. abdominopélvica), limitada pela abertura torácica superior acima, assoalho pélvico abaixo e paredes corporais no meio. SIN celom (2), celoma, coelom.
- **buccal c.,** vestíbulo da boca. SIN oral vestibule.
- **cleavage c.,** blastocele. SIN blastocele.
- **c. of concha** [TA], c. da concha; o espaço na porção inferior maior da concha abaixo da crista da hélice; forma o vestíbulo que leva ao meato acústico externo. SIN cavitas conchae [TA], cavum conchae*.
- **c.'s of corpora cavernosa,** cavernas dos corpos cavernosos. SIN cavernous spaces of corpora cavernosa, em space.
- **c.'s of corpus spongiosum,** cavernas do corpo esponjoso. SIN cavernous spaces of corporus spongiosum, em space.
- **cotyloid c.,** acetábulo. SIN acetabulum.
- **cranial c.** [TA], c. do crânio; o espaço no crânio ocupado pelo cérebro, seus revestimentos e líquido cefalorraquidiano. SIN cavitas cranii [TA], intracranial c.
- **crow c.,** cavidade da coroa. SIN cavitas coronae.
- **ectoplacental c.,** c. ectoplacentária. SIN epamniotic c.
- **ectotrophoblastic c.,** c. ectotrofoblástica; uma c. do desenvolvimento que aparece entre o trofoblasto e o ectoderma do disco embrionário em alguns mamíferos.
- **epamniotic c.,** c. epamniótica; c. ectoplacentária; c. do desenvolvimento existente em alguns mamíferos e produzida pela divisão do espaço pró-amniótico; está mais afastada do embrião que a c. amniótica em alguns mamíferos. SIN ectoplacental c.
- **epidural c.,** c. epidural. SIN epidural space.
- **glenoid c.,** c. glenóide. SIN mandibular fossa.
- **glenoid c. of scapula** [TA], c. glenóide da escápula; a cavidade na cabeça da escápula que recebe a cabeça do úmero para formar a articulação do ombro. SIN cavitas glenoidalis scapulae [TA], glenoid fossa (1).
- **greater peritoneal c.,** c. maior do peritônio. SIN peritoneal c.
- **head c.,** c. cefálica; a região cefálica nos embriões de vertebrados contendo os somitos modificados que dão origem aos músculos extrínsecos do olho.
- **idiopathic bone c.,** cisto ósseo idiopático. SIN solitary bone cyst.
- **inferior laryngeal c.,** c. infraglótica. SIN infraglottic c.
- **infraglottic c.** [TA], c. infraglótica; a parte da cavidade da laringe imediatamente abaixo da glote. SIN cavitas infraglottica [TA], aditus glottidis inferior, cavitas infraglotticum, cavum infraglotticum, inferior laryngeal c., infraglottic space.
- **intermediate laryngeal c.,** ádito da laringe; porção da c. da laringe situada entre as pregas vestibulares e as cordas vocais, com a qual se comunicam os ventrículos. SIN aditus glottidis superior.
- **intracranial c.,** c. do crânio. SIN cranial c.
- **laryngeal c.** [TA], c. da laringe; cavidade contínua acima com a faringe ao nível das pregas ariepigloticas e que se estende para baixo através da rima da glote até o espaço infraglótico. SIN cavitas laryngis [TA], c. of larynx, cavum laryngis.
- **c. of larynx,** c. da laringe. SIN laryngeal c.
- **lesser peritoneal c.,** bolsa omental. SIN omental bursa.
- **Meckel c.,** c. de Meckel. c. trigeminal. SIN trigeminal cave.
- **medullary c.** [TA], c. medular; a cavidade medular na diáfise de um osso longo. SIN cavitas medullaris [TA], cavum medullare.
- **c. of middle ear,** c. timpânica. SIN tympanic c.
- **nasal c.** [TA], c. nasal; a cavidade de cada lado do septo nasal, revestida por mucosa respiratória ciliada, que se estende das narinas, anteriormente, até a coana, posteriormente, comunicando-se com os seios paranasais através de seus orifícios na parede lateral, de onde também se projetam as três conchas; a lâmina cribriforme, através da qual passam os nervos olfatórios, forma o teto; o assoalho é formado pelo palato duro. SIN cavitas nasi [TA], cavum nasi.
- **nephrotomic c.,** c. nefrotômica. SIN nephrocele (2).
- **oral c.** [TA], c. oral; a região que consiste no vestíbulo da boca, na estreita fenda entre os lábios e a bochecha, e nos dentes e gengiva, além da cavidade oral propriamente dita. SIN cavitas oris [TA], cavum oris, mouth (1).
- **oral c. proper** [TA], c. própria da boca; o espaço entre os arcos dentários, limitado posteriormente pelo istmo da fauce (arco palatoglosso). SIN cavitas oris propria [TA].
- **orbital c.,** c. orbital. SIN orbit.
- **pelvic c.** [TA], c. pélvica; o espaço limitado lateralmente pelos ossos da pelve, acima pela abertura superior da pelve e abaixo pelo diafragma pélvico; contém as vísceras pélvicas. SIN cavitas pelvis [TA], cavitas pelvina*, cavum pelvis.
- **pericardial c.** [TA], **(1)** c. pericárdica; o espaço virtual entre as camadas parietal e visceral do pericárdio seroso; **(2)** no embrião, aquela parte do celoma primário que contém o coração; originalmente está em comunicação aberta com as cavidades pericardioperitoneais e, indiretamente, através delas, com a parte peritoneal do celoma. SIN cavitas pericardiaca [TA], cavum pericardii.
- **peritoneal c.** [TA], c. peritoneal; o interior do saco peritoneal, normalmente apenas um espaço virtual entre as camadas parietal e visceral do peritônio. SIN cavitas peritonealis [TA], cavum peritonei, greater peritoneal c.
- **perivisceral c.,** c. perivisceral; o espaço entre o ectoderma e o endoderma na gástrula. SIN primitive perivisceral c.
- **pharyngonasal c.,** nasofaringe. SIN nasopharynx.
- **c. of pharynx** [TA], c. da faringe; consiste em uma parte nasal (nasofaringe) contínua, anteriormente, com a cavidade nasal, recebendo as aberturas das tubas auditivas, uma abertura da parte oral (orofaringe), através da fauce para a cavidade oral, e uma parte laríngea (laringofaringe) que leva ao vestíbulo da laringe e ao esôfago. SIN cavitas pharyngis [TA], cavum pharyngis.
- **pleural c.,** [TA], c. pleural; o espaço virtual entre as camadas parietal e visceral da pleura. SIN cavitas pleuralis [TA], cavum pleurae, pleural space.
- **pleuroperitoneal c.,** c. pleuroperitoneal; aquela parte do celoma embrionário que depois se divide para dar origem às cavidades pleural e peritoneal.
- **primitive perivisceral c.,** c. perivisceral primitiva. SIN perivisceral c.
- **pulmonary c.,** c. pulmonar; uma das subdivisões bilaterais da cavidade torácica, situada de um lado do mediastino, revestida por pleura parietal e ocupada por um pulmão; o espaço existente quando é removido um pulmão. O termo não é sinônimo de c. pleural, que é um espaço entre as pleuras parietal e visceral normalmente vazio, à exceção de uma fina camada de líquido pleural e que circunda (mas não contém) o pulmão.
- **pulp c.** [TA], c. pulpar; a cavidade central de um dente que consiste na cavidade da coroa e no canal da raiz; contém a polpa dentária fibrovascular e é totalmente revestida por odontoblastos. SIN cavitas dentis [TA], cavitas pulparis*, c. of tooth, cavum dentis.
- **pulp c. of crown** [TA], c. pulpar da coroa; o espaço na coroa de um dente contínuo com o canal da raiz. SIN cavitas coronalis, cavum coronale.
- **Retzius c.,** c. de Retzius. SIN retropubic space.
- **segmentation c.,** c. de segmentação. SIN blastocele.

c. of septum pellucidum, c. do septo pelúcido; ventrículo de Duncan; quinto ventrículo; pseudocele; pseudoventrículo; ventrículo de Sylvius; ventrículo de Vieussens; ventrículos de Wenzel; espaço semelhante a uma fenda, cheio de líquido, de largura variável entre o septo transparente esquerdo e o direito, presente em menos de 10% dos cérebros humanos e que pode comunicar-se com o terceiro ventrículo. SIN cavum septum pellucidum [TA], Duncan ventricle, fifth ventricle, pseudocele, pseudoventricle, sylvian ventricle, ventricle of Sylvius, ventriculus quintus, Vieussens ventricle, Wenzel ventricle.

somite c., c. somítica. SIN myocele (2).

splanchnic c., c. esplâncnica; o celoma ou uma das cavidades do corpo dele derivadas. SIN visceral c.

subarachnoid c., espaço subaracnóideo, espaço leptomeníngeo. SIN subarachnoid space.

subdural c., espaço subdural. SIN subdural space.

subgerminal c., intestino primitivo. SIN primitive gut.

superior laryngeal c., vestíbulo da laringe. SIN vestibule of larynx.

thoracic c. [TA], c. torácica; o espaço nas paredes torácicas, limitado abaixo pelo diafragma e acima pelo pescoço. SIN cavitas thoracis [TA], cavum thoracis.

c. of tooth, c. pulpar. SIN pulp c.

trigeminal c., c. trigeminal; *termo oficial alternativo para trigeminal cave.

tympanic c. [TA], c. timpânica; câmara de ar no osso temporal que contém os ossículos; é revestida por mucosa e contínua com a tuba auditiva, anteriormente, e com o antro timpânico e as células aéreas da mastóide, posteriormente. SIN cavitas tympanica [TA], c. of middle ear, cavum tympani.

uterine c., c. of uterus [TA], c. do útero; o espaço no útero que se estende do canal cervical até as aberturas das tubas uterinas. SIN cavitas uteri [TA], cavum uteri.

visceral c., c. visceral. SIN splanchnic c.

ca·vo·gram (kā'vō-gram). Cavograma; angiograma da veia cava. SIN cavagram. [(vena) cava + G. *gramma*, escrita]

ca·vog·ra·phy (kā-vog'rā-fē). Cavografia. SIN venacavography.

ca·vo·sur·face (kā-vō-sur'fas). Cavossuperficial; relativo a uma cavidade e à superfície de um dente.

ca·vum, pl. **ca·va** (ka'vŭm, -vā) [TA]. Cavo; orifício; cavidade. SIN cavity. [L. neutro do adj. *cavus*, oco]

c. abdom'inis, cavidade abdominal. SIN abdominal cavity.
c. articula're, cavidade articular. SIN articular cavity.
c. con'chae, cavidade da concha; *termo oficial alternativo para cavity of concha.
c. corona'le, cavidade pulpar da coroa. SIN pulp cavity of crown.
c. den'tis, c. pulpar. SIN pulp cavity.
c. doug'lasi, fundo-de-saco de Douglas; escavação retouterina. SIN rectouterine pouch.
c. epidura'le, espaço extradural. SIN epidural space.
c. infraglot'ticum, c. infraglótica. SIN infraglottic cavity.
c. laryn'gis, c. da laringe. SIN laryngeal cavity.
c. mediastina'le, nome impróprio empregado algumas vezes para designar o mediastino.
c. medulla're, c. medular. SIN medullary cavity.
c. na'si, c. nasal. SIN nasal cavity.
c. o'ris, c. oral. SIN oral cavity.
c. pel'vis, c. pélvica. SIN pelvic cavity.
c. pericar'dii, c. pericárdica. SIN pericardial cavity.
c. peritone'i, c. peritoneal. SIN peritoneal cavity.
c. pharyn'gis, c. da faringe. SIN cavity of pharynx.
c. pleu'rae, c. pleural. SIN pleural cavity.
c. psalte'rii, ventrículo de Verga. SIN Verga ventricle.
c. ret'zii, espaco de Retzius, espaço retropúbico. SIN retropubic space. [A.A. Retzius]
c. sep'tum pellu'cidum [TA], c. do septo pelúcido. SIN cavity of septum pellucidum.
c. subarachnoid'eum, espaço subaracnóideo. SIN subarachnoid space.
c. subdura'le, c. subdural. SIN subdural space.
c. thora'cis, c. torácica. SIN thoracic cavity.
c. trigemina'le [TA], c. trigeminal. SIN trigeminal cave.
c. tym'pani, c. timpânica. SIN tympanic cavity.
c. u'teri, c. do útero. SIN uterine cavity.
c. ver'gae, ventrículo de Verga. SIN Verga ventricle.
c. vesicouteri'num, escavação vesicouterina. SIN vesicouterine pouch.

Cb Símbolo do colômbio.

C-band·ing. Bandeamento C. VER C-banding stain.

CBC Abreviatura de complete *blood count* (hemograma completo).

CBF Abreviatura de cerebral or coronary blood flow (fluxo sanguíneo cerebral ou coronário).

CBG Abreviatura de corticosteroid-binding *globulin* (globulina de ligação de corticosteróides).

Cbl Abreviatura de cobalamin (cobalamina).

Cbz Abreviatura de carbobenzoxy-(benzyloxycarbonyl) (carbobenzoxi-benziloxicarbonil).

C.C. Abreviatura de chief complaint (queixa principal), anotada na anamnese do paciente.

cc, c.c. Abreviatura de cubic *centimeter* (centímetro cúbico [cm³]).

CCA Abreviatura de chimpanzee coryza *agent* (vírus sincicial respiratório).

CCC Abreviatura de cathodal closure *contraction* (contração de fechamento catódico).

CCDM Abreviatura de *Control of Communicable Diseases Manual* (Manual de Controle de Doenças Transmissíveis).

CCK Abreviatura de cholecystokinin (colecistocinina).

CCNU Lomustina. SIN lomustine.

CCU Abreviatura de coronary care *unit* (unidade coronariana); critical care *unit* (unidade de terapia intensiva).

CD Abreviatura de curative *dose* (dose curativa); circular *dichroism* (dicroismo circular); cluster of differentiation (grupo de diferenciação).

CD 54. Molécula de adesão intercelular 1. VER intercellular adhesion *molecule*-1.

CD⁵⁰ 1. Abreviatura de curative *dose* (dose curativa). 2. No estudo de um agente terapêutico, a dose que cura 50% dos indivíduos testados.

Cd Símbolo do cádmio.

cd Símbolo de candela.

CDC Abreviatura de Centers for Disease Control and Prevention (Centro de Controle e Prevenção de Doenças); antes conhecido como Communicable Disease Center (Centro de Doenças Contagiosas).

CDE blood group. Grupo sanguíneo CDE. Ver grupo sanguíneo Rh, apêndice Grupos Sanguíneos.

cDNA Abreviatura de complementary DNA (DNA complementar), algumas vezes usada como cópia de DNA.

CDP Abreviatura de cytidine 5'-diphosphate (5'-difosfato de citidina).

CDP-cho·line Abreviatura de cytidine diphosphocholine (difosfocolina de citidina).

CDP-glyc·er·ide Abreviatura de cytidine diphosphoglyceride (difosfoglicerídio de citidina).

CDP-sug·ar Abreviatura de cytidine diphosphosugar (difosfoaçúcar de citidina).

Ce Símbolo do cério.

CEA Abreviatura de carcinoembryonic *antigen* (antígeno carcinoembrionário).

ce·bo·ceph·a·ly (sē-bō-sef'ā-lē). Cebocefalia; malformação da cabeça na qual as feições se assemelham às de um macaco, com defeito ou ausência do nariz e olhos muito próximos; parte do espectro da holoprosencefalia. [G. *kēbos*, macaco, + *kephalē*, cabeça]

⚠ **cec-.** VER ceco-.

ce·ca (sē'kā). Cecos; plural de cecum.

ce·cal (sē'kal). 1. Cecal; relativo ao ceco. 2. Que tem apenas uma abertura ou termina em um fundo-de-saco.

ce·cec·to·my (sē-sek'tō-mē). Cecectomia; tiflectomia; excisão do ceco. SIN typhlectomy. [ceco- + G. *ektomē*, excisão]

Cecil, Arthur Bond, urologista norte-americano, 1885–1967. VER Cecil *urethroplasty*.

ce·ci·tis (sē-sī'tis). Cecite; tiflite; inflamação do ceco. SIN typhlenteritis, typhlitis, typhloenteritis.

⚠ **ceco-, cec-.** O ceco. VER TAMBÉM typhlo- (1). Cf. typhlo-. [L. *caecum*, ceco, cego]

ce·co·co·los·to·my (sē'kō-kō-los'tō-mē). Cecocolostomia; formação de uma anastomose entre o ceco e o cólon.

ce·co·fix·a·tion (sē'kō-fik-sā'shŭn). Cecofixação; cecopexia. SIN cecopexy.

ce·co·il·e·os·to·my (sē'kō-il-ē-os'tō-mē). Cecoileostomia. SIN ileocecostomy.

ce·co·pexy (sē'kō-pek-sē). Cecopexia; fixação cirúrgica de um ceco móvel. SIN cecofixation, typhlopexy, typhlopexia. [ceco- + G. *pexis*, fixação]

ce·co·pli·ca·tion (sē'kō-pli-kā'shŭn). Cecoplicatura; redução cirúrgica do tamanho de um ceco dilatado pela formação de pregas ou dobras de sua parede. [ceco- + L. *plico*, pp. *-atus*, dobrar]

ce·cor·rha·phy (sē-kōr'ā-fē). Cecorrafia; sutura do ceco. SIN typhlorrhaphy. [ceco- + G. *rhaphē*, sutura]

ce·co·sig·moid·os·to·my (sē'kō-sig-moy-dos'tō-mē). Cecossigmoidostomia; formação de uma comunicação entre o ceco e o cólon sigmóide.

ce·cos·to·my (sē-kos'tō-mē). Cecostomia; formação cirúrgica de uma fístula cecal. SIN typhlostomy. [ceco- + G. *stoma*, boca]

ce·cot·o·my (sē-kot'ō-mē). Cecotomia; incisão do ceco. SIN typhlotomy. [ceco- + G. *tomē*, incisão]

ce·co·u·re·ter·o·cele (sē'cō-ū-rē'ter-ō-sēl). Cecoureterocele; uma ureterocele que se estende ao longo da uretra, algumas vezes até fora do meato uretral.

ce·cro·pins (sē-krō-pinz). Cecropinas; peptídeos antibacterianos que consistem em duas hélices α anfipáticas.

ce·cum, pl. **ce·ca** (sē'kŭm, sē'kā). [TA]. Ceco, pl. cecos. 1. O fundo-de-saco, com cerca de 6 cm de profundidade, situado abaixo do íleo terminal e que forma a primeira parte do intestino grosso. SIN blind gut, intestinum cecum, typhlon. 2. Qualquer estrutura semelhante que termina em um fundo-de-saco. SIN caecum. [L. neutro de *caecus*, cego]

cupular c. of the cochlear duct [TA], cúpula do ducto coclear; a extremidade superior cega do ducto coclear. SIN c. cupulare [TA], cupular blind sac, lagena (1).
c. cupula′re [TA], cúpula cega. SIN cupular c. of the cochlear duct.
intestinal c., ceco intestinal.
vestibular c. of the cochlear duct [TA], ceco vestibular do ducto coclear; a extremidade inferior do ducto coclear, que ocupa o recesso coclear no vestíbulo. SIN c. vestibulare [TA], vestibular blind sac.
c. vestibula′re [TA], ceco vestibular. SIN vestibular c. of the cochlear duct.
ce·dar leaf oil (sē′der). Óleo de folha de cedro; óleo obtido por destilação do vapor das folhas frescas da *Thuja occidentalis*; usado como repelente de insetos e contra-irritante, e em perfumaria. SIN thuja oil.
ce·dar wood oil. Óleo de cedro; óleo volátil obtido da madeira da *Juniperus virginiana* (família Pinaceae); usado como repelente de insetos, em perfumaria e como agente clarificante em microscopia.
Ced·e·cea (sed - e′sē - ā). Gênero do grupo Enterobacteriaceae que inclui as espécies *C. davisae* (a cepa típica), *C. lapagei* e *C. neteri*; esses microrganismos foram isolados nas vias respiratórias humanas, mas seu papel nas doenças ainda não foi definido.
Ceelen, Wilhelm, 1884–1964. VER C.-Gellerstedt *syndrome*.
cef·a·clor (sef′ā - klōr). Cefaclor; antibiótico semi-sintético de amplo espectro derivado da cefalosporina C; usado por via oral.
cef·a·drox·il (sef - ā - drok′sil). Cefadroxil; antibiótico semi-sintético de amplo espectro derivado da cefalosporina C; usado por via oral.
cef·a·man·dole nafate (sef - ā - man′dōl naf′āt). Nafato de cefamandol; antibiótico semi-sintético de amplo espectro derivado da cefalosporina C; usado por via injetável.
ce·faz·o·lin (se - faz′ō - lin). Cefazolina; cefalosporina de amplo espectro usada para tratar um amplo espectro de infecções graves; disponível como o sal sódico para administração intramuscular ou intravenosa.
ce·fon·i·cid di·so·di·um (se - fon′ī - sid). Cefonicida dissódica; cefalosporina de amplo espectro e ação prolongada estruturalmente relacionada ao cefamandol.
ce·fo·per·a·zone so·di·um (se - fō - per′ā - zōn). Cefoperazona sódica; antibiótico piperazina-cefalosporina semi-sintético.
ce·for·a·nide (se - fōr′ā - nīd). Ceforanida; antibiótico cefalosporina de amplo espectro e ação prolongada.
ce·fo·tax·ime so·di·um (se - fō - taks′ēm). Cefotaxima sódica; antibiótico cefalosporina de amplo espectro.
cef·o·te·tan di·so·di·um (sef′ō - te - tan). Cefotetan dissódico; antibiótico cefalosporina de amplo espectro.
ce·fox·i·tin so·di·um (se - fok′si - tin). Cefoxitina sódica; antibiótico semi-sintético derivado da cefamicina C, mas estrutural e farmacologicamente semelhante às cefalosporinas; usado por via injetável.
cef·taz·i·dime so·di·um (sef - taz′i - dēm). Ceftazidima sódica; antibiótico cefalosporina particularmente efetivo contra enterobactérias e espécies de *Pseudomonas*.
cef·ti·zox·ime so·di·um (sef - ti - zoks′ēm). Ceftizoxima sódica; antibiótico cefalosporina de amplo espectro semelhante à cefotaxima sódica.
cef·tri·ax·one di·so·di·um (sef - trī - aks′ōn). Cefitraxona dissódica; antibiótico cefalosporina semi-sintético de uso parenteral.
cel (sel). Cel; unidade de velocidade; 1 cm por segundo. [L. *celer*, rápido]
-cele. Tumefação; hérnia. [G. *kēlē*, tumor]
ce·len·ter·on (sē - len′ter - on). Celêntero. SIN primitive *gut*. [G. *koilos*, oco, + *enteron*, intestino]
cel·ery seed (sel′er - ē). Semente de aipo; o fruto maduro seco de *Apium graveolens* (família Umbelliferae); tem sido usado na dismenorréia e como sedativo.
Celestin, Felix, médico francês, *1900. VER C. *tube*.
ce·les·tine blue B (sē - les′tēn). [C.I. 51050]. Azul-celeste B; corante recomendado como substituto da hematoxilina quando esta não é disponível.
ce·li·ac (sē′lē - ak). Celíaco; relativo à cavidade abdominal. [G. *koilia*, abdome]
ce·li·a·gra (sē - lē - ag′rā). Celiagra; termo raramente usado para afecção dolorosa súbita do estômago ou de outros órgãos abdominais. [G. *koilia*, abdome, + *agra*, ataque]
celio-. O abdome. VER TAMBÉM celo- (3). [G. *koilia*, abdome]
ce·li·o·cen·te·sis (sē′lē - ō - sen - tē′sis). Celiocentese; termo raramente empregado para paracentese do abdome. [celio- + G. *kentēsis*, punção]
ce·li·o·my·al·gia (sē′lē - ō - mī - al′jē - ā). Celiomialgia; termo raramente usado para dor nos músculos abdominais. [celio- + G. *mys*, músculo, + *algos*, dor]
ce·li·o·my·o·si·tis (sē′lē - ō - mī - ō - sī′tis). Celiomiosite; inflamação dos músculos abdominais. [celio- + G. *mys*, músculo, + -*itis*, inflamação]
ce·li·o·par·a·cen·te·sis (sē′lē - ō - par - ā - sen - tē′sis). Celioparacentese; termo raramente usado para paracentese do abdome. [celio- + G. *parakentēsis*, punção para hidropisia]
ce·li·op·a·thy (sē - lē - op′ā - thē). Celiopatia; termo raramente usado para qualquer doença abdominal. [celio- + G. *pathos*, doença]
ce·li·or·rha·phy (sē - lē - ōr′ā - fē). Celiorrafia; sutura de uma ferida na parede abdominal. SIN laparorrhaphy. [celio- + G. *rhaphē*, sutura]
ce·li·os·co·py (sē - lē - os′kŏ - pē). Celioscopia. SIN peritoneoscopy. [celio- + G. *skopeō*, ver]
ce·li·ot·o·my (sē - lē - ot′ō - mē). Celiotomia; incisão transabdominal da cavidade peritoneal. SIN abdominal section, laparotomy (2), ventrotomy. [celio- + G. *tomē*, incisão]
vaginal c., c. vaginal; abertura da cavidade peritoneal através da vagina. SIN culdotomy (2).
ce·li·tis (sē - lī′tis). Celite; qualquer inflamação do abdome. [G. *koilia*, abdome, + -*itis*, inflamação]

CELL

cell (sel). **1.** Célula; a menor unidade de estrutura viva capaz de existência independente, composta de uma massa de protoplasma encerrada por membrana e contendo um núcleo ou nucleóide. As células são muito variáveis e especializadas em estrutura e função, embora todas devam, em algum estágio, replicar proteínas e ácidos nucleicos, utilizar energia e reproduzir-se. **2.** Uma pequena cavidade fechada ou parcialmente fechada; um compartimento ou receptáculo oco. **3.** Um recipiente de vidro, cerâmica ou outro material sólido dentro do qual ocorrem reações químicas, gerando eletricidade, ou são colocadas soluções para ensaios fotométricos. [L. *cella*, despensa, câmara]

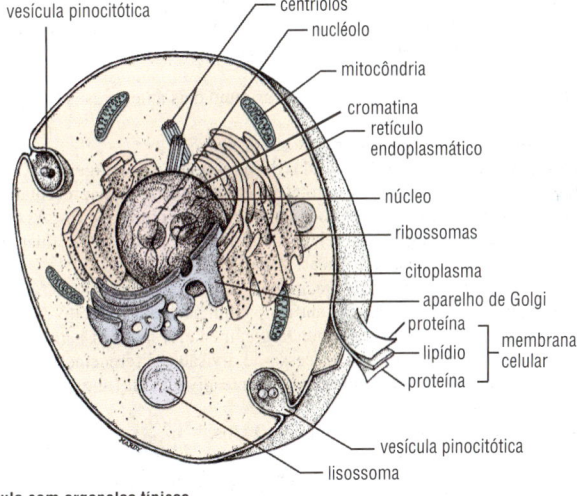

célula com organelas típicas

A c.'s, células alfa do pâncreas ou do lobo anterior da hipófise (adeno-hipófise).
absorption c., c. de absorção, elemento de absorção; pequena câmara de vidro com lados paralelos, na qual podem ser obtidos os espectros de absorção de soluções.
absorptive c.'s of intestine, células absortivas do intestino; células situadas na superfície das vilosidades do intestino delgado e na superfície luminal do intestino grosso caracterizadas por microvilosidades em sua superfície livre.
accessory c., c. acessória. SIN antigen-presenting c.'s.
acid c., c. ácida. SIN parietal c.
acidophil c., c. acidófila; c. cujo citoplasma ou grânulos se coram com corantes ácidos.
acinar c., c. acinar; qualquer c. secretora revestindo um ácino, sobretudo as células do pâncreas que fornecem suco pancreático e enzimas para distingui-las das células dos ductos e das ilhotas de Langerhans. SIN acinous c.
acinous c., SIN acinar c.
acoustic c., c. acústica; c. ciliar do órgão de Corti.
adipose c., c. adiposa, adipócito. SIN fat c.
adventitial c., c. adventícia. SIN pericyte.
air c.'s, células aéreas; **(1)** SIN pulmonary *alveolus*; **(2)** espaços no crânio que contêm ar.
air c.'s of auditory tube, células aéreas da tuba auditiva. SIN tubal air c.'s (of pharyngotympanic tube).
albuminous c., c. albuminosa; **(1)** SIN serous c.; **(2)** SIN zymogenic c.
algoid c., c. algóide; célula que se assemelha às células de algas, algumas vezes encontrada na diarréia crônica.
alpha c.'s of anterior lobe of hypophysis, células alfa do lobo anterior da hipófise; células acidófilas que constituem cerca de 35% das células do lobo

anterior. Há dois tipos: um que produz somatotropina, outro que produz pro-lactina.
alpha c.'s of pancreas, células alfa do pâncreas; células das ilhotas de Langerhans que secretam glucagon.
alveolar c., qualquer das células que revestem os alvéolos pulmonares, incluindo as células alveolares escamosas, as grandes células alveolares e os macrófagos alveolares. SIN pneumocyte.
amacrine c., c. amácrina; uma célula nervosa com dendritos ramificados curtos, mas que parecem não ter axônio; Cajal descreveu essas células na retina e deu nome a elas.
ameboid c., c. amebóide; uma célula como um leucócito, que possui movimentos amebóides, com capacidade de locomoção. SIN wandering c. SIN migratory c.
amniogenic c.'s, células amniogênicas; células a partir das quais se desenvolve o âmnio.
anabiotic c., c. anabiótica; célula capaz de ressuscitação após morte aparente; pressupõe-se que a existência de células tumorais anabióticas explique a recorrência de um câncer após um período assintomático muito longo depois da operação.
anaplastic c., c. anaplásica; (1) uma célula que voltou a um estado embrionário; (2) uma c. indiferenciada característica de neoplasias malignas.
angioblastic c.'s, células angioblásticas; aquelas células no embrião inicial a partir das quais se desenvolvem células sanguíneas primitivas e endotélio.
Anitschkow c., c. de Anitschkow. SIN cardiac histiocyte.
anterior c.'s, células etmoidais anteriores. SIN anterior ethmoidal c.'s.
anterior ethmoidal c.'s [TA], células etmoidais anteriores; o grupo anterior de células aéreas dos seios etmoidais; cada seio se comunica com o meato médio da cavidade nasal. SIN cellulae ethmoidales anteriores [TA], anterior c.'s, anterior ethmoidal air c.'s, anterior sinuses, sinus ethmoidales anteriores.
anterior ethmoidal air c.'s, células aéreas etmoidais anteriores. SIN anterior ethmoidal c.'s.
anterior horn c., neurônio motor. SIN motor neuron.
antigen-presenting c.'s (APC), células de apresentação de antígenos (CAA); células que processam antígenos proteicos em peptídeos e os apresentam na sua superfície em uma forma que pode ser reconhecida por linfócitos. As CAA incluem células de Langerhans, células dendríticas, macrófagos, células B e, em seres humanos, células T ativadas. SIN accessory c.
antigen-responsive c., c. sensível a antígenos. SIN antigen-sensitive c.
antigen-sensitive c., c. sensível a antígenos; um pequeno linfócito que, embora não seja uma célula ativada imunologicamente, responde a estímulo antigênico (imunogênico) por um processo de divisão e diferenciação que resulta na produção de células imunologicamente ativadas. SIN antigen-responsive c.
apolar c., c. apolar; um neurônio sem processos.
APUD c.'s, células APUD. VER APUD.
argentaffin c.'s, células argentafins; células que contêm grânulos que precipitam prata de uma solução de nitrato de prata amoniacal. VER TAMBÉM enteroendocrine c.'s.

argyrophilic c.'s, células argirófilas; células que se ligam a sais de prata, mas que precipitam prata apenas na presença de um agente redutor. VER TAMBÉM enteroendocrine c.'s.
Aschoff c., c. de Aschoff; grande componente celular de nódulos reumatóides no miocárdio com um núcleo característico e relativamente pouco citoplasma.
Askanazy c., c. de Askanazy. SIN Hürthle c.
astroglia c., c. da astróglia. SIN astrocyte.
atypical glandular c.'s of undetermined significance, células glandulares atípicas de importância indeterminada; o termo, no sistema Bethesda, para relatar diagnóstico citológico cervical e/ou vaginal descrevendo células que mostram diferenciação endometrial ou endocervical e exibem atipia nuclear que ultrapassa as alterações reativas ou reparadoras, mas não possuem aspectos definidos de adenocarcinoma invasivo. VER TAMBÉM Bethesda *system*.
atypical squamous c.'s of undetermined significance (ASCUS), células escamosas atípicas de importância indeterminada (CAASI); o termo usado no sistema Bethesda para relatar diagnóstico citológico cervical/vaginal descrevendo anormalidades celulares mais acentuadas que aquelas atribuíveis às alterações reativas, mas que, quantitativa ou qualitativamente, é insuficiente para um diagnóstico definitivo de lesão intra-epitelial escamosa (LIEE); pode refletir uma lesão benigna ou potencialmente séria. VER TAMBÉM Bethesda *system*, reactive *changes*, em *change*.
auditory receptor c.'s, células receptoras auditivas; células colunares no epitélio do órgão de Corti, que possuem pêlos (estereocílios) em suas extremidades apicais. VER Corti c.'s.
B c., (1) c. β do pâncreas ou do lobo anterior da hipófise; (2) SIN B lymphocyte.
balloon c., c. em balão; (1) c. degenerada incomumente grande com citoplasma de coloração pálida vacuolado ou reticulado, como na hepatite viral ou nas células epidérmicas degeneradas do herpes zoster; (2) uma grande forma de c. de nevos com abundante citoplasma não-corado, formado por degeneração vacuolar de melanossomas.
band c., c. em bastão; qualquer célula da série granulocítica (leucocítica) que tem um núcleo que poderia ser descrito como uma faixa curva ou espiralada, qualquer que seja o grau de entalhe, se o núcleo não estiver completamente segmentado em lobos unidos por um filamento. SIN band neutrophil, rod nuclear c., Schilling band c., stab c., stab neutrophil, staff c.
basal c., c. basal; c. da camada mais profunda do epitélio estratificado. SIN basilar c.
basaloid c., c. basalóide; c., geralmente da epiderme, semelhante a uma c. basal.
basilar c., c. basilar. SIN basal c.
basket c., (1) neurônio que emaranha suas ramificações axônicas terminais com o corpo celular de outro neurônio; (2) SIN smudge c.'s; (3) uma c. mioepitelial com processos ramificados observada em posição basal em relação às células secretoras de determinadas glândulas salivares e dos alvéolos da glândula lacrimal.
basophil c. of anterior lobe of hypophysis, c. basófila do lobo anterior da hipófise. SIN beta c. of anterior lobe of hypophysis.
beaker c., c. caliciforme. SIN goblet c.
Beale c., c. de Beale; uma c. ganglionar bipolar do coração com um prolongamento espiralado e outro reto.

células de apresentação de antígenos

captação do antígeno	endocitose por fagócitos (por células de Langerhans)	fagocitose	fagocitose	endocitose mediada por receptor	endocitose mediada por receptor
expressão de MHC classe II	constitutiva (+++)	indutível (−)	indutível (++)	constitutiva (++)	constitutiva (+++)
atividade coestimulante	constitutiva B7 (+++)	indutível B7 (−)	indutível B7 (++)	indutível B7 (−)	indutível B7 (++)
ativação de células T	células T inocentes células T efetoras células T de memória	(−)	células T efetoras células T de memória	células T efetoras células T de memória	células T inocentes células T efetoras células T de memória

MHC, complexo principal de histocompatibilidade; LPS, lipopolissacarídeo; IFN-γ, interferon gama.

Berger c.'s, células de Berger. SIN hilus c.'s.
berry c., c. morular, célula de Mott; uma hemácia crenada com espículas superficiais.
beta c. of anterior lobe of hypophysis, c. beta do lobo anterior da hipófise; uma célula de uma população de células funcionalmente diversas que contém grânulos basófilos e secretam hormônios como ACTH, lipotropina, tireotropina e as gonadotropinas. SIN basophil c. of anterior lobe of hypophysis.
beta c. of pancreas, c. beta do pâncreas; a c. predominante das ilhotas de Langerhans que secreta insulina.
Betz c.'s, células de Betz; grandes células piramidais na área motora do giro pré-central do córtex cerebral. SIN Bevan-Lewis c.'s.
Bevan-Lewis c.'s, células de Bevan-Lewis. SIN Betz c.'s.
bipolar c., c. bipolar; um neurônio que possui dois processos, como aqueles da retina ou os gânglios espiral e vestibular do oitavo nervo.
Bizzozero red c.'s, c. de Bizzozero; hemácias nucleadas no sangue humano.
blast c., blasto; c. precursora imatura; p. ex., eritroblasto, linfoblasto, neuroblasto. VER TAMBÉM -blast.
blood c., c. do sangue; uma das células do sangue, um leucócito ou eritrócito. SIN blood corpuscle.
Boll c.'s, células de Boll; células basais na glândula lacrimal.
bone c., c. óssea, osteócito. SIN osteocyte.
border c.'s, células limítrofes; células que formam o limite interno do órgão de Corti.
Böttcher c.'s, células de Böttcher; células da membrana basilar da cóclea.
Bowenoid c.'s, células de Bowen; células características da doença de Bowen; ceratinócitos intra-epidérmicos redondos, grandes e dispersos, com um núcleo hipercromático e citoplasma pálido.
bristle c., c. ciliada; c. pilosa do ouvido interno.
bronchic c.'s, células brônquicas. SIN pulmonary alveolus.
bronchiolar exocrine c., c. exócrina bronquiolar. SIN Clara c.
brood c., c.-fonte, célula-mãe. SIN mother c.
burr c., c. espiculada; hemácia crenada.
C c., c. C; **(1)** uma c. das ilhotas pancreáticas de cobaia; SIN gamma c. of pancreas. VER TAMBÉM medullary carcinoma of thyroid; **(2)** célula folicular da tireóide, redonda ou fusiforme, secretora de calcitonina; ultra-estruturalmente contém muitos grânulos neuroendócrinos que medem 60–550 nm; mais bem identificada imuno-histoquimicamente com anticorpos contra a calcitonina. SIN light c.'s of thyroid, parafollicular c.'s.
Cajal c., c. de Cajal; **(1)** SIN horizontal c. of Cajal; **(2)** SIN astrocyte.
caliciform c., c. caliciforme. SIN goblet c.
capsule c., c. da cápsula. SIN amphicyte.
carrier c., fagócito. SIN phagocyte.
cartilage c., condrócito. SIN chondrocyte.
castration c.'s, células de castração; células basófilas alteradas do lobo anterior da hipófise que se desenvolvem após castração; o corpo da célula é ocupado por um grande vacúolo que desloca o núcleo para a periferia, dando à c. o aspecto de um anel de sinete. SIN signet ring c.'s.
caterpillar c., histiócito cardíaco; célula de Anitschkow. SIN cardiac histiocyte.
centroacinar c., c. centroacinar; uma c. do ducto pancreático que ocupa a luz de um ácino; secreta bicarbonato e água, fornecendo um pH alcalino necessário para atividade enzimática no intestino.
chalice c., c. caliciforme. SIN goblet c.
chief c., c. principal; o tipo celular predominante de uma glândula.
chief c. of corpus pineale, c. principal do corpo pineal; pinealócito. SIN pinealocyte.
chief c. of parathyroid gland, c. principal da glândula paratireóide; uma c. clara arredondada com um núcleo central; secreta paratormônio.
chief c. of stomach, c. principal do estômago. SIN zymogenic c.
chromaffin c., c. cromafim; c. que se cora com sais crômicos, na medula supra-renal e paragânglios do sistema nervoso simpático.
chromophobe c.'s of anterior lobe of hypophysis, células cromófobas do lobo anterior da hipófise; células da adeno-hipófise desprovidas de grânulos acidófilos ou basófilos específicos quando coradas com corantes diferenciais comuns.
Clara c., c. de Clara; uma c. arredondada, em forma de clava, não-ciliada, que se projeta entre as células ciliadas no epitélio bronquiolar; acredita-se que tenha função secretora. SIN bronchiolar exocrine c.
Clarke c.'s, células de Clarke; grandes células multipolares características do núcleo torácico (núcleo de Clarke na lâmina VII) da medula espinhal.
Claudius c.'s, células de Claudius; células colunares no assoalho do ducto coclear externo ao órgão de Corti.
clear c., c. clara; **(1)** c. na qual o citoplasma parece vazio à microscopia óptica, como ocorre em determinadas células secretoras de glândulas sudoríparas écrinas e nas glândulas paratireóides quando o glicogênio não é corado; **(2)** qualquer célula, particularmente uma célula neoplásica, contendo abundante glicogênio ou outro material que não seja corado por hematoxilina ou eosina, de forma que o citoplasma celular é muito pálido em cortes corados rotineiramente.
cleavage c., blastômero. SIN blastomere.

cleaved c., c. clivada; c. com uma ou múltiplas fendas na membrana nuclear.
clonogenic c., c. clonogênica; c. que tem potencial de proliferar e originar uma colônia de células; algumas células-filhas de cada geração preservam esse potencial de proliferar.
clue c., c. indicadora; tipo de c. epitelial vaginal que parece granular e é revestida com microrganismos cocobacilares; observada na vaginose bacteriana.
cochlear hair c.'s, células pilosas cocleares; células de Corti; células sensoriais no órgão de Corti em contato sináptico com fibras sensoriais bem como fibras eferentes do nervo coclear (auditivo); a partir da extremidade apical de cada célula, estendem-se cerca de 100 estereocílios da superfície que fazem contato com a membrana tectorial. SIN Corti c.'s.
column c.'s, células colunares; neurônios na substância cinzenta da medula espinhal cujos axônios estão confinados no sistema nervoso central.
commissural c., c. comissural; neurônio cujo axônio passa para o lado oposto do neuroeixo. SIN heteromeric c.
compound granule c., c. granulosa composta. SIN gitter c.
cone c. of retina, cone da retina. SIN cone (2).
connective tissue c., c. do tecido conjuntivo; qualquer uma das células de formas variadas encontradas no tecido conjuntivo.
contrasuppressor c.'s, células contra-supressoras; subpopulação de células T, diferentes das células T auxiliares, que supostamente inibem a função da célula T supressora.
Corti c.'s, células de Corti. SIN cochlear hair c.'s
crescent c., c. em crescente, falciforme. SIN sickle c.
cytomegalic c.'s, células citomegálicas; células que contêm grandes corpúsculos de inclusão citomegálicos intranucleares e intracitoplasmáticos causados por citomegalovírus; um membro da família Herpesviridae.
cytotoxic c., c. citotóxica; **(1)** um subgrupo de linfócitos T CD8 que se ligam a outras células através do MHC classe I e são envolvidos na sua destruição. SIN T cytotoxic c.'s. **(2)** outras células do sistema imune capazes de destruir patógenos ou células aberrantes, isto é, macrófagos, células NK, células K.
cytotrophoblastic c.'s, células citotrofoblásticas; células-tronco (primordiais) que se fundem para formar o sinciciotrofoblasto sobrejacente das vilosidades placentárias. SIN Langhans c.'s (2).
D c., c. D. SIN delta c. of pancreas.
dark c.'s, células escuras; células das glândulas sudoríparas écrinas que possuem muitos ribossomas e grânulos secretores mucóides.
daughter c., célula-filha; uma das duas ou mais células formadas na divisão de uma célula-mãe.
Davidoff c.'s, células de Davidoff. SIN Paneth granular c.'s.
decidual c., c. decidual; uma c. do tecido conjuntivo ovóide, aumentada, encontrada no endométrio da gestante.
decoy c., célula chamariz; c. epitelial esfoliada benigna com núcleo picnótico observada em infecções urinárias; pode ser confundida com uma c. maligna.
deep c., c. profunda. SIN mesangial c.
Deiters c.'s, células de Deiters; **(1)** SIN phalangeal c.; **(2)** SIN astrocyte.
delta c. of anterior lobe of hypophysis, c. delta do lobo anterior da hipófise; um tipo celular que possui grânulos basófilos.
delta c. of pancreas, c. delta do pâncreas; c. das ilhotas que possui grânulos finos e contém somatostatina. SIN D c.
dendritic c., c. dendrítica; c. com origem na crista neural com processos extensos; desenvolve melanina precocemente.
Dogiel c.'s, células de Dogiel; os diferentes tipos celulares nos gânglios cefalorraquidianos.
dome c., c. em cúpula; uma das células superficiais arredondadas da camada peridérmica da epiderme fetal.
Downey c., c. de Downey; o linfócito atípico da mononucleose infecciosa.
dust c., macrófago alveolar. SIN alveolar macrophage.
effector c., c. efetora; leucócito diferenciado terminal que realiza uma ou mais funções específicas. VER TAMBÉM effector.
egg c., c.-ovo; o óvulo não fertilizado.
embryonic c., c. embrionária. SIN blastomere.
enamel c., c. de esmalte. SIN ameloblast.
end c., c. terminal; c. totalmente diferenciada; a c. madura de uma linhagem.
endodermal c., c. endodérmica; células embrionárias que formam o saco vitelino e dão origem ao epitélio dos tratos digestivo e respiratório e ao parênquima de glândulas associadas. SIN entodermal c.
endothelial c., c. endotelial; uma das células escamosas que formam o revestimento dos vasos sanguíneos e linfáticos e a camada interna do endocárdio. SIN endotheliocyte.
enterochromaffin c.'s, células enterocromafins. SIN enteroendocrine c.'s.
enteroendocrine c.'s, células enteroendócrinas; células dispersas por todo o trato digestivo, de vários tipos, e que parecem produzir pelo menos 20 diferentes hormônios gastrointestinais e neurotransmissores; contêm grânulos que podem ser argentafins ou argirófilos. SIN enterochromaffin c.'s, Kulchitsky c.'s.
entodermal c., c. entodérmica. SIN endodermal c.
ependymal c., c. ependimária; uma c. que reveste o canal central da medula espinal (de forma piramidal) ou um dos ventrículos cerebrais (de forma cubóide).

epidermic c., c. epidérmica; uma das células da epiderme.
epithelial c., c. epitelial; um dos muitos tipos de células que formam epitélio.
epithelial reticular c., c. reticular epitelial; uma das muitas células epiteliais ramificadas que, coletivamente, formam o estroma de sustentação para linfócitos no timo; acredita-se que produz timosina e outros fatores que controlam a função tímica.
epithelioid c., c. epitelióide; (1) uma c. não-epitelial que possui algumas características de epitélio; (2) grandes histiócitos mononucleares que possuem algumas características epiteliais, particularmente em áreas de inflamação granulomatosa onde são poligonais e possuem citoplasma eosinofílico.
erythroid c., c. eritróide; uma c. da série eritrocítica.
ethmoid c.'s, células etmoidais; células aéreas etmoidais; evaginações da mucosa dos meatos médio e superior da cavidade nasal para o labirinto etmoidal, formando múltiplos pequenos seios paranasais; são subdivididas em seios etmoidais anterior, médio e posterior. VER anterior ethmoidal c.'s, middle ethmoidal c.'s, posterior ethmoidal c.'s. SIN cellulae ethmoidales [TA], ethmoid air c.'s [TA], ethmoidal c.'s [TA], antra ethmoidalia, ethmoidal sinuses, sinus ethmoidales.
ethmoid air c.'s [TA], células aéreas etmoidais. SIN ethmoid c.'s.
ethmoidal c.'s [TA], células etmoidais. SIN ethmoid c.'s.
external pillar c.'s, células pilares externas. VER pillar c.'s.
exudation c., c. de exsudação. SIN exudation corpuscle.
Fañanás c., c. de Fañanás; astrócito especializado encontrado no córtex cerebelar.
fasciculata c., c. fasciculada; c. da zona fasciculada do córtex supra-renal que contém numerosas gotículas de lipídios devido à presença de corticosteróides.
fat c., c. adiposa; adipócito; uma c. do tecido conjuntivo distendida por um ou mais glóbulos de gordura, sendo o citoplasma geralmente comprimido em um invólucro delgado, com o núcleo em um ponto na periferia. SIN adipocyte, adipose c.
fat-storing c., c. armazenadora de gordura; c. multilocular cheia de gordura presente no espaço perissinusoidal no fígado. SIN lipocyte.
Ferrata c., c. de Ferrata. SIN hemohistioblast.
flame c., c. em chama; c. excretora ciliada, primitiva em trematóideos; o movimento dos cílios nessa c. na larva miracídio, dentro de um ovo de esquistossoma, indica viabilidade do ovo.
foam c.'s, células espumosas; células com citoplasma abundante, pálido, finamente vacuolado, geralmente histiócitos que fagocitaram ou acumularam material que se dissolve durante o preparo do tecido, principalmente lipídios. VER TAMBÉM lipophage.
follicular epithelial c., c. epitelial folicular; uma c. que reveste um folículo como o da glândula tireóide.
follicular ovarian c.'s, células foliculares ovarianas; células de um folículo ovariano que circundam o óvulo em desenvolvimento; formam o estrato granuloso do ovário e o *cumulus oophorus* (disco prolígero, ovígero).
foreign body giant c., célula gigante tipo corpo estranho; "célula" multinucleada ou sincício formado ao redor de partículas em reações inflamatórias crônicas, formada pela fusão de macrófagos.
formative c., c. formadora; célula da massa interna do blastocisto; coletivamente essas células dão origem ao embrião.
foveolar c.'s of stomach, células das fovéolas do estômago; células tecais das fossetas (fovéolas) gástricas.
fuchsinophil c., c. fucsinófila; c. com afinidade especial pela fucsina.
fusiform c.'s of cerebral cortex, células fusiformes do córtex cerebral; células fusiformes na sexta camada do córtex cerebral.
G c.'s, células G; células enteroendócrinas que secretam gastrina, encontradas basicamente na mucosa do antro pilórico do estômago.
gamma c. of pancreas, c. gama do pâncreas. SIN C c. (1).
ganglion c., c. ganglionar; originalmente, qualquer c. nervosa (neurônio); hoje, um neurônio cujo corpo celular está localizado fora dos limites do cérebro e da medula espinal, assim fazendo parte do sistema nervoso periférico; as células ganglionares são: 1) as células pseudo-unipolares dos nervos sensoriais espinais e cranianos (gânglios sensoriais ou sensitivos), ou 2) os neurônios motores multipolares periféricos que inervam as vísceras (gânglios viscerais ou autônomos). SIN gangliocyte.
ganglion c.'s of dorsal spinal root, células ganglionares da raiz dorsal da medula espinal; corpos de células nervosas pseudo-unipolares nos gânglios das raízes nervosas espinais dorsais; os nervos espinais sensoriais são compostos pelos ramos axonais periféricos dessas células ganglionares sensoriais, enquanto o ramo axonal central de cada uma dessas células entra na medula espinal como um componente da raiz dorsal.
ganglion c.'s of retina, células ganglionares da retina, as células nervosas da retina cujos processos (axônios) centrais formam o nervo óptico; seus processos periféricos formam sinapses com as células bipolares e, através delas, com os cones e bastonetes; esses corpos celulares são redondos ou em forma de cantil, e seu tamanho é bastante variável. VER TAMBÉM ganglionic *layer*.
Gaucher c.'s, células de Gaucher; células grandes, com vacuolações finas e uniformes derivadas do sistema reticuloendotelial, encontradas principalmente no baço, linfonodos, fígado e medula óssea de pacientes com doença de Gaucher; as células de Gaucher contêm querasina (um cerebrosídeo), que se acumula devido à ausência geneticamente determinada da enzima glicosilceramidase.
gemistocytic c., c. gemistocítica. SIN gemistocytic astrocyte.
germ c., c. germinativa. SIN sex c.
germinal c., c. da qual proliferam outras células.
ghost c., c.-fantasma; (1) uma célula morta na qual o contorno permanece visível, mas sem outras estruturas citoplasmáticas ou núcleo corável; (2) um eritrócito após a perda de sua hemoglobina.
giant c., célula gigante; uma c. de tamanho grande, freqüentemente com muitos núcleos.
Gierke c.'s, células de Gierke; células pequenas características da substância gelatinosa (lâmina II) do corno dorsal da medula espinal.
gitter c., célula granulosa composta; fagócito da micróglia cheio de lipídios comumente observado na borda de infartos cerebrais em cicatrização, uma conseqüência da fagocitose de lipídios por células cerebrais necróticas ou em degeneração. SIN compound granule c., gitterzelle. [Al. *Gitterzelle*, de *Gitter*, treliça, rede]
glia c.'s, células gliais. VER neuroglia.
glitter c.'s, leucócitos polimorfonucleares que se coram de azul-pálido com violeta genciana e contêm grânulos citoplasmáticos que exibem movimento browniano; observados no sedimento urinário e característicos de pielonefrite.
globoid c., c. globóide; grande c. de origem mesodérmica encontrada em grupos nos tecidos intracranianos na leucodistrofia de células globóides.
glomerulosa c., c. glomerulosa; uma célula da zona glomerulosa do córtex supra-renal que é a fonte de aldosterona; as células são dispostas em grupos esféricos ou ovais.
goblet c., c. caliciforme; c. epitelial que se torna distendida por um grande acúmulo de grânulos secretores mucosos em sua extremidade apical, conferindo-lhe o aspecto caliciforme. SIN beaker c., caliciform c., chalice c.

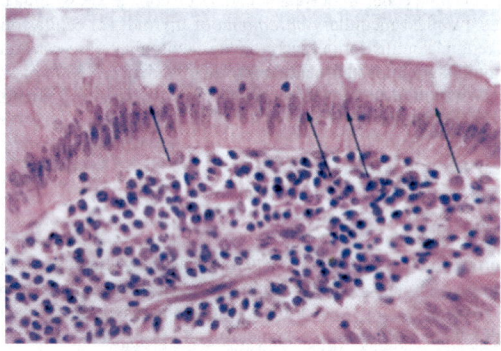

células caliciformes: fotomicrografia do epitélio intestinal mostrando células caliciformes únicas (setas) dispersas entre células absortivas

Golgi c.'s, células de Golgi. VER Golgi type I *neuron*, Golgi type II *neuron*.
Golgi epithelial c., c. epitelial de Golgi; célula glial encontrada no córtex cerebelar. VER Bergmann *fibers*, em *fiber*.
Goormaghtigh c.'s, células de Goormaghtigh. SIN juxtaglomerular c.'s.
granule c.'s, células granulosas; (1) pequenos corpos de neurônios nas camadas granulosas externa e interna do córtex cerebral; (2) pequenos corpos de neurônios na camada granulosa do córtex cerebelar.
granule c. of connective tissue, c. granulosa do tecido conjuntivo. SIN mast c.
granulosa c., c. da granulosa; uma c. da membrana granulosa que reveste o folículo ovariano vesicular, tornando-se uma célula lútea do corpo lúteo após a ovulação.
granulosa lutein c.'s, células luteínicas da granulosa; células derivadas da membrana granulosa de um folículo ovariano maduro que secretam estrogênio e progesterona, e formam o principal componente do corpo lúteo.
great alveolar c.'s, células alveolares grandes; pneumócitos granulares; células cubóides unidas às células alveolares pulmonares escamosas, possuindo em seu citoplasma corpúsculos lamelados (citossomas) que representam a fonte do surfactante que reveste os alvéolos. SIN granular pneumonocytes, type II c.'s.
guanine c., c. guanínica; célula cujo citoplasma contém cristais de guanina brilhantes.
gustatory c.'s, células gustativas. SIN taste c.'s.
gyrochrome c., c. girocrômica. VER gyrochrome.
hair c.'s, células ciliadas; células neuroepiteliais sensoriais presentes no órgão de Corti, na mácula e na crista do labirinto membranoso do ouvido, assim

como nas papilas gustativas; caracterizam-se pela presença de longos estereocílios ou cinocílios (ou ambos) que, à microscopia óptica, são observados como finos pêlos. VER TAMBÉM vestibular hair c.'s, cochlear hair c.'s, taste c.'s.
hairy c.'s, células pilosas; leucócitos de tamanho médio que possuem características de células reticuloendoteliais e múltiplas projeções citoplasmáticas (pêlos) na superfície celular, mas que podem ser um tipo de linfócito B; são encontradas na leucemia de células pilosas.
Haller c., c. de Haller; variante da célula aérea etmoidal que se desenvolve no assoalho da órbita adjacente ao óstio natural do seio maxilar. Uma c. de Haller doente pode obstruir o óstio e causar uma sinusite maxilar.
heart failure c., c. da insuficiência cardíaca; macrófago presente no pulmão, durante a insuficiência cardíaca esquerda, que, freqüentemente, transporta grandes quantidades de hemossiderina. VER TAMBÉM siderophore.
HeLa c.'s, células HeLa; as primeiras células malignas humanas cultivadas continuamente, derivadas do carcinoma cervical de uma paciente, Henrietta Lacks; usadas na cultura de vírus.
helmet c., c. em capacete; esquistócito em forma de capacete militar, observado na anemia hemolítica.
helper c.'s, células auxiliares. SIN T helper c.'s.
HEMPAS c.'s, células HEMPAS; os eritrócitos anormais da anemia diseritropoética congênita tipo II. VER HEMPAS.
Hensen c., c. de Hensen; uma das células de sustentação no órgão de Corti, ao lado da face externa das células de Deiters.
heteromeric c., c. heteromérica. SIN commissural c.
hilus c.'s, células hilares; células situadas no hilo ovariano que produzem androgênios; são consideradas equivalentes, no ovário, das células intersticiais do testículo. SIN Berger c.'s.
hobnail c., c. em tacha; célula característica de um adenocarcinoma de células claras; uma expansão redonda de citoplasma claro projeta-se para a luz dos túbulos neoplásicos, mas a parte basal da célula que contém o núcleo é estreita (assemelhando-se a uma tacha).
Hofbauer c., c. de Hofbauer; uma célula grande no tecido conjuntivo das vilosidades coriônicas; parece ser um tipo de fagócito.
horizontal c. of Cajal, c. horizontal de Cajal; pequena célula fusiforme encontrada na camada superficial do córtex cerebral com seu eixo longitudinal posicionado horizontalmente. SIN Cajal c. (1).
horizontal c.'s of retina, células horizontais da retina; células na parte externa da camada nuclear interna da retina, cujos eixos se situam mais ou menos paralelos à superfície. Acredita-se que unam os bastonetes de uma parte da retina aos cones de outra parte.
horny c., c. córnea. SIN corneocyte.
Hortega c.'s, células de Hortega. SIN microglia.
host c., c. hospedeira; uma célula (p. ex., uma bactéria) na qual um vetor pode ser propagado.
Hürthle c., c. de Hürthle; grande célula eosinofílica granular derivada do epitélio folicular da tireóide por acúmulo de mitocôndrias, p. ex., na doença de Hashimoto. SIN Askanazy c.
I c., c. I; fibroblasto cutâneo cultivado que contém inclusões ligadas à membrana; característica da mucolipidose II. SIN inclusion c.
immunologically activated c., c. imunologicamente ativada; imunócito que está em um estado elevado de reatividade capaz de produzir uma resposta imune.
immunologically competent c., c. imunologicamente competente; pequeno linfócito capaz de ser ativado imunologicamente por exposição a uma substância antigênica (imunogênica) para a respectiva célula; a ativação envolve a capacidade de produzir anticorpo ou a capacidade de participar da imunidade celular.
inclusion c., c. de inclusão. SIN I c.
indifferent c., c. indiferente; uma c. indiferenciada, não especializada.
inducer c., c. indutora; termo antigo para o subgrupo 1 das células T auxiliares.
innocent bystander c., c. espectadora inocente; a destruição de uma célula por um processo imune, embora tal célula não fosse o alvo direto.
intercapillary c., c. intercapilar. SIN mesangial c.
interdigitating reticulum c., c. reticular interdigitada; célula de apresentação do antígeno no paracórtex dos linfonodos, interagindo com linfócitos T.
internal pillar c.'s, células pilares internas. VER pillar c.'s.
interstitial c.'s, células intersticiais; **(1)** células situadas entre os túbulos seminíferos do testículo que secretam testosterona. SIN Leydig c.'s; **(2)** células derivadas da teca interna de folículos ovarianos atrésicos; assemelham-se às células luteais e são uma importante fonte de estrogênios; **(3)** células pineais semelhantes às células gliais com longos processos.
irritation c., c. irritativa. SIN Türk c.
islet c., c. das ilhotas; uma das células das ilhotas pancreáticas.
Ito c.'s, células de Ito; células contendo lipídios e que revestem os sinusóides hepáticos.
Jurkat c.'s, células de Jurkat; uma linhagem de células T freqüentemente empregadas em pesquisa imunológica, originalmente derivadas de um linfoma de Burkitt.

juvenile c., c. juvenil. SIN metamyelocyte.
juxtaglomerular c.'s, c. justaglomerulares; células localizadas no pólo vascular do corpúsculo renal que secretam renina e formam um componente do complexo justaglomerular; são células musculares lisas modificadas, basicamente, da arteríola aferente do glomérulo renal. SIN Goormaghtigh c.'s.
K c.'s, células K. SIN killer c.'s.
karyochrome c., c. cariocrômica. VER karyochrome.
keratinized c., c. queratinizada. SIN corneocyte.
killer c.'s, células destruidoras; células exterminadoras; células citotóxicas envolvidas em respostas imunes celulares anticorpo-dependentes; podem ser linfócitos T com receptores para a porção Fc das moléculas de IgG, e lisar ou lesar as células-alvo revestidas por IgG sem mediação do complemento. VER antibody-dependent cell-mediated *cytotoxicity*. SIN K c.'s, null c.'s (1).
Kulchitsky c.'s, células de Kulchitsky. SIN enteroendocrine c.'s.
Kupffer c.'s, células de Kupffer; células fagocíticas da série de fagócitos mononucleares encontradas na superfície luminal dos sinusóides hepáticos. SIN stellate c.'s of liver.
lacis c. (lah - sē′), c. *lacis*; c. mesangial extraglomerular; c. de Goormaghtigh; uma das células do aparelho justaglomerular encontrado no pólo vascular do corpúsculo renal. [Fr. *lacis*, rede].
Langerhans c.'s, células de Langerhans; **(1)** células claras dendríticas na epiderme, contendo grânulos distintos que aparecem em forma de bastonete ou raquete ao corte, mas que não possuem tonofilamentos, melanossomas e desmossomas; transportam receptores de superfície para imunoglobulina (Fc) e complemento (C3), e acredita-se que sejam células de fixação e processamento de antígenos de origem monocítica; participantes ativas na hipersensibilidade tardia cutânea. **(2)** Células observadas no granuloma eosinofílico e no linfoma dos pulmões.
Langhans c.'s, células de Langhans; **(1)** células gigantes multinucleadas observadas na tuberculose e em outras doenças granulomatosas; os núcleos são dispostos de forma arciforme na periferia das células. SIN Langhans-type giant c.'s. **(2)** Células citotrofoblásticas. SIN cytotrophoblastic c.'s.
Langhans-type giant c.'s, células gigantes do tipo Langhans. SIN Langhans c.'s (1).
LE c. c. LE; leucócito polimorfonuclear contendo um corpúsculo redondo amorfo que é um núcleo fagocitado de outra célula mais globulina antinuclear sérica (IgG) e complemento; formada *in vitro* no sangue de pacientes com lúpus eritematoso sistêmico. SIN lupus erythematosus c.
Leishman chrome c.'s, células crômicas de Leishman; leucócitos granulares basófilos observados no sangue circulante de algumas pessoas com febre hemoglobinúrica (hemoglobinúria malárica).
lepra c.'s, células da lepra; grandes fagócitos mononucleares distintos (macrófagos), com um citoplasma espumoso e, também, estruturas saculares mal coradas, resultantes da degeneração dessas células, observadas caracteristicamente em reações inflamatórias da lepra; a coloração indistinta resulta de numerosos bacilos da lepra situados muito próximos, que são álcool-ácido-resistentes e resistentes à coloração por métodos comuns.
Leydig c.'s, células de Leydig. SIN interstitial c.'s (1).
light c.'s of thyroid, células claras da tireóide. SIN C c. (2).
lining c., c. de revestimento. SIN littoral c.
Lipschütz c., c. de Lipschütz. SIN centrocyte (1).
littoral c., c. litorânea; as células que revestem os seios linfáticos dos linfonodos e dos seios sanguíneos da medula óssea. SIN lining c. [L. *littoralis*, litoral]
Loevit c., c. de Loevit; termo obsoleto para eritroblasto.
lupus erythematosus c., c. do lúpus eritematoso. SIN LE c.
luteal c., lutein c., c. luteínica; c. do corpo lúteo do ovário que é derivada das células granulosas do folículo pré-ovulatório; secreta progesterona e estrogênio.
lymph c., linfócito. SIN lymphocyte.
lymphoid c., c. linfóide; células leucocitárias do sistema imune.
M c., c. M. SIN microfold c.
macroglia c., c. da macróglia. SIN astrocyte.
malpighian c., c. de Malpighi; c. do estrato espinhoso da epiderme.
Marchand wandering c., c. migratória de Marchand; c. do sistema fagocítico mononuclear.
marrow c., c. da medula óssea; qualquer célula da medula óssea, principalmente células hematopoéticas.
Martinotti c., c. de Martinotti; pequena célula nervosa multipolar com dendritos ramificados curtos dispersos através de várias camadas do córtex cerebral; seu axônio ascende em direção à superfície do córtex.
mast c., mastócito; uma célula do tecido conjuntivo que contém grânulos secretores metacromáticos, basófilos, grosseiros; os grânulos contêm heparina, histamina e fator quimiotático de eosinófilos. Essas células estão envolvidas em reações de hipersensibilidade imediata e participam na regulação da composição da substância fundamental. SIN granule c. of connective tissue, labrocyte, mastocyte, tissue basophil.
mastoid c.'s [TA], células mastóides; numerosas cavidades intercomunicantes pequenas, no processo mastóide do osso temporal, que drenam para a mas-

tóide ou para o antro timpânico. SIN cellulae mastoideae [TA], mastoid air c.'s, mastoid sinuses.
mastoid air c.'s, células aéreas mastóideas. SIN mastoid c.'s.
memory B c.'s, células B de memória; linfócitos B que mediam a memória imunológica; permitem aumento da reação imunológica quando um organismo imunologicamente competente é reexposto a um antígeno.
memory T c.'s, células T de memória; linfócitos T que mediam a memória imunológica; permitem aumento da reação imunológica quando um organismo imunologicamente competente é reexposto a um antígeno.
Merkel tactile c., c. táctil de Merkel. SIN tactile *meniscus*.
mesangial c., c. mesangial; uma c. fagocítica no tufo capilar do glomérulo renal, interposta entre células endoteliais e a membrana basal na região central ou do pedículo do tufo. SIN deep c., intercapillary c.
mesenchymal c., c. mesenquimal; células fusiformes ou estreladas encontradas entre o ectoderma e o endoderma de embriões jovens; o formato das células no material fixado indica o fato de que, em vida, eles estavam se movendo de seu local de origem para áreas onde seriam reagregados e especializados; a maioria das células mesenquimais é derivada do mesoderma, mas, na região cefálica, também se desenvolvem a partir da crista neural ou ectoderma de superfície; são as células pluripotenciais mais surpreendentes do corpo do embrião, desenvolvendo-se em diferentes localizações em qualquer dos tipos de tecido conjuntivo ou de sustentação, músculo liso, endotélio vascular e células do sangue.
mesoglial c.'s, células mesogliais. SIN mesoglia.
mesothelial c., c. mesotelial; uma das células planas de origem mesodérmica formadoras da camada superficial das membranas serosas que revestem as cavidades corporais do abdome e tórax.
Mexican hat c., c. em sombreiro. SIN target c. (1).
Meynert c.'s, células de Meynert; células piramidais solitárias encontradas no córtex na região da fissura calcarina.
microfold c., células epiteliais intestinais especializadas encontradas em associação com os folículos linfóides nas placas de Peyer do íleo; caracterizadas por elaboradas invaginações da sua superfície apical que abrigam numerosos linfócitos e macrófagos; acredita-se que fagocitam antígenos e os apresentam às células linfóides subjacentes. SIN M c.
microglia c.'s, microglial c.'s, células da micróglia; células microgliais. SIN microglia.
middle c.'s, células etmoidais médias. SIN middle ethmoidal c.'s.
middle ethmoidal c.'s [TA], células etmoidais médias; o grupo médio de células aéreas dos seios etmoidais; cada seio se comunica com o meato médio da cavidade nasal. SIN cellulae ethmoidales mediae [TA], middle c.'s, middle ethmoidal air c.'s, middle ethmoidal sinuses, sinus ethmoidales mediae.
middle ethmoidal air c.'s, células aéreas etmoidais médias. SIN middle ethmoidal c.'s.
midget bipolar c.'s, células bipolares anãs; células bipolares, na camada nuclear interna da retina, que fazem sinapse com cones individuais na camada plexiforme externa; outras células bipolares maiores, na camada nuclear interna, fazem sinapse com os bastonetes e cones; os axônios de ambos os tipos fazem sinapse, na camada plexiforme interna, com os dendritos das células ganglionares.
migratory c., c. migratória. SIN ameboid c.
Mikulicz c.'s, células de Mikulicz; macrófagos espumosos contendo *Klebsiella rhinoscleromatis*; encontradas nos nódulos mucosos no rinoescleroma.
mirror-image c., c. em imagem espelhada; (1) uma c. cujos núcleos possuem características idênticas e estão posicionados no citoplasma de forma semelhante; (2) uma forma binucleada de célula de Reed-Sternberg freqüentemente encontrada na doença de Hodgkin; os núcleos gêmeos estão dispostos em relação a um plano imaginário entre si como um único núcleo com sua imagem espelhada.
mitral c.'s, células mitrais; grandes células nervosas no lobo olfatório do cérebro cujos dendritos fazem sinapse (nos glomérulos) com axônios das células receptoras olfatórias da mucosa nasal, e cujos axônios passam centralmente no trato olfatório até o córtex olfatório.
monocytoid c., c. monocitóide; c. que possui características morfológicas de um monócito, mas que não é um fagócito.
mossy c., c. musgosa; um dos dois tipos de células da neuróglia, que consistem em um corpo bastante grande com numerosos processos ramificados curtos.
mother c., c.-mãe; uma c. que, por divisão, dá origem a duas ou mais células-filhas. SIN brood c., metrocyte, parent c.
motor c., c. motora; neurônio cujo axônio inerva células efetoras periféricas como fibras musculares ou células glandulares.
mucoalbuminous c.'s, células mucoalbuminosas. SIN mucoserous c.'s.
mucoserous c.'s, células mucosserosas; células glandulares com características histológicas intermediárias entre células serosas e células mucosas. SIN mucoalbuminous c.'s, seromucous c.'s.
mucous c., c. mucosa; c. secretora de muco; p. ex., uma c. caliciforme.
mucous neck c., c. mucosa do colo; uma das células secretoras de mucina no colo de uma glândula gástrica.
Müller radial c.'s, células radiais de Müller. SIN Müller *fibers* (2), em *fiber*.

multipolar c., c. multipolar; uma célula nervosa com vários dendritos originados no corpo celular.
mural c., c. mural; c. não-endotelial encerrada na membrana basal dos capilares retinianos.
myeloid c., c. mielóide; especificamente, qualquer célula jovem que se transforma em um granulócito maduro do sangue, porém freqüentemente usada como sinônimo de célula da medula óssea.
myoepithelial c., c. mioepitelial; uma c. de origem ectodérmica, semelhante ao músculo liso, encontrada entre o epitélio e a membrana basal em vários órgãos, como as glândulas mamárias, sudoríparas e lacrimais.
myoid c.'s, células mióides; células achatadas de origem mesodérmica, semelhantes ao músculo liso, situadas imediatamente fora da lâmina basal do túbulo seminífero. SIN peritubular contractile c.'s.
Nageotte c.'s, células de Nageotte; células encontradas no líquido cefalorraquidiano, uma ou duas por milímetro cúbico em pessoas sadias, mas em números maiores em várias doenças.
natural killer c.'s, células destruidoras naturais; células exterminadoras naturais; células NK; grandes linfócitos granulares que não expressam marcadores de linhagem de células T ou B. Essas células possuem receptores Fc para IgG e podem destruir células-alvo utilizando citotoxicidade celular anticorpo-dependente. As células NK também podem usar perforina para destruir células na ausência de anticorpos. A destruição ocorre sem sensibilização prévia. SIN NK c.'s.
nerve c., c. nervosa. SIN neuron.
neurilemma c.'s, células do neurilema. SIN Schwann c.'s.
neuroendocrine c., c. neuroendócrina; (1) VER neuroendocrine (2); (2) SIN paraneurone.
neuroendocrine transducer c., c. transdutora neuroendócrina; uma c. endócrina que só libera seu produto hormonal para a corrente sanguínea ao receber um impulso nervoso.
neuroepithelial c.'s, células neuroepiteliais. SIN neuroepithelium.
neuroglia c.'s, células da neuróglia. VER neuroglia.
neurolemma c.'s, células do neurolema. SIN Schwann c.'s.
neurosecretory c.'s, células neurossecretoras; células nervosas, como as do hipotálamo, que produzem uma substância química (como um fator de liberação ou, mais raramente, um hormônio verdadeiro) que influencia a atividade de outra estrutura (p. ex., lobo anterior da hipófise). Ver também neurosecretion.
nevus c., nevócito; a c. de um nevo cutâneo pigmentado, que difere de um melanócito normal porque não possui dendritos. SIN nevocyte.
nevus c., A-type, nevócito tipo A; melanócitos na epiderme em nevos pigmentados, semelhantes às células epiteliais e freqüentemente contendo melanina.
nevus c., B-type, nevócito tipo B; melanócitos pequenos, geralmente não-pigmentados, na porção média da derme em nevos pigmentados.
nevus c., C-type, nevócito tipo C; melanócitos fusiformes não-pigmentados, na parte inferior da derme, em nevos pigmentados.
Niemann-Pick c., c. de Niemann-Pick. SIN Pick c.
NK c.'s, células destruidoras naturais, células NK. SIN natural killer c.'s.
nonclonogenic c., c. não-clonogênica; c. que não origina uma colônia de células (numerosas células geneticamente idênticas); pode sofrer duas ou mais divisões, mas todas as células-filhas são destinadas a morrer ou a diferenciar-se (perdendo todo o potencial para se dividir).
null c.'s, (1) células destruidoras naturais. SIN killer c.'s; (2) células nulas, grandes linfócitos granulares que não possuem marcadores de superfície ou proteínas associadas à membrana de linfócitos B ou T.
nurse c.'s, células nutrientes. SIN Sertoli c.'s.
oat c., pequena c.; c. em grão de aveia. SIN small c.
OKT c.'s, células OKT; termo antigo para células reconhecidas por anticorpos monoclonais contra antígenos do linfócito T; as células OKT-3 são linfócitos T como classe, porque compartilham um antígeno de diferenciação leucocitária comum; as células OKT-4 são células T auxiliares; as células OKT-8 são células T supressoras. OKT-4/OKT-8 expressa a razão entre células T auxiliares e supressoras, algumas vezes usada como medida do estado funcional do sistema imune e, portanto, base para o diagnóstico clínico e prognóstico. Atualmente é preferido o uso de designações CD. [célula *Ortho-Kung-T*]
olfactory c.'s, células olfatórias. SIN olfactory receptor c.'s.
olfactory receptor c.'s, células receptoras olfatórias; células nervosas muito finas, com grandes núcleos e encimadas por seis a oito longos cílios sensíveis no epitélio olfatório do teto do nariz; são receptores para o olfato. SIN olfactory c.'s, Schultze c.'s.
oligodendroglia c.'s, células da oligodendróglia. VER oligodendroglia.
Onodi c., c. de Onodi; uma variante de uma célula aérea etmoidal posterior em íntima relação com o nervo óptico imediatamente distal ao quiasma óptico.
Opalski c., c. de Opalski; uma c. glial caracteristicamente alterada nos gânglios da base e tálamo na degeneração hepatocerebral e na doença de Wilson.
osseous c., c. óssea. SIN osteocyte.
osteochondrogenic c., c. osteocondrogênica; uma das células indiferenciadas na camada interna do periósteo de um osso em desenvolvimento endocondral capaz de se transformar em um osteoblasto ou condroblasto.

osteogenic c., c. osteogênica; uma das células na camada interna do periósteo que forma tecido ósseo.
osteoprogenitor c., c. osteoprogenitora; c. mesenquimal que se diferencia em um osteoblasto. SIN preosteoblast.
oxyntic c., c. oxíntica. SIN parietal c.
oxyphil c., c. oxifílica; c. da glândula paratireóide cujo número aumenta com a idade; o citoplasma contém muitas mitocôndrias e cora-se pela eosina. Células semelhantes e tumores dessas células são encontrados nas glândulas salivares e na tireóide; nesta última, também é denominada célula de Hürthle.
P c., c. P; c. especializada característica com provável função marcapasso, encontrada no nodo S-A e na junção A-V.
packed human blood c.'s, concentrado de hemácias humanas, "papa" de hemácias; sangue total do qual foi retirado o plasma; pode ser preparado a qualquer momento durante o período de validade do sangue total do qual é obtido, mas não mais de 6 dias após a colheita do sangue se a separação do plasma e das células for realizada por centrifugação.
Paget c.'s, células de Paget; células epiteliais neoplásicas, relativamente grandes (células de carcinoma) com núcleos hipercromáticos e citoplasma abundante de coloração pálida; na doença de Paget da mama, essas células ocorrem no epitélio neoplásico nos ductos e na epiderme do mamilo, aréola e pele adjacente.
pagetoid c.'s, células pagetóides; melanócitos atípicos semelhantes às células de Paget, q.v., encontradas em alguns melanomas cutâneos do tipo disseminação superficial.
Paneth granular c.'s, células granulares de Paneth; células localizadas na base das glândulas intestinais do intestino delgado; contêm grandes grânulos refringentes acidófilos e podem produzir lisozima. SIN Davidoff c.'s.
parafollicular c.'s, células parafoliculares. SIN C c. (2).
paraganglionic c.'s, células paraganglionares; células do sistema nervoso simpático embrionário que se tornam células cromafins.
paraluteal c., c. paralútea. SIN theca lutein c.
paralutein c., c. paraluteínica. SIN theca lutein c.
parenchymal c., c. parenquimatosa. VER parenchyma.
parenchymatous c. of corpus pineale, c. parenquimatosa do corpo pineal, pinealócito. SIN pinealocyte.
parent c., c.-mãe. SIN mother c.
parietal c., c. parietal; uma das células das glândulas gástricas; situa-se sobre a membrana basal, coberta pelas células principais, e secreta ácido clorídrico, que chega à luz da glândula através de canais intracelulares e intercelulares finos (canalículos). SIN acid c., oxyntic c.
peptic c., c. péptica. SIN zymogenic c.
pericapillary c., c. pericapilar. SIN pericyte.
peripolar c., c. peripolar; c. granular localizada onde as cápsulas parietal e visceral do corpúsculo renal se encontram; parte da célula fica voltada para o espaço de filtração de Bowman.
perithelial c., c. peritelial. SIN pericyte.
peritubular contractile c.'s, células contráteis peritubulares. SIN myoid c.'s.
permissive c., c. permissiva; c. na qual a fase tardia da infecção viral sucede a fase inicial e a morte celular está associada à síntese maciça de vírus; p. ex., as células de macaco são permissivas para SV40.
pessary c., c. em pessário; hemácia na qual a hemoglobina desapareceu do centro, deixando apenas a periferia visível.
phalangeal c., c. falângica; as células de sustentação do órgão de Corti, fixadas à membrana basal e que recebem as células pilosas entre suas extremidades livres. VER TAMBÉM phalanx (2). SIN Deiters c.'s (1).
photo c., dispositivo eletrônico detector de luz usado para medir a transmissão de raios X através de um paciente para interrupção automática da exposição ou para calcular uma imagem digital.
photoreceptor c.'s, células fotorreceptoras; bastonetes e cones da retina.
physaliphorous c., células fisalíforas; células que possuem um citoplasma bolhoso ou vacuolado, p. ex., como as caracteristicamente observadas no cordoma.
Pick c., c. de Pick; célula mononuclear, arredondada ou poligonal, relativamente grande, com citoplasma espumoso, de coloração indistinta ou pálida, que contém numerosas gotículas de um fosfatídio, esfingomielina; essas células são amplamente distribuídas no baço e em outros tecidos, principalmente aqueles ricos em componentes reticuloendoteliais, em pacientes com doença de Niemann-Pick. SIN Niemann-Pick c.
pigment c., c. pigmentada; c. contendo grânulos de pigmento.
pigment c.'s of iris, células pigmentadas da íris; células do estroma da íris; em olhos escuros (mas não nos azuis), elas contêm grânulos de pigmento.
pigment c.'s of retina, células pigmentadas da retina; células na camada externa da retina que contêm grânulos de pigmentos.
pigment c. of skin, melanócito. SIN melanocyte.
pillar c.'s, células pilares; células que formam as paredes externa e interna do túnel no órgão de Corti. SIN Corti pillars, Corti rods, pillar c.'s of Corti, tunnel c.'s.
pillar c.'s of Corti, células pilares de Corti. SIN pillar c.'s.

pineal c.'s, células pineais; células do corpo pineal ou pinealócito.
plasma c., plasmócito; c. ovóide com núcleo excêntrico; o citoplasma é fortemente basófilo devido ao RNA abundante em seu retículo endoplasmático; os plasmócitos são derivados dos linfócitos B e são ativos na formação e secreção de anticorpos. SIN plasmacyte.
pluripotent c.'s, células pluripotentes; células primordiais que ainda podem diferenciar-se em vários tipos especializados de elementos teciduais; p. ex., células mesenquimais.
polar c., corpúsculo polar. SIN polar body.
polychromatic c., c. policromática; eritrócito primitivo na medula óssea, com material basófilo bem como hemoglobina (acidófila) no citoplasma. SIN polychromatophil c.
polychromatophil c., c. policromatófila. SIN polychromatic c.
posterior c.'s, células etmoidais posteriores. SIN posterior ethmoidal c.'s.
posterior ethmoidal c.'s [TA], células etmoidais posteriores; o grupo posterior de células aéreas dos seios etmoidais; cada seio se comunica com o meato superior da cavidade nasal. SIN cellulae ethmoidales posteriores [TA], posterior c.'s, posterior ethmoidal air c.'s, sinus ethmoidales posteriores.
posterior ethmoidal air c.'s, células aéreas etmoidais posteriores. SIN posterior ethmoidal c.'s.
pregnancy c.'s, células da gravidez; células cromófobas hipofisárias cujo número aumenta e que acumulam grânulos eosinofílicos durante a gravidez.
pregranulosa c.'s, células da pré-granulosa; células capsulares que circundam os óvulos primordiais no ovário embrionário; são derivadas do epitélio celômico.
prickle c., c. espinhosa; uma das células da camada espinhosa da epiderme; assim denominada devido aos artefatos de retração típicos observados em preparos histológicos, resultando em pontes intercelulares nos pontos de adesão por desmossomas. SIN spine c.
primary embryonic c., c. embrionária primária; em um embrião muito jovem, uma célula ainda capaz de se diferenciar.
primitive reticular c., c. reticular primitiva. SIN reticular c.
primordial c., c. primordial; c. de um grupo que constitui o primórdio de um órgão ou parte do embrião.
primordial germ c., c. germinativa primordial; a célula sexual indiferenciada mais primitiva, encontrada inicialmente fora da gônada. SIN gonocyte.
prolactin c., c. de prolactina. SIN mammotroph.
pseudo-Gaucher c., pseudocélula de Gaucher; plasmócito microscopicamente semelhante à célula de Gaucher, encontrado na medula óssea em alguns casos de mieloma múltiplo.
pseudounipolar c., c. pseudo-unipolar. SIN unipolar neuron.
pseudoxanthoma c., c. pseudoxantomatosa; células fagocíticas relativamente grandes (macrófagos) que contêm numerosos pequenos vacúolos lipídicos ou hemossiderina (ou ambos), em lesões hemorrágicas ou inflamatórias em organização.
pulpar c., c. pulpar; a c. macrofágica específica da substância esplênica.
Purkinje c.'s, células de Purkinje. SIN Purkinje cell layer.
pus c., piócito. SIN pus corpuscle.
pyramidal c.'s, células piramidais; neurônios do córtex cerebral que, em cortes perpendiculares à superfície cortical, exibem um formato triangular com um dendrito apical longo voltado para a superfície do córtex; também há dendritos laterais e um axônio basal que desce até camadas mais profundas.
pyrrol c., pyrrhol c., c. pirrólica; c. do sistema de macrófagos mononucleares que tem uma afinidade especial pelo azul-de-pirrol, captando o corante por um processo de pinocitose.
Raji c., c. de Raji; c. de uma linhagem cultivada de células linfoblastóides derivadas de um linfoma de Burkitt; possui muitos receptores para determinados componentes do complemento e, portanto, é adequada para uso na detecção de imunocomplexos. Expressa determinados receptores do complemento, bem como receptores Fc para imunoglobulina G.
reactive c., c. reativa. SIN gemistocytic astrocyte.
red blood c. (rbc, RBC), hemácia; eritrócito. SIN erythrocyte.
Reed c., c. de Reed. SIN Reed-Sternberg c.
Reed-Sternberg c., c. de Reed-Sternberg; grandes linfócitos transformados, provavelmente com origem nas células B, geralmente considerada patognomônica do linfoma de Hodgkin; uma c. típica tem um citoplasma acidófilo de coloração pálida e um ou dois grandes núcleos exibindo aglomeração marginal de cromatina e nucléolos profundamente acidófilos incomumente evidentes; a c. de Reed-Sternberg binucleada freqüentemente exibe uma forma espelhada (c. em imagem espelhada). SIN Reed c., Sternberg c., Sternberg-Reed c.
Renshaw c.'s, células de Renshaw; interneurônios inibidores inervados por colaterais de motoneurônios e que, por sua vez, formam sinapses com o mesmo motoneurônio e com motoneurônios adjacentes para exercer inibição; identificadas fisiologicamente e por técnica de injeção intracelular.
resting c., c. quiescente; c. que não está sofrendo mitose.
resting wandering c., macrófago fixo. SIN fixed macrophage.
restructured c., c. reestruturada; c. viável produzida por fusão de um carioplasto com um citoplasto.

reticular c., c. reticular; c. com processos que fazem contato com aqueles de outras células semelhantes para formar uma rede celular que envolve uma rede de fibras reticulares, constituindo o estroma de todos os órgãos linfóides, exceto o timo. SIN primitive reticular c.
reticularis c., c. reticular; c. da zona reticular da parte mais interna do córtex supra-renal.
reticuloendothelial c., c. reticuloendotelial; c. do sistema reticuloendotelial.
rhagiocrine c., macrófago. SIN macrophage.
Rieder c.'s, células de Rieder; mieloblastos anormais (12 a 20 μm de diâmetro) nos quais o núcleo pode ser ampla e profundamente entalhado (isto é, sugestivo de lobulação), ou pode realmente ser uma estrutura bi- ou multinucleada; essas células são observadas freqüentemente na leucemia aguda e, provavelmente, representam maturação mais rápida do núcleo que do citoplasma.
rod nuclear c., c. nuclear em bastão. SIN band c.
rod c. of retina, c. em bastonete da retina. SIN rod (2).
Rolando c.'s, células de Rolando; as células nervosas na substância gelatinosa de Rolando da medula espinhal.
rosette-forming c.'s, células formadoras de rosetas; termo geralmente usado para linfócitos T com uma afinidade por eritrócitos de carneiros e que, quando suspensos no soro, ligam-se a eritrócitos não-revestidos, não-sensibilizados em uma formação em roseta.
sarcogenic c., c. sarcogênica. SIN myoblast.
satellite c.'s, células satélites; células da neuróglia que circundam o corpo de uma célula ganglionar nos gânglios espinhais, cranianos e autônomos.
satellite c. of skeletal muscle, c. satélite do músculo esquelético; c. fusiforme alongada que ocupa depressões no sarcolema e entre o sarcolema e a lâmina basal; acredita-se que participe no reparo e na regeneração muscular mediante fusão com a fibra muscular adjacente. SIN sarcoplast.
scavenger c., c. removedora de detritos celulares; fagócito. SIN phagocyte.
Schilling band c., c. bastão de Schilling. SIN band c.
Schultze c.'s, células de Schultze. SIN olfactory receptor c.'s.
Schwann c.'s, células de Schwann; células de origem ectodérmica (crista neural) que compõem um envoltório contínuo ao redor de cada fibra nervosa de nervos periféricos; essas células são comparáveis às células da oligodendróglia do cérebro e da medula espinhal; como estas últimas, podem formar expansões membranosas que se enrolam em torno dos axônios e, assim, formar a bainha de mielina do axônio. SIN neurilemma c.'s, neurolemma c.'s.
segmented c., c. segmentada; leucócito polimorfonuclear amadurecido além da forma bastão, de modo que são observados dois ou mais lobos do núcleo.
sensitized c., c. sensibilizada; (1) c. que foi exposta ao antígeno ou opsonizada com anticorpos e/ou complemento; (2) pequena c. "comprometida" derivada, por divisão e diferenciação, de um linfócito em repouso; (3) uma c. que inclui uma c. bacteriana, que se combinou a anticorpo específico para formar um complexo capaz de reagir com componentes do complemento.
sensory c., c. sensorial; c. no sistema nervoso periférico que recebe impulsos aferentes (sensoriais); células receptoras sensoriais.
septal c., c. septal; uma c. redonda pálida dos pulmões nos septos entre os alvéolos pulmonares.
seromucous c.'s, células seromucosas. SIN mucoserous c.'s.
serous c., c. serosa; c., principalmente da glândula salivar, que secreta um líquido aquoso ou albuminoso diluído, em oposição a uma célula mucosa. SIN albuminous c. (1).
Sertoli c.'s, células de Sertoli; células alongadas, nos túbulos seminíferos, que envolvem as espermátides, proporcionando um microambiente que sustenta a espermiogênese; elas secretam proteína de ligação de androgênio e estabelecem a barreira hemato-testicular pela formação de zônulas de oclusão com as células de Sertoli adjacentes. SIN nurse c.'s.
sex c., c. sexual; um espermatozóide ou um óvulo. SIN germ c.
Sézary c., c. de Sézary; linfócito T atípico observado no sangue periférico na síndrome de Sézary; possui um grande núcleo convoluto e citoplasma escasso contendo vacúolos PAS-positivos.
shadow c.'s, células-fantasmas. SIN smudge c.'s.
sickle c., c. falciforme; drepanócito; eritrócito anormal, em forma de crescente, característico da anemia falciforme, resultante de uma anormalidade hereditária da hemoglobina (hemoglobina S) que causa diminuição da solubilidade com baixa tensão de oxigênio. SIN crescent c., drepanocyte, meniscocyte.
signet ring c.'s, células em anel de sinete. SIN castration c.
silver c., c. prateada; uma das muitas células observadas nas placas de esclerose múltipla, que possuem núcleos redondos ou ovais; o corpo da célula contém muitas partículas amarelas ou castanho-claras; as células são características da esclerose múltipla, mas são encontradas em outros distúrbios, incluindo sífilis.
skein c., reticulócito. SIN reticulocyte.
small c., pequena c.; c. grosseiramente fusiforme, curta, que contém um núcleo hipercromático, relativamente grande, freqüentemente observado em algumas formas de carcinoma broncogênico indiferenciado. SIN oat c.
small cleaved c., pequena c. clivada; c. linfóide, com origem na célula do centro folicular, que possui um núcleo de formato irregular com grumos de cromatina, ausência de nucléolos e uma ou mais fendas na membrana nuclear.

smudge c.'s, células-fantasma; leucócitos imaturos de qualquer tipo que sofreram ruptura parcial durante preparo de um esfregaço ou corte tecidual corado, devido à sua maior fragilidade; as células-fantasma são observadas em maior número na leucemia linfocítica crônica. SIN basket c. (2), Gumprecht shadows, shadow c.'s.
somatic c.'s, células somáticas; as células de um organismo, além das células germinativas.
sperm c., espermatozóide. SIN spermatozoon.
spider c., c. aracniforme; (1) SIN astrocyte; (2) uma célula em um rabdomioma do coração, com núcleo central e massa citoplasmática unida à parede celular por filamentos de citoplasma separados por áreas claras cheias de glicogênio.
spindle c., c. fusiforme; uma c. fusiforme, como aquelas das camadas mais profundas do córtex cerebral.
spine c., c. espinhosa. SIN prickle c.
splenic c.'s, células esplênicas; grandes células amebóides redondas (macrófagos) na polpa esplênica.
spur c., acantócito, hemácia espiculada com 5–10 projeções espinhosas de comprimentos variáveis, distribuídas irregularmente sobre a superfície celular; observada em pacientes com hepatopatia e abetalipoproteinemia.
squamous c., c. escamosa; c. epitelial plana, semelhante a uma escama.
squamous alveolar c.'s, células alveolares escamosas; células escamosas muito finas formadoras do epitélio gás-permeável que reveste os alvéolos pulmonares. SIN type I c.'s.
stab c., c. bastão. SIN band c.
staff c., c. bastão. SIN band c.
standard c., c. padrão, pilha padrão; uma c. elétrica que possui voltagem conhecida definida; usada para calibrar outras células elétricas.
stellate c.'s of cerebral cortex, células estreladas do córtex cerebral; pequenas células estreladas, na segunda e quarta camadas do córtex, e grandes células estreladas na parte mais profunda da terceira camada do córtex visual.
stellate c.'s of liver, células estreladas do fígado. SIN Kupffer c.'s.
stem c., c.-tronco; c. primordial; (1) qualquer célula precursora; (2) uma célula cujas células-filhas podem diferenciar-se em outros tipos celulares.
Sternberg c., c. de Sternberg. SIN Reed-Sternberg c.
Sternberg-Reed c., c. de Sternberg-Reed. SIN Reed-Sternberg c.
stichochrome c., VER stichochrome.
strap c., c. em fita; uma célula tumoral alongada, com largura uniforme, que pode mostrar estriações cruzadas; encontrada no rabdomiossarcoma.
supporting c., c. de sustentação. SIN sustentacular c.
suppressor c.'s, células supressoras; células do sistema imune que inibem ou ajudam a interromper uma resposta imune, p. ex., macrófagos supressores e células T supressoras.
surface mucous c.'s of stomach, células mucosas superficiais do estômago; células que revestem a superfície e as fovéolas gástricas; um produto mucoso ácido-resistente na extremidade apical de cada célula que, aparentemente, se difunde para fora para lubrificar e proteger a superfície mucosa. SIN theca c.'s of stomach.
sustentacular c., c. sustentacular; c. de sustentação; uma das células alongadas comuns, apoiadas sobre a membrana basal, que circundam as células especializadas mais curtas, servindo-lhes de suporte, em determinados órgãos, como o labirinto do ouvido interno ou o epitélio olfatório. SIN supporting c.
sympathetic formative c., c. formadora simpática; neuroblasto do sistema nervoso autônomo embrionário.
sympathicotropic c.'s, células simpaticotrópicas; grandes células epitelióides no hilo ovariano associadas a fibras nervosas não-mielinizadas.
sympathochromaffin c., c. simpatocromafin; o tipo celular na supra-renal embrionária da qual se originam as células ganglionares simpáticas e as células cromafins.
synovial c., c. sinoviais; células semelhantes a fibrotoplastos que formam 1–6 camadas epitelióides na membrana sinovial das articulações; acredita-se que forneçam proteoglicanas e ácido hialurônico para o líquido sinovial.
T c., c. T. SIN T lymphocyte.
Tγ c.'s, células Tγ; subgrupo de células T que possuem um receptor Fc para moléculas de imunoglobulina G.
Tμ c.'s, células Tμ; células T auxiliares que possuem um receptor Fc para moléculas de imunoglobulina M.
tactile c., c. táctil; uma das células epitelióides de um corpúsculo táctil. SIN touch c.
tanned red c.'s, eritrócitos submetidos a tratamento leve com substâncias químicas, como o ácido tânico, de forma que eles adsorvem aos seus antígenos solúveis de superfície; usados em testes de hemaglutinação.
target c., c. em alvo; (1) um eritrócito com um centro escuro circundado por uma faixa clara, que novamente é circundada por um anel mais escuro; assim, assemelha-se a um alvo de tiro; essas células são observadas em anemias de células em alvo ou após esplenectomia. SIN Mexican hat c.; (2) uma c. lisada por linfócitos T citotóxicos, como na rejeição do enxerto.
tart c., monócito com um núcleo engolfado no qual a estrutura ainda é bem preservada.

taste c.'s, células do paladar; células gustativas; células de coloração escura, em uma papila gustativa, que parecem possuir, estendendo-se até o poro gustativo, longas microvilosidades pilosas contendo vários microtúbulos muito próximos; as células gustativas fazem contato sináptico com as fibras nervosas sensoriais dos nervos facial, glossofaríngeo ou vago. SIN gustatory c.'s.
T cytotoxic c.'s (Tc), células T citotóxicas. SIN cytotoxic c. (1).
TDTH c.'s, um subgrupo funcional de células T auxiliares envolvidas nas reações de hipersensibilidade tardia.
tendon c.'s, células do tendão; células fibroblásticas alongadas dispostas em fileiras entre as fibras colágenas do tendão.
theca lutein c., c. luteínica da teca; c. secretora de esteróides do corpo lúteo que provém da teca interna do folículo ovariano no momento da ovulação e secreta progesterona sob o controle da prolactina. SIN paraluteal c., paralutein c.
theca c.'s of stomach, células tecais do estômago. SIN surface mucous c.'s of stomach.
T helper c.'s (Th), células T auxiliares; subgrupo de linfócitos que secretam várias citocinas reguladoras da resposta imune: *subgrupo 1*, que sintetizam gama interferon e interleucina 2 e estão envolvidas na imunidade celular; *subgrupo 2*, que sintetizam interleucinas 4, 5, 10, e estão envolvidas na síntese de imunoglobulina. SIN helper c.'s.
T helper subset 1 c.'s, células T auxiliares do subgrupo 1; um subgrupo de células T CD4+ que podem secretar interferon gama e IL-2 e são responsáveis pela imunidade celular.
T helper subset 2 c.'s, células T auxiliares do subgrupo 2; um subgrupo de células T CD4+ que sintetizam IL-4, IL-5 e IL-10 e facilitam a síntese de imunoglobulina.
Tiselius electrophoresis c., c. eletroforética de Tiselius; o recipiente especial em um aparelho de Tiselius que contém a solução a ser analisada eletroforeticamente.

subgrupos de células T *helper* (auxiliares)

subtipo TH	citocinas secretadas	principais efeitos imunológicos[1]
T_H1	IFNγ	ativam macrófagos
		promovem proliferação de células B e mudança de classe para IgG1
	IL-2	promoção, ativação de células T_H e T_C antígeno-específicas
	FNTβ	ativam macrófagos e neutrófilos
		promovem crescimento das células B e produção de imunoglobulina
T_H2	IL-4	quimioatração de linfócitos, mastócitos e basófilos
		promovem o crescimento de mastócitos e eosinófilos
		promovem proliferação de células B e mudança de classe para IgE e IgG4
		inibem a diferenciação de células T_H1
		inibem a produção de citocinas por macrófagos
	IL-5	promovem o crescimento e o desenvolvimento de eosinófilos
	IL-6	promovem o crescimento de células B e a produção de imunoglobulinas
	IL-10	inibem a produção de citocinas (incluindo IFNγ) pelas células T_H1, macrófagos e outras CAA
		inibem a diferenciação de células T_H1
		promovem o crescimento de células B e a produção de imunoglobulinas
	IL-13	iguais aos da IL-4

Abreviaturas: IFNγ = interferon gama; IL = interleucina; FNTβ = fator de necrose tumoral beta; CAA = célula de apresentação de antígeno.

[1] Apenas alguns efeitos pertinentes dessas citocinas são apresentados aqui. Todos os processos descritos são promovidos pela citocina, exceto afirmação em contrário.

Toker c., c. de Toker; c. epitelial com citoplasma claro encontrada em 10% dos mamilos normais; contém queratina 7, como as células do carcinoma de Paget, das quais tem de ser diferenciada citologicamente.
totipotent c., c. totipotente; c. pluripotente; c. indiferenciada capaz de se transformar em qualquer tipo de c. corporal.
touch c., c. táctil. SIN tactile c.
Touton giant c., c. gigante de Touton; c. xantomatosa em que os múltiplos núcleos se agrupam ao redor de uma ilhota de citoplasma não-espumoso.
transducer c., c. transdutora; qualquer c. que responda a um estímulo mecânico, térmico, fótico ou químico pela geração de um impulso elétrico sinapticamente transmitido a um neurônio sensorial em contato com a célula.
transitional c., c. de transição; qualquer célula considerada representante de uma fase do desenvolvimento de uma forma para outra.
tubal air c.'s (of pharyngotympanic tube) [TA], células aéreas da tuba auditiva; pequenas células aéreas ocasionais na parede inferior da tuba faringotimpânica, próximas do orifício timpânico, que se comunicam com a cavidade timpânica. SIN cellulae pneumaticae tubae auditivae [TA], air c.'s of auditory tube.
tufted c., c. em tufo; um tipo específico de célula do bulbo olfatório comparável à célula mitral do bulbo no que diz respeito às relações aferentes e eferentes, porém menor e de localização mais superficial.
tunnel c.'s, células do túnel. SIN pillar c.'s.
Türk c., c. de Türk; c. imatura, relativamente grande com determinadas características histológicas semelhantes às de um plasmócito, embora o padrão nuclear seja semelhante ao de um mieloblasto; encontrada no sangue circulante somente em condições patológicas. SIN irritation c., Türk leukocyte.
tympanic c.'s, [TA], células timpânicas; numerosas depressões em forma de sulcos, nas paredes da cavidade timpânica, comunicando-se com as células aéreas tubárias. SIN cellulae tympanicae [TA], tympanic air c.'s.
tympanic air c.'s, células aéreas timpânicas. SIN tympanic c.'s.
type I c.'s, células tipo I. SIN squamous alveolar c.'s.
type II c.'s, células tipo II. SIN great alveolar c.'s.
Tzanck c.'s, células de Tzanck; células epiteliais acantolíticas observadas no teste de Tzanck.
undifferentiated c., c. indiferenciada; c. primitiva que não assumiu as características morfológicas e funcionais que adquirirá mais tarde.
unipolar c., c. unipolar. SIN unipolar neuron.
vasoformative c., c. formadora de vaso. SIN angioblast (1).
veil c., c. velada; c. de véu; c. apresentadora de antígeno que possui processos citoplasmáticos semelhantes a um véu e circula no sangue e na linfa. SIN veiled c.'s (1).
veiled c.'s, células veladas; células de véu; **(1)** SIN veil c.; **(2)** VER Langerhan's c.'s.
vestibular hair c.'s, células pilosas vestibulares; células no epitélio sensorial da mácula e crista do labirinto membranoso do ouvido interno; fibras nervosas aferentes e eferentes do nervo vestibular terminam em sinapses com elas; a partir da extremidade apical de cada célula, estende-se um feixe de estereocílios e um cinocílio para dentro da membrana estacônica da mácula e para a cúpula das cristas.
Virchow c.'s, células de Virchow; **(1)** as lacunas no tecido ósseo que contêm os osteócitos; **(2)** termo obsoleto para designar os próprios osteócitos; **(3)** SIN corneal corpuscles, em corpuscle.
virus-transformed c., c. transformada por vírus; c. que foi geneticamente modificada em uma célula tumoral, sendo a modificação subseqüentemente transmitida para todas as células descendentes; células transformadas por vírus de RNA oncogênicos continuam a produzir vírus em alta concentração sem serem destruídas; células transformadas por vírus tumorais de DNA desenvolvem (juntamente com outras alterações) antígenos associados ao tumor e raramente produzem vírus.
visual receptor c.'s, células receptoras visuais; os bastonetes e cones da retina.
vitreous c., c. vítrea; c. observada na parte periférica do corpo vítreo que pode ser responsável pela produção de ácido hialurônico e, possivelmente, de colágeno. SIN hyalocyte.
wandering c., c. migratória. SIN ameboid c.
Warthin-Finkeldey c.'s, células de Warthin-Finkeldey; células gigantes com múltiplos núcleos superpostos, encontradas no tecido linfóide no sarampo, principalmente durante o estágio prodrômico.
wasserhelle c., c. clara da paratireóide. SIN water-clear c. of parathyroid.
water-clear c. of parathyroid, c. clara da paratireóide; tipo de célula principal, assim denominada porque o citoplasma contém muito glicogênio que não é preservado ou corado na preparação habitual. SIN wasserhelle c.
white blood c. (WBC), leucócito. SIN leukocyte.
WI-38 c.'s, células WI-38; as primeiras células humanas normais, derivadas do tecido pulmonar fetal, cultivadas continuamente. [*Wistar Institute*]
wing c., c. alada; uma das células poliédricas no epitélio da córnea sob a camada superficial.
yolk c.'s, células vitelinas; células embrionárias primitivas situadas entre o endoderma e o mesoderma; provavelmente dão origem ao endotélio dos vasos vitelinos.

zymogenic c., c. zimogênica; c. que secreta uma enzima; especificamente uma célula principal de uma glândula gástrica ou uma célula acinar do pâncreas. SIN albuminous c. (2), chief c. of stomach, peptic c.

cel·la, gen. e pl. **cel·lae** (sel′a, sel′e). Compartimento ou célula. [L. despensa ou compartimento]
  c. me′dia, célula média. SIN *pars* centralis ventriculi lateralis.
cel·lic·o·lous (se - lik′o - lŭs). Celícola; que vive dentro das células. [L. *cella*, células, + *colo*, morar em]
cel·lo·bi·ase (sel - o - bi′ās). Celobiase. SIN β-D-glucosidase.
cel·lo·bi·ose (sel - o - bi′ōs). Celobiose; dissacarídeo obtido da celulose e liquenina; uma glicose-β(1→4)-glicosídeo, diferindo da maltose apenas pela natureza da ligação glicosídica.
cel·lo·hex·ose (sel - o - heks′ōs). Celoexose. SIN D-glucose.
cel·loi·din (se - loy′din). Celoidina; solução de piroxilina em éter e álcool, usada para inclusão de amostras histológicas.
cel·lon (sel′on). Tetracloroetano. SIN tetrachloroethane.
cel·lo·na (sel - o′na). Atadura de celulose impregnada com gesso.
cel·lu·la, gen. e pl. **cel·lu·lae** (sel′u - la, - le). Célula. **1.** [NA]. Em anatomia macroscópica, um compartimento pequeno, mas macroscópico. SIN cellule. **2.** Em histologia, uma célula. [L. câmara pequena, dim. de *cella*]
  cel′lulae co′li, haustros do cólon. SIN *haustra* of colon, em *haustrum*.
  cel′lulae ethmoida′les [TA], células etmoidais. SIN ethmoid *cells,* em *cell.* VER TAMBÉM anterior ethmoidal *cells,* em *cell,* middle ethmoidal *cells,* em *cell,* posterior ethmoidal *cells,* em *cell.*
  cel′lulae ethmoidales anterio′res [TA], células etmoidais anteriores. SIN anterior ethmoidal *cells,* em *cell.*
  cel′lulae ethmoidales me′diae [TA], células etmoidais médias. SIN middle ethmoidal *cells,* em *cell.*
  cel′lulae ethmoidales posterio′res [TA], células etmoidais posteriores. SIN posterior ethmoidal *cells,* em *cell.*
  cel′lulae mastoid′eae [TA], células mastóideas. SIN mastoid *cells,* em *cell.*
  cel′lulae pneumat′icae tu′bae auditi′vae [TA], células pneumáticas da tuba auditiva. SIN tubal air *cells (of pharyngotympanic tube),* em *cell.*
  cel′lulae tympan′icae [TA], células timpânicas. SIN tympanic *cells,* em *cell.*
cel·lu·lar (sel′u - lar). Celular. **1.** Relativo a, derivado de, ou composto de células. **2.** Que possui numerosos compartimentos ou interstícios. [L. *cellula*, dim. de *cella*, despensa]
cel·lu·lar·i·ty (sel - u - lar′i - te). Celularidade; o grau, a qualidade ou a condição das células existentes.
cel·lu·lase (sel′u - lās). Celulase; endo-1,4-β-glicase; uma enzima que catalisa a hidrólise das ligações 1,4-β-glicosídio na celulose, liquenina e outros β-D-glucanos; encontrada em vários microrganismos no solo e nos tratos digestivos de herbívoros. Usada para produzir comprimidos digestivos e na remoção da celulose de alimentos para dietas especiais.
cel·lule (sel′ul). Célula. SIN cellula (1).
cel·lu·li·ci·dal (sel′u - li - si′dal). Celulicida; destrutivo para as células. [cellula + L. *caedo*, matar]
cel·lu·lif·u·gal (sel - u - lif′u - gal). Celulífugo; que se afasta de, ou que se estende em uma direção oposta a, uma célula ou corpo celular; designa determinadas células repelidas por outras células, ou processos que se estendem do corpo de uma célula. [cellula + L. *fugio*, fugir]
cel·lu·lin (sel′u - lin). Celulina. SIN cellulose.
cel·lu·lip·e·tal (sel - u - lip′e - tal). Celulípeto; que se move ou se estende em direção a uma célula ou corpo celular. [cellula + L. *peto*, buscar]
cel·lu·lite (sel′u - līt). Celulite. **1.** Termo coloquial para depósitos de gordura e tecido fibroso que causam ondulação da pele sobrejacente. **2.** SIN lipoedema.
cel·lu·li·tis (sel′u - li′tis). Celulite; inflamação do tecido conjuntivo frouxo subcutâneo (anteriormente denominado tecido celular).
  acute scalp c., c. aguda do couro cabeludo; inflamação profunda do couro cabeludo sem supuração.
  anaerobic c., c. anaeróbica; infecção dos tecidos moles subcutâneos por qualquer dentre várias bactérias anaeróbicas, geralmente uma cultura mista incluindo espécies de *Bacteroides,* cocos anaeróbicos e clostrídios.
  dissecting c., c. dissecante. SIN *perifolliculitis* abscedens et suffodiens.
  eosinophilic c., c. eosinofílica; celulite recorrente seguida por lesões cutâneas edematosas ou, algumas vezes, lesões urticariais papulares, anulares ou espirais; a pele e o tecido subcutâneo afetados são maciçamente infiltrados por eosinófilos e histiócitos, com pequenos focos necróticos dispersos (figuras de chama); de etiologia variada; algumas vezes sucede uma picada por artrópode. SIN Wells syndrome.
  gangrenous c., c. gangrenosa; infecção dos tecidos moles por microrganismos que provocam extensa necrose tecidual e oclusões vasculares locais; estreptococos, clostrídios e anaeróbios são causas conhecidas, porém a maioria dos casos recentes é polimicrobiana. SIN necrotizing c.
  necrotizing c., c. necrotizante. SIN gangrenous c.
  orbital c., c. orbitária; c. que envolve os tecidos posteriores ao septo orbitário.
  pelvic c., c. pélvica. SIN parametritis.
  periorbital c., c. periorbitária. SIN preseptal c.
  preseptal c., c. pré-septal; infecção envolvendo as camadas teciduais superficiais anteriores ao septo orbitário. SIN periorbital c.
cel·lu·los·an (sel′u - lo - san). Hemicelulose. SIN hemicellulose.
cel·lu·lose (sel′u - lōs). Celulose; um glucano linear B1→4, composto de resíduos celobiose, diferindo nesse aspecto do amido, que é constituído de resíduos maltose; forma a base das fibras vegetais e de madeira e é o composto orgânico mais abundante; útil para fornecer volume para a dieta. SIN cellulin. [L. *cellula*, célula, + -ose]
  c. acetate, acetato de c.; polímero comumente usado como meio de suporte para eletroforese.
  c. acetate phthalate, acetato ftalato de c.; um produto da reação do anidrido ftálico e um éster acetato parcial de c.; usado como agente de revestimento para comprimidos.
  carboxymethyl c., carboximetil c.; c. na qual alguns dos grupamentos OH são modificados para conter grupamentos $-CH_2-COOH$; usada na cromatografia em coluna. SIN CM-cellulose.
  *O***-diethylaminoethyl c.,** *O*-dietilaminoetil c.; c. à qual foram fixados grupamentos dietilaminoetil; usada na cromatografia por troca aniônica. SIN DEAE-cellulose.
  microcrystalline c., c. microcristalina; c. purificada, parcialmente despolimerizada, preparada por tratamento da α-celulose, obtida como uma polpa de material vegetal fibroso, com ácidos minerais; usada como diluente de comprimidos.
  oxidized c., c. oxidada; **(1)** ácido celulósico sob a forma de uma gaze absorvível; usado como hemostático em cirurgias onde não é possível realizar ligaduras (hemorragia capilar ou venosa de pequenos vasos) porque o ácido celulósico tem uma grande afinidade pela hemoglobina e produz um coágulo artificial; **(2)** uma substância absorvível estéril preparada pela oxidação de algodão contendo não menos de 16% e não mais de 22% de carboxil. VER TAMBÉM oxycellulose.
  TEAE-c., c. à qual foram fixados grupamentos trietilaminoetil; usada em cromatografia por troca iônica. SIN *O*-(triethylaminoethyl) c.
  *O***-(triethylaminoethyl) c.,** *O*-trietilaminoetil c. SIN TEAE-c.
cel·lu·los·ic ac·id (sel - u - los′ik). Ácido celulósico. VER oxidized *cellulose.*
celo-. 1. O celoma. [G. *koilōma,* oco (celoma)] **2.** Hérnia. [G. *kēlē,* hérnia]. **3.** O abdome. VER TAMBÉM celio-. [G. *koilia,* abdome]
ce·lom, ce·lo·ma (se′lom, se - lo′ma). Celoma. **1.** A cavidade entre o mesoderma esplâncnico e somático no embrião. **2.** SIN body *cavity.* [G. *koilōma,* oco]
  extraembryonic c., c. extra-embrionário; parte do celoma que se estende além dos limites do corpo embrionário.
ce·lom·ic (se - lom′ik). Celômico; relativo à cavidade corporal (body *cavity*).
ce·lo·phle·bi·tis (se - lo - fle - bi′tis). Celoflebite; inflamação de uma veia cava. SIN cavitis. [G. *koilos,* oco, + phlebitis]
ce·lo·scope (se′lo - skōp). Celoscópio; termo raramente usado para um dispositivo óptico para examinar uma cavidade do corpo. [G. *koilos,* oco, + *skopeō,* ver]
ce·los·co·py (se - los′ko - pe). Celoscopia; termo raramente usado para exame de qualquer cavidade do corpo com um instrumento óptico.
ce·lo·so·mia (se - lo - so′me - a). Celossomia; protrusão congênita das vísceras abdominais ou torácicas, geralmente com um defeito do esterno e das costelas, bem como das paredes abdominais. SIN kelosomia. [G. *kēlē,* hérnia, + *sōma,* corpo]
Ce·lo·vi·rus (sel′o - vi - rŭs). Adenovírus encontrado em galinhas.
ce·lo·zo·ic (se - lo - zo′ik). Celozóico; que habita qualquer uma das cavidades do corpo; aplicado a determinados protozoários parasitas, principalmente gregarinas. [G. *koilos,* oco, + *zoikos,* relativo a animais]
Celsius, Anders, astrônomo sueco, 1701–1744. VER Celsius *scale.*
Cel·si·us (C). Celsius. VER Celsius *scale.*
ce·ment (se - ment′) [TA]. Cemento. **1.** Camada de tecido mineralizado semelhante a osso que cobre a dentina da raiz e o colo de um dente, servindo para ancorar as fibras do ligamento periodontal. SIN cementum [TA], substantia ossea dentis, tooth **c. 2.** Cimento; em odontologia, material não-metálico usado para fins de vedação, enchimento ou restauração permanente ou temporária, feito pela mistura de componentes a uma massa plástica que se solidifica, ou como um selador aderente na fixação de várias restaurações dentárias dentro do dente ou sobre ele. [ver cementum]
  composite dental c., cimento dentário composto; um cimento dentário orgânico modificado pela inclusão de materiais inorgânicos tratados com um agente de acoplamento para ligá-los aos polímeros.
  copper phosphate c., cimento de fosfato de cobre; preparação dentária, a combinação de uma solução de ácido ortofosfórico com um cimento em pó (geralmente óxido de zinco) modificado com várias proporções de óxido de cobre.
  dental c., cimento dentário. VER cement (2).
  glass ionomer c., cimento de ionômero de vidro; cimento dentário produzido misturando um pó preparado a partir de um vidro de aluminossilicato de cálcio com uma solução aquosa de um ácido poliacrílico. [ion + -mer (1)]

inorganic dental c., cimento dentário inorgânico; cimento dentário que geralmente consiste em sais ou óxidos metálicos, os quais, quando misturados a um líquido específico, formam uma massa plástica que se solidifica.

intercellular c., cimento intercelular; substância adesiva hipotética outrora supostamente existente entre algumas células epiteliais.

modified zinc oxide-eugenol c., cimento de óxido de zinco e eugenol modificado; cimento dentário obtido pela mistura de óxido de zinco e eugenol com um ou mais aditivos.

organic dental c., cimento dentário orgânico; cimento dentário que consiste principalmente em polímeros sintéticos.

polycarboxylate c., cimento policarboxilado; pó contendo basicamente óxido de zinco misturado a um líquido contendo ácido poliacrílico que reage para formar uma massa cristalina dura após a colocação; quando usado para fixar aparelhos de metal aos dentes, tem o potencial de se ligar ao cálcio contido na estrutura do dente e, também, a qualquer metal contido no engate.

resin c., cimento de resina; um monômero ou um sistema monômero/polímero usado como agente de vedação dentária; usado na cimentação de restaurações ou braquetes ortodônticos aos dentes.

silicate c., cimento de silicato; material de enchimento dentário preparado misturando-se uma solução de ácido fosfórico modificada a um pó de vidro de flúor silicato de alumínio.

tooth c., cemento do dente. SIN cement (1). VER cement (2).

unmodified zinc oxide-eugenol c., cimento de óxido de zinco e eugenol não-modificado; cimento dentário obtido pela mistura de óxido de zinco e eugenol sem modificadores.

zinc phosphate c., cimento de fosfato de zinco; um pó, contendo basicamente óxido de zinco misturado a um líquido contendo ácido ortofosfórico para formar uma massa cristalina dura quando colocada, usado em odontologia como agente de vedação para restaurações metálicas e bandas ortodônticas, e como material de restauração temporário, ou uma base sob restaurações, particularmente em cavidades (cáries) profundas.

ce·men·ta·tion (sē - men - tā′shŭn). Cimentação. **1.** O processo de fixar partes por meio de um cimento. **2.** Em odontologia, a fixação de uma restauração aos dentes naturais por meio de um cimento.

ce·ment·i·cle (se - men′ti - kl). Cimentículo; um corpo esférico calcificado, composto de cimento situado livre na membrana periodontal, fixado ao cimento ou incrustado nele.

ce·ment·i·fi·ca·tion (se - men′ti - fi - kā′shŭn). Cementificação; produção metaplásica de cemento ou cementóide em um tecido conjuntivo menos diferenciado, p. ex., cementificação de um fibroma.

ce·ment·o·blast (se - men′tō - blast). Cementoblasto; célula de origem mesenquimal relacionada à formação da camada de cemento nas raízes dos dentes. [L. *cementum*, cemento, + G. *blastos*, germe]

ce·ment·o·blas·to·ma (se - men′tō - blas - tō′mă). Cementoblastoma; tumor odontogênico benigno de cementoblastos funcionais; apresenta-se como uma lesão mista radiotransparente-radiopaca fixada à raiz de um dente, e pode causar expansão do córtex ósseo ou estar associada a dor. SIN benign c., true cementoma.

benign c., c. benigno. SIN cementoblastoma.

ce·ment·o·cla·sia (se - men - tō - klā′zē - ă). Cementoclasia; destruição do cemento por cementoclastos. [L. *cementum*, cemento, + G. *klasis*, fratura]

ce·ment·o·clast (se - men′tō - klast). Cementoclasto; uma das células gigantes multinucleadas, idênticas aos osteoclastos, que estão associadas à reabsorção de cemento. [L. *cementum*, cemento, + G. *klastos*, quebrado]

ce·ment·o·cyte (se - men′tō - sīt). Cementócito; célula semelhante ao osteócito com numerosos processos, aprisionados em uma lacuna no cemento do dente. [L. *cementum*, cemento, + G. *kytos*, célula]

ce·ment·o·den·tin·al (se - men′tō - den′ti - năl). Cementodentário. SIN dentinocemental.

ce·men·to·gen·e·sis (se - men′to - jen′ē - sis). Cementogênese; o desenvolvimento do cemento sobre a dentina radicular de um dente. [cementum + G. *genesis*, produção]

ce·men·to·ma (se - men - tō′mă). Cementoma; termo inespecífico que se refere a qualquer tumor benigno produtor de cemento; são reconhecidos quatro tipos: 1) displasia periapical do cemento; 2) fibroma ossificante central; 3) cementoblastoma; 4) massa esclerótica de cemento. Quando o tipo não é especificado, o cementoma geralmente se refere à *displasia* (dysplasia) periapical do cemento. [L. *cementum*, cemento, + G. *-ōma*, tumor]

gigantiform c., c. gigantiforme; a ocorrência familiar de massas de cemento nas mandíbulas; herdado como uma característica autossômica dominante. VER TAMBÉM sclerotic cemental *mass*.

true c., c. verdadeiro. SIN cementoblastoma.

ce·men·tum (se - men′tŭm) [TA]. Cemento. SIN cement (1). [L. *caementum*, pedra áspera, não-polida, de *caedo*, cortar]

afibrillar c., c. afibrilar; c. que, à microscopia eletrônica, apresenta-se como material reticular elétron-denso, laminado, algumas vezes localizado sobre o esmalte do dente.

primary c., c. primário; c. que não possui cementócitos; pode cobrir toda a raiz do dente, mas freqüentemente está ausente no terço apical da raiz.

secondary c., c. secundário; c. que se forma na superfície do dente após a erupção; contém cementócitos.

ce·nes·the·sia (sē - nes - thē′zē - ă). Cenestesia; o sentido geral da existência corporal; a sensação causada pelo funcionamento dos órgãos internos. SIN coenesthesia. [G. *koinos*, comum, + *aisthēsis*, sensação]

ce·nes·the·sic, ce·nes·thet·ic (sē - nes - thē′zik, - sik; - thet′ik). Cenestésico; relativo à cenestesia.

△ **ceno-. 1.** Compartilhado em comum. [G. *koinos*, comum]. **2.** Novo, fresco. [G. *kainos*, novo]. **3.** Vazio (raro). VER TAMBÉM coeno-. [G. *kenos*, vazio]

ce·no·cyte (sē′nō - sīt). Cenócito; célula multinucleada ou hifa sem paredes transversais, característica das hifas ou zigomicetos. VER TAMBÉM nonseptate *mycelium*. SIN coenocyte. [G. *koinos*, comum, + *kytos*, célula]

ce·no·cyt·ic (sē - nō - sit′ik). Cenocítico; relativo a, ou que possui características de, um cenócito. SIN coenocytic.

cen·o·site (sē′nō - sīt). Cenósito; organismo comensal facultativo; que pode manter-se sozinho longe de seu hospedeiro habitual. [G. *koinos*, comum, + *sitos*, alimento]

ce·no·trope (sē′nō - trōp). Cenótropo; termo cientificamente mais preciso que o anterior "instinto", designativo do padrão de comportamento mostrado por todos os membros de um grande grupo que possuem o mesmo equipamento biológico e a mesma experiência. [G. *koinos*, comum, + *tropē*, desvio]

cen·sor (sen′sŏr). Censor; em teoria psicanalítica, a barreira psíquica que impede que emerjam na consciência determinados pensamentos e desejos, a não ser que estejam tão mascarados ou disfarçados a ponto de se tornarem irreconhecíveis. [L. juiz, crítico, de *censeo*, avaliar, julgar]

censoring (sen′sŏr - ing). Em epidemiologia, (1) perda de indivíduos de um estudo de acompanhamento por razões desconhecidas. (2) observações com valores desconhecidos a partir de uma extremidade de uma distribuição de freqüência, além de um limiar de medida.

cen·sus. Censo; contagem de uma população, originalmente para fins militares e de cobrança de impostos, agora com muitos outros objetivos; dados básicos sobre todas as pessoas — idade, sexo, ocupação, tipo de residência, etc. — são registrados no censo, que, freqüentemente, inclui também algumas informações sobre o estado de saúde. [L., de *censeo*, contar]

cen·ter (sen′ter) [TA]. Centro. **1.** O ponto médio de um corpo; em sentido amplo, o interior de um corpo. Centro de qualquer tipo, principalmente um centro anatômico. **2.** Um grupo de células nervosas que governam uma função específica. SIN centrum [TA]. [L. *centrum*; G. *kentron*]

active c., c. ativo; a parte de uma macromolécula na qual um substrato ou ligante, após se unir, produz atividade biológica; no caso de uma enzima, este é o centro catalítico, o local de uma enzima que catalisa a reação.

anospinal c., c. anoespinhal; c. na medula espinhal que controla a contração do esfíncter anal.

birthing c., c. de nascimento; uma unidade, geralmente em um hospital, que presta serviços de trabalho de parto e parto em um ambiente confortável, semelhante ao doméstico.

Broca c., c. de Broca; a parte posterior do giro frontal inferior do hemisfério esquerdo ou dominante, correspondendo aproximadamente à área 44 de Brodmann; Broca identificou essa região como um componente essencial dos mecanismos motores que controlam a fala articulada. SIN Broca area, Broca field, motor speech c.

Budge c., c. de Budge. SIN ciliospinal c.

catalytic c., c. catalítico. VER active c.

cell c., c. celular. SIN cytocentrum.

chondrification c., c. de condrificação; um local de formação inicial da cartilagem no corpo.

ciliospinal c., c. cilioespinhal; os neurônios motores pré-ganglionares, no primeiro segmento torácico da medula espinhal, que dão origem à inervação simpática que, finalmente, influencia o músculo dilatador das pupilares. SIN Budge c.

dentary c., c. dentário; c. de ossificação específico da mandíbula que dá origem à borda inferior de sua lâmina externa.

diaphysial c., c. diafisário; c. de ossificação primário na diáfise de um osso longo.

epiotic c., c. epiótico; o c. de ossificação da parte petrosa do osso temporal observado posterior ao canal semicircular posterior.

expiratory c., c. expiratório; a região do bulbo (medula oblonga) que é eletricamente ativa durante a expiração e onde a estimulação elétrica produz expiração ininterrupta.

feeding c., c. de alimentação; uma região da zona lateral do hipotálamo, cuja estimulação elétrica, no rato, desencadeia alimentação ininterrupta; a destruição da região causa anorexia prolongada.

germinal c. of Flemming, c. germinativo de Flemming; o centro de coloração clara em um nódulo linfático no qual as células predominantes são grandes linfócitos e macrófagos. SIN reaction c.

inspiratory c., c. inspiratório; a região do bulbo (medula oblonga) eletricamente ativa durante a inspiração e onde a estimulação elétrica produz uma inspiração ininterrupta.

Kerckring c., c. de Kerckring; um centro de ossificação independente ocasional no osso occipital; aparece na margem posterior do forame magno por volta da décima sexta semana de gestação. SIN Kerckring ossicle.

medullary c., c. semioval. SIN *centrum semiovale.*

microtubule-organizing c., c. organizador de microtúbulos; um *locus* nas células em intérfase e mitose, de onde se irradia a maioria dos microtúbulos; no centro desse centro está o centríolo; esse centro determina a polaridade dos microtúbulos celulares.

motor speech c., c. motor da fala. SIN Broca c.

ossific c., c. de ossificação. SIN ossification c.

c. of ossification, c. de ossificação. SIN ossification c. SIN centrum ossificationis [TA].

ossification c. [TA], c. de ossificação; o local de formação óssea inicial através do acúmulo de osteoblastos no tecido conjuntivo (ossificação membranosa) ou de destruição inicial da cartilagem antes do início da ossificação (ossificação endocondral). SIN c. of ossification, ossific c., point of ossification, punctum ossificationis.

primary c. of ossification, c. de ossificação primária. SIN primary ossification c. SIN centrum ossificationis primarium [TA].

primary ossification c. [TA], centro de ossificação primário; esse é o primeiro local onde o osso começa a se formar na diáfise de um osso longo ou no corpo de um osso irregular. SIN primary c. of ossification, primary point of ossification, punctum ossificationis primarium.

reaction c., c. de reação. SIN germinal c. of Flemming.

respiratory c., c. respiratório; a região no bulbo (medula oblonga) relacionada à integração de informações aferentes para determinar os sinais dos músculos respiratórios; os centros inspiratório e expiratório considerados juntos.

c. of ridge, c. da crista; a linha média bucolingual da crista residual.

c. of rotation, c. de rotação; ponto ou linha ao redor da qual se movem todos os outros pontos em um corpo. VER axis.

satiety c., c. da saciedade; termo que se refere à região do núcleo ventromedial no hipotálamo; a destruição dessa pequena região no rato leva à ingestão contínua de alimentos e à extrema obesidade.

secondary c. of ossification, c. de ossificação secundária. SIN secondary ossification c. SIN centrum ossificationis secundarium [TA].

secondary ossification c. [TA], c. de ossificação secundária; esse é o centro de formação óssea que aparece depois do centro de ossificação primária, geralmente na epífise. SIN punctum ossificationis secundarium, secondary c. of ossification, secondary point of ossification.

semioval c., c. semi-oval. SIN *centrum semiovale.*

sensory speech c., c. sensorial da fala. SIN Wernicke c.

speech c.'s, centros da fala; áreas do córtex cerebral envolvidas centralmente na função da fala; um está situado no giro frontal inferior esquerdo, um segundo centro nos giros supramarginal, angular e primeiro e segundo giros temporais. VER TAMBÉM Broca c., Wernicke c.

sphenotic c., c. esfenótico; um do par de centros de ossificação do osso esfenóide.

vasomotor c., c. vasomotor; área difusa da formação reticular na porção lateral do bulbo (medula oblonga) contendo neurônios que controlam o tônus vascular; consiste em áreas vasodepressoras e vasopressoras distintas.

vital c., c. vital; c. essencial para a vida; geralmente se refere aos centros localizados no bulbo (medula oblonga) necessários para a manutenção da respiração e da circulação.

Wernicke c., c. de Wernicke; a região do córtex cerebral considerada essencial à compreensão e à formulação da fala coerente e proposicional; compreende uma grande região dos lobos parietal e temporal, próxima ao sulco lateral do hemisfério cerebral esquerdo; corresponde aproximadamente às áreas de Brodmann 40, 39 e 22. SIN sensory speech c., Wernicke area, Wernicke field, Wernicke region, Wernicke zone.

Centers for Disease Control and Prevention (CDC), Centro de Controle e Prevenção de Doenças; o órgão federal responsável, nos EUA, pela erradicação, epidemiologia e educação sobre doenças sediado em Atlanta, Georgia, que compreende o *Center for Infectious Diseases* (Centro de Doenças Infecciosas), *Center for Environmental Health* (Centro de Saúde Ambiental), *Center for Health Promotion and Education* (Centro de Promoção de Saúde e Educação), *Center for Prevention Services* (Centro de Serviços de Prevenção), *Center for Professional Development and Training* (Centro de Desenvolvimento e Treinamento Profissional) e *Center for Occupational Safety and Health* (Centro de Segurança e Saúde Ocupacional). Anteriormente era conhecido como *Center for Disease Control* (Centro de Controle de Doenças) (1970), *Communicable Disease Center* (Centro de Doenças Transmissíveis) (1946).

cen·te·sis (sen-tē'sis). Centese; punção, principalmente quando usado como sufixo, como em paracentese. [G. *kentēsis*, punção, de *kenteō*, furar]

centi-(c). Prefixo utilizado nos sistemas SI e métrico para indicar um centésimo (10^{-2}). [L. *centum*, um centésimo]

cen·ti·bar (sen'ti-bar). Centibar; um centésimo de um bar.

cen·ti·grade (C) (sen'ti-grād). Centígrado. **1.** Base da escala de temperatura antiga na qual 100 graus separavam os pontos de liquefação e de fervura da água. VER Celsius *scale.* **2.** Um centésimo de um círculo, igual a 3,6° do círculo astronômico. [L. *centum*, um centésimo, + *gradus*, grau]

cen·ti·gram (sen'ti-gram). Centigrama; um centésimo de um grama; 0,15432358 grão.

cen·tile (sen'til). Centil; um centésimo. VER quantile. [L. *centum*, um centésimo, + *-ilis*, sufixo adj.]

cen·ti·li·ter (sen'ti-lē-ter). Centilitro; 10 ml; um centésimo de um litro; 162,3073 mínimos (EUA).

cen·ti·me·ter (cm) (sen'ti-mē-ter). Centímetro; um centésimo de um metro; 0,3937008 polegada.

cubic c. (cc, c.c.), c. cúbico (cm^3); um milésimo de um litro; 1 ml.

cen·ti·mor·gan (cM) (sen'ti-mōr-gan). Centimorgan (cM). VER morgan.

cen·ti·nor·mal (sen'ti-nōr-mal). Centinormal; um centésimo do normal; designa a concentração de uma solução.

cen·ti·pede (sen'ti-pēd). Centípode; artrópode predatório venenoso da ordem Chilopoda, caracterizado por um par de pernas por segmento possuidor de pernas. O veneno é injetado através do primeiro par de apêndices semelhantes a pernas, modificado em garras perfurantes; as picadas podem ser dolorosas e localmente necróticas, mas raramente são perigosas, exceto para crianças muito pequenas. Os gêneros encontrados nos EUA incluem *Scutigera, Lithobius, Scolopendra* e *Geophilus*. [L. *centum*, centena, + *pes* (*ped-*), pé]

cen·ti·poise (sen'ti-poyz). Centipoise; um centésimo de um poise.

cen·tra (sen'tră). Plural de centrum.

cen·trad (sen'trad). **1.** Em direção ao centro. **2.** Unidade de medida do poder de refração de um prisma; corresponde ao desvio de um raio de luz, cujo arco é 1/100 do raio do círculo, ou 0,57°.

cen·trage (sen'trāj). Centragem; a condição na qual os centros ópticos de todas as superfícies de reflexão e refração de um sistema óptico estão no mesmo eixo.

cen·tra·lis (sen-trā'lis). Central; no centro. [L.]

cen·tre mé·di·an de Luys (sen'tr mā-dē-an). Centro mediano de Luys. SIN centromedian *nucleus.* [Fr.]

cen·tren·ce·phal·ic (sen'tren-se-fal'ik). Centrencefálico; relativo ao centro do encéfalo.

cen·tri- (sen'tri). Forma combinante que indica centro.

centric (sen'trik). Cêntrico; que possui um centro (de um tipo ou número específico) ou que possui algo específico como seu centro (de interesse, foco, etc.). [G. *kentron*, centro]

cen·tric·i·put (sen-tris'i-put). Centricipúcio; a porção central da superfície superior do crânio, entre o occipúcio e o sincipúcio. [L. *centrum*, centro, + *caput*, cabeça]

cen·trif·u·gal (sen-trif'ū-găl). Centrífugo. **1.** Designa a direção da força que empurra um objeto para fora de um eixo de rotação. **2.** Algumas vezes, por analogia, designa também qualquer movimento para fora de um centro. Cf. eccentric (2). [L. *centrum*, centro, + *fugio*, fugir]

cen·trif·u·gal·i·za·tion (sen-trif'ū-găl-i-zā'shŭn). Centrifugação. SIN centrifugation.

cen·trif·u·gal·ize (sen-trif'ū-găl-īz). Centrifugar. SIN centrifuge (2).

cen·trif·u·ga·tion (sen-trif-ū-gā'shŭn). Centrifugação; submeter a sedimentação, por meio de uma centrífuga, sólidos suspensos em um líquido. SIN centrifugalization.

band c., SIN density gradient c.

density gradient c., c. por gradiente de densidade; ultracentrifugação de substâncias em soluções concentradas de sais de césio ou de sacarose; em equilíbrio, o meio exibe um gradiente de concentração (portanto, densidade) que aumenta na direção da força centrífuga e as substâncias de interesse se acumulam em camadas nos níveis de suas densidades. VER isopycnic *zone.* SIN band c., zone c.

zone c., c. por gradiente de densidade. SIN density gradient c.

cen·tri·fuge (sen'tri-fooj). Centrífuga. **1.** Aparelho por meio do qual partículas em suspensão em um líquido são separadas pelo movimento giratório do líquido, com a força centrífuga jogando as partículas para a periferia do recipiente girado. **2.** Centrifugar; submeter à ação giratória rápida, como em uma centrífuga. SIN centrifugalize.

cen·tri·lob·u·lar (sen-tri-lob'ū-lăr). Centrilobular; próximo ao, ou no centro de um, lóbulo, p. ex., do fígado.

cen·tri·ole (sen'trē-ōl). Centríolo; estruturas tubulares, medindo 150 nm por 300 a 500 nm, com uma parede que possui 9 microtúbulos triplos, geralmente observados como organelas pares situadas no citocentro; os centríolos podem ser múltiplos e numerosos em algumas células, como as células gigantes da medula óssea. [G. *kentron*, um ponto, centro]

anterior c., c. anterior. SIN proximal c.

distal c., c. distal; o centríolo no espermatozóide em desenvolvimento, a partir do qual se desenvolve o flagelo. SIN posterior c.

posterior c., c. posterior. SIN distal c.

proximal c., c. proximal; o c. situado em uma depressão na parede da porção posterior do núcleo do espermatozóide em desenvolvimento. SIN anterior c.

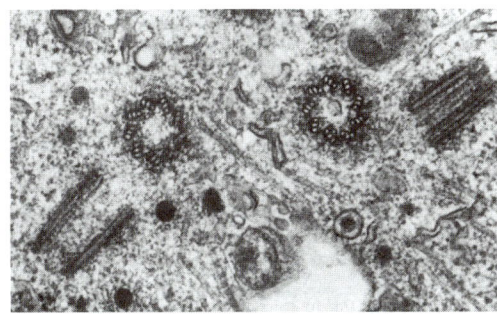

centríolo: micrografia eletrônica mostrando centríolos original e filho em um fibroblasto (90.000 ×)

cen·trip·e·tal (sen - trip'e - tal). Centrípeto. **1.** SIN afferent. **2.** Designa a direção da força que puxa um objeto em direção ao eixo de rotação. SIN axipetal. [L. *centrum*, centro, + *peto*, buscar]

centro-. Forma combinante que designa centro. [G. *kentron*]

cen·tro·blast (sen'trō - blast). Centroblasto; linfócito com um grande núcleo não-clivado. [centro- + G. *blastos*, germe]

Cen·tro·ces·tus (sen - trō - ses'tŭs). Gênero de trematódeos de peixe extremamente pequenos (família Heterophyidae) que podem provocar lesões intestinais semelhantes àquelas causadas por *Heterophyes heterophyes*. *C. formosana* foi descrito em seres humanos em Formosa. [G. *kentron*, ponto, centro, + *kestos*, cinto, ambas as palavras provenientes de *kenteō*, perfurar]

cen·tro·cyte (sen'trō - sīt). Centrócito. **1.** Célula cujo protoplasma contém grânulos simples e duplos, de vários tamanhos, coráveis por hematoxilina, observada em lesões do líquen plano. SIN Lipschütz cell. **2.** Um linfócito com um núcleo clivado. **3.** Uma célula B ativada, que não se divide e que expressa imunoglobulina da membrana. [centro- + G. *kytos*, célula]

cen·tro·ki·ne·sia (sen'trō - ki - nē'sē - ă). Centrocinesia; movimento excitado por um estímulo de origem central. [centro- + G. *kinēsis*, movimento]

cen·tro·ki·net·ic (sen'trō - ki - net'ik). Centrocinético. **1.** Relativo à centrocinesia. **2.** SIN excitomotor.

cen·tro·lec·i·thal (sen - trō - les'i - thăl). Centrolécito; designa um óvulo no qual o deutoplasma se acumula centralmente. [centro- + G. *lekithos*, vitelo]

cen·tro·mere (sen'trō - mēr). Centrômero. A constricção primária, não-corável de um cromossoma, que é o ponto de ligação da fibra fusiforme; proporciona o mecanismo de movimento do cromossoma durante a divisão celular; o centrômero divide o cromossoma em dois ramos, e sua posição é constante para um cromossoma específico, próximo de uma extremidade (acrocêntrico), próximo do centro (metacêntrico) ou entre (submetacêntrico). [centro- + G. *meros*, parte]

cen·tro·plasm (sen'trō - plazm). Centroplasma; a substância do citocentro. [centro- + G. *plasma*, coisa formada]

cen·tro·some (sen'trō - sōm). Centrossoma. SIN cytocentrum. [centro- + G. *sōma*, corpo]

cen·tro·sphere (sen'trō - sfēr). Centrosfera; o citoplasma especializado, freqüentemente na forma de gel, do citocentro. Contém os centríolos dos quais as fibras astrais (microtúbulos) se estendem durante a mitose. SIN astrocele, statosphere. [centro- + G. *sphaira*, bola, esfera]

cen·tro·stal·tic (sen - trō - stal'tik). Centrostáltico; relativo ao centro de movimento. [centro- + G. *stallein*, apresentar, extrair]

cen·trum, pl. **cen·tra** (sen'trŭm, sen'tră) [TA]. Centro. SIN center. [L. do G. *kentron*]

c. media'num, c. mediano. SIN centromedian *nucleus*.
c. medulla're, c. semi-oval. SIN c. semiovale.
c. ossificationis [TA], c. de ossificação. SIN center of ossification.
c. ossificationis primarium [TA], c. de ossificação primária. SIN primary center of ossification.
c. ossificationis secundarium [TA], c. de ossificação secundária. SIN secondary center of ossification.
c. ova'le, c. oval. SIN c. semiovale.
c. semiova'le, c. semi-oval; a grande massa de substância branca que compõe o interior do hemisfério cerebral; o nome refere-se ao formato geral desse centro branco em cortes horizontais do hemisfério. SIN c. medullare, c. ovale, medullary center, semioval center, Vicq d'Azyr c. semiovale, Vieussens c.
c. tendin'eum diaphrag'matis [TA], c. tendinoso do diafragma. SIN central *tendon* of diaphragm.
c. tendin'eum perine'i [TA], c. tendinoso do períneo. SIN central *tendon* of perineum.
c. of a vertebra, c. vertebral; **(1)** o centro de ossificação da massa central do corpo de uma vértebra; **(2)** corpo (*body*) da vértebra (em oposição aos arcos).
Vicq d'Azyr c. semiova'le, c. semi-oval de Vicq d'Azyr. SIN c. semiovale.
Vieussens c., c. de Vieussens. SIN c. semiovale.
Willis c. nervo'sum, c. nervoso de Willis. SIN celiac *ganglia*, em *ganglion*.

Cen·tru·roi·des (sen - tru - roy'dēz). Gênero de escorpiões norte-americanos, cujas espécies mais comuns são *C. gracilis*, escorpião-margarita; *C. vittatus*, escorpião com listra nas costas; e *C. sculpturatus*, escorpião esculpido mortal. VER TAMBÉM Scorpionida.

cen·tum (c) (sen'tum). Cem. [L. cem]

cen·u·ris, coe·nu·ris (se - nū'ris). Cenuro; cisticerco de tênia com múltiplos escóleces invertidos fixados à camada germinativa interna; produzido por cestódeos tenídeos do gênero *Multiceps*, tipicamente encontrado no cérebro ou tecidos de herbívoros, e o verme adulto no intestino de lobos, cães ou outros canídeos; foram descritos casos raros de infestação humana por cenuros. [G. *kenos*, vazio, + G. *uris*, cauda]

cen·u·ro·sis, ce·nu·ri·a·sis (sen - ū - rō'sis, sen - ū - rī'ă - sis). Cenurose; cenuríase; doença causada pela presença de um cisto de cenuro que, em ovinos, causa uma infestação cerebral conhecida como "modorra" devido à marcha cambaleante induzida no animal infectado; já foi descrita cenurose humana, mas é extremamente incomum, em contraste com a doença hidática. SIN coenurosis.

ce·pha·e·line (sef - a'ē - lēn). Cefaelina; um alcalóide da ipeca; emético e amebicida.

Ceph·a·e·lis (sef - ă - ē'lis). Gênero de plantas tropicais. SIN *Uragoga*. [G. *kephalē*, cabeça, + *eilō*, enrolar, embrulhar]

cephal-. VER cephalo-.

ceph·a·lad (sef'ă - lad). Na direção da cabeça. VER TAMBÉM cranial (1).

ceph·a·lal·gia (sef'al - al'jē - ă). Cefalalgia; cefaléia. SIN headache. [cephal- + G. *algos*, dor]

  benign coital c., c. benigna do coito. SIN coital *headache*.
  histaminic c., c. histamínica. SIN cluster *headache*.
  Horton c., c. de Horton. SIN cluster *headache*.

ceph·al·e·de·ma (sef'al - ĕ - dē'mă). Cefaledema; edema da cabeça.

ceph·a·le·mia (sef - ă - lē' - mē - ă). Cefalemia; congestão, ativa ou passiva, do cérebro. [cephal- + G. *haima*, sangue]

ceph·a·lex·in (sef - ă - lek'sin). Cefalexina; antibiótico de amplo espectro derivado da cefalosporina C.

ceph·al·he·ma·to·cele (sef'al - hē - mat'ō - sēl). Cefalematocele; um cefalematoma sob o pericrânio que se comunica com os seios durais. SIN cephalohematocele. [cephal- + G. *haima*, sangue, + *kēlē*, tumor]

ceph·al·he·ma·to·ma (sef'al - hē - mă - tō'mă). Cefalematoma; acúmulo de sangue devido a um derrame de sangue subperiósteo, freqüentemente em um recém-nascido, em virtude de traumatismo ao nascimento; diferente do *caput succedaneum*, no qual o derrame situa-se sobre o periósteo e consiste em soro. SIN cephalohematoma. [cephal- + G. *haima*, sangue, + -*ōma*, tumor]

ceph·al·hy·dro·cele (sef - ăl - hī'drō - sēl). Cefaloidrocele; acúmulo de líquido seroso ou aquoso sob o pericrânio. [cephal- + G. *hydōr*, água, + *kēlē*, tumor]

ce·phal·ic (se - fal'ik). Cefálico. SIN cranial (1).

ceph·a·lin (sef'ă - lin). Cefalina; termo anteriormente aplicado a um grupo de ésteres fosfatídicos semelhantes à lecitina, mas que contêm 2-etanolamina ou L-serina no lugar da colina; estes agora são conhecidos como fosfatidiletanolamina e fosfatidilserina. São amplamente distribuídos no corpo, principalmente no cérebro e na medula espinal, e são usados como hemostáticos locais e como reagentes nas provas de função hepática. SIN kephalin.

ceph·a·line (sef'ă - līn). Cefalina; designa membros da subordem de protozoários Cephalina (ordem Eugregarinida), caracterizados por corpos divididos em câmaras (protomerito anterior e deutomerito posterior, ou epimerito anterior, protomerito e deutomerito terminal); todos são parasitas de invertebrados.

ceph·a·li·tis (sef - ă - lī'tis). Cefalite; termo obsoleto para encefalite.

ceph·a·li·za·tion (sef'al - ĭ - zā'shŭn). Cefalização. **1.** Tendência evolutiva para que as funções importantes do sistema nervoso avancem no cérebro. **2.** Início e concentração da tendência de crescimento na extremidade anterior do embrião.

cephalo-, cephal-. Céfalo-, cefal-; cabeça. [G. *kephalē*]

ceph·a·lo·cau·dal (sef'ă - lō - kaw'dăl). Cefalocaudal; relativo à cabeça e à cauda, isto é, ao eixo longitudinal do corpo. [cephalo- + G. *cauda*, cauda]

ceph·a·lo·cele (sef'ă - lō - sēl). Cefalocele; protrusão de parte do conteúdo craniano, p. ex., meningocele, encefalocele. VER TAMBÉM encephalocele.

ceph·a·lo·cen·te·sis (sef'ă - lō - sen - tē'sis). Cefalocentese; introdução de uma agulha oca ou um trocarte e cânula no encéfalo para drenar ou aspirar um abscesso ou líquido de uma hidrocefalia. [cephalo- + G. *kentēsis*, punção]

ceph·a·lo·chord (sef'ă - lō - kōrd). Cefalocórdio; parte intracraniana do notocórdio no embrião.

ceph·a·lo·did·y·mus (sef'ă - lō - did'i - mŭs). Cefalodídimo; gêmeos conjugados fundidos, exceto na região cefálica; uma variedade de duplicidade anterior. VER conjoined *twins*, em *twin*. [cephalo- + G. *didymos*, gêmeo]

ceph·a·lo·di·pros·o·pus (sef'ă - lō - dī - pros'ō - pŭs). Cefalodiprosopo; gêmeos conjugados assimétricos com a cabeça do autosito carregando uma cabeça parasita reduzida. VER conjoined twins, em twin, diprosopus. [cephalo- + G. di-, dois, + prosōpon, face]

ceph·a·lo·dyn·ia (sef'ă-lō-din'ē-ă). Cefalodinia; cefaléia. [cephalo- + G. odynē, dor]

ceph·a·lo·gen·e·sis (sef'ă-lō-jen'ē-sis). Cefalogênese; formação da cabeça no período embrionário. [cephalo- + G. genesis, produção]

ceph·a·lo·gly·cin (sef'ă-lō-glī'sin). Cefaloglicina; antibiótico semi-sintético de amplo espectro produzido a partir da cefalosporina C.

ceph·a·lo·gram (sef'ă-lō-gram). Cefalograma. SIN cephalometric radiograph.

ceph·a·lo·gy·ric (sef'ă-lō-jī'rik). Cefalogírico; relativo à rotação da cabeça. [cephalo- + G. gyros, círculo]

ceph·a·lo·he·ma·to·cele (sef'ă-lō-hē-mat'ō-sēl). Cefaloematocele. SIN cephalhematocele.

ceph·a·lo·he·ma·to·ma (sef'ă-lō-hē-mă-tō'mă). Cefaloematoma. SIN cephalhematoma.

ceph·a·lo·he·mom·e·ter (sef'ă-lō-hē-mom'ē-ter). Cefalemômetro; instrumento que mostra o grau de pressão arterial intracraniana. [cephalo- + G. haima, sangue, + metron, medida]

ceph·a·lo·meg·a·ly (sef'ă-lō-meg'ă-lē). Cefalomegalia; aumento da cabeça. [cephalo- + G. megas, grande]

ceph·a·lom·e·lus (sef-ă-lom'ē-lŭs). Cefalômelo; indivíduo malformado com um membro acessório, semelhante a uma perna ou braço, que cresce da cabeça. [cephalo- + G. melos, membro]

ceph·a·lo·men·in·gi·tis (sef'ă-lō-men-in-jī'tis). Cefalomeningite; termo obsoleto para meningite. [cephalo- + G. mēninx (mēning-), membrana]

ceph·a·lom·e·ter (sef-ă-lom'ē-ter). Cefalômetro; instrumento usado para posicionar a cabeça de forma a obter radiografias laterais e póstero-anteriores reproduzíveis e orientadas. SIN cephalostat. [cephalo- + G. metron, medida]

ceph·a·lo·met·rics (sef-ă-lō-met'riks). Cefalometria; em cirurgia oral e ortodontia: 1. A medida científica dos ossos do crânio e face, utilizando uma posição fixa e reproduzível para exposição radiográfica lateral do crânio e dos ossos da face. VER TAMBÉM cephalometry. 2. Estudo científico das medidas da cabeça em relação a pontos de referências específicos; usado para avaliação do crescimento e desenvolvimento facial, incluindo perfil dos tecidos moles. [cephalo- + G. metron, medida]

ceph·a·lom·e·try (sef-ă-lom'ē-trē). Cefalometria; medidas científicas freqüentemente realizadas por meio de radiografia, da cabeça em vida, ou da cabeça de cadáveres sem remoção das partes moles, utilizando pontos de referência específicos e padronização suficiente para permitir resultados reproduzíveis. Comumente usada para documentar a idade com base no crescimento cefálico (como na ultra-sonografia obstétrica) ou para planejar ou medir o progresso na remodelagem cefálica (como em ortodontia). VER TAMBÉM craniometry, cephalometrics. [cephalo- + G. metron, medida]

ultrasonic c., c. ultra-sonográfica; medida da cabeça fetal por ultra-sonografia.

ceph·a·lo·mo·tor (sef'ă-lō-mō'ter). Cefalomotor; relativo aos movimentos da cabeça.

Ceph·a·lo·my·ia (sef'ă-lō-mī'yă). Nome anterior de *Oestrus*. [cephalo- + G. myia, mosca]

ceph·a·lont (sef'ă-lont). Cefalonte; estágio adulto de uma gregarina cefalina, um parasita esporozoário comumente encontrado em artrópodes e outros hospedeiros invertebrados. O corpo geralmente é dividido por um septo em um epimerito e protomerito anterior e um deuteromerito posterior; as gregarinas acefalinas não possuem um septo de divisão. [cephalo- + G. ōn (ont-), ser]

ceph·a·lop·a·gus (sef-ă-lop'ă-gŭs). Cefalópago; gêmeos conjugados com cabeças fundidas, mas o restante dos corpos separados. VER conjoined twins, em twin. VER TAMBÉM craniopagus, duplicitas posterior. [cephalo- + G. pagos, algo fixo]

ceph·a·lo·pel·vic (sef'ă-lō-pel'vik). Cefalopélvico; relativo ao tamanho da cabeça fetal em relação à pelve materna.

ceph·a·lo·pel·vim·e·try (sef'ă-lō-pel-vim'ē-trē). Cefalopelvimetria; medida radiográfica das dimensões da pelve e da cabeça fetal; a técnica foi em grande parte abandonada. SIN pelvicephalography, pelvocephalography. [cephalo- + pelvimetry]

ceph·a·lo·pha·ryn·ge·us (sef'ă-lō-fă-rin'jē-ŭs). Cefalofaríngeo. VER superior pharyngeal constrictor (muscle).

ceph·a·lor·i·dine (sef-ă-lōr'i-dēn). Cefaloridina; antimicrobiano de amplo espectro derivado da cefalosporina C.

ceph·a·lor·rha·chid·i·an (sef'ă-lō-ra-kid'ē-an). Cefalorraquidiano; relativo à cabeça e à coluna vertebral. [cephalo- + G. rhachis, espinha]

ceph·a·lo·spor·an·ic ac·id (sef'ă-lō-spōr-an'ik). Ácido cefalosporânico; o núcleo químico básico no qual se baseiam os derivados do antibiótico cefalosporina.

ceph·a·lo·spo·rin (sef'ă-lō-spōr'in). Cefalosporina; antibiótico produzido por um *Cephalosporium*, mas, após a descoberta do antibiótico, o nome Cephalosporium foi removido e o novo nome é Acremonium.

c. C, c. C; antibiótico cuja atividade é devida à porção ácido 7-aminocefalosporânico da molécula do ácido cefalosporânico; é efetiva contra bactérias Gram-positivas e Gram-negativas, porém é menos potente que a cefalosporina N. A adição de cadeias laterais produziu antibióticos de amplo espectro semi-sintéticos com maior atividade antibacteriana que a da cefalosporina C; a atividade antibiótica se deve à interferência com a síntese da parede celular bacteriana.

c. N, c. N; antibiótico ativo contra bactérias Gram-positivas e Gram-negativas, mas inativado pela penicilinase; à hidrólise produz penicilamina. SIN penicillin N, synnematin B.

c. P, c. P; antibiótico esteróide produzido por *Cephalosporium*, quimicamente relacionado aos ácidos fusídico e helvólico, que é ativo apenas contra bactérias Gram-positivas.

ceph·a·lo·spor·i·nase (sef'ă-lō-spōr'i-nās). Cefalosporinase. SIN β-lactamase.

Ceph·a·lo·spo·ri·um (sef'ă-lō-spō'rē-ŭm). Nome anterior de *Acremonium*.

ceph·a·lo·stat (sef'ă-lō-stat). Cefalostato. SIN cephalometer. [cephalo- + G. statos, estacionário]

ceph·a·lo·thin (sef-ă-lō'thin). Cefalotina; cefalosporina C quimicamente modificada, um antibiótico de amplo espectro.

ceph·a·lo·tho·rac·ic (sef'ă-lō-thō-ras'ik). Cefalotorácico; relativo à cabeça e ao tórax.

ceph·a·lo·tho·ra·cop·a·gus (sef'ă-lō-thōr-ă-kop'ă-gŭs). Cefalotoracópago; gêmeos conjugados com os corpos fundidos nas regiões cefálica e torácica. VER conjoined twins, em twin. [cephalo- + G. thorax, tórax, + pagos, algo fixo]

c. asym'metros, c. assimétrico. SIN c. monosymmetros.

c. disym'metros, c. dissimétrico; uma forma de c. com a cabeça fundida mostrando faces igualmente desenvolvidas e dirigidas lateralmente.

c. monosym'metros, c. monossimétrico; forma de c. na qual apenas uma das faces é bem desenvolvida. SIN c. asymmetros.

ceph·a·lo·tome (sef'ă-lō-tōm). Cefalótomo; instrumento anteriormente usado para cortar a cabeça do feto a fim de permitir sua compressão em casos de distocia. [cephalo- + G. tomē, corte]

ceph·a·lot·o·my (sef-ă-lot'ō-mē). Cefalotomia; operação anteriormente empregada para cortar a cabeça do feto.

ceph·a·lo·tox·in (sef'ă-lō-tok'sin). Cefalotoxina; veneno, que se acredita ser uma proteína, encontrado nas glândulas salivares de cefalópodos (octópodes). VER TAMBÉM eledoisin.

ceph·a·lo·tribe (sef'ă-lō-trīb). Cefalótribo; instrumento semelhante a um fórceps, com lâminas fortes e um cabo helicoidal, anteriormente usado para esmagar a cabeça fetal em casos de distocia. [G. tribō, esfregar, ferir]

ceph·a·my·cins (sef'ă-mī'sin). Cefamicina; família de antibióticos β-lactâmicos (semelhante à penicilina e cefalosporinas) produzida por várias espécies de *Streptomyces*.

ceph·a·pi·rin so·di·um (sef-ă-pī'rin). Cefapirina sódica; antibiótico semi-sintético de amplo espectro derivado da cefalosporina C; é usado por via injetável.

ceph·ra·dine (sef'ră-dēn). Cefradina; antibiótico semi-sintético de amplo espectro derivado da cefalosporina C; usado por via oral e injetável.

cep·tor (sep'ter, tōr). Receptor. SIN receptor (2). [L. capio, pp. captus, captar]

chemical c., receptor químico; receptor que inicia reações químicas em resposta aos estímulos apropriados.

contact c., receptor de contato; receptor nervoso na camada superficial da pele ou mucosa por meio do qual são recebidos impulsos gerados por impacto físico direto.

distance c., receptor a distância; mecanismo nervoso de um dos órgãos dos sentidos especiais por meio do qual o indivíduo é colocado em relação com o ambiente distante.

△ **-ceptor.** Forma combinante que designa captador, receptor. [L. capio, pp. captus, captar]

ce·ra (sē'ră). Cera. SIN wax (1). [L.]

ce·ra·ceous (se-rā'shŭs). Ceráceo; encerado. [L. cera, cera]

cer·am·i·dase (ser-am'i-dās). Ceramidase; uma enzima que hidrolisa as ceramidas em esfingosina e um ácido graxo; acilesfirgosina desacilase. A deficiência dessa enzima está associada à doença de Farber.

cer·a·mide (ser'ă-mīd). Ceramida; termo genérico para uma classe de esfingolipídio, derivados N-acil (ácido graxo) de uma base de cadeia longa ou esfingóide como esfinganina ou esfingosina; p. ex., $CH_3(CH_2)_{12}CH=CH-CHOH-CH(CH_2OH)-NH-CO-R$, onde R é o resíduo acil graxo, fixado, neste exemplo, à 4-esfingenina (esfingosina) na ligação amida. As ceramidas acumulam-se em indivíduos com doença de Farber.

c. dihexoside, c. diexosídio; o glicolipídio acumulado observado na lipidose glicolipídica.

c. lactosidase, c. lactosidase; enzima hidrolítica (uma β-galactosidase) que atua sobre ceramida lactosídio, produzindo glicosilceramida e galactose. A deficiência dessa enzima pode resultar em lipose de ceramida lactosídio. Cf. cytolipin.

c. lactoside, c. lactosídio; lactosilceramida que se acumula em indivíduos com lipose de ceramida lactosídio. Cf. cytolipin.

c. 1-phosphorylcholine, c. 1-fosforilcolina. SIN sphingomyelins.

c. saccharide, glicoesfingolipídio. SIN glycosphingolipid.

cer·a·sin (ser′ă-sin). Cerasina. SIN kerasin.
cerat-. VER kerat-.
ce·rate (sē′rāt). Cerato; preparação sólida untuosa raramente empregada, mais consistente que uma pomada, contendo cera suficiente para evitar sua liquefação quando aplicada à pele. [L. *cera*, cera]
cer·a·tin (ser′ă-tin). Ceratina; queratina. SIN keratin.
cerato-. VER kerato-.
cer·a·to·cri·coid (ser′ă-tō-krī′koyd). Ceratocricóide; relativo ao corno inferior da cartilagem tireóidea e à cartilagem cricóidea, ou à articulação cricotireóidea. SIN keratocricoid.
cer·a·to·hy·al (ser′ă-tō-hī′al). Ceratoióide; relativo a um dos cornos do osso hióide. SIN keratohyal.
Cer·a·to·phyl·li·dae (ser′ă-tō-fil′i-dē). Família de pulgas de mamíferos e aves, muitas das quais possuem uma ampla faixa de hospedeiros e servem como importantes vetores da peste, mantendo a infecção entre hospedeiros roedores selvagens e domésticos. Gêneros importantes incluem *Nosopsyllus* e *Ceratophyllus*. [G. *keras*, corno, + *phyllōdes*, como folhas]
Cer·a·to·phyl·lus (ser-ă-tof′-ă-lŭs). Gênero de pulgas (família Ceratophyllidae) encontradas em climas temperados; inclui importantes pulgas de aves domésticas, como *C. niger*, a pulga da galinha ocidental, e *C. gallinae*, a pulga da galinha oriental, embora essas pulgas tenham vários hospedeiros, incluindo seres humanos. [cerat- (kerat-) + G. *phyllon*, folha]
C. punjaten′sis, espécie de pulga abundante em roedores selvagens e domésticos na Índia; pode servir como agente de ligação entre roedores selvagens e seres humanos na transmissão da peste.
cer·car·ia, pl. **cer·car·i·ae** (ser-kā′rē-ă, -rē-ē). Cercária, pl. cercárias; larva de trematódeo, de vida livre na água, que emerge de seu hospedeiro caramujo; pode penetrar na pele de um hospedeiro final (como no caso do *Schistosoma* de seres humanos), encistar-se na vegetação (como a *Fasciola*) ou no peixe (como o *Clonorchis*), ou penetrar e encistar-se em vários hospedeiros artrópodes. O corpo e a cauda têm formatos muito variados, e a função especializada é adaptada às demandas específicas do ciclo vital de cada espécie. VER TAMBÉM sporocyst (1), redia. [G. *kerkos*, cauda]
cer·ci (ser′sī). Cercos. Plural de cercus.
cer·clage (sair-klazh′). Cerclagem. 1. Aproximar e unir as extremidades de um osso fraturado obliquamente com um anel ou com um fio circundante, bem apertado. 2. Cirurgia para descolamento da retina na qual a coróide e o epitélio pigmentar da retina são colocados em contato com a retina sensorial descolada por uma faixa que circunda a esclerótica posterior à inserção dos músculos retos oculares. 3. A realização de sutura com fio inabsorvível ao redor de um óstio cervical incompetente. [Fr. envolvimento, circundamento, enfaixamento]
cer·co·cys·tis (ser-kō-sis′tis). Cercocisto; forma especializada de larva cisticercóide de tênia que se desenvolve nas vilosidades de hospedeiros vertebrados, e não em hospedeiros invertebrados; p. ex., o c. de *Hymenolepis nana* em seu ciclo direto ou transmitido por ovos no ser humano. VER TAMBÉM cysticercus, cysticercoid. [G. *kerkos*, cauda, + *kystis*, bexiga]
cer·co·mer (ser′kō-mer). Cercômero; apêndice caudal de um cestódeo larvar, o estágio pró-cercóide de cestódeos pseudofilídeos; também pode ser encontrado nas larvas cisticercóides de cestódeos teniídeos, bem como em muitos himenolepídios (p. ex., *Hymenolepis nana*). Esse apêndice freqüentemente possui os ganchos originalmente usados pelo hexacanto em seu trajeto no hospedeiro intermediário no qual se desenvolve o estágio pró-cercóide ou outro estágio larvar. [G. *kerkos*, cauda, + *meros*, parte]
cer·co·mo·nad (ser-kō-mō′nad). Cercomonídeos; nome comum dos membros do gênero *Cercomonas*.
Cer·co·mo·nas (ser-kō-mō′nas). Gênero de protozoários flagelados de água doce e coprofílicos, no qual os membros possuem um flagelo anterior e um posterior. Já foram descritas espécies no intestino ou nas fezes do homem e de vários tipos de animais domésticos, mas geralmente pertencem a outros gêneros, como *Trichomonas* ou *Chilomastix*. [G. *kerkos*, cauda, + *monas* (*monad-*), unidade, mônada]
Cer·co·pi·the·coi·dea (ser′kō-pith-ē-koy′dē-ă). Uma das três superfamílias da subordem Anthropoidea; inclui pongídeos, macacos do Velho Mundo e o homem. [G. *kerkos*, cauda, + *pithēkos*, macaco]
Cer·co·pi·the·cus (ser-kō-pith-ē′kŭs). Gênero da família Cercopithecidae, representado por macacos de rabo longo e macacos africanos comuns.
cer·cus, gen. e pl. **cer·ci** (ser′kŭs, ker′kŭs; -sē, -kē). Cerco. 1. Estrutura rígida semelhante a um pêlo. 2. Um par de apêndices sensoriais especializados no 11.º segmento abdominal da maioria dos insetos. [L. Mod., do G. *kerkos*, cauda]
ce·rea flex·i·bil·i·tas (sē′rē-ă flek-si-bil′i-tas). "Flexibilidade cérea", na qual o membro permanece onde é colocado; freqüentemente observada na catatonia. [L.]
cer·e·bel·lar (ser-e-bel′ar). Cerebelar; relativo ao cerebelo.
cer·e·bel·lin (ser-ĕ-bel′in). Cerebelina; hexadecapeptídeo cerebelo-específico localizado nos pericários e dendritos das células de Purkinje cerebelares; usado como marcador para estudos de maturação do desenvolvimento neural da célula de Purkinje.
cer·e·bel·li·tis (ser-ĕ-bel-ī′tis). Cerebelite; termo obsoleto para inflamação do cerebelo.
cerebello-. O cerebelo. [L. *cerebrum*, cérebro, + *-ellum*, suf. dim.]
cer·e·bel·lo·len·tal (ser-e-bel′ō-len′tal). Cerebelolenticular; relativo ao cerebelo e ao cristalino do olho.
cer·e·bel·lo·med·ul·lary (ser-e-bel′ō-med′ū-lār-ē). Cerebelobulbar; relativo ao cerebelo e ao bulbo (medula oblonga).
cer·e·bel·lo·ol·i·vary (ser-e-bel′ō-ol′i-vār-ē). Cerebelo-olivar; relativo às conexões do cerebelo com a oliva inferior.
cer·e·bel·lo·pon·tine (ser-e-bel′ō-pon′tēn). Cerebelopontino; relativo ao cerebelo e à ponte; designa principalmente o recesso do cerebelo ou o ângulo entre essas duas estruturas.
cer·e·bel·lo·ru·bral (ser-e-bel′ō-roo′bral). Cerebelorrubro; relativo às conexões do cerebelo com o núcleo vermelho. [cerebello- + L. *ruber*, vermelho]
cer·e·bel·lum, pl. **ce·re·bel·la** (ser-e-bel′ŭm, -bel′ă) [TA]. Cerebelo, pl. cerebelos; a grande massa encefálica posterior, dorsal à ponte e ao bulbo (medula oblonga) e ventral ao tentório do cerebelo e à porção posterior do cérebro; consiste em dois hemisférios laterais unidos por uma porção média estreita, o verme. [L. dim. de *cerebrum*, cérebro]
cerebr-. VER cerebro-.
ce·re·bral (ser′ĕ-bral, sĕ-rē′bral). Cerebral; relativo ao cérebro.
cer·e·bra·tion (ser-ĕ-brā′shŭn). Cerebração; atividade dos processos mentais; pensamento. VER TAMBÉM mentation, cognition.
cerebri-. VER cerebro-.
cer·e·bri·form (se-rē′bri-form). Cerebriforme; semelhante às fissuras externas e convoluções do cérebro. [cerebri- + L. *forma*, formato, aspecto, natureza]
cer·e·bri·tis (ser-ĕ-brī′tis). Cerebrite; infiltrados inflamatórios focais no parênquima cerebral.
suppurative c., c. supurativa; inflamação (fleimão) do cérebro com supuração.
cerebro-, cerebr-, cerebri-. O cérebro. VER TAMBÉM encephalo-. [L. *cerebrum*, cérebro]
cer·e·bro·cu·pre·in (ser′ĕ-brō-koo′prē-in). Cerebrocupreína. SIN cytocuprein.
cer·e·bro·ma. Cerebroma. SIN encephaloma.
cer·e·bro·ma·la·cia (ser′ĕ-brō-mă-lā′shē-ă). Cerebromalacia. SIN encephalomalacia.
cer·e·bro·men·in·gi·tis (ser′ĕ-brō-men-in-jī′tis). Cerebromeningite. SIN meningoencephalitis.
cer·e·bron (ser′ĕ-bron). Cerebrona. SIN phrenosin.
cer·e·bron·ic ac·id (ser-ĕ-bron′ik). Ácido cerebrônico; constituinte dos cerebrosídeos cerebrais e outros glicolipídios. SIN phrenosinic acid.
cer·e·bro·path·ia (ser′ĕ-brō-path′ē-ă). Cerebropatia. SIN encephalopathy.
cer·e·brop·a·thy (ser-ĕ-brop′ă-thē). Cerebropatia. SIN encephalopathy.
cer·e·bro·phys·i·ol·o·gy (ser′ĕ-brō-fiz-ē-ol′ō-jē). Cerebrofisiologia; a fisiologia do cérebro.
cer·e·bro·scle·ro·sis (ser′ĕ-brō-skler-ō′sis). Cerebrosclerose; encefalosclerose; enrijecimento dos hemisférios cerebrais. [cerebro- + G. *sklērōsis*, enrijecimento]
cer·e·bro·side (ser′ĕ-brō-sīd). Cerebrosídeo; classe de glicoesfingolipídio; especificamente, uma monoglicosilceramida (monossacarídeo de ceramida), sendo o açúcar ligado à porção −CHOH- do esfingoide. Os cerebrosídeos são encontrados na bainha de mielina do tecido nervoso; p. ex., cerasina, nervona, oxinervona, frenosina, nomes também usados para o ácido graxo envolvido. O cerebrosídeo algumas vezes tem por prefixo glico-, galacto-, etc., no lugar da glicosilceramida correta, etc. Os ésteres sulfato dos cerebrosídeos estão entre os sulfatidatos.
c.-sulfatase, c. sulfatidase, c.-sulfatase, c.-sulfatidase; enzima que cliva o sulfato de um glicoesfingolipídio sulfatado (como um cerebrosídeo 3-sulfato).
cer·e·bro·si·do·sis (ser′ĕ-brō-sī-dō′sis). Cerebrosidose; uma lipidose como na doença de Gaucher (Gaucher *disease*).
cer·e·bro·spi·nal (ser′ĕ-brō-spī′nal, sĕ-rē′brō-). Cerebroespinal; relativo ao cérebro e à medula espinal. SIN encephalorrhachidian, encephalospinal.
cer·e·bro·ste·rol (ser′ĕ-brō-stēr′ol). Cerebrosterol; colesterol hidroxilado encontrado no cérebro e na medula espinal.
cer·e·brot·o·my (ser-ĕ-brot′ō-mē). Cerebrotomia; incisão do cérebro. [cerebro- + G. *tomē*, incisão]
cer·e·bro·vas·cu·lar (ser′ĕ-brō-vas′kū-lăr). Cerebrovascular; relativo ao suprimento sanguíneo para o cérebro, particularmente com referência a alterações histopatológicas.
cer·e·brum, pl. **ce·re·bra, ce·re·brums** (ser′ĕ-brŭm, sĕ-rē′brŭm; -bră; -brŭmz) [TA]. Cérebro; originalmente referia-se à maior parte do encéfalo, incluindo praticamente todas as partes dentro do crânio, exceto o bulbo (medula oblonga), a ponte e o cerebelo; agora, geralmente refere-se apenas às partes derivadas do telencéfalo e inclui principalmente os hemisférios cerebrais (córtex cerebral e gânglios da base). [L. cérebro]

cere·cloth (sēr'kloth). Gaze ou musselina de algodão impregnada com cera contendo um anti-séptico; usada em curativos cirúrgicos. [L. *cera*, cera]

Cerenkov, (Cherenkov) Pavel A., físico russo e Prêmio Nobel, *1904. VER C. *radiation.*

cer·e·sin (ser'ē - sin). Ceresina; mistura natural de hidrocarbonetos de alto peso molecular; substituto da cera de abelha, também usado em odontologia para impressões. SIN cerin, cerosin, earth war, mineral wax (2), purified ozokerite.

ce·rin (se'rin). Cerina. SIN *ceresin.*

Cer·i·thid·ea (ser - i - thid'ē - ā). Gênero de caramujos operculados (prosobrânquios) marinhos e de água salobra que servem como primeiro hospedeiro intermediário de muitos trematódeos. *C. cingulata* serve como hospedeiro para o *Heterophyes heterophyes* no Japão e Sudeste Asiático; *C. scalariformis* para cercárias que provocam a dermatite por cercária no sudeste dos EUA, da Flórida ao Texas.

ce·ri·um (Ce) (sēr'ē - ŭm). Cério; elemento metálico, n.° atômico 58, peso atômico 140,115. [de *Ceres*, o planetóide]

   c. oxalate, oxalato de c., uma mistura dos oxalatos de c., lantânio e outras terras raras; tem sido empregado no tratamento do vômito.

⌬ **cero-.** Cera. [L. *cera*, cera]

ce·roid (sē'royd). Ceróide; pigmento dourado ou amarelo-acastanhado, semelhante à cera, encontrado pela primeira vez em fígados fibróticos de ratos com deficiência de colina, e também presente em alguns dos fígados cirróticos (e determinados outros tecidos) de seres humanos. O ceróide é álcool-ácido-resistente, insolúvel em solventes lipídicos e, provavelmente, um tipo de lipofuscina, embora diferente das lipofuscinas verdadeiras por não se corar com o corante de redução férrica-ferricianeto de Schmorl; também exibe autofluorescência. Acumula-se na síndrome de Hermansky-Pudlak. [L. *cera*, cera, + G. *eidos*, aparência]

ce·ro·plas·ty (sē - rō - plas - tē) Ceroplastia; a fabricação de modelos de cera de peças anatômicas e anatomopatológicas ou de lesões cutâneas. [G. *kēros*, cera, + *plassō*, moldar]

cer·o·sin (ser'ō - sin). Cerosina. SIN *ceresin.*

ce·ro·tin·ic ac·id (ser - ō - tin'ik). Ácido cerotínico; um ácido graxo de cadeia longa encontrado em ceras naturais, na lanolina e em determinados lipídios.

cer·ti·fi·a·ble (ser - ti - fī'ă - bl). Interditável; diz-se de uma pessoa que exibe distúrbio do comportamento de gravidade suficiente para justificar hospitalização psiquiátrica involuntária.

cer·ti·fi·ca·tion (ser'ti - fi - kā'shŭn). **1.** Certificação; reconhecimento pela junta de uma especialidade médica do preenchimento bem-sucedido das exigências para reconhecimento como especialista. **2.** Interdição; o procedimento jurídico pelo qual um paciente é confinado em uma instituição psiquiátrica. **3.** Hospitalização psiquiátrica involuntária.

cer·ti·fied nurse-mid·wife (C.N.M.). Enfermeira-obstetriz; enfermeira que possui, no mínimo, graduação em enfermagem e educação avançada no tratamento de todo o ciclo de maternidade. A certificação é obtida através de um programa organizado de estudo e teste nacional pelo American College of Nurse-Midwives.

cer·ti·fy (ser'ti - fī). Internar um paciente em um hospital psiquiátrico de acordo com as leis do estado. [L. *certus*, certo, + *facio*, fazer]

ce·ru·le·an (se - roo'lē - ăn). Cerúleo; azul-celeste. SIN *blue*. [L. *caeruleus*, azul, de *caelum*, céu]

ce·ru·le·in (se - roo'lē - in). Ceruleína; decapeptídeo com atividade hipotensora; estimula o músculo liso e aumenta as secreções digestivas; tem estrutura semelhante à da colecistocinina e das gastrinas, mas é muito mais potente como estimulante da contração da vesícula biliar; também estimula a liberação de insulina. Inibe a biossíntese de ácidos graxos. [de *Cephalosporium caerulea*, da qual é isolada]

ce·ru·lo·plas·min (se - roo'lō - plaz - min). Ceruloplasmina; uma α-globulina azul, contendo cobre, do plasma sanguíneo, com um peso molecular de aproximadamente 122.000 e 6 ou 7 átomos de cobre por molécula; envolvida no transporte e na regulação do cobre, e pode reduzir o O_2 diretamente sem intermediários conhecidos; possui atividades ferroxidase e poliamina oxidase. A ceruloplasmina está ausente na doença de Wilson congênita. [L. *caeruleus*, azul-escuro]

ce·ru·men (sĕ - roo'men). Cerume; cerúmen; a secreção cérea (um sebo modificado), amarelo-acastanhada, de consistência mole das glândulas ceruminosas do meato auditivo interno. SIN ear wax, earwax. [L. *cera*, cera]

   c. inspissa'tum, inspissated c., c. espessado; cerume seco obstruindo o canal auditivo externo.

ce·ru·mi·nal (se - roo'mi - năl). Ceruminoso; relativo a cerúmen.

ce·ru·mi·no·lyt·ic (sĕ - roo'mi - nō - lit'ik). Ceruminolítico; uma das várias substâncias instiladas no canal auditivo externo para amolecer a cera. [cerumen, + G. *lysis*, afrouxamento]

ce·ru·mi·no·ma (se - roo - mi - nō'mă). Ceruminoma; tumor adenomatoso geralmente benigno das glândulas ceruminosas do canal auditivo externo.

ce·ru·mi·no·sis (se - roo - mi - nō'sis). Ceruminose; formação excessiva de cerúmen.

ce·ru·mi·nous (sĕ - roo'mi - nŭs). Ceruminoso; relativo ao cerúmen.

ce·ruse (sē'roos). Cerusa, alvaiade; carbonato de chumbo. SIN *lead carbonate*. [L. *cerussa*]

cer·veau iso·lé (ser - vō' ē - sō - lā'). Cérebro isolado; um animal com mesencéfalo transeccionado; respira espontaneamente, mas não responde; possui pupilas anormais (geralmente dilatadas) e um padrão de sono contínuo ao eletroencefalograma. Cf. encéphale isolé. [Fr. cérebro isolado]

cer·vi·cal (ser'vĭ - kal). Cervical; relativo ao pescoço, ou à cérvice, em qualquer sentido. SIN cervicalis. [L. *cervix* (*cervic*-), pescoço]

cer·vi·ca·lis (ser - vi - kā'lis). Cervical. SIN *cervical.*

   c. ascen'dens, c. ascendente; **(1)** SIN *iliocostalis cervicis* (*muscle*); **(2)** SIN *ascending cervical artery.*

cer·vi·cec·to·my (ser - vi - sek'tō - me). Cervicectomia; excisão do colo uterino. SIN trachelectomy. [cervix + G. *ektomē*, excisão]

cer·vi·ces (ser'vi - sēz). Plural de cérvix.

cer·vi·ci·tis (ser - vi - sī'tis). Cervicite; inflamação da mucosa, freqüentemente envolvendo também as estruturas mais profundas, do colo uterino. SIN trachelitis.

⌬ **cervico-.** Cérvice, ou colo, em qualquer sentido. [L. *cervix*, pescoço, colo]

cer·vi·co·brach·i·al (ser'vi - kō - brā'ke - ăl). Cervicobraquial; relativo ao pescoço e ao braço.

cer·vi·co·buc·cal (ser'vi - kō - bŭk'ăl). Cervicobucal; relativo à região bucal do colo de um dente pré-molar ou molar.

cer·vi·co·dyn·ia (ser'vi - kō - din'ē - ā). Cervicodinia; dor cervical. [cervico- + G. *odynē*, dor]

cer·vi·co·fa·cial (ser - vi - kō - fā'shăl). Cervicofacial; relativo ao pescoço e à face.

cer·vi·cog·ra·phy (ser - vi - kog'ră - fē). Cervicografia; técnica, equivalente à colposcopia para fotografar parte do colo uterino ou todo ele. [cervix + G. *graphō*, escrever]

cer·vi·co·la·bi·al (ser'vi - kō - lā'bē - ăl). Cervicolabial; relativo à região labial do colo de um dente incisivo ou canino.

cer·vi·co·lin·gual (ser'vi - kō - ling'gwăl). Cervicolingual; relativo à região lingual do colo de um dente.

cer·vi·co·lin·guo·ax·i·al (ser'vi - kō - ling'gwō - ak'sē - ăl). Cervicolinguoaxial; referente ao ângulo formado pela junção das paredes cervical (gengival), lingual e axial de uma cavidade.

cer·vi·co-oc·cip·i·tal (ser'vi - kō - ok - sip'i - tăl). Cervico-occipital; relativo ao pescoço e ao occipúcio.

cer·vi·co·plas·ty (ser'vi - kō - plas - tē). Cervicoplastia; cirurgia plástica do colo uterino ou do pescoço.

cervicoscopy. Cervicoscopia. SIN *visual inspection with acetic acid.*

cer·vi·co·tho·rac·ic (ser'vi - kō - thōr - as'ik). Cervicotorácico; relativo a: **1.** O pescoço e o tórax; **2.** A transição entre o pescoço e o tórax; **3.** A fusão de vértebras cervicais e torácicas.

cer·vi·cot·o·my (ser - vi - kot'ō - mē). Cervicotomia; incisão do colo uterino. SIN trachelotomy. [cervico- + G. *tomē*, incisão]

cer·vi·co·ves·i·cal (ser'vi - kō - ves'i - kăl). Cervicovesical; relativo ao colo do útero e à bexiga.

cer·vi·lax·in. Cervilaxina. SIN *relaxin.*

cer·vix, gen. **cer·vi·cis,** pl. **cer·vi·ces** (ser'viks, ser - vī'sis, - sēz) [TA]. Cérvice; colo. **1.** SIN *neck*. **2.** Qualquer estrutura semelhante ao pescoço. **3.** SIN *c. of uterus*. [L. colo]

   c. of the axon, colo do axônio; a porção constrita do axônio imediatamente antes do início da bainha de mielina.

   c. colum'nae posterio'ris, colo da coluna posterior; leve constricção da coluna cinzenta posterior da medula espinhal, observada ao corte transversal logo atrás da comissura cinzenta.

   c. den'tis [TA], colo dentário. SIN *neck of tooth.*

   strawberry c., colo em morango; eritema macular do colo uterino, característico da vaginite por *Trichomonas vaginalis*.

   c. of tooth, colo do dente; *termo oficial alternativo para *neck of tooth.*

   c. u'teri [TA], colo do útero. SIN *c. of uterus.*

   c. of uterus [TA], colo uterino; cérvice uterina; a parte inferior do útero que se estende do istmo do útero até a vagina. É dividida nas partes supravaginal e vaginal por sua passagem através da parede vaginal. SIN c. uteri [TA], cervix (3) [TA], neck of uterus, neck of womb.

   c. vesi'cae urina'riae [TA], colo vesical. SIN *neck of (urinary) bladder.*

ce·ryl (sēr'il). Cerila; o radical hidrocarboneto $C_{26}H_{53}$- do álcool cerílico (hexacosanol). SIN hexacosyl.

ce·sar·e·an (se - zā'rē - ăn). Cesariana; designa uma operação cesárea, que foi incluída sob a *lex cesarea*, lei romana (715 a.C.); não recebeu esse nome por ter sido realizada no nascimento de Julius Caesar (100 a.C.).

ce·si·um (Cs) (sē'zē - ŭm). Césio; elemento metálico, n.° atômico 55, peso atômico 132,90543; membro do grupo de metais alcalinos. O Cs[137] (meia-vida igual a 30,1 anos) é usado no tratamento de algumas neoplasias malignas. [L. *caesius*, cinza-azulado]

Cestan, Raymond, neurologista francês, 1872–1934. VER C.-Chenais *syndrome*.

Ces·to·da (ses-tō′dă). Subclasse de tênias (classe Cestoidea) que contém os membros típicos desse grupo, incluindo as tênias segmentadas que parasitam os seres humanos e os animais domésticos. SIN Eucestoda. [G. *kestos*, cinto]

Ces·to·dar·ia (sestō-dā′rē-ă). Subclasse da classe Cestoidea, representada por tênias que não possuem um escólex e não são segmentadas (monozóicas), em contraste com as tênias típicas da subclasse Cestoda; as larvas de Cestodaria (denominadas licóforas) caracteristicamente possuem 10 acúleos, em vez de seis. Acredita-se que as Cestodaria sejam tênias primitivas que parasitam o intestino e as cavidades celômicas de determinados peixes e alguns répteis.

ces·tode, ces·toid (ses′tōd, -toyd). Cestódeo; nome comum das tênias da classe Cestoidea ou suas subclasses, Cestoda e Cestodaria.

ces·to·di·a·sis (ses-tō-dī′ă-sis). Cestodíase; cestodiose; doença causada por infestação por um cestódeo.

Ces·toi·dea (ses-toy′dē-ă). As tênias, uma classe de vermes platelmintos caracterizados por ausência de um canal alimentar e, nas formas típicas (subclasse Cestoda), por um corpo segmentado com um escólex ou órgão de fixação em uma extremidade; os vermes adultos são parasitas vertebrados, geralmente encontrados no intestino delgado. [G. *kestos*, cinto, + *eidos*, forma]

ce·ta·ce·um (sē-tā′shē-ŭm). Espermacete; cetina. SIN spermaceti. [G. *kētos*, baleia]

cet·al·ko·ni·um chlo·ride (set′al-kō′nē-ŭm). Cloreto de cetalcônio; agente antibacteriano.

cet·hex·o·ni·um bro·mide (set-heks-ō′nē-ŭm). Brometo de cetexônio; anti-séptico.

ce·to·ste·a·ryl al·co·hol (se-tō-stē′ă-ril). Álcool cetoestearílico; componente do ingrediente do ungüento hidrofílico conhecido como cera emulsificante; uma mistura de álcoois alifáticos sólidos que consistem principalmente em álcoois estearílico e cetílico.

ce·trar·ia (sē-trā′rē-ă). Cetrária; musgo da Islândia; a planta seca, *Cetraria islandica* (família Parmeliaceae), um líquen, não um musgo, é usada como emoliente e como remédio popular para bronquite. SIN Iceland moss. [L. *caetra*, pequeno escudo espanhol (do formato de apotécios)]

ce·tri·mo·ni·um bro·mide (se-tri-mō′nē-ŭm). Brometo de cetrimônio; um anti-séptico.

ce·tyl (sē′til). Cetila; o radical univalente $C_{16}H_{33}–$ do álcool cetílico.

c. alcohol, álcool cetílico; o álcool de 16 carbonos que corresponde ao ácido palmítico, assim denominado porque é isolado entre os produtos da hidrólise do espermacete; é usado como auxiliar emulsificante e na preparação de bases de pomada "laváveis" (óleo em emulsões aquosas). SIN 1-hexadecanol, palmityl alcohol.

c. palmitate, palmitato de cetila; uma cera; o principal constituinte do espermacete.

ce·tyl·pyr·i·din·i·um chlo·ride (sē′til-pī-ri-din′ē-ŭm). Cloreto de cetilpiridínio; o monoidrato do sal quaternário da piridina e do cloreto de cetila; um detergente catiônico com ação anti-séptica contra bactérias não-formadoras de esporos.

ce·tyl·tri·meth·yl·am·mo·ni·um bro·mide (sē′til-trī-me′thil-ă-mō′nē-ŭm). Brometo de cetiltrimetilamônio; uma mistura de brometos de dodecil, tetradecil e hexadeciltrimetilamônio; um agente inodoro tenso-ativo, facilmente hidrossolúvel; desinfetante com forte ação bacteriostática, usado para a esterilização de instrumentos e utensílios.

cev·a·dil·la (se-vă-dil′ă). Cevadilha; cevadinha. SIN sabadilla. [Esp. dim. de *cebada*, cevada]

cev·a·dine (sev′ă-dēn). Cevadina; alcalóide presente nas sementes de *Schoenocaulon officinale* (*Sabadilla officinarum*), família Liliaceae; muito irritante para a pele e mucosas. VER TAMBÉM veratrine.

ce·vi·tam·ic ac·id (sev-i-tam′ik). Ácido cevitâmico. SIN ascorbic acid.

CF Abreviatura de citrovorum *factor* (fator citrovorum); coupling factor (fator de acoplamento).

Cf Símbolo do califórnio.

CFF Abreviatura de critical fusion frequency (freqüência de fusão crítica). VER critical flicker fusion *frequency*.

CG Abreviatura de chorionic *gonadotropin* (gonadotrofina coriônica); phosgene (fosgênio).

CGA Abreviatura de catabolite gene *activator* (ativador de gene de catabólitos).

cGMP GMPc; abreviatura de cyclic *guanosine* 3′,5′-monophosphate (3′,5′-monofosfato de guanosina cíclico).

CGP Abreviatura de chorionic "growth *hormone*-prolactin" (hormônio do crescimento-prolactina coriônico).

CGRP Abreviatura de calcitonin gene-related *peptide* (peptídeo relacionado ao gene da calcitonina).

CGS, cgs Abreviatura de centímetro-grama-segundo. VER centimeter-gram-second *system*, centimeter-gram-second *unit*.

CH Abreviatura de crown-heel *length* (comprimento cabeça-calcanhar).

Chaddock, Charles G., neurologista norte-americano, 1861–1936. VER C. *reflex, sign*.

Chadwick, James R., ginecologista norte-americano, 1844–1905. VER C. *sign*.

chae·ta (kē′tă). Cerda. SIN seta. [L. Mod. do G. *chaitē*, pêlo duro]

chafe (chāf). Esfoladura; causar irritação da pele por fricção. [Fr. *chauffer*, aquecer, do L. *calefacio*, tornar quente]

Chagas, Carlos, médico brasileiro, 1879–1934. VER C. *disease;* C.-Cruz *disease*.

cha·go·ma (sha-gō′mă). Chagoma; pequeno granuloma cutâneo causado pela multiplicação inicial do *Trypanosoma cruzi* (doença de Chagas).

chain (chān). Cadeia. **1.** Em química, uma série de átomos unidos por uma ou mais ligações covalentes. **2.** Em bacteriologia, um arranjo linear de células vivas que se dividiram em um plano e permanecem fixadas umas às outras. **3.** Uma série de reações. **4.** Em anatomia, uma série de estruturas ligadas, p. ex., c. de ossículos, c. ganglionar (chain *ganglia*, em *ganglion*). VER TAMBÉM sympathetic *trunk*. [L. *catena*]

A c., c. A; **(1)** o polipeptídeo mais curto constituinte da insulina contendo 21 resíduos aminoacil, começando com um resíduo glicil (terminação NH_2-); a insulina é formada pela ligação de uma c. A a uma c. B por duas ligações dissulfeto; a composição de aminoácidos da c. A é uma função da espécie; **(2)** em geral, um dos polipeptídeos em um complexo de múltiplas proteínas.

B c., c. B; **(1)** o polipeptídeo mais longo componente da insulina contendo 30 resíduos aminoacil, começando com um resíduo fenilalanil (terminação NH_2-); a insulina é formada pela ligação de uma c. B a uma c. A por duas ligações dissulfeto; a composição de aminoácidos da c. B é uma função da espécie; **(2)** a cadeia leve de uma imunoglobulina.

behavior c., c. de comportamento; comportamentos relacionados em uma série na qual cada resposta serve como um estímulo para a próxima resposta.

C c., c. C. SIN C-peptide.

cold c., c. fria; um sistema de proteção contra altas temperaturas ambientais para vacinas, soros e outras preparações biológicas termolábeis.

electron-transport c., c. transportadora de elétrons. SIN respiratory c.

ganglionic c., c. ganglionar. SIN sympathetic *trunk*.

heavy c., c. pesada; uma c. polipeptídica de alto peso molecular (cerca de 400–500 resíduos aminoacil), como as cadeias γ, α, μ, δ ou ε da imunoglobulina, determinando a classe e a subclasse da imunoglobulina. Essa cadeia também determina se o complemento pode ser ligado e se a cadeia pode atravessar a placenta. Há duas cadeias idênticas em cada imunoglobulina. SIN H chain.

J c., c. J; um glicopeptídeo, polipeptídeo rico em cisteína, ligado à IgA e IgM poliméricas; sua função é assegurar a polimerização correta das subunidades de IgA e IgM e ser secretado externamente. [*j*oining chain (cadeia de junção)]

L c., c. L; cadeia leve. SIN light c.

light c., c. leve; uma cadeia polipeptídica de baixo peso molecular (cerca de 200 resíduos aminoacil), como as cadeias κ ou λ na imunoglobulina. Há duas cadeias leves idênticas em cada monômero de imunoglobulina. SIN L c.

long c., c. longa; em bacteriologia, uma linha contínua com mais de oito células.

ossicular c., c. ossicular. SIN auditory ossicles, em ossicle.

respiratory c., c. respiratória; uma seqüência de reações de oxidação-redução com liberação de energia, por meio da qual elétrons são aceitos de compostos reduzidos e, finalmente, transferidos para o oxigênio, com formação de água. SIN cytochrome system, electron-transport c., electron-transport system.

short c., c. curta; em bacteriologia, um cordão de duas a oito células.

side c., c. lateral; **(1)** uma c. de átomos acíclicos ligados a um anel benzeno ou a qualquer composto de cadeia cíclica; **(2)** os átomos de um α-aminoácido além do grupamento α-carboxila, o grupamento α-amino, o α-carbono e o hidrogênio fixado ao α-carbono.

chain·ing (chān′ing). Encadeamento; comportamentos relacionados aprendidos em uma série na qual cada resposta serve como um estímulo para a resposta subseqüente.

cha·la·sia, cha·la·sis (kă-lā′zē-ă, -lā′sis). Calasia; inibição e relaxamento de qualquer contração muscular previamente mantida, geralmente de um grupo sinérgico de músculos. [G. *chalaō*, alargar]

cha·la·za (kă-lā′ză). **1.** Calázio. SIN chalazion. **2.** Calaza; ligamento suspensor da gema de um ovo de ave. [G. granizo; pequeno tubérculo, terçol (Galeno)]

cha·la·zi·on, pl. **cha·la·zia** (ka-lā′zē-on, -zē-ă). Calázio; granuloma inflamatório crônico de uma glândula meibomiana. SIN chalaza (1), meibomian cyst, tarsal cyst. [G. dim. de *chalaza*, terçol]

acute c., c. agudo. SIN hordeolum internum.

collar-stud c., c. em botão de colarinho; calázio que se estende através da placa társica anteriormente (calázio externo) e em direção à conjuntiva.

chal·cone (kal′kōn). Calcona; o composto original de uma série de pigmentos vegetais. Todos são flavonóides e tipicamente de cor amarela ou laranja. SIN benzalacetophenone.

chal·co·sis (kal-kō′sis). Calcose; intoxicação crônica pelo cobre. SIN chalkitis. [G. *chalkos*, cobre, latão]

c. len′tis, c. do cristalino; catarata causada por excesso de cobre intra-ocular. SIN copper cataract, sunflower cataract.

chal·i·co·sis (kal-i-kō′sis). Calicose; silicose; pneumoconiose causada pela inalação de poeira, inerente à ocupação de cortar pedras. SIN flint disease. [G. *chalix*, cascalho]

chalk (chawk). Giz; greda. SIN *calcium* carbonate. [L. *calx*]
   French c., giz de alfaiate. SIN talc.
   prepared c., greda preparada; carbonato de cálcio nativo purificado, geralmente moldado em cones; usado como adstringente leve e antiácido.
chal·ki·tis (kal-kī'tis). Calcite. SIN chalcosis. [G. *chalkos*, cobre, latão]
cha·lone (kā'lōn). Calônio; originalmente, um hormônio (p. ex., enterogastrona) que inibe, ao invés de estimular; atualmente, qualquer dos vários inibidores mitóticos (freqüentemente glicoproteínas) produzidos por um tecido e ativos apenas naquele tipo de tecido, independente da espécie; portanto, um inibidor mitótico tecido-específico reversível. [G. + *chalao*, relaxar, + *-ona*]
cha·ly·be·ate (kal-ib'ē-āt). Calibeado, ferruginoso; termo obsoleto para impregnado com ou contendo sais de ferro e para um agente terapêutico contendo ferro. [G. *chalyps (chalyb-)*, aço]
cham·ber (chām'ber) [TA]. Câmara; um compartimento ou espaço encerrado. VER TAMBÉM camera. [L. *camera*]
   altitude c., c. de altitude; uma câmara de descompressão para simular um ambiente de altitude elevada, particularmente sua baixa pressão barométrica. SIN high altitude c.
   anechoic c., c. anecóica; câmara destinada a absorver todo o som de forma a eliminar todos os ecos; usada para pesquisa de privação auditiva e sensorial.
   anterior c. of eyeball [TA], c. anterior do olho; o espaço entre a córnea anteriormente e a íris/pupila posteriormente, cheio de um líquido aquoso (humor aquoso) e que se comunica através da pupila com a câmara posterior. SIN camera anterior bulbi [TA], camera (1) [TA], camera oculi anterior, camera oculi major.
   aqueous c.'s, câmaras aquosas; as câmaras anterior e posterior do olho combinadas, que contêm o humor aquoso. VER anterior c. of eyeball, posterior c. of eyeball. VER TAMBÉM anterior *segment*.
   counting c., c. de contagem; aparelho para contar objetos microscópicos suspensos em líquido, como células e plaquetas no sangue total diluído ou bactérias em caldo de cultura. Consiste em uma lâmina de microscópio contendo uma cavidade rasa de profundidade uniforme, cujo assoalho é marcado com uma grade, a qual, quando fechada com uma lamínula, retém um volume preciso de líquido. Um cálculo baseado no número de elementos contados dentro das linhas da grade, na diluição do líquido e no volume da câmara de contagem permite uma estimativa da concentração de elementos no líquido antes da diluição. VER TAMBÉM hemocytometer.

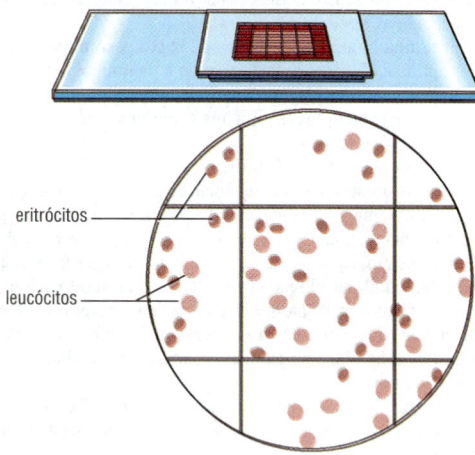

câmara de contagem de Zappert: (em cima) lâmina contendo câmara; (embaixo) imagem observada através do microscópio

   decompression c., c. de descompressão; c. para expor organismos a pressões abaixo da pressão atmosférica.
   c.'s of eyeball [TA], câmaras do olho; as cavidades do olho: câmaras anterior e posterior, cheias de humor aquoso, e a câmara vítrea, ocupada pelo vítreo. VER TAMBÉM anterior c. of eyeball, posterior c. of eyeball, postremal c. of eyeball. SIN camerae bulbi [TA].
   high altitude c., c. de altitude elevada. SIN altitude c.
   hyperbaric c., c. hiperbárica; c. que fornece pressões superiores à atmosférica, comumente usada para tratar a doença da descompressão e para fornecer oxigenação hiperbárica.
   ionization c., c. de ionização; c. para detectar a ionização do gás encerrado; usada para determinar a intensidade da radiação ionizante. VER TAMBÉM Geiger-Müller *counter*.
   posterior c. of eyeball, c. posterior do olho; o espaço anular, cheio de humor aquoso, entre a íris/pupila, anteriormente, e o cristalino e o corpo ciliar, posteriormente. SIN camera posterior bulbi [TA], camera oculi minor, camera oculi posterior.
   postremal c. of eyeball [TA], c. vítrea do olho; o grande espaço entre o cristalino e a retina; é ocupado pelo corpo vítreo. SIN camera postrema [TA], camera vitrea bulbi*, camera vitrea*, vitreous c.*, posterior segment of eyeball, vitreous camera, vitreous c. of eye.
   pulp c., c. pulpar; parte da cavidade pulpar que está contida na coroa ou no corpo do dente.
   relief c., c. de alívio; recesso na superfície de impressão de uma dentadura para reduzir ou eliminar a pressão da área específica da boca.
   Sandison-Clark c., c. de Sandison-Clark; c. que pode ser ajustada sobre um orifício perfurado em uma orelha de coelho, de forma que o tecido crescerá para preencher o defeito entre duas placas transparentes; se a distância entre as placas for pequena, o tecido vivo pode ser estudado microscopicamente.
   sinuatrial c., c. sinoatrial; a c. comum formada pelo átrio embrionário único e os cornos direito e esquerdo do seio venoso.
   vitreous c., c. vítrea; *termo oficial alternativo para postremal c. of eyeball.
   vitreous c. of eye, c. vítrea do olho. SIN postremal c. of eyeball.
   Zappert counting c., c. de contagem de Zappert; lâmina de vidro padronizada, especial, usada para contar células (principalmente eritrócitos e leucócitos) e outras partículas em um determinado volume de líquido; a porção central é estabelecida com precisão, de forma que a superfície uniformemente plana seja exatamente 0,1 mm mais baixa que as duas cristas paralelas sobre as quais pode ser colocada uma lamínula especial, uniformemente plana; linhas acuradamente demarcadas na porção central plana formam os limites de grupos de quadrados de áreas conhecidas, assim formando a base para determinar o volume de líquido no qual as células são contadas. As lâminas de vidro desse tipo são freqüentemente conhecidas como hemocitômetros.
Chamberlain, W. Edward, radiologista norte-americano, 1891–1947. VER C. *line*.
Chamberlen, Peter, obstetra inglês, 1560–1631. VER C. *forceps*.
cham·e·ce·phal·ic (kam-ĕ-se-fal'ik). Camecefálico; que tem a cabeça achatada; designa um crânio com um índice vertical ≤ 70; semelhante ao tapinocefálico. SIN chamecephalous. [G. *chamai*, no chão (baixo, atrofiado), + *kephalē*, cabeça]
cham·e·ceph·a·lous (kam-ĕ-sef'ă-lus). Camecéfalo. SIN chamecephalic.
cham·e·pro·sop·ic (kam'e-pro-sop'ik). Cameprosópico; que possui a face larga. [G. *chamai* (adv.), no chão (baixo, espalhado) + *prosōpikos*, facial]
cham·fer (sham'fer). Chanfro; arremate marginal no preparo de uma cavidade extracoronária de um dente que descreve uma curva de uma parede axial até à superfície cavitária. [do Fr. Ant. *chanfrein(t)*, borda biselada]
cham·o·mile (kam'o-mīl). Camomila; as flores da *Anthemis nobilis* (família Compositae); estomáquico. SIN camomile. [G. *chamaimēlon*, camomila, de *chamai*, no solo, + *mēlon*, maçã]
Champy, Christian, médico francês, *1885. VER C. *fixative*.
Chanarin, I., hematologista inglês do século XX. VER Dorfman-C. *syndrome*.
Chance, G.Q., radiologista inglês do século XX. VER C. *fracture*.
chan·cre (shan'ker). Cancro; a lesão primária da sífilis, que começa no local da infecção cutânea ou mucosa, após um intervalo de 10–30 dias, como uma pápula ou área de infiltração, de cor vermelho-escura, consistência dura e insensível; o centro geralmente sofre erosão ou se abre em uma úlcera que cicatriza lentamente após 4–6 semanas. A presença de *Treponema pallidum* ao exame em campo escuro é diagnóstica, exceto em úlceras orais, nas quais o *T. microdentium* está normalmente presente. SIN hard c., hard sore, hard ulcer, syphilitic ulcer (1). [Fr. indiretamente do L. *cancer*]
   hard c., c. duro. SIN chancre.
   mixed c., c. misto; ferida resultante da inoculação simultânea de um local com sífilis e cancróide.
   monorecidive c., c. monorrecidivo; c. que recorre no local de uma lesão previamente cicatrizada.
   c. re'dux, c. recidivante; um segundo cancro que ocorre em um indivíduo sifilítico, possivelmente uma reação alérgica sem a presença do espiroqueta específico.
   soft c., c. mole. SIN chancroid.
   sporotrichositic c., c. esporotricosítico; a lesão inicial no local da infecção cutânea na esporotricose.
   tularemic c., c. tularêmico; lesão primária, geralmente do dedo da mão, polegar ou mão, na tularemia.
chan·cri·form (shang'kri-form). Cancriforme; semelhante a um cancro.
chan·croid (shang'kroyd). Cancróide; uma úlcera infecciosa, dolorosa, irregular, no local da infecção por *Haemophilus ducreyi*, começando após um período de incubação de 3–7 dias; mais freqüente em homens; estreptobacilos Gram-negativos podem ser identificados pela coloração do material da úlcera. SIN soft chancre, soft sore, soft ulcer, venereal sore, venereal ulcer. [chancre + G. *eidos*, semelhança]
chan·croi·dal (shang-kroy'dăl). Cancróide; relativo a, ou da natureza de, um cancróide.
chan·crous (shang'krŭs). Cancroso; caracterizado pela presença de um cancro.
Chandler, Paul A., oftalmologista norte-americano, *1896. VER C. *syndrome*.

change (chănj). Modificação; alteração; em anatomopatologia, alteração estrutural de causa e importância incertas. SIN shift.
Armanni-Ebstein c., alteração de Armanni-Ebstein. SIN Armanni-Ebstein *kidney*.
Baggenstoss c., alteração de Baggenstoss; distensão dos ácinos pancreáticos por secreção proteinácea, observada na desidratação.
Crooke hyaline c., degeneração hialina de Crooke; substituição dos grânulos citoplasmáticos das células basófilas da hipófise anterior (adeno-hipófise) por material hialino homogêneo; um achado característico na síndrome de Cushing, mas geralmente ausente nas células de um adenoma basófilo. SIN Crooke hyaline degeneration.
fatty c., degeneração gordurosa. SIN fatty *metamorphosis*.
c. of life, mudança de vida; termo coloquial para (1) menopausa; (2) climatério.
reactive c.'s, alterações reativas; termo no sistema de classificação Bethesda, usado em laudos de diagnóstico citológico cervical/vaginal, que se refere a alterações de natureza benigna, associadas à inflamação (incluindo reparo típico), atrofia com inflamação, radiação, um dispositivo intra-uterino e outras causas inespecíficas. VER TAMBÉM Bethesda *system*, AGUS, LSIL, HSIL.
trophic c.'s, alterações tróficas; alterações resultantes da interrupção da inervação. VER TAMBÉM neurotrophic *atrophy*.

Changeux, Jean-Pierre, bioquímico francês do século XX. VER Monod-Wyman-Changeux *model*.

chan·nel (chan'el). Canal; passagem sulcada, em forma de canaleta ou ranhura. VER TAMBÉM canal. [L. *canalis*]
ion c., c. iônico; via de proteína macromolecular específica, com um "poro" aquoso, que atravessa a dupla camada lipídica da membrana plasmática de uma célula e mantém ou modula o potencial elétrico através dessa barreira, permitindo a entrada ou saída controlada de pequenos íons inorgânicos como Na^+, K^+, Cl^- e Ca^{2+}. É importante na propagação do potencial de ação em neurônios, mas também pode controlar a transdução de sinais extracelulares e a contração nas células musculares. Em geral, os canais iônicos são caracterizados por sua seletividade para determinados íons e sua regulação ou controle específico desses íons e sua sensibilidade específica a toxinas.
ligand-gated c., c. controlado por ligantes; uma classe de canais iônicos cuja permeabilidade iônica é regulada por receptores da membrana celular que respondem a sinais químicos extracelulares específicos.
transnexus c., canal transnexo; c. hidrofílico hexagonal de 15–20 Å capaz de transportar pequenos íons entre as células musculares cardíacas.
voltage-gated c., c. controlado por voltagem; uma classe de canais iônicos que se abrem e fecham em resposta à alteração no potencial elétrico através da membrana plasmática da célula; os canais de Na^+ controlados por voltagem são importantes para conduzir o potencial de ação ao longo dos processos da célula nervosa.

channelopathies (chan-el-op'ath-ēz). Distúrbios relacionados aos canais iônicos. SIN ion channel *disorders,* em *disorder*. [channel + G. *pathos*, doença]

Chantemesse, André, bacteriologista francês, 1851–1919. VER C. *reaction*.

cha·os (kā'os). Caos. **1.** Estado de desorganização total, que não tem atributos positivos. **2.** Um estado no qual não há relações causais. [G. vazio amorfo primitivo]
mathematical c., c. matemático; sistema dinâmico tão sensível a seu estado atual preciso (que, na prática, nunca será conhecido exatamente) que seu comportamento, embora determinista, é indistinguível do aleatório.

cha·o·tro·pic (kā-ō-trōp'ik). Caotrópico; pertinente ao caotropismo.

cha·o·tro·pism (kā-ō-trōp'izm). Caotropismo; a propriedade de determinadas substâncias, geralmente íons (p. ex., SCN^-, ClO_4^-, guanidínio), de romper a estrutura da água e, assim, promover a solubilidade de substâncias apolares em solventes polares (p. ex., água), o desdobramento de proteínas, a eluição, ou movimento através, de um meio cromatográfico de uma substância, do contrário firmemente ligada, etc. [G. *chaos*, desordem, confusão, + *tropē*, desvio]

CHAP Acrônimo para ciclofosfamida, uma hexametilmelamina, doxorrubicina (Adriamycin) e cisplatina, um esquema quimioterápico usado no tratamento do câncer ovariano.

cha·pe·rone (shap-ē-rōn). Acompanhante. **1.** Proteína necessária para o pregueamento e/ou montagem apropriada de outra proteína ou complexo de proteínas. **2.** Pessoa que acompanha um médico durante o exame de paciente do sexo oposto (ao do médico). [Ing. *escort, protector,* protetor, do Fr. *chaperon,* capuz, de *chape,* manto, do L.r. *cappa,* do L. *caput,* cabeça]

chap·pa (chap'pā). Doença caracterizada por nódulos subcutâneos, do tamanho de um ovo de pombo, que se rompem, liberam um material de aspecto gorduroso e formam úlceras; a erupção é precedida por fortes dores musculares e articulares. [Áfr. Ocid.]

chapped (chapt). Fissurado; que possui pele ou relativo à pele, principalmente das mãos, seca, descamativa e fissurada, devido à ação do frio ou à grande velocidade de evaporação da umidade da superfície cutânea. VER hand *eczema*. [I.M. *chap,* cortar, separar]

char·ac·ter (kar'ak-ter). Caráter, característica, traço; atributo em indivíduos sensível à análise formal e lógica e que pode ser usado como base de generalização sobre classes e outras afirmações que transcendem a individualidade. SIN characteristc (1). [G. *charakter,* traço característico, marca, de *charassō,* gravar]
acquired c., c. adquirido; um c. desenvolvido em um vegetal ou animal em virtude de influências ambientais durante a vida do indivíduo.
classifiable c., c. classificável; c. que permite a separação de indivíduos em classes distintas, mas não quantitativas, p. ex., tipos sanguíneos.
compound c., c. composto; c. herdado dependente de dois ou mais genes distintos.
denumerable c., c. enumerável; c. de classificação que também é contável (p. ex., número de filhos, número de dentes). SIN discrete c.
discrete c., c. distinto, bem definido. SIN denumerable c.
dominant c., c. dominante; c. hereditária determinada por um tipo de alelo. VER phenotype.
inherited c., c. hereditário; atributo distinto de um animal ou vegetal que é transmitido em um *locus* genético de geração para geração de acordo com a lei de Mendel. VER gene. SIN unit c.
mendelian c., c. mendeliano; c. hereditário sob o controle de um único *locus* (embora talvez modificado por genes em outros *loci*).
primary sex c.'s, características sexuais primárias; as glândulas sexuais, testículos ou ovários, e os órgãos sexuais acessórios.
recessive c., c. recessivo; característica hereditária determinada por um alelo apenas no estado homozigoto. VER *dominance* of traits.
secondary sex c.'s, características sexuais secundárias; aquelas características peculiares do homem ou da mulher que se desenvolvem na puberdade, p. ex., barba nos homens e mamas nas mulheres.
sex-linked c., características ligadas ao sexo; uma característica hereditária determinada por um gene ou um gonossoma. VER gene.
unit c., c. unitário. SIN inherited c.

char·ac·ter ar·mor. Armadura do caráter; padrão habitual de defesas organizadas contra a ansiedade.

char·ac·ter·is·tic (kar'ak-ter-is'tik). **1.** Característica, traço. SIN character. **2.** Característico; típico de um distúrbio específico.
receiver operating c. (ROC), característica de operação do receptor (COR); representação da sensibilidade de um teste diagnóstico como uma função de inespecificidade (1 − a especificidade). A curva de COR indica as propriedades intrínsecas do desempenho diagnóstico de um teste e pode ser usada para comparar os méritos relativos de procedimentos rivais.

char·ac·ter·i·za·tion (kar'ak-ter-i-zā'shŭn). Caracterização; o discernimento, descrição ou atribuição de traços de distinção.
denture c., c. dentária; modificação da forma e cor da base da dentadura e/ou dos dentes para produzir um aspecto mais natural.

cha·ras (char'as). Resina obtida das folhas maduras de variedades selecionadas de *Cannabis sativa*; usada para fumar.

char·bon (shar-bawn'). Antraz. SIN anthrax (2). [Fr. carvão]

char·coal (char'kōl). Carvão; carbono obtido por aquecimento ou queima da madeira com acesso de ar restrito. SIN carbo.
activated c., c. ativado; o resíduo da destilação destrutiva de vários materiais orgânicos, tratado para aumentar sua capacidade de adsorção; usado na diarréia, como antídoto em várias formas de envenenamento, e em processos de purificação em indústria e pesquisa. SIN medicinal c.
animal c., c. animal; c. produzido por combustão incompleta de tecidos animais, principalmente osso. SIN animal black, bone black, bone c.
bone c., c. ósseo. SIN animal c.
medicinal c., c. medicinal, carvão ativado. SIN activated c.
vegetable c., c. vegetal; c. obtido pela carbonização de tecidos vegetais, principalmente a madeira do salgueiro, faia, bétula ou carvalho. SIN wood c.
wood c., c. da madeira. SIN vegetable c.

Charcot, Jean M., neurologista francês, 1825–1893. VER C. *arteries, disease,* intermittent *fever, gait, joint, syndrome, triad, vertigo*; C.-Leyden *crystals,* em *crystal*; C.-Neumann *crystals,* em *crystal*; C.-Robin *crystals,* em *crystal*; C.-Böttcher *crystalloids,* em *crystalloid*; C.-Marie-Tooth *disease*; C.-Weiss-Baker *syndrome*; Erb-C. *disease*.

Chargaff, Erwin, bioquímico austro-norte-americano, *1905. VER C. *rule*.

charge trans·fer. Transferência de carga. VER charge transfer *complex*.

char·la·tan (shar'lă-tan). Charlatão; falso médico que diz curar doenças por procedimentos inúteis, remédios secretos e aparelhos diagnósticos e terapêuticos sem valor. SIN quack. [Fr., do It. *ciarlare,* palrar]

char·la·tan·ism (shar'lă-tan-izm). Charlatanismo; afirmação fraudulenta de conhecimentos médicos; tratamento de doenças sem o conhecimento de medicina ou autorização para sua prática. SIN quackery.

Charles, Jacques, físico francês, 1746–1823. VER C. *law*.

char·ley horse (char'lē hōrs). Dor localizada ou rigidez muscular após a contusão de um músculo. [gíria]

Charlton, Willy, médico alemão, *1889. VER Schultz-C. *phenomenon, reaction*.

Charnley, Sir John, cirurgião ortopédico inglês, 1911–1982. VER C. hip *arthroplasty*.

Charrière, Joseph F.B., fabricante de instrumentos francês, 1803–1876. VER C. *scale*.

chart. Tabela; gráfico; quadro. **1.** Registro de dados clínicos relacionados ao caso de um paciente. **2.** Curva. SIN curve (2). **3.** Em óptica, símbolos de tamanho graduado para medir a acuidade visual, ou tipos de prova para determinar a visão para longe ou perto. VER Snellen *test types*. [L. *charta*, folha de papiro]
  Amsler c., quadro de Amsler; um quadrado de 10 cm, dividido em quadrados de 5 mm, no qual se pode projetar um defeito no campo visual. SIN Amsler grid.
  isometric c., gráfico isométrico; gráfico que exibe três dimensões em uma superfície plana.
  Levey-Jennings c., gráfico de Levey-Jennings. SIN quality control c.
  Pickles c., gráfico de Pickles; representações diárias de novos casos de doença infecciosa usadas para mostrar o progresso de uma epidemia em uma população pequena, relativamente isolada.
  quality control c., gráfico de controle de qualidade; gráfico que ilustra os limites permissíveis de erro no desempenho de testes laboratoriais, sendo os limites um desvio definido em relação à média de um soro de controle, mais comumente ± 2 DP. VER TAMBÉM quality *control*. SIN Levey-Jennings c.
  Tanner growth c., gráfico de crescimento de Tanner; uma série de gráficos mostrando a distribuição dos parâmetros de desenvolvimento físico, como estatura, curvas de crescimento e espessura da prega cutânea, para crianças por sexo, idade e estágios de puberdade.
  Walker c., gráfico de Walker; sistema de representação dos tamanhos fetal e placentário relativos.

Charters, W.J., dentista norte-americano. VER C. *method*.

chart·ing. Registro clínico; fazer um registro, em forma de tabela ou gráfico, do progresso de um paciente. SIN clinical recording.

Chassaignac, Edouard P.M., cirurgião francês, 1804–1879. VER C. *space, tubercle*.

Chaudhry, Anand P. VER Gorlin-C.-Moss *syndrome*.

Chauffard, Anatole M.E., médico francês, 1855–1932. VER C. *syndrome*; Still-C. *syndrome*.

chaul·moo·gra oil (clawl - moo'grä). Óleo de chaulmogra; o óleo fixo obtido das sementes de *Taraktogenos kurzii* e *Hydnocarpus wightiana* (família Flacourtiaceae); anteriormente usado no tratamento da hanseníase. SIN gynocardia oil, hydnocarpus oil.

Chaussier, François, médico francês, 1746–1828. VER C. *line, sign*.

Chayes, Herman E.S., protodontista norte-americano, 1880–1933. VER C. *method*.

Ch.B. Abreviatura de *Chirurgiae Baccalaureus*, Bacharel em Cirurgia.

Ch.D. Abreviatura de *Chirurgiae Doctor*, Doutor em Cirurgia.

Cheadle, Walter B., pediatra inglês, 1835–1910. VER C. *disease*.

Cheatle, Sir George L., cirurgião inglês, 1865–1951. VER C. *slit*.

Δ check. Prova delta. SIN delta check.

check·bite (chek'bīt). Registro interoclusão. SIN interocclusal record.

check·er·ber·ry oil (chek'er - bār'ē). Óleo de gaultéria. SIN methyl salicylate.

Chédiak, Moisés, médico cubano do século XX. VER C.-Higashi *disease*; C.-Steinbrinck-Higashi *anomaly, syndrome*.

cheek (chēk). Bochecha; maçã-do-rosto; o lado da face que forma a parede lateral da boca. SIN bucca, gena, mala (1). [A.S. *ceáce*]

cheil-. VER cheilo-.

chei·lal·gia, chi·lal·gia (kī - lal'jē - ă). Queilalgia; dor no lábio. [cheil- + G. *algos*, dor]

cheil·lec·to·my, chi·lec·to·my (kī - lek'tō - mē). Queilectomia. **1.** Excisão de uma parte do lábio. **2.** Retirada de irregularidades ósseas na margem osteocondral de uma cavidade articular que interferem com os movimentos da articulação. [cheil- + G. *ektomē*, excisão]

cheil·ec·tro·pi·on, chil·ec·tro·pi·on (kī - lek - trō'pē - on). Queilectropia; eversão dos lábios ou de um lábio. [cheil- + G. *ektropos*, eversão]

chei·li·on (kī'lē - on). Quêilion; ponto cefalométrico localizado no ângulo da boca. [G. *cheilos*, lábios]

chei·li·tis, chi·li·tis (kī - lī'tis). Queilite; inflamação dos lábios ou de um lábio. VER TAMBÉM cheilosis. [cheil- + G. *-itis*, inflamação]
  actinic c., q. actínica. SIN solar c.
  angular c., q. angular; inflamação e fissura que se irradiam das comissuras da boca secundárias a fatores predisponentes como perda da dimensão vertical em usuários de dentaduras, deficiências nutricionais, dermatite atópica, ou infecção por *Candida albicans*. SIN angular stomatitis, commissural c., perlèche.
  commissural c., q. comissural. SIN angular c.
  contact c., q. de contato; inflamação dos lábios resultante do contato com um irritante primário ou alérgeno específico, incluindo ingredientes de batons. SIN c. venenata.
  c. exfoliati'va, q. esfoliativa; uma dermatite esfoliativa; pode estar relacionada à dermatite atópica ou à sensibilidade de contato.
  c. glandula'ris, q. glandular; distúrbio adquirido, de etiologia desconhecida, do lábio inferior, caracterizado por edema, ulceração, formação de crosta, hiperplasia de glândula mucosa, abscessos e trajetos fistulosos. SIN Baelz disease, myxadenitis labialis, Volkmann c.
  c. granulomato'sa, q. granulomatosa; edema crônico, difuso e mole dos lábios, de etiologia desconhecida, microscopicamente caracterizado por inflamação granulomatosa não-caseosa. VER TAMBÉM Melkersson-Rosenthal *syndrome*. SIN Meischer syndrome.
  impetiginous c., q. impetiginosa; piodermatite dos lábios com crostas amarelas devido à infecção por *Staphylococcus aureus* ou estreptococos.
  solar c., q. solar; atrofia da mucosa com ressecamento, formação de crosta e fissura da borda vermelha dos lábios em indivíduos idosos de pele clara, resultante da exposição crônica à luz solar; microscopicamente são observadas alterações displásicas (pré-malignas), análogas à ceratose solar. SIN actinic c.
  c. venena'ta, SIN contact c.
  Volkmann c., q. de Volkmann. SIN c. glandularis.

cheilo-, cheil-. Lábios. VER TAMBÉM chilo-, labio-. [G. *cheilos*, lábio]

chei·lo·gnath·o·glos·sos·chi·sis (kī'lō - nath'ō - glos - os'ki - sis). Queilognatoglossosquise; condição associada de fenda mandibular e do lábio inferior com língua bífida. [cheilo- + G. *gnathos*, mandíbula, + *glōssa*, língua, + *schisis*, fenda]

chei·lo·gnath·o·pal·a·tos·chi·sis (kī'lō - nath'ō - pal - ă - tos'ki - sis). Quilognatopalatosquise. SIN cheilognathouranoschisis.

chei·lo·gnath·o·u·ra·nos·chi·sis (kī - lō - nath'ō - ū - ră - nos'ki - sis). Quilognatouranosquise; fenda labial com fenda na mandíbula e no palato. SIN cheilognathopalatoschisis. [cheilo- + G. *gnathos*, mandíbula, + *ouranos*, céu (teto da boca), + *schisis*, fenda]

chei·lo·pha·gia, chi·lo·pha·gia (kī - lō - fā'jē - ă). Quilofagia; mordida dos lábios. [cheilo- + G. *phago*, comer]

chei·lo·plas·ty (kī'lō - plas - tē). Quiloplastia; termo antigo para designar cirurgia plástica dos lábios. [cheilo- + G. *plastos*, formado]

chei·lor·rha·phy (kī - lōr'ă - fē). Quilorrafia; sutura do lábio. [cheilo- + G. *rhaphē*, sutura]

chei·lo·sis, chi·lo·sis (kī - lō'sis). Quilose, queilose; condição caracterizada por descamação seca e fissura dos lábios, atribuída por alguns à deficiência de riboflavina e outras deficiências nutricionais. VER TAMBÉM cheilitis. [cheil- + G. *-osis*, condição]

chei·lot·o·my (kī - lot'ō - mē). Quilotomia; incisão no lábio. [cheilo- + G. *tomē*, incisão]

cheir-. VER cheiro-.

cheiralgia (kīr - al'jē - ă, - jya). Quiralgia; termo obsoleto para dor e parestesia na mão.
  c. paresthetica, q. parestésica; neuropatia por compressão do ramo superficial do nervo radial, caracterizada por dor e parestesia sobre o trajeto do nervo.

chei·rar·thri·tis (kī'rar - thrī'tis). Quirartrite; termo obsoleto para inflamação das articulações da mão. SIN chirarthritis. [cheir- + arthritis]

cheiro-, cheir-. Quiro; mão. VER TAMBÉM chiro-. [G. *cheir*, mão]

chei·rog·nos·tic (kī'rog - nos'tik). Quirognóstico; capaz de distinguir entre direita e esquerda, no que se refere às mãos ou ao lado do corpo tocado. SIN chirognostic. [cheiro- + G. *gnostikos*, perceptivo]

chei·ro·kin·es·the·sia (kī'rō - kin - es - thē'zē - ă). Quirocinestesia; a sensação subjetiva de movimento das mãos. SIN chirokinesthesia. [cheiro- + G. *kinēsis*, movimento, + *aisthēsis*, sensação]

chei·ro·kin·es·thet·ic (kī'rō - kin - es - thet'ik). Quirocinestésico; relativo à quirocinestesia.

chei·rol·o·gy, chi·rol·o·gy (kī'rol'ō - jē). Quirologia. SIN dactylology. [cheiro- + G. *logos*, palavra]

chei·ro·meg·a·ly, chi·ro·meg·a·ly (kī'rō - meg'ă - lē). Quiromegalia. SIN macrocheiria. [cheiro- + G. *megas*, grande]

chei·ro·po·dal·gia (kī'rō - pō - dal'jē - ă). Quiropodalgia; termo raramente usado para dor nas mãos e nos pés. SIN chiropodalgia. [cheiro- + G. *pous*, pé, + *algos*, dor]

chei·ro·pom·pho·lyx (kī - rō - pom'fō - liks). Quiroponfólix. SIN dyshidrosis. [cheiro- + G. *pompholyx*, bolha, de *pomphos*, vesícula]

chei·ro·spasm (kī'rō - spazm). Quiroespasmo; termo raramente usado para espasmo dos músculos da mão, como na cãibra dos escritores. SIN chirospasm. [cheiro- + G. *spasmos*, espasmo]

che·late (kē'lāt). **1.** Quelar; realizar quelação. **2.** Relativo à quelação. **3.** Quelato; complexo formado pela quelação.

che·la·tion (kē - lā'shun). Quelação; formação de complexo envolvendo um íon metálico e dois ou mais grupamentos polares de uma única molécula; assim, no heme, o íon Fe^{2+} é quelado pelo anel porfirina. A quelação pode ser usada para remover um íon da participação em regiões biológicas, como na quelação do Ca^{2+} do sangue pelo EDTA, que assim age como um anticoagulante. [G. *chēlē*, garra]

che·lic·era, pl. **che·lic·er·ae** (ke - lis'ī - ră, - ī - rē). Quelícera; um dos dois apêndices anteriores dos aracnídeos; em carrapatos e ácaros parasitas, as quelíceras são estruturas perfurantes e cortantes, e constituem importantes órgãos de alimentação. [G. *chēlē*, garra, + *keras*, corno]

chel·i·don (kel'ē - don). SIN cubital *fossa*. [G. *chelidōn*, andorinha, devido à semelhança com o formato de uma cauda de andorinha]

che·loid (kē'loyd). Quelóide. SIN keloid.

chem-. VER chemo-.

chem·ex·fo·li·a·tion (kem′eks-fō-lē-ā′shŭn). Quimioesfoliação; técnica quimiocirúrgica designada para remover cicatrizes de acne ou tratar alterações cutâneas crônicas causadas por exposição à luz solar. SIN chemical peeling.

chem·i·a·try (kem′i-ā-trē). Quimiatria; termo obsoleto para iatroquímica.

chem·i·cal (kem′i-kăl). Químico; relativo à química.

chem·i·co·cau·tery (kem′i-kō-kaw′ter-ē). Quimiocautério. SIN chemocautery.

chem·i·lu·mi·nes·cence (kem′ē-loo-min-es′ens). Quimioluminescência; luz produzida pela ação química, geralmente à temperatura ambiente ou abaixo desta. SIN chemoluminescence.

chem·i·o·tax·is (kem′ē-ō-taks′is). Quimiotaxia. SIN chemotaxis.

che·mise (shem-ēz′). Camisa; quadrado de gaze preso a um cateter que atravessa seu centro; usado para manter um tampão envolvendo um cateter inserido em uma lesão, como aquela resultante de uma ressecção perineal. [Fr. camisa]

chem·ist (kem′ist). Químico. **1.** Especialista ou perito em química. **2.** Farmacêutico (britânico).

chem·is·try (kem′is-trē). Química. **1.** A ciência relacionada com a composição atômica das substâncias, os elementos e suas interações, bem como com a formação, decomposição e propriedades das moléculas. **2.** As propriedades químicas de uma substância. **3.** Processos químicos. [G. *chēmeia*, alquimia]
analytic c., q. analítica; a aplicação da química à determinação e detecção da composição e identificação de substâncias específicas.
applied c., q. aplicada; a aplicação das teorias e princípios da química para fins práticos.
biologic c., bioquímica. SIN biochemistry.
clinical c., q. clínica; **(1)** a química da saúde e da doença humanas; **(2)** química relacionada ao tratamento de pacientes, como em um laboratório hospitalar.
ecologic c., q. ecológica; **(1)** química que se concentra nos efeitos das substâncias químicas produzidas pelo homem no meio ambiente, e também no desenvolvimento de agentes não-prejudiciais para o ambiente; **(2)** o estudo das interações moleculares entre espécies e entre as espécies e o ambiente.
epithermal c., q. epitérmica; denominada química do "átomo aquecido"; a ciência relacionada com as reações químicas dos átomos retraídos e radicais livres produzidos nos processos nucleares de baixa energia.
inorganic c., q. inorgânica; a ciência relacionada com substâncias que não envolvem moléculas contendo carbono.
macromolecular c., q. macromolecular; a química das macromoléculas (p. ex., proteínas, ácidos nucleicos) e polímeros (náilon, polietileno, etc.).
medicinal c., q. medicinal. SIN pharmaceutical c.
nuclear c., q. nuclear; a ciência relacionada com a química das reações e processos nucleares.
organic c., q. orgânica; ramo da química relacionado aos átomos ligados de forma covalente, centralizada em torno de compostos de carbono desse tipo; originalmente, e ainda incluindo, a química dos produtos naturais.
pharmaceutical c., q. farmacêutica; química medicinal em sua aplicação à análise, desenvolvimento, preparo e fabricação de drogas. SIN medicinal c., pharmacochemistry.
physiologic c., q. fisiológica. SIN biochemistry.
radiopharmaceutical c., q. radiofarmacêutica; a ciência relacionada com a marcação de fármacos com radionuclídeos.
synthetic c., q. sintética; a formação ou construção de compostos complexos pela união de outros mais simples.

chemo-, chem-. Química. [G. *chēmeia*, alquimia]

chemo·at·tract·ants (kem′ă-trak′tinz). Quimioatrativos; substâncias químicas que influenciam a migração das células. [chem- + attract + -i]

che·mo·au·to·troph (kem′ō-aw′tō-trōf, kē′mō). Quimioautótrofo; organismo que depende de substâncias químicas para obter energia e, principalmente, do dióxido de carbono como fonte de carbono. SIN chemolithotroph. [chemo- + G. *autos*, auto, + *trophikos*, nutrição]

che·mo·au·to·tro·phic (kem′ō-aw-tō-trof′ik, kē′mo-). Quimioautotrófico; relativo a um quimioautotrofo. SIN chemolithotrophic.

che·mo·bi·o·dy·nam·ics (kem′ō-bī-ō-dī-nam′iks, kē′mō-). Quimiobiodinâmica; estudo dedicado ao esclarecimento de correlações entre a constituição química de vários materiais e sua capacidade de modificar a função e a morfologia de sistemas biológicos. [chemo- + G. *bios*, vida, + *dynamis*, força]

che·mo·cau·tery (kem′ō-kaw-ter-ē, kē′mō-). Quimiocautério; qualquer substância que destrua tecidos após a aplicação. SIN chemical cautery, chemicocautery.

che·mo·cep·tor (kē′mō-sep-tŏr). Quimioceptor. SIN chemoreceptor.

che·mo·dec·to·ma (kem′ō-dek-tō′mă, kē′mō-). Quimiodectoma; tumor do corpo aórtico, tumor do corpo carotídeo, tumor do quimiorreceptor ou tumor do glomo jugular; paraganglioma não-cromafin; receptoma; neoplasia relativamente rara, em geral benigna, originada no tecido quimiorreceptor do corpo carotídeo, glomo jugular e corpos aórticos; consiste histologicamente em células hipercromáticas, arredondadas ou ovóides, que tendem a ser agrupadas em um padrão semelhante a um alvéolo com quantidade pequena a moderada de estroma fibroso e alguns canais vasculares grandes e com paredes finas. Cf. paraganglioma. SIN aortic body tumor, carotid body tumor, nonchromaffin paraganglioma. [chemo- + G. *dektēs*, receptor, de *dechomai*, receber, + *-oma*, tumor]

che·mo·dec·to·ma·to·sis (kem′ō-dek-tō-mă-to′sis, kē′mō-). Quimiodectomatose; múltiplos tumores de tecido perivascular do corpo carotídeo ou do tipo quimiorreceptor presumido, que foram descritos nos pulmões como neoplasias diminutas.

che·mo·dif·fer·en·ti·a·tion (kem′ō-dif-er-en-shē-ā′shŭn, kē′mō-). Quimiodiferenciação; diferenciação dos constituintes químicos celulares no embrião antes da citodiferenciação; algumas vezes reconhecível histoquimicamente. SIN invisible differentiation.

che·mo·het·er·o·troph (kem′ō-het′er-ō-trōf, kē′mō-). Quimioeterótrofo. SIN chemoorganotroph. [chem- + G. *heteros*, outro, + *trophē*, nutrição]

che·mo·het·er·o·troph·ic (kem′ō-het-er-ō-trof′ik, kē′mō-). Quimioeterotrófico. SIN chemoorganotrophic.

che·mo·im·mu·nol·o·gy (kem′ō-im-ū-nol′ō-jē, kē′mō-). Quimioimunologia; termo obsoleto para imunoquímica.

che·mo·kines (kē′mō-kinz). Quimiocinas; vários grupos compostos de citocinas polipeptídicas, geralmente de 8–10 kD, que são quimiocinéticas e quimiotáticas, estimulando o movimento e a atração dos leucócitos. SIN intercrines. [chemo- + G. *kineō*, colocar em movimento]

che·mo·ki·ne·sis (kem′ō-ki-nē′sis, kē′mō-). Quimiocinese; estimulação de um organismo por uma substância química. [chemo- + G. *kinēsis*, movimento]

che·mo·ki·net·ic (kem′ō-ki-net′ik, kē′mō-). Quimiocinético; referente à quimiocinese.

che·mo·lith·o·troph (kem′ō-lith′ō-trōf, kē′mō-). Quimiolitótrofo. SIN chemoautotroph.

che·mo·lith·o·tro·phic (kem′ō-lith-ō-trof′ik, kē′mō-). Quimiolitotrófico. SIN chemoautotrophic.

che·mo·lith·o·tro·phy (kem′ō-lith′ō-trōf-ē). Quimiolitotrofia; a utilização de compostos inorgânicos ou íons para obter equivalentes redutores e energia. [chemo- + G. *lithos*, cálculo, mineral, + *trophe*, nutrição]

che·mo·lu·mi·nes·cence (kem′ō-loo-min-es′ens, kē′mō-). Quimioluminescência. SIN chemiluminescence.

chem·ol·y·sis (kem-ol′i-sis). Quimiólise; decomposição química. [chemo- + G. *lysis*, dissolução]

che·mo·nu·cle·ol·y·sis (kem′ō-noo-klē-ol′i-sis, kē′mō-). Quimionucleólise; injeção de quimiopapaína no núcleo pulposo de um disco intervertebral. Uma opção para o tratamento de um núcleo pulposo herniado, p. ex., "disco deslizado".

che·mo·or·ga·no·troph (kem′ō-ōr′gă-nō-trōf, kē′mō-). Quimioorganótrofo; organismo que depende de substâncias químicas orgânicas como fonte de energia e carbono. SIN chemoheterotroph. [chemo- + G. *organon*, órgão, + *trophē*, nutrição]

che·mo·or·ga·no·tro·phic (kem′ō-ōr-gă-nō-trof′ik, kē′mō-). Quimioorganotrófico; relativo a um quimioorganótrofo. SIN chemoheterotrophic.

che·mo·pal·li·dec·to·my (kem′ō-pal-i-dek′tō-mē, kē′mō-). Quimiopalidectomia; destruição do globo pálido pela injeção de um agente químico. SIN chemopallidotomy. [chemo- + globus pallidus + G. *ektomē*, excisão]

che·mo·pal·li·do·thal·a·mec·to·my (kem′ō-pal′i-dō-thal-ă-mek′tō-mē, kē′mō-). Quimiopalidotalamectomia; destruição de partes do globo pálido e do tálamo por injeção de uma substância química. [chemo- + globus pallidus + thalamus + G. *ektomē*, excisão]

che·mo·pal·li·dot·o·my (kem′ō-pal-i-dot′ō-mē, kē′mō-). Quimiopalidotomia. SIN chemopallidectomy. [chemo- + globus pallidus + G. *tomē*, incisão]

chem·o·pre·ven·tion. Quimioprevenção; uso de drogas ou outros agentes para inibir o desenvolvimento ou a progressão de alterações malignas nas células.

che·mo·pro·phy·lax·is (kem′ō-prō′fi-lak′sis, kē′mō-). Quimioprofilaxia; prevenção de doença pelo uso de substâncias químicas ou fármacos.

che·mo·re·cep·tion (kēm-ō-rē-sep′shun). Quimiorrecepção; a capacidade de perceber substâncias químicas aromáticas ou que estimulem o paladar no ambiente. SIN chemosensation.

che·mo·re·cep·tive (kē-mō-rē-sep′tiv). Quimiorreceptivo; relativo à quimiorrecepção.

che·mo·re·cep·tor (kē′mō-rē-sep′tor). Quimiorreceptor; qualquer célula ativada por uma alteração em seu meio químico e que resulta em um impulso nervoso. Essas células podem ser 1) células "transdutoras" inervadas por fibras nervosas sensoriais (p. ex., as células receptoras gustativas das papilas gustativas; células no corpo carotídeo sensíveis a alterações no conteúdo de oxigênio e dióxido de carbono do sangue); ou 2) células nervosas propriamente ditas, como as células receptoras olfatórias da mucosa olfatória, e determinadas células do tronco cerebral que são sensíveis a alterações na composição do sangue ou do líquido cefalorraquidiano. SIN chemoceptor.

medullary c., q. bulbar; as células situadas na superfície ventrolateral do bulbo ou nas suas proximidades, estimuladas pela acidez local.
peripheral c., q. periférico; as células nos corpos carotídeo e aórtico estimuladas por alterações químicas na composição do sangue, como hipoxia.

che·mo·re·flex (kem-ō-rē′fleks, kē-mō-). Quimiorreflexo; reflexo iniciado pela estimulação de quimiorreceptores, p. ex., de um corpo carotídeo.

che·mo·re·sis·tance (kem′ō-rē-zis′tans, kē′mō-). Quimiorresistência; a resistência de bactérias ou células malignas à ação inibidora de determinadas substâncias químicas usadas no tratamento.

che·mo·re·sponse (kē-mō-rē-sponz′). Quimiorresposta; reação à estimulação química.

che·mo·sen·sa·tion (kē-mō-sen-sā′shun). Quimiopercepção. SIN chemoreception.

che·mo·sen·si·tive (kem-ō-sen′si-tiv, kē-mō-). Quimiossensível; capaz de perceber alterações na composição química do ambiente, p. ex., alterações no conteúdo de oxigênio e dióxido de carbono do sangue.

che·mo·se·ro·ther·a·py (kem′ō-sē-r′ō-thār-ă-pē, kē′mō-). Quimiossoroterapia; tratamento obsoleto de doença com uma combinação de drogas e soro.

che·mo·sis (kē-mō′sis). Quemose; edema da conjuntiva ocular, formando uma tumefação ao redor da córnea. [G. *chēmē*, um bocejo, a amêijoa (de sua concha aberta)]

chem·os·mo·sis (kem-os-mō′sis). Quimiosmose; reação química entre substâncias inicialmente separadas por uma membrana. [chem- + G. *ōsmos*, empurrão, impulso]

che·mo·stat (kem′ō-stat). Quimiostato; fermentador para crescimento microbiano no qual a razão entre o crescimento e a síntese de produtos secundários é controlada pela velocidade com que se adiciona um novo meio à cultura.

che·mo·sur·gery (kem′ō-ser-jer-ē, kē′mō-). Quimiocirurgia; excisão de tecido doente após ter sido fixado *in situ* por meios químicos.
Mohs c., q. de Mohs; técnica para remoção de tumores cutâneos com um mínimo de tecido normal, por necrose prévia com pasta de cloreto de zinco, mapeamento do local tumoral e excisão e exame microscópico de corte por congelamento de camadas horizontais de tecido, até que todo o tumor seja removido. Recentemente, a etapa preliminar de necrose química foi omitida. SIN microscopically controlled surgery, Mohs micrographic surgery, Mohs surgery.

che·mo·syn·the·sis (ke-m′ō-sin′thĕ-sis). Quimiossíntese. 1. Síntese química. 2. Quimiolitotrofia.

che·mo·tac·tic (kē-mō-tak′tik). Quimiotático; relativo à quimiotaxia.

che·mo·tax·is (kē-mō-tak′sis). Quimiotaxia. 1. Movimento de células ou organismos em resposta a substâncias químicas, pelo qual as células são atraídas (**quimiotaxia positiva**) ou repelidas (**quimiotaxia negativa**) por substâncias que possuem propriedades químicas. 2. A migração de leucócitos polimorfonucleares e macrófagos em direção a maiores concentrações de determinados fragmentos de complemento. SIN chemotaxis, chemotropism. [chemo- + G. *taxis*, arranjo ordenado]

che·mo·thal·a·mec·to·my (kem′ō-thal-ă-mek′tō-mē, kē′mō-). Quimiotalamectomia; destruição química de uma parte do tálamo, geralmente para alívio de dor ou discinesia. SIN chemothalamotomy. [chemo- + thalamus, + G. *ektomē*, excisão]

che·mo·thal·a·mot·o·my (kem′ō-thal-ă-mot′ō-mē, kē′mō-). Quimiotalamotomia. SIN chemothalamectomy.

che·mo·ther·a·peu·tic (kem′ō-thār-ă-pū′tik, kē′mō-). Quimioterapêutico; relativo à quimioterapia.

che·mo·ther·a·peu·tics (kem′ō-thār-ă-pū′tiks, kē′mō-). Quimioterapêutica; o ramo da terapêutica relacionado à quimioterapia.

che·mo·ther·a·py (kem′ō-thār-ă-pē, kē′mō-). Quimioterapia; tratamento de doença por meio de substâncias químicas ou drogas; geralmente usada em referência à doença neoplásica. VER TAMBÉM pharmacotherapy.
adjuvant c., q. adjuvante; q. administrada além do tratamento cirúrgico, a fim de reduzir o risco de recidiva local ou sistêmica.
combination c., poliquimioterapia; q. com mais de um fármaco, para tirar benefício de suas diferentes toxicidades.
consolidation c., q. de consolidação; ciclos repetitivos de tratamento durante o período pós-remissão imediato, usado principalmente para leucemia. SIN intensification c.
cytostatic c., q. citostática; q. que não permite proliferação de células tumorais, mas pode não destruir as células.
cytotoxic c., q. citotóxica; q. elaborada para destruir células tumorais.
induction c., q. de indução; uso da q. como medida inicial antes da cirurgia ou irradiação para tratamento de uma neoplasia maligna.
intensification c., q. de intensificação. SIN consolidation c.
salvage c., q. de salvamento; uso de q. em um paciente com recorrência de uma neoplasia maligna após tratamento inicial, na esperança de obter cura ou prolongar a vida. SIN salvage therapy.

che·mot·ic (kē-mot′ik). Quemótico; relativo a quemose.

che·mo·trans·mit·ter (kem-ō-trans′mit-er, kē-mō-). Quimiotransmissor; substância química produzida para se difundir através do espaço entre as células (sinapse) e causar respostas de neurônios ou células efetoras.

che·mo·troph (ke-mō-trōf). Quimiótrofo; organismo que obtém sua energia pela oxidação de nutrientes inorgânicos ou orgânicos (isto é, fontes químicas exógenas).

che·mot·ro·pism (kē-mot′rō-pi-zŭm). Quimiotropismo. SIN chemotaxis. [chemo- + G. *tropos*, direção, curso]

Chenais, Louis J., médico francês, 1872–1950. VER Cestan-C. *syndrome*.

Cheney, William D., radiologista norte-americano, *1918. VER C. *syndrome*.

che·no·de·ox·y·cho·lic ac·id (kē′nō-dē-oks-ē-kō′lik). Ácido quenodesoxicólico; importante ácido biliar em muitos vertebrados, geralmente conjugado à glicina ou taurina, que facilita a excreção de colesterol e a absorção de gordura; administrado para dissolver cálculos de colesterol. SIN chenodiol.

che·no·di·ol (kē-nō-dī′ol). Quenodiol. SIN chenodeoxycholic acid.

che·no·po·di·um (kē-nō-pō′dē-ŭm). Quenopódio; o fruto maduro seco do *Chenopodium ambrosoides* (família Chenopodiaceae), ambrósia-do-méxico, do qual se destila um óleo volátil usado como anti-helmíntico. SIN Jesuit tea, Mexican tea, wormseed (2). (G. *chēn*, ganso, + *pous* (*poud*-), pé]

Cherenkov, VER Cerenkov.

cher·ry juice (chăr′ē). Suco de cereja; o suco extraído do fruto fresco maduro do *Prunus cerasus*, contendo não menos de 1,0% de ácido málico; usado como agente aromatizante e como veículo para xaropes antitussígenos e outros preparados para administração oral.

che·rub·ism (che-r′ŭb-izm) [MIM*118400]. Querubismo; lesões hereditárias de células gigantes da mandíbula e maxilar, que surgem nos primeiros anos de vida; radiotransparências multiloculares e tumefação indolor simétrica progressiva da mandíbula e maxilar; bilateral; não há manifestações sistêmicas associadas. SIN fibrous dysplasia of jaws. [Hebr. *kerubh*, querubim]

chest. Tórax; peito; a parede anterior do tórax. VER TAMBÉM thorax. SIN pectus. [A.S. *cest*, caixa]
alar c., t. alar. SIN flat c.
barrel c., t. em tonel; tórax com formato permanente semelhante ao de um tonel, isto é, com aumento do diâmetro ântero-posterior, que é quase igual ao diâmetro lateral; geralmente com algum grau de cifose; observado em casos de enfisema.
flail c., t. instável; perda da estabilidade da caixa torácica após fratura do esterno e/ou das costelas; pode causar insuficiência respiratória.
flat c., t. plano; t. chato; tórax no qual o diâmetro ântero-posterior é menor que a média. SIN alar c., pterygoid c.
foveated c., funnel c., t. em funil. SIN *pectus* excavatum.
keeled c., t. em quilha. SIN *pectus* carinatum.
phthinoid c., t. ftinóide; t. tisicóide; um tórax estreito e longo, sendo as costelas inferiores mais oblíquas que o habitual, algumas vezes chegando quase até a crista do ílio, com as escápulas projetando-se para trás, o manúbrio esternal deprimido e o ângulo de Louis mais agudo que o normal; já foi considerado indicativo de tuberculose pulmonar.
pigeon c., t. de pombo. SIN *pectus* carinatum.
pterygoid c., t. pterigóide. SIN flat c.

Cheyne, John, médico escocês, 1777–1836. VER C.-Stokes *psychosis, respiration*.

chi (kī). Qui. 1. A 22.ª letra do alfabeto grego, χ. 2. Em química, designa o 22.º em uma série. 3. Símbolo para o ângulo diédrico entre o carbono α e as cadeias laterais de aminoácidos nos peptídeos e proteínas.

Chiari, Johann B., obstetra alemão, 1817–1854. VER C.-Frommel *syndrome*.

Chiari, Hans, patologista alemão, 1851–1916. VER Arnold-C. *deformity, malformation, syndrome*; C. *disease, net, syndrome,* II *syndrome*; C.-Budd *syndrome*; Budd-C. *syndrome*.

chi·asm (kī′azm). Quiasma. 1. Uma intersecção ou cruzamento de duas linhas. 2. [TA] Em anatomia, decussação ou cruzamento de dois feixes fibrosos, como tendões, nervos ou tratos. 3. Em citogenética, o local no qual dois cromossomas homólogos fazem contato (assim parecendo estar cruzados), permitindo a troca de material genético durante o estágio de prófase da meiose. SIN chiasma [TA]. [G. *chiasma*]
Camper c., q. de Camper. SIN tendinous c. of the digital tendons.
optic c. [TA], q. óptico; corpo quadrangular achatado na frente do túber cinéreo e infundíbulo, o ponto de cruzamento ou decussação dos axônios dos nervos ópticos; os axônios provenientes da retina nasal cruzam para o lado oposto, enquanto os axônios provenientes da retina temporal seguem diretamente em sentido caudal sem cruzar; alguns seguem transversalmente sobre a superfície posterior entre os dois tratos ópticos e outros seguem transversalmente sobre a superfície anterior entre os dois nervos ópticos. SIN chiasma opticum [TA], optic decussation.
tendinous c. of the digitasl tendons [TA], q. tendíneo dos tendões digitais; cruzamento dos tendões, a passagem dos tendões do músculo flexor profundo dos dedos (flexor longo dos dedos no pé) através do espaço deixado pela decussação das fibras dos tendões do flexor superficial dos dedos (flexor curto dos dedos no pé). SIN chiasma tendinum [TA], Camper c.

chi·as·ma, pl. **chi·as·ma·ta** (kī-az′mă, kī-az′mă-tă). [TA]. Quiasma. SIN chiasm. [G. *chiasma*, duas linhas que se cruzam, da letra *qui*, 3]
c. op′ticum [TA], q. óptico. SIN optic *chiasm*.

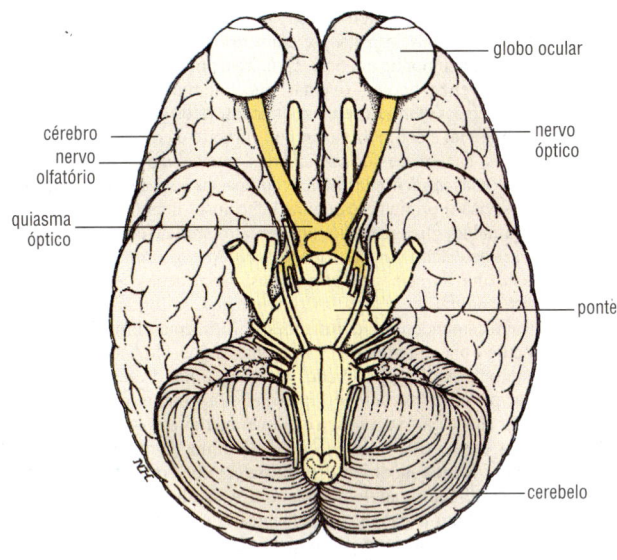

quiasma óptico

c. ten'dinum [TA], q. tendíneo. SIN tendinous *chiasm of the digital tendons*.
chi·as·ma·pexy (ki̅-as'mă-pek-se̅). Quiasmapexia; fixação cirúrgica do quiasma óptico. [G. *chiasma*, decussação, + *pēxis*, fixação]
chi·as·mat·ic (ki̅-az-mat'ik). Quiasmático; relativo a um quiasma.
chick·en·pox (chik'en-poks). Varicela; catapora. SIN varicella.
Chick-Martin test. Prova de Chick-Martin. Ver em test.
chi·cle (chik'el). Chicle. **1.** O suco leitoso, viscoso, parcialmente evaporado da *Manilkara zapotilla* (sapotácea), originária do oeste da Índia, México e América Central. **2.** Mistura de guta com álcoois triterpênicos. Usada na fabricação da goma de mascar. [Esp., do Nahuatl *chictli*]
Chievitz, Johan H., anatomista dinamarquês, 1850–1901. VER C. *layer, organ.*
chig·ger (chig'er). Ácaro trombiculídeo; larva de seis pernas das espécies de *Trombicula* e outros membros da família Trombiculidae; um estágio hematófago de ácaros que inclui os vetores da febre tsutsugamushi (tifo tropical).
chig·oe (chig'o̅). Bicho-do-pé; nome comum da *Tunga penetrans.*
chil-. VER chilo-.
Chilaiditi, Demetrius, radiologista austríaco, *1883. VER C. *syndrome.*
chil·blain (chil'bla̅n). Pérnio; eritema, prurido e queimação, principalmente nos dorsos dos quirodáctilos e pododáctilos, e nos calcanhares, nariz e orelhas, causados por constricção vascular pela exposição ao frio extremo (geralmente associado à umidade elevada); as lesões podem ser isoladas ou múltiplas e tornar-se vesiculares e ulceradas. SIN erythema pernio, perniosis. [chill + A.S. *blegen*, bolha]
CHILD VER CHILD *syndrome.*
child·bear·ing (chi̅ld'ba̅r-ing). Gravidez e parto.
child·birth (chi̅ld'berth). Parto; o processo de trabalho de parto e nascimento de uma criança. VER TAMBÉM birth, accouchement. SIN parturition.
child·hood (chi̅ld'hud). Infância; o período de vida entre a lactância e a puberdade.
chill. Calafrio. **1.** Sensação de frio. **2.** Sensação de frio com tremores e palidez, acompanhada por elevação da temperatura no interior do corpo; geralmente um sintoma de doença infecciosa devido à invasão do sangue por toxinas. SIN rigor (2). [A.S. *cele*, frio]
smelter's c.'s, calafrios do fundidor. SIN smelter's *fever.*
chilo-, chil-. Quilo-, quil-; lábios. VER TAMBÉM cheilo-. [G. *cheilos*, lábio]
chi·lo·mas·ti·gi·a·sis (ki̅'lo̅-mas-ti-gi̅'ă-sis). Quilomastigíase; quilomastose; infestação pelos protozoários flagelados do gênero *Chilomastix*, como *C. mesnili* do ceco humano. SIN chilomastosis.
Chi·lo·mas·tix (ki̅-lo̅-mas'tiks). Gênero de protozoários flagelados parasitas do intestino grosso do homem e outros primatas, e em muitos outros mamíferos, aves, anfíbios e répteis; comumente não é patogênico, mas uma espécie, *C. mesnili*, pode ser causa ocasional de diarréia em crianças. [chilo- + G. *mastix*, chicote]
chi·lo·mas·to·sis (ki̅'lo̅-mas-to̅'sis). Quilomastose. SIN chilomastigiasis.
Chi·lo·po·da (ki̅-lop'o̅-dă). Classe de centípedes (filo Arthropoda). [chilo- + G. *pous*, pé]
chi·lo·po·di·a·sis (ki̅'lo̅-po̅-di̅'ă-sis). Quilopodíase; invasão de uma das cavidades, principalmente a cavidade nasal, por uma espécie de Chilopoda.
chi·me·ra (ki̅-me̅r'ă, ki̅-). Quimera. **1.** Em embriologia experimental, o indivíduo produzido por enxerto de uma parte embrionária de um animal no embrião de outro, seja da mesma espécie ou de outra. **2.** Organismo que recebeu um transplante de tecido genética e imunologicamente diferente, como a medula óssea. **3.** Gêmeos dizigóticos que possuem tipos imunologicamente distintos de eritrócitos. **4.** Fusão proteica na qual duas proteínas diferentes são unidas por ligações peptídicas; geralmente produzida por engenharia genética. Os anticorpos quiméricos podem ter o fragmento Fab de uma espécie fundido ao fragmento Fc de outra. **5.** Qualquer fusão de macromolécula formada por duas ou mais macromoléculas de diferentes espécies ou de diferentes genes. [L. *Chimaera*, G. *Chimaira*, monstro mitológico (lit. uma cabra)]
radiation c., q. de radiação; indivíduo que foi submetido a irradiação corporal total a fim de reduzir a resposta imune contra células de doador e, portanto, possui as características imunológicas do hospedeiro e do doador após um enxerto de medula óssea de doador antigenicamente diferente.
chi·mer·ic (ki̅-me̅r'ik). Quimérico. **1.** Relativo a uma quimera. Cf. mosaicism. **2.** Composto de parte de origem diferente e aparentemente incompatíveis.
chi·me·rism (ki̅-me̅'r'izm). Quimerismo; o estado de ser uma quimera.
chim·pan·zee (chim-pan'ze̅, chim'pan-ze̅'). Chimpanzé; nome genérico dos macacos *Pan panisus* e *P. troglodytes*. [Dialeto africano.]
chin [TA]. Queixo; mento; a proeminência formada pela projeção anterior da mandíbula. SIN mentum [TA]. [A.S. *cin*]
double c., q. duplo. SIN buccula.
chi·ni·o·fon (ki-ni̅'e̅-o̅-fon). Quiniofon; mistura de ácido 7-iodo-8-hidroxi-quinolina-5-sulfônico e bicarbonato de sódio, usada no tratamento da disenteria amebiana.
chin·o·le·ine (chin'o̅-le̅-in). Quinoleína. SIN quinoline (1).
chip. Lasca; pequeno fragmento resultante de fratura, corte ou avulsão.
bone c.'s, lascas de osso; pequenos pedaços de osso esponjoso geralmente usados para preencher defeitos ósseos e promover reossificação.
chip-blow·er. Soprador de fragmentos; instrumento para soprar detritos ou secar uma cavidade dentária que está sendo escavada para obturação; consiste em um bulbo de borracha com bico metálico.
chi·ral (ki̅'ral). Designa um objeto, como uma molécula em uma determinada configuração ou conformação, que possui quiralidade. Uma molécula quiral não tem plano, eixo, nem centro de simetria.
chi·ral·i·ty (ki̅-ral'i-te̅). Quiralidade; a propriedade de não-superposição de um objeto com sua imagem especular; usado em química em relação aos isômeros estereoquímicos. [G. *cheir*, mão]
chi·rar·thri·tis (ki̅-rar-thri̅'tis). Quirartrite. SIN cheirarthritis.
chiro-, chir-. Quiro; a mão. VER TAMBÉM cheiro-. [G. *cheir*, mão]
chi·rog·nos·tic (ki̅-rog-nos'tik). Quirognóstico. SIN cheirognostic.
chi·ro·kin·es·the·sia (ki̅-ro̅-kin-es-the̅'ze̅-ă). Quirocinestesia. SIN cheirokinesthesia.
chi·ro·po·dal·gia (ki̅'ro̅-po̅-dal'je̅-ă). Quiropodalgia. SIN cheiropodalgia.
chi·rop·o·dist (ki̅'rop'o̅-dist). Quiropodista. SIN podiatrist. [chiro- + G. *pous*, pé]
chi·rop·o·dy (ki̅-rop'o̅-de̅). Quiropodia. SIN podiatry.
chi·ro·pom·pho·lyx (ki̅-ro̅-pom'fo̅-liks). Quiroponfólix. SIN dyshidrosis.
chi·ro·prac·tic (ki̅-ro̅-prak'tik). Quiroprático; sistema que, teoricamente, utiliza as forças de recuperação do corpo e a relação entre as estruturas músculo-esqueléticas e as funções do corpo, particularmente da coluna vertebral e do sistema nervoso, na restauração e manutenção da saúde. [chiro- + G. *praktikos*, eficiente]
chi·ro·prac·tor (ki̅-ro̅-prak'to̅r). Quiroprático; pessoa autorizada e diplomada para exercer a quiroprática.
Chiropsalmus. Gênero do filo invertebrado Cnidaria que inclui a vespa-do-mar.
C. quadrumanus, vespa-do-mar, a água-viva (medusa) mais venenosa que habita a costa dos Estados Unidos. VER TAMBÉM jellyfish. SIN box jelly, sea wasp.
Chi·rop·te·ra (ki̅-rop'ter-ă). Os morcegos, uma ordem de mamíferos placentários com distribuição mundial, caracterizada por uma modificação das patas anteriores que permite seu vôo. Podem emitir ultra-sons, que possibilita o seu deslocamento pelo eco, o encontro de insetos voadores e o afastamento de objetos no escuro. Embora a maioria seja insetívora, algumas espécies alimentam-se de néctar, frutas, peixes e sangue; as espécies hematófagas e insetívoras são importantes hospedeiros reservatórios de raiva. [chiro- + G. *pteron*, asa]
chi·ro·scope (ki̅'ro̅-sko̅p). Quiroscópio; instrumento haploscópico usado para coordenar mão e olho enquanto o paciente desenha; usado para treinamento da visão binocular. [chiro- + G. *skopeō*, ver]
chi·ro·spasm (ki̅'ro̅-spazm). Quiroespasmo. SIN cheirospasm.
chirurg. Abreviatura do L. *chirurgicalis*, cirúrgico.
chi·rur·geon (ki̅-rer'jon). Termo obsoleto para cirurgião. [G. *cheirourgos*, de *cheir*, mão, + *ergon*, trabalho]
chi·rur·gery (ki̅-rer'jer-e̅). Termo obsoleto para cirurgia. [G. *cheirourgia*]
chi·rur·gi·cal (ki̅-rer'ji-kăl). Termo obsoleto para cirúrgico. [L. *surgical*, de *chirurgia*, cirurgia, do G. *cheirourgia*, artesanato, de *cheir*, mão + *ergon*, trabalho]

chis·el (chiz′l). Cinzel; lâmina de extremidade cortante, com bisel único, com haste reta ou angulada, usada com pressão longitudinal ao longo do eixo do cabo para cortar ou separar a dentina e o esmalte.

   binangle c., c. biangulado; c. com haste angulada à qual se acrescenta um segundo ângulo a fim de colocar a borda cortante quase alinhada com o eixo do cabo, de forma a restabelecer o equilíbrio e evitar que gire em torno do eixo; usado quando é necessário angular o cinzel para se ter acesso.

chi-square (kī′skwār). Qui-quadrado; técnica estatística pela qual as variáveis são classificadas a fim de determinar se uma distribuição de escores é devida ao acaso ou a fatores experimentais.

chi·tin (kī′tin). Quitina; polímero linear de *N*-acetil-D-glucosamina, ligação β(1→4), com estrutura semelhante à da celulose e o segundo polissacarídeo mais abundante na natureza, sendo um componente da substância córnea no exoesqueleto de besouros, caranguejos, determinados microrganismos, etc., bem como em alguns vegetais e fungos.

chi·ti·nase (kī′ti-nās). Quitinase; enzima que catalisa a hidrólise aleatória de ligações β(1→4) na quitina (finalmente liberando *N*-acetil-D-glucosamina; algumas enzimas desse tipo exibem atividade de lisozima. SIN poly-β-glucosaminidase.

chi·tin·ous (kī′tin-us). Quitinoso; de, ou relativo à, quitina.

chi·to·bi·ose (kī′tō-bī′ōs). Quitobiose; unidade dissacarídica de repetição na quitina; difere da celobiose apenas pela presença de um grupamento *N*-acetilamino no carbono-2 no lugar do grupo hidroxila. Entretanto, a forma não-acetilada também é denominada quitobiose.

chi·to·sa·mine (kī-tō′sa-mēn). Quitosamina; D-glucosamina. VER glucosamine.

chi·u·fa (chē-oo′fä). Proctite e colite gangrenosa aguda, com febre alta, observada no sul da África e na América do Sul em grandes altitudes; em mulheres, pode haver acometimento da vulva e da vagina. SIN kanyemba.

CHL Abreviatura de crown-heel *length* (comprimento cabeça-tornozelo).

Chla·myd·ia (kla-mid′ē-ä). O único gênero da família Chlamydiaceae, incluindo todos os agentes dos grupos da psitacose–linfogranuloma–tracoma; as clamídias são bactérias esféricas ou ovóides, obrigatoriamente intracelulares, com um ciclo vital intracelular complexo; a forma infecciosa é o corpúsculo elementar, que penetra na célula do hospedeiro, multiplicando-se como o corpúsculo reticulado por fissão binária; a multiplicação ocorre em um vacúolo denominado corpúsculo de inclusão; a clamídia não possui peptidoglicana em suas paredes celulares; a espécie típica é *C. trachomatis*. Anteriormente denominada *Betsonia*. SIN *Chlamydozoon*. [G. *chlamys*, manto]

   C. pneumo'niae, espécie de bactéria isolada pela primeira vez em 1986 e atualmente reconhecida como uma causa comum de pneumonia, bronquite, rinossinusite e faringite em adultos e crianças. SIN TWAR.

   A *Chlamydia pneumoniae* é responsável por cerca de 25% dos casos de bronquite aguda e 10% dos casos de pneumonia adquirida na comunidade. Estudos recentes sugeriram que também pode participar na gênese da doença cardiovascular e da demência de Alzheimer de início tardio. Como a *C. trachomatis* e a *C. psittaci*, esse microrganismo algumas vezes causa miocardite e endocardite. Níveis elevados de anticorpos contra *C. pneumoniae* são encontrados em pessoas com infarto do miocárdio (IAM) e em pessoas que exibem formação significativa de ateroma à necrópsia, com freqüência significativamente maior que em grupos de controle. O microrganismo foi detectado por imunocitoquímica, reação da cadeia da polimerase e microscopia eletrônica em macrófagos e células musculares lisas de placas ateromatosas da aorta, artérias coronárias e artérias carótidas (amostras cirúrgicas e de necrópsia), mas não em artérias normais. A incidência de infecção aguda em pacientes com IAM, detectada por cultura da orofaringe, é maior que na população em geral. Uma revisão retrospectiva dos prontuários de pessoas com infarto agudo do miocárdio mostrou que era menor a probabilidade, em relação aos controles, de que tivessem sido tratados durante os 3 anos anteriores com tetraciclina ou quinolona, antibióticos ativos contra *C. pneumoniae*. Entretanto, até hoje os estudos prospectivos não mostraram associação entre a presença de anticorpo IgG contra *C. pneumoniae* e um aumento do risco de doença aterotrombótica. Os pesquisadores especularam que a infecção por *C. pneumoniae* pode ser um dos vários fatores capazes de iniciar alterações que culminam em aterosclerose, ou que a reinfecção pode deflagrar aterotrombose coronariana. Anticorpos contra *C. pneumoniae* também são encontrados em pessoas com hipertensão grave com incidência duas vezes maior que na população em geral. Além disso, o organismo foi detectado com freqüência muito maior na micróglia e astróglia do hipocampo e do córtex temporal em pessoas com doença de Alzheimer de início tardio que em cérebros normais.

   C. psi'ttaci, microrganismos bacterianos semelhantes à *C. trachomatis*, mas que formam microcolônias intracitoplasmáticas frouxamente unidas com até 12 μm de diâmetro, não produzem glicogênio em quantidade suficiente para ser detectado por corantes de iodo e não são suscetíveis à sulfadiazina. Várias cepas dessa espécie causam psitacose em seres humanos e ornitose em aves não-psitacídeas; pneumonite em bois, carneiros, porcos, gatos, cabras e cavalos; abortamento enzoótico em ovelhas; encefalomielite bovina esporádica, enterite em bezerros; clamidiose epizoótica em ratos almiscarados e lebres; encefalite no gambá; e conjuntivite no boi, carneiro e cobaia.

   C. tracho'matis, bactérias esféricas, imóveis, intracelulares obrigatórias; formam microcolônias intracitoplasmáticas compactas com até 10 μm de diâmetro que (por divisão) originam esférulas infecciosas com 0,3 μm ou mais de diâmetro, acumulam glicogênio por um período limitado em quantidade suficiente para ser detectado por coloração com iodo e, geralmente, são suscetíveis à sulfadiazina, tetraciclina e quinolonas; várias cepas dessa espécie causam tracoma, conjuntivite de inclusão e neonatal, linfogranuloma venéreo, pneumonite em camundongos, uretrite inespecífica, epididimite, cervicite, salpingite, proctite e pneumonia; principal agente de doenças bacterianas sexualmente transmitidas nos Estados Unidos; a espécie típica do gênero *Chlamydia*.

chla·myd·ia, pl. **chla·myd·i·ae** (kla-mid′ē-ä, -mid′ē-ē). Clamídia; termo vernacular usado para se referir a qualquer membro do gênero *Chlamydia*.

Chlam·y·di·a·ce·ae (kla-mid′ē-ā′sē-ē). Família da ordem Chlamydiales (anteriormente incluída na ordem Rickettsiales) que compreende os agentes do grupo psitacose–linfogranuloma–tracoma. A família contém pequenas bactérias cocóides, Gram-negativas, semelhantes às riquétsias, mas que diferem destas significativamente por possuírem um ciclo singular de desenvolvimento obrigatoriamente intracelular; as microcolônias intracitoplasmáticas dão origem a formas infecciosas por divisão. A classificação desses microrganismos anteriormente esteve em estado de mudança, mas agora eles pertencem a um único gênero, *Chlamydia*, o gênero típico da família.

chla·myd·i·al (kla-mid′ē-äl). Clamidial; relativo a, ou causado por, qualquer bactéria do gênero *Chlamydia*.

chla·myd·i·o·sis (klä-mid-ē-ō′sis). Clamidiose; termo geral para doenças causadas por espécies de *Chlamydia*. VER TAMBÉM ornithosis, psittacosis.

chlam·y·do·co·nid·i·um (klam′i-dō-kō-nid′ē-um). Clamidoconídio; conídio tálico que tem parede espessa e pode ser terminal ou intercalar. Observado em uma forma de reprodução assexuada. [G. *chlamys*, manto + conidium]

Chlam·y·do·phrys (kla-mid′ō-fris). Gênero de amebas encapsuladas, comumente encontradas como protozoários fecais. [G. *chlamys*, manto, + *ophrys*, cume]

Chlam·y·do·zo·on (klam′i-dō-zō′on). SIN *Chlamydia.*

chlo·as·ma (klō-az′mä). Cloasma; melanoderma ou melasma caracterizado pela ocorrência de extensas manchas castanhas, de formato e tamanho irregulares, na pele da face e de outros locais; as manchas faciais pigmentadas, se confluentes, também são denominadas máscara da gravidez e, na maioria das vezes, estão associadas à gravidez e ao uso de contraceptivos orais. VER TAMBÉM melasma. [[G. *chloazō*, tornar-se verde]

   c. bronzi'num, c. bronzeado; pigmentação cor de bronze, provavelmente produzida por desequilíbrio hormonal, que ocorre em áreas cada vez maiores na face, pescoço e tórax em pessoas expostas continuamente ao sol tropical; semelhante ao cloasma da zona temperada, mas intensificada devido à forte luz solar. SIN tropical mask.

chlo·phe·di·a·nol hy·dro·chlo·ride (klō-fē-dī′ä-nol). Cloridrato de clofedianol; agente antitussígeno quimicamente relacionado aos anti-histamínicos.

chlor-, chloro-. Clor-, cloro-. **1.** Forma combinante que significa verde. **2.** Forma combinante que indica associação com cloro. [G. *chloros*, verde]

chlor·a·ce·tic ac·id (klōr-ä-sē′tik). Ácido cloroacético. SIN chloroacetic acid.

chlor·ac·ne (klōr-ak′nē). Cloracne; erupção semelhante à acne causada por contato ocupacional, por inalação, ingestão ou através da pele, com determinadas substâncias cloradas (naftalenos e difenis) usadas como isolantes, inseticidas, fungicidas e herbicidas, incluindo o Agente Laranja; tampões ceratinosos (comedões) se formam nos orifícios pilossebáceos, e desenvolvem-se pápulas pequenas de tamanhos variados (2 a 4 mm). SIN tar acne.

chlo·ral (klōr′äl). Cloral; líquido oleoso fino com odor picante, formado pela ação do gás cloro sobre o álcool. SIN anhydrous c.

   anhydrous c., c. anidro. SIN chloral.

   c. betaine, c. betaína; o produto formado pelo hidrato de cloral e betaína; é lentamente hidrolisado no trato alimentar em hidrato de cloral; usado como hipnótico e sedativo.

   c. hydrate, hidrato de cloral; hipnótico, sedativo e anticonvulsivante; também é usado externamente como rubefaciente, anestésico e anti-séptico.

***m*-chlo·ral.** *m*-cloral; polímero do cloral obtido por contato prolongado com ácido sulfúrico; possui propriedades semelhantes às do hidrato de cloral. SIN metachloral, *p*-chloral, trichloral.

***p*-chlo·ral.** *p*-cloral. SIN *m*-chloral.

chlo·ral al·co·hol·ate. Alcoolato de cloral; complexo de cloral e etanol. Preparado por refluxo do tricloroacetaldeído (cloral) ou hidrato de cloral com álcool. Supostamente um constituinte ativo de uma "bebida batizada".

chlo·ral·ism (klōr′äl-izm). Cloralismo; uso habitual de compostos cloral como intoxicante, ou os sintomas conseqüentemente produzidos.

α-chlor·a·lose (klōr'ă-lōs). α-cloralose; conjugado de cloral e glicose usado como anestésico em animais de laboratório; não deprime tanto os reflexos cardiovasculares como a maioria dos outros agentes anestésicos.

chlor·am·bu·cil (klōr-am'bū-sil). Clorambucil; derivado da mostarda nitrogenada que deprime a proliferação e a maturação dos linfócitos. SIN chloraminophene, chloroambucil.

chlo·ra·mine B (klōr'ă-mēn). Cloramina B; substância anti-séptica atóxica usada na irrigação de feridas como substituto da cloramina T.

chlo·ra·mine T. Cloramina T; anti-séptico atóxico, porém forte, usado na irrigação de feridas e cavidades infectadas. SIN chlorazene.

chlor·am·i·no·phene (klōr-am'i-nō-fēn). Cloraminofeno. SIN chlorambucil.

chlor·am·i·phene (klōr-am'i-fēn). Cloramifeno. SIN clomiphene citrate.

chlor·am·phen·i·col (klōr-am-fen'i-kol). Cloranfenicol; antibiótico originalmente obtido do *Streptomyces venezuelae*. É efetivo contra vários microrganismos patogênicos, incluindo *Staphylococcus aureus, Brucella abortus*, bacilo de Friedländer e os microrganismos da febre tifóide, tifo e da febre maculosa das Montanhas Rochosas; ativo por via oral. Pode haver uma reação grave, resultando em lesão da medula óssea, com agranulocitose ou anemia aplásica. A síndrome do bebê cinzento pode ocorrer em recém-nascidos devido à ausência de glucoroniltransferase necessária para metabolizar o cloranfenicol.

c. acetyl transferase (CAT), c. acetiltransferase; enzima bacteriana freqüentemente usada como marcador para examinar o controle da expressão de genes eucarióticos.

c. palmitate, palmitato de cloranfenicol; mesma ação e uso do cloranfenicol; foi amplamente usado em suspensão para injeções pediátricas.

c. sodium succinate, succinato sódico de cloranfenicol; o derivado succinato sódico hidrossolúvel do cloranfenicol, adequado para administração parenteral; a atividade antibacteriana, os empregos e os efeitos colaterais são semelhantes aos da substância original.

chlo·rate (klō'āt). Clorato; sal do ácido clórico.

chlo·raz·a·nil (klō-raz'ă-nil). Clorazanil; um diurético.

chlo·ra·zene (klō'ră-zēn). Clorazeno. SIN chloramine T.

chlo·ra·zol black E (klor'ă-zol) [C.I. 30235]. Clorazol negro E; corante ácido, usado como corante para gordura e tecidos em geral, bem como para corar protozoários em esfregaços fecais ou em tecidos.

chlor·ben·zox·a·mine (klōr-ben-zok'să-mēn). Clorbenzoxamina; agente anticolinérgico. SIN chlorbenzoxyethamine.

chlor·ben·zox·y·eth·a·mine (klōr'ben-zok-sē-eth'ă-mēn). Clorbenzoxietamina. SIN chlorbenzoxamine.

chlor·bet·a·mide (klōr-bet'ă-mīd). Clorbetamida; um amebicida.

chlor·bu·tol (klōr-bū'tol). Clorbutol. SIN chlorobutanol.

chlor·cy·cli·zine hy·dro·chlo·ride (klōr-sik'li-zēn). Cloridrato de clorciclizina; um agente anti-histamínico H₁.

chlor·dane (klōr-dān). Clordano; hidrocarboneto clorado usado como inseticida; pode ser absorvido através da pele, com conseqüentes efeitos tóxicos graves: hiperexcitabilidade do sistema nervoso central, tremores, ausência de coordenação muscular, convulsões e morte; também causa lesão do fígado, rins e baço. É apenas levemente tóxico para animais.

chlor·dan·to·in (klōr-dan'tō-in). Clordantoína; um agente antifúngico tópico.

chlor·di·az·e·pox·ide hy·dro·chlo·ride (klōr'dī-az-ē-pok'sīd). Cloridrato de clordiazepóxido; o cloridrato de 7-cloro-2-metilamino-5-fenil-3*H*-1,4-benzodiazepina-4-óxido; ansiolítico. Um benzodiazepínico antigo.

chlor·e·mia (klōr-ē'mē-ă). Cloremia. **1.** SIN chlorosis. **2.** SIN hyperchloremia.

chlor·eth·ene ho·mo·pol·y·mer (klōr'eth-ēn). Homopolímero de cloreteno. SIN polyvinyl chloride.

chlor·gua·nide hy·dro·chlo·ride (klōr-gwah'nīd). Cloridrato de clorguanida. SIN chloroguanide hydrochloride.

chlor·hex·i·dine hy·dro·chlo·ride (klōr-hek'si-dēn). Cloridrato de clorexidina; um anti-séptico tópico.

chlor·hy·dria (klōr-hī'drē-ă). Cloridria. SIN hyperchlorhydria.

chlor·ic ac·id (klōr'ik). Ácido clórico; ácido de cloro pentavalente, HClO₃, existindo apenas em solução e como cloratos.

chlo·ride (klō'rīd). Cloreto; composto contendo cloro, em uma valência de −1, como nos sais do ácido clorídrico.

carbamylcholine c., c. de carbamilcolina; cloreto colinomimético que reage com os receptores muscarínicos e nicotínicos, ativando-os. É lentamente hidrolisado e, assim, seus efeitos são muito mais duradouros que os da acetilcolina. Usado clinicamente para estimular o músculo liso, como no íleo paralítico após a cirurgia.

chlor·i·dim·e·try (klōr-i-dim'e-trē). Cloridimetria; o processo de determinar a quantidade de cloretos no sangue ou na urina, ou em outros líquidos.

chlor·i·dom·e·ter (klōr-i-dom'e-ter). Cloridômetro; aparelho para determinar a quantidade de cloretos no sangue ou na urina, ou em outros líquidos.

chlor·i·du·ria (klōr-i-doo'rē-ă). Cloridúria. SIN chloruresis.

chlo·rin (klōr'in). Clorina; 2,3-diidroporfirina; 2,3-diidroporfirina; uma das estruturas básicas das clorofilas (para estrutura, ver porfirina). A adição da ponte de dois carbonos (ver estrutura da clorofila) à clorina produz forbina; a adição de cadeias laterais produz as forbidas, distinguidas por vários prefixos arbitrários (aqueles encontrados nas clorofilas são feo- e bacteriofeoforbida); a esterificação do grupo propiônico pelo fitil fornece as respectivas fitinas, e a adição de magnésio produz as clorofilas (fitinatos de magnésio). VER porphyrins.

chlo·ri·nat·ed (klōr'in-āt-ed). Clorado; que foi tratado com cloro.

chlor·in·da·nol (klōr-in'dă-nol). Clorindanol; um espermicida.

chlo·rine (Cl) (klōr'ēn). Cloro. **1.** Elemento gasoso, tóxico, esverdeado; n.° atômico 17, peso atômico 35,4527; halógeno usado como desinfetante e alvejante na forma de hipoclorito ou de água clorada, devido ao seu poder de oxidação. Um dos bioelementos. **2.** A forma molecular do c. (1), Cl₂ (dicloreto). [G. *chloros*, amarelo esverdeado]

chlo·rine group. Grupo do cloro; os halogênios.

chlor·i·o·dized (klōr-ī'ō-dīzd). Cloroiodado; que contém cloro e iodo.

chlor·i·o·dized oil. Óleo cloroiodado; óleo de amendoim clorado e iodado formado pela adição química de monocloreto de iodo; usado antigamente para radiografia dos seios da face e brônquios. SIN iodochlorol.

chlor·i·o·do·quin (klōr'ē-ō-dō'kwin). Cloriodoquina. SIN iodochlorhydroxyquin.

chlor·i·son·da·mine chlo·ride (klōr-i-son'dă-mēn). Cloreto de clorisondamina; composto de amônio quaternário com ação de bloqueio ganglionar semelhante à do hexametônio e pentolínio, porém mais potente; foi usado no tratamento da hipertensão grave, incluindo a fase maligna.

chlo·rite (klōr'īt). Clorito; sal do ácido cloroso; o radical ClO₂⁻.

chlor·mad·i·none ac·e·tate (klōr-mad'i-nōn). Acetato de clormadinona; derivado da progesterona associado a estrogênio como contraceptivo oral.

chlor·mer·od·rin (klōr-mer'od-rin). Clormerodrina; diurético mercurial quimicamente relacionado com a meralurida.

chlor·mez·a·none (klōr-mez'ă-nōn). Clormezanona; relaxante muscular e agente tranqüilizante com ações farmacológicas e empregos semelhantes aos do meprobamato.

chloro-. VER chlor-.

chlo·ro·a·ce·tic ac·id (klōr'ō-ă-sē'tik). Ácido cloroacético; um ácido acético no qual um ou mais dos átomos de hidrogênio são substituídos por cloro. De acordo com o número de átomos assim deslocados, o ácido é denominado monocloroacético (cloroacético), dicloroacético ou tricloroacético. SIN chloracetic acid.

chlo·ro·ac·e·to·phe·none (klōr'ō-as'ē-tō-fē'nōn). Cloroacetofenona; gás lacrimogêneo; usado em treinamentos e no controle de tumultos.

chlo·ro·am·bu·cil (klōr-ō-am'bū-sil). Clorambucil. SIN chlorambucil.

chlo·ro·a·ne·mia (klōr'ō-ă-nē'mē-ă). Cloroanemia. SIN chlorosis.

chlo·ro·az·o·din (klōr-ō-az'ō-din). Cloroazodina; agente bactericida usado como anti-séptico cirúrgico.

o-chlo·ro·benz·al·mal·o·no·ni·trile (or'thō-klōr'ō-ben-zal-ma-lon'ō-ni-tril). *o*-clorobenzalmalononitrilo; forte lacrimogêneo usado no controle de tumultos.

chlo·ro·bu·ta·nol (klōr-ō-bū'tă-nol). Clorobutanol; hipnótico sedativo e anestésico local; usado principalmente em preparações dermatológicas e como conservante em frascos de múltiplas doses para uso parenteral. SIN acetone chloroform, chlorbutol.

chlo·ro·cre·sol (klōr-ō-krē'sol). Clorocresol; usado como anti-séptico e desinfetante; é mais ativo em soluções ácidas que em soluções alcalinas.

chlo·ro·cru·o·rin (klōr-ō-kroo'or-in). Clorocruorina; pigmento esverdeado, semelhante à hemoglobina, encontrado em alguns vermes; contém uma porfirina que difere da protoporfirina por um grupamento formil no lugar do grupamento 2-vinil.

chlo·ro·eth·ane (klōr-ō-eth'ān). Cloroetano. SIN *ethyl* chloride.

chlo·ro·eth·yl·ene (klōr-ō-eth'i-lēn). Cloroetileno. SIN *vinyl* chloride.

chlo·ro·form (klōr'ō-form). Clorofórmio; anteriormente usado por via inalatória para produzir anestesia geral; também usado como solvente. SIN trichloromethane. [chlor(ine) + form(yl)]

acetone c., cloretona. SIN chlorobutanol.

chlo·ro·form·ism (klōr'ō-form-izm). Cloroformismo; inalação habitual de clorofórmio, ou os sintomas causados pela inalação.

chlo·ro·gua·nide hy·dro·chlo·ride (klōr-ō-gwah'nīd). Cloridrato de cloroguanida; agente antimalárico. SIN chlorguanide hydrochloride, proguanil hydrochloride.

chlo·ro·he·min (klōr-ō-hē'min). Cloremina. SIN hemin.

chlo·ro·ma (klō-rō'mă). Cloroma; distúrbio caracterizado pelo desenvolvimento de múltiplas massas verdes localizadas de células anormais (na maioria dos casos, mieloblastos), principalmente em relação ao periósteo do crânio, coluna vertebral e costelas; a evolução clínica é semelhante à da leucemia mielóide aguda, embora os tumores possam preceder os achados no sangue e na medula óssea; observada com maior freqüência em crianças e adultos jovens. VER TAMBÉM granulocytic *sarcoma*. [chloro- + *-ōma*, tumor]

***p*-chlo·ro·mer·cu·ri·ben·zo·ate (PCMB, *p*CMB, *p*-CMB)** (klōr'ō-mer'cūr-ē-ben'zō-āt). *p*-Cloromercuribenzoato; composto de mercúrio orgânico que reage com grupamentos −SH nas proteínas; um inibidor da ação daquelas proteínas (enzimas) que depende da reatividade de –SH. VER TAMBÉM *p*-mercuribenzoate.

chlo·ro·meth·ane (klōr-ō-meth′ān). Clorometano; refrigerante com propriedades anestésicas quando inalado; é hidrolisado em metanol. SIN methyl chloride.

chlo·rom·e·try (klo-rom′e-trē). Clorometria; a medida do conteúdo de cloro, ou o uso de técnicas analíticas envolvendo a liberação ou titulação do cloro.

chlo·ro·pe·nia (klōr-ō-pē′nē-ă). Cloropenia; deficiência de cloro. [chloro- + G. *penia*, escassez]

chlo·ro·per·cha (klōr-ō-per′chă). Cloropercha; solução de guta-percha em clorofórmio; usada em odontologia como agente para lutar (fechar com massa) o material de obturação de guta-percha à parede de um canal radicular preparado.

chlo·ro·phe·nol (klōr-ō-fē′nol). Clorofenol; um dentre vários produtos de substituição obtidos pela ação do cloro sobre o fenol; usado como anti-séptico.

o-**chlo·ro·phe·nol.** *o*-clorofenol; líquido anti-séptico, usado no tratamento do lúpus.

p-**chlo·ro·phe·nol.** *p*-clorofenol. SIN parachlorophenol.

chlo·ro·phen·o·thane (klōr-ō-fen′ō-thān). Clorofenotano. SIN dichlorodiphenyltrichloroethane.

chlo·ro·phyll (klōr′ō-fil). Clorofila; o complexo magnesiano do derivado forbina encontrado em organismos de fotossíntese; pigmentos vegetais verdes que absorvem a luz que, em plantas vivas, convertem a energia luminosa em energia de oxidação e redução, assim fixando CO_2 e emitindo O_2; as formas de ocorrência natural são clorofila *a*, *b*, *c* e *d*. VER TAMBÉM phorbin.

c. *a*, c. a; feofitinato *a* de magnésio(II) [(feofitinato *a*)-magnésio(II)]; o principal pigmento encontrado em todos os organismos de fotossíntese que emitem oxigênio (vegetais superiores e algas vermelhas e verdes).

c. *b*, c. b; (CH_3 na posição 7 substituído por CHO na estrutura da clorofila), feofitinato *b* de magnésio-(II) [(feofitinato *b*) magnésio(II)]; a clorofila geralmente característica de vegetais superiores (incluindo *Chlorophyta*, *Euglenaphyta* e algas verdes). Ausente em outros tipos de algas.

c. *c*, c. c; a clorofila presente em algas marrons, diatomáceas e flagelados. São conhecidas duas formas: c_1, na qual dois hidrogênios são perdidos do C-17 e C-18, assemelhando-se assim à fitoporfirina, e a cadeia lateral em C-17 torna-se um resíduo acrílico, $-CH=CH_2COOH$; c_2, na qual são observadas as mesmas alterações, mas são perdidos mais dois átomos de hidrogênio do grupamento etil em C-8, tornando-se um resíduo vinila semelhante àquele em C-3. As duas substâncias podem assim ser denominadas em termos de fitoporfirina: magnésio $3^1,3^2,17^1,17^2$-tetradesidro-13^2-(metoxicarbonil)fitoporfirinato e magnésio $3^1,3^2,8^1,8^2,17^1,17^2$-hexadesidro-$13^2$-(metoxicarbonil)-fitoporfirinato.

c. *d*, c. d; ($-CH=CH_2$ substituído por $-CO-CH_3$ na estrutura da clorofila), a clorofila encontrada em algas vermelhas (*Rhodophyceae*), juntamente com a clorofila *a*.

c. esterase, c. esterase. SIN chlorophyllase.

water-soluble c. derivatives, derivados hidrossolúveis da clorofila; o complexo cúprico de sais de sódio e/ou potássio da clorofila saponificada; usado topicamente para desodorização de lesões crônicas e para promover cicatrização de feridas.

chlo·ro·phyl·lase (klōr-ō-fil′-ās). Clorofilase; enzima hidrolisante reversível que catalisa a remoção do grupamento fitil de uma clorofila, deixando uma clorofilida. SIN chlorophyll esterase.

chlo·ro·phyl·lide, chlo·ro·phyl·lid (klōr′ō-fil-id). Clorofilídeo; aquilo que resta de uma molécula de clorofila quando é removido o grupamento fitil.

chlo·ro·pic·rin (klōr-ō-pik′rin). Cloropicrina; irritante pulmonar e gás lacrimogênio tóxico; também causa vômito, cólica e diarréia, e, portanto, é denominado gás do vômito. SIN nitrochloroform.

chlo·ro·plast (klōr′ō-plast). Cloroplasto; corpúsculo de inclusão celular vegetal que contém clorofila; presente nas células das folhas e talos jovens. Local de fotossíntese em vegetais superiores. [chloro- + G. *plastos*, formado]

chlo·ro·pred·ni·sone (klōr-ō-pred′ni-sōn). Cloroprednisona; antiinflamatório tópico.

chlo·ro·pro·caine hy·dro·chlo·ride (klōr-ō-prō′kān). Cloridrato de cloroprocaína; anestésico local com ação e emprego semelhantes aos do cloridrato de procaína.

chlo·rop·sia (klo-rop′sē-ă). Cloropsia; distúrbio no qual os objetos parecem ser verdes, como pode ocorrer na intoxicação por digitálicos. SIN green vision. [chloro- + G. *opsis*, visão]

chlo·ro·pyr·a·mine (klōr-ō-pir′ă-mēn). Cloropiramina; agente anti-histamínico H_1.

chlo·ro·quine (klōr′ō-kwīn). Cloroquina; agente antimalárico usado para tratamento e supressão do *Plasmodium vivax*, *P. malariae* e *P. falciparum*; disponível na forma de fosfato e sulfato. Não promove cura radical porque não tem efeito sobre os estágios exoeritrocíticos; cepas de *P. falciparum* resistentes à cloroquina desenvolveram-se no Sudeste Asiático, na África e na América do Sul. Também é usada na amebíase hepática e em determinadas doenças cutâneas, p. ex., lúpus eritematoso e líquen plano.

chlo·ro·sis (klōr-ō′sis). Clorose; termo raramente usado para designar uma forma de anemia microcítica hipocrômica (deficiência de ferro), caracterizada por grande redução da hemoglobina, desproporcional à diminuição do número de hemácias; observada principalmente em mulheres entre a puberdade e a terceira década, e geralmente associada a dietas deficientes em ferro e proteínas. SIN asiderotic anemia, chloremia (1), chloroanemia, chlorotic anemia, green sickness. [chloro- + G. *-osis*, distúrbio]

chlo·ro·then cit·rate (klōr′ō-then). Citrato de cloroteno; agente anti-histamínico.

chlo·ro·thi·a·zide (klōr-ō-thī′ă-zīd). Clorotiazida; diurético efetivo por via oral, que inibe a reabsorção tubular renal de sódio; usada no tratamento do edema causado por insuficiência cardíaca congestiva, hepatopatia, gravidez, tensão pré-menstrual e drogas; também utilizado como auxiliar no tratamento da hipertensão.

c. sodium, c. sódica; c. adequada para administração parenteral.

chlo·ro·thy·mol (klōr-ō-thī′mol). Clorotimol; antibacteriano para uso tópico. SIN chlorthymol.

chlo·rot·ic (klo-rot′ik). Clorótico; relativo a, ou que possui, os aspectos característicos da clorose.

chlo·ro·tri·an·i·sene (klōr′ō-trī-an′i-sēn). Clorotrianiseno; estrogênio sintético derivado do estilbeno, ativo por via oral.

chlo·rous (klōr′ŭs). Cloroso. 1. Relativo ao cloro. 2. Designa compostos de cloro nos quais sua valência é +3, p. ex., ácido cloroso.

chlo·rous ac·id. $HClO_2$; ácido cloroso; ácido que forma cloritos com bases.

β-chlo·ro·vi·nyl·di·chlo·ro·ar·sine (klōr′ō-vī′nil-dī-klōr′ō-ar′sēn). β-Clorovinildiclorarsina. SIN lewisite.

chlo·ro·zo·to·cin (klōr′ō-zō-tō-sin). Clorozotocina; composto de mostarda nitrogenada que é um composto cloroetilnitrosuréia usado na quimioterapia do câncer; um antineoplásico.

chlor·phen·e·sin (klōr-fen′ē-sin). Clorfenesina; agente antifúngico tópico.

c. carbamate, carbamato de c.; relaxante muscular esquelético no qual as ações são exercidas no sistema nervoso central.

chlor·phen·in·di·one (klōr-fen-in-dī′ōn). Clorfenidiona; anticoagulante quimicamente relacionado à fenidiona.

chlor·phen·ir·a·mine ma·le·ate (klōr-fen-ir′ă-mēn). Maleato de clorfeniramina; anti-histamínico H_1.

chlor·phe·nol red (klōr-fē′nol). Vermelho de clorfenol; indicador ácido-básico (PM 423, pK 6,0): amarelo em pH abaixo de 5,1; vermelho acima de 6,7.

chlor·phen·ox·a·mine (klōr-fen-ok′să-mēn). Clorfenoxamina; usada no tratamento do parkinsonismo idiopático, arteriosclerótico e pós-encefalítico, geralmente com administração concomitante de outros agentes antiparkinsonianos.

chlor·phen·ter·mine hy·dro·chlo·ride (klōr-fen′ter-mēn). Cloridrato de clorfentermina; amina simpaticomimética usada como anorexiante; assemelha-se à anfetamina.

chlor·pro·guan·il hy·dro·chlo·ride (klōr-prō′gwah-nil). Cloridrato de clorproguanil; o homólogo 3,4-dicloro da cloroguanida; usado para profilaxia causal e supressão da malária falcípara.

chlor·prom·a·zine (klōr-prō′ma-zēn). Clorpromazina; antipsicótico fenotiazínico com ações antiemética, antiadrenérgica e anticolinérgica.

c. hydrochloride, cloridrato de c.; clorpromazina adequada para administração oral, intramuscular e intravenosa.

chlor·prop·a·mide (klōr-prō′pă-mīd). Clorpropamida; agente hipoglicemiante efetivo por via oral química e farmacologicamente relacionado com a tolbutamida; usado no controle da hiperglicemia em pacientes selecionados com diabetes melito do adulto (tipo II).

chlor·pro·thix·ene (klōr-prō-thik′sēn). Clorprotixeno; antipsicótico do grupo tioxanteno; também possui atividades antiemética, adrenolítica, espasmolítica e anti-histamínica.

chlor·quin·al·dol (klōr-kwin′al-dol). Clorquinaldol; agente ceratoplásico, antibacteriano e antifúngico usado no tratamento das infecções cutâneas bacterianas e micóticas.

chlor·tet·ra·cy·cline (klōr′tet-ră-sī′klēn). Clortetraciclina; ativa contra grande variedade de microrganismos patogênicos, incluindo os estreptococos hemolíticos, estafilococos, bacilos tifóides e brucelas, bem como contra determinados vírus. Também disponível como cloridrato de clortetraciclina.

chlor·thal·i·done (klōr-thal′i-dōn). Clortalidona; diurético e anti-hipertensivo efetivo por via oral, usado no tratamento do edema associado à insuficiência cardíaca congestiva, insuficiência renal, cirrose hepática, gravidez e tensão pré-menstrual; causa aumento da excreção de sódio, cloreto, potássio e água.

chlor·then·ox·a·zin (klōr-then-ok′să-zin). Clortenoxazina; antipirético e analgésico.

chlor·thy·mol (klōr-thī′mol). Clortimol. SIN chlorothymol.

chlor·u·re·sis (klōr-ū-rē′sis). Clorurese; a excreção de cloreto na urina. SIN chloriduria, chloruria.

chlor·u·ret·ic (klōr-ū-ret′ik). Clorurético; relativo a um agente que aumenta a excreção de cloreto na urina, ou a esse efeito.

chlor·u·ria (klōr-ū′rē-ă). Cloruria. SIN chloruresis.

chlor·zox·a·zone (klōr-zok′sä-zōn). Clorzoxazona; relaxante muscular esquelético de ação central usado no tratamento do espasmo muscular doloroso causado por distúrbio músculo-esquelético.

cho·a·nae (kō′an-ă) [TA]. Cóano; a abertura da cavidade nasal para a nasofaringe de cada lado. SIN posterior nasal apertures*, isthmus pharyngonasalis, posterior nares, postnaris. [L. Mod. do G. *choanē*, funil]

  primary c., primitive c., c. primário, c. primitivo; abertura inicial das fossas nasais e do saco olfatório do embrião na parte rostral da cavidade oronasal primordial, antes da formação do palato secundário.

  secondary c., c. secundário; o c. definitivo que se abre para a nasofaringe, após o alongamento das cavidades nasais pela formação do palato secundário. SIN internal nostril.

cho·a·nal (kō′ă-năl). Coanal; relativo a um cóano.

cho·a·nate (kō′an-āt). Coanado; que possui um funil, isto é, com um anel ou colar.

cho·a·no·flag·el·late (kō′an-ō-flaj′ē-lāt). Coanoflagelado. SIN choanomastigote.

cho·a·noid (kō′ă-noyd). Coanóide; em forma de funil. SIN infundibuliform. [G. *choanē*, funil, + *eidos*, semelhança]

cho·a·no·mas·ti·gote (kō′an-ō-mas′ti-gōt). Coanomastigoto; termo, na rotina usado para descrever os estágios do desenvolvimento dos parasitas flagelados, que designa a forma em "grão de cevada" do flagelado do gênero *Crithidia*, caracterizado por um prolongamento em forma de colar que circunda a parte anterior e através do qual emerge o flagelo único. VER TAMBÉM amastigote, epimastigote, promastigote, trypomastigote. SIN choanoflagellate, collared flagellate. [G. *choanē*, funil, + *mastix*, chicote]

Cho·a·no·tae·nia in·fun·dib·u·lum (kō-ă-nō-tē′nē-ă). Espécie importante de tênias cosmopolitas de aves domésticas, presentes no intestino delgado e transmitidas por moscas domésticas e de estábulos; relacionada à *Dipylidium*, a tênia canina de poro duplo. [G. *choanē*, funil, + L., do G. *tainia*, tênia]

Chodzko re·flex. Reflexo de Chodzko. Ver em reflex.

choke (chōk). 1. Asfixiar; impedir a respiração por compressão ou obstrução da laringe ou traquéia; expressão comum para laringoespasmo. 2. Qualquer obstrução do esôfago em animais herbívoros por um corpo estranho parcialmente deglutido. [I.M. *choken*, do I. ant. *āceocian*]

chokes (chōks). Manifestação da doença descompressiva ou doença da altitude caracterizada por dispnéia, tosse e asfixia.

△ **chol-.** VER chole-.

cho·la·gog·ic (kō-lă-goj′ik). Colagogo. SIN cholagogue (2).

cho·la·gogue (kō′lă-gog). Colagogo. 1. Agente que promove o fluxo de bile para o intestino, principalmente em virtude de contração da vesícula biliar. 2. Relativo a esse agente ou efeito. SIN cholagogic. [chol- + G. *agōgos*, condutor]

cho·la·ic ac·id (kō-lā′ik). Ácido colaico. SIN taurocholic acid.

cho·lal·ic ac·id (kō-lal′ik). Ácido colálico. SIN cholic acid.

cho·lane, 5β-cho·lane (kō′lān). Colano, 5β-colano; hidrocarboneto original dos ácidos colânicos (ácidos cólicos); androstano com um grupamento –CH(CH₃)-CH₂CH₂CH₃ na posição 17. O 5α-colano algumas vezes é denominado alocolano. Quanto às estruturas, ver esteróides (steroids).

chol·a·ner·e·sis (kō-lă-ner′ē-sis). Colanerese; aumento da secreção de ácido cólico ou seus conjugados. [cholane + G. *hairesis*, captura]

cho·lan·ge·i·tis (kō′lan-jē-ī′tis). Colangeíte. SIN cholangitis.

chol·an·gi·ec·ta·sis (kō-lan-jē-ek′tă-sis). Colangectasia; dilatação dos ductos biliares, geralmente como seqüela de obstrução ou resultante da ausência congênita de uma parte da parede ductal. [chol- + G. *angeion*, vaso, + *ektasis*, dilatação]

chol·an·gi·o·car·ci·no·ma (kō-lan′jē-ō-kar-si-nō′mă). Colangiocarcinoma; um adenocarcinoma, basicamente nos ductos biliares intra-hepáticos, composto por ductos revestidos por células cubóides ou colunares que não contêm bile, com estroma fibroso abundante; geralmente não há cirrose.

chol·an·gi·o·en·ter·os·to·my (kō-lan′jē-ō-en-ter-os′tō-mē). Colangioenterostomia; anastomose cirúrgica do ducto biliar com o intestino.

chol·an·gi·o·fi·bro·sis (kō-lan′jē-ō-fī′brō′sis). Colangiofibrose; fibrose dos ductos biliares. [chol- + G. *angeion*, vaso, + fibrosis]

chol·an·gi·o·gas·tros·to·my (kō-lan′jē-ō-gas-tros′tō-mē). Colangiogastrostomia; formação de uma comunicação entre um ducto biliar e o estômago. [chol- + G. *angeion*, vaso, + *gastēr*, ventre, + *stoma*, boca]

chol·an·gi·o·gram (kō-lan′jē-ō-gram). Colangiograma; o registro radiológico dos ductos biliares obtido por colangiografia.

chol·an·gi·og·ra·phy (kō-lan-jē-og′ră-fē). Colangiografia; exame radiográfico dos ductos biliares com contraste. [chol- + G. *angeion*, vaso, + *graphō*, escrever]

  cystic duct c., c. do ducto cístico; radiografia do sistema biliar após introdução de contraste através do ducto cístico.

  intravenous c., c. intravenosa; c. dos ductos biliares opacificados por secreção hepática de um contraste injetado por via intravenosa.

  percutaneous c., c. percutânea; radiografia do sistema biliar após introdução de contraste por inserção de uma agulha através da pele, inferior à margem costal direita, até a substância hepática ou o interior da vesícula biliar.

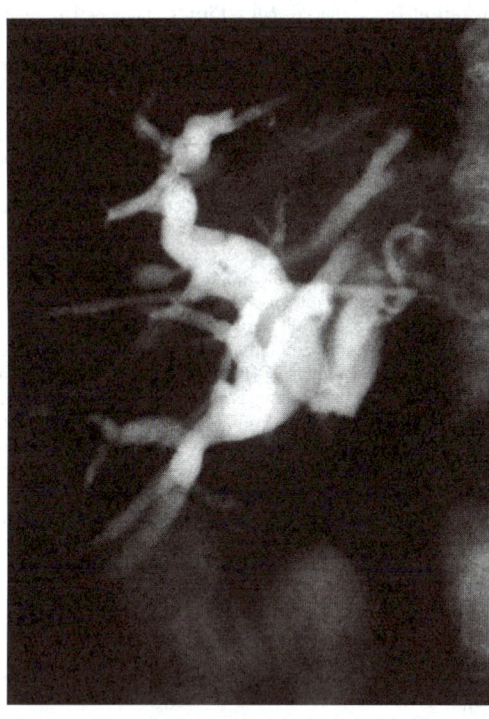

colangiografia transepática percutânea: mostrando obstrução do colédoco por tumor (área escura abaixo do centro da imagem)

  percutaneous transhepatic c. (PTHC), c. transepática percutânea; radiografia contrastada do sistema biliar realizada pela injeção de corante radiopaco através de uma agulha inserida por via percutânea até um ducto biliar intra-hepático.

chol·an·gi·ole (kō-lan′jē-ōl). Colangíolo; canalículo que ocorre entre um canalículo biliar e um ducto biliar interlobular. SIN canal of Hering. [chol- + G. *angeion*, vaso, + *-ole*, pequeno]

chol·an·gi·o·li·tis (kō-lan′jē-ō-lī′tis). Colangiolite; inflamação das pequenas radículas biliares ou colangíolos.

chol·an·gi·o·ma (kō-lan′jē-ō′mă). Colangioma; neoplasia originada no ducto biliar, principalmente no fígado; pode ser benigna ou maligna (colangiocarcinoma). [chol- + G. *angeion*, vaso, + *-oma*, tumor]

chol·an·gi·o·pan·cre·a·tog·ra·phy (kō-lan′jē-ō-pan-krē-ă-tog′ră-fē). Colangiopancreatografia; radiografia contrastada dos ductos biliares e pancreáticos após a injeção de contraste radiopaco.

  endoscopic retrograde c. (ERCP), c. retrógrada endoscópica; método de colangiopancreatografia utilizando um endoscópio para inspecionar e canular a ampola de Vater, com injeção de contraste para exame radiográfico dos ductos pancreáticos, hepáticos e colédoco.

chol·an·gi·os·co·py (kō-lan′jē-os′kŏ-pē). Colangioscopia; exame visual dos ductos biliares utilizando um endoscópio de fibra óptica. [chol- + G. *angeion*, vaso, + *skopeō*, examinar]

chol·an·gi·os·to·my (kō-lan-jē-os′tō-mē). Colangiostomia; formação de uma fístula para um ducto biliar. [chol- + G. *angeion*, vaso, + *stoma*, boca]

chol·an·gi·ot·o·my (ko-lan-ji-ot′o-mī). Colangiotomia; incisão de um ducto biliar. [chol- + G. *angeion*, vaso, + *tomē*, incisão]

chol·an·gi·tis (kō-lan-jī′tis). Colangite; inflamação de um ducto biliar ou de toda a árvore biliar. SIN angiocholitis, cholangeitis. [chol- + G. *angeion*, vaso, + *-itis*, inflamação]

  ascending c., c. ascendente. SIN c. lenta.

  c. lenta (len-tā′). c. lenta; infecção bacteriana discreta das vias biliares; algumas vezes causa de febre de origem indeterminada. SIN ascending c.

  primary sclerosing c., c. esclerosante primária; icterícia obstrutiva recorrente ou persistente, freqüentemente com colite ulcerativa, causada por fibrose obliterativa extensa dos ductos biliares extra-hepáticos ou intra-hepáticos; geralmente progride para cirrose, hipertensão porta e insuficiência hepática; mais comum em homens jovens.

  recurrent pyogenic c., c. piogênica recorrente; crises repetidas de c., mais comuns em asiáticos que vivem na Ásia, associadas a múltiplas estenoses e cálculos nos ductos biliares intra-hepáticos e extra-hepáticos.

cho·lan·ic ac·id (kō-lan′ik). Ácido colânico. SIN cholic acid.
cho·lan·o·poi·e·sis (kō′lan-ō-poy-ē′sis). Colanopoese; síntese hepática de ácido cólico ou seus conjugados, ou de sais biliares naturais. [chol- + G. *anō*, para cima, + *poiēsis*, produção]
cho·lan·o·poi·et·ic (kō′lan-ō-poy-et′ik). Colanopoético; relativo a, ou que promove, colanopoese.
chol·an·threne (kō-lan′thrēn). Colantreno; hidrocarboneto policíclico, um tanto carcinogênico, que é a estrutura original do 3 (ou 20)-metilcolantreno, altamente carcinogênico.
cho·las·cos (kō-las′kos). Colasco; termo raramente usado para indicar passagem de bile para a cavidade peritoneal livre. [chol- + G. *askos*, bolsa]
cho·late (kō′lāt). Colato; sal ou éster de um ácido cólico.
  c. ligase, c. ligase; enzima que converte o c., a coenzima A e o ATP em coloil-coenzima A, AMP e pirofosfato. SIN cholyl-coenzyme A synthetase.
  c. synthetase, c. thiokinase, c. sintetase, c. tiocinase; colato-CoA ligase.
♻ **chole-, chol-, cholo-.** Bile. Cf. bili-. [G. *cholē*]
cho·le·cal·cif·er·ol (kō′lē-kal-sif′er-ol). Colecalciferol; (5Z,7E)-(3S)-9,10-secocolesta-5,7,10(19)-trien-3-ol; formado por quebra da ligação 9,10 em 7-desidrocolesterol por irradiação ultravioleta, produzindo uma dupla ligação entre C-10 e C-19; provavelmente a vitamina D de origem animal encontrada na pele, no couro e nas penas de animais e aves expostos à luz solar, e também na manteiga, miolo, óleos de peixe e gema de ovo. SIN vitamina D_3. SIN calciol.
cho·le·chro·mo·poi·e·sis (kō′lē-krō-mō-poy-ē′sis). Colecromopoese; síntese de pigmentos biliares pelo fígado. [chole- + G. *chrōma*, cor, + *poiesis*, produção]
cho·le·cyst (kō′le-sist). Vesícula biliar, colecisto, colecíste. SIN gallbladder.
cho·le·cys·ta·gog·ic (kō′le-sis-ta-goj′ik). Colecistagógico; que estimula a atividade da vesícula biliar.
cho·le·cys·ta·gogue (kō-lē-sis′ta-gog). Colecistagogo; substância que estimula a atividade da vesícula biliar. [chole- + G. *kystis*, vesícula, + *agōgos*, guia]
cho·le·cys·tat·o·ny (kō-lē-sis-tat′ō-nē). Colecistatonia; atonia, fraqueza ou ausência de função da vesícula biliar. [chole- + G. *kystis*, vesícula, + *atonia*, atonia]
cho·le·cys·tec·ta·sia (kō′lē-sis-tek-tā′zē-ă). Colecistectasia; termo raramente usado para indicar dilatação da vesícula biliar. [chole- + G. *kystis*, vesícula, + *ektasis*, extensão]
ℹ **cho·le·cys·tec·to·my** (kō′lē-sis-tek′tō-mē). Colecistectomia; remoção cirúrgica da vesícula biliar. [chole- + G. *kystis*, vesícula, + *ektomē*, excisão]
cho·le·cyst·en·ter·os·to·my (kō′lē-sist-en-ter-os′tō-mē). Colecistenterostomia; formação de uma comunicação direta entre a vesícula biliar e o intestino. SIN enterocholecystostomy. [chole- + G. *kystis*, vesícula, + *enteron*, intestino, + *stoma*, boca]
cho·le·cyst·en·ter·ot·o·my (kō′lē-sist-en-ter-ot′ō-mē). Colecistenterotomia; formação de uma comunicação direta entre a vesícula biliar e o intestino. SIN enterocholecystostomy. [chole- + G. *kystis*, vesícula, + *enteron*, intestino, + *tomē*, corte]
cho·le·cys·tic (kō-lē-sis′tik). Colecístico; relativo ao colecisto, ou vesícula biliar.
cho·le·cys·tis (kō-lē-sis′tis). Vesícula biliar, colecisto, colecíste. SIN gallbladder. [chole- + G. *kystis*, vesícula]
cho·le·cys·ti·tis (kō′lē-sis-tī′tis). Colecistite; inflamação da vesícula biliar. [chole- + G. *kystis*, vesícula, + *-itis*, inflamação]
  acute c., c. aguda; inflamação e/ou necrose hemorrágica, com infecção, ulceração e infiltração neutrofílica variáveis da parede da vesícula biliar; geralmente causada por impactação de um cálculo no ducto cístico.
  chronic c., c. crônica; inflamação crônica da vesícula biliar, geralmente secundária à litíase, com infiltração linfocítica e fibrose que podem produzir espessamento acentuado da parede.
  emphysematous c., c. enfisematosa; c. devida à infecção por bactérias produtoras de gás, produzindo gás na vesícula biliar.
  xanthogranulomatous c., c. xantogranulomatosa; c. crônica com infiltração nodular visível por macrófagos, preenchidos por lipídios; pode estar associada à obstrução biliar por cálculos.
cho·le·cys·to·du·o·de·nos·to·my (kō-lē-sis′tō-doo-ō-dē-nos′tō-mē). Colecistoduodenostomia; estabelecimento de uma comunicação direta entre a vesícula biliar e o duodeno. SIN duodenocholecystostomy, duodenocystostomy (1). [chole- + G. *kystis*, vesícula, + L. *duodenum* + G. *stoma*, boca]
cho·le·cys·to·gas·tros·to·my (kō-lē-sis′tō-gas-tros′tō-mē). Colecistogastrostomia; estabelecimento de uma comunicação entre a vesícula biliar e o estômago. [chole- + G. *kystis*, vesícula, + *gastēr*, estômago, + *stoma*, boca]
cho·le·cys·to·gram (kō-lē-sis′tō-gram). Colecistograma; o registro radiográfico da estrutura e da função da vesícula biliar obtido por colecistografia.
cho·le·cys·tog·ra·phy (kō-lē-sis-tog′ra-fē). Colecistografia; estudo radiográfico da vesícula biliar após administração oral de um colecistopaco; ou visualização cintigráfica da vesícula biliar e dos ductos biliares centrais após administração de um radiofármaco secretado pelo fígado. SIN Graham-Cole test. [chole- + G. *kystis*, vesícula, + *grapho*, escrever]

cho·le·cys·to·il·e·os·to·my (kō-lē-sis′tō-il-ē-os′tō-mē). Colecistoileostomia; estabelecimento de uma comunicação entre a vesícula biliar e o íleo. [chole- + G. *kystis*, vesícula, + ileum, + G. *stoma*, boca]
cho·le·cys·to·je·ju·nos·to·my (kō-lē-sis′tō-jē-joo-nos′tō-mē). Colecistojejunostomia; estabelecimento de uma comunicação entre a vesícula biliar e o jejuno. [chole- + G. *kystis*, vesícula, + jejunum, + G. *stoma*, boca]
cho·le·cys·to·ki·nase (kō-lē-sis-tō-kī′nās). Colecistocinase; enzima que catalisa a hidrólise da colecistocinina.
cho·le·cys·to·ki·net·ic (kō′lē-sis′tō-ki-net′ik). Colecistocinético; que promove o esvaziamento da vesícula biliar.
cho·le·cys·to·ki·nin (CCK) (kō′lē-sis-tō-kī′nin). Colecistocinina; hormônio polipeptídico (o peptídeo humano possui 33 resíduos) liberado pela mucosa intestinal alta ao contato com o conteúdo gástrico; estimula a contração da vesícula biliar e a secreção de suco pancreático. VER TAMBÉM sincalide. SIN pancreozymin.
cho·le·cys·to·li·thi·a·sis (kō-lē-sis′tō-li-thī′ă-sis). Colecistolitíase; presença de um ou mais cálculos na vesícula biliar. [chole- + G. *kystis*, vesícula, + *lithos*, cálculo]
cho·le·cys·to·lith·o·trip·sy (kō-lē-sis′tō-lith′ō-trip-sē). Colecistolitotripsia; fragmentação de um cálculo biliar mais comumente pela aplicação de energia ultra-sônica aplicada por via transcutânea concentrada sobre o cálculo. [chole- + G. *kystis*, vesícula, + *lithos*, cálculo, + *tripsis*, fricção]
cho·le·cys·to·my (kō-lē-sis′tō-mē). Colecistomia. SIN cholecystotomy.
cho·le·cys·to·paque (kō-lē-sis′tō-pāk). Contraste radiográfico que opacifica a vesícula biliar após administração oral, em virtude de secreção hepática e concentração na vesícula biliar; usado em colecistografia.
cho·le·cys·top·a·thy (kō′lē-sis-top′ă-thē). Colecistopatia; doença da vesícula biliar.
cho·le·cys·to·pexy (kō-lē-sis′tō-pek-sē). Colecistopexia; sutura da vesícula biliar à parede abdominal. [chole- + G. *kystis*, vesícula, + *pēxis*, fixação]
cho·le·cys·tor·rha·phy (kō′lē-sis-tōr′ă-fē). Colecistorrafia; sutura de uma vesícula biliar incisada ou rota. [chole- + G. *kystis*, vesícula, + *rhaphē*, sutura]
cho·le·cys·to·so·nog·ra·phy (kō-lē-sis′tō-sō-nog′ră-fē). Colecistossonografia; exame ultra-sonográfico da vesícula biliar. [cholecysto- + sonography]
cho·le·cys·tos·to·my (kō′lē-sis-tos′tō-mē). Colecistostomia; estabelecimento de uma fístula para a vesícula biliar. [chole- + G. *kystis*, bexiga, + *stoma*, boca]
cho·le·cys·tot·o·my (kō′lē-sis-tot′ō-mē). Colecistotomia; incisão da vesícula biliar. SIN cholecystomy. [chole- + G. *kystis*, bexiga, + *tomē*, incisão]
  laparoscopic c., c. laparoscópica; técnica cirúrgica de invasividade mínima para remoção da vesícula biliar, na qual são usadas quatro ou cinco incisões pequenas (< 10 mm) para a introdução de um laparoscópio e vários instrumentos na cavidade abdominal, evitando assim a incisão tradicional.
cho·le·doch (kō′lē-dok). Colédoco. SIN bile duct (1). [G. *cholēdochos*, que contém bile, de *cholē*, bile, + *dechomai*, receber]
♻ **choledoch-.** VER choledocho-.
cho·le·doch·al (kō-lē-dok′al, kō-led′ō-kal). Relativo ao ducto colédoco.
cho·led·o·chec·to·my (kō-led-ō-kek′tō-mē). Coledocectomia; remoção cirúrgica de uma parte do colédoco. [cholecoch- + G. *ektomē*, excisão]
cho·led·o·chen·dy·sis (kō′led-ō-ken′dī-sis). Coledocotomia. SIN choledochotomy. [choledoch- + G. *endysis*, entrada em]
cho·led·o·chi·arc·tia (kō′led-ō-ki-ark′tē-ă). Coledoquiartia; termo obsoleto para indicar estenose do ducto biliar. [choledoch- + L. *artus* (impropriamente *arctus*), estreito]
cho·led·o·chi·tis (kō-led-ō-kī′tis). Coledoquite; inflamação do ducto colédoco. [choledoch- + G. *-itis*, inflamação]
♻ **choledocho-, choledoch-.** Colédoco-, coledoc-; o ducto colédoco (o ducto biliar comum). [G. *cholēdochos*, que contém bile, de *cholē*, bile, + *dechomai*, receber]
cho·led·o·cho·cho·led·o·chos·to·my (kō-led′ō-kō-kō-led′ō-kos′tō-mē). Coledococoledocostomia; união cirúrgia de porções divididas do ducto colédoco. [choledocho- + choledocho- + G. *stoma*, boca]
cho·led·o·cho·du·o·de·nos·to·my (kō-led′ō-kō-doo′ō-dē-nos′tō-mē). Coledocoduodenostomia; formação de uma comunicação, além da natural, entre o ducto colédoco e o duodeno. [choledocho- + duodenum + G. *stoma*, boca]
cho·led·o·cho·en·ter·os·tomy (kō-led′ō-kō-en-ter-os′tō-mē). Coledocoenterostomia; estabelecimento de uma comunicação, além da natural, entre o ducto colédoco e qualquer parte do intestino. [choledocho- + G. *enteron*, intestino, + *stoma*, boca]
cho·led·o·cho·je·ju·nos·to·my (kō-led′ō-kō-jē-joo-nos′tō-mē). Coledocojejunostomia; anastomose entre o ducto colédoco e o jejuno. [choledocho- + jejuno + G. *stoma*, boca]
cho·led·o·cho·lith (kō-led′ō-kō-lith). Coledocólito; cálculo no ducto colédoco. [choledocho- + G. *lithos*, cálculo]
cho·led·o·cho·li·thi·a·sis (kō-led′ō-kō-lith-ī′ă-sis). Coledocolitíase; presença de um cálculo no ducto colédoco.
cho·led·o·cho·li·thot·o·my (kō-led′ō-kō-li-thot′ō-mē). Coledocolitotomia; incisão do ducto colédoco para a extração de um cálculo. [choledocho- + G. *lithos*, cálculo, + *tomē*, incisão]

cho·led·o·cho·lith·o·trip·sy (kō-led′ō-kō-lith′ō-trip-sē). Coledocolitotripsia; fragmentação de um cálculo biliar no ducto colédoco por energia ultra-sônica transcutânea ou por laser direcionado por endoscopia. SIN choledocholithotrity. [choledocho- + G. *lithos*, cálculo, + *tripsis*, fricção]

cho·led·o·cho·li·thot·ri·ty (kō-led′ō-kō-li-thot′ri-tē). Coledocolitotritia. SIN choledocholithotripsy.

cho·led·o·cho·plas·ty (kō-led′ō-kō-plas-tē). Coledocoplastia; rearranjo dos tecidos do ducto colédoco. [choledocho- + G. *plastos*, formado]

cho·led·o·chor·rha·phy (kō-led-ō-kōr′ra-fē). Coledocorrafia; sutura de união das extremidades divididas do ducto colédoco. [choledocho- + G. *rhaphē*, sutura]

cho·led·o·chos·to·my (kō-led-ō-kos′tō-mē). Coledocostomia; estabelecimento de uma fístula para o ducto colédoco. [choledocho- + G. *stoma*, boca]

cho·led·o·chot·o·my (kō-led-ō-kot′ō-mē). Coledocotomia; incisão do ducto colédoco. SIN choledochendysis. [choledocho- + G. *tomē*, incisão]

cho·led·o·chous (kō-led′ō-kŭs). Aquilo que contém ou transporta bile.

cho·led·o·chus (kō-led′ō-kŭs). Colédoco. SIN bile duct (1). [ver choledoch]

cho·le·glo·bin (kō-lē-glō′bin). Coleglobina; composto pigmentado da globina e ferro porfirina (com um anel aberto devido à clivagem da ponte α-meteno por α-metil oxigenase); o primeiro intermediário na degradação da hemoglobina, posteriormente degradado sucessivamente em verdoemocromo, biliverdina e bilirrubina. SIN bile pigment hemoglobin, green hemoglobin, verdohemoglobin.

cho·le·he·ma·tin (kō-lē-hē′ma-tin). Colematina; pigmento vermelho na bile de animais herbívoros; derivado da clorofila e um produto da oxidação da hematina.

cho·le·he·mia (kō-lē-hē′mē-a). Colemia. SIN cholemia. [chole- + G. *haima*, sangue]

cho·le·ic (kō-lē-′ik). Coleico. SIN cholic.

cho·le·ic ac·ids. Ácidos coleicos; compostos de ácidos biliares e esteróis.

cho·le·lith (kō′lē-lith). Colélito. SIN gallstone. [chole- + G. *lithos*, cálculo]

cho·le·li·thi·a·sis (kō′lē-li-thī′a-sis). Colelitíase; presença de concreções na vesícula biliar ou ductos biliares. SIN chololithiasis.

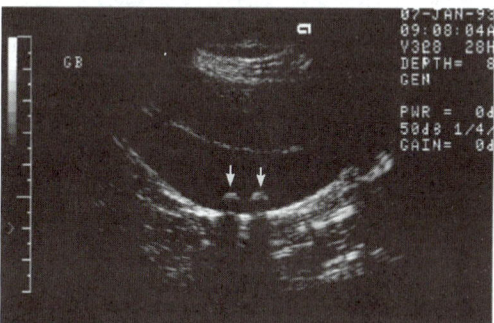

colelitíase: ultra-sonografia de dois cálculos na vesícula biliar

cho·le·li·thot·o·my (kō′lē-li-thot′ō-mē). Colelitotomia; remoção cirúrgica de um cálculo biliar. [chole- + G. *lithos*, cálculo, + *tomē*, incisão]

cho·le·lith·o·trip·sy (kō-lē-lith′ō-trip-sē). Colelitotripsia; termo raramente usado para o esmagamento de um cálculo biliar. [chole- + G. *lithos*, cálculo, + *tripsis*, fricção]

cho·le·li·thot·ri·ty (kō-lē-li-thot′ri-tē). Colelitotritia; termo raramente usado para o esmagamento de um cálculo biliar. [chole- + G. *lithos*, cálculo, + L. *tero*, pp. *tritus*, friccionar]

cho·lem·e·sis (kō-lem′e-sis). Colêmese; vômito de bile. [chole- + G. *emesis*, vômito]

cho·le·mia (kō-lē′mē-a). Colemia; presença de sais biliares no sangue circulante. SIN cholehemia. [chole- + G. *haima*, sangue]

cho·lem·ic (kō-lē′mik). Colêmico; relativo à colemia.

cho·le·path·ia (kō-lē-path′ē-a). Colepatia. **1.** Doença dos ductos biliares. **2.** Irregularidade nas contrações dos ductos biliares.
  c. spas′tica, c. espástica; contração espástica dos ductos biliares.

cho·le·per·i·to·ni·tis (kō′le-per-i-tō-nī′tis). Coleperitonite. SIN bile peritonitis.

cho·le·poi·e·sis (kō′lē-poy-ē′sis). Colepoese; formação de bile. SIN cholopoiesis. [chole- + G. *poiēsis*, produção]

cho·le·poi·et·ic (kō′lē-poy-et′ik). Colepoético; relativo à formação de bile.

chol·era (kol′er-a). Cólera; doença infecciosa epidêmica aguda causada pela bactéria *Vibrio cholerae*. Uma toxina solúvel, produzida no trato intestinal pela bactéria, ativa a adenilato ciclase da mucosa, causando secreção ativa de um líquido isotônico, que resulta em diarréia aquosa profusa, perda extrema de líquido e eletrólitos, bem como desidratação e colapso, mas sem alteração morfológica macroscópica da mucosa intestinal. SIN Asiatic c. [L. uma doença biliosa, do G. *cholē*, bile]

Asiatic c., c. asiática. SIN cholera.
  c. infan′tum, c. do lactente; termo antigo para designar uma doença de lactentes, caracterizada por vômitos, diarréia aquosa profusa, febre, prostração e colapso.
  c. mor′bus, c. mórbida; termo antigo para designar gastroenterite aguda grave de etiologia desconhecida, caracterizada por cólica intensa, vômitos e diarréia com fezes aquosas; outrora comum durante a estação do calor.
  pancreatic c., c. pancreática. SIN diarrhea pancreatica.
  c. sic′ca, c. seca; termo antigo para designar uma forma maligna de doença observada durante epidemias de cólera asiática nas quais há morte sem diarréia.
  typhoid c., c. tifóide; nome antigo para designar cólera (2) com manifestações predominantemente cerebrais, como confusão ou demência.

chol·er·a·gen (kol′er-a-jen). Coleráfeno; termo sugerido para um ou mais fator(es) produzido(s) durante o crescimento *in vitro* do vibrião da cólera e causa diarréia. [cholera + G. -*gen*, produtor]

chol·er·a·ic (kol′er-ā′ik). Colérico; relativo à cólera.

chol·er·a·phage (kol′er-a-fāj). Coleráfago; bacteriófago do *Vibrio cholerae*. [cholera- + G. *phagō*, comer]

cho·le·re·sis (kō-ler-ē′sis). Colerese; a secreção de bile, em oposição à expulsão de bile, pela vesícula biliar. [chole- + G. *hairesis*, captura]

cho·le·ret·ic (kol-er-et′ik). Colerético. **1.** Relativo à colerese. **2.** Um agente, geralmente um fármaco, que estimula o fígado a aumentar a secreção de bile.

chol·er·rhe·ic (kol-ĕ-rē′ik). Colerreico; designa diarréia secundária à não-absorção de sais biliares. [chole- + G. *hairesis*, captura]

chol·er·ic (kol′er-ik). Colérico. SIN bilious (3).

chol·er·i·form (kol′er-i-fōrm). Coleriforme; semelhante à cólera. SIN choleroid.

chol·er·i·gen·ic, chol·er·ig·en·ous (kol′er-i-jen′ik, -ij′en-ŭs). Colerigênico; colerígeno; que causa ou produz cólera.

chol·er·ine (kol′er-ēn). Colerina; forma leve de diarréia observada durante epidemias de cólera asiática.

chol·er·oid (kol′er-oyd). Coleróide. SIN choleriform.

cho·ler·rha·gia (kō-lē-rā′jē-a). Colerragia; fluxo substancial de bile. [chole- + G. *rhegnymi*, jorrar]

cho·ler·rha·gic (kō-lē-raj′ik). Colerrágico; que se refere ao fluxo de bile.

chol·e·scin·tig·ra·phy (kō-lē-sin-tig′ra-fē). Colecintigrafia; exame da vesícula biliar e dos ductos biliares por medicina nuclear; colecistografia por radionuclídios. [chole- + scintigraphy]

cho·les·tane (kō′les-tān). Colestano; o hidrocarboneto original do colesterol. Quanto à estrutura, ver esteróides (steroids).

cho·les·ta·nol (kō-les′tan-ol). Colestanol; que difere do colesterol na ausência da ligação dupla.

cho·les·tan·one (kō-les′tan-ōn). Colestanona; produto da oxidação do colestanol, que difere dele pela presença de um oxigênio cetônico no lugar do grupamento 3-hidroxila; um isômero da coprostanona.

cho·le·sta·sia, cho·le·sta·sis (kō-les-tā′sē-a, -les′tā-sis). Colestase; interrupção no fluxo de bile; a colestase devida à obstrução dos ductos biliares é acompanhada por formação de tampões de bile espessada nos pequenos ductos, canalículos no fígado e elevação da bilirrubina direta sérica e de algumas enzimas. [chole- + G. *stasis*, parada]

cho·le·sta·sis (-les′tā-sis). Colestase. VER cholestasia.
  intrahepatic cholestasis of pregnancy, colestase intra-hepática da gravidez; colestase intra-hepática com coloração biliar centrilobular sem células inflamatórias ou proliferação de células mesenquimais; clinicamente caracterizada por prurido e/ou icterícia; de causa desconhecida, mas associada a altos níveis de estrogênio. SIN cholestasis of pregnancy, cholestatic hepatosis icterus gravidarum, recurrent jaundice of pregnancy.
  cholestasis of pregnancy, c. da gravidez. SIN intrahepatic cholestasis of pregnancy.

cho·le·stat·ic (kō-les-tat′ik). Colestático; que tende a diminuir ou interromper o fluxo de bile.

cho·les·te·a·to·ma (kō-les-tē-a-tō′ma). Colesteatoma. **1.** Uma massa de epitélio de células escamosas queratinizadas e colesterol no ouvido médio, geralmente resultante de otite média crônica, com metaplasia escamosa ou extensão do epitélio escamoso para dentro a fim de revestir uma cavidade cística expansiva que pode envolver a mastóide e erodir o osso adjacente. **2.** Cisto epidermóide originado no sistema nervoso central em seres humanos ou animais. [cholesterol + G. *stear (steat-)*, sebo, + -*oma*, tumor]

cho·les·te·at·om·a·tous (kō-les-tē-a-tō′ma-tŭs). Colesteatomatoso; de, ou relativo a, colesteatoma.

cho·les·ten·one (kō-les′ten-ōn). Colestenona; uma desidrocolestanona, diferente da colestanona pela presença de uma ligação dupla entre os carbonos 4 e 5.

cho·les·ter·e·mia (kō-les-ter-ē′mē-ă). Colesteremia; a presença de quantidades aumentadas de colesterol no sangue. SIN cholesterinemia, cholesterolemia. [cholesterol + G. *haima*, sangue]

cho·les·ter·in·e·mia (kō-les′ter-in-ē′mē-ă). Colesterinemia. SIN cholesteremia.

cho·les·ter·in·o·sis (kō-les′ter-in-ō′sis). Colesterinose. SIN cholesterolosis.

cho·les·ter·i·nu·ria (kō-les′ter-i-noo′rē-ă). Colesterinúria. SIN cholesteroluria. [cholesterin + G. *ouron*, urina]

cho·les·ter·ol (kō-les′ter-ol). Colesterol; 5-colesten-3β-ol (colestano com uma ligação dupla 5,6 e um grupamento 3β-hidroxila); o esteróide mais abundante em tecidos animais, principalmente na bile e nos cálculos biliares, e presente nos alimentos, sobretudo em alimentos ricos em gorduras animais; circula no plasma associado a proteínas de várias densidades e tem uma participação importante na patogenia da formação do ateroma nas artérias. VER TAMBÉM lipoprotein.

cho·les·ter·ol·e·mia (kō-les′ter-ol-ē′mē-ă). Colesterolemia. SIN cholesteremia. [cholesterol + G. *haima*, sangue]

cho·les·ter·ol·o·gen·e·sis (kō-les′ter-ol-ō-jen′e-sis). Colesterologênese; a biossíntese de colesterol.

cho·les·ter·ol·o·sis (kō-les′ter-ol-ō′sis). Colesterolose. **1.** Condição resultante de um distúrbio do metabolismo dos lipídios, caracterizada por depósitos de colesterol no tecido, como na doença de Tangier. **2.** Cristais de colesterol na câmara anterior do olho, como na afacia com descolamento da retina associado. SIN cholesterinosis.

cho·les·ter·ol·u·ria (kō-les′ter-ol-oo′rē-ă). Colesterolúria; a excreção de colesterol na urina. SIN cholesterinuria.

cho·le·styr·a·mine (kō-les′tir-ă-mēn). Colestiramina; uma resina de troca aniônica usada para se ligar ao colesterol presente nos alimentos e, assim, impedir sua absorção sistêmica. Usada no tratamento da hipercolesterolemia. Pode se ligar a muitos fármacos ácidos no trato gastrointestinal e evitar sua absorção.

cho·le·u·ria (kō-lē-ū′rē-ă). Coleúria. SIN biliuria.

cho·lic (kō′lik). Cólico; relativo à bile. SIN choleic.

cho·lic ac·id. Ácido cólico; família de esteróides que compreende os ácidos (ou sais) biliares, geralmente na forma conjugada (p. ex., ácidos glicocólico e taurocólico). Quimicamente, os ácidos cólicos são ácidos colan-24-óicos (colânicos) (o C_{24} terminal do colano tornando-se um grupamento –COOH); biologicamente, os ácidos cólicos são derivados do colesterol (um derivado do colestano) e exibem vários graus de oxidação (grupamentos OH) e orientação nas posições 3, 7 e 12. São essas oxidações e orientações que distinguem os vários ácidos cólicos; p. ex., o ácido cólico é o ácido 3α,7α-12α-triidroxi-5β-colan-24-óico, o ácido desoxicólico é o ácido 3α,12α-diidroxi-5β-colânico. O ácido cólico é um detergente natural que ajuda na digestão de gorduras. SIN cholalic acid, cholanic acid.

cho·li·cele (kō′li-sēl). Colicele; aumento da vesícula biliar devido à retenção de líquidos. [G. *cholē*, bile, + *kēlē*, tumor]

cho·line (kō′lēn). Colina; íon (2-hidroxietil)trimetilamônio; encontrado na maioria dos tecidos animais na forma livre ou em combinação com lecitina (fosfatidilcolina), acetato (acetilcolina) ou citidina difosfato (citidina difosfocolina). Este é incluído no complexo de vitaminas B; como a acetilcolina (colina esterificada com ácido acético), é essencial para a transmissão sináptica. Vários sais de colina são usados na medicina. SIN lipotropic factor, transmethylation factor.

c. acetylase, c. acetilase. SIN c. acetyltransferase.
c. acetyltransferase, c. acetiltransferase; enzima que catalisa a condensação de colina e acetil-coenzima A, formando *O*-acetilcolina e coenzima A. SIN c. acetylase.
activated c., c. ativada. SIN cytidine diphosphocholine.
c. chloride, cloreto de colina; agente lipotrópico.
c. dihydrogen citrate, citrato diidrogenado de colina; agente lipotrópico.
c. esterase I, c. esterase I. SIN acetylcholinesterase.
c. esterase II, c. esterase II. SIN cholinesterase.
c. kinase, c. cinase; enzima que catalisa a formação de *O*-fosfocolina e ADP a partir de colina e ATP. SIN c. phosphokinase.
c. phosphatase, c. fosfatase. SIN *phospholipase* D.
c. phosphate cytidylyltransferase, c. fosfato citidililtransferase; enzima que catalisa uma etapa fundamental na biossíntese da lecitina: CTP + fosfocolina ↔ pirofosfato + CDP-colina.
c. phosphokinase, c. fosfocinase. SIN c. kinase.
c. phosphotransferase, c. fosfotransferase; enzima que catalisa a reação entre CDP-colina e 1,2-diacilglicerol para formar uma fosfatidilcolina e CMP (citidina monofosfato). A última etapa na biossíntese da lecitina.
c. salicylate, salicilato de colina; sal colínico do ácido salicílico; analgésico e antipirético (devido à fração salicilato).
c. theophyllinate, teofilinato de colina. SIN oxtriphylline.

cho·lin·er·gic (kol-in-er′jik). Colinérgico; relativo às células nervosas ou fibras que empregam acetilcolina como neurotransmissor. Cf. adrenergic. [choline + G. *ergon*, trabalho]

cho·lin·es·ter (kō′lin-es-ter). Coliéster; éster da colina; p. ex., acetilcolina.

cho·lin·es·ter·ase (kō-lin-es′ter-ās). Colinesterase; membro de uma família de enzimas capazes de catalisar a hidrólise das acilcolinas e algumas outras substâncias. Em mamíferos, encontrada na substância branca cerebral, no fígado, no coração, no pâncreas e no soro. Também é encontrada no veneno das cobras do gênero *Naja*. VER TAMBÉM acetylcholinesterase. SIN choline esterase II, nonspecific c., "s"-type c.

"e"-type c., c. do tipo "e". SIN acetylcholinesterase. ["e" como em eritrócito]
nonspecific c., c. inespecífica. SIN cholinesterase.
specific c., c. específica. SIN acetylcholinesterase.
"s"-type c., c. tipo "s". SIN cholinesterase. ["s" como em soro]
true c., c. verdadeira. SIN acetylcholinesterase.

cho·lin·es·ter·ase re·ac·ti·va·tor. Reativador da colinesterase; agente que reage diretamente com a enzima alquilfosforilada para liberar a unidade ativa; os agentes usados terapeuticamente para reativar formas fosforiladas de acetilcolinesterase são oximas, p. ex., diacetilmonoxima, monoisonitrosoacetona, 2-pralidoxima.

cho·lin·o·cep·tive (kō′lin-ō-sep′tiv). Colinoceptivo; relativo a locais químicos nas células efetoras aos quais a acetilcolina se une para exercer suas ações. Cf. adrenoceptive. [acetylcholine + L. *capio*, pegar]

cho·li·no·lyt·ic (kō′lin-ō-lit′ik). Colinolítico; que impede a ação da acetilcolina. [acetylcholine + G. *lysis*, afrouxamento]

chol·i·no·mi·met·ic (kol′i-nō-mi-met′ik). Colinomimético; que possui uma ação semelhante à da acetilcolina, a substância liberada por nervos colinérgicos; termo proposto para substituir o termo menos acurado, parassimpaticomimético. Cf. adrenomimetic. [acetylcholine + G. *mimētikos*, que imita]

cho·lin·o·re·ac·tive (kō′lin-ō-rē-ak′tiv). Colinorreativo; que responde à acetilcolina e substâncias correlatas.

chol·i·no·re·cep·tors (kol′i-nō-rē-sep′terz, -tōrz). Colinorreceptores. VER cholinergic *receptors*, em *receptor*.

cho·lis·tine sul·pho·meth·ate so·di·um (kō-lis′tēn sul-fō-meth′at). Sulfometato sódico de colistina. SIN colistimethate sodium.

cholo-. VER chole-.

chol·o·li·thi·a·sis (kol-ō-li-thī′ă-sis). Colelitíase. SIN cholelithiasis.

chol·o·pla·nia (kol-ō-plā′nē-ă). Coloplania; presença de sais biliares no sangue ou nos tecidos. [cholo- + G. *planē*, migração]

chol·o·poi·e·sis (kō-lō-poy-ē′sis). Colopoese. SIN cholepoiesis.

chol·or·rhea (kol-ō-rē′ă). Colorréia; termo obsoleto para indicar secreção excessiva de bile. [cholo- + G. *rhoia*, fluxo]

cho·los·co·py (kō-los′kō-pē). Coloscopia; termo raramente usado para designar colangioscopia. [cholo- + G. *skopeō*, ver]

chol·o·tho·rax (kō-lō-thōr′aks). Colotórax; bile na cavidade pleural.

cho·lo·yl (kō′lō-il). Coloíla; o radical do ácido cólico ou colato.

chol·ur·ia (kō-loo′rē-ă). Colúria. SIN biliuria. [G. *cholē*, bile, + *ouron*, urina]

cho·lyl-co·en·zyme A (kō′lil-kō-en′zīm). Colil-coenzima A; produto da condensação do ácido cólico e coenzima A; um intermediário na formação de sais biliares a partir dos ácidos biliares, como o ácido taurocólico a partir do ácido cólico.

c.-c. A synthetase, c.-c. A sintetase. SIN *cholate* ligase.

chon·dral (kon′dral). Condral. SIN cartilaginous. [G. *chondros*, cartilagem]

chon·dral·o·pla·sia (kon′dral-ō-plā′zē-ă). Condraloplasia; ocorrência de cartilagem em situações anormais no esqueleto ósseo. [G. *chondros*, cartilagem, + *allos*, outro, + *plasia*, formado]

chon·drec·to·my (kon-drek′tō-mē). Condrectomia; excisão de cartilagem. [G. *chondros*, cartilagem, + *ektomē*, excisão]

chon·dri·fi·ca·tion (kon′dri-fi-kā′shŭn). Condrificação; conversão em cartilagem. [G. *chondros*, cartilagem, + L. *facio*, fazer]

chon·dri·fy (kon′dri-fī). Condrificar; tornar cartilaginoso.

chondrio-. VER chondro-.

chon·dri·tis (kon-drī′tis). Condrite; inflamação da cartilagem. [G. *chondros*, cartilagem, + *-itis*, inflamação]

costal c., c. costocondrite. SIN costochondritis.

chondro-, chondrio-. Condro-, condrio-. **1.** Cartilagem ou cartilaginoso. **2.** Substância granular ou arenosa. [G. *condrion*, dim. de *chondros*, sêmola (grão grosseiramente moído), grão para moer, cartilagem]

chon·dro·blast (kon′drō-blast). Condroblasto; uma célula em divisão do tecido cartilaginoso em crescimento. SIN chondroplast. [chondro- + G. *blastos*, germe]

chon·dro·blas·to·ma (kon′drō-blas-tō-mă). Condroblastoma; tumor benigno originado nas epífises dos ossos longos, que consiste em tecido extremamente celular semelhante à cartilagem fetal.

chon·dro·cal·cin (kon′drō-kal-sin). Condrocalcina; proteína de peso molecular 69.000 que parece participar na mineralização do tecido rígido.

chon·dro·cal·ci·no·sis (kon′drō-kal-si-nō′sis). Condrocalcinose; calcificação da cartilagem. [chondro- + calcium + G. *-osis*, condição]

articular c., [MIM*118600], c. articular; doença caracterizada por depósitos de cristais de pirofosfato de cálcio livres de urato no líquido sinovial, cartilagem articular e tecidos moles adjacentes; causa várias formas de artrite, comu-

chon·dro·clast (kon′drō - klast). Condroclasto; célula multinucleada (célula gigante) envolvida na reabsorção da cartilagem calcificada; morfologicamente idêntica aos osteoblastos. [chondro- + G. *klastos*, quebrado em pedaços]

chon·dro·cos·tal (kon - drō - kos′tăl). Condrocostal. SIN costochondral. [chondro- + L. *costa*, costela]

chon·dro·cra·ni·um (kon - drō - krā′nē - ŭm). Condrocrânio; crânio cartilaginoso; as partes cartilaginosas do crânio em desenvolvimento. [chondro- + G. *kranion*, crânio]

chon·dro·cyte (kon′drō - sīt). Condrócito; célula cartilaginosa que não se divide; ocupa uma lacuna na matriz cartilaginosa. SIN cartilage cell. [chondro- + G. *kytos*, uma cavidade (célula)]

isogenous c.'s, condrócitos isógenos; clone de células cartilaginosas derivado de uma célula por divisão; ocorre em um grupo denominado nicho isógeno.

chon·dro·der·ma·ti·tis no·du·la·ris chron·i·ca he·li·cis (kon - drō - der - ma - tī′tis nod - ū - lar′is kron′i - kă hel′i - sis). Condrodermatite nodular crônica da hélice; nódulo (ou nódulos) doloroso(s), pequeno(s), crônico(s) e benigno(s) na hélice da orelha em idosos, que algumas vezes pode ulcerar e resulta do hábito de dormir sobre o lado afetado.

chon·dro·dys·pla·sia (kon′drō - dis - plā′zē - ă). [MIM*118650]. Condrodisplasia. SIN chondrodystrophy. [chondro- + G. *dys*, mau, + *plasis*, moldagem]

c. calcif′icans congen′ita [MIM*118650], c. calcificante congênita; herança autossômica dominante caracterizada por calcificações assimétricas e alterações ósseas displásicas, ocorrência menos freqüente de catarata congênita e ictiose em comparação com outras formas, e prognóstico relativamente bom. SIN Conradi disease, Conradi-Hünermann disease.

Nance-Sweeney c., c. de Nance-Sweeney. SIN chondrodystrophy with sensorineural deafness.

c. puncta′ta, c. pontilhada; distúrbio do desenvolvimento caracterizado por pontilhado epifisário, fendas coronais das vértebras, nanismo com encurtamento rizomélico dos membros, contraturas articulares, catarata congênita, ictiose e retardo mental. Existem formas autossômicas dominante e recessiva e ligadas ao X. SIN dysplasia epiphysialis punctata, hypoplastic fetal chondrodystrophy, stippled epiphysis.

rhizomelic c. punctata [MIM*215100], c. rizomélica pontilhada; condrodisplasia letal autossômica recessiva, causada por mutação no gene PEX 7 que codifica o receptor do sinal de orientação do peroxissoma tipo 2 (PTS2) no braço 6q do cromossoma.

chon·dro·dys·tro·phy (kon - drō - dis′trō - fē). Condrodistrofia; distúrbio no desenvolvimento dos primórdios cartilaginosos dos ossos longos, principalmente a região das placas epifisárias, resultando em interrupção do crescimento dos ossos longos e nanismo no qual os membros são anormalmente curtos, mas a cabeça e o tronco são praticamente normais; herança autossômica recessiva. SIN chondrodysplasia. [chondro- + G. *dys*, mau, + *trophē*, nutrição]

asphyxiating thoracic c., c. torácica asfixiante. SIN asphyxiating thoracic dystrophy.

asymmetric c., c. assimétrica. SIN enchondromatosis.

hereditary deforming c., c. deformante hereditária. (**1**) SIN hereditary multiple *exostoses*, em *exostosis*; (**2**) SIN enchondromatosis.

hypoplastic fetal c., c. fetal hipoplásica. SIN chondrodysplasia punctata.

myotonic c., c. miotônica; doença congênita rara que causa miotonia, hipertrofia muscular, anormalidades articulares e dos ossos longos e fraqueza. SIN Schwartz-Jampel disease.

c. with sensorineural deafness [MIM*215150], c. com surdez neurossensorial; displasia óssea caracterizada por nanismo, ponte nasal plana, fenda palatina, surdez neurossensorial, epífises grandes e achatamento dos corpos vertebrais; herança autossômica recessiva, causada por mutação no gene do colágeno tipo XI (COL11A2) no cromossomo 6p; existem formas dominantes. SIN Nance-Insley syndrome, Nance-Sweeney chondrodysplasia, OSMED, otospondylomegaepiphyseal dysplasia.

chon·dro·ec·to·der·mal (kon′drō - ek - tō - der′măl). Condroectodérmico; relativo à cartilagem derivada do ectoderma; p. ex., cartilagens branquiais que se desenvolveram a partir da crista neural.

chon·dro·fi·bro·ma (kon′drō - fi - brō′mă). Condrofibroma. SIN chondromyxoid fibroma.

chon·dro·gen·e·sis (kon - drō - jen′ĕ - sis). Condrogênese; formação de cartilagem. [chondro- + G. *genesis*, origem]

chon·dro·glos·sus (kon - drō - glos′ŭs). Condroglosso. VER chondroglossus *muscle*. [chondro- + G. *glossa*, língua]

chon·droid (kon′droyd). Condróide. **1.** Semelhante à cartilagem. SIN cartilaginoid. **2.** Cartilagem desenvolvida de forma não-característica, basicamente celular, com uma matriz basófila e cápsulas finas ou inexistentes. [chondro- + G. *eidos*, semelhança]

chon·dro·i·tin (kon - drō′i - tin). Condroitina; um (muco)polissacarídeo (proteoglicana) composto de resíduos alternados de ácido β-D-glucurônico e sulfato de N-acetil-D-galactosamina em ligações β(1-3) e β(1-4) alternadas; presente entre os constituintes da substância fundamental na matriz extracelular de tecido conjuntivo.

c. sulfate A, sulfato de condroitina A; condroitina com resíduos sulfúricos esterificando os grupamentos 4-hidroxila dos resíduos galactosamina; encontrado no tecido conjuntivo.

c. sulfate B, sulfato de condroitina B. SIN dermatan sulfate.

c. sulfate C, sulfato de condroitina C; condroitina com resíduos sulfúricos esterificando os grupamentos 6-hidroxila dos resíduos galactosamina.

chon·drol·o·gy (kon - drol′ō - jē). Condrologia; o estudo da cartilagem. [chondro- + G. *logos*, tratado]

chon·drol·y·sis (kon - drol′i - sis). Condrólise; desaparecimento da cartilagem articular devido à desintegração ou dissolução da matriz e células da cartilagem.

chon·dro·ma (kon - drō′mă). Condroma; neoplasia benigna derivada das células mesodérmicas que formam a cartilagem. [chondro- + G. -*ōma*, tumor]

extraskeletal c., c. extra-ósseo; condroma localizado nos tecidos moles, geralmente dos dedos das mãos e pés, não conectado ao osso ou periósteo subjacente.

juxtacortical c., c. justacortical. SIN periosteal c.

periosteal c., c. periosteal; condroma que se desenvolve a partir do periósteo ou do tecido conjuntivo periosteal. SIN juxtacortical c.

chon·dro·ma·la·cia (kon′drō - mă - lā′shē - ă). Condromalacia; amolecimento de qualquer cartilagem. [chondro- + G. *malakia*, amolecimento]

c. feta′lis, c. fetal; forma intra-uterina de condromalacia na qual o feto nasce morto com membros flexíveis.

generalized c., c. generalizada. SIN relapsing polychondritis.

c. of larynx, c. da laringe; presença de cartilagem laríngea mole, mais freqüente na epiglote de crianças pequenas. SIN laryngomalacia.

c. pate′llae, c. patelar; amolecimento da cartilagem articular da patela; pode causar patelalgia.

systemic c., c. sistêmica. SIN relapsing polychondritis.

chon·dro·ma·to·sis (kon′drō - mă - tō′sis). Condromatose; presença de múltiplos focos de cartilagem semelhantes a tumores.

synovial c., c. sinovial; condromatose ou nódulos osteocartilaginosos observados na membrana sinovial de uma articulação. SIN synovial osteochondromatosis.

chon·dro·ma·tous (kon - drō′mă - tŭs). Condromatoso; pertinente a, ou que apresenta as características de, um condroma.

chon·drome (kon′drōm). A informação genética contida em todas as mitocôndrias de uma célula. [mitochondria + -ome]

chon·dro·mere (kon′drō - mēr). Condrômero; unidade cartilaginosa do esqueleto axial fetal que se desenvolve em um único metâmero do corpo; uma vértebra cartilaginosa primordial juntamente com seu componente costal. [chondro- + G. *meros*, parte]

chon·dro·myx·o·ma (kon′drō - mik - sō′mă). Condromixoma. SIN chondromyxoid fibroma.

chon·dro·nec·tin (kon - drō - nek′tin). Condronectina; glicoproteína da matriz cartilaginosa que media a adesão de condrócitos ao colágeno tipo II. [chondro- + L. *necto*, ligar, + -in]

chon·dro·os·se·ous (kon - drō - os′ĕ - ŭs). Condrósseo; relativo à cartilagem e ao osso; seja como uma mistura dos dois tecidos ou como uma junção entre os dois, como a união de uma costela e sua cartilagem costal.

chon·dro·os·te·o·dys·tro·phy (kon′drō - os′tē - ō - dis′trō - fē). Condro-osteodistrofia; termo usado para designar um grupo de distúrbios dos ossos e cartilagem, que inclui síndrome de Morquio e condições semelhantes. SIN osteochondrodystrophia deformans, osteochondrodystrophy.

chon·drop·a·thy (kon - drop′ă - thē). Condropatia; qualquer doença da cartilagem. [chondro- + G. *pathos*, sofrimento]

chon·dro·pha·ryn·ge·us (kon′drō - făr - in - jē′ŭs). Condrofaríngeo. VER middle constrictor (*muscle*) of pharynx.

chon·dro·phyte (kon′drō - fit). Condrófito; massa cartilaginosa anormal que se desenvolve na superfície articular de um osso. [chondro- + G. *phytos*, crescimento]

chon·dro·plast (kon′drō - plast). Condroplasto. SIN chondroblast. [chondro- + G. *plastos*, formado]

chon·dro·plas·ty (kon′drō - plas - tē). Condroplastia; cirurgia plástica ou reparadora da cartilagem. [chondro- + G. *plastos*, formado]

chon·dro·po·ro·sis (kon′drō - pōr - ō′sis). Condroporose; condição da cartilagem na qual surgem espaços, sejam normais (no processo de ossificação) ou anormais. [chondro- + L. *porosus*, poroso]

chon·dro·sar·co·ma (kon′drō - sar - kō′mă). Condrossarcoma; neoplasia maligna derivada das células cartilaginosas, mais freqüente nos ossos pélvicos ou próximo das extremidades dos ossos longos, em pessoas de meia-idade e idosas; a maioria dos condrossarcomas surge *de novo*, mas alguns podem desenvolver-se em uma lesão cartilaginosa benigna preexistente.

chon·dro·sin, chon·dro·sine (kon′drō - sin). Condrosina; dissacarídio composto de uma molécula de ácido D-glucurônico e uma de D-galactosamina (condrosamina); um componente das condroitinas.

chon·dro·skel·e·ton (kon′drō-skel′ē-ton). Condroesqueleto; esqueleto formado de cartilagem hialina; p. ex., o esqueleto do embrião humano ou de determinados peixes adultos, como o tubarão ou a arraia.

chon·dro·ster·nal (kon-dro-ster′nal). Condroesternal. **1.** Relativo a uma cartilagem esternal. **2.** Relativo às cartilagens costais e ao esterno.

chon·dro·ster·no·plas·ty (kon-drō-ster′nō-plas-tē). Condroesternoplastia; correção cirúrgica de malformações do esterno.

chon·dro·tome (kon′drō-tōm). Condrótomo; bisturi muito duro usado para cortar cartilagem. SIN cartilage knife. [chondro- + G. *tomē*, cortar]

chon·drot·o·my (kon-drot′ō-mē). Condrotomia; divisão da cartilagem. [chondro- + G. *tomē*, corte]

chon·dro·tro·phic (kon-drō-trof′ik). Condrotrófico; que influencia a nutrição e, portanto, o desenvolvimento e crescimento da cartilagem. [chondro- + G. *trophē*, nutrição]

chon·dro·xi·phoid (kon-drō-zif′oyd). Condroxifóide; relativo à cartilagem xifóide ou ensiforme. [chondro- + G. *xiphos*, espada, + *eidos*, aspecto]

chon·drus (kon′drŭs). **1.** Cartilagem. SIN cartilage. **2.** A planta *Chondrus crispus*, *Fucus crispus* ou *Gigartina mamillosa* (família Gigartinaceae); demulcente em distúrbios crônicos e intestinais. SIN carragean (1), carragheen, Irish moss, pearl moss. [G. *chondros*, cartilagem]

CHOP Acrônimo para ciclofosfamida, doxorrubicina, vincristina e prednisona, um esquema quimioterápico para linfomas.

Chopart, François, cirurgião francês, 1743–1795. VER C. *amputation, joint*.

△ **chord-.** Cord-; cordão. VER TAMBÉM cord-. [G. *chordē*]

chor·da, pl. **chor·dae** (kōr′da, -dē) [TA]. Corda; cordão; estrutura tendinosa ou em forma de corda. VER TAMBÉM cord. [L., cord]

  c. arteriae umbilicalis [TA], cordão da artéria umbilical. SIN cord of umbilical artery.

  c. chirurgica'lis, categute cirúrgico. [L.]

  c. dorsa'lis, notocórdio. SIN notochord (2).

  false chordae tendineae [TA], cordas tendíneas falsas; cordas tendíneas que, ao contrário das cordas tendíneas verdadeiras, não se fixam aos folhetos das valvas atrioventriculares. Em vez disso, unem os músculos papilares entre si ou à parede ventricular (incluindo o septo interventricular), ou apenas passam entre dois pontos na parede ventricular (incluindo o septo). SIN chordae tendineae falsae [TA], chordae tendineae spuriae*, false tendinous cords*.

  c. mag'na, tendão do calcâneo. SIN calcaneal tendon.

  c. obli'qua membranae interosseae antebrachii [TA], c. oblíqua da membrana interóssea do antebraço. SIN oblique cord of interosseous membrane of forearm.

  c. spermat'ica, cordão espermático. SIN spermatic cord.

  c. spina'lis, medula espinal. SIN spinal cord.

  chordae tendineae cordis [TA], cordas tendíneas do coração. SIN chordae tendineae of heart.

  chordae tendineae falsae [TA], cordas tendíneas falsas. SIN false chordae tendineae.

  chor'dae tendin'eae of heart [TA], cordas tendíneas do coração; os filamentos tendíneos que seguem dos músculos papilares até os folhetos das valvas atrioventriculares (mitral e tricúspide). Com base em seu formato, posição ou área específica de fixação aos folhetos, foram descritos vários tipos: cordas em leque, cordas da zona rugosa, cordas de borda livre, cordas profundas e cordas basais. SIN chordae tendineae chordis [TA], tendinous cords*.

  chordae tendineae spuriae, cordas tendíneas falsas; *termo oficial alternativo para false chordae tendineae.

  c. tym'pani [TA], corda do tímpano; nervo que se origina do nervo facial no canal facial que atravessa o canalículo posterior da corda do tímpano até a cavidade timpânica, cruza sobre a membrana timpânica e o cabo do martelo, saindo através do canalículo anterior da corda do tímpano, na fissura petrotimpânica, para se unir ao ramo lingual do nervo mandibular na fossa infratemporal; conduz a sensação do paladar dos dois terços anteriores da língua e transporta fibras pré-ganglionares parassimpáticas até o gânglio submandibular, para inervação das glândulas salivares submandibular e sublingual. SIN cord of tympanum, parasympathetic root of submandibular ganglion, radix parasympathica ganglii submandibularis, tympanichord.

  c. umbilica'lis, cordão umbilical. SIN umbilical cord.

  c. vertebra'lis, notocórdio; termo obsoleto para notochord (2).

  c. voca'lis, pl. **chor'dae voca'les,** corda vocal. SIN vocal fold.

  chor'dae willis'ii, cordas de Willis. SIN Willis cords, em cord.

chord·al (kōr′dal). Cordal; relativo a qualquer corda ou cordão, principalmente à notocorda.

chor·da·me·so·derm (kōr-dă-mes′ō-derm). Corda mesodérmica; aquela parte do epiblasto de um embrião pequeno que tem a potencialidade de formar a notocorda e o mesoderma.

Chor·da·ta (kōr-dā′tă). O filo que inclui os vertebrados, definidos por possuírem: 1) um único cordão nervoso dorsal (o encéfalo e a medula espinal dos mamíferos); 2) uma haste cartilaginosa, a notocorda, que se forma dorsalmente ao intestino primitivo, no embrião incipiente, e é circundada e substituída pela coluna vertebral no subfilo vertebrado; 3) pela presença, em algum estágio do desenvolvimento, de fendas branquiais na faringe ou garganta. [L. *chorda*, do G. *chordē*, um cordão]

chor·date (kōr′dat). Cordado; animal do filo Chordata.

chor·dee (kōr-dē′). **1.** Ereção dolorosa do pênis na gonorréia ou na doença de Peyronie, com curvatura resultante da ausência de distensibilidade do corpo cavernoso uretral. SIN gryposis penis. **2.** Curvatura ventral do pênis, mais aparente à ereção, conforme observado na hipospádia. [Fr. cordado]

chor·di·tis (kōr-dī′tis). Cordite; inflamação de uma corda; geralmente da corda vocal. [G. *chordē*, corda, + *-itis*, inflamação]

  c. voca'lis infe'rior, c. vocal inferior; inflamação limitada principalmente à superfície inferior das cordas vocais e partes adjacentes. SIN chronic subglottic laryngitis.

chor·do·ma (kōr-dō′mă). Cordoma; neoplasia rara do tecido esquelético em adultos, derivada de porções persistentes da notocorda; composto de células dispostas em lóbulos, com abundante estroma mixóide; algumas células contêm vacúolos semelhantes a bolhas de sabão (células fisalíforas); mais freqüentemente na região do clivo ou da medula lombossacra. [(noto)chord + G. *-oma*, tumor]

chor·do·skel·e·ton (kōr-dō-skel′ē-ton). Cordoesqueleto; a parte do esqueleto embrionário que se desenvolve em conjunto com a notocorda.

cho·rea (kōr-ē′ă). Coréia; movimentos irregulares, espasmódicos, involuntários dos membros ou dos músculos faciais, freqüentemente acompanhados por hipotonia. A localização da lesão cerebral responsável não é conhecida. [L. do G. *choreia*, dança de coro, de *choros*, uma dança]

  c.-acanthocytosis, coréia-acantocitose; coréia familiar lentamente progressiva com deterioração mental associada, diminuição dos reflexos tendinosos profundos, atrofia bilateral dos núcleos putâmen e caudado e acantocitólise (aspecto espinhoso dos eritrócitos sanguíneos); o distúrbio tipicamente começa por volta do final da adolescência; em geral, a herança é autossômica recessiva. SIN acanthocytosis with c.

  acanthocytosis with c., acantocitose com coréia. SIN c.-acanthocytosis.

  acute c., c. aguda. SIN Sydenham c.

  benign familial c., c. familiar benigna; distúrbio do movimento raro, não-progressivo, caracterizado por coréia e atetose, que surge nos primeiros anos de vida e manifesta-se, freqüentemente, por ataxia da marcha e da coordenação dos membros superiores. O intelecto não é afetado. Provavelmente tem herança autossômica dominante com penetrância incompleta.

  chronic progressive c., c. progressiva crônica. SIN Huntington c.

  dancing c., c. dançante. SIN procursive c.

  degenerative c., c. degenerativa. SIN Huntington c.

  electric c., c. elétrica. **(1)** Distúrbio espasmódico progressivo fatal, possivelmente de origem malárica, ocorrendo principalmente na Itália; **(2)** uma forma grave de coréia de Sydenham, na qual os espasmos são rápidos e de caráter especialmente espasmódico.

  fibrillary c., c. fibrilar. SIN myokymia.

  c. gravida'rum, c. da gravidez; coréia de Sydenham que ocorre na gravidez.

  habit c., c. habitual. SIN tic.

  hemilateral c., c. hemilateral. SIN hemichorea.

  Henoch c., c. de Henoch. SIN spasmodic tic.

  hereditary c., c. hereditária. SIN Huntington c.

  Huntington c. [MIM*143100], c. de Huntington; distúrbio neurodegenerativo, com início geralmente na terceira ou quarta década de vida, caracterizado por coréia e demência; anatomopatologicamente, há atrofia bilateral acentuada do putâmen e da cabeça do núcleo caudado. A herança autossômica dominante com penetrância completa, causada por mutação associada à expansão da repetição dos trinucleotídios no gene de Huntington (DH) no cromossoma 4p. SIN chronic progressive c., degenerative c., hereditary c., Huntington disease.

  hysterical c., c. histérica; histeria de conversão na qual movimentos involuntários, rápidos e sem propósito (coreiformes) constituem a principal manifestação.

  juvenile c., c. juvenil. SIN Sydenham c.

  laryngeal c., c. laríngea; tique espasmódico envolvendo os músculos, resultando em uma fala hesitante, como na disfonia espasmódica.

  c. mi'nor, c. menor. SIN Sydenham c.

  Morvan c., c. de Morvan. SIN myokymia.

  posthemiplegic c., c. pós-hemiplégica. SIN posthemiplegic athetosis.

  procursive c., c. acelerada; c. festinante; c. dançante; uma forma na qual o paciente gira, corre para a frente ou realiza uma série de movimentos rítmicos de dança. SIN dancing c.

  rheumatic c., c. reumática. SIN Sydenham c.

  rhythmic c., c. rítmica; movimento padronizado na histeria de conversão.

  saltatory c., c. saltatória; movimentos dançantes rítmicos, como na c. acelerada.

  senile c., c. senil; distúrbio semelhante à c. de Sydenham, não associado à doença cardíaca ou demência, ocorrendo em pessoas idosas.

  Sydenham c., c. de Sydenham; c. pós-infecciosa que surge vários meses após uma infecção estreptocócica, com febre reumática subseqüente. A coréia envolve tipicamente os membros distais e está associada à hipotonia e labilidade emocional. A melhora ocorre em semanas ou meses e surgem exacerbações sem recorrência da infecção associada. SIN acute c., c. minor, juvenile c., rheumatic c., Sydenham disease.

cho·re·al (kōr-ē′al). Coreico; relativo à coréia.
cho·re·ic (kōr-ē′ik). Coreico; relativo a, ou da natureza da coréia.
cho·re·i·form (kōr-ē′i-form). Coreiforme. SIN choreoid.
△ **choreo-.** Coréia.
cho·re·o·ath·e·toid (kōr′ē-ō-ath′ē-toyd). Coreoatetóide; relativo a, ou caracterizado por, coreoatetose.
cho·re·o·ath·e·to·sis (kōr′ē-ō-ath-ē-tō′sis). Coreoatetose; movimentos anormais do corpo de padrões coreico e atetóide combinados. [choreo- + G. *athētos*, livre, + *-ōsis*, condição]
  congenital c., c. congênita. SIN double athetosis.
cho·re·oid (kōr′ē-oyd). Coreóide; coreiforme; semelhante à coréia. SIN choreiform.
△ **chorio-.** Corio-; qualquer membrana, principalmente a que envolve o feto. [G. *chorion*, membrana]
cho·ri·o·ad·e·no·ma (kō′rē-ō-ad-ē-nō′mă). Corioadenoma; neoplasia benigna do córion, principalmente com formação de mola hidatiforme.
  c. des′truens, c. destrutivo; mola hidatiforme na qual há um grau incomum de invasão do miométrio ou seus vasos sanguíneos, causando hemorragia, necrose e, ocasionalmente, ruptura do útero ou embolia de tecido molar para os pulmões; há proliferação acentuada do trofoblasto, mas também podem ser encontradas vilosidades avasculares. SIN invasive mole.
cho·ri·o·al·lan·to·ic (kō′rē-ō-al-an-tō′ik). Corioalantóico; pertinente à corioalantóide.
cho·ri·o·al·lan·to·is (kō′rē-ō-ă-lan′tō-is). Corioalantóide; membrana extra-embrionária formada pela fusão do alantóide com a serosa ou falso córion. Em mamíferos, forma a porção fetal da placenta; em embriões de aves é fundida à casca.
cho·ri·o·am·ni·o·ni·tis (kō′rē-ō-am′nē-ō-nī′tis). Corioamnionite; infecção envolvendo o córion, âmnion e líquido amniótico; geralmente, também há envolvimento das vilosidades placentárias e da decídua.
cho·ri·o·an·gi·o·ma (kō′rē-ō-an-jē-ō′mă). Corioangioma; tumor benigno dos vasos sanguíneos placentários (hemangioma), geralmente sem importância clínica; grandes tumores podem estar associados à insuficiência placentária e hidropisia fetal; em alguns casos, o estroma está edematoso e pode assemelhar-se ao tecido mixomatoso. VER TAMBÉM chorioangiosis. [chorion + angioma]
cho·ri·o·an·gi·o·ma·to·sis (kō′rē-ō-an′jē-ō′mă-tō′sis). Corioangiomatose. SIN chorioangiosis.
cho·ri·o·an·gi·o·sis (kō′rē-ō-an-jē-ō′sis). Corioangiose; aumento anormal do número de canais vasculares nas vilosidades placentárias; a corioangiose grave está associada a uma alta incidência de morte neonatal e grandes malformações congênitas. SIN chorioangiomatosis. [chorio- + G. *angeion*, vaso, + *-osis*, condição]
cho·ri·o·cap·il·la·ris (kō′rē-ō-kap-i-lā′ris). Coriocapilar. SIN capillary lamina of choroid.
cho·ri·o·car·ci·no·ma (kō′rē-ō-kar-si-nō′mă). Coriocarcinoma; neoplasia extremamente maligna, derivada de trofoblastos sinciciais placentários e citotrofoblastos, que forma lâminas e cordões irregulares, circundados por "lagos" irregulares de sangue; não são formadas vilosidades; as células neoplásicas invadem os vasos sanguíneos. Metástases hemorrágicas surgem relativamente cedo na evolução da doença, sendo freqüentemente encontradas nos pulmões, fígado, cérebro e vagina, bem como em vários outros órgãos pélvicos; o coriocarcinoma pode ocorrer após qualquer tipo de gravidez, principalmente a mola hidatiforme, e ocasionalmente origina-se em neoplasias teratóides dos ovários ou testículos. SIN chorioepithelioma.
cho·ri·o·cele (kō′rē-ō-sēl). Coriocele; hérnia do revestimento coróide do olho através de um defeito na esclerótica. [chorio- + G. *kēlē*, hérnia]
cho·ri·o·ep·i·the·li·o·ma (kō′rē-ō-ep-i-thē-lē-ō′mă). Corioepitelioma. SIN choriocarcinoma.
cho·ri·o·go·nad·o·tro·pin (kō′rē-ō-gon′ă-dō-trō-pin). Coriogonadotrofina. SIN chorionic gonadotropin.
△ **chorioid-, chorioido-.** Corioid, corioido-; para palavras iniciadas assim, e não encontradas aqui, ver choroid-, choroido-.
cho·ri·o·mam·mo·tro·pin (kō′rē-ō-mam′ō-trō-pin). Coriomamotropina. SIN human placental lactogen.
cho·ri·o·men·in·gi·tis (kō′rē-ō-men-in-jī′tis). Coriomeningite; uma meningite cerebral na qual há infiltração celular das meninges mais ou menos acentuada, freqüentemente com infiltração linfocítica dos plexos coróides, particularmente do terceiro e quarto ventrículos.
  lymphocytic c., c. linfocítica; uma forma de meningite viral que, geralmente, ocorre em adultos jovens durante os meses do outono e inverno. Causada por um vírus encontrado no camundongo doméstico comum. VER TAMBÉM lymphocytic choriomeningitis *virus*.
cho·ri·on (kō′rē-on). Córion; a membrana fetal mais externa, de múltiplas camadas, que consiste no mesoderma somático extra-embrionário, trofoblasto e, na superfície materna, em vilosidades banhadas por sangue materno; à medida que a gravidez progride, parte do cório se transforma na placenta fetal definitiva. SIN chorionic sac, membrana serosa (1). [G. *chorion*, membrana que envolve o feto]
  c. frondo'sum, c. frondoso; a parte do córion onde as vilosidades persistem, formando a parte fetal da placenta. SIN shaggy c.
  c. lae've, c. liso; a porção do córion da qual desaparecem as vilosidades nos estágios mais avançados da gravidez. SIN smooth c.
  previllous c., c. pré-viloso. SIN primitive c.
  primitive c., c. primitivo; o córion antes que suas vilosidades estejam bem-formadas. SIN previllous c.
  shaggy c., c. frondoso. SIN c. frondosum.
  smooth c., c. liso. SIN c. laeve.
cho·ri·on·ic (kō-rē-on′ik). Coriônico; relativo ao córion.
cho·ri·o·ret·i·nal (kō-rē-ō-ret′i-năl). Coriorretiniano; relativo ao revestimento coróide do olho e da retina. SIN retinochoroid.
cho·ri·o·ret·i·ni·tis (kō′rē-ō-ret′i-nī′tis). Coriorretinite. SIN retinochoroiditis.
  c. sclopeta'ria, c. esclopetária; proliferação de tecido fibroso na coróide e na retina em virtude de contusão da esclerótica por um projétil de arma de porte em alta velocidade. [L. *sclopetum*, arma de fogo de porte italiana do século XIV]
cho·ri·o·ret·i·nop·a·thy (kō′rē-ō-ret-i-nop′ă-thē). Coriorretinopatia; anormalidade primária da coróide com extensão para a retina. VER TAMBÉM choroidopathy.
cho·ris·ta (kō-ris′tă). Coristo; foco de tecido histologicamente normal, mas que não é normalmente encontrado no órgão ou estrutura em que está localizado; p. ex., tecido deslocado, durante o desenvolvimento, de seu local normal. Cf. choristoma. [G. *chōristos,* separado]
cho·ris·to·blas·to·ma (kō-ris′tō-blas-tō′mă). Coristoblastoma; neoplasia autônoma composta de células relativamente indiferenciadas de um coristoma. [choristoma + blastoma]
cho·ris·to·ma (kō-ris-tō′mă). Coristoma; massa formada por mau desenvolvimento de tecido de um tipo não encontrado normalmente no local. [G. *chōristos,* separado, + *-oma*]
cho·roid (ko′royd) [TA]. Coróide; a túnica vascular média do olho situada entre o epitélio pigmentar e a esclerótica. SIN choroidea [TA]. [G. *choroeidēs,* falsa leitura de *chorioeidēs,* semelhante a uma membrana]
cho·roi·dal (kō-roy′dăl). Coróide; relativo à coróide.
cho·roi·dea (kō-royd′ē-ă) [TA]. Coróide. SIN choroid. [ver choroid]
cho·roi·der·e·mia (kō-roy-der-ē′mē-ă) [MIM*303100]. Coroideremia; degeneração progressiva da coróide em homens, ocasionalmente em mulheres, começando com retinopatia pigmentar periférica, seguida por atrofia do epitélio pigmentar da retina e do coriocapilar, cegueira noturna, constricção progressiva dos campos visuais e, finalmente, cegueira completa; herança ligada ao X causada por mutação no gene da proteína-1 acompanhante Rab (REP1) em Xq; as mulheres heterozigotas exibem retinopatia pigmentar, mas sem defeito visual ou progressão periférica. SIN progressive choroidal atrophy, progressive tapetochoroidal dystrophy. [choroid + G. *erēmia,* ausência]
cho·roid·i·tis (kō-roy-dī′tis). Coroidite; inflamação da coróide. Cf. choriodopathy, chorioretinopathy. SIN posterior uveitis.
  anterior c., c. anterior; c. disseminada restrita à coróide periférica.
  areolar c., c. areolar; inflamação da coróide, com proeminente proliferação de pigmentos ocorrendo primeiro na região macular e, depois, mais na periferia.
  diffuse c., c. difusa; inflamação exsudativa disseminada da coróide com resolução progressiva de lesões antigas enquanto surgem novas lesões.
  disseminated c., c. disseminada; inflamação crônica da coróide, com múltiplos focos isolados.
  exudative c., c. exsudativa, freqüentemente com múltiplas lesões.
  juxtapupillary c., c. justapupilar; c. adjacente ao disco óptico.
  metastatic c., c. metastática; inflamação da coróide decorrente de êmbolos microbianos.
  multifocal c., c. multifocal; c. macular, peripapilar e periférica, freqüentemente designada histoplasmose ocular presumida.
  posterior c., c. posterior; c. disseminada restrita à coróide central.
  proliferative c., c. proliferativa; o tecido cicatricial denso produzido por coroidite grave.
  suppurative c., c. supurativa; inflamação purulenta da coróide.
  vitiliginous c., c. vitiliginosa. SIN bird shot retinochoroiditis.
△ **choroido-.** A coróide.
cho·roid·o·cy·cli·tis (kō-roy′dō-sī-klī′tis). Coroidociclite; inflamação do revestimento coróide e do corpo ciliar. [choroido- + G. *kyklos,* círculo]
cho·roi·dop·a·thy (kō-roy-dop′ă-thē). Coroidopatia; degeneração não-inflamatória da coróide.
  areolar c., c. areolar; degeneração pigmentar lentamente progressiva em pessoas jovens; caracterizada por focos pretos dispostos muito próximos e coalescentes no pólo posterior e na região macular. SIN central areolar choroidal atrophy, central areolar choroidal sclerosis.

central serous c., c. serosa central; descolamento da retina sensorial idiopático na mácula; mais comum em homens. SIN central angiospastic retinopathy, central serous retinopathy.

Doyne honeycomb c., c. alveolar de Doyne; termo obsoleto para macular *drusen*.

geographic c., c. geográfica. SIN serpiginous c.

helicoid c., c. helicóide. SIN serpiginous c.

myopic c., c. miópica; degeneração crônica da esclerótica e coróide com estafiloma posterior, associada à alta miopia.

serpiginous c., c. serpiginosa; anormalidade adquirida bilateral do epitélio pigmentar da retina e da coróide na qual o edema progressivo, múltiplo e irregular é seguido por cicatrizes atróficas em padrões lineares. SIN geographic c., helicoid c.

cho·roi·do·sis (ko' - roy - dō'sis). Coroidose; termo obsoleto para coroidopatia.

Chotzen, F., médico alemão do século XX. VER C. *syndrome*.

Christensen, Erna, neuropatologista dinamarquês, 1906–1967. VER C.-Krabbe *disease*.

Christian, Henry A., clínico norte-americano, 1876–1951. VER C. *disease, syndrome*; Hand-Schüller-C. *disease*; Weber-C. *disease*.

Christison, Sir Robert, médico escocês, 1797–1882. VER C. *formula*.

Christmas. Sobrenome de uma criança (Stephen Christmas) portadora da doença subseqüentemente denominada *doença de* Christmas; primeiro caso estudado em detalhes. VER Christmas *disease*, Christmas *factor*. VER TAMBÉM Christmas *factor, hemophilia* B.

△ **chrom-, chromat-, chromato-, chromo-.** Cor. [G. *chrōma*]

chro·maf·fin (krō'maf - in). Cromafim; que produz uma reação amarelo-acastanhada com sais de cromo; indica determinadas células na medula supra-renal e nos paragânglios. SIN chromaphil, chromatophil (3), chromophil (3), chromophile, pheochrome (1). [chrom- + L. *affinis*, afinidade]

chro·maf·fin·o·ma (krō - maf - in - ō'mă). Cromafinoma; neoplasia composta de células cromafins presentes na medula supra-renal, nos órgãos de Zuckerkandl ou nos paragânglios da cadeia simpática toracolombar; pode secretar catecolaminas. VER TAMBÉM pheochromocytoma. SIN chromaffin tumor.

chro·maf·fin·op·a·thy (krō'maf - in - op'ă - thē). Cromafinopatia; termo obsoleto para qualquer anormalidade do tecido cromafim, como na medula das supra-renais ou nos órgãos de Zuckerkandl. [chromaffin + G. *pathos*, sofrimento]

chro·man, chro·mane (krō'man, - mān). Cromano; unidade fundamental dos tocoferóides (vitamina E). VER TAMBÉM chromanol, chromene, chromenol.

chro·man·ol (krō'man - ol). Cromanol; 6-hidroxicromano (6-cromanol) é a unidade fundamental dos tocoferóides (vitamina E), tocóis e tocotrienóis, bem como do ubi-, toco- e filocromanol. VER TAMBÉM chroman, chromene, chromenol. SIN hydroxychroman.

chro·ma·phil (krō'mă - fil). Cromafil. SIN chromaffin.

△ **chromat-.** VER chrom-.

chro·mate (krō'māt). Cromato; sal do ácido crômico.

sodium c. Cr 51, cromato sódico Cr^{51}, cromo radioativo hexavalente aniônico na forma de cromato de sódio ($Na_2Cr^{51}O_4$) com uma meia-vida de 27,8 dias; usado para determinar o volume de hemácias circulantes e o tempo de sobrevida das hemácias.

chro·mat.ic (krō - mat'ik). Cromático; de, ou pertinente a, cor ou cores; produzido por, ou feito em, uma cor ou mais.

chro·ma·tid (krō'mă - tid). Cromátide; cada um dos dois filamentos formados por duplicação longitudinal de um cromossoma que se torna visível durante a prófase da mitose ou meiose; as duas cromátides são unidas pelo centrômero ainda não dividido; após a divisão do centrômero na metáfase e a separação das duas cromátides, cada cromátide torna-se um cromossoma. [G. *chrōma*, cor, + *-id* (2).]

chro·ma·tin (krō'ma - tin). Cromatina; o material genético do núcleo, consistindo em desoxirribonucleoproteína, que ocorre em duas formas durante a fase entre as divisões mitóticas: 1) como heterocromatina, presente como grumos condensados, facilmente coráveis; 2) como eucromatina, material disperso, levemente corado ou não-corado. Durante a divisão mitótica, a cromatina se condensa em cromossomas. [G. *chrōma*, cor]

heteropyknotic c., c. heteropicnótica. SIN heterochromatin.

oxyphil c., c. oxifila. SIN oxychromatin.

sex c., c. sexual; pequena massa condensada do cromossoma X inativado, geralmente situada logo dentro da membrana nuclear do núcleo em intérfase; o número de corpúsculos de cromatina sexual por núcleo é um menos o número de cromossomas X; portanto, homens normais e mulheres com a síndrome de Turner (XO) não possuem nenhum (cromatina sexual negativa), mulheres normais e homens com síndrome de Klinefelter (XXY) possuem um e mulheres XXX possuem duas massas de cromatina. Por razões técnicas, apenas cerca de metade das células em uma preparação exibem massas típicas. VER TAMBÉM Lyon *hypothesis*. SIN Barr chromatin body.

chro·ma·ti·nol·y·sis (krō'mă - ti - nol'i - sis). Cromatinólise. SIN chromatolysis.

chro·mat·i·nor·rhex·is (krō - mat'i - nō - rek'sis). Cromatinorrexe; fragmentação da cromatina. [chromatin- + G. *rhexis*, ruptura]

chro·ma·tism (krō'mă - tizm). Cromatismo. **1.** Pigmentação anormal. **2.** SIN chromatic aberration. [G. *chrōma*, cor]

△ **chromato-.** VER chrom-.

chro·ma·tog·e·nous (kro - mă - toj'ĕ - nŭs). Cromatógeno; que produz cor; que causa pigmentação. [chromato- + *-gen*, produtor]

chro·mat·o·gram (krō - mat'ō - gram). Cromatograma; o registro gráfico produzido por cromatografia.

chro·mat·o·graph (krō - mat'ō - graf). Cromatografar; realizar uma cromatografia.

chro·mat·o·graph·ic (krō'mat - ō - graf'ik). Cromatográfico; relativo à cromatografia.

chro·ma·tog·ra·phy (krō - mă - tog'ră - fē). Cromatografia; a separação de substâncias químicas e partículas (originalmente pigmentos vegetais e outras substâncias muito coloridas) por movimento diferencial através de um sistema de duas fases. A mistura de materiais a serem separados é percolada através de uma coluna ou folha de algum absorvente adequadamente escolhido (p. ex., um material de intercâmbio iônico); as substâncias menos absorvidas são menos retardadas e emergem mais cedo; aquelas mais fortemente absorvidas emergem mais tarde. SIN absorption c. [chromato- + G. *graphō*, escrever]

absorption c., c. de absorção. SIN chromatography.

adsorption c., c. de adsorção; c. na qual é obtida separação das substâncias pela diferença no grau de adsorção das substâncias a uma fase estacionária.

affinity c., c. de afinidade; c. onde o absorvente tem uma afinidade química única por um determinado componente da solução de passagem. SIN affinity. column.

column c., c. de coluna; forma de cromatografia de partição, adsorção, troca iônica ou afinidade, na qual uma fase é líquida (aquosa), fluindo para baixo em uma coluna cheia com a segunda fase, um sólido; as substâncias dissolvidas formam uma divisão entre as fases sólida e líquida, dependendo das condições químicas e físicas de cada fase; os solutos mais fortemente adsorvidos chegam ao fundo da coluna mais tarde que os solutos menos fortemente adsorvidos.

gas c., c. gasosa; procedimento cromatográfico no qual a fase móvel é uma mistura de gases ou vapores, separados no processo por sua adsorção diferencial em uma fase estacionária.

gas-liquid c. (GLC), c. líquido-gasosa; c. gasosa, com a fase estacionária sendo líquida, e não sólida.

gel filtration c., c. por filtração em gel. VER gel *filtration*.

high-performance liquid c. (HPLC), c. líquida de alto desempenho; tecnologia cromatográfica usada para separar e quantificar misturas de substâncias em solução. Uma amostra é injetada em um fluxo de solvente que segue através de uma coluna e detector. A separação durante a passagem através da coluna ocorre por absorção, partição, troca iônica ou exclusão de tamanho. A técnica é comumente usada em laboratórios para medir compostos orgânicos, incluindo hormônios esteróides, pesticidas e venenos, compostos tóxicos e carcinogênicos, além de drogas. SIN high-pressure liquid chromatography.

high-pressure liquid chromatography (HPLC), c. líquida de alta pressão. SIN high-performance liquid c.

ion exchange c., c. de troca iônica; c. na qual cátions ou ânions na fase móvel são separados por interações eletrostáticas com a fase estacionária. VER TAMBÉM anion exchange, cation exchange.

liquid-liquid c., c. líquida-líquida; c. na qual tanto a fase móvel quanto a fase estacionária (ou de movimento inverso) são líquidas, como na distribuição em contracorrente.

paper c., c. em papel; c. de partição na qual a fase em movimento é um líquido e a fase estacionária é papel.

partition c., c. de partição; a separação de substâncias semelhantes por divisões repetidas entre dois líquidos imiscíveis, de forma que as substâncias, na verdade, cruzam a divisão entre os líquidos em direções opostas; quando um dos líquidos está ligado como um filme sobre papel de filtro, o processo é denominado cromatografia de partição em papel ou cromatografia em papel.

reversed phase c., c. de fase invertida; forma de c. de partição na qual a fase estacionária é menos polar que a fase móvel.

thin-layer c. (TLC), c. em camada fina; c. através de uma camada fina de celulose ou material inerte semelhante, sustentado sobre uma lâmina de vidro ou plástico.

two-dimensional c., c. bidimensional; c. em papel na qual um ponto, localizado originalmente em um ângulo da folha, é orientado em uma direção ao longo de um lado da folha, após o que o papel é rodado 90° e dirigido, com outro solvente, na nova direção; os pontos resultantes são assim espalhados sobre todo o papel, produzindo um "mapa" ou "impressão digital". Também generalizada para incluir cromatografia seguida por eletroforese (ou vice-versa), cromatografia de coluna seguida por cromatografia em papel, etc.

chro·ma·toid (krō'mă - toyd). Cromatóide; substância refrátil composta de cromatina, considerada uma reserva alimentar não-glicogênica contida no citoplasma de determinados protozoários; observada em cistos de *Entamoeba histolytica* como barras arredondadas ou corpos cromatóides em contraste com a forma irregular dos corpos cromatóides nos cistos de *Entamoeba coli*. [chromato- + G. *eidos*, forma]

chro·mat·o·ki·ne·sis (krō′mă-tō-ki-nē′sis). Cromatocinesia; redistribuição da cromatina em várias formas. [chromato- + G. *kinēsis*, movimento]

chro·ma·tol·y·sis (krō-mă-tol′i-sis). Cromatólise; a desintegração dos grânulos de substância cromófila (corpúsculos de Nissl) em um corpo de célula nervosa, que pode ocorrer após exaustão da célula ou lesão de seu processo periférico; outras alterações consideradas parte da cromatólise incluem intumescência do pericário e deslocamento do núcleo de sua posição central para a periferia. SIN chromatinolysis, chromolysis, tigrolysis. [chromato- + G. *lysis*, dissolução]
  central c., c. central; c. associada a lesão axonal significativa. SIN retrograde c.
  retrograde c., c. retrógrada. SIN central c.
  transsynaptic c., c. transináptica. SIN transsynaptic *degeneration.*

chro·mat·o·lyt·ic (krō-mă-tō-lit′ik). Cromatolítico; relativo à cromatólise.

chro·ma·tom·e·ter (krō-mă-tom′e-ter). Cromatômetro. SIN colorimeter. [chromato- + G. *metron*, medida]

chro·mat·o·pec·tic (krō-mă-tō-pek′tik). Cromatopético; relativo a, ou que causa, cromatopexia. SIN chromopectic.

chro·mat·o·pex·is (krō-mă-tō-pek′sis). Cromatopexia; a fixação de líquido corante, isto é, à medida que o fígado funciona formando bilirrubina. SIN chromopexis. [chromato- + G. *pēxis*, fixação]

chro·mat·o·phil (krō-mat′ō-fil). 1. Cromatofílico. SIN chromophilic. 2. Cromatófilo. SIN chromophil (2). 3. Cromafim. SIN chromaffin.

chro·mat·o·phil·ia (krō-mă-tō-fil′ē-ă). Cromatofilia. SIN chromophilia.

chro·mat·o·phil·ic, chro·ma·toph·i·lous (krō-mă-tō-fil′ik, -tof′i-lŭs). Cromatofílico. SIN chromophilic.

chro·mat·o·pho·bia (krō-mă-tō-fō′bē-ă). Cromatofobia. SIN chromophobia.

chro·mat·o·phore (krō-mat′ō-fōr). Cromatóforo. 1. Um plastídio colorido, devido à presença de clorofila ou outros pigmentos, encontrado em determinadas formas de protozoários. 2. Melanófago; fagócito portador de pigmento encontrado principalmente na pele, mucosa e coróide do olho, e também em melanomas. 3. SIN chromophore. 4. Um plastídio colorido em vegetais; p. ex., cloroplastos, leucoplastos, etc. [chromato- + G. *phoros*, que carrega]

chro·mat·o·pho·ro·tro·pic (krō′mă-tō-fōr′ō-trop′ik). Cromatoforotrópico; designa a atração de cromatóforos pela pele ou outros órgãos. [chromatophore + G. *tropos*, volta]

chro.mat.o.plasm (krō′mă-tō-plazm). Cromatoplasma; a parte do citoplasma que contém pigmento.

chro·ma·top·sia (krō-mă-top′sē-ă). Cromatopsia; distúrbio no qual os objetos parecem estar anormalmente coloridos ou tingidos; designada de acordo com a cor vista: xantopsia, visão amarela; eritropsia, visão vermelha; cloropsia, visão verde; cianopsia, visão azul. SIN chromatic vision, clored vision, tinted vision. Cf. dyschromatopsia. [chromato- + G. *opsis*, visão]

chro·mat·o·some (krō-ma′tō-sōm). Cromatossoma; nucleossoma com uma proteína histona-1 ligada.

chro·ma·to·tro·pism (krō-mă-tot′rō-pizm). Cromatotropismo. 1. Alteração da cor. 2. O fenômeno de orientação em resposta à cor. [chromato- + G. *tropē*, volta]

chro·ma·tu·ria (krō-mă-too′rē-ă). Cromatúria; coloração anormal da urina. [chromato- + G. *ouron*, urina]

chrome (krōm). Cromo; principalmente como fonte de pigmento. [G. *chrōma*,

△ **-chrome.** Sufixo que indica relação com a cor. [G. *chrōma*, cor]

chro·mene (krō′men). Cromeno; 2*H*-1-benzopirano; unidade fundamental das tocoferolquinonas. VER TAMBÉM chroman, chromanol, chromenol.

chro·men·ol (krō′men-ol). Cromenol; 6-hidroxicromeno (6-cromenol) é a unidade fundamental das tocoferolquinonas (tocoferol oxidado) e plastocromenol-8. VER TAMBÉM chroman, chromanol, chromene. SIN hydroxychromene.

chrome red. Vermelho-cromo; cromato de chumbo básico.

chro·mes·the·sia (krō-mes-thē′zē-ă). Cromestesia. 1. A percepção da cor. 2. Condição na qual estímulos não-visuais, como o paladar ou o olfato, causam a percepção da cor. [G. *chrōma*, cor, + *aisthēsis*, sensação]

chrome yel·low [C.I. 77600]. Amarelo-cromo; pó amarelo fino usado em tintas e corantes. SIN lead chromate, Leipzig yellow, lemon yellow, Paris yellow.

chrom·hi·dro·sis (krōm-hī-drō′sis). Cromidrose; condição rara caracterizada pela excreção de suor contendo pigmento. SIN chromidrosis. [chrom- + G. *hidros*, suor]
  apocrine c., c. apócrina; excreção de suor colorido, geralmente preto, pelas glândulas apócrinas.

chro·mic ac·id (krō′mik). Ácido crômico; H_2CrO_4 ou $H_2Cr_2O_7$; forte agente oxidante formado pela dissolução de trióxido de cromo (CrO_3) em água. Foi usado em solução como anti-séptico tópico.

chro·mid·ia (krō-mid′ē-ă). Plural de chromidium.

chro·mid·i·a·tion (krō-mid-ē-ā′shŭn). Cromidiação. SIN chromidiosis.

chro·mid·i·o·sis (krō-mid-ē-ō′sis). Cromidiose; derrame de substância nuclear e cromatina para o protoplasma celular. SIN chromidiation.

chro·mid·i·um, pl. **chro·mid·ia** (krō-mid′ē-ŭm, -ē-ă). Cromídio, pl. cromídios; partícula ou estrutura basófila no citoplasma celular, rica em RNA, freqüentemente encontrada em células especializadas. [G. *chrōma*, cor, + *-idion*, sufixo diminutivo]

chro·mi·dro·sis (krō-mi-drō′sis). Cromidrose. SIN chromhidrosis.

chro·mi·um (Cr) (krō′mē-ŭm). Cromo; elemento metálico, n.º atômico 24, peso atômico 51,9961. Bioelemento essencial da dieta. O Cr^{51} (meia-vida de 27,70 dias) é usado como auxiliar no diagnóstico de muitos distúrbios (p. ex., perda de proteínas gastrointestinais). [G. *chrōma*, cor]
  c. trioxide, trióxido de cromo; CrO_3; ácido crômico, um agente oxidante forte usado como cáustico na remoção de verrugas e outros crescimentos pequenos na pele e genitália; o ácido hidratado, H_2CrO_4, forma sais de várias cores com potássio, chumbo e outras bases.

△ **chromo-.** VER chrom-.

Chro·mo·bac·te·ri·um (krō-mō-bak-tēr′ē-ŭm). Gênero de bactérias contendo bastonetes móveis, Gram-negativos. Esses microrganismos produzem um pigmento violeta (violaceína) e, algumas vezes, são patogênicos para o homem e outros animais. A espécie típica é *C. violaceum.*
  C. viola′ceum, espécie típica do gênero *C.*; é encontrado no solo e na água.

chro·mo·blast (krō′mō-blast). Cromoblasto; célula embrionária com potencial de se transformar em uma célula de pigmento. [chromo- + G. *blastos*, germe]

chro·mo·blas·to·my·co·sis (krō′mō-blas′tō-mī-kō′sis). Cromoblastomicose; micose crônica localizada da pele e dos tecidos subcutâneos caracterizada por lesões cutâneas tão rugosas e irregulares que se assemelham a uma couve-flor; causada por fungos dematiáceos como *Phialophora verrucosa, Exophiala (wangiella) dermatitidis, Fonsecaea pedrosoi, F. compacta* e *Cladosporium carrionii;* células fúngicas semelhantes a moedas de cobre formam corpos escleróticos arredondados no tecido, com hiperplasia epidérmica e microabscessos intra-epidérmicos. SIN chromomycosis. [chromo- + G. *blastos*, germe, + *mykē*, fungo, + *-osis*, condição]

chro·mo·cen·ter (krō′mō-sen-ter). Cromocentro. SIN karyosome.

chro·mo·cyte (krō′mō-sīt). Cromócito; qualquer célula pigmentada, como um eritrócito. [chromo- + G. *kytos*, célula]

chro·mo·gen (krō′mō-jen). Cromógeno. 1. Uma substância, sem cor definida própria, que pode ser transformada em um pigmento; indica especialmente o benzeno e seus homólogos, tolueno, xileno, quinona, naftaleno e antraceno, a partir dos quais são fabricadas as anilinas. 2. Um microrganismo que produz pigmento. 3. Uma substância, contendo um cromóforo, que é incolor se o cromóforo for removido.
  Porter-Silber c.'s, cromógenos de Porter-Silber; fenilidrazonas amarelas formadas pela reação de 17,21-diidroxi-20-oxosteróides com um reagente fenilidrazina-ácido sulfúrico; usados principalmente para determinar as concentrações plasmáticas de cortisol e o débito urinário de 17-hidroxicorticosteróides.

chro·mo·gen·e·sis (krō-mō-jen′e-sis). Cromogênese; produção de substância corante ou pigmento, freqüentemente através de uma reação catalisada por enzima. [chromo- + G. *genesis*, produção]

chro·mo·gen·ic (krō-mō-jen′ik). Cromogênico. 1. Designa um cromógeno. 2. Relativo à cromogênese.

chro·mo·gran·ins (krō′mō-gran-inz). Cromograninas; proteínas solúveis dos grânulos cromafins; a cromogranina A, uma glicoproteína ácida, corresponde a aproximadamente metade da quantidade total de proteínas da matriz do grânulo.

chro·mo·i·som·er·ism (krō′mō-ī-som′er-izm). Cromoisomerismo; isomerismo no qual os isômeros exibem cores diferentes.

chro·mo·lip·id (krō-mō-lip′id). Cromolipídio. SIN lipochrome (1).

chro·mol·y·sis (krō-mol′i-sis). Cromólise. SIN chromatolysis.

chro·mo·mere (krō′mō-mēr). Crômômero. 1. Um segmento condensado de um cromonema; faixas densamente coradas visíveis em cromossomas em determinadas condições. 2. SIN granulomere. [chromo- + G. *meros*, uma parte]

chro·mom·e·ter (krō-mom′e-ter). Cromômetro. SIN colorimeter.

chro·mo·my·co·sis (krō′mō-mī-kō′sis). Cromomicose. SIN chromoblastomycosis. [chromo- + G. *mykēs*, fungo, + *-osis*, condição]

chro·mone (krō′mōn). Cromona; 4*H*-1-benzopiran-4-ona; unidade fundamental de vários pigmentos vegetais e outras substâncias. VER TAMBÉM flavone, chromene, chroman.

chro·mo·ne·ma, pl. **chro·mo·ne·ma·ta** (krō-mō-nē′mă, -ma-tă). Cromonema; filamento espiralado, no qual estão situados os genes, que se estende por todo o comprimento de um cromossoma e exibe um teste de Feulgen intensamente positivo para DNA. SIN chromatic fiber. [chromo- + G. *nēma*, filamento]

chro·mo·nych·ia (krō-mō-nik′ē-ă). Cromoníquia; anormalidade na cor das unhas. [chromo- + G. *onyx (onych-)*, unha]

chro·mo·pec·tic (krō-mō-pek′tik). Cromopético. SIN chromatopectic.

chro·mo·pex·is (krō-mō-pek′sis). Cromopexia. SIN chromatopexis.

chro·mo·phil, chro·mo·phile (krō′mō-fil, krō′mō-fīl). Cromófilo. 1. SIN chromophilic. 2. Uma célula ou qualquer elemento histológico que se cora facilmente. SIN chromatophil (2). 3. SIN chromaffin. [chromo- + G. *phileō*, amar]

chro·mo·phil·ia (krō-mō-fil′ē-ă). Cromofilia; a propriedade possuída pela maioria das células que se coram facilmente com corantes apropriados. SIN chomatophilia. [chromo- + G. phileō, amar]

chro·mo·phil·ic, chro·moph·i·lous (krō-mō-fil′ik, -mof′i-lŭs). Cromofílico; cromófilo; que se cora facilmente; designa algumas células e estruturas histológicas. SIN chromatophil (1), chromatophilic, chromatophilous, chromphil (1), chromphile.

chro·mo·phobe (krō′mō-fōb). Cromófobo; resistente a colorações, que se cora com dificuldade ou não se cora; designa determinadas células desgranuladas no lobo anterior da hipófise. SIN chromophobic. [chromo- + G. phobos, medo]

chro·mo·pho·bia (krō-mō-fō′bē-ă). Cromofobia. **1.** Resistência a corantes por parte de células e tecidos. **2.** Aversão mórbida a cores. SIN chromatophobia. [chromo- + G. phobos, medo]

chro·mo·pho·bic (krō-mō-fō′bik). Cromofóbico. SIN chromophobe. [chromo- + phobos, medo]

chro·mo·phore (krō′mō-fōr). Cromóforo; o agrupamento atômico do qual depende a cor de uma substância. SIN chromatophore (3), color radical. [chromo- + G. phoros, que carrega]

chro·mo·phor·ic, chro·moph·o·rous (krō-mō-fōr′ik, -mof′ōr-ŭs). Cromofórico; cromóforo. **1.** Relativo a um cromóforo. **2.** Que produz ou transporta cor; designa determinados microrganismos.

chro·mo·pho·to·ther·a·py (krō′mō-phō′tō-thăr′ă-pē). Cromofototerapia. SIN chromotherapy. [chromo- + photo- + G. therapeia, tratamento clínico]

chro·mo·plast (krō′mō-plast). Cromoplasto; plastídio cheio de pigmentos carotenóides.

chro·mo·plas·tid (krō-mō-plas′tid). Cromoplastídio; plastídio pigmentado, contendo clorofila, formado em determinados protozoários. [chromo- + G. plastos, formado, + -id (2)]

chro·mo·pro·tein (krō-mō-prō′tēn). Cromoproteína; pertencente a um grupo de proteínas conjugadas, que consiste em uma combinação de pigmento (isto é, um grupo protético colorido) com uma proteína; p. ex., hemoglobina.

chro·mo·som·al (krō′mō-sō′măl). Cromossômico; relativo aos cromossomas.

chro·mo·some (krō′mō-sōm). Cromossoma; um dos corpúsculos (normalmente 46 em células somáticas dos seres humanos) no núcleo celular que possui os genes, tem a forma de um filamento de cromatina delicado durante a intérfase, contrai-se para formar um cilindro compacto segmentado em dois braços pelo centrômero, durante os estágios da metáfase e anáfase da divisão celular, e é capaz de reproduzir sua estrutura física e química através de sucessivas divisões celulares. Em bactérias e outros procariotas, o cromossoma não está encerrado em uma membrana nuclear e não sofre mitose. Os procariotas podem ter mais de um cromossoma. [chromo- + G. sōma, corpo]

cromossoma (conjunto)

n = haplóide			
2n = diplóide			
3n = triplóide		euplóide ou poliplóide	heteroplóide
4n = tetraplóide	anortoplóide		
5n = pentaplóide	ortoplóide		
6n = hexaplóide			
n + 1	= dissômico simples		
2n + 1	= trissômico simples	aneuplóide ou polissômico	
2n + 2 (igual)	= tetrassômico simples		
2n + 2 (dif.)	= trissômico duplo		

accessory c., c. acessório; cromossoma supranumerário que não é uma réplica exata de qualquer um dos cromossomas no complemento celular normal. SIN monosome (1), odd c., unpaired allosome, unpaired c.

acentric c., c. acêntrico; fragmento de um cromossoma que não possui centrômero e é incapaz de se fixar ao fuso mitótico, portanto, é incapaz de participar da divisão de um núcleo e é aleatoriamente distribuído nas células-filhas. SIN acentric fragment.

acrocentric c., c. acrocêntrico; cromossoma com o centrômero situado muito próximo de uma extremidade, de forma que o braço curto é muito pequeno, freqüentemente com um satélite.

bivalent c., c. bivalente; um par de cromossomas unidos temporariamente.

Christchurch c., c. de Christchurch; termo obsoleto que descreve um cromossoma acrocêntrico pequeno anormal (n.º 21 ou 22) com deleção completa ou quase completa do braço curto; encontrado em cultura de leucócitos, em alguns casos de leucemia linfocítica crônica e, também, em alguns parentes normais dos pacientes.

derivative c., c. derivado; cromossoma anômalo gerado por translocação. SIN translocation c.

dicentric c., c. dicêntrico; cromossoma com dois centrômeros que podem resultar de translocação recíproca.

double minute c.'s, cromossomas pequenos duplos; par de elementos extracromossomiais que não possuem centrômeros, freqüentemente associados a um gene de resistência a drogas.

fragile X c., c. X frágil; cromossoma X com um local frágil próximo da extremidade do braço longo, resultando no surgimento de um fragmento quase separado; só demonstrado em condições especiais de cultura; freqüentemente associado a retardo mental ligado ao X. VER Renpenning syndrome.

giant c., c. gigante; **(1)** SIN polytene c.; **(2)** lampbrush c.

heterotypical c., c. heterotípico; c. que faz par com um parceiro diferente, p. ex., os cromossomas X e Y.

homologous c.'s, cromossomas homólogos; membros de um único par de cromossomas.

lampbrush c., lamp-brush c., c. em escova de tubo de ensaio; **(1)** um grande cromossoma encontrado em ovócitos de determinados animais, caracterizado por muitas projeções laterais finas que produzem o aspecto de uma escova de tubo de ensaio. **(2)** área cromossomial com muitas voltas da cromatina de algumas espécies. SIN giant c. (2).

late replicating c., c. de replicação tardia; cromossoma (freqüentemente anômalo) mostrado, p. ex., por incorporação de um nucleotídio marcado, sofrendo duplicação tardia antes da mitose; anteriormente usado como forma de distinguir membros de um grupo de cromossomas.

marker c., c. marcador; cromossoma com características citologicamente distintas.

metacentric c., c. metacêntrico; c. com um centrômero posicionado centralmente que o divide em dois braços de comprimentos aproximadamente iguais.

mitochondrial c., c. mitocondrial; o componente DNA das mitocôndrias, cuja principal função é a síntese de trifosfato de adenosina e o controle da energia celular; o cromossoma contém cerca de 16.000 pares de bases dispostas em círculo. A herança é matrilínea, e a taxa de mutação é incomumente alta: como cada célula contém milhares de cópias, uma forma mutante pode assumir uma gradação quase contínua como em um processo galtoniano. A maioria das mutações conhecidas tem impacto sobre a cadeia respiratória.

nonhomologous c.'s, cromossomas não-homólogos; cromossomas que não são membros do mesmo par.

nucleolar c., c. nucleolar; c. regularmente associado a um nucléolo.

odd c., c. ímpar. SIN accessory c.

Philadelphia c. (Ph1), c. Filadélfia; um cromossoma 22 anormalmente encurtado, formado por translocação de uma parte do braço longo do cromossoma 22 para o cromossoma 9; encontrado em cultura de leucócitos de muitos pacientes com leucemia granulocítica crônica.

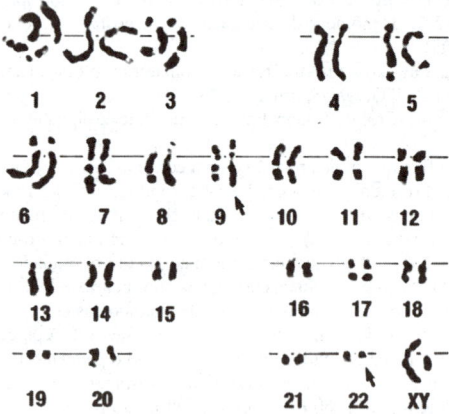

translocação do cromossoma Filadélfia: cariótipo de um paciente com leucemia granulocítica crônica mostrando a translocação do cromossoma Filadélfia, t(9:22)(q34;q11); o cromossoma Filadélfia é o cromossoma número 22

polytene c., c. politeno, estágio da divisão cromossomial que forma o c. gigante encontrado na glândula salivar de insetos dípteros; a grande largura é resultante de divisões repetidas do cromonema sem separação longitudinal subseqüente dos filamentos. SIN giant c. (1).

c. puffs, expansões cromossomiais; expansões de determinadas regiões dos cromossomas; locais de síntese de RNA.

ring c., c. em anel; c. com extremidades unidas para formar uma estrutura circular. A forma em anel é anormal no homem, mas a forma normal dos cro-

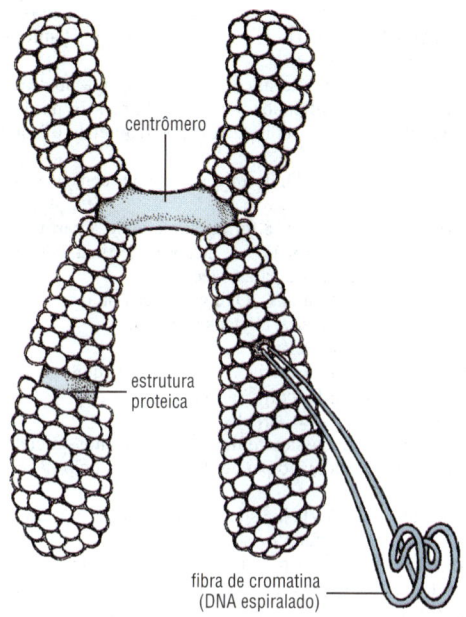

cromossoma

mossomas em determinadas bactérias.

sex c., c. sexual; o par de cromossomas responsáveis pela determinação do sexo. No homem e na maioria dos animais, os cromossomas sexuais são designados X e Y; as fêmeas possuem dois cromossomas X, e os machos, um cromossoma X e um Y. Em determinadas aves, insetos e peixes, os cromossomas sexuais são designados Z e W; os machos possuem dois cromossomas Z, e as fêmeas podem ter um cromossoma Z e um W, ou um Z e nenhum W. SIN gonosome.

submetacentric c., c. submetacêntrico; c. com o centrômero posicionado de forma a dividir o cromossoma em dois braços de comprimentos bem diferentes.

telocentric c., c. telocêntrico; c. com um centrômero terminal; esses cromossomas no homem são instáveis e surgem por erro de divisão ou quebra próximo ao centrômero, sendo geralmente eliminados em algumas divisões celulares.

translocation c., c. de translocação. SIN derivative c.

unpaired c., c. não-pareado. SIN accessory c.

W c., X c., Y c., Z c., c. W, c. X, c. Y, c. Z. VER sex c.'s.

c. walking, isolamento seqüencial de seqüências superpostas de DNA (isto é, clones); com esse procedimento podem ser transpostas grandes regiões do cromossoma. SIN overlap hybridization.

yeast artificial c.'s (YAC), c. artificial de levedura; seqüências de DNA de levedura que incorporaram fragmentos de DNA estranho muito grandes; o DNA recombinante é então introduzido na levedura por transformação; o uso de cromossomas artificiais de levedura permite a clonagem de grandes genes com suas seqüências reguladoras laterais.

chro·mo·some pair·ing. Pareamento cromossômico; o processo na sinapse pelo qual pares de cromossomas homólogos se alinham opostos uns aos outros antes de se separarem na formação da célula-filha; a aposição permite troca de material genético no *crossing-over*.

chro·mo·ther·a·py (krō-mō-thār′ă-pē). Cromoterapia; tratamento de doença por luz colorida. SIN chromophototherapy.

chro·mo·tox·ic (krō-mō-tok′sik). Cromotóxico; causado por uma ação tóxica sobre a hemoglobina, como na hipercromemia cromotóxica, ou resultante da destruição da hemoglobina.

chro·mo·trich·ia (krō-mō-trik′ē-ă). Cromotriquia; pêlos coloridos ou pigmentados. [chromo- + G. *thrix (trich-)*, pêlo]

chro·mo·trich·i·al (krō-mō-trik′ē-ăl). Cromotríquico; relativo à coloração do pêlo.

chro·mo·trope (krō′mō-trōp). Cromótropo; qualquer um dentre vários corantes que contêm ácido cromotrópico e que possuem a propriedade de passar de vermelho a azul na cromagem residual.

chro·mo·trope 2R [C.I. 16570]. Cromótropo 2R; corante ácido vermelho usado como contracorante e para coloração de hemácias em cortes.

chro·mo·trop·ic ac·id (krō′mō-trōp-ik). Ácido cromotrópico; usado como reagente e em cromotropos.

chro·nax·ia (krō-nak′sē-ă). Cronaxia. SIN chronaxie.

chro·nax·ie (krō′nak-sē). Cronaxia; medida da excitabilidade do tecido nervoso ou muscular; a menor duração de um estímulo elétrico efetivo que tem força igual a duas vezes a força mínima necessária para excitação. SIN chronaxia, chronaxis, chronaxy. [G. *chronos*, tempo, + *axia*, valor]

chro·nax·im·e·ter (krō-nak-sim′e-ter). Cronaxímetro; instrumento para medir cronaxia.

chro·nax·im·e·try (krō-nak′sim′e-trē). Cronaximetria; medida da cronaxia. [G. *chronos*, tempo, + *axia*, valor, + *metrein*, medir]

chro·nax·is (krō-nak′sis). Cronaxia. SIN chronaxie.

chro·naxy (krō′nak-sē). Cronaxia. SIN chronaxie.

chron·ic (kron′ik). Crônico. 1. Referente a um estado relativo à saúde, com longa duração. 2. Referente à exposição, prolongada ou de longo prazo, algumas vezes significando também baixa intensidade. 3. O *U.S. National Center for Health Statistics* define uma condição crônica como aquela com 3 meses de duração ou mais. [G. *chronos*, tempo]

chro·nic·i·ty (kron-is′i-tē). Cronicidade; o estado de ser crônico.

△ **chrono-.** Tempo. [G. *chronos*]

chro·no·bi·ol·o·gy (kron′ō-bī-ol′ō-jē). Cronobiologia; aspecto da biologia relacionado à cronologia dos eventos biológicos, principalmente fenômenos repetitivos ou cíclicos em organismos individuais. [chrono- + G. *bios*, vida, + *logos*, estudo]

chron·og·no·sis (kron-og-nō′sis). Cronognose; percepção da passagem do tempo. [chrono- + G. *gnōsis*, conhecimento]

chro·no·graph (kron′ō-graf). Cronógrafo; instrumento para medida gráfica e registro de breves períodos de tempo. [chrono- + G. *graphō*, registrar]

chro·nom·e·try (krō-nom′e-trē). Cronometria; medida de intervalos de tempo. [chrono- + G. *metron*, medida]

mental c., c. mental; estudo da duração de processos mentais e de comportamento.

chron·o·on·col·o·gy (kron′ō-on-kol′ō-jē). Cronooncologia; estudo da influência de ritmos biológicos sobre o crescimento neoplásico; também usado para descrever tratamento anticâncer com base na hora de administração da medicação. [G. *chronos*, tempo, + oncology]

chro·no·phar·ma·col·o·gy (kron′ō-far-ma-kol′ō-jē). Cronofarmacologia; ramo da cronobiologia relacionado aos efeitos dos fármacos sobre o momento de eventos e ritmos biológicos, e a relação entre o momento biológico e os efeitos dos fármacos.

chro·no·pho·bia (kron′ō-fō′bē-ă). Cronofobia; medo mórbido da duração ou imensidão do tempo.

chro·no·pho·to·graph (kron-ō-fō′tō-graf). Cronofotografia; fotografia pertencente a uma série a fim de mostrar as sucessivas fases de um movimento.

chro·no·ta·rax·is (kron′ō-tă-rak′sis). Cronotaraxia; distorção ou confusão do sentido de tempo. [chrono- + G. *taraxis*, confusão]

chronotherapy (krō′nō-ther′ă-pē). Cronoterapia; a prática de administrar fármacos em determinados horários do dia considerados ideais para aumentar a atividade ou reduzir a toxicidade. VER TAMBÉM chrono-oncology. [chrono- + therapy]

chro·no·tro·pic (kron′ō-trop′ik). Cronotrópico; que afeta a freqüência de movimentos rítmicos como os batimentos cardíacos.

chro·not·ro·pism (kron-ot′rō-pizm). Cronotropismo; modificação da freqüência de um movimento periódico, p. ex., o batimento cardíaco, através de alguma influência externa. [chrono- + G. *tropē*, volta, mudança]

negative c., c. negativo; retardo do movimento, particularmente da freqüência cardíaca.

positive c., c. positivo; aceleração do movimento, particularmente da freqüência cardíaca.

chro·o·coc·cals (krō-ō-kok-alz). Classe de cianobactérias na qual as células são solitárias ou formam colônias. [*Chroococcus*, do G. *chrōs, chroos*, cor, + *coccus*]

△ **chrys-, chryso-.** Ouro; corresponde ao L. auro-. [G. *chrysos*]

chry·san·the·mum-car·box·yl·ic ac·ids (kri-san′the-mum-kar-bok′si-lik). Ácidos crisântemo-carboxílicos; ácidos carboxílicos de ciclopropano substituídos em uma posição por dois grupamentos metila, o outro por 2-metil-1-propenil (ácido crisântemo-monocarboxílico) ou por 3-metoxi-2-metil-3-oxo-1-propenil (éster metil do ácido crisântemo-dicarboxílico); esses ácidos, esterificados com aletrolona ou piretrolona, são as aletrinas e piretrinas, respectivamente.

Chrys·a·o·ra (kris′-ă-ōr-a). Gênero do filo invertebrado Cnidaria que inclui a urtiga do mar.

C. quinquecirrha, a urtiga-do-mar, uma água-viva (medusa) que causa ardência moderada a intensa. VER TAMBÉM jellyfish. SIN sea nettle.

chrys·a·ro·bin (kris-ă-rō′bin). Crisarobina; extrato de pó-de-Goa; mistura complexa de produtos da redução do ácido crisofânico, emodina e éter monoetílico de emodina; usado localmente na dermatofitose, psoríase e eczema. [G. *chrysos*, ouro, + Ind. Bras. *araroba*, casca]

chrys·a·zine (kris′ă-zin). Crisazina. SIN danthron.

chry·si·a·sis (kri-sī′ă-sis). Crisíase; coloração cinza-azulada permanente da pele e das escleras, resultante da deposição de ouro nos macrófagos. SIN auriasis, aurothrocroderma. [G. *chrysos*, ouro]

chrys·o·cy·a·no·sis (kris′ō-sī-ă-nō′sis). Crisocianose; pigmentação da pele devida à reação ao uso terapêutico de sais de ouro.

chrys·oi·din (kris′oy-din) [C.I. 11270]. Crisoidina; corante (PM 249) feito de anilina, usado em histologia e como indicador (mudando de laranja para amarelo em pH 4,0 a 7,0); também empregado como substituto do castanho de Bismark. O citrato de crisoidina e o tiocianato de crisoidina são usados como anti-sépticos.

Chrys·o·my·ia (kris-ō-mī′ya). Gênero de moscas causadoras de miíase (família Calliphoridae) com adultos de tamanho médio e coloração metálica; inclui a larva da mosca do Velho Mundo, *C. bezziana* (algumas vezes denominada *Cochliomyia bezziana*), que é um invasor primário, comparável à *Cochliomyia hominivorax*, a mosca do Novo Mundo, enquanto a *C. megacephala* é um equivalente do Velho Mundo à *Cochliomyia macellaria*, sendo ambas invasoras secundárias ou saprofíticas. [G. *chrysos*, ouro, + *myia*, mosca]

Chrys·ops (kris′ops). Gênero de moscas da família Tabanidae, com cerca de 80 espécies norte-americanas, caracterizado por um padrão de asas manchadas; *C. discalis* é um vetor da *Francisella tularensis* nos Estados Unidos; *C. dimidiatus* e *C. silaceus* são os principais vetores da *Loa loa* no oeste da África. [G. *chrysos*, ouro, + *ōps*, olho]

Chrys·o·spo·ri·um par·vum (kris-ō-spōr′ē-ŭm par′vŭm). Nome antigo do *Emmonsia parva* (fungo).

chrys·o·ther·a·py (kris-ō-thăr′a-pē). Crisoterapia; auroterapia; tratamento de doenças pela administração de sais de ouro. SIN aurotherapy. [G. *chrysos*, ouro]

chunk·ing (chŭnk′ing). O processo, na memória de curto prazo, de combinar diferentes itens de informação de forma que ocupem o mínimo possível do espaço limitado na memória de curto prazo; p. ex., combinar, em um percepto, as quatro letras individuais que formam a palavra "gato".

Churg, Jacob, patologista norte-americano, *1910. Ver C.-Strauss *syndrome*.

chut·ta (chŭ′ta). Câncer do palato que se desenvolve em asiáticos que fumam charutos com a extremidade acesa dentro da boca. Uma associação semelhante foi descrita na América do Sul e na Sardenha.

Chvostek, Franz, cirurgião austríaco, 1834–1884. VER C. *sign*.

△ **chyl-.** VER chylo-.

chy·lan·gi·o·ma (kī-lan-jē-ō′ma). Quilangioma; massa de vasos lácteos dilatados, proeminentes e de vasos linfáticos intestinais maiores. [chyl- + G. *angeion*, vaso, + *-ōma*, tumor]

chy·la·que·ous (kī-lā′kwē-ŭs). Quiláceo; referente ao quilo aquoso. [chyl- + L. *aqua*, água]

chyle (kīl). Quilo; líquido branco ou amarelo-claro turvo, captado pelos vasos lácteos do intestino durante a digestão e transportado pelo sistema linfático através do ducto torácico para a circulação. O aspecto leitoso é devido à presença de quilomícrons na linfa. [G. *chylos*, suco]

chy·le·mia (kī-lē′mē-ă). Quilemia; a presença de quilo no sangue circulante. [chyl- + G. *haima*, sangue]

chy·li·dro·sis (kī-li-drō′sis). Quilidrose; sudorese de um líquido leitoso semelhante ao quilo. [chyl- + G. *hidrōs*, suor]

chy·li·fac·tion (kī-li-fak′shŭn). Quilificação. SIN chylopoiesis. [chyl- + L. *facio*, fazer]

chy·li·fac·tive (kī-li-fak′tiv). Quilificativo. SIN chylopoietic.

chy·lif·er·ous (kī-lif′er-ŭs). Quilífero; que conduz quilo. SIN chylophoric. [chyl- + L. *fero*, conduzir]

chy·li·fi·ca·tion (kī′li-fi-kā′shŭn). Quilificação. SIN chylopoiesis.

chy·li·form (kī′li-fōrm). Quiliforme; semelhante ao quilo.

△ **chylo-, chyl-.** Quilo. [G. *chylos*, suco]

chy·lo·cele (kī′lō-sēl). Quilocele; derrame de quilo na túnica vaginal propriamente dita e na cavidade da túnica vaginal testicular. [chylo- + G. *kēlē*, tumor] **parasitic c.,** q. parasitária. SIN elephantiasis scroti.

chy·lo·cyst (kī′lō-sist). Quilocisto. SIN cisterna chyli. [chylo- + G. *kystis*, bexiga]

chy·lo·me·di·as·ti·num (kī′lō-mē-dē-as-tī′nŭm). Quilomediastino; presença anormal de quilo no mediastino.

chy·lo·mi·cron, pl. **chy·lo·mi·cra, chy·lo·mi·crons** (kī-lō-mī′kron, -mī′kră, -mī′kronz). Quilomícron, quilomícrons; grande gotícula de lipídio (entre 0,8 e 5 nm de diâmetro) ou lipídio reprocessado sintetizado em células epiteliais do intestino delgado e contendo triacilglicerois, ésteres do colesterol e várias apolipoproteínas (p. ex., A-I, B-48, C-I, C-II, C-III, E); a menos densa (< 1,006 g/ml) das lipoproteínas plasmáticas, que funciona como veículo de transporte. [chylo- + G. *micros*, pequena]

chy·lo·mi·cro·ne·mia (kī′lō-mī-krō-nē′mē-ă). Quilomicronemia; a presença de quilomícrons, principalmente um número aumentado, no sangue circulante, como na hiperlipoproteinemia familiar tipo I. VER TAMBÉM familial chylomicronemia *syndrome*.

chy·lo·per·i·car·di·um (kī′lō-păr-i-kar′dē-ŭm). Quilopericárdio; derrame pericárdico leitoso resultante de obstrução do ducto torácico, por traumatismo ou de origem idiopática.

chy·lo·per·i·to·ne·um (kī′lō-păr-i-tō-nē′ŭm). Quiloperitônio. SIN chylous ascites.

chy·lo·phor·ic (kī-lō-fōr′ik). Quilofórico. SIN chyliferous. [chylo- + G. *phoros*, que carrega]

chy·lo·pleu·ra (kī-lō-ploor′ă). Quilopleura. SIN chylothorax.

chy·lo·pneu·mo·tho·rax (kī′lō-noo-mō-thōr′aks). Quilopneumotórax; quilo livre e ar no espaço pleural.

chy·lo·poi·e·sis (kī′lō-poy-ē′sis). Quilopoese; formação de quilo no intestino. SIN chylifaction, chylification. [chylo- + G. *poiesis*, produção]

chy·lo·poi·et·ic (kī′lō-poy-et′ik). Quilopoético; relativo à quilopoese. SIN chylifactive.

chy·lor·rhea (kī-lō-rē′ă). Quilorréia; o fluxo ou secreção de quilo. [chylo- + G. *rhoia*, fluxo]

chy·lo·sis (kī-lō′sis). Quilose; a formação de quilo a partir do alimento no intestino, sua digestão e absorção pela mucosa intestinal, bem como sua mistura com o sangue e transporte para os tecidos.

chy·lo·tho·rax (kī-lō-thōr′aks). Quilotórax; acúmulo de líquido quiloso no espaço pleural. SIN chylopleura, chylous hydrothorax.

chy·lous (kī′lŭs). Quiloso; relativo ao quilo.

chy·lu·ria (kī-loo′rē-ă). Quilúria; a eliminação de quilo na urina; uma forma de albidúria. [chyl- + G. *ouron*, urina]

chy·mase (kī′mās). Quimase. SIN chymosin.

chyme (kīm). Quimo; a massa semilíquida de alimentos parcialmente digeridos que passaram do estômago para o duodeno. SIN pulp (3) [TA], chymus. [G. *chymos*, suco]

chy·mi·fi·ca·tion (kī-mi-fi-kā′shŭn). Quimificação. SIN chymopoiesis. [G. *chymos*, suco, + L. *facio*, fazer]

chy·mo·pa·pa·in (kī′mō-pap-ā′in). Quimopapaína; uma cisteína proteinase semelhante à papaína em especificidade; em raras ocasiões, é usada para reduzir os discos intervertebrais deslocados como alternativa à cirurgia; usada como amaciante de carne. É a principal endopeptidase da papaia.

chy·mo·poi·e·sis (kī′mō-poy-ē′sis). Quimopoese; a produção de quimo; o estado físico do alimento (semilíquido) produzido pela digestão no estômago. SIN chymification. [G. *chymos*, suco, quimo, + *poiesis*, produção]

chy·mor·rhea (kī-mō-rē′ă). Quimorréia; fluxo de quimo. [G. *chymos*, suco, + *rhoia*, fluxo]

chy·mo·sin (kī′mō-sin). Quimosina; proteinase aspártica estruturalmente homóloga à pepsina, formada a partir da pró-quimosina; a enzima coaguladora do leite obtida da camada glandular do estômago de bezerros. Atua sobre uma ligação peptídica simples (–Phe–Met–) na κ-caseína. SIN chymase, pexin, rennase, rennet, rennin.

chy·mo·sin·o·gen (kī-mō-sin′ō-jen). Quimosinogênio. SIN prochymosin.

chy·mo·sta·tin (kī′mō-sta-tin). Quimostatina; oligopeptídeo conhecido por inibir proteases semelhantes à quimotripsina (p. ex., catepsinas A, B e D, e papaína).

chy·mo·tryp·sin (kī-mō-trip′sin). Quimotripsina; quimotripsina A ou B; uma proteína sérica do trato gastrointestinal que cliva preferencialmente ligações carboxila de aminoácidos hidrófobos, particularmente nos resíduos tirosil, triptofanil, fenilalanil e leucil; sintetizada no pâncreas como quimotripsinogênio, sendo, subseqüentemente, convertida em quimotripsina-π, δ e, finalmente, α por sucessivas clivagens dependentes de tripsina; proposta para uso no tratamento da inflamação e do edema associados a traumatismo e para facilitar a extração de catarata intracapsular. A q. A tem a especificidade supracitada, a q. B é homóloga à q. A e a q. C tem uma especificidade mais ampla (p. ex., atividade adicional sobre ligações carboxila de resíduos metionil, glutaminil e asparaginil).

chy·mo·tryp·sin·o·gen (kī′mō-trip-sin′ō-jen). Quimotripsinogênio; o precursor da quimotripsina. Convertido em π-quimotripsina pela ação da tripsina.

chy·mous (kī′mŭs). Quimoso; relativo ao quimo.

chy·mus (kī′mŭs). Quimo. SIN chyme.

chytide. Ruga cutânea.

Ci Abreviatura de curie.

Ciaccio, Carmelo, patologista italiano, 1877–1956. VER Ciaccio *stain*.

Ciaccio, Giuseppe V., anatomista italiano, 1824–1901. VER Ciaccio *glands*, em *gland*.

cib. Abreviatura do L. *cibus*, alimento.

ci·bo·pho·bia (sī-bō-fō′bē-ă). Cibofobia; temor de ingerir alimentos, ou aversão por alimentos. [L. *cibus*, alimento, + G. *phobos*, medo]

CIC Abreviatura de completely in the canal *hearing aid* (aparelho auditivo completamente no canal).

CIC Abreviatura de clean intermittent bladder *catheterization* (cateterismo vesical intermitente limpo).

cic·a·trec·to·my (sik-ă-trek′tō-mē). Cicatrectomia; excisão de uma cicatriz. [L. *cicatrix*, cicatriz, + G. *ektomē*, excisão]

cic·a·tri·ces (si-kā′tri-sēz). Plural de cicatrix.

cic·a·tri·cial (sik-ă-trish′ăl). Cicatricial; relativo a uma cicatriz.

cic·a·tri·cot·o·my, cic·a·tri·sot·o·my (sik′ă-trī′kot′ō-mē, -sot′ō-mē). Cicatricotomia; cicatrisotomia; corte em uma cicatriz. [L. *cicatrix*, cicatriz, + G. *tomē*, corte]

cic·a·trix, pl. **cic·a·tri·ces** (sik′ā-triks, si-kā′triks; sik-ā-trī′sēz). Cicatriz. [L.]

brain c., c. cerebral; cicatriz no cérebro resultante de lesão (gliose reativa), caracterizada por proliferação de elementos mesodérmicos (vasculares) e ectodérmicos (gliais). VER TAMBÉM isomorphous *gliosis*.

filtering c., c. filtrante. SIN filtering *bleb.*

meningocerebral c., c. meningocerebral; cicatriz e aderências envolvendo o cérebro e as meninges contíguas; tipicamente causada por traumatismo craniano.

vicious c., c. viciosa; c. que, por sua contração, causa uma deformidade.

cic·a·tri·zant (sik-at′ri-zant). Cicatrizante. **1.** Que causa ou favorece a cicatrização. **2.** Um agente com essa ação.

cic·a·tri·za·tion (sik′a-tri-za′shŭn). Cicatrização. **1.** O processo de formação de cicatriz. **2.** O fechamento de uma ferida processado não por primeira intenção.

ci·clo·pir·ox·ol·a·mine (sī-klō-pir′oks ol′a-mēn). Ciclopiroxolamina; agente antifúngico de amplo espectro usado no tratamento de várias infecções cutâneas por fungos e leveduras.

cic·u·tox·in (sik-ū-tok′sin). Cicutoxina; princípio tóxico presente na cicuta aquática, *Cicuta vitrosa* (família Umbelliferae); a ação farmacológica é semelhante à da picrotoxina.

-cide. Sufixo que designa um agente que mata (p. ex., inseticida), ou o ato de matar (p. ex., suicídio). [L. *-cida, -cidium*, de *caedo*, matar]

CIDP Abreviatura de chronic inflammatory demyelinating *polyneuropathy* (polineuropatia desmielinizante inflamatória crônica).

ci·gua·te·ra (sē′gwah-tār′a). Ciguatera; síndrome tóxica aguda, com características predominantemente gastrointestinais e neuromusculares induzidas pela ingestão da carne ou vísceras de vários peixes marinhos, do Caribe e dos recifes na região tropical do Pacífico, que contém ciguatoxina. [Esp. de *cigua*, caramujo-do-mar]

Casos esporádicos de ciguatera ocorrem ao longo da costa leste dos Estados Unidos, de Vermont ao sul da Flórida e nas Ilhas Virgens norte-americanas, Porto Rico e Havaí. Os surtos ocasionais resultam do consumo em grupo de grandes pescas de peixes contaminados. A condição provavelmente é subnotificada, muitos casos sendo erroneamente considerados como síndromes virais ou enjôo marítimo. A toxina lipossolúvel e termoestável é produzida pelo dinoflagelado *Gambierdiscus toxicus*, que é epífito nas algas vermelhas e marrons. Peixes herbívoros que procuram alimentos nas algas dos recifes consomem os flagelados e, por sua vez, são consumidos por peixes carnívoros; a toxina torna-se cada vez mais concentrada à medida que sobe na cadeia alimentar. As cabeças e vísceras dos peixes afetados contêm maiores concentrações que outras partes. Cerca de 400 espécies de peixes foram associadas à intoxicação humana, incluindo particularmente predadores, como cavala, barracuda, garoupa, moréia, vermelho, perca-do-mar, sororoca e barbeiro. O peixe contaminado tem aspecto, cheiro e gosto normais, e a ciguatoxina não é destruída pelo cozimento, secagem, salgadura ou congelamento. Os sinais e sintomas surgem 3–12 horas após a exposição (ocasionalmente em minutos) e incluem vômito e diarréia, mialgia, disestesia e parestesia dos membros e da região perioral, prurido, cefaléia, fraqueza e diaforese. Pode haver bradicardia e hipotensão. Já foram descritas algumas mortes causadas por paralisia respiratória. Os efeitos tóxicos geralmente desaparecem espontaneamente em cerca de 1 semana, mas os sintomas residuais podem persistir por meses. A exposição repetida pode aumentar a sensibilidade de um indivíduo à toxina. O diagnóstico é confirmado por identificação da toxina nas sobras do peixe ou no soro do paciente. O tratamento é puramente de suporte.

ci·gua·tox·in (sēg-wă-tok′sin). Ciguatoxina; saponina marinha de estrutura desconhecida, mas com a fórmula empírica $C_{35}H_{65}NO_8$; a substância tóxica causadora da ciguatera.

ci·la·stat·in so·di·um (sī-la-stat′in). Cilastatina sódica; inibidor da dipeptidase renal, desidropeptidase 1, usada, em conjunto com antibióticos metabolizados nos rins, para aumentar a resposta terapêutica ao antibiótico.

cili-. VER cilio-.

cil·ia (sil′ē-a). Cílios. Plural de cilium.

cil·i·ary (sil′ē-ar-ē). Ciliar. **1.** Relativo a quaisquer cílios ou processos ciliares, especificamente os cílios dos olhos. **2.** Relativo a determinadas estruturas do globo ocular. [L. Mod. *ciliaris*, relativo ou semelhante ao cílio, do L. *cilium*, cílio]

cil·i·a·stat·ic (sil-ē-a-stat′ik). Ciliostático; designa uma droga ou condição que lentifica ou interrompe o movimento dos cílios (geralmente usado em referência aos cílios da mucosa respiratória).

Ci·li·a·ta (sil-ē-ā′ta). Ciliados; antes considerados uma classe de protozoários cujos membros possuem cílios, ou estruturas deles derivadas, como cirros ou membranelas, mas agora posicionados no filo Ciliophora. Os membros típicos, como *Paramecium* ou *Balantidium coli* (parasita do homem), possuem dois núcleos distintos, um macronúcleo e um micronúcleo; apenas este último possui o material hereditário trocado na conjugação, uma forma de reprodução sexuada encontrada apenas nos ciliados. [L. *cilium*, cílio]

cil·i·at·ed (sil′ē-ā-ted). Ciliado; que possui cílios.

cil·i·ates (sil′ē-āts). Ciliados; nome comum para os membros da classe Ciliata.

cil·i·ec·to·my (sil-ē-ek′tō-mē). Ciliectomia. SIN cyclectomy.

cilio-, cili-. Cílios ou que significa ciliar, em qualquer sentido; cílios. [L. *cilium*, cílio]

cil·i·o·cy·toph·thor·ia (sil′ē-ō-sī-tō-thōr′ē-a). Ciliocitoftoria; tufos ciliares soltos (remanescentes do epitélio ciliado) que podem ser observados em vários líquidos corporais, principalmente amostras peritoneais, amnióticas e respiratórias; são móveis e podem ser confundidos com protozoários ciliados ou flagelados. [Pl. de ciliocytophthorium, de cilio- + cyto- + G. *phthora* corrupção, decaimento, + *-ium*, sufixo substantivo]

cil·i·o·gen·e·sis (sil′ē-ō-jen′ē-sis). Ciliogênese; a formação de cílios.

Ci·li·oph·o·ra (sil′ē-of′ō-ra). Cilióforos; filo de protozoários que inclui os muitos ciliados de vida livre e os suctórios sésseis; antes classificados como um subfilo do filo Protozoa. [cilio- + G. *phoros*, que carrega]

cil·i·o·ret·i·nal (sil′ē-ō-ret′i-năl). Ciliorretiniano; relativo ao corpo ciliar e à retina.

cil·i·o·scle·ral (sil′ē-ō-sklē′răl). Cilioescleral; relativo ao corpo ciliar e à esclerótica.

cil·i·o·spi·nal (sil′ē-ō-spī′nal). Cilioespinhal; relativo ao corpo ciliar e à medula espinhal; designa em particular o centro cilioespinhal (ciliospinal *center*).

cil·i·o·tox·ic·i·ty (sil′ē-ō-tok-sis′i-tē). Ciliotoxicidade; a característica de uma droga ou outra substância que compromete a atividade ciliar (geralmente se refere aos cílios da mucosa respiratória) (p. ex., fumaça dos derivados do tabaco).

cil·i·um, pl. **cil·ia** (sil′ē-ŭm, -ă). Cílio. **1.** [NA]. SIN eyelash. **2.** Extensão móvel de uma superfície celular, p. ex., de determinadas células epiteliais, contendo nove microtúbulos longitudinais duplos dispostos em um anel periférico, juntamente com um par central. [L. cílio]

Cil·lo·bac·te·ri·um (sil′ō-bak-tēr′ē-ŭm). Cilobactéria; gênero obsoleto de bactérias anaeróbicas, móveis, contendo bastonetes retos ou curvos, Gram-positivos.

ci·met·i·dine (si-met′i-dēn). Cimetidina; análogo e antagonista da histamina, usado para tratar úlcera péptica e distúrbios de hipersecreção por bloqueio de receptores H_2 da histamina, inibindo assim a secreção de ácido gástrico.

Ci·mex (sī′meks). Gênero de percevejos da família Cimicidae na ordem Hemiptera, com corpos chatos, castanho-avermelhados, sem asas, com olhos

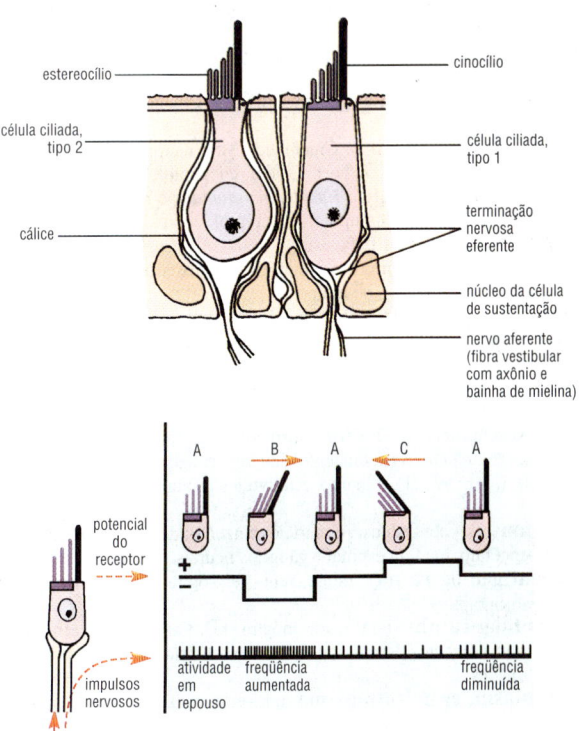

cílios: respostas excitatórias e inibitórias de estereocílios e cinocílios nas células ciliadas (tipos I e II) do aparelho vestibular à estimulação por movimento em direção oposta; (A) estado de repouso, (B) estimulação, (C) inibição

laterais proeminentes, bico triarticulado e odor característico proveniente das glândulas odoríferas torácicas; praga abundante nas residências humanas. Embora sua picada produza grupos lineares característicos de pápulas pruriginosas com um ponto hemorrágico central, o percevejo não é um vetor comprovado de doença humana, com a possível exceção da hepatite B. [L. *cimex*, percevejo, L. *lectulus*, leito]

C. hemipterus, percevejo freqüentemente encontrado nos trópicos.
C. lectularius, o percevejo comum.

Cimino, James E., nefrologista norte-americano, *1928. VER Brescia-C. *fistula*.

cIMP Abreviatura de cyclic inosine 3,5-monophosphate (3,5-monofosfato de inosina cíclico).

♻ **cin-.** VER cine-.

cin·an·es·the·sia (sin′an-es-thē′zē-ā). Cinanestesia. SIN kinanesthesia.

ci·nan·ser·in hy·dro·chlo·ride (si-nan′ser-in). Cloridrato de cinanserina; inibidor da serotonina.

cin·chol (sin′kol). Cincol. SIN β-sitosterol.

cin·cho·na (sin-kō′nä). Cinchona; a casca seca da raiz e do caule de várias espécies de *Cinchona*, gênero de árvores perenes (família Rubiaceae), nativa da América do Sul, mas cultivada em várias regiões tropicais. A casca cultivada contém 7 a 10% de alcalóides totais; cerca de 70% consistem em quinina. A cinchona contém mais de 20 alcalóides, dos quais dois pares de isômeros são mais importantes: quinina e quinidina, e cinchonidina e cinchonina. SIN bark (2), cinchona bark, Jesuits bark, Peruvian bark, quina, quinaquina, quinquina. [*Cinchona*, de Condessa de *Chinch'on*]

cin·chon·ic (sin-kon′ik). Cinchônico; relativo à cinchona.

cin·cho·nine (sin′kō-nēn). Cinchonina; alcalóide da quinolina preparado a partir da casca de várias espécies de *Cinchona*; agente tônico e antimalárico. Existem vários sais de cinchonina disponíveis.

cin·cho·nism (sin′kō-nizm). Cinchonismo; envenenamento por cinchona, quinina ou quinidina; caracterizado por zumbido, cefaléia, surdez e, ocasionalmente, choque anafilactóide. SIN quininism.

cin·cho·phen (sin′kō-fen). Cinchofeno; agente analgésico, antipirético e uricosúrico que pode produzir lesão hepática e lesões gástricas; usado em animais experimentais para produzir úlcera gástrica.

cin·cli·sis (sing′kli-sis). Cínclise; rápida repetição de um movimento, p. ex., piscar rápida e repetidamente. [G. *kinklizō*, balançar a cauda, mudar constantemente]

♻ **cine-, cin-.** Movimento, geralmente relativo a filmes. VER TAMBÉM kin-. [G. *kineō*, mover]

cin·e·an·gi·o·car·di·og·ra·phy (sin′ē-an′jē-ō-kar-dē-og′ră-fē). Cineangiocardiografia; filmes da passagem de um contraste através das câmaras cardíacas e dos grandes vasos.

cin·e·flu·o·rog·ra·phy (sin′ē-flōr-og′ră-fē). Cinefluorografia. SIN cineradiography.

cin·e·flu·o·ros·co·py (sin′ē-flōr-os′kō-pē). Cinefluoroscopia. SIN cineradiography.

cin·e·gas·tros·co·py (sin′ē-gas-tros′kō-pē). Cinegastroscopia; filmes de observações gastrocópicas.

cin·e·mat·ics (sin-ē-mat′iks). Cinemática. SIN kinematics.

cin·e·ole, cin·e·ol (sin′ē-ōl, -ol). Cineol; eucaliptol; expectorante estimulante obtido do óleo volátil do *Eucalyptus globulus* e de outras espécies de *Eucalyptus*. SIN cajeputol, cajuputol, eucalyptol.

cin·e·pho·to·mi·crog·ra·phy (sin′ē-fō′tō-mī-krog′ră-fē). Cinefotomicrografia; a produção de um filme de objetos microscópicos; freqüentemente se usa fotografia com lapso de tempo.

cin·e·plas·tics (sin-ē-plas′tiks). Cineplástica. SIN cineplastic amputation.

cin·e·ra·di·og·ra·phy (sin′ē-rā-dē-og′ră-fē). Cinerradiografia; radiografia de um órgão em movimento, p. ex., o coração, o trato gastrointestinal. SIN cinefluorography, cinefluoroscopy, cineroentgenography.

ci·ne·rea (si-nē′rē-ä). Cinéreo. 1. A substância cinzenta cerebral e outras partes do sistema nervoso. 2. Termo obsoleto para a camada do manto (mantle layer). [L. fem. de *cinereus*, cinzento, de *cinis*, cinzas]

ci·ne·re·al (si-nē′rē-ăl). Cinéreo; relativo à substância cinzenta do sistema nervoso.

ci·ner·i·tious (si-ner-ish′ŭs). Cinerício; cinzento; designa a substância cinzenta do encéfalo, medula espinal e gânglios neurais.

cin·e·roent·gen·og·ra·phy (sin′ē-rent-gen-og′ră-fē). Cinerradiografia. SIN cineradiography.

cin·e·seis·mog·ra·phy (sin′ē-sīz-mog′ră-fē). Cinessismografia; técnica para medir movimentos do corpo por registro fotográfico contínuo de tremores ou vibrações.

ci·ne·to·plasm, ci·ne·to·plas·ma (sin-et′ō-plazm, sin-et-ō-plaz′mä). Cinetoplasma. SIN kinetoplasm.

cin·gu·late (sin′gū-lāt). Cingulado; relativo a um cíngulo.

cin·gu·lec·to·my (sin-gū-lek′tō-mē). Cingulectomia. SIN cingulotomy. [cingulum + G. *ektomē*, excisão]

cin·gu·lot·o·my (sin-gū-lot′ō-mē). Cingulotomia; outrora, uma excisão cirúrgica uni ou bilateral da metade anterior do giro cingulado, mas agora realizada por destruição eletrolítica do giro cingulado anterior e do corpo caloso. SIN cingulectomy. [cingulum + G. *tomē*, corte]

cin·gu·lum, gen. **cin·gu·li,** pl. **cin·gu·la** (sin′gū-lŭm, -lē, -lä) [TA]. Cíngulo. 1. SIN girdle. 2. Feixe de fibras bem marcado que segue longitudinalmente na substância branca do giro do cíngulo; o feixe se estende da região da substância perfurada anterior para trás sobre a superfície dorsal do corpo caloso; atrás do esplênio deste último, curva-se para baixo e, depois, para a frente na substância branca do giro para-hipocampal; composto principalmente de fibras do núcleo talâmico anterior até os giros do cíngulo e para-hipocampal, também contém fibras de associação, que conectam esses giros ao córtex frontal, e suas várias subdivisões entre si. [L. cinto, de *cingo*, circundar]

c. den'tis [TA], c. do dente. SIN c. of tooth.

c. mem'bri inferior'is, c. dos membros inferiores; *termo oficial alternativo para pelvic girdle (cintura pélvica).

c. mem'bri superior'is, c. dos membros superiores; *termo oficial alternativo para pectoral girdle (cintura escapular).

c. pectorale [TA], c. peitoral. SIN pectoral girdle.

c. pelvici [TA], c. pélvico. SIN pelvic girdle.

c. of tooth [TA], c. do dente; uma crista em forma de U ou W na base da superfície lingual da coroa dos incisivos superiores e cúspides, os ramos laterais seguindo por uma curta distância ao longo dos ângulos da linha linguoproximal, a porção central logo acima da gengiva. SIN c. dentis [TA], basal ridge (2), lingual lobe.

cin·na·mal·de·hyde (sin-ă-mal′de-hīd). Cinamaldeído; principal constituinte do óleo de canela. SIN cinnamic aldehyde.

cin·na·mate (sin′ă-māt). Cinamato; sal ou éster do ácido cinâmico.

cin·nam·e·in (sin′am-ē-in). Cinameína. SIN benzyl cinnamate.

cin·na·mene (sin′ă-mēn). Cinameno. SIN styrene.

cin·nam·ic (si-nam′ik). Cinâmico; relativo ao cinamomo.

cin·nam·ic ac·id. Ácido cinâmico; obtido do óleo de cinamomo, bálsamo do Peru e bálsamo-de-tolu, ou do estoraque. Tem sido usado no lúpus como cosmético e em doenças infecciosas para promover leucocitose. SIN cinnamylic acid, phenylacrylic acid.

cin·nam·ic al·co·hol. Álcool cinâmico. SIN styrone.

cin·nam·ic al·de·hyde. Aldeído cinâmico. SIN cinnamaldehyde.

cin·na·mon (sin′ă-mon). Cinamomo; canela. 1. A casca seca do *Cinnamomum loureirri* Nees (família Lauraceae), casca aromática usada como especiaria e, na medicina, como adjuvante, antiflatulento e estomáquico aromático. SIN Saigon c. 2. A casca interna seca dos brotos de *Cinnamomum zeylanicum*. SIN Ceylon c. SIN cassia bark. SIN L. do G. *kinnamōmon*, cinamomo]

cassia c., cássia; *Cinnamomum cassia* Nees (família Lauraceae); fonte não-oficial da maior parte da canela encontrada nas lojas; a fonte do óleo de canela. SIN Chinese c.

Ceylon c., canela-do-Ceilão. SIN cinnamon (2).

Chinese c., canela chinesa. SIN cassia c.

Saigon c., canela de Saigon. SIN cinnamon (1).

cin·na·mon oil. Óleo de canela; o óleo volátil destilado do vapor das folhas e brotos de *Cinnamomum cassia*; contém não menos de 80% por volume dos aldeídos totais do óleo de canela. SIN cassia oil.

cin·na·myl·ic ac·id (sin-ă-mil′ik). Ácido cinamílico. SIN cinnamic acid.

cin·nar·i·zine (si-nar′i-zēn). Cinarizina; anti-histamínico H_1. SIN cinnipirine.

cin·nip·i·rine (si-nip′i-rēn). Cinipirina. SIN cinnarizine.

ci·no·cen·trum (sīn-ō-sen′trŭm). Cinocentro. SIN cytocentrum.

ci·nox·a·cin (si-noks′ä-sin). Cinoxacina; ácido orgânico sintético, quimicamente relacionado ao ácido nalidíxico, usado como antibacteriano para tratar infecções do trato urinário.

ci·nox·ate (si-nok′sāt). Cinoxato; filtro ultravioleta para aplicação tópica na pele.

ci·on (sī′on). Cíon; termo arcaico para úvula. [G. *kiōn*, pilar, a úvula]

cip·ro·flox·a·cin hy·dro·chlo·ride (sip-rō-floks′ä-sin). Cloridrato de ciprofloxacina; antibacteriano fluoroquinolona sintético de amplo espectro com atividade contra uma grande variedade de microrganismos Gram-negativos e Gram-positivos.

cir·an·tin (sir-an′tin). Cirantina. SIN hesperidin.

🛈 **cir·ca·di·an** (ser-kā′dē-ăn). Circadiano; relativo a variações ou ritmos biológicos com um ciclo de aproximadamente 24 horas. Cf. infradian, ultradian. [L. *circa*, cerca, + *dies*, dia]

cir·cel·lus (sir-sel′ŭs). Circelo; círculo pequeno. [L.]

c. veno'sus hypoglos'si, plexo venoso do canal do nervo hipogloso. SIN venous plexus of canal of hypoglossal nerve.

cir·cho·ral (ser-kō′ral). Circorário; que ocorre ciclicamente a intervalos de aproximadamente uma hora.

cir·ci·nate (ser′si-nāt). Circinado; circular; anular. [L. *circinatus*, tornado redondo, pp. de *circino*, fazer redondo, de *circinus*, um par de compassos]

cir·cle (ser′kl). Círculo. 1. [TA]. Em anatomia, uma estrutura ou grupo de estruturas anulares, formado por anastomose de artérias ou veias, mais ou menos conectados (comunicantes). 2. Uma linha ou processo com cada extremidade aproximadamente eqüidistante do centro. SIN circulus [TA]. [L. *circulus*]

arterial c. of cerebrum, c. arterial do cérebro. SIN cerebral arterial c.

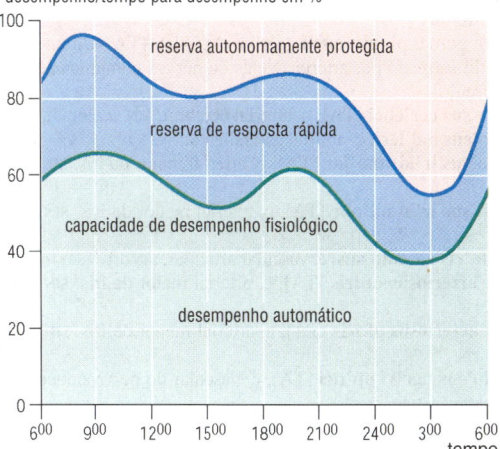

ritmo circadiano e capacidade de desempenho

---

articular vascular c., c. vascular articular. SIN articular vascular *plexus*; VER articular vascular *network*.
Carus c., c. de Carus. SIN Carus *curve.*
cerebral arterial c. [TA], c. arterial cerebral, polígono de Willis; o círculo de formato aproximadamente pentagonal de vasos na face ventral do encéfalo na área do quiasma óptico, hipotálamo e fossa interpeduncular; formado, seqüencialmente e na direção ântero-posterior, pela artéria comunicante anterior, pelas duas artérias cerebrais anteriores, pelas duas carótidas internas, pelas duas comunicantes posteriores e pelas duas artérias cerebrais posteriores. SIN circulus arteriosus cerebri [TA], arterial c. of cerebrum, c. of Willis.
closed c., c. fechado; circuito para administração de um anestésico inalatório em que há reinalação completa com absorção de dióxido de carbono.
defensive c., c. defensivo; termo obsoleto para o acréscimo de uma afecção secundária que limita ou interrompe o progresso da afecção primária, como se acredita ocorrer quando um pneumotórax se superpõe à tuberculose pulmonar, com o primeiro tendo um efeito terapêutico sobre o último.
greater arterial c. of iris, c. arterial maior da íris. SIN major arterial c. of iris.
Haller c., c. de Haller; **(1)** SIN vascular c. of optic nerve; **(2)** SIN areolar venous *plexus.*
Huguier c., c. de Huguier; anastomose ao redor do istmo uterino (junção do colo com o corpo) entre as artérias uterinas direita e esquerda.
least confusion c., menor c. de difusão; na configuração de raios que emergem de um sistema de lentes esferocilíndricas, o local onde os raios divergentes da primeira lente, que forma uma imagem linear, são balanceados por raios convergentes da segunda lente.
lesser arterial c. of iris, c. arterial menor da íris. SIN minor arterial c. of iris.
major arterial c. of iris, c. arterial maior da íris; círculo arterial na borda ciliar da íris. SIN circulus arteriosus iridis major [TA], major circulus arteriosus of iris [TA], greater arterial c. of iris.
minor arterial c. of iris, c. arterial menor da íris; círculo arterial próximo da margem pupilar da íris. SIN circulus arteriosus iridis minor [TA], minor circulus arteriosus of iris [TA], lesser arterial c. of iris.
Pagenstecher c., c. de Pagenstecher; no caso de um tumor abdominal livremente móvel, a massa é deslocada por toda a sua extensão, sendo sua posição marcada, na parede abdominal, periodicamente; quando esses pontos são unidos, forma-se um círculo, cujo centro marca o ponto de fixação do tumor.
Ridley c., c. de Ridley. SIN circular *sinus* (1).
rolling c., círculo rolante; mecanismo de replicação do DNA circular.
semi-closed c., c. semifechado; circuito para administração de um anestésico inalatório no qual a reinalação parcial com absorção de dióxido de carbono é combinada à perda, pelo circuito, de uma parte dos gases respirados através das válvulas.
vascular c., c. vascular; **(1)** o círculo ao redor da boca formado pelas artérias labiais inferior e superior; **(2)** SIN areolar venous *plexus.*
vascular c. of optic nerve [TA], c. vascular do nervo óptico; rede de ramos das artérias ciliares curtas na esclerótica ao redor do ponto de entrada do nervo óptico. SIN circulus vasculosus nervi optici [TA], circulus arteriosus halleri, circulus zinnii, Haller c. (1), Zinn corona, Zinn vascular c.
venous c. of mammary gland, c. venoso da glândula mamária. SIN areolar venous *plexus.*
vicious c., c. vicioso; a ação mutuamente aceleradora de duas doenças ou fenômenos independentes, ou de uma afecção primária e secundária.
Vieth-Müller c., c. de Vieth-Müller; um círculo geométrico que atravessa os centros ópticos de dois olhos pelo qual pontos adjacentes ao ponto de fixação,

ambos situados no círculo, teoricamente caem nos pontos correspondentes na retina.

c. of Willis, polígono de Willis. SIN cerebral arterial c.
Zinn vascular c., círculo vascular de Zinn; anel de Zinn; círculo vascular do nervo óptico. SIN vascular c. of optic nerve.

cir·cuit (ser′kit). Circuito; o trajeto ou curso do fluxo de casos ou correntes elétricas ou de outros tipos. [L. *circuitus*, que segue em círculo, de *circum*, ao redor, + *eo*, pp. *itus*, seguir]
anesthetic c., c. anestésico; equipamento usado durante anestesia inalatória para regular as concentrações de gases inalados; inclui uma bolsa reservatória e, geralmente, válvulas direcionais, tubos respiratórios e um removedor de dióxido de carbono.
Papez c., c. de Papez; uma longa cadeia de condução em circuito no prosencéfalo de mamíferos, que parte do hipocampo, atravessa o fórnice e segue até o corpo mamilar, de onde retorna ao hipocampo atravessando seqüencialmente os núcleos talâmicos anteriores, o giro do cíngulo e o giro para-hipocampal.
reverberating c., c. reverberante; teoria de condução periódica, através do córtex cerebral, de séries de impulsos que percorrem os circuitos neuronais.

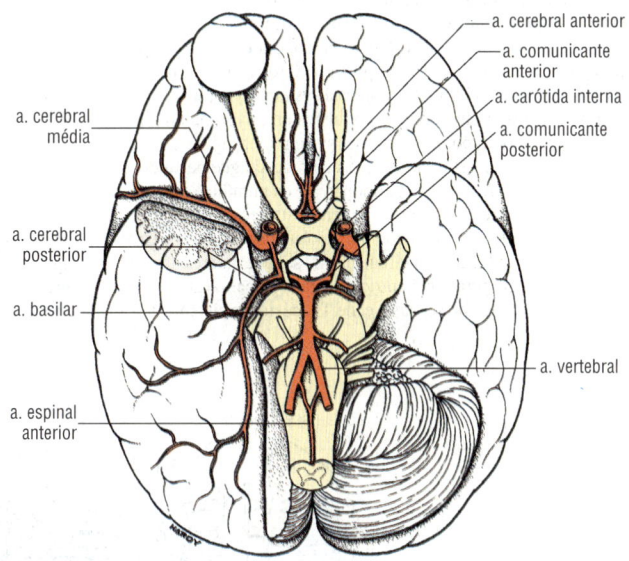

polígono de Willis: imagem de artérias na base do encéfalo

---

signal-processing c.'s, circuitos de processamento de sinal; o *hardware* eletrônico de aparelhos auditivos que permite a alteração na amplificação de várias faixas de freqüência do sinal acústico.

cir·cu·la·tion (ser - kū - lā′shŭn). Circulação; movimentos em círculo, ou em um trajeto circular, ou por um trajeto que leva de volta ao mesmo ponto; geralmente referente à circulação sanguínea, exceto especificação em contrário. [L. *circulatio*]
assisted c., c. assistida; aplicação de dispositivos externos para melhorar a pressão e/ou o fluxo no coração ou nas artérias.
blood c., c. sanguínea; o trajeto do sangue partindo do coração, atravessando artérias, capilares e veias para retornar ao coração.
capillary c., c. capilar; o trajeto do sangue através dos capilares.
collateral c., c. colateral; c. mantida em pequenos vasos que se anastomosam quando o vaso principal é obstruído.
compensatory c., c. compensatória; c. estabelecida em vasos colaterais dilatados quando o vaso principal da parte é obstruído.
cross c., c. cruzada; c. para um animal ou uma de suas partes, proveniente da circulação de outro animal.
embryonic c., c. embrionária; o plano básico da circulação de embriões jovens de mamíferos, inicialmente semelhante àquela em formas aquáticas, com um coração não-dividido e arcos aórticos visíveis na região branquial; à medida que a gestação progride, o arranjo dos grandes vasos sanguíneos torna-se mais semelhante ao de um adulto, mas o trajeto do sangue pelo coração, característico de um adulto, só pode ser atingido quando começa a respiração pulmonar ao nascimento.
enterohepatic c., c. êntero-hepática; c. de substâncias como os sais biliares que são absorvidos no intestino e transportados para o fígado, onde são secretados para a bile e entram novamente no intestino.
extracorporeal c., c. extracorpórea; circulação do sangue fora do corpo através de um aparelho que assume temporariamente as funções de um órgão, p. ex., através de um aparelho coração-pulmão ou rim artificial.

fetal c., c. fetal; a circulação que serve ao feto *in utero*, sendo o circuito placentário responsável pelo suprimento de oxigênio e nutrientes e pela eliminação de CO_2 e resíduos nitrogenados. VER TAMBÉM embryonic c.
greater c., c. maior. SIN systemic c.
hypophysial portal c., c. porta hipofisária. SIN portal hypophysial c.
hypothalamohypophysial portal c., c. porta hipotálamo-hipofisária. SIN portal hypophysial c.
lesser c., c. menor. SIN pulmonary c.
lymph c., c. linfática; a lenta passagem de linfa através dos vasos linfáticos e linfonodos.
placental c., c. placentária; a circulação de sangue através da placenta, durante a vida intra-uterina, que serve às necessidades do feto de oxigenação, absorção e excreção; também, a circulação materna através do espaço interviloso da placenta.
portal c., c. porta; **(1)** circulação sanguínea para o fígado proveniente do intestino delgado, da metade direita do cólon e do baço através da veia porta; algumas vezes especificada como a circulação porta hepática; **(2)** mais genericamente, qualquer parte da circulação sistêmica na qual o sangue que drena do leito capilar de uma estrutura flui através de um vaso maior ou de vasos maiores para suprir o leito capilar de outra estrutura antes de voltar ao coração; p. ex., o sistema porta hipotálamo-hipofisário.
portal hypophysial c., c. porta hipofisária; rede capilar que transporta hormônios hipofiseotrópicos do hipotálamo, onde são secretados para o sangue, para seus locais de ação na hipófise anterior. VER portal c., pituitary *gland*, hypothalamus. SIN hypophyseoportal system, hypophysial portal c., hypophysial portal system, hypophysioportal system, hypothalamohypophysial portal c., hypothalamohypophysial portal system (1).
pulmonary c., c. pulmonar; a passagem de sangue partindo do ventrículo direito, passando pela artéria pulmonar, até os pulmões, e retornando através das veias pulmonares para o átrio esquerdo. SIN lesser c.
Servetus c., c. de Servetus; epônimo obsoleto para designar a circulação pulmonar.
systemic c., c. sistêmica; a circulação de sangue através das artérias, capilares e veias do sistema geral, do ventrículo esquerdo para o átrio direito. SIN greater c.
thebesian c. (thē-bē′sē-an); c. de Thebesius; o sistema de veias menores no miocárdio.

cir·cu·la·to·ry (ser′kū-lă-tō-rē). Circulatório. **1.** Relativo à circulação. **2.** SIN sanguiferous.
cir·cu·lus, gen. e pl. **cir·cu·li** (ser′kū-lŭs, -lī). [TA]. Círculo. SIN circle. **2.** Um círculo formado por artérias, veias ou nervos comunicantes. [L. dim. de *circus*, círculo]
  c. arterio'sus cer'ebri [TA], c. arterial cerebral. SIN cerebral arterial *circle*.
  c. arterio'sus hal'leri, c. arterial de Haller. SIN vascular *circle* of optic nerve.
  c. arterio'sus ir'ids ma'jor [TA], c. arterial maior da íris. SIN major arterial *circle* of iris.
  c. arterio'sus ir'id mi'nor [TA], c. arterial menor da íris. SIN minor arterial *circle* of iris.
  c. articula'ris vasculo'sus, c. vascular articular. SIN articular vascular *plexus*.
  major c. arteriosus of iris [TA], c. arterial maior da íris. SIN major arterial *circle* of iris.
  minor c. arteriosus of iris [TA], c. arterial menor da íris. SIN minor arterial *circle* of iris.
  c. vasculo'sus ner'vi op'tici [TA], c. vascular do nervo óptico. SIN vascular *circle* of optic nerve.
  c. veno'sus hal'leri, c. venoso de Haller. SIN areolar venous *plexus*.
  c. veno'sus rid'leyi, c. venoso de Ridley. SIN circular *sinus* (1).
  c. zin'nii, c. de Zinn. SIN vascular *circle* of optic nerve.
circum-. Um movimento circular, ou uma posição circundando a parte indicada pela palavra a que se junta. VER TAMBÉM peri-. [L. ao redor]
cir·cum·a·nal (ser-kŭm-ā′nal). Circum-anal; perianal; que circunda o ânus. SIN perianal, periproctic.
cir·cum·ar·tic·u·lar (ser′kŭm-ar-tik′ū-lăr). Circum-articular; periarticular; que circunda uma articulação. SIN periarthric, periarticular. [circum- + L. *articulus*, articulação]
cir·cum·ax·il·lary (ser-kŭm-ak′si-lār-ē). Circum-axilar; ao redor da axila. SIN periaxillary.
cir·cum·bul·bar (ser-kŭm-bŭl′bar). Circumbulbar. SIN peribulbar.
cir·cum·cise (ser′kŭm-sīz). Circuncisar; remover o prepúcio ou outro tecido por incisão circunferencial (circuncisão).
cir·cum·ci·sion (ser-kŭm-sizh′ŭn). Circuncisão. **1.** Operação para remover

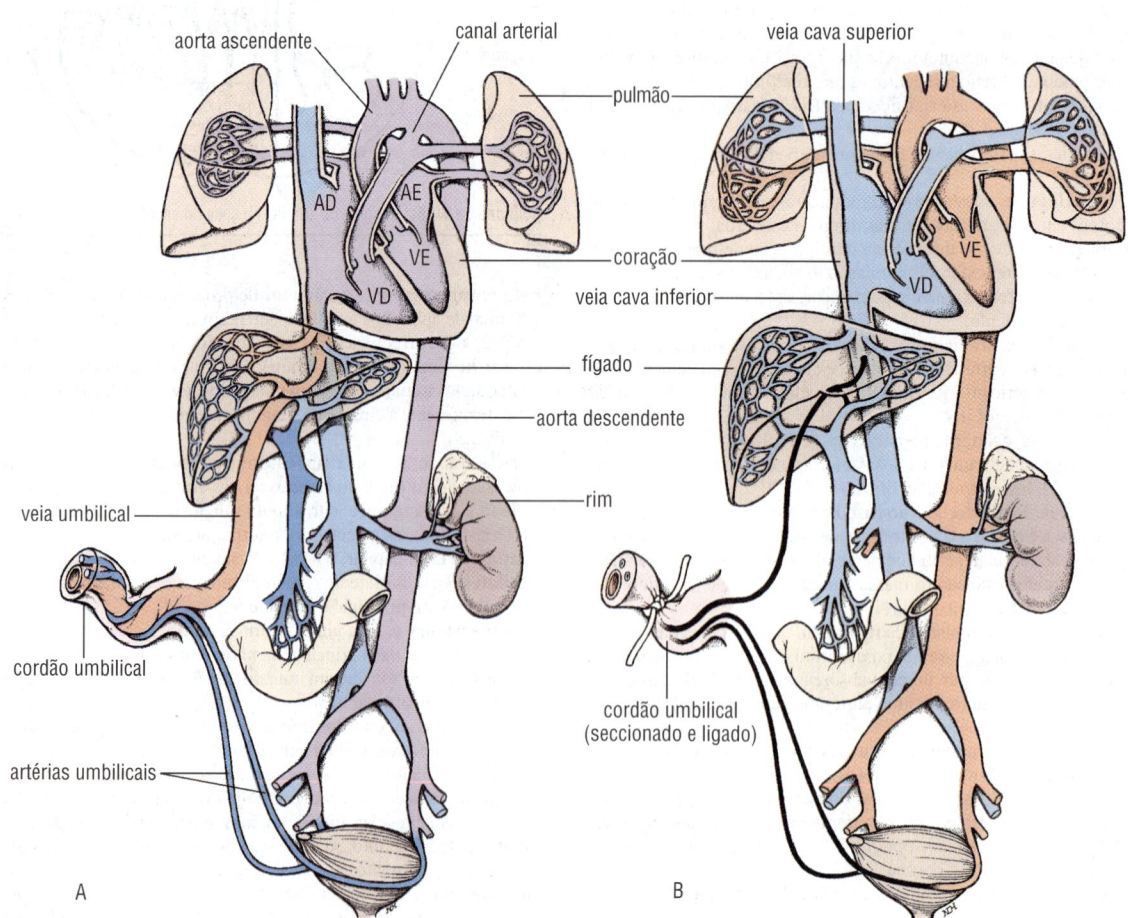

circulação fetal: (A) durante a gravidez, o oxigênio se difunde da circulação materna para a circulação fetal na placenta; o sangue oxigenado (vermelho) retorna para o feto através da veia umbilical; (B) após o nascimento, o cordão umbilical é seccionado e o sangue é oxigenado quando atravessa os pulmões; (AD) átrio direito, (AE) átrio esquerdo, (VE) ventrículo esquerdo, (VD) ventrículo direito

parte do prepúcio ou todo ele. **2.** Corte ao redor de uma parte anatômica (p. ex., a aréola mamária). SIN peritectomy (2). [L. *circumcido*, cortar ao redor, de *circum*, ao redor, + *caedo*, cortar]
female c., c. feminina; termo amplo que designa muitas formas de secção genital feminina, que varia da remoção do prepúcio clitoridiano até a remoção do clitóris, pequenos lábios e partes dos grandes lábios e infibulação; realizado por razões culturais, não-médicas.
cir·cum·cor·ne·al (ser-kŭm-kōr′nē-ăl). Circuncórneo. SIN pericorneal.
circumductio [TA], circundução. SIN circumduction.
cir·cum·duc·tion (ser-kŭm-dŭk′shŭn) [TA]. Circundução. **1.** Movimento circular de uma parte, p. ex., um membro. **2.** SIN cycloduction. SIN circumductio [TA]. [circum- + L. *duco*, pp. *ductus*, puxar]
cir·cum·fer·ence (c) (ser-kŭm′fer-ens) [TA]. Circunferência; o limite externo, particularmente de uma área circular. SIN circumferentia [TA]. [L. *circumferentia*, condução ao redor de]
articular c. of head of radius [TA], c. articular da cabeça do rádio; parte da cabeça do rádio que se articula com a incisura radial da ulna. SIN circumferentia articularis capitis radii [TA].
articular c. of head of ulna [TA], c. articular da cabeça da ulna; parte da cabeça da ulna que se articula com a incisura ulnar do rádio. SIN circumferentia articularis capitis ulnae [TA].
cir·cum·fer·en·tia (ser-kŭm-fer-en′shē-ă) [TA]. Circunferência. SIN circumference. [L. condução ao redor de]
c. articula′ris capitis ra′dii [TA], c. articular da cabeça do rádio. SIN articular *circumference* of head of radius.
c. articula′ris capitis ul′nae [TA], c. articular da cabeça da ulna. SIN articular *circumference* of head of ulna.
cir·cum·flex (ser′kŭm-fleks). Circunflexo; descreve um arco de um círculo ou aquele que dá a volta em torno de alguma coisa; designa várias estruturas anatômicas: artérias, veias, nervos e músculos. [circum- + L. *flexus*, dobrar]
cir·cum·gem·mal (ser-kŭm-jem′ăl). Circungemal; que circunda um corpo semelhante a um broto ou bulbo; designa um modo de terminação nervosa por fibrilas que circundam um bulbo terminal. SIN perigemmal. [circum- + L. *gemma*, broto]

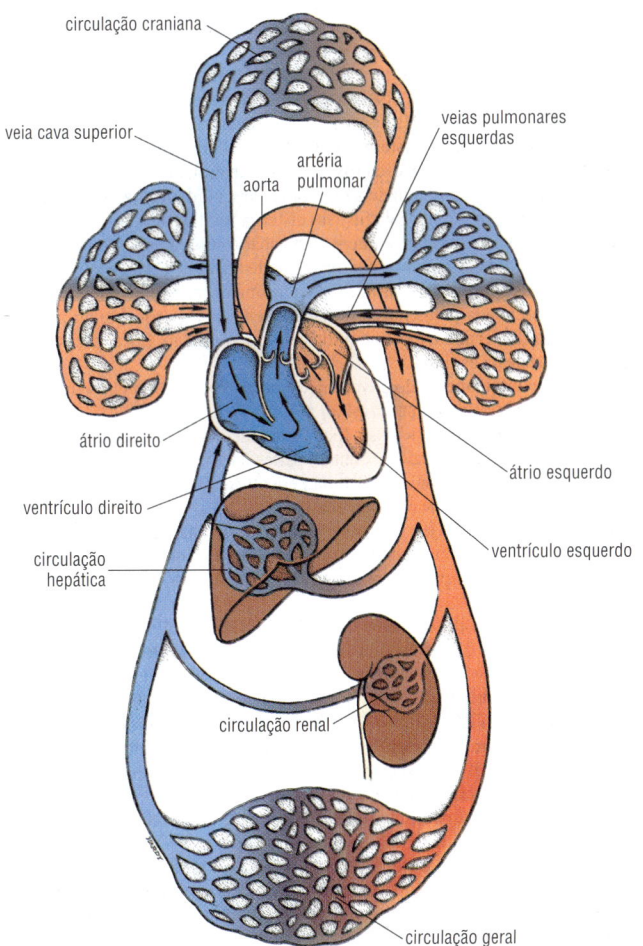

circulação pulmonar: através dos pulmões, do ventrículo direito para o átrio esquerdo
circulação sistêmica: através do corpo, do ventrículo esquerdo para o átrio direito

cir·cum·in·tes·ti·nal (ser′kŭm-in-tes′ti-năl). Circum-intestinal. SIN perienteric.
cir·cum·len·tal (ser-kŭm-len′tăl). Circunlenticular. SIN perilenticular.
cir·cum·man·dib·u·lar (ser′kŭm-man-dib′ū-lăr). Circumandibular; ao redor ou próximo da mandíbula.
cir·cum·nu·cle·ar (ser-kŭm-noo′klē-ăr). Circunuclear. SIN perinuclear.
cir·cum·oc·u·lar (ser-kŭm-ok′ū-lăr). Circum-ocular; ao redor do olho. SIN periocular, periophthalmic. [circum- + L. *oculus*, olho]
cir·cum·o·ral (ser-kŭm-ōr′ăl). Circum-oral. SIN perioral. [circum- + L. *os* (*oris*), boca]
cir·cum·or·bit·al (ser-kŭm-ōr′bi-tăl). Circum-orbitário; ao redor da órbita. SIN periorbital (2).
cir·cum·re·nal (ser-kŭm-rē′năl). Circunrenal. SIN perinephric. [circum- + L. *ren*, rim]
cir·cum·scribed (ser-kŭm-skrībd). Circunscrito; limitado por uma linha; limitado ou confinado. SIN circumscriptus. [circum- + L. *scribo*, escrever]
cir·cum·scrip·tus (ser-kŭm-skrip′tŭs). Circunscrito. SIN circumscribed. [L.]
cir·cum·stan·ti·al·i·ty (ser′kŭm-stan-shē-al′i-tē). Circunstancialidade; distúrbio no processo mental, voluntário ou involuntário, no qual a pessoa fornece uma quantidade excessiva de detalhes (circunstâncias), quase sempre tangenciais, elaborados e irrelevantes, para evitar fazer uma afirmação direta ou responder a uma pergunta; observada na esquizofrenia e em distúrbios obsessivos. Cf. tangentiality. [L. *circum-sto*, pr. p. *–stans*, estar em torno de]
cir·cum·val·late (ser-kŭm-val′āt). Circunvalado; indica uma estrutura circundada por uma parede, como as papilas circunvaladas (valadas) da língua. [circum- + L. *vallum*, parede]
cir·cum·vas·cu·lar (ser-kŭm-vas′kū-lăr). Circunvascular. SIN perivascular. [circum- + L. *vasculum*, vaso]
cir·cum·ven·tric·u·lar (ser′kŭm-ven-trik′ū-lăr). Circunventricular; ao redor ou na área de um ventrículo, como são os órgãos circunventriculares.
cir·cum·vo·lute (ser-kŭm-vol′oot). Circunvoluto; retorcido; enrolado em torno de. [L. *circum-volvo*, pp. *–volutus*, rodar em volta de]
cir·rhog·e·nous, cir·rho·gen·ic (sir-roj′e-nŭs, -rō-jen′ik). Cirrogênico; termo raramente usado para a propensão ao desenvolvimento de cirrose. [G. *kirrhos*, amarelo (fígado), + *-gen*, que produz]
cir·rhon·o·sus (sir-ron′ō-sŭs). Cirronose; doença do feto caracterizada anatomicamente por coloração amarela do peritônio e da pleura. [G. *kirrhos*, amarelo (fígado), + *nosos*, doença]
cir·rho·sis (sir-rō′sis). Cirrose; hepatopatia em estágio terminal caracterizada por lesão difusa das células parenquimatosas hepáticas, com regeneração nodular, fibrose e perturbação da arquitetura normal; associada à disfunção das células hepáticas e interferência com o fluxo sanguíneo no fígado, freqüentemente resultando em icterícia, hipertensão porta, ascite, e, finalmente, sinais bioquímicos e funcionais de insuficiência hepática. [G. *kirrhos*, amarelo (fígado), + *-osis*, condição]
alcoholic c., c. alcoólica; c. que freqüentemente se desenvolve no alcoolismo crônico, caracterizada em um estágio inicial por aumento do fígado devido à alteração gordurosa com fibrose leve e, mais tarde, por cirrose de Laënnec com contração do fígado.
biliary c., c. biliar; cirrose devida à obstrução biliar, que pode ser uma doença intra-hepática primária ou secundária à obstrução dos ductos biliares extra-hepáticos; esta última pode levar à colestase e proliferação em pequenos ductos biliares com fibrose, mas é raro haver perturbação acentuada do padrão lobular. VER TAMBÉM primary biliary c.
capsular c. of liver, c. capsular hepática. SIN Glisson c.
cardiac c., c. cardíaca; uma reação fibrótica extensa no fígado em virtude de pericardite constritiva crônica ou insuficiência cardíaca congestiva prolongada; a cirrose verdadeira com pontes fibrosas entre os lóbulos não é comum. SIN cardiac liver, congestive c., pseudocirrhosis, stasis c.
congestive c., c. congestiva. SIN cardiac c.
cryptogenic c., c. criptogênica; cirrose de etiologia desconhecida, sem história de alcoolismo ou hepatite aguda prévia.
fatty c., c. gordurosa; esteatose hepática; cirrose nutricional incipiente, principalmente em alcoólatras, na qual o fígado aumenta por alteração gordurosa, com leve fibrose.
Glisson c., c. de Glisson; peri-hepatite crônica com espessamento e subseqüente contração, resultando em atrofia e deformidade do fígado. SIN capsular c. of liver.
Hanot c., c. de Hanot. SIN primary biliary c.
juvenile c., c. juvenil. SIN chronic active *hepatitis.*
Laënnec c., c. de Laënnec; cirrose na qual os lóbulos hepáticos normais são substituídos por pequenos nódulos regenerativos, algumas vezes contendo gordura, separados por uma estrutura bastante regular de filamentos de tecido fibroso fino (fígado nodular); geralmente causada por alcoolismo. Pode causar grande comprometimento da função hepática, hipertensão porta com ascite e varizes esofágicas, bem como complicações potencialmente fatais. SIN portal c.
necrotic c., c. necrótica. SIN postnecrotic c.

cirrhosis 316 cistern

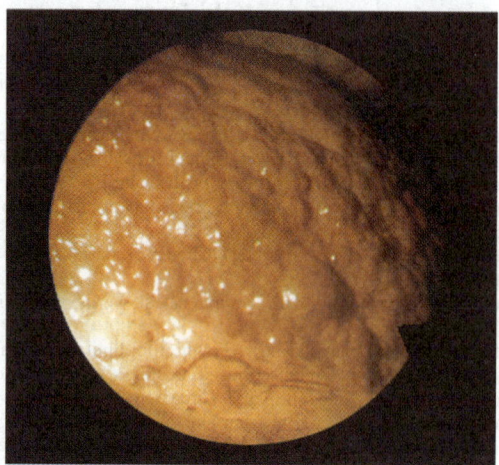

cirrose hepática: tipo micronodular (imagem laparoscópica)

nutritional c., c. nutricional; cirrose que ocorre em pessoas ou animais com deficiências alimentares gerais ou específicas; a deficiência de metionina e cistina pode causar alterações cirróticas em animais, mas não se sabe ao certo se a desnutrição humana causa cirrose ou apenas infiltração gordurosa reversível do fígado.

periportal c., c. periporta; cirrose hepática com faixas largas de fibrose circundando grandes segmentos do fígado, com nódulos regenerativos.

pigment c., c. pigmentar; cirrose resultante de depósitos excessivos de ferro no fígado, geralmente observada na hemocromatose.

pigmentary c., c. pigmentar, c. que resulta de depósitos exagerados de ferro no fígado, ocorre geralmente na hemocromatose.

pipe stem c., c. em haste de cachimbo; cirrose hepática com fibrose digitiforme predominantemente ao redor dos tratos portais, observada na esquistossomose. Causa hipertensão porta, mas raramente insuficiência hepática funcional.

portal c., cirrose porta. SIN Laënnec c.

posthepatitic c., c. pós-hepatite. SIN chronic active *hepatitis*.

postnecrotic c., c. pós-necrótica; cirrose caracterizada por necrose envolvendo lóbulos hepáticos inteiros, com colapso da estrutura reticular para formar grandes fibroses; os nódulos regenerativos também são grandes; pode ocorrer após necrose viral ou tóxica, ou ser decorrente de necrose isquêmica. SIN necrotic c.

primary biliary c., c. biliar primária; distúrbio que ocorre principalmente em mulheres de meia-idade, caracterizado por icterícia obstrutiva com hiperlipemia, prurido e hiperpigmentação da pele; não é observada obstrução de grandes ductos biliares ou proliferação de pequenos ductos biliares; o fígado mostra cirrose com acentuada infiltração porta por linfócitos e plasmócitos e, freqüentemente, por granulomas de células epitelióides; há anticorpos antimitocondriais séricos em 85–90% dos pacientes. SIN Hanot c.

pulmonary c., c. pulmonar; fibrose dos pulmões; geralmente fibrose pulmonar intersticial.

stasis c., c. de estase. SIN cardiac c.

syphilitic c., c. sifilítica; cirrose hepática que ocorre em virtude de sífilis terciária ou congênita.

toxic c., c. tóxica; cirrose hepática resultante de envenenamento crônico, como por chumbo ou tetracloreto de carbono.

cir·rhot·ic (sir - rot′ik). Cirrótico; relativo a, ou afetado por, cirrose ou fibrose avançada.

cir·ri (sir′ī). Plural de cirrus.

cir·rose, cir·rous (sir′ōs, sir′ŭs). Cirroso; relativo a, ou portador de, cirros.

cir·rus, pl. **cir·ri** (sir′rŭs, - rī). Cirro; estrutura formada por um grupo ou tufo de cílios fundidos, constituindo um dos órgãos sensoriais ou locomotores de alguns protozoários ciliados. [L. cacho]

cir·soid (ser′soyd). Cirsóide. SIN variciform. [G. *kirsos*, variz, + *eidos*, aspecto]

cir·som·pha·los (ser - som′fă - los). Cirsônfalo; termo raramente usado para *caput* medusae [G. *kirsos*, variz, + *omphalos*, umbigo]

cir·soph·thal·mia (ser - sof - thal′mē - ă). Cirsoftalmia; dilatação varicosa dos vasos sanguíneos conjuntivais. [G. *kirsos*, variz, + *ophthalmos*, olho]

CIS Abreviatura de *carcinoma* in situ.

♻ **cis-. 1.** Prefixo (em itálico) que significa deste lado, no lado próximo; oposto de *trans-*. **2.** Em genética, um prefixo que designa a localização de dois ou mais genes no mesmo cromossoma de um par homólogo, no acoplamento. **3.** Em química orgânica (em itálico), uma forma de isomerismo geométrico no qual grupos funcionais semelhantes estão fixados no mesmo lado do plano que inclui dois átomos de carbono fixos, adjacentes (p. ex., os grupamentos 2- e

3-OH da ribofuranose) em uma estrutura em anel. VER entgegen. **4.** Em química orgânica, uma forma de isomerismo geométrico em relação às ligações duplas carbono-carbono. Os grupamentos funcionais idênticos do mesmo lado da ligação dupla são *cis-*. Quando as quatro porções fixadas aos carbonos das ligações duplas são todas diferentes, deve ser seguida a nomenclatura E/Z. SIN zusammen (1). VER entgegen, zusammen. [L.]

cis·plat·in (sis′plă - tin). Cisplatina; agente quimioterápico com atividade antitumoral; a cisplatina liga-se ao DNA e interfere com a sua síntese; fortemente emetogênico.

cis·tern (sis′tern) [TA]. Cisterna. **1** [TA]. Qualquer cavidade ou espaço fechado que serve como reservatório, principalmente para quilo, linfa ou líquido cerebroespinhal. **2.** Um espaço ultramicroscópico que ocorre entre as membranas dos sacos achatados do retículo endoplasmático, o complexo de Golgi, ou as duas membranas do envoltório nuclear. SIN cisterna [TA]. [L. *cisterna*]

ambient c. [TA], c. ambiente; cisterna situada na face lateral do mesencéfalo e dorsalmente contínua com a cisterna do quadrigêmeo; a cisterna ambiente algumas vezes é definida como incluindo a cisterna do quadrigêmeo. SIN cisterna ambiens [TA].

basal c., c. basal. SIN interpeduncular c.

cerebellomedullary c., c. cerebelobulbar; a maior das cisternas subaracnóides entre o cerebelo e o bulbo; é dividida em uma c. cerebelobulbar posterior [TA], situada entre o cerebelo e a superfície dorsal do bulbo (também denominada cisterna magna), e uma cisterna cerebelobulbar lateral [TA], localizada entre o cerebelo e a face lateral do bulbo.

c. of chiasm, c. do quiasma. SIN chiasmatic c.

chiasmatic c. [TA], c. quiasmática; dilatação do espaço subaracnóide abaixo e anterior ao quiasma óptico. SIN cisterna chiasmatis [TA], c. of chiasm, c. chiasmatica.

chyle c., c. do quilo; *termo oficial alternativo para cisterna chyli.

c. of cytoplasmic reticulum, c. do retículo citoplasmático. VER cisterna.

c. of great cerebral vein, c. da veia magna do cérebro; *termo oficial alternativo para quadrigeminal c.

interpeduncular c. [TA], c. interpeduncular; dilatação do espaço subaracnóide rostral à ponte basilar e ventral e caudal aos corpos mamilares onde a membrana aracnóide se distende entre os dois lobos temporais acima da base do diencéfalo. VER interpeduncular *fossa*. SIN cisterna interpeduncularis [TA], basal c., cisterna basalis, cisterna cruralis, Tarin space.

c. of lamina terminalis [TA], c. da lâmina terminal; localizada imediatamente rostral à lâmina terminal. SIN cisterna laminae terminalis [TA].

lateral cerebellomedullary c. [TA], c. cerebelobulbar lateral. VER cerebellomedullary c. SIN cisterna cerebellomedullaris lateralis [TA].

c. of lateral cerebral fossa, c. da fossa cerebral lateral; uma expansão alongada do espaço subaracnóide onde a membrana aracnóide forma uma ponte sobre a abertura da fissura de Sylvius. SIN cisterna fossae lateralis cerebri [TA].

lumbar c. [TA], c. lombar; aumento do espaço subaracnóide entre o cone medular da medula espinhal (aproximadamente ao nível de L2) e a extremidade inferior do espaço subaracnóide e da dura-máter (aproximadamente ao nível de S2); ocupada pelas raízes dorsais e ventrais que constituem a cauda eqüina, pelo filo terminal e pelo líquido cefalorraquidiano. Local para punção lombar e anestesia espinhal.

c. of nuclear envelope, c. do envoltório nuclear. SIN cisterna caryothecae.

Pecquet c., c. de Pecquet. SIN cisterna chyli.

pericallosal c. [TA], c. pericalosa; localizada imediatamente adjacente a todo o comprimento do corpo caloso, contém partes da artéria pericalosa, um ramo da artéria cerebral anterior. SIN cisterna pericallosa [TA].

pontine c., c. pontina. SIN pontocerebellar c.

pontocerebellar c. [TA], c. pontocerebelar; localizada nas faces laterais da ponte em sua junção com o cerebelo, pode ser dividida em porções superior e inferior. SIN cisterna pontocerebellaris [TA], cisterna pontis, pontine c., prepontine c.

posterior cerebellomedullary c. [TA], c. cerebelobulbar posterior. VER cerebellomedullary c. SIN cisterna cerebellomedullaris posterior [TA], cisterna magna*.

prepontine c., c. pré-pontina. SIN pontocerebellar.

quadrigeminal c. [TA], c. quadrigeminal; uma expansão do espaço subaracnóide, localizada imediatamente dorsal ao teto do mesencéfalo, estendendo-se para a frente entre o corpo caloso e o tálamo; encerra as veias cerebrais internas que se unem caudalmente para formar a veia magna cerebral (veia de Galeno). SIN cisterna quadrigeminalis [TA], c. of great cerebral vein*, cisterna venae magnae cerebri*, Bichat canal, superior c.

subarachnoid c.'s [TA], cisternas subaracnóides; porções alargadas do espaço subaracnóide no crânio, onde a membrana aracnóide forma uma ponte sobre uma depressão na superfície cerebral. SIN cisternae subarachnoideae [TA].

superior c., c. superior. SIN quadrigeminal c.

Sylvian c., c. de Sylvius; o espaço subaracnóide associado ao sulco cerebral lateral (fissura de Sylvius); contém o segmento M1 da artéria cerebral média e a origem das artérias lenticuloestriadas, além de partes proximais da artéria cerebral média.

cis·ter·na, gen. e pl. **cis·ter·nae** (sis-ter′nă, -ter′nē) [TA]. Cisterna. SIN cistern. [L. uma cisterna subterrânea de água, de *cista*, caixa]
  c. am'biens [TA], c. ambiente. SIN ambient cistern.
  c. basa'lis, c. basal. SIN interpeduncular cistern.
  c. caryothe'cae, c. da carioteca; o espaço entre as membranas interna e externa do envoltório nuclear; pode ser contínuo em locais com cisternas do retículo endoplasmático. SIN cistern of nuclear envelope, perinuclear space.
  c. cerebellomedullaris lateralis [TA], c. cerebelobulbar lateral. SIN lateral cerebellomedullary cistern.
  c. cerebellomedulla'ris posterior [TA], c. cerebelobulbar posterior. SIN posterior cerebellomedullary cistern; VER cerebellomedullary cistern.
  c. chiasmatica [TA], c. quiasmática. SIN chiasmatic cistern.
  c. chias'matis [TA], c. quiasmática. SIN chiasmatic cistern.
  c. chy'li [TA], c. do quilo; saco dilatado na extremidade inferior do ducto torácico no qual se abrem o tronco intestinal e dois troncos linfáticos lombares; sua presença é inconstante e, quando presente, está localizada posteriormente à aorta, na face anterior dos corpos da primeira e segunda vértebras lombares. SIN chyle cistern*, ampulla chyli, chylocyst, Pecquet cistern, Pecquet reservoir, receptaculum chyli, receptaculum pecqueti.
  c. crura'lis, c. interpeduncular. SIN interpeduncular cistern.
  c. fos'sae latera'lis cer'ebri [TA], c. da fossa lateral do cérebro. SIN cistern of lateral cerebral fossa.
  c. interpeduncula'ris [TA], c. interpeduncular. SIN interpeduncular cistern.
  c. laminae terminalis [TA], c. da lâmina terminal. SIN cistern of lamina terminalis.
  c. lumbalis [TA], c. lombar. SIN lumbar cistern.
  c. mag'na, c. magna;*termo oficial alternativo para posterior cerebellomedullary cistern.
  c. pericallosa [TA], c. pericalosa. SIN pericallosal cistern.
  c. perilymphat'ica, c. perilinfática. SIN perilymphatic space.
  c. pon'tis, c. pontina. SIN pontocerebellar cistern.
  c. pontocerebellaris [TA], c. pontocerebelar. SIN pontocerebellar cistern.
  c. quadrigeminalis [TA], c. quadrigeminal. SIN quadrigeminal cistern; VER cistern of great cerebral vein.
  cisternae subarachnoideae [TA], cisternas subaracnóides. SIN subarachnoid cisterns, em cistern.
  subsurface c., c. subsuperficial; cisterna do retículo endoplasmático situada próximo da membrana plasmática; essas cisternas ocorrem principalmente nos corpos celulares dos neurônios.
  terminal cisternae, cisternas terminais; pares de túbulos do retículo sarcoplasmático orientados transversalmente, observados a intervalos regulares nas fibras musculares esqueléticas; formam uma tríade juntamente com um túbulo T intermediário.
  c. ve'nae mag'nae cer'ebri, c. da veia magna do cérebro; *termo oficial alternativo para quadrigeminal cistern.
cis·ter·nal (sis-ter′nal). Relativo a uma cisterna.
cis·tern·og·ra·phy (sis′tern-og′ră-fē). Cisternografia; o estudo radiográfico das cisternas basais do encéfalo após a introdução subaracnóidea de um contraste opaco ou de outro tipo, ou de um radiofármaco com um detector adequado. [cisterna + G. *graphō*, escrever]
  cerebellopontine c., c. cerebelopontina; o estudo radiográfico do ângulo cerebelopontino e das estruturas contíguas após a introdução de um contraste radiopaco no espaço subaracnóide.
  radionuclide c., c. por radionuclídeos; imagem cintigráfica das cisternas na base do cérebro após injeção subaracnóide de um radiofármaco emissor de raios gama.
cis·tron (sis′tron). Cístron. **1.** A menor unidade funcional de hereditariedade; um segmento de DNA cromossomial associado a uma única função bioquímica. Nos conceitos clássicos, um gene poderia consistir em mais de um cístron; em biologia molecular moderna, o cístron é essencialmente equivalente ao gene estrutural. **2.** A unidade genética definida pelo teste *cis/trans* [*cis* tr-ans + -on]
cis·ves·tism, cis·ves·ti·tism (sis-ves′tizm, -ves′ti-tizm). Cisvestismo; cisvestitismo; a prática de usar roupas impróprias para a sua posição ou condição social. Cf. transvestism. [L. *cis*, no lado próximo de, + *vestio*, vestir]
Ci·tel·lus (si-tel′ŭs). Nome anterior do gênero *Spermophilus*. [L. Mod.]
cito disp. Abreviatura do L. *cito dispensetur*, deixe-o ser aviado rapidamente.
cit·ral (sit′ral). Citral; um aldeído monoterpênico que consiste em ambos os isômeros geométricos encontrados nos óleos de limão, laranja, verbena e capim-limão; o citral-A é o trans-isômero e o citral-B é o cis-isômero (neral).
cit·rase, cit·ra·tase (sit′rās, -rā-tās). Citrase; citratase. SIN citrate lyase.
cit·rate (sit′rāt, sī′trāt). Citrato; um sal ou éster do ácido cítrico; os citratos são usados como anticoagulantes porque se ligam aos íons cálcio.
  c. aldolase, c. aldolase. SIN c. lyase.
  ATP c. (*pro*-3S)-lyase, ATP citrato (pro-3S)-liase; enzima que catalisa a reação de ATP, citrato e coenzima A para formar ADP, ortofosfato, oxaloacetato e acetil-CoA. Uma etapa importante na biossíntese de ácidos graxos. SIN citrate-cleavage enzyme.
  c. lyase, c. liase, *c. (pro*-3S)-liase; enzima que catalisa a clivagem de citrato em oxaloacetato e acetato na ausência de coenzima A. SIN citrase, citratase, c. aldolase.
  c. synthase, c. sintase; *c. (si)*-sintase; enzima que catalisa a condensação de oxaloacetato, água e acetil-Coa, formando citrato e coenzima A; uma etapa importante no ciclo do ácido tricarboxílico. SIN condensing enzyme, oxaloacetate transacetase.
cit·rat·ed (sit′rā-ted). Citratado; que contém um citrato; designa especificamente soro sanguíneo ou leite ao qual foi acrescentada uma solução de citrato de potássio e/ou de sódio.
cit·ric ac·id (sit′rik). Ácido cítrico; ácido 2-hidroxipropano-1,2,3-tricarboxílico; o ácido das frutas cítricas, amplamente distribuído na natureza e um intermediário fundamental no metabolismo intermediário.
cit·rin (sit′rin). Citrina. SIN *vitamin P*.
Cit·ro·bac·ter (sit′rō-bak-ter). Gênero de bactérias móveis (família Enterobacteriaceae) contendo bacilos Gram-negativos que usam o citrato como fonte de carbono; as células móveis são peritríquias. A fermentação da lactose por esses microrganismos é tardia ou ausente; eles produzem trimetilenoglicol a partir do glicerol. A espécie típica é *C. freundii*.
  C. amalona'tica, espécie de bactéria encontrada nas fezes, no solo, na água e no esgoto; isolada de amostras clínicas como patógeno oportunista. SIN *Levinea amalonatica*.
  C. diver'sus, espécie de bactéria encontrada nas fezes, no solo, na água, no esgoto e nos alimentos; isolada da urina, orofaringe, nariz, escarro e feridas; descrita em casos de meningite neonatal, onde freqüentemente é grave, resultando em formação de abscesso cerebral. SIN *C. koseri, Levinea diversus, Levinea malonatica*.
  C. freun'dii, espécie de bactéria encontrada na água, nas fezes e na urina; é um habitante do intestino normal, mas pode ser encontrada em infecções alimentares e em infecções das vias urinárias, da vesícula biliar, do ouvido médio e das meninges; é a espécie típica do gênero *C*.
  C. ko'seri, SIN *C. diversus*.
cit·ro·nel·la (sit-rō-nel′ă). *Cymbopogon (Andropogon) nardus* (família Gramineae); citronela; gramínea aromática do antigo Ceilão (agora Sri Lanka), da qual é destilado um óleo volátil (óleo de citronela) usado como perfume e repelente de insetos.
cit·ro·nel·lal (sit′-rō-nel′ăl). Citronelal; principal ingrediente volátil da grama-do-ceilão e do óleo de citronela. Usado em perfumes para sabão e como repelente de insetos.
ci·trul·line (sit′rul-ēn). Citrulina; N^5-(Aminocarbonil)-L-ornitina; α-amino-δ-ureidovalérico; 5-ureidonorvalina; aminoácido formado a partir da L-ornitina durante o ciclo da uréia, e também um produto na biossíntese do óxido nítrico; também encontrada na melancia (*Citrullus vulgaris*) e na caseína. Elevada em indivíduos com uma deficiência de argininossuccinato sintetase ou argininossuccinato liase.
cit·rul·li·ne·mia (sit′rul-i-nē′mē-ă) [MIM*215700]. Citrulinemia; distúrbio do ciclo da uréia no qual as concentrações de citrulina no sangue, na urina e no líquido cefalorraquidiano estão elevadas, devido à deficiência de argininossuccinato sintetase (ASS); manifesta-se clinicamente por letargia, vômito, intoxicação por amônia e retardo mental, e, em geral, tem início no primeiro ano de vida; herança autossômica recessiva, causada por mutação no gene da ASS no cromossoma 9 de alguns pacientes.
cit·rul·li·nu·ria (sit′rul-i-noo′rē-ă). Citrulinúria; aumento da excreção urinária de citrulina; uma manifestação de citrulinemia.
Civatte, Achille, dermatologista francês, 1877–1956. VER C. *bodies*, em *body; poikiloderma* of C.
Civinini, Filippo, anatomista italiano, 1805–1844. VER C. *canal, ligament, process*.
CJD Abreviatura de Creutzfeldt-Jakob *disease* (doença de Creutzfeldt-Jakob).
CK Abreviatura de *creatine* kinase (creatinoquinase).
Cl Símbolo do cloro.
clad·i·o·sis (klad-ē-ō′sis). Cladiose; dermatofitose semelhante à esporotricose, caracterizada por lesões verrucosas e linfangite ascendente; causada por *Scopulariopsis blochii*. VER *Scopulariopsis* [G. *klados*, ramo ou raiz, + -*osis*, condição]
Clado, Spiro, ginecologista francês, 1856–1905. VER C. *anastomosis, band, ligament, point*.
Cla·dor·chis wat·soni (kla-dōr′kis wat-sō′nī). Termo incorreto para *Watsonius watsoni*.
clad·o·spo·ri·o·sis (klad′ō-spō-rē-ō′sis). Cladosporiose; infecção por um fungo do gênero *Cladosporium*.
  cerebral c., c. cerebral; feoifomicose cerebral, uma micose cerebral geralmente causada por *Cladosporium trichoides* (*Xylohypha bantianum*).
Clad·o·spo·ri·um (klad-ō-spōr′i-ŭm). Gênero de fungos que possuem conidióforos dematiáceos ou de cor escura, com esporos ovais ou redondos, comumente isolados no solo ou em resíduos vegetais. [G. *klados*, ramo, + *sporos*, semente]
  C. carrion'ii, espécie de fungos que é uma causa da cromoblastomicose no homem.

C. cladosporioides, espécie causadora de infecção no local de um teste cutâneo em um paciente infectado pelo HIV.
C. wernec'kii, SIN *Exophiala werneckii.*
C. (Xylohypha) bantia'num, espécie de fungos que causa cladosporiose cerebral; provavelmente sinônimo de *C. trichoides.*

clair·voy·ance (klār - voy′ans). Clarividência; percepção de eventos objetivos (passados, presentes ou futuros) habitualmente não discerníveis pelos sentidos; um tipo de percepção extra-sensorial. [Fr.]

clam·ox·y·quin hy·dro·chlo·ride (klam - ok′si - kwin). Cloridrato de camoxiquina; um amebicida.

clamp (klamp). Pinça; instrumento para comprimir ou segurar uma estrutura. Cf. forceps. [I.M., do Hol. m. *klampe*]

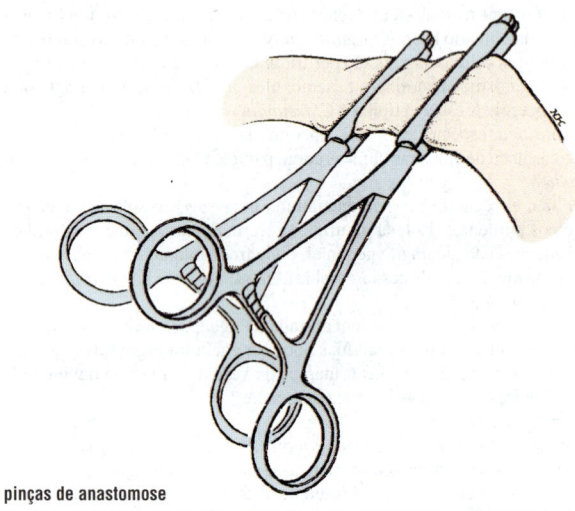

pinças de anastomose

Cope c., pinça de Cope; pinça usada na excisão do cólon e do reto.
Crafoord c., p. de Crafoord; pinça usada em cirurgias cardíacas, pulmonares e vasculares.
Crile c., p. de Crile; pinça para interrupção temporária do fluxo sanguíneo.
Fogarty c., p. de Fogarty; pinça com lâminas com suportes de borracha e superfícies serrilhadas para permitir uma preensão atraumática dos tecidos.
Gant c., p. de Gant; p. em ângulo reto usada em hemorroidectomia.
Gaskell c., p. de Gaskell; instrumento para esmagar o feixe atrioventricular em animais experimentais e, assim, produzir bloqueio atrioventricular.
gingival c., p. gengival; pedaço de metal em forma de espiral que circunda ou apreende o colo de um dente e moldado de forma a retrair o tecido gengival.
Kelly c., p. de Kelly; pinça hemostática curva, sem dentes, introduzida para cirurgia ginecológica.
Kocher c., p. de Kocher; pinça hemostática reta, pesada, com dentes entrelaçados na extremidade.
liver-shod c., pinça com dentes cobertos por tecido para minimizar a lesão de estruturas, como o intestino, quando a pinça é fechada.
Mikulicz c., p. de Mikulicz; pinça usada para esmagar paredes entre o cólon proximal e distal na colectomia em dois estágios.
Mixter c., p. de Mixter; uma pinça em ângulo reto.
Mogen c., p. de Mogen; um instrumento de circuncisão. [Estrela de Davi]
mosquito c., p.-mosquito; pequena pinça hemostática, reta ou curva, com ou sem dentes, usada para segurar tecidos delicados ou para hemostasia. SIN mosquito forceps.
Ochsner c., p. de Ochsner; pinça hemostática reta com dentes.
patch c., SIN *patch clamping.*
Payr c., p. de Payr; pinça grande, ligeiramente curva, usada em gastrectomia ou enterectomia.
Potts c., p. de Potts; uma pinça de fixação vascular, com dentes finos e múltiplas pontas, que causa traumatismo limitado do vaso enquanto o segura firmemente.
Rankin c., p. de Rankin; pinça de três lâminas usada na ressecção do cólon.
right angle c., p. em ângulo reto; uma pinça com uma curvatura de 90°, curta em sua extremidade, freqüentemente usada para dissecção ou passagem de ligaduras ao redor dos vasos.
rubber dam c., um dispositivo de metal semelhante a uma mola que circunda ou apreende o colo de um dente; é moldado de forma a evitar que um campo de látex com orifícios se solte do mesmo.
rubber-shod c., pequena pinça com ponta de borracha que mantém as suturas no lugar durante a cirurgia.

clamp con·nec·tion. Gancho de conexão; em fungos, uma hifa curta que ultrapassa um septo hifal e é fixada às duas células adjacentes ao septo; característica da maioria dos membros do filo Basidiomycetes.

cla·po·tage, cla·pote·ment (kla - pō - tahz′, kla - pōt - mawn′). Vascolejo; o som de "agitação de ondas" audível à sucussão de um estômago dilatado. [Fr.]

Clapton, Edward, médico inglês, 1830–1909. VER C. *line.*
Clara, Max, anatomista austríaco, 1899–1966. VER C. *cell.*
cla·rif·i·cant (kla - rif′i - kant). Clarificante; o agente que torna claro um líquido turvo. [L. *clarus,* claro, + *facio,* fazer]
clar·i·fi·ca·tion (klar′i - fi - kā′shŭn). Clarificação, purificação; o processo de tornar claro um líquido turvo. SIN lucidification.
Clark, Alonzo, farmacologista norte-americano, 1807–1887. VER C. weight *rule.*
Clark, Eliot R., anatomista norte-americano, 1881–1963. VER Sandison-C. *chamber.*
Clark, Leland, Jr., bioquímico norte-americano, *1918. VER C. *electrode.*
Clark, Wallace H., Jr., dermatopatologista norte-americano, *1924. VER C. *level.*
Clarke, Cecil. VER C.-Hadfield *syndrome.*
Clarke, Jacob A.L., anatomista inglês, 1817–1880. VER C. *column, nucleus.*
clas·mat·o·cyte (klaz - mat′o - sīt). Clasmatócito; termo obsoleto para macrófago. [G. *klasma,* fragmento, + *kytos,* cavidade (célula)]
clas·ma·to·sis (klaz - mă - tō′sis). Clasmatose; a extensão de processos semelhantes a pseudópodes em microrganismos unicelulares e células do sangue por plasmólise, e não por verdadeira formação de pseudópodes. [G. *klasma,* fragmento, + *-osis,* condição]
clasp. Grampo; gancho; braçadeira; fecho; garra; presilha. **1.** Parte de uma dentadura parcial removível que atua como um retentor direto e/ou estabilizador para a dentadura por circundar parcialmente um dente vizinho ou fazer contato com ele. **2.** Um retentor direto de uma dentadura parcial removível, geralmente consistindo em dois ramos unidos por um corpo que se conecta com um apoio oclusal; pelo menos um ramo do gancho geralmente termina na área inferior à protuberância (convergência gengival) do dente envolvido.
bar c., grampo em barra; **(1)** um grampo cujos ramos são extensões em barra de grandes conectores ou de dentro da base da dentadura; os ramos passam adjacentes aos tecidos moles e aproximam-se do ponto de contato sobre o dente em uma direção gengivo-oclusal; **(2)** um grampo que consiste em dois ou mais ramos distintos localizados opostos entre si sobre o dente; os ramos da barra originam-se da estrutura ou de um conector e podem atravessar os tecidos moles; um ramo (barra), o ramo de retenção, geralmente termina na área inferior à protuberância (convergência gengival) do dente; o outro, o ramo recíproco, termina na área superior à saliência (convergência oclusal). SIN Roach c.
circumferential c., grampo circunferencial; **(1)** grampo que circunda mais de 180° de um dente, incluindo ângulos opostos, e que, geralmente, toca o dente em toda a extensão do grampo, com pelo menos uma extremidade na área inferior à saliência (convergência gengival); **(2)** um grampo que consiste em dois braços circunferenciais, ambos originados do mesmo conector menor e localizados em superfícies opostas do dente vizinho.
continuous c., grampo contínuo. SIN continuous bar *retainer.*
extended c., grampo estendido; grampo que se estende de seu conector menor ao longo da superfície lingual e/ou facial de dois ou mais dentes.
Roach c., grampo de Roach. SIN bar c.

class (klas). Classe; na classificação biológica, a divisão imediatamente abaixo do filo (ou subfilo) e acima da ordem. [L. *classis,* uma classe, divisão]

clas·si·fi·ca·tion (klas′i - fi - kā′shŭn). Classificação; um arranjo sistemático em classes ou grupos baseado em características comuns observadas; uma forma de ordenar um grupo de fatos desconexos.
adansonian c., c. de Adanson; classificação dos organismos baseada na atribuição de pesos iguais a cada caráter do organismo; esse princípio tem sua maior aplicação em taxonomia numérica. [M. *Adanson*]
Angle c. of malocclusion, classificação de má oclusão de Angle; uma classificação de diferentes tipos de má oclusão, com base na relação mesiodistal dos molares permanentes após sua erupção e fechamento, e constituída por três classes: *Classe I:* relação normal entre o maxilar e a mandíbula, na qual a cúspide mesiobucal do primeiro molar maxilar se encaixa no sulco bucal do primeiro molar permanente mandibular; *Classe II:* relação distal da mandíbula, na qual a cúspide distobucal do primeiro molar permanente maxilar se encaixa no sulco bucal do primeiro molar mandibular, e ainda subclassificada como Divisão 1, labioversão dos dentes incisivos maxilares, e Divisão 2, linguoversão dos incisivos centrais maxilares, ambas podendo ser condições unilaterais; *Classe III:* relação mesial da mandíbula, na qual a cúspide mesiobucal do primeiro molar maxilar se encaixa na fresta entre o primeiro e o segundo molares permanentes mandibulares, subclassificada como uma condição unilateral.
Arneth c., c. de Arneth; uma classificação dos neutrófilos polimorfonucleares de acordo com o número de seus lobos nucleares. VER Arneth *stages,* em *stage.*
Astler-Coller c., c. de Astler-Coller; sistema de estadiamento que é uma modificação da classificação de Dukes para o câncer de cólon.
Bethesda c., c. de Bethesda. SIN Bethesda *system.*
Black c., c. de Black; uma classificação das cáries dentárias baseada na(s) superfície(s) do dente envolvida(s).

classificação de má oclusão de Angle	
classes	anomalias
I	relação normal do maxilar e mandibular; neutroclusão
II	relação distal da mandíbula; distoclusão
II div. 1	labioversão dos incisivos maxilares
div. 2	linguoversão dos incisivos centrais maxilares
	– "classe II pura"; oclusão distal sem anomalias dos dentes
	– classe II "direita" ou "esquerda": anomalias dos dentes nos lados direito ou esquerdo
III	relação mesial da mandíbula; mesioclusão

Caldwell-Moloy c., c. de Caldwell-Moloy; uma classificação das variações na pelve feminina, a saber, ginecóide, andróide, antropóide e platipelóide, com base no tipo dos segmentos posterior e anterior do estreito pélvico.
Cummer c., c. de Cummer; uma relação dos vários tipos de dentaduras parciais removíveis de acordo com a distribuição de retentores diretos.
DeBakey c., c. de DeBakey; consiste em três tipos: o Tipo I estende-se até o arco transverso e aorta distal, e o tipo II é limitado à aorta ascendente; as dissecções do tipo III começam na aorta descendente, estendendo-se o tipo IIIA em direção ao diafragma, e o tipo IIIB, abaixo dele.
Denver c., c. de Denver; um sistema para nomenclatura de cromossomas mitóticos humanos, baseado no comprimento e na posição do centrômero. [*Denver*, Colorado, onde foi feito o acordo]
Dukes c., c. de Dukes; classificação da extensão da invasão de um adenocarcinoma ressecado do cólon ou reto comumente modificada da seguinte forma: A (Dukes A), limitada à mucosa; B_1, para a muscular da mucosa; B_2, através da muscular da mucosa; C_1, limitada à parede intestinal, com metástases ganglionares; C_2, através da parede intestinal, com metástases ganglionares.
FAB c., c. FAB; c. franco-americano-britânica de leucemias agudas baseada no estudo das características microscópicas e citoquímica dos blastos; subdivide leucemias mielógenas agudas em 8 grupos (M_0-M_7) e leucemias linfoblásticas agudas em 3 grupos (L_1-L_3); amplamente usada na prática clínica. SIN French-American-British c.
French-American-British c., c. franco-americano-britânica. SIN FAB c.
Gell and Coombs C. (gel koomz), c. de Gell e Coombs; sistema de classificação que diferencia os 4 tipos de reações de hipersensibilidade: Tipo I: reações anafiláticas, Tipo II: reações citotóxicas, Tipo III: reações por imunocomplexos e Tipo IV: reações de hipersensibilidade celular/tardia.
International Labour Organization (ILO) C., c. da Organização Internacional do Trabalho; Classificação Internacional de Radiografias das Pneumoconioses de 1980 pela OIT; um sistema para descrição qualitativa e semiquantitativa dos achados nas radiografias de tórax causados por pneumoconiose, elaborada para estudos epidemiológicos; substitui as classificações de 1950, 1958, 1968 e 1971.
Jansky c., c. de Jansky; a classificação dos grupos sanguíneos humanos agora designados O, A, B e AB.
Kennedy c., c. de Kennedy; relação de várias formas de mandíbulas parcialmente edentadas de acordo com a distribuição dos dentes ausentes.
Kiel c., c. de Kiel; classificação do linfoma não-Hodgkin em baixo grau de malignidade (tipos linfocítico, linfoplasmocitóide, centrocítico e centroblástico-centrocítico) e alto grau de malignidade (centroblástico, linfoblástico de Burkitt ou células espiraladas e imunoblástico). SIN Lennert c.
Lancefield c., c. de Lancefield; classificação sorológica que divide os estreptococos hemolíticos em grupos (A a O) que têm uma relação definida com suas origens, baseada em testes de precipitação dependendo de substâncias grupo-específicas que são carboidratos; p. ex., o *Grupo A* contém cepas mais patogênicas para os seres humanos; *B*, cepas que causam mastite em vacas e presentes no leito normal, incluindo cepas da orofaringe e da vagina humanas; *C*, cepas de vários animais inferiores, incluindo algumas da orofaringe de bovinos e seres humanos; *D*, cepas do queijo e dos seres humanos; *E*, cepas do leite pasteurizado; *F*, cepas provenientes principalmente da orofaringe humana, associadas à amigdalite; *G*, cepas de seres humanos, algumas de macacos e cães; e *H*, *K* e *O*, cepas não-patogênicas algumas vezes provenientes das vias respiratórias humanas normais.
Lennert c., c. de Lennert. SIN Kiel c.
Lukes-Collins c., c. de Lukes-Collins; classificação de linfomas de acordo com a natureza imunológica da célula de origem, baseada em dados histológicos e clínicos.
multiaxial c., c. multiaxial; procedimento usado no DSM-III-R para diagnóstico de pacientes em cinco eixos: 1) existência de síndrome psiquiátrica; 2) história pregressa de distúrbios da personalidade e do desenvolvimento do paciente; 3) possíveis distúrbios clínicos não-mentais; 4) intensidade dos fatores de estresse psicossocial; 5) máximo nível de funcionamento adaptativo no último ano.
New York Heart Association c., uma classificação funcional para avaliar incapacidade cardiovascular. Classe I: pacientes com cardiopatia sem limitação da atividade física. A atividade habitual não causa sintomas. Classe II: pacientes com cardiopatia com discreta limitação da atividade; confortáveis em repouso. A atividade física habitual causa fadiga, palpitação, dispnéia ou angina. Classe III: pacientes com cardiopatia que provoca acentuada limitação da atividade: confortáveis em repouso. A atividade física menor que a habitual provoca sintomas. Classe IV: pacientes com cardiopatia resultando em incapacidade de realizar qualquer atividade física sem desconforto. Pode haver sintomas até mesmo em repouso.
Rappaport c., c. de Rappaport; uma classificação histológica de linfomas usada antes da disponibilidade dos métodos recentes para identificação de linfócitos B e T.
REAL c., c. REAL; classificação de linfoma publicada pela primeira vez em 1994 e baseada na correlação das características clínicas dos linfomas com sua histopatologia e imunofenótipo e genótipo de células neoplásicas; reúne as doenças linfoproliferativas em leucemia/linfoma crônico, linfoma ganglionar ou extraganglionar, linfoma/leucemia aguda, distúrbios dos plasmócitos e doença de Hodgkin. [*Revised European-American Lymphoma* classification (classificação Euro-Americana de Linfoma Revista)]
Runyon c., c. de Runyon; esquema de classificação para outras micobactérias, além do *Mycobacterium tuberculosis,* que divide as espécies em quatro categorias: 1) fotocromogênios, espécies que produzem um pigmento caroteno cuja cor varia do amarelo ao castanho quando cultivadas na presença de luz; 2) escotocromogênios, que produzem pigmento na presença ou na ausência de luz; 3) não-pigmentadas, que não produzem pigmento; e 4) de crescimento rápido, que crescem em meios sólidos em 5–10 dias em vez de 4–8 semanas. Essa classificação não tem importância clínica ou genética, mas continua tendo valor limitado na identificação de alguns microrganismos isolados na prática clínica.
Rye c., c. de Rye; classificação de doença de Hodgkin de acordo com os tipos predomínio linfocítico, nodular esclerosante, celularidade mista e depleção linfocítica. [*Rye*, NY, 1965]
Salter-Harris c. of epiphysial plate injuries, c. de Salter-Harris das lesões das placas epifisárias; classificação das lesões das placas epifisárias em cinco grupos (I a V), de acordo com o padrão de lesão da epífise, fise e/ou metáfise; a classificação correlaciona-se com diferentes prognósticos no tocante aos efeitos da lesão sobre o crescimento subseqüente e subseqüente deformidade da epífise.
Tessier c., c. de Tessier; uma classificação anatômica das fendas faciais, craniofaciais e laterofaciais que utiliza a órbita como a estrutura primária de referência. Há quinze localizações de fendas.
class switch. Mudança de classe; alteração no isotipo de anticorpo produzido após uma célula B ter encontrado um antígeno.
clas·tic (klas'tik). Clástico; que se separa em pedaços, ou que exibe uma tendência a se quebrar ou dividir. [G. *klastos*, quebrado]
clas·to·gen (klas'tō - jen). Clastógeno; um agente (p. ex., algumas substâncias químicas, raios X, luz ultravioleta) que causa quebras cromossomiais. [G. *klastos*, quebrado, + *genos*, nascimento]
clas·to·gen·ic (klas-tō-jen'ik). Clastogênico; relativo à ação de um clastógeno.
clath·rate (klath'rāt). Clatrato; tipo de composto de inclusão no qual pequenas moléculas são aprisionadas em uma rede de macromoléculas. [L. *clathrare*, pp. *–atus*, guarnecer com uma rede]
clath·rin (klath'rin). Clatrina; principal constituinte de uma rede poliédrica de proteínas que reveste as membranas (vesículas) e depressões revestidas das células eucarióticas, parecendo envolvida na secreção de proteínas. Essa proteína também ocorre nas vesículas sinápticas. [L. *clathri*, rede]
Clauberg, Karl W., bacteriologista alemão, *1893. VER C. *test, unit*.
Claude, Henri, psiquiatra francês, 1869–1945. VER C. *syndrome*.
clau·di·ca·tion (klaw - di - kā'shŭn). Claudicação; mancar, geralmente se refere à claudicação intermitente. [L. *claudicatio*, de *claudico*, mancar]
intermittent c., c. intermitente; condição causada por isquemia dos músculos; caracterizada por crises de incapacidade e dor, desencadeadas pela deambulação, principalmente nos músculos da panturrilha; entretanto, o distúrbio pode ocorrer em outros grupos musculares. SIN Charcot syndrome, myasthenia angiosclerotica.
neurogenic c., c. neurogênica; claudicação com lesão neurológica, geralmente associada à estenose raquiana lombar.
clau·di·ca·tory (klaw'di - kā - tōr - ē). Claudicatório; relativo a claudicação, principalmente claudicação intermitente.
Claudius, Friedrich M., anatomista alemão, 1822–1869. VER C. *cells*, em *cell*, *fossa*.

Clausen. J., médico dinamarquês. VER Dyggve-Melchior-Clausen *syndrome*.
claus·tra (klaws′tră). Claustros. Plural de claustrum.
claus·tral (klaws′trăl). Claustral; relativo ao claustro.
claus·tro·pho·bia (klaw-strō-fō′bē-ă). Claustrofobia; medo mórbido de permanecer em um local fechado. [L. *claustrum*, espaço fechado, + G. *phobos*, medo]
claus·tro·pho·bic (kalw-strō-fō′bik). Claustrofóbico; relativo a, ou que sofre de, claustrofobia.
claus·trum, pl. **claus·tra** (klaws′trŭm, klaws′tră). Claustro. **1.** Uma das diversas estruturas anatômicas semelhantes a uma barreira. **2.** [TA]. Uma lâmina fina, vertical, de substância cinzenta localizada próximo do putâmen, do qual está separada pela cápsula externa. O claustro consiste em duas partes: 1) uma parte insular e 2) uma parte temporal entre o putâmen e o lobo temporal. As células do claustro possuem conexões recíprocas com áreas sensoriais do córtex cerebral. [L. barreira]
  c. gut′turis, c. o′ris, c. oral; termo obsoleto para palato mole (soft *palate*).
  c. virgina′le, c. virginal; termo obsoleto para hímen (hymen).
clau·su·ra (klaw-soo′ră). Clausura. SIN atresia. [L. fechadura, ferrolho, de *claudo*, fechar]
cla·va (klā′vă). Clava. SIN gracile *tubercle*. [L. clava, bastão]
cla·val (klā′văl). Claval; relativo à clava.
cla·vate (klā′vāt). Claviforme; em forma de clava. [L. *clava*, clava]
Clav·i·ceps pur·pu·rea (klav′i-seps poor-poo′rē-ă). Fungo ascomiceto. VER ergot. [L. *clava*, clava, + *caput*, cabeça]
clav·i·cle (klav′i-kl) [TA]. Clavícula; um osso longo, duplamente curvo, que forma parte da cintura escapular (cíngulo do membro superior). Sua extremidade medial articula-se com o manúbrio do esterno na articulação esternoclavicular; sua extremidade lateral, com o acrômio da escápula na articulação acromioclavicular. SIN clavicula [TA], collar bone.
cla·vic·u·la, pl. **cla·vic·′u·lae** (klă-vik′oo-lă, -lī) [TA]. Clavícula. SIN clavicle. [L. *clavicula*, chave pequena, de *clavis*, chave]
cla·vic·u·lar (kla-vik′u-lăr). Clavicular; relativo à clavícula.
cla·vic·u·lus, pl. **cla·vic·u·li** (kla-vik′u-lŭs, -lī). Clavículo; uma das fibras colágenas perfurantes do osso. [L. Mod. dim. do L. *clavus*, cravo]
clav·u·lan·ic ac·id (kla-ū-lan′ik). Ácido clavulânico; um beta-lactâmico estruturalmente relacionado às penicilinas que inativa enzimas β-lactamase em microrganismos penicilina-resistentes; geralmente associado a penicilinas para potencializar e ampliar o espectro das penicilinas.
cla·vus, pl. **cla·vi** (klā′vŭs, -vī). Cravo; calo. **1.** Pequena calosidade cônica causada por pressão sobre uma proeminência óssea, geralmente sobre um artelho. SIN corn. [L. cravo, verruga, corno] **2.** Condição resultante da cicatrização de um granuloma do pé em framboesa, no qual o centro desaparece, deixando uma erosão. **3.** Sensação de que um prego está sendo enfiado na cabeça (*clavus hystericus*).
claw (klaw). Garra; unha afiada, delgada, geralmente curva, na pata de um animal. [L. *clavus*, cravo]
claw·foot (klaw′fut). Pé em garra; distúrbio do pé caracterizado por hiperextensão na articulação metatarsofalângica e flexão nas articulações interfalângicas, como uma contratura fixa.
claw·hand (klaw′hand). Mão em garra; atrofia dos músculos interósseos da mão com hiperextensão das articulações metacarpofalângicas e flexão das articulações interfalângicas; desenvolve-se em conseqüência de lesão do nervo, seja na medula espinhal ou ao nível do nervo periférico.
Claybrook, Edwin B., cirurgião norte-americano, 1871–1931. VER C. *sign*.
CLB Abreviatura de microrganismos *cyanobacterialike* (cianobactéria-símiles), *coccidialike* (coccídio-símiles) ou *Cryptosporidium-like* (*Cryptosporidium*-símiles), que agora foram identificados como coccídios no gênero *Cyclospora* (*C. cayetanensis*).
clean·ing (klēn′ing). Limpeza; em odontologia, um procedimento no qual são removidas as concreções dos dentes ou de uma prótese dentária. VER TAMBÉM dental *prophylaxis*.
  ultrasonic c., limpeza ultra-sônica; em odontologia, o uso de um ponto de vibração de alta freqüência para remover depósitos da estrutura do dente; também o processo de limpeza de dentaduras por colocação em um líquido especial, em um recipiente que gera vibrações de alta freqüência.
clear·ance (klēr′ans). **1.** Depuração (*C* com um subscrito indicando a substância removida). Remoção de uma substância do sangue, p. ex., por excreção renal, expressa em termos do fluxo de volume do sangue arterial ou plasma que conteria a quantidade de substância removida por unidade de tempo; medida em ml/min. A depuração renal de qualquer substância, exceto uréia ou água livre, é calculada como o fluxo de urina em ml/min multiplicado pela concentração urinária da substância dividida pela concentração plasmática arterial da substância; os valores normais humanos são comumente expressos por 1,73 m^2 de área de superfície corporal. **2.** Distância de separação; condição na qual os corpos podem passar um pelo outro sem impedimento, ou a distância entre os corpos. **3.** Remoção de algo de algum lugar; p. ex., "depuração de ácido esofágico" refere-se à remoção de algum ácido que tenha refluído do estômago para o esôfago, avaliado pelo tempo gasto para restabelecer o pH normal no esôfago.

  ***p*-aminohippurate c.,** depuração do *p*-amino-hipurato; uma boa medida do fluxo plasmático renal, que é levemente subestimada; quando uma baixa concentração plasmática de *p*-amino-hipurato (PAH) é mantida por infusão intravenosa, o rim extrai e excreta quase todo o PAH do plasma antes de ele chegar na veia renal.
  creatinine c., d. da creatinina; medida da depuração da creatinina endógena, usada para avaliar a taxa de filtração glomerular (TFG).
  endogenous creatinine c., d. da creatinina endógena; termo que distingue medidas baseadas na creatinina normalmente presente no plasma; como não é necessário infusão, pode ser obtido um valor médio pela coleta de urina durante um longo período, p. ex., 24 horas.
  exogenous creatinine c., d. da creatinina exógena; termo que distingue medidas baseadas na infusão intravenosa de creatinina para aumentar sua concentração plasmática e facilitar sua determinação química acurada.
  free water c., d. da água livre; o volume de água excretado na urina além daquele associado aos solutos excretados se a urina fosse isosmótica com o plasma; representa uma maior perda de água corporal que de soluto, tendendo a aumentar a osmolalidade corporal e tornando a urina hiposmótica. Ao contrário das outras depurações, é calculada subtraindo-se a depuração osmolal do volume real de urina excretado por minuto. Um valor negativo para a depuração de água livre representa o volume de água que o organismo "requisitou" do líquido tubular isosmótico para tornar a urina hiperosmótica e reduzir a osmolalidade corporal.
  interocclusal c., distância interoclusal; espaço interoclusal. SIN freeway *space*.
  inulin c., d. de inulina; uma medida acurada da taxa de filtração glomerular renal, porque a inulina é filtrada livremente com a água, e não é excretada nem reabsorvida pelas paredes do túbulo. A inulina não é um constituinte normal do plasma e precisa ser infundida continuamente para manter uma concentração plasmática constante e uma velocidade constante de excreção urinária durante a medida. Em um adulto normal, a depuração de inulina é de aproximadamente 120 ml/min (faixa 100–150) por 1,73 m^2 de superfície corporal.
  isotope c., d. de isótopo; a velocidade com que um isótopo é removido (geralmente por fluxo sanguíneo) de um tecido ou órgão como o cérebro.
  maximum urea c., d. máxima de uréia; a depuração de uréia quando o fluxo urinário ultrapassa 2 ml/min; o valor normal é de aproximadamente 75 ml sangue/min por 1,73 m^2 de superfície corporal.
  mucociliary c., limpeza mucociliar; o movimento do muco que recobre o epitélio respiratório pelo batimento dos cílios: movimento rápido e anterior (efetivo) e movimento lento, de retorno (recuperação).
  occlusal c., deslizamento oclusal; condição na qual as superfícies oclusais opostas podem deslizar umas sobre as outras sem qualquer projeção interveniente.
  osmolal c., d. osmolar; o volume de urina que seria excretado por minuto se os solutos urinários fossem acompanhados por água suficiente para tornar a urina isosmótica em relação ao plasma, isto é, de forma que a excreção de soluto não modificasse a osmolalidade dos líquidos corporais. Para seu cálculo, o volume de urina excretado por minuto é multiplicado pela osmolalidade urinária (geralmente medida pela depressão do ponto de congelamento) e dividida pela osmolalidade plasmática. A depuração osmolar é menor que o fluxo de urina real, quando a urina é hiposmótica, e é maior que esse fluxo quando a urina é hiperosmótica.
  standard urea c., d. padrão da uréia; o valor obtido quando a raiz quadrada do fluxo urinário (quando menor que 2 ml/min) é multiplicada pela concentração urinária de uréia e dividida pela concentração de uréia no sangue total; representa um ajuste empírico antigo para o efeito do baixo fluxo urinário sobre a excreção de uréia; algumas vezes é corrigida para o tamanho corporal pela divisão por alguma função de peso ou superfície corporal. Posteriormente, a concentração plasmática substituiu a concentração sanguínea no cálculo. O valor normal é de aproximadamente 54 ml/min por 1,73 m^2 em uma pessoa adulta. SIN Van Slyke formula.
  urea c., d. da uréia; o volume de plasma (ou sangue) que seria completamente depurado de uréia por excreção urinária em um minuto; originalmente calculado como o fluxo de urina multiplicado pela concentração urinária de uréia dividido pela concentração de uréia no sangue total, e não no plasma, representando a depuração da uréia sanguínea, e não a depuração da uréia plasmática.
clear·er (klēr′er). Clarificante; agente, usado em preparações histológicas, que é miscível tanto no líquido desidratante ou fixador como na substância de inclusão.
cleav·age (klēv′ij). **1.** Segmentação mitótica ou clivagem; série de divisões celulares mitóticas que ocorrem no ovo imediatamente após sua fertilização. SIN segmentation (2). VER TAMBÉM cleavage *division*. **2.** Cisão; divisão de uma molécula complexa em duas ou mais moléculas mais simples. SIN scission (2). **3.** Fendas lineares na pele que indicam a direção das fibras na derme. VER TAMBÉM tension *lines*, em *line*. **4.** Colo: depressão ou sulco mediano entre as mamas da mulher madura (coloquial).
  abnormal c. of cardiac valve, divisão anormal da válvula cardíaca; malformação congênita de um folheto valvular com um defeito que se estende a partir da margem livre.

adequal c., segmentação mitótica ou clivagem que resulta na formação de blastômeros de tamanhos aproximadamente iguais.
complete c., segmentação mitótica completa. SIN holoblastic c.
determinate c., segmentação mitótica ou clivagem determinada; c. que resulta em blastômeros capazes de se transformar apenas em uma estrutura embrionária específica.
discoidal c., segmentação mitótica ou clivagem discóide; c. meroblástica limitada à cicatrícula (pólo animal) do protoplasma de ovos ricos em vitelo, como os ovos telolécitos das aves.
enamel c., cisão do esmalte; a divisão do esmalte em um plano paralelo à direção dos bastões de esmalte.
equal c., segmentação mitótica ou clivagem igual; clivagem que produz blastômeros de tamanhos semelhantes.
equatorial c., c. equatorial; clivagem na qual o plano de divisão citoplasmática forma ângulos retos com o eixo do ovo.
holoblastic c., c. holoblástica; clivagem na qual os blastômeros são completamente separados; todo o ovo participa da divisão celular. SIN complete c., total c.
hydrolytic c., c. hidrolítica. SIN hydrolysis.
incomplete c., c. incompleta. SIN meroblastic c.
indeterminate c., c. indeterminada; clivagem que resulta em blastômeros com potências de desenvolvimento semelhantes, ambos capazes, quando isolados, de produzir um corpo embrionário inteiro.
meridional c., c. meridional; clivagem em um plano através do eixo do zigoto.
meroblastic c., c. meroblástica; separação incompleta dos blastômeros, com as divisões sendo limitadas à porção do ovo que não contém vitelo. SIN incomplete c.
phosphoroclastic c., c. fosfoclástica. SIN phosphorolysis.
progressive c., c. progressiva; em fungos, um tipo de esporulação no qual os planos de clivagem no citoplasma primeiro produzem protosporos e, depois, esporangiosporos em um esporângio.
pudendal c., fissura pudenda. SIN pudendal *cleft*.
subdural c., espaço subdural. SIN subdural *space*.
superficial c., c. superficial; c. meroblástica com as divisões limitadas ao citoplasma periférico (superficial) de um ovo centrolécito.
thioclastic c., c. tioclástica; a divisão de uma ligação de forma análoga à hidrólise ou fosfólise, mas com os elementos de um sulfeto de hidrogênio substituído (geralmente coenzima A) adicionados através da ruptura.
total c., c. total. SIN holoblastic c.
unequal c., c. desigual; c. que produz blastômeros de diferentes tamanhos nos dois pólos.
yolk c., c. vitelina; segmentação do vitelo.

cleav·er (klē′ver). Cutelo; faca pesada para cortar ou rachar.
enamel c., c. de esmalte; instrumento com uma haste pesada e uma lâmina muito curta, formando um ângulo de aproximadamente 90° com o eixo do cabo; usado com um movimento de cavar para retirar o esmalte das superfícies axiais de um dente na preparação de uma coroa.

cleft (kleft) [TA]. Fenda; fissura.
anal c., fissura anal. SIN intergluteal c.
branchial c.'s, fendas branquiais; uma série bilateral de aberturas semelhantes a fendas, na faringe, através das quais a água é colhida pelos animais aquáticos; nas paredes das fendas estão os filamentos vasculares das guelras, com a função de captar o oxigênio da água que atravessa as fendas; termo algumas vezes imprecisamente aplicado aos sulcos ectodérmicos branquiais dos embriões de mamíferos, que são homólogos rudimentares, imperfurados, das fendas branquiais completas. SIN gill c.'s.
cholesterol c., f. do colesterol; espaço causado pela dissolução dos cristais de colesterol em cortes de tecido incrustados em parafina.
complete posterior laryngeal c., f. laríngea posterior completa. VER laryngotracheoesophageal c.
facial c., f. facial; fenda resultante da união ou fusão incompleta de processos embrionários que, normalmente, se unem na formação da face, p. ex., fenda labial ou fenda palatina. SIN prosopoanoschisis.
first visceral c., primeira f. visceral. SIN hyomandibular c.
gill c.'s, fendas branquiais. SIN branchial c.'s.
gingival c., f. gengival; fissura associada à formação de bolsa e revestida por epitélio misto da gengiva e da bolsa.
gluteal c., f. glútea. SIN intergluteal c.
hyobranchial c., f. hiobranquial; a fenda caudal ao arco hióide do embrião.
hyomandibular c., f. hiomandibular; a fenda entre os arcos hióide e mandibular do embrião; o meato auditivo externo é desenvolvido a partir de sua porção dorsal. SIN first visceral c.
intergluteal c. [TA], f. interglútea; o sulco entre as nádegas. SIN crena analis [TA], crena ani*, crena interglutealis*, natal c.*, anal c., crena clunium, gluteal c.
interneuromeric c.'s, fendas interneuroméricas; fendas entre as elevações neuroméricas no segmentares no rombencéfalo primitivo.
Larrey c., f. de Larrey. SIN *trigonum* sternocostale.
laryngotracheoesophageal c., f. laringotraqueoesofágica; ausência de fusão da musculatura ou das lâminas cartilaginosas cricóides de intensidade variável: tipo 1, fenda submucosa dos músculos interaritenóides (conhecidos também como fenda laríngea posterior oculta ou fenda laríngea submucosa); tipo 2, fenda cricóide parcial (conhecida também como fenda laríngea posterior parcial); tipo 3, fenda cricóide total (conhecida também como fenda laringotraqueoesofágica ou fenda cricóide total); e tipo 4, extensão da fenda para o esôfago.
Maurer c.'s, manchas de Maurer. SIN Maurer *dots*, em *dot*.
median maxillary anterior alveolar c., fenda alveolar anterior maxilar mediana; defeito na linha média assintomático da crista anterior maxilar; o resultado da ausência de fusão ou desenvolvimento das metades laterais do palato.
natal c., f. interglútea; *termo oficial alternativo para intergluteal c.
oblique facial c., f. facial oblíqua. SIN prosoposchisis.
occult posterior laryngeal c., f. laríngea posterior oculta. VER laryngotracheoesophageal c.
partial cricoid c., fenda cricóide parcial. VER laryngotracheoesophageal c.
partial posterior laryngeal c., fenda laríngea posterior parcial. VER laryngotracheoesophageal c.
posterior laryngeal c., f. laríngea posterior; fenda laringotraqueoesofágica (tipos 2 ou 3).
pudendal c. [TA], f. pudenda; a fenda entre os lábios maiores do pudendo. SIN rima pudendi [TA], fissura pudendi, pudendal cleavage, pudendal slit, rima vulvae, urogenital c., vulvar slit.
residual c., f. residual; os remanescentes do divertículo hipofisário que ocorrem entre a porção distal e a porção intermediária; alguns animais apresentam uma luz distinta, mas, nos seres humanos, ela só existe durante o desenvolvimento pré-natal e, algumas vezes, em crianças pequenas. SIN residual lumen.
Schmidt-Lanterman c.'s, fendas de Schmidt-Lanterman. SIN Schmidt-Lanterman *incisures*, em *incisure*.
subdural c., f. subdural. SIN subdural *space*.
submucous laryngeal c., f. laríngea submucosa. VER laryngotracheoesophageal c.
synaptic c., f. sináptica; o espaço com cerca de 20 nm de largura entre o axolema e a superfície pós-sináptica. VER TAMBÉM synapse.
total cricoid c., f. cricóide total. VER laryngotracheoesophageal c.
urogenital c., f. urogenital. SIN pudendal c.
visceral c., f. visceral; qualquer fenda entre dois arcos branquiais (viscerais) no embrião.

cleid-. VER cleido-.
clei·dag·ra, cli·dag·ra (klī-dag′rä). Clidagra; cleidagra; termo raramente usado para uma dor forte e súbita na clavícula, semelhante à gota. [cleid- + G. *agra*, convulsão]
clei·dal (klī′dăl). Clidal; relativo à clavícula. SIN clidal.
cleido-, cleid-. A clavícula; também grafadas como clido-, clid-. [G. *kleis*, barra, ferrolho]
clei·do·cos·tal (klī-dō-kos′tăl). Clidocostal; relativo à clavícula e a uma costela. SIN clidocostal. [cleido- + L. *costa*, costela]
clei·do·cra·ni·al (klī′dō-krā′nē-ăl). Clidocranial; relativo à clavícula e ao crânio. SIN clidocranial. [G. *kleis*, clavícula, + *kranion*, crânio]
clei·dot·o·my (klī-dot′ō-mē). Clidotomia; corte da clavícula de um feto morto para realizar um parto vaginal. [cleido- + -tomy]
-cleisis. Fechamento. [G. *kleisis*, fechamento]
cleis·to·the·ci·um (klīs-tō-thē′sē-ŭm). Clistotécio; nos fungos, um ascocarpo fechado, com ascos dispersos aleatoriamente. [G. *kleistos*, fechado, + *thēkē*, caixa]
Cleland, W. Wallace, bioquímico norte-americano, *1930. VER C. *reagent*.
clem·as·tine (klem′as-tēn). Clemastina; meclastina; um anti-histamínico H₁. SIN meclastine.
cle·oid (klē′oyd). Cleóide; instrumento dentário com uma extremidade cortante elíptica e pontiaguda, usado na escavação de cáries ou esculturas de obturações e ceras. [A.S. *cle*, garra, + G. *eidos*, semelhança]
clep·to·par·a·site (klep-tō-par′ă-sīt). Cleptoparasita; parasita que se desenvolve na presa do seu hospedeiro. [G. *klepto*, roubar, + parasite]
Cléret, M. Francois, médico francês, 1876–1968. VER Launois-C. *syndrome*.
Clevenger, Shobal V., neurologista norte-americano, 1843–1920. VER C. *fissure*.
CLIA Abreviatura de Clinical Laboratory Improvement Amendments.
click (klik). Clique; som fraco e agudo.
ejection c., clique de ejeção; um som de ejeção em clique. VER sound.
mitral c., clique mitral; o estalido de abertura da válvula mitral.
systolic c., clique sistólico; um som agudo, em clique, ouvido durante a sístole cardíaca; quando auscultado no início da sístole, geralmente é um som de ejeção; no final da sístole, o clique geralmente significa insuficiência mitral, como na disfunção do aparelho valvar mitral quando apresenta prolapso para o átrio esquerdo durante a sístole (ver Barlow *syndrome*); raramente também pode ser devido a aderências pleuropericárdicas, ou a outros mecanismos extracardíacos.

click·ing (klik′ing). Ruído crepitante, às incursões da articulação temporomandibular, devido a um movimento assincrônico do disco e do côndilo.

clid-. VER clido-.

cli·dal (klī'dăl). Clidal. SIN cleidal.

cli·din·i·um bro·mide (klī-din'ē-ŭm). Brometo de clidínio; um anticolinérgico.

clido-, clid-. A clavícula. VER TAMBÉM cleido-. [G. *kleis*, barra, ferrolho]

cli·do·cos·tal (klī-dō-kos'tăl). Clidocostal. SIN cleidocostal.

cli·do·cra·ni·al (klī-dō-krā'nē-ăl). Clidocranial. SIN cleidocranial.

cli·ma·co·pho·bia (klī'mă-kō-fō'bē-ă). Climacofobia; medo mórbido de escadas ou de subir escadas. [G. *klimax*, escada, + *phobos*, medo]

cli·mac·ter·ic (klī-mak'ter-ik, klī-mak-ter'ik). **1.** Climatério; o período de alterações endócrinas, somáticas e psicológicas transitórias que ocorrem na transição para a menopausa. **2.** Um período crítico da vida. SIN climacterium. [G. *klimaktēr*, o degrau de uma escada]

cli·mac·ter·i·um (klī-mak-tēr'ē-ŭm). Climatério. SIN climacteric.

cli·ma·tol·o·gy (klī-mă-tol'ō-jē). Climatologia; o estudo do clima e sua relação com as doenças.

cli·ma·to·ther·a·py (klī'mă-tō-thār'ă-pē). Climatoterapia; tratamento de doenças por remoção do paciente para uma região com clima mais favorável para a recuperação.

cli·max (klī'maks). Clímax. **1.** O cume ou acme de uma doença; seu estágio de maior gravidade. **2.** SIN orgasm. [G. *klimax*, escada]

cli·mo·graph (klī'mō-graf). Climograma; diagrama que mostra o efeito do clima sobre a saúde. [G. *klima*, clima, + *grapho*, registrar]

clin·da·my·cin (klin-dă-mī'sin). Clindamicina; antibacteriano e antibiótico.

cline (klīn). Cline; relação sistemática entre a localização e as freqüências de alelos; as linhas que unem pontos de igual freqüência são denominadas isóclinas, e a direção da cline em qualquer ponto forma ângulos retos com uma linha isóclina. [G. *klinō*, inclinação]

clin·ic (klin'ik). Clínica. **1.** Instituição, edifício ou parte de uma construção onde são tratados os pacientes ambulatoriais. **2.** Uma instituição, edifício ou parte de uma construção onde é fornecida instrução médica para estudantes por meio de demonstrações na presença de doentes. **3.** Palestra ou simpósio sobre um tema relativo a doença. [G. *klinē*, leito]

clin·i·cal (klin'i-kl). Clínico. **1.** Relativo ao comportamento de um paciente ou à evolução da doença. **2.** Designa os sintomas e a evolução de uma doença, distintos dos achados laboratoriais de alterações anatômicas. **3.** Relativo a uma clínica. [G. *klinē*, leito, + -al]

Clin·i·cal Lab·o·ra·tory Im·prove·ment A·mend·ments (CLIA). Legislação federal e a equipe e procedimentos estabelecidos por ela sob a égide da Health Care Financing Administration (HCFA), para a supervisão e regulamentação de todos os procedimentos em laboratórios de análises clínicas nos EUA.

As Clinical Laboratory Improvement Amendments de 1988 (CLIA '88) foram aprovadas pelo Congresso em resposta às preocupações públicas com a qualidade dos testes laboratoriais, particularmente em laboratórios de consultórios médicos e na interpretação do esfregaço de Papanicolaou. Essa legislação colocou todos os 150.000 laboratórios de análises clínicas norte-americanos, incluindo laboratórios de consultórios médicos, sob normas uniformes. Um laboratório de análises clínicas é definido como qualquer unidade onde materiais colhidos do corpo humano são examinados com o objetivo de obter informações para o diagnóstico, prevenção ou tratamento de doença ou a avaliação da saúde. Os padrões aplicados à equipe e aos procedimentos laboratoriais baseiam-se na complexidade do teste e nos possíveis danos para o paciente. As normas regulamentadoras estabelecem procedimentos para aplicação e taxas para registro no CLIA, métodos de execução e supervisão, e sanções aplicáveis quando os laboratórios não atendem aos padrões. As normas regulamentadoras do CLIA definem três categorias de complexidade do teste: simples, moderada e alta. Existe uma subcategoria para microscopia realizada pelo médico no nível moderado de complexidade. Para testes de complexidade moderada ou alta, o laboratório precisa participar de um programa contínuo de avaliação de proficiência, por meio do qual um laboratório independente periodicamente submete amostras de composição conhecida para teste. A imposição e a implementação das normas regulamentadoras do CLIA causaram oposição, particularmente por parte de médicos que realizam testes no consultório. Os oponentes da legislação afirmam que, embora haja pouca ou nenhuma evidência demonstrável de que as normas do CLIA tenham resultado em melhora do atendimento dos pacientes, a regulamentação dos laboratórios em consultórios obstrui a capacidade dos médicos de atender às necessidades de seus pacientes. Os pacientes e os planos de saúde tiveram aumentos no custo dos testes laboratoriais devido às normas regulamentadoras do CLIA. Além disso, cerca de um terço dos médicos deixou de fazer alguns ou todos os exames no consultório em virtude do CLIA. Isso causou inconveniência e custo adicionais tanto para os pacientes quanto para os médicos. Particularmente para as crianças, pobres e idosos, a dificuldade de marcar consultas repetidas e de obedecer aos esquemas de monitorização diminui a qualidade do tratamento global do paciente. O recebimento tardio dos resultados pelos médicos diminui a obediência do paciente, causa atrasos ou erros no diagnóstico e exige a prescrição de tratamento antecipado, o que causa custo desnecessário e, em alguns casos, hospitalização desnecessária.

cli·ni·cian (klin-ish'ŭn). Um profissional de saúde que participa do tratamento dos pacientes, diferente daquele que trabalha em outras áreas.

clin·i·co·path·o·log·ic (klin'i-kō-path-ō-loj'ik). Clinicopatológico; relativo aos sinais e sintomas apresentados por um paciente, e também aos resultados dos estudos laboratoriais, pois estão relacionados aos achados no exame macroscópico e histológico do tecido por meio de biópsia e/ou necrópsia.

clino-. Uma inclinação (ascendente ou descendente) ou curva. [G. *klinō*, inclinar ou curvar)

cli·no·ce·phal·ic, cli·no·ceph·a·lous (klī-nō-se-fal'ik, -sef'ă-lŭs). Clinocefálico; clinocéfalo; relativo à clinocefalia.

cli·no·ceph·a·ly (klī'nō-sef'ă-lē). Clinocefalia; craniossinostose na qual a superfície superior do crânio é côncava, apresentando um perfil em forma de sela. SIN saddle head. [clino- + G. *kephalē*, cabeça]

cli·no·dac·ty·ly (klī'nō-dak'ti-lē). Clinodactilia; deflexão permanente de um ou mais dedos da mão. [clino- + G. *daktylos*, dedo]

cli·nog·ra·phy (klin-og'ră-fē). Clinografia; representação gráfica dos sinais e sintomas exibidos por um paciente. [G. *klinē*, leito, + *graphō*, escrever]

cli·noid (klī'noyd). Clinóide. **1.** Semelhante a uma cama com dossel. **2.** SIN clinoid process. [G. *klinē*, cama, + *eidos*, semelhança]

cli·o·quin·ol (klī-ō-kwin'ol). Clioquinol. SIN iodochlorhydroxyquin.

cli·ox·a·nide (klī-ok'să-nīd). Clioxanida; um anti-helmíntico.

clip (klip'). Grampo; clipe. **1.** Prendedor usado para segurar uma parte junto à outra. **2.** Fecho usado em um pequeno vaso.

wound c., grampo metálico ou dispositivo para aproximação cirúrgica de incisões cutâneas.

clith·ro·pho·bia (klith-rō-fō'bē-ă). Clitrofobia; temor mórbido de ser aprisionado. [G. *kleithron*, ferrolho, + *phobos*, temor]

clit·i·on (klit'ē-on). Clítio; ponto craniométrico no meio da parte mais alta do clivo no osso esfenóide. [G. *klitos*, declive]

clit·o·rid·e·an (klit'ō-ri-dē'an). Clitoridiano; relativo ao clitóris.

clit·o·ri·dec·to·my (klit'ō-ri-dek'tō-mē). Clitoridectomia; remoção do clitóris. [clitoris + G. *ektomē*, excisão]

clit·o·ri·di·tis (klit'o-ri-dī'tis). Clitoridite; inflamação do clitóris. SIN clitoritis. [clitoris + G. *–itis*, inflamação]

clit·o·ris, pl. **cli·to·ri·des** (klit'ō-ris, -tōr'i-dēz; klī'tō-ris) [TA]. Clitóris; um corpo cilíndrico, erétil, raramente com mais de 2 cm de comprimento, situado na porção mais anterior da vulva, que se projeta entre as extremidades ramificadas ou lâminas dos lábios menores do pudendo, que formam seu prepúcio e frênulo. Consiste em uma glande, um corpo e dois pilares, sendo o homólogo do pênis no homem, exceto por não ser perfurado pela uretra e não possuir um corpo esponjoso. [G. *kleitoris*]

clit·o·rism (klit'o-rizm). Clitorismo; ereção prolongada e geralmente dolorosa do clitóris; o análogo do priapismo.

clit·o·ri·tis (klit-ō-rī'tis). Clitorite. SIN clitoriditis.

clit·or·o·meg·a·ly (klit'ōr-ō-meg'ă-lē). Clitoromegalia; aumento do clitóris. [clitoris + G. *megas*, grande]

clit·or·o·plas·ty (klit'ō-rō-plas'tē). Clitoroplastia; qualquer procedimento de cirurgia plástica realizado no clitóris. [clitoris + G. *plastos*, formado]

cli·val (klī'văl). Clival; relativo ao clivo.

cli·vus, pl. **cli·vi** (klī'vŭs, -vē) [TA]. Clivo. **1.** Uma superfície em declive. **2** [TA]. A superfície inclinada do dorso da sela até o forame magno, composta de parte do corpo do esfenóide e parte da porção basal do osso occipital. SIN Blumenbach c. [L. inclinação]

Blumenbach c., c. de Blumenbach. SIN clivus (2).

c. ocula'ris, c. ocular; as paredes inclinadas da fóvea que levam à fovéola.

clo·a·ca (klō-ā'kă). Cloaca. **1.** Em embriões incipientes, a câmara revestida de endoderma na qual se esvaziam o intestino posterior e a alantóide. **2.** Em aves e monotremos, a câmara comum na qual se abrem o intestino posterior, a bexiga e os ductos genitais. [L. esgoto]

ectodermal c., c. ectodérmica; o proctódio do embrião.

endodermal c., c. endodérmica; porção terminal do intestino posterior interna à membrana cloacal do embrião.

persistent c., c. persistente; condição na qual a prega urorretal não dividiu a cloaca do embrião em porções retal e urogenital. SIN sinus urogenitalis, urogenital sinus (2).

clo·a·cal (klō-ā'kăl). Cloacal; relativo à cloaca.

clo·ba·zam (klō-bă-zam). Clobazam; um novo agente psicoterápico benzodiazepínico no qual os nitrogênios do anel heterocíclico estão nas posições 1,5-, e não nas posições 1,4- mais comuns; um ansiolítico.

clo·be·ta·sol pro·pi·o·nate (klō - bā′tă - sōl). Propionato de clobetasol; corticosteróide antiinflamatório geralmente usado em preparações tópicas.
clo·cor·to·lone (klō - kōr′tō - lōn). Clocortolona; corticosteróide antiinflamatório geralmente usado em preparações tópicas; disponível nas formas de acetato e pivalato.
clo·faz·i·mine (klō - faz′ĭ - mēn). Clofazimina; agente tuberculostático e leprostático.
clo·fen·a·mide (klō - fen′ă - mid). Clofenamida; um diurético. SIN monochlorphenamide.
clo·fi·brate (klō′fi - brāt). Clofibrate; agente antilipêmico que reduz os níveis plasmáticos de colesterol, triglicerídeos e ácido úrico; usado no tratamento da hipercolesterolemia e da aterosclerose.
clo·ges·tone ac·e·tate (klō - jes′tōn). Acetato de clogestona; um agente progestacional.
clo·ma·cran phos·phate (klō′mă - kran). Fosfato de clomacram; um tranqüilizante.
clo·me·ges·tone ac·e·tate (klō - me - jes′tōn). Acetato de clomegestona; agente progestacional.
clo·mi·phene cit·rate (klō′mi - fēn). Citrato de clomifeno; um análogo do estrogênio não-esteróide, clorotrianiseno; um estimulante da gonadotrofina hipofisária usado terapeuticamente para induzir ovulação; compete com o estrogênio ao nível hipotalâmico, interrompendo o sistema de retroalimentação negativo e resultando em aumento da secreção de gonadotrofina; seu uso freqüentemente resulta em múltiplos fetos. SIN chloramiphene.
clo·mip·ra·mine hy·dro·chlo·ride (klō - mip′ră - mēn). Cloridrato de clomipramina; um antidepressivo.
clo·nal (klō′năl). Clonal; relativo a um clone.
clo·na·ze·pam (klō - nā′zē - pam). Clonazepam; agente anticonvulsivante pertencente à classe dos benzodiazepínicos.
clone (klōn). **1.** Clone; uma colônia ou grupo de organismos (ou um organismo individual), ou uma colônia de células derivadas de um único organismo ou célula por reprodução assexuada, todos possuindo constituições genéticas idênticas. **2.** Clonar; produzir essa colônia ou indivíduo. **3.** Clone; uma pequena secção de DNA que foi copiada por meio de clonagem genética. VER cloning. **4.** Uma população homogênea de moléculas de DNA [G. *klōn,* uma tira, corte usado para propagação]
  cDNA c., c. de cDNA; um DNA duplo, que representa um mRNA, transportado em um vetor de clonagem.
  genomic c., c. genômico; uma célula com um vetor contendo um fragmento de DNA de um organismo diferente.
clo·nic (klon′ik). Clônico; relativo a, ou caracterizado por, clônus.
clon·ic·i·ty (klon - is′i - tē). Clonicidade; o estado de ser clônico.
clon·i·co·ton·ic (klon′i - kō - ton′ik). Clonicotônico; tanto clônico quanto tônico; diz-se de certas formas de espasmo muscular.
clo·ni·dine hy·dro·chlo·ride (klō′ni - dēn). Cloridrato de clonidina; um agente anti-hipertensivo com ações central e periférica; estimula os receptores adrenérgicos no cérebro, causando redução dos impulsos do sistema nervoso simpático; usado como adjunto para reduzir os sintomas de abstinência de drogas.

clon·ing (klōn′ing). Clonagem. **1.** Cultivo de uma colônia de células ou organismos geneticamente idênticos *in vitro*. **2.** Transplante de um núcleo de uma célula somática para um ovo, que então se transforma em um embrião; assim, muitos embriões idênticos podem ser gerados por reprodução assexuada. **3.** Com blastócitos, a divisão de um grupo de células através de microcirurgia e transferência da metade das células para uma zona pelúcida que teve seu conteúdo esvaziado. Os embriões resultantes, geneticamente idênticos, podem ser implantados em um animal para gestação. **4.** Técnica de DNA recombinante usada para produzir milhões de cópias de um fragmento de DNA. O fragmento é entrançado em um veículo de clonagem (isto é, plasmídeo, bacteriófago ou vírus animal). O veículo de clonagem penetra em uma célula bacteriana ou levedura (o hospedeiro), que então é cultivada *in vitro* ou em um hospedeiro animal. Em alguns casos, como na produção de drogas por engenharia genética, o DNA inserido é ativado e altera o funcionamento químico da célula hospedeira.

> A clonagem bem-sucedida de uma ovelha aparentemente normal e fértil mostrou as possibilidades da técnica, mas o anúncio de uma proposta de clonar um ser humano gerou controvérsia e ameaças de proibição legal. Os oponentes da clonagem humana desaprovam a criação experimental de embriões humanos que nunca teriam a oportunidade de implantação e cuja destruição final seria equivalente ao aborto. Muitos especialistas em bioética desaprovam até mesmo a implantação de um embrião humano criado artificialmente em um útero humano. Os que apóiam a pesquisa de clonagem temem que a proibição legal impeça investigações necessárias sobre reprodução humana e infertilidade. Em 1997, a *National Bioethics Advisory Commission*, após considerar as dimensões científicas e éticas da clonagem, recomendou uma proibição de toda a pesquisa sobre clonagem humana durante 5 anos. Dezenove países europeus assinaram um acordo proibindo a replicação genética artificial de seres humanos.

  A/T c., c. A/T; clonagem de fragmentos onde as únicas extremidades salientes (ou não-complementadas) são as bases A ou T; ocorre freqüentemente no uso de enzimas específicas para cortar ou produzir fragmentos de DNA.
  positional c., c. de posição. SIN reverse *genetics.*
clo·nism (klon′izm). Clonismo; um estado longo e contínuo de espasmos clônicos.
clo·no·gen·ic (klō - nō - jen′ik). Clonogênico; que se origina de, ou consiste em, um clone.
clon·o·graph (klon′ō - graf). Clonógrafo; instrumento para registrar os movimentos no espasmo clônico. [G. *klonos,* tumulto, + *graphō,* escrever]
clo·nor·chi·a·sis (klō - nōr - kī′ă - sis). Clonorquíase; uma doença causada pelo trematódeo *Clonorchis sinensis*, que afeta os ductos biliares distais dos seres humanos e de outros animais que se alimentam de peixe após a ingestão de peixe cru, defumado ou mal cozido ou camarão de água doce cru; a infestação inicial pode ser benigna, mas a infestação repetida ou crônica induz um distúrbio proliferativo e granulomatoso intenso. SIN clonorchiosis.
clo·nor·chi·o·sis (klō - nōr - ke - ō′sis). Clonorquiose. SIN clonorchiasis.
Clo·nor·chis si·nen·sis (klō - nōr′kis sī - nen′sis). O trematódeo hepático asiático, uma espécie de trematódeo (família Opisthorchiidae) que, no Extremo Oriente, infesta as vias biliares dos seres humanos e de outros animais que se alimentam de peixe; o peixe ciprinóide é o principal segundo hospedeiro intermediário, e vários caramujos operculados servem como primeiros hospedeiros intermediários. SIN *Opisthorchis sinensis*.
clo·nus (klō′nŭs). Clônus; uma forma de movimento caracterizada por contrações e relaxamentos de um músculo, ocorrendo em rápida sucessão e observada com, entre outras condições, espasticidade e alguns distúrbios convulsivos. VER TAMBÉM contraction. [G. *klonos,* tumulto]
  ankle c., c. do tornozelo; uma contração rítmica dos músculos da panturrilha após uma dorsiflexão passiva súbita do pé, estando a perna semifletida.
  toe c., c. do artelho; movimentos alternados de flexão e extensão do hálux após extensão forçada na articulação metatarsofalângica.
  wrist c., c. do punho; contrações e relaxamentos rítmicos dos músculos do antebraço excitados por uma extensão passiva forçada da mão.
clo·pam·ide (klō - pam′ĭd). Clopamida; diurético e anti-hipertensivo.
Cloquet, Hippolyte, anatomista francês, 1787–1840. VER C. *space*.
Cloquet, Jules G., anatomista francês, 1790–1883. VER C. *canal, hernia, septum;* proximal deep inguinal *lymph node*.
clor·az·e·pate (klōr - az′ē - pāt). Clorazepato; o sal mono ou dipotássico é usado como agente ansiolítico; uma pró-droga benzodiazepínica para o nordiazepam.
clor·pren·a·line hy·dro·chlo·ride (klōr - pren′ă - lēn). Cloridrato de clorprenalina; um broncodilatador. SIN isoprophenamine hydrochloride.
clos·trid·ia (klos - trid′ē - ă). Clostrídios. Plural de clostridium.
clos·trid·i·al (klos - trid′ē - ăl). Clostrídico; relativo a qualquer bactéria do gênero *Clostridium*.
clos·trid·i·o·pep·ti·dase A (klos - trid′ē - ō - pep′ti - dās). Clostridiopeptidase A. SIN *Clostridium histolyticum* collagenase.
clos·trid·i·o·pep·ti·dase B. Clostridiopeptidase B. SIN clostripain.

CLOSTRIDIUM

Clos·trid·i·um (klos - trid′ē - ŭm). Gênero de bactérias anaeróbias (ou anaeróbicas, aerotolerantes), formadoras de esporos, móveis (ocasionalmente imóveis) (família Bacillaceae) que contém bacilos Gram-positivos; as células móveis são peritríquias. Muitas das espécies são sacarolíticas e fermentativas, produzindo vários ácidos e gases e quantidades variáveis de produtos neutros; outras espécies são proteolíticas, algumas atacando proteínas com putrefação ou proteólise mais completa. Algumas espécies fixam o nitrogênio livre. Esses microrganismos algumas vezes produzem exotoxinas; geralmente são encontrados no solo e no trato intestinal de mamíferos, onde podem causar doença. A espécie típica é o *C. butyricum*. [G. *klōstēr,* fuso]
C. bifermen′tans, espécie bacteriana encontrada na carne pútrida e na gangrena gasosa; também comumente encontrada no solo, fezes e esgoto. Sua patogenicidade (devida sobretudo a uma toxina causadora de edema) varia de cepa para cepa.
C. botuli′num, espécie bacteriana amplamente encontrada na natureza e causa freqüente de intoxicação alimentar (botulismo) por carnes, frutas ou vegetais preservados que não foram apropriadamente esterilizados antes de serem enlatados. Os principais tipos, A a F, são caracterizados por neurotoxinas muito

potentes, antigenicamente distintas, mas farmacologicamente semelhantes, que só podem ser neutralizadas pela antitoxina específica; a toxina do grupo C contém pelo menos dois componentes; os casos registrados de botulismo humano foram causados principalmente pelos tipos A, B, E e F; o botulismo do lactente ocorre quando a colonização do trato gastrointestinal por *C. botulinum* resulta na absorção da toxina pela parede gastrointestinal; o tipo Cα causa botulismo em aves aquáticas domésticas e selvagens; Cβ e D estão associados a intoxicações no gado bovino. O tipo E geralmente está associado a derivados de peixe processados impropriamente.

C. butyr'icum, espécie bacteriana que ocorre no leite naturalmente coalhado, em vegetais amiláceos naturalmente fermentados e no solo; antes considerada não-patogênica, agora se sabe que inclui cepas produtoras de neurotoxinas; a espécie típica do gênero *C.*

C. cadav'eris, espécie bacteriana encontrada nas fezes humanas e no líquido pleural de um carneiro; não é patogênica para cobaias ou coelhos, mas foi uma causa rara de gangrena gasosa em seres humanos.

C. car'nis, espécie bacteriana encontrada em um coelho inoculado com solo; é patogênica para animais de laboratório, nos quais uma exotoxina provoca edema, necrose e morte.

C. chauvoe'i, espécie bacteriana que causa antraz sintomático (doença zoonótica) em bovinos e outros animais, e que produz uma exotoxina.

C. cochlear'ium, espécie bacteriana encontrada em feridas humanas de guerra e infecções sépticas; não é patogênica para cobaias.

C. difficile (di-fi'-sēl), espécie bacteriana encontrada nas fezes de seres humanos e animais. Coloniza recém-nascidos, que são poupados da doença diarreica induzida por toxina. Patogênica para os seres humanos, cobaias e coelhos; causa freqüente de colite e diarréia após o uso de antibiótico. Constatou-se que é uma causa de colite pseudomembranosa e está associada a várias doenças intestinais relacionadas à antibioticoterapia; também é a principal causa de diarréia hospitalar. [L. difícil]

C. fal'lax, espécie bacteriana encontrada em feridas de guerra, na apendicite e no antraz sintomático de carneiros; produz uma exotoxina fraca.

C. haemoly'ticum, espécie bacteriana encontrada em bovinos que estão morrendo de icteroemoglobinúria; é patogênica e tóxica para cobaias e coelhos e produz uma toxina hemolítica, instável.

C. histoly'ticum, espécie bacteriana encontrada em feridas de guerras, onde induz necrose tecidual; produz exotoxinas citolíticas que causam necrose local e descamação à injeção; não é tóxica se ingerida; é patogênica para pequenos animais de laboratório.

C. innomina'tum, espécie bacteriana encontrada em feridas de guerra sépticas e gangrenosas.

C. nigri'ficans, nome anterior da *Desulfotomaculum nigrificans*.

C. no'vyi, espécie bacteriana que consiste em três tipos A, B e C; o tipo A, de um caso de gangrena gasosa e da hepatite necrótica humana, produz γ-toxina (uma lecitinase hemolítica); B, da hepatite necrótica infecciosa de carneiros, produz β-toxina (uma lecitinase hemolítica); e C, encontrado na osteomielite bacilar de búfalos (*Bubalus bubalis*), não produz toxina. SIN *C. oedematiens*.

C. oedema'tiens, SIN *C. novyi.*

C. parabotuli'num, espécie bacteriana abrangendo os antes denominados *C. botulinum* tipos A e B; os tipos são identificados por testes de proteção com antitoxina de tipo conhecido; produz uma potente exotoxina e é patogênico para seres humanos e outros animais.

C. paraputri'ficum, espécie bacteriana encontrada nas fezes (principalmente de lactentes), gangrena gasosa e em culturas de líquidos e tecidos *postmortem*; não é patogênica para coelhos nem cobaias.

C. perfrin'gens, espécie bacteriana que é a principal causa de gangrena gasosa em seres humanos e uma causa de gangrena gasosa em outros animais, principalmente carneiros; também pode estar envolvida em enterite, apendicite e febre puerperal; é uma das causas mais comuns de intoxicação alimentar nos EUA. Esse microrganismo é encontrado no solo, na água, no leite, na poeira, no esgoto e no trato intestinal de seres humanos e outros animais. SIN *C. welchii*, gas bacillus, Welch bacillus.

C. ramo'sum, espécie bacteriana encontrada nas cavidades naturais dos seres humanos e de outros animais, bem como na água do mar e nas fezes; também é encontrada associada à mastoidite, otite, gangrena pulmonar, pleurisia pútrida, apendicite, infecções intestinais, balanite, abscesso hepático, osteomielite, septicemia e infecções urinárias. Já foi a espécie típica do obsoleto gênero *Ramibacterium*.

C. sep'ticum, espécie bacteriana encontrada no edema maligno de animais, em feridas de guerra humanas e em casos de apendicite; é patogênica para cobaias, coelhos, camundongos e pombos e produz uma exotoxina letal e hemolítica. SIN *Vibrion septique*, *Vibrio septicus*.

C. sordellii, cepa bacteriana que produz múltiplas toxinas, incluindo uma lecitinase, hemolisina e uma fibrinolisina, que resultam em edema e hipotensão potencialmente fatal, e infecções necróticas nos seres humanos. Está especialmente associada a infecção de feridas pós-traumáticas e pós-operatórias abdominais e ginecológicas; também causa tumefação inflamatória dos tecidos da cabeça de carneiros.

C. sphenoi'des, espécie bacteriana encontrada em feridas de guerra gangrenosas; não é patogênica para cobaias ou coelhos.

C. sporo'genes, espécie bacteriana encontrada no conteúdo intestinal, na gangrena gasosa e no solo; não é patogênica para cobaias ou coelhos, mas provoca tumefação local, temporária e leve.

C. ter'tium, espécie bacteriana encontrada em feridas, mas que não é patogênica para animais de laboratório.

C. tet'ani, espécie bacteriana que causa o tétano; produz uma potente exotoxina (neurotoxina) fortemente tóxica para os seres humanos e outros animais quando produzida nos tecidos ou injetada, mas não quando ingerida.

C. thermosaccharoly'ticum, espécie de bactérias termofílicas encontradas em latas com estufamento de ambas as extremidades que não cede à pressão dos dedos; não é patogênica para animais de laboratório.

C. welch'ii, SIN *C. perfringens.*

clos·trid·i·um, pl. **clos·trid·ia** (klos-trid'ē-ŭm,-ă). Clostrídio; termo vernacular usado para indicar qualquer membro do gênero *Clostridium*.

Clos·trid·i·um his·to·lyt·i·cum col·la·gen·ase. *Clostridium histolyticum* colagenase; uma enzima que catalisa a hidrólise do glicogênio, preferencialmente nas ligações peptídicas no lado amino de uma seqüência glicilprolil. SIN clostridiopeptidase A, collagenase A, collagenase I, microbial collagenase.

Clos·trid·i·um his·to·lyt·i·cum pro·tein·ase B. *Clostridium histolyticum* proteinase B. SIN clostripain.

clos·tri·pain (klos'tri-pān). Clostripaína; uma cisteína proteinase que divide preferencialmente no lado carboxil dos resíduos arginil e lisil. Também tem atividade esterase. SIN clostridiopeptidase B, *Clostridium histolyticum* proteinase B.

clo·sure (klō'zhŭr). Fechamento. **1.** A conclusão de uma via reflexa. **2.** O lugar de acoplamento entre estímulos no estabelecimento da aprendizagem condicionada. **3.** Atingir ou experimentar uma sensação de conclusão em uma tarefa mental.

flask c., fechamento do molde; em odontologia, o procedimento de unir as duas metades ou partes de um molde; os fechamentos experimentais do molde são fechamentos preliminares feitos para eliminar o excesso de material da dentadura e para garantir que esteja completamente preenchido; o fechamento final do molde é o último fechamento de um molde antes do endurecimento, após o acondicionamento experimental do molde com o material da base da dentadura.

velopharyngeal c., f. velofaríngeo; a aposição do palato mole e das paredes faríngeas superiores, como na deglutição e em alguns sons da fala.

clo·sy·late (klō'si-lāt). Closilato; contração aprovada pela USAN para o *p*-clorobenzenossulfonato.

clot (klot). Coágulo. **1.** Coagular, especialmente o sangue. **2.** Uma massa mole, não-rígida, insolúvel formada quando um líquido (p. ex., sangue ou linfa) se torna um gel. [I. ant. *klott*, grumo]

agonal c., c. agônico; trombose intravascular atribuída ao processo de morte.

antemortem c., c. antes da morte; coágulo sanguíneo encontrado à necrópsia, formado em qualquer uma das cavidades corporais ou dos grandes vasos antes da morte.

blood c., c. sanguíneo; a fase coagulada do sangue; a massa vermelha mole, coerente, gelatinosa, resultante da conversão do fibrinogênio em fibrina, assim aprisionando as hemácias (e outros elementos formados) no plasma coagulado.

chicken fat c., c. em gordura de galinha, coágulo formado *in vitro* ou *postmortem* a partir de leucócitos e plasma do sangue sedimentado.

currant jelly c., c. em gelatina de groselha; uma massa gelatinosa de hemácias e fibrina formada pela coagulação *in vitro* ou *postmortem* de sangue total ou sedimentado.

laminated c., c. laminado; c. formado em uma sucessão de camadas, como ocorre na evolução natural de um aneurisma.

passive c., c. passivo; c. formado em um saco aneurismático em consequência da cessação ou lentificação da circulação através do aneurisma.

postmortem c., c. *postmortem*; coágulo formado no coração ou nos grandes vasos após a morte.

clo·trim·a·zole (klō-trim'ă-zōl). Clotrimazol; agente antifúngico usado topicamente no tratamento de várias infecções por fungos e leveduras.

clot·tage (klot'ij). Termo obsoleto para designar o bloqueio de qualquer canal ou ducto por um coágulo sanguíneo.

Cloudman, Arthur M., zoólogo e patologista, *1901. VER C. *melanoma*.

clove oil (klōv). Óleo de cravo. SIN oil of clove.

clox·a·cil·lin so·di·um (klok-să-sil'in). Cloxacilina sódica; uma penicilina penicilinase-resistente.

clo·za·pine (klō'ză-pēn). Clozapina; um sedativo e antipsicótico tricíclico dibenzodiazepínico considerado atípico devido à baixa atividade antidopaminérgica central.

CLQ Abreviatura de cognitive laterality *quotient* (quociente de lateralidade cognitivo).

club·bing (klŭb´ing). Baqueteamento digital; condição que afeta os dedos das mãos e artelhos na qual a proliferação dos tecidos moles distais, principalmente dos leitos ungueais, resulta em espessamento e alargamento das extremidades dos dedos; as unhas são anormalmente curvas e os leitos ungueais excessivamente compressíveis, e a pele sobre elas é vermelha e brilhante. VER Hippocratic nails, em nail.
  hereditary c. [MIM*119900], b. digital hereditário; baqueteamento digital hereditário simples sem doença pulmonar ou outra doença progressiva associada, freqüentemente mais pronunciada nos homens; mais comum em pacientes negros; herança autossômica dominante. SIN acropachy.
club·foot (klŭb´fut). Pé torto. SIN *talipes* equinovarus.
club·hand (klŭb´hand). Mão torta; deformidade (angulação) congênita ou adquirida da mão, associada à ausência parcial ou completa do rádio ou da ulna; geralmente associada a deformidades intrínsecas na mão em variantes congênitas.
  radial c., mão torta radial; mão torta com desvio radial associado à ausência parcial ou completa do rádio.
  ulnar c., mão torta ulnar; mão torta com desvio ulnar associado à ausência parcial ou completa da ulna.
clump (klŭmp). Grumar; enfeixar; formar grumos, pequenas agregações ou grupos. [A.S. *clympre*, grumo]
clump·ing (klŭmp-ing). Aglutinação; a concentração em grupos de bactérias ou de outras células suspensas em um líquido.
clu·ne·al (kloo´nē-ăl). Glúteo; relativo às nádegas.
clu·nes (kloo´nēz). Nádegas. *termo oficial alternativo para buttocks. [pl. de L. *clunis*, nádega]
clu·pan·o·don·ic ac·id (kloo-pan´ō-don´ik). Ácido clupanodônico; um ácido graxo ω-3 com 22 carbonos e cinco ligações duplas; encontrado nos óleos de peixe e fosfolipídios no cérebro.

CLUSTER OF DIFFERENTIATION

cluster of differentiation. *Cluster* de diferenciação, grupo de diferenciação; moléculas da membrana celular usadas para classificar os leucócitos em subgrupos. As moléculas do CD são classificadas por anticorpos monoclonais. Há quatro tipos gerais: as proteínas transmembrana tipo I possuem sua extremidade COOH no citoplasma e sua extremidade NH₂ fora da célula; as proteínas transmembrana tipo II têm sua extremidade NH₂ no citoplasma e sua extremidade COOH fora da célula; as proteínas transmembrana tipo III atravessam a membrana plasmática mais de uma vez e, portanto, podem formar canais transmembrana; e as proteínas ancoradas por glicosilfosfatidilinositol (tipo IV), que estão presas à dupla camada lipídica por ancoragem ao glicosilfosfatidilinositol.
CD1a, uma proteína transmembrana tipo I, encontrada em timócitos, células de Langerhans, astrócitos cerebrais e células dérmicas, que está envolvida na apresentação não-clássica de antígenos ou é um receptor para um ligante ou hormônio indefinido; expressa em pacientes com leucemia linfoblástica aguda de células T, histiocitose X e timomas.
CD1b, uma proteína transmembrana tipo I, encontrada em timócitos corticais, células dérmicas e astrócitos cerebrais, que está envolvida na apresentação não-clássica de antígenos ou é um receptor para um ligante ou hormônio indefinido; expressa em pacientes com leucemia linfoblástica aguda de células T, linfoma de células T e timomas.
CD1c, uma proteína transmembrana tipo I, encontrada em timócitos corticais, células dérmicas e astrócitos cerebrais, que está envolvida na apresentação não-clássica de antígenos ou é um receptor para um ligante ou hormônio indefinido; expressa em pacientes com leucemia linfoblástica aguda de células T, leucemias linfocíticas crônicas de células B e células B na doença de imunodeficiência combinada grave.
CD2, uma proteína transmembrana tipo I, encontrada em timócitos, células T e algumas células *natural killer* (NK, destruidoras naturais), que atua como ligante para CD58 e CD59 e está envolvida na transdução de sinal e na adesão celular; expressa na leucemia linfoblástica aguda de células T e no linfoma de células T.
CD2r, uma proteína transmembrana tipo I, encontrada em células T e em algumas células *natural killer* (NK, destruidoras naturais), que não está relacionada aos locais de ligação para CD58 e CD59, expressa em células T ativadas em doenças auto-imunes.
CD3, uma proteína transmembrana tipo I, encontrada em células T, que forma a unidade de transdução de sinal para a célula T; expressa em pacientes com linfomas de células T.
CD4, uma proteína transmembrana tipo I, encontrada em células T *helper* (auxiliares)/indutoras, monócitos, macrófagos e células dendríticas, que está envolvida no reconhecimento de antígenos pela célula T, expressa na micose fungóide, síndrome de Sézary e linfomas de células T.
CD5, uma proteína transmembrana tipo I, encontrada em células T, timócitos e algumas células B, que é um ligante para CD72 e está envolvida na ativação ou adesão celular; expressa na leucemia linfocítica crônica de células B e no linfoma de células T.
CD6, uma proteína transmembrana tipo I, encontrada em células T, em timócitos medulares, alguns timócitos corticais, algumas células B e no cérebro. CD6 é fosforilada à ativação celular e, possivelmente, participa da transdução de sinal; expressa em algumas leucemias linfocíticas crônicas de células B.
CD7, uma proteína transmembrana tipo I, encontrada em timócitos, algumas células T, monócitos, células *natural killer* (NK, destruidoras naturais) e células-tronco (primordiais) hemopoéticas; expressa em pacientes com micose fungóide, alguns pacientes com linfoma linfoblástico agudo de células T e alguns pacientes com linfoma não-linfocítico agudo.
CD8, uma proteína transmembrana tipo I, encontrada em células T supressoras (citotóxicas), algumas células *natural killer* (NK, destruidoras naturais) e na maioria dos timócitos, que está envolvida no reconhecimento de antígenos das células T; expressa em alguns linfomas de células T e em leucemias de grandes linfócitos granulares.
CD9, uma proteína transmembrana tipo III, encontrada em plaquetas, megacariócitos, monócitos, pré-células B, eosinófilos, basófilos e células T ativadas; participa na transdução de sinal levando à ativação e agregação plaquetária; expressa em algumas leucemias linfocíticas agudas de células T e em algumas leucemias não-linfocíticas agudas.
CD10, uma proteína transmembrana tipo II, encontrada em células pré-B, células B do centro germinativo, alguns neutrófilos, células renais, precursores das células T e células epiteliais, que atua como uma metaloprotease zíncica que cliva ligações peptídicas no lado amino dos aminoácidos hidrofóbicos; expressa na leucemia linfocítica aguda e nos linfomas de células do centro folicular.
CD11a, uma proteína transmembrana tipo I, encontrada em linfócitos, neutrófilos, monócitos e macrófagos, que facilita a adesão celular e a ativação celular; expressa em linfomas.

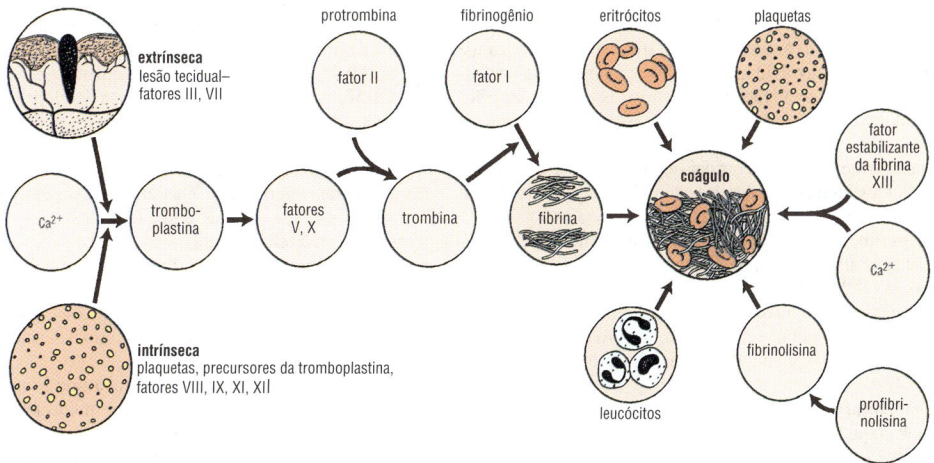

coagulação sanguínea

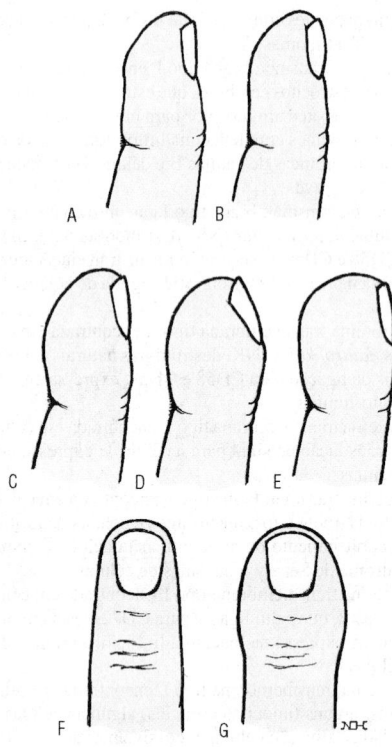

tipos de baqueteamento digital: (A) normal, (B) aumento da curvatura da unha, (C) baqueteamento leve, (D) tipo bico de papagaio, (E) tipo vidro de relógio, (F) normal, (G) tipo baqueta de tambor

CD11b, uma proteína transmembrana tipo I, encontrada em monócitos, macrófagos, granulócitos, algumas células B, células dendríticas e células *natural killer* (NK, destruidoras naturais), que facilita a adesão celular, a fagocitose e/ou a quimiotaxia; expressa em algumas leucemias linfocíticas crônicas de células B, na maioria das leucemias não-linfocíticas agudas e em algumas leucemias de células pilosas.

CD11c, uma proteína transmembrana tipo I, encontrada em monócitos, macrófagos, neutrófilos e algumas células B, que induz ativação celular e ajuda a deflagrar a explosão respiratória nos neutrófilos; expressa nas leucemias de células pilosas, leucemias não-linfocíticas agudas e em algumas leucemias linfocíticas crônicas de células B.

CDw12, uma proteína da membrana, encontrada em monócitos, neutrófilos e plaquetas; a função dessa porção não é conhecida.

CD13, uma proteína transmembrana tipo II, encontrada em células mielóides, que atua como uma metaloprotease de ligação do zinco, catalisando a remoção de aminoácidos da extremidade NH_2 dos peptídeos; expressa em alguns tipos de leucemia não-linfocítica aguda.

CD14, uma proteína transmembrana, encontrada em monócitos, macrófagos, neutrófilos, algumas células B e células dendríticas, que está envolvida na transdução do sinal que leva à explosão oxidativa e/ou síntese de fator de necrose tumoral α; expressa em alguns pacientes com leucemia não-linfocítica aguda e na leucemia linfocítica crônica de células B.

CD15, uma proteína transmembrana ancorada por fosfatidilinositol, encontrada em neutrófilos e que pode estar envolvida na fagocitose; expressa em pacientes com doença de Hodgkin, algumas leucemias linfocíticas crônicas de células B, leucemias linfoblásticas agudas e na maioria das leucemias não-linfocíticas agudas.

CD15s, uma proteína transmembrana, encontrada em neutrófilos, monócitos, células mielóides e algumas células T, que serve como o principal ligante para CD62E; expressa em carcinomas de células escamosas.

CD16, uma proteína transmembrana tipo I, encontrada em células *natural killer* (NK, destruidoras naturais) e macrófagos, que está envolvida no direcionamento da ativação das células NK.

CD16b, uma proteína ancorada por glicosilfosfatidilinositol presente em neutrófilos; deficiente em pacientes com hemoglobinemia paroxística noturna e expressa em leucemias linfocíticas granulares de grandes células e em leucemias de células *natural killer*.

CDw17, uma proteína transmembrana tipo I, encontrada em monócitos, neutrófilos e plaquetas que pode participar do acondicionamento do conteúdo de grânulos ou da exocitose.

CD18, uma proteína transmembrana tipo I, encontrada em linfócitos, neutrófilos, monócitos, macrófagos, algumas células B, células dendríticas e células *natural killer* (NK, destruidoras naturais), que parece ativa na transdução do sinal; expressa em alguns pacientes com leucemia linfocítica crônica de células B, na maioria dos pacientes com leucemia não-linfocítica aguda e em alguns pacientes com leucemia de células pilosas.

CD19, uma proteína transmembrana tipo I, encontrada em todas as células B e precursores das células B e em algumas células dendríticas foliculares, que atua como uma molécula acessória para transdução do sinal da célula B; expressa em todas as neoplasias de células B.

CD20, uma proteína transmembrana tipo III, encontrada em células B, que forma um canal de cálcio na parede celular, permitindo o influxo de cálcio necessário para ativação celular; expressa nos linfomas de células B, na leucemia de células pilosas e na leucemia linfocítica crônica de células B.

CD21, uma proteína transmembrana tipo I, encontrada em células B, células dendríticas foliculares, células epiteliais faríngeas e cervicais, alguns timócitos e algumas células T, que participa na transdução do sinal; expressa na leucemia de células pilosas, no linfoma de células B e em algumas leucemias linfocíticas agudas de células T.

CD22, uma proteína transmembrana tipo I, encontrada no citoplasma de células pré-B e na superfície de células B maduras, que facilita a transdução do sinal; expressa em pacientes com leucemias de células pilosas e em alguns pacientes com linfomas de células B.

CD22α, uma proteína transmembrana tipo I, encontrada em células B maduras, que facilita a adesão de células B a monócitos e hemácias.

CD22β, uma proteína transmembrana tipo I, encontrada em células B maduras, que facilita a adesão de células B às células T CD4-positivas.

CD23, uma proteína transmembrana tipo II, encontrada em células B maduras, monócitos, macrófagos ativados, eosinófilos, plaquetas e células dendríticas, que intensifica a captura e o processamento de antígeno associado à IgE.

CD24, uma proteína ancorada por glicosilfosfatidilinositol presente em células B, células pré-B, neutrófilos e alguns timócitos que podem participar da indução da proliferação e diferenciação das células B; expressa em pacientes com linfomas de células B e em alguns pacientes com leucemias linfocíticas crônicas de células B.

CD25, uma proteína transmembrana tipo I, presente em células T ativadas, células B ativadas, alguns timócitos, precursores mielóides e oligodendrócitos, que se associa à CD122 para formar um heterodímero que pode atuar como um receptor de grande afinidade para IL-2; expressa na maioria das neoplasias de células B, em algumas leucemias não-linfocíticas agudas e nos neuroblastomas.

CD26, uma proteína transmembrana tipo II, presente em células T maduras, algumas células B, membranas apicais das células epiteliais e endoteliais, rim, bordas em escova intestinais e canalículos biliares hepáticos, que se combina ao colágeno e se associa à adenosina desaminase.

CD27, uma proteína transmembrana tipo I, presente em células T maduras, timócitos medulares e algumas células B, que é um ligante para CD70 e serve como membro da família do fator de crescimento do nervo; expressa na leucemia linfocítica crônica.

CD28, uma proteína transmembrana tipo I, presente na maioria das células T CD4, em muitas células T CD8 e na maioria dos plasmócitos, que intensifica a transcrição e a estabilidade do RNA mensageiro da IL-2.

CD29, uma proteína transmembrana tipo I, presente em algumas células T auxiliares CD4, plaquetas e células dendríticas, que está envolvida na aderência entre células ou entre a célula e a matriz.

CD30, uma proteína transmembrana tipo I, presente em células T e B ativadas, que participaria da ativação e/ou diferenciação celular; expressa na doença de Hodgkin, em alguns linfomas de células T e nos linfomas anaplásicos de grandes células.

CD30I, uma proteína transmembrana tipo III, presente em células T ativadas e monócitos, que consegue induzir respostas diferenciais em células que expressam CD30, variando do crescimento à morte celular.

CD31, uma proteína transmembrana tipo I, presente em células mielóides, plaquetas, células endoteliais, células *natural killer* (NK, destruidoras naturais), monócitos e subgrupos de células T CD4-positivas, que atua como um transdutor co-sinal para macrófagos, induzindo explosão respiratória; é fundamental na transmigração de leucócitos através das junções intercelulares do endotélio vascular e media a agregação heterófila cálcio-dependente; expressa em células endoteliais neoplásicas.

CD32, uma proteína transmembrana tipo I, presente em monócitos, células B, neutrófilos, trofoblastos placentários e endotélio; atua como um transdutor de sinal para fagocitose mediada por IgG e explosão oxidativa de neutrófilos e monócitos; transduz um sinal inibitório nas células B e pode participar do transporte da IgG placentária.

CD33, uma proteína transmembrana tipo I, presente nas células mielóides e precursores mielóides; expressa em muitas leucemias não-linfoblásticas agudas e em algumas leucemias linfocíticas crônicas de células B.

CD34, uma proteína transmembrana tipo I, presente nas células mielóides e precursores mielóides, que participa da transdução de sinais; expressa em algumas leucemias não-linfocíticas agudas e em algumas leucemias linfocíticas agudas.

CD35, uma proteína transmembrana tipo I, presente em monócitos, granulócitos, células dendríticas, hemácias, algumas células T e podócitos glomerulares, que facilita a fagocitose e/ou ligação de imunocomplexos; expressa no tumor de Wilms.

CD36, uma proteína transmembrana, presente em monócitos, plaquetas, megacariócitos, veia umbilical, endotélio de pequenos vasos, reticulócitos e epitélio mamário, que pode ser envolvida na transdução de sinal; expressa em distúrbios mieloproliferativos.

CD37, uma proteína transmembrana tipo III, presente em células B maduras, algumas células T e monócitos, que participaria no transporte iônico; expressa em linfomas de células B, leucemia linfocítica crônica de células B e leucemia de células pilosas.

CD38, uma proteína transmembrana, presente em macrófagos, células dendríticas e células ativadas das linhagens de células *natural killer* (NK, destruidoras naturais), B e T, que pode facilitar a adesão das células B.

CD39, uma proteína transmembrana, presente em macrófagos, células dendríticas e células linfóides ativadas, que facilita a adesão das células B.

CD40, uma proteína transmembrana tipo I, presente em células B maduras, monócitos, células dendríticas e células epiteliais envolvidas na transdução de sinal, levando à ativação, proliferação, adesão e/ou diferenciação celular; expressa em leucemias linfocíticas crônicas de células B, linfomas e alguns carcinomas.

CD40l, uma proteína transmembrana tipo II, presente em células T CD4-positivas ativadas, algumas células T CD8-positivas ativadas e basófilos do sangue; um ligante para CD40 que induz ativação, proliferação e/ou diferenciação de células que expressam CD40.

CD41, uma proteína transmembrana tipo I, presente em plaquetas e megacariócitos, que serve como receptor para fibrinogênio, fibronectina, vitronectina, fator de von Willebrand e outros fatores e facilita a adesão e a agregação plaquetárias.

CD42, uma proteína transmembrana tipo I, presente em plaquetas e megacariócitos, que medeia a ligação das plaquetas aos vasos sanguíneos lesados.

CD43, uma proteína transmembrana tipo I, presente em timócitos, células T, granulócitos, monócitos, células *natural killer* (NK, destruidoras naturais), plaquetas, cérebro, células B ativadas, plasmócitos e células-tronco (primordiais) hematopoéticas, que serve como ligante para CD54 e facilita a adesão entre células; expressa em alguns mielomas e linfomas.

CD44, uma proteína transmembrana tipo I, presente em células T, células pré-B, monócitos, neutrófilos, substância branca do SNC, fibroblastos, músculo esquelético e timócitos medulares; facilita a ligação dos linfócitos aos vasos endoteliais e ajuda na adesão.

CD45, uma proteína transmembrana tipo I, presente em todas as células hematopoéticas, exceto eritrócitos, que ajuda na ativação celular; expressa em linfomas, leucemia linfocítica crônica de células B, leucemia de células pilosas e leucemia não-linfocítica aguda.

CD46, uma proteína transmembrana tipo I, presente em timócitos, células T, células B, células *natural killer* (NK, destruidoras naturais), monócitos, neutrófilos, plaquetas, células endoteliais, células epiteliais, fibroblastos, placenta e espermatozóides, que protege contra a lesão mediada pelo complemento.

CD47, uma proteína transmembrana sem especificidade tecidual, que está envolvida no fluxo de cátions na membrana.

CD48, uma proteína da membrana ancorada por glicosilfosfatidilinositol, presente nas células T, células B, timócitos, eosinófilos, neutrófilos, epitélio brônquico e glândula salivar, que participaria na transdução de sinais nas células T; ausente ou deficiente em pacientes com hemoglobinúria paroxística noturna.

CD49a, uma proteína transmembrana tipo I, presente em células T e B ativadas, monócitos, endotélio neurovascular e músculo liso, que forma um receptor para colágeno e laminina; expressa em melanomas.

CD49b, uma proteína transmembrana tipo I, presente em plaquetas, células T, células B, fibroblastos e células endoteliais envolvidas na adesão plaquetária do colágeno; pode ser expressa em melanomas.

CD49c, uma proteína transmembrana tipo I, presente em células B, glomérulo renal, tireóide e algumas membranas basais, que participaria da adesão intercelular; expressa na maioria das linhagens celulares cultivadas.

CD49d, uma proteína transmembrana tipo I, presente em células B e T, células *natural killer* (NK, destruidoras naturais), eosinófilos, monócitos, eritroblastos, timócitos e mioblastos, que facilita a adesão entre células e a migração de leucócitos e ajuda na ativação de linfócitos; expressa em melanomas.

CD49e, uma proteína transmembrana tipo I, presente em monócitos, neutrófilos, leucócitos, fibroblastos, plaquetas e mioblastos, que ajuda a formar um receptor para fibronectina e ativa o antiportador de sódio e hidrogênio; pode ter um papel acessório para a ativação de células T.

CD49f, uma proteína transmembrana tipo I, presente em plaquetas, macrófagos, monócitos, timócitos, células T e linhagens de células aderentes, que forma um receptor para invasão e laminina; expressa em algumas leucemias linfocíticas agudas.

CD50, uma proteína transmembrana tipo I, presente em timócitos, células B, monócitos e neutrófilos; envolvida na adesão intracelular.

CD51, uma proteína transmembrana tipo I, presente nas células endoteliais, monócitos, macrófagos, plaquetas, algumas células B, osteoclastos e células uterinas; participa na agregação plaquetária e/ou adesão de células endoteliais e na migração de monócitos.

CD52, uma proteína da membrana ancorada por glicosilfosfatidilinositol, presente em timócitos, células T, células B, alguns granulócitos, vesículas seminais, epidídimo e espermatozóides; participa na transdução de sinais.

CD53, uma proteína transmembrana tipo III, presente em leucócitos, plaquetas, osteoblastos e osteoclastos; contribui para a transdução de sinais gerados por CD2 nas células T e células *natural killer* (NK, destruidoras naturais), facilita o fluxo citoplasmático de cálcio nas células B, monócitos e granulócitos; e atua na ativação da explosão oxidativa de monócitos; expressa em neoplasias hematopoéticas e mielomas.

CD54, uma proteína transmembrana tipo I, presente em leucócitos e células endoteliais, e induzível em linfócitos, células dendríticas, ceratinócitos, condrócitos, fibroblastos e células epiteliais; atua como um ligante para CD11 e CD18 e ajuda na adesão intercelular.

CD55, uma proteína da membrana ancorada por glicosilfosfatidilinositol, presente em todas as células hematopoéticas e espermatozóides, que neutraliza a ativação do complemento; está ausente ou deficiente na hemoglobinúria paroxística noturna.

CD57, uma proteína da membrana, presente em células *natural killer* (NK, destruidoras naturais), algumas células T, algumas células B e monócitos de função desconhecida; expressa em leucemias de grandes linfócitos granulares.

CD58, uma proteína da membrana, presente em muitas células hematopoéticas e fibroblastos, que atua como ligante para CD2 e estaria envolvida na função das células T.

CD59, uma proteína da membrana ancorada por glicosilfosfatidilinositol, presente em muitas células hematopoéticas, endotélio vascular, células epiteliais e placenta, que inibe o ataque do complemento à membrana e estaria envolvida na transdução dos sinais das células T; ausente ou deficiente na hemoglobinúria paroxística noturna.

CDw60, uma proteína da membrana, presente em subgrupos de células T, alguns monócitos e plaquetas, que atuaria na transdução de sinais que leva à ativação celular; presente em linfomas de células T cutâneos.

CD61, uma proteína da membrana, presente em plaquetas, megacariócitos, células endoteliais, osteoclastos e células uterinas, que facilita a agregação e a adesão plaquetárias.

CD62e, uma proteína transmembrana tipo I, presente no endotélio, que facilita a adesão de neutrófilos, monócitos e algumas células T ao endotélio vascular; há maior expressão em locais de inflamação crônica.

CD62l, uma proteína transmembrana tipo I, presente em células B, células T, neutrófilos, timócitos, monócitos, eosinófilos, células progenitoras eritróides e mielóides, e células *natural killer* (NK, destruidoras naturais), que funciona como um receptor em linfonodo periférico e facilita a ligação ao endotélio em locais inflamatórios; encontrada em muitos leucócitos malignos.

CD62p, uma proteína transmembrana tipo I, presente em plaquetas ativadas, células endoteliais e megacariócitos, que facilita a adesão de monócitos e neutrófilos a plaquetas ativadas e a células endoteliais.

CD63, uma proteína transmembrana tipo III, presente em plaquetas ativadas, monócitos, macrófagos e nos grânulos secretores de células endoteliais vasculares e grânulos plaquetários densos; facilita a adesão ao endotélio ativado.

CD64, uma proteína transmembrana tipo I, presente em monócitos, megacariócitos e neutrófilos ativados, que atua como receptor de alta afinidade para IgG; presente em alguns casos de leucemia não-linfocítica aguda.

CDw65, uma proteína da membrana, presente em células mielóides e algumas células monocíticas, envolvida na transdução de sinal que leva à formação da explosão respiratória; presente em algumas leucemias não-linfocíticas agudas.

CD66a, uma proteína transmembrana tipo I, presente em neutrófilos, histiócitos, algumas células progenitoras mielóides e na borda em escova das células epiteliais colônicas, que facilita a adesão e a ativação neutrofílica; expressa na leucemia mielocítica crônica e em alguns casos de leucemia linfocítica aguda.

CD66b, uma proteína da membrana ancorada por glicosilfosfatidilinositol, presente em neutrófilos, que induz agregação e ativação; expressa na leucemia mielocítica crônica.

CD66c, uma proteína da membrana ancorada por glicosilfosfatidilinositol, presente em neutrófilos, que induz agregação e ativação; expressa na leucemia mielocítica crônica.

CD66d, uma proteína transmembrana tipo I, presente em neutrófilos, que facilita a adesão e a ativação de neutrófilos; expressa na leucemia mielocítica crônica.

CD66e, uma proteína ancorada por glicosilfosfatidilinositol, presente em tecidos derivados de todas as três camadas germinativas durante a embriogênese e as células epiteliais do cólon do adulto, que facilita a adesão cálcio-independente durante a embriogênese; expressa na maioria dos carcinomas de cólon e em outros carcinomas.

CD68, uma proteína transmembrana tipo I, presente em monócitos, macrófagos, osteoclastos, mastócitos, grânulos citoplasmáticos, plaquetas ativadas e grandes linfócitos; expressa nas células de Schwann do neuroma, em nervos que sofrem degeneração waleriana, em tumores das células mielóides e em linfomas anaplásicos e tumores epiteliais.
CD69, uma proteína transmembrana tipo II, presente em plaquetas, timócitos CD4-positivos ou CD8-positivos, linfócitos ativados e células T ativadas ou *natural killer* (NK, destruidoras naturais), que funciona como um transdutor de sinal, intensificando a ativação celular e/ou a agregação plaquetária.
CD70, uma proteína transmembrana tipo II, presente em células B ativadas e algumas células T ativadas, que intensifica a ativação das células T; expressa em células de Reed-Sternberg, alguns linfomas e tumores derivados da linhagem de monócitos.
CD71, uma proteína transmembrana tipo II, presente em células ativadas ou em proliferação, que facilita a captação celular de ferro; expressa em muitas leucemias agudas e alguns linfomas.
CD72, uma proteína transmembrana tipo II, presente em todas as células B e macrófagos, que participa na transdução de sinais ou adesão; expressa na leucemia linfoblástica aguda de células B, linfomas de células B e na leucemia linfocítica crônica de células B.
CD73, uma proteína da membrana ancorada por glicosilfosfatidilinositol, presente em algumas células B, algumas células T, timócitos, algumas células epiteliais e endoteliais, e células dendríticas; expressa na maioria das leucemias linfoblásticas agudas de células B, carcinomas de mama e leucemias de grandes leucócitos granulares.
CD74, uma proteína transmembrana tipo II, presente em células B, monócitos, células dendríticas e células T ativadas, que impede a ligação de peptídeos endógenos; expressa na leucemia linfocítica crônica de células B, leucemia de células pilosas e linfomas de grandes leucócitos granulares.
CDw75, uma proteína transmembrana tipo II, presente em células B maduras e algumas células T, que pode facilitar a adesão de células B; expressa em linfomas de células B com origem nas células foliculares.
CDw76, uma proteína da membrana, presente em células B maduras, algumas células T, melanócitos, células endoteliais, hepatócitos e células tubulares renais; expressa em linfomas de células B maduras e leucemias linfocíticas crônicas de células B.
CD77, uma proteína da membrana, presente em células B do centro germinativo, células dendríticas foliculares, endotélio e algumas células epiteliais, que atuaria como receptor para toxinas de *Escherichia coli* ou *Shigella dysenteriae*; expressa em linfomas de Burkitt e linfomas de células B com origem nas células do centro folicular.
CDw78, uma proteína da membrana, presente em células B e macrófagos teciduais, que estaria envolvida na transdução de sinais; expressa em algumas leucemias linfoblásticas agudas, linfomas de células B e algumas leucemias não-linfocíticas agudas.
CD79a, uma proteína transmembrana tipo I, presente nas células B, que medeia a transdução do sinal; expressa em neoplasias de células B maduras.
CD79b, uma proteína transmembrana tipo I, presente em células B, que medeia a transdução do sinal; expressa em tumores de células B e leucemias leucoblásticas agudas de células B.
CD80, uma proteína transmembrana tipo I, presente em células B ativadas, monócitos ativados, células dendríticas foliculares ativadas e algumas células T ativadas, que emite um sinal co-estimulador para células T durante a apresentação de antígenos; expressa em células linfoblastóides B.
CD81, uma proteína transmembrana tipo III, presente em muitos tipos celulares, incluindo linfócitos, que facilita a transdução do sinal; expressa em linfomas, leucemias, melanomas e neuroblastomas.
CD82, uma proteína transmembrana tipo III, presente nas células epiteliais, endotélio e linfócitos ativados, que participaria no fluxo de cálcio.
CD83, uma proteína transmembrana tipo I, presente em células dendríticas, células de Langerhans, células B e células reticulares interdigitadas, que participaria na apresentação de antígenos ou das interações celulares que sucedem a ativação dos linfócitos.
CDw84, uma proteína da membrana, presente em monócitos, células B iniciais, plaquetas, células B do centro germinativo, células B da zona do manto e linfócitos circulantes.
CD85, uma proteína da membrana, presente em plasmócitos, células B e monócitos.
CD86, uma proteína da membrana, presente em algumas células B do centro germinativo, células B ativadas por mitógenos e monócitos, que serve como ativador das células B; expressa em linfomas de grandes células anaplásicas, em células de Reed-Sternberg e em células B transformadas pelo vírus Epstein-Barr.
CD87, uma proteína da membrana ancorada por glicosilfosfatidilinositol, presente em células T ativadas, monócitos e neutrófilos ativados, que participa na ativação do plasminogênio da superfície celular; expressa em macrófagos em locais de inflamação.
CD88, uma proteína transmembrana tipo III, presente em neutrófilos, macrófagos, eosinófilos, mastócitos e células musculares lisas, que ajuda a deflagrar a quimiotaxia e auxilia na ativação celular, explosão respiratória e desgranulação; expressa em tumores monocitóides.
CD89, uma proteína transmembrana tipo I, presente em neutrófilos, monócitos, macrófagos e algumas células T e B, que ajuda na deflagração da explosão respiratória dos granulócitos; expressa em tumores monocitóides.
CDw90, uma proteína da membrana ancorada por glicosilfosfatidilinositol de função desconhecida, presente em pró-timócitos e no cérebro e em outros tecidos não-linfóides.
CD91, uma proteína da membrana, presente em monócitos e macrófagos, que facilitaria a endocitose.
CDw92, uma proteína da membrana, presente em neutrófilos, plaquetas e monócitos; de função desconhecida.
CD93, uma proteína da membrana, presente em neutrófilos, monócitos e células endoteliais; de função desconhecida.
CD94, uma proteína da membrana expressa em células *natural killer* (NK, destruidoras naturais) e algumas células T, que estimula a citólise das células *natural killer* e a liberação de fator de necrose tumoral.
CD95, uma proteína transmembrana tipo I, presente em células T e células mielóides, que induziria apoptose.
CD96, uma proteína transmembrana tipo I, presente em células T, células *natural killer* (NK, destruidoras naturais) e células B ativadas, expressa basicamente à ativação celular, sugerindo atividade de associação ao ligante.
CD97, uma proteína da membrana de função desconhecida, presente em monócitos e granulócitos maduros.
CD98, uma proteína transmembrana tipo II, presente em monócitos, células musculares cardíacas, células endoteliais, células T, células B e células *natural killer* (NK, destruidoras naturais), provavelmente envolvida na regulação dos fluxos de cálcio; aumentada nas células T em algumas doenças auto-imunes ou na hepatite crônica.
CD99, uma proteína transmembrana tipo I, presente em timócitos, linfócitos e células mielóides, envolvida em formações de rosetas com eritrócitos de carneiro.
CD99r, uma proteína transmembrana tipo I, semelhante à CD99, mas presente em células mielóides.
CD100, uma proteína da membrana, presente em células hematopoéticas, que pode induzir respostas proliferativas.
CDw101, uma proteína da membrana de função desconhecida, presente em neutrófilos, monócitos e algumas células T.
CD102, uma proteína transmembrana tipo I, presente em células endoteliais, plaquetas, monócitos, células dendríticas, subgrupos de linfócitos e em sinusóides esplênicos, que facilitaria a recirculação de células T de memória.
CD103, uma proteína transmembrana tipo I, presente em linfócitos intra-epiteliais intestinais, alguns leucócitos circulantes e algumas células T, que facilita a adesão aos epitélios; expressa na leucemia de células pilosas e em algumas leucemias linfocíticas crônicas de células B.
CD104, uma proteína transmembrana tipo I, presente em epitélios e timócitos, que facilita a adesão de células à matriz extracelular; expressa no carcinoma de células escamosas.
CD105, uma proteína transmembrana tipo II, presente no endotélio, pró-eritroblastos, monócitos e macrófagos ativados e células dendríticas foliculares, que participaria na adesão; expressa em células leucêmicas de origem linfóide B e mielóide.
CD106, uma proteína transmembrana tipo I, presente em células endoteliais ativadas, macrófagos, células dendríticas, estroma da medula óssea, mioblastos e miotúbulos, que facilita o recrutamento de leucócitos para locais de inflamação.
CD107a, uma proteína transmembrana tipo I, presente em plaquetas ativadas; é observado aumento de sua expressão na transformação de células com potencial metastático e em células embrionárias.
CD107b, uma proteína transmembrana tipo I, presente em plaquetas ativadas; é observado aumento de sua expressão na transformação de células com potencial metastático e em células embrionárias.
CDw108, uma proteína ancorada por glicosilfosfatidilinositol, de função desconhecida, presente em células T ativadas.
CDw109, uma proteína da membrana ancorada por glicosilfosfatidilinositol, de função desconhecida, presente em células T ativadas, plaquetas ativadas e células endoteliais.
CD115, uma proteína transmembrana tipo I, presente na placenta, macrófagos, monócitos e precursores de monócitos, envolvida na proliferação e diferenciação de monócitos e seus progenitores; expressa em coriocarcinomas.
CDw116, uma proteína transmembrana tipo I, presente em monócitos, granulócitos, células endoteliais, células dendríticas e fibroblastos, que estimula a proliferação e a diferenciação celulares; expressa no sarcoma osteogênico e nos carcinomas da mama e do pulmão.
CD117, uma proteína transmembrana tipo I, presente em progenitores hematopoéticos, mastócitos, melanócitos, espermatogônias, ovócitos e algumas células *natural killer* (NK, destruidoras naturais), que ajuda na transdução de sinal para linhagens celulares transfectadas; expressa em carcinomas do cólon.

CD120a, uma proteína transmembrana tipo I, presente em muitos tipos celulares, que tem uma elevada afinidade por fatores de necrose tumoral.
CD120b, uma proteína transmembrana tipo I, presente em muitos tipos de células, que apresenta uma elevada afinidade por fatores de necrose tumoral.
CDw121a, uma proteína transmembrana tipo I, presente em células T, timócitos, condrócitos, células sinoviais, células endoteliais, fibroblastos, ceratinócitos e hepatócitos, que ajuda na estimulação da proliferação e/ou ativação celulares.
CDw121b, uma proteína transmembrana tipo I, presente em células B, monócitos e macrófagos, que está envolvida na interação com interleucinas.
CDw122, uma proteína transmembrana tipo I, presente em células T ativadas, células B, monócitos e células *natural killer* (NK, destruidoras naturais), que pode formar complexos com CD25.
CD123, uma proteína transmembrana tipo I, presente em células-tronco (primordiais) pluripotentes e células progenitoras hematopoéticas comprometidas, envolvida na proliferação e/ou diferenciação celulares.
CDw124, uma proteína transmembrana tipo I, presente em células B maduras, células T, epitélio, precursores hematopoéticos e fibroblastos, que induz proliferação e/ou ativação celulares; expressa em linfomas e tumores pancreáticos, hepáticos e vesicais.
CD125, uma proteína transmembrana tipo I, presente em eosinófilos e basófilos, que estimula a proliferação e/ou diferenciação celulares.
CD126, uma proteína transmembrana tipo I, presente em plasmócitos, leucócitos, células epiteliais, fibroblastos, células neurais e hepatócitos, que estimula o crescimento e/ou diferenciação celulares; possível fator de crescimento para mielomas.
CDw127, uma proteína transmembrana tipo I, presente em precursores das células B, timócitos, células T maduras e monócitos, que induz crescimento e/ou diferenciação celulares.
CDw128, uma proteína transmembrana tipo III, presente em neutrófilos, basófilos, monócitos, ceratinócitos e algumas células T, que induz quimiotaxia e/ou ativação celulares; expressa em células de melanoma.
CD129, uma proteína transmembrana tipo I, presente em algumas células T, precursores mielóides e eritróides e em mastócitos, que induz crescimento e/ou diferenciação celulares; expressa na doença de Hodgkin, linfomas de grandes células e leucemia megacarioblástica.
CDw130, uma proteína transmembrana tipo I, presente na maioria dos leucócitos, células epiteliais, fibroblastos, hepatócitos e células neurais; interage com fatores inibidores da leucemia, interleucinas e outros fatores de proliferação celular.

---

clut·ter·ing (klŭt′er-ing) Distúrbio da fala, geralmente observado na infância, caracterizado por velocidade anormalmente rápida, perturbação da fluência, ritmo errático e má articulação, tornando difícil compreender o orador.
Clutton, Henry H., cirurgião inglês, 1850–1909. VER C. *joints,* em *joint.*
cly·sis (klī′sis). Clise. 1. Infusão de líquido, geralmente por via subcutânea, para fins terapêuticos. 2. Antigamente, um enema líquido; mais tarde, retirada de material de qualquer espaço ou cavidade corporal por meio de líquidos. [G. *klysis,* lavagem por um clister]
-clysis. Forma combinante que se refere a injeção ou enema. [G. *klysis,* lavagem por um clister]
clys·ter (klis′ter). Clister; termo antigo para enema. [G. *klystēr,* de *klyzō,* fut. *klysō,* retirar]
C.M. Abreviatura de *Chirurgiae Magister,* Mestre em Cirurgia.
CM- Símbolo do radical carboximetil.
Cm Símbolo de cúrio.
cM Abreviatura de centimorgan.
cm Abreviatura de centímetro; cm² para centímetro quadrado; cm³ para centímetro cúbico (cubic *centimeter*).
CMA Abreviatura de Certified Medical Assistant (Auxiliar Médico Certificado).
***p*-CMB** Abreviatura de *p*-cloromercuribenzoato.
cmc Abreviatura de critical micelle *concentration* (concentração micelar crítica).
CM-cel·lu·lose. SIN carboxymethyl *cellulose.*
CMG Abreviatura de cistometrograma.
CMI Abreviatura de cell-mediated *immunity* (imunidade celular).
CML 1. Abreviatura de linfocitotoxicidade celular. **2.** Acrônimo para chronic myelogenous *leukemia* (leucemia mielógena crônica).
CMO Abreviatura de calculated mean *organism* (organismo médio calculado).
CMP Símbolo de 5′-monofosfato de citidina (secundariamente, para qualquer monofosfato de citidina).
c-mpl. Um receptor da superfície celular em megacariócitos, plaquetas e células precursoras hematopoéticas CD34-positivas; parece ser o receptor para regulação da megacariocitopoese e produção plaquetária.
CMT Abreviatura de Certified Medical Transcriptionist (Transcritor Médico Certificado). VER medical transcriptionist.

CMV 1. Abreviatura de controlled mechanical *ventilation* (ventilação mecânica controlada); abreviatura de citomegalovírus. **2.** Uma associação de medicamentos antineoplásica, que consiste em cisplatina, metotrexato e vimblastina, usada no tratamento de neoplasias malignas da bexiga e outras.
cne·mi·al (ne′me-ăl). Cnêmio; relativo à perna, particularmente à porção tibial. [G. *knēmē,* perna]
cne·mis (nē′mis). A região tibial. [G. *knēmis* (*knēmid-*), perna]
cni·da, pl. **cni·dae** (nī′dă, nī′dē). Nematocisto. SIN nematocyst. [G. *knidē,* urtiga]
cni·do·cyst (nī′dō-sist). Nematocisto. SIN nematocyst.
Cnid·o·spora (nī-dō-spōr′ă). SIN Microspora. [G. *knidē,* urtiga, urtiga marinha, + *sporos,* semente]
Cni·do·spo·rid·ia (nī′dō-spō-rid′ēă). SIN Microsporida. [G. *knidē,* urtiga, marinha, + L. Mod., do G. *sporos,* semente]
C.N.M. Abreviatura de certified nurse-midwife (enfermeira-obstetriz).
CNS 1. Abreviatura de central nervous *system* (sistema nervoso central). **2.** Símbolo do radical tiocianato, CNS⁻ ou –CNS.
CO Símbolo de *carbon* monoxide (monóxido de carbono).
Co Símbolo de cobalto; coccígeo.
^{57}**Co** Símbolo de cobalto-57 (Co^{57}).
^{60}**Co** Símbolo de cobalto-60 (Co^{60}).
^{58}**Co** Símbolo de cobalto-58 (Co^{58}).
co-. VER con-.
CoA Abreviatura de coenzima A.
co·ac·er·vate (kō-as′er-vāt). Coacervato; um agregado de partículas coloidais separadas de uma emulsão (coacervação) pela adição de um terceiro componente (agente coacervante). [L. *coacervare,* pp. *–atus,* acumular em uma massa]
co·ac·er·va·tion (kō-as-er-vā′shŭn). Coacervação; formação de um coacervato.
co·ad·ap·ta·tion (kō′ad-ap-tā′shŭn). Coadaptação; a operação de seleção conjunta de dois ou mais *loci.*
co·ag·glu·ti·nation (kō-ă-gloo′tin-a′shŭn). Coaglutinação; agregação de partículas antigênicas ligadas com aglutininas de mais de uma especificidade.
co·ag·u·la (kō-ag′ū-lă). Plural de coagulum.
co·ag·u·la·ble (kō-ag′ū-lă-bl). Coagulável; capaz de ser coagulado.
co·ag·u·lant (kō-ag′ū-lant). Coagulante. **1.** Agente que causa, estimula ou acelera a coagulação, principalmente em relação ao sangue. **2.** SIN coagulative.
co·ag·u·late (kō-ag′ū-lāt). Coagular. **1.** Converter um líquido ou substância em solução em um sólido ou gel. **2.** Coagular; coalhar; transformar um líquido em sólido ou gel. [L. *coagulo,* pp. *–atus,* coagular]
co·ag·u·la·tion (kō-ag-ū-la′shŭn). Coagulação. 1. O processo de transformar um líquido em um sólido, referente principalmente ao sangue (isto é, coagulação sanguínea). **2.** Um coágulo. **3.** Transformação de um sol em um gel ou massa semi-sólida; p. ex., a coagulação da clara de um ovo por fervura. Em qualquer suspensão coloidal, a dispersão da fase contínua para fase dispersa é muito reduzida, levando assim à separação completa ou parcial da primeira; geralmente é um fenômeno irreversível, exceto se a natureza básica da substância for quimicamente alterada.
disseminated intravascular c. (DIC), c. intravascular disseminada (CID); síndrome hemorrágica que ocorre após a ativação descontrolada dos fatores da coagulação e de enzimas fibrinolíticas em todos os pequenos vasos sanguíneos; a fibrina é depositada, as plaquetas e os fatores da coagulação são consumidos e os produtos da degradação da fibrina inibem a polimerização da fibrina, resultando em necrose tecidual e hemorragia. VER TAMBÉM consumption *coagulopathy.*
co·ag·u·la·tive (kō-ag′ū-lă-tiv). Coagulativo; que causa coagulação. SIN coagulant (2).
co·ag·u·lop·a·thy (kō-ag-ū-lop′ă-thē). Coagulopatia; doença que afeta a coagulabilidade do sangue.
consumption c., c. de consumo; distúrbio no qual ocorrem reduções acentuadas das concentrações sanguíneas de plaquetas com exaustão dos fatores da coagulação no sangue periférico; freqüentemente usada como sinônimo de coagulação intravascular disseminada.
co·ag·u·lum, pl. **co·ag·u·la** (kō-ag′ū-lŭm,-lă). Coágulo; massa de consistência mole, não-rígida, insolúvel, formada quando um sol sofre coagulação. [L. um meio de coagulação, coalho]
co-alcoholic (kō-al-kō-hol′ik). Co-alcoólatra. **1.** A(s) pessoa(s) que permite(m) o alcoolismo através de atitudes como assumir responsabilidades para o alcoólatra, minimizar ou negar o problema com a bebida, ou explicar o comportamento do alcoólatra. **2.** Relativo ao co-alcoólatra ou ao co-alcoolismo. VER TAMBÉM splinting.
co-alcoholism (kō-al′kō-hol-izm). Co-alcoolismo; o conjunto de atitudes, atributos e comportamentos da pessoa que colabora com o alcoólatra, isso é necessário para alcançar um equilíbrio simbiótico entre alcoólatra e co-alcoólatra. VER TAMBÉM symbiosis.
co·a·les·cence (kō-ă-les′ens). Coalescência; fusão de partes originalmente separadas. SIN concrescence (1).
coal oil (kōl). Petróleo. SIN petroleum.

coagulopatia

algumas das causas mais importantes de coagulopatia de consumo (termo freqüentemente usado como sinônimo de coagulação intravascular disseminada)

aguda	subaguda/crônica
descolamento prematuro da placenta	abortamento séptico
embolia por líquido amniótico	toxemia da gravidez
reação hemolítica à transfusão	carcinoma (pulmão, próstata)
síndrome de Waterhouse-Friderichsen	síndrome de Kasabach-Merritt
sépsis por Gram-negativos	síndrome do feto morto
hiperpirexia maligna	pancreatite hemorrágica aguda
picada de cobra	leucemia aguda
leucemia promielocítica aguda	cirrose hepática descompensada
choque	
púrpura fulminante	

coal tar. Alcatrão; produto intermediário obtido durante a destilação destrutiva do carvão betuminoso; semi-sólido muito escuro de odor naftalênico característico e sabor forte, ardente; usado no tratamento de doenças cutâneas.

co·apt (kō'apt). Coaptar; juntar ou unir.

co·ap·ta·tion (kō-ap-tā'shŭn). Coaptação; união ou adaptação de duas superfícies; p. ex., as bordas de uma ferida ou as extremidades de um osso fraturado. [L. *co-apto*, pp. *–aptatus*, unir]

co·arct (kō-arkt'). Coarctar; restringir ou comprimir. SIN coarctate (1). [L. *co-arcto*, pp. *–arctatus*, comprimir]

co·arc·tate (kō-ark'tāt). **1.** Coarctar. SIN coarct. **2.** Coarctado; comprimido.

co·arc·ta·tion (kō-ark-tā'shŭn). Coarctação, coartação; constricção, estreitamento ou estenose.

  aortic c., c. aórtica; estreitamento congênito da aorta, geralmente localizado imediatamente distal à artéria subclávia esquerda (left subclavian *artery*), causando hipertensão dos membros superiores, sobrecarga ventricular esquerda e diminuição do fluxo sanguíneo para os membros inferiores e vísceras abdominais.

  reversed c., c. inversa; síndrome do arco aórtico na qual a pressão arterial nos braços é menor que nas pernas.

co·arc·tec·to·my (kō'ark-tek'tō-mē). Coarctectomia; excisão de uma coarctação (da aorta).

co·arc·tot·o·my (kō-ark-tot'ō-mē). Coarctotomia; divisão de um estreitamento. [coarct + G. *tome*, corte]

CoAS-, CoASH Símbolos para o radical coenzima A e coenzima A reduzida, respectivamente.

coat (kōt). Camada; revestimento; película, creme. **1.** O revestimento ou envoltório externo de um órgão ou uma parte. **2.** Uma das camadas de tecido membranoso ou de outros tecidos que forma a parede de um canal ou de um órgão oco. VER tunic.

  buffy c., creme leucocitário; a porção superior, mais leve, do coágulo sanguíneo (plasma coagulado e leucócitos), que ocorre quando a coagulação é retardada de forma que tenha havido tempo para as hemácias se sedimentarem; a porção de sangue centrifugado e anticoagulado que contém leucócitos e plaquetas. SIN crusta inflammatoria, crusta phlogistica, leukocyte cream.

  muscular c., camada muscular, *termo oficial alternativo para muscular *layer*.

  muscular c. of bronchi, c. muscular dos brônquios; *termo oficial alternativo para muscular *layer* of bronchi.

  muscular c. of colon, c. muscular do cólon; *termo oficial alternativo para muscular *layer* of colon.

  muscular c. of ductus deferens, c. muscular do ducto deferente, *termo oficial alternativo para muscular *layer* of ductus deferens.

  muscular c. of esophagus, c. muscular do esôfago; *termo oficial alternativo para muscular *layer* of esophagus.

  muscular c. of female urethra, c. muscular da uretra feminina; *termo oficial alternativo para muscular *layer* of female urethra.

  muscular c. of gallbladder, c. muscular da vesícula biliar; *termo oficial alternativo para muscular *layer* of gallbladder.

  muscular c. of intermediate part of male urethra, c. muscular da porção intermediária da uretra masculina; *termo oficial alternativo para muscular *layer* of prostatic urethra.

  muscular c. of large intestine, c. muscular do intestino grosso; *termo oficial alternativo para muscular *layer* of large intestine.

  muscular c. of male urethra, c. muscular da uretra masculina. SIN muscular *layer* of male urethra.

  muscular c. of pharynx, c. muscular da faringe; *termo oficial alternativo para muscular *layer* of pharynx.

  muscular c. of prostatic urethra, c. muscular da uretra prostática. SIN muscular *layer* of prostatic urethra.

  muscular c. of rectum, c. muscular do reto; *termo oficial alternativo para muscular *layer* of rectum.

  muscular c. of small intestine, c. muscular do intestino delgado; *termo oficial alternativo para muscular *layer* of small intestine.

  muscular c. of spongy part of male urethra, c. muscular da porção esponjosa da uretra masculina; *termo oficial alternativo para muscular *layer* of spongy (male) urethra.

  muscular c. of stomach, c. muscular do estômago; *termo oficial alternativo para muscular *layer* of stomach. VER TAMBÉM oblique *fibers* of muscular layer of stomach, em *fiber*.

  muscular c. of trachea, c. muscular da traquéia; *termo oficial alternativo para muscular *layer* of trachea.

  muscular c. of ureter, c. muscular do ureter; *termo oficial alternativo para muscular *layer* of ureter.

  muscular c. of urinary bladder, c. muscular da bexiga; *termo oficial alternativo para muscular *layer* of urinary bladder.

  muscular c. of uterine tube, c. muscular da tuba uterina; *termo oficial alternativo para muscular *layer* of uterine tube.

  muscular c. of uterus, c. muscular do útero. SIN myometrium.

  muscular c. of vagina, c. muscular da vagina; *termo oficial alternativo para muscular *layer* of vagina.

  sclerotic c., c. esclerótica. SIN sclera.

  serous c., c. serosa; *termo oficial alternativo para serosa.

  serous c. of peritoneum, c. serosa do peritônio; *termo oficial alternativo para serosa of peritoneum.

coat·ing (kōt'ing). Cobertura; camada de alguma substância espalhada sobre uma superfície.

  antireflection c., camada anti-reflexo; uma película de fluoreto de magnésio espalhada sobre uma lente para minimizar reflexos.

CoA trans·fer·as·es [EC 2.8.3.x]. CoA transferases; tiaforases; enzimas que transferem a CoA do acetil-CoA ou succinil-CoA para outros radicais acil.

Coats, George, oftalmologista britânico, 1876–1915. VER C. *disease*.

co·bal·a·min (Cbl) (kō-bal'ă-min). Cobalamina; termo geral para substâncias que contêm o núcleo dimetilbenzimidazolilcobamida da vitamina B_{12}.

  ATP c. adenoxyltransferase, ATP c. adenoxiltransferase; enzima que catalisa a reação de ATP, água e cobalamina para formar ortofosfato, pirofosfato e adenoxilcobalamina. A adenosilcobalamina é exigida pela metilmalonil-CoA mutase. A deficiência de ATP c. adenosiltransferase causará acidemia metilmalônica.

  c. concentrate, concentrado de cobalamina; o produto seco, parcialmente purificado, resultante do crescimento de culturas selecionadas de *Streptomyces* ou de outros microrganismos produtores de cobalamina; contém pelo menos 500 μg de cobalamina em cada grama.

co·balt (Co) (kō'bawlt). Cobalto; elemento metálico acinzentado, n.º atômico 27, peso atômico 58,93320; um bioelemento e constituinte da vitamina B_{12}; alguns de seus compostos são pigmentos, p. ex., azul cobalto. [Al. *kobalt*, duende ou espírito do mal]

co·balt-57 (^{57}Co). Cobalto-57 (Co^{57}); meia-vida, 271,8 dias; decai por captura eletrônica com emissão de raios gama de energia média (122,06 keV). Usado como método diagnóstico em alguns distúrbios metabólicos.

co·balt-58 (^{58}Co). Cobalto-58 (Co^{58}); emissor de pósitrons com meia-vida de 70,88 dias.

co·balt-60 (^{60}Co). Cobalto-60 (Co^{60}); meia-vida, 5,271 anos; emite partículas beta e raios gama energéticos; razão pela qual é usado em teleterapia de irradiação e em diagnóstico no lugar do rádio (radônio) e dos raios X. Também é usado como método diagnóstico em problemas relacionados à vitamina B_{12}.

co·bal·tous chlo·ride (kō-bawl'tŭs). Cloreto cobaltoso; usado no tratamento de vários tipos de anemia refratária para aumentar o hematócrito, a hemoglobina e a contagem de eritrócitos.

Cobb, Stanley, neuropatologista norte-americano, 1887–1968. VER C. *syndrome*.

co·bra (kō'bră). A maioria pertence ao gênero de serpentes extremamente venenosas, *Naja* (família Elapidae); são reconhecidas seis espécies, cinco africanas e uma asiática; o comportamento típico inclui movimentos do pescoço (capuz), elevação de um terço do corpo do solo e, em algumas espécies, o ato de cuspir veneno, que é basicamente neurotóxico. Também há outras que pertencem aos gêneros *Pseudohaje*, *Hemachatus* e *Ophiophagus*. [Port. cobra, do L. *coluber*, cobra]

co·bro·tox·in (kō'brō-tok-sin). Cobrotoxina; um polipeptídeo de 62 resíduos; a ação sobre as células é semelhante à da melitina porque promove a rup-

cobrotoxin / coccidium

tura das membranas; está sendo pesquisado seu uso como agente anti-reumático. SIN cobra toxin, direct lytic factor of cobra venom.

co·byr·ic ac·id (kō-bir'ik). Ácido cobírico; a hexamida do ácido cobirínico; uma parte da estrutura da vitamina B_{12}. SIN cobyrinamide, factor V_{1a}.

co·byr·in·a·mide (kō-bir-in'ă-mid). Cobirinamida. SIN cobyric acid.

co·byr·in·ic ac·id (kō-bir-in'ik). Ácido cobirínico; corrina com 8 grupamentos metil nas posições 1, 2, 5, 7, 12 (2), 15 e 17; grupamentos-CH_2COOH nas posições 2, 7 e 18; grupamentos-CH_2CH_2COOH nas posições 3, 8, 13 e 17; e cobalto divalente centralizado entre os quatro nitrogênios. As cadeias laterais ácidas são designadas, em ordem numérica, *a*, *b*, *c*, *d*, *e*, *f* e *g*. É uma parte da estrutura da vitamina B_{12}.

COC Abreviatura de cathodal opening *contraction* (contração de abertura catódica).

co·ca (kō'kă). Coca; as folhas secas da *Erythroxylon coca*, fornecendo não menos do que 0,5% de alcalóides solúveis em éter; a fonte da cocaína e de vários outros alcalóides. [América do Sul]

co·caine (kō-kān'). Cocaína; $C_{17}H_{21}NO_4$; benzoilmetilecgonina; alcalóide cristalino obtido das folhas da *Erythroxylon coca* (família Erythroxylaceae) e outras espécies de *Erythroxylon*, ou sintetizado a partir da ecgonina ou seus derivados; um potente estimulante do sistema nervoso central, vasoconstrictor e anestésico tópico, amplamente usado como euforiante e associado ao risco de graves efeitos físicos e mentais adversos.

O arbusto da coca é nativo da Bolívia e do Peru, onde, durante séculos, os nativos mascaram suas folhas juntamente com bolinhas calcárias ou cinzas vegetais para suportar a fome, a sede e a fadiga. Durante o século XIX, a cocaína foi amplamente usada em medicina como estimulante, antidepressivo e anestésico tópico, mas, devido ao seu forte potencial de induzir dependência, não é mais administrada sistemicamente. Sua popularidade como droga diminuiu um pouco com a disponibilidade das anfetaminas na década de 1920, mas ressurgiu na década de 1960. A cocaína geralmente é vendida na rua como o sal cloridrato, um pó fino branco geralmente conhecido como "coca", "branquinha", "neve", "pó" (nos Estados Unidos, "coke", "C", "snow", "flake" ou "blow"). Os traficantes de rua dissolvem-na ou adulteram com substâncias inertes como amido de milho, talco e açúcar, ou com drogas ativas como procaína e benzocaína. Na forma de pó, geralmente é "aspirada", embora também possa ser injetada ou absorvida pelas mucosas oral, vaginal ou retal. Pode-se preparar a cocaína na forma de um cigarro a partir do cloridrato (fumar "um baseado"). A produção da pasta básica de cocaína pura é perigosa porque emprega solventes altamente inflamáveis. A droga comumente denominada "crack" é uma forma bruta de pasta básica preparada a partir do cloridrato de cocaína com amônio ou bicarbonato de sódio e água. O produto endurecido resultante desse processo é quebrado em fragmentos irregulares denominados "pedras" (nos Estados Unidos, "rock", "ready rock", "french fries" ou "teeth"). O uso de "crack" nas ruas explodiu após sua introdução na década de 1980, causando aumentos das internações em pronto-socorros por superdosagem de cocaína, mortes relacionadas à droga e nascimento de bebês dependentes de cocaína.

A administração de cocaína provoca rapidamente euforia intensa, acompanhada por uma sensação de aumento da energia, alerta e autoconfiança e diminuição da necessidade de alimentos e sono. Há aumento da freqüência de pulso, pressão arterial e freqüência respiratória. Doses maiores podem causar comportamento bizarro ou violento, paranóia, dor torácica, tremores, convulsões, coma e morte por espasmo da artéria coronária ou parada respiratória. O "crack" fumado chega ao cérebro mais rapidamente que a cocaína inalada. Os efeitos de ambos desaparecem em menos de 30 minutos, sendo seguidos por depressão profunda, irritabilidade e fadiga ("bode do crack","*coke crash*"). O uso prolongado de cocaína causa sintomas crônicos, incluindo agitação, irritabilidade, depressão, insônia e uma psicose reversível caracterizada por paranóia, alucinações e delírios. A aspiração repetida de cocaína causa rinite, que pode culminar em perfuração do septo nasal. A cocaína não causa vício real porque não há desenvolvimento de tolerância; na verdade, alguns usuários regulares observam sensibilidade crescente aos seus efeitos físicos e psicológicos. Não obstante, pode haver desenvolvimento de dependência psicológica em menos de 2 semanas. A abstinência está associada a um desejo intenso de outra dose; a abstinência prolongada pode causar ansiedade, depressão e distúrbios do apetite e do sono.

crack c., "crack"; derivado da cocaína, geralmente fumado, resultando em um "barato" breve e intenso. O "crack" é relativamente barato e extremamente viciador. VER street *drug*.

c. hydrochloride, cloridrato de cocaína; sal hidrossolúvel usado para anestesia local do olho ou mucosas.

co·cain·i·za·tion (kō'kān-i-zā'shŭn). Cocainização; produção de anestesia tópica das mucosas pela aplicação de cocaína.

co·car·box·yl·ase (kō-kar-boks'i-lās). Cocarboxilase. SIN *thiamin pyrophosphate.*

co·car·cin·o·gen (kō-kar'si-nō-jen). Cocarcinógeno; substância que age simbioticamente com um carcinógeno na produção de câncer.

Coc·ca·ce·ae (kok-kā'sē-ē). Termo obsoleto para uma família de Eubacteriales que incluía todas as células esféricas dividindo-se em um (*Streptococcus*), dois (*Micrococcus*) ou três (*Sarcina*) planos, depois formando células, pares, tétrades, cubos ou estruturas maiores, ou cadeias. [G. *kokkos*, baga]

coc·cal (kok'ăl). Cocóide; relativo a cocos.

coc·ci (kok'sī). Plural de coccus.

Coc·cid·ia (kok-sid'ē-ă). Subclasse de protozoários importantes (classe Sporozoea, filo Apicomplexa) na qual os trofozoítas maduros são pequenos e tipicamente intracelulares; pode haver esquizogonia e esporogonia no mesmo hospedeiro, em contraste com as gregarinas (subclasse Gregarinia da classe Sporozoea), que possuem grandes trofozoítas extracelulares em vários invertebrados e não se reproduzem por esquizogonia. SIN Coccidiasina. [L. Mod., do G. *kokkos*, baga]

coc·cid·ia (kok-sid'ē-ă). Plural de coccidium.

coc·cid·i·al (kok-sid'ē-ăl). Coccídico; relativo aos coccídios.

Coc·ci·di·as·i·na (kok-sid'ē-ă-sī'nă). SIN Coccidia.

coc·cid·i·oi·dal (kok-sid-ē-oy'dăl). Coccidióidico; referente à doença ou ao microrganismo infeccioso da coccidioidomicose.

Coc·cid·i·oi·des (kok-sid-ē-oy'dēz). Gênero de fungos encontrado no solo das áreas semi-áridas do sudoeste dos Estados Unidos e em áreas menores na América Central e América do Sul, mas não foi encontrado em outros locais. A única espécie patogênica, *C. immitis*, causa coccidioidomicose. [coccidium + G. *eidos*, semelhança]

coc·cid·i·oi·din (kok-sid-ē-oy'din). Coccidioidina; solução estéril contendo os produtos derivados do crescimento do *Coccidioides immitis*; usado como teste intracutâneo, mais útil em termos diagnósticos em áreas não-endêmicas.

coc·cid·i·oi·do·ma (kok-sid'ē-oy-dō'mă). Coccidioidoma; lesão granulomatosa residual localizada benigna ou cicatriz no pulmão após coccidioidomicose primária.

coc·cid·i·oi·do·my·co·sis (kok-sid-ē-oy'dō-mī-kō'sis). Coccidioidomicose; micose sistêmica variável, benigna, grave ou algumas vezes fatal devido à inalação de artroconídios de *Coccidioides immitis*. Nas formas benignas da infecção, as lesões são limitadas às vias respiratórias superiores, pulmões e linfonodos próximos; em uma pequena percentagem de casos, a doença dissemina-se para outros órgãos viscerais, meninges, ossos, articulações e pele e tecidos subcutâneos. SIN Posadas disease. [coccidioides + G. *mykēs*, fungo, + *-osis*, condição]

disseminated c., c. disseminada; forma grave, crônica e progressiva de coccidioidomicose com disseminação do pulmão para outros órgãos. Os pacientes com essa doença geralmente apresentam imunocomprometimento significativo.

primary c., c. primária; uma doença comum no Vale de São Joaquim da Califórnia e em algumas outras áreas no sudoeste dos Estados Unidos, bem como na região Chaco da Argentina, causada por inalação dos artroconídios do *Coccidioides immitis*; início agudo de sintomas respiratórios acompanhados por febre, dores, mal-estar, artralgia, cefaléia e, ocasionalmente, uma erupção eritematosa ou papular incipiente; pode surgir eritema multiforme ou eritema nodoso. SIN desert fever, San Joaquin fever, San Joaquin Valley disease, San Joaquin Valley fever, valley fever.

primary extrapulmonary c., c. extrapulmonar primária; uma forma rara de coccidioidomicose que surge próximo de área de traumatismo local com nódulos firmes e indolores, ocorrendo em uma a duas semanas, acompanhada por adenopatia regional, com resolução espontânea em algumas semanas.

secondary c., c. secundária; lesões granulomatosas extrapulmonares progressivas ou disseminadas após coccidioidomicose primária. SIN coccidioidal granuloma.

subclinical c., c. subclínica; forma de coccidioidomicose que não faz o paciente procurar cuidados médicos porque os sintomas respiratórios são leves e autolimitados.

coc·cid·i·o·sis (kok-sid-ē-ō'sis). Coccidiose; nome coletivo de doenças causadas por qualquer espécie de coccídios; protozoonose comum e grave de muitas espécies de animais e aves domésticas e muitos animais selvagens mantidos em cativeiro; já foram descritas coccidiose intestinal e pulmonar em seres humanos com AIDS/SIDA.

coc·cid·i·o·stat (kok-sid'ē-ō-stat). Coccidiostático; agente químico geralmente acrescentado ao alimento de animais para inibir parcialmente ou retardar o desenvolvimento de coccidiose.

coc·cid·i·um, pl. **coc·cid·i·a** (kok-sid'ē-ŭm, -ē-ă). Coccídio; nome comum dado a parasitas protozoários (ordem Eucoccidiida) nos quais ocorre esquizogonia nas células epiteliais, geralmente no intestino, mas, em algumas espécies, nos ductos biliares e rim; o produto final da fusão sexual e diferenciação que ocorre no hospedeiro, o oocisto, geralmente passa para o solo nas fezes, sofre esporulação e, depois, atua como a forma infecciosa para outro hospedeiro. Os coccídios são parasitas na maioria das aves e mamíferos domésticos e selvagens, ocasionalmente em seres humanos, e são extremamente hospedeiro-específicos; a maioria não é patogênica, mas algumas espécies estão entre os patógenos mais graves e economicamente importantes, causando coccidiose em aves e mamíferos. VER *Isospora, Cryptosporidium.* [L. Mod. dim. de G. *kokkos*, baga]

coc·ci·nel·la (kok-sin-el′ä). Cochonilha, cochinilha. SIN cochineal.

coc·ci·nel·lin (kok-si-nel′in). Cochonilina; princípio corante derivado da cochonilha.

coc·co·bac·il·lary (kok′ō-bas′i-lār-ē). Cocobacilar. **1.** Relativo a um cocobacilo. **2.** Microrganismos que exibem formas cocóides, bacilares e intermediárias.

coc·co·ba·cil·lus (kok′ō-bā-sil′ŭs). Cocobacilo; um bastonete bacteriano curto, espesso, com formato de um coco oval ou ligeiramente alongado. [G. *kokkos*, baga]

coc·coid (kok′oyd). Cocóide; semelhante a um coco. [G. *kokkos*, baga, + *eidos*, semelhança]

coc·cu·lin (kok′ū-lin). Coculina. SIN picrotoxin.

coc·cus, pl. **coc·ci** (kok′ŭs, kok′sī). Coco. **1.** Bactéria de formato redondo, esferóide ou ovóide. **2.** SIN cochineal. [G. *kokkos*, baga]
   Neisser c., c. de Neisser. SIN *Neisseria gonorrhoeae.*
   Weichselbaum c., c. de Weichselbaum. SIN *Neisseria meningitidis.*

coc·cy·ceph·a·ly (kok′si-sef′ă-lē). Coccicefalia; malformação na qual o perfil cefálico sugere um bico. [G. *kokkyx*, cuco, + *kephalē*, cabeça)

coc·cy·dyn·ia (kok-sē-din′ē-ä). Coccidinia; dor na região coccígea. SIN coccygodynia, coccyodynia. [coccyx + G. *ŏdyne*, dor]

coc·cyg·eal (Co) (kok-sij′ē-äl). Coccígeo; relativo ao cóccix.

coc·cy·gec·to·my (kok-sē-jek′tō-mē). Coccigectomia; remoção do cóccix. [coccyx + G. *ektomē*, excisão]

coc·cyg·e·us Coccígeo. VER coccygeus *muscle.*

coc·cy·go·dyn·ia (kok′si-gō-din′ē-ä). Coccigodinia. SIN coccydynia. [coccyx + G. *odynē*, dor]

coc·cy·got·o·my (kok-sē-got′ō-mē). Coccigotomia; operação para liberar o cóccix de suas inserções. [coccyx + G. *tomē*, corte]

coc·cy·o·dyn·ia (kok′sē-ō-din′ē-ä). Cocciodinia. SIN coccydynia.

coc·cyx, gen. **coc·cy·gis,** pl. **coc·cy·ges** (kok′siks, -si-jis, -si-jēs) [TA]. Cóccix; pequeno osso na extremidade da coluna vertebral dos seres humanos, formado pela fusão de quatro vértebras rudimentares; articula-se acima com o sacro. SIN os coccygis [TA], coccygeal bone, tail bone. [G. *kokkyx*, cuco, o cóccix]

coch·i·neal (kotch′i-nēl) [C.I. 75470]. Cochonilha, cochinilha; os insetos fêmeas dessecados, *Coccus cacti*, encerrando as larvas jovens, ou o inseto fêmea dessecado, *Dactylopius coccus*, contendo ovos e larvas, dos quais é obtida a cochonilha; usada como agente de coloração e corante vermelho. SIN coccinella, coccus (2). [Esp. ant. *cochinilla*, tatuzinho, do G. *kokkinos*, baga]

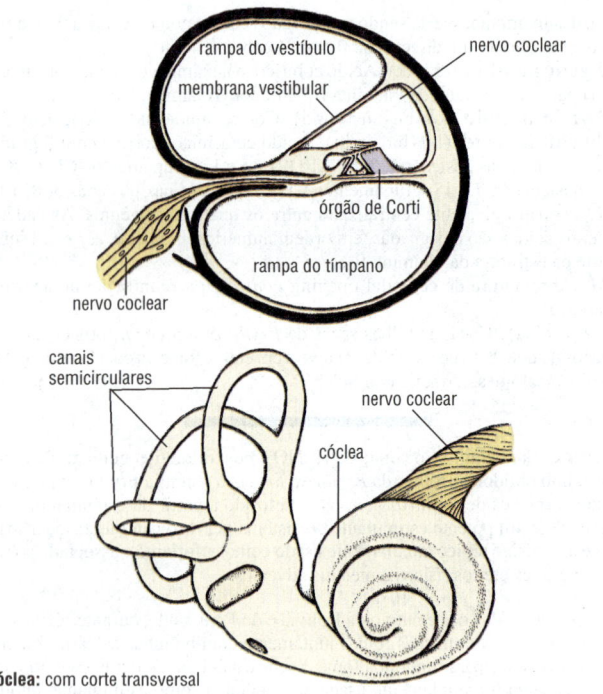

cóclea: com corte transversal

ℹ **co·chlea,** pl. **co·chle·ae** (kok′lē-ä, lē-ē) [TA]. Cóclea; uma cavidade cônica, na porção petrosa do osso temporal, que forma uma das divisões do labirinto ou ouvido interno. Consiste em um canal espiral que faz duas voltas e meia ao redor de um cerne de osso esponjoso, o modíolo; esse canal espiral da cóclea contém a cóclea membranosa ou ductus coclear, no qual se encontra o órgão espiral (de Corti). [L. concha de caramujo]
   membranous c., c. membranosa. SIN cochlear duct.

co·chle·ar (kok′lē-är). Coclear; relativo à cóclea.
   cochlear microphonic (kok′lē-är mī-krō-fon′ik), potencial coclear; potenciais bioelétricos produzidos pelas células pilosas do órgão de Corti em resposta ao som, que representam fielmente a freqüência e a intensidade da estimulação acústica. SIN cochlear potential, Wever-Bray phenomenon.

co·chle·a·re (kō-klē′ä, kok-lē-ä′rē). Uma colher. [L.]
   c. am′plum, uma colher de sopa cheia. [L.]
   c. mag′num, uma colher de sopa cheia. [L.]
   c. me′dium, uma colher de sobremesa cheia. [L.]
   c. mod′icum, uma colher de sobremesa cheia. [L.]
   c. par′vum, uma colher de chá cheia. [L.]

co·chle·ar·i·form (kok-lē-ar′i-fōrm). Cocleariforme; em forma de colher. [L. *cochleare*, colher, + *forma*, forma]

co·chle·ate (kok′lē-āt). Cocleado. **1.** Semelhante a uma concha de caramujo. **2.** Designa o aspecto de uma forma de placa de cultura. [L. *cochlea*, concha de caramujo]

coch·le·i·tis (kō-klē-ī′tis). Cocleíte; inflamação da cóclea. [cochlea + G. -*itis*, inflamação]

coch·le·o·sac·cu·lot·o·my (kok′lē-ō-sac-ū-lot′ō-mē). Cocleossaculotomia; operação para doença de Ménière realizada através da janela redonda para criar uma derivação (*shunt*) entre o ducto coclear e o sáculo.

coch·le·o·topic (kō-klē-ō-top′ik). Cocleotópico; referente à organização freqüência-responsiva das vias auditivas centrais no encéfalo. [cochlea + G. *topos*, lugar, + -*ic*]

co·chle·o·ves·tib·u·lar (kok′lē-ō-ves-tib′ū-lär). Cocleovestibular; relativo à cóclea e ao vestíbulo do ouvido.

Co·chli·o·my·ia (kok′lē-ō-mī′yä). Gênero de moscas varejeiras (família Calliphoridae) cujas larvas se desenvolvem em carne apodrecida ou carniças, ou em feridas ou úlceras.

   C. american′a, nome incorreto da *C. hominivorax.*
   C. homini′vorax, a larva de uma espécie que é uma peste grave em rebanhos do México à Argentina, sendo a causa primária de míases no hemisfério ocidental; atraída por sangue fresco, deposita ovos em feridas, picadas de carrapatos ou áreas úmidas intactas do corpo, e as larvas invadem tecidos vivos, causando míase grave e, freqüentemente, morte; sabe-se que ataca o homem, principalmente no nariz, embora também sejam atacadas as feridas, bem como os olhos e outras aberturas do corpo.

Cochrane, A.L., epidemiologista inglês, 1909–1988. VER C. *collaboration.*

co·cil·la·na (ko′sē-lah′nä). Cocilana; a casca seca da *Guarea rusbyi*, uma árvore boliviana, usada como expectorante na bronquite.

Cockayne, Edward A., médico inglês, 1880–1956. VER C. *disease, syndrome*; Weber-C. *syndrome.*

cock·tail (kok′tāl). Coquetel; uma mistura que inclui vários ingredientes ou drogas.
   Brompton c., c. Brompton; coquetel de morfina e cocaína geralmente usado para analgesia em pacientes com câncer terminal; as formulações variam, mas tipicamente há 15 mg de cloridrato de morfina e 10 mg de cloridrato de cocaína por 10 ml do coquetel. [*Brompton* Chest Hospital, London, England, onde foi desenvolvido]
   Philadelphia c., c. Filadélfia. SIN Rivers c.
   Rivers c., c. Rivers; uma infusão intravenosa lenta de 1.000 a 2.000 ml de glicose a 10% em solução salina isotônica à qual são adicionados cloridrato de tiamina e 25 unidades de insulina; usado no alcoolismo agudo. SIN Philadelphia c.

co·coa (kō′kō). Cacau; pó preparado a partir dos núcleos torrados das sementes maduras do *Theobroma cacao* (família Sterculiaceae); usado na preparação do xarope de cacau, um agente aromatizante. VER TAMBÉM cacao.

co·con·scious·ness (kō-kon′shŭs-nes). Co-consciência. **1.** Uma divisão da consciência em duas correntes. **2.** Consciência por uma personalidade dos pensamentos de outra personalidade no distúrbio dissociativo.

co·con·ver·sion (kō′kon-ver′shŭn). Co-conversão; a correção simultânea de dois locais no DNA durante a conversão genética.

△ **cocto-.** Prefixo indicando fervido ou modificado pelo calor. [L. *coctus*, cozido]

coc·to·la·bile (kok-tō-lā′bil, -bīl). Coctolábil; sujeito à alteração ou destruição quando exposto à temperatura de água fervente.

coc·to·sta·bile, coc·to·sta·ble (kok-tō-stā′bil, -bīl; -stā′bl). Coctoestável; resistente à temperatura da água fervente sem sofrer alteração ou destruição.

code (kōd). Código. **1.** Um conjunto de regras, princípios ou determinações éticas. **2.** Qualquer sistema projetado para fornecer informações ou facilitar a comunicação. **3.** Termo usado em hospitais para descrever uma emergência que exige membros da equipe treinados para a situação, como uma equipe de reanimação cardiopulmonar, ou o sinal para chamar essa equipe. **4.** Um sistema numérico para solicitar e classificar informações, p. ex., sobre categorias diagnósticas. [L. *codex*, livro]

ℹ **genetic c.,** c. genético; as informações genéticas transportadas pelas moléculas de DNA específicas dos cromossomas; especificamente, o sistema no qual

código genético					
1. Posição	2. Posição				3. Posição
	U(A)	C(G)	A(T)	G(C)	
U(A)	Phe	Ser	Tyr	Cys	U(A)
	Phe	Ser	Tyr	Cys	C(G)
	Leu	Ser	Fim	Fim	A(T)
	Leu	Ser	Fim	Trp	G(C)
C(G)	Leu	Pro	His	Arg	U(A)
	Leu	Pro	His	Arg	C(G)
	Leu	Pro	Gln	Arg	A(T)
	Leu	Pro	Gln	Arg	G(C)
A(T)	Ile	Thr	Asn	Ser	U(A)
	Ile	Thr	Asn	Ser	C(G)
	Ile	Thr	Lys	Arg	A(T)
	Met	Thr	Lys	Arg	G(C)
G(C)	Val	Ala	Asp	Gly	U(A)
	Val	Ala	Asp	Gly	C(G)
	Val	Ala	Glu	Gly	A(T)
	Val	Ala	Glu	Gly	G(C)

O denominado "léxico do código": mostra a relação de códons de mRNA (entre parênteses) com os aminoácidos codificados. As trincas são dispostas de acordo com as bases de ácido nucleico (A = adenina; C = citosina; G = guanina; T = timina; U = uracil; "Fim" (branco) indica códons de terminação da cadeia). As três cores indicam se os aminoácidos são hidrofóbicos (amarelo), hidrofílicos (azul) ou ambifílicos (rosa).

determinadas combinações de três nucleotídeos consecutivos (códon) em uma molécula de DNA controlam a inserção de um determinado aminoácido em locais equivalentes em uma molécula de proteína. O c. genético é quase universal em todos os reinos, procariótico, vegetal e animal. Há duas exceções conhecidas. Em protozoários ciliados, os códons AGA e AGG são lidos como sinais de terminação, e não como L-arginina. Isso também é válido para o código mitocondrial humano, que, além disso, usa AUA como código para L-metionina (em vez de isoleucina) e UGA para L-triptofano (em vez de um sinal de terminação).
soundex c., c. soundex; sistema soundex; uma seqüência de letras usadas para registrar nomes foneticamente, principalmente no encadeamento de registros.
co·deine (kō′dēn). Codeína; obtida do ópio, que contém 0,7 a 2,5%, mas geralmente produzida a partir da morfina. Usada como analgésico e antitussígeno; pode surgir dependência (física e psíquica), mas a codeína é menos propensa a causar vício que a morfina; a codeína é biotransformada em morfina, responsável pela maioria dos seus efeitos. SIN methylmorphine. [G. *kōdeia*, cabeça, cabeça de papoula]
Co·dex med·i·ca·men·tar·i·us (kō′deks med′i - ka - men - tār′ē - ŭs). O título oficial da Farmacopéia Francesa. [L. um livro sobre drogas]
cod·ing. Codificação; tradução de informações, p. ex., diagnósticos, respostas a questionários, em categorias numeradas para entrada em um sistema de processamento de dados.
place coding, codificação de lugar; codificação de freqüência determinada pela ativação do órgão de Corti da base até o ápice da cóclea em uma gradação com freqüências maiores, transmitidas de um local próximo à base, e freqüências menores de um local próximo ao ápice.
cod liv·er oil. Óleo de fígado de bacalhau; o óleo fixo, parcialmente desesterarinizado, extraído dos fígados frescos do bacalhau (*Gadus morrhuae*) e de outras espécies da família Gadidae, contendo vitaminas A e D; usado como fonte suplementar de vitaminas A e D.
Codman, Ernest Amory, cirurgião norte-americano, 1869–1940. VER C. *triangle, tumor.*
co·do·gen·ic (kō - dō - jen - ik). Codogênico; formado por um código; especificamente, o código genético.
co·dom·i·nant (kō - dom′i - nant). Co-dominante; em genética, designa um grau igual de dominância de dois genes, ambos sendo expressos no fenótipo do indivíduo; p. ex., os genes A e B do grupo sanguíneo ABO são co-dominantes; as pessoas com ambos são tipo AB.
co·don (kō′don). Códon; um grupo de três nucleotídeos consecutivos em um filamento de DNA ou RNA que fornece as informações genéticas para codificar um aminoácido específico que será incorporado a uma cadeia proteica ou servir como sinal de terminação. SIN triplet (3). [code + -on]
amber c., o códon de terminação UAG.
initiating c., códon iniciador; o trinucleotídeo AUG (ou algumas vezes GUG) que codifica o primeiro aminoácido nas seqüências proteicas, formilmetionina; o último freqüentemente é removido após a transcrição. SIN start c.
initiation c., c. de iniciação; uma seqüência de mRNA (ou ARNm) específica (geralmente AUG, mas algumas vezes GUG) que é o sinal para a adição de fMet-tRNA e o início da tradução.
nonsense c., c. de terminação. SIN termination c.
ochre c., o códon de terminação UAA.
opal c., c. de terminação UGA. SIN umber c.
punctuation c., c. finalizador ou de terminação. SIN termination c.
start c., c. de iniciação. SIN initiating c.
stop c., c. de terminação. SIN termination c.
termination c., c. de terminação; seqüência de trinucleotídeos (UAA, UGA ou UAG) que especifica o fim da tradução ou transcrição. Cf. amber c., ochre c., umber c. SIN nonsense c., punctuation c., stop c., termination sequence, termination signal.
umber c., o c. de terminação UGA. SIN opal c.
coe-. As palavras que começarem desse modo, e não forem encontradas aqui, devem ser procuradas em ce-.
co·ef·fi·cient (kō - ē - fish′ent). Coeficiente. **1.** A expressão da quantidade ou grau de qualquer qualidade de uma substância, ou do grau de alteração física ou química que normalmente ocorre nessa substância, sob determinadas condições. **2.** A razão ou fator que relaciona uma quantidade observada sob uma série de condições àquela observada em condições padronizadas, geralmente quando todas as variáveis são 1 ou uma simples potência de 10. [L. *co-* + *efficio* (*exfacio*), realizar]
absorption c., c. de absorção; (**1**) os mililitros de um gás em determinadas condições de temperatura e pressão que saturarão 100 ml de líquido; (**2**) a quantidade de luz absorvida ao atravessar 1 cm de uma solução molar de determinada substância, expressa como uma constante na lei de Beer-Lambert; Cf. specific absorption c.; (**3**) uma medida da taxa de diminuição da intensidade de um feixe de raios X em sua passagem através de uma substância, resultante de uma combinação de dispersão e conversão em outras formas de energia.
activity c. (γ), c. de atividade. VER activity (2).
biological c., c. biológico; termo raramente usado que designa a energia despendida pelo corpo em repouso.
Bunsen solubility c. (α), solubilidade de Bunsen; os mililitros de gás nas CNTP (condições normais de temperatura e pressão) dissolvidos por mililitro de líquido e pela pressão parcial atmosférica (760 mm Hg) do gás em qualquer temperatura predeterminada.
c. of consanguinity, c. de consangüinidade. SIN c. of inbreeding.
correlation c., c. de correlação; medida de associação que indica o grau com que duas variáveis possuem uma relação linear; esse coeficiente, representado pela letra r, pode variar entre +1 e −1; quando r = +1, há uma relação linear positiva perfeita na qual uma variável está diretamente relacionada com a outra; quando r = −1, há uma relação linear negativa perfeita entre as variáveis.
creatinine c., c. de creatinina; o número de miligramas de creatinina excretados diariamente por quilograma de peso corporal.
diffusion c., c. de difusão; a massa de material que se difunde através de uma unidade de área em uma unidade de tempo sob uma unidade de gradiente de concentração. SIN diffusion constant.
distribution c., c. de distribuição; a relação de concentrações de uma substância em duas fases imiscíveis em equilíbrio; a base de muitos procedimentos de separação cromatográficos. SIN partition c.
economic c., c. econômico; no crescimento e cultivo de microrganismos, a relação entre a massa produzida e o substrato consumido.
extinction c. (ε), c. de extinção. SIN specific absorption c.
extraction c., c. de extração; a percentagem de uma substância removida do sangue ou plasma em uma única passagem através de um tecido; p. ex., o c. de extração do ácido *p*-amino-hipúrico (PAH) no rim é a diferença entre as concentrações plasmáticas arterial e venosa renal de PAH, dividida pela concentração plasmática arterial de PAH.
filtration c., c. de filtração; uma medida da permeabilidade de uma membrana à água; especificamente, o volume de líquido filtrado na unidade de tempo através de uma unidade de área de membrana por unidade de diferença de pressão, levando em conta as pressões hidráulica e osmótica.
Hill c., c. de Hill; a inclinação da linha em um gráfico de Hill; uma medida do grau de cooperatividade. SIN Hill constant.
hygienic laboratory c., c. de higiene laboratorial. SIN Rideal-Walker c.
c. of inbreeding, c. de endogamia; a probabilidade de que a prole de um casamento consangüíneo seja homozigota para um alelo autossômico específico derivado de um ancestral comum. SIN c. of consanguinity.
isotonic c., c. isotônico; a quantidade de sais no plasma sanguíneo, ou a quantidade que deve ser adicionada à água destilada a fim de preparar uma solução isotônica.
c. of kinship, c. de parentesco; a probabilidade de que dois genes no mesmo *locus*, escolhidos aleatoriamente de dois indivíduos, sejam idênticos por descendência.

lethal c., c. letal; a concentração de desinfetante que mata bactérias a 20-25°C no menor período de tempo.

linear absorption c., c. de absorção linear; aquela fração de radiação ionizante absorvida em uma unidade de espessura de uma substância ou tecido. VER TAMBÉM absorption c. (3); Cf. attenuation.

Long c., c. de Long. SIN Long formula.

molar absorption c. (ε), c. de absorção molar; absorvência (de luz) ou densidade óptica por unidade de comprimento do trajeto (geralmente o centímetro) e por unidade de concentração (moles por litro); uma unidade fundamental em espectrofotometria. SIN absorbancy index (2), absorptivity (2), molar absorbancy index, molar absorptivity, molar extinction c.

molar extinction c., c. de extinção molar. SIN molar absorption c.

Ostwald solubility c. (Λ), os mililitros de gás dissolvidos por mililitro de líquido e por pressão parcial atmosférica (760 mm Hg) do gás em qualquer temperatura. Este difere do c. de solubilidade de Bunsen (α) porque a quantidade de gás dissolvido é expressa em termos de seu volume na temperatura da experiência, e não nas CNTP (condições normais de temperatura e pressão). Assim, $\lambda = \alpha (1 + 0{,}00367t)$, onde t = temperatura em graus Celsius.

oxygen utilization c., c. de utilização do oxigênio; o coeficiente de extração de oxigênio em qualquer tecido determinado.

partition c., c. de partição, c. de decomposição. SIN distribution c.

permeability c., c. de permeabilidade; um coeficiente associado à difusão simples através de uma membrana que é proporcional ao coeficiente de partição (decomposição) e ao coeficiente de difusão e inversamente proporcional à espessura da membrana.

phenol c., c. fenólico. SIN Rideal-Walker c.

Poiseuille viscosity c., c. de viscosidade de Poiseuille; uma expressão da viscosidade determinada pelo método do tubo capilar; o coeficiente $\eta = (\pi P r^4 / 8vl)$, onde P é a diferença de pressão entre a entrada e a saída do tubo, r o raio do tubo, l seu comprimento e v o volume de líquido administrado no tempo t. Se o volume estiver em centímetros cúbicos, o tempo em segundos, e l e r em centímetros, η estará em poise.

reflection c. (σ), c. de reflexão; medida da permeabilidade relativa de uma determinada membrana a um determinado soluto; calculado como a razão entre a pressão osmótica observada e aquela calculada a partir da lei de van't Hoff; também é igual a 1 menos a razão das áreas de poros efetivas disponíveis para o soluto e o solvente.

c. of relationship, c. de relacionamento; a probabilidade de que um gene presente em um cônjuge também esteja presente no outro e tenha a mesma origem.

reliability c., c. de confiabilidade; índice da consistência de medidas baseado freqüentemente na correlação entre escores obtidos no teste inicial e um reteste (confiabilidade do teste-reteste) ou entre escores em duas formas semelhantes do mesmo teste (confiabilidade forma-equivalente).

respiratory c., c. respiratório. SIN respiratory *quotient*.

Rideal-Walker c., c. de Rideal-Walker; valor que exprime o poder desinfetante de qualquer substância; é obtido dividindo-se o valor que indica o grau de diluição do desinfetante que mata um microrganismo em um determinado tempo pelo valor que indica o grau de diluição de fenol que mata o microrganismo no mesmo intervalo de tempo em condições semelhantes. SIN hygienic laboratory c., phenol c.

sedimentation c. (s), c. de sedimentação. SIN sedimentation *constant*.

selection c. (s), c. de seleção; a proporção de descendentes ou possíveis descendentes que não sobrevive à maturidade sexual; em geral é definido artificialmente pela expressão da aptidão de um fenótipo como uma fração da média ou adaptação ótima para fornecer a aptidão relativa, e subtraindo-se essa fração da unidade. Se o tamanho médio da família na população for de 3,2 e o do genótipo específico for 2,4, então a adaptação do fenótipo é de 2,4/3,2 = 0,75 e o coeficiente de seleção é 1 − 0,75 = 0,25.

specific absorption c. (a), c. de absorção específica; absorvência (da luz) por unidade de comprimento do trajeto (geralmente o centímetro) e por unidade de concentração da massa. Cf. molar absorption c. SIN absorbancy index (1), absorptivity (1), extinction c., specific extinction.

temperature c., c. de temperatura; modificação fracionada em qualquer propriedade física por aumento de um grau na temperatura.

ultrafiltration c., c. de ultrafiltração; o coeficiente de filtração de uma membrana semipermeável.

c. of variation (CV), c. de variação; a razão entre o desvio-padrão e a média.

velocity c., c. de velocidade; a velocidade de transformação de uma unidade de massa da substância em uma reação química.

c. of viscosity, c. de viscosidade; o valor da força por unidade de área necessário para manter uma unidade de velocidade relativa entre dois planos paralelos afastados em uma unidade de distância.

Coe·len·ter·a·ta (sē-len-tē-rā′tă). Um dos principais filos de invertebrados, ao qual pertencem formas como a medusa.

coe·len·ter·ate (sē-len′ter-at). Celenterados; nome comum de membros do filo Coelenterata.

coe·lom (sē′lom). Celoma. SIN body *cavity*.

co·en·es·the·sia (kō-en-es-thē′zē-ă). Cenestesia. SIN cenesthesia.

coeno-. Ter em comum. VER TAMBÉM ceno-. [G. *koinos*, comum]

coe·no·cyte (sē′nō-sit). Cenócito. SIN cenocyte.

coe·no·cyt·ic (sē-nō-sit′ik). Cenocítico. SIN cenocytic.

coe·nu·ro·sis (sē-noo-rō′sis). Cenurose. SIN cenurosis.

Coe·nu·rus (sē-noo′rŭs). Anteriormente nome genérico, agora usado para designar formas larvares de cestódeos tenióides nos quais uma bexiga é formada, com vários escóleces invaginados desenvolvendo-se em seu interior; diferente de um cisto hidático pela ausência de colônias de cistos-filhos, flutuando livremente, brotados na bexiga; larvas de *Coenurus* são encontradas em membros do gênero *Multiceps*. [G. *koinos*, comum, + *oura*, cauda]

C. cerebra'lis, as larvas cenuros da tênia *Multiceps multiceps*, encontradas no encéfalo e na medula espinhal de carneiros, cabras e outros ruminantes (alguns foram registrados em seres humanos); os adultos são encontrados no intestino de cães, raposas, coiotes e chacais.

C. seria'lis, as larvas cenuros da tênia *Multiceps serialis*, encontradas nos tecidos subcutâneos e intramusculares de coelhos e lebres (alguns foram registrados em seres humanos); os vermes adultos são encontrados no intestino de cães, raposas e chacais.

co·en·zyme (kō-en′zīm) Coenzima; uma substância (excluindo íons metálicos desacompanhados) que estimula a ação das enzimas ou é necessária para esta; as coenzimas têm menor tamanho molecular que as próprias enzimas, são dialisáveis e relativamente termoestáveis e, em geral, facilmente dissociáveis da porção proteica da enzima; várias vitaminas são precursoras das coenzimas. SIN cofactor (1).

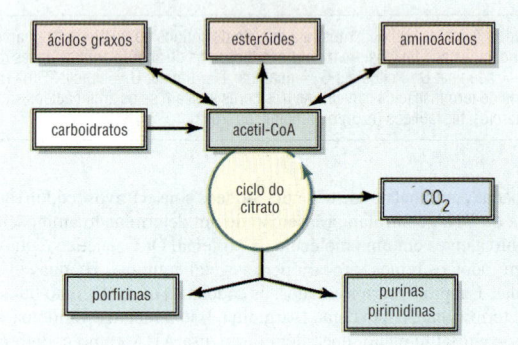

coenzima: posição central da acetilcoenzima A na troca de substâncias intermediárias

co·en·zyme A (CoA). Coenzima A; uma coenzima que contém ácido pantotênico, 3'-fosfato 5'-pirofosfato de adenosina e cisteamina; envolvida na transferência de grupamentos acila, notavelmente em transacetilações.

co·en·zyme F (kō-en′zīm). Coenzima F. SIN tetrahydrofolic acid.

co·en·zyme Q (CoQ, Q). Coenzima Q; quinonas com cadeias laterais isoprenóides (especificamente, ubiquinonas) que mediam a transferência de elétrons entre citocromo *b* e citocromo *c*; quimicamente semelhante às vitaminas E e K, e a outros tocoferóis, quinonas e tocóis.

co·en·zyme R. Coenzima R. SIN biotin.

coeur (koor). Coração. SIN heart. [Fr.]

c. en sabot (awn sah-bo′), c. em tamanco; a configuração radiográfica do coração na tetralogia de Fallot; o ápice elevado produz uma silhueta semelhante à de um tamanco de madeira. SIN sabot heart, wooden-shoe heart.

co·ev·o·lu·tion (kō-ev-ō-loo′shŭn). Coevolução; o processo pelo qual genes ou fragmentos de genes estão se modificando juntos, e não divergindo.

co·fac·tor (kō′fak′ter, tor). Co-fator. **1.** SIN coenzyme. **2.** Um átomo ou molécula essencial para a ação de uma grande molécula; p. ex., heme na hemoglobina, magnésio na clorofila. Os íons metálicos desacompanhados (solo) são considerados co-fatores para proteínas, mas não como coenzimas.

cobra venom c., c. do veneno de serpentes venenosas elapídeas; equivalente em ação ao C3B, o que significa que pode ativar a via alternativa do complemento.

molybdenum c. (mō-lib′dĕ-nŭm), c. do molibdênio; complexo de molibdênio e molibdopterina necessário para várias enzimas. Uma deficiência desse co-fator resultará em menor atividade da sulfito oxidase, xantina desidrogenase e aldeído oxidase, causando níveis elevados de sulfito, tiossulfito, xantina, etc.

platelet c. I, c. plaquetário I. SIN *factor* VIII.

platelet c. II, c. plaquetário II. SIN *factor* IX.

Coffey, Robert, cirurgião norte-americano, 1869–1933. VER C. *suspension*.

Coffin, Grange S., pediatra norte-americano, *1923. VER C.-Lowry *syndrome*; C.-Siris *syndrome*.

Cogan, David G., oftalmologista norte-americano, 1908–1993. VER C. *syndrome*; C.-Reese *syndrome*.

cog·ni·tion (kog-ni′shŭn). Cognição. **1.** Termo genérico que compreende as atividades mentais associadas ao raciocínio, aprendizado e memória. **2.** Qualquer processo em que se adquire conhecimento. [L. *cognitio*]

cog·ni·tive (kog′ni-tiv). Cognitivo; relativo à cognição.

co·he·sion (kō-hē′zhŭn). Coesão; a atração entre moléculas ou massas que as mantém unidas. [L. *co-haereo*, pp. *-haesus*, colar]

Cohnheim, Julius F., histologista, patologista e fisiologista alemão, 1839–1884. VER C. *area, field.*

co·ho·ba (kō-hō′bă). Cooba; substância alucinógena psicotomimética obtida da *Acacia niopo* (família Leguminosae), uma planta da América Central, *Piptadenia peregrina* e outros vegetais; entre seus constituintes estão a bufotenina e a dimetiltriptamina; usada em locais nativos como inalações ou enemas.

co·hort (kō′hort). Coorte. **1.** Componente da população nascido durante um determinado período e identificado por período de nascimento, de forma que suas características possam ser determinadas à medida que envelhece. **2.** Qualquer grupo designado seguido ou acompanhado durante um período, como em um estudo de coortes epidemiológico. [L. *cohors*, séquito, unidade militar]

coil (koyl). Bobina solenóide **1.** Uma espiral ou série de alças. **2.** Um objeto feito de fios enrolados em configuração espiral, usado em aplicações eletrônicas, ou uma alça de fio usada como antena. **3.** Uma alça espiral de fio usada para embolizar uma artéria ou obstruí-la.

detector c., b. detectora; bobina usada em ressonância magnética como antena para registrar emissões de radiofreqüência de núcleos estimulados, p. ex., bobina corporal, bobina cefálica.

random c., espiral aleatória, hélice aleatória; estrutura de uma macromolécula (tipicamente, um biopolímero) que se modifica com o tempo.

surface c., b. de superfície; bobina detectora aplicada diretamente a uma parte do corpo para ressonância magnética de alta resolução; freqüentemente uma aiça de metal.

coin-count·ing (koyn′kownt′ing). Contagem de moedas; movimento deslizante das extremidades do polegar e do indicador que ocorre na paralisia agitante.

co·in·te·grate. Co-integrada; estrutura resultante da transposição replicativa onde o transposon é duplicado.

co·i·tal (kō′i-tăl). Relativo ao coito.

Coiter (Koyter), Volcher, cirurgião e anatomista holandês, 1534–1576. VER C. *muscle.*

co·i·tion (kō-ish′ŭn). Coito. SIN coitus. [L. *co-eo*, pp. *-itus*, aproximar]

co·i·to·pho·bia (kō′i-tō-fō′bē-ă). Coitofobia; temor mórbido de relações sexuais. [L. *coitus*, relação sexual, + G. *phobos*, medo]

co·i·tus (kō′i-tŭs). Coito; união sexual entre macho e fêmea. SIN coition, copulation (1), pareunia, sexual intercourse. [L.]

c. interrup′tus, c. interrompido; interrupção da relação sexual antes de o homem ejacular.

c. reserva′tus, c. reservado; c. no qual a ejaculação é adiada ou suprimida.

Co·ker·o·my·ces (kō′ker-ō-mī′sēz). Gênero de fungo da ordem Mucorales; causa rara de doença no homem.

col (kol). Uma área crateriforme da mucosa oral interproximal unindo as papilas interdentárias lingual e bucal.

△ **col-.** VER con-.

co·la (kō′lă). Cola. **1.** SIN kola. **2.** [L.] percolar (forma imperativa).

col·chi·cine (kol′chi-sin) [USP]. Colchicina; alcalóide obtido do *Colchicum autumnale* (família Liliaceae); usada no tratamento crônico da gota. Inibe a formação de microtúbulos.

Col·chi·cum corm (kōl′chī-kum). Cormo de *Colchicum;* cormo seco de *Colchicum autumnale,* a origem botânica da colchicina, um alcalóide usado no tratamento da gota.

cold (kōld). **1.** Frio; baixa temperatura; a sensação produzida por uma temperatura notavelmente abaixo da temperatura a que se está acostumado ou de um nível confortável. **2.** Resfriado; termo popular para uma infecção viral que envolve as vias respiratórias superiores e é caracterizada por congestão das mucosas, secreção nasal aquosa e mal-estar generalizado, com duração de 3-5 dias. VER TAMBÉM rhinitis, coryza. SIN frigid (1).

head c., Rinite aguda SIN acute rhinitis.

rose c., polinose; febre do feno; rinite alérgica sazonal; rinite alérgica que ocorre na primavera e no início do verão.

cold-blood·ed (kōld-blŭd′ed). De sangue frio; pecilotérmico. SIN poikilothermic.

Coldman, Andrew James, epidemiologista canadense do século XX (1952–). VER Goldie-C. *hypothesis.*

Cole, Laurent, patologista francês, *1903. VER Benedict-Hopkins-C. *reagent.*

Cole, Rufus Ivory, médico norte-americano, 1872–1966.

Cole, Warren Henry, cirurgião, *1898. Co-desenvolvedor, com E.A. Graham, da colecistografia, descrita pela primeira vez em 1924. VER Graham-Cole *test.*

Cole-Cecil mur·mur. Sopro de Cole-Cecil. Ver em murmur.

co·lec·ta·sia (kō-lek-tā′zē-ă). Colectasia; distensão do cólon. [G. *kolon*, cólon, + *ektasis*, distensão]

col·ec·to·my (kō-lek′tō-mē). Colectomia; excisão de um segmento ou de todo o cólon. [G. *kolon*, cólon, + *ektomē*, excisão]

△ **coleo-.** Bainha, especificamente, a vagina. [G. *koleos*, bainha]

Co·le·op·te·ra (kō-lē-op′ter-ă). Ordem de insetos, os besouros, caracterizada por possuírem um par de asas duras, córneas, que se sobrepõem a um par de asas membranosas delicadas; é a maior das ordens de insetos, com o maior número de espécies de qualquer ordem animal ou vegetal. [G. *koleos*, bainha, + *pteron*, asa]

co·le·op·to·sis (kō-le-op′tō-sis). Coleoptose. SIN coloptosis.

co·le·ot·o·my (kol-e-ot′ō-mē). Coleotomia. SIN colpotomy. [G. *koleos*, bainha, + *tomē*, incisão]

co·les·ti·pol (kō-les′ti-pol). Colestipol; agente antilipêmico semelhante à colestiramina.

colet. Abreviatura do L. *coletur*, deixar filtrar, percolar.

co·li·bac·il·lo·sis (kō′li-bas-i-lō′sis). Colibacilose; doença diarreica causada pela bactéria *Escherichia coli*. Freqüentemente denominada colibacilose entérica.

co·li·ba·cil·lus, pl. **co·li·ba·cil·li** (kō′li-bă-sil′ŭs). Colibacilo. SIN *Escherichia coli.*

col·ic (kol′ik). **1.** Cólico; relativo ao cólon. **2.** Cólica, dor espasmódica no abdome. **3.** Cólica; em lactentes pequenos, paroxismos de dor gastrointestinal, com choro e irritabilidade, com várias causas, como deglutição de ar, perturbação emocional ou alimentação excessiva. [G. *kōlikos*, relativo ao cólon]

appendicular c., c. apendicular; dor em caráter de cólica que ocorre no início da apendicite aguda. SIN vermicular c.

biliary c., c. biliar; dor espasmódica intensa no hipocôndrio decorrente da impacção de um cálculo biliar no ducto cístico. SIN gallstone c., hepatic c.

copper c., cólica cúprica; afecção, semelhante à cólica plúmbica, que ocorre na intoxicação crônica pelo cobre.

Devonshire c., c. de Devonshire. SIN lead c.

gallstone c., c. biliar. SIN biliary c.

gastric c., c. gástrica; dor tipo cólica associada à gastrite ou úlcera péptica.

hepatic c., c. hepática. SIN biliary c.

infantile c., c. do lactente; episódios de dor abdominal causados por contração muscular anormal do intestino em lactentes.

lead c., c. plúmbica; dor abdominal em caráter de cólica intensa, com constipação, sintomática da intoxicação por chumbo. SIN Devonshire c., painter's c., Poitou c., saturnine c.

meconial c., c. meconial; dor abdominal de recém-nascidos.

menstrual c., c. menstrual; dor abdominal baixa, em caráter de cólica, associada à menstruação.

ovarian c., c. ovariana; dor abdominal baixa causada por torção de um ovário, como em um cisto ovariano.

painter's c., c. do pintor, cólica plúmbica. SIN lead c.

pancreatic c., c. pancreática; dor abdominal, em caráter de cólica intensa, semelhante à da cólica biliar, causada pela eliminação de um cálculo pancreático.

Poitou c., c. de Poitou, cólica plúmbica. SIN lead c.

renal c., c. renal; dor intensa em caráter de cólica, causada pela impacção ou passagem de um cálculo no ureter ou na pelve renal.

salivary c., c. salivar; crises periódicas de dor, na região de um ducto ou glândula salivar, acompanhada por tumefação aguda da glândula, que ocorre em casos de cálculo salivar.

saturnine c., c. saturnina, c. plúmbica. SIN lead c.

tubal c., c. tubária; dor abdominal baixa causada por contração espasmódica do oviduto excitado por um coágulo sanguíneo, outro irritante ou injeção de gás ou óleo.

ureteral c., c. ureteral; paroxismo de dor devido à obstrução aguda do ureter por um cálculo ou coágulo sanguíneo na maioria dos casos.

uterine c., c. uterina; cólicas dolorosas do músculo uterino que ocorrem algumas vezes no período menstrual, ou associada a doença uterina.

vermicular c., c. vermicular. SIN appendicular c.

zinc c., c. do zinco; c. zíncica; cólica resultante de intoxicação crônica pelo zinco.

col·i·ca (kol′i-kă). Cólica; uma artéria cólica. VER artery.

col·i·cin (kol′i-sin). Colicina; bacteriocina produzida por cepas de *Escherichia coli* e por outras enterobactérias (*Shigella* e *Salmonella*) que transportam os plasmídeos necessários. Muitas são tóxicas para cepas bacterianas relacionadas e ligam-se a receptores celulares específicos, interferindo com a função normal. [(*Escherichia*) *coli* + bacteriocina]

col·i·ci·nog·e·ny (kol′i-si-noj′ē-nē). Colicinogenia; propriedade bacteriana de produzir uma colicina.

col·icky (kol′i-kē). Colicativo; que designa a dor em cólica ou a ela se assemelha.

col·i·co·ple·gia (kol′i-kō-plē′jē-ă). Colicoplegia; intoxicação pelo chumbo caracterizada por cólica e paralisia. [G. *kolikos*, que sofre de cólica, + *plēgē*, parada]

co·li·my·cin (kō-li-mī'sin). Colimicina. SIN colistin.
col·in·e·ar·i·ty (kol'in-ē-ar'i-tē). Colinearidade. **1.** Deitado em linha reta. **2.** Os fenômenos em que a ordenação dos elementos correspondentes do DNA, do RNA dele transcrito e da seqüência de aminoácidos traduzida a partir do RNA é idêntica. [L. *collineo*, direcionar em uma linha reta]
co·li·pase (kō'lip-ās). Colipase; uma pequena proteína no suco pancreático essencial para a ação eficiente da lipase pancreática. Esse co-fator inibe a desnaturação de superfície da lipase. [co- + lipase]
co·li·phage (kō'li-fāj, kol'i-). Colífago; um bacteriófago com afinidade por uma ou outra cepa de *Escherichia coli*. Em geral, os colífagos, como outros bacteriófagos, são conhecidos por símbolos que só têm importância como forma de identificação laboratorial; outras notações, entretanto, identificam especificamente características variantes, p. ex., λdgal designa o prófago deficiente (colífago) λ, que transporta o gene bacteriano *gal* (galactose). [*(Escherichia) coli* + bacteriófago]
co·li·pli·ca·tion (kō'li-pli-kā'shŭn). Coliplicatura. SIN coloplication.
co·li·punc·ture (kō'li-pŭnk-choor). Colipunctura. SIN colocentesis.
co·lis·ti·meth·ate so·di·um (kō-lis-ti-meth'āt). Colistimetato sódico; contém o sal pentassódico do derivado penta (ácido metanossulfônico) da colistina A como principal componente, com uma pequena proporção do sal pentassódico do mesmo derivado da colistina B; antibiótico efetivo contra a maioria dos bacilos Gram-negativos (exceto *Proteus*), administrado por via intramuscular. VER TAMBÉM colistin sulfate, polymyxin. SIN cholistine sulphomethate sodium, colistin sulfomethate sodium.
co·lis·tin (kō-lis'tin). Colistina; colimicina; uma mistura de antibióticos polipeptídeos cíclicos de uma cepa de *Bacillus polymyxa*; separável em polimixinas. SIN colimycin.
c. sulfate, sulfato de colistina; o sal sulfato de uma substância antibacteriana produzida pelo crescimento de uma cepa de *Bacillus polymyxa*, que consiste basicamente em colistina A com pequenas quantidades de colistina B; é efetivo contra a maioria das bactérias Gram-negativas (exceto *Proteus*); administrado por via oral para ação antibacteriana intestinal. VER TAMBÉM colistimethate sodium, polymyxin.
c. sulfomethate sodium, sulfometato sódico de colistina. SIN colistimethate sodium.
co·li·tis (kō-lī'tis). Colite; inflamação do cólon. [G. *kōlon*, cólon, + *-itis*, inflamação]
amebic c., c. amebiana; inflamação do cólon na amebíase.
collagenous c., c. colágena; colite que ocorre principalmente em mulheres de meia-idade, caracterizada por diarréia aquosa persistente e um depósito de uma faixa de colágeno sob a membrana basal do epitélio de superfície do cólon.
c. cys'tica profun'da, c. cística profunda; cistos intramurais do intestino grosso contendo muco; o distúrbio pode ser confundido com carcinoma mucinoso, mas não é neoplásico.
c. cys'tica superficia'lis, c. cística superficial; forma de colite na qual há formação de cisto superficial no cólon.
granulomatous c., c. granulomatosa; alterações, idênticas àquelas da enterite regional, que envolvem o cólon.
hemorrhagic c., c. hemorrágica; cólicas abdominais e diarréia com sangue, sem febre, atribuídas a uma infecção autolimitada por uma cepa de *Escherichia coli*.
mucous c., c. mucosa; afecção da mucosa do cólon caracterizada por dor em caráter de cólica, constipação ou diarréia (algumas vezes alternadas) e eliminação de fragmentos e placas mucosas ou pseudomembranosas viscosas. SIN mucocolitis, myxomembranous c.
myxomembranous c., c. mixomembranosa. SIN mucous c.
pseudomembranous c., c. pseudomembranosa. SIN pseudomembranous enterocolitis.
ulcerative c., c. ulcerativa; doença crônica de causa desconhecida, caracterizada por ulceração do cólon e do reto, com hemorragia retal, abscessos das criptas mucosas, pseudopólipos inflamatórios, dor abdominal e diarréia; freqüentemente causa anemia, hipoproteinemia e desequilíbrio eletrolítico e, com menor freqüência, é complicada por peritonite, megacólon tóxico ou carcinoma do cólon.
uremic c., c. urêmica; colite caracterizada por hemorragias na mucosa, que ocorrem na insuficiência renal, possivelmente devido ao efeito irritante da amônia formada por decomposição da uréia aumentada nas secreções intestinais.
col·i·tose (kol'ī-tōs). Colitose; antígeno somático polissacarídico das espécies de *Salmonella*.
col·la (kol'ă). Colos. Plural de collum.
collaboration. Colaboração; cooperação.
Cochrane c., c. de Cochrane; uma rede mundial de epidemiologistas clínicos que revêem e publicam resultados de provas controladas randomizadas. O objetivo é fornecer melhores dados para uso na medicina baseada em evidências e estabelecer orientações para a prática clínica. VER TAMBÉM evidence-based *medicine*, clinical practice *guidelines*, em *guideline*.
col·la·cin (kol'lă-sin). Colacina; colágeno degenerado. SIN collastin.

col·la·gen (kol'lă-jen). Colágeno; a principal proteína (que constitui mais da metade das proteínas dos mamíferos) das fibras brancas de tecido conjuntivo, cartilagem e osso, que é insolúvel em água, mas pode ser transformada em gelatinas solúveis, facilmente digeríveis, por fervura em água, ácidos diluídos ou álcalis. É rica em resíduos glicila, L-alanil, L-prolil, e L-4-hidroxiprolil, mas pobre em enxofre e não possui resíduos L-triptofanil. Compreende uma família de moléculas geneticamente distintas, todas possuindo uma singular configuração helicoidal tripla de três subunidades polipeptídicas conhecidas como cadeias α; foram identificados pelo menos 13 tipos de colágeno, cada um com uma cadeia polipeptídica diferente. VER TAMBÉM collagen *fiber*. SIN ossein, osseine, ostein, osteine. [G. *koila*, cola, + *-gen*, que produz]
type I c., c. tipo I; o colágeno mais abundante, formando grandes fibrilas bem organizadas que possuem grande resistência à tração.
type II c., c. tipo II; colágeno peculiar da cartilagem, núcleo pulposo, notocorda e corpo vítreo; forma-se como delgadas fibrilas altamente glicosiladas.
type III c., c. tipo III; colágeno característico das fibras reticulares.
type IV c., c. tipo IV; forma menos nitidamente fibrilar de colágeno característica das membranas basais.
col·la·gen·ase (kol-ă'jĕ-nās). Colagenase; enzima proteolítica que atua sobre um ou mais tipos de colágeno.
microbial c., c. microbiana. SIN *Clostridium histolyticum* collagenase.
col·la·gen·ase A, col·la·gen·ase I. Colagenase A, colagenase I. SIN *Clostridium histolyticum* collagenase.
col·la·ge·na·tion (kol'ă-jĕ-nā'shŭn). Colagenação. SIN collagenization.
col·la·gen·ic (kol-ă-jen'ik). Colagênico. SIN collagenous.
col·lag·e·ni·za·tion (ko-laj'ĕ-ni-zā'shŭn). Colagenização. **1.** Substituição de tecidos ou fibrina por colágeno. **2.** Síntese de colágeno por fibroblastos. SIN collagenation.
col·lag·e·no·lyt·ic (ko-laj'ĕ-nō-lit'ik). Colagenolítico; que causa a lise do colágeno, gelatina e outras proteínas que contêm prolina. [collagen + G. *lysis*, que dissolve]
col·lag·e·no·sis (ko-laj-i-nō'sis). Colagenose. VER collagen *disease*.
reactive perforating c., c. reativa perfurante; distúrbio cutâneo raro caracterizado por extrusão de fibras de colágeno através da epiderme; geralmente começa no lactente ou na criança e apresenta-se clinicamente como pápulas umbilicadas recorrentes que desaparecem espontaneamente. O distúrbio pode ser hereditário ou adquirido; este último está associado ao diabetes melito e à insuficiência renal e difere da doença de Kyrle porque não há envolvimento folicular.
col·lag·e·nous (ko-laj'ĕ-nŭs). Colagenoso; que produz ou contém colágeno. SIN collagenic.
col·lapse (kō-laps'). Colapso. **1.** Condição de extrema prostração, semelhante ou idêntico ao choque hipovolêmico e que tem as mesmas causas. **2.** Um estado de profunda depressão física. **3.** Queda conjunta das paredes de uma estrutura. **4.** A falência de um sistema fisiológico. **5.** O definhamento de um órgão de sua estrutura adjacente, p. ex., colapso pulmonar. [L. *col-labor*, pp. *-lapsus*, cair junto]
absorption c., c. absortivo; colapso pulmonar devido à obstrução completa e rápida de um grande brônquio.
circulatory c., c. circulatório; falência da circulação, cardíaca ou periférica.
c. of dental arch, c. da arcada dentária; movimento dos dentes para ocupar um espaço que, normalmente, seria preenchido por outro dente (ausente), criando um posicionamento errado dos dentes adjacentes e opostos.
massive c., c. maciço; atelectasia relativamente súbita de todo um pulmão ou lobo.
pressure c., c. compressivo; colapso pulmonar devido à compressão externa do pulmão, como por um derrame pleural ou pneumotórax.
pulmonary c., c. pulmonar; atelectasia secundária causada por obstrução brônquica, derrame pleural ou pneumotórax, hipertrofia cardíaca ou aumento de outras estruturas adjacentes aos pulmões.
col·lar (kol'ăr). Colar; uma faixa, geralmente circundando o pescoço ou colo.
renal c., c. renal; no embrião, um anel de veias ao redor da aorta abaixo da origem da artéria mesentérica superior.
col·lar·ette (kol'er-et'). Colarete. **1.** A linha sinuosa, irregular na íris, que divide a zona pupilar central a partir da zona ciliar periférica e marca o local embrionário do círculo vascular menor atrofiado da íris. **2.** Escamas frágeis que envolvem os cílios na blefarite estafilocócica. SIN iris frill.
col·las·tin (kol-as'tin). Colastina. SIN collacin.
col·lat·er·al (ko-lat'er-ăl). Colateral. **1.** Indireto, subsidiário ou acessório ao objeto principal; lado a lado. **2.** Um ramo lateral de um axônio ou vaso sanguíneo.
col·lec·tins. Colectinas; família de moléculas que reconhecem e opsonizam micróbios durante a resposta pré-imune de um hospedeiro e podem ativar a via do complemento.
Colles, Abraham, cirurgião irlandês, 1773–1843. VER C. *fascia, fracture, ligament, space*.
Collet, Frédéric-Justin, otorrinolaringologista francês, 1870–1965.
col·lic·u·lec·to·my (ko-lik-ū-lek'tō-mē). Coliculectomia; excisão do colículo seminal.

col·lic·u·lus, pl. **col·lic·u·li** (ko-lik′u-lŭs, -lī) [TA]. Colículo; pequena elevação acima das partes vizinhas. [L. montículo, dim. de *collis*, monte]
  c. of arytenoid cartilage [TA], c. da cartilagem aritenóidea; a elevação da superfície ântero-lateral da cartilagem aritenóidea acima da fóvea triangular. SIN c. cartilaginis arytenoideae [TA].
  c. cartila′ginis arytenoi′deae [TA], c. da cartilagem aritenóidea. SIN c. of arytenoid cartilage.
  facial c. [TA], c. facial; porção proeminente da eminência medial, imediatamente rostral às estrias medulares na fossa rombóide; é formada pela curvatura interna do nervo facial e pelo núcleo abducente, ao redor do qual se curvam as fibras faciais. SIN c. facialis [TA], abducens eminence, eminentia abducentis, eminentia facialis, facial eminence, facial hillock.
  c. facia′lis [TA], c. facial. SIN facial c.
  c. infe′rior [TA], c. inferior. SIN inferior c.
  inferior c. [TA], c. inferior; a eminência ovóide, pareada, inferior, das lâminas do teto do mesencéfalo; recebe o menisco lateral e projeta-se, por meio do ramo do colículo inferior, até o corpo geniculado medial do tálamo, sendo, assim, uma estação intermediária essencial na via auditiva central. SIN c. inferior [TA], corpus quadrigeminum posterius, inferior nasal c., posterior quadrigeminal body.
  inferior nasal c., c. nasal inferior. SIN inferior c.
  seminal c. [TA], c. seminal; uma porção elevada da crista uretral na qual se abrem os dois ductos ejaculatórios e o utrículo prostático. SIN c. seminalis [TA], c. urethralis, seminal hillock, verumontanum.
  c. semina′lis [TA], c. seminal. SIN seminal c.
  superior c. [TA], c. superior; a maior eminência anterior arredondada, pareada, das lâminas do teto do mesencéfalo; as principais conexões aferentes das camadas superficiais são a retina e o córtex estriado; os impulsos para as camadas profundas do colículo são polimodais. Suas conexões eferentes são com a parte inferior do tronco cerebral e medula espinal (tratos tetobulbar e tetoespinal) e com o pulvinar e outros grupos celulares na parte caudal do tálamo; participa da via visual extrageniculada. As camadas do colículo superior, da região superficial para a profunda são: camada zonal (estrato zonal), camada cinzenta superficial (estrato cinzento superficial), camada óptica (estrato óptico), camada cinzenta intermediária (estrato cinzento intermediário), camada branca intermediária (estrato medular intermediário), camada cinzenta profunda (estrato cinzento profundo), camada branca profunda (estrato medular profundo). SIN c. superior [TA], anterior quadrigeminal body, corpus quadrigeminum anterius.
  c. supe′rior [TA], c. superior. SIN superior c.
  c. urethra′lis, c. uretral. SIN seminal c.
Collier, James S., médico inglês, 1870–1935. VER C. *tract, sign.*
col·li·ga·tion (kol-i-gā′shŭn). Coligação. **1.** Uma associação na qual os componentes são distinguíveis uns dos outros. **2.** A transformação de eventos isolados em uma experiência unificada. **3.** A formação de uma ligação covalente por meio de dois grupamentos que se combinam. [L. *cum*, junto, + *ligo*, ligar]
col·li·ga·tive (ko-lig′a-tiv). Coligativo. **1.** Dependente do número de partículas. **2.** Refere-se às propriedades de soluções que dependem apenas da concentração de substâncias dissolvidas, e não de sua natureza (p. ex., pressão osmótica, elevação do ponto de fervura, redução da pressão de vapor, depressão do ponto de congelamento).
col·li·ma·tion (kol-i-mā′shŭn). Colimação; o método, em radiologia, de restringir e confinar o feixe de raios X a uma determinada área e, em medicina nuclear, de restringir a detecção de radiações emitidas de uma determinada área de interesse. [L. *collineo*, orientar em linha reta]
col·li·ma·tor (kol′i-mā-ter). Colimador; um dispositivo de material com alto coeficiente de absorção usado em colimação.
Col·lins. VER Lukes-Collins *classification*, Treacher Collins *syndrome*.
col·li·ot·o·my (kol-ē-ot′o-mē). Coliotomia; termo obsoleto para lise de aderências. [G. *kolla*, cola, + *tomē*, incisão]
Collip, James B., endocrinologista canadense, 1892–1965. VER Noble-C. *procedure;* Anderson-C. *test.*
col·li·qua·tion (kol-i-kwā′shŭn). Coliquação. **1.** Descarga excessiva de líquido. **2.** Liquefação no processo de necrose. [L. *col-,* junto, + *liquo,* pp. *liquatus,* causar fusão]
col·liq·ua·tive (kōlik′wā-tiv). Coliquativo; indica ou é característico de coliquação.
Collis, John Leighton, cirurgião torácico inglês, *1911. VER C. *gastroplasty*; Collis-Nissen *fundoplication*; Collis-Belsey *fundoplication*; C.-Belsey *procedure.*
col·lo·di·on (ko-lō′dē-on). Colódio; líquido produzido pela dissolução de piroxilina ou algodão-pólvora em éter e álcool; à evaporação, deixa uma película contrátil brilhante; usado como protetor em cortes ou como veículo para a aplicação local de substâncias medicinais. SIN collodium. [L. Mod. *collodium,* do G. *kolla,* cola]
  blistering c., c. vesicatório. SIN cantharidal c.
  cantharidal c., c. vesicante; extrato pulverizado de clorofórmio de cantáridas em colódio flexível. SIN blistering c., c. vesicans.
  flexible c., c. flexível; uma mistura de cânfora, óleo de rícino e colódio, ou uma mistura de óleo de rícino, terebintina do Canadá e colódio, usada com o mesmo fim que o colódio, mas sua película possui a vantagem, para determinadas condições, de não se contrair.
  hemostatic c., c. hemostático. SIN styptic c.
  iodized c., c. iodado; uma solução de 5% de iodo em colódio flexível; um contra-irritante.
  salicylic acid c., c. de ácido salicílico; agente ceratolítico usado no tratamento de calosidades e verrugas.
  styptic c., c. estíptico; ácido tânico em colóide flexível; um adstringente e hemostático local. SIN hemostatic c., styptic colloid, xylostyptic ether.
  c. vesicans, c. vesicante. SIN cantharidal c.
col·lo·di·um (ko-lō′dē-ŭm). Colódio. SIN collodion. [G. *kolla,* cola, + *eidos,* aparência]
col·loid (ko′loyd). Colóide. **1.** Agregados de átomos ou moléculas em um estado finamente dividido (submicroscópico), dispersos em um meio gasoso, líquido ou sólido, e que resistem à sedimentação, difusão e filtração, diferindo assim dos precipitados. VER TAMBÉM hydrocolloide. **2.** Semelhante à cola. **3.** Material translúcido, amarelado, homogêneo com consistência de cola, menos líquido que mucóide ou mucinóide, encontrado nas células e tecidos em um estado de degeneração colóide. SIN colloidin. **4.** A secreção armazenada nos folículos da tireóide. Quanto aos colóides individuais não apresentados adiante, consulte o nome específico. [G. *kolla,* cola, + *eidos,* aparência]
  bovine c., c. bovino. SIN conglutinin.
  dispersion c., c. de dispersão. SIN dispersoid.
  emulsion c., c. de emulsão. SIN emulsoid.
  hydrophil c., hydrophilic c., c. hidrófilo. SIN emulsoid.
  hydrophobic c., c. hidrofóbico. SIN suspensoid.
  irreversible c., c. irreversível; c. instável; c. que não é novamente solúvel em água após secagem à temperatura ambiente. SIN unstable c.
  lyophilic c., c. liofílico. SIN emulsoid.
  lyophobic c., c. liofóbico. SIN suspensoid.
  protective c., c. protetor; colóide que tem o poder de evitar a precipitação de suspensóides sob a influência de um eletrólito.
  c. pseudomilium, pseudomílio colóide; mílio colóide. SIN colloid milium.
  reversible c., c. reversível; c. estável; colóide que é novamente solúvel em água após secar à temperatura ambiente. SIN stable c.
  stable c., c. estável. SIN reversible c.
  styptic c., c. estíptico. SIN styptic *collodion.*
  suspension c., c. de suspensão. SIN suspensoid.
  thyroid c., c. tireóideo; o material semilíquido que ocupa a luz dos folículos tireóideos; contém principalmente tireoglobulina.
  unstable c., c. instável. SIN irreversible c.
col·loi·dal (ko-loyd′ăl). Coloidal; indica ou é característico de um colóide.
col·loi·din (ko-loy′din). Coloidina. SIN colloid (3).
col·loid mil·i·um (kol′loyd mil′ē-ŭm). Milium colóide; pápulas amarelas que surgem na pele da cabeça e do dorso das mãos exposta ao sol, compostas de material colóide na derme semelhante a amilóide, mas com uma ultra-estrutura diferente. Há filamentos com menos de 2,0 nm de diâmetro, que podem ser uma forma de tecido elástico produzido por fibroblastos lesados de forma actínica. SIN colloid pseudomilium, elastosis colloidalis conglomerata. [L. *milium,* milho miúdo]
col·loi·do·cla·sia, col·loi·do·cla·sis (ko-loy-dō-klā′sē-ă, -sis). Coloidoclasia; termo obsoleto para ruptura do equilíbrio colóide no corpo. [colloid + G. *klasis,* fratura]
col·loi·do·clas·tic (ko-loy-dō-klas′tik). Coloidoclástico; termo obsoleto que indica coloidoclasia.
col·loi·do·gen (ko-loy′dō-jen). Coloidógeno; substância capaz de dar origem a uma solução ou suspensão coloidal.
col·lox·y·lin (ko-lok′si-lin). Coloxilina. SIN pyroxylin. [G. *kolla,* cola, + *xylinos,* lenhoso, de *xylon,* madeira]
col·lum, pl. **col·la** (kol′ŭm, kol′ă). Colo; *termo oficial alternativo para neck. [L.]
  c. anatom′icum hu′meri [TA], c. anatômico do úmero. SIN anatomical *neck* of humerus.
  c. chirur′gicum hu′meri [TA], c. cirúrgico do úmero. SIN surgical *neck* of humerus.
  c. cos′tae [TA], c. da costela. SIN neck of rib.
  c. den′tis, c. do dente. SIN neck of tooth.
  c. fem′oris [TA], c. do fêmur. SIN *neck* of femur.
  c. fib′ulae [TA], c. da fíbula. SIN *neck* of fibula.
  c. folli′culi pi′li, c. do folículo piloso. SIN *neck* of hair follicle.
  c. glan′dis [TA], c. da glande. SIN *neck* of glans.
  c. hu′meri, c. do úmero. VER anatomical *neck* of humerus, surgical *neck* of humerus.
  c. mal′lei [TA], c. do martelo. SIN *neck* of malleus.
  c. mandib′ulae [TA], c. da mandíbula. SIN *neck* of mandible.
  c. os′sis fem′oris, c. do fêmur. SIN *neck* of femur.

c. ra'dii [TA], c. do rádio. SIN *neck* of radius.
c. scap'ulae [TA], c. da escápula. SIN *neck* of scapula.
c. ta'li [TA], c. do tálus. SIN *neck* of talus.
c. vesicae, c. da bexiga; *termo oficial alternativo para *neck* of (urinary) bladder.
c. vesi'cae biliar'is [TA], c. da vesícula biliar. SIN *neck* of gallbladder.
c. vesi'cae fel'leae, c. da vesícula biliar; *termo oficial alternativo para *neck of gallbladder*.
col·lu·to·ri·um (kol-ū-tō′rē-ŭm). Colutório. SIN mouthwash. [L. Mod. de *col-luo*, pp. *-lutus*, lavar completamente]
col·lu·tory (kol′ū-tōr-ē). Colutório. SIN mouthwath. [L. *colluere*, enxaguar]
col·lyr·i·um (ko-lir′ē-ŭm). Originalmente, qualquer preparação para o olho; atualmente, um colírio (ou solução para lavar os olhos). [G. *kollyrion*, cataplasma, remédio para o olho]
colo-. O cólon (intestino). [G. *kolon*]
col·o·bo·ma (kol-ō-bō′mă). Coloboma; qualquer defeito, congênito, patológico ou artificial, principalmente do olho, devido ao fechamento incompleto da fissura óptica. [G. *koloboma*, lit., a parte retirada na mutilação, de *koloboō*, amputar, mutilar]
 c. of choroid, c. da coróide; defeito congênito da coróide e do epitélio pigmentar da retina, expondo a esclerótica; o defeito geralmente está situado abaixo do disco óptico na região da fissura fetal (coróide).
 Fuchs c., c. de Fuchs; crescente inferior congênito na coróide, na borda do disco óptico; não associado à miopia. SIN congenital conus.
 c. i'ridis, c. da íris; (1) retenção da fissura coróide, causando uma fenda congênita da íris, freqüentemente associada ao c. da coróide; (2) termo obsoleto para o defeito da íris resultante de uma iridectomia cirúrgica.
 c. len'tis, c. da lente; segmento do equador da lente desprovido de fibras zonulares, dando o aspecto de uma incisura.
 c. lo'buli, c. do lóbulo; fissura congênita do lóbulo da orelha.
 macular c., c. macular; defeito da retina central resultante da interrupção do desenvolvimento ou de inflamação intra-uterina da retina.
 c. of optic nerve, c. do nervo óptico; incisura congênita, na formação do nervo óptico, que aparece como uma escavação crateriforme no disco óptico. VER *optic pit*.
 c. palpebra'le, c. palpebral; incisura congênita na borda da pálpebra.
 c. of vitreous, c. do vítreo; entalhe congênito do corpo do vítreo por mesênquima; associado à miopia grave.
col·o·cen·te·sis (kō′lō-sen-tē′sis). Colocentese; punção do cólon com um trocarte ou bisturi para aliviar a distensão. SIN colipuncture, colopuncture. [colo- + G. *kentēsis*, punctura]
col·o·col·ic (kō-lō-kol′ik). Colocólico; do cólon para o cólon; diz-se de anastomose espontânea ou induzida entre duas partes do cólon.
col·o·co·los·to·my (kō′lō-kō-los′tō-mē). Cololostomia; estabelecimento de uma comunicação entre dois segmentos não-contínuos do cólon. [colo- + colo- + G. *stoma*, boca]
col·o·cynth (kol′ō-sinth). Coloquíntida; coloquinto, colocinto; o fruto seco e descascado da *Citrullus colocynthis* (família Cucurbitaceae), planta da costa arenosa do Mediterrâneo, um pouco semelhante à melancieira; antigamente usada como catártico e laxante. SIN bitter aplle. [G. *kolokynthē*, abóbora]
col·o·cys·to·plas·ty (kō-lō-sis′tō-plas-tē). Colocistoplastia; aumento da bexiga por fixação de um segmento do cólon a ela.
col·o·en·ter·i·tis (kō′lō-en-ter-ī′tis). Coloenterite. SIN enterocolitis.
col·o·hep·a·to·pexy (kō-lō-hep′ă-tō-pek′sē). Colo-hepatopexia; fixação do cólon ao fígado por aderências. [colo- + G. *hēpar* (*hēpat-*), fígado, + *pēxis*, fixação]
co·lol·y·sis (kō-lol′i-sis). Colólise; procedimento para liberar o cólon das aderências. [colo- + G. *lysis*, afrouxamento]
col·o·min·ic ac·id (kol-ō-min′ik). Ácido colomínico; polímero do ácido α(1,5)-*N*-acetilneuramínico; encontrado na *Escherichia coli*.
co·lon (kō′lon) [TA]. Cólon; a divisão do intestino grosso que se estende do ceco até o reto. [G. *kolon*]
 c. ascen'dens [TA], c. ascendente. SIN ascending c.
 ascending c. [TA], c. ascendente; a porção do cólon entre o orifício ileocecal e a flexura direita do cólon. SIN c. ascendens [TA].
 c. descen'dens [TA], c. descendente. SIN descending c.
 descending c. [TA], c. descendente; a parte do intestino grosso que se estende da flexura esquerda do cólon até a borda pélvica. SIN c. descendens [TA].
 giant c., c. gigante. SIN megacolon.
 iliac c., c. ilíaco; porção do cólon descendente que ocupa a fossa ilíaca esquerda, entre a crista ilíaca esquerda e a borda pélvica.
 irritable c., c. irritável; tendência à hiperperistalse colônica, algumas vezes associada a cólica e diarréia.
 lead-pipe c., c. em cano de chumbo, o cólon rígido e fibrosado da colite ulcerativa avançada. SIN stove-pipe c.
 c. pelvi'num, c. pélvico. SIN sigmoid c.
 sigmoid c. [TA], c. sigmóide; a parte do cólon que descreve uma curva em forma de S entre a borda pélvica e o terceiro segmento sacral; é contínuo com o reto. SIN c. sigmoideum [TA], c. pelvinum, flexura sigmoidea, sigmoid flexure.

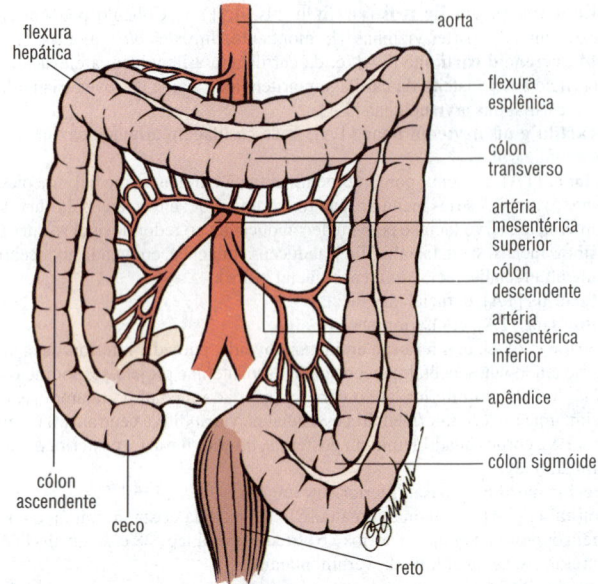

cólon: anatomia e suprimento sanguíneo

 c. sigmoi'deum [TA], c. sigmóide. SIN sigmoid c.
 spastic c., c. espástico; termo inespecífico usado para descrever manifestações como dor abdominal, flatulência e diarréia alternada com constipação, parecendo refletir o aumento da função muscular do cólon.
 stove-pipe c., cólon em cano de chumbo SIN lead-pipe c.
 transverse c. [TA], c. transverso; a parte do cólon entre as flexuras direita e esquerda. Pode estender-se um pouco transversalmente no abdome, porém, na maioria das vezes, curva-se centralmente, freqüentemente até níveis subumbilicais. SIN c. transversum [TA].
 c. transver'sum [TA], c. transverso. SIN transverse c.
co·lon·al·gia (ko-lon-al′jē-ă). Colonalgia; termo raramente usado para dor no cólon. [colon + G. *algos*, dor]
co·lon·ic (ko-lon′ik). Colônico; relativo ao cólon.
col·o·ni·za·tion (kol′on-i-zā′shŭn). Colonização. **1.** SIN innidiation. **2.** A formação de grupos populacionais compactos do mesmo tipo de microrganismo, como as colônias que se desenvolvem quando uma célula bacteriana começa a se reproduzir. **3.** Tratamento de determinadas passoas, p. ex., leprosos, pacientes mentais, em comunidades (colônias).
 genetic c., c. genética; propagação de um gene por um hospedeiro no qual esse gene foi introduzido, de forma natural ou artificial.
co·lon·o·gram (ko-lon′ō-gram). Colonograma; registro gráfico de movimentos do cólon.
co·lon·om·e·ter (kō′lō-nom′e-ter). Colonômetro; dispositivo para contar colônias bacterianas.
co·lon·op·a·thy (kō-lō-nop′ă-thē). Colonopatia; termo raramente usado para qualquer perturbação do cólon. SIN colopathy.
 fibrosing c., c. fibrosante; fibrose colônica observada em pacientes com fibrose cística, que se acredita ser causada por pancreatite.
co·lon·or·rha·gia (kō′lon-ō-rā′jē-ă). Colonorragia; termo raramente usado para colorragia.
co·lon·or·rhea (kō′lon-ō-rē′ă). Colonorréia. SIN colorrhea.
co·lon·o·scope (kō-lon′ō-skōp). Colonoscópio; endoscópio de fibra óptica flexível, longo.
co·lon·os·co·py (kō-lon-os′kō-pē). Colonoscopia; exame visual da superfície interna do cólon por meio de um colonoscópio. SIN coloscopy. [colon + G. *skopeō*, ver]
col·o·ny (kol′ō-nē). Colônia. **1.** Um grupo de células que crescem em uma superfície nutriente sólida, cada uma originando-se da multiplicação de uma célula individual; um clone. **2.** Um grupo de pessoas com interesses semelhantes, que vivem em um local ou área particular. [L. *colonia*, colônia]
 daughter c., c.-filha; colônia secundária que cresce sobre uma superfície de uma colônia mais antiga; é menor e pode ter características diferentes daquelas da colônia-mãe.
 filamentous c., c. filamentosa; em bafteriologia, uma colônia composta de longos filamentos entrelaçados, dispostos irregularmente.
 H c., c. H; uma colônia de microrganismos móveis que formam uma fina película de crescimento. Cf. O c. [Al. *Hauch*, respirar]
 lenticular c., c. lenticular; colônia bacteriana em forma de lentilha ou de uma lente duplo-convexa.

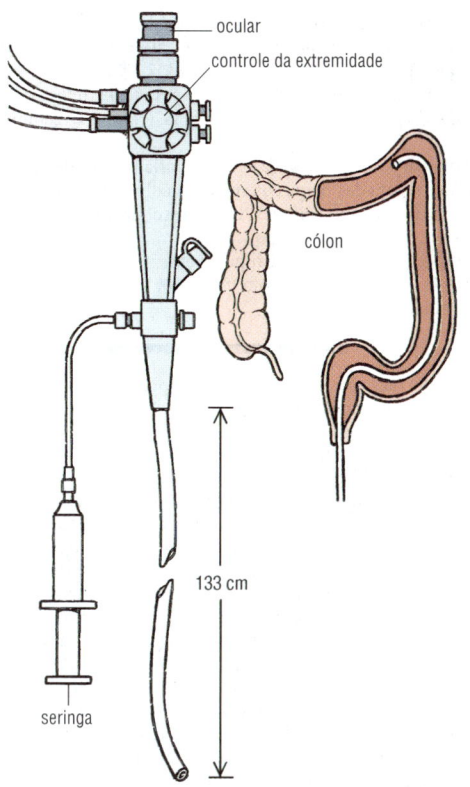

colonoscópio: com fibra óptica

mother c., c.-mãe; colônia que origina uma colônia secundária (uma colônia-filha), esta última crescendo sobre a superfície da primeira; a colônia-mãe é maior que a colônia-filha, e as características das colônias podem diferir.
mucoid c., c. mucóide; colônia mostrando crescimento viscoso ou pegajoso típico de um microrganismo que produz grandes quantidades de uma cápsula de carboidratos.
O c., c. O; crescimento de uma bactéria imóvel em colônias compactas, distintas, em contraste com uma película de crescimento produzida por algumas bactérias móveis. Cf. H c. [Al. *ohne Hauch,* sem respiração]
rough c., c. rugosa; colônia bacteriana com uma superfície achatada, granular; esse tipo de colônia geralmente está associado à perda da virulência em relação à das colônias lisas.
smooth c., c. lisa; colônia bacteriana com superfície arredondada e brilhante; esse tipo de colônia geralmente está associado a maior virulência que as colônias rugosas.
spheroid c., c. esferóide; colônia de protozoários na qual as células individuais são mantidas juntas em uma massa esférica consistente por meio de um material gelatinóide.
co·lop·a·thy (kō-lop′ă-thē). Colopatia. SIN colonopathy.
co·lo·pex·os·to·my (kō′lō-peks-os′tō-mē). Colopexostomia; termo raramente usado para estabelecimento de conexão entre a luz do cólon e a pele após a fixação do cólon à parede abdominal. [colo- + G. *pēxis,* fixação, + *stoma,* boca]
co·lo·pex·ot·o·my (kō′lō-peks-ot′ō-mē). Colopexotomia; termo raramente usado para incisão do cólon após sua fixação à parede abdominal. [colo- + G. *pēxis,* fixação, + *tomē,* incisão]
col·o·pexy (kol′ō-pek-sē). Colopexia; fixação de uma parte do cólon à parede abdominal. [colo- + G. *pēxis,* fixação]
co·lo·pho·ny (kō-lof′ō-nē). Colofônio, colofônia. SIN rosin. [*Colophōn,* cume, uma cidade na Jônia]
co·lo·pli·ca·tion (kō′lō-pli-kā′shŭn). Coloplicatura; redução da luz de um cólon dilatado fazendo-se pregas ou dobras em suas paredes. SIN coliplication. [colo- + L. Mod. *plica,* prega]
co·lo·proc·ti·tis (kō′lō-prok-tī′tis). Coloproctite; inflamação do cólon e do reto. SIN colorectitis, proctocolitis, rectocolitis. [colo- + G. *prōktos,* ânus (reto), + *-itis,* inflamação]
co·lo·proc·tos·to·my (kō′lō-prok-tos′tō-mē). Coloproctostomia; estabelecimento de uma comunicação entre o reto e um segmento descontínuo do cólon. SIN colorectostomy. [colo- + G. *prōktos,* ânus (reto), + *stoma,* boca]
co·lop·to·sis, co·lop·to·sia (kō-lop-tō′sis, -tō′sē-ă). Coloptose; deslocamento para baixo, ou prolapso, do cólon, principalmente da porção transversa. SIN coleoptosis. [colo- + G. *ptōsis,* queda]

co·lo·punc·ture (kō-lō-pŭnk′choor). Colopunctura; colocentese. SIN colocentesis.
col·or (kŭl′or). Cor. **1.** Característica da apresentação de objetos e fontes luminosas que pode ser especificada como matiz, luminosidade (brilho) e saturação. **2.** Parte visível (370–760 nm) do espectro eletromagnético, especificada como comprimento de onda, luminosidade e pureza. [L.]
complementary c.'s, cores complementares; pares de cores diferentes de luz que produzem luz branca quando combinadas.
confusion c.'s, cores de confusão; um conjunto de cores (geralmente de lãs coloridas), creme, amarelo-claro, azul-claro, cinza, marrom, verde, violeta, etc., usadas em testes para a cegueira de cores.
extrinsic c., c. extrínseca; cor aplicada à superfície externa de uma prótese dentária.
intrinsic c., c. intrínseca; a adição de pigmento colorido ao material de uma prótese dentária.
opponent c., c. oponente; pares de cores que compartilham canais coloridos na retina (vermelho-verde, azul-amarelo, preto-branco).
primary c., c. primária; as três cores dos pigmentos dos cones retinianos (vermelho, verde, azul) que podem ser combinadas para formar qualquer matiz.
pure c., c. pura; sensação visual produzida por luz de um comprimento de onda específico.
reflected c.'s, cores refletidas; aquelas cores observadas na luz que incide sobre uma superfície pigmentada.
saturated c., c. saturada; uma cor que contém uma quantidade mínima de pigmento branco.
simple c., c. primária. SIN primary c.
structural c., c. estrutural; cor criada por um efeito óptico (p. ex., através de interferência, refração ou difração). Muitos azuis de ocorrência natural pertencem a essa classe. Cf. natural *pigment.* SIN schemochromes.
tone c., timbre (de voz ou instrumento musical) ou qualidade de tom. SIN timbre.
co·lo·rec·tal (kol′ō-rek′tăl). Colorretal; relativo ao cólon e ao reto, ou a todo o intestino grosso.
co·lo·rec·ti·tis (kō′lō-rek′tī′tis). Colorretite. SIN coloproctitis.
co·lo·rec·tos·to·my (kō′lō-rek-tos′tō-mē). Colorretostomia. SIN coloproctostomy.
col·or·im·e·ter (kol-er-im′ē-ter). Colorímetro; dispositivo óptico para determinar a cor e/ou a intensidade da cor de um líquido. SIN chromatometer, chromometer.
Duboscq c., c. de Duboscq; aparelho antigo para medir a intensidade da tonalidade em um líquido mediante comparação com um líquido padrão; cilindros de vidro são imersos em cada uma das duas cubas, com um contendo líquido padrão e o outro o líquido a ser testado; ao olhar através dos cilindros, as tonalidades são igualadas elevando-se ou abaixando o cilindro em uma cuba, e a extensão da elevação ou abaixamento é indicada em uma escala que fornece a diferença exata de tonalidade.
col·or·i·met·ric (kol-er-i-met′rik). Colorimétrico; relativo à colorimetria.
col·or·im·e·try (kol-er-im′ē-trē). Colorimetria; procedimento para análise química quantitativa, baseado na comparação da cor apresentada em uma solução do material de prova com a de uma solução padrão; as duas soluções são observadas simultaneamente em um colorímetro, sendo quantificadas com base na absorção de luz.
col·or match. Correspondência de cores; o resultado do ajuste de mistura de cores até que todas as diferenças visualmente aparentes sejam mínimas.
co·lor·rha·gia (kō-lo-rā′jē-ă). Colorragia; secreção anormal proveniente do cólon. [colo- + G. *rhēgnymi,* jorrar]
co·lor·rha·phy (kō-lōr′ă-fē). Colorrafia; sutura do cólon. [colo- + G. *rhaphē,* sutura]
co·lor·rhea (kō-lo-rē′ă). Colorréia; termo raramente usado para diarréia, considerada decorrente de uma condição limitada ao cólon, ou que afeta principalmente este. SIN colonorrhea. [colo- + G. *rhoia,* fluxo]
col·or sol·id. Sólido de cor; distribuição esquemática de cor no espaço, sendo os atributos de tonalidade, saturação e brilho representados por coordenadas cilíndricas (semipolares).
col·or tri·an·gle. Triângulo de cor; gráfico no qual são representadas as coordenadas de cromaticidade.
co·los·co·py (kō-los′kō-pē). Coloscopia. SIN colonoscopy. [colo- + G. *skopeō,* ver]
co·lo·sig·moi·dos·to·my (kō′lō-sig-moy-dos′tō-mē). Colossigmoidostomia; estabelecimento de uma anastomose entre qualquer outra parte do cólon e o cólon sigmóide.
co·los·to·my (kō-los′tō-mē). Colostomia; estabelecimento de uma conexão artificial entre a luz do cólon e a pele. [colo- + G. *stoma,* boca]
co·los·tror·rhea (kō-los-tror-rē′ă). Colostrorréia; secreção anormalmente abundante de colostro. [colostrum, + G. *rhoia,* fluxo]
co·los·trous (kō-los′trŭs). Colostroso; que contém colostro.
co·los·trum (kō-los′trŭm). Colostro; líquido opalescente branco e fino, o primeiro leite secretado ao fim da gravidez; difere do leite secretado mais tarde por

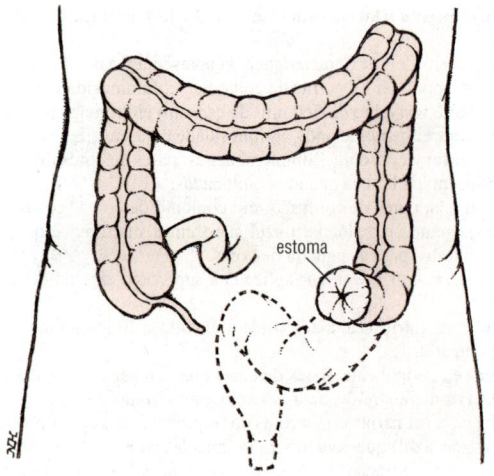

colostomia

conter mais lactalbumina e lactoproteína; o colostro também é rico em anticorpos que conferem imunidade passiva ao recém-nascido. SIN foremilk. [L.]

co·lot·o·my ((kō-lot′o-mē). Colotomia; incisão no cólon. [colo- + G. tomē, incisão]

Col·our In·dex. Publicação relacionada com a química de corantes, sendo cada corante apresentado identificado por um número C.I. (índice colorimétrico) de cinco dígitos, p. ex., o azul de metileno é C.I. 52015.

♻ **colp.** VER colpo-.

col·pa·tre·sia (kol-pa-trē′zē-ā). Colpatresia. SIN vaginal atresia. [colp- + G. atrētos, imperfurado]

col·pec·ta·sis, col·pec·ta·sia (kol-pek′tă-sis, -pek-tā′si-ă). Colpectasia; distensão da vagina. [colp- + G. aktasis, distensão]

col·pec·to·my (kol-pek′to-mē). Colpectomia. SIN vaginectomy. [colp- + G. ektomē, excisão]

♻ **colpo-, colp-.** A vagina. VER TAMBÉM vagino-. [G. kolpos, prega ou depressão]

col·po·cele (kol′pō-sēl). 1. Colpocele; uma hérnia que se projeta para a vagina. SIN vaginocele. 2. Colpoptose. SIN colpoptosis. [colpo- + G. kēlē, hérnia]

col·po·clei·sis (kol-pō-klī′sis). Colpoclise; operação para obliterar a luz da vagina. [colpo- + G. kleisis, fechamento]

col·po·cys·to·plas·ty (kol-pō-sis′tō-plas-tē). Colpocistoplastia; cirurgia plástica para reparar a parede vesicovaginal. [colpo- + G. kystis, bexiga, + plastos, formado]

col·po·cys·tot·o·my (kol′pō-sis-tot′o-mē). Colpocistotomia; incisão da bexiga através da vagina. [colpo- + G. kystis, bexiga, + tomē incisão]

col·po·cys·to·u·re·ter·ot·o·my (kol′pō-sis′tō-ū-rē-ter-ot′o-mē). Colpocistoureterotomia; incisão do ureter através da vagina e bexiga. [colpo- + G. kystis, bexiga, + oureter, ureter, + tomē, incisão]

col·po·dyn·ia (kol-pō-din′ē-ă). Colpodinia. SIN vaginodynia. [colpo- + G. odynē, dor]

col·po·hys·ter·ec·to·my (kol′pō-his-ter-ek′to-mē). Colpo-histerectomia. SIN vaginal hysterectomy. [colpo- + G. hystera, útero, + etomē, excisão]

col·po·hys·ter·o·pexy (kol-pō-his′ter-ō-pek-sē). Colpo-histeropexia; operação para fixação do útero realizada através da vagina. [colpo- + G. hystera, útero, + pēxis, fixação]

col·po·hys·ter·ot·o·my (kol′pō-his-ter-ot′o-mē). Colpo-histerotomia. SIN vaginal hysterotomy. [colpo- + G. hystera, útero, + tomē, incisão]

col·po·mi·cro·scope (kol-pō-mikrō-skōp). Colpomicroscópio; microscópio especial para exame visual direto do tecido cervical.

col·po·mi·cros·co·py (kol′pō-mī-kros′kō-pē). Colpomicroscopia; observação direta e estudo de células na vagina e no colo uterino ampliados in vivo, no tecido inalterado, por meio de um colpomicroscópio.

col·po·my·co·sis (kol′pō-mī-kō′sis). Colpomicose. SIN vaginomycosis.

col·po·my·o·mec·to·my (kol′pō-mī-ō-mek′tō-mē). Colpomiomectomia. SIN vaginal myomectomy. [colpo- + myoma + G. ektomē, excisão]

col·po·per·i·ne·o·plas·ty (kol′pō-pār-i-nē′ō-plas-tē). Colpoperineoplastia. SIN vaginoperineoplasty. [colpo- + perineum, + G. plastos, formado]

col·po·per·i·ne·or·rha·phy (kol′pō-pār-i-nē-ōr′ă-fē). Colpoperioneorrafia. SIN vaginoperineorrhaphy. [colpo- + perineum, + G. rhaphē, sutura]

col·po·pexy (kol′pō-pek-sē). Colpopexia. SIN vaginofixation. [colpo- + G. pēxis, fixação]

col·po·plas·ty (kol′pō-plas-tē). Colpoplastia. SIN vaginoplasty. [colpo- + G. plastos, formado]

col·po·poi·e·sis (kol′pō-poy-ē′sis). Colpopoese; construção cirúrgica de uma vagina. [colpo- + G. poiēsis, formação]

col·po·pto·sis, col·po·pto·sia (kol-pō-tō′sis, -tō-sē-ă; kol-pop-tō′sis). Colpoptose; prolapso das paredes vaginais. SIN colpocele (2). [colpo- + G. ptōsis, queda]

col·po·rec·to·pexy (kol-pō-rek′tō-pek-sē). Colporretopexia; reparo de um reto prolapsado por sutura à parede da vagina. [colpo- + rectum + G. pēxis, fixação]

col·por·rha·phy (kol-pōr′ă-fē). Colporrafia; reparo de ruptura da vagina por excisão e sutura das bordas da ruptura. [colpo- + G. rhaphē, sutura]

col·por·rhex·is (kol-pō-rek′sis). Colporrexe. SIN vaginal laceration. [colpo- + G. rhēxis, ruptura]

col·po·scope (kol′pō-skōp). Colposcópio; instrumento endoscópico que amplia células da vagina e do colo uterino in vivo para permitir observação direta e estudo desses tecidos.

col·pos·co·py (kol-pos′kō-pē). Colposcopia; exame da vagina e do colo uterino por meio de um endoscópio. [colpo- + G. skopeō, ver]

A colposcopia é usada principalmente para identificar áreas de displasia cervical em mulheres com esfregaços de Papanicolaou anormais e como ajuda em procedimentos de biópsia ou excisão, incluindo cauterização, crioterapia, vaporização com laser e excisão por alça eletrocirúrgica. O colposcópio é um instrumento fixo com iluminação própria e ampliação ajustável de 2× a 20× ou mais. É usado em conjunto com um espéculo vaginal padrão para examinar o colo uterino, particularmente a zona de transformação e a mucosa vaginal. Um filtro verde melhora a visualização dos vasos sanguíneos e a identificação de padrões vasculares anormais (pontilhado, mosaico ou atípico). A aplicação de solução de ácido acético a 5% acentua áreas com aumento da proteína celular e aumento da densidade nuclear, que tendem a representar áreas de alteração celular escamosa. A solução de Lugol (iodo-iodeto de potássio), que cora apenas células epiteliais escamosas com conteúdo normal de glicogênio, também pode ser aplicada para delinear o epitélio escamoso anormal. A biópsia cervical direcionada colposcopicamente é o procedimento de escolha após um esfregaço de Papanicolaou mostrando células escamosas atípicas de significado incerto, lesões intra-epiteliais escamosas de baixo ou alto grau, coilocitose, carcinoma in situ, ou carcinomas de maior grau.

col·po·spasm (kol′pō-spazm). Colpospasmo; contração espasmódica da vagina.

col·po·stat (kol′pō-stat). Colpostato; dispositivo para uso na vagina, como um aplicador de rádio, para tratamento do câncer cervical. [colpo- + G. statos, posto]

col·po·ste·no·sis (kol′pō-sten-ō′sis). Colpostenose; estreitamento da luz da vagina. [colpo- + G. stenōsis, estreitamento]

col·po·ste·not·o·my (kol′pō-sten-ot′ō-mē). Colpostenotomia; correção cirúrgica de uma colpostenose. [colpo- + G. stenōsis, estreitamento, + tomē, incisão]

col·po·sus·pen·sion (kol′pō-sus-pen′shun). Colpossuspensão; fixação por sutura do fórnice vaginal lateral ao ligamento de Cooper de cada lado, como uma modificação e aperfeiçoamento da suspensão uretrovesical de Marshall-Marchetti-Kranz padrão para incontinência urinária de esforço devida à cistocele. [colpo- + suspension]

col·pot·o·my (kol-pot′o-mē). Colpotomia; operação de secção na vagina. SIN coleotomy, vaginotomy. [colpo- + G. tomē, incisão]

col·po·u·re·ter·ot·o·my (kol′pō-ū-rē-ter-ot′o-mē). Colpoureterotomia; incisão de um ureter através da vagina. [colpo- + G. tomē, incisão]

col·po·xe·ro·sis (kol-pō-zē-rō′sis). Colpoxerose; ressecamento anormal da mucosa vaginal. [colpo- + G. xērōsis, ressecamento]

Col·ti·vi·rus (kol′tē-vī-rus). Gênero da família Reoviridae que causa a febre do carrapato do Colorado. [Colorado tick fever + virus]

Co·lu·bri·dae (kol-ū′bri-dē). Família de serpentes, em grande parte não-venenosas ou pouco venenosas, compreendendo mais de 1.000 espécies, encontrada na América do Norte, América do Sul, Ásia e África. [L. coluber, serpente]

co·lum·bi·um (Cb) (kol-ūm′bē-ūm). Colúmbio; nome antigo de nióbio. [Columbia, nome para América]

col·u·mel·la, pl. col·u·mel·lae (kol-oo-mel′ă, -mel′ē). Columela. 1. Uma coluna, ou uma pequena coluna. SIN columnella. 2. Em fungos, uma invaginação estéril de um esporângio, como nos Zygomycetes. [L. dim. de columna, coluna]
c. coch'leae, c. coclear. SIN modiolus of angle of mouth.
c. na'si, c. nasal; a margem inferior carnosa (terminação) do septo nasal.

col·umn (kol′um) [TA]. Coluna. 1. Uma parte ou estrutura anatômica na forma de um pilar ou funículo cilíndrico. VER TAMBÉM fascicle. 2. Um objeto (geralmente cilíndrico), massa ou formação vertical. SIN columna [TA]. [L. columna]
affinity c., c. de afinidade. SIN affinity chromatography.
anal c.'s [TA], colunas anais; número de cristas verticais na mucosa da metade superior do canal anal formado quando o calibre do canal é significativa-

mente reduzido em relação ao da ampola retal. SIN columnae anales [TA], Morgagni c.'s, rectal c.'s.

anterior c. [TA], c. anterior; a crista pronunciada, com orientação ventral, de substância cinzenta em cada metade da medula espinal; corresponde ao corno anterior ou ventral que aparece em cortes transversais da medula espinal, e contém os neurônios motores que inervam a musculatura óssea do tronco, pescoço e membros. VER TAMBÉM gray c.'s. SIN columna anterior [TA].

anterior gray c., c. cinzenta anterior. SIN central and lateral intermediate *substances,* em *substance.*

anterior c. of medulla oblongata, c. anterior do bulbo. SIN *pyramid* of medulla oblongata.

anterolateral c. of spinal cord, c. ântero-lateral da medula espinal. SIN lateral *funiculus.*

Bertin c.'s, colunas de Bertin. SIN renal c.'s.

branchial efferent c., c. eferente branquial. SIN special visceral efferent c.

Burdach c., c. de Burdach. SIN cuneate *fasciculus.*

Clarke c., c. de Clarke. SIN posterior thoracic *nucleus.*

dorsal c. of spinal cord, c. dorsal da medula espinal. SIN posterior c.

c. of fornix [TA], c. do fórnice; parte do fórnice que se curva para baixo, rostralmente ao tálamo dorsal e adjacente ao forame de Monro interventricular, continuando depois através do hipotálamo até o corpo mamilar; consiste basicamente em fibras originadas no hipocampo e subículo, a coluna do fórnice é a continuação direta do corpo do fórnice. SIN columna fornicis [TA], anterior pillar of fornix.

general somatic afferent c., c. aferente somática geral; no embrião, uma coluna de substância cinzenta no metencéfalo e na medula espinal, representada, no adulto, pelos núcleos sensoriais do nervo trigêmeo e células de retransmissão no corno dorsal.

general somatic efferent c., c. eferente somática geral; coluna de substância cinzenta no embrião, representada, no adulto, pelos núcleos dos nervos oculomotor, troclear, abducente e hipoglosso e por neurônios motores do corno ventral da medula espinal.

general visceral afferent c., c. aferente visceral geral; coluna de substância cinzenta no metencéfalo e na medula espinal do embrião, desenvolvendo-se no núcleo do trato solitário e nas células de retransmissão da medula espinal.

general visceral efferent c., c. eferente visceral geral; coluna de substância cinzenta no metencéfalo e medula espinal do embrião, representada, no adulto, pelo núcleo dorsal do vago, núcleos salivatórios superior e inferior e de Edinger-Westphal e neurônios motores viscerais da medula espinal.

Goll c., c. de Goll. SIN gracile *fasciculus.*

Gowers c., c. de Gowers. SIN anterior spinocerebellar *tract.*

gray c.'s, colunas cinzentas; as três massas de substância cinzenta, com formato semelhante a cristas (colunas anterior, posterior e intermediária), que se estendem longitudinalmente através do centro de cada metade lateral da medula espinal; em cortes transversais, essas colunas aparecem como cornos cinzentos e, portanto, são comumente denominadas corno ventral ou anterior, dorsal ou posterior, e lateral, respectivamente. SIN columnae griseae [TA].

intermediate c. [TA], c. intermédia; a região intermédia da substância cinzenta da medula espinal situada entre os cornos posterior e anterior. Essa área contém vários núcleos que, coletivamente, formam a lâmina espinal VIII [TA] de Rexed. Os núcleos da coluna intermediária, ou zona intermediária, são o núcleo intermediolateral no corno lateral, substância intermediária central, núcleo torácico posterior ou dorsal (núcleo de Clarke), substância intermediária lateral, núcleo intermediomedial, núcleos parassimpáticos sacrais [TA] (nuclei parasympathici sacrales [TA]), núcleo do nervo pudendo (nucleus nervi pudendi), partes da formação reticular espinal [TA] (formatio reticularis spinalis [TA]) e o núcleo medial anterior [TA] (nucleus medialis anterior [TA]). SIN columna intermedia [TA], intermediate region [TA], intermediate zone [TA].

intermediolateral cell c. of spinal cord, c. de células intermediolaterais da medula espinal. SIN intermediolateral *nucleus.*

lateral c., c. lateral; discreta protrusão da substância cinzenta da medula espinhal para o funículo lateral de cada lado, particularmente acentuada na região torácica, onde encerra neurônios motores pré-ganglionares da divisão simpática do sistema nervoso autônomo; corresponde ao corno lateral que aparece em cortes transversais da medula espinal. VER TAMBÉM gray c.'s. SIN columna lateralis, lateral c. of spinal cord.

lateral c. of spinal cord, c. lateral da medula espinal. SIN lateral c.

Lissauer c., c. de Lissauer. SIN dorsolateral *fasciculus.*

Morgagni c.'s, colunas de Morgagni. SIN anal c.'s.

posterior c. [TA], c. posterior; a crista acentuada, em sentido dorsolateral, de substância cinzenta em cada metade lateral da medula espinal, correspondente ao corno posterior ou dorsal que aparece em cortes transversais da medula espinal. SIN columna posterior [TA], dorsal c. of spinal cord, posterior c. of spinal cord (1).

posterior c. of spinal cord, c. posterior da medula espinal; **(1)** SIN posterior c.; **(2)** em linguagem clínica, o termo freqüentemente se refere ao funículo posterior da medula espinal.

rectal c.'s, colunas retais. SIN anal c.'s.

renal c.'s [TA], colunas renais; o prolongamento da substância cortical, separando as pirâmides renais. SIN columnae renales [TA], Bertin c.'s.

Rolando c., c. de Rolando; discreta crista de cada lado do bulbo relacionada ao núcleo trigêmeo e ao trato trigeminal descendente.

rugal c.'s of vagina, colunas vaginais. SIN vaginal c.'s.

Sertoli c.'s, colunas de Sertoli. VER Sertoli *cells,* em *cell.*

special somatic afferent c., c. aferente somática especial; coluna de substância cinzenta no metencéfalo do embrião, representada, no adulto, pelos núcleos dos nervos auditivo e vestibular.

special visceral efferent c., c. eferente visceral especial; coluna de substância cinzenta no metencéfalo do embrião, representada, no adulto, pelos núcleos trigeminal e facial e núcleo ambíguo. SIN branchial efferent c.

spinal c., c. vertebral. SIN vertebral c.

c. of Spitzka-Lissauer, c. de Spitzka-Lissauer. VER dorsolateral *fasciculus.*

Stilling c., c. de Stilling. SIN posterior thoracic *nucleus.*

Türck c., c. de Türck. SIN anterior corticospinal *tract.*

vaginal c.'s, colunas vaginais; duas discretas cristas longitudinais, anterior e posterior, na mucosa vaginal, cada uma caracterizada por várias pregas muscosas transversais. SIN columnae rugarum, rugal c.'s of vagina.

ventral white c. [TA], c. branca anterior. SIN white *commissure.*

vertebral c. [TA], c. vertebral; o conjunto de vértebras que se estendem do crânio até o cóccix, proporcionando sustentação e formando um envoltório ósseo flexível para a medula espinal. SIN columna vertebralis [TA], spine (2) [TA], backbone, dorsal spine, rachis, spina dorsalis, spinal c., vertebrarium.

co·lum·na, gen. e pl. **co·lum·nae** (ko-lŭm′nă, -nē) [TA]. Coluna. SIN column. [L.]

colum′nae ana′les [TA], colunas anais. SIN anal *columns,* em *column.*

c. ante′rior [TA], c. anterior. SIN anterior *column.*

colum′nae car′neae, colunas carnosas. SIN *trabeculae* carneae (of right and lef ventricles), em *trabecula.*

c. for′nicis [TA], c. do fórnice. SIN *column* of fornix.

colum′nae gris′eae [TA], colunas cinzentas. SIN gray *columns,* em *column.*

c. intermedia [TA], c. intermédia. SIN intermediate *column.*

c. latera′lis, c. lateral. SIN lateral *column.*

c. poste′rior [TA], c. posterior. SIN posterior *column.*

colum′nae rena′les [TA], colunas renais. SIN renal *columns,* em *column.*

colum′nae ruga′rum, colunas das rugas. SIN vaginal *columns,* em *column.*

c. vertebra′lis [TA], c. vertebral. SIN vertebral *column.*

co·lum·nel·la, pl. **col·um·nel·lae** (ko-lŭm-nel′ă, -nel′ē). Columela. SIN columella (1). [L. dim. de *columna,* coluna; outra forma de *columella*]

co·ly·pep·tic (kō-lē-pep′tik). Colipéptico; termo raramente usado para retardar a digestão. [G. *kōlyō,* impedir, + *pepsis,* digestão]

com-. VER con-.

co·ma (ko′mă). Coma. **1.** Estado de inconsciência profunda do qual não é possível despertar; pode ser devido à ação de uma substância tóxica ingerida ou

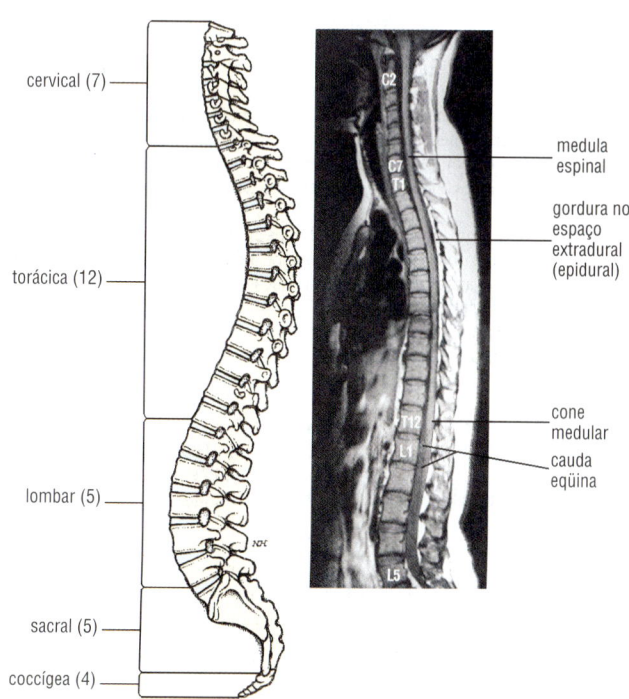

coluna vertebral: (esquerda) vista lateral da coluna completa, (direita) imagem de ressonância magnética sagital do atlas até a quinta vértebra lombar

formada no corpo, a traumatismo ou doença. [G. *kōma*, sono profundo, êxtase] **2.** Aberração de lentes esféricas; que ocorre em casos de incidência oblíqua (p. ex., a imagem de um ponto adquire um formato de cometa). [G. *kome*, cabelo] **3.** SIN coma *aberration.*

delayed c. after hypoxia, c. tardio após hipoxia; coma que se desenvolve alguns dias até 3 semanas após uma agressão hipóxica aguda; esta última geralmente foi suficientemente grave para causar um episódio inicial de coma, que cessou, e foi seguido por um intervalo transitório de aparente normalidade. SIN severe postanoxic encephalopathy.

diabetic c., c. diabético; coma que se desenvolve em casos graves e inadequadamente tratados de diabetes melito, sendo comumente fatal, exceto se for instituído tratamento adequado imediatamente; resulta da redução do metabolismo oxidativo do sistema nervoso central, que, por sua vez, é decorrente de cetoacidose grave e possivelmente, também da ação histotóxica dos corpos cetônicos e de distúrbios do equilíbrio hidroeletrolítico. SIN Kussmaul c.

hepatic c., c. hepático; coma que ocorre na insuficiência hepática avançada e nas derivações (*shunts*) portossistêmicas, causado por elevados níveis sanguíneos de amônia; os achados característicos incluem asterixe no estágio pré-coma e paroxismos de ondas trifásicas sincrônicas bilaterais ao EEG.

hyperosmolar (hyperglicemic) nonketotic c. (hī′per-os-mō-lār) coma hiperosmolar (hiperglicêmico) não-cetótico; complicação observada no *diabetes* melito na qual ocorre hiperglicemia muito acentuada (com níveis > 800 mg/dl), causando deslocamentos osmóticos da água nas células cerebrais e resultando em coma. Pode ser fatal ou causar lesão neurológica permanente. Não há cetoacidose nesses casos. SIN nonketotic hyperglycemia.

hypoglicemic c., c. hipoglicêmico; encefalopatia metabólica causada por hipoglicemia; geralmente observada em diabéticos e causada por excesso de insulina exógena.

hypoventilation c., c. da hipoventilação; coma observado na insuficiência pulmonar avançada e conseqüente hipoventilação. SIN CO_2 narcosis, hypoxic-hypercarbic encephalopathy, pulmonary encephalopathy.

Kussmaul c., c. de Kussmaul. SIN diabetic c.

metabolic c., c. metabólico; coma resultante de falência difusa do metabolismo neuronal, causada por anormalidades como distúrbios intrínsecos do metabolismo dos neurônios ou das células gliais, ou distúrbios extracerebrais que causam intoxicação ou desequilíbrios eletrolíticos.

thyrotoxic c., c. tireotóxico; c. que precede a morte no hipertireoidismo grave, como na crise tireotóxica ou tempestade tireóidea.

trance c., c. hipnótico. SIN lethargic *hypnosis.*

uremic c., c. urêmico; encefalopatia metabólica causada por insuficiência renal.

co·ma·tose (kō′mă-tōs). Comatoso; em estado de coma.

com·bi·na·tion (kom-bi-nā′shŭn). Combinação. **1.** O ato de combinar (isto é, juntando, unindo ou associando de outra forma) entidades distintas. **2.** O estado do que está assim combinado.

binary c., c. binária; o nome de uma espécie de bactérias que consiste em duas partes: um nome genérico e um epíteto específico.

new c., nova combinação; o novo nome que resulta da transferência de um microrganismo de um gênero para outro; o nome genérico muda, mas, na maioria dos casos, o epíteto específico permanece o mesmo.

com·bi·na·to·ri·al (kom′bin-ă-tor′ē-ăl). Combinatório; qualquer sistema que utiliza um agrupamento aleatório de componentes em quaisquer posições no arranjo linear de átomos, isto é, uma biblioteca combinatória de mutações poderia conter posições onde todas as quatro bases tivessem sido aleatoriamente inseridas.

com·bus·ti·ble (kom-bus′ti-bl). Combustível; capaz de combustão.

com·bus·tion (kom-bŭs′chŭn). Combustão; queima, a oxidação rápida de qualquer substância acompanhada pela produção de calor e luz. [L. *comburo*, pp. –*bustus*, queimar]

slow c., c. lenta. VER decay.

spontaneous c., c. espontânea; a ignição de uma massa de material por calor desenvolvido em seu interior pela oxidação das substâncias que o compõem sem ignição externa.

Comby, Jules, pediatra francês, 1853-1947. VER C. *sign.*

com·e·do, pl. **com·e·dos, com·e·do·nes** (kom′ē-do, kō-mē′dō; kom′ē-doz; kom-ē-dō′nēz). Comedão; infundíbulo do folículo piloso dilatado, cheio de escamas de queratina, bactérias, particularmente *Propionibacterium acnes*, e sebo; a lesão primária da acne vulgar. [L. glutão, de *com-edo,* comer]

closed c., c. fechado; um comedão com uma abertura estreita ou obstruída na superfície cutânea; os comedões fechados podem romper-se, produzindo uma reação inflamatória dérmica discreta. SIN whitehead (2).

open c., c. aberto; comedão com uma abertura larga na superfície cutânea, coberta com uma massa escurecida de resíduos epiteliais que contém melanina.

solar c., c. solar. VER Favre-Racouchot *disease.*

com·e·do·car·ci·no·ma (kō-mē′dō-kar-si-nō′mă). Comedocarcinoma; forma de carcinoma da mama ou outro órgão no qual tampões de células malignas necróticas podem ser espremidos dos ductos.

com·e·do·gen·ic (kom′ē-dō-jen′ik). Comedogênico; que tende a promover a formação de comedões. [comedo- + G. *genesis*, produção]

com·e·do·ne·cro·sis (kom′ē-dō-nek-rō′sis). Comedonecrose; tipo de necrose que ocorre em glândulas com inflamação luminal central com células desvitalizadas, geralmente ocorrendo na mama no carcinoma intraductal. [comedo + necrosis]

co·mes, pl. **com·i·tes** (kō′mēz, kom′i-tēz). Acompanhante, companheiro; vaso sanguíneo que acompanha outro vaso ou um nervo; as veias que acompanham uma artéria, freqüentemente em número de duas, são denominadas veias acompanhantes. [L. companheiro, de *com-*, junto, + *eo*, pp. *itus*, ir]

com·i·tance (kom′ē-tans). Comitância; característica do estrabismo na qual o desalinhamento dos olhos é mantido em todas as direções do olhar.

com·i·tant (komitant). Comitante; que possui comitância; em um estrabismo concomitante, o mesmo ângulo de desalinhamento dos olhos é mantido em todas as direções do olhar. SIN concomitant.

com·men·sal (kō-men′săl). Comensal. **1.** Relativo a, ou caracterizado por, comensalismo. **2.** Organismo que participa em comensalismo.

com·men·sal·ism (kō-men′săl-izm). Comensalismo; relação simbiótica na qual uma espécie obtém benefício e a outra não é prejudicada; p. ex., *Entamoeba coli* no intestino grosso humano. Cf. metabiosis, mutualism, parasitism. [L. *con-*, com, junto, + *mensa*, mesa]

epizoic c., c. epizóico. SIN phoresis (2).

com·mi·nut·ed (kom′i-noo-ted). Cominutivo; quebrado em vários pedaços; designa particularmente um osso fraturado. [L. *com-minuo*, pp. *-minutus*, tornar menor, quebrar em pedaços, de *minor*, menor]

com·mi·nu·tion (kom-i-noo′shŭn). Cominução; fragmentação.

com·mis·sura, gen. e pl., **com·mis·sur·ae** (kom-i-sūr′ă, -sūr′ē) [TA]. Comissura. SIN commissure. [L. união, sutura, de *committo*, enviar juntos, combinar]

c. alba anterior [TA], c. branca anterior. SIN white *commissure.*

c. al′ba posterior [TA], c. branca posterior. SIN white *commissure.*

c. ante′rior [TA], c. anterior. SIN anterior *commissure.*

c. ante′rior gris′ea, c. cinzenta anterior. VER *substantia* intermedia centralis.

c. bulbor′um [TA], c. dos bulbos. SIN *commissure* of bulbs.

c. cine′rea, aderência intertalâmica. SIN interthalamic *adhesion.*

c. colliculo′rum inferi′orum [TA], c. do colículo inferior. VER *commisure* of inferior colliculus.

c. colliculo′rum superio′rum [TA], c. do colículo superior. VER *commissure* of superior colliculus.

c. epithalamica, c. epitalâmica. SIN c. posterior.

c. for′nicis [TA], c. do hipocampo; a lâmina subcalosa triangular de fibras comissurais resultantes da convergência dos feixes direito e esquerdo do fórnice, que trocam numerosas fibras e curvam-se de volta, no fórnice contralateral, para terminar no hipocampo do lado oposto. SIN commissure of fornix [TA], hippocampi, delta fornicis, hippocampal commissure, psalterium, transverse fornix.

c. grisea posterior [TA], c. cinzenta posterior. VER gray *commissure.*

c. gris′ea, c. cinzenta. **(1)** SIN interthalamic *adhesion;* **(2)** VER *substantia* intermedia centralis.

c. grisea anterior, c. cinzenta anterior. VER gray *commissure.*

c. habenula′rum [TA], c. habenular; a conexão entre os núcleos habenulares direito e esquerdo; a decussação de fibras das duas estrias medulares, formando a porção dorsal do pedúnculo do corpo pineal. SIN habenular commissure [TA], commissure of habenulae.

c. hippocam′pi, c. do hipocampo. SIN c. fornicis.

c. labio′rum [TA], c. dos lábios. SIN *commissure* of lips.

c. labio′rum ante′rior [TA], c. anterior dos lábios do pudendo. SIN anterior labial *commissure.*

c. labio′rum poste′rior [TA], c. posterior dos lábios do pudendo. SIN posterior labial *commissure.*

c. lateralis palpebrum [TA], c. lateral das pálpebras. SIN lateral palpebral *commissure.*

c. medialis palpebrum [TA], c. medial das pálpebras. SIN medial palpebral *commissure.*

c. palpebra′rum latera′lis, c. lateral das pálpebras. SIN lateral palpebral *commissure.*

c. palpebra′rum media′lis, c. medial das pálpebras. SIN medial palpebral *commissure.*

c. poste′rior [TA], c. posterior; fina faixa de substância branca, cruzando de um lado a outro sobre a habênula do corpo pineal e sobre o ádito no aqueduto cerebral; é composta principalmente de fibras que conectam as regiões prétectais esquerda e direita e grupos celulares relacionados do mesencéfalo; dorsalmente, marca a junção do diencéfalo com o mesencéfalo. SIN c. epithalamica, posterior commissure.

c. supraop′tica dorsalis [TA], c. supra-óptica dorsal; as fibras comissurais situadas acima e atrás do quiasma óptico. SIN dorsal supraoptic commissure, Ganser commissure, Gudden commissure, Meynert commissure.

c. ventra′lis al′ba, c. branca anterior. SIN white *commissure.*

com·mis·sur·al (kom - i - sūr′al). Comissural; relativo a uma comissura.
com·mis·sure (kom′i - shūr) [TA]. Comissura. **1.** Ângulo do olho ou lábios. **2.** Feixe de fibras nervosas que passam de um lado ao outro no encéfalo ou na medula espinhal. SIN commissura [TA].
   anterior c. [TA], c. anterior; feixe redondo de fibras nervosas que cruzam a linha média do encéfalo próximo ao limite anterior do terceiro ventrículo. Consiste em uma parte anterior menor (pars anterior commissurae anterioris [TA]), cujas fibras seguem, em parte, para os bulbos olfatórios, e uma parte posterior maior (pars posterior commissurae anterioris [TA]), que conecta os lobos temporais esquerdo e direito. SIN commissura anterior [TA].
   anterior gray c. [TA], c. cinzenta anterior. VER gray c.
   anterior labial c. [TA], c. anterior dos lábios do pudendo; a junção dos lábios maiores do pudendo anteriormente, no monte do púbis. SIN commissura labiorum anterior [TA]
   anterior c. of the larynx, c. anterior da laringe; a junção das pregas vocais anteriormente na laringe.
   anterior white c. [TA], c. branca anterior. SIN white c.
   c. of bulbs [TA], c. dos bulbos; faixa mediana estreita que une as duas massas de tecido erétil (o bulbo do vestíbulo) de cada lado do óstio vaginal. SIN commissura bulborum [TA], c. of vestibular bulb, intermediate part of vestibular bulb, pars intermedia commissurae bulborum.
   c. of cerebral hemispheres, c. dos hemisférios cerebrais. SIN corpus callosum.
   dorsal supraoptic c., c. supra-óptica dorsal. SIN commissura supraoptica dorsalis.
   c. of fornix [TA], c. do hipocampo. SIN commissura fornicis.
   Ganser c., c. de Ganser. SIN commissura supraoptica dorsalis.
   gray c. [TA], c. cinzenta; faixas estreitas de substância cinzenta que atravessam a linha média dorsalmente ao canal central (c. cinzenta posterior [TA], commissura griesa posterior [TA]) e ventral ao canal central (c. cinzenta anterior [TA], commissura grisea anterior [TA]).
   Gudden c., c. de Gudden. SIN commissura supraoptica dorsalis.
   c. of habenulae, c. habenular. SIN commissura habenularum.
   habenular c. [TA], c. habenular. SIN commissura habenularum.
   hippocampal c., c. do hipocampo. SIN commissura fornicis.
   c. of inferior colliculus [TA], c. do colículo inferior; fibras nervosas na linha média entre os dois colículos inferiores, unindo os colículos e contendo algumas fibras originadas nos núcleos não-tectais.
   labial c. [TA], c. dos lábios; junção dos lábios superior e inferior que ocorre no ângulo da boca. VER TAMBÉM angle of mouth.
   lateral palpebral c. [TA], c. lateral das pálpebras; a união das pálpebras superior e inferior adjacente ao ângulo lateral. SIN commissura lateralis palpebrum [TA], commissura palpebrarum lateralis.
   c. of lips, c. dos lábios; a junção dos lábios lateral ao ângulo da boca. SIN commissura labiorum [TA], junction of lips.
   medial palpebral c. [TA], c. medial das pálpebras; a união das pálpebras superior e inferior adjacente ao ângulo medial. SIN commissura medialis palpebrum [TA], commissura palpebrarum medialis.
   Meynert c., c. de Meynert. SIN commissura supraoptica dorsalis.
   posterior c., c. posterior. SIN commissura posterior.
   posterior gray c. [TA], c. cinzenta posterior. VER gray c.
   posterior labial c. [TA], c. posterior dos lábios; discreta prega que une os lábios maiores do pudendo posteriormente, à frente do ânus. SIN commissura labiorum posterior [TA].
   posterior c. of the larynx, c. posterior da laringe. SIN interarytenoid fold.
   c. of superior colliculus [TA], c. do colículo superior; fibras nervosas que unem porções correspondentes e não-correspondentes dos dois colículos superiores através da linha média; pode conter fibras originadas fora do teto. SIN brachium colliculi superioris [TA].
   ventral white c., [TA], c. branca anterior. SIN white c.
   c. of vestibular bulb, c. do bulbo vestibular. SIN c. of bulbs.
   Wernekinck c., c. de Wernekinck; a decussação dos pedúnculos cerebelares antes de sua entrada no núcleo rubro do tegmento.
   white c., c. branca.; faixa estreita de substância branca que cruza a linha média da medula espinhal, dorsalmente ao canal central e à comissura cinzenta posterior (comissura branca posterior [TA]) e ventralmente ao canal central e à comissura cinzenta anterior (comissura branca anterior [TA]). SIN anterior white c. [TA], commissura alba anterior [TA], commissura alba posterior [TA], ventral white column [TA], ventral white c. [TA], commissura ventralis alba.
com·mis·sur·ot·o·my (kom′i - sūr - ot′ō - mē). Comissurotomia. **1.** Divisão cirúrgica de qualquer comissura, faixa fibrosa ou anel através de uma incisão ou ruptura, p. ex., insuflação por balão. **2.** SIN midline myelotomy.
   mitral c., c. mitral; abertura do óstio mitral estreitado para alívio de estenose mitral.
com·mit·ment (kŏ - mit′ment). Interdição; internação; alienação legal, por atestado ou voluntariamente, de um indivíduo em hospital ou instituição mental. [L. com-mitto, fornecer, consignar]
com·mom ve·hi·cle spread. Disseminação por veículo comum; disseminação de agente causador de doença de uma fonte que é comum àqueles que adquirem a doença, p. ex., água, leite, ar, seringa contaminada por agentes infecciosos ou nocivos.
com·mo·tio (kō - mō′shē - ō). Comoção; concussão. SIN concussion (2). [L. abalo, comoção, de commoveo, pp. -motus, colocar em movimento, agitar]
   c. cer'ebri, concussão cerebral. SIN brain concussion.
   c. re'tinae, concussão da retina; concussão da retina podendo causar edema leitoso, no pólo posterior, que desaparece após alguns dias.
com·mu·ni·ca·ble (kō - mūn′i - ka - bl). Transmissível; contagioso; capaz de ser transmitido; diz-se especialmente de uma doença.
com·mu·ni·cans, pl. **com·mu·ni·can·tes** (kō - mū′ni - kans, kō - mū - ni - kan′tēz). Comunicante; que liga ou une. [L. pret. pres. de communico, pp. -atus, compartilhar com alguém, tornar comum]
com·mu·ni·ca·tion (kō - mū - ni - kā′shŭn). Comunicação. **1.** Abertura ou passagem de união entre duas estruturas. **2.** Em anatomia, uma união ou junção de estruturas sólidas, fibrosas, p. ex., tendões e nervos. Utiliza-se incorretamente o termo anastomose como sinônimo. **3.** Informações ou idéias transmitidas de uma parte para outra. [L. communicatio]
   human c., c. humana; a produção e recepção de informações orais, escritas, por sinais ou gestos entre seres humanos; envolve o uso de símbolos conhecidos, como a linguagem recebida através dos sistemas auditivo, tátil, proprioceptivo e visual, e gerada através da voz e da fala, escrita, sinais manuais e gestos; algumas vezes, a comunicação entre seres humanos pode envolver os sentidos vestibular, olfativo e gustativo.
   simultaneous c., c. simultânea. SIN total c.
   total c., c. total; método para a educação de crianças surdas que usa uma combinação de linguagem dos sinais, alfabeto manual e comunicação oral. VER TAMBÉM oral auditory method, manual visual method, combined methods, em method. SIN simultaneous c.
com·mu·ni·ty (kō - mū′ni - tē). Comunidade; um determinado segmento de uma sociedade ou população.
   biotic c., c. biótica. SIN biocenosis.
   therapeutic c., c. terapêutica; centro de saúde comunitário ou sanatório especialmente estruturado, que proporciona um ambiente efetivo para mudanças comportamentais nos pacientes através de ressocialização e reabilitação.
com·mu·ni·ty men·tal health cen·ter. Centro comunitário de saúde mental; centro de tratamento mental localizado em uma área de captação vizinha próxima das casas dos pacientes, introduzido na década de 1960 através de nova legislação federal norte-americana; visava substituir os grandes hospitais estaduais, que geralmente estavam situados em áreas rurais distantes; suas características incluem oferta de uma série de serviços abrangentes por um ou mais membros das quatro profissões relacionadas à saúde mental, provimento de continuidade do tratamento, participação dos usuários nos centros, localização na comunidade para permitir fácil acesso, combinação de serviços diretos e indiretos ou preventivos, uso de pareceres centralizados no programa e, também, centralizados no caso, exigência de avaliação do programa e várias ligações com diversos serviços de saúde e humanos.
co·mor·bid·i·ty (kō - mōr - bid′i - tē). Co-morbidade; uma doença concomitante, mas não relacionada; termo geralmente usado em epidemiologia para indicar a coexistência de dois ou mais processos mórbidos. [co- + L. morbidus, doente]
com·pac·ta (kom - pak′tā). Estrato compacto. SIN stratum compactum.
com·pa·ges tho·ra·cis (kom - pā′jez thō - rā′sis). Caixa torácica. SIN thoracic cage.
com·par·a·scope (kom - par′ā - skōp). Comparoscópio; acessório para microscópio por meio do qual um observador pode comparar, direta e simultaneamente, os achados em dois preparados microscópicos. [L. comparo, comparar, + G. skopeō, ver]
com·par·ti·men·tum. Compartimento. SIN compartment.
   c. antebrachii anterius [TA], c. anterior do antebraço. SIN anterior compartment of forearm.
   c. antebrachii extensorum, c. extensor do antebraço; *termo oficial alternativo para posterior compartment of forearm.
   c. antebrachii flexorum, c. flexor do antebraço; *termo oficial alternativo para anterior compartment of forearm.
   c. antebrachii posterius [TA], c. posterior do antebraço. SIN posterior compartment of forearm.
   c. brachii anterius [TA], c. anterior do braço. SIN anterior compartment of arm.
   c. brachii extensorum, c. extensor do braço; *termo oficial alternativo para posterior compartment of arm.
   c. brachii flexorum [TA], c. flexor do braço; c. anterior do braço. SIN anterior compartment of arm.
   c. brachii posterius [TA], c. posterior do braço. SIN posterior compartment of arm.
   c. cruris, c. crural. SIN lateral compartment of leg.
   c. cruris anterius [TA], c. crural anterior; c. anterior da perna. SIN anterior compartment of leg.
   c. cruris extensorum, c. crural extensor; *termo oficial alternativo para anterior compartment of leg.

c. cruris fibularium, c. crural fibular; *termo oficial alternativo para lateral compartment of leg.
c. cruris flexorum, c. crural flexor; *termo oficial alternativo para posterior compartment of leg.
c. cruris laterale peroneorum [TA], c. crural lateral fibular; c. lateral da perna. SIN lateral compartment of leg.
c. cruris posterius [TA], c. crural posterior; c. posterior da perna. SIN posterior compartment of leg.
c. femoris adductorum, c. femoral adutor; *termo oficial alternativo para medial compartment of thigh.
c. femoris anterius [TA], c. anterior da coxa. SIN anterior compartment of thigh.
c. femoris extensorum [TA], c. femoral extensor; c. anterior da coxa. SIN anterior compartment of thigh.
c. femoris flexorum, c. femoral flexor; *termo oficial alternativo para posterior compartment of thigh.
c. femoris mediale [TA], c. medial da coxa. SIN medial compartment of thigh.
c. femoris posterius [TA], c. posterior da coxa. SIN posterior compartment of thigh.
compartment. Compartimento. **1.** Porção separada de um espaço maior; uma secção ou câmara distinta; os compartimentos dos membros são limitados, profundamente, por ossos e septos intermusculares e, superficialmente, por fáscia profunda e, em geral, não se comunicam com os outros compartimentos, daí uma infecção ou aumento anormal da pressão poder ser limitado a um compartimento; os músculos contidos nos compartimentos dos membros possuem funções e inervação semelhantes. **2.** Uma outra divisão, especificamente uma porção estrutural ou bioquímica de uma célula, separada do restante da célula. SIN compartimentum.
adductor c. of thigh, c. adutor da coxa; *termo oficial alternativo para medial c. of thigh.
anterior c. of arm [TA], c. anterior do braço; porção anterior do espaço encerrado pela fáscia braquial, separada do compartimento posterior pelo úmero e pelos septos intermusculares lateral e medial que se estendem a partir dele; contém músculos que produzem flexão, todos inervados pelo nervo musculocutâneo. SIN compartimentum brachii anterius [TA], compartimentum brachii flexorum [TA], flexor c. of arm*.
anterior c. of forearm [TA], c. anterior do antebraço; porção anterior do espaço encerrado pela fáscia do antebraço, separada do compartimento posterior pelo rádio e ulna e pela membrana interóssea interposta; os espaços são demarcados superficialmente pela borda subcutânea da ulna e pela artéria radial (pulso); contém os pronadores do antebraço, flexores do punho e flexores longos dos dedos, inervados pelos nervos mediano (principalmente) e ulnar; é incomum entre os compartimentos do membro, pois se comunica através do túnel do carpo com o espaço palmar médio. SIN compartimentum antebrachii anterius [TA], compartimentum antebrachii flexorum*, flexor c. of forearm*.
anterior c. of leg [TA], c. anterior da perna; porção anterior do espaço encerrado pela fáscia profunda da perna, separada do compartimento posterior pela tíbia e fíbula pela membrana interóssea interposta, e do compartimento lateral pelo septo intermuscular anterior; contém os dorsiflexores do pé e os extensores longos dos artelhos, todos inervados pelo nervo fibular profundo. SIN compartimentum cruris anterius [TA], compartimentum cruris extensorum*, extensor c. of leg*, dorsiflexor c. of leg.
anterior c. of thigh [TA], c. anterior da coxa; porção anterior do espaço encerrado pela fáscia lata, separada dos compartimentos medial e lateral pelos septos intermusculares medial e lateral, respectivamente; contém a diáfise do fêmur e os músculos que produzem flexão do quadril e/ou extensão do joelho, inervados pelo nervo femoral. SIN compartimentum femoris anterius [TA], compartimentum femoris extensorum [TA], extensor c. of thigh*, c. of thigh for extensors of knee, c. of thigh for flexors of hip.
dorsiflexor c. of leg, c. dorsiflexor da perna. SIN anterior c. of leg.
extensor c. of arm, c. extensor do braço; *termo oficial alternativo para posterior c. of arm.
extensor c. of forearm, c. extensor do antebraço; *termo oficial alternativo para posterior c. of forearm.
extensor c. of leg, c. extensor da perna; *termo oficial alternativo para anterior c. of leg.
extensor c. of thigh, c. extensor da coxa; *termo oficial alternativo para anterior c. of thigh.
fibular c. of leg, c. fibular da perna; *termo oficial alternativo para lateral c. of leg.
flexor c. of arm, c. flexor do braço; *termo oficial alternativo para anterior c. of arm.
flexor c. of forearm, c. flexor do antebraço; *termo oficial alternativo para anterior c. of forearm.
flexor c. of leg, c. flexor da perna; *termo oficial alternativo para posterior c. of leg.
flexor c. of thigh, c. flexor da coxa; *termo oficial alternativo para posterior c. of thigh.
lateral c. of leg [TA], c. lateral da perna; porção lateral do espaço encerrado pela fáscia profunda da perna, separada dos compartimentos anterior e posterior pelos septos intermusculares anterior e posterior da perna, respectivamente; contém os músculos que fazem a eversão do pé, inervados pelo fibular superficial. SIN compartimentum cruris laterale peroneorum [TA], compartimentum cruris fibularium*, fibular c. of leg*, peroneal c. of leg*, compartimentum cruris.
medial c. of thigh [TA], c. medial da coxa; porção medial do espaço encerrado pela fáscia lata, separada dos compartimentos anterior e posterior pelos septos intermusculares femorais medial e posterior, respectivamente; contém músculos que aduzem a coxa na articulação do quadril, todos inervados pelo nervo obturatório. SIN compartimentum femoris mediale [TA], adductor c. of thigh*, compartimentum femoris adductorum*.
nonplasmatic c., c. não-plasmático; compartimento circundado por uma única biomembrana (p. ex., vacúolos, lisossomas).
peroneal c. of leg, c. fibular da perna; *termo oficial alternativo para lateral c. of leg.
plantarflexor c. of leg, c. flexor plantar da perna. SIN posterior c. of leg.
plasmatic c., c. plasmático; compartimento circundado por uma membrana biológica dupla e contendo polinucleotídeos (p. ex., mitocôndrias).
posterior c. of arm [TA], c. posterior do braço; porção posterior do espaço encerrado pela fáscia braquial, separada do compartimento anterior pelo úmero e pelos septos intermusculares lateral e medial que dele se estendem; contém os músculos tríceps que estendem o antebraço na articulação do cotovelo e são inervados pelo nervo radial. SIN compartimentum brachii posterius [TA], compartimentum brachii extensorum*, extensor c. of arm*.
posterior c. of forearm [TA], c. posterior do antebraço; porção posterior do espaço encerrado pela fáscia do antebraço, separada do compartimento anterior pelo rádio e ulna e pela membrana interóssea interposta; os espaços são demarcados superficialmente pela borda subcutânea da ulna e da artéria radial (pulso); contém um músculo supinador do antebraço, extensores da mão no punho e extensores longos dos dedos, todos inervados pelo nervo radial. SIN compartimentum antebrachii posterius [TA], compartimentum antebrachii extensorum*, extensor c. of forearm*.
posterior c. of leg [TA], c. posterior da perna; porção posterior do espaço encerrado pela fáscia profunda da perna, separada do compartimento anterior pela tíbia e fíbula e pela membrana interóssea interposta, e do compartimento lateral pelo septo intermuscular posterior da perna; contém os músculos flexores plantares do pé e flexores longos dos artelhos, todos inervados pelo nervo tibial. SIN compartimentum cruris posterius [TA], compartimentum cruris flexorum*, flexor c. of leg*, plantarflexor c. of leg.
posterior c. of thigh [TA], c. posterior da coxa; porção posterior do espaço encerrado pela fáscia lata, separada dos compartimentos medial e anterior pelos septos intermusculares posterior e lateral, respectivamente; contém os músculos do jarrete (extensor da coxa na articulação do quadril e flexores da perna na articulação do joelho) e a cabeça curta do bíceps; todos inervados pelo nervo ciático (o primeiro pela porção do nervo tibial, o último pela porção do nervo fibular). SIN compartimentum femoris posterius [TA], compartimentum femoris flexorum*, flexor c. of thigh*, c. of thigh for extensors of hip joint, c. of thigh for flexors of knee.
c. of thigh for extensors of hip joint, c. da coxa para os extensores da articulação do quadril. SIN posterior c. of thigh.
c. of thigh for extensors of knee, c. da coxa para os extensores do joelho. SIN anterior c. of thigh.
c. of thigh for flexors of hip, c. da coxa para os flexores do quadril. SIN anterior c. of thigh.
c. of thigh for flexors of knee, c. da coxa para os flexores do joelho. SIN posterior c. of thigh.
com·part·men·ta·tion (kom - part′ment - ā′shŭn). Compartimentalização; a divisão de uma célula em regiões diferentes, do ponto de vista estrutural ou bioquímico.
com·pat·i·bil·i·ty (kom - pat - ī - bil′i - tē). Compatibilidade; a condição de ser compatível.
com·pat·i·ble (kom - pat′ī - bl). Compatível. **1.** Capaz de ser misturado sem sofrer alteração química destrutiva ou exibir antagonismo mútuo; diz-se dos elementos em uma mistura farmacêutica adequadamente formada. **2.** Designa a capacidade de duas entidades biológicas existirem juntas sem se anularem ou apresentarem efeitos prejudiciais sobre a função da outra; p. ex., sangue, tecidos ou órgãos que não causam reação quando transfundidos ou não causam rejeição quando transplantados. **3.** Designa relações satisfatórias entre duas ou mais pessoas como no trabalho ou casamento, ou em atividades sexuais. [L. *con-*, com, + *patior*, sofrer]
com·pen·sa·tion (kom - pen - sā′shŭn). Compensação. **1.** Processo pelo qual uma tendência de modificação em determinada direção é neutralizada por outra alteração de forma que a original não seja evidente. **2.** Um mecanismo inconsciente pelo qual se tenta superar deficiências reais ou imaginárias. [L. *compenso*, pp. *–atus*, contrabalançar, compensar]
attenuation c., c. de atenuação. SIN time-gain c.
depth c., c. de profundidade. SIN time-gain c.
gene dosage c., c. na dosagem de genes; o suposto mecanismo que ajusta os fenótipos ligados ao X de homens e mulheres para compensar o estado haplói-

de em homens e o estado diplóide em mulheres. Agora é amplamente atribuído à lionização que compensa a média da dose, mas não sua variância (quadrado do desvio padrão), que é maior em mulheres.

time-gain c. (TGC), c. de ganho temporal, em ultra-sonografia, um aumento no ganho do receptor com tempo para compensar a perda na amplitude do eco com a profundidade, geralmente devido à atenuação. SIN attenuation c., depth c., time compensation gain, time-compensated gain, time-varied gain control, time-varied gain.

com·pen·sa·to·ry (kom - pen′să - tōr - ē). Compensatório; que proporciona compensação; que supre uma deficiência ou perda.

com·pe·tence (kom′pĕ - tens). Competência. **1.** A qualidade de ser competente ou capaz de realizar uma função atribuída. **2.** O fechamento firme normal de uma válvula cardíaca. **3.** A capacidade de um grupo de células embrionárias responder a um indutor. **4.** A capacidade de uma célula (bacteriana) captar DNA livre, que pode levar à transformação. **5.** Em psiquiatria, a capacidade mental de distinguir o certo do errado e de administrar seus próprios interesses, ou de tomar parte na discussão em um processo legal. **6.** O estado de reatividade de uma célula, tecido ou organismo que permite responder a determinados estímulos. [Fr. *competence*, de L.L. *competentia*, congruência]

cardiac c., c. cardíaca; capacidade dos ventrículos de bombear o sangue que retorna para os átrios, de modo que a pressão arterial não aumente de forma anormal.

immunologic c., c. imunológica; capacidade de formar uma resposta imunológica.

com·pe·ti·tion (kom - pĕ - tish′un). Competição; o processo pelo qual a atividade ou presença de uma substância interfere com, ou suprime, a atividade de outra substância com afinidades semelhantes.

antigenic c., c. antigênica; competição que ocorre quando dois antígenos diferentes, cada um dos quais capaz de provocar uma resposta imunológica quando inoculado sozinho, são misturados e inoculados juntos; a resposta pode ser apenas a um, sendo a resposta ao outro ampla ou totalmente suprimida.

com·plaint (kom - plānt′). Queixa; um distúrbio, doença ou sintoma, ou a descrição dele. [Fr. ant. *complainte*, do L. *complango*, lamentar]

chief c., q. principal; o sintoma primário que um paciente declara como o motivo para procurar tratamento médico.

com·ple·ment (kom′plĕ - ment). Complemento; termo de Ehrlich para a substância termolábil, normalmente presente no soro, destrutiva para determinadas bactérias e outras células sensibilizadas por um anticorpo fixador de complemento específico. O complemento é um grupo de, pelo menos, 20 proteínas séricas distintas, cuja atividade é afetada por uma série de interações, resultando em clivagens enzimáticas a que podem seguir uma ou outra de, pelo menos, duas vias. No caso de hemólise imunológica (via clássica), o complexo compreende nove componentes (designados C1 a C9) que reagem em uma seqüência definida e cuja ativação geralmente é realizada pelo complexo antígeno-anticorpo; apenas os sete primeiros componentes estão envolvidos na quimiotaxia, e apenas os quatro primeiros estão envolvidos na aderência imunológica ou fagocitose, ou são fixados por conglutininas. Uma via alternativa (ver properdin *system*) pode ser ativada por outros fatores, além dos complexos antígeno-anticorpo, e envolve outros componentes, além de C1, C4 e C2, na ativação de C3. VER TAMBÉM *component* of complement. [L. *complementum*, aquele que completa, de *com-pleo*, preencher]

heparin c., c. heparina; o componente proteico da heparina no sangue.

c. pathways, vias do complemento; **(1)** a via do complemento clássica (geralmente iniciada por ligação de C1 a IgG ou do anticorpo IgM a C1) é um complexo de três subunidades: C1q, C1r e C1s. Após a ligação de C1q, C1r (um traço acima indica atividade enzimática) cliva C1s em C1s. C1s cliva C4 em C4a e C4b, e também C2 em C2a e C2b. C2b combina-se a C4b para formar C4b2b, que é uma C3 convertase. A C3 convertase cliva C3 em C3a e C3b. C3b une-se a C4bC2b para formar uma C5 convertase (também conhecida como C4b2b3b), que cliva C5 em C5a e C5b. Após C5b ser ligado à superfície celular, os componentes do complemento restantes (C6–C9), bem como C5b, formam o complexo de ataque à membrana (CAM). O CAM produz uma abertura na membrana celular. **(2)** Na via alternativa do complemento, C3b ligado à superfície une-se ao Fator B, que é clivado pelo Fator D em Ba e Bb. C3bBb é uma C3 convertase instável, exceto se a properdina (P) se ligar a ela para formar C3bBbP. A C3 convertase estável gera mais C3b. Quando um complexo de C3bBbC3b é formado, esta é a via alternativa C5 convertase. De C5b a C9, as vias clássica e alternativa são iguais. **(3)** Na via de ligação da lectina, a proteína ligadora de manose (PLM) inicia a via, que então usa componentes da via clássica do complemento. Alguns dos componentes "a" de ambas as vias possuem várias atividades biológicas, isto é, C3a é uma anafilatoxina.

com·ple·men·tar·i·ty (kom - plĕ - men - tār′i - tē). Complementaridade. **1.** O grau de pareamento de bases (A oposta a U ou T, G oposta a C) entre duas seqüências de moléculas de DNA e/ou RNA. **2.** O grau de afinidade, ou ajuste, de locais de combinação a antígeno e anticorpo.

com·ple·men·ta·tion (kom′plĕ - men - tā′shŭn). Complementação. **1.** Interação funcional entre dois vírus defeituosos, permitindo replicação em condições inibitórias para o vírus isolado. **2.** Interação entre duas unidades genéticas, sendo uma ou ambas deficientes, permitindo ao organismo que contém essas unidades funcionar normalmente, o que não seria possível se uma das unidades estivesse ausente.

intergenic c., c. intergênica; complementação entre fragmentos de material genético que regulam a mesma função, como uma via multienzimática, mas possuem defeitos em regiões de função genética distinta; essa complementação permite a síntese de um produto final normal.

intragenic c., c. intragênica; complementação entre fragmentos de material genético, cada um possuindo um defeito diferente no mesmo *locus*; o produto resultante de cada um é deficiente e não-funcional, mas os produtos defeituosos podem associar-se para produzir um produto que tem alguma atividade.

com·plex (kom′pleks). Complexo. **1.** Um conjunto organizado de sentimentos, pensamentos, percepções e memórias que podem ser parcialmente inconscientes e influenciar fortemente associações e atitudes. **2.** Em química, a combinação relativamente estável de duas ou mais substâncias em uma molécula maior sem ligação covalente. **3.** Um composto de estruturas químicas ou imunológicas. **4.** Uma entidade anatômica estrutural constituída por três ou mais partes inter-relacionadas. **5.** Termo informal usado para designar um grupo de estruturas individuais conhecidas ou consideradas anatômica, embriológica ou fisiologicamente relacionadas. [L. *complexus*, entrelaçado]

aberrant c., c. aberrante; complexo eletrocardiográfico anômalo, mais especificamente um complexo ventricular anormal causado por condução intraventricular anormal de um impulso supraventricular.

AIDS dementia c. (ADC), c. AIDS/SIDA-demência; c. demencial da AIDS/SIDA; c. de demência relacionado à AIDS/SIDA; encefalite por HIV-1 aguda ou crônica, a complicação neurológica mais comum nos estágios mais avançados de infecção por HIV; manifesta-se clinicamente por demência progressiva, acompanhada por anormalidades motoras. SIN AIDS dementia, HIV encephalopathy.

AIDS-related c. (ARC), c. relacionado à AIDS/SIDA; manifestações de AIDS/SIDA em pessoas que ainda não desenvolveram deficiência importante da função imune, caracterizada por febre com linfadenopatia generalizada, diarréia, emagrecimento, infecções oportunistas leves, citopenias.

amygdaloid c. [TA], corpo amigdalóide. SIN amygdaloid *body.*

anomalous c., c. anômalo; complexo no eletrocardiograma que difere significativamente do tipo fisiológico na mesma derivação.

antigen-antibody c., c. antígeno-anticorpo. VER immune c.

antigenic c., c. antigênico; composto de diferentes estruturas antigênicas, como uma célula ou bactéria, ou, por extensão, uma molécula contendo dois ou mais grupos determinantes de diferentes especificidades antigênicas.

apical c., c. apical; conjunto de estruturas anteriores que caracterizam um ou vários estágios do desenvolvimento de membros do filo de protozoários Apicomplexa; inclui as seguintes estruturas, visíveis à microscopia eletrônica: anel polar, conóide, róptrias, micronemas e túbulos subpeliculares.

atrial c., c. atrial; onda p no eletrocardiograma. SIN auricular c.

auricular c., c. auricular. SIN atrial p.

binary c., c. binário; complexo não-covalente de duas moléculas; freqüentemente, refere-se ao complexo enzima-substrato em uma reação catalisada por enzima. Cf. central c., Michaelis c. SIN enzyme-substrate c.

brain-wave c., c. de ondas cerebrais; uma combinação específica de atividade eletroencefalográfica rápida e lenta, que recorre com freqüência suficiente para ser identificada como um fenômeno distinto.

brother c., c. fraterno. SIN Cain c.

Cain c., c. fraterno, complexo de Cain; termo raramente usado para designar extrema inveja ou ciúme de um irmão, levando ao ódio. SIN brother c. [C. *Cain*, personagem bíblico]

Carney c., c. de Carney; condição autossômica dominante da síndrome de Cushing causada por inibição do receptor do ACTH mediada por imunoglobulina, mixomas cardíacos e cutâneos, lentigos, schwannomas melanóticos e tumores hipofisários e testiculares.

castration c., c. de castração; **(1)** medo de uma criança de ser lesada nos órgãos genitais pelo genitor do mesmo sexo como punição por culpa inconsciente de sentimentos edipianos; **(2)** fantasia de perda do pênis por uma mulher ou medo de sua perda real por um homem; **(3)** medo inconsciente de lesão por autoridades. SIN castration anxiety.

caudal pharyngeal c., c. faríngeo caudal; o corpo ultimobranquial associado à quarta bolsa faríngea e quinta bolsa faríngea transitória embrionárias.

central c., c. central; em uma reação catalisada por enzimas, o complexo estrutural da enzima e todos os substratos enzimáticos (ou a enzima com todos os produtos enzimáticos) equivalente ao complexo binário para uma enzima com um substrato. Cf. binary c., Michaelis c.

charge transfer c., c. de transferência de carga; **(1)** um complexo entre duas moléculas orgânicas no qual um elétron de uma (doadora) é transferido para a outra (aceptora), sendo distribuído geralmente por toda a molécula aceptora; a transferência subseqüente de um átomo de hidrogênio completa a redução do aceptor; esses complexos geralmente são muito coloridos e, assim, podem ser observados; **(2)** uma rede de pontes de hidrogênio no centro catalítico de algumas proteases. SIN charge transfer system.

Diana c., c. de Diana; termo raramente usado para designar idéias que levam à adoção de traços e comportamento masculino em uma mulher. [*Diana*, personagem mitológica L.]

diphasic c., c. difásico; complexo que consiste em deflexões positiva e negativa.

EAHF c., c. EAHF; combinação de alergias que consistem em *eczema*, *a*sma e febre do feno (*hay fever*).

Eisenmenger c., c. de Eisenmenger; a combinação de comunicação interventricular com hipertensão pulmonar e conseqüente derivação (*shunt*) direita-esquerda através do defeito, com ou sem cavalgamento da aorta associado. SIN Eisenmenger defect, Eisenmenger disease, Eisenmenger tetralogy.

Electra c., c. de Electra; equivalente feminino do complexo de Édipo no homem; termo usado para descrever conflitos não resolvidos durante a infância, em relação ao pai, que, subseqüentemente, influenciam as relações de uma mulher com homens. SIN father c. [*Electra*, filha de Agamemnon]

electrocardiographic c., c. eletrocardiográfico; deflexão ou grupo de deflexões no eletrocardiograma.

enzyme-substrate c., c. enzima-substrato. SIN binary c.

equiphasic c., c. eqüifásico. SIN isodiphasic c.

father c., c. paterno. SIN Electra c.

femininity c., c. de feminilidade; em psicanálise, o medo inconsciente, em meninos e homens, de castração pelas mãos da mãe, com conseqüente identificação com o agressor e desejo invejoso de mamas e vagina.

Ghon c., c. de Ghon. SIN Ghon *tubercle*.

Golgi c., c. de Golgi. SIN Golgi *apparatus*.

H-2 c., c. H-2; termo que designa genes do complexo principal de histocompatibilidade no camundongo.

---

histocompatibility c., c. de histocompatibilidade; família de cinqüenta ou mais genes, no sexto cromossoma humano, que codificam proteínas da superfície celular e participam da resposta imune.

Os genes de histocompatibilidade controlam a produção de proteínas nas membranas externas do tecido e das células do sangue, principalmente linfócitos, e são elementos essenciais no reconhecimento e na interação entre as células. As proteínas de superfície também determinam o nível e o tipo de resposta imune, estão envolvidas na apresentação de antígenos ao sistema imune e podem ter outras funções bioquímicas e imunológicas. No caso de aloenxertos, quanto maior a histocompatibilidade (isto é, quanto maior a semelhança entre antígenos do doador e da superfície celular do receptor), menor é a probabilidade de rejeição. Os principais determinantes de histocompatibilidade são os antígenos leucocitários humanos (HLA). A tipagem de HLA de um possível doador de medula óssea e um possível receptor de transplante é usada para prever rejeição do enxerto e doença enxerto-*versus*-hospedeiro.

HLA c., c. HLA; o principal complexo de histocompatibilidade em seres humanos. VER TAMBÉM human leukocyte *antigens*, em *antigen*.

immune c., imunocomplexo; antígeno combinado a anticorpo específico, ao qual o complemento também pode ser fixado, e que pode precipitar ou permanecer em solução. Freqüentemente associado à doença auto-imune.

inferiority c., c. de inferioridade; sentimento de inadequação expresso por timidez extrema, vergonha ou acanhamento, ou por reação compensatória de exibicionismo ou agressividade.

inferior olivary c. [TA], c. olivar inferior; os três núcleos que, coletivamente, formam o que é comumente denominado núcleo olivar inferior. Estes são o núcleo olivar principal (com suas lamelas dorsal, ventral e lateral) e os núcleos olivares acessório medial e acessório posterior (dorsal). VER TAMBÉM principal olivary *nucleus*. SIN complexus olivaris inferior [TA].

iron-dextran c., c. ferro-dextrano; solução coloidal de hidróxido férrico em complexo com dextrano parcialmente hidrolisado; usado no tratamento de anemias ferroprivas por injeção intramuscular.

isodiphasic c., c. isodifásico; complexo difásico cujas deflexões positiva e negativa são aproximadamente iguais. SIN equiphasic c.

j-g c., c. justaglomerular. SIN juxtaglomerular c.

Jocasta c., c. de Jocasta; termo raramente usado para designar a fixação libidinosa materna em um filho. [*Jocasta*, mãe e esposa de Édipo]

junctional c., c. juncional; a zona de fixação entre células epiteliais, que tipicamente consiste na zônula de oclusão, zônula de adesão e mácula aderente (desmossoma).

juxtaglomerular c., c. justaglomerular; complexo que consiste nas células justaglomerulares, que são células musculares lisas modificadas na parede da arteríola glomerular aferente e, algumas vezes, também na arteríola eferente; células *lacis* mesangiais extraglomerulares, localizadas no ângulo de reflexão da cápsula parietal para a visceral do corpúsculo renal; acredita-se que proporcione algum controle por retroalimentação do volume de líquido extracelular e da taxa de filtração glomerular. SIN j-g c., juxtaglomerular apparatus.

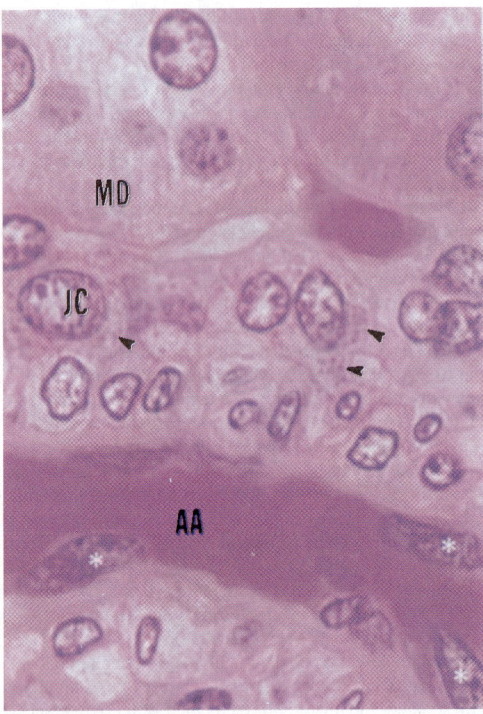

aparelho justaglomerular: rim de macaco; corte plástico, composto pela região da mácula densa (MD) do túbulo distal e células justaglomerulares (JC), células musculares lisas modificadas da arteríola glomerular aferente (AA); observar os grânulos (pontas de setas) nas células justaglomerulares e os núcleos (asteriscos) das células endoteliais que revestem a arteríola glomerular aferente; 1.325 ×

K c., c. K; ondas lentas frontocentrais difásicas, de grande amplitude no eletroencefalograma, relacionadas ao despertar do sono por um som; características dos estágios 2, 3 e 4 do sono.

α-keto acid dehydrogenase c., c. da α-cetoácido desidrogenase. VER α-*keto acid* dehydrogenase.

α-ketoglutarate dehydrogenase c., c. da α-cetoglutarato desidrogenase. SIN α-*ketoglutarate* dehydrogenase.

Lear c., c. de Lear; termo raramente usado para a fixação libidinosa de um pai em uma filha. [*Lear*, personagem de Shakespeare]

MAC c., c. de ataque à membrana (CAM). SIN membrane attack c.

major histocompatibility c. (MHC), c. principal de histocompatibilidade; um grupo de *loci* relacionados, coletivamente denominados c. H-2 no camundongo e c. HLA em seres humanos, que codifica os antígenos de histocompatibilidade da superfície celular e é o principal determinante do tipo tecidual e da compatibilidade do transplante. VER TAMBÉM human leukocyte *antigens*, em *antigen*.

mediator c., c. mediador; proteínas de coativação envolvidas na transcrição pela RNA polimerase de segmentos de DNA.

membrane attack c. (MAC), c. de ataque à membrana (CAM); complexo de componentes do complemento (C5–C9) que, quando ativado, liga-se à membrana de uma célula-alvo, penetrando-a com um resíduo hidrófobo exteriormente e um resíduo hidrófilo no interior da célula; isso permite a passagem de íons e água, edema da célula e lise subseqüente. SIN MAC c.

Meyenburg c., c. de Meyenburg; grupos de pequenos ductos biliares que ocorrem em fígados policísticos, separados das áreas portais.

Michaelis c., c. de Michaelis; complexo binário de uma enzima.

minor histocompatibility c. (MHC), c. menor de histocompatibilidade; genes fora do MHC presentes em vários cromossomas que codificam antígenos que contribuem para a rejeição do enxerto.

monophasic c., c. monofásico; complexo no eletrocardiograma totalmente negativo ou totalmente positivo.

multienzyme c., c. multienzimático; coleção estruturalmente distinta e ordenada de enzimas que, freqüentemente, catalisam etapas sucessivas de uma via metabólica (p. ex., complexo da piruvato desidrogenase).

Oedipus c., c. de Édipo; grupo evolutivamente distinto de idéias associadas, objetivos, impulsos sexuais e medos geralmente observados em meninos de 3 a 6 anos de idade: coincide com o pico da fase fálica do desenvolvimento psicossexual, o interesse sexual da criança se fixa basicamente no genitor do sexo oposto e é acompanhado por sentimentos agressivos em relação ao genitor do mesmo sexo; em teoria psicanalítica, é substituído pelo complexo de castração [*Oedipus*, personagem mitológica G.]

ostiomeatal c., c. ostiomeatal; ponto onde os seios frontal e maxilar normalmente drenam para a cavidade nasal; a obstrução produz inflamação dos seios paranasais afetados. SIN ostiomeatal unit.
persecution c., c. de perseguição; sensação de que as outras pessoas têm idéias maléficas contra o seu bem-estar.
primary c., c. primário. SIN Ranke c.
pyruvate dehydrogenase c., c. piruvato desidrogenase. VER *pyruvate* dehydrogenase.
QRS c., c. QRS; parte do eletrocardiograma que corresponde à despolarização de células cardíacas ventriculares.
Ranke c., c. de Ranke; as lesões típicas da tuberculose pulmonar primária, que consistem em um pequeno foco periférico de infecção (foco de Ghon), com envolvimento dos linfonodos hilares ou paratraqueais. SIN primary c.
ribosome-lamella c., c. ribossoma-lamela; inclusão citoplasmática cilíndrica composta de lâminas dispostas concentricamente alternadas com fileiras de ribossomas; característico da célula pilosa na reticuloendoteliose leucêmica.
Shone c., c. de Shone; lesão obstrutiva da válvula mitral com obstrução do trato de saída ventricular esquerdo e coarctação (coartação) da aorta.
sicca c., c. seco; ressecamento das mucosas, como dos olhos e boca, na ausência de uma doença do tecido conjuntivo como a artrite reumatóide.
spike and wave c., c. ponta-onda; padrão generalizado, sincrônico, observado no eletroencefalograma, que consiste em uma onda rápida e apiculada seguida por uma onda lenta; encontrado particularmente em pacientes com epilepsias generalizadas. Os complexos ponta-onda freqüentemente são caracterizados por sua freqüência, p. ex., ponta-onda lento, ponta-onda rápido.
superiority c., c. de superioridade; termo algumas vezes aplicado ao comportamento compensador, p. ex., agressividade, auto-afirmação, associado ao complexo de inferioridade.
superior olivary c., c. olivar superior; *termo oficial alternativo para superior olivary *nucleus.*
symptom c., c. sintomático; (**1**) VER syndrome; (**2**) VER complex (1).
synaptinemal c., c. sinaptonêmico; estrutura submicroscópica interposta entre os pares de cromossomas homólogos durante a sinapse. SIN synaptonemal c.
synaptonemal c., c. sinaptonêmico. SIN synaptinemal c.
Tacaribe c. of viruses, c. de vírus Tacaribe; grupo de arenavírus (Novo Mundo) que inclui os arbovírus antigenicamente relacionados Amapari, Junin, Latino, Machupo, Parana, Pichinde, Tacaribe e Tamiami.
ternary c., c. ternário; termo usado para descrever a combinação tripartida de, por exemplo, enzima–co-fator–substrato ou enzima–substrato$_1$–substrato$_2$ para uma enzima com múltiplos substratos, a forma ativa envolvida em muitas reações catalisadas por enzimas.
triple symptom c., síndrome de Behçet. SIN Behçet *syndrome.*
VATER c., c. de VATER; conjunto de defeitos *v*ertebrais, atresia *a*nal, fístula *t*raqueoesofágica com atresia *e*sofágica, e anomalias *r*enais e radiais; associado à anemia de Fanconi.
ventricular c., c. ventricular; as ondas QRST contínuas de cada batimento no eletrocardiograma.
ventrobasal c. [TA], núcleo ventrobasilar; a grande parte posterior do núcleo ventral do tálamo que recebe os lemniscos sensoriais somáticos (lemnisco medial, trato espinotalâmico, lemnisco trigeminal) e o lemnisco gustatório ascendente e se projeta, por sua vez, através da cápsula interna até o córtex do giro pós-central. Esse complexo de núcleos é somatotopicamente organizado e subdividido em um núcleo ventral póstero-lateral [TA] (nucleus ventralis posterolateralis [TA]), que representa a perna; um núcleo ventral posterior intermédio, que representa o braço; e um núcleo ventral póstero-medial [TA] (nucleus ventralis posteromedialis [TA]), que representa a face e um núcleo arqueado do tálamo, que recebe o lemnisco gustatório. SIN nuclei ventrobasales [TA], ventrobasal nuclei (complex) [TA], nucleus ventralis posterior thalami.

com·plex·ion (kom-plek′shŭn). Compleição; a cor, a textura e o aspecto geral da pele da face. [L. *complexio*, combinação, (depois) condição física]
com·plex·i·ty (kom-pleks′i-tē). Complexidade; o estado de consistir em muitas partes inter-relacionadas.
chemical c., c. química; o número de seqüências diferentes no DNA, conforme definido por cinética de hibridização.
com·plex·us (kom-plek′sŭs). Complexo; termo obsoleto para músculo semi-espinal da cabeça (semispinalis capitis *muscle*). [L. envolvimento, cerco]
c. olivaris inferior [TA], c. olivar inferior. SIN inferior olivary *complex.*
c. stimulans cordis [TA], sistema condutor do coração. SIN conducting *system* of heart.
com·pli·ance (kom-plī′ans). **1.** Complacência; medida da distensibilidade de uma câmara expressa como alteração do volume por unidade de alteração da pressão. **2.** Observância; a consistência e acurácia com que um paciente segue o esquema prescrito por um médico ou outro profissional de saúde. Cf. adherence (2), maintenance. **3.** Uma medida da facilidade com que uma estrutura ou substância pode ser deformada. Em medicina e fisiologia, geralmente uma medida da facilidade com que uma víscera oca (p. ex., pulmão, bexiga, vesícula biliar) pode ser distendida, *isto é,* a alteração de volume resultante da aplicação de uma diferença de pressão de uma unidade entre o interior e o exterior da víscera; a recíproca da elastância. [I.M. do Fr. ant., do L. *compleo*, realizar]
bladder c., c. vesical; alteração do volume vesical para uma determinada alteração na pressão; pode ser calculada a partir de uma curva de pressão-volume do citometrograma. SIN c. of bladder, detrusor c.
c. of bladder, c. da bexiga. SIN bladder c.
detrusor c., c. do detrusor. SIN bladder c.
dynamic c. of lung, c. dinâmica do pulmão; valor obtido quando a complacência pulmonar é avaliada durante a respiração, através da divisão do volume corrente pela diferença nas pressões transpulmonares instantâneas no final das incursões respiratórias, quando o fluxo nas vias aéreas é momentaneamente zero; esse valor difere acentuadamente da complacência estática quando as resistências e complacências não são uniformes em todo o pulmão (isto é, constantes de tempo diferentes).
c. of heart, c. do coração; a recíproca da rigidez passiva ou diastólica do ventrículo, mais comumente do ventrículo esquerdo; pode-se distinguir entre a complacência do músculo e a complacência das estruturas de sustentação, embora geralmente ambas sejam consideradas em conjunto (complacência da câmara); um coração hipertrofiado ou fibrosado apresentará uma parede rígida, isto é, diminuição da complacência.
specific c., c. específica; (**1**) a complacência de uma estrutura dividida por seu volume inicial; (**2**) mais especificamente, no caso dos pulmões, a complacência dividida pela capacidade residual funcional.
static c., c. estática; o valor obtido quando a complacência é medida em equilíbrio verdadeiro, isto é, na ausência de qualquer movimento.
thoracic c., c. torácica; aquela parte da complacência ventilatória total atribuível à complacência da caixa torácica.
ventilatory c., c. ventilatória; a soma da complacência dinâmica do pulmão e da complacência torácica.

com·pli·cat·ed (kom′pli-kā-ted). Complicado; que se tornou complexo; designa uma doença na qual há superposição de um processo ou evento mórbido, alterando sintomas e modificando sua evolução para pior. [L. *com-plico*, pp. *–atus*, embrulhar]
com·pli·ca·tion (kom-pli-kā′shŭn). Complicação; processo ou evento mórbido que ocorre durante uma doença e que não é parte essencial da doença, embora possa resultar dela ou ter causas independentes.
com·po·nent (kom-pō′nent). Componente; elemento que forma uma parte do todo. [L. *com-pono*, pp. *–positus*, colocar junto]
anterior c. of force, c. anterior de força; uma força que opera deslocando os dentes para a frente.
c. of complement (C), c. do complemento; qualquer uma das nove unidades de proteína distintas designadas C1 a C9. VER complement. VER TAMBÉM *complement* pathways.
c. of force, c. de força; (**1**) um dos fatores dos quais pode ser composta uma força resultante ou nos quais ela pode ser decomposta; (**2**) um dos vetores em que uma força pode ser decomposta.
c.'s of mastication, componentes da mastigação; os vários movimentos da mandíbula feitos durante o ato de mastigação, conforme determinado pelo sistema neuromuscular, articulações temporomandibulares, dentes e alimento mastigado; divididos, para fins de análise ou descrição, em componentes de abertura, fechamento, lateral esquerdo, lateral direito e ântero-posterior.
c.'s of occlusion, componentes de oclusão; os vários fatores envolvidos na oclusão, como a articulação temporomandibular, a neuromusculatura associada, os dentes e as estruturas de sustentação da dentadura.
plasma thromboplastin c. (PTC), c. de tromboplastina plasmática. SIN *factor* IX.
secretory c., c. secretor; cadeia polipeptídica encontrada em secreções externas (p. ex., lágrimas, saliva, colostro) associada às imunoglobulinas IgA e IgM. Também pode ocorrer na forma livre. A porção secretora é obtida por clivagem proteolítica do receptor da imunoglobulina nas células epiteliais.
com·pos·ite (kom-poz′-it). Composto; termo coloquial para materiais resinosos usados em odontologia restauradora. [L. *compositus*, reunir, de *compono*, reunir]
com·po·si·tion (kom-pō-zish′ŭn). Composição; em química, os tipos e números dos átomos que constituem uma molécula. [L. *compono*, arranjar]
base c., c. de bases; as proporções de quatro bases (adenina, citosina, guanina e timina ou uracil) presentes no DNA ou RNA; geralmente expressa como a percentagem (mol %) de G mais C.
modeling c., c. de modelagem. SIN modeling *plastic.*
com·pos men·tis (kom′pos men′tis). De mente sã; geralmente usado em sua forma oposta, *non compos mentis.* [L. dotado de mente; *compos*, que tem controle, + *mens* (ment-), mente]
com·pound (kom′pownd). Composto. **1.** Em química, substância formada pela união covalente ou eletrostática de dois ou mais elementos, em geral com características físicas totalmente diferentes de qualquer de seus componentes. **2.** Em farmácia, designa uma preparação que contém vários ingredientes. Quanto aos compostos não relacionados aqui, ver os nomes químicos ou farmacêuticos específicos. [através do Fr. ant., do L. *compono*]

componentes do complemento

componente	peso molecular (kD)	conc. sérica (µg/ml)	n.º de polipeptídeos	função
C1q	410	150	18	forma um complexo ligado ao Ca^{++} — $\overline{C1q\ C1r_2\ C1s_2}$; C1q liga-se à Ig complexada para ativar a via clássica
C1r	83	50	1	
C1s	83	50	1	
C4	210	550	3	moléculas da via clássica, ativadas por C1s para formar uma C3 convertase, $\overline{C4b.2a}$
C2	115	25	1	
C3	180	1.200	2	C3 ativo (C3b) opsoniza qualquer coisa a que se liga e ativa a via lítica. C3a causa desgranulação dos mastócitos e contração do músculo liso. iC3b, C3d, C3e e C3g são produtos da degradação de C3b
C5	180	70	2	C5b nas membranas inicia a via lítica. C5a é quimiotático para macrófagos e neutrófilos, causa contração do músculo liso, desgranulação dos mastócitos e aumento da permeabilidade capilar
C6	130	60	1	componentes da via lítica que se juntam na presença de C5b para formar o complexo de ataque da membrana e, assim, podem causar lise celular
C7	120	50	1	
C8	155	55	3	
C9	75	60	1	
B	95	200	1	B liga-se a C3b na presença de ativadores da via alternativa, a seguir é clivado por D, uma enzima sérica ativa para formar uma C3 convertase $\overline{C3b,Bb}$
D	25	10	1	
P (properdina)	185	25	4	estabiliza $\overline{C3b,Bb}$ para potencializar a atividade de alça de amplificação
MBL	540	1	18	liga-se aos carboidratos bacterianos
MASP	94	?	1	ativa C4 e C2
C4bp	550	250	7	C4bp liga-se a C4b, e H liga-se a C3b para agir como co-fatores para I, que cliva e inativa C3b e C4b
H(β_1H)	150	500	1	
I(C3bina)	100	30	2	
C1 inh	100	185	1	liga-se a $\overline{C1r_2}$ e $\overline{C1s_2}$ e os inativa
Proteína S (vitronectina)	83	505	1	liga-se a C5b-7, impede a fixação às membranas

acetone c., c. acetônico. SIN ketone *body.*
acyclic c., c. acíclico; composto orgânico no qual a cadeia não forma um anel. SIN aliphatic c., open chain c.
addition c., c. de adição; (**1**) precisamente, um complexo de duas ou mais moléculas completas no qual cada uma preserva sua estrutura fundamental e não são formadas nem quebradas ligações covalentes (p. ex., hidratos de sais, aduções); (**2**) genericamente, associação de ácidos com complexos orgânicos básicos (p. ex., aminas com HCl); (**3**) ainda mais livremente, adição de duas moléculas sem perda de qualquer átomo, mas formando novas ligações covalentes (p. ex., $CH_2=CH_2 + Br_2 \rightarrow BrCH_2—CH_2Br$).
alicyclic c.'s, compostos alicíclicos. VER cyclic c.
aliphatic c., c. alifático. SIN acyclic c.

APC c., c. APC; combinação de analgésicos em comprimido contendo aspirina (ácido acetilsalicílico), fenacetina e cafeína. Muito usado entre 1940 e 1960; constituintes originais de analgésicos populares vendidos sem receita médica. Atualmente é muito menos usado devido a preocupações com possível lesão renal causada por fenacetina.
aromatic c., c. aromático. VER cyclic c.
carbamino c., c. carbamínico; qualquer derivado do ácido carbâmico formado pela combinação de dióxido de carbono com um grupamento amino livre para formar um grupamento *N*-carboxi, –NH–COOH, como na hemoglobina, que forma carbaminoemoglobina.
closed chain c., c. de cadeia fechada. SIN cyclic c.
condensation c., c. de condensação; composto resultante da combinação de duas ou mais substâncias simples, com a divisão de alguma outra substância, como álcool ou água; p. ex., um peptídeo. Cf. conjugated c.
conjugated c., c. conjugado; composto formado pela união de dois compostos (como pela eliminação de água entre um álcool e um ácido orgânico para formar um éster) e facilmente convertido nos compostos originais (hidrólise). VER TAMBÉM conjugation (4); Cf. condensation c.
cyclic c., c. cíclico; qualquer composto no qual os átomos constituintes, ou qualquer parte deles, formam um anel. Usado principalmente em química orgânica onde: 1) numerosos compostos contêm anéis de átomos de carbono (compostos carbocíclicos) ou átomos de carbono mais um ou mais átomos de outros tipos (compostos heterocíclicos), geralmente nitrogênio, oxigênio ou enxofre; 2) os átomos no anel são todos do mesmo elemento (composto homocíclico ou isocíclico); 3) o anel é saturado ou contém ligações duplas não-conjugadas (composto alicíclico), o composto tem propriedades semelhantes ao composto acíclico correspondente (p. ex., o cicloexano assemelha-se ao hexano); 4) o anel contém ligações duplas conjugadas em uma alça fechada na qual há $4n + 2$ (onde n é o número inteiro) elétrons π removidos (regra de Hückel) (composto aromático; p. ex., benzeno, piridina), é mais estável que o anel saturado correspondente e exibe propriedades químicas incomuns características dele mesmo e não de outros tipos de anéis ou de compostos acíclicos. Esses compostos aromáticos possuem a capacidade de sofrer uma corrente anular induzida. SIN closed chain c., ring c.
genetic c., c. genético. SIN compound *heterozygote.*
glycosyl c., c. glicosil; o composto formado entre um açúcar e outra substância orgânica na qual o OH do grupamento redutor (hemiacetal) do primeiro é removido; p. ex., os nucleosídeos naturais, nos quais um N heterocíclico é ligado diretamente ao C-1 da ribose (ou desoxirribose) para produzir compostos ribosil. Cf. glycoside.
heterocyclic c., c. heterocíclico. VER cyclic c.
high-energy c.'s, compostos de alta energia; um grupamento de ésteres fosfóricos cuja hidrólise ocorre com uma transferência de energia livre padronizada de -5 a -15 kcal/mol (ou -20 a -63 kJ/mol) (em contraste com -1 a -4 kcal/mol, ou -4 a -17 kJ/mol) para ésteres fosfóricos simples como a glicose 6-fosfato ou α-glicerofosfatos, assim sendo capazes de provocar reações consumidoras de energia em células vivas ou sistemas reconstituídos fora das células; 5′-trifosfato de adenosina, em relação aos fosfatos β e γ, é o mais conhecido e considerado como a fonte de energia imediata para a maioria das sínteses metabólicas. Outros exemplos incluem anidridos ácidos, ésteres fosfóricos de enóis, derivados do ácido fosfâmico ($R–NH–PO_3H_2$), tioésteres acil (p. ex., da coenzima A), compostos de sulfônio ($R_3–S^+$) e ésteres aminoacil de porções ribosil. VER TAMBÉM high-energy *phosphates*, em *phosphate.*
homocyclic c., c. homocíclico. VER cyclic c.
impression c., c. de impressão. SIN modeling *plastic.*
inclusion c., c. de inclusão; o aprisionamento mecânico de pequenas moléculas em espaços entre outras moléculas; p. ex., a inclusão de moléculas de iodo por moléculas de amido para formar o bem conhecido "composto de adição" vermelho-a-preto.
inorganic c., c. inorgânico; composto no qual os átomos ou radicais consistem em outros elementos além do carbono e são tipicamente mantidos juntos por forças eletrostáticas, e não por ligações covalentes; freqüentemente são capazes de se dissociarem em íons nos solventes polares (p. ex., H_2O). Cf. organic c.
isocyclic c., c. isocíclico. VER cyclic c.
Kendall c.'s, compostos de Kendall; um grupo de corticosteróides. Composto A de Kendall (11-desidrocorticosterona), composto B de Kendall (corticosterona), composto E de Kendall (cortisona), composto F de Kendall (cortisol). SIN Kendall substance.
meso c.'s, mesocompostos; compostos contendo mais de um átomo de carbono assimétrico, com as configurações ao seu redor tão equilibradas que a molécula como um todo possui um plano de simetria, embora os átomos de carbono individuais não; esses compostos não são opticamente ativos; p. ex., ribitol, ácido múcico, *meso*-inositol, *meso*-cistina.
methonium c.'s, compostos de metônio; agentes que bloqueiam impulsos nos gânglios (p. ex., hexametônio) e são usados na hipertensão arterial, ou nas junções neuromusculares e são usados para paralisia neuromuscular em cirurgia (p. ex., decametônio).
modeling c., c. de modelagem. SIN modeling *plastic.*
nonpolar c., c. apolar; composto formado de moléculas que possuem uma distribuição simétrica de carga elétrica, de forma que não exigem pólos posi-

tivos ou negativos, e que não são ionizáveis em solução; p. ex., hidrocarbonetos. VER TAMBÉM organic c.
open chain c., c. de cadeia aberta. SIN acyclic c.
organic c., c. orgânico; composto formado de átomos (alguns dos quais são carbono) mantidos unidos por ligações covalentes (compartilhamento de elétrons). Cf. inorganic c.
polar c., c. polar; composto no qual a carga elétrica não é distribuída simetricamente, de forma que há separação de carga elétrica ou carga elétrica parcial e formação de pólos positivo e negativo definidos; p. ex., H_2O. Ver também inorganic c.
Reichstein c., c. de Reichstein. SIN Reichstein *substance*.
ring c., c. em anel. SIN cyclic c.
Wintersteiner c. F, c. F de Wintersteiner. SIN cortisone.
com·pre·hen·sion (kom - prē - hen′shŭn). Compreensão; conhecimento ou entendimento de um objeto, situação, evento ou afirmação verbal.
com·press (kom′pres). Compressa; chumaço de gaze ou de outro material usado para compressão local. [L. *com-primo*, pp. *-pressus*, pressionar juntos]
graduated c., c. graduada; camadas de tecido mais espesso no centro, tornando-se mais fino em direção à periferia.
wet c., c. úmida; gaze umedecida com solução salina ou anti-séptica.
com·pres·sion (kom - presh′ŭn). Compressão; pressionar junto; o ato de exercer pressão sobre um corpo de forma a aumentar sua densidade; a diminuição da dimensão de um corpo sob a ação de duas forças externas em sentidos opostos na mesma linha reta.
c. of brain, c. cerebral. SIN cerebral c.
cerebral c., c. cerebral; pressão sobre os tecidos intracranianos por um derrame de sangue ou líquor, um abscesso, uma neoplasia, uma fratura do crânio com afundamento ou edema cerebral. SIN c. of brain.
c. limiting, c. limitante; circuito de aparelho auditivo no qual a amplificação é reduzida quando há altos níveis sonoros de entrada.
c. of tissue, c. tecidual. SIN tissue *displaceability*.
wide dynamic range c., c. da faixa dinâmica ampla; circuito de aparelho auditivo no qual a amplificação é aumentada através da faixa de freqüência quando há baixos níveis sonoros de entrada.
com·pres·sor (kom - pres′er, - ōr). Compressor. **1.** Um músculo cuja contração causa compressão de qualquer estrutura. **2.** Um instrumento para comprimir uma parte, principalmente uma artéria, a fim de evitar perda de sangue. SIN compressorium.
c. urethrae [TA], compressor da uretra; parte do esfíncter uretral externo feminino com origem nos ramos isquiopúbicos, posteriores ao plano da uretra, que seguem anterior e medialmente para se fundirem com o músculo contralateral anterior à uretra, misturando-se a outras partes do músculo esfíncter externo da uretra (esfíncter uretrovaginal abaixo e esfíncter uretral acima). VER TAMBÉM external urethral *sphincter*.
c. ve′nae dorsa′lis pe′nis, c. da veia dorsal do pênis; variação do músculo bulboesponjoso na qual algumas fibras passam dorsais à veia dorsal do pênis; antigamente era considerada um componente importante no mecanismo de ereção. SIN Houston muscle.
com·pres·sor·i·um (kom - pres - ōr′ē - ŭm). Compressor. SIN compressor (2).
Compton, Arthur H., físico e prêmio Nobel norte-americano, 1892–1962. VER C. *effect*, scattering.
Compton scat·ter·ing. Dispersão de Compton. SIN Compton *effect*.
com·pul·sion (kom - pul′shŭn). Compulsão; pensamentos ou impulsos incontroláveis de realizar um ato, repetitivamente, como um mecanismo inconsciente de evitar idéias e desejos inaceitáveis que, por si próprios, geram ansiedade; a ansiedade manifesta-se plenamente se for impedida a realização do ato compulsivo; pode estar associado a pensamentos obsessivos. [L. *com-pello* pp., *-pulsus*, impelir, compelir]
com·pul·sive (kom - pŭl′siv). Compulsivo; influenciado por compulsão; de natureza constrangedora e irresistível.
com·put·er. Computador; dispositivo eletrônico programável que pode ser usado para armazenar e manipular dados a fim de realizar funções designadas; os dois componentes fundamentais são o *hardware*, isto é, o aparelho eletrônico real, e o *software*, isto é, as instruções ou o programa usado para realizar a função.
con-. Com, junto, em associação; aparece como com- antes de p, b ou m, como col- antes de l, e como co- antes de uma vogal; corresponde ao G. syn-. [L. *cum*, com, junto]
conA, con A Abreviatura de concanavalina A.
con·al·bu·min (kon - al - bū′min). Conalbumina; glicoproteína contendo D-manose e D-galactose, constituindo cerca de 12% do total de sólidos da clara de ovo. Liga-se aos íons ferro. SIN ovotransferrin.
con·a·nine (kon′ā - nēn). Conanina; alcalóide esteróide; pregnano com um grupamento metilimino unindo C-18 e C-20 (na configuração α). VER TAMBÉM conessine.
co·nar·i·um (kō - nā′rē - ŭm). Conário. SIN pineal *body*. [G. *kōnarion* (dim. de *kōnos*, cone), o corpo pineal]
co·na·tion (kō - nā′shŭn). Conação; tendência consciente para atuar intencionalmente, geralmente uma face do processo mental; historicamente alinhado com a cognição e o afeto, porém recentemente vem sendo usado com o sentido mais amplo de impulso, desejo, esforço proposital. [L. *conātio*, empreendimento, esforço]
co·na·tive (kon′ā - tiv). Conativo; pertinente a, ou caracterizado por, conação.
co·na·tus (kō - nah′tŭs, - nā′tŭs). Esforço; impulso; tendência; esforço para autopreservação e auto-afirmação. [L. tentativa]
con·cam·er·a·tion (kon - kam - er - ā′shŭn). Concameração; sistema de cavidades intercomunicantes. [L. *concameratio*, abóbada; de *concamero*, pp. *-atus*, abóbada sobre, de *camera*, abóbada]
con·ca·nav·a·lin A (conA, con A) (kon - kă - nav′ă - lin). Concanavalina A; fitomitógeno, extraído do feijão-de-porco (*Canavalia ensiformis*), que aglutina o sangue de mamíferos e reage com glicosanos; como outras fito-hemaglutininas, conA estimula os linfócitos T mais vigorosamente do que os linfócitos B.
con·ca·ta·mer (kon - kăt - ă - mer). Repetição linear de fragmentos de restrição. [*concat*enate + -mer]
con·cat·e·nate (kon - kat′ē - nāt). Concatenado; designa o arranjo de diversas estruturas, p. ex., linfonodos hipertrofiados, em uma fileira semelhante aos elos de uma corrente. [L. *concateno*, pp. *-atus*, unir, de *catena*, cadeia]
Concato, Luigi M., médico italiano, 1825–1882. VER C. *disease*.
con·cave (kon′kāv). Côncavo; que possui uma superfície deprimida ou oca. [L. *concavus*, arqueado ou abobadado]
con·cav·i·ty (kon - kav′i - tē). Concavidade; escavação ou depressão, com lados mais ou menos uniformemente curvos, em qualquer superfície.
con·ca·vo·con·cave (kon - kā′vō - kon′kāv). Côncavo-côncavo; bicôncavo. SIN biconcave.
con·ca·vo·con·vex (kon - kā′vō - kon′veks). Côncavo-convexo; côncavo em uma superfície e convexo na superfície oposta.
con·cen·tra·tion (c) (kon - sen - trā′shŭn). Concentração. **1.** Preparação produzida por extração de uma droga bruta, precipitação da solução e secagem. **2.** Aumento da quantidade de soluto em um determinado volume de solução por evaporação do solvente. **3.** A quantidade de uma substância por unidade de volume ou peso. Em fisiologia renal, símbolo U para concentração urinária, P para concentração plasmática; em fisiologia respiratória, símbolo C para quantidade por unidade de volume no sangue, F para concentração fracional (fração molar ou volume por volume) no gás seco; os subscritos indicam a localização e a espécie química. [L. *con-*, junto, + *centrum*, centro]
Baermann c., c. de Baermann; preparação baseada no princípio de que larvas de nematódeos ativas migrarão de uma amostra de fezes fresca, através de várias camadas de gaze, para a água de torneira, da qual as larvas podem ser isoladas por centrifugação.
buffy coat c., c. do creme leucocitário; centrifugação do sangue total contendo anticoagulante para obter uma camada leucocitária; os esfregaços de sangue para coloração podem ser preparados a partir dessa camada de células e examinados quanto à presença de parasitas (tripanossomas e leishmânias intracelulares).
critical micelle c. (cmc), c. crítica de micela; a concentração em que uma molécula anfipática (p. ex., um fosfolipídio) formará uma micela.
fecal c., c. fecal; preparação utilizando métodos de flutuação ou sedimentação para separar elementos parasitários de resíduos fecais.

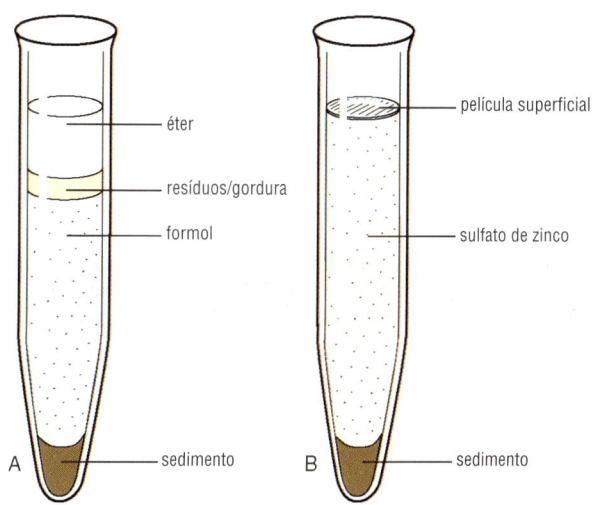

procedimentos de concentração fecal: várias camadas observadas nos tubos após centrifugação; (A) formol-éter (ou acetato etílico); (B) sulfato de zinco (a película superficial deve estar 2 a 3 mm distante da borda do tubo)

formalin-ether sedimentation c., c. de sedimentação em formol-éter; método de sedimentação para separar elementos parasitários de resíduos fecais através de centrifugação e uso de éter para reter os resíduos em uma camada separada dos parasitas.

formalin-ethyl acetate sedimentation c., c. de sedimentação no formol-acetato etílico; método de sedimentação para separar elementos parasitários de resíduos fecais através da centrifugação e do uso de acetato etílico (substituto do éter) para reter resíduos em uma camada separada dos parasitas.

gravity c., c. gravitacional; método para separar parasitas de resíduos através da sedimentação gravitacional de suspensões fecais.

M c., c. M; número máximo de células bacterianas que podem ser produzidas em uma unidade de volume de meio de crescimento.

mean corpuscular hemoglobin c. (MCHC), c. de hemoglobina corpuscular média (CHCM); Hb/Ht; a concentração de hemoglobina média, em um determinado volume de concentrado de hemácias, calculada a partir da hemoglobina presente e do hematócrito, em índices eritrocitários.

microhematocrit c., c. de micro-hematócrito; a centrifugação de sangue total, anticoagulado, utilizando tubos de micro-hematócrito, para obter um creme leucocitário contendo leucócitos; os esfregaços sanguíneos para coloração podem ser preparados a partir dessa camada de células e examinados à procura de parasitas (tripanossomas e leishmânias intracelulares).

minimal alveolar c., c. alveolar mínima; a concentração alveolar final de um anestésico inalatório que impede a resposta somática a um estímulo álgico em 50% dos indivíduos; índice de potência relativa de anestésicos inalatórios. SIN minimal anesthetic c.

minimal anesthetic c. (MAC), c. anestésica mínima. SIN minimal alveolar c.

minimal inhibitory c. (MIC), c. inibitória mínima; a menor concentração de antibiótico suficiente para inibir o crescimento bacteriano quando testada *in vitro*.

molar c., c. molar. VER molar (4).

normal c. (N), c. normal. VER normal (3).

zinc sulfate flotation c., c. de flutuação do sulfato de zinco; método que utiliza sulfato de zinco saturado para separar elementos parasitários de resíduos fecais através de diferenças na densidade relativa (peso específico); a maioria dos cistos de parasitas, oocistos, esporos, ovos e larvas pode ser encontrada na película superficial após a centrifugação.

con·cen·tric (kon-sen′trik). Concêntrico; que possui um centro comum, de forma que duas ou mais esferas, círculos ou segmentos de círculos estão dentro um do outro.

con·cept (kon′sept). Conceito. **1.** Uma idéia ou noção abstrata. **2.** Uma variável ou princípio explanatório em um sistema científico. SIN conception (1). [L. *conceptum*, algo compreendido, pp. neutro de *concipio*, receber, apreender]

no-threshold c., c. de não-limiar; c. segundo a qual o efeito biológico de radiação é proporcional à dose, mesmo para doses muito pequenas.

self-c., auto-imagem; avaliação do próprio indivíduo a seu respeito, incluindo autodefinição nos vários papéis sociais representados, incluindo avaliação do próprio estado em relação a uma única característica ou a muitas dimensões humanas, utilizando normas sociais ou pessoais como critérios.

con·cep·ti (kon-sep′ti). Conceptos; plural de conceptus.

con·cep·tion (kon-sep′shŭn). **1.** Conceito. SIN concept. **2.** Ato de formar uma idéia geral ou noção. **3.** Concepção; ato de conceber; a implantação do blastocisto no endométrio. [L. *conceptio*; ver concepto]

imperative c., conceito imperativo; conceito que não se origina por associação, mas surge espontaneamente e se recusa a ser abolido.

retained products of c., produtos retidos da concepção; fragmentos de tecido fetal, placentário ou das membranas que permanecem no útero após o parto ou abortamento, representando um aumento do risco de hemorragia ou infecção.

con·cep·tu·al (kon-sep′chŭ-ăl). Conceitual; relativo à formação de idéias, geralmente abstrações de ordem superior, a conceitos mentais.

con·cep·tus, pl. **con·cep·ti** (kon-sep′tŭs, -sep′ti). Concepto; o produto da concepção, isto é, embrião ou feto e membranas.

valores da concentração alveolar mínima (MAC) de anestésicos inalatórios, em ordem crescente de efetividade

	valores da MAC (% atm)	
	100% O₂	com 70% N₂O
halotano	0,75	0,29
isoflurano	1,15	0,50
sevoflurona	1,4–3,2	0,7–2,0
desflurona	6,0	3,0
N₂O	110	—

con·cha, pl. **con·chae** (kon′kă, kon′kē) [TA]. Concha; em anatomia, uma estrutura de formato comparável ao de uma concha, como a orelha ou pavilhão da orelha ou um osso turbinado do nariz. [L. concha]

c. of auricle [TA], c. da orelha; a grande cavidade ou assoalho da orelha, entre a porção anterior da hélice e a antélice; é dividida pelo pilar da hélice em cimba da concha, acima, e cavidade da concha, abaixo. SIN c. auriculae [TA], c. of ear.

c. auric′ulae [TA], c. da orelha. SIN c. of auricle.

c. bullosa, c. bolhosa; pneumatização anormal do turbinado médio que pode interferir com a ventilação normal dos óstios sinusais, podendo resultar em sinusite recorrente.

c. of ear, c. da orelha. SIN c. of auricle.

highest c., c. suprema; c. nasal suprema. SIN supreme nasal c.

inferior nasal c. [TA], c. nasal inferior; (**1**) lâmina óssea, esponjosa, fina, com margens curvas, na parede lateral da cavidade nasal, separando o meato médio do inferior; articula-se com os ossos etmóide, lacrimal, maxilar e palato; (**2**) a lâmina óssea acima e seu mucoperiósteo espesso contendo um extenso leito vascular cavernoso para troca de calor. SIN c. nasalis inferior [TA], inferior turbinated bone, turbinated body (2).

middle nasal c. [TA], c. nasal média; (**1**) a lâmina óssea, esponjosa, fina, média, com margens curvas, parte do labirinto etmoidal, que se projeta da parede lateral da cavidade nasal e separa o meato superior do meato médio; (**2**) a lâmina óssea acima e seu mucoperiósteo espesso contendo um leito vascular cavernoso para troca de calor. SIN c. nasalis media [TA], middle turbinated bone, turbinated body (2).

Morgagni c., c. de Morgagni. SIN superior nasal c.

c. nasa′lis infe′rior [TA], c. nasal inferior. SIN inferior nasal c.

c. nasa′lis me′dia [TA], c. nasal média. SIN middle nasal c.

c. nasa′lis supe′rior [TA], c. nasal superior. SIN superior nasal c.

c. nasa′lis supre′ma [TA], c. nasal suprema. SIN supreme nasal c.

Santorini c., c. santori′ni, c. de Santorini. SIN supreme nasal c.

sphenoidal conchae [TA], conchas esfenoidais; par de ossículos piramidais, cujas espinhas estão em contato com a lâmina medial do processo pterigóide, com as bases formando o teto da cavidade nasal. SIN conchae sphenoidales [TA], Bertin bones, Bertin ossicles, sphenoidal turbinated bones.

con′chae sphenoida′les [TA], conchas esfenoidais. SIN sphenoidal conchae.

superior nasal c. [TA], c. nasal superior; (**1**) a lâmina óssea, esponjosa, fina, superior, com margens curvas, parte do labirinto etmoidal, que se projeta da parede lateral da cavidade nasal e separa o meato superior do recesso esfenoetmoidal; (**2**) a lâmina óssea acima e seu mucoperiósteo espesso, que é menos vascularizado que o das conchas média e inferior. SIN c. nasalis superior [TA], Morgagni c., superior turbinated bone, turbinated body (2).

supreme c., c. suprema. SIN supreme nasal c.

supreme nasal c. [TA], c. nasal suprema; uma concha pequena freqüentemente presente na parte póstero-superior da parede nasal lateral; situa-se sobre o meato nasal supremo. SIN c. nasalis suprema [TA], fourth turbinated bone, highest c., highest turbinated bone, Santorini c., c. santorini, supraturbinal, supreme c., supreme turbinated bone, turbinated body (2).

con·choi·dal (kon-koy′dăl). Concoidal; conchoidal; conchóide; concóide; que tem o formato de uma concha; que possui convexidades e concavidades alternadas na superfície. [concha + G. *eidos*, aspecto]

con·com·i·tance (kon-kom′i-tăns). Concomitância; em esotropia, um olho acompanhando o outro em todas as incursões, como no estrabismo concomitante. [con- + L. *comito-*, pp. *-atus*, acompanhar]

con·com·i·tant. Concomitante. SIN comitant.

con·cor·dance (kon-kōr′dans). Concordância. **1.** Consenso nos tipos de dados que ocorrem em pares naturais. Por exemplo, em um traço como a esquizofrenia, um par de gêmeos idênticos é concordante se ambos forem afetados ou ambos não forem afetados; é discordante se apenas um deles for afetado. Da mesma forma, os pares poderiam ser gêmeos não-idênticos, ou irmãos, ou marido e mulher, etc. **2.** Um consenso negociado, compartilhado entre o médico e o paciente a respeito de esquema(s) de tratamento, desfechos e comportamentos; uma relação mais cooperativa que aquela baseada em obediência e desobediência. [L. *concordia*, consenso, harmonia]

con·cor·dant (kon-kōr′dant). Concordante; que designa ou exibe concordância.

con·cre·ment (kon′krē-ment). Concreção; depósito de material calcário em uma parte. [L. *con- cresco*, crescer junto]

con·cres·cence (kon-kres′ens). Concrescência. **1.** SIN coalescence. **2.** Em odontologia, a união das raízes de dois dentes adjacentes por cimento. [ver concrement]

con·cre·tio cor·dis (kon-krē′shē-ō kōr′dis). Extensa adesão entre as camadas parietal e visceral do pericárdio, com obliteração parcial ou completa da cavidade pericárdica. SIN internal adhesive pericarditis.

con·cre·tion (kon-krē′shŭn). Concreção; a formação de material sólido por agregação de unidades ou partículas distintas. [L. *cum*, junto, + *crescere*, crescer]

con·cret·i·za·tion (kon′krēt-i-ză′shŭn). Concretização; incapacidade de abstrair, com ênfase excessiva em detalhes específicos; observada em distúrbios mentais, como demência e esquizofrenia, e também normalmente em crianças. [L. *con-cresco*, pp. *-cretus*, crescer junto, endurecer]

con·cus·sion (kon-kŭsh′ŭn). Concussão. **1.** Pancada ou vibração violenta. **2.** Lesão de uma estrutura mole, como o cérebro, resultante de um golpe ou agitação violenta. SIN commotio. [L. *concussio*, de *con- cutio*, pp *-cussus*, agitar violentamente]

brain c., c. cerebral; síndrome clínica causada por forças mecânicas, geralmente traumáticas; caracterizada por comprometimento imediato e transitório da função neural, como alteração da consciência, perturbação da visão e equilíbrio, etc. SIN commotio cerebri.

spinal c., c. espinal. SIN spinal cord c.

spinal cord c., c. da medula espinal; lesão da medula espinal devido a um golpe na coluna vertebral, com disfunção transitória ou prolongada abaixo do nível da lesão. SIN spinal c.

con·den·sa·tion (kon-den-sā′shŭn). Condensação. **1.** Tornar mais sólido ou denso. **2.** Transformar um gás em líquido, ou um líquido em sólido. **3.** Em psicanálise, processo mental inconsciente no qual um símbolo substitui muitos outros. **4.** Em odontologia, o processo de colocar um material de enchimento em uma cavidade (cárie), utilizando tal força e direção para que não fiquem lacunas. [L. *con-denso*, pp. *-atus*, tornar espesso, condensar]

aldol c., c. aldol; formação de um aldol (um composto β-hidroxi carbonil) a partir de dois compostos carbonil; a reação inversa é uma clivagem aldol; a frutose 1,6-bifosfato aldolase catalisa essa reação.

Claisen c., c. de Claisen; a formação de um β-ceto éster a partir de dois ésteres, um dos quais possui um átomo de α-hidrogênio; a malato sintase, citrato sintase e ATP citrato liase catalisam essas reações.

con·dense (kon-dens′). Condensar; aumentar a densidade de; aplicado particularmente à inserção de amálgama de ouro ou prata em uma cavidade preparada em um dente.

con·dens·er (kon-den′ser). Condensador. **1.** Um aparelho para resfriar um gás em líquido, ou um líquido em sólido. **2.** Em odontologia, um instrumento manual ou motorizado usado para condensar um material, plástico ou não, na cavidade de um dente; variação de tamanhos e formatos permite a adaptação da massa ao contorno da cavidade. **3.** A lente simples ou composta de um microscópio que é usada para fornecer a iluminação necessária para visibilidade da amostra observada. **4.** SIN capacitor.

Abbé c., c. de Abbé; sistema de duas ou três lentes convexas e planoconvexas, acromáticas, de ângulo aberto, que podem ser deslocadas para cima ou para baixo sob a platina de um microscópio, regulando assim a concentração de luz (diretamente de uma lâmina ou refletida por um espelho) que atravessa o material a ser examinado na platina.

automatic c., c. automático. SIN automatic *plugger.*

cardioid c., c. cardióide; um tipo de condensador de campo escuro.

dark-field c., c. de campo escuro; aparelho para enviar luz refletida através do campo microscópico, de forma que o único objeto a ser examinado é iluminado, ficando o próprio campo escuro.

paraboloid c., c. paraboloide; um tipo de condensador de campo escuro.

con·di·tion (kon-dish′ŭn). Condicionar; condição. **1.** Treinar; submeter-se a condicionamento. **2.** Certa resposta produzida por um estímulo especificável ou emitido na presença de determinados estímulos com retribuição da resposta durante ocorrência prévia. **3.** Refere-se a várias classes de aprendizado no ramo comportamental da psicologia. [L. *conditio*, de *condico*, concordar]

fibrocystic c. of the breast, condição fibrocística da mama; condição benigna comum, em mulheres da terceira, quarta e quinta décadas de vida, caracterizada por formação, em uma ou ambas as mamas, de pequenos cistos contendo líquido que podem ser vistos como cistos azuis em forma de cúpula; associada à fibrose do estroma e a vários graus de hiperplasia epitelial intraductal e adenose esclerosante. SIN cystic hyperplasia of the breast.

con·di·tion·ing (kon-dish′ŭn-ing). Condicionamento; o processo de adquirir, desenvolver, educar, estabelecer, aprender ou treinar novas respostas em um indivíduo. Usado para descrever tanto o comportamento responsivo quanto o operante; em ambos os usos, refere-se a uma alteração da freqüência ou forma de comportamento em virtude da influência do ambiente.

assertive c., c. assertivo; c. positivo. SIN assertive *training.*

aversive c., c. aversivo. SIN aversive *training.*

avoidance c., c. de evitação; a técnica pela qual um organismo aprende a evitar estímulos desagradáveis ou punitivos por aprendizado da resposta antecipatória adequada para protegê-lo de estímulos adicionais desse tipo. Cf. escape c. SIN avoidance training.

classical c., c. clássico; forma de aprendizado, como nas experiências de Pavlov, na qual um estímulo previamente neutro torna-se um estímulo condicionado quando apresentado juntamente com um estímulo não-condicionado. Também denominado substituição do estímulo porque o novo estímulo provoca a resposta em questão. VER TAMBÉM respondent c. SIN stimulus substitution.

escape c., c. de escape; a técnica pela qual um organismo aprende a interromper estímulos desagradáveis ou punitivos através da execução de nova resposta apropriada que interrompe a liberação desses estímulos. Cf. avoidance c. SIN escape training.

higher order c., c. de primeira ordem; o uso de um estímulo previamente condicionado para condicionar outras respostas, de forma muito semelhante ao uso de estímulos não-condicionados.

instrumental c., c. instrumental; c. em que a resposta é um pré-requisito para alcançar algum objetivo; freqüentemente usado como sinônimo de condicionamento operante, mas alguns psicólogos fazem distinções entre esses dois termos.

operant c., c. operante; tipo de condicionamento desenvolvido por Skinner no qual o experimentador aguarda que a resposta a ser condicionada (emitida) ocorra espontaneamente, e, logo depois dela, o organismo recebe uma recompensa de reforço; após esse procedimento ser repetido muitas vezes, a freqüência de emissão da resposta desejada terá aumentado significativamente em relação à sua freqüência antes da experiência. VER TAMBÉM *schedules* of reinforcement, em *schedule*. SIN skinnerian c.

pavlovian c., c. de Pavlov. SIN respondent c.

respondent c., c. de Pavlov; um tipo de condicionamento, estudado pela primeira vez por I.P. Pavlov, no qual um estímulo previamente neutro (o som de um sino) produz uma resposta (salivação) em virtude de seu emparelhamento (associando-o contiguamente no tempo) várias vezes com um estímulo não-condicionado ou natural para aquela resposta (alimento mostrado a um cão faminto). SIN pavlovian c.

second-order c., c. de segunda ordem; o uso de um estímulo condicionado previamente bem-sucedido como o estímulo não-condicionado para condicionamento adicional.

skinnerian c., c. de Skinner. SIN operant c.

trace c., c. residual; condicionamento quando não há superposição temporal entre o estímulo do condicionamento e o estímulo não-condicionado.

con·dom (kon′dom). Preservativo; envoltório ou revestimento para o pênis ou vagina usado na prevenção da concepção ou da infecção durante o coito.

con·duc·tance (kon-dŭk′tans). Condutância. **1.** Medida de condutividade; a razão entre a corrente que flui através de um condutor e a diferença de potencial entre as extremidades do condutor; a condutância de um circuito é a recíproca de sua resistência. **2.** A facilidade com que um líquido ou gás entra em e flui através de um conduto, passagem de ar ou via respiratória; o fluxo por unidade de diferença de pressão.

con·duc·tion (kon-dŭk′shun). Condução. **1.** O ato de transmitir ou conduzir determinadas formas de energia, como calor, som ou eletricidade, de um ponto a outro, sem movimento evidente no corpo condutor. **2.** A transmissão de estímulos de vários tipos pelo protoplasma vivo. [L. *con- duco*, pp. *ductus*, levar, conduzir]

aberrant ventricular c., c. ventricular aberrante; condução intraventricular anormal de um batimento supraventricular, sobretudo quando os batimentos adjacentes são conduzidos normalmente. SIN ventricular aberration.

accelerated c., c. acelerada; qualquer aumento anormal da velocidade de condução; geralmente ocorre entre o átrio e os ventrículos, como nas síndromes de Wolff-Parkinson-White e Lown-Ganong-Levine; essas vias aceleradas formam a base de formas específicas de taquicardia de reentrada.

air c., c. aérea; em relação à audição, a transmissão de som para o ouvido interno, através do canal auditivo externo e das estruturas do ouvido médio.

anomalous c., c. anômala; condução de impulsos elétricos cardíacos através de qualquer via anormal.

antegrade c., c. anterógrada. SIN anterograde c.

anterograde c., c. anterógrada; condução na direção normal esperada entre quaisquer estruturas cardíacas. SIN antegrade c., forward c., orthograde c.

atrioventricular c. (AVC), AV c., c. atrioventricular (CAV), c. AV; condução anterógrada do impulso cardíaco dos átrios para os ventrículos através do nó AV ou qualquer via de condução anômala, representada, no eletrocardiograma, pelo intervalo PR. O tempo de condução PH vai do início da onda P ao primeiro componente de alta freqüência do eletrograma do feixe de His (normalmente 119 ± 38 ms); o tempo de condução A-H vai do início do primeiro componente de alta freqüência do eletrograma atrial ao primeiro componente de alta freqüência do eletrograma do feixe de His (normalmente 92 ± 38 ms); o tempo de condução P-A vai do início da onda P até o início do eletrograma atrial (normalmente 27 ± 18 ms).

avalanche c., c. em avalanche; a descarga de um impulso de um neurônio para um grande número de neurônios do mesmo sistema fisiológico, produzindo assim a liberação de uma quantidade muito grande de energia nervosa por um determinado estímulo.

bone c., c. óssea; em relação à audição, a transmissão do som para o ouvido interno através de vibrações aplicadas aos ossos do crânio. SIN osteophony.

concealed c., c. oculta; c. dissimulada; condução de um impulso através de uma parte do coração sem evidências diretas de sua presença no eletrocardiograma; a condução é deduzida apenas devido à sua influência sobre o ciclo cardíaco subseqüente.

decremental c., c. decrescente, condução com decremento; condução comprometida em uma parte de uma fibra devido à diminuição progressiva da resposta da porção não-excitada da fibra ao potencial de ação que chega até ela; manifesta-se por diminuição da velocidade de condução, da amplitude do potencial de ação e da extensão da propagação do impulso.

delayed c., c. tardia; bloqueio AV de primeiro grau. VER atrioventricular *block*, intraventricular *block*, bundle-branch *block*.
forward c., c. anterógrada. SIN anterograde c.
intraatrial c., c. intra-atrial; condução do impulso cardíaco através do miocárdio atrial, representada pela onda P no eletrocardiograma.
intraventricular c., c. intraventricular; condução do impulso cardíaco através do miocárdio ventricular, representada pelo complexo QRS no eletrocardiograma. O tempo de condução HR vai do início do primeiro componente de alta freqüência do eletrograma do feixe de His até o início do complexo QRS do eletrocardiograma de superfície (normalmente, 43 ± 12 ms); o tempo de condução HV vai do início do primeiro componente de alta freqüência do eletrograma do feixe de His até o início do eletrograma ventricular (normalmente, aproxima-se do intervalo HR, mas pode ser um pouco menor). SIN ventricular c.
nerve c., c. nervosa; a transmissão de um impulso ao longo de uma fibra nervosa.
orthograde c., c. ortógrada. SIN anterograde c.
Purkinje c., c. de Purkinje; condução do impulso cardíaco através do sistema de Purkinje.
retrograde VA c., c. VA retrógrada; condução retrógrada dos ventrículos ou do nodo AV para os átrios e através deles. SIN retroconduction, ventriculoatrial c., VA c.
saltatory c., c. saltatória; condução na qual o impulso nervoso salta de um nodo de Ranvier para o próximo.
sinoventricular c., c. sinoventricular; uma forma rara de condução do impulso sinusal durante paralisia do músculo atrial por hiperpotassemia. O impulso deixa o nodo sinoatrial e entra nos tratos internodais, rapidamente atingindo os tecidos juncionais, porém sem inscrever uma onda P devido à inativação das células musculares atriais.
supernormal c., c. supernormal. SIN supranormal c.
supranormal c., c. supranormal; transmissão de um impulso durante o breve período do ciclo cardíaco quando seria esperado que falhasse se ocorresse fora desse intervalo; considerado melhor que o esperado, e não melhor que o normal. Cf. supranormal *excitability*. SIN supernormal c.
synaptic c., c. sináptica; a condução de um impulso nervoso através de uma sinapse.
ventricular c., c. ventricular. SIN intraventricular c.
ventriculoatrial c. (VAC), VA c., c. ventriculoatrial (CVA); c. VA. SIN retrograde VA c.
con·duc·tiv·i·ty (kon - dŭk - tiv′i - tē). Condutividade. **1.** A capacidade de transmissão ou transporte de determinadas formas de energia, como calor, som e eletricidade, sem movimento perceptível do corpo condutor. **2.** A propriedade, inerente no protoplasma vivo, de transmitir um estado de excitação; p. ex, no músculo ou nervo.
hydraulic c., c. hidráulica; facilidade de filtração por pressão de um líquido através de uma membrana; especificamente, $Kf = \eta (\dot{Q}/A) (\delta x/\delta P)$, onde Kf = condutividade hidráulica, η = viscosidade do líquido filtrado, $\dot{Q}/A$ = volume de líquido filtrado por unidade de tempo e unidade de área, e $\delta x/\delta P$ = recíproca do gradiente de pressão através da membrana; as concentrações de soluto devem ser idênticas de ambos os lados da membrana. Também é aplicado mais livremente às medidas em uma membrana total de área e espessura desconhecidas com viscosidade do líquido desconhecida $(K = \dot{Q}/\delta P)$.
con·duc·tor (kon - dŭk′ter, - tōr). Condutor. 1. Uma sonda com um sulco ao longo do qual é passado um bisturi, abrindo um seio ou fístula; um guia sulcado. 2. Qualquer substância que possua condutividade.
con·duit (kon′doo - it). Conduto; um canal.
apical-aortic c., c. apical-aórtico; um conduto valvulado entre o ápice do VE e a aorta, usado no tratamento da obstrução do trato de saída do VE não tratável de outra forma.
ileal c., c. ileal; segmento isolado de íleo que serve como um substituto cutâneo para a bexiga, no qual podem ser implantados ureteres, cuja luz é ligada à pele; usado após cistectomia total ou outra perda da função vesical normal que exige derivação supravesical. SIN ileal bladder.
con·du·pli·cate (kon - doo′pli - kāt). Conduplicado; dobrado longitudinalmente sobre si mesmo. [L. *con-*, com, + *duplico*, pp. *–atus*]
con·du·pli·ca·to cor·pore (kon - doo - pli - kā′to kōr′pōr - ē). Condição em que o feto dobra-se sobre si mesmo na apresentação de ombro.
con·du·ran·go (kon - doo - rang′gō). Condurango; a casca do *Gonolobus condurango, Marsdenia condurango* (família Asclepiadaceae), um arbusto do Equador e do Peru; aromático amargo e adstringente. [Peru]
con·dy·lar (kon′di - lăr). Condilar; relativo a um côndilo.
con·dy·lar·thro·sis (kon′di - lar - thrō′sis). Condilartrose; uma articulação, como a do joelho, formada por superfícies condilares. [G. *kondylos*, côndilo, + *arthrōsis*, articulação]
con·dyle (kon′dīl) [TA]. Côndilo; uma superfície articular arredondada na extremidade de um osso. SIN condylus [TA].
balancing side c., c. do lado de balanceio; em odontologia, o côndilo mandibular no lado oposto ao que a mandíbula se move em uma incursão lateral.
c. of humerus [TA], c. do úmero; a extremidade distal do úmero, incluindo a tróclea, o capítulo e o olécrano, as fossas coronóide e radial. SIN condylus humeri [TA].
lateral c. [TA], c. lateral; o côndilo mais distante da linha média. SIN condylus lateralis [TA].
lateral c. of femur [TA], c. lateral do fêmur; o côndilo lateral é mais longo que o côndilo medial. SIN condylus lateralis femoris [TA].
lateral c. of tibia [TA], c. lateral da tíbia; o côndilo lateral é mais longo que o côndilo medial. SIN condylus lateralis tibiae [TA].
mandibular c., c. mandibular. SIN condylar *process* of mandible.
medial c. [TA], c. medial; côndilo mais próximo da linha média. SIN condylus medialis [TA].
medial c. of femur [TA], c. medial do fêmur; o côndilo mais curto e situado mais próximo da linha média. SIN condylus medialis femoris [TA].
medial c. of tibia [TA], c. medial da tíbia; o côndilo mais curto e situado mais próximo da linha média. SIN condylus medialis tibiae [TA].
occipital c. [TA], c. occipital; uma das duas facetas ovais alongadas na superfície inferior do osso occipital, uma de cada lado do forame magno, que se articula com o atlas. SIN condylus occipitalis [TA].
working side c., c. do lado de trabalho; em odontologia, o côndilo mandibular no lado para o qual a mandíbula se move em uma incursão lateral.
con·dy·lec·to·my (kon - di - lek′tō - mē). Condilectomia; excisão de um côndilo. [G. *kondylos*, côndilo, + *ektomē*, excisão]
con·dyl·i·on (kon - dil′ē - on). Condílio; um ponto na superfície lateral externa ou medial interna do côndilo mandibular. [G. *kondylion*, dim. de *kondylos*, côndilo]
con·dy·loid (kon′di - loyd). Condilóide; relativo, ou semelhante, a um côndilo. [G. *kondylōdēs*, como a proeminência de uma articulação, de *kondylos*, côndilo, + *eidos*, semelhança]
con·dy·lo·ma, pl. **con·dy·lo·ma·ta** (kon - di - lō′mă, - mah′tă). Condiloma; crescimento verrucoso no ânus ou na vulva, ou na glande do pênis. [G. *kondylōma*, protuberância]
c. acumina′tum, c. acuminado; crescimento verrucoso protruso contagioso na genitália externa ou no ânus, que consiste em crescimentos fibrosos cobertos por epitélio espesso, exibindo coilocitose, devido a contato sexual com infecção por papilomavírus humano (HPV); geralmente é benigno, embora tenha sido descrita degeneração maligna associada a tipos específicos de vírus. SIN genital wart, venereal wart.
flat c., c. plano; (1) SIN c. latum; (2) um condiloma do colo uterino ou de outro local causado por infecção pelo papilomavírus humano (HPV) e caracterizado, histologicamente, por coilocitose sem papilomatose.
giant c., c. gigante; um tipo de condiloma acuminado grande encontrado no ânus, na vulva ou saco prepucial do pênis de homens de meia-idade não circuncisados; tende a estender-se profundamente e a recorrer. VER TAMBÉM verrucous *carcinoma*.
c. la′tum, c. plano; erupção sifilítica secundária de pápulas de topo plano, que ocorrem em grupos, cobertas por uma camada necrótica de resíduos epiteliais, secretando um líquido seropurulento; são encontradas no ânus e em locais onde pregas cutâneas contíguas produzem calor e umidade. SIN flat c. (1), moist papule, mucous papule.
con·dy·lom·a·tous (kon - di - lō′mă - tŭs). Condilomatoso; relativo a um condiloma.
con·dy·lot·o·my (kon - di - lot′ō - mē). Condilotomia; divisão, sem remoção de um côndilo. [G. *kondylos*, côndilo, + *tomē*, incisão]
con·dy·lus (kon′di - lŭs) [TA]. Côndilo. SIN condyle. [L. do G. *kondylos*, a proeminência de qualquer articulação]
c. hu′meri [TA], c. do úmero. SIN condyle of humerus.
c. latera′lis [TA], c. lateral. SIN lateral condyle.
c. latera′lis fem′oris [TA], c. lateral do fêmur. SIN lateral condyle of femur.
c. latera′lis tib′iae [TA], c. lateral da tíbia. SIN lateral condyle of tibia.
c. media′lis [TA], c. medial. SIN medial condyle.
c. media′lis fem′oris [TA], c. medial do fêmur. SIN medial condyle of femur.
c. media′lis tibiae [TA], c. medial da tíbia. SIN medial condyle of tibia.
c. occipita′lis [TA], c. occipital. SIN occipital condyle.
cone (kōn). Cone. **1.** Superfície que une um círculo a um ponto situado em plano superior (contendo o círculo). **2.** O processo cônico, fotossensível, voltado para fora, de uma célula cônica essencial para a visão de precisão e a visão para cores; os cones são os únicos fotorreceptores na fóvea central e estão interpostos com números crescentes de bastonetes em direção à periferia da retina. SIN cone cell of retina. **3.** Cilindro metálico ou cone truncado, circular ou quadrado ao corte transversal, usado para confinar um feixe de raios X. SIN conus (1). [G. *kōnos*, cone]
antipodal c., c. antípoda; conjunto de raios astrais de uma célula em divisão, que se estendem do centríolo em direção oposta à placa equatorial.
arterial c., c. arterial. SIN conus arteriosus.
c. down, focalizar; confinar um feixe de raios X a uma região de interesse utilizando um colimador ou cone (3); coloquial, concentrar a atenção ou as atividades de alguém.

elastic c., c. elástico. SIN *conus* elasticus.

gutta-percha c., c. de guta-percha; material semi-rígido, em forma de cone, para enchimento de um canal radicular, composto de guta-percha e óxido de zinco.

Haller c.'s, cones de Haller. SIN *lobules* of epididymis, em *lobule*.

implantation c., c. de implantação. SIN *axon hillock*.

c. of light, c. de luz. SIN *light reflex* (3).

medullary c. [TA], c. medular. SIN *conus medullaris*.

nerve growth c., c. de crescimento nervoso; estrutura altamente móvel na borda anterior de um axônio em crescimento.

ocular c., c. ocular; o cone de luz no interior do bulbo do olho com a base formada pelos raios que entram através da pupila e o ápice focalizado na retina.

Politzer luminous c., c. luminoso de Politzer. SIN *light reflex* (3).

pulmonary c., c. pulmonar. SIN *conus arteriosus*.

retinal c.'s, cones retinianos. VER cone (2).

silver c., c. de prata; prata pura com formato cônico padrão, usado com cimento para obturar canais das raízes dos dentes.

theca interna c., c. da teca interna; espessamento cônico das células tecais de um folículo ovariano com seu ápice voltado para a superfície.

twin c., c.-gêmeo; dois cones retinianos fundidos.

vascular c.'s, cones vasculares. SIN *lobules* of epididymis, em *lobule*.

-cone. A cúspide de um dente no arco dental maxilar.

co·nes·si (ko-nes'e). Conessi; a casca da *Holarrhena antidysenterica* (família Apocynaceae), uma árvore indiana; usada como adstringente e no tratamento da disenteria e amebíase. SIN kurchi bark. [Índia Oriental]

co·nes·sine (kon'ĕ-sēn). Conessina; alcalóide esteróide derivado da *Holarrhena antidysenterica* (conessi); adstringente amarelo, usado no tratamento da disenteria amebiana e da tricomoníase vaginal. SIN neriine, wrightine.

co·nex·us, pl. **co·nex·us** (ko-nek'sŭs). Conexão. SIN *connection*. [L.]

c. intertendin'eus, c. intertendinosa. SIN *intertendinous connections* of extensor digitorum, em *connection*.

con·fab·u·la·tion (kon'fab-ū-lā'shŭn). Confabulação; a formulação de respostas bizarras e erradas, e uma presteza em fornecer uma resposta fluente, mas tangencial, sem qualquer relação com os fatos, a qualquer pergunta feita; observada na amnésia e na síndrome de Wernicke-Korsakoff. [L. *con-fabulor*, pp. *–fabulatus*, conversar, de *fabula*, narrativa]

con·fec·tio, gen. **con·fec·ti·o·nis,** pl. **con·fec·ti·o·nes** (kon-fek'shē-ō, -ō'nis, -ō'nēz). Electuário, eletuário. SIN *confection*. [L. de *conficio*, pp. *-fectus*, preparar]

con·fec·tion (kon-fek'shŭn). Electuário, eletuário; preparação farmacêutica que consiste em uma droga misturada a mel ou xarope; um sólido macio, algumas vezes usado como excipiente para massas de pílulas. SIN confectio, conserve, electuary. [L. *confectio*]

con·fer·tus (kon-fer'tŭs). Dispostos muito juntos; coalescentes. [L. *confercio*, pp. *-fertus*, abarrotar, de *farcio*, encher completamente, abarrotar]

con·fi·den·ti·al·i·ty (kon'fi-den-shē-al'i-tē). Sigilo; o direito protegido legalmente, conferido a (e dever exigido de) profissionais de saúde especificamente designados, de não revelar informações obtidas durante a consulta de um paciente. [L. *con-fido*, confiar, estar seguro]

con·fig·u·ra·tion (kon-fig-ū-rā'shŭn). Configuração. **1.** A forma geral de um corpo e suas partes. **2.** Em química, o arranjo espacial de átomos em uma molécula. A configuração de uma substância (p. ex., um açúcar) é o arranjo espacial único de seus átomos de forma que nenhum outro arranjo desses átomos pode ser superposto com correspondência completa, independentemente das alterações na conformação (isto é, torção ou rotação em ligações simples); a mudança de configuração exige ruptura e reunião das ligações, como nas transformações das configurações D em L dos açúcares. Cf. conformation.

cis c., *cis*; **(1)** VER cis- (4); **(2)** a propriedade de dois ou mais locais na mesma molécula de DNA.

con·fine·ment (kon-fīn'ment). Confinamento; reclusão; parto; dar à luz uma criança. [L. *confine* (neutro), limite, fronteira, de *con-* + *finis*, limite]

con·flict (kon'flikt). Conflito; tensão ou estresse experimentado por um organismo quando a satisfação de uma necessidade, um impulso, uma motivação ou um desejo é impedida pela presença de outras necessidades, impulsos ou motivações atraentes ou não.

approach-approach c., c. de aproximação-aproximação; uma situação de indecisão e vacilação quando um indivíduo se confronta com duas alternativas igualmente atraentes.

approach-avoidance c., c. de aproximação-evitação; situação de indecisão e vacilação quando o indivíduo se confronta com um único objeto ou acontecimento que apresenta tanto qualidades atraentes quanto sem atrativos.

avoidance-avoidance c., c. de evitação-evitação; situação de indecisão e vacilação quando o indivíduo se confronta com duas alternativas igualmente sem atrativos.

c. of interest, c. de interesses; conflito entre os interesses e as necessidades profissionais ou pessoais de um profissional de saúde e suas responsabilidades profissionais em relação a um paciente ou outro usuário.

interpersonal c., c. interpessoal; relativo a um conflito nas relações e trocas sociais entre as pessoas. Cf. intrapersonal c.

intrapersonal c., c. intrapessoal; conflito que ocorre apenas na dinâmica psicológica da mente do próprio indivíduo. VER intrapsychic.

role c., c. funcional; o dilema de um indivíduo que necessita representar dois papéis diferentes (p. ex., o cônjuge e o homem de negócios agressivo) que não podem ser facilmente harmonizados.

con·flu·ence (kon'floo-ĕns) [TA]. Confluência; um fluxo conjunto; união de duas ou mais correntes. SIN confluens [TA]. [L. *confluens*]

c. of sinuses [TA], c. dos seios; local de encontro, na protuberância occipital interna, dos seios sagital superior, reto e occipital, drenados pelos dois seios transversos da dura-máter. SIN confluens sinuum [TA].

con·flu·ens (kon-floo'enz) [TA]. Confluência. SIN *confluence, confluence*. [L.]

c. si'nuum [TA], c. dos seios. SIN *confluence* of sinuses.

con·flu·ent (kon'floo-ent). Confluente. **1.** Que une; que corre junto; designa determinadas lesões cutâneas que se fundem, formando uma placa; designa uma doença caracterizada por lesões que não são isoladas ou distintas entre si. **2.** Designa um osso formado pela fusão de dois ossos originalmente distintos. [L. *con-fluo*, fluir junto]

con·fo·cal (kon-fō'kal). Confocal; que tem os mesmos focos. VER confocal *microscope*.

con·for·ma·tion (kon-for-mā'shŭn). Conformação; a disposição espacial de uma molécula atingida por rotação de grupos em torno de ligações covalentes simples, sem romper quaisquer ligações covalentes; esta última restrição diferencia a conformação da configuração (como em anômeros e estereoisômeros relacionados), onde uma ou mais ligações tem de ser rompida na mudança de uma forma (configuração) para outra. A conformação é um dos aspectos mais importantes da química do açúcar, sendo básico para compreender as propriedades químicas dos açúcares. Cf. configuration.

boat c., c. em barco. VER Haworth conformational formulas of cyclic *sugars*.

envelope c., c. em envelope. VER Haworth conformational formulas of cyclic *sugars*.

con·form·er (kon-for'mer). Adaptador; um molde, geralmente de plástico, usado em reparo cirúrgico para manter espaço em uma cavidade ou para evitar fechamento por cicatrização de uma abertura artificial ou natural. [L. *conformo*, moldar]

con·found·ing. 1. Mistura; uma situação na qual os efeitos de dois ou mais processos não são separados; a distorção do efeito aparente de uma exposição em risco, produzida pela associação com outros fatores que podem influenciar o resultado. **2.** Uma relação entre os efeitos de dois ou mais fatores causais observados em um conjunto de dados, de forma que não é logicamente possível distinguir a contribuição de qualquer fator causador isolado para os efeitos observados.

con·fron·ta·tion (kon-fron-tā'shŭn). Confrontação; o ato do terapeuta, ou de outro paciente em um grupo terapêutico, de interpretar abertamente as resistências, atitudes, sentimentos ou efeitos de um paciente sobre o terapeuta, o grupo ou seu(s) membro(s).

con·fu·sion (kon-fū'zhŭn). Confusão; estado mental no qual as reações a estímulos ambientais são impróprias porque a pessoa se encontra aturdida, perplexa ou incapaz de se orientar. [L. *confusio*, que causa confusão]

con·fu·sion·al (kon-fū'zhŭn-ăl). Confusional; caracterizado por, ou pertinente a, confusão.

con·ge·ner (kon'jĕ-ner). Congênere. **1.** Uma dentre duas ou mais coisas do mesmo tipo, como entre animais ou vegetais, com relação à classificação. **2.** Um dentre dois ou mais músculos com a mesma função. [L. *con-*, com, + *genus*, raça]

con·ge·ner·ous (kon-jen'er-ŭs). Congêneres. **1.** Que possui a mesma função; designa determinados músculos que são sinérgicos. **2.** Derivado da mesma fonte, ou de natureza semelhante. VER congener.

con·gen·ic (kon-jen'ik). Congênico; relativo a uma raça endogâmica de animais produzidos por cruzamento repetido de uma linhagem genética com outra linhagem endogâmica (isogênica). [con- + G. *genos*, nascimento, + -ic]

con·gen·i·tal (kon-jen'i-tăl). Congênito; existente ao nascimento, refere-se a determinadas características mentais ou físicas, anomalias, malformações, doenças, etc., que podem ser hereditárias ou devidas a uma influência que ocorre durante a gestação até o momento do parto. SIN congenitus. [L. *congenitus*, nascido com]

con·gen·i·tus (kon-jen'i-tŭs). Congênito. SIN *congenital*. [L.]

con·gest·ed (kon-jes'ted). Congestionado; congesto; que contém um volume anormal de sangue; em um estado de congestão.

con·ges·tion (kon-jes'shŭn). Congestão; presença de um volume anormal de líquido nos vasos ou passagens de uma parte ou órgão; principalmente de sangue devido ao aumento do influxo ou à obstrução do efluxo. VER TAMBÉM hyperemia. [L. *congestio*, reunião, acúmulo, de *con-gero*, pp. *-gestus*, reunir]

active c., c. ativa; congestão devida a aumento do fluxo de sangue arterial para uma parte.

brain c., c. cerebral; aumento do volume do compartimento intravascular do cérebro; freqüentemente associado a edema cerebral. SIN encephalemia.
functional c., c. funcional; hiperemia que ocorre durante atividade funcional de um órgão. SIN physiologic c.
hypostatic c., c. hipostática; congestão devida ao acúmulo de sangue venoso em uma parte mais baixa. SIN hypostasis (2).
passive c., c. passiva; congestão causada por obstrução ou alentecimento da drenagem venosa, resultando em estagnação parcial do sangue nos capilares e vênulas.
physiologic c., c. fisiológica. SIN functional c.
venous c., c. venosa; enchimento excessivo e distensão das veias com sangue em virtude de obstrução mecânica ou insuficiência ventricular direita.
con·ges·tive (kon-jes′tiv). Congestivo; relativo à congestão.
con·glo·bate (kon-glō′bāt). Conglobado; formado em uma única massa arredondada. [L. *con-globo,* pp. *-atus,* reunir em um *globus,* globo]
con·glo·ba·tion (kon-glō-bā′shŭn). Conglobação; agregação de numerosas partículas em uma massa redonda.
con·glom·er·ate (kon-glom′ĕ-rāt). Conglomerado; composto de várias partes reunidas em uma massa. [L. *conglomero,* pp. *-atus,* rolar junto, de *glomus,* bola]
con·glu·ti·nant (kon-gloo′ti-nant). Conglutinante; adesivo, que promove o fechamento de uma ferida. [L. *con-glutino,* pp. *-atus,* unir com cola, de *gluten,* cola]
con·glu·ti·na·tion (kon-gloo-ti-nā′shŭn). Conglutinação. **1.** SIN adhesion (1). **2.** Aglutinação de complexo antígeno(eritrócito)-anticorpo-complemento por soro bovino normal (e alguns outros materiais colóides); o procedimento é uma forma de detectar anticorpo não-aglutinante.
con·glu·ti·nin (kon-gloo′ti-nin). Conglutinina; proteína sérica bovina que, quando absorvida por complexos eritrócito-anticorpo-complemento, causa a aglutinação dos mesmos; é comparativamente termoestável e parece dissociar-se quando diluída em soro fisiológico. SIN bovine colloid.
con·go·phil·ic (kon-gō-fil′ik). Congofílico; designa qualquer substância que adquire coloração por vermelho-Congo.
Con·go red (kong′gō) [C.I. 22120]. Vermelho-Congo; corante de algodão direto ácido, é absorvido por amilóide e induz fluorescência verde do amilóide em luz polarizada; usado como auxílio laboratorial no diagnóstico de amiloidose, como corante histológico e como indicador (pH 3,0, azul-violeta, a pH 5,0, vermelho) no teste para ácido clorídrico livre no conteúdo gástrico. VER Bennhold Congo red *stain.*
co·ni (kō′nī). Cones; plural de conus.
con·ic, con·i·cal (kon′ik, kon′i-kăl). Cônico; semelhante a um cone.
-conid. A cúspide de um dente na mandíbula.
co·nid·ia (ko-nid′ē-ă), Conídios; plural de conidium.
co·nid·i·al (ko-nid′ē-al). Conidial; relativo a um conídio.
Co·nid·i·o·bo·lus (ko-nid′ē-ō-bō′lŭs). Gênero de fungos que contém duas espécies, *C. coronatus* e *C. incongruus,* ambas causadoras de zigomicose (entomoftoramicose).
co·nid·i·og·e·nous (ko-nid-ē-oj′ĕ-nŭs). Conidiógeno; designa uma célula que dá origem a um conídio, p. ex., uma fiálide.
co·nid·i·o·phore (ko-nid′ē-ō-for). Conidióforo; uma hifa especializada que possui conídios em fungos. [conidium + G. *phoros,* que carrega]
Phialophore-type c., c. do tipo fialóforo; tipo de formação de esporo, característico do gênero *Phialophora,* no qual os conídios são formados endogenamente em conidióforos em forma de cantil, denominados fiálides.
co·nid·i·um, pl. **co·nid·ia** (ko-nid′ē-ŭm,-ē-ă). Conídio; um esporo assexuado de fungos produzidos externamente de várias maneiras. [L. Mod. dim. de G. *konis,* poeira]
co·ni·ine (kō′nē-ēn). Coniína; cicutina; o alcalóide ativo tóxico da cicuta; os sais bromidrato e cloridrato foram usados como antiespasmódicos; principal toxina da cicuta (*Conium maculatum*).
co·ni·o·fi·bro·sis (ko′nē-ō-fī-brō′sis). Coniofibrose; fibrose produzida por poeira, principalmente dos pulmões pela poeira inalada. [G. *konis,* poeira, + fibrose]
co·ni·o·lymph·sta·sis (kō′nē-ō-limf′stă-sis). Coniolinfoestase; estase de linfa causada por poeira, provavelmente por intervenção da fibrose. [G. *konis,* poeira, + linfa + G. *stasis,* parada]
co·ni·om·e·ter (kō-nē-om′ĕ-ter). Coniômetro; dispositivo para avaliar a quantidade de poeira no ar. [G. *konis,* poeira, + *metron,* medida]
co·ni·o·phage (kō′nē-ō-fāj). Coniófago. SIN alveolar macrophage. [G. *konis,* poeira, + *phagō,* comer]
co·ni·o·sis (kō-nē-ō′sis). Coniose; qualquer doença ou condição mórbida causada por poeira. [G. *konis,* poeira]
co·ni·ot·o·my (kō-nē-ot′ō-mē). Coniotomia; incisão do cone elástico da laringe. VER TAMBÉM cricothyrotomy.
co·ni·um (kō-nē′ŭm). Cicuta; o fruto verde seco da *Conium maculatum* (família Umbelliferae), também conhecido como funcho selvagem; tem sido usado como sedativo, antiespasmódico e anódino. SIN hemlock. [L. do G. *kōneion,* cicuta]

con·i·za·tion (kō-nī-zā′shŭn). Conização; excisão de um cone de tecido, p. ex., mucosa do colo uterino.
cautery c., c. por cautério; remoção de um cone de tecido endocervical com eletrocautério.
cold knife c., c. com bisturi frio; retirada de um cone de tecido endocervical com uma lâmina de bisturi fria de forma a preservar as características histológicas e evitar o ressecamento do tecido.

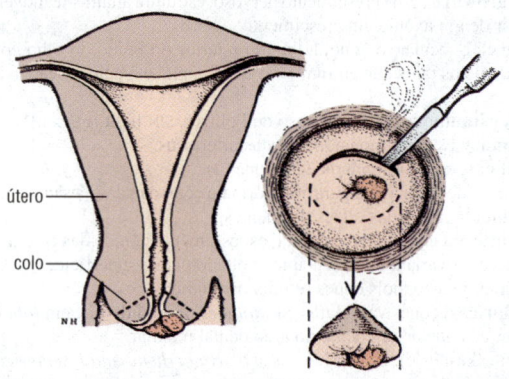

conização: processo maligno mostrado em vermelho, a linha tracejada mostra a extensão da ressecção

con·ju·gant (kon′joo-gant). Conjugante; membro de um par unido de organismos ou gametas que sofrem conjugação. VER TAMBÉM exconjugant. [L. *con-jugo,* unir]
con·ju·ga·ta (kon-joo-gā′tă) [TA]. Diâmetro; diâmetros conjugados da pelve. VER conjugate. [L. fem de *conjugatus,* pp. of *con-jugo,* unir]
c. anatomica [TA], diâmetro anatômico. SIN anatomical *conjugate.*
c. diagonal'is [TA], diâmetro diagonal. SIN diagonal *conjugate.*
c. externa [TA], diâmetro externo. SIN external *conjugate.*
c. recta [TA], diâmetro reto. SIN straight *conjugate.*
c. vera [TA], diâmetro verdadeiro. SIN true *conjugate.*
con·ju·gate (kon′joo-gāt) [TA]. **1.** Conjugado; unido ou pareado. SIN conjugated. **2.** Diâmetro; diâmetro conjugado da pelve. A distância entre quaisquer dois pontos especificados na periferia do canal pélvico. [L. *conjugatus,* unido. Ver conjugata]
anatomical c. [TA], diâmetro anatômico; medida da dimensão pélvica descrevendo a distância entre o promontório sacral e a borda inferior da sínfise púbica, determinada manualmente pela vagina ou por ultra-sonografia. É usado para extrapolar o diâmetro verdadeiro. SIN conjugata anatomica [TA].
diagonal c. [TA], diâmetro diagonal; a dimensão ântero-posterior da abertura superior da pelve que mede a distância clínica do promontório do sacro até a margem inferior da sínfise púbica. SIN conjugata diagonalis [TA], diagonal conjugate diameter, false c. (1).
effective c., diâmetro efetivo; o diâmetro interno medido da vértebra lombar mais próxima até a sínfise, na espondilolistese. SIN false c. (2).
external c. [TA], diâmetro externo; a distância em linha reta entre a depressão sob o último processo espinhoso das vértebras lombares e a borda superior da sínfise púbica. SIN conjugata externa [TA], external conjugate diameter.
false c., diâmetro falso; **(1)** SIN diagonal c.; **(2)** SIN effective c.
folic acid c., conjugado do ácido fólico; um folato com três moléculas de ácido glutâmico (pteropterina), em vez de uma, ou com sete (ácido pteroil-heptaglutâmico ou conjugado de vitamina B_c ou ácido fólico).
internal c., diâmetro interno. SIN median c.
median c. [TA], diâmetro mediano; distância do promontório do sacro até a borda posterior superior da sínfise púbica. SIN anteroposterior diameter of the pelvic inlet, conjugate axis, conjugate diameter of pelvic inlet, c. of pelvic inlet, internal c.
obstetric c., conjugado obstétrico; diâmetro verdadeiro. SIN true c.
obstetric c. of pelvic outlet, conjugado obstétrico da abertura inferior da pelve; o diâmetro da abertura inferior da pelve alongado pelo deslocamento posterior do cóccix.
c. of pelvic inlet, diâmetro da abertura superior da pelve; diâmetro mediano. SIN median c.
c. of pelvic outlet, diâmetro da abertura inferior da pelve; diâmetro reto. SIN straight c. VER TAMBÉM obstetric c. of pelvic outlet.
straight c. [TA], diâmetro reto; a distância da extremidade do cóccix até a borda inferior da sínfise púbica. SIN conjugata recta [TA], conjugate diameter of pelvic outlet, c. of pelvic outlet.
true c. [TA], diâmetro verdadeiro; o diâmetro que representa o menor diâmetro que a cabeça tem de atravessar ao descer para a abertura superior da pelve e

mede, determinado por raios X, a distância do promontório do sacro até um ponto na superfície interna da sínfise, alguns milímetros abaixo de sua margem superior. SIN conjugata vera [TA], obstetric conjugate diameter, obstetric c.

con·ju·gat·ed (kon′joo-gāt-ed). Conjugado. SIN conjugate (1).

con·ju·ga·tion (kon-jŭ-gā′shŭn). Conjugação. **1.** A união de dois organismos unicelulares ou dos gametas masculino e feminino de formas multicelulares, seguida por divisão da cromatina com a geração de duas novas células. **2.** Conjugação bacteriana realizada por contato simples, geralmente por meio de fímbrias especializadas através das quais genes de transferência e outros genes do plasmídeo são transferidos para bactérias receptoras. **3.** Reprodução sexuada entre protozoários ciliados, durante a qual dois indivíduos de tipos de união apropriada fundem-se ao longo de parte de seus comprimentos; seus macronúcleos degeneram, e os micronúcleos, em cada macronúcleo, dividem-se várias vezes (incluindo uma divisão meiótica); um dos pró-núcleos haplóides resultantes passa de cada conjugante para o outro e funde-se ao núcleo haplóide remanescente em cada conjugante; os organismos então se separam (tornando-se exconjugantes), sofrem reorganização nuclear e, subseqüentemente, dividem-se por mitose assexuada. **4.** A combinação, principalmente no fígado, de determinadas substâncias tóxicas formadas no intestino, drogas ou hormônios esteróides com ácido glucurônico ou sulfúrico; um meio pelo qual a atividade biológica de determinadas substâncias químicas é interrompida e as substâncias tornadas aptas para excreção. **5.** A formação de derivados glicil ou tauril dos ácidos biliares. **6.** Uma seqüência alternada de ligações químicas múltiplas e simples em uma substância química na qual há alguma deslocalização de π-elétrons. **7.** A união de duas substâncias. [L. *conjugo*, pp. *-jugatus*, unir]

con·junc·ti·va, pl. **con·junc·ti·vae** (kon-jŭnk-tī′vă, -vē) [TA]. Túnica conjuntiva; a mucosa que reveste a superfície anterior do bulbo do olho e a superfície posterior das pálpebras. SIN tunica conjunctiva [TA]. [L. fem. de *conjunctivus*, de *conjungo*, pp. *-junctus*, ligar]

bulbar c. [TA], túnica conjuntiva do bulbo; a parte da conjuntiva que cobre a superfície anterior da esclera e o epitélio da superfície da córnea. SIN tunica conjunctiva bulbi [TA], conjunctival layer of bulb.

palpebral c. [TA], túnica conjuntiva da pálpebra; a parte da conjuntiva que reveste a superfície posterior das pálpebras e é contínua com a conjuntiva bulbar nos fórnices conjuntivais. SIN tunica conjunctiva palpebrarum [TA], conjunctival layer of eyelids.

con·junc·ti·val (kon-jŭnk-tī′văl). Conjuntival; relativo à conjuntiva.

con·junc·tive (kon-jŭnk′tiv). Conjuntivo; que junta; que une; conectivo.

con·junc·ti·vi·plas·ty (kon-jŭnk-tī′vi-plas-tē). Conjuntivoplastia. SIN conjunctivoplasty.

con·junc·ti·vi·tis (kon-jŭnk-ti-vī′tis). Conjuntivite; inflamação da conjuntiva. SIN blennophthalmia (1).

actinic c., c. actínica. SIN ultraviolet keratoconjunctivitis.

acute contagious c., c. contagiosa aguda; termo obsoleto para designar uma conjuntivite aguda caracterizada por hiperemia intensa e abundante secreção mucopurulenta. SIN acute epidemic c., pinkeye.

acute epidemic c., c. epidêmica aguda. SIN acute contagious c.

acute hemorrhagic c., c. hemorrágica aguda; conjuntivite endêmica aguda específica com edema palpebral, lacrimejamento, hemorragias conjuntivais e folículos; geralmente causada por *Enterovirus* tipo 70.

acute viral c., c. viral aguda; inflamação epidêmica da conjuntiva caracterizada por folículos, principalmente no fórnice inferior; pode ser causada por adenovírus, herpesvírus e vírus da doença de Newcastle.

allergic c., c. alérgica; reação imunológica mediada por imunoglobulina E associada a prurido, eritema e lacrimejamento; é tipicamente sazonal e pode afetar até 10% da população.

angular c., c. angular; inflamação conjuntival bilateral subaguda, algumas vezes causada pelo bacilo *Moraxella*, caracterizada por eritema dos ângulos laterais e secreção viscosa e escassa que adere aos cílios. SIN Moraxella c.

arc-flash c., c. de arco voltaico. SIN ultraviolet keratoconjunctivitis.

c. ar′ida, c. seca. SIN xerophthalmia.

chemical c., c. química; inflamação conjuntival causada por irritantes químicos.

chronic c., c. crônica; hiperemia conjuntival, bilateral, persistente, com exsudação escassa; há tendência a remissão e exacerbação.

chronic follicular c., c. folicular crônica; inflamação indolente da conjuntiva, com folículos distintos, nos fórnices, que podem ser de natureza infecciosa, tóxica ou irritante.

cicatricial c., c. cicatricial; afecção ocular progressiva crônica que provoca fibrose da conjuntiva, primariamente, e da córnea seqüencialmente.

diphtheritic c., c. diftérica; inflamação conjuntival grave causada por *Corynebacterium diphtheriae* e caracterizada por uma membrana infiltrativa que, à remoção, deixa uma superfície desnuda. SIN membranous c.

follicular c., c. folicular; c. associada a tecido linfóide hipertrófico nos fórnices conjuntivais.

giant papillary c., c. papilar gigante; inflamação conjuntival caracterizada por grandes papilas e associada à sensibilização ao material antigênico presente na superfície de uma lente de contato.

gonococcal c., c. gonocócica; um tipo de conjuntivite hiperaguda, purulenta.

gonorrheal c., c. gonorreica. SIN gonorrheal ophthalmia.

granular c., c. granular. SIN trachomatous c.

hyperacute purulent c., c. purulenta hiperaguda; conjuntivite causada por *Neisseria gonorrhoeae* e caracterizada por edema e congestão da conjuntiva, edema das pálpebras e secreção purulenta.

inclusion c., c. de inclusão; conjuntivite folicular causada por *Chlamydia trachomatis*.

infantile purulent c., c. purulenta do lactente. SIN ophthalmia neonatorum.

larval c., c. larval; conjuntivite causada pela penetração de larvas no olho. VER ophthalmo-myiasis.

ligneous c., c. lígnea; c. lenhosa; conjuntivite caracterizada tipicamente por endurecimento lenhoso da conjuntiva do tarso superior, pseudomembranas esbranquiçadas e, em casos graves, opacidade da córnea; geralmente bilateral.

c. medicamento′sa, c. medicamentosa; conjuntivite causada por medicamento ou toxina instilada no saco conjuntival. SIN toxicogenic c.

membranous c., c. membranosa. SIN diphtheritic c.

molluscum c., c. por molusco; conjuntivite associada a lesões de molusco contagioso da pálpebra.

Moraxella c., c. por *Moraxella*. SIN angular c.

necrotic infectious c., c. infecciosa necrótica; inflamação necrótica, supurativa, unilateral da conjuntiva caracterizada por manchas brancas elevadas, dispersas, nos fórnices e na conjuntiva palpebral, e tumefação ipsolateral dos linfonodos pré-auriculares, parotídeos e submaxilares. SIN Pascheff c.

neonatal c., c. neonatal. SIN ophthalmia neonatorum.

Parinaud c., c. de Parinaud; inflamação necrótica crônica da conjuntiva caracterizada por grandes folículos avermelhados, irregulares, e por linfadenopatia regional.

Pascheff c., c. de Pascheff. SIN necrotic infectious c.

phlyctenular c., c. flictenular; conjuntivite circunscrita acompanhada pela formação de pequenos nódulos vermelhos de tecido linfóide (flictênulas) na conjuntiva. SIN phlyctenular ophthalmia.

pseudomembranous c., c. pseudomembranosa; reação inflamatória inespecífica caracterizada pelo surgimento, na conjuntiva, de uma placa fibrinosa coagulada que pode ser descolada do epitélio intacto.

purulent c., c. purulenta; inflamação violentamente aguda da conjuntiva, com pus abundante e tendência acentuada ao envolvimento da córnea.

simple c., c. simples; conjuntivite viral aguda, autolimitada e de curta duração.

snow c., c. da neve. SIN ultraviolet keratoconjunctivitis.

spring c., c. primaveril. SIN vernal c.

squirrel plague c., c. tularêmica; uma das causas da conjuntivite de Parinaud. SIN tularemic c., c. tularensis.

swimming pool c., c. da piscina; vermelhidão inespecífica do olho que pode ser causada por cloração da piscina, adenovírus e, raramente, *Chlamydia*.

toxicogenic c., c. toxicogênica. SIN c. medicamentosa.

trachomatous c., c. tracomatosa; infecção crônica da conjuntiva causada por *Chlamydia trachomatis*, caracterizada por folículos conjuntivais e subseqüente fibrose. VER TAMBÉM trachoma. SIN granular c.

tularemic c., c. tularen′sis, c. tularêmica. SIN squirrel plague c.

vernal c., c. vernal; inflamação conjuntival bilateral e crônica, com fotofobia e prurido intenso, que recorre sazonalmente durante o período de calor; caracterizada, na forma palpebral, por papilas arredondadas na conjuntiva da pálpebra superior e, na forma bulbar, por nódulos gelatinosos adjacentes ao limbo corneoescleral. SIN spring c., spring ophthalmia, vernal catarrh, vernal keratoconjunctivitis.

welder's c., c. do soldador. SIN ultraviolet keratoconjunctivitis.

con·junc·ti·vo·chal·a·sis (kon-jŭnk′ti-vō-kal′ă-sis). Conjuntivocalásia; condição na qual a *conjuntiva* do bulbo redundante cresce sobre a margem da pálpebra ou cobre o orifício inferior. [conjunctiva + G. *chalasis*, afrouxamento]

con·junc·ti·vo·dac·ry·o·cys·to·rhi·nos·to·my (kon-jŭnk′ti-vō-dak′rē-ō-sis′tō-rī-nos′tō-mē). Conjuntivodacriocistorrinostomia; procedimento para permitir drenagem lacrimal quando os canalículos estão fechados; são introduzidos tubos plásticos que se estendem do saco conjuntival, atravessam o saco lacrimal até o nariz; a abertura assim produzida. [conjunctiva + G. *dakryon*, lágrima, + *kystis*, saco, + *ris* (*rhin*-), nariz, + *stoma*, boca]

con·junc·ti·vo·dac·ry·o·cys·tos·to·my (kon-jŭnk′ti-vō-dak′rē-ō-sis-tos′to-mē). Conjuntivodacriocistostomia; **1.** Procedimento cirúrgico através da conjuntiva, que forma uma abertura para o saco lacrimal. **2.** A abertura assim formada. [conjunctiva + G. *dakryon*, lágrima + *kystis*, saco, + *stoma*, boca]

con·junc·ti·vo·plas·ty (kon-jŭnk-tī′vō-plas-tē, kon-jŭnk′ti-vō-). Conjuntivoplastia; cirurgia plástica da conjuntiva. SIN conjunctiviplasty.

con·junc·ti·vo·rhi·nos·to·my (kon-jŭnk′tī-vō-rī-nos′tō-mē). Conjuntivorrinostomia. **1.** Procedimento cirúrgico para construir uma passagem através da conjuntiva até a cavidade nasal. **2.** A abertura assim produzida. [conjunctiva + G. *ris* (*rhin*), nariz, + *stoma*, boca]

Conn, Harold J., microbiologista norte-americano, 1886–1975. VER Hucker-C. stain.

Conn, Jerome, médico norte-americano, *1907. VER C. *syndrome.*
con·nec·tins (kon - nek′tinz). Conectinas; termo coletivo para os componentes proteicos do citoesqueleto (tecido conjuntivo); originalmente descritas no músculo, mas posteriormente observadas nas membranas dos eritrócitos e de outras células.
con·nec·tion (kŏ - nek′shŭn). Conexão; união de elementos ou coisas; uma estrutura de conexão. SIN conexus, connexus.
    ambiguous atrioventricular c.'s, conexões atrioventriculares ambíguas; conexões nas quais metade da junção atrioventricular é conectada de forma concordante, e a outra metade, de forma discordante.
    anomalous pulmonary venous c.'s, total or partial, conexões venosas pulmonares anômalas, totais ou parciais; conexões nas quais algumas veias pulmonares ou todas elas se ligam ao átrio direito ou a uma de suas tributárias.
    atrioventricular c.'s, conexões atrioventriculares; as cinco formas distintas e separadas nas quais as câmaras atriais podem ser conectadas aos ventrículos são concordante, discordante, ambígua, entrada dupla e univentricular.
    concordant atrioventricular c.'s, conexões atrioventriculares concordantes; conexões nas quais as câmaras atriais conectam-se aos ventrículos morfologicamente apropriados.
    discordant atrioventricular c.'s, conexões atrioventriculares discordantes; conexões nas quais cada átrio está conectado a um ventrículo morfologicamente impróprio.
    double inlet atrioventricular c.'s, conexões atrioventriculares de entrada dupla; conexões nas quais os dois átrios estão conectados ao mesmo ventrículo.
    intertendinous c.'s of extensor digitorum [TA], conexões intertendíneas do músculo extensor dos dedos; faixas fibrosas que passam obliquamente entre os tendões divergentes do músculo extensor dos dedos no dorso da mão. SIN connexus intertendinei musculi extensoris digitorum [TA], conexus intertendineus, juncturae tendinum.
    marrow-mesenchyme c.'s, conexões medula óssea-mesênquima; continuações ininterruptas entre medula óssea e mesênquima da orelha média no feto e no recém-nascido.
    partial anomalous pulmonary venous c.'s, conexões venosas pulmonares anômalas parciais. VER anomalous pulmonary venous c.'s, total or partial.
    univentricular c.'s, conexões univentriculares; conexões nas quais uma das câmaras atriais está conectada a um ventrículo, mas a outra não tem conexão com a massa ventricular.
con·nec·tor (kŏ - nek′tor, - tōr). Conector; em odontologia, uma parte de uma dentadura (prótese dentária) parcial que une seus componentes.
    major c., c. principal; uma placa ou barra (barra lingual, barra palatina) usada para unir as bases de uma dentadura parcial.
    minor c., c. secundário; o elo conector (pino) entre o c. principal ou a base de uma dentadura parcial e outras unidades da prótese, como ganchos, retentores indiretos e resíduos oclusais.
    nonrigid c., c. não-rígido; um conector ou junta que não é rígida nem sólida. SIN stress-broken c., stress-broken joint.
    rigid c., c. rígido; c. que é sólido ou rígido, como uma junta soldada.
    stress-broken c., c. não-rígido. SIN nonrigid c.
Connell, F. Gregory, cirurgião norte-americano; 1875–1968. VER C. *suture.*
con·nex·in 26 (kon-eks′in). Conexina 26; a proteína da mácula comunicante (nexo), cujo gene (Cx26), quando sofre mutação, é responsável por uma grande parte dos casos de comprometimento auditivo não-sindrômico recessivo.
con·nex·ins, con·nex·ons (kon - neks′inz, - onz). Conexinas, conexonas; conjuntos proteicos complexos que atravessam a dupla camada lipídica da membrana plasmática e formam um canal contínuo com um diâmetro de poro de aproximadamente 1,5 nm; um par de conexinas de duas células adjacentes se une para formar um nexo (ou mácula comunicante) que une o espaço de 2-4 nm entre as células, resultando em acoplamentos elétrico e metabólico; um tipo de conexinas forma a mácula comunicante no coração e pode coordenar o batimento de todas as células musculares em uma região desse órgão.
con·nex·us (ko - nek′sŭs). Conexão. SIN connection. [L.]
    c. intertendin'ei musculi extensoris digitorum [TA], conexões intertendíneas do músculo extensor dos dedos. SIN intertendinous *connections* of extensor digitorum, em *connection.*
co·noid (kō′noyd). Conóide. **1.** Estrutura em forma de cone. **2.** Parte do complexo apical característico do subfilo dos protozoários, Apicomplexa; observado em esporozoítas, merozoítas ou outros estágios de desenvolvimento de esporozoários, e menos desenvolvido nos piroplasmas (famílias Babesiidae e Theileriidae). A função do conóide não é conhecida, mas acredita-se que seja uma organela de penetração na célula hospedeira, possivelmente auxiliada por uma forma projetável do conóide. [G. *kōnoeidēs,*, cônico]
    Sturm c., c. de Sturm; em óptica, o padrão de raios formados após a passagem através de uma combinação esferocilíndrica.
co·no·my·oi·din (kō - nō - mī′oy - din). Conomioidina; protoplasma contrátil na extremidade interna do segmento interno dos cones da retina; a motilidade é mais evidente em peixes e anfíbios, e pequena ou ausente em mamíferos. [G. *kōnos,* cone, + *mys,* músculo, + *eidos,* semelhança]

con·qui·nine (kon′kwi - nēn). Conquinina. SIN quinidine.
Conradi, Andrew, médico norueguês, 1809–1869. VER C. *line.*
Conradi, Erich, médico alemão do século XX. VER C. *disease.*
con·san·guin·e·ous (kon - sang - gwin′ē - ŭs). Consangüíneo; denotando consangüinidade. [L. *cum,* com, + *sanguis,* sangue: *consanguineus*]
con·san·guin·i·ty (kon - sang - gwin′i - tē). Consangüinidade; parentesco devido à ascendência comum. VER TAMBÉM relationship. [L. *consanguinitas,* relação sanguínea]
con·scious (con′shŭs). Consciente; cônscio. **1.** Que tem conhecimento ou percepção atual de si mesmo, de seus atos e do ambiente. **2.** Designa algo que ocorre com a atenção perceptiva do indivíduo, como um ato ou idéia consciente, distinto do automático ou instintivo. [L. *conscius,* conhecimento]
con·scious·ness (con′shŭs - nes). Consciência; o estado de estar consciente, ou perceber fatos físicos ou conceitos mentais; um estado de vigilância geral e responsividade ao ambiente; um sensório funcionante. [L. *con-scio,* conhecer, estar ciente de]
    clouding of c., turvação da consciência; estado no qual há embotamento mental e o paciente não está totalmente em contato com o ambiente.
    double c., c. dupla; condição na qual se vive em dois estados mentais aparentemente desconexos, estando, enquanto em um, inconsciente do outro ou dos atos realizados no outro. VER TAMBÉM dual *personality.*
    field of c., campo da c.; o conteúdo da consciência em um determinado momento.
con·sen·su·al (kon - sen′shoo - al). Consensual. **1.** Com consentimento; por consenso mútuo de todas as partes. **2.** Relativo a um reflexo produzido por estimulação indireta de um receptor, como a constricção pupilar em um olho quando o outro é estimulado por luz. [L. *con-sentio,* pp. *con-sensus,* concordar, sentir ao mesmo tempo + -al]
con·ser·va·tion (kon - ser - vā′shŭn). Conservação. **1.** Preservação de perda, lesão ou decomposição. **2.** Na teoria sensorimotora, a operação mental pela qual um indivíduo retém a idéia de um objeto após sua retirada no tempo e no espaço. [L. *conservatio,* preservação, manutenção]
    c. of energy, c. de energia; o princípio de que a quantidade total de energia, em um sistema fechado, permanece sempre igual, não havendo perda nem geração em qualquer processo químico ou físico ou na conversão de um tipo de energia em outro, dentro do referido sistema.
con·ser·va·tive (kon - ser′vă - tiv). Conservador; designa tratamento por procedimentos graduais, limitados ou bem estabelecidos, em oposição ao radical.
con·serve (kon′serv). Eletuário. SIN confection.
con·sol·i·dant (kon - sol′i - dant). Consolidante; substância que promove cicatrização ou união.
con·sol·i·da·tion (kon - sol - i - dā′shŭn). Consolidação; solidificação em uma massa densa firme; aplicado especialmente ao endurecimento inflamatório de um pulmão normalmente ventilado devido ao exsudato celular nos alvéolos pulmonares, como é observado comumente na pneumonia. [L. *consolido,* tornar espesso, condensar, de *solidus,* sólido]
con·spe·cif·ic (kon - spe - sif′ik). Co-específico; da mesma espécie. [L. *con-,* com, + específico]
con·spi·cu·i·ty (kon - spi - kū′i - tē). Conspicuidade; a visibilidade de uma estrutura de interesse em uma radiografia, uma função do contraste inerente da estrutura e da complexidade (ruído) da imagem adjacente.
con·stan·cy (kon′stan-sē). Constância; a qualidade de ser inalterado. [L. *constantia,* de *consto,* permanecer imóvel]
    color c., c. de cor; percepção inalterada da cor de um objeto apesar de modificações nas condições de iluminação ou observação.
    object c., c. de objeto; **(1)** a tendência de os objetos serem percebidos como inalterados, apesar de variações nas posições e condições nas quais os objetos são observados; p. ex., o formato de um livro é sempre percebido como um retângulo, independentemente do ângulo visual do qual é visto. **(2)** Em psicanálise, o investimento emocional relativamente durável em outra pessoa.
con·stant (kon′stănt). Constante; uma quantidade que, em determinadas condições, não varia com alterações no ambiente.
    association c., c. de associação; **(1)** em imunologia experimental, uma expressão matemática de interação hapteno-anticorpo: c. de associação média, K = [anticorpo ligado ao hapteno]/[anticorpo livre][hapteno livre]; **(2)** (K_a), a c. de equilíbrio envolvida na associação de dois ou mais compostos ou íons em um novo composto; a recíproca da constante de dissociação. SIN binding c.
    Avogadro c., c. de Avogadro. SIN Avogadro *number.*
    binding c., c. de ligação. SIN association c.
    decay c., c. de decaimento; a alteração fracional no número de átomos de um radionuclídeo que ocorre na unidade de tempo; a constante λ na equação para a fração (dN/N) do número de átomos (N) de um radionuclídeo que se desintegra no tempo dt, dN/N = -λdt. SIN disintegration c., radioactive c., transformation c.
    diffusion c., c. de difusão. SIN diffusion *coefficient.*
    disintegration c., c. de desintegração. SIN decay c.
    dissociation c. (K_d, K), c. de dissociação; a constante de equilíbrio envolvida na dissociação de um composto em dois ou mais compostos ou íons. A recíproca da constante de associação; *association c.* (2)

dissociation c. of an acid (K_d, K_a), c. de dissociação de um ácido; expressa pela equação geral $[H^+][A^-]/[HA] = K_a$, onde HA é o ácido não-dissociado.
dissociation c. of a base (K_b), c. de dissociação de uma base; expressa pela equação geral $[B^+][OH^-]/[BOH] = K_b$, onde BOH é a base não-dissociada.
dissociation c. of water, c. de dissociação da água; expressa pela equação $[H^+][OH^-] = K_w = 10^{-14}$ a 25°C.
equilibrium c. (K_{eq}), c. de equilíbrio; na reação $A + B \leftrightarrow C + D$ em equilíbrio (isto é, não há alteração final nas concentrações de A, B, C ou D), as concentrações dos quatro componentes estão relacionadas pela equação $K_{eq} = [C][D]/[A][B]$; K_{eq} é a constante de equilíbrio. Se qualquer componente na reação tiver um multiplicador (p. ex., $H_2 \leftrightarrow 2H$), esse multiplicador aparece como um expoente no cálculo de K (p. ex., $K_{eq} = [H]^2/[H_2]$). Quando essa equação é aplicada à ionização de uma substância em solução, K_{eq} é denominada constante de dissociação (K_d) e seu logaritmo negativo (base 10) é o pK_d. VER TAMBÉM Henderson-Hasselbach *equation*, mass-action *ratio*.
Faraday c. (F), c. de Faraday. VER faraday.
flotation c. (S_f), c. de flutuação; comportamento de sedimentação característico de uma fração lipoproteica de plasma em um campo centrífugo em um meio de densidade apropriada, atingido pela adição de um sal ou D_2O ao plasma. SIN negative S, Svedberg of flotation.
gas c. (R), c. dos gases; $R = 8,314 \times 10^7$ ergs K^{-1} mol^{-1} = 8,314 JK^{-1} mol^{-1}.
Hill c., c. de Hill. SIN Hill *coefficient*.
Michaelis c., c. de Michaelis; (1) a constante de dissociação verdadeira para o complexo binário enzima–substrato em uma reação catalisada por enzima de equilíbrio rápido com substrato único (geralmente simbolizado por K_s); (2) a concentração do substrato na qual é atingida metade da velocidade máxima real de uma reação catalisada por enzima (quando as velocidades são medidas na velocidade inicial e em situação de equilíbrio dinâmico); a razão das constantes de velocidade ($k_2 + k_3$)/k_1 na reação catalisada por enzima com substrato único: $E + S \leftrightarrow ES \leftrightarrow E$ + produtos onde E representa a enzima livre, S é o substrato e ES é o complexo binário central. A expressão para a constante de Michaelis será mais complexa em reações com múltiplos substratos. Uma constante de Michaelis aparente é uma constante determinada em condições que não estão rigorosamente em equilíbrio dinâmico e velocidade inicial ou que varia com a concentração de um ou mais co-substratos. VER Michaelis-Menten *equation*. SIN Michaelis-Menten c.
Michaelis-Menten c. (K_m), c. de Michaelis-Menten. SIN Michaelis c.
Newtonian c. of gravitation (G), c. newtoniana da gravitação; uma constante universal referente à força gravitacional, F, atraindo duas massas, m_1 e m_2, em direção uma à outra quando estão separadas por uma distância, r, na equação: $F = G(m_1 m_2 / r^2)$; tem o valor de $6,67259 \times 10^{-8}$ dina·cm^2·g^{-2} = $6,67259 \times 10^{-11}$·m^2·kg^{-1}·s^{-2} em unidades SI.
permeability c., c. de permeabilidade; uma medida da facilidade com que um íon consegue atravessar uma unidade de área de membrana impulsionado por uma diferença de 1,0 mol/l na concentração; geralmente expresso em centímetros por segundo. Cf. permeability *coefficient*.
Planck c. (h), c. de Planck; um c., $6,6260755 \times 10^{-34}$ J · s ou $6,6260755 \times 10^{-27}$ erg-segundos = $6,6260755 \times 10^{-34}$ J Hz^{-1}.
radioactive c. (Λ), c. radioativo. SIN decay c.
rate c.'s (k), constantes de velocidade; constantes de proporcionalidade iguais à velocidade inicial de uma reação dividida pela concentração do(s) reagente(s); p. ex., na reação $A \to B + C$, a velocidade da reação é igual a $-d[A]/dt = k_1[A]$. A constante de velocidade k_1 é uma constante de velocidade unimolecular, pois há apenas uma espécie molecular reagindo e possui unidades de tempo recíprocas (p. ex., s^{-1}). Para a reação inversa, $B + C \to A$, a velocidade é igual a $-d[B]/dt = d[A]/dt = k_2[B][C]$. A constante de velocidade k_2 é uma constante de velocidade bimolecular e tem unidades de concentração–tempo recíprocas (p. ex., M^{-1} s^{-1}). SIN velocity c.'s.
sedimentation c., c. de sedimentação; a constante s na equação de Svedberg para estimar o peso molecular de uma proteína a partir da velocidade de movimento em um campo centrífugo:

$$M = s \frac{RT}{D(1-\bar{V}_p)}$$

onde M é o peso molecular, R a constante do gás, T a temperatura absoluta, D a constante de difusão (em centímetros quadrados por segundo), $\bar{V}$ o volume específico parcial da proteína e ρ a densidade do solvente. A constante s, com dimensões de tempo por unidade de força do campo ($s = \frac{dr_b/dt}{\omega^2 r_0}$ onde r_b é a posição no momento t, r_0 é a posição no momento 0 e ω é a velocidade angular), geralmente situa-se entre 1×10^{-13} e 200×10^{-13} s. A unidade de Svedberg (S) é arbitrariamente estabelecida em 1×10^{-13} s e freqüentemente é usada para descrever a velocidade de sedimentação de macromoléculas; p. ex., 4S RNA. SIN sedimentation coefficient.
specificity c., c. de especificidade; razão entre a velocidade máxima (V_{max}) ou k_{cat} e o valor real de K_m para um substrato específico em uma reação catalisada por enzima.
time c., c. de tempo; a parte de um circuito que determina o intervalo no qual será calculada a média da velocidade dos eventos elétricos; em fisiologia pulmonar, os fatores que determinam a velocidade do fluxo nas vias aéreas.
transformation c., c. de transformação. SIN decay c.
velocity c.'s (k), constantes de velocidade. SIN rate c.'s.
con·stel·la·tion (kon-stel-ā'shŭn). Constelação; em psiquiatria, todos os fatores que determinam uma dada ação. [L.L. *constellatio*, de *cum*, junto, + *stella*, estrela]
con·sti·pate (kon'sti-pāt). Constipar; causar constipação.
con·sti·pat·ed (kon'sti-pāt-ed). Constipado; que sofre de constipação.
con·sti·pa·tion (kon-sti-pā'shŭn). Constipação; condição na qual os movimentos intestinais são raros ou incompletos. SIN costiveness. [L. *con-stipo*, pp. *-atus*, pressionar junto]
con·sti·tu·tion (kon-sti-too'shŭn). Constituição. **1.** A constituição física de um corpo, incluindo a forma de realização de suas funções, a atividade de seus processos metabólicos, a forma e o grau de suas reações a estímulos, e sua capacidade de resistência ao ataque de organismos patogênicos ou outras doenças. **2.** Em química, o número e o tipo de átomos na molécula e a relação que possuem entre si. [L. *constitutio*, constituição, disposição, de *constituo*, pp. *-stitutus*, estabelecer, de *statuo*, estabelecer]
con·sti·tu·tion·al (kon-sti-too'shŭn-ăl). Constitucional. **1.** Relativo à constituição de um corpo. **2.** Geral; relativo ao sistema como um todo; não local.
con·sti·tu·tive (kon-sti'too-tiv). Constitutivo. **1.** VER constitutive *enzyme*. **2.** Em genética, descritivo de um gene que é controlado por um promotor com atividade constante.
constric'tio [TA]. Constrição. SIN constriction (1).
  c. bronchoaortica esophagea, c. broncoaórtica do esôfago; *termo oficial alternativo para thoracic *constriction* of esophagus.
  c. diaphragmatica esophagea, c. diafragmática do esôfago; *termo oficial alternativo para diaphragmatic *constriction* of esophagus.
  c. partis thoracicae esophagea [TA], c. broncoaórtica do esôfago. SIN thoracic *constriction* of esophagus.
  c. pharyngoesophagealis [TA], c. faringoesofágica. SIN pharyngoesophageal *constriction*.
  c. phrenica esophagea [TA], c. diafragmática do esôfago. SIN diaphragmatic *constriction* of esophagus.
con·stric·tion (kon-strik'shŭn). Constrição. **1.** [TA] Uma porção normal ou anormalmente constrita de uma estrutura. SIN constrictio [TA]. VER TAMBÉM stricture, stenosis. **2.** O ato ou processo de ligar ou estreitar, tornando-se estreitado; a condição de estar constrito, comprimido. **3.** Uma sensação subjetiva de pressão ou tensão, como se o corpo, ou qualquer parte, estivesse firmemente amarrado ou comprimido. [L. *con-stringo*, pp. *-strictus*, contrair]
  broncho-aortic c., c. broncoaórtica; *termo oficial alternativo para thoracic c. of esophagus.
  diaphragmatic c. of esophagus [TA], c. diafragmática do esôfago; estreitamento normal do esôfago, demonstrado radiograficamente após radiografia de tórax com esôfago contrastado. Causada pela passagem de esôfago através do hiato esofágico do diafragma. SIN constrictio phrenica esophagea [TA], constrictio diaphragmatica esophagea*, inferior esophageal c.
  esophageal c.'s, c. esofágicas, três estreitamentos do esôfago, normalmente evidenciados em radiografias (após radiografia de tórax com esôfago contrastado). VER TAMBÉM pharyngoesophageal c., thoracic c. of esophagus, diaphragmatic c. of esophagus. SIN impressions of esophagus.
  inferior esophageal c., c. esofágica inferior; c. diafragmática do esôfago. SIN diaphragmatic c. of esophagus.
  middle esophageal c., c. esofágica média; c. broncoaórtica do esôfago. SIN thoracic c. of esophagus.
  pharyngoesophageal c. [TA], c. faringoesofágica; estreitamento normal do trato alimentar, demonstrado em radiografias de tórax com esôfago contrastado, na junção da faringe com o esôfago (nível vertebral C5) causado pela contração tônica ou ativa da parte cricofaríngea do músculo constritor inferior da faringe (esfíncter esofágico superior). VER TAMBÉM cricopharyngeal *part* of inferior constrictor (muscle) of pharynx. SIN constrictio pharyngoesophagealis [TA], upper esophageal c.
  primary c., constritor primário; o estreitamento entre os dois braços do cromossoma representado pelo centrômero.
  pyloric c., c. pilórico; sulco circular na face externa do intestino, na junção gastroduodenal sobre o esfíncter pilórico, assim demarcando o orifício pilórico.
  secondary c., c. secundário; estreitamento subsidiário do cromossoma associado, em alguns casos, com satélites, p. ex., os braços curtos de autossomas acrocêntricos.
  thoracic c. of esophagus [TA], c. broncoaórtica do esôfago; estreitamento normal do lado esquerdo do esôfago, demonstrado em radiografias de tórax com esôfago contrastado, ao nível vertebral de T4-T5, onde o esôfago é entalhado pelo brônquio-fonte esquerdo e o arco da aorta. SIN constrictio partis thoracicae esophagea [TA], broncho-aortic c.*, constrictio bronchoaortica esophagea*, middle esophageal c.
  upper esophageal c., c. esofágica superior; c. faringoesofágica. SIN pharyngoesophageal c.
  c.'s of ureter, constrições do ureter; estreitamentos fisiológicos normais do ureter observados em uma urografia excretora; o de posição mais alta ocorre

na origem do ureter na pelve renal; um segundo ocorre quando o ureter cruza os vasos ilíacos e a borda pélvica; o mais baixo ocorre quando o ureter penetra na parede vesical.

con·stric·tor (kon-strik′ter, -tōr). Constritor. **1.** Qualquer coisa que prende ou comprime uma parte. VER TAMBÉM inferior constrictor (*muscle*) of pharynx, middle constrictor (*muscle*) of pharynx, superior pharyngeal constrictor (*muscle*). **2.** Um músculo cuja ação é estreitar um canal; um esfíncter. [L. de *constringo*, contrair]

con·struct (kon′strukt). A combinação de um enxerto ósseo, instrumentação de metal, próteses e/ou cimento ósseo aplicada em um nível específico da coluna vertebral numa situação de instabilidade vertebral segmentar.

con·sul·tand (kon-sŭl′tand). Consulente, uma pessoa a respeito da qual o consultor genético fará previsões no tocante aos futuros filhos; não confundir com probando. [consult (pedir conselho) + L. *-andus*, sufixo gerundivo]

dummy c., c. simulado, uma pessoa na linha da descendência (desde o ancestral principal até o próprio consulente); para simplificar o problema, o c. simulado é analisado como se fosse o próprio consulente.

con·sul·tant (kon-sŭl′tant). Consultor. **1.** Médico ou cirurgião que não assume total responsabilidade por um paciente, mas atua como conselheiro, deliberando e aconselhando o médico ou cirurgião assistente. **2.** Membro da equipe hospitalar que não está de plantão, mas permanece de sobreaviso, a pedido do médico ou cirurgião responsável. [L. *consulto*, pp. *-atus*, deliberar, pedir conselho]

con·sul·ta·tion (kon-sŭl-tā′shŭn). Junta médica; encontro de dois ou mais médicos ou cirurgiões para avaliar a natureza e o progresso da doença em um determinado paciente e estabelecer o diagnóstico, prognóstico e/ou tratamento.

con·sump·tion (kon-sŭmp′shŭn). **1.** Consumo; o uso de alguma coisa, principalmente a velocidade em que é usada. **2.** Consunção; termo obsoleto para o desgaste dos tecidos do corpo, geralmente tuberculoso. [L. *con-sumo*, pp. *-sumptus*, consumir completamente, usar]

oxygen c. ($\dot{V}_{O_2}$), c. de oxigênio; **(1)** (Q_O ou Q_{O_2}); a velocidade com que o oxigênio é usado por um tecido; unidades: microlitros de oxigênio nas CNTP (condições normais de temperatura e pressão) usados por miligrama de tecido por hora; **(2)** ($\dot{V}_{O_2}$) (a velocidade com que o oxigênio do gás alveolar entra no sangue, igual, no estado de equilíbrio dinâmico, ao consumo de oxigênio pelo metabolismo tecidual em todo o corpo; unidades: mililitros de oxigênio CNTP usados por minuto ou mmol/min.

con·sump·tive (kon-sŭmp′tiv). Consumido; relativo a, ou que sofre de, consunção.

con·tact (kon′takt). Contato. **1.** O toque ou aposição de dois corpos. **2.** Uma pessoa que foi exposta a uma doença contagiosa. [L. *con- tingo*, pp. *-tactus*, tocar, pegar, de *tango*, tocar]

balancing c., c. de balanceio; **(1)** os contatos entre as dentaduras superior e inferior, no lado de balanceio ou mediotrusivo, para estabilizar as dentaduras; **(2)** os contatos entre as dentaduras superior e inferior, no lado oposto ao lado de trabalho ou laterotrusivo (ântero-posterior ou lateralmente), para fins de estabilizar as dentaduras; **(3)** os contatos entre dentes naturais ou artificiais superiores e inferiores no lado oposto ao lado de trabalho ou laterotrusivo. SIN balancing occlusal surface.

centric c., c. cêntrico. SIN centric occlusion.

deflective occlusal c., c. oclusal defletor; uma condição dos contatos dentários que desvia a mandíbula de um trajeto normal de fechamento para uma relação mandibular cêntrica. SIN cuspal interference, interceptive occlusal c., premature c.

initial c., c. inicial; **(1)** o primeiro encontro dos dentes opostos na elevação da mandíbula em direção ao maxilar; **(2)** o contato oclusal inicial de dentes opostos quando a mandíbula está fechada.

interceptive occlusal c., c. oclusal interceptivo. SIN deflective occlusal c.

premature c., c. prematuro. SIN deflective occlusal c.

proximal c., proximate c., c. proximal; a área onde as superfícies de dois dentes adjacentes no mesmo arco se tocam.

c. with reality, c. com a realidade; interpretação correta de fenômenos externos em relação às normas do meio social ou cultural.

working c.'s, contatos de trabalho; trabalho ou oclusão; contatos de dentes no lado da oclusão na direção em que a mandíbula se moveu. SIN working bite, working occlusion.

con·tac·tant (kon-tak′tănt). Contactante; qualquer um dentre um grupo heterogêneo de alérgenos que provocam manifestações de hipersensibilidade tardia por contato direto com a pele ou mucosa.

con·ta·gion (kon-tā′jŭn). Contágio. **1.** SIN contagium. **2.** Transmissão de infecção por contato direto, disseminação de gotículas ou objetos contaminados. O termo surgiu muito antes do desenvolvimento de idéias modernas de doença infecciosa e, desde então, perdeu muito de sua importância, sendo incluído sob o termo mais amplo de "doença transmissível". **3.** Produção, através de sugestão ou imitação, de uma neurose ou psicose em alguns membros de um grupo ou mais. [L. *contagio*; de *contingo*, tocar intimamente]

psychic c., c. psíquico; transmissão de um distúrbio nervoso ou psicológico menor por imitação, como na histeria de massas.

con·ta·gious (kon-tā′jŭs). Contagioso; relativo a contágio; infeccioso ou transmissível por contato com o doente ou suas secreções ou excreções frescas.

con·ta·gious·ness (kon-tā′jŭs-nes). Contagiosidade; a qualidade de ser contagioso.

con·ta·gium (kon-tā′jē-ŭm). O agente de uma doença infecciosa. SIN contagion (1). [L. um contato]

con·tain·ment. Confinamento, contenção; o conceito de erradicação regional ou global de doença transmissível, proposto por Fred Lowe Soper (1893–1977), em 1949, para a erradicação da varíola.

con·tam·i·nant (kon-tam′i-nant). Contaminante; uma impureza; qualquer material de natureza estranha associado a uma substância química, um princípio fisiológico ou um agente infeccioso.

con·tam·i·nate (kon-tam′i-nāt). Contaminar; causar ou resultar em contaminação. [L. *con-tamino*, misturar, corromper]

con·tam·i·na·tion (kon-tam-i-nā′shŭn). Contaminação. **1.** A presença de um agente infeccioso em uma superfície corporal; também sobre ou dentro de roupas, roupa de cama, brinquedos, instrumentos cirúrgicos ou curativos, ou outros objetos inanimados ou substâncias incluindo água, leite e alimento ou aquele próprio agente infeccioso. **2.** Em epidemiologia, a situação que existe quando uma população estudada para uma condição ou fator também possui outras condições ou fatores que modificam os resultados do estudo. **3.** Termo freudiano para uma fusão e condensação de significados de palavras, perceptos ou motivações para comportamento. **4.** A presença de material estranho que adultera ou torna impuro um material cuja composição é degradada. [L. *contamino*, pp. *-atus*, manchar, sujar]

con·tent (kon′tent). Conteúdo. **1.** Aquilo que está contido em algo, geralmente nesse sentido é usado no plural, *contents*. **2.** Em psicologia, a forma de um sonho, como é apresentado para a consciência. **3.** Uso ambíguo para concentração (3); p. ex., conteúdo sanguíneo de hemoglobina poderia significar tanto sua concentração quanto o produto de sua concentração pelo volume sanguíneo. [L. *contentus*, de *con- tineo*, pp. *-tentus*, manter junto, conter]

carbon dioxide c., c. de dióxido de carbono; o dióxido de carbono total disponível no soro ou plasma após a adição de ácido; determinado rotineiramente em laboratórios hospitalares como um componente dos perfis eletrolíticos.

GC c., c. GC; a quantidade de guanina e citosina em um ácido polinucleico, geralmente expressa em fração mol (ou percentagem) do total de bases; a temperatura de fusão desses biopolímeros varia com o c. GC.

latent c., c. latente; o significado oculto, inconsciente, de pensamentos ou ações, principalmente em sonhos ou fantasias.

manifest c., c. manifesto; aqueles elementos da fantasia e dos sonhos conscientemente disponíveis e relatados.

con·tig. Mapa físico de um cromossoma. VER contig *map*.

con·ti·gu·i·ty (kon-ti-gū′i-tē). Contigüidade. **1.** Contato sem continuidade real, p. ex., o contato dos ossos que formam uma sutura craniana. Cf. continuity. **2.** Ocorrência de dois ou mais objetos, eventos ou impressões mentais juntos no espaço (**c. espacial**) ou no tempo (**c. temporal**). [L. *contiguus*, contato, de *contingo*, tocar]

con·tig·u·ous (kon-tig′oo-ŭs). Contíguo; adjacente ou em contato real.

con·ti·nence (kon′ti-nens). Continência. **1.** A capacidade de reter urina e/ou fezes até o momento apropriado para sua eliminação. **2.** Moderação, temperança ou autocontrole em relação ao apetite, principalmente para o ato sexual. [L. *continentia*, de *con- tineo*, reter]

con·ti·nent (kon′ti-nent). Continente; que designa continência.

con·tin·ued (kon-tin′ūd). Contínuo; sem interrupção; diz-se particularmente de febre prolongada sem intervalos apiréticos, como febre tifóide, em comparação com os paroxismos de febre na malária. [L. *continuo*, unir, tornar contínuo]

con·ti·nu·i·ty (kon-ti-nu′i-tē). Continuidade; ausência de interrupção, uma sucessão de partes intimamente unidas, p. ex., a conjunção ininterrupta de células e estruturas que formam um osso único do crânio. Cf. contiguity. [L. *continuus*, contínuo]

con·tour (kon′toor). Contorno. **1.** O esboço de uma parte; a configuração superficial. **2.** Em odontologia, restaurar os contornos normais de um dente quebrado ou deformado, ou criar o formato ou configuração externa de uma prótese. [L. *con-* (intens.), + *torno*, virar (em um torno mecânico), de *tornus*, torno mecânico]

flange c., c. da borda; o desenho da borda de uma dentadura.

gingival c., c. gengival; o formato ou configuração da gengiva, seja natural ou artificial, ao redor dos colos dos dentes. SIN gum c.

gum c., c. gengival. SIN gingival c.

height of c., altura do contorno. VER *height* of contour.

△ **contra-.** Contra; oposto. VER TAMBÉM counter-. Cf. anti-. [L.]

con·tra·an·gle (kon′tră-ang′gl). Contra-ângulo. **1.** Um dos ângulos duplos ou triplos na haste de um instrumento por meio do qual a borda cortante ou ponta é levada até o eixo do cabo. **2.** Uma peça de extensão adicionada à extremidade de uma caneta dentária que, através de uma série de engrenagens, modifica o ângulo do eixo de rotação da broca em relação ao eixo da caneta.

con·tra·ap·er·ture (kon′tră-ap′er-choor). Contra-abertura. SIN counteropening.

con·tra·bev·el (kon′tră-bev′el). Bisel contrário; bisel localizado no lado oposto ao habitual.

con·tra·cep·tion (kon-tră-sep′shŭn). Contracepção; prevenção da concepção ou gravidez.

  emergency hormonal c., c. hormonal de emergência. SIN morning after *pill.* SIN postcoital c.

  postcoital c., c. pós-coital. SIN emergency hormonal c.

con·tra·cep·tive (kon-tră-sep′tiv). Contraceptivo. **1.** Agente para a prevenção da concepção. **2.** Relativo a qualquer medida ou agente designado para evitar a concepção. [L. *contra*, contra, + *conceptive*]

  barrier c., c. de barreira; dispositivo mecânico elaborado para evitar a penetração dos espermatozóides no óstio cervical; geralmente usado em combinação com um espermicida, isto é, diafragma vaginal.

  combination oral c., c. oral de associação; mistura de um esteróide com atividade progestacional e um estrogênio.

  intrauterine c. device, dispositivo contraceptivo intra-uterino. VER intrauterine contraceptive *devices*, em *device*.

  oral c., c. oral; preparação eficaz por via oral destinada a evitar a concepção.

con·tract. 1 (kon-trakt′). Contrair; encurtar; diminuir de tamanho; no caso do músculo, encurtar ou sofrer um aumento na tensão. **2** (kon-trakt′). Contrair; adquirir por contágio ou infecção. **3** (kon′trakt). Contrato; compromisso bilateral explícito entre o psicoterapeuta e o paciente para um curso definido de ação a fim de atingir o objetivo da psicoterapia. [L. *con-traho*, pp. –*tractus*, contrair]

con·trac·tile (kon-trak′til). Contrátil; que tem a propriedade de contrair.

con·trac·til·i·ty (kon-trak-til′i-tē). Contratilidade; a capacidade ou propriedade de uma substância, principalmente do músculo, de encurtar-se, tornar-se de tamanho reduzido ou desenvolver maior tensão.

  cardiac c., c. cardíaca; uma medida do desempenho da bomba cardíaca, o grau de encurtamento das fibras musculares quando ativadas por um estímulo independente de pré-carga e pós-carga.

con·trac·tion (C) (kon-trak′shŭn). Contração. **1.** Encurtamento ou aumento da tensão; designa a função normal do músculo. **2.** Retração ou redução do tamanho. **3.** Batimento cardíaco, como na contração prematura. Ver também entradas em beat. [L. *contractus*, contrair]

  after-c., pós-c.; VER aftercontraction.

  anodal closure c. (ACC, AnCC), c. de fechamento anódico; termo obsoleto para designar a contração momentânea de um músculo sob a influência do pólo positivo quando é estabelecido o circuito elétrico.

  anodal opening c. (AnOC, AOC), c. de abertura anódica; termo obsoleto para designar a contração momentânea de um músculo sob a influência do pólo positivo quando o circuito é aberto.

  automatic c., c. automática. SIN automatic *beat*.

  Braxton Hicks c., c. de Braxton Hicks; atividade miometrial rítmica que ocorre durante uma gravidez e que, geralmente, não é dolorosa.

  cathodal closure c. (CaCC, CCC), c. de fechamento catódico; termo obsoleto para designar a contração momentânea de um músculo sob a influência do pólo negativo quando é estabelecido um circuito elétrico.

  cathodal opening c. (CaOC, COC), c. de abertura catódica; termo obsoleto para designar a contração momentânea de um músculo sob a influência do pólo negativo quando o circuito é aberto.

  closing c., c. de fechamento; contração produzida no momento do fechamento do circuito quando se usa corrente contínua para estimular o músculo.

  escape c., batimento de escape. SIN escape *beat*.

  escape ventricular c., batimento ventricular de escape; um batimento de escape originado no ventrículo.

  fibrillary c.'s, contrações fibrilares; contrações que ocorrem espontaneamente em fibras musculares individuais; são observadas, comumente, alguns dias após lesão dos nervos motores que suprem o músculo, e esse tipo de atividade é distinguido da fasciculação, que está relacionada à ativação de unidades motoras.

  front-tap c., contração dos músculos da panturrilha quando se bate na superfície anterior da perna. SIN Gowers c.

  Gowers c., c. de Gowers. SIN front-tap c.

  hourglass c., c. em ampulheta; constrição da porção média de um órgão oco, como o estômago ou o útero grávido.

  hunger c.'s, contrações de fome; contrações fortes do estômago associadas a dores de fome.

  idiomuscular c., c. idiomuscular. SIN myoedema.

  isometric c., c. isométrica; desenvolvimento de força com comprimento constante da fibra muscular. Cf. isotonic c.

  isotonic c., c. isotônica; encurtamento com desenvolvimento de força constante. Cf. isometric c. SIN isotonic exercise.

  myotatic c., c. miotática; contração reflexa de um músculo esquelético que ocorre em virtude da estimulação dos receptores de estiramento do músculo, isto é, como parte de um reflexo miotático.

  opening c., c. de abertura; contração produzida no momento de abertura do circuito quando se usa corrente contínua para estimular o músculo ou o nervo motor.

  paradoxical c., c. paradoxal; uma contração tônica dos músculos tibiais anteriores quando se faz uma flexão dorsal passiva súbita do pé.

  postural c., c. postural; manutenção da tensão muscular (geralmente isométrica) suficiente para manter a postura.

  premature c., batimento prematuro. VER extrasystole.

  reflex detrusor c., c. reflexa do detrusor; função coordenada normal da bexiga com contrações mantidas da bexiga acompanhadas por relaxamento simultâneo dos mecanismos de saída esfincterianos para esvaziar a bexiga.

  tetanic c., c. tetânica. VER tetanus (2).

  tonic c., c. tônica; contração mantida de um músculo, empregada na manutenção da postura.

  uterine c., c. uterina; atividade rítmica do miométrio associada à menstruação, gravidez ou trabalho de parto.

con·trac·ture (kon-trak′choor). Contratura; encurtamento muscular estático devido a espasmo tônico ou fibrose, perda do equilíbrio muscular, estando os antagonistas paralisados, ou perda de movimento da articulação adjacente. [L. *contractura*, de *contraho*, contrair]

  Dupuytren c., c. de Dupuytren; uma doença da fáscia palmar que resulta em espessamento e encurtamento das faixas fibrosas na superfície palmar da mão e dedos, resultando em uma deformidade em flexão característica do quarto e quinto dedos.

  fixed c., c. fixa. SIN organic c.

  functional c., c. funcional; encurtamento muscular que cessa durante o sono ou anestesia geral, causada por contração muscular ativa prolongada.

  ischemic c. of the left ventricle, c. isquêmica do ventrículo esquerdo; contração irreversível do ventrículo esquerdo do coração, observada como complicação no período inicial da derivação cardiopulmonar e agora evitada por soluções cardioplégicas apropriadas. SIN myocardial rigor mortis, stone heart.

  organic c., c. orgânica; contratura geralmente devida a fibrose muscular e que persiste estando o indivíduo consciente ou inconsciente. SIN fixed c.

  Volkmann c., c. de Volkmann; contratura isquêmica resultante da necrose irreversível do tecido muscular, produzida por uma síndrome de compartimento; classicamente envolve os músculos flexores do antebraço.

con·tra·fis·su·ra (kon′tră-fi-shoor′ă). Contrafissura; fratura de um osso, como no crânio, em um ponto oposto ao local do traumatismo. [L. *contra*, contra, contrário, + *fissura*, fissura]

con·tra·in·di·cant (kon-tră-in′di-kant). Contra-indicante; que indica o contrário, isto é, que mostra que um método de tratamento que seria apropriado não é aconselhável por circunstâncias especiais de um determinado caso.

con·tra·in·di·ca·tion (kon-tră-in-di-kā′shŭn). Contra-indicação; qualquer sintoma ou circunstância especial que desaconselha o uso de um remédio ou a realização de um procedimento, geralmente devido ao risco.

con·tra·lat·er·al (kon-tră-lat′er-ăl). Contralateral; relativo ao lado oposto, como quando há dor ou paralisia do lado oposto ao da lesão. SIN heterolateral. [L. *contra*, oposto, + *latus*, lado]

  c. partner, parceiro contralateral; a estrutura correspondente do lado oposto.

con·trast (kon′trast). Contraste. **1.** Uma comparação na qual as diferenças são demonstradas ou realçadas. **2.** Em radiologia, a diferença entre as densidades de imagem de duas áreas é o contraste entre elas; esta é uma função do número de fótons de raios X transmitidos ou a intensidade dos sinais emitidos pelas duas regiões e a resposta do meio de registro. [L. *contra*, contra, + *sto*, pp. *status*, mostrar]

  simultaneous c., c. simultâneo; o realce da sensação visual de branco quando um objeto branco é colocado adjacente a um objeto preto; o objeto preto também parece mais preto em virtude da contigüidade do branco. As cores complementares adjacentes também parecem mais brilhantes; p. ex., o verde, assim como o vermelho, parece mais brilhante se essas duas cores são colocadas lado a lado.

  successive c., c. sucessivo; o efeito visual causado pela observação de um objeto colorido brilhante e, depois, uma superfície cinzenta; esta última parece tingida pela cor complementar do objeto. A observação de uma superfície da cor complementar do objeto, em vez de cinza, aumenta a intensidade da cor da superfície.

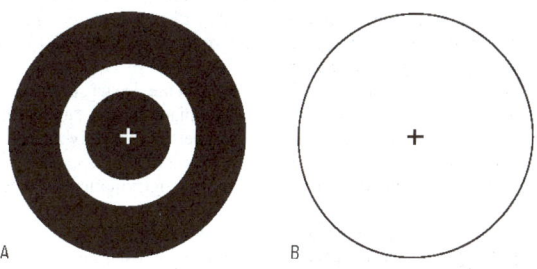

contraste sucessivo: observe a cruz branca em (A) por cerca de 30 segundos e, a seguir, olhe para a cruz preta em (B); a imagem de (A) que reaparece no campo branco de (B) é um contraste sucessivo

con·tre·coup (kawn-tr-koo′). Contragolpe; designa a forma de uma contrafissura, como no crânio, em um ponto oposto ao local do traumatismo. VER TAMBÉM contrecoup *injury* of brain. [Fr. contragolpe]

cont·rem. Abreviatura do L. *continuenter remedia*, continuar os medicamentos.

con·trol (kon-trōl′). **1.** Controlar; (v.), regular, conter, corrigir, restabelecer a normalidade. **2.** (s.) Controle; operações ou programas contínuos com o objetivo de reduzir uma doença. **3.** (s.) Membros de um grupo de comparação que diferem dos indivíduos de um estudo na experiência da doença ou alocação para um regime. **4.** (v.) Em estatística, ajustar ou levar em consideração influências estranhas. [L. Mediev. *contrarotulum*, um controle para verificar contribuições, do L. *rotula*, dim. de *rota*, roda]

autogenous c., controle autógeno; regulamentação pela ação de um produto genético no gene que codifica esse produto.

automatic gain c. (AGC), controle de ganho automático; característica de alguns aparelhos auditivos que reduz a amplificação em níveis de grande intensidade de entrada.

aversive c., controle aversivo; controle do comportamento de outro indivíduo pelo uso de meios psicologicamente nocivos; p. ex., tentar forçar melhores hábitos de estudo mediante suspensão da mesada de uma criança, ou negar o contato sexual se o parceiro não aceitar uma condição.

biologic c., controle biológico; controle de organismos vivos, incluindo vetores e reservatórios de doença, pelo uso de seus inimigos naturais (predadores, parasitas, competidores).

birth c., c. de natalidade; (**1**) restrição do número de filhos por meio de medidas contraceptivas; (**2**) projetos, programas ou métodos para controlar a reprodução, seja por aumento ou diminuição da fertilidade.

idiodynamic c., controle ioiodinâmico; impulsos nervosos do bulbo que preservam a condição trófica normal dos músculos.

negative c., controle negativo; regulamentação de uma atividade enzimática por um inibidor da enzima ou regulamentação de uma proteína por repressão da transcrição.

own c.'s, controles próprios; método de controle experimental no qual os mesmos indivíduos são usados em condições experimentais e de controle.

positive c., controle positivo; regulamentação de uma atividade enzimática por um ativador da enzima considerada. Também, regulamentação através da indução da biossíntese de uma proteína específica ou ativação do processamento de uma proteína.

quality c., controle de qualidade; o controle de erro analítico laboratorial por monitorização do desempenho analítico com soros de controle e manutenção do erro dentro de limites estabelecidos em torno dos valores de controle médios, mais comumente ± 2 DP (desvios-padrão).

reflex c., controle reflexo; impulsos nervosos transmitidos aos músculos para manter ação reflexa normal.

social c., controle social; a influência sobre o comportamento de uma pessoa exercida por outras pessoas ou pela sociedade como um todo; p. ex., através de padrões sociais apropriados, ostracismo ou leis criminais.

stimulus c., controle de estímulo; o uso de técnicas de condicionamento para colocar o comportamento-alvo de um indivíduo sob controle ambiental. VER classical *conditioning*.

synergic c., controle sinérgico; impulsos transmitidos do cerebelo que regulam a atividade muscular das unidades sinérgicas do corpo.

time-varied gain c. (TGC), compensação de ganho temporal. SIN time-gain compensation.

tonic c., controle tônico; impulsos nervosos que mantêm um tônus ou nível normal de atividade no músculo ou em outros órgãos efetores.

vestibulo-equilibratory c., c. vestibuloequilibrador; impulsos nervosos transmitidos dos canais semicirculares, sáculo e utrículo que servem para manter o equilíbrio do corpo.

Con·trol of Com·mun·i·ca·ble Dis·eases Manual **(CCDM).** Manual de Controle de Doenças Transmissíveis; o manual especializado, reconhecido internacionalmente, que está na 17.ª edição (2000), publicado pela American Public Health Association (Associação Americana de Saúde Pública).

con·tu·sion (kon-too′shŭn). Contusão; qualquer lesão mecânica (geralmente causada por um golpe) resultando em hemorragia sob a pele não-rompida. VER TAMBÉM bruise. [L. *contusio*, contusão]

brain c., c. cerebral; contusão do cérebro, geralmente de sua superfície, com extravasamento de sangue, mas sem ruptura da pia-aracnóide; a cicatrização resulta em uma área esclerótica deprimida superficial, possivelmente com incorporação das meninges. VER TAMBÉM brain *cicatrix*.

scalp c., c. do couro cabeludo; extravasamento de sangue intracutâneo ou subcutâneo sem ruptura macroscópica da pele.

con·u·lar (kon′u-lăr). Cônico; em forma de cone.

Co·nus (kō′nŭs). Gênero de moluscos que habitam as costas de algumas ilhas do Sul do Pacífico. Várias espécies, *C. geographus*, *C. textilis*, *C. aulicus*, *C. tulipa* e *C. marmoreus*, são venenosas, com sua picada ou espinho causando dor aguda, edema, parestesia, paralisia disseminada e, algumas vezes, coma e morte.

co·nus, pl. **co·ni** (kō′nŭs, -nī). Cone. **1** [TA]. SIN cone. **2.** Estafiloma posterior na coroidopatia miópica. [L. do G. *kōnos*, cone]

c. arterio'sus [TA], c. arterial; a porção esquerda ou ântero-superior, de paredes lisas, da cavidade do ventrículo direito do coração, que começa na crista supraventricular e termina no tronco pulmonar. SIN arterial cone, infundibulum (4), pulmonary cone, pulmonary c.

congenital c., c. congênito. SIN Fuchs *coloboma*.

distraction c., c. de tração; área cônica na qual o nervo óptico atravessa o canal da esclera em direção significativamente oblíqua.

c. elas'ticus [TA], c. elástico; porção mais espessa da membrana elástica da laringe, que se estende entre a cartilagem cricóide e os ligamentos vocais, sendo estes últimos realmente um espessamento da margem superior livre do cone elástico. SIN cricovocal membrane*, elastic cone.

co'ni epididym'idis, lóbulos do epidídimo; *termo oficial alternativo para lobules of epididymis, em lobule.

c. medulla'ris [TA], c. medular; a extremidade inferior afilada da medula espinal. SIN medullary cone [TA].

myopic c., c. miópico. SIN myopic *crescent*.

pulmonary c., c. pulmonar. SIN c. arteriosus.

supertraction c., c. de supertração; um cone ou anel amarelo-avermelhado na margem nasal do disco óptico, produzido por deslocamento do epitélio pigmentar da retina e da lâmina vítrea da coróide; ocorre na miopia avançada.

co'ni vasculo'si, cones vasculares. SIN lobules of epididymis, em lobule.

con·va·les·cence (kon-vă-les′ens). Convalescença; período entre o fim de uma doença e o restabelecimento do paciente até a saúde completa. [L. *convalesco*, fortalecer, de *valeo*, ser forte]

con·va·les·cent (kon-vă-les′ent). Convalescente. **1.** Em recuperação ou indivíduo que está se recuperando. **2.** Designa o período de convalescença.

con·val·lar·ia (kon-va-lār′-ē-ă). Convalária; flor, rizoma e raízes da *Convallaria majalis* (família Liliaceae), lírio-do-vale; eles contêm glicosídeos com ação semelhante à da digitálica (p. ex., convalatoxina). [L. *convallis*, vale fechado]

con·vec·tion (kon-vek′shŭn). Convecção; transmissão de calor em líquidos ou bases por movimento das partículas aquecidas, ou quando a camada de água no fundo de um recipiente aquecido sobe ou o ar quente em um cômodo ascende até o teto. [L. *con-veho*, pp. *–vectus*, transportar ou colocar junto]

con·ver·gence (kon-ver′jens). Convergência. **1.** A tendência de dois ou mais objetos para um ponto comum. **2.** A direção das linhas visuais para um ponto próximo. [L. *con'vergere*, inclinar junto]

accommodative c., c. acomodativa; o ângulo de convergência expresso em dioptrias; igual ao produto dos ângulos da convergência multiplicado pela distância interpupilar medida em centímetros.

amplitude of c., amplitude de c.; a distância entre o ponto próximo e o ponto remoto de convergência. SIN range of c.

angle of c., ângulo de c.; o ângulo que o eixo visual faz com a linha mediana quando se olha um objeto próximo.

far point of c., ponto remoto de c.; o ponto para o qual se dirigem as linhas visuais quando a convergência está em repouso.

near point of c., ponto próximo de c.; o ponto para o qual se dirigem as linhas visuais quando a convergência é máxima.

negative c., c. negativa; a pequena divergência dos eixos visuais quando a convergência está em repouso, como ao se observar o ponto distante ou durante o sono.

positive c., c. positiva; desvio interno dos eixos visuais mesmo quando a convergência está em repouso, como em casos de estrabismo convergente.

range of c., amplitude de c. SIN amplitude of c.

unit of c., unidade de c. VER meter *angle*.

con·ver·gent (kon-ver′jent). Convergente; que tende para um ponto comum.

con·ver·sion (kon-ver′zhŭn). Conversão. **1.** SIN transmutation. **2.** Um mecanismo de defesa inconsciente pelo qual a ansiedade gerada por um conflito inconsciente é convertida e expressa simbolicamente como um sintoma físico; transformação de uma emoção em uma manifestação física, como na histeria de conversão. VER conversion *hysteria*. **3.** Em virologia, a aquisição pelas bactérias de uma nova propriedade associada à presença de um profago. VER TAMBÉM lysogeny. [L. *con-verto*, pp. *–versus*, virar ao contrário, alterar]

con·ver·tase (kon′ver-tās). Convertase; proteases do complemento que convertem um componente em outro. VER *component* of complement.

con·ver·tin (kon-ver′tin). Convertina; forma ativa de fator VII designada VIIa.

con·vex (kon′veks, kōn-veks′). Convexo; aplicado a uma superfície que é uniformemente curvada para fora, o segmento de uma esfera. [L. *convexus*, abaulado, arqueado, convexo, de *con-veho*, juntar]

high c., c. alto; o segmento de uma esfera de raio curto.

low c., c. baixo; o segmento de uma esfera de raio longo.

con·vex·i·ty (kon-veks′i-tē). Convexidade. **1.** O estado de ser convexo. **2.** Uma estrutura convexa.

cortical c., c. cortical. SIN superolateral *surface* of cerebrum.

con·vex·o·ba·sia (kon-vek-sō-bā′sē-ă). Convexobasia; curvatura anterior do osso occipital. [L. *convexus*, curvo para fora, + *basis*, fundação]

con·vex·o·con·cave (kon-vek′sō-kon′kav). Convexo-côncavo; convexo em uma superfície e côncavo na superfície oposta.

con·vex·o·con·vex (kon-vek′sō-kon′veks). Convexo-convexo. SIN biconvex.

con·vo·lute (kon′vō-loot). Convoluto; enrolado junto, com uma parte sobre a outra; no formato de um rolo ou pergaminho. [L. con-volvo, pp. –volutus, rolar junto]

con·vo·lut·ed (kon′vō-loo-ted). Convoluto. SIN convolute.

con·vo·lu·tion (kon′vō-loo′shŭn). Convolução. **1.** Espiralamento ou enrolamento de um órgão. **2.** Especificamente, um giro do córtex cerebral ou cerebelar. [L. convolutio]

  angular c., c. angular. SIN angular gyrus.
  anterior c., giro pré-central. SIN precentral gyrus.
  ascending frontal c., c. pré-central. SIN precentral gyrus.
  ascending parietal c., c. parietal ascendente. SIN postcentral gyrus.
  callosal c., giro do cíngulo. SIN cingulate gyrus.
  cingulate c., c. do cíngulo. SIN cingulate gyrus.
  first temporal c., giro temporal superior. SIN superior temporal gyrus.
  hippocampal c., giro para-hipocampal. SIN parahippocampal gyrus.
  inferior frontal c., giro frontal inferior. SIN inferior frontal gyrus.
  inferior temporal c., giro temporal inferior. SIN inferior temporal gyrus.
  middle frontal c., giro frontal médio. SIN middle frontal gyrus.
  middle temporal c., giro temporal médio. SIN middle temporal gyrus.
  posterior central c., giro pós-central. SIN postcentral gyrus.
  second temporal c., giro temporal médio. SIN middle temporal gyrus.
  superior frontal c., giro frontal superior. SIN superior frontal gyrus.
  superior temporal c., giro temporal superior. SIN superior temporal gyrus.
  supramarginal c., giro supramarginal. SIN supramarginal gyrus.
  third temporal c., giro temporal inferior. SIN inferior temporal gyrus.
  transitional c., c. transicional. SIN transitional gyrus.
  transverse temporal c.'s, giros temporais transversos. SIN transverse temporal gyri, em gyrus.
  Zuckerkandl c., c. de Zuckerkandl. SIN subcallosal gyrus

con·vul·sant ((kon-vŭl′sant). Convulsivante; uma substância que causa convulsões. VER TAMBÉM eclamptogenic, epileptogenic.

con·vul·sion (kon-vŭl′shŭn). Convulsão. **1.** Espasmo violento ou série de contrações da face, tronco ou membros. **2.** SIN seizure (2). [L. convulsio, de convello, pp. –vulsus, rasgar]

  benign neonatal c.'s, convulsões neonatais benignas; epilepsia familiar, autolimitada, que começa com 2, 3 ou 6 dias de idade e melhora espontaneamente aos seis meses; herança autossômica dominante.
  clonic c., c. clônica; convulsão na qual as contrações são intermitentes, com os músculos contraindo-se e relaxando alternadamente.
  complex febrile c., c. febril complexa; uma convulsão febril prolongada (mais de 15 minutos de duração) ou associada a déficits neurológicos focais.
  febrile c., c. febril; convulsão breve, com menos de 15 minutos de duração, observada em um lactente ou uma criança pequena neurologicamente normal, associada a febre. SIN febrile seizure.
  hysterical c., hysteroid c., c. histérica, c. histeróide. VER hysteria.
  immediate posttraumatic c., c. pós-traumática imediata; uma convulsão que começa logo após um traumatismo.
  infantile c., c. do lactente; qualquer convulsão que ocorra na lactância (0-2 anos de idade).
  salaam c.'s, espasmos em salame; espasmos do lactente. SIN infantile spasm.
  tetanic c., c. tetânica. SIN tonic c.
  tonic c., c. tônica; uma convulsão na qual a contração muscular é mantida.

con·vul·sive (kon-vŭl′siv). Convulsivo; relativo a convulsões; caracterizado por, ou que causa, convulsões.

Cooke, A. Bennett, médico norte-americano, *1869. VER C. speculum.

Cooley, Denton, cirurgião cardiotorácico norte-americano, *1920, famoso por inventar muitos instrumentos cirúrgicos.

Cooley, Thomas B., pediatra norte-americano, 1871–1945. VER C. anemia.

Coolidge, William D., físico norte-americano, 1873–1975. VER C. tube.

Coomassie bril·liant blue R-250 [C.I. 42660]. Azul brilhante de Coomassie R-250; corante proteico geral usado em eletroforese devido à sua sensibilidade incomum. [originalmente, um nome comercial da Imperial Chemical; Coomassie (Kumasi), Gana]

Coombs, Carey F., médico inglês, 1879–1932. VER Carey C. murmur; C. murmur.

Coombs, Robin R.A., veterinário e imunologista inglês; *1921. VER Gell e C. reactions, em reaction; C. serum, test; direct C. test; indirect C. test.

Cooper, Sir Astley Paston, anatomista e cirurgião inglês, 1768–1841. VER C. fascia, hernia, herniotome, ligaments, em ligament; suspensory ligaments of C., em ligament.

co·op·er·a·tiv·i·ty. Cooperatividade; uma propriedade de determinadas proteínas (freqüentemente enzimas) nas quais as curvas de ligação ou curvas de saturação (ou, no caso de enzimas, uma representação de velocidades iniciais como uma função da concentração inicial de substrato, são não-hiperbólicas; sugere que a ligação de um ligante tem uma afinidade diferente em diferentes concentrações de ligantes. Tanto a alosteria quanto a histerese são modelos que exibirão cooperatividade. Cf. allosterism, hysteresis.

  negative c., c. negativa; cooperatividade na qual moléculas de ligante sucessivas parecem ligar-se com afinidade decrescente.
  positive c., c. positiva; cooperatividade na qual moléculas de ligante sucessivas parecem ligar-se com afinidade crescente.

Coo·pe·ria (koo-pē′rē-ă). Gênero de nematódeos delgados e pequenos (família Trichostrongylidae) que habitam o intestino delgado, raramente o abomaso (quarta câmara do estômago) de ruminantes; quando frescos, possuem cor rosa brilhante; só produzem efeitos graves quando presentes em grande número. Em animais parcialmente imunes, esses vermes são encerrados em nódulos na parede do intestino; são menos patogênicos em ovinos e caprinos que os tricostrôngilos Haemonchus, Ostertagia e Trichostrongylus.

  C. biso'nis, espécie encontrada em bovinos, ovinos, bisões e antílopes.
  C. curti'cei, espécie encontrada em ovinos, caprinos e veados silvestres na Europa, embora tenha distribuição cosmopolita.
  C. fiel'dingi, SIN C. punctata.
  C. oncoph'ora, espécie encontrada em bovinos e em ovinos domésticos e selvagens, mas raramente em cavalos; embora tenha distribuição mundial, é mais comum no norte dos Estados Unidos e no Canadá. SIN Strongylus radiatus, Strongylus ventricosus.
  C. pectina'ta, espécie encontrada em bovinos, ovinos, búfalo, dromedários e vários ruminantes selvagens; é comum no sul dos Estados Unidos.
  C. puncta'ta, espécie encontrada principalmente em bovinos, menos comumente em ovinos, búfalos e vários ruminantes selvagens; embora tenha distribuição mundial, é particularmente disseminada na América do Norte e comum no Havaí. SIN C. fieldingi.
  C. spatula'ta, espécie encontrada em bovinos e ovinos no sul dos Estados Unidos, Quênia, Austrália e Malásia.

co·or·di·nate. **1** (kō-ōr′di-nit). Coordenada; qualquer das escalas ou magnitudes que servem para definir a posição de um ponto. **2** (kō-ōr′di-nāt). Coordenar; realizar o ato de coordenação. [ver coordination]

co·or·di·na·tion (kō-ōr′di-nā′shun). Coordenação; o trabalho conjunto harmonioso, principalmente de vários músculos ou grupos musculares na execução de movimentos complicados. [L. co-, junto, + ordino, pp. –atus, arranjar, de ordo (ordin-), arranjo, ordem]

co·os·si·fi·ca·tion (kō-os′i-fi-kā′shŭn). Co-ossificação; estado de ser unido por formação óssea.

co·os·si·fy (kō-os′i-fī). Co-ossificar; unir em um osso. [L. co-, junto, + os, osso, + facio, fazer]

co·pai·ba (kō-pī′bă). Copaíba; a resina oleosa da Copaifera officinalis e outras espécies de Copaifera (família Leguminosae), uma planta sul-americana; o óleo de copaíba é usado como expectorante, diurético e estimulante. SIN balsam of copaiba. [Esp.]

COPD Abreviatura de chronic obstructive pulmonary disease (doença pulmonar obstrutiva crônica, DPOC).

Cope, Sir Vincent Z., cirurgião inglês, 1881–1974. VER C. clamp.

cope (kōp). **1.** Abóbada; cúpula; manto. A metade superior de um molde na arte da fundição; portanto, aplicável à porção superior ou cavidade de um molde para dentadura. **2.** Agüentar; enfrentar; ato que permite a uma pessoa ajustar-se às circunstâncias ambientais.

co·pe·pod (kō′pē-pod). Copépode; qualquer membro da ordem Copepoda.

Co·pep·o·da (kō-pep′ō-dă). Ordem de crustáceos de água marinha e fluvial, de vida livre, abundantes, de importância básica na cadeia alimentar aquática, tanto em ambientes marinhos quanto fluviais; algumas espécies são comumente denominadas pulgas-d'água. Alguns são ectoparasitas de vertebrados aquáticos de sangue frio e sangue quente; amiúde, os copépodes parasitas de peixes e baleias são muito modificados para penetração profunda na pele ou para aderência por ventosas e ganchos (p. ex., o piolho-dos-peixes, Argulus). Alguns copépodes (Cyclops, Dipatomus) são importantes como hospedeiros intermediários da tênia Diphyllobothrium latum e do nematódeo Dracunculus medinensis. [G. kōpē, remo, + pous (pod-), pé]

cop·ing (kōp′ing). **1.** Cobertura; revestimento ou capa metálica fina. **2.** Enfrentamento; método adaptativo ou bem-sucedido de lidar com situações individuais ou ambientais que envolvem estresse ou ameaça psicológica ou fisiológica.

  transfer c., cúpula de transferência; em odontologia, cobertura ou cúpula metálica, de resina acrílica ou outro material, usada para posicionar um molde em uma impressão.

co·pol·y·mer (kō′pol-i-mer). Copolímero; polímero no qual são combinados dois ou mais monômeros ou unidades básicas.

  c.-1, c.-1; sal acetato de uma mistura de polipeptídeos sintéticos compostos de quatro aminoácidos; usado para reduzir a taxa de recidiva da esclerose múltipla recidivante-remissiva.

cop·per (Cu) (kop′er). Cobre; elemento metálico, de n.° atômico 29, peso atômico 63,546; vários de seus sais são usados em medicina. Um bioelemento encontrado em várias proteínas. [L. cuprum, orig. Cyprium, de Cyprus, onde foi extraído]

c. arsenite, arsenito de c. SIN cupric arsenite.
c. bichloride, bicloreto de c. SIN cupric chloride.
c. chloride, cloreto de c. SIN cupric chloride.
c. citrate, citrato de c. SIN cupric citrate.
c. dichloride, bicloreto ou dicloreto de c. SIN cupric chloride.
c. sulfate, c. sulphate, sulfato de c. SIN cupric sulfate.
cop·per-64 (^{64}Cu). Cobre-64 (Cu^{64}); emissor de raios beta e positrons, com uma meia-vida de 12,82 h. Usado no estudo da doença de Wilson e em cintigrafias cerebrais para tumores.
cop·per-67 (^{67}Cu). Cobre-67 (Cu^{67}); emissor de raios beta e gama com uma meia-vida de 2,580 dias.
cop·per·as (kop′er - as). Vitríolo verde; melanterita; a forma comercial impura do sulfato ferroso.
cop·per·head (kop′er - hed). Trigonocéfalo; cobra venenosa do gênero *Agkistrodon* nos Estados Unidos.
cop·per pen·nies. Corpúsculos escleróticos. SIN sclerotic bodies, em body.
Coppet, Louis de, físico francês, 1841–1911. VER C. law.
co·pre·cip·i·ta·tion (kō - prē - sip - tā′shŭn). Co-precipitação; precipitação de antígeno não-ligado (livre) juntamente com um complexo antígeno-anticorpo; pode ocorrer particularmente quando um complexo solúvel é precipitado por um segundo anticorpo específico para o fragmento Fc da imunoglobulina do complexo.
cop·rem·e·sis (kop - rem′e - sis). Coprêmese. SIN fecal vomiting. [G. *kopros*, esterco, + *emesis*]
copro-. Sujeira, esterco, geralmente usado com referência a fezes. VER TAMBÉM scato-, sterco-. [G. *kopros*, esterco]
cop·ro·an·ti·bod·ies (kop′rō - an′ti - bod′ēz). Coproanticorpos; anticorpos encontrados no intestino e nas fezes; provavelmente são formados por plasmócitos na mucosa intestinal e consistem, principalmente, na classe IgA.
cop·ro·la·lia (kop - rō - lā′lē - ă). Coprolalia; utilização involuntária de palavras vulgares ou obscenas; observada na síndrome de Gilles de la Tourette. SIN coprophrasia. [copro- + G. *lalia*, falar]
cop·ro·lith (kop′rō - lith). Coprólito; fecalito. SIN fecalith. [copro- + G. *lithos*, cálculo]
co·prol·o·gy (kop - rol′ō - jē). Coprologia. SIN scatology (1). [copro- + G. *logos*, estudo]
cop·ro·ma (kop - rō′mă). Coproma. SIN fecaloma. [copro- + G. *-ōma*, tumor]
cop·ro·pha·gia (kop′rō - fā′jyă). Coprofagia; a ingestão de excremento. SIN coprophagy, scatophagy.
co·proph·a·gous (kō - prof′ă - gŭs). Coprófago; que se alimenta de excrementos.
co·proph·a·gy (kŏ - prof′ă - jē). Coprofagia. SIN coprophagia. [copro- + G. *phagō*, comer]
cop·ro·phil, cop·ro·phil·ic (kop′rō - fil, - fil′ik). Coprófilo; coprofílico. 1. Designa microrganismos presentes nas fezes. 2. Relativo à coprofilia. [ver coprophilia]
cop·ro·phile (kop′rō - fīl). Coprófilo; organismo que ingere as fezes de outros organismos.
cop·ro·phil·ia (kop - rō - fil′ē - ă). Coprofilia. 1. Atração de microrganismos por material fecal. 2. Em psiquiatria, uma atração mórbida por, e interesse em (com um elemento sexual), fezes. SIN mysophilia. [copro- + G. *philos*, predileção]
cop·ro·pho·bia (kop - rō - fō′bē - ă). Coprofobia; medo mórbido da defecação e das fezes. [copro- + G. *phobos*, medo]
cop·ro·phra·sia (kop - rō - frā′zē - ă). Coprofrasia. SIN coprolalia.
cop·ro·plan·e·sia (kop - rō - plan - ē′zē - ă). Coproplanesia; termo raramente usado para eliminação de fezes através de uma fístula ou ânus artificial. [copro- + G. *planēsis*,, viajante]
cop·ro·por·phyr·ia (kop′rō - pōr - fir′ē - ă). Coproporfiria; presença de coproporfirinas na urina, como na porfiria variegada.
hereditary c., c. hereditária; condição hereditária (autossômica dominante) de deficiência da coproporfirinogênio oxidase, resultando em superprodução de precursores da porfirina, levando a distúrbios neurológicos e fotossensibilidade.
cop·ro·por·phy·rin (kop - rō - pōr′fi - rin). Coproporfirina; um dos dois compostos porfirina encontrados normalmente nas fezes como produto da decomposição da bilirrubina (portanto, da hemoglobina); determinadas coproporfirinas estão elevadas em algumas porfirias. VER TAMBÉM porphyrinogens.
cop·ro·por·phy·rin·o·gen (kop′rō - pōr - fi - rin′ō - jen). Coproporfirinogênio. VER porphyrinogens.
c. oxidase, c. oxidase; enzima que catalisa uma etapa na biossíntese da porfirina, reagindo com o coproporfirinogênio III e O_2 para formar protoporfirinogênio IX e $2CO_2$. A deficiência dessa enzima resultará em coproporfiria hereditária.
cop·ro·stane (kop - ros′tān). Coprostano; o hidrocarboneto original do coprosterol.
3β·co·pros·ta·nol (kop - ros′tan - ol). 3β-coprostanol. SIN coprosterol.
epi-**co·pros·ta·nol.** *epi*-coprostanol; 5β-colestan-3α-ol; quanto à estrutura do colestano, ver steroids. SIN *epi*-coprosterol.

cop·ros·tan·one (kop - ros′tan - ōn). Coprostanona; 5β-colestan-3-ona, produto da oxidação do coprosterol.
cop·ro·sta·sis (kop - rō - stā′sis). Coprostase; termo raramente usado para impacção fecal. [copro- + G. *stasis*, estase]
cop·ros·ten·ol (kop - ros′ten - ol). Coprostenol. SIN allocholesterol.
co·pros·ter·ol (kop - ros′ter - ol). Coprosterol; 5β-colestan-3β-ol; o principal esterol das fezes produzido pela redução do colesterol por bactérias intestinais. Quanto à estrutura do coprostano e do colestano, ver steroids. SIN 3β-coprostanol, stercorin.
epi-**co·pros·ter·ol.** *epi*-coprosterol. SIN *epi*-coprostanol.
cop·ro·stig·mas·tane (kop - rō - stig - mas′tān). Coproestigmastano; o isômero 5β do estigmastano.
cop·ro·zoa (kop - rō - zō′ă). Coprozoário; protozoário que pode ser cultivado no material fecal, embora não viva necessariamente nas fezes no intestino. [copro- + G. *zōon*, animal]
cop·ro·zo·ic (kop - rō - zō′ik). Coprozóico; relativo a coprozoário.
cop·to·sis (kop - tō′sis). Coptose; estado de fadiga perpétua. [G. *kopto*, cansar, + *osis*, condição]
cop·u·la (kop′ū - la). 1. Em anatomia, uma parte estreita que une duas estruturas, p. ex., o corpo do osso hióide. 2. Tumefação formada durante o desenvolvimento inicial da língua pela porção medial do segundo arco branquial; é muito grande na eminência hipobranquial e não está presente na língua do adulto. 3. Termo obsoleto para zigoto. [L. ligação, elo]
His c., eminência de His. SIN hypobranchial *eminence*.
c. lin′guae, eminência lingual. SIN hypobranchial *eminence*.
cop·u·la·tion (kop - ū - lā′shŭn). Copulação; cópula. 1. SIN coitus. 2. Em protozoologia, a conjugação entre duas células que não se fundem, mas se separam após fertilização mútua; observada nos ciliófors, como em *Paramecium*. [L. *copulatio*, união]
copulines. Copulinas; substâncias que ocorrem nas secreções vaginais; homens que foram expostos a copulinas consideraram as mulheres mais atraentes, principalmente aquelas mulheres consideradas menos atraentes por controles testados com água. As copulinas de mulheres que ovulam (mas que não estão no período menstrual ou pré-menstrual) causaram um aumento da testosterona salivar nos homens.
CoQ Abreviatura de coenzima Q.
co·quille (kō - kēl′). Lentilha; lente esférica curva de espessura uniforme. [Fr.]
cor, gen. **cor·dis** (kōr, kor′dis) [TA]. Coração. SIN heart. [L.]
c. adipo′sum, c. adiposo. SIN fatty *heart* (2).
c. bilocula′re, c. bilocular; coração na qual os septos interatrial e interventricular estão ausentes ou incompletos.
c. bovi′num (kōrbō′vi - nŭm), c. de boi. SIN ox *heart*.
c. mo′bile, c. móvel; coração que se move indevidamente com as mudanças de posição corporal; associado a grandes defeitos ou ausência (congênita ou cirúrgica) do pericárdio. SIN movable heart.
c. pen′dulum, c. em pêndulo; uma forma extrema de coração móvel na qual o coração parece estar suspenso pelos grandes vasos. SIN pendulous heart.
c. pulmona′le, *cor pulmonale*; o *cor pulmonale* crônico é caracterizado por hipertrofia do ventrículo direito resultante de doença dos pulmões, exceto alterações pulmonares em doenças que afetam basicamente o lado esquerdo do coração e a artéria pulmonar, e excluindo-se cardiopatia congênita; o *cor pulmonale* agudo é caracterizado por dilatação e insuficiência do lado direito do coração devido a embolia pulmonar. Nos dois tipos ocorrem alterações características no eletrocardiograma, e, nos estágios mais avançados, geralmente há insuficiência cardíaca direita.
c. triatria′tum, c. triatriado; um coração com três câmaras atriais, sendo o átrio esquerdo subdividido por um septo transverso com uma única abertura pequena que separa as aberturas das veias pulmonares da valva mitral. SIN accessory atrium.
c. trilocula′re, c. trilocular; coração de três câmaras devido à ausência do septo interatrial ou interventricular.
c. trilocula′re biatria′tum, c. trilocular biatriado; ausência do septo interventricular.
c. trilocula′re biventricula′re, c. trilocular biventricular; ausência do septo interventricular.
cor·a·cid·i·um (kō - ră - sid′ē - ŭm). Coracídio; a primeira fase ciliada do embrião aquático do pseudófilo e outros cestódeos com ciclos aquáticos; dentro do embrióforo ciliado, há uma larva recurvada, o hexacanto, que se transforma no hospedeiro intermediário, geralmente um crustáceo aquático, no próximo estágio larvar, o procercóide.
cor·a·co·a·cro·mi·al (kōr′ă - kō - ă - krō′mē - ăl). Coracoacromial; relativo aos processos coracóide e acromial. SIN acromiocoracoid.
cor·a·co·bra·chi·a·lis (kōr′ă - kō - brā - kē - ā′lis). Coracobraquial; relativo ao processo coracóide da escápula e ao braço. VER TAMBÉM coracobrachialis *muscle*, coracobrachial *bursa*.
cor·a·co·cla·vic·u·lar (kōr′ă - kō - kla - vik′ū - lăr). Coracoclavicular; relativo ao processo coracóide e à clavícula. SIN scapuloclavicular (2).
cor·a·co·hu·mer·al (kōr′ă - kō - hū′mer′ăl). Coracoumeral; relativo ao processo coracóide e ao úmero.

cor·a·coid (kōr'ă - koyd) . Coracóide; de forma semelhante ao bico de corvo; designa um processo da escápula. [G. *korakōdes*, como o bico de corvo, de *korax*, rapina, + *eidos*, semelhança]

cor·al·lin (kōr'ă - lin) . Coralina. SIN aurin.
  yellow c., c. amarela; um sal sódico da aurina.

cord (kōrd) [TA]. **1.** Cordão; corda; em anatomia, qualquer estrutura longa semelhante a uma corda. Uma estrutura pequena, semelhante a uma corda, composta de algumas ou muitas fibras longitudinais, vasos, ductos ou combinações destes. VER TAMBÉM chorda. **2.** Em histopatologia, uma linhagem de células tumorais com apenas uma célula de largura. SIN fasciculus (2) [TA], funiculus [TA], funicle. [L. *chorda*, corda]

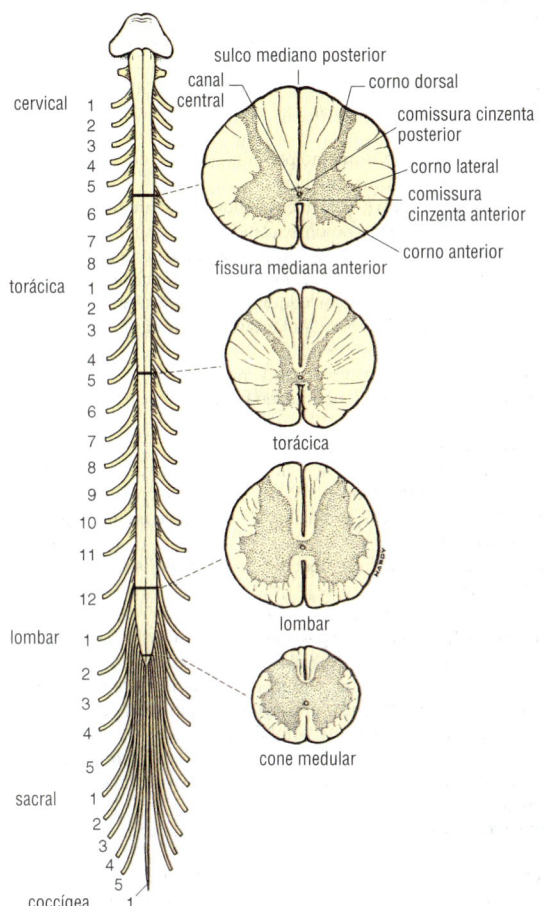

medula espinal: incluindo imagens em corte transversal mostrando variações regionais na substância cinzenta

Bergmann c.'s, cordões de Bergmann, estrias medulares do quarto ventrículo. SIN medullary *striae* of fourth ventricle, em *stria*.
Billroth c.'s, cordões de Billroth. SIN splenic c.'s.
condyle c., c. condilar. SIN condylar *axis*.
dental c., c. dentário; agregado de células epiteliais que formam o órgão rudimentar de esmalte.
false tendinous c.'s, cordas tendíneas falsas; *termo oficial alternativo para false *chordae* tendineae, em *chorda*.
false vocal c., corda vocal falsa; prega vestibular. SIN vestibular *fold*.
Ferrein c.'s, cordas de Ferrein. SIN vocal *fold*. VER vocal *fold*.
gangliated c., tronco simpático. SIN sympathetic *trunk*.
genital c., cordão genital; uma de um par de cristas mesenquimatosas que se projetam para a parte caudal do celoma de um embrião jovem e que contêm os ductos mesonéfrico e paramesonéfrico.
germinal c.'s, cordões germinativos; os cordões gonadais do ovário ou testículo embrionário. sin sex c.'s.
gonadal c.'s, cordões gonadais; colunas de células germinativas e foliculares que penetram centripetamente no córtex ovariano ou testicular embrionário.
gubernacular c., cordão gubernacular; o conteúdo do canal gubernacular, geralmente composto de remanescentes da lâmina dental e do tecido conjuntivo.
hepatic c.'s, cordões hepáticos; lâminas hepáticas observadas em cortes.
lateral c. of brachial plexus [TA], fascículo lateral do plexo braquial; no plexo braquial, o feixe de fibras nervosas, formadas pelas divisões anteriores dos troncos superior e médio, situado lateral à artéria axilar. Esse fascículo dá origem ao nervo peitoral lateral e termina dividindo-se no nervo musculocutâneo e na raiz lateral do nervo mediano. SIN fasciculus lateralis plexus brachialis [TA].
lymph c.'s, cordões linfáticos. SIN medullary c.'s (1).
medial c. of brachial plexus [TA], fascículo medial do plexo braquial; no plexo braquial, o feixe de fibras nervosas, formado pela divisão anterior do tronco inferior, situado medial à artéria axilar; dá origem ao nervo peitoral medial, aos nervos cutâneo medial do braço e cutâneo medial do antebraço, e termina dividindo-se na raiz medial do nervo mediano e nervo ulnar. SIN fasciculus medialis plexus brachialis [TA].
medullary c.'s, cordões medulares; **(1)** cordões do tecido linfóide denso entre os seios na medula de um linfonodo. SIN lymph c.'s. **(2)** rete c.'s.
nephrogenic c., cordão nefrogênico; um trato longitudinal dorsolateral de mesoderma intermédio; o primórdio dos túbulos mesonéfricos e metanéfricos.
nuchal c., cordão nucal; alça(s) de cordão umbilical ao redor do pescoço fetal, causando risco de hipoxia intra-uterina, sofrimento fetal ou morte.
oblique c. of interosseous membrane of forearm [TA], corda oblíqua da membrana interóssea do antebraço; uma faixa delgada que se estende da parte lateral do processo coronóide da ulna, distal e lateralmente ao rádio, imediatamente distal à tuberosidade bicipital. SIN chorda obliqua membranae interosseae antebrachii [TA], oblique ligament of elbow joint, round ligament of elbow joint, Weitbrecht c., Weitbrecht ligament.
omphalomesenteric c., cordão onfalomesentérico. SIN vitelline c.
posterior c. of brachial plexus [TA], fascículo posterior do plexo braquial; no plexo braquial, o feixe de fibras nervosas formado pelas divisões posteriores dos troncos superior, médio e inferior, situado posterior à artéria axilar; dá origem aos nervos subescapulares superior e inferior e toracodorsal, termina dividindo-se nos nervos axilar e radial. SIN fasciculus posterior plexus brachialis [TA].
psalterial c., estria vascular do ducto coclear. SIN *stria* vascularis of cochlear duct.
red pulp c.'s, cordões da polpa vermelha. SIN splenic c.'s.
rete c.'s, cordões de células primordiais (cordões medulares e cordões sexuais) nas gônadas embrionárias que se unem a alguns dos túbulos mesonéfricos e a partir dos quais se desenvolvem a rede testicular do homem e a rede ovariana da mulher. SIN medullary c.'s (2).
sex c.'s, cordões sexuais. SIN germinal c.'s.
spermatic c. [TA], cordão espermático; o cordão formado pelo ducto deferente e suas estruturas associadas que se estendem do anel inguinal profundo até o escroto, atravessando o canal inguinal. VER TAMBÉM *coverings* of spermatic cord, em *covering*. SIN funiculus spermaticus [TA], chorda spermatica, testicular c.
spinal c. [TA], medula espinal; a porção cilíndrica alongada do eixo cerebroespinal, ou sistema nervoso central, que está contida no canal espinal ou vertebral. SIN medulla spinalis [TA], chorda spinalis, spinal marrow.
splenic c.'s, cordões esplênicos; o tecido encontrado entre os seios venosos na polpa vermelha do baço. SIN Billroth c.'s, red pulp c.'s.
tendinous c.'s, cordas tendíneas; *termo oficial alternativo para chordae tendineae of heart, em *chorda*.
testicular c., cordões testiculares. SIN spermatic c.
testis c.'s, cordões testiculares; os cordões germinativos do testículo embrionário.
true vocal c., corda vocal verdadeira; prega vocal. SIN vocal *fold*.
c. of tympanum, corda do tímpano. SIN *chorda* tympani.
umbilical c., cordão umbilical; o pedículo de união definitivo entre o embrião ou feto e a placenta; ao nascimento, é composto basicamente de geléia de Wharton na qual estão incrustados os vasos umbilicais. SIN chorda umbilicalis, funiculus umbilicalis, funis (1).
c. of umbilical artery [TA], corda da artéria umbilical; a artéria umbilical obliterada que persiste como um cordão fibroso que segue para cima, ao longo da bexiga, até o umbigo. SIN chorda arteriae umbilicalis [TA], ligamentum umbilicale mediale, medial umbilical ligament.
vitelline c., cordão vitelino; um pedículo vitelino persistente na forma de um cordão sólido de tecido unindo o íleo ao umbigo. SIN omphalomesenteric c.
vocal c., corda vocal; prega vocal. SIN vocal *fold*.
Weitbrecht c., corda de Weitbrecht. SIN oblique c. of interosseous membrane of forearm.
Wilde c.'s, cordas de Wilde; impressões transversais no corpo caloso.
Willis c.'s, cordas de Willis; vários cordões fibrosos que cruzam o seio sagital superior. SIN chordae willisii.

cord-. VER chord-.
cor·date (kōr'dāt). Cordiforme; em forma de coração.
cor·dec·to·my (kor - dek'tō - mē). Cordectomia; excisão parcial ou total de uma corda vocal. [G. *chordē*, corda, + *ektomē*, excisão]
cor·dial (kōr'jŭl). Cordial; bebida aromática doce. [L. Mediev. *cordialis*, de *cor* (*cord*-), coração]
cor·di·a·nine (kor - dī'ă - nēn).Cordianina. SIN allantoin.

cor·di·form (kōr′di-fōrm). Cordiforme; em forma de coração. [L. *cor* (*cord*-), coração, + *forma*, forma]

cor·dis (kōr′dis). Cordial; do coração. [gen. de L. *cor*, coração]

diastasis c. (dī-as′tă-sis), diástase cardíaca; qualquer período de inatividade mecânica do coração, e particularmente dos ventrículos, que, em geral, surge normalmente durante freqüências cardíacas lentas quando os ventrículos completam seu enchimento precocemente e parecem estar inativos.

cor·do·cen·te·sis (cor-dō-cen-tē′sis). Cordocentese; coleta de amostra de sangue transabdominal do cordão umbilical fetal, realizada sob orientação ultra-sonográfica. SIN funipuncture. [cord + G. *kentēsis*, punção]

cor·don san·i·taire (kor-don′ san-i-tayr′). Barreira sanitária; a barreira erguida ao redor de um foco de infecção. [Fr., barreira sanitária]

cor·do·pexy (kōr′dō-pek-sē). Cordopexia. **1.** Fixação cirúrgica de qualquer cordão anatômico deslocado. **2.** Fixação lateral de uma ou ambas as cordas vocais para corrigir estenose glótica. [G. *chordē*, corda, + *pēxis*, fixação]

cor·dot·o·my (kōr-dot′ō-mē). Cordotomia. **1.** Qualquer operação na medula espinal. **2.** Divisão de tratos da medula espinal, que pode ser realizada por via percutânea (cordotomia estereotática) ou após laminectomia (cordotomia aberta) por várias técnicas, como incisão ou coagulação por radiofreqüência. **3.** Incisão através da porção membranosa da prega vocal para alargar a glote posterior na paralisia vocal bilateral. [G. *chordē*, corda, + *tomē*, corte]

anterolateral c., c. ântero-lateral; divisão do quadrante ântero-lateral da medula espinal para seccionar o trato espinotalâmico. SIN anterolateral tractotomy, spinal tractotomy, spinothalamic c.

open c., c. aberta. VER cordotomy (2).

posterior column c., c. da coluna posterior; divisão da coluna posterior da medula espinal.

spinothalamic c., c. espinotalâmica. SIN anterolateral c.

stereotactic c., c. estereotática. VER cordotomy (2).

Cor·dy·lo·bia (kōr-di-lō′bē-ă). Gênero de moscas varejeiras califorídeas. [G. *kordilē*, bordão, tumefação ou tumor]

C. anthropoph′aga, mosca tumbu da África, ao sul do Saara; uma espécie que causa uma miíase furuncular bolhosa; são acometidos muitos animais além do homem, principalmente cães domésticos, embora os ratos provavelmente sejam o principal reservatório da infestação humana.

cor·dy·lo·bi·a·sis (kōr′di-lō-bī′ă-sis). Cordilobíase; infestação de homens e animais por larvas de moscas do gênero *Cordylobia*. SIN African furuncular myiasis, tumbu dermal myiasis.

core (kōr). Núcleo; cerne; centro. **1.** A massa central de tecido necrótico em um furúnculo. **2.** Uma peça de metal, geralmente com um suporte no canal da raiz de um dente, projetada para reter uma coroa artificial. **3.** Um registro seccional, geralmente de gesso ou de um de seus derivados, das relações de partes, como os dentes, restaurações metálicas ou jaquetas. [L. *cor*, coração]

atomic c., núcleo atômico; o núcleo mais os elétrons sem valência.

central transactional c., o sistema de ativação reticular do cérebro.

△ **core-, coreo-, coro-.** A pupila (do olho). [G. *korē*, pupila]

co-receptor. Co-receptor; uma proteína da superfície celular que aumenta a sensibilidade do receptor do antígeno ao antígeno por ligação a outros ligantes.

B cell co-receptor, co-receptor da célula B; um complexo de três proteínas associadas ao receptor da célula B (CR2, CD19 e TAPA-1).

cor·ec·to·pia (kōr-ek-tō′pē-ă). Corectopia; localização excêntrica da pupila de forma que esta não esteja no centro da íris. [G. *korē*, pupila, + *ektopos*, deslocamento]

co·rel·y·sis (kō-rē-lī′sis). Corélise; termo raramente usado para liberação de aderências entre a cápsula do cristalino e a íris. [G. *korē*, pupila, + *lysis*, afrouxamento]

co·re·mi·um (kō-rē′mē-ŭm). Corêmio; aglomerado de conidióforos em forma de feixe. [G. *korēma*, sujeira, refugo]

△ **coreo-.** VER core-.

cor·e·o·plas·ty (kōr′ē-ō-plas-tē). Coreoplastia; o procedimento para corrigir uma pupila deformada, miótica ou ocluída. [G. *korē*, pupila, + *plassō*, formar]

cor·e·pexy (kōr′ē-pek-sē). Corepexia; sutura da íris para modificar o formato ou o tamanho da pupila.

purse-string c., c. em bolsa; sutura ao longo da margem pupilar e amarrada para diminuir uma pupila grande.

cor·e·praxy (kōr′ē-prak′sē). Corepraxia; procedimento para alargar uma pupila pequena. [G. *korē*, pupila, + *praxis*, ação]

laser c., c. com laser; o estroma da íris é aquecido com laser e a contratura do tecido da íris produzida aumenta a pupila.

mechanical c., c. mecânica; procedimento que aloja a margem pupilar no sulco de um dispositivo que, quando alargado, distende a borda pupilar para aumentar a pupila.

co·re·pres·sor (kō-rē-pres′or). Co-repressor; uma molécula, geralmente um produto de uma via metabólica específica, que se combina com um repressor produzido por um gene regulador e o ativa. O repressor ativado então se fixa a um gene operador e inibe a atividade dos genes estruturais. O mecanismo homeostático regula negativamente a produção de enzimas em sistemas enzimáticos repressíveis.

Corey, R. B., químico norte-americano, 1897–1971. VER Pauling-C. *helix*.

Cori, Carl F., bioquímico e prêmio Nobel tcheco-norte-americano, 1896–1984. VER C. *cycle, ester*.

Cori, Gerty Theresa, bioquímica e prêmio Nobel tcheca-norte-americana, 1896–1957. VER C. *disease*.

co·ria (kō′rē-ă). Plural de corium.

co·ri·an·der (kō-rē-an′der). Coriandro; o fruto maduro seco do *Coriandrum sativum* (família Umbelliferae); estimulante aromático leve e agente aromatizante.

co·ri·um, pl. **co·ria** (kō′rē-ŭm, -rē-ă). Córion; derme; *termo oficial alternativo para dermis. [L. pele, couro]

corn (kōrn). Calo. SIN clavus (1). [L. *cornu*, corno, casco]

asbestos c., calo do asbesto; uma lesão cutânea granulomatosa ou hiperceratótica no local de deposição de partículas de asbesto. SIN asbestos wart.

hard c., calo duro; a forma habitual de calo sobre uma articulação dos artelhos.

soft c., calo mole; calor formado por pressão entre dois artelhos, sendo a superfície macerada e de cor amarelada.

cor·nea (kōr′nē-ă). [TA]. Córnea; o tecido transparente que forma o sexto anterior da parede externa do olho, com um raio de 7,7 mm de curvatura em contraste com os 13,5 mm da esclera; consiste em epitélio escamoso estratificado contínuo com o epitélio da conjuntiva, substância própria, colágeno com arranjo bastante regular incrustado em mucopolissacarídeo, e uma camada interna de endotélio. É a principal estrutura refratária do olho. [L. fem. de *corneus*, córneo]

conical c., c. cônica; ceratocone. SIN keratoconus.

c. farina′ta, c. esfarinhada; pontilhado bilateral da parte posterior do estroma da córnea. SIN floury c.

floury c., c. esfarinhada. SIN c. farinata.

c. plana, c. plana; distúrbio congênito no qual a curvatura do arco da córnea é mais plana do que o normal, deixando o olho hiperópico.

c. uri′ca, c. úrica; deposição bilateral cristalina de uréia e urato de sódio no estroma da córnea.

c. verticilla′ta, c. verticilada; opacificações congênitas espirais na córnea. SIN Fleischer vortex.

cor·ne·al (kōr′nē-ăl). Corneano; relativo à córnea.

cor·ne·o·bleph·a·ron (kōr′nē-ō-blef′ă-ron). Corneobléfaro; aderência da margem palpebral à córnea. [cornea + G. *blepharon*, pálpebra]

cor·ne·o·cyte (kōr′nē-ō-sīt). Corneócito; a célula escamosa morta, cheia de queratina do estrato córneo. SIN horny cell, keratinized cell. [*cornea*, L. fem. de *corneus*, córneo, + G. *kytos*, célula]

cor·ne·o·scle·ra (kōr′nē-ō-sklēr′ă). Corneoesclera; a córnea e a esclera combinadas, quando consideradas como formando o revestimento externo do globo ocular.

cor·ne·o·scler·al (kōr′nē-ō-skēr′ăl). Corneoescleral; relativo à córnea e à esclera.

Corner, Edred M., cirurgião inglês, 1873–1950. VER C. *tampon*.

Corner, George W., anatomista norte-americano, 1889–1981. VER C.-Allen *test, unit*.

cor·ne·um (kōr′nē-ŭm). Córneo. VER *stratum* corneum epidermidis, *stratum* corneum unguis. [L., neutro de *corneus*, córneo, de *cornu*, corno]

cor·nic·u·late (kōr-nik′ū-lāt). Corniculado. **1.** Semelhante a um corno. **2.** Cornífero; que possui cornos ou apêndices em forma de corno. [L. *corniculatus*, que tem cornos]

cor·nic·u·lum (kōr-nik′ū-lŭm). Cornículo; pequeno corno. [L. dim. de *cornu*, corno]

c. laryn′gis, c. laríngeo. SIN corniculate cartilage.

cor·ni·fi·ca·tion (kōr-ni-fi-kā′shŭn). Cornificação. SIN keratinization. [L. *cornu*, corno, + *facio*, fazer]

cor·ni·fied (kōr′ni-fīd). Cornificado. SIN keratinized.

corn oil. Óleo de milho; óleo fixo refinado expresso do embrião da *Zea mays* (família Gramineae); um solvente. SIN maise oil.

corn·silk (kōrn′silk). Barba de milho. SIN zea.

corn smut (kōrn′smŭt). Fungo do milho. SIN *Ustilago maydis*.

cor·nu, gen. **cor·nus,** pl. **cor·nua** (kōr′noo, -nŭs, -noo-ă). Corno. **1.** [TA]. SIN horn. **2.** Qualquer estrutura composta de substância córnea. **3.** Uma das extensões coronais da polpa dental subjacente a uma cúspide ou lobo. **4.** As principais subdivisões do ventrículo lateral no hemisfério cerebral (corno frontal, corno occipital e corno temporal). VER TAMBÉM lateral *ventricle*. **5.** As principais divisões das colunas cinzentas da medula espinal (corno anterior, corno lateral, corno posterior). [L. corno]

c. ammo′nis, c. de Ammon. SIN Ammon *horn*.

c. ante′rius [TA], c. anterior. SIN anterior *horn*.

coccygeal c., c. coccígeo; dois processos que se projetam do dorso da base do cóccix para cima para se articularem com o corno sacral. SIN c. coccygeum [TA], coccygeal horn, cornua coccygealia.

cornua coccygea'lia, c. coccígeo. SIN coccygeal c.
c. coccygeum [TA], c. coccígeo. SIN coccygeal c.
c. cuta'neum, c. cutâneo. SIN cutaneous horn.
cornua of falciform margin of saphenous opening, corno da margem falciforme da abertura safena; pilar da margem falciforme do hiato safeno. VER inferior *horn* of falciform margin of saphenous opening, superior *horn* of falciform margin of saphenous opening.
c. frontale ventriculi lateralis [TA], c. frontal do ventrículo lateral. SIN cornua of lateral ventricle.
cornua of hyoid bone, c. do osso hióide. VER greater *horn* of hyoid bone, lesser *horn* of hyoid.
c. infe'rius [TA], c. inferior. SIN inferior horn.
c. infe'rius cartila'ginis thyroi'deae [TA], c. inferior da cartilagem tireóidea. SIN inferior *horn* of thyroid cartilage.
c. infe'rius mar'ginis falcifor'mis hia'tus saphe'ni [TA], pilar inferior da margem falciforme do hiato safeno. SIN inferior *horn* of falciform margin of saphenous opening.
c. infe'rius ventric'uli latera'lis [TA], c. inferior do ventrículo lateral. SIN inferior *horn* of lateral ventricle.
c. latera'le [TA], c. lateral. SIN lateral horn.
cornua of lateral ventricle, corno do ventrículo lateral. SIN c. frontale ventriculi lateralis [TA], c. occipitale ventriculi lateralis [TA], c. temporale ventriculi lateralis [TA]. VER anterior *horn* (1), inferior *horn*, posterior *horn*.
c. ma'jus os'sis hyoi'dei [TA], corno maior do hióide. SIN greater *horn* of hyoid bone.
c. mi'nus os'sis hyoi'dei [TA], corno menor do hióide. SIN lesser *horn* of hyoid.
c. occipitale ventriculi lateralis [TA], c. occipital do ventrículo lateral. SIN cornua of lateral ventricle.
c. posterius [TA], c. posterior. SIN posterior horn.
c. poste'rius ventric'uli latera'lis [TA], c. posterior do ventrículo lateral. SIN posterior *horn*.
sacral c. [TA], c. sacral; as partes mais caudais da crista sacral intermediária. De cada lado formam a margem lateral do hiato sacral e articulam-se com o corno coccígeo. SIN c. sacrale [TA], sacral horn*.
c. sacra'le [TA], c. sacral. SIN sacral c.
c. of spinal cord, c. da medula espinal. SIN posterior horn. VER anterior *horn* (2), lateral *horn*.
styloid c., c. estilóide. SIN lesser *horn* of hyoid.
c. supe'rius cartila'ginis thyroi'deae [TA], c. superior da cartilagem tireóidea. SIN superior *horn* of thyroid cartilage.
c. supe'rius margin'alis falcifor'mis [TA], pilar superior da margem falciforme. SIN superior *horn* of falciform margin of saphenous opening.
c. temporale ventriculi lateralis [TA], c. temporal do ventrículo lateral. SIN inferior *horn* of lateral ventricle, cornua of lateral ventricle.
cornua of thyroid cartilage, corno da cartilagem tireóidea. VER inferior *horn* of thyroid cartilage, superior *horn* of thyroid cartilage.
c. u'teri, c. do útero. SIN uterine horn.
cor·nua (kōr′noo-ă). Cornos. Plural de cornu.
cor·nu·al (kōr′noo-ăl). Córneo; relativo a um corno.
coro-. VER core-.
co·ro·na, pl. **co·ro·nae** (kō-rō′nă, -nē). [TA]. Coroa. SIN crown. [L. grinalda, coroa, do G. *korōnē*]
c. cap'itis, c. craniana; a parte mais alta da cabeça. SIN crown of head.
c. cilia'ris [TA], c. ciliar; a figura circular na superfície interna do corpo ciliar, formada pelos processos e pregas em conjunto. SIN ciliary crown, ciliary wreath.
c. clin'ica, c. clínica. SIN clinical crown.
c. den'tis, c. do dente. SIN crown of tooth.
c. glan'dis penis [TA], c. da glande do pênis. SIN c. of glans penis.
c. of glans penis [TA], c. da glande do pênis; a borda posterior proeminente da glande do pênis. SIN c. glandis penis [TA].
c. radia'ta, (1) [TA], c. radiada; uma massa de fibras em forma de leque na substância branca do córtex cerebral, composta pelas fibras amplamente irradiantes da cápsula interna; **(2)** uma única camada de células colunares derivadas da membrana prolígera, que se fixa à zona pelúcida do ovócito em um folículo secundário. SIN radiate crown.
c. seborrhe'ica, c. seborreica; uma faixa vermelha na linha de implantação do cabelo, ao longo da borda superior da fronte e têmporas, ocasionalmente observada na dermatite seborreica do couro cabeludo.
c. vene'ris, c. venérea; lesões sifilíticas papulares (erupção secundária) ao longo da margem anterior do couro cabeludo ou no dorso do pescoço. VER TAMBÉM *crown* of Venus.
Zinn c., c. de Zinn. SIN vascular *circle* of optic nerve.
cor·o·nad (kōr′ō-nad). Coronário; coronal; em direção a qualquer coroa.
cor·o·nal (kōr′ō-năl) [TA]. Coronal; relativo a uma coroa ou ao plano coronal. SIN coronalis [TA].
cor·o·na·le (kōr-ō-nā′lē). Coronal. **1.** SIN frontal bone. **2.** Um dos dois pontos mais separados na sutura coronal nos pólos do maior diâmetro frontal. [L. neutro de *coronalis*, relativo a uma *corona*, coroa]

cor·o·na·lis (kōr-ō-nā′lis) [TA]. Coronal. SIN coronal.
cor·o·na·ria (kōr-ō-nā′rē-ă). Coronária; uma artéria coronária, do coração.
cor·o·nar·ism (kōr′ō-nar-izm). Coronarismo. **1.** SIN coronary insufficiency. **2.** SIN angina pectoris. [coronary (artery) + -ism]
cor·o·na·ri·tis (kōr′ō-nă-rī′tis). Coronarite; inflamação da artéria ou artérias coronárias.
cor·o·nary (kōr′o-nar-ē). Coronário. **1.** Relativo, ou semelhante, a uma coroa. **2.** Circundando; designa várias estruturas anatômicas, p. ex., nervos, vasos sanguíneos, ligamentos. **3.** Especificamente, designa os vasos sanguíneos coronários do coração e, coloquialmente, a trombose coronária. [L. *coronarius*; de *corona*, coroa]
cafe c., c. do restaurante; colapso súbito ao comer que resulta da impacção de alimento fechando a glote; amiúde é erroneamente atribuído a doença coronariana.
Co·ro·na·vir·i·dae (kō-rō′nă-vir′i-dē). Uma família de vírus contendo RNA de filamento único com 3 ou 4 antígenos principais correspondendo a cada uma das principais proteínas virais; alguns vírus causam infecções respiratórias altas no homem semelhantes ao resfriado; outros causam infecções em animais (bronquite aviária infecciosa, encefalite suína, hepatite do camundongo, diarréia neonatal do bezerro e outras). Os vírus assemelham-se aos mixovírus, exceto pelas projeções em forma de pétalas que lembram o aspecto de coroa solar. Os virions possuem 120–160 nm de diâmetro, têm envoltório e são sensíveis ao éter. Acredita-se que os nucleopsídeos possuam simetria helicoidal; eles se desenvolvem no citoplasma e recebem seu envoltório ao brotarem em vesículas citoplasmáticas. Os Coronavirus e os Torovirus são os únicos gêneros reconhecidos. [L. *corona*, guirlanda, coroa]
Co·ro·na·vi·rus (kō-rō′nă-vī′rŭs). Gênero da família Coronaviridae que está associado a infecções respiratórias altas e, possivelmente, à gastroenterite no homem.
co·ro·na·vi·rus (kō-rō′nă-vī′rŭs). Coronavírus; qualquer vírus da família Coronaviridae.
cor·o·ner (kōr′on-er). Perito; médico-legista; um funcionário cujo dever é investigar mortes súbitas, suspeitas ou violentas para determinar a causa; em algumas comunidades, foi substituído pelo de examinador médico. [L. *corona*, coroa]
co·ro·ni·on (ko-rō′nē-on). Corônio; a extremidade do processo coronóide da mandíbula; um ponto craniométrico. SIN koronion. [G. *korōnē*, corvo]
cor·o·noid (kōr′ō-noyd). Coronóide; com formato semelhante ao bico de um corvo; designa determinados processos e outras partes dos ossos. [G. *korōnē*, corvo, + *eidos*, semelhante]
cor·o·noi·dec·to·my (kōr′ō-noy-dek′tō-mē). Coronoidectomia; remoção cirúrgica do processo coronóide da mandíbula. [coronoid + G. *ektomē*, excisão]
cor·po·ra (kōr′pōr-ă). Plural de corpus.
cor·po·re·al (kōr-pō′rē-ăl). Corpóreo; corporal; relativo ao corpo ou a um corpo.
cor·po·rin (kōr′pō-rin). Corporina; termo obsoleto para hormônio do corpo lúteo.
corpse (kōrps). Cadáver. SIN cadaver. [L. *corpus*, corpo]
corps ronds (kōr-ron′). Células redondas disceratóticas encontradas na epiderme, com uma massa basofílica central circundada por um halo claro; caracteristicamente encontradas na ceratose folicular. [Fr. *corps redondos*]
cor·pu·lence, cor·pu·len·cy (kōr′pū-lens, -len-sē). Corpulência. SIN obesity. [L. *corpulentia*, aumentativo de *corpus*, corpo]
cor·pu·lent (kōr′pū-lent). Corpulento. SIN obese.

CORPUS

cor·pus, gen. **cor·po·ris,** pl. **cor·po·ra** (kōr′pŭs, -pōr-is, -pōr-ă). [TA]. Corpo. **1.** SIN body. **2.** Qualquer corpo ou massa. **3.** A parte principal de um órgão ou outra estrutura anatômica, distinta da cabeça ou cauda. VER TAMBÉM body, diaphysis, soma. [L. corpo]
c. adipo'sum [TA], c. adiposo. SIN fat-pad.
c. adipo'sum buc'cae [TA], c. adiposo da bochecha. SIN buccal fat-pad.
c. adiposum fossae ischioanalis [TA], c. adiposo da fossa isquioanal. SIN fat *body* of ischiorectalis fossa.
c. adipo'sum fos'sae ischiorecta'lis, c. adiposo da fossa isquiorretal. SIN fat *body* of ischioanal fossa.
c. adipo'sum infrapatella're [TA], c. adiposo infrapatelar. SIN infrapatellar *fat-pad*.
c. adipo'sum or'bitae [TA], c. adiposo da órbita. SIN retrobulbar *fat*.
c. al'bicans, c. albicante; um corpo lúteo regredido caracterizado por fibrose progressiva e enrugamento do núcleo cicatricial com uma zona de luteína amorfa, entrelaçada, completamente hialinizada, circundando o tampão central de tecido cicatricial. SIN albicans (2), atretic c. luteum, c. candicans.
c. amygdaloi'deum [TA], c. amigdalóide. SIN amygdaloid *body*.

c. amyla'ceum, pl. **cor'pora amyla'cea,** corpúsculo amiláceo; um dentre vários pequenos corpos ovóides ou arredondados, algumas vezes laminados, semelhantes a um grão de amido e encontrados no tecido nervoso, na próstata e nos alvéolos pulmonares; sua importância histopatológica é pequena e, aparentemente, é derivado de células degeneradas ou secreções proteináceas. SIN amnionic corpuscle, amylaceous corpuscle, amyloid corpuscle, colloid corpuscle.
c. aor'ticum, c. aórtico. SIN paraaortic bodies, em body.
c. aran'tii, corpo de Arâncio; nódulos das válvulas semilunares. SIN nodules of semilunar cusps, em nodule.
cor'pora arena'cea, corpos arenosos; pequenas concreções calcárias no estroma da pineal e de outros tecidos do sistema nervoso central. SIN acervulus, brain sand, psammoma bodies (2).
atretic c. luteum, c. lúteo atrésico. SIN c. albicans.
c. atret'icum, c. atrésico. SIN atretic ovarian follicle.
cor'pora bigem'ina, corpos bigêmeos. SIN bigeminal bodies, em body.
c. callo'sum [TA], c. caloso; a grande placa comissural de fibras nervosas que interligam os hemisférios corticais (à exceção da maior parte dos lobos temporais, que são interligados pela comissura anterior). Situado no assoalho da fissura longitudinal e coberto de cada lado pelo giro do cíngulo, é arqueado de trás para diante e espesso em cada extremidade (esplênio [TA] e joelho [TA]), porém é mais fino em sua porção central longa (tronco [TA]); curva-se para trás por baixo de si mesmo no joelho, para formar o rostro [TA] do corpo caloso. SIN commissure of cerebral hemispheres.
c. can'dicans, c. albicante. SIN c. albicans.
corpora cavernosa recti, corpos cavernosos retos. SIN anal cushions, em cushion.
c. caverno'sum clitor'idis [TA], c. cavernoso do clitóris. SIN c. cavernosum of clitoris.
c. cavernosum of clitoris [TA], c. cavernoso do clitóris; uma das duas colunas paralelas de tecido erétil que formam o corpo do clitóris; elas divergem na raiz para formar os ramos do clitóris. SIN c. cavernosum clitoridis [TA], cavernous body of clitoris.
c. caverno'sum con'chae, plexo cavernoso das conchas. SIN cavernous (vascular) plexus of conchae.
c. caverno'sum pe'nis [TA], c. cavernoso do pênis; uma das duas colunas paralelas de tecido erétil que formam a parte dorsal do corpo do pênis; são separadas posteriormente, formando os ramos do pênis. SIN cavernous body of penis.
c. caverno'sum ure'thrae, c. cavernoso da uretra. SIN c. spongiosum penis.
c. cilia're [TA], c. ciliar. SIN ciliary body.
c. clavic'ulae [TA], c. da clavícula, diáfise da clavícula. SIN shaft of clavicle.
c. clitor'idis [TA], c. do clitóris. SIN body of clitoris.
c. coccy'geum [TA], c. do cóccix. SIN coccygeal body.
c. cos'tae [TA], c. da costela. SIN body of rib.
c. denta'tum, c. denteado; núcleo denteado. SIN dentate nucleus of cerebellum.
c. epididym'idis [TA], c. do epidídimo. SIN body of epididymis.
c. fem'oris, c. do fêmur, diáfise do fêmur. SIN shaft of femur.
c. fibro'sum, c. fibroso; a pequena massa cicatricial fibrosa no ovário formada após a atresia de um folículo ovariano; semelhante a um corpo albicante, porém menor.
c. fib'ulae [TA], c. da fíbula, diáfise da fíbula. SIN shaft of fibula.
c. fimbria'tum, c. fimbriado; **(1)** SIN fimbria hippocampi; **(2)** a extremidade externa do oviduto.
c. for'nicis [TA], c. do fórnice. SIN body of fornix.
c. gas'tricum [TA], c. gástrico. SIN body of stomach.
c. genicula'tum exter'num, c. geniculado externo. SIN lateral geniculate body.
c. genicula'tum inter'num, c. geniculado interno. SIN medial geniculate body.
c. genicula'tum latera'le [TA], c. geniculado lateral. SIN lateral geniculate body.
c. genicula'tum media'le [TA], c. geniculado medial. SIN medial geniculate body.
c. glan'dulae sudorif'erae, corpo das glândulas sudoríparas. SIN body of sweat gland.
c. hemorrhag'icum, c. hemorrágico; hematoma com um revestimento formado pela zona luteínica amarelo-brilhante; a reabsorção gradual dos elementos do sangue deixa uma cavidade cheia de líquido transparente, isto é, um cisto do corpo lúteo. SIN corpus luteum hematoma.
c. high'mori, c. highmoria'num, c. de Highmore. SIN mediastinum of testis.
c. hu'meri [TA], c. do úmero. SIN shaft of humerus.
c. incu'dis [TA], c. da bigorna. SIN body of incus.
c. juxtarestiforme, c. justarestiforme. SIN juxtarestiform body.
c. lin'guae [TA], c. da língua. SIN body of tongue.
c. lu'teum, c. lúteo; o corpo endócrino amarelo, com 1-1,5 cm de diâmetro, formado no ovário no local de um folículo ovariano roto imediatamente após a ovulação; há um estágio inicial de proliferação e vascularização antes da maturidade plena; depois, surge uma zona luteínica festonada e amarelo-brilhante, atravessada por trabéculas da teca interna contendo numerosos vasos sanguíneos; o corpo lúteo secreta estrogênio, como o folículo, e também progesterona. Se não houver gravidez, é denominado **falso corpo lúteo,** que sofre regressão progressiva para um corpo albicante. Se houver gravidez, é denominado **corpo lúteo verdadeiro,** que aumenta de tamanho, persistindo até o quinto ou sexto mês de gravidez antes da regressão. SIN yellow body.
c. luy'si, c. de Luys. SIN subthalamic nucleus.
c. mam'mae [TA], c. da mama. SIN body of breast.
c. mammilla're [TA], c. mamilar. SIN mammillary body.
c. mandib'ulae [TA], c. da mandíbula. SIN body of mandible.
c. maxil'lae [TA], c. da maxila. SIN body of maxilla.
c. medulla're cerebel'li [TA], c. medular do cerebelo; a substância branca interior do cerebelo.
c. metacarpale [TA], corpo do osso metacarpal. SIN shaft of metacarpal.
c. metatarsale [TA], c. (diáfise) do osso metatarsal. SIN shaft of metatarsal.
c. nu'clei cauda'ti [TA], c. do núcleo caudado. SIN body of caudate nucleus.
c. oliva're, c. olivar; oliva. SIN oliva.
c. os'is fem'oris [TA], c. do fêmur, diáfise do fêmur. SIN shaft of femur.
c. os'is hyoi'dei [TA], c. do hióide. SIN body of hyoid bone.
c. os'sis il'ii [TA], c. do ílio. SIN body of ilium.
c. os'sis isch'ii [TA], c. do ísquio. SIN body of ischium.
c. os'sis metacarpa'lis, c. do osso metacarpal; o corpo de um dos ossos metacarpais.
c. os'sis pu'bis [TA], c. do púbis. SIN body of pubis.
c. os'sis sphenoida'lis, c. do esfenóide. SIN body of sphenoid.
c. pampinifor'me, c. pampiniforme; epoóforo. SIN epoophoron.
c. pancrea'tis [TA], c. do pâncreas. SIN body of pancreas.
c. papilla're, camada papilar. SIN stratum papillare corii.
cor'pora para-aor'tica [TA], glomos aórticos. SIN paraaortic bodies, em body.
c. paratermina'le, c. paraterminal. SIN subcallosal gyrus.
c. pe'nis [TA], c. do pênis. SIN body of penis.
c. phalan'gis [TA], c. da falange. SIN shaft of phalanx.
c. pinea'le [TA], c. pineal. SIN pineal body.
c. pon'tobulba're, c. pontobulbar. SIN pontobulbar body.
cor'pora quadrigem'ina, corpos quadrigêmeos. SIN quadrigeminal bodies, em body. VER inferior colliculus, superior colliculus.
c. quadrigem'inum ante'rius, c. quadrigêmeo anterior. SIN superior colliculus.
c. quadrigem'inum poste'rius, c. quadrigêmeo posterior. SIN inferior colliculus.
c. ra'dii [TA], c. do rádio. SIN shaft of radius.
c. restifor'me [TA], c. restiforme, eminência restiforme. SIN restiform body.
c. spongio'sum pe'nis [TA], c. esponjoso do pênis; a coluna mediana de tecido erétil localizada entre os dois corpos cavernosos do pênis (e ventral aos mesmos); posteriormente, expande-se para o bulbo do pênis e, anteriormente, termina como a glande do pênis; é atravessado pela uretra. SIN c. cavernosum urethrae, spongy body of penis.
c. spongio'sum ure'thrae mulie'bris, c. esponjoso da uretra feminina; túnica esponjosa; a túnica submucosa da uretra feminina, contendo uma rede venosa que se insinua entre as túnicas musculares, conferindo-lhe uma natureza erétil.
c. ster'ni [TA], c. do esterno. SIN body of sternum.
c. stria'tum [TA], c. estriado. SIN striate body.
c. ta'li [TA], c. do tálus. SIN body of talus.
c. tib'iae [TA], c. da tíbia. SIN shaft of tibia.
c. trapezoid'eum [TA], c. do trapezóide. SIN trapezoid body.
c. triti'ceum, c. tritíceo. SIN triticeal cartilage.
c. ul'nae [TA], c. da ulna. SIN shaft of ulna.
c. un'guis [TA], c. da unha. SIN body of nail.
c. u'teri [TA], c. do útero. SIN body of uterus.
c. ver'tebrae [TA], c. vertebral. SIN vertebral body.
c. vesi'cae [TA], c. da bexiga. SIN body of bladder.
c. vesi'cae bilia'ris [TA], c. da vesícula biliar. SIN body of gallbladder.
c. vesi'cae fell'eae, c. da vesícula biliar; *termo oficial alternativo para body of gallbladder.
c. vit'reum [TA], c. vítreo. SIN vitreous body. VER TAMBÉM vitreous.

cor·pus·cle (kōr'pŭs-l). **1.** Corpúsculo; uma pequena massa ou corpo. **2.** Uma célula do sangue. SIN corpusculum. [L. *corpusculum*, dim. de *corpus*, corpo]
amnionic c., c. amniótico. SIN corpus amylaceum.
amylaceous c., amyloid c., c. amiláceo, c. amilóide. SIN corpus amylaceum.
articular c.'s, corpúsculos articulares; terminações nervosas encapsuladas nas cápsulas articulares. SIN corpuscula articularia.
axis c., axile c., c. axil; a porção central de um corpúsculo tátil.
basal c., c. basal. SIN basal body.
Bizzozero c., c. de Bizzozero. SIN platelet.
blood c., célula sanguínea. SIN blood cell.
bone c., osteócito SIN osteocyte.
bridge c., desmossoma. SIN desmosome.
bulboid c.'s, corpúsculos bulbóides. SIN Krause end bulbs, em bulb.

corpuscle 367 corpusculum

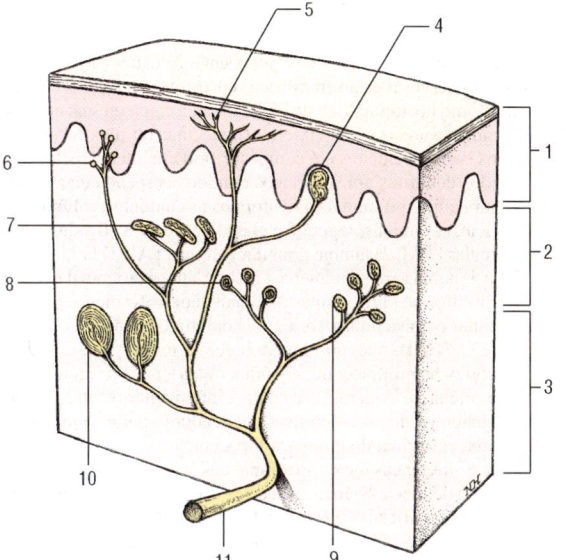

corpúsculos sensoriais: (4) c. de Meissner (tato), (5) terminação nervosa livre (dor), (6) disco de Merkel (tato leve), (7) c. de Ruffini (calor), (8) c. de Golgi (pressão leve), (9) c. de Krause (frio), (10) c. de Pacini (pressão forte), (11) fibra nervosa; e camadas cutâneas (1) epiderme (tato), (2) derme (temperatura), (3) tecido subcutâneo (pressão)

calcareous c.'s, corpúsculos calcários; massas arredondadas compostas de camadas concêntricas de carbonato de cálcio, características do tecido da tênia.
cement c., c. de cemento; um cementócito contido em uma lacuna ou cripta do cemento de um dente; um cementoblasto aprisionado.
chyle c., c. quiloso; célula com o mesmo aspecto de um leucócito, presente no quilo.
colloid c., c. colóide. SIN *corpus amylaceum.*
colostrum c., c. de colostro; um dos numerosos corpúsculos presentes no colostro; acredita-se que sejam leucócitos modificados contendo gotículas de gordura. SIN Donné c., galactoblast.
concentrated human red blood c., concentrado de hemácias humanas; preparado a partir de uma ou mais preparações de sangue humano total que não tenham mais de 14 dias e cada uma delas já tenha sido diretamente compatível com o sangue do provável receptor.
corneal c.'s, células de tecido conjuntivo encontradas entre as lâminas de tecido fibroso na córnea. SIN Toynbee c.'s, Virchow cells (3), Virchow c.'s.
Dogiel c., c. de Dogiel; uma terminação nervosa sensorial encapsulada.
Donné c., c. de Donné. SIN colostrum c.
dust c.'s, corpúsculos de poeira. SIN hemoconia.
Eichhorst c.'s, corpúsculos de Eichhorst; as formas globulares que ocorrem algumas vezes na poiquilocitose da anemia perniciosa.
exudation c., c. de exsudação; célula presente em um exsudato que ajuda na organização de novo tecido. SIN exudation cell, inflammatory c., plastic c.
genital c., c. genital; terminações nervosas encapsuladas especiais encontradas na pele da genitália e do mamilo. SIN corpuscula genitalia.
ghost c., c.-fantasma. SIN achromocyte.
Gluge c.'s, corpúsculos de Gluge; grandes piócitos contendo gotículas de gordura.
Golgi c., c. de Golgi. VER Golgi-Mazzoni c.
Golgi-Mazzoni c., c. de Golgi-Mazzoni; uma terminação nervosa sensorial encapsulada semelhante a um c. de Pacini, mas de estrutura mais simples.
Hassall concentric c.'s, corpúsculos concêntricos de Hassall. SIN thymic c.
inflammatory c., c. inflamatório. SIN exudation c.
lamellated c.'s, corpúsculos lamelados; pequenos corpos ovais na pele dos dedos das mãos, no mesentério, tendões e em outras partes, formados de camadas concêntricas de tecido conjuntivo com um cerne mole no qual corre o axônio de uma fibra nervosa, dividindo-se em várias fibrilas que terminam em expansões bulbosas; são sensíveis à pressão. SIN corpuscula lamellosa, pacinian c.'s, Vater c.'s, Vater-Pacini c.'s.
lymph c., lymphatic c., lymphoid c., linfócito; um tipo mononuclear de leucócito formado nos linfonodos e em outros tecidos linfóides, e também no sangue.
malpighian c.'s, corpúsculos de Malpighi; **(1)** SIN renal c; **(2)** SIN splenic lymph follicles, em follicle.
Mazzoni c., c. de Mazzoni; corpúsculo tátil aparentemente idêntico ao bulbo terminal de Krause. VER TAMBÉM Golgi-Mazzoni c.

Meissner c., c. de Meissner. SIN tactile c.
Merkel c., c. de Merkel. SIN tactile *meniscus.*
Mexican hat c., c. em sombrero. VER target cell *anemia.*
milk c., c. lácteo; uma das gotículas de gordura no leite.
molluscum c., c. do molusco. SIN molluscum *body.*
Negri c.'s, corpúsculos de Negri; termo obsoleto para Negri *bodies,* em *body.*
Norris c.'s, corpúsculos de Norris; hemácias descoradas que são invisíveis ou quase invisíveis no plasma sanguíneo, exceto se forem apropriadamente coradas.
oval c., c. oval. SIN tactile c.
pacchionian c.'s, corpúsculos de Pacchioni. SIN arachnoid *granulations,* em *granulation.*
pacinian c.'s, corpúsculos de Pacini. SIN lamellated c.'s.
pessary c., c. em pessário; uma hemácia alongada com hemoglobina concentrada na porção periférica.
phantom c., c.-fantasma. SIN achromocyte.
plastic c., c. plástico. SIN exudation c.
Purkinje c.'s, corpúsculos de Purkinje. SIN Purkinje cell *layer.*
pus c., piócito; um dos leucócitos polimorfonucleares que constituem a parte principal dos elementos formados no pus. SIN pus cell, pyocyte.
Rainey c.'s, corpúsculos de Rainey; esporos arredondados, ovóides ou falciformes ou bradizoítas, com 12–16 por 4–9 μm, encontrados nos cistos alongados (tubos de Miescher) do protozoário *Sarcocystis.*
red c., eritrócito. SIN erythrocyte.
renal c., c. renal; o tufo de capilares glomerulares e a cápsula glomerular que o encerra. SIN corpusculum renis, malpighian c.'s (1)
reticulated c., reticulócito. SIN reticulocyte.
Ruffini c.'s, corpúsculos de Ruffini; estruturas terminais sensoriais nos tecidos conjuntivos subcutâneos, que consistem em uma cápsula ovóide na qual a fibra sensorial termina com numerosos botões colaterais.
salivary c., um dos leucócitos presentes na saliva.
Schwalbe c., c. de Schwalbe. SIN taste *bud.*
shadow c., c.-fantasma. SIN achromocyte.
splenic c.'s, folículos esplênicos. SIN splenic lymph *follicles,* em *follicle.*
tactile c., c. tátil; um dos numerosos corpúsculos ovais encontrados nas papilas dérmicas da pele espessa, principalmente aquela dos dedos e artelhos; consiste em uma cápsula de tecido conjuntivo na qual as fibrilas axonais terminam ao redor de e entre uma pilha de células epitelióides cuneiformes; acredita-se que sejam mecanorreceptores para a sensibilidade tátil. SIN corpusculum tactus, Meissner c., oval c., touch c.
taste c., c. gustativo. SIN taste *bud.*
terminal nerve c.'s, corpúsculos nervosos terminais; termo genérico que designa terminações nervosas encapsuladas especializadas, como os corpúsculos articulares, bulbóides, genitais, lamelados e táteis, e o menisco tátil. SIN corpuscula nervosa terminalia.
third c., plaqueta. SIN platelet.
thymic c., c. tímico; pequenos corpos esféricos de células epiteliais queratinizadas e geralmente escamosas dispostas em um padrão concêntrico ao redor de grupos de linfócitos, eosinófilos e macrófagos em degeneração; encontrado na medula dos lóbulos do timo. SIN Hassall bodies, Hassall concentric c.'s, Virchow-Hassall bodies.
touch c., c. tátil. SIN tactile c.
Toynbee c.'s, corpúsculos de Toynbee. SIN corneal c.'s.
Traube c., c. de Traube. SIN achromocyte.
Tröltsch c.'s, corpúsculos de Tröltsch; espaços diminutos, semelhantes a corpúsculos, entre as fibras radiais da membrana do tímpano do ouvido.
Valentin c.'s, corpúsculos de Valentin; corpos pequenos, provavelmente amilóides, encontrados algumas vezes no tecido nervoso.
Vater c.'s, corpúsculos de Vater. SIN lamellated c.'s.
Vater-Pacini c.'s, corpúsculos de Vater-Pacini. SIN lamellated c.'s.
Virchow c.'s, corpúsculos de Virchow. SIN corneal c.'s.
white c., qualquer tipo de leucócito.
Zimmermann c., c. de Zimmermann. SIN platelet.
cor·pus·cu·la (kōr - pŭs′kū - lă). Plural de corpusculum.
cor·pus·cu·lar (kōr - pŭs′kū - lăr). Corpuscular; relativo a um corpúsculo.
cor·pus·cu·lum, pl. **cor·pus·cu·la** (kōr - pŭs′kū - lŭm, - kū - lă). Corpúsculo. SIN corpuscle.
corpus'cula articula'ria, corpúsculos articulares. SIN articular *corpuscles,* em *corpuscle.*
corpus'cula bulboi'dea, corpúsculos bulbóides. SIN Krause end *bulbs,* em *bulb.*
corpus'cula genita'lia, corpúsculos genitais. SIN genital *corpuscles,* em *corpuscle.*
corpus'cula lamello'sa, corpúsculos lamelados. SIN lamellated *corpuscles,* em *corpuscle.*
corpus'cula nervo'sa termina'lia, corpúsculos nervosos terminais. SIN terminal nerve *corpuscles,* em *corpuscle.*
c. re′nis, pl. **corpus'cula re'nis,** corpúsculo renal. SIN renal *corpuscle.*
c. tac′tus, pl. **corpus'cula tac'tus,** c. tátil. SIN tactile *corpuscle.*

cor·rec·tion (kō - rek'shŭn).Correção; o ato de reduzir uma falha; a eliminação de uma qualidade desfavorável.
  occlusal c., c. oclusal; **(1)** a correção da má oclusão, seja qual for o meio empregado; **(2)** eliminação da desarmonia dos contatos oclusais.
  spontaneous c. of placenta previa, c. espontânea da placenta prévia; a "migração" para cima da placenta, afastando-se do óstio interno graças às diferentes velocidades de crescimento dos segmentos superior e inferior do útero.
cor·rec·tive (kō - rek'tiv). Corretivo. **1.** Neutralização, modificação ou alteração do que é lesivo. **2.** Uma substância que modifica ou corrige um efeito indesejável ou prejudicial de outra substância. SIN corrigent. [L. *cor-rigo* (*conr-*), pp. -*rectus*, corrigir, de *rego*, manter reto]
cor·re·la·tion (kŏr - ĕ - lā'shŭn).Correlação. **1.** A relação mútua ou recíproca de dois ou mais itens ou partes. **2.** O ato de produzir essa relação. **3.** O grau em que variáveis se modificam juntas.
  product-moment c., c. produto-momento; um procedimento estatístico que fornece o coeficiente de correlação denominado r ($-1,00$ a $+1,00$) e envolve os valores reais, em vez de ordens (classe) das medidas.
  rank-difference c., c. de diferenças de postos; a relação entre séries pareadas de medidas, cada qual ordenada de acordo com a magnitude, que fornece um coeficiente conhecido como *rho;* o valor de *rho* varia de zero (ausência de relação) a +1,00 (relação perfeita).
Correra line. Linha de Correra; ver em line.
cor·re·spon·dence (kŏr - ĕ - spon'dens).Correspondência; em óptica, aqueles pontos em cada retina que possuem a mesma direção visual.
  abnormal c., c. anormal. SIN anomalous retinal c.
  anomalous retinal c., c. retiniana anômala; c. anormal; uma condição, freqüente no estrabismo, na qual os pontos retinianos correspondentes não possuem a mesma direção visual; a fóvea de um olho corresponde a uma área extrafoveal do outro. SIN abnormal c.
  dysharmonious retinal c., c. retiniana desarmônica; um tipo de correspondência retiniana anômala em que o ângulo da direção visual das duas retinas é diferente do ângulo objetivo do estrabismo.
  harmonious retinal c., c. retiniana harmoniosa; um tipo de correspondência retiniana anômala em que o ângulo da direção visual das duas retinas é igual ao ângulo objetivo do estrabismo.
Corrigan, Sir Dominic J., patologista e clínico irlandês, 1802–1880. VER C. *disease, pulse, sign.*
cor·ri·gent (kŏr'i - jent). Corretivo. SIN corrective.
cor·rin (kŏr'in).Corrina; o sistema cíclico de quatro anéis pirrólicos formando corrinóides, que são a estrutura central da vitamina B_{12} e compostos relacionados, diferindo da porfina (porfirina) porque dois dos anéis pirrólicos são diretamente ligados (C-19 a C-1). [de *core* (da molécula de vitamina B_{12})]
cor·rin·oid (kŏr'rin - oid). Corrinóide; composto contendo um anel corrina.
cor·rode (kō - rōd'). Corroer; causar, ou ser afetado por, corrosão.
cor·ro·sion (kō - rō'shŭn).Corrosão. **1.** Deterioração ou consumo gradual de uma substância por outra, principalmente por reação bioquímica ou química. Cf. erosion. **2.** O produto da corrosão, como a ferrugem. [L. *cor-rodo* (*conr-*), pp. –*rosus*, corroer]
cor·ro·sive (kō - rō'siv).Corrosivo. **1.** Que causa corrosão. **2.** Um agente que produz corrosão; p. ex., um ácido ou álcali forte.
cor·ru·ga·tor (kŏr'ŭ - gā - ter, - tōr).Corrugador; músculo que puxa a pele, enrugando-a. [L. *cor-rugo* (*conr-*), pp. –*atus*, enrugar, de *ruga*, uma ruga]

CORTEX

cor·tex, gen. **cor·ti·cis,** pl. **cor·ti·ces** (kōr'teks, - ti - sis, - ti - sēz).[TA]. Córtex; a porção externa de um órgão, como o rim, diferente da porção interna ou medular. [L. casca]
  adrenal c., c. supra-renal. SIN c. of suprarenal gland.
  agranular c., c. agranular. VER cerebral c.
  association c., c. de associação; termo genérico que designa as grandes expansões do córtex cerebral que não são sensoriais nem motoras no sentido habitual, mas estão envolvidas em estágios avançados de processamento das informações sensoriais, na integração multissensorial ou na integração sensorimotora. VER TAMBÉM cerebral c. SIN association areas.
  auditory c., c. auditivo; a região do córtex cerebral que recebe a radiação auditiva do corpo geniculado medial, um grupo de células talâmicas que recebem informações auditivas dos núcleos cocleares no rombencéfalo; corresponde aproximadamente às áreas 41 e 42 de Brodmann e está organizada tonotopicamente. SIN auditory area.
  cerebellar c., c. cerebelar; a fina camada superficial cinzenta do cérebro, que consiste em uma camada molecular externa (estrato molecular), uma camada única de células de Purkinje (a camada de células de Purkinje) e uma camada granular interna ou estrato granular. SIN c. cerebelli [TA].
  c. cerebel'li [TA], c. do cerebelo. SIN cerebellar c.
  cerebral c. [TA], c. cerebral; o manto celular cinzento (1–4 mm de espessura) que cobre toda a superfície do hemisfério cerebral dos mamíferos; caracterizado por uma organização laminar de componentes celulares e fibrosos de forma que suas células nervosas estão empilhadas em estratos definidos cujo número varia de um, como no arquicórtex do hipocampo, a cinco ou seis no neocórtex maior; a lâmina (camada) mais externa (molecular ou plexiforme) contém pouquíssimos corpos celulares e é composta, principalmente, pelas ramificações distais dos dendritos apicais longos emitidos perpendicularmente, até a superfície, por células piramidais e fusiformes nas lâminas profundas. Partindo da superfície, as lâminas, segundo a classificação de K. Brodmann, são: 1) lâmina molecular [TA]; 2) lâmina granular externa [TA]; 3) lâmina piramidal externa [TA]; 4) lâmina granular interna [TA]; 5) lâmina piramidal interna [TA]; e 6) lâmina multiforme [TA], muitas das quais são fusiformes. Essa organização multilaminar é típica do neocórtex (c. homotípico; isocórtex [TA] na terminologia de O. Vogt), que, no homem, cobre a maior parte do hemisfério cerebral. O córtex heterotípico, ou alocórtex (Vogt), mais primordial tem menos camadas celulares. Uma forma de córtex intermediário entre o isocórtex e o alocórtex, denominado justalocórtex (Vogt), cobre a parte ventral do giro do cíngulo e a área entorrinal do giro para-hipocampal.
  Com base nas diferenças locais no arranjo das células nervosas (citoarquitetura), Brodmann delineou 47 áreas, no córtex cerebral, que, em termos funcionais, podem ser classificadas em três categorias: córtex motor (áreas 4 e 6), caracterizado por uma lâmina granular interna pouco desenvolvida (lâmina agranular) e camadas de células piramidais proeminentes; córtex sensorial, caracterizado por uma lâmina granular interna proeminente (lâmina granular ou coniocórtex) e constituindo o córtex sensorial somático (áreas 1 a 3), o córtex auditivo (áreas 41 e 42) e o córtex visual (áreas 17 a 19); e córtex de associação, as grandes expansões remanescentes do córtex cerebral. SIN c. cerebri [TA], pallium [TA], brain mantle, mantle (2).
  c. cer'ebri [TA], c. cerebral. SIN cerebral c.
  deep c., c. profundo. SIN paracortex.
  dysgranular c., c. disgranular; a região do córtex cerebral que representa a transição entre o córtex agranular do giro pré-central e o córtex frontal granular (área 8 de Brodmann).
  fetal adrenal c., c. supra-renal fetal; uma extensa área da glândula supra-renal presente em primatas durante a vida fetal e por um curto período após o nascimento; localizado entre o córtex definitivo e a medula, contém grandes células secretoras de esteróides dispostas em um padrão reticular; a involução dessa zona em seres humanos é concluída em três meses após o nascimento. SIN androgenic zone (2), fetal reticularis (1), fetal zone, provisional c.
  frontal c., c. frontal; córtex do lobo frontal do hemisfério cerebral; **(1)** originalmente, toda a expansão cortical anterior ao sulco central, incluindo o córtex motor agranular e pré-motor (áreas 4 e 6 de Brodmann), o córtex disgranular (área 8) e o córtex frontal granular (pré-frontal) anterior a este último; **(2)** agora refere-se, com maior freqüência, ao córtex frontal granular (pré-frontal). SIN frontal area.
  c. glan'dulae suprarena'lis [TA], c. da glândula supra-renal. SIN c. of suprarenal gland.
  granular c., c. granular. VER cerebral c.
  c. of hair shaft, c. da diáfise pilosa; o principal componente estrutural da diáfise pilosa, composto de células queratinizadas fusiformes intimamente acondicionadas e revestidas pela cutícula pilosa.
  heterotypic c., c. heterotípico. SIN allocortex.

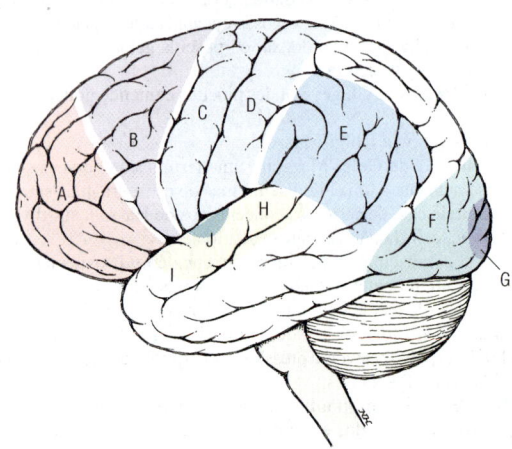

córtex cerebral: principais áreas funcionais: (A) inteligência biológica, (B) pré-motora, (C) somatomotora, (D) somatossensorial, (E) percepção corporal, (F) psíquica visual, (G) sensorial visual, (H) compreensão da fala, (I) psíquica auditiva, (J) sensorial auditiva

homotypic c., c. homotípico. SIN isocortex.
insular c., c. insular. SIN insula (1).
laminated c., c. laminado; neocórtex [TA] e alocórtex [TA].
c. of lens [TA], c. da lente; a parte mais macia, mais superficial da lente do olho que encerra a parte central do núcleo; seu poder de refração é inferior ao do núcleo. SIN c. lentis [TA].
c. len'tis [TA], c. da lente. SIN c. of lens.
c. of lymph node [TA], c. do linfonodo; a porção externa do linfonodo sob sua cápsula, que consiste em trabéculas fibrosas que separam massas de linfócitos densamente acondicionadas, dispostas em nódulos e separadas das trabéculas e cápsula por seios linfáticos. SIN c. nodi lymphatici [TA].
mastoid c., c. mastóideo; a lâmina óssea na superfície lateral do processo mastóide do osso temporal.
motor c., c. motor; a região do córtex cerebral que influencia, quase imediatamente, os movimentos da face, pescoço e tronco, e braço e perna; corresponde, aproximadamente, às áreas 4 e 6 de Brodmann do giro pré-central e às porções imediatamente adjacentes dos giros frontais superior e médio; seus efeitos sobre os neurônios motores que inervam a musculatura esquelética são mediados por fibras corticoespinais (trato piramidal) e fibras corticonucleares e são particularmente essenciais para a capacidade humana de realizar movimentos finamente graduados do braço e da perna. SIN excitable area, motor area, Rolando area.
c. no'di lymphat'ici [TA], c. do linfonodo. SIN c. of lymph node.
olfactory c., c. olfatório. SIN piriform c.
orbitofrontal c., c. orbitofrontal; o córtex cerebral que recobre a superfície basal dos lobos frontais. SIN fronto-orbital area.
ovarian c. [TA], c. do ovário; a camada do estroma ovariano situada imediatamente sob a túnica albugínea, composta de células de tecido conjuntivo e fibras, entre as quais há folículos primários e secundários (antrais) dispersos em vários estágios de desenvolvimento; a espessura do córtex varia de acordo com a idade da mulher, tornando-se mais fina com o passar dos anos. SIN c. ovarii [TA], c. of ovary.
c. ova'rii [TA], c. do ovário. SIN ovarian c.
c. of ovary, c. do ovário. SIN ovarian c.
parastriate c., c. paraestriado. VER visual c.
peristriate c., c. periestriado. VER visual c.
piriform c., c. piriforme; o córtex olfatório que corresponde à metade rostral do unco; recebendo suas principais vias aferentes do bulbo olfatório, é classificado como alocórtex. VER TAMBÉM cerebral c. SIN olfactory c., piriform area.
prefrontal c., c. pré-frontal. VER frontal c.
premotor c., c. pré-motor; termo um pouco mal definido que geralmente se refere ao córtex agranular da área 6 de Brodmann. SIN premotor area.
primary visual c., c. visual primário. VER visual c.
provisional c., c. provisório. SIN fetal adrenal c.
renal c. [TA], c. renal; parte do rim que consiste em lóbulos renais na zona externa sob a cápsula e, também, nos lóbulos das colunas renais que são extensões para dentro entre as pirâmides; contém os corpúsculos renais e os túbulos contornados proximal e distal. SIN c. renalis [TA].
c. rena'lis [TA], c. renal. SIN renal c.
secondary sensory c., c. sensorial secundário; região cortical que ocupa o opérculo parietal (lábio superior do sulco lateral) situado logo posterior à base do giro pós-central; como o córtex somático-sensorial primário do giro póscentral, essa região recebe impulsos sensoriais originados na face, no tronco e nos membros; as projeções para o córtex sensorial secundário provêm do complexo basal ventral (núcleos ventrais póstero-lateral e póstero-medial do tálamo) e do córtex somestésico primário.
secondary visual c., c. visual secundário. VER visual c.
sensory c., c. sensorial; outrora designava especificamente o córtex sensorial somático, mas agora é usado para designar coletivamente as regiões sensorial somática, auditiva, visual e olfatória do córtex cerebral.
somatic sensory c., somatosensory c., c. somatossensorial; a região do córtex cerebral que recebe a radiação sensorial somática do núcleo ventrobasal do tálamo; representa o mecanismo de processamento cortical primário para informações sensoriais originadas nas superfícies corporais (tato) e nos tecidos profundos, como o músculo, os tendões e as cápsulas articulares (propriocepção); corresponde, aproximadamente, às áreas 1, 2 e 3 de Brodmann no giro pós-central. SIN somesthetic area.
striate c., c. estriado. VER visual c.
supplementary motor c., c. motor suplementar; região a partir da qual, por estimulação elétrica, pode ser ativada a musculatura de todas as partes do corpo, da mesma forma que por estímulo do córtex motor do giro pré-central; a região corresponde aproximadamente à expansão da área 6 de Brodmann sobre a superfície medial do hemisfério cerebral; essa área tem, em grande parte, uma representação bilateral e está relacionada primariamente com atividades motoras tônicas e posturais.
suprarenal c., c. supra-renal. SIN c. of suprarenal gland.
c. of suprarenal gland [TA], c. da glândula supra-renal; a parte externa da glândula supra-renal, que consiste em três zonas de fora para dentro: zona glomerulosa, zona fasciculada e zona reticular; essa parte do córtex da glândula supra-renal produz hormônios esteróides como corticosterona, desoxicorticosterona e estrona. SIN c. glandulae suprarenalis [TA], adrenal c., suprarenal c.
temporal c., c. temporal. SIN temporal lobe.
tertiary c., c. terciário. SIN paracortex.
c. thymi [TA], c. do timo. SIN c. of thymus.
c. of thymus [TA], c. do timo; a parte externa de um lóbulo do timo; circunda a medula e é composto de massas de linfócitos aglomerados. SIN c. thymi [TA].
visual c., c. visual; a região do córtex cerebral que ocupa toda a superfície do lobo occipital e é composta pelas áreas 17–19 de Brodmann. A área 17 (também denominada córtex estriado ou área estriada porque a linha de Gennari é visível macroscopicamente em sua superfície) é o córtex visual primário, que recebe a radiação visual do corpo geniculado lateral do tálamo. As áreas adjacentes 18 (córtex ou área paraestriada) e 19 (córtex ou área periestriada) provavelmente estão envolvidas nas etapas subseqüentes de processamento de informações visuais; a área 18 é denominada córtex visual secundário. SIN visual area.

---

cor·tex·o·lone (kōr-teks'ō-lōn).Cortexolona; um hormônio mineralocorticóide do córtex da glândula supra-renal.
cor·tex·one (kōr-teks'ōn).Cortexona. SIN deoxycorticosterone.
Corti, Marquis Alfonso, anatomista italiano, 1822–1876. VER C. *arch, canal, cells,* em *cell, ganglion, membrane, organ, pillars,* em *pillar, rods,* em *rod,* auditory *teeth,* em *tooth; tunnel;* pillar *cells* of C., em *cell.*
cor·ti·cal (kōr'ti-kăl).Cortical; relativo a um córtex.
cor·ti·cal·i·za·tion (kōr'ti-kăl-i-zā'shŭn).Corticalização; em filogênese, a migração da função dos centros subcorticais para o córtex. SIN encephalization, telencephalization.
cor·ti·cal·os·te·ot·o·my (kōr'ti-kăl-os-tē-ot'ō-mē).Corticalosteotomia; uma osteotomia através do córtex, na base do segmento dentoalveolar, que serve para reduzir a resistência do osso à aplicação de forças ortodônticas.
cor·ti·cec·to·my (kōr-ti-sek'tō-mē).Corticectomia; remoção de uma porção específica do córtex cerebral. [cortic- + G. *ektomē*, excisão]
cor·ti·ces (kōr'ti-sēz).Plural de cortex.
cor·ti·cif·u·gal (kōr-ti-sif'ū-găl).Corticífugo. SIN corticofugal.
cor·ti·cip·e·tal (kōr-ti-sip'e-tăl). Corticípeto; que segue em direção à superfície externa; designa fibras nervosas que conduzem impulsos para o córtex cerebral. SIN corticoafferent. [L. *cortex*, córtex, casca, + *peto*, buscar]
cor·ti·co·af·fer·ent (kōr'ti-kō-af'er-ent).Corticoaferente. SIN corticipetal.
cor·ti·co·bul·bar (kōr'ti-kō-bŭl'bar).Corticobulbar. VER corticobulbar *fibers,* em *fiber,* corticonuclear *fibers,* em *fiber.*
cor·ti·co·cer·e·bel·lum (kor'ti-kō-ser-ĕ-bel'ŭm).Corticocerebelo. SIN neocerebellum.
cor·ti·co·ef·fer·ent (kōr'ti-kō-ef'er-ent).Corticoeferente. SIN corticofugal.
cor·ti·cof·u·gal (kōr'ti-kō-fū'găl).Corticífugo; que se afasta da superfície externa; designando principalmente fibras nervosas que conduzem impulsos a partir do córtex cerebral. SIN corticifugal, corticoefferent. [L. *cortex*, córtex, casca, + *fugio,* fugir]
cor·ti·coid (kōr'ti-koyd).Corticóide. **1.** Que possui uma ação semelhante àquela de um hormônio do córtex supra-renal. **2.** Qualquer substância que exibe essa ação. **3.** SIN corticosteroid.
cor·ti·co·me·di·al (kōr'ti-kō-mē'dē-ăl).Corticomedial; cortical e medial; especificamente usado para se referir a uma das duas principais divisões citológicas do complexo amigdalóide. VER *corpus* amygdaloideum.
cor·ti·co·ste·roid (kōr'ti-kō-stēr'oyd).Corticosteróide; um esteróide produzido pelo córtex supra-renal (isto é, corticóide supra-renal); um corticóide que contém um esteróide. SIN adrenocorticoid, corticoid (3), cortin.
cor·ti·cos·ter·one (kōr-ti-kos'ter-ōn).Corticosterona; um corticosteróide que induz alguma deposição de glicogênio no fígado, conservação de sódio e excreção de potássio; o principal glicocorticóide no rato.
cor·ti·co·tha·lam·ic (kōr'ti-kō-thal'ă-mik).Corticotalâmico; relativo ao córtex e ao tálamo; o termo é aplicado às fibras que se projetam do córtex cerebral até o tálamo, as fibras corticotalâmicas [TA].
cor·ti·co·troph (kōr'ti-kō-trof).Corticotrofo; célula da adeno-hipófise que produz hormônio adrenocorticotrófico (ACTH).
cor·ti·co·tro·pin (kōr'ti-kō-trō'pin).Corticotrofina. **1.** SIN adrenocorticotropic *hormone*. **2.** SIN β-corticotropin. [G. *tropē*, uma volta]
c.-zinc hydroxide, c. com hidróxido de zinco; corticotrofina purificada absorvida no hidróxido de zinco; os mesmos usos da cortitrofina, mas com uma duração prolongada de ação.
β-cor·ti·co·tro·pin. β-corticotrofina; β-corticotrofina degradada por ácido ou pepsina. SIN corticotropin (2).
Cor·ti·co·vir·i·dae (kōr'ti-kō-vir'i-dē). Nome de uma família de vírus bacterianos sem envoltório, sensíveis ao éter, de tamanho médio, com um capsídeo contendo lipídios e genoma de DNA circular, duplo filamentar (PM 5×10^6), responsável por cerca de 12% do peso do vírion.
Corticovirus. Único gênero da família Corticoviridae.
cor·ti·lymph (kōr'tē-limf).Cortilinfa; o líquido no túnel de Corti.

cor·tin (kōr′tin). Corticosteróide. SIN corticosteroid.
cor·ti·sol (kōr′ti - sol). Cortisol. SIN hydrocortisone.
  c. acetate, acetato de c. SIN hydrocortisone acetate.
cor·ti·sone (kōr′ti - sōn). Cortisona; um glicocorticóide que normalmente não é secretado em quantidades significativas pelo córtex supra-renal humano. Endogenamente, é provável que seja um metabólito da hidrocortisona, mas não possui atividade biológica até que seja convertido em hidrocortisona (cortisol); atua sobre o metabolismo dos carboidratos e influencia a nutrição e o crescimento dos tecidos conjuntivos (colágenos). Foi o primeiro glicocorticóide disponível para tratamento. SIN Wintersteiner compound F.
α-cor·tol (kōr′tol). α-Cortol; o enantiômero 5β do α-alocortol; um produto da redução da cortisona, presente na urina, que difere da cortisona porque os três grupamentos ceto são reduzidos a hidroxilas.
β-cor·tol. β-Cortol; α-cortol com um grupamento 20β-OH; o enantiômero 5β do β-alocortol, encontrado na urina.
α-cor·to·lone (kōr′tō - lōn). α-Cortolona; o enantiômero 5β da α-alocortolona; um produto da redução da cortisona, presente na urina, que difere da cortisona porque dois grupamentos ceto (nas posições 3 e 20) são reduzidos a hidroxilas.
β-cor·to·lone. β-Cortolona; α-cortolona com um grupamento 20β-OH; o enantiômero 5β da β-alocortolona, encontrada na urina.
co·run·dum (ko - run′dum). Coríndon; corindo; óxido de alumínio cristalino nativo. [Indu, *kurand*]
Corvisart des Marets, Baron Jean N., médico francês, 1755–1821. VER Corvisart *facies*.
co·rym·bi·form (kŏ - rim′bi - fōrm). Corimbiforme; designa a configuração aglomerada, semelhante a flores, das lesões cutâneas em doenças granulomatosas (p. ex., sífilis, tuberculose) [L. *corymbus*, aglomerado, grinalda]
cor·y·ne·bac·te·ria (kŏ - ri′nē - bak - tēr′ē - ă). Plural de corynebacterium.
cor·y·ne·bac·te·ri·o·phage (kŏ - ri′nē - bak - tēr′ē - ō - fāj). Corinebacteriófago; qualquer um dos bacteriófagos específicos para corinebactérias.
  β **c.**, c. β; um bacteriófago contendo DNA que induz toxigenicidade em cepas de *Corynebacterium diphtheriae* que são lisogênicas para seu prófago. SIN β phage.
Cor·y·ne·bac·te·ri·um (kŏ - ri′nē - bak - tēr′ē - ŭm). Gênero de bactérias imóveis (exceto alguns patógenos de plantas), aeróbias ou anaeróbias (família Corynebacteriaceae), que contém bastonetes de coloração irregular, Grampositivos, retos ou discretamente curvos, amiúde em forma de clava, em virtude de divisão por ruptura, exibindo uma disposição em estacas. Esses microrganismos são amplamente distribuídos na natureza. As espécies mais conhecidas são parasitas e patógenos de seres humanos e animais domésticos. A espécie típica é *C. diphtheriae*. [G. *coryne*, uma clava, + *bacterium*, pequeno bastonete]
  C. ac′nes, nome anterior do *Propionibacterium acnes.*
  C. amycolatum, espécie encontrada na flora cutânea normal, causa septicemia, freqüentemente associada a dispositivos de acesso venoso, e também foi isolada de infecções urinárias e abscessos de flora mista.
  C. diphthe′riae, espécie bacteriana que causa difteria e produz uma potente exotoxina que causa degeneração de vários tecidos, notavelmente do miocárdio, em seres humanos e animais experimentais, e catalisa a ADP-ribosilação do fator II de alongamento; as cepas virulentas desse microrganismo são lisogênicas; é comumente encontrada em membranas na faringe, laringe, traquéia e nariz em casos de difteria; também é encontrada na faringe e no nariz aparentemente saudáveis dos portadores, e algumas vezes na conjuntiva e em feridas superficiais; ocasionalmente, infecta as vias nasais e feridas de cavalos; é a espécie típica do gênero *C.* SIN Klebs-Loeffler bacillus, Loeffler bacillus.
  C. e′qui, SIN *Rhodococcus equi.*
  C. glucuronolyticum, espécie isolada de pacientes com infecções urinárias.
  C. haemoly′ticum, nome anterior do *Arcanobacterium haemolyticum.*
  C. hofman′nii, nome anterior do *C. pseudodiphtheriticum.*
  C. jeikeium, espécie associada à septicemia e lesões cutâneas em pacientes imunodeprimidos, particularmente associada a dispositivos de acesso venoso.
  C. matruchotii, espécie isolada em infecções mistas de amostras de olho humano.
  C. minutis′simum, espécie de bactéria que é um componente da flora cutânea normal, causa eritrasma em seres humanos.
  C. par′vum, nome anterior de *Propionibacterium acnes.*
  C. pseudodiphtherit′icum, espécie raramente patogênica encontrada em orofaringes normais. SIN Hofmann bacillus.
  C. stria′tum, espécie bacteriana encontrada no muco nasal e na orofaringe; também encontrada no úbere de vacas com mastite; patogênica para animais de laboratório; uma causa rara de infecção em pacientes imunodeprimidos.
  C. xero′sis, espécie de bactéria encontrada na conjuntiva normal e doente; não há evidências de que esse microrganismo seja patogênico.
cor·y·ne·bac·te·ri·um, pl. **cor·y·ne·bac·te·ria** (kŏ - ri′nē - bak - tēr′ē - ŭm, - ă). Corinebactéria; termo vernacular usado para se referir a qualquer membro do gênero *Corynebacterium.*

co·ry·za (kŏ - ri′ză). Coriza, rinite aguda. SIN acute rhinitis. [G.]
  allergic c., c. alérgica. SIN hay fever.
Co·ry·za·vi·rus (kŏ - ri′ză - vi′rŭs). Nome obsoleto de Rhinovirus.
cos·me·sis (koz - mē′sis). Preocupação na terapêutica com o aspecto do paciente; isto é, uma operação que melhora o aspecto. [G. *kosmēsis,* adorno, de *kosmēō,* ordenar, arranjar, adornar, de *kosmos,* ordem]
cos·met·ic (koz - met′ik). Cosmético. **1.** Relativo à cosmese. **2.** Relativo ao uso de cosméticos.
cos·met·ics (koz - met′iks). Cosmético; termo que descreve vários preparados aplicados à pele, aos lábios, ao cabelo e às unhas com o objetivo de embelezamento, de acordo com os ditames culturais.
cos·mid (koz′mid). Cosmídio; plasmídeo produzido por engenharia de recombinação, um DNA circular contendo, em ordem: uma origem plasmídica de replicação e um marcador de resistência medicamentosa, o local *cos* (extremidade coesiva) do bacteriófago λ e um fragmento de DNA eucariótico a ser clonado; os cosmídios são construídos para permitir clonagem de fragmentos com até 40.000 pares de bases de comprimento, sendo necessário um ou mais locais de restrição únicos para facilitar clonagem.
cos·mo·pol·i·tan (koz - mō - pol′i - tan). Cosmopolita; em ciências biológicas, um termo que indica distribuição mundial. [G. *kosmos,* universo, + *polis,* cidade-estado]
cos·ta, gen. e pl. **cos·tae** (kos′tă, - tē). **1.** [TA]. Costela [I-XII]. SIN rib [I-XII]. **2.** Bastão basal; uma organela de sustentação interna, semelhante a um bastão, que corre ao longo da base da membrana ondulante de certos parasitas flagelados, como o *Trichomonas.* SIN basal rod. [L.]
  c. cervica′lis [TA], costela cervical. SIN cervical rib.
  cos′tae fluctuan′tes [XI-XII], costelas flutuantes. SIN floating ribs [XI-XII], em rib [I-XII].
  cos′tae fluitan′tes, costelas flutuantes. SIN floating ribs [XI-XII], em rib [I-XII].
  c. lumbalis [TA], c. lombar. SIN lumbar rib.
  c. prima [I] [TA], primeira costela. SIN first rib [I].
  cos′tae spu′riae [VII-XII] [TA]. Costelas falsas. SIN false ribs, em rib [I-XII].
  cos′tae ve′rae [I-VII] [TA]. Costelas verdadeiras. SIN true ribs [I-VII], em rib [I-XII].
cos·tal (kos′tăl). Costal; relativo a uma costela.
cos·tal·gia (kos - tal′jē - ă). Costalgia. SIN pleurodynia. [L. *costa,* costela, + G. *algos,* dor]
cos·tec·to·my (kos - tek′tō - mē). Costectomia; excisão de uma costela. [L. *costa,* costela, + G. *ektomē,* excisão]
Costen, James B., otolaringologista norte-americano, 1895–1962. VER C. *syndrome.*
cos·ti·car·ti·lage (kos - ti - kar′ti - lij). Cartilagem costal. SIN costal cartilage.
cos·ti·form (kos′ti - fōrm). Costiforme; em forma de costela. [L. *costa,* costela, + *forma,* forma]
cos·tive (kos′tiv). Constipante; relativo a, ou que causa, constipação. [contração do L. *constipo,* comprimir]
cos·tive·ness (kos′tiv - ness). Constipação. SIN constipation.
△ **costo-.** As costelas. [L. *costa,* costela]
cos·to·cen·tral (kos - tō - sen′trăl). Costocentral. SIN costovertebral.
cos·to·chon·dral (kos - tō - kon′drăl). Costocondral; relativo às cartilagens costais. SIN chondrocostal.
cos·to·chon·dri·tis (kos′tō - kon - dri′tis). Costocondrite; inflamação de uma ou mais cartilagens costais, caracterizada por dor à palpação local e dor na parede torácica anterior que pode irradiar-se, porém sem o edema local típico da síndrome de Tietze. SIN costal chondritis. [costo- + G. *chondros,* cartilagem, + *-itis,* inflamação]
cos·to·cla·vic·u·lar (kos - tō - klă - vik′u - lăr). Costoclavicular; relativo às costelas e à clavícula.
cos·to·cor·a·coid (kos - tō - kōr′ă - koyd). Costocoracóide; relativo às costelas e ao processo coracóide da escápula.
cos·to·gen·ic (kos - tō - jen′ik). Costogênico; originado de uma costela.
cos·to·in·fe·ri·or (kos - tō - in - fēr′ē - ōr). Costoinferior; relativo às costelas inferiores.
cos·to·scap·u·lar (kos - tō - skap′u - lăr). Costoescapular; relativo às costelas e à escápula.
cos·to·sca·pu·la·ris (kos - tō - skap - u - lā′ris). Costoescapular. SIN serratus anterior (*muscle*).
cos·to·ster·nal (kos - tō - ster′năl). Costoesternal; relativo às costelas e ao esterno.
cos·to·ster·no·plas·ty (kos - tō - ster′nō - plas - tē). Costoesternoplastia; cirurgia para corrigir uma malformação da parede torácica anterior. [costo- + G. *sternon,* tórax, + *plastos,* formado]
cos·to·su·pe·ri·or (kos - tō - soo - pēr′ē - ōr). Costo-superior; relativo às costelas superiores.
cos·to·tome (kos′tō - tōm). Cóstotomo; instrumento, bisturi ou tesoura para cortar uma costela.
cos·tot·o·my (kos - tot′ō - mē). Costotomia; divisão de uma costela. [costo- + G. *tomē,* corte]

cos·to·trans·verse (kos-tō-trans-vers′). Costotransverso; relativo às costelas e aos processos transversais das vértebras que se articulam com elas. SIN transversocostal.

cos·to·trans·ver·sec·to·my (kos′tō-tranz-ver-sek′tō-mē). Costotransversectomia; excisão de uma porção proximal de uma costela e do processo transverso articulador.

cos·to·ver·te·bral (kos-tō-ver′tĕ-brăl). Costovertebral; relativo às costelas e aos corpos das vértebras torácicas com que se articulam. SIN costocentral, vertebrocostal (1).

cos·to·xi·phoid (kos-tō-zī′foyd). Costoxifóide; relativo às costelas e à cartilagem xifóide do esterno.

co·sub·strate (kō-sŭb′strāt). Co-substrato; o segundo ou outro substrato de uma enzima com múltiplos substratos; amiúde, refere-se especificamente à coenzima.

co·syn·tro·pin (kō-sin-trō′pin). Cosintropina; α^{1-24}- ou β^{1-24}-corticotropina; um agente corticotrófico sintético, que compreende os primeiros 24 resíduos aminoacil do ACTH humano, cuja seqüência é encontrada em várias outras espécies e que retém toda a atividade biológica do ACTH completo; os outros 15 resíduos diferem entre as espécies e conferem propriedades imunológicas específicas. SIN tetracosactide, tetracosactin.

Cotard, Jules, neurologista francês, 1840–1887. VER C. *syndrome*.

co·tar·nine (kō-tar′nēn). Cotarnina; um princípio alcalóide, $C_{12}H_{15}NO_4$, derivado da narcotina por oxidação; um adstringente. [anagrama de *narcotina*]

COTe Abreviatura de cathodal opening tetanus (tétano de abertura do catodo).

co·ti·nine (kō′ti-nēn). Cotinina; um dos principais produtos de desintoxicação da nicotina; eliminada rápida e completamente pelos rins. [anagrama de *nicotina*]

co·trans·la·tion·al (kō′tranz-lā′shun-ăl). Qualquer processo que envolva a maturação ou oferta de uma proteína que ocorre durante o processo de tradução.

co·trans·port (kō-trans′pōrt). Co-transporte; o transporte de uma substância através de uma membrana, acoplado ao transporte simultâneo de outra substância através da mesma membrana na mesma direção.

Cotte, Gaston, cirurgião francês, 1879–1951. VER C. *operation*.

Cotton, Frank A., químico norte-americano, *1930. VER C. *effect*.

cot·ton (kot′ŭn). Algodão; o revestimento branco, fofo e fibroso das sementes de uma planta do gênero *Gossypium* (família Malvaceae); amplamente usado em curativos cirúrgicos. [Árabe *qútun*]

absorbent c., a. absorvente; algodão do qual foi extraído todo o material gorduroso, de forma que ele absorve líquidos rapidamente.

purified c., a. purificado; algodão absorvente no qual os pêlos da semente de variedades de *Gossypium* e outras espécies afins são submetidos a remoção de impurezas aderidas, retirada da substância gordurosa, descoloramento e esterilização; usado em absorventes internos, tampões, etc.

soluble gun c., algodão-pólvora solúvel. SIN pyroxylin.

styptic c., a. estíptico; algodão absorvente umedecido com uma solução diluída de cloreto férrico e, depois, dessecado; aplicado localmente como hemostático.

cot·ton·pox (kot′ŭn-poks). Nome obsoleto para *variola* minor.

cot·ton·seed oil (kot′ŭn-sēd). Óleo de semente de algodão; o óleo fixo refinado obtido da semente de plantas cultivadas de diversas variedades de *Gossypium hirsutum* ou de outras espécies de *Gossypium* (família Malvaceae); um solvente.

Cotunnius (Cotugno), Domenico, anatomista italiano, 1736–1822. VER C. *aqueduct, canal, liquid, space: aqueductus* cotunnii; *liquor* cotunnii.

cot·y·le (kot′i-lē). Cótilo. 1. Qualquer estrutura em forma de cálice. 2. SIN acetabulum. [G. *kotylē*, qualquer coisa oca, a escavação ou encaixe de uma articulação]

cot·y·le·don (kot-i-lē′don). Cotilédone. 1. VER maternal c., fetal c. 2. Em vegetais, uma folha seminal, a primeira folha a nascer da semente. 3. Uma unidade placentária. VER maternal c. [G. *kotylēdon*, qualquer cavidade em forma de cálice]

fetal c., c. fetal; uma unidade da placenta fetal suprida pelos vasos de uma vilosidade-tronco; pode haver vários desses cotilédones entre dois septos placentários; tradicionalmente denominado cotilédone dos embriologistas.

maternal c., c. materno; uma unidade da placenta constituída de células trofoblásticas, tecido fibroso e vasos sanguíneos abundantes, que é visível macroscopicamente na superfície materna como um lobo de formato irregular circunscrito por uma fenda profunda e constituído de uma vilosidade-tronco com numerosas vilosidades ramificadas livres e vilosidades de ancoragem; os vasos placentários na placa coriônica suprem a vilosidade-tronco e seus ramos, permitindo a troca gasosa e metabólica através da camada trofoblástica com sangue materno no espaço interviloso; tradicionalmente denominado cotilédone dos médicos.

Cot·y·lo·gon·i·mus (kot-i-lō-gon′i-mŭs). Grupo de trematódeos heterofídeos, agora apropriadamente incluídos no gênero *Heterophyes*. [G. *kotylē*, cálice, + *gonimos*, produtivo]

cot·y·loid (kot′i-loyd). Cotilóide. 1. Em forma de cálice; caliciforme. 2. Relativo à cavidade cotilóide ou acetábulo. [G. *kotylē*, pequeno cálice, + *eidos*, aparência]

cough (kawf). 1. Tosse; passagem explosiva súbita de ar através da glote, que ocorre imediatamente à abertura da glote antes fechada, excitada por irritação mecânica ou química da traquéia ou dos brônquios, ou por compressão de estruturas adjacentes. 2. Tossir; forçar o ar através da glote por uma série de esforços respiratórios. [ecóico]

aneurysmal c., t. aneurismática; tosse causada por compressão do nervo laríngeo recorrente ou das outras estruturas próximas por um aneurisma aórtico.

brassy c., t. metálica; tosse em latido, metálica, alta, associada ao edema subglótico.

habit c., t. habitual; tosse persistente causada por um tique ou por causas psicológicas.

privet c., t. do alfeneiro; tosse alérgica observada na China durante os meses de maio e junho, supostamente causada por inalação do pólen de uma espécie de alfeneiro (*Lingustrum*); é análoga à febre do louro observada na Nova Inglaterra.

reflex c., t. reflexa; tosse excitada reflexamente por irritação em alguma parte distante, como a orelha ou o estômago.

weaver's c., t. do tecelão; termo usado para tosse, dispnéia e sensação de constricção do tórax, observada em pessoas que trabalham com fios embolorados.

whooping c., coqueluche. SIN pertussis.

cou·lomb (C, Q) (koo-lom′). Coulomb; a unidade de carga elétrica, igual a 3×10^9 unidades eletrostáticas; a quantidade de eletricidade fornecida por uma corrente de 1 A em 1 s, igual a 1/96.485 faraday. [CA de *Coulomb*, físico francês, 1736–1806]

cou·mar·a·none (koo-mar′ă-nōn). Cumaranona; $3(2H)$-benzofuranona; a base de muitos produtos vegetais, p. ex., aurona.

cou·mar·ic an·hy·dride (koo-mā′rik). Anidrido cumárico. SIN coumarin.

cou·ma·rin (koo′mă-rin). Cumarina. 1. Termo descritivo geral aplicado aos anticoagulantes e outras substâncias derivadas do dicumarol, um componente da fava-de-cheiro (fava-de-tonca, cumaru). 2. Um princípio neutro aromático obtido da fava-de-cheiro, *Dypterix odorata*, e produzido sinteticamente a partir do aldeído salicílico; é usado para disfarçar odores desagradáveis. SIN coumaric anhydride, cumarin. [*coumarou*, nome nativo da fava-de-cheiro]

cou·met·a·rol (koo-met′ă-rol). Cumetarol; um anticoagulante oral. SIN cumetharol, cumethoxaethane.

Councilman, William T., patologista norte-americano, 1854–1933. VER C. *body*.

Coun·cil·ma·nia (kown-sil-man′ē-ă). Termo genérico obsoleto para um grupo de amebas agora reconhecidas como *Entamoeba*. [W. *Councilman*]

coun·sel·ing (kown′sel-ing). Aconselhamento; relação profissional e atividade na qual uma pessoa procura ajudar outra a compreender e resolver seus problemas de ajuste; o fornecimento de conselhos, opiniões e instruções para orientar o julgamento ou a conduta de outra pessoa. VER psychotherapy. [L. *consilium*, deliberação]

genetic c., a. genético; o processo pelo qual um especialista em distúrbios genéticos fornece informações sobre o risco e o ônus clínico de um distúrbio ou distúrbios, a pacientes ou parentes em famílias com distúrbios genéticos, como uma ajuda para a tomada de decisões informadas e responsáveis sobre casamento, crianças, diagnóstico precoce e prognóstico.

marital c., a. conjugal; o processo pelo qual um conselheiro treinado ajuda casais a resolver problemas que surgem e perturbam o relacionamento; o marido e a mulher são atendidos pelo mesmo conselheiro em sessões separadas e conjuntas que enfocam problemas familiares imediatos.

pastoral c., a. pastoral; o uso de métodos psicoterápicos por membros do clero, membros de uma comunidade religiosa e/ou terapeutas leigos com paroquianos que buscam ajuda em problemas pessoais.

count (kownt). 1. Contagem; avaliação, enumeração ou cálculo. 2. Contar; enumerar ou avaliar.

Addis c., c. de Addis; enumeração quantitativa das hemácias, leucócitos e cilindros em uma amostra de urina de 12 horas; usada para acompanhar o progresso de uma doença renal conhecida.

Arneth c., c. de Arneth; a distribuição percentual de neutrófilos polimorfonucleares, baseada no número de lobos nos núcleos (de 1 a 5). VER TAMBÉM Arneth *index*.

blood c., c. sanguínea; hemograma. VER *blood* count.

CD4/CD8 c., c. CD4/CD8; a proporção entre linfócitos T auxiliares-indutores e linfócitos T citotóxicos-supressores no sangue periférico. A análise do subgrupo de células T é realizada por citometria de fluxo dos linfócitos após incubação com anticorpos monoclonais, marcados de forma fluorescente, contra o antígeno de superfície CD4 encontrado nas células T auxiliares-indutoras e no antígeno de superfície CD8 encontrado em células T citotóxicas-supressoras. Em pessoas saudáveis, a razão CD4/CD8 varia entre 1,6 e 2,2.

epidermal ridge c., c. de cristas epidérmicas; índice da freqüência de poros sudoríparos nas extremidades dos dedos por enumeração ao longo de uma série de linhas definidas arbitrariamente; um exemplo clássico de um traço galtoniano determinado quase exclusivamente por fatores genéticos.

filament-nonfilament c., c. filamento–não-filamento; contagem diferencial do número de neutrófilos que exibem divisão nuclear e aqueles que não exibem essa divisão.

total cell c., c. de células totais; número de células em uma determinada área ou volume.

viable cell c., c. de células viáveis; número de células em uma determinada área ou volume que estão se desenvolvendo.

count·er (kown′ter). Contador; um dispositivo que conta, geralmente cintilações.

automated differential leukocyte c., c. automático diferencial de leucócitos; instrumento que usa imageamento digital ou técnicas citoquímicas para diferenciar leucócitos.

electronic cell c., c. eletrônico de células; contador automático de células do sangue no qual as células que atravessam uma abertura alteram a resistência e são contadas como pulsos de voltagem, ou no qual as células que atravessam uma célula de fluxo defletem a luz; alguns tipos de contadores são capazes de realizar múltiplas medidas simultâneas em cada amostra de sangue; p. ex., contagem de leucócitos, contagem de hemácias, hemoglobina, hematócrito e índices eritrocitários.

Geiger-Müller c., c. Geiger-Müller; instrumento para medir a radioatividade por contagem da emissão de partículas radioativas; consiste em um cilindro metálico, negativamente carregado, em um tubo contendo um fio delgado, positivamente carregado, em seu centro; as radiações produzem ionização das moléculas de gás entre o cilindro e o fio, e resultam em uma descarga elétrica independente da energia da partícula ou do raio incidente.

proportional c., c. proporcional; um contador de Geiger-Müller que opera na faixa de voltagem e em condições nas quais a altura do pulso é proporcional à energia das partículas ou dos raios contados, tornando assim possível a discriminação entre partículas ou raios de diferentes energias.

scintillation c., c. de cintilação; instrumento usado para a detecção de radioatividade; a radiação é absorvida por um cintilador (um cristal ou um componente, como o POPOP, em solução) que emite pequenos lampejos de luz detectados por um fotocatodo. A emissão de elétrons resultante é amplificada por um fotomultiplicador e por um amplificador. SIN scintillometer, spinthariscope.

well c., cristal de cintilação com um orifício frontal para receber uma pequena amostra, mais detector e componentes eletrônicos associados.

whole-body c., c. de corpo inteiro; proteção e instrumentação, geralmente envolvendo mais de um detector, destinadas a avaliar a carga total do corpo de vários nuclídeos emissores de raios gama.

♻ **counter-.** Contra; oposto. VER TAMBÉM contra-. [L. *contra*, contra]

count·er·bal·anc·ing (kown′ter - bal′an - sing). Contrabalanceamento; um procedimento, em pesquisa comportamental, para distribuir influências indesejadas, mas inevitáveis, igualmente entre as diferentes condições experimentais ou indivíduos.

count·er·con·di·tion·ing (kown′ter - kon - dish′un - ing). Contracondicionamento; qualquer uma de um grupo de técnicas específicas de terapia comportamental, na qual é introduzida uma segunda resposta condicionada (p. ex., aproximar-se de uma cobra ou, até mesmo, tocá-la) com o objetivo expresso de contrapor-se ou anular uma resposta previamente condicionada ou aprendida (medo e evitação de cobras).

count·er·cur·rent (kown′ter - ker′ent). Contracorrente. **1.** Que flui em uma direção oposta. **2.** Uma corrente que flui em direção oposta à de outra.

count·er·cur·rent ex·chang·er. Cambiador contracorrente; um sistema no qual o calor ou as substâncias químicas se difundem passivamente através de uma membrana que separa as duas correntes, de forma que, em cada extremidade, o líquido que deixa um lado da membrana se assemelha, em temperatura ou composição, ao líquido que entra na outra; p. ex., as veias acompanhantes nos braços servem como cambiador contracorrente, com o sangue arterial servindo para reaquecer o sangue venoso mais frio.

count·er·cur·rent mul·ti·pli·er. Multiplicador de contracorrente; um sistema no qual a energia é usada para transportar material através de uma membrana que separa dois tubos de contracorrente unidos em uma extremidade, tomando a forma de um grampo de cabelo; por esse meio, pode-se obter uma concentração no líquido na curva do trampo, relativa aos líquidos de influxo e efluxo, que é muito maior do que aquela que o mecanismo de transporte produziria entre os dois lados da membrana em qualquer ponto; p. ex., as alças dos néfrons na medula renal atuam como multiplicadores de contracorrente.

count·er·die (kown′ter - dī). Contramolde; a imagem invertida de um molde, geralmente feita de um metal mais macio e com ponto de fusão mais baixo do que o do molde.

count·er·ex·ten·sion (kown′ter - eks - ten′shun). Contra-extensão. SIN countertraction.

count·er·im·mu·no·e·lec·tro·pho·re·sis (kown′ter - im′ū - nō - ē - lek′trō - fōr - ē′ - sis). Contraimunoeletroforese; uma modificação da imunoeletroforese na qual o antígeno (p. ex., soro contendo vírus da hepatite B) é colocado em depressões na placa de ágar-gel em direção ao catodo, e o antisoro é colocado em depressões em direção ao anodo; antígeno e anticorpo, movendo-se em direções opostas, formam precipitados na área entre as células onde se encontram em concentrações de proporções ideais.

count·er·in·ci·sion (kown′ter - in - sizh′un). Contra-incisão; uma segunda incisão na região de uma incisão primária destinada a aliviar a tensão do fechamento primário.

count·er·in·vest·ment (kown′ter - in - vest′ment). Contra-investimento. SIN anticathexis.

count·er·ir·ri·tant (kown - ter - ir′i - tan). Contra-irritante. **1.** Agente que causa irritação ou leve inflamação da pele a fim de aliviar sintomas de um processo inflamatório profundo. **2.** Relativo a, ou que produz, contra-irritação. Aumenta o fluxo sanguíneo para a área afetada.

count·er·ir·ri·ta·tion (kown′ter - ir - i - tā′shun). Contra-irritação; irritação ou inflamação leve (eritema, vesicação ou pustulação) da pele excitada a fim de aliviar sintomas de uma inflamação das estruturas mais profundas.

count·er·o·pen·ing (kown′ter - ō - pen - ing). Contra-abertura; uma segunda abertura, feita na parte inferior de um abscesso ou outra cavidade contendo líquido, que não está drenando satisfatoriamente através de uma abertura prévia. SIN contraaperture, counterpuncture.

count·er·pho·bic (kown - ter - fō′bik). Contrafóbico. **1.** Designa um estado de preferência real, por parte de uma pessoa fóbica, pela mesma situação que a pessoa teme. **2.** Oposto ao impulso fóbico, como no domínio contrafóbico de uma ação temida por meio da realização repetida da ação.

count·er·pul·sa·tion (kown′ter - pul - sā′shun). Contrapulsação; uma forma de ajudar o coração insuficiente por remoção automática do sangue arterial imediatamente antes e no decorrer da ejeção ventricular e sua devolução à circulação durante a diástole; um cateter com balão é introduzido na aorta e ativado por um mecanismo automático deflagrado pelo ECG.

intra-aortic balloon c., c. por balão intra-aórtico; insuflação e desinsuflação rítmica de um balão fixado a um cateter colocado na aorta distal à válvula aórtica para facilitar a ejeção durante a sístole e para limitar a regurgitação durante a diástole pela aplicação apropriada de pressões. Geralmente um tratamento de emergência para o choque cardiogênico ou para a angina intratável.

count·er·punc·ture (kown′ter - punk - choor). Contrapunção. SIN counteropening.

count·er·shock (kown′ter - shok). Contrachoque; um choque elétrico aplicado ao coração para interromper um distúrbio de seu ritmo.

cont·er·stain (kown′ter - stān). Contracorante; um segundo corante de outra cor, que possui afinidades por outros tecidos, células ou partes de células diferentes dos que captaram o corante primário, usado para tornar mais distintas as partes que captaram o primeiro corante.

count·er·trac·tion (kown - ter - trak′shun). Contratração; a resistência, ou movimento contrário, à tração de um membro: p. ex., no caso de tração da perna, a contratração pode ser realizada elevando-se os pés da cama de forma que o peso do corpo faça uma tração contra o peso preso ao membro. SIN counterextension.

count·er·trans·fer·ence (kown′ter - trans - fer′ens). Contratransferência; em psicanálise, a transferência de necessidades emocionais e conflitos das experiências passadas do analista (freqüentemente inconsciente) para o paciente ou as respostas emocionais atuais do analista à manifestação de transferência do paciente.

count·er·trans·port (kown - ter - tranz′pōrt). Contratransporte; o transporte de uma substância através de uma membrana, associado ao transporte simultâneo de outra substância através da mesma membrana na direção oposta.

coup de sa·bre (koo - dē - sahb′). Esclerodermia linear encontrada no couro cabeludo com alopecia cicatricial, na face ou na fronte. [Fr. golpe de sabre]

cou·ple (kŭ′pl). Copular; realizar coito; diz-se particularmente de animais inferiores.

cou·pling (kŭp′ling). Acoplamento. **1.** Geralmente resultante do pareamento repetido de um batimento sinusal normal com uma extra-sístole ventricular. **2.** VER coupling *phase*. **3.** Uma condição na qual um ou mais produtos de uma reação são os reagentes (ou substratos) subseqüentes de uma segunda reação.

constant c., acoplamento constante. SIN fixed c.

fixed c., acoplamento fixo; no qual são observadas várias extra-sístoles e o intervalo entre elas e o batimento normal precedente é constante. SIN constant c.

variable c., acoplamento variável; no qual são observadas várias extra-sístoles e o intervalo entre cada uma delas e o batimento sinusal precedente varia.

Courvoisier, Ludwig G., cirurgião francês, 1843–1918. VER C. *law, sign, gallbladder*.

cou·vade (koo - vahd′). Costume primitivo, em determinadas culturas, segundo o qual um homem apresenta dores de trabalho de parto quando sua mulher está em trabalho de parto, submetendo-se depois aos mesmos tabus e ritos de purificação. [Fr. *couver*, chocar]

Couvelaire, Alexandre, obstetra francês, 1873–1948. VER C. *uterus*.

cou·ver·cle (koo - ver′kl). Termo raramente usado para designar um coágulo externo, principalmente um coágulo sanguíneo formado no meio extravascular. [Fr. cobertura, tampa]

co·va·lent (kō - vāl′ent). Covalente; designa uma ligação interatômica caracterizada pelo compartilhamento de 2, 4 ou 6 elétrons.

cov·er·age. Cobertura; alcance; medida da extensão com que os serviços prestados cobrem a potencial necessidade desses serviços em uma comunidade;

aplicado especificamente a serviços como imunização nos países em desenvolvimento.

cov·er·ing (kŭv′er - ing). Cobertura; revestimento; uma camada circundante; algo que cobre ou encerra, formando uma camada externa. VER TAMBÉM tunica.
c.'s of spermatic cord, túnicas do cordão espermático; revestimentos do cordão espermático, incluindo as fáscias espermáticas externa e interna, músculo cremaster e fáscia cremastérica. SIN tunicae funiculi spermatici.

cov·er·slip (kŭv′er - slip). Lamínula. SIN cover glass.

cow (kow). **1.** Vaca (gíria); gerador de isótopos de vida curta baseado na decantação sucessiva ou em outro modo de separação ("ordenha") de um produto (filho) radioativo de vida curta de um genitor de vida mais longa; p. ex., Tc^{99m} de Mo^{99}, In^{113m} de Sn^{113}. **2.** A fêmea madura do gado doméstico (gênero *Bos*); também a fêmea madura de alguns outros animais como búfalo, elefante e baleia.

Cowden. Sobrenome da família em que a condição subseqüentemente conhecida como doença de Cowden (Cowden *disease*) foi descrita pela primeira vez.

Cowdry, Edmund Vincent, citologista norte-americano, 1888–1975. VER C. type A inclusion *bodies*, em *body*, type B inclusion *bodies*, em *body*.

cowl. VER caul.

Cowling rule. Regra de Cowling; ver em rule.

Cowper, William, anatomista inglês, 1666–1709. VER C. *cyst, gland, ligament*.

cow·per·i·an (kow - pēr′ē - an). Cowperiano; relativo a, ou descrito por, Cowper.

Cox, H.R., bacteriologista norte-americano, *1907.

coxa, gen. e pl. **cox·ae** (kok′să, -sē). [TA]. Coxa. **1.** SIN hip (1). **2.** SIN hip *joint*. [L.]

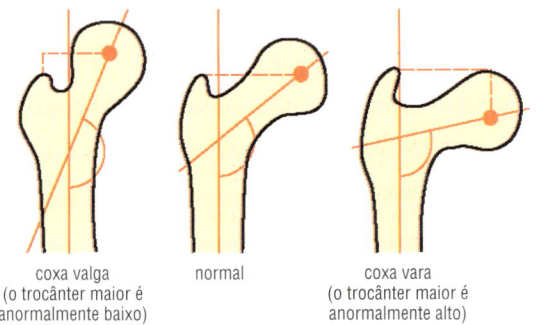

coxa valga, coxa vara: várias configurações do ângulo da articulação coxofemoral

coxa valga (o trocânter maior é anormalmente baixo) — normal — coxa vara (o trocânter maior é anormalmente alto)

c. adduc'ta, c. aduzida; c. vara. SIN c. vara.
false c. va'ra, c. vara falsa; aproximação da cabeça do fêmur da diáfise do fêmur, causada não por deformidade do colo do fêmur, mas pela curvatura da diáfise.
c. mag'na, c. magna; aumento e, freqüentemente, deformação da cabeça do fêmur; geralmente se refere a uma seqüela da doença de Legg-Calvé-Perthes ou osteoartrite.
c. pla'na, c. plana. SIN Legg-Calvé-Perthes *disease*.
c. val'ga, c. valga; alteração do ângulo produzido pelo eixo do colo do fêmur com o eixo da diáfise do fêmur, de forma que o ângulo é maior que 135°; o colo do fêmur se encontra em uma relação mais próxima da linha reta com a diáfise do fêmur.
c. va'ra, c. vara; alteração do ângulo formado pelo eixo do colo do fêmur com o eixo da diáfise do fêmur, de forma que o ângulo é menor que 135°; o colo do fêmur torna-se mais horizontal. SIN c. adducta.
c. va'ra lux'ans, c. vara com luxação; c. vara com luxação da cabeça do fêmur.

cox·al·gia (koks - al′jē - ă). Coxalgia. SIN coxodynia. [L. *coxa*, quadril, + G. *algos*, dor]

Cox·i·el·la (kok - sē - el′ă). Gênero de bactérias filtráveis (ordem Rickettsiales) contendo pequenas células Gram-negativas, pleomórficas, bacilares ou cocóides, observadas no meio intracelular no citoplasma de células infectadas, e, possivelmente, no meio extracelular em carrapatos infectados. Esses microrganismos não foram cultivados em meios acelulares; são parasitas em homens e em outros animais; a espécie típica é *C. burnetii*.
C. burnet'ii, espécie bacteriana que causa febre Q em seres humanos; é mais resistente que outras riquétsias e pode ser eliminada através de aerossóis, bem como vetores vivos. Pneumonia aguda e endocardite crônica também estão associadas a essa espécie. A espécie típica do gênero *Coxiella*.

cox·i·tis (koks - ī′tis). Coxite; coxartria; inflamação do quadril.

cox·o·dyn·ia (koks - ō - din′ē - ă). Coxalgia; dor na articulação coxofemoral. SIN coxalgia. [L. *coxa*, quadril, + G. *odynē*, dor]

cox·o·fem·o·ral (kok - sō - fem′o - răl). Coxofemoral; relativo ao osso do quadril e ao fêmur.

cox·o·tu·ber·cu·lo·sis (koks′ō - too - ber - kū - lō′sis). Coxotuberculose; tuberculose da articulação coxofemoral.

cox·sack·ie·vi·rus (kok - sak′ē - vī′rŭs). Vírus Coxsackie; grupo de picornavírus, incluídos no gênero Enterovirus, de formato icosaédrico, estáveis em pH ácido e com cerca de 28 nm de diâmetro, causando miosite, paralisia e morte em camundongos jovens, sendo responsáveis por várias doenças nos seres humanos, embora infecções inaparentes sejam comuns. São divididos antigenicamente em dois grupos, A e B, cada qual incluindo vários tipos sorológicos, p. ex., Enterovirus Coxsackie A1 a 24 e Enterovirus Coxsackie B1 a 6. Os vírus tipo A causam herpangina humana e doença mão-pé-e-boca; os vírus tipo B causam pleurodinia epidêmica; ambos os tipos de vírus podem causar meningite asséptica, miocardite e pericardite, além de diabetes juvenil de início agudo. [*Coxsackie*, N.Y., onde foi isolado pela primeira vez]

c.p. Abreviatura de chemically pure (quimicamente puro).

CPAP Abreviatura de continuous positive airway *pressure* (pressão positiva contínua nas vias aéreas).

CPEO Acrônimo para chronic progressive external *ophthalmoplegia* (oftalmoplegia externa progressiva crônica).

C-pep·tide. Peptídeo C; a cadeia de 30 aminoácidos que une as cadeias A e B de insulina na pró-insulina; removido na conversão da pró-insulina em insulina. SIN C chain.

CPK Abreviatura de *creatine* phosphokinase (creatinofosfoquinase).

CPM Abreviatura de continuous passive *motion* (movimentação passiva contínua).

cpm Abreviatura de counts per minute (contagens por minuto).

CPPD Abreviatura de calcium pyrophosphate deposition *disease* (doença por deposição de pirofosfato de cálcio).

CPPV Abreviatura de continuous positive pressure *ventilation* (ventilação com pressão positiva contínua).

CPR Abreviatura de cardiopulmonary *resuscitation* (reanimação cardiopulmonar).

cps Abreviatura de cycles per second (ciclos por segundo).

CR Abreviatura de conditioned *reflex* (reflexo condicionado); crown-rump *length* (comprimento cabeça–nádega); computed *radiography* (radiografia computadorizada).

Cr 1. Símbolo do cromo. **2.** Abreviatura de creatinina.

crab (krab). **1.** Caranguejo; um crustáceo, com muitas variedades comestíveis. **2.** Um inseto, o piolho do púbis, *Pthirus pubis*.

Crabtree, Herbert G., médico e bioquímico inglês do século XX. VER C. *effect*.

crack (krak). **1.** Fenda; fissura. **2.** VER crack *cocaine*. [gíria]
lacquer c.'s, fissuras na membrana de Bruch (Bruch *membrane*) observadas na miopia patológica.

crac·kle (krak′l). Estertor. SIN rale. [echoic]

cra·dle (krā′dl). Armação; estrutura usada para evitar que a roupa de cama entre em contato com um paciente. [I. M. *cradel*]

Crafoord, Clarence, cirurgião torácico sueco, 1899–1984. VER C. *clamp*.

Craig·ia (krā′gē - ă). Termo genérico obsoleto para um grupo de amebas agora reconhecidas como *Entamoeba*. [C. Craig]

Cramer, Friedrich, cirurgião alemão, 1847–1903. VER C. wire *splint*.

cramp (kramp). Cãibra. **1.** Espasmo muscular doloroso causado por contração tetânica prolongada. **2.** Espasmo muscular localizado relacionado ao uso ocupacional, qualificado de acordo com a ocupação do paciente; p. ex., c. da costureira, c. do escritor. [I.M. *crampe*, do Fr. ant., do Alemão]
heat c.'s, cãibras por calor; espasmos musculares induzidos por grande esforço em calor intenso, acompanhados por dor considerável; algumas vezes relacionados a deficiência de sal, hiperventilação ou abuso de álcool. SIN myalgia thermica.
intermittent c., c. intermitente. SIN tetany.
miner's c.'s, cãibras dos mineiros; cãibras causadas por perda excessiva de sal através da transpiração. SIN stoker's c.'s.
musician's c., c. dos músicos; uma distonia ocupacional que afeta aqueles que tocam instrumentos musicais, sendo geralmente denominada de acordo com o instrumento tocado.
pianist's c., piano-player's c., c. do pianista; distonia ocupacional que afeta os músculos dos dedos das mãos e antebraços em pianistas.
seamstress's c., c. da costureira; uma distonia ocupacional que ocorre nos dedos das mãos das mulheres que costuram.
shaving c., c. do barbeiro; distonia ocupacional que afeta as mãos e os dedos das mãos dos barbeiros.
stoker's c.'s, cãibras do foguista. SIN miner's c.'s.
tailor's c., c. do alfaiate; uma distonia ocupacional que afeta os antebraços e as mãos dos alfaiates.
typist's c., c. do datilógrafo; distonia ocupacional que afeta principalmente os músculos flexores longos das mãos dos datilógrafos.
violinist's c., c. do violinista; distonia ocupacional que acomete os dedos da mão que dedilha, ou, às vezes, do braço que segura o arco, em violinistas.

waiter's c., c. do garçom; distonia ocupacional caracterizada por espasmo dos músculos das costas e do braço dominante em garçons.

watchmaker's c., c. do relojoeiro; distonia ocupacional caracterizada por espasmo do músculo orbicular da pálpebra por manter a lente presa ao olho e espasmo dos músculos da mão por realizar os movimentos delicados do conserto de relógios.

writer's c., c. do escritor; distonia ocupacional que afeta principalmente os músculos do polegar e dos dois dedos adjacentes da mão que escreve, induzida pelo uso excessivo de um instrumento de escrita. SIN dysgraphia (2), graphospasm, scrivener's palsy.

Crampton, Charles Ward, médico norte-americano, *1877. VER C. *test*.
Crampton, Sir Philip, cirurgião irlandês, 1777–1858. VER C. *line, muscle*.
Crandall, Barbara F., médica norte-americana. VER Crandall *syndrome*.
♻ **crani-.** VER cranio-.
cra·nia (krā′nē-ă). Plural de cranium.
cra·ni·ad (krā′nē-ad). Cranial; situado mais próximo da cabeça em relação a um ponto de referência específico; oposto a caudal. VER TAMBÉM superior.
cra·ni·al (krā′nē-ăl). Cranial; craniano. **1** [TA]. Cranial, relativo ao crânio ou cabeça. SIN cranialis [TA], cephalic. VER TAMBÉM cephalad. **2.** SIN superior (2).
cra·ni·a·lis (krā-nē-ā′lis). [TA]. Cranial. SIN cranial (1).
cra·ni·am·phit·o·my (krā-nē-am-fit′ō-mē). Cranianfitomia; uma operação de descompressão na qual toda a circunferência da calvária é dividida. [G. *kranion*, crânio, + *amphi*, ao redor, + *tomē*, corte]
Cra·ni·a·ta (krā-nē-ā′tă). Os vertebrados. SIN Vertebrata. [L. Mediev. *cranium*, do G. *kranion*, crânio]
cra·ni·ec·to·my (krā-nē-ek′tō-mē). Craniectomia; excisão de uma parte do crânio, sem substituição do osso, p. ex., subtemporal ou suboccipital. [G. *kranion*, crânio, + *ektomē*, excisão]
 linear c., c. linear; excisão de uma tira de crânio contendo uma sutura prematuramente fundida.
♻ **cranio-, crani-.** O crânio. Cf. cerebro-. [G. *kranion*, crânio]
cra·ni·o·au·ral (krā′nē-ō-aw′răl). Cranioauricular; relativo ao crânio e à orelha.
cra·ni·o·cele (krā′nē-ō-sēl). Craniocele. SIN encephalocele. [cranio- + G. *kēlē*, hérnia]
cra·ni·o·ce·re·bral (krā′nē-ō-ser′ē-brăl). Craniocerebral; relativo ao crânio e ao cérebro.
cra·ni·o·cla·sia, cra·ni·o·cla·sis (krā-nē-ō-klā′sē-ă, krā-nē-ok′lă-sis). Cranioclasia; operação antigamente usada para esmagar o crânio fetal em casos de distocia. [cranio- + G. *klasis*, quebra]
cra·ni·o·clast (krā′nē-ō-klast). Cranioclasto; instrumento semelhante a um fórceps forte usado antigamente para esmagar e extrair a cabeça fetal após perfuração. [cranio- + G. *klaō*, quebrar em pedaços]
cra·ni·o·clei·do·dys·os·to·sis (krā′nē-ō-klī′dō-dis-os-tō′sis). Craniocleidodisostose. SIN cleidocranial dysostosis. [cranio- + G. *kleis*, clavícula, + dysostosis]
cra·ni·o·did·y·mus (krā′nē-ō-did′i-mŭs). Craniodídimo; gêmeos conjugados com corpos fundidos, mas com duas cabeças. VER conjoined *twins*, em *twin*. [cranio- + G. *didymos*, gêmeo]
cra·ni·o·fa·cial (krā′nē-ō-fā′shăl). Craniofacial; relativo à face e ao crânio.
cra·ni·o·fe·nes·tria (krā′nē-ō-fe-nes′trē-ă). Craniofenestria. SIN craniolacunia. [cranio- + L. *fenestra*, janela]
cra·ni·og·no·my (krā-nē-og′nō-mē). Craniognomia. SIN phrenology. [cranio- + G. *gnōmē*, julgamento]
cra·ni·o·graph (krā′-nē-ō-graf). Craniógrafo; instrumento de desenho para representar em escala os diâmetros e a configuração geral do crânio.
cra·ni·og·ra·phy (krā-nē-og′ră-fē). Craniografia; a arte de representar, por desenhos feitos a partir de medidas, a configuração do crânio e as relações de seus ângulos e pontos craniométricos. [cranio- + G. *graphō*, escrever]
cra·ni·o·la·cu·nia (krā′nē-ō-lă-koo′nē-ă). Craniolacunia; formação incompleta dos ossos da abóbada do crânio fetal, de forma que existem áreas não-ossificadas na calvária. SIN craniofenestria. [cranio- + L. *lacuna*, fenda]
cra·ni·ol·o·gy (krā-nē-ol′ō-jē). Craniologia; a ciência que estuda as variações no tamanho, formato e proporção do crânio, principalmente com as variações que caracterizam as diferentes raças de seres humanos. [cranio- + G. *logos*, estudo]
cra·ni·o·ma·la·cia (krā′nē-ō-mă-lā′shē-ă). Craniomalacia; amolecimento dos ossos do crânio. [cranio- + G. *malakia*, amolecimento]
 circumscribed c., c. circunscrita. SIN craniotabes.
cra·ni·o·me·nin·go·cele (krā′nē-ō-mē-ning′gō-sēl). Craniomeningocele; protrusão das meninges através de um defeito no crânio. [cranio- + G. *mēninx*, membrana, + *kēlē*, hérnia]
cra·ni·om·e·ter (krā-nē-om′ē-ter). Craniômetro; instrumento para medir os diâmetros do crânio.
cra·ni·o·met·ric (krā-nē-ō-met′rik). Craniométrico; relativo à craniometria.
cra·ni·om·e·try (krā-nē-om′ē-trē). Craniometria; medida do crânio seco, após remoção das partes moles, e estudo de sua topografia. [cranio- + G. *metron*, medida]

cra·ni·op·a·gus (krā-nē-op′ă-gŭs). Craniópago; gêmeos conjugados com crânios fundidos. VER conjoined *twins*, em *twin*. VER TAMBÉM janiceps, syncephalus. [cranio- + G. *pagos*, fixo]
 c. occipita′lis, c. occipital; gêmeos conjugados unidos na região occipital do crânio. SIN iniopagus.
 c. parasit′icus, c. parasita; variedade de craniópago na qual um feto tem forma rudimentar e parasita o outro. VER TAMBÉM epicomus.
cra·ni·op·a·thy (krā-nē-op′ă-thē). Craniopatia; qualquer doença dos ossos do crânio. [cranio- + G. *pathos*, sofrimento]
 metabolic c., c. metabólica. SIN Morgagni *syndrome*.
cra·ni·o·pha·ryn·ge·al (krā′nē-ō-fă-rin′jē-ăl). Craniofaríngeo; relativo ao crânio e à faringe.
cra·ni·o·pha·ryn·gi·o·ma (krā′nē-ō-fă-rin-jē-ō′mă). Craniofaringioma; uma neoplasia supra-selar, podendo ser cística, que se desenvolve a partir dos nichos de epitélio derivados da bolsa de Rathke; o padrão histológico, semelhante ao observado em adamantinomas, consiste em nichos de epitélio escamoso limitados por células dispostas radialmente; freqüentemente acompanhado por deposição de cálcio; algumas vezes tem uma arquitetura papilar microscopicamente. SIN Erdheim tumor, pituitary adamantinoma, pituitary ameloblastoma, Rathke pouch tumor, suprasellar cyst. [cranio- + *pharyngio* + -oma]
 ameloblastomatous c., c. ameloblastomatoso; uma forma de craniofaringioma semelhante a um ameloblastoma.
 cystic papillomatous c., c. papilomatoso cístico; uma forma de craniofaringioma caracterizada por grandes cistos dentro dos quais há crescimentos fungiformes irregulares de epitélio escamoso estratificado.
cra·ni·o·phore (krā′nē-ō-fōr). Crânióforo; um aparelho para segurar o crânio enquanto se medem seus ângulos e diâmetros. [cranio- + G. *phoros*, que suporta]
cra·ni·o·plas·ty (krā′nē-ō-plas-tē). Cranioplastia; uma operação para corrigir um defeito do crânio, como perfuração ou enxerto ósseo ou aplicação de material aloplástico. [cranio- + G. *plastos*, formado]
cra·ni·o·punc·ture (krā′nē-ō-pŭnk-choor). Craniopunção; punção do cérebro com fins exploratórios.
cra·ni·or·rha·chid·i·an (krā′nē-ō-ră-kid′ē-an). Craniorraquidiano. SIN craniospinal. [cranio- + G. *rhachis*, coluna vertebral]
cra·ni·or·rha·chis·chi·sis (krā′nē-ō-ră-kis′ki-sis). Craniorraquisquise; malformação congênita grave na qual há fechamento incompleto do crânio e da coluna vertebral. [cranio- + G. *rhachis*, coluna vertebral, + *schisis*, clivagem]
cra·ni·o·sa·cral (krā′nē-ō-sā′krăl). Craniossacral; designa as origens cranial e sacral da divisão parassimpática do sistema nervoso autônomo.
cra·ni·os·chi·sis (krā-nē-os′ki-sis). Cranioquise; malformação congênita na qual há fechamento incompleto do crânio. Geralmente acompanhado por defeito evidente do desenvolvimento do cérebro. [cranio- + G. *schisis*, clivagem]
cra·ni·o·scle·ro·sis (krā′nē-ō-skler-ō′sis). Crânioesclerose; espessamento do crânio. [cranio- + G. *sklēros*, duro, + -*osis*, condição]
cra·ni·os·co·py (krā-nē-os′kō-pē). Cranioscopia; exame do crânio no indivíduo vivo para fins craniométricos ou diagnósticos. [cranio- + G. *skopeō*, ver]
cra·ni·o·spi·nal (krā′nē-ō-spī′năl). Craniospinal; craniorraquidiano; relativo ao crânio e à coluna vertebral. SIN craniorrhachidian.
cra·ni·o·ste·no·sis (krā′nē-ō-sten-ō′sis). Crânioestenose; fechamento prematuro das suturas cranianas que resulta em malformação do crânio. [cranio- + G. *stenōsis*, estreitamento]
cra·ni·os·to·sis (krā′nē-os-tō′sis). Craniostose. SIN craniosynostosis. [cranio- + G. *osteon*, osso, + -*osis*, condição]
cra·ni·o·syn·os·to·sis (krā′nē-ō-sin′os-tō′sis). Craniossinostose; ossificação prematura do crânio e obliteração das suturas. As suturas específicas envolvidas determinam o formato resultante da cabeça malformada. SIN craniostosis.
cra·ni·o·tabes (krā′nē-ō-tā′bēz). Craniotabe; uma doença caracterizada por áreas de adelgaçamento e amolecimento nos ossos do crânio e alargamento das suturas e fontanelas. Geralmente de origem sifilítica ou raquítica. SIN circumscribed craniomalacia. [cranio- + L. *tabes*, debilitante]
cra·ni·o·tome (krā′nē-ō-tōm). Craniótomo; instrumento usado antigamente para perfurar e esmagar a cabeça fetal.
cra·ni·ot·o·my (krā-nē-ot′ō-mē). Craniotomia. **1.** Abertura para o crânio. **2.** Operação usada antigamente para perfuração da cabeça do feto, remoção do conteúdo e compressão do crânio vazio, quando o parto por meio natural era impossível. [cranio- + *tomē*, incisão]
 attached c., c. ligada; craniotomia com um segmento da calvária e tecidos moles fixados virados como um retalho para expor a cavidade craniana. SIN attached cranial section, osteoplastic c.
 detached c., c. livre; craniotomia com secção do crânio separado de suas fixações aos tecidos moles. SIN detached cranial section.
 osteoplastic c., c. osteoplástica. SIN attached c.
cra·ni·o·to·nos·co·py (krā′nē-ō-tō-nos′kō-pē). Craniotonoscopia; percussão auscultatória do crânio. [cranio- + G. *tonos*, tônus, + *skopeō*, examinar]
cra·ni·o·try·pe·sis (krā′nē-ō-trī-pē′sis). Craniotripese; trepanação do crânio. [cranio- + G. *trypēsis*, perfuração]

cra·ni·o·tym·pan·ic (krā′nē - ō - tim - pan′ik). Craniotimpânico; relativo ao crânio e ao ouvido médio.

cra·ni·um, pl. **cra·nia** (krā′nē - ŭm, - ă)[TA]. Crânio; os ossos da cabeça coletivamente. Em um sentido mais limitado, o neurocrânio, a caixa óssea que contém o cérebro, excluindo os ossos da face (viscerocrânio). SIN skull. [L. Mediev. do G. *kranion*]
  c. bif′idum, bifid c., c. bífido. SIN encephalocele.
  c. cerebra'le, cerebral c., c. cerebral. SIN neurocranium.
  c. viscera'le, visceral c., c. visceral. SIN viscerocranium.

crap·u·lent, crap·u·lous (krap′ŭ - lent, - lŭs). Crápula; termo raramente usado para bêbado; devido à intoxicação alcoólica. [L. *crapula*, embriaguez]

crash cart. Carrinho de parada; conjunto móvel de equipamento e suprimentos de emergência com o objetivo de estar imediatamente disponíveis para reanimação. Inclui medicação e também equipamento para desfibrilação, intubação, medicação intravenosa e instituição de acessos centrais.

cras·sa·men·tum (kras - a - men′tŭm). Espessamento. **1.** Termo antigo para coágulo sanguíneo (blood *clot*). **2.** Termo antigo para coagulum. [L. espessura, de *crassus*, espesso]

cra·ter (krā′ter). Cratera; a porção mais deprimida, geralmente central de uma úlcera.

cra·ter·i·form (krā - ter′i - fōrm). Crateriforme; escavado como uma tigela ou um pires. [L. *crater*, tigela, + *forma*, formato]

cra·ter·i·za·tion (krā - ter - i - zā′shŭn). Escavação de tecidos para fins terapêuticos. SIN saucerization.

craw-craw (kraw′kraw). Kra-kra; termo aplicado, na África Ocidental, a uma erupção cutânea papular pruriginosa, que pode causar ulceração; alguns casos são produzidos por *Onchocerca*.

Crawford, Brian H., físico inglês, *1906. VER Stiles-C. *effect*.

craz·ing (krā′zing). Fissuração; em odontologia, o surgimento de pequenas rachaduras na superfície de restaurações plásticas como materiais de enchimento, dentes de dentadura ou bases de dentadura.

cream (krēm). Creme. **1.** A camada superior gordurosa que se forma no leite em repouso ou que é separada dele por centrifugação; contém aproximadamente a mesma quantidade de açúcar e proteína que o leite, mas com 12 a 40% mais gordura. **2.** Qualquer líquido viscoso esbranquiçado semelhante a creme. **3.** Emulsão semi-sólida do tipo óleo em água ou água em óleo, comumente utilizada topicamente. [L. *cremor*, suco espesso, caldo]
  cleansing c., c. de limpeza; uma forma de creme usado para remover impurezas e cosméticos da pele.
  cold c., emulsão de água em óleo de vários óleos, ceras e água; a fórmula padrão, ungüento de água-de-rosas, contém óleo de amêndoas, água-de-rosas, espermacete, cera parafinada branca e borato de sódio; usado como creme de limpeza ou lubrificante.
  greaseless c., c. evanescente. SIN vanishing c.
  leukocyte c., c. leucocitário. SIN buffy *coat*.
  lubricating c., c. lubrificante; uma forma de creme usado como creme de massagem ou creme noturno; contém lanolina ou seus derivados.
  vanishing c., c. evanescente; uma emulsão de óleo em água contendo potássio, amônio ou estearato de sódio com água e mantendo, na forma emulsificada, mais ou menos ácido esteárico livre; também contém um ingrediente higroscópico, como o glicerol, e uma pequena quantidade de um ingrediente gorduroso; deixa uma película protetora, invisível, de ácido esteárico na pele. SIN greaseless c.

crease (krēs). Prega; uma linha ou depressão linear como a produzida por uma prega. VER TAMBÉM fold, groove, line.
  digital c., p. digital; um dos sulcos na superfície palmar de um dedo da mão, ao nível de uma articulação interfalângica. SIN digital flexion c., digital furrow.
  digital flexion c., p. digital. SIN digital c.
  ear lobe c., p. do lobo da orelha; prega diagonal encontrada em um ou ambos os lobos das orelhas, havendo uma possível relação com a doença coronariana em homens.
  flexion c., p. de flexão; uma prega permanente na pele na face flexora de uma articulação móvel.
  palmar c., p. palmar; qualquer uma das várias pregas de flexão normalmente encontradas na palma da mão, proximais às articulações metacarpofalângicas, porém em virtude de flexão nas mesmas.
  simian c., p. símia; p. simiesca; uma prega palmar transversa única formada por fusão das pregas palmares proximal e distal, assim denominada devido à sua semelhança com a prega de flexão transversa observada em alguns macacos; uma característica comum, mas não patognomônica, da síndrome de Down; também encontrada em 1% da população normal.
  Sydney c., p. de Sydney; uma variação da prega de flexão palmar transversa proximal que alcança a face ulnar da palma; associada à anemia linfocítica aguda nos primeiros anos de vida, embriopatia por rubéola e síndrome de Down. SIN Sydney line.

cre·a·ti·nase (krē′a - tī - nās). Creatinase; uma enzima que catalisa a hidrólise de creatina em sarcosina e uréia.

cre·a·tine (krē′a - tēn, tin). Creatina; *N*-(aminoiminometil)-*N*-metilglicina; ocorre na urina, algumas vezes como creatina, mas geralmente como creatinina, e nos músculos, geralmente como fosfocreatina. Elevada na urina de indivíduos com distrofia muscular.
  c. kinase (CK). Creatinoquinase (CK), uma enzima que catalisa a transferência reversível de fosfocreatina para ADP, formando creatina e ATP; importante na contração muscular. Determinadas isoenzimas estão elevadas no plasma após infarto do miocárdio. SIN phosphokinase.
  c. phosphate, fosfato de c. SIN phosphocreatine.
  c. phosphokinase (CPK), creatinofosfoquinase (CPK). SIN c. kinase.

cre·a·ti·ne·mia (krē′a - ti - nē′mē - ă). Creatinemia. A existência de concentrações anormais de creatina no sangue periférico. [creatine + G. *haima*, sangue]

cre·at·i·nin·ase (krē - at′i - nin - ās). Creatininase. Uma amido-hidrolase que catalisa a conversão de creatina em creatinina.

cre·at·i·nine (Cr) (krē - at′i - nēn, - nin). Creatinina; um componente da urina e o produto final do catabolismo da creatina; formada pela ciclização desfosforilativa não-enzimática da fosfocreatina para formar o anidrido interno da creatina.

cre·a·tin·u·ria (krē′a - ti - noor′ē - ă). Creatinúria; a excreção urinária de quantidades aumentadas de creatina. [creatine + G. *ouron*, urina]

Credé, Karl S.F., obstetra e ginecologista alemão, 1819–1892. VER C. *methods*, em *method*.

credentialing (krī - den′shal - ing). Credenciamento; revisão formal das qualificações de um profissional que se inscreveu para participar de um convênio ou plano de assistência médica. [*credential*, prova de autenticidade, do L. Med. *credentialis*, de *credo*, acreditar, + -ing]

creep (krēp). Deslocamento; qualquer deformação tempo-dependente que se desenvolve em um material ou um objeto em resposta à aplicação de uma força ou tensão.

cre·mas·ter (krē - mas′ter). Cremaster. VER cremasteric *fascia*, cremaster *muscle*. [G. *kremastēr*, um suspensor, no plural, os músculos que retraem os testículos, de *kremannymi*, pendurar]

crem·as·ter·ic (krem - as - ter′ik). Cremastérico; relativo ao músculo cremaster.

crem·no·cele (krem′nō - sēl). Cremnocele; uma protrusão do intestino para o lábio maior do pudendo. [G. *kremnos*, rochedo saliente, lábio do pudendo, + *kēlē*, hérnia]

crem·no·pho·bia (krem - nō - fō′bē - ă). Cremnofobia; temor mórbido de precipícios ou locais íngremes. [G. *kremnos*, precipício, + *phobos*, medo]

cre·na, pl. **cre·nae** (krē′na, krē′nē). Incisura; fenda; um corte em forma de V ou o espaço criado por esse corte; uma das incisuras nas quais as projeções opostas se encaixam nas suturas cranianas. [L. incisura]
  c. analis [TA], fenda interglútea. SIN intergluteal *cleft*.
  c. a'ni, fenda interglútea; *termo oficial alternativo para intergluteal cleft.
  c. clu'nium, SIN intergluteal *cleft*.
  c. cor'dis, sulco interventricular. **(1)** SIN anterior interventricular *sulcus*; **(2)** SIN posterior interventricular *sulcus*.
  c. interglutealis, fenda interglútea; *termo oficial alternativo para intergluteal *cleft*.

cre·nate, cre·nat·ed (krē′nāt, - nā - ted). Crenado; denteado; designa o contorno de uma hemácia enrugada, conforme se observa em uma solução hipertônica. [L. *crena*, incisura]

cre·na·tion (krē - nā′shŭn). Crenação; o processo de se tornar, ou de ser, crenado.

creno·cyte (krē′nō - sīt). Crenócito; uma hemácia com bordas serrilhadas, entalhadas. [L. *crena*, entalhe, + G. *kytos*, cavidade (célula)]

cre·no·cy·to·sis (krē′nō - sī - tō′sis). Crenocitose; a presença de crenócitos no sangue. [crenocyte + G. –*osis*, condição]

Cren·o·so·ma vul·pis (krē′nō - sō - ma vŭl′pis). Uma espécie de vermes pulmonares metastrôngilos de raposas, lobos, cães, guaxinins e outros pequenos carnívoros da Europa, Ásia e América do Norte; encontrados nos brônquios, causando bronquite. [G. *krēnē*, uma nascente (mineral), + *sōma*, corpo; L. *vulpes*, raposa]

cre·oph·a·gy, cre·oph·a·gism (krē - of′a - jē, krē - of′a - jizm). Creofagia; carnívoro; ato de comer carne. [G. *kreas*, carne, + *phagō*, comer]

cre·o·sol (krē′ō - sol). Creosol; um líquido aromático, discretamente amarelado, destilado do guáiaco ou do alcatrão de faia; um constituinte do creosoto. Cf. cresol.

cre·o·sote (krē′ō - sōt). Creosoto; mistura de fenóis (principalmente metilguaiacol, guaiacol e creosol) obtida durante a destilação do alcatrão da madeira, de preferência o derivado da faia; usado como desinfetante e preservativo da madeira. [G. *kreas*, carne, + *sōtēr*, preservativo]

crep·i·tant (krep′i - tant). Crepitante. **1.** Relativo a, ou caracterizado por, crepitação. **2.** Designa um ruído bolhoso fino (estertor) produzido pelo ar que penetra em um líquido no tecido pulmonar; ouvido na pneumonia e em alguns outros distúrbios. **3.** A sensação transmitida aos dedos da mão do examinador pelo gás ou ar nos tecidos subcutâneos.

crep·i·ta·tion (krep - i - tā′shŭn). Crepitação. **1.** Crepitação; a qualidade de um som bolhoso fino (estertor) que se assemelha ao ruído ouvido ao se esfregar cabelo entre os dedos da mão. **2.** A sensação percebida ao se colocar a mão sobre o local de uma fratura quando as extremidades quebradas do osso são movidas, ou sobre o tecido no qual existe gangrena gasosa. SIN bony crepitus. **3.** Ruído ou vibração produzida ao se esfregar o osso ou superfícies cartilaginosas degeneradas irregulares, como na artrite e em outros distúrbios. SIN crepitus (1). [ver crepitus]

crep·i·tus (krep′i-tūs). **1.** Crepitação. SIN crepitation. **2.** Flato; liberação ruidosa de gases do intestino. [L. de *crepo*, estrondo]

articular c., c. articular; o rangido de uma articulação, freqüentemente associado à osteoartrite.

bony c., c. óssea. SIN crepitation (2).

cres·cent (kres′ent). Crescente. **1.** Qualquer figura com a forma da lua em seu primeiro quarto, meia-lua. **2.** A figura formada pelas colunas cinzentas ou cornos ao corte transversal da medula espinal. **3.** SIN malarial c. [L. *cresco*, pp. *cretus*, crescer]

articular c., c. articular. SIN meniscus lens.

Giannuzzi c.'s, crescentes de Giannuzzi. SIN *serous demilunes*, em demilune.

glomerular c., c. glomerular; células endoteliais proliferadas que circundam parcialmente um glomérulo renal; ocorre na glomerulonefrite.

Heidenhain c.'s, crescentes de Heidenhain. SIN serous *demilunes*, em *demilune*.

malarial c., c. malárico; o(s) gametócito(s) masculino(s) ou feminino(s) do *Plasmodium falciparum*, cuja presença nas hemácias humanas é diagnóstica de malária falciparum. SIN crescent (3), sickle form.

myopic c., c. miópico; cone miópico; área em crescente, branca ou branco-acinzentada no fundo do olho, situada no lado temporal do disco óptico; causada por atrofia da coróide, permitindo que a esclera se torne visível. SIN myopic conus.

sublingual c., c. sublingual; a área em forma de crescente no assoalho da boca, formada pela parede lingual da mandíbula e parte adjacente do assoalho da boca.

cres·cen·tic (kres-sen′tik). Crescêntico; em forma de crescente.

cres·co·graph (kres′kō-graf).Crescógrafo; dispositivo para registrar o grau e a taxa de crescimento. [L. *cresco*, crescer, + G. *grapho*, desenhar ou escrever]

cre·sol (krē′sol). Cresol; mistura dos três cresóis isoméricos, *o*-, *m*- e *p*-cresol, obtidos do alcatrão. Suas propriedades são semelhantes às do fenol, porém é menos venenoso; usado como anti-séptico e desinfetante. SIN tricresol.

***m*-cre·sol.** *m*-cresol; anti-séptico local com maior poder germicida que o fenol e menor toxicidade para os tecidos; usado em desinfetantes e fumigantes; seu derivado acetato é usado como anti-séptico tópico e fungicida. SIN metacresol.

cre·so·lase (krē′sō-lās).Cresolase. SIN monophenol monooxygenase (1).

cre·sol red. Vermelho cresol; um indicador ácido-básico com valor de pK de 8,3; amarelo em pH < 7,4, vermelho em pH > 9,0.

CREST Acrônimo para calcinose, fenômeno de *R*aynaud, distúrbios da motilidade *e*sofágica, *e*sclerodactilia (*s*clerodactyly) e *t*elangiectasia. VER CREST *syndrome*.

CREST

crest (krest) [TA]. **1.** Crista; uma crista, principalmente uma crista óssea. VER TAMBÉM crista. **2.** Crina; pêlos compridos e flexíveis do pescoço de um animal macho, principalmente de um cavalo reprodutor ou touro. **3.** Penacho; penas no topo da cabeça de uma ave, ou escamas no ápice da cabeça de um peixe. SIN crista [TA]. [L. *crista*]

acoustic c., c. ampular. SIN ampullary c.

alveolar c., c. alveolar; **(1)** a porção do processo alveolar da maxila que se estende além da periferia dos encaixes dos dentes, situada interproximalmente; **(2)** o topo do processo alveolar residual.

c. of alveolar ridge, topo da crista alveolar; o cume da crista alveolar ou crista residual; a superfície contínua mais alta da crista, mas não necessariamente o centro desta.

ampullary c. [TA], c. ampular; uma elevação na superfície interna de cada ducto semicircular; filamentos do nervo vestibular atravessam a crista para alcançar as células pilosas em sua superfície; as células pilosas são cobertas pela cúpula, uma massa gelatinosa composta de proteínas e polissacarídeos. VER TAMBÉM *neuroepithelium* of ampullary crest. SIN crista ampullaris [TA], acoustic c., transverse septum (1).

ampullary c. (of semicircular ducts) [TA], c. ampular (dos ductos semicirculares); crista em formato de crescente que invagina para a luz das ampolas dos ductos semicirculares, possuindo epitélio sensorial sobre uma base de fibras nervosas e tecido conjuntivo. SIN crista ampullaris (ductuum semicircularium) [TA].

anterior lacrimal c. [TA], c. lacrimal anterior; uma crista vertical, na superfície lateral do processo frontal da maxila, que forma parte da borda medial da órbita. SIN crista lacrimalis anterior [TA].

arched c., c. arqueada da cartilagem aritenóidea. SIN arcuate c. of arytenoid cartilage.

arcuate c., c. arqueada da cartilagem aritenóidea. SIN arcuate c. of arytenoid cartilage.

arcuate c. of arytenoid cartilage [TA], c. arqueada da cartilagem aritenóidea; a crista, na superfície anterior da cartilagem aritenóidea, que separa a fóvea triangular da fóvea oblonga. SIN crista arcuata cartilaginis arytenoideae [TA], arched c., arcuate c.

articular c., c. articular. SIN intermediate sacral c.

basal c. of cochlear duct [TA], c. basilar do ducto coclear; extensão pronunciada da porção central do ligamento espiral que continua como a lâmina basilar. SIN crista basalaris ductus cochlearis [TA], crista spiralis ductus cochlearis*, spiral c. of cochelar duct*.

basilar c. of cochlear duct, c. basilar do ducto coclear; uma projeção interna do ligamento espiral da cóclea à qual está fixada a lâmina basilar que forma o assoalho do ducto coclear. SIN crista basilaris ductus cochlearis [TA].

c. of body of rib [TA], c. do corpo da costela; a margem inferior aguda do corpo de uma costela. SIN crista corporis costae [TA].

buccinator c., c. bucinadora; c. bucinatória; uma crista que segue da base do processo coronóide da mandíbula até a região do último dente molar; dá fixação à parte mandibular do músculo bucinador. SIN crista buccinatoria.

c. of cochlear opening, c. da janela da cóclea. SIN c. of round window.

conchal c. [TA], c. conchal da maxila; crista óssea que se articula com, ou dá fixação para, a concha nasal inferior. VER conchal c. of body of maxilla, conchal c. of palatine bone. SIN crista conchalis [TA], turbinated c.

conchal c. of body of maxilla [TA], c. conchal do corpo da maxila; crista da superfície nasal do corpo da maxila que se articula com a concha nasal inferior. SIN crista conchalis corporis maxillae [TA].

conchal c. of palatine bone [TA], c. conchal do palatino; a crista, na superfície nasal da parte perpendicular do osso palatino, à qual se fixa a concha nasal inferior. SIN crista conchalis ossis palatini [TA].

deltoid c., c. deltóide; tuberosidade para o músculo deltóide. SIN deltoid *tuberosity* (of humerus).

dental c., c. dental; a crista maxilar nos processos alveolares das maxilas no feto. SIN crista dentalis.

ethmoidal c. [TA], c. etmoidal, crista óssea que se articula com, ou proporciona inserção para, o osso etmóide, sobretudo a concha nasal média. VER ethmoidal c. of maxilla, ethmoidal of palatine bone. SIN crista ethmoidalis [TA].

ethmoidal c. of maxilla [TA], c. etmoidal da maxila; uma crista, na parte superior da superfície nasal do processo frontal da maxila, que dá fixação à porção anterior da concha nasal média. SIN crista ethmoidalis maxillae [TA].

ethmoidal c. of palatine bone [TA], c. etmoidal do palatino; uma crista, na superfície medial da parte perpendicular do osso palatino, ao qual a concha nasal média se fixa posteriormente. SIN crista ethmoidalis ossis palatini [TA].

external occipital c. [TA], c. occipital externa; uma crista que se estende da protuberância occipital externa até a borda do forame magno. SIN crista occipitalis externa [TA], linea nuchae mediana.

falciform c., c. falciforme. SIN transverse c. of internal acoustic meatus.

c. of fenestrae cochleae, c. da janela da cóclea. SIN c. of round window.

frontal c. [TA], c. frontal; uma crista que se origina no final do sulco sagital na superfície cerebral do osso frontal, terminando no forame ceco. SIN crista frontalis [TA].

ganglionic c., c. neural. SIN neural c.

gingival c., c. gengival. SIN gingival *margin*.

gluteal c., c. glútea. SIN gluteal *tuberosity*.

c. of greater tubercle [TA], c. do tubérculo maior; a crista, situada abaixo do tubérculo maior do úmero, na qual se insere o músculo peitoral maior. SIN crista tuberculi majoris [TA], bicipital ridges, pectoral ridge.

c. of head of rib [TA], c. da cabeça da costela; a crista que separa as superfícies articulares superior e inferior da cabeça de uma costela. SIN crista capitis costae [TA].

iliac c. [TA], c. ilíaca; a longa borda superior curva da asa do ílio. SIN crista iliaca [TA].

incisor c., c. incisiva; a parte frontal da crista nasal do processo palatino da maxila.

infratemporal c. of greater wing of sphenoid [TA], c. infratemporal da asa maior do esfenóide; uma crista rugosa que marca o ângulo de união das superfícies temporal e infratemporal da asa maior do esfenóide. SIN crista infratemporalis alaris majoris ossis sphenoidalis [TA], pterygoid ridge of sphenoid bone.

inguinal c., c. inguinal; uma elevação na parede corporal do embrião na abertura interna do canal inguinal; parte do gubernáculo do testículo se desenvolve em seu interior.

intermediate sacral c. [TA], c. sacral medial; cristas formadas pela fusão de processos articulares de todas as vértebras sacrais. SIN crista sacralis medialis [TA], articular c., crista sacralis intermedia.

internal occipital c. [TA], c. occipital interna; uma crista que vai da protuberância occipital interna até a margem posterior do forame magno, dando fixação à foice do cerebelo. SIN crista occipitalis interna [TA].

interosseous c., c. interóssea. SIN interosseous *border*.

intertrochanteric c. [TA], c. intertrocantérica; a crista arredondada que une os trocanteres maior e menor do fêmur, posteriormente, e marca a junção do colo com a diáfise do osso. SIN crista intertrochanterica [TA], trochanteric c.

interureteric c. [TA], prega interuretérica; uma prega de mucosa que se estende do óstio do ureter de um lado até o óstio do outro lado. SIN plica interureterica [TA], bar of bladder, interureteric fold, Mercier bar, plica ureterica, torus uretericus, ureteric fold.

lateral epicondylar c., c. epicondilar lateral. SIN lateral supraepicondylar ridge.

lateral sacral c. [TA], c. sacral lateral; cristas rugosas laterais aos forames sacrais; representam os processos transversos fundidos das vértebras sacrais. SIN crista sacralis lateralis [TA].

lateral supracondylar c., c. supracondilar lateral. SIN lateral supraepicondylar ridge.

c. of lesser tubercle [TA], c. do tubérculo menor; a crista, abaixo do tubérculo menor do úmero, na qual se insere o músculo redondo maior. SIN crista tuberculi minoris [TA], bicipital ridges.

marginal c. of tooth [TA], c. marginal do dente; as bordas arredondadas que formam as margens mesial e distal da face oclusal de um dente. SIN crista marginalis dentis [TA], marginal ridge.

medial epicondylar c., c. epicondilar medial. SIN medial supraepicondylar ridge.

medial c. of fibula [TA], c. medial da fíbula; uma crista de osso, na superfície posterior da fíbula, que separa a fixação do músculo tibial posterior daquela dos músculos flexor longo do hálux e sóleo. SIN crista medialis fibulae [TA].

medial supracondylar c., c. supracondilar medial. SIN medial supraepicondylar ridge.

median sacral c. [TA], c. sacral mediana; uma crista ímpar formada pelos processos espinhosos fundidos das quatro vértebras sacrais superiores. SIN crista sacralis mediana [TA].

c.'s of nail bed, cristas do leito ungueal. SIN crests of nail matrix, em crest.

c.'s of nail matrix [TA], c. da matriz da unha; as numerosas cristas longitudinais do leito ungueal distais à lúnula. SIN cristae matricis unguis.

nasal c. [TA], c. nasal; a crista, na linha média do assoalho da cavidade nasal, formada pela união dos ossos pareados maxilar e palatino; o vômer se fixa à crista. SIN crista nasalis [TA], semicrista incisiva.

nasal c. of horizontal plate of palatine bone [TA], c. nasal da lâmina horizontal do palatino; crista óssea de orientação superior (nasal), formada no encontro dos processos horizontais dos ossos palatinos direito e esquerdo, para fixação do septo nasal. SIN crista nasalis laminae horizontalis ossis palatini [TA].

nasal c. of palatine process of maxilla [TA], c. nasal do processo palatino da maxila; crista óssea de orientação superior (nasal), formada no encontro dos processos palatinos das maxilas direita e esquerda, para fixação do septo nasal. SIN crista nasalis processus palatini maxillae [TA].

c. of neck of rib [TA], c. do colo da costela; a margem superior bem definida do colo de uma costela. SIN crista colli costae [TA].

neural c., c. neural; células neuroectodérmicas originadas na face dorsal das pregas neurais ou tubo neural; essas células deixam o tubo ou as pregas neurais e diferenciam-se em vários tipos celulares, incluindo células ganglionares da raiz dorsal, células ganglionares autônomas, as células cromafins da medula supra-renal, células de Schwann, células dos gânglios sensoriais dos nervos cranianos 5, 9 e 10, parte das meninges, ou células pigmentares do tegumento. SIN ganglion ridge, ganglionic c.

obturator c. [TA], c. obturatória; uma crista que se estende do tubérculo púbico até a incisura do acetábulo, dando fixação ao ligamento pubofemoral da articulação coxofemoral. SIN crista obturatoria [TA].

c. of palatine bone, palatine c., c. do palatino. SIN palatine c. of horizontal process of palatine bone.

palatine c. of horizontal process of palatine bone [TA], c. palatina da lâmina horizontal do palatino; uma crista transversal próxima à borda posterior do palato ósseo, localizada na face inferior da lâmina horizontal do palatino. SIN crista palatina laminae horizontalis ossis palatini [TA], c. of palatine bone, palatine c., palatina.

c. of petrous part of temporal bone, c. da parte petrosa do osso temporal. SIN superior border of petrous part of temporal bone.

c. of petrous temporal bone, c. da parte petrosa do osso temporal. SIN superior border of petrous part of temporal bone.

posterior lacrimal c. [TA], c. lacrimal posterior; uma crista vertical, situada na superfície orbital do osso lacrimal, que, juntamente com a crista lacrimal anterior, limita a fossa para o saco lacrimal. SIN crista lacrimalis posterior [TA].

pubic c. [TA], c. púbica; a borda anterior rugosa do corpo do púbis, contínua lateralmente com o tubérculo púbico. SIN crista pubica [TA].

c. of round window [TA], c. da janela coclear; a borda da abertura da janela coclear à qual está fixada a membrana timpânica secundária. SIN crista fenestrae cochleae [TA], c. of cochlear opening, c. of fenestrae cochleae.

sacral c., c. sacral; uma das três cristas irregulares rugosas na superfície posterior do sacro; c. sacral mediana; cristas sacrais laterais. SIN crista sacralis [TA].

sagittal c., c. sagital; uma crista proeminente, ao longo da sutura sagital do crânio, presente em alguns animais em virtude do desenvolvimento do músculo temporal.

c. of scapular spine, c. da espinha da escápula; a borda subcutânea posterior da espinha da escápula que se expande, em sua parte medial, até uma área triangular uniforme.

sphenoidal c. [TA], c. esfenoidal; uma crista vertical, situada na linha média da superfície anterior do osso esfenóide, que se articula com a lâmina perpendicular do osso etmóide. SIN crista sphenoidalis [TA].

spiral c., c. espiral. SIN spiral ligament of cochlear duct.

spiral c. of cochlear duct, c. espiral do ducto coclear; *termo oficial alternativo para basal c. of cochlear duct.

c. of supinator muscle, c. do músculo supinador. SIN supinator c. (of ulna).

supinator c. (of ulna) [TA], c. do músculo supinador; a parte proximal da borda interóssea da ulna, na qual se origina uma parte do músculo supinador. SIN crista musculi supinatoris ulnae [TA], c. of supinator muscle.

supramastoid c. [TA], c. supramastóidea; a crista que forma a raiz posterior do processo zigomático do osso temporal. SIN crista supramastoidea [TA].

suprastyloid c. of radius [TA], c. supra-estilóidea do rádio; borda lateral do rádio distal que leva ao processo estilóide; local de inserção do músculo braquiorradial. SIN crista suprastyloidea radii [TA].

supraventricular c. [TA], c. supraventricular; a crista muscular interna que separa o cone arterial da parte remanescente da cavidade do ventrículo direito do coração. SIN crista supraventricularis [TA].

temporal c. of mandible [TA], c. temporal da mandíbula; crista, ao longo da face ântero-medial do processo coronóide e ramo superior da mandíbula, na qual se insere o músculo temporal. SIN crista temporalis mandibulae [TA].

terminal c., c. terminal. SIN crista terminalis of right atrium.

tibial c., c. tibial. SIN anterior border of tibia.

transverse c., c. transversa; (1) SIN transverse c. of internal acoustic meatus; (2) SIN crista transversalis.

transverse c. of internal acoustic meatus [TA], c. transversa do meato acústico interno; uma crista horizontal que divide o fundo do meato acústico interno em uma área superior e uma área inferior. Na primeira estão o intróito do canal facial e as aberturas para os ramos do nervo vestibular para o utrículo e para as ampolas dos canais semicirculares anterior e lateral. Neste último estão as aberturas para o nervo coclear e para os ramos do nervo vestibular para o sáculo e para a ampola do canal semicircular posterior. SIN crista transversa meatus acustici interni [TA], falciform c., transverse c. (1).

triangular c., c. triangular. SIN crista triangularis.

trigeminal c., c. trigeminal; a parte da crista neural cranial a partir da qual se desenvolve parte do gânglio do quinto nervo craniano.

trochanteric c., c. trocantérica. SIN intertrochanteric c.

turbinated c., c. turbinada. SIN conchal c.

urethral c. [TA], c. uretral; prega mucosa longitudinal na parede dorsal da uretra. VER urethral c. of female, urethral c. of male. SIN crista urethralis.

urethral c. of female [TA], c. uretral feminina; uma prega longitudinal visível de mucosa na parede posterior da uretra. SIN crista urethralis femininae [TA].

urethral c. of male [TA], c. uretral masculina; uma prega longitudinal, na parede posterior da uretra, que se estende da úvula da bexiga e atravessa a uretra prostática; proeminente em sua porção média é o colículo seminal. SIN crista urethralis masculinae [TA], crista phallica.

vertical c. of internal acoustic meatus [TA], c. vertical do meato acústico interno; crista óssea do fundo do meato acústico interno que separa a área vestibular superior da área facial acima da c. transversa mais proeminente, e a área vestibular inferior da área coclear abaixo da crista transversa. SIN crista verticalis meatus acustici interni [TA].

vestibular c. [TA], c. do vestíbulo; uma crista oblíqua, na parede interna do vestíbulo do labirinto, demarcando o recesso esférico acima e posteriormente. SIN crista vestibuli [TA], c. of vestibule.

c. of vestibule, c. do vestíbulo. SIN vestibular c.

vomerine c. of choana [TA], c. coanal do vômer; a borda posterior côncava do vômer e do epitélio respiratório sobrejacente que forma seu limite medial e separa os cóanos direito e esquerdo. SIN crista choanalis vomeris [TA].

cres·ta (kres′tā). Crista; pequena organela membranosa, característica de certos protozoários flagelados, próxima do escudo e observada no organismo vivo como uma estrutura de movimento independente. [L. *crispus*, tremor]

cres·yl·ate (kres′i-lāt). Cresilato; um sal de ácido cresílico, ou cresol.

cres·yl blue, cres·yl blue bril·liant (kres′il) [C.I. 51010]. Azul de cresil, azul de cresil brilhante; um corante de oxazina básico usado para corar o retículo em eritrócitos jovens (reticulócitos); também usado em coloração vital e como coloração seletiva para mucina epitelial da superfície gástrica e outros mucopolissacarídeos ácidos.

cres·yl echt, cres·yl fast vi·o·let. Cresil verdadeiro, cresil violeta; corante de oxazina básico metacromático, intimamente relacionado ao acetato de cresil violeta e usado para os mesmos fins.

cres·yl vi·o·let ac·e·tate. Acetato de cresil violeta; um corante de oxazina básico metacromático, usado como corante para núcleos e substância de Nissl; relacionado ao corante derivado alemão conhecido como cresil violeta verdadeiro.

cre·ta (krē'tä). Creta, greda. SIN calcium carbonate. [L. orig. adj. de *Creta*, Creta, isto é, terra cretense, greda]

cre·tin (krē'tin). Cretino; indivíduo com cretinismo. [Fr. *crétin*]

cre·tin·ism (krē'tin-izm). Cretinismo; termo obsoleto para hipotireoidismo congênito (congenital *hypothyroidism*). VER infantile *hypothyroidism*.

cre·tin·is·tic (krē'tin-is-tik). Cretinoso. SIN cretinous.

cre·tin·oid (krē'tin-oyd). Cretinóide; semelhante a um cretino; que apresenta sintomas semelhantes aos do cretinismo.

cre·tin·ous (krē'tin-ŭs). Cretinoso; relativo a cretinismo ou um cretino; afetado por cretinismo. SIN cretinistic.

Creutzfeldt, Hans Gerhard, neuropsiquiatra alemão, 1885–1964. VER Creutzfeldt-Jakob *disease*.

crev·ice (krev'is). Fenda; fissura; uma fenda ou pequena fissura longitudinal, principalmente em uma substância sólida. [Fr. *crevasse*]
   gingival c., fissura gengival. SIN gingival *sulcus*.

cre·vic·u·lar (krē-vik'ū-lār). **1.** Fissurado; relativo a qualquer fissura. **2.** Em odontologia, relativo principalmente à fissura ou sulco gengival.

CRF Abreviatura de corticotropin-releasing *factor* (fator liberador de corticotropina).

CRH Abreviatura de corticotropin-releasing *hormone* (hormônio liberador de corticotropina).

cri·bra (krī'brä, krib'rä). Plural de cribrum.

crib·rate (krib'rāt). Cribriforme. SIN cribriform.

cri·bra·tion (kri-brā'shŭn). Crivação; peneiração. **1.** Peneiração; passar através de uma peneira. **2.** Condição de ser crivado, esburacado ou perfurado muitas vezes.

crib·ri·form (krib'ri-form) [TA]. Cribriforme; semelhante a uma peneira; contém muitas perfurações. SIN cribrate, polyporous. [L. *cribrum*, peneira, + *forma*, forma]

cri·brum, pl. **cri·bra** (krī'brŭm, krib'rŭm; -brä, -ra). Lâmina cribriforme do osso etmóide. SIN cribriform *plate* of ethmoid bone. [L. peneira]

Cri·cet·i·nae (krī-sē'ti-nē). Subfamília de roedores (família Muridae) que inclui hamster e ratos nativos da América do Norte.

Cri·ce·tu·lus (kri-sē'tū-lŭs). Um dos quatro gêneros de hamsters; *C. griseus,* o hamster listrado nativo da Europa e da Ásia, é um reservatório de leishmaniose visceral.

Cri·ce·tus (kri-sē'tŭs). Um dos quatro gêneros de hamsters: *C. cricetus* é amplamente usado como animal para pesquisa.

Crick, Francis H.C., bioquímico inglês e Prêmio Nobel, *1916. VER Watson-C. *helix*.

cri·co·ar·y·te·noid (krī'kō-ar-i-tē'noyd). Cricoaritenóideo; relativo às cartilagens cricóidea e aritenóidea.

cri·co·ar·y·te·noi·de·us (krī-kō-ar-i-te-noy'dē-ŭs). Cricoaritenóideo. VER lateral cricoarytenoid (*muscle*), posterior cricoarytenoid (*muscle*).

cri·coid (krī'koyd). Cricóide; em forma de anel; designa a cartilagem cricóidea. [L. *cricoideus,* do G. *krikos,* anel, + *eidos,* forma]

cri·coi·dyn·ia (krī'koy-din'ē-ä). Cricoidinia; dor na cartilagem cricóidea. [cricoid + G. *odinē,* dor]

cri·co·pha·ryn·ge·al (krī'kō-fä-rin'jē-ăl). Cricofaríngeo; relativo à cartilagem cricóidea e à faringe; uma parte do músculo constrictor inferior da faringe. VER inferior constrictor (*muscle*) of pharynx.

cri·co·thy·roid (krī-kō-thī'royd). Cricotireóideo; relativo às cartilagens cricóidea e tireóidea.

cri·co·thy·roi·de·us (krī'kō-thī-roy'dē-ŭs). Cricotireóideo. VER cricothyroid *muscle*.

cri·co·thy·roi·dot·o·my (krī'kō-thī-roy-dot'ō-mē). Cricotireoidotomia. SIN cricothyrotomy.

cri·co·thy·rot·o·my (krī'kō-thī-rot'ō-mē). Cricotirotomia; incisão através da pele e da membrana cricotireóidea para alívio de obstrução respiratória; usada antes ou no lugar da traqueotomia em determinadas obstruções respiratórias de emergência. VER TAMBÉM coniotomy. SIN cricothyroidotomy, inferior laryngotomy, intercricothyrotomy. [cricoid + thyroid + G. *tomē,* incisão]

cri·cot·o·my (krī-kot'ō-mē). Cricotomia; divisão da cartilagem cricóidea, como na divisão cricóide, para aumentar a via aérea subglótica. [cricoid + G. *tomē,* incisão]

Crigler, John F., médico norte-americano, *1919. VER C.-Najjar *disease, syndrome*.

Crile, George W., cirurgião norte-americano, 1864–1943. VER C. *clamp*.

crim·i·nol·o·gy (krim-i-nol'ō-jē). Criminologia; o ramo da ciência que estuda as características físicas e mentais e o comportamento de criminosos. [L. *crimen,* crime, + G. *logos,* estudo]

crin·in (krin'in). Crinina; termo antigo para designar uma substância que estimula a produção de secreções por glândulas específicas. [G. *krino,* secretar, + -in]

crin·o·gen·ic (krin-ō-jen'ik). Crinogênico; que causa secreção; que estimula uma glândula a aumentar sua função. [G. *krino,* separar, + *-gen,* produzir]

crin·oph·a·gy (krin-of'ä-jē). Crinofagia; eliminação do excesso de grânulos secretores pelos lisossomas.

crip·pled (krip'ld). Incapaz; inválido; mutilado; designa uma pessoa que, devido a um defeito físico ou lesão, está parcial ou completamente incapacitada. [A.S. *creopan,* rastejar]

cri·sis, pl. **cri·ses** (krī'sis, sēz). Crise. **1.** Uma mudança súbita, geralmente para melhor, na evolução de uma doença aguda, em contraste com a melhora gradual por lise. **2.** Crise tabética; uma dor paroxística, em um órgão ou região do corpo circunscrita, que ocorre no curso da neurossífilis tabética. SIN tabetic c. **3.** Um ataque convulsivo. [G. *krisis,* uma separação, crise]
   addisonian c., c. addisoniana ou de Addison. SIN acute adrenocortical *insufficiency*.
   adolescent c., c. da adolescência; o turbilhão emocional que, freqüentemente, acompanha a adolescência.
   adrenal c., c. supra-renal. SIN acute adrenocortical *insufficiency*.
   anaphylactoid c., c. anafilactóide; **(1)** SIN anaphylactoid *shock*; **(2)** SIN pseudoanaphylaxis.
   blast c., c. blástica; uma alteração súbita do estado de um paciente com leucemia no qual as células do sangue periférico são quase exclusivamente blastos do tipo característico de leucemia; geralmente é acompanhada por uma diminuição do número de outros elementos formados do sangue, febre e deterioração clínica rápida.
   blood c., (1) o surgimento de um grande número de hemácias nucleadas no sangue periférico, acompanhado por reticulocitose e que ocorre na medula óssea "exaurida" na anemia perniciosa e na icterícia hemolítica; **(2)** leucocitose súbita, indicando uma mudança para melhor na evolução de uma doença hematológica grave.
   Dietl c., c. de Dietl; dor intermitente, algumas vezes com náuseas e vômitos, causada por obstrução proximal intermitente do ureter. Originalmente se acreditava que fosse causada por um rim móvel provocando acotovelamento do ureter com mudanças de posição. SIN incarceration symptom.
   febrile c., c. febril; o estágio, em uma doença febril, em que ocorre defervescência espontânea.
   gastric c., c. gástrica; uma crise, que geralmente dura vários dias, com forte dor abdominal ou ao redor da cintura, acompanhada por náuseas e vômitos e, algumas vezes, diarréia; ocorre na neurossífilis tabética.
   glaucomatocyclitic c., c. glaucomatociclítica; uma forma de glaucoma de ângulo aberto secundário monocular devido a ciclite leve recorrente.
   hemolytic c., c. hemolítica; hemólise maciça com anemia grave associada a doença hemolítica, como doença falciforme.
   identity c., c. de identidade; uma desorientação em relação à percepção de si mesmo, dos valores e do papel na sociedade, freqüentemente de início agudo e relacionada a um evento particular e significativo na vida de uma pessoa.
   laryngeal c., c. laríngea; um ataque de paralisia do músculo abdutor, ou espasmo do músculo adutor, da laringe, com dispnéia e respiração ruidosa, que ocorre na neurossífilis tabética.
   midlife c., c. da meia-idade; um ponto em uma seqüência de eventos, durante a meia-idade, no qual são avaliadas determinadas tendências de eventos prévios e subseqüentes na vida de uma pessoa, geralmente envolvendo um conjunto de insatisfações pessoais, profissionais ou sexuais.
   myasthenic c., c. miastênica; exacerbação grave, com risco de vida, das manifestações da miastenia grave (*myasthenia* gravis) que exige tratamento intensivo.
   myelocytic c., c. mielocítica; aumento temporário, mas visível e súbito, das células da série mielocítica no sangue circulante.
   ocular c., c. ocular; dor súbita e forte nos olhos.
   oculogyric crises, crises oculógiras; crises incapacitantes de desvio dos olhos para cima observada na encefalite letárgica e com o uso de agentes fenotiazínicos.
   otolithic c., c. otolítica; episódio de queda súbita sem perda da consciência, vertigem, distúrbios auditivos ou manifestações autônomas.
   salt-depletion c., c. de depleção de sal; doença grave resultante da perda de cloreto de sódio, geralmente na urina (isto é, nefrite perdedora de sal), no suor após exercício vigoroso em clima quente, ou em secreções intestinais, como na cólera. Pode ocorrer em virtude da doença de Addison ou crise de Addison; caracterizada por hipovolemia, hipotensão.
   sickle cell c., c. falciforme. VER sickle cell *anemia*.
   tabetic c., c. tabética. SIN crisis (2).
   therapeutic c., c. terapêutica; ponto crítico que leva a alteração positiva ou negativa no tratamento psiquiátrico.
   thyrotoxic c., thyroid c., c. tireotóxica; a exacerbação dos sinais e sintomas de hipertireoidismo; tireotoxicose grave; pode suceder choque, lesão ou tireoidectomia; caracterizada por pulso rápido (140–170/minuto), náuseas, diarréia, febre, emagrecimento, nervosismo extremo e aumento súbito da taxa metabólica; podem ocorrer coma e morte; ocasionalmente, todo o quadro clínico é de prostração profunda, fraqueza e colapso, sem a fase de hiperatividade muscular e taquicardia. SIN thyroid storm.
   vasoocclusive c., c. oclusiva vascular. SIN sickle cell *anemia*.
   visceral crises, crises viscerais; crises de dor epigástrica disseminada, forte, que ocorre em pacientes com neurossífilis tabética.

crispation

cris·pa·tion (kris - pā′shŭn). Crispação. **1.** Uma sensação de "arrepios" devido a pequenas contrações musculares fibrilares. **2.** Retração de uma artéria dividida ou de fibras musculares ou outros tecidos quando seccionados. [L. *crispo*, pp. *–atus*, encrespar]

CRISTA

cris·ta, pl. **cris·tae** (kris′tā, -tē). [TA]. Crista. SIN crest. [L. crista]
  c. ampulla′ris [TA], c. ampular. SIN ampullary crest.
  c. ampullaris (ductuum semicircularium) [TA], c. ampular (ducto semicircular). SIN ampullary crest (of semicircular ducts).
  c. arcua′ta cartila′ginis arytenoi′deae [TA], c. arqueada da cartilagem aritenóidea. SIN arcuate crest of arytenoid cartilage.
  c. basalaris ductus cochlearis [TA], c. basilar do ducto coclear. SIN basal crest of cochlear duct.
  c. basila′ris duc′tus cochlea′ris [TA], c. basilar do ducto coclear. SIN basilar crest of cochlear duct.
  c. buccinator′ia, c. bucinatória. SIN buccinator crest.
  c. cap′itis cos′tae [TA], c. da cabeça da costela. SIN crest of head of rib.
  c. choanalis vomeris [TA], c. coanal do vômer. SIN vomerine crest of choana.
  c. col′li cos′tae [TA], c. do colo da costela. SIN crest of neck of rib.
  c. concha′lis [TA], c. conchal. SIN conchal crest.
  c. concha′lis corporis maxil′lae [TA], c. conchal do corpo da maxila. SIN conchal crest of body of maxilla.
  c. concha′lis os′sis palati′ni [TA], c. conchal do palatino. SIN conchal crest of palatine bone.
  c. corporis costae [TA], c. do corpo da costela. SIN crest of body of rib.
  cris′tae cu′tis [TA], c. da pele. SIN dermal ridges, em ridge.
  c. denta′lis, c. dental. SIN dental crest.
  c. div′idens, c. divisória; a borda inferior livre do septo secundum, formando a margem superior do forame oval fetal; o limbo do forame oval.
  c. ethmoida′lis [TA], c. etmoidal. SIN ethmoidal crest.
  c. ethmoida′lis maxil′lae [TA], c. etmoidal da maxila. SIN ethmoidal crest of maxilla.
  c. ethmoida′lis os′sis palati′ni [TA], c. etmoidal do palatino. SIN ethmoidal crest of palatine bone.
  c. fenes′trae coch′leae [TA], c. da janela da cóclea. SIN crest of round window.
  c. fronta′lis [TA], c. frontal. SIN frontal crest.
  c. gal′li [TA], c. etmoidal; o processo mediano triangular do osso etmóide que se estende superiormente a partir da lâmina cribriforme; fornece inserção à foice do cérebro.
  c. glu′tea, c. glútea. SIN gluteal tuberosity.
  c. hel′icis, c. da hélice. SIN crus of helix.
  c. ili′aca [TA], c. ilíaca. SIN iliac crest.
  c. infratempora′lis alaris majoris ossis sphenoidalis [TA], c. infratemporal da asa maior do esfenóide. SIN infratemporal crest of greater wing of sphenoid.
  c. intertrochanter′ica [TA], c. intertrocantérica. SIN intertrochanteric crest.
  c. lacrima′lis ante′rior [TA], c. lacrimal anterior. SIN anterior lacrimal crest.
  c. lacrima′lis poste′rior [TA], c. lacrimal posterior. SIN posterior lacrimal crest.
  c. margina′lis dentis [TA], c. marginal do dente. SIN marginal crest of tooth.
  cris′tae ma′tricis un′guis, c. da matriz ungueal. SIN crests of nail matrix, em crest.
  c. media′lis fi′bulae [TA], c. medial da fíbula. SIN medial crest of fibula.
  cristae of mitochondria, cris′tae mitochondria′les, cristas mitocondriais; invaginações em forma de prateleira da membrana interna de uma mitocôndria.
  c. mus′culi supinato′ris ulnae [TA], c. do músculo supinador da ulna. SIN supinator crest (of ulna).
  c. nasa′lis [TA], c. nasal. SIN nasal crest.
  c. nasalis laminae horizontalis ossis palatini [TA], c. nasal da lâmina horizontal do palatino. SIN nasal crest of horizontal plate of palatine bone.
  c. nasalis processus palatini maxillae [TA], c. nasal do processo palatino da maxila. SIN nasal crest of palatine process of maxilla.
  c. obturato′ria [TA], c. obturatória. SIN obturator crest.
  c. occipita′lis exter′na [TA], c. occipital externa. SIN external occipital crest.
  c. occipita′lis inter′na [TA], c. occipital interna. SIN internal occipital crest.
  c. palati′na, c. palatina. SIN palatine crest of horizontal process of palatine bone.
  c. palatina laminae horizontalis ossis palatini [TA], c. palatina da lâmina horizontal do palatino. SIN palatine crest of horizontal process of palatine bone.
  c. phal′lica, c. fálica. SIN urethral crest of male.
  c. pu′bica [TA], c. púbica. SIN pubic crest.
  c. quar′ta, c. quarta; uma crista que se projeta para a extremidade posterior do ducto semicircular lateral do labirinto.
  c. sacra′lis [TA], c. sacral. SIN sacral crest.
  c. sacra′lis interme′dia, c. sacral medial. SIN intermediate sacral crest.
  c. sacra′lis latera′lis [TA], c. sacral lateral. SIN lateral sacral crest.
  c. sacralis medialis [TA], c. sacral medial. SIN intermediate sacral crest.
  c. sacra′lis median′a [TA], c. sacral mediana. SIN median sacral crest.
  c. sphenoida′lis [TA], c. esfenoidal. SIN sphenoidal crest.
  c. spira′lis, c. espiral. SIN spiral ligament of cochlear duct.
  c. spiralis ductus cochlearis, c. basilar do ducto coclear; *termo oficial alternativo para basal crest of cochlear duct.
  c. supracondyla′ris latera′lis, c. supra-epicondilar lateral; *termo oficial alternativo para lateral supraepicondylar ridge.
  c. supracondyla′ris media′lis, c. supra-epicondilar medial; *termo oficial alternativo para medial supraepicondylar ridge.
  c. supraepicondylaris lateralis [TA], c. supra-epicondilar lateral. SIN lateral supraepicondylar ridge.
  c. supraepicondylaris medialis [TA], c. supra-epicondilar medial. SIN medial supraepicondylar ridge.
  c. supramastoi′dea [TA], c. supramastóidea. SIN supramastoid crest.
  c. suprastyloidea radii [TA], c. supra-estilóidea do rádio. SIN suprastyloid crest of radius.
  c. supraventricula′ris [TA], c. supraventricular. SIN supraventricular crest.
  c. temporalis mandibulae [TA], c. temporal da mandíbula. SIN temporal crest of mandible.
  c. termina′lis, c. terminal. SIN c. terminalis of right atrium.
  c. terminalis atrii dextri [TA], c. terminal do átrio direito. SIN c. terminalis of right atrium.
  c. terminalis of right atrium [TA], c. terminal do átrio direito; uma crista vertical, na parede interior do átrio direito, situada à direita do seio da veia cava e que separa este do restante do átrio direito. SIN c. terminalis atrii dextri [TA], c. terminalis, tenia terminalis, terminal crest.
  c. transversa′lis [TA], c. transversal; uma crista, na superfície oclusal de um dente, formada pela união de duas cristas triangulares. SIN transverse ridge [TA], transverse crest (2).
  c. transver′sa meatus acustici interni [TA], c. transversa do meato acústico interno. SIN transverse crest of internal acoustic meatus.
  c. triangula′ris [TA], c. triangular do dente; uma crista que se estende do ápice de uma cúspide de um dente pré-molar ou molar em direção à parte central da superfície oclusal. SIN triangular ridge [TA], triangular crest.
  c. tuber′culi majo′ris [TA], c. do tubérculo maior. SIN crest of greater tubercle.
  c. tuber′culi mino′ris [TA], c. do tubérculo menor. SIN crest of lesser tubercle.
  c. urethra′lis [TA], c. uretral. SIN urethral crest.
  c. urethra′lis femini′nae [TA], c. uretral feminina. SIN urethral crest of female.
  c. urethra′lis masculi′nae [TA], c. uretral masculina. SIN urethral crest of male.
  c. verticalis meatus acustici interni [TA], c. vertical do meato acústico interno. SIN vertical crest of internal acoustic meatus.
  c. vestib′uli [TA], c. do vestíbulo. SIN vestibular crest.

cri·te·ri·on, pl. **cri·te·ria** (krī - tēr′ē - on, -ē - ă). Critério. **1.** Um padrão ou regra para julgamento; geralmente no plural (critérios), indicando um conjunto de padrões ou regras. **2.** Em psicologia, um padrão, como notas escolares, com o qual são comparados e confirmados os resultados dos testes de inteligência ou outros comportamentos avaliados. **3.** Uma lista de manifestações de uma doença ou distúrbio, que têm de estar presentes em um determinado número para justificar o diagnóstico em um determinado paciente. [G. *kritḗrion*, padrão]
Amsel criteria, critérios de Amsel; critérios para diagnóstico clínico de vaginose bacteriana; o diagnóstico é feito se três dos quatro critérios a seguir forem positivos: corrimento homogêneo, pH ≥ 4,8, presença de células indicadoras e odor de amina com a aplicação de KOH ao corrimento.
Hill's criteria of evidence, critérios de evidência de Hill; um conjunto de critérios epidemiológicos que ajudam a indicar se uma relação estatisticamente significativa, obtida em estudos epidemiológicos e outros, é uma relação causal. Os critérios são consistência, especificidade, solidez, relação dose–resposta, temporalidade, plausibilidade biológica, coerência e capacidade de confirmação experimental. A temporalidade é o único critério absoluto: a suposta causa tem de preceder o efeito.
Jones criteria, critérios de Jones; critérios (propostos por T.D. Jones em 1944 e modificados em 1965) usados para fazer o diagnóstico de febre reumática. Há cinco critérios maiores: cardite, poliartrite, coréia, eritema marginado e nódulos subcutâneos; os critérios menores incluem febre, artralgia, elevação da velocidade de hemossedimentação ou da proteína C reativa e intervalo PR prolongado ao ECG. O diagnóstico exige evidências de infecção recente por estreptococos β-hemolíticos do grupo A, mais dois critérios maiores e um menor, ou um critério maior e dois menores; os critérios de Jones revistos permitem o diagnóstico quando existe cardite indolente ou coréia sem outra causa, ou em pacientes com uma história prévia de febre reumática que possuem um critério maior e dois menores associados a uma infecção estreptocócica recente.
Spiegelberg criteria (para diagnóstico de gravidez ovariana), critérios de Spiegelberg; 1) o oviduto do lado afetado tem de estar intacto; 2) o saco amni-

ótico tem de ocupar a posição do ovário; 3) o saco amniótico tem de estar ligado ao útero pelo ligamento ovariano; e 4) é preciso que haja tecido ovariano na parede do saco amniótico.

Cri·thid·ia (kri - thid′ē - ă). Gênero de flagelados assexuados, monogenéticos, parasitas de insetos da família Trypanosomatidae. [L. Mod., do G. *krithidion*, dim. de *krithē*, cevada]

cri·thid·ia (kri - thid′ē - ă). Termo antigo para epigmastigota. [L. Mod. do G. *krithidion*, dim. de *krithē*, cevada]

crit·i·cal (krit - ĭ - kăl). Crítico. **1.** Que indica ou é da natureza de uma crise. **2.** Indica uma condição mórbida na qual pode haver morte. **3.** Em quantidade suficiente para constituir um momento decisivo.

CRL Abreviatura de crown-rump *length* (comprimento vértice–nádega).

CRM Abreviatura de certified reference *material* (material de referência registrado).

CRM Abreviatura de cross-reacting *material* (material de reação cruzada).

C.R.N.A. Abreviatura de certified registered *nurse* anesthetist (enfermeira com capacitação em anestesiologia).

cRNA Abreviatura de complementary ribonucleic acid (ácido ribonucleico complementar).

CRO Abreviatura de cathode ray *oscilloscope* (osciloscópio de raios catódicos).

Crocq, Jean, médico belga, 1868–1925. VER C. *disease.*

cro·cus (krō′kŭs). Croco; açafrão; os estigmas secos da *Crocus sativus* (*C. officinalis*) (família Iridaceae), antigamente usados, algumas vezes, na dispepsia flatulenta; também usado antigamente como antiespasmódico na asma e na dismenorréia e como corante e aromatizante. SIN saffron. [L. do G. *krokos*, croco, açafrão (feito com seus estigmas)]

Crohn, Burrill B., gastroenterologista norte-americano, 1884–1983. VER C. *disease.*

cro·mo·lyn so·di·um (krō′mō - lin). Cromoglicato sódico; usado para prevenção de crises asmáticas. Estabiliza as membranas dos mastócitos para evitar a liberação de leucotrienos e outras substâncias indutoras de broncoespasmo. SIN sodium cromoglycate.

Cronkhite, Leonard W., Jr., médico norte-americano, *1919. VER C.-Canada *syndrome.*

Crooke, Arthur, patologista inglês *1905. VER C. *granules,* em *granule,* hyaline *change,* hyaline *degeneration.*

Crookes, Sir William, físico e químico inglês, 1832–1919; ganhador do Prêmio Nobel de química em 1907. VER C. *glass*; C.-Hittorf *tube.*

Crosby, William Holmes, Jr., médico norte-americano, *1914. VER C. *capsule.*

cross (kros). **1.** Cruz; qualquer figura com o formato de uma cruz formada por duas linhas que se cruzam. SIN crux. **2.** Cruz do coração. SIN *crux of heart.* **3.** Cruzamento; um método de hibridização ou o híbrido assim produzido. [F. *croix,* L. *crux*]

  back c., cruzamento retrógrado; o cruzamento entre um animal homozigoto em um *locus* de interesse e um animal heterozigoto, comumente de mesma ascendência.

  double back c., c. duplamente retrógrado; acasalamento retrógrado em dois *loci* de interesse; tem especial valor e importância na análise de ligação.

  hair c.'s [TA], entrecruzamentos dos pêlos; figuras semelhantes a cruzes formadas por pêlos que crescem de duas direções que se encontram e depois se separam em uma direção perpendicular à orientação original. SIN cruces pilorum [TA].

  maltese c., c. de Malta; formação tétrade dos parasitas anulares iniciais no interior da hemácia observada na babesiose.

  Ranvier c.'s, cruzes de Ranvier; figuras pretas ou marrons, com o formato de uma cruz, que caracterizam os nodos de Ranvier ao corte longitudinal de um nervo corado por nitrato de prata.

  test c., c. de prova; em genética experimental, um acasalamento deliberado destinado a testar afirmações sobre o padrão de herança de um ou mais traços.

cross-bite (kros′bīt). Mordida cruzada; uma relação anormal de um ou mais dentes de um arco com o dente ou dentes opostos do outro arco causada por desvio labial, bucal ou lingual da posição do dente, ou por posição anormal da mandíbula.

cross·breed (kros′brēd). **1.** Híbrido. SIN hybrid. **2.** Hibridar, hibridizar, cruzar; produzir um híbrido.

cross·breed·ing (kros′brēd - ing). Hibridização, hibridação. SIN hybridization.

cross-dress·ing. Travestismo; vestir-se com roupas do sexo oposto. VER transvestism.

cross-eye (kros′ī). Estrabismo; grafia alternativa de crossed *eyes,* em *eye.*

cross·ing-over, cross.over (kros - ing - ō′ver, kros′ō - ver). Permuta; troca recíproca de material entre dois cromossomas pareados durante a meiose, resultando na transferência de um bloco de genes de cada cromossoma para seu homólogo. Ao contrário da recombinação genética [genetic recombination (2)], que é um fenômeno fenotípico, a permuta é genotípica. Qualquer número par de permutas entre dois *loci* anular-se-á fenotipicamente, e não haverá recombinação.

  somatic c.-o., permuta somática; permuta que ocorre durante a mitose de células somáticas, ao contrário da que ocorre na meiose.

  uneven c.-o., unequal c.-o., p. irregular, p. desigual; permuta que ocorre quando as rupturas não ocorrem em pontos precisamente homólogos em dois filamentos de cromátides e, portanto, resulta em duplicação localizada do material genético em uma cromátide e deleção complementar na outra.

cross-link (kros - lingk). Ligação cruzada; uma ligação covalente entre dois polímeros ou entre duas regiões diferentes do mesmo polímero.

cross-match·ing (kros′match - ing). Reação cruzada. **1.** Prova para detectar incompatibilidade entre doador e receptor de sangue, realizada antes da transfusão para evitar reações hemolíticas potencialmente letais entre as hemácias do doador e os anticorpos no plasma do receptor, ou o inverso; realizada misturando-se uma amostra de hemácias do doador com plasma do receptor (*reação cruzada principal*) e as hemácias do receptor com o plasma do doador (*reação cruzada secundária*). A incompatibilidade é indicada por aglutinação de hemácias e contra-indica o uso do sangue do doador. **2.** No alotransplante de órgãos sólidos (p. ex., rim), uma prova de identificação de anticorpos no soro de potenciais receptores de aloenxertos que reage diretamente com os linfócitos ou outras células de um possível doador de aloenxerto; a presença desses anticorpos geralmente, se não sempre, contra-indica a realização do transplante porque praticamente todos esses enxertos estarão sujeitos a um tipo de rejeição hiperagudo.

cross·over. Refere-se ao fenômeno de o som apresentado a um ouvido poder ser percebido no outro ouvido passando ao redor da cabeça por condução aérea ou através da cabeça por condução óssea.

cross-sec·tion. Corte transversal. **1.** Um corte transversal através de uma estrutura. **2.** A probabilidade de uma ativação [activation (5)] por uma reação nuclear quando um material é bombardeado por nêutrons, como na produção de radionuclídeos em uma bateria; unidade: barn (10^{-24} cm²/átomo).

cross-sec·tion·al. Síncrono. VER synchronic.

cross-taper (kros tā′per). Diminuição cruzada; uma prática em farmacoterapia de reduzir a dose de um medicamento e, simultaneamente, aumentar a dose de outro.

cross·way (kros′wā). Decussação; quiasma; o cruzamento de dois trajetos nervosos.

  sensory c., quiasma sensorial; a porção pós-lenticular do ramo posterior da cápsula interna do cérebro.

Crosti, A., dermatologista italiano do século XX. VER Gianotti-C. *syndrome.*

cro·ta·lid (krō′tă - lid). Crotalídeo; qualquer membro da família de cobras Crotalidae.

Cro·tal·i·dae (krō - tal′i - dē). Família de víboras do Novo Mundo, caracterizada pela presença de uma fosseta lacrimal termossensível, entre o olho e a narina de cada lado da cabeça, e presas anteriores, longas, ocas e móveis.

cro·ta·lin (krot′ă - lin). Crotalina; uma proteína do veneno da cascavel. [*Crotalus,* gênero de cascavéis]

cro·tal·ism (krō′tal - izm). Crotalismo. SIN crotalaria *poisoning.*

Cro·ta·lus (krot′ă - lŭs). Gênero de cascavéis (família Crotalidae) nativas da América do Norte, dotadas de grandes presas que são substituídas periodicamente, durante toda a vida, e de um veneno neurotóxico e hemolítico. As maiores espécies são as cascavéis dos estados sulinos (*C. adamanteus*) e dos estados do oeste (*C. atrox*); as menores são as cascavéis-anãs. [G. *krotalon,* uma cascavel, de *krotos,* ruído de chocalho]

cro·tam·i·ton (krō - tam′i - ton). Crotamiton; um sarcopticida para uso tópico na escabiose.

cro·taph·i·on (krō - taf′ē - on). Crotáfio; a extremidade da asa maior do esfenóide; um ponto em craniometria. [G. *krotaphos,* a região temporal da cabeça]

cro·ton·ase (krō′ton - ās). Crotonase. SIN enoyl-CoA hydratase.

cro·ton oil (krō′ton). Óleo de cróton; um óleo fixo extraído das sementes de *Croton tiglium* (família Euphorbiaceae), um arbusto das Índias Ocidentais; usado como purgativo irritante e, externamente, como contra-irritante e vesicante.

cro·to·nyl-ACP re·duc·tase (krō′to - nil). Crotonil-ACP redutase. SIN enoyl-ACP reductase.

cro·tox·in (krō - tok′sin). Crotoxina; a toxina do veneno da cascavel norte-americana. [*Crotalus* + toxina]

crot·tle (krot′el). Lecanora; orcela; urzela. SIN cudbear.

croup (kroop). Crupe. **1.** Obstrução aguda das vias aéreas superiores em lactentes e crianças caracterizada por tosse em ladrido com respiração difícil e ruidosa. **2.** Laringotraqueobronquite em lactentes e crianças pequenas causada por vírus parainfluenza 1 e 2. [Inglês da Escócia, provavelmente do A.S. *kropan,* chorar em voz alta]

croup·ous (kroo′p - ŭs). Crupal; relativo ao crupe; caracterizado por exsudação fibrinosa.

croupy (kroo′pē). Crupal; que possui as características de crupe, como uma tosse crupal.

Crouzon, Octave, médico francês, 1874–1938. VER C. *disease, syndrome.*

Crow, R.S., médico inglês. VER C.-Fukase *syndrome.*

crowd·ing (krowd′ing). Apinhamento, aglomerado; uma condição na qual os dentes estão apinhados, assumindo posições alteradas, como aglomeração, superposição, deslocamento em várias direções, torsiversão, etc.

Crowe, Samuel J., médico norte-americano, 1883–1955. VER C.-Davis mouth *gag*.

crown (krown) [TA]. Coroa. **1.** Qualquer estrutura, normal ou anormal, semelhante a, ou que sugere, uma coroa ou grinalda. **2.** Em odontologia, a parte de um dente que é coberta por esmalte, ou um substituto artificial para essa parte. SIN corona [TA]. [L. *corona*]
 anatomical c., c. anatômica. SIN c. of tooth.
 artificial c., c. artificial; uma restauração fixa da parte principal de toda a coroa de um dente natural; geralmente de ouro, porcelana ou resina acrílica.
 bell-shaped c., c. em forma de sino; a coroa de um dente que possui um contorno oclusogengival exagerado; os molares decíduos humanos exemplificam uma coroa em forma de sino.
 ciliary c., c. ciliar. SIN *corona* ciliaris.
 clinical c., c. clínica; a parte da coroa de um dente visível na cavidade oral. SIN corona clinica.
 c. of head, c. da cabeça. SIN *corona* capitis.
 jacket c., c. de jaqueta; uma coroa oca de resina acrílica, porcela fundida ou ouro moldado, combinações de ouro e acrílico ou ouro e porcelana; encaixa-se sobre o coto preparado da coroa natural.
 radiate c., c. radiada. SIN *corona* radiata.
 c. of tooth, c. do dente; a porção de um dente coberta por esmalte. SIN anatomical c., corona dentis.
 c. of Venus, c. de Vênus; lesões papulares da sífilis secundária na fronte, próximo à linha de implantação do cabelo.

crown·ing (krown′ing). Coroação. **1.** Preparo da coroa natural de um dente e revestimento da coroa preparada com um folheato de material dentário apropriado (molde de ouro ou metal não-precioso, porcelana, plástico ou combinações). **2.** O estágio do parto em que a cabeça fetal ultrapassou a saída pélvica e o maior diâmetro da cabeça está cercado pelo anel vulvar.

CRP Abreviatura de cAMP receptor *protein* (proteína receptora de AMPc); C-reactive *protein* (proteína C reativa).

CRT Abreviatura de cathode ray *tube* (tubo de raios catódicos).

cru·ces (kroo′sēz). Plural de crux.

cru·ci·ate (kroo′shē - āt). Cruciforme; que tem formato semelhante ou se assemelha a uma cruz. [L. *cruciatus*]

cru·ci·ble (kroo′si - bl). Cadinho; vaso usado como recipiente para reações ou fusões em alta temperatura. [L. Mediev. *crucibulum*, uma lâmpada noturna, depois, um cadinho]

cru·fo·mate (kroo′fō - māt). Crufomato; anti-helmíntico veterinário.

crunch (krunch). Rangido; som ouvido à ausculta torácica sincrônico com a contração cardíaca, indicando a presença de ar no mediastino. [onomatopeico]

cruor (kroo′or). Cruor; sangue coagulado. [L. sangue (que flui de uma ferida)]

cru·ra (kroo′ra). Plural de crus.

cru·ral (kroo′ral). Crural; relativo à perna ou à coxa, ou a qualquer parte que se assemelhe a uma perna ou ramo.

cru·re·us (kroo - rē′us). Músculo vasto intermédio. SIN vastus intermedius (*muscle*). [L. Mod.]

crus, gen. **cru·ris,** pl. **cru·ra** (kroos, kroo′ris, - rā) [TA]. Perna; pilar; ramo; pedúnculo. **1.** SIN leg. **2.** Qualquer estrutura anatômica semelhante a uma perna; geralmente (no plural) um par de fibras divergentes ou massas alongadas. VER TAMBÉM limb. [L.]
 ampullary crura of semicircular ducts, pilares membranáceos ampulares dos ductos semicirculares. SIN ampullary membranous *limbs* of semicircular ducts, em *limb*.
 anterior c. of stapes, ramo anterior do estribo. SIN anterior *limb* of stapes.
 c. ante′rius cap′sulae inter′nae [TA], ramo anterior da cápsula interna. SIN anterior *limb* of internal capsule.
 c. ante′rius stape′dis [TA], ramo anterior do estribo. SIN anterior *limb* of stapes.
 crura anthel′icis, ramos da antélice. SIN crura of antihelix.
 crura antihelicis [TA], ramos da antélice. SIN crura of antihelix.
 crura of antihelix [TA], ramos da antélice; duas cristas, inferior e superior, que limitam a fossa triangular, pelas quais a antélice começa na parte superior da orelha. SIN crura antihelicis [TA], crura anthelicis, leg of antihelix.
 crura of bony semicircular canals, pilares ósseos dos canais semicirculares. SIN bony *limbs* of semicircular canals, em *limb*.
 c. bre′ve incu′dis [TA], ramo curto da bigorna. SIN short *limb* of incus.
 c. cer′ebri [TA], base do pedúnculo cerebral; especificamente, o grande feixe de fibras nervosas corticífugas que segue longitudinalmente sobre a superfície ventral do mesencéfalo de cada lado da linha média; consiste em fibras que descem do córtex até o tegmento do tronco cerebral, substância cinzenta pontina e medula espinhal. VER TAMBÉM cerebral *peduncle, basis* pedunculi.
 c. clitor′idis [TA], ramo do clitóris. SIN c. of clitoris.
 c. of clitoris [TA], ramo do clitóris; a continuação de cada lado do corpo cavernoso do clitóris que diverge do corpo posteriormente e está fixada ao arco púbico. SIN c. clitoridis [TA].
 common c. of semicircular ducts, pilar membranáceo comum dos ductos semicirculares. SIN common membranous *limb* of semicircular ducts.
 c. cor′poris caverno′si pe′nis, ramo do corpo cavernoso do pênis. SIN c. of penis.
 c. dex′trum diaphrag′matis [TA], pilar direito do diafragma. SIN right c. of diaphragm.
 c. dex′trum fasci′culi atrioventricula′ris [TA], ramo direito do fascículo atrioventricular. SIN right *bundle* of atrioventricular bundle. VER TAMBÉM atrioventricular *bundle*.
 c. for′nicis [TA], pilar do fórnice; a parte do fórnice que sobe em uma curva para a frente, atrás do tálamo, para continuar para a frente como o corpo para o fórnice ventral ao corpo caloso. SIN c. of fornix [TA], posterior pillar of fornix.
 c. of fornix [TA], pilar do fórnice. SIN c. fornicis.
 c. hel′icis [TA], ramo da hélice. SIN c. of helix.
 c. of helix [TA], ramo da hélice; uma crista transversal que segue para trás a partir da hélice da orelha, dividindo a concha em uma porção superior (cimba) e uma porção inferior (cavidade da concha). SIN c. helicis [TA], crista helicis, limb of helix.
 c. inferius marginis falciformis hiatus sapheni, pilar inferior da margem falciforme do hiato safeno; *termo oficial alternativo para inferior *horn* of falciform margin of saphenous opening.
 lateral c., ramo lateral; ramo ou porção semelhante à perna de uma estrutura, mais distante da linha média. SIN c. laterale, lateral limb.
 c. latera′le, ramo lateral. SIN lateral c.
 c. latera′le an′uli inguina′lis superficia′lis [TA], pilar lateral do anel inguinal superficial. SIN lateral c. of the superficial inguinal ring.
 c. latera′le cartila′ginis ala′ris majo′ris [TA], ramo lateral da cartilagem alar maior. SIN lateral c. of the major alar cartilage of the nose.
 lateral c. of facial canal, pilar lateral do canal facial; segunda porção situada lateralmente, deslocada posteriormente, da parte horizontal do canal facial. VER horizontal *part* of facial canal. SIN lateral c. of horizontal part of the facial canal.
 lateral c. of horizontal part of the facial canal, pilar lateral da parte horizontal do canal facial. SIN lateral c. of facial canal. VER horizontal *part* of facial canal.
 lateral c. of the major alar cartilage of the nose [TA], ramo lateral da cartilagem alar maior do nariz; porção da cartilagem que se estende, lateral e posteriormente, com a forma de uma asa, dando suporte à asa do nariz e mantendo a narina pérvia. SIN c. laterale cartilaginis alaris majoris [TA].
 lateral c. of the superficial inguinal ring [TA], pilar lateral do anel inguinal superficial; porção da aponeurose do oblíquo externo que segue lateral ao anel inguinal superficial, fundindo-se com o ligamento inguinal e formando o limite lateral do anel. SIN c. laterale anuli inguinalis superficialis [TA].
 left c. of atrioventricular bundle, ramo esquerdo do fascículo atrioventricular. SIN left *bundle* of atrioventricular bundle.
 left c. of diaphragm [TA], pilar esquerdo do diafragma; a origem muscular do diafragma nas duas ou três vértebras lombares superiores que ascende à esquerda da aorta para alcançar o tendão central. SIN c. sinistrum diaphragmatis [TA].

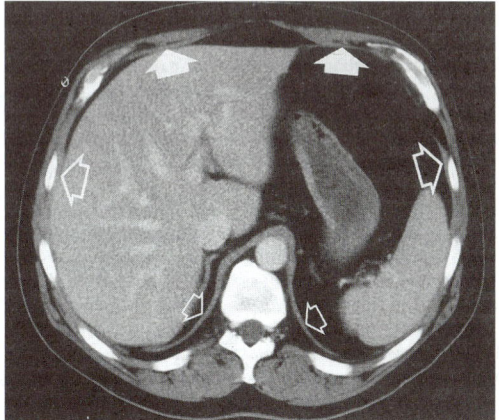

pilares do diafragma: anatomia normal à TC; imagem através da parte superior do abdome mostra os pilares do diafragma posteriormente (setas abertas pequenas), as origens costais do diafragma lateralmente (setas abertas grandes) e as origens cartilaginosas costais ântero-lateralmente (setas sólidas)

 long c. of incus, ramo longo da bigorna. SIN long *limb* of incus.
 c. lon′gum incu′dis [TA], ramo longo da bigorna. SIN lomb *limb* of incus.
 medial c. [TA], ramo medial; ramo ou porção semelhante a uma perna de uma estrutura mais próxima da linha média. SIN c. mediale [TA], medial limb.
 c. media′le [TA], ramo medial. SIN medial c.

c. media'le an'uli inguina'lis superficia'lis [TA], pilar medial do anel inguinal superficial. SIN medial c. of the superficial inguinal ring.
c. media'le cartila'ginis ala'ris major'is [TA], ramo medial da cartilagem alar maior. SIN medial c. of major alar cartilage of nose.
medial c. of facial canal, pilar medial do canal facial; primeira porção, posicionada medialmente, voltada anteriormente, da parte horizontal do canal facial. VER horizontal *part* of facial canal. SIN medial c. of the horizontal part of the facial canal.
medial c. of the horizontal part of the facial canal, pilar medial da parte horizontal do canal facial. SIN medial c. of facial canal. VER horizontal *part* of facial canal.
medial c. of major alar cartilage of nose [TA], ramo medial da cartilagem alar maior do nariz; porção da cartilagem que forma a porção ântero-inferior do septo cartilaginoso entre as narinas. SIN c. mediale cartilaginis alaris majoris [TA].
medial c. of the superficial inguinal ring [TA], pilar medial do anel inguinal superficial; porção da aponeurose do músculo oblíquo externo que segue medialmente ao anel inguinal superficial, formando o limite medial do anel. SIN c. mediale anuli inguinalis superficialis [TA].
cru'ra membrana'cea ampulla'ria duc'tuum semicircula'rium [TA], pilares membranáceos ampulares dos ductos semicirculares. SIN ampullary membranous *limbs* of semicircular ducts, em *limb*.
c. membrana'ceum commu'ne duc'tuum semicircula'rium [TA], pilar membranáceo comum dos ductos semicirculares. SIN common membranous *limb* of semicircular ducts.
c. membrana'ceum sim'plex duc'tus semicircula'ris [TA], pilar membranáceo simples dos ductos semicirculares. SIN simple membranous *limb* of semicircular duct.
cru'ra os'sea cana'lium semicircula'rium, pilares ósseos dos canais semicirculares. SIN bony *limbs* of semicircular canals, em *limb*.
c. pe'nis [TA], ramo do pênis. SIN c. of penis.
c. of penis, ramo do pênis; a porção posterior, afilada, do corpo cavernoso do pênis que diverge de seu parceiro contralateral para se fixar ao ramo isquiopúbico. SIN c. penis [TA], c. corporis cavernosi penis.
posterior c. of stapes, ramo posterior do estribo. SIN posterior *limb* of stapes.
c. poste'rius cap'sulae inter'nae [TA], ramo posterior da cápsula interna. SIN posterior *limb* of internal capsule.
c. poste'rius stape'dis [TA], ramo posterior do estribo. SIN posterior *limb* of stapes.
right c. of atrioventricular bundle, ramo direito do fascículo atrioventricular. SIN right *bundle* of atrioventricular bundle.
right c. of diaphragm [TA], pilar direito do diafragma; a origem muscular do diafragma dos corpos das três ou quatro vértebras lombares superiores que segue para cima e para a direita da aorta, em direção ao tendão central; o hiato esofágico é uma divisão das fibras do pilar direito para permitir a passagem do esôfago. SIN c. dextrum diaphragmatis [TA].
short c. of incus, ramo curto da bigorna. SIN short *limb* of incus.
simple c. of semicircular duct, pilar simples do ducto semicircular. SIN simple membranous *limb* of semicircular duct.
c. sinis'trum diaphrag'matis [TA], pilar esquerdo do diafragma. SIN left c. of diaphragm.
c. sinis'trum fasci'culi atrioventricula'ris, ramo esquerdo do fascículo atrioventricular. SIN left *bundle* of atrioventricular bundle. VER TAMBÉM atrioventricular *bundle*.
c. superius marginis falciformis hiatus sapheni, pilar superior da margem falciforme do hiato safeno. SIN superior *horn* of falciform margin of saphenous opening.
crus I (kroos). Lóbulo semilunar superior. SIN superior semilunar *lobule*.
crus II (kroos). Lóbulo semilunar inferior. SIN inferior semilunar *lobule*.
crush ((krŭsh). **1.** Esmagar; comprimir lesivamente entre dois corpos duros. **2.** Esmagamento; equimose ou contusão causada por pressão entre dois corpos sólidos. [Fr. Ant. *cruisir*]
crus·ot·o·my (kroos - ot'ō - mē). Crusotomia; uma tratotomia piramidal mesencefálica. [L. *crus,* perna, + G. *tomē,* incisão]
crust (krŭst). Crosta. **1.** Uma camada ou cobertura externa rígida; as crostas cutâneas freqüentemente são formadas por soro ou pus seco na superfície de uma vesícula ou pústula rota. **2.** Casca de ferida. SIN crusta. [L. *crusta*]
milk c., c. láctea. SIN *crusta* lactea.
crus·ta, pl. **crus·tae** (krŭs'tă, - tē). Crosta. SIN crust. [L.]
c. inflammato'ria, creme leucocitário. SIN buffy *coat*.
c. lac'tea, c. láctea; seborréia do couro cabeludo em um lactente. SIN milk crust.
c. phlogis'tica, creme leucocitário. SIN buffy *coat*.
Crus·ta·cea (krŭs - tā'shē - ă). Uma classe muito grande de animais aquáticos (filo Arthropoda) com um exoesqueleto quitinoso e apêndices articulados; p. ex., caranguejo, lagosta, pitu, camarão, isópodes, Ostracódeos e anfípodes. Alguns, como certos copépodes, são parasitas; outros servem como hospedeiros intermediários para vermes parasitas que causam doença em seres humanos e em vários outros vertebrados. VER TAMBÉM Copepoda. [L. *crusta,* crosta]

crutch (krŭtch). Muleta; acessório usado isoladamente ou em pares para ajudar a caminhar quando esse ato é prejudicado por uma incapacidade do membro inferior (ou tronco); transfere toda a sustentação de peso, ou parte dela, para os membros superiores. [A.S. *cryce*]
Cruveilhier, Jean, patologista e anatomista francês, 1791–1874. VER C. *fascia, fossa; fossa* navicularis Cruveilhier; C. *joint, ligaments,* em ligament, *plexus;* C.-Baumgarten *disease, murmur, sign, syndrome*.
crux, pl. **cru·ces** (krŭks, kroo'sēz). Cruz; uma junção ou cruzamento. SIN cross (1). [L.]
c. of heart, cruz do coração; a área de junção dos septos e paredes das quatro câmaras cardíacas. SIN cross (2).
cru'ces pilo'rum [TA], entrecruzamentos dos pêlos. SIN hair *crosses*, em *cross*.
Cruz, Oswaldo, médico brasileiro, 1872–1917. VER Chagas-C. *disease;* C. *trypanosomiasis*.
△ **cry-.** VER cryo-.
cry·al·ge·sia (krī - al - jē'zē - ă). Crialgesia; dor causada por frio. [G. *kryos,* frio, + *algos,* dor]
cry·an·es·the·sia (krī'an - es - thē'zē - ă). Crianestesia; incapacidade de perceber o frio.
cry·es·the·sia (krī - es - thē'zē - ă). Criestesia. **1.** Sensação subjetiva de frio. **2.** Sensibilidade ao frio. [G. *kryos,* frio, + *aisthēsis,* sensação]
cry for help. Pedido de socorro; telefonemas, anotações deixadas em locais visíveis e outros comportamentos que transmitem sofrimento extremo e possível consideração de suicídio.
△ **crymo-.** Frio. VER TAMBÉM cryo-, psychro-. [G. *krymos,* frio]
cry·mo·phil·ic (krī - mō - fil'ik). Crimófilo; criófilo; que prefere o frio; designa microrganismos que se desenvolvem melhor em baixas temperaturas. SIN cryophilic. [crymo- + G. *philos,* afeiçoado]
cry·mo·phy·lac·tic (krī'mō - fi - lak'tik). Crimofilático; criofilático; que resiste ao frio, diz-se de certos microrganismos que não são destruídos nem mesmo em temperaturas de congelamento. SIN cryphylactic. [crymo- + G. *phylaxis,* proteção contra]
△ **cryo-, cry-.** Frio. VER TAMBÉM crymo-, psychro-. [G. *kryos,* frio]
cry·o·an·es·the·sia (krī'ō - an - es - thē'zē - ă). Crioanestesia; aplicação localizada de frio como uma forma de produzir anestesia regional. SIN refrigeration anesthesia.
cry·o·bi·ol·o·gy (krī'ō - bī - ol'ō - jē). Criobiologia; o estudo dos efeitos das baixas temperaturas sobre organismos vivos.
cry·o·cau·tery (krī'ō - kaw'ter - ē). Criocautério; qualquer substância, como nitrogênio líquido ou neve de dióxido de carbono, ou um instrumento em baixa temperatura, cuja aplicação causa destruição tecidual por congelamento. SIN cold cauter.
cry·o·con·i·za·tion (krī'ō - kon - ī - zā'shŭn). Crioconização; congelamento de um cone de tecido endocervical *in vivo* com um criocautério.
cry·o·ex·trac·tion (krī'ō - ek - strak'shŭn). Crioextração; remoção de catarata pela adesão de uma sonda congeladora ao cristalino; raramente usada hoje.
cry·o·ex·trac·tor (krī'ō - ek - strak'tŏr, - tōr). Crioextrator; um instrumento, resfriado artificialmente, para extração do cristalino por congelamento ao contato.
cry·o·fi·brin·o·gen (krī'ō - fī - brin'ō - jen). Criofibrinogênio; tipo anormal de fibrinogênio encontrado muito raramente no plasma humano; é precipitado ao resfriamento, mas torna dissolver quando aquecido à temperatura ambiente.
cry·o·fi·brin·o·gen·e·mia (krī'ō - fī - brin'ō - je - nē'mē - ă). Criofibrinogenemia; a presença de criofibrinógenos no sangue.
cry·o·flu·o·rane (krī - ō - flōr'ān). Criofluorano; usado como refrigerante e propulsor de aerossol; pode ser irritante para as vias respiratórias e levemente narcótico.
cry·o·frac·ture (krīō - frak'choor). Criofratura. SIN freeze *fracture*. [cryo- + fracture]
cry·o·gen (krī'ō - jen). Criógeno; substância de congelação usada para produzir temperaturas muito baixas.
cry·o·gen·ic (krī - ō - jen'ik). Criogênico. **1.** Designa ou é característico de um criógeno. **2.** Relativo à criogenia.
cry·o·gen·ics (krī - ō - jen'iks). Criogenia; a ciência relacionada à produção e aos efeitos de temperaturas muito baixas, particularmente temperaturas na faixa do hélio líquido (< 4,25 K). [cryo- + G. *-gen,* que produz]
cry·o·glob·u·lin·e·mia (krī'ō - glob'ū - li - nē'mē - ă). Crioglobulinemia; presença de quantidades anormais de crioglobulina no plasma sanguíneo.
cry·o·glob·u·lins (krī - ō - glob'ū - linz). Crioglobulinas. **1.** Proteínas plasmáticas anormais (paraproteínas), agora agrupadas com as gamaglobulinas, caracterizadas por precipitação, gelificação ou cristalização quando o soro ou suas soluções são resfriadas; distinta das proteínas de Bence Jones por seu maior peso molecular (aproximadamente 200.000 em comparação com 35.000–50.000); podem surgir em pacientes com mieloma múltiplo. **2.** Qualquer globulina que forma um gel ou precipitado floculento ao ser resfriada.
cry·o·hy·drate (krī - ō - hī'drāt). Crioidrato; um sistema eutético de um sal e água.

cry·o·hy·poph·y·sec·to·my (krī'o - hī - pof'i - sek'to - me). Crioipofisectomia; destruição da hipófise pela aplicação de frio extremo. [cryo- + hypophysis + G. *ektomē*, excisão]

cry·ol·y·sis (krī - ol'i - sis). Criólise; destruição pelo frio. [cryo- + G. *lysis*, dissolução]

cry·om·e·ter (krī - om'ē - ter). Criômetro; dispositivo para medir temperaturas muito baixas. [cryo- + G. *metron*, medida]

cry·o·pal·li·dec·to·my (krī'o - pal - i - dek'to - me). Criopalidectomia; destruição do globo pálido pela aplicação de frio extremo. [cryo- + globo pálido + G. *ektomē*, excisão]

cry·op·a·thy (krī - op'a - thē). Criopatia. Uma condição mórbida na qual a exposição ao frio é um fator importante. SIN frigorism. [cryo + G. *pathos*, sofrimento]

cry·o·pexy (krī'o - pek - sē). Criopexia; na cirurgia do descolamento da retina, a "vedação" da retina sensorial ao epitélio pigmentar e à coróide por meio de uma sonda de congelamento aplicada à esclera. [cryo- + G. *pēxis*, fixação no lugar]

cry·o·phil·ic (krī - o - fil'ik). Criofílico. SIN crymophilic. [cryo- + G. *philos*, afeiçoado]

cry·o·phy·lac·tic (krī'o - fī - lak'tik). Criofilático. SIN crymophylactic.

cry·o·pre·cip·i·tate (krī'o - prē - sip'i - tāt). Crioprecipitado; precipitado que se forma quando um material solúvel é resfriado, principalmente em relação ao precipitado que se forma no plasma sanguíneo normal que foi submetido à precipitação por frio e que é rico em fator VIII.

cry·o·pre·cip·i·ta·tion (krī'o - prē - sip - i - ta'shun). Crioprecipitação; o processo de formar um crioprecipitado a partir da solução.

cry·o·pres·er·va·tion (krī'o - pres - er - va'shun). Criopreservação; manutenção da viabilidade de tecidos ou órgãos excisados em temperaturas extremamente baixas.

cry·o·probe (krī'o - prōb). Criossonda; instrumento usado em criocirurgia para aplicar frio extremo a uma área selecionada. [cryo- + L. *probo*, testar]

cry·o·pros·ta·tec·to·my (krī'o - pros - tā - tek'to - me). Crioprostatectomia; destruição da próstata por congelamento, utilizando-se uma criossonda especial. [cryo- + L. *prostata*, próstata, + G. *ektomē*, excisão]

cry·o·pro·tein (krī - o - pro'tēn). Crioproteína; uma proteína que precipita da solução, quando resfriada, e se dissolve novamente ao ser aquecida.

cry·o·pul·vi·nec·to·my (krī'o - pūl - vi - nek'to - me). Criopulvinectomia; destruição do núcleo pulvinar pela aplicação de frio extremo. [cryo- + pulvinar + G. *ektomē*, excisão]

cry·o·scope (krī'o - skōp). Crioscópio; instrumento para medir o ponto de congelamento.

cry·os·co·py (krī - os'ko - pē). Crioscopia; a determinação do ponto de congelamento de um líquido, geralmente sangue ou urina, em comparação com o da água destilada. SIN algoscopy. [cryo- + G. *skopeō*, examinar]

cry·o·spasm (krī'o - spazm). Criospasmo; espasmo produzido pelo frio. [cryo + G. *spasmos*, convulsão]

cry·o·stat (krī'o - stat). Criostato; câmara de congelamento. [cryo- + G. *statos*, situação]

cry·o·sur·gery (krī - o - ser'jer - ē). Criocirurgia; uma operação que usa temperatura de congelamento (atingida por nitrogênio líquido ou dióxido de carbono) como agente independente ou em um instrumento para destruir um tecido.

cry·o·thal·a·mec·to·my (krī'o - thal - a - mek'to - me). Criotalamectomia; destruição do tálamo pela aplicação de frio extremo. [cryo- + talamus + G. *ektomē*, excisão]

cry·o·ther·a·py (krī'o - thār'a - pē). Crioterapia; o uso do frio no tratamento de uma doença.

cry·o·tol·er·ant (krī - o - tol'er - ant). Criotolerante; tolerante a temperaturas muito baixas.

crypt (kript) [TA]. Cripta; uma depressão semelhante a uma cova ou recesso tubular. SIN crypta [TA].

anal c.'s, criptas anais. SIN anal *sinuses*, em *sinus*.

dental c., c. dental; o espaço ocupado pelo folículo dental.

enamel c., c. do esmalte; o espaço estreito, preenchido por mesênquima, entre a borda do dente e um órgão de esmalte. SIN enamel niche.

c.'s of Henle, criptas de Henle; invaginações da conjuntiva.

c.'s of iris, criptas da íris; (1) depressões próximas da margem pupilar da superfície anterior da íris. (2) espaços no estroma anterior da íris através dos quais o humor aquoso passa a cada movimento pupilar.

c.'s of Lieberkühn, criptas de Lieberkühn. SIN intestinal *glands*, em *gland*.

c.'s of Lieberkühn of large intestine, criptas de Lieberkühn do intestino grosso. SIN *glands* of large intestine, em *gland*.

c.'s of Lieberkühn of small intestine, criptas de Lieberkühn do intestino delgado. SIN *glands* of small intestine, em *gland*.

lingual c., c. lingual; uma depressão revestida por epitélio na tonsila lingual.

Morgagni c.'s, criptas de Morgagni. SIN anal *sinuses*, em *sinus*.

synovial c., c. sinovial; um divertículo da membrana sinovial de uma articulação.

tonsillar c., [TA], c. tonsilar; um dos diversos recessos profundos que se estendem a partir da superfície livre, onde se abrem na fossa tonsilar, para as tonsilas lingual, palatina, faríngea e tubária. SIN crypta tonsillaris [TA].

crypt-. VER crypto-.

cryp·ta, pl. **cryp·tae** (krip'tā, - tē) [TA]. Cripta. SIN crypt. [L. do G. *kryptos*, oculto]

c. tonsilla'ris, pl. **cryp'tae tonsilla'res** [TA], c. tonsilar. SIN tonsillar *crypt*.

cryp·tec·to·my (krip - tek'to - me). Criptectomia; excisão de uma cripta tonsilar ou outra. [crypt + G. *ektomē*, excisão]

cryp·ten·a·mine ac·e·tates, cryp·ten·a·mine tan·nates (krip - ten'a - mēn). Acetato de criptenamina, tanato de criptenamina; sais acetato ou tanato de alcalóides de um extrato não-aquoso de *Veratrum viride*, contendo os alcalóides hipotensores protoveratrinas A e B, germitrina, neogermetrina, germerina, germidina, jervina, rubijervina, isorrubijervina e germubida; usados como agentes anti-hipertensivos. VER TAMBÉM protoveratrine A and B.

cryp·tic (krip'tik). Críptico; escondido, oculto, larvado. [L. *kryptikos*]

cryp·ti·tis (krip - tī'tis). Criptite; inflamação de um folículo ou túbulo glandular, particularmente no cólon.

crypto-, crypt-. Oculto, obscuro; sem causa aparente. [G. *kryptos*, oculto, escondido]

cryptochrome (krip'to - krōm). Criptocromo; receptor flavoproteína da luz ultravioleta A envolvido na indução do ritmo circadiano em plantas, insetos e mamíferos.

cryp·to·coc·co·ma (krip'to - kok - o'mā). Criptococoma; um granuloma infeccioso, tipicamente no cérebro, mas também encontrado no pulmão e em outras partes, causado pelo *Cryptococcus neoformans*. [*Cryptococcus* (nome do gênero) + -oma]

cryp·to·coc·co·sis (krip'to - kok - o'sis). Criptococose; infecção aguda, subaguda ou crônica por *Cryptococcus neoformans*, que causa micose pulmonar, disseminada ou meníngea. A forma pulmonar pode melhorar espontaneamente em pessoas previamente normais, mas a disseminação para outros órgãos é fatal se não for tratada; a manifestação clínica mais comum é a meningite.

Cryp·to·coc·cus (krip - to - kok'us). Gênero de fungos leveduriformes que se reproduzem por brotamento. [crypto- + G. *kokkos*, bagas]

C. neofor'mans, espécie que causa criptococose em seres humanos e em outros mamíferos, particularmente a família do gato. As células são esféricas e se reproduzem por brotamento; uma característica proeminente é uma cápsula polissacarídica. *C. neoformans* var. *neoformans* tem distribuição mundial, e freqüentemente, pode ser isolado nos excrementos de pombos desgastados pelo tempo. *C. neoformans* var. *gattii* causa criptococose em climas subtropicais e tropicais. Essa variedade foi isolada na ramagem e na folha de espécies de eucalipto.

cryp·to·crys·tal·line (krip - to - kris'tā - lēn). Criptocristalino; que possui cristais diminutos.

Cryp·to·cys·tis trich·o·dec·tis (krip - to - sis'tis trī - ko - dek'tis). Nome dado antigamente à forma larvar da tênia do cachorro, *Dipylidium caninum*, denominada de acordo com os cisticercóides encontrados no piolho canino, *Trichodectes*. [crypto- + G. *kystis*, bexiga; tricho- + G. *dektēs*, mendigo]

cryp·to·did·y·mus (krip'to - did'i - mus). Criptodídimo; gêmeos conjugados, com o gêmeo parasita pouco desenvolvido e oculto no autósito maior. VER conjoined *twins*, em *twin*. [crypto- + G. *didymos*, gêmeo]

Cryp·to·gam·ia (krip - to - gam'ē - ā). Criptogamia; divisão não-taxonômica do reino vegetal, contendo todas as formas de vida vegetal que não se reproduzem por meio de sementes; são incluídos algas, bactérias, fungos, líquens, musgos, Hepáticas (planta criptogâmica da classe *Hepaticae*), samambaias, cavalinhas e licopódios. [crypto- + G. *gamos*, casamento]

cryp·to·gen·ic (krip - to - jen'ik). Criptogênico; de etiologia ou origem obscura, indeterminada, em contraste com fanerogênico. [crypto- + G. *genesis*, origem]

cryp·to·lith (krip'to - lith). Criptólito; concreção em um folículo glandular. [crypto- + G. *lithos*, cálculo]

cryp·to·men·or·rhea (krip'to - men - o - rē'ā). Criptomenorréia; ocorrência, a cada mês, dos sintomas gerais de menstruação sem qualquer fluxo de sangue, como em casos de hímen imperfurado. [crypto- + G. *mēn*, mês, + *rhoia*, fluxo]

cryp·toph·thal·mus, cryp·toph·thal·mia (krip - tof - thal'mus, - thal'mē - ā). Criptoftalmia; ausência congênita de pálpebras, com a pele seguindo de forma contínua da fronte para a bochecha sobre um olho rudimentar. [crypto- + G. *ophthalmos*, olho]

cryp·to·po·dia (krip - to - pō'dē - ā). Criptopodia; edema da parte inferior da perna e do pé, de forma que há grande distorção e a região plantar parece ser um coxim achatado. [crypto- + G. *pous*, pé]

cryp·to·pyr·role (krip - to - pir'ōl). Criptopirrol; 3-etil-2,4-dimetilpirrol; um dos derivados pirrólicos obtidos pela redução drástica do heme.

cryp·tor·chid (krip - tōr'kid). Criptórquio; relativo a, ou caracterizado por, criptorquidia. [crypto- + G. *orchis*, testículo]

cryp·tor·chi·dism (krip - tōr'ki - dizm). Criptorquidia. SIN cryptorchism.

cryp·tor·chism (krip - tōr'kizm). Criptorquidia; ausência de descida de um ou ambos os testículos. SIN cryptorchidism.

cryp·to·scope (krip'tō - skōp). Criptoscópio; termo obsoleto para um fluoroscópio de raios X simples. [G. *kryptos*, algo escondido, + *skopeō*, examinar]

cryp·to·spo·rid·i·o·sis (krip'tō - spō - rid - ē - ō'sis). Criptosporidiose; doença entérica causada por parasitas protozoários veiculados pela água do gênero *Cryptosporidium*; caracterizada histopatologicamente por atrofia e fusão das vilosidades intestinais e, clinicamente, por diarréia em seres humanos, bezerros, cordeiros e outros animais; a doença, em pessoas imunocompetentes, manifesta-se como uma diarréia autolimitada, enquanto, em pessoas imunodeprimidas, manifesta-se como uma diarréia grave e prolongada que pode ser fatal.

Cryp·to·spo·rid·i·um (krip'tō - spō - rid'ē - ŭm). Gênero de esporozoários coccídios (família Cryptosporiidae, subordem Eimeriina) que são patógenos importantes de bezerros e outros animais domésticos e parasitas oportunistas comuns dos seres humanos, que vicejam em condições de comprometimento da função imune; pode causar diarréia autolimitada em pessoas imunocompetentes.

  C. parvum, espécie de esporozoário que é causa importante de diarréia neonatal em bezerros e cordeiros; causa diarréia crônica, leve, autolimitada a grave, em seres humanos.

Cryp·to·stro·ma cor·ti·ca·le (krip - tō - strō'mă kōr - ti - kā'lē). Espécie de fungo que é um alérgeno comum, de crescimento abundante na casca de troncos de bordo empilhados; as pessoas que manipulam esses troncos inalam maciçamente esporos e desenvolvem pneumonite, bem como reações alérgicas, incluindo a doença da casca de bordo. [crypto- + G. *stroma*, leito]

cryp·to·tia (krip - tō'shē - ă). Criptotia; anormalidade rara, na qual a porção superior da orelha está escondida sob o couro cabeludo. [crypto- + G. *ōtos*, orelha]

cryp·to·xan·thin (krip - tō - zan'thin). Criptoxantina; (3R)-β,β-Caroten-3-ol; β-caroten-3-ol; carotenóide (especificamente, uma xantofila) que produz 1 mol de vitamina A por mol. Encontrada em muitas frutas e no morango, framboesa, amora, etc.

cryp·to·zo·ite (krip'tō - zō'īt). Criptozoíta; o estágio exoeritrocítico do plasmódio que se desenvolve diretamente a partir do esporozoíta inoculado pelo mosquito infectado; o desenvolvimento da primeira geração de merozoítas em tecidos de hospedeiros vertebrados ocorre no parênquima hepático. [crypto - + G. *zōē*, vida]

cryp·to·zy·gous (krip - toz'i - gŭs, - tō - zī'gŭs). Criptozigoso; que possui uma face estreita em comparação com a largura do crânio, de forma que, quando o crânio é visto de cima, os arcos zigomáticos não são visíveis. [crypto- + G. *zygon*, vitelo]

crys·tal (kris'tăl). Cristal; um sólido de formato regular e, para um determinado composto, ângulos característicos, formado quando um elemento ou composto se solidifica lentamente o suficiente, em virtude de congelamento a partir da forma líquida ou precipitação de solução, para permitir que as moléculas individuais assumam posições regulares entre si. [G. *krystallos*, gelo transparente, cristal]

  asthma c.'s, cristais da asma. SIN Charcot-Leyden c.'s.
  blood c.'s, hematoidina. SIN hematoidin.
  Böttcher c.'s, cristais de Böttcher; pequenos cristais observados microscopicamente no líquido prostático tratado com uma gota ou duas de solução de fosfato de amônio a 1%.
  Charcot-Leyden c.'s, cristais de Charcot-Leyden; cristais com o formato de pirâmides duplas alongadas, formados por eosinófilos, encontrados no escarro na asma brônquica e em outros exsudatos ou transudatos contendo eosinófilos. SIN asthma c.'s, Charcot-Neumann c.'s, Charcot-Robin c.'s, Leyden c.'s.
  Charcot-Neumann c.'s, cristais de Charcot-Neumann. SIN Charcot-Leyden c.'s.
  Charcot-Robin c.'s, cristais de Charcot-Robin. SIN Charcot-Leyden c.'s.
  chiral c., isômero estereoquímico; um cristal enantiomorfo, assimétrico, opticamente ativo.
  chlorohemin c.'s, cristais de cloroemina. SIN Teichmann c.'s.
  clathrate c., c. de clatrato; arranjo reticulado de moléculas de uma substância circundando moléculas de outra substância.
  ear c.'s, cristais auriculares. SIN otoliths.
  Florence c.'s, cristais de Florence; cristais rômbicos, castanhos, na interface entre uma gota de solução de Lugol e uma gota de líquido que contém sêmen; não é um teste específico para este último.
  hematoidin c.'s, cristais de hematoidina. SIN hematoidin.
  hydrate c., c. de hidrato; um dos vários arranjos microestruturais possíveis de moléculas de água baseados em forças intermoleculares; sugerido como envolvido no modo de ação de anestésicos inalatórios.
  knife-rest c., c. de fosfato de amônio e magnésio encontrado na urina alcalina.
  Leyden c.'s, cristais de Leyden. SIN Charcot-Leyden c.'s.
  Lubarsch c.'s, cristais de Lubarsch; cristais intracelulares no testículo semelhantes a cristais de esperma.
  sperm c., spermin c., c. de esperma, c. de espermina; um cristal de fosfato de espermina encontrado no sêmen; possivelmente idêntico aos cristais de Böttcher.
  Teichmann c.'s, cristais de Teichmann; cristais rômbicos de hemina; usados na detecção microscópica de sangue. VER hemin. SIN chlorohemin c.'s.
  thorn apple c.'s, cristais estramônio; cristais de urato de amônio com o formato de corpos arredondados com muitas pontas.
  twin c., c. gêmeo; dois cristais que crescem juntos ao longo de uma face comum.
  Virchow c.'s, cristais de Virchow; cristais amarelo-castanhos, âmbar ou laranja-queimado de hematoidina, freqüentemente observados no sangue extravasado nos tecidos.
  whetstone c.'s, cristais em pedra de amolar; cristais de xantina ocasionalmente observados na urina.

crys·tal·lin (kris'tă - lin). Cristalina; uma das várias proteínas hidrossolúveis encontradas no cristalino; são conhecidos os tipos alfa (uma proteína simples embrionária), beta e gama (baseados nas características de precipitação). Répteis e aves possuem uma δ-cristalina também. A ε-cristalina é idêntica à lactato desidrogenase (desidrogenase láctica).

  gamma c., c. gama; a forma de cristalina que se move mais lentamente à eletroforese.

crys·tal·line (kris'tă - lēn). Cristalino. **1.** Límpido; transparente. **2.** Relativo a um cristal ou cristais.

crys·tal·li·za·tion (kris'tăl - i - zā'shŭn). Cristalização; adoção de uma forma cristalina quando um vapor ou líquido é solidificado, ou um soluto se precipita da solução.

crys·tal·lo·gram (kris'tă - lō - gram). Cristalograma; fotografia produzida quando os raios X sofrem difração por um cristal. [G. *krystallos*, cristal + *gramma*, algo escrito]

crys·tal·log·ra·phy (kris - tăl - log'ră - fē). Cristalografia; o estudo do formato e da estrutura atômica dos cristais.

crys·tal·loid (kris'tăl - oyd). Cristalóide. **1.** Semelhante a um cristal, ou como tal. **2.** Um corpo que, em solução, consegue atravessar uma membrana semipermeável, ao contrário de um colóide, que não consegue fazê-lo.

  Charcot-Böttcher c.'s, cristalóides de Charcot-Böttcher; cristalóides fusiformes, com 10–25 μm de comprimento, encontrados nas células de Sertoli humanas.
  Reinke c.'s, cristalóides de Reinke; estruturas semelhantes a cristal, em forma de bastão, com extremidades pontiagudas ou arredondadas, presentes nas células intersticiais do testículo (células de Leydig) e ovário.

crys·tal·lo·pho·bia (kris'tăl - ō - fō'bē - ă). Cristalofobia. SIN hyalophobia. [G. *krystallon*, cristal, + *phobos*, medo]

crys·tal·lu·ria (kris - tă - loo'rē - ă). Cristalúria; a excreção de material cristalino na urina.

crys·tal vi·o·let (kris'tăl) [C.I. 42555]. Cristal violeta; substância que tem sido usada no tratamento externo de queimaduras, feridas e micoses da pele e mucosas, e, internamente, para tratamento de infestações por oxiúros e alguns trematódeos; usada também como corante para cromatina, amilóide, plaquetas no sangue, fibrina e neuróglia, e para diferenciação entre bactérias. SIN methylrosaniline chloride.

Cs Símbolo do césio.

CSD Abreviatura de catscratch *disease* (doença da arranhadura do gato).

C-sec·tion. Cesariana. VER cesarean *section*.

CSF Abreviatura de cerebrospinal *fluid* (líquido cefaloespinal); colony-stimulating *factors* (fatores estimulantes de colônias), em *factor*.

CSI. Abreviatura de Calculus Surface Index (Índice de Superfície do Cálculo).

CT Abreviatura de computed *tomography* (tomografia computadorizada).
  dynamic CT, TC dinâmica. SIN dynamic computed *tomography*.
  helical CT, TC helicoidal. SIN spiral computed *tomography*.
  spiral CT, TC helicoidal. SIN spiral computed *tomography*.

CTD Abreviatura de cumulative trauma *disorders* (distúrbios traumáticos cumulativos), em *disorder*.

Cte·no·ce·phal·i·des (tē - nō - se - fal'i - dēz). Gênero de pulgas. *C. canis* (pulga do cão) e *C. felis* (pulga do gato) são ectoparasitas quase universais de animais domésticos; atacam o homem quando esfomeados devido à ausência de animais domésticos. [G. *ketenōdes*, semelhante a uma amêijoa, + *kephalē*, cabeça]

CTL Abreviatura de cytotoxic T lymphocytes (linfócitos T citotóxicos).

CTP Abreviatura de cytidine 5'-triphosphate (5'-trifosfato de citidina).

Cu Símbolo do cobre.

^{67}Cu Símbolo do cobre-67 (Cu^{67}).

^{64}Cu Símbolo do cobre-64 (Cu^{64}).

cu·beb (kū'beb). Cubeba; o fruto seco, verde, quase completamente desenvolvido, da *Piper cubeba* (família Piperaceae), uma planta trepadeira das Índias Ocidentais, usado como estimulante, carminativo e irritante local; o óleo de cubeba tem sido usado como anti-séptico urinário leve. [Árabe e Hindu, *kababa*]

cu·bi·tal (kū'bi - tăl). Ulnar; relativo ao cotovelo ou à ulna.

cu·bi·tus, gen. e pl. **cu·bi·ti** (kū'bi - tŭs, - tī). [TA]. **1.** Cotovelo. SIN elbow (2). **2.** Ulna. SIN ulna. [L. cotovelo]

  c. val'gus, ulna valga; desvio do antebraço estendido para o lado externo (radial) do eixo do membro.
  c. va'rus, ulna vara; desvio do antebraço estendido para o lado interno (ulnar) do eixo do membro.

cu·boid, cu·boi·dal (kū'boyd, kū - boy'dăl). [TA]. Cubóide. **1.** Semelhante ao formato de um cubo. **2.** Relativo ao osso cubóide. [G. *kybos*, cubo, + *eidos*, semelhança]

cud·bear (kŭd'bār). Lecanora, orcela, urzela; agente corante vermelho-púrpura derivado do líquen *Ochrolechia tartarea* (família Lecanoraceae) e, devido aos princípios corantes da Roccellaceae, usado para tingir preparações farmacêuticas líquidas. SIN crottle.

cue (kū). Na teoria do condicionamento e aprendizado, um padrão de estímulos ao qual uma pessoa aprendeu ou está aprendendo a responder.
response-produced c.'s, estímulos produzidos por resposta; condicionamentos de estímulos sucessivos em uma cadeia de comportamentos, com cada resposta servindo para reforçar a resposta anterior e como um estímulo, ou condicionamento, para a próxima resposta. VER higher order *conditioning*, behavior *chain*.

cuff (kŭf). Manguito; qualquer estrutura semelhante a uma bainha.
musculotendinous c., manguito musculotendinoso. SIN rotator c. of shoulder.
perivascular c.'s, bainhas perivasculares. VER cuffing.
rotator c. of shoulder, manguito rotador do ombro; as faces anterior, superior e posterior da cápsula da articulação do ombro reforçada pelos tendões de inserção dos músculos *s*upra-espinal, músculo *i*nfra-espinal, redondo menor (*t*eres minor) e *s*ubescapular (SITS). SIN musculotendinous c.
vaginal c., cúpula vaginal; a porção do fórnice da vagina que permanece aberta para o peritônio após histerectomia.

cuff·ing (kŭf'ing). Embainhamento. **1.** Um acúmulo perivascular de vários leucócitos observados em doenças infecciosas, inflamatórias ou auto-imunes. **2.** Circundar uma estrutura com líquido ou células, como em uma bainha; nas radiografias de tórax, espessamento das paredes brônquicas à imagem. [I.M. *cuffe*, mitene]

cui·rass (kwē - rās'). Couraça; a superfície anterior do tórax em relação aos sintomas ou anormalidades. [Fr. *cuirasse*, couraça]
analgesic c., c. analgésica. SIN tabetic c.
tabetic c., c. tabética; uma zona analgésica ou hipoalgésica na região torácica proximal, encontrada na neurossífilis tabética. SIN analgesic c., Hitzig girdle.

cul-de-sac, pl. **culs-de-sac** (kool - de - sak'). Fundo-de-saco. **1.** Uma bolsa de fundo cego ou cavidade tubular fechada em uma extremidade; p. ex., divertículo; ceco. **2.** Escavação retouterina. SIN rectouterine *pouch*. [Fr. fundo de um saco]
conjunctival cul-de-sac, fórnice da conjuntiva. SIN conjunctival *fornix*.
Douglas cul-de-sac, fundo-de-saco de Douglas, escavação retouterina. SIN rectouterine *pouch*.
greater cul-de-sac, fundo gástrico. SIN *fundus* of stomach.
Gruber cul-de-sac, fundo-de-saco de Gruber; um divertículo lateral no espaço supra-esternal ao lado da extremidade medial da clavícula, atrás da fixação esternal do músculo esternocleidomastóideo.
lesser cul-de-sac, antro pilórico. SIN pyloric *antrum*.

cul·do·cen·te·sis (kŭl'dō - sen - tē'sis). Culdocentese; aspiração de líquido do fundo-de-saco (escavação retouterina) por punção do fórnice da vagina próximo à linha média entre os ligamentos uterossacros. [cul - de - sac + G. *kentēsis*, punção]

cul·do·plas·ty (kŭl'dō - plas - tē). Culdoplastia; cirurgia plástica para corrigir o relaxamento do fórnice posterior da vagina. [cul-de-sac + G. *plastos*, formado]

cul·do·scope (kŭl'dō - skōp). Culdoscópio; instrumento endoscópico usado na culdoscopia.

cul·dos·co·py (kŭl - dos'kō - pē). Culdoscopia; introdução de um endoscópio através da parede posterior da vagina, para examinar a bolsa retovaginal e as vísceras pélvicas. [cul - de - sac + G. *skopeō*, ver]

cul·dot·o·my (kŭl - dot'ō - mē). **1.** Culdotomia; corte através da parede posterior da vagina até o fundo-de-saco de Douglas. **2.** Laparotomia, celiotomia vaginal. SIN vaginal *celiotomy*. [cul - de - sac + G. *tomē*, incisão]

Cu·lex (kū'leks). Gênero de mosquitos (família Culicidae), que inclui mais de 2.000 espécies. Sobretudo tropical, mas de distribuição mundial; são vetores de várias doenças de seres humanos e de animais domésticos e selvagens, bem como de aves. [L. mosquito]
C. nigripalpus, espécie de mosquito que é um vetor da encefalite de St. Louis nos Estados Unidos.
C. pi'piens, um complexo de subespécies da abundante espécie politípica, o mosquito caseiro castanho ou mosquito de águas estagnadas dos climas temperados, que se reproduz comumente em águas estagnadas, principalmente em recipientes artificiais, e tem um ciclo de 5 a 6 dias em condições ideais; são encontradas formas intimamente relacionadas em áreas tropicais.
C. quinquefasciatus, espécie de mosquito que poderia servir como vetor da *Wuchereria bancrofti,* se essa infestação por filária fosse introduzida nos Estados Unidos.
C. restuans, espécie de mosquito que é um vetor secundário ou suspeito de encefalite eqüina oriental e encefalite eqüina ocidental nos Estados Unidos.
C. salinarius, espécie de mosquito que é um vetor secundário ou suspeito de encefalite eqüina oriental nos Estados Unidos.
C. tarsa'lis, espécie de mosquito que é um importante vetor dos vírus das encefalomielites eqüina de St. Louis e ocidental em cavalos, aves e seres humanos.

Cu·lic·i·dae (kū - lis'i - dē). Culicídeos; família de insetos (ordem Diptera) que abrange os mosquitos verdadeiros, todos incluídos na subfamília Culicinae.

cu·li·ci·dal (kū - li - sī'dăl). Culicida; um agente que destrói mosquitos [L. *culex,* mosquito, + *caedo,* destruir]

cu·li·cide (kū'li - sīd). Culicida; um agente que destrói mosquitos.

cu·lic·i·fuge (kū - lis'i - fooj). Culicífugo. **1.** Que afasta mosquitos. **2.** Agente que impede o mosquito de picar. [L. *culex,* mosquito + *fugo,* afastar]

Cu·li·coi·des (kū - li - koy'dēz). Gênero de diminutos mosquitos que picam ou mosquitos-pólvora, vetores de várias filárias humanas não-patogênicas (*Mansonella, Dipetalonema*), de *Onchocerca* em cavalos e bovinos, e de vários agentes virais de ovinos e aves domésticas. [L. *culex,* mosquito]
C. aus'teni, espécie que é um hospedeiro intermediário da filária *Mansonella perstans,* principalmente na África equatorial.
C. fu'rens, espécie que é um vetor da *Mansonella ozzardi,* nas Índias Ocidentais.
C. mil'nei, espécie que é um dos vetores da *Mansonella perstans* na África Ocidental.

Culiseta (kū - lis'ē - ta). Gênero de mosquitos (família Culicidae). São vetores de várias doenças em seres humanos e de animais domésticos e selvagens e aves.
C. inornata, espécie de mosquito que é um vetor secundário ou suspeito de encefalite eqüina oriental e da encefalite do Grupo California nos Estados Unidos.
C. melanura, espécie de mosquito que é o principal vetor endêmico do vírus da encefalomielite eqüina oriental; como essa espécie alimenta-se basicamente de aves, outros mosquitos (*Aedes* spp.) transmitem o vírus de aves para os seres humanos e cavalos.

Cullen, Thomas S., ginecologista norte-americano, 1868–1953. VER C. *sign*.

cul·men, pl. **cul·'mi·na** (kŭl'men) [TA]. Cúlmen; a porção proeminente anterior do montículo do verme do cerebelo; lóbulo do verme rostral à fissura primária; dividido em uma parte anterior [TA] (lóbulo IV de Larsell) e uma parte posterior [TA] (lóbulo V de Larsell). SIN lobulus culminis. [L. cume]

Culp, Ormond S., urologista norte-americano, 1910–1977. VER C. *pyeloplasty*.

cult (kŭlt). Culto; um sistema de crenças e rituais baseado em dogmas ou ensinamentos religiosos e caracterizado por devotos que estão prontos a obedecer, uma idealização irreal do líder, um abandono da ambição e dos objetivos pessoais e uma abstenção dos valores sociais tradicionais. [L. *cultus,* honraria, adoração]

cul·ti·va·tion (kŭl - ti - vā'shŭn). Cultivo. SIN culture. [L. Mediev. cultivo, pp. –atus, do L. colo, pp. cultus, cultivar]

cul·tur·al di·ver·si·ty. Diversidade cultural; a variedade inevitável de costumes, atitudes, práticas e comportamento existente entre grupos de indivíduos de diferentes etnias, raças ou nacionalidades que entram em contato.

cul·ture (kŭl'chŭr). Cultura. **1.** A propagação de microrganismos sobre ou em meio de diversos tipos. **2.** Uma massa de microrganismos sobre ou em um meio. **3.** A propagação de células de mamíferos, isto é, cultura de células. VER cell c. **4.** Conjunto de crenças, valores artísticos, históricos, características religiosas, costumes, etc., comuns a uma comunidade ou nação. SIN cultivation. [L. *cultura,* cultura, de *colo,* pp. *cultus,* cultivar]
batch c., c. de lote; uma técnica para produção em grande escala de micróbios ou produtos microbianos na qual, em um determinado momento, o fermentador é interrompido e a cultura avança gradualmente.
cell c., c. de células; a manutenção ou crescimento de células dispersas após a remoção do corpo, comumente sobre uma superfície de vidro imersa em líquido nutriente.
continuous c., c. contínua; técnica para produção de micróbios ou produtos microbianos na qual são fornecidos nutrientes continuamente para o fermentador.
discontinuous c., c. descontínua; técnica para produção de micróbios ou produtos microbianos na qual os microrganismos são cultivados em um sistema fechado até que um fator nutriente limite a velocidade.
elective c., c. eletiva; método de isolamento de microrganismos capaz de utilizar um substrato específico por incubação de um inóculo em um meio contendo o substrato; o meio geralmente contém substâncias, ou tem características, que inibem o crescimento de microrganismos indesejados. SIN enrichment c.
enrichment c., c. com enriquecimento. SIN elective c.
hanging-block c., c. em bloco pendente; a propagação de microrganismos em um cubo de meio de ágar solidificado que é inoculado, fixado a uma lamínula e invertido sobre uma câmara úmida ou lâmina escavada.
Harada-Mori filter paper strip c., c. em papel de filtro de Harada-Mori; uma combinação de papel de filtro, amostra fecal e água da torneira colocados em um tubo de centrífuga; proporciona um meio para a eclosão dos ovos e desenvolvimento das larvas dos nematódeos.
mixed lymphocyte c., c. de linfócitos mistos. VER mixed lymphocyte culture *test*.
monoxenic c., c. monoxênica; cultura de parasitas em associação com uma bactéria simples conhecida.
needle c., c. por agulha. SIN stab c.
neotype c., c. de neotipo. SIN neotype *strain*.

organ c., c. de órgãos; a manutenção ou crescimento de tecidos, primórdios de órgãos ou das partes de um órgão ou de todo um órgão *in vitro* de forma a permitir a diferenciação ou preservação da arquitetura ou função.

Petri dish c., c. em placa de Petri; uma combinação de papel de filtro, amostra fecal e água da torneira colocada em uma placa de Petri; proporciona um ambiente para a eclosão dos ovos e o desenvolvimento das larvas de nematódeos.

plastic envelope c., c. em saco plástico; método simplificado para transporte e cultura de amostras para o diagnóstico de infecção por *Trichomonas vaginalis*; o meio de cultura líquido é examinado microscopicamente através do saco, não sendo necessária coleta de amostra do meio por pipeta.

pouch c., c. em bolsa; sistemas de cultura em plástico para transporte de amostras, cultura e câmaras de exame para isolamento, crescimento e detecção de *Trichomonas vaginalis*.

pure c., c. pura; no sentido bacteriológico comum, uma cultura que consiste em uma única espécie e cepa de uma bactéria.

roll-tube c., c. em tubo rotatório; cultura em um tubo de meio que foi liquefeito e novamente solidificou enquanto o tubo girava; assim, o interior do tubo é revestido por uma fina camada de meio solidificado.

sensitized c., c. sensibilizada; cultura viva de um microrganismo ao qual é acrescentado um anti-soro específico; após a mistura é incubado por vários minutos (durante os quais o anticorpo no soro se combina aos microrganismos), o excesso de soro é removido por meio de centrifugação, lavado em soro fisiológico e novamente centrifugado; os microrganismos sensibilizados podem então ser novamente suspensos em solução salina fisiológica.

shake c., c. por agitação; cultura feita por inoculação em um meio de ágar ou gelatina liquefeita, distribuição completa do inóculo por agitação e, depois, permitindo a solidificação do meio no tubo em posição vertical.

slant c., c. inclinada; cultura feita sobre a superfície inclinada de um meio que foi solidificado em um tubo de ensaio inclinado em relação ao plano perpendicular, de forma a proporcionar maior área que a da luz do tubo. SIN slope c.

slope c., c. inclinada. SIN slant c.

smear c., c. em esfregaço; cultura obtida espalhando-se o material que se presume estar infectado sobre a superfície de um meio solidificado.

stab c., c. por punção; cultura por agulha; cultura produzida inserindo-se uma agulha com inóculo no centro de um meio sólido contido em um tubo de ensaio. SIN needle c.

stock c., c. de estoque; cultura de um microrganismo mantido apenas para conservar esse microrganismo em condição viável por subcultura (repique), quando necessário, em meio fresco.

streak c., c. em estria; cultura produzida fazendo-se leves riscos com uma agulha ou alça de inoculação sobre a superfície de um meio sólido.

tissue c., c. de tecido; a manutenção de tecido vivo após remoção do corpo, sendo colocado em um vaso com um meio nutritivo estéril.

type c., c.-tipo; uma cepa típica de microrganismo preservada em uma coleção de cultura como padrão.

xenic c., c. xênica; culturas de parasitas que crescem em associação com uma microbiota desconhecida. [G. *xenikos*, forasteiro, estrangeiro, de *xenos*, convidado, estrangeiro]

cum (kum). Com. [L.]

cu·ma·rin (kū'ma-rin). Cumarina. SIN coumarin.

cu·meth·a·rol (kū'-meth'a-rol). Cumetarol. SIN coumetarol.

cu·me·thox·a·eth·ane (kū-me-thoks'a-eth-ān). Cumetoxetano. SIN coumetarol.

Cummer, William E., dentista canadense, 1879–1942. VER C. *classification*, *guideline*.

cUMP Abreviatura de cyclic *uridine* 3',5'-monophosphate (3',5'-monofosfato de uridina [UMPc]).

cu·mu·la·tive (kū'mū-lă-tiv). Cumulativo; que tende a acumular, como determinadas drogas que podem ter um efeito cumulativo.

cu·mu·lus, pl. **cu·mu·li** (kū'mū-lŭs, -lī). Cúmulo; coleção ou pilha de células. [L. uma pilha]

c. **oöph'orus**, c. oóforo; disco prolígero; uma massa de células granulosas epiteliais que circundam o óvulo no folículo ovariano. SIN ovigerus, proligerous disk, proligerous membrane. [NA]

c. **ovar'icus**, c. ovariano; termo raramente usado para c. oöphorus.

cu·ne·ate (kū'nē-āt). Cuneiforme; em forma de cunha. [L. *cuneus*, cunha]

cu·ne·i·form (kū'nē-i-form). Cuneiforme; em forma de cunha. VER intermediate cuneiform (*bone*), lateral cuneiform (*bone*), medial cuneiform (*bone*).

cu·ne·o·cu·boid (kū'nē-ō-kū'boyd). Cuneocubóide; relativo aos ossos cuneiforme lateral e cubóide.

cu·ne·o·na·vic·u·lar (kū'-nē-ō-nă-vik'ū-lăr). Cuneonavicular; relativo aos ossos cuneiforme e navicular. SIN cuneoscaphoid.

cu·ne·o·scaph·oid (kū'-nē-ō-skaf'oyd). Cuneoescafóide. SIN cuneonavicular.

cu·ne·us, pl. **cu·nei** (kū'nē-ŭs, koo'nē-ī) [TA]. Cúneo; a região da face medial do lobo occipital de cada hemisfério cerebral limitada pela fissura parietooccipital e fissura calcarina. [L. cunha]

cu·nic·u·lus, pl. **cu·nic·u·li** (kū-nik'ū-lŭs, -lī). Cunículo; a escavação do ácaro da escabiose na epiderme. [L. coelho; uma passagem subterrânea]

cun·ni·lin·gus (kŭn-i-ling'gŭs). Cunilíngua; estimulação oral da vulva ou clitóris; um tipo de atividade sexual orogenital; ao contrário da felação, que é a estimulação oral do pênis. [L. *cunnus*, pudendo, + *lingo*, lamber]

Cun·ning·ham·el·la el·e·gans (kŭn-ing-ha-mel'a el'ĕ-ganz). Uma de várias espécies de fungos que podem causar mucormicose em seres humanos.

cun·nus (kŭn'ŭs). Vulva. SIN vulva. [L.]

cup (kŭp). **1.** Xícara; cálice; taça; escavação; uma estrutura escavada ou côncava, anatômica ou anormal. SIN poculum. **2.** Ventosa SIN cupping glass. [A.S. *cuppe*]

Diogenes c., cálice de Diógenes. SIN c. of palm.

dry c., ventosa seca; uma ventosa de vidro aplicada antigamente à pele íntegra, a fim de trazer o sangue para a região, mas sem removê-lo.

eye c., cálice ocular; pequeno receptáculo oval usado para aplicar um líquido à parte externa do olho.

glaucomatous c., escavação glaucomatosa; uma depressão profunda do disco óptico causada por glaucoma. SIN glaucomatous excavation.

ocular c., cúpula ocular. SIN optic c.

optic c., cúpula óptica; a cúpula de parede dupla formada pela invaginação da vesícula óptica embrionária; seu componente interno torna-se a camada sensorial da retina, e sua camada externa, a camada pigmentar. SIN caliculus ophthalmicus, ocular c.

c. of palm, a palma da mão quando contraída e aprofundada pela ação dos músculos de cada lado. SIN Diogenes c., poculum diogenis.

perilimbal suction c., ventosa de aspiração perilímbica; um dispositivo para aumentar a pressão intra-ocular por impedimento da circulação e do fluxo de humor aquoso do olho.

physiologic c., cálice fisiológico, escavação fisiológica. SIN depression of optic disk.

suction c., ventosa de aspiração; uma das ventosas de vidro de vários formatos, antigamente usada para produzir hiperemia local de acordo com o método de Bier.

wet c., ventosa úmida; uma ventosa de vidro aplicada antigamente a uma parte previamente escarificada ou incisada a fim de puxar e remover o sangue.

cu·po·la (koo'po-lă, kū') Cúpula. SIN cupula.

cupped (kŭpt). Escavado; feito em forma de cálice.

cup·ping (kŭp'ing). **1.** Escavação; formação de uma cavidade, ou escavação em forma de cálice. **2.** Aplicação de uma ventosa. VER TAMBÉM cup.

cu·pric (koo'prik, kū-). Cúprico; relativo ao cobre, particularmente ao cobre na forma de um íon positivo duplamente carregado.

cu·pric ac·e·tate, cu·pric ac·e·tate nor·mal. Acetato de cobre; acetato de cobre normal; estimulante local cáustico para úlceras.

cu·pric ar·se·nite. Arsenito de cobre; um pó cristalino verde, venenoso, obsoleto como agente medicinal; agora usado como inseticida e pigmento. SIN copper arsenite, Scheele green.

cu·pric chlo·ride. Cloreto de cobre; tem sido usado como anti-séptico no tratamento de suprimentos de água, tanques e piscinas. SIN copper bichloride, copper chloride, copper dichloride.

cu·pric cit·rate. Citrato de cobre; um sal de cobre usado como adstringente e anti-séptico. SIN copper citrate.

cu·pric sul·fate. Sulfato de cobre; um sal azul muito venenoso para algas; é um emético imediato e ativo, sendo usado como irritante, adstringente e fungicida. SIN copper sulfate, copper sulphate.

cu·pri·u·re·sis (koo'pri-ū-rē'sis, kū-). Cupriurese; a excreção urinária de cobre. [L. *cuprum*, cobre, + G. *ourēsis*, micção]

cu·pu·la, pl. **cu·pu·lae** (koo'poo-lă, -lē; kū'pū-lă) [TA]. Cúpula; uma estrutura em forma de cálice ou abóbada. SIN cupola. [L. dim. de *cupa*, cuba]

ampullary c., cúpula ampular. SIN c. ampullaris.

c. ampulla'ris [TA], cúpula ampular; massa gelatinosa localizada sobre as células pilosas das cristas ampulares dos ductos semicirculares; o movimento de líquido endolinfático causa o movimento da cúpula através das células pilosas da crista ampular. SIN c. ampullary c.

c. of cochlea, cúpula da cóclea. SIN cochlear c.

c. coch'leae [TA], cúpula da cóclea. SIN cochlear c.

cochlear c. [TA], cúpula da cóclea; o ápice da cóclea semelhante a uma abóbada. SIN c. cochleae [TA], c. of cochlea.

c. pleu'rae [TA], cúpula da pleura. SIN cervical pleura.

pleural c., cúpula da pleura; *termo alternativo oficial para cervical pleura.

cu·pu·lar (koo'poo-lăr, kū'pū-lăr). **1.** Cupular; relativo a uma cúpula. **2.** Cupuliforme; em forma de cúpula. SIN cupulate, cupuliform.

cu·pu·late (koo'poo-lāt, kū'pū-). Cupuliforme. SIN cupular (2).

cu·pu·li·form (koo'pū-li-form, kū'pū-). Cupuliforme. SIN cupular (2).

cu·pu·lo·gram (koo'poo-lō-gram). Cupulograma; uma representação gráfica da função vestibular em relação ao desempenho normal.

cu·pu·lo·lith·i·a·sis (koo'poo-lō-li-thī'a-sis, kū-). Cupulolitíase. SIN benign paroxysmal positional vertigo.

cu·rage (kū'rij, koo-rahzh'). Curagem; curetagem com o dedo da mão, em vez de cureta. [Fr. uma limpeza]

cu·ra·re (koo - rah′rē). Curare; um extrato de várias plantas, principalmente *Strychnos toxifera, S. castelnaei, S. crevauxii* e *Chondodendron tomentosum*, que provoca paralisia não-despolarizante do músculo esquelético após injeção intravenosa por bloqueio da transmissão na junção mioneural; usado clinicamente (p. ex., como cloreto de *d*-tubocurarina, iodeto de metocurina) para promover relaxamento muscular durante cirurgias. Freqüentemente classificado pelos vasos usados por índios do Amazonas e Orenoco para armazenamento. SIN arrow poison (1). [América do Sul]
calabash c., c. da cabaça (armazenado pelos índios em cabaças), curare de *Strychnos* sp.; contém ioimbina, indol e alcalóides do tipo estricnina.
pot c., curare de pote (curare armazenado em potes de barro), curare de *Chondodendron* sp.
tube c., curare de tubo (curare armazenado em tubos de bambu), curare de *Chondodendron* sp.; contém o alcalóide tubocurarina.
cu·ra·ri·form (koo - rar′i - form). Curariforme; designa uma substância que tem ação semelhante à do curare.
cu·rar·i·mi·met·ic (koo - rar′i - mī - met′ik). Curarimimético; que tem ação semelhante à do curare.
cu·ra·rine (kū′ră - rēn). Curarina; o princípio alcalóide do curare da cabaça.
cu·ra·ri·za·tion (kū - rah - ri - zā′shun). Curarização; indução de relaxamento muscular ou paralisia pela administração de curare ou substâncias relacionadas que possuem a capacidade de bloquear a transmissão do impulso nervoso na junção mioneural.
cur·a·tive (kū′ra - tiv). Curativo. **1.** Aquilo que cicatriza ou cura. **2.** Que tende a cicatrizar ou curar.
cur·cum·in (kur′koo - min). Curcumina; um pigmento amarelo das raízes e vagens de *Curcuma longa*; usado em doenças do fígado e biliares; encontrada no caril em pó; inibe a 5-lipoxigenase. SIN tumeric yellow.
curd (kerd). Coágulo; coalho; o coágulo do leite.
cure (kūr). **1.** Curar; tornar sadio. **2.** Cura; restabelecimento da saúde. **3.** Cura; um método ou curso especial de tratamento. VER dental *curing*. [L. *curo*, cuidar de]
cu·ret. Cureta. VER curette.
cu·ret·tage (kū - rĕ - tahzh′, koo-). Curetagem; uma raspagem, geralmente do interior de uma cavidade ou trato, para a remoção de novos crescimentos ou de outros tecidos anormais, ou para obter material para diagnóstico tecidual. SIN curettement.
periapical c., c. periapical; **(1)** retirada de um cisto ou granuloma de sua cripta óssea anormal, utilizando uma cureta; **(2)** a remoção de fragmentos de dentes e de resíduos dos alvéolos por ocasião da extração ou remoção subseqüente de seqüestros ósseos.
subgingival c., c. subgengival; remoção de tártaro subgengival, tecidos epitelial e de granulação ulcerados encontrados em bolsas periodontais. SIN apoxesis.
suction c., c. por sucção; uma forma de abortamento na qual o colo uterino é dilatado, se necessário, e os produtos da concepção removidos por uso de uma cânula acoplada a uma fonte de aspiração; técnica usada para concluir um abortamento incompleto espontâneo ou como uma forma de abortamento induzido. SIN dilation and suction.
cu·rette, cu·ret (kū - ret′, koo-). Cureta; instrumento em forma de alça, anel ou colher, com bordas afiadas e preso a um cabo em forma de bastão, usado para curetagem. [Fr.]
Hartmann c., c. de Hartmann; uma cureta, com um lado cortante, para a remoção de adenóides.
cu·rette·ment (kū - ret′ment, koo-). Curetagem. SIN curettage.
cu·rie (C, c, Ci) (kū′rē). Curie; unidade de medida de radioatividade, $3,70 \times 10^{10}$ desintegrações por segundo; antes definida como a radioatividade da quantidade de radônio em equilíbrio com 1 g de rádio; substituída pela unidade do SI, becquerel (1 desintegração por segundo). [Marie (1867-1934) e Pierre (1859-1906) *Curie*, químicos e físicos franceses e ganhadores do Prêmio Nobel]
cur·ing (kūr′ing). Cura. **1.** O ato de realizar uma cura. **2.** Um processo pelo qual algo é preparado para uso, como por aquecimento, envelhecimento, etc.
dental c., c. dentária; o processo pelo qual materiais plásticos tornam-se rígidos para formar uma base de dentadura, obturação, bandeja de impressão ou outro dispositivo.
cu·ri·um (Cm) (kū′rē - ŭm). Cúrio; elemento de n.º atômico 96, peso atômico 247,07, que não ocorre naturalmente na terra, mas foi produzido artificialmente, pela primeira vez, em 1944, por bombardeio de Pu^{239} com partículas alfa; o mais estável dos isótopos do cúrio é o Cm^{247}, com uma meia-vida de 15,6 milhões de anos. [ver curie]
Curling, Thomas B., cirurgião inglês, 1811–1888. VER stress *ulcer*.
cur·rent (ker′rĕnt). Corrente; uma corrente ou fluxo de líquido, ar ou eletricidade. [L. *currens*, part. pres. de *curro*, correr]
action c., c. de ação; corrente elétrica induzida nas fibras musculares quando estas são efetivamente estimuladas; normalmente é seguida por contração.
after-c., pós-corrente. VER aftercurrent.
alternating c. (AC), c. alternada; corrente que flui primeiro em uma direção e depois na outra; p. ex., corrente de 60 ciclos.
anodal c., c. anódica; corrente produzida nos tecidos sob o anodo quando o circuito é fechado.
ascending c., c. ascendente; a direção do fluxo de corrente em um nervo quando o anodo é posicionado perifericamente ao catodo, ao contrário da corrente descendente; a convenção usada é que a corrente flui do positivo para o negativo. SIN centripetal c.
axial c., c. axial; a porção central rapidamente móvel da corrente sanguínea em uma artéria.
centrifugal c., c. centrífuga. SIN descending c.
centripetal c., c. centrípeta. SIN ascending c.
d'Arsonval c., c. d'Arsonval. SIN high-frequency c.
demarcation c., c. de demarcação. SIN c. of injury.
descending c., c. descendente; a direção do fluxo da corrente em um nervo quando o catodo está posicionado perifericamente ao anodo, ao contrário da corrente ascendente. SIN centrifugal c.
direct c. (DC), c. contínua; corrente que flui apenas em uma direção; p. ex., aquela proveniente de uma bateria; algumas vezes denominada corrente galvânica. VER TAMBÉM galvanism.
electrotonic c., c. electrotônica. VER electrotonus.
galvanic c., c. galvânica. VER direct c., galvanism (1).
high-frequency c., c. de alta freqüência; corrente elétrica alternada com uma freqüência de 10.000 ciclos por segundo ou maior; não produz contrações musculares e não afeta os nervos sensoriais. SIN d'Arsonval c., Tesla c.
c. of injury, c. de lesão; a corrente gerada quando uma parte lesada de um nervo, músculo ou outro tecido excitável é conectada através de um condutor com a região não-lesada; o tecido lesado é negativo em relação ao não-lesado. SIN demarcation c.
labile c., c. lábil; corrente elétrica aplicada ao corpo por meio de eletrodos que são constantemente deslocados.
Tesla c., c. Tesla. SIN high-frequency c.
Curschmann, Heinrich, médico alemão, 1846–1910. VER C. *spirals*, em *spiral*.
curse (kers). Maldição; desgraça atribuída a um espírito maléfico.
Ondine c., maldição de Ondina; hipoventilação alveolar central idiopática, na qual há depressão do controle involuntário da respiração, mas o controle voluntário da ventilação não é comprometido. [*Ondine*, personagem da peça de J. Giraudoux, baseado em Undina, personagem da mitologia grega]
Curtis, Arthur H., ginecologista norte-americano, 1881–1955. VER Fitz-Hugh e C. *syndrome*.
cur·va·tu·ra, pl. **cur·va·tu·rae** (ker′vă - too′ră, - too′rē). Curvatura. SIN curvature. [L.]
c. primaria columnae vertebralis [TA], c. primária da coluna vertebral. SIN primary *curvature* of vertebral column.
curvaturae secondariae columnae vertebralis [TA], curvaturas secundárias da coluna vertebral. SIN secondary *curvatures* of vertebral column, em *curvature*.
c. ventric'uli ma'jor [TA], curvatura maior do estômago. SIN greater *curvature* of stomach.
c. ventric'uli mi'nor [TA], curvatura menor do estômago. SIN lesser *curvature* of stomach.
cur·va·ture (ker′vă - choor). Curvatura; um arqueamento ou flexura. VER angulation. SIN curvatura. [L. *curvatura*, de *curvo*, pp. –*atus*, arquear, curvar]
angular c., c. angular; deformidade com formação de giba, isto é, uma angulação aguda da coluna vertebral, que ocorre na doença de Pott. SIN Pott c.
anterior c., c. anterior; curvatura na qual uma parte mais distal ou cefálica é desviada anteriormente em relação ao plano anatômico coronal.
backward c., c. posterior; curvatura na qual uma parte mais distal ou cefálica é desviada posteriormente em relação ao plano anatômico coronal. SIN posterior c.
gingival c., c. gengival; o arredondamento da gengiva ao longo de sua linha de fixação ao colo de um dente.
greater c. of stomach [TA], c. maior do estômago; a borda do estômago à qual está fixado o omento maior. SIN curvatura ventriculi major [TA].
lateral c., c. lateral; curvatura na qual uma parte mais distal está desviada do plano sagital anatômico, produzindo alinhamento em valgo.
lesser c. of stomach [TA], c. menor do estômago; a borda direita do estômago à qual está fixado o omento menor. SIN curvatura ventriculi minor [TA].
occlusal c., c. oclusal. SIN *curve* of occlusion.
posterior c., c. posterior. SIN backward c.
Pott c., c. de Pott. SIN angular c.
primary c. of vertebral column [TA], c. primária da coluna vertebral; a curva ventralmente côncava da coluna vertebral fetal, conservada nas regiões torácica e sacral como as cifoses torácica e sacral. VER TAMBÉM kyphosis. SIN curvatura primaria columnae vertebralis [TA].
secondary c.'s of vertebral column [TA], curvaturas secundárias da coluna vertebral; curvas ventralmente convexas da coluna vertebral que se desenvolvem após o nascimento nas regiões cervical e lombar: as lordoses cervical e lombar. VER TAMBÉM lordosis. SIN curvaturae secondariae columnae vertebralis [TA].

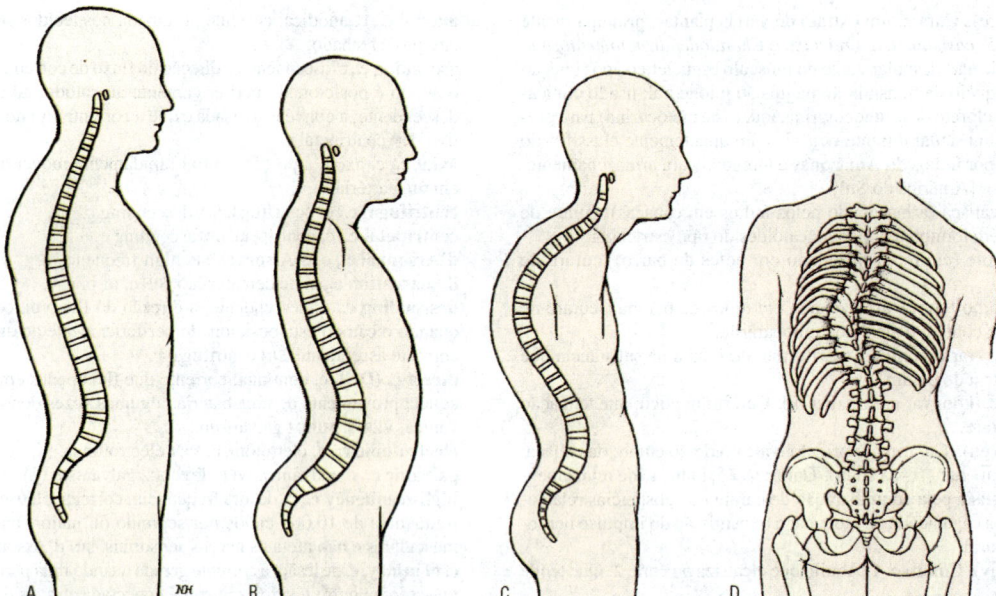

curvaturas da coluna vertebral: (A) normal, (B) lordose, (C) cifose, (D) escoliose

spinal c., c. vertebral. VER kyphosis, lordosis, scoliosis.
curve (kerv). Curva. **1.** Uma dobra ou linha contínua não-angular. **2.** Um gráfico ou representação gráfica, por meio de uma linha contínua que liga observações individuais, da evolução de uma atividade fisiológica, do número de casos de uma doença em um determinado período, ou de qualquer condição que também poderia ser apresentada por um quadro de figuras. SIN chart (2). [L. *curvo*, curvar]
active length-tension c., c. comprimento–tensão ativa; a relação entre tensão isométrica ativa e pré-carga (comprimento em repouso) para um músculo que se contrai.
alignment c., c. de alinhamento; a linha que atravessa o centro dos dentes lateralmente, na direção da curva do arco dentário.
anti-Monson c., c. anti-Monson. SIN reverse c.
Barnes c., c. de Barnes; curva correspondente, em geral, à curva de Carus, sendo o segmento de um círculo cujo centro é o promontório do sacro.
buccal c., c. bucal; a linha da arcada dentária desde o canino até o terceiro molar.
calibration c., c. de calibragem; a relação gráfica ou matemática entre as leituras obtidas em um processo analítico e a quantidade de analisado em uma calibragem. A relação freqüentemente é uma linha reta, e não uma curva.
Carus c., c. de Carus; uma linha curva imaginária obtida a partir de uma fórmula matemática, que supostamente indica a saída do canal pélvico. SIN Carus circle.
cephalic c., c. cefálica; curva que se adapta à da cabeça fetal, usada em referência ao formato do fórceps obstétrico.
characteristic c., c. característica; curva sensitométrica de filme radiográfico, uma representação da densidade do filme em comparação com o logaritmo da exposição relativa. SIN H and D c., Hunter and Driffield c.
compensating c., c. de compensação; a curvatura ântero-posterior e lateral no alinhamento das faces oclusais e margens incisais dos dentes artificiais; usada para desenvolver oclusão balanceada.
distribution c., c. de distribuição; um agrupamento sistemático de dados em classes ou categorias, de acordo com a freqüência de ocorrência de cada valor sucessivo ou faixas desses valores, resultando em um gráfico de uma distribuição de freqüência. SIN frequency c.
dose-response c., c. de dose–resposta; um gráfico que mostra a relação entre a dose de uma substância, agente infeccioso, etc., e a resposta biológica.
dye-dilution c., c. de diluição do corante; gráfico das concentrações séricas (diluições) de um corante, p. ex., azul de Evans, após sua injeção intravascular ou intracardíaca; útil no diagnóstico de desvios (*shunts*) cardíacos congênitos, na medida do débito cardíaco e na detecção de incompetência cardiovalvular. SIN indicator-dilution c.
epidemic c., c. epidêmica; um gráfico no qual o número de novos casos de uma doença é representado contra um intervalo de tempo para descrever uma epidemia ou surto específico.
flow-volume c., c. de fluxo–volume, volufluxograma; o gráfico produzido pela representação do fluxo instantâneo de gases respiratórios contra o volume pulmonar simultâneo, geralmente durante expiração forçada máxima.
force-velocity c., c. de força–velocidade; a relação entre velocidade isotônica de encurtamento e pós-carga de um músculo contrátil.
Frank-Starling c., c. de Frank-Starling. SIN Starling c.

frequency c., c. de freqüência. SIN distribution c.
Friedman c., c. de Friedman. SIN partogram.
gaussian c., c. de Gauss. SIN normal *distribution*.
growth c., c. de crescimento; uma representação gráfica da alteração no tamanho de um indivíduo ou uma população durante um período.
H and D c., c. H e D. SIN characteristic c.
Heidelberger c., c. de Heidelberger. SIN precipitation c.
Hunter and Driffield c., c. de Hunter e Driffield. SIN characteristic c.
indicator-dilution c., c. de diluição do indicador. SIN dye-dilution c.
intracardiac pressure c., c. de pressão intracardíaca; curva de pressão registrada no átrio ou ventrículo (curvas de pressão intra-atrial e intraventricular).
isovolume pressure-flow c., c. de pressão–fluxo isovolumétrica; a relação entre pressão transpulmonar e fluxo aéreo respiratório, expressa como função do volume pulmonar.
labor c., c. do trabalho de parto. SIN partogram.
logistic c., c. logística; uma curva em forma de S que representa o crescimento de uma população em uma área de limites fixos.
milled-in c.'s, curvas de oclusão. SIN milled-in *paths*, em *path*.
Monson c., c. de Monson; a curva de oclusão na qual cada cúspide e margem incisal toca, ou se adapta a, um segmento da superfície de uma esfera com 8 polegadas (~20,25 cm) de diâmetro, tendo seu centro na região da glabela.
muscle c., c. muscular. SIN myogram.
c. of occlusion, curvatura oclusal; **(1)** uma superfície curva que faz contato simultâneo com a porção principal das proeminências incisal e oclusal dos dentes existentes; **(2)** a curva de uma dentição na qual se localizam as superfícies oclusais. SIN occlusal cuvature.

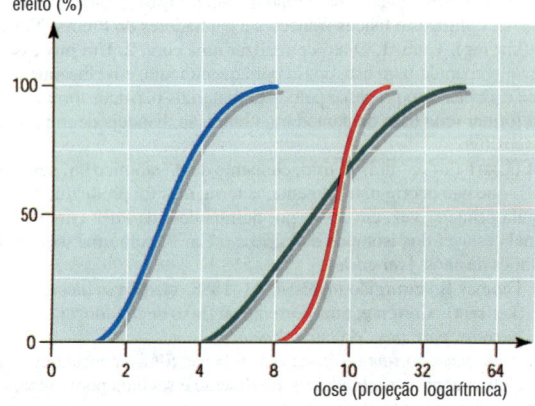

curva dose–resposta: uma dentre várias expressões

passive length-tension c., c. de comprimento–tensão passiva; a relação entre a tensão passiva e a pré-carga (comprimento em repouso) de um músculo em repouso.
Pleasure c., c. de Pleasure; uma curva oclusal que, quando vista em corte sagital, adapta-se a uma linha convexa para cima, exceto pelos últimos molares.
precipitation c., c. de precipitação; um gráfico da quantidade de precipitado formado em função da quantidade de antígeno acrescentado durante a titulação de um anticorpo com um antígeno. SIN Heidelberger c.
Price-Jones c., c. de Price-Jones; uma curva de distribuição dos diâmetros medidos de hemácias; situa-se à direita da curva normal (isto é, indicando maiores diâmetros) em casos de anemia perniciosa e outras formas em que há macrócitos, e à esquerda (isto é, indicando menores diâmetros) na deficiência de ferro e em outras formas de anemia microcítica.
probability c., c. de probabilidade; um gráfico da distribuição de Gauss (normal) que representa probabilidades relativas.
progress c., c. de progresso; uma representação gráfica de uma reação química ou catalisada por enzima na qual a concentração do produto ou do substrato, ou o complexo binário de armazenamento eletrostático, é representada contra o tempo.
pulse c., c. de pulso. SIN sphygmogram.
receiver operating characteristic c., c. de característica operacional do receptor; (1) uma representação da percentagem positiva verdadeira *versus* os resultados percentuais falso-positivos, geralmente em uma prova de um teste diagnóstico; (2) um meio gráfico de avaliar a capacidade de um teste de rastreamento de discriminar entre pessoas saudáveis e doentes. SIN ROC c.
reverse c., c. reversa; em odontologia; uma curva oclusal convexa para cima. SIN anti-Monson c.
ROC c., curva de característica operacional do receptor. SIN receiver operating characteristic c.
c. of Spee, c. de Spee; a curvatura anatômica do plano oclusal mandibular começando na extremidade da cúspide inferior e seguindo as cúspides bucais dos dentes posteriores, continuando até o molar terminal. SIN von Spee c.
Starling c., c. de Starling; um gráfico no qual o débito cardíaco ou o volume sistólico é representado contra a pressão diastólica final atrial ou ventricular média; com aumento do retorno venoso e da pressão atrial, o débito aumenta proporcionalmente até que aumentos adicionais sobrecarreguem o coração e o débito caia. SIN Frank-Starling c.
strength-duration c., c. de intensidade–duração; um gráfico que relaciona a intensidade de um estímulo elétrico à duração que deve ter para ser eficaz. SIN chronaxie, rheobase.
stress-strain c., c. de tensão–deformação; curva que mostra a razão entre deformação e carga durante o teste de um material sob tensão.
tension c., c. de tensão; a direção das trabéculas, no tecido ósseo esponjoso, que se forma como uma adaptação para resistir ao estresse.
Traube-Hering c.'s, curvas de Traube-Hering; oscilações lentas da pressão arterial que, geralmente, se estendem por vários ciclos respiratórios; relacionadas a variações do tônus vasomotor; variações rítmicas da pressão arterial. SIN Traube-Hering waves.
tuning c., curva de afinação; um gráfico de intensidade do limiar acústico em várias freqüências para um único neurônio.
volume-time c., c. de volume–tempo; volume de uma expiração representado contra o tempo. Esta é a curva básica gerada pela denominada "espirometria simples".
von Spee c., c. de von Spee. SIN c. of Spee.
whole-body titration c., c. de titulação do corpo inteiro; uma representação gráfica das alterações *in vivo*, no íon hidrogênio, $P_{A_{CO_2}}$ e bicarbonato, que ocorrem no sangue arterial em resposta a distúrbios ácido-básicos primários.
Cur·vu·la·ria (ker - vū - lā′rē - ā). Gênero de fungos de cor escura que crescem rapidamente em meios de cultura. Geralmente consideradas contaminantes, duas espécies, *C. lunata* e *C. geniculata*, estão entre as espécies capazes de produzir micetoma em seres humanos, ceratomicose, sinusite e feoifomicose.
Cushing, Harvey W., neurocirurgião norte-americano, 1869–1939. VER C. *basophilism, disease, syndrome, syndrome* medicamentosus, *effect, phenomenon, response,* pituitary *basophilism.*
Cushing, Hayward W., cirurgião norte-americano, 1854–1934. VER C. *suture.*
cush·ing·oid (kush′ing - oyd). Cushingóide; semelhante aos sinais e sintomas de doença ou síndrome de Cushing; fácies de lua cheia, obesidade com giba de búfalo, estriações, adiposidade, hipertensão, diabetes e osteoporose, geralmente causados por corticosteróides exógenos.
cush·ion (kush′ŭn). Coxim; em anatomia, qualquer estrutura semelhante a uma almofada.
anal c.'s, coxins anais; proeminências vasculares formadas por grupos de veias normalmente saculadas do plexo venoso retal superior, alimentadas por anastomoses arteriovenosas que causam seu ingurgitamento, estando geralmente situadas lateralmente à esquerda e ântero- e póstero-lateralmente do lado direito do canal anal. SIN cavernous bodies of anal canal, corpora cavernosa recti, hemorrhoidal c.'s, threshold pads of anal canal.
atrioventricular canal c.'s, coxins do canal atrioventricular; um par de montes de tecido conjuntivo embrionário recobertos por endotélio, projetando-se para o canal atrioventricular embrionário; um está localizado dorsalmente e o outro ventralmente, crescem juntos e se fundem um ao outro e à borda inferior do *septum primum*, dividindo o canal, originalmente único, em orifícios atrioventriculares direito e esquerdo. SIN endocardial c.'s.
endocardial c.'s, coxins endocárdicos. SIN atrioventricular canal c.'s.
c. of epiglottis, c. da epiglote. SIN epiglottic *tubercle.*
eustachian c., c. de Eustáquio. SIN *torus* tubarius.
hemorrhoidal c.'s, coxins hemorroidários. SIN anal c.'s.
levator c., c. do levantador. SIN *torus* levatorius.
Passavant c., c. de Passavant. SIN Passavant *ridge.*
pharyngoesophageal c.'s, coxins faringoesofágicos; plexos venosos nas paredes anterior e posterior da junção faringoesofágica. SIN pharyngoesophageal pads.
sucking c., c. sugador. SIN buccal *fat-pad.*
cusp (kŭsp) [TA]. **1.** Cúspide; em odontologia, uma elevação cônica que se origina na superfície de um dente a partir de um centro de calcificação independente. VER TAMBÉM dental *tubercle.* **2.** Válvula*; o folheto de uma das valvas cardíacas. SIN cuspis [TA]. [L. *cuspis,* ponta]
anterior c. of left atrioventricular valve, válvula anterior da valva atrioventricular esquerda; *termo oficial alternativo para anterior c. of mitral valve.
anterior c. of mitral valve [TA], válvula anterior da valva atrioventricular esquerda; a válvula posicionada ventralmente e a maior dentre as válvulas que se aproximam, durante a sístole ventricular, para fechar o óstio atrioventricular esquerdo; fixa-se à face septal do óstio. SIN cuspis anterior valvae atrioventricularis sinistrae [TA], anterior c. of left atrioventricular valve*, cuspis anterior valvae mitralis*.
anterior c. of right atrioventricular valve, válvula anterior da valva atrioventricular direita; *termo oficial alternativo para anterior c. of tricuspid valve.
anterior c. of tricuspid valve [TA], válvula anterior da valva atrioventricular direita; a válvula maior e de posição mais ventral dentre as três que se aproximam, durante a sístole ventricular, para fechar o óstio atrioventricular direito. SIN cuspis anterior valvae atrioventricularis dextrae [TA], anterior c. of right atrioventricular valve*, cuspis anterior valvae tricuspidalis*.
c. of Carabelli, cúspide de Carabelli; uma quinta cúspide encontrada nos primeiros molares maxilares, geralmente em posição lingual em relação à cúspide mesiolingual.
posterior c. of left atrioventricular valve, válvula posterior da valva atrioventricular esquerda; *termo oficial alternativo para posterior c. of mitral valve.
posterior c. of mitral valve [TA], válvula posterior da valva atrioventricular direita; a válvula de tamanho médio e situada mais dorsalmente das três válvulas que se aproximam, durante a sístole ventricular, para fechar o óstio atrioventricular direito. SIN cuspis posterior valvae atrioventricularis sinistrae [TA], cuspis posterior valvae mitralis*, posterior c. of left atrioventricular valve*.
posterior c. of right atrioventricular valve, válvula posterior da valva atrioventricular direita, *termo alternativo oficial para posterior c. of tricuspid valve.
posterior c. of tricuspid valve [TA], válvula posterior da valva tricúspide, a válvula de tamanho médio e de posição mais dorsal dentre as três que se aproximam durante a sístole ventricular para fechar o óstio atrioventricular direito. SIN cuspis posterior valvae atrioventricularis dextrae [TA], cuspis posterior valvae tricuspidalis*, posterior c. of right atrioventricular valve*.
semilunar c., válvula semilunar; um dos três segmentos semilunares que servem como as três válvulas de uma valva, impedindo a regurgitação no início da aorta; uma valva semelhante protege a entrada do tronco pulmonar; os segmentos são denominados, respectivamente, anterior, direito e esquerdo na valva pulmonar, e posterior, direito e esquerdo, na valva aórtica.
septal c. of right atrioventricular valve, válvula septal da valva atrioventricular direita; *termo oficial alternativo para septal c. of tricuspid valve.
septal c. of tricuspid valve [TA], válvula septal da valva atrioventricular direita; a válvula da valva tricúspide adjacente ao septo interventricular. SIN cuspis septalis valvae atrioventricularis dextrae [TA], cuspis septalis valvae tricuspidalis*, septal c. of right atrioventricular valve*.
talon c., cúspide em garra; uma cúspide anômala que se projeta lingualmente a partir do cíngulo dos incisivos permanentes. [Inglês garra, calcanhar, do Fr. ant., do L. *talus,* tornozelo]
c. of tooth [TA], cúspide do dente; uma elevação ou montículo na coroa de um dente que constitui uma parte da superfície oclusal. SIN cuspis dentis [TA], cuspis coronae.
cus·pad (kŭs′păd) Em direção à cúspide de um dente. [L. *ad,* para]
cus·pal (kŭs - pal). Cuspidal; relativo à cúspide.
cus·pid (kŭs′pid). **1.** Cuspidado; que possui apenas uma cúspide. SIN cuspidate. **2.** Dente canino. SIN canine *tooth* [L. *cuspis,* ponta]
cus·pi·date (kŭs′pi - dāt). Cuspidado. SIN cuspid (1).

---

*N.R.: Segundo a *Terminologia Anatômica Internacional* (2001), o termo cúspide deve ser substituído, quando se tratar de valvas, para válvula.

cus·pis, pl. **cus·pi·des** (kŭs′pis, kŭs′pi-dēz) [TA]. Cúspide, válvula. SIN cusp. [L. uma ponta]
  c. anterior valvae atrioventricularis dextrae [TA], válvula anterior da valva atrioventricular direita. SIN anterior cusp of tricuspid valve.
  c. anterior valvae atrioventricularis sinistrae [TA], válvula anterior da valva atrioventricular esquerda. SIN anterior cusp of mitral valve.
  c. anterior valvae mitralis, válvula anterior da valva atrioventricular esquerda; *termo oficial alternativo para anterior cusp of mitral valve.
  c. anterior valvae tricuspidalis, válvula anterior da valva atrioventricular direita; *termo oficial alternativo para anterior cusp of tricuspid valve.
  c. coro′nae, cúspide do dente. SIN cusp of tooth.
  c. den′tis [TA], cúspide do dente. SIN cusp of tooth.
  c. posterior valvae atrioventricularis dextrae [TA], válvula posterior da valva atrioventricular direita. SIN posterior cusp of tricuspid valve.
  c. posterior valvae atrioventricularis sinistrae [TA], válvula posterior da valva atrioventricular esquerda. SIN posterior cusp of mitral valve.
  c. posterior valvae mitralis, válvula posterior da valva atrioventricular esquerda; *termo oficial alternativo para posterior cusp of mitral valve.
  c. posterior valvae tricuspidalis, válvula posterior da valva atrioventricular direita; *termo oficial alternativo para posterior cusp of tricuspid valve.
  c. septa′lis val′vae atrioventricula′ris dex′trae [TA], válvula septal da valva atrioventricular direita. SIN septal cusp of tricuspid valve.
  c. septalis valvae tricuspidalis, válvula septal da valva atrioventricular direita; *termo oficial alternativo para septal cusp of tricuspid valve.
cu·sum (koo′sum). Acrônimo para soma cumulativa de uma série de medidas; usado basicamente na Grã-Bretanha.
cut (kŭt). Corte. **1.** Em biologia molecular, uma clivagem hidrolítica de duas ligações fosfodiéster opostas em um ácido nucleico de duplo filamento. Cf. nick. **2.** Seccionar ou dividir. **3.** Separar em frações. **4.** Termo informal para uma fração.
cu·ta·ne·o·mu·co·sal (kū-tā′nē-ō-mū-kō′sal). Cutâneo-mucoso. SIN mucocutaneous.
cu·ta·ne·ous (kū-tā′nē-ŭs). Cutâneo; relativo à pele. [L. cutis, pele]
cutch (kŭtch). Catechu; cato. SIN catechu nigrum.
cut·down (kŭt′down). Dissecção; dissecção de uma veia ou artéria para inserção de uma cânula ou agulha para a administração de líquidos intravenosos ou medicação, ou para medida da pressão. SIN venostomy.
Cu·te·reb·ra (kū-te-rē′brä). Gênero de gastrófilos cujos adultos são semelhantes a abelhões azuis ou pretos, cujas larvas comumente infestam roedores e lagomorfos (lebres e coelhos); as larvas transformam-se em grandes bernes espinhosos, geralmente no tecido conjuntivo subcutâneo do pescoço. Bernes semelhantes, provavelmente de outras espécies, não são incomuns em gatos e, algumas vezes, são encontrados em cães e em seres humanos. [L. cutis, pele, + *terebro*, perfurar, de *terebra*, escavador]
cu·ti·cle (kū′ti-kl). Cutícula. **1.** Uma camada fina externa, geralmente de natureza córnea. SIN cuticula (1). **2.** A camada, quitinosa em alguns invertebrados, presente na superfície das células epiteliais. **3.** SIN epidermis. [L. *cuticula*, dim. de *cutis*, pele]
  acquired c., acquired enamel c., c. adquirida, c. de esmalte adquirida. SIN acquired *pellicle*.
  dental c., c. dentária. SIN enamel c.
  enamel c., c. do esmalte; a cutícula do esmalte primária, que consiste em duas camadas extremamente finas (a camada interna transparente e sem estrutura, a externa celular), cobrindo toda a coroa dos dentes logo após a erupção e subseqüentemente desgastadas pela mastigação; é evidente, microscopicamente, como um material amorfo entre o epitélio de fixação e o dente. SIN adamantine membrane, cuticula dentis, dental c., membrana adamantina, Nasmyth c., Nasmyth membrane, skin of teeth.
  c. of hair, c. do pêlo. SIN cuticula pili.
  c. of nail, c. da unha; o prolongamento distal exposto da camada córnea da superfície profunda da prega ungueal proximal (eponíquio (2)), observada como uma "pele" fina sobreposta e aderida ao corpo da unha em sua porção proximal (a área da lúnula). É formada como um remanescente do eponíquio (1), que degenera no oitavo mês de gravidez.
  Nasmyth c., c. de Nasmyth. SIN enamel c.
  posteruption c., c. pós-erupção. SIN acquired *pellicle*.
  c. of root sheath, c. da bainha da raiz. SIN cuticula vaginae folliculi pili.
cu·tic·u·la, pl. **cu·tic·u·lae** (kū-tik′ū-lä, -lē). Cutícula. **1.** [NA]. SIN cuticle (1). **2.** SIN epidermis. [L. cuticle]
  c. den′tis, c. dentária. SIN enamel *cuticle*.
  c. pi′li, c. dos pêlos; uma camada de células semelhantes a ripas superpostas, que revestem o córtex piloso e servem para encerrar as células corticais do fio e fechar a haste do pêlo em seu folículo. SIN cuticle of hair.
  c. vagi′nae follic′uli pi′li, c. da bainha do folículo piloso; cutícula de células semelhantes a ripas, superpostas, revestindo o folículo piloso. SIN cuticle of root sheath.
cu·tin (kū′tin). Cutina; uma membrana animal, fina, especialmente preparada, usada como revestimento protetor para superfícies lesadas. [L. *cutis*, pele]

cu·tis (kū′tis) [TA]. Cútis; pele. SIN skin. [L.]
  c. anseri′na, pele arrepiada; contração dos músculos eretores dos pêlos, causada por frio, medo ou outro estímulo, que causa proeminência dos orifícios foliculares. SIN goose flesh, gooseflesh.
  c. lax′a [MIM*123700], c. flácida; pele frouxa. SIN dermatochalasis.
  c. marmora′ta, c. marmórea; mosqueamento róseo, fisiológico, normal da pele em lactentes, que persiste anormalmente em algumas crianças expostas ao frio.
  c. marmorata telangiectatica congenita, c. marmórea teleangiectásica congênita; malformação cutânea capilar-venosa com aspecto "marmóreo". SIN Van Lohuizen syndrome.
  c. rhomboida′lis nu′chae, c. romboidal da nuca; configurações sulcadas geométricas da pele do dorso do pescoço em virtude de exposição prolongada à luz solar com elastose solar.
  c. ve′ra, c. verdadeira. SIN dermis.
  c. ver′ticis gyra′ta, distúrbio congênito no qual a pele do couro cabeludo apresenta-se hipertrofiada e preguead, formando sulcos da parte anterior para a posterior; pode ser um componente da paquidermoperiostose.
cu·ti·za·tion (kū-ti-zā′shŭn). Cutização; a transição da mucosa para a pele nas margens cutâneo-mucosas.
cutpoint (kŭt′poynt). Limite; valor arbitrário em uma escala ordinal como a pressão arterial, além do qual os valores são considerados clinicamente anormais.
cu·vet, cu·vette (koo-vet′). Cubeta; pequeno recipiente ou cálice no qual são colocadas soluções para análise fotométrica.
Cuvier, Barão Georges L.C.F.D. de la, cientista francês, 1769–1832. VER C. *ducts*, em *duct, veins,* em *vein.*
CV Abreviatura de *coefficient* of variation (coeficiente de variação); cardiovascular (cardiovascular); closing *volume* (volume de fechamento).
CVA Abreviatura de cerebrovascular *accident* (acidente vascular cerebral).
CVP Abreviatura de central venous *pressure* (pressão venosa central).
CX Abreviatura de *phosgene* oxime (fosgênio oxima).
CxT Abreviatura de concentration × time (concentração × tempo). VER AUC.
♻ **cyan-.** VER cyano-.
cy·an·al·co·hols (sī-an-al′kō-holz). Cianoálcoois. SIN cyanohydrins.
cy·an·a·mide (sī-an′i-mīd). Cianamida; uma substância hidrossolúvel irritante e cáustica, H_2NCN ou $HN=C=NH$; termo freqüentemente usado para se referir à cianamida de cálcio.
cy·a·nate (sī′an-āt). Cianato; o radical –O–C≡N ou íon $(CNO)^-$.
cy·a·ne·mia (sī-a-ne′mē-a). Cianemia; termo obsoleto para cianose. [cyan- + G. *haima*, sangue]
cy·a·nide (sī′an-īd). Cianeto. **1.** O radical –CN ou íon $(CN)^-$. O íon é extremamente venenoso, formando ácido hidriociânico em água, e tem o odor de óleo de amêndoas; inibe as proteínas respiratórias (citocromos) a nível celular. **2.** Um sal de HCN ou uma molécula contendo ciano.
  c. methemoglobin, c. de metemoglobina. SIN cyanmethemoglobin.
cy·a·nid·e·non (sī-ā-nid′ē-non). Cianidenona. SIN luteolin.
cy·an·i·dol (sī′an-i-dol). Cianidol. SIN catechin.
cy·an·met·he·mo·glo·bin (sī′an-met-hē′mō-glō-bin). Cianometemoglobina; um composto relativamente atóxico de cianeto com metemoglobina, formado quando se administra azul de metileno em casos de envenenamento por cianeto. SIN cyanide methemoglobin.
♻ **cyano-, cyan-. 1.** Forma combinante que significa azul. **2.** Prefixo químico freqüentemente usado para designar compostos que contêm o grupamento cianeto, CN. [G. *kyanos*, substância azul-escura]
Cy·a·no·bac·te·ria (sī′ä-nō-bak-tēr′ē-ä). Uma divisão do reino Prokaryotae, que consiste em bactérias unicelulares ou filamentosas imóveis ou que possuem uma motilidade deslizante, reproduzem-se por divisão binária e realizam fotossíntese com a produção de oxigênio. Antigamente, essas bactérias azul-esverdeadas eram denominadas algas azul-esverdeadas. SIN Cyanophyceae.
cy·a·no·chro·ic, cy·an·och·rous (sī-an-ō-krō′ik, sī-an-ok′rŭs). Cianocróico. SIN cyanotic. [cyano- + G. *chroia*, cor]
cy·a·no·co·bal·a·min (sī-an-ō-kō-bal′ä-min). Cianocobalamina; um complexo de cianeto e cobalamina, como na vitamina B_{12}, no qual um grupamento cianeto ocupou a sexta posição coordenada do átomo de cobalto.
  radioactive c., c. radioativa; cianol[Co^{57}]cobalamina, ciano[Co^{58}]cobalamina, ou ciano[Co^{60}]cobalamina produzida pelo crescimento de determinados microrganismos em um meio contendo cobalto-57, cobalto-58 ou cobalto-60, usado na investigação da absorção e metabolismo de cianocobalamina (vitamina B_{12}).
cy·an·o·gen (sī-an′ō-jen). Cianogênio. **1.** Um composto de dois radicais ciano, NC–CN. **2.** Substâncias muito tóxicas (fórmula geral X-CN, onde X é um halógeno) usadas em sínteses químicas e como preservativos teciduais. Um exemplo é o brometo de cianogênio.
  c. chloride, CNCl; cloreto de cianogênio; líquido muito volátil; um veneno sistêmico usado como agente de advertência em fumigações com cianeto de hidrogênio.
cy·a·no·gen·ic (sī′an-ō-jen′ik). Cianogênico; capaz de produzir ácido cianídrico; diz-se de plantas como o sorgo–comum, sorgo–perene, a erva-do-bre-

jo e a cerejeira selvagem, que podem causar envenenamento por cianeto em animais herbívoros.

cy·a·no·hy·drins (sī'an - ō - hī'drinz). Cianoidrinas; R—CHOH—CN; compostos de adição de HCN e aldeídos. SIN cyanalcohols.

cy·an·o·phil, cy·an·o·phile (sī'an - ō - fīl, -fīl). Cianófilo; uma célula ou elemento que se cora diferencialmente de azul em um procedimento de coloração. [cyano- + G. *philos*, afinidade]

cy·a·noph·i·lous (sī - ă - nof'i - lŭs). Ciagnófilo; facilmente corável por um corante azul.

Cy·a·no·phy·ce·ae (sī'ă - nō - fī'sē - ē). Cianofíceas. SIN Cyanobacteria. [cyano- + G. *phykos*, alga marinha]

cy·a·no·pia (sī - ă - no'pē - ă). Cianopia. SIN cyanopsia.

cy·a·nop·sia (sī - ă - nop'sē - ă). Cianopsia; condição na qual todos os objetos parecem azuis; pode suceder temporariamente a extração de catarata. SIN blue vision, cyanopia. [cyano- + G. *opsis*, visão]

cy·a·nosed (sī'a - nōst). Cianótico. SIN cyanotic.

cy·a·no·sis (sī - ă - nō'sis). Cianose; coloração azulada ou púrpura-escuro da pele e mucosa devido à oxigenação deficiente do sangue, evidente quando a hemoglobina reduzida no sangue ultrapassa 5 g/100 ml. [G. cor azul-escura, de *kyanos*, substância azul]

compression c., c. por compressão; cianose acompanhada por edema e petéquias na cabeça, no pescoço e na parte superior do tórax, como um reflexo venoso resultante da forte compressão do tórax ou abdome; a conjuntiva e as retinas são afetadas de forma semelhante.

enterogenous c., c. enterógena; cianose aparente causada pela absorção de nitritos ou de outros materiais tóxicos do intestino com a formação de metemoglobina ou sulfemoglobina; a alteração da cor da pele é devida à cor chocolate da metemoglobina.

false c., c. falsa; cianose devida à presença de um pigmento anormal, como a metemoglobina, no sangue, e não resultante de deficiência de oxigênio.

hereditary methemoglobinemic c., c. metemoglobinêmica hereditária. SIN congenital methemoglobinemia.

late c., c. tardia; cianose causada por derivação (*shunt*) direita-esquerda, na cardiopatia congênita, que surge somente após insuficiência cardíaca. SIN cyanose tardive, tardive c.

c. ret'inae, c. da retina; congestão venosa da retina.

shunt c., c. por *shunt*; qualquer cor azul de toda a pele ou de uma região da pele ou mucosa causada por uma derivação (*shunt*) direita-esquerda que permite a passagem de sangue não-oxigenado para o lado esquerdo da circulação.

tardive c., c. tardia. SIN late c.

toxic c., c. tóxica; cianose causada por formação de metemoglobina resultante da ação de determinadas substâncias, p. ex., nitritos.

cy·a·not·ic (sī - ă - not'ik). Cianótico; relativo a, ou caracterizado por, cianose. SIN cyanochroic, cyanochrous, cyanosed.

cy·a·nu·ria (sī - ă - noo'rē - ă). Cianúria; a presença de urina azul. [cyano- + G. *ouron*, urina]

cy·a·nu·ric ac·id (sī - ă - noor'ik). Ácido cianúrico; um produto cíclico formado pelo aquecimento da uréia; usado industrialmente e como herbicida.

Cy·a·tho·sto·ma (sī - ă - thos'tō - mă). Ciatóstoma; gênero de vermes da traquéia e brônquios de aves domésticas da família de nematódeos Syngamidae. [G. *kyathos*, cálice, caliciforme, + *stoma*, boca]

C. bronchia'lis, espécie encontrada em gansos selvagens e patos, gansos e cisnes domésticos; encontrada na laringe, traquéia e brônquios e causa angústia e sintomas semelhantes aos produzidos pelo verme da traquéia das galinhas, *Syngamus trachea*; seu ciclo vital é considerado semelhante ao do *Syngamus trachea*.

Cy·a·tho·sto·mun (sī - ă - thos'tō - mŭn). Gênero de nematódeos estrongilóides (família Cyasthostomidae, antes parte da família Strongylidae); inclui muitos dos pequenos estrôngilos de cavalos antes colocados no gênero *Trichonema*, que foram variadamente divididos em vários gêneros e subgêneros. [ver *Cyathostoma*]

cy·ber·net·ics (sī - ber - net'iks). Cibernética. **1.** O estudo comparativo de computadores e do sistema nervoso humano, com o objetivo de explicar o funcionamento do cérebro. **2.** A ciência de controle e comunicação em sistemas vivos e não-vivos; caracteristicamente, o controle é governado por retroalimentação, isto é, por comunicação no sistema acerca da diferença entre o resultado real e o desejado, sendo a ação então modificada para minimizar essa diferença. VER TAMBÉM feedback. [G. *kybernētica*, coisas relativas ao controle ou orientação]

cy·brid (sī'brid). Cíbrido; célula com citoplasma de duas células diferentes em virtude da hibridização celular. [cell + hybrid]

cycl-. VER cyclo-.

cy·cla·mate (sī'klă - māt). Ciclamato; um sal ou éster do ácido ciclâmico; o de cálcio e o de sódio são edulcorantes artificiais não-calóricos.

cy·clam·ic ac·id (sī - klam'ik). Ácido ciclâmico; agente edulcorante, geralmente usado como ciclamado de sódio ou de cálcio. SIN cyclohexanesulfamic acid, cyclohexylsulfamic acid.

cy·cla·mide (sī'klă - mīd). Ciclamida. SIN glycyclamide.

cy·clan·de·late (sī - klan'de - lāt). Ciclandelato; antiespasmódico com ação semelhante à da papaverina; usado em doenças vasculares obliterativas e distúrbios vasoespásticos.

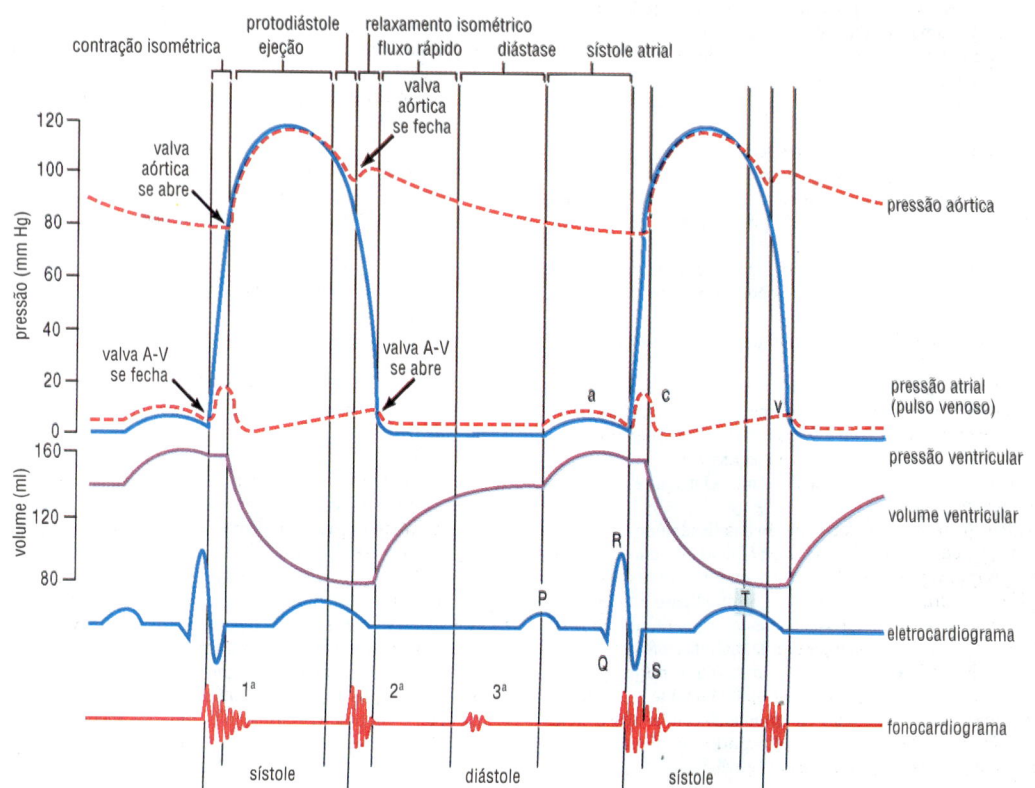

ciclo cardíaco: mostrando alterações nas pressões e nos volumes cardíacos, eletrocardiograma e fonocardiograma; A–V, atrioventricular

cy·clar·thro·di·al (sī - klar - thrō′dē - ăl). Ciclartrodial; relativo a uma ciclartrose.
cy·clar·thro·sis (sī - klar - thrō′sis). Ciclartrose; uma articulação capaz de realizar rotação. [cyclo - + G. *arthrōsis*, articulação]
cy·clase (sī′klās). Ciclase; nome descritivo aplicado a uma enzima que forma um composto cíclico; p. ex., adenilato ciclase.

CYCLE

cy·cle (sī′kl). Ciclo. **1.** Uma série recorrente de eventos. **2.** Um período de tempo recorrente. **3.** Compressão e rarefação sucessivas de uma onda, como uma onda sonora. [G. *kyklos*, círculo]
anovulatory c., c. anovulatório; um ciclo sexuado no qual não é liberado um óvulo.
brain wave c., c. de onda cerebral; o percurso completo (ascendente e descendente) de uma única onda, complexo ou impulso, como é observado em um eletroencefalograma.
carbon dioxide c., carbon c., c. do dióxido de carbono, c. do carbono; a circulação de carbono como CO_2 desde o ar expirado por animais e a deterioração da matéria orgânica até a vida vegetal, onde é sintetizado (através da fotossíntese) em material carboidrato, do qual, em virtude de processos catabólicos que ocorrem em toda a vida, é, afinal, novamente liberado para a atmosfera como CO_2.
cardiac c., c. cardíaco; o ciclo completo da sístole e da diástole cardíacas com os intervalos intermediários, ou começando com, qualquer evento na atividade cardíaca até o momento em que o mesmo evento é repetido.
cell c., c. celular; os eventos bioquímicos e estruturais periódicos que ocorrem durante a proliferação de células como em cultura tecidual; o ciclo é dividido em fases denominadas: G_0, Gap_1 (G_1), síntese (S_1), Gap_2 (G_2) e mitose (M). O período vai de uma divisão até a próxima. SIN mitotic c.
chewing c., c. de mastigação; um curso completo de movimento da mandíbula durante um único movimento mastigatório.
citric acid c., c. do ácido cítrico. SIN tricarboxylic acid c.
Cori c., c. de Cori; as fases no metabolismo dos carboidratos: 1) glicogenólise no fígado; 2) passagem de glicose para a circulação; 3) deposição de glicose nos músculos como glicogênio; 4) glicogenólise durante a atividade muscular e conversão em lactato, que é convertido em glicogênio no fígado. Também denominado ciclo do ácido láctico.
dicarboxylic acid c., c. do ácido dicarboxílico; **(1)** a parte do ciclo do ácido tricarboxílico que envolve os ácidos dicarboxílicos (ácidos succínico, fumárico, málico e oxaloacético); **(2)** um esquema cíclico no qual determinadas etapas do ciclo do ácido tricarboxílico são usadas com o ciclo do glioxilato; importante na utilização de ácido glioxílico em microrganismos.
endogenous c., c. endógeno; a porção de um ciclo vital de parasitas que ocorre no hospedeiro.
erythrocytic c., c. eritrocítico; a porção não-patogênica da fase vertebrada do ciclo vital de plasmódios que ocorre nos eritrócitos.
estrous c., a série de modificações fisiológicas uterinas, ovarianas e outras que ocorrem nos animais superiores, consistindo em proestro, estro, pós-estro e anestro.
exoerythrocytic c., ciclo exoeritrocitário, a porção não-patogênica da fase vertebrada do ciclo de vida dos plasmódios que ocorre nos hepatócitos, fora das células sanguíneas.
exogenous c., c. exógeno; a porção do ciclo vital de um parasita que ocorre fora do hospedeiro.
fatty acid oxidation c., c. de oxidação do ácido graxo; uma série de reações que envolvem compostos de acilcoenzima A, por meio das quais estes sofrem beta-oxidação e clivagem tioclástica, com a formação de acetil-coenzima A; a principal via do catabolismo dos ácidos graxos no tecido vivo.
forced c., c. forçado; um ciclo cardíaco (atrial ou ventricular) que é encurtado por um batimento forçado.
futile c., um ciclo de fosforilação e desfosforilação catalisado por duas enzimas que, normalmente, funcionam em duas vias metabólicas diferentes; o efeito final é a hidrólise de ATP e a produção de calor; p. ex., o ciclo resultante da ação desregulada da 6-fosfofrutocinase e frutose-1,6-bifosfatase no músculo; esses ciclos podem ser importantes na produção de calor, na regulação final de algumas vias e podem ser um fator na hipertermia maligna. SIN substrate c.
γ-glutamyl c., c. do γ-glutamil; uma via proposta para o transporte glutationa-dependente de determinados aminoácidos (mais notavelmente L-cistina, L-metionina e L-glutamina) e dipeptídeos em determinadas células; esse ciclo requer a formação de aminoácidos γ-glutamil e dipeptídeos γ-glutamil, bem como uma proteína para a translocação desses di- e triisopeptídeos para as células.
glycine-succinate c., c. da glicina-succinato; uma série de etapas metabólicas na qual a glicina é condensada com succinil-CoA e, depois, oxidada em CO_2 e

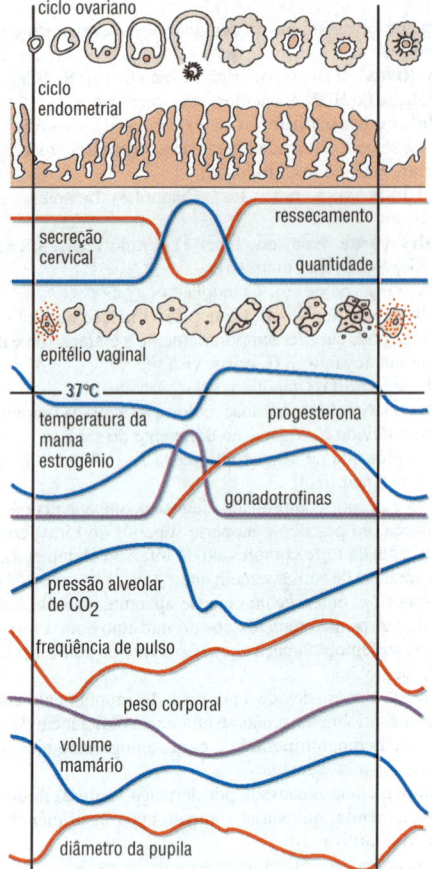

ciclo menstrual

H_2O com regeneração da succinil-CoA; importante na síntese do ácido δ-aminolevulínico e no metabolismo das hemácias. SIN Shemin c.
glyoxylic acid c., c. do ácido glioxílico; ciclo catabólico em vegetais e microrganismos como o do ácido tricarboxílico em animais; sua reação fundamental é a condensação de acetil-CoA com ácido glioxílico para ácido málico (análogo à condensação de acetil-CoA e ácido oxaloacético para formar ácido cítrico no ciclo do ácido tricarboxílico). SIN Krebs-Kornberg c.
gonadotrophic c. (gō′nad - ō - trōf′ik), c. gonadotrófico; uma série completa de desenvolvimento ovariano no inseto vetor desde o momento em que ele se alimenta de sangue até o momento em que são depositados os ovos totalmente desenvolvidos.
hair c., c. piloso; as fases cíclicas de crescimento (anágeno), regressão (catágeno) e quiescência (telógeno) na vida de um pêlo.
heterogonic life c., c. vital heterogônico; estágio de vida livre de um organismo (p. ex., *Strongyloides stercoralis*) que também possui um estágio de parasita.
homogonic life c., c. vital homogônico; estágio parasita do ciclo vital de um organismo (p. ex., *Strongyloides stercoralis*) que também possui um estágio de vida livre.
Krebs c., c. de Krebs. SIN tricarboxylic acid c.
Krebs-Henseleit c., Krebs ornithine c., Krebs urea c., c. de Krebs-Henseleit, c. da ornitina de Krebs, c. da uréia de Krebs. SIN urea c.
Krebs-Kornberg c., c. de Krebs-Kornberg. SIN glyoxylic acid c.
life c., c. vital; toda a história de vida de um organismo vivo.
masticating c.'s, ciclos de mastigação; os padrões de movimentos mandibulares formados durante a mastigação dos alimentos.
menstrual c., c. menstrual; o período no qual um óvulo amadurece, é ovulado e entra na luz uterina através das tubas uterinas; as secreções hormonais ovarianas realizam alterações endometriais de forma que, se houver fertilização, a nidação será possível; na ausência de fertilização, as secreções ovarianas diminuem, o endométrio descama e começa a menstruação; esse ciclo dura em média 28 dias, sendo designado como primeiro dia do ciclo aquele dia em que começa o fluxo menstrual.
mitotic c., c. mitótico. SIN cell c.
nitrogen c., a série de eventos na qual o nitrogênio da atmosfera é fixado, tornando-se assim disponível para a vida vegetal e animal, e depois é devolvido

para a atmosfera; as bactérias nitrificadoras convertem N_2 e O_2 em NO_2^- e NO_3^-, sendo este último absorvido por plantas e convertido em proteínas; quando o vegetal se decompõe, parte do nitrogênio é devolvida para a atmosfera e o restante é convertido por microrganismos em amônia, nitritos e nitratos; se os vegetais forem ingeridos, as excreções de animais ou a desintegração bacteriana devolvem o nitrogênio para o solo e o ar.

ornithine c., c. da ornitina. SIN urea c.

ovarian c., c. ovariano; o ciclo sexuado normal que inclui o desenvolvimento de um folículo ovariano (de Graaf), ruptura do folículo com liberação do óvulo e formação e regressão de um corpo lúteo.

pentose phosphate c., c. da pentose fosfato. SIN pentose phosphate *pathway*.

reproductive c., c. reprodutivo; o ciclo que começa com a concepção e se estende durante a gestação e o parto.

restored c., c. restaurado; um ciclo cardíaco atrial ou ventricular que sucede o ciclo de retorno e reassume o ritmo normal.

returning c., c. de retorno; um ciclo cardíaco atrial ou ventricular que começa com uma extra-sístole ou um batimento forçado.

Ross c., c. de Ross; o ciclo vital do plasmódio.

Shemin c., c. de Shemin. SIN glycine-succinate c.

substrate c., c. de substrato. SIN futile c.

succinic acid c., c. do ácido succínico; uma série de reações de oxidação-redução em que o ácido succínico e outros ácidos contendo quatro átomos de carbono (fumárico, málico, oxaloacético) tomam parte na oxidação do ácido pirúvico como parte do ciclo do ácido tricarboxílico. VER TAMBÉM dicarboxylic acid c.

tricarboxylic acid c., c. do ácido tricarboxílico; juntamente com a fosforilação oxidativa, a principal fonte de energia no organismo dos mamíferos e o objetivo do metabolismo dos carboidratos, gorduras e proteínas; uma série de reações, começando e terminando com o ácido oxaloacético, durante as quais um fragmento contendo dois carbonos é complexamente oxidado em dióxido de carbono e água com produção de 12 ligações de fosfato de alta energia. Assim denominado devido às quatro primeiras substâncias envolvidas (ácido cítrico, ácido *cis*-aconítico, ácido isocítrico e ácido oxalossuccínico) são todos ácidos tricarboxílicos; a partir do oxalossuccinato, os outros são, em ordem, α-cetoglutarato, succinato, fumarato, L-malato e oxaloacetato, que se condensa com a acetil-CoA (da degradação do ácido graxo) para formar citrato (ácido cítrico) novamente. SIN citric acid c., Krebs c.

urea c., c. da uréia; a seqüência de reações químicas, ocorridas basicamente no fígado, que resulta na produção de uréia; a reação fundamental é a hidrólise de L-arginina pela arginase em L-ornitina e uréia; a L-ornitina é então convertida em L-citrulina por uma reação de carbamoilação, depois em L-argininossuccinato por uma reação de aminação que envolve o ácido L-aspártico, e, finalmente, há uma etapa liase-dependente que gera arginina e fumarato. SIN Krebs-Henseleit c., Krebs ornithine c., Krebs urea c., ornithine c.

visual c., c. visual; a transformação de carotenóides envolvidos na descoloração e na regeneração do pigmento visual.

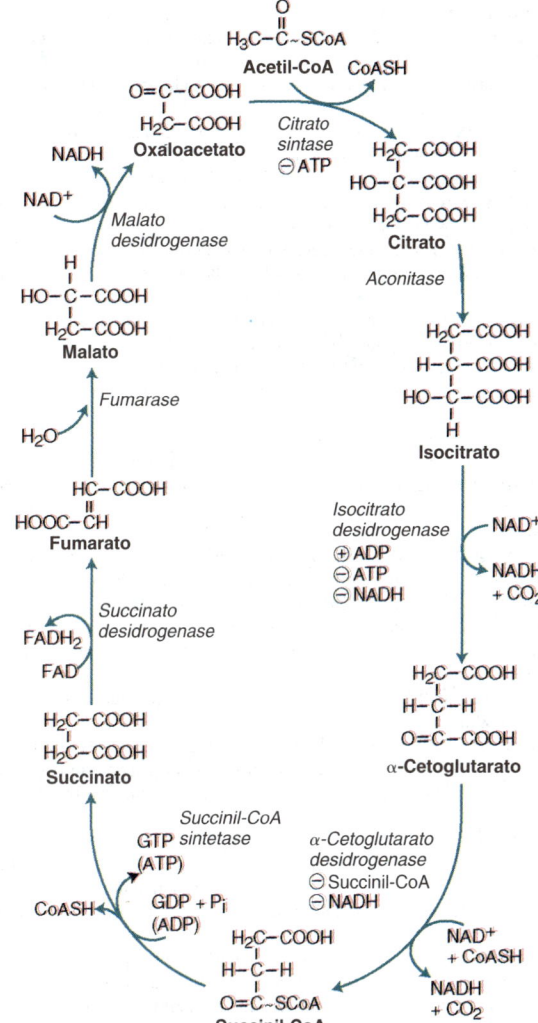

ciclo do ácido tricarboxílico (ciclo do ácido cítrico, ciclo de Krebs): + = ativador, − = inibidor, *termos em itálico* = nomes de enzimas, ~ = ligações de alta energia

cy·clec·to·my (sī - klek′tō - mē, sik - lek′tō - mē). Ciclectomia; excisão de uma parte do corpo ciliar. SIN ciliectomy. [cyclo- + G. *ektomē*, excisão]

cy·clen·ceph·a·ly, cy·clen·ce·pha·lia (sī - klen - sef′ă - lē, - se - fā′lē - ă). Cicloencefalia; condição em um feto malformado caracterizada por desenvolvimento insatisfatório e um grau variável de fusão dos dois hemisférios cerebrais. SIN cyclocephaly, cyclocephalia. [cyclo- + G. *enkephalos*, cérebro]

cy·cles per sec·ond (cps). Ciclos por segundo; o número de compressões e rarefações sucessivas por segundo de uma onda sonora. A designação preferida para essa unidade de freqüência é hertz.

cy·clic (sī′klik, sik′lik). Cíclico. **1.** Relativo a, ou característico de, um ciclo; que ocorre periodicamente, designando o curso dos sintomas em determinadas doenças ou distúrbios. **2.** Em química, contínuo, sem fim, como em um anel; designa um composto cíclico.

cy·clic AMP. AMP cíclico. SIN adenosine 3′,5′-cyclic monophosphate.

3′,5′-cy·clic AMP syn·the·tase. 3′,5′-AMP cíclico sintetase. SIN adenylate cyclase.

cy·clic GMP. GMP cíclico. SIN cyclic *guanosine* 3′,5′-monophosphate.

cyclin D. Ciclina D; proteína envolvida na progressão para divisão celular.

cy·cli·tis (sī - klī′tis). Ciclite; inflamação do corpo ciliar. [G. *kyklos*, círculo (corpo ciliar), + -*itis*, inflamação]

Fuchs heterochromic c., c. heterocrômica de Fuchs. SIN Fuchs syndrome.

heterochromic c., c. heterocrômica; ciclite inflamatória crônica na qual a íris do olho afetado sofre atrofia.

plastic c., c. plástica; inflamação do corpo ciliar e, geralmente, de todo o trato uveal, com exsudação fibrinosa para as câmaras anterior e vítrea.

purulent c., c. purulenta; inflamação supurativa do corpo ciliar.

cy·cli·zine hy·dro·chlo·ride (sī′kli - zēn). Cloridrato de ciclizina; um agente anti-histamínico H_1 útil na prevenção e no alívio da cinetose e dos sintomas causados por distúrbios vestibulares.

cy·cli·zine lac·tate. Lactato de ciclizina; um agente que tem o mesmo uso e ação que o cloridrato de ciclizina.

cyclo-, cycl-. **1.** Forma combinante relativa a um círculo ou ciclo; ou que designa uma associação com o corpo ciliar. **2.** Em química, uma forma combinante que indica uma molécula contínua, sem extremidade, ou a formação dessa estrutura entre duas partes de uma molécula. [G. *kyklos*, círculo]

cy·clo·ben·za·prine hy·dro·chlo·ride (sī - klō - ben′ză - prēn). Cloridrato de ciclobenzaprina; um relaxante muscular esquelético de ação central, usado para aliviar espasmos musculares agudos.

cy·clo·ceph·a·ly, cy·clo·ce·pha·lia (sī - klō - sef′ă - lē, - sē - fā′lē - ă). Ciclocefalia. SIN cyclencephaly. [cyclo- + G. *kephalē*, cabeça]

cy·clo·cho·roid·i·tis (sī′klō - kō - roy - dī′tis). Ciclocoroidite; inflamação do corpo ciliar e da coróide.

cy·clo·cry·o·ther·a·py (sī′klō - krī′ō - thār′ă - pē). Ciclocrioterapia; congelamento transescleral do corpo ciliar no tratamento do glaucoma.

cy·clo·cu·ma·rol (sīklō - kū′mă - rol). Ciclocumarol; anticoagulante 4-hidroxicumarina nº 63; substância anticoagulante sintética, relacionada à bis-hidroxicumarina.

cy·clo·des·truc·tive (sī′klō - dis - truk′tiv). Ciclodestrutivo; relativo a um procedimento designado para lesar o corpo ciliar a fim de reduzir a produção de líquido aquoso em pacientes com glaucoma. VER cyclocryotherapy, cyclodiathermy, cyclophotocoagulation.

cy·clo·di·al·y·sis (sī′klō - dī - al′i - sis). Ciclodiálise; estabelecimento de uma comunicação entre a câmara anterior e o espaço supracoroidal a fim de reduzir a pressão intra-ocular no glaucoma. [cyclo- + G. *dialysis*, separação]

cy·clo·di·a·ther·my (sī′klō - dī - ă - ther′mē). Ciclodiatermia; diatermia aplicada à esclera adjacente ao corpo ciliar no tratamento do glaucoma.

cy·clo·duc·tion (sī - klō - dŭk′shŭn). Ciclodução; rotação do olho ao redor de seu eixo visual. SIN circumduction (2) [TA], cyclotorsion. [cyclo- + L. *duco*, pp. *ductus*, retirar]

cy·clo·guan·il pam·o·ate (sī - klō - gwahn'il). Pamoato de cicloguanil; um agente antimalárico de ação prolongada que impede o crescimento ou a sobrevida dos parasitas pré-eritroeíticos e eritrocíticos.

cy·clo·hex·ane·sul·fam·ic ac·id (sī - klō - heks'an - sŭl - fam'ik). Ácido cicloexanossulfâmico. SIN cyclamic acid.

cy·clo·hex·i·mide (sī - klō - heks'i - mīd). Cicloeximida; um antibiótico obtido de determinadas cepas de *Streptomyces griseus*; usado em pesquisa bioquímica para inibir a síntese proteica *in vitro*; também é fungicida e repelente de ratos.

cy·clo·hex·yl·sul·fam·ic ac·id (sī - klō - hek'sil - sŭl - fam'ik). Ácido cicloexilsulfâmico. SIN cyclamic acid.

cy·cloid (sī'kloyd). Ciclóide; sugestivo de ciclotimia; termo aplicado a uma pessoa que tende a apresentar períodos de mudanças acentuadas de humor, mas dentro dos limites da normalidade. [cyclo + G. *eidos*, semelhante a]

cy·clol (sī'klol). Ciclol; um dipeptídeo cíclico que, supostamente, ocorre nas proteínas; ocorre em alguns dos alcalóides do ergot.

cy·clo·na·mine (sī - klo - nā'mēn). Ciclonamina. SIN ethamsylate.

cy·clo·ox·y·gen·ase (sī'klō - oks'ē - jen - ās). Ciclooxigenase. SIN *prostaglandin endoperoxide synthase*.

cy·clo·pea (sī - klō'pē - ā). Ciclopia. SIN cyclopia.

cy·clo·pe·an (sī - klō'pē - an). Ciclópico. SIN cyclopian.

cy·clo·pent·a·mine hy·dro·chlo·ride (sī - klō - pent'a - mēn). Cloridrato de ciclopentamina; uma amina simpaticomimética, com ação semelhante à da efedrina.

cy·clo·pen·tane (sī - klō - pen'tān). Ciclopentano; um hidrocarboneto de anel fechado que contém cinco átomos de carbono, isômero do penteno.

cy·clo·pen·ta[*a*]phen·an·threne (sī - klō - pen - ta[ā]fen'a - thrēn) Ciclopenta[a]fenantreno; fenantreno, em cujo lado *a* está fundido um fragmento de três carbonos; como o derivado peridro (saturado), é a estrutura básica dos esteróides.

cy·clo·pen·thi·a·zide (sī'klō - pen - thī'a - zīd). Ciclopentiazida; diurético benzotiadiazídico.

cy·clo·pen·to·late hy·dro·chlo·ride (sī - klō - pen'tō - lāt). Cloridrato de ciclopentolato; anticolinérgico, espasmolítico, usado em determinações de refração; produz cicloplegia e midríase; um agente atropínico com duração de ação curta.

cy·clo·pep·tide (sī - klō - pep'tīd). Ciclopeptídeo; um polipeptídeo que não possui grupamentos –NH$_2$ e –COOH na extremidade em virtude da combinação destes para formar outra ligação peptídica, produzindo um anel.

cy·clo·phen·a·zine hy·dro·chlo·ride (sī - klō - fen'a - zēn). Cloridrato de ciclofenazina; um tranqüilizante.

cy·clo·pho·ras·es (sī - klō - fōr'ās - ez). Cicloforases; o grupo de enzimas nas mitocôndrias que catalisam a oxidação completa do ácido pirúvico em dióxido de carbono e água; essencialmente, aquelas enzimas e coenzimas envolvidas no ciclo do ácido tricarboxílico.

cy·clo·pho·ria (sī - klō - fō'rē - ā). Cicloforia; tendência anormal de cada olho de rodar em torno de seu eixo ântero-posterior, sendo a rotação impedida por impulsos fusionais visuais. [cyclo- + G. *phora*, movimento]

cy·clo·phos·pha·mide (sī - klō - fos'fa - mīd). Ciclofosfamida; um agente alquilante com atividade antitumoral e empregos semelhantes aos da substância original, a mostarda nitrogenada (cloridrato de mecloretamina); também é supressor da atividade das células B e da produção de anticorpos, sendo usada no tratamento de doenças auto-imunes.

cy·clo·pho·to·co·ag·u·la·tion (sīklō - fō'tō - kō - ag - ū - lā'shŭn). Ciclofotocoagulação; fotocoagulação dos processos ciliares para reduzir a secreção de humor aquoso no glaucoma. [cyclo- + photocoagulation]

Cy·clo·phyl·li·dae (sī - klō - fil'i - dē). Ordem de tênias que inclui a maioria dos parasitas comuns dos seres humanos e dos animais domésticos. [cyclo- + G. *phyllon*, folha]

cy·clo·pia (sī - klō'pē - ā). Ciclopia; defeito congênito no qual as duas órbitas são unidas para formar uma cavidade única, contendo um olho, que, tipicamente, resulta da união dos primórdios ópticos direito e esquerdo; geralmente associada à holoprosencefalia ou cicloencefalia. SIN cyclopea, synophthalmia, synophthalmus. [G. *Kyklōps*, de *kyklos*, círculo, + *ōps*, olho]

cy·clo·pi·an (sī - klō'pē - an). Ciclópico; indica ciclopia ou é relativo a esta. SIN cyclopean.

cy·clo·ple·gia (sī - klō - plē'jē - ā). Cicloplegia; perda da força do músculo ciliar do olho; pode ser causada por desnervação ou por ação farmacológica. [cyclo- + G. *plēgē*, golpe]

cy·clo·ple·gic (sī - klō - plē'jik). Cicloplégico. **1.** Relativo à cicloplegia. **2.** Uma substância que paralisa o músculo ciliar e, portanto, a capacidade de acomodação.

cy·clo·pro·pane (sī - klō - prō'pān). Ciclopropano; um gás explosivo de odor característico; no passado, era amplamente usado para produzir anestesia geral. SIN trimethylene.

cy·clops (sī'klops). Ciclope; um indivíduo com ciclopia. SIN monoculus (1), monophthalmus, monops. [ver cyclopia]

cy·clo·ser·ine (sī - klō - ser'ēn). Cicloserina; antibiótico produzido por cepas de *Streptomyces orchidaceus* ou *S. garyphalus*, com um amplo espectro de atividade antibacteriana. SIN orientomycin.

cy·clo·sis (sī - klo'sis). Ciclose; o movimento do protoplasma e dos plastídeos contidos na célula do protozoário. [G., de *kykloō*, mover - se ao redor]

Cy·clo·spo·ra (sī - klō - spōr'ah). Gênero de parasitas coccídios semelhantes ao *Cryptosporidium* descritos em milípedes, répteis, insetívoros e em uma espécie de roedor. O gênero *Cyclospora* é caracterizado por oocistos ácido-resistentes com dois esporocistos, cada um com dois esporozoítas. Também é apontado como causa de uma diarréia humana comum, prolongada, mas auto-limitada em pacientes nas Américas, países do Caribe, Sudeste asiático e leste da Europa, previamente descrita como sendo causada por corpúsculos semelhantes a cianobactérias. SIN cyanobacteriumlike bodies.

C. cayetanensis, espécie que causa enterite com diarréia persistente; geralmente adquirida por ingestão de água ou alimentos contaminados.

cy·clo·spor·in A (sī - klō - spōr'in). Ciclosporina A. SIN cyclosporine.

cy·clo·spor·ine (sī - klō - spōr'ēn). Ciclosporina; um imunossupressor oligopeptídico cíclico produzido pelo fungo *Tolypocladium inflatum Gams*; usado para inibir a rejeição de órgãos transplantados. SIN cyclosporin A.

cy·clo·thi·a·zide (sī - klō - thī'a - zīd). Ciclotiazida; diurético e anti-hipertensivo.

cy·clo·thy·mia (sī - klō - thī'mē - ā). Ciclotimia; distúrbio mental caracterizado por acentuadas oscilações do humor, variando da depressão à hipomania, mas não no grau que ocorre no distúrbio bipolar. SIN cyclothymic disorder. [cyclo- + G. *thymos*, ira]

cy·clo·thy·mi·ac, cy·clo·thy·mic (sī - klō - thī'mē - ăk, - thī'mik). Ciclotímico; relativo à ciclotimia.

cy·clot·o·my (sī - klot'ō - mē). Ciclotomia; operação de secção do músculo ciliar. [cyclo- + G. *tomē*, incisão]

cy·clo·tor·sion (sī'klō - tōr'shun). Ciclotorção. SIN cycloduction.

cy·clo·tron (sī'klō - tron). Ciclótron; acelerador que produz íons de alta velocidade (p. ex., prótons e dêuterons), sob a influência de um campo magnético alternante, para bombardeio e ruptura de núcleos atômicos. Usado para produzir radionuclídeos emissores de pósitrons, clinicamente úteis. [cyclo- + G. *-tron*, sufixo instrumental]

cy·clo·tro·pia (sī - klō - trō'pē - ā). Ciclotropia; uma disparidade da posição ocular na qual um olho é rodado em torno de seu eixo visual, em relação ao outro olho. [cyclo- + G. *trope*, uma volta]

cy·clo·zo·o·no·sis (sī'klō - zō - ō - nō'sis). Ciclozoonose; uma zoonose que exige mais de um hospedeiro vertebrado (mas não invertebrado) para conclusão do ciclo vital; p. ex., vários cestódeos tenióides como *Taenia saginata* e *T. solium*, nos quais os seres humanos são hospedeiros obrigatórios; doença hidática, uma ciclozoonose na qual os seres humanos não são hospedeiros obrigatórios. [cyclo- + G. *zōon*, animal, + *nosos*, doença]

Cyd Símbolo de cytidine (citidina).

cy·e·sis (sī - ē'sis). Ciese; termo obsoleto para gravidez. [G. *kyēsis*]

cyl. Abreviatura de cylinder (cilindro), ou cylindrical *lens* (lente cilíndrica).

cyl·in·der (cyl., C) (sil'in - der). **1.** Uma lente cilíndrica (cylindrical *lens*). **2.** Cilindro; um molde renal em forma de cilindro ou bastão. **3.** Cilindro; recipiente metálico cilíndrico para gases armazenados sob alta pressão. [G. *kylindros*, cilindro]

Bence Jones c.'s, cilindros de Bence Jones; corpúsculos em forma de bastão ou cilindróides, discretamente irregulares, relativamente lisos, de material proteináceo viscoso no líquido das vesículas seminais.

crossed c.'s, cilindros cruzados; uma lente empregada em refração para determinar a potência e o eixo de uma lente cilíndrica para correção de astigmatismo; uma combinação de cilindros côncavos e convexos de potências semelhantes, cujos eixos formam um ângulo reto entre si.

Külz c., c. de Külz. SIN coma *cast*.

cyl·in·drax·is (sil - in - drak'sis). Cilindro-eixo; precursor histórico do termo axônio, baseado em uma interpretação da fibra nervosa mielinizada como um cilindro a partir do qual o axônio formou o eixo.

cy·lin·dri·cal (si - lin'dri - kăl). Cilíndrico; com o formato de um cilindro; referente a um cilindro.

cyl·in·dro·ad·e·no·ma (sil'in - drō - ad - ē - nō'mă). Cilindroadenoma. SIN cylindroma.

cyl·in·droid (sil'in - droyd). Cilindróide. SIN false *cast*. [G. *kylindrōdēs*, de *kylindros*, cilindro, + *eidos*, aspecto]

cyl·in·dro·ma (sil - in - drō'mă). Cilindroma; um tipo histológico de neoplasia epitelial, freqüentemente maligna, caracterizada por ilhotas de células neoplásicas incrustadas em um estroma hialino, que pode representar uma membrana basal espessa; pode se formar a partir de ductos das glândulas, principalmente nas glândulas salivares, pele e brônquios; nas glândulas salivares, também denominado carcinoma cístico adenóide. SIN cylindroadenoma. [G. *kylindros*, cilindro, *-oma*, tumor]

cyl·in·dru·ria (sil - in - droor'rē - ā). Cilindrúria; a presença de cilindros renais na urina.

cyl·lo·so·ma (sil - ō - sō'mă). Cilossoma; defeito congênito unilateral da parede abdominal inferior (eventração) com desenvolvimento defeituoso do membro inferior correspondente [G. *kyllos*, deformado, especialmente pé torto ou pernas tortas, + *sōma*, corpo]

cy·ma·rin (sī′mă - rin). Cimarina; K-estrofantina-α, um glicosídeo da cimarose presente nas sementes de *Strophanthus kombé*, a aglicona é estrofantina; um cardiotônico.

cym·ba con·chae (sim′bă kong′kē) [TA]. Cimba da concha; a parte menor e superior da orelha externa situada acima do ramo da hélice. [G. *kymbē*, a cavidade de um vaso, um cálice, bacia, barco]

cym·bo·ce·phal·ic, cym·bo·ceph·a·lous (sim-bō-se-fal′ik, -sef′ă-lus.) Cimbocefálico, cimbocéfalo; relativo à cimbocefalia.

cym·bo·ceph·a·ly (sim-bō-sef′ă-lē). Cimbocefalia. SIN scaphocephaly. [G. *kymbē*, a cavidade de um vaso, uma estrutura em forma de barco, + *kephalē*, cabeça]

cy·nan·thro·py (sī-nan′thrō-pē). Cinantropia; alucinação na qual o paciente late e rosna, imaginando-se um cão. [G. *kyōn*, cão, + *anthrōpos*, homem]

cy·no·ceph·a·ly (sī-nō-sef′ă-lē). Cinocefalia; cranioestenose em que o crânio se inclina para trás a partir das órbitas, produzindo uma semelhança com a cabeça de um cão. [G. *kyōn*, cão, + *kephalē*, cabeça]

cyn·o·dont (sī′nō-dont). Cinodonte. **1.** Um dente canino. **2.** Um dente que possui uma cúspide ou ponta. [G. *kyōn*, cão, + *odous* (odont-), dente]

cy·no·pho·bia (sī-nō-fō-bē-ă). Cinofobia; medo mórbido de cães. [G. *kyōn*, cão, + *phobos*, medo]

Cyon, Elie de, fisiologista russo, 1843–1912. VER C. nerve.

CYP. Abreviatura de enzimas do citocromo P450; geralmente seguida por um algarismo arábico, uma letra e outro algarismo arábico (p. ex., CYP 2D6). Essas enzimas são encontradas no interior do e sobre o retículo endoplasmático liso do fígado e de outras células, e são responsáveis por um grande número de reações de biotransformação de substâncias.

CYP 1A2, enzima microssomal, cujos substratos incluem teofilina, antidepressivos e tacrina. É inibida pelo suco de toranja (*grapefruit*) e quinolonas, e induzida pelo tabagismo, fenobarbital, fenitoína, rifampina e omeprazol.

CYP 2C9, enzima microssomal responsável pela oxidação do S-warfarin, da fenitoína e de muitos AINE. Os inibidores incluem antifúngicos azóis (p. ex., cetoconazol, itraconazol, metronidazol); induzida pela rifampina.

CYP 2C19, enzima microssomal parcialmente responsável pela oxidação de clomipramina, diazepam, propranolol, imipramina e omeprazol. Inibida pela fluoxetina, sertralina, omeprazol e ritinovir.

CYP 2D6, a isoenzima que metaboliza muitos antidepressivos, agentes antipsicóticos, bloqueadores beta-adrenérgicos e codeína. É inibida pela cimetidina e por vários antidepressivos e antipsicóticos.

CYP 2E1, enzima microssomal que participa da oxidação do etanol e do acetaminofeno. Inibida pelo dissulfiram e induzida pelo etanol e pela isoniazida (INH). Acredita-se que seja responsável pelo metabólito hepatotóxico do acetaminofeno.

CYP 3A, uma isoforma do citocromo P450 encontrada no trato gastrointestinal, bem como em células hepáticas e em outras células; os substratos incluem benzodiazepínicos, bloqueadores dos canais de cálcio, anti-histamínicos, hormônios esteróides e inibidores da protease. Inibida por antidepressivos, antifúngicos azóis, cimetidina e eritromicina. Induzida por fenobarbital, fenitoína, rifampina e carbamazepina.

cy·pri·do·pho·bia (sī′pri-dō-fō′bē-ă). Cipridofobia; medo mórbido de adquirir doença venérea ou de manter relações sexuais. [G. *Kypris*, Afrodite, + *phobos*, medo]

cy·pro·hep·ta·dine hy·dro·chlo·ride (sī-prō-hep′tă-dēn). Cloridrato de ciproeptadina; um potente antagonista da histamina e da serotonina, com ações anti-histamínica H₁ e antipruriginosa.

cy·pro·ter·one ac·e·tate (sī-prō′ter-ōn). Acetato de ciproterona; um esteróide sintético capaz de inibir os efeitos biológicos exercidos por hormônios androgênicos endógenos ou exógenos; um antiandrogênio.

Cys Símbolo de cisteína (meia-cistina) ou de seu mono ou dirradical.

CYST

cyst (sist). Cisto **1.** Uma vesícula. **2.** Um saco anormal contendo gás, líquido ou um material semi-sólido, com um revestimento membranoso. VER TAMBÉM pseudocyst. [G. *kystis*, bexiga, vesícula]

adventitious c., c. adventício. SIN pseudocyst (1).

allantoic c., c. alantóico. SIN urachal c.

alveolar hydatid c., c. hidático alveolar; cisto hidático de um tipo multiloculado, geralmente no fígado, causado por *Echinococcus multilocularis*, cujos adultos são encontrados em raposas; as larvas (hidátide alveolar) são encontradas principalmente em roedores microtinos, mas também em seres humanos, como os que preparam armadilhas de caça e outros que tratam de peles de raposas e outros carnívoros infectados; o crescimento se dá por brotamento exógeno e não é limitado por uma membrana laminada externa como no cisto hidático do *E. granulosus*; geralmente ocorrem necrose, cavitação, disseminação contígua e morte. SIN multilocular hydatid c., multiloculate hydatid c.

aneurysmal bone c., c. ósseo aneurismático; uma lesão osteolítica benigna solitária que se expande em um osso longo ou no interior de uma vértebra, consistindo em espaços cheios de sangue e separados por tecido fibroso contendo células gigantes multinucleadas; pode causar tumefação, dor e dor à palpação, além de comprometer a integridade estrutural do osso envolvido.

angioblastic c., c. angioblástico; tecido mesenquimal capaz de formar sangue no embrião.

apical periodontal c., c. periodontal apical; cisto odontogênico inflamatório derivado histogeneticamente de restos epiteliais de Malassez que circundam o ápice da raiz de um dente não-vital. SIN periapical c., radicular c., root end c.

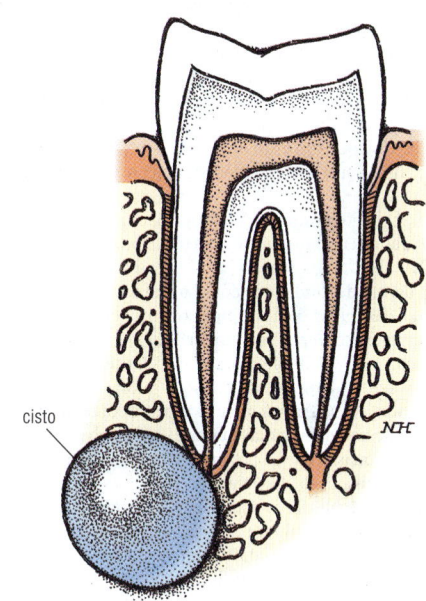

cisto periodontal apical

apoplectic c., c. apoplético; pseudocisto formado por sangue extravasado, como em um acidente vascular cerebral.

arachnoid c., c. aracnóide; cisto cheio de líquido revestido pela membrana aracnóide, freqüentemente situado próximo da face lateral da fissura de Sylvius; em geral de origem congênita. SIN leptomeningeal c.

Baker c., c. de Baker; uma coleção de líquido sinovial que escapou da articulação do joelho ou de uma bolsa e formou um novo saco revestido por líquido sinovial no espaço poplíteo; observado em doenças degenerativas ou em outras doenças articulares que produzem volumes aumentados de líquido sinovial.

Bartholin c., c. de Bartholin; cisto originado da glândula vestibular maior ou de seus ductos.

bile c., vesícula biliar. SIN gallbladder.

blood c., c. sanguíneo. SIN hemorrhagic c.

blue dome c., c. de cúpula azulada; **(1)** um dentre vários pequenos nódulos ou cistos azul-escuros no fórnice vaginal, causados por sangue menstrual retido na endometriose dessa região; **(2)** um cisto de retenção benigno da glândula mamária, na doença fibrocística, que contém um líquido pálido, discretamente amarelado, conferindo uma cor azul ao cisto quando observado através do tecido fibroso adjacente.

bone c., c. ósseo. VER solitary bone c.

botryoid odontogenic c., c. odontogênico botrióide; um tipo de cisto periodontal lateral que exibe um padrão de crescimento multilocular.

Boyer c., c. de Boyer. SIN subhyoid c.

branchial c., c. branquial; um cisto cervical originado da persistência embriológica dos sulcos branquiais ectodérmicos ou das bolsas faríngeas endodérmicas. SIN branchial cleft c.

branchial cleft c., c. da fenda branquial. SIN branchial c.

bronchogenic c., c. broncogênico; cisto revestido por epitélio colunar ciliado, considerado representante da diferenciação brônquica; pode haver músculo liso e glândulas mucosas.

bursal c., c. da bolsa; um cisto de retenção em uma bolsa.

calcifying and keratinizing odontogenic c., c. odontogênico calcificante e queratinizante. SIN calcifying odontogenic c.

calcifying odontogenic c., c. odontogênico calcificante; uma lesão mista radiotransparente-radiopaca das mandíbulas, que possui tanto características de uma neoplasia cística quanto de uma sólida; caracterizada microscopicamente por um revestimento epitelial que mostra uma camada de células basais colunares em paliçada, queratinização de células-fantasma, dentinóide e calcificação. SIN calcifying and keratinizing odontogenic c., Gorlin c.

cerebellar c., c. cerebelar; um cisto que, geralmente, ocorre na substância branca cerebelar lateral; freqüentemente é parte de um astrocitoma cerebelar.

chocolate c., c. de chocolate; cisto ovariano com hemorragia intracavitária e formação de um hematoma que contém sangue marrom antigo; freqüentemente observado na endometriose do ovário, mas algumas vezes com outros tipos de cistos.

choledochal c., c. do colédoco; cisto originado no ducto colédoco; geralmente torna-se aparente, no início da vida, como uma massa abdominal superior direita associada a icterícia.

chyle c., c. quiloso; uma dilatação circunscrita de um canal linfático do mesentério, que contém quilo.

colloid c., c. colóide; um cisto com conteúdo gelatinoso.

compound c., c. composto. SIN multilocular c.

corpora lutea c., c. do corpo lúteo; corpo lúteo persistente com formação de cisto.

Cowper c., c. de Cowper; um cisto de retenção de uma glândula bulbouretral.

daughter c., c.-filho; cisto secundário, geralmente múltiplo, derivado de um cisto-mãe.

dentigerous c., c. dentígero; cisto odontogênico derivado do epitélio de esmalte reduzido que circunda a coroa de um dente impactado ou incrustado. SIN follicular c. (2).

dermoid c., c. dermóide; tumor que consiste em estruturas ectodérmicas deslocadas ao longo das linhas de fusão embrionária, sendo a parede formada de tecido conjuntivo revestido por epitélio, incluindo anexos cutâneos e contendo queratina, sebo e pêlos. SIN dermoid tumor, dermoid (2).

dermoid c. of ovary, c. dermóide do ovário; teratoma cístico benigno comum do ovário, revestido, em sua maior parte, por pele e contendo pêlos e sebo, mas também geralmente contendo várias outras estruturas bem diferenciadas dentro de uma pequena massa que se projeta do tecido sólido para dentro.

distention c., c. de distensão. SIN retention c.

duplication c., c. de duplicação; malformação cística congênita fixada a, ou originada em, qualquer parte do canal alimentar, desde a base da língua até o ânus, que reproduz a estrutura do trato alimentar adjacente.

echinococcus c., c. equinocócico. SIN hidatid c.

endodermal c., c. endodérmico; cisto revestido por epitélio colunar; presumivelmente de origem dérmica.

endometrial c., c. endometrial; cisto resultante de implantação endometrial fora do útero, como na endometriose.

endothelial c., c. endotelial; cisto seroso cujo saco é revestido por endotélio.

enterogenous c., c. enterógeno; cisto mediastinal derivado de células seqüestradas do intestino anterior primitivo; pode ser classificado histologicamente como broncogênico, esofágico ou gástrico.

ependymal c., c. ependimário; distensão circunscrita de alguma porção do canal central da medula espinal ou dos ventrículos cerebrais. SIN neural c.

epidermal c., c. epidérmico; cisto formado por uma massa de células epidérmicas que, em virtude de traumatismo, foi empurrada sob a epiderme; o cisto é revestido por epitélio escamoso estratificado e contém camadas concêntricas de queratina. SIN implantation c., inclusion c. (1), inclusion dermoid.

epidermoid c., c. epidermóide; cisto esférico unilocular da derme, composto de queratina encistada e sebo; o cisto é revestido por um epitélio queratinizante semelhante à epiderme, derivado do infundíbulo folicular.

epithelial c., c. epitelial; cisto revestido por epitélio.

eruption c., c. de irrupção; forma de cisto dentígero nos tecidos moles em conjunto com um dente em irrupção; observado na crista alveolar de crianças.

extravasation c., c. por extravasamento; termo obsoleto para cisto hemorrágico.

exudation c., c. de exsudação; cisto resultante da distensão de uma cavidade fechada, como uma bolsa, por secreção excessiva de seu conteúdo líquido normal.

false c., c. falso. SIN pseudocyst (1).

fissural c., c. de fissura; um cisto derivado de remanescentes epiteliais aprisionados ao longo da linha de fusão de processos embrionários. SIN inclusion c. (2).

follicular c., c. folicular; (1) um folículo de Graaf cístico; (2) SIN dentigerous c.

Gartner c., c. de Gartner; um cisto do ducto principal nas estruturas vestigiais do para-oóforo no colo uterino ou parede vaginal ântero-lateral, que corresponde à porção sexual do mesonefro no homem.

gas c., c. gasoso; cisto com conteúdo gasoso, ao invés do conteúdo líquido ou pultáceo comum.

gingival c., c. gengival; um cisto derivado de remanescentes da lâmina dental situada na gengiva fixada, ocasionalmente produzindo erosão superficial da lâmina cortical do osso; a maioria está localizada na região cúspide–pré-molar.

globulomaxillary c. (glō′boo - lō - maks′il - lar - ē). c. globulomaxilar, um cisto de origem odontogênica encontrado entre as raízes dos dentes canino e incisivo lateral maxilar.

glomerular c., c. glomerular; cisto formado por dilatação da cápsula de Bowman, encontrado em casos raros de rins policísticos congênitos.

Gorlin c., c. de Gorlin. SIN calcifying odontogenic c.

granddaughter c., c.-neto; cisto terciário que, algumas vezes, se desenvolve em um cisto-filho, como no cisto hidático do *Echinococcus*.

hemorrhagic c., c. hemorrágico; cisto contendo sangue ou resultante do encapsulamento de um hematoma. SIN blood c., hematocele (1), hematocyst, sanguineous c.

hepatic c., c. hepático; c. congênito considerado originado de uma obstrução dos canalículos biliares; pode ser solitário, e seu tamanho pode variar de pequeno a enorme; também pode haver doença policística.

heterotrophic oral gastrointestinal c., c. gastrointestinal oral heterotrófico; cisto da cavidade oral, revestido por mucosa gástrica ou intestinal, decorrente de restos embrionários mal posicionados.

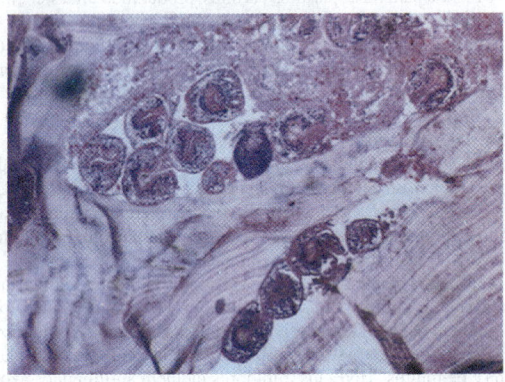

cisto hidático: corte contendo muitos proto-escóleces entre as camadas laminadas; hematoxilina e eosina, 32 ×

hydatid c., c. hidático; cisto formado no fígado, ou, menos freqüentemente, em outras partes, pelo estágio larvar do *Echinococcus*, principalmente em ruminantes; duas formas morfológicas causadas por *Echinococcus granulosus* são encontradas em seres humanos; o cisto hidático unilocular e o cisto hidático ósseo; uma terceira forma em seres humanos é o cisto hidático alveolar, causado por *Echinococcus multilocularis*. SIN echinococcus c., hydatid (1).

implantation c., c. de implantação. SIN epidermal c.

incisive canal c., c. do canal incisivo; cisto no canal incisivo, ou próximo dele, originado de proliferação de remanescentes epiteliais do ducto nasopalatino; o cisto embriológico maxilar mais comum. SIN median anterior maxillary c., nasopalatine duct c.

inclusion c., c. de inclusão; (1) SIN epidermal c.; (2) SIN fissural c.

junctional c., c. juncional; um cisto do testículo originado em estruturas que unem a rede do testículo ao epidídimo.

keratinous c., c. ceratinoso; um cisto epitelial contendo queratina.

Klestadt c., c. de Klestadt. SIN nasoalveolar c.

lacteal c., c. lácteo; um cisto de retenção na glândula mamária resultante do fechamento de um ducto lactífero. SIN milk c.

lateral periodontal c., c. periodontal lateral; cisto intra-ósseo, geralmente encontrado na região cúspide–pré-molar da mandíbula, derivado dos remanescentes da lâmina dental e representando o equivalente intra-ósseo do cisto gengival.

leptomeningeal c., c. leptomeníngeo. SIN arachnoid c.

lymphoepithelial c., c. linfoepitelial; um cisto cervical originado do epitélio da glândula salivar aprisionado em linfonodos durante a embriogênese. Também é observado na cavidade oral.

median anterior maxillary c., c. maxilar anterior mediano. SIN incisive canal c.

median palatal c., c. palatino mediano; um cisto embriológico localizado na linha média do palato duro.

median raphe c. of the penis, c. da rafe mediana do pênis; um cisto da rafe do pênis resultante do fechamento incompleto do sulco uretral, tornando-se clinicamente evidente na infância ou mais tarde.

meibomian c., c. de Meibomio; c. meibomiano. SIN chalazion.

milk c., c. lácteo. SIN lacteal c.

morgagnian c., c. de Morgagni. SIN vesicular *appendages* of epoophoron, em *appendage*.

mother c., c.-mãe; cisto hidático da camada interna, ou germinativa, a partir da qual se desenvolvem cistos secundários contendo escóleces (cistos-filhos); algumas vezes se desenvolvem cistos terciários (cistos-netos) no interior dos cistos-filhos; é mais freqüente no fígado, mas pode ser encontrado em outros órgãos e tecidos; os sintomas são os de um tumor da parte afetada. SIN parent c.

mucous c., c. mucoso; cisto de retenção resultante de obstrução no ducto de uma glândula mucosa. SIN mucocele (1).

multilocular c., c. multilocular; cisto contendo vários compartimentos formados por septos membranosos. SIN compound c.
multilocular hydatid c., multiloculate hydatid c., c. hidático multilocular. SIN alveolar hydatid c.
myxoid c., c. mixóide. SIN ganglion (2).
nabothian c., c. de Naboth; um cisto de retenção que se desenvolve quando uma glândula mucosa do colo uterino é obstruída; sem importância clínica. SIN nabothian follicle.
nasoalveolar c., c. nasoalveolar; um cisto de tecidos moles situado próximo da fixação da asa sobre o maxilar; provavelmente derivado da parte ânteroinferior do ducto nasolacrimal. SIN Klestadt c., nasolabial c.
nasolabial c., c. nasolabial. SIN nasoalveolar c.
nasopalatine duct c., c. do ducto nasopalatino. SIN incisive canal c.
necrotic c., c. necrótico; cisto devido a uma área encapsulada circunscrita de necrose com subseqüente liquefação do tecido morto.
neural c., c. neural. SIN ependymal c.
neurenteric c.'s, cistos neurentéricos; cistos paravertebrais, comumente conectados às meninges ou a uma parte do trato gastrointestinal, que se desenvolvem devido à separação incompleta do endoderma da notocorda durante o início da vida fetal; freqüentemente sintomáticos.
odontogenic c., c. odontogênico; cisto derivado do epitélio odontogênico. [odont + G. *genos*, nascimento, origem, + sufixo *–ic*, relativo a]
oil c., c. oleoso; cisto resultante da perda do revestimento epitelial de um cisto sebáceo, dermóide ou lácteo, ou da injeção subcutânea de material oleoso ou gorduroso.
omphalomesenteric c., c. onfalomesentérico; lesão cística encontrada no cordão umbilical, que provavelmente se desenvolve a partir de remanescentes do ducto onfalomesentérico no início da gestação. Pode ser diagnosticado por ultrasonografia pré-natal. SIN omphalomesenteric duct c.
omphalomesenteric duct c., c. do ducto onfalomesentérico. SIN omphalomesenteric c.
oophoritic c., c. ooforítico. SIN ovarian c.
osseous hydatid c., c. hidático ósseo; uma forma morfológica de cisto hidático causada por *Echinococcus granulosus* e encontrada nos ossos longos ou no arco pélvico dos seres humanos, se o embrião for filtrado no tecido ósseo; nesse local não há formação de membrana limitante, e o cisto cresce sem controle, produzindo estruturas esponjosas e induzindo fratura, seguindo-se disseminação para novos locais.
ovarian c., c. ovariano; tumor cístico do ovário, não-neoplásico (folicular, luteínico, de inclusão germinativa ou endometrial) ou neoplásico; geralmente restrito aos cistos benignos, isto é, cistadenoma seroso mucoso, ou cistos dermóides. SIN oophoritic c.
paraphysial c.'s, cistos parafisários; cistos originados de remanescentes vestigiais da paráfise; são a possível origem de alguns cistos colóides do terceiro ventrículo.
parasitic c., c. parasitário; cisto formado pelas larvas de um parasita metazoário, como um cisto hidático ou triquinótico.
parent c., c.-mãe. SIN mother c.
paroophoritic c., c. para-oofórico; cisto originado do para-oóforo.
parvilocular c., c. parvilocular; tumor composto de múltiplos cistos pequenos.
pearl c., c. em pérola; c. perolado; uma massa de células epiteliais introduzidas no interior do olho por uma lesão perfurante.
periapical c., c. periapical. SIN apical periodontal c.
phaeomycotic c., c. feomicótico; granuloma cístico subcutâneo causado por fungos pigmentados, geralmente solitário e localizado nas extremidades.
pilar c., c. piloso; um cisto comum da pele, principalmente do couro cabeludo, que contém sebo e queratina, e é revestido por células epiteliais estratificadas, de coloração pálida, derivadas do triquilema folicular.
piliferous c., c. pilífero; um cisto dermóide contendo pêlos.
pilonidal c., c. pilonidal. VER pilonidal *sinus*.
pineal c., c. pineal; cisto da glândula pineal; raramente tem importância clínica.
posttraumatic leptomeningeal c., c. leptomeníngeo pós-traumático; acúmulo cístico persistente de líquido cerebroespinal, com perda progressiva de osso e dura-máter, que ocorre no local de uma fratura anterior.
primordial c., c. primordial; cisto que se desenvolve no lugar de um dente através da degeneração cística do órgão do esmalte antes da formação de tecido odontogênico calcificado.
proliferating tricholemmal c., c. tricolêmico proliferativo. SIN pilar *tumor* of scalp.
proliferation c., proliferative c., proliferous c., c. de proliferação, c. proliferativo; um cisto-mãe contendo cistos-filhos; um cisto com formação tumoral em uma parte do saco.
protozoan c., c. de protozoário; forma infecciosa de muitos parasitas protozoários, como *Entamoeba histolytica*, *Giardia lamblia*, *Balantidium coli*, geralmente eliminada nas fezes e que possui um citoplasma bastante condensado e parede celular resistente.
pseudomucinous c., c. pseudomucoso; cisto que contém um líquido gelatinoso, antes considerado significativamente diferente da mucina, ocorrendo sobretudo no ovário.

radicular c., c. radicular. SIN apical periodontal c.
Rathke cleft c., c. da fenda de Rathke; um cisto intra-selar ou supra-selar revestido por epitélio cubóide derivado de remanescentes da bolsa de Rathke.
residual c., c. residual; a persistência de um cisto periodontal apical que permanece após extração do dente.
retention c., c. de retenção; cisto resultante de alguma obstrução do ducto excretor de uma glândula. SIN distention c., secretory c.
rete c. of ovary, c. da rede do ovário; cisto derivado dos cordões germinativos no hilo ovariano.
root end c., c. da extremidade da raiz. SIN apical periodontal c.
sanguineous c., c. sanguíneo. SIN hemorrhagic c.
sebaceous c., c. sebáceo. SIN pilar c.
secretory c., c. secretor. SIN retention c.
seminal vesical c., c. da vesícula seminal; um cisto, geralmente congênito, da vesícula seminal.
sequestration c., c. de seqüestro.
serous c., c. seroso; cisto contendo líquido seroso límpido, como um higroma.
simple bone c., c. ósseo simples. SIN solitary bone c.
solitary bone c., c. ósseo solitário; cisto unilocular contendo líquido seroso e revestido por uma fina camada de tecido conjuntivo, que geralmente ocorre na diáfise de um osso longo em uma criança. SIN idiopathic bone cavity, osteocystoma, simple bone c., traumatic bone c., unicameral bone c.
Stafne bone c., c. ósseo de Stafne. SIN lingual salivary gland *depression*.
static bone c., c. ósseo estático. SIN lingual salivary gland *depression*.
sterile c., c. estéril; cisto hidático sem cápsulas descendentes ou escóleces viáveis.
sublingual c., c. sublingual. SIN ranula (2).
sudoriferous c., c. sudorífero; cisto causado por bloqueio do ducto excretor das glândulas de Moll (Moll *glands*, em *gland*). SIN apocrine hidrocystoma.
suprasellar c., c. supra-selar. SIN craniopharyngioma.
surgical ciliated c., c. ciliado cirúrgico; cisto que se origina do epitélio do seio maxilar implantado ao longo de uma linha de entrada cirúrgica.
synovial c., c. sinovial. SIN ganglion (2).
Tarlov c., c. de Tarlov; cisto perineural encontrado nas radículas proximais da parte inferior da medula espinal; geralmente provoca sintomas.
tarry c., c. alcatroado; cisto ou coleção de sangue antigo que possui um aspecto alcatroado ou preto, pegajoso; geralmente causados por endometriose.
tarsal c., c. tarsal. SIN chalazion.
teratomatous c., c. teratomatoso; cisto contendo estruturas derivadas de todas as três camadas germinativas primárias do embrião.
thyroglossal duct c., thyrolingual c., c. do ducto tireoglosso, c. tireolingual; cisto na linha média do pescoço resultante do não-fechamento de um segmento do ducto tireoglosso.
Tornwaldt c., c. de Tornwaldt; inflamação ou obstrução da bolsa faríngea ou de uma fenda adenóide com a formação de um cisto que contém pus. SIN Tornwaldt disease.
traumatic bone c., c. ósseo traumático. SIN solitary bone c.
trichilemmal c., c. triquilêmico. SIN pilar c.
tubular c., c. tubular. SIN tubulocyst.
umbilical c., c. umbilical. SIN vitellointestinal c.
unicameral c., c. unicameral. SIN unilocular c.
unicameral bone c., c. ósseo unicameral. SIN solitary bone c.
unilocular c., c. unilocular; cisto que possui apenas um saco. SIN unicameral c.
unilocular hydatid c., c. hidático unilocular; a forma mais comum de cisto hidático no homem, causado por *Echinococcus granulosus* e encontrado no fígado, pulmões ou em qualquer outro local onde o embrião hexacanto possa se estabelecer se passar pelos filtros capilares hepático ou pulmonar; caracterizado por grandes formas, semelhantes a balões, revestidas internamente por uma membrana germinativa, e encerrado externamente em uma membrana laminada dentro de uma cápsula hospedeiro-parasita, cheio de líquido (líquido hidático) e escóleces infecciosos das tênias jovens (areia hidática).
urachal c., c. uracal; um cisto do úraco que pode comunicar-se com o umbigo ou com a bexiga, ou dar origem a uma tumefação na linha média. SIN allantoic c.
urinary c., c. urinário. SIN urinoma.
utricular c., c. do utrículo; dilatação da luz do utrículo; geralmente unilocular.
vitellointestinal c., c. vitelointestinal; pequeno tumor vermelho séssil ou pediculado no umbigo de um lactente; é devido à persistência de um segmento do ducto vitelointestinal. SIN umbilical c.
wolffian c., c. de Wolff; cisto situado nos ligamentos largos do útero e originado de quaisquer estruturas mesonéfricas.

cyst-. VER cysto-.
cys·ta·canth (sis′tă - kanth). Cistacanto; a larva completamente desenvolvida da Acanthocephala, infecciosa para o hospedeiro final e com uma probóscide totalmente formada e invertida, característica do verme adulto. [cyst- + G. *akantha*, espinho ou espinha]
cyst·ad·e·no·car·ci·no·ma (sist - ad′en - ō - kar - si - nō′mă). Cistadenocarcinoma; neoplasia maligna, derivada do epitélio glandular, na qual são forma-

dos acúmulos císticos de secreções retidas; as células neoplásicas apresentam vários graus de anaplasia e capacidade de invasão, e ocorrem extensão local e metástases; os cistadenocarcinomas desenvolvem-se freqüentemente nos ovários, onde são reconhecidos os tipos pseudomucoso e seroso.

cyst·ad·e·no·ma (sist′ad - ē - nō′ma). Cistadenoma; uma neoplasia histologicamente benigna, derivada do epitélio glandular, na qual são formados acúmulos císticos de secreções retidas; em alguns casos, partes consideráveis da neoplasia, ou mesmo toda a massa, podem ser císticas. SIN cystoadenoma.

papillary c. lymphomato'sum, c. papilar linfomatoso. SIN adenolymphoma.

cyst·al·gia (sist - al′jē - ă). Cistalgia; dor em uma bexiga ou vesícula, principalmente na bexiga urinária. [cyst- + G. *algos*, dor]

cys·ta·mine (sis′tă - mēn). Cistamina; decarboxicistina; forma-se quando a cistina é destilada. O dissulfeto da cisteamina.

cys·ta·thi·o·nase (sis - tă - thī′ō - nās). Cistationase. SIN cystathionine γ-lyase.

β-cys·ta·thi·o·nase. β-Cistationase. SIN cystathionine β-lyase.

γ-cys·ta·thi·o·nase. γ-Cistationase. SIN cystathionine γ-lyase.

cys·ta·thi·o·nine (sis - tă - thī′ō - nēn). Cistationina; o isômero L é um intermediário na conversão da L-metionina em L-cisteína; clivada por cistationases.

cys·ta·thi·o·nine β-ly·ase. Cistationina β-liase; enzima que catalisa a hidrólise da L-cistationina em piruvato, L-homocisteína e NH_3. VER TAMBÉM cystathionine γ-lyase. SIN β-cystathionase, cystine lyase.

cys·ta·thi·o·nine γ-ly·ase. Cistationina γ-liase; uma enzima hepática que exige o fosfato de piridoxal como coenzima e catalisa a hidrólise da L-cistationina em L-cisteína e 2-cetobutirato, liberando NH_3; também catalisa a formação de 2-cetobutirato a partir da L-homosserina, de piruvato (e NH_3 e H_2S) a partir da L-cisteína e de tiocisteína, piruvato e NH_3 a partir da cistina. Uma deficiência dessa enzima resulta em cistationinúria. Catalisa uma etapa no catabolismo da metionina e na biossíntese da cisteína. VER TAMBÉM cystathionine β-lyase. SIN cystathionase, cysteine desulfhydrase, cystine desulfhydrase, γ-cystathionase, homoserine deaminase, homoserine dehydratase.

cys·ta·thi·o·nine β-syn·thase. Cistationina β-sintase; enzima que catalisa a hidrólise reversível da L-cistationina em L-serina e L-homocisteína. Uma etapa na biossíntese da cisteína e no catabolismo da metionina. A deficiência dessa enzima leva a trombose vascular, luxação da lente do olho e desenvolvimento anormal. VER TAMBÉM cystathionine γ-synthase. SIN β-thionase, cysteine synthase, serine sulfhydrase.

cys·ta·thi·o·nine γ-syn·thase. Cistationina γ-sintase. SIN O-succinylhomoserine (thiol)-lyase.

cys·ta·thi·o·nin·u·ria (sis′tă - thī′ō - nin - oo′rē - ă). [MIM*219500]. Cistationinúria; distúrbio caracterizado por incapacidade de metabolizar a cistationina, normalmente devido à deficiência de cistationase, com alta concentração do aminoácido no sangue, tecido e urina; o retardo mental é um distúrbio associado; herança autossômica recessiva.

cys·te·a·mine (sis - tă′a - mēn). Cisteamina; composto sulfidril usado experimentalmente para produzir úlceras em ratos e como agente radioprotetor; antídoto para o acetaminofeno.

cys·tec·to·my (sis - tek′tō - mē). Cistectomia. **1.** Excisão da bexiga. **2.** Excisão da vesícula biliar (colecistectomia). **3.** Remoção de um cisto. [cyst- + G. *ektomē*, excisão]

Bartholin c., c. de Bartholin; remoção de um cisto de uma glândula vestibular principal. SIN vulvovaginal c.

partial c., c. parcial; remoção de uma parte ou de um segmento da bexiga.

radical c., c. radical; remoção de toda a bexiga, dos tecidos adiposos adjacentes e dos linfonodos regionais.

salvage c., c. de salvamento; remoção da bexiga após fracasso da quimio e radioterapia para neoplasia maligna.

total c., c. total; remoção de toda a bexiga.

vulvovaginal c., c. vulvovaginal. SIN Bartholin c.

cys·te·ic ac·id (sis - tā′ik). Ácido cisteico; um produto da oxidação da cisteína, e precursor da taurina e do ácido isetiônico. SIN 3-sulfoalanine.

cys·te·ine (C, Cys) (sis′tă - ēn). Cisteína; ácido amino-3-mercaptopropiônico; o isômero L é encontrado na maioria das proteínas; particularmente abundante na queratina.

c. desulfhydrase, c. dessulfidrase. SIN cystathionine γ-lyase.

c. synthase, c. sintase. SIN cystathionine β-synthase.

cys·te·ine sul·fin·ic ac·id (sis′tē - ēn - sul - fin′ik). Ácido cisteinossulfínico; um produto da oxidação natural da cisteína; um intermediário na formação da taurina (via ácido cisteico).

cys·tein·yl (sis′tēn - il). Cisteinil; radical aminoacil da cisteína.

△ **cysti-.** VER cysto-.

cys·tic (sis′tik). Cístico. **1.** Relativo à bexiga ou à vesícula biliar. **2.** Relativo a um cisto. **3.** Que contém cistos.

cys·ti·cer·coid (sis - ti - ser′koyd). Cisticercóide; tênia larvar semelhante a um cisticerco, mas que possui uma bexiga menor, contendo pouco ou nenhum líquido, na qual é encontrado o escólece da futura tênia adulta; a forma larvar é tipicamente encontrada em insetos hospedeiros intermediários. [cysti- + G. *kerkos*, cauda, + *eidos*, semelhança]

cys·ti·cer·co·sis (sis′ti - ser - kō′sis). Cisticercose. **1.** Doença causada por encistamento das larvas de cisticercos de algumas tênias (p. ex., *Taenia solium* ou *T. saginata*) nos tecidos subcutâneo, muscular ou do sistema nervoso central; a cisticercose tipicamente se desenvolve em suínos e bovinos, produzindo infestação da carne desses animais. Em seres humanos, resulta da eclosão de ovos de *Taenia solium* no intestino ou da ingestão acidental de ovos das fezes humanas; o encistamento no cérebro pode causar lesão neurológica grave, e o encistamento no olho (geralmente na câmara posterior) pode causar lesão oftálmica. **2.** Infestações larvárias em animais por outras larvas de vermes tenídeos. SIN cysticercus disease.

Cys·ti·cer·cus (sis - ti - ser′kŭs). Originalmente descrito como um gênero de cisticercos, sabendo-se agora tratar-se de larvas encistadas de várias tênias; entretanto, o nome do gênero foi mantido por conveniência ao se referir às formas encistadas larvares. VER cysticercus. SIN bladderworm. [G. *kystis*, bexiga, + *kerkos*, cauda]

C. bo'vis, a larva cisticerco da *Taenia saginata* em bovinos; a causa da infestação da carne bovina.

C. cellulo'sae, a larva cisticerco da *Taenia solium* em porcos; também é a causa da cisticercose humana.

cys·ti·cer·cus, pl. **cys·ti·cer·ci** (sis - ti - ser′kŭs - ser′sī). Cisticerco; a forma larvar de algumas espécies de *Taenia*, tipicamente encontrada nos músculos de hospedeiros intermediários mamíferos que servem como presa de diversos predadores; consiste em uma vesícula cheia de líquido na qual se desenvolve o escólece do cestódeo invaginado. VER TAMBÉM *Taenia saginata*, *Taenia solium*. [G. *kystis*, bexiga, + *kerkos*, cauda]

cys·ti·form (sis′ti - fōrm). Cistiforme. SIN cystoid (1).

ℹ **cys·tine** (sis′tīn). Cistina; 3,3′-ditiobis(ácido 2-aminopropiônico); o produto dissulfeto de duas cisteínas no qual dois grupos –SH se tornam um grupamento –S–S; se dois resíduos cisteinil nas cadeias polipeptídicas formarem uma ligação dissulfeto, então os dois polímeros apresentam ligação cruzada; algumas vezes ocorre como um depósito na urina, ou formando um cálculo vesical. Cf. *meso*-cystine. SIN dicysteine.

c. desulfhydrase, c. dessulfidrase. SIN cystathionine γ-lyase.

half c., meia-c.; refere-se à metade de uma molécula de cistina ou de um resíduo cistinil em uma proteína ou peptídeo.

c. lyase, c. liase. SIN cystathionine β-lyase.

***meso*-cys·tine.** *Meso*-cistina; isômero da cistina no qual a configuração em torno de um dos α-carbonos é D, em torno do outro, L, de forma que a molécula como um todo possui um plano de simetria e é opticamente inativa. Observe que a *meso*-cistina não é DL-cistina. A DL-cistina é uma mistura racêmica de DD-cistina e LL-cistina.

cys·ti·ne·mia (sis - ti - nē′mē - ă). Cistinemia; a presença de cistina no sangue. [cystine + G. *haima*, sangue]

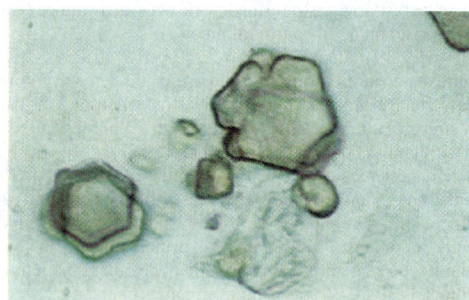

cistinose: imagem microscópica de cristais de cistina na urina

ℹ **cys·ti·no·sis** (sis - ti - nō′sis) [MIM*219800]. Cistinose; um distúrbio de armazenamento lisossômico com várias formas, todas de herança autossômica recessiva. A forma nefropática do início nos primeiros anos de vida é caracterizada por depósitos disseminados de cristais de cistina em todo o corpo, incluindo a medula óssea, a córnea e outros tecidos, com pequena elevação da cistina plasmática e cistinúria; associada a acentuada aminoacidúria generalizada, glicosúria, poliúria, acidose crônica, hipofosfatemia com raquitismo resistente à vitamina D e, freqüentemente, hipopotassemia; outras manifestações extra-renais incluem fotofobia e hipotireoidismo; devida a um defeito no transporte de cistina através das membranas lisossômicas causado por mutação no gene CTNS em 17p. Há uma forma mais leve com início na adolescência [MIM*219900] e uma com início na vida adulta sem lesão renal [MIM*219750]; estas duas últimas formas são consideradas alélicas à forma nefropática do início nos primeiros anos de vida. SIN cystine storage disease. [cystine + G. –*osis*, condição]

cys·ti·nu·ria (sis - ti - noo′rē - ă) [MIM*220100, *104614, *600918]. Cistinúria; excreção urinária excessiva de cistina, juntamente com lisina, arginina e ornitina, causada por defeito nos sistemas de transporte desses ácidos no rim e no intestino; algumas vezes, a função renal é comprometida por cristalúria de cistina e nefrolitíase. Há pelo menos três formas de cistinúria, que são distinguidas pela intensidade da excreção urinária de cistina em portadores obrigatórios, todos com herança autossômica recessiva. Os tipos I e II de cistinúria são distúrbios alélicos causados por mutação no gene 3 da família carreadora de soluto (SLC3A1), que é um gene transportador de aminoácidos no cromossoma 2q. O tipo III é causado por mutação em um *locus* separado. [cystine + G. *ouron*, urina]

cys·tin·yl (sis′tin - il). Cistinil; radical aminoacil da cistina.

cys·tis, pl. **cys·ti·des** (sis′tis, sis′ti - dēz). Cisto. VER cyst, pouch, sac. [G. *kystis*]
 c. fel′lea, vesícula biliar. SIN gallbladder.
 c. urina′ria, bexiga urinária. SIN urinary bladder.

cys·ti·stax·is (sis - ti - stak′sis). Cististaxe; termo obsoleto para gotejamento de sangue do revestimento epitelial da bexiga. [cysti- + G. *staxis*, gotejamento]

cys·ti·tis (sis - tī′tis). Cistite; inflamação da bexiga urinária. [cyst- + G. *–itis*, inflamação]
 bacterial c., c. bacteriana; inflamação vesical causada por bactérias.
 c. col′li, c. do colo; inflamação do colo vesical.
 c. cys′tica, c. cística; cistite glandular com a formação de cistos.
 emphysematous c., c. enfisematosa; inflamação da parede vesical causada por bactérias produtoras de gás, geralmente secundária ao diabetes melito.
 eosinophilic c., c. eosinofílica; inflamação vesical com muitos eosinófilos no sedimento urinário e também na parede vesical.
 follicular c., c. folicular; cistite crônica caracterizada por pequenos nódulos mucosos causados por infiltração linfocítica.
 c. glandula′ris, c. glandular; cistite crônica com metaplasia glandular do urotélio.
 hemorrhagic c., c. hemorrágica; inflamação vesical com hematúria macroscópica. Geralmente resultante de agressão química ou outra agressão traumática da bexiga (quimioterapia, radioterapia).
 incrusted c., c. incrustada; inflamação vesical com deposição de minerais inorgânicos sobre a parede luminal. Geralmente há evidência de inflamação crônica.
 interstitial c., c. intersticial; distúrbio inflamatório crônico de etiologia desconhecida envolvendo o epitélio e a muscular da bexiga, resultando em redução da capacidade vesical, alívio da dor por micção e sintomas irritativos vesicais graves. VER TAMBÉM Hunner *ulcer*.
 viral c., c. viral; inflamação vesical causada por infecção viral.

cysto-, cysti-, cyst-. Formas combinantes relacionadas a: **1.** A bexiga. **2.** O ducto cístico. **3.** Um cisto. Cf. vesico- [G. *kystis*, vesícula, bolsa]

cys·to·ad·e·no·ma (sis′tō - ad - ē - nō′mă). Cistoadenoma. SIN cystadenoma.

cys·to·car·ci·no·ma (sis′tō - kar - si - nō′mă). Cistocarcinoma; carcinoma no qual houve degeneração cística; termo erradamente usado, algumas vezes, em referência a cistoadenocarcinoma.

cys·to·cele (sis′tō - sēl). Cistocele; hérnia da bexiga geralmente para a vagina e o intróito. SIN vesicocele. [cysto- + G. *kēlē*, hérnia]

cys·to·chro·mos·co·py (sis′tō - krō - mos′kō - pē). Cistocromoscopia; exame do interior da bexiga após administração de um corante para ajudar na identificação ou estudo da função dos óstios ureterais. [cysto- + G. *chrōma*, cor, + *skopeō*, ver]

cys·to·du·o·de·nos·to·my (sis′tō - doo′ō - dē - nos′tō - mē). Cistoduodenostomia; drenagem de um cisto, geralmente pseudocisto pancreático, para o duodeno. SIN duodenocystostomy (2). [cysto- + duodenum, + G. *stoma*, boca]
 pancreatic c., c. pancreática; drenagem cirúrgica ou endoscópica de pseudocisto pancreático para o duodeno. SIN duodenocystostomy (3).

cys·to·en·ter·o·cele (sis - tō - en′ter - ō - sēl). Cistoenterocele; protrusão herniária de partes da bexiga e do intestino, geralmente para a vagina e intróito. [cysto- + G. *enteron*, intestino, + *kēlē*, hérnia]

cys·to·en·ter·os·to·my (sis - to - en - ter - os′tō - mē). Cistoenterostomia; drenagem intestinal de pseudocistos pancreáticos para alguma porção do trato intestinal, de preferência estômago, duodeno ou intestino delgado. [cysto- + G. *enteron*, intestino, + *stoma*, boca]

cys·to·e·pip·lo·cele (sis - tō - e - pip′lō - sēl). Cistoepiplocele; protrusão herniária de partes da bexiga e do omento. [cysto- + G. *epiploon*, omento, + *kēlē*, tumor]

cys·to·fi·bro·ma (sis′tō - fī - brō′mă). Cistofibroma; um fibroma no qual se formaram cistos ou focos semelhantes a cistos.

cys·to·gas·tros·to·my (sis′tō - gas - tros′tō - mē). Cistogastrostomia; drenagem de um pseudocisto pancreático para o estômago. [cysto- + G. *gastēr*, estômago, + *stoma*, boca]

cys·to·gram (sis′tō - gram). Cistograma; demonstração radiográfica da bexiga cheia com contraste.
 voiding c., c. miccional. SIN voiding cystourethrogram.

cys·tog·ra·phy (sis - tog′ră - fē). Cistografia; radiografia da bexiga após injeção de uma substância radiopaca. [cysto- + G. *graphō*, escrever]
 antegrade c., c. anterógrada; cistografia na qual o contraste entra na bexiga através dos ureteres ou cistotomia.

cys·toid (sis′toyd). Cistóide. **1.** Cistiforme; semelhante a um cisto. SIN cystiform, cystomorphous. **2.** Um tumor semelhante a um cisto, com conteúdo líquido, granular ou pulposo, mas sem uma cápsula. [cysto- + G. *eidos*, aspecto]

cys·to·je·ju·nos·to·my (sis′tō - jē - joo - nos′tō - mē). Cistojejunostomia; drenagem de um pseudocisto pancreático para o jejuno. [cysto- + jejunum, + G. *stoma*, boca]

cys·to·lith (sis′tō - lith). Cistólito. SIN vesical calculus. [cysto- + G. *lithos*, cálculo]

cys·to·li·thi·a·sis (sis′tō - li - thī′ă - sis). Cistolitíase; a presença de um cálculo vesical. SIN vesicolithiasis. [cysto- + G. *lithos*, cálculo, + *-iasis*, condição]

cys·to·lith·ic (sis - tō - lith′ik). Cistolítico; relativo a um cálculo vesical.

cys·to·lith·o·la·paxy (sis′tō - lith - ō - lă - paks - ē). Cistolitolapaxia; remoção de cálculos vesicais por esmagamento intravesical seguido por irrigação para remover fragmentos. [cysto- + G. *lithos*, cálculo, + *lapaxis*, esvaziamento]

cys·to·li·thot·o·my (sis′tō - li - thot′ō - mē). Cistolitotomia; remoção de um cálculo da bexiga através de uma incisão em sua parede. SIN vesical lithotomy. [cysto- + G. *lithos*, cálculo, + *tomē*, incisão]

cys·to·ma (sis - tō′mă). Cistoma; um tumor cístico; um novo crescimento contendo cistos. [cyst- + G. *-oma*, tumor]

cys·tom·e·ter (sis - tom′e - ter). Cistômetro; um dispositivo para estudar a função vesical por medida da capacidade, sensibilidade, pressão intravesical e urina residual. [cysto- + G. *metron*, medida]

cys·to·met·ro·gram (CMG) (sis - tō - met′rō - gram). Cistometrograma (CMG); um registro gráfico da pressão vesical em vários volumes. [cysto- + G. *metron*, medida, + *gramma*, escrito]

cys·to·me·trog·ra·phy (sis′tō - mē - trog′ră - fē). Cistometrografia. SIN cystometry.

cys·tom·e·try (sis - tom′e - trē). Cistometria; medida da relação pressão/volume da bexiga. SIN cystometrography. [ver cystometer]

cys·to·mor·phous (sis - tō - mōr′fŭs). Cistomorfo. SIN cystoid (1). [cysto- + G. *morphē*, forma]

cys·to·my·o·ma (sis′tō - mī - ō′mă). Cistomioma; um mioma no qual se desenvolveram cistos ou focos semelhantes a cistos.

cys·to·myx·o·ad·e·no·ma (sis - tō - mik′sō - ad - ē - ō′mă). Cistomixoadenoma; um adenoma no qual há cistos ou focos semelhantes a cistos associados a alteração mixomatosa no estroma.

cys·to·myx·o·ma (sis′tō - mik - sō′mă). Cistomixoma; um mixoma no qual se formaram cistos ou focos semelhantes a cistos.

cys·to·pan·en·dos·co·py (sis′tō - pan - en - dos′kō - pē). Cistopanendoscopia; inspeção do interior da bexiga e uretra por meio de endoscópios especialmente designados introduzidos de forma retrógrada através da uretra até o interior da bexiga. [cysto- + panendoscope]

cys·to·pa·ral·y·sis (sis - tō - pă - ral′i - sis). Cistoparalisia. SIN cystoplegia.

cys·to·pexy (sis′tō - pek - sē). Cistopexia; fixação cirúrgica da vesícula biliar ou da bexiga à parede abdominal ou a outras estruturas de sustentação. SIN ventrocystorrhaphy. [cysto- + G. *pēxis*, fixação]

cys·to·pho·tog·ra·phy (sis′tō - fō - tog′ră - fē). Cistofotografia; fotografia do interior da bexiga.

cys·to·plas·ty (sis′tō - plas - tē). Cistoplastia; qualquer cirurgia de reconstrução da bexiga. Cf. ileocystoplasty, colocystoplasty. [cysto- + G. *plastos*, formado]

cys·to·ple·gia (sis′tō - plē′jē - ă). Cistoplegia; paralisia da bexiga. SIN cystoparalysis. [cysto- + G. *plēgē*, golpe]

cys·to·pros·ta·tec·to·my (sis′tō - pros - tă - tek′tō - mē). Cistoprostatectomia; remoção cirúrgica simultânea da bexiga, próstata e vesículas seminais.

cys·to·py·e·li·tis (sis′tō - pī - el - ī′tis). Cistopielite; inflamação da bexiga e da pelve renal. [cysto- + G. *pyelos*, bacia (pelve), + *-itis*, inflamação]

cys·to·py·e·lo·ne·phri·tis (sis - tō - pī′el - ō - nef - rī′tis). Cistopielonefrite; inflamação da bexiga, da pelve renal e do parênquima renal. [cysto- + G. *pyelos*, vale (pelve), + *nephros*, rim, + *-itis*, inflamação]

cys·tor·rha·phy (sis - tōr′ă - fē). Cistorrafia; sutura de uma ferida ou defeito na bexiga. [cysto- + G. *rhaphē*, sutura]

cys·tor·rhea (sis′tō - rē - ă). Cistorréia; secreção mucosa da bexiga. [cysto- + G. *rhoia*, fluxo]

cys·to·sar·co·ma (sis′tō - sar - kō′mă). Cistossarcoma; um sarcoma no qual houve formação de cistos ou de focos semelhantes a cistos.
 c. phyllo′des, c. filodes; tumor filodes; um tumor fibroadenomatoso circunscrito ou infiltrativo que pode ser parcialmente cístico, da mama, próstata ou de outros órgãos, e benigno ou maligno; o estroma é celular e assemelha-se a um fibrossarcoma.

cys·to·scope (sis′tō - skōp). Cistoscópio; endoscópio tubular iluminado para exame do interior da bexiga. [cysto- + G. *skopeō*, examinar]

cys·tos·co·py (sis - tos′kō - pē). Cistoscopia; a inspeção do interior da bexiga por meio de um cistoscópio.

cys·to·spasm (sis′tō - spazm). Cistoespasmo; espasmo vesical; contração não-intencional e dolorosa da bexiga, freqüentemente sem micção.

cys·tos·to·my (sis - tos′tō - mē). Cistostomia; criação de uma abertura para a bexiga. SIN vesicostomy. [cysto- + G. *stoma*, boca]

cys·to·tome (sis'tō - tōm). Cistótomo. **1.** Instrumento para incisão da bexiga ou da vesícula biliar. **2.** Instrumento cirúrgico usado para incisar a cápsula de uma lente. SIN capsulotome.

cys·tot·o·my (sis - tot'ō - mē). Cistotomia; incisão ou punção da bexiga ou da vesícula biliar. SIN vesicotomy. [cysto- + G. *tomē*, incisão]
  suprapubic c., c. suprapúbica; abertura para a bexiga através de uma incisão ou punção acima da sínfise púbica.

cys·to·u·re·ter·i·tis (sis'tō - ū - rē - ter - ī'tis). Cistoureterite; inflamação da bexiga e de um ou ambos os ureteres.

cys·to·u·re·ter·o·gram (sis'tō - ū - rē'ter - ō - gram). Cistoureterograma; demonstração radiográfica da bexiga e dos ureteres.

cys·to·u·re·ter·og·ra·phy (sisto - oo - rē'ter - og'ra - fē). Cistouretrografia; radiografia da bexiga e dos ureteres.

cys·to·u·re·thri·tis (sis'tō - ū - rē - thrī'tis). Cistouretrite; inflamação da bexiga e da uretra.

cys·to·u·re·thro·cele (sis'tō - ū - rē'thrō - sēl). Cistouretrocele; hérnia da bexiga e uretra. [cysto- + urethra + G. *kēlē*, hérnia]

cys·to·u·re·thro·gram (sis - tō - ū - rēth'rō - gram). Cistouretrograma. SIN voiding c.
  micturating c., c. miccional. SIN voiding c.
  retrograde c., c. retrógrado; cistouretrograma realizado por injeção de contraste através do meato uretral ou da porção distal da uretra.
  voiding c. (VCUG), c. miccional; uma imagem radiológica feita durante a micção e com a bexiga e a uretra cheias de contraste para demonstrar a uretra. SIN cystourethrogram, micturating c., voiding cystogram.

cys·to·u·re·throg·ra·phy (sis'tō - ū'rē - throg'ra - fē). Cistouretrografia; radiografia da bexiga e da uretra durante a micção, após enchimento da bexiga com um contraste radiopaco, seja por injeção intravenosa, seja por cateterização retrógrada.

cys·to·u·re·thro·scope (sis - tō - ū - rē'thrō - skōp). Cistouretroscópio; instrumento que combina os usos de um cistoscópio e um uretroscópio, pelo qual tanto a bexiga quanto a uretra podem ser inspecionadas visualmente.

Cys·to·vir·i·dae (sis'tō - vir'i - dē). Nome provisório de uma família de vírus bacterianos monotípicos, cuja espécie típica é o fago Φ6. Os virions possuem 86 nm de diâmetro, são isométricos, possuem envoltórios lipídicos e são adsorvidos nas laterais dos pêlos das espécies de *Pseudomonas*. Os capsídeos possuem simetria cúbica, e os genomas possuem RNA filamentar duplo em três pedaços (PM 13×10^6). [G. *kystis*, bexiga]

cys·tyl·a·mi·no·pep·ti·dase (sis'til - a - mi - nō - pep'ti - dās). Cistilaminopeptidase; ocitocinase; uma enzima que degrada peptídeos contendo cistina, como a ocitocina.

Cyt Símbolo de cytosine (citosina).

cyt-. VER cyto-.

cy·ta·pher·e·sis (sī'ta - fē - rē'sis). Citaférese; procedimento no qual várias células podem ser separadas do sangue colhido e retidas, sendo o plasma e outros elementos formados retransfundidos para o doador. [cyt- + G. *aphairesis*, retirada]

cy·tar·a·bine (sī'tar - a - bēn). Citarabina. SIN arabinosylcytosine.

cy·tase (sī'tās). Citase; termo obsoleto, cunhado por Metchnikoff, para alexina ou complemento, que ele afirmava ser uma secreção digestiva do leucócito.

-cyte. Sufixo que significa célula. [G. *kytos*, uma cavidade (célula)]

cyt·i·dine (C, Cyd) (sī'ti - dēn). Citidina; um importante componente dos ácidos ribonucleicos. SIN 1-β-D-ribofuranosylcytosine, cytosine ribonucleoside.
  c. diphosphate choline, c. difosfato colina. SIN cytidine diphosphocholine.
  c. posphate, fofato de c. VER cytidylic acid.

cyt·i·dine 5'-di·phos·phate (CDP). 5'-difosfato de citidina; um éster, na posição 5', entre a citidina e o ácido difosfórico.

cyt·i·dine di·phos·pho·cho·line (CDP-cho·line) (sī'ti - dēn - dī'fos - fō - kō'lēn). Citidina difosfocolina (CDP-colina); intermediário na formação da fosfatidilcolina (lecitina) e esfingomielinas; formada pela ação da citidina 5'-trifosfato sobre a fosfocolina, ligando o grupamento fosfato de colina ao α-fosfato do 5'-trifosfato de citidina para produzir um pirofosfato. SIN activated choline, cytidine diphosphate choline.

cyt·i·dine di·phos·pho·glyc·er·ide (CDP-glyc·er·ide). (sī'ti - dēn dī'fos - fō - gli'cer - īd). Citidina difosfoglicerídeo (CDP-glicerídeo); um intermediário na formação de fosfolipídios (p. ex., cardiolipina) formado pela ação na CTP e 1,2-diacilgliceróis de uma citidil transferase, liberando CDP-glicerídeo e pirofosfato.

cyt·i·dine di·phos·pho·sug·ar (CDP-sug·ar). Citidina difosfoaçúcar (CAP- açúcar); uma forma ativada de um açúcar.

cyt·i·dine 5'-tri·phos·phate (CTP). 5'-trifosfato de citidina; um éster, na posição 5', entre a citidina e o ácido trifosfórico.

cyt·i·dyl·ic ac·id (sī - ti - dil'ik). Ácido citidílico; monofosfato de citidina (são possíveis cinco, dependendo do local de fixação do fosfato às hidroxilas do ribosil); um constituinte dos ácidos ribonucleicos.

cy·ti·sine (sit'ī - sin). Citisina; um agonista colinérgico nicotínico seletivo tóxico; um alcalóide da semente de *Laburnum anagyroides* e outras Leguminosae. Usada em estudos farmacológicos dos receptores colinérgicos nicotínicos no cérebro. SIN baptitoxine.

cyto-, cyt-. Uma célula. [G. *kytos*, uma cavidade (célula)]

cy·to·an·a·lyz·er (sī - tō - an'a - lī - zer). Citoanalisador; um aparelho óptico eletrônico que rastreia esfregaços contendo células suspeitas de malignidade. [cyto- + analyzer]

cy·to·ar·chi·tec·ton·ics (sī'tō - ar - ki - tek - ton'iks). Citoarquitetura. SIN cytoarchitecture. [cyto- + G. *architektonikē*, arquitetônico]

cy·to·ar·chi·tec·tur·al (sī - tō - ar - ki - tek'chŭr - al). Citoarquitetônico; relativo à citoarquitetura.

cy·to·ar·chi·tec·ture (sī'tō - ar'ki - tek - chŭr). Citoarquitetura; o arranjo das células em um tecido; p. ex., o arranjo dos corpos de células nervosas no cérebro, principalmente o córtex cerebral. SIN architectonics, cytoarchitectonics.

cy·to·bi·ol·o·gy (sī'tō - bī - ol'ō - jē). Citobiologia. SIN cytology.

cy·to·bi·o·tax·is (sī'tō - bī - ō - tak'sis). Citobiotaxia. SIN cytoclesis. [cyto- + G. *bios*, vida, + *taxis*, arranjo]

cy·to·cen·trum (sī - tō - sen'trŭn). Citocentro; uma zona de citoplasma contendo um ou dois centríolos, mas desprovida de outras organelas; geralmente situada próximo do núcleo de uma célula. SIN cell center, central body, centrosome, cinocentrum, kinocentrum, microcentrum. [cyto- + G. *kentron*, centro]

cy·to·chal·a·sins (sī - tō - kal'a - zinz). Citocalasinas; um grupo de substâncias derivadas de bolores que desagregam os microfilamentos da célula e interferem com a divisão do citoplasma, inibem o movimento celular e causam extrusão do núcleo; usadas para investigações em biologia celular [cyto- + G. *chalasis*, relaxante]

cy·to·chem·is·try (sī'tō - kem'is - trē). Citoquímica; o estudo da distribuição intracelular de substâncias químicas, locais de reação, enzimas, etc., freqüentemente por meio de reações de coloração, captação de isótopo radioativo, distribuição seletiva de metais em microscopia eletrônica ou outros métodos. SIN histochemistry.

cy·to·chrome (sī'tō - krōm). Citocromo; uma classe de hemoproteínas cuja principal função biológica é o transporte de elétrons e/ou hidrogênio em virtude de uma alteração da valência reversível do ferro heme. Os citocromos são classificados em quatro grupos (*a, b, c* e *d*) de acordo com as características espectroquímicas; existem muitas variantes, particularmente entre bactérias e em plantas verdes e algas, sendo uma variante do citocromo tipo *c* denominada citocromo *f*. O sistema mitocondrial dos citocromos fornece transporte eletrônico através da citocromo *c* oxidase até o oxigênio molecular, como aceptor terminal de elétrons (respiração). [cyto- + G. *chrōma*, cor]

cy·to·chrome aa_3. Citocromo aa_3. SIN cytochrome c. oxidase.

cy·to·chrome *b*. Citocromo *b*; um citocromo da cadeia respiratória. Uma deficiência desse citocromo leva à doença granulomatosa crônica.

cy·to·chrome b_5. Citocromo b_5; um citocromo no retículo endoplasmático que atua com várias oxigenases; uma deficiência desse citocromo resulta em uma forma de metemoglobinemia hereditária.

cy·to·chrome b_5 re·duc·tase. Citocromo b_5 redutase; uma flavoenzima que catalisa a redução da 2ferricitocromo b_5 em 2ferrocitocromo b_5 à custa de NADH; participa na dessaturação de ácidos graxos; sua deficiência pode levar à metemoglobinemia hereditária (tipo I, observada apenas no citosol eritrocitário; tipo II, deficiência em todos os tecidos; tipo III, deficiência em todas as células hematopoéticas).

cy·to·chrome *c*. Citocromo c; o citocromo móvel que transporta elétrons do Complexo III para o Complexo IV da cadeia respiratória.

cy·to·chrome *cd*. Citocromo *cd*. SIN cytochrome oxidase (*Pseudomonas*).

cy·to·chrome c_3 hy·dro·gen·ase. Citocromo c_3 hidrogenase; uma enzima hidrogenase que catalisa a redução do 2ferricitocromo c_3 por H_2 em 2ferrocitocromo c_3 e $2H^+$.

cy·to·chrome *c* ox·i·dase. Citocromo *c* oxidase; um citocromo do tipo *a*, contendo cobre, que catalisa a oxidação do 4ferrocitocromo *c* pelo oxigênio molecular em 4ferricitocromo *c* e $2H_2O$. Uma parte do Complexo IV da cadeia respiratória. Uma deficiência de um ou mais dos polipeptídeos desse complexo resulta em perda neuronal no cérebro, causando retardo psicomotor e doença neurodegenerativa. SIN cytochrome aa_3, indophenol oxidase, indophenolase.

cy·to·chrome *c* re·duc·tase. Citocromo *c* redutase. SIN NADH dehydrogenase.

cy·to·chrome c_2 re·duc·tase. Citocromo c_2 redutase. SIN NADPH-cytochrome c_2 reductase.

cy·to·chrome ox·i·dase (*Pseu·do·mo·nas*). Citocromo oxidase; enzima com ação idêntica à da citocromo *c* oxidase, mas que atua sobre o ferrocitocromo c_2. SIN cytochrome *cd*.

cy·to·chrome P-450$_{\text{SCC}}$. Citocromo P-450; colesterol monooxigenase (clivagem da cadeia lateral). [*450 nm*, a absorção máxima que exibe o citocromo reduzido associado ao monóxido de carbono]

cy·to·chrome per·ox·i·dase. Citocromo peroxidase; uma enzima hemoproteica que catalisa a reação entre H_2O_2 e 2ferrocitocromo *c* para produzir 2ferricitocromo *c* e $2H_2O$.

cy·to·chrome re·duc·tase. Citocromo redutase. SIN NADPH-ferrihemoprotein reductase.

cy·to·chy·le·ma (sī′tō - kī - lē′mă). Citoquilema; a porção mais líquida do citoplasma. [cyto- + G. *chylos*, suco]

cy·toc·i·dal (sī - tō - sī′dăl). Citocida; que causa a morte de células. [cyto- + L. *caedo*, matar]

cy·to·cide (sī′tō - sīd). Citocida; um agente que é destrutivo para as células. [cyto- + L. *caedo*, matar]

cy·toc·la·sis (si - tok′lă - sis). Citoclasia; fragmentação de células. [cyto- + G. *klasis*, quebra]

cy·to·clas·tic (sī - tō - klas′tik). Citoclástico; relativo à citoclasia.

cy·to·cle·sis (sī - tō - klē′sis). Citoclese; a influência de uma célula sobre outra. SIN biotaxis (2), cytobiotaxis. [cyto- + G. *klēsis*, chamada]

cy·to·cu·prein (sī - tō - koo′prē - in). Citocupreína; termo antigo para proteínas contendo cobre encontradas nos eritrócitos humanos e em outros tecidos. VER *superoxide* dismutase, ceruloplasmin. SIN cerebrocuprein, erythrocuprein, hemocuprein, hepatocuprein.

cy·to·cyst (sī′tō - sist). Citocisto; termo raramente usado para os remanescentes vesiculares da hemácia ou célula tecidual que encerra um esquizonte maduro. [cyto- + G., *kystis*, bexiga]

cy·to·di·ag·no·sis (sī′tō - dī - ag - nō′sis). Citodiagnóstico; diagnóstico do tipo e, quando possível, da causa de um processo mórbido por meio de estudo microscópico de células em um exsudato ou outra forma de líquido corporal.

cy·to·di·er·e·sis (sī′tō - dī - er′ē - sis). Citodiérese. SIN cytokinesis. [cyto- + G. *diairesis*, divisão]

cy·to·gene (sī′tō - jēn). Citogene. SIN plasmagene.

cy·to·gen·e·sis (sī - tō - jen′ē - sis). Citogênese; a origem e o desenvolvimento das células. [cyto- + G. *genesis*, origem]

cy·to·ge·net·i·cist (sī′tō - jē - net′i - sist). Citogeneticista; um especialista em citogenética.

cy·to·ge·net·ics (sī′tō - jē - net′iks). Citogenética; o ramo da genética que estuda a estrutura e a função da célula, principalmente os cromossomas.

A citogenética surgiu como fusão da citologia do século XIX com a genética do século XX, que passou a existir em 1903 com a articulação da teoria de herança cromossomial. O campo em desenvolvimento se interessava em detalhar o comportamento dos cromossomas e de suas subunidades funcionais, os genes, durante a reprodução, e em relacionar estatisticamente tal comportamento às características das células ou animais resultantes. A citogenética molecular moderna envolve o estudo microscópico de cromossomas que foram fixados em mitose e corados com vários agentes para delinear bandas características. Sondas de DNA podem ser aplicadas para localizar seqüências genéticas específicas. A cariotipagem é o arranjo de fotografias de cromossomas coradas em um formato padrão. As técnicas citogenéticas são usadas para pesquisa de erros congênitos do metabolismo e de aberrações genômicas, como a síndrome de Down, e para determinar o sexo em casos cuja anatomia é inconclusiva.

cy·to·gen·ic (sī - tō - jen′ik). Citogênico; relativo à citogênese.

cy·tog·e·nous (sī - toj′e - nŭs). Citógeno; que forma células.

cy·to·glu·co·pe·nia (sī′tō - gloo - kō - pē′nē - ă). Citoglicopenia; uma deficiência intracelular de glicose. [cyto- + G. *glucose* + G. *penia*, pobreza]

cy·toid (sī′toyd). Citóide; semelhante a uma célula. [cyto- + G. *eidos*, semelhança]

cy·to·ker·a·tin (sī - tō - ker - a - tĭnz). Citoqueratina. SIN keratin.

cy·to·kine (sī′tō - kīn). Citocina; qualquer das várias proteínas de baixo peso molecular, semelhantes a hormônios, secretadas por vários tipos celulares, que regulam a intensidade e a duração da resposta imune e medeiam a comunicação intercelular. VER interferon, interleukin, lymphokine, chemokines. Ver entradas nos vários fatores de crescimento. VER TAMBÉM interferon, interleukin, lymphokine. [cyto- + G. *kinēsis*, movimento]

As citocinas são produzidas por macrófagos, linfócitos B e T, mastócitos, células endoteliais, fibroblastos e células do estroma do baço, timo e medula óssea. São envolvidas na mediação da imunidade e da alergia e na regulação da maturação, do crescimento e da responsividade de determinadas populações celulares, algumas vezes incluindo as células que as produzem (atividade autócrina). Uma determinada citocina pode ser produzida por mais de um tipo de célula. Algumas citocinas estimulam ou inibem a ação de outras citocinas. As primeiras citocinas a serem identificadas foram denominadas de acordo com suas funções (p. ex., fator de crescimento de células T), mas essa nomenclatura tornou-se imprópria porque várias citocinas podem ter a mesma função, e a função de uma citocina pode variar com as circunstâncias de sua produção. Mais tarde, quando foi determinada a estrutura química de cada citocina, ela foi designada interleucina e recebeu um número (p. ex., interleucina-2 [IL-2], antes fator de crescimento das células T). As citocinas foram implicadas na geração e na recordação da memória de longo prazo e na concentração da atenção. Alguns dos efeitos degenerativos do envelhecimento podem ser devidos à perda progressiva da capacidade reguladora pelas citocinas. Como as citocinas derivadas do sistema imune (imunocitocinas) são citotóxicas, foram usadas contra alguns tipos de câncer.

c. network, rede de citocina; um grupo de citocinas que, juntas, modulam e regulam funções celulares fundamentais.

cy·to·ki·ne·sis (sī′tō - ki - nē′sis). Citocinese; alterações que ocorrem no citoplasma da célula fora do núcleo durante a divisão celular. SIN cytodieresis. [cyto- + G. *kinēsis*, movimento]

cy·to·lem·ma (sī - tō - lem′mă). Citolema. SIN cell membrane. [cyto- + G. *lemma*, casca]

cy·to·lip·in (sī - tō - lip′in). Citolipina; um glicoesfingolipídio, especificamente um oligossacarídeo ceramídico; **c. H,** uma lactosilceramida, pode exibir propriedades imunológicas em determinadas condições; **c. K** provavelmente é idêntico ao globosídeo. Cf. *ceramide* lactosidase.

cy·to·log·ic (sī - tō - loj′ik). Citológico; relativo à citologia.

cy·tol·o·gist (sī - tol′ō - jist). Citologista; especialista em citologia.

cy·tol·o·gy (sī - tol′ō - jē). Citologia; o estudo da anatomia, fisiologia, patologia e química da célula. SIN cellular biology, cytobiology. [cyto- + G. *logos*, estudo]

exfoliative c., c. esfoliativa; o exame, para fins diagnósticos, de células descamadas de uma neoplasia (ou outro tipo de lesão) e isoladas do sedimento do exsudato, secreções ou lavados teciduais (p. ex., escarro, secreção vaginal, lavados gástricos, urina). SIN cytopathology (2).

cy·tol·y·sin (sī - tol′i - sin). Citolisina; uma substância, isto é, um anticorpo que realiza destruição parcial ou completa de uma célula animal; pode exigir complemento. VER TAMBÉM perforin.

cy·tol·y·sis (sī - tol′i - sis). Citólise; a dissolução de uma célula. [cyto- + G. *lysis*, afrouxamento]

cy·to·ly·so·some (sī - tō - lī′sō - sōm). Citolisossoma; um tipo de lisossoma secundário que contém os remanescentes de mitocôndrias, ribossomas ou outras organelas. SIN autophagic vacuole.

cy·to·lyt·ic (sī - tō - lit′ik). Citolítico; relativo à citólise; que possui uma ação solvente ou destrutiva sobre as células.

cy·to·ma·trix (sī - tō - mā′triks). Citomatriz. SIN cytoplasmic matrix.

cy·to·me·ga·lic (sī - tō - meg′a - lik). Citomegálico; que designa, ou é caracterizado por, células significativamente aumentadas. [cyto- + G. *megas*, grande]

Cy·to·meg·a·lo·vi·rus (CMV) (sī - tō - meg′a - lō - vī′rŭs). Citomegalovírus (CMV); um grupo de vírus da família Herpesviridae que infectam seres humanos e outros animais, muitos dos vírus possuindo afinidade especial pelas glândulas salivares e causando aumento de células de vários órgãos, bem como desenvolvimento de inclusões características (olho de coruja) no citoplasma ou núcleo. A infecção intra-uterina do embrião pode resultar em malformação e morte fetal. São todos espécie-específicos e incluem vírus salivar, vírus da rinite por corpúsculos de inclusão de porcos, e outros. SIN visceral disease virus. [cyto- + G. *megas*, grande]

cy·to·mem·brane (sī - tō - mem′brăn). Citomembrana. SIN cell membrane.

cy·to·mere (sī′tō - mēr). Citômero; a estrutura que separa as partes do conteúdo de um grande esquizonte durante a esquizogonia, como em alguns dos esporozoários que sofrem divisão assexuada exoeritrocítica. Os citômeros são causados por invaginações complexas da superfície do esquizonte, que os isola; finalmente, os citômeros concluem o processo de brotamento na formação de grandes números de merozoítas. [cyto- + G. *meros*, parte]

cy·tom·e·ter (sī - tom′e - ter). Citômetro; lâmina de vidro padronizada, geralmente marcada, ou uma pequena câmara de vidro de volume conhecido, usada na contagem e na medição de células, principalmente células sanguíneas. [cyto- + G. *metron*, medida]

image c., c. de imagem; aparelho para medir vários testes qualitativos, como densidade de anticorpos.

cy·tom·e·try (sī - tom′e - trē). Citometria; a contagem de células, principalmente células sanguíneas, utilizando um citômetro ou hemocitômetro.

Feulgen c., c. de Feulgen; uma forma de citometria utilizando núcleos corados por Feulgen para caracterizar o padrão da cromatina e a distribuição nuclear do DNA das células.

flow c., c. de fluxo; método de medida da fluorescência de células coradas que estão em suspensão e fluindo através de um orifício estreito, geralmente em combinação com um ou dois lasers para ativar os corantes; usada para medir o tamanho, o número, a viabilidade e o conteúdo de ácido nucleico das células, com a ajuda do laranja de acridina, corante Feulgen fluorescente de Kasten, brometo de etídio, azul tripano e outros reagentes corantes selecionados. SIN flow cytophotometry.

cy·to·mi·cro·some (sī - tō - mī′krō - sōm). Citomicrossoma. VER microsome. [cyto- + G. *mikros*, pequeno, + *sōma*, corpo]

cy·to·mor·phol·o·gy (sī′tō - mōr - folō - jē). Citomorfologia; o estudo da estrutura das células.

citocinas e quimiocinas: peso molecular, fonte e função

citocinas humanas	PM (kDa)	fonte celular	principais funções
IL–1α	17,5	monócitos, MØ, células B, células T, células NK, células dendríticas	↑ febre e síntese de proteínas de fase aguda; ↑ ativação de timócitos e células T e crescimento, diferenciação e secreção de imunoglobulinas das células B
IL–1β	17,5	monócitos, MØ, células B, células T, células NK, células dendríticas	↑ febre e síntese de proteínas de fase aguda; ↑ ativação de timócitos e células T e crescimento, diferenciação e secreção de imunoglobulinas das células B
IL–2	15–20	células T	↑ crescimento e diferenciação de células T, células B e células NK
IL–3	14–30	células T, mastócitos e eosinófilos	↑ crescimento das células-tronco hematopoéticas e dos mastócitos
IL–4	15–19	células T, mastócitos e basófilos	↑ diferenciação das células B e células Th2; ↑ síntese de IgG_4 e IgE; ↓ célula Th1 pró-inflamatória e da função MØ
IL–5	homodímero 45	células T, mastócitos e eosinófilos	↑ crescimento e diferenciação de eosinófilos e células B (síntese de IgA)
IL–6	26	monócitos, MØ, células B, células T, células endoteliais vasculares	↑ síntese de proteínas de fase aguda; ↑ timócitos e ativação das células T; crescimento, diferenciação e produção de IgG das células B
IL–7	20–28	fibroblastos, células endoteliais e células T, CMO e células do estroma tímico	crescimento de pré-B; ↑ crescimento e diferenciação de pré-células T e células T maduras
IL–9	32–39	células T	↑ ativação de células T e mastócitos; ↑ expressão de IgE e IgC induzida por IL-4
IL–10	35–40	células T, células B B1 e MØ	↓ da função Th1, célula NK e Ø, incluindo síntese/liberação de citocinas; ↑ proliferação de células B e mastócitos
IL–11	23	fibroblastos e células do estroma da medula óssea	↑ crescimento dos megacariócitos (progenitores das plaquetas)
IL–12	heterodímero 35, 40 subunidades	células B e MØ	↑ produção de células NK, LTC e Th1; ↑ produção de IFN-γ por células NK e células T; ↑ atividade de células NK e da CCAD; coestimula a proliferação de células T
IL–13	9–17	células T	fator de crescimento para células B; ↑ síntese de IgM, IgE e IgG4; ↑ CD23 na membrana da célula B e da expressão do Ag classe II do MHC; ↓ funções dos monócitos/MØ incluindo síntese de citocinas pró-inflamatórias
IL–14	60	células dendríticas foliculares, células T	↑ proliferação de células B e da geração de células B de memória; ↓ síntese de imunoglobulinas
IL–15	14–15	monócitos, células epiteliais, músculo	↑ crescimento e diferenciação de células T
IL–16	17	células T, cérebro, timo, baço e pâncreas	quimiotático para células CD4, induz a proliferação de linhagens de células T
IL–17	homodímero 30–38	células T CD4	↑ células epiteliais, endoteliais e fibroblásticas para secretar IL-6, IL-8, FEC-GM
IL–18	18	monócitos/MØ	↑ produção de IFN-γ pelas células T; ↑ atividade NK
G-CSF	18–22	células do estroma da medula óssea e monócitos/MØ	↑ crescimento, diferenciação e ativação de precursores dos granulócitos e de granulócitos maduros
M-CSF	45–90	células T e monócitos/MØ	↑ crescimento, diferenciação e ativação de precursores dos macrófagos e de MØs maduros
GM-CSF	22	células T e monócitos/MØ	↑ crescimento, diferenciação e ativação de precursores dos granulócitos e granulócitos maduros e de MØs
TGF-β	homodímero 25	muitos tipos celulares, incluindo células T e monócitos/MØ	↑ produção de IgA e ativação de células T inocentes; ↓ ativação de monócitos e células T de memória; ativo no crescimento dos fibroblastos/cicatrização de feridas
IFN-γ	homodímero 40–70	células T e células NK	antiviral; ↑ função dos MØ e células NK; ↑ expressão do antígeno de superfície classes I e II do MHC
TNF-a	homotrímero 17	muitos tipos celulares, incluindo monócitos/MØ, células B, células T	expresso como homotrímero da superfície celular, também eliminado na forma solúvel por clivagem enzimática; ↑ febre e choque séptico; citotóxico para muitos tipos celulares tumorais

citocinas e quimiocinas: peso molecular, fonte e função (cont.)			
citocinas humanas	PM (kDa)	fonte celular	principais funções
LT-α (TNF-β)	homotrímero ou heterotrímero 20–25 subunidades	células T	(também conhecida como linfotoxina) secretada como homotrímero ou associada à LT-β e expressa como heterotrímero da superfície celular; envolvida na organogênese do tecido linfóide secundário
LIF	46	células T, linhagens mielomonocíticas	↑ síntese de proteínas de fase aguda; ↑ diferenciação dos MØs e da proliferação de células-tronco hematopoéticas
IL–8	6–8	muitos tipos celulares, incluindo monócitos, linfócitos e granulócitos	quimiotática e ativadora de neutrófilos promove angiogênese
GROα	7–11	monócitos, células epiteliais e endoteliais, e células tumorais, p. ex., melanoma	quimiotática e ativadora de neutrófilos promove angiogênese e crescimento de determinados tumores
IP-10	10–11	células endoteliais, monócitos e fibroblastos, e células do estroma tímico e esplênico	quimiotática para células T ativadas inibe a proliferação de células endoteliais
SDF-1	10	células do estroma, fígado, músculo	estimula o crescimento de pré-células B quimiotático para monócitos e células T
MIG	14–15	monócitos e macrófagos tratados com IFN-γ	quimiotático para linfócitos infiltrativos tumorais
MCP-1	11–17	muitos tipos celulares, incluindo monócitos/macrófagos, fibroblastos e determinados tumores	quimiotático de células T e induz quimiotaxia e ativação de monócitos
MCP-2	7,5–11	muitos tipos celulares, incluindo monócitos/macrófagos, fibroblastos e determinados tumores	quimiotático de células T e induz quimiotaxia e ativação de monócitos
MCP-3	11	muitos tipos celulares, incluindo monócitos/macrófagos, fibroblastos e determinados tumores	quimiotático de eosinófilos e células T; induz quimiotaxia e ativação de monócitos
MIP-1α	10	muitos tipos celulares, incluindo monócitos, linfócitos e células do estroma	quimiotático de monócitos e células T; inibe a proliferação de células-tronco hematopoéticas
MIP-1β	10	muitos tipos celulares, incluindo monócitos, linfócitos e células tumorais	quimiotático de monócitos e células T; inibe a proliferação de células-tronco hematopoéticas
RANTES	10	muitos tipos celulares, incluindo células T, monócitos, fibroblastos e determinadas linhagens de células tumorais	quimiotaxia de células T, monócitos e eosinófilos
eotaxina	8–9	células endoteliais, macrófagos alveolares, pulmão, intestino, coração, timo, baço, fígado, rim	quimiotaxia de eosinófilos
linfotactina	10	timócitos, células T ativadas	quimiotaxia de células T
I-309	10–16	células T, mastócitos	quimiotaxia de neutrófilos

abreviações

- ↑ = aumenta (estimula)
- ↓ = diminui (suprime)
- CMO = célula da medula óssea
- LTC = linfócitos T citotóxicos
- FEC-GM = fator estimulante de colônia de granulócitos-macrófagos
- IFN = interferon
- IL = interleucina
- LIF = fator inibidor de leucócitos
- LT = terminação longa
- MØ = macrófago
- MHC = complexo maior de histocompatibilidade
- MIP = proteína inibidora de macrófago
- células NK = células destruidoras naturais
- Th1 = célula auxiliar tipo 1
- Th2 = célula auxiliar tipo 2
- TNF = fator de necrose tumoral

cy·to·mor·pho·sis (sī′tō-mōr-fō′sis). Citomorfose; alterações que a célula sofre durante os vários estágios de sua existência. VER TAMBÉM prosoplasia. [cyto- + G. *morphōsis,* formação]

cy·to·path·ic (sī-tō-path′ik). Citopático; relativo a, ou que exibe, citopatia.

cy·to·path·o·gen·ic (sī′tō-path-ō-jen′ik). Citopatogênico; relativo a um agente ou substância que causa uma doença nas células, ao contrário das alterações histológicas; usado especialmente em referência aos efeitos observados em células em culturas teciduais.

cy·to·path·o·log·ic, cy·to·path·o·log·i·cal (sī′tō-pa-thō-loj′ik, -loj′i-kăl). Citopatológico. **1.** Designa alterações celulares na doença. **2.** Relativo à citopatologia.

cy·to·pa·thol·o·gist (sī′tō-pa-thol′ō-jist). Citopatologista; um médico, geralmente experiente em anatomia patológica, que é especialmente treinado e experiente em citopatologia.

cy·to·pa·thol·o·gy (sī′tō-pa-thol′ō-jē). Citopatologia. **1.** O estudo de alterações causadas por doença em células individuais ou em tipos celulares. **2.** SIN exfoliative *cytology.*

cy·top·a·thy (sī-top′a-thē). Citopatia; qualquer distúrbio de uma célula ou anomalia de qualquer de seus constituintes. [cyto- + G. *pathos,* doença]

cy·to·pemp·sis (sī-tō-pemp′sis). Citopempese. SIN transcytosis. [cyto- + G. *pempsis,* enviando através]

cy·to·pe·nia (sī-tō-pē′nē-ă). Citopenia; redução, isto é, hipocitose, ou ausência de elementos celulares no sangue circulante. [cyto- + G. *penia,* pobreza]

diagnóstico de citomegalovírus (CMV)	
histologia	fígado, rim, pulmão, glândulas salivares e outros órgãos
citologia	urina; corpúsculos de inclusão em células epiteliais, principalmente em crianças de até 3 meses; saliva
imunofluorescência	inclusões intranucleares e intracitoplasmáticas específicas em cortes teciduais
cultura viral	culturas teciduais de urina, culturas da orofaringe, linfócitos, secreção cervical, material de biópsia e necrópsia (esperma, leite materno)
tratamento de hibridização	separação do DNA celular do viral
evidências sorológicas de anticorpos	reação de ligação do complemento (RLC), hemaglutinação passiva, imunofluorescência, teste de neutralização em culturas teciduais, determinação de anticorpos IgM se houver suspeita de infecção ativa

cy·toph·a·gy (sī - tof′ă - jē). Citofagia; destruição de outras células por fagócitos. [cyto- + G. *phagō*, devorar]

cy·to·phan·ere (sī′tō - fă - nēr). Citofânero; uma espinha radial observada em determinados cistos de *Sarcocystis*, como em cistos teciduais de coelhos e carneiros. [cyto- + G. *phaneros*, visível, evidente, aberto]

cy·to·phar·ynx (sī′tō - far′inks). Citofaringe; uma organela encontrada em determinados flagelados e ciliados que serve como esôfago, através do qual o alimento passa do citóstoma para o interior da célula; o alimento é coletado em vacúolos alimentares, para o qual são secretadas enzimas digestivas.

cy·to·phil·ic (sī - tō - fil′ik). Citófilo. SIN cytotropic. [cyto- + G. *philos*, afinidade]

cy·to·pho·tom·e·try (sī′tō - fō - tom′ē - trē). Citofotometria; método para medir a absorção da luz monocromática p. estruturas microscópicas coradas (p. ex., cromossomas, núcleos, células inteiras) com a ajuda de uma célula fotoelétrica; também é usada para medir a luz emitida desses objetos por fluorescência em combinação com corantes de fluorocromo selecionados. [cyto- + G. *phōs*, luz + *metron*, medida]
  flow c., c. de fluxo. SIN flow *cytometry*.

cy·to·phy·lac·tic (sī′tō - fī - lak′tik). Citofilático; relativo à citofilaxia.

cy·to·phy·lax·is (sī′tō - fī - lak′sis). Citofilaxia; proteção de células contra agentes líticos. [cyto- + G. *phylaxis*, proteção]

cy·to·phy·let·ic (sī′tō - fī - let′ik). Citofilético; relativo à genealogia de uma célula. [cyto- + G. *phylē*, tribo]

cy·to·pi·pette (sī′tō - pi - pet′). Citopipeta; uma pipeta discretamente curva, de extremidade romba, geralmente feita de vidro e adaptada a um bulbo de borracha para produzir leve pressão negativa, visando à coleta de secreções vaginais para exame citológico.

cy·to·plasm (sī′tō - plazm). Citoplasma; a substância de uma célula, exclusiva do núcleo, que contém várias organelas e inclusões em um protoplasma coloidal. VER TAMBÉM protoplasm, hyaloplasm, cytosol. [cyto- + G. *plasma*, algo formado]
  ground-glass c., c. em vidro moído; citoplasma eosinofílico finamente granular, uniforme, observado nos hepatócitos de portadores do vírus da hepatite B, assim como nas células epidérmicas no ceratoacantoma.

cy·to·plas·mic (sī - tō - plaz′mik). Citoplasmático; relativo ao citoplasma.

cy·to·plas·mon (sī - tō - plaz′mon). A informação genética extranuclear total de uma célula eucariótica, excluindo a das mitocôndrias e dos plastídeos.

cy·to·plast (sī′tō - plast). Citoplasto; o citoplasma intacto vivo que permanece após enucleação celular. [cyto- + G. *plastos*, formado]

cy·to·poi·e·sis (sī - tō - poy - ē′sis). Citopoese; formação de células. [cyto- + G. *poiēsis*, formação]

cy·to·prep·a·ra·tion (sī′tō - prep - ă - rā′shŭn). Citopreparação; preparo laboratorial de uma amostra celular para exame citológico.

cy·to·py·ge (sī - tō - pī′jē). Citopígio; o orifício anal ("ânus" celular) encontrado em determinados protozoários estruturalmente complexos, como os ciliados que habitam o rume de herbívoros, através do qual é ejetado o excremento. [cyto- + G. *pygē*, nádegas]

cy·to·ryc·tes, cy·tor·rhyc·tes (sī - tō - rik′tēz). Citorictes; termo obsoleto para inclusion *bodies* (corpúsculos de inclusão), em *body*. [cyto- + G. *oryktēs*, cavador]

cytoscreener (sī′tō - skrēn′er). Citotecnólogo. SIN cytotechnologist.

cy·to·sides (sī′tō - sīdz). Citosídeos; dissacarídeos ceramídicos. VER glycosphingolipid.

cy·to·sine (Cyt) (sī′tō - sēn). Citosina; uma pirimidina encontrada em ácidos nucleicos.
  c. arabinoside (CA, AraC), c. arabinosídeo; **(1)** um nucleosídeo sintético usado como antimetabólito no tratamento de neoplasias; **(2)** termo incorreto para arabinosilcitosina.
  c. ribonucleoside, c. ribonucleosídeo. SIN cytidine.

cy·to·sis (sī - tō′sis). Citose. **1.** Um distúrbio no qual há mais que o número habitual de células, como na citose do líquido espinhal na leptomeningite aguda. **2.** Freqüentemente usado com um prefixo como forma de descrever determinados aspectos relativos às células; p. ex., isocitose, igualdade de tamanho; policitose, aumento anormal do número. [cyto- + G. –*osis*, condição]

cy·to·skel·e·ton (sī - tō - skel′ĕ - ton). Citoesqueleto; os tonofilamentos, queratina, desmina, neurofilamentos ou outros filamentos intermediários que servem como elementos citoplasmáticos de sustentação para enrijecer as células ou para organizar organelas intracelulares.

cy·to·smear (sī′tō - smēr). Esfregaço citológico. SIN cytologic *smear*.

cy·to·sol (sī′tō - sol). Citosol; citoplasma exclusivo da mitocôndria, retículo endoplasmático e outros componentes membranosos. [cyto- + "sol", abrev. de solúvel]

cy·to·sol·ic (sī - tō - so′lik). Citosólico; relativo ao, ou contido no, citosol.

cy·to·some (sī′tō - sōm). Citossoma. **1.** O corpo celular exclusivo do núcleo. **2.** Grânulo distinto encontrado nas grandes células alveolares (tipo II) do pulmão, que libera surfactante pulmonar nas superfícies alveolares. SIN multilamellar body. [cyto- + G. *sōma*, corpo]

cy·tos·ta·sis (sī - tos′tă - sis). Citostase; a lentificação do movimento e o acúmulo de células sanguíneas, principalmente leucócitos polimorfonucleares, nos capilares, como em uma região de inflamação; obstrução de um capilar em virtude de leucócitos acumulados. [cyto- + G. *stasis*, parada]

cy·to·stat·ic (sī - tō - stat′ik). Citostático; caracterizado por citostase.

cy·to·stome (sī′tō - stōm). Citoestoma; a "boca" celular de determinados protozoários complexos, geralmente com um esôfago curto ou citofaringe que leva o alimento para o organismo, onde é coletado em vacúolos alimentares, depois circula para dentro do organismo e, finalmente, é excretado através do citopígio. [cyto + G. *stoma*, boca]

cy·to·tac·tic (sī - tō - tak′tik). Citotático; relativo à citotaxia.

cy·to·tax·is, cy·to·tax·ia (sī - tō - tak′sis, - tak′sē - ă). Citotaxia; a atração (**c. positiva**) ou repulsão (**c. negativa**) de células entre si. [cyto- + G. *taxis*, arranjo]

cytotechnologist (sī′tō - tek - nol′ō - jist). Citotecnólogo; pessoa com treinamento especial em citopatologia, responsável pela triagem dos esfregaços de Papanicolaou e determinação de quais são negativos e quais necessitam ser revistos por um patologista. VER TAMBÉM Pap *smear*, Pap *test*. SIN cytoscreener.

cy·toth·e·sis (sī - toth′ĕ - sis). Citotese; reparo da lesão de uma célula; restauração de células. [cyto- + G. *thesis*, colocação]

cy·to·tox·ic (sī - tō - tok′sik). Citotóxico; prejudicial ou destrutivo para as células.

cy·to·tox·ic·i·ty (sī′tō - tok - sis′i - tē). Citotoxicidade; a qualidade ou estado de ser citotóxico.

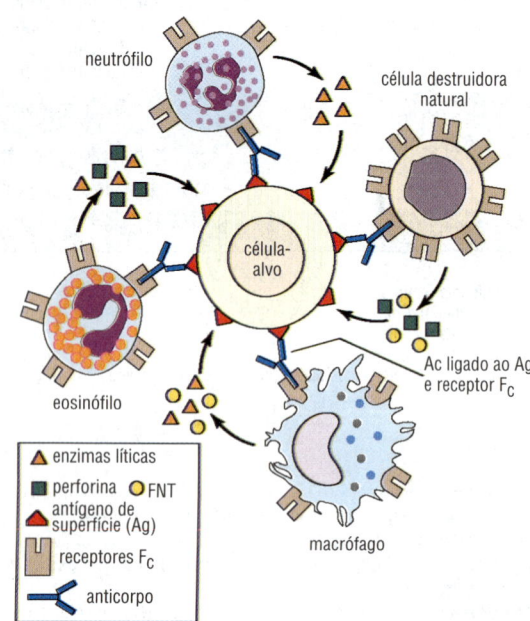

citotoxicidade celular anticorpo-dependente (CCAD): células citotóxicas inespecíficas são direcionadas para células-alvo específicas por ligação à região Fc do anticorpo ligado aos antígenos de superfície em células-alvo; várias substâncias (p. ex., enzimas líticas, fator de necrose tumoral (FNT), perforina) secretadas por células citotóxicas inespecíficas então medeiam a destruição de células-alvo

antibody-dependent cell-mediated c. (ADCC), c. celular anticorpo-dependente; uma forma de citotoxicidade mediada por células que funciona por ligação da região FC de anticorpos IgG aos receptores Fc em leucócitos. A região FAB do anticorpo liga-se à célula-alvo. A destruição da célula-alvo pode ser através de várias modalidades, p. ex., perforina, intermediários reativos do oxigênio, citocinas.
lymphocyte-mediated c., c. mediada por linfócitos; a atividade tóxica ou lítica de linfócitos, que pode ou não ser mediada por anticorpos. Os linfócitos T citotóxicos podem causar lise de células por produção de proteínas citolíticas como a perforina. As células B podem causar lise de células por ligação do anticorpo-complemento a uma célula-alvo. As células destruidoras naturais (NK, *natural killer*) são citotóxicas sem sensibilização prévia. VER TAMBÉM antibody-dependent cell-mediated c.
cy·to·tox·in (sī′tō - tok′sin). Citotoxina; substância específica, podendo ou não ser um anticorpo, que inibe ou impede as funções das células e/ou causa destruição destas. VER TAMBÉM perforin. [cyto- + G. *toxikon*, veneno]
vero c., verotoxina; uma citotoxina celular produzida pela *Escherichia coli* entero-hemorrágica que parece contribuir para a ocorrência de colite hemorrágica e síndrome hemolítico-urêmica. SIN Shigalike toxin.

cy·to·tro·pho·blast (sī - tō - trof′ō - blast). Citotrofoblasto; a camada interna do trofoblasto. SIN Langhans layer.
cy·to·tro·pic (sī - tō - trop′ik). Citotrópico; citofílico; que tem afinidade pelas células. SIN cytophilic.
cy·tot·ro·pism (sī - tot′rō - pizm). Citotropismo. **1.** Afinidade por células. **2.** Afinidade por células específicas, particularmente a capacidade dos vírus de localizar e lesar células específicas. [cyto- + G. *tropos*, volta]
cy·to·zo·ic (sī - tō - zō′ik). Citozóico; que vive em uma célula; designa alguns protozoários parasitas.
cy·to·zo·on (sī - tō - zō′on). Citozoon; uma célula ou organismo protozoário. [cyto- + G. *zōon*, animal]
cy·tu·ria (sī - too′rē - ā). Citúria; eliminação de células em número incomum na urina. [G. *kytos*, célula, + *ouron*, urina]
Czapek, Friedrich J.F., botânico tchecoslovaco, 1868–1921. VER C. solution *agar*; C.-Dox *medium*.
CZE Abreviatura de capillary zone *electrophoresis* (eletroforese de zona capilar).
Czerny, Vincenz, cirurgião alemão, 1842–1916. VER C. *suture;* C.-Lembert *suture*.

D

Δ, δ 1. Quarta letra do alfabeto grego, delta. **2.** Em química, designa uma ligação dupla, geralmente com um sobrescrito para indicar a posição em uma cadeia (Δ^5); aplicação de calor em uma reação (A $\xrightarrow{\Delta}$ B); ausência de tratamento térmico ($\cancel{\Delta}$); distância entre dois átomos em uma molécula; ou posição de um substituto localizado no quarto átomo a partir da carboxila ou outro grupamento funcional primário (δ); alteração (Δ), espessura (δ), desvio químico na RMN (δ).

D 1. Símbolo da potência da vitamina D do óleo de fígado de bacalhau, cujos múltiplos (5D, 100D, etc.) são usados para designar a potência da vitamina D do ergosterol (viosterol) irradiado ou outras substâncias; do deutério; da diidrouridina em ácidos nucleicos; da capacidade de difusão; do ácido aspártico; da diidrouridina; do coeficiente de difusão (diffusion *coefficient*) (em itálico). **2.** Em óptica, abreviatura de dioptria; de direita. **3.** Em eletrodiagnóstico, abreviatura de duração, sendo fechados o fluxo de corrente e o circuito. **4.** Em fórmulas dentárias, abreviatura para decíduo (2). **5.** Como subscrito, refere-se ao espaço morto (dead *space*). VER physiologic dead *space*. **6.** Linha D nos espectros de emissão de Na.

2,4-D Abreviatura de ácido (2,4-diclorofenoxi) acético.

d Símbolo de deci-; abreviatura de *dexter* [L.], direita; diâmetro; dia.

⚛ **D-.** Prefixo que indica que uma substância química está estericamente relacionada ao D-gliceraldeído, a base da nomenclatura estereoquímica. Cf. L-.

⚛ **d-.** Prefixo que indica que uma substância química é dextrorrotatória; deve ser evitado quando poderia ser usado (+) ou (−). Cf. *l*-.

⚛ **-d.** Sufixo que indica a presença de deutério em uma substância em concentrações acima do normal, assim marcando o composto; os subscritos (d_2, d_3, etc.) indicam o número desses átomos assim fortificados.

DA Abreviatura de developmental *age* (2) (idade de desenvolvimento).

Da Símbolo de dálton.

dA, dAdo Abreviatura de deoxyadenosine (desoxiadenosina).

da Símbolo de deca-.

Daae, Anders, médico norueguês, 1838–1910. VER D. *disease*.

DAB Abreviatura de cloridrato de 3'3-diaminobenzidina; na técnica de imunoperoxidase, usado para produzir um complexo colorido no local de atividade da peroxidase.

da·car·ba·zine (DTIC) (dā - kar'bă - zēn). Dacarbazina (DTIC); um agente antineoplásico usado no tratamento do melanoma maligno e do sarcoma.

⚛ **dacry-.** VER dacryo-.

dac·ry·ad·e·ni·tis (dak're - ad - ĕ - nī'tis). Dacrioadenite. SIN dacryoadenitis.

⚛ **dacryo-, dacry-.** Dacrio-, dacri-; lágrimas; saco ou ducto lacrimal. [G. *dakryon*, lágrima]

dac·ry·o·ad·e·ni·tis (dak - rē - ō - ad - ĕ - nī'tis). Dacrioadenite; inflamação da glândula lacrimal. SIN dacryadenitis. [dacryo- + G. *adēn*, glândula, + -*itis*, inflamação]

dac·ry·o·blen·nor·rhea (dak - rē - ō - blen - ō - rē'ă). Dacrioblenorréia; secreção crônica de muco de um saco lacrimal. [dacryo- + G. *blenna*, muco, + *rhoia*, fluxo]

dac·ry·o·cele (dak're - ō - sēl). Dacriocele. SIN dacryocystocele.

dac·ry·o·cyst (dak're - ō - sist). Dacriocisto. SIN lacrimal *sac*. [dacryo- + G. *kystis*, saco]

dac·ry·o·cys·tal·gia (dak'rē - ō - sis - tal'jē - ă). Dacriocistalgia; dor no saco lacrimal. [dacryocyst + G. *algos*, dor]

dac·ry·o·cys·tec·to·my (dak'rē - ō - sis - tek'tō - mē). Dacriocistectomia; remoção cirúrgica do saco lacrimal. [dacryocyst + G. *ektomē*, excisão]

ℹ **dac·ry·o·cys·ti·tis** (dak're - ō - sis - tī'tis). Dacriocistite; inflamação do saco lacrimal. [dacryocyst + G. -*itis*, inflamação]

dac·ry·o·cys·to·cele (dak're - ō - sis'tō - sēl). Dacriocistocele; aumento do saco lacrimal com líquido. SIN dacryocele. [dacryocyst + G. *kēlē*, hérnia]

dac·ry·o·cys·to·gram (dak're - ō - sis'tō - gram). Dacriocistograma; radiografia do aparelho lacrimal obtida após injeção de contraste a fim de determinar se existe obstrução e localizá-la; esse procedimento foi amplamente substituído pela TC e RM. [dacryocyst + G. *gramma*, escrito]

dac·ry·o·cys·to·rhi·nos·to·my (dak're - ō - sis'tō - rī - nos'tō - mē). Dacriocistorrinostomia; operação que produz uma anastomose entre o saco lacrimal e a mucosa nasal através de uma abertura no osso lacrimal. [dacryocyst + G. *rhis* (*rhin*-), nariz, + *stoma*, boca]

dac·ry·o·cys·tot·o·my (dak're - ō - sis - tot'ō - mē). Dacriocistotomia; incisão do saco lacrimal. [dacryocyst + G. *tomē*, incisão]

dac·ry·o·hem·or·rhea (dak're - ō - hem - ō - rē'ă). Dacrioemorréia; lágrimas com sangue. [dacryo- + G. *haima*, sangue, + *rhoia*, fluxo]

dac·ry·o·lith (dak're - ō - lith). Dacriólito; cálculo no aparelho lacrimal. SIN lacrimal calculus, ophthalmolith, tear stone. [dacryo- + G. *lithos*, cálculo]

Desmarres d.'s, dacriólitos de Desmarres. SIN Nocardia d.'s.

Nocardia d.'s, dacriólitos de Nocardia; pseudocálculos brancos, compostos de massas de espécies de *Nocardia* encontradas nos canalículos lacrimais. SIN Desmarres d.'s.

dac·ry·o·li·thi·a·sis (dak're - ō - li - thī'ă - sis). Dacriolitíase; a formação e a presença de dacriólitos.

dac·ry·on (dak're - on). Dácrio; o ponto de junção das suturas frontomaxilar e lacrimomaxilar na parede medial da órbita. Ver figura em craniometric *points*, em *point*. [G. lágrima]

dac·ry·ops (dak're - ops). Daciopo. **1.** Excesso de lágrimas no olho. **2.** Um cisto de um ducto da glândula lacrimal. [dacryo- + G. *ōps*, olho]

dac·ry·o·py·or·rhea (dak're - ō - pī - ō - rē'ă). Dacriopiorréia; secreção de lágrimas contendo leucócitos. [dacryo- + G. *pyon*, pus, + *rhoia*, fluxo]

dac·ry·or·rhea (dak're - ō - rē'ă). Dacriorréia; secreção excessiva de lágrimas. [dacryo- + G. *rhoia*, fluxo]

dac·ry·o·ste·no·sis (dak're - ō - ste - nō'sis). Dacrioestenose; estreitamento do ducto lacrimal. [dacryo- + G. *stenōsis*, estreitamento]

dac·ti·no·my·cin (dak'ti - nō - mī'sin). Dactinomicina; produzida por várias espécies de *Streptomyces* (p. ex., *S. parvulus*); um antibiótico antineoplásico usado especialmente no sarcoma de Ewing, rabdomiossarcoma e tumor de Wilms em crianças e doença trofoblástica em mulheres. VER TAMBÉM actinomycin. SIN actinomycin D.

dac·tyl (dak'til). Dáctilo. SIN digit. [G. *daktylos*]

⚛ **dactyl-.** VER dactylo-.

dac·ty·lal·gia (dak - ti - lal'jē - ă). Dactilalgia; dor nos dedos das mãos. SIN dactylodynia. [dactyl- + G. *algos*, dor]

Dac·ty·la·ria (dak - ti - lā're - ă). Gênero de fungos dematiáceos que habitam o solo. *D. gallopava* é um agente causador de feoifomicose em galinhas e perus. [G. *daktylos*, dedo]

dac·ty·li·tis (dak - ti - lī'tis). Dactilite; inflamação de um ou mais dedos das mãos.

  blistering distal d., d. distal bolhosa; infecção do coxim adiposo volar da falange distal do dedo da mão por estreptococos β-hemolíticos do grupo A.

  sickle cell d., d. falciforme. SIN hand-and-foot *syndrome*.

⚛ **dactylo-, dactyl-.** Dactilo-, dactil-; os dedos das mãos e (menos freqüentemente) os artelhos. VER entrada em digit. [G. *daktylos*, dedo]

dac·ty·lo·camp·sis (dak'ti - lō - kamp'sis). Dactilocampsia; flexão permanente dos dedos. [dactylo- + G. *kampsis*, flexão]

dac·ty·lo·camp·so·dyn·ia (dak'ti - lō - kamp'sō - din'ē - ă). Dactilocampsodinia; contração dolorosa de um ou mais dedos das mãos. [dactylo- + G. *kampsis*, flexão, + *odynē*, dor]

dac·ty·lo·dyn·ia (dak'ti - lō - din'ē - ă). Dactilodinia. SIN dactylalgia.

dac·ty·lo·gry·po·sis (dak'ti - lō - gri - pō'sis). Dactilogripose; contração dos dedos das mãos. [dactylo- + G. *grypōsis*, curvatura]

dac·ty·lol·o·gy (dak'ti - lol'ō - jē). Dactilologia; o uso do alfabeto de dedos para se comunicar. SIN cheirology, chirology. [dactylo- + G. *logos*, palavra]

dac·tyl·o·meg·a·ly (dak'til - ō - meg'ă - lē). Dactilomegalia. SIN megadactyly. [dactylo- + G. *megas*, grande]

dac·ty·los·co·py (dak - ti - los'kō - pē). Dactiloscopia; exame das marcas feitas pelas impressões das pontas dos dedos das mãos; empregada como método de identificação pessoal. VER Galton system of classification of *fingerprints*, em *fingerprint*. [dactylo- + G. *skopeō*, examinar]

dac·ty·lo·spasm (dak'ti - lō - spazm). Dactilospasmo; contração espasmódica dos dedos das mãos ou dos pés.

dac·ty·lus, pl. **dac·ty·li** (dak'ti - lŭs, - lī). Dáctilo. SIN digit. [G. *daktylos*]

dac·u·ro·ni·um (dak - ū - rō'nē - ŭm). Dacurônio; agente bloqueador neuromuscular esteróide não-despolarizante com início de ação mais rápido e duração mais curta que o pancurônio.

Da Fano, Corrado D., anatomista ítalo-americano, 1879–1927. VER Da F. *stain*.

DAG Abreviatura de diacylglycerol (diacilglicerol).

dag·ga (dag'ă). Daga; folhas de *Leonotis leonurus*, planta encontrada na África do Sul, onde é fumada como tabaco, com leve efeito sedativo; termo erroneamente aplicado ao haxixe indiano, *Cannabis sativa*. [termo aborígene]

Dagnini, Giuseppe, médico italiano, 1866–1928. VER Aschner-D. *reflex*.

DAH Abreviatura de disordered action of heart (ação cardíaca desordenada).

dah·lia (dal'yah). Corante violeta, cloreto de metil-trietil-amino-trifenilcarbinol. Também denominado violeta de Hoffman.

⚛ Formas Combinantes	☆ Termo oficial alternativo para a *Terminologia Anatomica*
ℹ Indica que o termo é ilustrado, ver Índice de Ilustrações	[MIM] Mendelian Inheritance in Man
SIN Sinônimo	I.C. Índice de Corantes
Cf. Comparar, confrontar	
[NA] *Nomina Anatomica*	**Termo de Alta Importância**
[TA] *Terminologia Anatomica*	

dah·lin. Dalina; inulina. SIN inulin. [de *dahlia*, em homenagem a *A. Dahl*, botânico sueco, 1751–1789]

dahll·ite (dah′līt). Podolito, dalita; um fosfato de cálcio de ocorrência natural, semelhante, em estrutura, às porções minerais dos ossos e dentes. SIN podolite.

dai·sy (dā′zē). Margarida-dos-campos; termo coloquial descritivo das formas segmentadas (merozoítas) do esquizonte maduro de *Plasmodium malariae*.

Dakin, Henry, químico norte-americano, 1880–1952. VER D. *fluid, solution;* D.-Carrel *treatment.*

Dale, Sir Henry Hallett, fisiologista inglês e ganhador do Prêmio Nobel, 1875–1968. VER D. *reaction;* D.-Feldberg *law;* Schultz-D. *reaction.*

Dalen, Johan A., oftalmologista sueco, 1866–1940. VER D.-Fuchs *nodules,* em *nodule.*

Dalgarno, Lynn, bióloga molecular australiana contemporânea.

Dalrymple, John, oculista inglês, 1803–1852. VER D. *sign.*

Dalton, John, químico, matemático e filósofo natural inglês, 1766–1844. VER D. *law;* D.-Henry *law;* daltonian; daltonism.

dal·ton (Da) (dawl′tŏn). Dálton; termo usado não-oficialmente para indicar uma unidade de massa igual a 1/12 da massa de um átomo de carbono-12, 1,0000 na escala de massa atômica; numericamente, mas não dimensionalmente, igual ao peso molecular ou da partícula (unidades de massa atômica). [J. *Dalton*]

dal·to·ni·an (dawl - tō′nē - ăn). Daltoniano. 1. Atribuído a, ou descrito por, John Dalton. 2. Relativo a daltonismo.

dal·ton·ism (dawl′tŏn - izm). Daltonismo; uma deficiência da visão para cores, principalmente deuteranomalia ou deuteranopia. [J. *Dalton*]

DALYs Abreviatura de disability-adjusted life *years,* em *year* (anos de vida ajustados à incapacidade).

DAM Abreviatura de diacetylmonoxime (diacetilmonoxima).

Dam, C.P. Henrik, bioquímico dinamarquês e ganhador do Prêmio Nobel, 1895–1976. VER D. *unit.*

dam. 1. Qualquer barreira ao fluxo de líquido. 2. Em cirurgia e odontologia, uma fina camada de borracha disposta de forma a impedir o acesso de líquido à parte operada. [A.S. *fordemman,* segurar, impedir]

post d., obturação palatal posterior. SIN posterior palatal *seal.*

rubber d. (1) Em cirurgia, delgadas tiras de borracha usadas como dreno ou barreira cirúrgica; (2) uma fina folha de borracha colocada sobre os dentes para isolá-los da cavidade oral.

damage. (1) Lesão, ferimento; (2) causar lesão a, agredir fisicamente.

diffuse alveolar damage, lesão alveolar difusa. SIN adult respiratory distress syndrome.

Dam·a·lin·ia (dam - ă - lin′ē - ă). Gênero de piolhos que contém muitas espécies encontradas em animais domésticos e selvagens; são todos extremamente hospedeiro-específicos, com uma espécie sendo limitada a cada espécie de mamífero. VER TAMBÉM *Bovicola, Trichodectes.*

dam·mar. Damar; resina que se assemelha ao copal, obtida de várias espécies de *Shorea* (família Dipterocarpaceae) nas Índias Orientais; usada, dissolvida em clorofórmio, para preparar amostras microscópicas. [Hindu *dāmar,* resina]

dam meth·yl·ase. Desoxiadenosina metilase; enzima responsável pela metilação de resíduos adenina em seqüências específicas. SIN deoxyadenosine methylase.

dAMP Abreviatura de deoxyadenylic acid (ácido desoxiadenílico).

damp. 1. Úmido. 2. Umidade atmosférica. 3. Ar impuro em uma mina; ar carregado com óxidos de carbono (exalação de gás tóxico, mofeta) ou com vários vapores de hidrocarboneto explosivos (grisu).

damp·ing. Amortecimento; levar um mecanismo a repousar com oscilação mínima, p. ex., em ecocardiografia, carga elétrica ou mecânica para reduzir a duração do eco, impulso transmissor e complexo transmissor. [I.M. *damp,* vapor venenoso]

Damus-Kaye-Stancel pro·ce·dure. Procedimento de Damus-Kaye-Stancel; ver em procedure.

Dana, Charles L., neurologista norte-americano, 1852–1935. VER D. *operation;* Putnam-D. *syndrome.*

da·na·zol (dā′nă - zol). Danazol; um supressor da hipófise anterior (adenohipófise) usado no tratamento da endometriose, doença fibrocística da mama e angioedema.

Dance, Jean B.H., médico francês, 1797–1832. VER D. *sign.*

dance (dans). Dança; movimentos involuntários relacionados à lesão cerebral.

hilar d., d. hilar; pulsações arteriais pulmonares vigorosas devidas a aumento do fluxo sanguíneo, freqüentemente observadas fluoroscopicamente em pacientes com derivações (*shunts*) esquerda-direita congênitas, principalmente comunicações interatriais.

Saint Anthony d., Saint Vitus d., Saint John d., d. de Santo Antônio, d. de São Vito, d. de São João; epônimos obsoletos para coréia de Sydenham (Sydenham *chorea*), em *chorea*.

dan·der. 1. Descamação fina da pele e do couro cabeludo. VER TAMBÉM dandruff. 2. Eflúvio normal de pêlo animal capaz de causar respostas alérgicas em pessoas atópicas.

dan·druff (dan′drŭf). Caspa; a presença, em quantidades variáveis, de escamas brancas ou acinzentadas no cabelo, devido à esfoliação excessiva ou esfarelada normal da epiderme. VER TAMBÉM seborrheic *dermatitis.* SIN pityriasis capitis, scurf, seborrhea sicca (2).

Dandy, Walter E., neurocirurgião norte-americano, 1886–1946. VER D. *operation;* D.-Walker *syndrome.*

Dane, D.S., virologista inglês do século XX. VER D. *particles,* em *particle.*

Dane stain. Coloração de Dane. Ver em stain.

Danforth, William Clark, ginecologista-obstetra norte-americano, 1878–1949. VER D. *sign.*

Danielssen, Daniel C., médico norueguês, 1815–1894. VER D. *disease;* D.-Boeck *disease.*

Danlos, Henri A., dermatologista francês, 1844–1912. VER Ehlers-D. *syndrome.*

DANS Abreviatura de ácido 1-dimetilaminonaftaleno-5-sulfônico; uma substância fluorescente verde usada em imuno-histoquímica para detectar antígenos.

dan·syl (Dns, DNS) (dan′sil). Dansil; o radical 5-dimetilaminonaftaleno-1-sulfonil; agente bloqueador dos grupamentos NH_2, usado na síntese de peptídeos.

dan·thron. Dantron; um laxante antraquinona. SIN chrysazine.

dan·tro·lene so·di·um (dan′trō - lēn). Dantroleno sódico; um relaxante muscular esquelético sintético, que atua diretamente sobre os músculos por desacoplamento dos eventos elétricos e mecânicos; também, o agente específico para a prevenção e o tratamento da hipertermia maligna.

Danysz, Jan, patologista polonês na França, 1860–1928. VER D. *phenomenon.*

DAPI Abreviatura de 4′6-diamidino-2-fenilindol.2HCl, uma sonda fluorescente para ADN. VER DAPI *stain.*

dap·sone (dap′sōn). Dapsona; antibiótico usado no tratamento da hanseníase e de determinadas doenças cutâneas, como a dermatite herpetiforme; é ativo contra o bacilo da tuberculose e usado no tratamento da coccidiose bovina e da mastite estreptocócica e, também, como agente de segunda linha na pneumonia por *Pneumocystis carinii*, uma doença comum em pessoas com AIDS/SIDA.

d′Arcet, Jean, químico francês, 1725–1801. VER d′A. *metal.*

Darier, Jean F., dermatologista francês, 1856–1938. VER D. *disease, sign.*

Darkschewitsch (Darkshevich), Liverij O., neurologista russo, 1858–1925. VER *nucleus* of D.

Darling, Samuel Taylor, médico norte-americano no Panamá, 1872–1925. VER D. *disease.*

Darrow red. Vermelho de Darrow; corante de oxazina básico usado como substituto do acetato de cresil violeta na coloração da substância de Nissl. [Mary A. *Darrow,* tecnóloga em coloração, norte-americana, 1894–1973]

d′Arsonval, Jacques Arsène, biofísico francês, 1851–1940. VER d′A. *current, galvanometer.*

dar·to·ic, dar·toid (dar - tō′ik, dar′toyd). Dartóico; dartóide, semelhante à túnica dartos em suas contrações involuntárias lentas. [G. *dartos,* esfolado]

dar·tos (dar′tōs). Túnica dartos. VER dartos *fascia.* [G. pelado ou esfolado, de *derō,* esfolar]

d. mulieb′ris, túnica dartos das mulheres; uma camada muito fina de músculo liso no tegumento dos lábios maiores do pudendo; menos desenvolvido que a túnica dartos do escroto.

Darwin, Charles R., biólogo e evolucionista inglês, 1809–1882. VER darwinian *ear;* darwinian *evolution;* darwinian *reflex;* darwinian *theory;* darwinian *tubercle.*

dar·win·i·an (dar - win′ē - an). Darwiniano; relativo, ou atribuído, a Darwin.

Das·y·proc·ta (das′ē - prok′tă). Gênero de roedores da família das cobaias, um hospedeiro reservatório do *Trypanosoma cruzi.* SIN agouti. [G. *dasyprōktos,* que possui nádegas peludas]

da·ta. Dados; fatos; elementos; múltiplos fatos (em geral, mas não necessariamente, empíricos) usados como base para inferência, testes, modelos, etc. A palavra está no plural e o verbo deve ser colocado no plural.

da·ta pro·cess·ing. Processamento de dados ou informações; conversão de informações brutas em uma forma passível de utilização ou armazenagem; análise estatística de dados por um programa de computador.

da·tum (dā′tŭm). Dado; fato; elemento; uma informação individual usada em um campo erudito. [L. *given,* de *do,* pp. *datum,* dar]

Da·tu·ra (dă - too′ră). Gênero de plantas solanáceas. Várias espécies (*D. arborea, D. fastuosa, D. ferox* e *D. sanguinea*) são usadas no Brasil, na Índia e no Peru para produzir inconsciência. As sementes contêm hioscina (escopolamina), um alcalóide com ação anticolinérgica semelhante à da atropina. [Hindu]

D. me′tel, D. fastuosa L. var. *alba;* uma espécie que contém escopolamina como seu principal alcalóide e traços de hiosciamina e atropina.

D. stramo′nium, estramônio; figueira-brava; figueira-do-inferno; espécie que é a principal fonte de estramônio. SIN Jamestown weed, jimson weed, stink weed, thorn apple.

da·tu·rine (da - too′rin, - rēn). Daturina. SIN hyoscyamine.

Daubenton (D'Aubenton), Louis J.M., médico francês, 1716–1799. VER D. *angle, line, plane*.

daugh·ter (daw'ter). Filha; em medicina nuclear, um isótopo resultante da desintegração de um radionuclídeo. VER daughter *isotope*, radionuclide *generator*. [I. ant. *dohtor*]

DES (diethylstilbestrol) daughter, filha do DES (dietilestilbestrol); a filha de uma mulher que recebeu dietilestilbestrol durante a gravidez; as filhas do DES correm risco de deformidade, adenose e outras alterações epiteliais da vagina e colo do útero, incluindo adenocarcinoma de células claras.

dau·no·my·cin (daw - nō - mī'sin). Daunomicina. SIN daunorubicin.

dau·no·ru·bi·cin (daw - nō - roo'bi - sin). Daunorrubicina; antibiótico do grupo rodomicina, obtido do *Streptomyces peucetius*; usado no tratamento da leucemia aguda; também usado em citogenética para produzir bandas cromossomiais do tipo Q. SIN daunomycin.

Davidoff, M. von, histologista alemão, †1904. VER D. *cells*, em *cell*.

Davidson, Edward C., cirurgião norte-americano, 1894–1933. VER D. *syringe*.

Daviel, Jacques, oculista francês, 1693–1762. VER D. *operation*, *spoon*.

Davies, J.N.P., patologista norte-americano, *1915. VER D. *disease*.

Davis, Hallowell, fisiologista norte-americano, 1896–1992. VER D. battery model of *transduction*.

Davis, John Staige, cirurgião norte-americano, 1872–1946. VER D. *graft*; Crowe-D. mouth *gag*.

Davis, David M., urologista norte-americano, *1886.

Davis in·ter·lock·ing sound. Sonda interligada de Davis. VER em sound.

Dawson, James R., patologista norte-americano, *1908. VER D. *encephalitis*.

Day, Richard H., médico norte-americano, 1813–1892. VER D. *test*.

Day, Richard L., pediatra norte-americano, *1905. VER Riley-D. *syndrome*.

daz·zling. Ofuscamento; a consequência da iluminação demasiado intensa para adaptação do olho; ao contrário do clarão, o ofuscamento é aliviado por óculos apropriadamente coloridos.

dB, db Abreviatura de decibel.

DBP Abreviatura de vitamin D-binding *protein* (proteína de ligação da vitamina D).

DC Abreviatura de direct *current* (corrente contínua).

D & C Abreviatura de dilatação e curetagem.

D.C. Abreviatura de Doctor of Chiropractic (Doutor em Quiroprática).

dCMP Abreviatura de deoxycytidylic acid (ácido desoxicitidílico).

DDA Abreviatura de dideoxyadenosine (didesoxiadenosina).

DDI Abreviatura de dideoxyinosine (didesoxiinosina).

d-dimer (dī'mer). Dímero d; um produto de degradação com ligação cruzada covalente, liberado do polímero de fibrina com ligação cruzada durante a fibrinólise mediada por plasmina; medidas laboratoriais desse produto feitas utilizando contas de látex ou ensaios ELISA podem ser usadas para identificar a presença de fibrinólise.

D.D.S. Abreviatura de Doctor of Dental Surgery (Doutor em Cirurgia Dentária).

DDT Abreviatura de dichlorodiphenyltrichloroethane, (diclorodifeniltricloroetano).

D & E 1. Abreviatura de dilation and evacuation (dilatação e esvaziamento). **2.** Abreviatura de *dilation* and extraction (dilatação e extração).

de-. 1. Distante de, cessação, sem; algumas vezes tem uma força intensiva. **2.** Para os nomes com esse prefixo não encontrados aqui, procurar a parte principal do nome. [L. *de*, de, distante]

de·a·cid·i·fi·ca·tion (dē - a - sid'i - fi - kā'shŭn). Desacidificação; a remoção ou neutralização de ácido.

de·ac·ti·va·tion (dē - ak - ti - vā'shŭn). Desativação; o processo de inativar ou de se tornar inativo.

de·ac·yl·ase (dē - as'il - ās). Desacilase. **1.** Membro da subclasse de hidrolases (EC classe 3), principalmente da subclasse de esterases, lipases, lactonases e hidrolases (EC subclasse 3.1). **2.** Qualquer enzima que catalisa a clivagem hidrolítica de um grupamento acil (R–CO–) em uma ligação éster; também inclui enzimas que clivam ligações amida (EC subclasse 3,5) e compostos acil semelhantes.

dead (ded). **1.** Morto; sem vida. VER TAMBÉM death. **2.** Amortecido.

DEAE-cel·lu·lose. DEAE-celulose. SIN *O-diethylaminoethyl cellulose*.

deaf (def). Surdo; que não ouve. [A.S. *deáf*]

de·af·fer·en·ta·tion (dē - af'er - en - tā'shŭn). Desaferenciação; perda dos estímulos nervosos sensoriais de uma parte do corpo, geralmente causado por interrupção das fibras sensoriais periféricas. [L. *de*, de, + afferent]

deaf·ness (def'nes). Surdez; termo geral que designa incapacidade de ouvir.

central d., s. central; surdez causada por distúrbio do sistema auditivo do tronco cerebral ou do córtex cerebral.

cortical d., s. cortical; surdez resultante de lesões bilaterais da área receptiva primária do lobo temporal.

hereditary d., s. hereditária. VER hereditary *hearing impairment*.

nerve d., neural d., s. nervosa, s. neural; termos usados anteriormente para s. sensorineural.

postlingual d., s. pós-lingual; comprometimento auditivo que ocorre após o desenvolvimento da fala e da linguagem.

surdez causada por displasias do desenvolvimento da cóclea

tipo de defeito do ouvido interno	características principais	alterações morfológicas
tipo Michel (1863)	aplasia completa	aplasia da porção petrosa do osso temporal ou do labirinto ósseo
tipo Mondini (1791)	hipoplasia grave do labirinto ósseo e membranoso	ausência de lâmina espiral na parte proximal da cóclea; alargamento do saco e ducto endolinfáticos; defeito do órgão de Corti
tipo Sceibe (1892)	aplasia do labirinto membranoso (cóclea e sáculo)	sáculo está alargado ou colapsado; o ducto coclear está alargado; o órgão de Corti é aplásico ou hipoplásico, com defeito das células de sustentação ou ciliadas

prelingual d., s. pré-lingual; comprometimento auditivo que ocorre antes do desenvolvimento da fala e da linguagem.

sudden d., s. súbita; perda auditiva sensorial profunda que se desenvolve em 24 horas ou menos; geralmente atribuída a uma infecção viral no ouvido interno.

word d., s. verbal. SIN auditory *aphasia*.

de·al·ba·tion (dē - al - bā'shŭn). Dealbação; branqueamento; o ato de branquear, clarear ou alvejar. [L. *de-albo*, pp. *-atus*, branquear]

de·al·co·hol·i·za·tion (dē - al'kō - hol - i - zā'shŭn). Desalcoolização; a retirada de álcool de um líquido; em técnica histológica, a retirada de álcool de uma amostra que foi previamente imersa nesse líquido.

de·al·ler·gize (dē - al'er - jīz). Desalergizar; termo obsoleto para dessensibilizar.

de·am·i·das·es (dē - am'i - dā - sez). Desamidases. SIN amidohydrolases.

de·am·i·da·tion, de·am·i·di·za·tion (dē - am - i - dā'shŭn, dē - am'i - di - zā'shŭn). Desamidação, desamidização; a remoção hidrolítica de um grupamento amida.

de·am·i·dize (dē - am'i - dīz). Desamidizar; realizar desamidação. SIN desamidize.

de·am·i·nas·es (dē - am'i - nā - sez) [EC 3.5.4.X]. Desaminases; enzimas que catalisam a hidrólise simples de ligações C–NH$_2$ de purinas, pirimidinas e pterinas, assim produzindo amônia (geralmente denominada em termos do substrato, p. ex., guanina desaminase, adenosina desaminase, AMP desaminase, pterina desaminase); geralmente não são usadas para desaminação de amidas acíclicas. As desaminases são distinguidas das amônia-liases (EC 4.3.1.x) porque estas últimas produzem insaturação no ponto de remoção do NH$_3$. SIN deaminating enzymes.

de·am·i·na·tion, de·am·i·ni·za·tion (dē - am - i - nā'shŭn, dē - am'i - ni - zā'shŭn). Desaminação; desaminização; remoção, geralmente por hidrólise, do grupamento NH$_2$ de um composto amino.

oxidative d., d. oxidativa; desaminação por enzimas que utiliza nucleotídeos flavina ou piridina (como FAD ou NAD$^+$).

de·am·in·ize (dē - am'i - nīz). Desaminizar; realizar desaminação.

Dean, Henry Trendley, dentista e epidemiologista norte-americano, 1893–1962. VER D. fluorosis *index*.

de·a·nol ac·et·a·mi·do·ben·zo·ate (dē'ă - nol as - ĕ - tam'i - dō - ben'zō - āt). Acetamidobenzoato de deanol; o sal ácido *p*-acetamidobenzóico do 2-dimetilaminoetanol; um estimulante do sistema nervoso central.

death (dĕth). Morte; a cessação da vida. Em organismos multicelulares inferiores, a morte é um processo gradual ao nível celular, porque os tecidos variam em sua capacidade de resistir à privação de oxigênio; em organismos superiores, é a cessação das funções integradas de tecidos e órgãos; em seres humanos, manifesta-se por desaparecimento dos batimentos cardíacos, ausência de respiração espontânea e morte cerebral. SIN mors. [A.S. *dēath*]

black d., m. negra; termo aplicado à epidemia mundial do século XIV, na qual diz-se que morreram 60 milhões de pessoas; as descrições indicam que se tratava da peste pneumônica.

brain d., m. cerebral. SIN cerebral d.

cerebral d., m. cerebral; síndrome clínica caracterizada pela perda permanente da função cerebral e do tronco cerebral, que se manifesta por ausência de responsividade a estímulos externos, ausência de reflexos cefálicos e apnéia. Um eletroencefalograma isoelétrico durante, no mínimo, 30 minutos, na ausência de hipotermia e intoxicação por depressores do sistema nervoso central, sustenta o diagnóstico. SIN brain d.

d. certificate, atestado de óbito; documento legal, oficial e registro essencial, assinado por médico autorizado ou outra autoridade designada, que inclui causa da morte, nome do morto, sexo, endereço, data da morte; podem ser incluídas outras informações, como, por exemplo, data e local de nascimento, ocupação; a causa imediata da morte é registrada na primeira linha do atestado, seguida pela condição ou condições que a causaram, com a causa subjacente na última linha; a causa subjacente é codificada e catalogada em publicações oficiais de mortalidade.
cot d., m. no berço. SIN sudden infant death *syndrome.*
crib d., m. no berço. SIN sudden infant death *syndrome.*
crude d. rate, taxa de mortalidade bruta. SIN death *rate.*
fetal d., m. fetal; morte antes da expulsão ou extração completa de um produto da concepção, independentemente da duração da gravidez. A morte fetal é considerada *precoce*, se ocorrer nas primeiras 20 semanas de gestação; *intermediária*, se ocorrer entre 21–28 semanas; e *tardia*, se ocorrer após 28 semanas.
genetic d., m. genética; morte do portador de um gene em qualquer idade antes de gerar um descendente vivo. Pode ser compatível com boa saúde e longa vida. VER TAMBÉM genetic *lethal.*
infant d., m. infantil; morte de um lactente nascido vivo no primeiro ano de vida.
local d., m. local; morte de uma parte do corpo ou de um tecido por necrose.
maternal d., m. materna; morte de uma mulher durante a gravidez ou nos primeiros 42 dias após o fim da gestação, independentemente da duração e do local da gravidez e da causa da morte; são reconhecidos dois períodos no intervalo de 42 dias: o primeiro período vai do 1.º ao 7.º dia; o segundo período vai do 8.º ao 42.º dia. As mortes maternas são ainda classificadas como: **m. materna direta,** morte resultante de complicações obstétricas da gestação, trabalho de parto ou puerpério, e de intervenções, omissões, tratamento incorreto ou uma cadeia de eventos causados por qualquer um destes; e **m. materna indireta,** morte obstétrica resultante de doença preexistente ou de doença que se desenvolve durante a gravidez, trabalho de parto ou puerpério; não é diretamente devida a causas obstétricas, mas a condições agravadas pelos efeitos fisiológicos da gravidez.
neonatal d., m. neonatal; morte de um lactente jovem, nascido vivo; classificada como: **m. neonatal precoce,** morte de um recém-nascido vivo que ocorre menos de 7 dias completos (168 horas) após o nascimento; **m. neonatal tardia,** morte de um recém-nascido vivo que ocorre após 7 dias completos de idade, mas antes de 28 dias completos.
perinatal d., m. perinatal; um termo inclusivo que se refere tanto a natimortos quanto a mortes neonatais.
programmed cell d., m. celular programada. SIN apoptosis.
somatic d., systemic d., m. somática, m. sistêmica; morte de todo o corpo; ao contrário da morte local.
sudden d., m. súbita; morte rápida e, em geral, inesperada; habitualmente por arritmia cardíaca ou infarto do miocárdio, mas também por qualquer causa de morte rápida, p. ex., embolia pulmonar, acidente vascular cerebral, ruptura de aneurisma aórtico, dissecção aórtica.

death-rat·tle (deth′rat′l). Estertor de morte; gorgolejo ou estertor respiratório na faringe ou traquéia de uma pessoa agonizante, causado pela perda do reflexo da tosse e acúmulo de muco.

Deaver, John Blair, cirurgião norte-americano, 1855–1931. VER D. *incision.*

Deaver, George G., fisiatra norte-americano, 1890-1973. VER D. *method.*

DeBakey, Michael Ellis, cirurgião cardíaco norte-americano, *1908. VER DeBakey *classification*, DeBakey *forceps.*

de·band·ing (dē - band′ing). Desconexão; retirada de aparelhos ortodônticos fixos.

de·bil·i·tant (dē - bil′i - tant). Debilitante. **1.** Que enfraquece; que causa debilidade. **2.** Termo obsoleto para um agente quelante ou que reprime a excitação. [L. *debilito*, enfraquecer, de *de*, neg., + *habilis*, capaz]

de·bil·i·tat·ing (dē - bil′i - tāt - ing). Debilitante; designa ou é característico de um processo mórbido que causa fraqueza.

de·bil·i·ty (dē - bil′i - tē). Debilidade; fraqueza. [L. *debilitas*, de *debilis*, fraco, de *de-* priv. + *habilis*, capaz]

debond (dē - bond′). Desconectar; separar um dispositivo dentário como uma faixa ortodôntica do dente ao qual foi fixado ou unido por uma resina. [de- + bond]

de·bouch (dē - boosh′). Desembocar; abrir ou esvaziar em outra parte. [Fr. *bouche*, boca]

dé·bouche·ment (dā - boosh - mon′). Desembocadura; abertura ou esvaziamento em outra parte. [Fr.]

Debré, Robert, pediatra e especialista em doenças infecciosas francês, 1882–1978. VER D. *phenomenon*; D.-Séméłaigne *syndrome*; Kocher-D.-Séméłaigne *syndrome.*

dé·bride·ment (dā - brēd - mon′). Desbridamento; excisão de tecido desvitalizado e de material estranho de uma ferida. [Fr. desbridar]

debris (de - brē). Resíduos; fragmentos; detrito; acúmulo inútil de diversas partículas; escória na forma de fragmentos. [Fr. *débris*, do Fr. ant. *desbrisier*, separar (de *des-* para baixo, distante, + *brisier*, romper), detritos, entulho]

particulate wear d., resíduos por desgaste; partículas microscópicas produzidas por atrito entre superfícies articulares em uma prótese articular total; os resíduos podem incluir partículas de metal, polietileno e cimento polimetilmetacrilato, bem como induzir osteólise.

de·bris·o·quine sul·fate (de′ - bris′ō - kwin). Sulfato de debrisoquina; agente anti-hipertensivo semelhante à guanetidina; também usado em estudos do metabolismo farmacológico.

debt (det). Débito; dívida; déficit; obrigação. [L. *debitum*, débito]
alactic oxygen d., débito de oxigênio aláctico; a parte do débito de oxigênio que não é o débito de oxigênio lactácido; durante a recuperação, os depósitos de ATP e fosfato de creatina precisam ser repostos por metabolismo oxidativo, e também é necessária uma pequena quantidade de oxigênio para restaurar os níveis normais de oxi-hemoglobina em todo o sangue circulante.
lactacid oxygen d., d. de oxigênio lactácido; a parte de um débito de oxigênio representada pela produção de ácido láctico por glicólise anaeróbica durante exercício e, portanto, pela necessidade de eliminá-lo por metabolismo oxidativo durante a recuperação.
oxygen d., d. de oxigênio; o oxigênio adicional, captado pelo organismo durante a recuperação do exercício, além das suas necessidades em repouso; algumas vezes é usado como sinônimo de déficit de oxigênio.

deca- (**da**). Prefixo usado nos sistemas SI e métrico para indicar múltiplos de 10. Também escrito deka-. [G. *deka*, dez]

dec·a·gram (dek′ā - gram). Decagrama; dez gramas.

de·cal·ci·fi·ca·tion (dē′kal - si - fi - kā′shŭn). Descalcificação. **1.** Remoção de cal ou sais de cálcio, principalmente fosfato tricálcico, dos ossos e dentes, seja *in vitro* ou *in vivo* em virtude de um processo mórbido. **2.** Precipitação de cálcio do sangue como pelo oxalato ou fluoreto, ou a conversão do cálcio sanguíneo em uma forma não-ionizada, como por citrato, assim impedindo ou retardando a coagulação. [L. *de-*, afastamento, + *calx* (*calc*-), cal, + *facio*, fazer]

de·cal·ci·fy (dē - kal′si - fī). Descalcificar; remover cal ou sais de cálcio, principalmente dos ossos ou dentes.

de·cal·ci·fy·ing (dē - kal′si - fī - ing). Descalcificante; indica um agente, medida ou processo que causa descalcificação.

dec·a·li·ter (dek′ā - lē - ter). Decalitro; dez litros.

de·cal·vant (dē - kal′vant). Decalvante; que remove os pêlos; que torna calvo. [L. *decalvare*, tornar calvo]

dec·a·me·ter (dek′ā - mē - ter). Decâmetro; dez metros.

dec·a·me·tho·ni·um bro·mide (dek - ā - me - thō′nē - ŭm). Brometo de decametônio; um bloqueador neuromuscular não-despolarizante sintético usado para produzir relaxamento muscular durante anestesia geral.

dec·a·mine (dek′ā - mēn). Decamina. SIN dequalinium acetate.

***n*-dec·ane** (dek′ān). *n*-Decano; um hidrocarboneto da parafina, CH_3–$(CH_2)_8$–CH_3.

de·can·nul·a·tion (dē - kan - ū - lā′shun). Descanulização; retirada planejada ou acidental de um tubo de traqueostomia.

***n*-dec·a·no·ic ac·id** (dek - ā - nō′ik). Ácido *n*-decanóico. SIN *n*-capric acid.

dec·a·no·in (dek - ā - nō′in). Decanoína. SIN caprin.

dec·a·nor·mal (dek - ā - nor′mal). Decanormal; termo raramente usado que designa a concentração de uma solução 10 vezes maior que o normal.

de·cant (dē - kant′). Decantar; retirar delicadamente a porção clara superior de um líquido, deixando o sedimento no vaso. [L. Mediev. *decantho*, de *de-* + *canthus*, o bico de um jarro, do G. *kanthos*, ângulo do olho]

de·can·ta·tion (dē - kan - tā′shŭn). Decantação; retirada da parte superior clara de um líquido, deixando um sedimento ou precipitado.

de·ca·pac·i·ta·tion (dē′kā - pas - i - tā′shŭn). Descapacitação; impedimento da capacitação dos espermatozóides e, portanto, da sua capacidade de fertilizar os óvulos. VER TAMBÉM decapacitation *factor.*

dec·a·pep·tide (dek′ā - pep′tīd). Decapeptídeo; um oligopeptídeo contendo 10 aminoácidos.

de·cap·i·tate (dē - kap′i - tāt). **1.** Decapitar; cortar a cabeça; especificamente, remover a cabeça de um feto para facilitar o parto em casos de distocia irremediável; cortar a cabeça de um animal no preparo para determinadas experiências fisiológicas; termo obsoleto. **2.** Decapitado; relativo a um animal experimental com a cabeça removida. [L. *de-*, para longe, + *caput*, cabeça]

de·cap·i·ta·tion (dē - kap - i - tā′shŭn). Decapitação; remoção de uma cabeça. VER decapitate.

de·cap·su·la·tion (dē - kap - soo - lā′shŭn). Descapsulação; incisão e remoção de uma cápsula ou membrana envolvente.
d. of kidney, d. renal; remoção ou desnudamento da cápsula renal.

de·car·bo·ni·za·tion (dē - kar′bon - i - zā′shŭn). Descarbonização; termo raramente usado que designa o processo de arterialização do sangue por oxigenação e remoção de dióxido de carbono nos pulmões.

de·car·box·yl·ase (dē - kar - boks′e - lās). Descarboxilase; qualquer enzima (EC 4.1.1.x) que remova uma molécula de dióxido de carbono de um grupamento carboxílico (p. ex., de um α-aminoácido, convertendo-o em uma amina).

de·car·box·yl·a·tion (dē′kar - boks - ē - lā′shŭn). Descarboxilação; uma reação que envolve a remoção de uma molécula de dióxido de carbono de um ácido carboxílico.

oxidative d., d. oxidativa; descarboxilação que exige a participação de coenzimas como NAD⁺, NADP⁺, FAD ou FMN.

de·cay (dē - kā′). 1. Decomposição; destruição de uma substância orgânica por combustão lenta ou oxidação gradual. 2. Putrefação. SIN putrefaction. 3. Deteriorar; sofrer combustão ou putrefação lenta. 4. Em odontologia, cárie. 5. Em psicologia, perda de informações registradas pelos sentidos e processadas na memória de curto prazo. VER TAMBÉM memory. 6. Decaimento; perda de radioatividade com o tempo; emissão espontânea de radiação e/ou partículas carregadas de um núcleo instável. [L. *de*, para baixo, + *cado*, cair]
  free induction d. (FID), decaimento da indução livre; em ressonância magnética, a curva de decaimento detectada pela bobina receptora após a aplicação de um pulso excitatório, sem pulsos adicionais.

de·cel·er·a·tion (dē - sel - er - ā′shŭn). Desaceleração. 1. O ato de desacelerar. 2. A taxa de diminuição da velocidade por unidade de tempo.
  early d., d. inicial; lentificação da freqüência cardíaca fetal no início da fase de contração uterina, denotando compressão da cabeça fetal.
  late d., d. tardia; qualquer bradicardia fetal transitória, cujo nadir ocorre após o pico da contração uterina. Pode representar insuficiência uteroplacentária.
  variable d., d. variável; bradicardia fetal transitória que, geralmente, denota compressão do cordão umbilical, podendo ocorrer em qualquer momento em relação a uma contração uterina.

de·cen·tra·tion (dē - sen - trā′shŭn). Descentralização; remoção do centro.

de·cer·e·brate (dē - ser′ē - brāt). 1. Descerebrar; causar descerebração. 2. Descerebrado; designa um animal assim preparado, ou um paciente cujo cérebro sofreu uma lesão que torna o paciente, em termos de comportamento neurológico, comparável a um animal descerebrado.

de·cer·e·bra·tion (dē - ser′ē - brā′shŭn). Descerebração; retirada do cérebro acima da borda inferior dos corpos quadrigêmeos, ou uma secção completa do encéfalo nesse nível ou um pouco abaixo.
  bloodless d., d. incruenta; destruição da função do cérebro por ligadura da artéria basilar aproximadamente no meio da ponte e nas artérias carótidas comuns no pescoço.

de·cer·e·brize (dē - ser′ē - brīz). Descerebrar; remover o cérebro.

de·chlo·ri·da·tion (dē′klor - i - dā′shŭn). Desclorização; descloretação; redução do cloreto de sódio nos tecidos e líquidos do corpo mediante redução de sua ingestão ou aumento de sua excreção. SIN dechlorination, dechloruration.

de·chlo·ri·na·tion (dē′klor - i - nā′shŭn). Desclorização. SIN dechloridation.

de·chlo·ru·ra·tion (dē′klor - oo - rā′shŭn). Descloretação. SIN dechloridation.

de·cho·les·ter·ol·i·za·tion (dē′kō - les′ter - ol - i - zā′shŭn). Descolesterolização; redução terapêutica da concentração de colesterol no sangue.

deci- (d). Prefixo usado no sistema SI e métrico para indicar um décimo (10⁻¹). [L. *decimus*, décimo]

dec·i·bel (dB, db) (des′i - bel). Decibel; um décimo de um bel; unidade para expressar a intensidade relativa do som em uma escala logarítmica. [L. *decimus*, décimo, + bel]

de·cid·ua (dē - sid′ū - ă). Decídua. SIN deciduous *membrane*. [L. *deciduus*, caindo (*membrana* qualificante, membrana, conhecimento]
  d. basa′lis, d. basal; a área de endométrio entre a vesícula coriônica implantada e o miométrio, que se transforma na parte materna da placenta. SIN d. serotina.
  d. capsula′ris, d. capsular; a camada de endométrio sobre a vesícula coriônica implantada; sofre atenuação progressiva, à medida que vesícula coriônica aumenta, e, no quarto mês, é comprimida contra a decídua parietal, sofrendo, a seguir, regressão rápida. SIN d. reflexa, membrana adventitia (2).
  ectopic d., d. ectópica; células deciduais que podem ser encontradas no colo uterino, no apêndice ou em outras áreas além do endométrio.
  d. menstrua′lis, d. menstrual; a mucosa suculenta do útero não-grávido no período menstrual.
  d. parieta′lis, d. parietal; a mucosa alterada que reveste a cavidade principal do útero grávido, além do local de fixação da vesícula coriônica. SIN d. vera.
  d. polypo′sa, d. polipposa; decídua parietal que exibe projeções polipóides da superfície endometrial.
  d. reflex′a, d. reflexa. SIN d. capsularis.
  d. seroti′na, d. serotina. SIN d. basalis.
  d. spongio′sa, d. esponjosa; a porção da decídua basal fixada ao miométrio.
  d. ve′ra, d. vera. SIN d. parietalis.

de·cid·u·al (dē - sid′ū - al). Decidual; relativo à decídua.

de·cid·u·ate (dē - sid′ū - āt). Deciduado; relativo aos mamíferos (p. ex., seres humanos, cães, roedores) que eliminam tecido uterino materno durante a expulsão da placenta no parto, ao contrário dos mamíferos não-deciduados (cavalo, porco). [VER deciduation]

de·cid·u·a·tion (dē - sid - ū - ā′shŭn). Deciduação; eliminação do tecido endometrial durante a menstruação. [L. *deciduus*, que cai]

de·cid·u·i·tis (dē - sid - ū - ī′tis). Deciduíte; inflamação da decídua.

de·cid·u·o·ma (dē - sid - ū - ō′mă). Deciduoma; uma massa intra-uterina de tecido decidual, provavelmente resultante de hiperplasia das células deciduais retidas no útero. SIN placentoma.
  Loeb d., d. de Loeb; massa de tecido decidual produzida no útero, na ausência de um óvulo fertilizado, por meio de estimulação mecânica ou hormonal.

de·cid·u·ous (dē - sid′ū - ŭs). Decíduo. 1. Não-permanente; designa aquilo que acabará por se desprender. 2. **(D)** (em fórmulas dentárias). Em odontologia, freqüentemente usado para designar a primeira dentição ou dentição primária. VER deciduous *tooth*. [L. *deciduus*, que cai]

dec·i·gram (des′i - gram). Decigrama; a décima parte de um grama.

dec·i·li·ter (des′i - lē - ter). Decilitro; a décima parte de um litro.

dec·i·me·ter (des′i - mē - ter). Decímetro; a décima parte de um metro.

dec·i·mor·gan (des′i - mōr - gan). Decimorgan. VER morgan.

dec·i·nor·mal (des - i - nōr′mal). Decinormal; um décimo do normal, indicando a concentração de uma solução.

decision. Decisão. 1. Ato ou efeito de decidir ou decidir-se; 2. Resolução após discussão ou exame prévio.
  limiting d., d. determinante; uma compreensão de si próprio atingida em virtude de resposta a um evento significativo ou traumático. VER TAMBÉM Time-Line *therapy*.

de·ci·sion tree. Árvore de decisão; escolhas alternativas disponíveis em cada estágio de decisão sobre como administrar um problema clínico, apresentada graficamente; em cada ramo ou nó de decisão, são mostradas as probabilidades de cada resultado (desfecho) que pode ser previsto; o valor relativo de cada resultado é descrito em termos de sua utilidade no que diz respeito à qualidade de vida, p. ex., conforme medido por probabilidade de morte, expectativa de vida ou ausência de incapacidade.

de Clerambault, G., psiquiatra francês, 1872–1934. VER de C. *syndrome*.

dec·lin·a·tor (dek′lin - ā - ter, -tōr). Declinador; um afastador que mantém certas estruturas afastadas durante uma operação.

de·clive (dē - klīv′) [TA]. Declive; a porção posterior descendente do montículo do verme do cerebelo; lóbulo do verme situado imediatamente caudal à fissura primária; lóbulo VI. SIN declivis, lobulus clivi. [L. *declivis*, inclinação descendente, de *clivus*, inclinação]

de·cli·vis (dē - klī′vis). Declive. SIN declive.

de·coc·tion (dē - kok′shŭn). Decocção. 1. O processo de fervura. 2. O nome farmacopeico de preparações feitas pela fervura de medicamentos vegetais brutos e, depois, filtradas, na proporção de 50 g da droga para 1.000 ml de água. SIN apozem, apozema. [L. *decoctio*, de *de-coquo*, pp. *-coctus*, ferver]

dé·colle·ment (dā - kŭl - mon′). Descolamento; termo raramente usado para separação cirúrgica de tecidos ou órgãos aderidos, normal ou anormalmente. [Fr. descolar]

de·com·pen·sa·tion (de′kom - pen - sā′shŭn). Descompensação. 1. Ausência de compensação na cardiopatia. 2. O surgimento ou exacerbação de um distúrbio mental devido à falha dos mecanismos de defesa.
  corneal d., d. corneal; edema da córnea resultante da incapacidade do endotélio córneo de manter a deturgescência.

de·com·pose (dē′kom - pōz). Decompor. 1. Separar um composto em seus componentes; desintegrar. 2. Deteriorar; putrefazer. [L. *de*, de, baixo, + *compono*, pp. *-positus*, colocar junto]

de.com·po·si·tion (dē′kom - pō - zish′ŭn). Decomposição. SIN putrefaction.

de·com·pres·sion (dē′kom - presh - ŭn). Descompressão; remoção de pressão. [L. *de*, de, baixo, + *com-primo*, pp. *- pressus*, pressionar junto]
  cardiac d., d. cardíaca; incisão do pericárdio ou aspiração de líquido do pericárdio para aliviar a pressão devida ao sangue ou outro líquido no saco pericárdico. SIN pericardial d.
  cerebral d., d. cerebral; remoção de um pedaço do crânio, com incisão da duramáter, para aliviar a pressão intracraniana.
  explosive d., d. explosiva. SIN rapid d.
  internal d., d. interna; remoção de tecido intracraniano, geralmente tumor, hematoma ou tecido cerebral; para aliviar a pressão.
  nerve d., d. nervosa; liberação de pressão sobre um tronco nervoso pela excisão cirúrgica de faixas constritivas ou alargamento de um canal ósseo.
  optic nerve sheath d., d. da bainha do nervo óptico; a abertura da bainha do nervo óptico para o espaço retrobulbar, por incisão ou fenestração da bainha. VER optic nerve sheath *fenestration*.
  orbital d., d. orbitária; remoção de uma parte da órbita óssea, geralmente superior (operação de Naffziger), lateral (operação de Krönlein) ou inferior (operação de Ogura).
  pericardial d., d. pericárdica. SIN cardiac d.
  rapid d., d. rápida; grande expansão súbita de gases devido a uma redução da pressão ambiente. SIN explosive d.
  spinal d., d. espinal; a remoção da pressão sobre a medula espinal criada por um tumor, cisto, hematoma, hérnia do núcleo pulposo, abscesso ou osso.
  suboccipital d., d. suboccipital; descompressão da fossa posterior por craniectomia occipital e abertura da dura-máter.
  subtemporal d., d. subtemporal; descompressão do cérebro por craniectomia temporal e abertura da dura-máter sobre a superfície ínfero-lateral do lobo temporal.
  trigeminal d., d. do trigêmeo; descompressão da raiz do nervo trigêmeo.

de·con·ges·tant (dē - kon - jes′tant). Descongestionante. 1. SIN decongestive. 2. Um agente que possui essa ação.

de·con·ges·tive (dē - kon - jes′tiv). Descongestivo; que possui a propriedade de reduzir o edema tecidual. SIN decongestant (1).

de·con·tam·i·na·tion (dē′kon - tam - i - nā′shŭn). Descontaminação; remoção ou neutralização de gás venenoso ou outros agentes prejudiciais do ambiente.

de·con·vo·lu·tion (dē - con - vō - loo′shŭn). Desconvolução; uma técnica matemática para solução de funções cuja entrada inclui sua saída; usada para resolver os elementos de imagem em tomografia computadorizada ou ressonância magnética. [de- + L. *convulutio*, enrolamento, de *convolvo*, enrolar-se]

de·cor·ti·ca·tion (dē - kor - ti - kā′shŭn). Decorticação. **1.** Remoção do córtex, ou camada externa, sob a cápsula de qualquer órgão ou estrutura. **2.** Uma operação para remoção do coágulo residual e/ou do tecido cicatricial recém-organizado que se forma após um hemotórax ou empiema negligenciado. [L. *decortico*, pp. *-atus*, retirar a casca, de *de*, de, + *cortex*, casca]
  cerebral d., d. cerebral; destruição do córtex cerebral, geralmente devido a anoxia.
  reversible d., d. reversível; perda temporária da função do córtex cerebral.

dec·re·ment (dek′rē - ment). **1.** Diminuição. **2.** Diminuição da velocidade de condução em determinado ponto; resultante de alteração das propriedades nesse ponto. VER TAMBÉM decremental *conduction*. [L. *decrementum*, de *decresco*, diminuir]

de·crep·i·ta·tion (dē - krep - i - tā′shŭn). Crepitação; o estalido de determinados sais quando aquecidos. [L. *de*, de, + *crepo*, pp. *crepitus*, crepitar]

de·cru·des·cence (dē - kroo - des′ens). Decrudescência; diminuição dos sintomas de uma doença. [L. *de*, de, + *crudesco*, agravar, de *crudus*, rude]

de·cu·bi·tal (dē - kū′bi - tăl). Decúbito; relativo a uma úlcera de decúbito.

de·cu·bi·tus (dē - kū′bi - tŭs). Decúbito. **1.** A posição do paciente na cama; p. ex., d. dorsal, d. lateral. VER decubitus *film*. **2.** Algumas vezes usado em referência a uma úlcera de decúbito (decubitus *ulcer*). [L. *decumbo*, deitar]
  Andral d., d. de Andral; posição adotada pelo paciente que se deita sobre o lado sadio em casos de pleurisia inicial.
  ventral d., d. ventral; úlceras de pressão (ulceração de decúbito) que ocorrem em localizações ventrais, como a parede abdominal ou a superfície anterior de um membro.

de·cur·rent (dē - kŭr′ent). Que se estende para baixo. [L. *de-curro*, pp. *-cursus*, correr para baixo]

de·cus·sate (dē′kŭ - sāt, dē - kŭs′āt). Decussar. **1.** Cruzar. **2.** Cruzado como os braços de um X. [L. *decusso*, pp. *-atus*, tomar a forma de um X, de *decussis*, uma grande moeda romana, de bronze (século II a.C.) de 10 unidades, marcada com um X para indicar sua denominação]

de·cus·sa·tio, pl. **de·cus·sa·ti·o·nes** (dē - kŭ - sā′shē - ō, - ō′nēz) [TA]. Decussação. **1.** Em geral, qualquer cruzamento ou interseção de partes. **2.** O entrecruzamento de dois feixes de fibras homônimos quando cada um cruza para o lado oposto do encéfalo no trajeto de sua subida ou descida através do tronco cerebral ou da medula espinal. SIN decussation. [L. (VER decussate)]
  d. bra'chii conjuncti'vi, d. dos pedúnculos cerebelares superiores. SIN *decussation* of superior cerebellar peduncles.
  d. fibrarum nervo'rum trochlear'ium [TA], d. das fibras do nervo troclear. SIN *decussation* of trochlear nerve fibers.
  d. fontina'lis, d. tegmentais. VER decussationes tegmentales.
  d. lemnisci mediales [TA], d. do lemnisco medial. SIN *decussation* of medial lemnisci.
  d. moto'ria, d. das pirâmides. SIN *decussation* of pyramids.
  d. pedunculo'rum cerebella'rium superio'rum [TA], d. dos pedúnculos cerebelares superiores. SIN *decussation* of superior cerebellar peduncles.
  d. pyram'idum [TA], d. das pirâmides. SIN *decussation* of pyramids.
  d. senso'ria, d. do lemnisco medial. SIN *decussation* of medial lemniscus.
  decussatio'nes tegmen'tales [TA], decussações tegmentais. SIN tegmental *decussations*, em *decussation*.
  d. tegmentalis anterior [TA], d. tegmental anterior. VER tegmental *decussations*, em *decussation*.
  d. tegmentalis posterior [TA], d. tegmental posterior. VER tegmental *decussations*, em *decussation*.

de·cus·sa·tion (dē - kŭ - sā′shŭn). Decussação. SIN decussatio. [L. *decussatio*]
  anterior tegmental d. [TA], d. tegmental anterior. VER tegmental d.'s (2).
  d. of brachia conjunctiva, d. dos pedúnculos cerebelares superiores. SIN d. of superior cerebellar peduncles.
  dorsal tegmental d. [TA], d. tegmental posterior. VER tegmental d.'s.
  d. of the fillet, d. do lemnisco medial. SIN d. of medial lemniscus.
  Forel d., d. de Forel. VER tegmental d.'s (2).
  fountain d., d. tegmentais. VER tegmental d.'s (1).
  Held d., d. de Held; o cruzamento de algumas fibras originárias dos núcleos cocleares para formar o lemnisco lateral.
  d. of medial lemniscus, d. do lemnisco medial; o entrecruzamento das fibras dos lemniscos mediais direito e esquerdo, que ascendem dos núcleos grácil e cuneiforme, imediatamente rostral ao nível da decussação dos tratos piramidais no bulbo. SIN decussatio lemnisci mediales [TA], decussatio sensoria, d. of the fillet, sensory d. of medulla oblongata.
  Meynert d., d. de Meynert. VER tegmental d.'s (1).

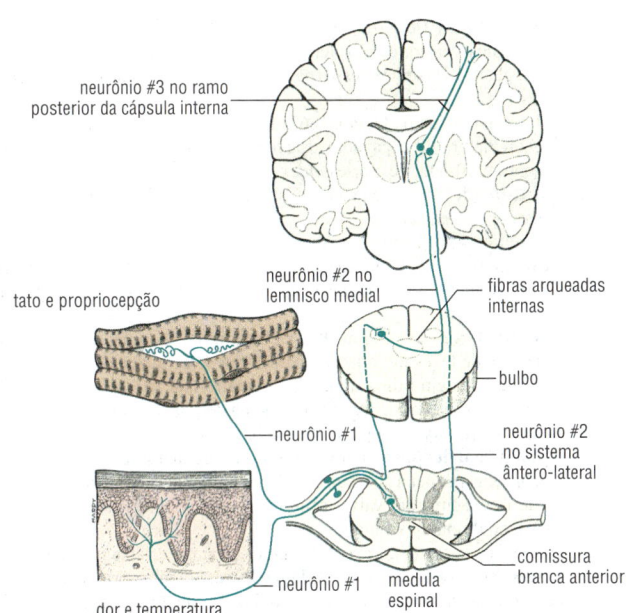

representação em diagrama das **decussações** de alguns tratos ascendentes; os neurônios de primeira ordem para o tato e propriocepção ascendem nas colunas posteriores para fazer sinapse em neurônios de segunda ordem no bulbo; os axônios desses neurônios de segunda ordem cruzam a linha média e ascendem até o tálamo através do lemnisco medial; os neurônios de primeira ordem para dor e temperatura entram no corno posterior para fazer sinapse em neurônios de segunda ordem aí localizados; os axônios desses neurônios de segunda ordem cruzam a linha média na comissura branca anterior e ascendem até o tálamo no sistema ântero-lateral; os neurônios de terceira ordem conectam o tálamo ao córtex cerebral

  motor d., d. das pirâmides. SIN d. of pyramids.
  optic d., d. óptica. SIN optic *chiasm*.
  posterior tegmental d. [TA], d. tegmental posterior. VER tegmental d.'s (1).
  d. of pyramids [TA], d. das pirâmides; o entrecruzamento dos feixes de fibras corticoespinais na região da borda inferior do bulbo. SIN decussatio pyramidum [TA], decussatio motoria, motor d.
  rubrospinal d., d. rubroespinal. VER tegmental d.'s (2).
  sensory d. of medulla oblongata, d. do lemnisco medial. SIN d. of medial lemniscus.
  d. of superior cerebellar peduncles [TA], d. dos pedúnculos cerebelares superiores; a decussação dos pedúnculos cerebelares superiores direitos no tegmento do mesencéfalo caudal. SIN decussatio pedunculorum cerebellarium superiorum [TA], decussatio brachii conjunctivi, d. of brachia conjunctiva, Wernekinck d.
  tectospinal d., d. tegmentais. VER tegmental d.'s (1).
  tegmental d.'s, decussações tegmentais; **(1)** a decussação tegmental posterior [TA] (dorsal tegmental decussation [TA], fountain d., Meynert's d.) é formada pelo cruzamento dos tratos tetospinal e tetobulbar direito e esquerdo; **(2)** a decussação tegmental anterior [TA] (ventral tegmental decussation [TA], Forel's decussation) é formada pelo cruzamento dos tratos rubrospinal e rubrobulbar; ambas as decussações estão localizadas no mesencéfalo. SIN decussationes tegmentales [TA].
  d. of trochlear nerve fibers [TA], d. das fibras do nervo troclear; o cruzamento dos dois nervos trocleares em sua saída através do véu medular anterior. SIN decussatio fibrarum nervorum trochlearium [TA].
  ventral tegmental d., d. tegmental ventral. VER tegmental d.'s (2).
  Wernekinck d., d. de Wernekinck. SIN d. of superior cerebellar peduncles.

de·cus·sa·ti·o·nes (dē - kŭs - ā - shē - ō′nēz). Decussações. Plural de decussatio.

de·den·ti·tion (dē - den - tish′ŭn). Desdentição; termo obsoleto que significa perda dos dentes.

de·dif·fer·en·ti·a·tion (dē - dif′er - en - shē - ā′shŭn). Desdiferenciação. **1.** O retorno das partes a um estado mais homogêneo. **2.** Anaplasia. SIN anaplasia.

de·do·la·tion (dē - dō - lā′shŭn). Decepação; ferida cortante produzida por um instrumento cortante que tangencia a superfície. [L. *de-dolo*, pp. *-atus*, decepars]

de·duc·tion (dē - dŭk′shŭn). Dedução; a derivação lógica de uma conclusão a partir de determinadas premissas. A conclusão será verdadeira se as premissas forem verdadeiras e o argumento dedutivo for válido. Cf. induction (9).

de-ef·fer·en·ta·tion (dē - ef - er - en - tā′shŭn). Desaferentação; perda das fibras nervosas motoras para uma área do corpo. [L. *de*, de, + efferent]

deep (dēp) [TA]. Profundo; situado em um nível mais profundo em relação a um ponto de referência específico. Cf. superficialis. SIN profundus [TA].

de·ep·i·car·di·al·i·za·tion (dē - ep - i - kar′dē - al - i - zā′shŭn). Desepicardialização; destruição cirúrgica obsoleta do epicárdio, geralmente pela aplicação de fenol, planejada (sem sucesso) para promover circulação colateral para o miocárdio.

Deetjen, Hermann, médico alemão, 1867–1915. VER D. *bodies,* em *body.*

def, DEF Abreviatura de decayed, extracted and filled tooth (dente cariado, extraído e obturado). VER def caries *index.*

de·fat·i·ga·tion (dē - fat - i - gā′shŭn). Cansaço; exaustão ou fadiga extrema. [L. *de-fatigo,* pp. *-atus,* cansar]

def·e·cate (def′ē - kāt). Defecar; realizar defecação.

def·e·ca·tion (def - ē - kā′shŭn). Defecação; a eliminação de fezes do reto. SIN motion (2), movement (3). [L. *defaeco,* pp. *-atus,* remover os resíduos, purificar]

de·fec·og·ra·phy (de - fē - kog′ra - fē). Defecografia; exame radiográfico do ato de defecação de fezes radiopacas. [defecation + G. *graphō,* escrever]

de·fect (dē′fekt). Defeito; uma imperfeição, malformação, disfunção ou ausência; um atributo de qualidade, ao contrário da deficiência, que é um atributo da quantidade. [L. *deficio,* pp. *–fectus,* falhar, faltar]

aortic septal d., aorticopulmonary septal d., d. septal aórtico, d. septal aorticopulmonar; uma pequena abertura congênita entre a aorta e a artéria pulmonar, cerca de 1 cm acima das valvas semilunares, p. ex., janela aorticopulmonar. SIN aorticopulmonary window.

atrial septal d., d. do septo interatrial; comunicação interatrial; um defeito congênito no septo entre os átrios, devido à falha do fechamento normal do forame *primum* ou *secundum;* pode envolver os coxins do canal atrioventricular; algumas vezes, há fortes evidências de herança autossômica dominante [MIM*108800]. Em grau variável, também é uma característica comum da síndrome de Ellis-van Creveld autossômica recessiva (Ellis-van Creveld *syndrome*) [MIM*225500] e da síndrome de Holt-Oram autossômica dominante (Holt-Oram *syndrome*) [MIM*142900].

atrial ventricular canal d., d. do canal atrioventricular; defeito causado por deficiência ou ausência de tecido septal imediatamente acima e abaixo do nível normal das valvas atrioventriculares, incluindo a região normalmente ocupada pelo septo A-V em corações com dois ventrículos. As valvas A-V são anormais em grau variável.

birth d., d. congênito; defeito presente ao nascimento.

congenital ectodermal d., d. ectodérmico congênito. SIN congenital ectodermal *dysplasia.*

coupling d., bócio familiar. VER familial *goiter.*

Eisenmenger d., d. de Eisenmenger. SIN Eisenmenger *complex.*

endocardial cushion d., d. do coxim endocárdico. SIN persistent atrioventricular *canal.*

fibrous cortical d., d. cortical fibroso; um defeito comum, medindo 1 a 3 cm, no córtex de um osso, mais comum na porção inferior da diáfise femoral de uma criança, preenchido por tecido fibroso. Por convenção, o *fibroma* não-osteogênico ou não-ossificante refere-se a lesões com mais de 3 cm de diâmetro. VER TAMBÉM nonossifying *fibroma.* SIN nonosteogenic fibroma.

filling d., d. de enchimento; deslocamento do contraste por uma lesão expansiva em um estudo radiográfico de uma víscera oca cheia de contraste, como um pólipo em um enema baritado (clister opaco); também é aplicado a defeitos na distribuição uniforme de radionuclídeo em um órgão, como uma metástase hepática em uma cintigrafia com colóide de enxofre marcado com Tc^{99m}.

Gerbode d., d. de Gerbode; um defeito na porção interventricular do septo membranoso, associado a uma comunicação entre o ventrículo direito e o átrio direito através de uma anormalidade na valva tricúspide.

iodide transport d., bócio familiar. VER familial *goiter.*

iodotyrosine deiodinase d., bócio familiar. VER familial *goiter.*

luteal phase d., d. da fase lútea; distúrbio caracterizado por secreção inadequada de progesterona durante a fase lútea do ciclo menstrual, com conseqüente infertilidade; função lútea subnormal comumente atribuída à secreção anormal de gonadotrofina hipofisária. SIN luteal phase deficiency.

metaphyseal fibrous cortical d., d. cortical fibroso metafisário; um pequeno defeito cortical fibroso localizado na metáfise de um osso longo.

organification d., bócio familiar. VER familial *goiter.*

osteoporotic marrow d. (os′tē - ō - pō - rō′tik). Defeito osteoporótico da medula óssea; defeito osteoporótico focal da medula óssea da mandíbula; um defeito radiotransparente focal composto de medula óssea normal.

postinfarction ventricular septal d., d. do septo interventricular pós-infarto; comunicação interventricular pós-infarto; um defeito no septo interventricular resultante da ruptura de um infarto agudo do miocárdio.

relative afferent pupillary d., d. pupilar aferente relativo. VER relative afferent *pupillary* defect.

salt-losing d., d. perdedor de sal; anormalidade tubular renal que causa perda de sódio na urina.

ventricular septal d., d. do septo interventricular; comunicação interventricular; defeito congênito no septo (membranoso ou muscular) entre os ventrículos cardíacos, geralmente resultante da falha de fechamento do forame interventricular pelo septo espiral.

de·fec·tive (dē - fek′tiv). Defeituoso; que designa ou exibe um defeito; imperfeito; uma falha da qualidade.

de·fem·i·na·tion (dē - fem - i - nā′shŭn). Desfeminização; um enfraquecimento ou perda das características femininas. [L. *de-,* afastamento, + *femina,* mulher]

de·fense (dē - fens′). Defesa; os mecanismos psicológicos usados para controlar a ansiedade, p. ex., racionalização, projeção. [L. *defendo,* repelir, afastar]

screen d., o uso de memórias ou afetos falsos ou incompletos para encobrir memórias e afetos reprimidos, mas associados.

ur-d.'s, Defesas primitivas. VER ur-defenses.

de·fen·sins (dē - fen′sinz). Defensinas; classe de antibióticos polipeptídicos básicos, encontrados em neutrófilos, que destroem bactérias por lesão da membrana. Esses peptídeos citotóxicos contêm 29-38 resíduos de aminoácidos. [L. *de-fendo,* pp. *de-fensum,* repelir, afastar, + *-in*]

def·er·ent (def′er - ent). Deferente; que leva para fora. [L. *deferens,* p. pres. de *defero,* levar embora]

def·er·en·tial (def - er - en′shăl). Deferencial, deferente; relativo ao ducto deferente.

def·er·en·ti·tis (def′er - en - tī′tis). Deferentite; inflamação do ducto deferente. SIN vasitis.

de·fer·ox·a·mine mes·y·late (de - fer - ok′să - mēn). Mesilato de deferoxamina; quelato usado no tratamento da intoxicação por ferro. SIN desferrioxamine mesylate.

de·fer·ves·cence (def - er - ves′ens). Defervescência; diminuição de uma temperatura elevada; diminuição da febre. [L. *de-fervesco,* cessar a fervura, de *de-* neg. + *fervesco,* começar a ferver]

de·fi·bril·la·tion (dē - fib - ri - lā′shŭn). Desfibrilação; a interrupção da fibrilação do músculo cardíaco (atrial ou ventricular) com restauração do ritmo normal, se bem-sucedida.

de·fi·bril·la·tor (dē - fib′ri - lā - ter). Desfibrilador. **1.** Qualquer agente ou medida, p. ex., um choque elétrico, que interrompe a fibrilação do músculo

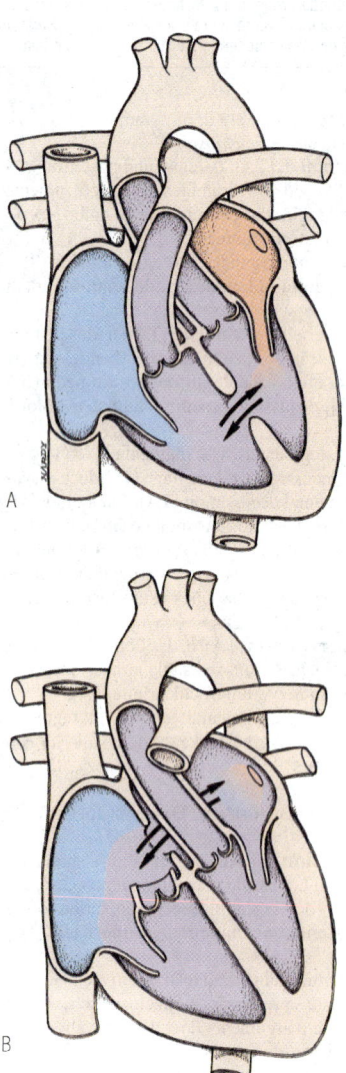

defeitos septais: (A) defeito interventricular, (B) defeito interatrial

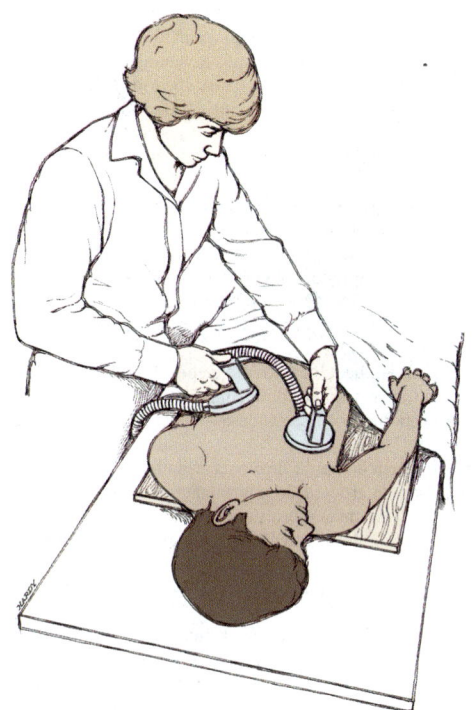

desfibrilação ventricular: colocação das pás

ventricular e restaura o batimento normal. **2.** O aparelho designado para administrar um choque elétrico desfibrilante.
external d., d. externo; um desfibrilador que administra seu choque desfibrilante através da parede torácica fechada.
de·fi·bri·na·tion (dē - fī - bri - nā′shŭn). Desfibrinação; retirada de fibrina do sangue, geralmente por meio de agitação constante enquanto o sangue é colhido em um recipiente com pérolas ou lascas de vidro.
de·fi·cien·cy (dē - fish′en - sē). Deficiência; uma quantidade insuficiente de algumas substâncias (como na deficiência alimentar ou na deficiência de hemoglobina na aplasia da medula óssea); organização (como na deficiência mental); atividade (como na deficiência enzimática ou redução da capacidade de transporte de oxigênio do sangue), etc., da qual a quantidade presente é de qualidade normal. VER TAMBÉM deficiency *disease*. [L. *deficio*, falhar, de *facio*, fazer]
adult lactase d., d. de lactase do adulto; início de deficiência de lactase, com conseqüente intolerância ao leite e má absorção na vida adulta. As formas hereditárias podem não se manifestar até a vida adulta; qualquer processo que lese as células do revestimento intestinal pode causar deficiência de lactase em adultos.
antitrypsin d., d. de antitripsina; a deficiência de α₁-antitripsina, um inibidor da protease (IP) sérica, está associada a enfisema e/ou cirrose hepática. Por focalização isoelétrica, foram identificadas numerosas variantes, com diferentes níveis de atividade normal; herança autossômica recessiva, causada por mutação no gene P1 no cromossoma 14q.
α₁-antitrypsin d., d. de α₁-antitripsina; ausência de um inibidor da proteinase sérica que pode causar paniculite não-supurativa nodular recidivante.
arch length d., d. do comprimento do arco; a diferença entre a circunferência disponível do arco dental e aquela necessária para acomodar os dentes sucedâneos em alinhamento adequado.
arginosuccinate lyase d., d. da arginosuccinato liase. SIN argininosuccinic aciduria.
arylsulfatase A d., d. da arilsulfatase A. SIN metachromatic *leukodystrophy*.
arylsulfatase B d., d. da arilsulfatase B. SIN Maroteaux-Lamy *syndrome*.
biotinidase d., d. de biotinidase; uma rara doença autossômica recessiva que causa perda do excesso de biotina; pode não haver manifestações clínicas, mas as manifestações extremas incluem convulsões, alopecia, dermatite, hipotonia, atrofia óptica, ataxia, retardo do desenvolvimento, deficiências auditivas e, às vezes, imunodeficiência; o traço tem uma prevalência de 1 em 60.000.
carnitine d., d. de carnitina; um distúrbio associado a muitos distúrbios da oxidação dos ácidos graxos. Os ácidos graxos são ligados à carnitina enquanto são transportados através da membrana mitocondrial interna; os erros nesse processo levam a problemas com a produção de energia; os pacientes podem apresentar episódios de hipoglicemia ou acidose metabólica, bem como miocardiopatia ou fraqueza muscular esquelética.

debrancher d., d. da enzima desramificadora. SIN brancher glycogen storage *disease*.
familial high density lipoprotein d., d. familiar de lipoproteína de alta densidade. SIN analphalipoproteinemia.
fructokinase d., d. de frutocinase. SIN essential *fructosuria*.
galactokinase d. [MIM*230200], d. de galactocinase; um erro congênito do metabolismo devido à deficiência congênita de galactocinase (GALK), resultando em aumento da concentração sanguínea de galactose (galactosemia), catarata, hepatomegalia e deficiência mental; herança autossômica recessiva, causada por mutação no gene GALK em 17q. A deficiência de galactose epimerase [MIM*230350] e a deficiência de galactose-1-fosfato uridil transferase [MIM*230400] produzem o mesmo quadro clínico.
glucose-6-phosphate dehydrogenase d., d. de glicose-6-fosfato desidrogenase; deficiência de glicose-6-fosfato desidrogenase, uma enzima importante para manter as concentrações celulares de nucleotídeos reduzidos. Um distúrbio ligado ao X com várias formas polimórficas pode causar várias anemias, incluindo favismo, anemia por sensibilidade à primaquina e a outras substâncias, anemia do recém-nascido e anemia hemolítica não-esferocítica crônica.
glucosephosphate isomerase d. [MIM*172400], d. de glicosefosfato isomerase; uma deficiência enzimática caracterizada por anemia hemolítica não-esferocítica crônica; herança autossômica recessiva. SIN phosphohexose isomerase d.
β-d-glucuronidase d., d. de β-d-glucuronidase; uma deficiência rara de β-d-glucuronidase; um distúrbio autossômico recessivo com várias formas alélicas, caracterizadas por metabolismo anormal dos mucopolissacarídeos, que causam deterioração mental progressiva, esplenomegalia e hepatomegalia e disostose múltipla. SIN mucopolysaccharidase.
glutathione synthetase d., d. de glutationa sintetase; erro congênito do metabolismo associado à excreção urinária maciça de 5-oxiprolina, níveis elevados de 5-oxiprolina no sangue e no líquido cerebroespinal, acidose metabólica grave, tendência à hemólise e distúrbio da função do sistema nervoso central. A deficiência de glutationa sintetase foi descrita como uma condição generalizada ou como uma deficiência restrita aos eritrócitos.
11-hydroxylase d., d. de 11-hidroxilase; um tipo de hiperplasia supra-renal congênita, com múltiplas manifestações, incluindo tipos hipertensivos e formas perdedoras de sal.
21-hydroxylase d., d. de 21-hidroxilase; uma forma de hiperplasia supra-renal congênita, com apresentações variáveis, incluindo os tipos virilizante simples, perdedor de sal e o não-clássico.
hypoxanthine guanine phosphoribosyltransferase d., d. de hipoxantina guanina fosforribosiltransferase; um distúrbio metabólico hereditário ligado ao sexo; a deficiência completa resulta em síndrome de Lesch-Nyhan; a deficiência incompleta está associada à artrite gotosa aguda e a cálculos renais.
immune d., imunodeficiência. SIN immunodeficiency.
immunity d., imunodeficiência. SIN immunodeficiency.
immunologic d., imunodeficiência. SIN immunodeficiency.
LCAT D., d. de LCAT; um distúrbio raro caracterizado por opacidades da córnea, anemia hemolítica, proteinúria, insuficiência renal e aterosclerose prematura, além de níveis muito baixos de atividade de lecitina colesterol aciltransferase (LCAT); resulta em acúmulo de colesterol não-esterificado no plasma e nos tecidos.
leukocyte adhesion d. (LAD), d. da adesão leucocitária; distúrbio hereditário (autossômico recessivo) no qual há um defeito do complexo de aderência CD18 que perturba a quimiotaxia. É caracterizada por infecções piogênicas bacterianas recorrentes e comprometimento da cicatrização de feridas.
long-chain 3-hydroxyacyl-CoA dehydrogenase d., d. da desidrogenase da 3-hidroxiacil-CoA de cadeia longa; um distúrbio da oxidação dos ácidos graxos; os pacientes podem apresentar episódios de hipoglicemia hipocetótica aguda (semelhante à encontrada na deficiência de MCAD), cardiomiopatia, fraqueza muscular e anormalidades hepáticas.
long-chain/very long-chain acyl-CoA dehydrogenase d., d. da desidrogenase da acil-CoA de cadeia longa/muito longa; um distúrbio da oxidação dos ácidos graxos em pacientes que não possuem a enzima desidrogenase da acil-CoA de cadeia muito longa; algumas vezes se manifesta como fraqueza, hipotonia, miocardiopatia, rabdomiólise e episódios de hipoglicemia durante jejum.
luteal phase d., d. da fase lútea. SIN luteal phase *defect*.
medium-chain acyl-CoA dehydrogenase d., d. da desidrogenase da acil-CoA de cadeia média; o distúrbio de oxidação dos ácidos graxos mais comum; apresenta-se como episódios agudos deflagrados por jejum prolongado por mais de 12-16 horas, com hipoglicemia, vômitos e letargia, que podem progredir para convulsões, coma ou colapso cardiopulmonar, geralmente se apresentando antes dos 3 anos de idade.
mental d., d. mental. SIN mental *retardation*.
muscle phosphorylase d., d. de fosforilase muscular; doença do depósito de glicogênio tipo V, que afeta o músculo, causada por deficiência de fosforilase muscular.
phosphohexose isomerase d., d. de fosfoexose isomerase. SIN glucosephosphate isomerase d.

placental sulfatase d., d. de sulfatase placentária; defeito enzimático na placenta que resulta em falha de conversão da 16α-hidroxidesidroepiandrosterona em estriol; as mulheres com esse distúrbio raramente entram em trabalho de parto espontâneo.
primary carnitine d., d. primária de carnitina; um defeito raro do metabolismo da carnitina devido a um defeito no transporte de carnitina; os pacientes podem apresentar hipoglicemia hipocetótica e desenvolver cardiomiopatia ou fraqueza muscular esquelética.
proximal femoral focal d. (PFFD), d. focal femoral proximal; defeito congênito no qual porções variáveis da extremidade superior do fêmur estão reduzidas ou ausentes.
pseudocholinesterase d. [MIM*177400], d. de pseudocolinesterase; um distúrbio autossômico dominante que se manifesta por respostas exageradas a substâncias comumente hidrolisadas pela pseudocolinesterase sérica (p. ex., succinilcolina); considerada como vinculada à produção de uma enzima variante que é menos ativa que a enzima normal na hidrólise de substratos apropriados, mas também anormalmente resistente aos efeitos das anticolinesterases, causada por mutação no gene E1 da pseudocolinesterase (CHE1) em 3q.
pyruvate kinase d. [MIM*266200], d. de piruvatocinase; um distúrbio no qual há deficiência de piruvatocinase nas hemácias; caracterizada por anemia hemolítica de grau variável de um paciente para outro; herança autossômica recessiva, causada por mutação no gene da piruvatocinase hepática e eritrocitária (PKLR) no cromossoma 1q.
riboflavin d., d. de riboflavina. VER ariboflavinosis.
secondary antibody d., d. de anticorpo secundária. SIN secondary *immunodeficiency.*
short-chain acyl-CoA dehydrogenase d., d. da desidrogenase de acil-CoA de cadeia curta; um distúrbio da oxidação dos ácidos graxos; os pacientes podem apresentar acidose crônica, retardo do crescimento, fraqueza muscular e retardo do desenvolvimento.
taste d. [MIM*171200], d. do paladar; redução ou ausência da capacidade de detectar um sabor amargo em um grupo de compostos, do qual a feniltiocarbamida é o protótipo, devido ao estado homozigoto de um alelo comum. VER TAMBÉM phenylthiourea.
def·i·cit (def′i-sit). Déficit; o resultado do consumo ou do uso de alguma coisa mais rápido que sua reposição ou substituição. [L. *deficio,* falhar]
base d., d. de base; diminuição na concentração total da base tampão do sangue, sinal indicativo de acidose metabólica ou de alcalose respiratória compensada.
oxygen d., d. de oxigênio; a diferença entre captação de oxigênio do organismo durante os estágios iniciais do exercício e durante um período semelhante de uma fase uniforme de exercício; algumas vezes considerado como a formação do débito de oxigênio.
pulse d., d. do pulso; **(1)** a ausência de ondas de pulso palpáveis em uma artéria periférica por um ou mais batimentos, como se observa freqüentemente na fibrilação atrial; **(2)** o número dessas ondas de pulso ausentes (geralmente expressas como freqüência cardíaca menos freqüência de pulso por minuto).
sleep d., d. de sono; ausência de tempo de sono ou ausência relativa de um dos estágios do sono, determinada por um estudo do sono.
def·i·ni·tion (def′i-nish′ŭn). Definição, poder resolutivo; em óptica, o poder de uma lente de permitir uma imagem nítida. VER TAMBÉM resolving *power.* [L. *de-finio,* pp. *-finitus,* limitar, de *finis,* limite]
de·flec·tion (dē-flek′shŭn). Deflexão. **1.** Deslocamento para um lado. **2.** No eletrocardiograma, um desvio da curva da linha de base isoelétrica; qualquer onda ou complexo do eletrocardiograma. [L. *deflecto,* pp. *-flexus,* curvar-se para o lado]
intrinsic d., d. intrínseca; com o eletrodo em contato direto com a fibra muscular, uma deflexão rápida negativa a partir do pico da última positividade, indicando que a frente de ativação alcançou o músculo subjacente.
intrinsicoid d., d. intrinsecóide; queda súbita a partir da última positividade, quando o eletrodo é colocado não diretamente sobre o músculo, mas a distância, como nas derivações torácicas unipolares em eletrocardiografia clínica.
de·flex·ion (dē′fleks-shŭn). Deflexão; termo usado para descrever a posição da cabeça fetal em relação à pelve materna na qual a cabeça está descendo em uma posição não-fletida ou estendida. [de- + L. *flexio,* flexão, de *flecto,* pp. *flexum,* flexionar]
def·lo·res·cence (de-flō-res′ens). Deflorescência; desaparecimento da erupção na escarlatina e em outros exantemas. [L. *de-floresco,* descolorir, murchar, de *flos* (*flor-*), flor]
de·flu·o·ri·da·tion (dē-flōr′i-dā′shŭn). Desfluoridização; remoção do excesso de fluoretos do suprimento de água de uma comunidade.
de·flu·vi·um (dē-flōō′vē-ŭm). Deflúvio. SIN defluxion. [L., de *de-fluo,* pp. *-fluxus,* fluir para baixo]
de·flux·ion (dē-flŭk′shŭn). Defluxo. **1.** Queda, como de cabelo. VER TAMBÉM effluvium. **2.** Fluxo descendente ou descarga de líquido. SIN defluvium. [L. *defluxio, de-fluo,* pp. *-fluxus,* fluir para baixo]
de·for·ma·bi·li·ty (dē-form′a-bil′i-tē). Deformabilidade; a capacidade de células, como os eritrócitos, de mudar de forma quando atravessam espaços estreitos, como a rede microvascular.
de·for·ma·tion (dē-fōr-mā′shŭn). Deformação. **1.** Desvio de forma do normal; especificamente, uma alteração do formato e/ou estrutura de uma parte antes normalmente formada. Ocorre após organogênese e freqüentemente envolve o sistema músculo-esquelético (p. ex., pé torto). **2.** Em reologia, a alteração no formato físico de uma massa por estresse aplicado. [L. *de-formo,* pp. *-atus,* deformar, de *forma,* forma]
de·form·ing (dē-form′ing). Deformante; que causa um desvio da forma normal.
de·for·mi·ty (dē-fōr′mi-tē). Deformidade; um desvio estrutural permanente do formato, tamanho ou alinhamento normais, resultando em desfiguramento; pode ser congênita ou adquirida. VER TAMBÉM deformation (1).
Åkerlund d., d. de Åkerlund; entalhe (incisura) com nicho do bulbo duodenal, como demonstrado radiograficamente.
Arnold-Chiari d. [MIM*207950], d. de Arnold-Chiari. SIN Arnold-Chiari *malformation.*
bell clapper d., d. em badalo; testículo e epidídimo livres da fixação posterior habitual da túnica vaginal, de forma que a túnica se insere em posição alta no cordão espermático, deixando a gônada mais propensa a sofrer torção.
boutonnière d., d. em botoeira; flexão da articulação interfalângica proximal com hiperextensão da articulação interfalângica distal do dedo, causada por separação do capuz extensor e protrusão da cabeça da falange proximal através da "casa de botão" resultante; pode ser causada por degeneração (artrite reumatóide) ou traumatismo.
contracture d., d. em contratura; deformidade de um membro sem alterações primárias perceptíveis do osso.
Erlenmeyer flask d., d. em frasco de Erlenmeyer; deformidade na extremidade distal do fêmur causada por uma falha do desenvolvimento da diáfise do osso até seu formato tubular normal, resultando em um osso largo por uma distância muito maior que o normal até a diáfise; encontrada na doença de Gaucher. [semelhança com um cantil de Erlenmeyer]
gunstock d., d. em coronha; uma forma de cúbito varo, resultante de fratura supracondilar ou condilar no cotovelo, na qual o eixo do antebraço estendido não é contínuo com o do braço, mas deslocado em direção à linha média.
Haglund d., d. de Haglund. SIN Haglund *disease.*
J-sella d., d. em J da sela turca; deformidade em forma de pêra ou em forma de J da sela turca causada por aumento da pressão sobre o osso esfenóide em crescimento; observada nas doenças por depósito de polissacarídeos.
keyhole d., d. em buraco de fechadura; ectrópio mucoso na borda posterior do ânus após esfincterotomia nesse local.
lobster-claw d., d. em garra de lagosta. VER ectrodactyly.
Madelung d., d. de Madelung; subluxação radioulnar distal devida à deficiência relativa do crescimento axial da face medial do terço distal do rádio, que, em conseqüência, está anormalmente inclinada em direção proximal e ulnar. SIN carpus curvus.
mermaid d., d. de sereia; membros de sereia. SIN sirenomelia.
parachute d., d. em pára-quedas. SIN parachute mitral *valve.*
reduction d., d. por redução; ausência ou atenuação congênita de uma ou mais partes do corpo; geralmente dos membros ou componentes dos membros.
silver-fork d., d. em dorso de garfo; deformidade semelhante à curva do dorso de um garfo observada na fratura de Colles (torção distal do rádio).
Sprengel d., d. de Sprengel; elevação congênita da escápula. SIN scapula elevata.
swan-neck d., d. em pescoço de cisne; hiperextensão da articulação interfalângica proximal com flexão da articulação interfalângica distal do dedo da mão.
torsional d., d. torcional; em ortopedia, uma deformidade causada por rotação anormal de uma parte de um membro em relação ao eixo longitudinal de todo o membro.
whistling d., d. em apito; deformidade causada por tecido insuficiente na borda inferior de uma fenda palatina reparada, produzindo o aspecto de apito.
Whitehead d., d. de Whitehead; ectrópio mucoso circunferencial no ânus após operação de Whitehead.
de·fur·fur·a·tion (dē-fer-fer-ā′shŭn). Desfurfuração; descamação da epiderme na forma de escamas finas. SIN branny desquamation. [L. *de,* distante de, + *furfur,* farelo]
de·gan·gli·on·ate (dē-gang′glē-on-āt). Desganglionar; privar de gânglios.
de·gen·er·a·cy (dē-jen′er-ă-sē). Degeneração. **1.** Condição caracterizada por deterioração de processos mentais, físicos ou morais. **2.** O fato de vários códons triplos diferentes codificarem o mesmo aminoácido. [L. *de,* de, + *genus,* (*gener-*), raça]
de·gen·er·ate 1 (dē-jen′er-āt). Degenerar; passar a um nível inferior de estado mental, físico ou moral; cair abaixo do tipo ou estado normal ou aceitável. **2** (dē-jen′ē-rāt). Degenerado; abaixo do normal ou aceitável; o que passou para um nível inferior.
de·gen·er·a·tio (dē-jen-er-ā′shē-ō). Degeneração. SIN degeneration. [L. *degenero,* pp. *-atus,* de *de,* de, + *genus,* raça]

DEGENERATION

de·gen·er·a·tion (dē - jen - er - āʹshŭn). Degeneração. **1.** Deterioração; que passa de um nível ou tipo mais alto para um inferior. **2.** Um agravamento das qualidades mentais, físicas ou morais. **3.** Uma anormalidade retrogressiva em células ou tecidos, em conseqüência do que suas funções freqüentemente são comprometidas ou destruídas; algumas vezes reversível; nos estágios iniciais, ocorre necrose. SIN retrograde metamorphosis. SIN degeneratio. [L. *degeneratio*]
adipose d., d. adiposa. SIN fatty d.
adiposogenital d., d. adiposagenital. SIN adiposogenital *dystrophy.*
age-related macular d., d. macular relacionada à idade; uma degeneração macular comum que começa com drusas na mácula e ruptura do pigmento, levando, algumas vezes, à perda acentuada da visão central.
amyloid d., d. amilóide; infiltração de amilóide entre células e fibras de tecidos e órgãos. SIN waxy d. (1)
angiolithic d., d. angiolítica; degeneração calcária das paredes dos vasos sangüíneos.
ascending d., d. ascendente; **(1)** degeneração retrógrada de uma fibra nervosa lesada; isto é, em direção à célula nervosa da fibra; **(2)** degeneração da medula espinal que começa em uma região e, depois, prossegue em direção cefálica.
atheromatous d., d. ateromatosa; acúmulo focal de material lipídico (ateroma) na íntima e na porção subíntima das artérias, finalmente resultando em espessamento fibroso ou calcificação.
axon d., d. axonal. SIN axonal d.
axonal d., d. axonal; um tipo de resposta da fibra nervosa periférica à agressão, na qual ocorre morte do axônio e subseqüente interrupção, com lesão secundária da bainha de mielina associada; causada por lesão focal das fibras nervosas periféricas; freqüentemente denominada degeneração waleriana. SIN axon d.
ballooning d., d. em balão; termo obsoleto para células que são infectadas por determinados vírus, resultando em tumefação visível da célula e vacuolação citoplasmática.
basophilic d., d. basófila; coloração azul dos tecidos conjuntivos quando se usa coloração pela hematoxilina-eosina; encontrada em condições como elastose solar.
calcareous d., d. calcária; em um sentido exato, não se trata de um processo degenerativo por si, mas da deposição de sais de cálcio insolúveis no tecido que sofreu degeneração e necrose, como na calcificação distrófica.
carneous d., d. carnosa. SIN red d.
caseous d., d. caseosa. SIN caseous *necrosis.*
colloid d., d. colóide; degeneração semelhante à degeneração mucóide na qual o material encontra-se espessado.
cone d., d. dos cones. SIN cone *dystrophy.*
corticobasal d., d. corticobasal; doença rara, progressiva, que envolve tanto o córtex cerebral quanto as estruturas extrapiramidais; clinicamente se manifesta como distúrbios dos movimentos voluntários e rigidez; as características histopatológicas incluem degeneração do córtex cerebral com neurônios em balão e degeneração da substância negra.
Crooke hyaline d., d. hialina de Crooke. SIN Crooke hyaline *change.*
descending d., d. descendente; **(1)** d. waleriana de uma fibra nervosa lesada; isto é, degeneração distal à lesão; **(2)** d. caudal ao nível de uma lesão da medula espinal.
disciform d., d. disciforme; neovascularização sub-retiniana foveal ou parafoveal, com separação da retina e hemorragia, levando finalmente a uma massa circular de tecido fibroso com perda acentuada da acuidade visual. SIN disciform macular d.
disciform macular d., d. macular disciforme. SIN disciform d.
ectatic marginal d. of cornea, d. marginal ectásica da córnea. SIN pellucid marginal corneal d.
elastoid d., d. elastóide; **(1)** SIN elastosis (2); **(2)** d. hialina do tecido elástico da parede arterial, observada durante a involução do útero.
elastotic d., d. elastótica. SIN elastosis (2).
familial pseudoinflammatory macular d. [MIM*136900], d. macular pseudo-inflamatória familiar; degeneração macular que ocorre durante a quinta década de vida, com desenvolvimento súbito de um escotoma central em um olho, seguido rapidamente por uma lesão semelhante no olho oposto; herança autossômica dominante. SIN Sorsby macular d.
fascicular d., d. fascicular; degeneração restrita a determinados fascículos de nervos ou músculos.
fatty d., d. gordurosa; esteatose; formação anormal de gotículas de gordura, microscopicamente visíveis, no citoplasma das células, em virtude de lesão. SIN adipose d., steatosis (2).
fibrinoid d., fibrinous d., d. fibrinóide, d. fibrinoso; processo que resulta em depósitos refringentes homogêneos, profundamente acidófilos, mal definidos, com algumas reações de coloração que se assemelham à fibrina, ocorrendo no tecido conjuntivo, nas paredes dos vasos sanguíneos e em outros locais.
fibrous d., d. fibrosa; não é uma degeneração por si, mas sim um processo reparador; as células e os focos de tecido previamente afetados por processos degenerativos e necrose são substituídos por tecido fibroso celular.
granular d., d. granular. SIN cloudy *swelling.*
granulovacuolar d., d. granulovacuolar; degeneração das células cerebrais do hipocampo em pessoas idosas, caracterizada por grânulos basófilos circundados por uma zona clara nos neurônios do hipocampo; é mais freqüente na doença de Alzheimer.
gray d., d. cinzenta; degeneração da substância branca da medula espinal, cujas fibras perdem suas bainhas de mielina e tornam-se mais escuras.
hepatolenticular d., d. hepatolenticular. SIN Wilson *disease (1).*
hyaline d., d. hialina; um grupo de vários processos degenerativos que afetam várias células e tecidos, resultando na formação de massas arredondadas ("gotículas") ou de faixas relativamente largas de substâncias homogêneas, translúcidas, refringentes e moderada a profundamente acidófilas; pode ocorrer no colágeno de tecido fibroso antigo, no músculo liso das arteríolas ou do útero, e como gotículas nas células do parênquima.
hyaloideoretinal d. [MIM*143200], d. hialóide retiniana; liquefação e destruição progressivas do humor vítreo com membranas pré-retinianas branco-acinzentadas, miopia, catarata, descolamento da retina e hiper e hipopigmentação; herança autossômica dominante. SIN Wagner disease, Wagner syndrome.
hydropic d., d. hidrópica. SIN cloudy *swelling.*
infantile neuronal d., d. neuronal infantil; distúrbio degenerativo de lactentes com perda neuronal disseminada no tálamo, cerebelo, ponte e medula espinal, semelhante à atrofia muscular do lactente.
liquefaction d., d. por liquefação; **(1)** necrose com amolecimento, como no tecido cerebral isquêmico; **(2)** dissolução da camada basal da epiderme por necrose de células dispersas com vacuolização, observada no líquen plano, no lúpus eritematoso e em outros distúrbios dermatológicos.
macular d., d. macular; qualquer degeneração ocular que afeta predominantemente o fundo posterior, porém mais comumente degeneração macular relacionada à idade.
Mönckeberg d., d. de Mönckeberg. SIN Mönckeberg *arteriosclerosis.*
mucinoid d., d. mucinóide; termo que inclui degeneração mucóide e colóide, sendo as alterações celulares essenciais semelhantes em ambas, e a única diferença é que, na degeneração colóide, a substância é mais firme e mais espessa que na degeneração mucóide, na qual esta é fina e semelhante a geléia.
mucoid d., d. mucóide; conversão de qualquer um dos tecidos conjuntivos em uma substância gelatinosa ou mucóide. SIN myxoid d., myxomatous d., myxomatosis (1).
mucoid medial d., d. mucóide da média. SIN cystic medial *necrosis.*
myelinic d., d. mielínica; formação de figuras de mielina no citoplasma das células, possivelmente por degradação ou hidratação de lipoproteína de organelas autodigeridas.
myopic d., d. miópica; associação de crescente do disco óptico, atrofia da coróide e do pigmento macular, neovascularização sub-retiniana, hemorragia e proliferação do pigmento na miopia maligna.
myxoid d., myxomatous d., d. mixóide, d. mixomatosa. SIN mucoid d.
neurofibrillary d., d. neurofibrilar; formação de fibras intracitoplasmáticas, argentofílicas, grosseiras, freqüentemente em novelos complexos nas células nervosas intracranianas. VER TAMBÉM Alzheimer *disease.*
Nissl d., d. de Nissl; doença do corpo celular que ocorre após transecção do axônio; caracterizada por dispersão do retículo endoplasmático granular, edema do soma e uma posição excêntrica do núcleo celular.
olivopontocerebellar d., d. olivopontocerebelar. SIN olivopontocerebellar *atrophy.*
parenchymatous d., d. parenquimatosa. SIN cloudy *swelling.*
pellucid marginal corneal d., d. marginal pelúcida da córnea; opacificação bilateral e vascularização da periferia da córnea, progredindo para a formação de um sulco e ectasia. SIN ectatic marginal d. of cornea.
primary neuronal d., d. neuronal primária. SIN Alzheimer *disease.*
primary pigmentary d. of retina, d. pigmentar primária da retina. SIN tapetoretinal d.
primary progressive cerebellar d., d. cerebelar progressiva primária; uma condição atáxica familiar relacionada à degeneração cerebelar.
pseudotubular d., d. pseudotubular; termo obsoleto para uma forma de degeneração observada nas glândulas supra-renais, principalmente de pacientes com doença infecciosa febril; as células enrugadas e depletadas de lipídios da zona fasciculada (e, algumas vezes, da zona glomerulosa) estão dispostas em um padrão circular em torno de espaços que podem estar vazios ou parcialmente cheios de fibrina, células necróticas ou material amorfo.
red d., d. vermelha; termo obsoleto para necrose, com coloração pela hemoglobina, que pode ocorrer em miomas uterinos, principalmente durante a gravidez; caracterizada por amolecimento e uma cor vermelha semelhante à da carne parcialmente cozida. SIN carneous d.
reticular d., d. reticular; edema epidérmico grave que resulta em bolhas multiloculares.

retrograde d., d. retrógrada; degeneração celular retrógrada com cromatólise dos corpos de Nissl e deslocamento periférico do núcleo da célula de origem de uma fibra nervosa lesada ou seccionada.
Salzmann nodular corneal d., d. nodular da córnea de Salzmann; nódulos grandes e proeminentes de um material opaco, sólido, que se projeta da superfície da córnea; algumas vezes ocorre em pessoas previamente afetadas por ceratite flictenular.
senile d., d. senil; o processo de involução que ocorre na velhice.
snail track d., d. em rastro de lesma; linha circunferencial de pontos brancos finos na periferia da retina associada a orifícios atróficos na retina.
Sorsby macular d., d. macular de Sorsby. SIN familial pseudoinflammatory macular d.
spheroidal d., d. esferóide. SIN climatic *keratopathy*.
spongy d. of infancy, d. esponjosa do lactente. SIN Canavan *disease*.
subacute combined d. of the spinal cord, d. combinada subaguda da medula espinal; um distúrbio subagudo ou crônico da medula espinal, como o que ocorre em determinados pacientes com deficiência de vitamina B_{12}, caracterizado por um grau leve a moderado de glicose associado a degeneração espongiforme das colunas posterior e lateral. SIN combined sclerosis, combined system disease, funicular myelitis (2), Putnam-Dana syndrome, vitamin B_{12} neuropathy.
tapetoretinal d. [MIM*272600], d. tapetorretinal; distúrbio hereditário da retina que afeta principalmente os fotorreceptores e o epitélio pigmentar da retina; pode ser uma manifestação da ataxia de Friedreich (Friedreich *ataxia*), doença de Refsum (Refsum *disease*) e abetalipoproteinemias. SIN primary pigmentary d. of retina.
Terrien marginal d., d. marginal de Terrien; uma forma de degeneração marginal pelúcida da córnea.
transsynaptic d., d. transináptica; atrofia das células nervosas após lesão dos axônios que fazem conexão sináptica com elas; observada principalmente no corpo geniculado lateral. SIN transneuronal atrophy, transsynaptic chromatolysis.
Türck d., d. de Türck; degeneração de uma fibra nervosa e sua bainha distal ao ponto de lesão ou corte do axônio; termo geralmente aplicado à degeneração no sistema nervoso central.
vacuolar d., d. vacuolar; formação de vacúolos não-lipídicos no citoplasma, na maioria das vezes devido ao acúmulo de água por edema turvo.
vitelliform d. [MIM*153700], d. viteliforme. SIN Best *disease*. SIN vitelliruptive d.
vitelliruptive d., d. viteliforme. SIN vitelliform d.
wallerian d., d. walleriana; as alterações degenerativas que o segmento distal de uma fibra nervosa periférica (axônio e mielina) sofre quando sua continuidade com seu corpo celular é interrompida por uma lesão focal.
waxy d., d. cérea; **(1)** SIN amyloid d.; **(2)** SIN Zenker d.
xerotic d., d. xerótica; fibrose da conjuntiva associada ao epitélio queratinizado.
Zenker d., d. de Zenker; termo obsoleto para uma forma de degeneração hialina grave ou necrose no músculo esquelético, que ocorre em infecções graves. SIN waxy d. (2).

---

de·gen·er·a·tive (dē - jen′er - ă - tiv). Degenerativo; relativo à degeneração.
de·glov·ing (dē - glov′ing). Desenluvamento. **1.** Exposição cirúrgica intra-oral da mandíbula anterior usada em várias cirurgias ortognáticas como genioplastia ou cirurgia alveolar mandibular. **2.** Exposição intra-oral do esqueleto facial médio em várias cirurgias do nariz e seios paranasais, particularmente para excisão de neoplasias. **3.** VER degloving *injury*.
deglut. Abreviatura de L. *deglutiatur*, deglutir.
de·glu·ti·tion (dē - gloo - tish′ŭn). Deglutição; o ato de deglutir. [L. *de-glutio*, deglutir]
de·glu·ti·tive (dē - gloo′ti - tiv). Deglutivo; relativo à deglutição.
Degos, Robert, dermatologista francês, *1904. VER D. *disease, syndrome;* Kohlmeier-D. *syndrome.*
deg·ra·da·tion (deg - ră - dā′shŭn). Degradação; a alteração de uma substância química em uma substância menos complexa. [L. *degradatus*, degradar]
de·gran·u·la·tion (dē - gran - ū - lā′shŭn). Desgranulação; desaparecimento ou perda de grânulos citoplasmáticos (lisossomas) de uma célula.
de·gree (dē - grē′). Grau. **1.** Uma das divisões na escala de um instrumento de medida, como um termômetro, barômetro, etc. VER apêndice de Escalas Térmicas Comparativas. VER scale. **2.** A 360.ª parte da circunferência de um círculo. **3.** Uma posição ou graduação em uma série graduada. **4.** Uma medida de lesão tecidual. [Fr. *degré;* L. *gradus,* degrau]
d.'s of freedom, graus de liberdade; em estatística, o número de comparações independentes que podem ser feitas entre os membros de uma amostra (p. ex., indivíduos, itens e resultados de testes, ensaios, condições); em uma tabela de contingência é o número de categorias de linha menos um multiplicado pelo número de categorias de colunas menos um.
de·gus·ta·tion (dē - gŭs - tā′shŭn). Degustação. **1.** O ato de saborear. **2.** O sentido do paladar. [L. *degustatio,* de *de-gusto,* pp. *-atus,* saborear]
de·hal·o·gen·ase (dē - hal′ō - jen - ās). Desalogenase; qualquer enzima (EC subclasse 3,8) que remove átomos de hidrogênio de halóides orgânicos.

Dehio, Karl K., médico russo, 1851–1927. VER D. *test.*
de·his·cence (dē - his′ens). Deiscência; uma ferida explosiva, subdividida ou fendida ao longo de linhas naturais ou de sutura. [L. *dehisco,* separar ou fender]
iris d., d. da íris; um defeito do olho caracterizado por múltiplos orifícios na íris.
root d., d. da raiz; uma perda do osso bucal ou lingual que se sobrepõe à porção da raiz de um dente, deixando a área coberta apenas por tecidos moles.
wound d., d. da ferida; ruptura de superfícies apostas de uma ferida.
de·hu·man·i·za·tion (dē - hū′măn - i - zā′shŭn). Desumanização; perda das características humanas; brutalização por meios mentais ou físicos; despojamento da auto-estima. [*de-* + *humanus,* humano, de *homo,* homem]
de·hy·drase (dē - hī′drās). Desidrase; nome antigo de desidratase.
de·hy·dra·tase (dē - hī′drā - tās). Desidratase; uma subclasse (EC 4.2.1.x) de liases (hidroliases) que removem H e OH como H_2O de um substrato, deixando uma ligação dupla, ou acrescentam um grupamento a uma ligação dupla pela eliminação de água de duas substâncias para formar uma terceira; o termo sintetase é usado, algumas vezes, quando é enfatizado o aspecto sintético da reação. Alguns nomes triviais de enzimas nessa subclasse possuem o termo genérico hidratase, enfatizando a reação inversa.
de·hy·drate (dē - hī′drāt). Desidratar. **1.** Extrair água de. **2.** Perder água. [L. *de,* de + G. *hydōr* (*hydr-*), água]
de·hy·dra·tion (dē - hī - drā′shŭn). Desidratação. **1.** Privação de água. SIN anhydration. **2.** Redução do conteúdo de água. **3.** SIN exsiccation (2). **4.** SIN desiccation.
absolute d., d. absoluta; déficit real de água determinado por uma diferença em relação ao normal ou em relação a um determinado conteúdo de água.
relative d., d. relativa; déficit de água relativo ao conteúdo de solutos que contribui para a pressão osmótica efetiva; um estado de aumento da pressão osmótica efetiva dos líquidos corporais.
voluntary d., d. voluntária; atraso ou déficit fisiológico que ocorre quando a sensação de sede não é suficientemente forte para produzir a reposição completa da perda hídrica, como na sudorese rápida.
dehydro-. Desidro; prefixo usado nos nomes dos compostos químicos que diferem de outros e de compostos mais familiares na ausência de dois átomos de hidrogênio; p. ex., ácido desidroascórbico, que se assemelha ao ácido ascórbico em todas as características estruturais, exceto por sua ausência de dois átomos de hidrogênio que existem na molécula de ácido ascórbico. Na nomenclatura sistemática, é preferível didesidro-, como sendo mais exato.
de·hy·dro·a·ce·tic ac·id (dē - hī′drō - ă - sē′tik). Ácido desidroacético; agente antimicrobiano usado como conservante em cosméticos.
L-de·hy·dro·a·scor·bic ac·id (dē - hī′drō - as - kōr′bik). Ácido L-desidroascórbico; a forma oxidada reversível do ácido ascórbico; é antiescorbútico, mas é convertido no corpo em ácido 2,3-diceto-L-gulônico, que não possui a atividade da vitamina C.
de·hy·dro·bil·i·ru·bin (dē - hī′drō - bil - ē - roo′bin). Desidrobilirrubina. SIN biliverdin.
de·hy·dro·cho·late (dē - hī - drō - kō′lāt). Desidrocolato; um sal ou éster do ácido desidrocólico.
7-de·hy·dro·cho·les·ter·ol (dē - hī′drō - kō - les′ter - ol). 7-desidrocolesterol; um zoosterol encontrado na pele e em outros tecidos animais que, ao ser ativado pela luz ultravioleta, torna-se anti-raquítico e passa a ser denominado colecalciferol (vitamina D_3). SIN provitamin D_3.
24-de·hy·dro·cho·les·ter·ol. 24-desidrocolesterol. SIN desmosterol.
de·hy·dro·cho·lic ac·id (dē - hī - drō - kol′ik). Ácido desidrocólico; tem um efeito estimulante sobre a secreção de bile pelo fígado (colerético) e aumenta a absorção de alimentos essenciais em estados associados à deficiência de formação de bile.
11-de·hy·dro·cor·ti·co·ster·one (dē - hī′drō - kōr - ti - ko - s′ter - ōn). 11-desidrocorticosterona; principalmente, um metabólito da corticosterona, encontrado no córtex supra-renal.
de·hy·dro·em·e·tine (dē - hī - drō - em′e - tēn). Desidroemetina; um derivado sintético da emetina; usado no tratamento da amebíase intestinal.
d. resinate, resinato de desidroemetina; um derivado da emetina.
dehydroepiandrosterone. Desidroepiandrosterona; agente esteróide relacionado a hormônios masculinos que foram defendidos como capazes de evitar as conseqüências fisiológicas do envelhecimento, sem estudos que mostrem seu benefício ou segurança.

---

de·hy·dro-3-ep·i·an·dros·ter·one (DHEA) (dē - hī′drō - ep - ē - an - dros′ter - ōn). Desidro-3-epiandrosterona; um esteróide secretado principalmente pelo córtex supra-renal, mas também pelo testículo; é o principal precursor dos 17-cetosteróides urinários. Fracamente androgênico, é metabolizado em delta-5-androstenediol, um hormônio com efeitos androgênicos e estrogênicos, e é um dos precursores da testosterona. Os níveis séricos estão elevados no virilismo supra-renal. Pode funcionar como neurotransmissor. SIN androstenolone, dehydroisoandrosterone.

A secreção de DHEA começa durante a vida fetal, alcança um pico na 3.ª década de vida e diminui continuamente a seguir; o nível aos 80 anos corresponde a apenas 10-20% do nível máximo. Essa diminuição foi especulativamente associada às alterações do envelhecimento. As formulações de DHEA são comercializadas como suplementos alimentares, embora essa substância não seja um nutriente nem um componente da cadeia alimentar humana. Encontrado em lojas de produtos naturais em cápsulas de 10, 25 e 50 mg, a propaganda afirma que a DHEA previne doenças degenerativas, incluindo aterosclerose, demência de Alzheimer e parkinsonismo, e outros efeitos do envelhecimento. Nenhum dos benefícios alegados foi demonstrado em grandes experiências clínicas randomizadas. A administração prolongada a mulheres após a menopausa foi associada à resistência à insulina, hipertensão e redução do LDL-colesterol. Uma análise de 16 preparações de DHEA por cromatografia líquida de alto desempenho mostrou uma variação do conteúdo de 0-150% da concentração indicada; apenas 7 produtos estavam entre os 90-110% esperados da concentração indicada.

de·hy·dro·gen·ase (dē - hī′drō - jen - ās). Desidrogenase; nome de classe das enzimas que oxidam substratos catalisando a remoção de hidrogênio dos metabólitos (doadores de hidrogênio) e transferindo-o para outras substâncias (aceptores de hidrogênio), que são assim reduzidas; a maioria das enzimas oxidativas (oxidorredutase, EC classe 1) realiza suas oxidações dessa forma.
 aerobic d., d. aeróbica; uma enzima (geralmente uma metaloflavoenzima) que catalisa a transferência de hidrogênio de algum metabólito para o oxigênio, formando peróxido de hidrogênio no processo; p. ex., xantina oxidase e outras em várias subclasses (p. ex., EC 1.1.3, 1.2.3, 1.7.3, 1.8.3, 1.10.3).
 anaerobic d., d. anaeróbica; uma enzima (geralmente uma piridinoenzima) que catalisa a transferência de hidrogênio de algum metabólito para alguma molécula aceptora (p. ex., NAD$^+$, citocromo) além do oxigênio; p. ex., lactato desidrogenases, isocitrato desidrogenases e outras na EC classe 1, excluindo-se aquelas apresentadas em desidrogenase aeróbica.
 α-keto acid d., d. α-cetoácida. VER α-*keto acid* dehydrogenase.
 Robison ester d., d. do éster de Robison. SIN glucose-6-phosphate dehydrogenase.

de·hy·dro·gen·ate (dē - hī′drō - jen - āt). Desidrogenar; submeter à desidrogenação.

de·hy·dro·gen·a·tion (dē - hī′drō - jen - ā′shŭn). Desidrogenação; retirada de um par de átomos de hidrogênio de um composto pela ação de enzimas (desidrogenases) ou outros catalisadores.

de·hy·dro·i·so·an·dros·ter·one (dē - hī′drō - ī - sō - an - dros′ter - ōn). Desidroisoandrosterona. SIN dehydro-3-epiandrosterone.

de·hy·dro·ret·i·nal·de·hyde (dē - hī′drō - ret - i - nal′dē - hīd). Desidrorretinaldeído; desidrorretinol com –CHO em vez de –CH$_2$OH no carbono terminal da cadeia lateral. SIN retinene-2, vitamin A$_2$ aldehyde.

de·hy·dro·ret·i·no·ic ac·id (dē - hī′drō - ret - i - nō′ik). Ácido desidrorretinóico; desidrorretinol com –COOH no lugar do –CH$_2$OH no carbono terminal da cadeia lateral.

de·hy·dro·ret·i·nol (dē - hī - drō - ret′i - nol). Desidrorretinol; retinol com uma ligação dupla adicional na posição 3-4 do anel cicloexano. SIN vitamin A$_2$.

de·hy·dro·sug·ars (dē - hī′drō - shug - erz). Desidroaçúcares. SIN anhydrosugars.

de·hyp·no·tize (dē - hip′nō - tīz). Desipnotizar; tirar do estado hipnótico.

de·im·i·nas·es (dē - im′i - nās - ez). Desiminases. SIN iminohydrolases.

de·in·sti·tu·tion·al·i·za·tion (dē′in - sti - too′shŭn - ăl - i - zā - shŭn). Desinstitucionalização; a alta de pacientes internados em um hospital mental para programas de tratamento em esquemas parciais e outros programas comunitários.

de·i·on·i·za·tion (de - ī′ - on - ī - zā′shŭn). Desionização; a produção de um estado livre de minerais pela remoção de íons.

Deiters, Otto F.K., anatomista alemão, 1834–1863. VER D. *cells,* em *cell,* terminal *frames,* em *frame, nucleus.*

dé·jà vou·lu (dā - zhă′voo - loo′). Já desejado; termo que designa um tipo de distúrbio da memória no qual o indivíduo acredita que seus desejos atuais são exatamente iguais aos desejos que já teve algum tempo antes.

dé·jà vu (dā - zhah - voo′). Já visto; sensação de ter estado em um lugar antes. VER déjà vu *phenomenon.* VER phenomenon. [Fr. já visto]

de·jec·ta (dē - jek′tă). Dejeto. SIN dejection (3). [L. neut, pl. de *de-jectus,* de *de-jicio,* jogar fora]

de·jec·tion (dē - jek′shŭn). **1.** Abatimento; depressão. SIN depression (4). **2.** Dejeção; evacuação; a eliminação de excremento. **3.** Dejeto; o material assim eliminado. SIN dejecta . [L. *dejectio,* de *de- jicio,* pp. *-jectus,* jogar fora]

Dejerine, Joseph J., neurologista parisiense, 1849–1917. VER D. *disease,* hand *phenomenon, reflex, sign;* D.- Roussy *syndrome*; D.- Sottas *disease*; D.- Klumpke *syndrome,* Landouzy-D. *dystrophy.*

Dejerine-Klumpke, Augusta, neurologista francesa (nascida nos EUA), 1859–1927. VER Klumpke *palsy*; Klumpke *paralysis*; Dejerine-Klumpke *palsy*; Dejerine-Klumpke *syndrome.*

♻ **deka-.** VER deca-.

Delafield, Francis, médico e patologista norte-americano, 1841–1915. VER D. *hematoxylin.*

de·lam·i·na·tion (dē - lam - i - nā′shŭn). Delaminação; divisão em camadas distintas. [L. *de,* de, + *lamina,* uma placa fina]

Delaney clause. Cláusula Delaney; uma cláusula da *Food Additive Amendment* da lei federal norte-americana, especificando que nenhuma substância que induza câncer em qualquer animal pode ser incorporada a alimentos. [James F. *Delaney,* congressista norte-americano]

de Lange, Cornelia, pediatra holandesa, 1871–1950. VER de L. *syndrome.*

Delbet, Pierre L.E., cirurgião francês, 1861–1925. VER D. *sign.*

Del Castillo, E.B., médico argentino do século XX. VER Del C. *syndrome.*

de-lead (dē - led′). Causar a mobilização e a excreção de chumbo depositado nos ossos e outros tecidos, como pela administração de um agente quelante.

del·e·te·ri·ous (del - ĕ - tēr′ē - ŭs). Deletério; lesivo; nocivo; prejudicial. [G. *dēlētērios,* de *dēleomai,* lesar]

de·le·tion (dē - lē′shŭn). Deleção; em genética, qualquer eliminação espontânea de parte do complemento genético normal, seja citogeneticamente visível (deleção cromossomial) ou encontrada por técnicas moleculares. [L. *deletio,* destruição]
 chromosomal d., d. cromossomial; perda microscopicamente evidente de parte de um cromossoma. VER TAMBÉM monosomy.
 gene d., d. genética; deleção de um segmento cromossomial pequeno demais para ser detectado citogeneticamente, deduzido do fenótipo em um *locus* específico.
 interstitial d., d. intersticial; deleção que não envolve as partes terminais de um cromossoma.
 nucleotide d., d. de nucleotídeo; deleção de um único nucleotídeo, que, em um gene transcrito, levará a uma mutação de deslocamento. SIN point d. (2).
 point d., d. de ponto; **(1)** deleção envolvendo uma perda submicroscópica de material genético pequena demais para ser resolvida por análise de ligação; **(2)** SIN nucleotide d.
 terminal d., d. terminal; deleção envolvendo a parte terminal de um cromossoma e levando a um término adesivo.

del·i·cate (del′i - kăt). Delicado; de fraco poder de resistência. [L. *delicatus,* suave, luxurioso, de *de,* de, + *lacio,* atrair, seduzir]

de·lim·i·ta·tion (dē - lim - i - tā′shŭn). Delimitação; demarcação; colocação de fronteiras ou limites; impedimento da disseminação de um processo mórbido no corpo ou de uma doença na comunidade. [L. *de-limito,* pp. *-atus,* limitar, de *limes,* fronteira]

del·i·quesce (del - i - kwes′). Deliqüescer; sofrer deliqüescência.

del·i·ques·cence (del - i - kwes′ens). Deliqüescência; tornar-se úmido ou líquido por absorção de água da atmosfera e, depois, dissolver-se na água absorvida; uma propriedade encontrada em alguns sais, como o CaCl$_2$. [L. *deliquesco,* fundir ou tornar líquido]

del·i·ques·cent (del - i - kwes′ent). Deliqüescente; designa um sólido capaz de sofrer deliqüescência.

de·li·ria (dē - lir′ē - ă). Delírios. Plural de delirium. VER delirium.

de·lir·i·ous (dē - lir′ē - ŭs). Delirante; em estado de delírio.

de·lir·i·um, pl. **de·li·ria** (dē - lir′ē - ŭm, dē - lir′ē - ă). Delírio; alteração do estado da consciência, consistindo em confusão, perturbação, desorientação, desordem do raciocínio e da memória, falha da percepção (delírios e alucinações), hiperatividade proeminente, agitação e hiperatividade do sistema nervoso autônomo; causado por vários distúrbios tóxicos, estruturais e metabólicos. [L. de *deliro,* estar louco, de *de-* + *lira,* trilho (isto é, sair do trilho)]
 acute d., d. agudo; delírio de início rápido, recente.
 alcohol withdrawal d., d. da abstinência alcoólica; delírio sofrido por um alcoólatra, causado pela interrupção abrupta do consumo de álcool.
 anxious d., d. ansioso; delírio em que o sintoma predominante é uma apreensão ou ansiedade incoerente.
 d. cor′dis, termo obsoleto para fibrilação atrial (atrial *fibrillation*).
 posttraumatic d., d. pós-traumático; delírio causado por uma lesão cerebral traumática estrutural.
 senile d., d. senil; delírio associado à demência senil.
 toxic d., d. tóxico; delírio causado pela ação de um veneno.
 d. tre′mens (DT), d. tremens; uma forma grave, algumas vezes fatal, de delírio causada por abstinência alcoólica após um período de intoxicação contínua. [L. pres. p. de *tremo,* tremor]

del·i·tes·cence (del - i - tes′ens). Delitescência; termo raramente usado para: **1.** Cessação súbita de sintomas; desaparecimento de um tumor ou de uma lesão cutânea. **2.** Período de incubação de uma doença infecciosa. [L. *delitesco,* ficar oculto]

de·liv·er (dē - liv′er). Libertar. **1.** Partejar; ajudar uma mulher no parto. **2.** Extrair de um espaço fechado, como o feto do útero, um objeto ou corpo estranho, p. ex., um tumor de sua cápsula ou vizinhança, ou o cristalino do olho em casos de catarata. [do. Fr. ant. do L. *de-* + *liber,* livre]

de·liv·ery (dē - liv′er - ē). Parto; passagem do feto e da placenta do canal genital para o mundo externo.

assisted cephalic d., parto cefálico assistido; extração de um feto em apresentação cefálica.

breech d., parto de nádegas; extração ou expulsão de um feto que se apresenta pelas nádegas ou pés.

forceps d., parto a fórceps; parto de uma criança assistido por meio de um instrumento projetado para segurar a cabeça fetal.

high forceps d., p. a fórceps alto; parto por fórceps aplicado à cabeça fetal antes da insinuação cefálica.

low forceps d., p. a fórceps baixo; parto por fórceps aplicado à cabeça fetal na estação $\geq$ +2 cm, e não no assoalho pélvico. Essa classificação de parto a fórceps pode ser com ou sem rotação da cabeça fetal.

midforceps d., p. a fórceps médio; parto por fórceps aplicado à cabeça fetal acima da estação +2, mas após sua insinuação.

outlet forceps d., p. a fórceps de saída; parto por fórceps aplicado à cabeça fetal quando esta chegou ao assoalho perineal e é visível entre as contrações.

perimortem d., p. pós-morte. SIN postmortem d.

postmortem d., p. pós-morte; extração do feto após a morte de sua mãe. SIN perimortem d.

premature d., p. prematuro; nascimento de um feto entre 20 e 37 semanas de gestação. VER TAMBÉM premature *birth*.

spontaneous cephalic d., p. cefálico espontâneo; expulsão não-assistida de um feto em apresentação cefálica.

del·le (del′eh). A porção central, mais clara, do eritrócito, observada em um esfregaço de sangue corado. [Al. *Delle*, região baixa, depressão]

del·len. Depressões; escavações rasas, em forma de pires, bem definidas, na margem da córnea, com cerca de 1,5 por 2 mm, devidas à desidratação localizada; também chamadas depressões de Fuchs. [Al. pl. de *Delle*, região baixa, depressão]

del·o·mor·phous (del - o - mōr′fŭs). Delomorfo; de forma definitiva; termo aplicado antigamente às células parietais das glândulas gástricas. [G. *delos*, manifesto, + *morphe*, forma]

de·louse (dē - lows′). Despiolhar; remover piolhos; livrar de infestação por piolhos; usado particularmente na profilaxia de doenças transmitidas por piolhos.

del·phi·nine (del′fin - ēn). Delfinina; alcalóide tóxico, derivado da aconina, da *Delphinium staphisagria*; assemelha-se à aconitina em sua ação e estrutura química.

Del·phin·i·um aja·cis (del - fin′ē - ŭm ā - jā′sis). Espécie de planta (família Ranuculaceae) que contém os alcalóides ajacina e ajaconina; as sementes maduras secas têm sido usadas externamente como um parasiticida na pediculose; raramente usada agora devido à sua toxicidade. SIN larkspur. [G. *delphinion*, espora]

del·ta (Δ) (del′tā). Delta. **1.** Quarta letra do alfabeto grego, Δ (maiúscula), δ (minúscula). **2.** Em anatomia, uma superfície triangular.

d. check, prova delta; uma comparação de valores consecutivos para um determinado teste em um arquivo laboratorial de um paciente usada para detectar alterações abruptas, geralmente produzida como parte de programas de controle de qualidade computadorizados. SIN Δ check.

d. for′nicis, d. do fórnice. SIN commissura fornicis.

Galton d., d. de Galton; **(1)** um triângulo mais ou menos bem demarcado, em uma impressão digital, de um lado ou de outro onde as cristas retas próximas da articulação da falange distal são sucedidas por arcos, alças ou espirais. VER TAMBÉM Galton system of classification of *fingerprints*, em *fingerprint*; **(2)** SIN triradius.

d. mesoscap′ulae, d., mesoscapular; a superfície triangular plana na extremidade vertebral da espinha da escápula, sobre a qual desliza o tendão para as fibras inferiores do músculo trapézio.

del·toid (del′toyd). Deltóide; semelhante à letra grega delta (Δ); triangular. [G. *deltoeidēs,* com o formato semelhante à letra *delta*]

de·lu·sion (dē - loo′zhŭn). Ilusão; uma crença falsa ou julgamento errado defendido com convicção apesar de evidências indiscutíveis contrárias. [L. *deludo*, pp. *-lusus*, enganar, trair, de *ludo*, representar]

d. of control, d. of being controlled, i. de controle, ilusão de ser controlado; uma ilusão na qual o indivíduo apresenta sentimentos, impulsos, pensamentos ou ações como não sendo seus próprios, mas como impostos por alguma força externa. SIN d. of passivity.

encapsulated d., i. encapsulada; ilusão geralmente relacionada a um tópico ou uma crença específica, mas que não impregna a vida ou o nível de funcionamento do indivíduo.

expansive d., i. de grandeza. SIN d. of grandeur.

d. of grandeur, i. de grandeza; ilusão na qual um indivíduo se julga possuidor de grande riqueza, inteligência, importância, poder, etc. SIN expansive d., grandiose d.

grandiose d., i. de grandeza. SIN d. of grandeur.

d. of negation, i. de negação; ilusão na qual um indivíduo imagina que o mundo e tudo que se relaciona com ele deixaram de existir. SIN nihilistic d.

nihilistic d., i. niilista. SIN d. of negation.

organic d.'s, i. orgânicas; falsas crenças apresentadas na ilusão associada à demência em conjunto com lesão traumática do cérebro, ou uma alteração orgânica no cérebro, como na síndrome de Alzheimer ou na intoxicação por cocaína ou outras drogas.

d. of passivity, i. de passividade. SIN d. of control.

d. of persecution, persecutory d., i. de perseguição; noção falsa de que o indivíduo está sendo perseguido; sintoma característico da esquizofrenia paranóide.

d. of reference, i. de referência; uma idéia delirante de que os eventos externos, etc., referem-se a si próprio.

somatic d., i. somática; ilusão que tem relação com uma lesão ou alteração inexistente de algum órgão ou parte do corpo; algumas vezes indistinguível da hipocondríase.

systematized d., i. sistematizada; ilusão logicamente construída a partir de uma premissa falsa e que incorpora um setor específico da vida do paciente.

unsystematized d., i. não-sistematizada; uma das ilusões de um grupo de ilusões aparentemente isoladas, desconexas.

de·lu·sion·al (dē - loo′zhŭn - al). Relativo a uma ilusão.

de·mand (dē - mand′). Demanda; a quantidade de uma substância, mercadoria ou serviço desejado ou necessário.

biochemical oxygen d. (BOD), d. bioquímica de oxigênio; a velocidade em que o oxigênio dissolvido é consumido por um organismo (freqüentemente, um microrganismo) ou uma cultura de células.

de·mar·ca·tion (dē - mar - kā′shŭn). Demarcação; estabelecimento de limites; uma fronteira. [Fr. do L. *de*, de, + L. Mediev. *marco*, marcar]

Demarquay, Jean N., cirurgião francês, 1814–1875. VER D. *sign*.

de·mas·cu·lin·iz·ing (dē - mas′kū - lin - īz′ing). Desmasculinizante; que priva das características masculinas ou inibe o desenvolvimento dessas características.

De·mat·i·a·ce·ae (dē - mat - ē - ā′sē - ē). Dematiáceas; família de fungos produtores de melanina, castanhos ou pretos, habitantes do solo, encontrados em vegetais em desintegração, madeira em decomposição e folhas no chão, e que inclui vários gêneros de coloração escura que causam cromoblastomicose em seres humanos, como *Exophiala, Phialophora, Fonsecaea* e *Cladosporium*.

de·mat·i·a·ceous (dē - mat - ē - ā′shŭs). Dematiáceo; denota conídios e/ou hifas escuros, geralmente castanhos ou pretos; usado freqüentemente para designar fungos de coloração escura.

deme (dēm). Demo; um grupo ou parentesco local, pequeno, altamente endogâmico. Cf. isolate. [G. *dēmos*, povo]

dem·e·car·i·um bro·mide (dem - ē - kar′ē - ŭm). Brometo de demecário; um potente inibidor da colinesterase usado no tratamento do glaucoma e da esotropia acomodativa; é estável em solução aquosa.

dem·e·clo·cy·cline (dem′ē - klō - sī′klēn). Demeclociclina; um antibiótico de amplo espectro excretado mais lentamente, e mais estável em ácidos e álcalis que outras formas de tetraciclinas; disponível como cloridrato.

dem·e·col·cine (dem - ē - kol′sēn). Demecolcina; alcalóide do *Colchicum autumnale* (família Liliaceae) quimicamente semelhante à colchicina, exceto pelo grupamento acetil ser substituído por um grupamento metil; usado no tratamento da gota e da leucemia, é considerado menos tóxico que a colchicina e tem uma ação sobre a mitose semelhante à da colchicina.

de·ment·ed (dē - ment′ed). Demente; que sofre de demência.

de·men·tia (dē - men′shē - ă). Demência; a perda, geralmente progressiva, das funções cognitiva e intelectual, sem comprometimento da percepção ou da consciência; causada por vários distúrbios, incluindo infecções graves e toxinas, porém mais comumente associada à doença cerebral estrutural. Caracterizada por desorientação, comprometimento da memória, do julgamento e da inteligência, e labilidade afetiva superficial. SIN amentia (2). [L. de *de-* priv. + *mens*, mente]

AIDS d., d. da AIDS/SIDA. SIN AIDS dementia *complex*.

Alzheimer d., d. de Alzheimer. SIN Alzheimer *disease*.

catatonic d., d. catatônica; demência com sintomas catatônicos.

dialysis d., d. da diálise. SIN dialysis encephalopathy *syndrome*.

epileptic d., d. epiléptica; demência que ocorre em um indivíduo afetado por epilepsia, e atribuída às convulsões prolongadas, à lesão epileptogênica ou aos agentes antiepilépticos.

hebephrenic d., d. hebefrênica; demência com sintomas hebefrênicos.

Lewy body d., d. do corpúsculo de Lewy. SIN diffuse Lewy body *disease*.

multi-infarct d., d. por múltiplos infartos. SIN vascular d.

paralytic d., d. paralítica; demência e paralisia resultantes de meningoencefalite sifilítica crônica. SIN d. paralytica.

d. paralytica, d. paralítica. SIN paralytic d.

posttraumatic d., d. pós-traumática; demência causada por lesão cerebral traumática.

d. prae′cox, d. precoce; qualquer uma pertencente ao grupo de distúrbios psicóticos conhecidos como esquizofrenias; termo usado outrora para descrever a esquizofrenia como uma condição isolada. [L. precocious]

presenile d., d. preseni′lis, d. pré-senil; **(1)** demência da doença de Alzheimer que se desenvolve antes dos 65 anos; **(2)** doença de Alzheimer. SIN Alzheimer *disease*.

primary d., d. primária; demência que ocorre independentemente como um distúrbio mental.

dementia

primary senile d., d. senil primária. SIN Alzheimer *disease*.
secondary d., d. secundária; demência crônica subseqüente e devida a uma psicose ou a algum outro processo mórbido subjacente.
senile d., d. senil; demência da doença de Alzheimer que se desenvolve após os 65 anos de idade.
toxic d., d. tóxica; demência causada por um agente exógeno.
vascular d., d. vascular; deterioração gradual das funções intelectuais com sinais neurológicos focais, em virtude de múltiplos infartos dos hemisférios cerebrais. SIN multi-infarct d.

de·meth·yl·ase (dē - meth'i - lās). Desmetilase. SIN methyltransferase.
de·meth·yl·a·tion. Desmetilação; a remoção enzimática de grupos metil.
♲ **demi-.** Demi-; metade, menor. VER TAMBÉM hemi-, semi-. [Fr. do L. *dimidius*, metade]
dem·i·gaunt·let (dem - ē - gawnt'let). Meia-luva; curativo em forma de luva para os dedos da mão e para a mão. [demi- + *gauntlet*, luva blindada, do I. médio, do Fr. antigo, do Alemão]
dem·i·lune (dem'ē - loon). Meia-lua. **1.** Um corpo pequeno com um formato semelhante ao de uma meia-lua ou um crescente. **2.** Termo freqüentemente usado para o gametócito do *Plasmodium falciparum*. [Fr. meia-lua]
  Giannuzzi d.'s, meias-luas de Giannuzzi. SIN serous d.'s.
  Heidenhain d.'s, meias-luas de Heidenhain. SIN serous d.'s.
  serous d.'s, meias-luas serosas; as células serosas na extremidade distal de uma unidade secretora tubuloalveolar, mucosa de determinadas glândulas salivares. SIN Giannuzzi crescents, Giannuzzi d.'s, Heidenhain crescents, Heidenhain d.'s.
de·min·er·al·i·za·tion (dē - min'er - āl - ī - zā'shŭn). Desmineralização; uma perda ou diminuição dos constituintes minerais do corpo ou de tecidos individuais, principalmente de osso.
dem·i·pen·ni·form (dem'ē - pen'i - fōrm). Semipeniforme. SIN semipennate.
Dem·o·dex (dem'ō - deks). Gênero de ácaros foliculares (família Demodicidae) diminutos (0,1-0,4 mm) que habitam a pele e geralmente são encontrados nas glândulas sebáceas e folículos pilosos dos mamíferos, incluindo os seres humanos. Alguns casos de blefarite em seres humanos foram atribuídos à infestação por *Demodex*; o uso de cremes faciais promove a infestação por *Demodex* em mulheres idosas, resultando em eritema facial com descamação folicular. [G. *dēmos*, ebo, + *dēx*, larva de caruncho]
  ***D. folliculo'rum*,** uma espécie muito comum, universalmente distribuída e, geralmente, não-patogênica de ácaro que habita os folículos pilosos e glândulas sebáceas dos seres humanos, comumente da face ao redor do nariz e da margem do couro cabeludo. SIN *Acarus folliculorum*.
de·mog·ra·phy (dē - mog'rā - fē). Demografia; o estudo das populações, principalmente em relação ao tamanho, densidade, fertilidade, taxa de mortalidade, taxa de crescimento, distribuição etária, migração e estatísticas vitais. [G. *demos*, povo, + *graphō*, escrever]
  dynamic d., d. dinâmica; um estudo do funcionamento de uma comunidade, incluindo registros estatísticos.
Demoivre, Abraham, matemático inglês, 1667–1754. VER D. *formula*.
de·mo·ni·ac (dē - mō'nē - ak). Demoníaco; arrebatado, perverso, como se possuído por espíritos malignos. [G. *daimōn*, um espírito]
dem·on·stra·tor (dem'on - strā - ter, - tōr). Demonstrador; assistente de um professor de anatomia, cirurgia, etc., que prepara a preleção através de dissecções ou reunião de pacientes, ou que instrui pequenas classes suplementares para as preleções regulares; um demonstrador corresponde, de modo geral, ao professor-agregado de uma universidade alemã. [L. *de-monstro*, pp. *-atus*, apontar]
De Morgan, Campbell, médico inglês, 1811–1876. VER De M. *spots*, em *spot*.
de·mor·phin·i·za·tion (dē - mōr'fin - i - zā'shŭn). Desmorfinização. **1.** Remoção da morfina de um opiáceo. **2.** Retirada gradual da morfina como método de vencer a dependência de morfina.
de Morsier, Georges, neurologista suíço do século XX. VER de M. *syndrome*.
de·mu·co·sa·tion (dē - mū - kō - sā'shŭn). Desmucosação; termo raramente usado para excisão ou retirada da mucosa de qualquer parte.
de·mul·cent (de - mŭl'sent). Demulcente. **1.** Suavizante; que alivia a irritação. **2.** Um agente, como uma mucilagem ou óleo, que suaviza e alivia a irritação, principalmente das mucosas. [L. *de-mulceo*, pp. *-mulctus*, acalmar suavemente, amolecer]
de Musset, Alfred. VER Musset.
de·my·e·li·na·tion, de·my·e·lin·i·za·tion (dē - mī'ē - li - nā'shŭn, dē - mī'ē - lin - i - zā'shŭn).Desmielinização; perda de mielina com preservação dos axônios ou dos tratos de fibras. A desmielinização central ocorre no sistema nervoso central (p. ex., a desmielinização observada na esclerose múltipla); a desmielinização periférica afeta o sistema nervoso periférico (p. ex., a desmielinização observada na síndrome de Guillain-Barré).
de·nar·co·tize (dē - nar'kō - tīz). Desnarcotizar; remover as propriedades narcóticas de um opiáceo; privar de propriedades narcóticas.
de·na·to·ni·um ben·zo·ate (dē - nā - tō'nē - ŭm). Benzoato de denatônio; um álcool desnaturante.
de·na·tur·a·tion (dē - na - tū - rā'shŭn). Desnaturação; o processo de tornar desnaturado.

de·na·tured (dē - nā'tŭrd). Desnaturado. **1.** Tornado antinatural ou modificado em relação ao normal em qualquer uma de suas características; freqüentemente aplicado a proteínas ou ácidos nucleicos aquecidos ou tratados de outra forma até o ponto de se alterarem as características estruturais terciárias. **2.** Adulterado, como por adição de metanol ao etanol.
den·dri·form (den'dri - fōrm). Dendriforme; em forma de árvore ou ramificado. SIN arborescent, dendritic (1), dendroid. [G. *dendron*, árvore, + L. *forma*, forma]
den·drite (den'drīt). Dendrito. **1.** Um dos dois tipos de processos protoplasmáticos ramificados da célula nervosa (sendo o outro o axônio). SIN dendritic process, dendron, neurodendrite, neurodendron. **2.** Uma estrutura arboriforme cristalina formada durante o congelamento de uma liga. [G. *dendritēs*, relativo a uma árvore]
  apical d., d. apical. SIN apical *process*.
den·drit·ic (den - drit'ik). Dendrítico. **1.** SIN dendriform. **2.** Relativo aos dendritos das células nervosas.
den·dro·gram (den'drō - gram). Dendrograma; uma figura arboriforme utilizada para representar graficamente uma hierarquia. [*dendron*, árvore, + *gramma*, um desenho]
den·droid (den'droyd). Dendróide. SIN dendriform. [G. *dendron*, árvore, + *eidos*, aparência]
den·dron. Dendrito. SIN dendrite (1). [G. uma árvore]
de·ner·vate (dē - ner'vāt). Desnervar; causar desnervação.
de·ner·va·tion (dē - ner - vā'shŭn). Desnervação; perda da inervação.
den·gue (den'gā). Dengue; uma doença de regiões tropicais e subtropicais que ocorre epidemicamente; é causada pelo vírus da dengue, um membro da família Flaviviridae. Há 4 tipos antigênicos, e estes são transmitidos por um mosquito do gênero *Aedes* (geralmente *A. aegypti*, mas freqüentemente *A. albopictus*). São reconhecidos quatro graus de gravidade: grau I, febre e sintomas constitucionais; grau II, grau I mais hemorragia espontânea (da pele, gengivas ou trato gastrointestinal); grau III, grau II mais agitação e insuficiência circulatória; grau IV, choque profundo. SIN Aden fever, bouquet fever, breakbone fever, dandy fever, date fever, dengue fever, dengue hemorrhagic fever, exanthesis arthrosia, polka fever, scarlatina rheumatica, solar fever (1). [Esp. corruptela da febre "dandy"]
  hemorrhagic d., d. hemorrágico; uma forma mais grave de dengue caracterizada por lesões cutâneas hemorrágicas, que explodiu em muitos surtos epidêmicos na bacia do Pacífico.
de·ni·al (dē - nī'al). Negação; um mecanismo de defesa inconsciente usado para aliviar a ansiedade por negação da existência de conflitos importantes, impulsos problemáticos, eventos, ações ou doença. SIN negation. [I. M., do Fr. ant., do L. *denegare*, negar]
den·i·da·tion (den - i - dā'shŭn). Desnidação; esfoliação da porção superficial da mucosa uterina; retirada da decídua menstrual. [L. *de*, + *nidus*, ninho]
de·ni·tra·tion (dē - nī - trā'shŭn). Desnitração. SIN denitrification.
de·ni·tri·fi·ca·tion (dē - nī'tri - fi - kā'shŭn). Desnitrificação. **1.** Retirada de nitrogênio de qualquer material ou composto químico; principalmente do solo, como por determinadas bactérias (desnitrificantes) que tornam o nitrogênio indisponível para o crescimento vegetal. **2.** Retirada de nitrogênio do solo pelo crescimento vegetal. SIN denitration.
de·ni·tri·fy (dē - nī'tri - fī). Desnitrificar; remover nitrogênio de qualquer material ou composto químico.
de·ni·tro·gen·a·tion (dē - nī'trō - jē - nā'shŭn). Desnitrogenação; eliminação de nitrogênio dos pulmões e tecidos corporais ao respirar gases desprovidos de nitrogênio.
Dennie, Charles Clayton, dermatologista norte-americano, 1883–1971. VER D.-Morgan *fold*; D. *line*.
de·nom·in·a·tor (dē - nōm'i - nā - tor). Denominador; a porção inferior de uma fração usada para calcular uma taxa ou razão; a população de risco no cálculo de uma taxa ou razão.
Denonvilliers, Charles P., cirurgião francês, 1808–1872. VER D. *aponeurosis, ligament*.
de novo (di - nō'vo). De novo; novamente; freqüentemente aplicado a vias bioquímicas específicas nas quais os metabólitos são recém-biossintetizados (p. ex., biossíntese de purina de novo). [L.]
dens, pl. **den·tes** (denz, den'tēz) [TA]. Dente. **1.** SIN tooth. **2.** Dente do áxis; um processo forte, semelhante a um dente, que se projeta para cima a partir do corpo do áxis, ou epistrofeu, ao redor do qual gira o atlas. SIN d. axis [TA], odontoid process of epistropheus, odontoid process. [L.]
  den'tes acus'tici [TA], dentes acústicos. SIN acoustic *teeth*.
  d. angula'ris, d. canino. SIN canine *tooth*.
  d. axis [TA], d. do áxis. SIN dens (2).
  d. bicus'pidus, pl. **den'tes bicus'pidi,** dentes bicúspides, dentes pré-molares. SIN premolar *tooth*.
  d. cani'nus, pl. **den'tes cani'ni** [TA], d. canino. SIN canine *tooth*.
  d. cuspida'tus, pl. **den'tes cuspida'ti,** dentes caninos. SIN canine *tooth*.
  d. decid'uus, pl. **den'tes deci'dui** [TA], d. decíduo. SIN deciduous *tooth*.

d. in den·te, dente invaginado; distúrbio embriológico na formação do dente resultante da invaginação do epitélio associada ao desenvolvimento da coroa na área destinada a tornar-se o espaço da polpa; após a calcificação, há invaginação de esmalte e dentina para o espaço da polpa, produzindo o aspecto radiográfico de um "dente dentro de um dente". SIN d. invaginatus.
d. incisi'vus, pl. **den'tes incisi'vi** [TA], d. incisivo. SIN incisor tooth.
d. invaginatus (denz in'va̅ - ge̅ - na̅' - tus). d. invaginado. SIN d. in dente. [L. Mediev. dobrado para dentro, do L. *vagina*, bainha]
d. lac'teus, d. de leite. SIN deciduous tooth.
d. molaris, pl. **den'tes mola'res** [TA], d. molar. SIN molar tooth. VER TAMBÉM molar.
d. molaris tertius [TA], terceiro dente molar. SIN third-year molar tooth.
d. per'manens, pl. **den'tes permanen'tes** [TA], d. permanente. SIN permanent tooth.
d. premola'ris, pl. **den'tes premola'res** [TA], d. pré-molar. SIN premolar tooth.
d. sapien'tiae, d. de siso. SIN third-year molar tooth. [L. *sapientia*, sabedoria]
d. seroti'nus, terceiro dente molar; *termo oficial alternativo para third-year molar tooth.
d. succeda'neus, d. permanente. SIN permanent tooth.

den·sim·e·ter (den - sim'e̅ - ter). Densímetro. SIN densitometer (1). [L. *densitas*, densidade, + G. *metron*, medida]

den·si·tom·e·ter (den - si - tom'e̅ - ter). Densitômetro. **1.** Também hidrômetro; instrumento para medir a densidade de um líquido. SIN densimeter. **2.** Instrumento para medir, em virtude da turvação relativa, o crescimento de bactérias em caldo; útil na análise microbiológica de nutrientes e antibióticos, estudos de bacteriófagos, etc. **3.** Instrumento para medir a densidade de componentes (p. ex., frações de proteínas) separados por eletroforese ou cromatografia, utilizando absorção ou reflexão de luz. **4.** Instrumento eletrônico para medir o enegrecimento de filme radiológico por exposição aos raios X; usado para sensitometria do filme, densitometria óssea, medida da função de dispersão da linha (microdensitômetro). **5.** Instrumento para medir a extensão de absorção ou reflexão da luz por um material. [L. *densitas*, densidade, + G. *metron*, medida]

den·si·tom·e·try (den - si - tom'e̅ - tre̅). Densitometria; procedimento que utiliza um densitômetro.

den·si·ty (ρ) (den'si - te̅). Densidade. **1.** A solidez de uma substância; a proporção entre a massa e a unidade de volume, geralmente expressa como g/cm³ (kg/m³ no sistema SI). **2.** A quantidade de eletricidade em uma determinada superfície ou em um determinado tempo por unidade de volume. **3.** Em física radiológica, a opacidade à luz de um filme radiográfico ou fotográfico exposto; quanto mais escuro o filme, maior é a densidade medida. **4.** Em radiologia clínica, uma área menos exposta em um filme, que corresponde a uma região de maior atenuação de raios X (radiopacidade) no indivíduo; quanto maior a quantidade de luz transmitida pelo filme, maior é a densidade do indivíduo; isso não é exatamente o oposto da definição anterior, pois um diz respeito à densidade do filme e o outro à densidade do indivíduo. [L. *densitas*, de *densus*, espesso]
bone d., d. óssea; medida quantitativa do conteúdo mineral do osso, usada como indicador de força estrutural do osso e como triagem de osteoporose.
buoyant d., d. de flutuação; a densidade que permite que uma substância flutue em algum líquido padrão.
count d., d. total, d. fotônica. SIN photon d.
flux d., d. de fluxo; **(1)** SIN flux (4); **(2)** a densidade do fluxo de partículas, a taxa de fluxo de partículas, ou a densidade de fluxo de energia, a taxa de fluxo de energia da intensidade. Cf. fluence.
incidence d., d. de incidência; a taxa de incidência pessoa–tempo.
optic d. (OD), d. óptica, absorvência. SIN absorbance.
photon d., d. de fóton, d. fotônica; o número de eventos contados e registrados em cintigrafia por centímetro quadrado ou por polegada quadrada da área de imagem. SIN count d.
spin d., d. de rotação (*spin*); o número de dipolos nucleares por unidade de volume.
vapor d., d. de vapor; a massa por unidade de volume de um vapor; como a densidade de vapor se modifica com a temperatura e pressão, é comumente expressa como peso específico, isto é, o peso do vapor dividido pelo peso de um igual volume de um gás de referência (p. ex., oxigênio ou hidrogênio) na mesma temperatura e pressão.

△ **dent-, denti-, dento-.** Dente; dental. VER TAMBÉM odonto-. [L. *dens*, dente]

den·tal (den'tal). Dental; relativo aos dentes. [L. *dens*, dente]

den·tal en·gine. Mecanismo dentário; a forma motora de um mandril dentário que causa sua rotação.

den·tal·gia (den - tal'je̅ - a̅). Dentalgia; dor de dente. SIN toothache. [L. *dens*, dente, + G. *algos*, dor]

den·tate (den'ta̅t). Denteado; entalhado; dentado. [L. *dentatus*, dentado]

den·ta·tec·to·my (den - ta̅ - tek'to̅ - me̅). Dentatectomia; destruição cirúrgica do núcleo denteado do cerebelo. [denteado (núcleo) + G. *ectome̅*, excisão]

den·ta·tum (den - ta̅'tum, den - tah'tum). Núcleo denteado do cerebelo. SIN dentate nucleus of cerebellum. [L. neut. of *dentatus*, denteado]

den·tes (den'te̅z). Dentes. Plural de dens. [L.]

△ **denti-.** VER dent-.

den·tia (den - te̅'a). Dentição; o processo de desenvolvimento ou erupção dos dentes. Também serve para indicar uma relação com os dentes. [dent- + sufixo -*ia*, condição, processo]
d. praecox (den - te̅'a pre̅ - coks). Dentição precoce; erupção prematura dos dentes. [L. prematuro]
d. tarda (den - te̅a' tar'da̅). Dentição tardia; erupção tardia dos dentes. [L. tardia]

den·ti·cle (den'ti - kl). Dentículo. **1.** SIN endolith. **2.** Uma projeção dentiforme de uma superfície dura. [L. *denticulus*, um dente pequeno]

den·tic·u·late, den·tic·u·lat·ed (den - tik'u̅ - lat, - lat - ed). Denticulado. **1.** Finamente denteado, entalhado ou serrilhado. **2.** Que possui dentes pequenos.

den·ti·form (den'ti - fo̅rm). Dentiforme; em forma de dente; cavilhado. VER TAMBÉM odontoid (1). [denti- + L. *forma*, forma]

den·ti·frice (den'ti - fris). Dentifrício; qualquer preparação usada na limpeza dos dentes, p. ex., um pó dentário, pasta de dente ou colutório. [L. *dentifricium*, de *dens*, dente, + *frico*, pp. *frictus*, esfregar]

den·tig·er·ous (den - tij'er - u̅s). Dentígero; originado de, ou associado a, um dente, como um cisto dentígero. [denti- + L. *gero*, manter]

den·ti·la·bi·al (den'ti - la̅'be̅ - a̅l). Dentilabial; relativo aos dentes e aos lábios. [denti- + L. *labium*, lábio]

den·ti·lin·gual (den - ti - ling'gwa̅l). Dentilingual; relativo aos dentes e à língua. [denti- + L. *lingua*, língua]

den·tin (den'tin). Dentina. SIN dentine. [L. *dens*, dente]
hereditary opalescent d., d. opalescente hereditária; **(1)** SIN dentinogenesis imperfecta; **(2)** SIN opalescent d.
hypersensitive d., d. hipersensível; dentina exposta, geralmente na porção cervical de um dente, dolorosa ao tato, a doces ou a alterações térmicas.
interglobular d., d. interglobular; matriz imperfeitamente calcificada de dentina situada entre os glóbulos calcificados próximos da periferia da dentina.
irregular d., irritation d., d. irregular; d. de irritação. SIN tertiary d.
opalescent d., d. opalescente; dentina geralmente associada a dentinogênese imperfeita. Confere um aspecto opalescente ou translúcido incomum aos dentes. SIN hereditary opalescent d. (2).
peritubular d., d. peritubular; uma camada eletrondensa de dentina observada adjacente ao processo odontoblástico.
primary d., d. primária; dentina que se forma até que a raiz esteja completa.
reparative d., d. reparadora. SIN tertiary d.
sclerotic d., d. esclerótica; dentina caracterizada por calcificação dos túbulos de dentina em virtude de lesão ou envelhecimento normal. SIN transparent d.
secondary d., d. secundária; dentina formada por função normal da polpa após a conclusão da formação da extremidade radicular.
tertiary d., d. terciária; dentina morfologicamente irregular em resposta a um irritante. SIN irregular d., irritation d., reparative d.
transparent d., d. transparente. SIN sclerotic d.
vascular d., d. vascular. SIN vasodentin.

den·ti·nal (den'ti - nal). Dentinário; relativo à dentina.

den·ti·nal·gia (den - ti - nal'je̅ - a̅). Dentinalgia; sensibilidade ou dor na dentina. [dentin + G. *algos*, dor]

den·tine (den'te̅n) [TA]. Dentina; o marfim que forma a massa do dente. Cerca de 20% é matriz orgânica, principalmente colágeno, com alguma elastina e uma pequena quantidade de mucopolissacarídeo; a fração inorgânica (70%) é principalmente hidroxiapatita, com algum carbonato, magnésio e fluoreto. A dentina é atravessada por um grande número de túbulos finos que seguem da cavidade pulpar para fora; dentro dos túbulos há processos oriundos dos odontoblastos. SIN dentinum [TA], dentin, ebur dentis, substantia eburnea.

den·tin·o·ce·ment·al (den'ti - no̅ - se - men'ta̅l). Dentinocementário; relativo à dentina e ao cemento dos dentes. SIN cementodentinal.

den·tin·o·e·nam·el (den'ti - no̅ - e̅ - nam'el). Amelodentinário; relativo à dentina e ao esmalte dos dentes. SIN amelodentinal.

den·tin·o·gen·e·sis (den'ti - no̅ - jen'e̅ - sis). Dentinogênese; o processo de formação da dentina no desenvolvimento dos dentes. [dentin + G. *genesis*, produção]
d. imperfec'ta [MIM*125490 & MIM*125500], d. imperfeita; um distúrbio autossômico dominante dos dentes caracterizado clinicamente por dentes cinza a amarelo-castanhos translúcidos, envolvendo tanto a dentição primária quanto a permanente; o esmalte fratura facilmente, deixando exposta a dentina, que sofre rápido atrito; nas radiografias, as câmaras e os canais da polpa parecem obliterados, e as raízes são curtas e grosseiras; algumas vezes ocorre associada à osteogênese imperfeita; herança autossômica dominante. SIN hereditary opalescent dentin (1).

den·ti·noid (den'ti - noyd). Dentinóide. **1.** Semelhante à dentina. **2.** SIN dentinoma. [dentin + G. *eidos*, semelhança]

den·ti·no·ma (den'ti - no̅'ma̅). Dentinoma; um tumor odontogênico benigno raro que consiste, microscopicamente, em dentina displásica e filamentos de epitélio em um estroma fibroso. SIN dentinoid (2). [dentin + G. *-oma*, tumor]

den·ti·num (den'ti - num) [TA]. Dentina. SIN dentine. [L. *dens*, dente]

den·tip·a·rous (den - tip′a - rŭs). Dentíparo; que produz dente. [denti- + L. *pario*, suportar]

den·tist. Dentista; um profissional legalmente qualificado de odontologia.

den·tis·try (den′tis - trē). Odontologia; a ciência de curar e a arte relacionada à estrutura e função do complexo orofacial, e à prevenção, diagnóstico e tratamento de deformidades, doenças e lesões traumáticas. SIN odontology, odontonosology.

community d., o. comunitária; odontologia de saúde pública, com uma base acadêmica, enfatizando a obrigação profissional de favorecer a prestação de prevenção, educação e cuidados com a população.

esthetic d., o. estética; campo da odontologia que cuida especialmente do aspecto da dentição alcançado através de seu arranjo, forma e cor.

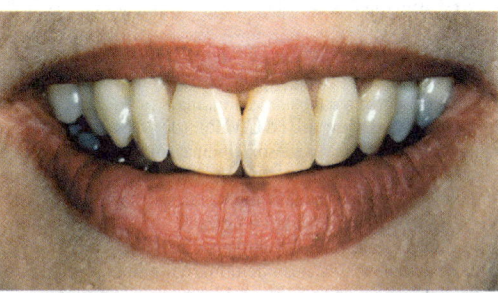

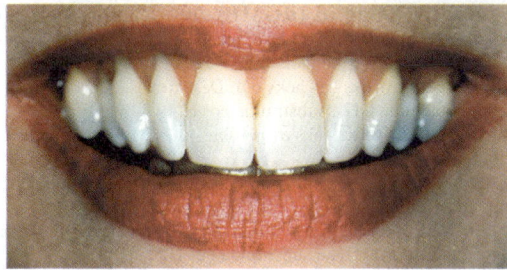

clareamento vital: de dentes naturais por razões estéticas; (em cima) antes; (embaixo) depois

forensic d., o. forense; **(1)** a relação e a aplicação de fatos dentários a problemas legais, como no uso dos dentes para identificar cadáveres; **(2)** a lei no que se refere à prática da odontologia. SIN dental jurisprudence, forensic odontology, legal d.

legal d., o. legal. SIN forensic d.

operative d., o. operatória; geralmente a restauração individual de dentes por meio de materiais metálicos ou não-metálicos. SIN restorative d.

pediatric d., o. pediátrica. SIN pedodontics.

preventive d., o. preventiva; uma filosofia e método de prática odontológica que busca evitar o início, a progressão e a recorrência de doença dental.

prosthetic d., o. protética. SIN prosthodontics.

public health d., o. de saúde pública; especialidade da odontologia relacionada com a prevenção e controle de doenças dentárias e promoção da saúde oral através de esforços comunitários organizados.

restorative d., o. restauradora. SIN operative d.

den·ti·tion (den - tish′ŭn). Dentição; os dentes naturais, considerados coletivamente, no arco dental; podem ser decíduos, permanentes ou mistos. [L. *dentitio*, dentição]

artificial d., d. artificial. SIN denture (1).

deciduous d., d. decídua. SIN deciduous *tooth*.

delayed d., d. tardia; erupção tardia dos dentes.

first d., primeira d. SIN deciduous *tooth*.

mandibular d., d. mandibular. SIN mandibular dental *arcade*.

maxillary d., d. maxilar. SIN maxillary dental *arcade*.

natural d., d. natural. VER dentition.

primary d., d. primária. SIN deciduous *tooth*.

retarded d., d. retardada; dentição na qual fenômenos de crescimento, como calcificação, alongamento e erupção, ocorrem mais tarde que na faixa média de variação normal em virtude de alguma disfunção metabólica sistêmica (p. ex., hipotireoidismo).

secondary d., d. secundária. SIN permanent *tooth*.

succedaneous d., d. sucedânea. SIN permanent *tooth*.

dento-. VER dent-.

den·to·al·ve·o·lar (den′to - al - vē′ō - lăr). Dentoalveolar; geralmente designa a porção do osso alveolar imediatamente em torno dos dentes; usado também para designar a unidade funcional dos dentes e do osso alveolar.

den·tode (den′tōd). Dentodo; reprodução exata de um dente em um molde montado gnatograficamente.

den·toid (den′toyd). Dentóide. SIN odontoid (1). VER TAMBÉM dentiform. [dent- + G. *eidos*, semelhança]

den·to·le·gal (den - tō - lē′gal). Dentolegal; relativo à odontologia e à lei. VER forensic *dentistry*.

den·to·li·va (den - tō - lī′vă). Termo raramente usado para oliva. [L. *dens*, dente, + *oliva*, oliva]

den·tu·lous (den′tū - lŭs). Que possui dentes naturais na boca.

den·ture (den′tūr). Dentadura. **1.** Um substituto artificial para dentes naturais ausentes e tecidos adjacentes. SIN artificial dentition. **2.** Algumas vezes usado para designar a dentição de animais.

bar joint d., d. de revestimento. SIN overlay d.

complete d., d. completa; prótese dentária que substitui a dentição natural perdida e estruturas associadas da maxila ou mandíbula. SIN full d.

design d., projeto da d.; uma visualização planejada da forma e da extensão de uma prótese dentária, feita após um estudo de todos os fatores envolvidos.

fixed partial d., d. parcial fixa; restauração de um ou mais dentes ausentes, que não pode ser facilmente removida pelo paciente ou dentista; está permanentemente fixada aos dentes naturais ou raízes, responsáveis pela sustentação primária do aparelho. SIN bridge (3), fixed bridge.

full d., d. completa. SIN complete d.

immediate d., d. imediata; uma dentadura completa ou parcial construída para inserção imediatamente após a remoção de dentes naturais. SIN immediate insertion d.

immediate insertion d., d. de inserção imediata. SIN immediate d.

implant d., d. de implante; uma dentadura que recebe sua estabilidade e retenção de uma subestrutura que está parcial ou totalmente implantada sob os tecidos moles da base da dentadura. VER TAMBÉM implant denture *substructure*, implant denture *superstructure*, subperiosteal *implant*.

interim d., d. provisória; prótese dentária usada por um curto intervalo de tempo por motivo de estética, mastigação, suporte oclusal ou conveniência, ou para condicionar o paciente a aceitar um substituto artificial para os dentes naturais perdidos até que possa ser feito um tratamento dentário protético mais definitivo. SIN provisional d., temporary d.

overlay d., d. de revestimento; dentadura completa sustentada por tecidos moles e dentes naturais que foram alterados de forma a permitir que a dentadura se encaixe sobre eles. Os dentes alterados podem ter sido adaptados por coroas curtas ou longas, diques ou barras de conexão. SIN bar joint d., hybrid prosthesis, overdenture, telescopic d.

partial d., d. parcial; prótese dentária que restaura um ou mais dentes naturais, porém não todos, e/ou partes associadas, e que é sustentada pelos dentes e/ou pela mucosa; pode ser removível ou fixa. SIN bridgework.

partial d., distal extension, d. parcial, extensão distal; dentadura parcial removível que é retida pelos dentes naturais apenas em uma extremidade dos segmentos basais dentários, e na qual uma parte da carga funcional é carregada pela crista residual.

provisional d., d. provisória. SIN interim d.

removable partial d., d. parcial removível; ponte removível; dentadura parcial que fornece dentes e estruturas associadas a uma mandíbula parcialmente edentada, e que pode ser facilmente removida da boca. SIN removable bridge.

telescopic d., d. telescópica, d. de revestimento. SIN overlay d.

temporary d., d. temporária. SIN interim d.

transitional d., d. transicional; dentadura parcial que serve como prótese temporária à qual serão acrescentados dentes à medida que mais dentes forem perdidos, e que será substituída depois das alterações teciduais pós-extração; uma dentadura transicional pode tornar-se uma dentadura provisória quando são removidos todos os dentes do arco dental.

treatment d., d. de tratamento; prótese dentária usada para tratamento ou condicionamento dos tecidos que servirão para sustentar e reter a base da dentadura.

trial d., d. de ensaio; conjunto de dentes artificiais fabricados de forma que possam ser colocados na boca do paciente para verificar a estética, fazer registro ou para qualquer outra operação considerada necessária antes da conclusão da dentadura. SIN wax model d.

wax model d., d. de modelo de cera. SIN trial d.

den·ture ser·vice. Serviços protéticos; aqueles procedimentos realizados no diagnóstico, construção e manutenção de substitutos artificiais para dentes naturais perdidos.

den·tur·ist (den′tūr - ist). Protético; técnico dentário que fabrica e ajusta dentaduras sem a supervisão de um dentista.

Denucé, Jean L.P., cirurgião francês, 1824–1889. VER D. *ligament*.

de·nu·cle·at·ed (dē - noo′klē - ā - ted). Desnucleado; privado de um núcleo.

de·nu·da·tion (den - ū - dā′shŭn). Desnudação; privar de uma camada de revestimento ou proteção; o ato de pôr a nu, como na remoção do epitélio de uma superfície. [L. *de-nudo*, pôr a nu, de *de*, de, + *nudus*, nu]

de·nude (dē′nood). Desnudar; realizar desnudação.

Denys, Joseph, bacteriologista belga, 1857–1932. VER D.-Leclef *phenomenon*.

de·o·dor·ant (dē - ō′der - ant). Desodorante. **1.** Que elimina ou mascara um cheiro, principalmente um cheiro desagradável. **2.** Um agente que possui essa ação; principalmente um cosmético combinado a um antitranspirante. SIN deodorizer. [L. *de-* priv. + *odoro*, pp. *-atus*, fornecer um odor para, de *odor*, cheiro]

de·o·dor·ize (dē - ō′der - īz). Desodorizar; usar um desodorante.

de·o·dor·iz·er (dē - ō′der - īz - er). Desodorizante. SIN deodorant (2).

de·on·tol·o·gy (dē - on - tol′ō - jē). Deontologia; o estudo da ética e dos deveres profissionais. [G. *deon* (*deont-*), aquilo que é obrigatório, pr. part., neutro de *dei*, (impers.) compete a, de *deō*, obrigar moralmente, + *logos*, estudo]

de·or·sum·duc·tion (dē - ōr′sŭm - dŭk′shŭn). Infradução; rotação de um olho para baixo. SIN infraduction. [L. *deorsum*, para baixo, + *duco*, levar]

de·os·si·fi·ca·tion (dē - os′i - fi - kā′shŭn). Desossificação; remoção dos constituintes minerais do osso. VER demineralization. [L. *de*, de, + *os*, osso, + *facio*, fazer]

de·ox·i·da·tion (dē′oks - i - dā′shŭn). Desoxidação; privar um composto químico de seu oxigênio.

de·ox·i·dize (dē - oks′i - dīz). Desoxidar; remover oxigênio de sua combinação química.

deoxy-. Desoxi-; prefixo de nomes químicos de substâncias para indicar substituição de um –OH por um H.

de·ox·y·a·den·o·sine (dA, dAdo) (dē - oks′ē - ă - den′ō - sēn). Desoxiadenosina; 2′-desoxirribosiladenina, um dos quatro principais nucleosídeos do ADN (sendo os outros a desoxicitidina, desoxiguanosina e timidina). O derivado 5′ também é um importante componente de uma forma de vitamina B_{12}. A desoxiadenosina acumula-se em indivíduos com doença por imunodeficiência combinada grave.

de·ox·y·a·den·o·sine meth·yl·ase. Desoxiadenosina metilase. SIN dam methylase.

5′-de·ox·y·ad·e·no·syl·co·bal·a·min (dē - oks′ē - ă - den - ō - sil - kō - bal′ă - min). 5′-desoxiadenosilcobalamina; uma forma coenzima ativa de vitamina B_{12}; necessária na conversão de metilmalonil-CoA em succinil-CoA. A deficiência de 5′-desoxiadenosilcobalamina resultará em acidemia metilmalônica.

de·ox·y·ad·e·nyl·ic ac·id (dAMP) (dē - oks′ē - ad - en - il′ik). Ácido desoxiadenílico; monofosfato de desoxiadenosina, um produto da hidrólise do ADN, diferente do ácido adenílico por conter desoxirribose no lugar da ribose. SIN adenine deoxyribonucleotide.

de·ox·y·bar·bi·tu·rate (dē - oks - ē - bar - bit′ŭr - āt). Desoxibarbiturato; um barbiturato que não possui o átomo de oxigênio na posição #2 no anel; exemplo de um desoxibarbiturato é o agente antiepiléptico, primidona. VER TAMBÉM barbiturate.

de·ox·y·cho·late (DOC) (dē - oks - ē - kō′lāt). Desoxicolato; um sal ou éster do ácido desoxicólico.

de·ox·y·cho·lic ac·id (dē - oks - ē - kō′lik). Ácido desoxicólico; ácido 7-desoxicólico; ácido 3α,12α-diidroxi-5β-colânico; um ácido biliar e colerético; usado em preparações bioquímicas como detergente.

de·ox·y·co·for·my·cin (dē′oks - ē - cō - fōr - mī′sin). Desoxicoformicina; um análogo da purina que atua como antimetabólito; potente inibidor da adenosina desaminase. Usado como agente antineoplásico. VER TAMBÉM pentostatin.

2-de·ox·y·co·for·my·cin. 2-desoxicoformicina. SIN pentostatin.

de·ox·y·cor·ti·cos·ter·one (DOC) (dē - oks′ē - kōr - ti - kos′ter - ōn). Desoxicorticosterona; um esteróide adrenocortical, principalmente um precursor da biossíntese da corticosterona, que ocasionalmente aparece nas secreções adrenocorticais; um potente mineralocorticóide sem atividade glicocorticóide considerável. SIN 21-hydroxyprogesterone, cortexone, deoxycortone, desoxycortone.

d. acetate, acetato de desoxicorticosterona; sal acetato usado para injeção intramuscular para terapia de reposição do esteróide adrenocortical.

d. pivalate, pivalato de desoxicorticosterona; sal pivalato do esteróide.

de·ox·y·cor·tone (dē - oks - ē - kōr′tōn). Desoxicortona. SIN deoxycorticosterone.

de·ox·y·cyt·i·dine (dē - oks - ē - sī′ti - dēn). Desoxicitidina; 2′-desoxirribosilcitosina, um dos quatro principais nucleosídeos do ADN (sendo os outros a desoxiadenosina, desoxiguanosina e timidina).

de·ox·y·cyt·i·dyl·ic ac·id (dCMP) (dē - oks′ē - sī - ti - dil′ik). Ácido desoxicitidílico; monofosfato de desoxicitidina, um produto da hidrólise do ADN.

de·ox·y·ep·i·neph·rine (dē - oks′ē - ep - i - nef′rēn). Desoxiepinefrina; uma amina simpaticomimética usada como vasoconstritor.

de·ox·y·gua·no·sine (dē - oks - ē - gwan′ō - sēn). Desoxiguanosina; 2′-desoxirribosilguanosina, um dos quatro principais nucleosídeos do ADN (sendo os outros a desoxiadenosina, desoxicitidina e timidina). Acumula-se em indivíduos com deficiência da fosforilase do nucleosídeo purina.

de·ox·y·gua·nyl·ic ac·id (dGMP) (dē - oks - ē - gwan - il′ik). Ácido desoxiguanílico; monofosfato de desoxiguanosina, um produto da hidrólise do ADN. SIN guanine deoxyribonucleotide.

de·ox·y·hex·ose (dē - oks - ē - heks′ōs). Desoxiexose; um desoxi-açúcar de 6 carbonos no qual uma OH é substituída por H.

de·ox·y·nu·cle·o·side (dē - oks′ē - noo′klē - ō - sīd). Desoxinucleotídeo. VER deoxyribonucleoside.

de·ox·y·nu·cle·o·tide (dē - oks′ē - noo′klē - ō - tīd). Desoxinucleotídeo. VER deoxyribonucleoside.

de·ox·y·pen·tose (dē - oks - ē - pen′tōs). Desoxipentose; um desoxi-açúcar de 5 carbonos no qual uma OH é substituída por H.

de·ox·y·ri·bo·al·dol·ase (dē - oks′ē - rī - bō - al′dō - lās). Desoxirriboaldolase. SIN deoxyribosephosphate aldolase.

de·ox·y·ri·bo·di·py·rim·i·dine pho·to·ly·ase (dē - oks′ē - rī′bō - dī - pī - rim′i - dēn). Desoxirribodipirimidina fotoliase; enzima no fermento que é ativada pela luz e, em consequência disso, consegue reverter uma reação fotoquímica prévia por clivagem do anel ciclobutano do dímero timina. SIN dipyrimidine photolyase, photoreactivating enzyme.

de·ox·y·ri·bo·nu·cle·ase (DNAse, DNAase, DNase) (dē - oks′ē - rī - bō - noo′klē - ās). Desoxirribonuclease; qualquer enzima (fosfodiesterase) que

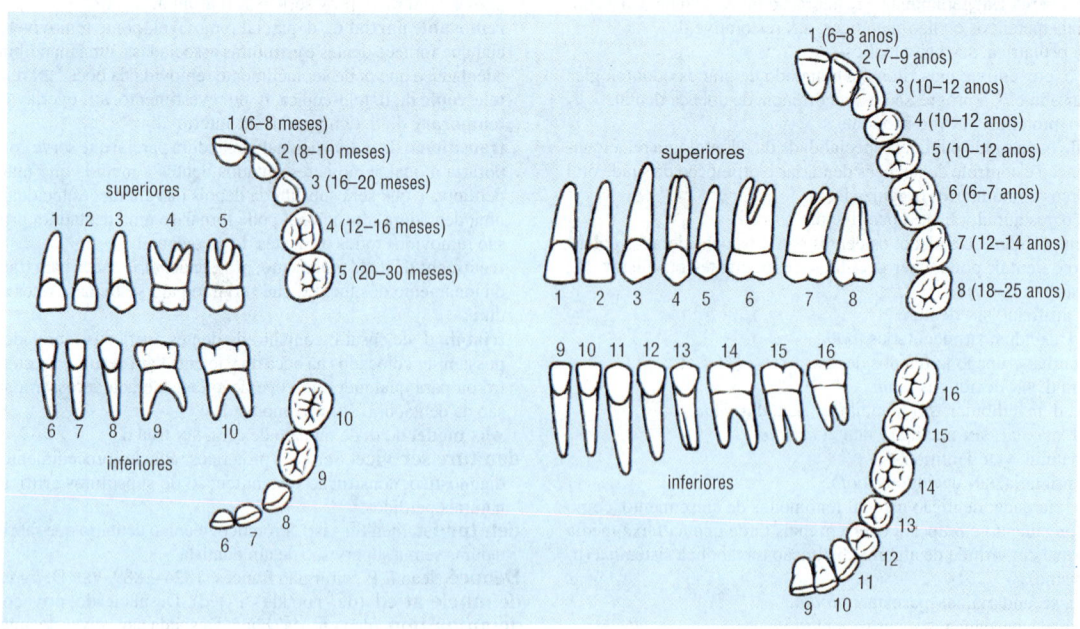

dentição decídua: esquerda; (1, 6) incisivo central; (2, 7) incisivo lateral; (3, 8) canino; (4, 9) primeiro molar; (5, 10) segundo molar

dentição permanente: direita; (1, 9) incisivo central; (2, 10) incisivo lateral; (3, 11) canino; (4, 12) primeiro bicúspide; (5, 13) segundo bicúspide; (6, 14) primeiro molar; (7, 15) segundo molar; (8, 16) terceiro molar

deoxyribonuclease (DNAse, DNAase, DNase) hidrolisa ligações fosfodiéster no ADN. VER TAMBÉM endonuclease, nuclease.
  acid d., d. ácida. SIN d. II.
  d. I, DNase I, d. I, DNase I; uma endonuclease que, basicamente, cliva o ADN de duplo filamento em uma mistura de oligodesoxirribonucleotídeos, cada um terminando em um 5'-fosfato; a estreptodornase é uma enzima semelhante. Em condições apropriadas, pode produzir interrupções em um filamento do ADN; usada na tradução de interrupções e no mapeamento de regiões hipersensíveis. SIN pancreatic d., thymonuclease.
  d. II, DNase II, d. II, DNase II; uma endonuclease que cliva os dois filamentos de ADN nativo (bem como o ADN de filamento único) para produzir uma mistura de oligodesoxinucleotídeos, cada um terminando em um 3'-fosfato. SIN acid d.
  pancreatic d., d. pancreática. SIN d. I.
  d. S₁, d. S₁. SIN endonuclease S₁ *Aspergillus.*
  spleen d., d. esplênica; nome antigo da micrococcal *endonuclease*.

de·ox·y·ri·bo·nu·cle·ic ac·id (DNA) (dē - oks'e - rī'bō - noo - klē'ic). Ácido desoxirribonucleico; (ADN); o tipo de ácido nucleico que contém desoxirribose como o componente açúcar e encontrado principalmente nos núcleos (cromatina, cromossomas) e nas mitocôndrias de células animais e vegetais, em geral ligado frouxamente à proteína (daí o termo desoxirribonucleoproteína); considerado o componente auto-reprodutor dos cromossomas e de muitos vírus, e o repositório de características hereditárias. Sua cadeia macromolecular linear consiste em moléculas de desoxirribose esterificadas com grupamentos fosfato entre os grupamentos 3'- e 5'-hidroxila; ligadas a essa estrutura estão as purinas adenina (A) e guanina (G), bem como as pirimidinas citosina (C) e timina (T). O ADN pode ser aberto ou circular, de filamento único ou duplo, e são conhecidas muitas formas, sendo a mais comum a de duplo filamento, na qual as pirimidinas e as purinas sofrem ligação cruzada através da ligação de hidrogênio no esquema A-T e C-G, colocando dois filamentos antiparalelos em uma hélice dupla. Os cromossomas são compostos de ADN de duplo filamento; o ADN mitocondrial é circular.
  A-DNA, uma forma de ADN na qual a hélice está orientada para a direita e o aspecto geral é curto e largo.
  antisense DNA, ADN anti-senso; ADN de orientação reversa; o filamento de ADN complementar ao que possui a mensagem genética e a partir do qual pode ser reconstruído. Uma seqüência de ADN complementar a uma porção de ARNm. Usado como potencial terapêutico para interromper a transcrição ou tradução de patógenos ou gene do hospedeiro impropriamente expresso.
  B-DNA, uma forma de ADN na qual a hélice está orientada para a direita e o aspecto geral é longo e fino.
  blunt-ended DNA, ADN de extremidade cega; ADN de duplo filamento no qual pelo menos uma das extremidades não possui bases sem par.
  competitor DNA, ADN competidor; ADN de um organismo de teste que é desnaturado e, depois, usado em experiências de hibridização *in vitro* nas quais compete com o ADN (homólogo) de um organismo de referência; usado para determinar a relação entre o organismo de teste e o organismo de referência.
  complementary DNA (cDNA), ADN complementar; **(1)** ADN de filamento único que é complementar ao ARN mensageiro; **(2)** ADN que foi sintetizado a partir do ARNm pela ação da transcriptase reversa.
  extrachromosomal DNA, ADN extracromossomial; ADN que ocorre naturalmente fora do núcleo (p. ex., ADN mitocondrial).

DNA fingerprinting, impressão digital do ADN, tipagem do ADN; identificação individual pelo ADN; técnica usada para comparar indivíduos por genotipagem molecular. O ADN isolado de uma amostra biológica é digerido e fracionado. A hibridização *Southern* com um ADN repetitivo marcado radioativamente produz um padrão auto-radiográfico único do indivíduo. SIN DNA profiling, DNA typing.
  Uma técnica desenvolvida em 1985 para comparar grupos de ADN pela localização de seqüências idênticas de nucleotídeos. As aplicações forenses da identificação individual pelo ADN baseiam-se na premissa de que não existem duas pessoas com constituições genéticas exatamente iguais. As características mais distintas do genoma de um indivíduo não são os próprios genes, mas o número variável de repetições consecutivas (VNTRs) que ocorrem entre os genes. Embora estas não transmitam informações genéticas, são bastante consistentes nas células de um indivíduo e muito variáveis de um indivíduo para outro. Na identificação digital pelo ADN, a amostra é dividida em fragmentos de nucleotídeos por tratamento com enzimas de restrição, sendo depois submetida à eletroforese em gel de forma a produzir um padrão característico de bandas. Sondas radioativas, compostas de seqüências curtas de nucleotídeos (10–15 pares de bases), então identificam locais de repetições consecutivas e hibridizam com elas. A comparação dos resultados de duas ou mais fontes de ADN revela seu grau de parentesco. A identificação individual pelo ADN oferece uma base estatística para avaliar a probabilidade de que amostras de sangue, cabelo, sêmen ou tecido sejam de uma determinada pessoa. Também oferece uma forma de determinar linhagens de seres humanos e animais. A *U.S. National Academy of Sciences* aprovou cautelosamente o uso de identificações individuais pelo ADN como evidência criminal, enquanto aguarda outras pesquisas e a padronização da técnica.

genomic DNA, ADN genômico; ADN que contém introns e exons.
junk DNA, ADN "lixo"; a porção do ADN que não é transcrita nem expressa, formando uma grande fração dos pares de bases do genoma humano; sua função não é conhecida.
DNA ligase, ADN ligase; enzima que leva à formação de uma ligação fosfodiéster em uma quebra de um filamento no ADN duplo; uma parte do sistema de reparo do ADN.
linker DNA, o ADN encontrado entre nucleossomas na cromatina; por não ser associado a proteínas tão fortemente quanto outras formas de ADN, é acessível à hidrólise pela exonuclease.
DNA nucleotidylexotransferase, ADN nucleotidilexotransferase; uma enzima que consegue catalisar a adição de um nucleotídeo, apresentado como um trifosfato de nucleosídeo, em um ADN ou polidesoxinucleotídeo semelhante; foi usada em estudos de recombinação do ADN para acrescentar nucleotídeos para formar caudas de homopolímero. SIN terminal addition enzyme, terminal deoxynucleotidyltransferase.
palindromic DNA, ADN palindrômico; um segmento de ADN no qual a seqüência é simétrica em torno de seu ponto médio.
DNA polymerase, ADN polimerase. VER nucleotidyltransferases.
DNA profiling, impressão digital do DNA. SIN DNA fingerprinting.
recombinant DNA, ADN recombinante; ADN alterado resultante da inserção na cadeia, por meios químicos, enzimáticos ou biológicos, de uma seqüência (uma cadeia total ou parcial de ADN) não originalmente (biologicamente) presente nessa cadeia.
repetitive DNA, ADN repetitivo; um segmento de ADN que consiste em um arranjo linear de múltiplas cópias da mesma seqüência de nucleotídeos.
satellite DNA, ADN satélite; ADN nas regiões satélites de cromossomas acrocêntricos.
sticky-ended DNA, ADN de extremidade coesiva; ADN de duplo filamento no qual um dos filamentos se projeta em relação ao outro (isto é, tem um número ímpar de bases) em uma extremidade ou mais.
DNA typing, tipagem do ADN. SIN DNA fingerprinting.
Z-DNA, uma forma de ADN na qual a hélice está orientada para a esquerda, e o aspecto geral é alongado e delgado.
zero time-binding DNA, ADN que se tornou a forma dupla no início de um processo de reassociação.

de·ox·y·ri·bo·nu·cle·o·pro·tein (DNP, Dnp) (dē - oks'e - rī - bō - noo'klē - ō - prō'tēn). Desoxirribonucleoproteína; o complexo de ADN e proteína no qual o ADN geralmente é encontrado após ruptura e isolamento celular.

de·ox·y·ri·bo·nu·cle·o·side (dē - oks'e - rī - bō - noo'klē - ō - sīd). Desoxirribonucleosídeo; um nucleosídeo componente do ADN que contém 2-desoxi-D-ribose; a produção da condensação da desoxi-D-ribose com purinas ou pirimidinas.

de·ox·y·ri·bo·nu·cle·o·tide (dē - oks'e - rī - bō - noo'klē - ō - tīd). Desoxirribonucleotídeo; um componente nucleotídeo do ADN que contém 2-desoxi-D-ribose; o éster fosfórico do desoxirribonucleosídeo; formado na biossíntese do nucleotídeo.

de·ox·y·ri·bose (dē - oks - ē - rī'bōs). Desoxirribose; uma desoxipentose, sendo a 2-desoxi-D-ribose o exemplo mais comum, que ocorre no ADN e é responsável por seu nome.
  d. phosphate, fosfato de desoxirribose. VER deoxyribonucleotide.

de·ox·y·ri·bose·phos·phate al·dol·ase (dē - oks'e - rī - bōs - fos'fāt). Desoxirribosefosfato aldolase; uma enzima que catalisa a clivagem de 2-desoxi-D-ribose 5-fosfato em D-gliceraldeído 3-fosfato e acetaldeído. SIN deoxyriboaldolase.

de·ox·y·ri·bo·side (dē - ok's - ē - rī'bō - sīd). Desoxirribosídeo; desoxirribose combinada através de seu átomo 1-O com um radical derivado de um álcool; não deve ser confundido com compostos desoxirribosil como os desoxirribonucleosídeos. Cf. deoxyribosyl.

de·ox·y·ri·bo·syl (dē - oks - ē - rī'bō - sil). Desoxirribosil; o radical formado a partir da desoxirribose por remoção da OH do carbono C-1; p. ex., desoxiadenosina. Cf. deoxyriboside.

de·ox·y·ri·bo·syl·trans·fer·as·es (dē - oks'e - rī'bō - sil - trans'fer - ās - es). Desoxirribosiltransferases; enzimas que catalisam a transferência de 2-desoxi-D-ribose a partir dos desoxirribosídeos para bases livres.

de·ox·y·ri·bo·tide (dē - oks - ē - rī'bō - tīd). Desoxirribotídeo; nome errôneo para desoxirribonucleotídeo ou derivado de desoxinucleotídeo, por analogia com nucleosídeo-nucleotídeo, pelo uso incorreto de desoxirribosídeo.

de·ox·y·ribo·vi·rus (dē - ok'se - vī'rūs). Desoxirribovírus. SIN DNA *virus.*

de·ox·y·thy·mi·dine (dT) (dē - oks'e - thi'mi - dēn). Desoxitimidina. SIN thymidine.

de·ox·y·thy·mi·dyl·ic ac·id (dTMP) (dē - oks′e - thī - mi - dil′ik). Ácido desoxitimidílico; um componente do ADN; original e adequadamente chamado ácido timidílico, mas o uso de desoxi- é menos ambíguo, uma vez que já se sabe da existência do ácido ribotimidílico. SIN thymine deoxyribonucleotide.

de·ox·y·ur·i·dine (dē - oks′e - ūr′i - dēn). Desoxiuridina; um derivado da uridina no qual um ou mais grupamentos hidroxila na porção ribose foram substituídos por um hidrogênio; p. ex., a 2′-desoxiuridina é um desoxinucleosídeo de ocorrência natural raro.

de·o·zon·ize (dē - ō′zō - nīz). Desozonizar; privar de ozônio.

de·pen·dence (dē - pen′dens). Dependência; a qualidade ou condição de contar com, ser influenciado por ou ser subserviente a uma pessoa ou objeto que reflete uma necessidade particular. [L. *dependeo*, pender de]
   anchorage d., d. de ancoragem; a necessidade de células normais de possuir uma superfície apropriada para se fixarem e, assim, crescerem em cultura.
   substance d., d. química; um padrão de sintomas comportamentais, fisiológicos e cognitivos que se desenvolve devido ao uso ou abuso de substâncias; geralmente indicado por tolerância aos efeitos da substância e por sintomas de abstinência que se desenvolvem quando é interrompido o uso da substância.

de·pen·den·cy (dē - pen′dens - ē). Dependência; o estado de ser dependente.
   pyridoxine d. with seizure, d. de piridoxina com convulsão; um distúrbio hereditário (autossômico recessivo) aparentemente associado à deficiência de glutamato descarboxilase tipo I cerebral; as convulsões podem ser controladas com vitamina B_6.

De·pen·do·vi·rus (dē - pen′dō - vī - rŭs). Dependovírus; um gênero de pequenos vírus de ADN de filamento único, defectivos, da família Parvoviridae, que dependem de adenovírus para replicação. SIN adeno-associated virus, adenosatellite virus. [L. *dependeo*, ser dependente de, + virus]

de·per·son·al·i·za·tion (dē - per′son - al - i - zā′shŭn). Despersonalização; um estado em que uma pessoa perde o sentido de sua própria identidade com relação a outras pessoas de sua família ou grupo, ou perde o sentido de sua própria realidade. SIN depersonalization syndrome.

de Pezzer, O., médico francês do século XIX. VER de P. *catheter*.

de·phas·ing. Defasagem; em ressonância magnética, após alinhamento por um pulso de radiofreqüência, a perda gradual de orientação dos núcleos atômicos magnéticos devido à transferência de energia molecular aleatória ou relaxamento.

de·phos·pho·ryl·a·tion (dē - fos′for - i - lā′shŭn). Desfosforilação; remoção de um grupamento fosfórico, em geral hidroliticamente e por ação enzimática, de um composto.

de·pig·men·ta·tion (dē - pig - men - tā′shŭn). Despigmentação; perda de pigmento, podendo ser parcial ou completa. VER TAMBÉM achromia (1).

dep·i·late (dep′i - lāt). Depilar; remover pêlos por qualquer meio. Cf. epilate. [L. *de-pilo*, pp. *-atus*, privar de pêlos, de *de-* neg. + *pilo*, crescer pêlos]

dep·i·la·tion (dep - i - lā′shŭn). Depilação. SIN epilation.

de·pil·a·to·ry (dē - pil′a - tō - rē). Depilatório. **1.** SIN epilatory (1). **2.** Um agente que causa a queda dos pêlos. SIN epilatory (2).
   chemical d., d. químico; substância depilatória aplicada topicamente.

de·ple·tion (dē - plē′shŭn). Depleção. **1.** A remoção de líquidos ou sólidos acumulados. **2.** Um estado de força reduzido devido ao excesso de descargas livres. **3.** Perda excessiva de um constituinte, geralmente essencial, do corpo, p. ex., sal, água, etc.
   salt d., d. de sal; perda excessiva de cloreto de sódio do organismo pela urina, suor, etc.; uma causa de desidratação secundária.
   water d., d. de água; redução do volume total de água no organismo; desidratação.

de·po·lar·i·za·tion (dē - pō′lar - i - zā′shŭn). Despolarização. **1.** Redução relativa da magnitude da polarização; nas células nervosas, a despolarização pode resultar de aumento da permeabilidade da membrana celular aos íons sódio. **2.** A destruição, neutralização ou mudança de direção da polaridade.
   dendritic d., d. dendrítica; a perda de uma carga elétrica negativa nos dendritos de uma célula nervosa.

de·po·lar·ize (dē - pō′lar - īz). Despolarizar; privar de polaridade.

de·pol·y·mer·ase (dē - pol′i - mer - ās). Despolimerase; nome usado originalmente, antes da compreensão da ação hidrolítica, para uma enzima que catalisa a hidrólise de uma macromolécula em componentes mais simples. VER nuclease.

de·pos·it (dē - poz′it). Depósito. **1.** Um sedimento ou precipitado. **2.** Um acúmulo anormal de material inorgânico em um tecido. [L. *de-pono*, pp. *-positus*, depositar]
   brickdust d., sedimento em pó de tijolo (silicato de alumínio e óxido de ferro). SIN sedimentum lateritium.

dep·ra·va·tion (dep′rā - vā′shŭn). Depravação. SIN depravity. [L. *depravatio*, de *depravo*, pp. *-atus*, corromper]

de·praved (dē - prāvd′). Depravado; deteriorado ou degenerado; corrupto. [L. *depravo*, corromper]

de·prav·i·ty (dē - prav′i - tē). Depravação; ato depravado ou a condição de ser depravado. SIN depravation.

de·pre·nyl (dē′pren - il). Deprenil; um inibidor da monoamina oxidase seletivo para a isozima tipo B. É usado como agente antiparkinsoniano. Não dá origem à crise hipertensiva que pode ocorrer quando inibidores da monoamina oxidase não-seletivos são usados em combinação com fontes alimentares de tiramina. SIN selegiline.

de·pres·sant (dē - pres′ant). Depressor. **1.** Que diminui o tônus ou a atividade funcional. **2.** Um agente que reduz a atividade nervosa ou funcional, como um sedativo ou anestésico. [L. *de-primo*, pp. *-pressus*, pressionar para baixo]

de·pressed (dē - prest′). Deprimido. **1.** Achatado de cima para baixo. **2.** Abaixo do nível normal ou do nível das partes adjacentes. **3.** Abaixo do nível funcional normal. **4.** Abatido; desanimado.

de·pres·sion (dē - presh′ŭn) [TA]. Depressão. **1.** Redução do nível de funcionamento. **2.** SIN excavation (1). **3.** Deslocamento de uma parte para baixo ou para dentro. **4.** Um estado mental temporário ou distúrbio mental crônico caracterizado por sentimentos de tristeza, solidão, desespero, baixa auto-estima e autocensura; os sinais associados incluem retardo psicomotor ou, menos freqüentemente, agitação, afastamento do contato social e estados vegetativos como perda do apetite e insônia. SIN dejection (1), depressive reaction, depressive syndrome. [L. *depressio*, de *deprimo*, pressionar para baixo]
   agitated d., d. agitada; depressão com excitação e agitação.
   anaclitic d., d. anaclítica; comprometimento do desenvolvimento físico, social e intelectual de um lactente após separação de sua mãe ou de um substituto da mãe; caracterizada por apatia, retraimento e anorexia.
   clinical d., d. clínica. SIN major d.
   endogenous d., d. endógena; qualquer distúrbio depressivo que ocorre na ausência de agentes precipitantes externos e que parece ter uma origem biológica. SIN endogenomorphic depression, nonreactive d.
   exogenous d., d. exógena; sinais e sintomas semelhantes aos da depressão endógena, mas os fatores precipitantes são sociais ou ambientais e externos ao indivíduo.
   involutional d., d. involutiva; depressão ou psicose que ocorre pela primeira vez nos anos involutivos (40 a 55 para mulheres, 50 a 65 para homens).
   lingual salivary gland d., d. da glândula salivar lingual; um entalhe na superfície lingual da mandíbula dentro do qual está uma parte da glândula submandibular; apresenta-se nas radiografias como uma radiotransparência ovóide bem circunscrita entre o canal mandibular e a borda inferior da mandíbula posterior. SIN Stafne bone cyst, static bone cyst.

---

   major d., d. maior; distúrbio mental caracterizado por depressão constante do humor, anedonia, distúrbios do sono e do apetite, e sentimentos de inutilidade, culpa e desesperança. Os critérios diagnósticos (*DSM-IV*) para um episódio de depressão maior incluem depressão do humor, redução significativa do interesse e/ou do prazer em praticamente todas as atividades, com duração de pelo menos 2 semanas. Além disso, devem existir 3 ou mais dos seguintes critérios: ganho ou perda de peso, aumento ou diminuição do sono, aumento ou diminuição do nível de atividade psicomotora, fadiga, sentimentos de culpa ou inutilidade, diminuição da capacidade de concentração e pensamentos recorrentes de morte ou suicídio. VER endogenous d., exogenous d., bipolar *disorder*. SIN clinical d., major depressive disorder.

   Aproximadamente 20 milhões de pessoas por ano sofrem de doença depressiva nos Estados Unidos. Cerca de 10% dos homens e 25% das mulheres apresentam depressão maior em algum momento de suas vidas, e 15–30% dessas pessoas cometem suicídio. O impacto negativo dessa doença sobre a economia dos Estados Unidos é estimado em 16 bilhões de dólares anuais. Os fatores de risco para depressão são abuso de drogas ou de álcool, doença física crônica, acontecimentos estressantes, isolamento social, história de maus-tratos físicos ou de abuso sexual e história familiar de doença depressiva. A depressão pode ser mascarada por abuso de drogas/fármacos. Em pessoas idosas pode ser confundida com demência senil, e vice-versa; as duas podem coexistir. Acredita-se que o distúrbio represente uma disfunção eletroquímica do sistema límbico, envolvendo distúrbios no metabolismo dos neurotransmissores dopamina e serotonina. Em pessoas com depressão familiar, o número de células gliais no córtex pré-frontal subgenicular é significativamente menor que em pessoas mentalmente saudáveis. O tratamento com psicofármacos, incluindo antidepressivos tricíclicos, inibidores seletivos da recaptação de serotonina (SSRIs), inibidores da monoamina oxidase (MAO) e outros, controla efetivamente a maioria dos casos de depressão clínica. A psicoterapia cognitiva demonstrou algum sucesso em reverter a depressão. Métodos refinados de eletroconvulsoterapia (ECT) têm sido usados com freqüência crescente desde a década de 1980, geralmente para casos que não respondem a outro tratamento. Mesmo na depressão grave, a taxa de resposta à ECT é de 80% ou mais. Essa forma de tratamento tem um início de ação mais rápido, causa menos efeitos colaterais que a farmacoterapia e é particularmente útil em pacientes idosos.

nonreactive d., d. não-reativa. SIN endogenous d.

d. of optic disk [TA], escavação do disco óptico; a escavação ou depressão normalmente presente no centro do disco óptico. SIN excavatio disci [TA], excavatio papillae, excavation of optic disk, physiologic cup, physiologic excavation.

pacchionian d.'s, depressões de Pacchioni. SIN granular *foveolae,* em *foveola.*

postdrive d., redução da freqüência cardíaca, freqüentemente com um bloqueio freqüência-dependente da condução AV e/ou VA após estimulação atrial rápida.

pterygoid d., d. pterigóide. SIN pterygoid *fovea.*

reactive d., d. reativa; um estado psicológico ocasionado diretamente por uma situação externa muito triste (freqüentemente a perda de uma pessoa querida), aliviada pela retirada da situação externa (p. ex., reunião com uma pessoa querida).

spreading d., d. alastrante; uma diminuição da atividade provocada por estimulação local do córtex cerebral e que se alastra lentamente por todo o córtex.

de·pres·sive (dē - pres′iv). Depressivo. **1.** Que empurra para baixo. **2.** Relativo a, ou que causa, depressão.

de·pres·sor (dē - pres′or). Depressor. **1.** Um músculo que aplana ou abaixa uma parte. **2.** Qualquer coisa que deprime ou retarda a atividade funcional. **3.** Um instrumento ou dispositivo usado para tirar determinadas estruturas do caminho durante uma operação ou exame. **4.** Um agente que diminui a pressão arterial. SIN hypotensor, vasodepressor (2). [L. *de-primo,* pp. *-pressus,* pressionar para baixo]

tongue d., abaixador de língua; instrumento com uma extremidade larga e plana, usado para pressionar a língua para baixo a fim de facilitar o exame da cavidade oral e da faringe.

dep·ri·va·tion (dep′ri - vā′shŭn). Privação; ausência, perda ou suspensão de algo necessário.

emotional d., p. emocional; falta de experiências interpessoais e/ou ambientais adequadas e apropriadas, geralmente nos primeiros anos de desenvolvimento.

sensory d., p. sensorial; diminuição ou ausência de estímulos externos habituais ou experiências de percepção, comumente resultando em sofrimento psicológico e funcionamento aberrante se persistir por muito tempo.

dep·si·pep·tide (dep′sē - pep′tid). Depsipeptídeo; um oligo ou polipeptídeo contendo uma ou mais ligações éster, bem como ligações peptídicas. VER TAMBÉM peptolide. [G. *deseō,* ligar, misturar, + peptide]

depth (depth). Profundidade; distância da superfície para baixo.

anesthetic d., p. anestésica; o grau de depressão do sistema nervoso central produzido por um anestésico geral; depende da potência do anestésico e da concentração em que é administrado.

focal d., d. of focus, p. focal; a maior distância em que um objeto pode ser movido e ainda manter uma imagem nítida. SIN penetration (3).

dep·tro·pine cit·rate (dep′trō - pēn). Citrato de deptropina; agente anti-histamínico com propriedades anticolinérgicas. SIN dibenzheptropine citrate.

de·pu·li·za·tion (dē - pū′li - zā′shŭn). Despulgação; destruição das pulgas, que transmitem o bacilo da peste de animais para seres humanos. [L. *de,* de, + *pulex* (*pulic-*), pulga]

dep·u·rant (dep′ū - rant). Depurante. **1.** Agente ou meio usado para realizar purificação. **2.** Agente que promove a excreção e a remoção de resíduos. [L. *de-* intens. + *puro,* pp. *-atus,* tornar puro]

dep·u·ra·tion (dep - ū - rā′shŭn). Depuração; purificação; remoção de resíduos ou excreções fétidas.

dep·u·ra·tive (dep′ū - ră - tiv). Depurativo; que tende a depurar; depurante.

de·qua·lin·i·um ac·e·tate (dē - kwah - lin′ē - ŭm). Acetato de dequalínio; um agente antimicrobiano. SIN decamine.

de·qua·lin·i·um chlo·ride. Cloreto de dequalínio; acetato de dequalínio, com o cloreto substituindo o acetato, usado como agente antimicrobiano basicamente em pastilhas para o tratamento de infecções da boca e da garganta.

de Quervain, Friedrich Joseph, cirurgião suíço, 1868–1940. VER de Q. *disease*; de Quervain *tenosynovitis*; de Q. *thyroiditis.*

der·a·del·phus (dār - ă - del′fŭs). Deradelfo; gêmeos conjugados com uma única cabeça e pescoço e corpos separados abaixo do nível torácico. VER conjoined *twins,* em *twin.* [G. *derē,* pescoço, + *adelphos,* irmão]

de·rail·ment (dē - rāl′ment). Descarrilamento; sintoma de um distúrbio mental em que a pessoa constantemente "sai dos trilhos" em seus pensamentos e linguagem (divagação); semelhante ao afrouxamento de associações.

der·an·en·ceph·a·ly, der·an·en·ce·pha·lia (dār - an′en - sef′ă - lē. - se - fā′lē - ă),Deranencefalia. **1.** Malformação congênita na qual não há cabeça, embora haja um pescoço rudimentar. **2.** Defeito do encéfalo e da parte superior da medula espinal. [G. *derē,* pescoço, + *an-,* priv., + *kephalē,* cabeça]

de·range·ment (dē - rānj′ment). Perturbação. **1.** Um distúrbio da ordem ou do arranjo regular. **2.** Termo raramente usado para um distúrbio mental. [Fr.]

Dercum, Francis X., neurologista norte-americano, 1856–1931. VER D. *disease.*

de·re·al·i·za·tion (dē - rē′ă - li - zā′shŭn). Desrealização; alteração da percepção do ambiente por um indivíduo de forma que coisas comumente familiares parecem estranhas, irreais ou bidimensionais.

de·re·ism (dē′rē - izm). Dereísmo; atividade mental fantasiosa em contraste com a realidade. [L. *de,* afastado, + *res,* coisa]

de·re·is·tic (dē - rē - is′tik). Dereístico; que vive na imaginação ou fantasia, com pensamentos incongruentes com a lógica ou a experiência.

der·en·ce·pha·lia (dār - en - se - fā′lē - ă). Derencefalia. SIN derencephaly.

der·en·ceph·a·lo·cele (dār - en - sef′ă - lō - sēl). Derencefalocele; na derencefalia, a protrusão do encéfalo rudimentar através de um defeito no canal vertebral cervical superior. [G. *derē,* pescoço, + *enkephalos,* encéfalo, + *kēlē,* hérnia]

der·en·ceph·a·ly (dār - en - sef′ă - lē). Derencefalia; raquisquise cervical e anencefalia, uma malformação que envolve uma abóbada craniana aberta com um encéfalo rudimentar geralmente empurrado em direção a vértebras cervicais bífidas. SIN derencephalia. [G. *derē,* pescoço, + *enkephalos,* encéfalo]

de·re·pres·sion (dē - rē - presh′ŭn). Desrepressão; mecanismo homeostático para regular a produção de enzimas em um sistema enzimático indutível: um indutor, geralmente um substrato de uma via enzimática específica, por combinação com um repressor ativo (produzido por um gene regulador), o desativa; a liberação do operador previamente reprimido é seguida por produção de enzimas.

der·i·va·tion (dār - i - vā′shŭn). **1.** Revulsão; a fonte ou processo de uma evolução. SIN revulsion. **2.** Derivação; o desvio de sangue ou de líquidos para uma parte para aliviar a congestão em outra. [L., *derivatio,* de *derivo,* pp. *-atus,* desviar, de *rivus,* corrente]

de·riv·a·tive (dē - riv′ă - tiv). Derivado; derivativo. **1.** Relativo a, ou que produz, derivação. **2.** Algo produzido por modificação de alguma coisa preexistente. **3.** Especificamente, um composto químico que pode ser produzido a partir de outra substância de estrutura semelhante em uma ou mais etapas, como na substituição de H por um grupamento alquil, acil ou amino.

derm-, derma-. A pele; corresponde ao L. cut-. VER entradas em cut. [G. *derma*]

der·ma·brad·er (derm′ă - brād - er). Dermabrasivo; dispositivo motorizado usado na dermabrasão.

der·ma·bra·sion (der - mă - brā′zhŭn). Dermabrasão; procedimento cirúrgico para retirar cicatrizes de acne (ou depressões na pele) com lixa, escovas rotatórias ou outros materiais abrasivos.

Der·ma·cen·tor (der - mă - sen′ter). Um gênero adornado, caracteristicamente marcado, de carrapatos rígidos (família Ixodidae) que possuem olhos e 11 festões; consiste em cerca de 20 espécies cujos membros comumente atacam cães, seres humanos e outros mamíferos. [derm- + G. *kentōr,* carrapato]

D. albopic′tus, o carrapato do inverno, uma espécie encontrada principalmente em cavalos, bois, alces e cervos no Canadá e no norte e oeste dos Estados Unidos; é um carrapato de hospedeiro único, mas os seres humanos algumas vezes são atacados ao retirar a pele de cervos ou vestir roupas feitas com essa pele.

D. anderso′ni, o carrapato da madeira; o vetor da febre maculosa das Montanhas Rochosas; também transmite tularemia e causa paralisia do carrapato; há marcas brancas e pretas características no grande escudo do macho.

D. margina′tus, uma espécie de carrapato encontrada em toda a Europa e o vetor da riquetsiose humana causada por *Rickettsia slovaca.*

D. occidenta′lis, o carrapato da costa do Pacífico, uma espécie encontrada em todos os herbívoros domésticos, cervos, cães, homens e outros animais na Califórnia e no Oregon.

D. reticula′tus, uma espécie comum que ataca carneiros, bois, cabras e cervos, causando por vezes problemas para os seres humanos; é encontrada na Europa, Ásia e América.

D. varia′bilis, o carrapato do cão americano, uma espécie que é uma praga comum de cães ao longo da costa leste dos Estados Unidos, um vetor da tularemia e o principal vetor da *Rickettsia rickettsii,* que causa febre maculosa das Montanhas Rochosas no centro e no leste dos Estados Unidos; também pode causar paralisia do carrapato.

Der·ma·coc·cus (der - ma - kok′us). Gênero de cocos aeróbicos, Gram-positivos encontrados na pele humana.

der′mad (der′mad). Em direção ao tegumento externo. [derm- + L. *ad,* para]

der·mal (der′măl). Dérmico; relativo à pele. SIN dermatoid (2).

Der·ma·nys·sus gal·li·nae (der - mă - nis′ŭs ga - lē′ - nē). O ácaro da galinha vermelha, parasita de galinhas, pombos e outras aves; algumas vezes ataca seres humanos e causa uma erupção pruriginosa, principalmente em indivíduos sensibilizados. SIN *Acarus gallinae.* [derm- + G. *nyssō,* puncionar; L. *gallina,* galinha]

dermat-. A pele. VER TAMBÉM derm-, dermato-, dermo-. [G. *derma*]

der·ma·tal·gia (der - mă - tăl′jē - ă). Dermatalgia; dor localizada, geralmente limitada à pele. SIN dermatodynia. [dermat- + G. *algos,* dor]

der·ma·ti·tis, pl. **der·ma·tit·i·des** (der - mă - tī′tis, - tit′i - dēz). Dermatite; inflamação da pele. [derm- + G. *-itis,* inflamação]

dermatitis

dermatite — divisão em tipos	
endógena	**dermatite de contato (ou exógena)**
atópica	irritação direta
	não-fotossensível
seborreica	fototóxica
numular	
dermatite crônica das mãos e dos pés	alérgica
	não-fotossensível
esfoliativa	fotoalérgica
dermatite de estase	
neurodermatite circunscrita	
prurido anal/vulvar	
erupção por drogas/fármacos	

actinic d., d. actínica. SIN photodermatitis.
d. aestiva'lis, d. estival; eczema recidivante durante o verão.
allergic contact d., d. de contato alérgica; uma reação alérgica tipo IV tardia da pele com vários graus de eritema, edema e vesiculação resultantes do contato cutâneo com um alérgeno específico. SIN contact allergy.
ancylostoma d., d. por ancilóstomos. SIN cutaneous larva migrans.
d. artefac'ta, d. artificial; lesões cutâneas auto-induzidas resultantes do hábito de esfregar, coçar ou arrancar pêlos, do fingimento de doença ou distúrbio mental. SIN factitial d., feigned eruption.
atopic d., d. atópica; dermatite caracterizada pelos fenômenos distintos de atopia, incluindo eczema do lactente e flexural. SIN atopic eczema.
berloque d., berlock d., d. de berloques; tipo de fotossensibilização que resulta em pigmentação castanho-escura à exposição à luz solar após aplicação de óleo de bergamota e de outros óleos essenciais presentes em perfumes e colônias.
blastomycetic d., d. blastomycot'ica, d. blastomicótica; blastomicose cutânea.
bubble gum d., d. por chiclete; dermatite de contato alérgica que se desenvolve ao redor dos lábios em crianças que mascam chiclete; causada por plásticos presentes na goma de mascar.
d. calor'ica, d. calórica. SIN erythema ab igne.
caterpillar d., d. de lagarta; dermatite de contato alérgica causada pela larva da mariposa de cauda marrom, lagarta, mariposa européia e outras lagartas. SIN caterpillar rash.
chemical d., d. química; dermatite de contato alérgica ou dermatite por irritação primária causada pela aplicação de substâncias químicas; geralmente caracterizada por eritema, edema e vesiculação do local exposto ou tocado e, em alguns casos, por acne ou distúrbios pigmentares.
d. combustio'nis, d. por combustão; inflamação da pele após uma queimadura.
contact d., d. de contato; uma dermatite mediada por linfócitos T (hipersensibilidade tipo IV) resultante do contato cutâneo com um alérgeno específico (dermatite de contato alérgica) ou irritante (dermatite de contato não-alérgica). SIN contact hypersensitivity (1).
contagious pustular d., d. pustular contagiosa. SIN orf virus.
cosmetic d., d. cosmética; erupção cutânea que resulta da aplicação de um cosmético; causada por sensibilização alérgica ou irritação primária.
diaper d., d. das fraldas; coloquialmente conhecida como erupção das fraldas; dermatite das coxas e nádegas resultante da exposição a urina e fezes nas fraldas dos lactentes. Antigamente atribuída à formação de amônia; a umidade, o crescimento bacteriano e a alcalinidade induzem juntos as lesões. VER TAMBÉM intertrigo. SIN diaper rash.
d. exfoliati'va infan'tum, d. exfoliati'va neonato'rum, d. esfoliativa neonatal; piodermite generalizada acompanhada por dermatite esfoliativa, com sintomas constitucionais, que afeta lactentes pequenos, podendo resultar de dermatite atópica, doença de Leiner ou síndrome da pele escaldada estafilocócica. SIN impetigo neonatorum (1).
exfoliative d., d. esfoliativa; eritema que se estende rapidamente, seguido, em alguns dias, por esfoliação generalizada com descamação da pele e associada, em alguns casos, a linfadenopatia ou perda de água e eletrólitos; pode ser uma reação farmacológica ou associada a várias dermatoses benignas, lúpus eritematoso ou linfoma, ou ser de causa indeterminada. SIN Wilson disease (2).
exudative discoid and lichenoid d., d. exsudativa discóide e liquenóide; dermatite que se assemelha a uma forma exsudativa de eczema numular; ocorre principalmente em homens judeus, com lesões ovais no pênis, tronco e face. SIN Sulzberger-Garbe disease, Sulzberger-Garbe syndrome.
factitial d., d. fictícia. SIN d. artefacta.
d. gangreno'sa infan'tum, d. gangrenosa infantil; uma erupção bolhosa ou pustular, de origem incerta, seguida por úlceras necróticas ou gangrena extensa em crianças com menos de 2 anos de idade; se não tratada, pode haver morte por infecção hematogênica, como abscesso hepático. SIN disseminated cutaneous gangrene, ecthyma gangrenosum, pemphigus gangrenosus (1).
d. herpetifor'mis, d. herpetiforme; uma doença cutânea crônica caracterizada por erupção pruriginosa simétrica de vesículas e pápulas, que ocorrem em grupos; as recidivas são comuns; associada à enteropatia sensível ao glúten e IgA juntamente com neutrófilos sob a epiderme da pele na lesão e perilesional. SIN Duhring disease.
d. hiema'lis, d. invernal. SIN winter itch.
infectious eczematoid d., d. eczematóide infecciosa; uma reação inflamatória da pele adjacente ao local de uma infecção piogênica; p. ex., otite purulenta, a área ao redor de uma colostomia ou infecção intranasal; acredita-se que se dissemine por auto-inoculação.
irritant contact d., d. de contato irritante; reações cutâneas que variam de eritema e descamação a queimaduras necróticas, resultantes de lesão não-imunológica por substâncias químicas em contato com a pele, imediata ou repetidamente.
mango d., d. da manga; uma dermatite de contato perioral resultante da sensibilização ao revestimento resinoso presente na casca da manga.
meadow d., meadow grass d., d. da campina; d. da grama; uma reação fotoalérgica ao contato com uma planta que contenha furocumarina na qual a configuração bizarra da erupção é a do padrão estriado do contato com a planta; freqüentemente ocorre após banho de sol.
d. medicamento'sa, d. medicamentosa. SIN drug eruption.
nickel d., d. por níquel; dermatite alérgica causada por contato com ou, em alguns casos, ingestão de níquel ou de outros metais que contenham níquel (p. ex., aço inoxidável).
d. nodo'sa, d. nodosa; uma erupção papular nas pernas, relacionada à oncocercose (q.v.).
d. nodula'ris necrot'ica, d. nodular necrótica; erupção recorrente de vesículas, pápulas e lesões papulonecróticas nas nádegas e nas superfícies extensoras dos membros, acompanhada por febre, dor de garganta, diarréia e eosinofilia; provavelmente uma variante da vasculite, pode ter intensidade e duração variáveis e crescentes e, algumas vezes, envolver o coração, os rins e o trato gastrointestinal. SIN Werther disease.
nummular d., d. numular. SIN nummular eczema.
papular d. of pregnancy, d. papular da gravidez; erupção papular intensamente pruriginosa do tronco e dos membros que ocorre durante a gravidez, sem toxicidade sistêmica; pode ser semelhante às pápulas urticariais pruriginosas e às placas da gravidez.
d. pediculoi'des ventrico'sus, d. por Pyemotes ventricosus. SIN straw itch.
primary irritant d., d. irritante primária; reação freqüentemente acumulativa de irritação causada pela exposição da pele a substâncias que são tóxicas para as células da epiderme ou do tecido conjuntivo; as lesões geralmente são eritematosas e papulares, mas podem ser purulentas ou necróticas, dependendo da natureza do material tóxico aplicado.
proliferative d., d. proliferativa SIN dermatophilosis.
rat mite d., d. do ácaro do rato; erupção de urticárias, pápulas ou vesículas causada pelo ácaro do rato.
d. re'pens, d. rastejante. SIN pustulosis palmaris et plantaris. [L. rastejante]
rhus d., dermatite de contato causada por exposição cutânea ao uroshiol de espécies de Toxicodendron (Rhus), como a hera, carvalho e sumagre venenosos.
sandal strap d., d. por tiras de sandália; dermatite de contato alérgica, nas superfícies dorsais dos pés, causada por tiras de sandália de borracha sintética ou aditivos da borracha natural.
schistosomal d., d. do esquistossoma; uma resposta de sensibilização à invasão cutânea repetida por cercárias de esquistossomas de aves, mamíferos ou seres humanos. SIN swimmer's itch, water itch (2).
seborrheic d., d. seborrhe'ica, d. seborreica; uma erupção macular descamativa comum que ocorre basicamente na face, couro cabeludo (caspa) e outras áreas de aumento da secreção das glândulas sebáceas, principalmente durante a lactância e após a puberdade; as lesões são cobertas por uma escama oleosa pouco aderente. A efetividade do tratamento com betaconazol apóia um papel etiológico da infecção por Pityrosporum ovale. SIN seborrheic eczema, Unna disease.
solar d., d. solar; dermatite em pessoas fotossensíveis causada por exposição aos raios solares.
stasis d., d. de estase; eritema e descamação dos membros inferiores devido ao comprometimento da circulação venosa, observados comumente em mulheres idosas ou secundariamente à trombose venosa profunda, com esta última apresentando início rápido e edema.
subcorneal pustular d., d. pustular subcórnea. SIN subcorneal pustular dermatosis.
traumatic d., d. traumática; qualquer dermatite causada por uma substância irritante ou por um agente físico.
d. veg'etans, d. vegetante; uma massa granulomatosa esponjosa benigna causada por infecção piogênica crônica. SIN pyoderma vegetans.

dermato-. VER derm-. [G. *derma*, pele]

der·mat·o·ar·thri·tis (der′mă - tō - ar - thrī′tis). Dermatoartrite; doença cutânea e artrite associadas.
  lipoid d., d. lipóide; uma reticuloistiocitose multicêntrica (multicentric *reticulohistiocytosis*).

Der·ma·to·bi·a (der - mă - tō′bē - ă). Gênero de moscas (família Oestridae) encontradas na América tropical. [dermato- + G. *bios*, forma de vida]
  D. cyaniven′tris, SIN *D. hominis.*
  D. hom′inis, uma espécie grande, azul, de asas castanhas, cujas larvas se desenvolvem em lesões abertas, semelhantes a furúnculos, na pele dos seres humanos, de muitos animais domésticos e de algumas aves. É um parasita bovino muito grave e lesivo, e freqüentemente ataca crianças pequenas nas Américas Central e do Sul. Seus ovos são depositados nas pernas ou abdome de outro inseto, como o mosquito; mais tarde, os ovos eclodem, quando estimulados por calor ou outros fatores, liberando as larvas do gastrófilo sobre a pele do hospedeiro do mosquito hematófago, e elas rapidamente invadem a pele para dar início à míiase. SIN *D. cyaniventris*, human botfly, skin botflies, warble botfly.

der·ma·to·bi·a·sis (der′mă - tō - bī′ă - sis). Dermatobíase; infestação de seres humanos e animais por larvas da mosca *Dermatobia hominis.* SIN human botfly myiasis.

der·mat·o·cel·lu·li·tis (der′mă - tō - sel - ū - lī′tis). Dermatocelulite; inflamação da pele e do tecido conjuntivo subcutâneo.

der·mat·o·cha·la·sis (der′mă - tō - kă - lā′sis). Dermatocalase; distúrbio congênito ou adquirido caracterizado por deficiência das fibras elásticas da pele, que pode pender em pregas; pode haver anomalias vasculares; a herança é autossômica dominante ou recessiva, esta última algumas vezes associada ao enfisema pulmonar e divertículos do trato alimentar ou bexiga. A forma dominante é causada por mutação no gene da elastina (ELN) em 7q. Também há uma forma ligada ao X que é devida à mutação no gene de Menkes (MNK), codificando a ATPase transportadora de cobre em Xq. SIN cutis laxa, generalized elastolysis, loose skin. [conjunctiva + G. *chalasis*, afrouxamento]

der·mat·o·co·ni·o·sis (der′mă - tō - kō - nī - o′sis). Dermatoconiose; dermatite ocupacional causada por irritação local por poeira. [dermato- + G. *konis*, poeira, + *-osis*, condição]

der·mat·o·cyst (der′mă - tō - sist). Dermatocisto; um cisto da pele.

der·mat·o·dyn·ia (der′mă - tō - din′ē - ă). Dermatodinia. SIN dermatalgia. [dermato- + G. *odyne*, dor]

der·mat·o·fi·bro·ma (der′mă - tō - fī - brō′mă). Dermatofibroma; um nódulo cutâneo benigno, de crescimento lento, que consiste em tecido fibroso celular mal demarcado encerrando capilares colapsados, com macrófagos dispersos pigmentados por hemossiderina e contendo lipídios. Os termos a seguir são considerados por alguns como sinônimos e, por outros, como variedades de dermatofibroma: hemangioma esclerosante, histiocitoma fibroso, fibrose subepidérmica nodular. SIN fibrous histiocytoma, sclerosing hemangioma (2)

der·mat·o·fi·bro·sar·co·ma pro·tu·ber·ans (der′mă - tō - fī′brō - sar - kō′mă prō - toō′ber - ans). Dermatofibrossarcoma protuberante; uma neoplasia dérmica, de crescimento relativamente lento, que consiste em um ou vários nódulos firmes, geralmente cobertos por pele vermelho-azulada escura, que tende a estar fixada a massas palpáveis; histologicamente, a neoplasia assemelha-se a um dermatofibroma celular com um padrão em forma de depósito acentuado; as metástases são incomuns, mas a incidência de recorrência é razoavelmente alta.
  pigmented d. p., d. p. pigmentado; variante incomum de dermatofibrossarcoma protuberante que contém melanócitos dendríticos intensamente pigmentados dispersos entre células fusiformes do tumor. SIN Bednar tumor, storiform neurofibroma.

der·ma·to·fi·bro·sis len·tic·u·lar·is dis·sem·i·na·ta (der′mă - tō - fī - brō′sis len - tik - ū - lā′ris di - sem - i - nā′tă) [MIM*166700]. Dermatofibrose lenticular disseminada; pequenas pápulas ou discos de tecido elástico dérmico aumentado que surgem no início da vida; quando também há osteopoiquilose, a condição é denominada osteodermatopoiquilose ou síndrome de Buschke-Ollendorf; herança autossômica dominante.

der·mat·o·glyph·ics (der′mă - tō - glif′iks). Dermatoglifo. **1.** As configurações dos padrões estriados característicos das superfícies volares da pele; na mão humana, o segmento distal de cada dedo possui três tipos de configurações: espiral, alça e arco. VER TAMBÉM fingerprint. **2.** A ciência ou estudo dessas configurações ou padrões. [dermato- + *glyphē*, trabalho entalhado]

der·mat·o·graph (der - mat′ō - graf). Dermatógrafo; a pápula linear produzida na pele no dermatografismo.

der·ma·tog·ra·phism (der - mă - tog′ră - fizm). Dermatografismo; uma forma de urticária na qual surgem pápulas no local e na configuração da aplicação da pressão ou fricção na pele. A linha branca resultante surge precocemente nas exacerbações da dermatite atópica. SIN autographism, factitious urticaria, skin writing. [dermato- + G. *grapho*, escrever]

der·ma·toid (der′mă - toyd). Dermatóide. **1.** Semelhante à pele. SIN dermoid (1). **2.** SIN dermal.

der·ma·tol·o·gist (der - mă - tol′ō - jist). Dermatologista; um médico que se especializa no diagnóstico e tratamento de doenças cutâneas e doenças sistêmicas relacionadas.

der·ma·tol·o·gy (der - mă - tol′ō - jē). Dermatologia; o ramo da medicina relacionado ao estudo da pele, doenças da pele e à relação entre lesões cutâneas e doença sistêmica. [dermato- + G. *logos*, estudo]

der·ma·tol·y·sis (der - mă - tol′i - sis). Dermatólise; afrouxamento ou atrofia da pele por doença; erroneamente usado como sinônimo de cútis flácida. SIN dermolysis. [dermato- + G. *lysis*, afrouxamento]

der·ma·to·ma (der - mă - tō′mă). Dermatoma; espessamento ou hipertrofia circunscrita da pele. [dermato- + G. *-oma*, tumor]

der·ma·tome (der′mă - tōm). Dermátomo. **1.** Instrumento para fazer cortes finos de epiderme/derme para enxerto, ou excisão de pequenas lesões. **2.** A parte dorsolateral de um somito embrionário. SIN cutis plate. **3.** A área de pele suprida por ramos cutâneos de um único nervo espinal; dermátomos adjacentes podem superpor-se. SIN dermatomal distribution, dermatomic area. [dermato- + G. *tomē*, corte]

der·mat·o·meg·a·ly (der′mă - tō - meg′ă - lē). Dermatomegalia; defeito congênito ou adquirido no qual a pele pende em pregas; pode ser parte de uma síndrome ou ocorrer isoladamente como cútis frouxa, dermatocalase ou dermatólise. [dermato- + G. *megas*, grande]

der·mat·o·mere (der′mă - tō - mēr). Dermatômero; uma área metamérica do tegumento embrionário. [dermato- + G. *meros*, parte]

der·mat·o·my·co·sis (der′mă - tō - mi - kō′sis). Dermatomicose; infecção da pele causada por dermatófitos, leveduras e outros fungos. Cf. dermatophytosis.
  d. ped′is, d. do pé, tinha do pé. SIN *tinea* pedis.

der·mat·o·my·o·ma (der′mă - tō - mi - ō′mă). Dermatomioma. SIN *leiomyoma* cutis. [dermato- + G. *mys*, músculo, + *-oma*, tumor]

der·mat·o·my·o·si·tis (der′mă - tō - mi - ō - sī′tis). Dermatomiosite; distúrbio progressivo caracterizado por fraqueza muscular proximal simétrica, com níveis séricos elevados de enzimas musculares e erupção cutânea, tipicamente um eritema vermelho-púrpura na face, e edema palpebral e dos tecidos periorbitais; o tecido muscular afetado mostra degeneração das fibras com reação inflamatória crônica; ocorre em crianças e adultos e, nestes últimos, pode estar associada a câncer visceral ou outros distúrbios do tecido conjuntivo. [dermato- + G. *mys*, músculo, + *-itis*, inflamação]

der·mat·o·neu·ro·sis (der′mă - tō - noo - rō′sis). Dermatoneurose; qualquer erupção cutânea devida a estímulos emocionais.

der·mat·o·no·sol·o·gy (der′mă - tō - nō - sol′ō - jē). Dermatonosologia; a ciência da nomenclatura e classificação das doenças de pele. [dermato- + G. *nosos*, doença, + *logos*, tratado]

der·mat·o·path·ia (der′mă - tō - path′ē - ă). Dermatopatia. SIN dermatopathy.
  d. pigmento′sa reticula′ris, d. pigmentosa reticular. SIN *livedo* reticularis.

der·mat·o·pa·thol·o·gy (der′mă - tō - pa - thol′ō - jē). Dermatopatologia; histopatologia da pele e do tecido subcutâneo, e estudo das causas de doença cutânea.

der·ma·top·a·thy (der′mă - top′ă - thē). Dermatopatia; qualquer doença da pele. SIN dermatopathia. [dermato- + G. *pathos*, que sofre]

Der·ma·toph·a·goi·des pter·o·nys·si·nus (der - mă - tof - ă - goy′dēz ter - ō - ni - sī′nŭs). Espécie comum de ácaros cosmopolitas encontrados na poeira doméstica e uma causa contribuinte comum de asma atópica. [dermato- + G. *phago*, comer; ptero- + G. *nysso*, picar, perfurar]

der·mat·o·phi·lo·sis (der′mă - tō - fi - lō′sis). Dermatofilose; dermatite exsudativa infecciosa de bovinos, ovinos, caprinos, eqüinos e outros animais (ocasionalmente seres humanos) causada pela bactéria *Dermatophilus congolensis*; é observada dermatofilose grave (algumas vezes fatal) em bovinos na África e no Caribe, invariavelmente associada a infestações pelo carrapato *Amblyomma variegatum*. SIN proliferative dermatitis, streptothrichosis, streptotrichiasis, streptotrichosis.

Der·ma·toph·i·lus con·go·len·sis (der - mă - tof′i - lŭs kon - gō - len′sis). Espécie de bactérias móveis, não-álcool-ácido-resistentes, aeróbicas ou anaeróbicas facultativas, Gram-positivas, que é o agente etiológico da dermatofilose; também causa dermatite proliferativa. [dermato- + G. *philos*, afinidade]

der·ma·to·pho·bia (der′mă - tō - fō′bē - ă). Dermatofobia; medo mórbido de adquirir uma doença cutânea. [dermatosis + G. *phobos*, medo]

der·mat·o·phy·lax·is (der′mă - tō - fi - lak′sis). Dermatofilaxia; proteção da pele contra agentes potencialmente prejudiciais; p. ex., infecção, luz solar excessiva, agentes nocivos. [dermato- + G. *phylaxis*, proteção]

der·mat·o·phyte (der′mă - tō - fīt). Dermatófito; um fungo que causa infecções superficiais da pele, pêlos e/ou unhas, isto é, tecidos queratinizados. As espécies de *Epidermophyton*, *Microsporum* e *Trichophyton* são consideradas dermatófitos, mas os agentes causadores da tinha versicolor, tinha nigra e candidíase cutânea não são classificados assim. [dermato- + G. *phyton*, planta]

der·mat·o·phy·tid (der - mă - tof′i - tid). Dermatofítide; uma manifestação alérgica de dermatofitose em um local distante daquele da infecção fúngica primária. As lesões, geralmente pequenas vesículas nas mãos e/ou braços, não possuem fungos e podem tornar-se extensas, cobrindo grandes áreas do corpo e causando desconforto extremo para o paciente. VER TAMBÉM -id (1), id *reaction*.

dermatophytosis 428 dermenchysis

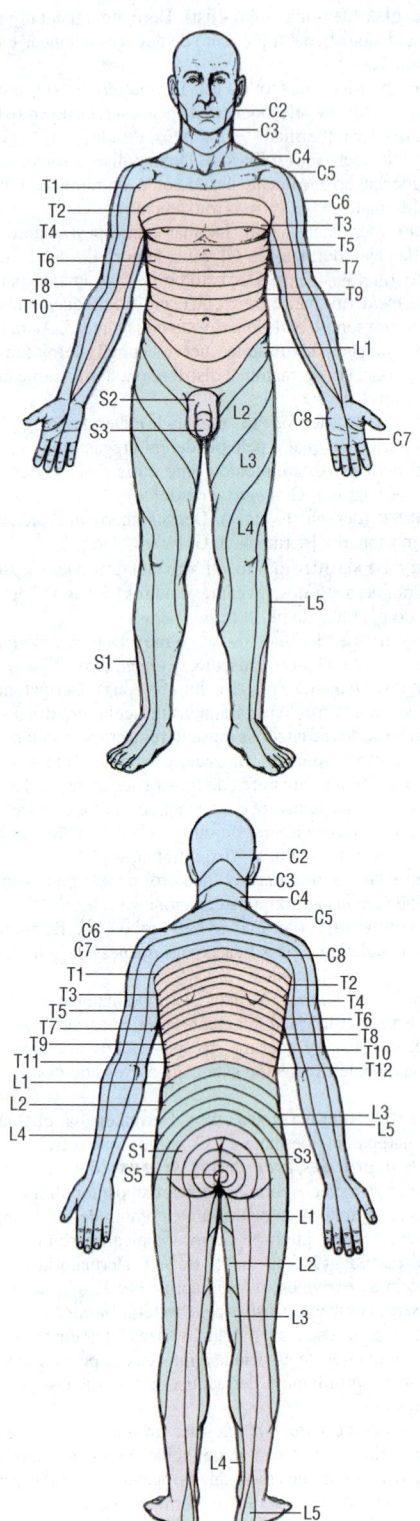

dermátomos

der·mat·o·phy·to·sis (der'mă - tŏ - fi - tō'sis). Dermatofitose; uma infecção dos pêlos, pele ou unhas causada por qualquer um dos dermatófitos. As lesões podem ocorrer em qualquer local do corpo e, na pele, são caracterizadas por eritema, pequenas vesículas papulares, fissuras e descamação. São locais comuns de infecção os pés (tinha do pé), unhas (onicomicose) e couro cabeludo (tinha da cabeça). Cf. dermatomycosis.

der·mat·o·pol·y·neu·ri·tis (der'mă - tō - pol'ē - noo - ri'tis). Dermatopolineurite. SIN acrodynia (2).

der·ma·tor·rha·gia (der'mă - tō - ră'jē - ă). Dermatorragia; hemorragia da pele ou para o interior da pele. [dermato- + G. rhḗgnymi, irromper]

der·ma·tor·rhea (der'mă - tō - rē'ă). Dermatorréia; secreção excessiva das glândulas sebáceas ou sudoríparas da pele. [dermato- + G. *rhoia*, fluxo]

der·ma·tor·rhex·is (der'mă - tō - rek'sis). Dermatorrexe; ruptura da pele; p. ex., como se observa nas estrias atróficas ou na síndrome de Ehlers-Danlos. [dermato- + G. *rhēxis*, ruptura]

der·ma·tos·co·py (der - mă - tos'kŏ - pē). Dermatoscopia; inspeção da pele, geralmente com o auxílio de uma lente de aumento ou por microscopia de epiluminescência (epiluminescence *microscopy*) (q.v.). [dermato- + G. *skopeō*, ver]

der·ma·to·sis, pl. **der·ma·to·ses** (der - mă - tō'sis, - sēz). Dermatose; termo inespecífico usado para designar qualquer anormalidade ou erupção cutânea. [dermato- + G. *-osis*, condição]
  acute febrile neutrophilic d., d. neutrofílica febril aguda; uma dermatose rara, predominante em mulheres, geralmente múltipla, na face, pescoço e membros superiores, em muitos casos acompanhada por conjuntivite, lesões da mucosa, febre, mal-estar, artralgia e neutrofilia no sangue periférico; a biópsia revela infiltrado polimorfonuclear da derme; ocorre remissão rápida com tratamento sistêmico com esteróides. SIN Sweet disease.
  ashy d., eritema distrófico crônico. SIN *erythema* dyschromicum perstans.
  Bowen precancerous d., d. pré-cancerosa de Bowen. SIN Bowen *disease*.
  chronic bullous d. of childhood, d. bolhosa crônica da infância; uma doença bolhosa rara, autolimitada, principalmente do tronco, regiões perioral e pélvica, com início na primeira década de vida, recorrências sucessivamente menos graves e remissão total na adolescência; é encontrado depósito linear de IgA na membrana basal epidérmica na pele envolvida e na pele normal. SIN linear IgA bullous disease in children.
  dermolytic bullous d., d. bolhosa dermolítica. SIN *epidermolysis* bullosa dystrophica.
  digitate d., d. digitada; parapsoríase em pequenas placas. VER *parapsoriasis* en plaque. SIN small plaque parapsoriasis.
  juvenile plantar d., d. plantar juvenil; dermatite dolorosa, ocorrendo basicamente em crianças, que faz com que a pele da região plantar pareça vitrificada e fissurada; pode estar associada a hiperidrose.
  lichenoid d., d. liquenóide; qualquer erupção cutânea crônica, caracterizada clinicamente por endurecimento e espessamento da pele com acentuação das marcas cutâneas e, microscopicamente, por infiltração linfocítica em faixa da derme papilar.
  d. medicamento'sa, d. medicamentosa. SIN drug *eruption*.
  d. papulo'sa ni'gra, d. papulosa negra; lesões papulares castanho-escuras, observadas em negros, na face e na região superior do tronco; histológica e clinicamente, assemelham-se a ceratoses seborreicas.
  pigmented purpuric lichenoid d., d. liquenóide purpúrica pigmentada; erupção constituída de pápulas liquenóides de pigmentação variada pela hemossiderina da púrpura associada; encontrada nas pernas, geralmente em homens com mais de 40 anos de idade. SIN Gougerot and Blum disease.
  progressive pigmentary d., d. pigmentar progressiva; púrpura crônica, principalmente das pernas em homens, que se dissemina para formar placas castanho-avermelhadas e eventualmente descritos como pontos em pimenta-de-caiena; associada, microscopicamente, a infiltração linfocítica perivascular, diapedese e hemossiderose. SIN Schamberg fever.
  radiation d., d. por irradiação; alterações cutâneas provocadas pela radiação ionizante, particularmente eritema no estágio agudo, perda de pêlos, temporária ou permanente, e alterações crônicas na epiderme e derme semelhantes à ceratose actínica, a partir da qual pode desenvolver-se carcinoma de células escamosas.
  subcorneal pustular d., d. pustular subcórnea; erupção anular crônica pruriginosa de vesículas e pústulas estéreis sob o estrato córneo. SIN Sneddon-Wilkinson disease, subcorneal pustular dermatitis.
  transient acantholytic d., d. acantolítica transitória; erupção papular pruriginosa, com acantólise suprabasal histológica, do tórax, com lesões dispersas nas faces dorsal e lateral dos membros, com duração de algumas semanas a vários meses; observada predominantemente em homens com mais de 40 anos. SIN Grover disease.

der·ma·to·ther·a·py (der'mă - tō - thăr'ă - pē). Dermatoterapia; tratamento de doenças cutâneas.

der·ma·to·thla·si·a (der'mă - tō - thlā'zē - ă). Dermatotlasia; um impulso incontrolável de apertar e ferir a pele. [dermato- + G. *thlasis*, contusão]

der·ma·to·tro·pic (der'mă - tō - trop'ik). Dermatotrópico; que possui afinidade pela pele. SIN dermotropic. [dermato- + G. *trŏpe*, desvio]

der·ma·to·zo·on (der'mă - tō - zō'on). Dermatozoário; animal parasita da pele. [dermato- + G. *zōon*, animal]

der·ma·to·zo·o·no·sis (der'mă - tō - zō - ō - nō'sis, - zō - on'ō - sis). Dermatozoonose; infestação da pele por um parasita de animais. [dermato- + G. *zōon*, animal, + *nosos*, doença]

der·ma·tro·phia, der·mat·ro·phy (der - mă - trō'fē - ă, der - mat'rŏ - fē). Dermatrofia; atrofia ou adelgaçamento da pele.

der·men·chy·sis (der - men'ki - sis). Dermenquise; termo raramente usado para administração subcutânea de remédios. [derm- + G. *enchysis*, derrame]

der·mis [TA]. Derme; uma camada de pele composta de uma camada superficial fina que apresenta interdigitação com a epiderme, camada papilar e camada reticular; contém vasos sanguíneos e linfáticos, nervos e terminações nervosas, glândulas e, exceto na pele glabra, folículos pilosos. SIN corium☆, cutis vera. [G. *derma*, pele]

dermo-. VER derm-. [G. *derma*, pele]

Der·mo·bac·ter (der - mō - bak′ter). Gênero bacteriano de bacilos imóveis, não-formadores de esporos, Gram-positivos, isolados da pele humana. O *Dermobacter hominis* foi associado a hemoculturas positivas.

der·mo·blast (der′mō - blast). Dermoblasto; uma das células mesodérmicas a partir das quais se desenvolve a derme. [dermo- + G. *blastos*, derme]

der·mo·cy·ma (der′mō - sī′mă). Dermocima; gêmeos conjugados desiguais, nos quais o parasita menor está incluído no tegumento do autósito. [dermo- + G. *kyma*, feto]

der·moid (der′moyd). Dermóide. **1.** SIN dermatoid (1). **2.** SIN dermoid cyst. [dermo- + G. *eidos*, semelhança]

   inclusion d., d. de inclusão. SIN epidermal cyst.

der·moi·dec·to·my (der - moy - dek′tō - mē). Dermoidectomia; termo raramente usado para remoção operatória de um cisto dermóide. [dermoid + G. *ektomē*, excisão]

der·mol·y·sis (der - mol′i - sis). Dermólise. SIN dermatolysis.

der·mo·ne·crot·ic (der′mō - nĕ - krot′ik). Dermonecrótico; relativo a qualquer aplicação ou doença que possa causar necrose da pele.

der·mop·a·thy (der - mop′a - thē). Dermopatia. SIN dermatopathy.

   diabetic d., d. diabética; pequenas máculas e pápulas das superfícies extensoras dos membros, mais comumente na região pré-tibial de diabéticos, que se tornam atróficas, hiperpigmentadas e, ocasionalmente, sofrem ulceração com fibrose; pode ser uma manifestação de microangiopatia.

der·mo·phle·bi·tis (der′mō - fle - bī′tis). Dermoflebite; inflamação das veias superficiais e da pele adjacente. [dermo- + G. *phleps*, veia, + *-itis*, inflamação]

der·mo·skel·e·ton (der - mō - skel′ĕ - ton). Dermoesqueleto. SIN exoskeleton (1).

der·mo·ste·no·sis (der′mō - stĕ - nō′sis). Dermoestenose; contração anormal da pele. [dermo- + G. *stenōsis*, estreitamento]

der·mo·tox·in (der - mō - tok′sin). Dermotoxina; substância produzida por um agente vivo, principalmente uma exotoxina formada por bactérias, sendo caracterizada por sua capacidade de causar alterações anormais na pele, p. ex., eritema, alterações degenerativas, necrose.

der·mo·trop·ic (der - mō - trop′ik). Dermotrópico. SIN dermatotropic.

der·mo·vas·cu·lar (der - mō - vas′kū - lăr). Dermovascular; relativo aos vasos sanguíneos da pele. [dermo- + L. *vasculum*, vaso pequeno]

der·o·did·y·mus (dār′ō - did′i - mŭs). Derodídimo. SIN dicephalus diauchenos. [G. *derē*, pescoço, + *didymos*, gêmeo]

de·ro·ta·tion (dē - rō - tā′shŭn). Rotação para trás. **1.** Uma rotação para trás. **2.** Em ortopedia, a correção de uma deformidade de rotação, fazendo-se voltar ou rodar a estrutura deformada para uma posição normal. [L. *de*, fora, + *rotatio*, rotação]

DES Abreviatura de diethylstilbestrol (dietilestilbestrol).

des-. Des-; em química, um prefixo que indica ausência de algum componente da parte principal do nome; amplamente substituído em inglês por "de-" (p. ex., desoxyribonucleic acid, dehydro-), mas mantido quando "de-" pode ser tomado por D- ou *d*-, como parte de "desmo-" (p. ex., desmosterol), e em termos como desoxycortone.

des·am·i·dize (dē - sam′i - dīz). Desamidizar. SIN deamidize.

De Sanctis, Carlo, psiquiatra italiano, *1888. VER De S.-Cacchione *syndrome*.

de·sat·u·rate (dē - sat′ū - rāt). Dessaturar; produzir dessaturação.

de·sat·u·ra·tion (dē′sat - ū - rā′shŭn). Dessaturação. **1.** O ato, ou o resultado do ato, de tornar algo menos completamente saturado; mais especificamente, a percentagem de locais de ligação total que permanecem vazios, p. ex., quando a hemoglobina apresenta 70% de saturação de oxigênio e nada mais, sua dessaturação é de 30%. Cf. saturation (5). **2.** O processo ou reação de remoção de dois átomos de hidrogênio de uma molécula, resultando na formação de uma ligação dupla.

Desault, Pierre-Joseph, cirurgião francês, 1744–1795. VER D. *bandage*.

Descartes (Cartesius), René, filósofo, matemático, fisiologista francês, 1596–1650. O fundador da filosofia moderna e proponente da escola mecanicista ou iatromatemática (mechanistic *school* or iatromathematical *school*). VER D. *law*.

Descemet, Jean, médico francês, 1732–1810. VER D. *membrane*.

des·ce·me·ti·tis (des′ĕ - mĕ - tī′tis). Descemetite; inflamação da membrana de Descemet.

des·ce·met·o·cele (des - ĕ - met′ō - sēl). Descemetocele; uma protrusão anterior da membrana de Descemet causada pela destruição da substância da córnea por infecção.

de·scen·dens (dē - sen′denz). Descendente. SIN descending. [L.]

   d. cervica′lis, d. cervical. SIN inferior root of ansa cervicalis.

   d. hypoglos′si, d. hipoglóssica. SIN superior root of ansa cervicalis.

de·scend·ing (dē - send′ing). Descendente; que segue para baixo ou em direção à periferia. SIN descendens. [L. *de-scendo*, pp. *–scensus*, descer, de *scando*, subir]

de·scen·sus (dē - sen′sŭs). Descida; queda de uma posição mais alta. VER TAMBÉM ptosis, procidentia. SIN descent (1). [L.]

   d. tes′tis, d. testicular; descida do testículo do abdome para o escroto durante o sétimo e o oitavo meses de vida intra-uterina.

   d. u′teri, d. uterina. SIN prolapse of the uterus.

   d. ventric′uli, gastroptose. SIN gastroptosis.

de·scent (dē - sent′). Descida. **1.** SIN descensus. **2.** Em obstetrícia, a entrada e a passagem da parte de apresentação do feto através do canal de parto. [L. descensus]

Deschamps, Joseph F.L., cirurgião francês, 1740–1824. VER D. *needle*.

de·sen·si·ti·za·tion (dē - sen′si - ti - zā′shŭn). Dessensibilização. **1.** A redução ou abolição da sensibilidade alérgica ou de reações ao antígeno específico (alérgeno). SIN antianaphylaxis. **2.** O ato de remover um complexo emocional. SIN hyposensitization.

   heterologous d., d. heteróloga; estimulação por um agonista que leva a um amplo padrão de ausência de resposta a estímulos adicionais por vários outros agonistas.

   homologous d., d. homóloga; perda de sensibilidade apenas à classe de agonista usada para dessensibilizar o tecido.

   systematic d., d. sistemática; um tipo de terapia comportamental para eliminar fobias ou ansiedades: o paciente e o terapeuta constroem uma lista de situações imaginárias que provocam a fobia, classificadas da que produz menor para a que produz maior ansiedade; o paciente então é treinado no relaxamento muscular profundo, sendo repetidamente instruído a imaginar-se na situação que produz menor ansiedade até que se sinta completamente relaxado ao fazê-lo; o procedimento é repetido para cada situação da lista até que o paciente desenvolva a capacidade de se sentir relaxado em qualquer das situações causadoras de ansiedade. A seguir, as situações imaginárias são substituídas por situações reais. SIN reciprocal inhibition (2).

de·sen·si·tize (dē - sen′si - tīz). Dessensibilizar. **1.** Reduzir ou remover qualquer forma de sensibilidade. **2.** Realizar dessensibilização (1). **3.** Em odontologia, eliminar ou reduzir a resposta dolorosa da dentina vital exposta a agentes irritantes ou a alterações térmicas.

de·ser·pi·dine (dē - ser′pi - dēn). Deserpidina; alcalóide éster isolado da *Rauwolfia canescens* (família Apocynaceae), com as mesmas ações e empregos da reserpina.

des·e·tope (dē′se - tōp). A parte da molécula de histocompatibilidade principal Classe II que interage com o antígeno. O termo desetope é derivado de seleção determinante. [*de*terminant *se*lection + -tope]

des·fer·ri·ox·a·mine mes·y·late (des′făr - ē - ok′să - mēn). Mesilato de desferrioxamina. SIN deferoxamine mesylate.

des·flu·rane (dés′floor′an). Desflurano; anestésico inalatório com características físicas que produzem rápida indução e recuperação da anestesia.

des·hy·dre·mia (des′hī - drē′mē - ă). Desidremia; hemoconcentração devida à perda de água do plasma sanguíneo. [L. *de-* distante de, + G. *hydor*, água, + *haima*, sangue + *-ia*]

des·ic·cant (des′i - kant). Dessecante. **1.** Secante; que causa ou promove o dessecamento. SIN desiccative. **2.** Um agente que absorve umidade; um agente secante. SIN desiccator (1). SIN exsiccant. [L. *de-sicco*, pp. *–siccatus*, dessecar]

des·ic·cate (des′i - kāt). Dessecar; secar completamente; tornar livre de umidade. SIN exsiccate.

des·ic·ca·tion (des - i - kā′shŭn). Dessecação; o processo de ser dessecado. SIN dehydration (4), exsiccation (1).

des·ic·ca·tive (des - i - kā′tiv). Dessecativo. SIN desiccant (1).

des·ic·ca·tor (des′i - kā - ter, tōr). Dessecador. **1.** SIN desiccant (2). **2.** Um aparelho, como um recipiente de vidro contendo cloreto de cálcio, ácido sulfúrico ou outro agente secante, no qual um material é colocado para secar.

   vacuum d., d. a vácuo; um dessecador que pode ser evacuado.

de·si·pra·mine hy·dro·chlo·ride (des - ip′ră - mēn). Cloridrato de desipramina; um derivado de dibenzazepina; um antidepressivo semelhante ao cloridrato de imipramina. Bloqueia seletivamente a recaptação da norepinefrina para os neurônios aminérgicos centrais.

des·lan·o·side (des - lan′ō - sīd). Deslanosídeo; um glicosídeo esteróide de ação rápida obtido a partir do lanatosídeo C (*Digitalis lanata*) por hidrólise alcalina; um cardiotônico.

desm-. VER desmo-.

Desmarres, Louis A., oftalmologista francês, 1810–1882. VER D. *dacryoliths*, em *dacryolith*; Desmarres *retractor*.

des·min (dez′minz). Desmina; proteínas encontradas em filamentos intermediários que co-polimerizam com a vimentina para formar constituintes do tecido conjuntivo, paredes celulares, filamentos, etc. Encontrada no disco Z das células musculares esqueléticas e cardíacas.

des·mi·tis (dez - mī′tis). Desmite; inflamação de um ligamento. [desm- + G. *-zeeitis*, inflamação]

desmo-, desm-. Conexão fibrosa; ligamento. [G. *desmos*, uma faixa]

des·mo·cra·ni·um (dez-mō-krā'nē-ŭm) [TA]. Desmocrânio; o primórdio mesenquimal do crânio.

des·mo·den·ti·um [TA]. Desmodente; as fibras colágenas, desde o cimento até o osso alveolar, que suspendem um dente em seu alvéolo; elas incluem fibras apicais, oblíquas, horizontais e da crista alveolar, indicando que a orientação das fibras varia em diferentes níveis. SIN desmodontium [TA], periodontal fiber*, periodontal ligament fibers.

des·mo·don·ti·um [TA]. Desmodonto. SIN desmodentium.

Des·mo·dus (dez'mō-dŭs). Gênero hematófago de quiróptero (ordem chiroptena), geralmente conhecido como morcego vampiro, encontrado em Trinidad, no México e nas Américas Central e do Sul; *D. artibaeus, D. rotundus* e *D. rufus*, três espécies encontradas em Trinidad e na América do Sul, são hospedeiros reservatórios do vírus da raiva. [desmo- + G. *odous*, dente]

des·mog·e·nous (dez-moj'ĕ-nŭs). Desmógeno; de origem ligamentosa ou no tecido conjuntivo; p. ex., designa uma deformidade causada por contração de ligamentos, fáscia ou cicatriz. [desmo- + G. *-gen*, que produz]

des·mog·ra·phy (dez-mog'ra-fē). Desmografia; descrição de, ou tratado sobre, os ligamentos. [desmo- + G. *grapho*, descrever]

des·moid (dez'moyd). Desmóide. **1.** Fibroso ou ligamentoso. **2.** Um nódulo ou massa relativamente grande de tecido conjuntivo cicatricial, incomumente firme, resultante da proliferação ativa de fibroblastos, mais freqüente nos músculos abdominais de mulheres que já tiveram filhos; os fibroblastos infiltram o músculo e a fáscia adjacentes. SIN abdominal fibromatosis, desmoid tumor. [desmo- + G. *eidos*, aparência, forma]

extra-abdominal d., d. extra-abdominal; tumor de consistência firme, profundo, mais freqüente nos ombros, tórax ou dorso de homens ou mulheres jovens, consistindo em tecido fibroso colágeno que infiltra o músculo adjacente; freqüentemente recorre, mas não metastatiza.

des·mo·las·es (dez'mō-lā'sez). Desmolases; termo antigo e inespecífico para enzimas que catalisam outras reações além daquelas que envolvem hidrólise; p. ex., aquelas que envolvem oxidação e redução, isomerização, a ruptura de ligações carbono-carbono.

des·mol·o·gy (dez-mol'ō-jē). Desmologia; o ramo da anatomia relacionado aos ligamentos. [desmo- + G. *logos*, estudo]

des·mop·a·thy (dez-mop'ă-thē). Desmopatia; qualquer doença dos ligamentos. [desmo- + G. *pathos*, que sofre]

des·mo·pla·sia (dez-mō-plā'zē-ă). Desmoplasia; hiperplasia de fibroblastos e formação desproporcional de tecido conjuntivo fibroso, principalmente no estroma de um carcinoma. [desmo- + G. *plasis*, moldagem]

des·mo·plas·tic (des-mō-plas'tik). Desmoplásico. **1.** Que causa ou forma aderências. **2.** Que causa fibrose no estroma vascular de uma neoplasia.

des·mo·pres·sin (des-mō-pres'in). Desmopressina; um análogo da vasopressina (hormônio antidiurético, ADH) que possui potente atividade antidiurética.

d. acetate, acetato de d.; um análogo sintético da vasopressina e um hormônio antidiurético.

des·mo·sine (dez'mō-sēn). Desmosina; um aminoácido de ligação cruzada formado a partir de resíduos lisil encontrados na elastina. [G. *desmos*, ligação, de *deō*, ligar, + *-ine*]

des·mo·some (dez'mō-sōm). Desmossoma; um local de adesão entre duas células epiteliais, consistindo em uma placa de fixação densa separada de uma estrutura semelhante, na outra célula, por uma fina camada de material extracelular. SIN bridge corpuscle, macula adherens. [desmo- + G. *sōma*, corpo]

des·mos·te·rol (dez-mos'ter-ol). Desmosterol; 5α-colesta-5,24-dieno-3β-ol; suposto intermediário na biossíntese de colesterol a partir do lanosterol através do zimosterol; acumula-se após administração prolongada de substâncias que interferem com a biossíntese do colesterol. SIN 24-dehydrocholesterol.

des·o·nide (des'ō-nīd). Desonida; um corticosteróide antiinflamatório usado em preparações tópicas.

des·ox·i·met·a·sone (des-ok-si-met'ă-sōn). Desoximetasona; um corticosteróide antiinflamatório usado em preparações tópicas.

desoxy-. VER deoxy-.

des·ox·y·cor·ti·cos·ter·one (des-oks-ē-kōr'ti-kos-ter-ōn). Desoxicorticosterona; um esteróide derivado do córtex supra-renal com forte atividade mineralocorticóide.

des·ox·y·cor·tone (des-oks-ē-kōr'tōn). Desoxicortona. SIN deoxycorticosterone.

de·spe·ci·a·tion (dē-spē'shē-ā'shŭn). **1.** Alteração ou perda das características da espécie. **2.** Remoção de propriedades antigênicas espécie-específicas de uma proteína estranha.

D'Éspine, Jean H.A., médico francês, 1846–1930. VER D. *sign*.

des·pu·ma·tion (des-pū-mā'shŭn). Despumação. **1.** A subida de impurezas para a superfície de um líquido. **2.** A retirada de impurezas da superfície de um líquido. [L. *de-spumo*, pp., *-atus*, escumar, de *spumo*, espumar, de *spuma*, espuma]

des·qua·mate (des'kwă-māt). Descamar; rasgar, descascar ou descamar, como o desprendimento da epiderme em escamas ou fragmentos, ou o desprendimento da camada externa de qualquer superfície. [L. *desquamo*, pp. *-atus*, descamar, de *squama*, escama]

des·qua·ma·tion (des-kwă-mā'shŭn). Descamação; o desprendimento da cutícula em escamas ou da camada externa de qualquer superfície.

branny d., d. esfarelada. SIN defurfuration.

des·qua·ma·tive (des-kwam'ă-tiv). Descamativo; relativo a, ou caracterizado por, descamação.

des·thi·o·bi·o·tin (des'thī-ō-bī'ō-tin). Destiobiotina; substância derivada da biotina pela remoção do átomo de enxofre; um precursor da biotina em bactérias e fungos; pode ser substituído pela biotina em alguns microrganismos, mas não tem efeito sobre, ou é inibitório para, o crescimento de outros.

de·stru·do (dē-stroo'dō). Destrudo; pulsão de morte; a energia associada ao instinto de morte ou destrutivo. [cunhado de forma análoga à *libido*, do L. *destruo*, destruir]

de·sulf·hy·dras·es (dē'sulf-hī'drā-sez). Dessulfidrases; enzimas ou grupos de enzimas que catalisam a remoção de uma molécula de H_2S ou H_2S substituído de um composto, como na conversão de cisteína em ácido pirúvico pela cisteína dessulfidrase (cistationina γ-liase). SIN desulfurases.

de·sul·fi·nase (dē-sul'fi-nās). Desulfinase; termo algumas vezes aplicado à enzima (aspartato-4-descarboxilase) removedora de sulfito de: 1) cisteinossulfinato, um intermediário na degradação da cisteína, produzindo alanina; 2) sulfinilpiruvato, outrora supostamente formado por desaminação da cisteinossulfinato, produzindo piruvato; a degradação do sulfinilpiruvato agora é considerada espontânea, não exigindo uma enzima.

De·sul·fo·to·ma·cu·lum (dē-sul-fō-tō-mak'ū-lŭm). Um gênero de bactérias bacilares (retas ou curvas), anaeróbicas, quimioorganotróficas, móveis, de coloração Gram-negativa, mas que possuem paredes celulares Gram-positivas. Encontradas no solo, no rúmen e em outras partes. A espécie típica é *D. nigrificans*.

D. nigrificans, uma espécie encontrada em alimentos deteriorados que exibem deterioração com "cheiro de enxofre" em virtude da produção de sulfeto de hidrogênio. Não é patogênica.

de·sul·fu·ras·es (dē-sul'fŭr-ās-ez). Dessulfurases. SIN desulfhydrases.

de·syn·chro·nous (de-sin'kron-ŭs). Assincrônico; ausência de sincronismo, como nas ondas cerebrais. [de- + G. *syn*, com + *chronos*, tempo]

DET Abreviatura de diethyltryptamine (dietiltriptamina).

det. Abreviatura de L. *detur*, dar. [deixar dar]

de·tach·ment (dē-tach'ment). Descolamento; separação; desligamento; insulamento; desapego. **1.** Sentimento ou emoção voluntária ou involuntária que acompanha um sentimento de separação do ambiente ou de associações normais. **2.** Separação de uma estrutura de sua sustentação.

exudative retinal d., descolamento exsudativo da retina; descolamento da retina sem rupturas retinianas, decorrente de doença inflamatória da coróide, tumores da retina e angiomatose retiniana.

retinal d., d. of retina, descolamento da retina; perda da aposição entre a retina sensorial e o epitélio pigmentar da retina. SIN detached retina, separation of retina.

rhegmatogenous retinal d., descolamento regmatoso da retina; separação da retina associada a ruptura, orifício ou laceração na retina sensorial.

vitreous d., descolamento do vítreo; separação do humor vítreo periférico da retina.

de·tec·tion (dē-tek'shŭn). Detecção. **1.** O ato da descoberta. **2.** Em cromatografia, visualização do material separado.

de·tec·tor (dē-tek'ter, -tōr). Detector; o componente de um instrumento laboratorial que detecta o sinal químico ou físico indicador da presença ou quantidade da substância de interesse.

solid-state d., d. de estado sólido; detector que usa um material cintilante cristalino em vez de uma câmara de ionização para detectar ou medir a radiação.

de·ter·gent (dē-ter'jent). Detergente. **1.** Que limpa. **2.** Um agente de limpeza ou de purificação, geralmente sais de bases ou ácidos alifáticos de cadeia longa (p. ex., compostos de amônio quaternário ou de ácido sulfônico) que, através de uma ação superficial que depende da existência de propriedades tanto hidrofílicas como hidrofóbicas, exercem efeitos de limpeza (dissolução de óleo) e antibacterianos; os derivados da acridina (p. ex., acriflavina, proflavina), bem como outros corantes (p. ex., verde brilhante, cristal violeta) possuem propriedades detergentes pelas mesmas razões. SIN detersive. [L. *de-tergeo*, pp. *-tersus*, remover esfregando]

anionic d.'s, detergentes aniônicos; detergentes, como sabões (sais metálicos alcalinos de ácidos graxos de cadeia longa), que possuem uma carga elétrica negativa em uma molécula semelhante a um lipídio e exercem um efeito antibacteriano limitado.

cationic d.'s, detergentes catiônicos; detergentes, como os sais amina ou compostos de amônio quaternário ou piridínio de ácidos graxos de cadeia longa, que possuem grupamentos positivamente carregados fixados às porções hidrofóbicas maiores.

zwitterionic d., d. zwitteriônico. SIN zwittergents.

de·te·ri·o·ra·tion (dē-tēr'i-ō-rā'shŭn). Deterioração; o processo ou condição de se tornar pior. [L. *deterior*, pior]

alcoholic d., d. alcoólica; demência que ocorre em pessoas cronicamente viciadas em álcool. VER chronic *alcoholism.*

senile d., d. senil; declínio lentamente progressivo da saúde física e mental, aparentemente devido a causas naturais resultantes dos processos de envelhecimento. VER Alzheimer *disease.*

de·ter·mi·nant (dē-ter′mi-nănt). Determinante; o fator que contribui para a geração de um traço. [L. *determans*, determinante, limitante]

allotypic d.'s, determinantes alotípicos; determinantes antigênicos de alotipos.

antigenic d., d. antigênico; o grupamento químico específico de uma molécula que determina especificidade imunológica. SIN determinant group.

disease d.'s, determinantes de doença; quaisquer variáveis que influenciam, direta ou indiretamente, a freqüência de ocorrência e/ou a distribuição de qualquer doença; essas variáveis incluem agentes mórbidos específicos, características do hospedeiro e fatores ambientais.

genetic d., d. genético; qualquer determinante antigênico ou característica de identificação, particularmente aqueles de alotipos. SIN genetic marker.

idiotypic antigenic d., d. antigênico idiotípico. SIN idiotope.

isoallotypic d.'s, determinantes isoalotípicos; determinantes genéticos que são tanto isotípicos quanto alotípicos porque aparecem em cadeias pesadas de todos os membros de, pelo menos, uma subclasse de imunoglobulina, mas também em cadeias pesadas de outra subclasse da mesma espécie.

mathematical d., d. matemático; operação algébrica formal nos termos de uma matriz quadrada de quantidades, fundamental para resolver múltiplas equações simultâneas e amplamente usada na análise de regressão, notavelmente em epidemiologia e genética quantitativa. Se o determinante for igual a zero, as equações não possuem solução precisa.

de·ter·mi·na·tion (dē-ter-mi-nā′shŭn). **1.** Definição; uma mudança, para melhor ou para pior, na evolução de uma doença. **2.** Propósito; um movimento geral para determinado ponto. **3.** Determinação; a medida ou estimativa de qualquer quantidade ou qualidade em investigação científica ou laboratorial. **4.** Conclusão; discernimento de um estado ou categoria (p. ex., no diagnóstico). **5.** Diferenciação; um processo, necessário e suficiente, no qual é causado um efeito. [L. *de-termino*, pp. *-atus*, limitar, determinar, de *terminus*, limite]

cell d., diferenciação celular; o processo pelo qual células embrionárias, previamente indiferenciadas, assumem uma característica de desenvolvimento específica. VER morphogenesis, induction, evocator.

sex d., determinação sexual; determinação do sexo de um feto *in utero* por identificação de cromossomas fetais.

de·ter·mi·nism (dē-ter′mi-nizm). Determinismo; a proposição de que todo comportamento é causado exclusivamente por influências genéticas e ambientais, sem componentes aleatórios e independentemente da vontade livre. [L. *determino*, limitar, de *terminus*, limite, + *-ism*]

psychic d., d. psíquico; em psicanálise, o conceito de que todos os fenômenos psicológicos e comportamentais resultam de causas antecedentes, que atuam inconscientemente.

de·ter·sive (dē-ter′siv). Detersivo. SIN detergent.

de·tox·i·cate (dē-tok′si-kāt). Desintoxicar; diminuir ou eliminar a qualidade venenosa de qualquer substância; reduzir a virulência de qualquer organismo patogênico. SIN detoxify. [L. *de*, de, + *toxicum*, veneno]

de·tox·i·ca·tion (dē-tok-si-kā′shŭn). Destoxificação; desintoxicação. SIN detoxification.

ammonia d., d. da amônia; a destoxificação da amônia e do íon amônio pela formação de sais de amônia, produtos específicos da excreção de nitrogênio ou L-glutamina.

de·tox·i·fi·ca·tion (dē-tok′si-fi-kā′shŭn). Destoxificação; desintoxicação. **1.** Recuperação dos efeitos tóxicos de uma substância. **2.** Eliminação das propriedades tóxicas de um veneno. **3.** Conversão metabólica de princípios farmacologicamente ativos em princípios farmacologicamente menos ativos. SIN detoxication.

de·tox·i·fy (dē-tok′si-fī). Destoxificar. SIN detoxicate.

de·tri·tion (dē-trish′ŭn). Desgastar pelo uso ou fricção. [L. *de-tero*, pp. *-tritus*, tirar esfregando.]

de·tri·tus (dē-trī′tŭs). Detrito; qualquer material quebrado, material cariado ou gangrenoso, cascalho, etc. [L. (ver detrition)]

de·tru·sor (dē-troo′ser, -sōr). Detrusor. **1.** Um músculo que tem a ação de expelir uma substância. **2.** VER detrusor (*muscle*). [L. *detrudo*, expelir]

de·tru·sor·rha·phy (dē-troo′-sor-a-fē). Detrussorrafia; procedimento no qual o músculo da bexiga (detrusor) é reconstruído ao redor da junção ureterovesical para formar uma válvula unidirecional competente. VER TAMBÉM ureteroneocystostomy. SIN extravesical reimplantation. [detrusor + G. *rhaphē*, bainha]

de·tu·mes·cence (dē-too-mes′ens). Detumescência; diminuição de um edema. [L. *de*, de, + *tumesco*, inchar, de *tumeo*, inchar]

de·tur·ges·cence (dē-toor-ges′ens). Deturgescência; o mecanismo pelo qual o estroma da córnea permanece relativamente desidratado. [L. *de*, de, + *turgesco*, começar a inchar]

deut-. VER deutero-.

deu·ten·ceph·a·lon (doo′ten-sef′ă-lon). Deutencéfalo; termo raramente usado para diencéfalo. [G. *deuteros*, segundo, + *enkephalos*, encéfalo]

deu·ter·a·nom·a·ly (doo′ter-ă-nom′ă-lē). Deuteranomalia; uma forma de tricromatismo anômalo devido a um defeito dos cones retinianos sensíveis ao verde. [G. *deuteros*, segundo, + *anomalia*, anomalia]

deu·ter·an·ope (doo′ter-ă-nōp). Deuterânope; pessoa afetada por deuteranopia.

deu·ter·an·o·pia (doo′ter-ă-nō′pē-ă). Deuteranopia; anormalidade congênita da retina na qual há dois, em vez de três, pigmentos no cone da retina (dicromatismo) e completa insensibilidade aos comprimentos de onda médios (verdes). [G. *deuteros*, segundo, + anopia]

deuterio-. Prefixo que indica "contendo deutério".

deu·te·ri·um (D) (doo-tē-r′ē-ŭm). Deutério. SIN hydrogen-2. [G. *deuteros*, segundo]

d. oxide, óxido de d., água pesada. SIN heavy water.

deutero-, deut-, deuto-. Formas combinantes que significam dois, ou segundo (em uma série); secundário. [G. *deuteros*, segundo)

deu·ter·o·my·ce·tes (du′ter-ō-mī-sē′tez). Deuteromicetos; membros da classe Deuteromycetes ou do filo Deuteromycota.

Deu·ter·o·my·cota (doo′ter-ō-mī-kō-ta). Um filo no qual a parte sexual (teleomorfa ou perfeita) do ciclo vital não foi descoberta; apenas a parte assexuada (anamorfa ou imperfeita) do ciclo vital foi descoberta. VER TAMBÉM Fungi Imperfecti.

deu·ter·on (doo′ter-on). Dêuteron; dêuton; o núcleo do hidrogênio-2, composto de um nêutron e um próton; ele assim possui a carga elétrica positiva única característica de um núcleo de hidrogênio. SIN deuton, diplon.

deu·ter·o·path·ic (doo′ter-ō-path′ik). Deuteropático; relativo a uma deuteropatia.

deu·ter·op·a·thy (doo-ter-op′ă-thē). Deuteropatia; uma doença ou sintoma secundário. [deutero- + G. *pathos*, que sofre]

deu·ter·o·plasm (doo′ter-ō-plazm). Deuteroplasma. SIN deutoplasm. [deutero- + G. *plasma*, algo formado]

deu·ter·o·por·phy·rin (doo′ter-ō-pōr′fi-rin). Deuteroporfirina; um derivado da porfirina semelhante às protoporfirinas, exceto pelas duas cadeias laterais vinil serem substituídas por hidrogênio.

deu·ter·o·some (doo′ter-ō-sōm). Deuterossoma; grânulos fibrosos esféricos densos encontrados na centrosfera e que atuam no desenvolvimento de centríolos ou corpúsculos basais. SIN procentriole organizer.

deu·ter·o·to·cia (doo′ter-ō-tō′se-ă). Deuterotocia; uma forma de partenogênese na qual a fêmea tem descendentes de ambos os sexos. SIN deuterotoky. [deutero- + G. *tokos*, parto]

deu·ter·ot·o·ky (doo-ter-ot′ō-kē). Deuterotoquia. SIN deuterotocia.

deuto-. VER deutero-.

deu·to·gen·ic (doo-tō-jen′ik). Deutogênico; de origem secundária após uma influência indutiva. [deuto- + G. *-gen*, produção]

deu·tom·er·ite (doo-tom′er-īt). Deutomerito; a porção nucleada posterior de um cefalonte fixado em um protozoário gregarino, separada por um septo ectoplásmico da porção anterior, ou protomerito. [deuto- + L. *meros*, parte]

deu·ton (doo′ton). Dêuteron; dêuton. SIN deuteron.

deu·to·nymph (doo′to-nimt). Deutoninfa; o terceiro estágio de um ácaro.

deu·to·plasm (doo′tō-plazm). Deutoplasma; o vitelo de um ovo meroblástico; o material não-vivo no citoplasma, principalmente aquele armazenado no ovo como alimento para o embrião em desenvolvimento, sendo os tipos mais comuns gotículas lipóides e grânulos vitelinos. SIN deuteroplasm. [deuto- + G. *plasma*, algo formado]

deu·to·plas·mic (doo-tō-plaz′mik). Deutoplásmico; relativo ao deutoplasma.

deu·to·plas·mi·gen·on (doo′tō-plaz-mi-jen′on). Deutoplasmígeno; aquilo que produz ou dá origem ao deutoplasma. [deutoplasm + G. *genos*, nascimento]

deu·to·plas·mol·y·sis (doo′tō-plaz-mol′i-sis). Deutoplasmólise; a desintegração do deutoplasma. [deutoplasm + G. *lysis*, dissolução]

Deutschländer, Carl E. W., cirurgião alemão, 1872–1942. VER D. *disease.*

DEV Abreviatura de duck embryo origin *vaccine* (vacina preparada com embrião de pato).

de·vas·cu·lar·i·za·tion (dē-vas′kū-lăr-i-zā′shŭn). Desvascularização; oclusão de todos os vasos sanguíneos, ou da maioria deles, para qualquer parte ou órgão. [L. *de*, distante, + *vasculum*, pequeno vaso, + *izo*, causar]

de·vel·op (dē-vel′op). Revelar; processar uma imagem fotográfica ou radiográfica exposta a fim de transformar a imagem latente em permanente. [Fr. ant. *desveloper*, revelar, de *voloper*, envolver]

de·vel·op·er (dē-vel′op-er). **1.** Fomentador um indivíduo ou procedimento que desenvolve ou fomenta algo. **2.** SIN eluent. **3.** Revelador; as substâncias químicas usadas para revelar um filme por redução das moléculas de halóide de prata fotoativadas para prata atômica. **4.** O fator (ou fatores) que faz com que uma célula, órgão ou organismo sofra uma série de alterações ordenadas.

de·vel·op·ment (dē-vel′op-ment). Desenvolvimento. **1.** O ato ou processo de progressão natural da maturação física e psicológica de um estágio prévio, inferior ou embrionário para um estágio posterior, mais complexo ou adulto. **2.** O processo de cromatografia.

cognitive d., d. cognitivo; o desenvolvimento evolutivo das funções intelectuais do lactente e da criança.
life-span d., d. durante toda a vida; desenvolvimento e domínio (ou perda) de diferentes habilidades biológicas, intelectuais, comportamentais e sociais em diferentes épocas da vida desde o período pré-natal até os períodos gerontológicos de crescimento.
psychosexual d., d. psicossexual; maturação e desenvolvimento das fases psíquica e de comportamento da sexualidade, desde o nascimento até a vida adulta, atravessando as fases oral, anal, fálica, de latência e genital.

Deventer, Hendrik van, obstetra holandês, 1651–1724. VER D. *pelvis*.

de·vi·ance (dē′vē-ans). Desvio. SIN deviation (3).

de·vi·ant (dē′vē-ant). Divergente **1.** Denotando desvio ou indicativo de desvio. **2.** Um indivíduo que exibe desvios, sobretudo sexuais.

de·vi·a·tion (dē-vē-ā′shŭn). **1.** Afastamento ou desvio do ponto ou trajeto normal. **2.** Uma anormalidade. **3.** Em psiquiatria e nas ciências comportamentais, um desvio de um padrão, papel ou regra aceita. SIN deviance. **4.** Uma medida estatística que representa a diferença entre um valor individual em um conjunto de valores e o valor médio nesse conjunto. [L. *devio*, afastar-se do caminho certo, de *de*, de, + *via*, caminho]
axis d., d. do eixo; deflexão do eixo elétrico do coração para a direita ou esquerda em relação ao normal. VER TAMBÉM left axis d., right axis d., axis. SIN axis shift.
conjugate d. of the eyes, d. conjugado dos olhos; **(1)** rotação dos olhos igual e simultaneamente na mesma direção, como ocorre normalmente; **(2)** uma condição na qual ambos os olhos estão virados para o mesmo lado em virtude de paralisia ou espasmo muscular.
dissociated horizontal d., d. horizontal dissociado; uma tendência freqüentemente associada a esotropia congênita reparada na qual um olho apresenta abdução, quando coberto, violando a lei de Herring (Herring *law*).
dissociated vertical d., d. vertical dissociado; uma tendência freqüentemente associada à esotropia congênita, na qual um olho apresenta elevação, abdução e torção externa, quando coberto, violando a lei de Herring (Herring *law*).
immune d., d. imunológico. SIN split *tolerance*.
d. to the left, d. para a esquerda. SIN *shift* to the left (1).
left axis d., d. do eixo elétrico para a esquerda; um eixo elétrico médio do coração que aponta para −30° ou mais negativo. VER hexaxial reference *system*.
primary d., d. primário; o desvio ocular observado na paralisia de um músculo ocular quando o olho não-paralisado é usado para fixação.
d. to the right, d. para a direita. SIN *shift* to the right (1).
right axis d., d. do eixo elétrico para a direita; um eixo elétrico médio do coração que aponta para a direita de + 90°. VER hexaxial reference *system*.
secondary d., d. secundário; desvio ocular observado na paralisia de um músculo ocular quando o olho paralisado é usado para fixação.
sexual d., d. sexual; prática sexual biologicamente atípica, considerada moralmente errada ou legalmente proibida. VER bestiality, pedophilia. SIN sexual perversion.
skew d., d. oblíquo; d. de ângulo; uma hipertropia na qual os olhos se movem igualmente em direções opostas; uma hipertropia adquirida, freqüentemente concomitante, que não se encaixa no padrão característico de lesão do nervo troclear ou de anormalidade do músculo ocular; freqüentemente causada por uma lesão do tronco cerebral ou cerebelar.
standard d. (SD, σ), d. padrão; **(1)** índice estatístico do grau de desvio da tendência central, isto é, da variabilidade em uma distribuição; a raiz quadrada da média dos quadrados dos desvios em relação à média; **(2)** medida da dispersão ou variação usada para descrever uma característica de uma distribuição de freqüência.

Devic, Eugène, médico francês, 1869–1930. VER D. *disease*.

de·vice (dē-vīs′). Dispositivo; mecanismo; um aparelho, geralmente mecânico, designado para realizar uma função específica, como uma prótese ou órtese. [I.M. do Fr. antigo *devis*, do L. *divisum*, dividido]
central-bearing d., d. de apoio central; em odontologia, um dispositivo que proporciona um ponto central de apoio, ou suporte, entre as bases superior e inferior de registro; consiste em um ponto de contato que está fixado a uma base e em uma placa fixada a outra, que proporciona a superfície sobre a qual o ponto de suporte repousa ou se move.
central-bearing tracing d., d. de traçado de apoio central; em odontologia, um dispositivo de apoio central usado para fazer um traçado e/ou para apoio entre as bases superior e inferior.
contraceptive d., d. contraceptivo; dispositivo usado para evitar gravidez; p. ex., diafragma oclusivo, preservativo, dispositivo intra-uterino.
intrauterine d.'s (IUD), dispositivos intra-uterinos (DIU); pedaços de plástico ou metal de vários formatos (p. ex., espiral, alça, "T" curvo) introduzidos no útero para exercer um efeito contraceptivo. SIN intrauterine contraceptive d.'s.
intrauterine contraceptive d.'s (IUCD), dispositivos contraceptivos intra-uterinos. SIN intrauterine d.'s.
left-ventricular assist d., d. de assistência ventricular esquerda; bomba mecânica introduzida em algum ponto na circulação para acompanhar a atividade do ventrículo esquerdo e, assim, reduzir sua carga.

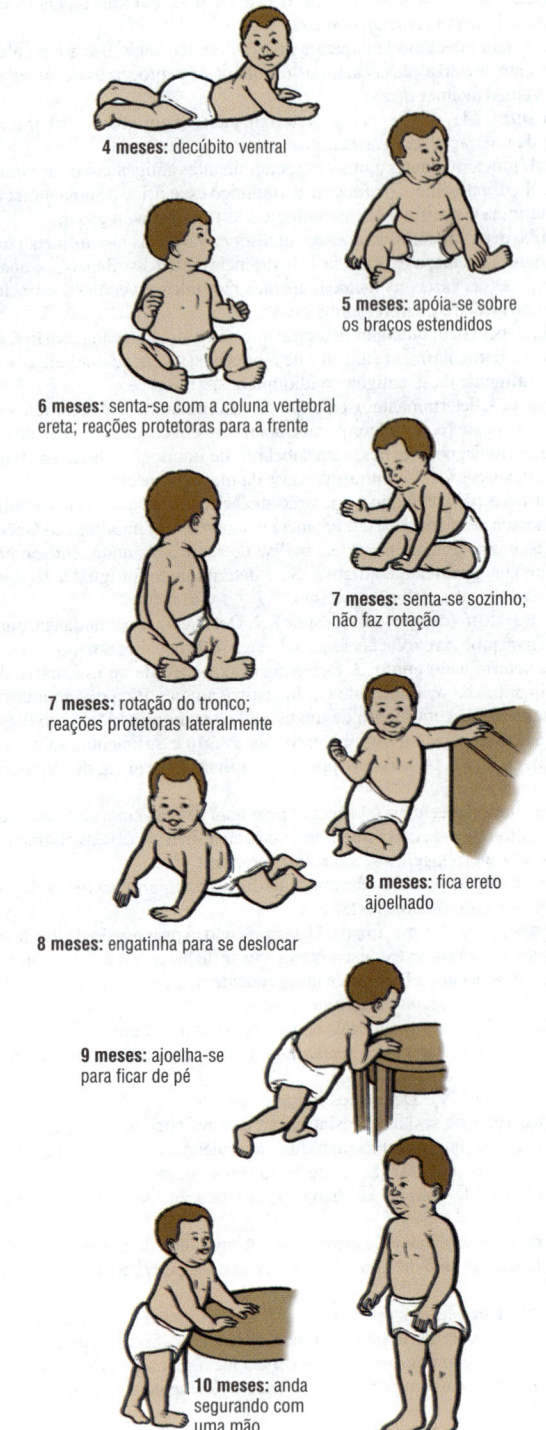

marcos do desenvolvimento

ventricular assist d., d. de assistência ventricular; qualquer dos vários dispositivos mecânicos que apóiam ou substituem a função de bombeamento do ventrículo esquerdo (DAVE) ou direito (DAVD). A extremidade de influxo da bomba está conectada ao ventrículo e a extremidade de efluxo à aorta (DAVE) ou à artéria pulmonar (DAVD). A maior parte do débito cardíaco, ou todo ele, é direcionada para o dispositivo a fim de dar tempo para a recuperação do músculo cardíaco lesado do paciente após infarto do miocárdio ou cirurgia cardíaca. Também usado como "uma ponte até o transplante", isto é, para manter o paciente cujo coração não se recuperará até que haja um doador de coração disponível.

de·vi·om·e·ter (dē-vē-om′ĕ-ter). Desviômetro; uma forma de estrabismômetro.

desenvolvimento motor, social e verbal e cognitivo da criança normal

idade	motor	área de habilidade social	verbal e cognitivo
2–3 meses	levanta a cabeça quando em decúbito ventral	sorri em resposta ao rosto humano ("sorriso social")	arrulha, balbucia
5–6 meses	vira-se na cama, senta sem ajuda	estabelece um vínculo com a pessoa que cuida dela, reconhece os pais	balbucia (repete um único som várias vezes)
7–11 meses	fica de pé se segurando	mostra medo em resposta a pessoas estranhas ("ansiedade na presença de estranhos")	imita sons, usa gestos
12–15 meses	caminha sem ajuda	teme a separação da pessoa que cuida dela ("ansiedade de separação")	diz a primeira palavra
16 meses–2,5 anos	sobe escada, rabisca uma folha de papel com lápis de cera	brinca sozinho, mostra negatividade (p. ex., a palavra favorita é "não")	fala em frases de duas palavras (p. ex., "Eu vou"), denomina partes do corpo e objetos
2,5–4 anos	anda de triciclo, despe-se e veste-se parcialmente sem ajuda; copia um círculo, linha ou cruz; identifica cores	brinca ao lado de outras crianças, mas não com elas ("brincadeira paralela"), pode passar grande parte do dia com outros adultos além dos pais (p. ex., pré-escola), desenvolve identidade sexual por volta dos 3 anos	usa frases completas (p. ex., "Posso fazer isso sozinho.")
4–6 anos	desenha uma pessoa em detalhes (p. ex., com os braços, pernas, corpo, olhos, cabelo), veste-se sozinho, salta usando pés alternados, amarra cadarços de sapatos aos 6 anos, copia um quadrado ou triângulo	brinca com outras crianças; pode ter amigos imaginários; tem curiosidade a respeito do corpo, brinca de "médico"; tem sentimentos românticos em relação ao genitor do sexo oposto ("a fase edipiana")	boa auto-expressão verbal (p. ex., conta histórias detalhadas)
6–11 anos	realiza atividades motoras complexas (p. ex., joga bola, anda de bicicleta, pula corda)	prefere brincar com crianças do mesmo sexo, é ativa e esforçada, desenvolve um senso moral de certo e errado, aprende a seguir regras, identifica-se com o genitor do mesmo sexo, mantém relacionamentos com outros adultos além dos pais (p. ex., professores, líderes de grupos)	desenvolve a capacidade de raciocínio lógico; compreende que os objetos possuem mais de uma propriedade (p. ex., podem ser de madeira e azuis); aprende a ler, escrever e calcular (estágio das "operações concretas de Piaget")
11–14 anos	tem maior força corporal, participa de esportes individuais e em equipe	mostra preocupação com papéis sexuais, imagem corporal e popularidade; continua a se separar da família; forma relações mais fortes com os colegas	desenvolve o raciocínio abstrato (início dos estágios de "operações formais" de Piaget) e a criatividade
14–17 anos	possui habilidades motoras semelhantes às do adulto	tem sentimentos de onipotência que a levam a assumir comportamento de risco (p. ex., não usar dispositivos contraceptivos, conduzir automóveis em alta velocidade)	continua o desenvolvimento à medida que a capacidade intelectual se aproxima de seu pico
17–20 anos	atinge o nível adulto de habilidades motoras	mostra preocupação com questões humanitárias, moralidade e autocontrole; pode ter uma crise de identidade que causa confusão de papéis (manifestada por comportamento criminal ou participação em cultos)	mostra desenvolvimento adicional do raciocínio matemático abstrato (p. ex., cálculo)

de·vi·tal·i·za·tion (dē-vī'tăl-i-zā'shŭn). Desvitalização. **1.** Privação de vitalidade ou das propriedades vitais. **2.** Em odontologia, o processo pelo qual a polpa do dente é destruída; p. ex., por meios químicos, infecção ou extirpação.

de·vi·tal·ize (dē-vī'tăl-īz). Desvitalizar; privar de vitalidade ou de propriedades vitais.

de·vi·tal·ized (dē-vī'tăl-īzd). Desvitalizado; desprovido de vida; morto.

dev·o·lu·tion (dev-ō-loo'shŭn). Involução; um processo contínuo de degeneração ou fragmentação, em contraste com a evolução. VER TAMBÉM involution, catabolism. [L. *de-volvo*, pp. *-volutus*, regredir]

Dewar, Sir James, químico inglês, 1842–1923. VER D. *flask*.

de Wecker, Louis H., médico francês, 1832–1906. VER de W. *scissors*.

dex·a·meth·a·sone (dek-să-meth'ă-sōn). Dexametasona; um potente análogo sintético do cortisol, com ação biológica semelhante; usado como antiinflamatório e como material de teste da função do córtex supra-renal.

dex·am·phet·a·mine (deks-am-fet'ă-mēn). Dexanfetamina. SIN dextroamphetamine sulfate.

d. sodium phosphate, fosfato sódico de dexanfetamina; o éster hidrossolúvel da dexanfetamina, com as mesmas ações e usos.

dex·brom·phen·ir·a·mine ma·le·ate (deks'brom-fen-ir'ă-mēn). Maleato de dexbronfeniramina; o isômero dextrorrotatório da bronfeniramina; um anti-histamínico.

dex·chlor·phen·ir·a·mine ma·le·ate (deks'klōr-fen-ir'ă-mēn). Maleato de dexclorfeniramina; o isômero dextrorrotatório da clofeniramina; um anti-histamínico.

dex·i·o·car·dia (deks-ē-ō-kar'dē-ă). Dexiocardia. SIN dextrocardia.

dex·pan·the·nol (deks-pan'thē-nol). Dexpantenol; ácido pantotênico com —CH₂OH substituindo a —COOH terminal; um agente colinérgico e uma fonte alimentar de ácido pantotênico. SIN panthenol, pantothenyl alcohol.

dex·ter (D) (deks'ter). Dextro; localizado no, ou relativo ao, lado direito. [L. de *dextra*, neut. *dextrum*]

dextr-. VER dextro-.

dex·trad (deks'trad). Em direção ao lado direito. [L. *dexter*, direita, + *ad*, para]

dex·tral (deks'trăl). Destrímano, dextrômano. SIN right-handed.

dex·tral·i·ty (deks-tral'i-tē). Dextralidade; destrimanismo; preferência pela mão direita ao realizar tarefas manuais.

dex·tran (deks'tran). Dextrana. **1.** Qualquer um dos vários polímeros da glico-

se hidrossolúveis, de alto peso molecular (PM médio 75.000; variando entre 1.000 e 40.000.000), produzidos pela ação de membros da família Lactobacillaceae e de alguns outros microrganismos sobre a sacarose; usada em solução de cloreto de sódio isotônica para o tratamento do choque, bem como na água destilada para o alívio do edema da nefrose; a dextrana de menor peso molecular (p. ex., PM 40.000) melhora o fluxo sanguíneo nas áreas de estase por redução da agregação celular. **2.** Poli(α-1,6-glicose); α-1,6-glucana com pontos de ramificação (1,2; 1,3; 1,4) e espaçamento dessas características da espécie; usado como substitutos ou expansores do plasma. VER dextransucrase.
d. 110, d. 110; dextrana (PM médio de 110.000) disponível na forma de solução a 5% em água ou soro fisiológico; usada como expansor do volume plasmático.
d. 40, d. 40; dextrana (PM médio de 40.000) usada como expansor do volume plasmático.
d. 70, d. 70; dextrana (PM médio de 70.000) usada como expansor de volume plasmático.
d. 75, d. 75; dextrana (PM médio de 75.000) usada como expansor do volume plasmático.
acid d., d. ácida; o produto do tratamento ácido e térmico da dextrana.
animal d., d. animal. SIN glycogen.
blue d., d. azul; dextrana de alto peso molecular contendo um corante clorotriazina azul, Azul Cibracon; usada para medir os volumes vazios em colunas de filtração com gel, bem como para verificar o recheio da coluna.
d. sulfate, sulfato de d.; o sal sódico de ésteres do ácido sulfúrico do polissacarídeo dextrana; contém não menos de 10 unidades por mg e não menos de 14% de sulfato; um anticoagulante.
dex·tran·ase (deks'tran-ās). Dextranase; enzima que hidrolisa ligações α-1,6-D-glicosídicas na dextrana; usada na prevenção de cáries.
dex·tran·su·crase (deks-tran-su'krās). Dextransacarase; uma glicosiltransferase que forma poli(α-1,6-D-glicosil), isto é, poliglicoses, dextranas ou α-glicanas, a partir da sacarose, liberando resíduos D-frutose.
dex·trase (deks'trās). Dextrase; termo inespecífico para o complexo de enzimas que converte dextrose (D-glicose) em ácido lático.
dex·tri·fer·ron (deks-tri-fer'on). Dextriferron; uma solução coloidal de hidróxido de ferro em complexo com a dextrina parcialmente hidrolisada, usada no tratamento da anemia ferropriva; é adequada para administração intravenosa e contém 20 mg de ferro por ml.
dex·trin (deks'trin). Dextrina; mistura de oligomoléculas (α-1,4-D-glicose) formadas durante a hidrólise enzimática ou ácida do amido, amilopectina ou glicogênio; na hidrólise adicional são convertidas em D-glicose. As dextrinas possuem peso molecular muito menor que as dextranas e, portanto, não são adequadas como expansores plasmáticos; a dextrina (geralmente a dextrina branca) é usada em preparações farmacêuticas. SIN starch gum.
acid d., d. ácida; o produto do tratamento ácido e térmico da dextrina.
limit d., d. limite; os fragmentos de polissacarídeos que permanecem no final (limite) da hidrólise exaustiva da amilopectina ou glicogênio por α-1,4-glicana maltoidrolase ou β-amilase, que não pode hidrolisar as ligações α-1,6 em pontos de ramificação; acumula-se em indivíduos com doença por depósito de glicogênio tipo III. SIN dextrin limit.
Schardinger d.'s, dextrinas de Schardinger; anéis cíclicos do monômero da glicose (geralmente 6 a 8) com ligação α-1,4; o resultado da ação do *Bacillus macerans* sobre o amido.
dex·tri·nase (deks'tri-nās). Dextrinase; qualquer das enzimas que catalisam a hidrólise de dextrinas; p. ex., amilo-1,6-glicosidase, dextrin dextranase.
limit d., d. limite; **(1)** SIN α-dextrin endo-1,6-α-glucosidase; **(2)** SIN oligo-α-1,6-glucosidase.
dex·trin dex·tran·ase. Dextrina dextranase; uma glicosiltransferase que transfere resíduos 1,4-α-D-glicosil, assim catalisando a síntese de dextranas (com ligações 1,6 entre unidades de monossacarídeos) a partir de dextrinas (com ligações 1,4) por transferência de glicose. SIN dextrin → dextran transglucosidase, dextrin 6-glucosyltransferase.
dex·trin → dex·tran trans·glu·co·si·dase. Dextrina → dextrana transglucosidase. SIN dextrin dextranase.
α-dex·trin en·do-1,6-α-glu·co·si·dase. α-dextrina endo-1,6-α-glicosidase; uma enzima com ação semelhante à da isoamilase; cliva as ligações 1,6-α-glicosídicas em pululan, amilopectina e glicogênio, e em dextrinas de limite de α e β-amilase da amilopectina e glicogênio. Cf. isoamylase. SIN limit dextrinase (1), pullulanase, R enzyme.
dex·trin 6-α-D-glu·co·si·dase. Dextrina 6-α-D-glucosidase. SIN amylo-1,6-glucosidase.
dex·trin 6-glu·co·syl·trans·fer·ase. Dextrina 6-glucosiltransferase. SIN dextrin dextranase.
dex·trin gly·co·syl·trans·fer·ase. Dextrina glicosiltransferase. SIN 4-α-D-glucanotransferase.
dex·trin lim·it. Dextrina limite. SIN limit *dextrin.*
dex·trin·o·gen·ic (deks'trin-ō-jen'ik). Dextrinogênico; capaz de produzir dextrina.
dex·tri·no·sis (deks-trin-ō'sis). Dextrinose. SIN glycogenosis.

debranching deficiency limit d., limit d., d. limítrofe por deficiência de ramificação. SIN type 3 *glycogenosis.*
dex·trin trans·gly·co·syl·ase. Dextrina transglicosilase. SIN 4-α-D-glucanotransferase.
dex·tri·nu·ria (deks-tri-noo'rē-ă). Dextrinúria; a eliminação de dextrina na urina.
dextro-, dextr-. 1. Prefixos que significam direita, em direção ao lado direito. **2.** Prefixos químicos que significam dextrorrotatório. [L. *dexter,* do lado direito].
dex·tro·am·phet·a·mine phos·phate (deks'trō-am-fet'ă-mēn). Fosfato de dextroanfetamina; mesmas ações e usos do sulfato de dextroanfetamina. SIN *d*-amphetamine phosphate.
dex·tro·am·phet·a·mine sul·fate. Sulfato de dextroanfetamina; de ação semelhante ao sulfato de anfetamina racêmico, porém mais estimulante para o sistema nervoso central; simpaticomimético e depressor do apetite. SIN *d*-amphetamine sulfate, dexamphetamine.
dex·tro·car·dia (deks'trō-kar'dē-ă). Dextrocardia; deslocamento do coração para a direita, seja como dextroposição, com deslocamento simples para a direita, seja como heterotaxia cardíaca, com transposição completa das cavidades direita e esquerda, resultando em um coração que é a imagem espelhada de um coração normal. SIN dexiocardia. [dextro- + G. *kardia,* coração]
corrected d., d. corrigida; deslocamento e rotação do coração para o lado direito do tórax, mas sem transposição especular das cavidades cardíacas. SIN dextroversion of the heart, false d., type 3 d.
false d., d. falsa. SIN corrected d.
isolated d., d. isolada; dextrocardia com transposição especular das câmaras cardíacas, mas sem deslocamento das vísceras abdominais. SIN type 2 d.
mirror image d., d. com imagem em espelho; inversão congênita esquerda-direita perfeita do coração, algumas vezes com outras anomalias congênitas, algumas vezes normal, exceto pela posição.
secondary d., d. secundária; dextroposição do coração por alguma doença dos pulmões, pleura ou diafragma. SIN type 4 d.
type 1 d., d. tipo 1. SIN d. with situs inversus.
type 2 d., d. tipo 2. SIN isolated d.
type 3 d., d. tipo 3. SIN corrected d.
type 4 d., d. tipo 4. SIN secondary d.
d. with si'tus inver'sus, d. com *situs inversus*; deslocamento do coração para o lado direito do tórax, com transposição especular das câmaras cardíacas juntamente com transposição das vísceras abdominais. SIN type 1 d.
dex·tro·car·di·o·gram (deks'trō-kar'dē-ō-gram). Dextrocardiograma; a parte do eletrocardiograma derivada do ventrículo direito.
dex·tro·ce·re·bral (deks'trō-ser'ē-brăl). Dextrocerebral; que possui um hemisfério cerebral direito dominante.
dex·troc·u·lar (deks-trok'ū-lăr). Dextrocular; termo raramente usado para indicar dominância ocular direita; designando aquele que prefere o olho direito no trabalho monocular, como microscopia. SIN right-eyed. [dextro- + L. *oculus,* olho]
dex·tro·cy·clo·duc·tion (deks'trō-sī-klō-dŭk'shŭn). Dextrociclodução; rotação do pólo superior da córnea para a direita. VER excycloduction. [dextro- + cyclo + L. *duco,* pp. *ductus,* conduzir]
dex·tro·duc·tion (deks-trō-dŭk'shŭn). Dextrodução; termo raramente usado para rotação de um olho para a direita. [dextro- + L. *duco,* pp. *ductus,* conduzir]
dex·tro·gas·tria (deks-trō-gas'trē-ă). Dextrogastria; condição na qual o estômago está deslocado para a direita; pode representar deslocamento simples ou *situs inversus*. Geralmente associada à dextrocardia. [dextro- + G. *gastēr,* estômago]
dex·tro·glu·cose (deks-trō-gloo'kōs). Dextroglicose. VER D-glucose.
dex·tro·gram (deks'trō-gram). Dextrograma; registro eletrocardiográfico em um animal experimental que representa a propagação do impulso através do ventrículo direito isolado.
dex·tro·gy·ra·tion (deks'trō-jī-rā'shŭn). Dextrorrotação; rotação para a direita. [dextro- + L. *gyro,* pp. *-atus,* girar em círculo, de *gyrus,* círculo]
dex·tro·man·u·al (deks-trō-man'ū-ăl). Destrímano, dextrômano. SIN right-handed. [dextro- + L. *manus,* mão]
dex·tro·meth·or·phan hy·dro·bro·mide (deks'trō-meth-or'fan hī-drō-brō'mīd). Bromidrato de dextrometorfano; um derivado sintético da morfina usado como agente antitussígeno. Inferior à codeína, mas aparentemente não há produção de dependência. Possui fraca ação depressora central.
dex·tro·mor·a·mide tar·trate (deks-trō-mōr'ă-mīd). Tartarato de dextromoramida; um analgésico narcótico química e farmacologicamente relacionado à metadona.
dex·trop·e·dal (deks-trop'ē-dăl). Dextropedal; designa aquele que usa a perna direita em relação à esquerda. SIN right-footed. [dextro- + L. *pes (ped-),* pé]
dex·tro·po·si·tion (deks'trō-pō-zi'shŭn). Dextroposição; localização ou origem anormal no lado direito de uma estrutura normalmente situada do lado esquerdo, p. ex., origem da aorta no ventrículo direito.
d. of the heart, d. do coração. VER dextrocardia.

dex·tro·pro·pox·y·phene hy·dro·chlo·ride (deks′trō - prō - pok′sē - fēn). Cloridrato de dextropropoxifeno. SIN propoxyphene hydrochloride.

dex·tro·pro·pox·y·phene nap·syl·ate. Napsilato de dextropropoxifeno. SIN propoxyphene napsylate.

dex·tro·ro·ta·tion (deks′trō - rō - tā′shŭn). Dextrorrotação; volta ou giro para a direita; particularmente, a rotação no sentido horário dado o plano de luz polarizada por soluções de determinadas substâncias opticamente ativas. Cf. levorotation.

dex·tro·ro·ta·to·ry (deks - trō - rō′ta - tōr - ē). Dextrorrotatório; designa dextrorrotação, ou determinados cristais ou soluções capazes dessa ação; como um prefixo químico, geralmente abreviado *d-*. Cf. levorotatory.

dex·trose (deks′trōs). Dextrose. VER D-glucose.

dex·tro·si·nis·tral (deks′trō - si - nis′tral). Dextrossinistro; da direita para a esquerda. [dextro- + L. *sinister*, esquerda]

dex·tro·thy·rox·ine so·di·um (deks - trō - thī - roks′ēn). Dextrotiroxina sódica; um agente anti-hipercolesterolêmico.

dex·tro·tor·sion (deks - trō - tōr′shŭn). Dextrotorção. **1.** Rotação para a direita. **2.** Em oftalmologia, um termo raramente usado para uma rotação conjugada do pólo superior de ambas as córneas para a direita. [dextro- + L. *torsio*, torção]

dex·tro·tro·pic (dek - trō - trop′ik). Dextrotrópico; que se volta para a direita. [dextro- + G. *tropos*, volta]

dex·tro·ver·sion (deks′trō - ver′zhŭn). Dextroversão. **1.** Versão para a direita. **2.** Em oftalmologia, uma rotação conjugada de ambos os olhos para a direita. [dextro- + L. *verto*, pp. *versus*, virar]

d. of the heart, d. do coração. SIN corrected *dextrocardia.*

d.f. Abreviatura de *degrees* of freedom (graus de liberdade), em *degree.*

df, DF Abreviatura de decayed and filled teeth (dentes cariados e obturados). SIN df caries *index.*

DFP Abreviatura de diisopropyl fluorophosphate (fluorofosfato de diisopropil).

dGlc Abreviatura de 2-deoxyglucose (2-desoxiglicose).

dGMP Abreviatura de deoxyguanylic acid (ácido desoxiguanílico).

DHAP Abreviatura de *dihydroxyacetone* phosphate (fosfato de diidroxiacetona).

Dharmendra an·ti·gen. Ver em antigen.

DHEA Abreviatura de dehydroepiandrosterone (desidroepiandrosterona).

DHEA Abreviatura de dehydro-3-epiandrosterone (desidro-3-epiandrosterona).

DHEAS Abreviatura do sulfate salt of dehydroepiandrosterone (sal sulfato de desidroepiandrosterona).

d'Herelle, Felix H., médico e bacteriologista canadense, 1873–1949. VER d'H. *phenomenon,* Twort-d'H. *phenomenon.*

DHF Abreviatura de dihydrofolic acid (ácido diidrofólico).

DHFR Abreviatura de dihydrofolate reductase (diidrofolato redutase).

D. Hy. Abreviatura de Doctor of Hygiene (Doutor em Higiene).

DI Abreviatura de dental *index* (índice dentário).

di-. Di-. **1.** Dois, duas vezes. **2.** Em química, freqüentemente usado no lugar de bis- quando não há probabilidade de confusão; p. ex., compostos dicloro-. Cf. bi-, bis-. [G. *dis*, dois]

dia-. Dia-; através, por toda a parte, completamente. [G. *dia*, através]

di·a·be·tes (dī - ā - bē′tēz). Diabetes; diabetes insípido ou diabetes melito, doenças que possuem em comum a poliúria; quando usado sem qualificação, refere-se ao diabetes melito. [G. *diabētēs,* um compasso, um sifão, diabetes]

adult-onset d., d. de início na vida adulta; diabetes melito não-insulino-dependente.

alimentary d., d. alimentar. SIN alimentary *glycosuria.*

alloxan d., d. por aloxana; diabetes melito experimental produzido em animais pela administração de aloxana, que lesa as células das ilhotas pancreáticas produtoras de insulina.

brittle d., d. lábil; diabetes melito em que há grandes flutuações das concentrações sanguíneas de glicose, difíceis de controlar.

bronze d., d. bronzeado; diabetes melito associado a hemocromatose, com depósitos de ferro na pele, fígado, pâncreas e outras vísceras, freqüentemente com lesão hepática grave e glicosúria. VER TAMBÉM hemochromatosis. SIN bronzed d., bronzed disease.

bronzed d., d. bronzeado. SIN bronze d.

calcinuric d., d. calcinúrico. SIN hypercalciuria.

chemical d., d. químico. SIN latent d.

galactose d., d. de galactose. SIN galactosemia.

gestational d., d. gestacional; intolerância aos carboidratos de gravidade variável com início ou diagnóstico durante a gravidez.

> O diabete gestacional ocorre em 3–6% de todas as gestações, e, embora tipicamente resolva após o parto, até 60% das mulheres com esse distúrbio acabam por desenvolver diabetes tipo 2. O diabetes que ocorre durante a gravidez aumenta o risco de pielonefrite materna e de algumas anomalias congênitas, além de, freqüentemente, estar associado a poliidrâmnio e macrossomia fetal, com conseqüente distocia. Recomenda-se que todas as gestantes sejam submetidas a triagem para diabetes gestacional entre a 24.ª e a 28.ª semana de gravidez por determinação do nível plasmático de glicose 1 hora após a administrçação oral de 50 g de glicose. Um nível acima de 140 mg/dl (7,8 mmol/l) é uma indicação para uma prova de tolerância à glicose em 3 horas. O diabetes gestacional geralmente pode ser tratado apenas com dieta, mas, algumas vezes, é necessário usar insulina.

growth-onset d., d. do início do crescimento. SIN insulin-dependent d. mellitus.

d. in'nocens, d. inocente; termo obsoleto para glicosúria renal (renal *glycosuria*).

d. insip'idus, d. insípido; excreção crônica de volumes muito grandes de urina pálida de baixa densidade, causando desidratação e sede extrema; comumente resulta da secreção inadequada de hormônio antidiurético hipofisário; as anormalidades urinárias podem ser imitadas em virtude da ingestão excessiva de líquido, como na polidipsia psicogênica. Existem vários tipos: central, neuro-hipofisária e nefrogênica. Foram descritas formas autossômicas dominantes [MIM*125700, *125800, *192340], ligadas ao X [MIM*304800 e *304900], e até mesmo forma autossômica recessiva [MIM*222000]. VER TAMBÉM nephrogenic d. insipidus.

insulin-dependent d. mellitus (IDDM), d. melito insulino-dependente; d. tipo I; diabete melito grave, freqüentemente lábil, que geralmente tem início abrupto durante as duas primeiras décadas de vida, mas que pode desenvolver-se em qualquer idade; caracterizada por polidipsia, poliúria, aumento do apetite, emagrecimento, baixos níveis plasmáticos de insulina e suscetibilidade à cetoacidose; destruição das células β pancreáticas mediada pelo sistema imune; são necessárias insulinoterapia e regulamentação alimentar. Termo declarado obsoleto pela *American Diabetes Association.* SIN growth-onset d., juvenile-onset d., type I d.

insulinopenic d., d. insulinopênico; qualquer forma de diabetes melito resultante da secreção inadequada de insulina.

d. intermit'tens, d. intermitente; diabetes melito no qual há períodos de metabolismo dos carboidratos relativamente normal seguidos por recidivas do estado diabético prévio.

juvenile d., d. juvenil; diabetes melito que surge em uma criança ou adolescente; freqüentemente fatal antes da descoberta da insulina, geralmente de início abrupto durante a primeira ou segunda década de vida; caracterizado por poliúria, polidipsia, emagrecimento; geralmente grave, insulino-dependente e propenso a períodos de cetoacidose; pode ser familiar, ocorrer após uma infecção viral como a caxumba; acredita-se que seja causado por destruição das ilhotas pancreáticas de origem imune ou induzida por vírus. SIN type I d. mellitus.

juvenile-onset d., d. juvenil. SIN insulin-dependent d. mellitus.

ketosis-prone d., d. propenso a cetose; o diabetes melito tipo I ou juvenil, no qual o tratamento inadequado leva ao desenvolvimento de cetoacidose.

ketosis-resistant d., d. resistente a cetose; diabetes melito tipo II ou do adulto, no qual raramente ocorrem episódios de cetoacidose.

latent d., d. latente; uma forma leve de diabetes melito na qual o paciente não apresenta sintomas, mas exibe algumas respostas anormais aos procedimentos diagnósticos, como uma alta concentração sanguínea de glicose em jejum ou redução da tolerância à glicose. Termo declarado obsoleto pela *American Diabetes Association.* SIN chemical d.

lipoatrophic d., d. lipoatrófico. SIN lipoatrophy.

lipogenous d., d. lipógeno; diabetes e obesidade combinados.

maturity-onset d., d. da maturidade; diabetes melito não-insulino-dependente.

maturity onset d. of youth, d. da maturidade no jovem; uma forma de diabetes melito relativamente leve, que não exige insulina e começa mais cedo que o habitual.

d. melli'tus (DM), d. melito; um distúrbio metabólico crônico no qual há comprometimento da utilização de carboidratos e aumento da utilização de lipídios e proteínas; é causado por uma deficiência absoluta ou relativa de insulina e caracterizado, em casos mais graves, por hiperglicemia crônica, glicosúria, perda de água e eletrólitos, cetoacidose e coma; as complicações em longo prazo incluem neuropatia, retinopatia, nefropatia, alterações degenerativas generalizadas nos grandes e pequenos vasos sanguíneos, e aumento da suscetibilidade a infecções. [L. adoçado com mel]

> O diabetes melito afeta pelo menos 16 milhões de americanos, figura como a sétima maior causa de morte nos Estados Unidos e custa à economia norte-americana mais de 100 bilhões de dólares anuais. Cerca de 95% das pessoas com DM possuem o tipo 2, no qual as células beta pancreáticas preservam algum potencial de produção de insulina, e o restante possui o tipo 1, no qual insulina exógena é necessária para so-

diabetes melito (DM): classificação etiológica
I. Diabetes melito primário (tipos 1 e 2)
II. Diabetes secundário
A. diabetes pancreático
– após pancreatectomia total ou parcial
– com destruição extensa do pâncreas
– através de tumor ou ferida
– pancreatite; hemocromatose
B. diabetes extrapancreático/endócrino
– com hipersomatotropismo (acromegalia)
– com hiperadrenalismo (síndrome de Cushing; síndrome de Conn, feocromocitoma)
– com hipertireoidismo
– com glucagonoma
C. diabetes fármaco-induzido
– (somatotropina; ACTH; adrenocortical [diabetes por esteróides]; hormônio tireoidiano)
– tiazídicos
III. Formas raras, excepcionais de diabetes p. ex., diabetes lipoatrófico (Lawrence); diabetes miatônico (Prader-Labhart-Willi); distúrbio dos receptores da insulina; DM com algumas síndromes genéticas

brevida em longo prazo. No DM tipo 1, que tipicamente causa sintomas antes dos 25 anos de idade, um processo auto-imune é responsável pela destruição das células beta. O DM tipo 2 é caracterizado por resistência à insulina nos tecidos periféricos, bem como por um defeito na secreção de insulina pelas células beta. A insulina regula o metabolismo dos carboidratos por mediação do transporte rápido de glicose e aminoácidos da circulação para o músculo e outras células teciduais, por promoção do armazenamento de glicose nos hepatócitos sob a forma de glicogênio, e pela inibição da gliconeogênese. O estímulo normal para a liberação de insulina do pâncreas é o aumento da concentração de glicose no sangue circulante, que, tipicamente, ocorre alguns minutos após uma refeição. Quando esse aumento produz uma resposta de insulina apropriada, de forma que o nível sanguíneo de glicose cai novamente, quando é absorvido pelas células, a tolerância à glicose é considerada normal. O fato central no diabetes melito é o comprometimento da tolerância à glicose em um grau capaz de ameaçar ou comprometer a saúde. Os critérios diagnósticos revistos para DM foram publicados pela *American Diabetes Association* em junho de 1997. Todos os critérios dependem da concentração de glicose no plasma venoso. O diagnóstico é confirmado quando quaisquer 2 testes realizados em dias diferentes produzem níveis nos limiares estabelecidos ou acima destes: no estado de jejum, 126 mg/dl (7,0 mmol/l); 2 horas após uma refeição (após administração de 75 g de glicose) ou, aleatoriamente, 200 mg/dl (11,1 mmol/l).

Reconhecido há muito tempo como um fator de risco independente para doença cardiovascular, o DM freqüentemente é associado a outros fatores de risco, incluindo distúrbios do metabolismo lipídico, obesidade, hipertensão e comprometimento da função renal. As recomendações atuais para o tratamento do DM enfatizam a educação e a individualização do tratamento. Estudos controlados mostraram que a manutenção rigorosa constante dos níveis plasmáticos de glicose em um nível mais próximo possível do normal reduz significativamente a incidência e a gravidade das complicações de longo prazo, particularmente complicações microvasculares (retinopatia, neuropatia e nefropatia). Esse controle envolve a limitação de carboidratos e de gordura saturada na dieta; monitorização da glicose sanguínea, incluindo autoteste pelo paciente e determinação periódica de hemoglobina glicosilada (Hb_{1AC}); e administração de insulina (sobretudo no DM tipo 1), fármacos que estimulam a produção endógena de insulina (no DM tipo 2), ou ambos. Alguns estudos sugerem que o risco de doença cardiovascular pode ser aumentado, em alguns pacientes, pelo tratamento intensivo do DM devido ao aumento do peso corporal, da pressão arterial, dos triglicerídeos e do colesterol total e do LDL-colesterol. Agentes farmacêuticos desenvolvidos durante a década de 1990 melhoraram o controle do DM mediante aumento da responsividade das células à insulina, neutralização da resistência à insulina e redução da absorção de carboidratos pós-prandial. Ver Também insulin resistance; alpha-reductase inhibitor.

metahypophysial d., d. meta-hipofisário; **(1)** diabetes melito causado por grandes quantidades de hormônio do crescimento hipofisário endógeno ou exógeno; **(2)** termo usado para designar a fase irreversível do diabetes melito na acromegalia.

Mosler d., d. de Mosler; inositúria com excreção de grandes volumes de água.
nephrogenic d. insipidus [MIM* 304800], d. insípido nefrogênico; d. insípido devido à incapacidade dos túbulos renais de responder ao hormônio antidiurético; herança ligada ao X, causada por mutação no gene receptor da vasopressina V2 (AVPR2) em Xq. Também há uma forma autossômica dominante [MIM* 125800], causada por mutação no gene aquaforina 2 (AQP2) em 12q. SIN vasopressin-resistant d.
non-insulin-dependent d. mellitus (NIDDM), diabetes melito não-insulinodependente; uma forma de diabetes melito freqüentemente leve, de início gradual, em geral acometendo pessoas obesas com mais de 35 anos; os níveis plasmáticos absolutos de insulina são normais ou altos, mas relativamente baixos em comparação com os níveis plasmáticos de glicose; a cetoacidose é rara, mas pode haver coma hiperosmolar; responde bem à regulação alimentar e/ou a agentes hipoglicemiantes orais, mas podem surgir complicações diabéticas e alterações degenerativas. Termo declarado obsoleto pela *American Diabetes Association*.
pancreatic d., d. pancreático; **(1)** diabetes melito demonstravelmente dependente de uma lesão pancreática; **(2)** diabetes após a retirada do pâncreas em um animal.
phlorizin d. (flō-rid′zin). d. florizínico. SIN phlorizin *glycosuria*.
phosphate d., d. de fosfato; secreção excessiva de fosfato na urina devido a um defeito na reabsorção tubular; geralmente parte de uma anormalidade mais generalizada, como a síndrome de Fanconi.
piqûre d., d. por punção. SIN puncture d. [Fr.]
pregnancy d., d. da gravidez. VER subclinical d.
puncture d., d. por punção; diabetes experimental produzido em animais por punção do assoalho do quarto ventrículo cerebral. SIN piqûre d.
renal d., d. renal. SIN renal *glycosuria*.
starvation d., d. por inanição; após jejum prolongado, glicosúria subseqüente à ingestão de carboidratos ou glicose devido à redução da secreção de insulina e/ou redução da taxa de metabolismo da glicose com redução da capacidade de formar glicogênio.
steroid d., d. por esteróides; diabetes melito produzido por doses farmacológicas de hormônios esteróides, particularmente glicocorticóides ou estrogênios; caracterizado por uma ou mais das manifestações típicas de diabetes melito.
steroidogenic d., d. esteroidogênico; tolerância anormal à glicose, freqüentemente diabetes melito evidente, induzido pelos efeitos metabólicos de hormônios esteróides do córtex supra-renal, como cortisona, ou análogos terapêuticos, como prednisona. O efeito pode ser temporário, resolvendo quando o tratamento com esteróides é interrompido, ou o diabetes melito pode persistir.
subclinical d., d. subclínico; uma forma de diabetes melito clinicamente evidente apenas em determinadas circunstâncias, como gravidez ou estresse extremo; as pessoas afetadas podem, com o tempo, apresentar formas graves da doença. Termo declarado obsoleto pela *American Diabetes Association*.
thiazide d., d. tiazídico; comprometimento do metabolismo dos carboidratos associado ao uso de diuréticos tiazídicos; são observadas manifestações graves em pessoas com diabetes melito, mas o comprometimento é leve ou ausente em não-diabéticos.
type I d., d. tipo I. SIN insulin-dependent d. mellitus.
type II d., d. tipo II; diabetes melito não-insulino-dependente.
type I d. mellitus, diabetes melito tipo I. SIN juvenile d.
vasopressin-resistant d., d. resistente à vasopressina. SIN nephrogenic d. insipidus.
di·a·bet·ic (dī-ă-bet′ik). Diabético. **1.** Relativo a, ou que sofre de, diabetes. **2.** Aquele que sofre de diabetes.
di·a·be·to·gen·ic (dī′ă-bet-ō-jen′ik, -bē-tō-jen′ik). Diabetogênico; que causa diabetes.
di·a·be·tog·en·ous (dī′ă-bē-toj′en-ŭs). Diabetógeno; causado pelo diabetes.
di·a·be·tol·o·gy (dī′ă-be-tol′ō-jē). Diabetologia; o campo da medicina relacionado ao diabetes.
di·a·cele (dī′ă-sēl). Diacele; termo raramente usado para terceiro ventrículo (third *ventricle*). [G. *dia-*, através, + *koilia*, cavidade]
di·ac·e·tal (dī-as′ĕ-tal). Diacetal. VER diacetyl.
di·ac·e·tate (dī-as′ĕ-tāt). Diacetato. **1.** SIN acetoacetate. **2.** Uma substância que contém dois resíduos acetato.
di·ac·e·te·mia (dī-as-ĕ-tē′mē-ă). Diacetemia; uma forma de acidose resultante da presença de ácido acetoacético (diacético) no sangue.
di·ac·e·ton·u·ria (dī-as-ĕ-tō-noo′rē-ă). Diacetonúria. SIN diaceturia.
di·ac·e·tu·ria (dī-as-ĕ-too′rē-ă). Diacetúria; a excreção urinária de ácido acetoacético (diacético). SIN diacetonuria.
di·a·ce·tyl, di·ac·e·tal (dī-as′ĕ-til, dī-as′ĕ-tal). Diacetil, diacetal; um líquido amarelo $(CH_3CO)_2$, que possui o odor pungente da quinona e transporta o aroma do café, vinagre, manteiga e outros alimentos; um produto intermediário da degradação dos carboidratos.
di·a·ce·tyl·cho·line (dī-as′ĕ-til-kō′lēn). Diacetilcolina. SIN succinylcholine.
di·a·ce·tyl·mon·ox·ime (DAM) (dī-as′ĕ-til-mon-ok′sīm). Diacetilmonoxima; uma 2-oxo-oxima que pode reativar a acetilcolinesterase fosforila-

da *in vitro* e *in vivo*; penetra na barreira hematoencefálica. Semelhante à 2-PAM.

di·a·ce·tyl·mor·phine (dī-as′ē-til-mōr′fēn). Diacetilmorfina. SIN heroin.

di·a·ce·tyl·tan·nic ac·id (dī-as′ē-til-tan′ik). Ácido diacetiltânico. SIN acetyltannic acid.

di·a·chron·ic (dī-ă-kron′ik). Diacrônico; sistematicamente observado com o decorrer do tempo nos mesmos indivíduos em oposição ao sincrônico ou transverso; as conclusões são equivalentes apenas quando há estabilidade rigorosa de todos os elementos. [dia- + G. *chronos*, tempo]

di·ac·id (dī-as′id). Diácido; indica uma substância que contém dois átomos de hidrogênio ionizáveis por molécula; mais genericamente, uma base capaz de se combinar com dois íons hidrogênio por molécula.

di·ac·la·sis, di·a·cla·sia (dī-ak′lă-sis, dī-ă-klā′zē-ă). Diáclase. SIN osteoclasis. [G. *diaklasis*, ruptura, de *dia*, através, + *klasis*, ruptura]

di·ac·ri·nous (dī-ak′ri-nŭs). Diácrino; que excreta por passagem simples através de uma célula glandular. [G. *diakrinō*, separar um do outro]

di·ac·ri·sis (dī-ak′ri-sis). Diácrise. SIN diagnosis. [G. *dia-*, através, + *krisis*, julgamento]

di·a·crit·ic, di·a·crit·i·cal (dī-ă-krit′ik, -krit′i-kăl). Diacrítico; que distingue; diagnóstico; que permite a distinção. [G. *diakritikos*, capaz de distinguir]

di·ac·tin·ic (dī′ak-tin′ik). Diactínico; que possui a propriedade de transmitir luz capaz de provocar reações químicas. [G. *dia*, através, + *aktis*, raio]

di·ac·yl·glyc·er·ol (DAG) (dī′as-il-glis′er-ol). Diacilglicerol; diglicerídeo; glicerol com duas porções acil esterificadas, seja 1,3-diacilglicerol ou 1,2-diacilglicerol; se os dois grupamentos acil forem diferentes, há quatro estereoisômeros possíveis; 1,2-diacilglicerol é um intermediário na síntese de triacilgliceróis e de lecitina; também serve como segundo mensageiro na estimulação da atividade da proteinocinase C.

d. acyltransferase, d. transferase; uma enzima, na biossíntese de gordura, que catalisa a transferência de uma porção acil da acil-CoA para 1,2-diacilglicerol, formando assim coenzima A livre e triacilglicerol.

d. lipase, d. lipase. SIN lipoprotein lipase.

di·ad (dī′ad). Díade. **1.** O túbulo transverso e uma cisterna nas fibras musculares cardíacas. **2.** SIN dyad (1).

di·ad·o·cho·ci·ne·sia (dī-ad′ō-kō-si-nē′zē-ă). Diadococinesia. SIN diadochokinesia.

di·ad·o·cho·ki·ne·sia, di·ad·o·cho·ki·ne·sis (dī-ad′ō-kō-ki-nē′zē-ă, -ki-nē′sis). Diadococinesia; a capacidade normal de colocar alternadamente um membro em posições opostas, como de flexão e extensão ou de pronação e supinação. SIN diadochocinesia. [G. *diadochos*, trabalho alternado, + *kinēsis*, movimento]

di·ad·o·cho·ki·net·ic (dī-ad′ō-kō-ki-net′ik). Diadococinético; relativo à diadococinesia.

di·ag·nose (dī-ag-nōs′). Diagnosticar; fazer um diagnóstico.

di·ag·no·sis (dī-ag-nō′sis). Diagnóstico; a determinação da natureza de uma doença, lesão ou defeito congênito. SIN diacrisis. [G. *diagnōsis*, decisão]

antenatal d., d. pré-natal. SIN prenatal d.

clinical d., d. clínico; diagnóstico feito a partir de um estudo dos sinais e sintomas de uma doença.

differential d., d. diferencial; a determinação de qual dentre duas ou mais doenças com sinais e sintomas semelhantes o paciente está sofrendo, por comparação sistemática e discriminação dos achados clínicos. SIN differentiation (2).

d. by exclusion, d. por exclusão; diagnóstico feito por exclusão daquelas doenças às quais pertencem apenas alguns sinais e sintomas dos pacientes, deixando uma doença como o diagnóstico mais provável, embora não haja testes nem achados definitivos que estabeleçam esse diagnóstico.

laboratory d., d. laboratorial; diagnóstico feito por estudo químico, microscópico, microbiológico, imunológico ou histopatológico de secreções, corrimento, sangue ou tecido.

neonatal d., d. neonatal; avaliação sistemática do recém-nascido à procura de evidências de doença ou malformações, e a conclusão alcançada.

pathologic d., d. histopatológico; um diagnóstico algumas vezes *postmortem*, feito a partir de um estudo anatômico e/ou histológico das lesões existentes.

physical d., d. físico; **(1)** um diagnóstico feito por meio de exame físico do paciente. **(2)** o processo de um exame físico.

prenatal d., d. pré-natal; diagnóstico que utiliza procedimentos disponíveis para o reconhecimento de doenças e malformações *in utero*, e a conclusão alcançada. SIN antenatal d.

di·ag·nos·tic (dī-ag-nos′tik). Diagnóstico. **1.** Relativo a ou que ajuda no diagnóstico. **2.** Que estabelece ou confirma um diagnóstico.

di·ag·nos·ti·cian (dī′-ag-nos-tish′an). Diagnosticista; profissional hábil em fazer diagnósticos; designação antiga dos especialistas em medicina interna.

***Diagnostic and Statistical Manual of Mental Disorders* (DSM).** *Manual Diagnóstico e Estatístico de Transtornos Mentais;* sistema de classificação, publicado pela *American Psychiatric Association*, que divide transtornos mentais reconhecidos em categorias claramente definidas baseadas em conjuntos de critérios objetivos. Representando uma visão majoritária (e não um consenso) de centenas de colaboradores e consultores, o DSM é amplamente reconhecido como padrão diagnóstico e muito usado para fins de notificação, codificação e estatística.

A primeira edição (1952), baseada na sexta revisão da *Classificação Internacional de Doenças (CID-6)*, tinha por objetivo promover uniformidade na denominação e notificação de distúrbios psiquiátricos. Continha definições de todos os distúrbios designados, mas não havia grupos de critérios diagnósticos. Enquanto sua classificação de transtornos mentais mostrava a influência da psicanálise freudiana, sua nomenclatura (p. ex., reação depressiva, reação de ansiedade, reação esquizofrênica) refletia as teorias de Adolf Meyer (1866–1950). A segunda edição (*DSM-II*, 1968) preservou a orientação psicanalítica, mas abandonou a terminologia "reação". A terceira edição (*DSM-III*, 1980) abandonou grande parte do pensamento rigorosamente psicodinâmico das edições anteriores e, pela primeira vez, forneceu critérios diagnósticos explícitos e introduziu um sistema multiaxial pelo qual diferentes aspectos da condição de um paciente poderiam ser avaliados separadamente. Em resumo, os eixos são: I, transtornos clínicos; II, transtornos de personalidade e retardo mental; III, transtornos clínicos gerais; IV, fatores de estresse psicossocial e ambiental; e V, nível geral de atuação. Uma versão revista da terceira edição (*DSM-IIIR*, 1987) incorporou vários aperfeiçoamentos e esclarecimentos. A quarta edição (*DSM-IV*) foi publicada em maio de 1994. É muito semelhante às suas duas precursoras em aspecto geral e, como elas, coordenada e parcialmente derivada da *CID-9*. Para muitos observadores, a modificação mais significativa no *DSM-IV* é a redenominação da categoria antes denominada "Síndromes e Transtornos Mentais Orgânicos" como "Delírio, Demência e Amnésia e Outros Transtornos Cognitivos", uma alteração da terminologia com o objetivo de evitar a implicação de que os transtornos mentais classificados em outras categorias não são orgânicos.

di·a·gram. Diagrama; uma representação gráfica simples de uma idéia ou objeto.

Dieuaide d., d. de Dieuaide. SIN triaxial reference *system*.

flow d., fluxograma; diagrama composto de blocos ligados por setas que representam etapas em um processo como a análise de decisão.

Venn d., d. de Venn; representação pictorial do quanto duas ou mais quantidades ou conceitos são mutuamente inclusivos e exclusivos.

di·a·ki·ne·sis (dī′ă-ki-nē′sis). Diacinese; estágio final da prófase na meiose I, na qual os quiasmas presentes durante o estágio diplóteno desaparecem, os cromossomas continuam a encurtar e o nucléolo e a membrana nuclear desaparecem. [G. *dia*, através, + *kinēsis*, movimento]

dial (dī′al, dīl). Mostrador; face de relógio ou de um instrumento semelhante à de um relógio. [L. *dies*, dia]

astigmatic d., m. astigmático; diagrama de linhas radiadas, utilizado para testar astigmatismo.

Di·a·lis·ter (dī-ăl-is′ter). Nome obsoleto para um gênero de bactérias, cuja espécie típica, *D. pneumosintes*, agora é colocada no gênero *Bacteroides*.

di·al·lyl (dī-al′il). Dialil; composto que contém dois grupamentos alil.

di·al·y·sance (dī-al′i-sans). Dialisância; o número de mililitros de sangue completamente depurado de qualquer substância por um rim artificial ou por

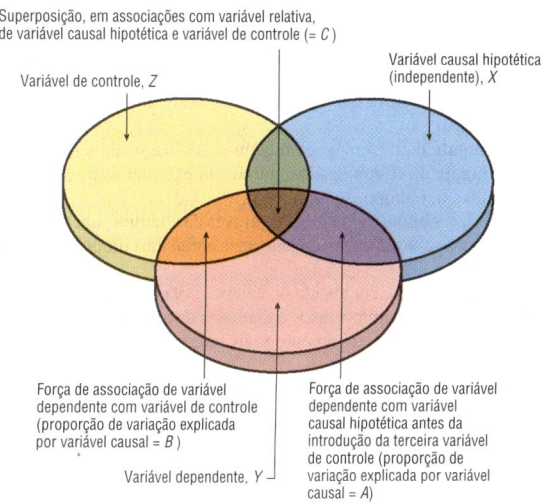

diagrama de Venn

dialysance

diálise peritoneal em uma unidade de tempo; as fórmulas de depuração convencionais são expressas em ml/min. [de dialysis]

di·al·y·sate (dī-al′i-sāt). Dialisado; a parte de uma mistura que atravessa uma membrana de diálise; o material que não atravessa é denominado retido. SIN diffusate.

di·al·y·sis (dī-al′i-sis). Diálise. 1. Uma forma de filtração para separar substâncias cristalóides de colóides (ou moléculas menores de maiores) em uma solução por interposição de uma membrana semipermeável entre a solução e o líquido de diálise; as substâncias cristalóides (menores) atravessam a membrana para o líquido de diálise do outro lado, os colóides não. 2. A separação de substâncias através de uma membrana semipermeável com base no tamanho da partícula e/ou dos gradientes de concentração. 3. Um método de função renal artificial. [G. uma separação, de *dialyo*, separar]

continuous ambulatory peritoneal d. (CAPD), d. peritoneal ambulatorial contínua; método de diálise peritoneal realizada em pacientes ambulatoriais com influxo e efluxo de dialisado durante atividades anormais.

equilibrium d., d. de equilíbrio; em imunologia, um método para a determinação de constantes de associação para reações hapteno-anticorpo em um sistema no qual as soluções de hapteno (dialisável) e anticorpo (não-dialisável) são separadas por membranas semipermeáveis. Como em equilíbrio a quantidade de hapteno livre será igual nos dois compartimentos de líquido, podem ser feitas determinações quantitativas de anticorpo ligado ao hapteno, anticorpo livre e hapteno livre.

extracorporeal d., d. extracorpórea; hemodiálise realizada através de um aparelho fora do corpo.

peritoneal d., d. peritoneal; retirada do corpo de substâncias solúveis e água por transferência através do peritônio, utilizando uma solução de diálise que é introduzida na e removida intermitentemente da cavidade peritoneal; a transferência de solutos difusíveis e água entre o sangue e a cavidade peritoneal depende do gradiente de concentração entre os dois compartimentos de líquido.

d. ret'inae, d. retiniana; separação congênita ou traumática da retina sensorial periférica do epitélio pigmentar da retina na *ora serrata*, freqüentemente causando um descolamento da retina. SIN retinodialysis.

di·a·lyze (dī′a-līz). Dialisar; realizar diálise; separar uma substância de uma solução por meio de diálise.

di·a·lyz·er (dī′a-lī-zer). Dialisador; o aparelho para realizar diálise; uma membrana usada em diálise.

di·a·mag·net·ic (dī′a-mag-net′ik). Diamagnético; que possui a propriedade de diamagnetismo.

di·a·mag·net·ism (dī-a-mag′ne-tizm). Diamagnetismo; a propriedade exibida por substâncias que possuem uma suscetibilidade magnética negativa muito pequena, produzida por moléculas nas quais todos os elétrons são pareados; um elétron não-pareado produz um movimento magnético, e, portanto, a molécula que o contém exibe paramagnetismo.

di·a·me·lia (dī-a-mē′lē-a). Diamelia; ausência de dois membros.

di·am·e·ter (dī-am′e-ter). Diâmetro. 1. Uma linha reta que une dois pontos opostos na superfície de um corpo mais ou menos esférico ou cilíndrico, ou no limite de uma abertura ou forame, atravessando o centro desse corpo ou abertura. 2. A distância medida ao longo dessa linha. [G. *diametros*, de *dia*, através, + *metron*, medida]

anteroposterior d. of the pelvic inlet, d. ântero-posterior da abertura superior da pelve. SIN median conjugate.

biparietal d., d. biparietal; o diâmetro da cabeça fetal entre as duas eminências parietais.

buccolingual d., d. bucolingual; o diâmetro da coroa de um dente medido da superfície bucal até a superfície lingual.

conjugate d. of pelvic inlet, d. conjugado da abertura superior da pelve. SIN median conjugate.

conjugate d. of pelvic outlet, d. conjugado da abertura inferior da pelve. SIN straight conjugate.

diagonal conjugate d., d. conjugado diagonal. SIN diagonal conjugate.

external conjugate d., d. conjugado externo. SIN external conjugate.

d. obli'qua [TA], d. oblíquo. SIN oblique d.

oblique d. [TA], d. oblíquo; uma medida através da abertura superior da pelve desde a articulação sacroilíaca de um lado até a eminência iliopectínea oposta. SIN d. obliqua [TA].

obstetric conjugate d., d. conjugado obstétrico. SIN true conjugate.

occipitofrontal d., d. occipitofrontal; o diâmetro da cabeça fetal desde a protuberância occipital externa até o ponto mais proeminente do osso frontal na linha média.

occipitomental d., d. occipitomental; o diâmetro da cabeça fetal desde a protuberância occipital externa até o ponto médio do queixo.

posterior sagittal d., d. sagital posterior; distância da junção sacrococcígea até o meio de uma linha imaginária entre as tuberosidades isquiáticas esquerda e direita.

suboccipitobregmatic d., d. suboccipitobregmático; o diâmetro da cabeça fetal desde o ponto posterior mais baixo do osso occipital até o centro da fontanela anterior.

total end-diastolic d. (TEDD), d. diastólico final total; diâmetro transversal do ventrículo esquerdo, incluindo as espessuras do septo e da parede posterior na diástole.

total end-systolic d. (TESD), d. sistólico final total; diâmetro transversal do ventrículo esquerdo, incluindo as espessuras do septo e da parede posterior na sístole.

trachelobregmatic d., d. traquelobregmático; o diâmetro da cabeça fetal desde o meio da fontanela anterior até o pescoço.

d. transver'sa [TA], d. transverso. SIN transverse d.

transverse d. [TA], d. transverso; o diâmetro transverso da abertura superior da pelve, medido entre as linhas terminais. SIN d. transversa [TA].

zygomatic d., d. zigomático; a maior largura do crânio nos arcos zigomáticos.

di·am·ide (dī′am-id, -īd). Diamida; um composto que contém dois grupamentos amida.

di·am·i·dines (dī-am′i-dēnz). Diamidinas; um grupo de substâncias que contêm dois grupamentos amidina; p. ex., estilbamidina, propamidina.

di·a·mine (dī′a-mēn, -min). Diamina; um composto orgânico contendo dois grupamentos amina por molécula; p. ex., etilenodiamina, $NH_2CH_2CH_2NH_2$.

d. oxidase, d. oxidase. SIN amine oxidase (copper-containing), amine oxidase (flavin-containing).

di·am·ni·ot·ic (dī-am-nē-ot′ik). Diamniótico; que possui dois sacos amnióticos.

Diamond, Louis K., médico norte-americano, 1902–1995. VER D.-Blackfan *anemia, syndrome*; Gardner-D. *syndrome;* Shwachman-Diamond *syndrome*.

di·am·tha·zole di·hy·dro·chlo·ride (dī-am′tha-zōl). Dicloridrato de diantazol; um agente antifúngico para uso tópico. SIN dimazole dihydrochloride.

di·an·dry, di·an·dria (dī′an-drē, dī-an′drē-a). Diandria; o fenômeno pelo qual um único óvulo é fertilizado por um espermatozóide diplóide e, portanto, produz um feto triplóide. Cf. digyny. [di- + G. *andros*, homem]

di·a·no·et·ic (dī′a-nō-et′ik). Dianético; pertinente à razão ou a outras funções intelectuais. [G. *dia*, através, + *noeō*, pensar]

di·a·pause (dī′a-pawz). Diapausa; um período de quiescência ou latência biológica com diminuição do metabolismo; um intervalo no qual o desenvolvimento é interrompido ou muito lentificado. [dia- + G. *pausis*, pausa]

embryonic d., d. embrionária; diapausa no curso da embriogênese; supõe-se que ocorre em casos de parto duplo e, possivelmente, de implante tardio.

di·a·pe·de·sis (dī′a-pe-dē′sis). Diapedese; a passagem de sangue, ou de qualquer de seus elementos formados, através das paredes intactas dos vasos sanguíneos. SIN migration (2). [G. *dia*, através, + *pēdēsis*, salto]

di·a·phan·og·ra·phy (dī-a-fa-nog′ra-fē). Diafanografia; exame de uma parte do corpo por transiluminação, particularmente para a detecção de câncer de mama. [G. *diaphanēs*, transparente, + *graphō*, escrever]

di·aph·a·nos·cope (dī-af′a-nō-skōp). Diafanoscópio; instrumento para iluminar o interior de uma cavidade a fim de determinar a transparência de suas paredes. SIN polyscope. [G. *diaphanēs*, transparente, + *skopeō*, examinar]

di·aph·a·nos·co·py (dī-af-a-nos′ko-pē). Diafanoscopia; exame de uma cavidade com um diafanoscópio.

di·a·phe·met·ric (dī′a-fē-met′rik). Diafemétrico; relativo à determinação do grau de sensibilidade tátil. [G. *dia*, através, + *haphē*, tato, + *metron*, medida]

di·a·phen hy·dro·chlo·ride (dī′a-fen). Cloridrato de diafeno; agente anti-histamínico com propriedades anticolinérgicas.

di·aph·o·rase (dī-af′ōr-ās). Diaforase; originalmente, uma série de flavoproteínas com atividade redutase nas mitocôndrias; atualmente, diidrolipoamida desidrogenase.

di·a·pho·re·sis (dī′a-fō-rē′sis). Diaforese. SIN perspiration (1). [G. *diaphorēsis*, de *dia*, através, + *phoreō*, carregar]

di·a·pho·ret·ic (dī-a-fō-ret′ik). Diaforético. 1. Relativo a, ou que causa, transpiração. 2. Um agente que aumenta a transpiração.

di·a·phragm (dī′a-fram). Diafragma. 1. A divisão musculomembranosa entre as cavidades abdominal e torácica. SIN diaphragma (2) [TA], interseptum, midriff, phren (1). 2. Um disco fino perfurado por uma abertura, usado em um microscópio, câmera ou outro instrumento óptico a fim de impedir a passagem dos raios de luz marginais, produzindo assim uma iluminação mais direta. 3. Um anel flexível coberto com uma folha abobadada de material elástico usado na vagina para evitar gravidez. 4. Em radiografia, uma grade (2) ou uma folha de chumbo com uma abertura. VER collimator. [G. *diaphragma*]

aperture d., d. de abertura; dispositivo metálico que limita a área do feixe que sai de um tubo de raios X.

Bucky d., d. de Bucky; em radiografia, um diafragma com uma grade móvel que evita sombras da grade. SIN Potter-Bucky d.

d. of mouth, d. da boca. SIN mylohyoid (*muscle*).

pelvic d., d. pélvico; o par de músculos levantador do ânus e coccígeo juntamente com a fáscia acima e abaixo deles. SIN d. of pelvis, diaphragma pelvis.

d. of pelvis, d. da pelve. SIN pelvic d.

Potter-Bucky d., d. de Potter-Bucky. SIN Bucky d.

d. sellae, d. da sela. SIN *diaphragma* sellae.

sellar d., d. da sela; *termo alternativo oficial para *diaphragma* sellae.

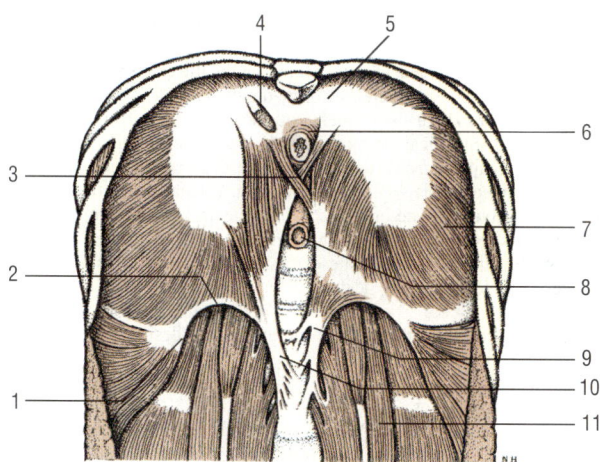

diafragma (superfície abdominal): (1) ligamento arqueado lateral, (2) ligamento arqueado medial, (3) ligamento arqueado mediano, (4) abertura da cava, (5) tendão central, (6) hiato esofágico com esôfago, (7) parte costal do diafragma, (8) hiato aórtico com aorta, (9) pilar esquerdo, (10) pilar direito, (11) músculos da parede abdominal posterior

d. of sella turcica, d. da sela turca. SIN *diaphragma sellae.*
urogenital d., d. urogenital; um conceito obsoleto de um folheto triangular, trilaminar de músculo e fáscia que cobre os ramos isquiopúbicos; composto pelos músculos esfíncter uretral e perineal transverso profundo (considerados músculos planos que formam um folheto contínuo), mais a membrana perineal, abaixo, e uma fáscia superior do diafragma, acima. Não há evidências desta última. O espaço que contém músculo entre as estruturas fasciais era denominado antigamente espaço perineal profundo. Os termos diafragma urogenital e espaço perineal profundo (deep perineal *space*) não são reconhecidos pela *Terminologia Anatômica* devido à compreensão mais acurada da morfologia, principalmente do esfíncter uretral. SIN diaphragma urogenitale.
di·a·phrag·ma, pl. **di·a·phrag·ma·ta** (dī-ă-frag'mă, -frag'mă-tă). [TA]. Diafragma. **1.** Uma fina divisão que separa regiões adjacentes. **2.** SIN diaphragm (1). [G. *diaphragma,* uma parede divisória, diafragma]
d. oris, d. oral. SIN mylohyoid (*muscle*).
d. pel'vis, d. pélvico. SIN pelvic *diaphragm.*
d. sel'lae [TA], d. da sela; uma prega da dura-máter que se estende transversalmente na sela turca e serve como teto da fossa hipofisária; é perfurada em seu centro para a passagem do infundíbulo. SIN sellar diaphragm*, diaphragm of sella turcica, diaphragm sellae, tentorium of hypophysis.
d. urogenita'le, d. urogenital. SIN urogenital *diaphragm.*
di·a·phrag·mal·gia (dī'ă-frag-mal'jē-ă). Diafragmalgia; termo raramente usado para designar dor no diafragma. SIN diaphragmodynia. [diaphragm + G. *algos,* dor]
di·a·phrag·mat·ic (dī'ă-frag-mat'ik). Diafragmático; relativo a um diafragma. SIN phrenic (1).
di·a·phrag·mat·o·cele (dī'ă-frag-mat'ō-sēl). Diafragmatocele; termo raramente usado para *hérnia* (hernia) diafragmática. [diaphragm + G. *kēlē,* hérnia]
di·a·phrag·mo·dyn·ia (dī'ă-frag-mō-din'ē-ă). Diafragmodinia. SIN diaphragmalgia. [diaphragm + G. *odynē,* dor]
di·aph·y·se·al (dī-ă-fiz'ē-ăl). Diafisário; relativo a uma diáfise. SIN diaphysial.
di·a·phy·sec·to·my (dī'ă-fi-sek'tō-mē). Diafisectomia; remoção parcial ou completa da diáfise de um osso longo. [diáfise + G. *ektomē,* excisão]
di·a·phys·i·al (dī-ă-fiz'ē-ăl). Diafisário; relacionado a diáfise. SIN diaphyseal.
di·aph·y·sis, pl. **di·aph·y·ses** (dī-af'i-sis, -sēz) [TA]. Diáfise; uma estrutura alongada semelhante a um bastão, como a parte de um osso longo entre as extremidades epifisárias. A diáfise de um osso longo, distinta das epífises, ou extremidades, e apófises, ou protuberâncias. SIN shaft [TA]. [G. um crescimento entre]
di·aph·y·si·tis (dī-af-i-sī'tis). Diafisite; inflamação da diáfise de um osso longo.
di·a·pi·re·sis (dī'ă-pī-rē'sis). Diapirese; passagem de partículas coloidais ou de outras partículas pequenas de material suspenso através das paredes não-rotas dos vasos sanguíneos. VER TAMBÉM diapedesis. [G. *diapeirō,* dirigir através, de *peirō,* perfurar]
di·a·pla·cen·tal (dī'ă-pla-sen'tăl). Diaplacentário; que atravessa ou "cruza" a placenta.
di·a·plex·us (dī-ă-plek'sŭs). Diaplexo; termo raramente usado para o plexo coróide (choroid *plexus*) do terceiro ventrículo. [G. *dia,* através, + L. *plexus,* pregueado]

di·ap·no·ic, di·ap·not·ic (dī-ap-nō'ik, -not'ik). Diapnóico, diapnótico. **1.** Relativo a, ou que causa, transpiração, principalmente transpiração insensível. **2.** Um leve sudorífico.
di·a·pop·hy·sis (dī-ă-pof'ĭ-sis). Diapófise, processo articular superior. SIN superior articular *process.*
Di·ap·to·mus (dī-ap'tō-mŭs). Gênero de crustáceos copépodes, o principal hospedeiro intermediário do *Diphyllobothrium latum* na América do Norte.
di·ar·rhea (dī-ă-rē'ă). Diarréia; eliminação intestinal anormalmente freqüente de material fecal semi-sólido ou líquido. [G. *diarrhoia,* de *dia,* através, + *rhoia,* fluxo]
cachectic d., d. caquética. d. da caquexia, diarréia que ocorre em pacientes com desgaste muscular acentuado. Geralmente decorrente de doença gastrointestinal subjacente.
choleraic. d. d. do verão. SIN summer d.
chronic bacillary d., d. bacilar crônica; diarréia prolongada que ocorre associada a infecção bacteriana, geralmente ocorrendo em pacientes com estase gastrointestinal, permitindo proliferação bacteriana no intestino com má absorção secundária. Ocorre na síndrome de alça cega após cirurgia intestinal, após vagotomia e, ocasionalmente, na esclerodermia ou diabetes.
Cochin China d., d. da Cochinchina; termo obsoleto para espru tropical (tropical *sprue*).
colliquative d., d. coliquativa; diarréia associada à eliminação excessiva de líquidos.
dientamoeba d., d. por *Dientamoeba*; uma diarréia considerada devida à infecção pelo flagelado *Dientamoeba fragilis*.
dysenteric d., d. disentérica; diarréia na disenteria bacilar ou amebiana.
fatty d., d. gordurosa; diarréia observada nas síndromes de má absorção, incluindo doença pancreática crônica, caracterizada por fezes fétidas, com aumento do conteúdo de gordura, que geralmente flutuam na água. SIN pimelorrhea.
flagellate d., d. por flagelados; diarréia causada por infecção pelo flagelado *Giardia lamblia.*
gastrogenous d., d. gastrógena; diarréia que pode ocorrer na aquilia gástrica, ou que é causada pela secreção excessiva de sucos gástricos e outros sucos intestinais.
lienteric d., d. lientérica; diarréia na qual aparecem alimentos não-digeridos nas fezes.
morning d., d. matinal; uma forma na qual ocorrem várias evacuações de fezes pastosas no início e no decorrer da manhã, permanecendo o intestino em repouso durante o restante do dia e da noite.
mucous d., d. mucosa; diarréia com a presença de muco considerável nas fezes.
nocturnal d., d. noturna; diarréia que ocorre principalmente à noite, geralmente associada à neuropatia autônoma diabética.
pancreatic d., d. pancreática. SIN d. pancreatica.
d. pancreatica (pan-krē-a'ti-kă), d. pancreática; diarréia caracterizada por ser grave, aquosa, secretora e hipopotassêmica; a maioria dos pacientes apresenta hipercalcemia e muitos hiperglicemia; resulta da secreção excessiva de VIP (peptídeo intestinal vasoativo) por um tumor das células das ilhotas pancreáticas. Algumas vezes denominada síndrome WDHA (WDHA *syndrome*). VER Verner-Morrison *syndrome,* WDHA *syndrome.* SIN pancreatic cholera, pancreatic d.
pancreatogenous d., d. pancreatogênica; diarréia na qual as fezes são volumosas, pálidas, fétidas, gordurosas e oleosas, em virtude da má absorção de gordura devido à deficiência da secreção de enzimas pancreáticas na pancreatite crônica.
serous d., d. serosa; diarréia caracterizada por fezes aquosas.
summer d., d. do verão; diarréia de lactentes em climas quentes, geralmente uma gastroenterite aguda devida à presença de *Shigella* ou *Salmonella.* SIN choleraic d.
toddler's d., fezes amolecidas recorrentes geralmente observadas em crianças saudáveis, de crescimento normal, entre 1 e 3 anos de idade, ocorrendo durante o dia; freqüentemente é devida à ingestão excessiva de líquido.
traveler's d., d. do viajante; diarréia de início súbito, freqüentemente associada a cólicas abdominais, vômito e febre, e que ocorre esporadicamente em viajantes, em geral durante a primeira semana de uma viagem; freqüentemente causada por cepas não-familiares de *Escherichia coli* enterotoxigênica.
tropical d., d. tropical. SIN tropical *sprue.*
di·ar·rhe·al, di·ar·rhe·ic (dī-ă-rē'ăl, -rē'ik). Diarreico; relativo à diarréia. SIN diarrhetic.
di·ar·rhe·tic. Diarreico. SIN diarrheal.
di·ar·thric (dī-ar'thrik). Diarticular; relativo a duas articulações. SIN biarticular, diarticular. [G. *di-,* dois, + *arthron,* articulação]
di·ar·thro·sis, pl. **di·ar·thro·ses** (dī-ar-thrō'sis, -sēz). Diartrose; *termo oficial alternativo para synovial *joint* (articulação sinovial). [G. articulação]
di·ar·tic·u·lar (dī-ar-tik'ū-lăr). Diarticular. SIN diarthric.
di·as·chi·sis (dī-as'ki-sis). Diásquise; inibição súbita da função produzida por um distúrbio focal agudo em uma parte do encéfalo afastada do local ori-

ginal de lesão, mas anatomicamente relacionada com ela através de tratos de fibras. [G. uma divisão]

di·a·scope (dī′ă-skōp). Diascópio; uma lâmina de vidro plana através da qual é possível examinar lesões cutâneas superficiais por meio de pressão. [G. *dia*, através, + *skopeō*, ver]

di·as·co·py (dī-as′kŏ-pē). Diascopia; exame de lesões cutâneas superficiais com um diascópio. [G. *dia*, através, + *skopeō*, ver]

di·a·stal·sis (dī-ă-stal′sis). Diastalse; o tipo de peristalse no qual uma região de inibição precede a onda de contração, como se observa no trato intestinal. [G. um arranjo]

di·a·stal·tic (dī-ă-stal′tik). Diastáltico; relativo à diastalse.

di·a·stase (dī′as-tās). Diástase; uma mistura, obtida do malte e que contém enzimas amilolíticas (principalmente α- e β-amilases), que converte o amido em dextrina e maltose; usada para tornar amidos solúveis, para ajudar na digestão de amidos, em determinados tipos de dispepsia, e para digerir o glicogênio em cortes histológicos. [Fr. do G. *diastasis*, separação, de *dia*, distante, + *histēmi*, fazer permanecer]

di·as·ta·sis (dī-as′tă-sis). Diástase. **1.** Qualquer separação simples de partes normalmente unidas. SIN divarication. **2.** A porção média da diástole quando o sangue entra no ventrículo lentamente ou deixa de entrar antes da sístole atrial. A diástase tem duração inversamente proporcional à freqüência cardíaca e está ausente em freqüências cardíacas muito altas. [G. uma separação]
   d. rec'ti, d. dos retos; separação dos músculos retos abdominais, afastando-se da linha média, algumas vezes observada durante ou após a gravidez.

di·as·ta·su·ria (dī-as-tās-ū′rē-ă). Diastasúria. SIN amylasuria.

di·a·stat·ic (dī-ă-stat′ik). Diastático; relativo a uma diástase.

di·a·ste·ma, pl. **di·a·ste·ma·ta** (dī′ă-stē′mă, -stē′mă-tă)([TA]. Diastema. **1.** Fissura ou abertura anormal em qualquer parte, principalmente se congênita. **2** [NA]. Espaço entre dois dentes adjacentes no mesmo arco dental. **3.** Fenda ou espaço entre o incisivo lateral maxilar e os dentes caninos, no qual o canino inferior é recebido quando a mandíbula se fecha; anormal em seres humanos, mas normal em cães e em muitos outros animais. [G. *diastēma*, um intervalo]

di·a·ste·ma·to·cra·nia (dī-ă-stē′mă-tō-krā′nē-ă). Diastematocrania; fissura sagital congênita do crânio. [G. *diastēma*, intervalo, + *kranion*, crânio]

di·a·ste·ma·to·my·e·lia (dī-ă-stē′mă-tō-mī-e′lē-ă). Diastematomielia; divisão sagital completa ou incompleta da medula espinal por um septo ósseo ou fibrocartilaginoso. [G. *diastēma*, intervalo, + *myelon*, medula óssea]

di·as·ter (dī′as-ter). Diáster. SIN amphiaster. [G. *di-*, dois, + *astēr*, estrela]

di·a·ste·re·o·i·so·mers (dī′ă-stār-ē-ō-ī′sō-merz). Diastereoisômeros; isômeros opticamente ativos que não são enantiomorfos (imagens especulares); p. ex., D-glicose e D-galactose.

di·as·to·le (dī-as′tō-lē). Diástole; dilatação pós-sistólica normal das cavidades cardíacas, durante a qual estas se enchem de sangue; a diástole atrial precede a diástole ventricular; a diástole de qualquer câmara alterna-se ritmicamente com a sístole ou contração da câmara. [G. *diastolē*, dilatação]
   atrial d., d. atrial; período de relaxamento e repolarização do músculo atrial.
   electrical d., d. elétrica; período do final da onda T ao início da próxima onda Q.
   gastric d., d. gástrica; uma fase de relaxamento da peristalse gástrica observada por fluoroscopia ou gastroscopia.
   late d., d. tardia. SIN presystole.
   ventricular d., d. ventricular; período de relaxamento e repolarização do músculo ventricular.

di·a·stol·ic (dī-ă-stol′ik). Diastólico; relativo à diástole.

di·as·tol·ogy (dī-as-tol′ō-jē). Diastologia; o estudo ou ciência da diástole cardíaca e seus componentes.

di·as·tro·phism (dī-as′trof-izm). Diastrofismo; distorção que ocorre em objetos em conseqüência de arqueamento. [G. *diastrophē*, de *diastrephein*, distorção]

di·a·tax·ia (dī′ă-tak′sē-ă). Diataxia; ataxia que afeta ambos os lados do corpo.
   cerebral d., d. cerebral; o tipo atáxico da paralisia cerebral congênita.

di·a·te·la (dī-ă-tē′lă). Diatela; termo raramente usado para tela coróide (*tela choroidea*) do terceiro ventrículo. [G. *dia*, através, entre, + L. *tela*, tela]

di·a·ther·mal (dī-ă-ther′mal). Diatérmico. SIN diathermic. [G. *dia*, através, + G. *thermē*, calor]

di·a·ther·man·cy (dī-ă-ther′man-sē). Diatermância; a condição de ser diatérmico.

di·a·ther·ma·nous (dī-ă-ther′man-ŭs). Diatérmano; permeável aos raios calóricos. SIN transcalent. [G. *dia-thermaino*, aquecer através, de *thermos*, quente]

di·a·ther·mic (dī-ă-ther′mik). Diatérmico; relativo a ou caracterizado ou afetado por diatermia. SIN diathermal.

di·a·ther·mo·co·ag·u·la·tion (dī-ă-ther′mō-kō-ag-ū-lā′shŭn). Diatermocoagulação. SIN surgical *diathermy.*

di·a·ther·my (dī′ă-ther-mē). Diatermia; elevação local da temperatura nos tecidos, produzida por corrente de alta freqüência, ondas ultra-sônicas ou radiação de microondas. SIN transthermia. [G. *dia*, através, + *thermē*, calor]
   medical d., d. clínica; diatermia leve que não causa destruição tecidual. SIN thermopenetration.
   short wave d., d. de onda curta; elevação terapêutica da temperatura tecidual por meio de uma corrente elétrica oscilante de freqüência extremamente alta (10–100 milhões Hz) e comprimento de onda curto de 3–30 metros.
   surgical d., d. cirúrgica; eletrocoagulação com um eletrocautério de alta freqüência, resultando em destruição tecidual local; geralmente usada para fechar vasos sanguíneos e interromper sangramento. SIN diathermocoagulation.
   ultrashortwave d., d. de onda ultracurta; diatermia de onda curta na qual o comprimento de onda é menor que 10 metros.

di·ath·e·sis (dī-ath′ĕ-sis). Diátese; o estado constitucional ou inato que predispõe a uma doença, grupo de doenças ou anomalia metabólica ou estrutural. [G. arranjo, condição]
   contractural d., d. contratural; termo antigo que designa uma tendência a apresentar contraturas na histeria.
   cystic d., d. cística; condição na qual há formação de múltiplos cistos no fígado, rins e outros órgãos.
   gouty d., d. gotosa; um estado de suscetibilidade a ataques de gota ou a desenvolvimento de tofos, geralmente associado a hiperuricemia ou hiperexcreção de urato na urina.
   spasmophilic d., d. espasmofílica; condição na qual há uma excitabilidade anormal dos nervos motores, demonstrada por uma tendência à tetania, laringospasmo ou convulsões generalizadas.

di·a·thet·ic (dī-ă-thet′ik). Diatético; relativo a uma diátese.

di·a·tom (dī′ă-tom). Diatomácea; membro de algas unicelulares microscópicas, cujos revestimentos compõem uma terra de infusórios sedimentar. [G. *diatomos*, cortado em dois]

di·a·to·ma·ceous (dī′ă-tō-mā′shŭs). Diatomáceo; relativo a diatomáceas ou a seus resíduos fósseis.

di·a·tom·ic (dī-ă-tom′ik). Diatômico. **1.** Designa uma substância com uma molécula composta de dois átomos. **2.** Designa qualquer íon ou agrupamento iônico composto apenas de dois átomos.

di·a·tor·ic (dī′ă-tor′ik). Diatórico. **1.** A abertura cilíndrica vertical formada na base de dentes de porcelana artificiais e que se estende até o corpo do dente, servindo como uma forma mecânica de fixação do dente à base da dentadura. **2.** Designa dentes que contêm um diatórico. [G. *diatoros*, perfurado]

di·a·tri·zo·ate. Diatrizoato; sal do ácido 3,5-diacetamido-2,4,6-triiodobenzóico. VER *sodium* diatrizoate.

di·az·e·pam (dī-az′ĕ-pam). Diazepam; um relaxante da musculatura esquelética, sedativo e ansiolítico; também usado como anticonvulsivante, particularmente no tratamento do estado de mal epiléptico, por via parenteral.

di·a·zines (dī′ă-zēnz). Diazinas; grupo de tuberculostáticos sintéticos, como a pirazina carboxamida e a piridazina-3-carboxamida.

di·az·in·on (dī-az′in-on). Diazinona; composto organofosforado que contém enxofre, usado como inseticida e inibidor da colinesterase.

⚠ **diazo-.** Prefixo que designa um composto que contém o grupamento $R-N=N-X$ ou $R=N_2$, onde X não é carbono (exceto pelo CN). Um exemplo é o diazometano, CH_2N_2. Cf. azo-. [G. *di-*, dois, + Fr. *azote*, nitrogênio]

di·az·o·tize (dī-az′ō-tīz). Diazotar; introduzir um grupamento diazo em um composto químico, geralmente através do tratamento de uma amina com ácido nitroso.

di·az·ox·ide (dī-ă-zok′sīd). Diazóxido; um agente anti-hipertensivo.

di·ba·sic (dī-bā′sik). Dibásico; que possui dois átomos de hidrogênio substituíveis; designando um ácido com dois átomos de hidrogênio ionizáveis.

di·ben·a·mine (dī-ben′ă-mēn). Dibenamina; antagonista inespecífico e irreversível em receptores alfa-adrenérgicos. Evita a vasoconstrição produzida pela epinefrina e norepinefrina e agentes semelhantes que causam vasoconstrição por uma ação sobre os receptores alfa-adrenérgicos.

di·benz·e·pin hy·dro·chlo·ride (dī-benz′ē-pin). Cloridrato de dibenzepina; um antidepressivo.

di·benz·hep·tro·pine cit·rate (dī-benz-hep′trō-pēn). Citrato de dibenzetropina. SIN deptropine citrate.

di·ben·zo·pyr·i·dine (dī-ben′zō-pir′i-dēn). Dibenzopiridina. SIN acridine.

di·ben·zo·thi·a·zine (dī-ben′zō-thī′ă-zēn). Dibenzotiazina. SIN phenothiazine.

di·benz·thi·one (dī-benz-thī′ōn). Dibenzotiona; um anti-séptico fúngico. SIN sulbentine.

Di·both·ri·o·ceph·a·lus (dī-both′rē-ō-sef′ă-lŭs). Nome antigo de *Diphyllobothrium*. [G. *di-*, dois, + *bothrion*, dim. de *bothros*, uma depressão, + *kephalē*, cabeça]
   D. la'tus, SIN Diphyllobothrium latum.

di·bro·mo·pro·pam·i·dine is·e·thi·o·nate (dī-brō′mō-prō-pam′i-dēn). Isetionato de dibromopropamidina; um anti-séptico.

di·brom·sa·lan (dī-brom′să-lan). Dibronsalam; um desinfetante.

di·bu·caine (dī′boo-kān). Dibucaína; anestésico local potente com uma ação de longa duração, usado por via injetável ou tópica na pele ou nas mucosas.

di·bu·caine hy·dro·chlo·ride (dī-bū′kān). Cloridrato de dibucaína; anestésico local potente (anestesia superficial e raquiana).

di·bu·caine num·ber (DN). Número da dibucaína; teste para diferenciação de uma ou de várias formas de pseudocolinesterases atípicas incapazes de inativar a succinilcolina em taxas normais; baseado na inibição percentual das enzimas pela dibucaína, a enzima normal tem um DN de 75 e mais, a enzima atípica heterozigota tem um DN de 40–70 e a enzima atípica homozigota tem um DN menor que 20. VER TAMBÉM fluoride number.

di·bu·to·line sul·fate (dī-bū′tō-lēn). Sulfato de dibutolina; um agente anticolinérgico usado como midriático, cicloplégico e antiespasmódico gastrointestinal.

di·bu·tyl phthal·ate (dī-bū′til thal′āt). Ftalato de butil; repelente de insetos.

DIC Abreviatura de disseminated intravascular *coagulation* (coagulação intravascular disseminada).

di·cac·o·dyl (dī-kak′ō-dil). Dicacodil. SIN cacodyl.

di·ce·lous (dī-sē′lŭs). Dicélico; que possui duas cavidades ou escavações em superfícies opostas. [G. *di-*, dois, + *koilos*, cavidade]

di·cen·tric (dī-sen′trik). Dicêntrico; referente a um cromossoma estrutural que possui dois centrômeros, um estado anormal.

di·ceph·a·lous (dī-sef′ă-lŭs). Dicéfalo; que possui duas cabeças.

di·ceph·a·lus (dī-sef′ă-lŭs). Dicéfalos; gêmeos conjugados simétricos com duas cabeças separadas. VER conjoined *twins*, em *twin*. SIN bicephalus, diplocephalus. [G. *di-*, dois, + *kephalē*, cabeça]
  d. di'auchenos, derodídimo; dicéfalo com pescoços separados. SIN derodidymus.
  d. di'pus dibra'chius, dicéfalo no qual há apenas dois braços e duas pernas para um corpo com dois eixos.
  d. di'pus tetrabra'chius, dicéfalo com duas pernas e quatro braços distintos.
  d. di'pus tribra'chius, dicéfalo com duas pernas e três braços.
  d. dip'ygus, anacatadídimo. SIN anakatadidymus. VER conjoined *twins*, em *twin*.
  d. mon'auchenos, dicéfalo no qual a união envolve a região cervical de forma que as duas cabeças estão sobre um único pescoço.

di·chei·lia, di·chi·lia (dī-kī′lē-ă). Diquelia; um lábio que parece ser duplo devido à presença de uma prega anormal de mucosa. [G. *di-*, dois, + *cheilos*, lábio]

di·chei·ria, di·chi·ria (dī-kī′rē-ă). Diqueria; duplicação completa ou incompleta da mão. VER TAMBÉM polydactyly. SIN diplocheiria, diplochiria. [G. *di-*, dois, + *cheir*, mão]

Di·chel·o·bac·ter no·do·sus. SIN Bacteroides nodosus.

di·chlo·ra·mine-T (dī-klōr′ă-mēn). Dicloramina-T; usado como anti-séptico em curativos cirúrgicos.

di·chlo·ride (dī-klōr′īd). Dicloreto; bicloreto; composto com uma molécula contendo dois átomos de cloro para um átomo de outro elemento.

di·chlo·ri·sone (dī-klōr′i-sōn). Diclorisona; agente antipruriginoso tópico.

di·chlo·ro·ben·zene (dī-klōr′ō-ben′zen). Diclorobenzeno; inseticida usado principalmente como repelente de traças.

di·chlo·ro·di·flu·o·ro·meth·ane (dī-klōr′ō-dī-floo-rō-meth′ān). Diclorodifluormetano; gás facilmente liquefeito utilizado como refrigerante e propelente de aerossol.

p,p'-**di·chlo·ro·di·phen·yl meth·yl car·bi·nol (DMC)** (dī-chlōr′ō-dī-fen′il).*p,p'*-diclorodifenilmetilcarbinol; composto sintético considerado efetivo como acaricida.

di·chlo·ro·di·phen·yl·tri·chlo·ro·eth·ane (DDT) (dī-chlōr′ō-dī-fen′il-trī-klōr-ō-eth′ān). Diclorodifeniltricloroetano; um inseticida que se tornou famoso durante e após a II Guerra Mundial. Durante um período, mostrou-se muito efetivo, mas as populações de insetos rapidamente desenvolveram tolerância a ele, e, por isso, perdeu muito de sua efetividade original; o emprego geral agora é amplamente desencorajado devido à toxicidade resultante da persistência ambiental desse agente. SIN chlorophenothane, dicophane.

di(2-chlo·ro·eth·yl)sul·fide. Di(2-cloroetil) sulfeto. SIN mustard *gas.*

di·chlo·ro·for·mox·ime. Dicloroformoxima. SIN phosgene oxime.

di·chlo·ro·hy·drin (dī-klōr-ō-hī′drin). Dicloroidrina; líquido incolor, inodoro, preparado por aquecimento de glicerina anidra com monocloreto de enxofre; um solvente de resinas. SIN dichloroisopropyl alcohol.

2,6-di·chlo·ro·in·do·phe·nol (dī-klōr′ō-in-dō-fē′nol). 2,6-diclorindofenol; um reagente para a análise química do ácido ascórbico que depende das propriedades redutoras deste último. É vermelho em solução ácida; na presença da vitamina C sofre redução e torna-se incolor, sendo a vitamina oxidada em ácido desidroascórbico. Com freqüência é denominado erroneamente diclorofenol-indofenol.

di·chlo·ro·i·so·pro·pyl al·co·hol (dī-klōr′ō-is-ō-prō′pil). Álcool dicloroisopropílico. SIN dichlorohydrin.

di·chlo·ro·phen (dī-klōr′ō-fen). Diclorofeno; usado topicamente como fungicida e bactericida, e, internamente, no tratamento de infestações por tênias de seres humanos e animais domésticos.

di·chlo·ro·phen·ar·sine hy·dro·chlo·ride (dī-klōr′ō-fen-ar′sēn). Cloridrato de diclorofenarsina; cloridrato de (3-amino-4-hidroxifenil)dicloroarsina, usado antigamente como anti-sifilítico arsenical.

2,6-di·chlo·ro·phe·nol·in·do·phe·nol (dī′klōr-ō-fē′nol-in-dō-fē′nol). 2,6-diclorofenol-indofenol; denominação errada do 2,6-dicloroindofenol.

(2,4-di·chlo·ro·phen·oxy) ace·tic ac·id (2,4-D). Ácido (2,4-diclorofenoxi) acético; um herbicida, mais tóxico para plantas dicotiledôneas de folhas largas (ervas daninhas) do que para as monocotiledôneas (cereais e gramíneas), usado com ácido (2,4,5-triclorofenoxi) acético como constituinte do Agente Laranja.

di·chlo·ro·vos (dī-klōr′ō-vos). Diclorovos. SIN dichlorvos.

di·chlor·phen·a·mide (dī-klōr-fen′ă-mīd). Diclorfenamida; uma anidrase carbônica com ações semelhantes àquelas da acetazolamida.

di·chlor·vos (dī-klōr′vos). Diclorvos; diclorovos; um anti-helmíntico usado em medicina veterinária e humana. SIN dichlorovos.

di·cho·ri·al, di·cho·ri·on·ic (dī-kō′rē-ăl, dī-kō-rē-on′ik). Dicoriônico; que mostra evidências de dois córions. [G. *di-*, dois, + chorion]

di·chot·ic (dī-kot′ik). Dicótico; dicotômico. **1.** SIN dichotomous. **2.** Apresentação simultânea de um som diferente a cada ouvido.

di·chot·o·mous (dī-kot′ō-mŭs). Dicotômico; indica ou se caracteriza por dicotomia. SIN dichotic (1).

di·chot·o·my (dī-kot′ō-mē). Dicotomia; divisão em duas partes. [G. *dichotomia*, um corte em dois, de *dicha*, em dois, + *tomē*, corte]

di·chro·ic (dī-krō′ik). Dicróico; relativo a dicroísmo.

di·chro·ism (dī′krō-izm). Dicroísmo; a propriedade de parecer possuir coloração diferente quando visto através da luz emitida e da luz transmitida. [G. *di-*, dois, + *chrōa*, cor]
  circular d. (CD), d. circular; a alteração da polarização circular para polarização elíptica da luz monocromática, polarizada circularmente na vizinhança imediata da faixa de absorção da substância que a luz atravessa. VER TAMBÉM Cotton *effect.*

di·chro·mat (dī′krō-mat). Dicromático; indivíduo com dicromatismo.

di·chro·mate (dī-krō′māt). Dicromato; bicromato; composto que contém o radical $CR_2O_7^=$.

di·chro·mat·ic (dī-krō-mat′ik). Dicromático. **1.** Que possui ou exibe duas cores. **2.** Relativo a dicromatismo (2).

di·chro·ma·tism (dī-krō′mă-tizm). Dicromatismo. **1.** O estado de ser dicromático (1). **2.** A anormalidade da visão em cores na qual existem apenas dois dos três pigmentos dos cones retinianos, como na protanopia, deuteranopia e tritanopia. SIN dichromatopsia. [G. *di-*, dois, + *chrōma*, cor]

di·chro·ma·top·sia (dī-krō-mă-top′sē-ă). Dicromatopsia. SIN dichromatism (2). [G. *di-*, dois, + *chrōma*, cor, + *opsis*, visão]

di·chro·mic (dī-krō′mik). Dicrômico; que possui, ou relativo a, duas cores.

di·chro·mo·phil, di·chro·mo·phile (dī-krō′mō-fil, dī-krō′mō-fīl). Dicromófilo; que assume coloração dupla; designa um tecido ou célula que aceita uma coloração tanto ácida quanto básica em diferentes partes. [G. *di-*, dois, + *chrōma*, cor, + *philos*, afinidade]

Dick, George Frederick, clínico norte-americano, 1881–1967. VER D. *method, test, test toxin.*

Dick, Gladys R.H., clínica norte-americana, 1881–1963. VER D. *method, test, test toxin.*

Dickens, Frank, bioquímico inglês, *1899. VER D. *shunt*; Warburg-Lipmann-D.-Horecker *shunt.*

di·clo·fen·ac (dī-clō′fen-ăk). Diclofenaco; um dos vários agentes antiinflamatórios não-esteróides usados no tratamento de distúrbios reumáticos, como artrite reumatóide; também usado na osteoartrite e em outros distúrbios. Atua impedindo a síntese de prostaglandina.

di·clox·a·cil·lin so·di·um (dī-klok-să-sil′in). Dicloxacilina sódica; uma penicilina semi-sintética resistente à penicilinase.

DICOM Abreviatura de Digital Imaging and Communications in Medicine, um padrão conjunto do *American College of Radiology* e da *National Equipment Manufacturers Association;* especifica entidades (ou objetos) e funções (ou serviços) para permitir a comunicação entre várias fontes de imagem e outros dispositivos de computador, como arquivos ou estações de trabalho. (*workstations*).

di·co·phane (dī′kō-fān). Dicófano. SIN dichlorodiphenyltrichloroethane.

di·co·ria (dī-kō′rē-ă). Dicoria. SIN diplocoria. [G. *di-*, dois, + *korē*, pupila]

di·cot·yl·ed·on. Dicotiledóne; planta (arbusto, erva ou árvore) cujas sementes consistem em dois cotilédones, isto é, a folha primária ou rudimentar do embrião de plantas com sementes.

di·cro·coe·li·o·sis (dī′krō-sē-li-ō′sis). Dicroceliose; infestação de animais e, raramente, de seres humanos por trematódeos do gênero *Dicrocoelium.*

Di·cro·coe·li·um (dik-rō-sē′lē-ŭm). Gênero de trematódeos digenéticos que habitam os ductos biliares e a vesícula biliar de herbívoros. A espécie *D. dentriticum* (trematódeo lancetado) raramente é encontrada nos seres humanos, mas é um parasita importante de carneiros em algumas localidades. [G. *dikroos*, bifurcado, + *koilia*, ventre]

di·crot·ic (dī-krot′ik). Dicrótico; relativo ao dicrotismo. [G. *dikrotos*, batimento duplo]

di·cro·tism (dī′krō-tizm). Dicrotismo; a forma do pulso na qual pode ser observado um batimento duplo em qualquer pulso arterial para cada batimento do coração; devido à acentuação da onda dicrótica. [G. *di-*, dois, + *krotos*, um batimento]

dicta- (dik´ta). Prefixo usado para designar duzentos. [G.]

dic·ty·o·ma (dik-tē-ō´ma). Dictioma; tumor benigno do epitélio ciliar com uma estrutura reticulada semelhante à retina embrionária. [G. *dikyton*, rede (retina), + *-oma*, tumor]

dic·ty·o·some (dik´tē-ō-sōm). Dictiossoma. SIN Golgi *apparatus*. [G. *diktyon*, rede, + *-some*]

dic·ty·o·tene (dik´tē-ō-tēn). Dictióteno; o estado de meiose no qual o desenvolvimento do ovócito é interrompido durante os vários anos entre o final da vida fetal e a menarca. [G. *diktyon*, rede, + *tainia*, faixa]

di·cu·ma·rol (dī-koo´ma-rol). Dicumarol; anticoagulante que inibe a formação de protrombina no fígado. Atua como antagonista da vitamina K; descoberto como o agente causador da deterioração do feno, que produzia hemorragia no gado bovino (doença do trevo-de-cheiro). SIN bishydroxycoumarin.

di·cy·clo·mine hy·dro·chlo·ride (dī-sī´klō-mēn). Cloridrato de diciclomina; agente anticolinérgico.

di·cys·te·ine (dī-sis´tēn). Dicisteína. SIN cystine.

di·dac·tic (dī-dak´tik). Didático; instrutivo; indica o ensino médico por conferências ou livros, para distingui-lo de demonstrações clínicas com pacientes ou exercícios laboratoriais. [G. *didaktikos*, de *didaskō*, ensinar]

di·dac·ty·lism (dī-dak´ti-lizm). Didactilismo; distúrbio congênito no qual o indivíduo possui apenas dois dedos em uma mão ou dois artelhos em um pé. [G. *di-*, dois, + *daktylos*, dedo ou artelho]

di·del·phic (dī-del´fik). Didélfico; que possui, ou relativo a, um útero duplo. [G. *di-*, dois, + *delphys*, útero]

Di·del·phis (dī-del´fis). Gênero de marsupiais, comumente denominados gambás, que servem como hospedeiros reservatórios de *Trypanosoma cruzi*. O *D. marsupialis* é a variedade norte-americana comum; *D. paraguayensis* é uma forma sul-americana. [G. *di-*, dois + *delphys*, útero]

di·de·ox·y·aden·o·sine (DDA) (dī´dē-oks´ē-ā-den´ō-sēn). Didesoxiadenosina; agente antiviral usado no tratamento da AIDS/SIDA, semelhante à DDC.

di·de·ox·y·cy·ti·dine (dī´dē-ok´-sē-sī´-ti-dēn). Didesoxicitidina; análogo do nucleosídeo pirimidina com atividade antiviral; usada no tratamento da AIDS/SIDA.

di·de·ox·y·in·o·sine (DDI) (dī´-dē-oks-ē-ī´-nō-sēn). Didesoxiinosina; agente antiviral; tem sido usada no tratamento da AIDS/SIDA.

DIDMOD Acrônimo para síndrome de Wolfram (Wolfram *syndrome*), que compreende *d*iabetes *i*nsípido, *d*iabetes *m*elito, atrofia *ó*ptica e surdez (*d*eafness).

didym-, didymo-. Didim-, dídimo-; o dídimo, testículo. [G. *didymos*, gêmeo]

did·y·mus (did´ē-mŭs). Dídimo. SIN testis. [G. *didymos*, a twin, pl. *didymoi*, testes]

-didymus. Gêmeo conjugado, com o primeiro elemento da palavra completa designando partes fundidas. VER TAMBÉM -dymus, -pagus. [G. *didymos*, gêmeo]

die (dī). Molde; em odontologia, a reprodução positiva da forma de um dente preparado em qualquer substância rígida adequada, geralmente em metal ou pedra artificial especialmente preparada. VER TAMBÉM counterdie.

dieb. alt. Abreviatura do L. *diebus alternis*, em dias alternados.

di·e·cious (dī-ē´shŭs). Diécio; designa animais ou plantas sexualmente distintos, sendo os indivíduos de um ou do outro sexo. [G. *di-*, dois, + *oikia*, casa]

Dieffenbach, Johann F., cirurgião alemão, 1792–1847.

Diego blood group, Di blood group. Grupo sanguíneo Diego. Ver Apêndice sobre Grupos Sanguíneos.

di·el (dī´el). Termo usado freqüentemente como sinônimo de diurno (2) ou circadiano. [irreg., do L. *dies*, dia]

di·el·drin (dī-el´drin). Dieldrina; hidrocarboneto clorado usado como inseticida; pode causar efeitos tóxicos em pessoas e animais expostos à sua ação por contato cutâneo, inalação ou contaminação alimentar.

di·e·lec·trog·ra·phy (dī-ē-lek-trog´ra-fē). Dieletrografia. SIN impedance plethysmography.

di·e·lec·trol·y·sis (dī´ē-lek-trol´i-sis). Dieletrólise. SIN electrophoresis.

Diels, Otto, químico alemão e ganhador do Prêmio Nobel, 1876–1954. VER D. *hydrocarbon*.

di·en·ceph·a·lo·hy·po·phy·si·al (dī-en-sef´ā-lō-hī-pō-fiz´ē-āl). Diencéfalo-hipofisário; relativo ao diencéfalo e à hipófise.

di·en·ceph·a·lon, pl. **di·en·ceph·a·la** (dī-en-sef´ā-lon, -sef´ā-lā) [TA]. Diencéfalo; a parte caudal do prosencéfalo, composta pelo epitálamo, tálamo e hipotálamo. [G. *dia*, através, + *enkephalos*, encéfalo]

die·ner (dē´ner). Servente; funcionário de laboratório que ajuda na limpeza; aplicado mais comumente a funcionários de laboratório que ajudam na realização de necropsias e na manutenção de necrotérios. [Alemão. *Diener*, servente]

di·en·es·trol (dī-en-es´trol). Dienestrol; um agente estrogênico. SIN estrodienol.

Di·ent·a·moe·ba frag·i·lis (dī-ent-ā-mē´bā fraj´i-lis). Uma espécie de pequenos flagelados semelhantes a amebas, anteriormente considerada uma ameba verdadeira, agora reconhecida como um ameboflagelado relacionado ao *Trichomonas*, parasita do intestino grosso de homens e de alguns macacos; pode ser não-patogênico, mas acredita-se que seja capaz de causar, algumas vezes, inflamação discreta com diarréia mucosa e distúrbio gastrointestinal em seres humanos.

di·er·e·sis (dī-er´ē-sis). Diérese. SIN *solution* of continuity. [G. *diairesis*, uma divisão]

di·e·ret·ic (dī-er-et´ik). Dierético. **1.** Relativo à diérese. **2.** Que divide; que ulcera; que corrói.

di·es·ter·ase (dī-es´ter-ās). Diesterase. VER phosphodiesterases.

di·es·trous (dī-es´trŭs). Diéstrico; relativo ao diestro.

di·es·trus (dī-es´trŭs). Diestro; um período de quiescência sexual interposto entre dois períodos de estro. [G. *dia*, entre, + *oistros*, desejo]

di·et (dī´et). Dieta. **1.** Alimentos e bebidas em geral. **2.** Uma orientação prescrita para comer e beber na qual a quantidade e o tipo de alimento, bem como o horário das refeições, são controlados para fins terapêuticos. **3.** Redução da ingestão calórica de forma a perder peso. **4.** Seguir qualquer dieta prescrita ou específica. [G. *diaita*, uma forma de vida; uma dieta]

acid-ash d., d. de resíduo ácido. SIN alkaline-ash d.

alkaline-ash d., d. de resíduo alcalino; dieta consistindo principalmente em frutas, vegetais e leite (com quantidades mínimas de carne, peixe, ovos, queijo e cereais), que, quando catabolisados, deixam um resíduo alcalino para ser excretado na urina. SIN acid-ash d., basic d.

balanced d., d. balanceada; dieta contendo os nutrientes essenciais com um suprimento razoável de todos os principais grupos alimentares.

basal d., d. basal; **(1)** dieta com um valor calórico igual à produção basal de calor e quantidades suficientes de nutrientes essenciais para atender às necessidades básicas; **(2)** em experiências com nutrição, uma dieta completa e adequada, exceto por um único constituinte (p. ex., uma vitamina, mineral ou aminoácido), cujo valor nutricional deve ser determinado, omitido por um período e os efeitos observados; o indivíduo é observado por um segundo período, durante o qual o ingrediente estudado é acrescentado à dieta.

basic d., d. básica. SIN alkaline-ash d.

bland d., d. branda; uma dieta regular que omite alimentos que irritam, mecânica ou quimicamente, o trato gastrointestinal.

BRAT d., d. BRAT; uma dieta limitada freqüentemente usada em regimes para gastroenterites agudas; acrônimo para *b*ananas, arroz (*r*ice), maçãs (*a*pples) (suco ou molho) e *t*orrada (*t*oast).

challenge d., d. de prova; dieta na qual uma ou mais substâncias específicas são incluídas para determinar se há uma reação anormal.

clear liquid d., d. líquida; dieta, freqüentemente usada no pós-operatório, que em geral consiste em água, chá, café, preparações com gelatina e em sopas ou caldos sem resíduos.

diabetic d., d. para diabetes; ajuste alimentar para pacientes com *diabetes* melito, com o objetivo de reduzir a necessidade de insulina ou de hipoglicemiantes orais e controlar o peso por ajuste da ingestão calórica e de carboidratos.

elimination d., d. de eliminação; uma dieta designada para detectar que ingrediente do alimento causa manifestações alérgicas no paciente; os itens alimentares aos quais o paciente pode ser sensível são afastados, separada e sucessivamente, da dieta até que se descubra o que causa os sintomas.

full liquid d., d. líquida completa; dieta que consiste apenas em líquidos, mas inclui sopas cremosas, sorvete e leite.

Giordano-Giovannetti d., d. de Giordano-Giovannetti; dieta designada para pacientes com insuficiência renal; fornece pequenas quantidades de proteína, basicamente na forma de aminoácidos essenciais, juntamente com derivados alfa-ceto de aminoácidos; a decomposição de proteínas no músculo esquelético é retardada, e, como as reações da transaminase são reversíveis, uma pequena proporção da amônia liberada pela decomposição da uréia é usada para síntese de aminoácidos não-essenciais. SIN Giovannetti d.

Giovannetti d., d. de Giovannetti. SIN Giordano-Giovannetti d.

gluten-free d., d. isenta de glúten; eliminação de todo o glúten do trigo, centeio, cevada e aveia da dieta; tratamento para enteropatia sensível ao glúten (doença celíaca). VER celiac *disease*.

gout d., d. para gota; dieta contendo uma quantidade mínima de bases purinas (carnes); fígado, rim e timo de vitela são especialmente excluídos e substituídos por laticínios, frutas e cereais; também são excluídas as bebidas alcoólicas. SIN purine-free d.

high-calorie d., d. hipercalórica; dieta que contém mais de 4.000 calorias por dia.

high-fat d., d. hiperlipídica; d. rica em lipídios; dieta contendo grandes quantidades de gordura.

high-fiber d., d. rica em fibras; dieta rica na parte não-digerível de plantas, que são as fibras. As fibras são encontradas nas frutas, vegetais, cereais integrais e legumes. As fibras insolúveis aumentam o volume fecal, reduzem o tempo de trânsito do alimento no intestino e reduzem a constipação e o risco de câncer de cólon. As fibras solúveis retardam a absorção de glicose, o que ajuda a controlar a glicemia no diabetes melito, e a absorção de lipídios, o que ajuda a controlar a hiperlipidemia. Recomendada no tratamento da doença diverticular do cólon.

Kempner d., d. de Kempner. SIN rice d.

ketogenic d., d. cetogênica; dieta rica em lipídios, pobre em carboidratos e com quantidade normal de proteínas, que causa cetose.
low-calorie d., d. hipocalórica; dieta de 1.200 calorias ou menos por dia.

low-fat d., d. hipolipídica; d. pobre em lipídios; uma dieta que contém uma proporção mínima de gordura.
    As dietas que contêm baixas quantidades de gordura e colesterol visam reduzir o risco de doença cardiovascular, especificamente aterosclerose. O *National Cholesterol Education Program* recomenda a manutenção de um nível de colesterol total não-superior a 200 mg/dl, com LDL-colesterol menor que 130 mg/dl e HDL-colesterol mínimo de 60 mg/dl. (De acordo com o *National Institutes of Health,* o LDL-colesterol, em pacientes com cardiopatia aterosclerótica, não deve ser maior que 100 mg/dl.) Cerca de metade dos norte-americanos adultos excedem esses limites de colesterol total e LDL-colesterol; para muitos, a razão é um distúrbio metabólico hereditário do metabolismo lipídico, não corrigível apenas por restrições alimentares. Uma dieta pobre em lipídios deve obter menos de 10% de suas calorias das gorduras saturadas (carnes, laticínios) e deve ser pobre em colesterol (< 300 mg/dia) e ácidos graxos trans (p. ex., óleos hidrogenados, como os encontrados na margarina dura ou gordura) e rica em cereais integrais, frutas e vegetais frescos, e legumes. As pessoas que seguem uma dieta extremamente pobre em gordura apresentam alguma reversão da aterosclerose, apesar da diminuição concomitante do HDL-colesterol. Uma dieta pobre em gordura também pode ajudar a reduzir o peso corporal ou a evitar ganho de peso, porque gorduras e óleos possuem mais que o dobro de calorias por grama que os carboidratos e as proteínas. Ver atherosclerosis; free radical.

low purine d., d. pobre em purinas; uma dieta pobre em precursores das purinas (como tecidos ricos em células com núcleos abundantes, como no fígado, vísceras, etc.) para minimizar a formação de ácido úrico. Útil no tratamento de pacientes com gota ou cálculos renais contendo urato.
low residue d., d. pobre em resíduos; dieta que deixa mínimos componentes não absorvidos no intestino, para minimizar o estresse funcional sobre o cólon.
low salt d., d. hipossódica; uma dieta com quantidades restritas de cloreto de sódio, útil no tratamento de alguns casos de hipertensão, insuficiência cardíaca e outras síndromes caracterizadas por retenção hídrica e/ou formação de edema.
macrobiotic d., d. macrobiótica; dieta que se alega promover longevidade, freqüentemente pela ênfase em produtos naturais e restrições de alimentos que não sejam cereais, bem como de líquidos.
Meulengracht d., d. de Meulengracht; programa nutricional para pacientes com úlcera péptica, contendo uma dieta relativamente completa, sem alimentos ácidos ou muito condimentados.
Minot-Murphy d., d. de Minot-Murphy; o uso de grandes quantidades de fígado cru no tratamento da anemia perniciosa (pernicious *anemia*). Os primeiros sucessos no tratamento dessa doença foram obtidos com essa dieta e levaram ao desenvolvimento de extrato hepático para tratamento.
Ornish prevention d.'s, dietas preventivas de Ornish; versões relaxadas da dieta de reversão de Ornish, que tem por objetivo evitar a doença coronariana. Essas dietas reduzem a gordura da dieta proporcionalmente ao nível sanguíneo de colesterol.
Ornish reversal d., d. de reversão de Ornish; dieta projetada por Dean Ornish, que apresenta evidências de que reverterá a doença coronariana. Consiste em 10% de calorias provenientes de gordura (principalmente poliinsaturada ou monoinsaturada, com 5 mg de colesterol por dia), 70–75% de carboidratos e 15–20% de proteínas.
purine-free d., d. isenta de purinas. SIN gout d.
purine-restricted d., d. com restrição de purinas. VER gout d.
rachitic d., d. raquítica; dieta que induzirá raquitismo em animais experimentais suscetíveis.
reducing d., d. redutora; dieta na qual o gasto calórico é maior que a ingestão calórica.
rice d., d. de arroz; dieta composta por arroz, frutas e açúcar, mais suplementos de vitamina e ferro, projetada por Kempner para tratamento da hipertensão. Em 2.000 calorias, a dieta contém 5 g ou menos de gordura, cerca de 20 g de proteínas, e não mais de 150 mg de sódio. SIN Kempner d.
Schmidt d., d. de Schmidt. SIN Schmidt-Strassburger d.
Schmidt-Strassburger d., d. de Schmidt-Strassburger; dieta obsoleta, designada para facilitar o exame das fezes em pacientes com diarréia, que consiste em leite, torrada seca, mingau de aveia, ovos, manteiga, pequenas quantidades de carne bovina e batata. SIN Schmidt d.
Sippy d., d. de Sippy; uma dieta usada antigamente nos estágios iniciais do tratamento da úlcera péptica, começando com leite e creme, a cada uma ou duas horas, para manter o ácido gástrico neutralizado, aumentando gradualmente para incluir cereais, ovos e biscoitos tipo *cracker,* após três dias, e purê de vegetais mais tarde.
smooth d., d. branda; dieta que contém poucas fibras; usada basicamente em doenças do cólon.
soft d., d. pastosa; uma dieta normal limitada a alimentos de consistência mole para os que têm dificuldade de mastigação ou deglutição; não há restrições quanto ao uso de temperos ou ao método de preparo dos alimentos.
subsistence d., d. de subsistência; uma dieta pobre que fornece apenas o suficiente para a subsistência.
Wilder d., d. de Wilder; dieta obsoleta, pobre em potássio, para o tratamento da doença de Addison (Addison *disease*).
di·e·tary (dī'ĕ-tār-ē). Dietético. **1.** Relativo à dieta.
Dieterle stain. Corante de Dieterle. Ver em stain.
di·e·tet·ic (dī'ĕ-tet'ik). Dietético. **1.** Relativo à dieta. **2.** Descritivo de alimento que, naturalmente ou através de processamento, tem um baixo conteúdo calórico.
di·e·tet·ics (dī-ĕ-tet'iks). Dietética; a aplicação prática de dieta na profilaxia e no tratamento de doenças.
di·eth·a·di·one (dī-eth-ă-dī'ōn). Dietadiona; um analéptico.
di·eth·a·nol·a·mine (dī-eth-ă-nol'ă-mēn). Dietanolamina; usada como emulsificante e como dispersante em cosméticos e fármacos. SIN diethylolamine.
di·eth·a·zine (dī-eth'ă-zēn). Dietazina; agente anticolinérgico.
di·eth·yl (dī-eth'il). Dietil; um composto contendo dois radicais etil.
5,5-di·eth·yl·bar·bi·tu·ric ac·id (dī-eth'il-bar-bi-tū'rik). Ácido 5,5-dietilbarbitúrico. SIN barbital.
di·eth·yl·car·bam·a·zine cit·rate (dī-eth'il-kar-bam'ă-zēn). Citrato de dietilcarbamazina; um microfilaricida efetivo, embora relativamente inefetivo contra as filárias adultas.
di·eth·yl·ene·di·a·mine (dī-eth'il-ēn-dī'ă-mēn). Dietilenodiamina. SIN piperazine.
1,4-di·eth·yl·ene di·ox·ide (dī-eth'il-ēn). Dióxido de 1,4-dietileno. SIN dioxane.
di·eth·yl·ene gly·col (dī-eth'il-ēn). Dietileno glicol; um solvente orgânico quimicamente relacionado ao etileno glicol. Após conversão metabólica, transforma-se em ácido oxálico, que é tóxico para o rim. Um líquido doce, viscoso, então usado para produzir o infame elixir de sulfanilamida, que causou a morte de mais de 100 crianças em 1937, levando à determinação que a FDA monitorizasse a segurança dos medicamentos.
di·eth·yl·ene·tri·a·mine pen·ta·a·ce·tic ac·id (DTPA) (dī-eth'il-ēn-trī'ă-mēn pen-ta-ă-sē'tik as'id). Ácido dietilenotriamina pentacético; importante agente quelante usado terapeuticamente (como no tratamento da intoxicação por chumbo) e em agentes diagnósticos contendo metal para estudo por ressonância magnética e cintigrafia nuclear.
di·eth·yl ether. Éter dietílico; solvente orgânico volátil, inflamável, antigamente muito usado em procedimentos cirúrgicos; foi usado como anestésico inalatório; as deficiências incluem: vapor irritante, início lento e fase de recuperação prolongada, risco de explosão. SIN ethyl ether, ethyl oxide, sulfuric ether.
di·eth·y·lol·a·mine (dī-eth-i-lol'ă-mēn). Dietilolamina. SIN diethanolamine.
di·eth·yl·pro·pi·on hy·dro·chlo·ride (dī-eth-il-prō'pē-on). Cloridrato de dietilpropiona; um agente simpaticomimético com ações semelhantes às da anfetamina e usado como supressor do apetite. Aumenta a pressão arterial e a freqüência cardíaca.
di·eth·yl·stil·bes·trol (DES) (dī-eth'il-stil-bes'trol). Dietilestilbestrol; composto estrogênico não-esteróide sintético. Algumas vezes usado como agente contraceptivo pós-coito para impedir a implantação do óvulo fertilizado. O primeiro carcinógeno transplacentário comprovado, responsável por um carcinoma vaginal de células claras tardio em filhas de mulheres que o tomaram durante a gravidez, quando se acreditava erroneamente que impedia a ameaça de abortamento. SIN stilbestrol.
di·eth·yl·tol·u·am·ide (dī-eth'il-tō-loo'ă-mīd). Dietiltoluamida; repelente de insetos.
di·eth·yl·tryp·ta·mine (DET) (dī-eth-il-trip'tă-mēn). Dietiltriptamina; agente alucinógeno semelhante à dimetiltriptamina.
di·e·ti·tian (dī-ĕ-tish'ŭn). Dietista, nutricionista; um especialista em dietética.
Dietl, Józef, médico polonês, 1804–1878. VER D. *crisis*.
Dieuaide di·a·gram. Diagrama de Dieuaide. Ver em diagram.
Dieulafoy, Georges, médico francês, 1839–1911. VER D. *erosion*.
di·far·ne·syl group (di-far'nē-sil). Grupamento difarnesílico; radical hidrocarboneto hexaisoprenóide, com uma cadeia aberta no carbono 30; ocorre como uma cadeia lateral na vitamina K_2.
di·fen·ox·in (dī-fen-ok'sin). Difenoxina; agente antidiarreico com ações semelhantes às do difenoxilato. SIN difenoxylic acid.

di·fen·ox·y·lic ac·id (dī-fen-ok′si-lik). Ácido difenoxílico. SIN difenoxin.

dif·fer·ence (dif′er-ens). Diferença; a magnitude ou grau pelo qual uma qualidade ou quantidade difere de outra do mesmo tipo.

   alveolar-arterial oxygen d., d. de oxigênio alvéolo-arterial; a diferença ou gradiente entre a pressão parcial de oxigênio nos espaços alveolares e no sangue arterial; $P_{(A-a)}O_2$. Normalmente, em adultos jovens, esse valor é menor que 20 mm Hg. VER TAMBÉM alveolar gas *equation*.

   arteriovenous carbon dioxide d., d. de dióxido de carbono arteriovenoso; a diferença do conteúdo de dióxido de carbono (em ml por 100 ml de sangue) entre o sangue arterial e venoso.

   arteriovenous oxygen d., d. de oxigênio arteriovenoso; a diferença do conteúdo de oxigênio (em ml por 100 ml de sangue) entre o sangue arterial e venoso.

   AV d., d. AV; abreviatura de diferença arteriovenosa da concentração de uma substância.

   cation-anion d., d. cátion-ânion. SIN anion *gap*.

   individual d.'s, diferenças individuais; em psicologia clínica, desvios individuais em relação à média do grupo ou entre si.

   light d., d. luminosa; (**1**) a diferença na sensibilidade luminosa dos dois olhos; (**2**) SIN brightness difference *threshold*.

   masking level d., d. do nível de mascaramento; técnica de comparação de respostas limiares com ruído de mascaramento apresentado em fase e fora de fase com o sinal de teste; a discriminação do mascaramento é normal e indica que a via auditiva do tronco cerebral está intacta.

   standard error of d., erro padrão de d.; índice estatístico da probabilidade de que uma diferença entre duas médias de amostras seja maior que zero.

dif·fer·en·tial (dif-er-en′shăl). Diferencial; relativo a, ou caracterizado por, uma diferença; que distingue. [L. *dif-fero*, separar, diferir, de *dis*, distante]

   threshold d., limiar de diferenciação. SIN differential *threshold*.

dif·fer·en·ti·at·ed (dif-er-en′shē-ā-ted). Diferenciado; que possui um caráter ou uma função diferente das estruturas adjacentes ou da forma original; diz-se de tecidos, células ou porções do citoplasma.

dif·fer·en·ti·a·tion (dif′er-en-shē-ā′shŭn). **1.** Diferenciação. A aquisição ou posse de uma ou mais características ou funções diferentes daquelas do tipo original. SIN specialization (2). **2.** Diagnóstico diferencial. SIN differential *diagnosis*. **3.** Remoção parcial de uma coloração de um corte histológico para acentuar as diferenças de coloração dos componentes teciduais.

   correlative d., d. de correlação; diferenciação devida à interação de diferentes partes de um organismo.

   echocardiographic d., d. ecocardiográfica; o processamento de um sinal de forma que o débito dependa da velocidade de alteração da entrada; p. ex., exibirá alterações de amplitude, mas reduzirá a duração da onda.

   invisible d., d. invisível. SIN chemodifferentiation.

   pressure pulse d., d. da pressão de pulso; o processamento de um sinal da pressão de pulso de forma que o débito dependa da velocidade de alterações da entrada, produzindo dP/dt (pressão) ou, para pulsos registrados de forma não-invasiva, dD/dt (velocidade de alteração do deslocamento).

dif·flu·ence (dif′loo-ens). Difluência; o processo de se tornar líquido. [L. *diffluo*, fluir em diferentes direções, dissolver]

dif·frac·tion (di-frak′shŭn). Difração; deflexão dos raios luminosos de uma linha reta ao passar pela borda de um corpo opaco ou ao ultrapassar um obstáculo do tamanho aproximado do comprimento de onda da luz. [L. *dif-fringo*, pp. *-fractus*, quebrar em pedaços]

dif·frac·tion grat·ing. Retículo de difração; um tipo de filtro composto de sulcos alinhados em uma fina camada de liga de alumínio e cobre sobre uma superfície de vidro; usado em espectrofotômetros para dispersar a luz em um espectro. VER monochromator.

dif·fu·sate (di-fū′zāt). Difundido; dialisado. SIN dialysate. [L. *dif-fundo*, pp. *-fusus*, verter em direções diferentes]

dif·fuse (di-fūs). **1** (di-fūz′). Difundir; disseminar; espalhar. **2** (di-fūs′). Difuso; disseminado; espalhado; não-restrito. [L. *dif-fundo*, pp. *-fusus*, verter em direções diferentes]

dif·fus·i·ble (di-fūz′i-bl). Difusível; capaz de se difundir.

dif·fu·sion (di-fū′zhŭn). Difusão. **1.** O movimento aleatório de moléculas ou íons, ou de pequenas partículas em solução ou suspensão, sob a influência de um movimento browniano (térmico) para uma distribuição uniforme em todo o volume disponível; o movimento é relativamente rápido nos líquidos e gases, porém é muito lento nos sólidos. **2.** Dispersão da luz.

   facilitated d., d. facilitada. VER facilitated *transport*.

   gel d., d. em gel; como no caso de provas de difusão da precipitina em gel nas quais os reagentes imunes se difundem em ágar. VER TAMBÉM immunodiffusion.

   passive d., d. passiva. VER facilitated *transport*.

di·flor·a·sone di·ac·e·tate (dī-flōr′ă-sōn). Diacetato de diflorasona; corticosteróide antiinflamatório usado em preparações tópicas.

di·flu·cor·to·lone (dī-floo-kōr′ti-lōn). Diflucortolona; um análogo sintético do esteróide glicocorticóide.

di·flu·ni·sal (dī-floo′ni-saul). Diflunisal; derivado do ácido salicílico com propriedades antiinflamatórias, analgésicas e antipiréticas, usado em distúrbios crônicos, como artrite reumatóide e osteoartrite.

di·ga·met·ic (dī-gă-met′ik). Digamético. SIN heterogametic.

di·gas·tric (dī-gas′trik). Digástrico. **1.** Que possui dois ventres; designa especialmente um músculo com duas partes carnosas separadas por uma parte tendinosa interposta. SIN biventral. VER digastric (*muscle*). **2.** Relativo ao músculo digástrico; designa uma fossa ou sulco com o qual está em relação e o nervo que supre seu ventre posterior. SIN digastricus (1). [G. *di-*, dois, + *gastēr*, ventre]

di·gas·tri·cus (dī-gas′tri-kŭs). Digástrico. **1.** SIN digastric. **2.** Designa o músculo digástrico (*musculus* digastricus). [L.]

Di·ge·nea (dī-jē′nē-a). Subclasse de vermes parasitas (classe Trematoda) caracterizada por um ciclo vital complexo, envolvendo estágios de desenvolvimento multiplicadores em um hospedeiro intermediário molusco, um estágio adulto em um vertebrado e, freqüentemente, envolvendo um outro hospedeiro de transporte ou um outro hospedeiro intermediário; inclui todos os trematódeos comuns de seres humanos e outros mamíferos. [G. *di-*, dois, + *genesis*, geração]

di·gen·e·sis (dī-jen′ē-sis). Digenesia; reprodução em padrões diferentes em gerações alternadas, como observado nos ciclos assexuado (invertebrado) e sexuado (vertebrado) de parasitas trematódeos digenéticos. [G. *di-*, dois, + G. *genesis*, geração]

di·ge·net·ic (dī-jĕ-net′ik). Digenético. **1.** Relativo a, ou caracterizado por, digenesia. SIN heteroxenous. **2.** Relativo ao trematódeo digenético.

DiGeorge, Angelo M., pediatra norte-americano, *1921. VER DiG. *syndrome*.

di·gest. Digerir. **1** (di-jest′, dī-). Amolecer por umidade e calor. **2** (di-jest′, dī-). Hidrolisar ou fragmentar em compostos químicos mais simples por meio de enzimas hidrolisantes ou ação química, como na ação das secreções do trato alimentar sobre o alimento. **3** (dī′jest). O material resultante da digestão ou hidrólise. [L. *digero*, pp. *-gestus*, forçar a separação, dividir, dissolver]

di·ges·tant (di-jes′tant, dī-). Digestivo. **1.** Que ajuda a digestão. **2.** Um agente que favorece ou auxilia o processo de digestão. SIN digestive (2).

di·ges·tion (di-jes′chŭn, dī-). Digestão. **1.** O processo de digerir. **2.** O processo mecânico, químico e enzimático pelo qual o alimento ingerido é convertido em material adequado para assimilação para a síntese de tecidos ou liberação de energia. [L. *digestio*. Ver digest]

   buccal d., d. bucal; parte da digestão realizada na boca; p. ex., a ação das amilases salivares.

   duodenal d., d. duodenal; aquela parte da digestão realizada no duodeno.

   gastric d., d. gástrica; parte da digestão, principalmente das proteínas, realizada no estômago pelas enzimas do suco gástrico. SIN peptic d.

   intercellular d., d. intercelular; digestão em uma cavidade por meio de secreções das células adjacentes, como a que ocorre nos metazoários.

   intestinal d., d. intestinal; parte da digestão realizada no intestino; afeta todos os alimentos: amidos, gorduras e proteínas.

   intracellular d., d. intracelular; digestão dentro dos limites de uma célula, como a que ocorre nos protozoários e em fagócitos.

   pancreatic d., d. pancreática; digestão no intestino pelas enzimas do suco pancreático.

   peptic d., d. péptica. SIN gastric d.

   primary d., d. primária; digestão no trato alimentar.

   salivary d., d. salivar; a conversão de amido em açúcar pela ação da amilase salivar.

   secondary d., d. secundária; a alteração no quilo realizada pela ação das células do corpo, na qual os produtos finais são assimilados no processo de metabolismo.

di·ges·tive (di-jes′tiv, dī-). Digestivo. **1.** Relativo à digestão. **2.** SIN digestant (2).

dig·it (dij′it) [TA]. Dedo, da mão ou do pé. VER TAMBÉM finger, toe. SIN digitus [TA], dactyl, dactylus. [L. *digitus*]

   binary d., dígito binário. SIN bit.

   clubbed d., d. em baqueta de tambor. VER clubbing.

   d.'s of foot, dedos do pé, artelhos, pododáctilo; *termo oficial alternativo para toe.

   primary d. of foot, hálux, primeiro pododáctilo. SIN great *toe* I.

dig·i·tal (dij′i-tăl). Digital; relativo, ou que se assemelha, a um dedo ou dedos ou uma impressão feita por eles; baseado na metodologia numérica.

dig·i·tal·in (dij-i-tal′in). Digitalina; mistura padronizada de glicosídeos digitálicos usada como cardiotônico no tratamento da insuficiência cardíaca congestiva.

   crystalline d., d. cristalina. SIN digitoxin.

Dig·i·tal·is (dij-i-tal′is, -ta′lis). Gênero de plantas florescentes perenes da família Schrophulariaceae. A *D. lanata*, uma espécie européia, e a *D. purpurea*, dedaleira, são as principais fontes de glicosídeos esteróides cardioativos usados no tratamento de algumas cardiopatias, particularmente da insuficiência cardíaca congestiva; também é usada no tratamento de taquiarritmias de origem atrial. SIN foxglove. [L. *digitalis*, relativo aos dedos; em alusão às flores semelhantes a dedos]

dig·i·tal·ism (dij′i-tal-izm). Digitalismo; os sinais e sintomas causados por envenenamento ou superdosagem (*overdose*) de digitálicos.

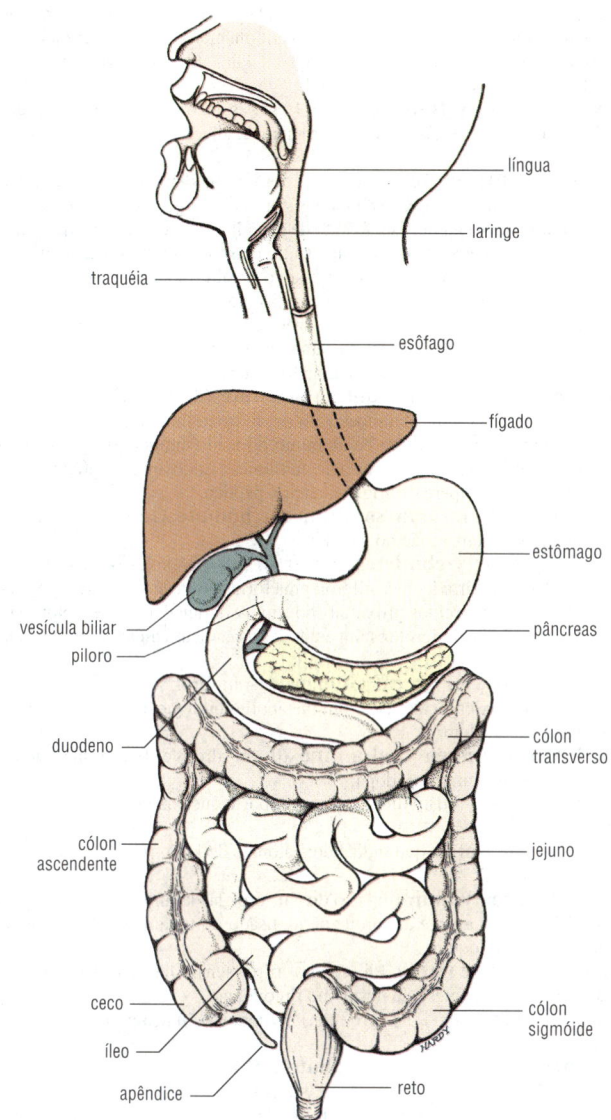

órgãos digestivos e estruturas associadas

---

dig·i·tal·i·za·tion (dij′i - tal - i - za′shŭn). Digitalização; administração de digitálicos por qualquer dos vários esquemas até que haja quantidades suficientes no organismo para produzir os efeitos terapêuticos.
dig·i·tate (dij′i - tāt). Digitado; caracterizado por vários processos ou impressões semelhantes a dedos. [L. *digitatus*, que possui dedos, de *digitus*, dedo]
dig·i·ta·tion (dij - i - tā′shŭn). Digitação; processo semelhante a um dedo. [L. Mod. *digitatio*]
dig·i·ta·ti·o·nes hip·po·cam·pi (dij - i - tā - shē - ō′nēz hip - ō - kam′pē). Digitações do hipocampo. SIN *foot* of hippocampus. [L. Mod. pl. de *digitatio*]
di·gi·ti (dij′i - tī). Dedos; plural de digitus. [L.]
dig·i·tin (dij′i - tin). Digitina. SIN digitonin.
dig·i·to·nin (dij - i - tō′nin). Digitonina. **1.** Um glicosídeo esteróide obtido da *Digitalis purpurea* que não tem ação cardíaca; usada como reagente na determinação dos níveis plasmáticos de colesterol e esteróides que possuem um grupamento 3-hidroxila em configuração beta. **2.** Uma mistura de quatro esteróides diferentes encontrada nas sementes da *Digitalis purpurea*; um forte veneno hemolítico. Pode atuar como detergentes aniônicos na solubilização de proteínas da membrana. SIN digitin.
dig·i·tox·i·gen·in (dij′i - toks′i - jen - in). Digitoxigenina; o aglicônio derivado da digitoxina; pode ser preparada por refluxo da digitoxina em uma mistura de água, álcool e ácido clorídrico.
dig·i·tox·in (dij - i - tok′sin). Digitoxina; um glicosídeo cardioativo obtido das folhas da *Digitalis purpurea*; é absorvido mais completamente pelo trato gastrointestinal que o digital. Eliminada sobretudo por metabolismo hepático. SIN crystalline digitalin.

dig·i·tox·ose (dij′i - toks′ōs). Digitoxose; a porção açúcar obtida por hidrólise ácida leve dos glicosídeos digitoxina, gitoxina e digoxina. A hidrólise produz 3 moles de digitoxose para cada mole do respectivo aglicônio.
D-dig·i·tox·ose (dij′i - toks′ōs). D-digitoxose; a porção carboidrato encontrada nos glicosídeos digitálicos; 2,6-didesoxi-D-*ribo*-hexose.
dig·i·tus, pl. **di·gi·ti** (dij′i - tŭs, - tī) [TA]. Dedo. SIN digit. [L.]
  d. anula′ris [TA], d. anular. SIN ring *finger*.
  d. auricula′ris, d. mínimo. SIN little *finger*.
  dig′iti hippocrat′ici, dedos hipocráticos; termo obsoleto para dedos em baqueta de tambor. VER clubbing.
  d. ma′nus [TA], d. da mão. SIN finger.
  d. (manus) me′dius [TA], d. médio da mão. SIN middle *finger*.
  d. (manus) min′imus [TA], d. mínimo da mão. SIN little *finger*.
  d. (manus) pri′mus, primeiro dedo da mão; *termo oficial alternativo para thumb.
  d. (manus) quartus IV, quarto dedo da mão; *termo oficial alternativo para ring *finger*.
  d. (manus) quin′tus [V], quinto dedo da mão. SIN little *finger*.
  d. (manus) secun′dus [II], segundo dedo da mão; *termo oficial alternativo para index *finger*.
  d. (manus) ter′tius [III], terceiro dedo da mão; *termo oficial alternativo para middle *finger*.
  d. ped′is [TA], d. do pé. SIN toe.
  d. (pedis) minimus [V] [TA], d. mínimo do pé. SIN little *toe* [V].
  d. pedis primus I, hálux; *termo oficial alternativo para great *toe* I.
  d. (pedis) quartus [IV] [TA], quarto dedo do pé. SIN fourth *toe* [IV].
  d. (pedis) quintus [V], quinto dedo do pé; *termo oficial alternativo para little *toe* [V].
  d. (pedis) secundus [II] [TA], segundo dedo do pé. SIN second *toe* [II].
  d. (pedis) tertius [III] [TA], terceiro dedo do pé. SIN third *toe* [III].
  d. val′gus, dedo valgo; desvio permanente de um ou mais dedos da mão em direção radial.
  d. va′rus, dedo varo; desvio permanente de um ou mais dedos da mão em direção ulnar.
di·glos·sia (dī - glos′ē - ă). Diglossia; distúrbio do desenvolvimento que resulta em uma divisão longitudinal da língua. VER bifid *tongue*. [G. *di-*, dois, + *glōssa*, língua]
di·glyc·er·ide li·pase (dī - glis′er - īd). Diglicerídeo lipase. SIN lipoprotein lipase.
di·gly·co·coll hy·dro·i·o·dide-io·dine (dī - glī′kō - kol hī - drō - ī′ō - dīd - ī′ō - dīn).Hidroiodeto-iodo de diglicocola; dois moles de hidroiodeto de diglicocola combinados a dois pesos atômicos de iodo; um agente antibacteriano usado na forma de comprimido para desinfetar a água que vai ser bebida.
di·gna·thus (dī - nath′ŭs). Dignato; um feto malformado com uma mandíbula dupla. SIN augnathus. [G. *di-*, dois, + *gnathos*, mandíbula]
di·gox·i·gen·in (dī - joks′ī - jen - in). Digoxigenina; o aglicônio da digoxina que se junta a 3 moles de digitoxose para formar o glicosídeo digoxina.
di·gox·in (di-jok′sin). Digoxina; um glicosídeo esteróide cardioativo obtido da *Digitalis lanata*. Eliminado sobretudo pelos rins.
Di Guglielmo, Giovanni, médico italiano, 1886–1961. VER Di G.'s *disease, syndrome*.
di·gy·ny, di·gyn·ia (dī′ji - nē, dī - jin′ē - ă). Diginia; fertilização de um óvulo diplóide por um espermatozóide, que resulta em um zigoto triplóide. Cf. diandry. [di- + G. *gynē*, mulher]
di·het·er·o·zy·gote (dī - het′er - ō - zī′gōt). Dieterozigoto; indivíduo heterozigoto em dois *loci* de interesse, principalmente na análise da ligação genética.
di·hy·brid (dī - hī′brid). Diíbrido; a prole dos mesmos genitores diferentes em duas características. [G. *di-*, dois, + L. *hybrida*, prole de uma porca domesticada com um porco selvagem]
di·hy·dral·a·zine (dī - hī - dral′ă - zēn). Diidralazina; agente anti-hipertensivo.
di·hy·drate (dī - hī′drāt). Diidrato; composto com duas moléculas de água de cristalização.
di·hy·dra·zone (dī - hī′dră - zōn). Diidrazona. SIN osazone.
♲ **dihydro-**. Diidro-; prefixo que indica a adição de dois átomos de hidrogênio. [G. *di*, dois, + *hydor*, água]
di·hy·dro·a·scor·bic ac·id (dī - hī′drō - as - kōr′bik). Ácido diidroascórbico. SIN L-gulonolactone.
di·hy·dro·bi·op·ter·in (dī - hī′drō - bī - op′ter - in). Diidrobiopterina; precursor da tetraidrobiopterina, um co-fator necessário para várias enzimas, incluindo a biossíntese de L-tirosina; a incapacidade de sintetizar diidrobiopterina pode resultar em uma forma de hiperfenilalaninemia maligna.
  d. reductase, d. redutase. SIN dihydropteridine reductase.
di·hy·dro·co·deine tar·trate (dī - hī - drō - kō′dēn). Tartarato de diidrocodeína; derivado analgésico da codeína, cuja potência equivale a um sexto da potência da morfina; um narcótico antitussígeno.
di·hy·dro·co·de·i·none (dī - hī - drō - kō′dēn - ōn). Diidrocodeinona; hidrocodona. SIN hydrocodone.

4,5α-di·hy·dro·cor·ti·sol (dī-hī-drō-kōr′ti-sol). 4,5α-diidrocortisol. SIN hydrallostane.

di·hy·dro·cor·ti·sone (dī-hī-drō-kōr′ti-sōn). Diidrocortisona; um metabólito da cortisona reduzido na ligação dupla 4,5.

di·hy·dro·er·go·cor·nine (dī-hī′drō-er-gō-kōr′nīn). Diidroergocornina; um alcalóide derivado do esporão do centeio preparado pela hidrogenação da ergocornina e menos tóxico que esta última. VER dihydroergotoxine mesylate.

di·hy·dro·er·go·cris·tine (dī-hī′drō-er-go-kris′ten). Diidroergocristina; derivado alcalóide do esporão do centeio preparado pela hidrogenação da ergocristina e menos tóxica que esta. VER dihydroergotoxine mesylate.

di·hy·dro·er·go·cryp·tine (dī-hī′drō-er-gō-krip′ten). Diidroergocriptina; derivado alcalóide do esporão do centeio preparado pela hidrogenação da ergocriptina e menos tóxica do que esta. VER dihydroergotoxine mesylate.

di·hy·dro·er·got·a·mine (dī-hī′drō-er-got′a-mēn). Diidroergotamina; um alcalóide derivado do esporão do centeio preparado pela hidrogenação da ergotamina; usado no tratamento da enxaqueca; menos tóxico e menos ocitócico que a ergotamina.

di·hy·dro·er·go·tox·ine mes·y·late (dī-hī′drō-er-gō-tok′sēn). Mesilato de diidroergotoxina; uma mistura de metanessulfato de diidroergocornina, metanessulfato de diidroergocristina e metanes-sulfato de diidroergocriptina; usado como bloqueador α-adrenérgico para alívio de insuficiência cardiovascular.

di·hy·dro·fo·late re·duc·tase (DHFR) (dī-hī-drō-fō′lāt). Diidrofolato redutase; uma enzima que oxida reversivelmente o tetraidrofolato em 7,8-diidrofolato com NADP$^+$. Uma enzima fundamental no metabolismo de um carbono; usada como indicador de resistência ao metotrexato. SIN 5,6,7,8-tetrahydrofolate dehydrogenase.

7,8-di·hy·dro·fo·lic ac·id (dī-hī-drō-fō′lik). Ácido 7,8-diidrofólico; intermediário entre o ácido fólico e o ácido 5,6,7,8-tetraidrofólico, com a oxidação deste último exigindo NADP+ e desidrofolato redutase.

dihydrogen. Diidrogênio. SIN hydrogen (2).

di·hy·dro·lip·o·am·ide S-ace·tyl·trans·fer·ase (dī-hī′drō-lip-ō-am′id ā-se-til-trans′fer-āz). Diidrolipoamida S-acetiltransferase; enzima que catalisa a transferência de um grupamento acetil de S^6-acetildiidrolipoamida para a coenzima A. Uma parte de muitos complexos enzimáticos (p. ex., complexo da piruvato desidrogenase). SIN lipoate acetyltransferase, thiotransacetylase A.

di·hy·dro·lip·o·am·ide de·hy·dro·gen·ase (dī-hī′drō-lip-ō-am′id dī-hī-dro′jen-āz). Diidrolipoamida desidrogenase; uma flavoenzima que oxida a diidrolipoamida à custa do NAD$^+$; completa a descarboxilação oxidativa do piruvato; uma parte de vários complexos enzimáticos (p. ex., complexo da α-cetoglutarato desidrogenase). A redução da atividade leva à perda neuronal no cérebro, resultando em retardo psicomotor. SIN coenzyme factor, lipoamide dehydrogenase, lipoamide reductase (NADH), lipoyl dehydrogenase.

di·hy·dro·li·po·ic ac·id (dī-hī′drō-lip-ō′ik). Ácido diidrolipóico; ácido lipóico reduzido, formado por clivagem da ligação –S–S– como resultado da aceitação de dois hidrogênios. Cf. lipoic acid.

di·hy·dro·mor·phi·none hy·dro·chlo·ride (dī-hī-drō-mor′fi-nōn). Cloridrato de diidromorfinona. SIN hydromorphone hydrochloride.

di·hy·dro·or·o·tase (dī-hī′drō-ōr-ō′tās). Diidro-orotase; uma enzima que catalisa o fechamento do anel do N-carbamoil-L-aspartato para formar L-5,6-diidro-orotato e água; uma enzima na biossíntese da pirimidina. SIN carbamoylaspartate dehydrase.

di·hy·dro·or·o·tate (dī-hī′drō-ōr-ō′tāt). Diidro-orotato; L-5,6-diidro-orotato; um intermediário na biossíntese das pirimidinas.

di·hy·dro·pter·i·dine re·duc·tase. Diidropteridina redutase; uma enzima que catalisa a formação reversível da tetraidrobiopterina a partir da diidrobiopterina utilizando NADPH; a deficiência dessa enzima pode resultar em hiperfenilaninemia maligna. SIN dihydrobiopterin reductase.

di·hy·dro·pte·ro·ic ac·id (dī-hī′drō-te-rō′ik). Ácido diidropteróico; intermediário na formação do ácido fólico; um composto de 6-hidroximetilpterina e ácido p-aminobenzóico, cuja combinação é inibida por sulfonamidas.

di·hy·dro·py·rim·i·dine de·hy·dro·gen·ase (dī-hī-drō′pi-rim′i-dēn dē-hī-dro′jen-āz). Diidropirimidina desidrogenase; enzima na biossíntese da pirimidina que reage a 5,6-diidrouracil com NADP$^+$ para formar uracil e NADPH; também age sobre a diidrotimina; a deficiência dessa enzima pode resultar em hiperuracil timinúria. SIN dihydrouracil dehydrogenase.

di·hy·dro·strep·to·my·cin (dī-hī′drō-strep-tō-mī′sin). Diidroestreptomicina; um antibiótico aminoglicosídeo com ação semelhante à da estreptomicina, mas com um maior risco de ototoxicidade.

di·hy·dro·ta·chys·ter·ol (dī-hī′drō-tā-kis′ter-ōl). Diidrotaquisterol. VER tachysterol.

di·hy·dro·tes·tos·ter·one (dī-hī′drō-tes-tos′ter-ōn). Diidrotestosterona. SIN stanolone.

di·hy·dro·ur·a·cil (dī-hī-drō-ūr′a-sil). Diidrouracil; 5,6-diidrouracil; um produto da redução do uracil e um dos intermediários do catabolismo do uracil.

di·hy·dro·ur·a·cil de·hy·dro·gen·ase. Diidrouracil desidrogenase. SIN dihydropyrimidine dehydrogenase.

di·hy·dro·ur·i·dine (hU, hu, D) (dī-hī-drō-ūr′i-dēn). Diidrouridina; uridina na qual a ligação dupla 5,6 foi saturada pela adição de dois átomos de hidrogênio; um raro constituinte de ácidos ribonucleicos de transferência.

△ **dihydroxy-.** Diidroxi-; prefixo que designa a adição de dois grupamentos hidroxila; como um sufixo, torna-se –diol.

di·hy·drox·y·ac·e·tone (dī′hī-drok-sē-as′e-tōn). Diidroxiacetona; $HOCH_2$-CO-CH_2OH; 1,3-diidroxi-2-propanona; glicerona; a cetose mais simples. SIN glycerulose.
  d. phosphate (DHAP), fosfato de d.; um dos intermediários na via glicolítica e na biossíntese de gordura; fosfato de glicerona.
  d. phosphate acyltransferase, fosfato de d. aciltransferase; enzima que catalisa uma etapa importante da biossíntese do plasmalogênio; um grupamento acil da acil-CoA é transferido para o fosfato de diidroxiacetona, produzindo coenzima A livre e fosfato de 1-acildiidroxiacetona.

2,8-di·hy·drox·y·ad·en·ine (dī-hī-drok′sē-ad′e-nēn). 2,8-diidroxiadenina; um produto menor insolúvel do catabolismo da adenina que está elevado em indivíduos com ausência de adenina fosforribosiltransferase.

di·hy·drox·y·a·lu·mi·num ami·no·ac·e·tate (dī-hī-drok′sē-a-loo′mi-num am′i-nō-as′e-tāt). Aminoacetato de diidroxialumínio; glicinato básico de alumínio, um sal básico de alumínio do ácido aminoacético contendo pequenas quantidades de hidróxido de alumínio e ácido aminoacético; usado como antiácido na hipercloridria e na úlcera péptica.

di·hy·drox·y·a·lu·mi·num so·di·um car·bon·ate. Carbonato sódico de diidroxialumínio; um antiácido gástrico.

1α,25-di·hy·drox·y·cho·le·cal·cif·er·ol (dī-hī-drok′sē-ko′lē-kal-si-i′fer-ol). 1α,25-diidroxicolecalciferol; uma forma ativa de vitamina D formada nos túbulos contorcidos proximais do rim. A deficiência do receptor para 1α,25-diidroxicolecalciferol resulta em todas as características da deficiência de vitamina D_3.

1,25-di·hy·drox·y·er·go·cal·cif·er·ol (dī-hī-drok′sē-er′gō-kal-sif′er-ol). 1,25-diidroxiergocalciferol; um metabólito biologicamente ativo da vitamina D_2. SIN ercalcitriol.

3,4-di·hy·drox·y·phen·yl·al·a·nine (dī-hī-droks′e-fen-il-al′a-nēn). 3,4-diidroxifenilalanina. SIN dopa.

di·i·o·dide (dī-ī′ō-dīd). Diiodeto; um composto que contém dois átomos de iodo por molécula.

△ **diiodo-.** Diiodo-; prefixo que indica dois átomos de iodo. [G. di, + ioeidēs, cor da flor violeta]

di·i·o·do·hy·drox·y·quin (dī-ī-ō′dō-hī-drok′si-kwin). Diiodoidroxiquina; $C_9H_5I_2NO$; um agente antiprotozoário, usado no tratamento da amebíase intestinal. SIN diodoquin.

di·i·o·do·ty·ro·sine (DIT) (dī′ī-ō-dō-tī′rō-sēn). Diiodotirosina; um intermediário na biossíntese do hormônio tireoidiano.

di·i·so·pro·mine (dī-ī-sō-prō′mēn). Diisopromina; um colagogo. SIN disopromine.

di·i·so·pro·pyl flu·o·ro·phos·phate (DFP) (dī-ī-sō-prō′pil flōr-ō-fos′fāt). Fluorofosfato de diisopropil. SIN isofluorphate.

di·i·so·pro·pyl im·i·no·di·ace·tic ac·id (DISIDA) (dī-ē-sō-prō′pil im′i-nō-dī-ā-sē-tik). Ácido diisopropil iminodiacético; radiofármaco marcado com Tc[99m], usado para colecintigrafia. SIN disofenin.

2,6-di·i·so·pro·pyl phe·nol. 2,6-Diisopropil fenol. SIN propofol.

2,3-di·ke·to-L-gul·on·ate. 2,3-Diceto-L-gulonato; um produto do catabolismo da vitamina C; formado a partir do L-desidroascorbato; não tem atividade de vitamina C.

di·ke·to·hy·drin·dyl·i·dene-di·ke·to·hy·drin·da·mine (dī-kē′tō-hī-drin-dil′i-dēn dī-kē′tō-hī-drind′a-mēn). Dicetoindridilideno-dicetoindridamina; o produto colorido formado na reação de um α-aminoácido e ninidrina (hidrato de tricetoidrindeno); uma reação usada no ensaio quantitativo de α-aminoácidos.

di·ke·tone (dī-kē′tōn). Dicetona; uma molécula contendo dois grupamentos carbonila; p. ex., acetilacetona ($CH_3COCH_2COCH_3$).

di·ke·to·pi·per·a·zines (dī-kē′tō-pī-per′a-zēnz). Dicetopiperazinas; uma classe de compostos orgânicos com estrutura de anel fechado formada a partir de dois α-aminoácidos pela união do grupamento α-amino de cada um ao grupamento carboxila do outro, com a perda de duas moléculas de água.

dil. Abreviatura de L. dilue, diluir, ou L. dilutus, diluído.

di·lac·er·a·tion (dī-las-er-ā′shun). Deslocamento de alguma parte de um dente em desenvolvimento, que então se desenvolve em sua nova relação, resultando em um dente com raiz(ízes) profundamente angular(es). [L. di-lacero, pp. laceratus, rasgar em pedaços, de lacer, lacerar]

di·la·tan·cy (dī-lā′tan-sē). Dilatância, plasticidade inversa; um aumento da viscosidade com aumento progressivo da velocidade de cisalhamento acompanhado por expansão volumétrica. [L. dilato, dilatar]

dil·a·ta·tion (dil-ā-tā′shun). Dilatação. SIN dilation.
  digital d., d. digital; uso do dedo ou da ponta do dedo da mão para aumentar um orifício ou abertura, como o aumento cirúrgico do orifício de uma valva mitral esclerosada.

dil·a·ta·tor (dil′ā-tā-ter, -tōr). Dilatador. SIN dilator.

di·late (dī′lāt). Dilatar; realizar ou sofrer dilatação.

di·la·tion (dī - lā′shŭn). Dilatação. **1.** Aumento fisiológico ou artificial de uma estrutura oca ou abertura. **2.** O ato de distender ou aumentar uma abertura ou a luz de uma estrutura oca. SIN dilatation. [L. *dilato*, pp. *dilatatus*, espalhar, dilatar]

   d. and extraction, d. e extração; forma de abortamento na qual o colo do útero é dilatado e o feto extraído em pedaços utilizando fórceps cirúrgico; técnica usada para concluir um abortamento espontâneo no segundo trimestre ou como forma de abortamento induzido.

   post-stenotic d., d. pós-estenótica; dilatação de uma artéria, mais comumente a artéria pulmonar ou a aorta, distal a uma área de estreitamento.

   d. and suction, d. e aspiração. SIN suction *curettage*.

   urethral d., d. uretral; aumento do calibre da uretra pela introdução de um dilatador.

di·la·tion and cu·ret·tage (D & C). Dilatação e curetagem; dilatação do colo do útero e curetagem do endométrio.

di·la·tion and evac·u·a·tion (D & E). Dilatação e evacuação; dilatação do colo do útero e retirada dos produtos da concepção.

di·la·tor (dī′lā - tĕr). Dilatador. **1.** Instrumento designado para aumentar uma estrutura oca ou abertura. **2.** Um músculo que abre um orifício. **3.** Uma substância que causa dilatação ou aumento de uma abertura ou da luz de uma estrutura oca. VER TAMBÉM bougie. SIN dilatator.

   Chevalier-Jackson d., d. de Chevalier-Jackson; dilatador esofágico que passa através de um endoscópio rígido.

   Hanks d., d. de Hanks; dilatadores uterinos feitos de metal sólido.

   Hegar d.'s, dilatadores de Hegar; uma série de velas cilíndricas de tamanho graduado usadas para dilatar o canal cervical.

   hydrostatic d., d. hidrostático; instrumento para dilatar estenoses esofágicas; é aplicada pressão líquida a uma área flexível do instrumento colocada no local da estenose para estabelecer uma pressão dilatadora uniforme.

   d. ir'idis, d. da íris. SIN dilator pupillae *muscle*.

   Kollmann d., d. de Kollmann; instrumento expansível metálico usado para dilatar estenoses uretrais.

   pneumatic d., d. pneumático; qualquer um dentre vários cateteres acoplados a balões distais que podem ser insuflados até as pressões desejadas para ultrapassar obstruções em vísceras ocas; usados com maior freqüência para romper o esfíncter esofágico inferior e tratar a acalásia.

   Pratt d.'s, dilatadores de Pratt; bastões metálicos cilíndricos de tamanhos graduados usados para dilatar o canal cervical.

   d. of pupil, d. da pupila. SIN dilator pupillae *muscle*.

   Walther d., d. de Walther; instrumento delicadamente curvo que se afunila em um diâmetro crescente, usado para dilatar a uretra feminina.

dil·do, dil·doe (dil′dō). Um pênis artificial; um objeto que tem o formato e o tamanho aproximado de um pênis ereto, comumente feito de madeira, plástico ou borracha; utilizado para o prazer sexual.

di·lem·ma. Dilema.

   masking dilemma, problema encontrado no estabelecimento de limiares da condução óssea na perda auditiva condutiva bilateral grave, no qual o grau de mascaramento do ouvido não-testado ultrapassa a atenuação interaural de forma que o mascaramento suficiente é excessivo.

dill oil. Óleo de endro; um óleo volátil destilado do fruto da *Anethum graveolens* (família Umbelliferae); um carminativo.

di·lox·a·nide fu·ro·ate (dī - lok′să - nīd fū′rō - āt). Furoato de diloxanida; um amebicida usado no tratamento da disenteria.

dil·ti·a·zem hy·dro·chlo·ride (dil - tī′ă - zem). Cloridrato de diltiazem; um agente bloqueador dos canais de cálcio usado como dilatador coronariano, antiarrítmico e anti-hipertensivo.

dil·u·ent. Diluente. **1.** Ingrediente em um medicamento que não possui atividade farmacológica, mas é farmaceuticamente necessário ou desejável. Nos comprimidos ou cápsulas pode ser lactose ou amido; é particularmente útil para aumentar o volume de fármacos potentes cuja massa é pequena demais para a fabricação ou administração. Pode ser um líquido para a dissolução de um agente ou agentes a serem injetados, ingeridos ou inalados. **2.** Designa aquilo que dilui; o agente diluidor.

di·lute (dil.) (dī - loot′). Diluir. **1.** Reduzir uma solução ou mistura em concentração, potência, qualidade ou pureza. **2.** Diluído; designa uma solução ou mistura assim realizada. [L. *di-luo*, dissolver, diluir]

di·lu·tion (dī - loo′shŭn). Diluição. **1.** O ato de ser diluído. **2.** Uma solução ou mistura diluída. **3.** Em técnicas microbiológicas, um método para contar o número de células viáveis em uma suspensão; uma amostra é diluída até o ponto no qual uma alíquota, quando cultivada, produza um número contável de colônias distintas.

dim. Abreviatura de L. *dimidius*, metade.

di·ma·zole di·hy·dro·chlo·ride (dī′mā - zōl). Diidrocloreto de dimazol. SIN diamthazole dihydrochloride.

di·ma·zon (dī - mā′zon). Dimazona; um composto azo presente em cristais vermelhos; usada com vaselina como pomada para estimular a proliferação celular epitelial e, assim, promover a cicatrização de feridas superficiais.

di·me·lia (dī - mē′lē - ă). Dimelia; duplicação congênita de todo um membro ou de uma parte dele. [G. *di-*, dois, + *melos*, membro]

di·men·hy·dri·nate (dī - men - hī′dri - nāt). Dimenidrinato; o sal 8-clorotecofilina do anti-histamínico difenidramina; usado para a prevenção da cinetose, como anti-histamínico e sedativo leve. Também usado no tratamento da doença de Parkinson, pois tem consideráveis propriedades anticolinérgicas.

di·men·sion (di - men′shŭn). Dimensão; escopo, tamanho, magnitude; designa, no plural, medidas lineares de comprimento, largura e altura.

   buccolingual d., d. bucolingual; o diâmetro ou dimensão de um dente pré-molar ou molar da superfície bucal até a superfície lingual.

   occlusal vertical d., d. vertical oclusal; a dimensão vertical da face quando os dentes ou as bordas de oclusão estão em contato na oclusão cêntrica; a *diminuição* da dimensão vertical oclusal pode resultar de modificação do formato do dente por atrito ou rangido, desvio dos dentes ou, em pacientes desdentados, por reabsorção das cristas residuais; o *aumento* pode resultar da modificação do formato do dente, posição do dente, altura das bordas de oclusão, rebaseamento ou realinhamento, ou dispositivos de oclusão.

   rest vertical d., d. vertical de repouso; a dimensão vertical da face com as mandíbulas em relação de repouso; a *diminuição* da dimensão vertical de repouso pode ou não acompanhar uma diminuição da dimensão vertical oclusal; pode ocorrer sem diminuição da dimensão vertical oclusal em pacientes com uma atividade preponderante da musculatura de fechamento da mandíbula, como em pacientes com tensão muscular muito aumentada ou nos mastigadores crônicos de goma de mascar; o *aumento* da dimensão vertical em repouso pode ou não acompanhar um aumento da dimensão vertical de oclusão; algumas vezes ocorre após a remoção de contatos oclusais remanescentes, talvez em virtude da remoção de estímulos reflexos nocivos.

   vertical d., d. vertical; uma medida vertical da face entre quaisquer dois pontos arbitrariamente selecionados, localizados convenientemente, um acima e outro abaixo da boca, geralmente na linha média. SIN vertical opening.

di·mer (dī′mer). Dímero; um composto ou uma unidade produzida pela combinação de duas moléculas semelhantes; no sentido mais rigoroso, sem perda de átomos (assim, o tetróxido de nitrogênio, N_2O_4, é o dímero do óxido de nitrogênio, NO_2), mas geralmente por eliminação de H_2O ou uma pequena molécula semelhante entre os dois (p. ex., um dissacarídeo), ou por associação não-covalente simples (como de duas moléculas idênticas de proteínas); ordens superiores de complexidade são denominadas trímeros, tetrâmeros, oligômeros e polímeros. [G. *di-*, dois, + *-mer*]

   pyrimidine d., d. de pirimidina; um produto da irradiação ultravioleta das pirimidinas nos ácidos nucleicos; mais freqüentemente dímeros de timidina.

   thymine d., d. de timina; um produto da irradiação ultravioleta da timina (livre no gelo ou ligado em ácidos nucleicos) no qual dois resíduos timina são ligados por formação de um anel ciclobutano envolvendo tanto C-5 quanto C-6 à custa das duas ligações duplas; são possíveis várias formas estereoisoméricas.

di·mer·cap·rol (dī - mer - kap′rol). Dimercaprol; agente quelante, desenvolvido como antídoto de lewisita e outros venenos arsenicais. Atua competindo pelo metal com os grupamentos −SH essenciais no sistema piruvato oxidase das células e forma, com o arsênico, um composto cíclico estável, relativamente atóxico, com o metal possuindo uma maior afinidade por ele que pelos grupamentos −SH das proteínas celulares; também usado como antídoto para o antimônio, bismuto, cromo, mercúrio, ouro e níquel. SIN antilewisite, British anti-Lewisite.

di·mer·cur·i·on (dī - mer′kūr - ī′on). Dimercúrio; o íon mercúrico, Hg^{2+}.

di·mer·ic (dī′mer - ik). Dimérico; que possui as características de um dímero.

dim·er·ous (dim′er - ŭs). Dímero; que consiste em duas partes. [G. *di-*, dois, + *meros*, parte]

di·met·a·crine tar·trate (dī - met′ă - krēn). Tartarato de dimetacrina; um antidepressivo.

di·meth·a·di·one (dī - meth - ă - dī′ōn). Dimetadiona; o metabólito ativo formado pela *N*-desmetilação da trimetadiona, um agente antiepiléptico do tipo oxazolidina-diona. Pode ser usado para medida *in vivo* do pH intracelular.

di·meth·i·cone (dī - meth′i - kōn). Dimeticona; um óleo de silicone que consiste em polímeros dimetilsiloxano, geralmente incorporados a uma base de vaselina ou a uma preparação não-gordurosa, sendo usado para proteção da pele normal contra vários irritantes cutâneos, principalmente industriais; também pode ser usado para evitar a dermatite das fraldas.

di·meth·in·dene ma·le·ate (dī - meth′in - dēn). Maleato de dimetindeno; anti-histamínico também usado como antipruriginoso.

di·me·this·ter·one (dī - me - this′ter - ōn). Dimetisterona; uma testosterona ou etisterona modificada; uma progestina sintética, efetiva por via oral, usada isoladamente ou associada ao etinil estradiol como agente contraceptivo.

di·meth·o·thi·a·zine mes·y·late (dī - meth - ō - thī′ă - zēn). Mesilato de dimetotiazina. SIN fonazine mesylate.

di·me·thox·a·nate hy·dro·chlo·ride (dī′me - thok′să - nāt). Cloridrato de dimetoxanato; agente antitussígeno não-narcótico, menos efetivo que a codeína.

di·me·thox·y·am·phet·a·mine (DMA). Dimetoxianfetamina; alucinógeno com propriedades semelhantes às da dietilamida do ácido lisérgico (*lysergic acid* diethylamide [LSD]).

2,5-di·me·thox·y-4-meth·yl·am·phet·a·mine (DOM). 2,5-dimetoxi-4-metilanfetamina; um agente alucinógeno quimicamente relacionado à anfetamina e à mescalina, uma droga ilícita.

di·meth·yl·al·lyl·py·ro·phos·phate (di - meth'il - ăl'lil - pī'rō - fos'fāt). Dimetilalilpirofosfato; um intermediário na biossíntese de esteróides e terpeno.

di·meth·yl·a·mi·no·az·o·ben·zene (dī - meth'il - ă - mē - nō - az - ō - ben'zēn) [C.I. 11160]. Dimetilaminoazobenzeno. SIN butter yellow.

di·meth·yl·ar·sin·ic ac·id (dī - meth'il - ar - sin'ik). Ácido dimetilarsínico. SIN cacodylic acid.

di·meth·yl·ben·zene (dī - meth - il - ben'zēn). Dimetilbenzeno. SIN xylol.

5,6-di·meth·yl·benz·im·id·a·zole (dī - meth'il - benz - ē - mid - a - zōl). 5,6-dimetilbenzimidazol; uma porção estrutural encontrada em uma das cobalaminas.

di·meth·yl·car·bi·nol (dī - meth - il - kar'bi - nol). Dimetilcarbinol. SIN isopropyl alcohol.

di·meth·yl-1-car·bo·me·thox·y-1-pro·pen-2-yl phos·phate. Fosfato de dimetil-1-carbometoxi-1-propeno-2-il; composto orgânico de fósforo usado como veneno sistêmico para a exterminação de pestes como ácaros, pulgões e moscas domésticas.

β,β-di·meth·yl·cys·teine (dī - meth - il - sis'tē - ēn). β,β-dimetilcisteína. SIN penicillamine.

di·meth·yl im·in·o·di·ace·tic ac·id (HIDA) (dī - meth'il im'i - nō - dī - ă - sē - tik). Ácido dimetil iminodiacético; radiofármaco marcado com Tc^{99m}, um agente inicial usado para colecintigrafia.

di·meth·yl ke·tone (dī - meth'il kē'tōn). Dimetil cetona. SIN acetone.

di·meth·yl mer·cu·ry (dī - meth - il - mer'kŭ - rē). Dimetil mercúrio; um contaminante de frutos-do-mar sintetizado em sedimentos a partir do mercúrio e de compostos químicos contendo mercúrio despejados em águas com vida marinha. O metilmercúrio é concentrado em formas de vida aquáticas e, assim, pode depositar-se em peixes usados para consumo humano. A causa provável da doença de Minimata, distúrbio teratogênico caracterizado por múltiplos defeitos congênitos. Um reagente inorgânico. VER TAMBÉM Minamata *disease.* SIN methylmercury.

di·meth·yl·phe·nol (dī - meth - il - fē'nol). Dimetilfenol. SIN xylenol.

di·meth·yl·phen·yl·pi·per·a·zin·i·um (DMPP) (dī - meth'il - fe - n'il - pi - pār - ă - zin'ē - um). Dimetilfenilpiperazínio; estimulante extremamente seletivo de células ganglionares autônomas; usado experimentalmente.

di·meth·yl phthal·ate (dī - meth'il thal'āt). Ftalato de dimetila; repelente de insetos.

di·meth·yl·pi·per·a·zine tar·trate (dī - meth'il - pi - pār'a - zēn). Tartarato de dimetilpiperazina; um diurético, também usado como solvente de ácido úrico.

di·meth·yl sul·fate. Sulfato de dimetila; substância química industrial (éster dimetil do ácido sulfúrico $(CH_3)_2SO_4$) usada na síntese como agente alquilante; causa nistagmo, convulsões e morte por complicações pulmonares.

di·meth·yl sulf·ox·ide (DMSO) (dī - meth'il). Sulfóxido de dimetila; Me$_2$SO; um solvente penetrante, que aumenta a absorção de agentes terapêuticos pela pele; um solvente industrial que foi proposto como analgésico efetivo e antiinflamatório na artrite e na bursite.

***N,N*-di·meth·yl·tryp·ta·mine (DMT)** (dī - meth'il - trip'tă - mēn). *N,N*-dimetiltriptamina; agente psicotomimético presente em diversos tabacos sul-americanos (p. ex., tabaco de cooba) e nas folhas da *Prestonia amazonica* (família Apocynaceae). Os efeitos são semelhantes aos do LSD, porém com início mais rápido, maior probabilidade de uma reação de pânico e menor duração (1 a 2 horas, "viagem de homem de negócios"); produz efeitos autônomos acentuados, incluindo um aumento significativo da pressão arterial.

di·meth·yl *d*-tu·bo·cu·ra·rine. Dimetil *d*-tubocurarina. SIN metocurine iodide.

di·meth·yl tu·bo·cu·ra·rine chlo·ride. Cloreto de dimetil *d*-tubocurarina; éter dimetílico do cloreto de *d*-tubocurarina; um relaxante da musculatura esquelética. VER tubocurarine chloride.

di·meth·yl tu·bo·cu·ra·rine io·dide. Iodeto de dimetil tubocurarina. SIN metocurine iodide.

di·me·tria (dī - mē'trē - ă). Dimetria; termo obsoleto para útero didelfo (*uterus didelphys*). [G. *di-*, dois, + *mētra*, útero]

Dimmer, Friedrich, oftalmologista austríaco, 1855–1926. VER D. *keratitis.*

di·mor·phic (dī - mōr'fik). Dimórfico. **1.** Em fungos, um termo que se refere ao crescimento e à reprodução em duas formas: mofo e levedura. SIN dimorphous (2). **2.** SIN dimorphous (1).

di·mor·phism (dī - mōr'fizm). Dimorfismo. **1.** Existência em dois formatos ou formas; designa uma diferença de forma cristalina exibida pela mesma substância, ou uma diferença na forma ou aspecto externo entre indivíduos da mesma espécie (p. ex., dimorfismo sexual). **2.** A ocorrência, em vegetais, de duas formas distintas de folhas ou outras partes na mesma planta. [G. *di-*, dois, + *morphe,* formato]

sexual d., d. sexual; as diferenças somáticas entre machos e fêmeas da mesma espécie, que surgem em conseqüência da maturação sexual; incluem as características sexuais secundárias, mas não se restringem a estas.

di·mor·phous (dī - mōr'fŭs). Dimórfico. **1.** Que possui a propriedade de dimorfismo. SIN dimorphic (2). **2.** SIN dimorphic (1).

dim·ple (dim'pl). **1.** Covinha; uma depressão natural, geralmente circular e de pequena área, no queixo, bochecha ou região sacral. **2.** Uma depressão de aspecto semelhante a uma covinha resultante de traumatismo ou da contração do tecido cicatricial. **3.** Produzir covinhas.

coccygeal d., fovéola coccígea. SIN coccygeal *foveola.*
postanal d., fovéola coccígea. SIN coccygeal *foveola.*

dimp·ling. 1. Produzir covinhas. **2.** Condição caracterizada pela formação de covinhas, naturais ou artificiais.

di·ner·ic (dī - ner'ik). Dinérico; relativo à interface entre dois líquidos mutuamente imiscíveis (p. ex., óleo e água) no mesmo recipiente. [di- + G. *nerōn,* água]

di·ni·tro·cel·lu·lose (dī - nī - trō - sel'ū - lōs). Dinitrocelulose. SIN pyroxylin.

4,6-di·ni·tro-*o*-cre·sol. 4,6-dinitro-*o*-cresol; inseticida usado contra ácaros na forma de *spray* ou pó; também usado como herbicida.

di·ni·tro·gen mon·ox·ide (dī - nī'trō - jen). Monóxido de dinitrogênio. SIN nitrous oxide.

2,4-di·ni·tro·phe·nol (DNP, Dnp) (dī - nī - trō - fē'nol). 2,4-dinitrofenol; N$_2$pH-OH; um corante tóxico, quimicamente relacionado ao nitrofenol (ácido pícrico), usado em estudos bioquímicos de processos oxidativos, onde desacopla a fosforilação oxidativa; também é um estimulante metabólico.

di·no·flag·el·late (dī - nō - flaj'ē - lāt). Dinoflagelado; um flagelado semelhante a um vegetal da subclasse Phytomastigophorea, da qual algumas espécies (p. ex., *Gonyaulax cantanella*) produzem uma potente neurotoxina que pode causar grave intoxicação alimentar após a ingestão de frutos-do-mar parasitados. [G. *dinos*, redemoinho, + L. *flagellum*, flagelo]

Dinoflagellida. Uma ordem no filo Sarcomastigophorea caracterizada pela presença de dois flagelos posicionados de forma a fazer com que o organismo se mova em espiral. Sua superfície externa é composta de placas contendo celulose, cujo tamanho e número variam com o gênero e espécie.

di·no·prost (dī'nō - prost). Dinoprost; um agente ocitócico. SIN prostaglandin F$_{2\alpha}$.
d. tromethamine, agente ocitócico. SIN prostaglandin F$_{2\alpha}$ tromethamine.

di·no·pros·tone (dī - nō - pros'tōn). Dinoprostona; agente ocitócico usado como abortivo. SIN prostaglandin E$_2$.

di·nu·cle·o·tide (dī - noo'klē - ō - tīd). Dinucleotídeo; um composto contendo dois nucleotídeos; p. ex., NAD$^+$, ApGp.

Di·oc·to·phy·ma (dī - ok - tō - fī'mă). Gênero de vermes nematódeos muito grandes que infestam o rim. [L. do G. *dionkoō*, distender, + *phyma*, crescimento]
D. rena'le, um grande nematódeo vermelho-sangue encontrado na pelve renal e na cavidade peritoneal do cachorro; muito comum em carnívoros selvagens, como a marta, mas raramente encontrado em seres humanos; o ciclo vital inclui sanguessugas ectoparasitárias do lagostim, que são então ingeridas por vários peixes e, finalmente, pelos seres humanos ou por qualquer dos vários outros hospedeiros mamíferos que comem peixe.

di·oc·to·phy·mi·a·sis (dī - ok'tō - fi - mī'a - sis). Dioctofimíase; infestação de animais e raramente de seres humanos pelo verme renal gigante *Dictophyma renale.*

di·oc·tyl cal·ci·um sul·fo·suc·ci·nate (dī - ok'til kal'sē - ŭm sŭl - fō - sŭk'si - nāt). Sulfossuccinato cálcico de dioctila. SIN docusate calcium.

di·oc·tyl so·di·um sul·fo·suc·ci·nate. Sulfossuccinato sódico de dioctila. SIN docusate sodium.

Di·o·don (dī'ō - don). Gênero de peixes baiacus-de-espinho, relacionados com o peixe-balão, baiacus e vários peixes da família Tetraodontidae. Embora o soprador comum seja amplamente ingerido como "borracho marinho" nos Estados Unidos, muitos sopradores, especialmente no Pacífico, são venenosos devido à presença de uma neurotoxina, tetrodotoxina, no fígado e no ovário. [G. *di-*, dois, + *odous* (*odont-*), dente]

di·o·done (dī'ō - dōn). Diodona. SIN iodopyracet.

di·o·do·quin (dī - ō'dō - kwin). Diodoquina. SIN diiodohydroxyquin.

Diogenes, de Sinope, filósofo grego, 412–323 a.C. VER D. *cup; poculum* diogenis.

-diol (dī'ol). –diol. **1.** Forma sufixa do prefixo diidroxi. **2.** Um membro de uma classe de substâncias que contêm dois grupamentos hidroxila.
gym-diol, gym-diol, composto no qual ambos os grupamentos hidroxila estão fixados ao mesmo átomo de carbono; um intermediário em muitas reações.

di·ol·a·mine (dī - ōl'ă - mēn). Diolamina; contração aprovada por USAN para dietanolamina.

di·op·ter (D) (dī - op'ter). Dioptria; a unidade do poder de refração das lentes, designando a recíproca do comprimento focal expresso em metros. [G. *dioptra*, um instrumento de nivelamento]
prism d. (p.d.), d. do prisma; a unidade de medida do desvio da luz ao atravessar um prisma, sendo uma deflexão de 1 cm a distância de 1 m.

di·op·trics (dī - op'triks). Dióptrico; o ramo da óptica relacionado com a refração da luz.

di·os·cin (dī - ōs - in). Dioscina; uma saponina esteróide encontrada em inhames (Dioscorea) e trílios.

di·ose (dī′ōs). Diose. SIN glycolaldehyde.

di·os·gen·in (dī′os-jen′in). Diosgenina; o aglicônio da dioscina, uma sapogenina derivada das saponinas dioscina e trilina encontradas nas raízes e plantas como o inhame; sua porção esteróide serve como fonte a partir da qual podem ser preparadas a pregnenolona e a progesterona.

di·otic (dī-ot′ik). Diótico; apresentação simultânea do mesmo som a cada ouvido. [di- + otic]

di·ov·u·lar (dī′ov-ū-lar). Diovular; relativo a dois óvulos. SIN biovular. [di- + L. Mod. *ovulum*, dim. do L. *ovum*, ovo]

di·ov·u·la·to·ry (dī-ō′vū-lă-tō′rē). Diovulatório; que libera dois óvulos em um ciclo ovariano.

di·ox·ane (dī-oks′ān). Dioxana; 1,4-dioxana; um líquido incolor usado como solvente para ésteres da celulose e em histologia como agente secante. SIN 1,4-diethylene dioxide.

di·ox·ide (dī-oks′īd). Dióxido; uma molécula que contém dois átomos de oxigênio; p. ex., dióxido de carbono, CO_2.

di·ox·in (dī-oks′in). Dioxina. **1.** Um anel que consiste em dois átomos de oxigênio, quatro grupamentos CH e duas ligações duplas; as posições dos átomos de oxigênio são especificadas por prefixos, como na 1,4-dioxina. **2.** Abreviatura de dibenzo[*b,e*][1,4]dioxina, que pode ser visualizada como um anidrido de duas moléculas de 1,2-benzenediol (pirocatecol), assim formando duas pontes de oxigênio entre duas porções benzeno, ou como uma 1,4-dioxina com um anel benzeno fundido para captar cada um dos dois grupamentos CH=CH. **3.** Um contaminante no herbicida, 2,4,5-T; é potencialmente tóxico, teratogênico e carcinogênico.

di·ox·y·ben·zone (dī-ok-sē-ben′zōn). Dioxibenzona; um filtro de luz ultravioleta para aplicação tópica na pele.

di·ox·y·gen·ase (dī-oks′ē-jen-ās). Dioxigenase; uma oxidorredutase que incorpora dois átomos de oxigênio (de uma molécula de O_2) ao substrato (reduzido).

D.I.P. Abreviatura de desquamative interstitial *pneumonia* (pneumonia intersticial descamativa).

dip. 1. Inclinação, colapso; inclinação descendente ou declive. **2.** Banho; preparado para revestir uma superfície por submersão, como para a destruição de parasitas cutâneos. [I.M. *dippen*]

Cournand d., colapso de Cournand; na pericardite constritiva, a rápida queda protodiastólica e reascensão da curva de pressão ventricular até um platô elevado (configuração em raiz quadrada).

di·pep·ti·dase (dī-pep′ti-dās). Dipeptidase; uma hidrolase que catalisa a hidrólise de um dipeptídeo em seus aminoácidos constituintes.

methionyl d., metionil d.; uma hidrolase que catalisa a hidrólise de um aminoácido L-metionil em L-metionina e um aminoácido.

di·pep·tide (dī-pep′tīd). Dipeptídeo; uma combinação de dois aminoácidos por meio de uma ligação peptídica (—CO—NH—).

di·pep·ti·dyl·car·box·y·pep·ti·dase (dī-pep′ti-dil). Dipeptidil carboxipeptidase. SIN peptidyl dipeptidase A.

di·pep·ti·dyl pep·ti·dase. Dipeptidil peptidase; uma hidrolase que ocorre em várias formas; d. p. I, dipeptidil transferase, que cliva dipeptídeos da extremidade amino dos polipeptídeos; d. p. II, com propriedades semelhantes àquelas da I, tem uma especificidade diferente e atua preferencialmente sobre os tripeptídeos; d. p. III atua sobre peptídeos mais longos.

di·pep·ti·dyl trans·fer·ase. Dipeptidil transferase; cliva dipeptídeos da extremidade amino dos polipeptídeos. VER dipeptidyl peptidase.

Di·pet·a·lo·ne·ma (dī-pet′a-lō-ne′mă). Gênero de nematódeos filariformes com espécies no homem e em muitos outros mamíferos; como outras filárias, produzem microfilárias no sangue ou nos líquidos teciduais, sendo encontrados os adultos no tecido conjuntivo profundo, membranas ou superfícies viscerais. [G. *di-*, dois, + *petalon*, folha, + *nēma*, filamento]

D. recondi'tum, espécie de filária encontrada em cães, transmitida por pulgas e piolhos, em contraste com a dirofilária canina, *Dirofilaria immitis*, que é transmitida por mosquitos.

D. streptocer'ca, nome antigo da *Mansonella streptocerca*.

di·phal·lus (dī-fal′ŭs). Difalia; anomalia congênita rara na qual o pênis apresenta duplicação parcial ou completa; podem ser simétricos, ou colocados um sobre o outro; freqüentemente há anomalias urogenitais ou outras anomalias associadas; ocorre quando há desenvolvimento de dois tubérculos genitais. Também pode estar associada a extrofia vesical e divisão do tubérculo genital. SIN bifid penis. [G. *di-*, dois, + *phallos*, pênis]

di·pha·sic (dī-fā′zik). Difásico; que ocorre em, ou caracterizado por, duas fases ou estágios.

di·phe·ma·nil meth·yl·sul·fate (dī-fē′mă-nil). Metilsulfato de difemanil; um agente anticolinérgico.

di·phem·e·thox·i·dine (dī-fem-ē-thok′si-dēn). Difemetoxidina; um agente anorexigênico.

di·phen·a·di·one (dī-fen-a-dī′ōn). Difenadiona; anticoagulante efetivo por via oral, com ações e usos semelhantes aos da bisidroxicumarina.

di·phen·an (dī′fen-ān, dī-fen′an). Difenano; usado como vermicida na oxiuríase.

di·phen·hy·dra·mine hy·dro·chlo·ride (dī-fen-hī′dră-mēn). Cloridrato de difenidramina; um anti-histamínico H_2 com propriedades anticolinérgicas e sedativas.

di·phen·i·dol (dī-fen′i-dol). Difenidol; antiemético.

o-di·phe·no·lase (dī-fen′ō-lās). o-difenolase; SIN catechol oxidase.

di·phe·nol ox·i·dase (dī-fen′ol). Difenol oxidase. SIN catechol oxidase.

di·phe·nox·y·late hy·dro·chlo·ride (dī-fen-ok′si-lāt). Cloridrato de difenoxilato; agente antidiarreico, quimicamente relacionado à meperidina, que inibe a contração rítmica da musculatura lisa; é pouco viciador. Semelhante à loperamida.

di·phen·yl (dī-fen′il). Difenil; líquido incolor; usado como agente de transferência de calor, freqüentemente como bifenis policlorados (PCB); como fungistático para laranjas (aplicado no interior dos contêineres em navios ou nos invólucros); e em sínteses orgânicas. Causa convulsões e depressão do sistema nervoso central. SIN biphenyl, phenylbenzene.

diphenyl-. Difenil-; prefixo que designa dois grupamentos fenil independentes fixados a um terceiro átomo ou radical, como na difenilamina.

di·phen·yl·chlor·ar·sine (dī-fen′il-klōr-ar′sēn). Difenilclorarsina; esternutatório, cuja inalação causa espirros violentos, tosse, salivação, cefaléia e dor retroesternal; um agente causador de vômitos comum usado no controle de multidões e tumultos.

di·phen·yl·cy·an·o·ar·sine (dī-fen′il-sī-an-ō-ar-sēn). Difenilcianoarsina; agente comum, causador de vômitos, usado no controle de multidões e tumultos.

di·phen·yl·en·i·mine (dī′fen-il-ēn′i-mēn). Difenilenimina. SIN carbazole.

di·phen·yl·hy·dan·to·in (dī′fen-il-hī-dan′tō-in). Difenilidantoína. VER phenytoin.

5,5-di·phen·yl·hy·dan·to·in (dī-fen′il-hī-dan′tō-in). 5,5-difenilidantoína. SIN phenytoin.

2,5-di·phen·yl·ox·a·zole (PPO) (dī′fen-il-oks′ā-zōl). 2,5-difeniloxazol; cintilador usado em medidas da radioatividade por contagem de cintilação líquida.

di·phen·yl·pyr·a·line hy·dro·chlo·ride (dī-fen-il-pir′ā-lēn). Cloridrato de difenilpiralina; anti-histamínico H_1 com ação e uso semelhantes aos da difenidramina.

di·phos·gene (dī-fos′jēn). Difosgênio; gás venenoso usado na I Guerra Mundial; também é discretamente lacrimejante.

di·phos·pha·tase (dī-fos′fa-tāz). Difosfatase. SIN pyrophosphatase.

inorganic diphosphatase, d. inorgânica. SIN inorganic *pyrophosphatase.*

di·phos·phate. Difosfato. SIN pyrophosphate.

di·phos·pho·thi·a·min (dī′fos-fō-thī′ă-min). Difosfotiamina. SIN thiamin pyrophosphate.

diph·the·ria (dif-thē-r′ēă). Difteria; doença infecciosa específica causada pela bactéria *Corynebacterium diphtheriae* e sua toxina extremamente potente; caracterizada por inflamação grave que pode formar um revestimento membranoso, com formação de exsudato fibrinoso espesso, da mucosa da faringe, do nariz e, algumas vezes, da árvore traqueobrônquica; a toxina produz degeneração nos nervos periféricos, no músculo cardíaco e em outros tecidos. A difteria tinha elevada taxa de fatalidade, principalmente em crianças, mas agora é rara devido à existência de uma vacina efetiva. [G. *diphthera*, couro]

cutaneous d., d. cutânea; uma úlcera superficial, em "saca-bocado", algumas vezes limitada ou seguida por uma bolha, resultante de infecção da pele por *Corynebacterium diphtheriae*; as manifestações sistêmicas são iguais às da difteria faríngea.

false d., d. falsa. SIN diphtheroid (1).

faucial d., d. da fauce; faringite grave que afeta as fauces, o local habitual afetado por infecção por *Corynebacterium diphtheriae*.

laryngeal d., d. laríngea; difteria que afeta a laringe, geralmente com asfixia causada por obstrução das vias aéreas pela membrana que se forma, com evolução fatal. SIN laryngotracheal d.

laryngotracheal d., d. laringotraqueal. SIN laryngeal d.

diph·the·ri·al, diph·the·rit·ic (dif-thē-r′ēăl, dif-thē-rit′ik). Diftérico; relativo à difteria, ou o exsudato membranoso característico dessa doença. SIN diphtheric.

diph·ther·ic. Diftérico. SIN diphtherial.

diph·the·roid (dif′thē-royd). Difteróide. **1.** Uma dentre várias infecções locais que sugerem difteria, mas causada por outros microrganismos além de *Corynebacterium diphtheriae*. SIN Epstein disease, false diphtheria, pseudodiphtheria. **2.** Qualquer microrganismo semelhante a *Corynebacterium diphtheriae*. [diphtheria + G. *eidos*, semelhança]

diph·the·ro·tox·in (dif′thēr-ō-tok′sin). Difterotoxina; a toxina da difteria.

di·phyl·lo·both·ri·a·sis (dī-fil′ō-both-rī′ă-sis). Difilobotríase; infestação pelo cestódeo *Diphyllobothrium latum*; a infestação humana é causada pela ingestão de peixe cru ou mal cozido infectado pela larva plerocercóide. Pode haver leucocitose e eosinofilia; se o verme estiver em posição suficientemente alta no canal alimentar, pode apropriar-se antecipadamente do suprimento de vitamina B_{12} ou impedir sua absorção, levando à anemia macrocítica hipercrômica semelhante à anemia perniciosa; todavia, esse distúrbio é raro, mesmo em áreas hiperendêmicas. SIN bothriocephaliasis.

Di·phyl·lo·both·ri·um (dī-fil-lō-both′rē-ŭm). Grande gênero de tênias (ordem Pseudophyllidea) caracterizado por um escólex espatulado com sulcos de sucção dorsais e ventrais ou bótrias. São encontradas várias espécies nos seres humanos, embora apenas uma, *D. latum*, tenha real importância. [G. *di-*, dois, + *phyllon*, folha, + *bothrion*, pequeno poço]

D. corda'tum, espécie encontrada em cães, mamíferos marinhos e, ocasionalmente, em seres humanos na Groenlândia.

D. dendriticum, forma adulta da tênia encontrada no intestino de aves que comem peixes; infesta os seres humanos.

D. hians, espécie de tênia encontrada em seres humanos no Japão.

D. houghtoni, tênia de cães e gatos; encontrada em seres humanos na China.

D. la'tum, a tênia do peixe, uma espécie que causa difilobotríase, encontrada em seres humanos e em mamíferos que se alimentam de peixe em muitas partes do norte da Europa, Japão e outras regiões da Ásia, e em populações escandinavas dos estados centro-setentrionais da América do Norte; freqüentemente tem 3 ou 4 mil segmentos, com largura maior que o comprimento; a cabeça possui bótrias típicas características do gênero. SIN *Dibothriocephalus latus*.

D. linguloi'des, SIN *Spirometra mansoni*.

D. man'soni, SIN *Spirometra mansoni*.

D. mansonoi'des, SIN *Spirometra mansonoides*.

D. nihonkaiense, espécie de tênia intimamente relacionada ao *Diphyllobothrium latum*; encontrada no Japão com números cada vez maiores de infestações humanas.

D. orcini, espécie de tênia encontrada em seres humanos no Japão.

D. pacificum, espécie de tênia encontrada em leões-marinhos; foi descrita como uma tênia humana adquirida de peixes marinhos; encontrada no Japão, Peru e Equador.

D. scoticum, espécie de tênia encontrada em seres humanos no Japão.

di·phy·o·dont (dī-fī′e-ō-dont). Difiodonte; que possui duas séries de dentes, como ocorre em seres humanos e na maioria dos outros mamíferos. [G. *di-*, dois, + *phyō*, produzir, + *odous* (*odont-*), dente]

di·pi·pro·ver·ine (dī-pī-prō′ver-ēn). Dipiproverina; antiespasmódico intestinal.

di·piv·e·frin hy·dro·chlo·ride (dī-piv′e-frin). Cloridrato de dipivefrina; uma pró-droga adrenérgica da epinefrina, usada na forma de gotas, no tratamento inicial para controle da pressão intra-ocular em portadores de glaucoma crônico de ângulo aberto.

dip·la·cu·sis (dip-lă-koo′sis). Diplacusia; percepção anormal do som, seja em ritmo ou em altura, de forma que um som é ouvido como dois. [G. *diplous*, duplo, + *akousis*, audição]

d. binaura'lis, d. biauricular; condição na qual o som é ouvido de forma diferente pelos dois ouvidos.

d. dysharmon'ica, d. desarmônica; condição na qual o mesmo som é ouvido com uma altura diferente em cada ouvido.

d. echo'ica, d. ecóica; condição na qual o som ouvido no ouvido afetado é repetido.

d. monaura'lis, d. monoauricular; condição na qual um som é percebido como dois no mesmo ouvido.

di·ple·gia (dī-plē′jē-ă). Diplegia; paralisia das partes correspondentes nos dois lados do corpo. SIN double hemiplegia. [G. *di-*, dois, + *plēgē*, ataque de paralisia]

congenital facial d., d. facial congênita. SIN Möbius *syndrome*.

facial d., d. facial; paralisia dos dois lados da face.

infantile d., d. infantil. SIN spastic d.

masticatory d., d. mastigatória; paralisia de todos os músculos da mastigação.

spastic d., d. espástica; um tipo de paralisia cerebral em que há espasticidade bilateral, sendo os membros inferiores afetados mais gravemente. Cf. flaccid *paralysis*. SIN Erb-Charcot disease (1), infantile d., Little disease, spastic spinal paralysis.

△ **diplo-.** Diplo-; duplo, duplicado. VER haplo-. [G. *diploos*, duplo]

dip·lo·al·bu·mi·nu·ria (dip′lō-al-bū-mi-noo′rē-ă). Diploalbuminúria; a coexistência de albuminúria nefrítica, ou anormal, e não-nefrítica, ou fisiológica.

dip·lo·ba·cil·lus (dip′lō-bă-sil′ŭs). Diplobacilo; duas células bacterianas em forma de bacilo unidas pelas extremidades. [diplo- + bacillus]

dip·lo·blas·tic (dip-lō-blas′tik). Diploblástico; formado de duas camadas germinativas. [diplo- + G. *blastos*, germe]

dip·lo·car·dia (dip-lō-kar′dē-ă). Diplocardia; anomalia na qual as metades esquerda e direita do coração são separadas em graus variáveis por uma fissura central. [diplo- + G. *kardia*, coração]

dip·lo·ceph·a·lus (dip-lō-sef′ă-lŭs). Diplocéfalo. SIN dicephalus.

dip·lo·chei·ria, dip·lo·chi·ria (dip′lō-kī′rē-ă). Diploquiria. SIN dicheiria. [diplo- + G. *cheir*, mão]

dip·lo·coc·ce·mia (dip-lō-kok-sē′mē-ă). Diplococcemia; a presença de diplococos no sangue; termo usado especialmente em referência à *Neisseria meningitidis* (meningococos) no sangue circulante.

dip·lo·coc·ci (dip′lō-kok′sī). Diplococos; plural de diplococcus.

dip·lo·coc·cin (dip-lō-kok′sin). Diplococcina; uma substância antibiótica cristalina isolada de culturas de cocos produtores de ácido lático presentes no leite ativo contra lactobacilos e determinados cocos Gram-positivos, mas inativo contra bactérias Gram-negativas.

Dip·lo·coc·cus (dip′lō-kok′ŭs). As espécies desse antigo gênero de bactérias agora são classificadas em outros gêneros. O *Diplococcus pneumoniae*, a espécie típica de *D.*, é um membro do gênero *Streptococcus*. VER *Neisseria*, *Peptococcus*, *Streptococcus*. [diplo- + G. *kokkos*, bago]

dip·lo·coc·cus, pl. **dip·lo·coc·ci** (dip′lō-kok′ŭs, -kok′sī). Diplococo. **1.** Células bacterianas esféricas ou ovóides unidas em pares. **2.** Nome comum de qualquer microrganismo que pertença ao antigo gênero bacteriano *Diplococcus*. [diplo- + G. *kokkos*, bago]

dip·lo·co·ri·a (dip-lō-kō′rē-ă). Diplocoria; a ocorrência de duas pupilas no olho. SIN dicoria. [diplo- + G. *korē*, pupila]

dip·loë (dip′lō-ē). [TA]. Díploe; a camada central de osso esponjoso entre as duas camadas de osso compacto, as tábuas externa e interna dos ossos chatos do crânio. [G. *diploē*, fem. de *diplous*, duplo]

dip·lo·gen·e·sis (dip-lō-jen′ĕ-sis). Diplogênese; produção de um feto duplo ou com algumas partes duplicadas. [diplo- + G. *genesis*, produção]

Dip·lo·go·nop·o·rus (dip′lō-gō-nop′o-rŭs). Gênero de tênias encontradas no Japão (*D. grandis*) e, provavelmente, também na Romênia (*D. brauni*) [diplo- + G. *gonos*, semente, + *poros*, poro]

di·plo·ic (dip-lō′ik). Diplóico; relativo à díploe.

dip·loid (dip′loyd). Diplóide; designa o estado de uma célula que contém dois conjuntos haplóides derivados do pai e da mãe, respectivamente; o complemento cromossomial normal de células somáticas (nos seres humanos, 46 cromossomas). [diplo- + G. *eidos*, semelhança]

dip·lo·kar·y·on (dip′lō-kar′ē-on). Diplocárion; um núcleo celular que contém quatro conjuntos haplóides; isto é, um núcleo tetraplóide. VER TAMBÉM polyploidy. [diplo- + G. *karyon*, núcleo]

dip·lo·mel·i·tu·ria (dip′lō-mel-i-too′rē-ă). Diplomelitúria; a ocorrência de glicosúria diabética e não-diabética no mesmo indivíduo. [diplo- + G. *meli*, mel, + *ouron*, urina]

dip·lo·my·e·lia (dip-lō-mī-e′lē-ă). Diplomielia; duplicação completa ou incompleta da medula espinal; pode ser acompanhada por um septo ósseo no canal vertebral. [diplo- + G. *myelon*, medula óssea]

dip·lon (dip′lon). Dêuteron. SIN deuteron.

dip·lo·ne·ma (dip-lō-nē′mă). Diplonema; a forma duplicada do filamento cromossomial visível no estágio diplóteno da meiose. [diplo- + G. *nēma*, filamento]

dip·lo·neu·ral (dip-lō-noo′răl). Diploneural; suprido por dois nervos de diferentes origens; diz-se de determinados músculos. [diplo- + G. *neuron*, nervo]

dip·lop·a·gus (dip-lop′a-gŭs). Diplópago; termo genérico para gêmeos conjugados, cada um com um corpo razoavelmente completo, embora possa haver um ou mais órgãos internos comuns. VER conjoined *twins*, em *twin*. [diplo- + G. *pagos*, algo fixo]

di·plo·pia (di-plō′pē-ă). Diplopia; a condição na qual um único objeto é percebido como dois objetos. SIN double vision. [diplo- + G. *ōps*, olho]

crossed d., d. cruzada; diplopia na qual a imagem vista pelo olho direito está à esquerda da imagem vista pelo olho esquerdo. SIN heteronymous d.

heteronymous d., d. heterônima. SIN crossed d.

homonymous d., d. homônima. SIN homonymous *images*, em *image*.

monocular d., d. monocular; uma imagem dupla ou uma imagem fantasma adicional produzida em um olho, quase sempre por uma aberração dos meios oculares; por exemplo, uma irregularidade corneana ou lenticular, um astigmatismo não-corrigido ou uma irregularidade do vítreo ou da retina. Se houver um processo semelhante nos dois olhos (diplopia monocular bilateral), isto é, a duplicação ainda existir com a oclusão de um dos olhos, o paciente pode ainda ver apenas duas imagens; a observação de múltiplas imagens (poliopia) é rara.

simple d., d. simples. SIN homonymous *images*, em *image*.

uncrossed d., d. não-cruzada. SIN homonymous *images*, em *image*.

dip·lo·po·dia (dip-lō-pō′dē-ă). Diplopodia; duplicação dos dedos do pé. [diplo- + G. *pous*, pé]

dip·lo·some (dip′lō-sōm). Diplossoma; alossomas pareados; o par de centríolos das células mamíferas. SIN paired allosome. [diplo- + G. *sōma*, corpo]

dip·lo·so·mia (dip-lō-sō′mē-ă). Diplosomia; condição na qual gêmeos que parecem funcionalmente independentes são unidos em um ou mais pontos. VER conjoined *twins*, em *twin*. [diplo- + G. *sōma*, corpo]

dip·lo·tene (dip′lō-tēn). Diplóteno; o estágio final da prófase na meiose, em que os cromossomas homólogos pareados começam a se repelir e a afastar-se, mas geralmente são mantidos unidos por quiasmas. Os quiasmas estão associados à quebra de duas cromátides, em pontos correspondentes, seguida por refusão das extremidades quebradas com troca de segmentos entre as cromátides; esta é considerada a base citológica para o cruzamento de genes. [diplo- + G. *tainia*, faixa]

di·po·dia (dī-pō′dē-ă). Dipodia. **1.** Anomalia do desenvolvimento que envolve duplicação completa ou incompleta de um pé. **2.** Em gêmeos conjugados e na sirenomielia, um grau de união que deixa dois pés evidentes. [G. *di-*, dois, + *pous* (*pod-*), pé]

di·pole (dī′pōl). Dipolo; um par de cargas elétricas separadas, uma positiva e outra negativa; ou um par de cargas parciais separadas. SIN doublet (2).

di·po·tas·si·um phos·phate (dī-pō-tas′ē-ŭm). Fosfato de dipotássio. SIN *potassium* phosphate.

di·pre·nor·phine (dī-pren′or-fēn). Diprenorfina; um antagonista narcótico semelhante à naloxona, porém mais potente.

di·pro·pyl·tryp·ta·mine (dī-prō-pil-trip′tă-mēn). Dipropiltriptamina; alucinógeno semelhante à dimetiltriptamina.

di·pro·so·pus (dī-pros′ō-pŭs, dī-prō-sō′pus). Diprosopo; gêmeos conjugados com fusão quase completa dos corpos e com membros normais. Pode haver duplicação parcial ou total da face. VER conjoined *twins*, em *twin*. [G. *di-*, dois + *prosōpon,* face]

dip·se·sis (dip-sē′sis). Dipsose; sede anormal ou excessiva, ou um desejo por formas incomuns de bebida. SIN dipsosis, morbid thirst. [G. *dipseō,* sede]

dip·so·gen (dip′sō-jen). Dipsógeno; um agente que provoca a sede. [G. *dipsa,* sede, + *-gen,* que produz]

dip·so·ma·nia (dip-sō-mā′nē-ă). Dipsomania; uma compulsão recorrente para ingerir bebidas alcoólicas em excesso. VER alcoholism. [G. *dipsa,* sede, + *mania,* loucura]

dip·so·sis (dip-sō′sis). Dipsose. SIN dipsesis. [G. *dipsa,* sede, + *-osis,* condição]

dip·so·ther·a·py (dip′sō-thār′ă-pē). Dipsoterapia; tratamento de determinadas doenças por abstenção, ao máximo possível, de líquidos.

Dip·tera (dip′ter-ă). Uma importante ordem de insetos (moscas e mosquitos de duas asas), incluindo muitos importantes vetores de doenças, como o mosquito, a mosca tsé-tsé, o mosquito-pólvora e o maruim. [G. *di-,* dois, + *pteron,* asa]

dip·ter·an (dip′ter-an). Díptero; designa insetos da ordem Diptera.

dip·ter·ous (dip′ter-ŭs). Diptérico; relativo a, ou característico da, ordem Diptera.

Di·pus sa·git·ta (dī′pŭs saj′i-tă). Pequeno roedor do sul da Rússia, que serve como vetor, através de pulgas, da *Yersinia pestis* (bacilo da peste). [G. *dipous,* jerboa, de dois pés; L. *sagitta,* seta]

di·py·gus (dī-pī′gŭs, dip′ē-gŭs). Dípigo; gêmeos conjugados com cabeça e tórax únicos e a pelve e os membros inferiores duplicados; quando a duplicação das partes inferiores é simétrica, geralmente é denominada duplicidade posterior. VER conjoined *twins,* em *twin.* [G. *di-,* dois, + *pyge,* nádegas]

dip·y·lid·i·a·sis (dip′i-li-dī′ă-sis). Dipilidíase; infestação de carnívoros e seres humanos pelo cestódeo *Dipylidium caninum.*

Dip·y·lid·i·um ca·ni·num (dip-i-lid′ē-ŭm kă-nī′nŭm). A espécie mais comum da tênia do cão, a tênia de poro duplo, cujas larvas são albergadas nas pulgas ou piolhos dos cães; o verme ocasionalmente infesta os seres humanos, principalmente crianças lambidas por cães recém-picados por pulgas infestadas. [G. *dipylos,* com duas entradas; L. neutro de *caninus,* relativo a *canis,* cão]

di·py·rid·am·ole (dī-pir-id′ă-mōl). Dipiridamol; dilatador coronariano que também possui uma fraca atividade de redução da agregação plaquetária; comumente usado no lugar do exercício para estudos da contratilidade miocárdica.

di·py·rim·i·dine pho·to·ly·ase (dī-pi-rim′i-dēn). Dipirimidina fotoliase. SIN deoxyribodipyrimidine photolyase.

di·py·rine (di-pī′rēn). Dipirina. SIN aminopyrine.

di·py·rone (dī-pī′rōn). Dipirona; analgésico, antiinflamatório e antipirético raramente usado nos EUA devido a uma alta incidência de agranulocitose. SIN methampyrone.

directive. Diretriz.

advance d., diretriz antecipada; documento legal que fornece instruções quanto ao tipo e grau de assistência médica a ser administrada no caso de o signatário do documento tornar-se mentalmente incompetente durante o curso de uma doença terminal, ou entrar em coma permanente (estado vegetativo persistente). Nos EUA foram aprovadas pelas Assembléias Legislativas dos vários estados as denominadas leis de Morte com Dignidade para proteger os direitos dos pacientes de recusar assistência médica, incluindo medidas terapêuticas para prolongamento da vida e paliativo na doença terminal, e também para esclarecer o papel dos médicos e protegê-los da acusação de eutanásia ou de suicídio assistido por médico quando interrompem esse tratamento, seguindo os desejos do paciente. Essas leis explicam detalhadamente as exigências rigorosas para o procedimento, incluindo a obrigatoriedade de que a assinatura de uma diretriz antecipada seja devidamente testemunhada, e torna mais fácil anular do que estabelecer uma diretriz antecipada. Quando a diretriz antecipada fornece instruções sobre os tipos de tratamento que o paciente deseja ou não receber, é conhecida como determinação em vida. Quando designa outra pessoa para tomar essas decisões, é conhecida como procuração para decisões relativas à saúde. Uma diretriz antecipada pode conter os dois tipos de instrução. Um agente que toma decisões terminais em nome de um paciente tem de seguir as instruções do paciente, interpretá-las, quando necessário, à luz da filosofia pessoal, das crenças religiosas e dos valores éticos do paciente, e com a devida consideração da probabilidade de que o paciente recupere a competência ou a saúde.

di·rec·tor (di-rek′ter, -tōr, dī-). **1.** Instrumento com sulcos suaves, usado com um bisturi para limitar a incisão de tecidos. SIN staff (2). **2.** Diretor; o chefe de um serviço ou de uma divisão de especialidade. [L. *dirigo,* pp. *-rectus,* dispor, colocar em ordem]

Di·ro·fi·la·ria (dī-rō-fi-lā′rē-ă). Gênero de filária (família Onchocercidae, superfamília Filarioidea); espécies de *D.* geralmente são encontradas em outros mamíferos, que não o homem, mas são conhecidos exemplos raros de infestação humana, como por *D. immitis.* [L. *dirus,* temível, + *filum,* filamento] *D. conjuncti'vae,* nome atribuído a filárias removidas de tumores e abscessos em vários locais em casos humanos, especialmente conjuntivas palpebrais e outros tecidos oculares, mas também tecidos subcutâneos de outros locais; provavelmente causada por várias espécies de origem animal. *D. im'mitis,* espécie de filária de cães e outros canídeos em regiões tropicais e subtropicais, encontrada principalmente no ventrículo direito e nas artérias pulmonares de cães; algumas vezes um grave patógeno em cães de corrida e de exibição, principalmente no sul dos Estados Unidos, onde são comuns os mosquitos vetores; *D. immitis* e seu hospedeiro canino foram usados para testar agentes quimioterápicos, e um extrato de *D. immitis* pode ser usado como antígeno intradérmico inespecífico no diagnóstico da filariose humana e em testes de fixação do complemento. VER TAMBÉM *Dipetalonema reconditum.* SIN heartworm.

di·ro·fi·la·ri·a·sis (dir′ō-fil-ă-rī′ă-sis). Dirofilaríase; dirofilariose; infestação de animais e, raramente, de seres humanos por nematódeos do gênero *Dirofilaria.*

dirt-eat·ing. Geofagia. SIN geophagia.

△ **dis-.** Em dois, separado; un-, não; muito. Cf. dys-. [L. separação]

dis·a·bil·i·ty (dis-ă-bil′i-tē). Incapacidade. **1.** De acordo com a *International Classification of Impairments, Disabilities and Handicaps* (Organização Mundial de Saúde), qualquer restrição ou ausência de capacidade de realizar uma atividade de uma forma ou dentro da amplitude considerada normal para um ser humano. O termo incapacidade reflete as consequências do comprometimento em termos de desempenho funcional e atividade do indivíduo; assim, as incapacidades representam distúrbios ao nível da pessoa. **2.** Comprometimento ou defeito de um ou mais órgãos ou membros.

developmental d., distúrbio de desenvolvimento; perda da função causada por eventos pré ou pós-natais na qual o distúrbio predominante se dá na aquisição de habilidades cognitivas, de linguagem, motoras ou sociais; p. ex., retardo mental, autismo, distúrbio do aprendizado e distúrbio de hiperatividade com déficit de atenção.

learning d., distúrbio do aprendizado; um distúrbio em um ou mais dos processos cognitivos básicos e psicológicos envolvidos na compreensão ou no uso da linguagem escrita ou falada; pode manifestar-se em comprometimento, relacionado à idade, da capacidade de ler, escrever, soletrar, falar ou realizar cálculos matemáticos.

di·sac·cha·rid·as·es (dī-sak′ă-rid-ās-ez). Dissacaridases; grupo de enzimas que catalisam a hidrólise dos dissacarídeos, produzindo dois monossacarídeos.

di·sac·cha·ride (dī-sak′ă-rīd). Dissacarídeo; produto da condensação de dois monossacarídeos por eliminação de água (geralmente entre uma OH alcoólica e uma OH hemiacetal); p. ex., sacarose, lactose, maltose.

dis·ag·gre·ga·tion (dis′ag-grē-gā′shŭn). Desagregação. **1.** Uma quebra em partes componentes. **2.** Incapacidade de coordenar várias sensações e incapacidade de compreender suas relações mútuas. [L. *dis-,* que separa, + *ag-grego* (*adg-*), pp. *-gregatus,* acrescentar algo]

dis·ar·tic·u·la·tion (dis-ar-tik-ū-lā′shŭn). Desarticulação; amputação de um membro através de uma articulação, sem cortar o osso. [L. *dis-,* afastado, + *articulus,* articulação]

dis·as·sim·i·la·tion (dis′ă-sim-i-lā′shŭn). Desassimilação; metabolismo destrutivo ou retrógrado. SIN dissimilation (1).

dis·as·so·ci·a·tion (dis′ă-sō-sē-ā′shŭn). Desassociação. SIN dissociation (1).

disc (disk). Disco. VER disk.

△ **disc-.** SIN disco-.

disc·ec·to·my (disk-ek′tō-mē). Discectomia; excisão, em parte ou no todo, de um disco intervertebral. SIN discotomy. [disco- + G. *ektomē,* excisão]

dis·charge (dis′charj). **1.** O que é emitido ou evacuado, como uma excreção ou secreção. **2.** A ativação ou deflagração de um neurônio.

after-d., pós-descarga. VER afterdischarge.

early d., alta precoce; alta de uma mulher e do recém-nascido do hospital nas primeiras 24 horas após um parto vaginal.

Dische, Zacharias, bioquímico austríaco norte-americano do século XX, 1895–1988. VER D. *reaction, reagent;* D.-Schwarz *reagent.*
dis·chro·na·tion (dis-krō-nā′shŭn). Dessincronização; distúrbio na percepção do tempo. [L. *dis-,* afastado, + G. *chronos,* tempo]
dis·ci (dis′kī). Discos; plural de discus.
dis·ci·form (dis′i-fōrm). Disciforme; em forma de disco.
dis·cis·sion (di-sish′ŭn). Discissão. **1.** Incisão ou corte através de uma parte. **2.** Em oftalmologia, abertura da cápsula e ruptura do córtex da lente com uma agulha-bisturi ou laser. [L. *di- scindo,* pp. *-scissus,* separar, dividir]
dis·ci·tis (dis-kī′tis). Discite; inflamação de um disco intervertebral ou espaço do disco freqüentemente relacionada a infecções. SIN diskitis.
♻ **disco-, disc-.** Disco; em forma de disco. [G. *diskos*]
dis·co·blas·tic (dis-kō-blas′tik). Discoblástico; designa uma discoblástula.
dis·co·blas·tu·la (dis′kō-blas′tū-lā). Discoblástula; uma blástula do tipo produzido pela clivagem discoidal meroblástica de um ovo com grande vitelo.
dis·co·gas·tru·la (dis′kō-gas′troo-lā). Discogástrula; uma gástrula do tipo formado após a clivagem discóide de um ovo com grande vitelo.
dis·co·gen·ic (dis′kō-gen′ik). Discogênico; designa um distúrbio que se origina no disco intervertebral ou a partir dele. [disco- + G. *genesis,* origem]
dis·coid (dis′koyd). **1.** Discóide; semelhante a um disco. **2.** Em odontologia, um instrumento escavador ou de escultura que possui uma lâmina circular com uma borda cortante na periferia. [disco- + G. *eidos,* aparência]
dis·con·ju·gate (dis-cŏn′joo-gāt). Desconjugado; que não tem ação pareada nem é unido; o oposto de conjugado. VER disconjugate *movement* of eyes. [L. *dis-,* afastado, + *jugatus,* unido]
dis·cop·a·thy (dis-kop′a-thē). Discopatia; doença de um disco, particularmente de um disco intervertebral. [disco- + G. *pathos,* doença]
  traumatic cervical d., d. cervical traumática; lesão caracterizada por fissura, laceração e/ou fragmentação de um disco cervical ou dos ligamentos adjacentes, com ou sem deslocamento de fragmentos contra a medula espinal, raízes nervosas ou ligamentos.
dis·co·pla·cen·ta (dis-kō-pla-sen′tă). Discoplacenta; uma placenta de formato discóide.
dis·cor·dance (dis-kōr′dans). Discordância. **1.** Dissociação de duas características nos membros de uma amostra populacional; usada como medida de dependência. **2.** Em genética, a presença de um determinado traço apenas em um membro de um par de gêmeos. Cf. concordance.
dis·cot·o·my (dis-kot′ō-mē). Discotomia. SIN discectomy. [disco- + G. *tomē,* incisão]
dis·crete (dis-krēt′). Distinto; separado; não-unido ou incorporado a outro; designa principalmente determinadas lesões cutâneas. [L. *dis- cerno,* pp. *-cretus,* separar]
dis·crim·i·na·tion (dis′krim-i-nā′shŭn). Discriminação; em termos de condicionamento, aquele que responde de forma diferencial, como quando um organismo apresenta uma resposta a um estímulo reforçado e uma resposta diferente a um estímulo não-reforçado. [L. *discrimino,* pp. *-atus,* separar]
dis·cus, pl. **dis·ci** (dis′kŭs, -kī). ([TA]. Disco. SIN lamella (2). [L. do G. *diskos,* disco]
  d. articula'ris [TA], d. articular. SIN articular *disk.*
  d. articula'ris acromioclavicula'ris [TA], d. articular acromioclavicular. SIN articular *disk* of acromioclavicular joint.
  d. articula'ris radioulna'ris distalis [TA], d. articular radioulnar distal. SIN articular *disk* of distal radioulnar joint.
  d. articula'ris sternoclavicula'ris [TA], d. articular esternoclavicular. SIN articular *disk* of sternoclavicular joint.
  d. articularis temporomandibularis [TA], d. articular temporomandibular. SIN articular *disk* of temporomandibular joint.
  d. interpu'bicus [TA], d. interpúbico. SIN interpubic *disk.*
  d. intervertebra'lis [TA], d. intervertebral. SIN intervertebral *disk.*
  d. lentifor'mis, termo raramente usado para designar o núcleo subtalâmico (subthalamic *nucleus*).
  d. ner'vi op'tici [TA], d. do nervo óptico. SIN optic *disk.*
  d. prolig·erus, d. prolígero; o ponto de fixação do cúmulo oóforo às células granulosas mais periféricas de um folículo antral.
dis·di·a·clast (dis-dī′ă-klast). Disdiaclasto; elemento duplamente refrativo no tecido muscular estriado. [G. *dis,* duas vezes, + *dia,* através, + *klastos,* quebrado]

DISEASE

dis·ease (di-zēz′). Doença. **1.** Interrupção, cessação ou distúrbio de função, sistema ou órgão do corpo. SIN illness, morbus, sickness. **2.** Distúrbio mórbido geralmente caracterizado por, pelo menos, dois destes critérios: agente(s) etiológico(s) reconhecido(s), grupo identificável de sinais e sintomas ou alterações anatômicas consistentes. VER TAMBÉM syndrome. **3.** Literalmente, "disease", o oposto de bem-estar (*ease*), quando algo está errado com uma função corporal. [Inglês *dis-* priv. + *ease,* bem-estar, conforto]
  aaa d., anemia endêmica no Egito antigo, atribuída, no Papiro de Ebers, à infestação intestinal por ancilóstomos; agora denominada ancilostomíase.
  ABO hemolytic d. of the newborn, d. hemolítica ABO do recém-nascido; eritroblastose fetal devida à incompatibilidade materno-fetal em relação a um antígeno do grupo sanguíneo ABO; o feto possui antígeno A ou B, que a mãe não apresenta, e esta produz anticorpo imune que causa lise das hemácias fetais.
  accumulation d., d. de acúmulo; doença caracterizada por acumulação anormal de um produto metabólico em algumas células e tecidos; os exemplos incluem as mucopolissacaridoses, lipoidoses.
  Acosta d., d. de Acosta. SIN altitude *sickness.*
  Adams-Stokes d., d. de Adams-Stokes. SIN Adams-Stokes *syndrome.*
  adaptation d.'s, doenças de adaptação; doenças que, teoricamente, caem no conceito de Selye da síndrome de adaptação geral.
  Addison d., d. de Addison. SIN chronic adrenocortical *insufficiency.*
  Addison-Biermer d., d. de Addison-Biermer. SIN pernicious *anemia.*
  akamushi d., d. de akamushi. SIN tsutsugamushi d.
  Albers-Schönberg d., d. de Albers-Schönberg. SIN osteopetrosis.
  Albright d., d. de Albright. SIN McCune-Albright *syndrome.*
  Alexander d., d. de Alexander; doença degenerativa do sistema nervoso central rara e fatal, que acomete lactentes, caracterizada por retardo psicomotor, convulsões e paralisia; a megaloencefalia está associada a alterações leucodistróficas disseminadas, principalmente nos lobos frontais.
  Almeida d., d. de Almeida. SIN paracoccidioidomycosis.
  Alpers d., d. de Alpers. SIN *poliodystrophia* cerebri progressiva infantilis.
  altitude d., d. da altitude. SIN altitude *sickness.*

ℹ **Alzheimer d.,** d. de Alzheimer; doença degenerativa progressiva do cérebro que causa comprometimento da memória e demência, manifestada por confusão, desorientação visuoespacial, incapacidade de calcular e deterioração do julgamento; podem ocorrer ilusões e alucinações. O distúrbio cerebral degenerativo mais comum, a doença de Alzheimer constitui 70% de todos os casos de demência. O início geralmente se dá no final da meia-idade, e tipicamente causa morte em 5 a 10 anos. SIN Alzheimer dementia, presenile dementia (2), dementia presenilis, primary neuronal degeneration, primary senile dementia.
  A doença de Alzheimer (DA) figura como a quarta causa de morte nos Estados Unidos, e seu custo anual para a nação é de quase 100 bilhões de dólares. O início é tipicamente insidioso, com deterioração progressiva da capacidade de aprender e reter informações. Ao recordar e repetir dados, o paciente comete erros de intrusão (inserção de palavras ou idéias irrelevantes) e recorre à confabulação. Há declínio da orientação e do julgamento; 50% dos pacientes apresentam depressão, 20% ilusões. Há agitação em 70%. Inúme-

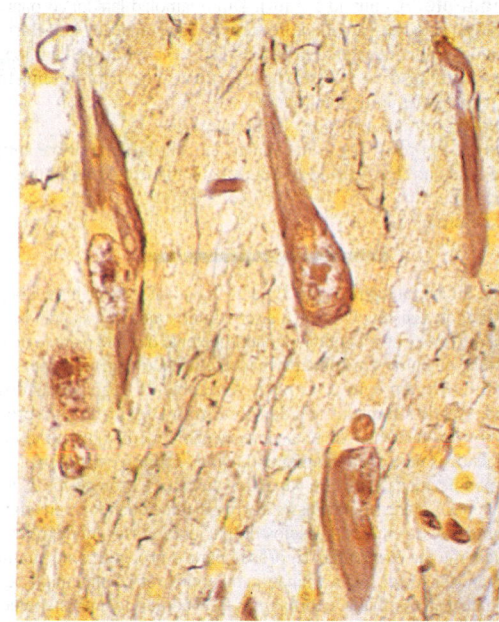

doença de Alzheimer: entrelaçados de neurofibrilas no citoplasma distendido de neurônios piramidais impregnados com prata

ros fármacos, incluindo muitos que não são considerados psicoativos, podem agravar os sintomas de DA; a depressão clínica pode mascarar a demência, e vice-versa. Os distúrbios do comportamento são as principais indicações para o uso de agentes psicotrópicos e contenções físicas, e influenciam significativamente a qualidade de vida dos idosos dementes. O exame neurológico pode ser praticamente normal, mas podem ocorrer mioclonia, bradicinesia, rigidez e convulsões na fase avançada da doença. A morte geralmente se deve a sepsis associada a infecção urinária ou pulmonar. Em estudos por imagens, podem-se observar evidências flagrantes de atrofia do córtex cerebral, com consequente aumento dos sulcos e ventrículos. Histologicamente, o córtex, o hipocampo e a amígdala exibem atrofia dos neurônios, com vacúolos citoplasmáticos e grânulos argentofílicos; distorção das neurofibrilas intracelulares (entrelaçados de neurofibrilas) devido à fosforilação excessiva das proteínas tau microtubulares; e placas compostas de massas argentofílicas granulares ou filamentosas com um cerne da forma de β-amilóide com 42 aminoácidos (Aβ42). A concentração de proteína tau no líquido cefalorraquidiano está aumentada, enquanto a de Aβ42 está diminuída. Corpúsculos de Lewy (inclusões eosinofílicas no citoplasma dos neurônios do SNC, considerados produtos da alteração do metabolismo dos neurofilamentos e reconhecidos como uma característica do parkinsonismo idiopático) são observados nos neurônios corticais de algumas pessoas com demência, incluindo DA. A demência associada aos corpúsculos de Lewy tende a surgir antes dos 60 anos de idade, progredir rapidamente e exibir características parkinsonianas (tremor, rigidez). Quase todas as pessoas com síndrome de Down que vivem além dos 40 anos de idade desenvolvem declínio cognitivo associado a achados histológicos típicos de DA. A idade avançada e uma história de traumatismo craniano também são fatores de risco para DA. Embora a maioria dos casos seja esporádica, cerca de 10% dos pacientes possuem uma história familiar de DA. A doença familiar, que frequentemente é caracterizada por início precoce e evolução rápida, foi relacionada a mutações de vários genes. Pelo menos metade dos pacientes com DA familiar de início precoce exibe mutações do gene pré-senilina-1 no cromossoma 14. Mutações do gene pré-senilina-2 no cromossoma 1 ou do gene da proteína precursora amilóide no cromossoma 21 foram encontradas em grupos menores com doença familiar. A doença familiar de início tardio foi relacionada a mutações no *locus* da apolipoproteína E (APOE) no cromossoma 19. Todas essas mutações estão associadas a aumento da produção de Aβ42. Já foi sugerido que a incorporação de proteínas pré-senilina aos neurônios programa-os para a morte através de apoptose. O declínio cognitivo na DA foi parcialmente atribuído à deficiência do neurotransmissor acetilcolina, e o tratamento com inibidores reversíveis da colinesterase (donezepil, galantamina, metrifonato, tacrina) tem melhorado a cognição e lentificado a progressão da demência em alguns pacientes. Muitos outros agentes (incluindo nicotina, extrato de ginkgo, vitamina E, selegilina, mesilatos ergolóides e ibuprofeno) têm mostrado pequena eficácia em alguns estudos. Evidências experimentais sugerem que a administração de estrogênio a mulheres pós-menopausa retarda o início e a progressão da DA não-familiar.

anarthritic rheumatoid d., d. reumatóide anartrítica; doença reumatóide sem artrite.
Anders d., d. de Anders. SIN *adiposis* dolorosa.
Andersen d., d. de Andersen. SIN type 4 *glycogenosis*.
antibody deficiency d., d. por deficiência de anticorpos. SIN antibody deficiency *syndrome*.
aortoiliac occlusive d., d. oclusiva aortoilíaca; obstrução da aorta abdominal e de seus principais ramos por aterosclerose.
Aran-Duchenne d., d. de Aran-Duchenne. SIN amyotrophic lateral *sclerosis*.
Australian X d., d. X australiana. SIN Murray Valley *encephalitis*.
autoimmune d., d. auto-imune; qualquer distúrbio no qual a perda de função ou destruição do tecido normal decorre de respostas imunes humorais ou celulares contra os constituintes teciduais do próprio corpo; pode ser sistêmica, como o lúpus eritematoso sistêmico, ou específica de um órgão, como a tireoidite.
aviator's d., d. dos aviadores; síndrome semelhante à doença da descompressão observada em ocupantes de aviões que chegam a altitudes muito grandes sem pressurização adequada da cabine. VER TAMBÉM decompression *sickness*.
Ayerza d., d. de Ayerza. SIN Ayerza *syndrome*.
Azorean d., d. dos Açores. SIN Machado-Joseph d.
Baelz d., d. de Baelz. SIN *cheilitis* glandularis.
Baló d., d. de Baló. SIN *encephalitis* periaxialis concentrica.
Baltic myoclonus d., d. mioclônica báltica; uma das epilepsias mioclônicas fotossensíveis familiares. Ao contrário da polimioclonia com corpúsculos de Lafora, no qual são observados corpúsculos de inclusão nas células cerebrais, o prognóstico frequentemente é favorável. Provavelmente é um distúrbio autossômico recessivo.
Bamberger d., d. de Bamberger; **(1)** SIN saltatory *spasm*; **(2)** SIN polyserositis.
Bamberger-Marie d., d. de Bamberger-Marie. SIN hypertrophic pulmonary *osteoarthropathy*.

Bang d., d. de Bang. SIN bovine *brucellosis*.
Banti d., d. de Banti. SIN Banti *syndrome*.
Barclay-Baron d., d. de Barclay-Baron. SIN vallecular *dysphagia*.
Barlow d., d. de Barlow. SIN infantile *scurvy*.
Barraquer d., d. de Barraquer. SIN progressive *lipodystrophy*.
Basedow d., d. de Basedow. SIN Graves d.
Batten d., d. de Batten; esfingolipidose cerebral (cerebral *sphingolipidosis*), tipo juvenil tardio. SIN ceroid lipofuscinosis.
Batten-Mayou d., d. de Batten-Mayou; esfingolipidose cerebral (cerebral *sphingolipidosis*), tipos do lactente e juvenil tardio.
Bazin d., d. de Bazin. SIN *erythema* induratum.
Bechterew d., d. de Bechterew. SIN *spondylitis* deformans.
Becker d., d. de Becker; uma obscura miocardiopatia sul-africana que causa insuficiência cardíaca congestiva rapidamente fatal e doença endomiocárdica mural idiopática.
Béguez César d., d. de Béguez César. SIN Chédiak-Higashi *syndrome*.
Behçet d., d. de Behçet. SIN Behçet *syndrome*.
Behr d., d. de Behr. SIN Behr *syndrome*.
Berger d., d. de Berger. SIN focal *glomerulonephritis*.
Bernard-Soulier d. (ber-nar'-sool-ya), d. de Bernard-Soulier; distúrbio autossômico recessivo de ausência ou diminuição das glicoproteínas da membrana plaquetária Ib, IX e V (o receptor para o fator VIII R). Essa deficiência pode levar a uma falha da ligação do fator de von Willebrand, causando hemorragia moderada.
Bernhardt d., d. de Bernhardt. SIN *meralgia* paresthetica.
Besnier·Boeck·Schaumann d., d. de Besnier-Boeck-Schaumann. SIN sarcoidosis.
Best d. [MIM*153700], d. de Best; degeneração macular autossômica dominante que começa durante os primeiros anos de vida. SIN vitelliform degeneration, vitelliform retinal dystrophy.
Bielschowsky d., d. de Bielschowsky; tipo de lipofuscinose de início nos primeiros anos de vida.
Biermer d., d. de Biermer. SIN pernicious *anemia*.
Binswanger d., d. de Binswanger; uma das causas de demência por múltiplos infartos, na qual há muitos infartos e lacunas na substância branca, com relativa preservação do córtex e dos gânglios da base. SIN Binswanger encephalopathy, encephalitis subcorticalis chronica, subcortical arteriosclerotic encephalopathy.
bird-breeder's d., d. do criador de pássaros. SIN bird-breeder's *lung*.
blinding d., oncocercose. SIN onchocerciasis.
Bloch-Sulzberger d., d. de Bloch-Sulzberger. SIN *incontinentia* pigmenti.
Blocq d., d. de Blocq. SIN astasia-abasia.
Blount d., d. de Blount; tíbia vara; pernas tortas não-raquíticas em crianças. SIN Blount-Barber d.
Blount-Barber d., d. de Blount-Barber. SIN Blount d.
blue d., febre maculosa das Montanhas Rochosas. SIN Rocky Mountain spotted *fever*.
Boeck d., d. de Boeck. SIN sarcoidosis.
Bornholm d., d. de Bornholm. SIN epidemic *pleurodynia*. [*Bornholm*, ilha dinamarquesa no mar Báltico onde a doença foi descrita pela primeira vez]
Bosin d., d. de Bosin. SIN subacute sclerosing *panencephalitis*.
Bouchard d., d. de Bouchard; dilatação miopática do estômago.
Bourneville d., d. de Bourneville. SIN tuberous *sclerosis*.
Bourneville-Pringle d., d. de Bourneville-Pringle; lesões faciais com esclerose tuberosa, descritas inicialmente como adenoma sebáceo, mas agora reconhecidas como angiomas.
Bowen d., d. de Bowen; uma forma de carcinoma intra-epidérmico caracterizada pelo desenvolvimento de pápulas róseas ou acastanhadas, de crescimento lento, ou placas erodidas recobertas por uma camada córnea espessada; microscopicamente, há disceratose com grandes células epidérmicas redondas com grandes núcleos e citoplasma pálido, dispersos em todos os níveis da epiderme. SIN Bowen precancerous dermatosis.
Brailsford-Morquio d., d. de Brailsford-Morquio. SIN Morquio *syndrome*.
brancher glycogen storage d., d. por depósito de glicogênio; tipo de doença por depósito de glicogênio, causada por deficiência de amilo-1,4-1,6-transglucosidase (enzima ramificadora). SIN brancher deficiency glycogenosis, debrancher deficiency.
Breda d., d. de Breda. SIN espundia.
Bright d., d. de Bright; nefrite não-supurativa com albuminúria e edema, associada, em casos fatais, a rins grandes e brancos; ou a hematúria e rins vermelhos; ou a rins granulados e contraídos, correspondentes aos estágios de glomerulonefrite agora denominados subagudo ou membranoso, agudo e crônico, respectivamente.
Brill d., d. de Brill. SIN Brill-Zinsser d.
Brill-Zinsser d., d. de Brill-Zinsser; reinfecção endógena associada ao "estado de portador" de pessoas que já tiveram tifo epidêmico; é uma doença razoavelmente leve e pode ser confundida com o tifo endêmico (murino); descrita pela primeira vez por Brill na cidade de Nova Iorque, mas só reconhecida como

uma forma recrudescente do tipo epidêmico após o trabalho de Zinsser. SIN Brill d., recrudescent typhus fever, recrudescent typhus.

Briquet d., d. de Briquet; neurose histérica, tipo conversão.

Brissaud d., d. de Brissaud. SIN tic.

broad beta d., hiperlipoproteinemia familiar tipo III.

Brodie d., d. de Brodie; **(1)** SIN Brodie *knee*; **(2)** neuralgia espinal histérica, que simula a doença de Pott, após um traumatismo.

bronzed d., d. bronzeada. SIN bronze *diabetes*. VER hemochromatosis.

Bruck d., d. de Bruck; doença caracterizada por osteogênese imperfeita, anquilose das articulações e atrofia muscular.

Brushfield-Wyatt d., d. de Brushfield-Wyatt; distúrbio familiar caracterizado por nevo unilateral, hemiplegia contralateral, hemianopsia, angioma cerebral e retardo mental; possivelmente uma variante da síndrome de Sturge-Weber. SIN nevoid amentia.

Buerger d., d. de Buerger. SIN *thromboangiitis* obliterans.

bulging eye d., oftalmomíase. SIN gedoelstiosis.

bulky d., termo usado para grandes tumores ou linfonodos; geralmente mais resistentes ao tratamento convencional. SIN bulky lymphadenopathy.

Bürger-Grütz d., d. de Bürger-Grütz; termo obsoleto para a hiperlipemia idiopática (idiopathic *hyperlipemia*).

Buschke d., d. de Buschke. SIN *scleredema* adultorum.

Busquet d., d. de Busquet; osteoperiostite dos ossos metatarsais, levando a exostoses no dorso do pé.

Byler d. [MIM*211600], d. de Byler; colestase intra-hepática progressiva, com início precoce de eliminação de fezes pastosas e fétidas, icterícia, hepatomegalia, nanismo e, ocasionalmente, morte; causada por um erro no metabolismo dos sais biliares conjugados; herança autossômica recessiva, causada por mutação no gene da colestase intra-hepática familiar 1 (FIC1) no cromossoma 18q. [*Byler*, uma família amish]

Caffey d., d. de Caffey. SIN infantile cortical *hyperostosis*.

caisson d. (kā′son), d. da descompressão. SIN decompression *sickness*. [Fr. *caisson* (de *caisse*, caixa) uma caixa ou cilindro impermeável, contendo ar sob alta pressão, usado na submersão de pilares estruturais]

calcium pyrophosphate deposition d. (CPPD), d. por depósito de pirofosfato de cálcio; uma artrite por depósito de cristais, que pode simular gota.

Calvé-Perthes d., d. de Calvé-Perthes. SIN Legg-Calvé-Perthes d.

Canavan d. [MIM*271900], d. de Canavan; doença degenerativa progressiva da lactância; afeta principalmente bebês judeus asquenazes; o início tipicamente se dá nos primeiros 3–4 meses de vida; caracterizada por megalencefalia, atrofia óptica, cegueira, regressão psicomotora, hipotonia e espasticidade; há aumento da excreção urinária de ácido *N*-acetilaspártico. A RM mostra aumento do cérebro, diminuição da atenuação da substância branca cerebral e cerebelar e ventrículos normais; anatomopatologicamente, há aumento do volume e do peso cerebrais e degeneração esponjosa na substância branca subcortical. Herança autossômica recessiva, causada por mutação do gene da aspartoaciclase A (ASPA) no cromossoma 17p em judeus e não-judeus afetados. VER TAMBÉM leukodystrophy. SIN Canavan sclerosis, Canavan-van Bogaert-Bertrand d., spongy degeneration of infancy.

Canavan-van Bogaert-Bertrand d., d. de Canavan-van Bogaert-Bertrand. SIN Canavan d.

Caroli d. [MIM*263200], d. de Caroli; dilatação cística congênita dos ductos biliares intra-hepáticos, algumas vezes associada a cálculos intra-hepáticos e obstrução biliar; pode ser uma parte do fenótipo da doença renal policística infantil.

Carrington d., d. de Carrington. SIN chronic eosinophilic *pneumonia*.

Carrión d., d. de Carrión. SIN Oroya *fever*.

Castleman d., d. de Castleman. SIN benign giant lymph node *hyperplasia*.

cat-bite d., d. da mordida de gato; provavelmente transmitida de ratos para gatos e, depois, para os homens. SIN cat-bite fever.

castscratch d. (CSD), d. da arranhadura de gato (DAG); infecção que causa adenopatia benigna crônica na maioria dos casos, principalmente em crianças e adultos jovens, geralmente associada a um arranhão ou mordida de gato. Na maioria dos casos é causada pela bactéria *Bartonella henselae*. A linfadenopatia geralmente resolve espontaneamente em alguns meses. A infecção pode causar outros sintomas clínicos, como febre de origem indeterminada, encefalite, microabscesso no fígado e baço e osteomielite. SIN benign inoculation lymphoreticulosis, benign inoculation reticulosis, catscratch fever, regional granulomatous lymphadenitis.

Uma lesão primária (tipicamente uma pápula solitária com 2–5 mm de diâmetro) desenvolve-se no local de inoculação em 50–95% dos casos, geralmente 1–2 semanas após a inoculação. Comumente segue-se linfadenopatia regional, em 75% dos pacientes envolvendo apenas um único linfonodo. Geralmente há dor à palpação do linfonodo, e cerca de 10% apresentam supuração. O estudo histopatológico de um linfonodo infectado mostra hiperplasia linfóide e formação de granuloma com áreas centrais de necrose estrelada contendo neutrófilos. Cerca de um terço dos pacientes apresenta sinais e sintomas sistêmicos transitórios, como febre, cefaléia, mal-estar ou erupção cutânea. Geralmente ocorre resolução espontânea da linfadenopatia em 6–12 semanas. A recuperação da DAG confere imunidade contra outros episódios. O *Centers for Disease Control* estima a incidência de DAG nos Estados Unidos em 2,5 casos por 100.000 pessoas por ano. A maioria dos pacientes tem menos de 21 anos, e os homens são mais afetados que as mulheres. Em 1988, uma bactéria denominada *Afipia felis* foi cultivada de linfonodos de pacientes com DAG e, durante certo período, foi considerada a causa da doença. Recentemente, estudos sorológicos mostraram que a *Bartonella henselae*, uma bactéria Gram-negativa, provavelmente é a causadora dos casos mais típicos de DAG. Algumas vezes, o microrganismo pode ser visualizado por coloração de prata de Warthin-Starry em linfonodos infectados. Existe um teste sérico com anticorpos imunofluorescentes. Os gatos são o principal reservatório da *Bartonella henselae*; 25–40% dos gatos clinicamente saudáveis nos Estados Unidos possuem anticorpos contra o organismo. Já se constatou que as pulgas transmitem infecção de um gato para outro. A maioria dos gatos infectados não adoece. Embora a DAG geralmente seja benigna e autolimitada, a infecção por *Bartonella henselae* ocasionalmente está associada a envolvimento grave ou sistêmico, incluindo síndrome oculoglandular de Parinaud (conjuntivite granulomatosa com linfadenite pré-auricular), encefalopatia, mielite, lesões osteolíticas, eritema nodoso, eritema marginado, púrpura trombocitopênica, anemia hemolítica auto-imune, artrite e pneumonia. Em pessoas imunodeprimidas, particularmente aquelas com AIDS/SIDA, a infecção por *Bartonella henselae* (talvez nem sempre associada a gatos) assume a forma de angiomatose bacilar (AB), na qual tumores nodulares constituídos de vasos sanguíneos densamente proliferativos surgem na pele, osso, cérebro, fígado, baço e outros tecidos. A antibioticoterapia não é recomendada na doença da arranhadura de gato não-complicada. A doxiciclina, ciprofloxacina e gentamicina podem ser usadas na encefalite ou na doença disseminada. Embora esses agentes costumem causar rápida melhora da angiomatose bacilar, a resposta da inflamação glandular e de outros sintomas da doença da arranhadura de gato é imprevisível.

celiac d., d. celíaca; doença que ocorre em crianças e adultos caracterizada por sensibilidade ao glúten, com inflamação crônica e atrofia da mucosa da porção superior do intestino delgado; as manifestações incluem diarréia, má absorção, esteatorréia e deficiências nutricionais e de vitaminas. SIN celiac sprue, celiac syndrome, gluten enteropathy.

cement d., d. do cimento; a osteólise que freqüentemente ocorre associada ao afrouxamento das substituições articulares totais do quadril cimentadas; as partículas microscópicas do cimento de polimetilmetacrilato induzem uma reação biológica por osteoclastos, que leva à reabsorção óssea e perda óssea progressiva.

central core d. [MIM*117000], d. do cerne; miopatia congênita caracterizada por hipotonia, retardo do desenvolvimento motor na lactância e fraqueza muscular não-progressiva ou lentamente progressiva; à biopsia, o cerne de fibras musculares é corado anormalmente, as miofibrilas são anormalmente compactas e há ausência virtual de mitocôndrias e retículo sarcoplasmático; histoquimicamente, os núcleos são desprovidos de atividade da enzima oxidativa, fosforilase e ATPase; herança autossômica dominante, freqüentemente subclínica, causada por mutação no gene receptor da rianodina-1 (RYR1) em 19q.

cerebrovascular d., d. cerebrovascular; termo geral para uma disfunção cerebral causada por uma anormalidade do suprimento sanguíneo cerebral.

Chagas d., d. de Chagas. SIN South American *trypanosomiasis*.

Chagas-Cruz d., d. de Chagas-Cruz. SIN South American *trypanosomiasis*.

α chain d., d. da cadeia alfa; termo vago ou indefinido; poderia ser usado para doença da cadeia pesada α (uma doença proliferativa de linfoplasmócitos, geralmente observada em homens mediterrâneos, caracterizada por envolvimento intestinal com esteatorréia, freqüentemente progressiva com evolução fatal) ou α talassemia (α *thalassemia*) (anormalidade genética na cadeia alfa globina da hemoglobina).

Charcot d., d. de Charcot. SIN amyotrophic lateral *sclerosis*.

Charcot-Marie-Tooth d., d. de Charcot-Marie-Tooth. SIN peroneal muscular *atrophy*.

Cheadle d., d. de Cheadle. SIN infantile *scurvy*.

Chédiak-Higashi d., d. de Chédiak-Higashi. SIN Chédiak-Higashi *syndrome*.

Chiari d., d. de Chiari. SIN Chiari *syndrome*.

Chicago d., d. de Chicago; termo obsoleto para designar a blastomicose norte-americana (North American *blastomycosis*).

cholesterol ester storage d. [MIM*278000], d. de depósito do éster de colesterol; lipidose causada por deficiência de atividade da lipase ácida lisossômica, resultando em acúmulo disseminado de ésteres do colesterol e triglicerídeos em vísceras com xantomatose, calcificação supra-renal, hepatoesplenomegalia, células espumosas na medula óssea e outros tecidos, e linfócitos vacuolados no sangue periférico; herança autossômica recessiva, causada por mutação do gene da lipase ácida lisossômica (LIPA) no cromossoma 10q. SIN cholesteryl ester storage d., Wolman d., Wolman xanthomatosis.

cholesteryl ester storage d., d. de depósito do éster de colesteril. SIN cholesterol ester storage d.

Christensen-Krabbe d., d. de Christensen-Krabbe. SIN *poliodystrophia* cerebri progressiva infantilis.

Christian d., d. de Christian; **(1)** SIN Hand-Schüller-Christian d.; **(2)** SIN relapsing febrile nodular nonsuppurative *panniculitis.*

Christmas d., doença de Christmas. SIN *hemophilia* B.

chronic active liver d., d. hepática ativa e crônica. SIN chronic *hepatitis.*

chronic granulomatous d., d. granulomatosa crônica; defeito congênito da destruição de bactérias fagocitadas por leucócitos polimorfonucleares, que não conseguem aumentar seu metabolismo de oxigênio, seja devido a defeito do citocromo [MIM*233710 e MIM*233690] ou a deficiência de outro fator específico [MIM*233700 e MIM*306400]. Conseqüentemente, há um aumento da suscetibilidade à infecção grave por microrganismos catalase-positivos; a herança geralmente é autossômica recessiva ou ligada ao X. SIN congenital dysphagocytosis, granulomatous d.

chronic hypertensive d., d. hipertensiva crônica; os efeitos cumulativos crônicos da elevação prolongada da pressão arterial sobre órgãos vitais, como o coração, o rim e o cérebro.

chronic obstructive pulmonary d. (COPD), d. pulmonar obstrutiva crônica (DPOC); termo geral usado para as doenças com estreitamento permanente ou temporário de pequenos brônquios, nas quais o fluxo expiratório forçado está lentificado, principalmente quando não se pode aplicar termo etiológico ou outro termo mais específico.

chylomicron retention d., d. de retenção de quilomícrons; distúrbio hereditário no qual a apolipoproteína B-48 é retida no intestino e está ausente no plasma; resulta em má absorção de gordura.

Coats d., d. de Coats. SIN exudative *retinitis.*

Cockayne d., d. de Cockayne. SIN Cockayne *syndrome.*

cold hemagglutinin d., d. por crioaglutinina; distúrbio associado à presença de auto-anticorpo hemaglutinante ativo *in vivo*, mas particularmente *in vitro* ou ativo apenas no frio; quando a concentração de anticorpo IgM é alta, pode haver aumento da viscosidade sérica, mas as manifestações clínicas (devidas à hemaglutinação) geralmente surgem após exposição ao frio; a hemólise geralmente é leve, mas pode ser intensa, resultando em anemia hemolítica auto-imune, tipo crioanticorpo. SIN cold agglutinin syndrome.

collagen d., collagen-vascular d., d. do colágeno, colagenose; grupo de doenças generalizadas que afetam o tecido conjuntivo e freqüentemente caracterizadas por necrose fibrinóide ou vasculite; em algumas doenças do colágeno, foi demonstrado auto-imunização, particularmente anticorpos antinucleares, e são encontrados imunocomplexos circulantes. O termo não é totalmente aceitável porque não há evidências de envolvimento primário do colágeno; "colágeno" já foi sinônimo de "tecido conjuntivo", em vez de descrever uma proteína fibrinosa específica nesse tecido. VER TAMBÉM connective-tissue d.

combined system d., d. sistêmica combinada. SIN subacute combined degeneration of the spinal cord.

communicable d., d. transmissível; qualquer doença transmissível por infecção ou contágio diretamente ou através de um vetor.

Concato d., d. de Concato. SIN polyserositis.

connective-tissue d., d. do tecido conjuntivo; grupo de doenças generalizadas que afetam o tecido conjuntivo, principalmente aquelas não herdadas como características mendelianas; a febre reumática e a artrite reumatóide foram inicialmente propostas como essas doenças, e foram acrescentadas outras doenças denominadas do colágeno.

Conradi d. [MIM*215100 & MIM*302950], d. de Conradi. SIN *chondrodysplasia* calcificans congenita.

Conradi-Hünermann d., d. de Conradi-Hünermann. SIN *chondrodysplasia* calcificans congenita.

contagious d., d. contagiosa; uma doença infecciosa transmissível por contato direto ou indireto; agora é usado como sinônimo de doença transmissível.

Cori d., d. de Cori. SIN type 3 *glycogenosis.*

Corrigan d., d. de Corrigan. SIN aortic *regurgitation.*

Cowden d. [MIM*158350], d. de Cowden; hipertricose e fibromatose gengival do lactente, acompanhadas por aumento pós-puberal fibradenomatoso da mama; as pápulas faciais são características de triquilemomas múltiplos. SIN multiple hamartoma syndrome.

Creutzfeldt-Jakob d. (CJD), d. Creutzfeldt-Jakob (DCJ); distúrbio neurológico progressivo, uma das encefalopatias espongiformes subagudas causadas por príons. As características clínicas da DCJ incluem uma síndrome cerebelar progressiva, incluindo ataxia, anormalidades da marcha e da fala e demência. Na maioria dos pacientes, essas manifestações são seguidas por movimentos involuntários (mioclonia) e pelo surgimento de um traçado eletroencefalográfico diagnóstico típico (supressão de salvas, que consiste em complexos de ondas agudas e lentas intermitentes sobre um fundo isoelétrico). A sobrevida média é de menos de 1 ano após o início dos sintomas. Não há alterações do LCR ou estas são inespecíficas. A atrofia cortical leve e a dilatação ventricular podem ser evidentes macroscopicamente. Ao exame microscópico, o achado característico é a encefalopatia espongiforme na substância cinzenta em todo o encéfalo e medula espinal. Também há perda neuronal acentuada e gliose, e pode haver desmielinização leve. As alterações ultra-estruturais incluem formação de vacúolos intracitoplasmáticos, a base do aspecto esponjoso. A DCJ ocorre em todo o mundo em uma taxa de aproximadamente 1-2 casos por milhão de pessoas por ano; em sua maioria, os casos são esporádicos, mas 10–12% são hereditários. A incidência máxima se dá entre 55 e 65 anos de idade; a doença é rara antes dos 30 anos. Casos de doença de Creutzfeldt-Jakob iatrogênica foram associados a transplantes de córnea, implantes de eletrodos, enxertos de dura-máter e administração de hormônio do crescimento humano. A DCJ é causada por uma proteína príon (uma isoforma anormal de proteína amilóide) que serve como fator de nucleação, induzindo anormalidades em outras proteínas. Essa proteína é detectável pelo *Western blot* no início da doença clínica. Outras doenças por príons, além da DCJ, incluem a síndrome de Gerstmann-Sträussler-Scheinker, insônia familiar fatal e kuru em seres humanos; *scrapie* (encefalopatia espongiforme contagiosa) em ovinos e caprinos; encefalopatia espongiforme bovina (doença da vaca louca) em bovinos e encefalopatias semelhantes e síndromes consumptivas em outras espécies. Todas essas doenças mostraram ser transmissíveis em animais de laboratório. VER TAMBÉM bovine spongiform *encephalopathy.*

Durante a década de 1990 foi descrito um número incomum de casos de doença de Creutzfeldt-Jakob em pessoas jovens na Grã-Bretanha. Esses pacientes exibiam ataxia, comprometimento da memória, demência e mioclonia. Além das alterações espongiformes características da DCJ, amostras de necrópsia desses pacientes mostraram placas amilóides incomuns com centros eosinofílicos densos extensamente distribuídos por todo o cérebro e cerebelo. Essas placas, visíveis com métodos de coloração de rotina, não foram observadas anteriormente na doença de Creutzfeldt-Jakob, mas assemelhavam-se às placas observadas no kuru. Além disso, esses pacientes não exibiam as alterações eletroencefalográficas características da DCJ clássica. Há suspeita de uma associação entre esse *cluster* regional de variante da doença de Creutzfeldt-Jakob e uma forma epizoótica de encefalopatia espongiforme bovina que afetou mais de 150.000 bovinos no Reino Unido entre 1986 e 1996. Entretanto, a revisão das estatísticas de mortalidade não mostra aumento da taxa de mortalidade por DCJ entre açougueiros, fazendeiros e veterinários na Inglaterra e Gales entre 1979 e 1996. VER TAMBÉM bovine spongiform *encephalopathy.*

Crigler-Najjar d., d. de Crigler-Najjar. SIN Crigler-Najjar *syndrome.*

Crocq d., d. de Crocq. SIN acrocyanosis.

Crohn d., d. de Crohn. SIN regional *enteritis.*

Crouzon d., d. de Crouzon. SIN Crouzon *syndrome.*

Cruveilhier-Baumgarten d., d. de Cruveilhier-Baumgarten. SIN Cruveilhier-Baumgarten *syndrome.*

Cushing d., d. de Cushing; hiperplasia supra-renal (síndrome de Cushing) causada por um adenoma basófilo da hipófise secretor de ACTH. SIN Cushing pituitary basophilism.

Cushing d. of the omentum, d. de Cushing do omento; obesidade central, associada a excesso de glicocorticóide, na qual células do estroma adiposo da gordura omental, mas não do tecido subcutâneo, podem gerar cortisol ativo a partir de cortisona inativa. Os pacientes apresentam aumento da produção de cortisol e da excreção urinária de cortisol, mas não há anormalidade no eixo hipotálamo–hipofisário–supra-renal.

cystic d. of the breast, d. cística da mama; distúrbio fibrocístico das mamas.

cysticercus d., cisticercose. SIN cisticercosis.

cystic d. of renal medulla [MIM*256100], d. cística da medula renal; presença de pequenos cistos na medula renal associados a anemia, depleção de sódio e insuficiência renal crônica. Existem dois tipos: 1) tipo autossômico recessivo fatal ou juvenil (também denominado nefroftise juvenil familiar), que começa em torno dos 10 anos de idade, com uma duração média de 6-8 anos; 2) tipo autossômico dominante ou do adulto. SIN microcystic d. of renal medulla.

cystine storage d., cistinose. SIN cystinosis.

cytomegalic inclusion d., d. de inclusão citomegálica; causada por citomegalovírus, um membro da família Herpesviridae; a presença de corpúsculos de inclusão no citoplasma e núcleos de células aumentadas de vários órgãos de recém-nascidos que morrem com icterícia, hepatomegalia, esplenomegalia, púrpura, trombocitopenia e febre; o distúrbio também ocorre, em todas as idades, como uma complicação de outras doenças nas quais os mecanismos imunes sofrem grande depressão, e foi encontrado incidentalmente no epitélio da glândula salivar, aparentemente como uma infecção localizada ou leve (doença por vírus da glândula salivar). SIN cytomegalovirus d., inclusion body d.

cytomegalovirus d., d. por citomegalovírus. SIN cytomegalic inclusion d.

Daae d., d. de Daae. SIN epidemic *pleurodynia.*

Danielssen d., d. de Danielssen. SIN anesthetic *leprosy.*
Danielssen-Boeck d., d. de Danielssen-Boeck. SIN anesthetic *leprosy.*
Darier d., d. de Darier. SIN *keratosis* follicularis.
Darling d., d. de Darling. SIN histoplasmosis.
Davies d., d. de Davies. SIN endomyocardial *fibrosis.*
decompression d., d. da descompressão. SIN decompression *sickness.*
deer-fly d., tularemia. SIN tularemia.
deficiency d., d. por deficiência; qualquer doença resultante de subnutrição ou da inadequação das calorias, proteínas, aminoácidos essenciais, ácidos graxos, vitaminas ou oligoelementos.
degenerative joint d., d. articular degenerativa. SIN osteoarthritis.
Degos d., d. de Degos. SIN malignant atrophic *papulosis.*
Dejerine d., d. de Dejerine. SIN Dejerine-Sottas d.
Dejerine-Sottas d., d. de Dejerine-Sottas; tipo familiar de polineuropatia sensorial desmielinizante que começa nos primeiros anos de vida e progride lentamente; clinicamente caracterizada por dor e parestesias nos pés, seguidas por fraqueza simétrica e debilitação das porções distais dos membros; uma das causas de "pernas de cegonha"; os pacientes cedo ficam presos à cadeira de rodas; os nervos periféricos apresentam aumento palpável e são indolores; anatomopatologicamente, é observada formação de bulbo de cebola nos nervos; espirais de processos de células de Schwann entrelaçados e superpostos que circundam os axônios desnudos; geralmente a herança é autossômica recessiva; também existe uma forma autossômica dominante; as duas formas podem ser causadas por mutações no gene 22 da proteína mielina periférica (PMP22) em 17q ou no gene zero da proteína mielina (MPZ) em 1q. SIN Dejerine d., hereditary hypertrophic neuropathy, progressive hypertrophic polyneuropathy.
demyelinating d., d. desmielinizante; termo genérico que designa um grupo de doenças, de causa desconhecida, nas quais há extensa perda da mielina no sistema nervoso central, como na esclerose múltipla e na doença de Schilder.
dense-deposit d., d. de depósito denso. VER membranoproliferative *glomerulonephritis.*
de Quervain d., d. de de Quervain; fibrose da bainha de um tendão do polegar. SIN radial styloid tendovaginitis.
Dercum d., d. de Dercum. SIN *adiposis* dolorosa.
Deutschländer d., d. de Deutschländer; tumor de um dos ossos metatarsais.
Devic d., d. de Devic. SIN *neuromyelitis* optica.
diffuse Lewy body d., d. difusa dos corpúsculos de Lewy; distúrbio cerebral degenerativo de pessoas idosas, caracterizado inicialmente por demência ou psicose progressiva e, subseqüentemente, por achados parkinsonianos, geralmente com rigidez acentuada; outras manifestações incluem movimentos involuntários, mioclonia, disfagia e hipotensão ortostática. No exame anatomopatológico são encontrados corpúsculos de Lewy difusamente nos núcleos do hipotálamo, prosencéfalo basal e tronco cerebral. SIN Lewy body dementia.
Di Guglielmo d., d. de Di Guglielmo; a forma aguda de mielose eritrêmica. SIN Di Guglielmo syndrome.
disappearing bone d., d. do desaparecimento ósseo; extensa descalcificação de um único osso; de causa desconhecida, algumas vezes associada a angioma. SIN Gorham d., Gorham syndrome.
diverticular d., d. diverticular; divertículos congênitos ou adquiridos sintomáticos de qualquer parte do trato gastrointestinal. Esses divertículos ocorrem em cerca de 15% da população, mas raramente causam sintomas.
dog d., d. do flebótomo. SIN phlebotomus *fever.*
dominantly inherited Lévi d., d. de Lévi com herança dominante. SIN snub-nose *dwarfism.*
Donohue d., d. de Donohue. SIN leprechaunism.
drug-induced d., d. induzida por medicamento, d. fármaco-induzida; reação tóxica a, ou condição mórbida resultante da, administração de um medicamento.
Dubois d., d. de Dubois. SIN Dubois *abscesses,* em *abscess.*
Duchenne d., d. de Duchenne. SIN Duchenne *dystrophy.*
Duchenne-Aran d., d. de Duchenne-Aran. SIN amyotrophic lateral *sclerosis.*
Duhring d., d. de Duhring. SIN *dermatitis* herpetiformis.
Dukes d., d. de Dukes. SIN *exanthema* subitum.
Duncan d. [MIM*308240], d. de Duncan. SIN X-linked lymphoproliferative *syndrome.* SIN lymphoproliferative syndrome.
Dupuytren d. of the foot, d. de Dupuytren do pé. SIN plantar *fibromatosis.*
Duroziez d., d. de Duroziez; estenose congênita da valva mitral.
Dutton d., d. de Dutton; febre recidivante africana, causada por *Borrelia duttonii* e transmitida pelo carrapato *Ornithodoros moubata.* SIN Dutton relapsing fever.
Eales d., d. de Eales; periflebite retiniana periférica que causa hemorragias retinianas ou intravítreo recorrentes em adultos jovens.
Ebstein d., d. de Ebstein. SIN Ebstein *anomaly.*
echinococcus d., equinococose. SIN echinococcosis.
Eisenmenger d., d. de Eisenmenger. SIN Eisenmenger *complex.*
elephant man's d., d. do homem elefante; (1) SIN Proteus *syndrome;* (2) SIN neurofibromatosis.
elevator d., d. do elevador; angústia respiratória que afeta pessoas que trabalham em elevadores de cereais, resultante da inalação de poeiras ou insetos.

emotional d., d. emocional. VER mental *illness.*
endemic d., d. endêmica; prevalência contínua de uma doença em uma população ou área específica. VER TAMBÉM endemic, enzootic.
Engelmann d., d. de Engelmann. SIN diaphysial *dysplasia.*
English sweating d., d. sudoreica inglesa; doença de natureza desconhecida que surgiu na Inglaterra e disseminou-se por toda a Europa em 1485, 1508 e 1528–30, caracterizada por sudorese intensa, prostração e elevada taxa de fatalidade. SIN sudor anglicus.
eosinophilic endomyocardial d., d. endomiocárdica eosinofílica; miocardiopatia restritiva associada a hiperprodução de eosinófilos e infiltração cardíaca pelos mesmos, clinicamente caracterizada por insuficiência ventricular diastólica e sistólica tardia. Algumas vezes associada à síndrome de Churg-Strauss ou à pericardite eosinofílica.
epidemic d., d. epidêmica; aumento significativo da prevalência de uma doença em uma população ou área específica, geralmente com uma causa ambiental, como um agente infeccioso ou tóxico.
Epstein d., d. de Epstein. SIN diphtheroid (1).
Erb d., d. de Erb. SIN progressive bulbar *paralysis.*
Erb-Charcot d., d. de Erb-Charcot; (1) SIN spastic *diplegia;* (2) SIN spastic *paraplegia.*
Erdheim d., d. de Erdheim. SIN cystic medial *necrosis.*
ergot alkaloid-associated heart d., cardiopatia associada aos alcalóides do esporão do centeio; cardiopatia causada por fibrose endomiocárdica que se estende até estruturas valvares, produzindo estenose e/ou regurgitação, associada ao uso de alcalóides do esporão do centeio.
Eulenburg d., d. de Eulenburg. SIN congenital *paramyotonia.*
exanthematous d., d. exantematosa. VER exanthema.
extramammary Paget d., d. de Paget extramamária; forma intra-epidérmica de adenocarcinoma mucinoso, mais comumente na região anogenital, que se apresenta como placas eritematosas nas pessoas idosas, podendo estar associadas a carcinoma das glândulas sudoríparas ou visceral regional. SIN Paget d. (3).
extrapiramidal d., d. extrapiramidal; termo geral para vários distúrbios causados por anormalidades dos gânglios da base ou determinados núcleos do tronco cerebral ou talâmicos; caracterizada por déficits motores, perda dos reflexos posturais, bradicinesia, tremor, rigidez e vários movimentos involuntários. SIN extrapyramidal motor system d.
extrapyramidal motor system d., d. do sistema motor extrapiramidal. SIN extrapyramidal d.
Fabry d. [MIM*301500], d. de Fabry; devida à deficiência de α-galactosidase e caracterizada por acúmulos anormais de glicolipídios neutros (p. ex., globotriasoilceramida) nas células endoteliais nas paredes dos vasos sanguíneos; os achados clínicos incluem angioceratomas nas coxas, nádegas e genitália, hipoidrose, parestesia nos membros, córnea verticilada e catarata subcapsular posterior rajada; a morte resulta de complicações renais, cardíacas ou vasculares cerebrais; herança recessiva ligada ao X causada por mutação do gene α-galactosidase (GLA) em Xq. SIN diffuse angiokeratoma, glycolipid lipidosis.
Fahr d., d. de Fahr; depósitos calcificados progressivos nas paredes dos vasos sanguíneos dos gânglios da base, em pessoas jovens ou de meia-idade; ocasionalmente associada a retardo mental e sintomas extrapiramidais.
Farber d., d. de Farber. SIN disseminated *lipogranulomatosis.*
Favre-Durand-Nicholas d., doença de Favre-Durand-Nicholas. SIN venereal *lymphogranuloma.*
Favre-Racouchot d., d. de Favre-Racouchot; comedões que surgem na pele lesada pelo sol devido à obstrução dos folículos pilossebáceos por elastose solar. SIN Favre-Racouchot syndrome, solar comedo.
Fazio-Londe d. [MIM*211500], d. de Fazio-Londe; paralisia bulbar progressiva que afeta o tronco cerebral; causada por degeneração motora; uma vari-

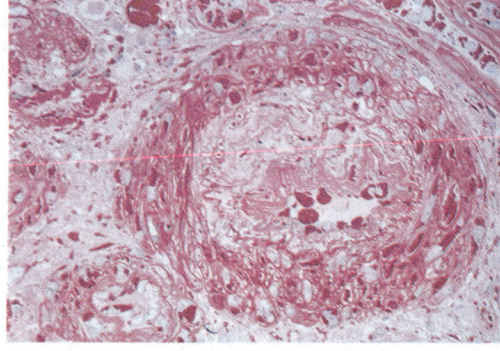

doença de Fabry: artéria exibindo acúmulo de gotículas de ácido periódico de Schiff (PAS)-positivas nas células musculares da túnica média; a túnica íntima mostra considerável espessamento; fixação de ósmio, coloração pelo ácido periódico de Schiff, 250 ×

ante da atrofia da musculatura paravertebral (q.v.).
Feer d., d. de Feer. SIN acrodynia (2).
femoropopliteal occlusive d., d. oclusiva femoropoplítea; obstrução das artérias femoral e poplítea por aterosclerose.
fibrocystic d. of the pancreas, d. fibrocística do pâncreas. SIN cystic *fibrosis*.
fifth d., quinta doença da infância, eritema infeccioso. SIN *erythema infectiosum*. [após escarlatina, sarampo, rubéola e quarta doença]
Filatov d., d. de Filatov. SIN Filatov-Dukes d.
Filatov-Dukes d., d. de Filatov-Dukes; doença infecciosa causadora de exantema da infância, de etiologia desconhecida. SIN Filatov d., parascarlatina, scarlatinella, scarlatinoid (2).
fish eye d., d. do olho de peixe; distúrbio hereditário que resulta em baixo HDL-colesterol e opacidades da córnea; também, baixa atividade de LCAT.
flax-dresser's d., d. do manipulador de linho; doença pulmonar obstrutiva crônica causada por inalação de partículas de linho bruto; uma forma de bissinose. VER TAMBÉM byssinosis.
Flegel d., d. de Flegel. SIN *hyperkeratosis* lenticularis perstans.
flint d., calicose. SIN chalicosis.
focal metastatic d., d. metastática focal; presença de uma única área de metástase de um tumor maligno ou infecção distante da lesão primária.
Folling d., d. de Folling. SIN phenylketonuria.
foot-and-mouth d. (FMD), d. do pé e boca, febre aftosa; doença extremamente infecciosa de ampla distribuição e grande importância econômica, que ocorre em bovinos, suínos, carneiros, caprinos e em todos os animais selvagens e domésticos de casco fendido, causada por um picornavírus (gênero Aphthovirus) e caracterizada por erupções vesiculares na boca, língua, cascos e úberes; os seres humanos raramente são afetados. SIN aftosa.
Forbes d., d. de Forbes. SIN type 3 *glycogenosis*.
Fordyce d., d. de Fordyce. SIN Fordyce *spots*, em *spot*.
Forestier d., d. de Forestier. SIN diffuse idiopathic skeletal *hyperostosis*.
Fothergill d., d. de Fothergill; **(1)** SIN trigeminal *neuralgia*; **(2)** SIN anginose *scarlatina*.
Fournier d., d. de Fournier; gangrena infecciosa envolvendo o escroto. SIN Fournier gangrene, syphiloma of Fournier.
fourth d., quarta d. da infância, exantema súbito. SIN *exanthema* subitum.
Fox-Fordyce d., d. de Fox-Fordyce; erupção pruriginosa crônica de pápulas secas e glândulas apócrinas rotas e distendidas, observada mais comumente em mulheres, com hiperceratose folicular dos mamilos, axilas e regiões pubiana e esternal. SIN apocrine miliaria.
Franklin d., d. de Franklin. SIN γ-heavy-chain d.
Freiberg d., d. de Freiberg; osteonecrose da cabeça do segundo metatarso. SIN Freiberg infarction.
Friend d., d. de Friend; leucemia do camundongo causada pelo vírus da leucemia de Friend, um membro da família Retroviridae.
functional d., d. funcional. SIN functional *disorder*.

functional cardiovascular d., d. cardiovascular funcional; eufemismo para sintomas cardiovasculares considerados psicogênicos. De forma mais geral, termo algumas vezes usado para designar função cardíaca anormal.
fusospirochetal d., d. fusoespiroquética; infecção da boca e/ou faringe associada a bacilos fusiformes e espiroquetas, comumente parte da flora normal da boca. VER TAMBÉM necrotizing ulcerative *gingivitis*.
Gairdner d., d. de Gairdner; ataques de angústia cardíaca acompanhados por apreensão. SIN angina pectoris sine dolore, angor pectoris (1).
Gamna d., d. de Gamna; uma forma de esplenomegalia crônica caracterizada por espessamento visível da cápsula e presença de múltiplos focos pequenos, crostiformes e castanhos (corpúsculos de Gamna-Gandy), que contêm ferro; esse distúrbio pode ser observado na esplenomegalia fibrocongestiva, na doença falciforme e em alguns exemplos de hemocromatose.
Gandy-Nanta d., d. de Gandy-Nanta; esplenomegalia siderótica, provavelmente a mesma que a doença de Gamna.
garapata d., d. do carrapato; febre do carrapato que ocorre na Espanha.
Garré d., d. de Garré. SIN sclerosing *osteitis*.

gastroesophageal reflux d. (GERD), d. por refluxo gastroesofágico (DRGE); síndrome causada por incompetência estrutural ou funcional do esfíncter esofágico inferior, que permite o fluxo retrógrado de suco gástrico ácido para o esôfago.

Embora a anormalidade subjacente na DRGE seja aparentemente congênita e irreversível, a incidência aumenta com a idade. Além do refluxo, a maioria dos casos envolve perturbação da motilidade gástrica e prolongamento do tempo de esvaziamento gástrico. Os sintomas incluem desconforto epigástrico e retroesternal recorrente, geralmente descrito como pirose, em conjunto com graus variáveis de eructação, náuseas, ânsia de vômito, tosse ou rouquidão. A DRGE é cada vez mais reconhecida como causa de irritação da orofaringe e tosse crônica. A incidência de DRGE em adultos com asma pode chegar a 80%. O distúrbio é mais comum em homens. A probabilidade de refluxo sintomático é aumentada por obesidade, gravidez, tabagismo, diabetes melito, esclerodermia e outras doenças do tecido conjuntivo. Os sintomas podem ser induzidos por decúbito, exercício vigoroso, levantamento de peso, tabagismo, grandes refeições ou consumo de álcool, chocolate, alimentos gordurosos e fármacos como teofilina, bloqueadores dos canais de cálcio e agentes anticolinérgicos. O refluxo de ácido pode causar esofagite péptica, formação de úlcera ou estenose esofágica. Alterações metaplásicas no epitélio escamoso esofágico, denominadas esôfago de Barrett, podem progredir para carcinoma. O diagnóstico é feito por anamnese, monitorização do pH esofágico, estudo radiográfico mostrando refluxo do bário deglutido e endoscopia para identificar ulceração ou estenose e permitir biópsia para excluir processos malignos. O tratamento inclui afastamento de causas conhecidas e administração de antiácidos, antagonistas H_2, agentes pró-cinéticos e inibidores da bomba de prótons.

Gaucher d., d. de Gaucher; distúrbio do armazenamento lisossômico devido a deficiência de glicocerebrosidase, resultando em acúmulo de glicocerebrosídeo; alta incidência em descendentes de judeus asquenazes; é mais grave em lactentes, caracterizada por hepatosplenomegalia, anormalidades hematológicas, lesões ósseas, manifestações neurológicas com ataxia, paraplegia espástica, convulsões e demência, além da presença de histiócitos característicos (células de Gaucher) nas vísceras; herança autossômica recessiva, causada por mutação no gene da glicocerebrosidase A (GBA) no cromossoma 1q. Há três formas principais: tipo I, juvenil não-cerebral [MIM*230800]; tipo II, juvenil cerebral [MIM*230900]; e tipo III, cerebral do adulto [MIM*231000]; as formas juvenis são mais graves. SIN cerebroside lipidosis.
Gerhardt-Mitchell d., d. de Gerhardt-Mitchell. SIN erythromelalgia.
Gerlier d., d. de Gerlier. SIN vestibular *neuronitis*.
gestational trophoblastic d., d. trofoblástica gestacional. SIN hydatidiform *mole*.
Gierke d., d. de Gierke. SIN type 1 *glycogenosis*.
Gilbert d., d. de Gilbert. SIN familial nonhemolytic *jaundice*.
Gilchrist d., d. de Gilchrist. SIN blastomycosis.
Gilles de la Tourette d., d. de Gilles de la Tourette. SIN Tourette *syndrome*.
Glanzmann d., d. de Glanzmann. SIN Glanzmann *thrombasthenia*.
glycogen-storage d., d. de depósito de glicogênio. SIN glycogenosis.
Goldflam d., d. de Goldflam. SIN *myasthenia* gravis.
Gorham d., d. de Gorham. SIN disappearing bone d.
Gougerot and Blum d., d. de Gougerot e Blum. SIN pigmented purpuric lichenoid *dermatosis*.
Gougerot-Sjögren d., d. de Gougerot-Sjögren. SIN Sjögren *syndrome*. [Sjögren, Henrik S.C.]
Gowers d., d. de Gowers; **(1)** SIN saltatory *spasm*; **(2)** uma forma distal de distrofia muscular progressiva.

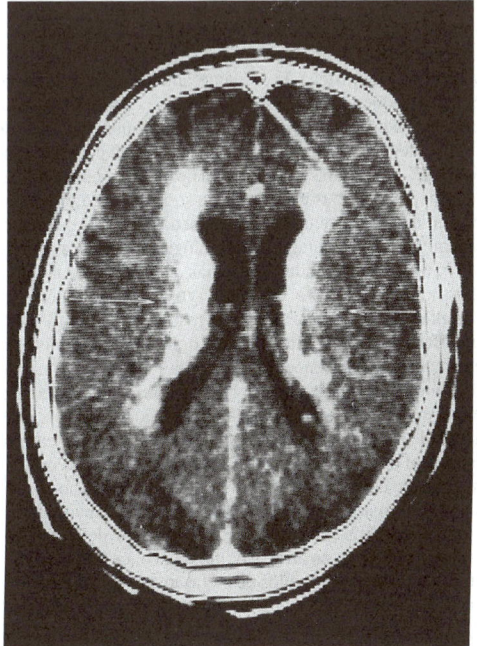

doença de Fahr: calcificação arteriosclerótica dos gânglios da base, dos dois lados (tomografia computadorizada)

graft versus host d., d. enxerto-*versus*-hospedeiro; reação de incompatibilidade (que pode ser fatal) em um indivíduo (hospedeiro) de baixa competência imunológica que recebeu tecido linfóide imunologicamente competente de um doador imunologicamente diferente; a reação, ou doença, é conseqüência da ação das células transplantadas contra os tecidos do hospedeiro que possuem um antígeno não encontrado no doador. Observada com maior freqüência após transplantes de medula óssea, a doença aguda ocorre após 7–30 dias, e a doença crônica, semanas a meses após o transplante, afetando, principalmente, o trato gastrointestinal, o fígado e a pele. SIN GVH d.
granulomatous d., d. granulomatosa. SIN chronic granulomatous d.
Graves d., d. de Graves; **(1)** bócio tóxico caracterizado por hiperplasia difusa da tireóide, uma forma de hipertireoidismo; a exoftalmia é um achado concomitante comum, mas não invariável; **(2)** disfunção da tireóide e todas as suas associações clínicas ou qualquer uma delas; **(3)** uma doença auto-imune órgão-específica da tireóide. VER thyrotoxicosis, Hashimoto *thyroiditis*, goiter, myxedema. SIN Basedow d., ophthalmic hyperthyroidism, Parry d.
Griesinger d., d. de Griesinger; febre biliar de Griesinger, uma forma grave de febre recidivante transmitida por piolhos, causada por *Borrelia recurrentis*, e que ocasiona febre alta, epistaxe, dispnéia, icterícia intensa, púrpura e esplenomegalia.
Grover d., d. de Grover. SIN transient acantholytic *dermatosis*.
GVH d., SIN graft versus host d.
Haff d., d. de Haff; rabdomiólise resultante de uma toxina não-identificada contida em alguns peixes, incluindo os peixes rodovalho e búfalo. [*Haff*, um braço do Mar Báltico no leste da Prússia]
Haglund d., d. de Haglund; proeminência anormal da face lateral póstero-superior do calcâneo. SIN Haglund deformity.
Hailey-Hailey d., d. de Hailey-Hailey. SIN benign familial chronic *pemphigus*.
Hallervorden-Spatz d., d. de Hallervorden-Spatz. SIN Hallervorden-Spatz *syndrome*.
Hallopeau d., d. de Hallopeau. SIN *pemphigus* vegetans (2).
Hamman d., d. de Hamman. SIN Hamman *syndrome*.
Hammond d., d. de Hammond. SIN athetosis.
hand-foot-and-mouth d., d. da mão-pé-e-boca; erupção exantematosa em crianças pequenas, que geralmente consiste em pequenas vesículas cinza-perolado dos dedos das mãos, dedos dos pés, regiões palmares e plantares, acompanhadas por vesículas e ulceração freqüentemente dolorosa da mucosa oral e da língua e por febre baixa; a doença dura 4–7 dias, sendo geralmente causada por vírus Coxsackie tipo A-16, já tendo sido identificados, porém, outros tipos.
Hand-Schüller-Christian d., d. de Hand-Schüller-Christian; a forma disseminada crônica da histiocitose de células de Langerhans. A tríade clássica de sinais consiste em diabetes insípido, exoftalmia e lesões ósseas compostas de histiócitos. SIN Christian d. (1), Christian syndrome, normal cholesteremic xanthomatosis, Schüller d., Schüller syndrome.
Hansen d., d. de Hansen. SIN leprosy.
Harada d., d. de Harada. SIN Harada *syndrome*.
Hartnup d. [MIM*234500], d. de Hartnup; distúrbio metabólico hereditário autossômico recessivo, caracterizado por aminoacidúria decorrente de defeito do transporte tubular renal de α-aminoácidos neutros; há aumento da excreção urinária de derivados do triptofano causado por defeito da absorção intestinal e degradação bacteriana de triptofano não-absorvido no intestino; as manifestações incluem erupção cutânea fotossensível, semelhante à pelagra, com ataxia cerebelar temporária. SIN Hartnup syndrome.
Hashimoto d., d. de Hashimoto. SIN Hashimoto *thyroiditis*.
heavy chain d., d. da cadeia pesada; termo usado para um grupo de doenças, as paraproteinemias, caracterizadas pela produção de imunoglobulinas ou fragmentos homogêneos, e associadas a distúrbios malignos da série de células plasmocíticas e linfóides. Já foram reconhecidos três tipos: doença da cadeia pesada γ, doença da cadeia pesada α e doença da cadeia pesada μ; cada uma é diagnosticada pelo achado do fragmento de cadeia pesada apropriado no soro e/ou na urina.
α-heavy-chain d., d. da cadeia pesada α; a forma mais comum da doença da cadeia pesada, caracterizada pelo achado, no soro, de uma proteína reativa com anti-soros contra cadeias α, mas não contra cadeias leves; as manifestações clínicas incluem diarréia, esteatorréia e má absorção grave.
γ-heavy-chain d., d. da cadeia pesada γ; doença da cadeia pesada caracterizada pelo achado, no soro e na urina, de um amplo pico protéico reativo com anti-soros contra cadeias γ e não-reativos com anti-soros contra cadeias leves; as manifestações comuns incluem anemia, linfocitose, eosinofilia, trombocitopenia, hiperuricemia, linfadenopatia e hepatosplenomegalia. SIN Franklin d.
μ-heavy-chain d., d. da cadeia pesada μ; a forma mais rara de doença da cadeia pesada, observada basicamente em pacientes com leucemia linfocítica crônica; o diagnóstico é feito por imunoeletroforese através do achado de um componente reativo com anti-soros contra cadeias μ, mas não contra cadeias leves.
Heck d., d. de Heck. SIN focal epithelial *hyperplasia*.

Heerfordt d., d. de Heerfordt. SIN uveoparotid *fever*.
hemoglobin C d., d. da hemoglobina C; o estado homozigoto da hemoglobina C.
hemoglobin H d., d. da hemoglobina H. VER *hemoglobin* H.
hemolytic d. of newborn, d. hemolítica do recém-nascido. SIN erythroblastosis fetalis.
hemorrhagic d. of the newborn, d. hemorrágica do recém-nascido; síndrome caracterizada por hemorragia interna ou externa espontânea, acompanhada por hipoprotrombinemia, discreta diminuição das plaquetas e elevação significativa dos tempos de sangramento e de coagulação, geralmente ocorrendo entre o terceiro e o sexto dias de vida e efetivamente tratada com vitamina K.
herring-worm d., anisaquíase. SIN anisakiasis.
Hers d., d. de Hers. SIN type 6 *glycogenosis*.
Hirschsprung d., d. de Hirschsprung. SIN congenital *megacolon*.
Hodgkin d., d. de Hodgkin; doença caracterizada por aumento crônico dos linfonodos, muitas vezes local no início e generalizado mais tarde, juntamente com aumento do baço, e, em geral, do fígado, sem leucocitose acentuada e, comumente, com anemia e febre contínua ou remitente (Pel-Ebstein); considerada uma neoplasia maligna de células linfóides de origem incerta (células de Reed-Sternberg), associada a infiltração inflamatória de linfócitos e eosinófilos e fibrose; pode ser classificada em tipo com predomínio linfocítico, esclerosante nodular, de celularidade mista e depleção linfocítica; uma doença semelhante ocorre em gatos domésticos. SIN Hodgkin lymphoma, lymphadenoma (2).
Hodgson d., d. de Hodgson; dilatação do arco aórtico associada à insuficiência da valva aórtica.
holoendemic d. (hol′ō-en-dem-ik), d. holoendêmica; uma doença para a qual um alto nível prevalente de infecção começa no início da vida e afeta a maior parte da população infantil, ou toda ela, levando a um estado de equilíbrio, de forma que a população adulta mostre evidências da doença com freqüência muito menor que as crianças.
hookworm d., ancilostomíase. VER ancylostomiasis, necatoriasis.
Huntington d. [MIM*143100], d. de Huntington. SIN Huntington *chorea*.
Hurler d., d. de Hurler. SIN Hurler *syndrome*.
Hurst d., d. de Hurst. SIN acute necrotizing hemorrhagic *encephalomyelitis*.
Hutchinson-Gilford d., d. de Hutchinson-Gilford. SIN progeria.
hyaline membrane d. of the newborn, d. da membrana hialina do recém-nascido; doença observada principalmente em recém-nascidos prematuros com angústia respiratória; caracterizada, no período *postmortem*, por atelectasia e ductos alveolares revestidos por uma membrana eosinofílica; também associada a quantidades reduzidas de surfactante pulmonar. SIN hyaline membrane syndrome, respiratory distress syndrome of the newborn.
hydatid d., d. hidática; infestação de seres humanos, ovinos e da maioria dos outros mamíferos herbívoros e onívoros por larvas da tênia *Echinococcus*.
hyperendemic d., d. hiperendêmica; doença que está constantemente presente em alta taxa de incidência e/ou prevalência e afeta igualmente todas as faixas etárias.
Iceland d., d. da Islândia. SIN epidemic *neuromyasthenia*.
I-cell d., d. da célula I. SIN *mucolipidosis* II.
idiopathic d., d. idiopática; doença de causa ou mecanismo desconhecido.
immune complex d., d. por imunocomplexo; categoria imunológica de doenças provocadas pela deposição de antígeno-anticorpo na rede microvascular. O complemento freqüentemente está envolvido e os produtos da decomposição do complemento atraem leucócitos polimorfonucleares para o local de deposição. A lesão tecidual freqüentemente é causada pelo processo de fagocitose "frustrada" por células polimorfonucleares. Vasculite ou nefrite é comum. O fenômeno de Arthus e a doença do soro são exemplos clássicos, mas muitos outros distúrbios, incluindo a maioria das doenças do tecido conjuntivo, podem pertencer a essa categoria imunológica; as doenças por imunocomplexo também podem ocorrer durante várias doenças de etiologia conhecida, como a endocardite bacteriana subaguda. VER TAMBÉM autoimmune d. SIN immune complex disorder, type III hypersensitivity reaction.
immunoproliferative small intestinal d., d. imunoproliferativa do intestino delgado; infiltração linfoplasmocítica difusa da mucosa proximal do intestino delgado e dos linfonodos mesentéricos, resultando em diarréia, emagrecimento, dor abdominal e baqueteamento dos dedos das mãos e dos pés; observada em pessoas pobres de países em desenvolvimento. SIN Mediterranean lymphoma.
inborn lysosomal d., d. lisossômica hereditária; distúrbio hereditário de uma ou mais enzimas de degradação normalmente localizadas nos lisossomas, levando ao acúmulo (armazenamento) de quantidades anormais de uma substância, p. ex. uma glicosaminoglicana, como na síndrome de Hurler (Hurler *syndrome*), ou de um lipopolissacarídeo, como na doença de Gaucher.
inclusion body d., d. de corpúsculos de inclusão. SIN cytomegalic inclusion d.
inclusion cell d., d. de células de inclusão. SIN *mucolipidosis* II.
industrial d., d. industrial; condição mórbida resultante da exposição a um agente liberado no ambiente por uma empresa comercial. Cf. occupational d.
infantile celiac d., d. celíaca infantil; enteropatia sensível ao glúten que surge na lactância, freqüentemente antes dos 9 meses de idade e caracterizada por início agudo, diarréia, dor abdominal e "atraso do desenvolvimento".

disease

infectious d., infective d., d. infecciosa; doença resultante da presença e atividade de um agente microbiano.

intercurrent d., d. intercorrente; uma nova doença que ocorre durante a evolução de outra doença, não relacionada ao processo mórbido primário.

interstitial d., d. intersticial; doença que ocorre principalmente na estrutura de tecido conjuntivo de um órgão, com o parênquima sofrendo secundariamente.

iron-storage d., d. de depósito de ferro; o armazenamento de excesso de ferro no parênquima de muitos órgãos, como na hemocromatose idiopática ou na hemossiderose por transfusão.

island d., d. da ilha. SIN tsutsugamushi d.

Itai-Itai d., d. de itai-itai; forma de envenenamento por cádmio descrita no povo japonês, caracterizada por disfunção tubular renal, osteomalacia, pseudofraturas e anemia por ingestão de frutos-do-mar contaminados ou outras fontes contendo cádmio.

Jaffe-Lichtenstein d., d. de Jaffe-Lichtenstein; termo obsoleto para displasia óssea fibrosa (fibrous *dysplasia* of bone).

Jansky-Bielschowsky d., d. de Jansky-Bielschowsky; esfingolipidose cerebral (cerebral *sphingolipidosis*), tipo juvenil inicial.

Jensen d., d. de Jensen. SIN retinochoroiditis juxtapapillaris.

jumping d., jumper d., d. saltitante; uma das síndromes de sobressalto anormais encontradas em partes isoladas do mundo, caracterizada por respostas muito exageradas, como saltar, agitar os braços e gritar, a estímulos mínimos. SIN jumping Frenchmen of Maine d., jumper d. of Maine.

jumping Frenchmen of Maine d., jumper d. of Maine, d. dos franceses saltitantes do Maine, d. saltitante do Maine. SIN jumping d.

Jüngling d., d. de Jüngling. SIN osteitis tuberculosa multiplex cystica.

Kashin-Bek d., d. de Kashin-Bek; forma de osteoartrose generalizada limitada a áreas da Ásia, incluindo o rio Urov; acredita-se que seja resultante da ingestão de trigo infectado pelo fungo *Fusarium sporotrichiella*.

Katayama d., d. de Katayama; fase aguda inicial de deposição de ovos da esquistossomose, uma síndrome toxêmica em infestações primárias maciças, raramente observada em casos crônicos. É considerada uma forma de doença por imunocomplexos do distúrbio semelhante à doença do soro. Descrita na esquistossomose japônica (*schistosomiasis* japonica), mas também observada em outras formas. SIN Katayama fever. [cidade do Japão onde a doença é comum]

Kawasaki d., d. de Kawasaki; vasculite sistêmica de origem desconhecida que ocorre basicamente em crianças com menos de 8 anos de idade. Os sinais e sintomas incluem uma febre com duração maior que 5 dias, erupção polimórfica, lábios eritematosos, secos, rachados; injeção conjuntival, edema das mãos e dos pés, irritabilidade, adenopatia e erupção descamativa perineal. Aproximadamente 20% dos pacientes não-tratados podem desenvolver aneurismas da artéria coronária. Quando a criança se recupera da doença, ocorrem trombocitose e descamação nas pontas dos dedos das mãos. SIN Kawasaki syndrome, mucocutaneous lymph node syndrome.

Kennedy d., d. de Kennedy; distúrbio recessivo ligado ao X caracterizado por atrofia muscular espinal e bulbar progressiva; as características associadas incluem degeneração distal dos axônios sensoriais e sinais de disfunção endócrina, incluindo diabetes melito, ginecomastia e atrofia testicular. SIN X-linked recessive bulbospinal neuronopathy.

Kienböck d., d. de Kienböck; osteonecrose do osso semilunar de etiologia desconhecida, embora possa ocorrer após traumatismo. SIN lunatomalacia.

Kikuchi d., d. de Kikuchi; linfadenite necrotizante de etiologia desconhecida, encontrada com maior freqüência em mulheres jovens no Japão, mas também em outras partes do mundo; o aumento dos linfonodos, associado à febre, cede espontaneamente.

Kimmelstiel-Wilson d., d. de Kimmelstiel-Wilson. SIN Kimmelstiel-Wilson *syndrome*.

Kimura d., d. de Kimura. SIN angiolymphoid *hyperplasia* with eosinophilia.

kinky-hair d., kinky hair d. [MIM*309400], d. do cabelo enroscado; erro congênito do metabolismo do cobre, com início algumas semanas após o nascimento; manifesta-se por cabelos curtos, escassos, pouco pigmentados e enroscados; atraso do desenvolvimento; desenvolvimento de convulsões; espasticidade e deterioração mental progressiva que leva à morte. Herança recessiva ligada ao X devida a um defeito do transporte de cobre, causada por mutação no gene Menkes (MNK), que codifica uma ATPase transportadora de cobre em Xq. SIN Menkes syndrome, trichopoliodystrophy.

Köhler d., d. de Köhler; osteonecrose do osso navicular do tarso ou da patela.

kok d., hiperecplexia SIN hyperekplexia.

Krabbe d., d. de Krabbe. SIN globoid cell *leukodystrophy*.

Kufs d., d. de Kufs; esfingolipidose cerebral (cerebral *sphingolipidosis*), tipo adulto.

Kugelberg-Welander d., d. de Kugelberg-Welander. SIN spinal muscular *atrophy*, type III.

Kussmaul d., d. de Kussmaul. SIN polyarteritis nodosa.

Kyasanur Forest d., d. da Kyasanur Forest; doença que ocorre em trabalhadores na Floresta de Kyasanur e em Mysore, Índia, causada por um flavivírus da família Flaviviridae, transmitido principalmente pelo *Haemaphysalis spinigera*, embora outros carrapatos também tenham sido envolvidos; os sinais e sintomas incluem febre, cefaléia, dor nas costas e nos membros, diarréia e hemorragia intestinal; não há sintomas relativos ao sistema nervoso central.

Kyrle d., d. de Kyrle. SIN hyperkeratosis follicularis et parafollicularis.

Lafora d., d. de Lafora. SIN Lafora body d.

Lafora body d. [MIM*254780], d. do corpúsculo de Lafora; uma forma de epilepsia mioclônica progressiva, que começa entre 6 e 19 anos de idade; caracterizada por convulsões tônico-clônicas generalizadas, mioclonia em repouso e em atividade, ataxia, demência e achados clássicos no EEG, incluindo poliponta e onda; há corpúsculos de inclusão citoplasmáticos basófilos em partes do cérebro, fígado e pele, bem como nas células ductais das glândulas sudoríparas. A morte geralmente ocorre nos 10 anos após o início do quadro; herança autossômica recessiva, causada por mutação no gene 2 da epilepsia mioclônica progressiva (EPM2A) no cromossoma 6q. SIN Lafora d.

Lane d., d. de Lane. SIN *erythema* palmare hereditarium.

L-chain d., d. da cadeia leve (L). SIN Bence Jones *myeloma*.

Legg-Calvé-Perthes d., Legg-Perthes d., Legg d., d. de Legg-Calvé-Perthes, d. de Legg-Perthes, d. de Legg; osteonecrose epifisária da extremidade superior do fêmur. SIN Calvé-Perthes d., coxa plana, osteochondritis deformans juvenilis, Perthes d., pseudocoxalgia, quiet hip d.

Legionnaires d., d. dos legionários; uma doença infecciosa aguda, causada por *Legionella pneumophila*, com sintomas prodrômicos gripais e febre alta que se eleva rapidamente, seguida por pneumonia grave e produção de escarro, geralmente não-purulento e, algumas vezes, confusão mental, alterações gordurosas hepáticas e degeneração tubular renal. Tem uma elevada taxa de caso-fatalidade; adquirida a partir da água contaminada, geralmente por aerossolização, e não por transmissão interpessoal. SIN legionellosis. [Convenção da Legião (*Legion*) Americana, 1976, na qual muitos delegados foram afetados]

Leigh d. [MIM*256000], d. de Leigh; encefalomielopatia subaguda que afeta lactentes, causando convulsões, espasticidade, atrofia óptica e demência; a causa genética é heterogênea; pode estar associada à deficiência de citocromo c oxidase ou NADH-ubiquinona oxidorredutase ou de outras enzimas envolvidas no metabolismo de energia. Já foram descritas heranças autossômica recessiva, recessiva ligada ao X e mitocondrial; foram identificadas mutações no gene surfeit-1 (SURF) [MIM*185620] no cromossoma 9, em uma subunidade de ATP sintase codificada por mtDNA [MIM*516060], na subunidade E1-alfa ligada ao X da piruvato desidrogenase [MIM*312170] e em várias subunidades do complexo mitocondrial I [MIM*161015 e MIM*620141]. SIN necrotizing encephalomyelopathy, necrotizing encephalopathy.

Leiner d., d. de Leiner. SIN *erythroderma* desquamativum.

Lenègre d., d. de Lenègre. SIN Lenègre *syndrome*.

lenticular progressive d., d. progressiva lenticular. SIN Wilson *disease*.

Leri-Weill d., d. de Leri-Weill. SIN dyschondrosteosis.

Letterer-Siwe d., d. de Letterer-Siwe; a forma disseminada aguda da histiocitose de células de Langerhans. SIN nonlipid histiocytosis.

Lev d., d. de Lev. SIN Lev *syndrome*.

Lindau d., d. de Lindau. SIN von Hippel-Lindau *syndrome*.

linear IgA bullous d. in children, d. bolhosa por IgA linear em crianças. SIN chronic bullous *dermatosis* of childhood.

Little d., d. de Little. SIN spastic *diplegia*.

Lobo d., d. de Lobo. SIN lobomycosis.

Löffler d., d. de Löffler. SIN Löffler *endocarditis*.

Lorain d., d. de Lorain. SIN idiopathic *infantilism*.

Lou Gehrig d., d. de Lou Gehrig. SIN amyotrophic lateral *sclerosis*.

Luft d. [MIM*238800], d. de Luft; doença metabólica devida ao desacoplamento relativo da fosforilação no músculo esquelético, causando miopatia e hipermetabolismo generalizado; uma miopatia mitocondrial.

lung fluke d., d. por trematódeos pulmonares; infestação pelo trematódeo pulmonar *Clonorchis sinensis*.

Lutz-Splendore-Almeida d., d. de Lutz-Splendore-Almeida. SIN paracoccidioidomycosis.

Lyell d., d. de Lyell. SIN staphylococcal scalded skin *syndrome*.

Lyme d., d. de Lyme; borreliose de Lyme; meningopolineurite por carrapatos; distúrbio inflamatório subagudo causado por infecção por *Borrelia burgdorferi*, espiroqueta não-piogênico transmitido pelo *Ixodes scapularis*, na parte leste dos Estados Unidos, e pelo *I. pacificus*, na parte oeste desse país; a lesão cutânea característica, eritema crônico migratório, geralmente é precedida ou acompanhada por febre, mal-estar, fadiga, cefaléia e rigidez cervical; pode haver manifestações neurológicas, cardíacas ou articulares semanas a meses depois. Acredita-se que as ninfas dos carrapatos sejam responsáveis por cerca de 90% da transmissão para seres humanos. As ninfas e as larvas alimentam-se principalmente no camundongo *Peromyscus leucopus*, enquanto o hospedeiro preferido dos adultos é o cervo. Os animais reservatórios infectados e os carrapatos não adoecem. Os sintomas articulares ou neurológicos residuais, que podem persistir por meses ou anos após a infecção inicial, provavelmente representam uma resposta imune ao microrganismo. Variações nas características clínicas ou na gravidade de um paciente para outro podem ser devidas a variações congênitas na resposta imune, talvez relacionadas ao sistema antigênico linfocítico humano. SIN Lyme borreliosis. [Lyme, CT, onde foi observada pela primeira vez]

Devido à cobertura da imprensa, a doença de Lyme é mais conhecida do que sua ocorrência justificaria. Menos de 18.000 casos são confirmados anualmente nos Estados Unidos. Geralmente é uma doença benigna, autolimitada, mesmo quando não-tratada. Estudos dos anticorpos em áreas endêmicas sugerem que até 50% das pessoas que contraem a infecção nunca apresentam sintomas. A taxa de caso-fatalidade é praticamente zero. O diagnóstico é essencialmente clínico. Os testes sorológicos para anticorpos contra *B. burgdorferi* são notoriamente insatisfatórios, tanto em sensibilidade quanto em especificidade. Em áreas não-endêmicas, resultados falso-positivos superam estatisticamente os resultados verdadeiro-positivos. O anticorpo IgM aparece e tem um pico relativamente tardio, de forma que metade dos pacientes é soronegativa durante o primeiro mês após o surgimento do exantema. A antibioticoterapia administrada cedo pode alterar ou evitar a resposta imune aguda esperada. O anticorpo IgG persiste por meses ou anos após a infecção e, portanto, não ajuda no diagnóstico da doença aguda. Devido ao quadro clínico inespecífico e variável e à não-fidedignidade das medidas diagnósticas laboratoriais, é inevitável que muitos casos de doença de Lyme não sejam diagnosticados e que, ao contrário, o diagnóstico muitas vezes seja feito erradamente. Um estudo que avalia os custos do diagnóstico errado da doença de Lyme constatou que 60% dos pacientes encaminhados a uma clínica de doença de Lyme nunca tiveram a doença e outros 19% apresentavam uma história pregressa de infecção, mas não de doença atual. O medicamento preferido é a doxiciclina, administrada por via oral durante várias semanas. A amoxicilina é a alternativa padrão para crianças e gestantes. A recuperação não confere imunidade contra futuros ataques; na verdade, em áreas hiperendêmicas, a taxa de reinfecção pode ser de até 20%. Os especialistas em doenças infecciosas não recomendam profilaxia com antibióticos após uma picada de carrapato, mesmo em áreas hiperendêmicas, nem aprovam tratamento de pessoas assintomáticas com evidências sorológicas de infecção passada. Uma vacina que consiste em proteína A da superfície externa (OspA) da *B. burgdorferi* sintetizada por uma cepa não-virulenta de *Escherichia coli* recombinante foi liberada em 1998. Os anticorpos induzidos pela vacina entram no carrapato quando este pica o indivíduo vacinado, e se ligam a quaisquer espiroquetas presentes, impedindo sua mobilização. Três doses da vacina administradas por um período de 12 meses conferem proteção de cerca de 80% contra a doença de Lyme. A vacina não é aprovada para pessoas com menos de 15 anos, e só é recomendada para aqueles que vivem ou trabalham em áreas hiperendêmicas.

lysosomal d., d. lisossômica; doença causada por funcionamento inadequado de uma enzima lisossômica; a maioria dessas doenças está associada a uma doença de depósito.
Machado-Joseph d. [MIM*109150], d. de Machado-Joseph; forma rara de ataxia hereditária, caracterizada por surgimento, no início da vida adulta, de doença espinocerebelar e extrapiramidal progressiva com oftalmoplegia externa, rigidez, sintomas de distonia rígida e, freqüentemente, amiotrofia periférica; encontrada predominantemente em pessoas de ascendência açoreana; herança autossômica dominante, causada por mutação da expansão de repetições de trinucleotídeos no gene Machado-Joseph (MJD1) em 14q. SIN Azorean d., Portuguese-Azorean d. [Sobrenomes de duas famílias estudadas nas principais descrições da doença.]
mad cow d., d. da vaca louca. SIN bovine spongiform *encephalopathy*.
Madelung d., d. de Madelung. SIN multiple symmetric *lipomatosis*.
Manson d., d. de Manson. SIN *schistosomiasis* mansoni.
maple bark d., pulmão dos cortadores de casca do bordo; pneumonite por hipersensibilidade causada por esporos de *Cryptostroma corticale* que crescem sob a casca de toras de bordo empilhadas.
maple syrup urine d. [MIM*248600], d. da urina em xarope de ácer (ou bordo); erro congênito do metabolismo causado por defeito da descarboxilação oxidativa de α-cetoácidos da leucina, isoleucina e valina; esses aminoácidos de cadeia ramificada existem no sangue e na urina em altas concentrações; as manifestações da doença incluem dificuldades de alimentação, retardo físico e mental, e urina com odor semelhante ao do xarope de bordo; é comum haver morte neonatal. Herança autossômica recessiva, causada por mutação da subunidade E1, E2 ou E4 do gene da desidrogenase de α-cetoácidos de cadeia ramificada (BCKDH) em 19q. Há várias formas diferenciadas pela subunidade do BCKDH que sofreu mutação. SIN branched chain ketoaciduria, branched chain kenonuria, ketoacidemia.

marble bone d., osteopetrose. SIN osteopetrosis.
Marburg d., d. de Marburg; infecção por um rabdovírus incomum composto de RNA e lipídios, provisoriamente colocado na família Filoviridae. O vírus é "pantrópico" e afeta a maioria dos sistemas orgânicos. A doença é caracterizada por erupção cutânea proeminente e hemorragias em muitos órgãos, e freqüentemente é fatal. Observada pela primeira vez em funcionários de laboratórios em Marburg, na Alemanha, expostos a macacos verdes africanos. Foi observada alguma transmissão interpessoal. Só devem ser feitas tentativas de isolar o vírus em laboratórios de alta segurança. SIN Marburg virus d.
Marburg virus d., d. do vírus de Marburg. SIN Marburg d.
Marchiafava-Bignami d., d. de Marchiafava-Bignami; distúrbio reconhecido basicamente por suas características anatomopatológicas, que consistem em desmielinização do corpo caloso e necrose laminar cortical envolvendo os lobos frontal e temporal. Ocorre predominantemente em alcoólatras crônicos, particularmente nos que bebem vinho.
Marfan d., d. de Marfan. SIN Marfan *syndrome*.
margarine d., d. da margarina; eritema multiforme causado por agente emulsificante usado na fabricação de margarina.
Marie-Strümpell d., d. de Marie-Strümpell. SIN ankylosing *spondylitis*.
Marion d., d. de Marion; obstrução congênita da uretra posterior.
Martin d., d. de Martin; periosteoartrite do pé causada por marcha excessiva.
McArdle d., d. de McArdle. SIN type 5 *glycogenosis*.
McArdle-Schmid-Pearson d., d. de McArdle-Schmid-Pearson. SIN type 5 *glycogenosis*.
mechanobullous d., epidermólise bolhosa. SIN *epidermolysis* bullosa. [G. *mechanē*, máquina, + bullous]
Meige d. [MIM*153200], d. de Meige; linfedema autossômico dominante com início por volta da puberdade.
Ménétrier d., d. de Ménétrier; hiperplasia da mucosa gástrica, seja mucóide ou glandular; este último tipo pode estar associado à síndrome de Zollinger-Ellison. SIN giant hypertrophy of gastric mucosa, hypertrophic gastritis, Ménétrier syndrome.
Ménière d., d. de Ménière; afecção caracterizada clinicamente por vertigem, náuseas, vômitos, zumbido e perda auditiva progressiva devida à hidropisia do ducto endolinfático. SIN endolymphatic hydrops, Ménière syndrome.
mental d., d. mental. VER mental *illness*.
Merzbacher-Pelizaeus d., d. de Merzbacher-Pelizaeus. SIN Pelizaeus-Merzbacher d.
metabolic d., d. metabólica; termo genérico para as doenças causadas por um processo metabólico anormal. Pode ser congênita, devida a uma anormalidade enzimática hereditária, ou adquirida, devida à doença de um órgão endócrino ou insuficiência funcional de um importante órgão metabólico como o fígado.
Meyenburg d., d. de Meyenburg. SIN relapsing *polychondritis*.
Meyer-Betz d., d. de Meyer-Betz. SIN myoglobinuria.
Mibelli d., d. de Mibelli. SIN porokeratosis.
microcystic d. of renal medulla, d. microcística da medula renal. SIN cystic d. of renal medulla.
micrometastatic d., d. micrometastática; a condição de um paciente submetido à remoção de todo o câncer clinicamente evidente, mas que apresenta a probabilidade de recorrência por metástases demasiado pequenas para serem aparentes.
microvillus inclusion d., atrofia congênita das microvilosidades intestinais; distúrbio que começa ao nascimento com diarréia aquosa persistente e má absorção potencialmente fatal associada a atrofia vilosa e hipoplasia das criptas no intestino delgado; a microscopia eletrônica mostra inclusões nas microvilosidades em enterócitos. SIN congenital microvillus atrophy.
Mikulicz d., d. de Mikulicz; edema benigno das glândulas lacrimais e, geralmente, também das glândulas salivares, em conseqüência de infiltração e substituição da estrutura glandular normal por tecido linfóide. VER TAMBÉM Mikulicz *syndrome*, Sjögren *syndrome*.
Milroy d. [MIM*153100], d. de Milroy; a forma congênita de linfedema autossômico dominante.
Minamata d., d. de Minamata; distúrbio neurológico causado por intoxicação por metil mercúrio; descrita pela primeira vez nos habitantes da Baía de Minamata, Japão, resultante da ingestão de peixes contaminados por mercúrio proveniente de lixo industrial. Caracterizada por perda sensorial periférica, tremores, disartria, ataxia e perda auditiva e visual.
miner's d., doença dos mineiros; **(1)** SIN ancylostomiasis, **(2)** SIN miner's *nystagmus*.
minimal-change d., d. de alterações mínimas. SIN lipoid *nephrosis*.
mixed connective-tissue d., d. mista do tecido conjuntivo; doença com características superpostas de várias doenças sistêmicas do tecido conjuntivo e com anticorpos séricos contra a ribonucleoproteína nuclear.
molecular d., d. molecular; doença na qual as manifestações são devidas a alterações da estrutura e da função molecular.
Mondor d., d. de Mondor; tromboflebite da veia toracoepigástrica da mama e da parede torácica.
Monge d., d. de Monge. SIN chronic mountain *sickness*.

Morgagni d., d. de Morgagni. SIN Adams-Stokes *syndrome.*
Morquio d., d. de Morquio. SIN Morquio *syndrome.*
Morquio-Ullrich d., d. de Morquio-Ullrich. SIN Morquio *syndrome.*
Morvan d., d. de Morvan. SIN syringomyelia.
motor neuron d. (MND), d. do neurônio motor; termo geral incluindo atrofia muscular espinal progressiva (do lactente, juvenil e do adulto), esclerose lateral amiotrófica, paralisia bulbar progressiva e esclerose lateral primária; freqüentemente, uma doença familiar. SIN motor system d.
motor system d., d. do sistema motor. SIN motor neuron d.
mountain d., mal da montanha; termo que pode significar doença da altitude aguda; também usado para designar a doença crônica caracterizada por baixa saturação de oxigênio da hemoglobina, decorrente da baixa pressão parcial de oxigênio no ar inspirado mais hipoventilação alveolar que se desenvolve em alguns indivíduos, principalmente nos idosos. A policitemia causa coloração rosada da pele, mas surge cianose aos mínimos esforços, juntamente com dispnéia, fadiga, cefaléia e torpor mental. Uma pessoa assim acometida volta ao normal logo após retornar a um local de menor altitude.
moyamoya d., *moyamoya*; distúrbio vascular cerebral que ocorre predominantemente em japoneses, nos quais os vasos da base do cérebro são ocluídos e revascularizados com uma fina rede de vasos; ocorre comumente em crianças pequenas, manifestando-se por convulsões, hemiplegia, retardo mental e hemorragia subaracnóide; o diagnóstico é feito pelo quadro angiográfico. [Jap. confuso]
Mucha-Habermann d., d. de Mucha-Habermann. SIN *pityriasis* lichenoides *et varioliformis acuta.*
multicore d., d. multinuclear; miopatia congênita não-progressiva caracterizada por fraqueza dos músculos proximais, degeneração multifocal das fibras musculares e áreas excêntricas de diminuição ou ausência de atividade enzimática oxidativa nos músculos.
Neumann d., d. de Neumann. SIN *pemphigus* vegetans (1).
neutral lipid storage d., d. de depósito de lipídios neutros. SIN Dorfman-Chanarin *syndrome.*
Newcastle d., d. de Newcastle; doença febril aguda e contagiosa de aves domésticas, semelhante à peste das aves, causada por um Paramyxovirus (vírus da doença de Newcastle) e caracterizada por alta infecciosidade e sintomas respiratórios e neurológicos; é facilmente transmissível para seres humanos, nos quais causa uma conjuntivite grave, mas transitória. SIN Ranikhet d. [*Newcastle* — upon — Tyne, Inglaterra, onde foi relatada pela primeira vez]
Nicolas-Favre d., d. de Nicolas-Favre. SIN venereal *lymphogranuloma.*
Niemann d., d. de Niemann. SIN Niemann-Pick d.
Niemann-Pick d. [MIM*257200], d. de Niemann-Pick; lipidose com acúmulo de esfingomielina em histiócitos no fígado, baço, linfonodos e medula óssea devido à deficiência de esfingomielinase; associada a hepatosplenomegalia, retardo físico e mental e manifestações neurológicas; manchas vermelho-cereja na mácula podem surgir posteriormente; é mais comum em lactentes judeus asquenazes e causa morte precoce; uma forma mais benigna pode ocorrer em adultos. Há diversas variantes: Tipo A, a forma clássica do lactente; Tipo B, a forma visceral; Tipo C, a forma juvenil; Tipo D, a variante de Nova Escócia; e Tipo E, a forma adulta; todas têm herança autossômica recessiva, sendo os Tipos A e B causados por mutação no gene da esfingomielinase ácida (SMPD) no cromossoma 11p. SIN Niemann d., sphingomyelin lipidosis.
Niemann-Pick C1 d. [MIM*257220], d. de Niemann-Pick C1 (NPC); distúrbio do armazenamento de lipídios hereditário raro, que afeta as vísceras e o sistema nervoso central, herdado de forma autossômica recessiva. Há dois tipos de doença, com as mesmas manifestações clínicas e anormalidades bioquímicas, resultando de anormalidades nos dois genes, NPC-1, o *locus* principal, e NPC-2, o *locus* menor; então dois tipos possuem fenótipos clínicos e bioquímicos idênticos. As células de pacientes com NPC são defeituosas na esterificação e liberação de colesterol dos lisossomas; ocorrem seqüestro lisossômico de colesterol derivado de LDL, incluindo infra-regulação tardia da captação de LDL e síntese *de novo*.
nil d., d. nula. SIN lipoid *nephrosis.*
nodular d., d. nodular; esofagostomíase em herbívoros e primatas, caracterizada por nódulos na parede do intestino grosso, ceco e, ocasionalmente, íleo; os nódulos são cheios de material caseoso e resultam da resposta do hospedeiro ao encistamento das larvas de espécies de *Oesophagostomum*.
Norrie d. [MIM*310600], d. de Norrie; massas bilaterais congênitas de tecido originadas na retina ou vítreo e semelhantes ao glioma (pseudoglioma), geralmente com atrofia da íris e desenvolvimento de catarata; retardo mental e surdez associados; herança recessiva ligada ao X, causada por mutação no gene da doença de Norrie (NDP) em Xp.
notifiable d., d. notificável; doença que, por exigências legais, deve ser notificada à saúde pública ou às autoridades veterinárias quando o diagnóstico é feito, devido à sua importância para a saúde humana ou animal. SIN reportable d.
oasthouse urine d. [MIM*250900], defeito metabólico hereditário autossômico recessivo na absorção de metionina, que é convertida por bactérias intestinais em ácido α-hidroxibutírico; caracterizada por diarréia, taquipnéia e excreção urinária acentuada de ácido α-hidroxibutírico (que causa um odor semelhante ao de um forno para secar lúpulo, malte ou tabaco). [*oast*, forno para secar lúpulo, malte ou tabaco]

occupational d., d. ocupacional; distúrbio mórbido resultante de exposição a um agente durante o desempenho habitual de uma profissão. Cf. industrial d.
Ofuji d., d. de Ofuji. SIN eosinophilic pustular *folliculitis.*
Oguchi d. [MIM*258100], d. de Oguchi; cegueira noturna não-progressiva congênita rara com coloração amarela ou cinza difusa do fundo de olho; após 2 ou 3 horas em total escuridão, o fundo de olho recupera a cor normal; herança autossômica recessiva, causada por mutação no gene arrestina (SAG) em 2q ou no gene rodopsina cinase (RHOK) em 13q.
Ollier d., d. de Ollier. SIN enchondromatosis.
Oppenheim d., d. de Oppenheim. SIN *amyotonia* congenita.
organic d., d. orgânica; doença na qual há alterações anatômicas ou fisiopatológicas em algum tecido ou órgão, ao contrário de um distúrbio funcional; particularmente de origem psicogênica.
Ormond d., d. de Ormond. SIN retroperitoneal *fibrosis.*
orphan d., d.-órfã; doença para a qual não foi desenvolvido tratamento devido à sua raridade (não afetando mais de 200.000 pessoas nos Estados Unidos). VER TAMBÉM orphan *products*, em *product*.
Osgood-Schlatter d., d. de Osgood-Schlatter; inflamação do centro de crescimento (apófise) que forma o tubérculo tibial. SIN apophysitis tibialis adolescentium, Schlatter d., Schlatter-Osgood d.
Osler d., d. de Osler. SIN *polycythemia* vera.
Osler-Vaquez d., d. de Osler-Vaquez. SIN *polycythemia* vera.
Otto d., d. de Otto; doença caracterizada por abaulamento do acetábulo para dentro da cavidade pélvica, resultando em protrusão da cabeça do fêmur; encontrada associada à artrite das articulações do quadril, geralmente artrite reumatóide. SIN Otto pelvis, protrusio acetabuli.
Owren d. [MIM*227400], d. de Owren; deficiência congênita de fator V, resultando em prolongamento do tempo de protrombina; há prolongamento constante dos tempos de sangramento e coagulação; herança autossômica recessiva causada por mutação no gene F5 no cromossoma 1q.
Paas d., d. de Paas; deformação óssea familiar caracterizada por coxa valga, patela dupla, encurtamento das falanges média e distal dos dedos das mãos e dos pés, deformidades dos cotovelos, escoliose e espondilite deformante das vértebras lombares; todas essas manifestações podem ser uni ou bilaterais.
Paget d., d. de Paget; (1) doença óssea generalizada, freqüentemente familiar, de pessoas idosas, com aumento da reabsorção e da formação ósseas, levando a espessamento e amolecimento dos ossos (p. ex., o crânio) e encurvamento dos ossos que sustentam o peso. SIN osteitis deformans. (2) doença de mulheres idosas, caracterizada por uma lesão infiltrada, um tanto eczematosa, que circunda e envolve o mamilo e a aréola, e associada ao câncer intraductal subjacente da mama e à infiltração da epiderme inferior por células malignas; (3) SIN extramammary Paget d.
Panner d., d. de Panner; osteonecrose epifisária do capítulo do úmero. SIN little league elbow.
paper mill worker's d., d. dos trabalhadores em fábrica de papel; alveolite alérgica extrínseca, causada pela polpa de madeira mofada contendo esporos de fungos *Alternaria*.
parasitic d., d. parasitária; doença causada pela presença e atividade vital de um parasita, ou como reação a um parasita.
Parkinson d., d. de Parkinson. SIN parkinsonism (1).
Parrot d., (1) pseudoparalisia de Parrot; pseudoparalisia em lactentes, devida à osteocondrite sifilítica; (2) SIN marasmus; (3) doença dos papagaios; psitacose. SIN psittacosis.
Parry d., d. de Parry. SIN Graves d.
Pavy d., d. de Pavy; albuminúria fisiológica cíclica ou recorrente.
pearl-worker's d., d. dos trabalhadores com madrepérola; hipertrofia inflamatória dos ossos que afeta os esmerilhadores de madrepérola.
Pel-Ebstein d., d. de Pel-Ebstein. SIN Pel-Ebstein *fever.*
Pelizaeus-Merzbacher d. [MIM*311601, *312080, *260600], d. de Pelizaeus-Merzbacher; uma leucodistrofia sudanófila com aspecto tigróide da mielina, resultante de desmielinização segmentar. Tipo I, clássico, nistagmo e tremor que surgem nos primeiros meses de vida, seguidos por desenvolvimento motor lento, algumas vezes com coreoatetose, espasticidade, atrofia óptica e convulsões, com morte no início da vida adulta, herança recessiva ligada ao X causada por mutação no gene da proteína proteolipídica (PLP) em Xq; também há uma forma autossômica recessiva; tipo 2, forma contralateral com morte em meses a anos após o nascimento, herança recessiva ligada ao X; tipo 3, de transição, com morte na primeira década; tipo 4, forma adulta associada a movimentos involuntários, ataxia e hiper-reflexia, mas sem nistagmo; herança autossômica dominante [MIM*169500]; tipo 5, formas variantes. A doença de Cockayne algumas vezes é incluída como uma sexta forma. SIN Merzbacher-Pelizaeus d.
Pellegrini d., d. de Pellegrini; densidade calcificada no ligamento colateral medial e/ou crescimento ósseo na face medial do côndilo medial do fêmur. SIN Pellegrini-Stieda d.
Pellegrini-Stieda d., d. de Pellegrini-Stieda. SIN Pellegrini d.
pelvic inflammatory d. (PID), d. inflamatória pélvica (DIP); inflamação supurativa aguda ou crônica das estruturas pélvicas femininas (endométrio, tubas uterinas, peritônio pélvico) devida à infecção por *Neisseria gonorrhoeae, Chlamydia trachomatis* ou outros microrganismos, tipicamente uma compli-

cação de infecção sexualmente transmitida do aparelho genital inferior, pode ser precipitada por menstruação, parto ou procedimentos cirúrgicos, incluindo abortamento; as complicações incluem abscesso tubo-ovariano, estenose tubária, com conseqüente infertilidade ou esterilidade e aumento do risco de gravidez ectópica, e aderências peritoneais.

periodic d., d. periódica; qualquer condição ou doença na qual os episódios tendem a recorrer a intervalos regulares; muitos desses casos são manifestações da febre familiar do Mediterrâneo; a causa da periodicidade geralmente é desconhecida.

Perthes d., d. de Perthes. SIN Legg-Calvé-Perthes d.

Pette-Döring d., d. de Pette-Döring. SIN nodular panencephalitis.

Peyronie d., d. de Peyronie; doença na qual placas ou filamentos de tecido fibroso denso que circundam o corpo cavernoso do pênis causam encurvamento do pênis e dor à ereção; algumas vezes associada à contratura de Dupuytren. SIN penile fibromatosis, van Buren d.

Pick d., d. de Pick; atrofia cerebral circunscrita progressiva; um tipo raro de distúrbio degenerativo cerebral que se manifesta basicamente como demência, na qual há surpreendente atrofia de partes dos lobos frontal e temporal. SIN Pick syndrome. [F. Pick]

pink d., d. rósea. SIN acrodynia (2).

Plummer d., d. de Plummer; epônimo algumas vezes aplicado ao hipertireoidismo resultante de um bócio nodular tóxico, geralmente não acompanhado por exoftalmia.

polycystic d. of kidneys, d. renal policística. SIN polycystic kidney.

polycystic liver d., d. hepática policística. SIN polycystic liver.

Pompe d., d. de Pompe. SIN type 2 glycogenosis.

Portuguese-Azorean d., d. portuguesa-açoreana. SIN Machado-Joseph d.

Posadas d., d. de Posadas. SIN coccidioidomycosis.

posttransplant lymphoproliferative d., d. linfoproliferativa pós-transplante; complicação do transplante de órgãos em crianças; caracterizada por uma síndrome semelhante à mononucleose, aumento das tonsilas e soroconversão para vírus Epstein-Barr.

Pott d., d. de Pott. SIN tuberculous spondylitis.

Potter d., d. de Potter. SIN Potter facies.

poultry handler's d., d. dos tratadores de aves domésticas; alveolite alérgica extrínseca semelhante ao pulmão dos tratadores de aves, causada por inalação de partículas das emanações de aves domésticas, como galinhas e perus.

primary d., d. primária; doença que se origina espontaneamente e não está associada nem é causada por uma doença, lesão ou evento prévio, mas que pode levar a uma doença secundária.

Pringle d., d. de Pringle. SIN adenoma sebaceum.

pseudo-Hurler d., pseudodoença de Hurler; gangliosidose G_{M1}. SIN infantile, generalized G_{M1} gangliosidosis.

pulseless d., d. sem pulso. SIN Takayasu arteritis.

Purtscher d., d. de Purtscher. SIN Purtscher retinopathy.

quiet hip d., d. de Legg-Calvé-Perthes. SIN Legg-Calvé-Perthes d.

ragpicker's d., d. do trapeiro. SIN pulmonary anthrax.

ragsorter's d., d. do trapeiro. SIN pulmonary anthrax.

Ranikhet d., d. de Ranikhet. SIN Newcastle d. [Ranikhet, cidade no norte da Índia]

rat-bite d., d. da mordida de rato. SIN rat-bite fever.

Rayer d., d. de Rayer. SIN biliary xanthomatosis.

Raynaud d., d. de Raynaud. SIN Raynaud syndrome.

reactive airway d., d. reativa das vias aéreas. SIN asthma.

Recklinghausen d. of bone, d. de Recklinghausen do osso. SIN osteitis fibrosa cystica.

Refsum d. [MIM*266500], d. de Refsum; distúrbio degenerativo raro devido a deficiência da α-hidroxilase do ácido fitânico; clinicamente caracterizada por retinite pigmentosa, ictiose, polineuropatia desmielinizante, surdez e sinais cerebelares; herança autossômica recessiva causada por mutação no gene que codifica a fitanoil-CoA hidrolase (PAHX ou PAYH) no cromossoma 10p. A doença de Refsum infantil [MIM*266510] é um comprometimento da função do peroxissoma com acúmulo de ácido fitânico, ácido pipecólico; herança autossômica recessiva, causada por mutação no gene PEX 1 em 7q. SIN heredopathia atactica polyneuritiformis, Refsum syndrome.

Reiter d., d. de Reiter. SIN Reiter syndrome.

reportable d., d. notificável. SIN notifiable d.

rhesus d., sensibilização da mãe, durante a gravidez, ao fator Rh presente no sangue fetal, levando à eritroblastose fetal.

rheumatic d., d. reumática. VER rheumatism.

rheumatic heart d., cardiopatia reumática; cardiopatia resultante da febre reumática, que se manifesta principalmente por anormalidades das valvas

rheumatoid d., d. reumatóide; artrite reumatóide (rheumatoid arthritis), que se refere particularmente a lesões não-articulares, como nódulos subcutâneos.

Ribas-Torres d., d. de Ribas-Torres; forma leve de varíola. VER TAMBÉM variola minor.

rice d., d. do arroz; beribéri, cujos primeiros episódios foram causados pela alimentação de pessoas com arroz sem casca (arroz polido), diminuindo o conteúdo de vitamina B_1 do arroz.

Riedel d., d. de Riedel. SIN Riedel thyroiditis.

Riga-Fede d., d. de Riga-Fede; ulceração do frênulo lingual em lactentes durante a dentição, relativa à abrasão do tecido contra os novos incisivos centrais.

Roger d., d. de Roger; anomalia cardíaca congênita que consiste em um defeito pequeno, isolado, assintomático, do septo interventricular, freqüentemente com um sopro alto e frêmito definido. SIN maladie de Roger.

Rokitansky d., d. de Rokitansky; **(1)** SIN acute massive liver necrosis; **(2)** SIN Chiari syndrome.

Romberg d., d. de Romberg. SIN facial hemiatrophy.

Rosai-Dorfman d., d. de Rosai-Dorfman. SIN sinus histiocytosis with massive lymphadenopathy.

Rougnon-Heberden d., d. de Rougnon-Heberden. SIN angina pectoris.

Roussy-Lévy d. [MIM*180800], d. de Roussy-Lévy; distúrbio de herança dominante que consiste em polineuropatia desmielinizante sensório-motora e tremor essencial coexistente. SIN Roussy-Lévy syndrome.

runt d., reação enxerto-versus-hospedeiro em camundongos, observada após injeção intravenosa de células esplênicas alogênicas em animais recém-nascidos. SIN wasting d.

salivary gland d., d. das glândulas salivares; distúrbio das glândulas salivares; isto é, síndrome de Sjögren (Sjögren syndrome).

salivary gland virus d., d. do vírus da glândula salivar. VER cytomegalic inclusion d.

Salla d. (sal'ya), d. de Salla; distúrbio autossômico recessivo no qual há defeito no transporte de ácido siálico livre através das membranas lisossômicas.

Sandhoff d. [MIM*268800], d. de Sandhoff; forma infantil da gangliosidose G_{M2}, caracterizada por um defeito na produção de hexosaminidases A e B; assemelha-se à doença de Tay-Sachs, mas ocorre predominantemente (se não exclusivamente) em crianças não-judias; acúmulo de glicosídeo e gangliosídeo G_{m2}, causado por mutação no gene da hexosaminidase B (HEX B) no cromossoma 5q.

sandworm d., erupção inflamatória da face interna da região plantar, observada em determinadas partes da Austrália, caracterizada por uma placa de eritema que se propaga em espirais e desaparece espontaneamente; provavelmente uma forma de erupção serpiginosa semelhante à larva migrans.

San Joaquin Valley d., SIN primary coccidioidomycosis.

Schenck d., d. de Schenck. SIN sporotrichosis.

Scheuermann d., d. de Scheuermann; osteonecrose epifisária de corpos vertebrais adjacentes na coluna torácica. SIN adolescent round back, juvenile kyphosis, osteochondritis deformans juvenilis dorsi.

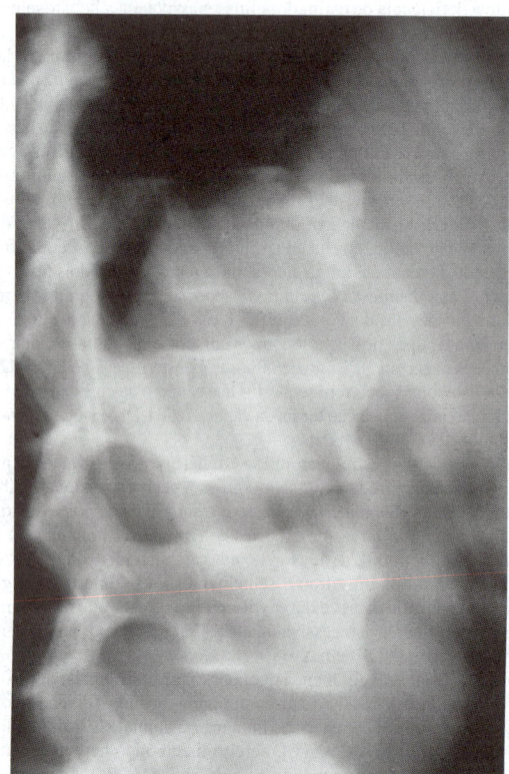

doença de Scheuermann: a necrose avascular de anéis apofisários dos corpos vertebrais é denominada doença de Scheuermann; na maioria das vezes não há cifose nem dor, e há envolvimento de poucos corpos vertebrais

Schilder d., d. de Schilder; termo usado para descrever pelo menos dois distúrbios diferentes descritos por Schilder: 1) Esclerose difusa ou encefalite periaxial difusa; distúrbio não-familiar que afeta basicamente crianças e adultos jovens, caracterizando-se por demência progressiva, distúrbios visuais, surdez, paralisia pseudobulbar e hemiplegia ou tetraplegia. A maioria dos pacientes morre alguns anos após o início; no exame anatomopatológico, há uma grande área assimétrica de destruição de mielina, algumas vezes envolvendo um hemisfério cerebral inteiro e tipicamente com extensão através do corpo caloso. 2) As leucodistrofias. SIN encephalitis periaxialis diffusa.

Schindler d. (shind′ler), d. de Schindler; distúrbio autossômico recessivo com atividade deficiente de α-N-acetilgalactosaminidase, resultando em acúmulo de glicoproteínas e de outros substratos depositados nos axônios terminais, basicamente na substância cinzenta.

Schlatter d., Schlatter-Osgood d., d. de Schlatter, d. de Schlatter-Osgood. SIN Osgood-Schlatter d.

Scholz d., d. de Scholz; epônimo antigo da forma juvenil de leucodistrofia metacromática.

Schüller d., d. de Schüller. SIN Hand-Schüller-Christian d.

Schwartz-Jampel d., d. de Schwartz-Jampel. SIN myotonic *chondrodystrophy.*

sclerocystic d. of the ovary, d. esclerocística do ovário. SIN polycystic ovary *syndrome.*

sea-blue histiocyte d. [MIM*269600], d. do histiócito azul-marinho; esplenomegalia e trombocitopenia leve, com histiócitos na medula óssea contendo grânulos citoplasmáticos que se coram de azul-brilhante; algumas vezes familiar; talvez uma lipidose; herança autossômica recessiva.

secondary d., d. secundária; **(1)** doença que sucede e resulta de uma doença, lesão ou evento anterior; **(2)** distúrbio consuntivo que sucede o transplante bem-sucedido de medula óssea para um hospedeiro irradiado letalmente; freqüentemente é grave e, em geral, associado a febre, anorexia, diarréia, dermatite e descamação. VER TAMBÉM graft versus host d.

self-limited d., d. autolimitada; processo mórbido que desaparece espontaneamente com ou sem tratamento específico.

Senear-Usher d., d. de Senear-Usher. SIN *pemphigus* erythematosus.

serum d., d. do soro. SIN serum *sickness.*

Sever d., d. de Sever; osteocondrose do calcanhar, provavelmente secundária a microfraturas ósseas onde o tendão de Aquiles se fixa à porção posterior do calcâneo; uma lesão por uso excessivo e uma causa comum de dor no calcanhar em crianças maiores. SIN calcaneal apophysitis.

sexually transmitted d. (STD), d. sexualmente transmitida (DST). VER venereal disease.

Shaver d., d. de Shaver. SIN bauxite *pneumoconiosis.*

shimamushi d., d. shimamushi. SIN tsutsugamushi d.

sickle cell d., anemia falciforme. SIN sickle cell *anemia.*

sickle cell C d. [MIM*141900], doença falciforme C; doença resultante de eritrócitos afoiçados (contendo hemoglobinas C e S) que surgem em resposta à diminuição da pressão parcial de oxigênio; caracterizada por anemia, crises devidas à hemólise ou oclusão vascular, úlceras de perna crônicas e deformidades ósseas, e infartos ósseos ou esplênicos.

sickle cell-thalassemia d., d. falciforme-talassemia; doença clinicamente semelhante à doença falciforme, na qual os indivíduos são heterozigotos mistos para o gene falciforme e para um gene da talassemia; cerca de 60–80% da hemoglobina é Hb S, até 20% Hb F e o restante Hb A. SIN microdrepanocytic anemia.

silo-filler's d., d. dos enchedores de silo; lesão pulmonar produzida por óxidos de nitrogênio pela silagem fresca; em sua forma aguda pode causar morte por edema pulmonar ou evoluir para uma doença pulmonar proliferativa subaguda ou crônica, algumas vezes levando à insuficiência pulmonar crônica.

Simmonds d., d. de Simmonds. SIN Sheehan *syndrome.*

Simons d., d. de Simons. SIN progressive *lipodystrophy.*

sixth d., sexta doença da infância. SIN *exanthema* subitum.

Sjögren d., d. de Sjögren. SIN Sjögren *syndrome.*

skinbound d., esclerodermia (geralmente aplicada ao envolvimento extenso).

slow virus d., d. por vírus lento; doença que tem uma evolução lenta, progressiva, que dura meses a anos, freqüentemente envolvendo o sistema nervoso central e, por fim, levando à morte; são exemplos visna e maedi em ovinos, causados por vírus do gênero Lentivirus (família Retroviridae), e a panencefalite esclerosante subaguda, aparentemente causada pelo vírus do sarampo. As encefalopatias espongiformes, incluindo kuru em seres humanos, *scrapie* em ovinos e a encefalopatia transmissível da marta, também podem ser classificadas como doenças por vírus lento, mas agora são consideradas doenças por príons.

Sneddon-Wilkinson d., d. de Sneddon-Wilkinson. SIN subcorneal pustular *dermatosis.*

specific d., d. específica; doença produzida pela ação de um microrganismo patogênico especial.

Spielmeyer-Sjögren d., d. de Spielmeyer-Sjögren; esfingolipidose cerebral (cerebral *sphingolipidosis*) do tipo juvenil tardio.

Spielmeyer-Stock d., d. de Spielmeyer-Stock; atrofia da retina na idiotia familiar amaurótica.

Spielmeyer-Vogt d., d. de Spielmeyer-Vogt; esfingolipidose cerebral (cerebral *sphingolipidosis*) do tipo juvenil tardio. SIN Vogt-Spielmeyer d.

stable d., d. estável; em oncologia, aumento menor que 25% ou diminuição menor que 50% no tamanho de todos os tumores.

Stargardt d. [MIM*248200], d. de Stargardt; *fundus flavimaculatus* iniciado com lesões maculares atróficas, causadas por mutação no gene transportador do cassete de ligação do ATP retina-específico (ABCR) em 1p.

startle d., hiperecplexia SIN hyperekplexia.

Steele-Richardson-Olszewski d., d. de Steele-Richardson-Olszewski. SIN progressive supranuclear *palsy.*

Steinert d., d. de Steinert. SIN myotonic *dystrophy.*

Still d., d. de Still; forma de artrite crônica juvenil (antigamente denominada artrite reumatóide juvenil) caracterizada por febre alta e sinais de doença sistêmica, que podem existir por semanas ou meses antes do início da artrite.

Stokes-Adams d., d. de Stokes-Adams. SIN Adams-Stokes *syndrome.*

stone-mason's d., silicose. SIN silicosis.

storage d., d. de depósito; termo genérico que inclui qualquer acúmulo de uma substância específica nos tecidos, geralmente devido à deficiência congênita de uma enzima necessária para metabolismo adicional da substância; p. ex., doenças de depósito de glicogênio.

Strümpell d., d. de Strümpell; **(1)** SIN *spondylitis deformans;* **(2)** SIN acute epidemic *leukoencephalitis.*

Strümpell-Marie d., d. de Strümpell-Marie. SIN ankylosing *spondylitis.*

Sturge-Weber d., d. de Sturge-Weber. SIN Sturge-Weber *syndrome.*

Sulzberger-Garbe d., d. de Sulzberger-Garbe. SIN exudative discoid and lichenoid *dermatitis.*

Sutton d., d. de Sutton. SIN *aphthae* major, em *aphtha.* [R.L. Sutton, Jr.]

Sweet d., d. de Sweet. SIN acute febrile neutrophilic *dermatosis.*

swineherd's d., d. do criador de porcos; leptospirose causada por uma leptospira que ocorre naqueles que cuidam de suínos, ou que abatem ou processam sua carne, caracterizada por dores em todo o corpo, febre, cefaléia, tonteira e náuseas.

swine vesicular d., d. vesicular dos suínos; doença contagiosa de suínos causada por um enterovírus suíno da família Picornaviridae, intimamente relacionado ao enterovírus humano Coxsackie B-5, sendo caracterizada por lesões vesiculares e erosões do epitélio da boca, narinas, focinho e pés; já foram descritas infecções humanas em trabalhadores de laboratório.

swollen belly d., doença fatal de lactentes infestados por *Strongyloides fuelleborni* subesp. *kellyi*; presente em áreas localizadas da Nova Guiné. SIN swollen belly syndrome.

Sydenham d., d. de Sydenham. SIN Sydenham *chorea.*

Sylvest d., d. de Sylvest. SIN epidemic *pleurodynia.*

systemic autoimmune d.'s, doenças auto-imunes sistêmicas; grupo de doenças do tecido conjuntivo caracterizadas pela presença de auto-anticorpos responsáveis por lesões teciduais mediadas imunopatologicamente; o lúpus eritematoso sistêmico é o protótipo.

systemic febrile d.'s, doenças febris sistêmicas; termo genérico para doenças caracterizadas por febre.

Takahara d., d. de Takahara. SIN acatalasia.

Takayasu d., d. de Takayasu. SIN Takayasu *arteritis.*

Tangier d., d. de Tangier. SIN analphalipoproteinemia. [uma ilha na Baía de Chesapeake, lar da família dos primeiros casos descritos]

Taussig-Bing d., d. de Taussig-Bing. SIN Taussig-Bing *syndrome.*

Taylor d., d. de Taylor; atrofia cutânea idiopática difusa.

Tay-Sachs d., d. de Tay-Sachs; doença de depósito lisossômico, resultante da deficiência de hexosaminidase A. O monossialogangliosídeo é armazenado em células neuronais centrais e periféricas. Os lactentes apresentam hiperacusia e irritabilidade, hipotonia e atraso no desenvolvimento de habilidades motoras. A cegueira com manchas vermelho-cereja na mácula e as convulsões são evidentes no primeiro ano de vida. A morte sobrevém em alguns anos. Transmissão autossômica recessiva; encontrada basicamente em populações judias. SIN infantile G_{M2} gangliosidosis.

Thiemann d., d. de Thiemann. SIN Thiemann *syndrome.*

third d., terceira doença da infância. SIN rubella.

Thomsen d., d. de Thomsen. SIN *myotonia* congenita.

Thygeson d., d. de Thygeson. SIN superficial punctate *keratitis.*

thyrocardiac d., d. tireocardíaca; cardiopatia resultante de hipertireoidismo.

thyrotoxic heart d., cardiopatia tireotóxica; sintomas, sinais e comprometimento fisiológico cardíacos devidos à hiperatividade da tireóide, em geral pela estimulação simpática excessiva.

Tommaselli d., d. de Tommaselli; hemoglobinúria e pirexia devidas à intoxicação por quinina.

Tornwaldt d., d. de Tornwaldt. SIN Tornwaldt *cyst.*

torsion d. of childhood, d. por torção da infância. SIN *dystonia* musculorum deformans.

Tourette d., d. de Tourette. SIN Tourette *syndrome.*

Trevor d., d. de Trevor. SIN tarsoepiphyseal *aclasis.*

tropical d.'s, doenças tropicais; doenças infecciosas e parasitárias endêmicas em regiões tropicais e subtropicais, incluindo doença de Chagas, leishmaniose, hanseníase, malária, oncocercíase, esquistossomose, doença do sono, febre amarela e outras; freqüentemente transmitidas pela água ou por insetos. VER TAMBÉM emerging *viruses*, em *virus*.

tsutsugamushi d., d. tsutsugamushi; doença infecciosa aguda, causada por *Rickettsia tsutsugamushi* e transmitida por *Trombicula akamushi* e *T. deliensis*, que ocorre em ceifadores de cânhamo em algumas partes do Japão; caracterizada por febre, edema doloroso das glândulas linfáticas, pequena crosta enegrecida na região genital, pescoço ou axila, e por erupção de grandes pápulas vermelho-escuras. SIN akamushi d., flood fever, inundation fever, island d., island fever, Japanese river fever, kedani fever, mite thyphus, scrub typhus, shimamushi d., tropical typhus, tsutsugamushi fever.

tunnel d., ancilostomíase. SIN ancylostomiasis.
Unna d., d. de Unna. SIN seborrheic *dermatitis*.
Unverricht d. [MIM*254800], d. de Unverricht; epilepsia mioclônica progressiva; um dos distúrbios degenerativos da substância cinzenta, caracterizados por mioclônus e convulsões generalizadas, com declínio neurológico e intelectual progressivo; início entre 8 e 13 anos de idade; herança autossômica recessiva, causada por mutação no gene da cistatina B (CSTB) em 21q22.
Urbach-Wiethe d., d. de Urbach-Wiethe. SIN lipoid *proteinosis*.
vagabond's d., d. dos vagabundos. SIN parasitic *melanoderma*.
vagrant's d., d. dos vadios. SIN parasitic *melanoderma*.
van Buren d., d. de van Buren. SIN Peyronie d.
Vaquez d., d. de Vaquez. SIN polycythemia vera.
venereal d., d. venérea; qualquer doença contagiosa adquirida por contato sexual; p. ex., sífilis, gonorréia, cancróide.
venoocclusive d. of the liver, d. venoclusiva do fígado; endoflebite obliterante de pequenas radículas da veia hepática, descrita em crianças jamaicanas, associada a ingestão de substâncias vegetais tóxicas no chá; causa ascite, que pode progredir para cirrose.
Vincent d., d. de Vincent. SIN necrotizing ulcerative *gingivitis*.
Virchow d., d. de Virchow. SIN megacephaly.
virus X d., d. do vírus X; termo antigo aplicado a várias doenças virais de etiologia obscura, p. ex., doença X australiana (encefalite de Murray Valley).
Vogt-Spielmeyer d., d. de Vogt-Spielmeyer. SIN Spielmeyer-Vogt d.
Voltolini d., d. de Voltolini; doença infecciosa do labirinto, que causa meningite em crianças pequenas.
von Economo d., d. de von Economo; encefalite única, provavelmente de origem viral, que sucedeu a pandemia de gripe de 1914–1918. Os sintomas incluíam oftalmoplegia e sonolência acentuada, e, em muitos sobreviventes, o desenvolvimento tardio de doença de Parkinson; a base do parkinsonismo pós-encefalítico. SIN encephalitis lethargica, polioencephalitis infectiva.
von Gierke d., d. de von Gierke. SIN type 1 *glycogenosis*.
von Recklinghausen d., d. de von Recklinghausen; neurofibromatose tipo 1. VER neurofibromatosis.
von Willebrand d. [MIM*193400], d. de von Willebrand; diátese hemorrágica caracterizada por tendência hemorrágica basicamente das mucosas, tempo de sangramento prolongado, contagem de plaquetas normal, retração do coágulo normal, deficiência parcial e variável de fator VIIIR e, possivelmente, um defeito morfológico das plaquetas; herança autossômica dominante com redução da penetrância e expressividade variável, causada por mutação no gene do fator de von Willebrand (FVW) em 12p. A doença de von Willebrand tipo III é um distúrbio mais grave, com redução significativa dos níveis de fator VIIIR. Há uma forma recessiva dessa doença [MIM*277480], que possui a propriedade significativa de representar uma mutação no mesmo *locus* da forma dominante.
Voorhoeve d., d. de Voorhoeve. SIN osteopathia striata.
Wagner d., d. de Wagner. SIN hyaloideoretinal *degeneration*.
wasting d., doença consuntiva. SIN runt d.
Weber-Christian d., d. de Weber-Christian; termo usado para casos de paniculite (*panniculitis*) não-supurativa nodular febril recidivante (q.v.) de causa indeterminada. SIN relapsing febrile nodular nonsuppurative *panniculitis*.
Wegner d., d. de Wegner. SIN syphilitic *osteochondritis*.
Weil d., d. de Weil; forma de leptospirose geralmente causada por *Leptospira interrogans* sorogrupo *icterohaemorrhagiae*, possivelmente adquirida por contato com a urina de ratos infectados; caracterizada clinicamente por febre, icterícia, dores musculares, congestão conjuntival e albuminúria; aglutininas aparecem regularmente no soro. SIN infectious icterus, infectious jaundice (1).
Werdnig-Hoffmann d., d. de Werdnig-Hoffmann. SIN spinal muscular *atrophy*, type I.
Werlhof d., d. de Werlhof; termo usado antigamente para designar a púrpura trombocitopênica idiopática (idiopathic thrombocytopenic *purpura*).
Wernicke d., d. de Wernicke. SIN Wernicke *syndrome*.
Werther d., d. de Werther. SIN *dermatitis* nodularis necrotica.
Wesselsbron d., d. de Wesselsbron. SIN Wesselsbron *fever*.
Whipple d., d. de Whipple; doença rara caracterizada por esteatorréia, freqüentemente linfadenopatia generalizada, artrite, febre e tosse; são encontrados muitos macrófagos "espumosos" na lâmina própria jejunal; causada por *Tropheryma whippleii*.

white spot d., SIN *morphea* guttata.
Whitmore d., d. de Whitmore. SIN melioidosis.
Wilkie d., d. de Wilkie. SIN superior mesenteric artery *syndrome*.
Wilson d. [MIM*277900], d. de Wilson; (1) distúrbio do metabolismo do cobre, caracterizado por cirrose hepática, degeneração dos gânglios da base, manifestações neurológicas e deposição de pigmento verde ou castanho-dourado na periferia da córnea; os níveis plasmáticos de cobre e ceruloplasmina estão diminuídos, a excreção urinária de cobre está aumentada e as quantidades de cobre no fígado, cérebro, rins e núcleo lenticular estão incomumente altas, enquanto a citocromo oxidase está reduzida; herança autossômica recessiva por mutação no gene da ATPase transportadora de cobre (ATP7B) no cromossoma 13q. SIN hepatolenticular degeneration. VER TAMBÉM Kayser-Fleischer *ring*; [S.A.K. Wilson] (2) SIN exfoliative *dermatitis*.
Winiwarter-Buerger d., d. de Winiwarter-Buerger. SIN *thromboangiitis* obliterans.
Wohlfart-Kugelberg-Welander d., d. de Wohlfart-Kugelberg-Welander. SIN spinal muscular *atrophy*, type III.
Wolman d., d. de Wolman. SIN cholesterol ester storage d.
woolsorter's d., d. dos selecionadores de lã; antraz pulmonar. SIN pulmonary *anthrax*.
Woringer-Kolopp d., d. de Woringer-Kolopp. SIN pagetoid *reticulosis*.
X d., d. X; uma das várias doenças virais de etiologia obscura.
X-linked lymphoproliferative d., d. linfoproliferativa ligada ao X. SIN X-linked lymphoproliferative *syndrome*.
yellow d., xantocromia. SIN xanthochromia.
Ziehen-Oppenheim d., d. de Ziehen-Oppenheim. SIN *dystonia* musculorum deformans.

dis·en·gage·ment (dis-en-gāj′ment). Desprendimento. **1.** O ato de soltar ou desembaraçar; no parto, o surgimento da cabeça na vulva. **2.** Ascensão da parte de apresentação da pelve após ultrapassar a abertura superior da pelve. [Fr.]

dis·e·qui·lib·ri·um (dis-ē′kwi-lib′rē-ŭm). Desequilíbrio; distúrbio ou ausência de equilíbrio.
  genetic d., d. genético; estado na composição genética de uma população que poderá mudar, durante a seleção, para um estado de equilíbrio ou absorção.
  linkage d., d. de união; estado que envolve dois *loci* nos quais a probabilidade de um gameta reunido não é igual ao produto das probabilidades dos genes constituintes. A diferença entre essas quantidades é o aumento do desequilíbrio; há muitas causas do desequilíbrio.

dis·flu·ency (dis-floo′en-sē). Incapacidade de produzir um fluxo uniforme de sons da fala no discurso articulado; o fluxo da fala é caracterizado por interrupções e repetições freqüentes. [dis- + fluency]

dis·flu·ent (dis-floo′ent). Sem fluência; relativo à disfluência.

dis·ger·mi·no·ma (dis-jer-mi-nō′mă). Disgerminoma. SIN dysgerminoma.

DISH Abreviatura de diffuse idiopathic skeletal *hyperostosis* (hiperostose óssea idiopática difusa.

dish. Prato; placa; recipiente raso, geralmente côncavo.
  Petri d., placa de Petri; placa pequena, rasa e circular, feita de vidro fino ou de plástico transparente com cobertura superposta, frouxamente adaptada, usada principalmente em microbiologia para o cultivo de microrganismos em meio sólido; freqüentemente é denominada placa.
  Stender d., recipiente de Stender; recipiente raso e plano usado na coloração de cortes.

dis·har·mo·ny (dis-har′mŏ-nē). Desarmonia. **1.** O estado de estar perturbado ou sem ordem. **2.** Em um sentido complexo, a ausência de uma relação matemática entre as freqüências do tom fundamental e seus sons harmônicos de forma que as freqüências dos sons harmônicos não são múltiplos de números inteiros ou parciais da freqüência do som fundamental. O efeito auditivo tem uma qualidade ruidosa ou desagradável, em oposição à música.
  occlusal d., d. oclusal; (1) contatos de superfícies oclusais opostas de dentes que não estão em harmonia com outros contatos dentários e com o controle anatômico e fisiológico da mandíbula; (2) oclusões que não coincidem com suas respectivas relações mandibulares. VER TAMBÉM deflective occlusal *contact*.

DISIDA Abreviatura de diisopropyl iminodiacetic acid (ácido diisopropil iminodiacético) ou disofenin (disofenina).

dis·im·pac·tion (dis′im-pak′shŭn). **1.** Afastamento de impacção em um osso fraturado. **2.** Remoção, geralmente manual, de um fecaloma.

dis·in·fect (dis-in-fekt′). Desinfetar; destruir microrganismos patogênicos em qualquer substância ou inibir seu crescimento e atividade vital.

dis·in·fec·tant (dis-in-fek′tănt). Desinfetante. **1.** Capaz de destruir microrganismos patogênicos ou de inibir sua atividade de crescimento. **2.** Um agente que possui essa propriedade.
  complete d., d. completo; desinfetante que destrói tanto as formas vegetativas quanto os esporos.
  incomplete d., d. incompleto; desinfetante que destrói apenas as formas vegetativas, deixando os esporos íntegros.

dis·in·fec·tion (dis-in-fek'shŭn). Desinfecção; destruição de microrganismos patogênicos ou de suas toxinas ou vetores por exposição direta a agentes químicos ou físicos.
  concurrent d., d. coordenada; aplicação de medidas desinfetantes logo que possível após a eliminação de material infeccioso do corpo de uma pessoa infectada, ou após contaminar objetos com esses materiais infecciosos.
  terminal d., d. terminal; aplicação de medidas desinfetantes após o paciente ter sido removido, p. ex., por morte, ou deixado de ser uma fonte de infecção.

dis·in·fes·ta·tion. Desinfestação; processo físico ou químico para destruir ou remover pequenas formas animais indesejáveis, particularmente artrópodes ou roedores, presentes na pessoa, na roupa ou no ambiente de um indivíduo ou animais domésticos.

dis·in·hi·bi·tion (dis'in-hi-bish'ŭn). Desinibição. **1.** Retirada de uma inibição, como por um processo tóxico ou orgânico. **2.** Retirada de um efeito inibitório por um estímulo, como quando um reflexo condicionado foi extinto, mas é restaurado por algum estímulo estranho.

dis·in·sec·tion, dis·in·sec·ti·za·tion (dis-in-sek'shŭn, dis'in-sek-ti-zā'shŭn). Desinsetização; afastamento de insetos de uma área. [L. *dis-*, afastado, + insect]

dis·in·te·gra·tion (dis-in-tĕ-grā'shŭn). Desintegração. **1.** Perda ou separação das partes componentes de uma substância, como no catabolismo ou no decaimento. **2.** Desorganização de processos psíquicos e comportamentais. [dis- + L. *integer*, inteiro, intacto]

dis·in·vag·i·na·tion (dis'in-vaj-i-nā'shŭn). Alívio de uma invaginação.

dis·junc·tion (dis-jŭnk'shŭn). Disjunção; a separação normal de pares de cromossomas na anáfase da meiose I ou II. [dis- + L. *junctio*, união, de *jungo*, pp. *junctum*, unir]

disk [TA]. Disco. **1.** Placa redonda, plana; qualquer estrutura circular aproximadamente plana. **2.** SIN lamella (2). **3.** Em odontologia, um pedaço circular de papel fino ou outro material, revestido por uma substância abrasiva, usado para cortar e polir dentes e obturações. [L. *discus*; G. *diskos*, disco]
  A d.'s, discos A. SIN A bands, em band.
  acromioclavicular d., d. acromioclavicular. SIN articular d. of acromioclavicular joint.
  Airy d., d. de Airy; a imagem de uma mancha circular formada por uma fonte luminosa puntiforme distante sobre a retina, devido à difração pela borda da abertura pupilar, onde o diâmetro da imagem diminui à medida que a abertura aumenta.
  anisotropic d.'s, discos anisotrópicos. SIN A bands, em band.
  articular d. [TA], d. articular; lâmina ou anel de fibrocartilagem fixado à cápsula articular e que separa as superfícies articulares dos ossos em uma distância variável, algumas vezes completamente; serve para adaptar duas superfícies articulares que não sejam totalmente congruentes. SIN discus articularis [TA], fibrocartilago interarticularis, fibroplate, interarticular fibrocartilage, intraarticular cartilage (1).
  articular d. of acromioclavicular joint [TA], d. da articulação acromioclavicular; o disco articular de fibrocartilagem geralmente encontrado entre a extremidade acromial da clavícula e a margem medial do acrômio. SIN discus articularis, acromioclavicularis [TA], acromioclavicular d., Weitbrecht cartilage.
  articular d. of distal radioulnar joint [TA], d. da articulação radioulnar distal; o disco que mantém unidas as extremidades distais do rádio e da ulna; está fixado por seu ápice a uma depressão entre o processo estilóide e a superfície distal da cabeça da ulna e, por sua base, à crista que separa a incisura ulnar da face carpal do rádio. SIN discus articularis radioulnaris distalis [TA], radioulnar d., radioulnar articular d., triangular cartilage, triangular d. of wrist, triquetrous cartilage (1).
  articular d. of sternoclavicular joint [TA], d. da articulação esternoclavicular; o disco fibrocartilaginoso que subdivide a articulação esternoclavicular em duas cavidades. SIN discus articularis sternoclavicularis [TA], sternoclavicular d., sternoclavicular articular d.
  articular d. of temporomandibular joint [TA], d. da articulação temporomandibular (ATM); a lâmina fibrocartilaginosa que separa a articulação em cavidades superior e inferior. SIN discus articularis temporomandibularis [TA], mandibular d., temporomandibular articular d.
  blastodermic d., d. blastodérmico; a agregação de blastômeros de um ovo telolécito após a clivagem.
  blood d., plaqueta. SIN platelet.
  Bowman d.'s, discos de Bowman; discos resultantes de segmentação transversa da fibra muscular estriada tratada com ácidos fracos, determinadas soluções alcalinas ou congelamento.
  Burlew d., d. de Burlew; aro de borracha impregnado com abrasivo usado em odontologia para polimento. SIN Burlew wheel.
  choked d., papiledema. SIN papilledema.
  ciliary d., d. ciliar. SIN orbiculus ciliaris.
  cone d.'s, discos do cone; discos membranosos de sacos achatados com cerca de 14 nm de espessura, observados no segmento externo dos cones da retina.
  cuttlefish d., d. de siba; círculo de papel ou plástico fino coberto com pó de osso de siba; usado, quando acoplado a um mandril e girado por uma caneta dentária, para polimento e acabamento de materiais dentários e dentes.
  diamond d., d. de diamante; disco de aço com a(s) superfície(s) de corte coberta(s) com finas lascas de diamante, para usar em canetas dentárias.
  embryonic d., d. embrionário. SIN germinal d.
  emery d.'s, d. de esmeril; discos de papel ou de outros materiais revestidos com pó de esmeril, usados para desgastar ou polir a superfície dos dentes ou obturações.
  germinal d., germ d., d. germinativo; d. embrionário; o ponto em um ovo telolécito onde o embrião começa a ser formado. SIN embryonic d., germinal area, area germinativa.
  H d., d. H. SIN H band.
  hair d., d. piloso; área ricamente inervada da pele, ao redor de um folículo piloso, que consiste em uma camada espessada de células epiteliais nas quais se ramificam terminações não-mielinizadas de um único axônio.
  Hensen d., d. de Hensen. SIN H band.
  herniated d., d. herniado; protrusão de um disco intervertebral degenerado ou fragmentado para o forame intervertebral, com possível compressão de uma raiz nervosa, ou para o canal vertebral, com possível compressão da cauda eqüina na região lombar ou da medula espinal em níveis mais altos. SIN protruded d., ruptured d.
  I d., d. I. SIN I band.
  intercalated d., d. intercalado; fixação intercelular especializada de músculo cardíaco que compreende junções comunicantes (nexos), fáscia aderente e, ocasionalmente, desmossomas.
  intermediate d., d. intermediário. SIN Z line.
  interpubic d., d. interpúbico. SIN interpubic disk.
  intervertebral d., d. intervertebral; disco interposto entre os corpos de vértebras adjacentes. É composto de uma parte fibrosa externa (anel fibroso) que circunda uma massa gelatinosa central (núcleo pulposo). SIN discus intervertebralis [TA], fibrocartilago intervertebralis, intervertebral cartilage.
  isotropic d., d. isotrópico. SIN I band.
  mandibular d., d. mandibular. SIN articular d. of temporomandibular joint.
  Merkel tactile d., d. tátil de Merkel. SIN tactile meniscus.
  Newton d., d. de Newton; disco que possui sete setores coloridos, cada um ocupando proporcionalmente o mesmo espaço que a cor primária correspondente no espectro; quando o disco é girado rapidamente, parece branco.
  optic d. [TA], d. do nervo óptico; área oval do fundo ocular desprovida de receptores para a luz, para onde os axônios da célula ganglionar da retina convergem para formar a cabeça do nervo óptico. SIN discus nervi optici [TA], blind spot (3), Mariotte blind spot, optic nerve head, optic papilla, papilla nervi optici, porus opticus.
  Placido da Costa d., d. de Plácido da Costa; ceratoscópio. SIN keratoscope.
  proligerous d., d. prolígero. SIN cumulus oöphorus.
  protruded d., d. protruso. SIN herniated d.
  Q d.'s, discos Q. SIN A bands, em band.
  radioulnar d., radioulnar articular d., d. radioulnar, d. articular radioulnar. SIN articular d. of distal radioulnar joint.
  Ranvier d.'s, discos de Ranvier; terminações nervosas táteis, de forma discóide, na pele.
  rod d.'s, discos do bastonete; discos membranosos de sacos achatados, com cerca de 14 nm de espessura, observados no segmento externo de bastonetes da retina.
  ruptured d., d. roto. SIN herniated d.
  sacrococcygeal d., d. sacrococcígeo; lâmina fina de fibrocartilagem interposta entre o sacro e o cóccix.
  sandpaper d.'s, discos de lixa; discos de papel revestidos com vários grãos de sílica; usados para desgaste ou polimento da superfície dos dentes ou de materiais dentários.
  stenopeic d., stenopaic d., d. estenopeico; disco metálico ou de outro material opaco com uma fenda estreita através da qual se pode olhar; usado como teste para astigmatismo.
  sternoclavicular d., sternoclavicular articular d., d. esternoclavicular, d. articular esternoclavicular. SIN articular d. of sternoclavicular joint.
  stroboscopic d., d. estroboscópico; disco giratório que produz imagens sucessivas de um objeto em movimento.
  tactile d., d. tátil. SIN tactile meniscus.
  temporomandibular articular d., d. articular temporomandibular. SIN articular d. of temporomandibular joint.
  transverse d., d. transverso; uma das faixas transversas escuras observadas ao exame microscópico de uma fibra muscular estriada.
  triangular d. of wrist, d. triangular do punho. SIN articular d. of distal radioulnar joint.
  Z d., d. Z. SIN Z line.

dis·ki·tis (dis-kī'tis). Discite. SIN discitis.

disko-. VER disco-.

dis·ko·gram (dis'kō-gram). Discograma; o registro gráfico, geralmente radiográfico, da discografia.

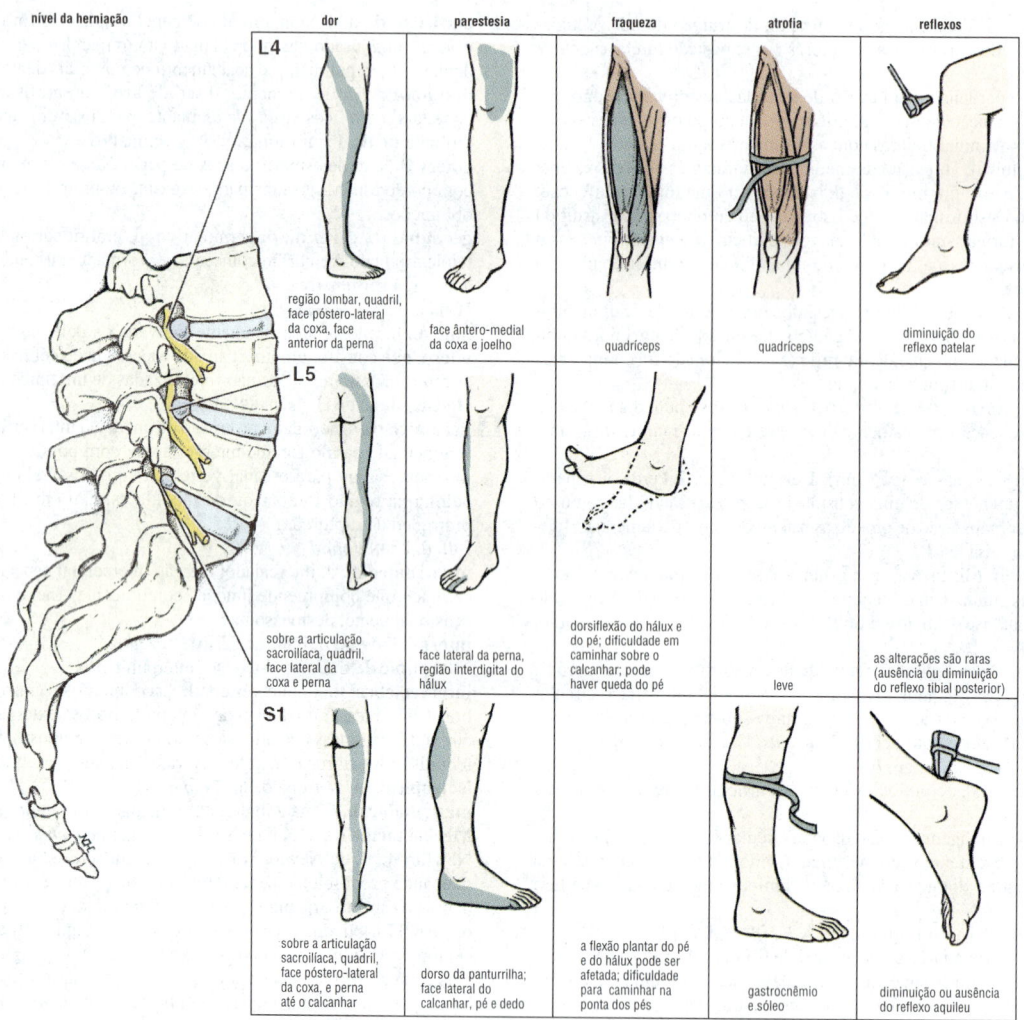

herniação de disco intervertebral

dis·kog·ra·phy (dis-kog′ră-fē). Discografia; historicamente, a demonstração radiográfica do disco intervertebral por injeção de contraste no núcleo pulposo. [disco- + G. *graphō*, escrever]
dis·lo·cate (dis′lō-kāt). Luxar; retirar da articulação.
dis·lo·ca·tio (dis-lō-kā′shē-ō). Luxação. SIN dislocation. [L.]
 d. erec′ta, l. ereta; luxação subglenóide do ombro na qual o úmero está em posição abduzida, com a cabeça do úmero deslocada para baixo.
dis·lo·ca·tion (dis-lō-kā′shŭn). Luxação; deslocamento de um órgão ou de qualquer parte; especificamente, um distúrbio ou perturbação da relação normal dos ossos em uma articulação. A direção da luxação é determinada pela posição da parte distal da articulação. SIN dislocatio, luxation (1). [L. *dislocatio*, de *dis-*, afastado, + *locatio*, localização]
 d. of articular processes, l. dos processos articulares; luxação completa de um ou de ambos os processos articulares, geralmente com acavalgamento do processo articular inferior da vértebra acima até uma posição anterior ao processo articular superior da vértebra abaixo. SIN locked facets.
 arytenoid d., l. aritenóide; separação da articulação cricoaritenóide com subluxação da cartilagem aritenóide. SIN arytenoid subluxation.
 closed d., l. fechada; luxação não complicada por uma ferida externa. SIN simple d.
 compound d., l. composta. SIN open d.
 fracture d., fratura-luxação; luxação associada a, ou acompanhada por, uma fratura de um dos ossos que formam a articulação.
 Kienböck d., l. de Kienböck; luxação do osso semilunar.
 open d., l. aberta; luxação complicada por uma ferida que se abre desde a superfície até a articulação afetada. SIN compound d.
 perilunar d., l. perilunar; luxação dos ossos carpais ao redor do semilunar, que permanece em sua posição anatômica normal em relação ao rádio; distinguir da luxação do semilunar, luxação de Kienböck.
 simple d., l. simples. SIN closed d.

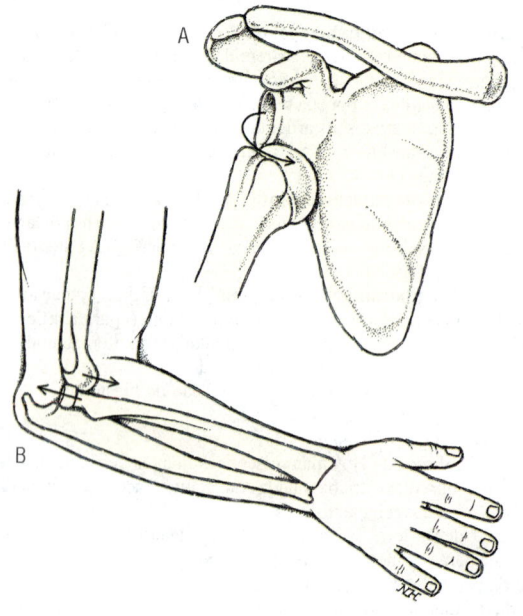

luxação: (A) luxação subglenóide do ombro, (B) luxação do cotovelo

dis·mem·ber (dis-mem′ber). Desmembrar. **1.** Amputar um braço ou perna. **2.** Dividir o corpo em partes.

dis·mu·tase (dis′mū-tās). Dismutase; nome genérico dado a enzimas que catalisam a reação de duas moléculas idênticas para produzir duas moléculas em diferentes estados de oxidação (p. ex., superóxido dismutase) ou de fosforilação (p. ex., glicose-1-fosfato fosfodismutase).

dis·mu·ta·tion (dis′mū-tā′shŭn). Dismutação; reação que envolve uma única substância, mas que gera dois produtos; p. ex., duas moléculas de acetaldeído podem reagir, produzindo um produto de oxidação (ácido acético) e um produto de redução (álcool etílico).

dis·o·bli·ter·a·tion (dis′ob-lit-er-ā′shŭn). Desobstrução; abertura de um canal anormalmente fechado.

di·so·fen·in (dī′sō-fen-in). Disofenina. SIN diisopropyl iminodiacetic acid.

di·so·mic (dī-sō′mik). Dissômico; relativo à dissomia.

di·so·my (dī′sō-mē). Dissomia. **1.** O estado de um indivíduo ou célula que possui dois membros de um par de cromossomas homólogos; o estado normal em seres humanos, em contraste com a monossomia e a trissomia. **2.** Um cromossoma anormal representado duas vezes em uma única célula. [G. *dis*, dois, + *sōma*, corpo]

di·so·pro·mine (di-sō-prō′mēn). Disopromina. SIN diisopromine.

di·so·pyr·a·mide (dī-sō-pir′ā-mīd). Disopiramida; um agente antiarrítmico semelhante à quinidina, com significativas propriedades anticolinérgicas.

dis·or·der (dis-ōr′der). Transtorno; distúrbio; perturbação da função e/ou da estrutura, resultante de uma falha genética ou embrionária no desenvolvimento ou de fatores exógenos como venenos, traumatismo ou doença.
  adjustment d.'s, transtornos de ajustamento; **(1)** um grupo de distúrbios mentais e comportamentais nos quais o desenvolvimento de sintomas está relacionado à existência de algum fator ambiental ou acontecimento estressante, sendo esperada sua remissão quando o estresse cessa; **(2)** um distúrbio cuja característica essencial é uma reação de inadaptação a um estresse psicológico identificável ou a um agente estressante, que ocorre semanas após o início do estresse e persiste por até seis meses; a natureza inadaptativa da reação é indicada por comprometimento da função ocupacional (incluindo escolar) ou das atividades sociais habituais ou relacionamentos com outras pessoas, ou por sintomas que excedem uma reação normal ou esperada ao estresse.
  affective d.'s, distúrbios afetivos ou da afetividade; um grupo de distúrbios mentais caracterizados por perturbação do humor.
  antisocial personality d., transtorno da personalidade anti-social; **(1)** padrão resistente e invasivo caracterizado por comportamento anti-social contínuo e crônico, com desrespeito e violação dos direitos e segurança alheios, começando antes dos 15 anos de idade; os sinais, nos primeiros anos de vida, incluem mentiras repetidas, furtos, belicosidade e vadiagem; na adolescência pode haver comportamento sexual precoce ou agressivo, ingestão excessiva de bebidas alcoólicas e uso de drogas ilícitas, com manutenção desse comportamento na vida adulta. **(2)** Diagnóstico do DSM que é estabelecido quando são atendidos os critérios especificados.
  anxiety d.'s, transtornos de ansiedade; grupo de doenças mentais inter-relacionadas, envolvendo reações de ansiedade em resposta ao estresse. Os tipos incluem: 1) ansiedade generalizada, sem dúvida a condição mais prevalente, que acomete um pouco mais as mulheres que os homens, principalmente entre 20 e 35 anos; 2) transtorno de pânico, no qual uma pessoa sofre repetidos ataques de pânico. Em torno de 2–5% dos norte-americanos sofrem desse mal, acometendo cerca de duas vezes mais mulheres que homens; 3) transtorno obsessivo-compulsivo, que acomete 2–3% da população norte-americana; 4) transtorno de estresse pós-traumático, mais freqüente entre veteranos combatentes ou sobreviventes de grandes traumatismos físicos; e 5) as fobias (p. ex., medo de cobras, multidões, confinamento, alturas, etc.), que afetam em menor escala cerca de uma em oito pessoas nos Estados Unidos. VER neurosis.
  articulation d.'s, distúrbios da articulação; erros na pronúncia, incluindo omissões, substituições, distorções e acréscimos de fonemas.
  Asperger d., transtorno de Asperger; **(1)** d. invasivo do desenvolvimento, caracterizado por comprometimento grave e persistente da interação social, e por padrões restritivos e repetitivos de comportamentos e interesses, comprometendo as áreas social e ocupacional, mas sem atrasos significativos no desenvolvimento da linguagem. **(2)** Um diagnóstico do DSM que é estabelecido quando são atendidos os critérios especificados.
  asthenic personality d., transtorno da personalidade astênica. SIN asthenic *personality*.
  attention deficit d., transtorno de déficit de atenção; distúrbio da atenção, organização e controle de impulsos que surge na infância e, algumas vezes, persiste até a vida adulta. Pode haver hiperatividade, mas esta não é necessária para o diagnóstico.
  attention deficit hyperactivity d., transtorno de déficit de atenção/hiperatividade; **(1)** distúrbio da infância e da adolescência que se manifesta em casa, na escola e em situações sociais, por graus impróprios de desatenção, impulsividade e hiperatividade para o desenvolvimento. **(2)** Um diagnóstico do DSM que é estabelecido quando são atendidos os critérios específicos. SIN hyperactive child syndrome.
  autistic d., transtorno autista; **(1)** uma forma grave de distúrbio invasivo do desenvolvimento. VER TAMBÉM autism, infantile *autism*; **(2)** um diagnóstico do DSM que é estabelecido quando são atendidos os critérios específicos. VER autism, infantile *autism*.
  avoidant d. of adolescence, transtorno de isolamento da adolescência. VER avoidant d. of childhood.
  avoidant d. of childhood, transtorno de isolamento da infância; distúrbio mental que ocorre na infância ou na adolescência caracterizado por afastamento excessivo do contato com pessoas não-familiares.
  avoidant personality d., transtorno da personalidade esquiva; **(1)** padrão inflexível e invasivo na vida adulta, caracterizado por hipersensibilidade a rejeição, humilhação, vergonha, sentimentos de inadequação que resultam em inibição social e relutância em iniciar relacionamentos, a menos que tenham fortes garantias de que serão aceitos sem críticas. **(2)** Um diagnóstico do DSM que é estabelecido quando são atendidos os critérios específicos. SIN avoidant personality.
  behavior d., transtorno do comportamento; termo genérico usado para designar doença mental ou disfunção psicológica, especificamente aquelas subclasses mentais, emocionais ou comportamentais para as quais não existem correlações orgânicas. VER antisocial personality d.
  bipolar d., transtorno bipolar; distúrbio afetivo caracterizado pela ocorrência de períodos alternados de euforia (mania) e depressão. SIN manic-depressive psychosis.
  body dysmorphic d., transtorno dismórfico corporal; **(1)** distúrbio psicossomático (somatiforme) caracterizado por preocupação com algum defeito imaginário no aspecto de uma pessoa de aparência normal. **(2)** Um diagnóstico do DSM que é estabelecido quando são atendidos os critérios específicos. SIN dysmorphophobia.
  borderline personality d., transtorno da personalidade limítrofe; **(1)** padrão permanente e invasivo que começa no adulto jovem e é caracterizado por impulsividade e imprevisibilidade, relações interpessoais instáveis, afetividade imprópria ou descontrolada, particularmente raiva, distúrbios de identidade, rápidas mudanças de humor, atos suicidas, automutilações, instabilidade profissional e conjugal, sentimentos crônicos de vazio ou tédio e intolerância à solidão. **(2)** Um diagnóstico do DSM que é estabelecido quando são atendidos os critérios específicos.
  character d., transtorno do caráter; termo antigo que se refere a um grupo de distúrbios do comportamento, agora substituído por um termo mais genérico, transtorno da personalidade.
  conduct d., transtorno de conduta; **(1)** distúrbio mental da infância ou adolescência caracterizado por um padrão persistente de violação das regras sociais e dos direitos alheios; as crianças com o distúrbio podem apresentar comportamento de agressividade física, crueldade com animais, vandalismo e roubo, juntamente com vadiagem, fraude e mentira. **(2)** Um diagnóstico do DSM que é estabelecido quando são atendidos os critérios específicos. VER antisocial personality d.
  conversion d., transtorno de conversão; **(1)** distúrbio mental no qual um conflito emocional inconsciente se expressa como uma alteração ou perda da função física, geralmente controlada pelo sistema nervoso voluntário. **(2)** Um diagnóstico do DSM que é estabelecido quando são atendidos os critérios específicos.
  cumulative trauma d.'s (CTD), distúrbios por traumatismos cumulativos; distúrbios crônicos envolvendo o tecido conjuntivo (músculos, tendões) e nervo, freqüentemente resultantes de atividades físicas ocupacionais. SIN repetitive strain d.'s, repetitive stress d.'s.
  cyclothymic d., transtorno ciclotímico. SIN cyclothymia.
  cyclothymic personality d., transtorno da personalidade ciclotímico. SIN cyclothymic *personality*.
  delusional d., distúrbio mental grave caracterizado pela presença de ilusões. As ilusões podem ser relacionadas a temas paranóides, grandiosos, somáticos ou eróticos.
  dependent personality d., transtorno da personalidade dependente; **(1)** padrão inflexível e invasivo na vida adulta, caracterizado por comportamento submisso e pegajoso e por dependência excessiva dos outros para atender às próprias necessidades emocionais, sociais ou econômicas. **(2)** Um diagnóstico do DSM que é estabelecido quando são atendidos os critérios específicos. SIN dependent personality.
  depersonalization d., transtorno de despersonalização; **(1)** distúrbio caracterizado por sentimentos persistentes ou recorrentes de estar distanciado dos próprios processos mentais ou do próprio corpo, como se o indivíduo fosse um autômato, um observador externo ou estivesse sonhando; o teste de realidade permanece intacto e há sofrimento clinicamente significativo. **(2)** Um diagnóstico do DSM que é estabelecido quando são atendidos os critérios específicos.
  dissociative d.'s, transtornos dissociativos; grupo de transtornos mentais caracterizados por distúrbios nas funções de identidade, memória, consciência ou percepção do ambiente; esse grupo inclui amnésia dissociativa (anteriormente, amnésia psicogênica), fuga dissociativa, transtorno dissociativo de identidade (anteriormente, transtorno de personalidade múltipla) e transtorno de despersonalização.

dissociative identity d., transtorno dissociativo de identidade; **(1)** transtorno no qual duas ou mais personalidades conscientes distintas prevalecem alternadamente na mesma pessoa, algumas vezes sem que uma personalidade esteja ciente da(s) outra(s). **(2)** Um diagnóstico do DSM que é estabelecido quando são atendidos os critérios específicos. SIN multiple personality.

dysthymic d., transtorno distímico; **(1)** perturbação crônica do humor caracterizada por depressão leve ou perda do interesse em atividades habituais. VER depression; **(2)** um diagnóstico do DSM que é estabelecido quando são atendidos os critérios específicos.

eating d.'s, transtornos alimentares; grupo de transtornos mentais que incluem anorexia nervosa, bulimia nervosa, pica e transtorno de ruminação do lactente.

emotional d., transtorno emocional. VER mental *illness*, behavior d.

erotomanic d., transtorno erotomaníaco; a falsa crença de que se é amado por outra pessoa como um astro do cinema ou um conhecido casual.

factitious d., transtorno factício; transtorno mental no qual o indivíduo intencionalmente produz sintomas de doença ou finge estar doente por razões psicológicas, e não para atingir objetivos ambientais.

familial bipolar mood d., transtorno do humor bipolar familiar; transtorno do humor bipolar que comumente tem herança autossômica dominante [MIM*125480] e, também, ocasionalmente ligado ao X [MIM*309200].

functional d., transtorno funcional; perturbação caracterizada por sintomas físicos sem base orgânica conhecida ou detectável. VER behavior d., neurosis. SIN functional disease, functional illness.

gender identity d.'s, transtornos da identidade sexual; **(1)** transtorno mental em crianças, adolescentes ou adultos caracterizado por forte e persistente identificação com o sexo oposto, que se manifesta por insistência do indivíduo de que ele é, ou deseja ser, do sexo oposto; esse transtorno envolve desconforto persistente com o próprio sexo atribuído ou com o próprio papel sexual, de forma que há sofrimento clinicamente significativo ou comprometimento funcional, que freqüentemente leva à adoção, em graus variáveis, do papel do sexo oposto. **(2)** Um diagnóstico do DSM que é estabelecido quando são atendidos os critérios específicos. VER TAMBÉM transsexualism.

generalized anxiety d., transtorno de ansiedade generalizada; **(1)** episódios crônicos e repetidos de reações de ansiedade; um transtorno psicológico no qual as manifestações proeminentes são ansiedade ou medo mórbido e pavor acompanhados de alterações autônomas. **(2)** Um diagnóstico do DSM que é confirmado quando são atendidos os critérios especificados. VER anxiety.

grandiose type of paranoid d., transtorno paranóide de grandeza; delírio no qual a pessoa acredita que possui algum grande talento ou conhecimento não reconhecido, ou que fez uma descoberta importante, esforçando-se para obter reconhecimento público ou oficial.

histrionic personality d., transtorno histriônico da personalidade; **(1)** padrão de comportamento persistente e invasivo na vida adulta, caracterizado por emotividade excessiva, dramática e superficial; comportamento de busca de atenção; e necessidade de aprovação e reafirmação, começando nos primeiros anos de vida e presente em vários contextos. **(2)** Um diagnóstico do DSM que é estabelecido quando são atendidos os critérios específicos. SIN hysterical personality d., hysterical personality.

hysterical personality d., transtorno da personalidade histérica. SIN histrionic personality d.

identity d., transtorno da identidade; perturbação mental na qual o indivíduo tem sofrimento intenso em relação a própria capacidade de harmonizar aspectos da sua personalidade em um sentido aceitável e coerente de individualidade.

immune complex d., doença por imunocomplexo. SIN immune complex *disease*.

immunoproliferative d.'s, distúrbios imunoproliferativos; distúrbios nos quais há proliferação contínua de células do sistema imune que pode resultar em anormalidades das γ-globulinas, como na leucemia linfocítica crônica, "macroglobulinemias" e mieloma múltiplo.

impulse control d., transtorno do controle dos impulsos; grupo de transtornos mentais caracterizados por incapacidade de uma pessoa de resistir a um impulso de realizar algum ato prejudicial para si própria ou para os outros; inclui o jogo patológico, a pedofilia, a cleptomania, a piromania, a tricotilomania e os transtornos explosivos intermitentes e isolados.

induced psychotic d., transtorno psicótico induzido; transtorno mental grave produzido por um agente tóxico como uma droga ou alucinógeno. VER psychosis.

intermittent explosive d., transtorno explosivo intermitente; **(1)** distúrbio que pode começar nos primeiros anos de vida, ou após traumatismo craniano em qualquer idade, caracterizado por atos repetidos de comportamento violento e agressivo em pessoas normais sob outros aspectos; esse comportamento é significativamente desproporcional ao evento que o provoca. **(2)** Um diagnóstico do DSM que é estabelecido quando são atendidos os critérios específicos. SIN dyscontrol, episodic dyscontrol syndrome.

internet addiction d., transtorno de dependência da internet; suposta síndrome clínica envolvendo dispêndio excessivo de tempo "surfando na rede"; sem critérios ou etiologia claramente definidos.

ion channel d.'s, distúrbios dos canais iônicos; várias doenças, a maioria hereditária e de natureza episódica, causadas por disfunção dos canais de cálcio, cloreto, potássio ou sódio do nervo ou músculo; as miotonias hereditárias e as paralisias periódicas estão incluídas nessa categoria; a herança geralmente é dominante, sendo o defeito primário devido a mutações do gene que codifica o *locus* 7q32, 17q ou 1q31-32. SIN channelopathies.

isolated explosive d., transtorno explosivo isolado; transtorno do controle de impulsos, caracterizado por um único episódio de incapacidade de resistir a um ato violento, orientado externamente, que teve grande impacto sobre os outros.

jealous type of paranoid d., transtorno paranóide do tipo ciumento; a falsa crença de que o cônjuge ou amante é infiel, levando a confrontos repetidos, ou a tomada de medidas extraordinárias para intervir na infidelidade imaginada.

late luteal phase dysphoric d., distúrbio disfórico do final da fase lútea; transtorno disfórico pré-menstrual. SIN premenstrual *syndrome*.

LDL receptor d., distúrbio do receptor da LDL; anormalidade da eliminação de LDL do plasma devido à anormalidade na atividade do seu receptor; causa hipercolesterolemia.

lymphoplasmacellular d.'s, distúrbios linfoplasmocitários; termo usado em referência a um grupo de distúrbios que incluem plasmocitoma, mieloma múltiplo, linfoma linfoplasmacítico, linfoma MALT e amiloidose.

major depressive d., transtorno depressivo maior. SIN major *depression*.

major mood d., transtorno maior do humor. VER bipolar d., affective *psychosis*, endogenous *depression*, dysthymia, manic-depressive d.

manic-depressive d., transtorno maníaco-depressivo; termo obsoleto para transtorno bipolar.

mental d., transtorno mental; síndrome psicológica ou padrão de comportamento associado a sofrimento subjetivo e/ou comprometimento objetivo. VER TAMBÉM mental *illness*, behavior d.

mitochondrial d.'s, distúrbios mitocondriais; grupo de distúrbios hereditários diversos causados por mutação genética do DNA mitocondrial; inclui a miopatia de fibras vermelhas anfractuosas; oftalmoplegia externa progressiva; síndrome de Leigh; epilepsia mioclônica com miopatia de fibras vermelhas anfractuosas (MERRF); miopatia mitocondrial, encefalopatia, lactacidose e acidente vascular cerebral (MELAS); e neuropatia óptica de Lieber.

mood d.'s, transtornos do humor; grupo de transtornos mentais envolvendo um transtorno do humor, acompanhado por uma síndrome maníaca ou depressiva, parcial ou completa, que não é causada por qualquer outro transtorno mental. O humor refere-se a uma emoção prolongada que perturba toda a vida psíquica; geralmente envolve depressão ou exaltação; p. ex., episódio maníaco, episódio depressivo maior, transtornos bipolares e transtorno depressivo (ver cada um em entradas separadas).

multiple personality d., transtorno de personalidade múltipla; termo antigo para transtorno dissociativo de identidade.

narcissistic personality d., transtorno da personalidade narcisista; **(1)** padrão invasivo na vida adulta de autocentralização, auto-importância, ausência de empatia por outras pessoas, sentimento de que a vida lhe deve algo e a consideração de que os outros são basicamente objetos para atender às próprias necessidades, que se manifesta em vários contextos. **(2)** Um diagnóstico do DSM que é estabelecido quando são atendidos os critérios específicos.

neuropsychologic d., transtorno neuropsicológico; disfunção cerebral, decorrente de qualquer causa física, que se manifesta por alterações do humor, do comportamento, da percepção, da memória, da cognição ou do julgamento e/ou psicofisiologia.

neurotic d., transtorno neurótico. SIN neurosis.

obsessive-compulsive d., transtorno obsessivo-compulsivo; **(1)** tipo de transtorno de ansiedade cuja característica essencial é a presença de obsessões recorrentes, idéias, pensamentos, impulsos ou imagens persistentes e impertinentes ou compulsões (comportamentos repetitivos, significativos e intencionais realizados em resposta a uma obsessão), suficientemente graves para causar grande sofrimento, perda de tempo ou interferir significativamente com a rotina normal, funcionamento ocupacional ou atividades ou relacionamentos sociais habituais do indivíduo. **(2)** Um diagnóstico do DSM que é estabelecido quando são atendidos os critérios específicos. VER TAMBÉM obsessive-compulsive personality d.

obsessive-compulsive personality d., transtorno da personalidade obsessivo-compulsiva; **(1)** padrão invasivo na vida adulta, caracterizado por perfeccionismo inatingível; preocupação com regras, detalhes e organização; tentativas absurdas de controlar as outras pessoas; dedicação excessiva ao trabalho; e reflexão até o ponto de indecisão, à custa da flexibilidade, abertura e eficiência. **(2)** Um diagnóstico do DSM que é estabelecido quando são atendidos os critérios específicos. SIN compulsive personality, obsessive personality, obsessive-compulsive personality.

oppositional d., transtorno opositivo. SIN oppositional defiant d.

oppositional defiant d., transtorno desafiador e opositivo; **(1)** transtorno da infância ou da adolescência caracterizado por um padrão recorrente de comportamento negativista, hostil e desobediente para com as figuras de autoridade. **(2)** Um diagnóstico do DSM que é estabelecido quando são atendidos os critérios específicos. SIN oppositional d.

organic mental d., transtorno mental orgânico; anormalidade psicológica, cognitiva ou comportamental, associada a disfunção cerebral transitória ou permanente, geralmente caracterizada pela presença de uma síndrome cerebral orgânica.

overanxious d., transtorno de excesso de ansiedade; transtorno mental da infância ou adolescência caracterizado por preocupação excessiva e comportamento temeroso não relacionado especificamente à separação ou devido a estresse recente, agora incluído no transtorno de ansiedade generalizada.

panic d., transtorno de pânico; ataques de pânico recorrentes e imprevisíveis. VER generalized anxiety d.

paranoid d., transtorno paranóide. SIN persecutory type of paranoid d.

paranoid personality d., transtorno da personalidade paranóide; (1) transtorno da personalidade menos debilitante que o transtorno paranóide ou o transtorno delirante; a característica essencial é uma tendência invasiva e injustificada, que começa no início da vida adulta e apresenta-se em diversos contextos, de interpretar erroneamente as ações alheias como deliberadamente exploradoras, prejudiciais, humilhantes ou ameaçadoras. (2) Um diagnóstico do DSM que é estabelecido quando são atendidos os critérios específicos. SIN paranoid personality.

persecutory type of paranoid d., transtorno paranóide do tipo persecutório; um dos tipos mais comuns de transtornos paranóides, envolve um único tema ou série de temas relacionados, como estar sendo vítima de uma conspiração, fraude, espionagem, perseguição, envenenamento ou intoxicação com drogas, estar sendo alvo de comentários maliciosos, de molestamento ou obstrução em sua busca de objetivos de longo prazo; pequenas desfeitas podem ser exageradas e tornar-se o foco de um sistema de ilusões. VER paranoia; Cf. paranoid personality d. SIN paranoid d.

personality d., transtorno da personalidade; designação genérica para um grupo de transtornos do comportamento caracterizados por padrões inadaptativos arraigados e permanentes de experiência interna subjetiva e desvio do comportamento, do estilo de vida e do ajuste social, cujos padrões podem manifestar-se em comprometimento do julgamento, do afeto, do controle de impulsos e do relacionamento interpessoal.

pervasive developmental d., transtorno invasivo do desenvolvimento; grupo de transtornos mentais do lactente, da criança ou do adolescente, caracterizados por distorções na aquisição das múltiplas funções psicológicas básicas necessárias para a elaboração de habilidades sociais, habilidades de linguagem e imaginação; também é caracterizado por restrição ou estereotipia das atividades e interesses. VER TAMBÉM Rett *syndrome*, Asperger d.

plasma iodoprotein d., distúrbio da iodoproteína plasmática. VER familial goiter.

posttraumatic stress d., transtorno de estresse pós-traumático; (1) desenvolvimento de sintomas característicos após um evento psicologicamente traumático que, geralmente, está fora da faixa de experiência humana habitual; os sintomas incluem diminuição da responsividade a estímulos ambientais, várias disfunções autônomas e cognitivas e disforia. (2) Um diagnóstico do DSM que é estabelecido quando são atendidos os critérios específicos.

premenstrual dysphoric d., transtorno disfórico pré-menstrual; (1) padrão invasivo que ocorre durante a última semana da fase lútea na maioria dos ciclos menstruais durante pelo menos um ano, com remissão alguns dias após o início da fase folicular, com alguma combinação de depressão do humor, labilidade do humor, grande ansiedade ou irritabilidade; vários sintomas físicos específicos e comprometimento funcional significativo; a intensidade dos sintomas é comparável à daqueles observados em um episódio depressivo maior, distinguindo esse transtorno da síndrome pré-menstrual, muito mais complexa. VER TAMBÉM premenstrual *syndrome*; (2) conjunto específico de critérios no DSM, proposto para fins de pesquisa adicional.

psychogenic pain d., transtorno doloroso psicogênico; transtorno no qual a principal queixa é a dor desproporcional aos achados objetivos, e que está relacionada a fatores psicológicos.

psychosomatic d., psychophysiologic d., transtorno psicossomático, transtorno psicofisiológico; transtorno caracterizado por sintomas físicos de origem psíquica, geralmente envolvendo um único sistema orgânico inervado pelo sistema nervoso autônomo; as alterações fisiológicas e orgânicas são decorrentes de um distúrbio mantido.

psychotic d., transtorno psicótico. SIN psychosis.

reactive attachment d., transtorno de apego reativo; (1) transtorno mental do lactente ou da criança pequena, caracterizado por perturbação das relações sociais; atribuído ao recebimento de cuidados flagrantemente anormais. (2) Um diagnóstico do DSM que é estabelecido quando são atendidos os critérios específicos.

REM behavior d., transtorno do comportamento REM; transtorno caracterizado por ausência da atonia dos músculos voluntários, que normalmente ocorre no sono REM.

repetitive strain d.'s, distúrbios por traumatismos cumulativos. SIN cumulative trauma d.'s.

repetitive stress d.'s, distúrbios por traumatismos cumulativos. SIN cumulative trauma d.'s.

rumination d., transtorno de ruminação; (1) transtorno mental que ocorre no lactente, caracterizado por regurgitação repetida dos alimentos acompanhada por perda de peso ou ausência de ganho de peso. (2) Um diagnóstico do DSM que é estabelecido quando são atendidos os critérios específicos.

schizoid personality d., transtorno da personalidade esquizóide; (1) padrão inflexível e invasivo de comportamento na vida adulta, caracterizado por isolamento social, frieza emocional ou altivez ou restrição e indiferença às outras pessoas. (2) Um diagnóstico do DSM que é estabelecido quando são atendidos os critérios específicos. SIN schizoid personality.

schizophreniform d. (skiz′ō-fren′ĭ-form), transtorno esquizofreniforme; (1) transtorno cujas características essenciais são idênticas às da esquizofrenia, com a exceção de que a duração, incluindo as fases prodrômica, ativa e residual, é menor que seis meses. (2) Um diagnóstico do DSM que é estabelecido quando são atendidos os critérios específicos.

schizotypal personality d., transtorno da personalidade esquizotípica; (1) padrão inflexível e invasivo de comportamento na vida adulta, caracterizado por desconforto e reduzida capacidade para relacionamentos íntimos, distorções cognitivas ou perceptivas e comportamento excêntrico. (2) Um diagnóstico do DSM que é estabelecido quando são atendidos os critérios específicos. SIN schizotypal personality.

seasonal affective d. (SAD), transtorno afetivo sazonal; perturbação depressiva do humor que ocorre aproximadamente no mesmo período, ano após ano, e apresenta remissão espontânea no mesmo período a cada ano. O tipo mais comum é a depressão de inverno, sendo caracterizada por hipersonia matinal, diminuição da energia, aumento do apetite, ganho ponderal e desejo por carboidratos. Tudo desaparece na primavera.

separation anxiety d., transtorno de ansiedade de separação; (1) transtorno mental que ocorre na infância, caracterizado por ansiedade excessiva quando a criança é separada de alguém a quem é apegada, geralmente um dos genitores. (2) Um diagnóstico do DSM que é estabelecido quando são atendidos os critérios específicos.

sexual d.'s, transtornos sexuais; grupo de transtornos do comportamento e psicofisiológicos nos quais há variabilidade sintomática da função sexual, incluindo o comportamento erotizado associado à atividade sexual (as parafilias) ou aos distúrbios do desejo, excitação e orgasmo.

shared psychotic d., transtorno psicótico compartilhado. SIN *folie à deux*.

sleep terror d., terror noturno. VER night terrors.

somatization d., transtorno de somatização; (1) transtorno mental caracterizado por apresentação de uma história clínica complicada e de sintomas físicos referentes a vários sistemas orgânicos, porém sem causa orgânica detectável ou conhecida. VER conversion, hysteria, Briquet *syndrome*; (2) um diagnóstico do DSM que é estabelecido quando são atendidos os critérios específicos.

somatoform d., transtorno somatiforme; grupo de transtornos no qual os sintomas físicos sugerem distúrbios físicos para os quais não há achados orgânicos demonstráveis ou mecanismos fisiológicos conhecidos, e para os quais há evidências positivas ou forte presunção de que os sintomas estão relacionados a fatores psicológicos, p. ex., histeria, transtorno de conversão, hipocondria, transtorno doloroso, transtorno de somatização, transtorno dismórfico corporal e síndrome de Briquet.

substance abuse d.'s, transtornos de abuso de substâncias; grupo de transtornos mentais no qual o comportamento mal-adaptado e as alterações biológicas estão associados ao uso regular de álcool, drogas e substâncias relacionadas, que afetam o sistema nervoso central e resultam em incapacidade de atender a importantes obrigações pessoais e sociais.

substance dependence d., transtorno de dependência de substância; padrão mal-adaptado de uso de álcool, drogas ou outras substâncias, com tolerância e/ou sintomas de abstinência, comportamento de busca da droga e fracasso na interrupção do uso, com prejuízo das atividades sociais, interpessoais e ocupacionais.

substance-induced organic mental d.'s, transtornos mentais orgânicos induzidos por substâncias; transtornos mentais causados pelo uso de drogas, p. ex., cocaína, álcool, etc.

thought d., transtorno do pensamento. SIN thought process d.

thought process d., transtorno do pensamento; sintoma referente à função intelectual na esquizofrenia, que se manifesta por irrelevância e incoerência na expressão verbal, variando do simples bloqueio e leve circunstancialidade à total incoerência. SIN thought d.

triple repeat d.'s, distúrbios do códon; grupo de distúrbios hereditários nos quais uma mutação genética em um cromossoma específico produz uma forma anormal de proteína terminada por uma cadeia longa de repetições de aminoácidos glutamato; inclui doença de Huntington, doença de Kennedy, doença de Machado-Joseph, distrofia miotônica, síndrome do X frágil e algumas doenças espinocerebelares.

visceral d., distúrbio visceral; termo obsoleto usado em referência a distúrbio psicossomático.

dis·or·ga·ni·za·tion (dis-ōr′gan-ĭ-zā′shŭn). Desorganização; destruição de um órgão ou tecido com consequente perda funcional.

dis·o·ri·en·ta·tion (dis'or-ē-en-tā'shŭn). Desorientação; perda do sentido de familiaridade com o meio circundante (tempo, lugar e pessoa); perda da própria orientação.

dis·par·ate (dis'pa-rāt). Díspar; desigual; diverso; dessemelhante. [L. *disparo*, pp. *-atus*, separar, de *paro*, preparar]

dis·par·i·ty (dis-par'i-tē). Disparidade; desigualdade; a condição de ser díspar. [L. *dispar*, dessemelhante]
  fixation d., d. de fixação; o grau de heteroforia possível na presença de fusão.
  retinal d., d. retiniana; a pequena diferença nas imagens retinianas decorrente da separação lateral dos dois olhos que estimula a visão estereoscópica.

dis·pen·sa·ry (dis-pen'ser-ē). Dispensário. **1.** Consultório médico, especialmente o consultório de um profissional que avia medicamentos. **2.** A sala do farmacêutico em um hospital, onde os medicamentos são fornecidos com prescrição médica. **3.** Departamento ambulatorial de um hospital. [L. *dis-penso*, pp. *-atus*, distribuir por peso, de *penso*, pesar]

Dis·pen·sa·to·ry (dis-pen'sa-tō-rē). Dispensatório; trabalho originalmente com o objetivo de ser um comentário sobre a Farmacopéia, mas que agora é mais que um suplemento desse trabalho, que contém uma avaliação das fontes, forma de preparo, ação fisiológica e empregos terapêuticos da maioria dos agentes, oficiais e não-oficiais; usado no tratamento de doenças.[L. *dispensator*, administrador, intendente; ver dispensary]

dis·pense (dis-pens'). Aviar; preparar medicamento e outras necessidades para o enfermo; preparar uma prescrição médica.

di·sper·my, di·sperm·ia (dī'sper-mē, dī-sperm'ē-ā). Dispermia; penetração de dois espermatozóides em um óvulo.

dis·per·sal (dis-per'săl). Dispersão. SIN dispersion (1).
  flash d., d. instantânea; a propriedade de rápida desintegração de um comprimido quando colocado sobre a língua.

dis·perse (dis-pers'). Dispersar; dissipar, causar desaparecimento de, espalhar, diluir.

dis·per·sion (dis-per'zhŭn). Dispersão. **1.** O ato de dispersar ou de ser dispersado. SIN dispersal. **2.** Incorporação das partículas de uma substância na massa de outra, incluindo soluções, suspensões e dispersões coloidais (soluções). **3.** Especificamente, o que geralmente é denominado solução coloidal (colloidal *solution*). **4.** A extensão ou grau com que valores de uma distribuição de freqüência estatística estão dispersos em torno de uma média ou valor mediano. [L. *dispersio*]
  coarse d., suspensão coloidal. SIN suspension (4).
  colloidal d., d. coloidal. SIN colloidal *solution*.
  molecular d., d. molecular; dispersão na qual a fase dispersa consiste em moléculas individuais; se as moléculas forem menores que o tamanho coloidal, o resultado é uma solução verdadeira.
  optic rotatory d. (ORD), d. óptica rotatória; a modificação da rotação óptica com o comprimento de onda da luz polarizada monocromática incidente; o deslocamento da primeira de zero para a faixa de absorção é conhecido como efeito Cotton (Cotton *effect*).
  temporal d., d. temporal; repolarização assincrônica das fibras miocárdicas que predispõe a fluxo de corrente anormal e ritmos ectópicos (principalmente com bradiarritmias ou taquiarritmias ventriculares).

dis·per·si·ty (dis-per'si-tē). Dispersidade; grau de redução das dimensões das partículas na formação de colóide.

dis·per·soid (dis-per'soyd). Dispersóide; solução coloidal na qual a fase dispersa pode ser concentrada por centrifugação. SIN dispersion colloid, molecular dispersed solution.

di·spi·reme (dī-spī'rēm). Dispirema; o entrelaçamento da cromatina dupla na telófase da mitose. [G. *di-*, duas vezes, + *speirēma*, espiral, convolução]

dis·place·a·bil·i·ty (dis-plās-ā-bil'i-tē). Deslocabilidade; a capacidade de, ou suscetibilidade ao, deslocamento.
  tissue d., d. tecidual; a propriedade dos tecidos que permite que seja deslocado de uma posição ou forma inicial ou relaxada. SIN compression of tissue.

dis·place·ment (dis-plās'ment). Deslocamento. **1.** Retirada da localização ou posição normal. **2.** O acréscimo a um líquido (particularmente um gás) em um recipiente aberto de um outro de maior densidade, por meio do qual o primeiro é expelido. **3.** Em química, uma alteração na qual um elemento, radical ou molécula é substituído por outro, ou no qual um elemento troca cargas elétricas com outro por redução ou oxidação. **4.** Em psiquiatria, a transferência de impulsos de uma expressão para outra, como o da luta para o diálogo.
  affect d., d. de afeto; um desvio dos sentimentos em relação a um objeto que, originalmente, o despertara para algum objeto associado.
  mesial d., d. mesial. SIN mesioversion.
  tissue d., d. tecidual; a modificação na forma ou posição dos tecidos em virtude da pressão.

display.
  differential d., exibição diferencial; o uso de tecnologias baseadas na RT-PCR para amplificar o mRNA de células ou tecidos específicos e, depois, compará-los diretamente com o mRNA amplificado de outra célula ou tecido.

dis·pro·por·tion (dis-prō-pōr'shŭn). Desproporção; ausência de proporção ou simetria.
  cephalopelvic d., d. cefalopélvica; condição na qual a cabeça fetal é grande demais para atravessar a pelve materna.

Disse, Josef, anatomista alemão, 1852–1912. VER D. *space*.

dis·sect (di-sekt', dī-). Dissecar. **1.** Cortar afastando ou separar os tecidos do corpo para estudo. **2.** Em uma cirurgia, separar as diferentes estruturas ao longo das linhas naturais por divisão da estrutura de tecido conjuntivo. [L. *disseco*, pp. *-sectus*, cortar em partes]

dis·sec·tion (di-sek'shŭn, dī-). Dissecção; o ato de dissecar. SIN anatomy (3) [TA], necrotomy (1).
  aortic d., d. aórtica; processo anormal, caracterizado por separação da túnica média da aorta, que leva à formação de um aneurisma dissecante. Classificada de acordo com a localização da seguinte forma: o tipo I envolve a aorta ascendente, o arco transverso e a aorta distal; o tipo II é limitado à aorta ascendente; o tipo III estende-se distalmente na aorta descendente, geralmente a partir de um ponto inicial imediatamente distal à artéria subclávia esquerda.
  functional neck d., d. cervical funcional; cirurgia para remover metástases para os linfonodos cervicais; difere de uma dissecção cervical radical pela preservação de qualquer uma das seguintes estruturas: o músculo esternocleidomastóideo, o nervo acessório espinal e a veia jugular interna. SIN limited neck d.
  limited neck d., d. cervical limitada. SIN functional neck d.
  radical neck d., d. cervical radical; cirurgia para a remoção de metástases para os linfonodos cervicais na qual é removido todo o tecido entre as fáscias cervicais superficial e profunda, desde a mandíbula até a clavícula. VER TAMBÉM functional neck d.

dis·sec·tor (dis-ek'ter). **1.** Aquele que disseca. **2.** Um guia por escrito para dissecção. **3.** Instrumento para dissecar.

dis·sem·i·nat·ed (di-sem'i-nā'ted). Disseminado; amplamente disperso por todo um órgão, tecido ou corpo. [L. *dissemino*, pp. *-atus*, espalhar a semente, de *semen* (*-min-*), semente]

dis·sep·i·ment (di-sep'i-ment). Septo; tecido de separação, divisão ou septo. [L. *dis- sepio*, pp. *-septus*, dividir por uma cerca]

dis·sim·i·la·tion (di-sim-i-lā'shŭn). **1.** Dissimilação. SIN disassimilation. **2.** SIN catabolism.

dis·sim·u·la·tion (di-sim-ū-lā'shŭn). Dissimulação; esconder a verdade sobre uma situação, particularmente sobre um estado de saúde ou durante um exame do estado mental, como por uma pessoa que finge ou alguém com doença fictícia. [L. *dissimulatio*, de *dissimulo*, fingir, de *dis*, afastado, + *simillis*, mesmo]

dis·so·ci·a·tion (di-sō-sē-ā'shŭn, -shē-ā'shŭn). Dissociação. **1.** Separação, ou uma dissolução de relações. SIN disassociation. **2.** A modificação de um composto químico complexo em outro mais simples por qualquer reação lítica, por ionização, heterólise ou homólise. **3.** Uma separação inconsciente de um grupo de processos mentais do restante, resultando no funcionamento independente desses processos e na perda das associações habituais; p. ex., separação entre afeto e cognição. VER multiple *personality*. **4.** Estado usado como parte essencial de uma técnica para cura em psicologia e psicoterapia, p. ex. em hipnoterapia ou na técnica de programação neurolingüística de terapia da linha do tempo. VER TAMBÉM Time-Line *therapy*. **5.** A translocação entre um grande cromossoma e um pequeno cromossoma supranumerário. **6.** Separação dos componentes nucleares de um dicárion heterocariocítico. [L. *dis-socio*, pp. *-atus*, separar, de *socius*, parceiro, aliado]
  albuminocytologic d., d. albuminocitológica; aumento da proteína no líquido cefalorraquidiano sem aumento da contagem de células, característico da síndrome de Guillain-Barré; também está associada a bloqueio espinal e à neoplasia intracraniana, sendo observada nas fases tardias da poliomielite.
  atrial d., d. atrial; batimento mutuamente independente dos dois átrios ou de partes dos átrios.
  atrioventricular d. (AVD), AV d., d. atrioventricular, d. AV; **(1)** qualquer situação na qual átrios e ventrículos são ativados e se contraem independentemente, como no bloqueio AV completo; **(2)** mais especificamente, a dissociação entre átrios e ventrículos que resulta da lentificação do marcapasso atrial ou da aceleração do marcapasso ventricular em freqüências quase iguais (raramente iguais), cada uma despolarizando sua própria câmara, assim interferindo com a despolarização pelo outro (interferência-dissociação).
  complete atrioventricular d., complete AV d., d. atrioventricular completa, d. AV completa; dissociação AV não interrompida por capturas ventriculares. SIN complete AV block (2), third degree AV block.
  electromechanical d., d. eletromecânica; persistência da atividade elétrica no coração sem contração mecânica assistida; freqüentemente é um sinal de ruptura cardíaca. SIN pulseless electrical activity.
  incomplete atrioventricular d., incomplete AV d., d. atrioventricular incompleta, d. AV incompleta; dissociação AV interrompida por capturas ventriculares.
  interference d., d. por interferência; a operação simultânea de dois focos marcapassos cardíacos distintos, não-associados, causados por interferência (um fenômeno fisiológico normal) devido à transformação de seus respectivos territórios em refratários para o outro. Geralmente é indicada dissociação atrioventricular, com as frequências sendo muito próximas, com a frequência atrial

um pouco menor que a do marcapasso no controle dos ventrículos. A captura em qualquer direção, geralmente do ventrículo pelo átrio, na dissociação incompleta. SIN d. by interference.

d. by interference, d. por interferência. SIN interference d.

isorhythmic d., d. isorrítmica; dissociação AV caracterizada por freqüências atriais e ventriculares iguais ou muito semelhantes.

light-near d., d. luz-perto. SIN *pupillary* light-near dissociation.

longitudinal d., d. longitudinal; dissociação entre câmaras cardíacas paralelas, como entre um átrio e o outro ou entre um ventrículo e o outro, em contraste com a dissociação entre átrios e ventrículos.

pupillary light-near d., dissociação pupilar luz-perto. VER *pupillary* light-near dissociation.

sleep d., d. do sono. SIN sleep *paralysis.*

syringomyelic d., d. siringomielínica; perda da sensibilidade álgica e térmica com relativa preservação da sensibilidade táctil, relacionada a uma cavidade na porção central da medula espinal que interrompe a decussação das fibras nervosas.

tabetic d., d. tabética; perda da sensibilidade proprioceptiva com preservação da sensibilidade álgica e térmica devido a envolvimento das colunas posteriores da medula espinal.

visual-kinetic d., d. visuocinética; o processo de programação neurolingüística de remover uma sinestesia da experiência interna de uma pessoa. VER TAMBÉM neurolinguistic *programming.*

dis·solve (di-zolv′). Dissolver; modificar ou causar modificação de uma forma sólida para uma forma dispersa por imersão em um líquido de propriedades adequadas. [L. *dis-solvo,* pp. *-solutus,* afrouxar, dissolver]

dis·so·nance (di′sŏ-nans). Dissonância; em psicologia social e teoria da atitude, estado aversivo que surge quando um indivíduo tem ciência mínima da inconsistência ou conflito dentro de si mesmo. VER cognitive dissonance *theory*. [L. *dissonus,* discordante, confuso]

cognitive d., d. cognitiva; estado motivacional, estudado por psicólogos sociais e clínicos, que existe quando as atitudes, as percepções e o estado de dissonância relacionados de uma pessoa são incompatíveis entre si, p. ex., odiar negros, mas admirar Martin Luther King.

dis·sym·me·try (di-sim′ĕ-trē). Dissimetria. SIN asymmetry. [dis- + symmetry]

dis·tad (dis′tad). Distal; em direção à periferia; em direção distal.

dis·tal (dis′tăl) [TA]. Distal. **1.** Situado fora do centro do corpo, ou do ponto de origem; aplicado especificamente à extremidade ou parte distante de um membro ou órgão. **2.** Em odontologia, distante do plano sagital mediano da face, seguindo a curvatura do arco dental. SIN distalis [TA]. [L. *distalis*]

dis·ta·lis (dis-tā′lis) [TA]. Distal. SIN distal.

dis·tance (dis′tans). Distância; a medida do espaço entre dois objetos. [L. *distantia,* de *di-sto,* manter afastado, estar distante]

focal d., d. focal; a distância do centro de uma lente até seu foco.

infinite d., d. infinita; o limite da visão a distância; os raios que penetram nos olhos, a partir de um objeto, são praticamente paralelos. SIN infinity.

interarch d., d. interarco; **(1)** a distância vertical entre os arcos maxilar e mandibular em condições de dimensões verticais, que têm de ser especificadas; **(2)** a distância vertical entre as cristas maxilar e mandibular. SIN interalveolar space, interridge d.

interocclusal d., d. interoclusal; a distância vertical entre as superfícies oclusais opostas, pressupondo a relação em repouso se não houver menção em contrário. SIN interocclusal rest space (1). **(2)** SIN freeway *space.*

interridge d., d. intercristas. SIN interarch d.

large interarch d., d. interarco grande; uma grande distância entre os arcos maxilar e mandibular; também pode indicar uma dimensão vertical excessiva. SIN open bite (1).

pupillary d., d. pupilar; a distância entre o centro de cada pupila; os principais pontos de referência em medida para o ajuste de armações de óculos e lentes.

reduced interarch d., d. interarco reduzida; dimensão vertical de oclusão que resulta em uma distância interoclusal excessiva, quando a mandíbula está em posição de repouso, e em uma distância intercrista reduzida quando os dentes estão em contato.

small interarch d., d. interarco pequena; uma distância pequena entre os arcos maxilar e mandibular. SIN close bite.

sociometric d., d. sociométrica; algum grau mensurável de percepção mútua ou social, aceitação e compreensão; hipoteticamente, a maior distância sociométrica está associada a maior falta de acurácia na avaliação de uma relação (p. ex., é mais fácil compreender e lidar com um nativo que com um estrangeiro).

dis·ten·si·bil·i·ty (dis-ten-si-bil′i-tē). Distensibilidade; capacidade de ser distendido ou estirado. [L. *dis- tendo,* estender]

dis·ten·tion, dis·ten·sion (dis-ten′shŭn). Distensão; o ato ou estado de ser distendido ou estirado. VER TAMBÉM dilation. [L. *dis-tendo,* estender]

dis·ti·chi·a·sis (dis′ti-kī′ă-sis). Distiquíase; uma fileira congênita, anormal, acessória de cílios. [G. *di-* duplo, + *stichos,* fileira]

dis·till (dis-til′). Destilar; extrair uma substância por destilação.

dis·til·late (dis′ti-lāt). Destilado; o produto da destilação.

dis·til·la·tion (dis-ti-lā′shŭn). Destilação; volatilização de um líquido por calor e subseqüente condensação do vapor; uma forma de separar o volátil do não-volátil, ou o mais volátil do menos volátil, parte de uma mistura líquida. [L. *de-(di-)stillo,* pp. *-atus,* gotejar]

destructive d., d. destrutiva. SIN dry d.

dry d., d. seca; submissão de uma substância orgânica ao calor em um recipiente fechado, de forma que não haja oxigênio e a combustão seja impedida, com o objetivo de realizar sua decomposição com liberação de constituintes voláteis e formação de novas substâncias. SIN destructive d.

fractional d., d. fracionada; destilação de uma substância líquida em graus variáveis de calor, pela qual os componentes de diferentes pontos de fervura são coletados separadamente.

molecular d., d. molecular; destilação em alto vácuo, com o objetivo de tornar possível o uso de baixas temperaturas para minimizar a lesão de moléculas termolábeis que seriam decompostas por fervura em maiores temperaturas.

dis·to·buc·cal (dis-tō-bŭk′al). Distobucal; relativo às superfícies distal e bucal de um dente; designa o ângulo formado por sua junção.

dis·to·buc·co·oc·clu·sal (dis′tō-bŭk′ō-ō-koo′sal). Distobucoclusal; relativo às superfícies distal, bucal e oclusal de um dente bicúspide ou molar; designa particularmente o ângulo formado pela junção dessas superfícies.

dis·to·buc·co·pul·pal (dis′tō-bŭk′ō-pŭl′pal). Distobucopulpar; relativo ao ângulo triedro formado pela junção de uma parede distal, bucal e pulpar de uma cavidade.

dis·to·cer·vi·cal (dis-tō-ser′vi-kăl). Distocervical; relativo ao ângulo formado pela junção das paredes distal e cervical (gengival) de uma cavidade classe V.

dis·to·clu·sal (dis-tō-kloo′sal). Distoclusal. **1.** Relativo a, ou caracterizado por, distoclusão. **2.** Designa uma cavidade composta ou restauração envolvendo as superfícies distal e oclusal de um dente. **3.** Designa o ângulo formado pelas paredes distal e oclusal de uma cavidade classe V. SIN disto-occlusal.

dis·to·clu·sion (dis-tō-kloo′zhŭn). Distoclusão; má oclusão na qual o arco mandibular se articula com o arco maxilar em uma posição distal ao normal; na classificação de Angle, uma má oclusão classe II. SIN distal occlusion (2).

dis·to·gin·gi·val (dis-tō-jin′ji-val). Distogengival; relativo à junção da superfície distal com a linha gengival de um dente.

dis·to·in·ci·sal (dis′tō-in-sī′zal). Distoincisal; relativo ao ângulo diedro formado pela junção das paredes distal e incisal de uma cavidade classe V em um dente anterior.

dis·to·la·bi·al (dis-tō-lā′bē-al). Distolabial; relativo às superfícies distal e labial de um dente; designa o ângulo formado por sua junção.

dis·to·la·bi·o·pul·pal (dis′tō-lā′bē-ō-pŭl′pal). Distolabiopulpar; relativo ao ângulo triedro formado pela junção das paredes distal, labial e pulpar da parte incisal de uma cavidade classe V (mesioincisal).

dis·to·lin·gual (dis-tō-ling′gwal). Distolingual; relativo às superfícies distal e lingual de um dente; designa o ângulo formado por sua junção.

dis·to·lin·guo·oc·clu·sal (dis′tō-ling′gwō-ō-kloo′zal). Distolinguoclusal; relativo às superfícies distal, lingual e oclusal de um dente bicúspide ou molar; designa especialmente o ângulo formado pela junção dessas superfícies.

Dis·to·ma (dis′tō-mă). Termo obsoleto para vários trematódeos digenéticos, agora designados como outros gêneros; p. ex., *Fasciola, Fasciolopsis, Paragonimus, Opisthorchis, Clonorchis, Dicrocoelium, Heterophyes* e *Schistosoma.* SIN *Distomum.* [G. *di-,* dois, + *stoma,* boca]

dis·to·mi·a·sis, dis·to·ma·to·sis (dis′tō-mī′ă-sis, -mă-tō′sis). Distomíase, distomatose; presença, em qualquer órgão ou tecido, de trematódeos digenéticos antes classificados como Distoma ou Distomum; em geral, infecção por qualquer trematódeo parasita.

hemic d., esquistossomose. SIN schistosomiasis.

pulmonary d., paragonimíase. SIN paragonimiasis.

dis·to·mo·lar (dis-tō-mō′lar). Distomolar; dente supranumerário localizado na região posterior ao terceiro molar.

Dis·to·mum (dis′tō-mŭm). SIN *Distoma.*

dis·to·oc·clu·sal (dis′tō-ō-kloo′sal). Distoclusal. SIN distoclusal.

dis·to·oc·clu·sion (dis′tō-ō-kloo′zhŭn). Distoclusão. SIN distal *occlusion* (1).

dis·to·place·ment (dis′tō-plās-ment). Distoposição. SIN distoversion.

dis·to·pul·pal (dis-tō-pŭl′pal). Distopulpar; relativo ao ângulo diedro formado pela junção das paredes distal e pulpar de uma cavidade.

dis·tor·tion (dis-tōr′shŭn). Distorção. **1.** Em psiquiatria, um mecanismo de defesa que ajuda a reprimir ou disfarçar pensamentos inaceitáveis. **2.** Em impressões dentárias, a deformação permanente do material de impressão após o registro de um molde. **3.** Deturpação do formato normal. **4.** Em oftalmologia, ampliação desigual de um campo de visão. [L. *distortio,* de *dis-torqueo,* arrancar]

barrel d., d. em barril; imagem irregular produzida quando a ampliação periférica é maior que a ampliação axial. VER Petzval *surface.*

parataxic d., d. parataxica; uma atitude em relação à outra pessoa baseada em uma avaliação distorcida, geralmente devido a uma identificação muito próxima daquela pessoa com figuras emocionalmente significativas do passado do paciente.

pincushion d., d. em alfineteira; imagem irregular produzida quando a ampliação axial é maior que a ampliação periférica. VER Petzval *surface*.

dis·to·ver·sion (dis'tō-ver-zhun). Distoversão; posicionamento anômalo de um dente distal ao normal, em uma direção posterior após a curvatura do arco dental. SIN distoplacement.

dis·tract·i·bil·i·ty (dis-trak-tĭ-bil'i-tē). Transtorno da atenção na qual a mente é facilmente desviada por ocorrências inconseqüentes; observada na mania e no transtorno de déficit de atenção.

dis·trac·tion (dis-trak'shŭn). **1.** Distração, dificuldade ou impossibilidade de concentração ou fixação da mente. **2.** Força aplicada a uma parte do corpo para separar fragmentos ósseos ou superfícies articulares. [L. *dis-traho*, pp. *-tractus*, puxar em direções diferentes]

dis·tress (dis-tres'). Sofrimento ou angústia física ou mental. [L. *distringo*, separar]

 fetal d., sofrimento fetal. SIN nonreassuring fetal *status*.

dis·tri·bu·tion (dis-tri-bū'shŭn). Distribuição. **1.** A passagem dos ramos das artérias ou nervos até os tecidos e órgãos. **2.** A área na qual terminam os ramos de uma artéria ou de um nervo, ou a área suprida por essa artéria ou nervo. **3.** Os números relativos de indivíduos em cada uma das várias categorias ou populações como em diferentes amostras etárias, sexuais e ocupacionais. VER frequency d. **4.** Divisão. **5.** O padrão de ocorrência de uma substância dentro de ou entre células, tecidos, organismos ou grupos taxonômicos. [L. *distribuo*, pp. *-tributus*, distribuir, de *tribus*, uma tribo]

 Bernoulli d., d. de Bernoulli; a distribuição da probabilidade associada a dois desfechos mutuamente exclusivos e exaustivos, p. ex., morte ou sobrevida.

 binomial d., d. binomial; **(1)** uma distribuição de probabilidade associada a dois desfechos mutuamente exclusivos, p. ex., a existência ou a ausência de um sinal clínico; **(2)** o possível arranjo do número de sucessos nas evoluções a partir de um número fixo, *n*, de provas de Bernoulli independentes; as probabilidades associadas a cada um constituem um processo binomial de ordem *n*.

 chi-square d. (kī), d. qui-quadrado; diz-se que uma variável tem uma distribuição qui-quadrado com *K* graus de liberdade se for distribuída como a soma dos quadrados de variáveis aleatórias independentes *K*, cada uma das quais possui uma distribuição normal (de Gauss) com média zero e variação um. A distribuição qui-quadrado é a base para muitas variações do teste do qui-quadrado, talvez o teste mais usado para determinar a significância estatística em biologia e medicina.

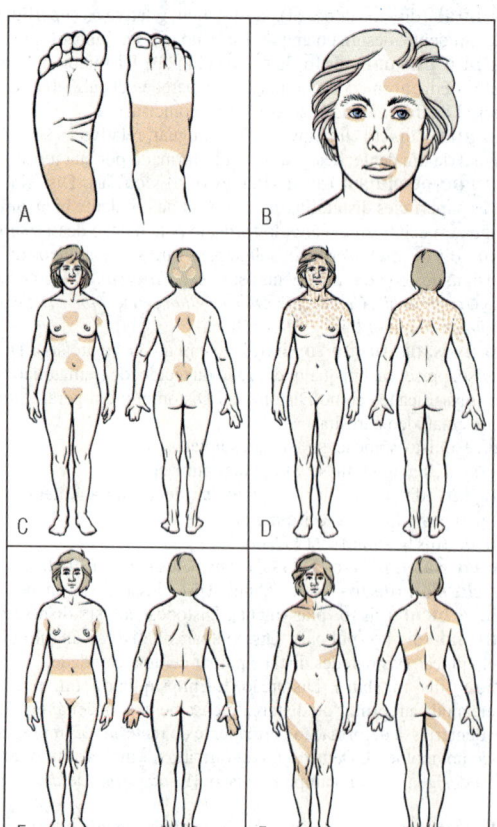

distribuição anatômica de distúrbios cutâneos comuns: (A) dermatite de contato (sapatos); (B) dermatite de contato (cosméticos, perfumes, brincos); (C) dermatite seborreica; (D) acne; (E) escabiose; (F) herpes zoster

 countercurrent d., d. contracorrente; método de separação de duas ou mais substâncias por distribuição repetida entre duas fases líquidas imiscíveis que se deslocam uma contra a outra, em direções opostas; uma forma de cromatografia líquido-líquido.

 dermatomal d., d. em dermátomos. SIN dermatome (3).

 epidemiological d., d. epidemiológica. VER histogram.

 exponential d., d. exponencial; o tempo decorrido até o fracasso de um processo em risco constante.

 f d., d. de f; a distribuição da razão de duas quantidades independentes, cada uma delas distribuída como uma variância em amostras normalmente distribuídas. Assim designada em homenagem ao estatístico e geneticista inglês R.A. Fisher.

 frequency d., d. de freqüência; descrição estatística de dados brutos em termos do número ou da freqüência de itens caracterizados por cada uma de uma série ou faixa de valores de uma variável contínua.

 gaussian d., d. de Gauss. SIN normal d.

 lognormal d., d. lognormal; se uma variável y for tal que x = log y, diz-se que possui uma distribuição lognormal; esta é uma distribuição assimétrica.

 multinomial d., distribuição da probabilidade associada à classificação de cada amostra de indivíduos em uma dentre várias categorias mutuamente exclusivas e exaustivas.

 normal d., d. normal; distribuição de freqüência campanular específica, que os estatísticos consideram como representante da infinita população de medidas a partir das quais foi colhida uma amostra; caracterizada por dois parâmetros, a média (x) e o desvio padrão (σ), na equação. SIN gaussian curve, gaussian d.

 Poisson d., d. de Poisson; **(1)** distribuição descontínua importante no trabalho estatístico e definida pela equação $p(x) = e^{-\mu} \mu^x / x!$, onde *e* é a base de logaritmos naturais, *x* é a seqüência de números inteiros, μ é a média e *x*! representa o fatorial de *x*; **(2)** uma função da distribuição usada para descrever a ocorrência de eventos raros, ou a distribuição por amostragem de contagens isoladas em um período de tempo ou espaço contínuo.

 skew d., d. assimétrica; uma distribuição de freqüência assimétrica; em biologia e medicina, geralmente é uma distribuição lognormal.

 t d., d. t; a distribuição do quociente de variáveis aleatórias independentes, cujo numerador é um valor normal padronizado e o denominador a raiz quadrada positiva do quociente de um valor com distribuição qui-quadrado e seu número de graus de liberdade.

dis·tri·chi·a·sis (dis-tri-kī'ă-sis). Distriquíase; crescimento de dois pêlos em um único folículo. [G. *dis*, duplo, + *thrix* (*trich*-), pêlo]

dis·trix (dis'triks). Distriquia; divisão dos fios de cabelo em suas pontas. [G. *dis*, duas vezes, + *thrix*, pêlo]

dis·tro·pin. Distropina. SIN dystrophin.

dis·tur·bance (dis-ter'bans). Distúrbio; desvio de, interrupção de ou interferência com um estado normal.

 emotional d., mental d., d. emocional, d. mental. VER mental *illness*, behavior *disorder*.

di·sulf·am·ide (dī-sulf'ă-mīd). Dissulfamida; um diurético.

di·sul·fate (dī-sŭl'fāt).. Dissulfato; molécula que contém dois sulfatos.

di·sul·fide (dī-sŭl'fīd). Dissulfeto. **1.** Molécula que contém dois átomos de enxofre para cada átomo do elemento de referência, p. ex., CS_2, dissulfeto de carbono. **2.** Um composto que contém o grupamento –S–S–, p. ex., cistina.

 asymmetric d., d. assimétrico. SIN mixed d.

 mixed d., d. misto; dissulfeto que não é simétrico em ambos os lados da ligação –S–S–; p. ex., o dissulfeto formado entre a coenzima A e a glutationa ou entre a cisteína e a coenzima A ou glutationa. SIN asymmetric d.

 symmetric d., d. simétrico; dissulfeto que é simétrico em ambos os lados da ligação –S–S–; isto é, dissulfeto formado a partir de compostos idênticos contendo tiol; p. ex., cistina, dissulfeto de glutationa.

di·sul·fi·ram (dī-sŭl'fi-ram). Dissulfiram; antioxidante que interfere com a degradação metabólica normal do álcool no corpo, resultando em aumento das concentrações de acetaldeído no sangue e nos tecidos. Usado no tratamento do alcoolismo crônico; quando é consumida uma pequena dose de álcool, há uma reação desagradável. Também é usado como quelante no envenenamento por cobre e níquel. SIN tetraethylthiuram disulfide.

DIT Abreviatura de diiodotirosina (diiodotyrosine).

di·ter·penes (dī-ter'pēnz). Diterpênicos; hidrocarbonetos ou seus derivados contendo quatro unidades isopreno, assim contendo 20 átomos de carbono e quatro grupamentos metil ramificados; p. ex., vitamina A, retineno, aconitina.

di·thi·az·a·nine io·dide (dī-thī-az'ă-nēn). Iodeto de ditiazanina; anti-helmíntico de amplo espectro, efetivo contra *Strongyloides*.

di·thi·o·thre·i·tol (dī-thē'ō-thrē-tol). Ditiotreitol; doador de grupamentos tiol usados em estudos bioquímicos e farmacológicos. SIN Cleland reagent.

di·thra·nol (dith'ră-nol). Ditranol. SIN anthralin.

Dittrich, Franz, patologista alemão, 1815–1859. VER D. *plugs*, em *plug*, *stenosis*.

di·u·re·sis (dī-ū-rē'sis). Diurese; excreção de urina; comumente designa a produção de volumes incomumente grandes de urina. [G. *dia*, completamente, + *ourēsis*, micção]

alcohol d., d. alcoólica; diurese após a ingestão de bebidas alcoólicas; parcialmente devida à inibição da secreção de hormônio antidiurético pela neuro-hipófise.
osmotic d., d. osmótica; diurese devida a alta concentração de substâncias osmoticamente ativas nos túbulos renais (p. ex., uréia, sulfato de sódio), que limitam a reabsorção de água.
water d., d. hídrica; diurese após a ingestão de água; devida à redução da secreção do hormônio antidiurético pela neuro-hipófise em resposta à diminuição da pressão osmótica do sangue.
di·u·ret·ic (dī-ū-ret′ik). Diurético. **1.** Que promove a excreção de urina. **2.** Um agente que aumenta o volume de urina excretada.
cardiac d., d. cardíaco; diurético que age aumentando a função cardíaca e, assim, melhorando a perfusão renal.
direct d., d. direto; diurético cujo efeito primário é sobre a função tubular renal.
indirect d., d. indireto; diurético que atua aumentando a função cardíaca ou o estado de hidratação.
loop d., d. de alça; classe de agentes diuréticos (p. ex., furosemida, ácido etacrínico) que atuam inibindo a reabsorção de sódio e cloreto, não apenas nos túbulos proximais e distais, mas também na alça de Henle.
mercurial d.'s, diuréticos mercuriais; diuréticos contendo mercúrio orgânico (p. ex., Mercuhydrin) que promovem perda renal significativa de sal e água. Figuram dentre os primeiros agentes diuréticos potentes usados no tratamento da insuficiência cardíaca congestiva, mas agora obsoletos.
osmotic d.'s, diuréticos osmóticos; substâncias, como o manitol, que, por seus efeitos osmóticos, retêm água durante a formação da urina e, assim, diluem os eletrólitos na urina, tornando a reabsorção menos eficiente; eles promovem a eliminação de água e eletrólitos na urina.
potassium sparing d.'s, diuréticos poupadores de potássio; agentes diuréticos que, ao contrário da maioria dos diuréticos, retêm potássio; são exemplos o triantereno e a amilorida. Freqüentemente associados a diuréticos que promovem a perda de sódio e potássio. Usados na hipertensão e na insuficiência cardíaca congestiva.
di·ur·nal (dī-er′nal). Diurno. **1.** Relativo às horas do período do dia; oposto de noturno. **2.** Repetido uma vez a cada 24 horas, p. ex., uma variação diurna ou um ritmo diurno. Cf. circadian. [L. *diurnus*, do dia]
di·va·lence, di·va·len·cy (dī-vā′lens, dī-vā′len-sē). Divalência. SIN bivalence.
di·va·lent (dī-vā′lent, div′ă). Divalente. SIN bivalent (1).
di·val·pro·ex so·di·um (dī-val′prō-eks). Divalproex sódico; ácido pentanóico, 2-propil-, sal sódico (2:1); anticonvulsivante usado em crises de ausência e em distúrbios convulsivos relacionados. Derivado do ácido valpróico.
di·var·i·ca·tion (dī′var-i-kā′shŭn). Divaricação. SIN diastasis (1). [L. *divaricare*, separar em pedaços]
di·ver·gence (dī-ver′jens). Divergência. **1.** Movimento ou deslocamento em direções diferentes. **2.** O afastamento de ramos do neurônio para formar sinapses com vários outros neurônios. [L. *di-*, afastado, + *vergo*, inclinar]
di·ver·gent (dī-ver′jent). Divergente; que se move em direções diferentes; que se irradia.
di·ver·tic·u·la (dī-ver-tik′ū-lă). Divertículos. Plural de diverticulum.
di·ver·tic·u·lar (dī-ver-tik′ū-lăr). Diverticular; relativo a um divertículo.
di·ver·tic·u·lec·to·my (dī′ver-tik-ū-lek′tō-mē). Diverticulectomia; excisão de um divertículo.
di·ver·tic·u·li·tis (dī′ver-tik-ū-lī′tis). Diverticulite; inflamação de um divertículo, principalmente das pequenas bolsas na parede do cólon, que se enchem de matéria fecal estagnada e inflamam; raramente, pode causar obstrução, perfuração ou hemorragia.
di·ver·tic·u·lo·ma (dī′ver-tik-ū-lō′mă). Diverticuloma; desenvolvimento de uma massa granulomatosa na parede do cólon. [diverticulum + G. *-oma*, tumor]
di·ver·tic·u·lo·pexy (dī-ver-tik′ū-lō-pek-sē). Diverticulopexia; cirurgia para obliterar um divertículo sem ressecá-lo, geralmente fixando a extremidade a uma estrutura próxima de forma que o divertículo não se encha mais. [diverticulum + G. *pēxis*, fixação]
di·ver·tic·u·lo·sis (dī′ver-tik-ū-lō′sis). Diverticulose; presença de vários divertículos intestinais, comuns na meia-idade; as lesões são divertículos de pulsão adquiridos.
di·ver·tic·u·lum, pl. **di·ver·tic·u·la** (dī-ver-tik′ū-lŭm, ū-lă) [TA]. Divertículo; uma abertura em forma de bolsa ou saco de um órgão tubular ou sacular, como o intestino ou a bexiga. [L. *deverticulum* (ou *di-*), um desvio, de *deverto*, desviar]
allantoenteric d., d. alantoentérico. SIN allantoic d.
allantoic d., d. alantóico; saculação do intestino posterior, revestida por endoderma, que representa o primórdio do alantóide; na maioria dos amniotas, cresce para dentro do celoma extra-embrionário; em seres humanos, a parte distal da luz alantóica é rudimentar, não se estendendo além do pedículo corporal. SIN allantoenteric d.
diverticula ampul′lae duc′tus deferen′tis [TA], d. da ampola do ducto deferente. SIN diverticula of ampulla of ductus deferens.

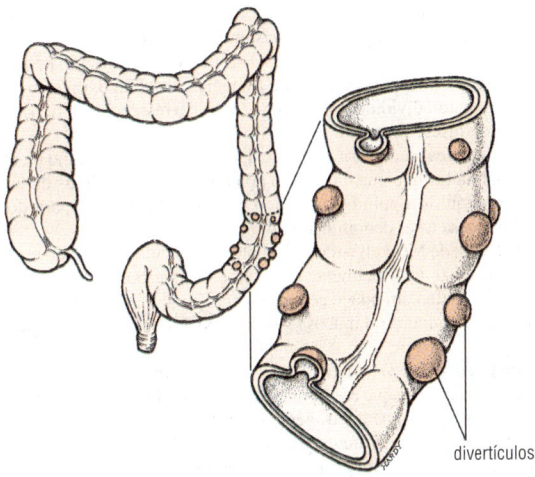

diverticulose: observada em um segmento do cólon descendente

caliceal d., d. caliceal; distensão congênita ou adquirida de um cálice renal que o torna suscetível à formação de cálculo. VER TAMBÉM Fraley *syndrome*.
cervical d., d. cervical; um divertículo no pescoço derivado da retenção de parte de uma das bolsas faríngeas (endodérmicas) ou de sulcos branquiais (ectodérmicos) do embrião.
diverticula of colon, divertículos do cólon; divertículos que são herniações da mucosa e da submucosa através das fibras da grande camada muscular (muscular própria) do cólon ou entre essas fibras. Geralmente múltiplos, ocorrem em 50% das populações ocidentais acima dos 70 anos de idade, porém são muito menos comuns em outras populações. Podem causar hemorragia e episódios de inflamação grave. SIN colonic diverticula.
colonic diverticula, divertículos colônicos. SIN diverticula of colon.
diverticula of ampulla of ductus deferens [TA], divertículos da ampola do ducto deferente; as saculações irregulares da parte ampular do ducto deferente próximas ao seu fim no ducto ejaculatório. SIN diverticula ampullae ductus deferentis [TA].
duodenal d., d. duodenal; divertículo do duodeno, freqüentemente de grande tamanho, que ocasionalmente é encontrado projetando-se do duodeno próximo da papila duodenal.
epiphrenic d., d. epifrênico; divertículo que se origina logo acima da junção cardioesofágica e geralmente se projeta para o lado direito do mediastino inferior.
false d., d. falso; divertículo do intestino que atravessa um defeito na parede muscular do intestino e, assim, não inclui uma camada de músculo em sua parede.
Heister d., d. de Heister. VER *bulb* of jugular vein.
hypopharyngeal d., d. hipofaríngeo. SIN pharyngoesophageal d.
Kommerell d., d. de Kommerell; não é um divertículo verdadeiro, mas uma tumefação bulbar na origem da artéria subclávia esquerda devida a um rema-

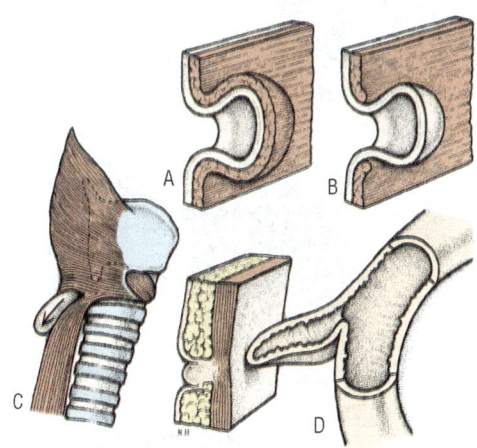

divertículo: (A) divertículo verdadeiro (inclui todas as camadas da parede); (B) divertículo falso do íleo (inclui apenas a mucosa); (C) divertículo de Zenker do esôfago; (D) divertículo de Meckel do íleo

nescente do quarto arco aórtico esquerdo; as síndromes de compressão por anel vascular associadas envolvem persistência do arco aórtico direito; a artéria subclávia esquerda pode passar atrás do esôfago; o divertículo pode ser suficientemente grande para comprimir a traquéia e o esôfago, mesmo após o anel vascular ter sido dividido, e pode ser necessário ressecção ou fixação à parede torácica ou fáscia vertebral.

laryngotracheal d., d. laringotraqueal; divertículo do assoalho da extremidade caudal da faringe que dá origem ao epitélio e às glândulas da laringe, traquéia, brônquios e pulmões. Quando esse divertículo se separa do intestino anterior, passa a ser denominado tubo.

Meckel d., d. de Meckel; o remanescente do pedículo vitelino do embrião, que, quando persiste anormalmente como um saco ou bolsa cega no adulto, está localizado no íleo um pouco acima do ceco; pode estar fixado ao umbigo e, se o revestimento incluir a mucosa gástrica, pode haver ulceração péptica e hemorragia.

metanephric d., d. metanéfrico; saculação da porção caudal do ducto mesonéfrico de cada lado, que cresce em sentido cefalodorsal para fazer contato com as massas de tecido metanefrogênico (blastemas néfricos) e dar origem ao revestimento epitelial do ureter e da pelve e aos ductos coletores do rim.

Nuck d., d. de Nuck. SIN *processus* vaginalis *of peritoneum*.

pancreatic diverticula, divertículos pancreáticos; os brotos endodérmicos ventrais e dorsais do intestino anterior embrionário que constituem os primórdios do parênquima pancreático.

Pertik d., d. de Pertik; recesso faríngeo anormalmente profundo.

pharyngoesophageal d., d. faringoesofágico; divertículo mais comum do esôfago; divertículo de pulsão que se desenvolve entre o músculo constritor faríngeo inferior e o músculo cricofaríngeo. SIN hypopharyngeal d., Zenker d.

pituitary d., d. hipofisário; evaginação tubular de ectoderma do estomódio do embrião; cresce dorsalmente em direção ao processo infundibular do diencéfalo, em torno do qual cria uma massa caliciforme, dando origem à parte distal e à parte justaneural da hipófise. SIN craniopharyngeal canal, hypophyseal pouch, Rathke d., Rathke pocket, Rathke pouch.

pulsion d., d. de pulsão; divertículo formado por pressão do interior, freqüentemente causando herniação da mucosa através da muscular.

Rathke d., d. de Rathke. SIN pituitary d.

thyroid d., thyroglossal d., d. da tireóide, d. tireoglosso; o broto endodérmico do assoalho da faringe embrionária; o primórdio do parênquima da tireóide.

tracheobronchial d., d. traqueobrônquico; o primórdio pulmonar endodérmico que dará origem ao revestimento epitelial do trato respiratório. SIN lung bud.

traction d., d. de tração; divertículo formado pela tração de aderências constritoras, ocorrendo principalmente no terço distal do esôfago, decorrente de linfadenite tuberculosa hilar ou mediastinal.

true d., d. verdadeiro; termo que designa um divertículo que inclui todas as camadas da parede a partir da qual se projeta.

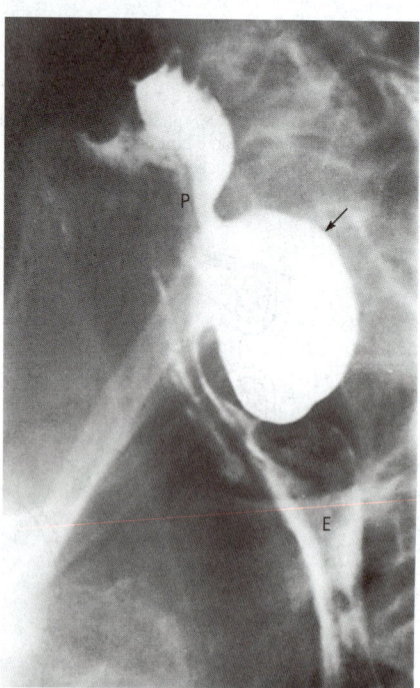

divertículo faringoesofágico (seta): radiografia contrastada, incidência lateral; observar a aspiração de contraste; P = faringe, E = esôfago

urethral d., d. uretral; saculação da parede uretral, seja por um defeito congênito ou, mais comumente, em virtude de inflamação penetrante crônica.

ventricular d., d. ventricular; evaginação congênita do ventrículo direito ou esquerdo.

vesical d., d. vesical; divertículo da parede vesical; pode ser verdadeiro ou falso.

Zenker d., d. de Zenker. SIN pharyngoesophageal d.

di·vic·ine (dī'vis-ēn). Divicina; base com propriedades alcalóides presente na *Lathyrus sativus*, que é responsável, ao menos em parte, pela ação venenosa desta última. VER lathyrism.

divisio. Divisão SIN division.

d.'s anteriores plexus brachialis [TA], divisões anteriores do plexo braquial. SIN anterior *divisions* of (trunks of) brachial plexus, em *division*.

d. autonomica systematis nervosi peripherici [TA], d. autônoma do sistema nervoso periférico. SIN autonomic *division* of nervous system.

d. lateralis dextra hepatis [TA], d. lateral direita do fígado. SIN right lateral *division* of liver.

d. lateralis sinistra, d. lateral esquerda do fígado; *termo oficial alternativo para left *lobe* of liver.

d. lateralis sinistra hepatis [TA], d. lateral esquerda do fígado. SIN left lateral *division* of liver.

d. medialis dextra hepatis [TA], d. medial direita do fígado. SIN right medial *division* of liver.

d. medialis sinistra hepatis [TA], d. medial esquerda do fígado. SIN left medial *division* of liver.

d.'s posteriores plexus brachialis [TA], divisões posteriores do plexo braquial. SIN posterior *divisions* of (trunks of) brachial plexus, em *division*.

di·vi·sion (di-vizh'ŭn). Divisão; uma separação em duas partes ou mais. VER TAMBÉM ramus.

anterior primary d., d. primária anterior. SIN anterior *ramus* of spinal nerve.

anterior d.'s of (trunks of) brachial plexus [TA], divisões anteriores do plexo braquial; parte dos troncos superior, médio e inferior do plexo braquial destinada a inervar os compartimentos anteriores ou flexores do membro superior. SIN divisiones anteriores plexus brachialis [TA].

autonomic d. of nervous system [TA], d. autônoma do sistema nervoso; a parte do sistema nervoso que representa a inervação motora dos músculos lisos, do músculo cardíaco e das células glandulares. Consiste em dois componentes fisiológica e anatomicamente distintos, mutuamente antagonistas; as partes simpática e parassimpática. Nessas duas partes, a via de inervação consiste em uma seqüência sináptica de dois neurônios motores, um dos quais está situado na medula espinal ou no tronco cerebral como o neurônio pré-sináptico (pré-ganglionar), cujo axônio fino, mas mielinizado (fibra pré-sináptica (pré-ganglionar), emerge com um nervo espinal ou craniano que sai e faz sinapse com um ou mais dos neurônios pós-sinápticos (pós-ganglionares ou, mais especificamente, ganglionares) que compõem os gânglios autônomos; as fibras pós-sinápticas não-mielinizadas, por sua vez, inervam os músculos lisos, o músculo cardíaco ou as células glandulares. Os neurônios pré-sinápticos da parte simpática estão situados na coluna celular intermediolateral dos segmentos torácicos e dos dois segmentos lombares superiores da substância cinzenta espinal; os da parte parassimpática compõem os núcleos motores viscerais (eferentes viscerais) do tronco cerebral, bem como a coluna lateral do segundo ao quarto segmento sacral da medula espinal. Os gânglios da parte simpática são os gânglios paravertebrais do tronco simpático e os gânglios pré-vertebrais ou colaterais lombares e sacrais; os da parte parassimpática situam-se próximo do órgão a ser inervado ou como gânglios intramurais no interior do próprio órgão, exceto na cabeça, onde há quatro gânglios parassimpáticos distintos (ciliar, ótico, pterigopalatino e submandibular). A transmissão de impulso do neurônio pré-sináptico para o pós-sináptico é mediada pela acetilcolina nas partes simpática e parassimpática; classicamente se diz que a transmissão da fibra pós-sináptica para os tecidos efetores viscerais é feita pela acetilcolina na parte parassimpática e pela noradrenalina na parte simpática; evidências recentes sugerem a existência de outras classes não-colinérgicas, não-adrenérgicas de fibras pós-sinápticas. SIN divisio autonomica systematis nervosi peripherici [TA], pars autonomica systematis nervosi peripherici [TA], autonomic part of peripheral nervous system*, autonomic nervous system, involuntary nervous system, systema nervosum autonomicum, vegetative nervous system, visceral motor system, visceral nervous system.

cleavage d., d. por clivagem; a rápida divisão mitótica do zigoto com diminuição do tamanho das células individuais ou blastômeros e a formação de uma mórula. VER TAMBÉM cleavage (1).

conjugate d., d. conjugada; divisão simultânea de núcleos haplóides, como nos Basidiomycota.

craniosacral d. of autonomic nervous system, d. craniossacral do sistema nervoso autônomo. SIN parasympathetic *part* of autonomic division of peripheral nervous system.

direct nuclear d., d. nuclear direta. SIN amitosis.

equatorial d., d. equatorial; divisão nuclear na qual cada cromossoma se divide igualmente.

indirect nuclear d., d. nuclear indireta. SIN mitosis.

lateral d. of left liver, lobo esquerdo do fígado; *nome oficial alternativo para left *lobe* of liver.

left lateral d. of liver [TA], lobo esquerdo do fígado; no esquema cirúrgico para subdividir o fígado, a parte situada à esquerda do plano aproximadamente vertical da veia hepática esquerda e que inclui os segmentos posterior esquerdo e ântero-lateral (segmentos hepáticos II e III); corresponde ao lobo anatômico esquerdo do fígado, e assim é demarcado externamente pelo ligamento falciforme, na superfície diafragmática, e pelas fissuras para o ligamento venoso e ligamento redondo na superfície visceral. SIN divisio lateralis sinistra hepatis [TA].

left medial d. of liver [TA], d. medial esquerda do fígado; no esquema cirúrgico para subdividir o fígado, a parte situada entre os planos aproximadamente verticais das veias hepáticas esquerda e média, incluindo o segmento medial esquerdo (segmento hepático IV); na superfície diafragmática, é aproximadamente o terço esquerdo do lobo anatômico direito do fígado; na superfície visceral, sua porção inferior corresponde ao lobo quadrado. SIN divisio medialis sinistra hepatis [TA].

meiotic d., d. meiótica. SIN meiosis.

mitotic d., d. mitótica. SIN mitosis.

multiplicative d., d. multiplicativa; reprodução, por divisão simultânea, de uma célula-mãe em várias células-filhas. Se o processo ocorre sem fertilização da célula-mãe, ou encistamento, as células-filhas são denominadas merozoítas; caso se transformem em um cisto, e geralmente após a fertilização, são denominados esporozoítas.

posterior primary d., d. primária posterior. SIN posterior *ramus* of spinal nerve.

posterior d.'s of (trunks of) brachial plexus [TA], divisões (troncos) posteriores do plexo braquial; parte dos troncos superior, médio e inferior do plexo braquial que inerva os compartimentos posterior ou extensor do membro superior. SIN divisiones posteriores plexus brachialis [TA].

reduction d., d. redutora. SIN *reduction* of chromosomes.

Remak nuclear d., d. nuclear de Remak. SIN amitosis.

right lateral d. of liver [TA], d. lateral direita do fígado; no esquema cirúrgico para subdividir o fígado, a parte situada à direita do plano aproximadamente vertical da veia hepática direita, incluindo os segmentos anterior direito e póstero-lateral (segmentos hepáticos VI e VII); é aproximadamente o terço direito do lobo anatômico direito do fígado. SIN divisio lateralis dextra hepatis [TA].

right medial d. of liver [TA], d. medial direita do fígado; no esquema cirúrgico para subdividir o fígado, a parte situada entre os planos aproximadamente verticais das veias hepáticas direita e média, incluindo os segmentos anterior direito e póstero-medial (segmentos hepáticos V e VIII); é aproximadamente o terço médio do lobo anatômico direito do fígado. SIN divisio medialis dextra hepatis [TA].

div.in p.aeg. Abreviatura do L. *divide in partes aequales*, dividir em partes iguais.

di·vulse (di - vŭls′). Divulsionar; romper. [L. *divello*, pp. *di-vulsus*, afastar]

di·vul·sion (di - vŭl′shŭn). Divulsão. **1.** Remoção de uma parte por ruptura. **2.** Dilatação forçada das paredes de uma cavidade ou canal.

di·vul·sor (di - vŭl′ser, -sōr). Divulsor; instrumento para dilatação forçada da uretra ou de outro canal ou cavidade.

Dix. M.R., otologista inglês do século XX. VER Dix-Hallpike *maneuver*.

di·xyr·a·zine (dī - zir′a - zēn). Dixirazina; composto fenotiazina usado como antipsicótico.

di·zy·got·ic, di·zy·gous (di′zī - got′ik, dī - zī′gŭs). Dizigótico; relativo a gêmeos provenientes de dois zigotos distintos, isto é, que possuem a mesma relação genética que irmãos, mas compartilhando um meio intra-uterino comum. [G. *di*, dois, + *zygotos*, unido]

diz·zi·ness (diz′i - nes). Tonteira; termo impreciso comumente usado para descrever vários sintomas, tais como síncope, vertigem, desequilíbrio. VER TAMBÉM vertigo. [A.S. *dyzig*, tolo]

djen·kol·ic ac·id (jeng - kol′ik). Ácido djencólico; *S,S*′-metilenobiscisteína; um aminoácido contendo enxofre, que se assemelha à cistina, mas com uma ponte metileno entre os dois átomos de enxofre; muito insolúvel. [*djenkol*, feijão no qual foi isolado pela primeira vez]

DL-. Prefixo (letras maiúsculas pequenas) para designar uma substância que consiste em quantidades iguais dos dois enantiomorfos, D e L; substitui o antigo *dl-* como uma definição mais exata da estrutura.

***dl*-nar·co·tine** (nar′kō - tēn). *dl*-narcotina. SIN gnoscopine.

DM Abreviatura de adamsita; diabetes melito (*diabetes* mellitus); sopro diastólico (diastolic *murmur*); dopamina.

DMA Abreviatura de dimetoxianfetamina (dimethoxyamphetamine).

DMARD Acrônimo para disease modifying antirheumatic *drugs* (agentes antirreumáticos modificadores de doença), em *drug*.

DMC Abreviatura de *p,p*′,-diclorodifenil metil carbinol (*p,p*′, -dichlorodiphenyl methyl carbinol).

D.M.D. Abreviatura de Doctor of Dental Medicine (Doutor em Medicina Odontológica).

dmfs, DMFs Abreviatura de dentes cariados, ausentes e obturados. VER TAMBÉM dmfs caries *index*.

DMPP Abreviatura de dimetilfenilpiperazínio) (dimethylphenylpiperazinium).

DMSA VER TC^{99m}-ácido dimercaptossuccínico (^{99m}Tc-dimercaptosuccinic acid).

DMSO Abreviatura de dimetil sulfóxido (dimethyl sulfoxide).

DMT Abreviatura de *N,N* -dimetiltriptamina (*N,N*-dimethyltryptamine).

DN Abreviatura de número de dibucaína (dibucaine number).

DNA Abreviatura de deoxyribonucleic acid (ácido desoxirribonucleico). Para termos que possuem essa abreviatura, ver subentradas em deoxyribonucleic acid.

DNA diagnostics. Diagnóstico por DNA. SIN genetic *testing*. VER DNA markers, familial *screening*, prenatal *screening*.

dnaG Primase. SIN primase.

DNA markers. Marcadores de DNA; segmentos de DNA cromossomial sabidamente ligados a traços ou doenças hereditárias. Embora os próprios marcadores não causem os distúrbios, eles existem em conjunto com os genes responsáveis e são transmitidos com eles. Alguns marcadores, polimorfismos do comprimento do fragmento de restrição, consistem em segmentos de DNA que podem ser identificados em auto-radiografias (produzidas após digestão do DNA por enzimas de restrição e segregação dos fragmentos resultantes através de eletroforese em gel).

DNAse, DNAase, DNase Abreviaturas de desoxirribonuclease (deoxyribonuclease).

DNP, Dnp 1. Abreviatura de 2,4 - dinitrofenol (2,4-dinitrophenol). **2.** Abreviatura de desoxirribonucleoproteína (deoxyribonucleoprotein).

DNR Abreviatura de "do not resuscitate" (não reanimar).

Dns, DNS Abreviaturas de dansil (dansyl).

D.O. Abreviatura de Doctor of Osteopathy (Doutor em Osteopatia).

DOA Abreviatura de dead on arrival (morto ao chegar).

do·bu·ta·mine (dō - bū′tā - mēn). Dobutamina; derivado sintético da dopamina caracterizado por propriedades inotrópicas proeminentes, mas com propriedades cronotrópicas e arritmogênicas fracas; um agente cardiotônico.

DOC Abreviatura de desoxicorticosterona (deoxycorticosterone), desoxicolato (deoxycholate).

d'Ocagne, Philbert M., matemático francês, 1862–1938. VER d'O, *nomogram*.

***n*-doc·o·sa·no·ic ac·id** (do′kō - san - ō′ik). Ácido *n*-docosanóico. SIN behenic acid.

doc·tor (dok′ter). Doutor. **1.** Título conferido por uma universidade a alguém que acompanhou um curso prescrito de estudo, ou fornecido como título de distinção; como doutor em medicina, leis, filosofia, etc. **2.** Médico, especialmente um a que foi conferido o grau de M.D. (doutor em medicina) por uma universidade ou escola de medicina. [L. professor, de *doceo*, pp. *doctus*, ensinar]

doc·trine (dok′trin). Doutrina; sistema particular de princípios ensinados ou defendidos. [L. *doceo*, ensinar]

Arrhenius d., d. de Arrhenius; a teoria de dissociação eletrolítica (1887) que se tornou a base de nossa compreensão moderna dos eletrólitos; em uma solução eletricamente condutiva (p. ex., ácido, base ou sal) existem íons livres antes

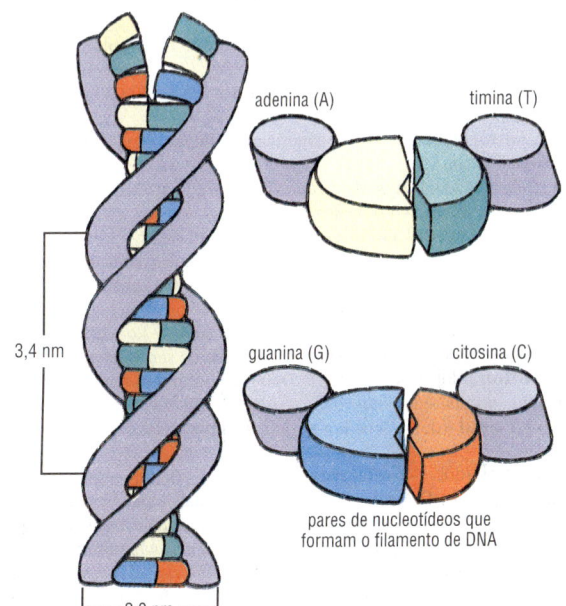

DNA (ácido desoxirribonucleico)

da eletrólise, e a proporção de moléculas dissociadas em íons pode ser calculada a partir de medidas da condutividade elétrica, bem como da pressão osmótica. SIN Arrhenius law.

humoral d., d. humoral; a teoria grega antiga de quatro humores corporais (sangue, biles amarela e preta, e fleuma) que determinavam a saúde e a doença. Os humores foram associados aos quatro elementos (ar, fogo, terra e água), que, por sua vez, correspondiam a uma das qualidades (quente, frio, seco e úmido). Uma mistura apropriada e equilibrada dos humores caracterizava a saúde do corpo e da mente; um desequilíbrio resultava em doença. Também se supunha que era preciso determinar o temperamento do corpo ou da mente, p. ex., sanguíneo (sangue), colérico (bile amarela), melancólico (bile preta) ou fleumático (fleuma). SIN fluidism, humoralism, humorism.

Monro d., d. de Monro; doutrina que afirma que a cavidade craniana é uma caixa rígida fechada e que, portanto, uma alteração no volume de sangue intracraniano só pode ocorrer através do deslocamento ou substituição do líquido cefalorraquidiano. SIN Monro-Kellie d.

Monro-Kellie d., d. de Monro-Kellie. SIN Monro d.

doc·u·sate cal·ci·um (dok'ū - sāt). Docusato cálcico; agente ativo na superfície, utilizado no tratamento da constipação como emoliente fecal não-laxante. SIN dioctyl calcium sulfosuccinate.

doc·u·sate so·di·um. Docusato sódico; agente ativo na superfície, utilizado como agente dispersante em preparações aplicadas topicamente. Após a administração oral, reduz a tensão superficial do trato gastrointestinal e é usado no tratamento da constipação como agente umidificante e emoliente fecal. SIN dioctyl sodium sulfosuccinate.

do·de·cane (dō'dĕ - kān). Dodecano; n-$C_{12}H_{26}$; hidrocarboneto saturado, não-ramificado, reto, contendo 12 átomos de carbono; o 12.° membro da série alcalina que começa com o metano.

n-**do·dec·a·no·ic ac·id** (dō - dek'ă - nō - ik). Ácido *n*-dodecanóico. SIN lauric acid.

do·dec·an·o·yl-CoA syn·the·tase (dō - dek'an - ō - il - kō - ā sin'the - tās). Dodecanoil-CoA sintetase. SIN long-chain fatty acid-CoA ligase.

do·de·car·bo·ni·um chlo·ride (dō - dĕ - kar - bō'nē - um). Cloreto de dodecarbônio; um anti-séptico.

do·de·cyl (dō'dĕ – sil). Dodecil; o radical do dodecano.
  d. gallate, galato de dodecil; um antioxidante.
  d. sulfate, sulfato de dodecil. VER *sodium* dodecyl sulfate.

Döderlein, Albert, S.G., obstetra alemão, 1860–1941. VER D. *bacillus*.

Doerfler, Leo G., audiologista norte-americano, *1919. VER D.-Stewart *test*.

Dogiel, Alexander S., histologista russo, 1852–1922. VER D. *corpuscle*.

Dogiel, Jan von, anatomista e fisiologista russo. 1830–1905. VER D. *cells* em *cell*.

dog·ma. Dogma; teoria ou crença formalmente afirmada, definida e considerada verdadeira.
  central d., d. central; a proposição de que, enquanto as informações genéticas são transferidas dos pais para os filhos através da duplicação do DNA, no interior da célula, as informações genéticas são transferidas do DNA para o mRNA (transcrição) e, depois, para proteínas (tradução); proposto por Francis Crick.

dog·mat·ic (dog - mat'ik). Dogmático. VER dogmatic *school*. [G. *dogmatikos*, relativo a opiniões; *d. iatroi*, médicos que seguem princípios gerais; de *dogma*, uma opinião]

dog·ma·tist (dog'mă - tist). Dogmatista; seguidor da escola dogmática (dogmatic *school*).

Döhle, Karl G. P., histologista e patologista alemão, 1855–1928. VER D. *bodies*, em *body*, *inclusions*, em *inclusion*.

Doisy, Edward A., bioquímico norte-americano e Prêmio Nobel, 1893–1986. VER Allen-D. *test*, *unit*.

dol (dōl). Dol; unidade de medida da dor. [L. *dolor*, dor]

dolicho-. Dolico-; longo. [G. *dolichos*]

dol·i·cho·ce·phal·ic, dol·i·cho·ceph·a·lous (dol - i - kō - sĕ - fal'ik, - sef'ă - lŭs). Dolicocefálico, dolicocéfalo; que possui uma cabeça desproporcionalmente longa; designa um crânio com um índice cefálico abaixo de 75. SIN dolichocranial. [dolicho- + G. *kephalĕ*, cabeça]

dol·i·cho·ceph·a·ly, dol·i·cho·ceph·a·lism (dol - i - kō - sef'ă - lē, sef'ă - lizm). Dolicocefalia, dolicocefalismo; a condição de ser dolicocéfalo.

dol·i·cho·co·lon (dol - i - kō - kō'lon). Dolicocólon; um cólon intestinal de comprimento anormal. [dolicho- + G. *kōlon*, cólon]

dol·i·cho·cra·ni·al (dol - i - kō - krā'nē - ăl). Dolicocraniano. SIN dolichocephalic.

dol·i·cho·fa·cial (dol - i - kō - fā'shăl). Dolicofacial. SIN dolichoprosopic.

dol·i·chol (dol'i - kol). Dolicol; poliisoprenos nos quais o membro terminal é saturado e oxidado em um álcool, geralmente fosforilado e freqüentemente glicosilado; encontrado no retículo endoplasmático, mas não nas membranas mitocondriais ou plasmáticas; os níveis urinários estão elevados em distúrbios que exibem perfis cutâneos, retais ou cerebrais anormais à microscopia eletrônica de biopsias.
  d. phosphate, fosfato de dolicol; um intermediário na glicosilação de proteínas e lipídios; contém 11-24 unidades isopreno; um produto da via da isoprenilação; participa da formação de fixações glicosilfosfatidilinositol de proteínas nas biomembranas.

dol·i·cho·pel·lic, dol·i·cho·pel·vic (dol - i - kō - pel'ik, - pel'vik). Dolicopélvico; que possui uma pelve desproporcionalmente longa; designa uma pelve com um índice pélvico acima de 95. [dolicho- + G. *pellis*, bacia (pelve)]

dol·i·cho·pro·sop·ic, dol·i·cho·pro·so·pous (dol - i - kō - pros - ō'pik, - kō - pros'ō - pŭs). Dolicoprosópico; dolicofacial; que possui uma face desproporcionalmente longa. SIN dolichofacial. [dolicho- + G. *prosōpikos*, facial]

dol·i·cho·sten·o·me·lia (dol'i - kō - sten'ō - mē'lē - ă). Dolicoestenomelia; biotipo corporal estreito que, como a aracnodactilia, é uma característica comum de vários tipos de distúrbios hereditários do tecido conjuntivo. [dolicho- + G. *stenos*, estreito, + *melos*, membro]

dol·i·cho·u·ran·ic, dol·i·chu·ran·ic (dol'i - kō - ū - ran'ik, dol - ik - ū-). Dolicourânico; que possui um palato longo, com um índice palatino menor que 110. [dolicho- + G. *ouranos*, abóbada do palato]

Doll, Richard, epidemiologista inglês, *1912. VER Armitage-D. *model*.

do·lor (dō'lŏr). Dor, como um dos quatro sinais de inflamação (dor, calor, rubor, tumor) enunciados por Celsus. [L.]
  d. cap'itis, d. de cabeça; cefaléia, principalmente aquela devida a alterações no couro cabeludo ou nos ossos, e não nas estruturas intracranianas.

do·lo·rif·ic (dō - lōr - if'ik). Dolorífico; doloroso; que causa dor.

do·lo·rim·e·try (dō - lō - rim'ē - trē). Dolorimetria; a medida da dor. [L. *dolor*, dor, + G. *metron*, medida]

do·lor·ol·o·gy (dō - lōr - ol'ō - jē). Dolorologia; o estudo e o tratamento da dor. [L. *dolor*, dor, + G. *logos*, estudo]

DOM Abreviatura de 2,5-dimetoxi-4-metilanfetamina (2,5-dimethoxy-4-methylamphetamine).

do·main (dō - mān'). Domínio. **1.** Unidade homóloga de aproximadamente 110–120 aminoácidos, cujos grupamentos constituem as cadeias leves e pesadas da molécula de imunoglobulina; cada um tem uma função específica. A cadeia leve (L) tem dois domínios: um na região variável e outro na região constante da cadeia; a cadeia pesada (H) tem quatro a cinco domínios, dependendo da classe de imunoglobulina: um na região variável e os outros na região constante. **2.** Uma região de uma proteína que possui alguma característica física ou papel distintivo. **3.** Uma estrutura globular, independentemente pregueada, composta de uma porção de uma cadeia polipeptídica. Um domínio pode interagir com outro domínio; pode estar associado a uma função específica. Os domínios podem variar em tamanho. [Fr. *domaine*, de L. *dominium*, propriedade, domínio]
  dinucleotide d., d. do dinucleotídeo. SIN dinucleotide *fold*.

Dombrock blood group. Grupo sanguíneo de Dombrock. VER apêndice sobre Grupos Sangüíneos.

dome. Cúpula.
  d. of pleura, c. pleural; *termo oficial alternativo para cervical *pleura*.

do·mes·tic vi·o·lence. Violência doméstica; lesão intencional infligida, praticada por e contra membro(s) da família; os tipos incluem violência conjugal, maus-tratos infantis e abuso sexual, incluindo incesto. Vários tipos de violência, como o abuso sexual, também acontecem fora da unidade familiar. A *American Medical Association*, como organizações semelhantes em outros países, publicou notas de aconselhamento para os médicos sobre a detecção e o tratamento da violência doméstica.

dom·i·cil·i·at·ed (dō - mi - sil'ē - āt - ed). Domiciliado; estado de íntima associação de um organismo em moradias ou atividades humanas, de forma que ocorre domesticação parcial, levando à dependência do organismo de associação contínua com o ambiente humano; isso freqüentemente resulta na transformação do organismo domiciliado em uma praga nociva, um vetor ou um hospedeiro intermediário de doença humana. [L. *domicilium*, residência]

dom·i·nance (dom'i - nans). Dominância; o estado de ser dominante.
  cerebral d., d. cerebral; o fato de um hemisfério cerebral ser dominante sobre o outro e exercer maior influência sobre determinadas funções; o hemisfério cerebral esquerdo geralmente é dominante no controle da fala, linguagem e processamento analítico, bem como da matemática, enquanto o hemisfério direito (geralmente não-dominante) processa conceitos espaciais e de linguagem relacionados a determinados tipos de imagens visuais; a preferência pelo uso de uma das mãos (pessoas destras possuem dominância cerebral esquerda) é considerada um exemplo geral de dominância cerebral.
  false d., falsa dominância. SIN quasidominance.
  genetic d., d. genética; designa um padrão de herança de um traço mendeliano autossômico devido a um gene que sempre se manifesta fenotipicamente; geralmente, o fenótipo no homozigoto é mais grave que no heterozigoto, mas os detalhes dependem do critério de fenotipagem usado.
  d. of traits, d. de traços; uma expressão da aparente relação fisiológica existente entre dois ou mais genes que podem ocupar o mesmo *locus* cromossomial (alelos). Em um *locus* específico, há três possíveis combinações de dois genes alelos, *A* e *a*; dois homozigotos (*AA* e *aa*) e um heterozigoto (*Aa*). Se um indivíduo heterozigoto apresenta apenas a característica hereditária determinada pelo gene *A*, mas não *a*, diz-se que *A* é dominante e *a* recessivo; nesse caso, *AA* e *Aa*, embora sejam genótipos diferentes, devem exibir fenótipo indistinguí-

vel. Se *AA, Aa* e *aa* puderem ser distinguidos uns dos outros, *A* e *a* são codominantes.

dom·i·nant (dom′i - nant). Dominante. **1.** Que regulamenta ou controla. **2.** Em genética, designa um alelo possuído por um dos genitores de um híbrido que é expresso neste último para a exclusão de um alelo contrastante (o recessivo) do outro genitor. [L. *dominans*, p. pres. de *dominor*, regulamentar, de *dominus*, mestre, de *domus*, casa]

do·mi·o·dol (dō - mē′ō - dol). Domiodol; forma orgânica de iodo associada ao glicerol; usado como mucolítico/expectorante.

do·mi·phen bro·mide (dō′mi - fen). Brometo de domifeno; um anti-séptico.

dom·per·i·done (dom - per′i - dōn). Domperidona; antagonista da dopamina (como a clorpromazina) com propriedades antieméticas.

Donath, Julius, médico alemão, 1870–1950. VER D.-Landsteiner *phenomenon*, cold *autoantibody*; Landsteiner-D. *test*.

Donders, Franz C., oftalmologista holandês, 1818–1889. VER D. *law, pressure; space* of D.

Don Juan (don wän). Em psiquiatria, termo usado para designar homens com hiperatividade sexual compulsiva ou romântica, geralmente com uma sucessão de parceiras. [lendário nobre espanhol]

Don Juan·ism (don wän′izm). VER Don Juan.

Donnan, Frederick G., físico-químico inglês, 1870–1956. VER D. *equilibrium*; Gibbs-D. *equilibrium*.

Donné, Alfred, médico francês, 1801–1878. VER D. *corpuscle*.

Donohue, William L., patologista pediátrico canadense, 1906–1984. VER D. *disease*.

do·nor (dō′ner). Doador. **1.** Indivíduo do qual é retirado sangue, tecido ou um órgão para transplante. **2.** Uma substância que transferirá um átomo ou um radical para um aceptor; p. ex., a metionina é um doador de metila; a glutationa é um doador de glutamil. **3.** Um átomo que facilmente libera elétrons para um aceptor; p. ex., nitrogênio, que doará ambos os elétrons para um reservatório compartilhado para formação de uma ligação coordenada. [L. *dono*, pp. *donatus*, doar, dar]

hydrogen d., d. de hidrogênio; metabólito do qual o hidrogênio é retirado (por um sistema desidrogenase) e transferido por um transportador para outro metabólito, que assim é reduzido.

universal d., d. universal; na classificação dos grupos sanguíneos, uma pessoa que pertence ao grupo O; isto é, cujos eritrócitos não contêm aglutinogênio A nem B e, portanto, não são aglutinados pelo plasma contendo uma dessas isoaglutininas comuns (ou ambas).

Donovan, Charles, cirurgião irlandês, 1863–1951. VER D. *bodies*, em *body*; Leishman-D. *body*.

Doose, H., pediatra e epileptologista alemão do século XX. VER D. *syndrome*.

do·pa, DO·PA, Do·pa (dō′pä). Dopa; intermediário no catabolismo da L-fenilalanina e L-tirosina, e na biossíntese da norepinefrina, epinefrina; e melanina; a forma L, levodopa, é biologicamente ativa. VER dopa *reaction*. SIN 3,4-dihydroxyphenylalanine.

alpha methyl d., alfa metil d. SIN methyldopa.

d. decarboxylase, d. descarboxilase. SIN aromatic D-amino acid decarboxylase.

decarboxylated d., d. descarboxilada. SIN dopamine.

d. oxidase, d. oxidase; nome provisório dado às enzima(s) que catalisa(m) a formação de melaninas a partir da dopa; agora parece que as monofenol monooxigenases contendo cobre e/ou catecol oxidases são responsáveis pela oxidação de L-tirosina em dopa e dopa quinona.

d. quinone, d. quinona; produto de oxidação da dopa e um intermediário na formação de melanina a partir da tirosina.

L-dopa. L-dopa. SIN levodopa.

do·pa·mine (DM) (dō′pä - mēn). Dopamina; intermediário no metabolismo da tirosina e precursor da norepinefrina e epinefrina; representa 90% das catecolaminas; sua presença no sistema nervoso central e localização nos gânglios basais (núcleos caudado e lentiforme) sugerem que a dopamina tem outras funções. A depleção de dopamina produz doença de Parkinson (Parkinson *disease*). SIN 3-hydroxytyramine, decarboxylated dopa.

d. hydrochloride, cloridrato de dopamina; uma amina biogênica e transmissor natural, usada como agente vasopressor para tratamento do choque.

do·pa·mine β-hy·drox·y·lase. Dopamina β-hidroxilase. SIN dopamine β-monooxygenase.

do·pa·mine β-mon·o·ox·y·gen·ase. Dopamina β-monoxigenase; enzima contendo cobre que catalisa a oxidação de ácido ascórbico e 3,4-diidroxifeniletilamina simultaneamente por O_2 para produzir norepinefrina, desidroascorbato e água; uma etapa crucial no metabolismo das catecolaminas. A enzima é estimulada pelo fumarato. SIN dopamine β-hydroxylase.

do·pa·min·er·gic (dō′pä - min - er′jik). Dopaminérgico; relativo às células ou fibras nervosas que empregam dopamina como seu neurotransmissor. [dopamina + G. *ergon*, trabalho]

dope (dōp). **1.** Entorpecente; narcótico; estimulante; qualquer substância, estimulante ou depressora, administrada devido ao seu efeito temporário, ou usada habitualmente ou por vício. **2.** Administrar ou tomar tal droga. [Holandês, *doop*, molho]

dop·ing (dōp′ing). Doping; a administração de substâncias estranhas a um indivíduo; freqüentemente usado em referência a atletas que tentam aumentar a força física e psicológica.

Doppler, Johann Christian, matemático e físico austríaco, 1803-1853. VER D. *echocardiography, effect, phenomenon, shift, ultrasonography*.

Dop·pler. Instrumento diagnóstico que emite um feixe de ultra-som para o corpo; o ultra-som refletido pelas estruturas em movimento modifica sua freqüência (efeito Doppler). Útil no diagnóstico das doenças vasculares periférica e cardíaca.

do·ra·pho·bia (dō - rä - fō′bē - ä). Dorafobia; medo mórbido de tocar a pele ou o pêlo de animais. [G. *dora*, couro, pele, + *phobos*, medo]

Dorello, P., anatomista italiano, *1872. VER D. *canal*.

Dorendorf, H., médico alemão, *1866. VER D. *sign*.

Dorfman, Maurice L., dermatologista israelense do século XX. VER D.-Chanarin *syndrome*.

Döring, G., neurologista alemão do século XX. VER Pette-D. *disease*.

dor·nase (dōr′nās). Dornase; contração obsoleta de desoxirribonuclease. VER TAMBÉM streptodornase.

pancreatic d., d. pancreática; preparação estabilizada de desoxirribonuclease a partir do pâncreas bovino; usada por inalação na forma de aerossóis para reduzir secreções mucopurulentas espessas em determinadas infecções broncopulmonares.

Dorno, Carl, climatologista suíço, 1865–1942.

do·ro·ma·ni·a (dō - rō - mā′nē - ä). Doromania; desejo anormal de dar presentes. [G. *dōron*, presente, + *mania*, insanidade]

dor·sa (dōr′sä). Dorsos. Plural de dorsum.

dor·sab·dom·i·nal (dōr - sab - dom′i - nal). Dorsoabdominal; relativo ao dorso e ao abdome.

dor·sad (dor′sad). Dorsal; em direção ao dorso. [L. *dorsum*, dorso, + *ad*, para]

dor·sal (dōr′säl). [TA]. Dorsal. **1.** Relativo às costas ou a qualquer dorso. SIN tergal. **2.** SIN posterior (2). **3.** Em anatomia veterinária, relativo à superfície posterior ou superior de um animal. Freqüentemente usado para indicar a posição de uma estrutura em relação a outra; isto é, mais próximo da superfície posterior do corpo. **4.** Termo antigo que significa torácico, em um sentido limitado; p. ex., vértebras dorsais. [L. Mediev. *dorsalis*, de *dorsum*, dorso]

dor·sa·lis (dōr - sā′lis) [TA]. Dorsal. SIN posterior (2). [L.]

Dorset, Marion, bacteriologista norte-americano, 1872–1935. VER D. culture egg *medium*.

dor·si·duct (dōr′si - dŭkt). Dorsiduzir; puxar para trás ou para as costas. [L. *dorsum*, dorso, + *duco*, pp. *ductus*, puxar]

dor·si·flex·ion (dōr - si - flek′shŭn). Dorsiflexão; movimento para cima (extensão) do pé ou seus dedos ou da mão ou seus dedos.

dor·si·scap·u·lar (dōr′si - skap′ū - lär). Dorsiescapular; relativo à superfície dorsal da escápula.

dor·si·spi·nal (dōr′si - spī′nal). Dorsiespinal; relativo à coluna vertebral, especialmente à sua superfície dorsal.

dor·so·ceph·a·lad (dōr′sō - sef′ä - lad). Dorsocefálico; em direção ao occipúcio, ou parte posterior da cabeça. [L. *dorsum*, dorso, + G. *kephalē*, cabeça, + L. *ad*, para]

dor·so·lat·er·al (dōr - sō - lat′er - äl). Dorsolateral; relativo ao dorso e ao lado.

dor·so·lum·bar (dōr - sō - lŭm′bar). Dorsolombar; referente ao dorso na região das vértebras torácicas inferiores e lombares superiores.

dor·so·ven·trad (dōr - sō - ven′trad). Dorsoventral; da face dorsal em direção à ventral.

dor·sum, gen. **dor·si,** pl. **dor·sa** (dōr′sŭm, - sī, - sä). [TA]. **1.** Dorso; a parte posterior do corpo. **2.** A superfície superior ou posterior, ou as costas de qualquer parte. SIN tergum. [L. dorso]

d. ephip′pii, dorso da sela. SIN d. sellae.

d. of foot [TA], d. do pé; a superfície posterior ou superior do pé. SIN d. pedis [TA].

d. of hand [TA], d. da mão; o dorso da mão; superfície da mão oposta à palma.

d. lin′guae [TA], d. da língua. SIN d. of tongue.

d. ma′nus [TA], d. da mão. SIN dorsum of hand.

d. na′si [TA], d. do nariz. SIN d. of nose.

d. of nose [TA], d. do nariz; a crista externa do nariz, voltada para frente e para cima. SIN d. nasi [TA].

d. pe′dis [TA], d. do pé. SIN d. of foot.

d. of penis [TA], d. do pênis; a face do pênis oposta à da uretra. SIN d. penis [TA].

d. pe′nis [TA], d. do pênis. SIN d. of penis.

d. scap′ulae, d. da escápula; a superfície posterior da escápula.

d. sel′lae [TA], d. da sela; porção quadrada de osso no corpo do esfenóide posterior à sela turca ou fossa hipofisária. SIN d. ephippii.

d. of tongue [TA], d. da língua; a superfície superior da língua dividida pelo sulco terminal nos dois terços anteriores, a parte pré-sulcal, e um terço posterior, a parte pós-sulcal. SIN d. linguae [TA].

dos·age (dō′sij). Dosagem. **1.** A administração de medicamento ou de outro agente terapêutico em quantidades prescritas. **2.** A determinação da dose apropriada de um remédio. Cf. dose. **3.** Em medicina nuclear, a quantidade de radiofármaco administrada.

dose (dōs). Dose. **1.** A quantidade de uma substância ou outro remédio a ser administrada ou aplicada em dose única ou em quantidades fracionadas em um determinado período. Cf. dosage (2). **2.** Em medicina nuclear, quantidade de energia absorvida por unidade de massa de material irradiado (dose absorvida). VER TAMBÉM dosage (3). [G. *dosis*, uma administração]

absorbed d., d. absorvida; a quantidade de energia absorvida por unidade de massa de material irradiado no local alvo; em radioterapia, a unidade usada antigamente para a dose absorvida era o rad (100 ergs/g); a unidade atual (SI) é o gray (1 J/kg ou 100 rad).

air d., dose de exposição. SIN exposure d.

bone marrow d., d. para a medula óssea; a dose cumulativa recebida pelo órgão formador de sangue, decorrente de irradiação terapêutica ou precipitação radioativa; a dose leucemogênica presumida.

booster d., d. de reforço; dose administrada em algum momento após uma dose inicial para reforçar o efeito, diz-se geralmente de antígenos para a produção de anticorpos.

cumulative d., d. cumulativa; a dose total resultante de repetidas exposições da mesma parte do corpo ou de todo o corpo à radio ou quimioterapia.

curative d. (CD, CD^{50}), d. curativa; **(1)** a quantidade de qualquer substância necessária para a cura de uma doença ou que corrigirá as manifestações de deficiência de um fator específico na dieta; **(2)** dose efetiva de substâncias aplicadas terapeuticamente. VER TAMBÉM CD^{50}. SIN therapeutic d.

daily d., d. diária; a quantidade total de um remédio a ser tomada em 24 horas.

depth d., d. de profundidade; a dose de radiação a uma distância sob a superfície, incluindo radiação secundária ou dispersão, em relação à dose na superfície.

divided d., d. dividida; fração definida do total de uma dose; administrada repetidamente a curtos intervalos de forma que a dose completa seja tomada no período especificado, geralmente um dia. SIN fractional d.

effective d. (ED), d. efetiva; **(1)** a dose que produz um efeito específico; quando seguida por subscrito (geralmente "ED$_{50}$", designa a dose que tem esse efeito sobre uma determinada percentagem (p. ex., 50%) dos animais de prova; ED$_{50}$ é a dose efetiva mediana; **(2)** em proteção radiológica, a soma das doses equivalentes em todos os tecidos e órgãos do corpo ponderada para os efeitos teciduais da radiação. A unidade SI de dose efetiva é o sievert (Sv) (=100 rem). **(3)** Em radiologia diagnóstica, se um paciente que pesa *W* absorve *A* joules de energia, e a razão derivada experimentalmente de dose efetiva para energia absorvida em um espectro antropomórfico com massa *M* é *R*, então a dose efetiva é A·R·M/W. Essa fórmula resulta em um maior valor para crianças apesar de sua menor absorção de radiação.

epilation d., d. epilatória; a quantidade mínima de radiação suficiente para causar perda dos pêlos, geralmente em 10 a 14 dias.

equianalgesic d., d. eqüianalgésica; a razão qualitativa entre potência real em miligramas de analgésicos comparáveis necessária para atingir o efeito terapêutico equivalente.

equivalent d., d. equivalente; em proteção radiológica, a dose absorvida média por um tecido ou órgão e ponderada para a qualidade do tipo de radiação. A unidade da dose equivalente é o sievert.

erythema d., d. eritematosa; a quantidade mínima de raios X ou outra forma de radiação suficiente para produzir eritema; historicamente, essa dose era indicada pelo medidor de Sabouraud como a matriz B, de Holzknecht como 5(5H), de Hampson como 4, e de Kienbock como 10.

exit d., d. de saída; a dose de exposição à radiação que sai de um corpo, oposta à porta de entrada.

exposure d., d. de exposição; a dose de radiação, expressa em roentgens, administrada em um ponto no ar livre. SIN air d.

fractional d., d. fracionada. SIN divided d.

gonad d., d. gonadal; a dose de exposição das gônadas masculinas ou femininas, geralmente por irradiação secundária incidental em irradiação diagnóstica ou terapêutica, ou por irradiação de todo o corpo. SIN gonadal d.

gonadal d., d. gonadal. SIN gonad d.

initial d., d. inicial. SIN loading d.

integral d., d. integral; a energia total absorvida pelo corpo, o produto da massa de tecido irradiado pela dose absorvida; unidade, o rad-grama (= 100 erg).

L d.'s, doses L; grupo de termos que indicam a atividade ou potência relativa da toxina diftérica; as doses L são distintamente diferentes da dose letal mínima (DLM) e da dose mínima de reação, visto que as duas últimas representam os efeitos diretos da toxina, enquanto as doses L referem-se à potência combinada da toxina com antitoxina específica. ["L" para L. *limes*, limite, fronteira]

L$^+$ d., L$_+$ d., d. L$^+$, d. L$_+$; alternativas para L†, a dose mortal limite (*limes tod dose*) de toxina diftérica, isto é, a menor quantidade de toxina que, quando misturada a uma unidade de antitoxina e injetada por via subcutânea em uma cobaia de 250 g, causa morte do animal em 96 horas (baseado na média em uma série); teoricamente, poder-se-ia esperar que a diferença entre as doses L+ e L$_0$ fossem idênticas a 1 DLM (dose letal mínima), mas isso não ocorre na prática; em vários filtrados tóxicos, a diferença pode variar de algumas até mais de 100 DLM, indicando que a combinação toxina–antitoxina *não* é uma união química firme que ocorre em proporções constantes.

lethal d. (LD), d. letal (DL); a dose de uma preparação química ou biológica (p. ex., uma exotoxina bacteriana ou uma suspensão de bactérias) que, provavelmente, causa morte; esta varia de acordo com o tipo de animal e a via de administração; quando seguida por um subscrito (geralmente "DL$_{50}$" ou dose letal mediana), designa a dose que, provavelmente, causará a morte em uma determinada percentagem (p. ex., 50%) dos animais de prova; a dose letal mediana é DL$_{50}$, a dose letal absoluta é DL$_{100}$ e a dose letal mínima é DL$_{05}$.

Lf d., L$_f$ d., d. Lf, d. L$_f$; a dose limite de floculação da toxina diftérica, isto é, a menor quantidade de toxina que, quando misturada a uma unidade de antitoxina, produz a floculação mais rápida no teste de Ramon (*in vitro*); em geral, a d. L$_f$ é um pouco menor que a d. L$_r$.

Lo d., L$_o$ d., d. Lo, d. L$_o$; a dose nula limite da toxina diftérica, isto é, a maior quantidade de toxina que, quando misturada a uma unidade de antitoxina e injetada por via subcutânea em uma cobaia de 250 g, não produz reação reconhecível na média de uma série; na verdade, a d. L$_0$ geralmente é registrada como a que causa edema local quase imperceptível na área da inoculação.

loading d., d. inicial, d. de ataque; dose comparativamente grande administrada no início do tratamento para que uma substância comece a produzir seu efeito, sobretudo quando a depuração desta é lenta, e exige um longo período para atingir níveis sanguíneos estáveis sem uma dose inicial elevada. SIN initial d.

Lr d., L$_r$ d., d. Lr, d. L$_r$; a dose de reação limite da toxina diftérica, isto é, a menor quantidade de toxina que, quando misturada a uma unidade de antitoxina e injetada por via intracutânea na pele raspada de uma cobaia suscetível, produz uma reação positiva mínima e inflamação localizada na região da injeção; a d. L$_r$ aproxima-se muito da d. L$_0$, como seria esperado, visto que um pequeno excesso de toxina não-neutralizada resulta em uma reação.

maintenance d., d. de manutenção. VER maintenance drug *therapy*.

maximal d., d. máxima; a maior quantidade de uma substância ou procedimento físico que um adulto pode receber com segurança.

maximal permissible d., d. máxima permissível. VER maximum permissible d.

maximum permissible d. (MPD), d. máxima permissível; definida pela Comissão Internacional de Proteção Radiológica (*International Commission on Radiological Protection*) como a maior dose de radiação que, à luz do conhecimento presente, não deve causar lesão corporal detectável nas pessoas em qualquer momento de sua vida. Essa dose tem sido reduzida a cada relatório da Comissão. A DMP é apresentada em termos de exposição aguda ou crônica de todo o corpo ou de órgãos, sistemas ou regiões do corpo, e é diferente para pessoas submetidas a exposição ocupacional e para o público em geral.

maximum tolerated d., d. máxima tolerada; dose que produz toxicidade de grau 3 (grave) ou de grau 4 (com risco de vida) em 30% ou menos dos pacientes testados.

median effective dose (ED$_{50}$), d. efetiva mediana (DE$_{50}$). VER effective d.

minimal d., d. mínima; a menor quantidade de uma substância ou procedimento físico que produzirá um efeito fisiológico desejado em um adulto.

minimal infecting d. (MID), d. infectante mínima (DIM); a menor quantidade de material infeccioso que, regularmente, causa infecção; geralmente expressa como D.I.$_{50}$, a quantidade que causa infecção em 50% de uma série adequada de animais ou células (culturas de células).

minimal lethal d. (MLD, mld), d. letal mínima (DLM, dlm); **(1)** a dose mínima de uma substância tóxica ou agente infeccioso que é letal, conforme analisado em vários animais experimentais (p. ex., a menor quantidade de toxina diftérica que, na média, mata uma cobaia de 250 g em 96 horas após inoculação subcutânea); quando seguida por um subscrito (geralmente "DLM$_{50}$"), designa a dose mínima letal para uma determinada percentagem (p. ex., 50%) dos animais assim examinados; **(2)** LD$_{05}$. VER lethal d.

minimal reacting d. (MRD, mrd), d. mínima de reação (DRM; a dose mínima de uma substância tóxica causadora de uma reação cutânea em uma série de animais de laboratório suscetíveis; o ensaio baseia-se no desenvolvimento de uma característica inflamação focal, "padrão", mínima, mas definida (congestão e edema, enduração, alterações degenerativas e descamação de células epidérmicas).

optimum d., d. ótima; a dose de uma substância ou radiação que produzirá o efeito desejado com mínima probabilidade de sintomas indesejáveis.

preventive d., d. preventiva; a menor quantidade de qualquer substância que evitará a ocorrência de sintomas de uma doença ou as conseqüências da ausência de um determinado fator na dieta.

sensitizing d., d. sensibilizante; em anafilaxia experimental, o inóculo antigênico que torna um animal suscetível (sensível) ao choque anafilático após um inóculo subseqüente (dose de choque) do mesmo antígeno (anafilactogênio).

shocking d., d. de choque; em anafilaxia experimental, o inóculo de antígeno que causa choque anafilático em um animal sensibilizado por um inóculo prévio (dose sensibilizante) do mesmo antígeno.

skin d., d. cutânea; a dose absorvida de radiação aplicada à superfície cutânea.

therapeutic d., d. terapêutica, dose curativa. SIN curative d.

tissue culture infectious d. (TCID$_{50}$, TCD$_{50}$), d. infecciosa de cultura de tecidos; a quantidade de um agente citopatogênico, como um vírus, que produzirá um efeito citopático em 50% das culturas inoculadas.

tolerance d., d. de tolerância; a maior dose de um remédio que pode ser aceita sem a produção de sintomas nocivos.

dos·im·e·ter (do̅-sim′ĕ-ter). Dosímetro; aparelho para medir radiação, principalmente raios X. [G. *dosis*, dose, + *metron*, medida]

do·sim·e·try (do̅-sim′ĕ-tre̅). Dosimetria; medida da exposição à radiação, principalmente raios X ou raios gama; cálculo da dose de radiação emitida por radionuclídeos administrados internamente.

thermoluminescence d., d. por termoluminescência; o cálculo de uma dose de radiação por medida da emissão de luz após aquecimento de um material absorvente especial (p. ex., fluoreto de lítio) colocado no feixe de radiação; a emissão de luz é proporcional ao grau de exposição à radiação.

X-ray d., d. de raios X. SIN roentgenometry.

dot (dot). Um pequeno ponto.

Gunn d.'s, manchas de Gunn; minúsculos pontos brancos ou amarelados, muito brilhantes, geralmente observados na parte posterior do fundo do olho; não são anormais.

Horner-Trantas d.'s, máculas de Horner-Trantas; infiltrados celulares brancos evanescentes que ocorrem na forma bulbar de ceratoconjuntivite primaveril.

Maurer d.'s, granulações de Maurer; precipitados finamente granulares ou partículas citoplasmáticas irregulares que, em geral, são observados difusamente nas hemácias infestadas pelos trofozoítas de *Plasmodium falciparum*, algumas vezes por trofozoítas de *P. malariae*; raramente observadas em esfregaços sanguíneos de *P. falciparum* porque seus trofozoítas raramente são encontrados no sangue periférico. SIN Maurer clefts.

Mittendorf d., ponto de Mittendorf; pequeno ponto visível na face posterior da cápsula da lente ao exame oftalmológico; representa um remanescente do sistema vascular hialóide primitivo.

Schüffner d.'s, granulações de Schüffner; granulações finas, redondas, vermelhas ou amarelo-avermelhadas (pela coloração de Romanovsky) caracteristicamente observadas em eritrócitos infestados pelo *Plasmodium vivax* e *P. ovale*, mas não encontradas comumente em infestações por *P. malariae* e *P. falciparum*. SIN Schüffner granules.

Trantas d.'s, nódulos de Trantas; nódulos vermelho-acinzentados, pálidos, desiguais, de aspecto gelatinoso, na conjuntiva do limbo, na conjuntivite primaveril.

Ziemann d.'s, pontilhado de Ziemann; pontilhado fino observado nos eritrócitos na malária causada por *P. malariae*. SIN Ziemann stippling.

dot·age (do̅′tij). Decrepitude; a deterioração das faculdades mentais anteriormente íntegras, comum na idade avançada.

dou·blet (dŭb′let). **1.** Dubleto, par de lentes; combinação de duas lentes para corrigir a aberração cromática e esférica. **2.** dipolo. SIN dipole. **3.** Par; qualquer seqüência de dois nucleotídeos em um filamento polinucleotídeo. **4.** Bipolar; um par de picos ou linhas em um espectro situados próximos.

Wollaston d., prisma de Wollaston; combinação de duas lentes planoconvexas, na ocular de um microscópio, destinada a corrigir a aberração cromática.

douche (doosh). **1.** Ducha; uma corrente de água, gás ou vapor direcionada contra uma superfície ou projetada para uma cavidade. **2.** Chuveiro; instrumento para administrar uma ducha. **3.** Duchar; aplicar uma ducha. [Fr. de *doucher*, despejar]

Douglas, Beverly, cirurgiã norte-americana, 1891–1975.

Douglas, Claude G., fisiologista inglês, 1882–1963. VER D. *bag*.

Douglas, James, anatomista escocês em Londres, 1675–1742. VER D. *abscess, cul-de-sac, fold, line, pouch; cavum* douglasi.

Douglas, John C., obstetra irlandês, 1777–1850. VER D. *mechanism*.

dove·tail (dŭv′tāl). Rabo-de-andorinha, ensambladura; porção alargada da preparação de uma cavidade geralmente estabelecida para aumentar a configuração de retenção e resistência.

dow·el (dow′l). Pino, cavilha. **1.** Pino de ouro fundido ou metal pré-formado colocado em um canal radicular a fim de proporcionar retenção de uma coroa. **2.** Pino de metal pré-formado colocado em molde de cobre para permitir fixação do molde. **3.** Pino ou bastão que alinha ou une duas estruturas encaixando-se em orifícios em ambas; pinos de vários materiais são usados em cirurgia ortopédica e odontologia. **4.** SIN dowel *graft*.

Down, John Langdon H., médico inglês, 1828–1896. VER D. *syndrome*.

Downey, Hal, hematologista norte-americano, 1877–1959. VER D. *cell*.

down·growth (doun-gro̅th). Algo que cresce para baixo; o processo de crescimento para baixo.

epithelial d., a invasão da parte interior do olho pelo epitélio superficial em conseqüência de uma ferida ocular penetrante.

down-reg·u·la·tion. Infra-regulação; desenvolvimento de um estado refratário ou tolerante após administração repetida de uma substância ativa farmacológica ou fisiologicamente; freqüentemente acompanhada por diminuição inicial da afinidade dos receptores pelo agente e uma subseqüente diminuição do número de receptores.

Downs, William B., ortodontista norte-americano, 1899–1966. VER D. *analysis*.

Dox, Arthur W., químico norte-americano, *1882. VER Czapek-D. *medium*.

dox·a·cu·ri·um chlo·ride (doks′a - koo′re̅ - um). Cloreto de doxacúrio; bloqueador neuromuscular não-despolarizante, semelhante ao pancurônio, porém sem efeitos colaterais cardiovasculares.

dox·a·pram hy·dro·chlo·ride (doks′ă - pram). Cloridrato de doxapram; estimulante do sistema nervoso central, defendido, mas raramente usado, como estimulante respiratório em anestesia.

dox·a·zo·cin (doks′a - zo̅ - sin). Doxazocina; agente anti-hipertensivo que bloqueia seletivamente o subtipo α₁ (pós-juncional) dos receptores α-adrenérgicos; possui ações farmacológicas semelhantes às da prazocina. Impede os efeitos de elevação da pressão arterial da norepinefrina, fenilefrina e outros agonistas em receptores α₁ vasculares.

dox·e·pin hy·dro·chlo·ride (dok′se̅ - pin). Cloridrato de doxepina; agente antidepressivo.

dox·o·phyl·line (doks′o̅ - fil′in). Doxofilina; substância semelhante à teofilina usada, embora raramente nos Estados Unidos, como broncodilatador na asma e na doença pulmonar obstrutiva crônica (DPOC).

dox·o·ru·bi·cin (dok′so̅ - roo′bi - sin). Doxorrubicina; antibiótico antineoplásico isolado do *Streptomyces peucetius*; também usado em citogenética para produzir bandas cromossomiais do tipo Q. SIN adriamycin.

dox·y·cy·cline (dok - se̅ - si′kle̅n). Doxiciclina; antibiótico de amplo espectro.

dox·yl·a·mine suc·ci·nate (dok - sil′ă - me̅n). Succinato de doxilamina; anti-histamínico. SIN mereprine.

Doyère, Louis, fisiologista francês, 1811–1863. VER D. *eminence*.

Doyle, J.B., ginecologista norte-americano, *1907. VER D. *operation*.

Doyne, Robert Walter, oftalmologista inglês, 1857–1916. VER D. honeycomb *choroidopathy*.

D.P. Abreviatura de Doctor of Podiatry (Doutor em Podiatria).

D.P.H. Abreviatura de Department of Public Health (Departamento de Saúde Pública); Doctor of Public Health (Doutor em Saúde Pública); Diploma of Public Health (Diploma em Saúde Pública).

D.P.M. Abreviatura de Doctor of Podiatric Medicine (Doutor em Medicina Podiátrica).

DPT. Abreviatura de diphtheria-pertussis-tetanus (vaccine), difteria-coqueluche-tétano (vacina). VER diphtheria toxoid, tetanus toxoid e pertussis *vaccine*.

DR Abreviatura de digital *radiography* (radiografia digital).

Dr. Abreviatura de doctor (doutor).

dr Abreviatura de dram (dracma).

drachm (dram). Dracma. SIN dram. [G. *drachme̅*, antigo peso grego, equivalente a aproximadamente 60 g]

dra·cun·cu·li·a·sis, dra·cun·cu·lo·sis (dra - kŭng - kū - li′ă - sis, - kū - lo̅′sis). Dracunculíase; infestação por *Dracunculus medinensis*.

Dra·cun·cu·lus (dra - kŭng′kū - lŭs). Gênero de nematódeos (superfamília Dracunculoidea) que possuem algumas semelhanças com filárias verdadeiras; entretanto, os adultos são maiores (as fêmeas medem até 1 m), e o hospedeiro intermediário é um crustáceo de água doce, e não um inseto. [L. dim. de *draco*, serpente]

D. lova, termo antigo incorreto para *Loa loa*.

D. medinen'sis, espécie de nematódeos que infestam a pele, com 30 a 120 cm de comprimento, outrora erroneamente classificados como *Filaria*; os vermes adultos vivem em qualquer local no corpo de seres humanos e vários mamíferos semi-aquáticos; as fêmeas migram ao longo dos planos fasciais até os tecidos subcutâneos, onde se formam úlceras crônicas incômodas na pele; quando o hospedeiro entra na água, as larvas saem das úlceras, de onde se projetam as cabeças das fêmeas; essas larvas, se ingeridas por espécies de *Cyclops*, transformam-se na fase infecciosa no hospedeiro intermediário; o homem e vários animais contraem a infestação acidentalmente ao beberem água contaminada por *Cyclops* infestados. Popularmente conhecidos como "verme da Guiné", "filária de Medina" e freqüentemente mencionados na literatura hebraica como

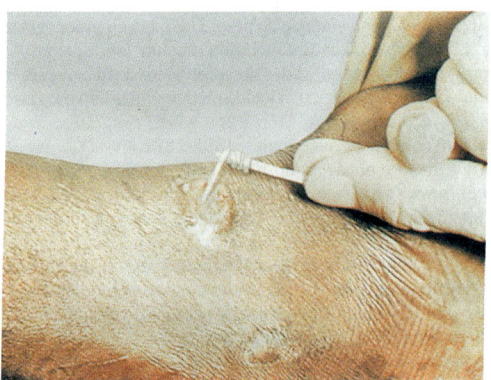

Dracunculus medinensis: verme adulto sendo removido enrolado em um bastão

a "serpente de fogo" que flagelava os israelitas na Antiguidade. [L. de Medina]

D. oc'uli, termo antigo incorreto para *Loa loa*.

D. persa'rum, termo antigo para *D. medinensis*. [L. dos persas]

draft. 1. Corrente de ar em um espaço fechado. **2.** Dose; a quantidade de medicamento líquido prescrito em dose única. SIN draught.

drag. 1. A face inferior ou impressa de um molde de dentadura. **2.** Arrasto; qualquer tendência de um objeto em movimento de deslocar outra coisa junto.

solvent d., arrasto por solvente; a influência exercida por um fluxo de solvente através de uma membrana sobre o movimento simultâneo de um soluto através da membrana.

dra·gée (dra - zhā′). Drágea; pílula ou cápsula revestida de açúcar. [Fr.]

Dragendorff, Georg J.N., médico e químico farmacêutico alemão, 1836–1898. VER D. *test*.

Drager, Glenn A., neurologista norte-americano, *1917. VER Shy-D. *syndrome*.

Dräger, Heinrich, fabricante alemão de aparelhos respiratórios industriais e de mergulho e de aparelhos para anestesia, 1847–1917. VER D. *respirometer*.

drain (drān). **1.** Drenar; remover líquido de uma cavidade à medida que este se forma, p. ex., para drenar um abscesso. **2.** Dreno; dispositivo, geralmente no formato de um tubo ou pavio, para remover líquido à medida que este se acumula em uma cavidade, principalmente uma cavidade de ferida. [A.S. *drehnian*, drenar]

cigarette d., d. em cigarro; mecha de gaze enrolada em material fino, flexível, semelhante à borracha, que permite drenagem capilar.

Mikulicz d., d. de Mikulicz; dreno feito com várias tiras de gaze mantidas unidas por uma única camada de gaze.

Penrose d., d. de Penrose; dreno de borracha macia, tubular.

stab d., d. por incisão; dreno introduzido em uma cavidade através de punção feita em uma parte inferior distante da ferida cirúrgica, destinado a evitar infecção da ferida.

sump d., d. bitubular; dreno consistindo em um tubo externo aberto para o exterior, com um tubo menor em seu interior que está preso a uma bomba de sucção; ambos possuem múltiplas perfurações que permitem a passagem de líquido e ar através do tubo de sucção.

drain·age (drān′ij). Drenagem; retirada contínua de líquidos de uma ferida ou de outra cavidade.

capillary d., d. capilar; drenagem por meio de uma mecha de gaze ou outro material.

closed d., d. fechada; drenagem de uma cavidade corporal através de um sistema impermeável à água ou ar. Cf sump *drain*.

dependent d., d. gravitacional; drenagem da parte mais baixa para um receptáculo colocado em um nível mais baixo que a estrutura drenada. SIN downward d.

downward d., d. gravitacional. SIN dependent d.

infusion-aspiration d., d. por infusão–aspiração; tipo de drenagem na qual antibióticos são infundidos continuamente numa cavidade ao mesmo tempo em que o líquido está sendo drenado (aspirado) da cavidade.

open d., d. aberta; drenagem que permite a entrada de ar.

postural d., d. postural; drenagem usada na bronquiectasia e em abscessos pulmonares. O corpo do paciente é posicionado de forma que a traquéia fique inclinada para baixo e abaixo da área torácica afetada.

suction d., d. por aspiração; drenagem fechada de uma cavidade, com um aspirador acoplado ao tubo de drenagem.

through d., drenagem obtida pela passagem de um tubo perfurado, aberto nas duas extremidades, através de uma cavidade; além disso, a cavidade pode ser lavada por uma solução passada através do tubo.

tidal d., d. corrente; drenagem da bexiga por meio de um aparelho de enchimento e esvaziamento intermitente.

Wangensteen d., d. de Wangensteen; drenagem contínua por aspiração através de um tubo gástrico ou duodenal de demora.

dram (dr). Dracma; uma unidade de peso: 1/8 onça; 60 grãos (gr), medida de farmácia; 1/16 onça, peso avoirdupois. SIN drachm. [ver drachm]

drape (drāp). **1.** Cobrir outras partes do corpo além da que vai ser examinada ou operada. **2.** Campo cirúrgico; o tecido ou material usado para isso. [I.M. do L.L. *drappus*, tecido]

Draper, John William, químico inglês, 1811–1882. VER D. *law*.

draught (draft). Corrente de ar; dose. SIN draft.

draw-sheet (draw′shēt). Traçado; lençol estreito colocado transversalmente sobre o leito e debaixo do paciente para ajudar a movimentá-lo ou a trocar a roupa de cama suja.

dream (drēm). Sonho; atividade mental durante o sono na qual eventos, pensamentos, emoções e imagens são vividos como se fossem reais.

anxiety d., s. de ansiedade; um sonho (ou pesadelo) no qual o medo mórbido e a ansiedade formam uma parte importante.

wet d., orgasmo fisiológico verdadeiro durante o sono, incluindo, em homens, uma ejaculação noturna geralmente associada a um sonho de contexto sexual.

dream-work. Em psicanálise, o processo pelo qual se efetua a mudança do conteúdo latente para o manifesto de um sonho.

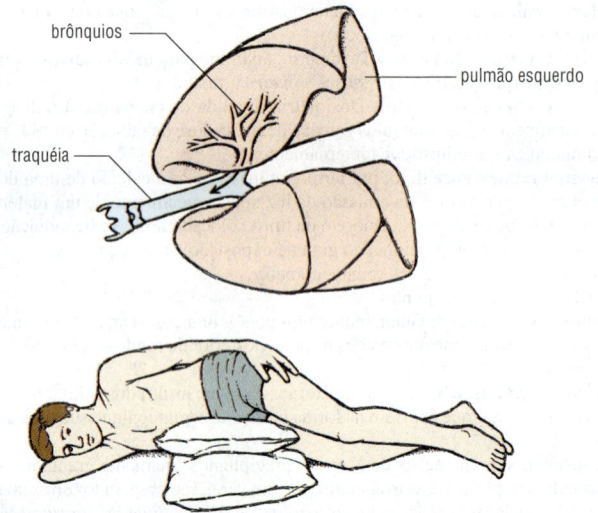

drenagem postural do pulmão esquerdo

Drechs·lera (dresh′ler - ă). Gênero sapróbico de fungos, freqüentemente isolados no laboratório de análises clínicas, caracterizado por conídios fixados a um conidióforo em ziguezague. A maioria das espécies desse gênero que causam feoifomicose em seres humanos, gatos e cavalos foi transferida para os gêneros *Bipolaris* ou *Exserohilum*.

Dreifuss, Fritz E., *1926. VER Emery-D. muscular *dystrophy*.

drep·a·nid·i·um (drep - ă - nid′ē - ŭm). Drepanídio; forma jovem falciforme ou em crescente de uma gregarina. [G. *drepane*, foice]

drep·a·no·cyte (drep′ă - nō - sīt). Drepanócito. SIN sickle *cell*. [G. *drepane*, foice, + *kytos*, cavidade (célula)]

drep·a·no·cyt·ic (drep′ă - nō - sit′ik). Drepanocítico; relativo, ou semelhante, a uma célula falciforme.

dress·er (dres′er). Na Grã-Bretanha, um auxiliar de cirurgia cuja obrigação primária é colocar bandagens e fazer curativo das feridas.

dress·ing (dres′ing). Curativo; o material aplicado, ou a própria aplicação de material, a uma ferida para proteção, absorção, drenagem, etc.

adhesive absorbent d., c. absorvente adesivo; curativo individual estéril que consiste em uma compressa absorvente simples fixada a uma tira de tecido revestida com um adesivo sensível à pressão.

antiseptic d., c. anti-séptico; curativo estéril de gaze impregnada com anti-séptico.

bolus d., c. amarrado. SIN tie-over d.

dry d., c. seco; gaze ou outro material seco aplicado a uma ferida.

fixed d., c. fixo; curativo endurecido com uma substância que produz imobilização quando seca.

Lister d., c. de Lister; o primeiro tipo de curativo anti-séptico, de gaze impregnada com ácido carbólico.

occlusive d., c. oclusivo; curativo que fecha hermeticamente uma ferida.

pressure d., c. compressivo; curativo por meio do qual se exerce pressão na área coberta para evitar o acúmulo de líquido nos tecidos subjacentes; usado mais comumente após enxerto cutâneo e no tratamento de queimaduras.

tie-over d., c. amarrado; curativo feito sobre um enxerto cutâneo ou outra ferida suturada e fixado por fios de sutura deixados com comprimento suficiente para isso. SIN bolus d.

water d., c. úmido; aplicação de gaze ou outro material que é mantido umedecido com água ou solução salina esterilizada.

wet-to-dry d., curativo aplicado umedecido com solução salina e que se deixa secar antes de remover.

Dressler, William, médico norte-americano, 1890–1969. VER D. *beat*, *syndrome*.

Dreyer, Georges, patologista inglês, 1873–1934. VER D. *formula*.

DRG Abreviatura de diagnosis-related *group* (agrupamento de classificações diagnósticas).

drib·ble (dri′bl). **1.** Babar. **2.** Pingar, gotejar, como a urina de uma bexiga distendida.

drift. Desvio; flutuação. **1.** Movimento gradual, como o afastamento de uma posição original. **2.** Alteração gradual do valor de uma variável aleatória com o tempo em virtude de vários fatores, alguns aleatórios e alguns efeitos sistemáticos de tendência, manipulação, etc.

antigenic d., desvio antigênico; o processo de alterações "evolutivas" na estrutura molecular do DNA/RNA em microrganismos durante sua passagem de um hospedeiro para outro; pode ser devido à recombinação, deleção ou inser-

ção de genes, mutações pontuais ou combinações desses eventos; leva à alteração (em geral lenta e progressiva) da composição antigênica, e, portanto, das respostas imunológicas de indivíduos e populações à exposição ao microrganismo em questão; comum com o vírus influenza.
   genetic d., desvio genético; alteração nas freqüências de traços genéticos ou freqüências de alelos durante gerações.
   pure random d., desvio aleatório simples; aquele que possui apenas componentes aleatórios com um valor médio igual a zero e ausência de efeitos sistemáticos. O movimento browniano em um recipiente imóvel mostra desvio aleatório puro, mas, no Mississippi, mostra uma tendência constante de seguir a jusante.

drift·ing. Movimento ao acaso de um dente para uma posição de maior estabilidade.

drifts (drifts). Desvios; movimentos oculares lentos de maior amplitude que os movimentos de fixação do olhar. SIN drift movements.

drill. 1. Perfurar; fazer um orifício em um osso ou outra substância rígida. **2.** Broca; trépano; instrumento para fazer ou alargar um orifício no osso ou no dente. [Holandês Médio *drillen*, perfurar]
   bur d., broca. VER bur.
   dental d., caneta dentária; instrumento elétrico giratório, no qual podem ser introduzidas pontas de corte. VER TAMBÉM handpiece.

drill-out. Escavação; escavar.
   cochlear d.-o., escavação coclear; implantação de eletrodos em uma cóclea na qual a luz da rampa do tímpano foi obliterada pela deposição de osso novo devido ao processo inflamatório no labirinto; a parede coclear e o osso novo são escavados de forma que os eletrodos possam ser posicionados próximo dos neurônios remanescentes da divisão auditiva do 8.º nervo craniano.

Drinker, Philip, higienista industrial norte-americano, 1893–1972. VER D. *respirator*.

drip. Gotejar; gotejamento. **1.** Deixar cair uma gota de cada vez. **2.** Um fluxo em gotas.
   alkaline milk d., gotejamento de leite alcalino; mistura variável de bicarbonato de sódio em leite integral, gotejada no estômago através de um pequeno tubo oral ou nasal para produzir acloridria constante; tratamento, agora obsoleto, para determinadas úlceras.
   intravenous d., gotejamento intravenoso; a introdução lenta, porém contínua, de soluções por via intravenosa, uma gota de cada vez.
   Murphy d., gotejamento de Murphy. SIN proctoclysis.
   postnasal d., gotejamento pós-nasal; termo usado algumas vezes para descrever a sensação de secreção mucóide ou mucopurulenta na região posterior das narinas.

drive. Pulsão, impulso. **1.** Em psicanálise, uma ânsia irresistível básica. **2.** Em psicologia, classificada como inata (p. ex., fome) ou aprendida (p. ex., acumulação) e apetitiva (p. ex., fome, sede, sexo) ou aversiva (p. ex., medo, dor, luto). VER TAMBÉM motive, motivation.
   acquired d.'s, pulsões adquiridas. SIN secondary d.'s.
   exploratory d., p. exploratória; a pulsão típica de crianças pequenas e de alguns animais para investigar o não-familiar ou desconhecido.
   learned d., p. aprendida. SIN motive (1).
   meiotic d., impulso meiótico; aptidão diferencial em homens e mulheres.
   physiological d.'s, pulsões fisiológicas; aquelas pulsões, como fome e sede, derivadas das necessidades biológicas de um organismo. SIN primary d.'s.
   primary d.'s, pulsões primárias. SIN physiological d.'s.
   secondary d.'s, pulsões secundárias; aquelas pulsões não diretamente relacionadas às necessidades biológicas; uma pulsão secundária pode ser aprendida como derivação de uma pulsão primária, caso em que freqüentemente é denominada motivo. SIN acquired d.'s.

driv·ing (drīv'ing). Impulso, excitação; a indução de uma freqüência no eletroencefalograma por estimulação sensorial nessa freqüência.
   photic d., i. fótico; fenômeno EEG normal no qual a freqüência da atividade registrada sobre as regiões parieto-occipitais depende da freqüência do *flash* durante a estimulação fótica.

drom·o·ma·nia (drom - ō - mā'nē - ă). Dromomania; impulso incontrolável de passear ou viajar. [G. *dromos*, corrida, + *mania*, insanidade]

dro·mo·stan·o·lone pro·pi·o·nate (drō - mos'tan- ō - lōn, drō - mō - stan'ō - lōn). Propionato de dromostanolona; agente antineoplásico.

dro·nab·i·nol (drō - nab'i - nol). Dronabinol; a principal substância psicoativa presente na *Cannabis sativa*; usado terapeuticamente como antinauseante para controlar as náuseas e vômitos associados à quimioterapia do câncer. VER TAMBÉM tetrahydrocannabinol.

drop. 1. Gotejar, cair ou ser preparado ou vertido em glóbulos (pílulas pequenas). **2.** Um glóbulo líquido. **3.** Gota, volume de líquido considerado como unidade de dosagem, equivalente no caso da água a aproximadamente 1 mínimo (0,06161 ml). VER TAMBÉM drops. **4.** Pastilha, preparado sólido na forma globular, geralmente para ser dissolvido na boca. [A.S. *droppan*]
   enamel d., nódulo de esmalte. SIN enameloma.
   hanging d., gota pendente; gota de líquido na superfície inferior da lâmina para exame microscópico.

dro·per·i·dol (drō - per'i - dol). Droperidol; agente butirofenona usado em neuroleptanalgesia e medicação pré-anestésica; a farmacologia é semelhante à do haloperidol; bloqueador de receptores de dopamina. Exibe efeitos antieméticos.

dropfoot. Queda do pé. VER footdrop.

drop·let (drop'let). Gotícula; gota minúscula, como uma partícula de umidade eliminada pela boca ao tossir, espirrar ou falar; estas podem transmitir infecções para outras pessoas pelas vias aéreas. [drop + *-let*, sufixo dim.]

drop·per. Conta-gotas. SIN instillator.

drops. Gotas; termo popular usado para um medicamento tomado em doses medidas por gotas, geralmente uma tintura, ou aplicado por gotejamento, como um colírio.
   eye d., colírio. VER eyewash, ophthalmic *solutions*, em *solution*.
   knock-out d., "Boa-noite, cinderela"; nome popular dado ao alcoolato de cloral administrado com intenção criminal para produzir inconsciência rapidamente; é formado adicionando-se hidrato de cloral à cerveja ou a alguma bebida alcoólica mais forte.
   nose d., gotas nasais; preparação líquida para administração intranasal com conta-gotas, sendo usada, na maioria das vezes, para descongestão nasal, mas também para qualquer outra indicação apropriada.
   stomach d., gotas estomacais; tônico estomacal, em geral tintura de genciana, usado isoladamente ou com outros estomáquicos.

drop·si·cal (drop'si - kăl). Hidrópico. SIN hydropic.

drop·sy (drop'sē). Hidropisia, anasarca; termo antigo para edema generalizado, na maioria das vezes associado a insuficiência cardíaca. [G. *hydrōps*]
   abdominal d., ascite. SIN ascites.
   cardiac d., anasarca cardíaca; edema devido à insuficiência cardíaca.
   epidemic d., anasarca epidêmica; doença que causa epidemias ocasionais na Índia e nas Ilhas Maurício; caracterizada por edema, anemia, angiomatose eruptiva e febre leve; pode estar associada a deficiência nutricional.
   famine d., anasarca da inanição; edema que ocorre na hipoproteinemia decorrente de baixa ingestão proteica observada na inanição de um grande grupo populacional.
   nutritional d., anasarca nutricional; edema devido à hipoproteinemia secundária à desnutrição.
   d. of pericardium, derrame pericárdico. SIN pericardial *effusion*.

drown·ing. Afogamento; morte nas 24 horas seguintes a imersão em líquido, seja por anoxia ou parada cardíaca causada por redução extrema súbita da temperatura (síndrome de imersão). VER TAMBÉM near d.
   dry d., a. seco; afogamento por asfixia em um indivíduo cujos reflexos laríngeos são fortes, resultando em espasmo que impede a inalação de água; estaria associado à maior taxa de recuperação.
   near d., quase-afogamento; sobrevida inicial após imersão em líquido; a vítima morreria mais de 24 horas depois, p. ex., por SARA (síndrome de angústia respiratória do adulto).
   secondary d., a. secundário; edema pulmonar com conseqüente asfixia, resultante de hipoxia e aumento da permeabilidade dos capilares pulmonares, que ocorre em pacientes imersos em água e que a aspiraram.

drows·i·ness (drow'zē - nes). Sonolência; estado de comprometimento da consciência associado a um desejo ou tendência para dormir.

Dr.P.H. Abreviatura de Doctor of Public Health (Doutor em Saúde Pública).

drug (drŭg). **1.** Agente terapêutico, fármaco, medicamento, droga; qualquer substância, além de alimento, usada na prevenção, diagnóstico, alívio, tratamento ou cura de uma doença. Quanto aos tipos ou classificações das doenças, ver o nome específico. VER TAMBÉM agent. **2.** Drogar; administrar ou tomar uma droga, geralmente indicando uma quantidade excessiva ou um narcótico. **3.** Droga; termo genérico dado a qualquer substância, estimulante ou depressora, que possa causar hábito ou vício, principalmente um narcótico. [I.M. *drogge*]
   addictive d., qualquer droga (substância) que crie um certo grau de euforia e tenha forte potencial viciante.
   crude d., substância bruta; uma preparação não-refinada, geralmente de origem vegetal, encontrada nas formas intata, quase-intata, fragmentada e em pó.
   disease modifying antirheumatic d.'s, agentes anti-reumáticos modificadores da doença; agentes que aparentemente alteram o curso e a progressão da artrite reumatóide, em oposição às substâncias de ação mais rápida, que suprimem a inflamação e reduzem a dor, mas não impedem a erosão da cartilagem ou osso ou a incapacidade progressiva.
   d. holiday, interrupção temporária do tratamento; intervalo durante o qual um paciente cronicamente medicado pára de tomar a medicação; usado para permitir alguma recuperação das funções normais, para manter a sensibilidade ao agente e para reduzir a probabilidade de efeitos colaterais.
   nonsteroidal anti-inflammatory d.'s (NSAID), antiinflamatórios não-esteróides(AINE); um grande número de agentes com ações antiinflamatórias (e também geralmente analgésicas e antipiréticas); os exemplos incluem ácido acetilsalicílico (AAS), acetaminofeno, diclofenaco, indometacina, cetorolaco, ibuprofeno e naproxeno. Faz-se um contraste com os compostos esteróides (como a hidrocortisona ou a prednisona) que possuem atividade antiinflamatória.

orphan d.'s, agentes órfãos. SIN orphan *products*, em *product*.
psychedelic d., droga psicodélica, alucinógeno. SIN hallucinogen.
psychodysleptic d., droga psicodisléptica, alucinógeno. SIN hallucinogen.
psycholytic d., droga psicolítica, alucinógeno. SIN hallucinogen.
psychotomimetic d., droga psicotomimética, alucinógeno. SIN hallucinogen.
psychotropic d., agente psicotrópico; qualquer substância que afete a mente.
recreational d., droga ilícita. SIN street d.
scheduled d., medicação controlada; substâncias que pertencem a qualquer das cinco classes do *Controlled Substances Act* (1970). VER TAMBÉM controlled *substance*.
street d., droga ilícita; substância controlada usada para fins não-medicinais. Essas drogas compreendem várias anfetaminas, anestésicos, barbitúricos, opiáceos e substâncias psicoativas, e muitas são derivadas de fontes naturais (p. ex., as plantas *Papaver somniferum, Cannabis sativa, Amanita pantherina, Lophophora williamsii*). Os nomes usados na gíria incluem *acid* (LSD, dietilamida do ácido lisérgico), *angel dust* (fenciclidina), *coke* (cocaína), *downers* (barbitúricos), *grass* (maconha), *hash* (haxixe, tetraidrocanabinol concentrado), *magic mushrooms* (psilocibina) e *speed* (anfetaminas). Durante a década de 1980, surgiu uma nova classe de "drogas planejadas", em sua maioria análogos de substâncias psicoativas com o objetivo de escapar da regulamentação do *Controlled Substances Act*. Também o crack, uma forma de cocaína potente, para ser fumada, emergiu como um importante problema de saúde pública. Nos Estados Unidos, historicamente, o uso ilegal de drogas como cocaína, maconha e heroína obedece a ciclos. SIN recreational d.
drug-fast. Resistente a medicamentos, fármaco-resistente; relativo a microrganismos que resistem ou se tornam tolerantes a um agente antibacteriano.
drug.gist (drŭg'ist).Boticário; termo antigo comum para farmacêutico.
drug in·ter·ac·tions. Interações medicamentosas; o resultado farmacológico, seja desejável ou indesejável, de agentes que interagem com outras substâncias, com agentes químicos fisiológicos endógenos (p. ex., IMAO com epinefrina), com componentes da dieta e com substâncias químicas usadas em testes diagnósticos ou os resultados desses testes.
drum, drum·head (drŭm, drŭm'hed). Membrana timpânica. SIN tympanic *membrane*.
Drummond, Sir David, médico inglês, 1852–1932. VER *artery* of D.; D. *sign*.
drunk·en·ness (drŭnk'en - nes).Embriaguez; intoxicação, geralmente alcoólica. VER TAMBÉM acute *alcoholism*.
sleep d., embotamento da sensibilidade; um estado de semivigília no qual a faculdade de orientação está latente, e, sob a influência de impressões opressivas semelhantes a pesadelos, a pessoa pode tornar-se ativamente excitada e violenta. SIN somnolentia (2).
dru·sen (droo'sen). Drusas; pequenas estruturas brilhantes observadas na retina e no disco óptico. [Alemão pl. de *Druse*, nódulo pétreo, geode]
basal laminar d., drusas laminares basais; lesões pequenas, redondas, translúcidas, com 25–75 μm de diâmetro, que representam espessamento nodular da membrana basal do epitélio pigmentar da retina (retinal pigment *epithelium*), freqüentemente com descolamento focal sobrejacente do epitélio pigmentar da retina da membrana de Bruch (Bruch *membrane*). SIN cuticular d.
basal linear d., drusas lineares basais; depósitos de colágeno bem espaçados, localizados entre a membrana plasmática (plasma *membrane*) e a membrana basal (basement *membrane*) do epitélio pigmentar (pigment *epithelium*) da retina.
cuticular d., drusa cuticular. SIN basal laminar d.
exudative d., drusas exsudativas; acúmulos de material amorfo e granular, processos citoplasmáticos e fibras curvas entre a membrana basal do epitélio pigmentar da retina e a zona colágena interna da membrana de Bruch (Bruch *membrane*); os tipos de drusas exsudativas incluem a drusa dura e a drusa mole. SIN typical d.
hard d., d. dura; tipo de drusa exsudativa ou típica que se apresenta oftalmoscopicamente como nódulos amarelos, distintos, caracterizados histopatologicamente por acúmulos bem definidos de material hialino nas zonas colágenas interna e externa da membrana de Bruch (Bruch *membrane*).
intrapapillary d., d. intrapapilar. SIN d. of the optic nerve head.
d. of the macula, d. da mácula; excrescências da membrana de Bruch que produzem uma janela no epitélio pigmentar da retina e são uma característica da degeneração retiniana macular relacionada à idade. SIN macular d.
macular d., d. macular. SIN d. of the macula.
d. of the optic nerve head, d. da cabeça do nervo óptico; massas acelulares calcárias, laminadas, basófilas, semelhantes a cristais na cabeça do nervo óptico, anteriores à lâmina cribriforme, que podem simular papiledema e/ou causar defeitos do campo visual. SIN intrapapillary d.
soft d., d. mole; tipo de drusa exsudativa que se apresenta oftalmoscopicamente como lesões amarelas placóides, caracterizadas histopatologicamente por descolamentos serosos localizados do epitélio pigmentar da retina (retinal pigment *epithelium*) da membrana de Bruch (Bruch *membrane*).
typical d., d. típica. SIN exudative d.
dry ice (drī īs).Gelo seco. SIN *carbon* dioxide snow.
ds Abreviatura de double-stranded (de duplo filamento).

DSA Abreviatura de digital subtraction *angiography* (angiografia de subtração digital).
DSM Abreviatura de *Diagnostic and Statistical Manual of Mental Disorders* (Manual Diagnóstico e Estatístico de Transtornos Mentais).
DT Abreviatura de *delirium* tremens (*delirium tremens*).
dT Abreviatura de deoxythymidine (desoxitimidina).
DTaP Abreviatura de diphtheria, tetanus, and acellular pertussis vaccine (vacina contra difteria, tétano e coqueluche acelular).
DT-di·aph·o·rase. DT-diaforase. SIN *NADPH* dehydrogenase (quinone).
dTDP Abreviatura de thymidine 5′-diphosphate (5′-difosfato de timidina).
dTDP-sug·ars. dTDP-açúcares; açúcares ou derivados do açúcar ligados à dTDP.
DTH Abreviatura de delayed-type hypersensitivity (hipersensibilidade do tipo tardio).
dThd Abreviatura de thymidine (timidina).
DTIC Abreviatura de dacarbazine (dacarbazina).
dTMP Abreviatura de deoxythymidylic acid (ácido desoxitimidílico); thymidine 5′-monophosphate (5′-monofosfato de timidina).
DTP Abreviatura de distal *tingling* on percussion (formigamento distal à percussão); diphtheria toxoid, tetanus toxoid, and pertussis *vaccine* (vacina com toxóide diftérico, toxóide tetânico e coqueluche); e coquetel de meperidina (Demerol), clorpromazina (Thorazine) e prometazina (Phenergan), algumas vezes usado como sedativo.
DTPA Abreviatura de diethylenetriamine pentaacetic acid (ácido dietilenotriamina pentacético).
DTR Abreviatura de deep tendon *reflex* (reflexo tendinoso profundo).
dTTP Abreviatura de thymidine 5′-triphosphate (5′-trifosfato de timidina).
du·al·ism (doo'ăl - izm). Dualismo. **1.** Em química, uma teoria, apresentada por Berzelius, de que todo composto, não importando o número de elementos que o formam, tem duas partes, uma eletricamente negativa, a outra positiva; ainda aplicável, com modificação, a compostos polares, mas inaplicável a compostos apolares. **2.** Em hematologia, o conceito de que as células do sangue têm duas origens, isto é, linfogênica e mielogênica. **3.** A teoria de que a mente e o corpo são dois sistemas distintos, de naturezas independentes e diferentes. [L. *dualis*, relativo a dois, de *duo*, dois]
Duane, Alexander, oftalmologista norte-americano, 1858–1926. VER D. *syndrome*.
Dubin, I. Nathan, patologista norte-americano, 1913–1980. VER D.-Johnson *syndrome*.
DuBois, Eugene F., fisiologista norte-americano, 1882–1959. VER DuB. *formula*; Aub-DuB. *table*.
Dubois, Paul A., obstetra francês, 1795–1871. VER D. *abscesses*, em *abscess, disease*.
du·boi·sine (doo - boy'sēn). Duboisina; alcalóide obtido das folhas de *Duboisia myoporoides* (família Solanaceae). VER hyoscyamine.
Du Bois-Reymond, Emil H., fisiologista alemão, 1818–1896. VER Du Bois-Reymond *law*.
Duboscq, Jules, óptico (opticista) francês, 1817–1886. VER D. *colorimeter*.
Dubowitz, Victor, pediatra sul-africano-inglês, *1931. VER D. *score*.
Dubreuil-Chambardel, Louis, dentista francês, 1879–1927. VER Dubreuil-Chambardel *syndrome*.
Duchenne, Guillaume B.A., neurologista francês, 1806–1875. VER D. *disease, sign;* D.-Aran *disease;* Aran-D. *disease;* D.-Erb *paralysis;* D. *dystrophy*.
Duckworth, Sir Dyce, médico inglês, 1840–1928. VER D. *phenomenon*.
Ducrey, Augusto, dermatologista italiano, 1860–1940. VER D. *bacillus, test*.

DUCT

duct (dŭkt) [TA]. Ducto; estrutura tubular que dá saída à secreção de uma glândula ou órgão, capaz de conduzir líquido. VER TAMBÉM canal. SIN ductus [TA]. [L. *duco*, pp. *ductus*, levar]
aberrant d.'s, ductos aberrantes. SIN aberrant *ductules*, em *ductule*.
aberrant bile d.'s, ductos biliares aberrantes; pequenos ductos ocasionalmente presentes nos ligamentos hepáticos ou originados na superfície do fígado.
accessory pancreatic d. [TA], d. pancreático acessório; o ducto excretor da cabeça do pâncreas; um ramo do qual se une ao ducto pancreático, e o outro se abre independentemente no duodeno na papila duodenal menor. SIN ductus pancreaticus accessorius [TA], Bernard canal, Bernard d., ductus dorsopancreaticus, Santorini canal, Santorini d.
alveolar d., d. alveolar; **(1)** a parte das vias respiratórias distal ao bronquíolo respiratório; nele têm origem os sacos alveolares e alvéolos; **(2)** o menor dos ductos intralobulares na glândula mamária, no qual se abrem os alvéolos secretores. SIN ductulus alveolaris.
amnionic d., d. amniótico; a abertura transitória entre as pregas seroamnióticas em aves logo antes de se fundirem para formar a rafe seroamniótica.

anal d.'s, ductos anais; ductos curtos revestidos por epitélio colunar simples ou estratificado que se estende das válvulas anais até os seios anais.
arterial d., canal arterial. SIN *ductus* arteriosus.
Bartholin d., d. de Bartholin. SIN major sublingual d.
Bellini d.'s, ductos de Bellini. SIN papillary d.'s.
Bernard d., d. de Bernard. SIN accessory pancreatic d.
bile d., (1) d. colédoco; ducto formado pela união dos ductos hepático e cístico; drena para a papila duodenal. SIN ductus choledochus [TA], choledoch d., choledoch, choledochus, common bile d. (2) d. biliar; qualquer dos ductos que conduzem bile entre o fígado e o intestino, incluindo os ductos hepático, cístico e colédoco, um ducto formado pela união dos ductos hepático e cístico; drena para a papila duodenal. SIN ductus biliaris [TA], biliary d.
biliary d., d. biliar. SIN bile d. (2).
Blasius d., d. de Blasius. SIN parotid d.
Botallo d., d. de Botallo. SIN *ductus* arteriosus.
bucconeural d., d. bucconeural. SIN craniopharyngeal d.
d. of bulbourethral gland [TA], d. da glândula bulbouretral; o ducto longo e fino de cada lado, que desce através da fáscia inferior do diafragma urogenital para entrar no bulbo do pênis e segue 2 ou 3 cm para a frente antes de terminar na uretra. SIN ductus glandulae bulbourethralis [TA].
canalicular d.'s, ductos canaliculares; (1) ductos lactíferos. SIN lactiferous d.'s; (2) dúctulos biliares. SIN biliary *ductules*, em *ductule*.
carotid d., d. carotídeo. SIN *ductus* caroticus.
cervical d., d. cervical. VER cervical *diverticulum*.
choledoch d., d. colédoco. SIN bile d. (1).
cochlear d. [TA], d. coclear; tubo membranoso espiral suspenso na cóclea, situado entre e separando a rampa do vestíbulo e a rampa do tímpano; começa por uma extremidade cega, o ceco vestibular, no recesso coclear do vestíbulo, terminando em outra extremidade cega, o ceco cupular, na cúpula da cóclea; contém endolinfa e comunica-se com o sáculo através do ducto de união; o órgão espiral (de Corti), o órgão receptor neuroepitelial para audição, ocupa o assoalho do ducto. SIN ductus cochlearis [TA], Löwenberg canal, Löwenberg scala, membranous cochlea, scala media.
common bile d., d. colédoco. SIN bile d. (1).
common hepatic d. [TA], d. hepático comum; a parte do sistema ductal biliar formada pela confluência dos ductos hepáticos direito e esquerdo. Na porta do fígado recebe o ducto cístico, tornando-se o ducto colédoco. SIN ductus hepaticus communis [TA], hepatocystic d.
craniopharyngeal d., d. craniofaríngeo; a parte tubular fina do divertículo hipofisário; o pedículo da bolsa de Rathke. SIN bucconeural d., hypophysial d.
Cuvier d.'s, ductos de Cuvier; termo obsoleto para as veias cardinais comuns.
cystic d. [TA], d. cístico; o ducto que sai da vesícula biliar; ele se une ao ducto hepático para formar o ducto colédoco. SIN ductus cysticus [TA], cystic gall d.
cystic gall d., d. cístico. SIN cystic d.
deferent d., d. deferente. SIN *ductus* deferens.
efferent d., d. eferente. SIN efferent *ductules* of testis, em *ductule*.

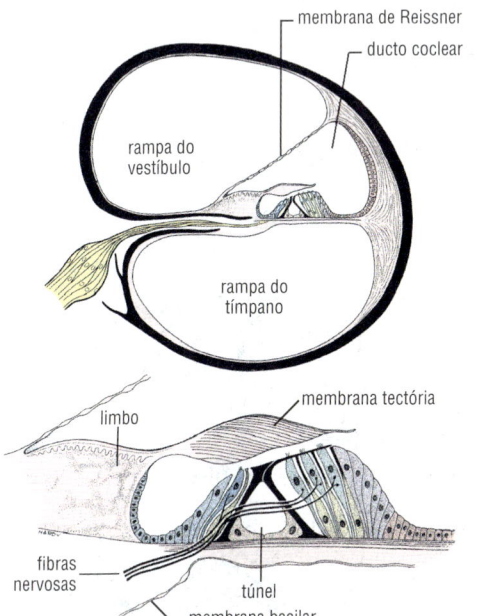

ducto coclear e órgão espiral: corte transversal mostrando fibras e células nervosas (amarelo), células de sustentação (púrpura), células de Hensen (vermelho), estrias vasculares (verde), células ciliadas externas (azul-escuro), células ciliadas internas (preto)

ejaculatory d. [TA], d. ejaculatório; o ducto formado pela união do ducto deferente ao ducto excretor da vesícula seminal, que se abre para a uretra prostática. SIN ductus ejaculatorius [TA], spermiduct (2).
endolymphatic d. [TA], d. endolinfático; pequeno canal membranoso que une o sáculo e o utrículo do labirinto membranáceo, atravessando o aqueduto do vestíbulo e terminando em uma extremidade cega destilada, o saco endolinfático, na superfície posterior da porção petrosa do osso temporal sob a duramáter. SIN ductus endolymphaticus [TA].
d. of epididymis [TA], d. do epidídimo; tubo contorcido no qual se abrem os dúctulos eferentes e que termina no ducto deferente. SIN ductus epididymidis [TA].
excretory d., d. excretor; ducto que leva a secreção de uma glândula ou um líquido de qualquer reservatório. SIN ductus excretorius.
excretory d.'s of lacrimal gland, ductos excretores da glândula lacrimal; os múltiplos (6–10) ductos excretores da glândula lacrimal que se abrem no fórnice superior da conjuntiva. SIN ductuli excretorii glandulae lacrimalis, excretory ductules of lacrimal gland.
excretory d. of seminal gland [TA], d. excretor da glândula seminal; a passagem que vai de uma vesícula seminal até o ducto ejaculatório. SIN ductus excretorius vesiculae seminalis [TA], excretory d. of seminal vesicle*.
excretory d. of seminal vesicle, d. excretor da glândula seminal; *termo oficial alternativo para excretory d. of seminal gland.
frontonasal d., d. frontonasal; a passagem que desce a partir do seio frontal para se abrir no infundíbulo etmoidal.
galactophorous d.'s, ductos galactóforos. SIN lactiferous d.'s.
gall d., termo obsoleto para bile d (ducto biliar).
Gartner d., d. de Gartner. SIN longitudinal d. of epoöphoron.
genital d., d. genital. SIN genital *tract*.
guttural d., tuba auditiva. SIN pharyngotympanic (auditory) *tube*.
hemithoracic d., d. hemitorácico; ducto torácico acessório, geralmente drenando para o ducto torácico, mas algumas vezes drenando independentemente para a veia subclávia direita. SIN ductus hemithoracicus.
Hensen d., d. de Hensen. SIN *ductus* reuniens.
hepatic d., d. hepático. VER common hepatic d., right hepatic d., left hepatic d.
hepatocystic d., d. hepático comum. SIN common hepatic d.
Hoffmann d., d. de Hoffmann. SIN pancreatic d.
hypophysial d., d. hipofisário. SIN craniopharyngeal d.
incisive d. [TA], d. incisivo; ducto rudimentar raro, ou protrusão da mucosa para o canal incisivo, de cada lado da extremidade anterior da crista nasal. SIN ductus incisivus [TA].
intercalated d.'s, ductos intercalados; os pequenos ductos glandulares, como as glândulas salivares e o pâncreas, que saem dos ácinos; são revestidos por células cúbicas baixas.
interlobar d., d. interlobar; ducto que drena a secreção do lobo de uma glândula e é formado pela junção de vários ductos interlobulares.
interlobular d., d. interlobular; qualquer ducto que sai de um lóbulo de uma glândula, sendo formado pela junção dos ductos intralobulares.
intralobular d., d. intralobular; ducto situado em um lóbulo de uma glândula.
jugular d., d. jugular. SIN jugular lymphatic *trunk*.
lactiferous d.'s [TA], ductos lactíferos; um dos ductos, em número de 15 a 20, que drenam os lobos da glândula mamária; eles se abrem no mamilo. SIN ductus lactiferi [TA], canalicular d.'s (1), galactophore, galactophorous canals, galactophorous d.'s, mamillary d.'s, mammary d.'s, milk d.'s, tubuli galactophori, tubuli lactiferi.
left d. of caudate lobe of liver [TA], d. esquerdo do lobo caudado do fígado; tributário do ducto hepático esquerdo que drena bile da metade esquerda do lobo caudado. SIN ductus lobi caudati sinister hepatis [TA].
left hepatic d. [TA], d. hepático esquerdo; o ducto que drena bile da metade esquerda do fígado, incluindo o lobo quadrado e a parte esquerda do lobo caudado. SIN ductus hepaticus sinister [TA].
longitudinal d. of epoöphoron [TA], d. longitudinal do epoóforo; vestígio rudimentar do ducto mesonéfrico na mulher no qual se abrem os túbulos do epoóforo; está localizado no ligamento largo do útero, paralelo à parte lateral da tuba uterina, e nas paredes laterais do colo do útero e da vagina. SIN ductus longitudinalis epoöphori [TA], ductus deferens vestigialis, Gartner canal, Gartner d.
Luschka d.'s, ductos de Luschka; estruturas tubulares, semelhantes a glândulas, na parede da vesícula biliar, sobretudo na parte coberta por peritônio.
lymphatic d., d. linfático; um dos dois grandes canais linfáticos, ducto linfático direito ou ducto torácico.
major sublingual d. [TA], d. sublingual maior; o ducto que drena a porção anterior da glândula sublingual; abre-se na papila sublingual. SIN ductus sublingualis major [TA], Bartholin d.
mamillary d.'s, ductos lactíferos. SIN lactiferous d.'s.
mammary d.'s, ductos lactíferos. SIN lactiferous d.'s.
mesonephric d., d. mesonéfrico; ducto no embrião que drena os túbulos mesonéfricos; no homem, torna-se o ducto deferente; na mulher, torna-se rudimentar. VER TAMBÉM longitudinal d. of epoöphoron. SIN ductus mesonephricus, wolffian d.

metanephric d., d. metanéfrico; a porção tubular delgada do divertículo metanéfrico; o primórdio do revestimento epitelial do ureter. VER epoophoron, longitudinal d. of epoöphoron.
milk d.'s, ductos lactíferos. SIN lactiferous d.'s.
minor sublingual d.'s [TA], ductos sublinguais menores; de 8–20 pequenos ductos da glândula salivar sublingual que se abrem para a boca na superfície da prega sublingual, alguns se unem aos ductos submandibulares. SIN ductus sublinguales minores [TA], Rivinus d.'s, Walther canals, Walther d.'s.
Müller d., müllerian d., d. de Müller. SIN paramesonephric d.
nasal d., d. nasal. SIN nasolacrimal d.
nasolacrimal d. [TA], d. lacrimonasal; a passagem que segue do saco lacrimal para baixo de cada lado até a porção anterior do meato nasal inferior, através do qual as lágrimas são conduzidas até a cavidade nasal. SIN ductus nasolacrimalis [TA], nasal d.
nephric d., d. néfrico. SIN pronephric d.
omphalomesenteric d., d. onfalomesentérico; termo obsoleto para yolk *stalk*.
pancreatic d. [TA], d. pancreático; o ducto excretor do pâncreas que atravessa a glândula da cauda até a cabeça, onde drena para o duodeno na papila duodenal maior. SIN ductus pancreaticus [TA], Hoffmann d., Wirsung canal, Wirsung d.
papillary d.'s, ductos papilares; os maiores ductos excretores retos na medula e papilas renais cujas aberturas formam a área cribriforme que se abre para um cálice menor; são uma continuação dos túbulos coletores. SIN Bellini d.'s.
paramesonephric d., d. paramesonéfrico; um dos dois tubos embrionários que se estendem ao longo do mesonefro aproximadamente paralelos ao ducto mesonéfrico e drenam para a cloaca; na mulher, as partes superiores dos ductos formam as tubas uterinas, enquanto as partes inferiores se fundem para formar o útero e parte da vagina; no homem, vestígios dos ductos formam o utrículo prostático e o apêndice do testículo. SIN ductus paramesonephricus, Müller d., müllerian d.
paraurethral d.'s [TA], ductos paraurentais; ductos inconstantes que seguem ao longo da lateral da uretra feminina, e que conduzem a secreção mucóide das glândulas de Skene para o vestíbulo. SIN ductus paraurethrales [TA], d.'s of Skene glands, Schüller d.'s.
parotid d. [TA], d. parotídeo; o ducto da parótida que se abre da bochecha para o vestíbulo da boca oposto ao colo do segundo dente molar superior. SIN ductus parotideus [TA], Blasius d., Stensen d., Steno d.
Pecquet d., d. de Pecquet. SIN thoracic d.
perilymphatic d., d. perilinfático. SIN cochlear *aqueduct*.
pharyngobranchial d.'s, ductos faringobranquiais. VER *ductus* pharyngobranchialis III, *ductus* pharyngobranchialis IV.
pronephric d., d. pronéfrico; o ducto do pronefro. SIN nephric d.
prostatic d's., ductos prostáticos. SIN prostatic *ductules*, em *ductule*.
right d. of caudate lobe of liver [TA], d. direito do lobo caudado do fígado; o ducto biliar da metade direita do lobo caudado, tributário do ducto hepático direito. SIN ductus lobi caudati dexter hepatis [TA].
right hepatic d. [TA], d. hepático direito; o ducto que conduz a bile da metade direita do fígado e da parte direita do lobo caudado para o ducto hepático comum. SIN ductus hepaticus dexter [TA].
right lymphatic d. [TA], d. linfático direito; um dos dois vasos linfáticos terminais, um tronco curto, com cerca de 2 cm de comprimento, formado pela união do vaso linfático jugular direito e dos vasos dos linfonodos do membro superior direito, parede torácica e ambos os pulmões; situa-se à direita da raiz do pescoço e drena para a veia braquiocefálica direita. Freqüentemente, não é formado ducto linfático direito, com os vasos que normalmente contribuem para sua formação entrando, independentemente, no sistema venoso. SIN ductus lymphaticus dexter [TA], ductus thoracicus dexter*.
Rivinus d.'s, ductos de Rivinus. SIN minor sublingual d.'s.
saccular d. [TA], d. sacular; porção sacular do ducto utriculossacular; estende-se entre o sáculo e o ducto endolinfático. VER TAMBÉM utriculussaccular d. SIN ductus saccularis [TA].
salivary d., d. salivar. SIN striated d.
Santorini d., d. de Santorini. SIN accessory pancreatic d.
Schüller d.'s, ductos de Schüller. SIN paraurethral d.'s.
secretory d., d. secretor. SIN striated d.
semicircular d.'s [TA], ductos semicirculares; três pequenos tubos membranosos nos canais semicirculares ósseos situados no labirinto ósseo e que formam alças de aproximadamente dois terços de um círculo. Os três ductos semicirculares: d. semicircular anterior [TA] (ductus semicircularis anterior [TA]), lateral semicircular d. [TA] (ductus semicircularis lateralis [TA]) e posterior semicircular d. [TA] (ductus semicircularis posterior [TA]) situam-se em planos formando ângulos retos entre si e se abrem para o vestíbulo por cinco aberturas, sendo uma destas comum aos ductos anterior e lateral. Cada ducto possui uma ampola em uma extremidade dentro da qual terminam os filamentos do nervo vestibular. SIN ductus semicirculares [TA].
seminal d., d. seminal; qualquer um dos ductos que conduzem o sêmen do epidídimo para a uretra, ducto deferente ou ducto ejaculatório. SIN gonaduct (1).
d.'s of the Skene glands, ductos das glândulas de Skene. SIN paraurethral d.'s.
spermatic d., d. espermático. SIN *ductus* deferens.
Stensen d., Steno d., d. de Stensen, d. de Steno. SIN parotid d.
striated d., d. estriado; tipo de ducto intralobular encontrado em algumas glândulas salivares que modifica o produto secretor; seu nome provém da extensa invaginação da membrana basal. SIN salivary d., secretory d.
subclavian d., d. subclávio. SIN subclavian lymphatic *trunk*.
submandibular d. [TA], d. submandibular; o ducto da glândula salivar submandibular; abre-se na papila sublingual próximo do frênulo da língua. SIN ductus submandibularis [TA], ductus submaxillaris, submaxillary d., Wharton d.
submaxillary d., d. submaxilar. SIN submandibular d.
sudoriferous d., d. sudorífero. SIN d. of sweat glands.
sweat d., d. sudoríparo. SIN d. of sweat glands.
d. of sweat glands, d. das glândulas sudoríparas; a porção superficial da glândula sudorípara que atravessa o córion e a epiderme, abrindo-se na superfície pelo poro sudoríparo. SIN ductus sudoriferus, sudoriferous d., sweat d.
testicular d., d. testicular. SIN *ductus* deferens.
thoracic d. [TA], d. torácico; o maior vaso linfático no corpo, que começa na cisterna do quilo aproximadamente ao nível da segunda vértebra lombar; a parte abdominal se estende para cima para atravessar a abertura aórtica do diafragma, onde se torna a parte torácica e cruza o mediastino posterior para formar o arco do ducto torácico e drenar para o ângulo venoso esquerdo (origem da veia braquicefálica). SIN ductus thoracicus [TA], Pecquet d., van Horne canal.

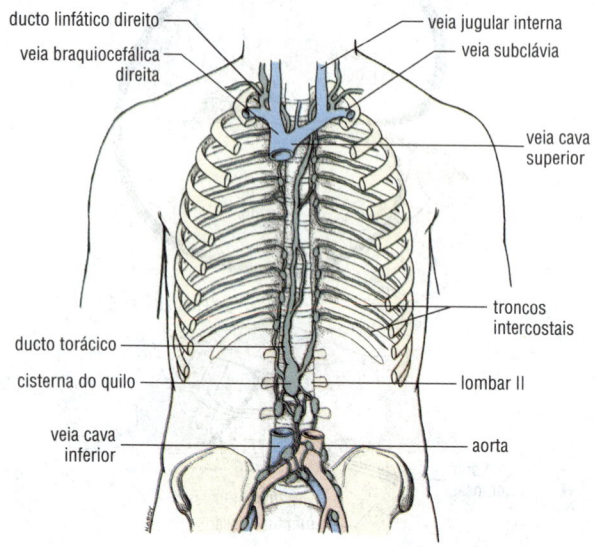

ductos lacrimais

ductos torácico e linfático direito: também são mostrados linfonodos e vasos linfáticos profundos

thyroglossal d. [TA], d. tireoglosso; tubo endodérmico transitório no embrião, que leva tecido formador de tireóide em sua extremidade caudal; normalmente, o ducto desaparece após a tireóide ter se deslocado para sua localização definitiva no pescoço; seu ponto de origem é regularmente marcado na raiz da língua do adulto pelo forame cego; ocasionalmente, sua regressão incompleta resulta na formação de cistos ao longo de seu trajeto embrionário. VER TAMBÉM pyramidal *lobe* of thyroid gland. SIN ductus thyroglossus [TA], thyrolingual d.
thyrolingual d., d. tireolingual. SIN thyroglossal d.
umbilical d., d. umbilical. SIN yolk *stalk*.
uniting d., d. de união. SIN *ductus* reuniens.
utricular d. [TA], d. utricular; porção utricular do d. utriculossacular; estende-se entre o utrículo e o ducto endolinfático. VER TAMBÉM utriculosaccular d. SIN ductus utricularis [TA].
utriculosaccular d. [TA], d. utriculossacular; ducto que conecta a face interna do utrículo ao ducto endolinfático por uma curta distância de sua origem no sáculo. SIN ductus utriculosaccularis [TA], Böttcher canal.
vitelline d., vitellointestinal d., d. vitelino; d. vitelointestinal. SIN yolk *stalk*.
Walther d.'s, ductos de Walther. SIN minor sublingual d.'s.
Wharton d., d. de Wharton. SIN submandibular d.
Wirsung d., d. de Wirsung. SIN pancreatic d.
wolffian d., d. de Wolff. SIN mesonephric d.

duc·tal (dŭk′tăl). Ductal; relativo a um ducto.
duc·tile (dŭk′tĭl). Dúctil; designa a propriedade de um material que pode ser dobrado, esticado (como um fio) ou deformado de outra forma sem se romper. [L. *ductilis*, capaz de ser guiado ou tracionado]
duc·tion (dŭk′shŭn). Ducção; ducção. **1.** O ato de levar, trazer ou conduzir. **2.** Em oftalmologia, rotações oculares em relação a um olho; geralmente designando também a direção do movimento ocular; p. ex., rotação em direção ao nariz, adução; em direção à têmpora, abdução; para cima, supra ou sursundução; para baixo, infradução; do pólo superior da córnea, ciclodução; do pólo superior de uma córnea para fora, exciclodução; do pólo superior de uma córnea para dentro, inciclodução. [L. *duco*, levar]
forced d., d. forçada; manobra para determinar se há obstrução mecânica no olho; segurando com a pinça um músculo ocular, faz-se uma tentativa de mover passivamente o globo ocular na direção da rotação restrita. SIN passive d.
passive d., d. passiva. SIN forced d.
duct·less (dŭkt′les). Sem ducto; que não possui ducto; designa algumas glândulas que possuem apenas secreção interna.
duc·tu·lar (dŭk′too-lăr). Ductular; relativo a um dúctulo.
duc·tule (dŭk′tool). Dúctulo; um pequeno ducto. SIN ductulus.
aberrant d.'s [TA], dúctulos aberrantes; os divertículos superiores ou inferiores do epidídimo. SIN ductuli aberrantes [TA], aberrant ducts, ductus aberrantes, vasa aberrantia.
biliary d.'s, dúctulos biliares; os ductos excretores do fígado que unem os ductos interlobulares ao ducto hepático direito (ou esquerdo). SIN canalicular ducts (2), ductuli biliferi, ductus biliferi, tubuli biliferi.
efferent d.'s of testis [TA], dúctulos eferentes do testículo; 12-14 pequenos ductos seminais que vão do testículo até a cabeça do epidídimo. SIN ductuli efferentes testis [TA], efferent duct, vas efferens (3).
excretory d.'s of lacrimal gland, dúctulos excretores da glândula lacrimal. SIN excretory *ducts* of lacrimal gland, em *duct*.
inferior aberrant d. [TA], d. aberrante inferior; túbulo estreito, espiralado, freqüentemente unido à primeira parte do ducto deferente ou à parte inferior do ducto do epidídimo. SIN ductulus aberrans inferior [TA], Haller vas aberrans.
interlobular d.'s, dúctulos interlobulares; dúctulos biliares que ocupam os canais portais nos lóbulos hepáticos e que se abrem para os dúctulos bilíferos. SIN ductuli interlobulares.
prostatic d.'s [TA], dúctulos prostáticos; cerca de 20 pequenos canais que recebem a secreção prostática dos túbulos glandulares e a expelem através de aberturas de cada lado da crista uretral na parede posterior da uretra. SIN ductuli prostatici [TA], ductus prostatici, prostatic ducts.
superior aberrant d. [TA], d. aberrante superior; divertículo da cabeça do epidídimo. SIN ductulus aberrans superior [TA].
transverse d.'s of epoöphoron [TA], dúctulos transversos do epoóforo; uma série de 10–15 túbulos curtos que se abrem para o ducto longitudinal do epoóforo e representam vestígios do ducto mesonéfrico. SIN ductuli transversi epoöphori [TA], tubuli epoöphori.
duc·tu·lus, pl. **duc·tu·li** (dŭk′too-lŭs, -too-lī). Dúctulo. SIN ductule. [L. Mod. dim. de L. *ductus*, ducto]
d. aberrans infe′rior [TA], d. aberrante inferior. SIN inferior aberrant *ductule*.
d. aberrans supe′rior [TA], d. aberrante superior. SIN superior aberrant *ductule*.
ductuli aberran′tes [TA], dúctulos aberrantes. SIN aberrant *ductules*, em *ductule*.
d. alveola′ris, pl. **duc′tuli alveola′res,** d. alveolar. SIN alveolar *duct*.
duc′tuli bilif′eri, dúctulos bilíferos. SIN biliary *ductules*, em *ductule*.
ductuli efferen′tes tes′tis [TA], dúctulos eferentes do testículo. SIN efferent *ductules* of testis, em *ductule*.
duc′tuli excreto′rii glan′dulae lacrima′lis, dúctulos excretores da glândula lacrimal. SIN excretory *ducts* of lacrimal gland, em *duct*.
duc′tuli interlobula′res, dúctulos interlobulares. SIN interlobular *ductules*, em *ductule*.
duc′tuli paroöph′ori, dúctulos paraoóforos; remanescentes tubulares do mesonefro embrionário que formam o paraoóforo. SIN tubuli paroöphori.
duc′tuli prostat′ici [TA], dúctulos prostáticos. SIN prostatic *ductules*, em *ductule*.
duc′tuli transver′si epoöph′ori [TA], dúctulos transversos do epoóforo. SIN transverse *ductules* of epoöphoron, em *ductule*. VER TAMBÉM epoophoron.

DUCTUS

duc·tus, gen. e pl. **duc·tus** (dŭk′tŭs) [TA]. Ducto. SIN duct. [L. que leva, de *duco*, pp. *ductus*, levar]
d. aber′rantes, d. aberrante. SIN aberrant *ductules*, em *ductule*.
d. arterio′sus, canal arterial; vaso fetal que une a artéria pulmonar esquerda à aorta descendente; nos primeiros dois meses após o nascimento, normalmente se transforma em um cordão fibroso, o ligamento arterial; a perviedade pós-natal persistente é uma deficiência cardiovascular corrigível. SIN arterial canal, arterial duct, Botallo duct.
d. biliaris [TA], d. biliar. SIN bile *duct* (2).
d. bilif′eri, d. bilífero. SIN biliary *ductules*, em *ductule*.
d. carot′icus, d. carótico; parte da aorta dorsal embrionária entre pontos de junção com as artérias do terceiro e quarto arcos; desaparece no início do desenvolvimento. SIN carotid duct.
d. choled′ochus [TA], d. colédoco. SIN bile *duct* (1).
d. cochlea′ris [TA], d. coclear. SIN cochlear *duct*.
d. cys′ticus [TA], d. cístico. SIN cystic *duct*.
d. def′erens [TA], d. deferente; o ducto secretor do testículo, que vai do epidídimo, do qual é a continuação, até a uretra prostática, onde termina como o ducto ejaculatório. SIN deferent canal, deferent duct, spermatic duct, spermiduct (1), testicular duct, vas deferens.
d. def′erens vestigia′lis, d. deferente vestigial. SIN longitudinal *duct* of epoöphoron.
d. diverticulum, d. diverticular. SIN ductal *aneurysm*.
d. dorsopancreat′icus, d. pancreático acessório. SIN accessory pancreatic *duct*.
d. ejaculato′rius [TA], d. ejaculatório. SIN ejaculatory *duct*.
d. endolymphat′icus [TA], d. endolinfático. SIN endolymphatic *duct*.
d. epididym′idis [TA], d. do epidídimo. SIN *duct* of epididymis.
d. excreto′rius, d. excretor. SIN excretory *duct*.
d. excretorius glandulae vesiculosae [TA], d. excretor da glândula seminal. SIN ductus excretorius vesiculae seminalis.
d. excreto′rius vesic′ulae semina′lis [TA], d. excretor da glândula seminal. SIN excretory *duct* of seminal gland.
d. glan′dulae bulbourethra′lis [TA], d. da glândula bulbouretral. SIN *duct* of bulbourethral gland.
d. hemithorac′icus, d. hemitorácico. SIN hemithoracic *duct*.
d. hepat′icus commu′nis [TA], d. hepático comum. SIN common hepatic *duct*.
d. hepat′icus dex′ter [TA], d. hepático direito. SIN right hepatic *duct*.
d. hepat′icus sinis′ter [TA], d. hepático esquerdo. SIN left hepatic *duct*.
d. incisi′vus [TA], d. incisivo. SIN incisive *duct*.
d. lactif′eri [TA], ductos lactíferos. SIN lactiferous *ducts*, em *duct*.
d. lingua′lis, d. lingual; uma depressão na superfície superior da língua no ápice do sulco terminal; ela marca o ponto de origem do ducto tireoglosso do embrião; conhecido mais comumente como o forame cego.
d. lo′bi cauda′ti dex′ter hepatis [TA], d. direito do lobo caudado do fígado. SIN right *duct* of caudate lobe of liver.
d. lo′bi cauda′ti sinis′ter hepatis [TA], d. esquerdo do lobo caudado do fígado. SIN left *duct* of caudate lobe of liver.
d. longitudina′lis epoöph′ori [TA], d. longitudinal do epoóforo. SIN longitudinal *duct* of epoöphoron. VER TAMBÉM epoöphoron.
d. lymphat′icus dex′ter [TA], d. linfático direito. SIN right lymphatic *duct*.
d. mesoneph′ricus, d. mesonéfrico. SIN mesonephric *duct*. VER TAMBÉM longitudinal *duct* of epoöphoron.
d. nasolacrima′lis [TA], d. lacrimonasal. SIN nasolacrimal *duct*.
d. pancreat′icus [TA], d. pancreático. SIN pancreatic *duct*.
d. pancreat′icus accesso′rius [TA], d. pancreático acessório. SIN accessory pancreatic *duct*.
d. paramesoneph′ricus, d. paramesonéfrico. SIN paramesonephric *duct*.
d. paraurethra′les [TA], ductos paraauretrais. SIN paraurethral *ducts*, em *duct*.
d. parotid′eus [TA], d. parotídeo. SIN parotid *duct*.
patent d. arterio′sus, persistência do canal arterial (PCA). VER d. arteriosus.
d. perilymphat′icus, aqueduto da cóclea. SIN cochlear *aqueduct*.
d. pharyngobranchia′lis III, d. faringobranquial III; comunicação estreita entre a terceira bolsa branquial e a faringe no embrião.

d. pharyngobranchia'lis IV, d. faringobranquial IV, comunicação estreita entre a quarta bolsa branquial e a faringe no embrião.
d. prostat'ici, dúctulos prostáticos. SIN prostatic *ductules*, em *ductule*.
d. reun'iens [TA], d. de união; tubo membranoso curto que vai da extremidade inferior do sáculo até o ducto coclear do labirinto membranáceo. SIN canaliculus reuniens, canalis reuniens, Hensen canal, Hensen duct, uniting canal, uniting duct.
d. saccularis [TA], d. sacular. SIN saccular *duct*.
d. semicircula'res [TA], ductos semicirculares. SIN semicircular *ducts*, em *duct*.
d. sublingua'les mino'res [TA], ductos sublinguais menores. SIN minor sublingual *ducts*, em *duct*.
d. sublingua'lis ma'jor [TA], d. sublingual maior. SIN major sublingual *duct*.
d. submandibula'ris [TA], d. submandibular. SIN submandibular *duct*.
d. submaxilla'ris [TA], d. submaxilar. SIN submandibular *duct*.
d. sudorif'erus, d. sudorífero. SIN duct of sweat glands.
d. thorac'icus [TA], d. torácico. SIN thoracic *duct*.
d. thorac'icus dex'ter, d. torácico direito; *termo oficial alternativo para right lymphatic *duct*.
d. thyroglos'sus [TA], d. tireoglosso. SIN thyroglossal *duct*.
d. utricularis [TA], d. utricular. SIN utricular *duct*.
d. utric'ulosaccula'ris [TA], d. utriculosacular. SIN utriculosaccular *duct*.
d. veno'sus, d. venoso; no feto, a continuação da veia umbilical esquerda através do fígado até a veia cava inferior; após o nascimento, sua luz é obliterada, formando o ligamento venoso.
d. veno'sus aran'tii, termo raramente usado para d. venosus.

Duddell, Benedict, oculista inglês do século XVIII. VER D. *membrane*.
Duffy blood group. Grupo sanguíneo de Duffy. Ver apêndice de Grupos Sanguíneos.
Dugas, Louis A., médico norte-americano, 1806–1884.
Duhring, Louis A., dermatologista norte-americano, 1845–1913. VER D. *disease*.
Dührssen, Alfred, ginecologista-obstreta alemão, 1862–1933. VER D. *incisions*, em *incision*.
Duke, William Waddell Duke, patologista norte-americano, 1883–1945. VER D. bleeding time *test*.
Dukes, Clement, médico inglês, 1845–1925. VER D. *disease*; Filatov-D. *disease*.
Dukes, Cuthbert E., patologista inglês, 1890–1977. VER D. *classification*.
dul·cin (dŭl'sĭn). Dulcina; tem sido usada como substituta para o açúcar, sendo 200 vezes mais doce que o açúcar de cana. Devido à hidrólise em aminofenol, pode produzir um efeito prejudicial quando usada durante longos períodos.
dul·cite, dul·ci·tol, dul·cose (dŭl'sĭt, -si'tol, -kōs). Dulcita, dulcitol, dulcose; galactitol.
dull (dŭl). Obtuso; deprimido; sem fio; cego; apático; inerte; vago; impreciso; surdo; não-afiado nem agudo, em qualquer sentido; qualificando um instrumento cirúrgico, a ação da mente, a dor, um som (principalmente a nota de percussão), etc. [I.M. *dul*]
dull·ness, dul·ness (dŭl'nes). Macicez; o caráter do som obtido por percussão sobre uma parte sólida incapaz de ressoar; geralmente aplicado a uma área contendo menos ar que aquelas que conseguem ressoar.
shifting d., m. móvel, m. de decúbito; sinal de líquido peritoneal livre no qual a macicez à percussão muda de lugar, geralmente de um lado para o outro, quando o paciente é virado de um lado para outro.
Dulong, Pierre L, químico francês, 1785–1838. VER D.-Petit *law*.
dum·my (dŭm'ē). Dente artificial em uma prótese dentária parcial fixa. SIN pontic.
Dumontpallier, Alphonse, médico francês, 1827–1899. VER D. *pessary*.
dump·ing (dŭmp'ing). Despejar; descarregar; esvaziar. SIN dumping *syndrome*.
Duncan, James M., ginecologista escocês, 1826–1890. VER Duncan *folds*, em *fold*, Duncan *mechanism*, Duncan *placenta*, Duncan *ventricle*.
Duncan. Sobrenome dos primeiros pacientes estudados afetados pelo que agora é conhecido como doença de Duncan (Duncan *disease*).
Dunn, Richard L. VER Lison-D. *stain*.
du·o·crin·in (doo-ō-krĭn'ĭn). Duocrinina; suposto hormônio gastrointestinal liberado pelo contato do conteúdo gástrico com o intestino e que estimula a atividade secretora das glândulas duodenais (glândulas de Brunner). [duodenum + G. *krinō*, secretar, + -in]
du·o·de·nal (doo'ō-dē'năl, doo-od'ĕ-năl). Duodenal; relativo ao duodeno.
du·o·de·nec·to·my (doo-ō-dē-nek'tō-mē). Duodenectomia; excisão do duodeno. [duodenum + G. *ektomē*, excisão]
du·o·de·ni·tis (doo-od-ē-nī'tis). Duodenite; inflamação do duodeno.
♲ **duodeno-.** Forma combinante relativa ao duodeno. [L. *duodenum*, scil., *digitorum* largura de 12 dedos]
du·o·de·no·cho·lan·gi·tis (doo-ō-dē'nō-kō-lan-jī'tis). Duodenocolangite; inflamação do duodeno e do ducto colédoco. [duodeno- + G. *cholē*, bile, + *angeion*, vaso, + -itis, inflamação]

du·o·de·no·cho·le·cys·tos·to·my (doo-ō-dē'nō-kō-lē-sis-tos'tō-mē). Duodenocolecistostomia. SIN cholecystoduodenostomy. [duodeno- + G. *cholē*, bile, + *kystis*, bexiga, + *stoma*, boca]
du·o·de·no·cho·led·o·chot·o·my (doo-ō-dē'nō-kō-led-ō-kot'ō-mē). Duodenocoledocotomia; incisão do ducto colédoco e da porção adjacente do duodeno. [duodeno- + G. *cholèdochus*, ducto colédoco, + *tomē*, incisão]
du·o·de·no·cys·tos·to·my (doo-ō-dē'nō-sis-tos'tō-mē). Duodenocistostomia. **1.** SIN cholecystoduodenostomy. **2.** SIN cystoduodenostomy. **3.** SIN pancreatic *cystoduodenostomy*.
du·o·de·no·en·ter·os·to·my (doo-ō-dē'nō-en-ter-os'tō-mē). Duodenoenterostomia; estabelecimento de comunicação entre o duodeno e outra parte do trato intestinal. [duodeno- + G. *enteron*, intestino, + *stoma*, boca]
du·o·de·no·je·ju·nos·to·my (doo-ō-dē'nō-jē-joo-nos'tō-mē). Duodenojejunostomia; formação cirúrgica de uma comunicação artificial entre o duodeno e o jejuno. [duodeno- + jejunum, + G. *stoma*, boca]
du·o·de·nol·y·sis (doo-ō-dē-nol'i-sis). Duodenólise; incisão de aderências no duodeno. [duodeno- + G. *lysis*, lise, liberação]
du·o·de·nor·rha·phy (doo-ō-dē-nōr'ă-fē). Duodenorrafia; sutura de uma ruptura ou incisão no duodeno. [duodeno- + G. *rhaphē*, sutura]
du·o·de·nos·co·py (doo-ō-dē-nos'kō-pē). Duodenoscopia; inspeção do interior do duodeno através de um endoscópio. [duodeno- + G. *skopeō*, examinar]
du·o·de·nos·to·my (doo-ō-dē-nos'tō-mē). Duodenostomia; estabelecimento de uma fístula para o duodeno. [duodeno- + G. *stoma*, boca]
du·o·de·not·o·my (doo-ō-dē-not'ō-mē). Duodenotomia; incisão do duodeno. [duodeno- + G. *tomē*, incisão]
🛈 **du·o·de·num,** gen. **du·o·de·ni,** pl. **du·o·de·na** (doo-ō-dē'nŭm, doo-od'ĕ-nŭm; -od'ĕ-nă, -dē'nă). [TA]. Duodeno; a primeira divisão do intestino delgado, com cerca de 25 cm ou 12 dedos transversos (daí seu nome) de comprimento, que se estende do piloro até a junção com o jejuno ao nível da primeira ou segunda vértebra lombar do lado esquerdo. É dividido na parte superior, cuja primeira parte é a ampola; a parte descendente, na qual se abrem os ductos colédoco e pancreático, a parte horizontal (inferior) e a parte ascendente, terminando na junção duodenojejunal. [L. Mediev. do L. *duodeni*, doze]
du·o·vi·rus (doo'ō-vī'rŭs). Duovírus. SIN rotavirus.
du.plex (doo'pleks). Dúplex; que possui duas funções. VER duplex *ultrasonography*.
du·pli·ca·tion (doo-pli-kā'shŭn). **1.** Duplicação. VER TAMBÉM reduplication. **2.** Inclusão de duas cópias do mesmo material genético em um genoma; uma etapa importante na diversificação de genomas, como na evolução das cadeias de hemoglobina (não-alelas) a partir de um ancestral comum. SIN gene d. [L. *duplicatio*, duplicação, de *duplico*, duplicar]
d. of chromosomes, d. cromossomial; aberração cromossomial resultante de cruzamento desigual ou troca de segmentos entre dois cromossomas homólogos; um cromossoma do par perde um pequeno segmento, enquanto o outro ganha esse segmento; o cromossoma que ganhou o segmento sofreu duplicação, enquanto seu homólogo sofreu deleção. VER *hemoglobin* Lepore.
gene d., d. genética. SIN duplication (2).
du·pli·ci·tas (doo-plis'i-tahs). Duplicidade; duplicação de uma parte. [L. duplicação, de *duplex* (*duplic*-), duas vezes]

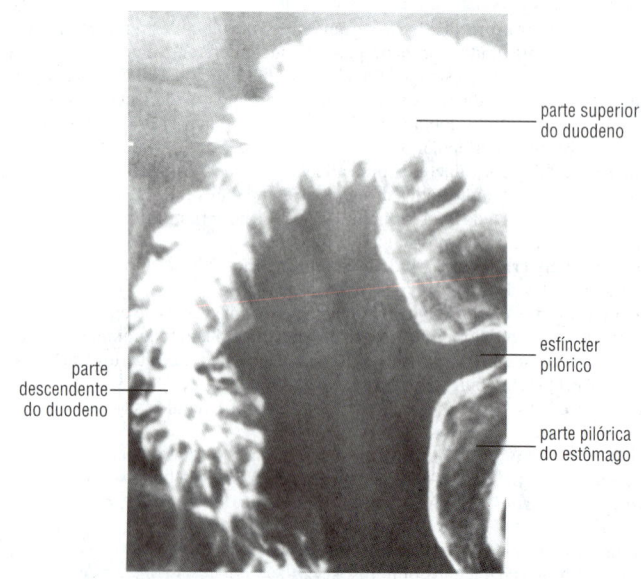

duodeno: radiografia após ingestão de bário

d. ante′rior, d. anterior; gêmeos conjugados nos quais há dois tórax e duas cabeças e uma pelve única com um par de membros inferiores. VER conjoined *twins,* em *twin.* VER TAMBÉM cephalodidymus, ileadelphus, iliadelphus. SIN catadidymus.

d. poste′rior, d. posterior; gêmeos conjugados nos quais há apenas uma cabeça e a parte superior do tronco é única, com nádegas e pernas duplicadas. VER conjoined *twins,* em *twin.* VER TAMBÉM dipygus. SIN anadidymus, ileadelphus, iliadelphus.

Dupré, cirurgião e anatomista parisiense do século XVII. VER D. *muscle.*

Dupuytren, Baron Guillaume, cirurgião e patologista cirúrgico francês, 1777–1835. VER D. *amputation, canal, contracture, disease* of the foot, *fascia, fracture, hydrocele, sign, suture, tourniquet.*

du·ra (doo′rā). [TA]. Dura-máter. SIN dura mater. [L. fem. de *durus,* duro]

d. mater cranialis [TA], d.m., parte encefálica. SIN cranial *dura mater.*

dur·a·en·ceph·a·lo·syn·gi·o·sis (door′a - en - sef′a - lō - sin - anj - ē - ō′sis). Dura-encefalo-sinangiose; transposição cirúrgica da artéria temporal superficial com a aponeurose epicrânica fixada à dura subjacente, com probabilidade de revascularização cerebral; usada mais comumente na síndrome moyamoya. SIN encephaloduroarteriosynangiosis.

du·ral (doo′rāl). Dural; relativo à dura-máter. SIN duramatral.

du·ra mat·er (doo′rā mā′ter) [TA]. Dura-máter (d.m.); paquimeninge (distinta da leptomeninge, a pia-máter e a aracnóide combinadas); membrana fibrosa, firme, que forma o revestimento externo do sistema nervoso central. SIN dura [TA], pachymeninx [TA]. [L. mãe dura, tradução incorreta do Ar. *umm al - jāfiyah,* proteção ou revestimento firme]

d.m. of brain, dura-máter, parte encefálica. SIN cranial d.m.

cranial d.m. [TA], d.m., parte encefálica; a dura-máter intracraniana, que consiste em duas camadas: a *camada periosteal* externa, que normalmente sempre adere ao periósteo dos ossos da abóbada craniana; e a *camada meníngea* interna, que, na maioria dos locais, se funde à externa. As duas camadas se separam para acomodar vasos meníngeos e grandes seios venosos (durais). A camada meníngea também é envolvida na formação das várias pregas de dura-máter, como a foice do cérebro e a tenda do cerebelo, sendo comparável e contínua com a dura-máter da medula espinal. O espaço peridural craniano é então um espaço criado como artefato entre o osso e o periósteo/camada periosteal da dura-máter combinados, que surge apenas em virtude de processos patológicos ou traumáticos, e não é contínuo com nem comparável ao espaço epidural vertebral. SIN dura mater cranialis [TA], d.m. encephali*, cerebral part of dura mater, d.m. of brain.

d.m. enceph′ali, d.m., parte encefálica; *termo oficial alternativo para cranial d.m.

spinal d.m. [TA], d.m., parte espinal; membrana forte com apenas uma camada, comparável à, e contínua com a, camada meníngea da d.m. intracraniana do encéfalo (no forame magno). Ao contrário da d.m., parte encefálica, não adere às estruturas ósseas de revestimento (vértebras) nem ao seu periósteo, estando separada deste último por um espaço considerável, o espaço epidural vertebral — um espaço verdadeiro que contém o plexo venoso vertebral interno incrustado em uma matriz de gordura epidural. SIN d.m. spinalis [TA], d.m. of spinal cord, endorrhachis, theca vertebralis.

d.m. of spinal cord, d.m., parte espinal. SIN spinal d.m.

d.m. spina′lis [TA], d.m., parte espinal. SIN spinal d.m.

du·ra·ma·tral (doo - rā - ma̱′trāl). Dural. SIN dural.

Duran-Reynals, Francisco, bacteriologista norte-americano, 1899–1958. VER Duran-Reynals permeability *factor.*

du·ra·plas·ty (doo′rā - plas - tē). Duraplastia; cirurgia de reconstrução na dura-máter aberta que envolve um fechamento primário ou secundário com outro tecido mole (p. ex., músculo, fáscia, aloenxerto de dura-máter). [dura (mater) + G. *plastos,* formado]

du·ra·tion (D) (doo - rā′shŭn). Duração; um período contínuo de tempo.

half amplitude pulse d., d. do pulso de meia-amplitude; o tempo, em milissegundos, necessário para uma onda alcançar metade de sua magnitude completa.

pulse wave d., d. do pulso; o intervalo entre o início e o fim de uma onda de pulso.

Dürck, Hermann, patologista alemão, 1869–1941. VER D. *nodes,* em *node.*

dur. dolor. Abreviatura do L. *duarte dolare,* enquanto persistir a dor.

Duret, Henri, neurocirurgião francês, 1849–1921. VER D. *lesion, hemorrhage.*

Durham, Arthur E., cirurgião inglês, 1834–1895. VER D. *tube.*

Duroziez, Paul L., médico francês, 1826–1897. VER D. *disease, murmur, sign.*

DUSN Acrônimo para diffuse unilateral subacute *neuroretinitis* (neurorretinite subaguda unilateral difusa).

dUTP Abreviatura de deoxyuridine 5-triphosphate (desoxiuridina 5-trifosfato)

Dutton, Joseph Everett, médico inglês, 1877–1905. VER D. *disease,* relapsing *fever.*

Duverney, Guichaud Joseph, anatomista francês, 1648–1730. VER D. *fissures,* em *fissure, gland, muscle.*

dwarf (dwōrf). Anão; pessoa de tamanho anormalmente pequeno com desproporção entre as partes do corpo. VER dwarfism. [A.S. *dweorh*]

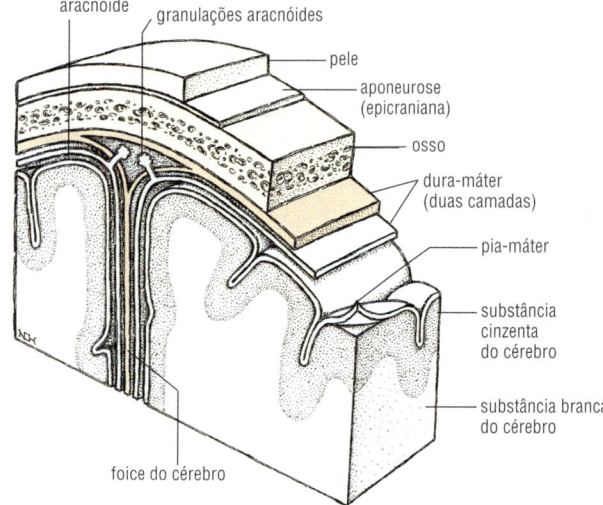

dura-máter: e estruturas associadas do couro cabeludo, crânio e meninges (vista coronal)

hypophysial d., anão hipofisário; nanismo resultante de deficiência da produção de hormônio do crescimento causada por anormalidade hipotalâmica ou hipofisária. SIN pituitary d.

hypothyroid d., anão hipotireóideo; nanismo associado à ausência de função tireóidea.

pituitary d., anão hipofisário. SIN hypophysial d.

dwarf·ism (dwōrf′izm). Nanismo; condição ou grupo de condições nas quais a altura da pessoa está abaixo do 3.º percentil.

achondroplastic d., nanismo acondroplásico. VER achondroplasia.

acromelic d., nanismo acromélico. SIN acromesomelic d.

acromesomelic d., nanismo acromesomélico; forma de nanismo de membros curtos, caracterizada por nariz chato e encurtamento especialmente notável do segmento distal dos membros, isto é, os antebraços e pernas, dedos das mãos e dos pés; herança autossômica recessiva. SIN acromelic d., acromesomelia.

aortic d., nanismo aórtico; subdesenvolvimento da estatura física associado à estenose aórtica grave.

asexual d., nanismo assexual; nanismo no qual o desenvolvimento sexual do adulto é deficiente.

ateliotic d., nanismo ateliótico. SIN panhypopituitarism.

camptomelic d., nanismo camptomélico; nanismo com encurtamento dos membros inferiores devido à curvatura para a frente do fêmur e da tíbia.

chondrodystrophic d., nanismo condrodistrófico. VER chondrodystrophy.

deprivation d., nanismo por privação; baixa estatura devida à privação emocional. SIN psychosocial d.

diastrophic d. [MIM*222600], nanismo diastrófico. SIN diastrophic *dysplasia.*

disproportionate d., nanismo desproporcional; nanismo caracterizado por encurtamento mais significativo dos membros ou do tronco; quando há envolvimento primário dos membros, o encurtamento pode predominar nos segmentos proximais (rizomelia), segmentos médios (mesomelia) ou segmentos distais (acromelia); geralmente resulta de displasias ósseas intrínsecas hereditárias.

Fröhlich d., nanismo de Fröhlich; nanismo com síndrome de Fröhlich.

Hunter-Thompson d. [MIM*201250], nanismo de Hunter-Thompson; forma grave de nanismo acromesomélico, caracterizada por encurtamento dos segmentos distais dos membros; os membros inferiores apresentam acometimento mais grave que os membros superiores; freqüentemente associado a luxações dos cotovelos, joelhos e quadris. Herança autossômica recessiva, causada por mutações no gene da proteína morfogenética 1 derivada da cartilagem (CDMP1) no cromossoma 20q.

hypothyroid d., nanismo hipotireóideo. SIN infantile *hypothyroidism.*

infantile d., nanismo infantil. SIN infantilism (1.).

Laron type d., nanismo do tipo Laron; nanismo associado a ausência ou níveis muito baixos de somatomedina C (fator de crescimento insulino-símile I) ou anormalidades na atividade do receptor.

lethal d., nanismo letal; nanismo que leva à morte intra-uterina ou neonatal.

Lorain-Lévi d., nanismo de Lorain-Lévi. SIN pituitary d.

mesomelic d., nanismo mesomélico; nanismo com encurtamento dos antebraços e das pernas.

metatropic d. [MIM*250600], nanismo metatrópico; displasia óssea caracterizada por nanismo desproporcional no qual o tronco é longo em relação aos membros ao nascimento, mas sofre inversão dessa proporção com subseqüen-

te desenvolvimento, com cifoescoliose acentuada e progressiva; há alargamento metafisário dos ossos longos, a pelve tem formato de alabarda e o cóccix é longo, resultando em um apêndice sacral; herança autossômica recessiva.
micromelic d., nanismo micromélico; nanismo com membros anormalmente curtos ou pequenos.
panhypopituitary d., nanismo por pan-hipopituitarismo; o tipo I é um distúrbio autossômico recessivo com deficiência de hormônio do crescimento humano, ACTH, FSH, etc., que possui desenvolvimento sexual tardio, hipotireoidismo e insuficiência supra-renal; o tipo II é semelhante, mas é um distúrbio ligado ao X.
phocomelic d., nanismo focomélico; nanismo no qual as diáfises dos ossos longos são anormalmente curtas ou as partes intermediárias dos membros estão ausentes.
physiologic d., nanismo fisiológico; nanismo caracterizado por desenvolvimento normal em uma velocidade muitíssimo menor em relação à do desenvolvimento de outros membros da mesma família, raça ou de outras raças. SIN primordial d., true d.
pituitary d., nanismo hipofisário; uma forma rara de nanismo causada pela ausência de uma hipófise anterior funcional; pode estar presente ao nascimento ou desenvolver-se durante os primeiros anos de vida. SIN Lorain-Lévi d., Lorain-Lévi infantilism, Lorain-Lévi syndrome, pituitary infantilism.
primordial d., nanismo primordial. SIN physiologic d.
proportionate d., nanismo proporcional; nanismo caracterizado por encurtamento simétrico dos membros e do tronco; geralmente resulta de anormalidades químicas, endócrinas, nutricionais ou não-ósseas.
psychosocial d., nanismo psicossocial. SIN deprivation d.
rhizomelic d., nanismo rizomélico; uma das síndromes de condrodisplasia pontilhada (q.v.), autossômica recessiva, com distúrbios variáveis de queratinização cutânea e anormalidades faciais, cardíacas, ópticas e do sistema nervoso central variáveis; também há pontilhado epifisário. Há múltiplos defeitos enzimáticos, incluindo nos peroxissomas, e os lactentes afetados não se desenvolvem e, geralmente, morrem durante o primeiro ano de vida.
Robinow d., nanismo de Robinow. SIN Robinow syndrome.
Seckel d., nanismo de Seckel. SIN Seckel syndrome.
senile d., nanismo senil; nanismo caracterizado por anomalias craniofaciais com aspecto progeróide.
sexual d., nanismo sexual; nanismo com desenvolvimento sexual normal.
Silver-Russell d., nanismo de Silver-Russell. SIN Silver-Russell syndrome.
snub-nose d. [MIM*127100], nanismo de nariz arrebitado; nanismo caracterizado por baixo peso ao nascimento, nariz arrebitado e constituição atarracada; herança autossômica dominante. Há um fenótipo autossômico recessivo semelhante [MIM*223600]. SIN dominantly inherited Lévi disease.
thanatophoric d., nanismo tanatofórico; nanismo letal caracterizado por micromelia, ossos longos arqueados, cabeça aumentada, corpos vertebrais achatados e hipotonia muscular; a ausência de ventilação pulmonar causa dificuldades respiratórias com cianose, que causa morte nas primeiras horas ou dias após o nascimento.
true d., nanismo verdadeiro. SIN physiologic d.
Dwyer, Frederick, cirurgião ortopédico inglês, 1920–1975. VER D. *osteotomy.*
Dy Símbolo de dysprosium (dispróprio).
dy·ad (dī′ad). Díade. **1.** Um par. SIN diad (2). **2.** Em química, um elemento bivalente. **3.** Um par de pessoas em uma situação de interação, p. ex., paciente e terapeuta, marido e mulher. **4.** O cromossoma duplo resultante da divisão de uma tétrade durante a meiose. **5.** Duas unidades tratadas como uma. **6.** Um par de células resultantes da primeira divisão meiótica. [G. *dyas*, o número dois, dualidade]
dy·clo·nine hy·dro·chlo·ride (dī′klō - nēn). Cloridrato de diclonina; anestésico local tópico.
dy·dro·ges·ter·one (dī - drō - jes′ter - ōn). Didrogesterona; esteróide sintético, derivado da retroprogesterona, com efeitos progestacionais.
dye (dī). Corante; um corante ou material de coloração; uma substância que consiste em grupamentos cromóforo e auxocromo fixados a um ou mais anéis benzeno, sendo sua cor devida ao cromóforo e suas afinidades de coloração ao auxocromo. Os corantes são usados para coloração intravital de células vivas, coloração de tecidos e microrganismos, como anti-sépticos e germicidas, e alguns como estimulantes do crescimento epitelial. Quanto aos corantes individuais, ver os nomes específicos. Termo comumente, mas impropriamente, usado para contraste radiográfico. [A.S. *deah, deag*]
acidic d.'s, corantes ácidos; corantes que se ionizam em solução para produzir íons negativamente carregados ou ânions; consistem em sais sódicos de fenóis e corantes de ácido carboxílico; suas soluções tendem a ser neutras ou discretamente alcalinas; são exemplos a eosina e o azul de anilina.
acridine d.'s, corantes acridina; derivados da substância acridina, que está intimamente relacionada ao xanteno; importantes como fluorocromos em histologia, citoquímica e quimioterapia; os exemplos incluem acriflavina, laranja de acridina e quinacrina-mostarda.
azin d.'s, corantes azina; corantes derivados da fenazina que incluem importantes corantes histológicos, como vermelho neutro, azocarmina G e safranina O.
azo d.'s, corantes azo; corantes nos quais o grupamento azo é o cromóforo e une anéis benzeno ou naftaleno; incluem um grande número de corantes biológicos, como o vermelho Congo e o óleo vermelho O; também usado clinicamente para promover o crescimento epitelial no tratamento de úlceras, queimaduras e outras feridas; muitos possuem ação anticoagulante.
azocarmine d.'s, corantes de azocarmim; corantes que produzem uma cor vermelho-púrpura escura como corantes histológicos.
basic d.'s, corantes básicos; corantes que se ionizam em solução para produzir íons positivamente carregados ou cátions; o grupamento auxocromo é uma amina que pode formar um sal com um ácido como o HCl; as soluções geralmente são um pouco ácidas; os exemplos incluem fucsina básica e azul de toluidina O.
chlorotriazine d.'s, corantes clorotriazina; corantes que contêm uma ou mais porções clorotriazina que reagem com polissacarídeos.
diphenylmethane d.'s, corantes difenilmetano; corantes nos quais o carbono central que une dois grupamentos fenil não possui um grupameto amino ou imino; o cromóforo é o anel quinóide; uma formulação alternativa é como uma cetonimida; o exemplo mais comum é a auramina O.
ketonimine d.'s, corantes cetonimina; corantes nos quais o cromóforo é o =C=NH unido a dois anéis benzeno; são acrescentados grupamentos alquilamino na posição para- ao carbono de metano em ambos os anéis. O membro mais importante para fins biológicos é a auramina O; uma formulação alternativa é como um corante difenilmetano.
natural d.'s, corantes naturais; corantes obtidos de animais ou vegetais; os exemplos incluem carmim, obtido da cochinilha no inseto fêmea dessecado *Dactylopius coccus* da América Central, e hematoxilina, extraído da casca do pau-campeche *Haematoxylon campechianum* na região do Caribe.
nitro d.'s, corantes nitro; corantes nos quais o cromóforo é $-NO_2$, que é tão ácido que todos os corantes desse grupamento são do tipo ácido; exemplos importantes na coloração citoplasmática são ácido pícrico e amarelo naftol S.
oxazin d.'s, corantes oxazina; semelhantes aos corantes azina, porém um dos átomos N conectantes é substituído por O; os representantes mais importantes são o azul de cresil brilhante, a orceína, o litmo e o violeta de cresil.
rosanilin d.'s, corantes rosanilina; vários corantes triaminotrifenilmetano ou misturas deles freqüentemente vendidos com o nome de fucsina básica; os corantes rosanilina diferem de outros corantes trifenilmetano porque os grupamentos amino não são substituídos, e podem ter grupamentos metil introduzidos diretamente nos anéis benzeno; os quatro corantes possíveis são pararrosanilina, rosanilina, nova fucsina e magenta II.
salt d., c. salino. SIN neutral stain.
synthetic d.'s, corantes sintéticos; compostos orgânicos originalmente derivados do alcatrão; atualmente produzidos por síntese a partir do benzeno e seus derivados; os exemplos incluem a eosina, o azul de metileno e a fluoresceína.
thiazin d.'s, corantes tiazina; semelhantes aos corantes azina, exceto por um dos átomos N conectantes ser substituído por S; incluem muitos corantes biológicos importantes, principalmente em hematologia, p. ex., azure A, azure B e azul de metileno.
triphenylmethane d.'s, corantes trifenilmetano; grupo de corantes que inclui pararrosanilina, bem como muitos outros usados em histologia e citologia; empregados como corantes nucleares, citoplasmáticos e do tecido conjuntivo; importantes em histoquímica como no preparo do reagente de Schiff.
xanthene d.'s, corantes xanteno; derivados do composto xanteno; incluem as pironinas, rodaminas e fluoresceínas.
Dyggve, Holger, pediatra dinamarquês, 1913–1984. VER D.-Melchior-Clausen *syndrome.*
-dymus. -dimo. **1.** Sufixo a ser combinado com raízes numéricas; p. ex., dídimo, trídimo, tetradimo. **2.** Algumas vezes é a forma reduzida de -didymus. [G. *-dymos*, dobra]
dy·nam·ics (dī - nam′iks). Dinâmica. **1.** A ciência de movimento em resposta a forças. **2.** Em psiquiatria, usado como contração de psicodinâmica. **3.** Nas ciências comportamentais, qualquer das numerosas influências intrapessoais e interpessoais ou fenômenos associados ao desenvolvimento da personalidade e processos interpessoais. [G. *dynamis*, força]
group d., d. de grupo; termo usado para representar o estudo de aspectos fundamentais do comportamento de um grupo, p. ex., motivos, atitudes; está relacionado com a mudança do grupo, e não com características estáticas.
dynamo-. Forma combinante que indica força, energia. [G. *dynamis*, força]
dy·na·mo·gen·e·sis (dī′na - mō - jen′e - sis). Dinamogênese; a produção de força, principalmente de energia muscular ou nervosa. SIN dynamogeny. [dynamo- + G. *genesis*, produção]
dy·na·mo·gen·ic (dī′na - mō - jen′ik). Dinamogênico; que produz energia ou força, principalmente energia ou atividade nervosa ou muscular.
dy·na·mog·e·ny (dī - na - moj′e - nē). Dinamogenia. SIN dynamogenesis.
dy·nam·o·graph (dī - nam′ō - graf). Dinamógrafo; instrumento para registrar o grau de força muscular. [dynamo- + G. *graphō*, escrever]
dy·na·mom·e·ter (dī - na - mom′e - ter). Dinamômetro; instrumento para medir o grau de força muscular. SIN ergometer. [dynamo- + G. *metron*, medida]
dy·nam·o·scope (dī - nam′ō - skōp). Dinamoscópio; estetoscópio modificado para ausculta dos músculos. [dynamo- + G. *skopeō*, examinar]

dy·na·mos·co·py (dī - nă - mos′kō - pē). Dinamoscopia; ausculta de um músculo em contração.

dy·na·therm (dī′nă - therm). Aparelho de diatermia; aparelho usado para induzir diatermia. [G. *dynamis*, força, + *thermē*, calor]

dyne (dīn). Dina; a unidade de força no sistema CGS, substituído no sistema SI pelo newton (1 N = 10^5 dinas), que dá a um corpo de 1 g de massa uma aceleração de 1 cm/s²; expressa como F (dinas) = m (gramas) × a (cm/s²). [G. *dynamis*, força]

dyn·ein (dīn′ēn). Dineína; proteína associada a estruturas móveis, que exibe atividade de adenosina trifosfatase; forma "braços" nos túbulos externos de cílios e flagelos. Funciona como um motor molecular. VER TAMBÉM tubulin, dynein *arm*. [dyne + protein]

dy·nor·phin (dī′nōr - fin). Dinorfina; ligante opióide endógeno que atua como agonista em receptores opiáceos. Neuropeptídeo extremamente potente, amplamente distribuído, que possui 17 resíduos aminoácidos e contém leu⁵-encefalina como sua seqüência NH₂-terminal.

dy·phyl·line (dī - fil′in). Difilina; exibe ações vasodilatadora periférica e broncodilatadora características de outros compostos da teofilina.

dys-. Dis; mau, difícil; oposto de eu-. Cf. dis-. [G.]

dys·a·cou·sia, dys·a·cu·sia (dis - ă - kū′sē - ă). Disacusia SIN dysacusis.

dys·a·cu·sis (dis - ă - kū′sis). Disacusia. **1.** Qualquer comprometimento da audição envolvendo dificuldade em processar detalhes de som, ao contrário de qualquer perda de sensibilidade ao som. **2.** Dor ou desconforto no ouvido decorrente da exposição ao som. SIN dysacousia, dysacusia. [dys- + G. *akousis*, audição]

dys·ad·ap·ta·tion (dis′ad - ap - tā′shŭn). Inadaptação; incapacidade da retina e da íris de se acomodarem bem a intensidades luminosas variáveis.

dys·an·ti·graph·ia (dis′an - tē - graf′ē - ă). Disantigrafia; forma de agrafia na qual o indivíduo é incapaz de copiar material escrito ou impresso. [dys- + G. *antigraphō*, escrever para trás]

dys·a·phia (dis - ā′fē - ă, dis - af′ē - ă). Disafia; comprometimento do sentido do tato. [dys- + G. *haphē*, tato]

dys·a·phic (dis - ā′fik). Disáfico; relativo ao comprometimento da sensibilidade de tátil.

dys·ar·te·ri·ot·o·ny (dis - ar - tēr - ē - ot′ō - nē). Disarteriotonia; pressão sanguínea anormal, seja muito alta ou muito baixa. [dys- + G. *artēria*, artéria, + *tonos*, tensão]

dys·ar·thria (dis - ar′thrē - ă). Disartria; transtorno da fala devido a estresse emocional, lesão cerebral ou paralisia, ausência de coordenação ou espasticidade dos músculos usados para a fala. SIN dysarthrosis (1). [dys- + G. *arthroō*, articular]
ataxic d., d. atáxica; disartria causada por lesões cerebelares.
hyperkinetic d., d. hipercinética; disartria causada por coréia e mioclônus.
hypokinetic d., d. hipocinética; disartria causada pelos tipos rígidos de doença extrapiramidal (extrapyramidal *disease*).
lower motor neuron d., disartria do neurônio motor inferior; disartria causada por disfunção dos núcleos motores e da porção inferior da ponte ou bulbo, ou de outras conexões neurais, centrais e periféricas aos músculos da articulação.
rigid d., d. rígida. SIN spastic d.
spastic d., d. espástica; disartria causada por lesões ao longo dos tratos corticobulbares. SIN rigid d.

dys·ar·thric (dis - ar′thrik). Disártrico; relativo à disartria.

dys·ar·thro·sis (dis - ar - thrō′sis). Disartrose. **1.** SIN dysarthria. **2.** Malformação de uma articulação. **3.** Uma falsa articulação. [dys- + G. *arthrōsis*, articulação]

dys·au·to·no·mia (dis′aw - tō - nō′mē - ă). Disautonomia; funcionamento anormal do sistema nervoso autônomo. [dys- + G. *autonomia*, autocontrole]
familial d. [MIM*223900], d. familiar; síndrome congênita com distúrbios específicos do sistema nervoso e aberrações da função do sistema nervoso autônomo, como indiferença à dor, diminuição do lacrimejamento, deficiência da homeostasia vasomotora, incoordenação motora, reações cardiovasculares lábeis, hiporreflexia, episódios freqüentes de pneumonia brônquica, hipersalivação com aspiração e dificuldade à deglutição, hiperêmese, instabilidade emocional e intolerância a anestésicos; herança autossômica recessiva. Mapeado no cromossoma humano 9q31-q33. SIN Riley-Day syndrome.

dys·ba·rism (dis′bar - izm). Disbarismo; termo genérico para o complexo de sintomas resultantes da exposição a pressão barométrica reduzida ou alterada, incluindo todos os efeitos fisiológicos resultantes dessas alterações, com exceção de hipoxia, e incluindo os efeitos da descompressão rápida. [dys- + G. *baros*, peso]

dys·ba·sia (dis - bā′zē - ă). Disbasia. **1.** Dificuldade na marcha. **2.** Marcha difícil ou distorcida observada em pessoas com determinados distúrbios mentais. [dys- + G. *basis*, passo]
d. angiosclerot'ica, d. angiospas'tica, d. angiosclerótica, d. angioespástica; termos obsoletos que significam dificuldade intermitente na marcha devido a causas vasculares periféricas.
d. lordot'ica progressi'va, d. lordótica progressiva; afecção caracterizada por lordoscoliose da porção inferior da coluna vertebral, que ocorre quando o paciente fica de pé ou caminha e geralmente desaparece quando o paciente se deita. SIN torsion neurosis.

dys·be·ta·lip·o·pro·tei·ne·mia (dis - bā′tă - lip - ō - prō′tēn - ē′mē - ă). Disbetalipoproteinemia. SIN type III familial hyperlipoproteinemia.

dys·bo·lism (dis′bō - lizm). Disbolismo; metabolismo anormal, mas não necessariamente mórbido, como na alcaptonúria. [dys- + G. *bolē* (*metabolē*). + *-ismos*, metabolismo]

dys·bu·lia (dis - boo′lē - ă). Disbulia; fraqueza ou incerteza de vontade. [dys- + G. *boulē*, vontade]

dys·bu·lic (dis - boo′lik). Disbúlico; relativo a, ou caracterizado por, disbulia.

dys·cal·cu·lia (dis - kal - kū′lē - ă). Discalculia; dificuldade na realização de problemas matemáticos simples; comumente observada em lesões do lobo parietal. [dys- + L. *calculo*, calcular, de *calculus*, seixo, contador]

dys·ce·pha·lia (dis - sē - fā′lē - ă). Discefalia; malformação da cabeça e da face. SIN dyscephaly. [dys- + G. *kephalē*, cabeça]
d. mandib'ulo-oculofacia'lis [MIM*234100], d. mandíbulo-oculofacial; síndrome de anomalias ósseas da calvária, face e mandíbula, com braquignatia, nariz curvo e estreito, além de múltiplos defeitos oculares, incluindo microftalmia, microcórnea e catarata, freqüentemente com alopecia sobre as suturas cranianas, alopecia areata ou ausência de sobrancelhas. O padrão de herança ainda não foi decidido. SIN Hallermann-Streiff syndrome, Hallermann-Streiff-François syndrome, mandibulo-oculofacial syndrome, oculomandibulodyscephaly, oculomandibulofacial syndrome, progeria with cataract, progeria with microphthalmia.

dys·ceph·a·ly (dis - sef′ă - lē). Discefalia. SIN dyscephalia.

dys·chei·ral, dys·chi·ral (dis - kī′ral). Relativo à disquiria.

dys·chei·ria, dys·chi·ria (dis - kī′rē - ă). Disquiria; perturbação da sensibilidade na qual, embora não haja perda de sensibilidade aparente, o paciente é incapaz de dizer que lado do corpo foi tocado (aquiria), ou refere-se ao lado errado (aloquiria), ou a ambos os lados (sinquiria). [dys- + G. *cheir*, mão]

dys·che·zia (dis - kē′zē - ă). Disquezia; dificuldade na defecação [dys- + G. *chezō*, defecar]

dys·chon·dro·gen·e·sis (dis - kon - drō - jen′ē - sis). Discondrogênese; desenvolvimento anormal da cartilagem. [dys- + G. *chondros*, cartilagem, + *genesis*, produção]

dys·chon·dro·pla·sia (dis - kon - drō - plā′zē - ă). Discondroplasia. SIN enchondromatosis. [dys- + G. *chondros*, cartilagem, + *plasis*, formação]
d. with hemangiomas, d. com hemangiomas. SIN Maffucci syndrome.

dys·chon·dros·te·o·sis (dis′kon - dros - tē - ō′sis) [MIM*127300]. Discondrosteose; displasia óssea, mais grave em mulheres e com um predomínio feminino, caracterizada por arqueamento do rádio, luxação dorsal da porção distal da ulna com limitação do movimento do cotovelo e do punho (a deformidade do punho é denominada deformidade de Madelung) e nanismo mesomélico; herança dominante, causada por mutação no gene homeobox de baixa estatura (SHOX) na região pseudo-autossômica de Xp. A displasia mesomélica de Langer, a forma homozigota de discondrosteose, também é causada por mutações homozigotas no gene SHOX. SIN Leri pleonosteosis, Leri-Weill disease, Leri-Weill syndrome. [dys- + G. *chondros*, cartilagem, + *osteon*, osso, + *-osis*, condição]

dys·chroia, dys·chroa (dis - kroy′ă, - krō′ă). Má aparência; despigmentação cutânea. [dys- + G. *chroia, chroa*, cor]

dys·chro·ma·top·sia (dis′krō - mă - top′sē - ă). Discromatopsia; condição na qual a capacidade de perceber as cores não é totalmente normal. Cf. anomalous *trichromatism*, dichromatism, monochromatism, chromatopsia. [dys- + G. *chrōma*, cor, + *opsis*, visão]

dys·chro·ma·to·sis (dis - krō - mă - tō′sis). Discromatose; anomalia assintomática da pigmentação que ocorre em japoneses; pode ser localizada ou difusa. [dys- + G. *chrōma*, cor, + *-osis*, condição]

dys·chro·mia (dis - krō′mē - ă). Discromia; qualquer anormalidade na cor da pele.

dys·ci·ne·sia (dis′si - nē′zē - ă). Discinesia. SIN dyskinesia.

dys·con·trol (dis - kon - trōl′). Descontrole. SIN intermittent explosive *disorder*.

dys·co·ria (dis - kō′rē - ă). Discoria; anormalidade no formato da pupila. [dys- + G. *korē*, pupila do olho]

dys·cra·sia (dis - krā′zē - ă). Discrasia. **1.** Estado geral mórbido resultante da presença de material anormal no sangue, geralmente aplicado a doenças que afetam as células do sangue ou as plaquetas. **2.** Termo antigo que indica doença. [G. mau temperamento, de dys- + *krasis*, mistura]
blood d., d. sanguínea; estado mórbido do sangue; geralmente se refere a elementos celulares anormais de caráter permanente.

dys·cra·sic, dys·crat·ic (krā′sik, krat′ik). Discrásico; relativo a, ou afetado por, discrasia.

dys·di·ad·o·cho·ki·ne·sia, dys·di·ad·o·cho·ci·ne·sia (dis - dī - ad′ō - kō - ki - nē′zē - ă). Disdiadococinesia; comprometimento da capacidade de realizar rapidamente movimentos alternantes. [dys- + G. *diadochos*, trabalhando em turnos, + *kinēsis*, movimento]

dys·di·a·do·cho·ki·ne·sis (dis′dī - ad - ō - kō - ki - nē′sis). Adiadococinesia SIN adiadochokinesis.

dys·e·mia (dis - ē′mē - ă). Disemia; qualquer condição anormal ou doença do sangue. [dys- + G. *haima*, sangue]

dys·en·ce·pha·lia splanch·no·cys·ti·ca (dis'en - se - fā'lē - ā splangk - nō - sis'ti - ka) [MIM*249000]. Disencefalia esplancnocística; síndrome de malformação, letal no período neonatal e caracterizada por retardo do crescimento intra-uterino, fronte inclinada, encefalocele occipital, anomalias oculares, fenda palatina, polidactilia, rins policísticos e outras malformações; herança autossômica recessiva. Mapeado no cromossoma humano 17q21-q24. SIN Meckel syndrome, Meckel-Gruber syndrome.

dys·en·ter·ic (dis - en - tār'ik), Disentérico; relativo a, ou que sofre de, disenteria.

dys·en·tery (dis - en - tār - ē). Disenteria; doença caracterizada por evacuações aquosas freqüentes, em geral com sangue e muco, e acompanhada clinicamente por dor, tenesmo, febre e desidratação. [G. *dysenteria*, de *dys-*, mau, + *entera*, intestino]
  amebic d., d. amebiana; diarréia resultante de inflamação ulcerativa do cólon, causada principalmente por infecção por *Entamoeba histolytica*; pode ser leve ou grave e pode estar associada a infecção amebiana de outros órgãos.
  bacillary d., d. bacilar; infecção por *Shigella dysenteriae, S. flexneri* ou outros microrganismos.
  balantidial d., d. balantidiana; tipo de colite que se assemelha em muitos aspectos à disenteria amebiana; causada pelo parasita ciliado *Balantidium coli*.
  bilharzial d., esquistossomose; disenteria devida à infecção por *Schistosoma mansoni, S. haematobium* ou *S. japonicum*.
  fulminating d., d. fulminante. SIN malignant d.
  helminthic d., d. helmíntica; disenteria causada por infestação por vermes parasitas.
  malignant d., d. maligna; disenteria na qual os sinais e sintomas são intensamente agudos, levando a prostração, colapso e, freqüentemente, morte. SIN fulminating d.
  viral d., d. viral; diarréia aquosa abundante, atribuída a infecção viral.

dys·er·e·thism (dis - er'ē - thizm). Diseretismo; condição de resposta lenta aos estímulos. [dys- + G. *erethismos*, irritação]

dys·er·gia (dis - er'jē - ā). Disergia; ausência de atividade harmônica entre os músculos envolvidos na execução de qualquer movimento voluntário específico. [dys- + G. *ergon*, trabalho]

dys·es·the·sia (dis - es - thē'zē - ā). Disestesia. **1.** Comprometimento da sensibilidade, quase chegando à anestesia. **2.** Condição na qual uma sensação desagradável é produzida por estímulos comuns; causada por lesões das vias sensoriais, periféricas ou centrais. **3.** Sensações anormais experimentadas na ausência de estimulação. [G. *dysaisthēsia*, de *dys-*, difícil, + *aisthēsis*, sensação]

dys·fi·brin·o·ge·ne·mia (dis'fī - brin'ō - jē - nē'mē - ā) [MIM*134820]. Disfibrinogenemia; distúrbio autossômico dominante de fibrinogênios qualitativamente anormais de vários tipos; cada tipo recebe o nome da cidade na qual foi descoberto o fibrinogênio anormal. Os exemplos incluem: 1) Amsterdam, Bethesda II, Cleveland, Los Angeles, Saint Louis, Zurich I e II: principal defeito, agregação de monômeros da fibrina; prolongamento do tempo de protrombina; efeito inibitório sobre a coagulação normal; assintomático; 2) Bethesda I e Detroit: principal defeito, liberação de fibrinopeptídeo; prolongamento do tempo de trombina; efeito inibitório sobre a coagulação normal; sangramento anormal; 3) Baltimore: principal defeito, liberação de fibrinopeptídeos; prolongamento do tempo de trombina; ausência de efeito inibitório sobre a coagulação normal; hemorragia e trombose; 4) Leuven: principal defeito, agregação questionável dos monômeros da fibrina; prolongamento do tempo de protrombina; pequeno efeito inibitório sobre a coagulação normal; sangramento anormal; 5) Metz: principal defeito não-descrito; tempo de trombina infinito; efeito inibitório sobre a coagulação normal não-descrito; sangramento anormal; 6) Nancy: principal defeito, agregação de monômeros de fibrina; leve efeito inibitório sobre a coagulação normal; assintomático; 7) Oklahoma: principal defeito não-descrito; tempo de trombina normal; ausência de efeito sobre a coagulação normal; sangramento anormal; 8) Oslo: principal defeito não-descrito; tempo de trombina encurtado; efeito sobre a coagulação normal não-descrito; trombose anormal; 9) Parma: principal defeito não-descrito; tempo de trombina infinito; ausência de efeito inibitório sobre a coagulação normal; sangramento anormal; 10) Paris I: principal defeito não-descrito; tempo de trombina infinito; efeito inibitório sobre a coagulação normal; assintomático; 11) Paris II: principal defeito não-relatado; efeito inibitório sobre a coagulação normal; assintomático; 12) Troyes: principal defeito não-descrito; tempo de trombina prolongado; efeito inibitório sobre a coagulação normal não-descrito; assintomático; 13) Vancouver: principal defeito não-descrito; tempo de trombina prolongado; ausência de efeito sobre a coagulação normal; sangramento anormal; 14) Wiesbaden: principal defeito, agregação de monômeros da fibrina; tempo de trombina prolongado; efeito inibitório sobre a coagulação normal; hemorragia e trombose.

dys·func·tion (dis - funk'shŭn). Disfunção; função anormal ou difícil.
  constitutional hepatic d., d. hepática constitucional. SIN familial nonhemolytic jaundice.
  dental d., d. dentária; funcionamento anormal das estruturas dentárias.
  minimal brain d., d. cerebral mínima. VER attention deficit *disorder*.
  papillary muscle d., d. do músculo papilar; comprometimento da função de um músculo papilar, geralmente devido a isquemia ou infarto, com conseqüente incompetência da valva mitral (raramente tricúspide). SIN papillary muscle syndrome.
  phagocyte d. (fā'gō - sit), d. de fagócitos; distúrbio da função fagocítica.
  placental d., d. placentária. SIN dysmature (3).
  psychosexual d., sexual d., d. psicossexual, d. sexual; transtorno da função sexual, p. ex., impotência, ejaculação precoce, anorgasmia, considerada de etiologia psicológica, e não física.
  sphincter of Oddi d., d. do esfíncter de Oddi; anormalidade estrutural ou funcional do esfíncter de Oddi que interfere com a drenagem do ducto colédoco ou pancreático. SIN biliary dyskinesia.
  temporomandibular joint d. (TMD, TMJ), d. da articulação temporomandibular (ATM); comprometimento crônico da função da articulação temporomandibular. VER temporomandibular *arthrosis*, myofascial pain-dysfunction *syndrome*.

dys·gam·ma·glob·u·lin·e·mia (dis - gam'ā - glob'ū - li - nē'mē - ā). Disgamaglobulinemia; anormalidade da imunoglobulina, um distúrbio da percentagem de distribuição das γ-globulinas ou deficiência seletiva de uma ou mais imunoglobulinas.

dys·gen·e·sis (dis - jen'ē - sis). Disgenesia; distúrbio do desenvolvimento. [dys- + G. *genesis*, geração]
  cortical d., d. cortical. SIN cortical *dysplasia*.
  gonadal d., d. gonadal; distúrbio do desenvolvimento gonadal, do qual foram identificados vários tipos e graus, incluindo aplasia ou agenesia gonadal, gônadas rudimentares, defeito congênito das gônadas e hermafroditismo verdadeiro; apenas algumas vezes as características da genitália externa, dos ductos genitais e do desenvolvimento sexual secundário estão relacionadas unicamente a um determinado tipo de disgenesia gonadal. A **XO gonadal d.** (d. gonadal XO) consiste em monossomia do X com gônada em fita, e não um ovário verdadeiro, sendo observada principalmente na síndrome de Turner; a **XX gonadal d.** (d. gonadal XX) é um distúrbio autossômico recessivo, com cariótipo feminino, gônadas em fita e amenorréia primária, mas sem características corporais de síndrome de Turner; a **XY gonadal d.** (d. gonadal XY) é um distúrbio ligado ao X associado a um cariótipo masculino e a um biotipo feminino, gônadas em fita e ausência de características sexuais secundárias.
  iridocorneal mesenchymal d., d. mesenquimal iridocorneana; disgenesia da córnea e da íris, produzindo anomalias pupilares, embriotoxona posterior e glaucoma secundário, parcialmente resultante de desenvolvimento anômalo do mesênquima ocular.
  seminiferous tubule d., d. do túbulo seminífero; termo raramente usado para um distúrbio no qual os túbulos seminíferos exibem uma citoarquitetura anormal e extensa hialinização; os testículos são pequenos, e são formados poucos espermatozóides; o biotipo pode ser eunucóide, e pode haver ginecomastia; a eliminação urinária de gonadotrofina geralmente é alta, e a incidência de deficiência e doença mentais está aumentada; a cromatina sexual pode ser masculina ou feminina, e a secreção de andrógenio varia de subnormal a normal. É uma característica constante da síndrome de Klinefelter (Klinefelter *syndrome*), e o termo pode ser usado como sinônimo desta. SIN germinal aplasia.
  testicular d. [MIM*305700], d. testicular; distúrbio congênito da estrutura e da função dos túbulos seminíferos, resultando em infertilidade masculina; o defeito na espermatogênese pode ser incompleto, como na interrupção da maturação ou descamação prematura, ou a espermatogênese pode estar completamente ausente, como na síndrome apenas das células de Sertoli.

dys·gen·ic (dis - jen'ik). Disgênico; que se aplica a fatores que possuem um efeito prejudicial sobre qualidades hereditárias, físicas ou mentais.

dys·ger·mi·no·ma (dis - jer - mi - nō'mā). Disgerminoma; neoplasia maligna do ovário (equivalente ao seminoma testicular), composta de células germinativas gonadais indiferenciadas e mais freqüente em pacientes com menos de 20 anos. As neoplasias são cinza-amareladas e de consistência firme; contêm focos de necrose e hemorragia, e tendem a ser encapsuladas; caracteristicamente, disseminam-se por meio dos vasos linfáticos, mas também ocorrem metástases disseminadas. SIN disgerminoma. [dys- + L. *germen*, broto, + G. -*ōma*, tumor]

dys·geu·sia (dis - goo'sē - ā). Disgeusia; distorção ou perversão na percepção de um sabor. Pode haver uma percepção desagradável quando há um sabor normalmente agradável, ou a percepção pode ocorrer na ausência de um sabor (alucinação gustativa). SIN parageusia. [dys- + G. *geusis*, paladar]

dys·gna·thia (dis - nath'ē - ā). Disgnatia; qualquer anormalidade que se estende além dos dentes e inclui a maxila e/ou a mandíbula [dys- + G. *gnathos*, mandíbula]

dys·gnath·ic (dis - nath'ik). Disgnático; relativo a, ou caracterizado por, anormalidade da maxila e da mandíbula.

dys·gno·sia (dis - nō'sē - ā). Disgnosia; qualquer distúrbio cognitivo, isto é, qualquer doença mental. [G. *dysgnōsia*, dificuldade de conhecimento]

dys·gon·ic (dis - gon'ik). Disgônico; termo usado para indicar que o crescimento de uma cultura bacteriana é lento e relativamente deficiente; usado principalmente em referência ao crescimento de culturas do bacilo da tuberculose bovina (*Mycobacterium bovis*). VER TAMBÉM eugonic. [dys- + G. *gonikos*, relativo a semente ou descendência]

dys·graph·ia (dis - graf′ē - ā). Disgrafia. **1.** Dificuldade em escrever. **2.** Cãibra do escritor SIN writer's cramp. [dys- + G. *graphē*, escrita]

dys·hem·a·to·poi·e·sis (dis - hē′ma - tō - poy - ē′sis). Disematopoese; formação deficiente do sangue. SIN dyshemopoiese. [dys- + G. *haima (haimat-)*, sangue, + *poiēsis*, formação]

dys·hem·a·to·poi·et·ic (dis - hē′ma - tō - poy - et′ik). Disematopoético; relativo a, ou caracterizado por, disematopoese. SIN dyshemopoietic.

dys·he·mo·poi·e·sis (dis - hē′mō - poy - ē′sis). Disemopoese. SIN dyshematopoiesis.

dys·he·mo·poi·et·ic (dis - hē′mō - poy - et′ik). Disemopoético. SIN dyshematopoietic.

dys·hid·ria (dis - hid′rē - ā). Disidria. SIN dyshidrosis.

dys·hi·dro·sis (dis - i - drō′sis). Disidrose; erupção vesicular ou vesicopustular de múltiplas causas, que ocorre basicamente nas superfícies volares das mãos e dos pés; as lesões disseminam-se perifericamente, mas tendem a exibir desaparecimento central. SIN cheiropompholyx, chiropompholyx, dyshidria, dyshidrotic eczema, pompholyx. [dys- + G. *hidrōs*, suor]

dysjunction. Disjunção; uma separação de partes ou estruturas normalmente unidas; clivagem.
  Le Fort III craniofacial d., d. craniofacial Le Fort III. SIN craniofacial dysjunction *fracture*.

dys·kar·y·o·sis (dis - kar - ē - ō′sis). Discariose; maturação anormal observada em células esfoliadas que possuem citoplasma normal, mas núcleos hipercromáticos, ou distribuição irregular da cromatina; pode ser seguida pelo desenvolvimento de uma neoplasia maligna. [dys- + G. *karyon*, núcleo, + *-ōsis*, condição]

dys·kar·y·ot·ic (dis - kar - ē - ot′ik). Discariótico; relativo a, ou caracterizado por, discariose.

dys·ker·a·to·ma (dis - ker - ā - tō′mā). Disceratoma; tumor cutâneo que exibe disceratose. [dys- + G. *keras*, corno, + *-oma*, tumor]
  warty d., d. verrucoso; tumor solitário benigno da pele, geralmente do couro cabeludo, face ou pescoço, com um tampão ceratótico central; parece originar-se de um folículo piloso e, microscopicamente, assemelha-se a uma lesão de ceratose folicular, porém é maior, com crescimento mais extenso para o epitélio. SIN isolated dyskeratosis follicularis.

dys·ker·a·to·sis (dis′ker - ā - tō′sis). Disceratose. **1.** Queratinização prematura de células epiteliais individuais que não alcançaram a camada superficial queratinizante; as células disceratóticas geralmente se tornam arredondadas e podem separar-se das células adjacentes e desprender-se. **2.** Epidermalização do epitélio conjuntival e córnea. **3.** Distúrbio da queratinização. [dys- + G. *keras*, corno, + *-osis*, condição]
  benign d., d. benigna; disceratose que pode ocorrer em doenças congênitas e bolhosas da pele.
  d. congen'ita [MIM*305000], d. congênita; distrofia ungueal, leucoplasia oral e pigmentação reticular da pele, atrofia testicular com anemia, progredindo mais comumente para pancitopenia; herança recessiva ligada ao X, causada por mutação do gene DKC1 que codifica a discenina em Xq.
  intraepithelial d. [MIM*127600], d. intra-epitelial; distúrbio autossômico dominante que consiste em lesões esponjosas brancas na mucosa bucal, no assoalho da boca, na face lateral ventral da língua, na gengiva e no palato. Placas gelatinosas transitórias se formam sobre a córnea, o que pode produzir cegueira temporária.
  isolated d. follicula'ris, d. folicular isolada. SIN warty *dyskeratoma*.

dys·ker·a·tot·ic (dis′ker - ā - tot′ik). Disceratótico; relativo a, ou caracterizado por, disceratose.

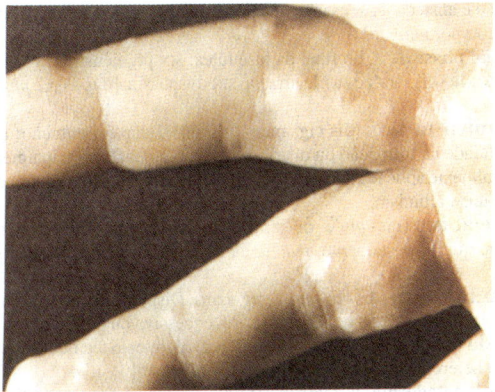

disidrose: observar vesículas situadas profundamente nas faces laterais e flexurais dos dedos das mãos

dys·ki·ne·sia (dis - ki - nē′zē - ā) [MIM*242650]. Discinesia; dificuldade em realizar movimentos voluntários. Termo geralmente usado em relação a vários distúrbios extrapiramidais. SIN dyscinesia. [dys- + G. *kinēsis*, movimento]
  biliary d., d. biliar. SIN sphincter of Oddi *dysfunction*.
  extrapyramidal d.'s, discinesias extrapiramidais; movimentos involuntários anormais atribuídos a estados patológicos de uma ou mais partes do corpo estriado e caracterizados por movimentos automáticos, estereotipados, não-supressíveis que só cessam durante o sono; p. ex., doença de Parkinson; coréia; atetose; hemibalismo.
  lingual-facial-buccal d., d. tardia. SIN tardive d.
  tardive d., d. tardia; movimentos involuntários dos músculos faciais e da língua, freqüentemente persistentes, que se desenvolvem como complicação tardia de algum tratamento neuroléptico, provavelmente com antipsicóticos típicos. SIN lingual-facial-buccal d.
  tracheobronchial d., d. traqueobrônquica; degeneração do tecido elástico e conjuntivo dos brônquios e da traquéia.

dys·ki·ne·sis. Discinesia. SIN dyskinesia.
  ciliary dyskinesis, discinesia ciliar; **(1)** ausência ou comprometimento do movimento ciliar, que ocorre como um distúrbio primário ou secundário. VER TAMBÉM Kartagener *syndrome*; **(2)** associada a infecções recorrentes nas vias respiratórias.

dys·ki·net·ic (dis - ki - net′ik). Discinético; que designa ou é característico de discinesia.

dys·lex·ia (dis - lek′sē - ā). Dislexia; comprometimento da capacidade de leitura com um nível de competência abaixo do esperado com base no nível de inteligência do indivíduo e na presença de visão normal e reconhecimento das letras e reconhecimento normal do significado de figuras e objetos. SIN incomplete alexia. [dys- + G. *lexis*, palavra, frase]

dys·lex·ic (dis - lek′sik). Disléxico; relativo a, ou caracterizado por, dislexia.

dys·lo·gia (dis - lō′jē - ā). Dislogia; comprometimento da fala e do raciocínio em virtude de um distúrbio mental. [dys- + G. *logos*, fala, raciocínio]

dys·ma·se·sis (dis - mā - sē′sis). Dismasese; dificuldade na mastigação. [dys- + G. *masēsis*, mastigação]

dys·ma·ture (dis′ma - tūr). Dismaturo. **1.** Designa deficiência do desenvolvimento ou da maturação; freqüentemente indicando anormalidades estruturais e/ou funcionais. **2.** Em obstetrícia, designa um feto cujo peso ao nascimento é impropriamente baixo para sua idade gestacional. **3.** Desenvolvimento imaturo da placenta de forma que haja anormalidade da função. SIN placental *dysfunction*.

dys·ma·tu·ri·ty (dis′mā - choor - i - tē). Dismaturidade; síndrome de um recém-nascido com relativa ausência de gordura subcutânea, enrugamento cutâneo, unhas proeminentes nas mãos e nos pés, e tingimento da pele do lactente e das membranas placentárias por mecônio; freqüentemente associada a pós-maturidade ou a insuficiência placentária.

dys·me·lia (dis - mē′lē - ā). Dismelia; anormalidade congênita caracterizada por ausência ou encurtamento dos membros. VER amelia, phocomelia. [dys- + G. *melos*, membro]

dys·men·or·rhea (dis - men - ōr - ē′ā). Dismenorréia; menstruação difícil e dolorosa. SIN menorrhalgia. [dys- + G. *mēn*, mês, + *rhoia*, fluxo]
  functional d., d. funcional, d. primária. SIN primary d.
  mechanical d., d. mecânica; dismenorréia devida à obstrução à eliminação do sangue menstrual, como na estenose cervical. SIN obstructive d.
  membranous d., d. membranosa; dismenorréia acompanhada por esfoliação da decídua menstrual.
  obstructive d., d. obstrutiva, d. mecânica SIN mechanical d.
  ovarian d., d. ovariana; forma de dismenorréia secundária devida à doença de um ovário.
  primary d., d. primária; dismenorréia devida a um distúrbio funcional, e não a inflamação, novos crescimentos ou fatores anatômicos. SIN functional d.
  secondary d., d. secundária; dismenorréia devida a inflamação, infecção, tumor ou fatores anatômicos.
  spasmodic d., d. espasmódica; dismenorréia acompanhada por contrações dolorosas do útero.
  tubal d., d. tubária; forma de dismenorréia secundária devida a estenose ou a outra condição anormal das tubas de Falópio.
  ureteric d., d. ureteral; forma de dismenorréia secundária caracterizada por dor devida ao espasmo do ureter que ocorre na época da menstruação.
  uterine d., d. uterina; forma de dismenorréia secundária resultante de doença do útero.
  vaginal d., d. vaginal; forma de dismenorréia secundária devida a obstrução ou a outra condição anormal da vagina.

dys·met·ria (dis - mē′trē - ā, - met′rē - ā). Dismetria; um aspecto da ataxia, com comprometimento da capacidade de controlar a distância, a força e a velocidade de um ato. Geralmente usado para descrever anormalidades do movimento causadas por distúrbios cerebelares. VER TAMBÉM hypermetria, hypometria. [dys- + G. *metron*, medida]
  ocular d., d. ocular; anormalidade dos movimentos oculares na qual os olhos "ultrapassam" um objeto ao tentar focalizá-lo.

dys·mor·phia (dis-mōr'fē-ă). Dismorfismo. SIN dysmorphism.
dys·mor·phism (dis-mōr'fizm). Dismorfismo; anormalidade do formato. SIN dysmorphia. [G. *dysmorphia*, imperfeição da forma]
dys·mor·pho·gen·e·sis (dis'mōr-fō-jen'ē-sis). Dismorfogênese; o processo de formação anormal do tecido. [dys- + G. *morphē*, forma, + *genesis*, produção]
dys·mor·phol·o·gy (dis-mōr-fol'ō-jē). Dismorfologia; termo genérico para o estudo ou tema do desenvolvimento anormal da forma tecidual. Um ramo da genética clínica. [dys- + G. *morphē*, forma, + *logos*, estudo]
dys·mor·pho·pho·bia (dis'mōr-fō-fō'bē-ă). Dismorfofobia. SIN body dysmorphic *disorder*. [dys- + G. *morphē*, forma, + *phobos*, medo]
dys·my·e·li·na·tion (dis-mī-ē-li-nā'shŭn). Desmielinização; deposição imprópria ou ruptura da bainha de mielina de uma fibra nervosa, causada por metabolismo anormal da mielina.
dys·my·o·to·nia (dis-mī-ō-tō'nē-ă). Dismiotonia; tonicidade muscular anormal (hiper- ou hipo-). VER dystonia. [dys- + G. *mys*, músculo, + *tonos*, tensão, tônus]
dys·nys·tax·is (dis-nis-tak'sis). Disnistaxe; condição em que o indivíduo desperta com facilidade e a qualidade do sono é comprometida. SIN light sleep. [dys- + G. *nystaxis*, sonolência]
dys·o·don·ti·a·sis (dis'ō-don-tī'ă-sis). Disodontíase; dificuldade ou irregularidade na erupção dos dentes. [dys- + G. *odous*, dente, + *-iasis*, condição]
dys·on·to·gen·e·sis (dis'on-tō-jen'ē-sis). Disontogênese; deficiência do desenvolvimento embrionário. [dys- + G. *on*, ser, + *genesis*, origem]
dys·on·to·ge·net·ic (dis'on-tō-jē-net'ik). Disontogenético; caracterizado por disontogênese.
dys·o·rex·ia (dis-ō-rek'sē-ă). Disorexia; diminuição ou perversão do apetite. [dys- + G. *orexis*, apetite]
dys·os·mia (dis-oz'mē-ă). Disosmia; distorção ou perversão da percepção de um odor; pode haver uma percepção desagradável na presença de um odor normalmente agradável, ou a percepção pode ocorrer quando não há odor (alucinação olfativa). SIN parosmia, parosphhresia. [dys- + G. *osmē*, cheiro]
dys·os·te·o·gen·e·sis (dis-os-tē-ō-jen'ē-sis). Disosteogênese; formação óssea defeituosa. SIN dysostosis. [dys- + G. *osteon*, osso, + *genesis*, produção]
dys·os·to·sis (dis-os-tō'sis). Disostose. SIN dysosteogenesis. [dys- + G. *osteon*, osso, + *-osis*, condição]
   acrofacial d., d. acrofacial; disostose mandibulofacial associada a malformação dos membros como defeito do rádio e dos polegares, e sinostose radioulnar. VER TAMBÉM Treacher Collins *syndrome*. SIN acrofacial syndrome.
   cleidocranial d., clidocranial d. [MIM*119600], d. cleidocraniana; distúrbio do desenvolvimento caracterizado por ausência ou hipoplasia das clavículas, crânio em forma de caixa com suturas abertas, bossa frontal, ossos wormianos, capacidade de opor os ombros e ausência de dentes; herança autossômica dominante, causada por mutação no gene do fator de transcrição (CBFA1), que codifica o fator de ligação central, domínio *runt* subunidade alfa 1 em 6p. Há uma forma autossômica recessiva [MIM*216330]. SIN cleidocranial dysplasia, clidocranial dysplasia, craniocleidodysostosis.
   craniofacial d. [MIM*123500], d. craniofacial. SIN Crouzon *syndrome*.
   mandibuloacral d. [MIM*248370], d. mandibuloacral; distúrbio autossômico recessivo caracterizado por mandíbula hipoplásica, apinhamento dentário, acroosteólise, rigidez articular e atrofia da pele das mãos e pés; as clavículas são hipoplásicas, as suturas cranianas são largas e há múltiplos ossos wormianos.
   mandibulofacial d., d. mandibulofacial; síndrome variável de malformações basicamente de derivados do primeiro arco branquial; caracterizada por fissuras palpebrais inclinadas para fora e para baixo, com incisuras ou colobomas no terço externo das pálpebras inferiores, defeitos ósseos ou hipoplasia dos ossos malares e do zigoma, hipoplasia da mandíbula, macrostomia com palato alto ou fenda palatina e má posição e má oclusão dos dentes, orelhas externas malformadas e de implantação baixa, crescimento atípico dos pêlos, e algumas depressões ou fendas entre a boca e a orelha. VER TAMBÉM Treacher Collins *syndrome*. SIN mandibulofacial dysostosis syndrome, mandibulofacial dysplasia.
   metaphysial d., d. metafisária; rara anormalidade do desenvolvimento do esqueleto na qual as metáfises de ossos tubulares são expandidas por depósitos de cartilagem.
   d. mul'tiplex, d. múltipla; padrão específico de alterações radiográficas observadas em muitos distúrbios do armazenamento de lisossomas.
   orodigitofacial d., d. orodigitofacial. SIN orofaciodigital *syndrome*.
   otomandibular d., d. otomandibular; hipoplasia da mandíbula, freqüentemente com malformação da articulação temporomandibular, associada a malformações da orelha, mas não a malformações oculares ou defeitos malares. SIN otomandibular syndrome.
   peripheral d. [MIM*170700], d. periférica; disostose dos ossos metacarpais, acompanhada por características faciais variáveis; possivelmente herança autossômica dominante.
dys·pal·lia (dis-pal'ē-ă). Dispalia; distorção do desenvolvimento do pálio cerebral. [dys- + L. *pallium*, manto]

dys·pa·reu·nia (dis-pa-roo'nē-ă). Dispareunia; ocorrência de dor durante a relação sexual. [dys- + G. *pareunos*, deitar ao lado de, de *para*, ao lado de, *eunē*, cama]
dys·pep·sia (dis-pep'sē-ă). Dispepsia; comprometimento da função gástrica ou "perturbação gástrica" devida a algum distúrbio do estômago; caracterizada por dor epigástrica, algumas vezes queimação, náuseas e eructação gasosa. SIN gastric indigestion. [dys- + G. *pepsis*, digestão]
   acid d., d. ácida; dispepsia associada ao excesso de acidez gástrica.
   adhesion d., d. por aderência; dor, dispepsia e outros sintomas que, supostamente, resultam de aderências perigástricas.
   atonic d., d. atônica; dispepsia com comprometimento do tônus nas paredes musculares do estômago. SIN functional d. (1).
   fermentative d., d. fermentativa; dispepsia acompanhada por fermentação do conteúdo gástrico, que geralmente ocorre na dilatação gástrica.
   flatulent d., d. flatulenta; dispepsia com eructações freqüentes do ar engolido, algumas vezes sem doença orgânica subjacente.
   functional d., d. funcional; **(1)** d. atônica, SIN atonic d.; **(2)** d. nervosa, SIN nervous d.
   nervous d., d. nervosa; dispepsia associada a nervosismo, tensão ou ansiedade. SIN functional d. (2).
   reflex d., d. reflexa; dispepsia funcional excitada por irritação reflexa decorrente de doença em outro local além do estômago ou intestino.
dys·pep·tic (dis-pep'tik). Dispéptico; relativo a, ou que sofre de, dispepsia.
dys·pha·gia, dys·pha·gy (dis-fā'jē-ă, dis'fā-jē). Disfagia; dificuldade para deglutir. VER TAMBÉM aglutition. [dys- + G. *phago*, comer]
   d. luso'ria, disfagia atribuída à compressão pela artéria subclávia direita, que se origina anormalmente da aorta descendente e passa por trás do esôfago. [cunhado a partir do L. *lusus naturae*, um esporte da natureza]
   d. nervo'sa, nervous d., d. nervosa. SIN esophagism.
   sideropenic d., d. sideropênica. SIN Plummer-Vinson *syndrome*.
   vallecular d., d. valecular; disfagia causada por alimento que se aloja em uma valécula acima da epiglote. SIN Barclay-Baron disease.
dys·pha·go·cy·to·sis (dis-fag'ō-sī-tō'sis). Disfagocitose; perturbação da fagocitose, principalmente pela incapacidade das células de ingerir e digerir bactérias.
   congenital d., d. congênita. SIN chronic granulomatous *disease*.
dys·pha·sia (dis-fā'zē-ă). Disfasia; comprometimento da produção da fala e incapacidade de dispor as palavras de forma compreensível; causada por uma lesão adquirida do cérebro. SIN dysphrasia. [dys- + G. *phasis*, que fala]
dys·phe·mia (dis-fē'mē-ă). Disfemia; perturbação da fonação, articulação ou audição devida a déficits emocionais ou mentais. [dys- + G. *phēmē*, fala]
dys·pho·nia (dis-fō'nē-ă). Disfonia; alteração da produção da voz. [dys- + G. *phōnē*, voz]
   abductor spasmodic d., d. espasmódica abdutora; forma respiratória de disfonia espasmódica causada por abertura excessiva e longa das cordas vocais para fonemas surdos que se estendem para vogais.
   adductor spasmodic d., d. espasmódica adutora; forma de disfonia espasmódica na qual o fechamento excessivo das cordas vocais afeta o início e a manutenção da fonação.
   d. pli'cae ventricula'ris, d. das pregas ventriculares; fonação com as faixas ventriculares, e não com as cordas vocais.
   spasmodic d., d. espasmódica; contração espasmódica dos músculos intrínsecos da laringe, excitados pela tentativa de fonação, que produz subtipos adutores ou abdutores, causada por um distúrbio do sistema nervoso central. Uma forma localizada de distúrbio do movimento. SIN d. spastica, spastic d.
   spastic d., d. espástica. SIN spasmodic d.
   d. spas'tica, d. espástica. SIN spasmodic d.
dys·pho·ria (dis-fōr'ē-ă). Disforia; humor de insatisfação geral, agitação, depressão e ansiedade; sensação de aborrecimento ou desconforto. [dys- + G. *phora*, comportamento]
   late luteal phase d., d. do final da fase lútea. SIN premenstrual *syndrome*.
dys·phra·sia (dis-frā'zē-ă). Disfrasia. SIN dysphasia. [dys- + G. *phrasis*, que fala]
dys·pig·men·ta·tion (dis'pig-men-tā'shŭn). Despigmentação; qualquer anormalidade na formação ou distribuição do pigmento, principalmente cutâneo; geralmente aplicada à redução anormal da pigmentação (despigmentação). VER TAMBÉM albinism.
dys·pin·e·al·ism (dis-pin'ē-ăl-izm). Dispinealismo; termo obsoleto para a síndrome que, supostamente, resulta da deficiência da secreção da glândula pineal.
dys·pi·tu·i·tar·ism (dis-pi-too'i-ter-izm). Dispituitarismo; o complexo de fenômenos devidos à secreção hipofisária excessiva ou deficiente.
dys·pla·sia (dis-plā'zē-ă). Displasia; desenvolvimento tecidual anormal. VER TAMBÉM heteroplasia. [dys- + G. *plasis*, moldagem]
   anhidrotic ectodermal d. [MIM*305100], d. ectodérmica anidrótica; distúrbio caracterizado por ausência ou deficiência das glândulas sudoríparas, nariz em sela, hiperpigmentação ao redor dos olhos, dentes malformados ou ausentes, cabelo ralo, unhas displásicas, pele lisa e finamente enrugada, sindactilia,

ausência de tecido mamário e, ocasionalmente, retardo mental; herança recessiva ligada ao X, causada por mutação no gene ED1 no cromossoma Xq. Também há uma forma autossômica recessiva [MIM*224900]. SIN hypohidrotic ectodermal d.

anterofacial d., anteroposterior facial d., anteroposterior d., d. ântero-facial, d. facial ântero-posterior, d. ântero-posterior, crescimento anormal da face ou do crânio em direção ântero-posterior, conforme observação e medida com cefalograma.

asphyxiating thoracic d. [MIM*208500], d. torácica asfixiante. SIN asphyxiating thoracic *dystrophy.*

branchiootorenal d., d. brânquio-oto-renal; distúrbio autossômico dominante que se manifesta por cistos branquiais, pólipos ou seios cutâneos pré-auriculares, anomalias do ouvido e malformações renais. SIN BOR syndrome.

bronchopulmonary d., d. broncopulmonar; insuficiência pulmonar crônica observada basicamente em lactentes nascidos prematuramente; definida clinicamente como necessidade persistente de oxigênio suplementar com 1 mês de idade e tipicamente observada em lactentes que necessitaram de ventilação com pressão positiva.

cerebral d., d. cerebral; desenvolvimento anormal do telencéfalo.

cervical d., d. cervical; displasia do colo uterino, atipia epitelial envolvendo parcial ou completamente a espessura do epitélio escamoso cervical, mais freqüente em mulheres jovens; parece regredir freqüentemente, mas pode progredir para carcinoma durante um longo período; a displasia grave pode ser microscopicamente indistinguível do carcinoma *in situ.*

chondroectodermal d. [MIM*225500], d. condroectodérmica; tríade de condrodisplasia, displasia ectodérmica e polidactilia, com defeitos cardíacos congênitos em mais da metade dos pacientes; herança autossômica recessiva. Mapeamento no cromossoma humano 4p16. SIN Ellis-van Creveld syndrome.

cleidocranial d., clidocranial d., d. cleidocraniana. SIN cleidocranial *dysostosis.*

cochlear d., d. coclear; ausência de desenvolvimento completo da cóclea óssea.

congenital ectodermal d., d. ectodérmica congênita; desenvolvimento incompleto da epiderme e dos anexos cutâneos; a pele é lisa e sem pêlos, a face é anormal, e os dentes e as unhas podem ser afetados; a sudorese pode ser deficiente. SIN congenital ectodermal defect.

congenital hip d., d. congênita do quadril. SIN developmental hip d.

cortical d., d. cortical; desorganização por malformação da citoarquitetura do córtex em relação aos neurônios. SIN cortical dysgenesis, neuronal migration abnormality.

craniocarpotarsal d., d. craniocarpotársica. SIN craniocarpotarsal *dystrophy.*

craniodiaphysial d. [MIM*218300], d. craniodiafisária; pequena estatura, espessamento dos ossos do crânio com esclerose e alargamento diafisário de ossos tubulares; herança autossômica recessiva. Também pode haver uma forma autossômica dominante [MIM 122860].

craniometaphysial d., d. craniometafisária; síndrome de displasia metafisária associada a esclerose acentuada e supercrescimento de ossos do crânio (leontíase óssea) e a hipertelorismo.

dentin d., d. da dentina; distúrbio hereditário dos dentes, envolvendo tanto a dentição primária quanto a permanente, no qual a morfologia clínica e a cor dos dentes são normais, mas, radiologicamente, os dentes exibem raízes curtas [MIM 125400], obliteração das câmaras pulpares e canais, e mobilidade e esfoliação prematura; herança autossômica dominante. Em outro tipo de displasia, os dentes são opalescentes [MIM 125420].

developmental hip d., d. congênita do quadril; anormalidade congênita na qual os quadris de um recém-nascido sofrem luxação facilmente; a etiologia é complexa, com contribuição de fatores mecânicos, familiares, hormonais e de apresentação ao nascimento; o predomínio feminino é de 9:1. SIN congenital hip d.

diaphysial d., d. diafisária; aumento fusiforme simétrico, progressivo, das diáfises dos ossos longos, caracterizado pela formação de novo osso periosteal e endosteal em excesso e pela conversão irregular desse osso cortical em osso esponjoso; a anemia não ocorre como regra, como na osteopetrose. SIN Engelmann disease.

diastrophic d. [MIM*222600], d. diastrófica; displasia óssea caracterizada por escoliose, "polegar do carona" devido ao encurtamento do primeiro osso metacarpal, fenda palatina, orelha malformada com calcificação, condrite, encurtamento do tendão de Aquiles, pé torto e achados radiográficos característicos; herança autossômica recessiva, causada por mutação no gene transportador de sulfato da displasia diastrófica (DTDST) no cromossoma 5q. SIN diastrophic dwarfism.

ectodermal d., d. ectodérmica; defeito congênito dos tecidos ectodérmicos, incluindo a pele e seus anexos; associada a displasia dos dentes e hipertermia. VER anhidrotic ectodermal d., hidrotic ectodermal d.

enamel d., d. do esmalte. SIN *amelogenesis* imperfecta.

d. epiphysea'lis mul'tiplex, d. epifisária múltipla. SIN multiple epiphyseal d.

d. epiphysia'lis hemime'lia, d. epifisária hemimélica. SIN tarsomegaly.

d. epiphysia'lis puncta'ta, d. epifisária pontilhada. SIN *chondrodysplasia* punctata.

epithelial d., d. epitelial; distúrbio da diferenciação de células epiteliais que podem regredir, permanecer estáveis ou progredir para carcinoma invasivo.

faciodigitogenital d., d. faciodigitogenital; síndrome de hipertelorismo ocular, narinas antevertidas, lábio superior largo, escroto em bolsa de sela ou xale, umbigo protruso e frouxidão dos ligamentos que resulta em joelho recurvado, pés planos e dedos hiperextensíveis; a forma ligada ao X [MIM*305400] é causada por mutação no gene FGD1 em Xp; também existem formas autossômica dominante [MIM*100050] e recessiva [MIM*227300]. SIN Aarskog-Scott syndrome.

familial white folded d., d. pregueada branca familiar. SIN white sponge *nevus.*

fibromuscular d., d. fibromuscular; doença não-aterosclerótica idiopática que causa estenose das artérias, geralmente das artérias renais, e hipertensão; duas variedades são hiperplasia fibromuscular e fibrose perimuscular.

fibrous d. of bone, d. fibrosa do osso; distúrbio da manutenção do osso medular no qual o osso que sofre lise fisiológica é substituído por proliferação anormal de tecido fibroso, resultando em distorção e expansão assimétrica do osso; pode ser limitada a um único osso (displasia fibrosa monostótica) ou envolver múltiplos ossos (displasia fibrosa poliostótica).

fibrous d. of jaws, d. fibrosa da mandíbula. SIN cherubism.

florid osseous d., cemental d., d. óssea florida, d. do cemento. SIN sclerotic cemental *mass.*

hidrotic ectodermal d. [MIM*129500], d. ectodérmica hidrótica; distrofia congênita das unhas e do cabelo com espessamento das unhas e cabelos ralos ou ausentes; freqüentemente associada à ceratodermia das regiões palmares e plantares; a função dos dentes e das glândulas sudoríparas é normal; herança autossômica dominante.

hypohidrotic ectodermal d., d. ectodérmica hipoidrótica. SIN anhidrotic ectodermal d.

mandibulofacial d., d. mandibulofacial. SIN mandibulofacial *dysostosis.*

McKusick metaphyseal d., d. metafisária de McKusick. SIN cartilage-hair *hypoplasia.*

metaphysial d., d. metafisária; anormalidade que ocorre quando o novo osso nas metáfises dos ossos longos não sofre remodelagem para a estrutura tubular normal; as extremidades dos ossos longos parecem ser expandidas e poróticas, com córtex fino; pode haver supercrescimento associado dos ossos do crânio (craniometafysial d.).

Mondini d., d. de Mondini; anomalia congênita do labirinto ótico ósseo e membranáceo caracterizada por cóclea aplásica e deformidade do vestíbulo e canais semicirculares, com perda parcial ou completa da função auditiva e vestibular; pode estar associada a otorréia espontânea de líquido cefalorraquidiano, resultando em meningite. VER TAMBÉM Mondini *hearing impairment.*

monostotic fibrous d., d. fibrosa monostótica; displasia fibrosa de um único osso. SIN localized osteitis fibrosa, osteitis fibrosa circumscripta.

mucoepithelial d. [MIM*158310], d. mucoepitelial; doença de desprendimento das células epiteliais, caracterizada por lesões mucosas vermelhas, ao redor dos orifícios, na mucosa oral, nasal, vaginal, uretral, anal, vesical e conjuntival, com catarata, ceratose folicular, alopecia não-cicatricial, infecções pulmonares freqüentes, pneumotórax e, algumas vezes, *cor pulmonale*; herança autossômica dominante.

multiple epiphyseal d. (EDM), d. epifisária múltipla; distúrbio das epífises caracterizado por dificuldade para caminhar, dor e rigidez das articulações, dedos das mãos curtos e grossos e, freqüentemente, baixa estatura; nas radiografias, as epífises são irregulares e mosqueadas, os centros de ossificação surgem tardiamente e podem ser múltiplos, mas as vértebras são normais. Há pelo menos 3 formas de herança autossômica dominante: EDM1 [MIM*132400], devida à mutação no gene da proteína da matriz oligomérica da cartilagem (COMP) no cromossoma 19p; EDM2 [MIM*600304], devida à mutação no gene do colágeno tipo IX (COL9A2) em 1p; e EDM3 [MIM*600969], que está ligada a um *locus* desconhecido. Também há uma forma autossômica recessiva [MIM*226900]. SIN d. epiphysealis multiplex.

neuronal intestinal d., d. intestinal neuronal. SIN neuronal *hyperplasia.*

oculoauriculovertebral d., OAV d. [MIM*257700], d. oculoauriculovertebral; síndrome caracterizada por dermóides epibulbares, apêndices pré-auriculares, micrognatia e anomalias vertebrais e de outros tipos. SIN Goldenhar syndrome, OAV syndrome.

oculodentodigital d. [MIM*164200], d. oculodentodigital; microftalmia, coloboma ou anomalias da íris associadas a malformação e mau posicionamento dos dentes e a anomalias dos dedos das mãos, incluindo sindactilia, campilodactilia ou ausência de falanges; herança autossômica dominante. Também há uma forma recessiva na qual a manifestação ocular é mais grave [MIM*257850].

oculovertebral d., d. oculovertebral; microftalmia, colobomas ou anoftalmia com órbita pequena, face "torta" devido à displasia unilateral do maxilar, macrostomia com dentes malformados e má oclusão, malformações vertebrais e costelas ramificadas e hipoplásicas. SIN oculovertebral syndrome, Weyers-Thier syndrome.

odontogenic d., d. odontogênica. SIN odontodysplasia.

ophthalmomandibulomelic d. [MIM*164900], d. oftalmomandibulomélica; distúrbio autossômico dominante com turvação da córnea e múltiplas anormalidades da mandíbula e dos membros.

otospondylomegaepiphyseal d., d. otoespondilomegaepifisária. SIN *chondrodystrophy* with sensorineural deafness.
periapical cemental d., d. do cemento periapical; condição benigna, indolor, não-neoplásica das mandíbulas, que ocorre quase exclusivamente em mulheres negras de meia-idade; as lesões geralmente são múltiplas, na maioria das vezes envolvendo dentes anteriores mandibulares vitais, circundam os ápices das raízes, e inicialmente, são radiotransparentes (e tornam-se mais opacas à medida que amadurecem). SIN periapical osteofibrosis.
polyostotic fibrous d., d. fibrosa poliostótica; a ocorrência de lesões de displasia fibrosa em múltiplos ossos, comumente de um lado do corpo; pode ocorrer com áreas de pigmentação e disfunção endócrina (síndrome de McCune-Albright). SIN multifocal osteitis fibrosa, osteitis fibrosa disseminata.
pseudoachondroplastic spondyloepiphysial d., d. espondiloepifisária pseudo-acondroplásica. SIN pseudoachondroplasia.
retinal d., d. retiniana; crescimento exagerado de tecido glial que compensa a aplasia dos elementos sensoriais.
septooptic d., d. do septo óptico; hipoplasia congênita do nervo óptico associada a anomalias cerebrais da linha média. SIN de Morsier syndrome.
skeletal d.'s, displasias ósseas; grupo heterogêneo de distúrbios (mais de 120 tipos), cada um deles resultando em numerosos distúrbios do sistema ósseo e a maioria incluindo nanismo. VER TAMBÉM chondrodystrophy.
spondyloepiphyseal d., d. espondiloepifisária; grupo de distúrbios caracterizados por deficiência do crescimento da coluna vertebral, com achatamento das vértebras ou platispondilia, ausência de ossificação das epífises, nanismo com tronco curto e encurtamento dos membros e, algumas vezes, com outras malformações; já foram descritas herança autossômica dominante [MIM*183900 e MIM*184100], autossômica recessiva [MIM*208230 e MIM*271600] e recessiva ligada ao X [MIM*313400].
spondyloepiphyseal d. congenita (SEDC) [MIM*183900], d. espondiloepifisária congênita; displasia óssea caracterizada por nanismo com tronco curto e membros curtos, ossificação tardia dos ramos do púbis e das epífises femoral e tibial, achatamento dos corpos vertebrais, miopia, descolamento da retina e fenda palatina; herança autossômica dominante causada por mutação no gene do colágeno tipo II (COL2A1) em 12q.
spondyloepiphyseal d. tarda, d. espondiloepifisária tardia; displasia óssea de início posterior, geralmente na segunda década de vida, caracterizada por baixa estatura, achatamento das vértebras, envolvimento epifisário com fusão óssea da articulação do quadril, osteoartrite prematura e achados radiográficos distintos. Existem formas autossômica dominante [MIM*184100] e recessiva ligada ao X [MIM*313400].
ventriculoradial d., d. ventriculorradial; síndrome congênita que consiste em uma comunicação interventricular com ausência do polegar ou do rádio associada.

dys·plas·tic (dis - plas'tik). Displásico; relativo a, ou caracterizado por, displasia.
dysp·nea (disp - nē'ă). Dispnéia; dificuldade ou angústia respiratória subjetiva, geralmente associada a doença do coração ou dos pulmões; ocorre normalmente durante esforço físico intenso ou em grandes altitudes. [G. *dyspnoia*, de *dys-*, mau, + *pnoē*, respiração]
cardiac d., d. cardíaca; falta de ar de origem cardíaca.
exertional d., d. aos esforços; falta de ar excessiva após exercício.
expiratory d., d. expiratória; dificuldade com a fase expiratória da respiração, freqüentemente devida à obstrução da laringe ou grandes brônquios, como por um corpo estranho.
functional d., d. funcional; falta de ar sem doença subjacente aparente.
nocturnal d., d. noturna; dispnéia que ocorre à noite, algumas horas após se deitar. Ocorre na insuficiência cardíaca e resulta da reabsorção de água de áreas mais baixas após a remoção do efeito da gravidade, causando hipervolemia, agravando a insuficiência ventricular esquerda.
paroxysmal nocturnal d., d. paroxística noturna; dispnéia aguda que aparece subitamente à noite, geralmente despertando o paciente; causada por congestão pulmonar com ou sem edema pulmonar, que resulta de insuficiência cardíaca esquerda após mobilização de líquido das áreas inferiores ao se deitar.
Traube d., d. de Traube; epônimo obsoleto para dispnéia inspiratória, com expansão torácica máxima e um ritmo respiratório lento.
dysp·ne·ic (disp - nē'ik). Dispneico; "sem fôlego"; relativo a, ou que sofre de, dispnéia.
dys·prax·ia (dis - prak'sē - ă). Dispraxia; funcionamento comprometido ou doloroso de qualquer órgão. [dys- + G. *praxis*, ato]
dys·pro·si·um (Dy) (dis - prō'sē-ŭm). Disprósio; elemento metálico da série dos lantanídeos (terras-raras), número atômico 66, peso atômico 162,50. [G. *dysprositos*, difícil de alcançar]
dys·pro·tein·e·mia (dis - prō'tēn - ē'mē - ă). Disproteinemia; anormalidade das proteínas plasmáticas, geralmente das imunoglobulinas.
dys·pro·tein·e·mic (dis - prō - tēn - ē'mik). Disproteinêmico; relativo à disproteinemia.
dys·ra·phism, dys·raph·ia (dis'ră - fizm, dis - raf'ē - ă). Disrafismo, disrafia; fusão defeituosa, especialmente das pregas neurais, resultando em um estado disráfico ou defeito do tubo neural. [dys- + G. *rhaphē*, sutura]

spinal d., d. espinal; termo genérico usado para descrever um conjunto de anormalidades congênitas que inclui defeitos nas vértebras e coluna ou raízes nervosas subjacentes.
dys·rhyth·mia (dis - rith'mē - ă). Disritmia; distúrbio do ritmo. Ver também entradas em ritmo. Cf. arrhythmia. [dys- + G. *rhythmos*, ritmo]
cardiac d., arritmia cardíaca; qualquer anormalidade da freqüência, regularidade ou seqüência da ativação cardíaca.
electroencephalographic d., d. eletroencefalográfica; traçado de ondas cerebrais difusamente irregular.
esophageal d., d. esofágica; motilidade anormal das camadas musculares da parede esofágica, como a que ocorre no espasmo esofágico.
paroxysmal cerebral d., d. cerebral paroxística; eletroencefalograma difusamente anormal, freqüentemente observado na epilepsia.
dys·som·nia (dis - som'nē - ă). Dissonia; distúrbio do sono normal ou do padrão rítmico.
dys·spon·dy·lism (dis - spon'di - lizm). Dispondilismo; anormalidade do desenvolvimento da medula espinal ou da coluna vertebral. [dys- + G. *spondylos*, vértebra]
dys·sta·sia (dis - stā'sē - ă). Distasia; dificuldade em ficar de pé. SIN dystasia. [dys- + G. *stasis*, estar de pé]
dys·stat·ic (dis - tat'ik). Distático; caracterizado pela dificuldade em se manter de pé.
dys·syl·la·bia (dis - il - lā'bē - ă). Dissilabia. SIN syllable-stumbling. [dys- + G. *syllabē*, sílaba]
dys·syn·er·gia (dis - in - er'jē - ă). Dissinergia; um aspecto da ataxia, no qual um ato não é realizado de forma tranqüila ou acurada devido à ausência de associação harmoniosa de seus vários componentes; geralmente usado para descrever anormalidades do movimento causadas por distúrbios cerebelares. [dys- + G. *syn*, com, + *ergon*, trabalho]
d. cerebellaris myoclonica, d. cerebelar mioclônica; distúrbio familiar que começa no final da segunda infância, caracterizado por ataxia cerebelar progressiva, mioclônus de ação e preservação do intelecto. Provavelmente tem múltiplas causas, com as anormalidades mitocondriais sendo uma delas. SIN dentatorubral cerebellar atrophy with polymyoclonus.
detrusor sphincter d., d. do esfíncter detrusor; distúrbio da relação normal entre a contração da bexiga (detrusor) e o relaxamento do esfíncter durante esforços miccionais voluntários ou involuntários.
dys·tas·ia. Distasia. SIN dysstasia.
dys·tel·e·pha·lan·gy (dis - tel'ē - fă - lan'jē). Distelefalangia; encurtamento da falange distal do dedo mínimo. [dys- + G. *telos*, extremidade, + falange]
dys·thy·mia (dis - thī'mē - ă). Distimia; distúrbio crônico do humor que se manifesta como depressão durante a maior parte do dia, na maioria das vezes acompanhado por alguns dos seguintes sintomas: diminuição do apetite ou ingestão excessiva de alimentos, insônia ou hipersonia, diminuição da energia ou fadiga, baixa auto-estima, diminuição da concentração, dificuldade em tomar decisões e sentimentos de desesperança. VER mood *disorders*, em *disorder*, endogenous *depression*, exogenous *depression*. [dys- + G. *thymos*, mente, emoção]
dys·thy·mic (dis - thī'mik). Distímico; relativo à distimia.
dys·to·cia (dis - tō'sē - ă). Distocia; parto difícil. [G. *dystokia*, de *dys-*, difícil, + *tokos*, parto]
arrest of active phase d., distocia com interrupção da fase ativa; interrupção da dilatação cervical adicional por mais de 2 horas após o trabalho de parto ter entrado na fase ativa (geralmente definida como contração ativa com dilatação cervical de pelo menos 4 cm); as causas incluem contrações uterinas inadequadas e desproporção cefalopélvica.
arrest of descent d., distocia com interrupção da descida; incapacidade do feto de descer após uma hora no segundo estágio, apesar do esforço materno; tipicamente causada por esforço materno inadequado, má posição fetal ou tamanho fetal.
fetal d., d. fetal; distocia devida a uma anormalidade do feto.
maternal d., d. materna; distocia causada por uma anormalidade ou problema físico na mãe.
placental d., d. placentária; retenção ou eliminação difícil da placenta.
shoulder d., d. do ombro; interrupção do trabalho de parto normal após o desprendimento da cabeça por impacção da porção anterior do ombro contra a sínfise púbica.
dys·to·nia (dis - tō'nē - ă). Distonia; estado de tonicidade anormal (hipo ou hipertonicidade) em qualquer dos tecidos, resultando em comprometimento do movimento voluntário. [dys- + G. *tonos*, tensão]
d. lenticula'ris, d. lenticular; distonia resultante de uma lesão do núcleo lenticulado.
d. musculo'rum defor'mans, d. muscular deformante; distúrbio genético, ambiental ou idiopático, que geralmente começa na infância ou na adolescência, caracterizando-se por contrações musculares que distorcem a coluna vertebral, os membros, os quadris e, algumas vezes, os músculos supridos por nervos cranianos. Os movimentos anormais são aumentados por excitação e, ao menos inicialmente, abolidos pelo sono. A musculatura é hipertônica, quando

em atividade, e hipotônica quando em repouso. As formas hereditárias geralmente começam com postura involuntária do pé ou da mão (forma autossômica recessiva [MIM*224500]), ou do pescoço ou tronco (forma autossômica dominante [MIM*128100]); as duas formas podem progredir para produzir contorções de todo o corpo. SIN torsion disease of childhood, torsion d., Ziehen-Oppenheim disease.
torsion d., d. de torção. SIN d. musculorum deformans.
dys·ton·ic (dis-ton′ik). Distônico; relativo à distonia.
dys·to·pia (dis-tō′pē-ă). Distopia; posição defeituosa ou anormal de uma parte ou órgão. SIN allotopia, malposition. [dys- + G. *topos*, lugar]
   pituitary d., d. hipofisária; ausência de união da neuro-hipófise e adeno-hipófise.
dys·top·ic (dis-top′ik). Distópico; pertinente a, ou caracterizado por, distopia.
VER TAMBÉM ectopic.
dys·tro·phia (dis-trō′fē-ă). Distrofia. SIN dystrophy. [L. do G. *dys-*, mau, + *trophē*, nutrição]
   d. adipo′sogenita′lis, d. adiposogenital. SIN adiposogenital *dystrophy*.
   d. brevicol′lis, condição caracterizada por sintomas de distrofia adiposogenital associados a encurtamento deformante do pescoço, mas sem sinostose das vértebras cervicais (como ocorre na síndrome de Klippel-Feil).
   d. myoton′ica, distrofia miotônica. SIN myotonic *dystrophy*.
   d. un′guium, distrofia ungueal; distrofia das unhas.
dys·tro·phic (dis-trof′ik). Distrófico; pertinente ou relacionado à distrofia.
dys·tro·phin (dis-trō′fin). Distrofina; proteína encontrada no sarcolema dos músculos normais; não existe nos indivíduos com distrofia muscular pseudo-hipertrófica nem em outras formas de distrofia muscular; sua função seria a de ligação do citoesqueleto da célula muscular à proteína extracelular. SIN distropin, dystrophin.
dys·tro·phy (dis′trō-fē). Distrofia; alterações progressivas que resultariam da nutrição deficiente de um tecido ou órgão. SIN dystrophia [dys + G. *trophē*, nutrição]
   adiposogenital d., d. adiposogenital; distúrbio caracterizado basicamente por obesidade e hipogonadismo hipogonadotrófico em meninos adolescentes; o nanismo é raro e, quando presente, acredita-se que reflita hipotireoidismo. Pode haver perda visual, anormalidades do comportamento e diabetes insípido. O termo síndrome de Fröhlich freqüentemente é usado como sinônimo desse distúrbio. Embora o caso original envolvesse um tumor primário, acredita-se que a maioria dos casos resulte de disfunção hipotalâmica em áreas que regulam o apetite e o desenvolvimento gonadal. As causas mais comuns são neoplasias hipofisárias e hipotalâmicas. SIN adiposis orchica, adiposogenital degeneration, adiposogenital syndrome, dystrophia adiposogenitalis, Fröhlich syndrome, hypophysial syndrome, hypothalamic obesity with hypogonadism, Launois-Cléret syndrome.
   adult foveomacular retinal d., d. retiniana foveomacular do adulto; distúrbio autossômico dominante que se apresenta na quinta década de vida com diminuição discreta da visão e lesão amarela, redonda, subfoveal com uma mancha hiperpigmentada central.
   adult pseudohypertrophic muscular d. [MIM*310200.0002], d. muscular pseudo-hipertrófica do adulto. SIN Becker muscular d.
   anterior corneal d., d. corneana anterior; opacificação da córnea com envolvimento do epitélio, membrana basal (basement *membrane*) ou membrana de Bowman da córnea (Bowman *membrane* of the cornea).
   asphyxiating thoracic d. [MIM*208500], d. torácica asfixiante; hipoplasia hereditária do tórax associada a anormalidade óssea pélvica. SIN asphyxiating thoracic chondrodystrophy, asphyxiating thoracic dysplasia, Jeune syndrome, thoracic-pelvic-phalangeal d.
   Becker muscular d., d. muscular de Becker; distúrbio muscular hereditário de início tardio, geralmente na segunda ou terceira década de vida, que afeta os músculos proximais com característica pseudo-hipertrofia das panturrilhas; possui características clínicas semelhantes às da distrofia muscular de Duchenne, porém é muito mais leve e não tem uma genética letal; herança recessiva ligada ao X, e tanto a distrofia de Becker quanto a de Duchenne são causadas por mutação no gene da distrofina em Xp. Cf. Duchenne d. SIN adult pseudohypertrophic muscular d., Becker-type tardive muscular d.
   Becker-type tardive muscular d., d. muscular tardia tipo Becker. SIN Becker muscular d.
   central areolar choroidal d., d. coroidal areolar central; distúrbio progressivo autossômico dominante de perda visual com áreas bem demarcadas de atrofia do epitélio pigmentar da retina (retinal pigmental *epithelium*) e coriocapilar.
   central cloudy corneal d. of François, d. corneana turva central de François; opacificação autossômica dominante do estroma corneano central que consiste em áreas poligonais turvas.
   central crystalline corneal d. of Snyder, d. corneana cristalina central de Snyder; opacificação autossômica dominante do estroma corneano central por cristais policromáticos em forma de agulha.
   childhood muscular d., d. muscular da infância. SIN Duchenne d.
   Cogan d., d. de Cogan. SIN map-dot-fingerprint d.
   cone d., d. dos cones; anormalidade da retina na qual há grave deficiência da percepção da cor e ocorrem alterações típicas no eletrorretinograma. VER achromatopsia. SIN cone degeneration.

cone-rod retinal d., d. retiniana dos cones-bastonetes; distúrbio que afeta mais os cones que os bastonetes da retina, caracterizado por diminuição da visão central e da visão colorida.
congenital hereditary endothelial d., d. endotelial hereditária congênita; distúrbio com herança dominante ou recessiva caracterizado por córnea turva e espessa ao nascimento ou no período neonatal.
corneal d. [MIM*217600], d. corneana; opacificação central da córnea, geralmente bilateral, simétrica, envolvendo predominantemente as camadas epitelial, do estroma ou endotelial, freqüentemente em um padrão típico; herança autossômica recessiva.
craniocarpotarsal d. [MIM*193700], d. craniocarpotarsal; síndrome caracterizada por características faciais específicas com olhos afundados, hipertelorismo, filtro longo, nariz pequeno e boca pequena e enrugada (como se estivesse assobiando) e malformações com desvio ulnar das mãos, camptodactilia, talipes eqüinovaro e defeitos do osso frontal; herança autossômica dominante. SIN craniocarpotarsal dysplasia, Freeman-Sheldon syndrome, whistling face syndrome.
Duchenne d., d. de Duchenne; a distrofia muscular infantil mais comum, que geralmente se inicia antes dos 6 anos. Caracterizada por fraqueza simétrica e desgaste, primeiro, dos músculos pélvicos e crurais e, depois, dos músculos peitorais e dos membros superiores proximais; pseudo-hipertrofia de alguns músculos, principalmente da panturrilha; envolvimento cardíaco; algumas vezes retardo mental leve; evolução progressiva e morte precoce, geralmente na adolescência. Herança ligada ao X (afeta os homens e é transmitida pelas mulheres). SIN childhood muscular d., Duchenne disease, pseudohypertrophic muscular d.
Emery-Dreifuss muscular d., d. muscular de Emery-Dreifuss; tipo geralmente benigno de distrofia muscular que surge na infância ou no início da vida adulta. A fraqueza começa nos músculos do cíngulo do membro superior e nos músculos proximais dos membros superiores, propagando-se para o cíngulo do membro inferior e para os músculos distais dos membros inferiores. Freqüentemente ocorrem contraturas dos músculos flexores do cotovelo, flexores do pescoço e da panturrilha; não há pseudo-hipertrofia muscular nem retardo mental. É comum haver miocardiopatia. Distúrbio hereditário ligado ao X, não-alelo à distrofia muscular de Duchenne.
facioscapulohumeral muscular d. [MIM*158900], d. muscular facioescapuloumeral; distúrbio hereditário muito variável, que surge na infância ou na adolescência, caracterizado por fraqueza e debilitação, algumas vezes assimétrica, principalmente dos músculos da face, cíngulo do membro superior, braços e, posteriormente, cíngulo do membro inferior e pernas; herança autossômica dominante. sin facioscapulohumeral atrophy, Landouzy-Dejerine d.
Favre d., d. de Favre. SIN vitreotapetoretinal d.
fingerprint d., d. em impressão digital; condição na qual se observam linhas paralelas finas em uma área de configuração de impressão digital na camada epitelial basal e na membrana basal do epitélio corneano. VER TAMBÉM map-dot-fingerprint d.
fleck d. of cornea [MIM*121850], d. mosqueada da córnea; ocorrência bilateral de manchas sutis no estroma corneano; as manchas variam em tamanho e formato, possuindo margens nítidas e centros claros; pode haver fotofobia; herança autossômica dominante.
Fuchs endothelial d., d. endotelial de Fuchs; distrofia corneana comum com herança autossômica dominante, caracterizada por ceratopatia em gota com perda do endotélio e edema progressivo da córnea.
gelatinous droplike corneal d., d. corneana gelatinosa semelhante a gotas; distúrbio autossômico recessivo, bilateral, caracterizado por depósitos de amilóide elevados, semelhantes a amoras, envolvendo o epitélio e o estroma anterior da córnea.
granular corneal d., d. granular da córnea; distúrbio autossômico dominante caracterizado por depósitos hialinos no estroma da córnea.
Groenouw corneal d., d. corneana de Groenouw; (1) tipo granular de distrofia da córnea, com herança autossômica dominante [MIM*121900], causada por mutação no gene do fator de transformação do crescimento, beta-induzido (TGFB1) que codifica a ceratoepitelina no cromossomo 5q; (2) tipo macular progressivo de distrofia da córnea, caracterizado por opacidades pontilhadas e episódios de fotofobia, erosão da córnea e sensação de corpo estranho; herança autossômica recessiva.
gutter d. of cornea, d. sulcada da córnea; sulco marginal geralmente situado cerca de 1 mm abaixo do limbo; e, algumas vezes, bilateral. SIN keratoleptynsis (1).
hereditary epithelial d., d. epitelial hereditária. SIN Meesman d.
hypertrophic d., d. hipertrófica. SIN squamous cell *hyperplasia.*
infantile neuroaxonal d., d. neuroaxonal infantil; distúrbio familiar, raro, dos primeiros anos de vida, que se manifesta como deterioração psicomotora progressiva, aumento dos reflexos, sinal de Babinski, hipotonia e cegueira progressiva. No exame anatomopatológico são encontrados esferóides eosinofílicos de axoplasma edemaciado em vários núcleos do sistema nervoso central.
Landouzy-Dejerine d., d. de Landouzy-Dejerine. SIN facioscapulohumeral muscular d.
lattice corneal d. [MIM*122200], d. reticulada da córnea; distrofia da córnea causada por acúmulo localizado de amilóide em um padrão reticular; manifes-

ta-se na puberdade e é lentamente progressiva até a perda final da visão; herança autossômica dominante, causada por mutação no gene do fator de transformação do crescimento beta-induzido (TGFB1) que codifica a ceratoepitelina em 5q.
Leyden-Möbius muscular d., d. muscular de Leyden-Möbius. SIN limb-girdle muscular d.
limb-girdle muscular d. [MIM*253600], d. muscular do cíngulo dos membros; grupo de distrofias musculares, provavelmente de natureza heterogênea. O início geralmente se dá na infância ou no início da vida adulta, e ambos os sexos são afetados. Caracterizada por fraqueza e debilitação, geralmente simétricas, dos músculos do cíngulo do membro inferior e/ou dos músculos do cíngulo do membro superior, mas não dos músculos faciais. Não há pseudo-hipertrofia muscular, envolvimento cardíaco nem retardo mental. Já foram descritas heranças autossômicas dominante e recessiva. SIN Leyden-Möbius muscular d., pelvofemoral muscular d., scapulohumeral muscular d.
macular corneal d., d. macular da córnea; distúrbio autossômico recessivo caracterizado por depósitos de glicosaminoglicanas no estroma da córnea.
macular retinal d., d. macular da retina; grupo de distúrbios que envolvem predominantemente a porção posterior do fundo do olho, causados pela degeneração da camada sensorial da retina, epitélio pigmentar da retina, membrana de Bruch, coróide ou uma combinação desses tecidos. VER Stargardt *disease*, Best *disease*.
map-dot-fingerprint d., d. em impressões digitais; distrofia em impressões digitais, acompanhada por padrões semelhantes a mapas e inclusões epiteliais microcísticas. SIN Cogan d.
Meesman d. [MIM*122100], d. de Meesman; distrofia epitelial caracterizada por cistos e opacidades progressivas no epitélio corneano, com início no primeiro ano de vida; herança autossômica dominante com penetração incompleta. SIN hereditary epithelial d.
microcystic epithelial d., d. epitelial microcística; cistos intra-epiteliais, simétricos, bilaterais, na área central da córnea de mulheres saudáveis, sem predisposição hereditária.
mucopolysaccharide keratin d., d. de queratina mucopolissacarídica; achado histológico, observado no epitélio superficial da hiperplasia fibrosa inflamatória oral, que consiste em acúmulos de material eosinofílico homogêneo na camada espinhosa superficial.
muscular d., d. muscular; termo genérico que designa vários distúrbios degenerativos progressivos, hereditários, que afetam os músculos esqueléticos e, freqüentemente, também outros sistemas orgânicos. SIN myodystrophy, myodystrophia.
myotonic d. [MIM*160900], distrofia miotônica; a distrofia muscular mais comum em adultos, caracterizada por fraqueza muscular progressiva e debilitação de alguns dos músculos supridos por nervos cranianos, bem como os músculos distais dos membros; outras características clínicas incluem miotonia, catarata, hipogonadismo, anormalidades cardíacas e calvície frontal; geralmente surge na terceira década de vida; herança autossômica dominante causada por expansão de repetições de trinucleotídeos anormais no gene da proteinocinase da distrofia miotônica (DMPK) no cromossoma 19q. Esse distúrbio exibe antecipação (aumento da gravidade em gerações sucessivas devido à amplificação sucessiva das repetições de trinucleotídeos); a forma congênita grave é quase sempre limitada à prole de mulheres afetadas. SIN dystrophia myotonica, myotonia atrophica, myotonia dystrophica, Steinert disease.
neuroaxonal d., d. neuroaxonal; distúrbio raro que começa no segundo ano de vida e evolui inexoravelmente; caracterizado clinicamente por dificuldade de marcha, fraqueza e arreflexia, posteriormente surgindo achados corticoespinais e pseudobulbares, cegueira, perda da apreciação da dor e deterioração mental; no exame anatomopatológico, são encontrados esferóides eosinofílicos de axoplasma edemaciado em vários núcleos centrais; herança autossômica recessiva.
oculopharyngeal d., d. oculofaríngea; forma de oftalmoplegia (*ophthalmoplegia*) externa progressiva crônica, que geralmente se apresenta na meia-idade ou na velhice, com ptose crônica e/ou dificuldade para deglutir. Muitos pacientes acometidos têm ascendência franco-canadense.
pattern retinal d., d. retiniana padrão; espectro de doenças autossômicas dominantes que afetam o epitélio pigmentar da retina (retinal pigment *epithelium*), causando perda visual leve a moderada.
pelvofemoral muscular d., d. muscular pélvico-femoral. SIN limb-girdle muscular d.
posterior corneal d., d. posterior da córnea; opacificação com envolvimento primário do endotélio da córnea.
posterior polymorphous corneal d., d. polimorfa posterior da córnea; distúrbio autossômico dominante caracterizado por anormalidades vesiculares e lineares do endotélio corneano; algumas vezes causa edema da córnea.
pre-Descemet corneal d., d. corneana pré-Descemet; opacificação com envolvimento primário do estroma posterior da córnea.
progressive tapetochoroidal d., d. tapetocoroidal progressiva. SIN choroideremia.
pseudohypertrophic muscular d., d. muscular pseudo-hipertrófica. SIN Duchenne d.
reflex sympathetic d. (RSD), d. simpática reflexa; dor persistente difusa, geralmente em um membro, amiúde associada a distúrbios vasomotores, alterações tróficas e limitação ou imobilidade articular; freqüentemente sucede alguma lesão local. VER TAMBÉM causalgia. SIN shoulder-hand syndrome, sympathetic reflex d.
Reis-Bücklers corneal d., d. corneana de Reis-Bücklers; distúrbio autossômico dominante da membrana de Bowman (Bowman *membrane*) da córnea, caracterizado por opacidade reticular associada a erosões recorrentes da córnea.
ringlike corneal d. [MIM*121900], d. anular da córnea; opacidades filiformes do estroma anterior da córnea, com início agudo, doloroso, seguido por diminuição da visão; herança autossômica dominante, causada por mutationina, o gene do fator de transformação do crescimento beta-induzido (TGFB1) que codifica o ceratoepitélio no cromossoma 5q.
scapulohumeral muscular d., d. muscular escapuloumeral. SIN limb-girdle muscular d.
stromal corneal d., d. do estroma corneano; opacificação com envolvimento da camada média da córnea.
sympathetic reflex d., d. reflexa simpática. SIN reflex sympathetic d.
thoracic-pelvic-phalangeal d., d. toracopelvicofalângica. SIN asphyxiating thoracic d.
twenty-nail d., d. das 20 unhas; surgimento de cristas longitudinais em todas as unhas; observada na alopecia circunscrita e no líquen plano.
vitelliform retinal d., d. retiniana vitelliforme. SIN Best *disease*.
vitreotapetoretinal d. [MIM*268100], d. vitreotapetorretiniana; retinosquise central e periférica bilateral, autossômica recessiva, com degeneração pigmentar da retina, atrofia coriorretiniana, degeneração do vítreo e cegueira noturna. SIN Favre d.
vortex corneal d., d. verticilado da córnea; padrão espiralado de células epiteliais da córnea anormalmente pigmentadas, observado na doença de Fabry (Fabry *disease*) e em resposta a determinados medicamentos (incluindo cloroquina, clorpromazina e amiodarona).
vulvar d., d. vulvar; espectro de erupções vulvares que consistem em pápulas atróficas brancas, incluindo líquen escleroso e atrófico, hiperplasia de células escamosas (distrofia hipertrófica), ou uma combinação destes (distrofia mista). VER TAMBÉM *lichen* sclerosus et atrophicus.
dystropin. Distrofina. SIN dystrophin.
dys·tro·py (dis'trō-pē). Distropia; comportamento anormal ou excêntrico. [dys- + G. *tropos*, desvio]
dys·u·ria (dis-ū'rē-ă). Disúria; dificuldade ou dor à micção. SIN dysury. [dys- + G. *ouron*, urina]
dys·u·ric (dis-ū'rik). Disúrico; relativo a, ou que sofre de, disúria.
dys·u·ry (dis'ū-rē). Disúria. SIN dysuria.
dys·ver·sion (dis-ver'zhŭn). Rotação em qualquer direção, menor que a inversão; particularmente da cabeça do nervo óptico (*situs inversus* do disco óptico). [dys- + L. *verto*, girar]

E

ε **1.** Quinta letra do alfabeto grego, epsilon. **2.** Símbolo de molar absorption *coefficient* (coeficiente de absorção molar) ou de extinction *coefficient* (coeficiente de extinção). Quanto aos termos que começam com esse prefixo, VER o termo específico. **3.** Em química, designa a posição de um substituto localizado no quinto átomo do grupamento carboxila ou de outro grupamento funcional primário. Quanto a termos que começam com esse prefixo, ver o termo específico.

E 1. Símbolo de exa-; extraction *ratio* (taxa de extração); glutamic acid (ácido glutâmico); *energy* (energia); electromotive *force* (força eletromotriz); glutamyl (glutamil); internal *energy* (energia interna). **2.** Como subscrito, refere-se ao expired *gas* (gás expirado); símbolo obsoleto de einsteinium (einstênio).

E_0^*, E^0, E_h Símbolos para potencial de oxidation-reduction potential (oxirredução).

E_2 Símbolo de estradiol (estradiol).

E_1 Símbolo de estrone (estrona).

Ē Abreviatura de *entgegen* (alemão, oposto).

E_a Abreviatura de *energy* of activation (energia de ativação).

e Símbolo de carga elétrica elementar; base do logaritmo natural ou neperiano (2,71828...). É o limite de $1 + (1/n!)$.

EAE Abreviatura de experimental allergic *encephalitis* (encefalite alérgica experimental).

Eagle, Harry, médico e biólogo celular norte-americano, 1905–1992. VER E. basal *medium*, minimum essential *medium*.

Eagle, Watt W., otorrinolaringologista norte-americano do século XX.

Eales, Henry, oftalmologista inglês, 1852–1913. VER E. *disease*.

ear (ēr) [TA]. Orelha; o órgão da audição; composta pela **orelha externa**, que inclui a orelha e o meato acústico, ou auditivo, externo; a **orelha média** ou cavidade timpânica, com seus ossículos; e a **orelha interna** ou labirinto, que inclui os canais semicirculares, o vestíbulo e a cóclea. VER TAMBÉM auricle. SIN auris [TA]. [A.S. *eáre*]

Aztec e., o. asteca; orelha sem o lóbulo.

bat e., o. de morcego. SIN lop-ear.

bladder e., o. vesical; protrusão de parte da bexiga para o canal inguinal proximal; freqüentemente observada em CUM (cistouretrografia miccional) pediátrica e raramente tem importância clínica.

Blainville e.'s, orelhas de Blainville; assimetria no tamanho ou no formato das orelhas.

boxer's e., o. de boxeador, o. em couve-flor. SIN cauliflower e.

Cagot e. (kă-gō′), o. de Cagot; orelha sem lóbulo. [um povo dos Pirineus, entre os quais são comuns os estigmas físicos]

cauliflower e., o. em couve-flor; espessamento e endurecimento da orelha, com distorção dos contornos após extravasamento de sangue nos seus tecidos. SIN boxer's e.

darwinian e., o. de Darwin; orelha na qual a borda superior não é enrolada para formar a hélice, mas se projeta para cima como uma borda plana, angulosa.

dog e., o. de cachorro; ângulo redundante de pele, geralmente resultante de aproximação inadequada das bordas cutâneas no fechamento de uma ferida, deixando uma protuberância excessiva ou um pedaço triangular de tecido.

external e., o. externa. SIN auris externa. VER TAMBÉM auricle, external acoustic *meatus*, pinna.

glue e., otite média de "cola"; inflamação da orelha média com líquido mucóide causada por obstrução crônica da tuba auditiva.

internal e., o. interna. SIN auris interna. VER TAMBÉM labyrinth.

lop e., o. pendente. SIN outstanding e. VER lop-ear.

middle e., o. média. SIN auris media. VER TAMBÉM tympanic *cavity*.

Morel e., o. de Morel; orelha grande, malformada, proeminente, com sulcos obliterados e bordas afiladas.

Mozart e., o. de Mozart; deformidade da orelha quando os dois ramos da antélice e o ramo da hélice são fundidos, produzindo saliência da parte superior da orelha. [Wolfgang Amadeus Mozart, 1756–1791, compositor, que se diz ter sido portador dessa deformidade]

outstanding e., o. proeminente; protrusão excessiva da orelha em relação à cabeça, geralmente devido à ausência de desenvolvimento da prega da antélice. SIN lop e., protruding e.

protruding e., o. protrusa. SIN outstanding e.

scroll e., o. em espiral; deformidade da orelha externa na qual a orelha está enrolada para frente.

Stahl e., o. de Stahl; orelha externa deformada, na qual a fossa oval e a porção

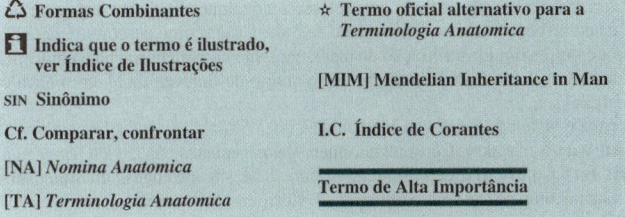

⌒ **Formas Combinantes**

🅸 **Indica que o termo é ilustrado, ver Índice de Ilustrações**

SIN **Sinônimo**

Cf. Comparar, confrontar

[NA] *Nomina Anatomica*

[TA] *Terminologia Anatomica*

☆ Termo oficial alternativo para a *Terminologia Anatomica*

[MIM] Mendelian Inheritance in Man

I.C. Índice de Corantes

Termo de Alta Importância

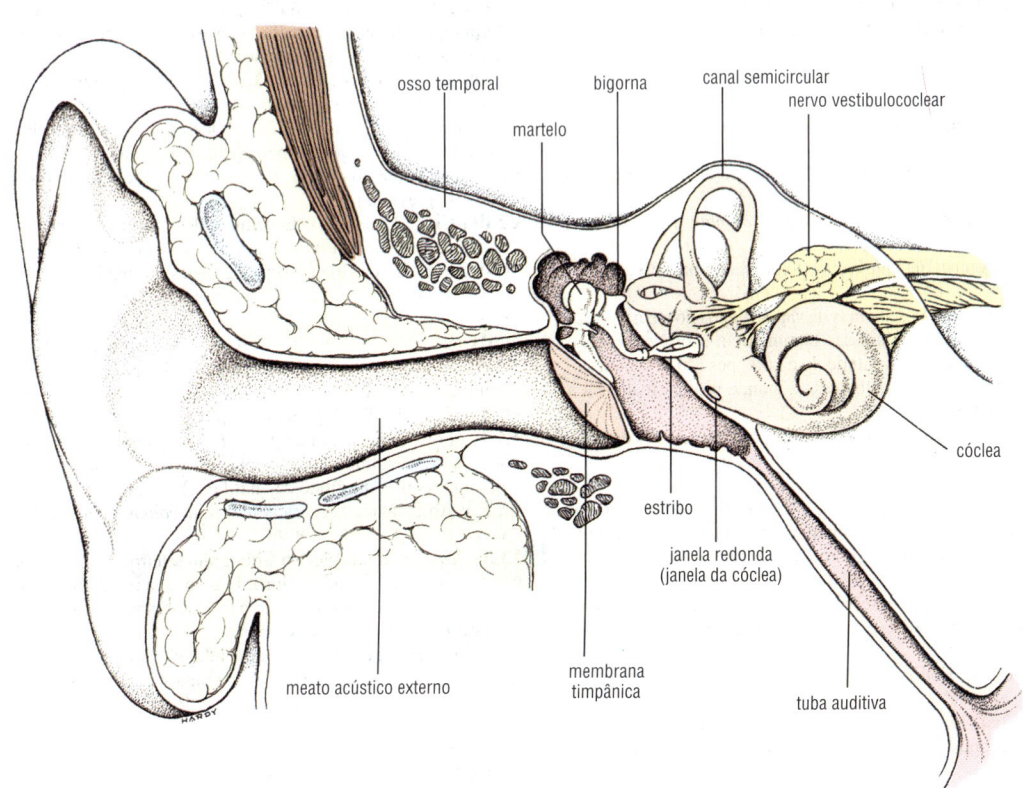

orelha

superior da escafa são cobertas pela hélice; antigamente era considerada um estigma de degeneração constitucional.
  swimmer's e., o. de nadadôr; otite externa. SIN *otitis* externa.
  telephone e., o. de telefone; perda auditiva induzida por ruído causada por exposição à estática nos telefones.
  Wildermuth e., o. de Wildermuth; orelha na qual a hélice está virada para trás e a antélice é proeminente.
ear·ache (ēr'āk). Otalgia; dor no ouvido. SIN otalgia, otodynia.
ear·drum (ēr'drŭm). Tímpano; a orelha média. Cf. tympanic *membrane.* SIN tympanum.
Earle, Wilton R., patologista norte-americano, 1902–1964. VER E. L. *fibrosarcoma, solution.*
ear·piece (ēr - pēs). Audiofone; fone de ouvido; parte de um aparelho introduzido no canal auditivo externo para levar o som até a orelha.
ear·plug (ēr'plŭg). Termo genérico que designa dispositivos oclusivos no canal auditivo externo para proteção contra perda auditiva induzida por ruído ou para evitar a entrada de água na orelha. VER TAMBÉM hearing *protectors,* em *protector.*
earth (ĕrth). Terra. **1.** Solo; o material macio da terra, ao contrário da rocha e da areia. **2.** Um mineral facilmente pulverizado. **3.** Um óxido insolúvel de alumínio ou de alguns outros elementos caracterizados por elevado ponto de fusão. [A.S. *eorthe*]
  alkaline e.'s, terras alcalinas. VER alkaline earth *elements,* em *element.*
  diatomaceous e., t. diatomácea; pó feito de material diatomáceo dessecado; usado como agente filtrante, adsorvente e abrasivo em muitas operações químicas.
  fuller's e., t. de pisoeiro; **(1)** variedade amorfa de caulim de composição variada, contendo um silicato de magnésio e alumínio. O nome é derivado de um processo antigo de limpeza ou de "enchimento" da lã para remover óleo e partículas de sujeira com uma pasta aquosa de terra ou argila. **(2)** argila refinada usada algumas vezes como pó secante ou aplicada molhada como água como forma de emplastro. Atualmente refere-se a qualquer argila que possa ser usada como descorante no refinamento de óleo. Usada como descorante para óleos e outros líquidos, filtração de meio, enchimento para borracha e em formulações agrícolas. [de *fulling,* processo antigo de limpeza da lã, com terra ou argila]
  rare e.'s, terras-raras. VER lanthanides.
ear·wax (ēr'wăks). Cerume; cerúmen. SIN cerumen.
eat (ēt). Comer. **1.** Ingerir alimento sólido. **2.** Mastigar e engolir qualquer substância como se faz com o alimento. **3.** Corroer. [A.S. *etan*]
Eaton, Lee M., neurologista norte-americano, 1905-1958. VER E.-Lambert *syndrome.*
Eaton, Monroe A., microbiologista norte-americano, *1904. VER E. *agent.*
E.B., EB Abreviatura de elementary *bodies* (1), em *body.*
Ebbinghaus, Hermann, alemão, 1850–1909. VER E. *test.*
Eberth, Karl J., médico alemão, 1835–1926. VER E. *bacillus, lines,* em *line, perithelium.*
Ebner, Victor von. VER von Ebner.
e·bo·na·tion (ē - bō - nā'shŭn). Remoção de fragmentos ósseos livres de uma ferida. [L.]
ébran·le·ment (ā - brahn - la - mon'). Torção do pedículo de um pólipo para causar atrofia. [Fr.]
Ebstein, Wilhelm, médico alemão, 1836–1912. VER E. *anomaly, disease, sign;* Armanni-E. *change, kidney;* Pel-E. *disease, fever.*
EBT Abreviatura de electron beam *tomography* (tomografia com feixe de elétrons).
eb·ul·lism (ĕb'ŭ - lĭzm). Formação de bolhas de vapor d'água nos tecidos produzidas por uma redução extrema da pressão barométrica; ocorre se o corpo for exposto a pressões acima de uma altitude de 63.000 pés (20.000 metros), ou se um mergulhador subir rapidamente de uma grande profundidade até a superfície. [L. *ebullire,* ferver]
ebur (ē'bŭr). Tecido semelhante ao marfim em seu aspecto externo ou estrutura. [L. ivory]
  e. den'tis, dentina. SIN dentine.
eb·ur·na·tion (ē - bŭr - nā'shŭn). Eburnação; alteração do osso subcondral exposto na doença articular degenerativa, na qual este é convertido em uma substância densa com uma superfície lisa como o marfim. SIN bone sclerosis. [L. *eburneus,* de marfim]
  e. of dentin, e. da dentina; condição observada na interrupção da cárie dentária, em que a dentina descalcificada é lustrada e adquire um aspecto polido, freqüentemente de cor castanha.
ebur·ne·ous (ē - bŭr'nē - ŭs). Ebúrneo; semelhante ao marfim, principalmente na cor.
ebur·ni·tis (ē - bŭr - nī'tĭs). Eburnite; aumento da densidade e da dureza da dentina, podendo ocorrer após a exposição da dentina. [L. *eburneus,* de marfim, + G. *-itis,* inflamação]
EBV Abreviatura do Epstein-Barr *virus* (vírus Epstein-Barr).
EC Abreviatura de *Enzyme Commission of the International Union of Biochemistry,* usado em conjunto com um número único para definir uma enzima específica na lista da *Enzyme Commission [Enzyme Nomenclature]* (1984); p. ex., EC 1.1.1.1 define uma desidrogenase alcoólica e EC 2.6.1.1 define a aspartato aminotransferase, também conhecida como transaminase glutâmico-oxalacética (TGO).
△ **ec-.** Fora de, longe de. [G.]
E-cad·her·rin (ē - cad - hēr'in). E-caderina. SIN uvomorulin.
écar·teur (ā - kar - tēr'). Um tipo de afastador. [Fr. *écarter,* separar]
ecau·date (ē - kaw'dāt). Sem cauda. [L. *e-* priv. + *cauda,* cauda]
ec·bo·line (ĕk'bō - lēn). Ecbolina. SIN ergotoxine.
ec·cen·tric (ĕk - sĕn'trĭk). Excêntrico. **1.** Anormal ou peculiar em idéias ou comportamento. SIN erratic (1). **2.** Procedente de um centro. Cf. centifugal (2). **3.** SIN peripheral. [G. *ek,* fora, + *kentron,* centro]
ec·cen·tro·chon·dro·pla·sia (ĕk - sĕn'trō - kon - drō - plā'zē - ă). Excentrocondroplasia; desenvolvimento epifisário anormal a partir de centros excêntricos de ossificação. [G. *ek,* fora, + *kentron,* centro, + *chondros,* cartilagem, + *plasis,* moldagem]
ec·cen·tro·pi·e·sis (ĕk - sĕn'trō - pī - ē'sĭs). Excentropiese; pressão exercida de dentro para fora. [G. *ek,* fora, + *kentron,* centro, + *piesis,* pressão]
ec·chon·dro·ma (ĕk - kon - drō'mă). Econdroma. **1.** Neoplasia cartilaginosa que se origina como hipertrofia da cartilagem posicionada normalmente, como uma massa que se protrai da superfície articular de um osso, ao contrário do encondroma. **2.** Um econdroma que rompeu através da diáfise de um osso e se tornou pediculado. SIN ecchondrosis. [G. *ek,* de, + *chondros,* cartilagem, + *-oma,* tumor]
ec·chon·dro·sis (ĕk - kon - drō'sĭs). Econdrose. SIN ecchondroma.
ec·chor·do·sis phy·sa·li·phor·'a (ĕk - kor - dō'sĭs fĭz - ăl - ē - for' - mē - ă). Resto de notocorda do clivo craniano que pode formar um pequeno tumor.
ec·chy·mo·ma (ĕk - i - mō'mă). Equimoma; pequeno hematoma após uma contusão. [G. *ek,* fora, + *chymos,* suco, + *-oma,* tumor]
ℹ **ec·chy·mo·sis** (ĕk - i - mō'sĭs). Equimose; placa púrpura causada por extravasamento de sangue para a pele, diferindo das petéquias apenas em tamanho (> 3 mm de diâmetro). [G. *ekchymōsis,* equimose, de *ek,* fora, + *chymos,* suco]
  bilateral medial orbital e.'s, equimoses orbitais mediais bilaterais. SIN racoon *eyes,* em *eye.*
  Tardieu e.'s, manchas de Tardieu; petéquias e/ou equimoses subpleurais e subpericárdicas, observadas nos tecidos de pessoas que foram estranguladas, ou asfixiadas de outra forma. SIN Tardieu petechiae, Tardieu spots.
ec·chy·mot·ic (ĕk - i - mot'ĭk). Equimótico; relativo a uma equimose.
Eccleston. VER Paget-Eccleston *stain.*
ec·crine (ĕk'rĭn). Écrino. **1.** SIN exocrine (1). **2.** Designa o fluxo de suor das glândulas sudoríparas não-conectadas aos folículos pilosos. [G. *ek-krino,* secretar]
ec·cri·nol·o·gy (ĕk - rĭ - nol'ō - jē). Ecrinologia; o ramo da fisiologia e da anatomia que estuda as secreções e as glândulas secretoras (exócrinas). [G. *ek-krino,* secretar, + *logos,* estudo]
ec·cri·sis (ĕk'rĭ - sĭs). Écrise. **1.** A remoção de produtos residuais. **2.** Qualquer produto residual; excremento. [G. separação]
ec·crit·ic (ĕ - krit'ĭk). Ecrítico. **1.** Que promove a expulsão de substâncias residuais. **2.** Agente que promove excreção.
ec·cy·e·sis (ĕk - sī - ē'sĭs). Ecciese. SIN ectopic *pregnancy.* [G. *ek,* fora, + *kyesis,* gravidez]
ec·dem·ic (ĕk - dem'ĭk). Ecdêmico; designa uma doença trazida de fora para uma região. [G. *ekdēmos,* estranho; do lar, de *dēmos,* povo]
ec·dys·i·asm (ĕk - diz'ē - azm). Ecdisiasmo; tendência mórbida de se despir para causar desejo sexual em outros. [do G. *ekdyō,* remover as próprias roupas]
ec·dy·sis (ĕk'dĭ - sĭs). Ecdise; descamação, desprendimento ou mudança de pele como um fenômeno necessário para permitir o crescimento em artrópodes e renovação da pele em anfíbios e répteis. [G. *ekdysis,* descamação]
ec·dys·ist (ĕk - dĭs - ĭst). Ecdisita; pessoa que realiza ecdisiasmo.
ECF Abreviatura de extracellular *fluid* (líquido extracelular).
ECF-A Abreviatura de eosinophil chemotactic *factor* of anaphylaxis (fator quimiotático eosinofílico da anafilaxia).
ECFV Abreviatura de extracellular fluid *volume* (volume de líquido extracelular).
ℹ **ECG** Abreviatura de electrocardiogram (eletrocardiograma).
ec·go·nine (ĕk'gō - nēn, - nĭn). Ecgonina; a parte importante da molécula da cocaína; um anestésico tópico; base de muitos alcalóides da coca.
  ecgonine e., SIN benzoylecgonina.
Echid·noph·a·ga gal·li·na·cea (ĕk - id - nof'ă - gă gal - i - nā'sē - ă). A pulga firmemente aderente, que é uma praga séria de aves domésticas na América subtropical; freqüentemente ataca também mamíferos domésticos e seres humanos.
△ **echin-.** VER echino-.
echi·nate (ĕk'ĭ - nāt). Equinado. SIN echinulate.
△ **echino-, echin-.** Equino-, equin-, equini-; espinhoso. [G. *echinos,* ouriço, ouriço-do-mar]

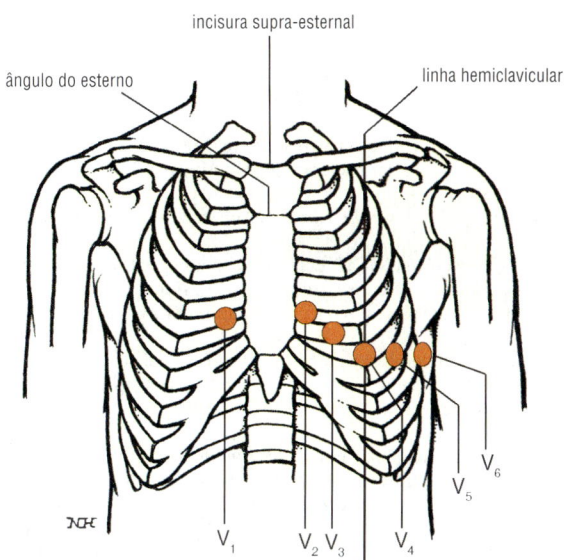

posicionamento das derivações do ECG: pontos de reparo para posicionamento das derivações torácicas

---

Echi·no·chas·mus (ē - kī - nō - kaz′mŭs). Gênero de trematódeos digenéticos (família Echinostomatidae), particularmente comum em aves pernaltas e que se alimentam de peixes; a espécie *E. perfoliatus* var. *japonicus* é descrita como um parasita intestinal raro dos seres humanos no Japão. [echino- + G. *chasma*, boca aberta]

echi·no·coc·ci·a·sis (ē - kī′nō - kok - sē′ă - sis). Equinococose. SIN echinococcosis.

echi·no·coc·co·sis (ē - kī′nō - kok - kō′sis). Equinococose; infecção por *Echinococcus*; a infecção larvar é denominada doença hidática (hydatid *disease*). SIN echinococciasis, echinococcus disease.

Echi·no·coc·cus (ē - kī′nō - kok′ŭs). Gênero de cestódeos teníedos muito pequenos, com dois a cinco segmentos nos vermes adultos; os adultos são encontrados em vários carnívoros, mas não em seres humanos; as larvas, na forma de cistos hidáticos, são encontradas no fígado e em outros órgãos de ruminantes, porcos, cavalos, roedores e, em determinadas circunstâncias epidemiológicas, de seres humanos (p. ex., pastores de ovinos que vivem com seus cães infectados). [echino- + G. *kokkos*, coco]

E. granulo'sus, tênia hidática, uma espécie na qual os adultos infectam o cão e a forma larvar (cistos hidáticos ósseos e uniloculares) infecta ovinos e outros ruminantes, porcos e cavalos; também pode ocorrer em seres humanos, dando origem a um grande cisto no fígado ou em outros órgãos e tecidos.

E. multilocula'ris, espécie de tênia que ocorre, nas regiões temperadas do norte e árticas, na forma adulta, em raposas; a larva (cisto hidático alveolar) é encontrada no fígado de roedores microtinos e no homem; produz um cisto proliferativo, freqüentemente de crescimento lento, no fígado que, em seres humanos, geralmente é fatal.

E. voge'li, espécie descrita em florestas tropicais úmidas do Panamá e do norte da América do Sul, que causa uma forma policística de doença hidática humana intermediária entre a doença hidática cística e a alveolar; o ciclo típico envolve cães domésticos e selvagens como hospedeiros da tênia adulta, e roedores como a paca (*Cuniculus paca*) como o hospedeiro intermediário da forma cística.

echi·no·cyte (ek′i - nō - sīt). Equinócito; hemácia crenada. [echino- + G. *kytos*, célula]

echi·no·derm (e - kī′nō - derm). Membro do filo Echinodermata.

Echi·no·der·ma·ta (e - kī - nō - der′mă - tă). Filo de Metazoa que inclui estrelas-do-mar, ouriços-do-mar, lírios-do-mar e outras classes. Todos, exceto os pepinos-do-mar (Holothuroidea), possuem uma forma básica radialmente simétrica e a maioria possui um endoesqueleto calcário com espinhos externos. Eles habitam o fundo do mar, alguns próximos da costa, outros em águas profundas. [echino- + G. *derma*, pele]

Echi·no·rhyn·chus (e - kī - nō - ring′kŭs). Gênero de vermes acantocefalídeos (cabeça com espinhos) que, originalmente, incluía espécies agora contidas nos gêneros *Macracanthorhynchus*, *Gigantorhynchus* e outros. [echino- + G. *rhynchos*, tromba]

ech·i·no·sis (ek - i - nō′sis). Equinose; condição na qual as hemácias perderam seus contornos uniformes, tornando-se semelhantes a um cavalo-marinho ou ouriço-do-mar. [echino- + G. *-osis*, condição]

Echi·no·sto·ma (ē - kī - nō - stō′mă, ek - i - nos′tō - mă). Gênero de trematódeos digenéticos (família Echinostomatidae) com espinhos orais característicos; amplamente distribuída e parasita de uma grande variedade de aves e mamíferos hospedeiros; foram descritas várias espécies em seres humanos no Sudeste Asiático. [echino- + G. *stoma*, boca]

E. iloca'num, espécie descrita em seres humanos nas Filipinas.

E. malay'anum, espécie tipicamente encontrada no porco, mas ocasionalmente descrita em seres humanos na Malásia; a infecção resulta da ingestão de caramujos infectados por cistos (metacercárias).

echi·no·sto·mi·a·sis (ē - kī′nō - stō - mī′ă - sis). Equinostomíase; infecção de aves e mamíferos, incluindo seres humanos, por trematódeos do gênero *Echinostoma*.

echin·u·late (e - kin′ū - lāt). Equinado; espinhoso; coberto por pequenos espinhos. SIN echinate. [L. mod. *echinulus*, dim. do L. *echinus*, ouriço]

Ech·is (ek′is, ē′kis). A víbora de escamas serrilhadas, um gênero de cobras pequenas (< 1 m), irritáveis e alertas que possuem veneno altamente tóxico; são responsáveis por muitos casos de picadas de cobra com muitas fatalidades. [G. *echis*, víbora]

ech·o (ek′ō). Eco. **1.** Som reverberante algumas vezes ouvido durante a ausculta torácica. **2.** Em ultra-sonografia, o sinal acústico recebido de estruturas dispersivas ou reflexivas ou o padrão correspondente de luz em um TRC (tubo de raios catódicos) ou ultra-sonograma. **3.** Em ressonância magnética, o sinal detectado após um pulso de inversão. [G.]

atrial e., e. atrial; reativação elétrica do átrio por um impulso retrógrado que retorna do nó A–V enquanto o impulso anterógrado continua até o ventrículo; caracterizado, eletrocardiograficamente, por um par de ondas P encerrando um complexo QRS, sendo a segunda onda P de polaridade oposta (geralmente invertida na derivação II), indicando que é o inverso (a via retrógrada) da via da primeira onda P (a via anterógrada).

navigator e., método de sincronização (*gating*) respiratória q.v., usado em ressonância magnética (magnetic resonance *imaging*) para limitar o artefato causado pelo movimento respiratório; um sinal é derivado do topo do diafragma, e os dados da imagem só são colhidos quando esta se encontra em uma faixa selecionada.

nodus sinuatrialis e., NS e., e. do nó sinoatrial, e. NS; batimento sinusal pós-ectópico que ocorre antes do que seria esperado em relação ao intervalo de descarga do nó sinusal precedente; isto é, o intervalo após um batimento prematuro de origem supraventricular é menor que a duração comum do ciclo entre batimentos sinusais, enquanto, habitualmente, seria esperado que o intervalo fosse maior que a duração do ciclo.

e. planar, e. plano; método de ressonância magnética que permite rápida aquisição de imagem durante decaimento por indução livre, utilizando gradientes de radiofreqüência rapidamente oscilantes e tecnicamente difíceis.

spin e., spin-eco; técnica comumente usada para recuperar sinais de relaxamento T1 e T2 em ressonância magnética, utilizando-se um pulso de inversão de 180° na seqüência de pulso para compensar a perda de magnetização transversa causada por heterogeneidade do campo magnético.

ech·o·a·cou·sia (ek′ō - ă - koo′zē - ă). Ecoacusia; distúrbio subjetivo da audição no qual um som parece ser repetido. [echo + G. *akouō*, ouvir]

ech·o·a·or·tog·ra·phy (ek′ō - ā - ōr - tog′ră - fē). Ecoaortografia; aplicação de técnicas de ultra-sonografia ao diagnóstico e estudo da aorta. [echo + aortography]

ech·o·car·di·o·gram (ek - ō - kar′dē - ō - gram). Ecocardiograma; o registro obtido por ecocardiografia. VER ultrasonography.

ech·o·car·di·og·ra·phy (ek′ō - kar - dē - og′ră - fē). Ecocardiografia; o uso de ultra-som no estudo do coração e dos grandes vasos e no diagnóstico de lesões cardiovasculares. SIN ultrasonic cardiography, ultrasound cardiography. [echo + cardiography]

contrast e., e. contrastada; a injeção de contraste de altos refletores de eco (p. ex., bolhas) para definir uma câmara ou delinear um desvio no coração.

cross-sectional e., e. bidimensional. SIN two-dimensional e.

Doppler e., e. Doppler; uso de técnicas de ultra-sonografia Doppler para aumentar a ecocardiografia bidimensional, permitindo que as velocidades sejam registradas na imagem ecocardiográfica. VER duplex *ultrasonography*, Doppler *ultrasonography*.

M-mode e., e. modo M. VER M-mode.

real-time e., e. em tempo real. SIN two-dimensional e.

sector e., e. setorial; ecocardiografia bidimensional com um transdutor estacionário.

stress e., e. com esforço; monitorização ecocardiográfica de um estímulo circulatório, geralmente exercício.

transesophageal e., e. transesofágica; registro do ecocardiograma de um transdutor engolido pelo paciente até distâncias predeterminadas no esôfago e no estômago.

transthoracic e., e. transtorácica; a ecocardiografia padrão registrada em "janelas" ecocardiográficas na parede torácica, incisura jugular ou epigástrio.

two-dimensional e., e. bidimensional; ecocardiografia na qual uma imagem é reconstruída a partir dos ecos estimulados e detectados por um arranjo linear ou por transdutores móveis. SIN cross-sectional e., real-time e.

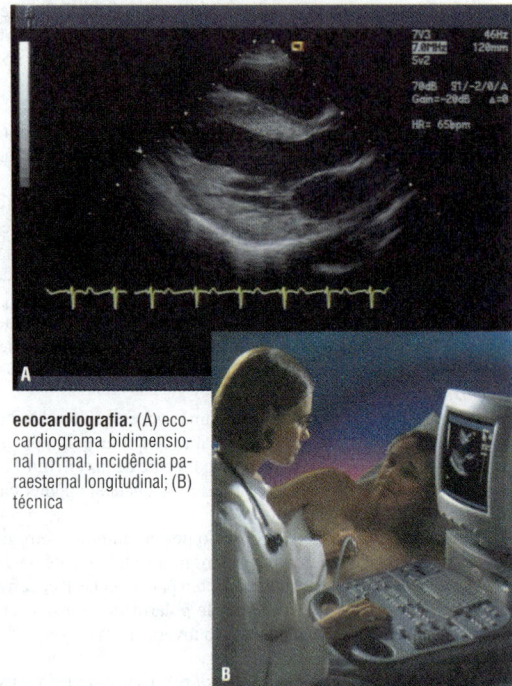

ecocardiografia: (A) ecocardiograma bidimensional normal, incidência paraesternal longitudinal; (B) técnica

ech·o·en·ceph·a·log·ra·phy (ek′ō-en-sef-a-log′ra-fē). Ecoencefalografia; o uso de ultra-som refletido no diagnóstico de processos intracranianos. [echo + encephalography]

echo-free (ek′ō-frē). Anecóico. SIN anechoic.

ech·o·gen·ic (ek-ō-jen′ik). Ecogênico; relativo a uma estrutura ou meio (p. ex., tecido) que possui ecos internos. Cf. hypoechoic (hipoecóico), hyperechoic (hiperecóico) e anechoic (anecóico), que se referem, respectivamente, a escassez, abundância e ausência de ecos exibidos na imagem de uma estrutura.

ech·o·gram (ek′ō-gram). Ecograma; registro obtido utilizando técnicas de reflexão acústica em qualquer um dos vários modos de exibição, principalmente um ecocardiograma. VER TAMBÉM ultrasonogram. [echo + G. *gramma*, diagrama]

echog·ra·pher (e-kog′ra-fer). Ecografista. SIN ultrasonographer.

ech·o·graph·ia (ek-ō-graf′ē-a). Ecografia; forma de agrafia em que uma pessoa não consegue escrever espontaneamente, mas consegue fazê-lo por meio de ditado ou cópia. [echo + G. *graphō*, escrever]

echog·ra·phy (e-kog′ra-fē). Ecografia. SIN ultrasonography. [echo + G. *graphō*, escrever]

ech·o·la·lia (ek-ō-lā′lē-a). Ecolalia; repetição involuntária, semelhante a um papagaio, de uma palavra ou frase que acabou de ser dita por outra pessoa. Geralmente observada na esquizofrenia. SIN echo reaction, echo speech, echophrasia. [echo + G. *lalia*, forma de fala]

ech·o·lo·ca·tion (ek′ō-lō-kā′shŭn). Ecolocalização; termo aplicado ao método pelo qual os morcegos orientam seu vôo e evitam objetos sólidos. Esses animais emitem sons agudos que, embora sejam inaudíveis para os seres humanos, são ouvidos pelos próprios morcegos como sons refletidos (ecos) de objetos no seu caminho.

ech·o·mo·tism (ek′ō-mō′tizm). Ecomotismo. SIN echopraxia. [echo + L. *motio*, movimento]

e·chop·a·thy (e-kop′a-thē). Ecopatia; forma de psicopatologia, geralmente associada à esquizofrenia, na qual as palavras (ecolalia) ou ações (ecopraxia) de outra pessoa são imitadas e repetidas. [echo + G. *pathos*, que sofre]

e·choph·o·ny, ech·o·pho·nia (ē-kof′ō-nē, ek-ō-fō′nē-a). Ecofonia; duplicação do som da voz ouvida algumas vezes durante a ausculta torácica. [echo + G. *phōnē*, voz]

ech·o·phra·sia (ek-ō-frā′zē-a). Ecofrasia. SIN echolalia. [echo + *phrasis*, fala]

ech·o·prax·ia (ek′ō-prak′sē-a). Ecopraxia; imitação involuntária de movimentos feitos por outra pessoa. VER echopathy. SIN echomotism. [echo + G. *praxis*, ação]

ech·o·scope (ek′ō-skōp). Ecoscópio; instrumento para exibir ecos por meio de pulsos ultra-sônicos em um osciloscópio para demonstrar estruturas situadas em locais profundos do corpo. [echo + G. *skopeō*, ver]

ech·o·thi·o·phate io·dide (ek-ō-thī′ō-fāt). Iodeto de ecotiofato; potente composto organofosforado e inibidor da colinesterase, usado no olho no tratamento do glaucoma.

Ec·ho·vi·rus 28 (ek′ō-vī′rŭs). Vírus ECHO 28; reclassificado como Rhinovirus tipo 1.

ech·o·vi·rus (ek′ō-vī-rŭs). Vírus ECHO. SIN ECHO *virus*.

Eck, Nikolai V., fisiologista russo, 1849–1917. VER E. *fistula*; reverse E. *fistula*.

Ecker, Alexander, anatomista alemão, 1816–1887. VER E. *fissure*.

Ecker, Enrique Eduardo, bacteriologista norte-americano, 1887–1966. VER Rees-E. *fluid*.

ec·la·bi·um (ek-lā′bē-ŭm). Eclábio; eversão de um lábio. [G. *ek*, fora, + L. *labium*, lábio]

ec·lamp·sia (ek-lamp′sē-a). Eclâmpsia; ocorrência de uma ou mais convulsões não-atribuíveis a outros distúrbios cerebrais, como epilepsia ou hemorragia cerebral, em um paciente com pré-eclâmpsia. [G. *eklampsis*, resplendor para diante]

puerperal e., e. puerperal; convulsões e coma associados à hipertensão, edema ou proteinúria que ocorrem em uma mulher após o parto.

superimposed e., e. superposta; convulsões que ocorrem em uma mulher com pré-eclâmpsia superposta.

ec·lamp·tic (ek-lamp′tik). Eclâmptico; relativo à eclâmpsia.

ec·lamp·to·gen·ic, ec·lamp·tog·e·nous (ek-lamp-tō-jen′ik, -tog′ē-nŭs). Eclamptogênico; que causa eclâmpsia.

ec·lec·tic (ek-lek′tik). Eclético; que retira de diferentes fontes o que parece ser o melhor ou mais desejável. [G. *eklektikos*, que seleciona, de *ek*, fora, + *lego*, selecionar]

ec·lec·ti·cism (ek-lek′ti-sizm). Ecleticismo. **1.** Um sistema atualmente extinto de medicina que defendeu o uso de plantas nativas para obter curas específicas de determinados sinais e sintomas. **2.** Sistema de medicina praticado por médicos gregos e romanos antigos que não eram filiados a uma seita médica, mas que adotavam a prática e o ensino que consideravam o melhor de outros sistemas.

♻ **eco-.** Eco-; o ambiente. [G. *oikos*, casa, lar, habitação]

eco·en·do·cri·nol·o·gy (ē′kō-en′dō-kri-nol′ō-jē). Ecoendocrinologia; o estudo das interações de sistemas endócrinos com o ambiente.

ECoG Abreviatura de electrocorticography (eletrocorticografia).

ec·o·log·i·cal fal·la·cy. Falácia ecológica; a tendenciosidade (viés) que pode ocorrer devido a uma associação observada entre variáveis em um nível agregado não representa necessariamente uma associação que existe em um nível individual; um erro de inferência devido à incapacidade de distinguir entre diferentes níveis de organização.

e·col·o·gy (ē-kol′o-jē). Ecologia; o ramo da biologia relacionado com o complexo total de inter-relações entre organismos vivos, englobando as relações de organismos entre si, com o ambiente e com todo o equilíbrio energético em determinado ecossistema. SIN bioecology, bionomics (2). [eco- + G. *logos*, estudo]

human e., e. humana; as relações das pessoas com seu ambiente total (biológico e social).

landscape e., e. da paisagem; estudo dos efeitos recíprocos do padrão espacial sobre os processos ecológicos.

econ·a·zole (e-kōn′a-zōl). Econazol; agente antifúngico de amplo espectro usado no tratamento da dermatofitose dos pés e de infecções fúngicas correlatas.

Economo. VER von Economo.

econ·o·my (ē-kon′ō-mē). Economia; sistema; o corpo considerado como um agregado de órgãos em funcionamento. [G. *oikonomia*, administração da casa, de *oikos*, casa, + *nomos*, uso, lei]

ec·o·spe·cies (ē-kō-spē′shēz). Ecoespécies; duas ou mais populações de uma espécie isoladas por barreiras ecológicas, teoricamente capazes de trocar genes e produzir híbridos, mas parcialmente separadas uma da outra por diferenças no *habitat* ou no comportamento.

ec·o·sys·tem (ē′kō-sis-tem). Ecossistema. **1.** A unidade fundamental em ecologia, compreendendo os organismos vivos e os elementos não-vivos que interagem em uma região definida. **2.** Uma biocenose (comunidade biótica) e seu biótopo. SIN ecological system.

parasite-host e., e. parasita-hospedeiro. SIN parasitocenose.

ec·o·tax·is (ē-kō-tak′sis). Ecotaxia; migração de linfócitos "residentes" do timo e da medula óssea para tecidos que possuem um microambiente apropriado. [eco- + G. *taxis*, ordem, arranjo]

écou·vil·lon (ā-koo-vē-yōhn′). Escovilhão; escova com cerdas firmes para a limpeza de feridas ou abrasão do interior de uma cavidade. [Fr. escova de limpeza]

ECP Abreviatura de eosinophil cationic *protein* (proteína catiônica de eosinófilos).

ec·phy·ma (ek-fī′ma). Ecfima; crescimento ou protuberância verrucosa. [G. uma erupção espinhosa]

ECS Abreviatura de eletrocerebral silence (silêncio eletrocerebral).

ec·sta·sy (ek′sta-sē). Êxtase; exaltação mental e/ou uma experiência arrebatadora. [G. *ekstasis*, admiração]

ec·stat·ic (ek-stat′ik). Extasiado; relativo a, ou caracterizado por, êxtase.

ec·stro·phe (ek'strō-fē). Extrofia. SIN exstrophy.
ECT Abreviatura de electroconvulsive *therapy* (terapia eletroconvulsiva), electroshock *therapy* (terapia por eletrochoque).
ect-. VER ecto-.
ec.tad (ek'tad). Para fora. [G. *ektos*, fora, + L. *ad*, para]
ec·tal (ek'tal). Externo. [G. *ektos*, fora]
ec·ta·sia, ec·ta·sis (ek-tā'zē-ă, ek'tă-sis). Ectasia; dilatação de uma estrutura tubular. [G. *ektasis*, estiramento]
  annuloaortic e., e. anuloaórtica; dilatação supravalvar da aorta, envolvendo tanto sua parede quanto o anel valvar, que, entretanto, permanece de menor diâmetro que a parede dilatada distal; muitos casos estão relacionados à síndrome de Marfan. SIN aortoannular e.
  aortoannular e., SIN annuloaortic e.
  e. cor'dis, e. do coração; dilatação do coração.
  corneal e., e. corneana. SIN keratoectasia.
  diffuse arterial e., e. arterial difusa; aumento espontâneo com dilatação dos vasos.
  familial aortic e. (ek'tă-zē-ă). e. aórtica familiar. SIN familial aortic ectasia *syndrome*.
  hypostatic e., e. hipostática; dilatação de um vaso sanguíneo, geralmente uma veia, em uma porção mais baixa do corpo, como nas veias varicosas da perna.
  mammary duct e., e. do ducto mamário; dilatação dos ductos mamários por resíduos lipídicos e celulares em mulheres idosas; a ruptura dos ductos pode resultar em inflamação granulomatosa e infiltração por plasmócitos. VER TAMBÉM plasma cell *mastitis*.
  scleral e., e. escleral. SIN sclerectasia.
  e. ventric'uli paradox'a, e. ventricular paradoxal. SIN hourglass *stomach*.
-ectasia, -ectasis. Dilatação; expansão. [G. *ektasis*, estiramento]
ec·tat·ic (ek-tat'ik). Ectático; relativo a, ou caracterizado por, ectasia.
ec·ten·tal (ek-ten'tăl). Ectental; relativo ao ectoderma e ao endoderma; designa a linha onde essas duas camadas se unem. SIN ectoental. [G. *ektos*, fora, + *entos*, dentro]
ect·eth·moid (ekt-eth'moyd). Ectetmóide. SIN ethmoidal *labyrinth*. [G. *ektos*, fora, + ethmoid]
ec·thy·ma (ek-thī'mă). Ectima; infecção piogênica da pele iniciada por estreptococos β-hemolíticos e caracterizada por crostas aderentes sob as quais ocorre ulceração; as úlceras podem ser únicas ou múltiplas e curam com formação de cicatriz. [G. uma pústula]
  contagious e., e. contagiosa. SIN orf.
  e. gangreno'sum, e. gangrenosa. SIN dermatitis gangrenosa infantum.
ec·ti·ris (ek-tī'ris). Ectíris; a camada externa da íris. [G. *ektos*, fora, + iris]
ecto-, ect-. Ecto-, ect-; externo; do lado de fora. VER TAMBÉM exo-. [G. *ektos*, fora]
ec·to·an·ti·gen (ek-tō-an'ti-jen). Ectoantígeno; qualquer toxina ou outro elemento excitante da formação de anticorpos, separado ou que pode ser separado de sua fonte. SIN exoantigen.
ec·to·blast (ek'tō-blast). Ectoblasto. **1.** SIN ectoderm. **2.** Conforme usado por alguns embriologistas experimentais, a camada celular externa original a partir da qual são formadas as camadas germinativas primárias; nesse sentido, é sinônimo de epiblasto. **3.** Uma parede celular. [ecto- + G. *blastos*, germe]
ec·to·car·dia (ek-tō-kar'dē-ă). Ectocardia; deslocamento congênito do coração. SIN exocardia. [ecto- + G. *kardia*, coração]
ec·to·cer·vi·cal (ek'tō-ser'vi-kăl). Ectocervical; relativo à parte vaginal do colo do útero revestida por epitélio escamoso estratificado.
ec·to·chor·oi·dea. Ectocoróide. SIN suprachoroid lamina of sclera.
ec·to·cor·nea (ek-tō-kōr'nē-ă). Ectocórnea; a camada externa da córnea.
ec·to·crine (ek'tō-krin). Ectócrino. **1.** Relativo a substâncias, sintetizadas ou produzidas por decomposição de organismos, que afetam a vida vegetal. **2.** Uma substância com propriedades ectócrinas. **3.** Um ectormônio. Cf. endocrine, exocrine. [ecto- + G. *krinō*, separar]
  ecological e., e. ecológico; substância química que sofre biossíntese em uma espécie e que exerce um efeito sobre a função de outra espécie através de mecanismos do ambiente externo; p. ex., a biossíntese de vitaminas por ruminantes e sua subseqüente ingestão por outros animais. VER TAMBÉM ectohormone.
ec·to·cyst (ek'tō-sist). Ectocisto; a camada externa de um cisto hidático. [ecto- + G. *kystis*, vesícula]
ec·to·derm (ek'tō-derm). Ectoderma; a camada externa de células no embrião, após estabelecimento das três camadas germinativas primárias (ectoderma, mesoderma, endoderma), a camada germinativa em contato com a cavidade amniótica. SIN ectoblast (1). [ecto- + G. *derma*, pele]
  amnionic e., e. amniótico; camada interna do âmnion contínua com o ectoderma corporal.
  chorionic e., e. coriônico. SIN trophoblast.
  epithelial e., e. epitelial; a parte do ectoderma que se separa do neuroectoderma aproximadamente na quarta semana de vida embrionária; a epiderme e seus derivados especializados se desenvolvem dele. SIN superficial e.
  extraembryonic e., e. extra-embrionário; derivado do epiblasto fora do corpo do embrião.
  superficial e., e. superficial. SIN epithelial e.

ec·to·der·mal (ek-tō-der'măl). Ectodérmico; relativo ao ectoderma. SIN ectodermic.
ec·to·der·ma·to·sis (ek'tō-der-mă-tō'sis). Ectodermatose. SIN ectodermosis.
ec·to·der·mic (ek-tō-der'mik). Ectodérmico. SIN ectodermal.
ec·to·der·mo·sis (ek'tō-der-mō'sis). Ectodermose; distúrbio de qualquer órgão ou tecido desenvolvido a partir do ectoderma. SIN ectodermatosis.
ec·to·en·tad (ek-tō-en'tad). De fora para dentro.
ec·to·en·tal (ek-tō-en'tăl). Ectoental. SIN ectental.
ec·to·en·zyme (ek-tō-en'zīm). Ectoenzima. **1.** Uma enzima excretada externamente e que atua fora do organismo. **2.** Uma enzima que está fixada à superfície externa da membrana plasmática de uma célula.
ec·to·eth·moid (ek-tō-eth'moyd). Ectoetmóide. SIN ethmoidal *labyrinth*.
ec·tog·e·nous (ek-toj'e-nŭs). Ectógeno. SIN exogenous. [ecto- + G. *-gen*, que produz]
ec·to·hor·mone (ek'tō-hōr-mōn). Ectormônio; mediador químico para-hormonal de importância ecológica que é secretado principalmente por um organismo (geralmente um invertebrado) para seu ambiente imediato (ar ou água); pode alterar o comportamento ou a atividade funcional de um segundo organismo, freqüentemente da mesma espécie que o que secreta o ectormônio. VER TAMBÉM ecological *ectocrine*.
ec·to·mere (ek'tō-mēr). Ectômero; um dos blastômeros envolvidos na formação de ectoderma. [ecto- + G. *meros*, parte]
ec·to·me·rog·o·ny (ek'tō-mĕ-rog'o-nē). Ectomerogonia; a produção de merozoítas na reprodução assexuada de esporozoários parasitas na superfície de esquizontes e de blastóforos, ou por invaginação para o esquizonte, em contraste com a endomerogonia; a ectomerogonia foi observada em várias espécies de *Eimeria*. [ecto- + G. *meros*, parte, + *gonē*, geração]
ec·to·mes·en·chyme (ek-tō-mes'en-kīm). Ectomesênquima. SIN mesectoderm (2). [ecto- + G. *mesos*, meio, + *enkyma*, infusão]
ec·to·morph (ek'tō-mōrf). Ectomorfo; tipo corporal cu constituição física (biotipo ou somatotipo) em que predominam os tecidos originados do ectoderma; de um ponto de vista morfológico, os membros predominam sobre o tronco. SIN longitype. [ecto- + G. *morphē*, forma]
ec·to·mor·phic (ek-tō-mōrf'ik). Ectomórfico; relativo a, ou que possui as características de, um ectomorfo.
-ectomy. Ectomia; remoção de uma estrutura anatômica. VER TAMBÉM -tomy. [G. *ektomē*, excisão]
ec·top·a·gus (ek-top'ă-gŭs) Ectópago; gêmeos conjugados nos quais os corpos são unidos lateralmente. VER conjoined *twins*, em twin. [ecto- + G. *pagos*, algo fixo]
ec·to·par·a·site (ek-tō-par'ă-sīt). Ectoparasita; parasita que vive na superfície do corpo do hospedeiro.
ec·to·par·a·sit·i·cide (ek'tō-par-ā-sit'i-sīd). Ectoparasiticida; agente aplicado diretamente ao hospedeiro para destruir ectoparasitas. [ectoparasite + L. *caedo*, matar]
ec·to·par·a·sit·ism (ek'tō-par'ă-sī-tizm). Ectoparasitismo. SIN infestation.
ec·to·per·i·to·ni·tis (ek'tō-păr-i-tō-nī'tis). Ectoperitonite; inflamação com início na camada mais profunda do peritônio, a que está próxima das vísceras ou da parede abdominal.
ec·to·phyte (ek'tō-fīt). Ectófito; vegetal parasita da pele. [ecto- + G. *phyton*, planta]
ec·to·pia (ek-tō'pē-ă). Ectopia; deslocamento congênito ou má posição de qualquer órgão ou parte do corpo. SIN ectopy, heterotopia (1). [G. *ektopos*, fora do lugar, de *ektos*, fora, + *topos*, lugar]
  e. cloa'cae, e. da cloaca. SIN cloacal *exstrophy*.
  e. cor'dis, e. do coração; condição congênita na qual o coração é exposto na parede torácica devido a uma anomalia do desenvolvimento do esterno e do pericárdio.
  crossed renal e., e. renal cruzada; rim ectópico localizado no lado oposto (contralateral) da linha média em relação à sua inserção ureteral na bexiga. Na maioria dos casos, as duas porções renais são fundidas (ectopia fundida cruzada).
  crossed testicular e., e. testicular cruzada; testículo que cruzou a linha média para se unir ao testículo contralateral no canal inguinal ou hemiescroto contralateral.
  e. len'tis, e. da lente do olho; deslocamento da lente do olho. SIN dislocation of lens.
  e. lentis et pupillae, e. da lente do olho e da pupila; distúrbio caracterizado por corectopia e um cristalino subluxado e luxado.
  e. mac'ulae, e. da mácula; condição na qual uma mácula é deslocada de forma que as duas fóveas não estão mais em pontos retinianos correspondentes. SIN heterotopia maculae.
  e. pupil'lae congen'ita, e. pupilar congênita; deslocamento da pupila presente ao nascimento.
  e. re'nis, e. renal; deslocamento do rim.
  e. tes'tis, e. do testículo. SIN testis e.
  testis e., e. do testículo; testículo em posição anômala fora do trajeto normal de descida. SIN e. testis, parorchidium.

ectopia

  thoracoabdominal e. cordis, e. cardíaca toracoabdominal. SIN *pentalogy* of Cantrell.
  ureteral e., e. ureteral; interrupção anormal do ureter na bexiga, uretra ou fora do trato urinário.
  e. vesi'cae, e. vesical. SIN *exstrophy* of the bladder.
ec·top·ic (ek - top'ik). Ectópico. **1.** Fora do lugar; diz-se de um órgão que não está em sua posição apropriada, ou de uma gravidez que ocorre fora da cavidade uterina. SIN aberrant (3), heterotopic (1). **2.** Em cardiologia, designa um batimento cardíaco que tem sua origem em algum foco anormal; que se desenvolve a partir de um outro foco fora do nodo sinoatrial. [ver ectopia]
ec·to·pla·cen·tal (ek'tō - pla - sen'tal). Ectoplacentário. **1.** Fora, além ou ao redor da placenta; em primatas, refere-se especialmente às partes do trofoblasto não envolvidas diretamente na formação da placenta. **2.** Em roedores, refere-se à parte de crescimento ativo do trofoblasto envolvida na formação da placenta.
ec·to·plasm (ek'tō - plazm). Ectoplasma; o citoplasma periférico, mais viscoso, de uma célula; contém microfilamentos, mas não possui outras organelas. SIN exoplasm. [ecto- + G. *plasma*, algo formado]
ec·to·plas·mat·ic, ek·to·plas·mic, ek·to·plas·tic (ek - tō - plas - mat'ik - plas'mik, - plas'tik). Ectoplasmático, ectoplásmico, ectoplástico; relativo ao ectoplasma.
ec·to·py (ek'tō - pē). Ectopia. SIN ectopia.
ec·to·ret·i·na (ek'tō - ret'i - nā). Ectorretina. SIN pigmented *layer* of retina.
ec·to·sarc (ek'tō - sark). Ectossarco; a membrana externa, ou ectoplasma, de um protozoário. [ecto- + G. *sarx*, carne]
ec·tos·co·py (ek - tos'kō - pē). Ectoscopia; método obsoleto de diagnóstico de doença de qualquer dos órgãos internos pelo estudo dos movimentos da parede abdominal ou do tórax causados por fonação. [ecto- + G. *skopeō*, examinar]
ec·tos·te·al (ek - tos'tē - āl). Ectósteo; relativo à superfície externa de um osso. [ecto- + G. *osteon*, osso]
ec·tos·to·sis (ek - tos - tō'sis). Ectostose; ossificação da cartilagem sob o pericôndrio, ou formação de osso sob o periósteo. [ecto- + G. *osteon*, osso, + *-osis*, condição]
ec·to·thrix (ek'tō - thriks) Ectótrico; bainha de esporos (conídios) na face externa de um pêlo. [ecto- + G. *thrix*, pêlo]
ec·to·tox·in (ek - tō - tok'sin). Ectotoxina. SIN exotoxin.
ec·to·zo·on (ek - tō - zō'on). Ectozoário; animal parasita que vive na superfície do corpo. [ecto- + G. *zōon*, animal]
♻ **ectro-.** Ectro-; ausência congênita de uma parte. [G. *ektrōsis*, malogro]
ec·tro·chei·ry, ec·tro·chi·ry (ek - trō - kī'rē). Ectroquiria; ausência total ou parcial de uma mão. [ectro- + G. *cheir*, mão]
ec·tro·dac·ty·ly, ec·tro·dac·tyl·ia, ec·tro·dac·tyl·ism (ek - trō - dak'ti - lē, - dak - til'i - ā, - dak'ti - lizm). Ectrodactilia; ausência congênita, parcial ou completa, de um ou mais dedos das mãos ou dos pés. Existem diversas formas e o padrão de herança pode ser autossômico dominante com penetração reduzida [MIM*183600 e MIM*183802], autossômico recessivo [MIM*225290 e MIM*225300] ou ligado ao X [MIM*313350]. [ectro- + G. *daktylos*, dedo]
ec·tro·gen·ic (ek - trō - jen'ik). Ectrogênico; relativo a ectrogenia.
ec·trog·e·ny (ek - troj'e - nē). Ectrogenia; ausência ou defeito congênito de qualquer parte do corpo. [ectro- + G. *-gen*, que produz]
ec·tro·me·lia (ek - trō - mē'lē - ā). Ectromelia. **1.** Hipoplasia ou aplasia congênita de um ou mais membros. **2.** Uma doença de camundongos causada pelo vírus da ectromelia, um membro da família *Poxviridae*; caracterizada por perda gangrenosa dos pés e de áreas necróticas nos órgãos internos; em colônias de camundongos de laboratórios, geralmente resulta em altas taxas de mortalidade. [ectro- + G. *melos*, membro]
ec·tro·mel·ic (ek - trō - mel'ik). Ectromélico; relativo a, ou caracterizado por, ectromelia.
ec·tro·pi·on, ec·tro·pi·um (ek - trō'pē - on, - pē - ŭm). Ectrópio; uma rotação externa da margem de uma parte, p. ex., de uma pálpebra. [G. *ek*, fora, + *tropē*, volta]
  atonic e., e. atônico; ectrópio da pálpebra inferior após paralisia do músculo orbicular do olho. SIN flaccid e., paralytic e.
  cicatricial e., e. cicatricial; ectrópio das pálpebras após queimaduras, lacerações ou infecção cutânea.
  flaccid e., e. flácido. SIN atonic e.
  paralytic e., e. paralítico. SIN atonic e.
  spastic e., e. espástico; ectrópio da pálpebra inferior em virtude de irritação ocular e/ou contração do músculo orbicular do olho.
  e. u'veae, e. da úvea; eversão do epitélio posterior pigmentado da íris na margem pupilar.
ec·trop·o·dy (ek - trop'ō - dē). Ectropodia; ausência total ou parcial de um pé. [ectro- + G. *pous*, pé]
ec·tro·syn·dac·ty·ly (ek'trō - sin - dak'ti - lē). Ectrossindactilia; anormalidade congênita caracterizada por ausência de um ou mais dedos e fusão de outros. [ectro- + G. *syn*, junto, + *daktylos*, dedo]
ec·tyl·u·rea (ek'til - ū - rē'ā). Ectiluréia; sedativo obsoleto leve usado no tratamento da tensão nervosa e da ansiedade.

ec·type (ek'tīp). Ectipo; somatotipo extremo, como ectomorfo (longilíneo) ou endomorfo (braquilíneo). [G. *ek*, fora, + *typos*, modelo]
ec·u·re·sis (ek - ū - rē'sis). Ecurese; condição na qual a excreção urinária e a ingestão de água provocam desidratação absoluta do corpo. VER TAMBÉM emuresis. [G. *ek*, fora, + *ourēsis*, micção]
ec·ze·ma (ek'zē - mā, eg'zē - mā, eg - zē'mā). Eczema; termo genérico para designar condições inflamatórias da pele, particularmente com vesiculação no estágio agudo, tipicamente eritematosas, edematosas, papulares e crostosas; seguido freqüentemente por liquenificação e descamação, algumas vezes por escurecimento do eritema e, raramente, hiperpigmentação; freqüentemente acompanhado por sensações de prurido e queimação; as vesículas se formam por espongiose intra-epidérmica; amiúde hereditário e associado a rinite alérgica e asma. [G. de *ekzeō*, ferver]
  allergic e., e. alérgico; erupção macular, papular ou vesicular decorrente de uma reação alérgica, p. ex., dermatite de contato.
  atopic e., e. atópico. SIN atopic *dermatitis*.
  baker e., e. do padeiro; eczema alérgico devido ao contato com farinha, fermento ou outros ingredientes manuseados pelos padeiros.
  chronic e., e. crônico. SIN lichenoid e.
  dyshidrotic e., e. disidrótico. SIN dyshidrosis.
  e. erythemato'sum, e. eritematoso; forma seca de eczema caracterizada por extensas áreas de eritema com descamação.
  flexural e., e. flexural; eczema da pele nas dobras do cotovelo, joelho, punho, etc., associado a atopia, que persiste durante toda a infância.
  hand e., e. das mãos; eczema que afeta de forma predominante e persistente as mãos; de múltiplas causas, incluindo alérgica, industrial, irritante, disidrótica, bacteriana e mecanismos atópicos; diferenciado das fissuras das mãos pela existência de vesiculação ou espongiose.
ℹ **e. herpet'icum,** e. herpético; condição febril causada por disseminação cutânea de herpesvírus tipo I, mais comum em crianças, que consiste em uma erupção difusa de vesículas que rapidamente se tornam pústulas umbilicadas; clinicamente indistinguível de uma vacínia generalizada. Os dois podem ser distinguidos por microscopia eletrônica ou demonstração de corpos de inclusão nos esfregaços, que são intranucleares no eczema herpético e intracitoplasmáticos no eczema da vacínia. SIN pustulosis vacciniformis acuta.
  infantile e., e. do lactente; eczema em lactentes; o aspecto clínico varia de acordo com o mecanismo causador dominante, p. ex., hipersensibilidade de contato, candidíase, atopia, seborréia, ou uma combinação incluindo intertrigo e dermatite das fraldas.
  e. intertri'go, e. do intertrigo. VER intertrigo.
  lichenoid e., e. liquenóide; espessamento da pele com linhas cutâneas acentuadas no eczema. SIN chronic e.
  nummular e., e. numular; placas de eczema distintas, em forma de moedas. SIN nummular dermatitis.
  e. papulo'sum, e. papuloso; dermatite caracterizada pela erupção de pápulas escoriadas avermelhadas isoladas ou agregadas.
  e. parasit'icum, e. parasitário; erupção eczematosa precipitada por infestação por parasitas.
  e. pustulo'sum, e. pustuloso; um estágio posterior de eczema vesicular no qual as vesículas foram infectadas secundariamente; as lesões são cobertas por crostas purulentas.
  seborrheic e., e. seborreico. SIN seborrheic *dermatitis*.
  stasis e., e. de estase; erupção eczematosa das pernas causada ou agravada por estase vascular.
  tropical e., e. tropical; eczema que ocorre em placas nas superfícies extensoras dos membros; de ocorrência comum e etiologia desconhecida.
  e. tylot'icum, e. tilótico; disidrose hiperceratótica.
  varicose e., e. varicoso; eczema que ocorre em áreas nas quais a pele foi comprometida por varicosidades.
  e. verruco'sum, e. verrucoso; eczema com hiperceratose; eczema liquenificado crônico.
  e. vesiculo'sum, e. vesiculoso; dermatite caracterizada pela erupção de vesículas sobre placas eritematosas que se rompem e exsudam soro.
  weeping e., e. úmido; dermatite eczematosa, úmida.
  winter e., e. de inverno; eczema resultante da evaporação acelerada da umidade (incluindo perdas insensíveis pelo suor) da superfície cutânea; ocorre na forma de placas secas rachadas, em geral nas extremidades, mas, não raramente, também no tronco, em qualquer estação, em circunstâncias (ocupacionais, ambientais) de dessecamento excessivamente rápido da pele.
ec·zem·a·ti·za·tion (ek - zem'ā - ti - zā'shŭn). Eczematização. **1.** Formação de uma erupção semelhante a eczema. **2.** Ocorrência de eczema secundário a uma dermatose preexistente.
ec·ze·ma·toid (ek - zem'ā - toyd). Eczematóide; de aspecto semelhante ao do eczema.
ec·ze·ma·tous (ek - zem'ā - tŭs). Eczematoso; caracterizado por, ou semelhante ao, eczema.
ED Abreviatura de effective *dose* (dose efetiva); ethyldichloroarsine (etildicloroarsina).

ED₅₀ Abreviatura de median effective dose (dose efetiva mediana).
ed·ath·a·mil (ē - dath′a - mil). Edatamil. SIN ethylenediaminetetraacetic acid.
EDC Abreviatura de estimated date of confinement (data estimada do parto). VER Nägele *rule*.
e·de·a (e - dē′a). Edéia; a genitália externa. [G. *aidoia*, genitais]

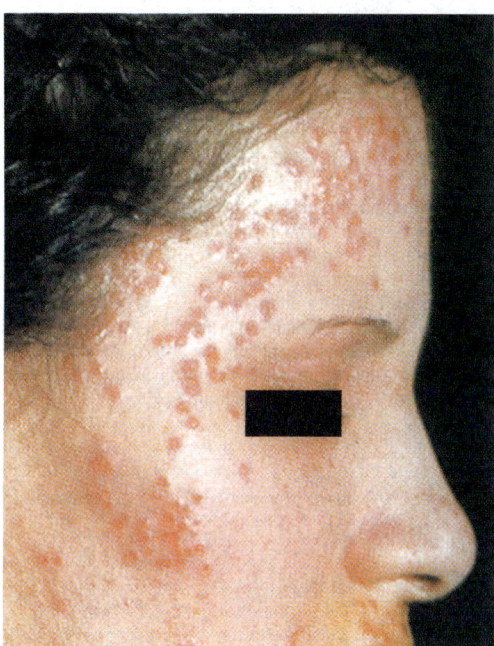

eczema herpético

ede·ma (e - dē′ma). Edema; acúmulo de volume excessivo de líquido aquoso nas células ou tecidos intercelulares. [G. *oidēma*, edema]
  ambulant e., e. deambulatório; edema que se forma nas pernas durante períodos de marcha.
  angioneurotic e., e. angioneurótico. SIN angioedema.

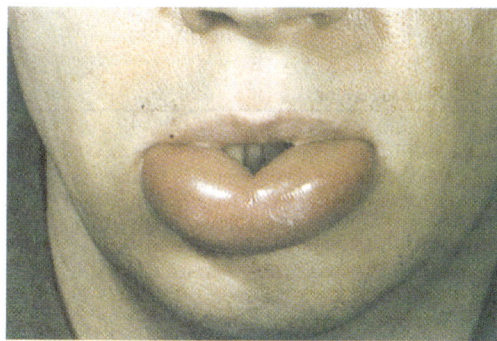

edema angioneurótico: observado no lábio inferior

  Berlin e., e. de Berlin; edema da retina após traumatismo não-penetrante do globo do olho.
  blue e., e. azul; o edema e a cianose de um membro na paralisia histérica.
  brain e., e. cerebral. SIN cerebral e.
  brawny e., e. sem cacifo; e. não-depressível. SIN nonpitting e.
  brown e., e. marrom; edema pulmonar associado a congestão passiva crônica.
  bullous e., e. bolhoso; aspecto avermelhado, edemaciado, do orifício ureteral na parede vesical, freqüentemente observado em cálculos ureterais distais ou na tuberculose do ureter.
  bullous e. vesi′cae, e. bolhoso da bexiga; uma área proeminente de edema focal, envolvendo o epitélio vesical, que consiste em massas elevadas de tecido edematoso ou grupos de vesículas cheias de líquido claro; freqüentemente associado a inflamação crônica ou irritação secundária das tubas uterinas, corpos estranhos ou inflamação perivesical.
  cachectic e., e. caquético; eczema que ocorre em doenças caracterizadas por definhamento e hipoproteinemia; devido à baixa pressão oncótica plasmática. SIN marantic e.
  cardiac e., e. cardíaco; edema resultante de insuficiência cardíaca congestiva.
  cerebral e., e. cerebral; tumefação cerebral devida ao aumento do volume do compartimento extravascular causado pela captação de água nos neurópilos e na substância branca. VER TAMBÉM brain *swelling*. SIN brain e.
  cystoid macular e., e. macular cistóide; eczema do pólo posterior do olho secundário à permeabilidade anormal dos capilares na retina sensorial central.
  dependent e., e. de declive; aumento clinicamente detectável do volume de líquido extracelular localizado em uma área em declive, como de um membro, caracterizado por edema ou cacifo.
  gestational e., e. gestacional; ocorrência de acúmulo generalizado e excessivo de líquido nos tecidos com cacifo maior que 1+ após 12 horas de repouso no leito, ou de um ganho ponderal de 2,5 kg ou mais em 1 semana devido à influência da gravidez.
  e. glot′tidis, e. de glote; edema da laringe.
  heat e., e. de calor; edema causado por temperatura externa excessivamente alta.
  hereditary angioneurotic e. (HANE) [MIM*106100], e. angioneurótico hereditário; forma relativamente rara de edema caracterizada por surgimento, em geral na adolescência, de eritema seguido por edema, envolvendo as vias respiratórias altas ou gastrointestinal, associada a uma deficiência de inibidor da C1 esterase ou uma forma funcionalmente inativa do inibidor. Há duas formas clinicamente indistinguíveis: tipo I, no qual o nível sérico de inibidor da C1 esterase é baixo (até 30% do normal), e tipo II, no qual o nível é normal ou elevado. Há ativação descontrolada de componentes iniciais do complemento e a produção de um fator semelhante à cinina que induz o angioedema; pode haver morte por edema das vias respiratórias altas e asfixia. A herança é autossômica dominante, causada por mutação no gene inibidor da C1-esterase (C1NH) no cromossoma 11q.
  hydremic e., e. hidrêmico; termo obsoleto para o edema que ocorre em estados caracterizados por hidremia acentuada.
  infantile acute hemorrhagic e. of the skin, e. hemorrágico agudo cutâneo do lactente; uma forma geralmente benigna de vasculite cutânea, caracterizada por púrpura equimótica, freqüentemente em um padrão de roseta, e edema inflamatório em lactentes.
  inflammatory e., e. inflamatório; edema causado por derrame de líquido nos tecidos moles que circundam um foco inflamatório.
  lymphatic e., e. linfático; edema causado por estase nos canais linfáticos.
  marantic e., e. marântico. SIN cachectic e.
  menstrual e., e. menstrual; retenção de água e aumento de peso, que ocorrem no decorrer ou antes da menstruação.
  e. neonato′rum, e. neonatal; edema difuso, firme e comumente fatal, que ocorre no recém-nascido, geralmente começando nas pernas e propagando-se para cima.
  nephrotic e., e. nefrótico; edema resultante de disfunção renal.
  noninflammatory e., e. não-inflamatório; edema de causas mecânicas ou outras causas, não caracterizado por inflamação ou congestão.
  nonpitting e., e. sem cacifo; e. não-depressível; edema dos tecidos subcutâneos que não pode ser facilmente deprimido por compressão. Geralmente decorrente de uma anormalidade metabólica, como aumento do conteúdo de glicosaminoglicana, como o que ocorre na doença de Graves (Graves *disease*) (mixedema pré-tibial) ou na fase inicial da esclerodermia. SIN brawny e.
  nutritional e., e. nutricional; forma de edema devido a ingestão proteica insuficiente, resultando em hipoproteinemia e baixa pressão oncótica plasmática.
  periodic e., e. periódico. SIN angioedema.
  pitting e., e. depressível; e. com cacifo; edema que mantém por um tempo a depressão produzida por pressão.
  premenstrual e., e. pré-menstrual. VER menstrual e.
  pulmonary e., e. pulmonar; edema pulmonar geralmente resultante de estenose mitral ou insuficiência ventricular esquerda.
  salt e., e. salino; edema causado por ingestão excessiva ou retenção de cloreto de sódio.
  solid e., e. sólido; infiltração dos tecidos subcutâneos por material mucóide, como no mixedema.
  Yangtze e., e. de Yangtze. SIN gnathostomiasis.
edem·a·ti·za·tion (e - dem′a - ti - zā′shŭn). Edematização; que torna edemaciado.
edem·a·tous (e - dem′ă - tŭs). Edematoso; caracterizado por edema.
eden·tate (ē - den′tāt). Edentado, edêntulo. SIN edentulous. [L. *edentatus*]
eden·tu·lous (ē - den′tū - lŭs). Desdentado; sem dentes, edêntulo; que perdeu os dentes naturais. SIN edentate. [L. *edentulus*, desdentado]
edes·tin (ē - des′tin). Edestina; globulina hexamérica derivada do grão do óleo de rícino, semente de cânhamo e outras sementes. Mantém o crescimento de animais na ausência de outras proteínas alimentares.
ed·e·tate (ed′e - tāt). Edetato; contração aprovada pela USAN para etilenodiaminatetraacetato, o ânion do ácido etilenodiaminotetraacético; vários edetatos

são usados como agentes quelantes para transportar cátions para dentro (p. ex., edetato férrico de sódio como transportador do íon ferro) ou para fora (p. ex., edetato de sódio para a remoção de íons cálcio ou metais pesados).

ed·e·tate cal·ci·um di·so·di·um. Edetato de cálcio dissódico; nome contraído para um sal de etilenodiaminotetraacetato, um agente usado como quelante de chumbo e de alguns outros metais pesados. Disponível em várias formas: dissódico, sódico e trissódico.

edet·ic ac·id (ē - det′ik). Ácido edético. SIN ethylenediaminetetraacetic acid.

edge (ej). Margem; borda; uma linha na qual termina uma superfície. VER TAMBÉM border, margin.

 cutting e., borda cortante; **(1)** o ângulo ativo afiado, biselado, em forma de bisturi de um instrumento dental manual; **(2)** SIN incisal *margin*.
 denture e., borda da dentadura. SIN denture *border*.
 incisal e., borda incisal. SIN incisal *margin*.
 leading e., borda dianteira; a parte inicial de uma onda.
 shearing e., borda de corte. SIN incisal *margin*.

Edinger, Ludwig, anatomista alemão, 1855–1918. VER E.-Westphal *nucleus*.

edis·y·late (e - dis′i - lāt). Edisilato; contração aprovada pela USAN para 1,2-etanodissulfonato, $O_3S(CH_2)_2SO_3^-$.

Edlefsen, Gustav J.F., médico alemão, 1842–1910. VER E. *reagent*.

EDM Abreviatura de multiple epiphyseal *dysplasia* (displasia epifisária múltipla).

Edman, Pehr, cientista australiano, 1916–1977. VER E. *method, reagent*.

EDRF Acrônimo para endothelium-derived relaxing *factor* (fator de relaxamento derivado do endotélio), agora conhecido como óxido nítrico (nitric oxide).

Edridge-Green, Frederick W., oftalmologista inglês, 1863–1953. VER Edridge-Green *lamp*.

ed·ro·pho·ni·um chlo·ride (ed - rō - fō′nē - ŭm). Cloreto de edrofônio; antagonista competitivo de curta duração de relaxantes do músculo esquelético (derivados do curare e tritiodeto de galamina) e uma anticolinesterase, usado como antídoto para agentes curariformes, como um agente diagnóstico na miastenia grave e na crise miastênica.

EDS Abreviatura de Ehlers-Danlos *syndrome* (síndrome de Ehlers-Danlos).

EDSS Abreviatura de expanded disability status *scale* (escala expandida de incapacidade).

EDTA Abreviatura de ethylenediaminotetraacetic acid (ácido etilenodiaminotetraacético).

educt (ē′dŭkt). Extrato.

edul·co·rant (e - dŭl′kō - rant). Edulcorante; adoçante.

edul·co·rate (e - dŭl′kō - rāt). Edulcorar; adoçar ou tornar menos acre. [L. *e*-intensivo, + *dulcoro*, adoçar, de *dulcor*, doçura, de *dulcis*, doce]

Edwards, James Hilton, médico e geneticista inglês, *1928. VER E. *syndrome*.

Edwards, M.L., médico norte-americano, *1906. VER Carpentier-Edwards *valve*; Starr-Edwards *valve*.

Ed·ward·si·el·la (ed′ward - sē - el′lă). Gênero de bactérias Gram-negativas, anaeróbicas facultativas (família Enterobacteriaceae) que contêm bastonetes móveis, peritríquios, não-encapsulados. A espécie típica é *E. tarda*, ocasionalmente isolada das fezes de homens saudáveis e daqueles com diarréia, do sangue de seres humanos e outros animais, e da urina humana. *E. tarda* é um agente etiológico da gastroenterite em seres humanos. As duas outras espécies desse gênero são *E. hoshinae* e *E. ictaluri*.

EEE Abreviatura de eastern equine *encephalomyelitis* (encefalomielite eqüina ocidental).

EEG Abreviatura de electroencephalogram (eletroencefalograma); electroencephalography (eletroencefalografia).

eel (ēl). Enguia; qualquer dentre vários peixes serpentiformes, sem escamas. [I.m. *ele*, do. I. ant. *ael*]
 vinegar e., *Turbatrix aceti*. SIN *Turbatrix aceti*.

EENT Abreviatura de eye, ear, nose and throat (olho, orelha, nariz e garganta). VER TAMBÉM ENT.

ef·face·ment (e - făs′ment). Apagamento; o adelgaçamento do colo imediatamente antes ou no decorrer do trabalho de parto.

ef·fect (e - fekt′). Efeito; o resultado ou a conseqüência de uma ação. [L. *efficio*, pp. *effectus*, realizar, de *facio*, fazer]
 abscopal e., e. abscopal; reação produzida após irradiação, mas que ocorre fora da zona de absorção da radiação.
 additive e., e. aditivo; efeito no qual duas ou mais substâncias ou ações usadas em combinação produzem um efeito total, igual à soma aritmética dos e. individuais.
 after-e., pós-efeito. VER aftereffect.
 Anrep e., e. Anrep; pequeno efeito inotrópico positivo transitório de aumentos abruptos das pressões aórtica e ventricular esquerda sistólicas relacionado à recuperação de isquemia subendocárdica transitória (p. ex., resposta da pressão arterial ao frio).
 Arias-Stella e., fenômeno de Arias-Stella. SIN Arias-Stella *phenomenon*.
 autokinetic e., e. autocinético; em psicologia, o aparente movimento de um ponto de luz pequeno e fixo, que está sendo observado em um quarto escuro.
 Bernoulli e., e. de Bernoulli; a diminuição da pressão de um líquido que ocorre na conversão de energia potencial em energia cinética quando o movimento do líquido é acelerado, de acordo com a lei de Bernoulli; aplicado em aspiradores de água, atomizadores e umidificadores nos quais um gás é acelerado através da extremidade de um orifício estreito, cheio de líquido.
 Bohr e., e. Bohr; a influência exercida pelo dióxido de carbono sobre a curva de dissociação do oxigênio do sangue; isto é, a curva é desviada para a direita, o que significa uma aparente redução na afinidade da hemoglobina pelo oxigênio. Cf. Haldane e.
 Bowditch e., e. Bowditch; auto-regulação homeométrica da função cardíaca induzida por modificação da freqüência cardíaca.
 Circe e., e. Circe; um efeito observado na catálise enzimática na qual a difusão acelerada do substrato ocorre através de forças de atração do local ativo da enzima.
 clasp-knife e., fenômeno do canivete; sinal do canivete. SIN clasp-knife *spasticity*.
 Compton e., e. Compton, dispersão Compton; na absorção de radiação eletromagnética de energia média, uma diminuição da energia dos fótons de bombardeamento com o deslocamento de um elétron orbital, geralmente de uma órbita externa. SIN Compton scattering.
 Cotton e., e. Cotton; o deslocamento positivo e negativo a partir do zero da rotação da luz monocromática plano-polarizada e a transformação da luz monocromática polarizada circularmente em luz polarizada elipticamente na vizinhança imediata da faixa de absorção da substância que a luz atravessa. VER TAMBÉM optic rotatory *dispersion*, circular *dichroism*.

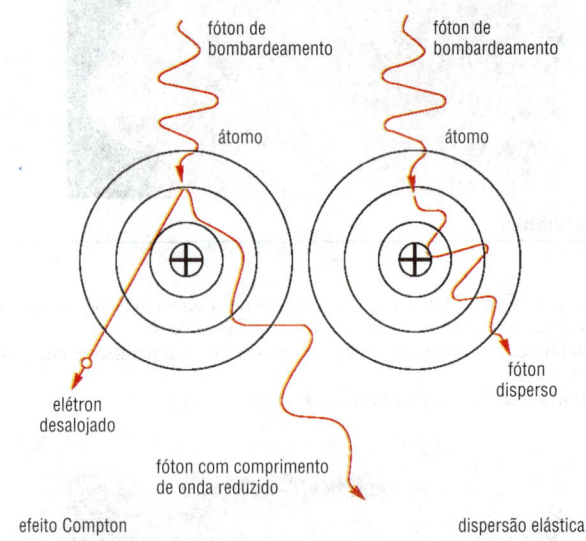

efeito Compton e dispersão elástica

 Crabtree e., e. Crabtree; inibição da respiração celular de sistemas isolados por altas concentrações de glicose; um "recíproco" do efeito Pasteur; devido, em parte, à inibição da hexocinase por níveis elevados de glicose 6-fosfato. Cf. Pasteur e.
 cumulative e., e. cumulativo; a condição na qual a administração repetida de uma droga pode produzir efeitos que são mais acentuados que os produzidos pela primeira dose. SIN cumulative action.
 Cushing e., fenômeno de Cushing. SIN Cushing *phenomenon*.
 cytopathic e., e. citopático; alterações degenerativas nas células (principalmente em cultura tecidual) associadas à multiplicação de determinados vírus; quando, em cultura tecidual, a disseminação do vírus é restrita por uma camada de ágar (ou outra substância adequada), o efeito citopático pode levar à formação de placa.
 Doppler e., e. Doppler; uma alteração na freqüência observada quando a fonte sonora e o observador estão em movimento relativo, afastando-se ou aproximando-se um do outro. VER TAMBÉM Doppler *shift*. SIN Doppler phenomenon.
 electrophonic e., e. eletrofônico; a sensação de audição produzida quando uma corrente alternada de freqüência e magnitude adequadas é passada de uma fonte externa através da cabeça de uma pessoa.
 experimenter e.'s, efeitos do experimentador; a influência do comportamento, dos traços de personalidade ou das expectativas do experimentador em relação aos resultados da própria pesquisa. VER double blind *study*.
 Fahraeus-Lindqvist e., e. Fahraeus-Lindqvist; a diminuição da viscosidade aparente que ocorre quando se faz uma suspensão, como o sangue, fluir por um tubo de menor diâmetro; observado em tubos com diâmetro menor que, aproximadamente, 0,3 mm. SIN sigma e.

Fenn e., e. Fenn; o aumento da liberação de calor em um músculo estimulado quando realiza trabalho mecânico; o calor liberado aumenta proporcionalmente a distância de encurtamento do músculo e proporcionalmente à tensão que ele deve desenvolver (p. ex., o peso que levanta) durante o encurtamento; assim, a energia química aumentada é consumida tanto para liberar o maior calor quanto para realizar maior trabalho mecânico.

first-pass e., metabolismo de primeira passagem. SIN first-pass *metabolism*.

flash-lag e., e. de arrasto; o aparente arrasto, atrás de um objeto em movimento, de uma parte dele que se acende rapidamente.

founder e., e. fundador; uma freqüência extraordinariamente alta de um gene em determinada população derivada de um pequeno grupo de ancestrais não-representativos.

gene dosage e., e. de dosagem de genes; em alelos codominantes, a relação mais ou menos linear entre o valor fenotípico e o número de genes de um tipo substituído por outro.

generation e., e. de geração; variação do estado de saúde decorrente dos diferentes fatores causadores de doença aos quais cada geração sucessiva nascida é exposta durante a vida.

Haldane e., e. Haldane; promoção da dissociação de dióxido de carbono no sangue por um aumento da oxigenação de hemoglobina.

halo e., e. halo: (1) o efeito (geralmente benéfico) que a conduta, a atenção e os cuidados de um profissional têm sobre um paciente durante uma consulta médica, independentemente do procedimento ou serviços médicos envolvidos na consulta; (2) a influência sobre uma observação da percepção pelo observador das características do indivíduo observado (além das características em estudo), ou a influência da recordação ou conhecimento do observador de achados em uma ocasião anterior.

Hawthorne e., e. de Hawthorne; o efeito (geralmente positivo ou benéfico) de ser estudado sobre as pessoas estudadas; seu conhecimento do estudo freqüentemente influencia seu comportamento. [cidade em Illinois; local da usina Western Electric]

healthy worker e., e. do trabalhador saudável; fenômeno observado inicialmente em estudos de doenças ocupacionais; os trabalhadores geralmente exibem menores taxas de mortalidades que a população em geral porque as pessoas doentes e incapacitadas não são contratadas.

hyperchromic e., e. hipercrômico; aumento da absortividade (ou extinção) em determinado comprimento de onda da luz por uma solução ou substância devido a alterações estruturais em uma molécula.

hypochromic e., e. hipocrômico; fenômeno no qual uma molécula individual, contendo vários cromóforos, tem certa absortividade (ou densidade óptica) em determinado comprimento de onda menor que a soma das densidades ópticas dos cromóforos individuais (naquele mesmo comprimento de onda).

Mach e., e. de Mach; o surgimento de uma linha clara ou escura em uma radiografia onde há uma interface côncava ou convexa no paciente, uma forma óptica fisiológica de realce da borda. VER TAMBÉM Mach *band*.

e. modifier, e. modificador; fator que modifica o efeito de um suposto fator causal em estudo; p. ex., a idade é um modificador do efeito em muitas situações.

nuclear Overhauser e. (NOE), e. nuclear Overhauser; efeito observado em ressonância magnética nuclear no qual há uma interação com o vizinho mais próximo através do espaço.

Orbeli e., e. Orbeli; a fadiga de um músculo estimulado por seu nervo (isto é, indiretamente) é reduzida por estimulação concomitante das fibras simpáticas para o músculo; acredita-se que seja causado pela difusão de norepinefrina a partir das fibras adrenérgicas que inervam os vasos sanguíneos no músculo.

oxygen e., e. do oxigênio; aumento da radiossensibilidade celular por uma alta concentração de oxigênio e, inversamente, diminuição da radiossensibilidade em um ambiente hipóxico.

Pasteur e., e. Pasteur; a inibição da fermentação pelo oxigênio, observada pela primeira vez por Pasteur; não observada, ou apenas discretamente observada, em tumores malignos. Cf. Crabtree e.

photechic e., e. Russell; a capacidade de um agente, que não a luz, produzir uma imagem latente que possa ser revelada em uma emulsão de filme fotográfico. SIN Russell e.

photoelectric e., e. fotoelétrico; (1) a perda de elétrons da superfície de um metal quando exposto à luz; (2) uma forma de interação da radiação com a matéria na qual toda a energia do fóton incidente é absorvida, com expulsão de um fotoelétron e radiação característica pelo preenchimento da vaga em outra órbita; como a absorção de energia por grama de tecido é proporcional ao cubo do número atômico, essa forma é importante em radiografia diagnóstica.

piezoelectric e., e. piezoelétrico; a propriedade de determinados materiais cristalinos ou cerâmicos de emitir eletricidade quando deformados e de se deformarem quando atravessados por uma corrente elétrica, um mecanismo de interconversão de energia elétrica e acústica; um transdutor de ultra-som envia e recebe energia acústica utilizando esse efeito.

position e., e. de posição; uma modificação na expressão fenotípica de um ou mais genes devido a uma alteração em sua localização física em relação a outros genes; pode resultar de modificação na estrutura do cromossoma ou do cruzamento.

Purkinje e., fenômeno de Purkinje. SIN Purkinje *phenomenon*.

quantal e., e. quântico; efeito que só pode ser expresso em termos binários, como presente ou ausente.

Raman e., e. Raman; modificação na freqüência sofrida por luz monocromática dispersa na passagem através de uma substância transparente cujas características determinam o grau de modificação, produzindo um espectro no qual a faixa de comprimento de onda incidente é flanqueada por pequenas faixas satélites com maiores e menores comprimentos de onda.

Rivero-Carvallo e., e. Rivero-Carvallo; aumento inspiratório do sopro sistólico na insuficiência tricúspide; a característica que distingue a insuficiência tricúspide da insuficiência mitral.

Russell e., e. Russell. SIN photechic e.

second gas e., e. do segundo gás; quando é inspirada uma concentração constante de um anestésico, como o halotano, o aumento da concentração alveolar é acelerado pela administração concomitante de óxido nitroso, porque a absorção alveolar deste último cria uma pressão intrapulmonar subatmosférica potencial que causa aumento do influxo traqueal.

sigma e., e. sigma. SIN Fahraeus-Lindqvist e.

Somogyi e., e. Somogyi; no diabetes, um fenômeno de rebote de hiperglicemia reativa em resposta a um período anterior de hipoglicemia relativa que aumentou a secreção de agentes hiperglicêmicos (epinefrina, norepinefrina, glucagon, cortisol e hormônio do crescimento); descrito em pacientes diabéticos que receberam insulina em excesso e desenvolveram hipoglicemia noturna não-diagnosticada, tornando-os hiperglicêmicos (sugerindo insulina insuficiente) quando examinados na manhã seguinte.

Staub-Traugott e., e. Staub-Traugott; em pessoas normais, uma diminuição do nível sanguíneo de glicose que sucede uma segunda dose oral de glicose administrada cerca de 30 minutos após a primeira.

Stiles-Crawford e., e. Stiles-Crawford; a luz que entra através do centro da pupila produz um maior efeito visual que a luz que entra obliquamente.

synergistic e., e. sinérgico. SIN synergism.

Tyndall e., fenômeno de Tyndall. SIN Tyndall *phenomenon*.

Venturi e., e. Venturi; termo aplicado à operação de um tubo de Venturi e sistemas semelhantes.

Wedensky e., e. Wedensky; efeito reforçador relativamente prolongado que sucede a aplicação de um choque ou estímulo máximo a uma preparação neuromuscular durante o qual um estímulo subliminar, em geral pequeno demais para provocar uma resposta, produzirá uma resposta; uma redução relativamente longa do limiar de excitabilidade após um choque máximo.

Wolff-Chaikoff e., e. Wolff-Chaikoff. SIN Wolff-Chaikoff *block*.

Zeeman e., e. Zeeman; a divisão de linhas espectrais em três ou mais linhas simétricas quando a fonte luminosa é submetida a um campo magnético.

ef·fec·tive·ness. Efetividade. **1.** Medida da acurácia ou do sucesso de uma técnica diagnóstica ou terapêutica quando realizada em um ambiente clínico médio. Cf. efficacy. **2.** O quanto um tratamento atinge seus objetivos pretendidos.

relative biologic e. (RBE), e. biológica relativa; fator usado para comparar o efeito biológico de doses absorvidas de diferentes tipos e energias de radiação ionizante. É determinada pela razão entre uma dose absorvida da radiação específica em questão e a dose absorvida de uma radiação de referência necessária para produzir um efeito biológico idêntico em um organismo, órgão ou tecido específico.

ef·fec·tor (e - fek'tŏr, -tōr). Efetor. **1.** Termo cunhado por C. Sherrington para designar um tecido periférico que recebe impulsos nervosos e reage por contração (músculo), secreção (glândula) ou descarga elétrica (órgão elétrico de determinados peixes ósseos). **2.** Uma pequena molécula metabólica que, por combinação com um gene repressor, deprime a atividade de um óperon. **3.** Uma pequena molécula que se liga a uma proteína e, assim, altera a atividade dessa proteína. **4.** Substância, técnica, procedimento ou indivíduo que causa um efeito. [L. produtor]

ef·fem·i·na·tion (e - fem - i - nā′shŭn). Efeminação; aquisição de características femininas, seja fisiologicamente como parte do amadurecimento feminino, ou patologicamente por indivíduos de ambos os sexos. [L. *ef-femino*, pp. *-atus*, tornar feminino, de *ex*, fora, + *femina*, mulher]

ef·fer·ent (ef'er - ent). Eferente; que conduz (líquido ou um impulso nervoso) de determinado órgão, ou parte deste, para fora; p. ex., as conexões eferentes de um grupo de células nervosas, vasos sanguíneos eferentes, ou o ducto excretor de um órgão. [L. *efferens*, de *effero*, conduzir para fora]

gamma e., e. gama; o axônio fino de um neurônio motor gama que inerva as fibras musculares intrafusais de um fuso muscular.

ef·fer·vesce (ef - er - ves′). Efervescer; ferver ou formar bolhas que ascendem, em grande número, até a superfície de um líquido como no desenvolvimento de CO_2 a partir de uma solução aquosa quando a pressão é reduzida. [L. *effervesco*, borbulhar, de *ferveo*, fazer ferver]

ef·fer·ves·cent (ef - er - ves′ent). Efervescente. **1.** Fervente; borbulhante. **2.** Que causa efervescência, como um pó efervescente. **3.** Que tende a efervescer quando liberado de pressão, como uma solução efervescente.

ef·fi·ca·cy (ef′ĭ - ka - sē). Eficácia; o quanto uma intervenção, procedimento, esquema ou serviço específico produz um resultado benéfico em condições ideais. Cf. effectiveness. [L. *efficacia*, de *ef-ficio*, realizar, executar]

ef·fi·cien·cy (e - fish'en - sē). Eficiência. **1.** A produção do efeito ou dos resultados desejados com desperdício mínimo de tempo, dinheiro, esforço ou habilidade. **2.** Uma medida de efetividade; especificamente, o trabalho útil realizado dividido pela energia utilizada.
  quantum e., e. quântica. SIN quantum yield.
  visual e., e. visual; classificação usada no cálculo da compensação para lesões oculares industriais, incorporando medidas de acuidade central, campo visual e motilidade ocular.

ef·fleu·rage (e - fler - ahz'). Um movimento de golpes na massagem. [Fr. *effleurer*, tocar levemente]

ef·flo·resce (e - flōr - es'). Eflorescer; tornar-se pulverizado por perda da água de cristalização quando exposto a uma atmosfera seca. [L. *ef-floresco* (*exf-*), florir, de *flos* (*flor-*), flor]

ef·flo·res·cent (e - flōr - es'ent). Eflorescente; designa um corpo cristalino que se transforma gradualmente em um pó, por perda de sua água de cristalização, quando exposto a uma atmosfera seca.

ef·flu·vi·um, pl. **ef·flu·via** (e - floo'vē - ŭm, - ē - ă). Eflúvio; perda de pêlos. VER TAMBÉM defluxion (1). [L. fluxo de saída, de *ef-fluo*, fluir para fora]
  anagen e., e. anagênico; súbita queda de pêlos difusa que ocorre na quimioterapia ou radioterapia para câncer; geralmente é reversível quando termina o tratamento.
  telogen e., e. telogênico; queda transitória aumentada de fios de cabelo normais por desenvolvimento prematuro da fase telogênica em folículos anagênicos, resultante de vários tipos de estresse, p. ex., parto, choque, uso de medicamentos ou interrupção do uso de um contraceptivo oral, febre e dieta com emagrecimento acentuado.

ef·fort (ef'ert). Esforço; emprego deliberado de força física ou mental.
  distributed e., e. distribuído; em psicologia, aprendizado que envolve pequenas unidades de trabalho e períodos de repouso intercalados, ao contrário do aprendizado massificado no qual o indivíduo trabalha continuamente até dominar a habilidade.

ef·fuse (ef - ūz'). Difuso, derramado; fino e amplamente espalhado; designa o caráter de crescimento em uma superfície de uma cultura bacteriana. [L. *effundo*, pp. *-fusus*; verter, derramar]

ef·fu·sion (e - fū'zhŭn). Efusão; derrame. **1.** A saída de líquido dos vasos sanguíneos ou linfáticos para os tecidos ou para uma cavidade. **2.** Acúmulo do líquido derramado. [L. *effusio*, derrame]
  complex pleural e., derrame pleural complexo; derrame pleural sem infecção real, mas com sinais de inflamação significativa (p. ex., pH baixo, glicose baixa, desidrogenase láctica elevada, muitos leucócitos).
  joint e., derrame articular; aumento do líquido na cavidade sinovial de uma articulação.
  loculated pleural e., derrame pleural loculado; derrame pleural limitado a uma ou mais cavidades fixas no espaço pleural.
  middle-ear e., derrame da orelha média; condição na qual o ar na orelha média foi substituído por líquido seroso ou mucóide em conseqüência de otite média. SIN secretory otitis media, serous otitis media.
  parapneumonic e., derrame parapneumônico; derrame pleural associado à pneumonia.
  pericardial e., derrame pericárdico; aumento do líquido no saco pericárdico; pode causar comprometimento circulatório por compressão do coração; na maioria das vezes é causado por inflamação, infecção, neoplasia maligna e uremia. SIN dropsy of pericardium.
  pleural e., derrame pleural; aumento do líquido no espaço pleural; pode causar dispnéia por compressão pulmonar e/ou aumento da pressão intratorácica, resultando em desvio do mediastino e aumento do trabalho respiratório; um derrame transudativo possui baixo conteúdo proteico e geralmente é devido a insuficiência cardíaca, uremia ou hipoalbuminemia; um derrame exsudativo tem alto conteúdo proteico e celular e, na maioria das vezes, é decorrente de inflamação, neoplasia maligna ou infecção; um derrame pleural infectado é um empiema; um derrame pleural associado à pneumonia é um derrame parapneumônico; um derrame pleural sem infecção real, mas com sinais de inflamação significativa (p. ex., pH baixo, glicose baixa, desidrogenase láctica [LDH] alta, muitos leucócitos), é um derrame pleural complexo e freqüentemente está associado à pneumonia; um derrame pleural loculado não se desloca livremente no espaço pleural, mas fica confinado a uma ou mais cavidades fixas. SIN hydrothorax.
  subpulmonic e., d. subpulmonar; acúmulo de líquido no espaço pleural, localizado radiograficamente, em sua maior parte, entre o diafragma e a superfície basal do pulmão.

eflor·ni·thine hy·dro·chlo·ride (ē - flōr'ni - thēn). Cloridrato de eflornitina; medicamento órfão antineoplásico e antiprotozoário usado no tratamento da pneumonia por *Pneumocystis carinii* na AIDS/SIDA e da doença do sono por *Trypanosoma brucei gambiense*.

EGD Abreviatura de esophagogastroduodenoscopy (esofagogastroduodenoscopia).

eges·ta (ē - jes'tă). Egesta, excreção; resíduos alimentares não-absorvidos que são eliminados pelo trato digestivo. [L. *e-gero*, pp. *-gestus*, conduzir para fora, expelir]

EGF Abreviatura de epidermal growth *factor* (fator de crescimento epidérmico).

EGFR Abreviatura de epidermal growth factor *receptor* (receptor do fator de crescimento epidérmico).

egg (eg). Ovo; a célula, ou gameta sexual feminino; após a fertilização e a fusão dos pró-núcleos, torna-se um zigoto, e não mais um ovo. Em répteis e aves, o ovo possui uma camada protetora, membranas, albumina e vitelo para a nutrição do embrião. VER TAMBÉM oocyte, ovum. [A.S. *aeg*]
  centrolecithal e., ovo centrolécito; um ovo no qual o vitelo está concentrado próximo ao centro da célula ovo, como ocorre em muitos insetos.
  homolecithal e., ovo homolécito; um ovo no qual a quantidade total de vitelo é pequena e distribuída de forma bastante uniforme em todo o citoplasma. SIN isolecithal e.
  isolecithal e., ovo isolécito. SIN homolecithal e.
  microlecithal e., ovo microlécito; um ovo contendo uma pequena quantidade de deutoplasma.
  telolecithal e., ovo telolécito; ovo que contém uma quantidade relativamente grande de deutoplasma concentrado no pólo abapical; p. ex., ovos de répteis e aves.

egg clus·ter. Um dos grupos de células resultantes da rotura dos cordões gonadais no córtex ovariano; esses grupos posteriormente se transformam em folículos ovarianos primários.

Egger, Fritz, clínico suíço, 1863–1938. VER E. *line*.

Eggleston, Cary, médico norte-americano, 1884–1966. VER E. *method*; Bradbury-Eggleston *syndrome*.

egg·shell. Casca de ovo; o revestimento calcário do ovo de uma ave.

eglan·du·lous (ē - glan'doo - lŭs). Eglanduloso; destituído de glândulas. [L. *e*, sem, + gland ou glandula]

Eglis glands. Glândulas de Eglis; VER em gland.

e·go (ē'gō). Ego; eu; em psicanálise, um dos três componentes do aparelho psíquico na estrutura freudiana, sendo os outros dois o id e o superego. Embora o ego tenha alguns componentes conscientes, muitas de suas funções são aprendidas e automáticas. Ele ocupa uma posição entre as pulsões primárias (princípio de prazer) e as demandas do mundo externo (princípio de realidade), e, portanto, desempenha o papel mediador entre a pessoa e a realidade externa, realizando as funções importantes de perceber as necessidades próprias (*self*), tanto físicas quanto psicológicas, e as qualidades e atitudes do ambiente. Avalia, coordena e integra essas percepções de tal forma que as demandas internas possam ser ajustadas às exigências externas, e também é responsável por determinadas funções defensivas para proteger a pessoa contra as demandas do id e do superego. [L. eu]

ego-al·ien (ē'gō - ā'lē - en). Egodistônico. SIN ego-dystonic.

ego·bron·choph·o·ny (ē'gō - brong - kof'ō - nē). Egobroncofonia; egofonia com broncofonia. [G. *aix* (*aig-*), cabra, + *bronchos*, brônquio, + *phōnē*, voz]

ego·cen·tric (ē - gō - sen'trik). Egocêntrico; caracterizado por concentração extrema da atenção em si mesmo, isto é, autocentrado. Cf. allocentric. SIN egotropic. [ego + G. *kentron*, centro]

ego·cen·tric·i·ty (ē'gō - sen - tris'i - tē). Egocentricidade; a condição de ser egocêntrico.

ego-dys·ton·ic (ē'gō - dis - ton'ik). Egodistônico; repugnante à divergência dos objetivos do ego e necessidades psicológicas relacionadas do indivíduo (p. ex., um pensamento obsessivo ou comportamento compulsivo); o oposto de egossintônico. SIN ego-alien. [ego + G. *dys*, mau, + *tonos*, tensão]

ego-ideal. Ideal do eu; ideal do ego; em psicanálise, um ideal, mais ou menos consciente, de excelência pessoal para o qual o indivíduo se empenha, e que é derivado de uma imagem composta das características pessoais de um genitor, de uma figura pública ou de uma ou mais pessoas que ele admira.

ego·ma·nia (ē - gō - mā'nē - ă). Egomania; autocentrismo, auto-estima ou autocontentamento extremos. [ego + G. *mania*, mania]

ego·phon·ic (ē - gō - fon'ik). Egofônico; relativo à egofonia.

egoph·o·ny (ē - gof'ō - nē). Egofonia; qualidade interrompida peculiar dos sons da voz, como o balido de uma cobra, ouvido aproximadamente no nível superior do líquido em casos de pleurisia com derrame. SIN caprilóquism, tragophonia, tragophony. [G. *aix*, (*aig-*), cabra, + *phōnē*, voz]

ego-syn·ton·ic (ē'gō - sin - ton'ik). Egossintônico; aceitável para os objetivos do ego e as necessidades psicológicas relacionadas do indivíduo (p. ex., um delírio); o oposto de egodistônico. [ego- + G. *syn*, junto, + *tonos*, tensão]

ego·tro·pic (ē - gō - trop'ik). Egocêntrico. SIN egocentric. [ego + G. *tropē*, mudança]

EGTA Abreviatura de ethyleneglycotetraacetic acid (ácido etilenoglicotetraacético).

EHEC Abreviatura de enterohemorrhagic *Escherichia coli* (*Escherichia coli* êntero-hemorrágica).

Ehlers, Edward L., dermatologista dinamarquês, 1863–1937. VER E.-Danlos *syndrome*.

Ehrenritter, Johann, anatomista austríaco, †1790. VER E. *ganglion.*
Ehret, Heinrich, médico alemão, *1870. VER E. *phenomenon.*
Ehrlich, Paul, bacteriologista, imunologista alemão e Prêmio Nobel, 1854–1915. VER *Ehrlichia*; E. *anemia, inner body, phenomenon, postulate,* diazo *reagent, theory*; E.-Türk *line.* VER entradas em stain; reaction.
Ehr·lich·ia (er - lik´ē - à). Gênero de pequenas bactérias Gram-negativas, freqüentemente pleomórficas, cocóides ou elipsóides, imóveis (ordem Rickettsiales), encontradas isoladas ou em inclusões compactas nos leucócitos circulantes de mamíferos; as espécies são os agentes etiológicos da erliquiose e são transmitidas por carrapatos. A espécie típica é *E. canis.* [P. *Ehrlich*]
E. ca´nis, a espécie bacteriana que causa a doença transmitida por carrapatos erliquiose canina (transmitida pelo carrapato *Rhipicephalus sanguineus*); é a espécie típica do gênero *E.* Ocasionalmente, causa infecção transmitida por carrapatos em seres humanos.
E. chaffee´nsis, espécie bacteriana descrita recentemente, associada à erliquiose humana; infecta os monócitos dos seres humanos e é transmitida pelo carrapato vetor, *Amblyomma americanum,* o carrapato Lone Star (estrela solitária).
E. equi, espécie bacteriana que causa erliquiose granulocítica humana; observada nos estados do Meio-Atlântico, sul da Nova Inglaterra e sul do Meio-Oeste, e é transmitida por carrapatos (*Ixodes*).
E. phagocytophila, espécie bacteriana que causa erliquiose granulocítica humana; também causa febre transmitida por carrapatos no gado bovino; observada nos estados do Meio-Atlântico, sul da Nova Inglaterra e sul do Meio-Oeste dos EUA, e é transmitida por carrapatos (*Ixodes*).
E. ristic´ii, a espécie bacteriana que causa erliquiose monocítica eqüina.
E. sennet´su, a espécie bacteriana que causa febre de Sennetsu em seres humanos. SIN *Rickettsia sennetsu.*
Ehr·lic·hi·eae. Membros da família Rickettsiaceae; parasitas intracelulares obrigatórios dos leucócitos do sangue periférico.

ehr·lich·i·o·sis (er - lik - ē - ō´sis). Erliquiose; infecção pelas riquétsias leucocíticas do gênero *Ehrlichia*; em seres humanos é causada principalmente por *E. sennetsu,* que produz manifestações semelhantes às da febre maculosa das Montanhas Rochosas.

> As espécies de *Ehrlichia* foram reconhecidas há muito tempo como causas de doença hemorrágica febril de gravidade variável em animais, incluindo cães e cavalos. A infecção humana por *E. sennetsu,* limitada ao Extremo Oriente, é uma doença semelhante à mononucleose. O primeiro caso humano de erliquiose no hemisfério ocidental foi descrito em 1986. Desde então, foram reconhecidas duas formas distintas da doença em seres humanos, cada uma associada a uma espécie diferente de *Ehrlichia* e a um grupo diferente de carrapatos vetores. Mais de 90% dos pacientes relatam picadas por vários carrapatos. Ainda não foi identificado um reservatório animal, mas suspeita-se de roedores e cervos. Após um período de incubação de 1–4 semanas, a infecção começa como uma doença febril inespecífica, com calafrios, sudorese, cefaléia e dores articulares e musculares. Um quarto dos pacientes apresenta erupção cutânea inespecífica transitória não relacionada ao local da picada do carrapato. As complicações sistêmicas podem envolver as vias respiratórias (dor de garganta, tosse, infiltrados pulmonares, síndrome de angústia respiratória aguda), o sistema digestivo (náuseas, vômitos, dor abdominal, hemorragia gastrointestinal) ou o fígado (80% têm hepatite). Outras complicações possíveis incluem meningite, pericardite, insuficiência renal e coagulação intravascular disseminada. Estudos iniciais dessas infecções, baseados em populações com doença mais visível e facilmente identificável, superestimaram as taxas de fatalidade. Com o tratamento, a taxa de caso-fatalidade nas duas formas de erliquiose provavelmente não ultrapassa 1%. A erliquiose granulocítica humana é clinicamente indistinguível da erliquiose monocítica humana, mas, na primeira, as mórulas são encontradas nos neutrófilos, e não nos monócitos, e a doença é um pouco mais grave. Nas duas formas de erliquiose, a tecnologia de reação em cadeia da polimerase é o teste sorológico mais sensível e específico. A tetraciclina e a doxiciclina são altamente eficazes na interrupção da progressão de ambas as formas de erliquiose humana. Como outros agentes, incluindo o cloranfenicol, não se mostraram efetivos, as tetraciclinas são usadas até mesmo em crianças, para as quais geralmente são contra-indicadas devido ao risco de manchar os dentes e suprimir o crescimento ósseo. O tratamento freqüentemente é iniciado quando há suspeita, enquanto se aguarda a confirmação do diagnóstico clínico por teste sorológico. A farmacoterapia é mantida por 14 dias.

human e., e. humana; forma de erliquiose que se apresenta clinicamente como uma doença febril aguda indiferenciada, caracterizada por febre, calafrios, diarréia e cefaléia, após picada(s) de carrapato, provavelmente pelo carrapato Lone Star (estrela solitária), *Amblyomma americanum.* Geralmente é causada por *Ehrlichia chaffeensis.* Descrita pela primeira vez em 1987. (Considerada, predominantemente, uma forma monocítica de erliquiose.)
human granulocytic e. (HGE), e. granulocítica humana; doença infecciosa aguda caracterizada por febre, calafrios, cefaléia, dores articulares e musculares, e, algumas vezes, por envolvimento respiratório, gastrointestinal, hepático ou outro envolvimento sistêmico; descrita pela primeira vez em 1994, nos estados do nordeste e norte do Meio-Oeste e na Califórnia; o agente causador pode ser distinguido apenas por estudos moleculares de *Ehrlichia equi,* a causa da erliquiose eqüina. O carrapato do cervo, *Ixodes scapularis,* é o principal vetor, e a incidência máxima se dá no mês de julho. Estudos hematológicos mostram redução do número de hemácias, leucócitos e plaquetas. Grupos de microrganismos em desenvolvimento denominados mórulas podem ser observados em neutrófilos em esfregaços de sangue corados, mas as provas sorológicas são mais sensíveis.
human monocytic e. (HME), e. monocítica humana; doença infecciosa aguda caracterizada por febre, calafrios, cefaléia, dor muscular e articular, e envolvimento respiratório, gastrointestinal e sistêmico variável; estudos hematológicos mostram redução do número de hemácias, leucócitos e plaquetas. O achado de grupos de organismos em desenvolvimento, denominados mórulas, no citoplasma de monócitos em um esfregaço corado do sangue periférico, estabelece o diagnóstico, mas sua detecção freqüentemente é difícil. As provas sorológicas mostram anticorpos contra *Ehrlichia chaffeensis,* microrganismo muito semelhante ao agente da erliquiose canina, *E. canis.* Essa doença foi amplamente limitada ao sudeste e ao centro-sul dos Estados Unidos. O carrapato Lone Star (estrela solitária) (*Amblyomma americanum*) e o carrapato *Dermacentor variabilis* são os principais vetores, e a incidência é maior entre os meses de abril e setembro, durante o pico de atividade desses carrapatos.
Eichhorst, Hermann L., médico suíço, 1849–1921. VER E. *corpuscles,* em *corpuscle, neuritis.*
Eicken, Karl von, laringologista alemão, 1873–1960. VER E. *method.*
***n*-ei·co·sa·no·ic ac·id** (ī´kō - sā - nō´ik). Ácido *n*-eicosanóico. SIN arachidic acid.
ei·co·sa·noids (ī´kō - sā - noydz). Eicosanóides; as substâncias fisiologicamente ativas derivadas do ácido araquidônico, isto é, as prostaglandinas, leucotrienos e tromboxanos; sintetizadas por uma via em cascata. [G. *eicosa-,* vinte, + *eidos,* forma]
9-ei·co·se·no·ic ac·id (ī´kō - sē - nō´ik). Ácido 9-eicosenóico. SIN gadoleic acid.
ei·det·ic (ī - det´ik). Eidético; idético. **1.** Relativo à capacidade de visualização e memória para objetos vistos anteriormente, que atinge seu máximo em crianças de 8 a 10 anos. **2.** Uma pessoa que possui essa capacidade em alto grau. [G. *eidon,* visto (aoristo de verbo)]
EIEC Abreviatura de enteroinvasive *Escherichia coli* (*Escherichia coli* enteroinvasiva).
Ei·ken·el·la cor·ro·dens (ī - ke - nel´ă kōr - rō´denz). Espécie de bactérias imóveis, em forma de bastonete, Gram-negativas, facultativamente anaeróbicas, que, caracteristicamente, deprime o ágar sob suas colônias; faz parte da flora normal da cavidade oral humana adulta, mas pode ser um patógeno oportunista, em cultura pura ou mista, particularmente em hospedeiros imunodeprimidos. [M. *Eiken,* 1958]
ei·ko·nom·e·ter (ī - kō - nom´ē - ter). Eiconômetro. **1.** Instrumento para determinar o poder de ampliação de um microscópio, ou o tamanho de um objeto microscópico. **2.** Instrumento para determinar o grau de aniseiconia. [G. *eikon,* imagem, + *metron,* medida]
ei·loid (ī´loyd). Eilóide; semelhante a uma bobina ou rolo. [G. *eilō,* rolar para cima, + *eidos,* aparência]
Eimer, Gustav Heinrich Theodor, zoólogo alemão, 1843–1898.
Ei·me·ri·i·dae (ī - mēr - ī´i - dē). Família de coccídios esporozoários; são gêneros importantes *Eimeria* e *Isospora,* sendo as infecções por *Eimeria* as mais comuns e mais graves em animais domésticos. [ver *Eimeria*]
Einarson gal·lo·cy·a·nin-chrome al·um stain. Ver em stain.
ein·stein (īn´stīn). Einstein; unidade de energia igual a 1 mol quantum e, por conseguinte, a $6,0221367 \times 10^{23}$ quanta. O valor de einstein, em kJ, depende do comprimento de onda. [A. *Einstein,* físico teórico naturalizado americano, nascido na Alemanha, e prêmio Nobel, 1879–1955]
ein·stein·i·um (Es) (īn - stīn´ē - ŭm). Einstênio; elemento transurânico preparado artificialmente, n.º atômico 99, peso atômico 252,0; possui muitos isótopos, todos radioativos (Es^{252} possui a maior meia-vida conhecida, 1,29 ano).
Einthoven, Willem, fisiologista holandês e prêmio Nobel, 1860–1927. VER E. *equation, law,* string *galvanometer, triangle.*
Eisenlohr, Carl, médico alemão, 1847–1896.
Eisenmenger, Victor, médico alemão, 1864–1932. VER E. *complex, defect, disease, syndrome, tetralogy.*
ei·sod·ic (ī - sod´ik). Eisódico; termo raramente usado para aferente. [G. *eis,* dentro, + *hodos,* caminho]
ejac·u·late (ē - jak´ū - lāt). **1.** Ejacular; expelir subitamente. **2.** Ejaculado; sêmen expelido na ejaculação. [ver ejaculation]
ejac·u·la·tion (ē - jak - ū - lā´shŭn). Ejaculação; o processo que resulta em

propulsão de sêmen dos ductos genitais e uretra para o exterior; causado pelas contrações rítmicas dos músculos que circundam os órgãos genitais internos e os músculos isquiocavernoso e bulbocavernoso, resultando em aumento da pressão sobre o sêmen nas glândulas genitais internas e na uretra interna. [L. *eiaculo*, pp. *-atus*, projetar]

    premature e., ejaculação precoce; durante o ato sexual, a chegada muito rápida ao clímax e ejaculação no homem em relação aos seus próprios desejos ou aos desejos de sua parceira.

    retrograde e., e. retrógrada; passagem do sêmen ejaculado para a bexiga; observada em doença neurológica, diabetes e, ocasionalmente, após cirurgia da próstata.

ejac·u·la·to·ry (ē-jak′ū-lā-tōr-ē). Ejaculatório; relativo a uma ejaculação.

ejec·ta (ē-jek′tā). Ejeto. SIN ejection (2). [L. neut. pl. de *ejectus*, pp. de *ejicio*, expelir]

ejec·tion (ē-jek′shŭn). Ejeção. **1.** O ato de dirigir ou atirar pela força física interna. **2.** Aquilo que é ejetado. SIN ejecta. [L. *ejectio*, de *ejicio*, expulsar]

ejec·tor (ē-jek′tor, -tōr). Ejetor; um dispositivo usado para expelir (ejetar) uma substância à força.

    saliva e., e. de saliva; tubo de aspiração oco, perfurado, usado na evacuação de saliva ou resíduos líquidos da cavidade oral. SIN dental pump, saliva pump.

EJP Abreviatura de excitatory junction *potential* (potencial da junção excitatória).

Ejrup, Erick, clínico sueco do século XX. VER E. *maneuver*.

⚠ **eka-.** Eca; prefixo usado para designar um elemento não-descoberto ou recém-descoberto da tabela periódica, antes que seja dado um nome apropriado e oficial pelos especialistas; p. ex., eca-ósmio, agora plutônio. [Sânscrito *eka*, um]

Ekbom, Karl A., neurologista sueco, *1907. VER E. *syndrome*.

EKG Abreviatura de electrocardiogram (eletrocardiograma).

eki·ri (ē-kī′rī). Uma forma tóxica, aguda, de disenteria em lactentes, observada no Japão e causada por *Shigella sonnei*. [Japão]

EKY Abreviatura de electrokymogram (eletroquimograma).

elab·o·ra·tion (ē-lab′or-ā′shŭn). Elaboração; o processo de resolução em detalhes por trabalho e estudo. [L. *e-laborō*, pp. *-atus*, trabalhar, esforçar, de *labor*, labuta, elaborar]

    secondary e., e. secundária; o processo mental que ocorre parcialmente durante o sonho e parcialmente durante a recordação ou descrição de um sonho, por meio do qual o conteúdo latente (relativamente desorganizado e psicologicamente doloroso) do sonho é disposto em ordem mais coerente e lógica, resultando no conteúdo manifesto do sonho; um aspecto do trabalho do sonho.

Elae·oph·o·ra schnei·deri (ē-lē-of′ō-rā schnī′der-ī). Verme sanguíneo do carneiro; uma espécie de nematódeo que causa dermatose filariana. [L. mod. *elaea*, de G. *elaia*, oliva, + *agnos*, carneiro, + *phoros*, manter]

el·a·id·ic ac·id (el-ā-id′ik). Ácido elaídico; *trans*-isômero monobásico insaturado do ácido oleico; encontrado na gordura de ruminantes. Cf. oleic acid.

elai·o·path·ia (el′ā-ō-path′ē-ā). Eleopatia. SIN eleopathy. [G. *elaion*, óleo, + *pathos*, que sofre]

E-LAM Abreviatura de endothelial-leukocyte adhesion *molecule* (molécula de adesão leucócito-endotelial).

el·a·pid (el′ā-pid). Elapídeo; qualquer membro da família de cobras Elapidae.

Elap·i·dae (ē-lap′i-dē). Família de cobras muito venenosas caracterizada por um par de presas comparativamente curtas, permanentemente eretas, profundamente sulcadas na frente da boca. Há mais de 150 espécies, incluindo as serpentes naja, krait, mamba e coral. [G. *elops*, uma serpente]

elas·tance (ē-las′tans). Elastância, o inverso da capacitância; medida da tendência de uma estrutura de retornar à sua forma original após a remoção de uma força deformante. Em medicina e fisiologia, geralmente é uma medida da tendência de uma víscera oca (p. ex., pulmão, bexiga, vesícula biliar) de retornar às suas dimensões originais após a retirada de uma força distensiva ou compressiva, com a pressão de retração resultante de uma unidade de distensão ou compressão da víscera; a recíproca da complacência. A relação entre elasticidade e elastância é da mesma natureza que aquela entre a capacidade indutiva específica de um material de isolamento e a capacitância de um condensador específico feito desse material.

elas·tase (ē-las′tās). Elastase; uma serina proteinase que hidrolisa a elastina; já foram identificadas outras enzimas semelhantes à elastase (p. ex., elastase pancreática [pancreatopeptidase E] e elastase leucocitária [elastase lisossômica ou neutrofílica]) com diferentes seqüências e parâmetros cinéticos; todos possuem especificidades razoavelmente amplas.

elas·tic (ē-las′tik). Elástico. **1.** Que tem a propriedade de voltar ao formato original após ser distendido, comprimido, curvado ou distorcido de outra forma. **2.** Uma faixa de borracha ou plástico usada em ortodontia como uma fonte primária ou auxiliar de força para movimentar os dentes. O termo geralmente é modificado por um adjetivo para descrever a direção da força ou a localização dos pontos de união terminais. [G. *elastreō*, forma épica de *elaunō*, dirigir, empurrar]

    intermaxillary e., e. intermaxilar; material usado para proporcionar tração elástica entre os dentes superiores e inferiores.

    vertical e., e. vertical; material elástico usado em uma direção perpendicular ao plano oclusal, unindo um arame em arco ao outro e geralmente usado para melhorar a intercuspidação.

elas·ti·ca (ē-las′ti-kā). **1.** Elástica; a camada elástica na parede de uma artéria. **2.** Tecido elástico. SIN elastic *tissue*.

elas·ti·cin (ē-las′ti-sin). Elasticina. SIN elastin.

elas·tic·i·ty (ē-las-tis′i-tē). Elasticidade; a qualidade ou condição de ser elástico.

    physical e. of muscle, e. física do músculo; a qualidade do músculo que lhe permite ceder ao estiramento físico passivo.

    physiologic e. of muscle, e. fisiológica do músculo; a qualidade biológica, exclusiva do músculo, de ser capaz de se modificar e retornar ao tamanho sob controle neuromuscular.

    total e. of muscle, e. total do músculo; o efeito combinado da elasticidade física e fisiológica do músculo.

elas·tin (ē-las′tin). Elastina; uma mucoproteína fibrosa, elástica, amarela, que é a principal proteína do tecido conjuntivo de estruturas elásticas (p. ex., grandes vasos sanguíneos, tendões, ligamentos, etc.); o precursor da elastina é a pró-elastina. SIN elasticin.

elas·to·fi·bro·ma (ē-las′tō-fī-brō′mā). Elastofibroma; massa de crescimento lento, não-encapsulada, de tecido fibroso, colágeno, pouco celular e tecido elástico; geralmente ocorre no tecido adiposo subescapular de pessoas idosas. [G. *elastos*, abatido, + L. *fibra*, *-oma*, tumor]

elas·toi·din (ē-las′toy-din). Elastoidina; um colágeno complexo.

elas·tol·y·sis. Elastólise; dissolução das fibras elásticas. [elasto- + G. *lysis*, afrouxamento, de *luō*, afrouxar]

    generalized e., e. generalizada. SIN dermatochalasis.

elas·to·ma (ē-las-tō′mā). Elastoma; um depósito de tecido elástico semelhante a um tumor.

    juvenile e., e. juvenil; nevo de tecido conjuntivo caracterizado pelo aumento do número e do tamanho das fibras elásticas. VER TAMBÉM osteodermatopoikilosis.

    Miescher e., e. de Miescher; grupos circinados de pápulas hiperceratóticas que se tornam deslocadas, deixando uma pequena depressão sanguínea; associado ao pseudoxantoma elástico.

elas·tom·e·ter (ē-las-tom′e-ter). Elastômetro; dispositivo para medir a elasticidade de qualquer corpo ou dos tecidos animais.

elas·to·mu·cin (ē-las-tō-mū′kin). Elastomucina; a mucoproteína de tecido conjuntivo; p. ex., elastina.

elas·tor·rhex·is (ē-las-tō-rek′sis). Elastorrexe; fragmentação de tecido elástico na qual os filamentos ondulados normais parecem fragmentados e aglomerados, assumindo uma coloração basófila. [G. *rhēxis*, ruptura]

elas·to·sis (ē-las-tō′sis). Elastose. **1.** Alteração degenerativa do tecido elástico. **2.** Degeneração das fibras colágenas, com alteração das propriedades de coloração, que passam a ser semelhantes ao tecido elástico. SIN elastoid degeneration (1), elastotic degeneration.

    e. colloida'lis conglomera'ta, e. coloidal conglomerada. SIN colloid milium.

    e. dystroph'ica, e. distrófica. SIN angioid *streaks*, em *streak*.

    e. per'forans serpigino'sa, e. perfurante serpiginosa; grupos circinados de pápulas ceratóticas assintomáticas; a epiderme está espessada ao redor de um tampão central de tecido elástico dérmico que é expulso através da epiderme.

    solar e., e. solar; elastose observada histologicamente na pele exposta ao sol de pessoas idosas ou daquelas portadoras de lesão actínica crônica.

ela·tion (ē-lā′shŭn). Elação; o sentimento ou expressão de excitação ou alegria; se prolongada e imprópria, uma característica da mania. [L. *elatio*, de *effero*, pp. *e-latus*, levantar]

e·laun·in (ē-law′nin). Elaunina; um componente das fibras elásticas formado a partir da deposição de elastina entre fibras de oxitalana; encontrado no tecido conjuntivo da derme, particularmente em associação com as glândulas sudoríparas. [G. *elaunō*, guiar]

Elaut, Leon J.S., patologista belga do século XX. VER E. *triangle*.

el·bow (el′bō). Cotovelo. **1.** A região do membro superior entre o braço e o antebraço que circunda a articulação do cotovelo, em especial posteriormente. **2.** A articulação entre o braço e o antebraço. SIN cubitus (1) [TA], ancon. **3.** Um corpo angular semelhante a um cotovelo fletido. [A.S. *elnboga*]

    little league e., SIN Panner *disease*.

    Little Leaguer's e., e. do jogador de beisebol juvenil; epicondilite medial; epicondilite do epicôndilo medial na origem dos músculos flexores do antebraço; relacionada ao arremesso de bola e geralmente observada em crianças ou adolescentes.

    miner's e., c. do mineiro; inflamação com distensão da bolsa do olécrano por líquido.

    nursemaid's e., c. da babá; subluxação da cabeça do rádio do ligamento anular causada pela tração súbita da mão com o cotovelo esticado e o antebraço pronado. SIN Malgaigne luxation.

    tennis e., c. de tenista; epicondilite lateral do úmero; inflamação crônica na origem dos músculos extensores do antebraço no epicôndilo lateral do úmero, em virtude de esforço incomum ou repetitivo (não necessariamente por jogar tênis). SIN epicondylalgia externa, lateral humeral epicondylitis.

el·bowed (el'bōd). Acotovelado; angular.

el·der, el·'der flow·ers. Sabugueiro; flores de sabugueiro. SIN sambucus.

electro-. Eletro-; elétrico, eletricidade. [G. *ēlektron,* âmbar (no qual se pode gerar eletricidade estática por fricção)]

elec·tro·an·al·ge·sia (ē - lek'trō - an - al - jē'zē - ā). Eletroanalgesia; analgesia induzida pela passagem de uma corrente elétrica.

elec·tro·a·nal·y·sis (ē - lek'trō - ā - nal'i - sis). Eletroanálise; análise quantitativa de metais por eletrólise.

elec·tro·an·es·the·sia (ē - lek'trō - an - es - thē'zē - ā). Eletroanestesia; anestesia produzida por uma corrente elétrica.

elec·tro·ax·on·og·ra·phy (ē - lek'trō - ak - son - og'rā - fē). Eletroaxonografia. SIN axonography.

elec·tro·bi·os·co·py (ē - lek'trō - bī - os'kō - pē). Eletrobioscopia; termo raro para uso de eletricidade como uma forma de determinar se há ou não vida. [electro- + G. *bios,* vida, + *skopeō,* examinar]

elec·tro·car·di·o·gram (ECG, EKG) (ē - lek - trō - kar'dē - ō - gram). Eletrocardiograma; registro gráfico das correntes de ação integradas do coração obtido com o eletrocardiógrafo, apresentado como modificações da voltagem com o passar do tempo. [electro- + G. *kardia,* coração, + *gramma,* desenho]
  concordant changes e., e. de alterações concordantes; a presença de mais de uma alteração da onda, todas na mesma direção (polaridade).
  discordant changes e., e. de alterações discordantes; a presença de mais de uma alteração da onda, cada uma com uma direção (polaridade) diferente.
  scalar e. (skăl'ar), e. escalar; o registro das derivações eletrocardiográficas que pode ser exibido em um plano do corpo, ao contrário do vetocardiograma, no qual a exibição é feita em dois planos ou mais.
  unipolar e., e. unipolar; eletrocardiograma feito com o eletrodo explorador colocado no tórax, sobre a região do coração ou em um único membro, sendo o eletrodo indiferente (potencial "zero") a terminação central.

elec·tro·car·di·o·graph (ē - lek - trō - kar'dē - ō - graf) Eletrocardiógrafo; instrumento de registro do potencial das correntes elétricas que atravessam o coração.

elec·tro·car·di·og·ra·phy (ē - lek'trō - kar - dē - og'rā - fē). Eletrocardiografia. **1.** Método de registro das correntes elétricas que atravessam o músculo cardíaco. **2.** O estudo e a interpretação de eletrocardiogramas.
  fetal e., e. fetal; registro do eletrocardiograma do feto *in utero.*
  precordial e., e. precordial; registro de sinais eletrocardiográficos na parede anterior esquerda do tórax; convencionalmente são usadas seis posições de eletrodos, mas pode ser usado qualquer número de eletrodos.

elec·tro·car·di·o·pho·no·gram (ē - lek'trō - kar - dē - ō - fōn'ō - gram). Eletrocardiofonograma; registro obtido por eletrocardiofonografia.

elec·tro·car·di·o·pho·nog·ra·phy (ē - lek'trō - kar - dē - ō - fō - nog'rā - fē). Eletrocardiofonografia; método de registro elétrico dos sons cardíacos. [electro- + G. *kardia,* coração, + *phōnē,* som, + *graphō,* escrever]

elec·tro·cau·ter·i·za·tion (ē - lek'trō - caw'ter - i - zā'shŭn). Eletrocauterização; cauterização por passagem de corrente de alta freqüência através do tecido ou por um dispositivo metálico eletricamente aquecido.

elec·tro·cau·tery (ē - lek'trō - caw'ter - ē). Eletrocautério. **1.** Instrumento para orientar uma corrente de alta freqüência através de uma área local de tecido. **2.** Instrumento cauterizador metálico aquecido por uma corrente elétrica. SIN electric cautery.

elec·tro·ce·re·bral in·ac·tiv·i·ty·Inatividade elétrica cerebral. SIN electrocerebral silence.

elec·tro·ce·re·bral si·lence (ECS) (ē - lek'trō - ser - ē'brăl sī'lens). Silêncio eletrocerebral; encefalograma plano ou isoelétrico; um eletroencefalograma sem atividade cerebral por 2 μv de pares de eletrodos colocados simetricamente distantes 10 ou mais centímetros, e com resistência intereletrodo entre 100 e 10.000 ohms; se for obtido esse registro por 30 minutos em um adulto com morte cerebral clínica e se forem excluídas intoxicação por drogas, hipotermia e hipotensão recente, é apoiado o diagnóstico de morte cerebral. SIN electrocerebral inactivity, flat electroencephalogram, isoelectric electroencephalogram.

elec·tro·chem·i·cal (ē - lek'trō - kem'i - kăl). Eletroquímico; designa reações químicas envolvendo eletricidade e os mecanismos envolvidos.

elec·tro·co·ag·u·la·tion (ē - lek'trō - kō - ag - ŭ - lā'shŭn). Eletrocoagulação; coagulação produzida por um eletrocautério.

elec·tro·co·chle·o·gram (ē - lek'trō - kok'lē - ō - gram). Eletrococleograma; o registro obtido por eletrococleografia.

elec·tro·co·chle·og·ra·phy (ē - lek'trō - kok - lē - og'rā - fē). Eletrococleografia; medida dos potenciais elétricos gerados na orelha interna em virtude de estimulação sonora. [electro- + L. *cochlea,* concha de caramujo, + G. *graphō,* escrever]

elec·tro·con·trac·til·i·ty (ē - lek'trō - kon - trak - til'i - tē). Eletrocontratilidade; a força de contração do tecido muscular em resposta a um estímulo elétrico.

elec·tro·con·vul·sive (ē - lek'trō - kon - vŭl'siv). Eletroconvulsivo; designa uma resposta convulsiva a um estímulo elétrico. VER electroshock *therapy.*

elec·tro·cor·ti·co·gram (ē - lek - trō - kōr'ti - kō - gram). Eletrocorticograma; registro da atividade elétrica derivado diretamente do córtex cerebral.

elec·tro·cor·ti·cog·ra·phy (ECoG) (ē - lek'trō - kōr - ti - kog'rā - fē). Eletrocorticografia; a técnica de registro da atividade elétrica do córtex cerebral por meio de eletrodos colocados diretamente sobre ele.

elec·tro·cute (ē - lek'trō - kūt). Eletrocutar; causar morte pela passagem de uma corrente elétrica através do corpo. [electro- + execute]

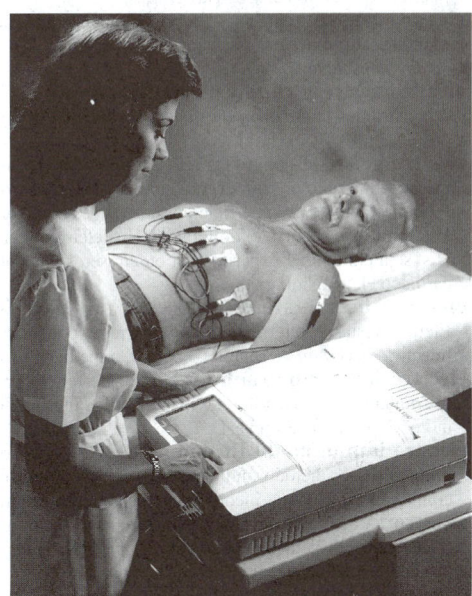
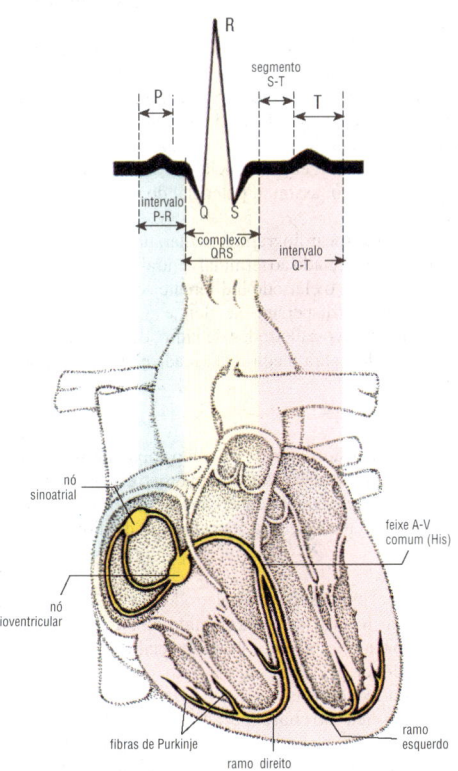

eletrocardiografia (ECG): (esquerda) eletrocardiograma em repouso; (direita) uma imagem elétrica do coração é representada por deflexões positivas e negativas em um gráfico, marcado com as letras P, Q, R, S e T, correspondente aos eventos do ciclo cardíaco

elec·tro·cu·tion (ē-lek-trō-kū'shŭn). Eletrocução; morte causada por eletricidade. VER electrocute. SIN electrothanasia.

elec·tro·cys·tog·ra·phy (ē-lek'trō-sis-tog'ra-fē). Eletrocistografia; registro de correntes ou alterações elétricas no potencial elétrico da bexiga.

elec·trode (ē-lek'trōd). Eletrodo. **1.** Dispositivo para registrar um dos dois membros de um circuito elétrico; um dos dois pólos de uma bateria elétrica ou da extremidade dos condutores conectados a ele. **2.** Uma terminação elétrica especializada para determinada reação eletroquímica. [electro- + G. *hodos*, forma]

  active e., e. ativo; pequeno eletrodo cujo efeito excitador é usado para estimular ou registrar potenciais de uma área localizada. SIN exciting e., localizing e., therapeutic e.

  calomel e., e. de calomelano; eletrodo no qual o fio é conectado, através de um reservatório de mercúrio, a uma pasta de cloreto mercuroso (Hg_2Cl_2, calomelano) em uma solução de cloreto de potássio coberto por mais solução de cloreto de potássio; comumente usado como eletrodo de referência.

  carbon dioxide e., e. de dióxido de carbono; eletrodo de vidro em uma película de solução de bicarbonato coberta por uma fina membrana plástica permeável ao dióxido de carbono, mas impermeável à água e aos eletrólitos; a pressão de dióxido de carbono de uma amostra de gás ou líquido equilibra-se rapidamente através da membrana e é medida em termos do pH resultante da solução de bicarbonato, percebido pelo eletrodo de vidro; comumente usado para análise de CO_2 em amostras de sangue arterial. SIN Severinghaus e.

  central terminal e., e. terminal central; em eletrocardiografia, um eletrodo no qual as conexões dos três membros (braço direito, braço esquerdo e perna esquerda) são unidas e levam ao eletrocardiógrafo para formar o eletrodo indiferente, teoricamente em potencial zero para o sistema.

  Clark e., e. de Clark; eletrodo de oxigênio que consiste na extremidade de um fio de platina exposto a uma fina camada de eletrólito coberta por uma membrana plástica permeável ao oxigênio, mas não à água ou ao eletrólito. Quando se aplica uma determinada voltagem, o oxigênio é destruído na superfície da platina; o fluxo de corrente então é proporcional à velocidade com que o oxigênio consegue se difundir da amostra de gás ou líquido fora da membrana para a superfície de platina. Trata-se, portanto, de uma medida da pressão de oxigênio na amostra; comumente usado para medir a pressão de oxigênio em amostras de sangue arterial.

  dispersing e., e. dispersor. SIN indifferent e.

  exciting e., e. ativo. SIN active e.

  exploring e., e. explorador; eletrodo colocado sobre um tecido excitável, ou próximo a ele; em eletrocardiografia unipolar, o eletrodo é colocado sobre o tórax na região do coração e forma um par com um eletrodo indiferente.

  glass e., e. de vidro; um globo de vidro de paredes finas que contém uma solução tampão padronizada, quinidrona, e um fio de platina; quando imerso em uma solução desconhecida, surge uma diferença de potencial que varia com o pH da solução desconhecida; essa diferença pode ser calculada para fornecer o pH; usado em medidores de pH.

  hydrogen e., e. de hidrogênio; o padrão final de referência em todas as determinações de pH, limitado e tecnicamente difícil de usar, que consiste em um pedaço de platina esponjosa preta, parcialmente imersa em uma solução em um pequeno tubo de vidro; o tubo acima da solução é preenchido com gás hidrogênio que é borbulhado através da solução e absorvido pela platina; o eletrodo que mede o potencial entre H_2 e H^+, cujo potencial "padrão" (1 atmosfera, 1 molar) é considerado igual a zero; assim, o potencial do eletrodo de hidrogênio mede $[H^+]$ ou o pH.

  indifferent e., e. indiferente; em eletrocardiografia unipolar, um eletrodo distante colocado em um membro ou conectado ao terminal central e pareado com um eletrodo explorador; supõe-se que o eletrodo indiferente contribua pouco ou nada para o registro resultante. SIN dispersing e., silent e.

  ion-selective e.'s, eletrodos íon-seletivos; eletrodos de vidro, de troca de íons líquidos ou no estado sólido, usados, para medir a atividade eletrolítica e de íons cálcio nos líquidos biológicos.

  localizing e., e. localizador. SIN active e.

  negative e., e. negativo. SIN cathode.

  oxidation-reduction e., e. de oxidação-redução; eletrodo capaz de medir o potencial de oxidação-redução (oxirredução). VER quinhydrone e. SIN redox e.

  oxygen e., e. de oxigênio; eletrodo que, geralmente, consiste em uma alça de platina ou gotas de mercúrio, usado para medir a concentração de dioxigênio em uma solução.

  positive e., e. positivo. SIN anode.

  quinhydrone e., e. de quinidrona; um dos diversos eletrodos de oxidação-redução nos quais a razão das duas formas (quinona-quinidrona), determinada pela concentração de íon hidrogênio, estabelece um potencial que pode ser medido e convertido em um valor de pH (falha em pH > 8).

  redox e., e. redox. SIN oxidation-reduction e.

  reference e., e. de referência; um eletrodo com expectativa de ter um potencial constante, como um eletrodo de calomelano, e usado com outro eletrodo para completar um circuito elétrico através de uma solução; p. ex., quando um eletrodo de referência é usado com um eletrodo de vidro para medida do pH, alterações na voltagem entre os dois eletrodos podem ser atribuídas aos efeitos do pH apenas sobre o eletrodo de vidro.

  resectoscope e., ressectoscópio eletrocirúrgico; eletrodo de alça que permite a remoção de tecido bem como cauterização da superfície desnuda; usado na ablação do endométrio.

  rollerball e., e. de rolamento; um eletrodo esférico que desliza como um rolo de pintura sobre o tecido superficial, cauterizando-o; usado na ablação do endométrio.

  Severinghaus e., e. de Severinghaus. SIN carbon dioxide e.

  silent e., e. indiferente. SIN indifferent e.

  therapeutic e., e. terapêutico. SIN active e.

elec·tro·der·mal (ē-lek'trō-der'măl). Eletrodérmico; relativo às propriedades elétricas da pele, geralmente referindo-se à alteração da resistência. [electro- + G. *derma*, pele]

elec·tro·des·ic·ca·tion (ē-lek'trō-des-i-kā'shŭn). Eletrodessecação; destruição de lesões ou fechamento de vasos sanguíneos (geralmente da pele, mas também de superfícies disponíveis de mucosa) por corrente elétrica monopolar de alta freqüência. [electro- + L. *desicco*, dessecar]

elec·tro·di·ag·no·sis (ē-lek'trō-dī-ag-nō'sis). Eletrodiagnóstico. **1.** O uso de dispositivos eletrônicos para fins diagnósticos. **2.** Por convenção, os estudos realizados no laboratório de EMG, isto é, estudos da condução nervosa e exame por eletrodo com agulha (EMG propriamente dita). SIN electroneurography. **3.** Determinação da natureza de uma doença através da observação de alterações na atividade elétrica. SIN evoked electromyography.

elec·tro·di·al·y·sis (ē-lek'trō-dī-al'i-sis). Eletrodiálise; em um campo elétrico, a retirada de íons de moléculas e partículas maiores. Cf. electroosmosis.

elec·tro·en·ceph·a·lo·gram (EEG) (ē-lek'trō-en-sef'ă-lō-gram). Eletroencefalograma; o registro obtido por meio do eletroencefalógrafo.

  flat e., e. isoelétrico. SIN electrocerebral silence.

  isoelectric e., e. isoelétrico. SIN electrocerebral silence.

elec·tro·en·ceph·a·lo·graph (ē-lek'trō-en-sef'ă-lō-graf). Eletroencefalógrafo; sistema para registro dos potenciais elétricos cerebrais derivados de eletrodos fixados ao couro cabeludo. [electro- + G. *encephalon*, encéfalo, + *graphō*, escrever]

elec·tro·en·ceph·a·log·ra·phy (EEG) (ēlek'trō-en-sef'ă-log'ră-fē). Eletroencefalografia; registro dos potenciais elétricos captados por um eletroencefalógrafo.

elec·tro·en·dos·mo·sis (ē-lek'trō-en-dos-mō'sis). Eletroendosmose; endosmose produzida por meio de um campo elétrico.

elec·tro·focus·ing (ē-lek'trō-fō-kus-ing). Eletrofocalização; o processo de separar macromoléculas ou pequenas moléculas através de eletroforese em um gradiente de pH.

elec·tro·gas·tro·gram (ē-lek'trō-gas'trō-gram). Eletrogastrograma; o registro obtido com o eletrogastrógrafo.

elec·tro·gas·tro·graph (ē-lek'trō-gas'trō-graf). Eletrogastrógrafo; instrumento usado em eletrogastrografia. [electro- + G. *gastēr*, estômago, + *graphō*, escrever]

elec·tro·gas·trog·ra·phy (ē-lek'trō-gas-trog'ră-fē). Eletrogastrografia; o registro dos fenômenos elétricos associados à secreção e motilidade gástrica.

elec·tro·gram (ē-lek'trō-gram). Eletrograma. **1.** Qualquer registro em papel ou filme feito por um evento elétrico. **2.** Em eletrofisiologia, um registro feito diretamente da superfície por derivações unipolares ou bipolares.

  His bundle e. (HBE), e. do feixe de His; eletrograma registrado no feixe de His, seja em animal experimental ou em seres humanos durante cateterismo cardíaco eletrofisiológico.

elec·tro·he·mo·sta·sis (ē-lek'trō-hē-mos'tă-sis, -hē-mō-stā'sis). Eletroemostasia; interrupção da hemorragia por meio de um eletrocautério. [electro- + G. *haima*, sangue, + *stasis*, impedir]

elec·tro·hys·ter·o·graph (ē-lek'trō-his'ter-ō-graf). Eletroisterógrafo; instrumento que registra a atividade elétrica uterina. [electro- + G. *hystera*, útero, + *graphō*, escrever]

elec·tro·im·mu·no·dif·fu·sion (ē-lek'trō-im'ū-nō-di-fū'zhŭn). Eletroimunodifusão; método imunoquímico que combina separação eletroforética com imunodifusão por incorporação de anticorpo ao meio de suporte.

elec·tro·ky·mo·gram (EKY) (ē-lek-trō-kī'mō-gram). Eletroquimograma; técnica obsoleta para fazer um registro gráfico dos movimentos cardíacos produzidos pelo eletroquimógrafo.

elec·tro·ky·mo·graph (ē-lek-trō-kī'mō-graf). Eletroquimógrafo; aparelho obsoleto para registrar, a partir de alterações na silhueta cardíaca, os movimentos do coração e dos grandes vasos; consiste em um fluoroscópio, um tubo de raios X e um tubo fotomultiplicador juntamente com um eletrocardiógrafo.

elec·trol·y·sis (ē-lek-trol'i-sis). Eletrólise. **1.** Decomposição de um sal ou de outra substância química por meio de uma corrente elétrica. **2.** Destruição dos folículos pilosos por meio de eletricidade galvânica. [electro- + G. *lysis*, dissolução]

elec·tro·lyte (ē-lek'trō-līt). Eletrólito. **1.** Qualquer substância que, em solu-

eletroencefalograma

| tipo de onda | forma | freqüência por segundo | amplitude em µV | variações fisiológicas do potencial |||
| | | | | no EEG em vigília || no EEG durante o sono |
				adulto	criança	todas as idades
beta	～	14–30	5–50	proeminente frontal e pré-central, em grupos	raramente proeminente	beta-atividade ("fusos") sinal de sono leve
alfa	WWW	8–13	20–120	atividade predominante	atividade predominante, a partir de 5 anos	não é um sinal de sono
teta	ww	4–7	20–100	constante, não-proeminente	atividade predominante, de 18 meses a 5 anos	sinal normal de sono
delta	∪∪	0,5–3	5–250	não-proeminente	atividade predominante até 18 meses	sinal concomitante de sono profundo
gama	—	31–60	–10	leis que determinam o predomínio e a localização não são completamente conhecidas		

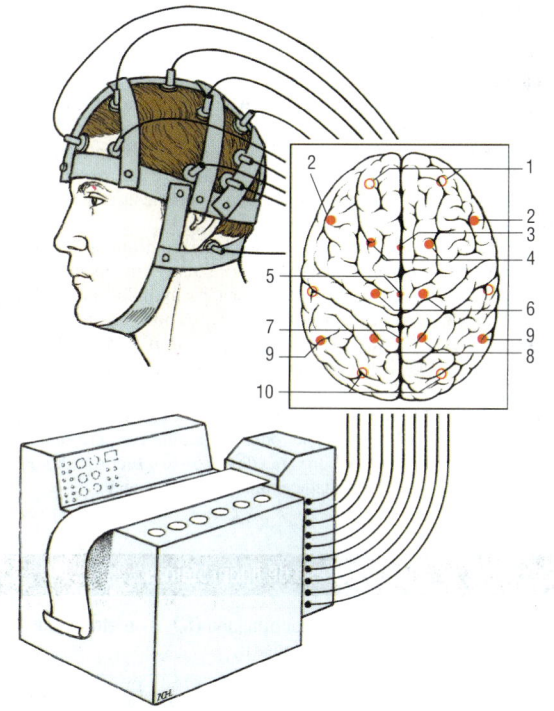

eletroencefalografia: o detalhe mostra as derivações usadas, (1) frontal, (2) temporal (frontel), (3) bregma, (4) pré-central, (5) vértice, (6) central, (7) lambda, (8) parietal, (9) temporal (posterior), (10) occipital

ção ou na forma liquefeita, conduz eletricidade e é decomposta (eletrolisada) por ela. **2.** Uma substância ionizável em solução. [electro- + G. *lytos*, solúvel]
amphoteric e., e. anfotérico; e. que pode dar ou receber um íon hidrogênio e, assim, comportar-se como ácido ou como base. SIN ampholyte.
elec·tro·lyt·ic (ē-lek-trō-lit′ik). Eletrolítico; que se refere a, ou é causado por, eletrólise.
elec·tro·lyze (ē-lek′trō-līz). Eletrolisar; decompor quimicamente por meio de uma corrente elétrica.
elec·tro·lyz·er (ē-lek′trō-līz-er). Eletrolisador; aparelho obsoleto para o tratamento de estenoses, fibromas, etc., por eletrólise.
elec·tro·mag·net (ē-lek-trō-mag′net). Eletromagneto; eletroímã; barra de ferro maleável tornada magnética por uma corrente elétrica ao seu redor.

elec·tro·mas·sage (ē-lek′trō-mas-sazh′). Eletromassagem; massagem combinada à aplicação de eletricidade.
elec·tro·mic·tu·ra·tion (ē-lek′trō-mik-too-rā′shŭn). Eletromicção; estimulação elétrica do cone medular para esvaziar a bexiga de paraplégicos. [electro- + L. *micturio*, micção]
e·lec·tro·morph (ē-lek′trō-mōrf). Eletromorfo; forma mutante de uma proteína, fenotipicamente distinta por sua mobilidade eletroforética. [electro- + G. *morphē*, forma, formato]
elec·tro·mo·til·i·ty (ē-lek′trō-mō-til′i-tē). Eletromotilidade; a motilidade das células pilosas externas auditivas em resposta à estimulação elétrica.
elec·tro·my·o·gram (EMG) (ē-lek-trō-mī′ō-gram). Eletromiograma (EMG); representação gráfica das correntes elétricas associadas à ação muscular.
elec·tro·my·o·graph (ē-lek-trō-mī′ō-graf). Eletromiógrafo; instrumento para registro de correntes elétricas geradas em um músculo ativo.
elec·tro·my·og·ra·phy (ē-lek′trō-mī-og′rǎ-fē). Eletromiografia (EMG). **1.** O registro de atividade elétrica gerada no músculo para fins diagnósticos; podem ser usados eletrodos de registro de superfície e com agulha, embora se costume empregar este último, de forma que o procedimento também é denominado exame por eletrodo em agulha. **2.** Termo que compreende todo estudo eletrodiagnóstico realizado no laboratório de EMG, incluindo não apenas o exame com eletrodo em agulha, mas também os estudos de condução nervosa. [electro- + G. *mys*, músculo, + *graphō*, escrever]
  evoked e., e. evocada. SIN electrodiagnosis.
elec·tron (β-) (ē-lek′tron). Elétron; uma das partículas subatômicas com carga elétrica negativa situada na órbita do núcleo positivo, em um dos vários níveis de energia denominados camadas; estima-se que possua 1/1836,15 da massa de um próton; quando emitido do interior do núcleo de uma substância radioativa, o elétron é denominado partícula β. Um núcleo e seus elétrons constituem um átomo. VER TAMBÉM shell. [electro- + -on]
  Auger e., e. de Auger; elétron expulso de uma órbita por interação fotoelétrica com um fóton emitido quando outro elétron, em uma órbita de maior energia, passa de um nível de energia maior para um menor; o elétron de Auger recua com energia igual à radiação característica menos a diferença nas energias de ligação da camada. VER photoelectric *effect*, transition e.
  conversion e., e. de conversão; um elétron de conversão interna.
  emission e., e. de emissão; uma partícula beta resultante de decaimento radioativo.
  internal conversion e., e. de conversão interna; um elétron semelhante a um elétron de Auger, liberado de uma das órbitas do átomo quando ativado por um raio gama do núcleo desse átomo; o elétron possui energia cinética igual à transição de energia final da desintegração.
  positive e., e. positivo. SIN positron.
  transition e., e. de transição; um elétron que passa de um nível de energia para outro para ocupar uma vaga em uma camada, com a emissão de radiação característica.
  valence e., e. de valência; um dos elétrons que tomam parte em reações químicas de um átomo.

elec·tro·nar·co·sis (ē-lek'trō-nar-kō'sis). Eletronarcose; produção de insensibilidade à dor pelo uso de corrente elétrica.

elec·tro·neg·a·tive (ē-lek-trō-neg'a-tiv). Eletronegativo. **1.** Relativo a, ou carregado com, eletricidade negativa. **2.** Referente a um elemento cujos átomos não-carregados tendem a ionizar por adição de elétrons, tornando-se assim ânions (p. ex., oxigênio, flúor, cloro).

elec·tro·neu·rog·ra·phy (ē-lek'trō-noo-rog'ra-fē). Eletroneurografia. SIN electrodiagnosis (2).

elec·tro·neu·rol·y·sis (ē-lek'trō-noo-rol'i-sis). Eletroneurólise; destruição do tecido nervoso por eletricidade.

elec·tro·neu·ro·my·og·ra·phy (ē-lek'trō-noor'ō-mī-og'ra-fē). Eletroneuromiografia. SIN electrodiagnosis (2).

elec·tron·ic (ē-lek-tron'ik). Eletrônico. **1.** Relativo a elétrons. **2.** Designa dispositivos ou sistemas que utilizam o fluxo de elétrons em um vácuo, gás ou semicondutor.

elec·tron-volt (eV, ev). Elétron-volt; a energia conferida a um elétron por um potencial de 1 V; igual a $1,60218 \times 10^{-12}$ erg no sistema CGS, ou $1,60218 \times 10^{-19}$ J no sistema SI.

elec·tro·nys·tag·mog·ra·phy (ENG) (ē-lek'trō-nis'tag-mog'ra-fē). Eletronistagmografia (ENG); método de nistagmografia baseado em eletrooculografia; são colocados eletrodos cutâneos nos cantos externos, para registrar nistagmo horizontal, ou acima e abaixo de cada olho para nistagmo vertical. [electro- + nystagmus + G. *graphō*, escrever]

elec·tro·oc·u·lo·gram (ē-lek'trō-ok'ū-lō-gram). Eletrooculograma; registro de correntes elétricas em eletrooculografia.

elec·tro·oc·u·log·ra·phy (EOG) (ē-lek'trō-ok'ū-log'ra-fē). Eletrooculografia; oculografia na qual eletrodos colocados sobre a pele adjacente aos olhos medem alterações no potencial de repouso entre a parte anterior e a parte posterior do globo ocular quando os olhos se movem; um teste elétrico sensível para detecção de disfunção do epitélio pigmentar da retina.

elec·tro·ol·fac·to·gram (EOG) (ē-lek'trō-ol-fak'tō-gram). Eletroolfatograma; onda eletronegativa de potencial que ocorre na superfície do epitélio olfatório em resposta à estimulação por um odor. SIN osmogram, Ottoson potential.

elec·tro·os·mo·sis (ē-lek'trō-os-mō'sis). Eletroosmose; a difusão de uma substância através de uma membrana em um campo elétrico. Cf. electrodialysis.

elec·tro·para·cen·te·sis (ē-lek'tro-par'a-sen-tē'sis). Eletroparacentese; retirada de líquido, como do olho, com um instrumento ativado eletricamente.

elec·tro·pher·o·gram (ē-lek-trō-fer'ō-gram). Eletroferograma; o padrão densitométrico ou colorimétrico obtido em papel de filtro ou em fitas porosas semelhantes sobre as quais as substâncias foram separadas por eletroforese; também pode referir-se às próprias fitas. SIN electrophoretogram, ionogram, ionopherogram.

elec·tro·phil, elec·tro·phile (ē-lek'trō-fil, -fil). Eletrófilo. **1.** O átomo ou agente que atrai elétron em uma reação orgânica. Cf. nucleophil. **2.** Relativo a um eletrófilo. SIN electrophilic. [electro- + G. *philos*, que tem afinidade]

elec·tro·phil·ic (ē-lek-trō-fil'ik). Eletrofílico. SIN electrophil (2).

elec·tro·pho·bia (ē-lek-trō-fō'bē-a). Eletrofobia; medo mórbido de eletricidade. [electro- + G. *phobos*, medo]

elec·tro·pho·re·sis (ē-lek-trō-fōr'ē-sis). Eletroforese; o movimento de partículas em um campo elétrico em direção a um pólo elétrico (anodo ou catodo); usado para separar e purificar biomoléculas. VER TAMBÉM electropherogram. SIN dielectrolysis, ionophoresis, phoresis (1). [electro- + G. *phorēsis*, que conduz]

capillary zone e. (CZE), e. de zona capilar; método para separar moléculas de forma extremamente rápida com base em sua mobilidade eletroforética.

carrier e., e. em suporte; eletroforese realizada sobre um suporte (como papel, gel de poliacrilamida, etc.).

disk e., e. em disco; modificação da eletroforese em gel na qual é introduzida uma descontinuidade (pH, tamanho do poro do gel) próximo à origem para produzir uma lâmina (disco) dos materiais separados; as faixas de separação preservam seu formato discóide enquanto atravessam o gel.

free e., e. livre; eletroforese de substâncias colocadas em uma solução em tubo em forma de U.

gel e., e. em gel; eletroforese através de um gel, geralmente um tubo cilíndrico ou sobre uma placa que consiste em um gel de composição uniforme.

isoenzyme e., e. de isoenzimas; separação eletroforética de enzimas séricas; a separação da desidrogenase láctica e creatinofosfocinase é comumente usada para diagnóstico de infarto agudo do miocárdio.

lipoprotein e., e. de lipoproteínas; separação eletroforética das lipoproteínas plasmáticas.

polyacrylamide gel e. (PAGE), e. em gel de poliacrilamida; gel formado por ligação cruzada da acrilamida, usada para a separação de proteínas ou de ácidos nucleicos. Essas substâncias são separadas com base no tamanho e na carga elétrica.

pulsed-field gel e., e. em gel de campo pulsado. SIN pulse-field gel e.

pulse-field gel e., e. em gel de campo pulsado; eletroforese em gel na qual, após o início da migração eletroforética, a corrente é brevemente interrompida e reaplicada em uma orientação diferente; permite a purificação de longas moléculas de DNA. SIN pulsed-field gel e.

thin-layer e. (TLE), e. em camada fina; migrações eletroforéticas (separações) através de uma camada fina de material inerte, como celulose, sobre uma lâmina de vidro ou plástico.

elec·tro·pho·ret·ic (ē-lek'trō-phōr-et'ik). Eletroforético; relativo à eletroforese, como uma separação eletroforética. SIN ionphoretic.

elec·tro·pho·ret·o·gram (ē-lek'trō-fōr-et'ō-gram). Eletroforetograma; eletroferograma. SIN electropherogram.

elec·tro·phren·ic (ē-lek'trō-fren'ik). Eletrofrênico; designa estimulação elétrica do nervo frênico geralmente em seu ponto motor no pescoço. VER TAMBÉM electrophrenic *respiration*.

elec·tro·phys·i·ol·o·gy (ē-lek'trō-fiz-ē-ol'ō-jē). Eletrofisiologia; o ramo da ciência relacionado aos fenômenos elétricos que estão associados a processos fisiológicos. Os fenômenos elétricos são proeminentes em neurônios e efetores.

elec·tro·por·a·tion (ē-lek'trō-pōr-ā-shŭn). Eletroporação; técnica pela qual se aplica um breve choque elétrico às células; orifícios momentâneos se abrem brevemente na membrana plasmática, permitindo a entrada de macromoléculas (p. ex., uma forma de introduzir DNA novo em uma célula).

elec·tro·pos·i·tive (ē-lek-trō-pos'i-tiv). Eletropositivo. **1.** Relativo a, ou carregado com, eletricidade positiva. **2.** Referente a um elemento cujos átomos tendem a perder elétrons; p. ex., sódio, potássio, cálcio.

elec·tro·punc·ture (ē-lek-trō-pŭnk'choor). Eletropunção; passagem de uma corrente elétrica através de eletrodos em agulha que perfuram os tecidos.

elec·tro·ra·di·ol·o·gy (ē-lek'trō-rā-dē-ol'ō-jē). Eletrorradiologia; termo obsoleto para o uso de eletricidade e raios X no tratamento.

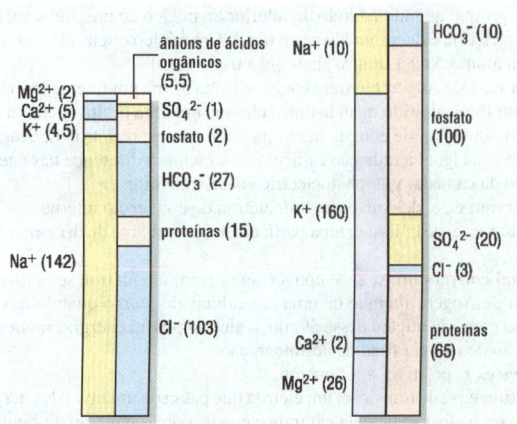

eletroferograma: do plasma sanguíneo (esquerda) e do líquido intracelular (direita); os níveis de concentração iônica são apresentados entre parênteses (em mmol/l)

S_f	D	ultracentrifugado (S_f) densidade (D)	eletroforese
$-4 - 10^4$	$-0,94$	① quilomícrons	
-400	$-0,98$	VLDL (lipoproteínas de densidade muito baixa)	② pré-β-lipoproteínas
-20	$-1,006$	LDL (lipoproteínas de baixa densidade)	③ β-lipoproteínas
-0	$-1,063$ $-1,210$	HDL (lipoproteínas de alta densidade)	④ α-lipoproteínas

eletroforese de lipoproteínas

grupos de lipoproteínas no sangue normal; beta e pré-beta lipoproteínas são invertidas na separação eletroforética (S_f = unidade Svedberg = unidade de flotação)

elec·tro·ra·di·om·e·ter (ē-lek′trō-rā-dē-om′e-ter). Eletrorradiômetro; eletroscópio modificado designado para a diferenciação da energia radiante. [electro- + L. *radius*, raio, + G. *metron*, medida]

elec·tro·ret·i·no·gram (ERG) (ē-lek′trō-ret′i-nō-gram). Eletrorretinograma; registro das correntes de ação retinianas produzidas na retina por um estímulo luminoso adequado. [electro- + retina + G. *gramma*, algo escrito]

elec·tro·ret·i·nog·ra·phy (ē-lek′trō-ret′i-nog′ra-fē). Eletrorretinografia; o registro e o estudo das correntes de ação retinianas.

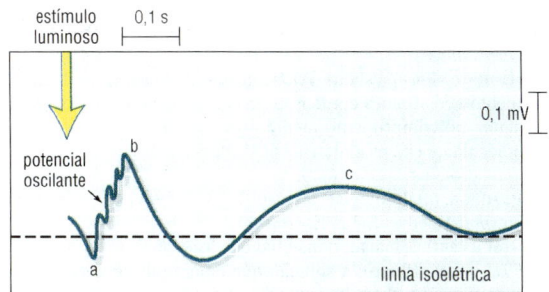

eletrorretinografia: eletrorretinograma com ondas a, b e c

elec·tro·scis·sion (ē-lek′trō-si-shŭn). Eletrocisão; divisão de tecidos por meio de um bisturi eletrocautério. [electro- + L. *scissio*, divisão, de *scindo*, dividir]

elec·tro·scope (ē-lek′trō-skōp). Eletroscópio; instrumento para a detecção de cargas elétricas ou ionização de gás por raios β ou raios X; consiste em duas tiras de folha de ouro, suspensas de um condutor isolado e encerradas em um recipiente hermeticamente fechado, vistas com um microscópio de pequeno aumento. [electro- + G. *skopeō*, examinar]

elec·tro·shock (ē-lek′trō-shok). Eletrochoque. VER electroshock *therapy*.

elec·tro·sol (ē-lek′trō-sol). Metal coloidal. SIN colloidal metal.

elec·tro·spec·trog·ra·phy (ē-lek′trō-spek-trog′ra-fē). Eletroespectrografia; o registro, o estudo e a interpretação de padrões de onda eletroencefalográficos.

elec·tro·spi·no·gram (ē-lek-trō-spī′nō-gram). Eletroespinograma; o registro obtido por eletroespinografia.

elec·tro·spi·nog·ra·phy (ē-lek′trō-spī-nog′ra-fē). Eletroespinografia; o registro de atividade elétrica espontânea da medula espinal.

elec·tro·ste·nol·y·sis (ē-lek′trō-stē-nol′i-sis). Eletroestenólise; a precipitação de metais nos poros das membranas no decorrer da eletrólise.

elec·tro·steth·o·graph (ē-lek′trō-steth′ō-graf). Eletroestetógrafo; instrumento que amplifica ou registra os sons respiratórios e cardíacos do tórax. [electro- + G. *stēthos*, tórax, + *graphō*, registrar]

elec·tro·stric·tion (ē-lek-trō-strik′shŭn). Eletrostrição. 1. A contração no volume em uma solução proteica durante a proteólise devido à formação de novos grupos com carga elétrica. 2. A alteração reversível nas dimensões de uma substância ou material quando um campo elétrico é aplicado a ele.

elec·tro·sur·gery (ē-lek-trō-ser′jer-ē). Eletrocirurgia; divisão de tecidos por corrente de alta freqüência aplicada localmente com um instrumento metálico ou agulha. VER TAMBÉM electrocautery. SIN electrotomy.

elec·tro·tax·is (ē-lek-trō-tak′sis). Eletrotaxia; reação de protoplasma vegetal ou animal a um anodo ou catodo. VER TAMBÉM tropism. SIN electrotropism, galvanotaxis, galvanotropism. [electro- + G. *taxis*, disposto de forma ordenada]

   negative e., e. negativa; eletrotaxia pela qual um organismo é atraído em direção a um anodo ou repelido de um catodo.

   positive e., e. positiva; eletrotaxia pela qual um organismo é atraído em direção a um catodo ou repelido de um anodo.

elec·tro·tha·na·sia (ē-lek′trō-thā-nā′zē-ā). Eletrotanásia. SIN electrocution. [electro- + G. *thanatos*, morte]

elec·tro·ther·a·peu·tics, elec·tro·ther·a·py (ē-lek′trō-thar-ā-pū′tiks, -thar′a-pē). Eletroterapêutica, eletroterapia; uso da eletricidade no tratamento de doenças.

elec·tro·therm (ē-lek′trō-therm). Eletrotermo; folha flexível de bobinas de resistência usadas para aplicação de calor à superfície do corpo. [electro- + G. *thermē*, calor]

elec·tro·tome (ē-lek′trō-tōm). Eletrótomo; bisturi elétrico.

elec·tro·tomy (ē-lek-trot′ō-mē). Eletrotomia. SIN electrosurgery. [electro- + G. *tomē*, incisão]

elec·tro·ton·ic (ē-lek-trō-ton′ik). Eletrotônico; relativo a eletrotônus.

elec·trot·o·nus (ē-lek-trot′ō-nŭs). Eletrotônus; alterações na excitabilidade e condutividade em uma célula nervosa ou muscular causadas pela passagem de uma corrente elétrica constante. VER TAMBÉM catelectrotonus, anelectrotonus. SIN galvanotonus (1). [electro- + G. *tonos*, tensão]

elec·trot·ro·pism (ē-lek-trot′rō-pizm, ē-lek-trō-trō′pizm). Eletrotropismo. SIN electrotaxis. [electro- + G. *tropē*, mudança]

elec·tu·ar·y (ē-lek′choo-ā-rē). Eletuário. SIN confection. [G. *eleikton*, medicamento que derrete na boca, de *ekleichō*, lamber]

el·e·doi·sin (el-ē-doy′sin). Eledoisina; toxina undecapeptídica formada na glândula de veneno de cefalópodes do gênero *Eledone* e causa vasodilatação e contração do músculo liso extravascular.

ele·i·din (ē-lē′i-din). Eleidina; queratina refrativa e que se cora fracamente presente nas células do estrato lúcido na epiderme palmar e plantar.

el·e·ment (el′e-ment). Elemento. 1. Uma substância composta de átomos de apenas um tipo, isto é, de número atômico (protônico) idêntico, que, portanto, não podem ser decompostos em dois ou mais elementos e que podem perder suas propriedades químicas apenas por união com algum outro elemento ou por uma reação nuclear que modifica o número de prótons. 2. Uma estrutura ou entidade indivisível. 3. Uma entidade funcional, freqüentemente exógena, dentro de uma bactéria, como um elemento extracromossomial [L. *elementum*, um rudimento, início]

   actinide e.'s, elementos actínicos. SIN actinides.

   alkaline earth e.'s, elementos alcalino-terrosos; aqueles elementos da família Be, Mg, Ca, Sr, Ba e Ra cujos hidróxidos são extremamente ionizados e, portanto, alcalinos em solução aquosa.

   amphoteric e., e. anfotérico; um ou mais elementos cujos óxidos se unem com a água para formar hidróxidos que podem agir como ácidos ou bases (p. ex., alumínio).

   anatomical e., e. anatômico; qualquer unidade anatômica, como uma célula. SIN morphologic e.

   copia e.'s, elementos de cópia; um elemento genético móvel com organização de seqüência semelhante à de um retrovírus.

   electronegative e., e. eletronegativo; elemento cujos átomos possuem uma tendência a aceitar elétrons e formar íons negativos (p. ex., oxigênio, enxofre, cloro).

   electropositive e., e. eletropositivo; elemento cujos átomos possuem uma tendência a perder elétrons e formar íons positivos (p. ex., sódio).

   extrachromosomal e., extrachromosomal genetic e., e. extracromossomial, e. genético extracromossomial. SIN plasmid.

   fold-back e.'s, tipo de e. transponível que possui longas repetições invertidas, de forma que, quando é desnaturado, são formadas alças.

   labile e.'s, e. lábeis; células teciduais, como as do epitélio, tecido conjuntivo, etc., que continuam a multiplicar-se por mitose durante a vida do indivíduo.

   long interspersed e.'s (LINES), e. longos e dispersos; seqüências repetitivas longas no DNA com repetições terminais observadas no DNA dos seres humanos e camundongos.

   morphologic e., e. morfológico. SIN anatomical e.

   neutral e., e. neutro; e. do grupo zero da tabela periódica que compreende os gases nobres: He, Ne, Ar, Kr, Xe, Rn.

   noble e., e. nobre. SIN noble metal.

   P e.'s, e. P; uma classe de e. transponíveis na *Drosophila* responsáveis pela disgenesia híbrida; utilizados como ferramentas para introduzir genes em novas localizações no genoma.

   picture e., e. de imagem. VER pixel.

   rare earth e.'s, e. terras-raras. SIN lanthanides.

   short interspersed e.'s (SINES), elementos curtos e dispersos; seqüências extremamente repetitivas de DNA com cerca de 300 pares de bases de comprimento que ocorrem aproximadamente a cada 3.000–5.000 pares de bases (pb) no genoma.

   trace e.'s, oligoelementos; e. presentes em quantidades mínimas no corpo, muitas das quais são essenciais no metabolismo ou para a fabricação de compostos essenciais; p. ex., Zn, Se, V, Ni, Mg, Mn. SIN microelements, microminerals.

   transposable e., e. transponível; seqüência de DNA que pode mudar de posição no genoma; o evento de transposição pode envolver tanto recombinação quanto replicação, produzindo duas cópias do pedaço móvel de DNA; a inserção desses fragmentos de DNA pode romper a integridade do gene-alvo, possivelmente causando ativação de genes latentes, deleções, inversões e várias aberrações cromossomiais. VER TAMBÉM transposon.

   volume e., e. de volume. VER voxel.

eleo-. Óleo. VER TAMBÉM oleo-. [G. *elaion*, azeite de oliva]

el·e·o·ma (el-ē-ō′mä). Eleoma. SIN lipogranuloma. [G. *elaion*, óleo, + *-oma*, tumor]

el·e·om·e·ter (el-ē-om′e-ter). Eleômetro. SIN oleometer. [G. *elaion*, óleo, + *metron*, medida]

el·e·op·a·thy (el-ē-op′a-thē). Eleopatia; condição rara na qual há edema mole das articulações, atribuída ao depósito adiposo após uma contusão; ou, possivelmente, uma condição resultante da injeção de óleo de parafina como forma de simulação de doença. SIN elaiopathia.

el·e·o·stear·ic ac·id (el-ē-ō-stē′a-rik, -stēr′ik). Ácido eleosteárico; um ácido graxo de 18 carbonos com três ligações duplas (nos carbonos 9, 11 e 13); isomérico com o ácido linolênico; encontrado em gorduras vegetais.

el·e·o·ther·a·py (el - ē - ō - thār′a - pē). Oleoterapia. SIN oleotherapy. [G. *elaion*, óleo]

el·e·phan·ti·a·sis (el - ē - fan - tī′a - sis). Elefantíase; hipertrofia, edema e fibrose da pele e do tecido subcutâneo, principalmente dos membros inferiores e da genitália associada a hidrocele, ou aumento de um membro, geralmente causado por obstrução crônica dos vasos linfáticos, na maioria das vezes resultante de anos de infecção pela filária *Wuchereria bancrofti* ou *Brugia malayi*. VER TAMBÉM filariasis. SIN elephant leg. [G. de *elephas*, elefante]
  congenital e., e. congênita; aumento congênito de um ou mais membros ou de outras partes devido à dilatação dos linfáticos. VER TAMBÉM entradas em hereditary *lymphedema*, congenital type.
  gingival e., e. gengival; hiperplasia fibrosa da gengiva.
  e. neuromato′sa, e. neuromatosa; aumento de um membro devido à neurofibromatose difusa da pele e do tecido subcutâneo.
  e. scro′ti, e. do escroto; edema castanho do escroto em virtude de obstrução linfática crônica. SIN lymph scrotum, parasitic chylocele.
  e. telangiecto′des, e. telangiectóide; hipertrofia da pele e dos tecidos subcutâneos acompanhada por, e dependente de, dilatação dos vasos sanguíneos.
  e. vul′vae, e. da vulva. SIN chronic hypertrophic *vulvitis*.

el·e·va·tion (el - ē - vā′shŭn) [TA]. Toro, protuberância. SIN torus (1).
  e. of levator palati, t. do levantador. SIN *torus* levatorius.
  tactile e.'s [TA], tórulos tácteis; pequenas áreas na pele das regiões palmares e plantares, especialmente ricas em terminações nervosas sensoriais. SIN toruli tactiles [TA].

el·e·va·tor (el′ē - vā - tĕr). Elevador. **1.** Instrumento para erguer uma parte afundada, como o fragmento afundado de osso na fratura do crânio, ou para elevação de tecidos de sua fixação ao osso. **2.** Alavanca para raiz; elevador para raiz; instrumento cirúrgico usado para luxar e remover dentes e raízes que não podem ser agarrados pelas pontas do fórceps, ou para afrouxar dentes e raízes antes da aplicação do fórceps. SIN dental lever. [L. de *e-levo*, pp. *-atus*, levantar]
  periosteal e., rugina; um instrumento usado para separar o periósteo do osso. SIN rugine (1).
  screw e., e. de rosca; instrumento dentário com extremidade afilada utilizado para extrair a raiz de um dente quebrado.

elim·i·nant (ē - lim′i - nant). Evacuante. **1.** Um evacuante que promove a excreção ou a remoção de detritos. **2.** Um agente que aumenta a excreção.

elim·i·na·tion (ē - lim - i - nā′shŭn). Eliminação; expulsão; remoção de resíduos do corpo; livrar-se de qualquer coisa. [L. *elimino*, pp. *-atus*, esvaziar, de *limen*, limiar]
  carbon dioxide e. (VCO_2), e. de dióxido de carbono; a velocidade de passagem do dióxido de carbono do sangue para o gás alveolar, que, no estado de equilíbrio dinâmico, é igual à produção metabólica de dióxido de carbono pelo metabolismo tecidual em todo o corpo; unidades: ml/min nas CNTP (condições normais de temperatura e pressão) ou mmol/min.

elin·gua·tion (ē - ling - gwā′shŭn). Elinguação. SIN glossectomy. [L. *e*, fora, + *lingua*, língua]

el·i·nin (el′i - nin). Elinina; fração lipoproteica de hemácias que contém os fatores Rh e A e B.

ELISA Abreviatura de enzyme-linked immunosorbent *assay* (ensaio imunossorvente ligado a enzima).

elix·ir (ē - lik′sĕr). Elixir; líquido hidroalcoólico claro, adocicado, para uso oral; os elixires contêm substâncias flavorizantes e são usados como veículos ou para o efeito terapêutico dos agentes medicinais ativos. [L. med., do Árabe, *al-iksir*, a pedra filosofal]
  phenobarbital e., e. de fenobarbital; mistura hidroalcoólica (12–15% de álcool), colorida, de sabor agradável, que contém 20 mg de fenobarbital por 5 ml (uma colher de chá cheia); útil na administração do fenobarbital a crianças ou a pessoas com dificuldade para engolir comprimidos; usado como anticonvulsivante e sedativo.

Ellik, Milo, urologista norte-americano, *1905. VER E. *evacuator*.
Elliot, John W., cirurgião norte-americano, 1852–1925. VER E. *position*.
Elliot, Robert Henry, oftalmologista inglês, 1864–1936. VER E. *operation*.
Elliott, Thomas R., médico inglês, 1877–1961. VER E. *law*.

el·lip·sis (ē - lip′sis). Elipse; omissão de palavras ou idéias, deixando o todo para ser completado pelo leitor ou ouvinte. [G. *ek-*, fora, + *leipsis*, que deixa]

el·lip·soid (ē - lip′soyd). Elipsóide. **1.** Condensação esférica ou fusiforme de macrófagos fagocíticos em um estroma reticular que reveste a parede dos capilares arteriais esplênicos pouco antes de liberarem seu sangue nos cordões da polpa vermelha. **2.** A extremidade externa do segmento interno dos bastonetes e cones da retina. **3.** Que possui o formato de uma elipse ou oval. SIN sheath of Schweigger-Seidel. [G. *ellips*, oval, + *eidos*, forma]

el·lip·to·cy·to·sis (ē - lip′tō - si - tō′sis). Eliptocitose; distúrbio hematológico no qual 50–90% das hemácias têm a forma de bacilos e eliptócitos; freqüentemente associada a uma anemia hemolítica. Há várias formas autossômicas dominantes [MIM*130500, MIM*130600 e MIM*179650], com uma forma ligada ao grupo sanguíneo Rh, causada por mutação no gene que codifica a banda de proteína da membrana eritrocitária 4.1 (EPB41) no cromossoma 1p, enquanto a forma não-ligada é devida à mutação no gene da alfa-espectrina em 1q, ou no gene da beta-espectrina em 14q, ou no gene da banda 3 em 17q. Há uma forma autossômica recessiva [MIM*225450] conhecida. SIN ovalocytosis.

Ellis, Richard W.B., médico inglês, 1902–1966. VER E.-van Creveld *syndrome*.
Ellison, Edwin H., médico norte-americano, 1918–1970. VER Zollinger-E. *syndrome, tumor*.
Ellsworth, Read McLane, médico norte-americano, 1899–1970. VER E.-Howard *test*.
Eloesser, Leo, cirurgião torácico norte-americano, 1881–1976. VER Eloesser *flap*; E. *procedure*.

elon·ga·tion (ē - lon - gā′shŭn). Alongamento. **1.** O aumento das medidas de comprimento após fratura em tensão no comprimento medido, expresso em percentagem do comprimento medido original. **2.** O alongamento de uma macromolécula; p. ex., na síntese de ácidos graxos de cadeia longa ou na síntese de uma proteína.

Elschnig, Anton, oftalmologista alemão, 1863–1939. VER E. *pearls*, em *pearl*, *spots*, em *spot*; Koerber-Salus-E. *syndrome*.

el·u·ant (el′ū - ant). Eluante; o material que foi eluído.

el·u·ate (el′ū - āt). Eluato; a solução que emerge de uma coluna ou papel cromatográfico. VER TAMBÉM elution.

el·u·ent (el′ū - ent). Eluente; a fase móvel da cromatografia. VER TAMBÉM elution. SIN developer (2), elutant.

elu·tant (ē - loo′tant). Eluente. SIN eluent.

elute (ē - loot′). Eluir; realizar uma eluição, fracionar. SIN elutriate.

elu·tion (ē - loo′shŭn). Eluição. **1.** A separação, por lavagem, de dois sólidos. **2.** A remoção, por meio de um solvente adequado, de um material de outro que é insolúvel naquele solvente, como na cromatografia em coluna. **3.** A remoção de anticorpos absorvidos à superfície do eritrócito. SIN elutriation. [L. *e-luo*, pp. *lutus,* lavar]
  gradient e., e. por gradiente; eluição em cromatografia em coluna na qual se usa uma mudança de pH ou de concentração iônica para separar substâncias.

elu·tri·ate (ē - loo′trē - āt). Eluir. SIN elute.

elu·tri·a·tion (ē - loo - trē - ā′shŭn). Eluição. SIN elution. [L. *elutrio*, pp. *-atus*, lavar, decantar, de *e-luo*, lavar]

elytro-. A vagina. VER TAMBÉM colpo-, vagino-. [G. *elytron*, bainha (vagina)]
em-. VER en-.

EMA Abreviatura de epithelial membrane *antigen* (antígeno da membrana epitelial).

ema·ci·a·tion (ē - mā - sē - ā′shŭn). Emaciação; definhamento; tornar-se anormalmente magro por perda extrema de massa muscular e tecido adiposo. SIN wasting (1). [L. *e-macio*, pp. *-atus*, tornar magro]

emac·u·la·tion (ē - mak - ū - lā′shŭn). Retirada de manchas ou outras marcas da pele. [L. *emaculo*, pp. *-atus*, livrar de manchas, de *e-*, fora, + *macula*, mancha]

em·a·na·tion (em - ă - nā′shŭn). Emanação. **1.** Qualquer substância que se desprende ou é emitida de uma fonte ou origem; exalação. **2.** A radiação emitida por um elemento radioativo. [L. *e-mano*, pp. *-atus*, exalar]
  actinium e., e. de actínio; radônio-219. VER emanon.
  radium e., e. de rádio; radônio-222. VER emanon.
  thorium e., e. de tório; radônio-220. VER emanon.

em·a·na·to·ri·um (em′ă - nă - tōr′ē - ŭm). Emanatório; instituição onde, anteriormente, se administrava a radioterapia agora considerada perigosa (utilizando águas radioativas e a inalação de emanações de rádio).

eman·ci·pa·tion (ē - man - si - pā′shŭn). Emancipação; em embriologia, a delimitação de uma área específica em um campo formador de órgãos, dando formato definido e limites ao primórdio do órgão.

em·a·non (em′ă - non). Termo obsoleto usado antigamente para designar coletivamente todos os isótopos do radônio, quando o termo radônio era restrito ao isótopo radônio-222, o intermediário de ocorrência natural da série radioativa do urânio-238; assim denominado porque os nomes originais do radônio-219, radônio-220 e radônio-222 eram, respectivamente, "emanação de actínio", "emanação de tório" e "emanação de rádio". [L. *emano*, exalar, + *-on*]

em·a·no·ther·a·py (em′ă - nō - thār′ă - pē) Emanoterapia; tratamento obsoleto de várias doenças por meio da emanação de rádio (radônio) ou outra emanação.

emar·gi·nate (ē - mar′ji - nāt). Emarginado; entalhado; com margem denteada. SIN notched. [L. *emargino*, privar de sua borda, de *e-* priv. + *margo* (*margin-*), margem]

emar·gi·na·tion (ē - mar′ji - nā′shŭn). Emarginação, chanfradura. SIN notch.

emas·cu·la·tion (ē - mas - kū - lā′shŭn). Emasculação; castração do homem por retirada dos testículos e/ou pênis. SIN eviration (1). [L. *emasculo*, pp. *-atus*, castrar, de *e-* priv. + *masculus*, masculino]

EMB Abreviatura de eosin-methylene blue (eosina-azul de metileno). VER eosin-methylene blue *agar*.

Em·ba·dom·o·nas (em - bă - dom′ō - nas, em′bă - dō - mō′nas). Nome antigo de *Retortamonas*. [G. *embadon*, superfície, + *monas*, unidade, mônada]

em·balm (em‑bahlm′). Embalsamar; tratar um corpo morto com bálsamos ou outras substâncias químicas para evitar sua deterioração. [L. *in*, dentro de, + *balsamum*, bálsamo]

Embden, Gustav G., bioquímico alemão, 1874–1933. VER E. *ester*; Robison‑E. *ester*; E.‑Meyerhof *pathway*; E.‑Meyerhof‑Parnas *pathway*.

em·bed (em‑bed′). Incrustar; circundar uma amostra patológica ou histológica com uma substância de consistência firme e, algumas vezes, dura, como parafina, cera, celoidina ou uma resina, a fim de tornar possível fazer cortes finos para exame microscópico. SIN imbed.

em·be·lin (em′be‑lin). Embelina; o princípio ativo do fruto seco da *Embelia ribes* e *E. robusta* (família Myrsinaceae); tem sido usado como tenicida.

em·boite·ment (awm‑bwaht‑mawn′). Encaixamento. SIN preformation theory. [Fr., encaixamento]

em·bo·le (em′bō‑lē). **1.** Redução da luxação de um membro. SIN embolia. **2.** Formação da gástrula por invaginação da blástula. SIN emboly. [G. *embolē*, inserção]

em·bo·lec·to·my (em‑bō‑lek′tō‑mē). Embolectomia; remoção de um êmbolo. [G. *embolos*, um tampão (êmbolo) + *ektomē*, excisão]

em·bo·le·mia (em‑bō‑lē′mē‑ă). Embolemia; a presença de êmbolos no sangue circulante.

em·bo·li (em‑bō‑lī). Êmbolos; plural de embolus.

em·bo·lia (em‑bō′lē‑ă). Redução da luxação de um membro. SIN embole (1).

em·bol·ic (em‑bol′ik). Embólico; relativo a um êmbolo ou à embolia.

em·bol·i·form (em‑bol′i‑fōrm). Emboliforme; com o formato de um êmbolo. [G. *embolos*, tampão (êmbolo), + L. *forma*, forma]

em·bo·lism (em′bō‑lizm). Embolia; obstrução ou oclusão de um vaso por um êmbolo. [G. *embolisma*, pedaço ou fragmento; lit. algo introduzido]

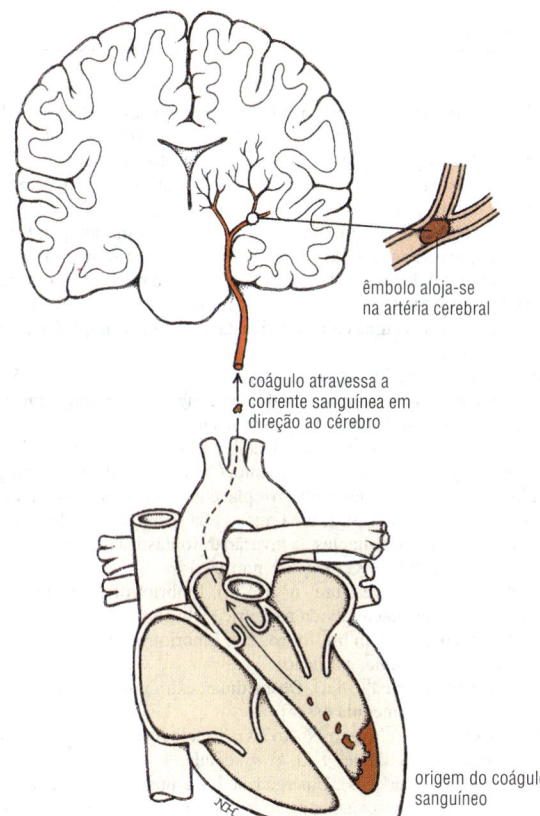
embolia

air e., e. gasosa; e. causada por bolhas de ar no sistema vascular; a e. gasosa venosa pode resultar da introdução de ar através de cateteres intravenosos, principalmente cateteres centrais, e geralmente tem de ser significativa para bloquear o fluxo sanguíneo pulmonar e causar sintomas; a e. gasosa arterial geralmente também é iatrogênica, causada por derivação (*bypass*) cardiopulmonar ou outras intervenções intravasculares, raramente após lesão pulmonar penetrante; um pequeno volume de ar arterial pode causar morte por bloqueio das artérias coronárias e/ou cerebrais; pequenas bolhas introduzidas no sistema venoso também podem causar sintomas se chegarem ao lado arterial. Cf. paradoxical e. SIN gas e.

amnionic fluid e., e. por líquido amniótico; obstrução e constrição dos vasos sanguíneos pulmonares por líquido amniótico que entra na circulação materna, causando choque obstétrico. VER TAMBÉM amnionic fluid *syndrome*.

atheromatous e., e. ateromatosa. SIN cholesterol e.

bland e., e. leve; e. por material não‑séptico simples.

bone marrow e., e. por medula óssea; obstrução de um vaso por medula óssea, geralmente após fratura de um osso.

cellular e., e. celular; e. decorrente de uma massa de células oriundas de um tecido em desintegração.

cholesterol e., e. de colesterol; e. por resíduos lipídicos de um depósito ateromatoso ulcerado, geralmente de uma grande artéria para pequenos ramos arteriais; geralmente é pequena e raramente causa infarto. SIN atheromatous e.

cotton-fiber e., e. por fibras de algodão; e. por fibras de algodão de gaze estéril usada na administração de medicação ou transfusão intravenosa; pode se formar como granulomas de corpo estranho em pequenas artérias pulmonares.

crossed e., e. cruzada. SIN paradoxical e.

direct e., e. direta; e. que ocorre na direção da corrente sanguínea.

fat e., e. gordurosa; a ocorrência de glóbulos de gordura na circulação após fraturas de um osso longo, em queimaduras, no parto e associados à degeneração gordurosa do fígado; na maioria das vezes, os êmbolos bloqueiam os vasos pulmonares ou cerebrais quando surgem sintomas referíveis a uma dessas regiões ou a ambas. SIN oil e.

gas e., e. gasosa. SIN air e.

hematogenous e., e. hematogênica; e. que ocorre através de um vaso sanguíneo.

infective e., e. infecciosa. SIN pyemic e.

lymph e., lymphogenous e., e. linfática, e. linfogênica; e. que ocorre em um vaso linfático.

miliary e., e. miliar; e. que ocorre simultaneamente em vários capilares. SIN multiple e. (1).

multiple e., e. múltipla; **(1)** E. miliar. SIN miliary e.; **(2)** embolia causada pela retenção de inúmeros pequenos êmbolos.

obturating e., e. obturadora; fechamento completo da luz de um vaso por êmbolos.

oil e., e. gordurosa. SIN fat e.

paradoxical e., e. paradoxal; **(1)** obstrução de uma artéria sistêmica por um êmbolo originado no sistema venoso que atravessa um defeito de septos cardíacos, persistência do forame oval ou outra derivação para o sistema arterial; **(2)** obstrução por um êmbolo minúsculo que atravessa os capilares pulmonares do sistema venoso para o arterial. SIN crossed e.

pulmonary e., e. pulmonar; embolia das artérias pulmonares, na maioria das vezes por fragmentos que se desprendem de trombos de uma veia da perna ou pélvica, comumente quando a trombose sucedeu uma cirurgia ou um período de confinamento ao leito.

pyemic e., e. piêmica; e. infecciosa; obstrução de uma artéria por um êmbolo que se solta de um foco de supuração. SIN infective e.

retinal e., e. retiniana; e. de uma artéria da retina.

retrograde e., e. retrógrada; e. de uma veia por um êmbolo transportado em uma direção oposta à da corrente sanguínea normal, após ter sido desviado para uma veia menor. SIN venous e.

riding e., e. por acavalgamento. SIN straddling e.

saddle e., e. em sela; uma e. por acavalgamento em qualquer bifurcação vascular, p. ex., e. da aorta que oclui as duas artérias ilíacas comuns.

straddling e., e. a cavaleiro; e. que ocorre na bifurcação de uma artéria e que bloqueia ambos os ramos de forma mais ou menos completa. SIN riding e.

tumor e., e. tumoral; e. por tecido neoplásico transportado a partir de um tumor e que pode crescer como uma metástase.

venous e., e. venosa. SIN retrograde e.

em·bo·li·za·tion (em′bol‑i‑zā′shŭn). Embolização. **1.** A formação e a liberação de um êmbolo para a circulação. **2.** Introdução terapêutica de várias substâncias na circulação para ocluir vasos, seja para interromper ou evitar hemorragia, para desvitalizar uma estrutura, tumor ou órgão por oclusão de seu suprimento sanguíneo, ou para reduzir o fluxo sanguíneo para uma malformação arteriovenosa.

em·bo·lo·my·cot·ic (em′bō‑lō‑mī‑kot′ik). Embolomicótico; relativo a, ou causado por, um êmbolo infeccioso. [G. *embolos*, êmbolo, + *mykēs*, fungo]

em·bo·lo·ther·a·py (em‑bō‑lō‑thăr′ă‑pē). Emboloterapia; oclusão de artérias por introdução de coágulos sanguíneos, esponja de gelatina absorvível (Gelfoam®), espirais, balões, etc., com um cateter angiográfico; usada para controlar hemorragia inoperável ou para tratamento pré‑operatório de neoplasias muito vascularizadas. [G. *embolos*, êmbolo, + *therapeia*, tratamento médico]

em·bo·lus, pl. **em·bo·li** (em′bō‑lŭs, ‑lī). **1.** Êmbolo; um tampão, composto de um trombo ou vegetação que se desprende, massa de bactérias ou outro corpo estranho, ocluindo um vaso. **2.** Núcleo emboliforme. SIN emboliform nucleus. [G. *embolos*, tampão, cunha ou rolha]

catheter e., e. por cateterismo; agregados de plaquetas e fibrinas espiralados em forma de vermes, produzidos durante cateterismo vascular, originando‑se no cateter ou em seu fio condutor; embolização do próprio cateter.

em·bo·ly (em'bō-lē). Formação da gástrula por invaginação da blástula. SIN embole (2).

em·bouche·ment (ahm-boosh-mon'). Embocadura; a abertura de um vaso sanguíneo para outro. [Fr.]

em·bra·sure (em-brā'shoor). Em odontologia, uma abertura que se alarga para fora ou para dentro; especificamente, o espaço adjacente à área de contato interproximal que se alarga em direção ao lado facial, gengival, lingual, oclusal ou incisal. [Fr. abertura em uma parede para canhão]
   buccal e., espaço existente no lado facial da área de contato interproximal entre dentes posteriores adjacentes.
   gingival e., espaço existente cervical à área de contato interproximal entre dentes adjacentes.
   incisal e., espaço existente na face incisal da área de contato interproximal entre dentes anteriores adjacentes.
   labial e., e. labial; espaço existente no lado facial da área de contato interproximal entre dentes anteriores adjacentes.
   lingual e., espaço existente na face lingual da área de contato interproximal entre dentes adjacentes.
   occlusal e., espaço existente na face oclusal das áreas de contato interproximais entre dentes posteriores adjacentes.

em·bro·ca·tion (em-brō-kā'shŭn). Embrocação; termo raramente usado para linimento ou para a aplicação de um linimento. [G. *embrochē*, fomentação]

embry-. VER embryo-.

em·bryo (em'brē-ō). Embrião. **1.** Organismo nos estágios iniciais do desenvolvimento. **2.** Em seres humanos, o organismo em desenvolvimento desde a concepção até, aproximadamente, o fim do segundo mês; os estágios do desenvolvimento desse período até o nascimento são comumente designados fetais. **3.** Uma planta primordial dentro de uma semente. [G. *embryo*, de *en*, em, + *bryō*, inchar]
   heterogametic e., e. heterogamético; embrião masculino com cariótipo XY.
   hexacanth e., e. hexacântico; o embrião das tênias da subclasse Cestoda, como a *Taenia saginata*, caracterizado por três pares de ganchos usados para penetração através do intestino de um hospedeiro intermediário. SIN oncosphere e.
   homogametic e., e. homogamético; embrião feminino com cariótipo XX.
   oncosphere e., e. oncosférico. SIN hexacanth e.
   presomite e., e. pré-somítico; embrião antes do surgimento do primeiro par de somitos, que são evidentes cerca de 20–21 dias após a fertilização em seres humanos.
   previllous e., e. pré-vilosidade; o embrião de um mamífero placentário antes da formação de vilosidades coriônicas.

embryo-, embry-. Embrio, embri-; o embrião. [G. *embryon*, embrião]
   em·bry·o·blast (em'brē-ō-blast). Embrioblasto. SIN inner cell mass. [embryo- + G. *blastos*, germe]
   em·bry·o·car·dia (em'brē-ō-kar'dē-ă). Embriocardia; condição na qual a cadência dos sons cardíacos se assemelha à do feto, com a primeira e a segunda bulhas semelhantes e uniformemente espaçadas; um sinal de doença miocárdica grave. SIN pendulum rhythm, tic-tac rhythm, tic-tac sounds. [embryo- + G. *kardia*, coração]
   em·bry·o·gen·e·sis (em'brē-ō-jen'ĕ-sis). Embriogênese; fase do desenvolvimento pré-natal envolvida no estabelecimento da configuração característica do corpo embrionário; em seres humanos, a embriogênese geralmente é considerada como se estendendo do final da segunda semana, quando o disco embrionário é formado, ao fim da oitava semana, após a qual o concepto geralmente passa a ser chamado de feto. [embryo- + G. *genesis*, origem]
   em·bry·o·gen·ic, em·bry·o·ge·net·ic (em-brē-ō-jen'ik, -jĕ-net'ik). Embriogênico, embriogenético; que produz um embrião; relativo à formação de um embrião.
   em·bry·og·e·ny (em-brē-oj'ĕ-nē). Embriogenia; a origem e o crescimento do embrião.
   em·bry·oid (em'brē-oyd). Embrióide. SIN embryonoid.
   em·bry·ol·o·gist (em-brē-ol'ō-jist). Embriologista; aquele que se especializa em embriologia.
   em·bry·ol·o·gy (em-brē-ol'ōjē). Embriologia; ciência da origem e do desenvolvimento do organismo a partir da fertilização do óvulo até o final da oitava semana. Algumas vezes engloba todos os estágios da vida pré-natal. [embryo- + G. *logos*, estudo]
   em·bry·o·ma (em-brē-ō'mă). Embrioma. SIN embryonal tumor.
   em·bry·o·mor·phous (em'brē-ō-mōr'fŭs). Embriomorfo. **1.** Relativo à formação e à estrutura do embrião. **2.** Aplicado a estruturas ou tecidos do corpo semelhantes àquelas no embrião, ou restos embrionários. [embryo- + G. *morphē*, formato]
   em·bry·o·nal (em'brē-ō'năl). Embrionário; relativo a um embrião. SIN embryonate (1).
   em·bry·o·nate (em'brē-ō-nāt). Embrionado. **1.** SIN embryonal. **2.** Que contém um embrião. **3.** Impregnado.
   em·bry·on·ic (em-brē-on'ik). Embriônico; de, relativo a, ou na condição de um embrião.
   em·bry·on·i·form (em-brē-on'i-fōrm). Embrioniforme. SIN embryonoid.
   em·bry·on·i·za·tion (em'brē-on-i-zā'shŭn). Embrionização; reversão de uma célula ou tecido para uma forma embrionária.
   em·bry·o·noid (em'brē-ō-noyd). Embrionóide; semelhante a um embrião ou a um feto. SIN embryoid, embryoniform. [embryo- + G. *eidos*, aparência]
   em·bry·o·ny (em'brē-ō-nē). Embrionia; a formação de um embrião.
   em·bry·op·a·thy (em-brē-op'ă-thē). Embriopatia; condição mórbida do embrião ou feto. SIN fetopathy. [embryo- + G. *pathos*, doença]
   em·bry·o·phore (em'brē-ō-fōr). Embrióforo; membrana ou parede ao redor do embrião hexacântico de tênias, formando a porção interna da casca do ovo. No gênero *Taenia*, o e. é excepcionalmente espesso, com estriações radiais que formam uma estrutura extremamente protetora; no gênero *Diphyllobothrium*, o e. é ciliado e reforça o ciclo de vida aquático deste e de outros cestódeos pseudofilídios. VER TAMBÉM coracidium. [embryo- + G. *phoros*, que possui]

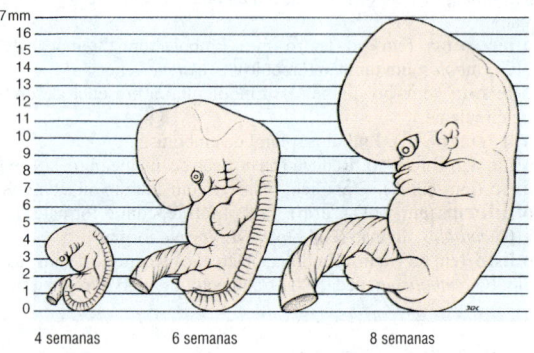

embriões humanos

   em·bry·o·plas·tic (em-brē-ō-plas'tik). Embrioplásico. **1.** Que produz um embrião. **2.** Relativo à formação de um embrião. [embryo- + G. *plassō*, formar]
   em·bry·ot·o·my (em-brē-ot'ō-mē). Embriotomia; qualquer cirurgia mutilante do feto para tornar possível sua remoção quando o parto é impossível por meios naturais. [embryo- + G. *tomē*, que corta]
   em·bry·o·tox·ic·i·ty (em'brē-ō-tok-sis'i-tē). Embriotoxicidade; danos ao embrião que podem resultar em morte, retardo do crescimento ou desenvolvimento anormal de uma parte que pode afetar sua estrutura ou função.
   em·bry·o·tox·on (em'brē-ō-tok'son). Embriotoxo; opacidade congênita da periferia da córnea, uma característica da osteogênese imperfeita. [embryo- + G. *toxon*, arco]
      anterior e., e. anterior. SIN arcus senilis.
      posterior e., e. posterior; anormalidade congênita comum caracterizada por um anel de Schwalbe branco e proeminente.
   em·bry·o·troph (em'brē-ō-trof). Embriotrofo. **1.** Material nutritivo fornecido ao embrião durante o desenvolvimento. Cf. hemotroph, histotroph. **2.** Nos estágios de implantação de mamíferos placentários decíduos, o líquido adjacente à vesícula blastodérmica; uma mistura da secreção das glândulas uterinas, resíduos celulares resultantes da invasão trofoblástica do endométrio e plasma exsudado. [embryo- + G. *trophē*, nutrição]
   em·bry·o·tro·phic (em'brē-ō-trof'ik). Embriotrófico; relativo a qualquer processo ou agência envolvida na nutrição do embrião.
   em·bry·ot·ro·phy (em'brē-ot'rō-fē). Embriotrofia; a nutrição do embrião. [embryo- + G. *trophē*, nutrição]

emed·ul·late (ē-med'ŭ-lāt). Desmedular; extrair qualquer medula óssea. [L. *e-*, de, + *medulla*, medula óssea]

emei·o·cy·to·sis (ē'mē-ō-si-tō'sis). Emeiocitose. SIN exocytosis (2). [L. *emitto*, enviar para diante, + G. *kytos*, célula, + *-osis*, condição]

emer·gence (ē-mer'jens). Emergência. **1.** Recuperação da função normal após um período de inconsciência, principalmente aquela associada a um anestésico geral. **2.** VER property e.
   property e., e. de propriedade; propriedades em um sistema complexo que não existem nas partes componentes, p. ex., simetria; isto é, em uma hierarquia ecológica, as populações possuem propriedades não-expressas por um indivíduo ou por uma comunidade.

emer·gen·cy (ē-mer'jen-sē). Emergência; a condição de um paciente que exige tratamento imediato. [L. *e-mergo*, pp. *-mersus*, elevar, emergir, de *mergo*, mergulhar]

emer·gent (ē-mer'jent). Emergente. **1.** Que surge de forma súbita e inesperada; exigindo julgamento rápido e ação imediata. **2.** Que sai, deixando uma cavidade ou outra parte.

Emery, Alan E. H., médico inglês contemporâneo. VER E.-Dreifuss muscular *dystrophy*.

em·ery (em'er-ē). Esmeril; um abrasivo contendo óxido de alumínio e ferro. [Fr. ant. *emeri*, do L. ant. *smericulum*, do G. *smiris*]

em·e·sis (em′ĕ-sis). **1.** Êmese, vômito; SIN vomiting. **2.** Forma combinante, usada como sufixo, para vômito. [G. de *emeō*, vomitar]

emet·ic (ĕ-met′ik). Emético. **1.** Relativo a ou que causa vômito. **2.** Um agente que causa vômito; p. ex., xarope de ipeca. [G. *emetikos*, que produz vômito, de *emeō*, vomitar]

em·e·tine (em′ĕ-tēn). Emetina; o principal alcalóide da ipeca, usado como emético; seus sais são usados na amebíase; disponível na forma de cloridrato.

em·e·to·ca·thar·tic (em′ĕ-tō-kă-thar′tik). Emetocatártico. **1.** Tanto emético como catártico. **2.** Agente que causa vômito e limpeza da parte inferior do intestino.

eme.to.gen.ic. Emetogênico; que possui a capacidade de induzir êmese (vômito), uma propriedade comum de agentes anticâncer, narcóticos e amorfina.

e·me·to·ge·nic·i·ty. Emetogenicidade; a propriedade de ser emetogênico.

EMF Abreviatura de electromotive *force* (força eletromotriz).

EMG Abreviatura de electromyogram (eletromiograma).

△ **-emia.** Sangue. [G. *haima*]

emic·tion (ē-mik′shŭn). Termo raramente usado para micção.

em·i·gra·tion (em-i-grā′shŭn). Emigração; a passagem de leucócitos através do endotélio e da parede de pequenos vasos sanguíneos. [L. *e-migro*, pp. *-atus*, emigrar]

EMINENCE

em·i·nence (em′i-nens) [TA]. Eminência; área circunscrita elevada acima do nível geral da superfície adjacente, particularmente sobre uma superfície óssea. SIN eminentia [TA]. [L. *eminentia*]

abducens e., colículo facial. SIN facial *colliculus.*

arcuate e. [TA], e. arqueada do temporal; proeminência na superfície anterior da porção petrosa do osso temporal, indicando a posição do canal semicircular superior. SIN eminentia arcuata [TA].

articular e. of temporal bone, tubérculo articular do temporal. SIN articular *tubercle* of temporal bone.

canine e., proeminência do canino; elevação no maxilar que corresponde ao encaixe do dente canino. SIN canine proeminence.

collateral e. [TA], e. colateral; elevação longitudinal do assoalho do trígono colateral do ventrículo lateral do cérebro, entre o hipocampo e o *calcar avis*, causada pela proximidade do assoalho da fissura colateral. SIN eminentia collateralis [TA].

e. of concha [TA], e. da concha; a proeminência, na superfície craniana da orelha, que corresponde à concha. SIN eminentia conchae [TA], apophysis conchae.

cruciate e., e. cruciforme do occipital. SIN cruciform e.

cruciform e. [TA], e. cruciforme do occipital; elevação óssea semelhante a uma cruz, na face interna da porção escamosa do osso occipital, formada pela intersecção do sulco dos seios transversos e crista do occipital interna, com a protuberância occipital interna no centro da "cruz". SIN eminentia cruciformis [TA], cruciate e.

deltoid e., tuberosidade para o músculo deltóide. SIN deltoid *tuberosity* (of humerus).

Doyère e., e. de Doyère; a área discretamente elevada da superfície da fibra muscular estriada que corresponde ao local da placa terminal motora (motor *endplate*).

facial e., colículo facial. SIN facial *colliculus.*

forebrain e., e. do prosencéfalo. SIN frontonasal *prominence.*

frontal e., túber frontal; *termo oficial alternativo para frontal *tuber.*

genital e., e. genital; em embriões muito pequenos, a elevação mediana vagamente delineada imediatamente cefálica ao proctódio; sua parte central transforma-se no tubérculo genital.

hypobranchial e., e. hipobranquial; elevação mediana no assoalho da faringe embrionária caudal ao tubérculo ímpar; funde-se lateralmente à parte ventral do segundo e terceiro branquiais, e, neste último, o desenvolvimento é incorporado na raiz da língua. SIN copula linguae, His copula.

hypoglossal e., trígono do nervo hipoglosso. SIN hypoglossal *trigone.*

hypothenar e. [TA], e. hipotenar; a massa carnosa na face medial da palma da mão. SIN hypothenar (1) [TA], eminentia hypothenaris,* antithenar, hypothenar prominence.

ileocecal e., papila ileal. SIN ileal *papilla.*

iliopectineal e., e. iliopúbica. SIN iliopubic e.

iliopubic e. [TA], e. iliopúbica; elevação arredondada na superfície superior do osso do quadril na junção do ílio e do ramo superior do púbis. SIN eminentia iliopubica [TA], iliopectineal e.

intercondylar e. [TA], e. intercondilar; elevação na extremidade proximal da tíbia entre as duas superfícies articulares. SIN eminentia intercondylaris [TA], eminentia intercondyloidea, intercondyloid e., spinous process of tibia.

intercondyloid e., e. intercondilar. SIN intercondylar e.

maxillary e., tuberosidade maxilar. SIN maxillary *tuberosity.*

medial e., e. medial; termo originalmente usado para descrever uma elevação longitudinal da fossa rombóide que se estende por todo o comprimento do rombencéfalo, sendo constituído de elevações específicas como o colículo facial e os trígonos dos nervos hipoglosso e vago; agora usado para descrever apenas a elevação medial no assoalho do quarto ventrículo imediatamente rostral ao colículo facial, com as outras elevações sendo designadas separadamente. SIN eminentia medialis, eminentia teres, funiculus teres, round e.

median e. [TA], e. mediana; o segmento inferior, pouco proeminente, do infundíbulo do hipotálamo, imediatamente proximal ao pedículo hipofisário; a região é caracterizada pelos tufos capilares das artérias infundibulares, das quais se origina o sistema venoso porto-hipotalâmico-hipofisário. SIN eminentia mediana.

olivary e., oliva. SIN oliva.

omental e. of pancreas [TA], túber omental do pâncreas; saliência na superfície anterior do corpo do pâncreas à esquerda dos vasos mesentéricos superiores. SIN tuber omentale pancreatis [TA], omental tuber.

orbital e. of zygomatic bone, tubérculo orbital do osso zigomático. SIN orbital *tubercle* (of zygomatic bone).

parietal e., túber parietal; *termo oficial alternativo para parietal *tuber.*

pyramidal e., e. piramidal. SIN eminentia pyramidalis.

radial e. of wrist, e. radial do punho; eminência plana, algo grande, no lado radial da face palmar do punho, devida ao tubérculo do escafóide e ao tubérculo do trapézio. SIN eminentia carpi radialis.

restiform e., corpo restiforme. SIN restiform *body.*

round e., e. medial. SIN medial e.

e. of scapha [TA], e. da escafa; a proeminência, na superfície craniana da orelha, correspondente à escafa. SIN eminentia scaphae [TA].

thenar e. [TA], e. tenar; a massa carnosa na superfície lateral da palma da mão; a palma radial. SIN eminentia thenaris, thenar proeminence.

thyroid e., e. tireóidea. SIN laryngeal *prominence.*

e. of triangular fossa of auricle [TA], e. da fossa triangular da orelha; a proeminência, na superfície craniana da orelha, correspondente à fossa triangular. SIN eminentia fossae triangularis auricularis [TA], agger perpendicularis, eminentia triangularis.

ulnar e. of wrist, e. ulnar do punho; eminência menor que a radial, no lado ulnar da face palmar do punho, devido à presença do osso pisiforme. SIN eminentia carpi ulnaris.

em·i·nen·tia, pl. **em·i·nen·ti·ae** (em-i-nen′shē-ă, -shē-ē) [TA]. Eminência. SIN eminence. [L. prominence, de *e-mineo*, projetar]

e. abducen′tis, colículo facial. SIN facial *colliculus.*

e. arcua′ta [TA], e. arqueada do temporal. SIN arcuate *eminence.*

e. articula′ris os′sis tempora′lis, tubérculo articular do temporal. SIN articular *tubercle* of temporal bone.

e. car′pi radia′lis, e. radial do punho. SIN radial *eminence* of wrist.

e. car′pi ulna′ris, e. ulnar do punho. SIN ulnar *eminence* of wrist.

e. collatera′lis [TA], e. colateral. SIN collateral *eminence.*

e. con′chae [TA], e. da concha. SIN eminence of concha.

e. crucifor′mis [TA], e. cruciforme do occipital. SIN cruciforme *eminence.*

e. facia′lis, colículo facial. SIN facial *colliculus.*

e. fos′sae triangula′ris auricula′ris [TA], e. da fossa triangular da orelha. SIN eminence *of triangular fossa of auricle.*

e. fronta′lis, túber frontal; *termo oficial alternativo para frontal *tuber.*

e. hypoglos′si, trígono do nervo hipoglosso. SIN hypoglossal *trigone.*

e. hypothena′ris, e. hipotenar; *termo oficial alternativo para hypothenar *eminence.*

e. iliopu′bica [TA], e. iliopúbica. SIN iliopubic *eminence.*

e. intercondyla′ris [TA], e. intercondilar. SIN intercondylar *eminence.*

e. intercondyloi′dea, e. intercondilar. SIN intercondylar *eminence.*

e. maxil′lae, e. maxilar. SIN maxillary *tuberosity.*

e. media′lis, e. medial. SIN medial *eminence.*

e. media′na, e. mediana. SIN median *eminence.*

e. orbita′lis (os′sis zygoma′tici), tubérculo orbital (do osso zigomático). SIN orbital *tubercle* (of zygomatic bone).

e. parieta′lis, túber parietal; *termo oficial alternativo para parietal *tuber.*

e. pyramida′lis [TA], e. piramidal; uma projeção cônica posterior à janela vestibular no ouvido médio; é oca e contém o músculo estapédio. SIN pyramid of tympanum, pyramidal eminence, pyramis tympani.

e. restifor′mis, corpo restiforme. SIN restiform *body.*

e. sca′phae [TA], e. da escafa. SIN eminence of scapha.

e. sym′physis, tubérculo mentual (da mandíbula). SIN mental *tubercle* (of mandible).

e. te′res, e. medial. SIN medial *eminence.*

e. thena′ris, e. tenar; *termo oficial alternativo para thenar *eminence.*

e. triangula′ris, e. da fossa triangular da orelha. SIN eminence of triangular fossa of auricle.

va'gi e., trígono do nervo vago. SIN vagal (nerve) trigone.
em·i·o·cy·to·sis (ē'mē-ō-sī-tō'sis). Emiocitose. SIN exocytosis (2). [L. *emitto,* enviar para diante, + G. *kytos,* célula, + *-osis,* condição]
em·is·sar·i·um (em-i-sā'rē-ŭm). Veia emissária. SIN emissary *vein.* [L. saída, de *e-mitto,* pp. *-missus,* enviar]
  e. condyloid'eum, veia emissária condilar. SIN condylar emissary *vein.*
  e. mastoid'eum, v. e. mastóidea. SIN mastoid emissary *vein.*
  e. occipita'le, v. e. occipital. SIN occipital emissary *vein.*
  e. parieta'le, v. e. parietal. SIN parietal emissary *vein.*
em·is·sary (em'i-sār-ē). **1.** Emissário; relativo a, ou que proporciona, uma saída ou dreno. **2.** Veia emissária. SIN emissary *vein.* [ver emissarium]
emis·sion (ē-mish'ŭn). Emissão; ejaculação; expulsão vigorosa; geralmente refere-se a uma descarga dos órgãos genitais internos masculinos para a uretra interna; o conteúdo dos órgãos, incluindo os espermatozóides, o líquido prostático e o líquido da vesícula seminal, mistura-se, na uretra interna, com muco proveniente das glândulas bulbouretrais para formar o sêmen. [L. *emissio,* de *e-mitto,* enviar]
  characteristic e., radiação característica. SIN characteristic *radiation.*
  continuous otoacoustic e., e. otoacústica contínua; uma forma de emissão otoacústica evocada na qual a emissão possui a mesma freqüência que o estímulo e persiste pelo mesmo tempo que o estímulo.
  distortion-product otoacoustic e., e. otoacústica por produtos de distorção; uma forma de emissão otoacústica evocada na qual é produzida uma terceira freqüência quando são usados dois tons puros como estímulo.
  evoked otoacoustic e., e. otoacústica evocada; uma forma resultante da estimulação acústica, ao contrário da emissão otoacústica espontânea.
  otoacoustic e., e. otoacústica; som que emana do ouvido e que pode ser registrado por pequenos microfones colocados no canal auditivo externo, parecendo ser produzido pelas células ciliadas externas da cóclea. As emissões otoacústicas ocorrem espontaneamente e podem ser evocadas por estímulos acústicos; são mais proeminentes em mulheres que em homens, e são particularmente fortes em lactentes. Indicativas da integridade das células ciliares auditivas, são medidas para rastrear comprometimento auditivo em recém-nascidos.
  transient evoked otoacoustic e., e. otoacústica evocada transitória; uma forma na qual a duração da resposta é limitada.
emis·siv·i·ty (ē-mi-siv'i-tē). Emissividade; a emissão de raios caloríficos; um "corpo negro" perfeito tem uma emissividade de 1; uma superfície metálica extremamente polida teria uma e. apenas de 0,02.
EMIT Abreviatura de enzyme-multiplied *immunoassay* technique (técnica de imunoensaio multiplicado por enzima).
Emmet, Thomas A., ginecologista norte-americano, 1828–1919. VER E. *needle, operation.*
em·me·tro·pia (em-ē-trō'pē-ă). Emetropia; o estado de refração do olho no qual raios paralelos, quando o olho está em repouso, são focalizados exatamente sobre a retina. [G. *emmetros,* de acordo com a medida, + *ōps,* olho]
em·me·tro·pic (em-ē-trop'ik). Emetrópico; pertinente a, ou caracterizado por, emetropia.
em·me·trop·i·za·tion (em'ē-trōp-i-zā'shŭn). Emetropização; o processo pelo qual a refração do segmento ocular anterior e o comprimento axial do olho tendem a equilibrar-se para produzir emetropia.
Emmonsia. Gênero de Fungos Imperfeitos (Fungi Imperfecti) sapróbicos da família Moniliaceae; também chamado *Haplosporangium.*
  E. parva var. crescens, a principal espécie fúngica que causa adiaspiromicose em animais e o único agente de adiaspiromicose humana; a infecção é adquirida por inalação de conídios do fungo que cresce no solo.
  E. parva var. parva, uma espécie fúngica que causa adiaspiromicose em animais.
Em·mon·si·el·la cap·su·la·ta (e-mon-sī-el'ă kap-soo-lā'tă). SIN Ajellomyces capsulatum.
em·o·din (em'ō-din). Emodina; substância cristalina (catártico) encontrada no ruibarbo, na senna, na cáscara sagrada e em outras substâncias purgantes. SIN archin, frangulic acid.
emol·lient (ē-mol'ē-ent). Emoliente. **1.** Calmante para a pele ou mucosa. **2.** Um agente que amacia a pele ou alivia a irritação da pele ou mucosa. SIN malactic. [L. *emolliens,* p. pres. de *e- mollio, emollire,* amaciar]
emo·tion (ē-mō'shŭn). Emoção; forte sentimento, estado mental vigilante, ou estado intenso de impulso ou inquietação, que pode ser voltado para um objeto definido, e é evidenciado tanto em alterações do comportamento quanto psicológicas, com manifestações do sistema nervoso autônomo associadas. [L. *e-moveo,* pp. *-motus,* sair, agitar]
emo·tion·al (ē-mō'shŭn-ăl). Emocional; relativo a, ou caracterizado por, uma emoção.
emo·ti·o·vas·cu·lar (ē-mō'shē-ō-vas'kū'ler). Vásculo-emocional; relativo a alterações vasculares, como palidez e rubor, causadas por emoções de vários tipos.
em·pasm, em·pas·ma (em'pazm, em-paz'mă). Termo obsoleto, empasma; um polvilho. [G. *empasma,* de *em-passo,* borrifar]

tipos de enfisema	
1. enfisema centrilobular/centriacinar	inicia-se próximo ao bronquíolo terminal no centro do lóbulo (também denominado enfisema acinar proximal)
2. enfisema panlobular/panacinar	afeta todo o pulmão da periferia para dentro (também denominado enfisema generalizado)
3. enfisema localizado	um, ou poucos, locais de destruição alveolar, circundados por arquitetura pulmonar normal (também denominado enfisema bolhoso, acinar distal ou parasseptal)
4. enfisema perifocal	ocorre na vizinhança de lesões focais ou fibrose (também denominado enfisema paracicatricial ou irregular)

em·path·ic (em-path'ik). Empático; relativo a, ou caracterizado por, empatia.
em·pa·thize (em'pă-thīz). Sentir empatia em relação a outra pessoa; colocar-se no lugar do outro.
em·pa·thy (em'pă-thē). Empatia. **1.** A capacidade de perceber, intelectual e emocionalmente, as emoções, os sentimentos e as reações que outra pessoa está apresentando e de comunicar efetivamente aquela compreensão do indivíduo. Cf. sympathy (3). **2.** A antropomorfização ou humanização de objetos e o sentimento de si próprio como parte deles. [G. *en* (em), em, + *pathos,* sentimento]
  generative e., e. generativa; a experiência interna de compartilhar e compreender o estado psicológico momentâneo de outra pessoa.
em·per·i·po·le·sis (em-păr'i-pō-lē'sis). Emperipolese; penetração ativa de uma célula por outra, que permanece intacta; observada em culturas teciduais nas quais leucócitos penetraram em macrófagos e, subseqüentemente, saíram. [G. *en* (em), dentro, + *peri,* ao redor, + *poleomai,* vagar]
em·phrax·is (em-frak'sis). Enfraxia. **1.** Uma obstrução da abertura da glândula sudorípara. **2.** Uma impacção. [G. uma obstrução]
em·phy·se·ma (em-fizē'mă). Enfisema. **1.** Presença de ar nos interstícios do tecido conjuntivo de uma parte. **2.** Uma condição pulmonar caracterizada por aumento além do normal do tamanho dos espaços aéreos distais ao bronquíolo terminal (aquelas partes que contêm alvéolos), com alterações destrutivas em suas paredes e redução do seu número. A manifestação clínica é dispnéia aos esforços, devido ao efeito combinado (em vários graus) de redução da superfície alveolar para troca gasosa e colapso das pequenas vias aéreas com aprisionamento do gás alveolar em expiração; isso faz com que o tórax seja mantido na posição de inspiração ("tórax em barril"), com expiração prolongada e aumento do volume residual. Freqüentemente, mas não necessariamente, há sintomas de bronquite crônica coexistentes. Duas variedades estruturais são e. panlobular (panacinar) e enfisema centrilobular (centriacinar); os enfisemas paracicatricial, parasseptal e bolhoso também são comuns. SIN pulmonary e. [G. insuflação do estômago, etc. de *en,* em, + *physēma,* sopro, de *physa,* fole]
  alveolar duct e., e. do ducto alveolar; e. no qual o envolvimento primário se dá nos ductos alveolares e bronquíolos respiratórios, ao contrário do enfisema panacinar.
  bullous e., e. bolhoso; e. no qual os espaços aéreos aumentados têm 1 a vários centímetros de diâmetro, freqüentemente visíveis em radiografias do tórax. Os sacos de ar de paredes finas, sob tensão, comprimem o tecido pulmonar, sejam eles isolados ou múltiplos; algumas vezes é sensível à ressecção cirúrgica com melhora da função pulmonar.
  centriacinar e., e. centriacinar. SIN centrilobular e.
  centrilobular e., e. centrilobular; e. que afeta a porção central dos lóbulos pulmonares secundários, ao redor do bronquíolo central, tipicamente envolvendo a parte superior dos pulmões ou lobos; pode estar relacionado à inflamação dos bronquíolos e aos efeitos da poeira inalada, que se aglomera próximo dos bronquíolos respiratórios; observado na pneumoconiose dos mineiros de carvão e em moradores assintomáticos de áreas urbanas (forma leve). SIN centriacinar e.
  compensating e., compensatory e., e. compensatório; aumento da capacidade aérea de uma parte do pulmão quando outra parte está consolidada, retraída ou é incapaz de realizar sua função respiratória; os alvéolos estão distendidos, mas não há destruição das paredes alveolares e, portanto, não é um e. verdadeiro, como este termo é definido agora.
  congenital lobar e., e. lobar congênito; causa comum de angústia respiratória neonatal, que geralmente envolve o lobo superior esquerdo.
  cutaneous e., e. cutâneo. SIN subcutaneous e.

diffuse obstructive e., e. obstrutivo difuso; o principal componente da doença pulmonar obstrutiva crônica.
ectatic e., e. com ectasia; doença obstrutiva das vias aéreas com áreas de dilatação dos ácinos alveolares. Observado basicamente em associação com deficiência hereditária de α_1-antitripsina. VER panlobular e.
familial e., e. familiar; enfisema hereditário associado à grande deficiência de α_1-antitripsina. Pode ocorrer como uma característica isolada [MIM*130700, 130710] ou com cútis flácida (*cutis* laxa) e anemia hemolítica (hemolytic *anemia*) [MIM*235360].
gangrenous e., gangrena gasosa. SIN gas gangrene.
generalized e., e. generalizada. SIN panlobular e.
increased markings e., e. com aumento da trama pulmonar; termo aplicado à doença pulmonar obstrutiva mista na qual os achados radiográficos de enfisema coexistem com imagens não-vasculares, provavelmente relacionadas à inflamação brônquica.
interlobular e., e. interlobular; enfisema intersticial nos septos de tecido conjuntivo entre os lóbulos pulmonares.
interstitial e., e. intersticial; (1) presença de ar nos tecidos pulmonares conseqüente à ruptura das células aéreas; (2) presença de ar ou gás no tecido conjuntivo.
intestinal e., e. intestinal. SIN pneumatosis cystoides intestinalis.
irregular e., e. irregular; enfisema que não exibe relação consistente com qualquer parte do ácino; sempre associado à fibrose.
mediastinal e., e. mediastinal. SIN pseudomediastinum.
panacinar e., e. panacinar. SIN panlobular e.
panlobular e., e. panlobular; enfisema que afeta todas as partes do lóbulo pulmonar secundário, tipicamente envolvendo a parte inferior do pulmão e freqüentemente associado a deficiência de α_1-antitripsina. SIN generalized e., panacinar e.

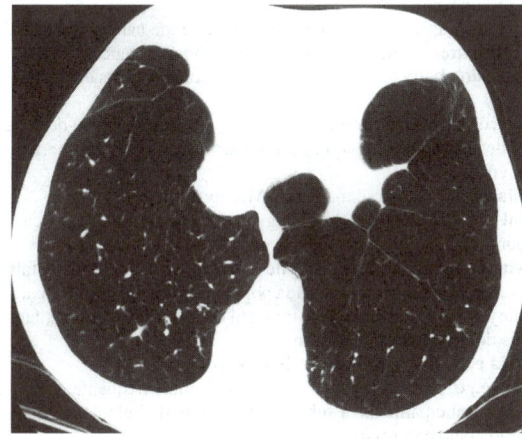

enfisema panlobular: TC de alta resolução dos lobos inferiores mostra destruição uniforme dos lóbulos pulmonares secundários

paracicatricial e., e. paracicatricial; dilatação dos espaços aéreos terminais adjacentes a uma cicatriz no pulmão. VER TAMBÉM paraseptal e.
paraseptal e., e. parasseptal; enfisema envolvendo a periferia dos lóbulos pulmonares. SIN scar e.
pulmonary e., e. pulmonar. SIN emphysema (2).
scar e., e. cicatricial. SIN paraseptal e.
senile e., e. senil; enfisema decorrente da atrofia fisiológica da idade avançada.
subcutaneous e., e. subcutâneo; a presença de ar ou gás nos tecidos subcutâneos. SIN aerodermectasia, cutaneous e., pneumoderma, pneumohypoderma.
subgaleal e., e. subgaleal; acúmulo de ar ou gás entre a camada interna do couro cabeludo e o crânio.
surgical e., e. cirúrgico; enfisema subcutâneo por gás aprisionado nos tecidos por uma operação ou lesão, freqüentemente observado após insuflação de dióxido de carbono durante procedimentos laparoscópicos.
unilateral lobar e., e. lobar unilateral; lobo (ou pulmão) radiograficamente hipertransparente secundário à bronquiolite obliterante, com aprisionamento de ar. SIN MacLeod syndrome, Swyer-James syndrome (1), Swyer-James-MacLeod syndrome.
em·phy·sem·a·tous (em-fi-sem′ă-tŭs). Enfisematoso; relativo a, ou afetado por, enfisema.
em·pir·ic (em-pir′ik). 1. Empírico. SIN empirical. 2. Empirista; membro de uma escola de médicos greco-romanos, no final do período antes de Cristo e nos primeiros anos depois de Cristo, que confiavam e baseavam sua prática apenas na experiência, evitando toda a especulação, teoria ou raciocínio abstrato; estavam pouco preocupados com as causas ou com a correlação de sintomas a fim de obter uma compreensão verdadeira de uma doença, embora considerassem o conhecimento básico, a fisiologia, a patologia e a anatomia inúteis e sem valor prático. 3. Moderno: teste de uma hipótese por observação cuidadosa, ou seja, com base racional na experiência. [ver empírico]
em·pir·i·cal (em-pir′i-kăl). Empírico. 1. Fundamentado na experiência prática, e não apenas no raciocínio, mas não estabelecido cientificamente, ao contrário do racional (rational) (1). 2. Relativo a um empirista (empiric) (2). 3. Baseado no teste de observação cuidadosa de uma hipótese; racional. SIN empiric (1). [G. *empeirikos,* de *empeiria,* experiência, de *en,* em, + *peira,* uma prova]
em·pir·i·cism (em-pir′i-sizm). Empirismo; observação da experiência como um guia prático ou para o uso terapêutico de qualquer remédio.
em·por·i·at·rics (em-pōr-ē-at′riks). Emporiatria; a especialidade da medicina de viagem, que lida com doenças que os viajantes podem adquirir, principalmente nos trópicos. [G. *emporion,* mercado, de *emporos,* viajante, mercador, + *(technē) iatrikē,* arte médica]
em·pros·thot·o·nos (em′pros-thot′ō-nŭs). Emprostótono; contração tetânica dos músculos flexores, curvando o dorso com concavidade para a frente. [G. *emprosthen,* para a frente, + *tonos,* tensão]
em·py·ec·to·my (em-pī-ek′tō-mē). Empiectomia; ressecção de um empiema e de sua cápsula.
em·py·e·ma (em-pī-ē′mă, -pi-ē′mă). Empiema; pus em uma cavidade corporal; quando usado sem qualificação, refere-se especificamente ao piotórax. [G. *empyēma,* supuração, de *en,* em, + *pyon,* pus]
e. benig′num, e. benigno. SIN latent e.
e. of gallbladder, e. da vesícula biliar; colecistite aguda grave com inflamação purulenta da vesícula biliar.
latent e., e. latente; a presença de pus em uma cavidade, particularmente um dos seios acessórios, sem sintomas subjetivos. SIN e. benignum.
loculated e., e. loculado; piotórax no qual aderências pleurais formam uma ou mais bolsas contendo pus.
mastoid e., e. mastoidite. SIN mastoiditis.
e. necessita′tis, e. da necessidade; uma forma de piotórax na qual o pus extravasa para o exterior, produzindo um abscesso subcutâneo que, finalmente, se rompe através da pele; pode resultar em recuperação espontânea sem exigir cirurgia.
e. of the pericardium, pericardite purulenta. SIN purulent pericarditis.
pneumococcal e., e. pneumocócico; infecção da cavidade pleural por *Streptococcus pneumoniae,* o pneumococo, com formação de pus.
pulsating e., e. pulsátil; uma coleção de pus grande e tensa na cavidade pleural, através da qual as pulsações cardíacas são transmitidas para a parede torácica.
streptococcal e., e. estreptocócico; exsudação purulenta para a cavidade pleural causada por infecção por *Streptococcus hemolyticus.*
em·py·e·mic (em-pī-ē′mik). Empiêmico; relativo a empiema.
em·py·e·sis (em-pī-ē′sis). Empiese; erupção pustular. [G. supuração]
em·py·o·cele (em′pī-ō-sēl). Empiocele; hidrocele supurativa; uma coleção de pus no escroto. [G. *en,* em, + *pyon,* pus, + *kēlē,* tumor]
em·py·reu·ma (em-pī-roo′mă). Empireuma; odor característico emitido por substâncias orgânicas quando carbonizadas ou submetidas a destilação destrutiva em recipientes fechados. [G. um fogo apagado]
emu Abreviatura de electromagnetic *unit* (unidade eletromagnética).
emul·gent (ē-mŭl′jent). Emulgente; indica um processo de filtração, extração ou purificação. [L. *e- mulgeo,* pp. *-mulsus,* extrair, drenar]
emul·si·fi·er (ē-mŭl′si-fī-er). Emulsificador; um agente, como a goma arábica ou a gema de ovo, usado para fazer uma emulsão de um óleo fixo. Sabões, detergentes, esteróides e proteínas podem agir como emulsificadores; eles estabilizam sistemas bifásicos de fases oleosa e aquosa.
emul·si·fy (ē-mŭl′si-fī). Emulsificar; fazer na forma de uma emulsão.
emul·sin (ē-mŭl′sin). Emulsina. 1. Preparação ou fermento derivado de amêndoas, que contém β-glucosidase. 2. Algumas vezes usada como sinônimo de β-glucosidase.
emul·sion (ē-mŭl′shŭn). Emulsão; sistema contendo dois líquidos imiscíveis no qual um é disperso, na forma de glóbulos muito pequenos (fase interna), por todo o outro (fase externa) (p. ex., óleo em água (leite) ou água em óleo (maionese)). [L. mod. de *e-mulgeo,* pp. *-mulsus,* extrair ou drenar]
emul·sive (ē-mŭl′siv). Emulsivo. 1. Designa uma substância que pode ser transformada em emulsão. 2. Designa uma substância, como uma mucilagem, pela qual uma gordura ou resina pode ser emulsificada. 3. Que torna suave ou maleável. 4. Que fornece um óleo fixo sob pressão.
emul·soid (ē-mŭl′soyd). Emulsóide; uma dispersão coloidal na qual as partículas dispersas são mais ou menos líquidas e exercem uma determinada atração sobre, e adsorvem, uma determinada quantidade de líquido na qual estão suspensas. SIN emulsion colloid, hydrophil colloid, hydrophilic colloid, lyophilic colloid.

em·u·re·sis (em-ū-rē′sis). Emurese; condição na qual a excreção urinária e a ingestão de água produzem uma hidratação absoluta do corpo. VER TAMBÉM ecuresis. [G. *en* (*em*), em, + *ourēsis*, micção]

emyl·ca·mate (e-mil′ka-māt, em-il-kam′āt). Emilcamato; um sedativo leve, usado para controlar a tensão e a ansiedade e para aliviar a dor e o espasmo muscular.

en-. Em; usa-se em- antes de b, p ou m. [G.]

en·al·a·pril·at (ē-nal′a-pril-āt). Enalaprilato; o metabólito ativo do enalapril, um inibidor da ECA (enzima conversora do angiotensinogênio) usado no tratamento da hipertensão e da insuficiência cardíaca congestiva.

enal·a·pril ma·le·ate (e-nal′a-pril). Maleato de enalapril; uma pró-droga do enalaprilato, um inibidor da enzima de conversão da angiotensina usado como anti-hipertensivo e no tratamento da insuficiência cardíaca congestiva.

enam·el (ē-nam′el) [TA]. Esmalte; a substância dura brilhante que cobre a porção exposta do dente. Em sua forma madura, é composto de uma porção inorgânica constituída de 90% de hidroxiapatita e 6–8% de carbonato de cálcio, fluoreto de cálcio e carbonato de magnésio; o restante constituindo uma matriz orgânica de proteína e glicoproteína; estruturalmente, é constituída de bastões orientados, cada um consistindo em uma pilha de pequenos bastões encerrados em uma bainha prismática orgânica. SIN enamelum [TA], substantia adamantina, substantia vitrea. [I. m. do Fr. *enamailer*, aplicar esmalte, de *en*, sobre, + *amil*, esmalte, do Alemão]

dwarfed e., e. nanóide. SIN nanoid e.

interrod e., e. interbastão; esmalte que ocupa o espaço entre os bastões de esmalte e serve para uni-los.

mottled e., e. mosqueado; alterações na estrutura do esmalte devidas à ingestão excessiva de flúor durante a formação do dente; seu aspecto varia de pequenas opacidades brancas a manchas amarelas e pretas.

nanoid e., e. nanóide; uma condição de adelgaçamento anormal do esmalte. SIN dwarfed e.

whorled e., e. convoluto; esmalte no qual os bastões assumem um trajeto espiral ou torcido.

en·am·el·ins. Enamelinas; uma classe de proteínas que formam a matriz orgânica do esmalte dental maduro. [enamel + -in]

enam·el·o·blast (en-am′el-ō-blast). Ameloblasto. SIN ameloblast.

enam·el·o·gen·e·sis (ē-nam′el-ō-jen′ē-sis). Amelogênese. SIN amelogenesis.

e. imperfec′ta, a. imperfeita. SIN *amelogenesis* imperfecta.

enam·el·o·ma (ē-nam-el-ō′ma). Pérola de esmalte; uma anomalia do desenvolvimento na qual há um pequeno nódulo de esmalte abaixo da junção cemento-esmalte, geralmente na bifurcação dos dentes molares. SIN enamel drop, enamel nodule, enamel pearl.

enam·e·lum (ē-nam′e-lŭm) [TA]. Esmalte. SIN enamel.

enan·thal (ē-nan′thăl). Enantal. SIN heptanal.

enan·thate (e-nan′thāt). Enantato; contração aprovada pela USAN para heptanoato, $CH_3(CH_2)_5COO^-$.

en·an·them, en·an·the·ma (en-an′them, en-an-thē′ma). Enantema; uma erupção da mucosa, principalmente a que ocorre em conjunto com um dos exantemas. [G. *en*, em, + *anthēma*, erupção, de *antheō*, florescer]

enantio-. Forma combinante que significa oposto ou invertido. [G. *enantios*, oposto]

en·an·ti·o·mer (ē-nan′tē-ō-mer). Enantiômero; um membro de um par de moléculas que são imagens especulares que não podem ser superpostas; nenhuma das moléculas possui um plano interno de simetria. SIN optic antipode. [enantio- + G. *meros*, parte]

en·an·ti·o·mer·ic (ē-nan′tē-ō-mer′ik). Enantiomérico; relativo a enantiômero.

en·an·ti·om·er·ism (ē-nan-tē-om′er-izm). Enantiomerismo; em química, isomerismo no qual as moléculas em sua configuração estão relacionadas entre si como um objeto e sua imagem especular (enantiômeros) e, consequentemente, não podem ser superpostas; o enantiomerismo acarreta atividade óptica, com ambos os enantiômeros (em quantidades idênticas) girando o plano de luz polarizada igualmente, mas em direções opostas.

en·an·ti·o·morph (ē-nan′tē-ō-mōrf). Enantiomorfo; um enantiômero sob a forma cristalina.

en·an·ti·o·mor·phic (ē-nan′tē-ō-mōr′fik). Enantiomórfico. **1.** Relativo a dois objetos, sendo cada um deles a imagem especular do outro. **2.** Em química, relativo aos isômeros cujas atividades ópticas possuem igual magnitude, mas sinais opostos. SIN enantiomorphous. [enantio- + G. *morphē*, forma]

en·an·ti·o·mor·phism (ē-nan′tē-ō-mōr′fizm). Enantiomorfismo; a relação de dois objetos de formas semelhantes, mas que não podem ser superpostos, como as duas mãos ou um objeto e sua imagem especular. [enantio- + G. *morphē*, forma]

en·an·ti·o·mor·phous (ē-nan′tē-ō-mōr′fŭs). Enantiomórfico. SIN enantiomorphic.

en·ar·thro·di·al (en-ar-thrō′dē-al). Enartrodial; relativo a uma enartrose.

en·ar·thro·sis (en-ar-thrō′sis). Enartrose, articulação esferóidea; *termo oficial alternativo para ball and socket *joint*. [G. *en-arthrōsis*, uma articulação onde a esfera está profundamente localizada dentro da cavidade]

en bloc (ahn blok). Em bloco; como um todo; usado em referência a técnicas de necropsia nas quais os órgãos viscerais são removidos em grandes blocos, permitindo que o dissector preserve a continuidade da arquitetura do órgão durante a dissecção subseqüente. [Fr., em bloco]

en·cai·nide hy·dro·chlo·ride (en-kā′nīd). Cloridrato de encainida; um antiarrítmico.

en·cap·su·lat·ed (en-kap′soo-lā-ted). Encapsulado; encerrado em uma cápsula ou bainha. SIN encapsuled.

en·cap·su·la·tion (en-kap-soo-lā′shŭn). Encapsulação; encerramento em uma cápsula ou bainha. [L. *in* + capsula, dim. de *capsa*, caixa]

en·cap·suled (en-kap′soold). Encapsulado. SIN encapsulated.

en·car·di·tis (en-kar-dī′tis). Endocardite. SIN endocarditis.

en·ce·li·tis, en·ce·li·i·tis (en-sē-lī′tis, -lē-ī′tis). Encelite; termo obsoleto para designar a inflamação de qualquer víscera abdominal. [G. *en*, em, + *koilia*, ventre, + *-itis*, inflamação]

encephal-. VER encephalo-.

en·ceph·a·lal·gia (en-sef-ă-lal′jē-ă). Encefalalgia, cefaléia. SIN headache. [encephalo- + G. *algos*, dor]

en·céph·ale iso·lé (ahn-saf-al′ē-sō-lā′). Cérebro isolado; animal com transecção da porção caudal do bulbo e com respiração mantida artificialmente; ele permanece alerta, tem ciclos de sono–vigília, reações pupilares normais e um eletroencefalograma normal. Cf. cerveau isolé. [Fr. cérebro isolado]

en·ceph·a·le·mia (en-sef-ă-lē′mē-ă). Encefalemia, congestão cerebral. SIN brain congestion. [encephalo- + G. *haima*, sangue]

en·ce·phal·ic (en′se-fal′ik). Encefálico; relativo ao encéfalo, ou às estruturas situadas dentro do crânio.

en·ceph·a·lit·ic (en-sef-ă-lit′ik). Encefalítico; relativo à encefalite.

en·ceph·a·li·tis, pl. **en·ceph·a·lit·i·des** (en-sef-ă-lī′tis, en-sef-ă-lit′i-dēz). Encefalite; inflamação do encéfalo. [G. *enkephalos*, encéfalo, + *-itis*, inflamação]

acute hemorrhagic e., e. hemorrágica aguda; e. de caráter apoplectóide decorrente de extravasamento de sangue. SIN e. hemorrhagica.

acute inclusion body e., e. aguda com corpúsculo de inclusão. SIN herpes simplex e.

acute necrotizing e., e. necrotizante aguda; uma forma aguda de e. caracterizada por destruição do parênquima cerebral; causada por vírus herpes simples e outros vírus.

Australian X e., e. australiana X. SIN Murray Valley e.

bacterial e., e. bacteriana; e. de etiologia bacteriana. SIN e. pyogenica, purulent e., suppurative e.

bunyavirus e., e. por buniavírus; e. de início abrupto, com forte cefaléia frontal e febre baixa a moderada, causada por membros do gênero Bunyavirus (família Bunyaviridae); as infecções também ocorrem em roedores, lagomorfos e animais domésticos. SIN California e.

California e., e. da Califórnia. SIN bunyavirus e.

coxsackie e., e. por vírus Coxsackie; e. viral, mais freqüente em lactentes e envolvendo principalmente a substância cinzenta do bulbo e da medula espinal, causada pelo enterovírus Coxsackie B humano.

Dawson e., e. de Dawson. SIN subacute sclerosing *panencephalitis*.

epidemic e., e. epidêmica; e. viral que ocorre de forma epidêmica, como a e. B japonesa, a de St. Louis e a e. letárgica.

equine e., e. eqüina. SIN equine *encephalomyelitis*.

experimental allergic e. (EAE), e. alérgica experimental. SIN experimental allergic *encephalomyelitis*.

Far East Russian e., e. do extremo oriente russo; e. transmitida pelo carrapato (subtipo oriental).

e. hemorrhag′ica, e. hemorrágica. SIN acute hemorrhagic e.

herpes e., e. herpética. SIN herpes simplex e.

herpes simplex e., e. por vírus herpes simples; a e. aguda mais comum, causada por HSV-1; afeta pessoas de qualquer idade; envolve preferencialmente as porções ínfero-mediais do lobo temporal e as porções orbitais dos lobos frontais; ao exame histopatológico, nos estágios agudos, há necrose hemorrágica grave associada a corpúsculos de inclusão eosinofílicos intranucleares nos neurônios e nas células gliais. SIN acute inclusion body e., herpes e.

hyperergic e., e. hiperérgica; e. resultante de uma reação alérgica imunológica do sistema nervoso a estímulos antigênicos.

Ilhéus e., e. de Ilhéus; e. causada pelo vírus Ilhéus (gênero Flavivirus) e endêmica no leste do Brasil e em outras partes das Américas do Sul e Central; transmitida por mosquitos.

inclusion body e., e. com corpúsculos de inclusão. SIN subacute sclerosing *panencephalitis*.

Japanese B e., e. B japonesa; e. ou encefalomielite epidêmica do Japão, da Rússia siberiana e de outras partes da Ásia; causada pelo vírus da encefalite B japonesa (gênero Flavivirus) e transmitida por mosquitos; pode ocorrer como uma infecção subclínica, assintomática, mas pode causar uma meningoencefalite aguda. SIN e. japonica, Russian autumn e.

e. japon'ica, e. japonesa B. SIN Japanese B e.
lead e., e. plúmbica. SIN lead encephalopathy.
e. lethar'gica, e. letárgica. SIN von Economo disease.
Mengo e., e. de Mengo; e. que ocorre na África, causada pela cepa Mengo do vírus da encefalomiocardite, um membro dos Picornaviridae.
Murray Valley e., e. do Vale de Murray; e. grave, com alta taxa de mortalidade, que ocorre no Vale de Murray, na Austrália; a doença é mais grave em crianças, sendo caracterizada por cefaléia, febre, mal-estar, sonolência ou convulsões e rigidez de nuca; pode haver lesão cerebral extensa; é causada pelo vírus da encefalite do Vale de Murray (gênero Flavivirus). SIN Australian X disease, Australian X e.
necrotizing e., e. necrotizante; qualquer e. na qual ocorre necrose cerebral extensa, p. ex., encefalomielite hemorrágica necrotizante aguda.
e. neonato'rum, e. neonatal; encefalite do recém-nascido, descrita por R. Virchow como caracterizada pela presença de células repletas de lipídios no encéfalo.
e. periaxia'lis concen'trica, e. periaxial concêntrica; encefalite clinicamente semelhante à adrenoleucodistrofia, mas, ao exame histopatológico, caracterizada por glóbulos ou círculos concêntricos de desmielinização da substância branca cerebral separados por tecido normal. SIN Baló disease.
e. periaxialis diffusa, e. periaxial difusa. SIN Schilder disease.
postvaccinal e., e. pós-vacinal. SIN postvaccinal encephalomyelitis.
Powassan e., e. de Powassan; doença aguda de crianças, cujo quadro clínico varia de doença febril indiferenciada a encefalite; causada pelo vírus de Powassan, um membro da família Flaviviridae, e transmitida por carrapatos ixodídeos; mais freqüente no Canadá.
purulent e., e. purulenta. SIN bacterial e.
e. pyogen'ica, e. piogênica. SIN bacterial e.
Rasmussen e., e. de Rasmussen; e. na qual são encontrados anticorpos contra um receptor do glutamato estimulante no SNC; talvez auto-imune. SIN Rasmussen syndrome.
Russian autumn e., e. japonesa B. SIN Japanese B e.
Russian spring-summer e. (Eastern subtype), e. da primavera-verão russa (subtipo oriental); e. transmitida por carrapato, cujo vírus pertence à família Flaviviridae.
Russian spring-summer e. (Western subtype), e. da primavera-verão russa (subtipo ocidental). SIN tick-borne e. (Central European subtype).
Russian tick-borne e., e. russa transmitida por carrapato. SIN tick-borne e. (Eastern subtype).
secondary e., e. secundária; termo coletivo para designar as encefalites pós-infecciosas, pós-exantema e pós-vacinal.
subacute inclusion body e., e. subaguda com corpúsculo de inclusão. SIN subacute sclerosing panencephalitis.
e. subcortical'is chron'ica, e. subcortical crônica. SIN Binswanger disease.
suppurative e., e. supurativa. SIN bacterial e.
tick-borne e. (Central European subtype), e. transmitida por carrapato (subtipo da Europa Central); meningoencefalite transmitida por carrapato causada por um flavivírus intimamente relacionado ao vírus causador do tipo do Extremo Oriente; é transmitida pelo *Ixodes ricinus*, também por leite cru infectado, principalmente leite de cabra. SIN biundulant meningoencephalitis, Central European tick-borne fever, diphasic milk fever, Russian spring-summer e. (Western subtype).
tick-borne e. (Eastern subtype), e. transmitida por carrapato (subtipo Oriental); uma forma grave de encefalite causada por um flavivírus (família Flaviviridae) e transmitida por carrapatos (*Ixodes pertulcatus* e *I. ricinus*). SIN Russian tick-borne e.
van Bogaert e., e. de van Bogaert. SIN subacute sclerosing panencephalitis.
varicella e., e. da varicela; e. que ocorre como uma complicação da varicela.
vernal e., e. primaveril; e. transmitida por carrapato (subtipo Oriental).
woodcutter's e., e. dos cortadores de madeira; e. transmitida por carrapato (subtipo oriental).
en·ceph·a·li·to·gen (en-sef′ă-li′tō-jen). Encefalitógeno; um agente que provoca encefalite, particularmente com referência ao antígeno que produz encefalomielite alérgica experimental. [encephalitis + G. -gen, que produz]
en·ceph·a·li·to·gen·ic (en-sef′ă-li-tō-jen′ik). Encefalitogênico; que produz encefalite; tipicamente por mecanismos hipersensíveis. VER encephalitogen.
En·ceph·a·li·to·zo·on (en-sef′ă-li-tō-zō′on). Gênero de parasitas protozoários, antes considerados parte da família Toxoplasmatidae, classe Sporozoea, mas agora reconhecidos como membros do filo de protozoários Microspora, família Nosematidae. *E. cuniculi* é considerado o parasita microsporo primário de mamíferos, comumente encontrado no encéfalo e nos túbulos renais de roedores e carnívoros, e causando nosematose em coelhos. [encephalitis + G. *zōon*, animal]
E. cuniculi, infecção críptica comum da maioria dos mamíferos e de algumas aves, transmitida pelo alimento contaminado por urina e por via transplacentária. Já foi descrita infecção humana disseminada entre indivíduos imunoprimidos. A infecção lactente observada por diagnóstico sorológico sugere infecção assintomática disseminada em regiões tropicais.

E. hellem, espécie de *E.* descrita em infecções oftálmicas humanas, causando ceratopatia pontilhada e ulceração da córnea em pacientes com AIDS/SIDA.
E. intestinale, microsporídio que causa diarréia, descrito em pacientes infectados por HIV; a doença pode ser localizada no trato gastrointestinal ou pode disseminar-se por via intravascular.
E. intestinalis, uma espécie de *E.* descrita no músculo humano; foram descritos pouquíssimos casos. Antes denominada *Septata intestinale*.
en·ceph·a·li·za·tion (en-sef′ă-li-zā′shŭn). Encefalização. SIN corticalization.
encephalo-, encephal-. Encefalo-, encefal-; o encéfalo. Cf. cerebro-. [G. *enkephalos*, encéfalo]
en·ceph·a·lo·cele (en-sef′ă-lō-sēl). Encefalocele; abertura congênita no crânio com herniação da substância encefálica. SIN craniocele, cranium bifidum, bifid cranium. [encephalo- + G. *kēlē*, hérnia]
basal e., e. basal; defeito no assoalho do crânio com a herniação de tecido encefálico, algumas vezes associado ao coloboma (*coloboma*) do nervo óptico.
en·ceph·a·lo·cys·to·cele. Encefalocistocele. SIN hydrencephalocele.
en·ceph·a·lo·dur·o·ar·te·ri·o·syn·an·gi·o·sis (en-sef′ă-lō-door-ō-ar-tēr′-ē-ō-sin-anj-ē-ō′sis). Encefaloduroarteriossinangiose. SIN duraencephalosynangiosis.
en·ceph·a·lo·dyn·ia (en-sef′ă-lō-din′ē-ă). Encefalodinia. SIN headache. [encephalo- + G. *odynē*, dor]
en·ceph·a·lo·dys·pla·sia (en-sef′ă-lō-dis-plā′zē-ă). Encefalodisplasia; qualquer anormalidade congênita do encéfalo. [encephalo- + G. *dys*, mau, + *plastos*, formado]
en·ceph·a·lo·gram (en-sef′ă-lō-gram). Encefalograma; o registro obtido por encefalografia. [encephalo- + G. *gramma*, desenho]
en·ceph·a·log·ra·phy (en-sef-ă-log′ră-fē). Encefalografia; técnica obsoleta de representação radiográfica do encéfalo. VER pneumoencephalography. [encephalo- + G. *graphō*, escrever]
gamma e., e. gama; visualização do encéfalo pela administração de pequenas quantidades de radiofármacos emissores de raios gama; o termo pode ser usado para designar vários estudos específicos (p. ex., cintigrafia da perfusão cerebral, imagem do neuroceptor cerebral), dependendo do radiofármaco usado.
en·ceph·a·loid (en-sef′ă-loyd). Encefalóide; semelhante à substância cerebral; designa um carcinoma de consistência mole, semelhante à encefálica, com referência aos aspectos macroscópicos. [encephalo- + G. *eidos*, semelhança]
en·ceph·a·lo·lith (en-sef′ă-lō-lith). Encefalólito; uma concreção no encéfalo ou em um de seus ventrículos. SIN cerebral calculus. [encephalo- + G. *lithos*, cálculo]
en·ceph·a·lol·o·gy (en-sef-ă-lol′ō-jē). Encefalologia; o ramo da medicina que lida com o encéfalo em todas as suas relações. [encephalo- + G. *logos*, estudo]
en·ceph·a·lo·ma (en-sef-ă-lō′mă-lā′shē-ă). Encefaloma; herniação da substância encefálica. SIN cerebroma.
en·ceph·a·lo·ma·la·cia (en-sef′ă-lō-mă-lā′shē-ă). Encefalomalacia; amolecimento anormal do parênquima cerebral freqüentemente devido a isquemia ou infarto. SIN cerebromalacia. [encephalo- + G. *malakia*, amolecimento]
en·ceph·a·lo·men·in·gi·tis (en-sef′ă-lō-men-in-jī′tis). Encefalomeningite. SIN meningoencephalitis. [encephalo- + G. *mēninx*, membrana, + *-itis*, inflamação]
en·ceph·a·lo·me·nin·go·cele (en-sef′ă-lō-me-ning′gō-sēl). Encefalomeningocele. SIN meningoencephalocele. [encephalo- + G. *mēninx*, membrana, + *kēlē*, hérnia]
en·ceph·a·lo·men·in·gop·a·thy (en-sef′ă-lō-men-in-gop′ă-thē). Encefalomeningopatia. SIN meningoencephalopathy.
en·ceph·a·lo·mere (en-sef′ă-lō-mēr). Encefâlomero. SIN neuromere. [encephalo- + G. *meros*, uma parte]
en·ceph·a·lom·e·ter (en-sef-ă-lom′ĕ-ter). Encefâlometro; aparelho para indicar no crânio a localização dos centros corticais. [encephalo- + G. *metron*, medida]
en·ceph·a·lo·my·e·li·tis (en-sef-ă-lō-mī′ĕ-lī′tis). Encefalomielite; inflamação do encéfalo e da medula espinal. [encephalo- + G. *myelon*, medula óssea, + *-itis*, inflamação]
acute disseminated e., e. disseminada aguda; um distúrbio desmielinizante agudo do sistema nervoso central, no qual há desmielinização focal em todo o encéfalo e medula espinal. Esse processo é comum na encefalomielite pós-infecciosa, pós-exantema e pós-vacinal.
acute necrotizing hemorrhagic e., e. hemorrágica necrotizante aguda; distúrbio desmielinizante fulminante do sistema nervoso central que afeta principalmente crianças e adultos jovens. Quase sempre precedida por uma infecção respiratória, caracterizada pelo início abrupto de febre, cefaléia, confusão e rigidez de nuca, logo seguida por convulsões focais, hemiplegia ou tetraplegia, achados referentes ao tronco cerebral e coma; o LCR (líquido cefalorraquidiano) mostra evidências de um processo inflamatório; causada por destruição maciça da substância branca de um ou de ambos os hemisférios, freqüen-

temente acompanhada por destruição semelhante da substância branca do tronco encefálico e dos pedúnculos cerebrais; de etiologia desconhecida. SIN acute hemorrhagic leukoencephalitis, acute necrotizing hemorrhagic leukoencephalitis, Hurst disease.

e. associated with carcinoma, e. associada a carcinoma. SIN paraneoplastic encephalomyelopathy.

benign myalgic e., e. miálgica benigna. SIN epidemic neuromyasthenia.

eastern equine e. (EEE), e. eqüina oriental; uma forma de e. eqüina transmitida por mosquito, observada no leste dos Estados Unidos e causada pelo vírus da encefalite eqüina oriental, uma espécie de Alphavirus que pertence à família Togaviridae; a febre inicial e a viremia são seguidas por sinais de envolvimento do sistema nervoso central (excitação, depois sonolência, paralisia e morte); a incidência de infecção clínica em seres humanos é baixa, mas a taxa de fatalidade pode ser alta.

epidemic myalgic e., e. miálgica epidêmica. SIN epidemic neuromyasthenia.

equine e., e. eqüina; doença viral aguda, freqüentemente fatal, de cavalos e mulas transmitida por mosquitos e caracterizada por distúrbios do sistema nervoso central; nos Estados Unidos, essa doença é tipicamente causada por um dentre três alfavírus, e as doenças resultantes são designadas encefalomielites eqüina ocidental, eqüina oriental e eqüina venezuelana; esses vírus pertencem à família Togaviridae e também podem causar doença neurológica em seres humanos. SIN equine encephalitis.

experimental allergic e., e. alérgica experimental; encefalite alérgica desmielinizante produzida pela injeção de tecido cerebral, geralmente com um adjuvante. SIN experimental allergic encephalitis.

granulomatous e., e. granulomatosa; e. na qual ocorrem granulomas.

herpes B e., e. por vírus herpes B; doença freqüentemente letal de seres humanos causada por infecção com um herpesvírus de macaco normalmente latente.

mouse e., e. do camundongo; encefalomielite causada pelo vírus da encefalomielite do camundongo (uma espécie de Enterovirus) que não é patogênica em macacos ou no homem, mas ataca colônias de camundongos e causa uma paralisia flácida, geralmente dos membros posteriores.

postvaccinal e., e. pós-vacinal; um tipo grave de encefalomielite que pode suceder a vacinação contra raiva. SIN postvaccinal encephalitis.

Venezuelan equine e. (VEE), e. eqüina venezuelana; forma de e. eqüina transmitida por mosquitos, encontrada em regiões da América do Sul, Panamá e Trinidad, causada pelo vírus da encefalomielite eqüina venezuelana (uma espécie de Alphavirus na família Togaviridae) e caracterizada por menor envolvimento do sistema nervoso central do que ocorre na encefalomielite eqüina oriental ou ocidental; febre, diarréia e depressão são comuns; em seres humanos, há febre e cefaléia intensa após um período de incubação de 2–5 dias, e, em alguns casos, houve envolvimento do sistema nervoso central.

viral e., virus e., e. viral; encefalomielite causada por um vírus neurotrópico.

western equine e. (WEE), e. eqüina ocidental; e. eqüina encontrada no oeste dos Estados Unidos e em partes da América do Sul, transmitida por mosquitos e causada pelo vírus da encefalomielite eqüina ocidental (uma espécie de Alphavirus da família Togaviridae); a infecção é semelhante, porém mais leve que a e. eqüina oriental em seres humanos e, como regra geral, não é aparente, mas alguns casos com envolvimento do sistema nervoso central foram fatais.

zoster e., e. zoster; inflamação do encéfalo e da medula espinal causada pelo vírus varicela-zoster, um membro da família Herpesviridae.

en·ceph·a·lo·my·e·lo·cele (en-sef′a-lō-mī′e-lō-sēl). Encefalomielocele; defeito congênito do crânio, geralmente na região occipital, e das vértebras cervicais com herniação das meninges e do tecido neural. [G. *enkephalos*, encéfalo, + *myelon*, medula óssea, + *kēlē*, hérnia]

en·ceph·a·lo·my·e·lo·neu·rop·a·thy (en-sef′a-lō-mī′e-lō-noo-rop′a-thē). Encefalomieloneuropatia; uma doença que acomete o encéfalo, a medula espinal e os nervos periféricos.

en·ceph·a·lo·my·e·lop·a·thy (en-sef′a-lō-mī-e-lop′a-thē). Encefalomielopatia; qualquer doença que acometa o encéfalo e a medula espinal. [G. *enkephalos*, encéfalo, + *myelon*, medula óssea, + *pathos*, que sofre]

carcinomatous e., e. carcinomatosa. SIN paraneoplastic e.

epidemic myalgic e., e. miálgica epidêmica; doença superficialmente semelhante à poliomielite, caracterizada por envolvimento difuso do sistema nervoso associado a mialgia.

necrotizing e. [MIM*256000], e. necrotizante. SIN Leigh *disease*.

paracarcinomatous e., e. paracarcinomatosa. SIN paraneoplastic e.

paraneoplastic e., e. paraneoplásica; e. como um efeito distante do carcinoma, na maioria das vezes carcinoma pulmonar de pequenas células; caracterizada por substancial perda das células nervosas, que pode ser difusa, mas freqüentemente predomina em partes específicas do sistema nervoso central, particularmente nos lobos límbicos, bulbo, cerebelo e substância cinzenta da medula espinal. SIN carcinomatous e., encephalomyelitis associated with carcinoma, paracarcinomatous e.

subacute necrotizing e. (SNE), e. necrotizante subaguda; um distúrbio fatal raro, basicamente de crianças, tendo início agudo e crônico, que se manifesta basicamente como disfunção do tronco cerebral, com ataxia, paralisias dos nervos cranianos, paralisia pseudobulbar, hemiplegia ou quadriplegia, deterioração mental e movimentos involuntários; foram constatadas deficiências de piruvato desidrogenase ou citocromo C oxidase em alguns pacientes; no exame histopatológico, há necrose simétrica disseminada envolvendo grande parte do tronco encefálico; essas alterações são semelhantes às observadas na encefalopatia de Wernicke.

en·ceph·a·lo·my·e·lo·ra·dic·u·li·tis (en-sef′a-lō-mī′e-lō-rā-dik′u-lī-tis). Encefalomielorradiculite. SIN encephalomyeloradiculopathy.

en·ceph·a·lo·my·e·lo·ra·dic·u·lop·a·thy (en-sef′a-lō-mī′e-lō-rā-dik′u-lop-ā-thē). Encefalomielorradiculopatia; processo mórbido que envolve o encéfalo, a medula espinal e as raízes espinais. SIN encephalomyeloradiculitis.

en·ceph·a·lo·my·o·car·di·tis (en-sef′a-lō-mī′o-kar-dī′tis). Encefalomiocardite; encefalite e miocardite associadas; freqüentemente causadas por uma infecção viral, como na poliomielite.

en·ceph·a·lon, pl. **en·ceph·a·la** (en-sef′a-lon, la) [TA]. Encéfalo; a parte do eixo cerebroespinal contida no crânio, composta do prosencéfalo, mesencéfalo e rombencéfalo. [G. *enkephalos*, encéfalo, de *en*, em, + *kephalē*, cabeça]

en·ceph·a·lo·path·ia (en-sef′a-lō-path′ē-a). Encefalopatia. SIN encephalopathy.

en·ceph·a·lop·a·thy (en-sef′a-lop′a-thē). Encefalopatia; qualquer distúrbio do encéfalo. SIN cerebropathia, cerebropathy, encephalopathia, encephalosis. [encephalo- + G. *pathos*, que sofre]

bilirubin e., e. por bilirrubina. SIN kernicterus.

Binswanger e., e. de Binswanger. SIN Binswanger *disease*.

bovine spongiform e. (BSE), e. espongiforme bovina (EEB); doença do gado bovino descrita pela primeira vez em 1986, na Grã-Bretanha; caracterizada clinicamente por comportamento apreensivo, hiperestesia e ataxia, e, histologicamente, por alterações espongiformes na substância cinzenta do tronco encefálico; causada por um príon, como as encefalopatias espongiformes de outros animais (p. ex., *scrapie*) e dos seres humanos (doença de Creutzfeldt-Jakob). VER Creutzfeldt-Jakob *disease*. SIN mad cow disease.

Em meados da década de 90, foi descrito um número incomum de casos de doença de Creutzfeldt-Jakob (DCJ) em pessoas com menos de 30 anos de idade na Grã-Bretanha. Esses pacientes exibiam manifestações clínicas típicas, mas não as alterações EEG características da DCJ, e amostras de necrópsia mostraram placas amilóides incomuns semelhantes às do kuru, mas não observadas antes na DCJ. Esses casos de variante da doença de Creutzfeldt-Jakob (V-DCJ) foram especulativamente associados a uma encefalopatia espongiforme epizoótica ou bovina (doença da vaca louca) que matou mais de 150.000 bois no Reino Unido entre 1986 e 1996. Embora a ligação entre EEB e V-DCJ não possa ser confirmada com base nos dados existentes, a simples possibilidade dessa ligação já levou ao desenvolvimento de recomendações para ajudar a reduzir ou evitar a ocorrência de EEB no gado bovino em todo o mundo. Não há evidências das atividades de supervisão norte-americanas nem dos estudos científicos que indiquem a existência de EEB nos Estados Unidos. Desde 1990, testes laboratoriais feitos em amostras de cérebros do gado bovino com sinais referentes ao SNC não mostraram evidências de EEB. Desde julho de 1989, o Departamento de Agricultura norte-americano proibiu a importação de carne e derivados bovinos do Reino Unido. De acordo com as estatísticas de mortalidade, a incidência anual de DCJ nos Estados Unidos permaneceu estável em aproximadamente 1 caso por milhão de pessoas entre 1979 e 1994. Consultores da OMS condenaram a prática de alimentar o gado com ração derivada de carne e osso de ruminantes e exigiram a adoção de medidas para garantir que nenhuma parte de qualquer animal com sinais de uma encefalopatia espongiforme entre em qualquer cadeia alimentar humana ou animal. Leite, laticínios, gelatina e banha são considerados seguros.

demyelinating e., e. desmielinizante; perda idiopática extensa das bainhas de mielina no encéfalo, como ocorre na leucodistrofia.

hepatic e., e. hepática. SIN portal-systemic e.

HIV e., e. por HIV. SIN AIDS dementia *complex*.

hypernatremic e., e. hipernatrêmica; derrames subaracnóides e subdurais em lactentes com desidratação hipernatrêmica.

hypertensive e., e. hipertensiva; encefalopatia metabólica causada por edema cerebral difuso; ocorre após a elevação abrupta da pressão arterial em um paciente hipertenso crônico.

hypoxic-hypercarbic e., e. hipóxica-hipercárbica. SIN hypoventilation *coma*.

hypoxic ischemic e., e. isquêmica hipóxica; lesão encefálica permanente devida à ausência de oxigênio ou fluxo sangüíneo adequado para o encéfalo.

lead e., e. plúmbica; encefalopatia metabólica, causada pela ingestão de compostos de chumbo e observada sobretudo nos primeiros anos de vida; é caracterizada, ao exame histopatológico, por edema cerebral extenso, condição esponjosa, neurocitólise e alguma inflamação reativa; as manifestações clínicas incluem convulsões, delírio e alucinações. VER TAMBÉM lead *poisoning*. SIN lead encephalitis, saturnine e.

metabolic e., e. metabólica; coma ou seus precursores resultantes de uma anormalidade difusa do metabolismo neuronal ou das células gliais cerebrais. A encefalopatia metabólica primária é causada por qualquer um dos distúrbios cerebrais degenerativos que culminam em coma; a encefalopatia metabólica secundária ocorre quando o metabolismo encefálico é perturbado por distúrbios extracerebrais que causam intoxicação, desequilíbrios eletrolíticos ou deficiências nutricionais, p. ex., doença hepática ou renal ou venenos exógenos.

necrotizing e., e. necrotizante. SIN Leigh *disease*.

palindromic e., e. palindrômica; uma forma relativamente leve que tende a recidivar.

pancreatic e., e. pancreática; encefalopatia metabólica associada a necrose pancreática extensa.

portal-systemic e., e. portossistêmica, e. hepática; e. associada à cirrose hepática, atribuída à passagem de substâncias nitrogenadas tóxicas da circulação porta para a circulação sistêmica; as manifestações cerebrais podem incluir coma. SIN hepatic *e*.

progressive subcortical e., e. subcortical progressiva. SIN progressive multifocal *leukoencephalopathy*.

pulmonary e., e. pulmonar. SIN hypoventilation *coma*.

recurrent e. [MIM*130950], e. recorrente; forma progressiva de e. que ocorre em jovens membros da mesma família; caracterizada por cefaléia, vertigem, ataxia do tronco, sonolência e torpor, comprometimento da fala, movimentos coreico-atetóides, e, algumas vezes, convulsões; provavelmente herança autossômica dominante.

saturnine e., e. saturnina. SIN lead e.

severe postanoxic e., e. pós-anóxica grave. SIN delayed *coma* after hypoxia.

spongiform e., e. espongiforme; e. caracterizada por vacuolização nas células nervosas e gliais.

subacute spongiform e., e. espongiforme subaguda; uma forma de encefalopatia espongiforme associada a um "vírus lento", que até hoje não foi descrito adequadamente; é contagiosa e tem uma evolução rapidamente progressiva, fatal; p. ex., doença de Creutzfeldt-Jakob, kuru, síndrome de Gerstmann-Sträussler, scrapie. VER prion.

subcortical arteriosclerotic e., e. arteriosclerótica subcortical. SIN Binswanger *disease*.

thyrotoxic e., e. tireotóxica; e. metabólica que ocorre em casos graves de tireotoxicose.

traumatic e., e. traumática; e. resultante de lesão estrutural do encéfalo.

traumatic progressive e., e. progressiva traumática; lesão encefálica progressiva crônica resultante de múltiplos traumatismos encefálicos, p. ex., demência pugilística.

Wernicke e., e. de Wernicke. SIN Wernicke *syndrome*.

Wernicke-Korsakoff e., e. de Wernicke-Korsakoff. VER Wernicke *syndrome*, Korsakoff *syndrome*.

en·ceph·a·lo·py·o·sis (en-sef′a-lo-pi-o′sis). Encefalopiose; termo arcaico para inflamação purulenta do encéfalo. [encephalo- + G. *pyosis*, supuração]

en·ceph·a·lor·rha·chid·i·an (en-sef′a-lo-ra-kid′e-an). Encefalorraquidiano. SIN cerebrospinal. [encephalo- + G. *rhachis*, coluna vertebral]

en·ceph·a·los·chi·sis (en-sef-a-los′ki-sis). Encefalosquise; ausência congênita do fechamento da parte rostral do tubo neural. [encephalo- + G. *schisis*, fissura]

en·ceph·a·lo·scle·ro·sis (en-sef′a-lo-skler-o′sis). Encefaloesclerose; esclerose, ou endurecimento, do encéfalo. VER TAMBÉM cerebrosclerosis. [encephalo- + G. *sklerosis*, endurecimento]

en·ceph·a·lo·scope (en-sef′a-lo-skop). Encefaloscópio; qualquer instrumento usado para ver o interior de um abscesso encefálico ou de outra cavidade cerebral através de uma abertura no crânio. [encephalo- + G. *skopeo*, ver]

en·ceph·a·los·co·py (en-sef-a-los′ko-pe). Encefaloscopia; exame do encéfalo ou da cavidade de um abscesso cerebral por inspeção direta.

en·ceph·a·lo·sis. Encefalose. SIN encephalopathy.

en·ceph·a·lo·spi·nal (en-sef′a-lo-spi′nal). Encefaloespinal. SIN cerebrospinal.

en·ceph·a·lo·tome (en-sef′a-lo-tom). Encefalótomo; instrumento para uso na realização de encefalotomia.

en·ceph·a·lot·o·my (en-sef-a-lot′o-me). Encefalotomia; dissecção ou incisão do encéfalo. [encephalo- + G. *tome*, incisão]

en·chon·dral (en-kon′dral). Encondral. SIN intracartilaginous.

en·chon·dro·ma (en-kon-dro′ma). Encondroma; crescimento cartilaginoso benigno que começa na cavidade medular de um osso originalmente formado a partir da cartilagem; os e. podem distender a cortical, principalmente de ossos pequenos, e podem ser solitários ou múltiplos (endocondromatose). [L. mod. do G. *en*, em, + *chondros*, cartilagem, + *-oma*, tumor]

en·chon·dro·ma·to·sis (en-kon′dro-ma-to′sis) [MIM*166000 *225795]. Encondromatose; distúrbio raro caracterizado por proliferação hamartomatosa de cartilagem nas metáfises de vários ossos, na maioria das vezes das mãos e pés, causando distorção do crescimento em comprimento e fraturas patológicas; pode haver desenvolvimento de condrossarcoma. Quando a e. está associada a hemangiomas nas regiões cutâneas ou viscerais, a condição é denominada síndrome de Maffucci (Maffucci *syndrome*). A maioria dos casos é esporádica, mas alguns têm herança autossômica dominante com penetrância reduzida. SIN asymmetric chondrodystrophy, dyschondroplasia, hereditary deforming chondrodystrophy (2), Ollier disease.

en·chon·drom·a·tous (en-kon-dro′ma-tus). Encondromatoso; relativo a, ou que possui, os elementos de encondroma.

en·clave (en-klav, ahn-klahv′). Inclusão; massa destacada de tecido encerrada em tecido de outro tipo; observada sobretudo no caso de massas isoladas de tecido glandular destacadas da glândula principal. [Fr. do L. *clavis*, chave]

en·cod·ing (en-kod′ing). Codificação; o primeiro estágio no processo de memória, seguido por armazenamento e retirada, envolvendo processos associados à recepção ou breve registro de estímulos através de um ou mais dos sentidos e modificação daquela informação; um processo de decaimento ou perda dessa informação (um tipo de esquecimento) ocorre rapidamente, exceto se os dois estágios subseqüentes, armazenamento e recuperação, forem ativados.

en·cop·re·sis (en-ko-pre′sis). Encoprese; a eliminação repetida, geralmente involuntária, de fezes em locais impróprios (p. ex., roupa). [G. *enkopros*, cheio de fezes]

en·cra·ni·al (en-kra′ne-al). Endocraniano. SIN endocranial.

en·cra·ni·us (en-kra′ne-us). Encrânio; em gêmeos conjugados, uma forma de inclusão fetal na qual o parasita menor vive parcial ou totalmente dentro da cavidade craniana do autósito maior. [G. *en*, em, + *kranion*, crânio]

encu Acrônimo para equivalent *normal child unit* (unidade equivalente da criança normal), aquelas informações de qualquer fonte (análise de ligação, fenótipos parentais e colaterais, bioquímica do estado de portador, etc.) que terão o mesmo impacto sobre a probabilidade de, em uma prole habitual, um consulente ser portador de um traço autossômico dominante; p. ex., cada criança normal contribui com um encu. Cf. ensu.

en·cyst·ed (en-sis′ted). Encistado; encapsulado por um saco membranoso. [G. *kystis*, bexiga]

en·cyst·ment (en-sist′ment). Encistamento; a condição de ser ou se tornar encistado.

end. Uma extremidade, ou o ponto mais distante de uma extremidade.

acromial e. of clavicle [TA], e. acromial da clavícula; a extremidade lateral achatada da clavícula que se articula com o acrômio e está fixada ao processo coracóide pelos ligamentos conóide e trapezóide. SIN extremitas acromialis claviculae [TA], acromial extremity of clavicle.

distal e., e. distal; a extremidade posterior de um aparelho odontológico. SIN heel (3) [TA].

fixed e. [TA], e. fixa; para determinado movimento, a extremidade de um osso que é mantida imóvel (em conseqüência de fixação muscular), enquanto a outra extremidade do osso (a extremidade móvel) se movimenta em resposta à atividade do músculo ou gravidade. SIN punctum fixa [TA].

mobile e. [TA], e. móvel; para determinado movimento, a extremidade de um osso que se move em resposta à atividade muscular ou gravidade, enquanto a outra extremidade do osso (a extremidade fixa) é mantida imóvel (em virtude de fixação muscular). SIN punctum mobile [TA].

sternal e. of clavicle, e. esternal da clavícula; a extremidade medial alargada da clavícula que se articula com o manúbrio esternal. SIN extremitas sternalis claviculae [TA], sternal extremity of clavicle.

end-. VER endo-.

end·a·del·phos (end′a-del′fos). Endadelfo; gêmeos conjugados desiguais nos quais o membro parasita está incluído no corpo do hospedeiro. [end- + G. *adelphos*, irmão]

End·a·moe·ba (end′a-me′ba). Gênero de amebas parasitas em invertebrados; originalmente descrito em baratas. [endo- + G. *amoibe*, alteração]

end·an·gi·i·tis, end·an·ge·i·tis (end-an-je-i′tis). Endangeíte; inflamação da túnica íntima de um vaso sanguíneo. SIN endoangiitis, endovasculitis. [endo- + G. *angeion*, vaso, + *-itis*, inflamação]

e. obliterans, e. obliterante; inflamação da túnica íntima de um vaso com conseqüente oclusão de sua luz.

end·a·or·ti·tis (end′a-or-ti′tis). Endaortite; inflamação da túnica íntima da aorta. SIN endo-aortitis.

end·ar·ter·ec·to·my (end-ar-ter-ek′to-me). Endarterectomia; excisão de depósitos ateromatosos juntamente com o endotélio doente e a túnica média ou a maior parte da túnica média de uma artéria de forma a deixar um revestimento liso, que consiste principalmente na adventícia. [endo- + artery + G. *ektome*, excisão]

carotid e., e. carotídea; excisão de material oclusivo, incluindo a túnica íntima e a maior parte da túnica média, da artéria carótida.

coronary e., e. coronariana; excisão de material oclusor, incluindo a túnica íntima e a maior parte da túnica média, da artéria coronária.

end·ar·te·ri·tis (end′ar-ter-i′tis). Endarterite; inflamação da túnica íntima de uma artéria. SIN endoarteritis.

bacterial e., e. bacteriana; implantação e crescimento de bactérias com for-

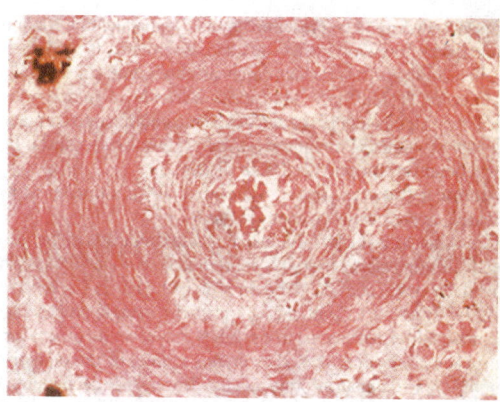

endangiite: observe o estreitamento da luz do vaso por espessamento fibroso

mação de vegetações na parede arterial, como pode ocorrer em um canal arterial persistente ou em uma fístula arteriovenosa.
  e. defor'mans, e. deformante; endarterite com placas ateromatosas e depósitos calcários.
  e. oblit'erans, obliterating e., e. obliterante; um grau extremo de endarterite proliferativa fechando a luz arterial. SIN arteritis obliterans, obliterating arteritis.
  e. prolif'erans, proliferating e., e. proliferante; endarterite crônica acompanhada por um aumento acentuado do tecido fibroso na túnica íntima.
end·au·ral (end - aw'răl). Endaural; dentro da orelha. [endo- + L. *auris*, orelha]
end·brain. Telencéfalo. SIN telencephalon.
end-brush (end'brŭsh). Telodendro. SIN telodendron.
end-bulb. Bulbo terminal. VER end *bulb*.
end-di·a·stol·ic (end'dī - ă - stol'ik). Diastólico final, telediastólico. **1.** Que ocorre no fim da diástole, imediatamente antes da próxima sístole, como na pressão diastólica final. **2.** Que interrompe os momentos finais da diástole, quase prematuro, como na extra-sístole diastólica final.
endectocide. Endectocida; uma substância efetiva contra endoparasitas e ectoparasitas, p. ex., o antibiótico macrolídeo avermectina. VER TAMBÉM ivermectin. [*endo*parasite + *ecto*parasite + -cide]
en·de·mia (en - dē'mē - ă). Endemia; termo obsoleto para uma doença endêmica.
en·dem·ic (en-dem'ik). Endêmico; designa um padrão temporal de ocorrência da doença em uma população na qual a doença ocorre com regularidade previsível apenas com flutuações relativamente pequenas em sua freqüência com o decorrer do tempo. Cf. epidemic, sporadic. SIN enzootic. [G. *endēmos*, nativo, de *en*, em, + *dēmos*, o povo]
en·dem·o·ep·i·dem·ic (en - dem'ō - ep - i - dem'ik). Endemoepidêmico; designa um grande aumento temporário do número de casos de uma doença endêmica.
end·er·gon·ic (en-der-gon'ik). Endergônico; referente a uma reação química que ocorre com absorção de energia do meio ambiente (isto é, uma alteração positiva na energia livre de Gibbs). Cf. exergonic. [endo- + G. *ergon*, trabalho]
en·der·mic, en·der·mat·ic (en-der'mik, en-der-mat'ik). Endérmico; dentro ou através da pele; designa um método de tratamento, como por inunção; o remédio produz seu efeito constitucional quando absorvido através da superfície cutânea à qual é aplicado. [G. *en*, em, + *derma* (*dermat*-), pele]
en·der·mo·sis (en - der - mō'sis). Endermose; qualquer doença eruptiva da mucosa.
end-feet. Terminações axônicas. SIN axon *terminals,* em *terminal.*
end-gut. Intestino posterior. SIN hindgut.
end·ing. Terminação. **1.** Um fim ou conclusão. **2.** Uma t. nervosa.
  annulospiral e., t. anulospiral; um dentre dois tipos de t. nervosa sensorial associada a um fuso neuromuscular (sendo o outro a terminação em ramalhete de flores); após entrar no fuso muscular, a fibra se divide em dois ramos planos, semelhantes a fitas, que se enrolam em anéis ou espirais ao redor das fibras musculares intrafusais. SIN annulospiral organ.
  calyciform e., caliciform e., t. caliciforme; uma t. sináptica em relação a determinadas células pilosas neuroepiteliais da orelha interna.
  epilemmal e., t. epilêmica; uma t. nervosa em íntima relação com a superfície externa do sarcolema.
  flower-spray e., t. em ramalhete de flores; um dos dois tipos de t. nervosa sensitiva associada ao fuso neuromuscular (sendo o outro a terminação anulospiral); nesse tipo, os ramos da fibra se espalham sobre a superfície das fibras intrafusais como um ramalhete de flores. SIN flower-spray organ of Ruffini.
  free nerve e.'s, terminações nervosas livres; uma forma de t. periférica de fibras nervosas sensoriais na qual os filamentos terminais acabam livremente no tecido. SIN terminationes nervorum liberae.
  grape e.'s, terminações em parreira; um termo autodescritivo aplicado às terminações sinápticas nas extremidades dos ramos axonais curtos, semelhantes a pedículos.
  hederiform e., t. hederiforme; um tipo de t. sensorial livre na pele.
  nerve e., t. nervosa; qualquer uma das t. especializadas das fibras nervosas sensoriais ou motoras periféricas. VER motor *endplate*, corpuscle, bulb.
  sole-plate e., placa terminal motora. SIN motor *endplate.*
  synaptic e.'s, terminações sinápticas. SIN axon *terminals,* em *terminal.*
Endo, Shigeru, bacteriologista japonês, 1869–1937. VER E. *agar, medium.*
endo-, end-. Prefixos que indicam dentro, interno, que absorve ou que contém. VER TAMBÉM ento-. [G. *endon*, dentro]
en·do·ab·dom·i·nal (en'dō - ab - dom'i - năl). Endoabdominal; dentro do abdome.
en·do·am·y·lase (en'dō - am'il - ās). Endoamilase; uma glucanoidrolase que atua nas ligações glicosídicas internas (p. ex., α-amilase).
en·do·an·eu·rys·mo·plas·ty (en'dō - an - ū - riz'mō - plas - tē). Endoaneurismoplastia. SIN aneurysmoplasty.
en·do·an·eu·rys·mor·rha·phy (en'dō - an - ū - riz - mōr'ă - fē). Endoaneurismorrafia. SIN aneurysmoplasty. [endo- + G. *aneurysma,* aneurisma, + *rhaphē,* sutura]
en·do·an·gi·i·tis (en'dō - an - jē - ī'tis). Endoangiite. SIN endangiitis.
en·do·a·or·ti·tis (en'dō - ā - ōr - tī'tis). Endoaortite. SIN endaortitis.
en·do·ap·pen·di·ci·tis (en'dō - ă - pen - di - sī'tis). Endoapendicite; inflamação catarral simples, limitada de forma mais ou menos rigorosa à superfície mucosa do apêndice vermiforme.
en·do·ar·te·ri·tis (en'dō - ar - ter - ī'tis). Endoarterite. SIN endarteritis.
en·do·aus·cul·ta·tion (en'dō - aws - kŭl - tā'shŭn). Endoausculta; ausculta dos órgãos torácicos, principalmente do coração, por meio de um tubo estetoscópico introduzido no esôfago ou no coração.
en·do·bag. Endossaco. SIN endosac.
en·do·ba·si·on (en'dō - bā'sē - on). Endobásio; um ponto cefalométrico e craniométrico localizado na linha média no ponto mais posterior da borda anterior do forame magno no contorno do forame; situa-se discretamente posterior e interno ao básio.
en·do·bi·ot·ic (en - dō - bī - ot'ik). Endobiótico; que vive como um parasita no hospedeiro.
en·do·bron·chi·al (en - dō - brong'kē - ăl). Endobrônquico. SIN intrabronchial.
en·do·car·di·ac, en·do·car·di·al (en - dō - kar'dē - ak, - dē - ăl). Endocardíaco. **1.** SIN intracardiac. **2.** Relativo ao endocárdio.
en·do·car·di·og·ra·phy (en'dō - kar - dē - og'ră - fē). Endocardiografia; eletrocardiografia com o eletrodo explorador dentro das câmaras cardíacas. VER TAMBÉM intracardiac *catheter.*
en·do·car·dit·ic (en'dō - kar - dit'ik). Endocardítico; relativo à endocardite.
en·do·car·di·tis (en'dō - kar - dī'tis). Endocardite; inflamação do endocárdio. SIN encarditis.
  abacterial thrombotic e., e. trombótica abacteriana. SIN nonbacterial thrombotic e.
  acute bacterial e., e. bacteriana aguda; um tipo de e. bacteriana grave causada por organismos piogênicos, tais como estreptococos hemolíticos ou estafilococos.
  atypical verrucous e., e. verrucosa atípica. SIN Libman-Sacks e.
  bacterial e., e. bacteriana; endocardite causada pela invasão direta de bactérias, e que leva à deformidade e destruição das válvulas. Dois tipos são endocardite bacteriana aguda e endocardite bacteriana subaguda.
  cachectic e., e. caquética. SIN nonbacterial thrombotic e.
  e. chorda'lis, e. das cordas tendíneas; endocardite que afeta particularmente as cordas tendíneas.
  constrictive e., e. constritiva; espessamento do endocárdio devido a inflamação de qualquer origem que restringe o relaxamento diastólico de um ou de ambos os ventrículos, produzindo insuficiência ventricular diastólica, p. ex., endocardite fibroplástica de Löffler.
  infectious e., infective e., e. infecciosa; e. causada por infecção por microrganismos.
  isolated parietal e., e. parietal isolada; espessamento fibroso do endocárdio ventricular esquerdo sem envolvimento valvar.
  Libman-Sacks e., e. de Libman-Sacks; e. verrucosa algumas vezes associada ao lúpus eritematoso disseminado. SIN atypical verrucous e., Libman-Sacks syndrome, nonbacterial verrucous e.
  Löffler e., e. de Löffler; e. parietal constritiva fibroplásica com eosinofilia, uma e. de causa obscura caracterizada por insuficiência cardíaca congestiva progressiva, múltiplos êmbolos sistêmicos e eosinofilia. SIN Löffler disease, Löffler syndrome (2).
  Löffler parietal fibroplastic e., e. fibroplásica parietal de Löffler; esclerose do endocárdio associada a numerosos eosinófilos.
  malignant e., e. maligna; e. bacteriana aguda, geralmente secundária à supuração em outra parte e que tem um curso fulminante. SIN septic e.

marantic e., e. marântica; e. trombótica não-bacteriana associada ao câncer e a outras doenças debilitantes. Cf. terminal e.
mural e., e. mural; inflamação do endocárdio envolvendo as paredes das câmaras cardíacas.
mycotic e., e. micótica; endocardite causada por infecção fúngica.
nonbacterial thrombotic e., e. trombótica não-bacteriana; lesões endocárdicas verrucosas que ocorrem nos estágios terminais de muitas doenças infecciosas e consuntivas crônicas. SIN abacterial thrombotic e., cachectic e., terminal e., thromboendocarditis.
nonbacterial verrucous e., e. verrucosa não-bacteriana. SIN Libman-Sacks e.
polypous e., e. poliposa; e. bacteriana com formação de massas pediculadas de fibrina ou trombos fixados às valvas ulceradas.
rheumatic e., e. reumática; envolvimento endocárdico como parte da cardiopatia reumática, reconhecido clinicamente por envolvimento valvar; no estágio agudo, pode haver pequenas vegetações de fibrina ao longo das linhas de fechamento das valvas, com subseqüente espessamento fibroso e encurtamento dos folhetos.
septic e., e. séptica. SIN malignant e.
subacute bacterial e. (SBE), e. bacteriana subaguda; endocardite de menor gravidade que a endocardite bacteriana aguda.
terminal e., e. terminal. SIN nonbacterial thrombotic e.
valvular e., e. valvar; inflamação limitada ao endocárdio das valvas.
vegetative e., verrucous e., e. vegetativa, e. verrucosa; e. associada à presença de coágulos de fibrina (vegetações) que se formam nas superfícies ulceradas das valvas.

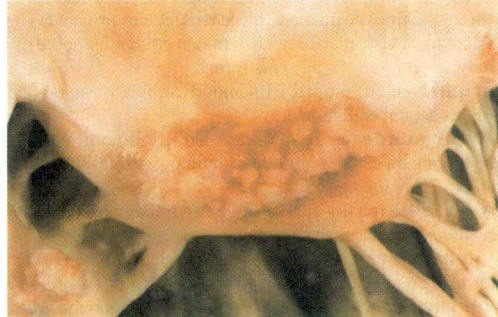

endocardite vegetativa: (mostrada aqui na valva mitral)

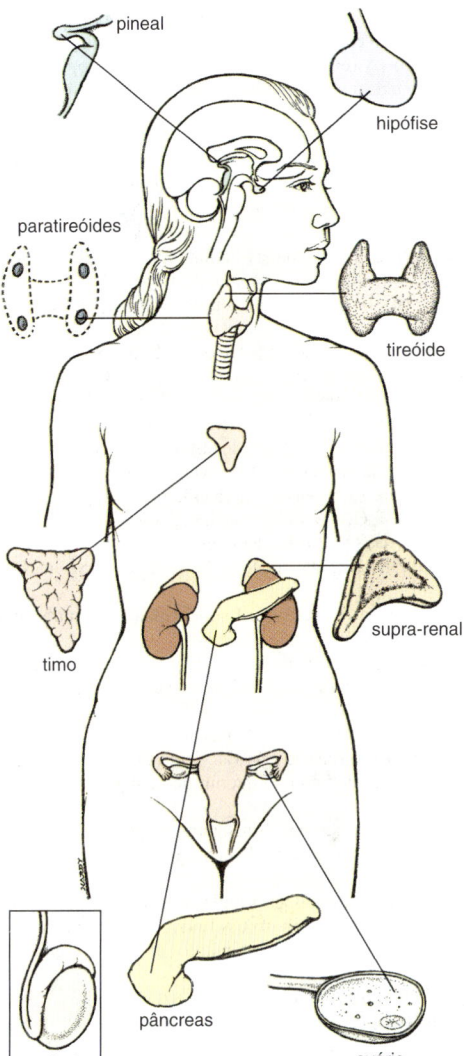

sistema endócrino: mostrando vários órgãos endócrinos

en·do·car·di·um, pl. **en·do·car·dia** (en - dō - kar′dē - ŭm, - ē - ă) [TA]. Endocárdio; a túnica mais interna do coração, que inclui o endotélio e o tecido conjuntivo subendotelial; na parede atrial, também há músculo liso e numerosas fibras elásticas. [endo- + G. *kardia*, coração]
en·do·ce·li·ac (en - dō - sē′lē - ak). Endocelíaco; dentro de uma das cavidades corporais. [endo- + G. *koilia*, cavidade, ventrículo]
en·do·cer·vi·cal (en′dō - ser′vi - kăl). Endocervical. **1.** Dentro de qualquer cérvice, especificamente dentro da cérvice uterina. SIN intracervical. **2.** Relacionado à endocérvice.
en·do·cer·vi·ci·tis (en′dō - ser - vi - sī′tis). Endocervicite; inflamação do epitélio colunar do colo uterino.
en·do·cer·vix (en - dō - ser′viks). Endocérvice; a mucosa do canal cervical.
en·do·chon·dral (en - dō - kon′drăl). Endocondral. SIN intracartilaginous. [endo- + G. *chondros*, cartilagem]
en·do·co·ag·u·la·tion (en - dō - kō - ag - oo - lā′shun). Endocoagulação. SIN thermocoagulation.
en·do·co·li·tis (en′dō - kō - lī′tis). Endocolite; inflamação catarral simples do cólon.
en·do·cra·ni·al (en - dō - krā′nē - ăl). Endocranial. **1.** Dentro do crânio. **2.** Relativo ao endocrânio. SIN encranial, entocranial.
en·do·cra·ni·um (en′dō - krā′nē - ŭm). Endocrânio; a membrana de revestimento do crânio, ou dura-máter do encéfalo. SIN entocranium.
en·do·crine (en′dō - krin). Endócrino. **1.** Que secreta internamente, na maioria das vezes para a circulação sistêmica; de, ou relativo a, essa secreção. Cf. paracrine. **2.** A secreção interna ou hormonal de uma glândula sem ducto. **3.** Designa uma glândula que fornece uma secreção interna. [endo- + G. *krinō*, separar]
en·do·cri·nol·o·gist (en′dō - kri - nol′ō - jist). Endocrinologista; aquele que se especializa em endocrinologia.
en·do·cri·nol·o·gy (en′dō - kri - nol′ō - jē). Endocrinologia; a ciência e a especialidade médica relacionadas às secreções internas ou hormonais e suas relações fisiológicas e patológicas. [endocrine + G. *logos*, estudo]
en·do·cri·no·ma (en′dō - kri - nō′mă). Endocrinoma; termo obsoleto para um tumor com tecido endócrino que conserva a função do órgão de origem, geralmente em grau excessivo.
en·do·crin·o·path·ic (en′dō - kri - nō - path′ik). Endocrinopático; relativo a, ou que sofre de, uma endocrinopatia.
en·do·cri·nop·a·thy (en′dō - kri - nop′a - thē). Endocrinopatia; distúrbio na função de uma glândula endócrina e suas conseqüências. [endocrine + G. *pathos*, doença]
en·do·cri·no·ther·a·py (en′dō - kri - nō - thār′a - pē). Endocrinoterapia; tratamento de doença pela administração de extratos de glândulas endócrinas. [endocrine + G. *therapeia*, tratamento médico]
en·do·cy·clic (en - dō - sī′klik, - sik′lik). Endocíclico; dentro de um ciclo ou anel; p. ex., os seis átomos de carbono do anel benzeno no tolueno. Cf. exocyclic.
en·do·cyst (en′dō - sist). Endocisto; a camada interna de um cisto hidático.
en·do·cys·ti·tis (en′dō - sis - tī′tis). Endocistite; termo obsoleto para inflamação do revestimento epitelial da bexiga. [endo- + G. *kystis*, bexiga, + -*itis*, inflamação]
en·do·cy·to·sis (en′dō - sī - tō′sis). Endocitose; internalização de substâncias do meio extracelular através da formação de vesículas a partir da membrana plasmática. Há duas formas: (a) fase líquida (pinocitose) e (b) mediada por receptor. VER TAMBÉM phagocytosis. Cf. exocytosis (2). [endo- + G. *kytos*, célula, + -*osis*, condição]
en·do·derm (en′dō - derm). Endoderma; a camada mais interna das três camadas germinativas primárias do embrião (ectoderma, mesoderma, endoderma); dele deriva o revestimento epitelial do trato intestinal primitivo e o componente epitelial das glândulas e outras estruturas (p. ex., sistema respiratório inferior) que se desenvolvem como crescimentos do tubo intestinal. SIN entoderm. [endo- + G. *derma*, pele]

en·do·di·a·scope (en′dō-dī′a-skōp). Endodiascópio; um tubo de raios X que pode ser colocado em uma cavidade do corpo; um dispositivo arcaico.

en·do·di·as·co·py (en′dō-dī-as′kō-pē). Endodiascopia; visualização radiológica por meio de um endodiascópio; um procedimento arcaico. [endo- + G. *dia*, através, + *skopeō*, ver]

en·do·don·tia (en-dō-don′shē-a). Endodontia. SIN endodontics.

en·do·don·tics (en-dō-don′tiks). Endodontia; campo da odontologia relacionado com a biologia e patologia da polpa dental e dos tecidos periapicais, e com a prevenção, diagnóstico e tratamento de doenças e lesões nesses tecidos. SIN endodontia, endodontology. [endo- + G. *odous*, dente]

en·do·don·tist (en-dō-don′tist). Endodontista; aquele que se especializa na prática da endodontia. SIN endodontologist.

en·do·don·tol·o·gist (en′dō-don-tol′ō-jist). Endodontologista. SIN endodontist.

en·do·don·tol·o·gy (en′dō-don-tol′ō-jē). Endodontologia. SIN endodontics.

en·do·dy·o·cyte (en′dō-dī′ō-sīt). Endodiócito. **1.** Trofozoíta formado por endodiogenia. **2.** SIN merozoite. [endo- + G. *dys*, dois, + *kytos*, célula]

en·do·dy·og·e·ny (en′dō-dī-oj′e-nē). Endodiogenia; processo de desenvolvimento assexuado observado em determinados coccídios, como *Toxoplasma* e *Frenkelia*, no qual não ocorre divisão nuclear separada, como na esquizogonia; as duas filhas se desenvolvem internamente no genitor, sem conjugação nuclear. [endo- + G. *dys*, dois, + *genesis*, criação]

en·do·en·ter·i·tis (en′dō-en-ter-ī′tis). Endoenterite; termo obsoleto para inflamação da mucosa intestinal. [endo- + G. *enteron*, intestino, *-itis*, inflamação]

en·do·en·zyme (en-dō-en′zīm). Endoenzima. **1.** SIN intracellular *enzyme*. **2.** Enzima que catalisa uma endo-hidrólise.

en·do·e·soph·a·gi·tis (en′dō-ē-sof-a-jī′tis). Endoesofagite; termo obsoleto para inflamação do revestimento interno do esôfago.

en·do·far·a·dism (en-dō-far′a-dizm). Endofaradismo; aplicação de uma corrente elétrica alternada no interior de qualquer cavidade do corpo. VER fulguration.

en·do·gal·va·nism (en-dō-gal′van-izm). Endogalvanismo; aplicação de uma corrente elétrica direta no interior de qualquer cavidade do corpo. VER fulguration.

en·dog·a·my (en-dog′a-mē). Endogamia; reprodução por conjugação entre células-irmãs, os descendentes de uma célula original. [endo- + G. *gamos*, casamento]

en·do·gas·tric (en-dō-gas′trik). Endogástrico; dentro do estômago.

en·do·gas·tri·tis (en′dō-gas-trī′tis). Endogastrite; termo obsoleto para designar inflamação da mucosa do estômago. [endo- + G. *gastēr*, estômago, + *-itis*, inflamação]

en·do·gen·ic (en-dō-jen′ik). Endógeno. SIN endogenous.

en·do·ge·note (en-dō-jē′nōt). Endogenota; em genética microbiana, o genoma da célula receptora. [endo- + genote]

en·dog·e·nous (en-doj′ē-nŭs). Endógeno; que se origina, ou é produzido, dentro do organismo ou de uma de suas partes. SIN endogenic. [endo- + G. *-gen*, produção]

endo·glin (en′dō-glin). Endoglina; uma proteína, na superfície das células endoteliais, que se liga ao fator transformador do crescimento β (TGF-β).

en·do·gnath·i·on (en-dog-nath′ē-on, en-dō-nā′thē-on). Endognátio; a parte medial dos dois segmentos que constituem o osso incisivo. VER mesognathion. [endo- + G. *gnathos*, mandíbula]

en·do·her·ni·ot·o·my (en′dō-her-nē-ot′ō-mē). Endo-herniotomia; procedimento obsoleto para fechamento, por fios de sutura, do revestimento interior de um saco herniário.

en·do·in·tox·i·ca·tion (en′dō-in-tok-si-kā′shŭn). Endointoxicação; intoxicação por uma toxina endógena.

en·do·la·ryn·ge·al (en′dō-la-rin′jē-al). Endolaríngeo; dentro da laringe.

En·do·li·max (en-dō-lī′maks). Gênero de pequenas amebas não-patogênicas parasitas do intestino grosso dos seres humanos e de outros animais. [endo- + G. *leimax*, uma campina ou jardim]

en·do·lith (en′dō-lith). Endólito; corpo calcificado encontrado na câmara pulpar de um dente; pode ser composto de dentina irregular (dentículo verdadeiro) ou devido à calcificação ectópica de tecido pulpar (dentículo falso). SIN denticle (1), pulp calcification, pulp calculus, pulp nodule, pulp stone. [endo- + G. *lithos*, pedra]

en·do·lymph (en′dō-limf) [TA]. Endolinfa; o líquido contido no labirinto membranáceo da orelha interna; a endolinfa tem composição semelhante à do líquido intracelular (o potássio é o principal íon positivo). SIN endolympha [TA], Scarpa fluid, Scarpa liquor.

en·do·lym·pha (en′dō-lim′fa) [TA]. Endolinfa. SIN endolymph. [endo- + L. *lympha*, um líquido claro]

en·do·lym·phic (en-dō-lim′fik). Endolínfico; relativo à endolinfa.

en·do·me·rog·o·ny (en′dō-me-rog′ō-nē). Endomerogonia; produção de merozoítas na reprodução assexuada de protozoários esporozoários por um processo que se origina no interior do esquizonte (em contraste com a ectomerogonia); observada em espécies de *Eimeria*. [endo- + G. *meros*, parte, + *gonē*, geração]

en·do·me·tria (en-dō-mē′trē-a). Endométrios; plural de endometrium.

en·do·me·tri·al (en-dō-mē′trē-al). Endometrial; relativo a, ou composto de, endométrio.

en·do·me·tri·oid (en-dō-mē′trē-oyd). Endometrióide; microscopicamente semelhante ao tecido endometrial.

en·do·me·tri·o·ma (en′dō-mē-trē-ō′ma). Endometrioma; massa circunscrita de tecido endometrial ectópico na endometriose. [endometrium + *-oma*, tumor]

en·do·me·tri·o·sis (en′dō-mē-trē-ō′sis). Endometriose; ocorrência ectópica de tecido endometrial, freqüentemente formando cistos que contêm sangue alterado. SIN endometrial implants. [endometrium + *-osis*, condição]

en·do·me·tri·tis (en′dō-mē-trī′tis). Endometrite; inflamação do endométrio. [endometrium + *-itis*, inflamação]
  decidual e., e. decidual; inflamação da mucosa decidual do útero grávido.
  e. dis'secans, e. dissecante; endometrite com ulceração e esfoliação da mucosa.

en·do·me·tri·um, pl. **en·do·me·tria** (en′dō-mē′trē-ŭm, -trē-a) [TA]. Endométrio; a mucosa que forma a camada interna da parede uterina; consiste em um epitélio colunar simples e uma lâmina própria que contém glândulas uterinas tubulares simples. A estrutura, a espessura e o estado do endométrio sofrem alteração significativa com o ciclo menstrual. SIN tunica mucosa uteri [TA]. [endo- + G. *mētra*, útero]
  Swiss cheese e., e. em queijo suíço. SIN simple endometrial *hyperplasia*.

en·do·me·tro·pic (en′dō-mē-trop′ik). Endometrópico; indica um estímulo externo capaz de produzir uma resposta do útero, especificamente do endométrio. [endo- + G. *mētra*, útero, + *tropē*, volta]

en·do·mi·to·sis (en′dō-mī-tō′sis). Endomitose. SIN endopolyploidy.

en·do·morph (en′dō-mōrf). Endomorfo; tipo ou construção constitucional (biotipo ou somatotipo) no qual prevalecem os tecidos originados no endoderma; de um ponto de vista morfológico, o tronco predomina sobre os membros. SIN brachytype. [endo- + G. *morphē*, forma]

en·do·mor·phic (en′dō-mōr′fik). Endomórfico; relativo a, ou que possui as características de, um endomorfo.

en·do·mo·tor·sonde (en′dō-mō′tor-sond′). Endomotorsonda; cápsula radiotelemétrica para estudar o interior do trato gastrointestinal. [endo- + L. *motor*, motor, + Fr. *sonde*, sonda]

En·do·my·ce·ta·les (en′dō-mī-sē-ta′lēz). Ordem de Ascomycota que inclui as leveduras. SIN Saccharomycetales.

en·do·my·o·car·di·al (en′dō-mī-ō-kar′dē-al). Endomiocárdico; relativo ao endocárdio e ao miocárdio.

en·do·my·o·car·di·tis (en′dō-mī′ō-kar-dī′tis). Endomiocardite; inflamação do endocárdio e do miocárdio; endêmica no leste da África.

en·do·my·o·me·tri·tis (en′dō-mī-ō-mē-trī′tis). Endomiometrite; sépsis envolvendo os tecidos uterinos. [endo- + G. *mys*, músculo, + *mētra*, útero, + *-itis*, inflamação]

en·do·mys·i·um (en′dō-miz′ē-ŭm, -mis′ē-ŭm) [TA]. Endomísio; a bainha de tecido conjuntivo fina que circunda uma fibra muscular. [endo- + G. *mys*, músculo]

en·do·neu·ri·um (en-dō-noo′rē-ŭm) [TA]. Endoneuro; a estrutura de sustentação de tecido conjuntivo mais interna dos troncos nervosos, que circunda fibras nervosas mielinizadas e não-mielinizadas; consiste principalmente em substância fundamental, colágeno e fibroblastos; com o perineuro e o epineuro, forma o estroma do nervo periférico. SIN Henle sheath, sheath of Key and Retzius. [endo- + G. *neuron*, nervo]

en·do·nu·cle·ase (en-dō-noo′klē-ās). Endonuclease; uma enzima (fosfodiesterase) que cliva as ligações fosfodiéster internas em uma molécula de DNA, assim produzindo fragmentos de DNA de vários tamanhos. Cf. exonuclease.
  micrococcal e., e. micrócica; uma enzima, produzida por um membro do gênero *Micrococcus*, que cliva ácidos nucleicos em oligonucleotídeos terminando em 3′-fosfatos. SIN micrococcal nuclease, spleen e., spleen phosphodiesterases.
  nucleate e., e. nucleada. SIN endonuclease *Serratia marcescens*.
  restriction e., e. de restrição; uma de muitas e. isoladas de bactérias que clivam ou hidrolisam (cortam) cadeias de DNA com duplo filamento estranhas em locais de reconhecimento específicos definidos por seqüências de DNA; essas endonucleases tornaram-se dispositivos laboratoriais padronizados para fazer cortes específicos no DNA como uma primeira etapa na dedução de seqüências, sendo algumas vezes denominadas "bisturis químicos"; geralmente são designadas por uma abreviação de três ou quatro letras do nome do organismo do qual foram isoladas (p. ex., EcoB de *Escherichia coli*, cepa B). SIN restriction enzyme.
  single-stranded nucleate e., e. nuclear monofilamentar; endonuclease S_1 *Aspergillus*.
  spleen e., e. esplênica. SIN micrococcal e.

en·do·nu·cle·ase S_1 *As·per·gil·lus*. Endonuclear nuclear monofilamentar; uma enzima que cliva RNA ou DNA em mono- ou oligonucleotídeos de extremidade 5′; prefere ácidos polinucleicos monofilamentares. SIN deoxyribonuclease S_1.

en·do·nu·cle·ase Ser·ra·tia mar·ces·cens. Endonuclease *Serratia marcescens*; uma nuclease (uma oligonucleotidoidrolase nuclear) que forma oligonucleotídeos que terminam em 5′-fosfatos de RNA e DNA; hidrolisa tanto ácidos polinucleicos de duplo filamento como os monofilamentares. SIN nucleate endonuclease.

en·do·nu·cle·o·lus (en′dō - noo - klē′ō - lŭs). Endonucléolo; um pequeno ponto não-corável próximo do centro de um nucléolo.

en·do·par·a·site (en - dō - par′a - sit). Endoparasita; um parasita que vive no corpo de seu hospedeiro.

en·do·pep·ti·dase (en - dō - pep′ti - dās). Endopeptidase; enzima que catalisa a hidrólise de uma cadeia peptídica em pontos centrais da cadeia, não-próximos das extremidades; p. ex., pepsina, tripsina. Cf. exopeptidase. SIN proteinase.

en·do·per·i·ar·te·ri·tis (en′dō - pār′i - ar - ter - i′tis). Endoperiarterite. SIN panarteritis. [endo- + G. *peri*, ao redor, + arteritis]

en·do·per·i·car·di·ac (en′dō - pār - ē - kar′dē - ak). Endopericardíaco. SIN intrapericardiac.

en·do·per·i·my·o·car·di·tis (en′dō - pār′i - mī′ō - kar - dī′tis). Endoperimiocardite; inflamação simultânea do músculo cardíaco e do endocárdio e pericárdio. SIN pancarditis. [endo- + G. *peri*, ao redor, + *mys*, músculo, + *kardia*, coração, + -*itis*, inflamação]

en·do·per·i·to·ni·tis (en′dō - pār′i - tō - nī′tis). Endoperitonite; inflamação superficial do peritônio.

en·do·per·ox·ide (en′dō - per - ok′sīd). Endoperóxido; um grupamento peróxido (–O–O–) unindo dois átomos que fazem parte de uma molécula maior.

en·do·phle·bi·tis (en′dō - fle - bī′tis). Endoflebite; inflamação da túnica íntima de uma veia. [endo- + G. *phleps* (*phleb*-), veia, + -*itis*, inflamação]

en·doph·thal·mi·tis (en - dof - thal - mī′tis). Endoftalmite; inflamação dos tecidos no bulbo do olho. [endo- + G. *ophthalmos*, olho, + -*itis*, inflamação]
 granulomatous e., e. granulomatosa; uma inflamação crônica, difusa dos tecidos intra-oculares.
 e. ophthal′mia nodo′sa, e. oftalmia nodosa; endoftalmite decorrente de pêlos de lagarta intra-oculares. VER *ophthalmia* nodosa.
 e. phacoanaphylac′tica, e. facoanafilática; inflamação do trato uveal em virtude de sensibilização pelo córtex da lente do olho; simula a oftalmia simpática.

en·doph·thal·mo·do·ne·sis (en′dof - thal - mō - dō - nē′sis). Endoftalmodonese; tremor de qualquer estrutura intra-ocular, principalmente de uma lente implantada (pseudofacodonese). [endo- + ophthalmo- + G. *doneō*, agitar]

en·do·phyte (en′dō - fīt). Endófito; um parasita vegetal que vive dentro de outro organismo. [endo- + G. *phyton*, planta]

en·do·phyt·ic (en - dō - fit′ik). Endofítico. **1.** Relativo a um endófito. **2.** Referente a um tumor invasivo, infiltrativo.

en·do·plasm (en′dō - plazm). Endoplasma; a parte interna ou medular do citoplasma, ao contrário do ectoplasma, que contém as organelas celulares. SIN entoplasm.

en·do·plas·mic (en′dō - plas′mik). Endoplásmico; referente ao endoplasma.

en·do·plast (en′dō - plast). Endoplasto; nome antigo de endossoma. [endo- + G. *plastos*, formado]

en·do·plas·tic (en - dō - plas′tik). Endoplásico; relativo ao endoplasma.

en·do·po·lyg·e·ny (en′dō - pō - lij′e - nē). Endopoligenia; reprodução assexuada na qual mais de dois descendentes são formados dentro do organismo original, e na qual ocorrem duas ou, possivelmente, mais divisões nucleares antes que comece a formação do merozoíto; uma forma de brotamento interno observada no *Toxoplasma gondii*. Cf. endodyogeny. [endo- + G. *polys*, muitos, + *genesis*, criação]

en·do·pol·y·ploid (en - dō - pol′ē - ployd). Endopoliplóide; relativo à endopoliploidia.

en·do·pol·y·ploi·dy (en - dō - pol′ē - ploy - dē). Endopoliploidia; o processo ou estado de duplicação do conteúdo de DNA dos núcleos sem formação de fuso ou citocinese associada, resultando em um núcleo poliplóide. SIN endomitosis. [endo- + G. polyploidy]

en·do·re·du·pli·ca·tion (en′dō - rē - doo′pli - kā′shŭn). Endorreduplicação; uma forma de poliploidia ou polissomia por reduplicação dos cromossomos, dando origem a cromossomas de quatro filamentos na prófase e na metáfase.

en·dor·phin·er·gic (en′dōr - fin - er′jik). Endorfinérgico; relativo às células ou fibras nervosas que utilizam uma endorfina como neurotransmissor. [endorphin- + G. *ergon*, trabalho]

en·dor·phins (en - dōr - finz). Endorfinas; peptídeos opióides originalmente isolados do encéfalo, mas agora encontrados em muitas partes do corpo; no sistema nervoso, as endorfinas se ligam aos mesmos receptores a que se ligam os opiáceos exógenos. Já foram isoladas várias endorfinas (p. ex., α, β e γ) que variam não apenas em suas propriedades físicas e químicas, mas também na ação fisiológica. VER TAMBÉM enkephalins. [de *endogenous morphine*]

en·dor·rha·chis (en - dō - ra′kis). Endorraque. SIN spinal *dura mater*. [endo- + G. *rhachis*, a coluna vertebral]

en·do·sac (en′dō - sak). Endossaco; um saco ou bolsa usado em cirurgia laparoscópica no qual o tecido é colocado para facilitar a remoção ou a fragmentação. SIN endobag.

en·do·sal·pin·gi·o·sis (en′dō - sal - pin - jē′ō′sis). Endossalpingiose; mucosa aberrante no ovário ou em outra parte, que consiste em mucosa tubária ciliada sem estroma do tipo endometrial.

en·do·sal·pin·gi·tis (en′dō - sal - pin - jī′tis). Endossalpingite; inflamação da membrana de revestimento das tubas auditivas ou uterinas. [endo- + G. *salpinx* (*salping*-), tuba, + -*itis*, inflamação]

en·do·sal·pinx (en′dō - sal′pinks). Endossalpinge; a mucosa da tuba de Falópio. [endo- + G. *salpinx*, tuba]

en·do·sarc (en′dō - sark). Endossarco; o endoplasma de um protozoário. SIN entosarc. [endo- + G. *sarx* (*sark*-), carne]

en·do·scope (en′dō - skōp). Endoscópio; instrumento para exame do interior de um canal ou víscera oca. [endo- + G. *skopeō*, examinar]
 flexible e., e. flexível; instrumento óptico iluminado que conduz as imagens de volta até o observador através de um feixe flexível de pequenas (cerca de 10 μm) fibras transparentes. É usado para inspecionar partes internas do corpo. Esses instrumentos geralmente são equipados com mecanismos de direção e podem ter outras aberturas para permitir a introdução de instrumentos de coleta de amostra e/ou operatórios ao longo de seu eixo até o local interno. VER TAMBÉM fiberoptics. SIN fiberscope.

en·dos·co·pist (en - dos′kō - pist). Endoscopista; especialista treinado no uso de um endoscópio.

en·dos·co·py (en - dos′kō - pē). Endoscopia; exame do interior de um canal ou víscera oca por meio de um instrumento especial, como um endoscópio. [ver endoscope]
 peroral e., e. peroral; exame visual de partes internas do corpo por introdução de um instrumento (endoscópio) através da boca; os exemplos incluem esofagoscopia, gastroscopia, broncoscopia.
 virtual e., e. virtual; dados de tomografia computadorizada reconstruídos em 3 dimensões para fornecer informações semelhantes àquelas obtidas por endoscopia.

en·do·skel·e·ton (en - dō - skel′e - tŏn). Endoesqueleto; a estrutura óssea interna do corpo; o esqueleto em seu contexto habitual, distinto do exoesqueleto.

en·do·some (en′dō - sōm). Endossoma; um corpo mais ou menos central no núcleo vesicular de determinados protozoários Feulgen-negativos (DNA-) (p. ex., tripanossomas, amebas parasitas e fitoflabelados), com a cromatina (DNA₊) situada entre a membrana nuclear e o endossoma. Cf. nucleolus. [endo- + G. *sōma*, corpo]

en·do·son·og·ra·phy (en′dō - sō - nog′rā - fē). Endossonografia; ultra-sonografia na qual é utilizado um transdutor de ultra-som montado sobre, ou introduzido através de, um endoscópio de fibra óptica.

en·do·so·nos·co·py (en - dō - son′ō - skō - pē). Endossonoscopia; estudo ultrasonográfico realizado por transdutores inseridos no corpo como sondas em miniatura no esôfago, na uretra, na bexiga, na vagina ou no reto.

en·do·sperm (en′dō - sperm). Endosperma; tecido de armazenamento encontrado em muitas sementes que nutrem o embrião de uma planta.

en·do·spore (en′dō - spōr). Endósporo. **1.** Um corpo resistente formado no interior das células vegetativas de algumas bactérias, particularmente aquelas que pertencem aos gêneros *Bacillus* e *Clostridium*. **2.** Um esporo fúngico originado dentro de uma célula ou dentro da extremidade tubular de um esporóforo, como na esférula do *Coccidioides immitis*. [endo- + G. *sporos*, semente]

en·dos·te·al (en - dos′tē - al). Endosteal; relativo ao endósteo.

en·dos·te·i·tis, en·dos·ti·tis (en′dos - tē - ī′tis, en′dos - tī′tis). Endosteíte; inflamação do endósteo ou da cavidade medular de um osso. SIN central osteitis (2), perimyelitis. [endo- + G. *osteon*, osso, + -*itis*, inflamação]

en·dos·te·o·ma (en - dos′tē - ō′ma). Endosteoma; uma neoplasia benigna do tecido ósseo na cavidade medular de um osso. SIN endostoma. [endo- + G. *osteon*, osso, + -*ōma*, tumor]

en·do·steth·o·scope (en - dō - steth′o - skōp). Endostetoscópio; um tubo estetoscópico usado em endoausculta. [endo- + G. *stēthos*, tórax, + *skopeō*, examinar]

en·dos·te·um (en - dos′tē - ŭm) [TA]. Endósteo; uma camada de células que reveste a superfície interna do osso na cavidade medular central. SIN medullary membrane, perimyelis. [endo- + G. *osteon*, osso]

en·dos·to·ma (en - dō - stō′ma). Endostoma. SIN endosteoma.

en·do·ten·din·e·um (en′dō - ten - din′ē - ŭm). Endotendíneo; o tecido conjuntivo fino que circunda fascículos secundários de um tendão. [endo- + L. *tendon*, tendão, + -*eus*, adj.; o todo, em sua forma neutra, usado como substantivo]

en·do·the·li·a (en - dō - thē′lē - a). Endotélios; plural de endothelium.

en·do·the·li·al (en - dō - thē′lē - al). Endotelial; relativo ao endotélio.

en·do·the·lin. Endotelina; um peptídeo de 21 aminoácidos originalmente derivado das células endoteliais. É um vasoconstritor extremamente potente. Já foram identificados três produtos genéticos diferentes: endotelina 1, endotelina 2 e endotelina 3; estes são encontrados no encéfalo, rim e endotélio (endotelina 1), intestino (endotelina 2) e intestino e glândula supra-renal (endotelina 3).

en·do·the·li·o·cyte (en - dō - thē′lē - ō - sīt). Endoteliócito. SIN endothelial *cell*.

en·do·the·li·oid (en - dō - thē′lē - oyd). Endotelióide; semelhante ao endotélio.

en·do·the·li·o·ma (en′dō - thē - lē - ō′ma). Endotelioma; termo genérico que designa um grupo de neoplasias, particularmente tumores benignos, derivadas do tecido endotelial de vasos sanguíneos ou canais linfáticos; os endoteliomas podem ser benignos ou malignos. [endothelium + -oma, tumor]

en·do·the·li·o·sis (en'dō - the̅ - le̅ - ō'sis). Endoteliose; proliferação de endotélio.

en·do·the·li·um, pl. **en·do·the·li·a** (en - dō - the̅'le̅ - um, -le̅ - ă) [TA]. Endotélio; uma camada de células planas que revestem principalmente os vasos sanguíneos e linfáticos e o coração. [endo- + G. *the̅le̅*, mamilo]

e. of anterior chamber [TA], e. da câmara anterior; uma camada única de grandes células escamosas que recobre a superfície posterior da córnea. SIN e. posterius corneae [TA], e. camerae anterioris.

e. cam'erae anterio'ris, SIN e. of anterior chamber.

e. posterius corneae [TA], e. posterior da córnea. SIN e. of anterior chamber.

en·do·ther·mic (en - dō - ther'mik). Endotérmico; designa uma reação química durante a qual o calor (entalpia) é absorvido. Cf. exothermic (1). [endo- + G. *therme̅*, calor]

en·do·thrix (en'dō - thriks). Endotrix; esporos fúngicos (conídios) que invadem o interior de um fio de cabelo; não há bainha externa visível de esporos, como no caso do ectotrix. [endo- + G. *thrix*, cabelo]

en·do·tox·e·mia (en'dō - tok - se̅'me̅ - ă). Endotoxemia; presença, no sangue, de endotoxinas que, se derivadas de bactérias bacilares Gram-negativas, podem causar um fenômeno de Shwartzman generalizado, com choque.

en·do·tox·ic (en - dō - tok'sik). Endotóxico; designa uma endotoxina.

en·do·tox·i·co·sis (en'dō - tok - si - kō'sis). Endotoxicose; envenenamento por uma endotoxina.

en·do·tox·in (en - dō - tok'sin). Endotoxina. **1.** Uma toxina bacteriana que não é liberada livremente para o meio adjacente, ao contrário da exotoxina. **2.** As complexas macromoléculas de fosfolipídios-polissacarídeos que são parte da parede celular de várias cepas relativamente avirulentas, bem como virulentas, de bactérias Gram-negativas. As toxinas são relativamente termoestáveis, menos potentes que a maioria das exotoxinas, menos específicas, e não formam toxóides; à injeção, podem causar um estado de choque e, em doses menores, febre e leucopenia seguidas por leucocitose; possuem a capacidade de produzir os fenômenos de Shwartzman e de Sanarelli-Shwartzman. SIN intracellular toxin.

en·do·tra·che·al (en'dō - trā'ke̅ - ăl). Endotraqueal; dentro da traquéia.

en·do·u·rol·o·gy (en - dō - ūr - ol'ō - je̅). Endourologia; procedimentos cirúrgicos genitourinários (diagnósticos e terapêuticos) realizados através de instrumentos. Estes podem ser cistoscópicos, pelviscópicos, celioscópicos, laparoscópicos, percutâneos ou ureteroscópicos.

en·do·vac·ci·na·tion (en'dō - vak - si - nā'shŭn). Endovacinação; administração oral de vacinas.

en·do·vas·cu·li·tis (en'dō - vas'kū - li'tis). Endovasculite. SIN endangiitis.

hemorrhagic e., e. hemorrágica; hiperplasia endotelial e medial dos vasos sanguíneos placentários com trombose, fragmentação e diapedese das hemácias, resultando em natimortos ou em distúrbios do desenvolvimento fetal.

en·do·ve·nous (en - dō - ve̅'nŭs). Endovenoso. SIN intravenous.

end-piece. Peça terminal; a parte terminal da cauda de um espermatozóide, que consiste no axonema e na membrana flagelar.

end·plate, end-plate (end'plăt). Placa terminal; a terminação de uma fibra nervosa motora em relação a uma fibra muscular esquelética.

motor e., placa terminal motora; a grande e complexa formação terminal por meio da qual o axônio de um neurônio motor estabelece contato sináptico com uma fibra (célula) muscular estriada; vários ramos terminais de um axônio motor terminam em formações terminais sinápticas irregulares claviformes, que estão acomodadas em uma depressão única, do tipo calha, na superfície da fibra muscular; a membrana pós-sináptica, o sarcolema que forma o fundo da depressão, está muito aumentada na área superficial por invaginações profundas que fazem saliência para o citoplasma subjacente da fibra muscular; o intervalo subsináptico entre a membrana plasmática das terminações axônicas e o sarcolema é preenchido por uma substância amorfa; a fenda é fechada em direção à superfície pela bainha de Schwann, que se separa dos axônios à medida que estes últimos entram na fenda, e, assim, forma uma cobertura sobre esta; a pequena saliência dessa placa de fechamento corresponde à eminência de Doyère. SIN sole-plate ending.

end-tid·al (end - ti'dăl). Corrente final; ao fim de uma expiração normal.

en·dy·ma (en'di - mă). Epêndima. SIN ependyma. [G. peça de roupa]

E.N.E. Abreviatura de ethylnorepinephrine (etilnorepinefrina).

-ene. Sufixo aplicado a um nome químico que indica a presença de uma ligação dupla carbono-carbono; p. ex., propeno (propano insaturado, $CH_3–CH=CH_2$). [G. *ene̅*, sufixo adjetivo feminino]

ene·di·ol (ēn - dī'ol). Enediol; a distribuição atômica –C(OH)=C(OH)– produzida por migração de prótons do CH de um grupamento –CHOH que está fixado a um grupamento –CO– ao oxigênio do grupamento –CO– (geralmente induzido por álcalis), dando origem aos átomos de carbono duplamente ligados (o grupamento-ene), cada um possuindo um grupamento –CHOH (um diol); um caso especial de enolização.

en·e·ma (en'e̅ - mă). Enema; uma injeção retal para limpar o intestino ou para administrar drogas ou alimento. [G.]

air contrast e., e. contrastado com ar, clister opaco duplo; enema com duplo contraste radiográfico no qual é introduzido ar após o revestimento do cólon com uma suspensão de bário densa. SIN air contrast barium e., double contrast e.

air contrast barium e., e. baritado contrastado com ar. SIN air contrast e.

analeptic e., e. analéptico; um enema de 500 ml de água morna com meia colher de chá de sal de cozinha.

barium e., e. baritado, clister opaco; um tipo de enema contrastado; administração de suspensão de sulfato de bário, um meio radiopaco, para estudo radiográfico e fluoroscópico do trato intestinal inferior.

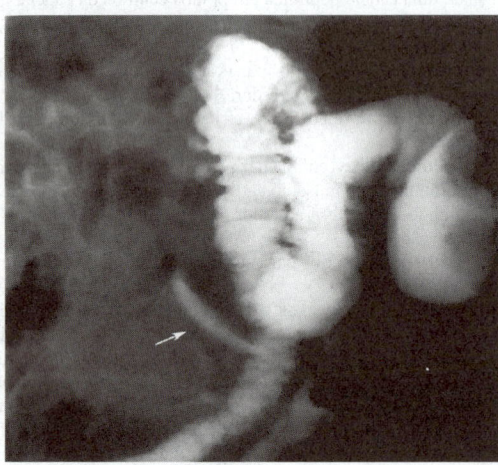

enema baritado: radiografia do cólon mostrando divertículo roto (seta)

blind e., e. cego; a introdução, no reto, de um tubo de borracha para facilitar a expulsão de flatos.

contrast e., e. contrastado; enema utilizando sulfato de bário ou um contraste hidrossolúvel.

double contrast e., e. com duplo contraste. SIN air contrast e.

flatus e., e. de flatos; um enema de sulfato de magnésio em glicerina e água morna.

high e., e. elevado; um enema instilado até um ponto alto no cólon. SIN enteroclysis (1).

Hypaque e., e. com Hypaque (diatrizoato de meglumina); enema com contraste radiográfico hidrossolúvel, seja diatrizoato ou outro.

nutrient e., e. nutritivo; injeção retal de alimento pré-digerido.

oil retention e., e. de retenção de óleo; injeção retal de óleo mineral, introduzido sob baixa pressão e retido por várias horas antes de ser expelido, para amolecer as fezes.

small bowel e., e. do intestino delgado; exame radiográfico do intestino delgado, por enchimento retrógrado a partir do intestino grosso cheio de contraste. Cf. enteroclysis, small bowel *series*.

soapsuds e., e. de espuma de sabão; enema de sabão fragmentado ou em pó em água morna.

turpentine e., e. de terebintina; um enema de terebintina e azeite de oliva em espuma de sabão.

en·e·ma·tor (en - ē - mā'ter, -tōr). Enemador; dispositivo usado para administrar um enema.

en·e·mi·a·sis (en - ē - mī'ă - sis). Enemíase; o uso de enemas.

en·er·get·ics (en - er - jet'iks). Energética; o estudo das mudanças de energia envolvidas em reações físicas e químicas e nos sistemas em geral.

en·er·gy (en'er - jē). Energia; a aplicação de força; a capacidade de realizar trabalho, assumindo as formas de energia cinética, energia potencial, energia química, energia elétrica, etc. SIN dynamic force. [G. *energeia*, de *en*, em, + *ergon*, trabalho]

e. of activation (E_a), e. de ativação; energia que tem de ser acrescentada àquela já possuída por uma molécula ou moléculas a fim de iniciar uma reação; geralmente expressa na equação de Arrhenius relacionando uma constante de velocidade à temperatura absoluta.

binding e., e. de ligação; energia que seria liberada de um núcleo atômico específico formado através da combinação de prótons e nêutrons individuais. SIN fusion e.

chemical e., e. química; energia liberada ou absorvida por uma reação química, p. ex., oxidação de carbono, ou absorvida na formação de uma substância química.

free e. (F), e. livre; uma função termodinâmica simbolizada como F, ou G (energia livre de Gibbs), $= H – TS$, onde H é a entalpia de um sistema, T a temperatura absoluta e S a entropia; as reações químicas prosseguem esponta-

ÍNDICE DAS PRANCHAS ANATÔMICAS

CONTEÚDO

Prancha 1: Crânio, Vista Anterior
Prancha 2: Esqueleto da Cabeça e Pescoço, Vista Lateral
Prancha 3: Musculatura da Cabeça e Pescoço, Vista Lateral
Prancha 4: Artérias da Cabeça e Pescoço, Vista Lateral
Prancha 5: Anatomia Superficial da Cabeça e Pescoço, Vista Lateral
Prancha 6: Anatomia da Cabeça e Pescoço, Vista Mediossagital
Prancha 7: Encéfalo, Vista Lateral
Prancha 8: Esqueleto, Vista Lateral
Prancha 9: Esqueleto, Vista Anterior
Prancha 10: Artérias do Tórax e Abdome, Vista Anterior
Prancha 11: Focos de Ausculta
Prancha 12: Musculatura do Tórax e Abdome, Vista Anterior
Prancha 13: Esqueleto, Vista Posterior
Prancha 14: Musculatura do Dorso, Vista Posterior
Prancha 15: Esqueleto do Membro Superior, Vista Anterior
Prancha 16: Artérias do Membro Superior, Vista Anterior
Prancha 17: Nervos do Membro Superior, Vista Anterior
Prancha 18: Musculatura do Tórax e do Membro Superior, Vista Lateral
Prancha 19: Esqueleto do Membro Inferior, Vista Anterior
Prancha 20: Artérias do Membro Inferior, Vistas Anterior e Posterior
Prancha 21: Nervos do Membro Inferior, Vistas Anterior e Posterior
Prancha 22: Musculatura do Membro Inferior, Vistas Lateral e Medial
Prancha 23: Sistema Respiratório, Vista Anterior
Prancha 24: Sistema Digestivo, Vista Anterior
Prancha 25: Sistema Linfático, Vista Anterior
Prancha 26: Sistemas Urogenitais Masculino e Feminino, Vista Mediossagital
Prancha 27: Coração, Vista Anterior

ÍNDICE

A

Acrômio, A9, A12, A14
Acrômio da escápula, A18
Ampola do ducto lactífero, A12
Anel inguinal superficial, A12
Ângulo
 da mandíbula, A1, A2
 do esterno, A8, A9, A10
 inferior da escápula, A9
 venoso esquerdo, A25
Ânus, A26
Aorta
 abdominal, A10
 arco da, A27
 ascendente, A10
 torácica, A10
Ápice, A23
Ápice da bexiga, A26
Aponeurose epicrânica, A5, A6
Arco
 da aorta, A10, A27
 palmar profundo, A16
 palmar superficial, A16
 zigomático, A2
Artéria/Artérias
 alveolar interna, A4
 auricular posterior, A4, A5
 axilar, A4, A10, A16
 braquial, A16
 braquial profunda, A16
 braquiocefálica, A4, A10, A27
 bucal, A4
 carótida comum, A4
 carótida comum direita, A10
 carótida comum esquerda, A27
 carótida externa, A4
 carótida interna, A4
 cervical ascendente, A4, A10
 cervical profunda, A4
 cervical superficial, A4
 cervical transversa, A4, A10
 circunflexa anterior do úmero, A16
 circunflexa femoral lateral, A20
 circunflexa femoral medial, A20
 circunflexa ilíaca profunda, A10
 circunflexa ilíaca superficial, A12
 circunflexa posterior do úmero, A16
 colateral média, A16
 colateral radial, A16
 colateral ulnar inferior, A16
 colateral ulnar superior, A16
 cone arterial, A27
 coronária direita, A27
 digitais palmares comuns, A16
 digitais palmares próprias, A16
 dorsal da escápula, A4, A10
 epigástrica inferior, A10
 epigástrica superior, A10, A12
 facial, A4
 facial transversa, A4, A5
 femoral, A10, A12
 ilíaca comum, A10, A22
 ilíaca externa, A10, A22
 ilíaca interna, A10, A22
 iliolombar, A10
 inferior medial do joelho, A22
 infra-orbital, A4, A5
 7.ª intercostal anterior, A10
 9.ª intercostal posterior, A10
 intercostal suprema, A4
 interóssea anterior, A16
 interóssea comum, A16
 interóssea posterior, A16
 labial inferior, A4
 labial superior, A4
 lingual, A4
 2.ª lombar, A10
 maxilar, A4
 mentual, A4
 mesentérica inferior, A10
 mesentérica superior, A10
 musculofrênica, A10
 obturatória, A22
 occipital, A4, A5
 oftálmica, A4
 primeira intercostal posterior, A4
 pulmonar esquerda, A27
 radial, A16, A18
 radial do indicador, A16
 ramo descendente da artéria circunflexa femoral lateral, A20
 ramos da (artéria) pulmonar (direita), A27
 recorrente radial, A16
 recorrente ulnar anterior, A16
 recorrente ulnar posterior, A16
 renal direita, A10
 renal esquerda, A10
 sacral lateral, A22
 sacral média, A10
 subclávia, A16
 subclávia direita, A4
 subclávia esquerda, A10, A27
 subcostal, A10
 subescapular, A4, A16
 superior medial do joelho, A22
 supra-escapular, A4, A10
 supra-orbital, A4, A5
 supratroclear, A4
 temporal superficial, A4, A5
 testicular esquerda, A10
 tireóidea inferior, A4, A10
 tireóidea superior, A4
 torácica inferior, A4, A10
 torácica lateral, A16
 torácica superior, A16
 ulnar, A16
 umbilical, A22
 vertebral, A4, A10
 zigomático-orbital, A4, A5
Articulação(ões)
 acromioclavicular, A15
 calcaneocubóidea, A19, A20
 carpometacarpais, A15
 carpometacarpal do polegar, A15
 do cotovelo, A15
 do joelho, A19, A20
 do ombro, A15
 do quadril, A19, A20
 esternoclavicular, A15
 interfalângicas, A19, A20
 interfalângicas proximais, A15
 metacarpofalângicas, A15
 radiocarpal, A15
 radioulnar distal, A15
 radioulnar proximal, A15
 sacroilíaca, A19, A20
 talocrural, A19, A20
 tarsometatarsais, A19, A20
 temporomandibular, A2
 tibiofibular distal, A19, A20
 tibiofibular proximal, A19, A20
 umerorradial, A15
 umeroulnar, A15
Asa maior
 do esfenóide, A2
 do osso esfenóide (face orbital), A1
 do osso esfenóide (face temporal), A1
Atlas, A6, A8
Átrio do coração, A27
Aurícula direita, A27
Áxis, A6, A8

B

Baço, A24
Bainha do músculo reto do abdome, lâmina anterior, A12
Bexiga, A26
Bregma, A2
Brônquio
 principal direito, A23
 principal esquerdo, A23
Bulbo, A6, A7

Imagens anatômicas fornecidas por:

adam.com™

A.D.A.M.
Softwere, Inc.
1600 River Edge Parkway
Suite 800
Atlanta, GA 30328
(770) 980-0888
www.adam.com

C

C1, A8
C1 (Atlas), A2
C2, A8
C2 (Áxis), A2
Cabeça
 curta do músculo bíceps femoral, A22
 lateral do músculo tríceps braquial, A18

longa do músculo bíceps braquial, A18
longa do músculo bíceps femoral, A22
medial do músculo gastrocnêmio, A22
Cabeça da fíbula, A19, A20
Cabeça do fêmur, A19, A20
Calcâneo, A13, A19, A20
Calvária, A6
Canal
anal, A26
óptico, A1
Capítulo, A15
Cápsula sinovial da articulação do joelho, A22
Carina da traquéia, A23
Cartilagem
cricóidea, A6, A23
10.ª costal, A9
tireóidea, A6, A23
Cavidade
nasal, A23, A24
oral, A24
Ceco, A24
Cerebelo, A6, A7
Cisterna do quilo, A25
Cisterna magna, A6
Clavícula, A9, A12, A13, A15, A17, A18
Clitóris, A26
Cóano, A23
Cóccix, A8, A9, A13
Colo
ascendente, A24
descendente, A24
sigmóide, A24
transverso, A24
Colo do fêmur, A19, A20
Colo do útero, A26
Concha
nasal inferior, A6, A23
nasal inferior e média, A1
nasal média, A6, A23
nasal superior, A6, A23
Côndilo
lateral, A19, A20
medial, A19, A20
Confluência dos seios, A6
Cordas tendíneas, A27
Corpo caloso, A6
Corpo cavernoso, A26
Corpo esponjoso do pênis, A26
Corpo, A26
da mandíbula, A1, A2
de C6, A6
de L3, A8
do esterno, A8, A9, A12
do púbis, A19, A20
mamilar, A6
pineal, A6
Costela
1.ª, A2, A9, A13, A15
11.ª, A9
12.ª, A9
Couro cabeludo, A6
Crânio, A13
Crista
ilíaca, A8, A9, A14, A19, A20, A22

púbica, A9
supraventricular, A27
Cubóide, A19, A20
Cuneiforme
intermédio, A19
lateral, A19
medial, A19

D

Diafragma, A23, A24
urogenital, A26
Ducto
ejaculatório, A26
parotídeo, A5
Ducto deferente, A26
Duodeno, A24
Dura-máter, A6

E

Encéfalo, A23, A24
Epicôndilo
lateral, A15
lateral do úmero, A18
medial, A15
Epidídimo, A26
Epiglote, A6
Escápula, A13, A15
Escroto, A26
Esfíncter externo do ânus, A26
Esôfago, A24
Espinha
ilíaca ântero-inferior, A8, A19, A20
ilíaca ântero-superior, A8, A9, A12, A19, A20
nasal anterior da maxila, A1, A2
Espinha da escápula, A18
Esterno, A15
Estômago, A24

F

Falange
distal, A15, A19, A20
média, A15, A19, A20
proximal, A15, A19, A20
Falanges, A13
Faringe, A23
Fáscia
aponeurose toracolombar, A14
espermática externa, A12
profunda, A12
profunda do pênis, A12
Fascículo
funículo espermático, A12, A26
funículos da medula espinal, A6, A7
lateral, A17
medial, A17
posterior, A17
Fêmur, A13, A19, A20
Fibras intercrurais da aponeurose do músculo oblíquo externo do abdome, A12
Fíbula, A13, A19, A20
Fissura

horizontal do pulmão direito, A23
oblíqua do pulmão direito, A23
oblíqua do pulmão esquerdo, A23
Focos de ausculta das valvas, A11
Forame
infra-orbital, A1
mentual, A1
sacral posterior, A8
supra-orbital, A1
Fórnice, A6
anterior da vagina, A26
posterior da vagina, A26
Fossa
coronóidea, A15
ilíaca, A19, A20
incisiva, A6
navicular, A26
Fundo, A26

G

Giro
angular, A7
frontal inferior, A7
frontal médio, A7
frontal superior, A7
pós-central, A7
pré-central, A7
supramarginal, A7
temporal médio, A7
temporal superior, A7
Glabela, A1, A2
Glande do pênis, A26
Glândula
hipófise, A6
parótida, A5
próstata, A26
submandibular, A5

H

Hiato do triângulo deltopeitoral, A12
Hipófise, A6

I

Íleo, A24
Ílio, A13
Incisura
jugular, A9
pré-occipital, A7
Intestino
delgado, A24
grosso, A24
Ísquio, A13, A19, A20

J

Jejuno, A24

L

Lábio maior do pudendo, A26
Lábio menor do pudendo, A26
Lâmina do teto, A6

Lâmina terminal, A6
Laringe, A6, A23, A24
Laringofaringe, A23, A24
Ligamento arterial, A27
Ligamento nucal, A6
Ligamento(s)
falciforme do fígado, A24
inguinal, A9, A12
longitudinal posterior, A6
patelar, A22
sacroespinal, A22
suspensor, A12
suspensor do pênis, A12, A26
umbilical mediano, A26
Linfonodos
aórticos laterais, A25
ilíacos comuns, A25
ilíacos externos, A25
ilíacos internos, A25
inguinais profundos, A25
sacrais, A25
Língua, A24
Linha alba, A12
Lobo
direito do fígado, A24
esquerdo do fígado, A24
frontal, A7
inferior do pulmão direito, A23
inferior do pulmão esquerdo, A23
médio do pulmão direito, A23
occipital, A7
parietal, A7
superior do pulmão direito, A23
superior do pulmão esquerdo, A23
temporal, A7
Lóbulo
parietal inferior, A7
parietal superior, A7

M

Maléolo
lateral, A19, A20
medial, A19, A20
Mamilo, A12
Mandíbula, A6
Manúbrio do esterno, A8, A9, A12, A15
Margem
inferior da mandíbula, A1
medial da escápula, A9
Margem
costal, A8, A9, A12
infra-orbital, A1
supra-orbital, A1
Margem falciforme do hiato safeno, A12
Maxila, A2
Maxila (corpo), A1
Meato
acústico externo, A2, A5
Mesencéfalo, A6
Músculo(s)
abaixador do ângulo da boca, A3
abaixador do lábio inferior, A3
abdutor longo do polegar, A18
adutor do polegar, A18

adutor longo, A22
adutor magno, A22
ancôneo, A18
auricular anterior, A3
auricular posterior, A3
auricular superior, A3
braquial, A18
braquiorradial, A18
bulboesponjoso, A26
cabeça lateral do gastrocnêmio, A22
constritor da faringe, A6
da parede anterior do abdome, A26
deltóide, A3, A12, A14, A18
epicrânico, A3
escaleno anterior, A3
esplênio da cabeça, A3, A14
esternocleidomastóideo, A3, A5, A12, A14, A18
extensor curto do polegar, A18
extensor dos dedos, A18
extensor longo do polegar, A18
extensor radial curto do carpo, A18
extensor radial longo do carpo, A18
extensor ulnar do carpo, A18
fibular longo, A22
genioglosso, A6
genio-hióideo, A6
glúteo máximo, A22
glúteo médio, A22
grácil, A22
infra-espinal, A14, A18
1.º interósseo dorsal, A18
latíssimo do dorso, A14, A18, A22
levantador da escápula, A3, A14
levantador do ânus, A26
levantador do lábio superior, A3
masseter, A3
mentual, A3
milo-hióideo, A6
músculo papilar posterior, A27
nasal, A3
oblíquo externo do abdome, A12, A14, A18, A22
oblíquo interno do abdome, A22
obturador interno, A22
orbicular da boca, A3
papilar anterior, A27
papilar septal (medial), A27
peitoral maior, A3, A12, A18
piriforme, A22
platisma, A3, A12
redondo maior, A14, A18
redondo menor, A14, A18
reto femoral, A22
risório, A3
sartório, A12, A22
semi-espinal da cabeça, A14
semimembranáceo, A22
semitendíneo, A22
serrátil anterior, A12, A18
temporal, A3
temporoparietal, A3
tensor da fáscia lata, A22
tibial anterior, A22
trapézio, A3, A5, A12, A14, A18
tríceps braquial, cabeça longa, A14
vasto lateral, A22
vasto medial, A22
zigomático maior, A3
zigomático menor, A3

N

Nasofaringe, A23, A24
Navicular, A19, A20
Nervo(s)
  acessório espinal, A5
  auricular magno, A5
  auricular maior, A14
  auriculotemporal, A5
  axilar, A17
  cervical transverso, A5
  clúnio superior, A14
  clúnios médios, A14
  cutâneo femoral lateral, A12, A14, A21
  cutâneo lateral do antebraço, A17, A18
  femoral, A12, A21
  fibular comum, A21, A22
  fibular profundo, A21
  fibular superficial, A21
  glúteo inferior, A21
  glúteo superior, A21
  ilio-hipogástrico, A21
  ilioinguinal, A21
  infra-orbital, A5
  infratroclear, A5
  interósseo anterior, A17
  isquiático, A21
  mediano, A17
  mentual, A5
  musculocutâneo, A17
  nervo cutâneo femoral posterior, A21
  obturatório, A21
  occipital maior, A5
  occipital menor, A5, A14
  3.ª occipital, A5, A14
  palmares comuns do nervo mediano, A17
  palmares comuns do nervo ulnar, A17
  palmares digitais próprios, A17
  peitoral lateral, A17
  peitoral medial, A17
  plantar lateral, A21
  plantar medial, A21
  radial, A17
  radial profundo, A17
  radial superficial, A17
  safeno, A21, A22
  subcostal, A21
  supraclavicular intermédio, A5
  supraclavicular lateral, A14
  supraclavicular medial, A5
  supraclavicular posterior, A5
  supra-orbital, A5
  supratroclear, A5
  sural, A21
  sural lateral, A21
  sural lateral superficial, A22
  sural medial, A21
  tibial, A21
  trigêmeo, A7
  ulnar, A17
  zigomaticofacial, A5

O

Olécrano, A18
Oliva inferior, A7
Omento menor, A24
Orofaringe, A23, A24
Osso(s)
  carpais, A13, A15
  do quadril, A13, A19, A20
  frontal, A2
  lacrimal, A1
  metacarpais, A15
  metatarsais, A13, A19, A20
  nasal, A1, A2
  occipital, A2
  parietal, A1, A2
  tarsais, A13
  temporal, A1, A2
  zigomático, A1, A2
Óstio
  da vagina, A26
  do ureter, A26
  faríngeo da tuba auditiva, A6, A23

P

Palato
  duro, A23, A24
  mole, A6, A23, A24
Pâncreas, A24
Parte
  abdominal do ducto torácico, A25
  cervical do ducto torácico, A25
  escamosa do osso frontal, A1
  orbital do músculo orbicular do olho, A3
  orbital do osso frontal, A1
  palpebral do músculo orbicular do olho, A3
  torácica do ducto torácico, A25
Pata anserina, A22
Patela, A19, A20, A22
Pele, A6
Pênis, A26
Periósteo, A6
Plexo
  braquial, A17
  corióideo do terceiro ventrículo, A6
  lombar, A21
  sacral, A21
Pólo
  frontal, A7
  occipital, A7
  temporal, A7
Ponte, A6, A7
Prega
  salpingofaríngea, A6
  salpingopalatina, A6
  vestibular, A6
  vocal, A6, A23

Processo
  alveolar da mandíbula, A1
  coracóide da escápula, A9, A15
  espinhoso de L5, A8
  espinhoso de S1, A8
  espinhoso de T3, A8
  frontal da maxila, A1
  mastóide, A2
  transverso de C5, A8
  transverso de T10, A8
  xifóide, A9
  zigomático do osso frontal, A1
Processo axilar da mama, A12
Promontório do sacro, A9
Protuberância
  mentual, A1, A2
  occipital externa, A2
Púbis, A13

Q

Quiasma óptico, A6

R

Rádio, A13, A15, A17
Ramo(s)
  ascendente da artéria braquial profunda, A16
  bucal do nervo facial, A5
  carpal palmar da artéria ulnar, A16
  cervical do nervo facial, A5
  cutâneo anterior do nervo intercostal, A12
  cutâneo lateral de T4–T11, A14
  cutâneo lateral do nervo ilio-hipogástrico, A14
  cutâneo lateral do nervo intercostal, A12
  cutâneo lateral do nervo subcostal, A14
  cutâneo lateral dos ramos dorsais dos nervos espinais T7–T12, A14
  cutâneo medial dos ramos dorsais dos nervos espinais C4–C8, A14
  cutâneo medial dos ramos dorsais dos nervos espinais T1–T6, A14
  cutâneos anteriores do nervo femoral, A21
  da mandíbula, A1, A2
  dorsal do nervo occipital maior, A14
  dos nervos espinais, A21
  esternocleidomastóideo da artéria occipital, A4
  frontal da artéria frontal superficial, A5
  frontal da artéria temporal superficial, A4
  mandibular do nervo facial, A5
  nasal externo do nervo infra-orbital, A5
  palmar superficial da artéria radial, A16
  parietal da artéria temporal superficial, A4, A5

perfurante da artéria torácica interna, A10, A12
perineal do nervo cutâneo femoral posterior, A21
profundo da artéria ulnar, A16
superior do púbis, A19, A20
temporal do nervo facial, A5
ventral dos nervos espinais, A14
zigomático do nervo facial, A5
Recesso
esfenoetmoidal, A6
faríngeo, A6
Região da orofaringe, A6
Retináculo
dos músculos extensores, A18
lateral da patela, A22
medial da patela, A22
Reto, A24, A26

S

S5, A8
Sacro, A8, A13, A19, A20, A26
Seio
esfenoidal, A6, A23
frontal, A6, A23
occipital, A6
reto, A6
sagital superior, A6
transverso do pericárdio, A27
Septo
intermuscular lateral, A18
nasal, A1
Septo pelúcido, A6
Sínfise
mentual, A1
púbica, A9, A22, A26
Sulco
calcarino, A7
central, A7
frontal inferior, A7
frontal superior, A7
intertubercular, A9
intraparietal, A7
lateral, A7
parietooccipital, A7
pós-central, A7
pré-central, A7
semilunar, A7

temporal inferior, A7
temporal superior, A7
Sulco intertubercular, A15
Superfície
medial do lobo frontal, A6
medial do lobo occipital, A6
medial do lobo parietal, A6
Sutura
coronal, A1, A2
esfenofrontal, A1
esfenoparietal, A1
esfenozigomática, A1
frontolacrimal, A1
frontomaxilar, A1
frontonasal, A1
frontozigomática, A1
intermaxilar, A1
internasal, A1
lambdóidea, A2
nasomaxilar, A1
zigomaticomaxilar, A1

T

Tabaqueira anatômica, A18
Tálamo, A6
Tálus, A19, A20
Tecido conjuntivo subcutâneo, A6
Tendão
central do diafragma, A23
do músculo grácil, A22
do músculo quadríceps femoral, A22
do músculo sartório, A22
do músculo semitendíneo, A22
Testículo, A26
Tíbia, A13, A19, A20
Tonsila faríngea, A6
Toro tubário, A6, A23
Trabécula
septal, A27
septomarginal, A27
Traquéia, A6, A23
Trato iliotibial, A14, A22
Triângulo de ausculta, A14
Triângulo lombar, A14
Trocanter
maior, A19, A20
menor, A19, A20

Tróclea, A15
Tronco
braquiocefálico, A27
broncomediastinal esquerdo, A25
celíaco, A10
costocervical, A4, A10
inferior, A17
jugular, A25
linfático direito, A25
lombossacro, A21
médio, A17
pulmonar, A27
subclávio esquerdo, A25
superior, A17
tireocervical, A4, A10
toracoacromial, A10
Tubérculo
carótico de C6, A2, A8
ilíaco, A9
maior, A9, A15
menor, A9, A15
mentual, A1
púbico, A9
Tuberosidade da tíbia, A19, A20

U

Ulna, A13, A15, A17
Umbigo, A12
Úmero, A13, A15, A17
Ureter, A26
Uretra, A26
Útero, A26
Úvula, A6

V

Vagina, A26
Valva(s)
aórtica, A11
atrioventricular direita, A27
focos de ausculta das, A11
localização da, A11
mitral, A11
pulmonar, A11, A27
tricúspide, A11, A27
Veia cava
inferior, A25, A27
superior, A25, A27

Veia(s)
auricular posterior, A5
basílica, A12
braquiocefálica direita, A25
braquiocefálica esquerda, A25, A27
cefálica, A12
cervical superficial, A12
circunflexa ilíaca superficial, A12
epigástrica superior, A12
facial, A5
femoral, A12
genicular medial inferior, A22
genicular medial superior, A22
jugular anterior, A5, A12
jugular externa, A5, A12, A18
jugular interna esquerda, A25
obturatória, A12
retromandibular, A5
sacral lateral, A22
safena magna, A12
subclávia esquerda, A25
supra-orbital, A5
temporal superficial, A5
toracoepigástrica, A12
zigomático-orbital, A5
Ventre
frontal do músculo epicrânio, A3
occipital do músculo epicrânio, A3
Ventrículo
3.º, A6
4.º, A6
Vértebra, C7, A8
Vértebra proeminente, A8
Vértebras
cervicais, A13
lombares, A13
torácicas, A13
Vesícula biliar, A24
Vesícula seminal, A26
Vestíbulo da cavidade nasal, A23
Vestíbulo da cavidade oral, A24
Vestíbulo da vagina, A26

neamente na direção que envolve uma diminuição final na energia livre do sistema (isto é, $\Delta G < 0$).

fusion e., e. de fusão. SIN binding e.

Gibbs e. of activation, e. de ativação de Gibbs; a energia de Gibbs que tem de ser acrescentada àquela já possuída por uma molécula ou moléculas a fim de iniciar uma reação.

Gibbs free e. (G), e. livre de Gibbs. VER free e.

Helmholtz e. (A), e. de Helmholtz; energia equivalente à energia interna menos a contribuição da entropia (TS).

internal e. (U), e. interna; energia de um sistema medida pelo calor absorvido do meio adjacente ao sistema e o trabalho realizado no sistema pelo meio adjacente.

kinetic e. (K), e. cinética; a energia do movimento.

latent e., e. latente. SIN potential e.

nuclear e., e. nuclear; energia emitida no decorrer de uma reação nuclear ou armazenada na formação de um núcleo atômico.

nutritional e., e. nutricional. SIN trophodynamics.

e. of position, e. potencial. SIN potential e.

potential e., e. potencial; a energia existente em um corpo em virtude de sua posição ou estado de existência, que não está sendo exercida no momento. SIN e. of position, latent e.

psychic e., e. psíquica; em psicanálise, uma força mental hipotética, análoga do conceito físico de energia, que possibilita e vitaliza a atividade psicológica de um indivíduo. VER TAMBÉM libido. SIN psychic force.

radiant e., e. radiante; energia contida nos raios luminosos ou qualquer outra forma de radiação.

solar e., e. solar; energia derivada da luz solar.

total e., e. total; a soma das energias cinética e potencial.

en·flu·rane (en - floor'ān). Enflurano; um potente anestésico inalatório volátil, não-inflamável e não-explosivo.

ENG Abreviatura de electronystagmography (eletronistagmografia).

en·gage·ment (en - gāj'ment). Insinuação; em obstetrícia, o mecanismo pelo qual o diâmetro biparietal da cabeça fetal penetra o plano da abertura superior da pelve.

en·gas·tri·us (en - gas'trē - ŭs). Engástrio; gêmeos conjugados diferentes nos quais o parasita menor está total ou parcialmente fora do abdome do autósito maior. [G. *en*, em, + *gastēr*, ventre]

Engelmann, Guido, cirurgião alemão, *1876. VER E. *disease*.

Engelmann, Theodor W., fisiologista alemão, 1843–1909. VER E. basal *knobs*, em *knob*.

en·gi·neer·ing (en - jin - ēr'ing). Engenharia; a aplicação prática de princípios físicos, mecânicos e matemáticos.

biomedical e., e. biomédica; aplicação de princípios de engenharia para obter soluções de problemas biomédicos.

dental e., e. dentária; aplicação dos princípios da engenharia à odontologia.

genetic e., e. genética; manipulação interna de material genético básico de um organismo para modificar a hereditariedade biológica ou produzir peptídeos de alta pureza, como hormônios ou antígenos.

Englisch, Josef, médico austríaco, 1835–1915. VER E. *sinus*.

en·globe (en - glōb'). Englobar; abranger por um corpo esferóide; diz-se da ingestão de bactérias e outros corpos estranhos pelos fagócitos.

en·globe·ment (en - glōb'ment). Englobamento; o processo de inclusão por um corpo esferóide, como por um fagócito.

en·gorged (en - gōrjd'). Congestionado; ingurgitado; cheio por completo; distendido com líquido. VER TAMBÉM congested, hyperemic. [Fr. ant. do L. mediev. *gorgia*, garganta, passagem estreita, do L. *gurges*, remoinho]

en·gorge·ment (en - gōrj'ment). Ingurgitamento; distensão por líquido ou outro material. VER TAMBÉM congestion, hyperemia.

en·gram (en'gram). Engrama; na hipótese mnemônica, uma alteração física ou traço de memória feito no sistema nervoso central de um organismo em virtude de experiência ou da repetição de estímulos. [G. *en*, em, + *gramma*, marca]

en·graph·ia (en - graf'ē - ă). Engrafia; a formação de engramas.

en grappe (ahn-grap'). Em cacho; designa o arranjo agrupado, semelhante a um cacho de uva, de microconídios de determinados dermatófitos. [Fr. *en*, em, + *grappe*, cacho de uvas]

en·hance·ment (en-hans'ment). Realce; acentuação; intensificação. **1.** O ato de aumentar. **2.** Em imunologia, o prolongamento de um processo ou evento por supressão de um processo de oposição.

acoustic e., intensificação acústica; manifestação de aumento da amplitude do eco que retorna de regiões além de um objeto, como um cisto cheio de líquido, que causa pequena ou nenhuma atenuação do feixe de ultra-som. Cf. acoustic *shadow*.

contrast e., realce por contraste; a administração intravenosa de contraste iodado hidrossolúvel, o que aumenta o número de TC do acúmulo vascular, bem como algumas lesões (particularmente no encéfalo), devido ao extravasamento anormal para o interstício; a propriedade de mostrar aumento da radiopacidade pela concentração do contraste.

edge e., realce da borda; uso do processamento de imagem analógica ou digital para aumentar o contraste de cada interface; equivalente ao uso de um filtro de passagem alta.

immunologic e., reforço imunológico. SIN immunoenhancement.

ring e., realce anular; em tomografia computadorizada, quando um círculo brilhante aparece em uma imagem feita após injeção de contraste, característico da localização do contraste na parede de um abscesso.

en·hanc·ers. Intensificadores; elementos genéticos importantes na função de um promotor específico. [I.m. *enhaucen*, elevação, aumento, do Fr. ant. *enhaucier*, do L. ant. *inalto*, de *altus*, alto, + *-er*, agente sufixo]

en·keph·a·lin·er·gic (en - kef'ă - lin - er'jik). Encefalinérgico; relativo às células ou fibras nervosas que empregam uma encefalina como seu neurotransmissor. [enkephalin + G. *ergon*, trabalho]

en·keph·a·lins (en - kef'ă - linz). Encefalinas; endorfinas pentapeptídicas, encontradas em muitas partes do encéfalo, que se ligam a sítios receptores específicos, alguns dos quais podem ser receptores opiáceos relacionados à dor; consideradas neurotransmissores endógenos e analgésicos que não viciam. A metencefalina é Tyr-Gly-Gly-Phe-Met; a leuencefalina tem Leu no lugar de Met; a pró-encefalina tem Pro no lugar de Met.

en·large·ment (en-larj'ment) [TA]. Aumento. **1.** Um aumento de tamanho; uma tumefação, um aumento ou uma proeminência anatômica. **2.** Uma intumescência ou tumefação. SIN intumescentia [TA], intumescence (1).

cervical e. [TA], intumescência cervical; uma tumefação fusiforme da medula espinal que se estende da terceira vértebra cervical até a segunda vértebra torácica, com espessura máxima oposta à quinta ou sexta vértebra cervical, decorrente da inervação do membro superior. SIN intumescentia cervicalis [TA], cervical e. of spinal cord.

cervical e. of spinal cord, intumescência cervical da medula espinal. SIN cervical e.

choroid e. [TA], glomo corióideo; a porção aumentada do plexo corióideo localizada no átrio do ventrículo lateral; pode tornar-se parcialmente calcificado com a idade. VER TAMBÉM choroid *glomus*. SIN glomus choroideum [TA], choroid glomus, choroid skein.

gingival e., aumento gengival; crescimento exagerado (localizado ou difuso) de tecido gengival, de natureza inespecífica. VER TAMBÉM gingival *hyperplasia*.

lumbosacral e. [TA], intumescência lombossacral; uma tumefação fusiforme da medula espinal que começa ao nível da décima vértebra torácica e afila-se até o cone medular, com espessura máxima oposta à última vértebra torácica, decorrente da inervação do membro inferior. SIN intumescentia lumbosacralis [TA], lumbosacral e. of spinal cord.

lumbosacral e. of spinal cord, intumescência lombossacral da medula espinal. SIN lumbosacral e.

tympanic e. [TA], intumescência timpânica; uma tumefação, não-ganglionar, no ramo timpânico do nervo glossofaríngeo; é considerada possivelmente semelhante ao glomo carótico. VER TAMBÉM tympanic *ganglion*. SIN intumescentia tympanica [TA], tympanic intumescence.

e. of the vestibular aqueduct, intumescência do aqueduto do vestíbulo; comprometimento auditivo hereditário recessivo, associado a um grande aqueduto do vestíbulo.

-enoic. Sufixo que indica um ácido não-saturado. [-ene + -ic]

enol (ē'nol). Enol; um composto que possui um grupamento hidroxila (álcool) fixado a um átomo de carbono ligado duplamente (etilênico) (–CH=CH–(OH)–); adequadamente grafado em itálico quando fixado, como um prefixo ou infixo, a um nome completo; p. ex., enol piruvato (*enol* pyruvate); fosfoenolpiruvato (phospho*enol*pyruvate); geralmente em equilíbrio com seu tautômero ceto. [-ene + -ol]

eno·lase (ē'nol - ās). Enolase; enzima que catalisa a desidratação reversível de 2-fosfo-D-glicerato em fosfoenolpiruvato (phospho*enol*pyruvate) e água; uma etapa na glicólise e na gliconeogênese; existem várias isozimas; exige íon magnésio e é inibida por F⁻. SIN phosphopyruvate hydratase.

neuron-specific e., e. neurônio-específica; uma isoenzima da enolase presente em neurônios e células gliais; corantes para essa enzima são usados freqüentemente no diagnóstico diferencial de tumores neuronais ou neuroendócrinos.

eno·li·za·tion (ē'nol - i - zā'shŭn). Enolização; conversão de uma forma ceto em uma forma enol; p. ex., $CH_3-CO-COOH \rightarrow CH_2=C(OH)COOH$.

enol **py·ru·vate** (ē - nol - pī'roo - vāt). Enol piruvato; $CH_2=C(OH)-COO^-$, a forma de piruvato encontrada no fosfoenolpiruvato (fosfato de enol piruvato) biologicamente como na forma livre.

en·oph·thal·mia (en - of - thal'mē - ă). Enoftalmia. SIN enophthalmos.

en·oph·thal·mos (en'of-thal'mos). Enoftalmia; recuo do bulbo do olho para dentro da órbita. SIN enophthalmia. [G. *en*, em, + *ophthalmos*, olho]

en·or·gan·ic (en - ōr - gan'ik). Enorgânico; termo raramente usado que designa aquilo que ocorre como característica inata de um organismo.

en·os·to·sis (en - os - tō'sis). Enostose; uma massa de tecido ósseo proliferativo dentro de um osso. [G. *en*, em, + *osteon*, osso, + *-osis*, condição]

en·o·yl (ēn'ō - il). Enoil; o radical acil de um ácido alifático insaturado. [-ene + -oyl]

en·o·yl-ACP re·duc·tase. Enoil-ACP redutase; uma enzima que catalisa a hidrogenação de acil-ACP (onde ACP é uma proteína transportadora de acil) se associa a 2,3-desidroacil-ACPs, com NAD⁺ como aceptor de hidrogênio; importante no metabolismo de ácidos graxos. SIN crotonyl-ACP reductase.

en·o·yl-ACP re·duc·tase (NADPH). Enoil-ACP redutase (NADPH); uma enzima que realiza a mesma reação que a enoil-ACP (onde ACP é a proteína transportadora de acil) redutase, mas com NADP⁺ como aceptor de hidrogênio. SIN acyl-ACP dehydrogenase, acyl-ACP reductase.

en·o·yl-CoA hy·dra·tase. Enoil-CoA hidratase; Δ²-eEoil-CoA hidratase; uma enzima que catalisa uma reação reversível entre uma L-3-hidroxiacil-CoA e uma 2,3- (ou 3,4-) *trans*-enoil-CoA na degradação de ácidos graxos. SIN crotonase, enoyl hydrase.

eno·yl-CoA re·duc·tase. Enoil-CoA redutase. SIN *acyl-CoA* dehydrogenase (NADPH).

2-en·o·yl-CoA re·duc·tase. 2-enoil-CoA redutase; acil-CoA desidrogenase (NADP⁺).

en·o·yl hy·dra·se. Enoil hidrase. SIN enoyl-CoA hydratase.

E.N.S. Abreviatura de ethylnorepinephrine (etilnorepinefrina).

en·si·form (en′si-fōrm). Ensiforme. SIN xiphoid. [L. *ensis*, espada, + *forma*, aparência]

en·sis·ter·num (en′sis-ter′nŭm). Ensisterno. SIN xiphoid *process*. [L. *ensis*, espada, + sternum]

ensu Acrônimo de *e*quivalent *n*ormal *s*on *u*nit (unidade equivalente do filho normal), as informações de qualquer fonte (ligação, portador, fenótipo, etc.) que terão o mesmo impacto sobre a probabilidade condicional de uma consulente ser portadora de um traço ligado ao X como é um filho normal; cada filho normal contribui com um ensu. Cf. encu.

ENT Abreviatura de ears, nose e throat (orelhas, nariz e garganta). VER otorhinolaryngology.

ent-. VER ento-.

en·tac·tin (ent-ak′tin). Entactina; uma glicoproteína que se liga à laminina e ao colágeno tipo IV na lâmina basal do glomérulo renal e é um importante fator de fixação celular; a entactina é uma proteína de ligação do cálcio sulfatado. SIN nidogen.

en·tad. Em direção ao interior. [G. *entos*, dentro, + L. *ad*, para]

en·tal (en′tal). Relativo ao interior; interno. [G. *entos*, dentro]

ent·am·e·bi·a·sis (ent-ă-mē-bī′ă-sis). Entamebíase; infecção por *Entamoeba histolytica*. VER amebiasis, amebic *dysentery*.

Ent·a·moe·ba (ent-ă-mē′bă). Gênero de amebas parasitas na cavidade oral, do ceco e do intestino grosso dos seres humanos e de outros primatas e em muitos mamíferos domésticos e selvagens e em aves; com a exceção da *E. histolytica*, membros do gênero parecem ser habitantes relativamente inofensivos do hospedeiro. [G. *entos*, dentro, + *amoibē*, alteração]

E. bucca′lis, nome anterior da *E. gingivalis*.

E. chattoni, espécie que não provoca sintomas; mais freqüente em macacos, mas algumas vezes foi identificada em seres humanos; os cistos são uninucleados.

E. co′li, espécie não-patogênica de ameba que ocorre no intestino grosso do homem, de outros primatas, cães e, possivelmente, porcos; freqüentemente é confundida com *E. histolytica*, mas distinguida por detalhes nucleares e pelo número de núcleos e forma de cromatóides no cisto.

E. dispar, espécie não-patogênica que ocorre no intestino grosso de seres humanos; anteriormente considerada *E. histolytica*, a *E. dispar* agora é considerada uma espécie distinta; é não-patogênica e não está associada a amebíase sintomática em seres humanos. Morfologicamente assemelha-se à *E. histolytica*; entretanto, nunca foram encontradas hemácias ingeridas nos trofozoítas.

E. gingiva′lis, uma espécie de ameba encontrada na cavidade oral do homem, de outros primatas, cães e gatos; em seres humanos, freqüentemente está associada à má higiene oral e a suas doenças resultantes.

E. hartman′ni, espécie de ameba encontrada no intestino grosso de seres humanos, de outros primatas e cães; agora considerada uma espécie distinta, não-patogênica e menor que a *E. histolytica*, mas indistinguível desta; anteriormente denominada a "pequena raça" de *E. histolytica*.

E. histoly′tica, espécie de ameba que é o único patógeno distinto do gênero, a denominada "grande raça" da *E. histolytica*, causando disenteria tropical ou amebiana em seres humanos e, também, em cães (os seres humanos são o reservatório das infecções caninas). Em seres humanos, o microrganismo pode penetrar nos tecidos epiteliais do cólon, causando ulceração (disenteria amebiana); em uma pequena proporção desses casos, o microrganismo pode alcançar o fígado pela corrente sanguínea porta e produzir abscessos (amebíase hepática); em alguns casos, pode então se disseminar para outros órgãos, como os pulmões, encéfalo, rim ou pele e, freqüentemente, ser fatal. VER TAMBÉM *E. dispar*.

E. moshkov′skii, espécie de ameba muito semelhante à *E. histolytica*, provavelmente não-infecciosa para o homem, mas uma causa de dificuldades diagnósticas, pois foi isolada de esgotos humanos e pode ser responsável por resultados falso-positivos em testes de efluentes vegetais de esgoto.

E. polecki, espécie de ameba comumente encontrada nos intestinos de porcos; também parasita macacos, bovinos, caprinos, ovinos e cães; também encontrada em seres humanos, onde não produz sintomas; a importância clínica está na possibilidade de confundir o organismo com *E. histolytica*.

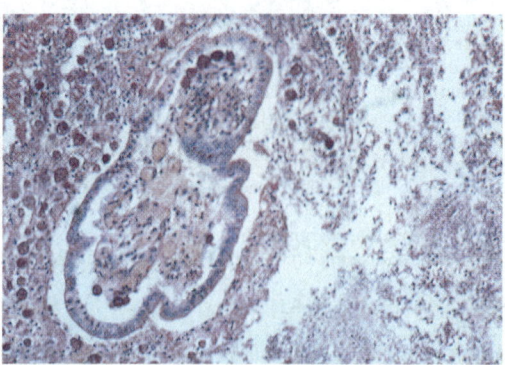

Entamoeba histolytica: muitos trofozoítas são observados em uma lesão ulcerativa do cólon; coloração pelo ácido periódico de Schiff; 80 ×

enter-. VER entero-.

en·ter·al (en′ter-ăl). Enteral; dentro, ou através, do intestino ou trato gastrointestinal, particularmente distinto de parenteral. [G. *enteron*, intestino]

en·ter·al·gia (en-ter-al′jē-ă). Enteralgia; enterodinia; dor abdominal intensa associada a espasmo do intestino. SIN enterdynia, enterodynia. [entero- + G. *algos*, dor]

en·ter·a·mine (en-ter-am′ēn). Enteramina. SIN serotonin.

en·ter·dy·nia (en-ter-din′ē-ă). Enterodinia. SIN enteralgia.

en·ter·ec·ta·sis (en-ter-ek′tă-sis). Enterectasia; termo obsoleto para dilatação do intestino. [entero- + G. *ektasis*, estiramento]

en·ter·ec·to·my (en-ter-ek′tō-mē). Enterectomia; ressecção de um segmento do intestino. [entero- + G. *ektomē*, excisão]

en·ter·el·co·sis (en-ter-el-kō′sis). Enterelcose; termo obsoleto para ulceração do intestino. [entero- + G. *helkos*, úlcera]

en·ter·ic (en-ter′ik). Entérico; relativo ao intestino. [G. *enterikos*, de *entera*, intestino]

en·ter·i·tis (en-ter-ī′tis). Enterite; inflamação do intestino, especialmente do intestino delgado. [entero- + G. *-itis*, inflamação]

e. anaphylac′tica, e. anafilática; inflamação hemorrágica e necrotizante que se desenvolve no íleo (e também no cólon) de cães sensibilizados quando eles são alimentados com uma segunda dose do material sensibilizante. SIN chronic anaphylaxis.

chronic cicatrizing e., e. cicatrizante crônica. SIN regional e.

diphtheritic e., e. diftérica; enterite com a formação de uma membrana ou de uma falsa membrana. VER TAMBÉM pseudomembranous *enterocolitis*.

granulomatous e., e. granulomatosa. SIN regional e.

human eosinophilic e., e. eosinofílica humana; inflamação eosinofílica segmentar do trato gastrointestinal em seres humanos; o agente etiológico suspeito é o *Ancylostoma caninum*; os indicadores laboratoriais são eosinofilia e aumento da IgE.

mucomembranous e., e. mucomembranosa; afecção da mucosa intestinal caracterizada por constipação ou diarréia (algumas vezes alternadas), cólica e eliminação de fragmentos pseudomembranosos ou moldes incompletos do intestino. SIN mucoenteritis (2).

e. necrot′icans, e. necrótica; enterite com necrose da parede intestinal causada por *Clostridium welchii*.

phlegmonous e., e. flegmonosa; inflamação aguda grave do intestino, com parede intestinal edemaciada infiltrada com pus.

e. polypo′sa, e. poliposa; enterite associada à formação de pólipo.

pseudomembranous e., e. pseudomembranosa. SIN pseudomembranous *enterocolitis*.

regional e., e. regional; enterite crônica subaguda, de causa desconhecida, envolvendo o íleo terminal e, com menor freqüência, outras partes do trato gastrointestinal; caracterizada por úlceras profundas segmentares que podem causar fístulas, e estreitamento e espessamento do intestino por fibrose e infiltração linfocítica, com granulomas tuberculóides não-caseificados que também podem ser encontrados em linfonodos regionais; os sinais e sintomas incluem febre, diarréia, cólica abdominal e emagrecimento. SIN chronic cicatrizing e., Crohn disease, distal ileitis, regional ileitis, terminal ileitis, granulomatous e.

tuberculous e., e. tuberculosa; a tuberculose entérica pode ser causada por tuberculose bovina contraída pela ingestão de leite não-pasteurizado ou pela deglutição de bacilos da tuberculose expectorados de lesões cavitárias no pulmão; pode ocorrer na ausência de tuberculose pulmonar óbvia.

entero-, enter-. Entero-, enter-; o intestino. [G. *enteron*, intestino]

en·ter·o·a·nas·to·mo·sis (en′ter-ō-an-as-tō-mō′sis). Enteroanastomose. SIN enteroenterostomy.

en·ter·o·an·the·lone (en-ter-ō-an′thē-lōn). Enteroantelona. SIN enterogastrone.

PRANCHA 1: CRÂNIO, VISTA ANTERIOR

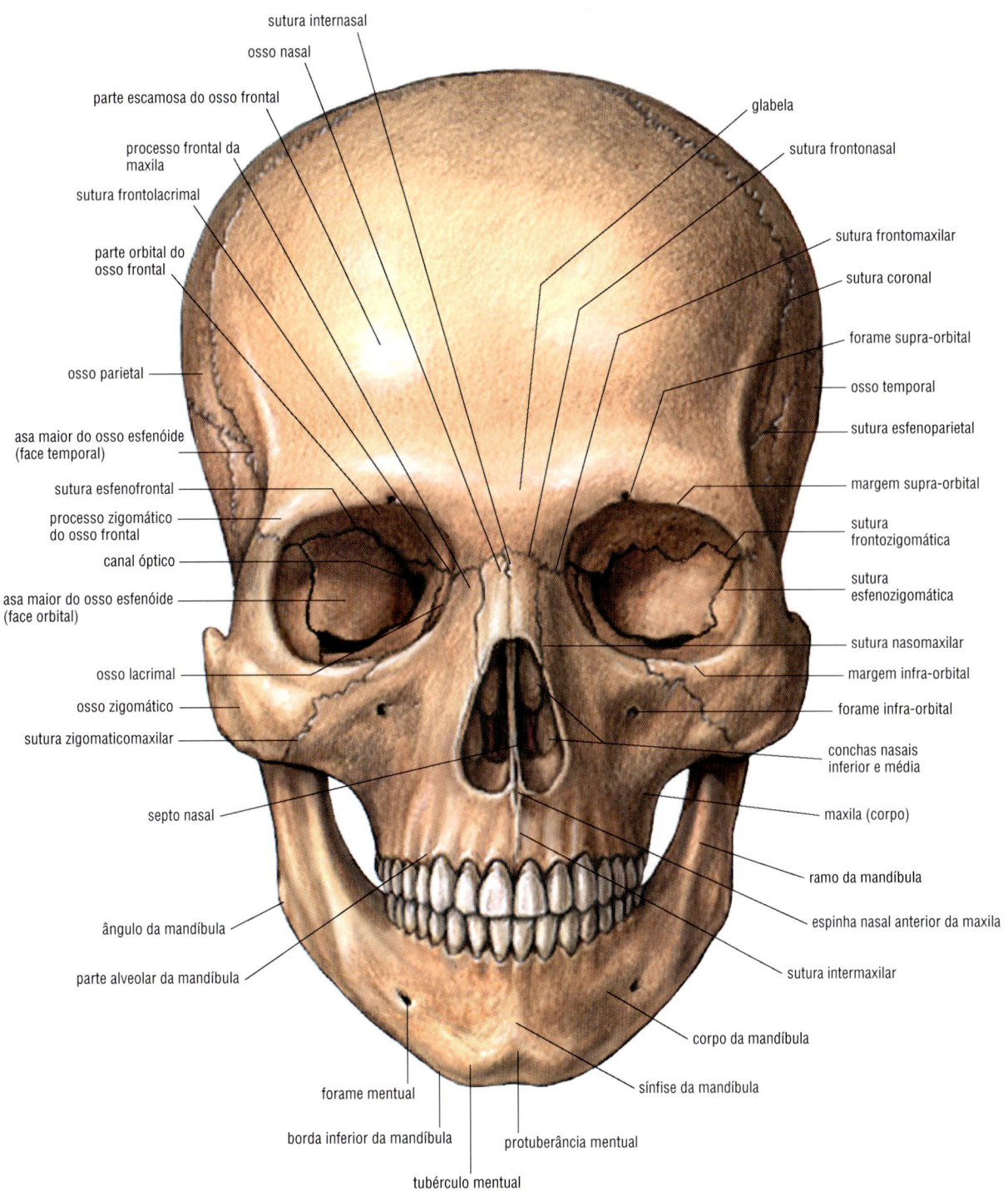

PRANCHA 2: ESQUELETO DA CABEÇA E PESCOÇO, VISTA LATERAL

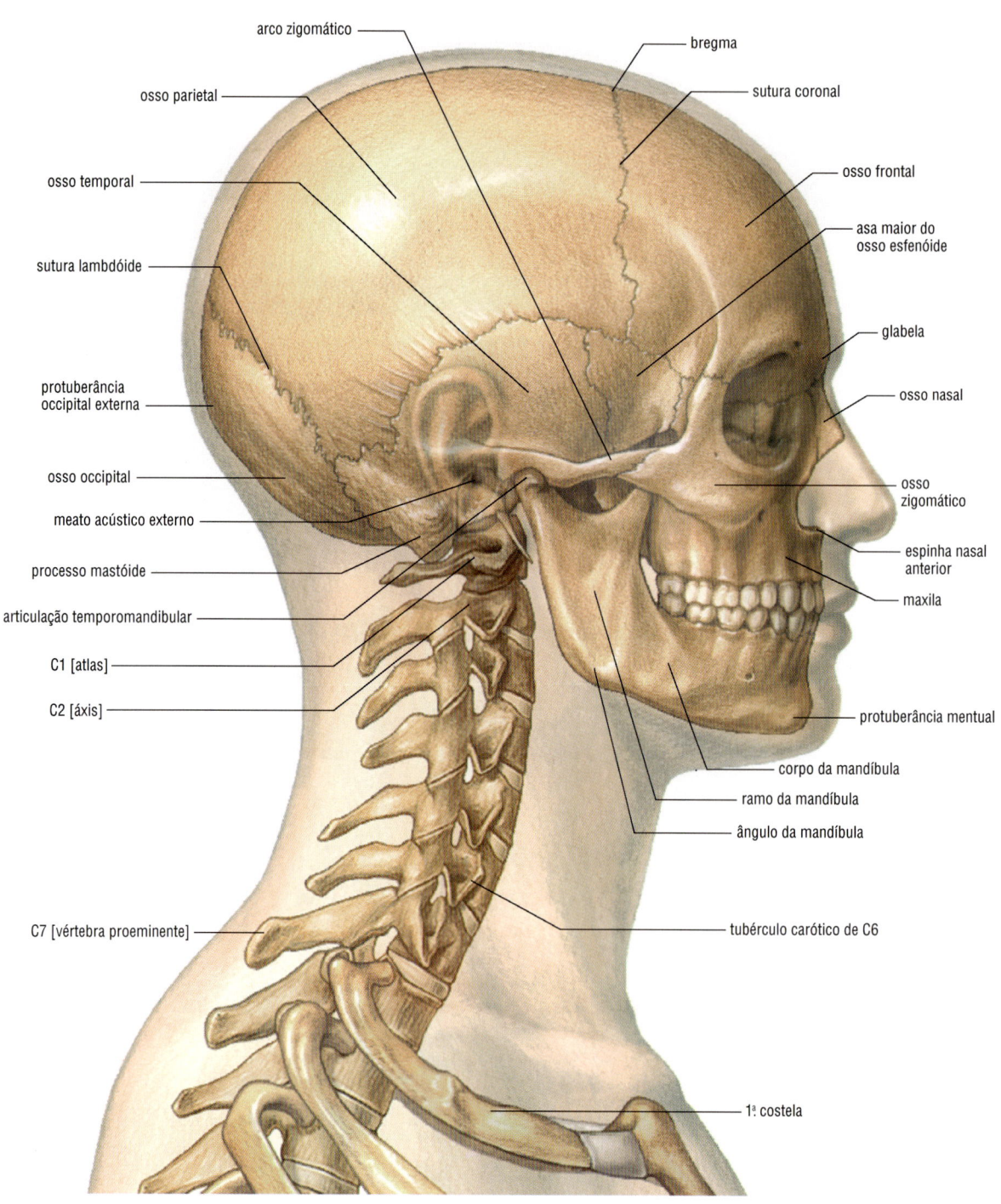

PRANCHA 3: MUSCULATURA DA CABEÇA E PESCOÇO, VISTA LATERAL

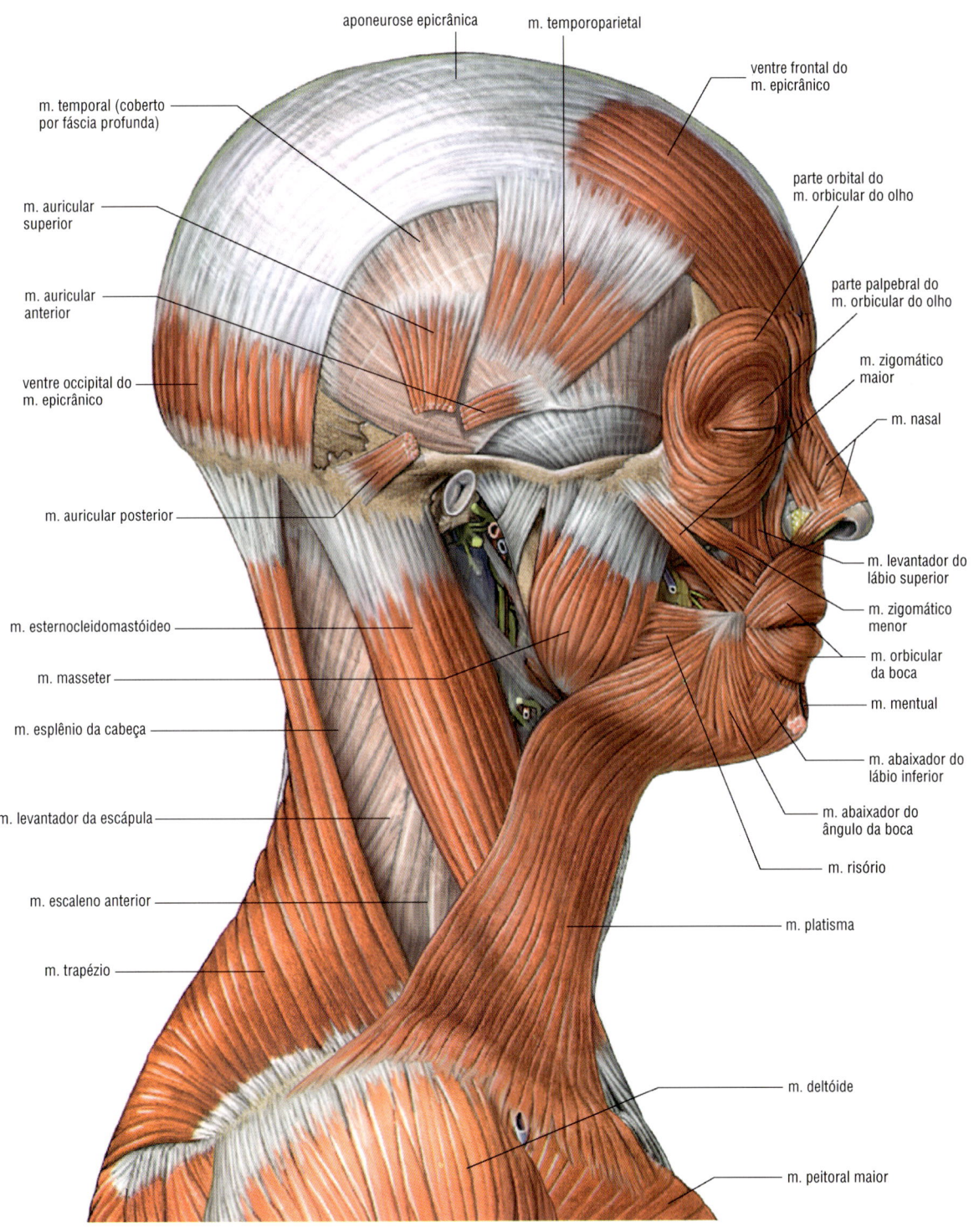

PRANCHA 4: ARTÉRIAS DA CABEÇA E PESCOÇO, VISTA LATERAL

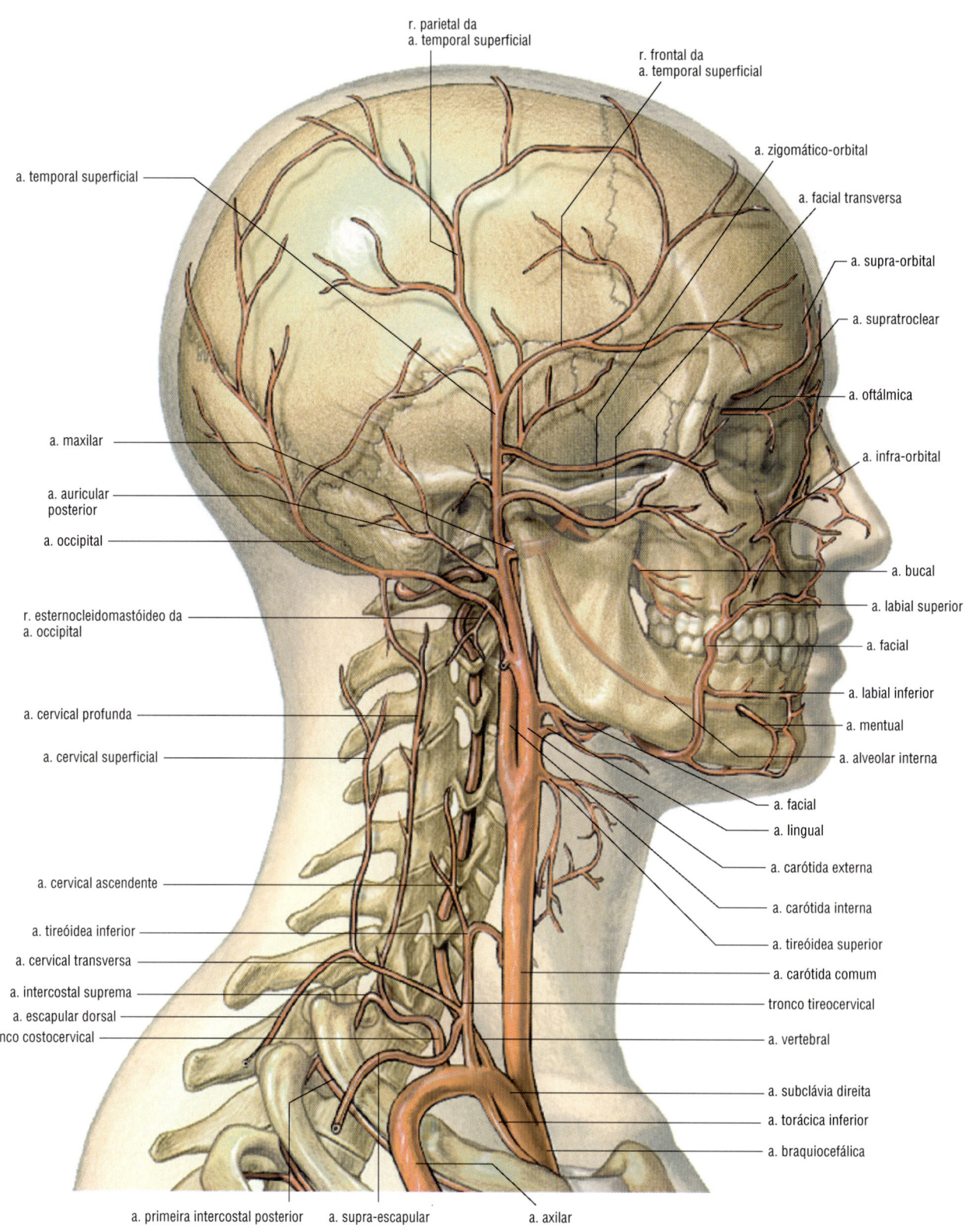

PRANCHA 5: ANATOMIA SUPERFICIAL DA CABEÇA E PESCOÇO, VISTA LATERAL

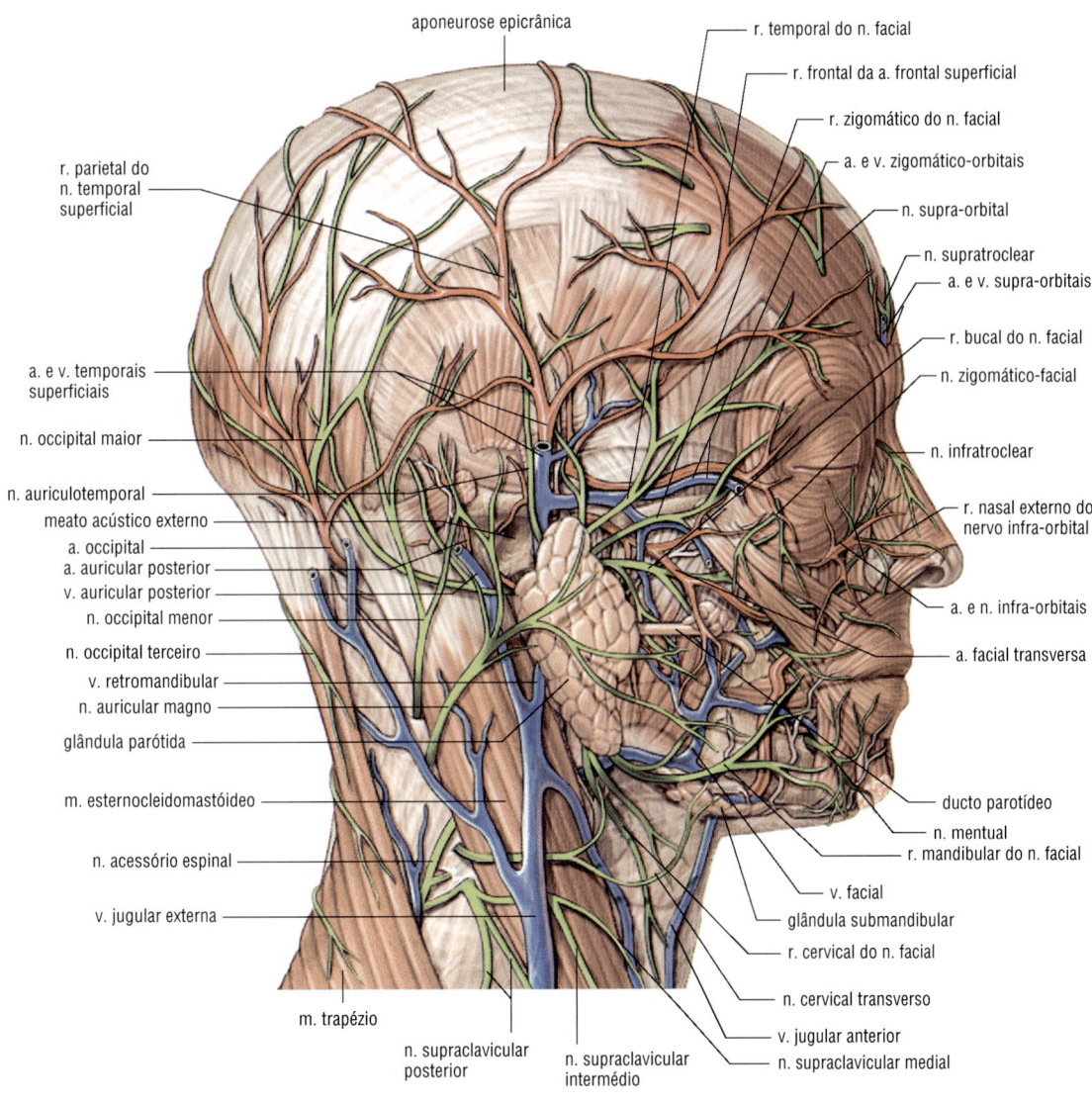

PRANCHA 6: ANATOMIA DA CABEÇA E PESCOÇO, VISTA MEDIOSSAGITAL

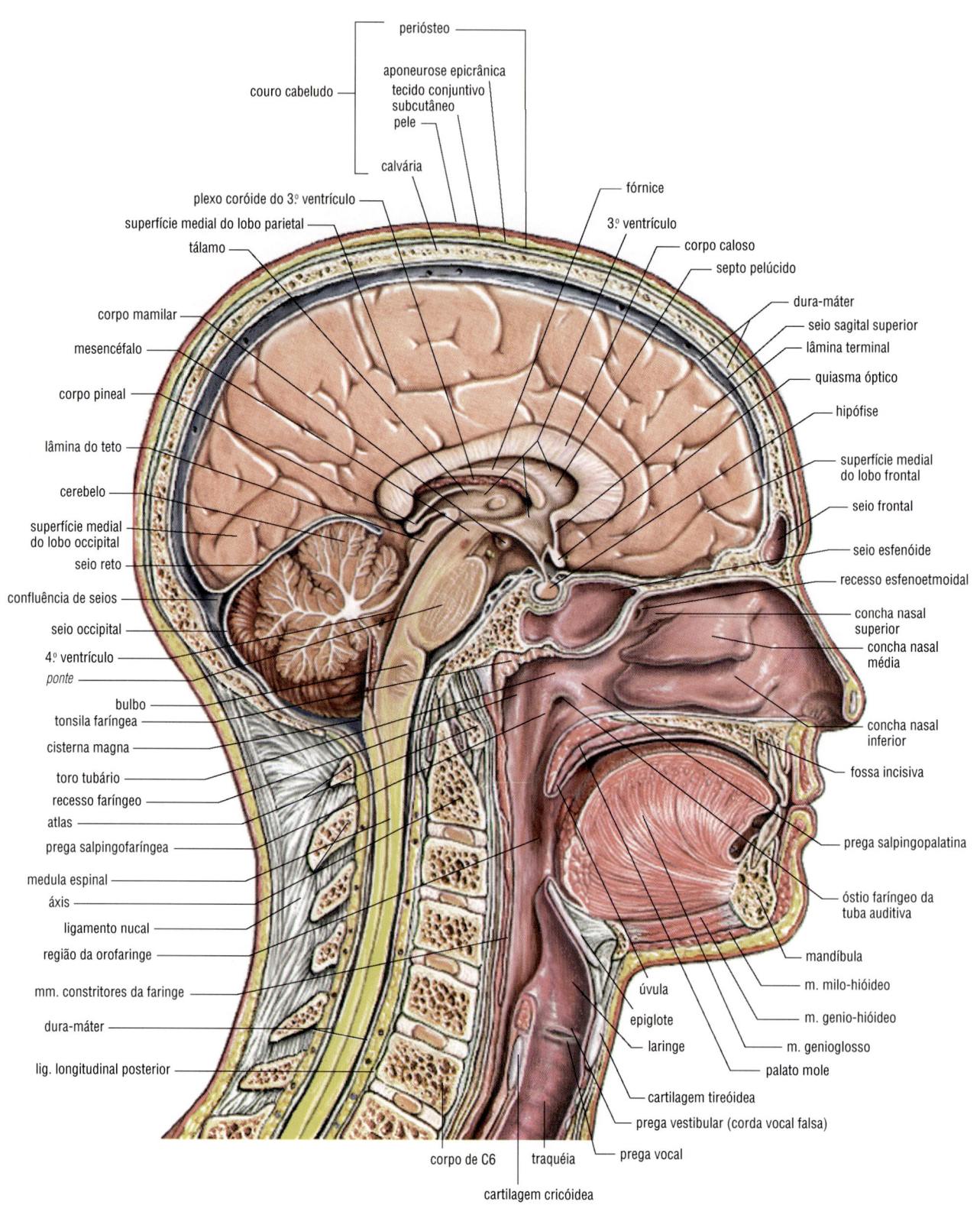

PRANCHA 7: ENCÉFALO, VISTA LATERAL

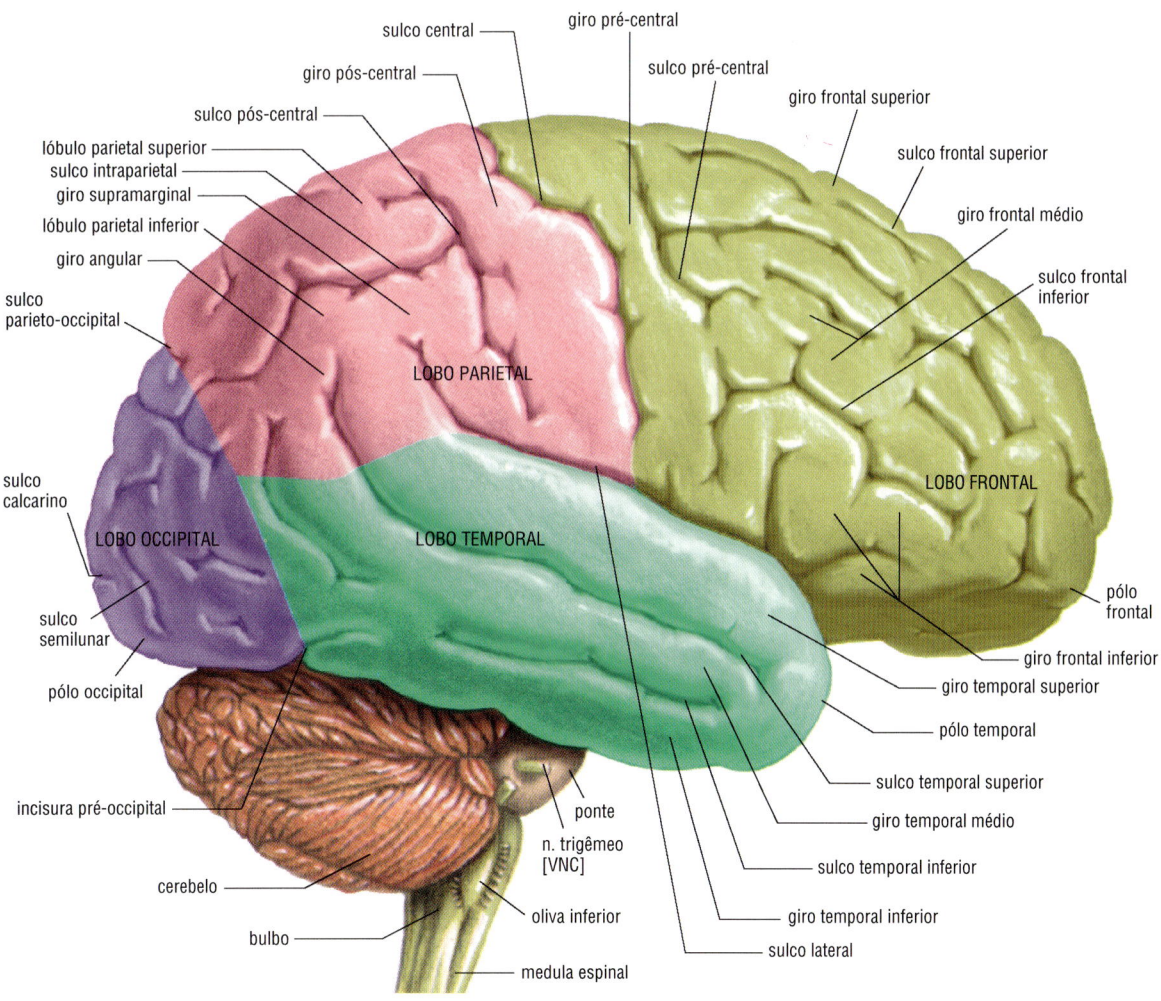

PRANCHA 8: ESQUELETO, VISTA LATERAL

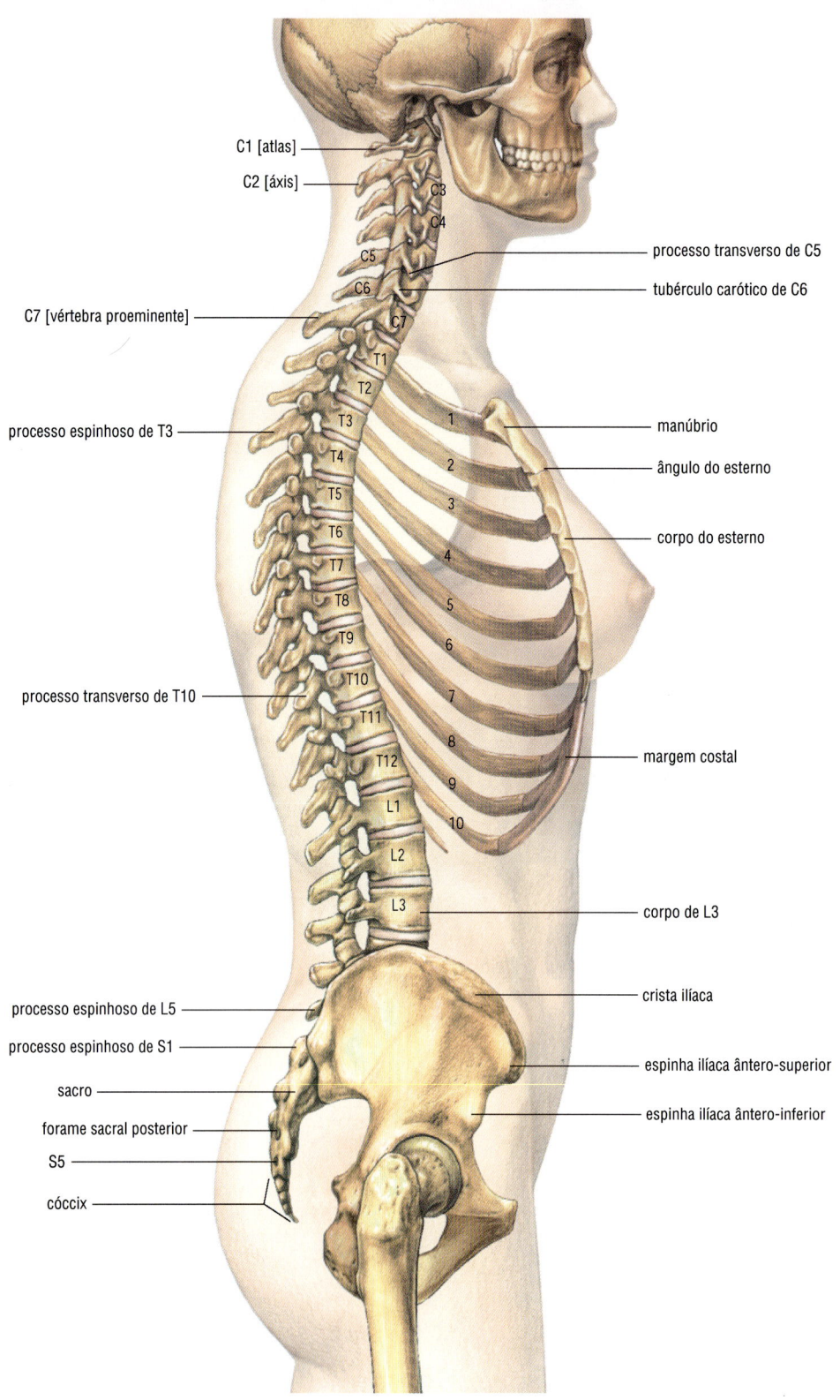

PRANCHA 9: ESQUELETO, VISTA ANTERIOR

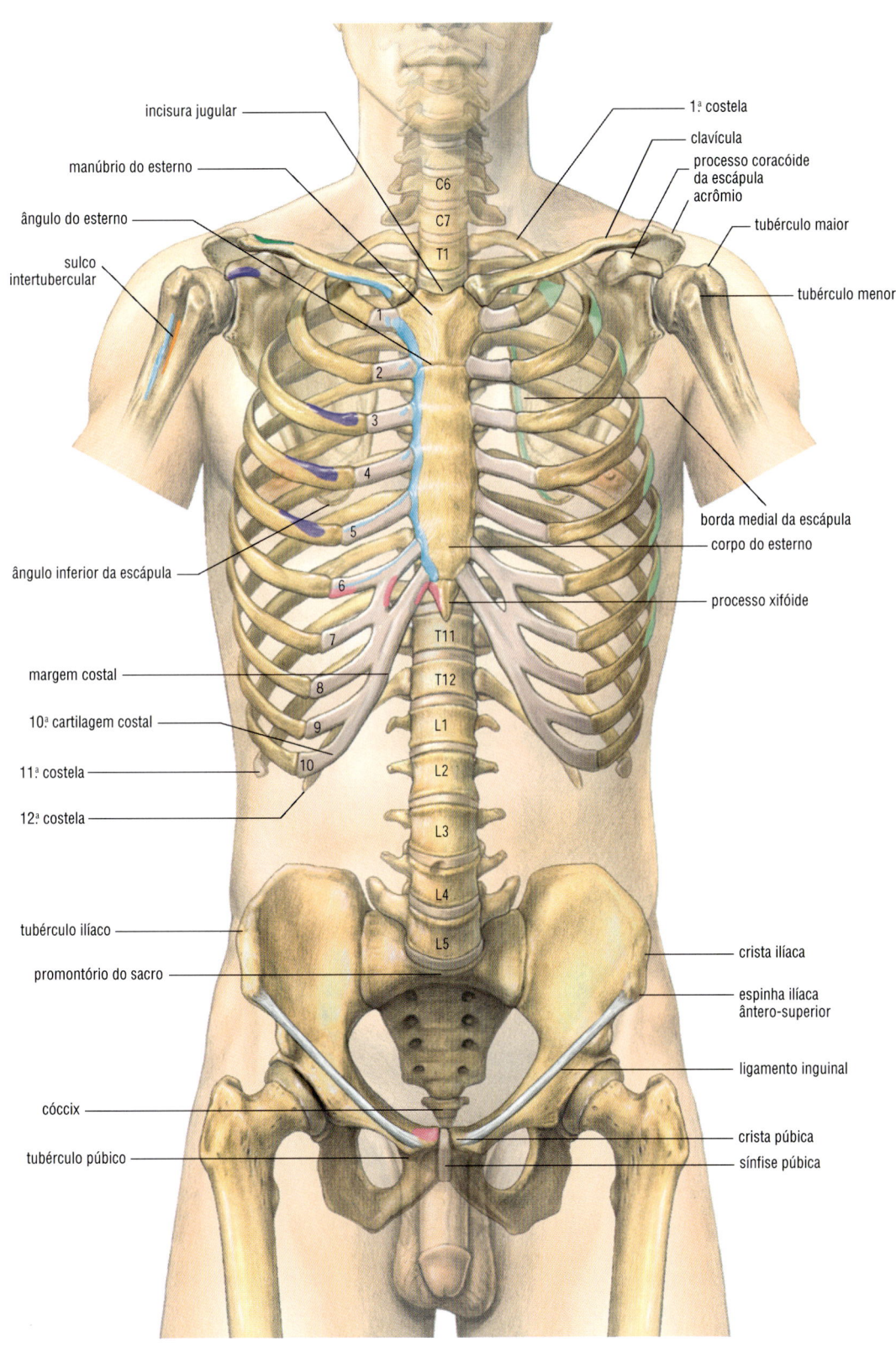

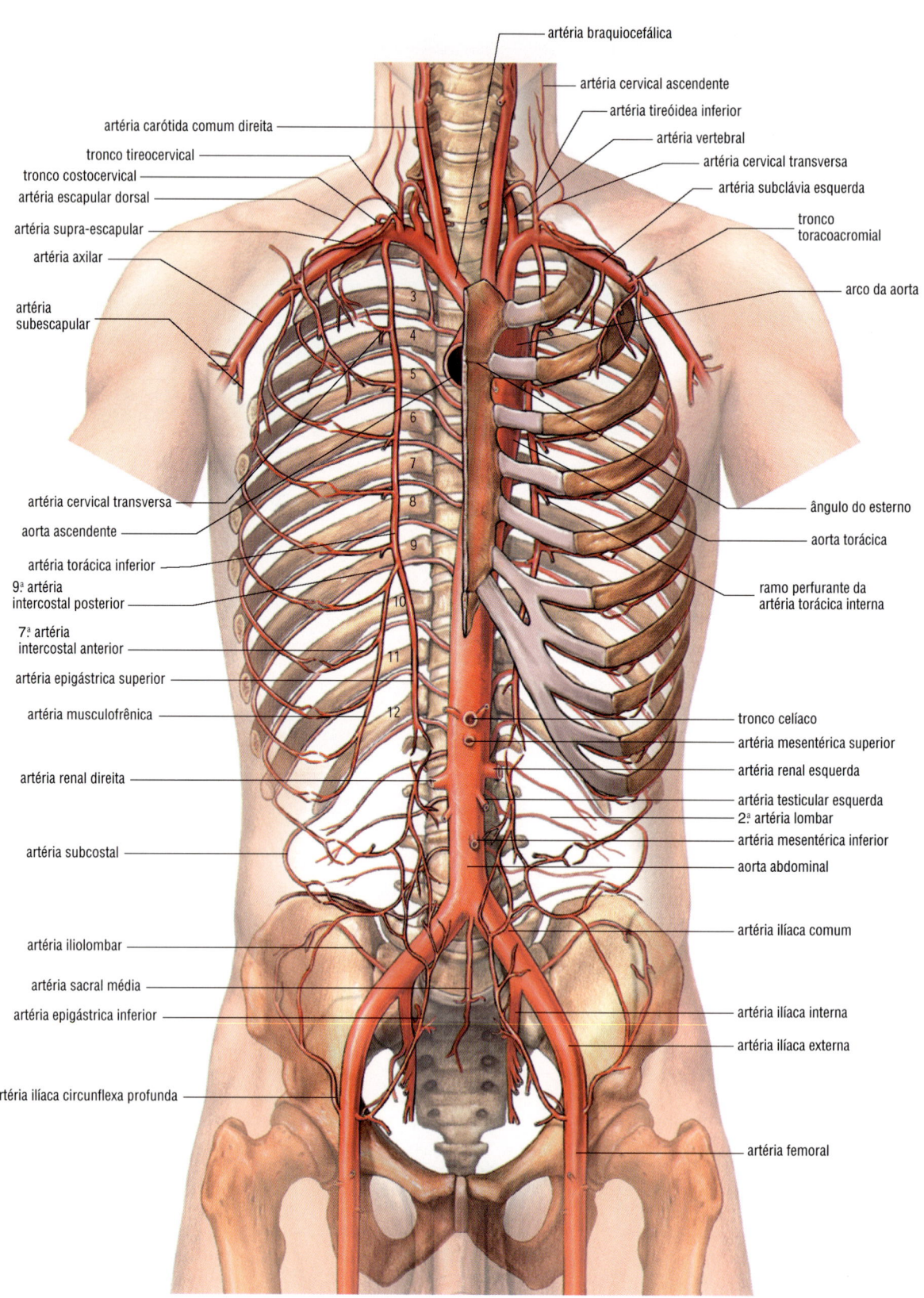

PRANCHA 11: FOCOS DE AUSCULTA

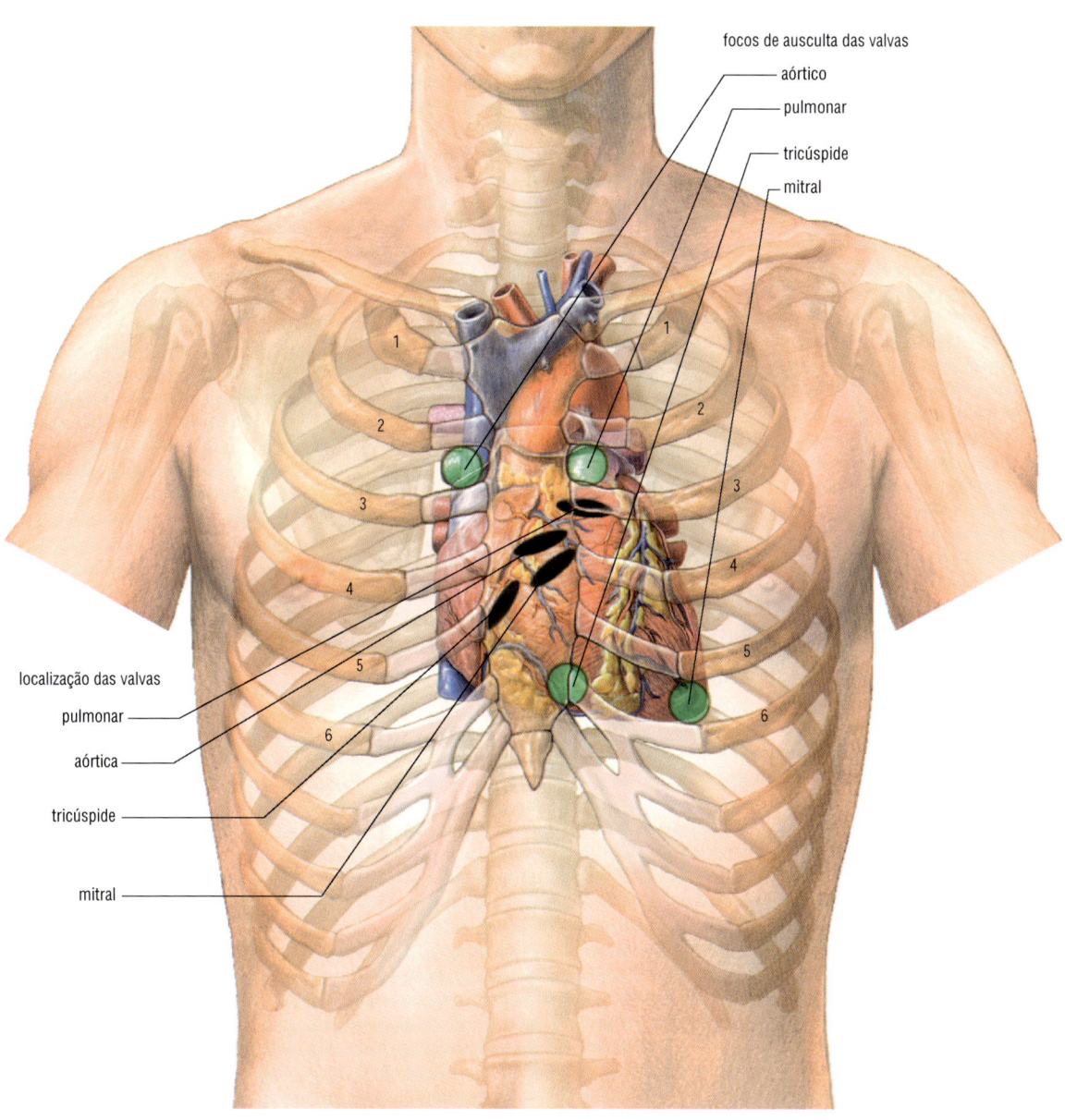

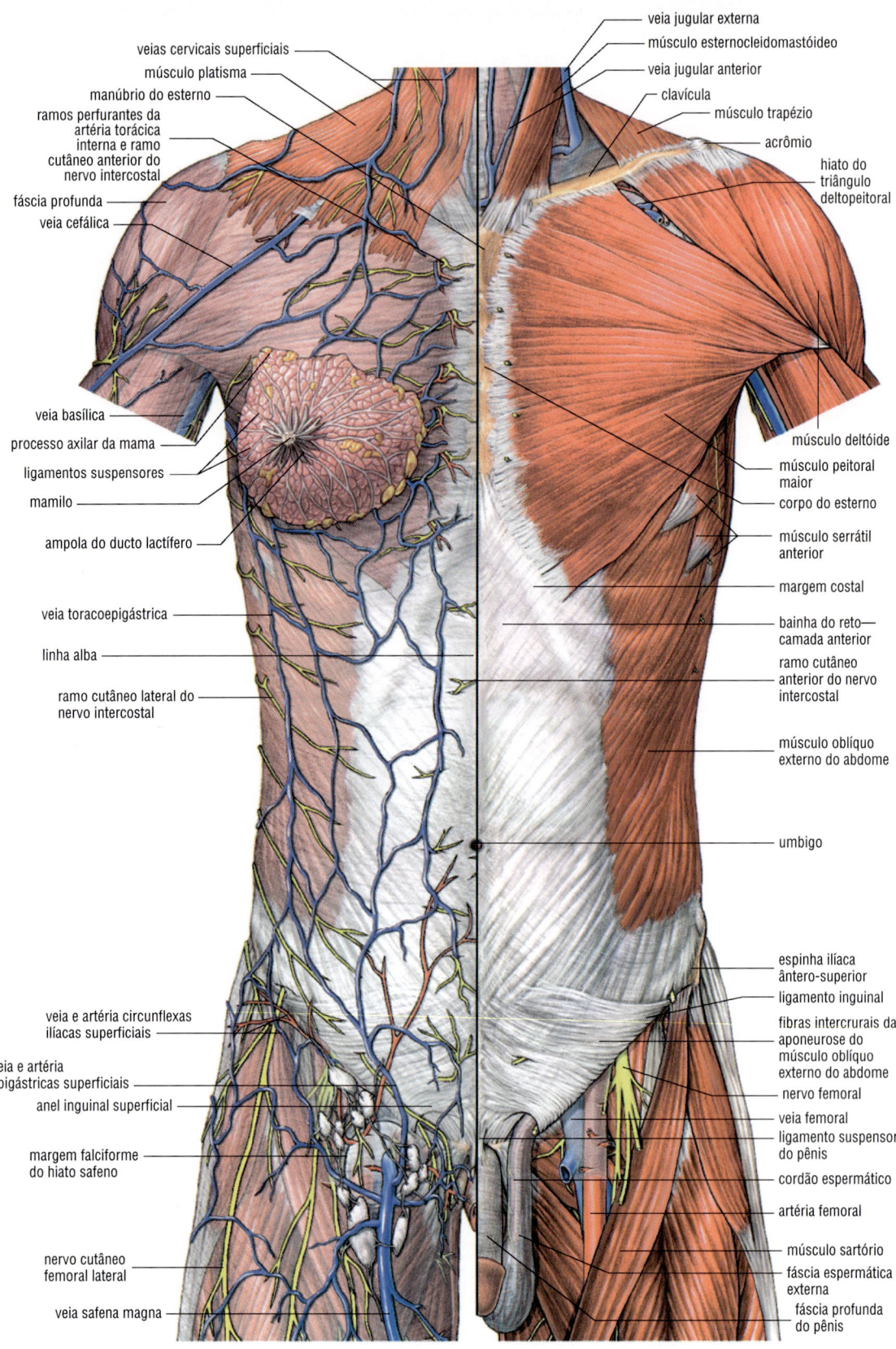

PRANCHA 13: ESQUELETO, VISTA POSTERIOR

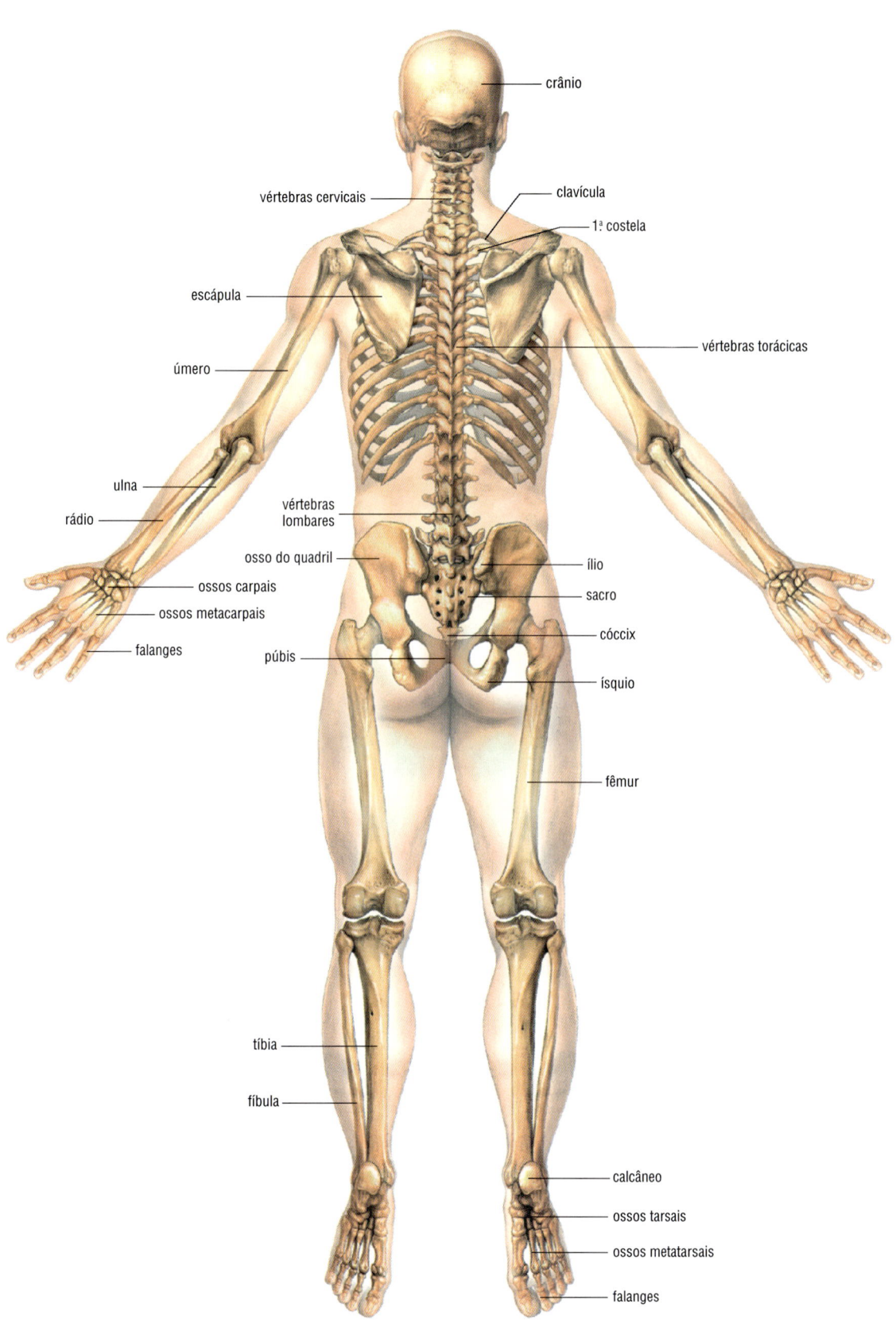

PRANCHA 14: MUSCULATURA DO DORSO, VISTA POSTERIOR

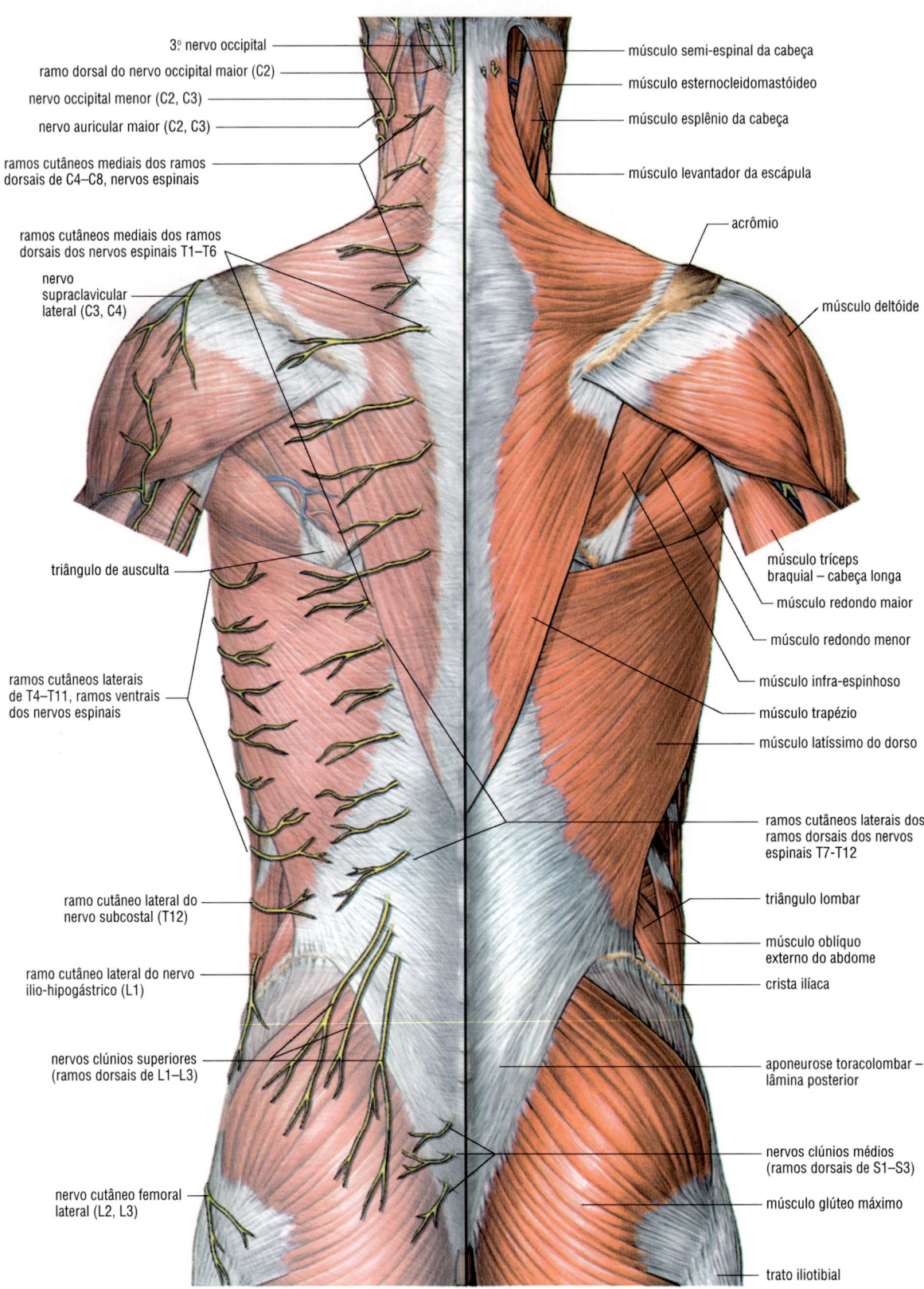

PRANCHA 15: ESQUELETO DO MEMBRO SUPERIOR, VISTA ANTERIOR

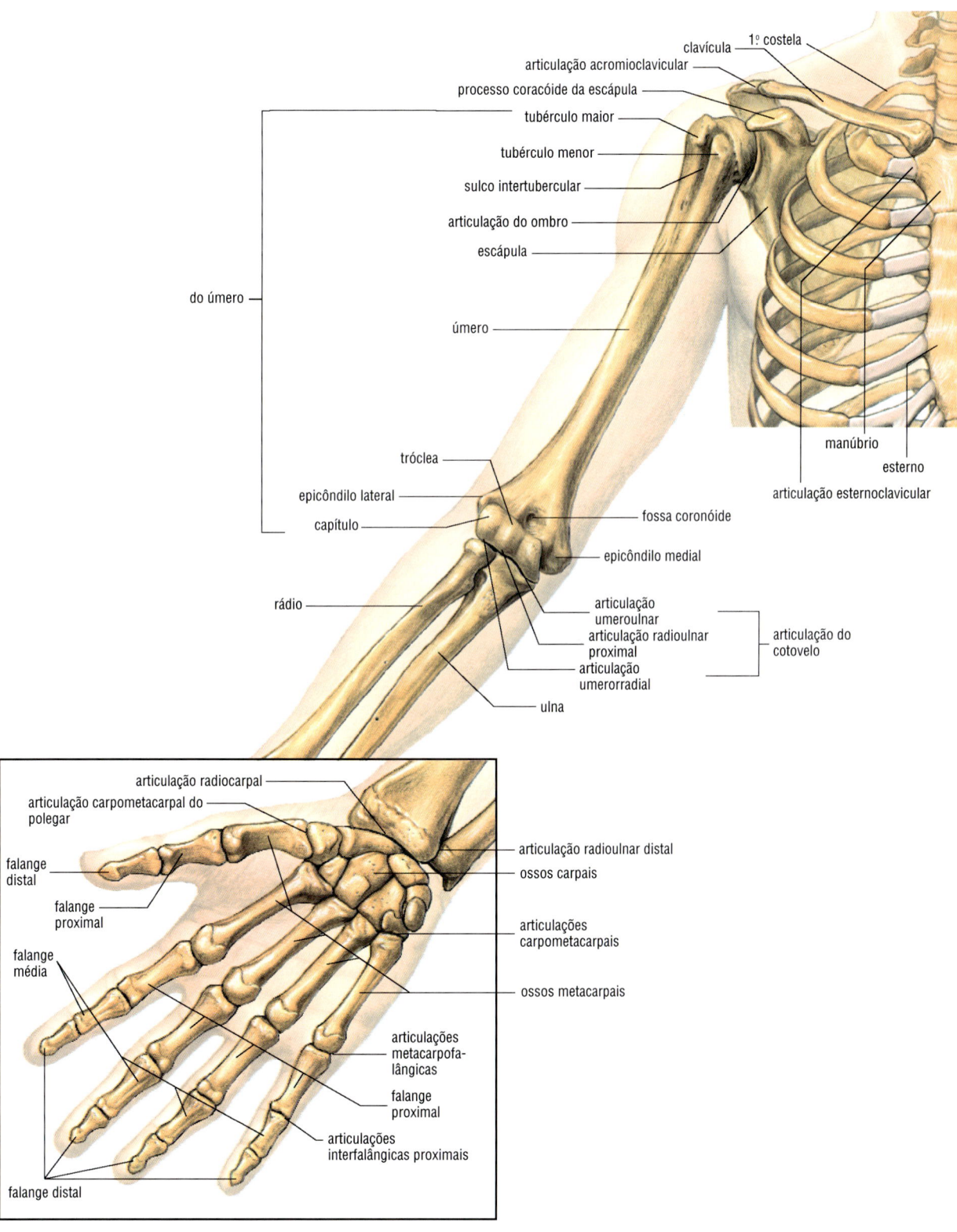

PRANCHA 16: ARTÉRIAS DO MEMBRO SUPERIOR, VISTA ANTERIOR

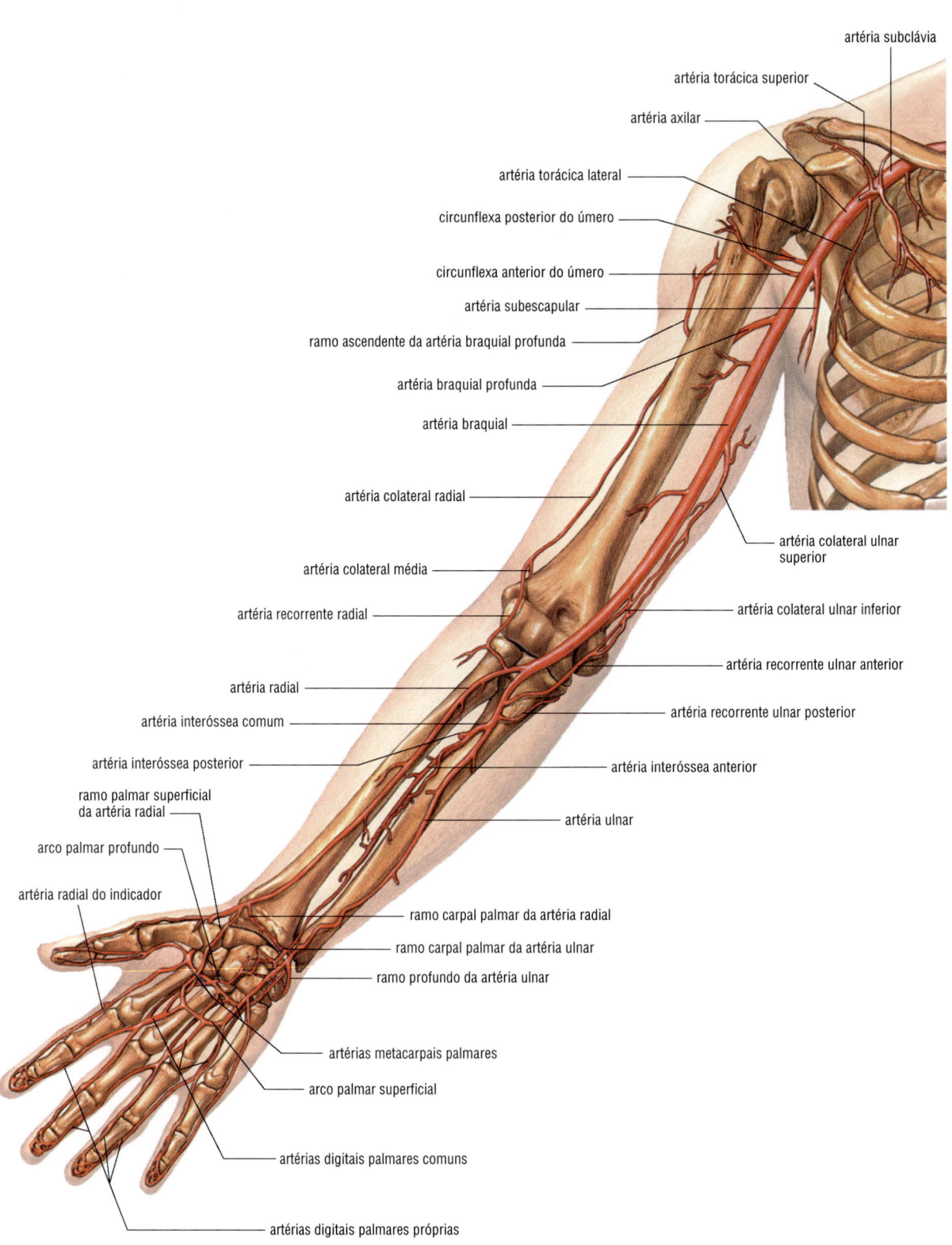

PRANCHA 17: NERVOS DO MEMBRO SUPERIOR, VISTA ANTERIOR

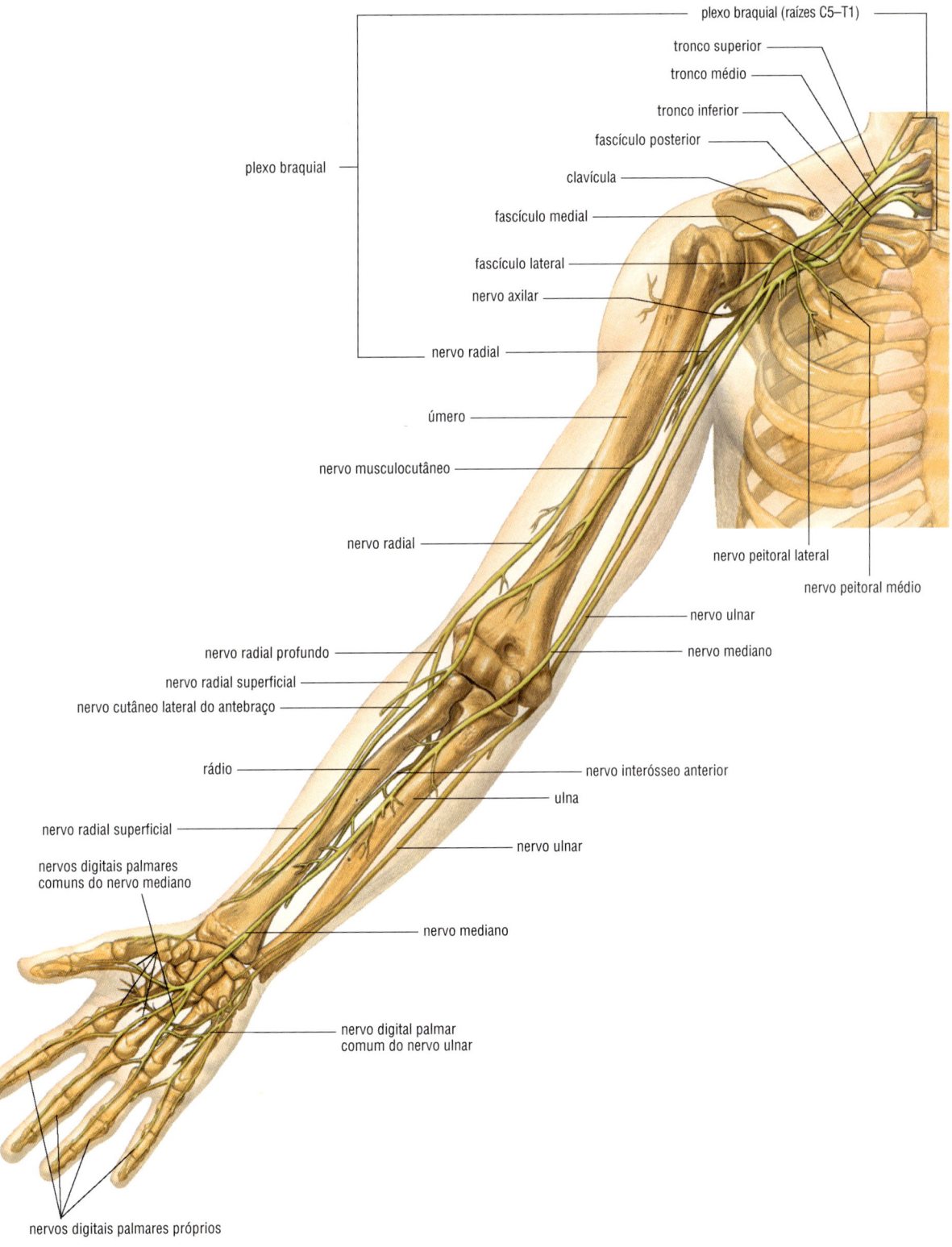

PRANCHA 18: MUSCULATURA DO TÓRAX E DO MEMBRO SUPERIOR, VISTA LATERAL

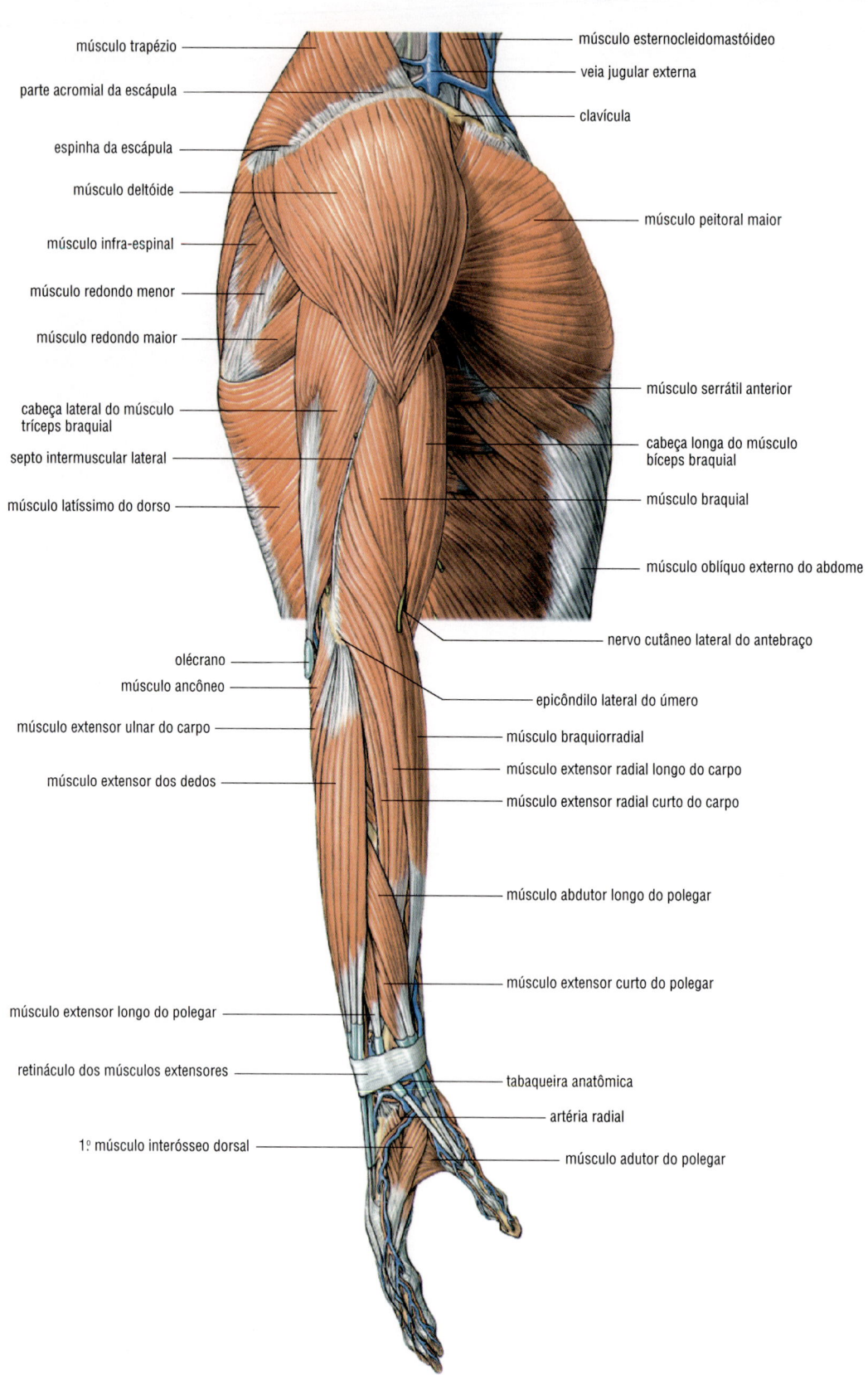

PRANCHA 19: ESQUELETO DO MEMBRO INFERIOR, VISTA ANTERIOR

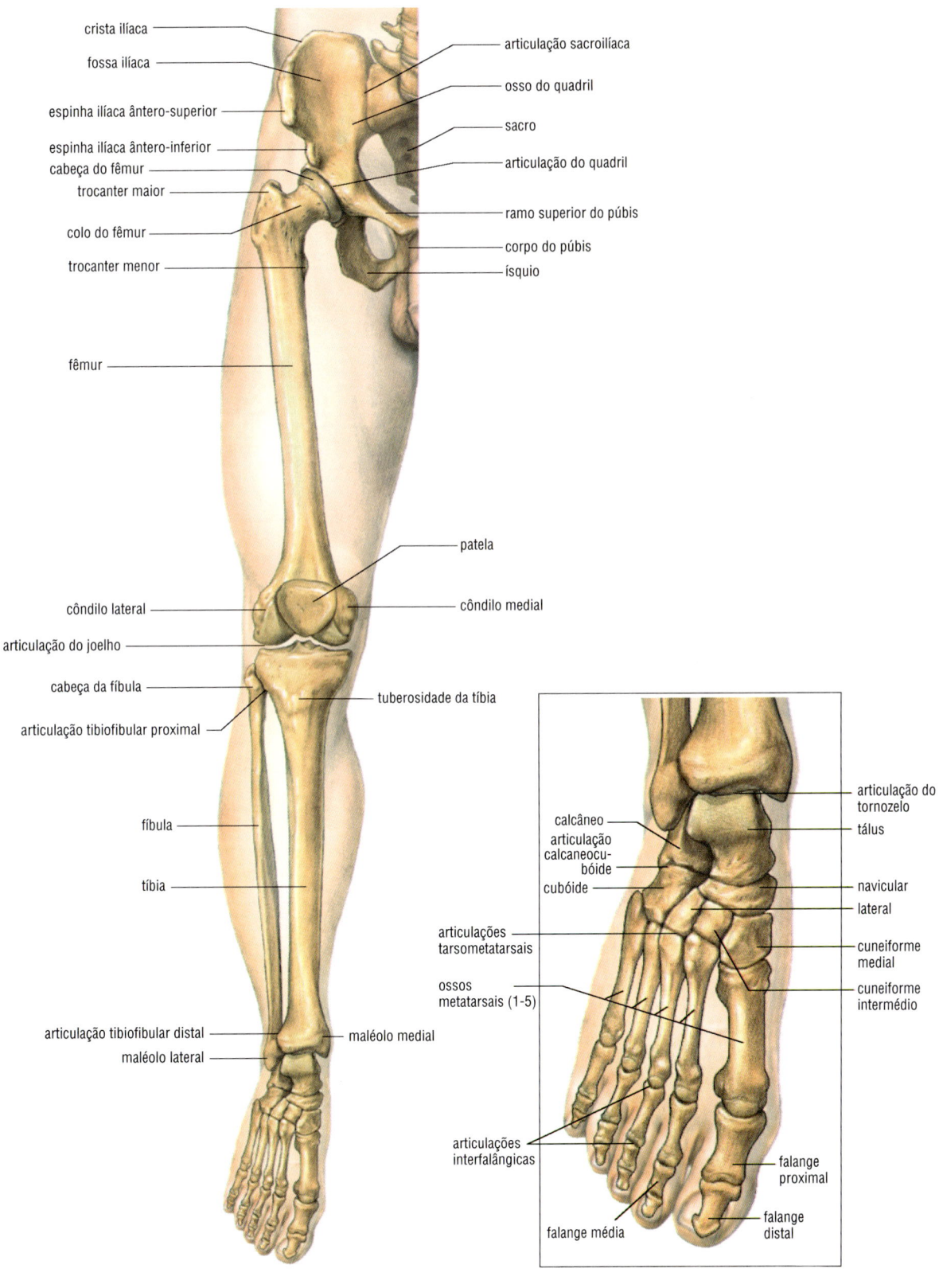

PRANCHA 20: ARTÉRIAS DO MEMBRO INFERIOR, VISTAS ANTERIOR E POSTERIOR

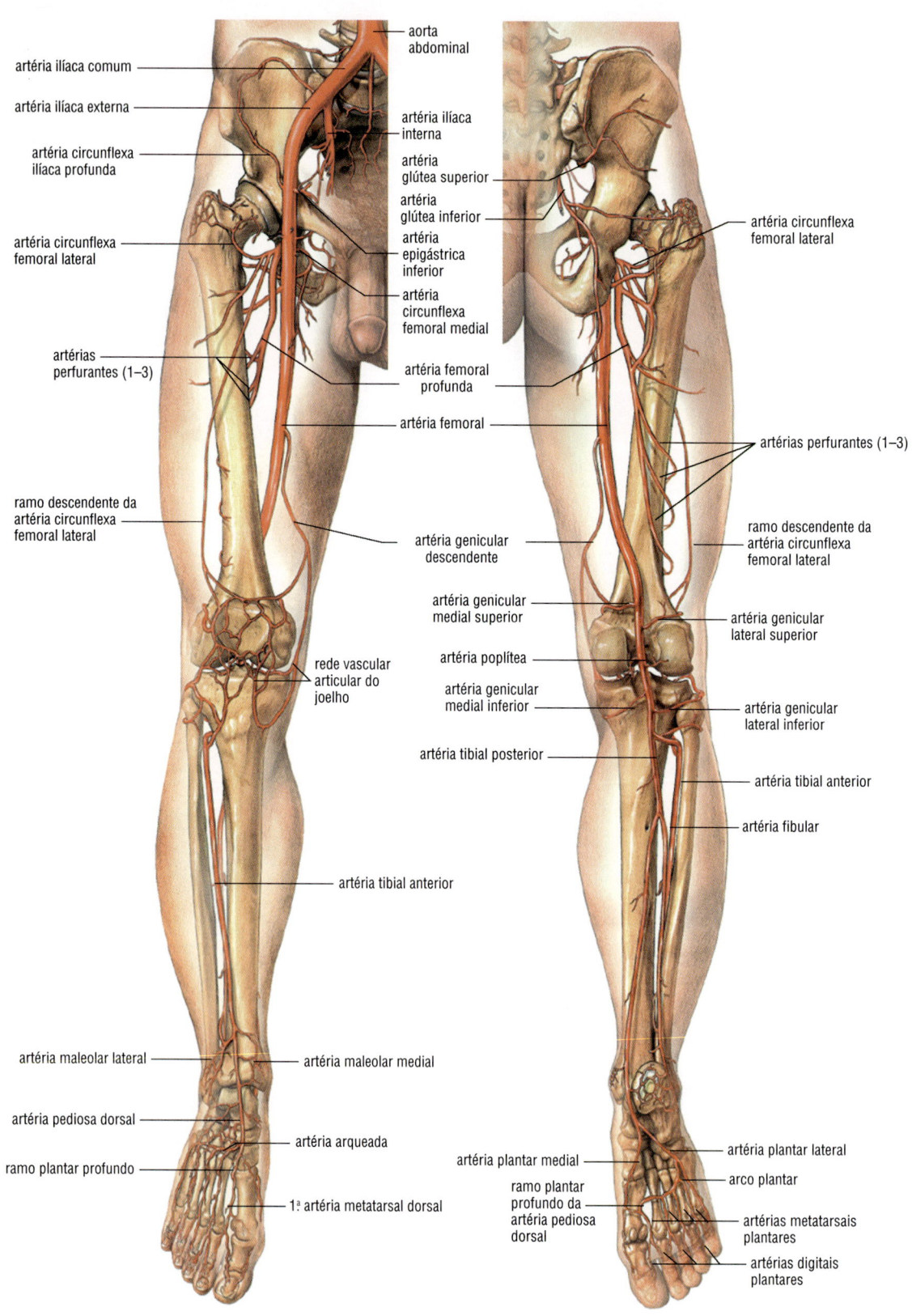

PRANCHA 21: NERVOS DO MEMBRO INFERIOR, VISTAS ANTERIOR E POSTERIOR

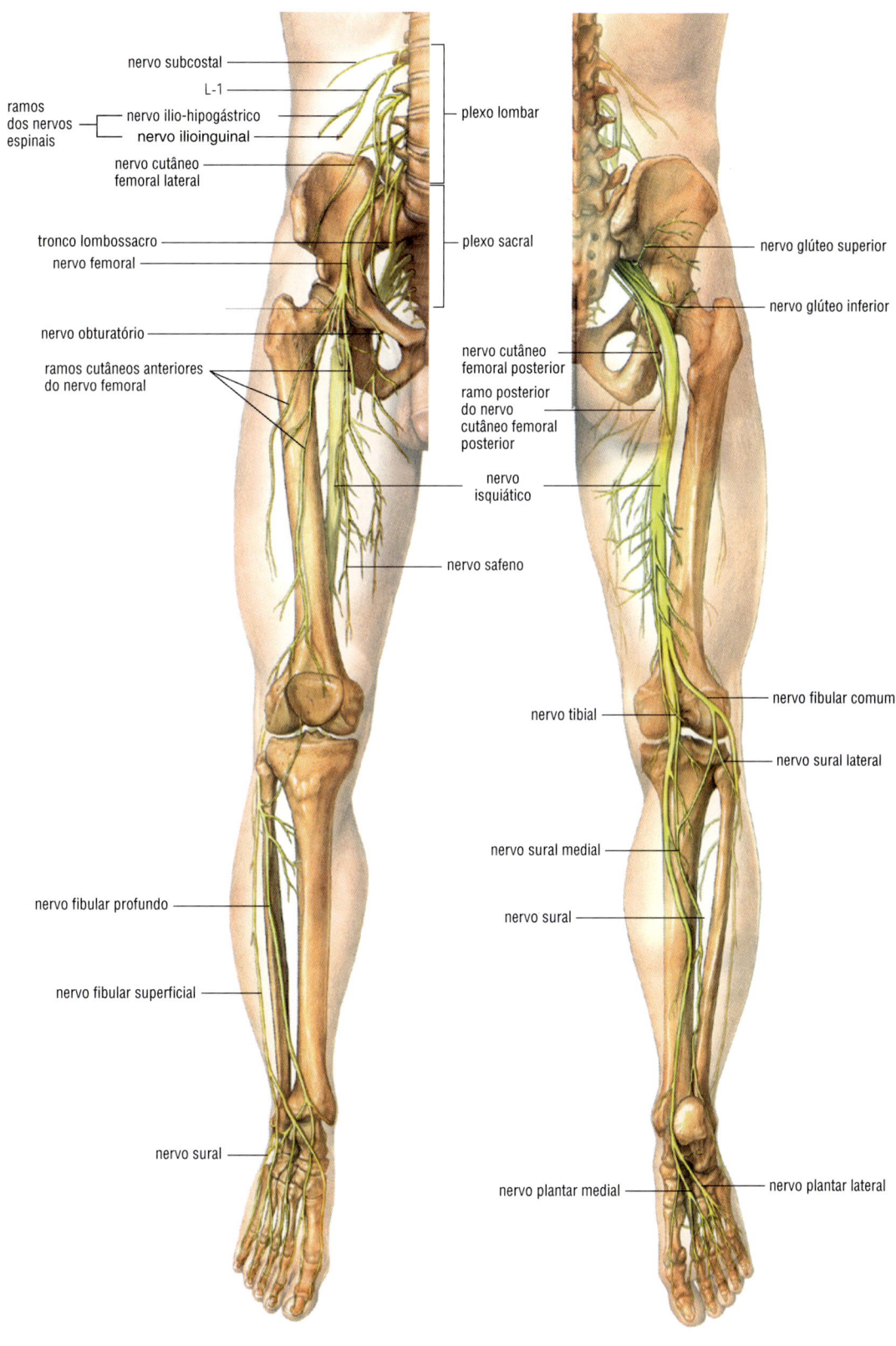

PRANCHA 22: MUSCULATURA DO MEMBRO INFERIOR, VISTAS LATERAL E MEDIAL

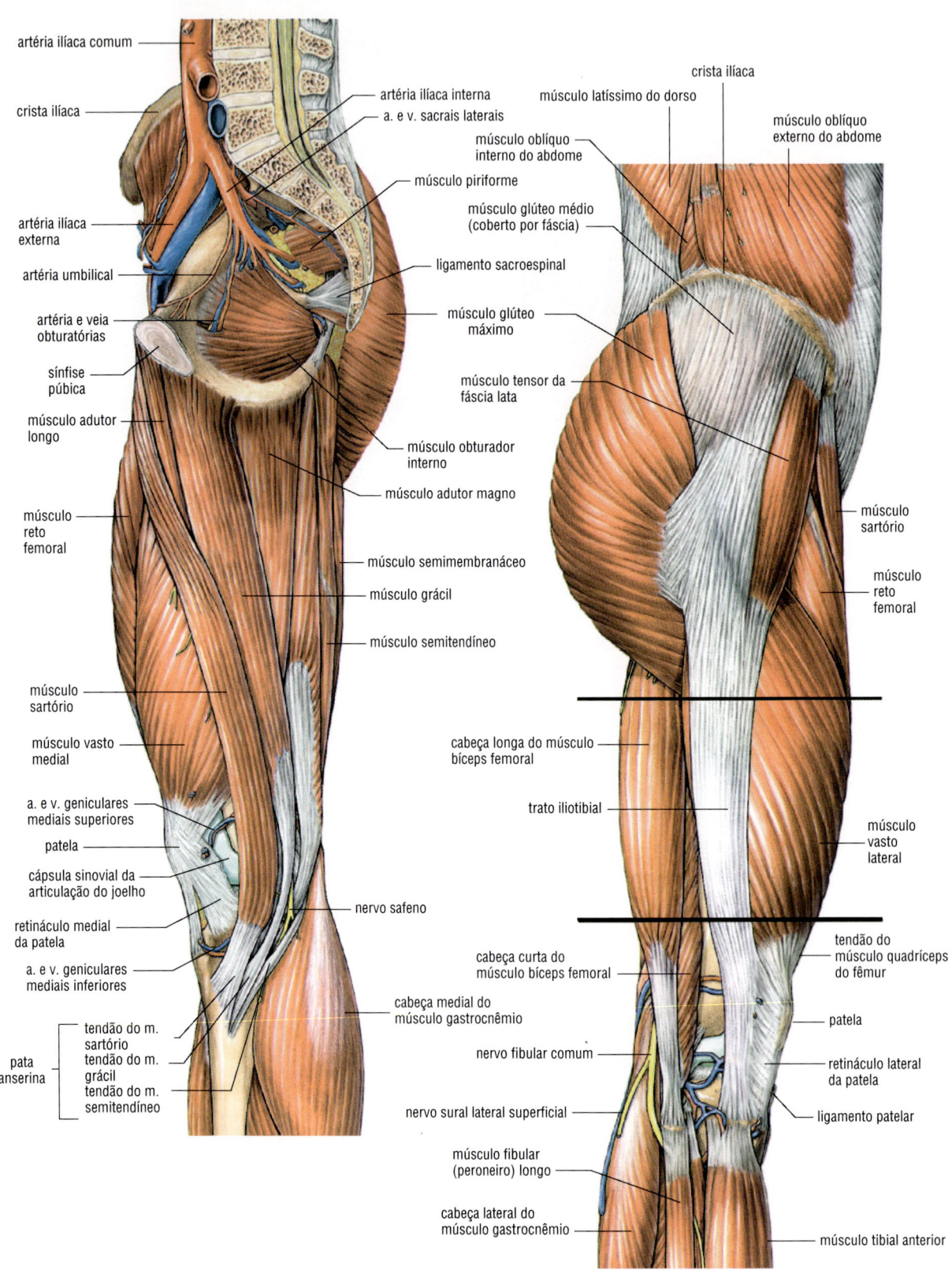

PRANCHA 23: SISTEMA RESPIRATÓRIO, VISTA ANTERIOR

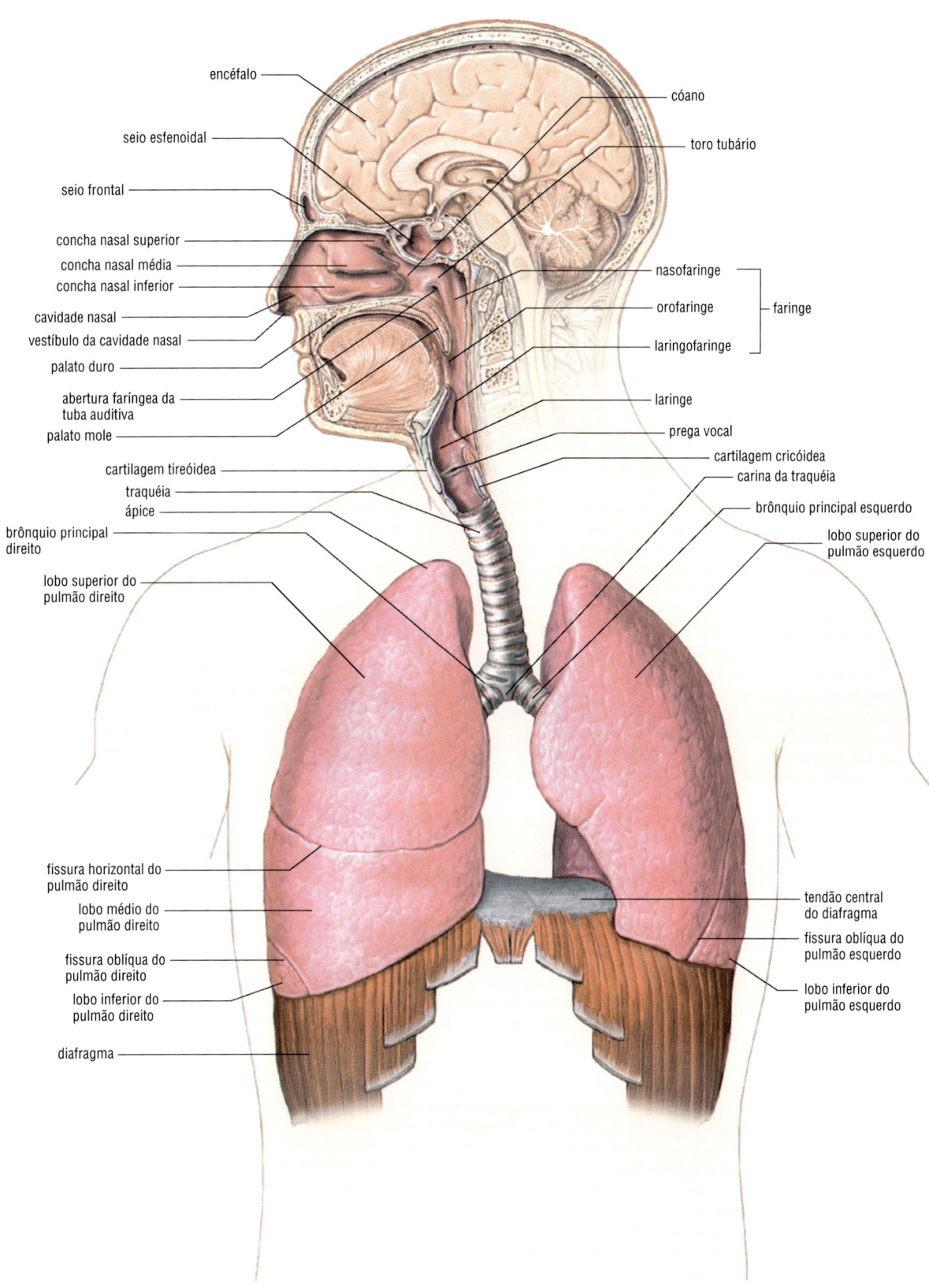

PRANCHA 24: SISTEMA DIGESTIVO, VISTA ANTERIOR

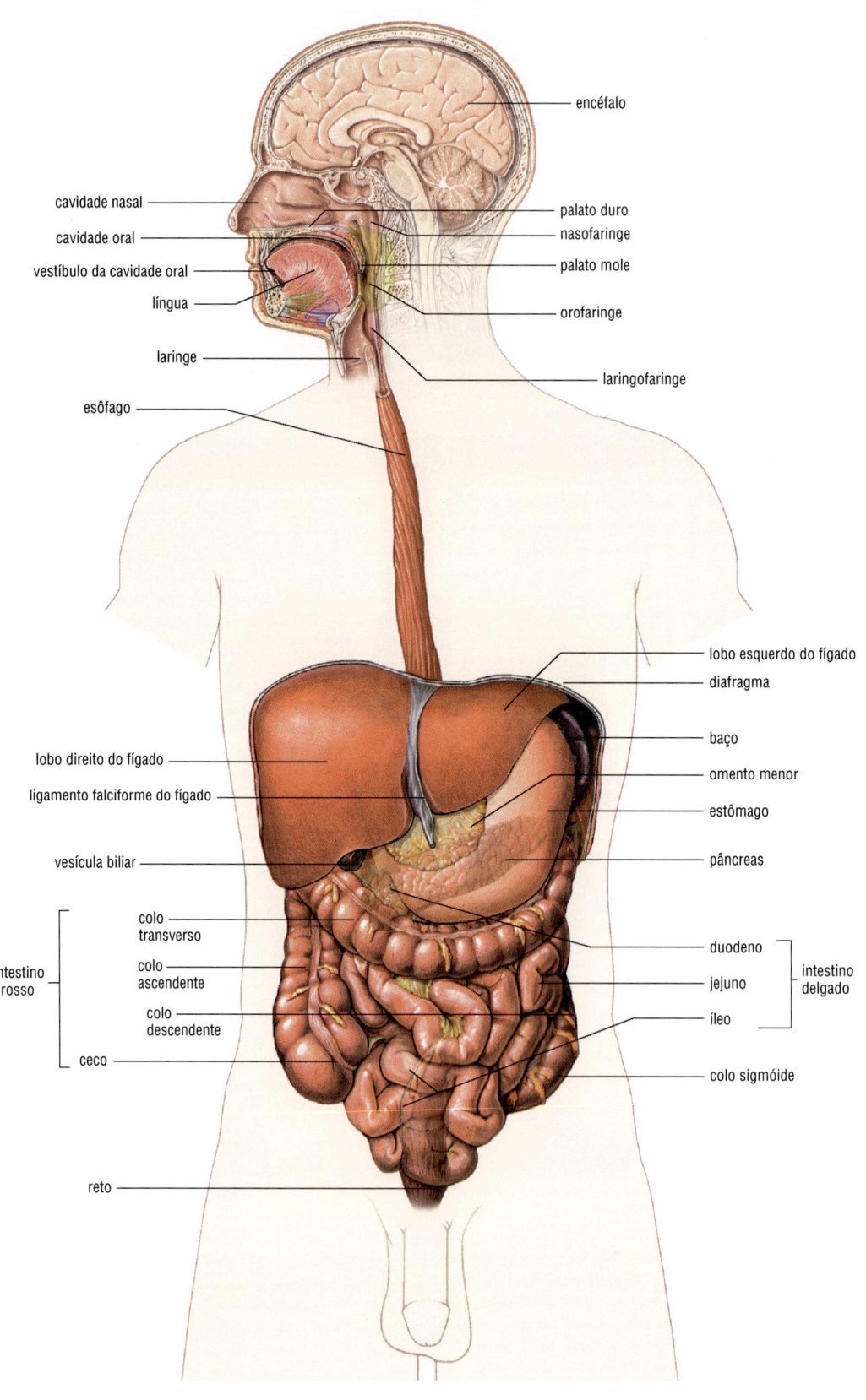

PRANCHA 25: SISTEMA LINFÁTICO, VISTA ANTERIOR

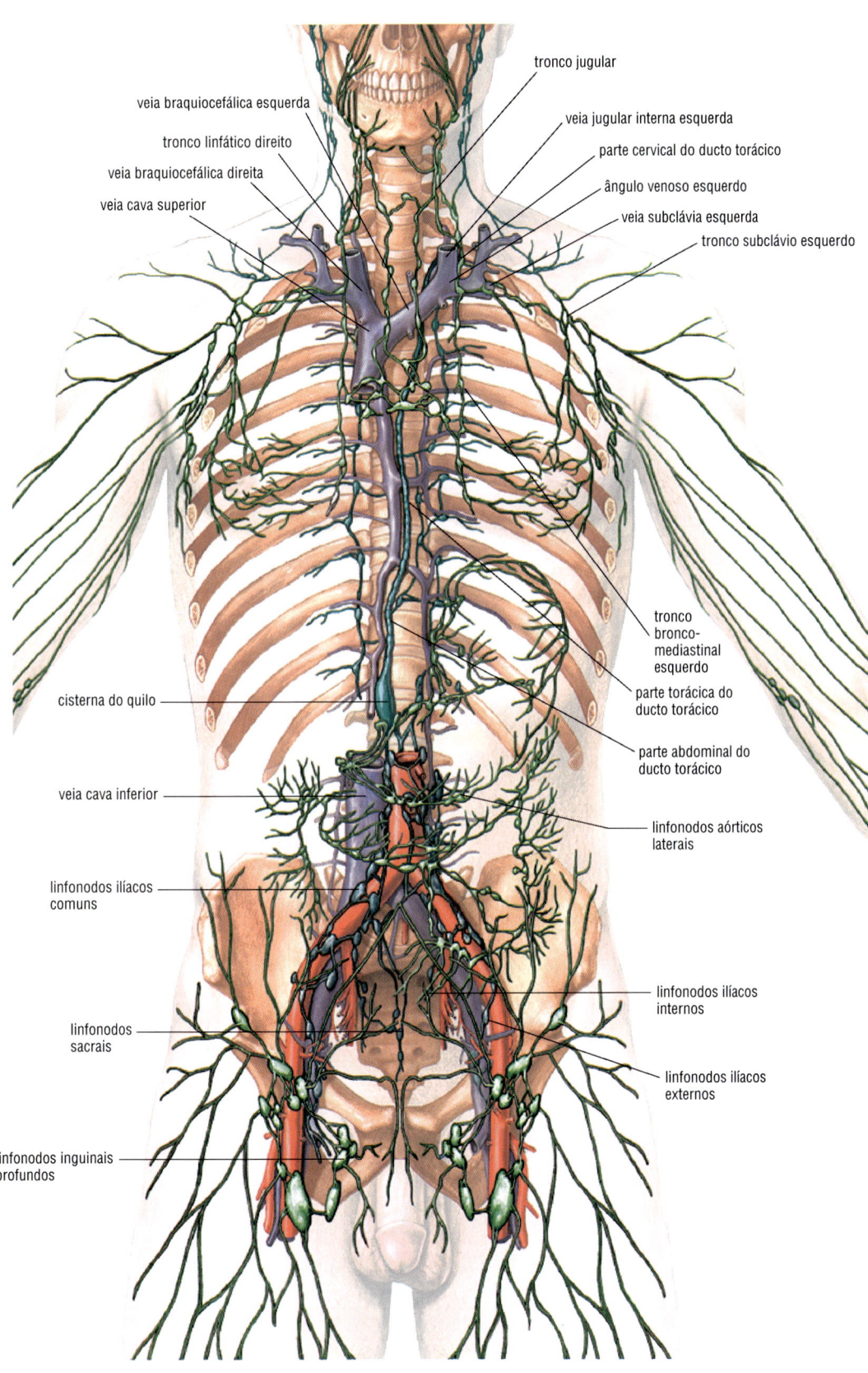

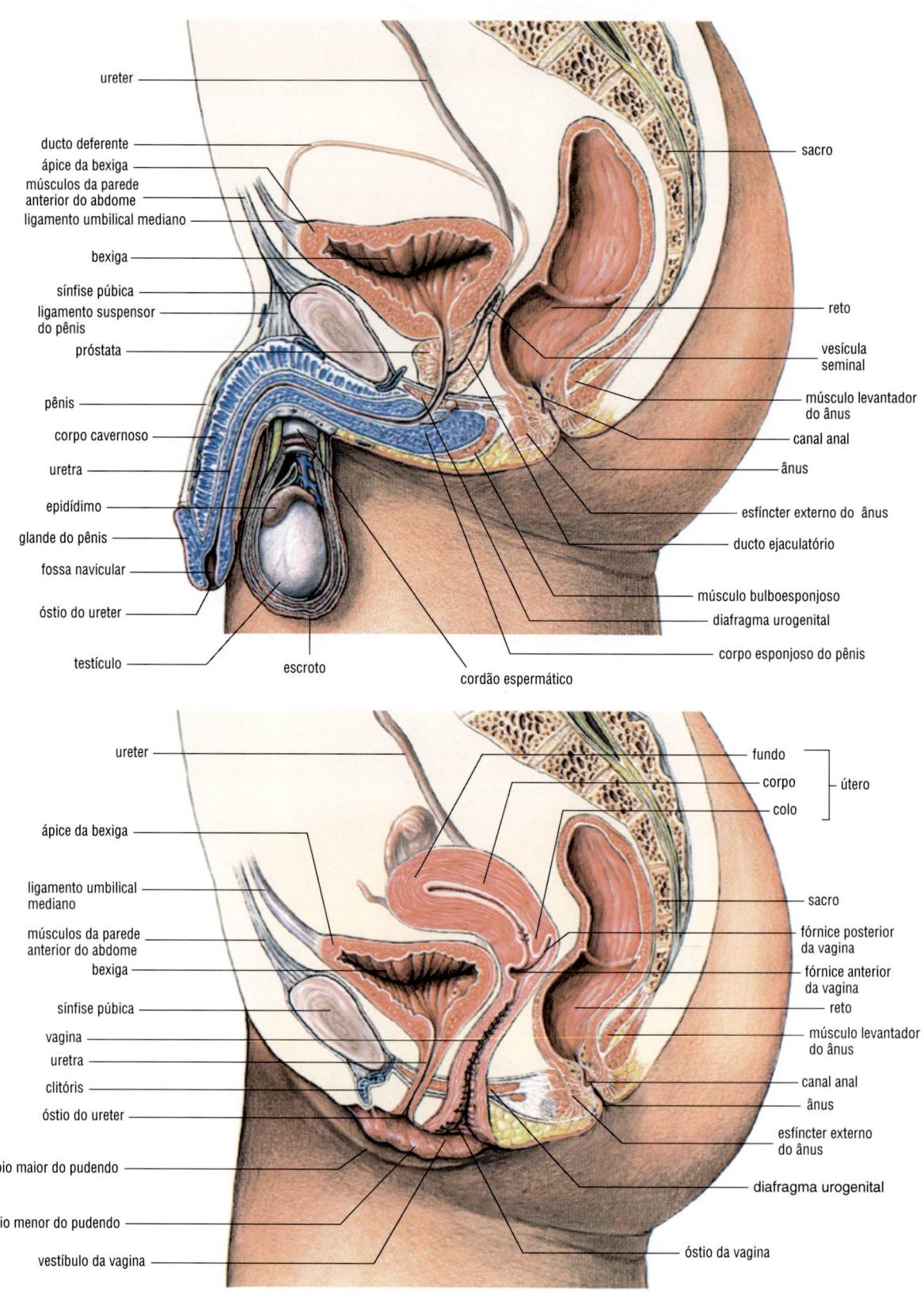

PRANCHA 27: VISTA ANTERIOR DO CORAÇÃO COM VENTRÍCULO DIREITO ABERTO

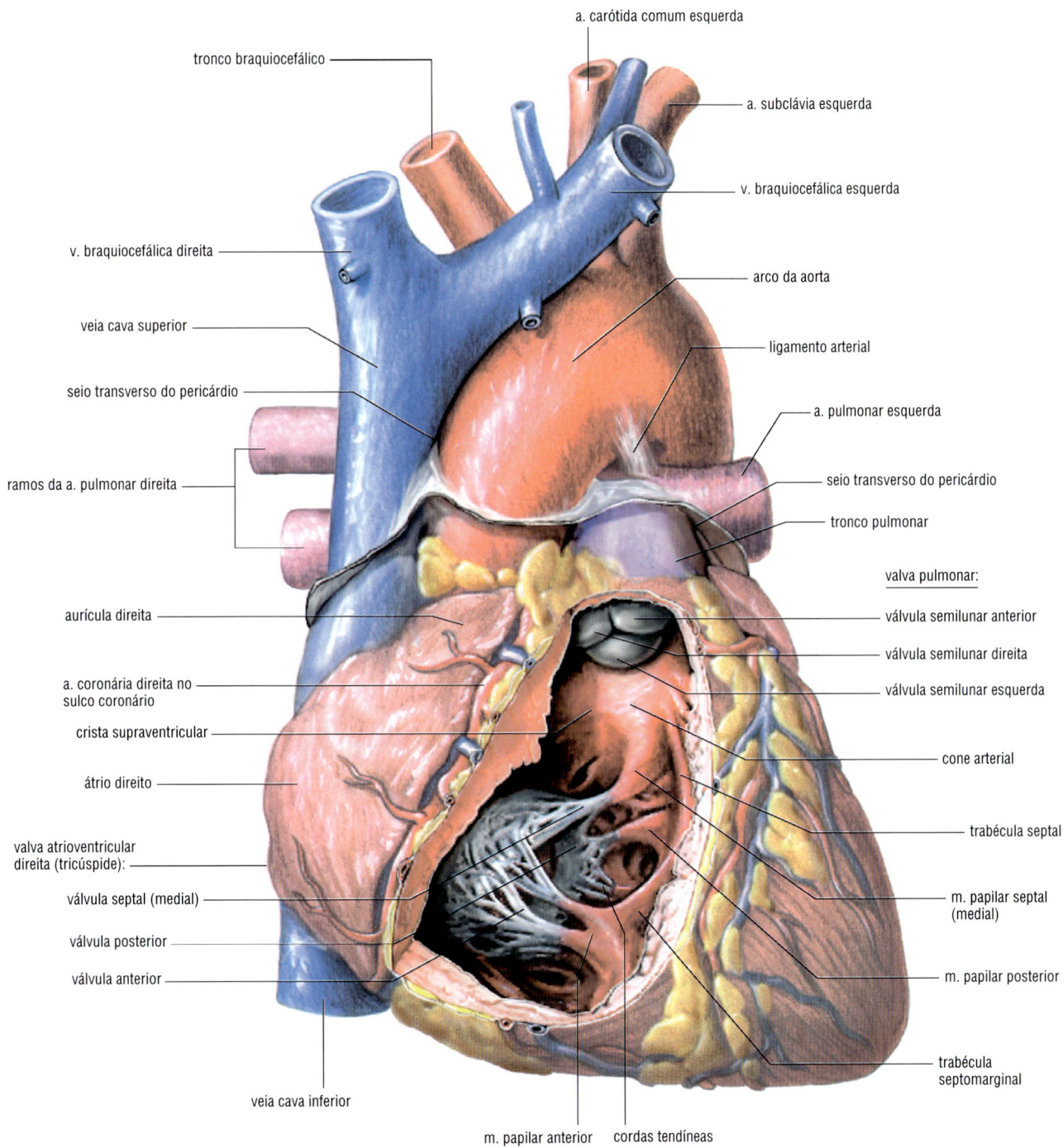

En·ter·o·bac·ter (en'ter-ō-bak'ter). Gênero de bactérias aeróbicas, facultativamente anaeróbicas, não-formadoras de esporos, móveis (família Enterobacteriaceae) que contêm bacilos Gram-negativos. As células são peritríquias, e algumas cepas possuem células encapsuladas. A glicose é fermentada com produção de ácido e gás. O teste de Voges-Proskauer geralmente é positivo. A gelatina é lentamente liquefeita pelas formas mais comuns (*E. cloacae*). Esses microrganismos são encontrados nas fezes de seres humanos e de outros animais, e no esgoto, no solo, na água e em laticínios; reconhecido como agente de infecções hospitalares comuns das vias urinárias, pulmões ou sangue; algo resistentes aos antibióticos. Esse gênero, caracteristicamente, adquire resistência rapidamente, em parte devido à presença de β-lactamases indutíveis; a espécie típica é *E. cloacae*.
  E. aerog'enes, espécie bacteriana encontrada na água, no solo, no esgoto, nos laticínios e nas fezes de seres humanos e de outros animais. Microrganismos previamente identificados como cepas móveis de *Aerobacter aerogenes*, agora são classificados nessa espécie. SIN *Klebsiella mobilis*.
  E. cloa'cae, espécie bacteriana encontrada nas fezes de seres humanos e de outros animais e no esgoto, no solo e na água; algumas vezes é encontrada na urina e no pus e em outras amostras de animais; é a espécie típica do gênero *E*. Uma causa grave de infecção hospitalar.
  E. sakazakii, espécie bacteriana particularmente associada à meningite neonatal adquirida em berçários.
en·ter·o·bac·te·ria (en'ter-ō-bak-tēr'ē-ā). Enterobactérias; plural de enterobacterium.
En·ter·o·bac·te·ri·a·ce·ae (en'ter-ō-bak-tēr-ē-ā'sē-ē). Uma família de bactérias aeróbicas, facultativamente anaeróbicas, não-formadoras de esporos (ordem Eubacteriales) contendo bacilos Gram-negativos. Algumas espécies são imóveis, e existem formas imóveis de espécies móveis; as células móveis são peritríquias. Esses microrganismos crescem bem em meios de cultura artificiais. Eles reduzem nitratos a nitritos e utilizam a glicose de forma fermentativa com a produção de ácido ou de ácido e gás. A indofenol oxidase não é produzida por esses microrganismos. Eles não liquefazem o alginato, e o pectato só é liquefeito por membros de um gênero, *Pectobacterium*. Essa família inclui muitos parasitas animais e alguns parasitas vegetais que causam mela, cecídio e decomposição. Alguns desses microrganismos ocorrem como saprófitas, que decompõem materiais vegetais contendo carboidratos. O gênero típico é a *Escherichia*.
en·ter·o·bac·te·ri·um, pl. **en·ter·o·bac·te·ria** (en'ter-ō-bak-tēr'ē-um,-ā). Enterobactéria; um membro da família Enterobacteriaceae.
en·ter·o·bi·a·sis (en'ter-ō-bī'a-sis). Enterobíase; infecção por *Enterobius vermicularis*, o oxiúro humano.
En·ter·o·bi·us (en-ter-ō'bī-us). Gênero de vermes nematódeos, outrora incluídos no gênero *Oxyuris*, que inclui os oxiúros (*E. vermicularis*) de seres humanos e outros primatas. [entero- + G. *bios*, vida]
en·ter·o·cele (en'ter-o-sēl). Enterocele. **1.** Uma protrusão herniária através de um defeito na bolsa retovaginal ou vesicovaginal. [entero- + G. *kēlē*, hernia] **2.** Cavidade abdominal. SIN abdominal cavity. [entero- + G. *koilia*, uma cavidade] **3.** Uma hérnia intestinal. [ver 1]
  partial e., e. parcial. SIN parietal hernia.
en·ter·o·cen·te·sis (en'ter-ō-sen-tē'sis). Enterocentese; punção do intestino com uma agulha oca (trocarte e cânula) para retirar substâncias. [entero- + G. *kentēsis*, punção]
en·ter·o·cho·le·cys·tos·to·my (en'ter-ō-kō-lē-sis-tos'tō-mē). Enterocolecistostomia. SIN cholecystenterostomy. [entero- + G. *cholē*, bile, + *kystis*, vesícula, + *stoma*, boca]
en·ter·o·cho·le·cys·tot·o·my (en'ter-ō-kō-lē-sis-tot'ō-mē). Enterocolecistotomia. SIN cholecystenterostomy. [entero- + G. *cholē*, bile, + *kystis*, vesícula, + *tomē*, corte]
enterocidal (en-ter-ō-sī'dal). Enterocida; agente que mata parasitas residentes no trato gastrointestinal.
en·ter·o·clei·sis (en-ter-ō-klī'sis). Enterocleise; oclusão da luz do canal alimentar. [entero- + G. *kleisis*, fechamento]
  omental e., e. omental; uso do omento para ajudar no fechamento de uma abertura no intestino.
en·ter·o·cly·sis (en-ter-o-k'li-sis). Enteróclise. **1.** Enema alto. SIN high enema. **2.** Em radiografia do intestino delgado, enchimento por introdução de meio de contraste através de um cateter avançado até o duodeno ou jejuno. [entero- + G. *klysis*, lavagem]
  radiologic e., e. radiológica; método de obter imagens do duodeno e do intestino delgado por intubação do duodeno e instilação de bário diluído; também conhecida como enema do intestino delgado.
en·ter·o·coc·cem·ia (en'ter-ō-kok-sēm'ē-ah). Enterococcemia; uma doença hematogênica, que algumas vezes leva à septicemia, causada por membros dos estreptococos do grupo D, *Enterococcus faecalis* ou *Enterococcus faecium*.
En·ter·o·coc·cus (en'ter-ō-kok'us). Gênero de bactérias anaeróbicas facultativas, geralmente imóveis, não-formadoras de esporos, Gram-positivas (família Streptococcaceae), anteriormente classificadas como parte do gênero *Streptococcus*. Encontrado no trato intestinal de seres humanos e animais, os enterococos causam infecções intra-abdominais, de feridas e das vias urinárias. A espécie típica é *E. faecalis*. *E. faecium* também é clinicamente significativo, devido à sua tendência a desenvolver resistência a antibióticos.
  E. faecalis, espécie bacteriana encontrada nas fezes humanas e nos intestinos de muitos animais de sangue quente; ocasionalmente encontrada em infecções urinárias e em lesões sanguíneas e cardíacas em casos de endocardite subaguda; uma importante causa de infecção hospitalar, principalmente associada a patógenos Gram-negativos. SIN *Streptococcus faecalis*.
  E. faecium, a segunda espécie mais comum desse gênero isolada em infecção humana; essa espécie tem baixo nível de resistência à ampicilina, e, nos Estados Unidos e em outros países onde a vancomicina é usada freqüentemente, cepas resistentes vêm surgindo rapidamente como causas de infecções hospitalares; em casos de septicemia em pacientes imunodeprimidos, as taxas de fatalidade podem ser maiores que 50%.
en·ter·o·coc·cus, pl. **en·ter·o·coc·ci** (en'ter-ō-kok'us,-kok'sī). Enterococo; um estreptococo que habita o trato intestinal. [entero- + G. *kokkos*, baga]
en·ter·o·co·li·tis (en'ter-ō-kō-lī'tis). Enterocolite; inflamação da mucosa de maior ou menor extensão dos intestinos delgado e grosso. SIN coloenteritis. [entero- + G. *kolon*, cólon, + *-itis*, inflamação]
  antibiotic e., e. antibiótica; enterocolite causada por administração oral de antibióticos de amplo espectro, resultante do crescimento exagerado de estafilococos resistentes ao antibiótico ou leveduras e fungos, quando os microrganismos Gram-negativos fecais normais são suprimidos, resultando em diarréia ou enterocolite pseudomembranosa.
  necrotizing e., e. necrotizante; extensa ulceração e necrose do íleo e do cólon em prematuros no período neonatal; possivelmente devido à isquemia intestinal perinatal e à invasão bacteriana.
  pseudomembranous e., e. pseudomembranosa; enterocolite com formação e eliminação de material pseudomembranoso nas fezes; é mais comum como seqüela de antibioticoterapia; causada por uma exotoxina necrolítica produzida pelo *Clostridium difficile*. SIN pseudomembranous colitis, pseudomembranous enteritis.
  regional e., e. regional; as alterações da enterite regional envolvendo o cólon e o intestino delgado.
en·ter·o·co·los·to·my (en'ter-ō-kō-los'tō-mē). Enterocolostomia; estabelecimento de uma nova comunicação entre o intestino delgado e o cólon. [entero- + G. *kolon*, cólon, + *stoma*, boca]
en·ter·o·cyst (en'ter-ō-sist). Enterocisto; um cisto da parede intestinal. SIN enterocystoma. [entero- + G. *kystis*, vesícula]
en·ter·o·cys·to·cele (en'ter-ō-sis'tō-sēl). Enterocistocele; uma hérnia da parede intestinal e vesical. [entero- + G. *kystis*, bexiga, + *kēlē*, hérnia]
en·ter·o·cys·to·ma (en'ter-ō-sis-tō'mā). Enterocistoma. SIN enterocyst.
En·ter·o·cy·to·zo·on (en'ter-ō-sī'tō-zō'on). Gênero do filo de protozoários Microspora, todos os quais são parasitas intracelulares obrigatórios, formadores de esporos.
  E. bieneusi, agente de microsporidiose, que infecta basicamente o intestino delgado, principalmente em indivíduos imunodeprimidos. É o microsporídio descrito com maior freqüência em pacientes com AIDS/SIDA, nos quais foi implicado na diarréia crônica e no emagrecimento; o tratamento sugerido foi com octreotídeo e albendazol. VER TAMBÉM microsporidia.
en·ter·o·dyn·ia (en'ter-ō-din'ē-ā). Enterodinia. SIN enteralgia. [entero- + G. *odynē*, dor]
en·ter·o·en·ter·os·to·my (en'ter-ō-en-ter-os'tō-mē). Enteroenterostomia; estabelecimento de uma nova comunicação entre dois segmentos de intestino. SIN enteroanastomosis, intestinal anastomosis.
en·ter·o·gas·tri·tis (en'ter-ō-gas-trī'tis). Enterogastrite. SIN gastroenteritis. [entero- + G. *gastēr*, ventre, + *-itis*, inflamação]
en·ter·o·gas·trone (en'ter-ō-gas'trōn). Enterogastrona; um hormônio, obtido da mucosa intestinal, que inibe a secreção e a motilidade gástricas; a secreção de enterogastrona é estimulada por exposição da mucosa duodenal a lipídios da dieta. Alguns dos efeitos atribuídos à enterogastrona podem ser decorrentes do peptídeo insulinotrópico glicose-dependente. SIN anthelone E, enteroanthelone.
en·ter·og·e·nous (en-ter-oj'ē-nus). Enterógeno; de origem intestinal. [entero- + G. *-gen*, que produz]
en·ter·o·graph (en'ter-ō-graf). Enterógrafo; instrumento designado para uso em enterografia.
en·ter·og·ra·phy (en-ter-og'rā-fē). Enterografia; a realização de um registro gráfico definindo a atividade muscular intestinal. [entero- + G. *graphō*, escrever]
en·ter·o·hep·a·ti·tis (en'ter-ō-hep-ā-tī'tis). Enteroepatite; inflamação do intestino e do fígado. [entero- + G. *hēpar* (*hēpat*-), fígado, + *-itis*, inflamação]
en·ter·o·hep·a·to·cele (en'ter-ō-hep'ā-tō-sēl). Enteroepatocele; hérnia umbilical congênita contendo intestino e fígado. VER omphalocele. [entero- + G. *hēpar* (*hēpat*-), fígado, + *kēlē*, hérnia]
en·ter·oi·dea (en-ter-oy'dē-ā). Enteróide; febres decorrentes da infecção causada por qualquer bactéria intestinal, incluindo as febres entéricas (tifóide e paratifóide A e B) e as febres parentéricas. [entero- + G. *eidos*, semelhança]

en·ter·o·ki·nase (en′ter-ō-ki′nās). Enterocinase. SIN enteropeptidase.
en·ter·o·ki·ne·sis (en′ter-ō-ki-nē′sis). Enterocinese; contração muscular do canal alimentar. VER TAMBÉM peristalsis. [entero- + G. *kinēsis*, movimento]
en·ter·o·ki·net·ic (en′ter-ō-ki-net′ik). Enterocinético; relativo a, ou que produz, enterocinese.
en·ter·o·lith (en′ter-ō-lith). Enterólito; um cálculo intestinal formado de camadas de sabões e fosfatos terrosos circundando um cerne formado por algum corpo rígido, como um caroço de fruta engolido ou outra substância não-digerível. [entero- + G. *lithos*, pedra]
en·ter·o·li·thi·a·sis (en′ter-ō-li-thī′ā-sis). Enterolitíase; presença de cálculos no intestino.
en·ter·ol·o·gy (en-ter-ol′ō-jē). Enterologia; o ramo da ciência médica que estuda especialmente o trato intestinal. [entero- + G. *logos*, estudo]
en·ter·ol·y·sis (en-ter-ol′i-sis). Enterólise; divisão de aderências intestinais. [entero- + G. *lysis*, dissolução]
en·ter·o·meg·a·ly, en·ter·o·me·ga·lia (en′ter-ō-meg′ā-lē, -ō-me-gā′lē-ā). Enteromegalia. SIN megaloenteron. [entero- + G. *megas*, grande]
en·ter·o·me·nia (en-ter-ō-mē′nē-ā). Enteromenia; menstruação vicariante devida à presença de tecido sensível aos efeitos do estrogênio/progesterona no intestino. [entero- + G. *emmēnos*, mensalmente]
en·ter·o·mer·o·cele (en′ter-ō-mēr′ō-sēl). Enteromerocele; termo raramente usado para hérnia femoral (femoral *hernia*) [entero- + G. *mēros*, coxa, + *kēlē*, hérnia]
en·ter·om·e·ter (en-ter-om′ē-ter). Enterômetro; instrumento usado na medida do diâmetro do intestino. [entero- + G. *metron*, medida]
En·te·ro·mo·nas (en′ter-ō-mō′nas, en-ter-om′ō-nas). Gênero de protozoários flagelados. Uma espécie desse gênero, *E. hominis*, é encontrada como residente não-patogênico raro do intestino grosso humano. [entero- + G. *monas*, mônada]
en·ter·o·my·co·sis (en′ter-ō-mī-kō′sis). Enteromicose; doença intestinal de origem fúngica. [entero- + G. *mykēs*, fungo, + *-osis*, condição]
en·ter·o·pa·re·sis (en′ter-ō-pa-rē′sis, -par′i-sis). Enteroparesia; termo raramente usado para um estado de diminuição ou ausência de peristalse com flacidez dos músculos das paredes intestinais. [entero- + G. *paresis*, afrouxamento, relaxamento]
en·ter·o·path·o·gen (en′ter-ō-path′ō-jen). Enteropatógeno; organismo capaz de causar doença no trato intestinal.
en·ter·o·path·o·gen·ic (en′ter-ō-path-ō-jen′ik). Enteropatogênico; capaz de produzir doença no trato intestinal.
en·ter·op·a·thy (en-ter-op′ā-thē). Enteropatia; uma doença intestinal. [entero- + G. *pathos*, sofrimento]
  gluten e., e. por glúten, doença celíaca. SIN celiac disease.
  protein-losing e., e. perdedora de proteínas; aumento da perda fecal de proteínas séricas, principalmente albumina, causando hipoproteinemia.
en·ter·o·pep·ti·dase (en′ter-ō-pep′ti-dās). Enteropeptidase; uma glicoenzima proteolítica intestinal da mucosa duodenal que converte tripsinogênio em tripsina (remove um hexapeptídeo do tripsinogênio). SIN enterokinase.
en·ter·o·pex·y (en′ter-ō-pek-sē). Enteropexia; fixação de um segmento do intestino à parede abdominal. [entero- + G. *pēxis*, fixação]
en·ter·o·ple·gia (en′ter-ō-plē′jē-ā). Enteroplegia; termo raramente usado para íleo adinâmico (adynamic *ileus*). [entero- + G. *plēgē*, ataque]
en·ter·o·proc·tia (en′ter-ō-prok′shē-ā). Enteroproctia; termo raramente usado para designar a existência de um ânus artificial, como por uma colostomia. [entero- + G. *prōktos*, ânus]
en·ter·op·to·sis, en·ter·op·to·sia (en′ter-ō-tō′sis, -tō′sē-ā). Enteroptose; descida anormal dos intestinos na cavidade abdominal, geralmente associada à queda das outras vísceras. [entero- + G. *ptōsis*, queda]
en·ter·op·tot·ic (en′ter-ō-tot′ik). Enteroptótico; relativo a, ou que sofre de, enteroptose.
en·ter·o·re·nal (en′ter-ō-rē′nāl). Enterorrenal; relativo aos intestinos e aos rins.
en·ter·or·rha·gia (en′ter-ō-rā′jē-ā). Enterorragia; hemorragia no trato intestinal. [entero- + G. *rhēgnymi*, rompimento]
en·ter·or·rha·phy (en-ter-ōr′ā-fē). Enterorrafia; sutura do intestino. [entero- + G. *rhaphē*, sutura]
en·ter·or·rhex·is (en′ter-ō-rek′sis). Enterorrexe; termo raramente usado para ruptura do intestino. [entero- + G. *rhēxis*, ruptura]
en·ter·o·scope (en′ter-ō-skōp). Enteroscópio; um espéculo para examinar o interior do intestino em casos cirúrgicos. [entero- + G. *skopeō*, ver]
en·ter·o·sep·sis (en′ter-ō-sep′sis). Enterossépsis; sépsis que ocorre no canal alimentar, ou é derivada dele. [entero- + G. *sēpsis*, putrefação]
en·ter·o·spasm (en′ter-ō-spazm). Enterospasmo; peristalse aumentada, irregular e dolorosa. [entero- + G. *spasmos*, espasmo]
en·ter·o·sta·sis (en-ter-os′tā-sis). Enterostase; estase intestinal; um retardo ou interrupção da passagem do conteúdo intestinal. SIN intestinal stasis. [entero- + G. *stasis*, parada]
en·ter·o·ste·no·sis (en′ter-ō-sten-ō′sis). Enterostenose; estreitamento da luz intestinal. [entero- + G. *stenōsis*, estreitamento]

en·ter·os·to·my (en-ter-os′tō-mē). Enterostomia; uma conexão entre segmentos do intestino ou uma fístula para o intestino através da parede abdominal. [entero- + G. *stoma*, boca]

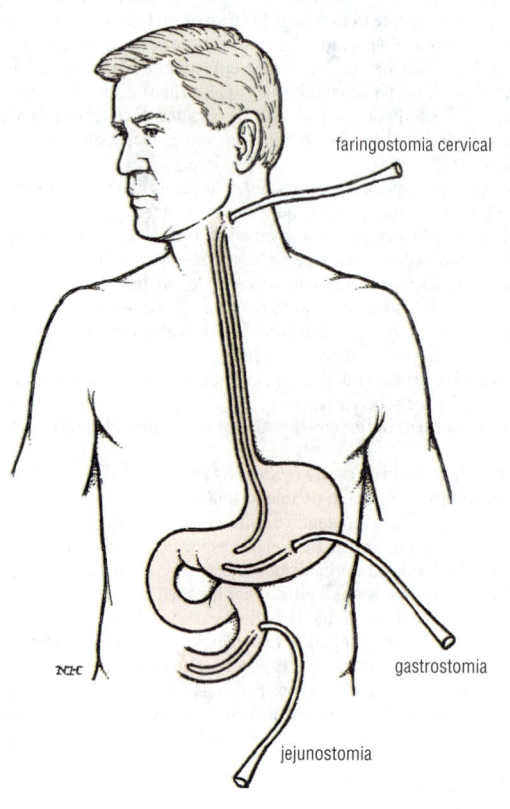

enterostomia

  double e., e. dupla; enterostomia na qual as aberturas proximal e distal do intestino dividido são suturadas à parede abdominal.
en·ter·o·tome (en′ter-ō-tōm). Enterótomo; instrumento para realizar incisão no intestino, principalmente na criação de um ânus artificial. [entero- + G. *tomē*, corte]
en·ter·ot·o·my (en-ter-ot′ō-mē). Enterotomia; incisão no intestino.
en·ter·o·tox·i·ca·tion (en′ter-ō-tok-si-kā′shŭn). Enterotoxicação. SIN autointoxication.
en·ter·o·tox·i·gen·ic (en′ter-ō-tok-si-jen′ik). Enterotoxigênico; designa um organismo que contém ou produz uma toxina específica para células da mucosa intestinal.
en·ter·o·tox·in (en′ter-ō-tok′sin). Enterotoxina; uma citotoxina específica para as células da mucosa intestinal.
  ***Clostridium perfringens* e.,** e. do *Clostridium perfringens*; uma toxina produzida pelo *Clostridium perfringens* que altera a permeabilidade da membrana.
  cytotonic e., e. citotônica; uma e. que causa alterações morfológicas na célula-alvo, mas não a mata.
  ***Escherichia coli* e.,** e. da *Escherichia coli*; e. produzida por determinadas cepas (sorotipos) de *Escherichia coli*, aparentemente associada a um plasmídeo transferível.
  staphylococcal e., e. estafilocócica; uma exotoxina solúvel produzida por algumas cepas de *Staphylococcus aureus*, e uma causa de intoxicação alimentar.
en·ter·o·tox·ism (en′ter-ō-tok′sizm). Enterotoxismo. SIN autointoxication.
en·ter·o·tro·pic (en′ter-ō-trop′ik). Enterotrópico; atraído por, ou que afeta o, intestino. [entero- + G. *tropikos*, volta]
En·te·ro·vi·rus (en′ter-ō-vī′rŭs). Um grande e diverso grupo de vírus (família Picornaviridae) que inclui poliovírus tipos 1 a 3, vírus Coxsackie A e B, vírus ECHO e os enterovírus identificados desde 1969 e designados por meio de números. Eles são habitantes transitórios do canal alimentar e estáveis em pH baixo.
en·ter·o·zo·ic (en′ter-ō-zō′ik). Enterozóico; relativo a um enterozoário.
en·ter·o·zo·on (en′ter-ō-zō′on). Enterozoário; animal parasita do intestino. [entero- + G. *zōon*, animal]
ent·ge·gen (*E*) (ent′ge-gen). Termo usado quando os dois grupamentos superiores, fixados aos diferentes átomos em uma ligação dupla, geralmente uma

ligação dupla carbono-carbono, estão em lados opostos da ligação dupla (portanto, análogo a *trans-*). Também usado quando esses grupamentos estão em lados opostos de uma estrutura anular. [Alemão oposto]

en·thal·py (H) (en'thal-pē). Entalpia; conteúdo de calor, simbolizado por *H*; uma função termodinâmica, definida como *E* + *PV*, na qual *E* é a energia interna de um sistema, *P*, a pressão e *V*, o volume; o calor de uma reação, medido em pressão constante, é ΔH. SIN heat (4). [*enthalpō*, aquecer]

en·the·si·tis (en-thē-sī'tis). Entesite; condição que ocorre na inserção de músculos, onde a concentração recorrente da força muscular provoca inflamação com uma forte tendência à fibrose e calcificação. [G. *enthetos*, implantado, + *-itis*, inflamação]

en·the·so·path·ic (en-thē-sō-path'ik). Entesopático; que designa, ou é característico de, entesopatia.

en·the·sop·a·thy (en-thē-sop'a-thē). Entesopatia; um processo patológico que ocorre no local de inserção de tendões musculares e ligamentos nos ossos ou cápsulas articulares. [G. *en*, em, + *thesis*, colocação, + *pathos*, que sofre]

en·thla·sis (en'thlā-sis). Entalasia; fratura com afundamento do crânio. [G. entalhe, de *en*, em, + *thlaō*, esmagar]

en thyrse (ahn tirs'). Em tirso; microconídios de alguns dermatófitos dispostos isoladamente ao longo de ambos os lados de uma hifa. [Fr. do G. *en-*, em, + *thyrsos*, talo, bastão]

en·tire (en-tīr'). Inteiro; ileso; contínuo; que possui uma margem ou borda contínua uniforme sem entalhes ou projeções; designa uma margem, como a de uma colônia bacteriana.

en·ti·ty (en'ti-tē). Entidade; uma coisa independente; aquele que contém em si mesmo todas as condições essenciais para a individualidade; aquele que forma, em si mesmo, um todo completo; clinicamente, designa uma doença ou condição separada ou distinta. [L. *ens* (*ent-*), sendo, p. pres. de *esse*, ser]

ento-, ent-. Ento-, ent-; interno, ou dentro. VER TAMBÉM endo-. [G. *entos*, dentro]

en·to·blast (en'tō-blast). Entoblasto; nucléolo celular. [ento- + G. *blastos*, germe]

en·to·cele (en'tō-sēl). Entocele; uma hérnia interna. [ento- + G. *kēlē*, hérnia]

en·to·cho·roi·dea (en'tō-kō-roy'dē-ā). Entocoróide, lâmina capilar da coróide. SIN capillary lamina of choroid. [ento- + G. *chorioeidēs*, coróide]

en·to·cone (en-tō-kōn). Entocone; a cúspide mesiolingual de um dente molar maxilar. [ento- + G. *kōnos*, cone]

en·to·co·nid (en-tō-kō'nid). Entoconídio; a cúspide posterior interna de um dente molar mandibular. [ento- + G. *kōnos*, cone]

en·to·cor·nea (en-tō-kōr'nē-ā). Entocórnea. SIN posterior limiting lamina of cornea.

en·to·cra·ni·al (en'tō-krā'nē-āl). Entocranial. SIN endocranial.

en·to·cra·ni·um (en'tō-krā'nē-ŭm). Entocrânio. SIN endocranium.

en·to·derm (en'tō-derm). Entoderma. SIN endoderm. [ento- + G. *derma*, pele]

en·to·ec·tad (en-tō-ek'tad). De dentro para fora. [G. *entos*, dentro, + *ektos*, sem, + L. *ad*, para]

En·to·lo·ma si·nu·a·tum (en-tō-lō'mā sī-nū-ā'tum). Uma espécie de cogumelo capaz de produzir micetismo gastrointestinal.

en·to·mi·on (en-tō'mē-on). Entômio; a ponta do ângulo mastóide do osso parietal. [G. *entomē*, entalhe]

en·to·mol·o·gy (en-tō-mol'ō-jē). Entomologia; a ciência que estuda os insetos. [G. *entomon*, inseto, + *logos*, estudo]

en·to·mo·pho·bia (en'tō-mō-fō'bē-ā). Entomofobia; medo mórbido de insetos. [G. *entomon*, inseto, + *phobos*, medo]

Entomophthora (en-tō-mof'thor-ā). SIN Conidiobolus.
E. coronata, gênero de fungo reclassificado como *Conidiobolus*, a causa da conidiobolomicose.

Entomophthorales (en-tō-mof'thor-al'ēz). Ordem da classe de fungos Zygomycetes. Os gêneros incluem *Conidiobolus*, que causa uma inflamação granulomatosa crônica da mucosa nasal e dos seios paranasais (conidiobolomicose) e *Basidiobolus*, que causa um granuloma subcutâneo crônico (basidiobolomicose). Quando a conidiobolomicose e a basidiobolomicose são consideradas juntas, são denominadas entomoftoramicose.

en·to·moph·tho·ra·my·co·sis (en-tō-mof'thō-ra-mī-kō'sis). Entomoftoramicose; doença causada por fungos dos gêneros *Basidiobolus* ou *Conidiobolus*; os tecidos subcutâneos ou paranasais são invadidos por hifas não-septadas largas que são circundadas por material eosinofílico. Uma forma de zigomicose. VER zygomycosis. [Entomophthorales (nome da ordem) + G. *mykēs*, fungo, + *-osis*, condição]
e. basidiobo'lae, e. por *Basidiobolus*; ficomise subcutânea causada pelo fungo *Basidiobolus ranarum*, caracterizada pelo desenvolvimento de granulomas fibróticos subcutâneos, de consistência firme, planos, que não ulceram; algumas vezes, as lesões podem estender-se até os músculos e linfonodos e outros tecidos profundos; a doença é encontrada na Indonésia, em Uganda e em outros países africanos tropicais, mas foi observada na América tropical; uma forma de zigomicose. SIN subcutaneous phycomycosis.
e. conidiobo'lae, e. por *Conidiobolus*; uma zigomicose causada por *Conidiobolus coronatus*, caracterizada por grandes pólipos nasais e granulomas da cavidade nasal; foi descrita no Texas, na Índia Ocidental, na África e na América do Sul; uma forma de zigomicose.

En·to·mo·pox·vi·rus (en'tē-mō-poks-vī'rŭs). O gênero de vírus (família Poxviridae) que compreende os poxvírus de insetos; parecem não se multiplicar em vertebrados. [G. *entomom*, inseto]

en·top·ic (en-top'ik). Entópico; colocado dentro; que ocorre ou está situado no lugar normal; oposto a ectópico. [G. *en*, dentro, + *topos*, lugar]

en·to·plasm (en'tō-plasm). Entoplasma, endoplasma. SIN endoplasm.

ent·op·tic (en-top'tik). Entóptico; dentro do bulbo do olho; que ocorre ou está situado no lugar normal; oposto a ectópico. [ento- + G. *optikos*, relativo à visão]

en·to·ret·i·na (en-tō-ret'i-nā). Entorretina; as camadas da retina desde a plexiforme externa até a camada de fibras nervosas inclusive. SIN Henle nervous layer.

en·to·sarc (en'tō-sark). Entossarco. SIN endosarc.

En·to·zoa (en-tō-zō'ā). Nome não-taxonômico para o ramo do reino Animalia cujos membros possuem uma cavidade ou trato digestivo; inclui todos os vertebrados e as formas invertebradas superiores. [ento- + G. *zōon*, animal]

en·to·zo·al (en-tō-zō'al). Entozoário; relativo aos entozoários.

en·to·zo·on, pl. **en·to·zoa** (en-tō-zō'on, -ā). Entozoário; parasita animal cujo *habitat* é qualquer dos órgãos ou tecidos internos. [ento- + G. *zōon*, animal]

en·trails (en'trālz). Entranhas; as vísceras de um animal.

en·tro·pi·on, en·tro·pi·um (en-trō'pē-on, -pē-ŭm). Entrópio. **1.** Inversão ou virada para dentro de uma parte. **2.** A inversão da margem de uma pálpebra. [G. *en*, em, + *tropē*, virada]
atonic e., e. atônico; e. que sucede a perda de tônus do músculo orbicular do olho ou de elasticidade da pele.
cicatricial e., e. cicatricial; e. que sucede a fibrose da conjuntiva palpebral.
spastic e., e. espástico; e. decorrente da contratura excessiva do músculo orbicular do olho.

en·tro·pi·on·ize (en-trō'pē-on-īz). Entropionizar; inverter uma parte.

en·tro·py (S) (en'tri-pē). Entropia; a fração de calor (energia) não-disponível para a realização de trabalho, geralmente porque (em uma reação química) foi usada para aumentar o movimento aleatório dos átomos ou moléculas no sistema; assim, a entropia é uma medida da casualidade ou desordem. A entropia ocorre na equação da energia livre de Gibbs (*G*): $\Delta G = \Delta H - T\Delta S$ (ΔH, alteração na entalpia ou conteúdo de calor; *T*, temperatura absoluta; ΔS, alteração na entropia). VER TAMBÉM second law of thermodynamics. [G. *entropia*, uma volta em direção à]

en·ty·py (en'ti-pē). Entipia; um tipo de gastrulação observada em alguns embriões mamíferos pequenos nos quais o endoderma cobre o ectoderma embrionário e amniótico; parte do trofoblasto pré-placentário também pode ser coberta. [G. *entypē*, padrão]

enu·cle·ate (ē-noo'klē-āt). Enuclear; remover totalmente; descascar como uma noz, como na remoção de um olho de sua cápsula ou um tumor de seu tecido adjacente comprimido.

enu·cle·a·tion (ē-noo-klē-ā'shŭn). Enucleação. **1.** Remoção de toda uma estrutura (como o bulbo de um olho ou tumor), sem ruptura, como se tira o miolo de uma noz. **2.** Remoção ou destruição do núcleo de uma célula. [L. *enucleo*, remover a casca, de *e*, fora, + *nucleus*, noz, núcleo]

en·u·re·sis (en-ū-rē'sis). Enurese; eliminação ou extravasamento involuntário de urina. [G. *en-oureō*, urinar em]
diurnal e., e. diurna; incontinência durante o período de vigília.
nocturnal e., e. noturna; incontinência urinária durante o sono. SIN bed-wetting.

en·ve·lope (en'vĕ-lōp). Invólucro, envoltório; em anatomia, uma estrutura que encerra ou cobre.
corneocyte e., envoltório corneócito; uma camada eletrondensa, com 10–15 nm de espessura, de proteína extremamente cruzada na superfície citoplasmática da membrana celular de corneócitos epidérmicos; é bastante resistente a agentes proteolíticos. SIN subplasmalemmal dense zone.
nuclear e., envoltório nuclear; a membrana dupla no limite do nucleoplasma; possui poros regularmente espaçados cobertos por um complexo de poros nucleares em forma de disco e um espaço ou cisterna com cerca de 150 Å de largura entre as duas camadas; a membrana externa é contínua com o retículo endoplasmático periodicamente. SIN caryotheca, karyotheca, nuclear membrane.
viral e., envoltório viral; a estrutura ou o revestimento externo que encerra os nucleocapsídios de alguns vírus que amadurecem por brotamento através da membrana celular; pode conter lipoproteínas.

en·ven·om·a·tion (en-ven-ō-mā'shŭn). Envenenamento; o ato de injetar um material venenoso (veneno) por picada, espinho, mordida ou outro aparelho venenoso.

en·vi·ron·ment (en-vī'ron-ment). Meio; meio ambiente; a reunião de todas as condições e influências externas que afetam a vida e o desenvolvimento de um organismo. Pode ser dividido em físico, biológico, social, cultural, etc., qualquer um deles ou todos podem influenciar o estado de saúde da população. [Fr. *environ*, ao redor]

en·vy (en′vē). Inveja; sentimento de descontentamento ou ciúme de uma pessoa, resultante da comparação com outra pessoa.
    penis e., i. do pênis; o conceito psicanalítico de que a mulher inveja as características ou capacidades masculinas, sobretudo a posse de um pênis.
en·zo·ot·ic (en - zō - ot′ik). Enzoótico. SIN endemic. [G. *en*, em, + *zōon*, animal]
en·zy·got·ic (en - zī - got′ik). Enzigótico; derivado de um único óvulo fertilizado; designa gêmeos assim derivados. [G. *eis* (*en*), um, + *zygote*]
en·zy·mat·ic (en - zī - mat′ik). Enzimático; relativo a uma enzima. SIN enzymic.
en·zyme (en′zīm). Enzima; uma proteína que atua como catalisador para induzir alterações químicas em outras substâncias, enquanto ela mesma permanece aparentemente inalterada pelo processo. As enzimas, com exceção daquelas descobertas há muito tempo (p. ex., pepsina, emulsina), geralmente são designadas acrescentando-se –ase ao nome do substrato sobre o qual a enzima atua (p. ex., glicosidase), à substância ativada (p. ex., hidrogenase) e/ou ao tipo de reação (p. ex., oxidorredutase, transferase, hidrolase, liase, isomerase, ligase ou sintetase — sendo estes os seis principais grupos nas Recomendações para Nomenclatura Enzimática da *International Union of Biochemistry*). Quanto às enzimas individuais não apresentadas a seguir, ver o nome específico. SIN organic catalyst (1). [G. + L. *en*, em, + *zyme*, fermento]
    acetyl-activating e., e. ativadora de acetil. SIN *acetyl-CoA* ligase.
    acyl-activating e., e. ativadora de acil; **(1)** SIN long-chain fatty acid-CoA ligase; **(2)** SIN butyrate-CoA ligase.
    adaptive e., e. adaptativa. SIN induced e.
    allosteric e., e. alostérica; uma enzima que exibe a propriedade de alosterismo.
    amino acid activating e., e. ativadora de aminoácidos. SIN *aminoacyl-tRNA* synthetases.
    angiotensin-converting e. (ACE), e. de conversão da angiotensina (ECA). SIN peptidyl dipeptidase A.
    antitumor e., e. antitumoral; uma enzima que estimula a degradação de um metabólito específico que não pode ser sintetizado por células tumorais, inibe a síntese de um metabólito necessário por células tumorais, ou inibe a utilização de DNA tumor-específica; p. ex., asparaginase.
    autolytic e., e. autolítica; enzima capaz de causar lise da célula que a forma.
    branching e., e. ramificadora. SIN 1,4-α-D-glucan-branching enzyme.
    β-carotene-cleavage e., e. de clivagem do β-caroteno. SIN β-carotene 15,15′-dioxygenase.
    citrate-cleavage e., e. de clivagem do citrato. SIN ATP *citrate* (*pro-3S*)-*lyase*.
    cold-sensitive e., e. sensível ao frio; enzima que perde sua estabilidade quando a temperatura é reduzida.
    condensing e., e. condensadora. SIN *citrate* synthase.
    constitutive e., e. constitutiva; enzima constantemente produzida pela célula, independentemente das condições de crescimento. Cf. induced e.
    cooperative e., e. cooperativa; enzima que exibe a propriedade de cooperatividade.
    D e., e. D. SIN 4-α-D-glucanotransferase.
    deamidizing e.'s, enzimas de desamidização. SIN amidohydrolases.
    deaminating e.'s, enzimas de desaminação. SIN desaminases.
    debranching e.'s, enzimas desramificadoras; enzimas que produzem destruição de ramos no glicogênio; outrora consideradas uma única enzima, agora se sabe tratar-se de uma mistura de transferases (4-α-D-glucanotransferase) e hidrolases (amilo-1,6-glicosidase). SIN debranching factors.
    digestive e.'s, enzimas digestivas; **(1)** enzimas utilizadas no sistema digestivo; **(2)** enzimas que são hidrolases de macromoléculas (p. ex., amilases, proteinases).
    disproportionating e., 4-α-D-glicanotransferase. SIN 4-α-D-glucanotransferase.
    extracellular e., e. extracelular; uma enzima que realiza suas funções fora da célula; p. ex., as várias enzimas digestivas. SIN exoenzyme.
    heat-stable e., e. termoestável. SIN thermostable e.
    hydrolyzing e.'s, hidrolases. SIN hydrolases.
    immobilized e., e. imobilizada; uma enzima que foi ligada, em geral de forma covalente, a uma matriz orgânica ou inorgânica insolúvel ou que foi encapsulada.
    induced e., inducible e., e. induzida, e. indutível; **(1)** uma enzima que pode ser detectada em uma cultura em crescimento de microrganismos, após a adição de uma substância específica (indutora) ao meio de cultura, mas não era detectável antes da adição e pode agir sobre o indutor. Um protótipo é a β-galactosidase da *Escherichia coli*, sintetizada após a adição de vários galactosídeos, sejam ou não bons substratos. Cf. constitutive e.; **(2)** qualquer enzima que tenha sua taxa de biossíntese aumentada devido à presença do substrato ou de alguma outra entidade molecular. SIN adaptive e.
    intracellular e., e. intracelular; uma enzima que realiza suas funções dentro da célula que a produz; a maioria das enzimas é intracelular. SIN endoenzyme (1).
    Kornberg e., e. de Kornberg; DNA polimerase I da *Escherichia coli*.
    malate-condensing e., malato sintase. SIN *malate* synthase.
    malic e., malato desidrogenase. SIN *malate* dehydrogenase.
    marker e., e. marcadora; enzima usada para identificar um tipo celular específico, uma organela celular ou um componente celular.

as principais enzimas digestivas

enzima	fonte da enzima	ação digestiva
ação das enzimas que digerem carboidratos		
ptialina (amilase salivar)	glândulas salivares	amido → dextrina, maltose, glicose
amilase	pâncreas	amido → dextrina, maltose, glicose dextrina → maltose, glicose
maltase	mucosa intestinal	maltose → glicose
sacarose	mucosa intestinal	sacarose → glicose, frutose
lactase	mucosa intestinal	lactose → glicose, galactose
ação das enzimas que digerem proteínas		
pepsina	mucosa gástrica	proteína → polipeptídeos
tripsina	pâncreas	proteínas e polipeptídeos → polipeptídeos, dipeptídeos, aminoácidos
aminopeptidase	mucosa intestinal	polipeptídeos → dipeptídeos, aminoácidos
dipeptidase	mucosa intestinal	dipeptídeos → aminoácidos
ação das enzimas que digerem a gordura (triglicerídeo)		
lipase faríngea	mucosa faríngea	triglicerídeos → ácidos graxos, diglicerídeos, monoglicerídeos
esteapsina	mucosa gástrica	triglicerídeos → ácidos graxos, diglicerídeos, monoglicerídeos
lipase pancreática	pâncreas	triglicerídeos → ácidos graxos, diglicerídeos, monoglicerídeos

    membrane e., e. da membrana; uma enzima presente ou incrustada em uma membrana biológica.
    methionine-activating e., metionina adenosiltransferase. SIN *methionine* adenosyltransferase.
    new yellow e., nova e. amarela; nome antigo da D-aminoácido oxidase encontrada em leveduras, uma flavoenzima; assim denominada para distinguir-se da antiga enzima amarela de Warburg. Cf. *amino acid* oxidases.
    old yellow e., antiga e. amarela. SIN *NADPH* dehydrogenase.
    P e., e. P. SIN phosphorylase.
    pantoate-activating e., e. ativadora de pantoato. SIN *pantothenate* synthetase.
    phosphorylase-rupturing e. (PR e.), fosforilase fosfatase. SIN *phosphorylase* phosphatase.
    photoreactivating e. (PR e.), e. fotorreativadora. SIN deoxyribodipyrimidine photolyase.
    PR e., abreviatura de phosphorylase-rupturing e. (fosforilase fosfatase); photoreactivating e. (e. fotorreativadora).
    Q e., e. Q; enzima ramificadora de 1,4-α-glicana em vegetais.
    R e., e. R. SIN α-dextrin endo-1,6-α-glucosidase.
    reducing e., e. redutase. SIN reductase.
    repair e., e. de reparo; uma enzima que pode catalisar o reparo do DNA lesado; p. ex., DNA ligase.
    repressible e., e. repressível; enzima produzida continuamente, exceto se a produção for reprimida por excesso de um inibidor (co-repressor). VER TAMBÉM inactive *repressor*.
    respiratory e., e. respiratória; uma enzima tecidual que é parte de um sistema de oxidação-redução que realiza a conversão de substratos em CO_2 e H_2O e a transferência dos elétrons removidos para O_2.
    restriction e., e. de restrição. SIN restriction *endonuclease*.
    RNA e., e. de RNA. SIN ribozyme.
    Schardinger e., e. de Schardinger. SIN *xanthine* oxidase.
    splitting e.'s, enzimas de fragmentação; enzimas que, como as aldolases, catalisam a conversão de uma molécula em duas moléculas menores sem a adição ou subtração de quaisquer átomos.

enzyme | **epicanthus**

T e., e. T; 1,4-α-D-glicana 6-α-D-glucosiltransferase.
terminal addition e., e. de adição terminal. SIN DNA nucleotidylexotransferase.
thermostable e., e. termoestável; enzima que não é facilmente sujeita à destruição ou alteração pelo calor. SIN heat-stable e.
thiol e., e. tiol; enzima cuja atividade depende de um grupamento tiol livre.
transferring e.'s, enzimas de transferência, transferases. SIN transferases.
Warburg old yellow e., antiga e. amarela de Warburg. SIN NADPH dehydrogenase. VER TAMBÉM new yellow e., yellow e.
Warburg respiratory e., e. respiratória de Warburg. SIN Atmungsferment.
yellow e., e. amarela. SIN flavoenzyme. VER TAMBÉM Warburg old yellow e., new yellow e.
En·zyme Com·mis·sion. Comissão de Enzimas. VER EC.
en·zy·mic (en - zī′mik). Enzimático. SIN enzymatic.
en·zy·mol·o·gist (en - zī - mol′ō - jist). Enzimologista; um especialista em enzimologia.
en·zy·mol·o·gy (en - zī - mol′ō - jē). Enzimologia; o ramo da química que estuda as propriedades e ações das enzimas. [enzyme + G. *logos*, estudo]
en·zy·mol·y·sis (en - zī - mol′ĭ - sis). Enzimólise. 1. A divisão ou clivagem de uma substância em partes menores por meio de ação enzimática. 2. Lise pela ação de uma enzima. [enzyme + G. *lysis*, dissolução]
en·zy·mop·a·thy (en - zī - mop′ă - thē). Enzimopatia; qualquer distúrbio da função enzimática, incluindo deficiência genética ou defeito em enzimas específicas. [enzyme + G. *pathos*, doença]
EOG Abreviatura de electrooculography (eletrooculografia); electroolfactogram (eletroolfatograma).
eo·sin (ē′ō - sin). Eosina; derivado da fluoresceína usado como corante ácido fluorescente para colorações e contracolorações citoplasmáticas em histologia e nas colorações sanguíneas do tipo Romanovsky. [G. ēōs, amanhecer]
  e. B, e. B; o sal dissódico de 4′,5′-dibromo-2′,7′-dinitrofluoresceína. SIN acid red 91, e. I bluish. [C.I. 45400]
  e. I bluish, e. I azulada. SIN e. B.
  e. y, e. Y, e. Y; o sal dissódico de 2′,4′,5′,7′-tetrabromofluoresceína. SIN acid red 87, e. yellowish. [C.I. 45380]
  e. yellowish, e. amarelada. SIN e. y.
eo·sin·o·cyte (ē - ō - sin′ō - sīt). Eosinócito, eosinófilo. SIN eosinophilic leukocyte.
eo·sin·o·pe·nia (ē′ō - sin - ō - pē′nē - ă). Eosinopenia; a presença de eosinófilos em número anormalmente pequeno no sangue periférico. SIN hypoeosinophilia. [eosino(phil) + G. *penia*, escassez]
eo·sin·o·phil, eo·sin·o·phile (ē - ō - sin′ō - fil, - fīl). Eosinófilo. SIN eosinophilic leukocyte. [eosin + G. *philos*, afinidade]
eo·sin·o·phil·ia (ē′ō - sin - ō - fil′ē - ă). Eosinofilia. SIN eosinophilic leukocytosis.
  simple pulmonary e., e. pulmonar simples; infiltrados pulmonares observados como sombras migratórias transitórias na radiografia do tórax, acompanhados por eosinofilia sanguínea; freqüentemente assintomática, mas pode haver tosse, febre e dispnéia; a maioria dos casos é devida a helmintíases, principalmente por *Ascaris lumbricoides*; alguns casos ocorrem após administração de drogas. SIN Löffler syndrome (1).
  tropical e., e. tropical; eosinofilia associada a tosse e asma, causada por infecção por filárias oculta sem evidências de microfilaremia, mais freqüente na Índia e no Sudeste Asiático.
eo·sin·o·phil·ic (ē - ō - sin - ō - fil′ik). Eosinofílico; que se cora facilmente com corantes eosina; designa esses elementos celulares ou teciduais.
eo·sin·o·phil·u·ria (ē - ō - sin′ō - fil - ū′rē - ă). Eosinofilúria; presença de eosinófilos na urina.
eo·sin·o·tac·tic (ē′ō - sin - ō - tak′tik). Eosinotático; que exerce uma força de atração ou repulsão sobre células eosinofílicas. [eosino(phile) + G. *taktikos*, em arranjo ordenado]
eo·sin·o·tax·is (ē′ō - sin - ō - tak′sis). Eosinotaxia; movimento de eosinófilos com referência a um estímulo que os atrai ou repele.
eo·so·pho·bia (ē - ō - sō - fō′bē - ă). Eosofobia; temor mórbido do amanhecer. [G. ēōs, amanhecer, + *phobos*, medo]
EP Abreviatura de endogenous *pyrogen* (pirógeno endógeno).
epac·tal (ē - pak′tăl). Epactal, supranumerário. SIN supernumerary. [G. *epaktos*, importado, de *epagō*, trazer para cima ou para dentro]
ep·am·ni·ot·ic (ep′am - nē - ot′ik). Epamniótico; sobre ou acima do âmnio. [G. *epi*, sobre, + *amnion*]
ep·ar·te·ri·al (ep′ar - tēr - ē - ăl). Epaterial; sobre ou superior a uma artéria. [G. *epi*, sobre, + *artēia*, artéria]
ep·ax·i·al (ep - ak′sē - ăl). Epaxial; acima ou atrás de qualquer eixo, como o eixo espinhal ou o eixo de um membro. [G. *epi*, sobre, + L. *axis*, eixo]
EPEC Abreviatura de enteropathogenic *Escherichia coli* (*Escherichia coli* enteropatogênica).
ep·en·dy·ma (ep - en′di - mă)[TA]. Epêndima; a membrana celular que reveste o canal central da medula espinal e os ventrículos cerebrais. SIN endyma. [G. *ependyma*, um revestimento superior]
ep·en·dy·mal (ep - en′di - măl). Ependimário; relativo ao epêndima.

ep·en·dy·mi·tis (ep - en - di - mī′tis). Ependimite; inflamação do epêndima.
ep·en·dy·mo·blast (ep - en′di - mō - blast). Ependimoblasto; uma célula ependimária embrionária. [ependyma + G. *blastos*, germe]
ep·en·dy·mo·blas·to·ma (ep - en′di - mō - blas - tō′mă). Ependimoblastoma; uma neoplasia glial do sistema nervoso central, que ocorre tipicamente na infância; o protótipo das células tumorais assemelha-se ao ependimoblasto. [ependymoblast + G. *-ōma*, tumor]
ep·en·dy·mo·cyte (ep - en′di - mō - sīt). Ependimócito; uma célula ependimária. [ependyma + G. *kytos*, célula]
ep·en·dy·mo·ma (ep - en - di - mō′mă). Ependimoma; um glioma derivado de células ependimárias relativamente indiferenciadas, que representa cerca de 1–3% de todas as neoplasias intracranianas; os ependimomas ocorrem em todas as faixas etárias e podem originar-se do revestimento de qualquer ventrículo ou, mais comumente, do canal central da medula espinal; histologicamente, as células neoplásicas tendem a ser dispostas radialmente em torno dos vasos sanguíneos, aos quais estão fixadas por processos fibrilares.
  myxopapillary e., e. mixopapilar; ependimoma de crescimento lento do filo terminal, mais freqüente em adultos jovens, que consiste em células cubóides em distribuição papilar ao redor de um centro vascular mucinoso.
eph·apse (ef′aps). Efapse; um lugar onde dois ou mais processos de células nervosas (axônios, dendritos) se tocam sem formar um contato sináptico típico; pode haver alguma forma de transmissão neural nesses locais de contato não-sináptico. [G. *ephapsis*, contato]
eph·ap·tic (e-fap′tik). Efáptico; relativo a uma efapse.
ephe·bic (ē - fē′bik). Efébico; termo raramente empregado relativo ao período de puberdade ou a um jovem. [G. *ephēbikos*, relativo à juventude, de *hēbē*, juventude]
eph·e·bol·o·gy (ef - ē - bol′ō - jē). Efebologia; termo raramente usado para o estudo das alterações morfológicas e outras alterações que incidem na puberdade. [G. *ephēbos*, puberdade, + *logos*, estudo]
ephed·ra (ē - fed′răh). Éfedra; *Ephedra equisetina* (família Gnetaceae). Ma Huang; a fonte vegetal do alcalóide efedrina. Nativa da China e da Índia, possui de 0,75 a mais de 1% de efedrina; também contém um pouco de pseudo-efedrina.
ephed·rine (ē - fed′rin, ef′ē - drin). Efedrina; um alcalóide obtido das folhas da *Ephedra equisetina*, *E. sinica* e outras espécies (família Gnetaceae), ou produzido sinteticamente; um agente adrenérgico (simpaticomimético) com ações semelhantes à da adrenalina; usado como broncodilatador, midriático, agente pressor e vasoconstritor tópico. Geralmente os sais usados são cloridrato de efedrina e sulfato de efedrina.
ephe·lis, pl. **ephe·li·des** (ef - ē′lis - ef - ē′li - dēz). Efélide; sarda. SIN freckle. [G.]
epi-. Epi-; sobre, a seguir, ou subseqüente a. [G.]
ep·i·an·dros·ter·one (ep′i - an - dros′ter - ōn). Epiandrosterona; isômero inativo (3β ao invés de 3α) da androsterona; encontrado na urina e no tecido testicular e ovariano. SIN isoandrosterone.
ep·i·bati·dine (ep′ī - băt′tī - dīn). Epibatidina; um alcalóide tóxico extraído da pele de uma rã sul-americana, *Epipedobates tricolor*. Aparentemente derivada de insetos específicos consumidos na bacia Amazônica. O extrato bruto era usado como veneno de flecha por caçadores nativos; exerce analgesia por outro mecanismo que não a ativação de receptores opiáceos ou inibição da ciclooxigenase.
ep·i·blast (ep′i-blast). Epiblasto; dá origem ao ectoderma, mesoderma e endoderma do embrião propriamente dito. [epi- + G. *blastos*, germe]
ep·i·blas·tic (ep-i-blas′tik). Epiblástico; relativo a epiblasto.
ep·i·bleph·a·ron (ep′i - blef′ă - ron). Epibléfaro; uma prega cutânea horizontal congênita próxima da margem palpebral, causada por inserção anormal das fibras musculares. Na pálpebra superior, simula blefarocalasia; na pálpebra inferior, causa inversão dos cílios para dentro. [epi- + G. *blepharon*, pálpebra]
epib·o·ly, epib·o·le (ē - pib′ō - lē). Epibolia. 1. Um processo envolvido na gastrulação de ovos telolécitos na qual, em virtude do crescimento diferencial, algumas das células do protoderma se movem sobre a superfície em direção aos lábios do blastoporo. 2. Crescimento de epitélio na cultura de um órgão para circundar o tecido mesenquimal subjacente. [G. *epibolē*, vestir ou espalhar]
ep·i·bul·bar (ep - i - būl′bar). Epibulbar; sobre um bulbo de qualquer tipo; especificamente, sobre o bulbo do olho.
ep·i·can·thus (ep - i - kan′thŭs). Epicanto. SIN palpebronasal fold. [epi- + G. *kanthos*, canto]
  e. inver·sus, e. inverso; uma prega cutânea em forma de crescente da pálpebra inferior no canto interno; freqüente na blefaroptose congênita.
  e. palpebra·lis, e. palpebral; epicanto originado da pálpebra superior acima da porção tarsal e estendendo-se até a porção inferior da órbita.
  e. supracilia·ris, e. supraciliar; epicanto originado na região dos supercílios e que se estende em direção ao saco lacrimal.
  e. tarsa·lis, e. do tarso; epicanto originado na prega tarsal e que desaparece na pele próxima do canto interno.

ep·i·car·dia (ep-i-kar′dē-ă). Epicárdia. SIN abdominal *part* of esophagus. [epi- + G. *kardia*, coração]
ep·i·car·di·al (ep-i-kar′dē-ăl). Epicárdico. **1.** Relativo à epicárdia. **2.** Relativo ao epicárdio.
ep·i·car·di·um (ep-i-kar′dē-ŭm). Epicárdio; *termo oficial alternativo para visceral *layer* of serous pericardium.* [epi- + G. *kardia*, coração]
ep·i·chord·al (ep-i-kōr′dăl). Epicórdico; na face dorsal do notocórdio; aplicável particularmente à parte do encéfalo que se desenvolve dorsal à parte cefálica do notocórdio. [epi- + G. *chordē*, corda]
ep·i·cil·lin (ep-i-sil′in). Epicilina; antibiótico beta-lactâmico semi-sintético relacionado à penicilina; um antibacteriano.
ep·i·co·mus (ep-i-kō′mŭs, ē-pik′ō-mŭs). Epícomo; gêmeos conjugados desiguais nos quais o parasita menor é unido ao autósito maior no topo da cabeça. VER conjoined *twins*, em *twin*. [epi- + G. *komē*, cabelo da cabeça]
ep·i·con·dy·lal·gia (ep′i-kon-di-lal′jē-ă). Epicondilalgia; dor em um epicôndilo do úmero ou nos tendões ou músculos que nele se originam. [epicondyle + G. *algos*, dor]
 e. exter′na, e. externa. SIN tennis *elbow*.
ep·i·con·dyle (ep-i-kon′dīl) [TA]. Epicôndilo; projeção de um osso longo próxima da extremidade articular, acima do côndilo ou sobre este. SIN epicondylus [TA]. [epi- + G. *kondylos*, junta]
 lateral e. of femur [TA], e. lateral do fêmur; o epicôndilo situado na face lateral da extremidade distal do osso. SIN epicondylus lateralis femoris [TA], epicondylus lateralis ossis femoris, lateral femoral tuberosity.
 lateral e. of humerus [TA], e. lateral do úmero; o epicôndilo situado na face lateral da extremidade distal do osso. SIN epicondylus lateralis humeri [TA].
 medial e. of femur [TA], e. medial do fêmur; o epicôndilo situado proximal ao côndilo medial. SIN epicondylus medialis ossis femoris, medial femoral tuberosity.
 medial e. of humerus [TA], e. medial do úmero; o epicôndilo situado proximal e medial ao côndilo. SIN epicondylus medialis humeri [TA], epitrochlea.
ep·i·con·dy·li (ep-i-kon′di-lī). Epicôndilos; plural de epicondylus.
ep·i·con·dyl·i·an (ep-i-kon-dil′ē-an). Epicondiliano. SIN epicondylic.
ep·i·con·dyl·ic (ep-i-kon-dil′ik). Epicondílico; relativo ao epicôndilo ou à parte acima de um côndilo. SIN epicondylian.
ep·i·con·dy·li·tis (ep′i-kon-di-lī′tis). Epicondilite; inflamação de um epicôndilo.
 lateral humeral e., e. umeral lateral. SIN tennis *elbow*.
ep·i·con·dy·lus, pl. **ep·i·con·dy·li** (ep-i-kon′di-lŭs, -lī) [TA]. Epicôndilo. SIN epicondyle. [L.]
 e. lateralis femoris [TA], e. lateral do fêmur. SIN lateral *epicondyle* of femur.
 e. latera′lis hu′meri [TA], e. lateral do úmero. SIN lateral *epicondyle* of humerus.
 e. latera′lis os′sis fem′oris, e. lateral do fêmur. SIN lateral *epicondyle* of femur.
 e. medialis femoris [TA], e. medial do fêmur. SIN medial *epicondyle* of femur.
 e. media′lis hu′meri [TA], e. medial do úmero. SIN medial *epicondyle* of humerus.
 e. media′lis os′sis fem′oris, e. medial do fêmur. SIN medial *epicondyle* of femur.
ep·i·cor·a·coid (ep-i-kōr′ă-koyd). Epicoracóide; sobre o processo coracóide ou acima deste.
ep·i·cra·ni·al. Epicrânico; epicraniano; relativo ao epicrânio.
ep·i·cra·ni·um (ep-i-krā′nē-ŭm). Epicrânio; o músculo, a aponeurose e a pele que cobrem o crânio. [epi- + G. *kranion*, crânio]
ep·i·cra·ni·us. Epicrânico. VER epicranius (*muscle*).
ep·i·cri·sis (ep-i-krī′sis). Epicrise; uma crise secundária; uma crise que interrompe uma recrudescência de sintomas mórbidos após uma crise primária.
ep·i·crit·ic (ep-i-krit′ik). Epicrítico; o aspecto da sensibilidade somática que permite a discriminação e a localização topográfica de estímulos táteis e térmicos mais sutis. Cf. protopathic. [G. *epikritikos*, adjudicatório, de *epi*, sobre, + *krinō*, separar, julgar]
ep·i·cys·ti·tis (ep′i-sis-tī′tis). Epicistite; inflamação do tecido celular ao redor da bexiga. [epi- + G. *kystis*, bexiga, + *-itis*, inflamação]
ep·i·cyte (ep′i-sīt). Epícito; uma membrana celular, principalmente de protozoário; a camada externa do citoplasma em gregarinas. [epi- + G. *kytos*, célula]
ep·i·dem·ic (ep-i-dem′ik). Epidemia; a ocorrência, em uma comunidade ou região, de casos de uma doença, comportamento específico relacionado à doença ou outros eventos relacionados à saúde claramente acima da expectativa normal; a palavra também é usada para descrever surtos de doença em animais ou vegetais. Cf. endemic, sporadic. [epi- + G. *dēmos*, o povo]
 behavioral e., e. comportamental; uma epidemia que se origina em padrões comportamentais (em contraste com microrganismos invasores); os exemplos incluem mania de dança medieval, episódios de pânico por aglomeração.
 point e., e. de ponta; uma epidemia onde ocorre um agrupamento acentuado de casos de doença em um período muito curto (em alguns dias ou mesmo horas) devido à exposição de pessoas ou animais a uma fonte comum de infecção, como alimento ou água.
ep·i·dem·ic·i·ty (ep′i-dem-is′i-tē). Epidemicidade; o estado de doença prevalente na forma epidêmica.
ep·i·de·mi·og·ra·phy (ep′i-dem-ē-og′ră-fē). Epidemiografia; um tratado descritivo de doenças epidêmicas ou de qualquer epidemia específica. [G. *epidēmios*, epidemia, + *graphē*, escrito]
ep·i·de·mi·ol·o·gist (ep-i-dē-mē-ol′ō-jist). Epidemiologista; um investigador que estuda a ocorrência de doença ou outras condições, estados ou eventos relacionados à saúde em populações específicas; aquele que pratica epidemiologia; o controle da doença geralmente também é considerado uma atribuição do epidemiologista.
ep·i·de·mi·ol·o·gy (ep-i-dē-mē-ol′ō-jē). Epidemiologia; o estudo da distribuição e dos fatores determinantes de estados ou eventos relacionados à saúde em populações específicas, e a aplicação deste estudo para controle dos problemas de saúde. [G. *epidēmios*, epidemia, + *logos*, estudo]
 clinical e., e. clínica; o campo relacionado à aplicação de princípios epidemiológicos em uma situação clínica.
 genetic e., e. genética; o ramo da epidemiologia que estuda o papel dos fatores genéticos e suas interações com fatores ambientais na ocorrência de doença em várias populações.
 molecular e., e. molecular; o uso em estudos epidemiológicos de técnicas de biologia molecular como a tipagem de DNA.
ep·i·derm, ep·i·der·ma (ep′i-derm, ep-i-der′mă). Epiderme. SIN epidermis.
ep·i·der·mal, ep·i·der·mat·ic (ep-i-der′măl, -der-mat′ik). Epidérmico; relativo à epiderme. SIN epidermic.
ep·i·der·mal·i·za·tion (ep-i-der′mal-i-zā′shŭn). Epidermalização. SIN squamous *metaplasia*.
ep·i·der·mic (ep-i-der′mik). Epidérmico. SIN epidermal.
ep·i·der·mi·do·sis (ep′i-der-mi-dō′sis). Epidermidose. SIN epidermosis.
ep·i·der·mis, pl. **ep·i·der·mi·des** (ep-i-derm′is, -derm′i-dēz) [TA]. Epiderme. **1.** A porção epitelial superficial da pele (cútis). A epiderme espessa das regiões palmares e plantares contém os seguintes estratos (a partir da superfície): estrato córneo (camada de queratina), estrato lúcido (camada clara), estrato granuloso (camada granular), estrato espinhoso (camada de células espinhosas) e estrato basal (camada de células basais); em outras partes do corpo, o estrato lúcido pode estar ausente. **2.** Em botânica, a camada mais externa de células nas folhas e as partes jovens de plantas. SIN cuticle (3), cuticula (2), epiderm, epiderma. [G. *epidermis*, a pele externa, de *epi*, sobre, + *derma*, pele]
ep·i·der·mi·tis (ep-i-der-mī′tis). Epidermite; inflamação da epiderme ou das camadas superficiais da pele.
ep·i·der·mo·dys·pla·sia (ep-i-der′mō-dis-plā′zē-ă). Epidermodisplasia; deficiência do crescimento ou desenvolvimento da epiderme. [epidermis + G. *dys-*, mau, + *plasis*, moldagem]
 e. verrucifor′mis [MIM*226400], e. verruciforme; doença hereditária rara com numerosas verrugas planas nas mãos e nos pés, em pacientes com defeitos hereditários da imunidade celular e aumento da suscetibilidade a infecções pelo papilomavírus humano; algumas vezes há desenvolvimento de carcinoma cutâneo. Há um componente genético na etiologia, mas o padrão de herança é incerto no momento.
ep·i·der·moid (ep-i-der′moyd). Epidermóide. **1.** Semelhante à epiderme. **2.** Um colesteatoma ou outro tumor cístico originado de células epidérmicas aberrantes. [epidermis + G. *eidos*, aparência]
ep·i·der·mol·y·sis (ep′i-der-mol′i-sis). Epidermólise; condição na qual a epiderme está frouxamente fixada ao cório, esfoliando-se facilmente ou formando bolhas. [epidermis + G. *lysis*, afrouxamento]
 e. bullo′sa [MIM*131800], e. bolhosa; grupo de doenças cutâneas não-inflamatórias crônicas hereditárias no qual grandes bolhas e erosões resultam de pequeno traumatismo mecânico; uma forma localizada nas mãos e nos pés é denominada síndrome de Weber-Cockayne (Weber-Cockayne *syndrome*), de herança autossômica dominante causada por mutação no gene que codifica a queratina-5 (KRT5) no cromossoma 12q ou o gene da queratina-14 (KRT14) em 17q. SIN mechanobullous disease.
 e. bullosa, dermal type, e. bolhosa, tipo dérmico. SIN e. bullosa dystrophica.
 e. bullo′sa dystroph′ica [MIM*131705], e. bolhosa distrófica; forma de epidermólise bolhosa na qual ocorre fibrose após a separação de toda a epiderme, com formação de bolhas; sua herança é autossômica dominante (surgindo no lactente ou na criança) ou traço recessivo (presente ao nascimento ou surgindo nos primeiros meses de vida); esta última inclui os tipos letal e não-letal; tanto a forma dominante quanto a recessiva são causadas por mutação no gene para o colágeno tipo VII (COL7A1) no cromossoma 3p. SIN dermolytic bullous dermatosis, e. bullosa, dermal type.
 e. bullosa, epidermal type (bu′lō-să), e. bolhosa, tipo epidérmico. SIN e. bullosa simplex.
 e. bullosa, junctional type, e. bolhosa, tipo juncional. SIN e. bullosa lethalis.
 e. bullo′sa letha′lis [MIM*226700], e. bolhosa letal; uma forma de epidermólise bolhosa caracterizada por lesões crostosas periorais e perinasais per-

sistentes e que não cicatrizam, com bolhas freqüentes na mucosa oral e na traquéia, mas não nas regiões palmares e plantares, complicada por sépsis dérmica e perda de proteínas e eletrólitos séricos, levando à morte; herança autossômica recessiva, causada por mutação em qualquer um dos três polipeptídeos distintos da laminina-5: alfa-3 (LAMA3) no cromossoma 18q; beta-3 (LAMB3) e gama-2 (LAMC2) em 1q ou no gene que codifica a integrina; beta-4 (ITGB4) em 17q. SIN e. bullosa, junctional type, Herlitz syndrome.

e. bullo'sa sim'plex [MIM*131900], e. bolhosa simples; epidermólise bolhosa na qual as lesões cicatrizam rapidamente sem fibrose; a formação de bolha é intra-epidérmica e a microscopia revela vacuolação das células basais e dissolução das tonofibrilas; é mais freqüente nos pés de adultos após traumatismo não-costumeiro, como longas marchas; herança autossômica dominante causada por mutação no gene da queratina-5 (KRT5) no cromossoma 12q ou no gene da queratina-14 (KRT14) em 17q. SIN e. bullosa, epidermal type.

Ep·i·der·mo·phy·ton (ep'i - der - mof'i - ton, - der'mō - fī'ton). Gênero de fungos, separados por Sabouraud do *Trichophyton* com base no fato de que nunca invadem os folículos pilosos, cujos macroconídios são claviformes e de paredes lisas. A única espécie, *E. floccosum*, é uma espécie antropofílica que é uma causa comum de tinha dos pés e tinha inguinal. [epidermis + G. *phyton*, planta]

ep·i·der·mo·sis (ep - i - der - mō'sis). Epidermose; doença cutânea que afeta apenas a epiderme. SIN epidermidosis.

ep·i·der·mot·ro·pism (ep - i - der - mot'rō - pizm). Epidermotropismo; movimento em direção à epiderme, como na migração de linfócitos T para a epiderme na micose fungóide. [epidermis + G. *tropē*, uma volta]

ep·i·di·a·scope (ep - i - dī'a - skōp). Epidiascópio, retroprojetor; um projetor pelo qual as imagens são refletidas por um espelho através de uma lente, ou lentes, em uma tela, utilizando luz refletida para objetos opacos e luz transmitida para objetos translúcidos ou transparentes. SIN overhead projector. [epi- + G. *dia*, através, + *skopeō*, ver]

ep·i·did·y·mal (ep - i - did'i - mal). Epididimal; relativo ao epidídimo.

ep·i·did·y·mec·to·my (ep'i - did - i - mek'tō - mē). Epididimectomia; remoção cirúrgica do epidídimo. [epididymis + G. *ektomē*, excisão]

ep·i·did·y·mis, gen. **ep·i·did·y·mi·dis**, pl. **ep·i·did·y·mi·des** (ep - i - did'i - mis, - di - dim'i - dis, - di - dim'i - dēz) [TA]. Epidídimo; uma estrutura alongada conectada à superfície posterior do testículo, consistindo em cabeça, corpo e cauda, que se vira agudamente sobre si mesma para se tornar o ducto deferente; o principal componente é o ducto muito contorcido do epidídimo, que, na cauda e no início do ducto deferente, é um reservatório para espermatozóides. O epidídimo transporta, armazena e amadurece espermatozóides entre o testículo e o ducto deferente (*vas deferens*). SIN parorchis. [L. mod. do G. *epididymis*, de *epi*, sobre, + *didymos*, gêmeo, no pl. testículos]

ca'put e., cabeça do epidídimo. SIN head of epididymis.
cau'da e., cauda do epidídimo. SIN tail of epididymis.
cor'pus e., corpo do epidídimo. SIN body of epididymis.

ep·i·did·y·mi·tis, pl. **epididymiditides** (ep - i - did - i - mī'tis). Epididimite; inflamação do epidídimo.

ep·i·did·y·mo-or·chi·tis (ep - i - did'i - mō - ōr - kī'tis). Epididimorquite; inflamação simultânea do epidídimo e do testículo. [epididymis + G. *orchis*, testículo]

ep·i·did·y·mo·plas·ty (ep - i - did'i - mō - plas - tē). Epididimoplastia; reparo cirúrgico do epidídimo. [epididymis + G. *plastos*, formado]

ep·i·did·y·mot·o·my (ep'i - did - i - mot'ō - mē). Epididimotomia; incisão do epidídimo, como no preparo para epididimovasostomia ou para drenagem de material purulento. [epididymis + G. *tomē*, corte]

ep·i·did·y·mo·vas·ec·to·my (ep - i - did'i - mō - va - sek'tō - mē). Epididimovasectomia; remoção do epidídimo e do ducto deferente (*vas deferens*), geralmente proximal à sua entrada no canal inguinal. [epididymis + vasectomy]

ep·i·did·y·mo·va·sos·to·my (ep - i - did'i - mō - va - sos'tō - mē). Epididimovasostomia; anastomose cirúrgica do ducto deferente (*vas deferens*) ao epidídimo. [epididymis + vasostomy]

ep·i·du·ral (ep - i - doo'ral). Epidural; peridural; extradural; sobre (ou fora) da dura-máter. SIN peridural.

ep·i·du·rog·ra·phy (ep - i - doo - rog'ra - fē). Epidurografia; visualização radiográfica do espaço extradural após a instilação regional de um contraste radiopaco; técnica obsoleta.

ep·i·es'tri·ol (ep - i - es'trē - ol). Epiestriol. VER estriol.

ep·i·fas'cial (ep - i - fash'ē - al). Epifascial; sobre a superfície de uma fáscia, designa um método de injeção de drogas pelo qual a solução é depositada sobre a fáscia lata, em vez de ser injetada no parênquima muscular.

ep·i·gas·tral·gia (ep'i - gas - tral'jē - ā). Epigastralgia; dor na região epigástrica. [epigastrium + G. *algos*, dor]

ep·i·gas·tric (ep-i-gas'trik). Epigástrico; relativo ao epigástrio.

ep·i·gas·tri·um (ep - i - gas'trē - um) [TA]. Epigástrio. SIN epigastric region. [G. *epigastrion*]

ep·i·gas·tri·us (ep - i - gas'trē - ūs). Epigástrios; gêmeos conjugados desiguais nos quais o parasita menor está fixado ao autósito maior na região epigástrica. VER conjoined twins, em twin.

ep·i·gen·e·sis (ep - i - jen'ē - sis). Epigênese. **1.** Desenvolvimento da descendência de um zigoto. Cf. preformation *theory*. **2.** Controle da expressão da atividade dos genes sem alteração da estrutura genética. [epi- + G. *genesis*, criação]

ep·i·ge·net·ic (ep'i - je - net'ik). Epigenético; relativo à epigênese.

ep·i·glot·tic, ep·i·glot·tid·e·an (ep - i - glot'ik, ep - i - glo - tid'ē - an). Epiglótico; relativo à epiglote.

ep·i·glot·ti·dec·to·my (ep'i - glot - i - dek'tō - mē). Epiglotidectomia; excisão da epiglote. [epiglottis + G. *ektomē*, excisão]

ep·i·glot·ti·di·tis (ep'i - glot - i - dī'tis). Epiglotidite. SIN epiglottitis.

ep·i·glot·tis (ep - i - glot'is) [TA]. Epiglote; uma lâmina de cartilagem elástica em forma de folha, coberta por mucosa, na raiz da língua, que serve como uma válvula de desvio sobre a abertura superior da laringe durante o ato de deglutição; ela fica ereta quando estão sendo engolidos líquidos, mas é passivamente curvada sobre a abertura quando são engolidos alimentos sólidos. [G. *epiglōttis*, de *epi*, sobre, + *glōttis*, a abertura da traquéia]

bifid e., e. bífida; malformação congênita na qual os lados direito e esquerdo da epiglote não são unidos; associada a estridor e aspiração no recém-nascido devido à fenda entre os dois lados da epiglote para a glote.

ep·i·glot·ti·tis (ep - i - glot - ī'tis). Epiglotite; inflamação da epiglote que pode causar obstrução respiratória, principalmente em crianças; freqüentemente causada por infecção por *Haemophilus influenzae* tipo b. SIN epiglottiditis.

epig·na·thus (e - pig'nā - thus). Epignatos; gêmeos conjugados desiguais nos quais o parasita menor, incompleto, está ligado ao autósito maior pela mandíbula. VER conjoined *twins*, em *twin*. [epi- + G. *gnathos*, mandíbula]

ep·i·hy'al (ep - i - hī'al). Epiial; acima do arco hióide.

ep·i·hy'oid (ep - i - hī'oyd). Epiióide; sobre o osso hióide; designa determinadas glândulas tireóides acessórias acima do músculo gênio-hióideo.

ep·i·ker·a·to·phak·ia (ep'i - ker'a - tō - phak'ē - ā). Epiceratofaquia; modificação de erro de refração por aplicação de uma córnea de doador à superfície anterior da córnea do paciente, da qual foi removido o epitélio. SIN epikeratophakic keratoplasty. [epi- + G. *keras*, corno, + *phakos*, lente]

ep·i·ker·a·to·pros·the·sis (ep'i - ker'a - tō - pros'thē - sis). Epiceratoprótese; uma lente de contato aplicada ao estroma da córnea para substituir o epitélio. [epi- + G. *keras*, corno, + *prosthesis*, um acréscimo]

ep·i·la·mel·lar (ep'i - la - mel'ar). Epilamelar; sobre uma membrana basal ou acima desta. [epi- + L. *lamella*, dim. de *lamina*, uma placa de metal fina]

ep·i·late (ep'i - lāt). Epilar; depilar; extrair um pêlo; remover o pêlo de uma parte por extração forçada, eletrólise ou afrouxamento na raiz por meios químicos. Cf. depilate. [L. *e*, fora, + *pilus*, um pêlo]

ep·i·la·tion (ep - i - lā'shun). Epilação; o ato ou o resultado da remoção de pêlos. SIN depilation.

epil·a·to·ry (e - pil'a - tō - rē). Epilatório; depilatório. **1.** Que possui a propriedade de remover pêlos; relativo à epilação. SIN depilatory (1), psilotic (2). VER TAMBÉM decalvant. **2.** SIN depilatory (2).

ep·i·lem·ma (ep - i - lem'ā). Epilema; a bainha de tecido conjuntivo de fibras nervosas próximo de seu término. [epi- *lemma*, casca]

ep·i·lep·i·do·ma (ep'i - lep - i - dō'mā). Epilepidoma; tumor resultante da hiperplasia do tecido derivado do epiblasto verdadeiro. [epi- + G. *lepis*, revestimento exterior + *-ōma*, tumor]

ep·i·lep·sia (ep - i - lep'sē - ā). Epilepsia. SIN epilepsy. [G.]

e. partia'lis contin'ua, e. parcial contínua; **(1)** uma forma de epilepsia caracterizada por contrações musculares clônicas repetitivas com ou sem grandes convulsões; **(2)** estado de mal epiléptico motor parcial simples do córtex de Rolando, freqüentemente com características mioclônicas; **(3)** um tipo de convulsão observado comumente na encefalite de Rasmussen. SIN Kojewnikoff epilepsy.

ep·i·lep·sy (ep'i - lep'sē). Epilepsia; distúrbio crônico caracterizado por disfunção encefálica paroxística devido à descarga neuronal excessiva e, em geral, associado a alguma alteração da consciência. As manifestações clínicas do ataque podem variar de anormalidades complexas do comportamento, incluindo convulsões generalizadas ou focais a crises momentâneas de comprometimento da consciência. Esses estados clínicos foram submetidos a várias classificações, nenhuma universalmente aceita até hoje, e, conseqüentemente, as terminologias usadas para descrever os diferentes tipos de ataque ainda são puramente descritas e não-padronizadas; são variavelmente baseadas 1) nas manifestações clínicas da convulsão (motora, sensorial, reflexa, psíquica ou vegetativa), 2) no substrato anatomopatológico (hereditário, inflamatório, degenerativo, neoplásico, traumático ou criptogênico), 3) na localização da lesão epileptogênica (regiões de Rolando, temporal, diencefálica) e 4) no período da vida no qual ocorrem os ataques (noturno, diurno, menstrual, etc.). SIN convulsive state, epilepsia, falling sickness. [G. *epilēpsia*, convulsão]

anosognosic e., e. anosognóstica; epilepsia caracterizada por ataques dos quais a pessoa não toma conhecimento. SIN anosognosic seizures.

automatic e., e. psicomotora. SIN psychomotor e.

autonomic e., e. autônoma; episódios de disfunção autônoma provavelmente devidos à irritação diencefálica. SIN diencephalic e., vasomotor e., vasovagal e.

benign childhood e. with centrotemporal spikes, e. benigna da infância com pontas centrotemporais; uma síndrome de epilepsia específica que começa na infância e remite na adolescência, caracterizada por convulsões motoras parciais simples noturnas ou por convulsões tônico-clônicas generalizadas. O EEG mostra pontas centrotemporais ativadas pelo sono e um padrão de base normal sob outros aspectos.

centrencephalic e., e. centrencefálica; termo impreciso que se refere à epilepsia caracterizada, eletroencefalograficamente, por descargas sincrônicas bilaterais e, clinicamente, por crises de ausência ou por convulsões tônico-clônicas generalizadas.

childhood absence e., crise de ausência infantil; síndrome de epilepsia generalizada caracterizada pelo início de crises de ausência na infância, tipicamente aos seis ou sete anos. Há uma forte predisposição genética e as meninas são afetadas com maior freqüência que os meninos. O EEG revela atividade ponta-onda de 3 Hz generalizada sobre um fundo normal. O prognóstico de remissão é bom se o paciente não apresentar também convulsões tônico-clônicas generalizadas. VER TAMBÉM absence. SIN petit mal e., pyknolepsy.

childhood e. with occipital paroxysms, e. infantil com paroxismos occipitais; uma síndrome de epilepsia benigna caracterizada por freqüentes pontas occipitais, amiúde ativadas pelo fechamento do olho. Possui uma semiologia convulsiva que inclui manifestações visuais; nem sempre há remissão mais tarde.

complex precipitated e., e. precipitada complexa; uma forma de epilepsia reflexa iniciada por estímulos sensoriais especializados, p. ex., determinados padrões visuais.

cortical e., e. cortical. SIN focal e.
cryptogenic e., e. criptogênica. SIN generalized tonic-clonic seizure.
diencephalic e., e. diencefálica. SIN autonomic e.
early posttraumatic e., e. pós-traumática precoce; convulsões que começam uma semana após traumatismo craniano grave.

eating e., e. induzida por comida; convulsões epilépticas, freqüentemente generalizadas, provocadas por uma refeição; um tipo de epilepsia reflexa.

focal e., e. focal; epilepsia de várias etiologias caracterizada por convulsões focais ou convulsões tônico-clônicas generalizadas secundariamente. Os sintomas ictais freqüentemente estão relacionados à região encefálica onde a convulsão começa focalmente. SIN cortical e., local e., localization-related e. (2), partial e.

frontal lobe e., e. do lobo frontal; uma epilepsia relacionada à localização, com convulsões originadas no lobo frontal. Existem várias síndromes clínicas, dependendo da localização exata das convulsões e da semiologia clínica do tipo da convulsão. As epilepsias do lobo frontal foram divididas em várias síndromes específicas, incluindo a síndrome de convulsões motoras suplementares, convulsões do cíngulo, convulsões da região polar frontal anterior, convulsões frontais orbitais, convulsões dorsolaterais, convulsões operculares e convulsões do córtex motor.

generalized e., e. generalizada; uma importante categoria de síndromes epilépticas caracterizadas por um ou mais tipos de convulsões generalizadas.

generalized tonic-clonic e., e. tônico-clônica generalizada. SIN generalized tonic-clonic seizure.

grand mal e., e. do tipo grande mal; designação antiga para epilepsia caracterizada por convulsão tônico-clônica generalizada (generalized tonic-clonic seizure).

idiopathic e., e. idiopática; (1) epilepsia sem causa evidente; termo freqüentemente usado para descrever as epilepsias genéticas; (2) e. tônico-clônica generalizada. SIN generalized tonic-clonic seizure.

intractable e., e. intratável; epilepsia não controlada adequadamente por medicação. SIN pharmacoresistent e.

jacksonian e., e. jacksoniana. SIN jacksonian seizure.

juvenile absence e., crise de ausência juvenil; uma síndrome epiléptica generalizada com início por volta da puberdade, caracterizada por crises de ausência e convulsões tônico-clônicas generalizadas. O EEG freqüentemente mostra um padrão ponta-onda generalizado de 3 Hz.

juvenile myoclonic e., e. mioclônica juvenil; uma síndrome epiléptica que, tipicamente, começa no início da adolescência, sendo caracterizada por contrações mioclônicas no início da manhã que podem progredir para uma convulsão tônico-clônica generalizada. Um distúrbio genético: algumas famílias tiveram ligação genética com o cromossoma 6. O EEG é caracterizado por polipontas e ondas generalizadas em 4–6 Hz.

Kojewnikoff e., e. de Kojewnikoff. SIN epilepsia partialis continua.
laryngeal e., e. laríngea; uma forma de epilepsia reflexa precipitada por tosse.
local e., e. local. SIN focal e.
localization-related e., e. relacionada com localização; (1) SIN myoclonus e.; (2) SIN focal e.
major e., e. maior. SIN generalized tonic-clonic seizure.
masked e., e. mascarada; uma forma de epilepsia caracterizada por crises atônicas (crises de queda) e tônicas ou tônico-clônicas em crianças com déficits neurológicos (hemiplégicas, atáxicas, etc.) e retardo mental; caracterizada, no EEG, por descargas de pontas e ondas (2/s); geralmente progride apesar da medicação.

matutinal e., e. matutina, uma forma de e. que ocorre ao despertar.
myoclonic astatic e., e. astática mioclônica, uma variante do pequeno mal caracterizada por crises tônicas ou tônico-clônicas em crianças com déficits neurológicos (hemiplegia, ataxia, etc.) e retardo mental; caracterizada no EEG por pontas-ondas (2/s); geralmente evolui apesar da medicação.

myoclonus e. [MIM*159800 e MIM*220300], e. mioclônica; um grupo clinicamente diverso de síndromes de epilepsia, algumas benignas, outras progressivas. Muitas são hereditárias com herança mitocondrial mendeliana e não-mendeliana. Todas são caracterizadas pela ocorrência de mioclônus, que pode ser limitado ou predominar na condição. As síndromes específicas incluem síndrome mioclônica com mancha vermelho-cereja, lipofuscinose ceróide, epilepsia mioclônica com fibras vermelhas rotas e mioclônus báltico. SIN localization-related e. (1).

nocturnal e., e. noturna; uma síndrome epiléptica caracterizada apenas por convulsões noturnas.

occipital lobe e., e. do lobo occipital; uma epilepsia relacionada com a localização na qual as convulsões se originam no lobo occipital. Os sintomas comumente incluem anormalidades visuais durante as convulsões.

parietal lobe e., e. do lobo parietal; uma epilepsia relacionada com a localização na qual as convulsões se originam no lobo parietal. A semiologia da convulsão pode envolver anormalidades da sensibilidade.

partial e., e. parcial. SIN focal e.
pattern-sensitive e., e. de padrão; uma forma de epilepsia reflexa precipitada pela visão de certos padrões.
petit mal e., e. do tipo pequeno mal. SIN childhood absence e.
pharmacoresistent e., e. fármaco-resistente. SIN intractable e.
photogenic e., e. fotogênica; uma forma de epilepsia reflexa precipitada pela luz.

posttraumatic e., e. pós-traumática; estado convulsivo subseqüente e etiologicamente relacionado a um traumatismo craniano; com lesão encefálica que se manifesta clinicamente ou é determinada por exames especiais como a tomografia computadorizada. Para se pressupor uma relação causal, é preciso que o indivíduo não tenha história de epilepsia prévia, doença cerebral e traumatismo encefálico prévio. As crises devem ter se iniciado, dependendo da gravidade da ferida, 3 meses a 2 anos após o traumatismo alegado e ser de um tipo compatível com o local da lesão e com as anormalidades EEG.

primary generalized e., e. generalizada primária; epilepsia sem evidências de doença do sistema nervoso central focal ou multifocal. As convulsões são generalizadas desde o início, tanto pelo EEG quanto por critérios clínicos. Freqüentemente uma forma genética pura de epilepsia. VER TAMBÉM generalized tonic-clonic seizure.

procursive e., e. procursiva; uma crise psicomotora iniciada pelo ato de rodopiar ou correr.

psychomotor e., e. psicomotora; crises com elaborados e múltiplos componentes sensoriais, motores e/ou psíquicos, sendo a característica comum uma turvação ou perda da consciência e amnésia em relação ao evento; as manifestações clínicas podem assumir a forma de automatismos; explosões emocionais de humor, ira ou demonstração de medo; distúrbios motores ou psíquicos; ou pode estar relacionada a qualquer esfera da atividade humana. Eletroencefalograficamente, a crise é caracterizada por descargas em ponta no lobo temporal, principalmente durante o sono. VER TAMBÉM procursive e., visceral e., uncinate e. SIN automatic e.

reflex e., e. reflexa; convulsões induzidas por estimulação periférica; p. ex., audiogênica, laríngea, fotogênica ou outro estímulo. SIN sensory precipitated e.

rolandic e., e. rolândica; uma forma autossômica dominante, benigna, de epilepsia que ocorre em crianças, caracterizada clinicamente por interrupção da fala, contrações musculares do lado da face e do braço, e descargas epilépticas eletroencefalográficas. [Luigi Rolando]

secondary generalized e., e. generalizada secundária; um grupo de síndromes epilépticas de etiologias diversas, com envolvimento cerebral difuso ou multifocal. Os pacientes tipicamente possuem vários tipos de convulsões generalizadas, incluindo convulsões tônicas, atônicas, mioclônicas, de ausência atípica e tônico-clônicas generalizadas. Também pode haver convulsões parciais. Uma síndrome clássica é a síndrome de Lennox-Gastaut. SIN symptomatic e.

sensory e., e. sensorial; epilepsia focal iniciada por um fenômeno somatossensorial.

sensory precipitated e., e. sensorial precipitada. SIN reflex e.
sleep e., e. do sono; termo incorreto para narcolepsia.
somnambulic e., e. sonambúlica; automatismo pós-ictal no qual o paciente caminha ou corre exibindo comportamento natural do qual ele não se recorda subseqüentemente.

startle e., e. do sobressalto; e. do susto; forma de epilepsia reflexa precipitada por ruídos súbitos.

supplementary motor area e., e. da área motora suplementar; uma síndrome epiléptica relacionada com a localização na qual as convulsões se originam da área motora suplementar do lobo frontal mesial. A semiologia da convulsão típica inclui movimentos tônicos bilaterais súbitos, vocalização e preservação da consciência. As crises freqüentemente são noturnas.

symptomatic e., e. sintomática. SIN secondary generalized e.
temporal lobe e., e. do lobo temporal; epilepsia relacionada com a localização, com convulsões originadas no lobo temporal, mais comumente o lobo temporal mesial. A patologia mais comum é a esclerose do hipocampo. SIN uncinate fit.
tonic e., e. tônica; uma crise na qual o corpo fica rígido.
tornado e., e. em furacão; tipo de epilepsia focal ou convulsão parcial com uma aura de vertigem acentuada e uma sensação de estar sendo puxado para o espaço.
uncinate e., e. uncinada; forma de epilepsia psicomotora ou convulsão parcial complexa iniciada por um estado de sonhos e alucinações do olfato e do paladar, geralmente resultante de uma lesão temporal medial. SIN uncinate attack.
vasomotor e., e. vasomotora. SIN autonomic e.
vasovagal e., e. vasovagal. SIN autonomic e.
visceral e., e. visceral; epilepsia, geralmente psicomotora, na qual as crises são iniciadas por sintomas ou sensações viscerais; a maioria dos casos tem seu foco no lobo temporal.
e. with grand mal seizures on awakening, e. com convulsões do tipo grande mal ao despertar; síndrome epiléptica generalizada, caracterizada por início na segunda década de vida, tipicamente com convulsões tônico-clônicas generalizadas, a maioria das quais ocorre logo após o despertar (independentemente da hora do dia), exacerbadas pela privação do sono. Há uma predisposição genética e o EEG mostra um dos vários padrões generalizados de descargas interictais; é comum haver fotossensibilidade.
e. with myoclonic absences, e. mioclônica com crises de ausências; forma de epilepsia generalizada caracterizada por crises de ausência, acentuadas contrações clônicas rítmicas bilaterais, freqüentemente associadas a contração tônica, e um padrão de ponta-onda de 3 Hz no EEG. O início geralmente se dá por volta dos sete anos, sendo os homens afetados com maior freqüência.

ep·i·lep·tic (ep-i-lep'tik). Epiléptico; relativo a, caracterizado por, ou que sofre de epilepsia.
ep·i·lep·ti·form (ep-i-lep'ti-form). Epileptiforme. SIN epileptoid.
ep·i·lep·to·gen·ic, ep·i·lep·tog·e·nous (ep-i-lep-tō-jen'ik, ep-i-lep-toj'e-nŭs). Epileptogênico; que causa epilepsia.
ep·i·lep·toid (ep-i-lep'toyd). Epileptóide; semelhante à epilepsia; designa determinadas convulsões, principalmente de natureza funcional. SIN epileptiform. [G. *epilēpsia*, convulsão, epilepsy, + *eidos*, semelhança]
ep·i·loia (ep-i-loy'ă). Epilóia. SIN tuberous sclerosis.
ep·i·man·dib·u·lar (ep-i-man-dib'ū-lar). Epimandibular; sobre a mandíbula. [epi- + L. *mandibulum*, mandíbula]
ep·i·mas·ti·cal (ep-i-mast'i-kăl). Epacmástico; que aumenta gradualmente até atingir um pico e, depois, diminui; diz-se de uma febre. [G. *epakmastikos*, que chega a um pico]
ep·i·mas·ti·gote (ep-i-mas'ti-gōt). Epimastigota; termo que substitui "estágio de crítidia", para evitar confusão com os flagelados parasitas de insetos do gênero *Crithidia*. No estágio epimastigota, o flagelo origina-se do cinetoplasto ao longo do núcleo e emerge da extremidade anterior do organismo; há uma membrana ondulada. [epi- + G. *mastix*, chicote]
ep·i·men·or·rha·gia (ep-i-men-ō-rā'jē-ă). Epimenorragia; menstruação prolongada e profusa que ocorre a qualquer momento, sendo porém mais freqüente no início e no fim da vida menstrual.
ep·i·men·or·rhea (ep-i-men'ō-rē'ă). Epimenorréia; menstruação muito freqüente, que ocorre a qualquer momento, mas sobretudo no início e no fim da vida menstrual.
ep·i·mer (ep'i-mer). Epímero; uma das duas moléculas (que possui mais de um centro quiral) diferindo apenas na configuração espacial em torno de um único átomo quiral; p. ex., α-D-glicose e α-D-galactose (em relação ao carbono-4). VER sugars. Cf. anomer. [epi- + G. *meros*, parte]
ep·i·mer·ase (ep'i-mer-ās)[EC 5.1]. Epimerase; uma classe de enzimas que catalisam alterações epiméricas.
ep·i·mere (ep'i-mēr). Epímero; a parte dorsal do miótomo. VER myotome (3). [epi- + G. *meros*, parte]
ep·im·er·ite (ep-i-mēr'īt). Epimerito; a estrutura de ancoragem semelhante a um gancho na extremidade anterior de um esporozoário gregarino cefalina; é deixado incrustado nos tecidos quando o restante do cefalonte é solto na luz do intestino do hospedeiro invertebrado. [epi- + G. *meros*, parte]
ep·i·mi·cro·scope (ep-i-mī'krō-skōp). Epimicroscópio; um microscópio com um condensador construído ao redor da objetiva; usado para a investigação de pequenas amostras opacas, ou apenas um pouco translúcidas. SIN opaque microscope.
ep·i·mor·pho·sis (ep'i-mor-fō'sis). Epimorfose; regeneração de uma parte de um organismo por crescimento na superfície de corte. [epi- + G. *morphē*, formato]
ep·i·mys·i·ot·o·my (ep'i-mis-ē-ot'ō-mē). Epimisiotomia; incisão da bainha de um músculo. [epimysium + G. *tomē*, corte]
ep·i·mys·i·um (ep-i-mis'ē-ŭm) [TA]. Epimísio; o envoltório de tecido conjuntivo fibroso que circunda um músculo esquelético. SIN perimysium externum. [epi- + G. *mys*, músculo]

ep·i·neph·rine (ep'i-nef'rin). Epinefrina; adrenalina; uma catecolamina que é o principal neuro-hormônio da medula supra-renal da maioria das espécies; também é secretada por neurônios. O isômero L é o estimulante mais potente (simpaticomimético) de receptores α- e β-adrenérgicos, resultando em aumento da freqüência cardíaca e da força de contração, vasoconstrição ou vasodilatação, relaxamento do músculo liso bronquiolar e intestinal, glicogenólise, lipólise e outros efeitos metabólicos; usada no tratamento da asma brônquica, distúrbios alérgicos agudos, glaucoma de ângulo aberto, parada cardíaca e bloqueio atrioventricular, e como vasoconstritor tópico e local. Os sais geralmente usados são cloridrato de epinefrina e bitartarato de epinefrina, sendo este último usado com maior freqüência em preparações tópicas. SIN adrenaline. [epi- + G. *nephros*, rim, + -ine]
ep·i·neph·ros (ep-i-nef'ros). Epinefro. SIN suprarenal gland. [epi- + G. *nephros*, rim]
ep·i·neu·ral (ep-i-noo'răl). Epineural; sobre o arco neural de uma vértebra.
ep·i·neu·ri·al (ep-i-noo'rē-ăl). Epineural; relativo ao epineuro.
ep·i·neu·ri·um (ep-i-noo'rē-ŭm) [TA]. Epineuro; a estrutura de sustentação mais externa de troncos nervosos periféricos, que consiste em uma condensação de tecido conjuntivo areolar; subdividida em camadas que circundam todo o tronco nervoso (epineuro epifascicular) e camadas que se estendem entre os fascículos do nervo (epineuro interfascicular). Com o endoneuro e o perineuro, o epineuro compõe o estroma nervoso periférico. [epi- + G. *neuron*, nervo]
epifascicular e., e. epifascicular; a porção do epineuro que circunda todo o tronco nervoso, ao contrário do epineuro epifascicular, que segue para baixo entre os fascículos nervosos.
ep·i·o·nych·i·um (ep-i-ō-nik'ē-ŭm). Epioníquio. SIN eponychium.
ep·i·ot·ic (ep'i-ot'ik, -ō'tik). Epiótico; um dos componentes da cápsula ótica de alguns vertebrados; no mamífero, a parte petrosa do osso temporal incorpora os vários elementos óticos observados em vertebrados inferiores. [epi- + G. *ous*, orelha]
ep·i·pas·tic (ep-i-pas'tik). Epipástico. **1.** Utilizável como talco. **2.** Um talco. [G. *epi-passō*, polvilhar]
ep·i·per·i·car·di·al (ep'i-per-i-kar'dē-ăl). Epipericárdico; sobre o pericárdio ou ao seu redor.
ep·i·phar·ynx (ep'i-far'ingks). Epifaringe. SIN nasopharynx. [G. *epi*, sobre, + *pharynx*]
ep·i·phe·nom·e·non (ep'i-fē-nom'ē-non). Epifenômeno; um sintoma que surge no decorrer de uma doença, que não é habitual, e não está necessariamente associado à doença.
epiph·o·ra (ē-pif'ō-ră). Epífora; hiperfluxo de lágrimas sobre a bochecha, devido à drenagem imperfeita pelas vias condutoras de lágrimas. SIN tearing, watery eye (1). [G. um fluxo súbito, de *epi*, sobre, + *pherō*, conduzir]
atonic e., e. atônica; epífora decorrente da fraqueza do músculo orbicular do olho.
ep·i·phren·ic, ep·i·phre·nal (ep'i-fren'ik, -frē'năl). Epifrênico; sobre o diafragma ou acima dele. [epi- + G. *phrēn*, diafragma]
ep·i·phys·i·al, epiph·y·se·al (ep-i-fiz'ē-ăl). Epifisário; relativo a uma epífise.
epiph·y·si·od·e·sis (ep'i-fiz-ē-od'ē-sis). Epifisiodese. **1.** União prematura da epífise com a diáfise, resultando em cessação do crescimento. **2.** Procedimento cirúrgico que destrói, parcial ou totalmente, uma epífise e pode incorporar um enxerto ósseo para produzir fusão da epífise ou cessação prematura de seu crescimento; geralmente é realizado para igualar o comprimento da perna. [epiphysis + G. *desis*, ligação]
epiph·y·si·ol·y·sis (ep-i-fiz-ē-ol'i-sis). Epifisiólise; afrouxamento ou separação, parcial ou completa, de uma epífise da metáfise de um osso. [epiphysis + G. *lysis*, afrouxamento]
ep·i·phys·i·op·a·thy (ep-i-fiz-ē-op'ă-thē). Epifisiopatia; qualquer distúrbio de uma epífise dos ossos longos. [epiphysis + G. *pathos*, que sofre]
epiph·y·sis, pl. **epiph·y·ses** (ep'i-sis, -sēz)[TA]. Epífise; parte de um osso desenvolvida a partir de um centro de ossificação distinto daquele da diáfise e separado inicialmente desta última por uma camada de cartilagem. [G. uma excrescência, de *epi*, sobre, + *physis*, crescimento]
atavistic e., e. atávica; osso independente filogeneticamente, mas que agora está fundido a outro osso, p. ex., o processo coracóide da escápula.
e. cer'ebri, e. cerebral. SIN pineal body.
pressure e., e. de pressão; um centro secundário de ossificação na extremidade articular de um osso longo.
stippled e., e. pontilhada. SIN chondrodysplasia punctata.
traction e., e. de tração; um centro secundário de ossificação no local de fixação de um tendão.
epiph·y·si·tis (e-pif-i-sī'tis). Epifisite; inflamação de uma epífise.
ep·i·pi·al (ep'i-pī'ăl). Epipial; sobre a pia-máter.
epiplo-. Epiplo-; omento. VER TAMBÉM omento-. [G. *epiploon*]
epip·lo·cele (e-pip'lō-sēl). Epiplocele: termo raramente usado para hérnia do omento. [epiplo- + G. *kēlē*, hérnia]
ep·i·plo·ic (ep'i-plō'ik). Epiplóico. SIN omental.

epip·lo·on (e‑pip′lō‑on). Epíploo; epíploon. SIN greater omentum. [G.]

epipodophyllotoxin (ĕp‑ē‑pō‑dō‑ fī′lō‑tosk′in, –fil′ō‑toks′in). Epipodofilotoxina; produto natural que inibe a topoisomerase II. VER TAMBÉM etoposide. [epi‑ + *Podophyllum*, gênero de origem botânica, + toxin]

ep·i·pter·ic (ep′i‑ter′ik). Epiptérico; na vizinhança do ptério.

ep·i·py·gus (ep‑i‑pī′gŭs). Epípigo; gêmeos conjugados desiguais nos quais o parasita menor, incompleto, está fixado à nádega do autósito maior. VER pygomelus, conjoined *twins*, em *twin*. [epi‑ + G. *pygē*, nádegas]

D-ep·i·rham·nose (ep‑i‑ram′nōz). D-epirranose; 6-desoxi-D-glicose; ocorre em vegetais e bactérias em combinação com diacilglicerol e freqüentemente é sulfatada (em C-6) em glicolipídios. SIN quinovose.

ep·i·scle·ra (ep′i‑sklĕr′ă). Esclera; o tecido conjuntivo entre a esclera e a conjuntiva. [epi‑ + sclera]

ep·i·scle·ral (ep‑i‑sklĕr′ăl). Escleral. **1.** Sobre a esclera. **2.** Relativo à episclera.

ep·i·scle·ri·tis (ep‑i‑skle‑rī′tis). Esclerite; inflamação do tecido conjuntivo escleral. VER TAMBÉM scleritis.

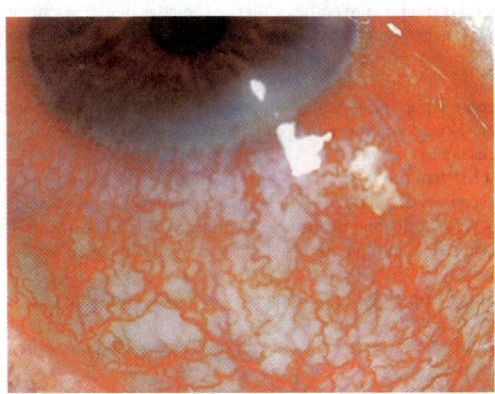

esclerite: na artrite reumatóide

e. multinodula'ris, e. multinodular; esclerite com muitos nódulos próximos do limbo córneo-escleral.

nodular e., e. nodular; esclerite com focos de inflamação localizada nos tecidos esclerais.

e. periodi'ca fu'gax, e. periódica fugaz; esclerite transitória difusa com tendência a recidivar a intervalos regulares. SIN subconjunctivitis.

episio-. Episio-; vulva. VER TAMBÉM vulvo-. [G. *episeion*, região pubiana]

ep·i·si·o·per·i·ne·or·rha·phy (e‑piz′ē‑ō‑per′i‑nē‑ōr′ă‑fē, e‑pis′). Episioperineorrafia; reparo de uma incisão ou ruptura do períneo e laceração da vulva ou reparo de uma incisão cirúrgica da vulva e do períneo. [episio‑ + G. *perinaion*, períneo, + *rhaphē*, sutura]

ep·i·si·o·plas·ty (e‑piz′ē‑ō‑plas‑tē, e‑pis′). Episioplastia; cirurgia plástica da vulva. [episio‑ + G. *plastos*, formado]

ep·i·si·or·rha·phy (e‑piz‑i‑ōr′ră‑fē, e‑pis‑). Episiorrafia; reparo de uma laceração da vulva ou de uma episiotomia. [episio‑ + G. *rhaphē*, sutura]

ep·i·si·o·ste·no·sis (e‑piz′i‑ō‑stē‑nō′sis, e‑pis′). Episioestenose; estreitamento do orifício vulvar. [episio‑ + G. *stenōsis*, estreitamento]

ep·i·si·ot·o·my (e‑piz‑ē‑ot′ō‑mē, e‑pis‑). Episiotomia; incisão cirúrgica da vulva para evitar laceração no momento do parto ou para facilitar a cirurgia vaginal. SIN vaginoperineotomy. [episio‑ + G. *tomē*, incisão]

ep·i·so·de (ep′i‑sōd). Episódio; um importante evento ou série de eventos que ocorrem no decorrer de eventos contínuos, p. ex., um episódio de depressão.

acute schizophrenic e., e. esquizofrênico agudo. SIN acute *schizophrenia.*

e. of care, todos os serviços prestados a um paciente com problemas clínicos durante um período específico de tempo, ao longo de um *continuum* de assistência em um sistema integrado.

manic e., e. de mania; manifestação de um importante distúrbio do humor no qual há um período distinto durante o qual o humor predominante do indivíduo é elevado, expansivo ou irritável, e há sintomas associados da fase excitada ou maníaca do distúrbio bipolar. VER affective *disorders*, em *disorder*, endogenous *depression*.

ep·i·some (ep′i‑sōm). Epissoma; um elemento extracromossomial (plasmídeo) que pode integrar-se ao cromossoma bacteriano do hospedeiro ou replicar-se e atuar de forma estável quando fisicamente separado do cromossoma. [epi‑ + G. *sōma*, corpo (cromossoma)]

resistance-transferring e.'s, epissomas de transferência de resistência. SIN resistance *plasmids*, em *plasmid*.

ep·i·spa·di·as (ep‑i‑spā′dē‑ăs). Epispádia; malformação na qual a uretra se abre no dorso do pênis; freqüentemente associada à extrofia da bexiga. [epi‑ + G. *spaō*, rasgar-se, estriar]

balanitic e., e. balanítica; posição excessivamente proximal do meato no dorso da glande do pênis.

coronal e., e. coronal; posição excessivamente proximal do meato no sulco coronal.

penile e., e. peniana; posição proximal do meato uretral no dorso do corpo do pênis.

penopubic e., e. penopubiana; posição do meato uretral na junção da base do pênis e na parte inferior da parede abdominal.

ep·i·spi·nal (ep‑i‑spī′năl). Epiespinal; sobre a coluna vertebral ou a medula espinal, ou sobre qualquer estrutura semelhante à coluna vertebral.

ep·i·sple·ni·tis (ep‑i‑splē‑nī′tis). Episplenite; inflamação da cápsula esplênica.

epis·ta·sis (e‑pis′tă‑sis). Epístase. **1.** A formação de uma película ou espuma na superfície de um líquido, principalmente urina em repouso. **2.** Interação fenotípica de genes não-alélicos. **3.** Uma forma de interação genética na qual um gene mascara ou interfere com a expressão fenotípica de um ou mais genes em outros *loci*; o gene cujo fenótipo é expresso é dito "epistático", enquanto o fenótipo alterado ou suprimido é dito "hipostático". SIN epistasy. [G. scum; epi‑ + G. *stasis*, estase]

epis·ta·sy (e‑pis′tă‑sē). Epistase. SIN epistasis.

ep·i·stat·ic (ep‑is‑tat′ik). Epistático; relativo a epistase.

ep·i·stax·is (ep′i‑stak′sis). Epistaxe; hemorragia nasal. SIN nasal hemorrhage, nosebleed. [G. de *epistazō*, sangrar no nariz, de *epi*, sobre, + *stazō*, gotejar]

renal e., e. renal; hematúria sem lesão detectável.

epis·te·mol·o·gy (ē‑pis′tō‑mol′ō‑gē). Epistemologia; o estudo do conhecimento e das regras de evidências envolvidas. Tradicionalmente, um ramo da filosofia, agora está passando a ser usado também como uma disciplina incorporada em, e em alguns aspectos peculiar a, campos individuais de cultura (medicina, ciência, história, etc.).

epis·te·mo·phil·i·a (ē‑pis′tē‑mō‑fil′ē‑ă). Epistemofilia; amor, particularmente excessivo, pelo conhecimento. [G. *epistēmē*, conhecimento, + *philos*, afeição]

ep·i·ster·nal (ep‑i‑ster′năl). Esternal. **1.** Sobre o esterno. **2.** Relativo ao episterno.

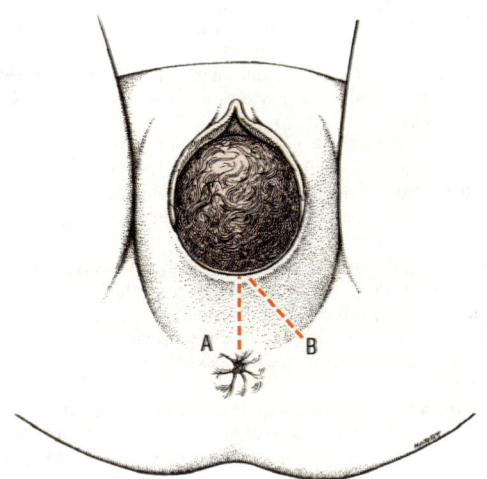

episiotomia: (A) mediana e (B) mediolateral

ep·i·ster·num (ep‑i‑ster′nŭm). Episterno. SIN manubrium of sternum. [epi‑ + L. *sternum*, tórax]

ep·i·stro·phe·us (ep‑i‑strō′fē‑ŭs). Epistrofeu. SIN axis (5). [G. o pivô]

ep·i·tar·sus (ep‑i‑tar′sŭs). Epitarso; uma prega de conjuntiva que se origina na superfície tarsal da pálpebra e desaparece na pele próxima ao ângulo medial do olho. [epi‑ + G. *tarsos*, esteira plana, borda da pálpebra]

ep·i·taxy (ep‑i‑tak′sē). Epitaxia; o crescimento de um cristal em uma ou mais orientações específicas no substrato de outro tipo de cristal, com um ajuste geométrico preciso entre as redes em contato; observada nas camadas alternadas de diferente composição em cálculos renais e da vesícula biliar, indicando uma alteração abrupta da composição durante a formação. [epi‑ + G. *taxis*, arranjo]

ep·i·ten·din·e·um (ep′i‑ten‑din′ē‑ŭm). Epitendíneo; a bainha fibrosa branca que envolve um tendão. SIN epitenon. [L.]

epit·e·non (ē‑pit′ē‑non, ep‑i‑ten′on). Epitendão. SIN epitendineum.

17-ep·i·tes·tos·ter·one (ep′i‑tes‑tos′ter‑ōn). 17-Epitestosterona; epímero

17α da testosterona; um esteróide biologicamente inativo encontrado nos testículos e ovários; pode ser um metabólito da 4-androsteno-3,17-diona e um precursor do 17α-estradiol.

ep·i·thal·a·mus (ep′i-thal′ă-mŭs) [TA]. Epitálamo; uma pequena área dorsomedial do tálamo correspondente à habênula e a suas estruturas associadas: estria medular do tálamo, glândula pineal e comissura habenular. [epi- + thalamus]

ep·i·tha·lax·i·a (ep′i-thă-lak′sē-ă). Epitalaxia; descamação de qualquer epitélio superficial, mas especialmente daquele que reveste o intestino. [epithelium + G. *allaxis*, troca]

ep·i·the·lia (ep-i-thē′lē-ă). Epitélios; plural de epithelium.

ep·i·the·li·al (ep-i-thē′lē-ăl). Epitelial; relativo a, ou que consiste em, epitélio.

ep·i·the·li·al·i·za·tion (ep-i-thē′lē-ăl-i-zā′shŭn). Epitelização; formação de epitélio sobre uma superfície desnuda. SIN epithelization.

ep·i·the·li·o·cyte (ep-i-thē′lē-ō-sīt). Epiteliócito; uma célula epitelial de cultura de tecido *in vitro*. [epithelium + G. *kytos*, célula]

ep·i·the·li·o·fi·bril (ep-i-thē′lē-ō-fī′bril). Epiteliofibrila. SIN tonofibril.

ep·i·the·li·o·glan·du·lar (ep-i-thē′lē-ō-glan′dū-lăr). Epitelioglandular; relativo ao epitélio glandular.

ep·i·the·li·oid (ep-i-thē′lē-oyd). Epitelióide; semelhante ao epitélio, ou que possui algumas das suas características. [epithelium + G. *eidos*, semelhança]

ep·i·the·li·o·lyt·ic (ep-i-thē′lē-ō-lit′ik). Epiteliolítico; destrutivo para o epitélio.

ep·i·the·li·o·ma (ep′i-thē-lē-ō′mă). Epitelioma. **1.** Uma neoplasia epitelial ou hamartoma da pele, principalmente com origem nos anexos cutâneos. **2.** Termo obsoleto para designar um carcinoma da pele derivado de células escamosas, basais ou anexiais. [epithelium + G. -*ōma*, tumor]
  e. adenoi′des cys′ticum, e. adenóide cístico. SIN trichoepithelioma.
  basal cell e., e. de células basais, e. basocelular. SIN basal cell carcinoma.
  Borst-Jadassohn type intraepidermal e., e. intra-epidérmico de Borst-Jadassohn; lesões pré-cancerosas clinicamente sugestivas de ceratose actínica ou seborreica, com nichos de queratinócitos imaturos ou anormais na epiderme.
  e. cunicula′tum, e. cuniculado; carcinoma verrucoso encontrado raramente na região plantar, formando uma massa verrucosa de crescimento lento que pode invadir profundamente, mas que raramente metastatiza.
  Malherbe calcifying e., e. calcificante de Malherbe. SIN pilomatrixoma.
  malignant ciliary e., e. ciliar maligno; hiperplasia maligna do epitélio ciliar com envolvimento freqüente da camada pigmentada. SIN adult medulloepithelioma.
  multiple self-healing squamous e. [MIM*132800], e. escamoso autocicatrizante múltiplo; múltiplos tumores cutâneos, mais freqüentes na cabeça, cada um semelhante a um carcinoma escamoso bem diferenciado ou ceratoacantoma; tumores individuais resolvem-se espontaneamente após vários meses, deixando cicatrizes deprimidas profundas, com bordas crenadas irregulares, geralmente sendo substituídos por outros novos tumores; herança autossômica dominante.
  sebaceous e., e. sebáceo; tumor benigno do epitélio glandular sebáceo no qual predominam células germinativas ou basalóides pequenas.

ep·i·the·li·om·a·tous (ep-i-thē-lē-ō′mă-tŭs). Epiteliomatoso; relativo ao epitelioma.

ep·i·the·li·op·a·thy (ep′i-thē-lē-op′ă-thē). Epiteliopatia; doença que envolve o epitélio. [epithelium + G. *pathos*, que sofre]
  acute multifocal placoid pigment e., e. pigmentar placóide multifocal aguda; doença aguda que se manifesta por rápida perda da visão, e lesões placóides, multifocais, de cor creme, do epitélio pigmentar da retina (retinal pigment *epithelium*); resolve com restauração da visão.

ep·i·the·li·o·sis (ep-i-thē-lē-ō′sis). Epiteliose; proliferação de células epiteliais, como se observa nos ductos mamários na doença fibrocística.

ep·i·the·li·o·tro·pic (ep-ē-thē′lē-ō-trō′pik). Epiteliotrópico; que possui afinidade pelo epitélio.

ep·i·the·li·um, pl. **ep·i·the·lia** (ep-i-thē′lē-ŭm, -ă) [TA]. Epitélio; a camada avascular puramente celular que cobre todas as superfícies livres, cutâneas, mucosas e serosas, incluindo as glândulas e outras estruturas delas derivadas. [G. *epi*, sobre, + *thēlē*, mamilo, termo aplicado originalmente à pele fina que cobre os mamilos e à camada papilar da borda dos lábios]
  anterior e. of cornea, e. anterior da córnea; o e. escamoso estratificado que cobre a superfície externa da córnea; é liso, geralmente consiste em cinco camadas de células e contém muitas terminações nervosas livres. SIN e. anterius corneae.
  e. ante′rius cor′neae, e. anterior da córnea. SIN anterior e. of cornea.
  Barrett e., e. de Barrett; e. esofágico colunar observado na síndrome de Barrett (Barrett *syndrome*).
  ciliated e., e. ciliado; qualquer e. que possui cílios móveis na superfície livre.
  columnar e., e. colunar; e. formado de uma única camada de células prismáticas cuja altura é maior que a largura. SIN cylindrical e.
  crevicular e., e. crevicular; o e. escamoso estratificado que reveste a face interna da parede de tecidos moles do sulco gengival. SIN sulcular e.
  cuboidal e., e. cubóide; e. simples com células que parecem cubos em um corte vertical, mas são poliédricas à observação superficial.
  cylindrical e., e. cilíndrico. SIN columnar e.
  e. duc′tus semicircula′ris, e. do ducto semicircular. SIN e. of semicircular duct.
  enamel e., e. do esmalte; as várias camadas do órgão do esmalte que permanecem na superfície do esmalte após concluída a sua formação. SIN reduced enamel e.
  external dental e., external enamel e., e. dental externo, e. do esmalte externo; as células cubóides da camada externa do órgão odontogênico de um dente em desenvolvimento.
  germinal e., e. germinativo; uma camada cubóide de e. peritoneal que cobre as gônadas, antes considerado a origem das células germinativas.
  gingival e., e. gengival; e. escamoso estratificado que sofre algum grau de queratinização e cobre a gengiva livre e fixa.

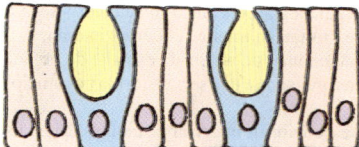
epitélio colunar do intestino

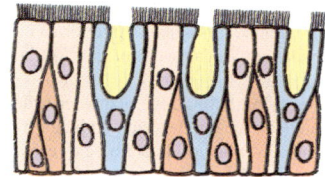
epitélio colunar ciliado pseudo-estratificado

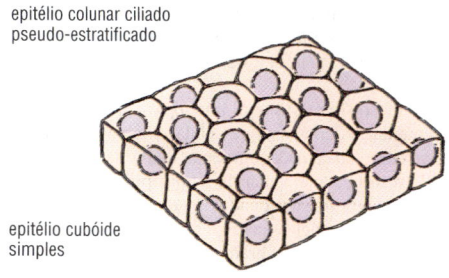
epitélio cubóide simples

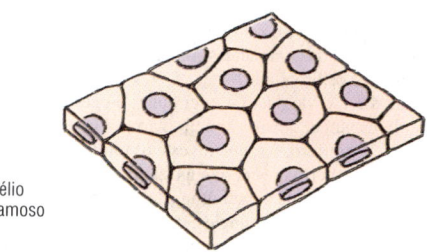
epitélio escamoso

tipos de epitélio

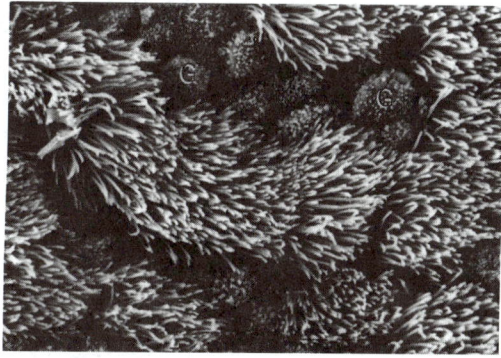

epitélio ciliado: micrografia eletrônica de varredura da superfície luminal de um brônquio; as células não-ciliadas são as células caliciformes (G); os cílios das muitas células ciliadas ocupam o restante da micrografia

glandular e., e. glandular; e. composto de células secretoras.
inner dental e., inner enamel e., e. dental interno; e. do esmalte interno; a camada epitelial colunar de matriz do esmalte do órgão odontogênico de um dente em desenvolvimento, que se transforma nos ameloblastos produtores de esmalte.
junctional e., e. juncional; um colar de células epiteliais fixadas à superfície do dente e ao tecido conjuntivo subepitelial encontrado na base do sulco gengival. SIN epithelial attachment of Gottlieb, epithelial attachment.
laminated e., e. estratificado. SIN stratified e.
e. of lens, e. da lente do olho; a camada de células cubóides situadas sobre a superfície anterior da lente cristalina no interior da cápsula da lente do olho. No equador, as células se alongam e dão origem às fibras da lente. SIN e. lentis.
e. lentis, e. da lente. SIN e. of lens.
mesenchymal e., e. mesenquimal; o e. plano derivado das células mesenquimais que reveste alguns espaços de tecido conjuntivo como a câmara anterior do olho, os espaços perilinfáticos da orelha e os espaços subdural e subaracnóide.
muscle e., e. muscular. SIN myoepithelium.
olfactory e., e. olfatório; um e. do tipo pseudo-estratificado que contém células olfatórias, receptoras, nervosas, cujos axônios se estendem até o bulbo olfatório do encéfalo.
pavement e., e. escamoso simples. SIN simple squamous e.
pigment e., e. pigmentar; e. composto de células contendo grânulos de pigmento ou melanina, como na camada pigmentar da retina ou da íris.
pigment e. of optic retina, e. pigmentar da retina óptica. VER retina.
pseudostratified e., e. pseudo-estratificado; um e. que, ao exame superficial, parece estratificado porque os núcleos celulares estão em diferentes níveis, mas no qual todas as células tocam a membrana basal, sendo, portanto, classificado como um epitélio simples.
reduced enamel e., e. do esmalte. SIN enamel e.
respiratory e., e. respiratório; o epitélio ciliado pseudo-estratificado que reveste a porção condutora das vias aéreas, incluindo parte da cavidade nasal e da laringe, a traquéia e os brônquios.
e. of semicircular duct, e. do ducto semicircular; o e. escamoso simples dos ductos semicirculares. SIN e. ductus semicirculares.
seminiferous e., e. seminífero; o e. que reveste os túbulos contorcidos do testículo onde ocorrem a espermatogênese e a espermiogênese.
simple e., e. simples; um e. que possui uma camada de células.
simple squamous e., e. escamoso simples; e. composto de uma única camada de células achatadas, semelhantes a escamas, como o mesotélio, o endotélio e o encontrado nos alvéolos pulmonares. SIN pavement e.
stratified e., e. estratificado; um tipo de e. composto de uma série de camadas, cujas células variam em tamanho e formato. É denominado mais especificamente de acordo com o tipo de células na superfície, p. ex., e. escamoso estratificado, e. colunar estratificado, e. colunar ciliado estratificado. SIN laminated e.
stratified ciliated columnar e., e. colunar ciliado estratificado; um e. que consiste em várias camadas de células, com as células mais profundas sendo poliédricas e as células superficiais sendo colunares com cílios móveis, como o que reveste o esôfago fetal.
stratified squamous e., e. escamoso estratificado; um e. que consiste em várias camadas de queratina contendo células nas quais as células superficiais são achatadas e semelhantes a escamas e as células mais profundas são poliédricas. Os filamentos de queratina tornam-se progressivamente mais abundantes em direção à superfície, podendo, nas superfícies secas do corpo, consistir em uma camada de corneócitos mortos.
sulcular e., e. sulcular. SIN crevicular e.
surface e., e. superficial; (1) uma camada de células epiteliais celômicas que recobre as cristas gonádicas; (2) o revestimento mesotelial do ovário definitivo.
transitional e., e. de transição; um epitélio pseudo-estratificado muito distensível, com grandes células superficiais poliplóides, que são cubóides no estado relaxado, mas largas e escamosas no estado distendido; encontrado no rim, no ureter e na bexiga.
ep·i·the·li·za·tion (ep-i-thē-li-zā'shun). Epitelização. SIN epithelialization.
ep·i·them (ep'i-them). Epitema; uma aplicação externa, como um cataplasma, mas não um emplastro ou linimento. [G. *epithēma*, cobertura]
ep·i·thet (ep'i-thet). Epíteto; termo ou nome que qualifica. [G. *epithetos*, adicionado, de epi- + *tithēmi*, colocar]
specific e., e. específico; em bacteriologia, a segunda parte do nome de uma espécie; não é, por si só, um nome; o nome de uma espécie bacteriana consiste em duas partes: o nome genérico e o epíteto específico.
shared e., e. compartilhado. SIN susceptibility cassette.
ep·i·tox·oid (ep-i-tok'soyd). Epitoxóide; um toxóide que tem menos afinidade por antitoxina específica do que pela toxina.
ep·i·trich·i·al (ep-i-trik'ē-ăl). Epitriquial; relativo ao epitríquio.

ep·i·trich·i·um (ep-i-trik'ē-ŭm). Epitríquio. SIN periderm. VER dome *cell*. [epi- + G. *trichion*, dim. de *thrix* (*trich*-), pêlo]
ep·i·troch·lea (ep-i-trok'lē-ă). Epitróclea. SIN medial *epicondyle* of humerus. [epi- + L. *trochlea*, polia, bloco, contr. do G. *trochilia*]
ep·i·troch·le·ar (ep-i-trok'lē-ar). Epitroclear; relativo à epitróclea.
ep·i·tu·ber·cu·lo·sis (ep'i-too-ber-kū-lō'sis). Epituberculose; a ocorrência de tumefação de linfonodos ou infiltração pulmonar em uma área próxima de um foco de tuberculose pulmonar ou de glândulas brônquicas aumentadas.
ep·i·tym·pan·ic (ep-i-tim-pan'ik). Epitimpânico; acima, ou na parte superior, da cavidade ou membrana timpânica.
ep·i·tym·pa·num (ep'i-tim'pa-num). Epitímpano. SIN epitympanic *recess*.
ep·i·typh·li·tis (ep'ī-tif-lī'tis). Epitiflite; inflamação dos tecidos ao redor ou próximo do ceco. VER appendicitis. [epi- + G. *typhlon*, ceco, + -itis, inflamação]
ep·i·zo·ic (ep-i-zō'ik). Epizóico; que vive como um parasita na superfície cutânea.
ep·i·zo·ol·o·gy (ep'i-zō-ol'ō-jē). Epizoologia. SIN epizootiology. [epi- + G. *zōon*, animal, + *logos*, estudo]
ep·i·zo·on, pl. **ep·i·zoa** (ep-i-zō'on, -zō'ă). Epizoário; um parasita animal que vive na superfície do corpo. [epi- + G. *zōon*, animal]
ep·i·zo·ot·ic (ep'i-zō-ot'ik). Epizoótico. **1.** Designa um padrão temporal de ocorrência de doença em uma população animal na qual a doença ocorre com uma freqüência claramente superior à freqüência esperada nessa população durante determinado período. **2.** Uma epidemia de doença em uma população animal. [epi- + G. *zōon*, animal]
ep·i·zo·ot·i·ol·o·gy (ep'i-zō-ot'ē-ol'ō-jē). Epizootiologia; epidemiologia de doenças em populações de animais. SIN epizoology. [epi- + G. *zōon*, animal, + *logos*, estudo]
éplu·chage (ā-ploo-shazh'). Desbridamento; termo raramente usado para a remoção de todo o tecido contaminado em feridas infectadas. [F. limpeza]
EPN Um organofosforado - contendo enxofre-anticolinesterase usado como inseticida e acaricida.
EPO Abreviatura de *exclusive provider organization* (*organização provedora de serviços exclusiva*).
epo·e·tin al·fa (ē-pō'ē-tin). Epoetina alfa; eritropoetina, um potente estimulante da síntese de hemácias. Freqüentemente usada em pacientes com anemia e naqueles submetidos a transplantes renais e a tratamento com AZT.
ep·o·nych·ia (ep-ō-nik'ē-ă). Eponíquia; infecção envolvendo a prega ungueal proximal.
ep·o·nych·i·um (ep-ō-nik'ē-ŭm) [TA]. Eponíquio. **1.** A camada de epiderme fina, condensada, rica em eleidina, que precede e, inicialmente, cobre a lâmina ungueal no embrião. Normalmente degenera no oitavo mês, exceto na base ungueal, onde permanece como a cutícula da unha. **2** [NA]. A camada córnea da epiderme superposta e em contato direto com a raiz da unha, proximalmente, ou com as laterais da lâmina ungueal, lateralmente, formando a superfície inferior da parede ungueal ou pregas ungueais. SIN hidden nail skin, perionychium. **3.** A pele fina aderida à unha em sua porção proximal. SIN epionychium. [G. *epi*, sobre, + *onyx* (*onych*-), unha]
ep·o·nym (ep'ō-nim). Epônimo; o nome de uma doença, estrutura, operação ou procedimento, geralmente derivado do nome da pessoa que a descobriu ou descreveu primeiro. [G. *epōnymos*, denominado segundo]
ep·o·nym·ic (ep-ō-nim'ik). **1.** Eponímico; relativo a um epônimo. **2.** Um epônimo.
ep·o·oph·o·ron (ep'ō-of'ō-ron). Epoóforo; uma coleção de túbulos rudimentares na mesossalpinge entre o ovário e a tuba uterina; composto de duas porções, o ducto longitudinal do epoóforo e os dúctulos transversos do epoóforo, são os vestígios de túbulos da porção média do mesonefro e o homólogo dos dúctulos aberrantes e do ducto proximal do epidídimo no homem. SIN corpus pampiniforme, organ of Rosenmüller, pampiniform body. [epi- + G. *ōophoros*, condutor de ovos]
epo·prost·en·ol, epo·prost·en·ol so·di·um (e-pō-prost'en-ol). Epoprostenol, epoprostenol sódico. SIN prostacyclin.
epor·nit·ic (ep'or-nit'ik). Epornítico; referente a um surto de doença em uma população de aves. [epi- + G. *ornithos*, ave + -ic]
ep·ox·y (ē-pok'sē). Epóxi; termo químico que descreve um átomo de oxigênio ligado a dois átomos de carbono ligados

$$-\mathrm{CH}-\mathrm{CH}-$$
$$\diagdown \mathrm{O} \diagup$$

Geralmente, qualquer éter cíclico, mas freqüentemente é aplicado a um anel de três membros; especificamente, um anel de três membros é um oxirano, um anel de quatro membros é um oxetano, um anel de cinco membros é um oxolano e um anel de seis membros é um oxano; os oxiranos são comumente produzidos a partir de perácidos que agem sobre alquenos. Os epóxis são importantes intermediários químicos e a base das resinas epóxi (polímeros) formadas a partir de monômeros epóxi.
2,3-epox·y·squa·lene (ē-pok'sē-skwā'lēn). 2,3-epoxiesqualeno; um derivado oxirano do esqualeno; um precursor de todos os esteróides.

Epple, August, colaborador de Leonard S. Fosdick. VER Fosdick-Hansen-E. *test.*

EPR Abreviatura de electron paramagnetic *resonance* (ressonância paramagnética eletrônica).

EPS Abreviatura de exophthalmos-producing *substance* (substância produtora de exoftalmia).

ep·si·lon (ep′si-lon). Épsilon; quinta letra do alfabeto grego, ε.

EPSP Abreviatura de excitatory postsynaptic *potential* (potencial pós-sináptico excitatório).

Epstein, Alois, pediatra alemão, 1849–1918. VER E. *disease, pearls,* em *pearl, sign, symptom.*

Epstein, Michael Anthony, virologista inglês, *1921. VER E.-Barr *virus.*

epu·lis (ep - ū′lis). Epúlide; uma massa gengival exofítica inespecífica. [G. *epoulis,* abscesso da gengiva]
  congenital e. of newborn, e. congênita do recém-nascido; tumor nodular benigno congênito da crista alveolar, de histogênese desconhecida; histologicamente, é composto de grandes células com um citoplasma granular semelhante ao de um tumor de células granulares (mioblastoma).
  e. fissura'tum, e. fissurada. SIN inflammatory fibrous *hyperplasia.*
  giant cell e., e. de células gigantes. SIN giant cell *granuloma.*
  e. gravida'rum, e. gravídica; granuloma piogênico gengival que se desenvolve durante a gravidez.
  pigmented e., e. pigmentada. SIN melanotic neuroectodermal *tumor* of infancy.

ep·u·loid (ep′u - loyd). Epulóide; massa gengival semelhante a uma epúlide.

Eq, eq Abreviatura de equivalent.

equa·tion (ē - kwā′zhŭn). Equação; uma afirmação que expressa a qualidade de duas coisas, geralmente com o uso de símbolos matemáticos ou químicos. [L. *aequare,* tornar igual]
  alveolar gas e., e. de gás alveolar; a equação que define a relação em estado de equilíbrio dinâmico entre a pressão de oxigênio alveolar e a pressão barométrica, composição do gás inspirado, pressão alveolar de dióxido de carbono e razão de troca respiratória; a equação é usada em várias formas, dependendo de quais suposições de simplificação são aceitáveis para diferentes aplicações.
  Arrhenius e., e. de Arrhenius; uma equação que relaciona a velocidade da reação química (k) à temperatura absoluta (T) pela equação: $d(\ln k)/dT) = \Delta E_a/RT^2$, onde E_a é a energia de ativação e R é a constante de gás universal.
  Bohr e., e. de Bohr; uma equação para calcular o espaço morto respiratório considerando-se que o gás expirado dos pulmões é uma mistura de gás do espaço morto e gás alveolar, isto é, o volume do espaço morto dividido pelo volume corrente é igual à diferença entre a composição dos gases alveolar e expirado misto, dividida pela diferença entre a composição dos gases alveolar e inspirado; a composição do gás pode ser expressa em quaisquer unidades consistentes de concentração ou pressão parcial de oxigênio ou dióxido de carbono.
  chemical e., e. química; uma equação na qual, em um lado, estão os reagentes e, no outro, os produtos de uma reação química; as duas metades podem ser separadas por um sinal de igual ou por setas.
  constant field e., e. de campo constante. SIN Goldman e.
  Einthoven e., e. de Einthoven. SIN Einthoven *law.*
  Gay-Lussac e., e. de Gay-Lussac; a equação química geral para fermentação alcoólica; $C_6H_{12}O_6 = 2CO_2 + 2CH_3CH_2OH$.
  Gibbs-Helmholtz e., e. de Gibbs-Helmholtz; (1) uma equação que expressa a relação em uma célula galvânica entre a energia química transformada e a força eletromotriz máxima que pode ser obtida. (2) $\Delta G = \Delta H - T[\partial \Delta G/\partial T]_P$, onde ΔG é a alteração na energia livre de Gibbs, ΔH é a alteração na entalpia, T é a temperatura absoluta e P é a pressão.
  Goldman e., e. de Goldman; uma equação derivada para prever potenciais de membrana em termos da permeabilidade da membrana aos íons e suas concentrações de cada lado. SIN constant field e., Goldman-Hodgkin-Katz e., GHK e.
  Goldman-Hodgkin-Katz e., GHK e., e. de Goldman-Hodgkin-Katz, e. GHK. SIN Goldman e.
  Henderson-Hasselbalch e., e. de Henderson-Hasselbalch; uma fórmula que relaciona o valor do pH de uma solução ao valor do pK_a do ácido na solução e a razão das concentrações do ácido e da base conjugada: $pH = pK_a + \log([A^-]/[HA])$, onde $[A^-]$ é a concentração da base conjugada e $[HA]$ é a concentração do ácido protonado. Para o sistema tampão bicarbonato no sangue, $pH = pK' + \log\text{-}([HCO_3^-]/[CO_2])$. O valor de pK' para o plasma sanguíneo é 6,10 e inclui a primeira constante de dissociação de H_2CO_3, a relação entre $[H_2CO_3]$ e $[CO_2]$ e outras correções. A pressão parcial de CO_2 multiplicada por sua solubilidade no plasma a 38°C (0,0301 mM/mm Hg) é comumente substituída por $[CO_2]$; p. ex., quando a concentração plasmática de bicarbonato é de 24 mEq/L e a P_{CO_2} é de 40 mm Hg, o valor do pH é de $6,10 + \log(24/0,0301 \times 40) = 7,40$.
  Henri-Michaelis-Menten e., e. de Henri-Michaelis-Menten. SIN Michaelis-Menten e.
  Hill e., e. de Hill; a equação $y(1-y) = [S]^n/K_d$, onde y é o grau fracional de saturação, $[S]$ é a concentração de ligante, n é o coeficiente de Hill e K_d é a constante de dissociação para o ligante. O coeficiente de Hill é uma medida da cooperatividade da proteína; quanto maior o valor, maior é a cooperatividade. Esse coeficiente não pode ser maior que o número de locais de ligação. Para a curva de ligação da hemoglobina ao oxigênio, é usada uma constante de associação, K_a, e a equação se torna $y/(1-y) = K_a[S]^n$. Para hemoglobina humana, $n = 2,5$. Cf. Hill *plot.*
  Hüfner e., e. de Hüfner; uma equação que expressa a relação entre a dissociação de mioglobina e a pressão parcial de oxigênio: $([MBO_2]/[Mb]) = (K \times pO_2)$.
  Lineweaver-Burk e., e. de Lineweaver-Burk; um rearranjo da equação de Michaelis-Menten, $1/v = 1/V_{máx} + (K_m/V_{máx})(1/[S])$, onde v é a velocidade da reação, $V_{máx}$ é a velocidade máxima, K_m é a constante de Michaelis e $[S]$ é a concentração de substrato. Cf. double-reciprocal *plot.*
  Michaelis-Menten e., e. de Michaelis-Menten; uma equação de velocidade inicial para uma reação com substrato único, não-cooperativa, catalisada por enzima, relacionando a velocidade inicial à concentração inicial de substrato; $v = V_{máx}[S]/(K_m + [S])$, onde v é a velocidade inicial da reação, $V_{máx}$ é a velocidade máxima, $[S]$ é a concentração inicial de substrato e K_m é a constante de Michaelis. Equações semelhantes podem ser derivadas para condições nas quais o produto está presente e para enzimas de múltiplos substratos. SIN Henri-Michaelis-Menten e.
  Nernst e., e. de Nernst; a equação que relaciona o potencial de equilíbrio dos eletrodos às concentrações iônicas; a equação que relaciona o potencial elétrico e o gradiente de concentração de um íon através de uma membrana permeável em equilíbrio: $E = [RT/nF][\ln(C_1/C_2)]$, onde E = potencial, R = constante de gás absoluto, T = temperatura absoluta, n = valência, F = o Faraday, $\ln$ = o logaritmo natural, e C_1 e C_2 são as concentrações iônicas nos dois lados; em soluções não-ideais, a concentração deve ser substituída pela atividade. VER TAMBÉM activity (2).
  personal e., e. pessoal; um pequeno erro de julgamento, resposta perceptual ou ação peculiar ao indivíduo e tão constante que geralmente é possível levá-la em conta ao aceitar as declarações ou conclusões da pessoa, assim chegando à exatidão aproximada; observada em pessoas cujo trabalho envolve leituras de eventos no tempo, como navegadores e controladores de tráfego aéreo.
  rate e., e. de velocidade; expressão matemática para uma reação química, radioquímica ou catalisada por enzima.
  Rayleigh e., e. de Rayleigh; uma razão entre vermelho e verde necessária a cada observador para se igualar ao amarelo espectral. SIN Rayleigh test.
  Svedberg e., e. de Svedberg. VER sedimentation *constant.*
  van't Hoff e., e. de van't Hoff; (1) equação para pressão osmótica de soluções diluídas. VER van't Hoff *law*; (2) para qualquer reação, $d(\ln K_{eq})/d(1/T)$ é igual a $-\Delta H/R$, onde K_{eq} é a constante de equilíbrio, T a temperatura absoluta, R a constante de gás universal e ΔH a alteração na entalpia; assim, a representação de $\ln K_{eq}$ vs. $1/T$ permite a determinação de ΔH.

equa·tor (ē - kwā′ter) [TA]. Equador; uma linha que circunda um corpo globular, eqüidistante em todos os pontos dos dois pólos; a periferia de um plano que corta uma esfera no ponto médio de, e formando ângulos retos com, seu eixo. [L. mediev. *aequator,* do L. *aequo,* tornar igual]
  e. bul'bi oc'uli [TA], e. do bulbo do olho. SIN e. of eyeball.
  e. of eyeball [TA], e. do bulbo do olho; uma linha imaginária que circunda o bulbo do olho eqüidistante dos pólos anterior e posterior. SIN e. bulbi oculi [TA].
  e. of lens [TA], e. da lente do olho; a periferia da lente do olho situada entre as duas camadas da zônula ciliar. SIN e. lentis [TA].
  e. len'tis [TA], e. da lente do olho. SIN e. of lens.

equa·to·ri·al (ē - kwā - tō′rē - al). Equatorial; situado, como o equador da Terra, eqüidistante de cada extremidade.

equi·ax·i·al (ē′kwi - ak′sē - ăl). Equiaxial; que possui eixos de comprimentos iguais.

equi·ca·lor·ic (ē′kwi - kă - lōr′ik). Equicalórico; igual em valor calórico. VER TAMBÉM isodynamic. [L. *aequus,* igual, + *calor,* calor]

eq·ui·len·in (ek-wi-len′in). Equilenina; um esteróide fracamente estrogênico isolado da urina de éguas prenhes. [L. *equa,* égua]

equil·i·bra·tion (ē′kwi - li - brā′shŭn, - i -). Equilibração, compensação. 1. O ato de manter um equilíbrio. 2. O ato de expor um líquido, p. ex., sangue ou plasma, a um gás em determinada pressão parcial até que as pressões parciais do gás dentro e fora do líquido sejam iguais. 3. Em odontologia, modificação das formas oclusais dos dentes por trituração, com o objetivo de igualar a força de oclusão, produzindo contatos oclusais simultâneos, ou harmonizar as relações das cúspides. 4. Em cromatografia, a saturação da fase estacionária com o vapor do solvente de eluição a ser usado.

equi·lib·ri·um (ē - kwi - lib′rē - ŭm). Equilíbrio. 1. A condição de estar uniformemente balanceado; um estado de repouso entre duas ou mais forças antagonistas que se neutralizam com precisão. 2. Em química, um estado de repouso aparente criado por duas reações que prosseguem em direções opostas em igual velocidade; em equações químicas, algumas vezes é indicado por duas setas opostas (↔) em vez do sinal de igual. SIN dynamic e. VER TAMBÉM equilibrium *constant.* [L. *aequilibrium,* uma posição horizontal, de *aequus,* igual, + *libra,* um equilíbrio]
  acid-base e., e. ácido-básico. SIN acid-base *balance.*

Donnan e., e. de Donnan; quando uma membrana semipermeável ou seu equivalente (p. ex., um permutador de íons sódio) separa uma substância não-difusível, como proteína, de substâncias difusíveis, os ânions e cátions difusíveis são distribuídos nos dois lados da membrana de forma que 1) os produtos de suas concentrações sejam iguais, e 2) a soma dos ânions difusíveis e não-difusíveis de cada lado da membrana seja igual à soma das concentrações de cátions difusíveis e não-difusíveis; a distribuição desigual de íons difusíveis assim produzida cria uma diferença potencial através da membrana (potencial de membrana). SIN Gibbs-Donnan e.
dynamic e., e. dinâmica. SIN equilibrium (2).
genetic e., e. genético; a condição de um sistema genético dinâmico no qual as várias taxas de modificação entre todos os possíveis pares de partes são tais que a composição é invariável.
Gibbs-Donnan e., e. de Gibbs-Donnan. SIN Donnan e.
Hardy-Weinberg e., e. de Hardy-Weinberg; aquele estado no qual a estrutura genética da população se adapta à previsão da lei de Hardy-Weinberg; não é uma equação estável, embora possa ser aproximada para uma grande população em cruzamento. SIN random mating e.
homeostatic e., e. homeostático. VER homeostasis.
nitrogenous e., e. nitrogenado; uma condição na qual a quantidade de nitrogênio excretada do corpo é igual àquela ingerida com o alimento; equilíbrio nutritivo no que se refere à proteína.
nutritive e., e. nutritivo; condição na qual há um perfeito equilíbrio entre a ingestão e a excreção de material nutritivo, de forma que não haja ganho nem perda de peso. SIN physiologic e.
physiologic e., e. fisiológico. SIN nutritive e.
radioactive e., e. radioativo; uma situação (não um equilíbrio verdadeiro) na qual um átomo específico está sendo produzido pela decomposição radioativa de um precursor enquanto este está se decompondo; as duas decomposições se equivalem de tal forma que, após um período, a razão de radioatividade entre o produto e o precursor é constante com o tempo.
random mating e., e. de cruzamento aleatório. SIN Hardy-Weinberg e.
secular e., e. secular; tipo de equilíbrio radioativo no qual a meia-vida do radioisótopo precursor (original) é bem maior que a do produto (descendente) a ponto a radioatividade do produto tornar-se igual à do precursor com o tempo.
stable e., e. estável; equilíbrio no qual, após cada pequena perturbação, tende a haver restauração do estado original.
transient e., e. transitório; tipo de equilíbrio radioativo no qual a meia-vida do radioisótopo original é maior que a do produto de forma que a razão entre as atividades do precursor e do produto se torna constante à medida que elas diminuem com o tempo.
unstable e., e. instável; equilíbrio no qual a resposta a uma pequena perturbação tenderá a aumentar a perturbação (p. ex., um processo de *feedback* registrado de ordem zero).
eq·ui·lin (ek′wi-lin). Equilina; um esteróide estrogênico presente na urina de éguas grávidas. [L. *equa*, égua]
equi·mo·lar (ē-kwi-mō′ler). Equimolar; que contém um número igual de moles ou que possui a mesma molaridade, como em duas ou mais substâncias.
equi·mo·lec·u·lar (ē′kwi-mō-lek′u-ler). Equimolecular; que contém um número igual de moléculas ou entidades moleculares, como em duas ou mais soluções.
e·quine (ē′kwīn). Eqüino; relativo a, derivado de, ou semelhante ao cavalo, mula, asno ou outros membros do gênero *Equus*. [L. *equinus*, de *equus*, cavalo]
equi·no·val·gus (ē-kwī-nō-val′gus, ek′wi-nō-). Equinovalgo. SIN talipes equinovalgus.
equi·no·var·us (ē-kwī-nō-vā′rus, ek′wi-nō-). Eqüinovaro. SIN talipes equinovarus.
equi·tox·ic (ē-kwi-tok′sik). Equitóxico; de toxicidade equivalente.
equiv·a·lence, equiv·a·len·cy (ē-kwiv′ă-lens, -len-sē). Equivalência. **1.** A propriedade de um elemento ou radical de se combinar com ou deslocar, em proporção definida e fixa, outro elemento ou radical em um composto. **2.** O ponto em um teste de precipitina no qual o anticorpo e o antígeno são apresentados em proporções ideais. [L. *aequus*, igual, + *valentia*, valência]
equiv·a·lent (Eq, eq) (ē-kwiv′ă-lent). Equivalente. **1.** Igual em qualquer aspecto. **2.** Aquilo que é igual em tamanho, peso, força ou em qualquer outra qualidade a alguma outra coisa. **3.** Que possui a capacidade de equilibrar ou neutralizar um ao outro. **4.** Que possui valências iguais. **5.** SIN gram e. [ver equivalence]
combustion e., e. de combustão; o valor calórico de um grama de carboidrato ou gordura oxidado fora do corpo.
gold e., e. de ouro; uma unidade de força dos colóides protetores; o número de miligramas de colóide protetor apenas suficiente para evitar a precipitação de 10 ml de uma solução de ouro a 0,0053–0,0058% pela ação de 1 ml de uma solução de cloreto de sódio a 10%. SIN gold number.
gram e., e. -grama; **(1)** o peso em gramas de um elemento que se combina a ou substitui 1 g de hidrogênio; **(2)** o peso atômico ou molecular em gramas de um átomo ou grupo de átomos envolvidos em uma reação química dividido pelo número de elétrons doados, captados ou compartilhados pelo átomo ou grupo de átomos no decorrer dessa reação; **(3)** o peso de uma substância contida em 1 L de uma solução 1 N; uma variante de (1). SIN combining weight, equivalent weight, equivalent (5).
Joule e. (J), e. de Joule; o equivalente dinâmico do calor; o trabalho convertido em calor que aumentará a temperatura de 1 libra de água em 1°F é 778 pé-libras; em unidades métricas, 1 caloria, que eleva a temperatura de 1 g de água em 1°C, igual a 4,184 × 10^7 dina-centímetros, ou 4,184 J.
lethal e., e. letal; **(1)** a combinação de efeitos seletivos que possuem, em média, o mesmo impacto sobre a composição dos genes que a morte; p. ex., dois portadores com risco de morte de 50% seriam o equivalente letal de um portador com risco de 100%; **(2)** na população, a genética de equivalente letal de traços recessivos é expressa como o dobro da soma do número esperado de mortes atribuíveis à carga genética; **(3)** expressão usada da carga genética de genes recessivos no estado heterozigoto que, se em estado homozigoto, causaria morte ou um risco de morte. O número esperado de mortes por todos esses genes é expresso no equivalente.
metabolic e. (MET), e. metabólico; o custo de oxigênio do gasto energético medido em repouso em decúbito dorsal (1 MET = 3,5 ml O$_2$ por kg de peso corporal por minuto); múltiplos do MET são usados para estimar o custo de oxigênio da atividade, p. ex., 3–5 MET para trabalho leve; mais de 9 MET para trabalho pesado.
nitrogen e., e. de nitrogênio; o teor de nitrogênio da proteína; usado no cálculo da decomposição proteica no corpo a partir do nitrogênio excretado na urina, com 1 de nitrogênio sendo considerado como originado em 6,25 g de proteína catabolizada.
starch e., e. do amido; o oxigênio consumido na combustão de determinado peso de gordura em comparação com aquele consumido na combustão de igual peso de amido; o número é aproximadamente 2,38, aquele para o amido sendo considerado como 1.
toxic e., e. tóxico; a quantidade de toxina ou outro veneno por quilograma de peso corporal necessária para matar um animal.
ER Abreviatura de endoplasmic *reticulum* (retículo endoplasmático).
Er Símbolo de erbium (érbio).
erad·i·ca·tion. Erradicação; referindo a doença, é a interrupção de toda transmissão de infecção por extermínio do agente infeccioso através de vigilância e controle; foi conquistada a erradicação global da varíola, a erradicação regional da malária e, talvez, em alguns lugares, a do sarampo.
Eranko, Eino, anatomista finlandês, 1924–1984. VER E. fluorescence *stain*.
Erb, Wilhelm H., neurologista alemão, 1840–1921. VER E. *disease, palsy, paralysis;* E.-Charcot *disease;* Duchenne-E. *paralysis*.
ERBF Abreviatura de effective renal blood *flow* (fluxo sanguíneo renal efetivo).
er·bi·um (Er) (er′bē-ŭm). Érbio; um elemento pertencente à família das terras-raras (lantanídeos), de número atômico 68, peso atômico 167,26. [de Ytterby, um povoado da Suécia]
er·cal·cid·i·ol (er-kal-sid′ē-ol). Ercalcidiol. SIN 25-hydroxyergocalciferol.
er·cal·ci·ol (er-kal′sē-ol). Ercalciol. SIN ergocalciferol.
er·cal·cit·ri·ol (er-kal-sit′rē-ol). Ercalcitriol. SIN 1,25-diidroxiergocalciferol.
ERCP Abreviatura de endoscopic retrograde *cholangiopancreatography* (colangiopancreatografia retrógrada endoscópica).
Erdheim, Jakob, médico austríaco, 1874–1937. VER E. *disease, tumor*.
Erdmann, Hugo, químico alemão, 1862–1910. VER E. *reagent*.
erec·tile (ē-rek′til). Erétil; capaz de ereção.
erec·tion (ē-rek′shŭn). Ereção; a condição do tecido erétil quando cheio de sangue, que então se torna rígido e inflexível; designa particularmente esse estado do pênis. [L. *erectio*, de *erigo*, pp. *erectus*, erguer]
erec·tor (ērek′tor, -tōr). Eretor. **1.** Que eleva ou produz ereção. **2.** Designa especificamente determinados músculos que possuem essa ação. SIN arrector. [L. mod.]
er·e·mo·pho·bia (er′ē-mō-fō′bē-ă). Eremofobia; temor mórbido de locais desertos ou de solidão. [G. *erēmia*, solidão, + *phobos*, medo]
er·eu·tho·pho·bi·a (er′oo-tho-fō′bē-ă). Ereutofobia; temor mórbido de corar. [G. *ereuthos*, corar, + *phobos*, medo]
ERG Abreviatura de electroretinogram (eletrorretinograma).
erg. A unidade de trabalho no sistema CGS; o trabalho realizado por 1 dina atuando sobre 1 cm, 1 g cm^2 s^{-2}; no sistema SI, 1 erg é igual a 10^{-7} J. [G. *ergon*, trabalho]
er·ga·sia (er-gā′zē-ă). Ergasia. **1.** Qualquer forma de atividade, particularmente mental. **2.** O total de funções e reações de um indivíduo. [G. trabalho]
er·ga·si·o·pho·bia (er-gas′ē-ō-fō′bē-ă). Ergasiofobia; aversão ao trabalho de qualquer tipo. [G. *ergasia*, trabalho, + *phobos*, medo]
er·gas·the·nia (er-gas-thē′nē-ă). Ergastenia; termo raramente usado para designar debilidade ou quaisquer sintomas mórbidos devidos a esforço excessivo. [G. *ergasia*, trabalho, + *asthenia*, fraqueza, doença]
er·gas·to·plasm (er-gas′tō-plazm). Ergastoplasma. SIN granular endoplasmic *reticulum*. [G. *ergastēr*, homem de trabalho, + *plasma*, algo formado]
erg·ine (erg′ēn). Ergina. SIN lysergic acid amide.

ergo-. Ergo-; trabalho. [G. *ergon*]

er·go·ba·sine (er-gō-bā′sēn). Ergobasina. SIN ergonovine.

er·go·cal·cif·er·ol (er′gō-kal-sif′er-ol). Ergocalciferol; ergosterol ativado, a vitamina D de origem vegetal; origina-se da irradiação ultravioleta do ergosterol, que é clivado na ligação 9,10 e desenvolve uma ligação dupla entre C-10 e C-19; usado na profilaxia e no tratamento da deficiência de vitamina D. SIN calciferol, ercalciol, viosterol, vitamin D_2.

er·go·cor·nine (er-gō-kōr′nēn). Ergocornina; um alcalóide isolado do esporão do centeio.

er·go·cris·tine (er′gō-kris′tēn). Ergocristina; um alcalóide isolado do esporão do centeio.

er·go·cryp·tine (er-gō-krip′tēn). Ergocriptina; um alcalóide isolado do esporão do centeio.

er·go·dy·nam·o·graph (er′gō-dī-nam′ō-graf). Ergodinamógrafo; instrumento para registrar tanto o grau de força muscular quanto o trabalho realizado pela contração muscular. [ergo- + G. *dynamis*, força, + *graphō*, escrever]

er·go·es·the·si·o·graph (er′gō-es-thē′zē-ō-graf). Ergoestesiógrafo; um aparelho para registrar graficamente a aptidão muscular, conforme mostrado na capacidade de neutralizar resistências variáveis. [ergo- + G. *aisthēsis*, sensação, + *graphō*, registrar]

er·go·gen·ic (er-gō-jen′ik). Ergogênico; que tende a aumentar o trabalho.

er·go·graph (er′gō-graf). Ergógrafo; instrumento para registrar a quantidade de trabalho realizada por contrações musculares, ou a amplitude da contração. [ergo- + G. *graphō*, escrever]

  Mosso e., e. de Mosso; instrumento que consiste em polias, pesos e uma alavanca registradora, usado para obter um registro gráfico da flexão de um dedo, da mão ou do braço.

er·go·graph·ic (er-gō-graf′ik). Ergográfico; relativo ao ergógrafo e ao registro feito por ele.

er·go·lines (er′gō-linz). Ergolinas; uma classe de drogas com proeminentes ações agonistas ou antagonistas sobre os receptores da dopamina. Os agentes pertencentes a esse grupo incluem a bromocriptina, pergolida e lisurida.

er·gom·e·ter (er-gom′e-ter).. Ergômetro. SIN dynamometer. [ergo- + G. *metron*, medida]

er·go·met·rine (er-gō-met′rēn). Ergometrina. SIN ergonovine.

  e. maleate, maleato de e. SIN ergonovine maleate.

er·go·nom·ics (er-gō-nom′iks). Ergonomia; ramo da ecologia que estuda fatores humanos no projeto e na operação de máquinas e do ambiente físico. [ergo- + G. *nomos*, lei]

er·go·no·vine (er-gō-nō′vēn, -vin). Ergonovina; um alcalóide do esporão do centeio; sua hidrólise produz ácido D-lisérgico e L-2-aminopropanol; estimula as contrações uterinas. SIN ergobasine, ergometrine, ergostetrine.

  e. maleate, maleato de e.; potente agente ocitócico; essa ação é mais proeminente, e outras ações do esporão do centeio (vasoconstrição, estimulação do sistema nervoso central, bloqueio adrenérgico, etc.) são menos proeminentes que a dos outros alcalóides do esporão do centeio; efetivo por via oral e parenteral. SIN ergometrine maleate.

er·go·sine (er′gō-sēn, -sin). Ergosina; um alcalóide do esporão do centeio com ações semelhantes às da ergotamina.

er·gos·ter·in (er-gos′ter-in). Ergosterina. SIN ergosterol.

er·gos·ter·ol (er-gos′ter-ol). Ergosterol; a mais importante das pró-vitaminas D_2; a radiação ultravioleta converte o ergosterol em lumisterol, taquisterol e ergocalciferol; principal esterol em leveduras, no esporão do centeio e em fungos. SIN ergosterin.

er·go·stet·rine (er-gō-stet′rēn, -rin). Ergostetrina. SIN ergonovine.

er·got (er′got). Esporão do centeio; o estágio resistente, que resiste ao inverno, do fungo ascomicetoso parasita *Claviceps purpurea*, um patógeno do centeio que transforma sua semente em uma massa compacta, semelhante a um esporão, de pseudotecido fúngico (o esclerócio) contendo cinco ou mais pares opticamente isoméricos de alcalóides. Os isômeros levorrotatórios induzem contrações uterinas, controlam hemorragia e aliviam alguns distúrbios vasculares localizados (enxaqueca). VER TAMBÉM ergotism. SIN rye smut. [Fr. ant. *argot*, esporão do galo]

  corn e., *Ustilago maydis.* SIN *Ustilago maydis.*

er·got·a·mine (er-got′a-mēn). $C_{33}H_{35}N_5O_5$; um alcalóide oriundo do esporão do centeio, usado para alívio da enxaqueca; é um potente estimulante da musculatura lisa, sobretudo dos vasos sanguíneos e do útero, e provoca bloqueio adrenérgico (sobretudo dos receptores α); e. hidrogenada, diidroergotamina, é menos tóxica e tem menos efeitos colaterais. Também disponível como tartarato de e.

er·got·am·i·nine (er-got-am′i-nēn). Ergotaminina, um isômero da ergotamina, mas praticamente inerte.

er·go·thi·o·ne·ine (er′gō-thī-ō-nē′in). Ergotioneína; a betaína de um derivado da histidina contendo enxofre, presente no sangue e em outros tecidos de mamíferos e no esporão do centeio. SIN thiolhistidylbetaine, thioneine.

er·got·ism (er′got-izm). Ergotismo; envenenamento por uma substância tóxica contida no esclerócio do fungo, *Claviceps purpura*, que cresce no centeio; caracterizado por necrose das extremidades (gangrena) devida à contração do leito vascular periférico. VER TAMBÉM ergot *poisoning*. SIN Saint Anthony fire (1).

er·go·tox·ine (er′gō-tok′sēn, -sin). Ergotoxina; uma mistura de alcalóides obtidos do esporão do centeio, que consiste em 1:1:1 de ergocristina, ergocornina e ergocriptina, mais tóxica que outros alcalóides do esporão do centeio naturais e semi-sintéticos; um potente estimulante da musculatura lisa, particularmente dos vasos sanguíneos e do útero, e produz bloqueio adrenérgico (principalmente dos receptores alfa). SIN ecboline.

er·go·tro·pic (er′gō-trop′ik). Ergotrópico; o termo introduzido por W.R. Hess para designar os mecanismos e o estado funcional do sistema nervoso que favorecem a capacidade do organismo de gastar energia, diferente dos mecanismos trofotrópicos que promovem repouso e reconstituição das reservas de energia. Em geral, o equilíbrio entre mecanismos nervosos ergotrópicos e trofotrópicos corresponde, em grande parte, ao equilíbrio entre as subdivisões simpática e parassimpática do sistema nervoso autônomo. [ergo- + G. *tropos*, uma volta]

er·i·o·dic·ty·on (ār′ē-ō-dik′tē-on). Erva-santa; as folhas secas de *Eriodictyon californicum* (família Hydrophyllaceae); o extrato líquido e o xarope foram usados como expectorante e flavorizante para mascarar o sabor de substâncias amargas. SIN mountain balm, yerba santa.

eris·o·phake (e-ris′ō-fāk). Erisofaco; instrumento cirúrgico designado para segurar a lente do olho por sucção na extração da catarata; agora raramente usado. [G. *erysis*, extração, + *phakos*, lentilha]

Erlenmeyer, Emil, químico alemão, 1825–1909. VER E. *flask*, flask *deformity*.

erode (ē-rōd′). Erodir. **1.** Causar, ou ser afetado, por erosão. **2.** Remover por ulceração. [L. *erodo*, corroer]

erog·e·nous (ē-roj′e-nŭs). Erógeno; capaz de produzir excitação sexual quando estimulado. [G. *eros*, amor, + *genos*, nascimento]

eros (ē′ros, ār′os). eros; em psicanálise o princípio vital que representa todos os instintos direcionados para a procriação e a vida. Ver também instinct. Cf. thanatos. [G. *amor*]

erose (ē-rōs). Irregular, desigual; denotando uma borda ou margem que é irregularmente denteada ou serrilhada, como se fosse roída ou mordida; termo usado sobretudo em referência a colônias bacterianas. [L. *erodo*, pp. *erosus*, arrancar]

ero·sion (ē-rō′zhŭn). Erosão. **1.** Um desgaste ou um estado de estar desgastado, como por atrito ou pressão. Cf. corrosion. **2.** Uma úlcera superficial, no estômago e no intestino, uma úlcera limitada à mucosa, sem penetração da muscular da mucosa. **3.** O desgaste de um dente por ação química ou por abrasivo; quando a causa é desconhecida, é denominada erosão idiopática. SIN odontolysis. [L. *erosio*, de *erodo*, corroer]

  Dieulafoy e., e. de Dieulafoy; gastroenterite ulcerativa aguda que complica a pneumonia, possivelmente causada por superprodução de hormônios esteróides supra-renais.

  recurrent corneal e., e. recorrente da córnea; vesiculação repetida seguida por esfoliação do epitélio da córnea.

ero·sive (ē-rō-siv). Erosivo. **1.** Que tem a propriedade de erodir ou desgastar. **2.** Um agente que causa erosão.

erot·ic (ē-rot′ik). Erótico; libidinoso; relativo à paixão sexual; capaz de produzir excitação sexual. [G. *erōtikos*, relativo ao amor, de *erōs*, amor]

er·o·tism, erot·i·cism (er′o-tizm, ē-rot′i-sizm). Erotismo; uma condição de excitação sexual.

  anal e., e. anal; experiência prazerosa centrada na defecação e em atividades relacionadas associadas à região anal, principalmente durante a fase anal em crianças de 1 a 3 anos.

er·o·ti·za·tion (er′ō-ti-zā′shŭn). Erotização; um processo no qual um objeto ou ação é tornado sexualmente excitante. SIN libidinization.

ero·to·gen·e·sis (er′ō-tō-jen′ē-sis). Erotogênese; a origem ou gênese de impulsos sexuais. [G. *erōs*, amor, + *genesis*, origem]

ero·to·gen·ic (er′ō-tō-jen′ik). Erotogênico; capaz de causar excitação ou estimulação sexual. [G. *erōs*, amor, + -*gen*, produção]

ero·to·ma·nia (er′ō-tō-mā′nē-ă). Erotomania. **1.** Inclinação excessiva ou mórbida de pensamentos e comportamentos eróticos. **2.** O efeito alucinatório de que a pessoa está envolvida em um relacionamento com outra, geralmente inatingível. [G. *erōs*, amor, + *mania*, mania]

ero·to·path·ic (er′o-tō-path′ik). Erotopático; relativo à erotopatia.

er·o·top·a·thy (er-ō-top′a-thē). Erotopatia; qualquer anormalidade do impulso sexual. [G. *erōs*, amor, + *pathos*, que sofre]

ero·to·pho·bia (er′ō-tō-fō′bē-ă). Erotofobia; aversão mórbida ao pensamento de amor sexual e à sua expressão física. [G. *erōs*, amor, + *phobos*, medo]

ERP Abreviatura de early receptor *potential* (potencial de receptor precoce).

ERPF Abreviatura de effective renal plasma *flow* (fluxo plasmático renal efetivo).

er·rat·ic (ē-rat′ik). Errático. **1.** SIN eccentric (1). **2.** Designa sintomas que variam em intensidade, freqüência ou localização. [L. *erro*, pp. *erratus*, vaguear]

er·ror (er′ōr). Erro. **1.** Um defeito na estrutura ou função. **2.** Em bioestatística:

1) uma decisão errada, como na hipótese de teste ou classificação por uma função discriminante; 2) a diferença entre o valor verdadeiro e o valor observado de uma variável, atribuída ao acaso ou a uma leitura errada por um observador. **3.** Resultados falso-positivos e falso-negativos em um estudo dicotômico. **4.** Uma crença falsa ou errada; em ciências biomédicas e outras ciências, há muitas variedades de erro, p. ex., devido à tendenciosidade (viés), medidas não-acuradas ou defeito dos instrumentos.
alpha e., e. alfa. SIN e. of the first kind.
beta e., e. beta. SIN e. of the second kind.
experimental e., e. experimental; o erro total de medida atribuído à realização de uma observação empírica. É comumente expresso como o desvio padrão de experiências repetidas. Pode haver muitos componentes, incluindo aqueles no procedimento de amostragem, as medidas, a escolha não-criteriosa de um modelo, tendenciosidade do observador, etc.
e. of the first kind, e. do primeiro tipo; em um teste de Neyman-Pearson de uma hipótese estatística, a probabilidade de rejeitar a hipótese nula quando esta é verdadeira. SIN alpha e., type I e.
inborn e.'s of metabolism, erros congênitos do metabolismo; grupo de distúrbios, cada um dos quais envolve um distúrbio de uma única enzima, de origem genética e operando desde o nascimento; os efeitos são atribuíveis ao acúmulo do substrato sobre o qual a enzima normalmente atua (p. ex., fenilcetonúria), à deficiência do produto da enzima (p. ex., albinismo), ou ao metabolismo forçado através de uma via auxiliar (p. ex., oxalúria).
interobserver e., e. interobservador; as diferenças entre interpretações de dois ou mais indivíduos que fazem observações do mesmo fenômeno.
intraobserver e., e. intra-observador; as diferenças entre interpretações de um indivíduo que faz observações do mesmo fenômeno em diferentes momentos.
residual e., e. residual; a discrepância estimada entre o dado medido real e o valor calculado após um modelo ter sido ajustado ao conjunto de dados por um avaliador.
e. of the second kind, e. do segundo tipo; em um teste de Neyman-Pearson de uma hipótese estatística, a probabilidade de aceitar a hipótese nula quando esta é falsa; o complemento da eficiência do teste. SIN beta e., type II e.
technical e., e. técnico; aquele componente de erro experimental devido à realização da experiência e, em princípio, estimado por determinações repetidas em alíquotas da mesma amostra.
type I e., e. tipo I. SIN e. of the first kind.
type II e., e. tipo II. SIN e. of the second kind.
er·ta·cal·ci·ol (er - tă - kal'sē - ol). Ertacalciol. VER tachysterol.
er·u·bes·cence (er - oo - bes'ens). Enrubescimento; vermelhidão da pele. [L. *erubescere*, avermelhar]
eru·cic ac·id (ē - roo'sik). Ácido erúcico; um ácido graxo insaturado de 22 carbonos presente nas sementes da flor de sangue (agrião mexicano) e de várias espécies de *Cruciferae* (nabo, mostarda preta e goiveiro); considerado tóxico para o músculo cardíaco.
eruc·ta·tion (ē - rŭk - tā'shŭn). Eructação; a eliminação de gás ou de um pequeno volume de líquido ácido do estômago através da boca. SIN belching, ructus. [L. *eructo*, pp. *-atus*, eructar]
erup·tion (ē - rŭp'shŭn). Erupção. **1.** Um brotamento, particularmente o surgimento de lesões na pele. **2.** Uma dermatose cutânea ou mucosa de desenvolvimento rápido, sobretudo quando surge como manifestação local de um dos exantemas; uma erupção é caracterizada, de acordo com a natureza da lesão, como macular, papular, vesicular, pustular, bolhosa, nodular, eritematosa, etc. **3.** A passagem de um dente através do processo alveolar e perfuração das gengivas. [L. *e-rumpo*, pp. *-ruptus*, irromper]
accelerated e., e. acelerada; padrão de erupção dentária cronologicamente avançada em comparação com o padrão médio de erupção dentária; a erupção do primeiro dente ocorre em uma idade mais jovem que a média, e os intervalos de tempo entre as erupções dentárias subseqüentes são menores que a média.
butterfly e., e. em borboleta. SIN butterfly (2).
clinical e., e. clínica; desenvolvimento da coroa de um dente que pode ser observado clinicamente.
continuous e., e. contínua; a erupção de um dente na boca e seu movimento contínuo em uma direção vertical.
creeping e., e. serpiginosa. SIN cutaneous *larva migrans.*
delayed e., e. tardia; padrão de erupção dentária cronologicamente tardio em comparação com o padrão médio de erupção dentária; a erupção do primeiro dente ocorre em uma idade mais avançada que a média, e os intervalos entre as erupções dentárias subseqüentes são maiores que a média.
drug e., e. medicamentosa; farmacodermia; qualquer erupção causada pela ingestão, injeção ou inalação de um medicamento, sendo, na maioria das vezes, resultante de sensibilização alérgica; as reações às drogas aplicadas à superfície cutânea geralmente não são designadas como erupção medicamentosa, mas como dermatite de contato. SIN dermatitis medicamentosa, dermatosis medicamentosa, medicinal e.
feigned e., e. fictícia. SIN *dermatitis* artefacta.
fixed drug e., e. medicamentosa fixa; um tipo de e. medicamentosa que recorre no mesmo local (ou locais) após a administração de determinada substância; as lesões geralmente consistem em máculas intensamente eritematosas e purpúreas, bem demarcadas, e algumas vezes em vesículas herpéticas; as áreas afetadas sofrem involução gradual, mas se agravam e aumentam com uma nova administração do medicamento agressor e podem tornar-se hiperpigmentadas.
iodine e., e. de iodo; e. acneiforme ou folicular ou lesão granulomatosa causada por uma reação à administração sistêmica de iodo ou iodeto.
Kaposi varicelliform e., e. variceliforme de Kaposi; uma complicação atualmente rara do herpes simples ou da vacínia superposta à dermatite atópica, com vesículas e vesiculopápulas generalizadas e febre alta.
medicinal e., e. medicamentosa. SIN drug e.
passive e., e. passiva; a e. contínua aparente dos dentes, na verdade resultante de regressão das gengivas e da crista óssea.
polymorphous light e., e. polimorfa lumínica; e. papular pruriginosa comum que surge em poucas horas e dura até vários dias na pele exposta à luz ultravioleta de ondas curtas (UVB); microscopicamente se observam edema subepidérmico e infiltração linfocítica perivascular profunda.
seabather's e., e. do banho de mar; erupção cutânea pruriginosa atribuída a hipersensibilidade ao veneno da larva de uma espécie de água-viva (*Linuche unguiculata*).
e. sequestrum (sē'kwes - trum), e. de seqüestro; espícula óssea sobrejacente à fossa oclusal central de um molar permanente em erupção.
serum e., e. sérica; urticária observada na doença do soro.
surgical e., e. cirúrgica; a exposição de um dente incluso para permitir sua erupção adicional para a cavidade oral por remoção cirúrgica dos tecidos moles, osso e, algumas vezes, dentes sobrejacentes.
erup·tive (ē - rŭp'tiv). Eruptivo; caracterizado por erupção.
ERV Abreviatura de expiratory reserve *volume* (volume de reserva expiratório).
er·y·sip·e·las (er - i - sip'ē - las). Erisipela; celulite cutânea superficial, aguda, específica, causada por estreptococos β-hemolíticos e caracterizada por erupções quentes, vermelhas, edematosas, endurecidas e bem definidas; geralmente acompanhada por sinais e sintomas constitucionais graves. [G. de *erythros*, vermelho + *pella*, pele]
ambulant e., e. migratória. SIN e. migrans.
e. inter'num, e. interna; e. erisipelatosa na vagina, útero e peritônio, que ocorre no puerpério.
e. mi'grans, e. migratória; uma forma amplamente disseminada, que envolve toda a face ou superfície do corpo. SIN ambulant e., wandering e.
e. per'stans facie'i, e. persistente da face; erupção vermelho-escura, crônica de e. da face.
phlegmonous e., e. flegmonosa; uma forma caracterizada por invasão dos tecidos subcutâneos, com a formação de abscessos profundos.
e. pustulo'sum, e. pustulosa; desenvolvimento de pústulas sobre a área da erisipela.
surgical e., e. cirúrgica; e. causada por infecção da ferida após um procedimento cirúrgico.
swine e., e. suína; uma doença destrutiva de suínos, que ocorre nas formas aguda e crônica, causada por *Erysipelothrix rhusiopathiae*.
wandering e., e. migratória. SIN e. migrans.
er·y·sip·e·loid (er - i - sip'ē - loyd). Erisipelóide; uma celulite específica, geralmente autolimitada, da mão causada por *Erysipelothrix rhusiopathiae;* apresenta-se como eritema cutâneo escuro, com configuração em diamante no local da ferida sofrida ao manusear peixe ou carne, e pode tornar-se generalizada, com placas de eritema e bolhas e, algumas vezes, toxemia grave. SIN blubber finger, crab hand, pseudoerysipelas, seal fingers, whale fingers. [G. *erysipelas* + *eidos*, semelhança]
Er·y·sip·e·lo·thrix (ār - i - sip'ē - lō - thriks, - si - pel'ō - thriks). Gênero de bactérias (família Corynebacteriaceae) imóveis, Gram-positivas, em forma de bastonetes e que tendem a formar filamentos longos; as células mais velhas tendem a tornar-se Gram-negativas. Produzem ácido, mas não gás, a partir da glicose. São facultativamente anaeróbicas e catalase-negativas. Os membros desse gênero infectam mamíferos, aves e peixes. A espécie típica é a *E. rhusiopathiae*. [erysipelas + G. *thrix*, pêlo]
E. insidio'sa, SIN *E. rhusiopathiae.*
E. rhusiopath'iae, uma espécie que causa erisipela suína, erisipelóide humana, poliartrite não-supurativa em cordeiros e septicemia em camundongos, e comumente infecta pessoas que manuseiam peixes; é a espécie típica do gênero *E*. SIN *E. insidiosa.*
er·y·sip·e·lo·tox·in (ār - i - sip'ē - lō - tok'sin). Erisipelotoxina; toxina produzida por tipos de *Streptococcus pyogenes* (estreptococos hemolíticos do grupo A); a causa bacteriana da erisipela.
er·y·the·ma (er - i - thē'mă). Eritema; vermelhidão devida à dilatação capilar. [G. *erythēma*, rubor]
e. ab ig'ne, e. *ab igne;* e. calórico; erupção macular, pigmentada, reticulada, observada freqüentemente na região pré-tibial em padeiros, foguistas e outros expostos a fontes de calor radiante. SIN dermatitis calorica, e. caloricum, toasted shins.

acrodynic e., e. acrodínico. SIN acrodynia (2).
e. annula're, e. anular; lesões redondas ou anulares.
e. annula're centrif'ugum, e. anular centrífugo; erupção eritematosa recorrente, expansiva, crônica, que consiste em pequenas e grandes lesões anulares, com escamas marginais escassas e claras no centro, geralmente de causa desconhecida. SIN e. figuratum perstans.
e. annula're rheumat'icum, e. anular reumático; uma variante do e. multiforme associada à febre reumática.
e. arthrit'icum epidem'icum, e. artrítico epidêmico. SIN Haverhill fever.
e. calor'icum, e. calórico. SIN e. ab igne.
e. chron'icum mi'grans, e. crônico migratório; um anel eritematoso elevado com bordas endurecidas que avançam à área central clara, irradiando-se do local de uma picada de carrapato e persistindo por 2–16 semanas; a lesão cutânea característica da doença de Lyme, causada pelo espiroqueta *Borrelia burgdorferi*, que pode ser identificada por PCR em biopsias.
e. circina'tum, e. circinado; e. multiforme no qual as lesões são agrupadas de forma mais ou menos circular.
cold e., e. do frio; erupção cutânea caracterizada por eritema e prurido, causada por exposição ao frio.
e. dyschro'micum per'stans, e. discrômico persistente; lesões maculares discretamente elevadas, cinza ou vermelhas, de tamanhos variados, que tendem a coalescer no tronco e nas porções proximais dos membros, comumente em latino-americanos de pele escura; causa desconhecida. SIN ashy dermatosis.
e. eleva'tum diu'tinum, e. elevado diuturno; erupção simétrica crônica rara de nódulos achatados de cor rosa ou púrpura, que ocorre em placas nas nádegas, tendões de Aquiles e extensores dos punhos, cotovelos e joelhos, tornando-se essas áreas fibróticas e, finalmente, retraídas. As lesões iniciais mostram vasculite necrotizante com depósitos fibrinóides ou lipídicos nas paredes dos vasos.
e. exfoliati'va, e. esfoliativo. SIN keratolysis exfoliativa.
e. figura'tum per'stans, e. figurado persistente. SIN e. annulare centrifugum.
e. gyra'tum, e. figurado; eritema circinado no qual as várias lesões anulares se superpõem.
e. indura'tum, e. indurado; nódulos subcutâneos duros recorrentes que, freqüentemente, se rompem e formam úlceras necróticas, geralmente nas panturrilhas e, com menor freqüência, nas coxas ou nos braços de mulheres de meia-idade; estão associados a alterações eritrocianóticas no clima frio; embora microscopicamente granulomatosas e necrotizantes, as lesões são estéreis; mas os testes cutâneos tuberculínicos geralmente são positivos e a amplificação por reação da cadeia da polimerase freqüentemente é positiva para DNA do complexo de *Mycobacterium tuberculosis*. SIN Bazin disease, nodular tuberculid.
e. infectio'sum, e. infeccioso; exantema infeccioso leve da infância, caracterizado por erupção maculopapular eritematosa, que resulta em erupção facial reticulada ou aspecto de "face esbofeteada". A infecção também pode ser acompanhada por febre e artrite; causada pelo parvovírus B 19. SIN fifth disease.
e. intertri'go, intertrigo. VER intertrigo.
e. kerato'des, e. ceratóide; ceratodermia com uma borda eritematosa.
macular e., e. macular. SIN roseola.
e. margina'tum, e. marginado; uma variante do e. multiforme observada na febre reumática; ocasionalmente tem uma configuração que sugere a designação eritema migratório (língua geográfica).
e. multifor'me, e. multiforme; erupção aguda de máculas, pápulas ou vesículas subepidérmicas que apresentam um aspecto multiforme, sendo a lesão característica um alvo ou íris na face dorsal das mãos e antebraços; sua origem pode ser alérgica, incluindo sensibilidade a medicamentos, ou pode ser causada por herpes simples; a erupção, embora geralmente seja autolimitada (p. ex., multiforme menor), pode ser recorrente ou ter uma evolução grave, algumas vezes com morte (p. ex., síndrome multiforme maior ou de Stevens-Johnson).
e. multifor'me bullo'sum, e. multiforme bolhoso. SIN Stevens-Johnson syndrome.
e. multifor'me exudati'vum, e. multiforme exsudativo. SIN Stevens-Johnson syndrome.
e. multifor'me ma'jor, e. multiforme maior. SIN Stevens-Johnson syndrome.
necrolytic migratory e., e. migratório necrolítico; dermatite eritematosa, descamativa e, algumas vezes, bolhosa e erosiva, que ocorre irregularmente em placas principalmente na parte inferior do tronco, nádegas, períneo e coxas; associada a emagrecimento, anemia, estomatite e elevação do glucagon plasmático em tumores das células das ilhotas (glucagonoma) do pâncreas. VER TAMBÉM glucagonoma syndrome.
e. neonato'rum, e. neonatal. SIN e. toxicum neonatorum.
e. nodo'sum, e. nodoso; paniculite caracterizada pela súbita formação de nódulos dolorosos nas superfícies extensoras dos membros inferiores, com lesões autolimitadas, mas que tendem a recorrer; associado a artralgia e febre; pode ser resultante de sensibilidade a medicamentos ou associada à sarcoidose e a várias infecções. As biopsias profundas revelam paniculite septal com infiltração por linfócitos e células gigantes multinucleadas dispersas. SIN nodal fever.
e. nodo'sum lepro'sum, e. nodoso da lepra; um tipo agudo de reação lepromatosa com envolvimento sistêmico generalizado e nódulos cutâneos e subcutâneos profundos e dolorosos em face, coxas e braços; geralmente observado em casos não-diagnosticados, não-tratados ou negligenciados de hanseníase. Podem ser observados imunocomplexos e bacilos de Hansen fragmentados, escassos nas lesões.
e. nodo'sum mi'grans, e. nodoso migratório. SIN subacute migratory panniculitis.
e. nuchae, e. nucal. SIN Unna nevus.
e. palma're heredita'rium [MIM*133000], e. palmar hereditário; condição hereditária, que pode ser precipitada pela gravidez, caracterizada por eritema simétrico assintomático das regiões palmares; herança autossômica dominante. SIN Lane disease.
e. papula'tum, e. papuloso; a forma papular do e. multiforme.
e. paratrim'ma, e. devido à estase sobre pontos de pressão.
e. per'nio, e. pérnio. SIN chilblain.
e. per'stans, e. persistente; provavelmente uma forma crônica de eritema multiforme na qual as recidivas são tão persistentes que a erupção é quase permanente.
scarlatiniform e., e. scarlatinoi'des, e. escarlatiniforme; e. escarlatinóide; erupção macular eritematosa acompanhada por leves sintomas constitucionais e seguida por descamação.
e. sim'plex, e. simples; rubor ou eritema da pele causado por uma reação tóxica ou por um fenômeno neurovascular.
e. sola're, e. solar. SIN sunburn.
symptomatic e., e. sintomático; termo geral aplicado a vários e. associados a doença sistêmica, febres, estados alérgicos, etc.
e. tox'icum, e. tóxico; um exantema inócuo, autolimitado, de causa desconhecida, que ocorre em recém-nascidos.
e. tox'icum neonato'rum, e. tóxico neonatal; erupção idiopática transitória comum de eritema, pequenas pápulas e, ocasionalmente, pústulas cheias de leucócitos eosinofílicos sobrejacentes a folículos pilosos do recém-nascido. SIN e. neonatorum.
e. tubercula'tum, e. tuberculoso; eritema multiforme no qual as pápulas são grandes.
er·y·them·a·tous (er-i-them′a-tŭs, thē′mă-tŭs). Eritematoso; relativo a, ou caracterizado por, eritema.
er·y·ther·mal·gia (er′i-ther-mal′jē-ă). Eritermalgia. SIN erythromelalgia.
erythr-. Eritr-. VER erythro-.
er·y·thral·gia (ar-i-thral′jē-ă). Eritralgia; eritema doloroso da pele. VER TAMBÉM erythromelalgia. [erythro- + G. *algos*, dor]
ery·thras·ma (er-i-thraz′mă). Eritrasma; erupção de placas castanho-avermelhadas bem circunscritas, principalmente nas axilas e regiões inguinais, devida à presença de *Corynebacterium minutissimum* no estrato córneo. [G. *erythraino*, avermelhar]
eryth·re·de·ma (ē-rith-rē-dē′mă). Eritredema. SIN acrodynia (2). [erythro- + G. *oidēma*, edema]
er·y·thre·mia (er-i-thrē′mē-ă). Eritremia. SIN polycythemia vera. [erythro- + G. *haima*, sangue]
altitude e., e. de altitude. SIN chronic mountain sickness.
er·y·thris·tic (er-i-thris′tik). Rufo. SIN rufous.
er·y·thrite (ē-rith-rīt). Eritrita. SIN erythritol.
eryth·ri·tol (ē-rith′ri-tol). Eritritol; o álcool de açúcar de 4 carbonos obtido pela redução da eritrose, notável por seu poder adoçante (duas vezes maior que o da sacarose); encontrado em líquens, algas e fungos. SIN erythrite, erythrol.
eryth·ri·tyl tet·ra·ni·trate (ē-rith′ri-til tet-ră-nī′trăt). Tetranitrato de eritritil; vasodilatador usado na angina de peito e na hipertensão. SIN erythrol tetranitrate, tetranitrol.
erythro-, erythr-. Eritro-, eritr-. **1.** Forma combinante que designa vermelho ou hemácia; correspondente ao L. rub-. **2.** Indica a estrutura da eritrose em um açúcar maior; usado dessa forma em itálico (p. ex., 2-desoxi-D-*eritro*-pentose). [G. *erythros*, vermelho]
eryth·ro·blast (ē-rith′rō-blast). Eritroblasto; originalmente, um termo que designava todas as formas de hemácias humanas que contêm um núcleo, tanto patológicas (isto é, megaloblásticas) quanto normais (p. ex., normoblásticas). A série patológica ou megaloblástica é observada na recidiva da anemia perniciosa. O termo megaloblasto também é usado para indicar a primeira geração de células na série de hemácias que pode ser distinguida das células endoteliais precursoras; portanto, com esse uso, megaloblasto designa tanto uma célula normal quanto uma anormal. Na *série eritroblástica* de maturação, podem ser reconhecidos quatro estágios: 1) pró-eritroblasto, 2) eritroblasto basófilo, 3) eritroblasto policromático e 4) eritroblasto ortocromático. Na *série megaloblástica* de maturação, são observados estágios semelhantes aos encontrados na série normoblástica: 1) pró-megaloblasto, 2) megaloblasto basófilo, 3) megaloblasto policromático e 4) megaloblasto ortocromático. Na *série normal* de maturação, após perda do núcleo, os eritrócitos jovens são denominados *reticulócitos*; essas células podem ser reconhecidas com colorações supravitais como azul de cresil brilhante; finalmente, os reticulócitos tornam-se eritrócitos, ou hemácias maduras. SIN erythrocytoblast. [erythro- + G. *blastos*, germe]

eryth·ro·blas·te·mia (ē-rith′rō-blas-tē′mē-ă). Eritroblastemia; a presença de hemácias nucleadas no sangue periférico. [erythroblast + G. *haima*, sangue]

eryth·ro·blas·to·pe·nia (ē-rith′rō-blas-tō-pē′nē-ă). Eritroblastopenia; deficiência primária de eritroblastos na medula óssea, observada na anemia aplásica. [erythroblast + G. *penia*, pobreza]

transient e. of childhood, e. transitória da infância; distúrbio de causa desconhecida, com anemia normocítica, normocrônica grave, mas transitória, que tipicamente ocorre entre 6 meses e 3 anos de idade; freqüentemente sucede uma doença viral e, em geral, resolve em 1–2 meses.

eryth·ro·blas·to·sis (ē-rith′rō-blas-tō′sis). Eritroblastose; a presença de eritroblastos em número considerável no sangue. [erythroblast + -*ōsis*, condição]
fetal e., e. fetal. SIN e. fetalis.
e. feta'lis, e. fetal; anemia hemolítica grave que, na maioria dos casos, resulta do desenvolvimento, em uma mãe Rh-negativa, de anticorpos anti-Rh em resposta ao fator Rh presente no sangue fetal (Rh-positivo); é caracterizada por muitos eritroblastos na circulação e, freqüentemente, por edema generalizado (hidropisia fetal) e aumento do fígado e do baço; a doença algumas vezes é causada por anticorpos contra outros antígenos além do Rh. SIN anemia neonatorum, congenital anemia, fetal e., hemolytic anemia of newborn, hemolytic disease of newborn, neonatal anemia, Rh antigen incompatibility.

eryth·ro·blas·tot·ic (ē-rith′rō-blas-tot′ik). Eritroblastótico; pertinente à eritroblastose, principalmente eritroblastose fetal.

eryth·ro·cat·al·y·sis (ē-rith′rō-kă-tal′i-sis). Eritrocatálise; fagocitose das hemácias. [erythro- + G. *katalysis*, dissolução]

eryth·ro·chro·mia (ē-rith′rō-krō′mē-ă). Eritrocromia; coloração vermelha. [erythro- + G. *chrōma*, cor]

eryth·ro·cla·sis (er-i-throk′lă-sis). Eritroclasia; fragmentação das hemácias. [erythro- + G. *klasis*, quebra]

eryth·ro·clas·tic (ē-rith′rō-klas′tik). Eritroclástico; relativo à eritroclasia; destrutivo para as hemácias.

eryth·ro·cu·pre·in (ē-rith′rō-koo′prē-in). Eritrocupreína. SIN cytocuprein.

eryth·ro·cy·a·no·sis (ē-rith′rō-sī-ă-nō′sis). Eritrocianose; uma condição observada em meninas e mulheres jovens na qual a exposição dos membros ao frio faz com que se tornem edemaciados e vermelho-escuros; resulta da exposição direta a temperaturas baixas, mas não-congelantes. [erythro- + G. *kyanos*, azul, + -*ōsis*, condição]

🅘 **eryth·ro·cyte** (ē-rith′rō-sīt). Eritrócito; uma hemácia madura. SIN red blood cell, red corpuscle. [erythro- + G. *kytos*, célula]

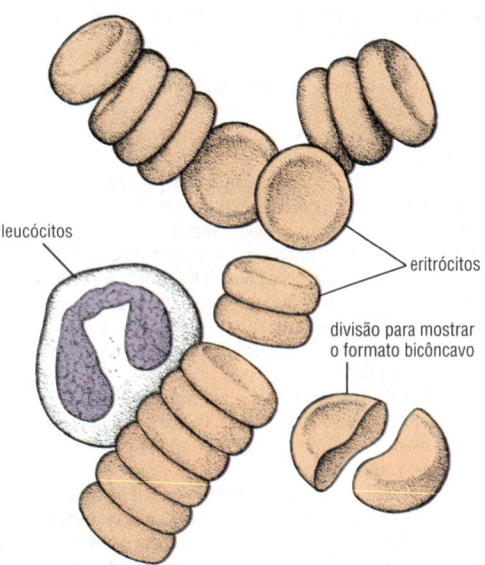

eritrócitos: hemácias agrupadas empilhadas (como pilhas de moedas)

eryth·ro·cy·the·mia (ē-rith′rō-sī-thē′mē-ă). Eritrocitemia. SIN polycythemia. [erythro- + G. *kytos*, célula, + *haima*, sangue]

eryth·ro·cyt·ic (ē-rith-rō-sit′ik). Eritrocítico; relativo a um eritrócito.

eryth·ro·cy·to·blast (ē-rith-rō-sī′tō-blast). Eritrocitoblasto. SIN erythroblast. [erythro- + G. *kytos*, célula, + *blastos*, germe]

eryth·ro·cy·tol·y·sin (ē-rith′rō-sī-tol′i-sin). Eritrocitolisina. SIN hemolysin (1).

eryth·ro·cy·tol·y·sis (ē-rith′rō-sī-tol′i-sis). Eritrocitólise. SIN hemolysis. [erythrocyte + G. *lysis*, afrouxamento]

eryth·ro·cy·tom·e·ter (ē-rith′rō-sī-tom′ē-ter). Eritrocitômetro; instrumento para contar as hemácias; Hayden usou este termo para designar um instrumento para medir o diâmetro das hemácias. [erythrocyte + G. *metron*, medida]

eryth·ro·cy·to·pe·nia (ē-rith′rō-sī-tō-pē′nē-ă). Eritrocitopenia. SIN erythropenia.

eryth·ro·cy·to·poi·e·sis (ē-rith′rō-sī′tō-poy-ē′sis). Eritrocitopoese. SIN erythropoiesis.

eryth·ro·cy·tor·rhex·is (ē-rith′rō-sī-tō-rek′sis). Eritrocitorrexia; uma eritrocitólise parcial na qual partículas de protoplasma escapam das hemácias, que então sofrem crenação e deformação. SIN erythrorrhexis. [erythrocyte + G. *rhēxis*, ruptura]

eryth·ro·cy·tos·chi·sis (ē-rith′rō-sī-tos′ki-sis). Eritrocitosquise; fragmentação das hemácias em pequenas partículas morfologicamente semelhantes a plaquetas. [erythrocyte + G. *schisis*, divisão]

eryth·ro·cy·to·sis (ē-rith′rō-sī-tō′sis). Eritrocitose; policitemia, particularmente aquela que ocorre em resposta a algum estímulo conhecido.

eryth·ro·cy·tu·ria (ē-rith′rō-sī-too′rē-ă). Eritrocitúria; hemácias na urina.

eryth·ro·de·gen·er·a·tive (ē-rith′rō-de-jen′er-ă-tiv). Eritrodegenerativo; relativo a, ou caracterizado por, degeneração das hemácias.

eryth·ro·der·ma (ē-rith-rō-der′mă). Eritrodermia; designação específica para eritema intenso e geralmente disseminado da pele causado por dilatação dos vasos sanguíneos, freqüentemente precedendo ou associado à esfoliação. SIN erythrodermatitis. [erythro- + G. *derma*, pele]
bullous congenital ichthyosiform e. (ik-thē-os′ē-form). e. ictiosiforme congênita bolhosa; e. difuso e erosão da pele ao nascimento, com subseqüente descamação, tendendo a melhorar mais tarde, caracterizada por hiperceratose epidermolítica generalizada e herança autossômica dominante. VER TAMBÉM epidermolytic *hyperkeratosis*. SIN generalized epidermolytic hyperkeratosis, ichthyismus hystrix, ichthyosis hystrix.
congenital ichthyosiform e., e. ictiosiforme congênita; genodermatose caracterizada por eritema crônico difuso e formação de escamas, podendo ser dividida em formas bolhosa e não-bolhosa.
e. desquamati'vum, e. descamativa; dermatite seborreica grave, extensa, com dermatite esfoliativa, linfadenopatia generalizada e diarréia no recém-nascido; freqüentemente ocorre em crianças subnutridas e caquéticas. SIN Leiner disease.
nonbullous congenital ichthyosiform e., e. ictiosiforme congênita não-bolhosa; eritrodermia ou uma película de colódio ao nascimento, geralmente sem melhora durante a infância, caracterizada por proliferação de ceratinócitos epidérmicos com acúmulo de lipídios; herança autossômica recessiva.
e. psoriat'icum, e. psoriática; extensa dermatite esfoliativa simulando psoríase.
Sézary e., e. de Sézary. SIN Sézary syndrome.

eryth·ro·der·ma·ti·tis (ē-rith′rō-der-mă-tī′tis). Eritrodermatite. SIN erythroderma.

eryth·ro·dex·trin (ē-rith′rō-deks′trin). Eritrodextrina; uma forma parcialmente digerida de dextrina identificada por sua reação colorida com o iodo (isto é, torna-se vermelho).

eryth·ro·don·tia (ē-rith-rō-don′shē-ă). Eritrodontia; coloração avermelhada dos dentes, como a que pode ocorrer na porfiria. [erythro- + G. *odous*, dente]

eryth·ro·gen·e·sis im·per·fec·ta (ē-rith-rō-jen′ē-sis im-per-fek′tă). Eritrogênese imperfeita. SIN congenital hypoplastic anemia.

eryth·ro·gen·ic (ē-rith-rō-jen′ik). Eritrogênico. **1.** Que produz a cor vermelha, como uma erupção ou uma sensação de cor vermelha. **2.** Referente à formação de hemácias. [erythro- + -*gen*, que produz]

eryth·ro·go·ni·um, pl. **eryth·ro·go·nia** (ē-rith-rō-gō′nē-ŭm, -nē-ă). Eritrogônia; o precursor de um eritrócito; ocasionalmente refere-se ao tecido eritropoético como um todo. [erythro- + G. *gonē*, geração]

er·y·throid (er′i-throyd, ē-rith′royd). Eritróide; de cor avermelhada.

er·y·throid·in (er′i-thrōy′din). Eritroidina; um antagonista colinérgico nicotínico que, ao contrário da maioria dos membros desse grupo de agentes, é uma amina terciária e, portanto, entra no sistema nervoso central.

eryth·ro·ker·a·to·der·mia (ē-rith′rō-kār-ă-tō-der′mē-ă) [MIM*133190]. Eritroceratodermia; síndrome neurocutânea caracterizada por placas eritematosas papuloescamosas com início logo após o nascimento; mais tarde surgem ataxia, nistagmo, disartria e diminuição dos reflexos tendíneos profundos; a e. progressiva simétrica tem herança autossômica dominante e não envolve as regiões palmares nem as plantares. [erythro- + G. *keras*, corno, + *derma*, pele, + -*ia*, condição]
e. varia'bilis [MIM*133200], e. variável; dermatose caracterizada por placas hiperceratóticas de configuração geográfica bizarra, associada a áreas eritrodérmicas cujo tamanho, formato e posição podem variar significativamente de um dia para outro; os pêlos, as narinas e os dentes não são afetados; o início geralmente se dá no primeiro ano de vida; herança autossômica dominante ou recessiva, causada por mutationina, o gene conexina que codifica a proteína da mácula comunicante (nexus) beta-3 (GJB3) em 1p.

eryth·ro·ki·net·ics (ē - rith′rō - ki - net′iks). Eritrocinética; uma consideração da cinética dos eritrócitos, desde sua geração até sua destruição; os estudos eritrocinéticos algumas vezes são feitos em casos de anemia para avaliar o equilíbrio entre a produção e a destruição de eritrócitos. [erythro- + G. *kinēsis*, movimento]

er·y·throl (er′i - throl). Eritrol. SIN erythritol.
  e. tetranitrate, tetranitrato de e. SIN erythrityl tetranitrate.

eryth·ro·leu·ke·mia (ē - rith′rō - loo - kē′mē - ă). Eritroleucemia; proliferação neoplásica simultânea de tecidos eritroblásticos e leucoblásticos.

eryth·ro·leu·ko·sis (ē - rith′rō - loo - kō′sis). Eritroleucose; condição semelhante à leucemia na qual o tecido eritropoético é afetado além do tecido leucopoético.

er·y·throl·y·sin (er - i - throl′i - sin). Eritrolisina, hemolisina. SIN hemolysin (1).

er·y·throl·y·sis (er - i - throl′i - sis). Eritrólise, hemólise. SIN hemolysis.

eryth·ro·mel·al·gia (ē - rith′rō - mel - al′jē - ă). Eritromelalgia. **1.** Distúrbio raro, mais comum na meia-idade, caracterizado por crises paroxísticas de forte dor em queimação, vermelhidão, hiperalgesia e sudorese, envolvendo um ou mais membros, geralmente os dois pés; as crises podem ser deflagradas por calor, sendo geralmente aliviadas pelo frio e pela elevação dos membros. **2.** Dor pulsátil e em queimação paroxística na pele, freqüentemente precipitada por esforço ou calor, afetando as mãos e os pés, associada a lesão vermelho-escura mosqueada nas partes com aumento da temperatura cutânea; associada a, e freqüentemente precedendo, distúrbios mieloproliferativos e outros distúrbios. SIN erythermalgia, Gerhardt-Mitchell disease. [erythro- + G. *melos*, membro, + *algos*, dor]

eryth·ro·me·lia (ē - rith - rō - mē′lē - ă). Eritromelia; eritema idiopático difuso e atrofia da pele dos membros inferiores. [erythro- + G. *melos*, membro]

eryth·ro·my·cin (ē - rith - rō - mī′sin). Eritromicina; antibiótico macrolídeo obtido de culturas de uma cepa de *Streptomyces erythraeus* encontrada no solo; é ativo contra *Corynebacterium diphtheriae* e várias outras espécies de *Corynebacterium*, estreptococos hemolíticos do grupo A, *Streptococcus pneumoniae* e *Bordetella pertussis*; as bactérias Gram-positivas geralmente são mais suscetíveis à sua ação que as bactérias Gram-negativas, embora *Neisseria* e *Brucella* sejam suscetíveis à sua ação. Disponível na forma de estolato, etilcarbonato, etilsuccinato, gluceptato, lactobionato, estearato e sais; ativa contra *Legionella* e *Mycoplasma pneumoniae*. Freqüentemente prescrita como substituto em pacientes alérgicos à penicilina.
  e. estolate, estolato de e.; um sal do antibiótico macrolídeo eritromicina.
  e. glucoheptonate, glucoeptonato de e.; um sal do antibiótico macrolídeo eritromicina.
  e. propionate, propionato de e.; um sal do antibiótico macrolídeo eritromicina.
  e. stearate, estearato de e.; um sal do antibiótico macrolídeo eritromicina.

er·y·thron (er′i - thron). Éritron; a massa total de hemácias circulantes e a parte do sistema hematopoético da qual são derivadas.

eryth·ro·ne·o·cy·to·sis (ē - rith′rō - nē - ō - sī - tō′sis). Eritroneocitose; a presença, na circulação periférica, de formas regenerativas de hemácias. [erythrocyte + G. *neos*, novo, + *kytos*, célula, + *-osis*, condição]

eryth·ro·pe·nia (ē - rith - rō - pē′nē - ă). Eritropenia; deficiência do número de hemácias. SIN erythrocytopenia. [erythrocyte + G. *penia*, escassez]

eryth·ro·pha·gia (ē - rith - rō - fā′jē - ă). Eritrofagia; destruição fagocítica das hemácias. [erythrocyte + G. *phagō*, comer, + *-ia*]

eryth·ro·phag·o·cy·to·sis (ē - rith′rō - fag′ō - sī - tō′sis). Eritrofagocitose; fagocitose de eritrócitos.

eryth·ro·phil (ē - rith′rō - fil). Eritrófilo. **1.** Que se cora facilmente com corantes vermelhos. SIN erythrophilic. **2.** Uma célula ou elemento tecidual que se cora de vermelho. [erythro- + G. *philos*, afinidade]

eryth·ro·phil·ic (ē - rith - rō - fil′ik). Eritrofílico. SIN erythrophil (1).

eryth·ro·phore (ē - rith′rō - fōr). Eritróforo; um cromatóforo que contém grânulos de pigmento vermelho ou castanho. SIN allophore. [erythro- + G. *phoros*, que conduz]

eryth·ro·pla·kia (ē - rith - rō - plā′kē - ă). Eritroplaquia; uma lesão vermelha, aveludada, semelhante a uma placa, de mucosa que, freqüentemente, representa alteração maligna. [erythro- + G. *plax*, placa]

eryth·ro·pla·sia (ē - rith - rō - plā′zē - ă). Eritroplasia; eritema e displasia do epitélio. [erythro- + G. *plassō*, formar]
  e. of Queyrat, e. de Queyrat; termo obsoleto para carcinoma *in situ* da glande do pênis.

eryth·ro·poi·e·sis (ē - rith′rō - poy - ē′sis). Eritropoese; a formação de hemácias. SIN erythrocytopoiesis. [erythrocyte + G. *poiēsis*, produção]

eryth·ro·poi·et·ic (ē - rith′rō - poy - et′ik). Eritropoético; relativo a, ou caracterizado por, eritropoese.

eryth·ro·poi·e·tin (ē - rith - rō - poy′ē - tin). Eritropoetina; uma proteína contendo ácido siálico que promove a eritropoese por estímulo da formação de pró-eritroblastos e liberação de reticulócitos da medula óssea; é formada pelo rim e pelo fígado e, possivelmente, por outros tecidos, podendo ser detectada no plasma e na urina humanos. SIN erythropoietic hormone (2), hematopoietin, heopoietin.

eryth·ro·pros·o·pal·gia (ē - rith′rō - pros - ō - pal′jē - ă). Eritroprosopalgia; distúrbio semelhante à eritromelalgia, mas com a dor e a vermelhidão ocorrendo na face. [erythro- + G. *prosōpon*, face, + *algos*, dor]

eryth·rop·sia (ē - rith - rop′sē - ă). Eritropsia; anormalidade da visão na qual todos os objetos parecem tintos de vermelho. SIN red vision. [erythro- + G. *ōps*, olho]

eryth·ro·pyk·no·sis (ē - rith′rō - pik - nō′sis). Eritropicnose; alteração das hemácias para desenvolver os denominados "corpúsculos bronzeados", sob a influência do parasita da malária. [erythro- + G. *pyknos*, denso]

er·y·thror·rhex·is (er′i - thrō - rek′sis, ē - rith - rō - rek′sis). Eritrorrexia. SIN erythrocytorrhexis. [erythrocyte + G. *rhēxis*, ruptura]

er·y·throse (ē - rith′rōs). Eritrose; uma aldotetrose epimérica com a treose. O D-isômero participa do metabolismo intermediário.
  e. 4-phosphate, 4-fosfato de eritrose; um derivado fosforilado da eritrose que serve como importante intermediário na via da pentose fosfato.

eryth·ro·sin B (ē - rith′rō - sin) [C.I. 45430]. Eritrosina B; tetraiodofluoresceína, um corante ácido vermelho fluorescente, usado como contracorante em histologia e como indicador fluorescente.

er·y·throx·y·line (er - i - throk′si - lēn). Eritroxilina; nome dado à cocaína por seu descobridor, Gaedeke, em 1855.

eryth·ru·lose (ē - rith′roo - lōs). Eritrulose; o análogo 2-ceto da eritrose; a única cetotetrose.

er·y·thru·ria (er - i - throo′rē - ă). Eritrúria; a eliminação de urina vermelha. [erythro- + G. *ouron*, urina]

Es Símbolo do einsteinium (einstênio).

Esbach, Georges H., médico francês, 1843–1890. VER E. *reagent*.

es·cape (es - kāp′). Escape; termo usado para descrever a situação em que um marcapasso falha ou a condução AV falha e outro marcapasso, geralmente inferior, assume a função de controle por um ou mais batimentos.
  junctional e., e. juncional; escape com a junção AV como marcapasso.
  ventricular e., e. ventricular; escape com um foco ventricular ectópico como marcapasso.

es·char (es′kar). Escara; uma crosta espessa, coagulada, ou tecido necrosado que se desenvolve após uma queimadura térmica ou após cauterização química ou física da pele. [G. *eschara*, lareira, ferida produzida por queimação]

es·char·ec·to·my (es′kar - rek - tō - mē). Escarectomia; excisão completa ou parcial de uma escara, geralmente após uma queimadura.

es·cha·rot·ic (es - kă - rot′ik). Escarótico; cáustico ou corrosivo. [G. *escharōtikos*]

es·cha·rot·o·my (es - kă - rot′ō - mē). Escarotomia; incisão cirúrgica em uma escara (derme necrótica) para reduzir a constrição, principalmente após uma queimadura de terceiro grau circunferencial de um membro ou do tórax. [eschar + G. *tomē*, incisão]

Esch·e·rich·ia (esh - ē - rik′ē - ă). Gênero de bactérias aeróbicas, facultativamente anaeróbicas, contendo bacilos Gram-negativos curtos, móveis ou não. As células móveis são peritríquias. A glicose e a lactose são fermentadas com produção de ácido e gás. Esses microrganismos são encontrados nas fezes; alguns são patogênicos para os seres humanos, causando enterite, peritonite, cistite, etc. É o gênero típico da família Enterobacteriaceae. A espécie típica é a *E. coli*. [T. Escherich, pediatra e bacteriologista alemão, 1857–1911]

E. co′li, espécie encontrada normalmente no intestino dos seres humanos e de outros vertebrados, encontra-se amplamente distribuída na natureza, e é uma causa freqüente de infecções do trato urogenital e de meningite neonatal e diarréia em lactentes; cepas enteropatogênicas (sorotipos) de *E. coli* causam diarréia por enterotoxina, cuja produção parece estar associada a um epissoma transferível; a espécie típica do gênero. SIN colibacillus, colon bacillus.

enterohemorrhagic *E. coli* **(EHEC)**, *E. coli* êntero-hemorrágica; cepas êntero-hemorrágicas de *E. coli*, comumente do sorotipo 0157:H7; produz uma toxina semelhante à produzida pela *Shigella*; associada à lesão do epitélio, isquemia do intestino e necrose do cólon. Aparentemente responsável por uma forma hemorrágica de colite sem febre, que pode ser muito grave; transmitida basicamente por carne bovina e de aves contaminada. Também pode causar anemia hemolítica microangiopática, insuficiência renal e a síndrome hemolítico-urêmica.

enteroinvasive *E. coli* **(EIEC)**, *E. coli* enteroinvasiva; cepa enteroinvasiva de *E. coli* que penetra na mucosa intestinal e se multiplica nas células epiteliais do cólon, resultando em alterações da mucosa semelhantes às observadas na shigelose. Essa cepa causa uma doença diarreica grave, que pode assemelhar-se à shigelose, exceto pela ausência de vômito e pela menor duração da doença.

enteropathogenic *E. coli* **(EPEC)**, *E. coli* enteropatogênica; cepa enteropatogênica de *E. coli*; os microrganismos aderem à mucosa do intestino delgado e produzem alterações características nas microvilosidades. Essa cepa produz doenças gastrointestinais sintomáticas, algumas vezes graves, sobretudo em recém-nascidos e crianças pequenas; tipicamente produz toxinas, uma das quais é termolábil, semelhante àquela produzida pelo *Vibrio cholerae*, e a outra termoestável.

enterotoxigenic *E. coli* **(ETEC)**, *E. coli* enterotoxigênica; cepa enterotoxigênica de *E. coli*; fixa-se à mucosa do duodeno ou do intestino delgado proxi-

mal, onde forma toxinas termoestáveis e termolábeis que ativam a adenilato ciclase, causando diarréia aquosa. Responsável por 40–70% dos casos de diarréia dos viajantes; transmitida principalmente por fezes humanas. A causa mais importante de diarréia em lactentes que vivem em áreas tropicais.
E. freun'dii, nome anterior de *Citrobacter freundii.*

es·cor·cin, es·cor·cin·ol (es-kōr'sin, -sin-ol). Escorcina, escorcinol; um pó marrom derivado da esculetina, substância derivada da esculina; usada para a detecção de defeitos na córnea e na conjuntiva, que são marcados por uma coloração vermelha.

es·cu·la·pi·an (es-kū-lā'pē-ăn). Esculapiano, relativo a Esculápio. SIN aesculapian.

es·cu·lent (es'kū-lent). Esculento; alimentício; que serve de alimento. [L. *esculentus,* comestível]

es·cu·lin (es'kū-lin). Esculina; glicosídeo da casca da castanha-da-índia; usada como protetor para queimadura solar. SIN aesculin. [L. *aesculus,* o carvalho italiano]

es·er·i·dine (es-er'i-dēn). Eseridina; alcalóide da semente da *Physostigma;* agente parassimpaticomimético. SIN eserine aminoxide, eserine oxide.

es·er·ine (es'er-ēn). Eserina. SIN physostigmine.
  e. aminoxide, aminóxido de e. SIN eseridine.
  e. oxide, óxido de e. SIN eseridine.
  e. salicylate, salicilato de e. SIN physostigmine salicylate.

⟁ **-esis.** –ese; condição, ação ou processo. [G. *-esis,* condição ou processo]

Esmarch, Johann F.A. von, cirurgião alemão, 1823–1908. VER E. *tourniquet.*

es·mo·lol hy·dro·chlo·ride (es'mō-lol). Cloridrato de esmolol; um bloqueador β-adrenérgico de ação breve.

es·o·de·vi·a·tion (es'ō-dē-vē-ā'shŭn). Esodesvio. 1. SIN esophoria. 2. SIN esotropia.

es·od·ic (e-sod'ik). Aferente. SIN afferent. [G. *esō,* para dentro, + *hodos,* caminho]

esoph·a·gal·gia (ē-sof-ă-gal'jē-ă). Esofagalgia; esofagodinia; termo raramente usado para designar a dor no esôfago. [esophagus + G. *algos,* dor]

esoph·a·ge·al (ē-sof'ă-jē'ăl, ē'-so-fajē'-ăl). Esofágico; relativo ao esôfago.

e·soph·a·gec·to·my (ē-sof-ă-jek'tō-mē). Esofagectomia; excisão de todo o esôfago, ou de qualquer parte dele. [esophagus + G. *ektomē,* excisão]
  Ivor Lewis e., e. de Ivor Lewis; abordagem comumente usada para esofagectomia via laparotomia e toracotomia direita, com anastomose intratorácica.
  three-incision e., e. por três incisões; esofagectomia via incisões de laparotomia, torácica direita e cervical.
  transhiatal e., e. trans-hiatal; ressecção do esôfago por uma incisão cervical acima e acesso trans-hiatal através de uma incisão abdominal abaixo.
  transthoracic e., e. transtorácica; ressecção do esôfago através de uma incisão de toracotomia.

esoph·a·gi (ē-sof'ă-jī, -gī). Esôfagos; plural de esophagus.

esoph·a·gism (ē-sof'ă-jizm). Esofagismo; espasmo esofágico que causa disfagia. SIN dysphagia nervosa, nervous dysphagia.

esoph·a·gi·tis (ē-sof-ă-jī'tis). Esofagite; inflamação do esôfago.
  reflux e., peptic e., e. de refluxo, e. péptica; inflamação do terço inferior do esôfago por regurgitação do conteúdo gástrico ácido, geralmente devida à disfunção do esfíncter esofágico inferior; os sintomas incluem dor subesternal, "pirose" e regurgitação de suco ácido.

esoph·a·go·car·di·o·plas·ty (ē-sof'ă-gō-kar'dē-ō-plas-tē). Esofagocardioplastia; um procedimento de revisão do esôfago e da extremidade cárdica do estômago.

esoph·a·go·cele (ē-sof'ă-gō-sēl). Esofagocele; protrusão da mucosa do esôfago através de uma laceração da túnica muscular. [esophagus + G. *kēlē,* hérnia]

esoph·a·go·dyn·ia (ē-sof'ă-gō-din'ē-ă). Esofagodinia. SIN esophagalgia. [esophagus + G. *odynē,* dor]

esoph·a·go·en·ter·os·to·my (ē-sof'ă-gō-en-ter-os'tō-mē). Esofagoenterostomia; formação cirúrgica de uma comunicação direta entre o esôfago e o intestino. [esophagus + G. *enteron,* intestino, + *stoma,* boca]

esoph·a·go·gas·trec·to·my (ē-sof'ă-gō-gas-trek'tō-mē). Esofagogastrectomia; remoção de uma parte do terço inferior do esôfago e da parte proximal do estômago.

esoph·a·go·gas·tro·a·nas·to·mo·sis (ē-sof'ă-gō-gas'trō-ă-nas-tō-mō'sis). Esofagogastroanastomose. SIN esophagogastrostomy.

esoph·a·go·gas·tro·du·o·de·nos·co·py (EGD) (ē-sof'ă-gō-gas'trō-doo'ō-den-os-kō-pē). Esofagogastroduodenoscopia; exame endoscópico do esôfago, estômago e duodeno, geralmente realizado utilizando um instrumento de fibra óptica.

esoph·a·go·gas·tro·my·ot·o·my (ē-sof'ă-gō-gas'trō-mī-ot'ō-mē). Esofagogastromiotomia. SIN esophagomyotomy.

esoph·a·go·gas·tro·plas·ty (ē-sof'ă-gō-gas'trō-plas-tē). Esofagogastroplastia. SIN cardioplasty.

esoph·a·go·gas·tros·to·my (ē-sof'ă-gō-gas-tros'tō-mē). Esofagogastrostomia; anastomose do esôfago ao estômago, geralmente após esofagogastrectomia. SIN esophagogastroanastomosis, gastroesophagostomy. [esophagus + G. *gastēr,* estômago, + *stoma,* abertura]

esoph·a·go·gram (e-sof'ă-gō-gram). Esofagograma. SIN esophagram.

esoph·a·gog·ra·phy (ē-sof-ă-gog'ră-fē). Esofagografia; radiografia do esôfago utilizando contraste radiopaco deglutido ou injetado; a técnica de obtenção de um esofagograma. [esophagus + G. *graphō,* escrever]

esoph·a·gol·o·gy (ē-sof'ă-gol'ō-gē). Esofagologia; estudo da estrutura, da fisiologia e das doenças do esôfago. [esophagus + g. *logos,* estudo]

esoph·a·go·ma·la·cia (ē-sof'ă-gō-ma-lā'shē-a). Esofagomalacia; amolecimento das paredes do esôfago. [esophagus + G. *malakia,* amolecimento]

esoph·a·go·my·ot·o·my (ē-sof'ă-gō-mī-ot'ō-mē). Esofagomiotomia; divisão longitudinal da camada muscular até a submucosa da porção inferior da parede esofágica; algumas fibras musculares do cárdia também podem ser divididas. SIN cardiomyotomy, esophagogastromyotomy. [esophagus + G. *mys,* músculo, + *tomē,* incisão]

esoph·a·go·plas·ty (ē-sof'ă-gō-plas-tē). Esofagoplastia; procedimento cirúrgico de revisão da parede do esôfago. [esophagus + G. *plastos,* formado]

esoph·a·go·pli·ca·tion (ē-sof'ă-gō-pli-kā'shun). Esofagoplicatura; redução do tamanho de um esôfago dilatado ou de uma bolsa no esôfago, através de dobras longitudinais ou pregueamento de sua parede. [esophagus + L. *plico,* preguear]

esoph·a·go·pto·sis, esoph·a·go·pto·sia (ē-sof'ă-gō-tō'sis, -tō'sē-ă). Esofagoptose; relaxamento e queda das paredes do esôfago. [esophagus + G. *ptōsis,* queda]

esoph·a·go·scope (ē-sof'ă-gō-skōp). Esofagoscópio; endoscópio para inspeção do interior do esôfago. [esophagus + G. *skopeō,* examinar]

esoph·a·gos·co·py (ē-sof-ă-gos'kō-pē). Esofagoscopia; inspeção do interior do esôfago por meio de um endoscópio. [esophagus + G. *skopeō,* examinar]

esoph·a·go·spasm (ē-sof'ă-gō-spazm). Esofagoespasmo; espasmo das paredes esofágicas.

esoph·a·go·ste·no·sis (ē-sof'ă-gō-stē-nō'sis). Esofagoestenose; estenose ou estreitamento geral do esôfago. [esophagus + G. *stenōsis,* estreitamento]

esoph·a·go·sto·mi·a·sis (ē-sof'ă-gō-stō-mī'ă-sis). Esofagostomíase. SIN oesophagostomiasis. [esophagus + G. *stoma,* abertura, + *-iasis,* condição]

esoph·a·gos·to·my (ē-sof-ă-gos'tō-mē). Esofagostomia; formação cirúrgica de uma abertura diretamente no esôfago, de fora para dentro. [esophagus + G. *stoma,* abertura]

esoph·a·got·o·my (ē-sof-ă-got'ō-mē). Esofagotomia; incisão através da parede do esôfago. [esophagus + G. *tomē,* incisão]

esoph·a·gram (ē-sof'ă-gram). Esofagograma; registro radiográfico de esofagografia contrastada ou com bário. SIN esophagogram.

ℹ **esoph·a·gus,** pl. **esoph·a·gi** (ē-sof'ă-gŭs, -gī; -jī) [TA]. Esôfago; a porção do canal digestivo entre a faringe e o estômago. Tem cerca de 25 cm de comprimento e consiste em três partes: a parte cervical, da cartilagem cricóide até a abertura superior do tórax; a parte torácica, da abertura superior do tórax até o diafragma; e a parte abdominal, abaixo do diafragma até o óstio cárdico do estômago. [G. *oisophagos,* esôfago]

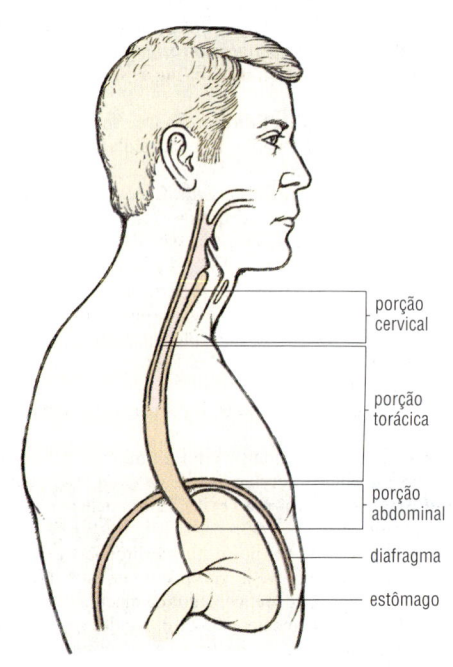

esôfago

Barrett e., e. de Barrett. SIN Barrett *syndrome*.
es·o·pho·ria (es - o͞ - fo͞'re - ă). Esoforia; tendência dos olhos de se virarem para dentro, evitada pela visão binocular. SIN esodeviation (1). [G. *eso͞*, para dentro, + *phora*, condução]
es·o·phor·ic (es - o͞ - fŏr'ik). Esofórico; relativo a, ou caracterizado por, esoforia.
es·o·tro·pia (es - o͞ - tro͞'pē - ă). Esotropia; a forma de estrabismo na qual os eixos visuais convergem; pode ser paralítica ou concomitante, monocular ou alternada, acomodativa ou não-acomodativa. SIN convergent squint, convergent strabismus, esodeviation (2), internal squint. [G. *eso͞*, para dentro, + *tropē*, virar]
  A-pattern e., e. de padrão A; estrabismo convergente maior no olhar para cima que no olhar para baixo.
  basic e., e. básica. SIN nonaccommodative e.
  consecutive e., e. consecutiva; esotropia que sucede a correção cirúrgica de exotropia.
  cyclic e., e. cíclica; estrabismo convergente periódico que, freqüentemente, ocorre a cada 48 horas. SIN alternate day strabismus.
  mixed e., e. mista; tipo de esotropia em que concorrem fatores acomodativos e não-acomodativos.
  nonaccommodative e., e. não-acomodativa; tipo de esotropia não-influenciada por correção de erro de refração. SIN basic e.
  nonrefractive accomodative e., e. acomodativa não-refrativa; tipo de esotropia em que uma anormalidade do mecanismo acomodativo de convergência não é eliminada por correção do erro de refração.
  refractive accommodative e., e. acomodativa refrativa; tipo de esotropia eliminada por correção de erro de refração hipermétrope.
  V-pattern e., e. de padrão V; estrabismo convergente maior no olhar para baixo que no olhar para cima.
  X-pattern e., e. de padrão X; convergência decrescente a partir da posição primária tanto no olhar para cima como para baixo.
es·o·tro·pic (es - o͞ - trop'ik). Esotrópico; relativo a, ou caracterizado por, esotropia.
ESP Abreviatura de extrasensory *perception* (percepção extra-sensorial).
es·pun·dia (es - poon'dē - ă). Espúndia; um tipo de leishmaniose americana causada por *Leishmania braziliensis* que afeta as mucosas, sobretudo nas regiões nasal e oral, resultando em alterações flagrantemente destrutivas; particularmente no Brasil, onde uma proporção significativa das pessoas infectadas por *L. braziliensis* desenvolve esse distúrbio; pode metastatizar a partir de úlceras originalmente encontradas em outras partes do corpo. SIN Breda disease, bubas braziliana. [Esp. do L. *spongia*, esponja]
es·qui·nan·cea (es - kwi - nan'sē - ă). Esquinância; sensação de sufocação causada por edema inflamatório na garganta, como na amigdalite ou na faringite supurativa. [Fr. *esquinancie*, amigdalite]
ESR Abreviatura de erythrocyte sedimentation *rate* (velocidade de hemossedimentação); electron spin *resonance* (ressonância com rotação de elétrons).
es·sence (es'ens). Essência. **1.** A verdadeira característica ou substância de um corpo. **2.** Um elemento. **3.** Um extrato líquido. **4.** Uma solução alcoólica do óleo volátil de uma planta. **5.** Qualquer substância volátil responsável pelo odor ou sabor do organismo (geralmente uma planta) que o produz; por extensão, perfumes ou flavorizantes sintéticos. [L. *essentia*, de *esse*, ser]
  essence of rose, e. de rosas. SIN oil of rose.
es·sen·tial (e - sen'shăl). Essencial. **1.** Necessário, indispensável (p. ex., aminoácidos essenciais, ácidos graxos essenciais). **2.** Característico de. **3.** Determinante. **4.** De etiologia desconhecida. **5.** Relativo a uma essência (p. ex., óleo essencial). **6.** SIN intrinsic.
Esser, Johannes F.S., cirurgião holandês, 1877–1946.
Essick, C., anatomista norte-americano do século XX. VER E. cell *bands*, em band.
Essig splint. Imobilização ou tala de Essig. Ver em splint.
es·taz·o·lam (ēs - taz' - o͞ - lam). Estazolam; benzodiazepínico com propriedades sedativas/hipnóticas.
es·ter (es'ter). Éster; composto orgânico que contém o grupamento —X(O)—O—R (X = carbono, enxofre, fósforo, etc.; R = radical de um álcool), formado pela eliminação de H₂O entre a —OH de um grupamento ácido e a —OH de um grupamento álcool; geralmente escrita como no acetato de etil (do ácido acético e álcool etílico), CH₃CO—OC₂H₅ ou CH₃COOC₂H₅.
  carboxylic acid e., e. do ácido carboxílico; especificamente, um éster derivado de um ácido carboxílico e um álcool; R—CO—R'
  Cori e., e. de Cori. SIN D-glucose 1-phosphate.
  Embden e., e. de Embden; hexose fosfato; uma mistura de D-glicose 6-fosfato e D-frutose 6-fosfato; importante na compreensão do metabolismo do açúcar.
  Harden-Young e., e. de Harden-Young; D-frutose 1,6-bifosfato; intermediário importante no metabolismo do açúcar.
  Neuberg e., e. de Neuberg. SIN fructose 6-phosphate.
  Robison e., e. de Robison. SIN D-glucose 6-phosphate.
  Robison-Embden e., e. de Robison-Embden. SIN D-glucose 6-phosphate.
  sugar e., e. do açúcar; éster de um açúcar com um ácido orgânico ou inorgânico; p. ex., D-glicose 6-fosfato.
  thiol e., e. tiol; éster formado a partir de um ácido carboxílico e um tiol (isto é, RCO—S'), p. ex., acetil-coenzima A.
es·ter·ase (es'ter - ās). Esterase; termo genérico para enzimas (EC classe 3.1, hidrolases) que catalisam a hidrólise de ésteres.
  C1 e., e. C1; subunidade do primeiro componente do complemento (C1) envolvido na ativação da via clássica.
es·ter·i·fi·ca·tion (es'ter'i - fi - kā'shŭn). Esterificação; o processo de formação de um éster, como na reação de etanol e ácido acético para formar acetato de etil.
Estes, William L., Jr., cirurgião norte-americano, 1885–1940. VER E. *operation*.
es·the·ma·tol·o·gy (es - thē - mă - tol'o͞ - jē). Estematologia; a ciência relacionada aos sentidos e órgãos dos sentidos. [G. *aisthēma*, percepção, + *logos*, estudo]
es·the·sia (es - thē'zē - ă). Estesia. **1.** SIN perception. **2.** SIN sensitivity (2). [G. *aisthēsis*, sensação]
es·the·sic (es - thē'sik). Estésico; relativo à percepção mental da existência de qualquer parte do corpo. [G. *aisthēsis*, sensação]
esthesio-. Estesio-. **1.** Sensação, percepção. [G. *aesthēsis*, percepção da sensação]
es·the·si·od·ic (es - thē - zē - od'ik) Estesiódico; que conduz impressões sensoriais. SIN esthesodic. [esthesio- + G. *hodos*, forma]
es·the·si·o·gen·e·sis (es - thē'zē - o͞ - jen'ē - sis). Estesiogênese; a produção de sensação, principalmente de eretismo nervoso. [esthesio- + G. *genesis*, origem]
es·the·si·o·gen·ic (es - thē - zē - o͞ - jen'ik). Estesiogênico; que produz uma sensação.
es·the·si·og·ra·phy (es - thē - zē - og'ră - fē). Estesiografia. **1.** Descrição dos órgãos do sentido e do mecanismo de sensibilidade. **2.** Mapeamento na superfície cutânea das áreas de sensibilidade tátil e de outras formas de sensibilidade. [esthesio- + G. *graphē*, escrito]
es·the·si·ol·o·gy (es - thē - zē - ol'o͞ - jē). Estesiologia; a ciência que estuda os fenômenos sensoriais. [esthesio- + G. *logos*, estudo]
es·the·si·om·e·ter (es - the - zē - om'e - ter) Estesiômetro; instrumento para determinar o estado da sensibilidade tátil e de outras formas de sensibilidade. SIN tactometer. [esthesio- + G. *metron*, medida]
es·the·si·om·e·try (es - thē - zē - om'e - trē). Estesiometria; medida do grau de sensibilidade tátil ou de outro tipo.
es·the·si·o·neu·ro·blas·to·ma (es - thē'zē - o͞ - noor'o͞ - blas - to͞'mă). Estesioneuroblastoma; neoplasia de células neuronais imaturas, pouco diferenciadas, supostamente originárias de precursores neuroepiteliais. [esthesio- + neuroblastoma]
  olfactory e., e. olfatório. SIN olfactory neuroblastoma.
es·the·si·o·neu·ro·cy·to·ma (es - thē'zē - o͞ - nur'o͞ - sī - to͞'mă). Estesioneurocitoma; uma neoplasia composta de células semelhantes a neurônios, quase maduras, supostamente originadas de um gânglio espinal ou craniano. [esthesio- + G. neurocytoma]
es·the·si·o·phys·i·ol·o·gy (es - thē'zē - o͞ - fiz - ē - ol'o͞ - jē). Estesiofisiologia; a fisiologia da sensibilidade e dos órgãos do sentido.
es·the·si·os·co·py (es - thē - zē - os'ko͞ - pē). Estesioscopia; exame do grau e da extensão da sensibilidade tátil e de outros tipos. [esthesio- + G. *skopeo͞*, ver]
es·the·sod·ic (es'thē - zod'ik). Estesódico. SIN esthesiodic.
es·thet·ic (es - thet'ik). **1.** Relativo à sensibilidade. **2.** Estético; relativo à estética (isto é, beleza). [G. *aisthēsis*, sensibilidade]
es·thet·ics (es - thet'iks). Estética; o ramo da filosofia que estuda a arte e a beleza, principalmente os seus componentes.
  denture e., **(1)** o efeito cosmético produzido por uma prótese dentária; **(2)** as qualidades envolvidas na aparência de determinada restauração.
es·ti·mate (es'ti - māt). Estimativa. **1.** Uma medida ou declaração sobre o valor de alguma quantidade que se sabe, acredita ou supõe incorporar algum grau de erro. **2.** O resultado da aplicação de qualquer estimador a uma amostra aleatória de dados. Não é uma variável aleatória, mas a percepção de uma quantidade fixa, e não tem variância, embora comumente também forneça uma estimativa da variância do estimador. (Não deve ser confundida com um estimador, que é um preceito para obter uma estimativa.) [L. *aestimo*, pp. *aestimatum*, estimar]
  Kaplan-Meier estimate, e. de Kaplan-Meier; método não-paramétrico de compilar tabelas de vida ou de sobrevida, que combina probabilidades calculadas de sobrevida com estimativas para permitir observações expurgadas (censuradas); usada principalmente em estudos de sobrevida de câncer e de doenças crônicas semelhantes.
es·ti·ma·tion (es - ti - mā'shŭn). Estimativa; qualquer procedimento estatístico não-trivial que atribui a uma quantidade desconhecida (parâmetro) um valor plausível com base em dados apropriados e pertinentes colhidos em uma amostra aleatória adequada.
es·ti·ma·tor (es'ti - mā - tor). Estimador; ordem para obter uma estimativa de uma amostra aleatória de dados. Um estimador é um procedimento, não um

resultado, e, portanto, é uma variável aleatória e tem uma variância. P. ex., um estimador do peso médio de homens adultos pode consistir na ordem "Some os pesos de 100 homens e divida por 100". O resultado (a estimativa) variará de uma amostra para outra, mas a resposta não será uma variável aleatória.
least squares e., e. por mínimos quadrados; a ordem "Atribuir ao parâmetro desconhecido o valor que minimiza a média dos quadrados dos erros residuais".
maximum likelihood e., e. de máxima verossimilhança; "Atribuir ao parâmetro desconhecido o valor que maximiza a probabilidade para a amostra". Para muitos problemas, esse procedimento é ótimo.

es·ti·val (es'ti-val). Estival; referente ao ou que ocorre no verão. SIN aestival. [L. *aestivus*, verão (adj.)]

es·ti·va·tion (es-ti-va'shŭn). Estivação; viver durante o verão em um estado quiescente, entorpecido. Cf. hibernation.

es·ti·vo·au·tum·nal (es'ti-vō-aw-tŭm'năl). Estivo-outonal; relativo ao ou que ocorre no verão e no outono. [L. *aestivus*, verão (adj.) + *autumnalis*, outonal]

Estlander, Jakob A., cirurgião finlandês, 1831–1881. VER E. *flap*.

es·tra·di·ol (E₂) (es-tra-dī'ol). Estradiol; β-estradiol; 17β-estradiol; o estrogênio natural mais potente em mamíferos, formado pelo ovário, placenta, testículo e, possivelmente, pelo córtex supra-renal; as indicações terapêuticas do estradiol são aquelas típicas de um estrogênio. O α-estradiol (17α-estradiol), exibe atividade biológica consideravelmente menor. O estradiol é usado no tratamento de distúrbios menstruais, problemas da menopausa, etc. SIN estrogenic hormone, oestradiol.
  e. benzoate, benzoato de e.; ésteres de ácido graxo do 17β-estradiol geralmente dissolvidos em óleo para injeção; esses ésteres exibem ação mais prolongada que o esteróide não-esterificado.
  e. cypionate, cipionato de e.; possui as mesmas ações e usos que o estradiol, mas tem ação prolongada; administrado em óleo por injeção intramuscular.
  e. dipropionate, dipropionato de e.; um estrogênio natural esterificado para uso parenteral.
  ethinyl e., etinil estradiol. SIN ethynyl e.
  ethynyl e., etinil e.; derivado semi-sintético do 17β-estradiol; ativo por via oral, com meia-vida longa, está entre os mais potentes compostos estrogênicos conhecidos; usado em preparações contraceptivas orais. SIN ethinyl e.
  e. undecylate, undecilato de e.; estrogênio natural esterificado para uso parenteral.
  e. valerate, valerato de e.; mesmas ações e usos do estradiol, mas com ação prolongada; administrado no óleo de gergelim por injeção intramuscular.

es·tra·gon oil (es'tra-gon). Óleo de estragão. SIN tarragon oil.

es·tra·mus·tine phos·phate so·di·um (es-tra-mŭs'tēn). Fosfato sódico de estramustina; agente antineoplásico que combina as ações do estrogênio e da mostarda nitrogenada no tratamento do carcinoma da próstata.

es·trane (es'trān). Estrano; hidrocarboneto original hipotético dos compostos estrogênicos (esteróides) cujos nomes começam com "estr-" (estradiol, estrona, estriol); concebido para estabelecer uma nomenclatura sistemática.

es·tra·tri·ene (es-tra-trī'ēn). Estratrieno; o estrano triplamente insaturado hipotético, que é o núcleo da maioria dos esteróides estrogênicos naturais em animais.

es·trin (es'trin). Estrina. SIN estrogen.

es·tri·ol (es'trē-ol). Estriol; metabólito estrogênico do estradiol, geralmente o metabólito estrogênico predominante encontrado na urina (principalmente durante a gravidez); epímeros em C-16 e/ou C-17 são conhecidos como 16-epiestriol, etc. SIN folliculin hydrate, oestriol, trihydroxyestrin.

es·tro·die·nol (es-trō-dē'nol). Estrodienol. SIN dienestrol.

es·tro·gen (es'trō-jen). Estrogênio; termo genérico que designa qualquer substância, natural ou sintética, que exerce efeitos biológicos característicos dos hormônios estrogênicos como o 17β-estradiol. Os e. são produzidos pelo ovário, placenta, testículos e, possivelmente, pelo córtex supra-renal, e também por determinadas plantas; eles estimulam as características sexuais secundárias e exercem efeitos sistêmicos, como crescimento e maturação dos ossos longos; são usados terapeuticamente em qualquer distúrbio atribuível à deficiência de estrogênio ou sensível à estrogenioterapia, como distúrbios menstruais e problemas da menopausa. Eles controlam o ciclo menstrual. São usados em determinados tratamentos de distúrbios coronarianos em mulheres. SIN estrin, oestrogen. [G. *oistrus*, estrus, + *-gen*, que produz]
  catechol e., e. catecol; qualquer derivado 2-hidroxilado de um estrogênio; eles, com seus derivados metilados, podem representar até metade de todos os metabólitos de e. excretados.
  conjugated e., e. conjugado; uma preparação amorfa de formas conjugadas, hidrossolúveis, naturais de estrogênios mistos obtidos na urina de éguas grávidas (e. eqüino conjugado); o principal e. presente no sulfato de estrona sódico; adequado para administração parenteral, oral e tópica, e usado em condições que respondem à estrogenioterapia.
  esterified e.'s, e. esterificados; uma mistura dos sais sódicos de ésteres sulfato de substâncias estrogênicas; usados na estrogenioterapia oral.

es·tro·gen·ic (es-trō-jen'ik). Estrogênico. **1.** Que desencadeia o estro em animais. **2.** Que possui uma ação semelhante à do estrogênio.

es·trone (E₁) (es'trōn). Estrona; um metabólito do 17β-estradiol, comumente encontrado na urina, nos ovários e na placenta; tem atividade biológica consideravelmente menor que o hormônio original. SIN follicular hormone, folliculin, keratohydroxyestrin, oestrone.

es·trous (es'trŭs). Estrual; relativo ao estro. SIN estrual.

es·tru·al (es'troo-ăl). Estrual. SIN estrous.

es·trus (es'trŭs). Estro; a parte ou fase do ciclo sexual de animais fêmeas caracterizada por desejo de permitir o coito; os animais exibem sinais comportamentais e outros sinais facilmente detectáveis durante esse período. SIN heat (3). [G. *oistros*, desejo louco]
  postpartum e., e. pós-parto; estro com ovulação e produção de corpo lúteo que ocorre em alguns animais (p. ex., foca) imediatamente após o nascimento da cria.

esu Abreviatura de electrostatic *unit* (unidade eletrostática).

ESWL Abreviatura de electrohydraulic shock wave *lithotripsy* (litotripsia por ondas de choque eletro-hidráulicas); extracorporeal shock wave *lithotripsy* (litotripsia por ondas de choque extracórpreas).

es·y·late (es'ĭ-lāt). Esilato; contração aprovada pela USAN para o etanossulfonato, CH₃CH₂SO₃⁻.

Et Abreviatura de ethyl (etil).

eta (āt'a). Eta; a sétima letra do alfabeto grego. **1.** Em química, designa a posição distante sete átomos do grupamento carboxila ou outro grupamento funcional primário. **2.** Símbolo de viscosidade.

et·a·fed·rine hy·dro·chlo·ride (et-ă-fed'rĕn). Cloridrato de etafedrina; um agente simpaticomimético.

etaf·e·none (e-taf'ē-nōn). Etafenona; vasodilatador coronariano.

etam·sy·late (e-tam'si-lāt). Etansilato. SIN ethamsylate.

état (ā-tah'). Uma condição ou estado. [Fr. estado]
  e. criblé (ā-tah'kri-blā), e crivoso; em neuropatologia, um termo que descreve atrofia perivascular do tecido cerebral, produzindo lacunas. [Fr. crivo]
  e. mamelonné, e. mamelonado; termo obsoleto para designar a condição da mucosa gástrica na inflamação crônica, quando esta apresenta muitas projeções nodulares. [Fr. nodoso, tuberculoso]

ETEC Abreviatura de enterotoxigenic *Escherichia coli* (*Escherichia coli* enterotoxigênica).

eth·ac·ri·dine lac·tate (eth-ak'ri-dēn). Lactato de etacridina; anti-séptico para tratamento de feridas. SIN acrinol.

eth·a·cry·nate so·di·um (eth-ă-kri'nāt). Etacrinato sódico; sal sódico do ácido etacrínico para uso parenteral.

eth·a·cryn·ic ac·id (eth-ă-krin'ik). Ácido etacrínico; uma cetona insaturada derivada do ácido ariloxiacético; um potente diurético de alça e um anti-hipertensivo fraco.

eth·a·di·one (eth-ă-dī'ōn). Etadiona; um anticonvulsivante.

eth·am·bu·tol hy·dro·chlo·ride (eth-am'boo-tol). Cloridrato de etambutol; tuberculostático efetivo contra microrganismos resistentes a outros agentes; uma reação grave é o comprometimento visual que, entretanto, parece ser reversível. Associado a outros medicamentos antituberculosos para retardar ou evitar o surgimento de cepas resistentes dos bacilos da tuberculose.

etha·mi·van (eth-am'i-van). Etamivan; estimulante do sistema nervoso central e analéptico, já foi usado como agente auxiliar no tratamento de depressão respiratória grave causada por barbitúricos e retenção de dióxido de carbono.

eth·a·mox·y·tri·phe·tol (eth-ă-moks'ē-tri-fē'tol). Etamoxitrifetol; o antiestrogênio prototípico que inibe os efeitos do estrogênio em seus receptores celulares específicos; os dois antiestrogênios com mais ampla relação estrutural são o citrato de clomifeno e o tamoxifeno.

etham·sy·late (e-tham'si-lāt). Etansilato; agente hemostático. SIN cyclonamine, etamsylate.

eth·a·nal (eth'ă-nal). Etanal. SIN acetaldehyde.

eth·ane (eth'ān). Etano; CH₃CH₃; um constituinte de gases naturais e "engarrafados".

eth·ane·di·a·mine (eth-ān-dī'ă-mēn). Etanodiamina. SIN ethylenediamine.

eth·a·no·ic ac·id (eth-ă-nō'ik). Ácido etanóico. SIN acetic acid.

eth·a·nol (eth'an-ol). Etanol. SIN alcohol (2).

eth·a·nol·a·mine (eth-an-ol'ă-mēn). Etanolamina; usada para preparar oleato de etanolamina, um agente esclerosante.

eth·a·nol·a·mine·phos·pho·trans·fer·ase (eth-ă-nol'ă-mēn-fos-fō-trans'fer-ās). Etanolaminafosfotransferase; uma transferase que catalisa a reação da CDP-etanolamina com um 1,2-diacilglicerol para produzir CMP e uma fosfotidiletanolamina; uma etapa fundamental na biossíntese dos fosfolipídios. SIN phosphorylethanolamine glyceridetransferase.

eth·av·e·rine hy·dro·chlo·ride (eth-av'ē-rēn, eth-ă-ver'ēn). Cloridrato de etaverina; um relaxante do músculo liso. SIN ethylpapaverine hydrochloride.

eth·chlor·vy·nol (eth-klōr'vī-nol). Eticlorvinol; um hipnótico obsoleto.

eth·en·yl (eth'en-il). Etenil. SIN vinyl.

eth·en·yl·ben·zene (eth-en-il-ben'zēn). Etenilbenzeno, estireno. SIN styrene.

eth·en·yl·ene (eth-en'il-ēn). Vinileno. SIN vinylene.

ether (ē′ther). Éter. **1.** Qualquer composto orgânico no qual dois átomos de carbono são independentemente ligados a um átomo de oxigênio comum, assim contendo o grupamento —C—O—C—. VER TAMBÉM epoxy. **2.** Livremente usado para designar o éter dietílico ou um éter anestésico, embora um grande número de éteres tenha propriedades anestésicas. Quanto aos éteres individuais, ver o nome específico. [G. *aithēr*, o ar puro superior]
  anesthetic e., e. anestésico; designação geral para muitos éteres.
  glycol e.'s, éteres de glicol; substâncias químicas como o éter monometílico de etilenoglicol e éter monoetílico de etilenoglicol; são teratógenos que induzem atrofia testicular em animais.
  solvent e., e. solvente; forma bastante pura de éter ($C_4H_{10}O$), mas não suficientemente pura para anestesia; usado como solvente.
  xylostyptic e., e. xilostíptico. SIN styptic *collodion*.

ethe·re·al (ē-thēr′ē-ăl). Etéreo. **1.** Relativo ao ou que contém éter. **2.** Dissolvido em um éter. [G. *aitherios*, etéreo, de *aithēr*, o ar superior].

ether·i·fi·ca·tion (ē-ther′i-fi-kā′shŭn). Eterificação; conversão de um álcool em um éter.

ether·i·za·tion (ē′ther-i-zā′shŭn). Eterização; administração de éter dietílico para produzir anestesia.

ethi·a·zide (e-thī′ă-zīd). Etiazida; um diurético.

eth·i·cal (eth′i-kăl). Ético; relativo à ética; em conformidade com as regras que governam a conduta pessoal e profissional.

eth·ics (eth′iks). Ética; o ramo da filosofia que lida com a distinção entre certo e errado, com as consequências morais das ações humanas. [G. *ethikos*, originário dos costumes, de *ethos*, costume]
  medical e., é. médica; os princípios da conduta profissional adequada relativos aos direitos e deveres do médico, dos pacientes e dos colegas de profissão, bem como às ações do médico no tratamento dos pacientes e no relacionamento com suas famílias.

eth·i·dene (eth′i-dēn). Etideno. SIN ethylidene.

ethid·i·um (eth-id′ē-ŭm). Etídio. SIN homidium bromide.

ethid·i·um bro·mide (e-thid′ē-ŭm). Brometo de etídio; um fluorocromo sensível que se liga ao DNA; usado em citoquímica e eletroforese.

ethin·drone (e-thin′drōn). Etindrona. SIN ethisterone.

eth·i·nyl (e-thī′nil). Etinil. SIN ethynyl.
  e. trichloride, tricloreto de e. SIN trichloroethylene.

eth·i·nyl·es·tre·nol (eth′i-nil-es′tre-nol). Etinilestrenol. SIN lynestrenol.

eth·i·o·dized oil (eth-ī′ō-dīzd). Óleo etiodado; meio radiopaco usado antigamente para linfangiografia e histerossalpingografia.

eth·i·on·am·ide (eth′i̇̄on-ă-mīd). Etionamida; medicamento antituberculoso de segunda linha. Os efeitos colaterais são comuns, as manifestações mais comuns são gastrointestinais.

ethi·o·nine (e-thī′ō-nēn). Etionina; um análogo e antagonista da metionina, que difere na presença de um grupamento *S*-etil no lugar do grupo *S*-metil.

ethis·ter·one (e-this′ter-ōn). Etisterona; esteróide semi-sintético efetivo por via oral, que tem efeitos biológicos semelhantes aos da progesterona. SIN ethindrone, pregneninolone.

ethmo-. Etmo-; forma combinante que designa: **1.** Etmóide. **2.** O osso etmóide. [G. *ēthmos*, crivo]

eth·mo·cra·ni·al (eth-mō-krā′nē-ăl). Etmocraniano; relativo ao osso etmóide e ao crânio como um todo.

eth·mo·fron·tal (eth-mō-fron′tăl). Etmofrontal; relativo aos ossos etmóide e frontal.

eth·moid (eth′moyd) [TA]. Etmóide. VER ethmoid *bone*. SIN os ethmoidale [TA]. [G. *ēthmos*, crivo, + *eidos*, semelhança]

eth·moi·dal (eth-moy′dăl). Etmoidal; etmóideo; semelhante a um crivo.

eth·moi·da·le (eth-moy-da′lē). Etmoidal; ponto cefalométrico na fossa anterior do crânio localizado no ponto sagital mais baixo da lâmina cribriforme do osso etmóide.

eth·moi·dec·to·my (eth-moy-dek′tō-mē). Etmoidectomia; remoção completa ou parcial da mucosa de revestimento e das divisões ósseas entre os seios etmoidais. [ethmo- + G. *ektomē*, excisão]

eth·moid·i·tis (eth-moy-dī′tis). Etmoidite; inflamação dos seios etmoidais.

eth·mo·lac·ri·mal (eth-mō-lak′ri-măl). Etmolacrimal; relativo aos ossos etmóide e lacrimal.

eth·mo·max·il·lary (eth-mō-mak′si-lā-rē). Etmomaxilar; relativo aos ossos etmóide e maxilar.

eth·mo·na·sal (eth-mō-nā′săl). Etmonasal; relativo aos ossos etmóide e nasal.

eth·mo·pal·a·tal (eth-mō-pal′ă-tăl). Etmopalatino; relativo aos ossos etmóide e palatino.

eth·mo·sphe·noid (eth-mō-sfē′noyd). Etmoesfenóide; relativo aos ossos etmóide e esfenóide.

eth·mo·tur·bi·nals (eth-mō-ter′bi-nalz). Etmoturbinados; as conchas do osso etmóide; as conchas superior e média; algumas vezes existe uma terceira, a concha suprema.

eth·mo·vo·mer·ine (eth′mō-vō′mer-in). Etmovomerino; relativo ao osso etmóide e ao vômer.

eth·nic group (eth′nik). Grupo étnico; grupo social caracterizado por uma tradição social e cultural distinta mantida de geração a geração, história e origem comuns e um sentimento de identificação com o grupo; os membros do grupo possuem características distintas em seu modo de vida, experiências comuns e, freqüentemente, uma herança genética comum; essas características podem ser refletidas em sua vivência de saúde e doença.

eth·no·cen·trism (eth-nō-sen′trizm). Etnocentrismo; a tendência de avaliar outros grupos de acordo com os valores e padrões do próprio grupo étnico, particularmente com a convicção de que o próprio grupo étnico é superior aos outros grupos. [G. *ethnos*, raça, tribo, + *kentron*, centro de um círculo]

eth·nol·o·gy (eth-nol′ō-jē). Etnologia; a ciência que compara a cultura e/ou as raças humanas; antropologia cultural.

eth·no·phar·ma·col·o·gy (eth′nō-farm-ă-kol′ō-jē). Etnofarmacologia; o estudo das diferenças na resposta a drogas baseado em etnicidades variadas; farmacogenética.

eth·o·hep·ta·zine cit·rate (eth-ō-hep′tă-zēn). Citrato de etoeptazina; um analgésico obsoleto.

eth·o·hex·a·di·ol (eth′ō-hek-să-dī′ol, -hek-sā′dī-ol). Etoexadiol; usado como repelente de insetos.

ethol·o·gist (ē-thol′ō-jist). Etologista; especialista em etologia.

ethol·o·gy (ē-thol′ō-jē). Etologia; o estudo do comportamento animal. [G. *ethos*, caráter, hábito, + *logos*, estudo]

eth·o·mox·ane (eth-ō-mok′sān). Etomoxano; agente ansiolítico. SIN ethoxybutamoxane.

eth·o·phar·ma·col·o·gy (eth′ō-far-mă-kol′ō-jē). Etofarmacologia; o estudo dos efeitos dos medicamentos sobre o comportamento, baseado na observação e na descrição de elementos espécie-específicos (atitudes e posturas durante encontros sociais). VER TAMBÉM pharmacogenetics. [G. *ethos*, caráter, hábito, + pharmacology]

eth·o·pro·pa·zine hy·dro·chlo·ride (eth-ō-prō′pă-zēn). Cloridrato de etopropazina; um agente anticolinérgico com alguma atividade bloqueadora anti-histamínica e bloqueadora ganglionar. SIN profenamine hydrochloride.

eth·o·sux·i·mide (eth-ō-sŭk′si-mīd). Etossuximida; anticonvulsivante usado no controle da epilepsia com ausência (pequeno mal); algumas vezes há lesão da medula óssea e anemia aplásica.

eth·o·to·in (eth-ō-tō′in). Etotoína; anticonvulsivante usado no tratamento da epilepsia tônico-clônica generalizada.

eth·o·tri·mep·ra·zine (eth′ō-trī-mep′ră-zēn). Etotrimeprazina. SIN etymemazine.

ethox·a·zene hy·dro·chlo·ride (e-thok′să-zēn). Cloridrato de etoxazeno; um composto azo.

eth·oxy (e-thok′sē). Etoxi; o radical monovalente, CH_3CH_2O—.

eth·ox·y·bu·ta·mox·ane (eth-ok′si-bū-tă-mok′sān). Etoxibutamoxano. SIN ethomoxane.

eth·ox·y·zol·a·mide (eth-ok-sē-zol′ă-mīd). Etoxizolamida; diurético relacionado, química e farmacologicamente, à acetazolamida.

eth·yl (Et) (eth′il). Etila; o radical hidrocarboneto, CH_3CH_2—.
  e. alcohol, álcool etílico. SIN alcohol (2).
  e. aminobenzoate, aminobenzoato de etila. SIN benzocaine.
  e. biscoumacetate, biscoumacetato de etila; anticoagulante quimicamente relacionado à bisidroxicumarina e ao warfarin.
  e. butyrate, butirato de etila; usado em perfumaria.
  e. carbamate, carbamato de etila. SIN urethan.
  e. chloride, cloreto de etila; líquido explosivo muito volátil (pressurizado); quando vaporizado sobre a pele, produz anestesia local por congelamento superficial, mas também é um potente anestésico inalatório. SIN chloroethane.
  e. formate, formiato de etila; líquido volátil, inflamável, usado como fumegante, larvicida agrícola e fungicida; também usado como flavorizante.
  e. oleate, oleato de etila; veículo alternativo em injeções de acetato de desoxicorticosterona, menaftona, etc.
  e. oxide, óxido de etila. SIN diethyl ether.
  e. salicylate, salicilato de etila; o éster do ácido salicílico do álcool etílico, com a mesma ação que o salicilato de metila.

eth·yl·ate (eth′i-lāt). Etilato; substância na qual o hidrogênio do grupamento hidroxila do etanol é substituído por um átomo metálico, geralmente sódio ou potássio; p. ex., C_2H_5ONa, etilato de sódio.

eth·yl·benz·tro·pine (eth′il-benz-trō′pēn). Etilbenzatropina; agente anticolinérgico.

eth·yl·cel·lu·lose (eth-il-sel′ŭ-lōs). Etilcelulose; um éter etílico da celulose, usado no revestimento de comprimidos.

eth·yl·di·chlo·ro·ar·sine (ED) (eth′il-dī-klōr-ō-ar′sēn). Etildicloroarsina; $C_2H_5AsCl_2$; agente vesicante usado na I Guerra Mundial; irritante para as vias respiratórias.

eth·yl·ene (eth′i-lēn). Etileno; constituinte explosivo do gás de iluminação comum; acelera o amadurecimento de frutas.
  e. oxide, óxido de etileno; fumegante, usado para esterilização a frio de instrumentos cirúrgicos. SIN oxirane.
  e. tetrachloride, tetracloreto de etileno. SIN tetrachlorethylene.

eth·yl·ene·di·a·mine (eth'i-lēn-dī'ă-mēn). Etilenodiamina; líquido incolor volátil de odor amoniacal e sabor cáustico; o dicloridrato é usado como acidificante da urina. Combinada à teofilina para produzir aminofilina, um sal hidrossolúvel adequado para administração intravenosa ou retal. SIN ethanediamine.

eth·yl·ene·di·a·mine·tet·ra·a·ce·tic ac·id (EDTA) (eth'il-ēn-dī'ă-mēn-tet-ră-ă-sē'tik). Ácido etilenodiaminotetracético; agente quelante usado para remover cátions multivalentes de soluções como quelatos, e empregado em pesquisa bioquímica para retirar Mg^{2+}, Fe^{2+}, etc., de reações afetadas por esses íons. Na forma de sal sódico, usado como abrandador da água, para estabilizar drogas rapidamente decompostas na presença de traços de íons metálicos, e como anticoagulante; na forma de sal sódico de cálcio, usado para retirar o rádio, o chumbo, o estrôncio, o plutônio e o cádmio do tecido duro, formando compostos solúveis não-ionizados estáveis, que são excretados pelos rins. Cf. EGTA. SIN edathamil, edetic acid.

eth·yl·ene di·bro·mide. Etilenodibrometo; composto usado em gasolinas antidetonantes. Causa forte irritação cutânea; pode produzir bolhas. A inalação causa lesões pulmonares tardias. A exposição prolongada também pode resultar em lesão hepática e renal. Pode ser um carcinógeno humano.

eth·yl·ene gly·col. Etilenoglicol. VER glycol (2).

eth·yl·es·tre·nol (eth-il-es'tre-nol). Etilestrenol; esteróide anabólico semi-sintético, eficaz por via oral.

eth·yl ether. Éter etílico. SIN diethyl ether.

eth·yl green. Verde de etila. SIN brilliant green.

eth·yl·i·dene (eth-il'i-dēn). Etilideno; etideno; o radical $CH_3CH=$. SIN ethidene.

eth·yl·i·dyne (eth-il'i-dīn). Etilidina; o radical $CH_3C≡$.

eth·yl·mor·phine hy·dro·chlo·ride (eth-il-mōr'fēn). Cloridrato de etilmorfina; o éster etílico da morfina; antiespasmódico, antitussígeno e analgésico narcótico, usado localmente como linfagogo irritante na doença catarral crônica da orelha média, rinite atrófica e doenças oculares dolorosas (irite, úlcera da córnea, etc.).

eth·yl·nor·ep·i·neph·rine (E.N.E., E.N.S.) (eth'il-nōr-ep-i-nef'rin). Etilnorepinefrina; simpaticomimético, usado na asma; não eleva a pressão arterial.

eth·yl·pa·pav·er·ine hy·dro·chlo·ride (eth'il-pa-pav'er-ēn). Cloridrato de etilpapaverina. SIN ethaverine hydrochloride.

eth·yl·par·a·ben (eth-il-par'ă-ben). Etilparabeno; preservativo antifúngico.

eth·yl·phen·yl·eph·rine hy·dro·chlo·ride (eth'il-fen-il-ef'rēn). Cloridrato de etilfenilefrina. SIN etilefrine hydrochloride.

eth·yl·stib·a·mine (eth-il-stib'ă-mēn). Etilestibamina; composto orgânico sintético do antimônio.

ethy·no·di·ol (ē-thī-nō-dī'ol). Etinodiol; esteróide semi-sintético, efetivo por via oral, com efeitos biológicos muito semelhantes aos da progesterona; além disso, é fracamente estrogênico e androgênico; administrado em associação com um estrogênio como contraceptivo oral.

e. diacetate, diacetato de e.; agente antifertilidade, geralmente usado em combinação com o mestranol.

ethy·nyl (e-thī'nil). Etinil; o radical monovalente $HC≡C-$. SIN acetenyl, ethinyl.

eti·do·caine (e-tī'dō-kān). Etidocaína; anestésico local.

eti·dro·nate di·so·di·um (e-ti-drō'nāt). Etidronato dissódico; droga que afeta a reabsorção óssea, usada no tratamento da doença de Paget, ossificação heterotópica e hipercalcemia da malignidade.

eti·dron·ic ac·id (e-ti-dron'ik). Ácido etidrônico; usado como regulador do cálcio, geralmente na forma do sal etidronato dissódico.

et·il·ef·rine hy·dro·chlo·ride (et-il-ef'rin). Cloridrato de etilefrina; amina simpaticomimética vasopressora. SIN ethylphenylephrine hydrochloride.

♻ **etio-.** Etio-. **1.** Prefixo usado com (p. ex.) colano para indicar substituição da cadeia lateral C-17 por H; assim, etiocolano é o isômero 5β do androstano. **2.** Forma combinante que significa causa. [G. *aitia*, causa]

eti·o·cho·lan·o·lone (ē'tē-ō-kō-lan'ō-lōn). Etiocolanolona; metabólito de hormônios adrenocorticais e testiculares, e um importante 17-cetosteróide urinário; causa febre quando administrada a seres humanos.

eti·o·gen·ic (ē'tē-ō-jen'ik). Etiogênico; de natureza causal. [G. *aitis*, causa, + *genesis*, produção]

eti·o·lat·ed (ē'tē-ō-lāt-ed). Etiolado; sujeito a, ou caracterizado por, etiolamento.

eti·o·la·tion (ē-tē-ō-lā'shŭn). Etiolamento. **1.** Palidez resultante da ausência de luz, como em pessoas confinadas devido a doença ou aprisionamento, ou em plantas descoradas por serem privadas de luz. **2.** O processo de descoramento ou empalidecimento por supressão da luz. [Fr. *étioler*, estiolar, branquear]

eti·o·log·ic (ē'tē-ō-loj'ik). Etiológico; relativo a etiologia.

eti·ol·o·gy (ē-tē-ol'ō-jē). Etiologia. **1.** A ciência e o estudo das causas das doenças e seu modo de ação. Cf. pathogenesis. **2.** A ciência das causas, causalidade; em uso comum, causa. [G. *aitia*, causa, + *logos*, tratado, discurso]

eti·o·path·ic (ē'tē-ō-path'ik). Etiopático; referente a lesões específicas relacionadas com a causa de uma doença. [G. *aitia*, causa, + pathology]

eti·o·pa·thol·o·gy (ē'tē-ō-pă-thol'ō-jē). Etiopatologia, consideração da causa de um estado ou achado anormal. [G. *aitia*, causa, + pathology]

eti·o·por·phy·rin (ē'tē-ō-pōr'fi-rin). Etioporfirina; um derivado da porfirina caracterizado pela presença, em cada um dos quatro anéis pirróis, de um grupamento metila e um grupamento etila; assim, pode haver quatro formas isoméricas.

eti·o·tro·pic (ē'tē-ō-trop'ik). Etiotrópico; voltado contra a causa; designa um remédio que atenua ou destrói o fator causador de uma doença. [G. *aitia*, causa, + *tropē*, volta]

eto·fam·ide (ē-tō'fă-mīd). Etofamida; amebicida intraluminal semelhante ao teclozano e à diloxanida.

etom·i·date (ē-tom'i-dāt). Etomidato; potente hipnótico intravenoso usado em anestesia.

eto·po·side (e-tō-pō'sīd). Etoposídeo; derivado semi-sintético da podofilotoxina; inibidor mitótico usado no tratamento de tumores testiculares refratários, câncer pulmonar de pequenas células e outros cânceres.

etor·phine (et-ōr-fēn). Etorfina; analgésico narcótico que possui uma potência cerca de 1.000 vezes maior que a da morfina; usada em dardos tranqüilizantes.

et·o·zo·lin (et-ō-zō'lin). Etozolina; diurético.

ETP Abreviatura de electron transport *particles* (partículas transportadoras de elétrons) em *particle*.

etret·i·nate (e-tret'i-nāt). Etretinato; retinóide usado no tratamento da psoríase recalcitrante grave.

et·y·mem·a·zine (et-i-mem'ă-zēn). Etimemazina; anti-histamínico. SIN ethotrimeprazine.

Eu Símbolo do europium (európio).

♻ **eu-.** Eu-; bom, bem; oposto de dis-, caco-. [G.]

eu·al·leles (ū'ă-lēlz). Eualelos; genes que sofreram diferentes substituições de nucleotídeos na mesma posição. Cf. heteroalleles.

Eu·bac·te·ri·a·les (ū'bak-tē-rē-ā'lēz). Nome obsoleto para uma ordem de bactérias que continham células rígidas, indiferenciadas, simples, que eram esféricas ou bastonetes retos. A ordem continha espécies móveis (peritríquias) e imóveis, Gram-negativas e Gram-positivas, e formadoras de esporos e não-formadoras de esporos. Continha 13 famílias: Achromobacteriaceae, Azotobacteriaceae, Bacillaceae, Bacteroidaceae, Brevibacteriaceae, Brucellaceae, Corynebacteriaceae, Enterobacteriaceae, Lactobacillaceae, Micrococcaceae, Neisseriaceae, Propionibacteriaceae e Rhizobacteriaceae.

Eu·bac·te·ri·um (ū'bak-tēr'ē-ŭm). Gênero que contém mais de 40 espécies de bactérias anaeróbicas, não-formadoras de esporos, imóveis, contendo bastonetes Gram-positivos retos ou curvos que geralmente ocorrem isoladamente, em pares ou em cadeias curtas. Geralmente esses microrganismos atacam carboidratos. Podem ser patogênicos e raramente estão associados a sépsis intra-abdominal em seres humanos. A espécie típica é *E. limosum*.

E. aerofa'ciens, espécie bacteriana raramente encontrada no intestino de seres humanos; patogênica para camundongos.

E. combe'si, espécie bacteriana do solo florestal encontrada em uma área então denominada África Ocidental Francesa; não é patogênica para cobaias ou camundongos. Antigamente era denominada *Cillobacterium combesi*.

E. contor'tum, espécie bacteriana encontrada em casos de apendicite gangrenosa pútrida e nos intestinos.

E. crispa'tum, nome antigo de *Lactobacillus crispatus*.

E. filamento'sum, nome antigo de *Clostridium ramosum*.

E. len'tum, espécie bacteriana comumente encontrada nas fezes de pessoas normais; causa ocasional de septicemia e infecções hospitalares.

E. limo'sum, espécie bacteriana encontrada nas fezes humanas e, provavelmente, nas fezes de outros animais de sangue quente. A espécie típica do gênero.

E. minu'tum, espécie bacteriana raramente encontrada no intestino de lactentes (leite materno); originalmente encontrada em um caso de diarréia do lactente; é patogênica para camundongos.

E. monilifor'me, espécie bacteriana raramente encontrada nas vias respiratórias de seres humanos; é patogênica para cobaias, causando morte em oito dias. Antigamente era denominada *Cillobacterium moniliforme*.

E. par'vum, espécie bacteriana encontrada no intestino grosso de um cavalo e em um caso de apendicite aguda; raramente encontrada no intestino de potros e seres humanos, e não é patogênica para animais de laboratório.

E. poeciloi'des, espécie bacteriana raramente encontrada no intestino de seres humanos; originalmente encontrada em um caso de oclusão intestinal; é patogênica para cobaias e coelhos.

E. pseudotortuo'sum, espécie bacteriana encontrada em um caso de apendicite aguda, purulenta; raramente encontrada no intestino.

E. quar'tum, espécie bacteriana encontrada em casos de diarréia do lactente; encontrada no intestino de crianças, mas é algo incomum.

E. quin'tum, espécie bacteriana encontrada em casos de diarréia do lactente; patogênica para cobaias.

E. recta'le, espécie bacteriana encontrada em associação com uma úlcera retal; encontrada no reto.

E. ten'ue, espécie bacteriana isolada das fezes de cães; sua patogenicidade é desconhecida; antigamente era denominada *Cillobacterium tenue*.

E. tortuo'sum, espécie bacteriana raramente encontrada no intestino de seres humanos.

eu·bi·ot·ics (ū-bī-ot'iks). Eubiótica; a ciência de viver de forma sadia. [eu- + G. *biotikos*, relativo à vida]

eu·caine (ū'kān). Eucaína; anestésico local.

eu·ca·lyp·tol (ū-kă-lip'tol). Eucaliptol. SIN cineole.

eu·ca·lyp·tus (ū-kă-lip'tŭs). Eucalipto; as folhas secas do *Eucalyptus globulus* (família Myrtaceae), a goma azul ou a árvore da febre australiana.

e. oil, óleo de e.; o óleo volátil destilado com vapor das folhas frescas de *Eucalyptus*; contém pelo menos 70% de eucaliptol; usado como anti-séptico e expectorante em pastilhas para tosse e vaporizadores aromáticos.

eu·cap·nia (ū-kap'nē-ă). Eucapnia; um estado no qual a pressão arterial de dióxido de carbono é ótima. VER TAMBÉM normocapnia. [eu- + G. *kapnos*, vapor]

eu·car·y·ote (ū-kar'ē-ōt). Eucarioto. SIN eukaryote. [eu- + G. *karyon*, cerne, núcleo]

eu·car·y·ot·ic (ū-kar-ē-ot'ik). Eucariótico. SIN eukaryotic.

eu·ca·sin (ū-kā'sin). Eucasina; caseinato de amônio preparado pela passagem do gás amoníaco sobre a caseína seca finamente pulverizada; acrescentada como alimento concentrado ao caldo de carne, chocolate, etc.

eu·cat·ro·pine hy·dro·chlo·ride (ū-kat'rō-pēn). Cloridrato de eucatropina; não produz anestesia, dor, nem aumento da pressão intra-ocular.

Eu·ces·to·da (ū-ses-tō'dă). SIN Cestoda.

eu·chlor·hy·dria (ū-klōr-hi'drē-ă). Eucloridria; condição na qual o ácido clorídrico livre é encontrado em quantidade normal no suco gástrico. [eu- + cholohydric (acid) + -ia]

eu·cho·lia (ū-kō'lē-ă). Eucolia; estado normal da bile em relação ao volume e qualidade. [eu- + G. *cholē*, bile]

eu·chro·mat·ic (ū-krō-mat'ik). Eucromático. **1.** SIN orthochromatic. **2.** Característico da eucromatina.

eu·chro·ma·tin (ū-krō'mă-tin). Eucromatina; as partes de cromossomas que, durante a interfase, são filamentos dispersos não-espiralados e não-corados por corantes habituais; metabolicamente ativa, ao contrário da heterocromatina inerte.

eu·chro·mo·some (ū-krō'mō-sōm). Eucromossoma. SIN autosome.

Eucoleus (ū-kō'lē-us). Um dos três gêneros de nematódeos tricurídeos, comumente denominados *Capillaria*.

eu·cor·ti·cal·ism (ū-kōr'ti-kăl-izm). Eucorticalismo; funcionamento normal do córtex supra-renal.

eu·cra·sia (ū-krā'zhē-ă). Eucrasia. **1.** Termo obsoleto para homeostasia. **2.** Termo obsoleto para uma condição de redução da suscetibilidade aos efeitos adversos de determinados medicamentos, alimentos, etc. [G. *eukrasia*, bom temperamento, de *eu*, bem, + *krasis*, mistura]

eu·cu·pine (ū'koo-pēn). Eucupina. SIN euprocin hydrochloride.

eu·di·a·pho·re·sis (ū-dī'ă-fō-rē'sis). Eudiaforese; sudorese livre normal. [eu- + G. *diaphorēsis*, transpiração]

eu·dip·sia (ū-dip'sē-ă). Eudipsia; sede moderada comum. [eu- + G. *dipsa*, sede]

Eu·flag·el·la·ta (ū-flaj'ĕ-lā'tă). Termo antigo para designar os protozoários flagelados agora incluídos no subfilo Mastigophora.

eu·gen·ic (ū-jen'ik). Eugênico; relativo a eugenia.

eu·gen·ic ac·id. Ácido eugênico. SIN eugenol.

eu·gen·ics (ū-jen'iks). Eugenia. **1.** Práticas e políticas, como de seleção do parceiro ou de esterilização, que tendem a melhorar as qualidades inatas da descendência e da espécie humana. **2.** Práticas e aconselhamento genético voltados para prever deficiências e doenças genéticas. SIN orthogenics. [G. *eugeneia*, nobreza de nascimento, de *eu*, bem, + *genesis*, produção]

eu·gen·ism (ū'jen-izm). Eugenismo; a crença de que a espécie humana pode ser aperfeiçoada através de cruzamentos seletivos.

eu·ge·nol (ū'je-nol). Eugenol; obtido do óleo de cravo; usado em odontologia com óxido de zinco como analgésico e como base para materiais de impressão; também usado em perfumaria como substituto do óleo de cravo. SIN eugenic acid.

Eu·gle·na (ū-glē'nă). Gênero disseminado de flagelados da água doce, de vida livre, fotossensibilizadores (família Euglinidae). [eu- + G. *glēnē*, bulbo do olho]

E. grac'ilis, espécie abundante, algumas vezes usada na determinação das concentrações de vitamina B_{12} no soro e na urina em vários tipos de anemia.

E. vir'idis, espécie que habita águas estagnadas, freqüentemente em grande número.

Eu·gle·ni·dae (ū-glē'ni-dē). Família de flagelados verdes (fitomônadas) (subfilo Mastigophora, classe Phytomastigophorea).

eu·glob·u·lin (ū-glob'ū-lin). Euglobulina; a fração da globulina sérica solúvel em soluções salinas isotônicas e menos solúvel em solução de $(NH_4)_2SO_4$ que a fração pseudoglobulina.

eu·gly·ce·mia (ū-glī-sē'mē-ă). Euglicemia; concentração sanguínea normal de glicose. SIN normoglycemia. [eu- + G. *glykys*, doce, + *haima*, sangue]

eu·gly·ce·mic (ū-glī-sē'mik). Euglicêmico; que designa, é característico de, ou promove euglicemia. SIN normoglycemic.

eu·gna·thia (ū-nā'thē-ă, -nath'ē-ă). Eugnatia; anormalidade limitada aos dentes e às suas sustentações alveolares imediatas. SIN eugnathic anomaly. [eu- + G. *gnathos*, mandíbula]

eu·gno·sia (ū-nō'sē-ă). Eugnosia; capacidade normal de sintetizar estímulos sensoriais. [eu- + G. *gnōsis*, percepção]

eu·gon·ic (ū-gon'ik). Eugônico; termo usado para indicar que o crescimento de uma cultura bacteriana é rápido e relativamente exuberante; usado especialmente em referência ao crescimento de culturas do bacilo da tuberculose humana (*Mycobacterium tuberculosis*). VER TAMBÉM dysgonic. [G. *eugonos*, produtivo, de *eu*, bem, + *gonos*, semente, descendência]

Eu·gre·ga·rin·i·da (ū'greg-ă-rin'i-dă). Ordem das gregarinas (subclasse Gregarinia), que se reproduzem apenas por esporogonia, na qual não há esquizogonia; são parasitas de anelídeos e artrópodes. [eu- + L. *gregarius*, gregário]

eu·hy·dra·tion (ū-hī-drā'shŭn). Euidratação; estado normal de conteúdo de água corporal; ausência de hidratação ou desidratação absoluta ou relativa.

Eu·kar·y·o·tae, Eu·car·y·o·tae (ū-kar-ē-ō'tē). Eucariotos; super-reino de organismos caracterizados por células eucarióticas; membros acelulares (reino Protoctista) são caracterizados por uma única unidade eucariótica; membros mais complexos (multicelulares) foram designados para os reinos Fungi, Plantae e Animalia.

eu·kar·y·ote (ū-kar'ē-ōt). Eucarioto. **1.** Uma célula contendo um núcleo ligado à membrana com cromossomas de DNA, RNA e proteínas, na maioria das vezes grandes (10–100 μm), com a divisão celular envolvendo uma forma de mitose da qual participam os fusos mitóticos (ou algum arranjo de microtúbulos); há mitocôndrias, e, nas espécies que realizam fotossíntese, são encontrados plastídeos; os ondulipódios (cílios ou flagelos) possuem organização 9+2 complexa de tubulina e várias proteínas. A presença de uma célula do tipo eucariota caracteriza os quatro reinos acima da Monera ou nível procarioto de complexidade: Protoctista, Fungi, Plantae e Animalia, combinados no super-reino Eukaryotae. **2.** Nome comum de membros do Eukaryotae. SIN eucaryote. [eu- + G. *karyon*, cerne, núcleo]

eu·kar·y·ot·ic (ū'kar-ē-ot'ik). Eucariótico; relativo a, ou característico de, um eucarioto. SIN eucaryotic.

eu·ker·a·tin (ū-kār'ă-tin). Euqueratina; queratina dura presente no cabelo, lã, chifre, unhas, etc.

eu·ki·ne·sia (ū-ki-nē'zē-ă). Eucinesia; movimento normal. [eu- + G. *kinēsis*, movimento]

Eulenburg, Albert, neurologista alemão, 1840–1917. VER E. *disease*.

eu·mel·a·nin (ū-mel'ă-nin). Eumelanina; o tipo mais abundante de melanina humana, encontrada na pele e no cabelo de pessoas morenas e negras; polímeros de ligação cruzada de 5,6-diidroxindóis, geralmente ligados a proteínas; os níveis estão diminuídos em alguns tipos de albinismo. [eu- + G. *melos* (melan-), preto]

eu·mel·a·no·some (ū-mel'ă-nō-sōm). Eumelanossoma. SIN melanosome.

eu·me·tria (ū-mē'trē-ă). Eumetria; graduação da intensidade de impulsos nervosos para atender às necessidades. [G. moderação, generosidade de medida]

eu·mor·phism (ū-mōr'fizm). Eumorfismo; preservação da forma natural de uma célula. [eu- + G. *morphē*, forma]

eu·my·cetes (ū-mī-sē'tēz). Eumicetos; os fungos verdadeiros. [eu- + G. *mykēs*, fungo]

eumycetoma (oo-mī-set-ō'mă). Eumicetoma; micetoma causado por fungos. Cf. actinomycetoma.

Eu·my·ce·to·zo·ea (ū'mī-sē-tō-zō'ē-ă). Eumicetozoários; formas animais microscópicas, freqüentemente conhecidas como animais do lodo, que consistem em uma massa semilíquida irregular de protoplasma ameboide multinucleada; embora sejam agrupados como uma classe da superclasse Rhizopoda (subfilo Sarcodina), algumas das formas de micetozoários são muito semelhantes a determinadas espécies de pseudomicetos e, algumas vezes, são classificados como membros dos Myxomycetes, os fungos do lodo. VER TAMBÉM Proteomyxidia. [eu- + G. *mykēs* (mykēt-), fungo, + *zōon*, animal]

eu·nuch (ū'nŭk). Eunuco; indivíduo do sexo masculino cujos testículos foram removidos ou nunca se desenvolveram. [G. *eunouchos*, camareiro, de *eunē*, cama, + *eklō*, ter]

eu·nuch·ism (ū'nŭk-izm). Eunuquismo. **1.** O estado de ser um eunuco; ausência dos testículos ou ausência de desenvolvimento ou funcionamento das gônadas, com conseqüente ausência de função reprodutiva e sexual e de desenvolvimento de características sexuais secundárias. **2.** SIN eunuchoidism.

eu·nuch·oid (ū'nŭ-koyd). Eunucóide; semelhante a, ou que possui as características gerais de, um eunuco; geralmente indica o tipo físico de um homem que sofreu hipogonadismo antes da puberdade. [G. *eunouchos*, eunuco, + *eidos*, semelhante]

eu·nuch·oi·dism (ū'nŭ-koyd-izm). Eunucoidismo; estado no qual os testículos estão presentes, mas não funcionam normalmente; pode ter origem gonadal ou hipofisária. SIN eunuchism (2), male hypogonadism.

hypergonadotropic e., e. hipergonadotrópico; eunucoidismo de origem gonadal, comumente acompanhado por níveis aumentados de gonadotropinas hipofisárias no sangue e na urina, como na síndrome de Klinefelter (Klinefelter *syndrome*).
hypogonadotropic e., e. hipogonadotrópico. SIN hypogonadotropic *hypogonadism.*
eu·os·mia (ū-oz'mē-ă). Euosmia. **1.** Um odor agradável. **2.** Olfato normal. [eu- + G. *osmē*, odor]
eu·pan·cre·a·tism (ū-pan'krē-ă-tizm). Eupancreatismo; o estado da função digestiva pancreática normal.
eu·pa·ral (ū'pa-răl). Euparal; um meio para montar amostras histológicas, composto de sandaraca, eucaliptol, paraldeído, cânfora e salicilato de fenila.
Eu·pa·ryph·i·um (ū-pa-rif'ē-ŭm) Gênero de trematódeos não-patogênicos (família Echinostomatidae), com várias espécies descritas no intestino dos seres humanos. [eu- + G. *paryphē*, uma borda]
eu·pav·er·in (ū-pav'ĕ-rin). Eupaverina; relaxante do músculo liso.
eu·pep·sia (ū-pep'sē-ă). Eupepsia; boa digestão. [G. de *eu*, bem + *pepsis*, digestão]
eu·pep·tic (ū-pep'tik). Eupéptico; que digere bem; que tem uma boa digestão.
eu·pep·tide (ū-pep'tīd). Eupeptídeo; um peptídeo que contém ligações peptídicas normais (entre grupamentos α-carboxila e grupos α-amino). Cf. isopeptide, peptide. [G. *eu-*, normall, habitual + peptide]
eu·phen·ics (ū-fē'niks). Eufenia; modificação do ambiente interno ou externo de um indivíduo de forma a evitar ou modificar a expressão fenotípica de um defeito genético, sem modificar o genótipo ou a herança. [eu- + G. *phainō*, demonstrar]
Eu·phor·bia pi·lu·lif·e·ra (ū-fōr'bē-ă pil-ū-lif'er-ă). Espécie de planta (família Euphorbiaceae); a erva seca tem sido usada na asma, coriza e outras afecções respiratórias, na angina de peito e como antiespasmódico. SIN asthma-weed (2).
eu·pho·ret·ic (ū-fō-ret'ik). Euforizante. SIN euphoriant.
eu·pho·ria (ū-fōr'ē-ă). Euforia; uma sensação de bem-estar, comumente exagerada e não necessariamente bem fundamentada. [eu- + G. *pherō*, suportar]
eu·pho·ri·ant (ū-fōr'ē-ant). Euforizante. **1.** Que possui a capacidade de produzir uma sensação de bem-estar. **2.** Agente que tem essa capacidade. SIN euphoretic.
eu·pla·sia (ū-plā'zē-ă). Euplasia; o estado de células ou tecidos que é normal ou característico daquele tipo específico. [eu- + G. *plassō*, formar]
eu·plas·tic (ū-plas'tik). Euplástico. **1.** Relativo à euplasia. **2.** Que cicatriza facilmente e bem. [G. *euplastos*, facilmente moldado; *eu*, bem, + *plastos*, formado]
eu·ploid (ū'ployd). Euplóide; relativo à euploidia.
eu·ploidy (ū'ploy-dē). Euploidia; o estado de uma célula que contém séries haplóides completas. [eu- + G. *-ploos*, -multiplicado]
eup·nea (ūp-nē'ă). Eupnéia; respiração fácil e livre; o tipo observado em um indivíduo normal em condições de repouso. [G. *eupnoia*, de *eu*, bem, + *pnoia*, respiração]
eu·prax·ia (ū-prak'sē-ă). Eupraxia; capacidade normal de realizar movimentos coordenados. [eu- + G. *praxis*, realização]
eu·pro·cin hy·dro·chlo·ride (ū'prō-sin). Cloridrato de euprocina; um derivado da quinina. SIN eucupine.
Eu·proc·tis (ū-prok'tis). Gênero de mariposa. Os pêlos do casulo e da lagarta da espécie *E. chrysorrhoea*, a mariposa de cauda castanha, causam a dermatite da lagarta. [eu- + G. *prōktos*, parte traseira]
eu·rhyth·mia (ū-rith'mē-ă). Eurritmia; relações corporais harmoniosas dos órgãos distintos. [eu- + G. *rhythmos*, ritmo]
eu·ro·pi·um (Eu) (ū-rō'pē-ŭm). Európio; elemento do grupo das terrasraras (lantanídeos), número atômico 63, peso atômico 151,965. [L. *Europa*, Europa]
△ **eury-.** Amplo, largo; oposto de esteno-. [G. *eurys*, largo]
euryblepharon (ū-rē-blef'ă-ron). Euribléfaro; anomalia congênita caracterizada por saculação da face lateral da pálpebra inferior distante do olho. [eury- + G. *blepharon*, pálpebra]
eu·ry·ce·phal·ic, eu·ry·ceph·a·lous (ū'rē-se-fal'ik, -sef'ă-lŭs). Euricefálico, euricéfalo; que possui uma cabeça anormalmente larga; algumas vezes usado em referência a uma cabeça braquicefálica. [eury- + G. *kephalē*, cabeça]
eu·ryg·nath·ic (ū-rig-nath'ik). Eurignático; que possui uma mandíbula larga. SIN eurygnathous.
eu·ryg·na·thism (ū-rig'nă-thizm). Eurignatismo; a condição de possuir uma mandíbula larga. [eury- + G. *gnathos*, mandíbula]
eu·ryg·na·thous (ū-rig'nă-thŭs). Eurignato. SIN eurygnathic.
eu·ry·on (ū'rē-on). Êurio; a extremidade, de qualquer lado, do maior diâmetro transverso da cabeça; ponto usado em craniometria. [G. *eurys*, largo]
eu·ry·op·ic (ū-rē-ōp'ik). Euriópico; de olhos afastados. VER blepharodiastasis. [eury- + G. *ops*, olho]

eu·ry·so·mat·ic (ū'rē-sō-mat'ik). Eurissomático; que possui um corpo atarracado. [eury- + G. *soma*, corpo]
eu·scope (ū'skōp). Euscópio; instrumento para mostrar em uma tela uma imagem aumentada de um microscópio. [eu- + G. *skopeō*, ver]
Eu·sim·u·li·um (ū-si-mū'lē-ŭm). SIN *Simulium.* [eu- + L. *simulo*, simular]
eu·sta·chi·an (ū-stā'shŭn, ū-stā'kē-ăn). De Eustáquio; descrito por, ou atribuído a, Eustáquio.
Eustachio, Bartolommeo E., anatomista italiano, 1524–1574. VER eustachian *catheter*, eustachian *cushion*, eustachian *tonsil*, *tuba* eustachiana, eustachian *tube*, eustachian *tuber*, eustachian *valve*.
eu·sta·chi·tis (ū-stā-kī'tis). Inflamação da mucosa da tuba de Eustáquio (tuba auditiva).
eus·the·nia (ū-sthē'nē-ă). Eustenia; força normal. [eu- + G. *sthenos*, força]
eu·stron·gyl·oi·des (ū-stron-jil'oy-dēz). Eustrongilóide; nematódeo encontrado em peixes, anfíbios e répteis; infecções humanas, que se manifestam por sintomas gastrointestinais, são raras e estão relacionadas ao consumo de peixe cru; as larvas são vermelho-rosadas.
Eu·stron·gy·lus (ū-stron'ji-lŭs). Nome antigo de *Dioctophyma*. [eu- + G. *strongylos*, arredondado]
eu·sys·to·le (ū-sis'tō-lē). Eussistolia; uma condição na qual a sístole cardíaca é normal em força e tempo. [eu- + systole]
eu·sys·tol·ic (ū-sis-tol'ik). Eussistólico; relativo à eussistolia.
eu·tec·tic (ū-tek'tik). Eutético. **1.** Facilmente fundido; indica especificamente misturas de algumas substâncias químicas que possuem um menor ponto de fusão que qualquer um de seus ingredientes individuais; p. ex., um sólido, como o mentol, que, quando triturado com outro sólido da mesma classe, como a cânfora, se une a ele para formar um líquido, e a mistura possui um ponto de fusão menor que o de seus componentes. **2.** A liga que congela em uma temperatura constante; o mínimo da série. [eu- + G. *tēxis*, fundir]
eu·tha·na·sia (ū-thă-nā'zē-ă). Eutanásia. **1.** Uma morte indolor, silenciosa. **2.** Causar a morte intencional de uma pessoa com uma doença incurável ou dolorosa, como um ato de piedade. [eu- + G. *thanatos*, morte]
eu·then·ics (ū-then'iks). Eutenia; a ciência relacionada com o estabelecimento de condições de vida ideais para vegetais, animais ou seres humanos, principalmente através de provisões e ambiente adequados. [G. *eutheneō*, prosperar]
eu·ther·a·peu·tic (ū'thăr-ă-pū'tik). Euterapêutico; que possui excelentes propriedades curativas.
Eu·the·ria (ū-thē'rē-ă). Subclasse de mamíferos, excluindo os monotremados e marsupiais, que possuem uma placenta através da qual os conceptos são nutridos. [eu- + G. *thērion*, animal]
eu·ther·mic (ū-ther'mik). Eutérmico; em uma temperatura ideal. [eu- + G. *thermos*, quente]
eu·thy·mia (ū-thī'mē-ă). Eutimia. **1.** Alegria; paz e tranqüilidade mental. **2.** Moderação do humor, que não é maníaco nem depressivo. [eu- + G. *thymos*, mente]
eu·thy·mic (ū-thī'mik). Eutímico; relativo à ou caracterizado por, eutimia.
eu·thy·roid·ism (ū-thī'roy-dizm). Eutireoidismo; uma condição na qual a tireóide está funcionando normalmente, com secreção em quantidade e de constituição apropriadas.
eu·thy·scope (ū'thi-skōp). Eutiscópio; um oftalmoscópio modificado, raramente usado hoje, em que o local de fixação excêntrica pode ser ofuscado por uma luz brilhante enquanto a fóvea verdadeira é simultaneamente coberta por um disco opaco; usado em pleóptica. [G. *euthys*, reto, + *skopeō*, ver]
eu·thys·co·py (ū-this'kō-pē). Eutiscopia; exame com o eutiscópio.
eu·ton·ic (ū-ton'ik). Eutônico. SIN normotonic (1). [eu- + G. *tonos*, tônus]
eu·tri·cho·sis (ū-tri-kō'sis). Eutricose; crescimento normal de cabelo sadio. [eu- + G. *thrix*, cabelo]
eu·tro·phia (ū-trō'fē-ă). Eutrofia; estado de nutrição e crescimento normais. SIN eutrophy. [G. de *eu*, bem, + *trophē*, nutrição]
eu·tro·phic (ū-trof'ik). Eutrófico; relativo a, caracterizado por, ou que promove eutrofia.
eu·tro·phy (ū'trō-fē). Eutrofia. SIN eutrophia.
eu·vo·lia (ū-vō'lē-ă). Euvolia; conteúdo ou volume de água normal de determinado compartimento; p. ex., euvolia extracelular.
eV, ev Abreviatura de electron-volt (elétron-volt).
evac·u·ant (ē-vak'ū-ant). Evacuante. **1.** Que promove excreção, principalmente do intestino. **2.** Um agente que aumenta a excreção, principalmente um catártico.
evac·u·ate (ē-vak'ū-āt). Evacuar; realizar evacuação. [L. *e-vacuo*, pp. *-vacuatus*, esvaziar]
evac·u·a·tion (ē-vak-ū-ā'shŭn). Evacuação. **1.** Retirada de material, principalmente de resíduos do intestino por defecação. **2.** SIN stool (2). **3.** Retirada de ar de um recipiente fechado; produção de vácuo.
evac·u·a·tor (ē-vak'ū-ā-tŏr). Evacuador; um evacuador mecânico; instrumento para a remoção de líquido ou de pequenas partículas de uma cavidade corporal, ou de fezes impactadas do reto.
Ellik e., e. de Ellik; instrumento especial com receptáculo de vidro, bulbo de

látex ou plástico e tubulação flexível, usado para evacuar fragmentos de tecido, coágulos de sangue ou cálculos da bexiga.

evag·i·na·tion (ē-vaj-i-nā′shŭn). Evaginação; protrusão de alguma parte ou órgão de sua posição normal. [L. *e*, fora, + *vagina*, bainha]

eval·u·a·tion. Avaliação; apreciação objetiva, sistemática, da relevância, efetividade e impacto de atividades à luz de objetivos específicos.

ev·a·nes·cent (ev-ā-nes′ent). Evanescente; de curta duração. [L. *e*, fora, + *vanesco*, desaparecer]

Evans, Herbert M., anatomista e fisiologista norte-americano, 1882–1971. VER Evans blue.

Evans, Robert S., médico norte-americano, 1912–1974. VER E. *syndrome*.

Evans blue [C.I. 23860]. Azul de Evans; corante diazo usado para a determinação do volume sanguíneo com base na diluição de uma solução padrão do corante no plasma após sua injeção intravenosa; liga-se a proteínas e também é usado como corante vital para acompanhar a difusão através das paredes dos vasos sanguíneos. SIN azovan blue.

e·vap·o·rate (ē-vap′or-āt). Evaporar; causar ou sofrer evaporação. SIN volatilize.

evap·o·ra·tion (ē-vap-ō-ra′shŭn). Evaporação. **1.** Uma mudança da forma de líquido para a forma de vapor. **2.** Perda de volume de um líquido por conversão em vapor. SIN volatilization. [L. *e*, fora, + *vaporo*, emitir vapor]

eva·sion (ē-vā′zhŭn). Evasão; o ato de escapar, evitar ou imitar.
   macular e., e. macular. SIN *horror fusionis.*

event. Evento; ocorrência.
   sentinel e., e. sentinela; tipo de indicador clínico usado para monitorizar e avaliar a qualidade do tratamento, incluindo eventos que exigem atenção imediata.

even·tra·tion (ē′ven-trā′shŭn). Eventração. **1.** Protrusão do omento e/ou do intestino através de uma abertura na parede abdominal. SIN evisceration (4). **2.** Remoção do conteúdo da cavidade abdominal. [L. *e*, fora, + *venter*, ventre]
   e. of the diaphragm, e. do diafragma; elevação extrema de uma metade ou de uma parte do diafragma, que geralmente é atrófico e anormalmente fino.

ever·sion (ē-ver′zhŭn). Eversão; reviramento para fora, como da pálpebra ou do pé. [L. *e-everto*, pp. *-versus*, virar]

evert (ē-vert′). Everter; virar para fora. [L. *e-verto*, virar]

ev·i·ra·tion (ev-i-rā′shŭn, ē-vī-rā′shŭn). Eviração. **1.** Emasculação; castração. SIN *emasculation.* **2.** Perda ou ausência das características masculinas, com aquisição de características femininas; um tipo de efeminação. **3.** Crença delirante de um homem de que se tornou uma mulher. [L. *e*, fora, + *vir*, homem]

evis·cer·a·tion (ē-vis-er-ā′shŭn). Evisceração. **1.** Exenteração. SIN *exenteration.* **2.** O processo pelo qual o tecido ou os órgãos que geralmente residem em uma cavidade corporal são deslocados para fora dessa cavidade, em geral através de uma ruptura traumática da parede da cavidade; p. ex., evisceração do intestino. **3.** Remoção do conteúdo do bulbo do olho, deixando a esclera e, algumas vezes, a córnea. **4.** SIN *eventration (1).* [L. *eviscero*, desentranhar]

evis·cer·o·neu·rot·o·my (ē-vis′er-ō-noo-rot′ō-mē). Evisceroneurotomia; evisceração do olho com divisão do nervo óptico. [L. *eviscero*, desentranhar, + G. *neuron*, nervo, + *tomē*, corte]

evo·ca·tion (ev-ō-kā′shŭn, ē-vō-kā′shŭn). Evocação; indução de um tecido específico, produzida pela ação de um evocador durante a embriogênese. [L. *evoco*, pp. *evocatus*, evocar]

evo·ca·tor (ev′ō-kā-ter, -tōr). Evocador; um fator no controle da morfogênese na fase inicial de um embrião.

ev·o·lu·tion (ev-ō-loo′shŭn). Evolução. **1.** Um processo contínuo de mudança de um estado, condição ou forma para outro. **2.** Um distanciamento progressivo entre o genótipo e o fenótipo em uma linha de descendência. **3.** A liberação de um gás ou calor no decorrer de uma reação química ou enzimática. [L. *e-volvo*, pp. *-volutus*, estender]
   biologic e., e. biológica; a doutrina que afirma que todas as formas de vida animal ou vegetal são provenientes de alterações graduais de formas mais simples e, finalmente, de organismos unicelulares. SIN organic e.
   chemical e., e. química; a teoria do processo pelo qual a vida se originou da matéria inorgânica.
   coincidental e., e. concomitante. SIN concerted e.
   concerted e., e. concomitante; a capacidade de dois genes relacionados de evoluírem juntos, embora constituindo um único *locus*. SIN coincidental e.
   convergent e., e. convergente; o desenvolvimento evolutivo de estruturas semelhantes em duas ou mais espécies, amiúde muito diferentes filogeneticamente, em resposta a semelhanças do ambiente; p. ex., as estruturas semelhantes a asas em insetos, aves e mamíferos voadores.
   darwinian e., e. darwiniana; a proposição de que a filogenia de todas as espécies é completamente atribuível aos efeitos combinados da variação aleatória (mutação) nos genótipos dos membros de uma linhagem, em virtude da influência de acidentes não-dirigidos, com conseqüências para seus fenótipos, e da influência da sobrevida preferencial (embora não certa) daqueles fenótipos resultantes mais adequados para sobreviver no ambiente contemporâneo. O sistema proposto sobrevive principalmente devido aos fatores genéticos que conservam avidamente a ontogenia da linhagem.
   divergent e., e. divergente; o processo pelo qual uma espécie ou produto genético dá origem a dois ou mais produtos diferentes.
   emergent e., e. emergente; surgimento de uma propriedade em um sistema complexo, p. ex., organismo, que só poderia ter sido prevista com dificuldade, ou que talvez não poderia ter sido prevista, a partir do conhecimento e da compreensão das alterações individuais do genótipo consideradas separadamente.
   organic e., e. orgânica. SIN biologic e.
   saltatory e., e. saltatória; a teoria de que a evolução de uma nova espécie, a partir de uma espécie antiga pode ocorrer como um grande salto, tal como uma grande repadronização de cromossomas, ao invés de haver um acúmulo gradual de pequenos passos ou mutações. Cf. emergent e.
   spontaneous e., e. espontânea; o parto, sem auxílio, de um feto em posição transversa.

evul·sion (ē-vŭl′shŭn). Evulsão; arrancamento ou extração violenta. Cf. avulsion. [L. *evulsio*, de *e-vello*, pp. *-vulsus*, arrancar]

Ewart, William, médico inglês, 1848–1929. VER E. *procedure, sign*.

Ewing, James, patologista norte-americano, 1866–1943. VER E. *sarcoma, tumor*.

Ewing, James H., patologista, 1798–1827. VER E. *sign*.

Ewin·gel·la (oo′ing-el′ah). Gênero recém-nomeado de bactérias (família Enterobacteriaceae) que geralmente são móveis, produzem ácido, mas não gás, a partir da glicose, usam citrato como fonte de carbono e não produzem sulfeto de hidrogênio com açúcar triplo; a espécie típica é *E. americana*, encontrada nas vias respiratórias humanas e isolada de casos de septicemia, geralmente associada a sépsis polimicrobiana.

ex-. Ex-; fora de, saindo de, afastando-se de. [L. e G. fora de]

exa- (E). Exa-; prefixo usado nos sistemas SI e métrico para designar um quintilhão (10^{18}).

ex·ac·er·ba·tion (eg-zas-er-bā′shŭn, -ek-sas-). Exacerbação; agravamento de uma doença ou de qualquer um de seus sinais ou sintomas. [L. *exacerbo*, pp. *-atus*, agravar, aumentar, de *acerbus*, amargo]

ex·al·ta·tion (eks′al-tā′shŭn). Exaltação; declaração, discurso ou comunicação que transmitem um grande nível de satisfação, prazer e alegria.

ex·am·i·na·tion (eg-zam-i-nā′shŭn). Exame, análise, pesquisa; qualquer investigação ou inspeção feita para fins de diagnóstico; geralmente qualificada pelo método usado.

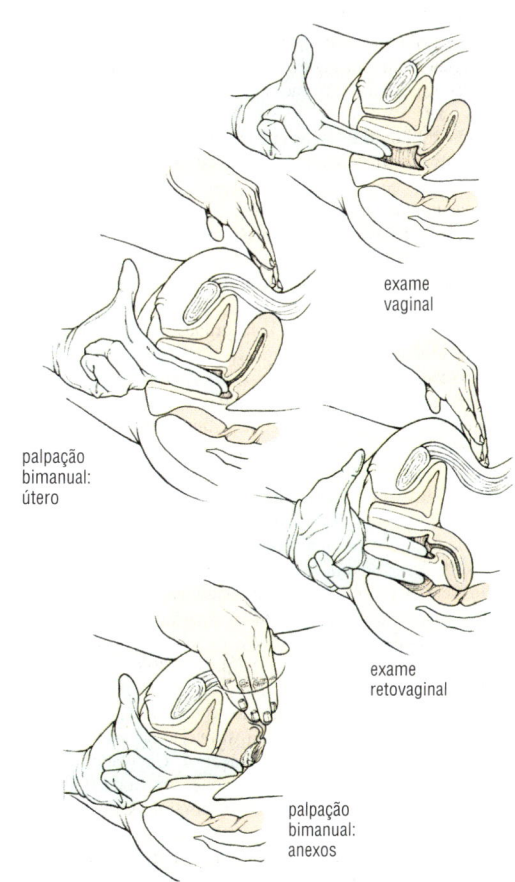

exame vaginal

palpação bimanual: útero

exame retovaginal

palpação bimanual: anexos

exame pélvico

cytologic e., e. citológico; exame microscópico de células, principalmente para diagnóstico de doença.
direct wet mount e., e. direto a fresco; revisão microscópica em aumentos pequeno (100×) e grande (400×) seco de uma amostra de fezes fresca e em solução fisiológica para detectar parasitas, incluindo trofozoítas protozoários móveis.
EMG e., e. por EMG; **(1)** parte do exame eletrodiagnóstico que usa eletrodos em agulha (sentido limitado); **(2)** sinônimo de todo exame eletrodiagnóstico, incluindo não apenas o exame com eletrodos em agulha (eletromiograma propriamente dito), mas também os estudos de condução nervosa (sentido amplo).
fecal e., e. de fezes; revisão microscópica de preparações a fresco diretas, métodos de concentração e esfregaços corados permanentes para isolar e identificar parasitas de amostras de fezes.
ova and parasite e., pesquisa de ovos e parasitas; uma ampla revisão de uma amostra de fezes, utilizando preparações diretas a fresco, preparações concentradas a fresco e esfregaços corados permanentes, para o isolamento e a identificação de parasitas protozoários e helmintos em estágios como trofozoítas, cistos, oocistos, esporos, ovos e larvas.
Papanicolaou e., e. de Papanicolaou, e. preventivo ginecológico. VER Pap *test*.
permanent stained smear e., esfregaço permanente corado; revisão microscópica, com ampliação (1.000×) em imersão em óleo, de amostras de fezes submetidas a coloração tricrômica, hematoxilina férrica e outras desse tipo; usado basicamente para trofozoítas, cistos, oocitos e esporos de trofozoítas.
physical e., e. físico; exame por meios como inspeção visual, palpação, percussão e ausculta a fim de obter informações para diagnóstico.
postmortem e., e. *postmortem*. SIN autopsy.
ex·am·in·er (eg - zam′in - er). Examinador; aquele que realiza um exame. [L. *examino*, pesar, examinar]
medical e., e. médico; **(1)** um médico que examina uma pessoa e relata a condição física dessa pessoa ao acompanhante ou indivíduo a cujo pedido foi feito o exame. **(2)** Nos estados ou municípios nos quais foi abolido o cargo de médico legista, um médico indicado para investigar todos os casos de morte súbita, violenta ou suspeita.
ex·an·them (eg - zan′them). Exantema. SIN exanthema.
ex·an·the·ma (eg - zan - thē′ma). Exantema; erupção cutânea que ocorre como manifestação de uma doença aguda por vírus ou cocos, como na escarlatina ou no sarampo. SIN exanthem. [G. efflorescence, uma erupção, de *anthos*, flor]
Boston e., e. de Boston; doença viral semelhante ao exantema súbito, com o surgimento do e. se houver, após cessar a febre; é causado pela cepa 16 do vírus ECHO. [Boston é o nome da cidade em que ocorreu uma epidemia]
epidemic e., e. epidêmico. SIN epidemic *polyarthritis*.
keratoid e., e. ceratóide; sinal que ocorre no estágio secundário da bouba: placas de descamação fina, clara, furfurácea, irregularmente dispersas nos membros e no tronco.
e. su′bitum, e. súbito; uma doença de lactentes e crianças pequenas, causada pelo herpesvírus-6, caracterizada por início súbito com febre que dura vários dias (algumas vezes com convulsões) e seguida por um e. macular fino (algumas vezes maculopapular) que surge em algumas horas a um dia após cessar a febre. SIN Dukes disease, fourth disease, pseudorubella, roseola infantilis, roseola infantum, sixth disease.
ex·an·them·a·tous (eg - zan - them′ā - tŭs). Exantematoso; relativo a um exantema.
ex·an·the·sis (eg - zan - thē′sis). **1.** Uma erupção cutânea ou exantema. **2.** O surgimento de uma erupção. [G.]
e. arthro′sia, dengue. SIN dengue.
ex·an·thrope (ek′zan - thrōp). Exantropia; uma causa externa de doença, que não se origina no corpo. [G. *ex*, fora de, + *anthrōpos*, homem]
ex·an·throp·ic (ek - zan - throp′ik). Exantrópico; que se origina fora do corpo humano.
ex·ar·te·ri·tis (eks - ar - ter - ī′tis). Exarterite. SIN periarteritis.
ex·cal·a·tion (eks - kā - lā′shŭn). Ausência, supressão ou ausência de desenvolvimento de uma dentre uma série de estruturas, como um dedo ou uma vértebra. [G. *ex*, de, + *chalaō*, diminuir, liberar]
ex·ca·va·tio (eks - kā - vā′shē - ō). Escavação. SIN excavation (1). [L. de *excavo*, pp. *-cavatus*, escavar, de *ex*, fora, + *cavus*, cavidade]
e. dis′ci [TA], e. do disco óptico. SIN depression of optic disk.
e. papil′lae, e. da papila. SIN depression of optic disk.
e. rectouteri′na [TA], e. retouterina. SIN rectouterine *pouch*.
e. rectovesica′lis [TA], e. retovesical. SIN rectovesical *pouch*.
e. vesicouteri′na [TA], e. vesicouterina. SIN vesicouterine *pouch*.
ex·ca·va·tion (eks - kā - vā′shŭn). Escavação. **1.** Cavidade, bolsa ou recesso natural; uma área afundada ou deprimida. SIN depression (2) [TA], excavatio. **2.** Uma cavidade formada artificialmente ou em virtude de um processo patológico.
atrophic e., e. atrófica; um exagero da escavação normal ou fisiológica do disco óptico causada por atrofia do nervo óptico.
glaucomatous e., e. glaucomatosa. SIN glaucomatous *cup*.
e. of optic disk, e. do disco óptico. SIN depression of optic disk.
physiologic e., e. fisiológica. SIN depression of optic disk.
ex·ca·va·tor (eks′cā - vā - tor, - tor). Escavador. **1.** Um instrumento, como uma grande colher ou cureta, usado para raspar o tecido patológico. **2.** Em odontologia, um instrumento, geralmente uma pequena colher ou cureta, para limpar e moldar uma cavidade cariada, preparando-a para obturação.
hatchet e., e. em forma de machadinha. VER hatchet.
hoe e., e. em forma de enxada; escavador dental de bisel único, com a lâmina em ângulo com o eixo do cabo e a borda cortante perpendicular ao plano do ângulo.
ex·ce·men·to·sis (ek′se - men - tō′sis). Excementose; proliferação nodular de cemento na superfície da raiz de um dente.
ex·cen·tric (ek - sen′trik). Excêntrico; forma alternativa de eccentric (2,3).
ex·cess (ek′ses). Excesso; o que está em quantidade maior que a habitual ou especificada.
antibody e., e. de anticorpos; em uma prova de precipitação, a presença de anticorpos em uma quantidade maior que a necessária para combinar com todos os antígenos presentes. VER prozone.
antigen e., e. de antígeno; **(1)** em uma prova de precipitação, a presença de antígeno não-combinado acima do necessário para se combinar a todos os anticorpos; a precipitação pode ser inibida porque a presença de excesso de antígeno dá origem a complexos antígeno-anticorpo solúveis; **(2)** *in vivo*, a interação antígeno-anticorpo resultante com esse excesso de antígenos pode dar origem a imunocomplexos, que têm um potencial de induzir lesão celular; poderia ser tolerogênio.
base e., excesso de base; medida de alcalose metabólica, geralmente prevista pelo nomograma de Siggaard-Andersen; a quantidade de ácido forte que teria sido adicionada por unidade de volume de sangue total para titulá-lo até o pH 7,4, a 37°C, e em uma pressão de dióxido de carbono de 40 mm Hg.
convergence e., e. de convergência, a condição na qual uma esoforia ou esotropia é maior para a visão de objetos próximos do que para objetos distantes.
negative base. e., e. de bases negativas; uma medida de acidose metabólica, geralmente deduzida a partir do nomograma; a quantidade de álcalis fortes que tem de ser adicionada por unidade de volume de sangue total para que o pH deste seja 7,4 a 37°C numa pressão de dióxido de carbono de 40 mm Hg.
ex·change (eks - chānj′). Troca; substituição; substituir uma coisa por outra, ou o ato dessa substituição.
sister chromatid e., troca de cromátides-irmãs; a troca durante a mitose de material genético homólogo entre cromátides-irmãs; aumentada em virtude de fragilidade cromossômica desordenada devida a fatores genéticos ou ambientais. VER recombination.
ex·cip·i·ent (ek - sip′ē - ent). Excipiente; substância mais ou menos inerte adicionada em uma prescrição como diluente ou veículo, ou para dar forma ou consistência quando o remédio é administrado na forma de comprimido; p. ex., xarope simples, gomas vegetais, pó aromático, mel e vários elixires. [L. *excipiens*; p. pres. de *ex-cipio*, retirar]
ex·cise (ek - sīz′). Excisar; seccionar. VER TAMBÉM resect.
ex·ci·sion (ek - sizh′ŭn). Excisão. **1.** Ressecção; o ato de seccionar; a remoção cirúrgica parcial ou completa de uma estrutura ou órgão. SIN resection (3). **2.** Exérese; em biologia molecular, um evento de recombinação no qual um elemento genético é removido. SIN exeresis. [L. *excido*, seccionar]

loop e., e. por alça; técnica cirúrgica ginecológica diagnóstica e terapêutica para remoção de células displásicas do colo uterino. SIN loop electrosurgical excision procedure, loop resection.

> Nesse procedimento, realizado em consultório, é usada uma pequena alça metálica para ressecar zonas visíveis de epitélio anormal do colo uterino. Assim como os procedimentos de cauterização, criocirurgia e com laser de CO_2, a excisão por alça é uma forma simples e barata de remover células displásicas. Ao contrário desses procedimentos, obtém uma amostra, de forma que se possa estudar a lesão histologicamente e avaliar a integridade de sua remoção. Inicialmente, o colo uterino é preparado com ácido acético e soluções de iodo para realçar a demarcação de áreas anormais. Sob anestesia local e visualização colposcópica, as lesões são rapidamente seccionadas em sua parte inferior com um eletrodo em alça descartável. O risco de complicações (hemorragia, dor pós-operatória intensa, infecção, estenose cervical) é baixo. A taxa de sucesso do procedimento de excisão eletrocirúrgica por alça, definida pela ausência de evidências citológicas, histológicas ou colposcópicas de anormalidade 4–48 meses após o tratamento, é de 80–90%. Embora a excisão por alça não cure a infecção pelo papilomavírus humano (HPV), oferece excelente prognóstico em displasias induzidas por HPV, através da ressecção do epitélio da zona de transformação, que é mais suscetível a essas alterações. O procedimento não é apropriado na displasia grave ou no carcinoma *in situ*, que são tratados por conização cervical.

ex·cit·a·bil·i·ty (ek - sī′ta - bil′i - tē). Excitabilidade; que possui a capacidade de ser excitável.

supranormal e., e. supranormal; no final da terceira fase do potencial de ação cardíaco, o limiar de estimulação bem-sucedido cai abaixo (isto é, menos negativo que) do nível necessário para produzir excitação durante o restante da fase de diástole, de forma que um estímulo subliminar comum torna-se efetivo. Cf. supranormal *conduction*.

ex·cit·a·ble (ek-sī′tă-bl). Excitável. **1.** Capaz de responder rapidamente a um estímulo; que tem possibilidade de excitação sexual. Cf. irritable. **2.** Em neurofisiologia, que se refere a um tecido, célula ou membrana capaz de sofrer excitação em resposta a um estímulo adequado.

ex·cit·ant (ek-sī′tănt). Excitante. SIN stimulant. [L. *excito*, pp. *-atus*, p. pres. *-ans*, despertar]

ex·ci·ta·tion (ek-sī-tā′shŭn). Excitação. **1.** O ato de aumentar a rapidez ou a intensidade dos processos físicos ou mentais. **2.** Em neurofisiologia, a resposta tudo-ou-nada completa de um nervo ou músculo a um estímulo adequado, que comumente inclui propagação da excitação ao longo das membranas da célula ou células envolvidas. VER TAMBÉM stimulation.

anomalous atrioventricular e., e. atrioventricular anômala; batimento atrial ectópico conduzido para o ventrículo.

ex·cit·a·to·ry (ek-sī′tă-tō-rē). Excitatório; que tende a produzir excitação.

ex·cite·ment (ek-sīt′ment). Excitamento; estado emocional que, algumas vezes, é caracterizado por seu potencial de atividade impulsiva ou mal controlada.

catatonic e., e. catatônico; estado catatônico excitado observado em um dos transtornos esquizofrênicos. VER catatonia.

manic e., e. maníaco; estado mental excitado observado em um transtorno bipolar (maníaco-depressivo), caracterizado por hiperatividade, loquacidade, vôo da imaginação, linguagem comprimida, grandiosidade e, algumas vezes, delírios de grandeza. VER mania, manic-depressive. SIN acute mania.

ex·ci·to·glan·du·lar (ek-sī′tō-glan′dū-lăr). Excitoglandular; que aumenta a atividade secretora de uma glândula.

ex·ci·to·met·a·bol·ic (ek-sī′tō-met-ă-bol′ik). Excitometabólico; que aumenta a atividade dos processos metabólicos.

ex·ci·to·mo·tor (ek-sī′tō-mō′ter). Excitomotor; que causa ou aumenta a rapidez do movimento. SIN centrokinetic (2).

ex·ci·to·mus·cu·lar (ek-sī′tō-mŭs′kū-lăr). Excitomuscular; que causa atividade muscular.

ex·ci·tor (ek-sī′ter, -tōr). Excitante. SIN stimulant (2).

ex·ci·to·se·cre·to·ry (ek-sī′tō-sē-krē′tō-rē). Excitossecretor; que estimula a secreção.

ex·ci·to·tox·ic (ek-sī′-tō-tok-sik). Excitotóxico; que possui a propriedade de excitar e, depois, intoxicar células ou tecidos; os exemplos incluem lesão e morte de nervos produzidas por glutamato. [excite + G. *toxikon*, tóxico]

ex·ci·to·tox·ins (ek-sī′tō-toks′ins). Excitotoxinas; toxinas que se ligam a determinados receptores (p. ex., alguns receptores do glutamato) e podem causar morte neuronal; as excitotoxinas podem estar envolvidas na lesão cerebral associada a acidentes vasculares cerebrais.

ex·clave (eks-klāv′). Uma porção afastada, isolada de uma glândula ou outra parte, como a tireóide ou pâncreas; uma glândula acessória. [L. *ex*, fora, + *-clave*, (em enclave)]

ex·clu·sion (eks-kloo′zhŭn). Exclusão; impedimento; desligamento da porção principal. [L. *ex- cludo*, pp. *-clusus*, fechar]

allelic e., e. alélica; em cada célula de um indivíduo heterozigoto em um *locus* autossômico, a supressão não-preferencial da manifestação fenotípica de um ou outro dos alelos; desse modo, o fenótipo do corpo é mosaico. Cf. lyonization.

e. of pupil, e. da pupila. SIN seclusion of *pupil*.

exclusive provider organization (EPO). Organização de profissionais exclusivos, Medicina de Grupo; um plano de assistência gerenciada no qual os usuários devem receber tratamento de profissionais afiliados; o tratamento realizado fora da rede aprovada deve ser pago pelos pacientes. VER TAMBÉM managed *care*.

ex·con·ju·gant (eks-kon′joo-gant). Exconjugante; membro de um par conjugado de protozoários ciliados após separação e antes da divisão mitótica subseqüente de cada um dos exconjugantes. VER TAMBÉM conjugant, conjugation (3). [ex- + L. *conjugo*, unir]

ex·co·ri·ate (eks-kō′rē-āt). Escoriar; arranhar ou desnudar de outra forma a pele por meios físicos.

ex·co·ri·a·tion (eks-kō′rē-ā′shŭn). Escoriação; marca de arranhadura; interrupção linear da superfície cutânea, geralmente coberta com crostas de sangue ou serosas. [L. *excorio*, esfolar, despir, de *corion*, pele, couro]

neurotic e., e. neurótica; escoriação auto-induzida repetida, com ou sem lesões cutâneas subjacentes, associada a problemas comportamentais compulsivos ou neuróticos.

ex·cre·ment (eks′krē-ment). Excremento; material residual ou qualquer excremento eliminada do corpo; p. ex., fezes. [L. *ex- cerno*, pp. *-cretus*, separar]

ex·cre·men·ti·tious (eks′krē-men-tish′us). Excrementício; relativo a qualquer excremento.

ex·cres·cence (eks-kres′ens). Excrescência; qualquer saliência de uma superfície. [L. *ex- cresco*, pp. *-cretus*, crescer]

Lambl e.'s, e. de Lambl; pequenas projeções pontiagudas das bordas das válvulas da aorta de importância desconhecida.

ex·cre·ta (eks-krē′tă). Excreções. SIN excretion (2). [L. neut. pl. de *excretus*, pp. de *ex-cerno*, separar]

ex·crete (eks-krēt′). Excretar; separar do sangue e expulsar; realizar excreção.

ex·cre·tion (eks-krē′shŭn). Excreção. **1.** O processo pelo qual o resíduo não-digerido dos alimentos e as escórias do metabolismo são eliminados, substâncias são removidas para regular a composição dos líquidos e tecidos corporais, ou substâncias são expelidas para realizar funções em uma superfície externa. **2.** O produto de um tecido ou órgão que é material a ser eliminado do corpo. SIN excreta. Cf. secretion. [ver excrement]

ex·cre·to·ry (eks′krĕ-tō-rē). Excretor; relativo à excreção.

ex·cur·sion (eks-ker′zhŭn). Excursão; qualquer movimento de um ponto a outro, geralmente com a idéia implícita de retornar novamente à posição original.

lateral e., e. lateral; movimento da mandíbula para o lado direito ou esquerdo.

protrusive e., e. protrusiva; movimento da mandíbula para uma posição anterior à posição central.

retrusive e., e. retrusiva; o leve movimento posterior e de retorno da mandíbula entre a posição de fechamento e uma posição discretamente posterior.

ex·cy·clo·duc·tion (ek-sī-klō-dŭk′shŭn). Excicloducção; uma cicloducção na qual o pólo superior da córnea é rodado para fora (lateralmente). [ex- + cyclo- + L. *duco*, pp. *ductus*, levar]

ex·cy·clo·pho·ria (ek-si-klō-fō′rē-ă). Excicloforia; uma cicloforia na qual os pólos superiores de cada córnea tendem a rodar lateralmente. [ex- + cyclo- + G. *phora*, condução]

ex·cy·clo·tor·sion (eks′sī-klō-tōr′shun). Exciclotorção. SIN extorsion (1). [ex- + cyclo- + L. *torqueo*, pp. *torsus*, torcer]

ex·cy·clo·tro·pia (eks′sī-klō-trō′pē-ă). Exciclotropia; uma ciclotropia na qual os pólos superiores das córneas são rodados para fora (lateralmente) em relação um ao outro. [ex- + cyclo- + G. *tropē*, volta]

ex·cy·clo·ver·gence (eks-sī-klō-ver′jens). Exciclovergência; rotação do pólo superior da córnea para fora. [ex- + cyclo- + L. *vergo*, curvar, inclinar]

ex·cys·ta·tion (ek-sis-tā′shŭn). Excistação; remoção de um cisto; designa a ação de determinados organismos encistados ao escapar de seu invólucro.

ex·duc·tion (eks-dŭk′shŭn). Exdução. SIN lateroduction. [ex- + L. *duco*, pp. *ductus*, levar]

ex·e·mia (ek-sē′mē-ă). Exemia; condição, como no choque, na qual uma porção considerável do sangue é removida da circulação principal, mas permanece nos vasos sangüíneos de determinadas áreas onde está estagnada. [G. *ex*, fora de, + *haima*, sangue]

ex·en·ce·pha·lia (eks′en-se-fā′lē-ă). Exencefalia. SIN exencephaly.

ex·en·ce·phal·ic (eks′en-se-fal′ik). Exencefálico; relativo à exencefalia. SIN exencephalous.

ex·en·ceph·a·lo·cele (eks′en-sef′ă-lō-sēl). Exencefalocele; herniação do encéfalo. [*ex*, fora, + G. *enkephalos*, encéfalo, + *kēlē*, tumor]

ex·en·ceph·a·lous (eks-en-sef′ă-lŭs). Exencefálico. SIN exencephalic.

ex·en·ceph·a·ly (eks-en-sef′ă-lē). Exencefalia; condição na qual o crânio está defeituoso com o encéfalo exposto ou protruso. SIN exencephalia. [G. *ex*, fora, + *enkephalos*, encéfalo]

ex·en·ter·a·tion (eks-en-ter-ā′shŭn). Exenteração; remoção de órgãos e tecidos internos, geralmente a remoção radical do conteúdo de uma cavidade corporal. SIN evisceration (1). [G. *ex*, fora, + *enteron*, intestino]

anterior pelvic e., e. pélvica anterior; remoção da bexiga, partes inferiores do ureter, vagina, útero, anexos e linfonodos adjacentes; é necessária uma derivação urinária.

orbital e., e. da órbita; remoção de todo o conteúdo da órbita.

pelvic e., e. pélvica; remoção de todos os órgãos e estruturas adjacentes da pelve; geralmente realizada para ablação cirúrgica de câncer da bexiga, colo uterino e reto.

posterior pelvic e., e. pélvica posterior; remoção da vagina, útero, anexos, reto, ânus e linfonodos adjacentes; é necessária uma colostomia.

total pelvic e., e. pélvica total; remoção da bexiga, partes inferiores do ureter, vagina, útero, anexos, reto, ânus e linfonodos adjacentes; é necessário realizar colostomia e derivação urinária. SIN Brunschwig operation.

ex·en·ter·i·tis (eks-en-ter-ī′tis). Exenterite; inflamação do revestimento peritoneal do intestino. [G. *exō*, do lado de fora, + enteritis]

ex·er·cise (ek′ser-sīz). Exercício. **1.** *Ativo:* exercício corporal com o objetivo de restaurar a saúde de órgãos e funções ou de mantê-los sadios. **2.** *Passivo:* movimento dos membros sem esforço do paciente.

isometric e., e. isométrico; exercício que consiste em contrações musculares sem movimento das partes envolvidas do corpo.

isotonic e., e. isotônico. SIN isotonic *contraction*.

Kegel e.'s, exercícios de Kegel; contração e relaxamento alternados dos músculos perineais para tratamento da incontinência urinária de esforço.

ex·er·e·sis (ek-ser′ĕ-sis). Exérese. SIN excision. [G. *exairesis*, retirar, de *haireō*, segurar]

ex·er·gon·ic (ek-ser-gon′ik). Exergônico. **1.** Referente a uma reação química que ocorre com uma carga negativa na energia livre de Gibbs. Cf. endergonic. **2.** Qualquer processo que possa produzir trabalho. [exo- + G. *ergon*, trabalho]

ex·flag·el·la·tion (eks-flaj-ē-lā′shŭn). Exflagelação; a extrusão de microgametas semelhantes a flagelos rapidamente ondulantes dos microgametócitos; no caso de parasitas da malária humana, isso ocorre no sangue ingerido pelo vetor anofelino apropriado alguns minutos após sua ingestão pelo mosquito. SIN polymitus.

ex·fo·li·a·tion (eks-fō-lē-ā′shŭn). Esfoliação. **1.** Separação e eliminação de células superficiais de um epitélio ou de qualquer superfície tecidual. **2.** Descamação da camada córnea da epiderme, que varia de pequenas quantidades ao desprendimento de todo o tegumento. **3.** Perda de dentes decíduos após a perda fisiológica da estrutura da raiz. [L. mod. do L. *ex*, fora, + *folium*, folha]
e. of lens, e. da lente do olho; separação em camadas da cápsula da lente; pode ocorrer se os olhos forem expostos a calor intenso.

ex·fo·li·a·tive (eks-fō′lē-ā-tiv). Esfoliativo; caracterizado por esfoliação, descamação ou escamação abundante. [L. mod. *exfoliativus*]

ex·ha·la·tion (eks-ha-lā′shŭn). Exalação. **1.** Expiração. SIN expiration (1). **2.** Emanação de gás ou vapor. **3.** Qualquer gás ou vapor exalado ou emitido. [L. *ex-halo*, pp. *-halatus*, expirar]

ex·hale (eks′hāl). Exalar. **1.** Expirar. SIN expire (1). **2.** Emitir um gás ou vapor ou odor.

ex·haus·tion (eg-zos′chŭn). Exaustão. **1.** Fadiga extrema; incapacidade de responder a estímulos. **2.** Remoção de conteúdo; utilização de todo o suprimento de alguma coisa. **3.** Extração dos constituintes ativos de uma droga por tratamento com água, álcool ou outro solvente. [L. *ex-haurio*, pp. *-haustus*, extrair, esvaziar]
heat e., e. pelo calor; forma de reação ao calor caracterizada por prostração, fraqueza e colapso, resultante de desidratação grave.

ex·hi·bi·tion·ism (ek-si-bish′ŭn-izm). Exibicionismo; compulsão mórbida de expor uma parte do corpo, principalmente os órgãos genitais, com o objetivo de provocar interesse sexual no observador.

ex·hi·bi·tion·ist (ek-si-bish′ŭn-ist), exibicionista; a pessoa que pratica exibicionismo.

ex·hil·a·rant (eg-zil′ar-ant). Hilariante; estimulante; mentalmente estimulante. [L. *ex-hilaro*, pp. *-atus*, p. pres. *-ans*, alegrar]

ex·is·ten·tial (eg-zi-sten′shăl). Existencial; relativo a um ramo da filosofia, o existencialismo, que diz respeito à busca pelo significado da própria existência, que foi estendido para psicoterapia existencial (existential *psychotherapy*). [L. *existentia*, existência]

ex·i·tus (eks′i-tus). Saída; escape; morte. [L. de *ex-eo*, pp. *-itus*, sair]

Exner, Siegmund, fisiologista austríaco, 1846–1926. VER Call-E. *bodies*, em *body*; E. *plexus*.

⌂ **exo-**. Exo-; exterior, externo ou para fora. VER TAMBÉM ecto-. [G. *exō*, fora]

ex·o·am·y·lase (ek-sō-am′il-ās). Exoamilase; uma glicanoidrolase que atua sobre uma ligação glicosídica próxima de uma extremidade do polissacarídeo; p. ex., β-amilase.

ex·o·an·ti·gen (ek-sō-an′ti-jen). Exoantígeno. SIN ectoantigen.

ex·o·car·dia (ek-sō-kar′dē-ă). Exocardia. SIN ectocardia.

ex·o·crine (ek′sō-krin). Exócrino. **1.** Designa secreção glandular liberada em uma superfície apical ou luminal. SIN eccrine (1). **2.** Designa uma glândula que secreta externamente através de ductos excretores. [exo- + G. *krinō*, separar]

ex·o·cy·clic (ek-sō-sī′klik, -sik′lik). Exocíclico; relativo a átomos ou grupos fixados a uma estrutura cíclica, mas que não são cíclicos; p. ex., o grupo metila do tolueno. Cf. endocyclic.

ex·o·cy·to·sis (ek′sō-sī-tō′sis). Exocitose. **1.** O surgimento de células inflamatórias migratórias na epiderme. **2.** O processo pelo qual são liberados grânulos ou gotículas secretoras de uma célula; a membrana ao redor do grânulo se funde com a membrana celular, que se rompe, e a secreção é liberada. SIN emeiocytosis, emiocytosis. Cf. endocytosis. [exo- + G. *kytos*, célula, + *-osis*, condição]

ex·o·de·vi·a·tion (ek′sō-dē-vē-ā′shŭn). Exodesvio. **1.** SIN exophoria. **2.** SIN exotropia.

ex·o·don·tia (ek-sō-don′shē-ă). Exodontia; o ramo da prática odontológica relacionado à extração de dentes. [exo- + G. *odous*, dente]

ex·o·don·tist (ek-sō-don′tist). Exodontista; aquele especializado na extração de dentes.

ex·o·en·zyme (ek-sō-en′zim). Exoenzima. SIN extracellular *enzyme*.

ex·og·a·my (ek-sog′ă-mē). Exogamia; reprodução sexuada por meio da conjugação de dois gametas de diferentes ascendências, como em determinadas espécies de protozoários. [exo- + G. *gamos*, casamento]

ex·o·gas·tru·la (eks-ō-gas′troo-lă). Exogástrula; embrião anormal no qual o intestino primitivo foi evertido.

ex·o·ge·net·ic (ek′sō-je-net′ik). Exogenético. SIN exogenous.

ex·o·ge·note (ek-sō-je′nōt). Exogenoto; em genética microbiana, o fragmento de material genético que foi transferido de um doador para o receptor e, sendo homólogo a uma região do genoma original do receptor (endogenoto), produz, na região homóloga, uma condição análoga à diploidia. [exo + genote]

ex·og·e·nous (eks-oj′ē-nŭs). Exógeno; que se origina ou é produzido fora do organismo. SIN ectogenous, exogenetic. [exo- + G. *-gen*, produção]

exo-1,4-α-D-glu·co·si·dase. Exo-1,4-α-D-glicosidase; uma hidrolase que remove resíduos terminais de α-D-glicose com ligação 1,4 das extremidades não-redutoras das cadeias, com liberação de β-D-glicose. SIN acid maltase, amyloglucosidase, γ-amilase, glucoamylase.

ex·o·lev·er (ek′sō-lē′ver). Exoalavanca; uma alavanca modificada para a extração de raízes dentárias. [exo- + L. *levare*, levantar]

ex·om·pha·los (eks-om′fă-lŭs). Exonfalia. **1.** Protrusão do umbigo. SIN exumbilication (1). **2.** SIN umbilical *hernia*. **3.** SIN omphalocele. [G. *ex*, fora, + *omphalos*, umbigo]

ex·on (ek′son). Exon; parte de um DNA que codifica um segmento do RNA mensageiro maduro a partir desse DNA e, portanto, é expressa ("traduzida") em proteína) no ribossoma. [ex- + on]

ex·on shuf·fle. Rearranjo de exons; a variação nos padrões pelos quais o RNA pode produzir diversos grupos de exons a partir de um único gene.

ex·o·nu·cle·ase (ek-sō-noo′klē-ās). Exonuclease; uma nuclease que libera um nucleotídeo de cada vez, de forma seriada, começando em uma extremidade de um polinucleotídeo (ácido nucleico); várias foram preparadas a partir da *Escherichia coli*, designadas exonucleases I e II, etc.; a exonuclease III, que remove nucleotídeos das extremidades 3′ do DNA, é usada no seqüenciamento do DNA. Cf. endonuclease.

ex·o·pep·ti·dase (ek-sō-pep′ti-dās). Exopeptidase; enzima que catalisa a hidrólise do aminoácido terminal de uma cadeia peptídica; p. ex., carboxipeptidase. Cf. endopeptidase.

Ex·o·phi·a·la (ek-sō-fī′ă-lă). Gênero de fungos patogênicos que possuem conidióforos dematiáceos com aneloconídios de uma ou duas células. Causam micetoma ou feoifomicose; em casos de micetoma, surgem grânulos pretos nos abscessos subcutâneos; em casos de feoifomicose, são encontradas hifas hialinas ou castanhas nos tecidos. [*exo* + G. *phialē*, um vaso plano e largo]
E. jeansel′mei, espécie de fungo encontrada em casos de micetoma ou feoifomicose.
E. wernec′kii, espécie de fungo que causa a ceratofitose negra (tinea nigra). SIN *Cladosporium werneckii*.

ex·o·pho·ria (ek′sō-fō′rē-ă). Exoforia; tendência dos olhos de se desviarem para fora quando a fusão é suspensa. SIN exodeviation (1). [exo- + G. *phora*, condução]

ex·o·phor·ic (ek-sō-fōr′ik). Exofórico; relativo à exoforia.

ex·oph·thal·mic (ek-sof-thal′mik). Exoftálmico; relativo à exoftalmia; caracterizado por proeminência do bulbo do olho.

ex·oph·thal·mom·e·ter (ek-sof-thal-mom′ē-ter). Exoftalmômetro; instrumento para medir a distância entre o pólo anterior do olho e um ponto de referência fixo, freqüentemente o osso zigomático. SIN orthometer, proptometer, statometer. [exophthalmos + G. *metron*, medida]

ⓘ **ex·oph·thal·mos, ex·oph·thal·mus** (ek-sof-thal′mos). Exoftalmia; protrusão de um ou de ambos os bulbos do olho; pode ser congênita e familiar, ou causada por patologia, como um tumor retroorbitário (geralmente unilateral) ou doença da tireóide (geralmente bilateral). SIN proptosis. [G. *ex*, fora, + *ophthalmos*, olho]
endocrine e., e. endócrina; exoftalmia associada a distúrbios da tireóide. VER Graves *ophthalmopathy*, Graves *orbitopathy*.
malignant e., e. maligna; protrusão progressiva, inexorável dos bulbos dos olhos.

ex·o·phyte (ek′sō-fīt). Exófito; parasita vegetal exterior ou externo. [exo- + G. *phyton*, planta]

ex·o·phyt·ic (ek-sō-fit′ik). Exofítico. **1.** Relativo a um exófito. **2.** Designa uma neoplasia ou lesão que cresce para fora de uma superfície epitelial.

ex·o·plasm (ek′sō-plazm). Exoplasma. SIN ectoplasm.

ex·o·se·ro·sis (ek′sō-se-rō′sis). Exosserose; exsudação serosa da superfície cutânea, como no eczema ou em escoriações.

ex·o·skel·e·ton (ek-sō-skel′ē-tŏn). Exoesqueleto. **1.** Partes duras, como cabelo, dentes, unhas, penas, cascos, escamas, etc., desenvolvidas a partir da epiderme em vertebrados. SIN dermoskeleton. **2.** Envoltório quitinoso externo de um inseto, ou o revestimento quitinoso ou calcário de alguns crustáceos e outros invertebrados.

ex·o·spore (ek′sō-spōr). Exósporo; um esporo exógeno, não-encerrado em um esporângio. [exo- + G. *sporos*, semente]

ex·o·spo·ri·um (ek-sō-spō′rē-um). Exospório; o invólucro externo de um esporo.

ex·os·tec·to·my (ek-sos-tek′tō-mē). Exostectomia; remoção de uma exostose. SIN exostosectomy. [exostosis + G. *ektomē*, excisão]

ex·os·to·sec·to·my (ek-sos-tō-sek′tō-mē). Exost. SIN exostectomy.

ⓘ **ex·os·to·sis**, pl. **ex·os·to·ses** (eks-os-tō′sis, -sēz). Exostose; uma projeção óssea coberta por cartilagem, originada em qualquer osso que se desenvolve da cartilagem. VER TAMBÉM osteochondroma. SIN hyperostosis (2), poroma (2). [exo- + G. *osteon*, osso, + *-osis*, condição]
e. bursa′ta, e. da bolsa; exostose originada na superfície articular de um osso e coberta por cartilagem e por um saco sinovial.

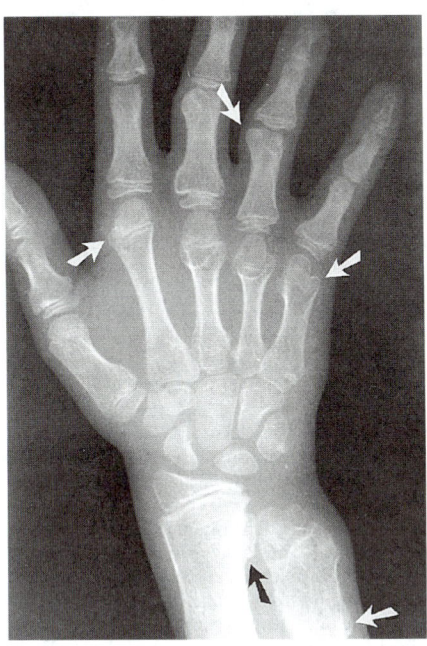

exostose: vários osteocondromas pequenos (setas)

e. cartilagin'ea, e. cartilaginosa; condroma ossificado originado na epífise ou na superfície articular de um osso.
hereditary multiple exostoses [MIM*133700], exostoses múltiplas hereditárias; um distúrbio do crescimento ósseo endocondral no qual múltiplos osteocondromas dos ossos longos, em geral benignos, surgem durante a infância, comumente com encurtamento do rádio e da fíbula; o crânio não é envolvido; os efeitos adversos geralmente são mecânicos, mas é raro haver degeneração maligna; herança autossômica dominante com heterogeneidade genética, sendo alguns casos decorrentes de mutação no gene exostose-1 (EXT1) em 8q. SIN hereditary deforming chondrodystrophy (1), multiple e., osteochondromatosis.
ivory e., e. ebúrnea; tumor pequeno, redondo, ebúrneo, que se origina de um osso, geralmente de um dos ossos do crânio.
multiple e., e. múltipla. SIN hereditary multiple exostoses.
solitary osteocartilaginous e., e. osteocartilaginosa solitária. SIN osteochondroma.
subungual e., e. subungueal; crescimentos ósseos dolorosos que elevam a unha do hálux ou dos dedos da mão em pessoas jovens.
ex·o·ter·ic (ek - sō - tār'ik). Exotérico; de origem externa; que se origina fora do organismo. [G. *exōterikos*, externo]
ex·o·ther·mic (ek - sō - ther'mik). Exotérmico. **1.** Designa uma reação química durante a qual é emitido calor (isto é, entalpia). Cf. endothermic. **2.** Relativo ao calor externo do corpo. [exo- + G. *thermē*, calor]
ex·o·tox·ic (ek - sō - tok'sik). Exotóxico. **1.** Relativo a uma exotoxina. **2.** Relativo à introdução de um veneno ou toxina exógena.
ex·o·tox·in (ek - sō - tok'sin). Exotoxina; substância prejudicial, específica, solúvel, antigênica, geralmente termolábil, produzida por algumas bactérias Gram-positivas ou Gram-negativas; é formada dentro da célula, mas é liberada para o meio onde é rapidamente ativa em quantidades extremamente pequenas; a maioria das exotoxinas é de natureza proteica (PM 70.000-900.000) e pode ter a porção tóxica da molécula destruída por calor, armazenamento prolongado ou substâncias químicas; a forma atóxica, mas antigênica, é um toxóide. SIN ectotoxin, extracellular toxin.
ex·o·tro·pia (ek'sō - trō'pē - ā). Exotropia; aquele tipo de estrabismo no qual os eixos visuais divergem; pode ser paralítico ou concomitante, monocular ou alternante, constante ou intermitente. SIN divergent squint, divergent strabismus, exodeviation (2), external squint, wall-eye (1). [exo- + G. *tropē*, volta]
A-pattern e., e. A; estrabismo divergente maior no olhar para baixo do que para cima.
basic e., e. básica; exotropia na qual o estrabismo é igual na visão para perto e para longe.
divergence excess e., e. por excesso de divergência; exotropia na qual o estrabismo é notavelmente maior na visão para longe que na visão para perto.
divergence insufficiency e., e. por insuficiência de divergência; exotropia na qual o estrabismo é notavelmente maior na visão para perto que na visão para longe.
V-pattern e., e. V; estrabismo divergente maior no olhar para cima que no olhar para baixo.
X-pattern e., e. X; divergência crescente da posição primária tanto no olhar para cima quanto para baixo.
ex·pan·sion (eks - pan'shŭn). Expansão. **1.** Aumento do tamanho, como o aumento do tórax ou dos pulmões. **2.** A extensão de qualquer estrutura, como um tendão. **3.** Uma extensão; uma área ampla. [L. *ex-pando*, pp. *-pansus*, estender]
clonal e. (klō'nal), e. clonal; produção de células-filhas, todas provenientes de uma única célula.
extensor e., e. extensora. SIN extensor digital e.
extensor digital e., e. digital extensora; aponeurose tendínea triangular, incluindo o tendão do extensor dos dedos centralmente, os tendões interósseos de cada lado e um tendão lumbrical lateralmente. Cobre a face dorsal da articulação metacarpofalangiana e a falange proximal. SIN dorsal hood, extensor aponeurosis, extensor e.
hygroscopic e., e. higroscópica; **(1)** expansão devida à absorção de umidade; **(2)** em moldes dentários, a adição de água à superfície do revestimento do molde durante a fixação para aumentar o tamanho da matriz.
perceptual e., e. perceptiva; desenvolvimento de uma capacidade de reconhecer e interpretar estímulos sensitivos através de associações com estímulos semelhantes anteriores; a expansão perceptiva por relaxamento das defesas é um objetivo da psicoterapia.
setting e., e. de consolidação; o aumento das dimensões que ocorre concomitantemente ao endurecimento de vários materiais, como o gesso.
wax e., e. de cera; em odontologia, um método de expansão dos modelos de cera para compensar a contração do ouro durante o processo de moldagem.
ex·pan·sive·ness (ek - span'siv - nes). Expansividade; um estado de otimismo, loquacidade e reatividade.
ex·pec·ta·tion. Expectativa; em teoria da probabilidade e estatística, a média verdadeira ou o valor esperado (da distribuição de uma amostra).
ex·pec·ta·tion of life. Expectativa de vida; o número médio de anos que se espera que viva um indivíduo de determinada idade se for mantida a taxa de mortalidade atual; uma abstração estatística baseada nas taxas de mortalidade existentes específicas para a idade.
e. o. l. at age x, e. de vida na idade x; o número médio de anos adicionais que uma pessoa de idade x viveria se fossem mantidas as tendências atuais de mortalidade, com base em taxas de mortalidade específicas para a idade em determinado ano.
e. o. l. at birth, e. de vida ao nascimento; o número médio de anos de vida que se pode esperar para um recém-nascido, se forem mantidas as tendências de mortalidade atuais.
ex·pect·ed. Esperado; em teoria de probabilidade e estatística, sinônimo de média ou distribuição; não precisa ser um valor provável nem mesmo possível. Por exemplo, o número esperado de crianças em famílias completas pode ser 2,53, mas esse não é um tamanho possível de qualquer família real.
ex·pec·to·rant (ek - spek'tō - rānt). Expectorante. **1.** Que promove secreção da mucosa das vias aéreas ou facilita sua expulsão. **2.** Agente que aumenta a secreção brônquica e facilita sua expulsão. [L. *ex*, fora, + *pectus*, tórax]
ex·pec·to·rate (ek - spek'tō - rāt). Expectorar; cuspir; rejeitar saliva, muco ou outro líquido da boca.
ex·pec·to·ra·tion (ek - spek - tō - rā'shŭn). Expectoração. **1.** Muco e outros líquidos formados nas vias aéreas e nas digestivas altas (a boca) e expelidos por tosse. VER TAMBÉM sputum (1). **2.** O ato de cuspir; expelir da boca saliva, muco e outro material das vias aéreas ou vias digestivas altas. SIN spitting.
prune-juice e., e. em suco de ameixa. SIN prune-juice *sputum.*
ex·pe·ri·ence (ek - spēr'ē - ens). Experiência; o sentimento de emoções e sensações, em oposição ao pensamento; envolvimento no que está acontecendo, e não reflexão abstrata sobre um evento ou um encontro interpessoal. [L. *experientia*, de *experior*, tentar]
corrective emotional e., e. emocional corretiva; reexposição em circunstâncias favoráveis a uma situação emocional com a qual uma pessoa não conseguia lidar no passado.
ex·per·i·ment (eks - per'i - ment). Experimento; experiência; ensaio; teste. **1.** Um estudo no qual o investigador altera intencionalmente um ou mais fatores, em condições controladas, a fim de estudar os efeitos desse ato. **2.** Em ressonância magnética nuclear, o termo aplicado a uma seqüência de pulso. [L. *experimentum*, de *experior*, testar, tentar]
Carr-Purcell e., e. de Carr-Purcell; em ressonância magnética, a técnica spin-eco múltipla.
control e., e. controlado; experimento usado para conferir outro, verificar o resultado ou mostrar o que teria ocorrido se o fator em estudo tivesse sido omitido. VER TAMBÉM control, control *animal*.
delayed reaction e., e. de reação tardia; método para medir a memória: o estímulo é apresentado e retirado antes que o organismo tenha tempo de responder a ele; o intervalo durante o qual o estímulo está ausente, considerando-se que o organismo responda corretamente, é uma indicação da extensão da memória.
double blind e., e. duplo-cego, e. com dupla incógnita; experimento realizado em que nem o experimentador, nem os pacientes sabem quem faz parte do

grupo-controle; evita tendenciosidade (viés) nos resultados registrados. VER TAMBÉM double-masked e.

double-masked e., e. duplo-mascarado; ensaio duplo-cego realizado sem que o paciente ou o observador conheçam a identidade do controle ou a variável.

factorial e.'s, experimentos fatoriais; um projeto experimental no qual duas ou mais séries de tratamentos são tentadas em todas as combinações.

hertzian e.'s, experimentos de Hertz; experimentos que demonstram que a indução eletromagnética é propagada em ondas, análogas às ondas luminosas, mas que não afetam a retina.

Mariotte e., e. de Mariotte; experimento no qual uma pessoa mira fixamente com um olho (estando o outro fechado) um ponto preto em um cartão, no qual também está marcada uma cruz preta; quando o cartão é aproximado ou afastado do olho, a determinada distância a cruz torna-se invisível, mas aparece novamente quando o cartão continua a se mover; isso prova a ausência de fotorreceptores no local onde o nervo óptico entra no olho.

pulse-chase e., experimento no qual uma enzima, uma via metabólica, uma cultura de células, etc., interage com uma breve adição (pulso) de uma substância marcada, seguida por sua remoção e substituição (afastamento) por um excesso da substância não-marcada.

Scheiner e., e. de Scheiner; uma demonstração de acomodação; através de dois pequenos orifícios em um cartão, separados por uma distância menor que o diâmetro da pupila, o paciente olha para uma agulha; a uma curta distância do olho, a agulha parece dupla; à medida que é afastada do olho, é encontrado um ponto onde parece única, e, além desse ponto, permanece única para o olho emétrope, mas para o olho míope logo se torna novamente dupla.

ex·pi·ra·tion (eks-pi-rā'shŭn). Expiração. **1.** SIN exhalation (1). **2.** Morte. [L. *expiro*, ou *ex-spiro*, pp. *-atus*, expirar]

ex·pi·ra·to·ry (ek-spī'ra-tō-rē). Expiratório; relativo à expiração.

ex·pire (ek-spīr'). Expirar. **1.** SIN exhale (1). **2.** Morrer.

ex·plant (eks'plant). Explante; tecido vivo transferido de um organismo para um meio artificial de cultura.

ex·plan·ta·tion (eks-plan-tā'shŭn). Explantação; o ato de transferir um explante.

ex·plo·ra·tion (eks-plōr-ā'shŭn). Exploração; exame ativo, geralmente envolvendo um procedimento cirúrgico, para determinar o estado de uma cavidade corporal a fim de auxiliar o diagnóstico. [L. *ex-ploro*, pp. *-ploratus*, explorar]

ex·plor·a·to·ry (eks-plōr'ă-tōr-ē). Exploratório; relativo a, ou com o propósito de, exploração.

ex·plor·er (ek'splōr'er). Explorador; uma sonda pontiaguda usada para investigar superfícies dentárias naturais ou restauradas a fim de detectar cáries ou outros defeitos.

ex·plo·sion (eks-plō'zhŭn). Explosão; aumento súbito e violento de volume acompanhado por ruído e liberação de energia, como por uma alteração química, reação nuclear ou escape de gases ou vapores sob pressão. [L. *explosio*, de *explodo*, afastar por movimento súbito]

ex·pose (eks-pōz'). Expor; realizar ou sofrer exposição. [Fr. ant. *exposer*, do L. *ex-pono*, pp. *ex-positum*, exibir, expor]

ex·po·sure (eks-pō'zhoor). Exposição. **1.** Demonstração, revelação, exibição ou facilitação do acesso. **2.** Em odontologia, perda da estrutura dentária rígida que cobre a polpa dentária em virtude de cáries, manipulação ou trauma. **3.** Proximidade e/ou contato com a fonte de um agente patológico de tal forma que possa haver transmissão efetiva do agente ou efeitos prejudiciais. **4.** A quantidade de um fator a qual um grupo ou um indivíduo foi exposto, em contraste com a dose, a quantidade que entra ou que interage com o organismo.

ex·press (eks-pres'). Espremer; comprimir. [L. *ex-premo*, pp. *-pressus*, espremer]

ex·pres·sion (eks-presh'ŭn). Expressão. **1.** Ato de espremer; expelir por pressão. **2.** Mobilidade das feições conferindo um significado emocional particular à face. SIN facies (3) [TA]. **3.** Qualquer ato realizado por um indivíduo. **4.** Algo que manifesta outra coisa. **5.** O ato de permitir a apresentação de informações. **6.** Uma função matemática que consiste em uma combinação de constantes, variáveis, outras funções e operações matemáticas.

differential gene e., e. gênica diferencial; expressão gênica que responde a sinais ou estímulos; um meio de controle gênico; p. ex., os efeitos de determinados hormônios sobre a biossíntese de proteínas.

gene e., e. gênica; **(1)** o efeito detectável de um gene; **(2)** surgimento de um traço hereditário; por diversas razões genéticas (p. ex., caráter recessivo, hipóstase, parastase) e ambientais (a ausência de estímulos pertinentes), um gene pode não ser expresso. Nessas circunstâncias, não terá impacto sobre a evolução de Darwin.

integrated rate e., e. de velocidade integrada; equação de uma reação química ou catalisada por enzima para toda a curva de progresso.

e. library, biblioteca de expressão; coleção de plasmídeos ou fagos contendo uma amostra representativa de DNAc ou fragmentos genômicos construídos de tal forma que serão transcritos e traduzidos pelo organismo hospedeiro (geralmente bactérias).

ex·pres·siv·i·ty (eks-pres-siv'i-tē). Expressividade; em genética clínica, a intensidade com que um gene se manifesta.

ex·pul·sive (eks-pŭl'siv). Expulsivo; que tende a expelir. [L. *ex-pello*, pp. *-pulsus*, fazer sair, expulsar]

ex·qui·site (eks-kwiz'it). Agudo; extremamente intenso, pungente; diz-se de dor espontânea ou à palpação de uma parte. [L. *exquiro*, pp. *exquisitus*, procurar]

ex·san·gui·nate (ek-sang'gwi-nāt). Exsanguinar. **1.** Remover ou retirar o sangue circulante; tornar exangue. **2.** SIN exsanguine. [L. *ex*, fora, + *sanguis*, (*-guin*), sangue]

ex·san·gui·na·tion (ek-sang'gwi-nā'shŭn). Exsanguinação; remoção de sangue; que torna exangue.

ex·san·guine (ek-sang'gwin). Exangue; sem sangue. SIN exsanguinate (2).

ex·sect (ek-sekt'). Termo raramente usado que significa excisar. [L. *ex- seco*, pp. *-sectus*, extirpar]

ex·sec·tion (ek-sek'shŭn). Termo raramente usado que significa excisão.

Exserohilum (eks'er-ō-hī'lum). Gênero de fungos; causa de feoifomicose humana.

ex·sic·cant (ek-sik'ant). Exsicante. SIN desiccant.

ex·sic·cate (ek'si-kāt). Exsicar. SIN desiccate.

ex·sic·ca·tion (ek-si-kā'shŭn). Exsicação. **1.** SIN desiccation. **2.** A retirada de água de cristalização. SIN dehydration (3). [L. *ex sicco*, pp. *siccatus*, secar]

ex·so·ma·tize (ek-sō'ma-tīz). Exsomatizar; remover do corpo. [G. *ex*, fora de, + *sōma*, corpo]

ex·sorp·tion (ek-sōrp'shŭn). Exsorpção; movimento de substâncias do sangue para a luz intestinal. [L. *ex*, fora, + *sorbeo*, sugar]

ex·stro·phy (ek'strō-fē). Extrofia; eversão congênita de um órgão oco. SIN ecstrophe. [G. *ex*, fora, + *strophē*, uma volta]

e. of bladder, e. da bexiga; abertura congênita na parede anterior da bexiga e na parede abdominal à sua frente, com exposição da parede posterior da bexiga. SIN ectopia vesicae.

cloacal e., e. da cloaca; anomalia congênita com duas unidades vesicais extrofiadas separadas por um segmento de intestino extrofiado, geralmente o ceco, recebendo o íleo superiormente e continuando distalmente até o microcólon, que termina cegamente. Pode haver diversas variantes de perturbação anatômica. SIN ectopia cloacae.

ex·tend (eks-tend'). Estender; retificar um membro para diminuir ou extinguir o ângulo formado por flexão; colocar o segmento distal de um membro em tal posição que seu eixo seja contínuo com o do segmento proximal. [L. *ex- tendo*, pp. *-tensus*, estender]

ex·ten·sion (eks-ten'shŭn) [TA]. Extensão. **1.** O ato de colocar a porção distal de uma articulação em continuidade (embora apenas paralela) com o eixo longitudinal da porção proximal. **2.** Tração exercida sobre um membro em direção distal. **3.** Termo obsoleto para tração. [L. *extensio*, extensão]

Buck e., Tração de Buck. SIN Buck traction.

primer e., e. do iniciador; técnica para determinar a região 5' não-traduzida de uma molécula de RNA específica. Usa um oligonucleotídeo complementar à seqüência de RNA conhecida como iniciador da síntese de DNAc através da transcriptase reversa.

ridge e., e. da crista; cirurgia intra-oral para aprofundar os sulcos labial, bucal e/ou lingual; é realizada para aumentar a altura intra-oral da crista alveolar a fim de ajudar a retenção de uma dentadura.

skeletal e., e. óssea. SIN skeletal traction.

ex·ten·sor (eks-ten'ser,-sōr) [TA]. Extensor; um músculo cuja contração causa o movimento de uma articulação, com o membro ou o corpo assumindo assim uma posição mais reta, ou ficando a distância entre as partes proximal e distal à articulação aumentada ou estendida; o antagonista de um flexor. VER muscle. [L. aquele que estende, de *ex-tendo*, estender]

ex·te·ri·or (eks-tē'rē-ōr). Exterior; fora; externo. [L.]

ex·te·ri·or·ize (eks-tēr'ē-ōr-īz). Exteriorizar. **1.** Orientar os interesses, pensamentos ou sentimentos de um paciente canalizando-os para fora, para algum objetivo ou finalidade definida. **2.** Expor um órgão, temporariamente, para observação ou, permanentemente, para fins de experimentação. **3.** Fixação de um segmento intestinal com suprimento sangüíneo intacto à face externa da parede abdominal.

ex·tern (eks'tern). Externo; um estudante avançado ou recém-formado que auxilia no tratamento clínico ou cirúrgico de pacientes hospitalizados; outrora, alguém que vivia fora da instituição. [F. *externe*, do lado de fora, estudante externo]

ex·ter·nal (eks-ter'năl) [TA]. Externo; do lado de fora ou mais distante do centro; freqüentemente usado de forma errada para significar lateral. SIN externus [TA]. [L. *externus*]

ex·ter·nus (eks-ter'nŭs) [TA]. Externo. SIN external.

ex·ter·o·cep·tive (eks'ter-ō-sep'tiv). Exteroceptivo; relativo aos exteroceptores; designa a superfície do corpo que contém os órgãos terminais adaptados para receber impressões ou estímulos externos. [L. *ex-terus*, do lado de fora + *capere*, trazer]

ex·ter·o·cep·tor (eks'ter-ō-sep'ter, -tōr). Exteroceptor; um dos órgãos terminais periféricos dos nervos aferentes, na pele ou mucosa, que respondem à estimulação por agentes externos. [L. *ex-terus*, externo, + *receptor*, receptor]

ex·tinc·tion (eks-tingk'shŭn). Extinção. **1.** Em psicologia, modificação do

comportamento ou condicionamento clássico ou operacional, uma diminuição progressiva da freqüência de uma resposta que não é reforçada positivamente; a suspensão de reforços conhecidos por manter um comportamento indesejável. VER conditioning. 2. SIN absorbance. [L. *extinguo*, extinguir]
specific e., e. específica. SIN specific absorption *coefficient.*
visual e., e. visual. SIN pseudo-*hemianopia.*
ex·tin·guish (eks-ting′gwish). Extinguir. 1. Abolir; debelar uma chama (fogo); destruir. 2. Em psicologia, abolir progressivamente uma resposta previamente condicionada. VER conditioning. [L. *extinguo*, apagar, debelar]
ex·tir·pa·tion (eks-tir-pā′shŭn). Extirpação; remoção parcial ou completa de um órgão ou de um tecido doente. [L. *extirpo*, erradicar, de *stirps*, um pedículo, raiz]
Exton, William G., médico norte-americano, 1876–1943. VER E. *reagent.*
ex·tor·sion (eks-tōr′shŭn). 1. Rotação conjugada dos pólos superiores de cada córnea para fora. SIN excyclotorsion. 2. Rotação externa de um membro ou de um órgão. [L. *extorsio*, de *ex- torqueo*, rodar para fora]
ex·tor·tor (eks-tōr′ter, -tōr). Um rotador externo.
△ **ex·tra-.** Extra-; sem, fora de [L.]
ex·tra·ar·tic·u·lar (eks-trā-ar-tik′ū-lăr). Extra-articular; fora de uma articulação.
ex·tra·ax·i·al (eks-trā-aks′ē-ăl). Extra-axial; fora do eixo; aplicado a lesões intracranianas que não se originam no encéfalo.
ex·tra·buc·cal (eks-trā-bŭk′ăl). Extrabucal; fora ou que não é parte da bochecha.
ex·tra·bul·bar (eks-trā-bul′bar). Extrabulbar; fora de, ou não relacionado a, qualquer bulbo, como o bulbo da uretra ou o bulbo (medula oblonga).
ex·tra·cal·i·ce·al (eks′trā-kă-lis′ē-ăl). Extracalicial; fora de um cálice.
ex·tra·cap·su·lar (eks-trā-kap′soo-lăr). Extracapsular; fora da cápsula articular.
ex·tra·car·pal (eks-trā-kar′păl). Extracarpal. 1. Fora do carpo, que não possui relação com ele. 2. No lado externo do carpo.
ex·tra·cel·lu·lar (eks-trā-sel′ū-lăr). Extracelular; fora das células.
ex·tra·chro·mo·som·al (eks′trā-krō-mō-sōm′ăl). Extracromossomial; fora ou separado de um cromossoma.
ex·tra·cor·po·re·al (eks′trā-kōr-pō′rē-ăl). Extracorpóreo; fora do corpo ou de qualquer "corpo" anatômico, ou não relacionado com essas estruturas.
ex·tra·cor·pus·cu·lar (eks′trā-kōr-pus-kū-lăr). Extracorpuscular; fora dos corpúsculos, principalmente dos corpúsculos sanguíneos.
ex·tra·cra·ni·al (eks-trā-krā′nē-ăl). Extracraniano; fora da cavidade craniana.
ex·tract. 1 (ek′strakt). Extrato; preparação concentrada de uma droga obtida por remoção dos constituintes ativos da droga com solventes adequados, evaporando todo ou quase todo o solvente e ajustando a massa ou pó residual ao padrão prescrito. 2. (ek-strakt′). Extrair; remover parte de uma mistura com um solvente. 3. Realizar extração. [L. *ex-traho*, pp. *-tractus*, retirar]
alcoholic e., e. alcoólico; extrato sólido obtido por extração dos princípios de uma substância solúveis em álcool, seguida pela evaporação do álcool.
allergenic e., e. alergênico; extrato (geralmente contendo proteína) de várias fontes, p. ex., alimento, bactéria, pólen e semelhantes, suspeitos de ação específica no estímulo de manifestações de alergia; pode ser usado para teste cutâneo ou dessensibilização. SIN allergic e.
allergic e., e. alérgico. SIN allergenic e.
belladonna e., e. de beladona; extrato pulverizado das folhas e/ou raízes de *Atropa belladonna*; usado para formular várias apresentações farmacêuticas. Contém os alcalóides da beladona (atropina e escopolamina) e tem sido usado no tratamento de úlceras, diarréia e parkinsonismo.
Büchner e., e. de Büchner; um extrato acelular de leveduras, como o preparado por Eduard e Hans Büchner, tendo sido observado que catalisa a fermentação alcoólica; essa observação praticamente eliminou o "vitalismo" como sendo responsável por reações químicas biológicas e iniciou os primórdios da bioquímica moderna (enzimologia).
equivalent e., e. equivalente; um extrato líquido com a mesma potência, peso a peso, que o medicamento original. SIN valoid.
fluid e., e. líquido. VER fluidextract.
hydroalcoholic e., e. hidroalcoólico; extrato sólido obtido por extração dos princípios solúveis da droga com álcool e água, seguida por evaporação da solução.
liquid e., e. líquido. SIN fluidextract.
pollen e., e. do pólen; líquido obtido por extração da proteína do pólen de plantas usado para teste diagnóstico ou tratamento.
ex·tract·ant (ek-strak′tant). Extrator; agente usado para isolar ou extrair uma substância de uma mistura ou combinação de substâncias, dos tecidos ou de uma droga bruta.
ex·trac·tion (ek-strak′shŭn). Extração. 1. Luxação e remoção de um dente de seu alvéolo. 2. A separação de material (soluto) em um solvente. 3. A porção ativa de uma droga; a produção de um extrato. 4. Remoção cirúrgica por tração. 5. Remoção do feto do útero ou vagina no fim da gravidez ou próximo do fim, seja manualmente ou com instrumentos. 6. Remoção por aspiração do produto da concepção antes da falha menstrual. [L. *ex-traho*, pp. *-tractus*, ex-trair]
Baker pyridine e., e. de piridina de Baker; tratamento com piridina quente dos tecidos fixados na solução de Bouin diluída, usado para extrair fosfolipídios desses tecidos como um controle na coloração histoquímica desse material.
breech e., e. pélvica; extração obstétrica do bebê pelas nádegas.
partial breech e., e. pélvica parcial; parto pélvico assistido pelo obstetra com desprendimento espontâneo do feto até o nível do umbigo.
podalic e., e. podálica; extração obstétrica do bebê pelos pés.
serial e., e. seriada; extração seletiva de determinados dentes decíduos e/ou permanentes durante os primeiros anos do desenvolvimento dental, geralmente com a extração final dos primeiros ou, ocasionalmente, segundos pré-molares para incentivar o ajuste autônomo do apinhamento moderado a intenso dos dentes anteriores; pode ou não exigir tratamento ortodôntico subseqüente.
spontaneous breech e., e. pélvica espontânea; parto de um feto em apresentação pélvica com extração completa de todo o corpo fetal do útero.
total breech e., pélvica total, parto de um feto na apresentação pélvica com e. completa de todo o corpo fetal do útero.
ex·trac·tives (ek-strak′tivs). Extrator; substâncias presentes em tecidos vegetais ou animais que podem ser isoladas por tratamento sucessivo com solventes e recuperadas pela evaporação da solução.
ex·trac·tor (ek-strak′ter, tōr). Extrator; instrumento para uso na retirada ou tração de qualquer parte natural, como um dente ou corpo estranho.
vacuum e., e. a vácuo; aparelho para tracionar a cabeça de um feto por meio de um capuz macio preso por vácuo.
ex·tra·cys·tic (eks-trā-sis′tik). Extracístico; fora da, ou não relacionado à, vesícula biliar ou bexiga ou qualquer tumor cístico.
ex·tra·du·ral (eks-trā-doo′răl). Extradural. 1. Situado no lado externo da dura-máter. 2. Não ligado à dura-máter.
ex·tra·em·bry·on·ic (eks′trā-em-brē-on′ik). Extra-embrionário; situado fora do corpo embrionário; p. ex., as membranas envolvidas na proteção e nutrição do embrião e que são descartadas por ocasião do nascimento, sem ser incorporadas em seu organismo.
ex·tra·ep·i·phy·si·al (eks′trā-ep-i-fiz′ē-ăl). Extra-epifisário; não relacionado ou unido a uma epífise.
ex·tra·gen·i·tal (eks′trā-jen′i-tăl). Extragenital; situado fora, distante dos órgãos genitais, ou que não tem relação com esses órgãos.
ex·tra·he·pat·ic (eks-trā-he-pat′ik). Extra-hepático; situado fora do fígado ou que não tem relação com esse órgão.
ex·tra·lig·a·men·tous (eks-trā-lig-ă-men′tŭs). Extraligamentar; situado fora de, ou não relacionado com, um ligamento.
ex·tra·mal·le·o·lus (eks-trā-mal-ē′ō-lŭs). Extramaléolo. SIN lateral *malleolus.*
ex·tra·med·ul·lary (eks-trā-med′ū-lăr-ē). Extramedular; extrabulbar; fora de, ou não relacionado com, qualquer medula, especialmente a medula oblonga (bulbo).
ex·tra·mi·to·chon·dri·al (eks-trā-mī-tō-kon′drē-al). Extramitocondrial; fora da mitocôndria.
ex·tra·mu·ral (eks-trā-mū′răl). Extramural; fora da estrutura da parede de uma parte. [extra- + L. *murus*, parede]
ex·tra·ne·ous (eks-trā′nē-ŭs). Estranho; fora do organismo e não pertencente a ele. [L. *extraneus*]
ex·tra·nu·cle·ar (eks-trā-noo′klē-er). Extranuclear; localizado fora, ou não envolvendo um núcleo celular.
ex·tra·oc·u·lar (eks-trā-ok′ū-lăr). Extra-ocular; adjacente, mas fora do bulbo do olho.
ex·tra·o·ral (eks-trā-o′răl). Extra-oral; fora da cavidade oral; externamente à cavidade oral. Em seu emprego habitual também inclui qualquer coisa externa aos lábios e bochechas.
ex·tra·ov·u·lar (eks′trā-ov′ū-lăr, ōv′ū-lăr). Extra-ovular; fora do ovo; existência após a eclosão do ovo, como em répteis e aves.
ex·tra·pap·il·lary (eks-trā-pap′i-lā-rē). Extrapapilar; não ligado a qualquer estrutura papilar.
ex·tra·pa·ren·chy·mal (eks′trā-pă-reng′ki-măl). Extraparenquimatoso; não relacionado com o parênquima de um órgão.
ex·tra·per·i·ne·al (eks-trā-per-i-ne′al). Extraperineal; não ligado ao períneo.
ex·tra·per·i·os·te·al (eks-trā-per-ē-os′tē-ăl). Extraperiosteal; não ligado, ou não relacionado ao periósteo.
ex·tra·per·i·to·ne·al (eks-trā-per-i-tō-nē′ăl). Extraperitoneal; fora da cavidade peritoneal.
ex·tra·phys·i·o·log·ic (eks′trā-fiz-ē-ō-loj′ik). Extrafisiológico; fora do domínio da fisiologia; mais que fisiológico e, portanto, patológico.
ex·tra·pla·cen·tal (eks-trā-pla-sen′tăl). Extraplacentário; não relacionado à placenta.
ex·tra·pros·tat·ic (eks-trā-pros-tat′ik). Extraprostático; fora ou independente da próstata.
ex·tra·psy·chic (eks-trā-fiz′ik). Extrapsíquico; designa a dinâmica psico-

lógica que ocorre na mente em associação com as trocas do indivíduo com outras pessoas ou eventos. Cf. intrapsychic.

ex·tra·pul·mo·nary (eks-tră-pŭl'mō-nār-ē). Extrapulmonar; fora dos pulmões ou que não possui relação com esses órgãos.

ex·tra·py·ram·i·dal (eks-tră-pi-ram'i-dăl). Extrapiramidal; fora do trato piramidal. VER extrapyramidal motor *system*.

ex·tra·sen·so·ry (eks-tră-sen'sōr-ē). Extra-sensorial; fora ou além dos sentidos habituais; não limitado aos sentidos, como na percepção extra-sensorial (extrasensory *perception*).

ex·tra·se·rous (eks-tră-sē'rŭs). Extra-seroso; fora de uma cavidade serosa.

ex·tra·so·mat·ic (eks-tră-sō-mat'ik). Extra-somático; fora do corpo ou não relacionado a ele.

ex·tra·sys·to·le (eks-tră-sis'tō-lē). Extra-sístole; termo inespecífico para designar um batimento ectópico de qualquer fonte no coração. SIN premature beat, premature systole.
  atrial e., e. atrial; complexo prematuro do coração que se origina de um foco atrial ectópico. SIN auricular e.
  atrioventricular e., e. atrioventricular. SIN junctional e.
  auricular e., e. atrial. SIN atrial e.
  interpolated e., e. interpolada; extra-sístole ventricular ou atrial que, em vez de ser seguida por uma pausa compensatória ou não-compensatória, fica entre dois ciclos sinusais consecutivos.
  junctional e., e. juncional; batimento prematuro originado na junção AV e que leva à contração simultânea ou quase simultânea dos átrios e ventrículos. SIN atrioventricular e.
  return e., e. de retorno; uma forma de ritmo recíproco no qual o impulso originado no ventrículo ascende em direção aos átrios, mas, antes de alcançá-los, é refletido de volta para os ventrículos, a fim de produzir uma segunda contração ventricular.
  supraventricular e., e. supraventricular; extra-sístole que se origina em um centro acima do ventrículo, isto é, que se origina no átrio ou na junção AV.
  ventricular e., e. ventricular; um complexo ventricular prematuro.

ex·tra·tar·sal (eks-tră-tar'săl). Extratarsal. **1.** Fora, que não possui relação com o tarso. **2.** Na face externa do tarso.

ex·tra·tra·che·al (eks-tră-trā'kē-ăl). Extratraqueal; fora da traquéia.

ex·tra·tub·al (eks-tră-too'băl). Extratubário; fora de qualquer tuba; especificamente, fora da tuba auditiva (de Eustáquio) ou da uterina (de Falópio).

ex·tra·u·ter·ine (eks-tră-ū'ter-in). Extra-uterino; fora do útero.

ex·tra·vag·i·nal (eks-tră-vaj'i-năl). Extravaginal; fora da vagina.

ex·trav·a·sate (eks-trav'ă-sāt). Extravasar. **1.** Exsudar ou sair de um vaso para os tecidos, referente ao sangue, linfa ou urina. **2.** Extravasado; a substância exsudada. SIN extravasation (2), suffusion (4). [L. *extra*, fora de, + *vas*, vaso]

ex·trav·a·sa·tion (eks-trav'ă-sā'shŭn). Extravasamento. **1.** O ato de extravasar. **2.** SIN extravasate (2). [extra- + L. *vas*, vaso]

ex·tra·vas·cu·lar (eks-tră-vas'kū-lăr). Extravascular; fora dos vasos sanguíneos ou linfáticos, ou de qualquer vaso sanguíneo especial.

ex·tra·ven·tric·u·lar (eks-tră-ven-trik'ū-lăr). Extraventricular; fora de qualquer ventrículo, especialmente de um dos ventrículos do coração.

ex·tra·ver·sion (eks-tră-ver'zhŭn, -shŭn). Extroversão. SIN extroversion.

ex·tra·vert (eks'-tră-vert). Extroverter. SIN extrovert.

ex·tra·vi·su·al (ek-stră-vizh'oo-ăl). Extravisual; fora do campo de visão, ou além do espectro visível.

ex·trem·i·tal (eks-trem'i-tăl). Extremo; relativo a uma extremidade. VER TAMBÉM distal.

ex·trem·i·tas (eks-trem'i-tas) [TA]. Extremidade. SIN extremity. VER limb. [L. de *extremus*, último, externo]
  e. acromia'lis clavic'ulae [TA], e. acromial da clavícula. SIN acromial end of clavicle.
  e. ante'rior splenica [TA], pólo anterior do baço. SIN anterior extremity of spleen.
  e. infe'rior [TA], e. inferior, pólo inferior. SIN inferior pole.
  e. infe'rior ren'is [TA], pólo inferior do rim. SIN inferior pole of kidney.
  e. infe'rior tes'tis [TA], pólo inferior do testículo. SIN lower pole of testis.
  e. poste'rior splenica [TA], pólo posterior do baço. SIN posterior extremity of spleen.
  e. sterna'lis clavic'ulae [TA], e. esternal da clavícula. SIN sternal end of clavicle.
  e. supe'rior [TA], e. superior, pólo superior. SIN superior pole.
  e. supe'rior ren'is [TA], pólo superior do rim. SIN superior pole of kidney.
  e. supe'rior tes'tis [TA], pólo superior do testículo. SIN upper pole of testis.
  e. tuba'ria ovar'ii [TA], e. tubária do ovário. SIN tubal extremity of ovary.
  e. uteri'na ovar'ii [TA], e. uterina do ovário. SIN uterine extremity of ovary.

ex·trem·i·ty (eks-trem'i-tē) [TA]. Extremidade; uma das extremidades de uma estrutura alongada ou pontiaguda. Incorretamente utilizado com o significado de membro. VER TAMBÉM limb, end, pole. SIN extremitas [TA].
  acromial e. of clavicle, e. acromial da clavícula. SIN acromial end of clavicle.
  anterior e. of caudate nucleus, e. anterior do núcleo caudado; cabeça do núcleo caudado. SIN head of caudate nucleus.
  anterior e. of spleen [TA], pólo anterior do baço; a extremidade anterior do baço (extremitas anterior splenis [NA]). SIN extremitas anterior splenica [TA].
  inferior e., pólo inferior; **(1)** *termo oficial alternativo para inferior *pole*; **(2)** incorreta mas comumente usado como sinônimo de membro inferior (lower limb).
  inferior e. of kidney, pólo inferior do rim; *termo oficial alternativo para inferior *pole* of kidney.
  lower e., membro inferior. SIN lower limb.
  posterior e. of spleen [TA], pólo posterior do baço; a extremidade posterior do baço (extremitas posterior splenis [NA]). SIN extremitas posterior splenica [TA].
  sternal e. of clavicle, e. esternal da clavícula. SIN sternal end of clavicle.
  superior e., pólo superior; **(1)** *termo oficial alternativo para superior *pole*; **(2)** incorreta mas comumente usado como sinônimo de membro superior (upper limb).
  superior e. of kidney, pólo superior do rim; *termo oficial alternativo para superior *pole* of kidney.
  tubal e. of ovary [TA], e. tubária do ovário; a extremidade lateral arredondada do ovário, geralmente voltada para o infundíbulo da tuba uterina. SIN extremitas tubaria ovarii [TA], lateral pole.
  upper e., membro superior. SIN upper limb.
  upper e. of fibula, cabeça da fíbula. SIN head of fibula.
  uterine e. of ovary [TA], e. uterina do ovário; a extremidade medial arredondada do ovário, geralmente voltada para o útero. SIN extremitas uterina ovarii [TA], medial pole of ovary.

ex·trin·sic (eks-trin'sik). Extrínseco; que se origina fora da parte em que foi encontrado ou sobre a qual age; designa especialmente um músculo, como os músculos extrínsecos da mão. [L. *extrinsecus*, de fora]

ex·tro·gas·tru·la·tion (eks'trō-gas-troo-lā'shŭn). Extrogastrulação; evaginação do material do intestino primitivo durante a gastrulação, em vez da invaginação normal, em consequência de alguma manipulação natural ou experimental do embrião em desenvolvimento ou do seu ambiente.

ex·tro·ver·sion (eks'trō-ver'zhŭn, -shŭn). Extroversão. **1.** Versão para fora. **2.** Uma característica que envolve as relações sociais, como as praticadas por um extrovertido. SIN extraversion. [incorretamente formada do L. *extra*, fora, + *verto*, pp. *versus*, virar]

ex·tro·vert (eks'trō-vert). Extrovertido; uma pessoa gregária cujos principais interesses estão fora de si próprio, e que é socialmente autoconfiante e se envolve nos afazeres de outros. Cf. introvert. SIN extravert.

ex·trude (eks-trood'). Expulsar; expelir; protrair.

ex·tru·sion (eks-troo'zhŭn). Extrusão. **1.** Empurrar ou forçar a saída de uma posição normal. **2.** A erupção excessiva ou migração de um dente além de sua posição oclusal normal.
  e. of a tooth, e. de um dente; alongamento de um dente; movimento de um dente em uma direção oclusal ou incisal.

ex·tu·bate (eks'too-bāt). Extubar; remover um tubo.

ex·tu·ba·tion (eks'too-bā'shŭn). Extubação; remoção de um tubo de um órgão, estrutura ou orifício; especificamente, a remoção do tubo após intubação. [L. *ex*, fora, + *tuba*, tubo]

ex·u·ber·ant (ek-zoo'ber-ănt). Exuberante; designa proliferação ou crescimento excessivo, como de um tecido ou granulação. [L. *exubero*, abundar, ser abundante]

ex·u·date (eks'oo-dāt). Exsudato; qualquer líquido que exsudou de um tecido ou de seus capilares, mais especificamente em virtude de traumatismo ou inflamação (p. ex., pus peritoneal na peritonite, ou o exsudato que forma uma crosta sobre uma escoriação cutânea), caso em que é caracteristicamente rico em proteínas e leucócitos. Cf. transudate. SIN exudation (2). [L. *ex*, fora, + *sudo*, suar]

ex·u·da·tion (eks-oo-dā'shŭn). Exsudação. **1.** O ato ou processo de exsudar. **2.** SIN exudate.

ex·ud·a·tive (eks-oo'dă-tiv). Exsudativo; relativo ao processo de exsudação ou a um exsudato.

ex·ude (ek-zood'). Exsudar; de modo geral, gotejamento ou saída gradual de uma estrutura ou tecido do corpo; mais especificamente, restrito a um líquido ou semi-sólido que assim o faz e pode tornar-se incrustado ou infectado devido à lesão ou inflamação. [L. *ex*, fora, + *sudo*, suar]

ex·ul·cer·ans (eks-ŭl'ser-anz). Ulcerante.

ex·um·bil·i·ca·tion (eks'ŭm-bil-i-kā'shŭn). Exumbilicação. **1.** SIN exomphalos (1). **2.** SIN umbilical hernia. **3.** SIN omphalocele. [L. *ex*, fora, + *umbilicus*, umbigo]

ex vi·vo (ex vē'vo). Refere-se ao uso ou posicionamento de um tecido ou célula, após retirada de um organismo, enquanto o tecido ou as células permanecem viáveis. [L. do vivo]

eye (ī) [TA]. Olho. **1.** O órgão da visão, que consiste no bulbo e no nervo óptico. SIN oculus [TA]. **2.** A área do olho, incluindo pálpebras e outros órgãos acessórios do olho; o conteúdo da órbita (comum). [A.S. *ēage*]
  amaurotic cat e., o. de gato amaurótico; um reflexo amarelo da pupila em casos de retinoblastoma ou pseudoglioma.

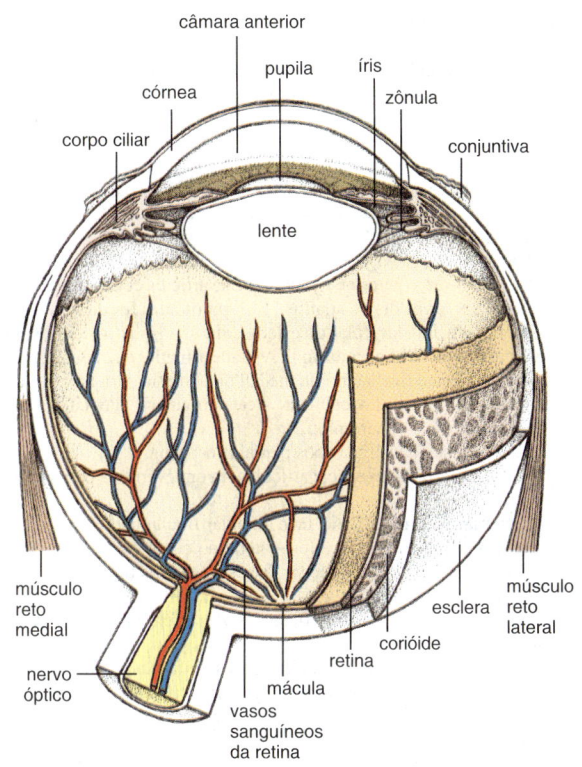

olho

câmara anterior · pupila · íris · zônula · conjuntiva · córnea · corpo ciliar · lente · músculo reto lateral · esclera · coroide · retina · mácula · vasos sanguíneos da retina · nervo óptico · músculo reto medial

aphakic e., o. afácico; olho cuja lente está ausente.
artificial e., o. artificial; disco curvo de vidro ou plástico opaco, contendo uma imitação de íris e pupila no centro, inserido sob as pálpebras e sustentado pelo conteúdo orbitário após evisceração ou enucleação; pode ser adquirido pronto ou feito sob medida.
black e., o. preto; equimose palpebral e do tecido vizinho.
blear e., blefarite ciliar; blefarite acompanhada por secreção viscora que tende a causar aderência das margens palpebrais. SIN lippitude, lippituto.
bleary e., o. lacrimejante; olho dolorido, lacrimejante, com um aspecto embaçado e, por extensão, diminuição da visão.
compound e., o. composto; o olho dos artrópodes, mais desenvolvido em insetos e crustáceos; o olho consiste em um grupo de elementos visuais funcionalmente relacionados (omatídios) cujas superfícies corneanas formam coletivamente um segmento de uma esfera.
crossed e.'s, estrabismo. SIN strabismus.
cyclopian e., cyclopean e., o. ciclópico. VER cyclopia.
dark-adapted e., o. adaptado à escuridão; olho que esteve na escuridão ou semi-escuridão e sofreu regeneração de rodopsina (púrpura visual), o que o torna mais sensível à iluminação reduzida. SIN scotopic e.
dominant e., o. dominante; olho habitualmente usado em tarefas monoculares. SIN master e.
epiphysial e., o. epifisário. SIN pineal e.
exciting e., o. excitante; o olho lesado na oftalmia simpática.
fixing e., o. fixador; o olho, em casos de estrabismo, que está voltado para o objeto fitado.
hare's e., lagoftalmia. SIN lagophthalmia.
light-adapted e., o. adaptado à luz; olho que foi exposto à luz, com descoramento da rodopsina (púrpura visual) e insensibilidade à baixa iluminação. SIN photopic e.
Listing reduced e., o. reduzido de Listing; uma representação que simplifica cálculos de imagem retiniana: raio da superfície de refração anterior, 5,1 mm; comprimento total, 20 mm; distância do ponto nodal até a retina, 15 mm.
master e., o. dominante. SIN dominant e.
parietal e., o. parietal. SIN pineal e.
phakic e., o. fácico; olho que contém a lente natural.
photopic e., o. fotópico. SIN light-adapted e.
pineal e., o. pineal; olho fotorreceptor, não-formador de imagem, situado na linha média ou próximo dela em alguns crustáceos e vertebrados inferiores; homólogo à glândula pineal em formas superiores. SIN epiphysial e., parietal e.
raccoon e.'s, olhos de guaxinim; equimose bilateral na região periorbitária; sugere uma fratura da base do crânio e também pode ser observada no neuroblastoma. SIN bilateral medial orbital ecchymoses.
reduced e., o. reduzido; desenho simplificado do sistema óptico ocular, representado como possuindo uma única superfície refrativa e um índice uniforme de refração; um modelo baseado nesse conceito é usado em retinoscopia e oftalmoscopia.
schematic e., o. esquemático; a representação do sistema óptico de um olho normal ideal no qual são representados as curvaturas e os índices de refração dos elementos refrativos e suas distâncias intermediárias.
scotopic e., o. escotópico. SIN dark-adapted e.
shipyard e., o. de estaleiro. SIN epidemic keratoconjunctivitis virus.
squinting e., o. estrábico; o olho, em casos de estrabismo, que não está voltado para o objeto fitado.

acomodação do olho

diminuição da capacidade de acomodação relacionada à idade (em dioptrias [Δ]) para pessoas de visão normal

8 anos – 13,8 Δ	40 anos – 5,8 Δ
16 anos – 12,0 Δ	48 anos – 2,5 Δ
24 anos – 10,2 Δ	56 anos – 1,25 Δ
32 anos – 8,2 Δ	64 anos – 1,1 Δ

sympathizing e., o. simpatizante; o olho não lesado na oftalmia simpática que, posteriormente, é envolvido no processo patológico.
watery e., (1) Epífora. SIN epiphora: **(2)** lacrimejamento excessivo.
web e., Pterígio. SIN pterygium (1).
eye·ball (ī'bawl) [TA]. Bulbo do olho; o olho propriamente dito sem os anexos. SIN bulbus oculi [TA], bulb of eye, globe of eye.
eye·bank. Banco de olhos; um lugar onde as córneas de olhos removidas após a morte são preservadas para subseqüente ceratoplastia.
eye·brow [TA]. Supercílio; a linha crescente de pêlos na borda superior da órbita. SIN supercilium.
eye·glass·es. Óculos. SIN spectacles.
eye·grounds (ī'growndz). Fundo do olho; o fundo do olho observado com o oftalmoscópio.
eye·lash. Cílio; um dos pêlos que se projetam da margem palpebral. SIN cilium (1).
ectopic e., c. ectópico; a condição na qual os cílios crescem da pálpebra em outro local além da margem palpebral. SIN canities poliosis.
piebald e., cílios no piebaldismo; feixe isolado de cílios brancos entre cílios normalmente pigmentados. SIN canities circumscripta, ciliary poliosis.
eye·lid [TA]. Pálpebra; uma das duas pregas móveis que cobrem a frente do bulbo do olho quando fechadas; formada por um núcleo fibroso (placa tarsal) e pelas partes palpebrais do músculo orbicular do olho cobertas por pele na região anterior, superficial e revestida por conjuntiva na superfície posterior, profunda; a contração rápida das fibras musculares contidas faz o olho piscar; ambas possuem uma margem fixa (orbitária) e uma margem livre, esta última separada centralmente pela fissura palpebral, unida nas comissuras lateral e medial das pálpebras e possuindo cílios, as aberturas das glândulas tarsais e ciliares e (medialmente) os pontos lacrimais. SIN palpebra [TA], blepharon, lid.
inferior e. [TA], p. inferior; a pálpebra inferior, menor e menos móvel; um ligamento controlador do músculo reto inferior estende-se até ela, puxando a pálpebra para baixo quando o olhar é dirigido para cima. SIN palpebra inferior [TA], lower e.,* lower lid.
lower e., p. inferior; *termo oficial alternativo para inferior e.
superior e. [TA], p. superior; a pálpebra superior, maior e mais móvel que cobre a maior parte da superfície anterior do bulbo do olho, incluindo a córnea, quando fechada; uma parte da glândula lacrimal e a aponeurose do músculo levantador da pálpebra superior estendem-se até ela, o músculo abrindo e fechando o olho e realizando elevação adicional quando o olhar é voltado para cima. SIN palpebra superior [TA], upper e.,* upper lid.
third e., terceira pálpebra. SIN plica semilunaris of conjunctiva (2).
upper e., p. superior; *termo oficial alternativo para superior e.
eye·piece (ī'pēs). Ocular; a lente composta na extremidade do tubo do microscópio mais próxima do olho; amplia a imagem feita pela objetiva.
eye·spot. Ocelo. **1.** Uma mancha colorida ou um plastídeo (cromatóforo) em um organismo unicelular. **2.** SIN ocellus (1).
eye·stone. Pequena concha lisa ou outro objeto introduzido sob a pálpebra para retirar um corpo estranho.
eye·strain. Fadiga visual; astenopia. SIN asthenopia.
eye·wash. Colírio; solução oftálmica; uma solução calmante usada para lavar os olhos.

F

F 1. Símbolo de concentração fracionária (fractional concentration), seguido por subscritos, que indicam a localização e a espécie química; Fahrenheit; farad; fertilidade (fertility); campo visual (visual *field*); flúor (fluorine); folato (folate); geração filial e (filial *generation*), seguido por algarismos subscritos, que indicam combinações específicas; fenilalanina (phenylalanine); razão de variância (variance *ratio*). **2.** Abreviatura de foco (focus [1]); escala francesa (French *scale*).

F Símbolo de faraday, constante de Faraday (Faraday *constant*), força (force); energia livre (free *energy*).

f Símbolo de femto-; freqüência respiratória (respiratory *frequency*); volatilidade (fugacity); formil (formyl); forma fumarose (geralmente após o símbolo do monossacarídeo).

F.A.A.N. Abreviatura de *Fellow of the American Academy of Nursing*.

FAB Abreviatura de *French-American-British* (classificação de leucemias agudas). VER FAB *classification*.

Fab. VER Fab *fragment*.

fa·bel·la (fa-bel′lă). Fabela; osso sesamóide no tendão da cabeça lateral do músculo gastrocnêmio. [L. mod. dim. de *faba*, fava]

Faber, Knud H., médico dinamarquês, 1862–1956. VER F. *anemia, syndrome*.

fa·bism (fā′bizm). Favismo. SIN favism. [L. *faba*, fava]

fab·ri·ca·tion (fab-ri-kā′shŭn). Confabulação; ato de contar histórias falsas como se fossem verdadeiras; p.ex., a simulação de sintomas ou doença, ou o fingimento de uma resposta ou um cálculo incorretos durante um exame do estado mental ou psicológico.

Fabricius (Fabrizzi), Girolamo (Hieronymus ab Aquapendente), anatomista e embriologista italiano, 1537–1619. VER *bursa* fabricii; F. *ship*.

Fabry, Johannes, dermatologista alemão, 1860–1930. VER F. *disease*.

F.A.C.C.P. Abreviatura de *Fellow of the American College of Chest Physicians*.

F.A.C.D. Abreviatura de *Fellow of the American College of Dentists*.

face (fās) [TA]. Face. **1.** A porção frontal da cabeça; o rosto, incluindo os olhos, o nariz, a boca, a testa, as bochechas e o queixo; exclui as orelhas. SIN facies (1) [TA]. **2.** SIN surface.
  bird f., face de pássaro. SIN brachygnathia.
  cow f., f. bovina. SIN *facies* bovina.
  dish f., f. côncava. SIN *facies* scaphoidea.
  frog f., f. de sapo; o aspecto produzido pelo alargamento do nariz, que ocorre em certos casos de pólipos nasais.
  hippocratic f., f. hipocrática. SIN hippocratic *facies*.
  masklike f., f. de máscara. SIN Parkinson *facies*.
  moon f., f. de lua cheia; a face redonda, geralmente vermelha, com grande queixada, observada na doença de Cushing ou no hiperadrenocorticalismo exógeno.
  moon shaped f., f. de lua cheia. SIN moon *facies*.
  superolateral f. of cerebral hemisphere [TA], f. súpero-lateral do hemisfério cerebral. SIN superolateral *surface* of cerebrum.

face-bow. Arco facial; dispositivo que se assemelha a um compasso, utilizado em odontologia para registrar a relação entre os maxilares e as articulações temporomandibulares (ATM); o registro pode ser então utilizado para orientar um molde da maxila em relação ao eixo de abertura e fechamento do articulador. SIN hinge-bow.
  adjustable axis f., arco facial de eixo ajustável, um compasso cujas extremidades podem ser ajustadas para permitir a localização do eixo de rotação da mandíbula. SIN kinematic f.
  kinematic f., arco facial cinemático. SIN adjustable axis f.

face-lift. Cirurgia plástica da face, ritidectomia. SIN rhytidectomy.

fac·et, fa·cette (fas′et, fă-set′) [TA]. Face, fóvea. **1.** Pequena área lisa em um osso ou outra estrutura firme. **2.** Área desgastada em um dente, produzida pela mastigação ou trituração. [Fr. *facette*]
  acromial f. of clavicle [TA], face articular acromial da clavícula; uma faceta pequena e oval, na extremidade lateral da clavícula, para articulação com o acrômio. SIN facies articularis acromialis claviculae [TA], acromial articular facies of clavicle, acromial articular surface of clavicle.
  articular f., face articular; superfície articular relativamente pequena de um osso, especialmente de uma vértebra.
  articular f. of head of fibula [TA], face articular da cabeça da fíbula; a superfície circular plana na cabeça da fíbula para articulação com a faceta correspondente no côndilo lateral da tíbia. SIN facies articularis capitis fibulae [TA].
  articular f. of head of rib [TA], face articular da cabeça da costela; superfície articular na cabeça de uma costela que se articula com o corpo de uma vértebra. SIN facies articularis capitis costae [TA].
  articular f. of lateral malleolus [TA], face articular do maléolo lateral da fíbula; a superfície, na face medial do maléolo lateral, que se articula com o tálus. SIN facies articularis malleoli lateralis fibulae [TA], malleolar articular surface of fibula.
  articular f. of medial malleolus [TA], face articular do maléolo medial da fíbula; faceta articular na superfície lateral do maléolo medial para articulação com o tálus; ela é contínua com a superfície articular inferior da tíbia. SIN facies articularis malleoli medialis tibiae [TA], malleolar articular surface of tibia.
  articular f. of radial head [TA], fóvea articular da cabeça do rádio; depressão no topo (superfície superior) da cabeça do rádio para articulação com o capítulo do úmero. SIN fovea articularis capitis radii [TA], articular pit of head of radius, fovea of radial head.
  articular f. of tubercle of rib [TA], face articular do tubérculo da costela; faceta oval na parte ínfero-medial do tubérculo de uma costela para articulação com uma faceta no processo transverso de uma vértebra. SIN facies articularis tuberculi costae [TA].
  f. (of atlas) for dens [TA], fóvea do dente; faceta circular, na superfície (interna) posterior do arco anterior do atlas, que se articula com o processo odontóide do áxis. SIN fovea dentis atlantis [TA], pit of atlas for dens.
  clavicular f., incisura clavicular do esterno. SIN clavicular *notch* of sternum.
  clavicular articular f. of acromion [TA], face articular da clavícula do acrômio; faceta pequena e oval na borda medial do acrômio para articulação com a extremidade lateral da clavícula. SIN facies articularis clavicularis acromii [TA], articular surface of acromion.
  corneal f., depressão da córnea após perda de estroma.
  costal f.'s, faces costais; superfície articular em uma vértebra para articulação com uma costela.
  fibular articular f. of tibia [TA], face articular fibular da tíbia; a faceta articular circular e plana na porção ínfero-lateral do côndilo lateral da tíbia para articulação com a cabeça da fíbula. SIN facies articularis fibularis tibiae [TA], fibular articular surface of tibia.
  inferior articular f. of atlas, superfície articular inferior do atlas. SIN inferior articular *surface* of atlas.
  inferior costal f. [TA], fóvea costal inferior; semifaceta, na margem inferior do corpo de uma vértebra, que se articula com a cabeça de uma costela. SIN fovea costalis inferior [TA], inferior costal pit.
  lateral malleolar f. of talus [TA], face maleolar lateral do tálus; a superfície da tróclea do tálus que se articula com o maléolo lateral da fíbula. SIN facies malleolaris lateralis tali [TA], lateral malleolar surface of talus.
  Lenoir f., f. de Lenoir; a superfície articular medial da patela.
  locked f.'s, luxação de processos articulares. SIN *dislocation* of articular processes.
  medial malleolar f. of talus [TA], face maleolar medial do tálus; a superfície da tróclea do tálus que se articula com o maléolo medial da tíbia. SIN facies malleolaris medialis tali [TA].
  f. (on talus) for calcaneonavicular part of bifurcate ligament [TA], face articular (no tálus) da parte calcaneonavicular do ligamento bifurcado; pequena face, na margem lateral da superfície articular navicular, que entra em contato com a superfície medial da parte medial do ligamento bifurcado. SIN facies articularis partis calcaneonavicularis ligamenti bifurcati tali [TA].
  f. (on talus) for plantar calcaneonavicular ligament [TA], face articular (no tálus) do ligamento calcaneonavicular plantar; porção mais inferior da superfície articular da cabeça do tálus que entra em contato com (repousa sobre) o ligamento calcaneonavicular plantar. SIN facies ligamenti calcaneonavicularis plantaris tali [TA].
  posterior articular f. of dens [TA], face articular posterior do dente do áxis; a face, na superfície posterior do dente do áxis, que se articula com o ligamento transverso do atlas. SIN facies articularis posterior dentis [TA], posterior articular surface of dens.
  sternal f. of clavicle [TA], face articular esternal da clavícula; a superfície oval, na extremidade esternal da clavícula, que se articula com o disco fibrocartilaginoso da articulação esternoclavicular. SIN facies articularis sternalis claviculae [TA], sternal articular surface of clavicle.
  superior articular f. of atlas, superfície articular superior do atlas. SIN superior articular *surface* of atlas.
  superior costal f. [TA], fóvea costal superior; semifaceta, na margem superior do corpo de uma vértebra, que se articula com a cabeça de uma costela; uma única costela articula-se com a fóvea costal inferior e também com a fóvea costal superior da vértebra adjacente. SIN fovea costalis superior [TA], superior costal pit.

◇ Formas Combinantes
🔲 Indica que o termo é ilustrado, ver Índice de Ilustrações
SIN Sinônimo
Cf. Comparar, confrontar
[NA] *Nomina Anatomica*
[TA] *Terminologia Anatomica*

☆ Termo oficial alternativo para a *Terminologia Anatomica*
[MIM] Mendelian Inheritance in Man
I.C. Índice de Corantes
Termo de Alta Importância

superior f. of trochlear of talus [TA], face superior da tróclea do tálus; a superfície da tróclea do tálus em contato com a superfície articular inferior da tíbia. SIN facies superior tali [TA], superior surface of talus.
transverse costal f. [TA], fóvea costal transversa; faceta no processo transverso de uma vértebra para articulação com o tubérculo de uma costela. SIN fovea costalis processus transversi [TA], costal pit of transverse process.
fac·e·tec·to·my (fas-ē-tek'tō-mē). Facetectomia; excisão de uma faceta. [faceta + G. *ektomē*, excisão]
fa·cial (fā'shăl). Facial; relativo à face. SIN facialis.
fa·ci·a·lis (fā-shē-ā'lis). Facial. SIN facial. [L.]
♲ **-facient**. -faciente; causador; quem ou o que produz algo. [L. *facio*, fazer]

FACIES

fa·ci·es, pl. **fa·ci·es** (fā'shē-ēz, fash'-ēz) [TA]. **1.** [TA]. Face. SIN face (1). **2.** [NA]. Superfície. SIN surface. **3.** Expressão. SIN expression (2). [L.]
acromial articular f. of clavicle, face articular acromial da clavícula. SIN acromial facet of clavicle.
adenoid f., face adenóide; aparência da criança com hipertrofia das adenóides: boca aberta e, freqüentemente, apatia, associadas a um nariz afilado com narinas estreitas.
f. antebrachia'lis ante'rior, região anterior do antebraço. SIN anterior region of forearm.
f. antebrachia'lis poste'rior, região posterior do antebraço. SIN posterior region of forearm.
f. ante'rior [TA], superfície anterior. SIN anterior surface.
f. ante'rior antebra'chii, região anterior do antebraço. SIN anterior region of forearm.
f. ante'rior bra'chii, região anterior do braço. SIN anterior region of arm.
f. ante'rior cor'neae [TA], superfície anterior da córnea. SIN anterior surface of cornea.
f. ante'rior cor'poris maxil'lae [TA], superfície anterior da maxila. SIN anterior surface of maxilla.
f. ante'rior cru'ris, região anterior da perna. SIN anterior region of leg.
f. ante'rior glan'dulae suprarena'lis [TA], superfície anterior da glândula supra-renal. SIN anterior surface of suprarenal gland.
f. ante'rior ir'idis [TA], superfície anterior da íris. SIN anterior surface of iris.
f. ante'rior latera'lis cor'poris hu'meri, superfície ântero-lateral (da diáfise) do úmero. SIN anterolateral surface of (shaft of) humerus.
f. ante'rior len'tis [TA], superfície anterior da lente do olho. SIN anterior surface of lens.
f. ante'rior media'lis cor'poris hu'meri, superfície ântero-medial da diáfise do úmero. SIN anteromedial surface of shaft of humerus.
f. ante'rior mem'bri inferio'ris [TA], superfície anterior do membro inferior. SIN anterior surface of lower limb.
f. ante'rior palpebra'rum, superfície anterior da pálpebra. SIN anterior surface of eyelids.
f. ante'rior par'tis petro'sae os'sis tempora'lis [TA], superfície anterior da parte petrosa do osso temporal. SIN anterior surface of petrous part of temporal bone.
f. ante'rior patel'lae [TA], superfície anterior da patela. SIN anterior surface of patella.
f. ante'rior pros'tatae [TA], superfície anterior da próstata. SIN anterior surface of prostate.
f. ante'rior ra'dii [TA], superfície anterior do rádio. SIN anterior surface of radius.
f. ante'rior re'nis [TA], superfície anterior do rim. SIN anterior surface of kidney.
f. ante'rior ul'nae [TA], superfície anterior da ulna. SIN anterior surface of ulna.
f. anterior uteri [TA], superfície anterior do útero. SIN anterior surface of uterus.
f. anteroinfe'rior corporis pancrea'tis [TA], superfície ântero-inferior do pâncreas. SIN anteroinferior surface of pancreas.
f. anterolateralis cartilaginis arytenoideae [TA], superfície ântero-lateral da cartilagem aritenóidea. SIN anterolateral surface of arytenoid cartilage.
f. anterolatera'lis cor'poris hu'meri [TA], superfície ântero-lateral (da diáfise) do úmero. SIN anterolateral surface of (shaft of) humerus.
f. anteromedia'lis cor'poris hu'meri [TA], superfície ântero-medial da diáfise do úmero. SIN anteromedial surface of shaft of humerus.
f. anterosuperioris corporis pancrea'tis [TA], superfície ântero-superior do corpo do pâncreas. SIN anterosuperior surface of body of pancreas.
f. antoni'na, face antonina; expressão facial causada por alteração nas pálpebras e no segmento anterior do olho; encontrada na lepra.

aortic f., face aórtica; aspecto pálido e amarelado da pessoa com incompetência da valva aórtica; inespecífica.
f. approxima'lis de'ntis, superfície aproximal do dente. SIN approximal surface of tooth.
f. articula'ris [TA], superfície articular. SIN articular surface.
f. articula'ris acromia'lis clavic'ulae [TA], face articular acromial da clavícula. SIN acromial facet of clavicle.
f. articula'ris ante'rior den'tis [TA], face articular anterior do dente do áxis. SIN anterior articular surface of dens.
f. articula'ris arytenoi'dea cricoi'deae [TA], superfície articular aritenóidea da cricóide. SIN arytenoidal articular surface of cricoid.
f. articula'ris calca'nea ta'li [TA], face articular calcânea do tálus. SIN calcaneal articular surface of talus.
f. articula'ris cap'itis cos'tae [TA], face articular da cabeça da costela. SIN articular facet of head of rib.
f. articula'ris cap'itis fib'ulae [TA], face articular da cabeça da fíbula. SIN articular facet of head of fibula.
f. articula'ris car'pi ra'dii [TA], face articular carpal do rádio. SIN carpal articular surface of radius.
f. articula'ris cartila'ginis arytenoi'deae [TA], face articular da cartilagem aritenóidea. SIN articular surface of arytenoid cartilage.
f. articula'ris clavicularis acro'mii [TA], face articular clavicular do acrômio. SIN clavicular articular facet of acromion.
f. articula'ris cuboi'dea ossis calca'nei [TA], face articular do cubóide no calcâneo. SIN articular surface on calcaneus for cuboid bone.
f. articula'ris fibula'ris tib'iae [TA], face articular fibular da tíbia. SIN fibular articular facet of tibia.
f. articula'ris fossae mandibularis os'sis tempora'lis [TA], face articular da fossa mandibular do osso temporal. SIN articular surface of mandibular fossa of temporal bone.
f. articula'ris infe'rior atlan'tis [TA], face articular inferior do atlas. SIN inferior articular surface of atlas.
f. articula'ris infe'rior tib'iae [TA], face articular inferior da tíbia. SIN inferior articular surface of tibia.
f. articula'ris malle'oli lateralis fib'ulae [TA], face articular do maléolo lateral da fíbula. SIN articular facet of lateral malleolus.
f. articula'ris malle'oli media'lis tib'iae [TA], face articular do maléolo medial da tíbia. SIN articular facet of medial malleolus.
f. articula'ris navicula'ris ta'li [TA], face articular navicular do tálus. SIN navicular articular surface of talus.
f. articularis partis calcaneonavicularis ligamenti bifurcati tali [TA], face articular (no tálus) da parte calcaneonavicular do ligamento bifurcado. SIN facet (on talus) for calcaneonavicular part of bifurcate ligament.
f. articula'ris patel'lae [TA], face articular da patela. SIN articular surface of patella.
f. articula'ris poste'rior den'tis [TA], face articular posterior do dente do áxis. SIN posterior articular facet of dens.
f. articula'ris sterna'lis clavic'ulae [TA], face articular esternal da clavícula. SIN sternal facet of clavicle.
f. articula'ris supe'rior atlan'tis [TA], face articular superior do atlas. SIN superior articular surface of atlas.
f. articula'ris supe'rior tib'iae [TA], face articular superior da tíbia. SIN superior articular surface of tibia.
f. articula'ris talaris ante'rior calcanei [TA], face articular talar anterior do calcâneo. SIN anterior talar articular surface of calcaneus.
f. articula'ris tala'ris calca'nei [TA], face articular talar do calcâneo. SIN talar articular surfaces of calcaneus, em surface.
f. articula'ris talaris media calcanei [TA], f. articular talar média do calcâneo. SIN middle talar articular surface of calcaneus.
f. articularis talaris posterior calca'nei [TA], f. articular talar posterior do calcâneo. SIN posterior talar articular surface (of calcaneus).
f. articula'ris thyroi'dea cricoi'deae [TA], f. articular tireóidea da cartilagem cricóidea. SIN thyroid articular surface of cricoid (cartilage).
f. articula'ris tuber'culi cos'tae [TA], f. articular do tubérculo da costela. SIN articular facet of tubercle of rib.
f. auricula'ris os'sis il'ii [TA], f. auricular do ílio. SIN auricular surface of ilium.
f. auricula'ris os'sis sac'ri [TA], f. auricular do sacro. SIN auricular surface of sacrum.
f. bovi'na, face bovina; f. observada no hipertelorismo ocular; típica de disostose craniofacial. SIN cow face.
f. brachia'lis ante'rior, f. anterior do braço. SIN anterior region of arm.
f. brachia'lis poste'rior, f. posterior do braço. SIN posterior region of arm.
f. cerebra'lis, f. cerebral. SIN cerebral surface.
cherubic f., face de querubim; f. característica observada no querubismo; encontrada também na glicogenose, particularmente no tipo 2.
f. co'lica sple'nis [TA], f. cólica do baço. SIN colic impression of spleen.
f. contac'tus den'tis, f. de contato do dente. SIN approximal surface of tooth.
Corvisart f., f. de Corvisart; f. característica observada na insuficiência cardí-

aca ou na regurgitação aórtica; f. edemaciada, purpúrea e cianótica, associada a olhos brilhantes e pálpebras inchadas; inespecífica.
f. costa'lis [TA], f. costal. SIN costal surface.
f. costa'lis pulmo'nis [TA], f. costal do pulmão. SIN costal surface of lung.
f. costa'lis scap'ulae [TA], f. costal da escápula. SIN costal surface of scapula.
f. crura'lis ante'rior, f. anterior da perna. SIN anterior region of leg.
f. crura'lis poste'rior, f. posterior da perna. SIN posterior region of leg.
f. cubita'lis ante'rior, f. cubital anterior. SIN anterior region of elbow.
f. cubita'lis poste'rior, f. cubital posterior. SIN posterior region of elbow.
f. diaphragmat'ica [TA], f. diafragmática. SIN diaphragmatic surface.
f. digita'lis dorsa'lis (manus et pedis) [TA], f. dorsal dos dedos (da mão e do pé). SIN dorsal surface of digit (of hand or foot).
f. digita'lis palma'ris, f. palmar dos dedos das mãos. SIN palmar surfaces of fingers, em surface.
f. digita'lis planta'ris, f. plantar dos dedos dos pés. SIN plantar surface of toe.
f. digita'lis ventra'lis, f. ventral dos dedos das mãos. SIN palmar surfaces of fingers, em surface.
f. dista'lis den'tis [TA], f. distal do dente. SIN distal surface of tooth.
f. doloro'sa, face dolorosa; expressão facial de uma pessoa infeliz, doente ou com dor.
f. dorsa'lis [TA], f. dorsal. SIN dorsal surface.
f. dorsa'lis os'sis sac'ri [TA], f. dorsal do sacro. SIN dorsal surface of sacrum.
f. dorsa'lis scap'ulae, f. dorsal da escápula. SIN posterior surface of scapula.
elfin f., face do elfo; f. caracterizada por nariz curto e arrebitado, boca larga, olhos bem espaçados e bochechas pletóricas; a f. pode estar associada à hipercalcemia, à estenose aórtica supravalvar e ao retardo mental.
f. exter'na [TA], f. externa. SIN external surface.
f. exter'na os'sis fronta'lis [TA], f. externa do frontal. SIN external surface of frontal bone.
f. exter'na os'sis parieta'lis [TA], f. externa do parietal. SIN external surface of parietal bone.
f. facia'lis den'tis, f. facial do dente. SIN vestibular surface of tooth.
f. femora'lis ante'rior, f. femoral anterior. SIN anterior region of thigh.
f. femora'lis poste'rior, f. femoral posterior. SIN posterior region of thigh.
f. gas'trica sple'nis [TA], f. gástrica do baço. SIN gastric impression on spleen.
f. glu'tea os'sis il'ii [TA], f. glútea do ílio. SIN gluteal surface of ilium.
hippocratic f., f. hippocra'tica, face hipocrática; expressão sofrida da face, com olhos fundos, bochechas e têmporas deprimidas, lábios relaxados e tez acinzentada; f. observada em pessoas moribundas, após uma doença grave e prolongada. SIN hippocratic face.
hound-dog f., face de sabujo; aparência facial na cútis laxa, com a pele da face frouxa, pendendo em dobras.
Hutchinson f., face de Hutchinson; expressão facial peculiar causada pela ptose palpebral e pelos olhos imóveis na oftalmoplegia externa.
f. infe'rior hemispherii cerebelli [TA], f. inferior do hemisfério cerebelar. SIN inferior surface of cerebellar hemisphere.
f. infe'rior hemispherii cer'ebri [TA], f. inferior dos dois hemisférios cerebrais, considerados como uma unidade. SIN f. medialis et inferior hemispherii cerebri.
f. infe'rior lin'guae [TA], f. inferior da língua. SIN inferior surface of tongue.
f. infe'rior par'tis petro'sae os'sis tempora'lis [TA], f. inferior da parte petrosa do temporal. SIN inferior surface of petrous part of temporal bone.
f. inferolatera'lis pros'tatae [TA], f. ínfero-lateral da próstata. SIN inferolateral surface of prostate.
f. infratemporalis alaris majoris ossis sphenoidalis [TA], f. infratemporal da asa maior do osso esfenóide. SIN infratemporal surface of greater wing of sphenoid.
f. infratempora'lis corporis maxil'lae [TA], f. infratemporal do corpo da maxila. SIN infratemporal surface of (body of) maxilla.
f. interloba'res pulmo'nis, f. interlobares do pulmão. SIN interlobar surfaces of lung, em surface.
f. inter'na [TA], f. interna. SIN internal surface.
f. inter'na os'sis fronta'lis [TA], f. interna do frontal. SIN internal surface of frontal bone.
f. inter'na os'sis parieta'lis [TA], f. interna do parietal. SIN internal surface of parietal bone.
f. intestina'lis u'teri [TA], f. intestinal do útero. SIN intestinal surface of uterus.
f. latera'lis [TA], f. lateral. SIN lateral surface.
f. latera'lis bra'chii, f. lateral do braço. SIN lateral surface of arm.
f. latera'lis cru'ris, f. lateral da perna. SIN lateral surface of leg.
f. latera'lis digi'ti ma'nus, f. lateral do dedo da mão. SIN lateral surface of finger.
f. latera'lis dig'iti pe'dis, f. lateral do dedo do pé. SIN lateral surface of toe.
f. latera'lis fib'ulae [TA], f. lateral da fíbula. SIN lateral surface of fibula.
f. latera'lis mem'bri inferio'ris, f. lateral do membro inferior. SIN lateral surface of lower limb.
f. latera'lis os'sis zygomat'ici [TA], f. lateral do zigomático. SIN lateral surface of zygomatic bone.
f. latera'lis ova'rii [TA], f. lateral do ovário. SIN lateral surface of ovary.

f. latera'lis tes'tis [TA], f. lateral do testículo. SIN lateral surface of testis.
f. latera'lis tib'iae [TA], f. lateral da tíbia. SIN lateral surface of tibia.
leonine f., face leonina. SIN leontiasis.
f. ligamenti calcaneonavicularis plantaris tali [TA], f. articular do ligamento calcaneonavicular plantar do tálus. SIN facet (on talus) for plantar calcaneonavicular ligament.
f. lingua'lis den'tis [TA], f. lingual do dente. SIN lingual surface of tooth.
f. luna'ta acetab'uli [TA], f. semilunar do acetábulo. SIN lunate surface of acetabulum.
f. malleola'ris latera'lis ta'li [TA], f. maleolar lateral do tálus. SIN lateral malleolar facet of talus.
f. malleola'ris media'lis ta'li [TA], f. maleolar medial do tálus. SIN medial malleolar facet of talus.
f. masticato'ria, superfície mastigatória. SIN denture occlusal surface.
f. maxilla'ris alaris majoris ossis sphenoidalis [TA], f. maxilar da asa maior do esfenóide. SIN maxillary surface of greater wing of sphenoid bone.
f. maxilla'ris os'sis palati'ni, f. maxilar do palatino. SIN maxillary surface of palatine bone.
f. media'lis [TA], f. medial. SIN medial surface.
f. media'lis cartilag'inis arytenoi'deae [TA], f. medial da cartilagem aritenóidea. SIN medial surface of arytenoid cartilage.
f. media'lis dig'iti pe'dis [TA], f. medial dos artelhos. SIN medial surface of toes.
f. media'lis fib'ulae [TA], f. medial da fíbula. SIN medial surface of fibula.
f. media'lis hemispherii cer'ebri [TA], f. medial do hemisfério cerebral. SIN medial surface of cerebral hemisphere.
f. media'lis ova'rii [TA], f. medial do ovário. SIN medial surface of ovary.
f. media'lis pulmo'nis, f. medial do pulmão, face mediastinal do pulmão. SIN mediastinal surface of lung.
f. media'lis tes'tis, f. medial do testículo. SIN medial surface of testis.
f. media'lis tib'iae, f. medial da tíbia. SIN medial surface of tibia.
f. media'lis ul'nae, f. medial da ulna. SIN medial surface of ulna.
f. mediastinalis pulmonis [TA], f. mediastinal do pulmão. SIN mediastinal surface of lung.
f. mesia'lis den'tis [TA], f. mesial do dente. SIN mesial surface of tooth.
mitral f., face mitral; bochechas rosadas, levemente coradas, de pacientes portadores de valvopatia mitral; inespecífica.
moon f., face de lua cheia; arredondamento da face devido à deposição aumentada de gordura nas porções laterais observado em pacientes com hiperadrenocorticalismo, tanto de origem endógena (p.ex., doença de Cushing) como exógena, tal como ocorre no uso terapêutico de agentes semelhantes à cortisona.
myasthenic f., face miastênica; expressão facial observada na miastenia grave, provocada pela queda das pálpebras e dos cantos da boca e pela fraqueza dos músculos da face.
myopathic f., face miopática; aparência facial de alguns pacientes com miopatias e miastenia grave, consistindo em ptose palpebral bilateral e incapacidade para elevar os cantos da boca devido à fraqueza muscular.
f. nasa'lis maxil'lae [TA], f. nasal da maxila. SIN nasal surface of maxilla.
f. nasa'lis os'sis palati'ni [TA], f. nasal do palatino. SIN nasal surface of palatine bone.
f. occlusa'lis den'tis [TA], f. oclusal dos dentes. SIN denture occlusal surface.
f. orbita'lis [TA], f. orbital. SIN orbital surface.
f. palati'na la'minae horizonta'lis os'sis pala'tini [TA], f. palatina da lâmina horizontal do palatino. SIN palatine surface of horizontal plate of palatine bone.
f. palmares digitorum [TA], f. palmar dos dedos das mãos. SIN palmar surfaces of fingers, em surface.
f. pancreatica splenica [TA], f. pancreática do baço.
Parkinson f., face de Parkinson; f. sem expressão ou semelhante a uma máscara, característica do parquinsonismo (1). SIN masklike face.
f. patella'ris fem'oris [TA], f. patelar do fêmur. SIN patellar surface of femur.
f. pelvi'ca os'sis sa'cri [TA], f. pélvica do sacro. SIN pelvic surface of sacrum.
f. poplit'ea fem'oris [TA], f. poplítea do fêmur. SIN popliteal surface of femur.
f. poste'rior [TA], f. posterior. SIN posterior surface.
f. poste'rior cartilag'inis arytenoi'deae [TA], f. posterior da cartilagem aritenóidea. SIN posterior surface of arytenoid cartilage.
f. poste'rior cor'neae [TA], f. posterior da córnea. SIN posterior surface of cornea.
f. poste'rior corporis hu'meri [TA], f. posterior da diáfise do úmero. SIN posterior surface of shaft of humerus.
f. poste'rior cru'ris, f. posterior da perna. SIN posterior region of leg.
f. poste'rior fib'ulae [TA], f. posterior da fíbula. SIN posterior surface of fibula.
f. poste'rior glan'dulae suprarena'lis [TA], f. posterior da glândula suprarenal. SIN posterior surface of suprarenal gland.
f. poste'rior ir'idis [TA], f. posterior da íris. SIN posterior surface of iris.
f. poste'rior len'tis [TA], f. posterior da lente. SIN posterior surface of lens.
f. poste'rior mem'bri inferio'ris, f. posterior do membro inferior. SIN posterior surface of lower limb.

f. poste'rior palpebra'rum [TA], f. posterior da pálpebra. SIN posterior surface of eyelids.
f. poste'rior pancrea'tis [TA], f. posterior do pâncreas. SIN posterior surface of pancreas.
f. poste'rior par'tis petro'sae os'sis tempora'lis [TA], f. posterior da parte petrosa do temporal. SIN posterior surface of petrous part of temporal bone.
f. poste'rior pros'tatae [TA], f. posterior da próstata. SIN posterior surface of prostate.
f. poste'rior ra'dii [TA], f. posterior do rádio. SIN posterior surface of radius.
f. poste'rior re'nis [TA], f. posterior do rim. SIN posterior surface of kidney.
f. posterior scapulae [TA], f. posterior da escápula. SIN posterior surface of scapula.
f. poste'rior tib'iae [TA], f. posterior da tíbia. SIN posterior surface of tibia.
f. poste'rior ul'nae [TA], f. posterior da ulna. SIN posterior surface of ulna.
Potter f., face de Potter; face característica observada na agenesia renal bilateral e em outras malformações renais graves, que apresenta hipertelorismo ocular, baixa implantação das orelhas, queixo recuado e achatamento do nariz. VER TAMBÉM Potter syndrome. SIN Potter disease.
f. pulmona'les cor'dis dextra/sinistra [TA], f. pulmonar direita/esquerda do coração. SIN right/left pulmonary surfaces of heart, em surface.
f. rena'lis glan'dulae suprarena'lis [TA], f. renal da glândula supra-renal. SIN renal surface of suprarenal gland.
f. rena'lis lie'nis, f. renal do baço; * termo oficial alternativo para renal impression of spleen.
f. rena'lis sple'nis [TA], f. renal do baço. SIN renal impression of spleen.
f. sacropelvi'na os'sis il'ii [TA], f. sacropélvica do ílio. SIN sacropelvic surface of ilium.
f. scaphoi'dea, face escafóide; malformação facial caracterizada por fronte protuberante, maxila e nariz deprimidos e queixo proeminente. SIN dish face.
f. sternocosta'lis cor'dis [TA], f. esternocostal do coração. SIN sternocostal surface of heart.
f. supe'rior hemisphe'rii cerebel'li, f. superior do hemisfério cerebelar. SIN superior surface of cerebellar hemisphere.
f. supe'rior ta'li [TA], f. superior do tálus. SIN superior facet of trochlear of talus.
f. superolatera'lis hemispherii cer'ebri [TA], f. súpero-lateral do hemisfério cerebral. SIN superolateral surface of cerebrum.
f. symphysia'lis [TA], f. sinfisial. SIN symphysial surface of pubis.
f. tempora'lis [TA], f. temporal. SIN temporal surface.
f. urethra'lis pe'nis [TA], f. uretral do pênis. SIN urethral surface of penis.
f. vesica'lis u'teri [TA], f. vesical do útero. SIN vesical surface of uterus.
f. vestibula'ris den'tis [TA], f. vestibular do dente. SIN vestibular surface of tooth.
f. viscera'lis hep'atis [TA], f. visceral do fígado. SIN visceral surface of liver.
f. viscera'lis sple'nis [TA], f. visceral do baço. SIN visceral surface of the spleen.
VER TAMBÉM colic impression of spleen, gastric impression on spleen, renal impression of spleen.

fa·cil·i·ta·tion (fă-sĭl′ĭ-tā′shŭn). Facilitação; exacerbação ou reforço de um reflexo ou outra atividade nervosa pela chegada de outros impulsos excitatórios ao centro do reflexo. [L. facilitas, de facilis, fácil]
Wedensky f., f. de Wedensky; chegada de um impulso a uma zona bloqueada, aumentando a excitabilidade do nervo além do bloqueio e indicando que a preparação neuromuscular distal ao bloqueio foi modificada, embora o estímulo intensificador não seja conduzido através da zona bloqueada.
fac·ing (fās′ĭng). Revestimento; material da cor do dente (geralmente de plástico ou porcelana), utilizado para ocultar a superfície bucal ou labial de uma coroa de metal, a fim de dar a aparência externa de um dente natural.
facio-. Facio-; face. VER TAMBÉM prosopo-. [L. facies]
fa·ci·o·lin·gual (fā′shē-ō-lĭng′gwăl). Faciolingual; relativo à face e à língua, indicando freqüentemente uma paralisia que afeta essas partes.
facioplasty (fā′shē-ō-plas-tē). Facioplastia; cirurgia plástica que envolve a face. [facio- + G. plastos, formado]
fa·ci·o·ple·gia. (fā′shē-ō-plē′jē-ă). Facioplegia. SIN facial paralysis. [facio- + G. plēgē, um golpe]
F.A.C.N.M. Abreviatura de Fellow of the American College of Nuclear Medicine.
F.A.C.N.P. Abreviatura de Fellow of the American College of Nuclear Physicians.
F.A.C.O.G. Abreviatura de Fellow of the American College of Obstetricians and Gynecologists.
F.A.C.P. Abreviatura de Fellow of the American College of Physicians ou of Prosthodontists.
F.A.C.R. Abreviatura de Fellow of the American College of Radiology.
FACS Abreviatura de fluorescence-activated cell sorter (separador de células ativado por fluorescência).
F.A.C.S. Abreviatura de Fellow of the American College of Surgeons.
F.A.C.S.M. Abreviatura de Fellow of the American College of Sports Medicine.
F-ac·tin. Actina F. Ver em actin.
fac·ti·tious (fak-tĭsh′ŭs). Factício; artificial; auto-induzido; que não ocorre naturalmente. [L. factitius, produzido por arte, de facio, fazer]

FACTOR

fac·tor (fak′ter). Fator. **1.** Uma das causas contribuintes de qualquer ação. **2.** Um dos componentes que, por multiplicação, compõem um número ou uma expressão. **3.** SIN gene. **4.** Uma vitamina ou outro elemento essencial. **5.** Um evento, uma característica ou outra entidade definível que produz uma mudança em um estado de saúde. **6.** Uma variável absoluta e independente utilizada para identificar, por meio de códigos numéricos, a adesão a um grupo qualitativamente identificável; por exemplo, o superpovoamento é um fator na transmissão de doenças. [L. autor, causador, de facio, fazer]
f. I, f. I; f. convertido a fibrina por ação da trombina no processo de coagulação do sangue. VER TAMBÉM fibrinogen.
f. II, f. II; glicoproteína convertida a trombina pelo fator Xa, pelas plaquetas, pelos íons cálcio e pelo fator V no processo de coagulação do sangue. VER TAMBÉM prothrombin.
f. IIa, f. IIa; trombina. SIN thrombin.
f. III, f. III; f. tecidual ou tromboplastina no processo de coagulação do sangue; inicia a via extrínseca ao reagir com o f. VII e com o cálcio para formar o f. VIIa. VER thromboplastin.
f. IV, f. IV; os íons cálcio no processo de coagulação do sangue.
f. V, f. V; f. do processo de coagulação do sangue, também conhecido como: proacelerina (Owren), f. lábil ou f. lábil do plasma (Quick), globulina aceleradora do plasma (Ware e Seegars), trombogênio (Nolf), protromboquinase (Milstone), f. de conversão de protrombinas plasminas (Stefanini), componente A da protrombina (Quick), acelerador da protrombina (Fantl e Nance), co-fator da tromboplastina (Honorato) e f. acelerador. O f. V não tem ação enzimática própria, mas participa da via comum da coagulação do sangue ligando o f. Xa à superfície das plaquetas. A deficiência desse f. leva a uma rara tendência hemorrágica, conhecida como para-hemofilia ou hipoproacelerinemia, com herança autossômica recessiva; indivíduos hererozigotos são identificados pelo reduzido nível de f. V, sem apresentar, contudo, tendência a hemorragias. SIN accelerator f., labile f., plasma accelerator globulin, plasma labile f., plasmin prothrombins conversion f., proaccelerin, prothrombokinase, thrombogene.
f. V$_{1a}$, f. V$_{1a}$, ácido cobírico. SIN cobyric acid.
f. V$_a$, f. V$_a$; acelerina no processo de coagulação do sangue.
f. VII, f. VII; f. do processo de coagulação do sangue, conhecido também como: proconvertina (Owren), convertina, acelerador da conversão da protrombina sérica (de Vries, Alexander), f. estável (Stefanini), co-fator V (Owren), protrombinogênio (Quick), cotromboplastina (Mann e Hurn), acelerador sérico (Jacox). O f. VII forma um complexo com a tromboplastina tecidual e com o cálcio para ativar o f. X. Sabe-se que o f. VII está envolvido: 1) na deficiência congênita de f. VII, com púrpura e sangramento de mucosas, herança autossômica recessiva; 2) na deficiência adquirida de f. VII associada à deficiência de vitamina K, período neonatal e administração de agentes protrombinopênicos; 3) no excesso adquirido de f. VII em alguns pacientes com tromboembolia. O f. VII acelera a conversão de protrombina em trombina na presença de tromboplastina tecidual, cálcio e f. V. SIN proconvertin, prothrombinogen, stable f.
f. VIII, f. VIII; f. do processo de coagulação do sangue, conhecido também como: f. anti-hemofílico A (Brinkhous), globulina anti-hemofílica (1) (Patek e Taylor), globulina A anti-hemofílica (Cramer), f. anti-hemofílico plasmática (Ratnoff), f. da tromboplastina plasmática A (Aggeler), componente tromboplástico do plasma (Shinowara), tromboplastinogênio (Quick), protromboquinase (Feissly), co-fator plaquetário (Johnson), plasmoquinina (Laki), trombocatilisina (Leggenhager) e acelerador da conversão da protrombina pró-sérica. O f. VIII participa da coagulação sanguínea formando um complexo com o f. IXa, plaquetas e cálcio e catalisando enzimaticamente a ativação do f. X. A deficiência de f. VIII está associada à hemofilia A clássica. O **f. VIII:C** é o componente coagulante do f. VIII que, em pessoas normais, circula no plasma ligado ao **f. VIIIR** (f. de von Willebrand), a proteína plasmática relacionada ao f. VIII, uma grande glicoproteína sintetizada pelas células endoteliais e pelos megacariócitos e que circula no plasma, onde se liga às artérias que perderam seus revestimentos de células endoteliais, criando uma superfície à qual as plaquetas aderem. Os distúrbios envolvendo o f. VIIIR formam um grupo heterogêneo de anormalidades denominado doença de von Willebrand. A deficiência desse f. pode prejudicar o processo de coagulação do sangue. SIN antihemophilic f. A, antihemophilic globulin A, antihemophilic globulin (1), plasma thromboplastin f., platelet cofactor I, prothrombokinase.

f. IX, f. IX; f. do processo de coagulação do sangue, conhecido também como: f. de Christmas (Biggs e Macfarlane), componente da tromboplastina plasmática (Aggeler), globulina B anti-hemofílica (Cramer), f. da tromboplastina plasmática B (Aggeler), f. plasmático X (Shulman), f. anti-hemofílico B e co-fator plaquetário II. O f. IX é necessário para a formação da tromboplastina intrínseca do sangue e afeta a quantidade formada (e não a velocidade de formação). Sua forma ativa, o f. IXa (EC 3.4.21.22), é uma serina proteinase que converte o f. X em f. Xa por meio da ruptura de uma ligação arginina-isoleucina. A deficiência do f. IX causa a hemofilia B. SIN antihemophilic f. B, antihemophilic globulin B, Christmas f., plasma f. X, plasma tromboplastin component, plasma thromboplastin f. B, platelet cofactor II.

f. X, f. X; f. do processo de coagulação do sangue, conhecido também como: f. de Stuart, f. de Stuart-Prower, protrombase e protrombinase. Sua forma ativa, o f. Xa (EC 3.4.21.6), é formada a partir do f. X por meio de proteólise limitada e auxilia a conversão da protrombina em trombina. A deficiência de f. X prejudica a coagulação sanguínea. SIN prothrombinase, Stuart f., Stuart-Prower f.

f. X for *Haemophilus*, hemina. SIN hemin.

f. XI, f. XI; f. do processo de coagulação do sangue, conhecido também como antecedente da tromboplastina plasmática, um componente do sistema de contato que é absorvido do plasma e do soro por vidro e superfícies semelhantes. Sua forma ativa, o f. XIa (EC 3.4.21.27), é uma serina proteinase que converte o f. IX em f. IXa. A deficiência do f. XI resulta em tendência hemorrágica e é causada por um gene autossômico recessivo. SIN plasma thromboplastin antecedent.

f. XII, f. XII; f. do processo de coagulação do sangue, conhecido também como f. de contato e f. de Hageman. Quando ativado pelo contato com o vidro ou outro agente para a sua forma ativa, o f. XIIa (EC 3.4.21.38), uma serina proteinase, ativa os fatores VII e XI e converte o f. XI em f. XIa, sua forma ativa. A deficiência de f. XII acarreta prolongamento significativo do tempo de coagulação do sangue venoso, porém apenas raramente provoca tendência hemorrágica; a deficiência é causada por um gene autossômico recessivo. SIN glass f., Hageman f.

f. XIII, f. XIII; f. do processo de coagulação do sangue, conhecido também como: f. estabilizador da fibrina, f. de Laki-Lorand e f. L-L. É catalisado pela trombina à sua forma ativa, o f. XIIIa, que se liga de forma cruzada a subunidades do coágulo de fibrina para formar fibrina insolúvel. SIN fibrin-stabilizing f., L-L f., Laki-Lorand f.

f. 3, f. 3; **(1)** nome operacional dado a um produto natural, incompletamente caracterizado, que contém selênio e que, em quantidades diminutas, impede a lesão hepática por deficiência de vitamina E em ratos; **(2)** f. III do grupo da vitamina B_{12}, 5-hidroxibenzimidazol, análogo dos componentes nucleotídeos B_{12} habituais.

ABO f.'s, fatores ABO; ver Apêndice de Grupos Sanguíneos.

accelerator f., f. V. SIN f. V.

acetate replacement f., ácido lipóico. SIN lipoic acid.

adrenal weight f., f. do peso da supra-renal; substância postulada de origem adeno-hipofisária, responsável pela manutenção do peso do córtex da supra-renal.

adrenocorticotropic releasing f., f. liberador do hormônio adrenocorticotrópico; hormônio produzido pelo hipotálamo que induz a hipófise a secretar o hormônio adrenocorticotrópico.

angiogenesis f., f. da angiogênese; substância de peso molecular (PM) de 2.000 a 20.000, secretada pelos macrófagos, que estimula a neovascularização na cicatrização de feridas ou no estroma de tumores.

animal protein f. (APF), f. da proteína animal. SIN vitamin B_{12}.

antialopecia f., f. antialopecia. SIN inositol.

antianemic f., f. antianemia. SIN vitamin B_{12}.

antiangiogenesis f., f. antiangiogênese; uma de várias moléculas capazes de inibir a angiogênese.

antiberiberi f., f. antiberibéri. SIN thiamin.

anti–black-tongue f., f. antipelagra. SIN nicotinic acid.

anticomplementary f., f. anticomplementar; fator que interfere com a ação ou função de seu complemento.

antidermatitis f., f. antidermatite. SIN pantothenic acid.

antihemophilic f. A (AHF), f. anti-hemofílico A. SIN f. VIII.

antihemophilic f. B, f. anti-hemofílico B. SIN f. IX.

antihemorrhagic f., f. anti-hemorrágico. SIN vitamin K.

antineuritic f., f. antineurítico. SIN thiamin.

antinuclear f. (ANF), f. antinuclear; f. presente no soro — em geral, anticorpos — com forte afinidade por determinadas proteínas nucleares e detectado pela técnica do anticorpo fluorescente; presente no lúpus eritematoso, na artrite reumatóide e em outras condições auto-imunes; pode também ser encontrado, em níveis mais baixos, nos indivíduos normais.

antipellagra f., f. antipelagra. SIN nicotinic acid.

antipernicious anemia f. (APA), f. antianemia perniciosa; **(1)** SIN vitamin B_{12}; **(2)** especificamente, a cianocobalamina.

antisterility f., f. antiesterilidade. SIN vitamin E (2).

atrial natriuretic f. (ANF), f. natriurético atrial; antigo nome do f. natriurético extraído dos átrios cardíacos. Por se saber agora que se trata de um peptídeo, o termo não é mais utilizado.

f. B, f. B. VER complement pathways.

B_T f., f. B_T. SIN carnitine.

bacteriocin f.'s, fatores de bacteriocinas. SIN bacteriocinogenic plasmids, em plasmid.

B cell differentiating f., f. diferenciador das células B. SIN interleukin-4.

B cell differentiation/growth f.'s, fatores de crescimento/diferenciação das células B; várias substâncias, tais como interleucina 4, 5 e 6, geralmente obtidas a partir do sobrenadante de culturas de células T. Essas substâncias são necessárias para o crescimento, maturação e diferenciação das células B em plasmócitos ou células B de memória.

B cell stimulatory f. 2, f. 2 estimulador de células B. SIN interleukin-6.

bifidus f., f. bífido; substância não-identificada, associada ao *Lactobacillus bifidus*, sp. *pennsylvanicus*, presente no leite de mamíferos.

biotic f.'s, fatores bióticos; fatores ou influências ambientais resultantes das atividades de organismos vivos, em contraste com aqueles resultantes de fatores climáticos, geológicos ou outros.

Bittner milk f., f. lácteo de Bittner. SIN mammary tumor virus of mice.

branching f., f. ramificador; enzima 1,4-α-glucano-ramificadora.

C f.'s, fatores C. SIN coupling f.'s.

CAMP f., f. de CAMP. VER CAMP test.

capillary permeability f., f. de permeabilidade capilar. SIN vitamin P.

Castle intrinsic f., f. intrínseco de Castle. SIN intrinsic f.

Christmas f., f. de Christmas. SIN f. IX.

citrovorum f. (CF), f. citrovorum. SIN folinic acid.

clearing f.'s, fatores depuradores; lipases lipoproteicas que aparecem no plasma durante a lipemia e catalisam a hidrólise de triglicerídeos apenas quando estes últimos estão ligados a proteínas e quando existe um aceptor (p. ex., albumina sérica), "limpando", dessa forma, o plasma.

clotting f., f. de coagulação; qualquer um dos vários componentes do plasma envolvidos no processo de coagulação do sangue. SIN coagulation f.

coagulation f., f. de coagulação. SIN clotting f.

cobra venom f., f. do veneno de cobras do gênero *Naja*; componente do veneno de *Naja* capaz de ativar a via alternativa do complemento.

coenzyme f., diidro lipoamida desidrogenase. SIN dihydrolipoamide dehydrogenase.

colony-stimulating f.'s (CSF), fatores estimuladores de colônias (FEC); um grupo de fatores de crescimento – glicoproteínas – que regula a diferenciação das células mielóides. Essas substâncias agem de modo autócrino ou parácrino sobre as células da medula óssea; parecem agir sinergicamente de forma complexa e pouco conhecida, tendo a capacidade de atuar sobre várias linhagens de células progenitoras e influenciar a função da célula madura.

complement chemotactic f., f. quimiotático do complemento; o complexo ativado do quinto, sexto e sétimo componentes do complemento – C 5a, C 3a, C 5b, 6, 7 –, que induz quimiotaxia no caso de leucócitos polimorfonucleares.

complement f. I, f. I do complemento; uma glicoproteína heterodimérica; sua deficiência leva à ativação descontrolada de C3.

corticotropin-releasing f. (CRF), f. liberador de corticotropina. SIN corticotropin-releasing hormone.

coupling f.'s, fatores de acoplamento; proteínas que restauram a capacidade fosforilativa às mitocôndrias que a perderam, isto é, que se tornaram "desacopladas", de modo que a oxidação e o transporte de elétrons não produzem mais ATP. São geralmente denominados fator de acoplamento F_1, f. de acoplamento F_2, etc. SIN C f.'s.

f. D, f. D. VER complement pathways.

debranching f.'s, fatores desramificadores. SIN debranching enzymes, em enzyme.

decapacitation f., f. de descapacitação; f. que se acredita estar presente no líquido epididimário e no plasma seminal e que impede a capacitação dos espermatozóides.

diabetogenic f., f. diabetogênico; termo raramente utilizado para um f. presente em extratos não-purificados do lobo anterior da hipófise que provoca alterações degenerativas nas células das ilhotas pancreáticas e causa diabetes permanente.

diffusing f., hialuronidase. SIN hyaluronidase (1).

direct lytic f. of cobra venom, f. lítico direto de veneno de cobras *Naja*. SIN cobrotoxin.

Duran-Reynals permeability f., Duran-Reynals spreading f., f. de permeabilidade de Duran-Reynals, f. de dispersão de Duran-Reynals, hialuronidase. SIN hyaluronidase (1).

elongation f., f. de alongamento; proteínas que catalisam o prolongamento de cadeias de peptídeos durante a biossíntese proteica. SIN transfer f. (3).

endothelial relaxing f. (en′dō - thē′li - al) f. de relaxamento do endotélio; óxido nítrico, que age como neurotransmissor e é produzido por macrófagos ativados. Consegue destruir células tumorais, parasitas e bactérias intracelulares.

endothelium-derived relaxing f. (EDRF), f. de relaxamento derivado do endotélio; uma substância difusível produzida por células endoteliais que causa relaxamento da musculatura lisa vascular; óxido nítrico (NO).

eosinophil chemotactic f. of anaphylaxis (ECF-A), f. quimiotático para eosinófilos da anafilaxia (FQE-A); peptídeo (PM 500 a 600) quimiotático para leucócitos eosinófilos e liberado por mastócitos rompidos.

epidermal growth f. (EGF), f. de crescimento epidérmico; proteína antigênica termoestável isolada de glândulas submaxilares de camundongos machos; quando injetada em animais recém-nascidos, acelera a abertura das pálpebras e a erupção dos dentes, estimula o crescimento e a queratinização da epiderme e, em doses maiores, inibe o crescimento do corpo e o desenvolvimento de pêlos e provoca esteatose hepática.

erythrocyte maturation f., f. de maturação de eritrócitos. SIN *vitamin* B_{12}.

essential food f.'s, fatores essenciais da alimentação; aquelas substâncias necessárias na dieta: certos aminoácidos e ácidos graxos insaturados, vitaminas, minerais essenciais, etc.

extrinsic f., f. extrínseco; vitamina B_{12} alimentar.

fermentation *Lactobacillus casei* f., f. de fermentação do *Lactobacillus casei*. SIN pteropterin.

fertility f., f. de fertilidade. SIN F *plasmid*.

fibrin-stabilizing f., f. estabilizador da fibrina. SIN f. XIII.

filtrate f., f. filtrado; antiga designação do ácido pantotênico.

Fitzgerald f., f. de Fitzgerald. SIN high molecular weight *kininogen*.

Flaujeac f., f. de Flaujeac. SIN high molecular weight *kininogen*.

Fletcher f., f. de Fletcher. SIN prekallikrein.

G f., fator G; **(1)** a única variância comum ou o f. que é comum (ou seja, intercorrelaciona-se empiricamente com) a diferentes testes de inteligência (em geral); **(2)** substância exigida para o crescimento de um organismo específico.

glass f., f. de contato. SIN f. XII.

glucose tolerance f., f. de tolerância à glicose; complexo hidrossolúvel que contém cromo e nicotinato, necessário para a tolerância normal à glicose.

f. Gm, f. Gm; f. que determina alguns dos alotipos das imunoglobulinas humanas; encontrado somente nas cadeias γ de IgG (γ-globulina).

gonadotropin-releasing f., f. liberador de gonadotropina. SIN gonadoliberin (1).

granulocyte colony-stimulating f. (G-CSF) (gran′oo-lō-sīt), f. estimulador de colônias de granulócitos (FEC-G); glicoproteínas sintetizadas por várias células que estimulam a produção de neutrófilos a partir de células-tronco (primordiais) hematopoéticas. VER TAMBÉM colony-stimulating f.'s.

granulocyte-macrophage colony-stimulating f. (GM-CSF) (gran′oo-lō-sit-mak′rō-fāj). f. estimulador de colônias de granulócitos e macrófagos (FEC-GM); glicoproteína secretada por macrófagos ou por células do estroma ósseo e que age como um fator de crescimento de células progenitoras mielóides, tais como granulócitos, macrófagos e eosinófilos. VER TAMBÉM colony-stimulating f.'s.

growth f.'s, fatores de crescimento; substâncias naturais, produzidas pelo corpo (hormônios) ou obtidas de alimentos (vitaminas, minerais), que promovem o crescimento e o desenvolvimento, direcionando a maturação e a diferenciação celulares e mediando a manutenção e o reparo dos tecidos; alterações nos fatores de crescimento podem estar envolvidas em neoplasias benignas e malignas.

growth hormone-releasing f. (GHRF, GH-RF), f. liberador do hormônio de crescimento. SIN somatoliberin.

f. H, f. H; **(1)** antiga designação da biotina; **(2)** precursor ou análogo da vitamina B_{12}; **(3)** glicoproteína que regula a atividade do fator C3b do complemento; sua deficiência resulta na falta de inibição da via hemolítica alternativa, levando à ativação e ao consumo contínuos do fator C3 (síndrome hemolítico-urêmica).

Hageman f., f. de Hageman. SIN f. XII.

HG f., f. HG. SIN glucagon.

histamine-releasing f., f. liberador de histamina; uma linfocina produzida por linfócitos estimulados por antígenos que induz a liberação de histamina pelos basófilos.

human antihemophilic f., f. anti-hemofílico humano; concentrado liofilizado de f. VIII, obtido a partir de plasma humano normal fresco; utilizado como agente hemostático na hemofilia. SIN antihemophilic globulin (2), human antihemophilic fraction.

hyperglycemic-glycogenolytic f. (HGF), f. glicogenolítico e hiperglicemiante. SIN glucagon.

impact f., f. de impacto; expressão matemática da freqüência com que artigos originais de determinada revista médica são citados em outras revistas médicas.

inhibition f., f. de inibição. SIN migration-inhibitory f.

initiation f. (IF), f. de iniciação; uma de várias proteínas solúveis envolvidas no início da síntese de ARN ou proteína.

insulinlike growth f. (IGF), f. de crescimento insulino-símile (antes designado somatomedina C), é a somatomedina mais importante para o crescimento pós-natal; é produzido no fígado, no rim, no músculo, na hipófise, no sistema digestório e nos condrócitos. O IGF-I é uma proteína básica (PM 7.600) que circula ligada a seis diferentes proteínas transportadoras de IGF (IGF-BP). Essas proteínas aumentam a meia-vida de circulação do IGF-I para 3–18 h, quando comparada a meia-vida de 20–30 min do hormônio livre. A produção tecidual local do IGF-I/SM-C, sobretudo nos ossos, seria importante na mediação do crescimento através de seus efeitos parácrinos. SIN somatomedins.

intrinsic f. (IF), f. intrínseco; uma mucoproteína relativamente pequena (PM ≅ 50.000), secretada pelas células cervicais das glândulas gástricas e necessária para a absorção adequada de vitamina B_{12} e de outras cobalaminas; sua deficiência causa anemia perniciosa. SIN Castle intrinsic f.

f. Inv, f. Inv; antiga designação dos alótipos Km de um f. de imunoglobulinas humanas; encontrado nas cadeias κ.

ischemia-modifying f.'s, fatores modificadores de isquemia; vários fatores que participam na determinação da magnitude da necrose associada a um acidente vascular cerebral; incluem viscosidade e osmolalidade do sangue, a pressão sanguínea e a anatomia das artérias intracranianas e do pescoço.

labile f., f. lábil. SIN f. V.

***Lactobacillus bulgaricus* f. (LBF),** f. do *Lactobacillus bulgaricus*, panteteína. SIN pantetheine.

***Lactobacillus casei* f.,** f. do *Lactobacillus casei*, ácido fólico. SIN folic acid (2).

Laki-Lorand f., f. de Laki-Lorand. SIN f. XIII.

LE f.'s, fatores LE; imunoglobulinas antinucleares no plasma de pessoas com lúpus eritematoso disseminado, associadas a testes LE-positivos.

lethal f., f. letal. VER genetic *lethal*.

leukemia inhibitory f., f. inibidor de leucemia; uma linfocina que inibe a migração de neutrófilos.

leukocytosis-promoting f., f. promotor de leucocitose; substância obtida por Menkin a partir de exsudatos inflamatórios; estimula a leucocitose.

leukopenic f., f. leucopênico; princípio obtido por Menkin a partir de exsudatos inflamatórios; produz leucopenia quando injetado em animais normais.

lipotropic f., f. lipotrópico, colina. SIN choline.

liver filtrate f., f. do filtrado hepático; antiga designação do ácido pantotênico.

liver *Lactobacillus casei* f., ácido fólico. SIN folic acid (2).

L-L f., f. L-L. SIN f. XIII.

luteinizing hormone/follicle-stimulating hormone-releasing f. (LH/FSH-RF), f. liberador do hormônio folículo estimulante/hormônio luteinizante. SIN gonadoliberin (2).

luteinizing hormone-releasing f. (LH-RF, LRF), f. liberador do hormônio luteinizante; antiga designação do luteinizing hormone-releasing *hormone*.

lymph node permeability f. (LNPF), f. de permeabilidade do linfonodo; uma substância, liberada por linfócitos estimulados ou lesados, que aumenta a permeabilidade capilar e o acúmulo de células mononucleares.

macrophage-activating f. (MAF) (mak′rō-fāj), f. ativador de macrófagos; uma linfocina, derivada basicamente de células T CD4$^+$, que induz a ativação dos macrófagos. O principal f. ativador de macrófagos é o interferon gama. Em camundongos, a interleucina-4 também age como um f. ativador de macrófagos (FAM).

macrophage colony-stimulating f. (M-CSF), f. estimulador de colônias de macrófagos (FEC-M); f. de crescimento – glicoproteína – que leva determinada linhagem de células a proliferar e amadurecer em macrófagos. VER TAMBÉM colony-stimulating f.'s.

maize f., zeatina. SIN zeatin.

mammotropic f., f. mamotrópico, prolactina. SIN prolactin.

maturation f., vitamina B12. SIN *vitamin* B_{12}.

megakaryocyte growth and development f., f de crescimento e desenvolvimento de megacariócitos. SIN thrombopoietin.

melanotropin-releasing f. (MRF), f. liberador de melanotropina. SIN melanoliberin.

mesodermal f., f. mesodérmico; uma proteína que consegue estimular a formação de primórdios de rim e músculo em embriões.

migration-inhibitory f. (MIF), f. inibidor da migração; substância solúvel e não-dialisável, produzida por linfócitos sensibilizados (isto é, linfócitos de um animal sensibilizado) quando expostos ao antígeno específico, que causa aderência e inibição da migração de macrófagos. SIN inhibition f.

milk f., f. lácteo, vírus do tumor mamário de camundongos. SIN mammary tumor *virus* of mice.

monocyte-derived neutrophil chemotactic f. (MDNCF), f. quimiotático para neutrófilos derivados de monócitos. SIN interleukin-8.

mouse antialopecia f., inositol. SIN inositol.

müllerian inhibiting f., f. inibidor mülleriano. SIN müllerian inhibiting *substance*.

müllerian regression f., müllerian duct inhibitory f., f. de regressão mülleriano, f. inibidor do ducto mülleriano; substância não-esteróide, originada no testículo fetal, que atua unilateralmente, inibindo o desenvolvimento dos ductos paramesonéfricos (müllerianos) e agindo junto com a testosterona para promover o desenvolvimento do ducto deferente e de estruturas correlatas.

multicolony-stimulating f. (multi-CSF), f. estimulador de múltiplas colônias. SIN interleukin-3.

myocardial depressant f. (MDF), f. depressor do miocárdio; f. tóxico presente no choque e que prejudica a contratilidade cardíaca; provavelmente um peptídeo liberado na subperfusão da área esplâncnica por ocasião da liberação de enzimas proteolíticas pelo pâncreas.

natural killer cell stimulating f., f. estimulador de células destruidoras naturais; antiga designação da interleucina-12.

nephritic f., f. nefrítico; proteína sérica (possivelmente um auto-anticorpo IgG), encontrada em alguns pacientes com glomerulonefrite membranoproliferativa e hipocomplementemia, que, juntamente com os co-fatores da via alternativa de ativação do complemento, realiza a clivagem do terceiro componente do complemento (C3).

nerve growth f. (NGF), f. de crescimento de nervos; proteína (PM ≅ 26.000) que controla o desenvolvimento de neurônios simpáticos pós-ganglionares e, possivelmente, também de células ganglionares sensoriais (raiz dorsal) em mamíferos; fatores semelhantes, porém não-idênticos, foram isolados de venenos de várias espécies de cobras; o f. foi isolado de glândulas submaxilares de camundongos machos e, quando injetado em animais recém-nascidos, os gânglios simpáticos tornam-se hiperplásicos e hipertróficos; estimula a síntese de ácidos nucleicos e proteínas.

neural f., f. neural; proteína que pode induzir a formação de tecido notocordial em embriões.

neutrophil-activating f., f. ativador de neutrófilos. SIN interleukin-8.

neutrophil chemotactant f. (noo'trō-fil kē'mō-tak-tant), f. quimiotático para neutrófilos. SIN interleukin-8.

nuclear f.-κB, fator nuclear κB; um f. de transcrição associado à produção de citocinas.

osteoclast activating f., f. ativador de osteoclastos; uma linfocina que estimula a reabsorção óssea e inibe a síntese de colágeno ósseo.

Ψ f., f. Ψ. SIN psi f.

f. P, f. P; substância química (postulada por T. Lewis), formada nos músculos esquelético ou cardíaco isquêmicos, tida como responsável pela dor da claudicação intermitente e da angina do peito. SIN substance P of Lewis.

P f., f. P; VER grupo sanguíneo P, em Apêndice de Grupos Sanguíneos.

pellagra-preventing f. (p-p f.), f. preventivo da pelagra. SIN nicotinic acid.

plasma labile f., f. lábil do plasma. SIN f. V.

plasma thromboplastin f. (PTF), f. tromboplastina plasmática. SIN f. VIII.

plasma thromboplastin f. B, f. tromboplastina plasmática B. SIN f. IX.

plasma f. X, f. plasmático X. SIN f. IX.

plasmin prothrombins conversion f. (PPCF), f. de conversão de protrombinas plasminas. SIN f. V.

platelet f. 3, f. plaquetário 3; um fator da coagulação do sangue derivado das plaquetas; trata-se, quimicamente, de uma lipoproteína fosfolipídica que atua juntamente com determinados fatores tromboplastina plasmática na conversão de protrombina em trombina.

platelet-activating f. (PAF), f. ativador de plaquetas. SIN platelet-aggregating f.

platelet-aggregating f. (PAF), f. agregador de plaquetas (FAP); mediador fosfolipídico da agregação plaquetária, da inflamação e da anafilaxia. É produzido em resposta a estímulos específicos por vários tipos celulares, incluindo neutrófilos, basófilos, plaquetas e células endoteliais. Já foram identificadas diversas espécies moleculares do FAP, que variam quanto ao comprimento da cadeia lateral O-alquila. É um importante mediador da broncoconstrição. SIN platelet-activating f.

platelet-derived growth f. (PDGF), f. de crescimento derivado das plaquetas; um f. encontrado nas plaquetas que é mitogênico para as células da região de uma ferida, p.ex., produzindo proliferação endotelial; glicoproteína catiônica mitogênica para fibroblastos, células da musculatura lisa e células gliais. O principal f. sérico necessário ao crescimento e à proliferação de células derivadas do mesênquima em culturas de tecidos.

platelet tissue f., f. tecidual plaquetário. SIN thromboplastin.

p-p f., ácido nicotínico; abreviatura de pellagra-preventing f (fator de prevenção da pelagra).

predisposing f.'s, fatores predisponentes; fatores relacionados à personalidade, a situações e a outros fatores que motivam e guiam um indivíduo a tomar determinadas atitudes relacionadas com o seu bem-estar físico e psíquico.

prolactin-inhibiting f., f. inibidor da prolactina; dopamina, uma substância que inibe a secreção de prolactina pela porção anterior da glândula hipófise.

properdin f. B, f. B da properdina; proteína sérica normal (PM ≅ 95.000) e um dos componentes do sistema da properdina; combina-se com C3b para formar a C3 convertase da via alternativa.

properdin f. D, f. D da properdina; uma α-globulina sérica normal (PM ≅ 25.000) necessária ao sistema da properdina para clivar o fator B em Ba e Bb. Bb combina-se com C3b para formar a C3 convertase da via alternativa do complemento.

protein f., f. proteico; f. (6,25) pelo qual o teor de nitrogênio de uma proteína é multiplicado para se obter a quantidade dessa proteína.

psi f., f. psi; uma proteína responsável pela iniciação específica da reação catalisada pela RNA polimerase nos locais promotores de genes. SIN Ψ f.

pyruvate oxidation f., f. de oxidação do piruvato. SIN lipoic acid.

quality f. (QF), f. de qualidade; f. pelo qual as doses de radiação absorvidas são multiplicadas para se obter, para fins de proteção à radiação, um valor que expressa a efetividade biológica aproximada da dose absorvida. Cf. RBE, relative biologic *effectiveness*.

ρ f., f. ρ. SIN rho f.

R f.'s, fatores R. SIN resistance *plasmids*, em *plasmid*.

radiation weighting f., f. de ponderação da radiação; em radioproteção, um f. que pondera a dose absorvida de radiação de energia e tipo específicos segundo seu efeito em tecidos. VER equivalent *dose*, relative biologic *effectiveness*, quality f.

releasing f. (RF), f. liberador; (1) substâncias, geralmente de origem hipotalâmica, capazes de acelerar a secreção de determinado hormônio pela hipófise anterior; (2) fatores necessários na fase de término tanto da biossíntese de RNA como da biossíntese de proteínas. SIN termination f., liberins, releasing hormone, statins.

resistance f.'s, fatores de resistência. SIN resistance *plasmids*, em *plasmid*.

resistance-inducing f. (RIF), f. indutor de resistência; agente encontrado em embriões de pintos normais que interfere na multiplicação do vírus do sarcoma aviário; trata-se de um vírus da leucose antigenicamente relacionado com o vírus do sarcoma aviário.

resistance-transfer f., f. de transferência de resistência; a porção do plasmídeo contendo genes que conferem resistência, p.ex., a antibióticos.

Rh f., f. Rh; antígeno do sistema do grupo sanguíneo Rh. Ver Apêndice de Grupos Sanguíneos. SIN Rhesus f.

Rhesus f., f. Rhesus; ver Apêndice de Grupos Sanguíneos. SIN Rh f.

rheumatoid f.'s (RF), fatores reumatóides; anticorpos existentes no soro de indivíduos com artrite reumatóide. Esses fatores são auto-anticorpos das classes IgM, IgG e IgA. O f. mais comum é IgM e o que geralmente é dosado. Fatores reumatóides também são encontrados em outras doenças auto-imunes e em algumas doenças infecciosas.

rho f., f. rho; f. de término que libera o RNA a partir do molde DNA; uma proteína bacteriana que é uma helicase dependente de ATP. SIN ρ f.

risk f., f. de risco; uma característica estatisticamente, mas nem sempre causalmente, associada a um risco aumentado de morbidade ou mortalidade, p.ex., o tabagismo como f. de risco para doença cardíaca.

σ f., f. σ. SIN sigma f.

S f., f. S; as variáveis individuais ou os subgrupos empiricamente muito pequenos de intercorrelações ou variância comum, encontrados em diferentes testes de inteligência (específico).

secretor f., f. secretor; a capacidade de secretar antígenos do grupo sanguíneo ABO na saliva e em outros líquidos do corpo, controlada por um par de genes alelos denominados *Se* e *se* (ou *S* e *s*), sendo *Se* o fenótipo dominante com relação a *se*; a saliva de genótipos *SeSe* e *Sese* contém as substâncias A, B ou H do grupo sanguíneo encontradas em seus eritrócitos; a saliva de não-secretores (genótipo *sese*) não contém substâncias do grupo sanguíneo; testes para avaliar a secreção de ABH são úteis em ligação genética e estudos de populações; o fenômeno secretor está também intimamente associado ao grupo sanguíneo de Lewis.

sex f., f. sexual. SIN F *plasmid*.

sigma f., f. sigma; f. que inibe a ligação inespecífica do DNA da RNA polimerase, bem como auxilia a identificação do ponto de partida da transcrição; promove a ligação da RNA polimerase a locais específicos de iniciação. SIN σ f.

slow-reacting f. of anaphylaxis (SRF-A), f. de reação lenta da anafilaxia. SIN slow-reacting *substance*.

SLR f., *Streptococcus lactis* **R f.,** f. SLR, f. R do *Streptococcus lactis*. SIN rhizopterin.

somatotropin release-inhibiting f. (SRIF, SIF), f. inibidor da liberação de somatotropina. SIN somatostatin.

somatotropin-releasing f. (SRF), f. liberador de somatotropina. SIN somatoliberin.

spreading f., hialuronidase. SIN hyaluronidase (1).

stable f., f. estável. SIN f. VII.

stem cell f., f. estimulador de células primordiais (células-tronco); uma citocina que promove o crescimento das células primordiais hematopoéticas e sua diferenciação em várias linhagens celulares.

stringent f., f. limitante; o produto de um gene (uma enzima) que é vital à resposta celular de produção diminuída de ribossomos em consequência da carência de aminoácidos. VER TAMBÉM stringent *response*.

Stuart f., Stuart-Prower f., f. de Stuart, f. de Stuart-Prower. SIN f. X.

sun protection f. (SPF), f. de proteção solar (FPS); a proporção da dose mínima de raios ultravioleta necessária para provocar eritema com ou sem filtro solar; os filtros solares muito efetivos têm FPS ≥ 15.

T-cell growth f., f. de crescimento das células T; designação obsoleta da interleucina-2.

T-cell growth f.-1, fator 1 de crescimento das células T; designação obsoleta da interleucina-2.

T-cell growth f.-2, fator 2 de crescimento das células T; designação obsoleta da interleucina-4.

termination f., f. de término. SIN releasing f. (2).

testis-determining f. (TDF), f. de desenvolvimento dos testículos; o produto de um gene do braço curto do cromossoma Y, responsável pela formação dos testículos.

thymic lymphopoietic f., f. linfopoético do timo; glicoproteína (PM ≅ de 12.000) extraída do timo; esse(s) hormônio(s) produzido(s) pelo timo confere(m) competência imunológica às células timo-dependentes e induze(m) linfopoese.

thyroid-stimulating hormone-releasing f. (TSH-RF), f. liberador do hormônio tireoestimulante. SIN thyroliberin.

thyrotropin-releasing f. (TRF), f. liberador de tireotropina; antiga designação para thyrotropin-releasing *hormone*.

tissue f., f. tecidual, tromboplastina. SIN thromboplastin.

tissue weighting f., f. de ponderação tecidual; em radioproteção, um f. que pondera a dose equivalente em determinado órgão ou tecido em função de sua contribuição relativa para os efeitos deletérios totais que resultam da irradiação uniforme de todo o corpo. VER effective *dose*.

transfer f., f. de transferência; **(1)** o gene de transferência de um plasmídeo de conjugação, especialmente do plasmídeo de resistência; **(2)** um extrato dialisável obtido dos leucócitos de uma pessoa com sensibilidade do tipo tardio e que, após ser injetado na pele de uma pessoa não-sensível, transfere a sensibilidade específica para o receptor; **(3)** SIN elongation f.

transforming f., f. transformador; o DNA responsável pela transformação bacteriana.

transforming growth f.'s (TGF), fatores transformadores do crescimento; dois fatores de crescimento polipeptídicos: o f. α, obtido de meios de cultura condicionados de células transformadas ou tumorais, estimula o crescimento de muitas células epidérmicas e epiteliais, e o f. β, obtido do rim e de plaquetas, controla a proliferação celular e a diferenciação em muitos tipos celulares.

transforming growth f. α (TGFα), f. transformador do crescimento α; uma citocina produzida por células tumorais e células transformadas que está associada ao crescimento e à diferenciação. É também produzida em tecidos normais durante a embriogênese e em determinados tecidos adultos.

transforming growth f. β (TGFβ), f. transformador do crescimento β; uma citocina reguladora com propriedades multifuncionais que podem intensificar ou inibir muitas funções celulares, interferindo inclusive na produção de outras citocinas e aumentando a deposição de colágeno. Tem múltiplos subtipos e é produzida por plaquetas e macrófagos, embora possa ser produzida por muitos outros tipos de células.

transmethylation f., f. de transmetilação, colina. SIN choline.

tumor angiogenic f. (TAF), f. de angiogênese tumoral (FAT); uma substância liberada por tumores sólidos que induz a formação de novos vasos sanguíneos para suprir o tumor.

tumor necrosis f. (TNF), f. de necrose tumoral (FNT). SIN cachectin.

tumor necrosis f.-α, fator de necrose tumoral α; uma citocina pleotrópica amplamente sintetizada por todo o sistema genital feminino.

tumor necrosis f.-β, fator de necrose tumoral β; uma citocina produzida pelas células T CD4 e CD8, após exposição a um antígeno.

uncoupling f.'s fatores de desacoplamento. SIN uncouplers.

von Willebrand f., f. de von Willebrand. VER f. VIII.

W f., f. W, biotina. SIN biotin.

Williams f., f. de Williams, cininogênio de alto peso molecular. SIN high molecular weight *kininogen*.

---

fac·to·ri·al (fak-tōr′ē-ăl). Fatorial (n!). **1.** Pertinente a um fator ou fatores estatísticos. **2.** De um número inteiro, o número inteiro multiplicado sucessivamente por números inteiros menores até o número 1; p.ex., 5! é igual a 5 × 4 × 3 × 2 × 1 = 120.

fac·ul·ta·tive (fak-ŭl-tā′tiv). Facultativo; capaz de viver sob mais de um conjunto específico de condições ambientais; que possui uma via alternativa.

fac·ul·ty (fak′ŭl-tē). Faculdade; uma capacidade natural ou especializada de um organismo vivo.

FAD Abreviatura de flavina adenina dinucleotídeo (*flavin* adenine dinucleotide).

Faget, Jean C., médico francês, 1818–1884. VER F. *sign*.

Fahr, Theodore, médico alemão, 1877–1945. VER F. *disease*.

Fahraeus, Robert (Robin) Sanno, patologista sueco, 1888–1968. VER F.-Lindqvist *effect*.

Fahrenheit (F), Gabriel D., físico teuto-holandês, 1686–1736. VER Fahrenheit *scale*.

fail·ure (fāl′ūr). Insuficiência; estado de insuficiência, falência ou mau desempenho.

backward heart f., i. cardíaca retrógrada; conceito (outrora considerado mutuamente exclusivo da i. cardíaca anterógrada) que afirma resultarem os fenômenos da i. cardíaca congestiva do ingurgitamento passivo das veias, causado por aumento "retrógrado" da pressão proximal às câmaras cardíacas insuficientes. Cf. forward heart f.

cardiac f., i. cardíaca. SIN heart f. (1).

congestive heart f., i. cardíaca congestiva. SIN heart f. (1).

coronary f., i. coronariana; i. coronariana aguda.

electrical f., insuficiência elétrica; condição na qual a i. cardíaca é secundária a um distúrbio do impulso elétrico.

forward heart f., i. cardíaca anterógrada; um conceito (outrora considerado mutuamente exclusivo de i. cardíaca retrógrada) que afirma resultarem os fenômenos da i. cardíaca congestiva do débito cardíaco inadequado e, especialmente, da conseqüente inadequação do fluxo sanguíneo renal que leva à retenção de sódio e água. Cf. backward heart f.

heart f., i. cardíaca; **(1)** inadequação do coração como bomba, de modo que não é possível manter a circulação do sangue, levando ao desenvolvimento de congestão e edema nos tecidos; SIN cardiac f., cardiac insufficiency, congestive heart f., myocardial insufficiency. VER TAMBÉM forward heart f., backward heart f., right ventricular f., left ventricular f.; **(2)** as síndromes clínicas resultantes incluem dispnéia ou edema não-depressível, hepatomegalia dolorosa à palpação, turgência jugular e estertores pulmonares em várias combinações.

high output f., i. de alto débito; i. cardíaca na qual, apesar da relativa falência do miocárdio e da conseqüente i. cardíaca congestiva, o débito cardíaco é mantido em níveis normais ou acima do normal, como se observa às vezes no enfisema, na tireotoxicose, etc.

left-sided heart f., i. cardíaca esquerda; incapacidade das câmaras esquerdas do coração de manter sua carga circulatória, com aumento correspondente da pressão na circulação pulmonar, geralmente com congestão pulmonar e, por fim, edema pulmonar. SIN left ventricular f.

left ventricular f., i. ventricular esquerda. SIN left-sided heart f.

low output f., i. de baixo débito; i. cardíaca na qual o débito cardíaco está abaixo do normal, como se observa geralmente na i. resultante de coronariopatia, cardiopatia hipertensiva ou valvopatia cardíaca.

pacemaker f., falência do marcapasso; incapacidade do marcapasso artificial em gerar ou transmitir estímulos efetivos para o miocárdio.

power f., falência de bomba. SIN pump f.

premature ovarian f., i. ovariana prematura. SIN premature *menopause*.

pump f., i. da bomba, falência da bomba; termo utilizado para enfatizar o defeito mecânico do coração como bomba; no infarto agudo do miocárdio, falência de bomba significa insuficiência cardíaca congestiva, edema pulmonar ou choque cardiogênico. Cf. electrical f. SIN power f.

pure autonomic f., i. autônoma pura; doença neurológica degenerativa esporádica de início no adulto, que se manifesta principalmente como hipotensão ortostática e síncope, sem defeitos neurológicos a não ser uma evidente disfunção do sistema nervoso autônomo; provavelmente causada por degeneração seletiva de neurônios nos gânglios simpáticos, com desnervação da vasculatura dos músculos lisos e das glândulas supra-renais. SIN Bradbury-Eggleston syndrome.

renal f., i. renal; perda da função renal, tanto aguda quanto crônica, que resulta em azotemia e síndrome urêmica.

respiratory f., i. respiratória; perda da função pulmonar, tanto aguda quanto crônica, que resulta em hipoxemia e hipercapnia; via final comum para uma miríade de doenças respiratórias.

right ventricular f., i. ventricular direita; i. cardíaca congestiva manifestada por turgência jugular, hepatomegalia e edema postural devido à falência do ventrículo direito como bomba.

secondary f., i. secundária; **(1)** disfunção de um órgão como resultado de doença preexistente em outro local; **(2)** responsividade cada vez menor a um fármaco após uma resposta satisfatória inicial, que ocorre geralmente vários meses depois do início do tratamento.

f. to thrive, retardo no crescimento e desenvolvimento; condição na qual o crescimento e o ganho de peso de um lactente estão muito abaixo dos níveis normais para a idade.

faint (fānt). **1.** Extremamente fraco; ameaçado de síncope. **2.** Um episódio de síncope. VER TAMBÉM syncope. [I. m., do Fr. ant. *feindre*, fingir]

fal·cate (fal′kāt). Falcato. SIN falciform.

fal·ces (fal′sēz). Foices; plural de falx (foice).

fal·cial (fal′shăl). Falcial; relativo à foice do cerebelo ou à foice do cérebro. SIN falcine.

fal·ci·form (fal′si-fōrm). Falciforme; que tem a forma de um crescente ou de uma foice. SIN falcate. [L. *falx*, foice, + *forma*, forma]

fal·cine (fal′sēn). Falcial. SIN falcial.

fal·cu·la (fal′kū-lă). Fálcula. SIN *falx* cerebelli. [L. dim. de *falx*]

fal·cu·lar (fal′kū-lăr). Falcular. **1.** Que se parece com uma foice. **2.** Relativo à foice do cerebelo ou à foice do cérebro.

fal·lo·pi·an (fa-lō′pē-an). Falopiano; descrito por, ou atribuído a, Fallopius.

Fallopio, VER Fallopius.

Fallopius (Fallopio), Gabriele, anatomista italiano, 1523–1562. VER fallopian *aqueduct*; fallopian *arch*; fallopian *canal*; fallopian *hiatus*; fallopian *ligament*; fallopian *neuritis*; fallopian *pregnancy*; fallopian *tube*; *aqueductus* fallopii; *tuba* fallopiana; fallopian *tube*.

Fallot, Étienne-Louis A., médico francês, 1850–1911. VER *pentalogy* of F.; F. *tetrad*, *triad*; *trilogy* of F.

false neg·a·tive (fawls neg′ă-tiv). Falso-negativo. **1.** Resultado de teste que, erroneamente, exclui um indivíduo de um grupo diagnóstico ou de referência específico. **2.** Indivíduo cujos resultados de testes o excluem de um grupo di-

false negative

agnóstico específico ao qual ele pertence de fato. **3.** Termo utilizado para indicar um resultado falso-negativo. VER false-negative *result*.

fal·se pos·i·tive (fawls pos′i-tiv). Falso-positivo. **1.** Resultado de teste que erroneamente designa um indivíduo para um grupo diagnóstico ou de referência específico; deve-se sobretudo a métodos de avaliação insuficientemente exatos. **2.** Indivíduo cujos resultados de testes o incluem em um grupo diagnóstico específico, embora ele não pertença de fato a esse grupo. **3.** Termo utilizado para indicar um resultado falso-positivo. VER false-positive *result*.

fal·set·to (fal-set′tō). Falsete; termo descritivo de fonação em uma freqüência anormalmente alta. [It., de *falso*, falso, + *-etto*, dim. sufixo]

fal·si·fi·ca·tion (fawl′si-fi-kā′shŭn). Falsificação; ato deliberado de deturpação com a finalidade de enganar. VER Munchausen *syndrome*. [L. *falsus*, falso, + *facio*, fazer]

    retrospective f., f. retrospectiva; distorção inconsciente de experiências passadas com a finalidade de ajustar-se às necessidades psicológicas atuais.

falx, pl. **fal·ces** (falks, fal′sēz). [TA]. Foice; estrutura com forma de foice. [L. foice]

    f. aponeurot′ica, f. aponeurótica. SIN inguinal f.
    cerebellar f., f. do cerebelo; *termo oficial alternativo para f. cerebelli.
    f. cerebel′li [TA], f. do cerebelo; curto processo da dura-máter que se projeta para a frente a partir da crista occipital interna abaixo do tentório; ocupa a fissura cerebelar posterior e a valécula e bifurca-se abaixo em dois ramos divergentes que passam de cada lado do forame magno. SIN cerebellar f.*, falcula.
    cerebral f., f. do cérebro; *termo oficial alternativo para f. cerebri.
    f. cer′ebri [TA], f. do cérebro; prega em forma de foice da dura-máter na fissura longitudinal entre os dois hemisférios cerebrais; liga-se, anteriormente, à crista etmoidal do osso etmóide e, caudalmente, à superfície superior do tentório. SIN cerebral f.*.
    inguinal f. [TA], f. inguinal; tendão comum de inserção dos músculos transverso e oblíquo interno na crista púbica e no tubérculo púbico e na linha iliopectínea; é freqüentemente mais muscular do que aponeurótico e pode estar mal desenvolvido; forma a parede posterior do canal inguinal medial. SIN f. inguinalis [TA], conjoint tendon*, tendo conjunctivus*, conjoined tendon, f. aponeurotica, inguinal aponeurotic fold.
    f. inguina′lis [TA], f. inguinal. SIN inguinal f.
    f. sep′ti, f. do septo. SIN valve of foramen ovale.

fa·mil·i·al (fa-mil′ē-ăl). Familial; que afeta mais membros de uma mesma família do que pode ser atribuído ao acaso, geralmente em um único grupo com ascendentes em comum; comumente utilizado, embora incorretamente, para significar genético. [L. *familia*, família]

fa·mil·i·al neu·ro·vis·cer·o·lip·i·do·sis. Neurovisceolipidose familial. SIN infantile, generalized G$_{M1}$ *gangliosidosis*.

fam·i·ly (fam′i-lē). Família. **1.** Grupo de duas ou mais pessoas unidas por laços sanguíneos, adotivos ou maritais ou lei comum equivalente. **2.** Na classificação biológica, um grupamento taxonômico localizado no nível intermediário entre a ordem e a tribo ou gênero. **3.** Grupo de substâncias estruturalmente relacionadas. **4.** Grupo de proteínas com seqüência e perfis farmacológicos e/ou de registro característicos. [L. *familia*]

    alu f., f. Alu; conjunto de seqüências dispersas do genoma humano que apresenta locais de clivagem Alu em cada extremidade.
    alu-equivalent f., f. Alu-equivalente; conjunto de seqüências do genoma de mamíferos que está relacionado à f. Alu humana.
    cancer f., grupo de parentes unidos por laços sanguíneos do qual várias pessoas tiveram câncer; o modo de agregação pode ser genético e homogêneo, como ocorre na polipose familial do cólon; variado, como ocorre na neurofibromatose; ou devido à exposição comum a um agente carcinogênico ou oncogênico, como um vírus.
    extended f., f. estendida; grupo de pessoas que engloba membros de várias gerações, unidos por laços sanguíneos, adotivos, maritais ou equivalentes.
    gene f., f. gênica; grupo de genes que apresentam seqüências semelhantes.
    nuclear f., f. nuclear; em genética, dois genitores e sua progênie em comum.

fa·mo·ti·dine (fa-mō′ti-dēn). Famotidina; antagonista da histamina H$_2$ utilizado no tratamento de úlceras duodenais para reduzir a secreção de ácido clorídrico.

fam·o·tine hy·dro·chlo·ride (fam′ō-tēn). Cloridrato de famotina; agente antiviral.

Fañanás, J., médico espanhol. VER F. *cell*.

Fanconi, Guido, pediatra suíço, 1892–1979. VER F. *anemia, pancytopenia, syndrome*.

fang. Presa. **1.** Dente longo ou presa, geralmente um canino. **2.** Dente oco de uma cobra através do qual o veneno é expelido. [A.S. *fōhan*, agarrar]

fan·go (fang′gō). Fango; lama das fontes termais de Battaglio, na Itália, aplicada externamente para tratar o reumatismo e outras doenças das articulações e dos músculos. [It. lama]

Fan·nia (fan′ē-ă). Gênero de moscas da família Muscidae. Entre as espécies, incluem-se *F. canicularis* (a menor mosca doméstica), comumente observada nas cozinhas ou próximo a alimentos, que se assemelha à *Musca domestica* (a mosca doméstica comum), porém um pouco menor e com três listras marrons no tórax, e *F. scalaris* (a mosca das latrinas), que comumente deposita seus ovos em fezes líquidas de seres humanos e de animais e é distinguida da *F. canicularis* pelas duas listras marrons em seu tórax.

fan·ta·sy (fan′tă-sē). Fantasia; imagens mais ou menos coerentes, como em sonhos e devaneios, porém não-restritas pela realidade. SIN phantasia. [G. *phantasia*, idéia, imagem]

FAP Abreviatura de familial adenomatous *polyposis* (polipose adenomatosa familiar).

Farabeuf, Louis H., cirurgião francês, 1841–1910. VER F. *amputation, triangle*.

far·ad (F) (fa′rad). Farad; unidade prática de capacidade elétrica; a capacidade de um condensador que possui uma carga de 1 coulomb sob uma força eletromotriz de 1 V. [M. *Faraday*]

Faraday, Michael, físico e químico inglês, 1791–1867. VER farad; faraday; F. *constant, laws*, em *law*.

far·a·day (F), Fa·ra·day (fa′ră-dā). Faraday; 96.485,309 coulombs por mol, a eletricidade necessária para reduzir um equivalente de um íon monovalente. [M. *Faraday*]

far·a·dism (fa′ră-dizm). Faradismo; eletricidade (indução) farádica.
    surging f., f. ondulante; corrente de amplitude gradualmente crescente e decrescente, obtida pela interposição de uma resistência rítmica a uma corrente alternada produzida pela bobina de indução.

far·a·di·za·tion (fa′rad-i-zā′shŭn). Faradização; aplicação terapêutica da corrente elétrica farádica (induzida).

fa·ra·do·con·trac·til·i·ty (fa′ră-dō-kon′trak-til′i-tē). Contratilidade farádica; contratilidade dos músculos sob o estímulo de uma corrente elétrica farádica (induzida).

fa·ra·do·mus·cu·lar (fa′ră-dō-mŭs′kū-lăr). Faradomuscular; relativo à ação de aplicar uma corrente elétrica farádica (induzida) diretamente em um músculo.

far·a·do·pal·pa·tion (fa′ră-dō-pal-pā′shŭn). Faradopalpação; estesiometria por meio de um eletrodo pontiagudo através do qual uma corrente alternada fraca passa para um eletrodo indiferente.

far·a·do·ther·a·py (fa′ră-dō-thār′ă-pē). Faradoterapia; tratamento de doença ou de paralisia por meio de corrente elétrica farádica (induzida).

Farber, Sidney, patologista pediátrico norte-americano, 1903–1973. VER F. *disease, syndrome*.

far·cy (far′sē). Farcinose. **1.** Doença linfática do gado causada pela *Nocardia farcinica*. **2.** Forma cutânea do mormo. [L. *farcio*, encher]

far·del (far′del). Fardo; a penalidade total mensurável a que se fica sujeito como resultado da ocorrência de uma doença genética em um indivíduo; uma de duas principais considerações quantitativas nos aspectos prognósticos do aconselhamento genético, sendo a outra o risco de ocorrência. O f. avalia de forma aproximada a duração e a gravidade de uma penalidade, isto é, a integral da função intensidade-tempo total; p.ex., a cegueira para as cores tem uma baixa intensidade de penalidade ao longo da vida, a anencefalia causa angústia intensa por um curto período de tempo, a doença de Alzheimer é intermediária quanto a esses dois fatores, porém o f. é maior. [I. m., do Fr. ant., do Ar. *fardah*, fardo]

far·fa·ra (far′far-ă). Fárfara, folhas de tussilagem; as folhas secas de *Tussilago farfara* (família Compositae); um demulcente. [L. *farfarus*, fárfara, tussilagem]

fa·ri·na (fă-rē′nă). Farinha ou alimento preparado a partir de grãos de cereais, tais como *Avena sativa* (aveia) ou *Triticum sativum* (trigo); utilizada como alimento amiláceo. [L.]
    f. avenae (fă-rē′nă ā-vē-nă), farinha de aveia.
    f. tritici (fă-rē′nă trit′ĭ-sē), farinha de trigo.

far·i·na·ceous (far-i-nā′shŭs). Farináceo. **1.** Relativo à farinha. **2.** Amiláceo.

α-far·ne·sene (far′nĕ-sēn). α-farneseno; hidrocarboneto de cadeia aberta e reta composto por três unidades isopreno; uma das quatro formas isoméricas é encontrada na casca das maçãs.

β-far·ne·sene. β-farneseno; um dos dois isômeros (*trans*) presentes no feromônio de alarme de alguns afídeos, bem como em vários óleos essenciais.

far·ne·sene al·co·hol. Álcool de farneseno. SIN farnesol.

far·ne·sol (far′nĕ-sol). Farnesol; um grupamento difarnesil presente na cadeia lateral da vitamina K$_2$ e que compõe o esqualeno; encontrado no óleo de citronela; um álcool sesquiterpênico. SIN farnesene alcohol.

far·nes·yl py·ro·phos·phate (far′nĕ-sil pi′rō-fos′făt). Pirofosfato de farnesil; o derivado pirofosforil do farnesol; um intermediário importante na síntese de esteróides, dolicol, ubiquinona, proteínas preniladas e heme a.

far·no·qui·none (far′nō-kwin′ōn). Farnoquinona. SIN menaquinone-6.

Farnsworth, Dean, oficial naval norte-americano, 1902–1959. SIN F.-Munsell color *test*.

Farr, William, estatístico médico inglês, 1807–1883. VER F. *laws*, em *law*.

Farrant mount·ing flu·id. Líquido de montagem de Farrant. VER em *fluid*.

Farre, Arthur, ginecologista e obstetra inglês, 1811–1887. VER F. *line*.

far·sight·ed·ness (far′sīt′ed-nes). Hipermetropia. SIN hyperopia.

Fas. Fas; receptor presente em células que se liga ao Fas-ligante para induzir apoptose. VER TAMBÉM Fas *ligand*.

FASCIA

fas·cia, pl. **fas·ci·ae**, **fas·ci·as** (fash′ē-ă, -ē-ē) [TA]. Fáscia; lâmina de tecido fibroso que envolve o corpo por baixo da pele; envolve também músculos e grupos de músculos e separa suas diversas camadas ou grupos. [L. uma faixa ou um filete]
f. abdominalis parietalis, f. parietal do abdome; *termo oficial alternativo para extraperitoneal f.
Abernethy f., f. de Abernethy; camada de tecido areolar subperitoneal em frente à artéria ilíaca externa. VER iliac f.
f. adhe'rens, f. aderente; ampla junção intercelular no disco intercalado do músculo cardíaco que fixa os filamentos de actina.
anal f., f. inferior do diafragma da pelve. SIN inferior f. of pelvic diaphragm.
antebrachial f. [TA], f. antebraquial; f. contínua com a f. braquial; forma duas faixas espessas, os retináculos extensor e flexor, na região do punho. SIN f. antebrachii [TA], deep f. of forearm, f. of forearm.
f. antebra'chii [TA], f. antebraquial. SIN antebrachial f.
f. axilla'ris [TA], f. axilar. SIN axillary f.
axillary f. [TA], f. axilar; a f. perfurada que forma o assoalho da axila. É contínua com as fáscias peitoral e clavipeitoral, anteriormente, com a f. braquial, lateralmente, e com a f. dos músculos latíssimo do dorso e serrátil anterior posterior e medialmente. SIN f. axillaris [TA].
bicipital f., aponeurose bicipital. SIN bicipital aponeurosis.
brachial f. [TA], f. do braço; a f. profunda do braço; é contínua proximalmente com a f. peitoral e com a f. que recobre o deltóide; é contínua distalmente com a f. antebraquial. SIN f. brachii [TA], deep f. of arm.
f. bra'chii [TA], f. do braço. SIN brachial f.
broad f., f. profunda da coxa. SIN deep f. of thigh.
f. buc'copharyn'gea [TA], f. bucofaríngea. SIN buccopharyngeal f.
buccopharyngeal f. [TA], f. bucofaríngea; f. que recobre a camada muscular da faringe e continua para a frente sobre o músculo bucinador. SIN f. buccopharyngea [TA].
Buck f., f. de Buck. SIN f. of penis.
f. bul'bi, bainha fascial do bulbo do olho. SIN fascial sheath of eyeball.
Camper f., f. de Camper. SIN fatty layer of subcutaneous tissue of abdomen.
f. cervica'lis [TA], f. cervical. SIN (deep) cervical f.
f. cervicalis profunda, f. cervical profunda. SIN (deep) cervical f.
f. cine'rea, giro fasciolar. SIN fasciolar gyrus.
clavipectoral f. [TA], f. clavipeitoral; f. que se estende entre o processo coracóide, a clavícula e a parede torácica. Inclui a f. muscular que envolve os músculos subclávio e peitoral menor e, também, a forte membrana (membrana costocoracóidea) formada no espaço entre eles e o ligamento suspensor da axila. A f. clavipeitoral (e os músculos que ela envolve) constitui a parede anterior profunda da axila. SIN f. clavipectoralis [TA].
f. clavipectora'lis [TA], f. clavipeitoral. SIN clavipectoral f.
f. clitor'idis [TA], f. do clitóris. SIN f. of clitoris.
f. of clitoris [TA], f. do clitóris; tecido fibroso comparável à f. do pênis. SIN f. clitoridis [TA].
Colles f., f. de Colles. SIN subcutaneous tissue of perineum.
Cooper f., f. de Cooper. SIN cremasteric f.
cremasteric f. [TA], f. cremastérica; revestimento intermediário do funículo espermático, formado por delicado tecido conectivo e por fibras musculares derivadas do músculo oblíquo interno (músculo cremaster). VER TAMBÉM aponeurosis of internal oblique muscle. SIN f. cremasterica [TA], Cooper f., Scarpa sheath.
f. cremaster'ica [TA], f. cremastérica. SIN cremasteric f.
cribriform f. [TA], f. cribriforme; a parte da f. superficial da coxa que reveste o hiato safeno. SIN f. cribrosa [TA], Hesselbach f.
f. cribro'sa [TA], f. cribosa. SIN cribriform f.
crural f., f. crural. SIN deep f. of leg.
f. cru'ris [TA], f. da perna. SIN deep f. of leg.
Cruveilhier f., f. de Cruveilhier. SIN subcutaneous tissue of perineum.
dartos f. [TA], túnica dartos; camada de tecido muscular liso no tegumento do escroto. VER TAMBÉM dartos muliebris, dartos muscle. SIN tunica dartos [TA], superficial f. of scrotum*, membrana carnosa, tunica carnea.
deep f., f. profunda; membrana fibrosa fina, destituída de gordura, que envolve os músculos, separa os diversos grupos musculares e os músculos individuais, forma bainhas para os nervos e vasos, torna-se especializada ao redor das articulações para formar ou reforçar ligamentos, envolve diversos órgãos e glândulas e une todas as estruturas em uma massa firme e compacta. A Terminologia Anatomica [TA] recomenda que os termos "fáscia superficial" e "fáscia profunda" não sejam utilizados de forma genérica, sem especificações, por causa da variação de seus significados no âmbito internacional. Os termos recomendados são "tecido subcutâneo [TA] (tela subcutanea)", no lugar de fáscia superficial, e "fáscia muscular" ou "fáscia visceral" (fascia musculorum ou fascia viscera[is]) no lugar de fáscia profunda. SIN f. profunda.
deep f. of arm, f. profunda do braço. SIN brachial f.
(deep) cervical f. [TA], f. cervical (profunda); f. do pescoço; divide-se em uma camada externa ou de revestimento (lâmina superficial), que circunda o pescoço e envolve os músculos trapézio e esternocleidomastóideo, uma camada média ou pré-traqueal em relação aos músculos infra-hióideos e uma camada profunda ou pré-vertebral relacionado aos músculos axiais e às vértebras. SIN f. cervicalis [TA], deep f. of neck, f. cervicalis profunda.
deep f. of forearm, f. profunda do antebraço. SIN antebrachial f.
deep f. of leg [TA], f. da perna; é contínua com a f. lata e fixa-se proximalmente à patela, ao ligamento patelar, ao tubérculo e aos côndilos da tíbia e à cabeça da fíbula; na extremidade distal, espessa-se para formar os retináculos flexor e extensor. SIN f. cruris [TA], crural f., f. of leg.
deep f. of neck, f. cervical. SIN (deep) cervical f.
deep f. of penis, f. do pênis. SIN f. of penis.
deep perineal f., f. do períneo; *termo oficial alternativo para perineal f.
deep f. of thigh, f. lata; a forte f. e profunda da coxa, que envolve os músculos da coxa e que se espessa lateralmente, formando o trato iliotibial. SIN f. lata [TA], broad f.
f. denta'ta hippocam'pi, f. denteada do hipocampo. SIN dentate gyrus.
dentate f., giro dentado. SIN dentate gyrus.
f. diaphrag'matis pel'vis infe'rior [TA], f. inferior do diafragma da pelve. SIN inferior f. of pelvic diaphragm.
f. diaphrag'matis urogenita'lis infe'rior, membrana do períneo; designação obsoleta da perineal membrane.
dorsal f. of foot [TA], f. dorsal do pé; f. que envolve os tendões extensores dos artelhos e se funde com o retináculo extensor inferior. SIN f. dorsalis pedis [TA].
dorsal f. of hand [TA], f. dorsal da mão; f. profunda do dorso da mão, contínua proximalmente com o retináculo extensor. SIN f. dorsalis manus [TA].
f. dorsa'lis ma'nus [TA], f. dorsal da mão. SIN dorsal f. of hand.
f. dorsa'lis pe'dis [TA], f. dorsal do pé. SIN dorsal f. of foot.
Dupuytren f., f. de Dupuytren. SIN palmar aponeurosis.
endoabdominal f. [TA], f. endoabdominal; (1) SIN extraperitoneal f.; (2) termo utilizado genericamente para incluir não só a f. extraperitoneal parietal, mas também a f. visceral na cavidade abdominopélvica. SIN f. endoabdominalis [TA].
f. endoabdominalis [TA], f. endoabdominal. SIN endoabdominal f.
endopelvic f., f. endopélvica; *termo oficial alternativo para parietal pelvic f.
f. endopelvina, f. parietal da pelve; *termo oficial alternativo para parietal pelvic f.
endothoracic f. [TA], f. endotorácica; f. extrapleural que reveste a parede do tórax; estende-se sobre a cúpula da pleura (como a membrana suprapleural) e também forma uma delgada camada entre o diafragma e a pleura (f. frenicopleural). Essa camada areolar frouxa forma um plano cirúrgico extrapleural. SIN f. endothoracica [TA].
f. endothora'cica [TA], f. endotorácica. SIN endothoracic f.
external spermatic f. [TA], f. espermática externa; o revestimento fascial externo do funículo espermático; é contínua, no anel inguinal superficial, com a f. que reveste o músculo oblíquo externo. VER TAMBÉM aponeurosis of external oblique muscle. SIN f. spermatica externa [TA].
f. of extraocular muscles, f. dos músculos extrínsecos do bulbo de olho. SIN muscular f. of extraocular muscle.
extraperitoneal f. [TA], f. extraperitoneal; plano fascial constituído principalmente por tecido areolar frouxo entre o peritônio parietal e as fáscias muscular interna (f. do iliopsoas e lâmina interna da f. toracolombar) e transversal da parede do corpo; sua qualidade e quantidade variam consideravelmente, sendo muito espessa e gordurosa posteriormente, como f. pararrenal em torno dos rins, e delgada e fibrosa anteriormente, sob a linha alba na parede abdominal anterior. SIN endoabdominal f. (1) [TA], parietal abdominal. [TA], f. abdominalis parietalis*, f. subperitonealis, subperitoneal f.
f. extraperitonealis [TA], f. extraperitoneal. SIN extraperitoneal f.
f. of forearm, f. do antebraço. SIN antebrachial f.
Gallaudet f., f. de Gallaudet. SIN perineal f.
Gerota f., f. de Gerota. SIN renal f.
Godman f., f. de Godman; extensão da camada pré-traqueal da f. cervical para dentro do tórax e sobre o pericárdio.
Hesselbach f., f. de Hesselbach. SIN cribriform f.
hypothenar f., f. hipotenar; porção ulnar mais delgada da f. palmar que recobre os músculos hipotenares, formando um teto para o compartimento hipotenar da palma. VER TAMBÉM palmar f.
iliac f. [TA], f. ilíaca; a f. que cobre os músculos ilíaco e psoas, contínua com a f. transversal, ântero-lateralmente, e com a bainha femoral inferiormente. SIN pars iliaca fasciae iliopsoaticae [TA], f. ilíaca.
f. ili'aca, f. ilíaca. SIN iliac f.
iliopectineal f., f. iliopectínea; f. formada pela união das fáscias que cobrem os músculos ilíaco e pectíneo, que revestem o assoalho da fossa iliopectínea. VER iliopectineal arch.
inferior f. of pelvic diaphragm [TA], f. inferior do diafragma da pelve; a f.

que cobre a face inferior dos músculos levantador do ânus e coccígeo. SIN f. diaphragmatis pelvis inferior [TA], anal f.
inferior f. of urogenital diaphragm, membrana do períneo; designação obsoleta da perineal *membrane*.
f. in'fraspina'ta, f. infra-espinal. SIN infraspinous f.
infraspinatus f., f. infra-espinal. SIN infraspinous f.
infraspinous f. [TA], f. infra-espinal; f. fixada às bordas da fossa infra-espinal e que cobre o músculo infra-espinal; é contínua com a f. que cobre o deltóide. SIN f. infraspinata, infraspinatus f.
infundibuliform f., f. infundibuliforme. SIN internal spermatic f.
intercolumnar fasciae, fibras intercrurais. SIN intercrural *fibers* of superficial ring, em *fiber*.
internal spermatic f. [TA], f. espermática interna; revestimento interno do funículo espermático, contínuo, acima do anel inguinal profundo, com a f. transversal. SIN f. spermatica interna [TA], infundibuliform f., tunica vaginalis communis.
interosseous f., f. interóssea; a f. que cobre os músculos interósseos da mão ou do pé; consiste em uma camada dorsal e em uma camada palmar ou plantar.
f. investiens [TA], f. de revestimento. SIN investing *layer*.
f. investiens perinei superficialis, membrana do períneo; *termo oficial alternativo para perineal f.
investing f., camada de revestimento da fáscia cervical. SIN investing *layer* of cervical fascia.
lacrimal f., f. lacrimal; parte da periórbita que forma uma ponte através da fossa ou do saco lacrimal.
f. la'ta [TA], f. lata. SIN deep f. of thigh.
f. of leg, f. da perna. SIN deep f. of leg.
lumbodorsal f., aponeurose toracolombar. SIN thoracolumbar f.
masseteric f. [TA], f. massetérica; a f. que recobre a superfície lateral do músculo masseter. SIN f. masseterica [TA].
f. massete'rica [TA], f. massetérica. SIN masseteric f.
middle cervical f., camada pré-traqueal da fáscia cervical. SIN pretracheal *layer* of cervical fascia.
muscular f. [TA], f. muscular; uma membrana fibrosa relativamente delgada, desprovida de gordura, que reveste os músculos, diretamente sobre suas superfícies, separando os vários grupos musculares e os músculos individuais. A *Terminologia Anatomica* [TA] recomenda que os termos "fáscia superficial" e "fáscia profunda" não sejam utilizados de forma genérica, sem mais especificações, por causa da variação de seus significados no âmbito internacional. Os termos recomendados são "tecido subcutâneo [TA] (tela subcutanea)" no lugar de fáscia superficial e "fáscia muscular" ou "fáscia visceral" (fascia musculorum ou fascia viscera[is]) no lugar de fáscia profunda.
muscular f. of extraocular muscle [TA], f. dos músculos extrínsecos do bulbo do olho; a parte da f. orbital que envolve os músculos extra-oculares; é delgada na parte posterior, porém torna-se mais espessa onde é contínua com a bainha bulbar; as bainhas fasciais dos quatro músculos retos são unidas por uma membrana intermuscular. SIN f. muscularis musculorum bulbi [TA], f. of extraocular muscles, fascial sheaths of extraocular muscles.
f. muscula'ris muscu'lo'rum bul'bi [TA], f. dos músculos extrínsecos do bulbo do olho. SIN muscular f. of extraocular muscle.
f. musculi quadrati lumborum, camada anterior da aponeurose toracolombar; *termo oficial alternativo para anterior *layer* of thoracolumbar fascia.
f. nu'chae [TA], f. da nuca. SIN nuchal f.
nuchal f. [TA], f. da nuca; f. que envolve os músculos posteriores do pescoço. SIN f. nuchae [TA].
obturator f. [TA], f. obturatória; parte da f. da pelve que recobre o músculo obturador interno. SIN f. obturatoria [TA], f. of obturator internus.
f. obturato'ria [TA], f. obturatória. SIN obturator f.
f. of obturator internus, f. obturatória. SIN obturator f.
orbital fasciae, fáscias orbitais; estruturas fasciais da órbita, consistindo na periórbita, no septo orbital, na f. muscular e na bainha fascial do globo ocular. SIN fasciae orbitales.
fas'ciae orbita'les, fáscias orbitais. SIN orbital fasciae.
palmar f., f. palmar; a f. profunda da palma da mão, cujas porções lateral e medial mais delgadas são as fáscias tenar e hipotenar, e a parte central espessa — a aponeurose palmar —, que forma o teto do compartimento central da palma. VER TAMBÉM palmar *aponeurosis*.
parietal abdominal f. [TA], f. extraperitoneal. SIN extraperitoneal f.
parietal pelvic f. [TA], f. parietal da pelve; incluindo a f. obturatória, recobre os músculos que passam do interior da pelve para a coxa. SIN f. pelvis parietalis [TA], endopelvic f.*, f. endopelvina*.
parotid f. [TA], f. parotídea; a parte da f. de revestimento do pescoço que envolve a glândula parótida e se fixa (acima) ao arco zigomático. SIN f. parotidea [TA], fibrous capsule of parotid gland, parotid sheath.
f. parotid'ea [TA], f. parotídea. SIN parotid f.
parotideomasseteric f., f. parotidomassetérica; uma membrana densa que recobre as superfícies lateral e medial da glândula parótida, sendo contínua, anteriormente, com a f. que recobre o músculo masseter. VER parotid f., masseteric f. SIN f. parotideomasseterica.
f. parotideomasseter'ica, f. parotidomassetérica. SIN parotideomasseteric f.
pectoral f. [TA], f. peitoral; a f. que cobre o músculo peitoral maior; fixa-se ao esterno e à clavícula; é contínua, lateral e inferiormente, com as fáscias do ombro, da axila e do tórax. SIN f. pectoralis [TA].
f. pectora'lis [TA], f. peitoral. SIN pectoral f.
pelvic f. [TA], f. da pelve; tem componentes visceral e parietal: f. visceral da pelve e f. parietal da pelve. SIN f. pelvis [TA], f. pelvica*.
f. pelvica, f. da pelve; *termo oficial alternativo para pelvic f.
f. pel'vis [TA], f. da pelve. SIN pelvic f.
f. pel'vis parieta'lis [TA], f. parietal da pelve. SIN parietal pelvic f.
f. pel'vis viscera'lis [TA], f. visceral da pelve. SIN visceral pelvic f.
f. pe'nis [TA], f. do pênis. SIN f. of penis.
f. of penis [TA], f. do pênis; uma camada profunda que envolve os três corpos eréteis do pênis. SIN f. penis [TA], Buck f., deep f. of penis, f. penis profunda.
f. pe'nis profun'da, f. do pênis. SIN f. of penis.
f. pe'nis superficia'lis, tecido subcutâneo do pênis. SIN subcutaneous *tissue* of penis.
perineal f., f. do períneo; f. que envolve intimamente os músculos superficiais do períneo (músculos isquiocavernoso, bulboesponjoso e transverso superficial do períneo); na parte anterior, funde-se ao ligamento suspensor do pênis/clitóris e continua-se com a f. profunda, cobrindo o músculo oblíquo externo do abdome e a bainha do reto. SIN f. perinei [TA], deep perineal f.*, f. investiens perinei superficialis*, superficial investing f. of perineum*, Gallaudet f.
f. perine'i [TA], f. do períneo. SIN perineal f.
f. perine'i superficia'lis, tecido superficial do períneo. SIN subcutaneous *tissue* of perineum.
perirenal f., f. renal. SIN renal f.
pharyngobasilar f. [TA], f. faringobasilar; camada fibrosa da parede da faringe, situada entre as camadas mucosa e muscular; fixa-se (acima) à parte basilar do osso occipital e à parte petrosa do osso temporal. Essa camada e a mucosa que a reveste formam a parede da faringe não-muscular (abóbada faríngea) acima do músculo constritor superior da faringe. SIN f. pharyngobasilaris [TA], aponeurosis pharyngea, tela submucosa pharyngis.
f. pharyngobasila'ris [TA], f. faringobasilar. SIN pharyngobasilar f.
phrenicopleural f. [TA], f. frenicopleural; camada delgada da f. endotorácica localizada entre a pleura diafragmática e o diafragma. SIN f. phrenicopleuralis [TA].
f. phrenicopleura'lis [TA], f. frenicopleural. SIN phrenicopleural f.
plantar f., f. plantar; compreende uma parte central espessa – a aponeurose plantar – que cobre o compartimento central da sola do pé, e as partes medial e lateral, mais finas, que recobrem os músculos do hálux e do dedo mínimo (compartimentos), respectivamente.
popliteal f., f. poplítea; f. que recobre a fossa poplítea, contínua com a f. lata, superiormente, e com a f. da perna, inferiormente.
Porter f., f. de Porter, camada pré-traqueal da f. cervical. SIN pretracheal *layer* of cervical fascia.
prececocolic f. [TA], f. pré-cecocólica; parte irregular da f. endoabdominal que cruza o ceco na sua parte anterior, às vezes estendendo-se superiormente sobre uma parte do cólon ascendente. SIN f. prececocolica [TA].
f. prececocolica [TA], f. pré-cecocólica. SIN prececocolic f.
presacral f. [TA], f. pré-sacral; camada da f. endopélvica que passa entre o sacro e o reto, formando o limite anterior do espaço fascial pré-sacral (retroretal), no qual está engastado o plexo nervoso hipogástrico. SIN f. presacralis [TA], lamina retrorectalis fasciae endopelvicae, retrorectal lamina of endopelvic fascia, retrorectal lamina of hypogastric sheath.
f. presacralis [TA], f. pré-sacral. SIN presacral f.
pretracheal f., camada pré-traqueal da f. cervical. SIN pretracheal *layer* of cervical fascia.
prevertebral f., camada pré-vertebral da f. cervical. SIN prevertebral *layer* of cervical fascia.
f. profun'da, f. profunda. SIN deep f.
f. pros'tatae [TA], f. da próstata. SIN f. of prostate.
f. of prostate, f. da próstata; condensação da f. visceral da pelve que envolve a próstata. SIN f. prostatae [TA].
rectosacral f. [TA], f. retossacral; fusão da f. visceral do reto e da f. endopélvica pré-sacral na superfície posterior do reto. SIN f. rectosacralis [TA], mesoprocton.
f. rectosacralis [TA], f. retossacral. SIN rectosacral f.
rectovesical f., septo retovesical. SIN rectovesical *septum*.
renal f. [TA], f. renal; a condensação do tecido fibroareolar e da gordura que circundam o rim para formar uma bainha para o órgão. SIN f. renalis [TA], Gerota capsule, Gerota f., perirenal f.
f. rena'lis [TA], f. renal. SIN renal f.
Scarpa f., f. de Scarpa. SIN membranous *layer* of subcutaneous tissue of abdomen.
semilunar f., f. aponeurose do músculo bíceps braquial. SIN bicipital *aponeurosis*.

Sibson f., f. de Sibson. SIN suprapleural *membrane*.
f. spermat'ica exter'na [TA], f. espermática externa. SIN external spermatic f.
f. spermat'ica inter'na [TA], f. espermática interna. SIN internal spermatic f.
subperitoneal f., f. extraperitoneal. SIN extraperitoneal f.
f. subperitonea'lis, f. extraperitoneal. SIN extraperitoneal f.
subsartorial f., septo intermuscular anteromedial. SIN anteromedial intermuscular *septum*.
superficial f., tecido subcutâneo. SIN subcutaneous *tissue*.
superficial investing f. of perineum, f. perineal; *termo oficial alternativo para perineal f.
f. superficia'lis, tecido superficial. SIN subcutaneous *tissue*.
superficial f. of penis, tecido subcutâneo do pênis. SIN subcutaneous *tissue* of penis.
superficial f. of perineum, tecido subcutâneo do períneo. SIN subcutaneous *tissue* of perineum.
superficial f. of scrotum, túnica dartos; *termo oficial alternativo para dartos f.
f. supe'rior diaphrag'matis pel'vis [TA], f. superior do diafragma da pelve. SIN superior f. of pelvic diaphragm.
superior f. of pelvic diaphragm [TA], f. superior do diafragma da pelve; a f. que cobre a superfície superior dos músculos levantador do ânus e pubococcígeo. SIN f. superior diaphragmatis pelvis [TA].
temporal f. [TA], f. temporal; a f. que cobre o músculo temporal; é composta de duas camadas: a lâmina superficial e a lâmina profunda; ambas se fixam acima da linha temporal superior, porém divergem na parte inferior, fixando-se nas superfícies lateral e medial do arco zigomático. SIN f. temporalis [TA], temporal aponeurosis.
f. tempora'lis [TA], f. temporal. SIN temporal f.
f. thoracolumba'lis [TA], aponeurose toracolombar. SIN thoracolumbar f.
thoracolumbar f. [TA], aponeurose toracolombar; dá origem aos músculos oblíquo interno e transverso do abdome; apresenta três camadas: posterior, média e anterior – as camadas posterior e média circundam os músculos eretores da espinha lombar, e as camadas média e anterior circundam o músculo quadrado lombar. SIN f. thoracolumbalis [TA], lumbodorsal f., thoracolumbar aponeurosis.
Toldt f., f. de Toldt; continuação da f. de Treitz, atrás do corpo do pâncreas.
f. transversa'lis [TA], f. transversal. SIN transversalis f.
transversalis f., f. transversal; f. que reveste a parede abdominal ânterolateral, entre a superfície interna da musculatura abdominal e o peritônio. SIN f. transversalis [TA].
Treitz f., f. de Treitz; f. localizada atrás da cabeça do pâncreas.
triangular f., ligamento inguinal reflexo. SIN reflected inguinal *ligament*.
f. triangula'ris abdom'inis, ligamento inguinal reflexo. SIN reflected inguinal *ligament*.
Tyrrell f., septo retovesical. SIN rectovesical *septum*.
umbilical f. [TA], f. umbilical; a camada fascial delgada interposta entre a f. transversal e a f. umbilicovesical. Estende-se entre os ligamentos umbilicais mediais, desde o umbigo e até a frente da bexiga, e forma o limite posterior do espaço retropúbico. SIN umbilical prevesical f.
f. umbilicalis [TA], f. umbilical. SIN umbilical f.
umbilical prevesical f., f. umbilical. SIN umbilical f.
umbilicovesical f., f. umbilicovesical; uma camada fascial delgada que se estende entre os ligamentos umbilicais mediais e é contínua com a f. que envolve a bexiga.
vastoadductor f., septo intermuscular anteromedial. SIN anteromedial intermuscular *septum*.
visceral f. [TA], f. visceral; uma membrana fibrosa e delgada que envolve diversos órgãos e glândulas, ora ligando estruturas, ora formando divisões entre elas. A *Terminologia Anatomica* [TA] recomenda que os termos "fáscia superficial" e "fáscia profunda" não sejam utilizados de forma genérica, sem especificações, por causa da variação de seus significados no âmbito internacional. Os termos recomendados são "tecido subcutâneo [TA] (tela subcutanea)" no lugar de fáscia superficial e "fáscia muscular" ou "fáscia visceral" (fascia musculorum ou fascia viscera[is]) no lugar de fáscia profunda.
visceral pelvic f. [TA], f. visceral da pelve; f. que recobre os órgãos pélvicos e envolve os vasos e nervos localizados no espaço subperitoneal. SIN f. pelvis visceralis [TA].
Zuckerkandl f., f. de Zuckerkandl; a camada posterior da f. renal.

fas·cial (fash′e - ăl). Fascial; relativo a qualquer fáscia.
fas·ci·cle (fas′i-kl). Fascículo; faixa ou feixe de fibras, geralmente de fibras musculares ou nervosas; um trato de fibras nervosas. SIN fasciculus (1) [TA].
anterior f. of palatopharyngeus (muscle) [TA], f. anterior do músculo palatofaríngeo; parte mais espessa do músculo do arco palatofaríngeo que avança entre os músculos levantador e tensor do véu palatino para se fixar na borda posterior do palato duro e na aponeurose palatina; ao fazê-lo, algumas fibras cruzam a linha média e interdigitam-se com as fibras do músculo contralateral. SIN fasciculus anterior musculi palatopharyngei [TA].
muscle f., f. muscular; feixe de fibras musculares circundadas por perimísio.
nerve f., f. nervoso; feixe de fibras nervosas circundadas pelo perineuro.
posterior f. of palatopharyngeus muscle [TA], f. posterior do músculo palatofaríngeo; porção mais delgada do músculo do arco palatofaríngeo, que se origina na região da linha média, onde suas fibras se interdigitam com as da parte contralateral, passando então posteriormente ao músculo levantador do véu palatino para se juntarem à camada longitudinal da musculatura faríngea; age como um tipo de esfíncter, reduzindo o calibre do istmo das fauces no arco palatofaríngeo. SIN fasciculus posterior musculi palatopharyngei [TA], musculus sphincter palatopharyngeus*, palatopharyngeal sphincter*, pharyngeal ridge, sphincter of the pharyngeal isthmus, velopharyngeal sphincter.
fas·cic·u·lar (fa - sik′u - lăr). Fascicular; relativo ou pertencente a um fascículo; disposto em fascículos ou feixes. SIN fasciculate, fasciculated.
fas·cic·u·late, fas·cic·u·lat·ed (fa - sik′u - lāt, - lā - ted). Fascicular, fasciculado. SIN fascicular.
fas·cic·u·la·tion (fa - sik′u - lā′shŭn). Fasciculação. **1.** Arranjo em fascículos. **2.** Contrações involuntárias ou tremores de grupos (fascículos) de fibras musculares, uma forma mais grosseira de contração muscular do que a fibrilação.
fas·cic·u·li (fa - sik′u - lī). Fascículos; plural de fasciculus.

FASCICULUS

fas·cic·u·lus, gen. e pl. **fas·cic·u·li** (fă - sik′u - lŭs, fă - sik′u - lī) [TA]. Fascículo. **1.** SIN fascicle. **2.** SIN cord. **3.** SIN bundle. [L. dim. de *fascis*, feixe]
f. anterior musculi palatopharyngei [TA], fascículo anterior do músculo palatofaríngeo. SIN anterior *fascicle* of palatopharyngeus (muscle).
anterior f. proprius [TA], f. próprio anterior. SIN fasciculi proprii.
anterior pyramidal f., trato corticospinal anterior. SIN anterior corticospinal *tract*.
arcuate f.; (1) f. longitudinal superior. SIN superior longitudinal f.; **(2)** f. unciforme. SIN unciform f.
f. at'rioventricula'ris [TA], f. atrioventricular. SIN atrioventricular *bundle*.
Burdach f., f. de Burdach, f. cuneiforme. SIN cuneate f.
calcarine f., f. calcarino; um grupo de fibras de associação curtas sob a fissura calcarina do lobo occipital do cérebro.
central tegmental f., f. tegmental central. SIN central tegmental *tract*.
f. cir'cumoliva'ris pyram'idis, f. circum-olivar da pirâmide; um feixe anômalo de fibras nervosas na superfície anterior do bulbo que emerge da pirâmide e se curva para a frente e dorsalmente sobre o pólo inferior da oliva; é interpretado de modo variado como um feixe aberrante de fibras pontocerebelares, ou de fibras corticopontinas.
f. corticospina'lis ante'rior, trato corticospinal anterior. SIN anterior corticospinal *tract*.
f. corticospina'lis latera'lis, trato corticospinal lateral. SIN lateral corticospinal *tract*.
cuneate f. [TA], f. cuneiforme; a maior subdivisão lateral do funículo posterior. SIN f. cuneatus [TA], Burdach column, Burdach f., Burdach tract, cuneate funiculus, wedge-shaped f.
f. cunea'tus [TA], f. cuneiforme. SIN cuneate f.
dorsal longitudinal f. [TA], f. longitudinal posterior; um feixe de fibras nervosas delgadas e pouco mielinizadas que une, reciprocamente, a zona periventricular do hipotálamo com as partes ventrais da substância cinzenta central do mesencéfalo. SIN f. longitudinalis posterior [TA], Schütz bundle, tract of Schütz.
dorsolateral f. [TA], trato póstero-lateral; um feixe longitudinal de delgadas fibras não-mielinizadas e pouco mielinizadas que recobre o ápice do corno posterior da substância cinzenta espinal, composto de fibras radiculares posteriores e de fibras de associação curtas que interligam segmentos vizinhos do corno posterior. SIN posterolateral tract [TA], tractus dorsolateralis [TA], tractus posterolateralis [TA], dorsolateral tract*, f. dorsolateralis, f. marginalis, Lissauer bundle, Lissauer column, Lissauer f., Lissauer marginal zone, Lissauer tract, marginal f., Spitzka marginal tract, Spitzka marginal zone, Waldeyer tract, Waldeyer zonal layer.
f. dorsolatera'lis [TA], trato póstero-lateral. SIN dorsolateral f.
Flechsig fasciculi, fascículos de Flechsig; o f. próprio anterior [TA] e o f. próprio lateral [TA]. VER fasciculi proprii.
Foville f., f. de Foville, estria terminal. SIN terminal *stria*.
fronto-occipital f., f. occipitofrontal. SIN occipitofrontal f.
gracile f. [TA], f. grácil; a menor subdivisão medial do funículo posterior. SIN f. gracilis [TA], funiculus gracilis, Goll column, posterior pyramid of the medulla, slender f., tract of Goll.
f. grac'ilis [TA], f. grácil. SIN gracile f.
hooked f., f. unciforme. SIN unciform f.
inferior longitudinal f. [TA], f. longitudinal inferior; um feixe bem delineado de fibras de associação longas que percorre todo o comprimento dos lobos tem-

poral e occipital do cérebro, seguindo, em parte, paralelamente ao corno inferior do ventrículo lateral. SIN f. longitudinalis inferior [TA].
inferior occipitofrontal f. [TA], f. occipitofrontal inferior. VER occipitofrontal f.
interfascicular f. [TA], f. interfascicular. SIN semilunar f.
f. interfascicularis [TA], f. interfascicular. SIN semilunar f.
intersegmental fasciculi, fascículos próprios. SIN fasciculi proprii.
f. latera'lis plex'us brachia'lis [TA], f. lateral do plexo braquial. SIN lateral cord of brachial plexus.
lateral f. proprius [TA], f. próprio lateral. SIN fasciculi proprii.
lateral pyramidal f., trato corticospinal lateral. SIN lateral corticospinal tract.
lenticular f. [TA], f. lenticular; fibras eferentes do núcleo pálido que cruzam a cápsula interna e penetram entre o núcleo subtalâmico e a zona incerta; unem-se para formar o fascículo talâmico. VER TAMBÉM lenticular loop. SIN f. lenticularis [TA].
f. lenticula'ris [TA], f. lenticular. SIN lenticular f.
Lissauer f., f. de Lissauer. SIN dorsolateral f.
fasci'culi longitudina'les ligamen'ti crucifor'mis atlan'tis [TA], fascículos longitudinais do ligamento cruciforme do atlas. SIN longitudinal bands of cruciform ligament of atlas, em band.
fascic'uli longitudina'les pon'tis, fascículos longitudinais da ponte. SIN longitudinal pontine fasciculi.
f. longitudina'lis infe'rior [TA], f. longitudinal inferior. SIN inferior longitudinal f.
f. longitudina'lis media'lis [TA], f. longitudinal medial. SIN medial longitudinal f.
f. longitudina'lis posterior [TA], f. longitudinal posterior. SIN dorsal longitudinal f.
f. longitudina'lis supe'rior [TA], f. longitudinal superior. SIN superior longitudinal f.
longitudinal pontine fasciculi, fascículos longitudinais da ponte; os feixes maciços de fibras corticofugas que passam longitudinalmente através da parte ventral da ponte; são compostos de fibras corticorreticulares, tetopontinas, corticopontinas, corticonucleares (corticobulbares) e corticospinais. SIN fasciculi longitudinales pontis, longitudinal pontine bundles.
macular f., f. macular; conjunto de fibras do nervo óptico que se liga diretamente à mácula lútea. SIN f. macularis.
f. macula'ris, f. macular. SIN macular f.
mammillotegmental f. [TA], f. mamilotegmentar; um pequeno feixe de fibras que, a partir do corpo mamilar, avança dorsalmente por uma curta distância junto ao fascículo mamilotalâmico e, em seguida, desce o tronco cerebral até alcançar os núcleos tegmentais dorsal e ventral do mesencéfalo. SIN f. mammillotegmentalis [TA].
f. mammillotegmenta'lis [TA], f. mamilotegmentar. SIN mammillotegmental f.
mammillothalamic f. [TA], f. mamilotalâmico; um feixe espesso e compacto de fibras nervosas que, a partir de cada corpo mamilar, desce até terminar no núcleo anterior do tálamo. SIN f. mammillothalamicus, f. thalamomammillaris, mamillothalamic tract, Vicq d' Azyr bundle.
f. mammillothalamicus, f. mamilotalâmico. SIN mammillothalamic f.
marginal f., trato póstero-lateral. SIN dorsolateral f.
f. margina'lis, trato póstero-lateral. SIN dorsolateral f.
media'lis plex'us brachia'lis [TA], f. medial do plexo braquial. SIN medial cord of brachial plexus.
f. medialis telencephali [TA], f. medial do telencéfalo. SIN medial forebrain bundle.
medial longitudinal f. [TA], f. longitudinal medial; um feixe longitudinal de fibras que se estende desde o limite superior do mesencéfalo até os segmentos cervicais da medula espinal, localizado próximo à linha média e ventralmente à substância cinzenta central; é composto, em grande parte, de fibras provenientes dos núcleos vestibulares, ascendendo estas até os neurônios motores que inervam os músculos oculares externos (núcleos abducente, troclear e oculomotor) e descendendo até os segmentos da medula espinal que inervam a musculatura do pescoço. SIN f. longitudinalis medialis [TA], Collier tract, medial longitudinal bundle, posterior longitudinal bundle.
f. of Meynert, f. de Meynert, trato habenulointerpeduncular. SIN retroflex f.
oblique pontine f., f. oblíquo da ponte; um feixe de fibras da superfície ventral da ponte que se dirige da porção mesial anterior para fora e para trás. SIN f. obliquus pontis, oblique bundle of pons.
f. obli'quus pon'tis, f. oblíquo da ponte. SIN oblique pontine f.
occipitofrontal f., f. occipitofrontal; fibras de associação, compostas por feixes superior (fascículo occipitofrontal superior [TA]) e inferior (fascículo occipitofrontal inferior [TA]) que se estendem desde o lobo occipital até o lobo frontal do hemisfério cerebral. SIN fronto-occipital f.
f. occip'itofronta'lis, f. occipitofrontal. VER occipitofrontal f.
f. occipitofrontalis inferior [TA], f. occipitofrontal inferior. VER occipitofrontal f.
f. occipitofrontalis superior [TA], f. occipitofrontal superior. VER occipitofrontal f.

oval f., f. interfascicular. VER semilunar f.
f. pedun'culomammilla'ris, f. pedunculomamilar. SIN peduncle of mammillary body.
pedunculomammillary f., f. pedunculomamilar. SIN peduncle of mammillary body.
perpendicular f., f. perpendicular; feixe de fibras de associação que corre verticalmente e interliga regiões dos lobos temporal, occipital e parietal.
f. posterior musculi palatopharyngei [TA], fascículo posterior do músculo palatofaríngeo. SIN posterior fascicle of palatopharyngeus muscle.
f. poste'rior plex'us brachia'lis [TA], f. posterior do plexo braquial. SIN posterior cord of brachial plexus.
posterior f. proprius [TA], f. próprio posterior. SIN fasciculi proprii.
proper fasciculi, fascículos próprios. SIN fasciculi proprii.
fascic'uli pro'prii, fascículos próprios; (fascículo próprio anterior [TA], fascículo próprio lateral [TA], fascículo próprio posterior [TA]); sistema de fibras de associação espinospinais ascendentes e descendentes da medula espinal, que se localiza nos funículos anterior, lateral e posterior na interface substância cinzenta–substância branca. SIN anterior f. proprius [TA], lateral f. proprius [TA], posterior f. proprius [TA], ground bundles, intersegmental fasciculi, lateral proprius bundle, proper fasciculi.
f. pro'prius ante'rior [TA], f. próprio anterior; feixe fundamental da coluna anterior da medula espinal. VER fasciculi proprii. SIN anterior ground bundle.
f. pro'prius latera'lis [TA], f. próprio lateral. VER fasciculi proprii.
f. pyramida'lis ante'rior, trato corticospinal anterior. SIN anterior corticospinal tract.
f. pyramida'lis latera'lis, f. piramidal lateral. SIN lateral corticospinal tract.
retroflex f. [TA], trato habenulointerpeduncular; um feixe compacto de fibras que se origina na habênula e segue ventralmente até o núcleo interpeduncular na base do mesencéfalo; parte de suas fibras ultrapassa esse núcleo e termina nos núcleos da rafe do tegmento caudal do mesencéfalo. SIN f. retroflexus [TA], habenulointerpeduncular tract, habenulopeduncular tract [TA], tractus habenulointerpeduncularis [TA], f. of Meynert, habenulopeduncular tract, retroflex bundle of Meynert.
f. retroflex'us [TA], trato habenulointerpeduncular. SIN retroflex f.
f. rotun'dus, trato solitário. SIN solitary tract.
round f., trato solitário. SIN solitary tract.
rubroreticular fasciculi, fascículos rubrorreticulares; feixes de fibras que ligam o núcleo rubro aos núcleos pontino e reticular do mesencéfalo. SIN fasciculi rubroreticulares.
fasciculi rubroreticula'res, fascículos rubrorreticulares. SIN rubroreticular fasciculi.
semilunar f. [TA], f. interfascicular; um feixe compacto composto de ramos descendentes das fibras da raiz posterior, localizado próximo ao limite entre os fascículos grácil e cuneiforme da medula espinal cervical e torácica; corresponde ao f. septomarginal, trato de Hoche ou área oval de Flechsig no segmento espinal lombar, e ao triângulo de Philippe-Gombault no segmento espinal sacral; como estes, o feixe somente pode ser demonstrado nos casos de desmielinização resultantes de lesões nas raízes dorsais. SIN f. interfascicularis [TA], interfascicular f. [TA], f. semilunaris*, comma bundle of Schultze, comma tract of Schultze.
f. semiluna'ris, f. interfascicular; *termo oficial alternativo para semilunar f.. VER semilunar f.
septomarginal f. [TA], f. septomarginal. VER semilunar f. SIN f. septomarginalis [TA].
f. septomargina'lis [TA], f. septomarginal. SIN septomarginal f.
slender f., f. grácil. SIN gracile f.
f. solita'rius, trato solitário. SIN solitary tract.
solitary f., trato solitário. SIN solitary tract.
subcallosal f., f. subcaloso; feixe de fibras nervosas delgadas que corre longitudinalmente sob o corpo caloso, no ângulo entre este último e o núcleo caudado; forma uma continuação anterior do tapete do lobo temporal e parece ser constituído, em grande parte, por fibras que se projetam do córtex cerebral para o núcleo caudado. SIN f. subcallosus for superior occipitofrontal fasciculus*.
f. subcallo'sus for superior occipitofrontal fasciculus, f. subcaloso para fascículo occipitofrontal superior, *termo oficial alternativo para subcallosal f.
subthalamic f. [TA], f. subtalâmico; fibras nervosas que cruzam a cápsula interna entre o núcleo subtalâmico e o globo pálido; contém fibras palidossubtalâmicas e subtalamopálidas. SIN f. subthalamicus [TA].
f. subthalamicus [TA], f. subtalâmico. SIN subthalamic f.
superior longitudinal f. [TA], f. longitudinal superior; o longo feixe de fibras de associação, situado lateralmente ao centro oval do hemisfério cerebral, que une os lobos frontal, occipital e temporal; as fibras partem do lobo frontal, atravessam o opérculo até a extremidade posterior do sulco lateral, onde muitas delas se irradiam para o lobo occipital, e outras giram para baixo e para a frente ao redor do putame e passam para as porções anteriores do lobo temporal. SIN f. longitudinalis superior [TA], arcuate f. (1).
superior occipitofrontal f. [TA], f. occipitofrontal superior. VER occipitofrontal f.

thalamic f. [TA], f. talâmico; fibras nervosas que formam um feixe composto, contendo fibras cerebelotalâmicas (cruzadas) e palidotalâmicas (não-cruzadas), que se insinuam entre o tálamo e a zona incerta do subtálamo. VER TAMBÉM *fields* of Forel, em *field*. SIN f. thalamicus [TA].
   f. thalam'icus [TA], f. talâmico. SIN thalamic f.
   f. thal'amomammilla'ris, f. mamilotalâmico. SIN mammillothalamic f.
   transverse fasciculi [TA], fascículos transversos. SIN fasciculi transversi.
   fascic'uli transver'si [TA], fascículos transversos; as fibras dirigidas transversalmente nas partes distais das aponeuroses palmar e plantar. SIN transverse fasciculi [TA].
   unciform f., uncinate f. [TA], f. uncinado do telencéfalo; uma longa faixa de fibras de associação, que une reciprocamente os lobos frontal e temporal dos hemisférios cerebrais, segue caudalmente através da substância branca do lobo frontal, curva-se agudamente no sentido ventral sob o tronco da fissura de Sylvius e, por fim, espalha-se para o córtex da metade anterior dos giros temporais superior e médio. SIN f. uncinatus [TA], arcuate f. (2), frontotemporal tract, hooked f., temporofrontal tract.
   uncinate f. of cerebellum [TA], f. unciforme do cerebelo; fibras eferentes fastigiais que se cruzam no cerebelo e descem sobre a superfície lateral do pedúnculo cerebelar superior; essas fibras terminam, em grande parte, nos núcleos vestibulares e na formação reticular da ponte e medula oblonga. SIN f. uncinatus cerebelli [TA], hooked bundle of Russell, uncinate bundle of Russell, uncinate f. of Russell.
   uncinate f. of Russell, f. unciforme de Russell, f. unciforme do cerebelo. SIN uncinate f. of cerebellum.
   f. uncina'tus [TA], f. uncinado. SIN unciform f.
   f. uncinatus cerebelli [TA], f. unciforme do cerebelo. SIN uncinate f. of cerebellum.
   wedge-shaped f., f. cuneiforme. SIN cuneate f.

fas·ci·ec·to·my (fash-ē-ek'tō-mē). Fasciectomia; excisão de faixas de fáscia. [fascia + G. *ektomē*, excisão]
fas·ci·i·tis (fas-ē-ī'tis, fash-). Fascite, fasciite. **1.** Inflamação da fáscia. **2.** Proliferação reativa de fibroblastos na fáscia. SIN fascitis.
   eosinophilic f., f. eosinófila; induração e edema dos tecidos conectivos dos membros, aparecendo geralmente após esforço físico; associada a velocidade de hemossedimentação (VHS) elevada, IgG elevada e eosinofilia. SIN Shulman syndrome.

   group A streptococcal necrotizing f., f. necrosante por estreptococos do grupo A; complicação tóxica grave e freqüentemente fulminante de infecção por estreptococos β-hemolíticos do grupo A, na qual a fáscia superficial e o tecido muscular subjacente são rapidamente destruídos.

> Durante a década de 1990, ocorreu uma elevação na incidência de doença sistêmica aguda causada por cepas de *Streptococcus pyogenes* produtoras de toxinas. Como ocorre na síndrome do choque tóxico estafilocócica, as síndromes estreptocócicas mediadas por toxinas são caracterizadas por evolução rápida, choque e toxicidade multissistêmica desproporcionais às evidências locais de infecção. A incidência de fasciite necrosante causada por estreptococos aumentou significativamente em 1994, tanto nos Estados Unidos quanto na Europa. Acredita-se que essa doença seja a mesma "escarlatina maligna" que ocorreu há um século. Na fasciite necrosante, os estreptococos localizados em uma ferida na pele, geralmente em um dos membros, invadem e destroem os músculos subjacentes e outros tecidos moles. A pele do membro afetado apresenta eritema, formação de bolhas e, freqüentemente, anestesia causada por destruição de nervos sensoriais. O rápido alastramento da infecção ao longo dos planos fasciais e a necrose liquefativa disseminada são acompanhados por febre alta, intensa dor local, choque e outras evidências de toxicidade sistêmica. Os objetivos do tratamento da fasciite necrosante estreptocócica consistem na inibição e destruição dos patógenos, na reversão do choque e da toxicidade sistêmica e na conservação da estrutura e da função. O tratamento inclui hidratação intravenosa e medidas de suporte agressivas, bem como a administração de penicilina, clindamicina ou outros antibióticos apropriados. (A resistência aos antibióticos não tem sido um problema na síndrome do choque tóxico estreptocócica.) Na fasciite necrosante, o desbridamento ou a amputação podem salvar vidas. Culturas de material da orofaringe de contactantes são recomendadas para identificar possíveis fontes de nova infecção por estreptococos toxigênicos virulentos.

   necrotizing f., f. necrosante; infecção rara nos tecidos moles, envolvendo basicamente a fáscia superficial e causando extensa destruição dos tecidos circundantes; a evolução é freqüentemente fulminante e pode envolver todos os componentes dos tecidos moles, incluindo a pele; ocorre geralmente no pós-operatório, após traumatismos mínimos e nos casos de abscessos ou úlceras cutâneas que receberam cuidados inadequados. VER TAMBÉM group A streptococcal necrotizing f.
   nodular f., f. nodular; rápida proliferação tumoriforme de fibroblastos, considerada não-neoplásica, acompanhada de leve exsudação inflamatória, que ocorre na fáscia; a fibrose pode infiltrar o tecido circundante, porém não progride indefinidamente, nem ocorre metástase. SIN pseudosarcomatous f.
   parosteal f., f. periosteal; forma rara de f. nodular que surge no periósteo e que pode estar associada a formação óssea cortical reativa.
   plantar f., f. plantar; inflamação da fáscia plantar que causa dor no pé ou no calcanhar.
   proliferative f., f. proliferativa; nódulo subcutâneo benigno de crescimento rápido, caracterizado por proliferação de fibroblastos e de células gigantes basofílicas, algo semelhantes às células ganglionares.
   pseudosarcomatous f., f. pseudo-sarcomatosa. SIN nodular f.

fascio-. Fascio-; uma fáscia. [L. *fascia*, uma faixa ou um filete]
fas·ci·od·e·sis (fas-ē-od'e-sis, fas-). Fasciodese; ligadura (sutura) cirúrgica de uma fáscia a outra fáscia ou a um tendão. [fascio- + G. *desis*, união]
Fas·ci·o·la (fa-sē'ō-lă, fa-sī'ō-lă). Gênero de grandes trematódeos hepáticos digenéticos e foliformes de mamíferos (família Fasciolidae, classe Trematoda). [L. dim. de *fascia*, uma faixa]
   F. gigan'tica, espécie semelhante à *F. hepatica*, porém de tamanho maior, encontrada em herbívoros, especialmente na África, onde também infesta seres humanos.
   F. hepat'ica, trematódeo hepático comum que habita os ductos biliares de ovinos e bovinos; os hospedeiros intermediários são caramujos aquáticos do gênero *Lymnaea* ou de gêneros correlatos; depois que as cercárias abandonam os caramujos, encistam-se junto a plantas aquáticas, por meio das quais têm acesso ao tubo intestinal; esse trematódeo raramente é encontrado em seres humanos, nos quais pode causar lesão biliar considerável.

fas·ci·o·la, pl. **fas·ci·o·lae** (fa-sē'ō-lă, fa-sī'ō-lă; -ō-lē). Fascíola; uma pequena faixa ou grupo de fibras. [L. dim. de *fascia*, faixa, filete]
   f. cine'rea, giro fasciolar. SIN fasciolar gyrus.
fas·ci·o·lar (fa-sē'ō-lăr, fa-sī'). Fasciolar; relativo ao giro fasciolar.
fas·ci·o·li·a·sis (fas'ē-ō-lī'ă-sis, fa-sī'ō-lī'ă-sis). Fasciolíase; infestação por uma espécie de *Fasciola*.
fas·ci·o·lid (fa-sē'ō-lid, fa-sī'). Fasciolídeo; membro da família Fasciolidae.
fas·ci·o·lop·si·a·sis (fas'ē-ō-lop-sī'ă-sis, fa-sī'ō-). Fasciolopsíase; parasitação por qualquer dos trematódeos do gênero *Fasciolopsis*.
Fas·ci·o·lop·sis (fas'ē-ō-lop'sis, fa-sī'ō-). Gênero de trematódeos fasciolídeos muito grandes e intestinais. [*Fasciola* + G. *opsis*, forma, aparência]
   F. bus'ki, o grande trematódeo intestinal; uma espécie encontrada nos intestinos de seres humanos da Ásia oriental e meridional; transmitido pela ingestão de castanhas-d'água ou de outra vegetação contaminada por metacercárias infestantes.
   F. rathoui'si, espécie relatada na China, em alguns casos, no intestino e no fígado; trata-se possivelmente da *F. buski*.
fas·ci·or·rha·phy (fash-ē-ōr'ă-fē). Fasciorrafia; sutura de uma fáscia ou aponeurose. SIN aponeurorrhaphy. [fascio- + G. *rhaphē*, sutura]
fas·ci·ot·o·my (fash-ē-ot'ō-mē). Fasciotomia; incisão através de uma fáscia; utilizada no tratamento de certas doenças e lesões, quando existe edema significativo ou é prevista a sua formação, podendo comprometer o fluxo sangüíneo; a f. pode ser combinada a embolectomia no tratamento da embolia arterial aguda. [fascio- + G. *tomē*, incisão]
fas·ci·tis (fa-sī'tis). Fascite, fasciite. SIN fasciitis.
fast. 1. Durável; resistente a mudanças; termo aplicado a microrganismos corados que não podem ser descorados. VER TAMBÉM acid-fast. **2.** Jejum. [A.S. *foest*, firme, fixo]
fast green FCF [I.C. 42053]. Corante ácido de arilmetano amplamente utilizado em histologia e citologia e menos sujeito ao desvanecimento do que o verde-claro FCF, substituindo-o em muitos procedimentos; utilizado como corante citoquímico quantitativo para histonas em pH alcalino, após a extração com ácido de DNA e, também, em eletroforese como corante de proteínas.
fas·tid·i·ous (fas-tid'ē-ŭs). Fastidioso; em bacteriologia, que tem exigências nutricionais complexas.
fas·ti·ga·tum (fas-ti-gā'tŭm). Núcleo do fastígio. SIN fastigial *nucleus*. [L. *fastigatus*, pontiagudo]
fas·tig·i·um (faz-tij'ē-ŭm). Fastígio. **1.** [TA]. Ápice do teto do quarto ventrículo do cérebro, um ângulo formado pelos véus bulbares superior e inferior, que se estende para dentro da substância do verme. **2.** O acme ou período de desenvolvimento pleno de uma doença. [L. cume, como o de um espigão; uma extremidade pontiaguda]
fast·ness (fast'nes). Resistência; estado de tolerância exibido por bactérias frente a uma droga ou outro agente. VER fast.
fat. 1. Tecido adiposo. SIN adipose *tissue*. **2.** Gordo; termo comum para obeso. **3.** Gordura; material semi-sólido, gorduroso, encontrado em tecidos animais e

em muitas plantas, composto de uma mistura de ésteres de glicerol; junto com os óleos, constituem os homolipídios. **4.** Um triacilglicerol ou uma mistura de triacilgliceróis. [A.S. *faet*]

brown f., gordura castanha; tecido termogênico composto de células que contêm numerosas gotículas de gordura; massas lobulares encontradas nas regiões interescapular e mediastinal e em outros locais; embora encontrada mais freqüentemente em certos animais hibernantes, essa g. é também encontrada em porcos, roedores e em recém-nascidos humanos. SIN brown adipose tissue, hibernating gland, interscapular gland, interscapular hibernoma, multilocular adipose tissue, multilocular f.

multilocular f., g. multilocular. SIN brown f.

neutral f., g. neutra; triéster de ácidos graxos e glicerol (isto é, triacilglicerol).

paranephric f. [TA], g. paranéfrica, a gordura perirrenal. SIN adipose capsule, capsula adiposa renis, fatty renal capsule, perirenal fat capsule.

retrobulbar f. [TA], g. retrobulbar; a massa de gordura armazenada na órbita que contribui para o suporte do globo ocular. SIN corpus adiposum orbitae [TA], orbital fat body*, fat body of orbit, orbital fat-pad.

saturated f., g. saturada. VER saturated *fatty acid*.

split f., ácidos graxos livres, após sofrerem redução pela ação de lipases, gorduras neutras ou fosfolipídios.

unilocular f., g. unilocular; tecido adiposo no qual a gordura existe em uma única gotícula nos adipócitos. SIN white f. (2).

unsaturated f., g. insaturada. VER unsaturated *fatty acid*.

white f., (1) SIN adipose *tissue*; **(2)** SIN unilocular f.

fa·tal (fā′tăl). Fatal; pertinente a ou que causa a morte; que indica sobretudo a inevitabilidade da morte. [L. *fatalis*, do ou pertencente ao destino]

fa·tal·i·ty (fă - tal′i - tē). Fatalidade. **1.** Condição, doença ou desastre que termina em morte. **2.** Caso individual de morte.

fate. Destino; resultado final.

prospective f., d. provável; desenvolvimento normal de qualquer parte do ovo ou do embrião, sem interferências.

fat·i·ga·bil·i·ty (fat′i - gă - bil′i - tē). Fatigabilidade; condição na qual a fadiga é facilmente induzida.

fa·ti·ga·ble (făt′i - gă - bl) Fatigável; que se cansa diante de esforço muito leve. [L. *fatigabilis*, facilmente cansado, de *fatigo*, cansar(-se)]

fa·tigue (fă - tēg′). Fadiga. **1.** Estado que se segue a um período de atividade mental ou física, caracterizado por capacidade diminuída para o trabalho e eficiência reduzida de realização, geralmente acompanhado por sensação de cansaço, sonolência ou irritabilidade; pode também sobrevir quando, por qualquer motivo, o gasto de energia ultrapassa os processos restauradores e pode estar restrito a um único órgão. **2.** Sensação de tédio e lassidão causadas pela ausência de estimulação, monotonia ou falta de interesse no ambiente circundante [Fr., do L. *fatigo*, cansar(-se)]

auditory f., f. auditiva; alteração temporária do limiar de sensibilidade após exposição ao som.

battle f., f. de batalha; termo utilizado para indicar doença psiquiátrica resultante do estresse de batalha. SIN shell shock.

functional vocal f., f. vocal funcional. SIN phonasthenia.

fat·pad [TA]. Coxim adiposo; acúmulo de tecido adiposo algo encapsulado. SIN corpus adiposum [TA], fat body*.

Bichat f.-p., bola de Bichat. SIN buccal f.-p.

buccal f.-p., coxim adiposo da bochecha; massa encapsulada de gordura localizada na bochecha no lado externo do músculo bucinador e especialmente acentuada no lactente; acredita-se que o corpo adiposo reforça e sustenta a bochecha durante o ato de sugar. SIN corpus adiposum buccae [TA], Bichat f.-p., Bichat protuberance, fat body of cheek, sucking cushion, sucking pad, suctorial pad.

Imlach f.-p., coxim adiposo de Imlach; gordura que cerca o ligamento redondo do útero no canal inguinal.

infrapatellar f.-p. [TA], coxim adiposo infrapatelar; massa gordurosa que ocupa a área entre o ligamento da patela e a prega sinovial infrapatelar da articulação do joelho. SIN corpus adiposum infrapatellare [TA], infrapatellar fat body.

ischiorectal f.-p., coxim adiposo isquiorretal. SIN fat *body* of ischioanal fossa.

orbital f.-p., gordura retrobulbar. SIN retrobulbar *fat*.

fat·ty (făt′ē). Oleoso ou gorduroso; relativo, em qualquer sentido, à gordura.

fat·ty ac·id. Ácido graxo; qualquer ácido derivado de gorduras por hidrólise (p.ex., ácidos oleico, palmítico ou esteárico); qualquer ácido orgânico monobásico de cadeia longa; acumulam-se em doenças associadas aos peroxissomas.

activated f. a., a. g. ativado; éster tiol da acil-coenzima A gordurosa.

diethenoid f. a., a. g. dietenóide; a. g. que contém duas ligações duplas, p.ex., ácido linoleico.

essential f. a., a. g. essencial; a. g. considerado essencial do ponto de vista nutricional; p.ex., ácido linoleico, ácido linolênico.

ω-3 f. a.'s, a. g. ω-3; classe de a. g. que possui uma ligação dupla no terceiro carbono a partir da porção metila; supostamente atuam na diminuição dos níveis de colesterol e LDL. SIN omega-3 f. a.'s.

omega-3 f. a.'s, a. g. ômega-3. SIN ω-3 f. a.'s.

saturated f. a., a. g. saturado; a. g. cuja cadeia de átomos de carbono não contém ligações etilênicas ou outras ligações insaturadas entre os átomos de carbono (p.ex., ácido esteárico e ácido palmítico); é chamado saturado por não ser mais capaz de absorver hidrogênio.

f. a. synthase complex, complexo ácido graxo sintase; complexo de multienzimas que catalisa a formação de palmitato a partir de acetil-coenzima A, malonil-coenzima A e NADPH.

f. a. thiokinase, ácido graxo tiocinase (tioquinase); **(1)** cadeia longa: ligase do ácido graxo de cadeia longa-CoA; **(2)** cadeia média: butirato-CoA ligase.

unesterified free f. a. (FFA, UFA), a. g. livre não-esterificado; a. g. livres que são encontrados no plasma como conseqüência de lipólise no tecido adiposo, ou quando triacilgliceróis plasmáticos são levados para os tecidos.

unsaturated f. a., a. g. insaturado; a. g. cuja cadeia de carbono apresenta uma ou mais ligações duplas ou triplas (p.ex., ácido oleico, com uma ligação dupla na molécula, e ácido linoleico, com duas); denomina-se insaturado por ser capaz de absorver hidrogênio adicional.

fau·ces, gen. **fau·ci·um** (faw′sēz, faw′sē - ŭm) [TA]. Fauces; espaço entre a cavidade da boca e a faringe, limitado pelo palato mole e pela base da língua. VER TAMBÉM *isthmus* of fauces. SIN oropharyngeal passage. [L. a garganta]

fau·cial (faw′shăl). Faucal; relativo a fauce.

fau·na (faw′nă). Fauna; as formas animais de um continente, uma região, uma localidade ou um *habitat*. [L. mod. relativo à *Fauna*, irmã de *Faunus*, uma deidade rural]

fa·ve·o·late (fă - vē′ō - lāt). Faveolado, faviforme; marcado por pequenas depressões.

fa·ve·o·lus, pl. **fa·ve·o·li** (fă - vē′ō - lŭs, - ō - lī). Favéolo; pequena cova ou depressão. [L. mod. dim. de *favus*, favo de mel]

fa·vic chan·de·liers (fā′vik shan - dĕ - lērz′). Candelabros fávicos; hifas especializadas de fungos que se apresentam curvas, ramificadas e assemelhando-se a chifres galhados, formadas pelos patógenos *Trichophyton schoenleinii* e *T. concentricum*.

fa·vid (fā′vid). Fávide; reação alérgica na pele observada em pacientes com favo.

fa·vism (fā′vizm). Favismo; condição aguda, observada principalmente na Itália, que ocorre após a ingestão de certas espécies de favas, p.ex., *Vicia faba*, ou inalação do pólen de sua flor; caracteriza-se por febre, cefaléia, dor abdominal, anemia grave, prostração e coma; ocorre em certos indivíduos com deficiência eritrocítica genética de glicose-6-fosfato desidrogenase. A exposição ao acaso a *Vicia faba*, pelo seu impacto sobre o fenótipo da glicose-6-fosfato desidrogenase, afeta a expressão do gene, um exemplo de penetrância incompleta. SIN fabism. [Ital. *favismo*, de *fava*, fava]

Favre, Maurice J., médico francês, 1876–1954. VER Gamna-F. *bodies*, em *body*; Nicolas-F. *disease*, Goldmann-Favre syndrome.

Favre dys·tro·phy. Distrofia de Favre. VER em dystrophy.

fa·vus (fā′vŭs, fah′vŭs). Favo; tipo grave e persistente de tinha crônica do couro cabeludo e das unhas, com fibrose e formação de crostas denominadas escútulas, causada por três dermatófitos diferentes, *Trichophyton schoenleinii* (mais comum), *T. violaceum* e *Microsporum gypseum*; ocorre mais freqüentemente nos países do Mediterrâneo, no sudeste da Europa, no sul da Ásia e no norte da África. SIN crusted ringworm, honeycomb ringworm, tinea favosa. [L. favo de mel]

Fc. VER Fc *fragment*.

F.C.A.P. Abreviatura de *Fellow of the College of American Pathologists*.

F.C.C.P. Abreviatura de *Fellow of the College of Chest Physicians*.

Fd Abreviatura de ferredoxin (ferredoxina).

FDA Abreviatura de *Food and Drug Administration of the United States Department of Health and Human Services*.

FDNB Abreviatura de fluoro-2,4-dinitrobenzene (fluoro-2,4-dinitrobenzeno).

FDP Abreviatura de fibrin/fibrinogen degradation *products* (produtos da degradação da fibrina/fibrinogênio), em *product*.

Fe Símbolo do ferro. [L. *ferrum*, ferro]

^{52}Fe Símbolo do ferro-52.

^{55}Fe Símbolo do ferro-55.

^{59}Fe Símbolo do ferro-59.

fear (fēr). Temor; apreensão; medo; alarme; por existir um estímulo identificável, o temor é diferenciado da ansiedade, que não apresenta um estímulo facilmente identificável. [A.S. *faer*]

fea·tures (fē′choorz). Características; as várias partes da face, testa, olhos, nariz, boca, queixo, bochechas e orelhas, que lhe conferem individualidade e seu caráter. [através do Fr. ant., do L. *factura*, feitura, de *facio*, fazer]

feb·ri·cant (feb′ri-kant). Febricitante. SIN febrifacient.

fe·bric·u·la (fē - brik′ū - lă). Febrícula; febre contínua simples; febre branda de curta duração, de origem indefinida e sem nenhuma patologia característica. [L. dim. de *febris*, febre]

feb·ri·fa·cient (feb - ri - fā′shĕnt). Febricitante; **1.** Que causa ou favorece o desenvolvimento de febre. SIN febriferous, febrific. **2.** Qualquer agente que produz febre. VER TAMBÉM pyrogenic. SIN febricant. [L. *febris*, febre, + *facio*, fazer]

fe·brif·er·ous (fē-brif′er-ŭs). Febricitante. SIN febrifacient (1). [L. *febris*, febre, + *fero*, levar, + *-ous*]

fe·brif·ic (fē-brif′ik). Febricitante. SIN febrifacient (1).

fe·brif·u·gal (fē-brif′u-găl). Febrífugo, antipirético (1). SIN antipyretic (1).

feb·ri·fuge (feb′ri-fūj). Febrífugo, antipirético (2.) SIN antipyretic (2). [L. *febris*, febre, + *fugo*, pôr em fuga]

feb·rile (feb′ril, feb′brīl). Febril; que indica febre ou se relaciona com ela. SIN feverish (1), pyrectic, pyretic.

fe·bris (fē′bris). Febre. SIN fever. [L.]
 f. melitensis (fē′bris mel-ĭ-ten′sis). Brucelose; infecção por *Brucella melitensis*. VER TAMBÉM *Brucella melitensis*.
 f. undulans (fē′bris ŭn-doo-lanz′), f. ondulante, brucelose. SIN brucellosis.

fe·cal (fē′kăl). Fecal; relativo às fezes.

fe·ca·lith (fē′kă-lith). Fecalito; massa dura consistindo em fezes ressecadas. SIN coprolith, stercolith. [L. *faeces*, fezes, + G. *lithos*, pedra]

fe·cal·oid (fē′kă-loyd). Fecalóide; semelhante a fezes. [L. *faeces*, fezes, + G. *eidos*, semelhança]

fe·ca·lo·ma (fē′kă-lō-mă). Fecaloma; acúmulo de fezes ressecadas no cólon ou no reto, dando a impressão de um tumor abdominal. SIN coproma, fecal tumor, scatoma, stercoroma.

fe·ca·lu·ria (fē′kă-loo′rē-ă). Fecalúria; mistura de fezes com urina, eliminada pela uretra de pessoas com uma fístula que une o trato intestinal ao sistema urinário baixo, freqüentemente observada de forma mais dramática pela eliminação de flatos através da uretra. [L. *faeces*, fezes, + G. *ouron*, urina]

fe·ces (fē′sēz). Fezes; a matéria eliminada pelo intestino durante a defecação, consistindo em resíduos não digeridos de alimentos, epitélio, muco intestinal, bactérias e escórias alimentares. SIN stercus. [L., pl. de *faex* (*faec-*), sedimento]

Fechner, Gustav T., físico alemão, 1801–1887. VER Weber-F. *law*; F.-Weber *law*.

fec·u·lent (fek′u-lent). Feculento; sujo. [L. *faeculentus*, cheio de excremento, de *faeces*, sedimento, fezes]

fe·cund (fē′kŭnd, fek′ŭnd). Fecundo. SIN fertile (1). [L. *fecundus*, fértil]

fec·un·date (fē′kŭn-dāt). Fecundar; impregnar; tornar fértil. [L. *fecundo*, pp. *-atus*, tornar fecundo, fertilizar]

fec·un·da·tion (fē-kŭn-dā′shŭn). Fecundação; o ato de tornar fértil. VER TAMBÉM fertilization, impregnation.

fec·un·di·ty (fē′kŭn′di-tē). Fecundidade; capacidade de produzir uma prole viva.

Fede, Francesco, médico italiano, 1832–1913. VER Riga-F. *disease*.

feed·back (fēd′bak). Retroalimentação. **1.** Em dado sistema, o retorno, como entrada, de parte da saída, como um mecanismo regulatório; p. ex., a regulação de um forno por um termostato. **2.** Explicação para o aprendizado de habilidades motoras: estímulos sensoriais causados por contrações musculares modulam a atividade do sistema motor. **3.** O sentimento desencadeado pela reação de outra pessoa para consigo. VER biofeedback.
 auditory f., r. auditiva; som indesejado que surge em um sistema de amplificação de som, quando o microfone capta o som do alto-falante; um problema importante no uso de aparelhos para surdez.
 negative f., r. negativa; o que ocorre quando o sinal ou a percepção do sinal de retorno causa uma redução da amplificação.
 positive f., r. positiva; o que ocorre quando o sinal ou o sentido do sinal de retorno causa um aumento da amplificação ou leva à instabilidade.
 tubuloglomerular f., r. túbulo-glomerular; mecanismo de controle do fluxo sanguíneo que atua nos rins e que limita as alterações na taxa de filtração glomerular.

feed·ing (fēd′ing). Alimentação; que alimenta ou nutre.
 fictitious f., a. fictícia. SIN sham f.
 forced f., forcible f., a. forçada; (1) dar alimento líquido por meio de um tubo nasal introduzido até o estômago; (2) forçar uma pessoa a comer mais alimento do que o desejado. SIN forced alimentation.
 gastric f., a. gástrica; introduzir nutrientes diretamente no estômago por meio de um tubo inserido através da nasofaringe e do esôfago, ou diretamente através da parede abdominal.
 nasal f., a. nasal; nutrir por meio de um tubo flexível introduzido através das vias nasais até o estômago.
 sham f., a. falsa; procedimento utilizado no estudo da fase psíquica da secreção gástrica: em experimentos com cães, o alimento, após ser ingerido, não penetra no estômago, saindo por uma fístula esofágica feita no pescoço; a mastigação e deglutição de alimento provocam secreção abundante de suco gástrico. SIN fictitious f.

feel·ing (fēl′ing). Sentimento. **1.** Qualquer tipo de experiência consciente de sensação. **2.** A percepção mental de um estímulo sensorial. **3.** Qualidade de qualquer estado mental ou humor que permite reconhecê-los como prazerosos ou desprazerosos. **4.** Sensação corpórea que está correlacionada com determinada emoção.

Feer, Emil, pediatra suíço, 1864–1955. VER F. *disease*.

FEF Abreviatura de forced expiratory *flow* (fluxo expiratório forçado).

Fehling, Hermann von, químico alemão, 1812–1885. VER F. *reagent, solution*.

Feil, André, médico francês, *1884. VER Klippel-F. *syndrome*.

Feiss, Henry O., cirurgião ortopedista norte-americano do século XX. VER F. *line*.

FEL Abreviatura de familial erythrophagocytic lymphohistiocytosis (linfo-histiocitose enterofagocítica familiar).

fel·bam·ate (fel′bă-māt). Felbamato; agente anticonvulsivante/antiepiléptico quimicamente relacionado com o meprobamato; útil nas crises epilépticas parciais complexas.

Feldberg, Wilhelm, fisiologista britânico, 1900–1993. VER Dale-F. *law*.

Feldman, Harry Alfred, epidemiologista norte-americano, 1914–1986. VER Sabin-F. dye *test*.

Fe·li·dae (fē′li-dē). Família de Carnivora, que abrange os gatos domésticos e os selvagens, tais como leões e tigres. [L. *felis*, gato]

fe·line (fē′līn). Felino; pertencente ou relacionado aos gatos. [L. *felis*, gato]

Felix, Arthur, bacteriologista polonês, 1887–1956. VER Weil-F. *reaction, test*.

fel·la·tio (fē-lā′shē-ō). Felação; estimulação oral do pênis; um tipo de atividade sexual orogenital; em contraste com cunilíngua, que é a estimulação oral da vulva ou do clitóris. SIN irrumation. [L.]

fel·o·dip·ine (fē-lō′di-pēn). Felodipina; agente bloqueador de cálcio da classe diidroperidina, que se assemelha à nifedipina.

fel·on (fel′on). Panarício. SIN whitlow. [I. m. *feloun*, maligno]

Fel·son. Benjamin, radiologista norte-americano, 1913–1988. VER silhouette *sign* of Felson.

felt·work. **1.** Rede fibrosa. **2.** Plexo cerrado de fibrilas nervosas. VER neuropil.

Felty, Augustus R., médico norte-americano, 1895–1963. VER F. *syndrome*.

fel·y·pres·sin (fel-i-pres′in). Felipressina; vasopressina [Phe^2, Lys^8]; lisina vasopressina com L-fenilalanina na posição 2. SIN octapressin.

fe·male (fē′māl). Fêmea; em zoologia, relativo ao gênero que concebe os seres ou carreia os ovos.
 genetic f., f. genética; (1) a criatura com cariótipo feminino normal, incluindo dois cromossomas X; (2) a criatura com núcleos celulares que contêm corpúsculos de Barr (cromatina sexual), normalmente ausentes em machos.
 XO f., f. XO; a fêmea genética na síndrome de Turner, cujo critério para a identificação do sexo é a evidência macroscópica da genitália externa.
 XXX f., f. XXX. VER triple X *syndrome*.

fem·i·ni·za·tion (fem′i-ni-zā′shŭn). Feminização; desenvolvimento de características femininas externas em um macho.
 testicular f., f. testicular. SIN complete androgen insensitivity syndrome. VER testicular feminization *syndrome*.

fem·o·ral (fem′o-răl). Femoral; relativo ao fêmur ou à coxa.

fem·o·ro·cele (fem′o-ro-sēl). Femorocele. SIN femoral *hernia*. [L. *femur*, coxa, + G. *kēlē*, hérnia]

fem·o·ro·tib·i·al (fem′o-rō-tib′ē-ăl). Femorotibial; relativo ao fêmur e à tíbia.

⚠ **femto-** (f). fento- (f); prefixo utilizado pelo sistema métrico e SI para indicar um submúltiplo de um quadrilhão de avos (10^{-15}). [Dinamarquês e norueguês *femten*, quinze]

fe·mur, gen. **fe·mo·ris,** pl. **fem·o·ra** (fē′mŭr, fem′o-ris, -ă) [TA]. Fêmur. **1.** SIN thigh. **2.** Osso longo da coxa que se articula, proximalmente, com o osso do quadril e, distalmente, com a tíbia e patela. [L. coxa]

fen·bu·fen (fen-boo′fen). Fenbufeno; agente antiinflamatório não-esteróide que se assemelha ao ibuprofeno.

fen·ca·mine (fen′kă-mēn). Fencamina; estimulante do sistema nervoso central.

fen·clo·fen·ac (fen-klō′fen-ak). Fenclofenaco; antiinflamatório não-esteróide utilizado no tratamento de doenças das articulações; similar ao diclofenaco.

fen·clo·nine (fen′klō-nēn). Fenclonina; um inibidor da serotonina.

Fendt, H., dermatologista austríaco do século XIX. VER cutaneous *pseudolymphoma*; Spiegler-F. *sarcoid*.

fe·nes·tra, pl. **fe·nes·trae** (fe-nes′tră, -trē). Janela. **1** [TA]. Abertura anatômica, freqüentemente fechada por uma membrana. **2.** Abertura deixada em um aparelho gessado ou outra forma de curativo fixo, a fim de permitir o acesso a uma ferida ou à inspeção da parte. **3.** A abertura em uma das lâminas de um fórceps obstétrico. **4.** Abertura lateral, na bainha de um instrumento endoscópico, que permite uma visão lateral ou manobras operativas. **5.** Aberturas na parede de um tubo, cateter ou trocarte destinadas a promover melhor fluxo de ar ou líquidos. SIN window (1) [TA]. [L. janela]
 f. of the cochlea, j. da cóclea. SIN round *window*.
 f. coch′leae [TA], j. da cóclea. SIN round *window*.
 f. nov-ova′lis, j. neo-oval; abertura artificial através da cápsula ótica para dentro do canal semicircular lateral, ligando o labirinto membranáceo ao antro mastóideo, produzida durante a cirurgia de fenestração.
 f. ova′lis, j. do vestíbulo. SIN oval *window*.
 f. rotun′da, j. da cóclea. SIN round *window*.
 f. of the vestibule, j. do vestíbulo. SIN oval *window*.
 f. vestib′uli, j. do vestíbulo. SIN oval *window*.

fen·es·trat·ed (fen′es-trā′ted). Fenestrado; que possui janelas ou aberturas semelhantes a janelas.

fen·es·tra·tion (fen - es - tra′shŭn). Fenestração. **1.** Presença de aberturas ou janelas em uma parte. **2.** Fazer aberturas em um curativo, para permitir a inspeção das partes. **3.** Em odontologia, uma perfuração cirúrgica do mucoperiósteo e do processo alveolar, a fim de expor a extremidade da raiz de um dente para permitir a drenagem do exsudato tecidual.
   optic nerve sheath f., f. da bainha do nervo óptico; abertura de uma janela, na dura-máter da bainha do nervo óptico, para aliviar papiledema e evitar perda adicional de fibras do nervo óptico.
   tracheal f., f. traqueal; procedimento cirúrgico que visa a criação de uma abertura mucocutânea epitelizada desde o pescoço até a traquéia.
fen·eth·yl·line hy·dro·chlo·ride (fen - eth′ ĭ - lēn). Cloridrato de fenetilina; agente analéptico.
fen·flur·a·mine hy·dro·chlo·ride (fen - floo′rā - mēn). Cloridrato de fenfluramina; agente anorexígeno.
Fenn, Wallace Osgood, fisiologista norte-americano, 1893–1971. VER F. *effect.*
fen·nel (fen′l). Funcho, erva-doce; semente de funcho, o fruto maduro e seco de variedades cultivadas de *Foeniculum vulgare* (família Umbelliferae), erva nativa do sul da Europa e da Ásia; diaforético e carminativo; óleo volátil destilado a partir do fruto e utilizado como aromatizante. [através do Fr. ant., do L. *faeniculum,* funcho, dim. de *faenum,* feno]
fen·o·pro·fen cal·ci·um (fen - ō - prō′fen). Fenoprofeno cálcico; analgésico antiinflamatório utilizado para tratar dor leve a moderada e osteoartrite; semelhante ao ibuprofeno.
fen·o·ter·ol (fen′ō - ter′ōl). Fenoterol; broncodilatador agonista β₂, utilizado em inalação.
fen·pip·ra·mide (fen - pip′rā - mĭd). Fempipramida; agente antiespasmódico.
fen·ta·nyl cit·rate (fen′tă - nĭl). Citrato de fentanila; analgésico narcótico de curta duração, cerca de 100 vezes mais potente do que a morfina, utilizado como analgésico suplementar em anestesia geral.
fen·ti·clor (fen′tĭ - klōr). Fenticlor; agente antiinfeccioso tópico.
fen·u·greek (fen′ū - grēk). Feno-grego; planta anual, natural do oeste da Ásia, cultivada na África e em partes da Europa; as sementes mucilaginosas são utilizadas como alimento e na preparação de temperos culinários (*curry*). [L. *faenum graecum,* feno grego, de *faenum,* feno, + *Graecus,* grego]
Fenwick, Edwin Hurry, urologista britânico, 1856–1944. VER F.-Hunner *ulcer.*
fer·al (fer′ĭl). Feroz; relativo a um animal selvagem e não-domesticado.
Féréol, Louis Felix Henri, médico francês, 1825–1891.
Ferguson, J. K. W., obstetra do século XX. VER F. *reflex.*
Fergusson, Sir William, cirurgião escocês, 1808–1877. VER F. *incision.*
fer·ment (fer-ment′). **1.** Fermentar; causar ou sofrer fermentação. **2.** Fermento; agente que causa fermentação. [L. *fermentum,* levedura]
fer·ment·a·ble (fer - ment′ă - bl). Fermentável; capaz de sofrer fermentação.
fer·men·ta·tion (fer - men - tā′shŭn). Fermentação. **1.** Mudança química induzida em um composto orgânico complexo pela ação de uma enzima, através da qual a substância é dividida em compostos mais simples. **2.** Em bacteriologia, o catabolismo anaeróbico de substratos com a produção de energia e compostos menores; o mecanismo da f. não envolve uma cadeia respiratória ou um citocromo, e, portanto, o oxigênio não é o aceptor final de elétrons como ocorre na oxidação. [L. *fermento,* pp. *-atus,* fermentar, de L. *fermentum,* fermento]
   acetic f., acetous f., f. acética; f., que ocorre no vinho e na cerveja, através da qual o álcool é oxidado a ácido acético (vinagre).
   alcoholic f., f. alcoólica; formação anaeróbica de etanol e CO_2 a partir da D-glicose. Cf. Gay-Lussac *equation.*
   amylic f., f. amílica; f. da batata, do milho ou de outra substância amilácea, por meio da qual o óleo fúsel é produzido.
   lactic acid f., f. do ácido láctico; produção de ácido láctico no leite ou em outros meios que contenham carboidratos, causada pela presença de qualquer uma das várias bactérias do ácido láctico.
fer·ment·a·tive (fer - ment′ă - tĭv). Fermentativo; que produz ou tem a capacidade de produzir fermentação.
fer·ment·er (fer-ment′er). Fermentador; grande recipiente utilizado em culturas de microrganismos.
fer·mi·um (Fm) (fer′mē - ŭm). Férmio; elemento radioativo produzido artificialmente em 1955, com número atômico 100 e massa atômica 257,095; o Fm^{257} apresenta a meia-vida mais longa já conhecida (100,5 dias) desse elemento transurânico. [E. *Fermi,* físico ítalo-americano, laureado com um Prêmio Nobel, 1901–1954]
Fernandez re·ac·tion. Reação de Fernandez. Ver em reaction.
Fernbach, Auguste, microbiologista francês, 1860–1939. VER F. *flask.*
fern·ing. Termo utilizado para descrever o padrão de arborização produzido pelo muco cervical secretado no meio do ciclo que, ao se cristalizar, assemelha-se a uma folha de samambaia (fern) ou de palmeira.
fer·ra·tin (fer′ă - tĭn). Ferratina; agente hematínico.
fer·re·dox·ins (fer - ĕ - dok′sĭnz). Ferredoxinas; proteínas que contêm complexos ferro-enxofre e que apresentam atividade carreadora de elétrons, porém nenhuma função clássica de enzima. As ferredoxinas são encontradas em vegetais verdes, algas, bactérias anaeróbicas e nas mitocôndrias do córtex da glândula supra-renal e do músculo cardíaco. Estão envolvidas em diversas reações de oxidação-redução em organismos vivos (p.ex., fixação de nitrogênio).
Ferrein, Antoine, anatomista francês, 1693–1769. VER F. *canal, cords,* em *cord, foramen, ligament, pyramid, tube, vasa* aberrantia, em *vas; processus* ferreini.
ferri-. Ferri-; prefixo que indica a presença de um íon férrico em um composto. [L. *ferrum,* ferro]
fer·ric (fer′ik). Férrico; relativo ao ferro, em particular, indicando um sal que contém átomo de ferro com a valência mais alta (tripla), Fe^{3+}.
fer·ric am·mo·ni·um cit·rate. Citrato férrico de amônio; composto utilizado na anemia hipocrômica; é relativamente livre de ação adstringente e irritante.
fer·ric am·mo·ni·um cit·rate, green. Citrato férrico de amônio, verde; composto utilizado na anemia hipocrômica.
fer·ric am·mo·ni·um cit·rate am·mo·ni·um sul·fate. Sulfato férrico de amônio; agente adstringente e estíptico. SIN ammonium ferric sulfate, ferric alum, iron alum.
fer·ric chlo·ride. Cloreto férrico; agente adstringente e estíptico.
fer·ric fruc·tose. Frutose férrica; frutose com potássio e ferro; agente hematínico.
fer·ric glyc·er·o·phos·phate. Glicerofosfato férrico; agente tônico e fonte de ferro.
fer·ric hy·drox·ide. Hidróxido férrico; composto antigamente utilizado na forma recém-preparada, como antídoto para o envenenamento por arsênio.
fer·ric ox·ide. Óxido férrico; composto utilizado como corante.
fer·ric phos·phate. Fosfato férrico; composto utilizado como alimento e como suplemento alimentar.
   soluble f. p., fosfato férrico solúvel; f. f. com citrato de sódio; agente hematínico.
fer·ric sul·fate. Sulfato férrico; persulfato, tersulfato ou sesquissulfato de ferro; agente adstringente e estíptico.
fer·ri·cy·a·nide (fe - rĭ - sī′ă - nĭd, fer - ē-). Ferricianeto; o ânion $Fe(CN)_6^{3-}$.
fer·ri·cy·to·chrome (fe - rĭ - sī′tō - krōm, fer - ē-). Citocromo férrico; citocromo que contém ferro (férrico) oxidado.
fer·ri·heme (fe′rĭ - hēm, fer′ē-). Heme férrico. SIN hematin.
   f. chloride, cloreto de heme férrico. SIN hemin.
fer·ri·he·mo·glo·bin (fer′ĭ - hē - mō - glō′bĭn, fer′ē-). Hemoglobina férrica. SIN methemoglobin.
fer·ri·por·phy·rin (fe - rĭ - pōr′fĭ - rĭn, fer - ē-). Porfirina férrica; composto formado por um íon férrico e por uma porfirina; p.ex., protoporfirina férrica (hemina).
   f. chloride, cloreto de porfirina férrica, hemina. SIN hemin.
fer·ri·pro·to·por·phy·rin (fer′ĭ - prō - tō - pōr′fĭ - rĭn, fer′ē-). Protoporfirina férrica. SIN hemin.
fer·ri·tin (fer′ĭ - tĭn, fer′ā-). Ferritina; complexo ferro-proteína que contém até 23% de ferro, formado pela união de íons férricos com apoferritina; é encontrado na mucosa intestinal, no baço, na medula óssea, nos reticulócitos e no fígado e regula o armazenamento e o transporte do ferro da luz intestinal para o plasma.
ferro-. Ferro-; prefixo que indica a presença de ferro metálico ou do íon divalente. Fe^{2+}. [L. *ferrum,* ferro]
fer·ro·che·la·tase (far - ō - kē′lă - tās). Ferroquelatase; liase que catalisa a hidrólise ácida reversível do heme, formando protoporfirina IX e ferro ferroso livre; inibida pelo chumbo; a deficiência de f. causa protoporfiria eritropoética.
fer·ro·cho·li·nate (far′ō - kō′li - nāt). Ferrocolinato; quelato de citrato de colina de ferro, utilizado, por via oral, na prevenção e no tratamento de anemias por deficiência de ferro.
fer·ro·cy·a·nide (far - ō - sī′ă - nĭd). Ferrocianeto; composto que contém o ânion $Fe(CN)_6^{4-}$.
fer·ro·cy·to·chrome (far - ō - sī′tō - krōm). Citocromo ferroso; citocromo que contém ferro reduzido (ferroso).
fer·ro·heme (far′ō- hēm). Heme. SIN heme.
fer·ro·ki·net·ics (far - ō - ki - net′iks). Ferrocinética; o estudo do metabolismo do ferro, utilizando ferro radioativo. [L. *ferrum,* ferro, + G. *kinēsis,* movimento]
fer·ro·por·phy·rin (far - ō - pōr′fĭ - rĭn). Porfirina ferrosa; o composto formado por um íon ferroso e por uma porfirina; p.ex., protoporfirina ferrosa (heme).
fer·ro·pro·teins (far - ō - prō′tēnz). Ferroproteínas; proteínas que contêm ferro em um grupamento prostético; p.ex., heme, citocromos.
fer·ro·pro·to·por·phy·rin (far′ō - prō - tō - pōr′fĭ - rĭn). Protoporfirina ferrosa. SIN heme.
fer·ro·so·fer·ric (far - ō′sō - far′ik). Ferrosoférrico; que indica uma combinação de um composto ferroso com um composto férrico, como em Fe_3O_4.
fer·ro·ther·a·py (far′ō - thăr′ă - pē). Ferroterapia; uso terapêutico do ferro. [L. *ferrum,* ferro]
fer·rous (far′ŭs). Ferroso; relativo ao ferro, em particular, indica um sal que contém um átomo de ferro com sua valência mais baixa, Fe^{2+}. [L. *ferreus,* feito de ferro]

fer·rous cit·rate. Citrato ferroso; composto que ocorre em várias formas, duas delas sendo o citrato ácido monoferroso monoidratado e o dicitrato triferroso decaidratado; agente hematínico.

fer·rous fu·ma·rate. Fumarato ferroso; fumarato de ferro; agente hematínico.

fer·rous glu·co·nate. Gluconato ferroso; gluconato de ferro; agente hematínico.

fer·rous lac·tate. Lactato ferroso; lactato de ferro; agente hematínico.

fer·rous suc·ci·nate. Succinato ferroso; succinato de ferro; agente hematínico.

fer·rous sulfate. Sulfato ferroso. SIN iron *sulfate.*
  dried f. s., sulfato ferroso desidratado; agente hematínico.

fer·ru·gi·na·tion (fe-roo′ji-nā′shŭn). Acúmulo de depósitos minerais que contêm ferro nas paredes de pequenos vasos sanguíneos e na área de um neurônio morto. [L. *ferrugo,* ferrugem]

fer·ru·gi·nous (fe-roo′ji-nŭs). Ferruginoso. **1.** Que contém ferro; associado ao ou que contém ferro. **2.** Da cor da ferrugem. [L. *ferrugineus,* ferrugem, da cor da ferrugem]

fer·rule (fer′ool). Virola; argola ou anel de metal utilizado ao redor da coroa ou da raiz de um dente. [corruptela através do Fr. ant. e do L. mediev., do L. *viriola,* um pequeno bracelete]

Ferry, Erwin S., físico norte-americano, 1868–1956. VER F.-Porter *law.*

fer·tile (fer′til). **1.** Fértil; frutífero; capaz de conceber e dar à luz um ser. SIN fecund. **2.** Impregnado; fertilizado. [L. *fertilis,* de *fero,* dar à luz]

fer·til·i·ty (fer-til′i-tē). Fertilidade; produção real de prole viva, ou seja, não inclui natimortos.

fer·til·i·za·tion (fer′til-i-zā′shŭn). Fertilização; o processo que se inicia com a penetração do oócito secundário pelo espermatozóide e se completa com a fusão dos pró-núcleos masculino e feminino.
  in vitro **f. (IVF),** f. *in vitro*; processo (geralmente múltiplo) pelo qual óvulos são colocados em um meio ao qual se adiciona esperma para que ocorra a fecundação; o zigoto produzido dessa forma é, então, introduzido no útero, permitindo-se que se desenvolva até o termo.
  in vivo **f.,** f. *in vivo*; f. de um ovo maduro na porção distal da tuba uterina de uma fêmea doadora fértil (não em um meio artificial), para subseqüente transferência não-cirúrgica para uma fêmea receptora infértil.

fer·til·i·zin (fer-til′i-zin). Fertilizina; complexo formado por polissacarídeo ácido e aminoácido, associado à membrana do gameta feminino de vários organismos; fornece grupamentos receptores que aglutinam espermatozóides e os ligam aos óvulos.

Fer·u·la (făr′oo-lă). Gênero de plantas da família Umbelliferae. *F. assafoetida, F. rubricaulis* e *F. foetida* fornecem a assa-fétida; *F. galbaniflua* e *F. rubricaulis,* o gálbano; e *F. sumbul,* o sumbul. [L. planta gigante]

fer·ves·cence (fer-ves′ens). Fervescência; aumento da febre. [L. *fervesco,* começar a ferver, de *ferveo,* ferver]

FESS Abreviatura de functional endoscopic sinus *surgery* (cirurgia endoscópica funcional dos seios).

fes·ter. Supurar; inflamar-se. **1.** Formar pus ou putrefazer-se. **2.** Tornar-se inflamado. [L. *fistula*]

fes·ti·nant (fes′ti-nant). Festinante; rápido; que tem pressa; que acelera. [L. *festino,* acelerar]

fes·ti·na·tion (fes-ti-nā′shŭn). Festinação. SIN festinating *gait.* [L. *festino,* acelerar]

fes·toon (fes-toon′). Festão. **1.** Entalhe localizado no material da base de uma dentadura para estimular o contorno do tecido natural que está sendo substituído pela dentadura. **2.** Característica peculiar de certas espécies de carrapatos duros (com escudo), que consiste em pequenas áreas retangulares separadas por sulcos ao longo da margem posterior do dorso, tanto de machos como de fêmeas. [através do Fr. do L. *festum,* festival, daí decorações festivas]
  gingival f., f. gengival; aumento de volume em forma de arco das margens da gengiva.

fes·toon·ing (fes-toon′ing). Festonado, provido de festões; ondulante, como o padrão das papilas dérmicas localizadas embaixo de uma vesícula subepidérmica.

FET Abreviatura de forced expiratory *time* (tempo expiratório forçado).

fe·tal (fē′tăl). Fetal. **1.** Relativo a um feto. **2.** Nome dado ao ser em desenvolvimento dentro do útero após a oitava semana.

fe·tal·ism (fē′tăl-izm). Fetalismo; presença de certas estruturas ou características fetais no corpo após o nascimento.

fe·tal re·tic·u·la·ris (fē′tăl re-tik-ū-lā′ris). **1.** SIN fetal adrenal *cortex.* **2.** SIN androgenic *zone* (2). **3.** SIN X *zone* (2).

fe·ta·tion (fē-tā′shŭn). Fetação, gravidez. SIN pregnancy.

fe·ti·cide (fē′ti-sīd). Feticida; destruição do embrião ou do feto no interior do útero. [L. *fetus* + *caedo,* matar]

fet·id (fet′id, fē′tid). Fétido; que exala mau cheiro. [L. *foetidus*]

fet·ish (fet′ish, fē′tish). Fetiche; objeto inanimado ou parte não-sexual de um corpo ao qual se atribuem qualidades mágicas ou eróticas. [Fr. *fétiche,* do L. *factitius,* feito com arte, artificial]

fet·ish·ism (fet′ish-izm, fē′tish-). Fetichismo; ato de venerar ou utilizar para estimulação e gratificação sexual o que é considerado como um fetiche.

fe·to·glob·u·lins (fē-tō-glob′ū-linz). Fetoglobulinas; um grupo de proteínas com função desconhecida encontradas no sangue fetal. A α-f. ocorre em pequena quantidade em adultos normais e em quantidade maior no feto e na gestante, principalmente no segundo trimestre de gravidez; níveis elevados são também detectados em adultos com doença hepática e neoplasias.

fe·tog·ra·phy (fē-tog′ră-fē). Fetografia; radiografia do feto *in utero*, utilizando contraste; uma técnica obsoleta. Cf. amniography. [L. *fetus* + G. *graphō,* escrever]

fe·tol·o·gy (fē-tol′ō-jē). Fetologia. SIN maternal-fetal *medicine.* [L. *fetus* + G. *logos,* estudo]

fe·tom·e·try (fē-tom′e-trē). Fetometria; estimativa do tamanho do feto, principalmente de sua cabeça, antes do parto. [L. *fetus,* + G. *metron,* medida]

fe·top·a·thy (fē-top′a-thē). Fetopatia. SIN embryopathy. [L. *fetus* + G. *pathos,* sofrimento, doença]
  diabetic f., f. diabética; f. resultante de diabetes materno, que pode causar macrossomia e morte fetal.

fe·to·pla·cen·tal (fē′tō-pla-sen′tăl). Fetoplacentário; relativo ao feto e à sua placenta.

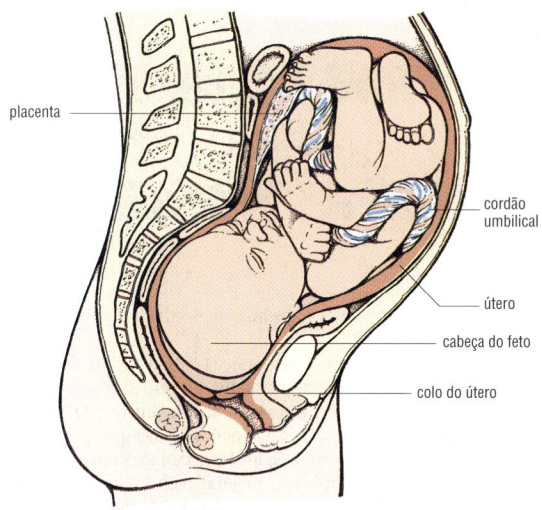

feto: (antes do parto)

fe·to·pro·teins (fē-tō-prō′tēnz). Fetoproteínas; proteínas fetais encontradas em pequena quantidade nos adultos nas seguintes formas: α**-f.** (AFP) eleva-se no sangue materno durante a gravidez e, quando detectada por amniocentese, é um importante indicador de defeitos do tubo neural (aberto). É também utilizada como um marcador tumoral em adultos (ver definição adiante); β**-f.,** embora seja uma proteína do fígado fetal, tem sido detectada em pacientes adultos com doença hepática; γ**-f.** é encontrada em várias neoplasias. VER TAMBÉM fetoglobulins.
  α **f.,** proteína normalmente produzida durante a 12.ª e a 15.ª semanas de gestação, diminuindo a seguir; porém aparece no sangue em certos tumores, tais como carcinomas embrionários do testículo e ovário, hepatoma e, menos freqüentemente, em pacientes com carcinomas de pâncreas, estômago, cólon ou pulmão. Quando presente, é um marcador útil no acompanhamento de um tumor.

fe·tor (fē′tor). Fedor; odor muito desagradável. [L. um cheiro desagradável, de *feteo,* feder]
  f. hepat′icus, hálito hepático; odor característico percebido no hálito de pessoas com doença hepática grave; causado por substâncias aromáticas voláteis que se acumulam no sangue e na urina devido a falha no metabolismo hepático. SIN liver breath.
  f. o′ris, halitose. SIN halitosis.

fe·to·scope (fē′tō-skōp). Fetoscópio. **1.** Endoscópio de fibra óptica utilizado em fetologia. **2.** Estetoscópio projetado para ouvir os sons do coração do feto.

fe·tos·co·py (fē-tos′kō-pē). Fetoscopia; uso de um endoscópio de fibra óptica para visualizar o feto e a superfície fetal da placenta por via transabdominal e, também, para coletar sangue fetal da veia umbilical para o diagnóstico pré-natal de doenças fetais.

fe·tu·in (fē-too′in). Fetuína; globulina de baixo peso molecular que consiste quase na totalidade da globulina do sangue fetal. [fetus + -in]

fe·tus, pl. **fe·tus·es** (fē′tŭs, fē′tŭs-ez). Feto. **1.** Nome dado à cria ainda não nascida de um animal vivíparo após o período embrionário. **2.** [NA]. Em seres humanos, o produto da concepção a partir do final da oitava semana de gestação até o momento do nascimento. [L. prole]

| desenvolvimento do feto ||||
semana de gravidez	comprimento (em cm)	peso (em g)	alterações específicas observadas
12.ª	7,5–10		membros em forma de cotos e diferenças sexuais visíveis; presença de abertura anal e sobrancelhas
16.ª	16		corpo completamente formado; pálpebras fechadas e fundidas; pele muito vermelha; lanugem na testa e no queixo; início da articulação do esqueleto, das estruturas dentárias e da formação do sangue no fígado
20.ª	25		*Vernix caseosa* sobre a testa e queixo; mecônio; ceco descendente em processo de rotação intestinal; há enzimas digestivas; formação de sangue na medula
24.ª	30–32		lanugem em todo o corpo; presença de epiderme nas regiões palmares e plantares
28.ª	35–40	1.000	capacidade para viver fora do útero; panículo adiposo incompleto; caretas faciais; cabelo com 0,5 cm de comprimento; migração dos testículos; abertura das pálpebras; voz chorosa
32.ª	46	1.800	aumento da *vernix caseosa*; pele vermelha
36.ª	51	2.500	aumento do panículo adiposo; as unhas alcançam a extremidade dos dedos; voz forte
40.ª	49–53	3.200	completamente desenvolvido

f. in fe'tu, condição na qual um pequeno e malformado feto está contido dentro de outro feto.
harlequin f., f. arlequim; forma autossômica recessiva grave de bebê-colódio em um recém-nascido, geralmente prematuro; trata-se de uma forma de eritrodermia ictiosiforme caracterizada pelo encapsulamento do corpo por placas, freqüentemente fissuradas, marrom–acinzentadas que se assemelham às placas de uma armadura, deformidade grotesca da face com eversão dos lábios e gangrena das falanges terminais; em geral, o óbito ocorre em alguns dias, embora o tratamento com o 13-*cis*-ácido retinóico tenha sido bem-sucedido em alguns casos. SIN ichthyosis fetalis (1).
impacted f., f. impactado; f. que, por causa de seu grande tamanho ou por estreitamento do canal pélvico, está comprimido, incapaz de avançar ou recuar espontaneamente.
f. papyra'ceus, f. papiráceo; o feto gêmeo que morreu e foi achatado contra a parede uterina pelo crescimento do f. vivo.
f. sanguinolentis (san - gwi'nō - len'tis), f. morto que se tornou macerado.
Feulgen, Robert, citoquímico e bioquímico do ácido nucleico, alemão, 1884–1955. Foi o primeiro a detectar o DNA em células por meio de um teste citoquímico específico. VER Feulgen *cytometry*.
FEV Abreviatura de forced expiratory *volume* (volume expiratório forçado), escrita com subscrito, indicando o intervalo de tempo em segundos.

FEVER

fe·ver (fē'ver). Febre; resposta fisiológica complexa a doença, mediada por citocinas pirogênicas e caracterizada por elevação na temperatura central, produção de reagentes de fase aguda e ativação dos sistemas imunes. SIN febris, pyrexia. [A.S. *fefer*]
absorption f., f. de absorção; elevação da temperatura que ocorre freqüentemente após o parto, sem outros sintomas inconvenientes, provavelmente devido à absorção da secreção uterina através de abrasões na parede vaginal.
acclimating f., f. de aclimatação; aumento de temperatura acompanhado de mal-estar e resultante de trabalho realizado em ambiente muito quente.
Aden f., f. de Aden, dengue SIN dengue.
aestivoautumnal f., malária falciparum. SIN falciparum *malaria*.
African hemorrhagic f., f. hemorrágica africana; f. hemorrágica associada aos vírus Marburg e Ebola, morfologicamente similares, porém antigenicamente distintos, bem como a numerosos vírus que causam doenças semelhantes. VER TAMBÉM viral hemorrhagic f.
African tick f., f. africana transmitida por carrapato, f. hemorrágica da Criméia Congo. SIN Crimean-Congo hemorrhagic f.
African tick-bite f., f. africana transmitida pela picada de carrapato; doença febril causada pela bactéria *Rickettsia africae*, encontrada no sul da África e caracterizada por manchas escuras (*taches noires*) nos locais das picadas dos carrapatos *Amblyomma* infectados e linfadenopatia.
algid pernicious f., f. perniciosa álgida; ataque de malária perniciosa no qual o paciente apresenta manifestações de colapso e choque.
ardent f., f. ardente; termo às vezes empregado para a hiperpirexia que ocorre na f. intermitente da malária. SIN heat apoplexy (2).
Argentinean hemorrhagic f., f. hemorrágica argentina; forma de f. hemorrágica encontrada na América do Sul, aparentemente transmitida pelo contato de roedores com os seres humanos e causada pelo vírus Junin, um membro da família Arenaviridae.
artificial f., f. artificial. SIN pyretotherapy.
aseptic f., f. asséptica; f. acompanhada de mal-estar causada pela absorção de tecido morto, porém não infectado, que ocorre após um ferimento.
Assam f., f. de Assam, leishmaniose visceral. SIN visceral *leishmaniasis*.
Australian Q f., f. Q australiana; variedade da f. Q encontrada na Austrália; infecção contagiosa aguda causada pela riquétsia *Coxiella burnetii*, transmitida por carrapatos e enzoótica em animais da Austrália, principalmente em mamíferos marsupiais (nesóquias).
autumn f., f. outonal; **(1)** f. semelhante ao dengue e que ocorre no final do verão na Índia. SIN seven-day f. (1). **(2)** SIN hasamiyami.
benign tertian f., f. terçã benigna, malária virax. SIN vivax *malaria*.
bilious remittent f., f. biliosa remitente; **(1)** termo antigo da f. recidivante; **(2)** vômitos "biliosos" observados na malária e associados a aumento acentuado da bilirrubina sérica.
black f., f. maculosa das Montanhas Rochosas. SIN Rocky Mountain spotted f.
blackwater f., f. hemoglobinúrica; hemoglobinúria resultante de hemólise grave que ocorre na malária *falciparum*. SIN malarial *hemoglobinuria*.
blue f., f. maculosa das Montanhas Rochosas. SIN Rocky Mountain spotted f.
Bolivian hemorrhagic f., f. hemorrágica boliviana; doença similar à f. hemorrágica argentina, porém causada pelo vírus Machupo, um membro da família Arenaviridae.
bouquet f., dengue. SIN dengue.
boutonneuse f., f. botonosa, f. maculosa mediterrânea. SIN Mediterranean spotted f.
brass founder's f., f. dos vapores metálicos; doença ocupacional, caracterizada por sinais e sintomas semelhantes aos da malária e causada pela inalação de partículas e vapores de óxidos metálicos. Os vapores são formados pela evaporação a temperaturas muito elevadas e condensação no ar em finas partículas. SIN brass founder's ague, foundryman's f., metal fume f., zinc fume f.
Brazilian hemorrhagic f., f. hemorrágica brasileira, f. maculosa brasileira. SIN Brazilian spotted f.
Brazilian purpuric f., f. purpúrica brasileira, f. maculosa brasileira. SIN Brazilian spotted f.

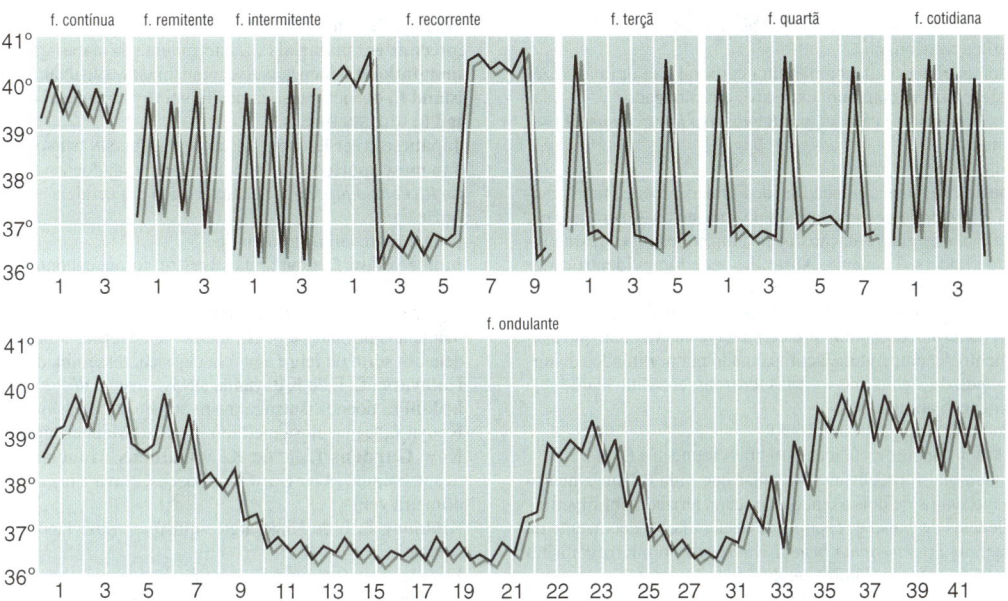

febre: as unidades no eixo horizontal correspondem a dias

Brazilian spotted f., f. maculosa brasileira; sepse fulminante que, em geral, se inicia com conjuntivite, caracterizada por lesões cutâneas purpúricas e por uma alta taxa de mortalidade; acredita-se que seja causada pelo *Haemophilus aegyptius*. SIN Brazilian hemorrhagic f., Brazilian purpuric f.
breakbone f., f. quebra-ossos, dengue. SIN dengue.
Bunyamwera f., f. Bunyamwera; doença febril humana encontrada na África, causada pelo vírus Bunyamwera (família Bunyaviridae) e transmitida por mosquitos culicídeos.
Burdwan f., f. Burdwan, leishmaniose visceral. SIN visceral *leishmaniasis*.
Bwamba f., f. Bwamba; doença febril humana encontrada na África, causada por um vírus da família Bunyaviridae e transmitida por mosquitos.
cachectic f., leishmaniose visceral. SIN visceral *leishmaniasis*.
camp f., f. de acampamento; (1) qualquer doença febril epidêmica que afeta grupos de pessoas em um acampamento; (2) termo obsoleto para tifo (typhus).
canicola f., f. canícola; doença humana, causada pelo sorotipo *canicola* da *Leptospira interrogans* e transmitida pela urina contaminada, geralmente de cães, mas raramente de bovinos e suínos.
catarrhal f., f. catarral; termo antigo para o grupo de doenças do sistema respiratório que engloba o resfriado comum, a gripe e as pneumonias lobular e lobar.
cat-bite f., f. da mordedura de gato; doença da mordedura do gato. SIN cat-bite *disease*.
catheter f., f. do cateter uretral. SIN urinary f.
catscratch f., f. por arranhadura de gato; doença da arranhadura do gato. SIN catscratch *disease*.
Central European tick-borne f., f. da Europa Central transmitida por carrapato. SIN tick-borne *encephalitis* (Central European subtype).
cerebrospinal f., meningite meningocócica. SIN meningococcal *meningitis*.
Charcot intermittent f., f. intermitente de Charcot; calafrios, dor no quadrante superior direito do abdome e icterícia, associados a obstrução intermitente do ducto comum por cálculos.
childbed f., f. puerperal. SIN puerperal f.
Colorado tick f., f. do Colorado transmitida por carrapato; infecção causada pelo vírus da f. do Colorado transmitida por carrapato e, aos seres humanos, pelo *Dermacentor andersoni*; as manifestações são leves, não ocorre erupção cutânea, a febre não é excessiva e a doença raramente, ou nunca, leva à morte.
Congolian red f., tifo murino. SIN murine *typhus*.
continued f., f. contínua; termo obsoleto para uma doença acompanhada de febre contínua, sem a intermitência que ocorre, p.ex., na malária. O termo foi utilizado em muitos casos de f. tifóide e também englobou muitos tipos de doenças febris.
cotton-mill f., bissinose. SIN byssinosis.
Crimean f., f. da Criméia, f. maculosa mediterrânea. SIN Mediterranean spotted f.
Crimean-Congo hemorrhagic f., f. hemorrágica da Criméia-Congo; forma de f. hemorrágica — diferente da f. hemorrágica de Omsk, encontrada na parte central da Rússia – transmitida por espécies do carrapato *Hyalomma* e causada pelo vírus da f. hemorrágica da Criméia-Congo, um membro da família Bunyaviridae; os cavalos são o principal reservatório da infecção humana, caracterizada por início abrupto, febre alta, cefaléia, mialgia, lesões hemorrágicas petequiais disseminadas pelo corpo, sangramento gastrointestinal e alta taxa de mortalidade. SIN African tick f.
dandy f., dengue. SIN dengue.
date f., dengue. SIN dengue.
deer-fly f., tularemia. SIN tularemia.
dehydration f., f. por desidratação. SIN thirst f.
dengue f., dengue. SIN dengue.
dengue hemorrhagic f., dengue. SIN dengue.
desert f., coccidioidomicose primária. SIN primary *coccidioidomycosis*.
digestive f., f. digestiva; um leve aumento da temperatura corporal que ocorre durante o período da digestão.
diphasic milk f., encefalite transmitida por carrapato (subtipo da Europa Central). SIN tick-borne *encephalitis* (Central European subtype).
double quotidian f., f. cotidiana dupla; tipo de malária caracterizado por dois paroxismos de diários de f..
drug f., f. medicamentosa; f. resultante de reação alérgica a uma droga e que desaparece rapidamente com a interrupção da mesma.
Dumdum f., leishmaniose visceral. SIN visceral *leishmaniasis*.
Dutton relapsing f., f. recidivante de Dutton. SIN Dutton *disease*.
Ebola hemorrhagic f., f. hemorrágica por vírus Ebola. SIN hemorrhagic f.
elephantoid f., f. elefantóide; linfangite e elevação da temperatura corporal que marcam o início da elefantíase endêmica (filariose).
enteric f., f. entérica; (1) f. tifóide. SIN typhoid f.; (2) o grupo que engloba as febres tifóide e paratifóide.
entericoid f., f. que não é a paratifóide nem a tifóide, mas que se assemelha à f. tifóide.
ephemeral f., f. efêmera; episódio febril que dura, no máximo, um ou dois dias.
epidemic hemorrhagic f., f. hemorrágica epidêmica; condição caracterizada por início agudo com cefaléia, calafrios, febre alta, sudorese, sede, fotofobia, coriza, tosse, mialgia, artralgia e dor abdominal acompanhada de náuseas e vômitos; essa fase dura de três a seis dias e é seguida por hemorragias capilares e no interstício renal, edema, oligúria, azotemia e choque; a maioria dos tipos é causada por numerosos vírus, entre eles os togavírus, os arenavírus, os flavivírus e os buniavírus e transmitida por roedores. SIN hemorrhagic f. with renal syndrome, Songo f.
epimastical f., f. epacmástica; f. que se eleva de forma constante até atingir o acme, quando, então, declina em crise ou lise.
eruptive f., f. maculosa mediterrânea. SIN Mediterranean spotted f.
essential f., f. essencial; f. que não está associada a uma doença infecciosa conhecida.
exanthematous f., f. exantemática; f. acompanhada de exantema.
exsiccation f., f. por desidratação. SIN thirst f.
falciparum f., malária *falciparum*. SIN falciparum *malaria*.
familial Mediterranean f., f. familiar do Mediterrâneo. SIN familial paroxysmal *polyserositis*.
Far East hemorrhagic f., f. hemorrágica do Extremo Oriente; infecção trans-

mitida por carrapatos contaminados com *Rickettsia sibirica*, encontrada principalmente na Sibéria e na Mongólia.
fatigue f., f. por fadiga; elevação da temperatura corporal que dura às vezes vários dias, após esforço físico contínuo, excessivo e prolongado.
field f., f. do campo; leptospirose causada por *Leptospira interrogans*. **(1)** SIN harvest f.; **(2)** SIN mud f.
five-day f., f. de cinco dias; SIN trench f.
Flinders Island spotted f., f. maculosa da Ilha de Flinders; doença febril causada pela bactéria *Rickettsia honei*, encontrada no sudeste da Austrália e caracterizada por cefaléia, mialgia e erupção cutânea maculopapular. [Denominada de f. da Ilha de Flinders, Tasmânia, Austrália, onde foram identificados os primeiros casos da doença]
flood f., f. fluvial, doença tsutsugamushi. SIN tsutsugamushi *disease*.
food f., f. alimentar; distúrbio, observado principalmente na infância, que consiste em súbito aumento de temperatura, acompanhado por acentuados distúrbios digestivos, durando de alguns dias a várias semanas; acredita-se que seja uma forma de intoxicação alimentar.
Fort Bragg f., f. do Forte Bragg. SIN pretibial f.
foundryman's f., f. dos vapores metálicos. SIN brass founder's f.
Gambian f., f. de Gâmbia; f. recidivante irregular que dura de um a quatro dias, apresentando intervalos de dois a cinco dias, caracterizada por hipertrofia do baço e freqüências de pulso e respiratória aceleradas; é decorrente da presença, no sangue, do *Trypanosoma brucei gambiense*, o microrganismo patogênico da doença do sono de Gâmbia ou da África Ocidental.
glandular f., mononucleose infecciosa. SIN infectious *mononucleosis*.
Haverhill f., f. de Haverhill; infecção causada pelo *Streptobacillus moniliformis*, caracterizada, no início, por calafrios e febre alta (que gradualmente diminui), seguidos por artrite, em geral das articulações maiores e da coluna vertebral, e por uma erupção cutânea que surge principalmente sobre as articulações e nas superfícies extensoras dos membros; o termo "f. de Haverhill" é utilizado para indicar infecções causadas pelo *Streptobacillus moniliformis* que não estão associadas a mordedura de rato, mas que resultam da ingestão de alimento ou água contaminada. SIN erythema arthriticum epidemicum. [*Haverhill*, Massachusetts, onde uma epidemia ocorreu em 1926]
harvest f., f. do ceifeiro; causada por *Leptospira interrogans*. SIN field f. (1).
hay f., f. do feno; forma de atopia caracterizada por inflamação irritativa aguda das mucosas dos olhos e das vias aéreas superiores, acompanhada por coceira e profusa secreção aquosa, geralmente sem elevação de temperatura, seguida ocasionalmente por bronquite e asma; o episódio reaparece anualmente, na mesma época do ano ou quase na mesma época do ano, na primavera, no verão ou no final do verão e outono, e resulta de uma reação alérgica ao pólen de árvores, gramíneas, sementes, flores, etc. SIN allergic coryza.
hematuric bilious f., f. biliosa hematúrica; hematúria resultante de lesões renais causadas pelo hematozoário da malária, o *Plasmodium falciparum*.
hemoglobinuric f., f. hemoglobinúrica. SIN malarial *hemoglobinuria*.
hemorrhagic f., f. hemorrágica; síndrome que ocorre em cerca de 20 a 40% das infecções causadas por vários vírus diferentes das famílias Arenaviridae (f. de Lassa, f. hemorrágica boliviana, f. hemorrágica argentina), Bunyaviridae (f. hemorrágica da Criméia-Congo), Flaviviridae (dengue, f. hemorrágica de Omsk), Filoviridae (f. por vírus Ebola, doença causada pelo vírus Marburg), etc. Alguns tipos de f. hemorrágica são transmitidos por carrapatos, outros tipos são transmitidos por mosquitos e alguns tipos parecem ser zoonoses; as manifestações clínicas são f. alta, petéquias disseminadas pelo corpo, sangramento gastrointestinal e em outros órgãos, hipotensão e choque; o dano ao rim pode ser grave, principalmente na f. hemorrágica coreana, e sinais neurológicos podem aparecer, principalmente nos tipos argentino e boliviano. Cinco tipos de febre hemorrágica são transmitidos de pessoa para pessoa: f. hemorrágica boliviana, f. de Lassa, f. por vírus Ebola, doença causada pelo vírus Marburg e f. hemorrágica da Criméia-Congo. VER TAMBÉM epidemic hemorrhagic f. SIN Ebola hemorrhagic f.
hemorrhagic f. with renal syndrome, f. hemorrágica com síndrome renal. SIN epidemic hemorrhagic f.
hepatic intermittent f., f. hepática intermitente; paroxismos de f. semelhantes a calafrios que ocorrem em pacientes com um ou mais cálculos no ducto colédoco.
herpetic f., f. herpética; doença de curta duração, aparentemente infecciosa, caracterizada por calafrios, náuseas, elevação da temperatura, dor de garganta e por erupção herpética na face e em outras áreas; a infecção primária é causada pelo vírus do herpes simples.
hospital f., tifo epidêmico. SIN epidemic *typhus*.
icterohemorrhagic f., f. íctero-hemorrágica; infecção causada pelo sorotipo conhecido como *icterohemorrhagiae* da *Leptospira interrogans*, caracterizada por febre, icterícia, lesões hemorrágicas, azotemia e manifestações do sistema nervoso central. SIN leptospirosis icterohemorrhagica.
Ilhéus f., f. de Ilhéus; doença febril causada pelo vírus Ilhéus, um vírus do gênero Flavivirus, e transmitida por um mosquito. VER TAMBÉM Ilhéus *encephalitis*.
inanition f., f. de inanição. SIN thirst f.

induced f., f. induzida. SIN pyretotherapy.
intermittent malarial f., f. intermitente da malária. VER intermittent *malaria*.
inundation f., doença tsutsugamushi. SIN tsutsugamushi *disease*.
island f., doença tsutsugamushi. SIN tsutsugamushi *disease*.
jail f., tifo. SIN typhus.
Japanese river f., doença tsutsugamushi. SIN tsutsugamushi *disease*.
Japanese spotted f., f. maculosa japonesa; doença febril causada pela bactéria *Rickettsia japonica* e caracterizada por cefaléia e exantema; encontrada no Japão.
jungle f., malária. SIN malaria.
jungle yellow f., f. amarela silvestre; forma encontrada na América do Sul e transmitida pelo *Aedes leucocelaenus* e por vários mosquitos que habitam no topo das árvores e pertencem ao gênero *Haemagogus*; é transmitida habitualmente aos primatas e ocasionalmente aos seres humanos, nos quais desencadeia um surto de febre amarela clássica, disseminado pelo *Aedes aegypti*.
Katayama f., f. de Katayama. SIN Katayama *disease*.
kedani f., doença tsutsugamushi SIN tsutsugamushi *disease*.
Kenya f., f. maculosa mediterrânea. SIN Mediterranean spotted f.
Kew Gardens f., f. de Kew Gardens; riquetsiose variceliforme. SIN rickettsialpox. [*Kew Gardens*, Queens, Nova York, onde a f. foi relatada pela primeira vez]
Kinkiang f., f. de Kinkiang; esquistossomose japônica. SIN schistosomiasis *japonica*.
Korean hemorrhagic f., f. hemorrágica coreana; forma de f. hemorrágica epidêmica causada pelo vírus Hantaan. SIN Manchurian hemorrhagic f.
Lassa f., f. de Lassa; forma grave de f. hemorrágica epidêmica extremamente fatal; identificada pela primeira vez em Lassa, Nigéria; é causada pelo vírus Lassa, um membro da família Arenaviridae, e caracterizada por f. alta, dor de garganta, dores musculares intensas, erupção cutânea com hemorragias, cefaléia, dor abdominal, vômitos e diarréia; o rato *Mastomys natalensis* com polimastia atua como reservatório, porém a transmissão de pessoa-a-pessoa também é comum. SIN Lassa hemorrhagic f.
Lassa hemorrhagic f., f. hemorrágica de Lassa. SIN Lassa f.
laurel f., f. do louro; afecção da mesma natureza que a f. do feno, que ocorre no período de florescência do loureiro.
malarial f., f. da malária. VER malaria.
malignant tertian f., f. terçã maligna, malaria falciparum. SIN falciparum *malaria*.
Malta f., f. de Malta, brucelose. SIN brucellosis.
Manchurian f., f. da Manchúria; f. muito semelhante ao tifo que ocorre de setembro a dezembro no sul da Manchúria; o patógeno provável é a *Rickettsia manchuriae*.
Manchurian hemorrhagic f., f. hemorrágica da Manchúria. SIN Korean hemorrhagic f.
Marseilles f., f. de Marselha, f. maculosa mediterrânea. SIN Mediterranean spotted f.
marsh f., malária. SIN malaria.
Mediterranean f., **(1)** SIN brucellosis; **(2)** SIN familial paroxysmal *polyserositis*.
Mediterranean erythematous f., f. eritematosa do Mediterrâneo; forma de f. maculosa mediterrânea que causa vermelhidão cutânea; seu curso e outros sintomas podem ser semelhantes àqueles da f. exantemática do Mediterrâneo. VER *Rickettsia conorii*.
Mediterranean exanthematous f., f. exantemática do Mediterrâneo. VER boutonneuse f.
Mediterranean spotted f., f. maculosa do Mediterrâneo; infecção transmitida por carrapatos contaminados com *Rickettsia conorii* e encontrada na África, na Europa, no Oriente Médio e na Índia; é conhecida por diferentes nomes em diferentes locais, p.ex., f. de Marselha, f. da Criméia, tifo da Índia transmitido por carrapato e f. queniana. As duas formas da infecção são: a f. exantemática do Mediterrâneo (q.v.), que se manifesta como erupções cutâneas; e a f. eritematosa do Mediterrâneo (q.v.), que se manifesta como vermelhidão cutânea. VER *Rickettsia conorii*. SIN boutonneuse f., Crimean f., eruptive f., fièvre boutonneuse, Indian tick typhus, Kenya f., Marseilles f., tick typhus.
meningotyphoid f., f. meningotifóide; f. tifóide caracterizada por sintomas de irritação ou inflamação das meninges cerebrais ou espinais.
metal fume f., f. dos vapores metálicos. SIN brass founder's f.
Mexican spotted f., f. maculosa das Montanhas Rochosas. SIN Rocky Mountain spotted f.
miliary f., f. miliar; **(1)** doença infecciosa caracterizada por sudorese abundante e formação de sudâminas que ocorria antigamente em epidemias graves; **(2)** SIN miliaria.
milk f., f. do leite; **(1)** elevação discreta de temperatura que se segue ao parto, considerada resultante do início da secreção de leite mas que, provavelmente, corresponde à f. de absorção; **(2)** doença metabólica afebril que ocorre logo após o parto no gado bovino leiteiro, caracterizada por hipocalcemia e que se manifesta por perda da consciência e paralisia geral.
mill f., bissinose. SIN byssinosis.

miniature scarlet f., reação que consiste em febre, náuseas, vômitos e erupção cutânea escarlatiforme transitória que aparece em um indivíduo suscetível, quando recebe uma injeção contendo a toxina do *Streptococcus pyogenes*. [L. *minio*, pp. *atus*, colorir com *minium*, vermelho brilhante]
monoleptic f., f. monoléptica; f. contínua que apresenta apenas um paroxismo. Cf. polyleptic f.
Mossman f., f. de Mossman; f. observada principalmente entre cortadores de cana-de-açúcar no Distrito de Mossman, em North Queensland, Austrália, e causada por uma leptospira.
mud f., f. da lama; leptospirose causada por *Leptospira interrogans*; (outrora acreditava-se que fosse causada pelo sorovariante grippotyphosa); ocorre no verão e no final do outono na Alemanha e na Rússia; transmitida pelo camundongo *Microtus arvalis*.
mumu f., f. de mumu; termo samoano para elephantoid f.
nanukayami f., f. de nanukayami; forma de leptospirose encontrada no Japão e causada por uma leptospira habitualmente encontrada no rato do campo ou no arganaz. SIN nanukayami.
nine mile f., f. Q. SIN Q f.
nodal f., eritema nodoso. SIN erythema nodosum.
North Queensland tick f., f. de North Queensland transmitida por carrapato; forma leve de tifo transmitida por carrapatos, caracterizada por escaras, adenopatia, erupção cutânea e febre e causada por *Rickettsia australis*; acredita-se que seja transmitida pelo carrapato *Ixodes holocyclus*.
Omsk hemorrhagic f., f. hemorrágica de Omsk; forma de febre hemorrágica epidêmica, encontrada na região central da Rússia, causada pelo vírus da f. hemorrágica de Omsk — um membro da família Flaviviridae — e transmitida pelos carrapatos *Dermacentor*; está associada a sintomas e hemorragias gastrointestinais e a pouco ou nenhum envolvimento do sistema nervoso central.
o'nyong-nyong f., f. de O'nyong-nyong; doença semelhante ao dengue, causada pelo vírus O'nyong-nyong, um membro da família Togaviridae, e transmitida por um mosquito; caracteriza-se por dor nas articulações e notável linfadenopatia, seguidas de erupção maculopapular na face, que se estende para o tronco e para os membros e que desaparece após vários dias, sem descamação.
Oropouche f., f. de Oropouche; doença febril aguda causada por uma espécie de Bunyavirus.
Oroya f., f. de Oroya; forma aguda, febril, generalizada, endêmica e sistêmica de bartonelose; caracterizada por febre alta, dores reumáticas, anemia grave e progressiva e albuminúria. SIN Carrión disease.
Pahvant Valley f., f. do Vale de Pahvant, tularemia. SIN tularemia.
paludal f., f. palustre, malária. SIN malaria.
pappataci f., f. papataci, f. do flebótomo. SIN phlebotomus f.
paratyphoid f., f. paratifóide; doença infecciosa aguda com sintomas e lesões que se assemelham aos da f. tifóide, embora de caráter mais brando; está associada à presença do microrganismo paratifóide do qual pelo menos três variedades (tipos A, B e C) foram descritas. SIN paratyphoid.
parenteric f., f. paraentérica; uma de um grupo de febres que se assemelham clinicamente à f. tifóide e às f. paratifóides A e B, porém são causadas por bactérias que diferem especificamente daquelas de qualquer uma dessas doenças.
parrot f., psitacose. SIN psittacosis.
Pel-Ebstein f., f. de Pel-Ebstein; febre remitente encontrada na doença de Hodgkin. SIN Pel-Ebstein disease.
periodic f., f. periódica; termo obsoleto introduzido para descrever os episódios de febre intermitente observados em uma doença que, posteriormente, foi identificada e denominada de familial Mediterranean f. (f. mediterrânea familiar).
Persian relapsing f., f. recidivante persa; f. recidivante transmitida por carrapatos; é encontrada no Oriente Médio, causada pela *Borrelia persica* e transmitida pelo *Ornithodoros tholozani* e, possivelmente, pelo *Ornithodoros lahorensis*.
pharyngoconjunctival f., f. faringoconjuntival; doença que geralmente ocorre de forma epidêmica, caracterizada por febre, faringite e conjuntivite e causada por vários tipos de adenovírus.
Philippine hemorrhagic f., f. hemorrágica filipina; infecção grave com manifestações hemorrágicas, causada por arbovírus e que apresenta uma taxa de mortalidade considerável; é provavelmente adquirida pela picada do mosquito transmissor do vírus da dengue; encontrada em áreas urbanas tropicais e subtropicais do Sudeste Asiático, do sul do Pacífico, da Austrália, das Américas Central e do Sul e das ilhas do Caribe.
phlebotomus f., f. por flebótomos; doença infecciosa, mas não contagiosa, encontrada na Península dos Bálcãs e em outras regiões do sul da Europa, causada por vários vírus da família Bunyaviridae, aparentemente inoculados pela picada do mosquito-pólvora *Phlebotomus papatasii*; os sinais e sintomas assemelham-se aos da dengue, mas são menos graves e de duração mais curta. SIN dog disease, pappataci f., Pym f., sandfly f., three-day f.
pinta f., termo utilizado no México para a f. maculosa das Montanhas Rochosas.
polka f., dengue. SIN dengue.
polyleptic f., f. poliléptica; f. na qual são observados dois ou mais paroxismos; p.ex., a f. que ocorre na varíola, a f. recidivante e a f. intermitente. Cf. monoleptic f.
polymer fume f., f. dos vapores de polímeros; doença ocupacional caracterizada por febre, dor no peito e tosse, sendo causada pela inalação dos vapores desprendidos pela queima de um plástico, o politetrafluoretileno.
pretibial f., f. pré-tibial; doença branda observada pela primeira vez entre os militares do Forte Bragg, na Carolina do Norte, e caracterizada por f. moderada, prostração, esplenomegalia e erupção cutânea localizada na face anterior das pernas; causada pelo sorotipo *autumnalis* da *Leptospira interrogans*. SIN Fort Bragg f.
protein f., f. causada por proteína; f. produzida pela administração de proteína estranha, como a do leite.
puerperal f., f. puerperal; sépsis pós-parto acompanhada de elevação na temperatura que ocorre 24 horas após o parto e antes do 11.º dia de pós-parto. SIN childbed f., puerperal sepsis.
Pym f., f. de Pym, f. por flebótomos. SIN phlebotomus f.
pyogenic f., f. piogênica, piemia. SIN pyemia.
Q f., f. Q; doença causada pela riquétsia *Coxiella burnetii* e que se propaga entre ovinos e bovinos, nos quais não provoca sintomas; as infecções humanas ocorrem como resultado de contato não apenas com esses animais, mas também com outros seres humanos infectados, ar e poeira contaminados, hospedeiros que atuam como reservatórios silvestres e outras fontes. SIN nine mile f. [*Q* de "query", palavra inglesa para "pergunta, dúvida, ponto de interrogação", porque o agente etiológico não era conhecido]
quartan f., f. quartã, malária malariae. SIN malariae *malaria*.
quintan f., f. quintã, f. das trincheiras. SIN trench f.
quotidian f., f. cotidiana, malária cotidiana. SIN quotidian *malaria*.
rabbit f., tularemia. SIN tularemia.
rat-bite f., f. por mordedura de rato; denominação comum para duas doenças bacterianas associadas à mordedura de rato, sendo uma delas causada pelo *Streptobacillus moniliformis* (p.ex., f. de Haverhill) e a outra causada pelo *Spirillum minus* (p.ex., sodoku); ambas as doenças são caracterizadas por f. recidivante, calafrios, cefaléia, artralgia, linfadenopatia e erupção cutânea maculopapulosa nos membros. SIN rat-bite disease, sodoku, sokosho.
recrudescent typhus f., doença de Brill-Zinsser, tifo recrudescente. SIN Brill-Zinsser *disease*.
recurrent f., f. recorrente, f. recidivante. SIN relapsing f.
red f., red f. of the Congo, tifo murino. SIN murine *typhus*.
relapsing f., f. recidivante; doença infecciosa aguda causada por uma de várias cepas de *Borrelia*, caracterizada por numerosos ataques febris que duram cerca de seis dias, separados entre si por intervalos apiréticos com aproximadamente a mesma duração; o microrganismo é encontrado no sangue durante os períodos febris, mas não durante os intervalos, estando seu desaparecimento associado a anticorpos específicos e anticorpos previamente estimulados. Existem duas variedades epidemiológicas: 1) aquela transmitida por piolhos, encontrada principalmente na Europa, no norte da África e na Índia e causada por cepas de *Borrelia recurrentis*; 2) aquela transmitida por carrapatos, encontrada na África, na Ásia e nas Américas do Norte e do Sul e causada por várias espécies de *Borrelia*, sendo cada uma dessas espécies transmitida por uma espécie diferente de carrapato, *Ornithodoros*. SIN bilious typhoid of Griesinger, recurrent f., spirillum f., typhinia.
remittent f., f. remitente; padrão de febre no qual a temperatura varia durante cada período de 24 horas, mas nunca alcança o valor normal. A maioria dessas febres é remitente, e o padrão não é característico de nenhuma doença, embora, durante o século XIX, o termo tenha sido considerado um diagnóstico.
remittent malarial f., f. remitente da malária. VER remittent *malaria*.

rheumatic f., f. reumática; síndrome subaguda febril que surge após uma infecção por estreptococo β-hemolítico do grupo A (em geral, faringite) e é mediada por uma resposta imune ao microrganismo; é mais freqüentemente encontrada em crianças e adultos jovens; caracteriza-se por f., miocardite (que causa taquicardia e, às vezes, insuficiência cardíaca aguda), endocardite (com incompetência valvar, seguida de cura com fibrose) e poliartrite migratória; nódulos subcutâneos, eritema marginado e coréia de Syndenham podem ser observados, porém com menor freqüência; recaídas podem ocorrer após uma reinfecção por estreptococos.

> Os critérios para o diagnóstico da febre reumática aguda foram publicados por Jones em 1944. Os esquemas para a prevenção dos ataques inicial e recorrente e os parâmetros terapêuticos permanecem basicamente inalterados há décadas. Embora a febre reumática aguda tenha deixado de ser um problema de saúde pública importante nos Estados Unidos, sua incidência ainda é alta nos países em desenvolvimento. Na Índia, por exemplo, onde os serviços médicos não conseguiram acompanhar o ritmo da urbanização e da industrialização, 250.000 novos casos são diagnosticados anualmente em crianças em idade escolar. Nos Estados Unidos, a incidência de febre reumática, que declinou de forma constante

durante muitas décadas após o advento do tratamento da faringite estreptocócica com antibióticos, começou a aumentar novamente no final da década de 1980 e durante a década de 1990, com alguns grupos urbanos apresentando um aumento de 10 vezes na incidência. Historicamente, a febre reumática é uma doença que afeta crianças pertencentes às classes socioeconômicas mais baixas. Em alguns grupos novos, a maioria das vítimas era de adultos e, quando crianças eram afetadas, freqüentemente pertenciam a famílias das classes média e alta. Cerca de 75% dos pacientes negaram qualquer história recente de dor de garganta, e alguns daqueles que apresentavam uma história pregressa de faringite estreptocócica tinham sido tratados com antibióticos. As manifestações cardíacas e articulares da febre reumática são consideradas fenômenos autoimunes, resultantes de um fator reumatogênico que foi postulado, porém nunca isolado. Sabe-se que a patogenicidade dos estreptococos está associada à presença de uma proteína M na membrana celular, que é também responsável pela aparência rugosa da superfície dos microrganismos ao exame microscópico e pela produção de colônias mucóides no ágar-sangue. Os microrganismos implicados em vários grupos novos de febre reumática pertencem a cepas mucóides, sobretudo os sorotipos M 3 e M 18. O uso generalizado dos antibióticos nos últimos anos, nem sempre adequado ou justificado pelo conhecimento médico atual, pode ter causado o ressurgimento da febre reumática ao favorecer o aumento e a disseminação de cepas virulentas de estreptococos, ou ao reduzir a capacidade de certas populações para elaborar uma resposta imune contra eles. Atualmente, as autoridades em doenças infecciosas estão reavaliando o diagnóstico e o tratamento da infecção estreptocócica, particularmente no que diz respeito às provas rápidas para a detecção do antígeno estreptocócico e aos esquemas medicamentosos aprovados para o tratamento da faringite estreptocócica aguda e, conseqüentemente, para a profilaxia da febre reumática. VER Jones *criteria* (critérios de Jones), em *criterion*.

---

rice-field f., f. dos campos de arroz; doença febril que afeta os trabalhadores dos campos de arroz, descrita no Vale do Pó, na Itália, e em Sumatra; causada por *Leptospira interrogans* VER TAMBÉM field f.
Rift Valley f., f. do Vale de Rift; doença endêmica fatal que afeta carneiros e é causada pelo vírus da f. do Vale de Rift — um membro da família Bunyaviridae — patogênico tanto para seres humanos como para bovinos e que provoca, nos seres humanos, uma f. de tipo indeterminado; é transmitida por mosquitos e por contato direto. [*Vale de Rift*, no Quênia]
Rocky Mountain spotted f., f. maculosa das Montanhas Rochosas; doença infecciosa aguda com alta taxa de mortalidade, caracterizada por cefaléia frontal e occipital, dor lombar intensa, mal-estar, f. contínua e moderadamente alta e erupção cutânea nos punhos, regiões palmares, tornozelos e regiões plantares do segundo ao quinto dia, espalhando-se, posteriormente, para todas as partes do corpo; ocorre na primavera, principalmente no sudeste dos Estados Unidos e na região das Montanhas Rochosas, embora seja também endêmica em outras áreas dos Estados Unidos, em regiões do Canadá, no México e na América do Sul; o microrganismo patogênico é a *Rickettsia rickettsii*, transmitida por duas ou mais espécies de carrapatos do gênero *Dermacentor*; nos Estados Unidos, é disseminada pelo *D. andersoni*, nos estados do oeste, e pelo *D. variabilis* (um carrapato de cães), nos estados do leste. SIN black f., black measles (2), blue disease, blue f., Mexican spotted f., São Paulo f., Tobia f.
Roman f., f. romana; f. terçã maligna ou estivooutonal, encontrada, no passado, na Campagna e na cidade de Roma; é causada pelo *Plasmodium falciparum*.
Ross River f., f. do Rio Ross. SIN epidemic polyarthritis.
sakushu f., f. sakushu. SIN hasamiyami.
Salinem f., f. de Salinem; infecção causada pela *Leptospira pyrogenes*, descrita em Salinem. SIN Salinem infection.
salt f., f. do sal; elevação da temperatura de um lactente após injeção retal de uma solução salina. VER TAMBÉM thirst f.
sandfly f., f. transmitida pelo mosquito-pólvora. SIN phlebotomus f.
San Joaquin f., f. de São Joaquim. SIN primary *coccidioidomycosis*.
San Joaquin Valley f., f. do Vale São Joaquim. SIN primary *coccidioidomycosis*.
São Paulo f., f. maculosa das Montanhas Rochosas. SIN Rocky Mountain spotted f.
scarlet f., escarlatina. SIN scarlatina.
Schamberg f., f. de Schamberg. SIN progressive pigmentary *dermatosis*.
Sennetsu f., f. de Sennetsu; doença humana encontrada no oeste do Japão, causada pela riquétsia *Ehrlichia sennetsu* e caracterizada por febre, mal-estar, anorexia, dor nas costas e linfadenopatia.
septic f., septicemia. SIN septicemia.
seven-day f., f. de sete dias. **(1)** SIN autumn f. (1); **(2)** SIN hasamiyami.
shin bone f., f. das trincheiras. SIN trench f.
ship f., tifo. SIN typhus.
shoddy f., f. dos trapos; doença febril que atinge os trabalhadores de fábricas antigas e empoeiradas, caracterizada por tosse, dispnéia e cefaléia; causada pela inalação de poeira.
simian hemorrhagic f., f. hemorrágica dos símios; doença altamente fatal que afeta macacos, causada pelo vírus da f. hemorrágica dos símios e caracterizada por febre, edema facial, anorexia, adipsia, petéquias cutâneas, diarréia, hemorragias e morte.
Sindbis f., f. de Sindbis; doença febril que afeta os seres humanos, encontrada na África, na Austrália e em outros países e caracterizada por artralgia, erupção cutânea e mal-estar; é causada pelo vírus Sindbis, um membro da família Togaviridae, e transmitida por mosquitos culicídeos.
slime f., infecção por leptospiras acompanhada de icterícia; provavelmente causada pela *Leptospira icterohemorrhagica*.
slow f., f. lenta; f. contínua de longa duração.
smelter's f., f. do fundidor de metal; f. dos vapores de metal que afeta os trabalhadores de caldeiras de fundição de zinco. SIN smelter's chills, smelter's shakes.
snail f., esquistossomose. SIN schistosomiasis.
solar f., (1) SIN dengue; **(2)** SIN sunstroke.
Songo f., f. de Songo. SIN epidemic hemorrhagic f.
South African tick-bite f., f. da África do Sul transmitida pela picada de carrapato; f. semelhante ao tifo encontrada na África do Sul, causada pela *Rickettsia rickettsii* e geralmente caracterizada por uma escara inicial e adenite regional, seguidas por rigidez muscular e erupção cutânea maculopapulosa no quinto dia, freqüentemente acompanhadas de graves sintomas referentes ao sistema nervoso central.
spirillum f., f. recidivante. SIN relapsing f.
spotted f., f. maculosa; tifo transmitido por carrapatos, causado pela *Rickettsia rickettsii* e encontrado nas Américas do Norte e do Sul e na Sibéria.
steroid f., f. por esteróides; f. aparentemente causada por concentrações plasmáticas elevadas de certos esteróides pirogênicos; pode ser produzida pela administração de etiocolanolona.
symptomatic f., f. sintomática. SIN traumatic f.
syphilitic f., f. sifilítica; elevação de temperatura freqüentemente presente nos estágios iniciais da roséola, na sífilis secundária.
tertian f., f. terçã. SIN vivax *malaria*.
therapeutic f., f. terapêutica. SIN pyrotherapy.
thermic f., termoplegia. SIN heatstroke.
thirst f., f. por desidratação; elevação de temperatura observada em lactentes após redução da ingestão de líquidos, diarréia ou vômitos; é provavelmente causada pela redução da água corporal, com diminuição da perda de calor por evaporação; uma condição análoga é observada em adultos, quando esforço físico contínuo é realizado na vigência de desidratação. SIN dehydration f., exsiccation f., inanition f.
three-day f., f. por flebótomo. SIN phlebotomus f.
Tobia f., f. de Tobia. SIN Rocky Mountain spotted f.
traumatic f., f. por traumatismo; elevação de temperatura que surge após um ferimento traumático. SIN symptomatic f., wound f.
trench f., f. das trincheiras; f. incomum causada pela riquétsia *Bartonella quintana* e transmitida pelo piolho *Pediculus humanus*; surgiu pela primeira vez na forma de uma epidemia durante a guerra de trincheiras, que ocorreu na Primeira Guerra Mundial; é caracterizada por início súbito de calafrios e f., mialgia (principalmente nas costas e pernas), cefaléia e mal-estar geral que dura caracteristicamente cinco dias, podendo ocorrer recidiva. SIN five-day f., quintan f., shin bone f.
trypanosome f., estágio febril da doença do sono.
tsutsugamushi f., tsutsugamushi. SIN tsutsugamushi *disease*.
typhoid f., f. tifóide; doença infecciosa aguda causada pela *Salmonella typhi* e caracterizada por f. contínua que aumenta na primeira semana, formando uma curva semelhante a degraus, intensa depressão física e mental, erupções cutâneas maculosas cor-de-rosa no tórax e abdome, timpanismo, constipação no início, diarréia e, às vezes, hemorragia intestinal e perfuração do intestino; a duração média é de quatro semanas, embora formas frustas e recaídas não sejam incomuns; as lesões localizam-se principalmente nos folículos linfáticos dos intestinos (placas de Peyer), nos gânglios mesentéricos e no baço; os títulos de anticorpos do teste de Widal elevam-se durante a infecção, e culturas de sangue e urina inicialmente positivas tornam-se negativas, resultando, em geral, em imunidade. SIN abdominal typhoid, enteric f. (1), typhoid (2).
undifferentiated type f.'s, febres de tipo indeterminado; termo atribuído a doenças resultantes de infecção por vírus — que pertenciam antigamente ao grupo dos arbovírus, patogênicos para os seres humanos nos quais a única manifestação constante é a febre; erupção cutânea, linfadenopatia e artralgia (isoladas ou em combinação) podem ocorrer em alguns indivíduos, mas não em outros; alguns vírus podem produzir infecções nas quais uma f. de tipo indeterminado é a única manifestação, enquanto outros vírus podem produzir, em algumas pessoas, somente uma f. indeterminada e, em outras, uma f. semelhante, seguida por manifestações secundárias, tais como f. hemorrágica ou encefalite.

undulant f., f. ondulante, brucelose. SIN brucellosis. [que se refere à aparência ondulante da longa curva de temperatura]
undulating f., f. ondulante, brucelose. SIN brucellosis.
f. of unknown origin, f. de origem indeterminada; f. (temperatura > 38,3°C ou 101°F) sem causa conhecida após investigação intensiva. Os critérios exatos para o uso do termo variam, principalmente com relação à duração da f. e à extensão da investigação clínica; em geral, uma f. com duração maior do que uma semana (alguns autores preferem 2 a 3 semanas) e investigação minuciosa — realizada em paciente internado ou em, pelo menos, três consultas ambulatoriais — que inclui anamnese detalhada, exame físico e testes laboratoriais, tais como culturas, estudos sorológicos e procedimentos invasivos para a realização de biópsia e/ou culturas, conforme indicado por sinais clínicos ou considerações epidemiológicas.
urethral f., f. do cateter uretral; SIN urinary f.
urinary f., f. do cateter uretral; elevação de temperatura, geralmente suave e transitória, que surge após cateterização da uretra ou após a eliminação de coágulos sanguíneos ou cálculos. SIN catheter f., urethral f.
urticarial f., f. esquistossomose japônica. SIN *schistosomiasis japonica.*
uveoparotid f., f. uveoparotídea; hipertrofia crônica das glândulas parótidas e inflamação do trato uveal acompanhadas por f. contínua prolongada e de baixa intensidade; reconhecida atualmente como uma forma de sarcoidose. SIN Heerfordt disease.
Uzbekistan hemorrhagic f., f. hemorrágica ubequistanesa; f. de origem viral encontrada na região central da Ásia e provavelmente transmitida pelo *Hyalomma anatolicum.*
valley f., f. coccidioidomicose primária. SIN primary *coccidioidomycosis.*
Venezuelan hemorrhagic f., f. hemorrágica venezuelana; doença febril causada pelo vírus Guanarito, na Venezuela, e caracterizada por cefaléia, artralgia, faringite, leucopenia, trombocitopenia e manifestações hemorrágicas.
viral hemorrhagic f., f. hemorrágica viral; doença epidêmica caracterizada por febre, mal-estar, dor muscular, sintomas do sistema respiratório, vômitos e diarréia; epistaxe, hemoptise, hematêmese e hemorragias subconjuntivais ocorrem nos casos graves; em alguns pacientes ocorrem erupções cutâneas e tremores por todo o corpo; doença causada por vários vírus diferentes, pertencentes às famílias Arenaviridae, Bunyaviridae, Flaviviridae, Filoviridae, etc. VER TAMBÉM hemorrhagic f.
vivax f., malária vivax. SIN vivax *malaria.*
Wesselsbron f., doença de Wesselsbron; doença transmitida por mosquitos, que afeta seres humanos e ovinos, causada pelo vírus Wesselsbron — um membro da família Flaviviridae — e caracterizada por abortamento e morte de cordeiros em ovinos, e por febre, cefaléia, dores musculares e erupção cutânea discreta em seres humanos. SIN Wesselsbron disease. [*Wesselsbron*, cidade da África do Sul, onde o agente patogênico foi isolado pela primeira vez]
West African f., hemoglobinúria da malária. SIN malarial *hemoglobinuria.*
West Nile f., doença febril causada pelo vírus West Nile — um membro da família Flaviviridae — e caracterizada por cefaléia, febre, erupção cutânea maculopapular, mialgia, linfadenopatia e leucopenia; disseminada por mosquitos *Culex* a partir de um reservatório em aves.
wound f., f. por traumatismo. SIN traumatic f.
Yangtze Valley f., f. do Vale Yangtze, esquistossomose japônica. SIN *schistosomiasis* japonica.
yellow f., f. amarela; hepatite viral tropical transmitida por mosquitos, causada pelo vírus da f. amarela — um membro da família Flaviviridae — com uma forma urbana, transmitida pelo *Aedes aegypti*, e uma forma rural silvestre, transmitida por diversos mosquitos do grupo *Haemagogus*, que se contaminam ao picar mamíferos que habitam em árvores; caracteriza-se clinicamente por febre, pulso lento, albuminúria, icterícia, congestão da face e hemorragias, principalmente hematêmese; costumava ocorrer na forma de epidemia, principalmente em cidades portuárias, sobretudo no final do verão, com uma taxa de mortalidade que variava de 20 a 40% dos casos; a recuperação é acompanhada de imunidade à reinfecção.
Zika f., f. por Zika; doença aguda, provavelmente transmitida por mosquitos, que se assemelha clinicamente à dengue; é causada pelo vírus *Zika*, um membro da família Flaviviridae.
zinc fume f., f. dos vapores do zinco. SIN brass founder's f.

fe·ver·ish (fē′ver-ish). Febril. **1.** SIN febrile. **2.** Que tem febre.
FF Abreviatura de filtration *fraction* (fração de filtração).
FFA Abreviatura de unesterified free *fatty acid* (ácido graxo livre não-esterificado).
FFP Abreviatura de fresh frozen *plasma* (plasma congelado fresco).
F.F.R. Abreviatura de *Fellow of the Faculty of Radiologists* (Reino Unido).
FGAR Abreviatura de *N*-formylglycinamide ribotide (*N*-formilglicinamida ribotídeo).
FH₄ Abreviatura de tetrahydrofolic acid (ácido tetra-hidrofólico). VER 5,6,7,8-tetrahydrofolate dehydrogenase, tetrahydrofolate methyltransferase.

FIBER

fi·ber (fī′ber) [TA]. Fibra; fio ou filamento delgado. **1.** Estruturas filamentosas extracelulares, tais como as fibras colágenas e elásticas do tecido conectivo. **2.** Axônio de célula nervosa e sua bainha formada por uma célula glial ou por uma célula de Schwann. **3.** Células alongadas, filiformes, tais como as células musculares e as células epiteliais que compõem a parte principal da lente do olho. **4.** Nutrientes de uma dieta que não são digeridos pelas enzimas do sistema gastrointestinal. SIN fibra [TA], fibre. [L. *fibra*]
A f.'s, fibras A; fibras nervosas mielínicas encontradas em nervos somáticos, com 1 a 22 μm de diâmetro; conduzem impulsos nervosos a uma velocidade que varia de 6 a 120 m/s.
accelerator f.'s, fibras aceleradoras; fibras nervosas simpáticas pós-ganglionares que se originam nos gânglios cervicais superior, médio e inferior do tronco simpático e conduzem impulsos nervosos para o coração, aumentando a rapidez e a força dos batimentos cardíacos. SIN augmentor f.'s.
adrenergic f.'s, fibras nervosas que transmitem impulsos nervosos para outras células nervosas, músculos lisos ou células glandulares por meio de uma substância transmissora semelhante à epinefrina: a norepinefrina (noradrenalina).
afferent f.'s, fibras aferentes; fibras que conduzem impulsos para um gânglio ou para um centro nervoso localizados no cérebro ou na medula espinal.
alpha f.'s, fibras alfa; grandes fibras nervosas somáticas motoras ou proprioceptivas com uma velocidade de condução de impulsos que varia de 80 a 120 m/s.
anastomosing f.'s, anastomotic f.'s, fibras anastomosantes; fibras individuais que passam de um tronco nervoso ou feixe muscular para outro.
anterior external arcuate f.'s, [TA], fibras arqueadas externas anteriores. VER external arcuate f.'s.
arcuate f.'s, fibras arqueadas; fibras nervosas ou tendinosas que passam sob a forma de um arco de uma parte para outra. VER arcuate f.'s of cerebrum, external arcuate f.'s, internal arcuate f.'s.
arcuate f.'s of cerebrum [TA], fibras arqueadas do cérebro; fibras de associação curtas que ligam giros adjacentes no córtex cerebral. SIN fibrae arcuatae cerebri [TA].
argyrophilic f.'s, fibras argirófilas; fibras do tecido conectivo reticular que reagem com sais de prata e tornam-se pretas ao microscópio.
association f.'s, fibras de associação; fibras nervosas que interligam subdivisões do córtex cerebral do mesmo hemisfério ou segmentos diferentes da medula espinal no mesmo lado. SIN endogenous f.'s, intrinsic f.'s.
astral f.'s, fibras astrais; fibras (fibrilas) que se irradiam da centrosfera em direção à periferia da célula sob o microscópio óptico; ao microscópio eletrônico, as fibras aparecem como microtúbulos. Cf. kinetochore f.'s, polar f.'s.
augmentor f.'s, fibras aceleradoras. SIN accelerator f.'s.
autonomic nerve f.'s [TA], fibras nervosas autônomas; qualquer uma das fibras nervosas pré e/ou pós-sinápticas que, em conjunto, compõem as partes simpática e parassimpática da divisão autônoma do sistema nervoso periférico. SIN neurofibrae autonomicae [TA], visceral motor f.'s.
B f.'s, fibras B; fibras mielínicas de nervos autônomos com diâmetro ≤ 2 μm e que conduzem impulsos a uma velocidade que varia de 3 a 15 m/s.
Bergmann f.'s, fibras de Bergmann; fibras filamentosas da glia que cruzam o córtex cerebelar perpendicularmente à superfície.
beta f.'s, fibras beta; fibras nervosas que possuem uma velocidade de condução que varia de 40 a 70 m/s.
bulbar corticonuclear f.'s [TA], fibras corticonucleares do bulbo; fibras nervosas que se projetam dos córtex sensoriais somáticos e motores até os núcleos de retransmissão sensoriais e motores do bulbo, tais como o núcleo do nervo hipoglosso, o núcleo do nervo acessório e os núcleos grácil e cuneiforme. VER corticonuclear f.'s. SIN fibrae corticonucleares bulbi [TA].
C f.'s, fibras C; fibras amielínicas, com 0,4 a 1,2 μm de diâmetro, que conduzem impulsos nervosos de 0,7 a 2,3 m/s.
cerebellohypothalamic f.'s, fibras cerebelo-hipotalâmicas; fibras nervosas que se originam em células dos núcleos cerebelares e se projetam, via pedúnculo cerebelar superior, para o hipotálamo contralateral, principalmente para as áreas dorsal, lateral e posterior e para o núcleo dorsomedial.
cerebelloolivary f.'s [TA], fibras cerebeloolivares; axônios de neurônios localizados nos núcleos cerebelares que saem através do pedúnculo cerebelar superior, cruzam a decussação e descem associados ao trato tegmental central. Dependendo de sua origem, essas fibras terminam em um dos núcleos olivares acessórios, ou no núcleo olivar principal; partem dos núcleos interpostos anterior e posterior para os núcleos olivares acessório posterior e acessório medial, respectivamente; do núcleo cerebelar medial para o núcleo olivar acessório medial; e do núcleo cerebelar lateral para o núcleo olivar principal. SIN fibrae cerebelloolivares [TA].
cerebellospinal f.'s, fibras cerebelospinais; fibras que se originam nos núcleos cerebelares do fastígio e interposto (principalmente o posterior) e descem

para o lado contralateral da medula espinal. VER fastigiospinal f.'s.
cholinergic f.'s, fibras colinérgicas; fibras nervosas que transmitem impulsos para outras células nervosas, fibras musculares ou células glandulares por meio de uma substância transmissora, a acetilcolina.
chromatic f., cromonema. SIN chromonema.
circular f.'s, fibras circulares; as fibras circulares do músculo ciliar. SIN fibrae circulares [TA], Müller f.'s (1), Müller muscle (2), Rouget muscle.
climbing f.'s, fibras trepadeiras; fibras nervosas, localizadas no córtex cerebelar, que fazem sinapse nas pequenas ramificações lisas dos dendritos das células de Purkinje.
collagen f., collagenous f., f. colágena; f. individual cujo diâmetro varia de menos de 1 μm até cerca de 12 μm e é composta por fibrilas; as fibras, geralmente dispostas em feixes, apresentam algumas ramificações e um comprimento indefinido; quimicamente, a f. é formada por uma glicoproteína — colágeno — que produz gelatina sob fervura; constituem-se no principal elemento do tecido conectivo irregular, dos tendões, das aponeuroses e da maioria dos ligamentos e está presente na matriz da cartilagem e do tecido ósseo. SIN white f. (2).
commissural f.'s, fibras comissurais; fibras nervosas que cruzam a linha média e unem duas partes ou regiões correspondentes do sistema nervoso.
cone f., f. do cone; uma parte da célula do cone da retina; a **f. interna do cone** é uma parte delgada da célula do cone, semelhante a um axônio, que se estende do corpo celular até o pedículo, localizado no estrato plexiforme externo da retina; na fóvea externa, onde as células do cone são muito alongadas, elas se estreitam até uma **f. externa do cone**, localizada entre o segmento interno e o corpo celular.
corticobulbar f.'s, fibras corticobulbares; termo antigamente utilizado para descrever as projeções que partem dos córtex sensorial e motor para núcleos do rombencéfalo — que inervam a musculatura da face, a língua e as maxilas — e algumas fibras para os núcleos de retransmissão do rombencéfalo; o termo foi substituído por: fibras corticonucleares do bulbo (para o bulbo), fibras corticonucleares da ponte (para a ponte) e fibras corticonucleares do mesencéfalo (para o mesencéfalo). VER cada entrada separadamente.
corticomesencephalic f.'s [TA], fibras corticomesencefálicas; axônios que se originam no córtex cerebral e terminam em estruturas mesencefálicas, tais como o teto, a substância negra e o tegmento. SIN fibrae corticomesencephalicae [TA].
corticonuclear f.'s, fibras corticonucleares; termo descritivo em referência às fibras que se originam em uma estrutura cortical (cerebral e cerebelar) e se dirigem a grupos de células subcorticais; são compostas pelas fibras corticonucleares do bulbo [TA], as fibras corticonucleares da ponte [TA] e as fibras corticonucleares do mesencéfalo [TA]; fibras corticonucleares do cerebelo (axônios das células de Purkinje que se dirigem para os núcleos do cerebelo). SIN fibrae corticonucleares [TA].
corticopontine f.'s [TA], fibras corticopontinas; fibras que compõem o trato corticopontino (corticopontine *tract*). SIN fibrae corticopontinae [TA].
corticoreticular f.'s [TA], fibras corticorreticulares; fibras corticofugais distribuídas pela formação reticular do mesencéfalo e do rombencéfalo. VER TAMBÉM corticonuclear f.'s. SIN fibrae corticoreticulares [TA].
corticorubral f.'s [TA], fibras corticorrubrais; fibras nervosas que se projetam do córtex cerebral (principalmente das regiões pré-central e pré-motora) até o núcleo rubro do mesencéfalo. SIN fibrae corticorubrales [TA].
corticospinal f.'s [TA], fibras corticospinais. SIN pyramidal f.'s.
corticothalamic f.'s, fibras corticotalâmicas; termo geral que designa as fibras nervosas originadas em qualquer área do córtex cerebral e que terminam nos núcleos do tálamo.
cuneocerebellar f.'s [TA], fibras cuneocerebelares. SIN cuneocerebellar *tract.*
cuneospinal f.'s [TA], fibras cuneospinais; axônios que se originam no núcleo cuneiforme do bulbo e descem ipsolateralmente pelo fascículo cuneiforme para terminar principalmente no corno posterior da medula espinal nos níveis cervical e torácico alto. SIN fibrae cuneospinales [TA].
delta f.'s, fibras delta; fibras nervosas com velocidades de condução da ordem de 8 a 30 m/s.
dentatorubral f.'s, fibras dentatorrubrais; fibras nervosas que partem do núcleo denteado do cerebelo e se projetam, através do pedúnculo cerebelar superior e da decussação, até o núcleo rubro contralateral do mesencéfalo. SIN fibrae dentatorubrales.
dentatothalamic f.'s, fibras dentatotalâmicas; fibras nervosas que se projetam do núcleo denteado do cerebelo até o tálamo contralateral, através do pedúnculo cerebelar superior (e da decussação); penetram no tálamo como um componente do fascículo talâmico.
dentinal f.'s, dental f.'s, fibras dentinárias; (**1**) os prolongamentos das células pulpares, os odontoblastos, que se estendem radialmente através da dentina até a junção da dentina com o esmalte (amelodentinária) e que estão contidos dentro dos túbulos dentinários. SIN Tomes f.'s. (**2**) fibras colágenas delgadas intertubulares que, juntamente com a substância de base da dentina infiltrada com sais de cálcio, constituem a matriz da dentina.
depressor f.'s, fibras depressoras; fibras nervosas sensoriais que apresentam terminações nervosas sensíveis à pressão, localizadas na parede de certas artérias e capazes de ativar a região do tronco encefálico responsável pela diminuição da pressão, quando estimuladas pela elevação da pressão intra-arterial.
dietary f., f. dietéticas; polissacarídeos e lignina vegetais resistentes à hidrólise pelas enzimas digestivas do homem.
efferent f.'s, fibras eferentes; fibras que conduzem impulsos para tecidos efetores (músculos liso, cardíaco e estriado e glândulas) localizados na periferia; as fibras que saem de um grupo de células específico (p.ex., fibras eferentes da parte basilar da ponte), utilizado como referência para um grupo de células.
elastic f.'s, fibras elásticas; fibras cujo diâmetro varia de 0,2 a 2 μm, podendo, contudo, ser maior em alguns ligamentos; ramificam-se e anastomosam-se para formar redes e fundem-se para criar membranas fenestradas; as fibras e membranas são compostas por microfibrilas com cerca de 10 nm de largura e uma substância amorfa que contém elastina. SIN yellow f.'s.
enamel f.'s, fibras do esmalte. SIN *prismata* adamantina, em *prisma.*
endogenous f.'s, fibras endógenas, fibras de associação. SIN association f.'s.
exogenous f.'s, fibras exógenas, fibras de associação; fibras nervosas por meio das quais determinada região do sistema nervoso central é ligada a outras regiões; o termo aplica-se tanto para as conexões de fibras aferentes como para as eferentes.
external arcuate f.'s, fibras arqueadas externas; incluem: 1) fibras arqueadas externas posteriores [TA], que partem de células do núcleo cuneiforme acessório ou lateral e se dirigem para o cerebelo; 2) fibras arqueadas externas anteriores [TA], que partem dos núcleos arqueados localizados na base do bulbo e passam ao redor da superfície lateral do bulbo; ambas penetram no cerebelo como componentes do corpo restiforme do pedúnculo cerebelar inferior. SIN fibrae arcuatae externae.
fastigiobulbar f.'s, fibras fastigiobulbares; fibras nervosas que se projetam dos núcleos do fastígio do cerebelo até o tronco cerebral; fibras cruzadas e não-cruzadas que terminam principalmente nos núcleos vestibulares e reticulares e no núcleo olivar acessório medial.
fastigiospinal f.'s, fibras fastigiospinais; fibras cruzadas descendentes que se originam no núcleo do fastígio do cerebelo e terminam na substância cinzenta da medula espinal no nível cervical e, possivelmente, em níveis mais baixos.
frontopontine f.'s [TA], fibras frontopontinas; grupo grande de fibras que partem do lobo frontal do hemisfério cerebral, principalmente do giro pré-central, descem pela cápsula interna, compõem mais caudalmente a parte medial dos pilares do cérebro, através da qual se estendem caudalmente, indo terminar na substância cinzenta (núcleos da ponte) da parte ventral da ponte. VER TAMBÉM corticopontine *tract.* SIN fibrae frontopontinae [TA].
gamma f.'s, fibras gama; fibras nervosas com velocidade de condução de 15 a 40 m/s. VER TAMBÉM gamma *efferent.*
Gerdy f.'s, fibras de Gerdy. SIN superficial transverse metacarpal *ligament.*
gracilespinal f.'s [TA], fibras gracilespinais; axônios que partem de neurônios do núcleo grácil do bulbo e descem ipsolateralmente pelo fascículo grácil, indo terminar principalmente no corno posterior da medula espinal, nos níveis torácico baixo e lombossacral. SIN fibrae gracilispinales [TA].
Gratiolet f.'s, fibras de Gratiolet. SIN optic *radiation.*
gray f.'s, fibras cinzentas. SIN unmyelinated f.'s.
hypothalamocerebellar f.'s, fibras hipotalamocerebelares; fibras nervosas que se originam de células localizadas no hipotálamo e se projetam para o córtex cerebelar e para os núcleos cerebelares.
hypothalamospinal f.'s [TA], fibras hipotalamoespinais; grupo de fibras que se origina principalmente no núcleo paraventricular e nas áreas hipotalâmicas lateral e posterior, desce ipsolateralmente através do tronco cerebral ventrolateral e para dentro do funículo lateral da medula espinal e termina em conexão com os neurônios do núcleo intermediolateral. SIN fibrae hypothalamospinales [TA].
inhibitory f.'s, fibras inibitórias; fibras nervosas que inibem a atividade das células nervosas com as quais têm conexões sinápticas, ou do tecido efetor no qual terminam (músculo liso, músculo cardíaco, glândulas).
intercolumnar f.'s, fibras intercrurais do anel superficial. SIN intercrural f.'s of superficial ring.
intercrural f.'s of superficial ring [TA], fibras intercrurais do anel superficial; fibras arqueadas horizontais que passam pelo ligamento inguinal através dos pilares medial e lateral do anel inguinal superficial. SIN fibrae intercrurales anuli inguinalis superficialis [TA], intercolumnar fasciae, intercolumnar f.'s.
internal arcuate f.'s [TA], fibras arqueadas internas; fibras que partem dos núcleos grácil e cuneiforme, seguem um trajeto curvilíneo através da linha média do bulbo e formam o lemnisco medial contralateral; o termo pode também designar outras fibras, tais como aquelas do trato olivocerebelar que arqueiam através da substância do bulbo e podem cruzar a decussação sensitiva. SIN fibrae arcuatae internae [TA].
intrafusal f.'s, fibras intrafusais; fibras musculares presentes dentro de um fuso neuromuscular.
intrathalamic f.'s [TA], fibras intratalâmicas; fibras que partem de um núcleo do tálamo dorsal e terminam em outro. SIN fibrae intrathalamicae [TA].
intrinsic f.'s, fibras intrínsecas, de associação. SIN association f.'s.
James f.'s, fibras de James; conexões entre o átrio e o feixe de His consideradas como a base da síndrome do intervalo P-R curto; essas fibras devem ser

distinguidas dos controvertidos tratos internodais do átrio, às vezes referidos como "tratos de James". SIN James tracts.

kinetochore f.'s, fibras do cinetocoro; fibras do fuso mitótico, presas ao centrômero, que se estendem em direção aos pólos. Cf. astral f.'s, polar f.'s.

Korff f.'s, fibras de Korff; fibras argirófilas que passam entre os odontoblastos na periferia da polpa do dente e se difundem dentro da dentina.

Kühne f., fibras de Kühne; f. muscular artificial produzida pelo enchimento do intestino de um inseto com uma cultura de mixomicetos; utilizada para demonstrar a contratilidade do protoplasma.

f.'s of lens, fibras da lente; células alongadas, de origem ectodermal, que formam a substância da lente cristalina do olho. SIN fibrae lentis.

long association f.'s [TA], fibras de associação longas; fibras nervosas que interligam lobos ou giros do córtex cerebral de um mesmo hemisfério que não são imediatamente adjacentes um ao outro; fibras nervosas que unem segmentos não-contínuos e de um mesmo lado da medula espinal; fibras que interligam pontos distantes. SIN fibrae associationes longae [TA].

longitudinal pontine f.'s [TA], fibras longitudinais da ponte. VER longitudinal pontine *fasciculi*, em *fasciculus*. SIN fibrae pontis longitudinales [TA].

Mahaim f.'s, fibras de Mahaim; fibras paraespecíficas que se originam no nó A-V, no feixe de His ou nos ramos de feixes e se inserem no miocárdio ventricular; são vias potenciais para arritmias reentrantes. SIN nodoventricular f.'s.

medullated nerve f., f. nervosa mielinizada. SIN myelinated nerve f.

meridional f.'s of ciliary muscle [TA], fibras meridionais do músculo ciliar; as fibras longitudinais do músculo ciliar. SIN fibrae meridionales muscularis ciliaris [TA].

mesencephalic corticonuclear f.'s [TA], fibras corticonucleares do mesencéfalo; fibras nervosas que se projetam principalmente do córtex motor até os núcleos motores do mesencéfalo, tais como o oculomotor e o troclear; os estímulos são transmitidos em cadeia pelos núcleos adjacentes a esses núcleos motores. VER corticonuclear f.'s. SIN fibrae corticonucleares mesencephali [TA].

mossy f.'s, fibras musgosas; fibras nervosas intensamente ramificadas, localizadas no córtex cerebelar, que terminam em formações de rosetas e fazem sinapses com os dendritos das células granulares.

motor f.'s, fibras motoras; fibras nervosas transmissoras de impulsos que ativam as células efetoras, p. ex., em músculo ou tecido glandular.

Müller f.'s, fibras de Müller; **(1)** SIN circular f.'s; **(2)** células neurogliais de sustentação da retina que percorrem toda a espessura da retina, indo do estrato limitante interno até as bases das células dos cones e bastonetes, onde formam uma série de complexos juncionais. SIN Müller radial cells, sustentacular f.'s of retina.

myelinated nerve f., f. nervosa mielinizada; axônio envolvido por uma bainha de mielina formada pelas células da oligodendróglia (no cérebro e na medula espinal) e pelas células de Schwann (nos nervos periféricos). SIN medullated nerve f.

Nélaton f.'s, fibras de Nélaton. SIN Nélaton *sphincter*.

nerve f., f. nervosa; axônio de uma célula nervosa, embainhado por células da oligodendróglia no cérebro e na medula espinal e por células de Schwann nos nervos periféricos.

nodoventricular f.'s, fibras nodoventriculares. SIN Mahaim f.'s.

nonmedullated f.'s, fibras não-mielinizadas. SIN unmyelinated f.'s.

nuclear bag f., f. do saco nuclear; o maior tipo de fibra muscular intrafusal presente em um fuso neuromuscular; contém um agregado central de núcleos (saco nuclear).

nuclear chain f., f. da cadeia nuclear; o menor e mais numeroso tipo de fibra muscular intrafusal presente em um fuso neuromuscular; contém uma única fileira de núcleos centralmente posicionados.

nucleocortical f.'s, fibras corticonucleares; termo geral utilizado para as projeções que partem de um núcleo e se dirigem para uma estrutura cortical suprajacente; termo empregado de modo específico para designar os axônios de células de núcleos cerebelares que se projetam para o córtex cerebelar (fibras nucleocorticais do cerebelo), onde terminam como fibras musgosas.

oblique f.'s of muscular layer of stomach [TA], fibras oblíquas da camada muscular do estômago; fibras musculares lisas da camada mais interna da túnica muscular do estômago; as fibras estão presentes principalmente na extremidade cardíaca do estômago e espalham-se sobre as superfícies anterior e posterior. SIN fibrae obliquae tunicae muscularis [TA].

occipitopontine f.'s [TA], fibras occipitopontinas; grupo de fibras que se origina no lobo occipital do hemisfério cerebral e desce pela cápsula interna e pela parte lateral dos pilares do cérebro até os núcleos pontinos da parte basilar da ponte. VER TAMBÉM corticopontine *tract*. SIN fibrae occipitopontinae [TA].

occipitotectal f.'s [TA], fibras occipitotetais; fibras que se originam nas regiões visuais do lobo occipital e passam, através da parte retrolentiforme da cápsula interna, até o teto, onde terminam principalmente no colículo superior. SIN fibrae occipitotectales [TA].

olivocochlear f.'s, trato olivococlear. VER olivocochlear *tract*.

olivospinal f.'s, fibras olivospinais; feixe delgado de fibras nervosas localizado na zona periférica do funículo lateral da medula espinal, composto mais provavelmente de fibras espinoolivares do que de fibras olivospinais. SIN fibrae olivospinales [TA], Helwig bundle.

osteocollagenous f.'s, fibras osteocolágenas; fibras colágenas delgadas localizadas na matriz do tecido ósseo.

osteogenetic f.'s, fibras osteogênicas; fibras localizadas na camada osteogênica do periósteo.

parietopontine f.'s [TA], fibras parietopontinas; conjunto de fibras que se origina no lobo parietal do hemisfério cerebral, desce pela cápsula interna e pela parte lateral dos pilares do cérebro e termina nos núcleos pontinos da parte ventral da ponte. VER TAMBÉM corticopontine *tract*. SIN fibrae parietopontine [TA].

pectinate f.'s, músculo pectíneo. SIN pectinate *muscles*, em *muscle*.

perforating f.'s, fibras perfurantes; feixes de fibras colágenas que penetram na lamela circunferencial externa do osso ou no cemento dos dentes. SIN Sharpey f.'s.

periodontal f., f. periodontal; *termo oficial alternativo para desmodentium.

periodontal ligament f.'s, fibras do ligamento periodontal. SIN desmodentium.

periventricular f.'s [TA], fibras periventriculares; conjunto heterogêneo de finas fibras nervosas, localizadas na substância cinzenta periventricular do hipotálamo, a continuação caudal do conjunto é formada pelo fascículo longitudinal dorsal. SIN fibrae periventriculares [TA].

pilomotor f.'s, fibras pilomotoras; fibras nervosas que inervam os músculos eretores dos folículos pilosos responsáveis pela piloereção.

polar f.'s, fibras polares; fibras do fuso mitótico que se estendem dos dois pólos do fuso em direção ao equador. Cf. astral f.'s, kinetochore f.'s.

pontine corticonuclear f.'s [TA], fibras corticonucleares da ponte; fibras nervosas que se projetam dos córtex sensorial e motor até os núcleos retransmissores sensoriais e motores localizados no tegmento da ponte, tais como os núcleos do nervo facial, do abducente e do trigêmeo; as fibras podem ser diretas ou retransmitidas pelos núcleos reticulares adjacentes. VER corticonuclear f.'s. SIN fibrae corticonucleares pontis [TA].

pontocerebellar f.'s [TA], fibras pontocerebelares; fibras que partem dos núcleos da parte basilar da ponte e cruzam a linha média (há uma projeção não-cruzada), penetram no cerebelo pelo pedúnculo cerebelar médio e terminam como fibras musgosas no córtex cerebelar. SIN fibrae pontocerebellares [TA].

postcommissural f.'s [TA], fibras pós-comissurais; fibras localizadas na coluna do fórnice que passam caudalmente (posteriormente) até a comissura anterior para penetrarem nos núcleos mamilares; a parte maior da coluna do fórnice. SIN fibrae postcommissurales [TA].

posterior external arcuate f.'s [TA], fibras arqueadas externas posteriores. VER external arcuate f.'s.

postganglionic f.'s, fibras pós-ganglionares; f. cujo corpo celular está localizado em um gânglio autônomo (motor) e cujo processo periférico termina em músculo liso, músculo cardíaco ou epitélio glandular; estão associadas às partes simpática e parassimpática do sistema nervoso autônomo.

postganglionic nerve f. [TA], f. nervosa pós-ganglionar. VER postganglionic.

precollagenous f.'s, fibras pré-colágenas; fibras argirófilas imaturas.

precommissural f.'s [TA], fibras pré-comissurais; fibras localizadas na coluna do fórnice que passam rostralmente (anteriormente) até a comissura anterior para penetrarem nos núcleos septais. SIN fibrae precommissurales [TA].

preganglionic f.'s, fibras pré-ganglionares; f. cujo corpo celular está localizado em um núcleo autônomo na medula espinal ou no tronco cerebral e cujo axônio termina em um gânglio autônomo (motor); encontradas em nervos que transportam fibras simpáticas ou parassimpáticas.

preganglionic nerve f.'s, fibras nervosas pré-ganglionares. VER preganglionic. SIN neurofibrae preganglionicae.

pressor f.'s, fibras pressoras; fibras nervosas sensoriais cuja estimulação causa vasoconstrição e elevação da pressão sanguínea.

pretectoolivary f.'s [TA], fibras pré-tetoolivares; fibras que se originam nos núcleos pré-tetais e se projetam principalmente para o núcleo olivar acessório medial ipsolateral. SIN fibrae pretectoolivares [TA].

projection f.'s, fibras de projeção; fibras nervosas que ligam o córtex cerebral a outros centros localizados no cérebro ou na medula espinal; fibras que partem de células localizadas no sistema nervoso central e se dirigem para locais distantes.

Prussak f.'s, fibras de Prussak; fibras elásticas e do tecido conectivo que limitam a parte flácida da membrana timpânica.

Purkinje f.'s, fibras de Purkinje. SIN subendocardial *branches* of atrioventricular bundles, em *branch*.

pyramidal f.'s, fibras piramidais; fibras que compõem o trato corticospinal. VER TAMBÉM corticospinal *tract*. SIN corticospinal f.'s [TA], fibrae corticospinales [TA], fibrae pyramidales.

raphespinal f.'s, fibras rafespinais; fibras nervosas que se originam nas células dos núcleos escuro, pálido e magno da rafe da ponte e do bulbo e terminam na substância cinzenta da medula espinal; fibras envolvidas na inibição descendente de impulsos nociceptivos no corno dorsal (posterior); contém serotonina.

red f.'s, fibras vermelhas; fibras vermelhas do músculo estriado que são ricas em sarcoplasma, mioglobina e mitocôndrias; possuem um diâmetro menor e contraem-se mais lentamente do que as fibras brancas.

| grupos de fibras nervosas ||||||
diâmetro da fibra	histologia	grupos de fibras		velocidade de condução	função
1–22 μm			α	80–120 m/s	impulsos motores, impulsos aferentes de fusos musculares e órgãos tendinosos
			β	60 m/s	impulsos tácteis da pele
3–20 μm	fibras espessas com bainhas de mielina relativamente espessas	A	γ	40 m/s	impulsos eferentes para partes contráteis de fibras musculares intrafusais
			δ	20 m/s	impulsos mecanorrreceptores; sensações de frio, calor e dor da pele (rápidas)
1–3 μm	fibras delgadas ou bainhas de mielina delgadas	B		10 m/s	fibras autônomas pré-ganglionares
1 μm	fibras sem bainha	C		1 m/s	fibras autônomas pós-ganglionares e fibras aferentes do tronco simpático, impulsos de mecanorreceptores, receptores de frio e calor (lentos)

Reissner f., f. de Reissner; f. semelhante a um bastonete, altamente refrativa, que corre caudalmente a partir do órgão subcomissural por toda a extensão do canal central do tronco cerebral e da medula espinal.
Remak f.'s, fibras de Remak. SIN unmyelinated f.'s.
reticular f.'s, fibras reticulares; fibras colágenas (tipo III) que formam o estroma do tecido conectivo frouxo característico dos tecidos embrionários, do mesênquima, da polpa vermelha do baço, do córtex e da medula dos linfonodos e dos compartimentos hematopoéticos da medula óssea e correspondem a uma parte significativa das fibras colágenas da pele, dos vasos sanguíneos, da membrana sinovial, do tecido uterino e do tecido de granulação; caracterizam-se pela organização das fibras — que formam uma malha reticular de filamentos finos — e pela afinidade pela prata e pelos corantes do ácido periódico de Schiff.
Retzius f.'s, fibras de Retzius; as fibras rígidas das células de Deiters.
rod f., f. do bastonete; parte da célula do bastonete da retina que se estende para ambos os lados a partir do corpo celular; a fibra interna do bastonete termina em uma extremidade sináptica localizada no estrato plexiforme externo.
Rosenthal f., f. de Rosenthal; massa eosinofílica oval ou alongada considerada um processo modificado de um astrócito; encontrada em grande número em certos astrocitomas de crescimento lento e em áreas de gliose reativa crônica.
rubroolivary f.'s [TA], fibras rubroolivares; axônios que partem de células da parte parvocelular do núcleo rubro, descem ipsolateralmente como um componente do trato tegmental central e terminam principalmente no núcleo olivar principal. SIN fibrae rubroolivares [TA].
Sappey f.'s, fibras de Sappey; fibras musculares não-estriadas localizadas nos ligamentos controladores do globo ocular.
Sharpey f.'s, fibras de Sharpey. SIN perforating f.'s.
short association f.'s [TA], fibras de associação curtas; fibras nervosas que podem interligar lobos ou giros adjacentes do córtex cerebral do mesmo hemisfério ou segmentos contínuos da medula espinal do mesmo lado; fibras que interligam pontos próximos ou adjacentes. SIN fibrae associationes breves [TA].
skeletal muscle f.'s, fibras musculares esqueléticas; células contrácteis multinucleadas que variam de menos de 10 até 100 μm de diâmetro e de menos de 1 mm até vários centímetros de comprimento; a f. é composta de sarcoplasma e miofibrilas transversalmente estriadas, que, por sua vez, são compostas de miofilamentos; os músculos esqueléticos humanos são uma mistura de fibras vermelhas, brancas e intermediárias.
somatic nerve f.'s [TA], fibras nervosas somáticas; fibras aferentes e eferentes distribuídas pelo lado externo das cavidades do corpo, isto é, pelas paredes; a maioria das fibras somáticas aferentes conduz impulsos que estimulam a sensação consciente; todas as fibras somáticas eferentes estimulam músculos somáticos (voluntários/estriados/esqueléticos). SIN neurofibrae somaticae [TA].
spindle f., f. fusiforme. VER mitotic *spindle*.
spinocuneate f.'s, fibras espinocuneiformes; axônios que se originam em células localizadas no corno posterior, nos níveis cervical e torácico superior da medula espinal, ascendem ipsolateralmente pelo fascículo cuneiforme e terminam no núcleo cuneiforme. Constituem uma parte do sistema pós-sináptico–coluna dorsal. SIN fibrae spinocuneatae [TA].
spinogracile f.'s [TA], fibras espinográceis; axônios que se originam de neurônios localizados no corno posterior, nos níveis torácico baixo e lombossacral da medula espinal, ascendem ipsolateralmente pelo fascículo grácil e terminam no núcleo grácil. Constituem uma parte do sistema pós-sináptico–coluna dorsal. SIN fibrae spinograciles [TA].
spinohypothalamic f.'s [TA], fibras espino-hipotalâmicas; axônios que se originam na substância cinzenta da medula espinal, ascendem como parte do trato ântero-lateral e terminam no hipotálamo. SIN fibrae spinohypothalamicae [TA].
spinomesencephalic f.'s [TA], fibras espinomesencefálicas; grupo composto de fibras que viajam pelo lemnisco espinal (trato ântero-lateral) e terminam no mesencéfalo; o grupo inclui as fibras espinotetais [TA], até as camadas mais profundas do colículo superior, e as fibras espinoperiaquedutais [TA], que terminam na substância cinzenta periaquedutal. SIN fibrae spinomesencephalicae [TA].
spinoolivary f.'s [TA], fibras espinoolivares; fibras que partem da medula espinal e ascendem basicamente pelo mesmo lado para terminar nos núcleos acessórios do complexo olivar inferior. SIN fibrae spinoolivares [TA].
spinoperiaqueductal f.'s [TA], espinoperiaquedutais; axônios que se originam em corpos celulares do corno posterior, ascendem como parte do trato ântero-lateral contralateral e terminam na substância cinzenta periaquedutal do mesencéfalo; estão envolvidos nas vias descendentes para a supressão da dor. VER TAMBÉM spinomesencephalic f.'s. SIN fibrae spinoperiaqueductales [TA].
spinoreticular f.'s [TA], fibras espinorreticulares; fibras nervosas que se originam na medula espinal e terminam na formação reticular do tronco cerebral; algumas fibras ascendem como parte do trato ântero-lateral. SIN fibrae spinoreticulares [TA], spinoreticular tract [TA].
spinotectal f.'s [TA], fibras espinotetais; axônios que se originam em corpos celulares localizados no corno posterior, cruzam a comissura branca anterior, ascendem como parte do trato ântero-lateral e terminam nas camadas mais profundas do colículo superior. VER TAMBÉM spinomesencephalic f.'s. SIN fibrae spinotectales [TA].
stress f.'s, fibras de estresse; feixes longos de microfilamentos compostos de actina; acredita-se que estejam envolvidos na fixação de células de uma cultura ao substrato e também na determinação da forma de células, tais como os fibroblastos; podem estar envolvidos na mobilidade celular.
striatonigral f.'s, fibras estriadonigrais. SIN strionigral f.'s.
strionigral f.'s, fibras estriadonigrais; fibras nervosas que se originam nas células do caudado e do putame e terminam principalmente na parte reticular da substância negra; essas fibras utilizam GABA e substância P. SIN striatonigral f.'s.
sudomotor f.'s, fibras sudomotoras; fibras nervosas simpáticas pós-ganglionares e colinérgicas que inervam as glândulas sudoríparas.
sustentacular f.'s of retina, fibras sustentaculares da retina. SIN Müller f.'s (2).
T f., f. T; f. que se ramifica em ângulos retos para a direita e para a esquerda; termo utilizado para descrever os padrões de ramificação dos axônios das células granulares localizados na camada molecular do cerebelo.
tautomeric f.'s, fibras tautoméricas; fibras nervosas da medula espinal que não se estendem além dos limites do segmento da medula espinal no qual elas se originaram.
tectoolivary f.'s [TA], fibras tetoolivares; fibras que se originam nas camadas profundas do colículo superior e se projetam até o núcleo olivar acessório medial contralateral. SIN fibrae tectoolivares [TA].
tectopontine f.'s [TA], fibras tetopontinas; fibras que partem do teto do me-

sencéfalo e terminam nos núcleos ipsolaterais da parte basilar da ponte e no núcleo reticular do tegmento. SIN fibrae tectopontinae [TA].

tectoreticular f.'s [TA], fibras tetorreticulares; fibras que se originam no colículo superior e se projetam bilateralmente para a formação reticular, principalmente para a formação reticular do mesencéfalo. SIN fibrae tectoreticulares [TA].

temporopontine f.'s [TA], fibras temporopontinas; grupo de fibras que se origina no córtex cerebral do lobo temporal, sobretudo nos giros temporal superior e temporal médio, acompanha a parte sublentiforme da cápsula interna para dentro da margem lateral do pilar do cérebro, por onde desce até terminar nos núcleos pontinos na parte basilar da ponte. VER TAMBÉM corticospinal *tract*. SIN fibrae temporopontinae [TA].

thalamocortical f.'s, fibras talamocorticais; termo geral que designa as fibras nervosas que partem dos núcleos do tálamo e se projetam para o córtex cerebral, onde terminam.

Tomes f.'s, fibras de Tomes. SIN dentinal f.'s (1).

transseptal f.'s, fibras transeptais; fibras não-elásticas que percorrem cada um dos dentes sobre as cristas dos alvéolos.

transverse pontine f.'s [TA], fibras transversais da ponte; fibras que partem dos núcleos da ponte, cruzam a decussação e penetram no cerebelo como pedúnculos cerebelares médios. SIN fibrae pontis transversae [TA].

unmyelinated f.'s, fibras não-mielinizadas; f. que não apresentam revestimento de mielina (SNC); axônios sem revestimento; no SNP, são representados por todos os axônios que repousam em canais dentro de uma única célula de Schwann (unidade da célula de Schwann); f. de condução lenta. SIN gray f.'s, nonmedullated f.'s, Remak f.'s.

vasomotor f.'s, fibras vasomotoras; fibras viscerais eferentes pós-ganglionares que inervam os músculos lisos das paredes dos vasos.

visceral motor f.'s, fibras viscerais motoras. SIN autonomic nerve f.'s.

Weitbrecht f.'s, fibras de Weitbrecht. SIN retinaculum of articular capsule of hip.

white f., (1) fibras musculares brancas de mamíferos; essas fibras apresentam um diâmetro maior do que o das fibras vermelhas, menos mioglobina, sarcoplasma e mitocôndrias e contraem-se mais rapidamente; **(2)** SIN collagen f.

yellow f.'s, fibras elásticas. SIN elastic f.'s.

zonular f.'s [TA], fibras zonulares; fibras delicadas que se dirigem do equador da lente para o corpo ciliar, conhecidas em conjunto como zônula ciliar. SIN fibrae zonulares [TA].

---

fi·ber·op·tic (fī - ber - op′tik). Fibróptico; relativo à fibra óptica.

fi·ber·op·tics (fī - ber - op′tiks). Fibróptica; sistema óptico no qual a imagem é conduzida através de um feixe compacto de fibras transparentes, flexíveis e com pequeno diâmetro.

fi·ber·scope (fī′ber - skōp). Fibroscópio. SIN flexible *endoscope*.

fibr-. VER fibro-.

fi·bra, pl. **fi·brae** (fī′brä, fī′brē) [TA]. Fibra. SIN fiber, fiber. [L.]

fi'brae arcua'tae cer'ebri [TA], fibras arqueadas do cérebro. SIN arcuate *fibers* of cerebrum, em *fiber*.

fi'brae arcua'tae exter'nae, fibras arqueadas externas. SIN external arcuate *fibers*, em *fiber*.

fibrae arcuatae externae anteriores [TA], fibras arqueadas externas anteriores. VER external arcuate *fibers*, em *fiber*.

fibrae arcuatae externae posteriores [TA], fibras arqueadas externas posteriores. VER external arcuate *fibers*, em *fiber*.

fi'brae arcua'tae inter'nae [TA], fibras arqueadas internas. SIN internal arcuate *fibers*, em *fiber*.

fibrae associationes breves [TA], fibras de associação curtas. SIN short association *fibers*, em *fiber*.

fibrae associationes longae [TA], fibras de associação longas. SIN long association *fibers*, em *fiber*.

fibrae cerebelloolivares [TA], fibras cerebeloolivares. SIN cerebelloolivary *fibers*, em *fiber*.

fi'brae circula'res [TA], fibras circulares. SIN circular *fibers*, em *fiber*.

fibrae corticomesencephalicae [TA], fibras corticomesencefálicas. SIN corticomesencephalic *fibers*, em *fiber*.

fi'brae corticonuclea'res [TA], fibras corticonucleares. SIN corticonuclear *fibers*, em *fiber*.

fibrae corticonucleares bulbi [TA], fibras corticonucleares do bulbo. SIN bulbar corticonuclear *fibers*, em *fiber*.

fibrae corticonucleares mesencephali [TA], fibras corticonucleares do mesencéfalo. SIN mesencephalic corticonuclear *fibers*, em *fiber*.

fibrae corticonucleares pontis [TA], fibras corticonucleares da ponte. SIN pontine corticonuclear *fibers*, em *fiber*.

fi'brae corticopon'tinae [TA], fibras corticopontinas. SIN corticopontine *fibers*, em *fiber*.

fi'brae corticoreticula'res [TA], fibras corticorreticulares. SIN corticoreticular *fibers*, em *fiber*.

fibrae corticorubrales [TA], fibras corticorrubrais. SIN corticorubral *fibers*, em *fiber*.

fi'brae corticospina'les [TA], fibras corticospinais. SIN pyramidal *fibers*, em *fiber*.

fibrae cuneocerebellares [TA], fibras cuneocerebelares. SIN cuneocerebellar *tract*.

fibrae cuneospinales [TA], fibras cuneospinais. SIN cuneospinal *fibers*, em *fiber*.

fi'brae dentatorubra'les, fibras dentadorrubrais. SIN dentatorubral *fibers*, em *fiber*.

fibrae frontopontinae [TA], fibras frontopontinas. SIN frontopontine *fibers*, em *fiber*.

fibrae gracilispinales [TA], fibras gracilespinais. SIN gracilespinal *fibers*, em *fiber*.

fibrae hypothalamospinales [TA], fibras hipotalamoespinais. SIN hypothalamospinal *fibers*, em *fiber*.

fi'brae intercrura'les anuli inguinalis superficialis [TA], fibras intercrurais do anel inguinal superficial. SIN intercrural *fibers* of superficial ring, em *fiber*.

fibrae intrathalamicae [TA], fibras intratálmicas. SIN intrathalamic *fibers*, em *fiber*.

fi'brae len'tis, fibras da lente. SIN fibers of lens, em *fiber*.

fi'brae meridiona'les muscularis ciliaris [TA], fibras meridionais do músculo ciliar. SIN meridional *fibers* of ciliary muscle, em *fiber*.

fi'brae obli'quae tunicae muscularis [TA], fibras oblíquas da túnica muscular. SIN oblique *fibers* of muscular layer of stomach, em *fiber*.

fibrae occipitopontinae [TA], fibras occipitopontinas. SIN occipitopontine *fibers*, em *fiber*.

fibrae occipitotectales [TA], fibras occipitotetais. SIN occipitotectal *fibers*, em *fiber*.

fibrae olivospinales [TA], fibras olivospinais. SIN olivospinal *fibers*, em *fiber*.

fibrae parietopontinae [TA], fibras parietopontinas. SIN parietopontine *fibers*, em *fiber*.

fi'brae periventricula'res [TA], fibras periventriculares. SIN periventricular *fibers*, em *fiber*.

fibrae pontis longitudinales [TA], fibras longitudinais da ponte; SIN longitudinal pontine *fibers*, em *fiber*. VER longitudinal pontine *fasciculi*, em *fasciculus*.

fi'brae pon'tis transver'sae [TA], fibras transversais da ponte. SIN transverse pontine *fibers*, em *fiber*.

fibrae pontocerebellares [TA], fibras pontocerebelares. SIN pontocerebellar *fibers*, em *fiber*.

fibrae postcommissurales [TA], fibras pós-comissurais. SIN postcommissural *fibers*, em *fiber*.

fibrae precommissurales [TA], fibras pré-comissurais. SIN precommissural *fibers*, em *fiber*.

fibrae pretectoolivares [TA], fibras pré-tetoolivares. SIN pretectoolivary *fibers*, em *fiber*.

fi'brae pyramida'les, fibras piramidais. SIN pyramidal *fibers*, em *fiber*.

fibrae rubroolivares [TA], fibras rubroolivares. SIN rubroolivary *fibers*, em *fiber*.

fibrae spinocuneatae [TA], fibras espinocuneiformes. SIN spinocuneate *fibers*, em *fiber*.

fibrae spinograciles [TA], fibras espinográceis. SIN spinogracile *fibers*, em *fiber*.

fibrae spinohypothalamicae [TA], fibras espino-hipotalâmicas. SIN spinohypothalamic *fibers*, em *fiber*.

fibrae spinomesencephalicae [TA], fibras espinomesencefálicas. SIN spinomesencephalic *fibers*, em *fiber*.

fibrae spinoolivares [TA], fibras espinoolivares. SIN spinoolivary *fibers*, em *fiber*.

fibrae spinoperiaqueductales [TA], fibras espinoperiaquedutais. SIN spinoperiaqueductal *fibers*, em *fiber*.

fibrae spinoreticulares [TA], fibras espinorreticulares. SIN spinoreticular *fibers*, em *fiber*.

fibrae spinotectales [TA], fibras espinotetais. SIN spinotectal *fibers*, em *fiber*.

fibrae tectoolivares [TA], fibras tetoolivares. SIN tectoolivary *fibers*, em *fiber*.

fibrae tectopontinae [TA], fibras tetopontinas. SIN tectopontine *fibers*, em *fiber*.

fibrae tectoreticulares [TA], fibras tetorreticulares. SIN tectoreticular *fibers*, em *fiber*.

fibrae temporopontinae [TA], fibras temporopontinas. SIN temporopontine *fibers*, em *fiber*.

fi'brae zonula'res [TA], fibras zonulares. SIN zonular *fibers*, em *fiber*.

fibrates (fī′brāts). Fibratos, ácidos fíbricos. SIN fibric acids.

fi·bre (fī′ber). Fibra. SIN fiber.

fi·bre·mia (fī - brē′mē - ă). Fibremia; termo obsoleto para denominar a presença de fibrina no sangue que causa trombose ou embolismo. SIN inosemia (2). [fibrin + G. *haima*, sangue]

fibric acids. Ácidos fíbricos; drogas estruturalmente relacionadas com o clofibrato e utilizadas no tratamento da hipercolesterolemia e da hipertrigliceridemia. SIN fibrates.

fi·bril (fi′bril). Fibrila; uma fibra diminuta ou um componente de uma fibra. SIN fibrilla. [L. mod. *fibrilla*]
  anchoring f.'s, fibrilas de ancoragem; fibrilas colágenas que se inserem na lâmina basal da epiderme, fixando-a à derme subjacente.
  collagen f.'s, fibrilas colágenas. SIN unit f.'s.
  muscular f., f. muscular, miofibrila. SIN myofibril.
  subpellicular f., microtúbulo subpelicular. SIN subpellicular *microtubule*.
  unit f.'s, fibrilas colágenas; as fibrilas que compõem uma fibra colágena, com um comprimento que varia de 20 a 200 nm, um diâmetro médio de cerca de 100 nm (substancialmente maiores nos tendões) e estriações transversais com um comprimento médio de cerca de 64 nm. SIN collagen f.'s.

fi·bril·la, pl. **fi·bril·lae** (fī-bril′ă, -ē). Fibrila. SIN fibril. [L. mod. dim. de L. *fibra*, uma fibra]

fi·bril·lar, fi·bril·lary (fi′bri-lăr, -lar-ē). Fibrilar. **1.** Relativo a uma fibrila. **2.** Relativo às contrações ou aos espasmos rápidos das fibras ou dos pequenos grupos de fibras do músculo esquelético ou cardíaco. SIN filar (1).

fi·bril·late (fi′bri-lāt). Fibrilar. **1.** Fazer fibrilar ou tornar-se fibrilante. **2.** SIN fibrillated. **3.** Estar em um estado de fibrilação (3).

fi·bril·lat·ed (fi′bri-lā-ted). Fibrilar; composto de fibrilas. SIN fibrillate (2).

fi·bril·la·tion (fī-bri-lā′shŭn, fib-ri-). Fibrilação. **1.** A condição de ser fibrilar. **2.** A formação de fibrilas. **3.** Contrações ou espasmos extremamente rápidos de fibrilas musculares, porém não do músculo como um todo. **4.** Espasmos vermiculares, geralmente lentos, de fibras musculares individuais; ocorre comumente nos átrios ou ventrículos do coração, bem como nas fibras do músculo esquelético recentemente desnervadas.
  atrial f., auricular f., f. atrial; condição na qual as contrações rítmicas normais dos átrios cardíacos são substituídas por espasmos irregulares e rápidos da parede muscular; os ventrículos respondem irregularmente ao bombardeamento arrítmico proveniente dos átrios. SIN ataxia cordis.
  ventricular f., f. ventricular; movimentos fibrilares rápidos, grosseiros ou delicados do músculo ventricular que substituem a contração normal.

fi·bril·lin (fi′bril-in). Fibrilina; proteína microfibrilar encontrada no tecido conectivo e com ampla distribuição pelo corpo; seu peso molecular (PM) é de cerca de 350.000. Há boas evidências de que a síndrome de Marfan é causada por mutações na f. [MIM*134797]. [L. mod. *fibrilla*, fibril, + -in]

fi·bril·lo·flut·ter (fib′ril-ō-flut′er). Fibrilo-*flutter*. SIN impure *flutter*.

fi·bril·lo·gen·e·sis (fi′bril-ō-jen′ē-sis). Fibrilogênese; desenvolvimento de finas fibrilas (como visto por meio do microscópio eletrônico), normalmente presentes no interior das fibras colágenas do tecido conectivo.

fi·brin (fi′brin). Fibrina; proteína filamentosa e elástica derivada do fibrinogênio, que, sob a ação da trombina, libera os fibrinopeptídeos A e B durante o processo de coagulação do sangue; um dos componentes dos trombos, das vegetações e dos exsudatos inflamatórios agudos, tais como os encontrados na difteria e na pneumonia lobar. [L. *fibra*, fibra]

fi·brin·ase (fi′brin-ās). **1.** Fibrinase; antigo nome do *factor* XIII (fator XIII). **2.** Plasmina. SIN plasmin.

⚠ **fibrino-.** Fibrina. [L. *fibra*, fibra]

fi·bri·no·cel·lu·lar (fi′bri-nō-sel′ū-lăr). Fibrinocelular; composto de fibrina e células, como ocorre em certos tipos de exsudatos resultantes de inflamação aguda.

fi·brin·o·gen (fī-brin′ō-jen). Fibrinogênio; globulina do plasma sanguíneo, convertida em fibrina pela ação da trombina e na presença de íons cálcio, a fim de produzir a coagulação do sangue; a única proteína coagulável do plasma sanguíneo dos vertebrados; mostra-se ausente na afibrinogenemia e defeituosa na disfibrinogenemia.
  human f., f. humano; f. preparado a partir de plasma humano normal; coagulante (fator de coagulação) utilizado como auxiliar no tratamento da hipofibrinogenemia aguda, congênita e crônica adquirida.

fi·brin·og·e·nase (fī-brin′ō-je-nās). Fibrinogenase, trombina. SIN thrombin.

fi·brin·o·ge·ne·mia (fi-brin′ō-jĕ-nē′mē-ă). Fibrinogenemia. SIN hyperfibrinogenemia.

fi·bri·no·gen·e·sis (fi′bri-nō-jen′ē-sis). Fibrinogênese; formação ou produção de fibrina.

fi·bri·no·gen·ic, fi·bri·nog·e·nous (fi′brin-ō-jen′ik, fi′bri-noj′ē-nŭs). Fibrinogênico; **1.** Relativo ao fibrinogênio. **2.** Que produz fibrina.

fi·brin·o·gen·ol·y·sis (fi-brin′ō-jen-ol′i-sis). Fibrinogenólise; inativação ou dissolução do fibrinogênio no sangue. [fibrinogen + G. *lysis*, dissolução]

fi·brin·o·gen·o·pe·nia (fi-brin′ō-jen-ō-pē′nē-ă). Fibrinogenopenia; concentração de fibrinogênio no sangue menor do que a normal. [fibrinogen + G. *penia*, escassez]

fi·brin·oid (fi′bri-noyd). Fibrinóide. **1.** Que se assemelha à fibrina. **2.** Material homogêneo, proteináceo, intensa ou brilhantemente acidófilo, que: 1) é freqüentemente formado nas paredes dos vasos sanguíneos e no tecido conectivo de pacientes com certas doenças, tais como lúpus eritematoso disseminado, poliarterite nodosa, esclerodermia, dermatomiosite e febre reumática; 2) é, às vezes, observado nas feridas em cicatrização, nas úlceras pépticas crônicas, na placenta, nas arteríolas necróticas da hipertensão maligna e em outras condições. [fibrin + G. *eidos*, semelhança]

fi·bri·no·ki·nase (fi′brin-ō-ki′nās). Fibrinocinase; nome proposto para a enzima que converte o plasminogênio em plasmina; denominada subseqüentemente de urocinase, porém agora chamada de *ativador* de plasminogênio. VER plasminogen *activator*. SIN fibrinolysokinase.

fi·bri·nol·y·sin (fī-brin-ō-li′sin). Fibrinolisina, plasmina. SIN plasmin.
  streptococcal f., estreptoquinase. SIN streptokinase.

fi·bri·nol·y·sis (fī-bri-nol′i-sis). Fibrinólise. **1.** Hidrólise da fibrina. **2.** O processo de dissolução da fibrina nos coágulos sanguíneos. [fibrino- + G. *lysis*, dissolução]

fi·bri·no·ly·so·ki·nase (fi′brin-ō-li-sō-ki′nās). Fibrinolisocinase; SIN fibrinokinase.

fi·bri·no·lyt·ic (fi-brin-ō-lit′ik). Fibrinolítico; que indica, é caracterizado por ou causa fibrinólise.

fi·brin·o·pep·tide (fi′brin-ō-pep′tid). Fibrinopeptídeo; um de dois peptídeos (A e B) liberados das terminações amino-terminais das cadeias 2α- (ou Aα) e 2β- (ou Bβ) do fibrinogênio pela ação da trombina, a fim de formar fibrina; tem efeito vasoconstritor.

fi·bri·no·pu·ru·lent (fi-bri-nō-pū′roo-lent). Fibrinopurulento; relativo ao pus ou exsudato purulento que contém uma quantidade relativamente grande de fibrina.

fi·bri·nos·co·py (fi-bri-nos′kō-pē). Fibrinoscopia; exame químico e físico da fibrina de exsudatos, coágulos sanguíneos, etc. [fibrino- + G. *skopeō*, visão]

fi·brin·ous (fi′brin-ŭs). Fibrinoso; relativo a ou composto de fibrina.

fi·bri·nu·ria (fi-bri-noo′rē-ă). Fibrinúria; eliminação de urina que contém fibrina. [fibrin + G. *ouron*, urina]

⚠ **fibro-, fibr-.** Fibra. [L. *fibra*]

fi·bro·ad·e·no·ma (fi′brō-ad-ĕ-nō′mă). Fibroadenoma; neoplasia benigna, derivada do epitélio glandular, na qual há um estroma evidente de fibroblastos em proliferação e elementos do tecido conectivo; normalmente encontrada no tecido mamário.
  giant f., f. gigante; f. grande e benigno encontrado principalmente nas adolescentes.
  intracanalicular f., f. intracanalicular; f. de mama formado por nódulos de tecido fibroso que invaginam e comprimem os ductos.
  pericanalicular f., f. pericanalicular; f. da mama que consiste em um número elevado de pequenos ductos circundados por faixas concêntricas de tecido fibroso.

fi·bro·ad·i·pose (fi-brō-ad′i-pōz). Fibroadiposo; relativo a ou que contém estruturas fibrosas e gordurosas. SIN fibrofatty.

fi·bro·a·re·o·lar (fi′brō-ă-rē′ō-lăr). Fibroareolar; que indica tecido conectivo de natureza fibrosa e areolar.

fi·bro·blast (fi′brō-blast). Fibroblasto; célula estrelada ou fusiforme e com processos citoplasmáticos, encontrada no tecido conectivo e capaz de formar fibras colágenas; um f. inativo é, às vezes, denominado fibrócito.

fi·bro·blas·tic (fi-brō-blas′tik). Fibroblástico; relativo aos fibroblastos.

fi·bro·car·ti·lage (fi-brō-kar′ti-lij). Fibrocartilagem; tipo de cartilagem que contém fibras colágenas tipo I visíveis; aparece como uma transição entre os tendões e ligamentos ou ossos. SIN fibrocartilago.
  basilar f., f. basilar. SIN basilar *cartilage*.
  circumferential f., f. circunferencial; anel de f. situado ao redor da extremidade articular de um osso, servindo para aprofundar a cavidade da articulação. VER TAMBÉM acetabular *labrum*, glenoid *labrum* of scapula.
  external semilunar f., menisco lateral. SIN lateral *meniscus*.
  interarticular f., f. interarticular, disco articular. SIN articular *disk*.
  internal semilunar f. of knee joint, menisco medial. SIN medial *meniscus*.
  interpubic f., f. interpúbica; *termo oficial alternativo para interpubic *disk*.
  semilunar f., menisco. VER lateral *meniscus*, medial *meniscus*.
  stratiform f., f. estratiforme; camada de f. situada no fundo de um sulco em um osso, através da qual passa um tendão.

fi·bro·car·ti·lag·i·nous (fi′brō-kar-ti-laj′i-nŭs). Fibrocartilaginoso; relativo a ou composto de fibrocartilagem.

fi·bro·car·ti·la·go (fi′brō-kar-ti-lā′gō). Fibrocartilagem. SIN fibrocartilage.
  f. basa′lis, f. basilar. SIN basilar *cartilage*.
  f. interarticula′ris, f. interarticular, disco articular. SIN articular *disk*.
  f. interpubica, f. interpúbica; *termo oficial alternativo para interpubic *disk*.
  f. intervertebra′lis, f. intervertebral. SIN intervertebral *disk*.

fi·bro·cel·lu·lar (fi-brō-sel′ū-lăr). Fibrocelular; fibroso e celular.

fi·bro·chon·dri·tis (fi-brō-kon-dri′tis). Fibrocondrite; inflamação de uma fibrocartilagem.

fi·bro·chon·dro·ma (fi′brō-kon-drō′mă). Fibrocondroma; neoplasia benigna de tecido cartilaginoso na qual há uma quantidade relativamente incomum de estroma fibroso.

fi·bro·con·ges·tive (fi′brō-kon-jes′tiv). Fibrocongestivo; termo às vezes utilizado para indicar a condição geral de um órgão ou tecido no qual uma congestão persistente, aguda ou crônica, causou degeneração e necrose de células e substituição por elementos do tecido conectivo, como ocorre na esplenomegalia congestiva crônica.

fi·bro·cys·tic (fī - brō - sis′tik). Fibrocístico; relativo a ou caracterizado pela presença de fibrocistos.

fi·bro·cyte (fī′brō - sīt). Fibrócito; designação às vezes aplicada a um fibroblasto inativo. [fibro- + G. *kytos*, célula]

fi·bro·dys·pla·sia (fī′brō - dis - plā′zē - ă). Fibrodisplasia; desenvolvimento anormal do tecido conectivo fibroso.
  f. ossif′icans progressi′va [MIM*135100], f. ossificante progressiva; transtorno generalizado do tecido conectivo no qual há ossificação ectópica com substituição de tendões, fáscias e ligamentos por osso; doença genética letal transmitida por herança autossômica dominante. VER TAMBÉM fibrous *dysplasia* of bone.

fi·bro·e·las·tic (fī′brō - ē - las′tik). Fibroelástico; composto de fibras colágenas e elásticas.

fi·bro·e·las·to·sis (fī′brō - ē - las - tō′sis). Fibroelastose; proliferação excessiva de tecido fibroso composto de fibras colágenas e elásticas.
  endocardial f., endomyocardial f., f. endocárdica, f. endomiocárdica; **(1)** condição congênita caracterizada por espessamento do endocárdio da parede do ventrículo esquerdo (principalmente por tecido fibroso e elástico), espessamento e malformação de valvas cardíacas, alterações subendocárdicas no miocárdio e hipertrofia do coração; os principais sinais e sintomas são cianose, dispnéia, anorexia e irritabilidade; **(2)** SIN endomyocardial *fibrosis.*

fi·bro·ep·i·the·li·o·ma (fī′brō - ep - i - thē - lē - ō′mă). Fibroepitelioma; tumor de pele composto por tecido fibroso entremeado por faixas anastomosantes delgadas de células basais da epiderme que envolvem cistos de queratina; pode dar origem ao carcinoma de células basais do tipo nodular. SIN Pinkus tumor.

fi·bro·fat·ty (fī - brō - fat′ē). Fibroadiposo. SIN fibroadipose.

fi·bro·fol·lic·u·lo·ma (fī - brō - fŏ - lik - ū - lō′mă). Fibrofoliculoma; pequenos hamartomas papulares da bainha fibrosa do folículo piloso, com extensões sólidas de epitélio do infundíbulo folicular; fibrofoliculomas múltiplos podem ter origem familial.

fi·bro·gen·e·sis (fī - brō - jen′ē - sis). Fibrogênese; produção ou desenvolvimento de fibras.

fi·bro·gli·o·sis (fī′brō - glī - ō′sis). Fibrogliose; reação celular que ocorre dentro do cérebro, geralmente em resposta a um traumatismo penetrante, na qual tanto astrócitos como fibroblastos participam e que culmina em uma cicatriz fibrosa e glial. [fibro- + G. *glia*, cola, + *-osis*, condição]

fi·broid (fī′broyd). Fibróide. **1.** Que se parece com ou é composto de fibras ou tecido fibroso. **2.** Termo antigo para certos tipos de leiomioma, principalmente aqueles encontrados no útero. **3.** SIN fibroleiomyoma. [fibro- + G. *eidos*, semelhança]

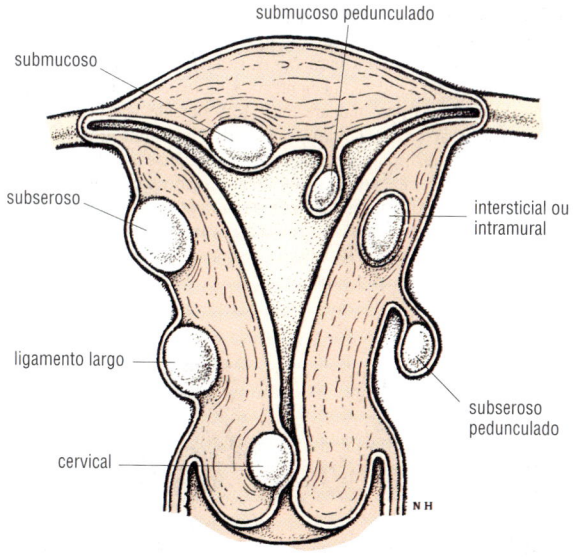

fibróides (localização)

fi·broid·ec·to·my (fī - broy - dek′tō - mē). Fibroidectomia, miomectomia. SIN myomectomy. [fibroid + G. *ektomē*, excisão]

fi·bro·in (fī′brō - in). Fibroína; proteína branca e insolúvel que forma o principal componente (70%) da teia de aranha e da seda.

fi·bro·lei·o·my·o·ma (fī - brō - lī′ō - mī - ō′mă). Fibroleiomioma; leiomioma contendo tecido fibroso colágeno não-neoplásico que pode torná-lo duro; o f. surge geralmente no miométrio, e a proporção de tecido fibroso aumenta com a idade. SIN fibroid (3), leiomyofibroma.

fi·bro·li·po·ma (fī - brō - li - pō′mă). Fibrolipoma; lipoma com um estroma abundante de tecido fibroso. SIN lipoma fibrosum.

fi·bro·ma (fī - brō′mă). Fibroma; neoplasia benigna derivada do tecido conectivo fibroso. [fibro- + G. *-oma*, tumor]
  ameloblastic f., f. ameloblástico; tumor odontogênico misto benigno, caracterizado por proliferação neoplásica dos componentes epiteliais e mesenquimais do broto do dente, sem a produção de tecido dentário duro; apresenta-se clinicamente como uma radiolucência indolor e de crescimento lento, que ocorre mais comumente na mandíbula de crianças e adolescentes.
  aponeurotic f., f. aponeurótico; f. recorrente, não-metastático, porém infiltrativo e que sofre calcificação, observado mais freqüentemente nas regiões palmares de pessoas jovens como um pequeno nódulo duro não aderido à pele suprajacente.
  cementoossifying f., f. cemento-ossificante; forma de f. que apresenta cementículos e osso rodeado por osteoblastos em estroma moderadamente celular.
  central ossifying f., f. ossificante central; tumor fibroósseo benigno, indolor, de crescimento lento, expansível e bem delimitado das maxilas e da mandíbula, derivado das células do ligamento periodontal; apresenta-se inicialmente como uma radiolucência que se torna progressivamente mais opaca, enquanto o tumor amadurece.
  chondromyxoid f., f. condromixóide; tumor ósseo benigno e pouco comum, encontrado mais freqüentemente na tíbia de adolescentes e adultos jovens; é composto de tecido mixóide lobulado com raros focos condróides. SIN chondrofibroma, chondromyxoma.
  concentric f., f. concêntrico; neoplasia benigna, na verdade um leiomioma, que ocupa toda a circunferência da parede do útero.
  desmoplastic f., f. desmoplástico; tumor fibroso benigno do osso que afeta crianças e adultos jovens; pode causar destruição da parte cortical do osso.
  giant cell f., f. de células gigantes; tumor da mucosa oral composto de tecido conectivo fibroso com fibroblastos grandes, estrelados e multinucleados; apresenta uma histologia similar à da papila retrocúspide, da pápula fibrosa do nariz, da pápula perolada do pênis e do fibroma ungueal.
  irritation f., f. irritativo; nódulo de crescimento lento da mucosa oral composto por tecido fibroso coberto por epitélio e resultante de irritação mecânica por dentaduras, restaurações, mordeduras na bochecha, etc.
  f. mol′le, acrocórdone. SIN skin tag.
  f. mol′le gravida′rum, molusco fibroso da gravidez; pólipos cutâneos que se desenvolvem em mulheres durante a gravidez e freqüentemente desaparecem após o parto.
  f. myxomato′des, f. mixomatóide, mixofibroma. SIN myxofibroma.
  nonossifying f., f. não-ossificante; foco osteolítico loculado de tecido fibroso celular, que expande discretamente um osso, encontrado, em geral, próximo à extremidade de um osso longo em crianças maiores; semelhante ao defeito fibroso cortical (fibrous cortical *defect*), embora maior.
  nonosteogenic f., f. não-osteogênico. SIN fibrous cortical *defect.*
  odontogenic f., f. odontogênico; tumor odontogênico raro encontrado em tecidos moles ou como uma lesão óssea central. O tumor é composto por tecido conectivo fibroso, epitélio odontogênico e, às vezes, calcificação.
  peripheral ossifying f., f. ossificante periférico; proliferação gengival reativa e focal, derivada histologicamente de células do ligamento periodontal, que em geral se desenvolve em resposta a irritantes locais (placa e tártaro); consiste microscopicamente em um estroma fibroso celular hiperplásico que sustenta depósitos de osso, cemento e calcificação distrófica.
  periungual f., f. periungueal; múltiplos nódulos lisos e firmes formados nas pregas ungueais, freqüentemente com mais de 10 mm de comprimento, que surge durante ou após a puberdade em alguns pacientes com esclerose tuberosa.
  rabbit f., f. de Shope. SIN Shope f.
  recurring digital f. of childhood, f. digital recorrente da infância; nódulos múltiplos, fibrosos e de cor de carne encontrados na face extensora das falanges terminais de dedos adjacentes de lactentes e crianças pequenas e que, freqüentemente, recidivam após tentativa de excisão; não metastatizam e podem regredir espontaneamente em dois ou três anos; são compostos de células em fuso que contêm inclusões citoplasmáticas e considerados como derivados de miofibrilas. SIN infantile digital fibromatosis.
  Shope f., f. de Shope; tumor de tecido conectivo de coelho causado por um poxvírus do gênero *Leporipoxvirus* e considerado por Shope como transmissível por suspensões de células ou por filtrados de Berkefeld; está associado à mixomatose e é utilizado na Europa como fonte de vacina para proteger contra o vírus mixoma. SIN rabbit f.
  telangiectatic f., f. telangiectásico; neoplasia benigna de tecido fibroso na qual existem numerosos canais vasculares, pequenos e grandes, freqüentemente dilatados. SIN angiofibroma.

fi·bro·ma·toid (fī - brō′mă - toyd). Fibromatóide; foco, nódulo ou massa (de fibroblastos em proliferação) que se assemelha a um fibroma, porém não é considerado como neoplásico.

fi·bro·ma·to·sis (fī′brō - mă - tō′sis). Fibromatose. **1.** Condição caracterizada por múltiplos fibromas que apresentam distribuição relativamente ampla. **2.** Hiperplasia anormal de tecido fibroso.
  abdominal f., f. abdominal. SIN desmoid (2).
  aggressive infantile f., f. agressiva da infância; a contraparte infantil dos tumores desmóides abdominais ou extra-abdominais, caracterizados por nódulos subcutâneos firmes que crescem rapidamente em qualquer parte do corpo, invadem localmente e recidivam, porém não metastatizam.
  f. col'li, f. cervical; massa fibrosa encontrada na porção média do músculo esternocleidomastóideo; a massa pode ser um hematoma resultante de trauma ao nascimento e pode causar torcicolo.
  congenital generalized f. [MIM*228550], f. generalizada congênita; tumores fibrosos múltiplos, subcutâneos e viscerais, presentes ao nascimento; distúrbio raro, freqüentemente fatal na primeira semana de vida, embora às vezes ocorra remissão espontânea; é provável que seja uma herança autossômica recessiva.
  gingival f., f. gengival; f. que pode estar associada a tricodiscomas. Várias formas genéticas são conhecidas e todas são autossômicas dominantes [MIM*135300, *135400, *135500, *135550].
  infantile digital f., f. digital infantil. SIN recurring digital *fibroma* of childhood.
  juvenile hyalin f. [MIM*228600], f. hialina juvenil; distúrbio raro, deformante, da cabeça e do pescoço, transmitido por herança recessiva, no qual se observam tumores e nódulos cutâneos generalizados em crianças sem distúrbio mental; as lesões consistem em fibroblastos separados por estroma hialino eosinófilo, composto principalmente por glicosaminoglicanas. SIN systemic hyalinosis.
  juvenile palmo-plantar f., f. palmoplantar juvenil; f. que acomete crianças do nascimento até a adolescência; apresenta-se como um nódulo único, pobremente delimitado, na eminência tenar ou hipotenar ou cobrindo o calcâneo na parte média da região plantar.
  palmar f., f. palmar; proliferação fibroblástica nodular, encontrada na fáscia palmar de uma ou de ambas as mãos, que precede a contratura de Dupuytren ou está associada a esta.
  penile f., f. peniana. SIN Peyronie *disease*.
  plantar f., f. plantar; proliferação fibroblástica nodular, encontrada na fáscia plantar de um ou de ambos os pés; raramente é associada a contratura. SIN Dupuytren disease of the foot.
fi·bro·ma·tous (fī - brō′mă - tŭs). Fibromatoso; relativo a ou da natureza de um fibroma.
fi·bro·mec·to·my (fī - brō - mek′tō - mē). Fibromectomia, miomectomia. SIN myomectomy.
fi·brom·e·ter (fī′brō - mē′ter). Fibrômetro; instrumento que mede a formação do coágulo (como em coagulograma *in vitro*) por meio da detecção mecânica do coágulo por uma sonda em movimento.
fi·bro·mus·cu·lar (fī′brō - mŭs′kū - lăr). Fibromuscular; tanto fibroso como muscular; que se refere aos tecidos fibroso e muscular.
fi·bro·my·al·gia (fī - brō - mī - al′ja). Fibromialgia; síndrome caracterizada por dor crônica de origem musculoesquelética, porém com causa incerta. O *American College of Rheumatology* estabeleceu critérios diagnósticos que incluem: dor em ambos os lados do corpo, tanto acima quanto abaixo da cintura, com uma distribuição axial (coluna cervical, torácica ou lombar ou face anterior do tórax); além disso, é preciso que haja pontos dolorosos à palpação em, pelo menos, 11 dos 18 locais especificados. SIN fibromyalgia syndrome.
fi·bro·my·ec·to·my (fī′brō - mī - ek′tō - mē). Fibromiectomia; excisão de um fibromioma.
fi·bro·my·o·ma (fī′brō - mī - ō′mă). Fibromioma; um leiomioma que contém uma quantidade relativamente abundante de tecido fibroso.
fi·bro·my·o·si·tis (fī′brō - mī - ō - sī′tis). Fibromiosite; inflamação crônica de um músculo, acompanhada de proliferação ou hiperplasia de tecido conectivo. [fibro- + G. *mys*, músculo, + *-itis*, inflamação]
fi·bro·myx·o·ma (fī′brō - mik - sō′mă). Fibromixoma; mixoma que contém uma quantidade relativamente abundante de fibroblastos maduros e tecido conectivo. [fibro- + G. *myxa*, muco, + *-ōma*, tumor]
fi·bro·nec·tins (fī - brō - nek′tins). Fibronectinas; glicoproteínas multifuncionais de alto peso molecular encontradas na membrana da superfície das células, no plasma sanguíneo e em outros líquidos corporais. Acredita-se que as fibronectinas atuem como moléculas adesivas, semelhantes a ligantes, que participam na inibição por contato; são também conhecidas como proteína LETS (*l*arge *e*xternal *t*ransformation *s*ensitive), que é reduzida após ocorrer a transformação celular. SIN zetaprotein. [L. *fibra*, fibra, + *nexus*, interconexão]
  plasma f., fibronectina plasmática; α$_2$-glicoproteína circulante que age como uma opsonina, mediando a depuração reticuloendotelial e dos macrófagos de microagregados de fibrina, resíduos de colágeno e partículas bacterianas, e protegendo a perfusão microvascular e a drenagem linfática.
fi·bro·neu·ro·ma (fī′brō - noo - rō′mă). Fibroneuroma, neurofibroma. SIN neurofibroma.
fi·bro·os·te·o·ma (fī′brō - os - tē - ō′mă). Fibroosteoma; osteoma no qual as células neoplásicas formadoras de osso estão situadas em um estroma relativamente abundante de tecido fibroso.

fi·bro·pap·il·lo·ma (fī′brō - pap - i - lō′mă). Fibropapiloma; papiloma caracterizado por uma quantidade evidente de tecido conectivo fibroso na base e que forma os núcleos nos quais as células epiteliais neoplásicas estão agrupadas.
fi·bro·pla·sia (fī - brō - plā′zē - ă). Fibroplasia; produção de tecido fibroso que, geralmente, implica um crescimento anormal de tecido fibroso não-neoplásico. [fibro- + G. *plasis*, uma moldura]
  retrolental f., retinopatia da prematuridade. SIN *retinopathy* of prematurity.
fi·bro·plas·tic (fī - brō - plas′tik). Fibroplásico; que produz tecido fibroso. [fibro- + G. *plastos*, formado]
fi·bro·plate (fī′brō - plāt). Disco articular. SIN articular *disk*.
fi·bro·pol·y·pus (fī - brō - pol′i - pŭs). Pólipo fibroso; pólipo composto principalmente de tecido fibroso.
fi·bro·re·tic·u·late (fī′brō - re - tik′ū - lāt). Fibrorreticular; relativo ao tecido fibroso ou que consiste em uma rede de tecido fibroso.
fi·bro·sa. Fibroso.
  pericardium fibrosa [TA], pericárdio fibroso. VER pericardium.
fi·bro·sar·co·ma (fī′brō - sar - kō′mă). Fibrossarcoma; neoplasia maligna derivada do tecido fibroso profundo, caracterizada por feixes de fibroblastos imaturos em proliferação, dispostos em um padrão característico em ziguezague com formação variável de colágeno e que tende a invadir localmente e metastatizar por meio da corrente sanguínea.
  ameloblastic f., f. ameloblástico; tumor odontogênico radiolucente, de crescimento rápido, doloroso e destrutivo, que em geral se origina de alterações malignas no componente mesenquimal de um fibroma ameloblástico preexistente. SIN ameloblastic sarcoma.
  Earle L f., f. de Earle L; f. transplantável, derivado do tecido subcutâneo de um camundongo da linhagem C3H, que cresceu em cultura de tecido na qual foi adicionado 20-metilcolantreno.
  infantile f., f. infantil; f. de crescimento rápido, mas que raramente metastatiza; em geral aparece nos membros durante o primeiro ano de vida.
fi·brose (fī - brōs′). Fibrosar; formar tecido fibroso.
fi·bro·se·rous (fī - brō - sē′rŭs). Fibrosseroso; composto de tecido fibroso com uma superfície serosa; que indica qualquer membrana serosa.
fi·bro·sis (fī - brō′sis). Fibrose; formação de tecido fibroso como um processo reparativo ou reativo, em oposição à formação de tecido fibroso como um constituinte normal de um órgão ou tecido.
  African endomyocardial f., f. endomiocárdica africana; f. das camadas internas do miocárdio que, freqüentemente, afeta o endocárdio, causando limitações diastólicas ao coração; nativa da África Oriental.
  congenital f. of the extraocular muscles [MIM*135700], f. congênita dos músculos oculomotores; distúrbio autossômico dominante associado à blefaroptose e à ausência de movimentos oculares.
  cystic f., cystic f. of the pancreas [MIM*219700], f. cística, f. cística do pâncreas; distúrbio metabólico congênito no qual as secreções das glândulas exócrinas são anormais; o muco apresenta-se excessivamente viscoso, causando a obstrução das vias de passagem (que incluem os ductos pancreático e biliar, intestinos e brônquios), e as concentrações de sódio e cloreto do suor mostram-se elevadas durante toda a vida do paciente; os sintomas geralmente aparecem na infância e incluem íleo meconial, crescimento deficiente, apesar de o apetite ser normal, malabsorção e fezes volumosas e fétidas, bronquite crônica com tosse, pneumonia recorrente, bronquiectasia, enfisema, baqueteamento digital e depleção de sal, quando a temperatura está elevada. O mapeamento genético detalhado e a biologia molecular foram realizados por meio de genética reversa; trata-se de herança autossômica recessiva causada por mutação no gene regulador da condutância da f. cística (CFTR) no cromossoma 7q. SIN Clarke-Hadfield syndrome, fibrocystic disease of the pancreas, mucoviscidosis, viscidosis.

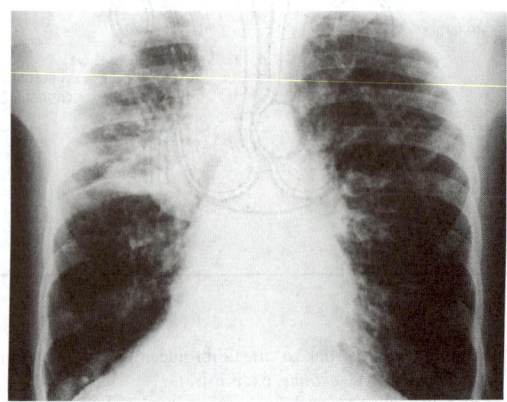

fibrose cística: alterações características do estágio final da fibrose cística são mostradas, inclusive espessamento da parede dos brônquios, bronquiectasia e atelectasia persistente

endocardial f., f. endocárdica; fibrose ou colagenose do endocárdio. SIN endocardial sclerosis.

endomyocardial f., f. endomiocárdica; espessamento do endocárdio ventricular por f., que envolve o miocárdio subendocárdico e, às vezes, as valvas atrioventriculares, acompanhada de trombose mural, levando à falência ventricular direita e esquerda progressiva, com insuficiência mitral e tricúspide; acomete adultos e é endêmica em algumas regiões da África. SIN Davies disease, endocardial fibroelastosis (2), endomyocardial fibroelastosis.

idiopathic interstitial f., f. intersticial idiopática. SIN idiopathic pulmonary f.

idiopathic pulmonary f. (IPF), f. pulmonar idiopática; processo inflamatório, que varia de agudo a crônico, ou f. intersticial do pulmão de etiologia desconhecida associados a colagenoses. SIN chronic fibrosing alveolitis, cryptogenic fibrosing alveolitis, fibrosing alveolitis, Hamman-Rich syndrome, idiopathic interstitial f.

interstitial pulmonary f., f. pulmonar intersticial; inclui tanto a f. pulmonar idiopática quanto a f. pulmonar associada a doença do tecido conectivo e a outras doenças primárias conhecidas.

leptomeningeal f., f. da leptomeninge; reação fibrosa que ocorre dentro do espaço subaracnóideo; é, às vezes, uma seqüela de meningite infecciosa ou química. VER TAMBÉM adhesive *arachnoiditis*.

mediastinal f., f. mediastinal; f. que pode obstruir a veia cava superior, as artérias e as veias pulmonares e os brônquios; é causada mais freqüentemente pela histoplasmose; a tuberculose e outras condições desconhecidas são causas menos comuns. SIN fibrosing mediastinitis, idiopathic fibrous mediastinitis.

nodular subepidermal f., f. subepidérmica nodular. VER dermatofibroma.

oral submucous f., f. da submucosa da boca; condição pré-cancerosa da mucosa oral e dos tratos respiratório e digestivo superiores, encontrada caracteristicamente em indianos.

pericentral f., f. pericentral; f. que ocorre ao redor das veias centrais nos lóbulos hepáticos.

perimuscular f., f. perimuscular; f. encontrada na média externa das artérias, em geral nas artérias renais de mulheres jovens, onde causa estenose segmental e hipertensão; um tipo de displasia fibromuscular. SIN subadventitial f.

pipestem f., f. que apresenta uma forma característica de cachimbo e se forma ao redor das veias porta hepáticas em alguns casos de infecção maciça e prolongada por *Schistosoma mansoni*; acredita-se que seja induzida pelo grande número de ovos de esquistossomas nos tecidos hepáticos. SIN Symmers clay pipestem f., Symmers f.

replacement f., f. de substituição; formação de tecido fibroso, que ocupa áreas onde diversas outras células e tecidos sofreram atrofia, degeneração ou necrose.

retroperitoneal f., f. retroperitoneal; f. de estruturas retroperitoneais e do tecido conectivo que, freqüentemente, envolve e obstrui os ureteres; a causa é, em geral, desconhecida. SIN idiopathic fibrous retroperitonitis, Ormond disease, periureteritis plastica.

subadventitial f., f. subadventícia. SIN perimuscular f.

Symmers clay pipestem f., Symmers f., f. de Symmers. SIN pipestem f.

fi·bro·si·tis (fī-brō-sī′tis). Fibrosite. 1. Inflamação do tecido fibroso. 2. Termo utilizado para indicar dor, inflamação ou rigidez musculares generalizadas, com múltiplos focos sensíveis (pontos-gatilho); a etiologia é desconhecida. SIN muscular rheumatism. [fibro- + G. -*itis*, inflamação]

cervical f., f. cervical. SIN posttraumatic neck *syndrome*.

fi·bro·tho·rax (fī-brō-thō′raks). Fibrotórax; fibrose do espaço pleural.

fi·brot·ic (fī-brot′ik). Fibrótico; relativo a, ou caracterizado por, fibrose.

fi·brous (fī′brŭs). Fibroso; composto de ou que contém fibroblastos e, também, as fibrilas e fibras do tecido conectivo formado por tais células.

fi·bro·xan·tho·ma (fī′brō-zan-thō′mă). Fibroxantoma; neoplasia fibro-histiocítica.

atypical f., f. atípico; tumor cutâneo, solitário, freqüentemente ulcerado, pequeno e geralmente benigno, composto de histiócitos espumosos, células fusiformes e células bizarras gigantes; é, em geral, encontrado na pele exposta de pessoas idosas; microscopicamente, o f. atípico assemelha-se muito ao histiocitoma fibroso maligno, porém origina-se na derme.

fib·u·la (fib′ū-lă). [TA]. Fíbula; o menor dos dois ossos da perna, situado lateralmente; não é um osso sustentador de peso e se articula com a tíbia, acima, e com a tíbia e o tálus, abaixo. SIN calf bone, calf-bone (1), perone, peroneal bone. [L. *fibula* (contr. de *figibula*), aquele que fixa, prende, um fecho, uma fivela, de *figo*, fixar, prender]

fib·u·lar (fib′ū-lăr). Fibular; relativo à fíbula. SIN fibularis, peroneal. [L. *fibularis*]

fib·u·la·ris (fib-ū-lā′ris). Fibular. SIN fibular. [L. mod.]

fib·u·lo·cal·ca·ne·al (fib′ū-lō-kal-kā′nē-ăl). Calcaneofibular; relativo à fíbula e ao calcâneo.

fi·cain (fī-kān). Ficaina. SIN ficin (2).

fi·cin (fī′sin). Ficina. 1. Cisteína endopeptidase isolada de figos (*Ficus carica, globata* e *doliaria*); utilizada na indústria como proteína digestiva; possui uma ampla especificidade a substratos proteicos; agente anti-helmíntico. 2. O látex não processado e seco do *Ficus* spp. SIN ficain.

Fick, Adolf, médico alemão, 1829–1901. VER F. *method, principle*.

FID Abreviatura de free induction *decay* (decaimento de indução livre).

Fiedler, Carl L.A., médico alemão, 1835–1921. VER F. *myocarditis*.

field (fēld). Campo; área definida de superfície plana, considerada em relação a algum objeto específico. [A.S. *feld*]

auditory f., c. auditivo; espaço incluído dentro dos limites de audição de um som definido, como o produzido por um diapasão.

Broca f., c. de Broca. SIN Broca *center*.

Cohnheim f., c. de Cohnheim. SIN Cohnheim *area*.

f. of consciousness, c. da consciência. VER field of *consciousness*.

f. of fixation, c. de fixação; em oftalmologia, a distância angular ao redor da qual a linha de fixação pode ser girada.

f.'s of Forel, campos de Forel; três regiões circunscritas e ricas em mielina localizadas no subtálamo e conhecidas como campos H (de Haubenfelder); 1) campo H_1, que corresponde ao fascículo talâmico, um estrato de fibras horizontais situado na junção entre o subtálamo e o tálamo suprajacente; é composto por fibras palidotalâmicas e cerebelotalâmicas (*brachium conjunctivum*) e está separado do campo H_2, localizado mais ventralmente, pela zona incerta; 2) campo H_2, formado pelo fascículo lenticular e arqueia-se sobre a margem dorsal do núcleo subtalâmico; é composto, em grande parte, por fibras palidotalâmicas; 3) campo H_3 ou campo pré-rúbrico, um campo grande, de substância branca e cinzenta entremeada, imediatamente rostral ao núcleo rubro, que une os campos H_1 e H_2 ao redor da margem medial da zona incerta; sua substância cinzenta forma o núcleo pré-rubral. VER TAMBÉM lenticular *loop*. SIN campi foreli, tegmental f.'s of Forel.

free f., c. livre; (c. espaço tridimensional) em um meio homogêneo e isotrópico, sem limites; na prática, um c. no qual os efeitos dos limites são insignificantes.

H f.'s, campos H. VER f.'s of Forel.

individuation f., c. de individuação; c. dentro do qual um organizador consegue produzir o rearranjo de tecidos primordiais de tal forma que um embrião completo seja formado.

involved f., c. comprometido; no tratamento por radiação, a área ocupada por um tumor.

magnetic f., c. magnético; a esfera de influência de um magneto.

microscopic f., c. microscópico; área dentro da qual objetos são visíveis através de oculares e objetivas de microscópio de diversos graus de aumento.

nerve f., c. nervoso; a distribuição regional de terminais nervosos.

prerubral f., c. pré-rúbrico. VER f.'s of Forel.

sound f., c. de som; ambiente no qual ondas sonoras são propagadas. SIN acoustical surround.

tegmental f.'s of Forel, campos tegmentais de Forel. SIN f.'s of Forel.

visual f. (F), c. visual; área visualizada por um dos olhos sem a realização de movimento; é freqüentemente medida por meio de um arco (perímetro) localizado a 330 mm de distância do olho.

Wernicke f., c. de Wernicke. SIN Wernicke *center*.

Fielding, George H., anatomista britânico, 1801–1871. VER F. *membrane*.

Field rap·id stain. Corante rápido de Field. VER em stain.

field-vole (fēld-vōl). Arganaz do campo; espécie de camundongo silvestre (*Microtus montebelloi*) que é hospedeiro natural da *Leptospira hebdomadis*, o microrganismo causador de um tipo de leptospirose que se assemelha à mononucleose infecciosa.

Fiessinger, Noël Armand, médico francês, 1881–1946. VER F.-Leroy-Reiter *syndrome*.

fièv·re (fē-evr′). Febre; termo francês para febre.

f. boutonneuse (fē-evr′ boo-ton-nŭz′), f. botonosa. SIN Mediterranean spotted *fever*.

fig. Figo; o fruto parcialmente seco do *Ficus carica* (família Moraceae); utilizado como alimento, laxante suave e demulcente. [L. *ficus*; A.S. *fic*]

FIGLU Abreviatura de formiminoglutamic acid (ácido formiminoglutâmico).

fig·u·ra·tus (fig-ū-rā′tŭs). Figurado; termo descritivo de certas lesões da pele. [L. *figuro*, pp. -*atus*, formar, moldar]

fig·ure (fig′ūr). Figura; símbolo. 1. Uma forma ou formato. 2. Uma pessoa que representa os aspectos essenciais de uma função em particular (p.ex., um patrão, que é visto como a figura de um pai, ou uma professora, que é vista como a figura de uma mãe). 3. Uma forma, um contorno ou uma representação de um objeto ou de uma pessoa. [L. *figura*, de *fingo*, formar, moldar]

authority f., f. da autoridade; pessoa real ou projetada em uma posição de poder; os pais, a polícia e o chefe/patrão são figuras autoritárias para algumas pessoas; durante a fase de transferência da psicanálise, o psicanalista torna-se uma f. autoritária.

flame f., f. em forma de chama; pequena área de necrose dérmica ou subcutânea com coloração eosinófila intensa dos feixes de colágeno; observada nas lesões da celulite eosinofílica.

fortification f.'s, espectro de fortificação. SIN fortification *spectrum*.

mitotic f., f. mitótica; a aparência microscópica de uma célula que sofre mitose; uma célula cujos cromossomas são visíveis ao microscópio óptico.

myelin f., f. de mielina; arranjo enrolado ou em espiral de uma dupla camada de lipídios dentro de uma célula, que se assemelha superficialmente à bainha de mielina dos nervos; é observado pelo microscópio eletrônico no citoplasma ou como inclusões dentro de mitocôndrias e de vacúolos autofágicos, onde podem representar artefatos da fixação de lipídios. SIN myelin body.

Purkinje f.'s, figuras de Purkinje; sombras de vasos da retina, observadas como linhas escuras sobre um campo avermelhado, quando a luz penetra no olho através da esclera e não da pupila.

fig·ure and ground. Figura e fundo; o aspecto da percepção no qual o que é percebido é separado em pelo menos duas partes, cada uma com diferentes atributos, mas que se influenciam mutuamente. A figura é a mais distinta; o fundo, o menos nítido; p.ex., um pássaro ou uma árvore (figura) vistos contra o céu (fundo).

fi·la (fī′lă). Filos; plural de filum. [L.]

fi·la·ceous (fī-lā′shŭs). Filamentoso. SIN filamentous. [L. *filum*, um fio]

fil·ag·grin (fĭl-ag′grĭn). Filagrina; principal proteína do grânulo ceratoialino, composta principalmente pelos resíduos L-histidil, lisil e arginil (proteínas básicas do estrato córneo). Agrega os filamentos intermediários de ceratina e promove a formação das ligações dissulfídicas. [*fil*ament + *aggr*egat*in*g.]

fil·a·men, filamin (fĭl′ă-men). Filamina; proteína de alto peso molecular que se liga à actina e compõe parte da estrutura filamentar intracelular das células fibroblásticas; sua distribuição nas células é resultante de sua interação com a actina polimerizada.

fil·a·ment (fĭl′ă-ment). **1.** Filamento. SIN filamentum. **2.** Filamentar; em bacteriologia, uma forma fina semelhante a um fio, não-segmentada ou segmentada e sem constrições. [L. *filamentum*, de *filum*, um fio]

actin f., f. de actina; um dos elementos contráteis encontrados nas fibras musculares e em outras células; no músculo esquelético, os filamentos de actina apresentam cerca de 5 nm de largura e 100 μm de comprimento e estão fixados aos filamentos Z. SIN thin f.

axial f., f. axial; f. central de um flagelo ou cílio; ao microscópio eletrônico, é visto como um complexo formado por nove pares de microtúbulos periféricos e um par central de microtúbulos. SIN axonema (2).

cytokeratin f.'s, filamentos de citoqueratina. SIN keratin f.'s.

intermediate f.'s, filamentos intermediários; classe de filamentos proteicos rígidos (que inclui os filamentos de queratina, neurofilamentos, desmina e vimentina) com 8 a 10 nm de espessura e compõem parte do citoesqueleto do citoplasma da maioria das células eucarióticas; recebem essa denominação por apresentarem uma espessura intermediária, quando comparados aos filamentos de actina e aos microtúbulos.

keratin f.'s, filamentos de queratina; classe de filamentos intermediários que formam uma rede dentro das células epiteliais e se ancoram aos desmossomas, transmitindo, dessa forma, resistência à tração ao tecido. SIN cytokeratin f.'s.

myosin f., f. de miosina; um dos elementos contráteis encontrados nas fibras musculares lisas, esqueléticas e cardíacas; no músculo esquelético, o f. tem cerca de 10 nm de espessura e 1,5 μm de comprimento. SIN thick f.

parabasal f., f. parabasal; termo antigamente utilizado para rhizoplast.

pial f., f. pial; *termo oficial alternativo para pial part of filum terminale.

root f.'s, filamentos radiculares. SIN radicular *fila*, em *filum*.

spermatic f., um espermatozóide, especialmente a cauda de um espermatozóide.

thick f., f. de miosina. SIN myosin f.

thin f., f. de actina. SIN actin f.

Z f., filamento Z; a delgada estrutura em ziguezague, encontrada na linha Z das fibras musculares esqueléticas, na qual os filamentos de actina estão fixados.

fil·a·men·tous (fĭl-ă-men′tŭs). Filamentoso. **1.** Estrutura semelhante a um fio. SIN filiform (1). **2.** Composto de filamentos ou de estruturas semelhantes a fios. SIN filaceous, filar (2).

fil·a·men·tum, pl. **fil·a·men·ta** (fĭl-ă-men′tŭm, -tă). Filamento; fibrila, fibra delgada ou estrutura semelhante a um fio. SIN filament (1). [L.]

fi·lar (fī′lăr). **1.** Fibrilar. SIN fibrillar. **2.** Filamentoso. SIN filamentous. [L. *filum*, um fio]

Fi·lar·i·a (fĭ-lar′ē-ă). Antigo gênero dos nematódeos que, atualmente, são classificados em vários gêneros e espécies da família Onchocercidae; p.ex., *Wuchereria bancrofti* (*F. bancrofti, F. diurna* ou *F. nocturna*), *Brugia malayi* (*F. malaya*), *Onchocerca volvulus* (*F. volvulus*), *Mansonella perstans* (*F. perstans* ou *F. sanguinis hominis*), *M. streptocerca, M. ozzardi* (*F. demarquayi* ou *F. ozzardi*), *Loa loa* (*F. extraocularis, F. lentis, F. loa* ou *F. oculi humani*) e *Dracunculus medinensis* (*F. medinensis*). VER TAMBÉM filaria.

fi·lar·ia, pl. **fi·lar·i·ae** (fĭ-lar′ē-ă, -ē-ē). Filária; nome comum dado a nematódeos da família Onchocercidae que, quando adultos, vivem no sangue, nos líquidos tissulares, nos tecidos ou nas cavidades do corpo de muitos vertebrados. As fêmeas põem ovos parcialmente embrionados; os embriões libertam-se dos ovos e circulam pelo sangue ou pelos líquidos tissulares na forma de microfilárias; quando as microfilárias são ingeridas por um artrópode sugador de sangue adequado, as formas larvais desenvolvem-se; posteriormente, quando o artrópode se alimenta novamente de sangue, larvas infectantes podem ser depositadas sobre a pele de outro hospedeiro vertebrado. [L. *filum*, um fio]

fi·lar·i·al (fĭ-lā′rē-ăl). Relativo a uma filária (ou filárias), incluindo as microfilárias.

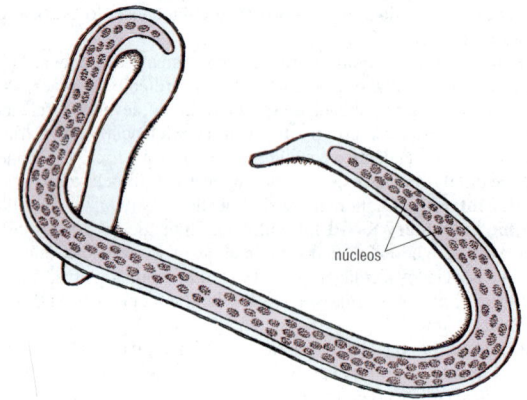

filária (microfilária de *Wuchereria bancrofti*)

fil·a·ri·a·sis (fĭl-ă-rī′ă-sĭs). Filaríase; a presença de filárias nos tecidos do corpo, no sangue (microfilariemia) ou nos líquidos tissulares, encontrada em regiões tropicais e subtropicais; os vermes vivos provocam pouca reação tecidual, que pode ser assintomática. A morte dos vermes adultos, contudo, provoca inflamação granulomatosa e fibrose permanente, que causam obstrução dos vasos linfáticos de densas cicatrizes hialínicas localizadas nos tecidos subcutâneos; a conseqüência mais grave é a elefantíase ou paquidermia.

bancroftian f., f. bancroftiana; f. causada pela *Wuchereria bancrofti*.

Brug f., f. de Brug; infecção pela filária *Brugia malayi*, que causa adenite, febre, linfangite e, às vezes, elefantíase; ocorre primariamente no Sudeste Asiático, na Indonésia, na China, no Japão, na Coréia e nas Filipinas.

periodic f., f. periódica; forma de f. na qual as microfilárias aparecem no sangue periférico a intervalos regulares de 24 horas; é, em geral, uma referência à periodicidade noturna da filaríase bancroftiana.

fi·lar·i·ci·dal (fĭ-lar-ĭ-sī′dăl). Filaricida; que é mortal para as filárias.

fi·lar·i·cide (fĭ-lar′ĭ-sīd). Filaricida; agente que mata as filárias. [filaria + L. *caedo*, matar]

fi·lar·i·form (fĭ-lar′ĭ-fōrm). Filarióide. **1.** Que se assemelha às filárias ou a outros tipos de pequenos vermes nematódeos. VER TAMBÉM filariform *larva*. **2.** Fino ou semelhante a um fio de cabelo.

Fil·a·ri·i·cae (fĭ-lar′ē-ĭ-sē). SIN Filarioidea.

Fi·lar·i·oi·dea (fĭ-lar′ē-oy′dē-ă). Superfamília de nematódeos que parasitam muitas espécies de animais, incluindo os seres humanos; engloba as famílias Filariidae, Diplotraenidae, Onchocercidae e Stephanofilariidae. VER *Filaria*. VER TAMBÉM *Dipetalonema, Dirofilaria, Loa loa, Mansonella, Onchocerca, Wuchereria* e *Brugia*. SIN Filariicae.

Filatov, Nil F., pediatra russo, 1847–1902. VER F. *disease*.

Filatov, Vladimir P., oftalmologista russo, 1875–1956. VER F. *flap*; F.-Gillies *flap*.

file (fĭl). Lima; ferramenta para alisar, amolar ou cortar.

Hedström f., l. de Hedström; lima grosseira de canal radicular semelhante a uma grosa.

periodontal f., l. periodontal; instrumento com um conjunto de cristas ou pontos dispostos em fileiras sobre a superfície, utilizado para raspar ou remover cálculos dentários.

root canal f., l. para canais; instrumento de aço, pontiagudo e flexível, utilizado para raspar as paredes internas do canal radicular.

fil·i·al (fĭl′ē-ăl). Filial; que indica a relação da prole para com seus pais. VER filial *generation*. [L. *filialis*, de *filius*, filho, *filia*, filha]

fi·li·form (fĭl′ĭ-fōrm). Filiforme. **1.** SIN filamentous (1). **2.** Em bacteriologia, que denota um crescimento plano ao longo da linha de inoculação feita na forma de esfregaço ou picada. [L. *filum*, fio]

fi·li·form ad·na·tum. Blefarocoloboma. SIN ankyloblepharon.

fil·i·o·pa·ren·tal (fĭl′ē-ō-pă-ren′tăl). Filioparental; relativo ao relacionamento entre uma criança e seus pais. [L. *filius*, filho, + *parens*, pais, de *pario*, parir]

fil·let (fĭl′et). **1.** Lemnisco. SIN lemniscus. **2.** Faixa, banda, laço ou fita utilizados para tracionar uma parte do feto. [Fr. *filet*, uma fita, faixa]

lateral f., lemnisco lateral. SIN lateral *lemniscus*.

medial f., lemnisco medial. SIN medial *lemniscus*.

fill·ing (fĭl′ing). Obturação; termo leigo para uma restauração dentária.

film (fĭlm). **1.** Filme; folha fina de material flexível coberta com uma substância sensível à luz ou aos raios X e utilizada para tirar fotografias ou fazer radiografias. **2.** Película; camada ou cobertura delgada. **3.** Uma radiografia (coloquial).

absorbable gelatin f., película gelatinosa absorvível; lâmina delgada de gela-

tina, não-antigênica, absorvível e insolúvel em água, obtida após a secagem de uma solução de gelatina-formaldeído colocada em placas; utilizada no fechamento e reparo de defeitos em membranas, tais como a dura-máter e a pleura; sofre absorção em 1 a 6 meses.
bitewing f., "bite-wing"; embalagem especial de f. radiográfico que permite que uma lingüeta da embalagem do filme seja mantida entre as superfícies oclusais dos dentes.
decubitus f., radiografia de decúbito; radiografia exposta com a pessoa em decúbito e denominada de acordo com o lado que está mais próximo do filme. SIN right or left lateral decubitus f.
horizontal beam f., radiografia com feixe horizontal; radiografia feita com o eixo central das ondas de raios X paralelo ao solo, permitindo, assim, revelar níveis hidroaéreos.
latitude f., f. de latitude. SIN wide-latitude f.
panoramic x-ray f., radiografia panorâmica; em odontologia, uma radiografia feita para fornecer uma visão panorâmica das arcadas dentárias superior e inferior inteiras, bem como das articulações temporomandibulares.
plain f., radiografia simples; radiografia feita sem o uso de contraste.
precorneal f., película pré-corneal; película protetora com 7 a 9 nm de espessura, composta de uma camada oleosa externa, uma intermediária aquosa e uma interna mucoproteica. SIN tear f.
right or left lateral decubitus f., radiografia em decúbito lateral direito ou esquerdo. SIN decubitus f.
scout f., radiografia simples preliminar; radiografia feita antes que o contraste seja administrado, como a radiografia preliminar de uma angiografia, de uma urografia ou de um exame gastrointestinal com o uso de contraste baritado. SIN scout radiograph.
f. speed, velocidade do f.; a relativa sensibilidade da emulsão do f. à luz ou à exposição à radiação; a velocidade é inversamente proporcional à resolução dos detalhes.
spot f., *spot*; radiografia feita durante um exame sob fluoroscopia com um dispositivo fixado ao fluoroscópio.
tear f., película lacrimal. SIN precorneal f.
wide-latitude f., f. de latitude ampla; f. que não mostra grandes diferenças de contraste com diferenças na exposição; a inclinação das *curvas* H e D é baixa. SIN latitude f.
film chang·er. Trocador de filmes; dispositivo que move o filme para estudos radiográficos exigindo exposições rápidas e seriadas aos raios X, tais como a angiografia. SIN rapid f. c., serial f. c.
rapid f. c., t. de filmes rápido. SIN film changer.
serial f. c., t. de filmes seriado. SIN film changer.
Fil·mer, David L., bioquímico norte-americano, *1932. VER Adair-Koshland-Némethy-Filmer *model*; Koshland-Némethy-Filmer *model*.
fil·o·po·dia (fil - ō - pō′dē - ă). Filopódios; plural de filopodium.
fil·o·po·di·um, pl. **fil·o·po·dia** (fī - lō - pō′dē - ŭm, - ă). Filópode; pseudópode delgado e filamentoso encontrado em certas amebas de vida livre. [L. *filum*, fio, + G. *pous*, pé]
fi·lo·pres·sure (fī - lō - presh′ŭr). Pressão temporária realizada sobre um vaso sanguíneo por uma ligadura, que é removida quando o fluxo de sangue cessa. [L. *filum*, fio]
fi·lo·var·i·co·sis (fī′lō - var- ē - kō′sis). Uma série de dilatações observadas ao longo do trajeto do axônio de uma fibra nervosa. [L. *filum*, fio, + *varix*, dilatação de uma veia]
Fil·o·vi·ri·dae (fī′lō - vī′rā - dā). Família de vírus RNA de filamento simples, sentido negativo e filamentoso com um nucleocapsídeo envolto por um envelope. Antigamente, esses vírus pertenciam à família Rhabdoviridae e estão associados à febre hemorrágica. O reservatório natural desses vírus não é conhecido. VER Ebola *virus*. [L. *filum*, fio, + virus]
Fil·o·vi·rus (fī′lō - vī - rŭs). Gênero da família Filoviridae que inclui os vírus Marburg e Ebola.
fil·ter (fil′ter). **1.** Filtro; substância porosa através da qual um líquido ou gás é passado, a fim de separá-lo de matéria particulada ou impurezas e, assim, esterilizá-lo. SIN filtrum. **2.** Filtrar; utilizar ou submeter à ação de um f. **3.** Filtro; em radiologia diagnóstica ou terapêutica, uma tela feita com um ou mais metais — tais como o alumínio e o cobre — que, quando colocada na frente do feixe de raios X ou gama, permite a passagem de uma proporção maior de radiação de energia mais alta e a atenuação da radiação de energia mais baixa e menos desejável, aumentando a energia média ou endurecendo o feixe. **4.** Dispositivo utilizado em análise espectrofotométrica para isolar um segmento do espectro. **5.** Algoritmo matemático aplicado a dados de imagens com o propósito de aumentar a qualidade da imagem, geralmente por meio da supressão ou do aumento das freqüências espaciais altas. **6.** Circuito ou dispositivo eletrônico passivo que permite seletivamente a passagem de certos sinais elétricos. **7.** Dispositivo colocado na veia cava inferior para impedir o embolismo pulmonar por coágulo proveniente dos membros inferiores. Existem muitos tipos. [L. mediev. *filtro*, pp. *-atus*, filtrar através de feltro, de *filtrum*, feltro]
bandpass f., f. de passagem de faixa, f. de passagem de sintonia; dispositivo que permite a passagem de uma faixa limitada de freqüências.
Berkefeld f., f. de Berkefeld; f. para bactérias utilizado em 1891 e feito de terra conhecida como "Kieselguhr", nome tirado de uma mina em Hanover, Alemanha, onde foi encontrada. As fontes de águas subterrâneas dessa mina apresentavam uma cor azul-clara, fato que sugeriu o uso da terra como filtro. [Berkefeld, nome do proprietário da mina]
bird's nest f., f. em "ninho de ave"; f. para a veia cava inferior constituído por uma malha de fios metálicos.
Greenfield f., f. de Greenfield; f. para a veia cava que apresenta várias hastes dispostas em forma de um guarda-chuva.
high-pass f., f. de alta freqüência, f. de passagem alta; dispositivo ou material que permite a passagem de sinais de alta freqüência, enquanto atenua os demais sinais.

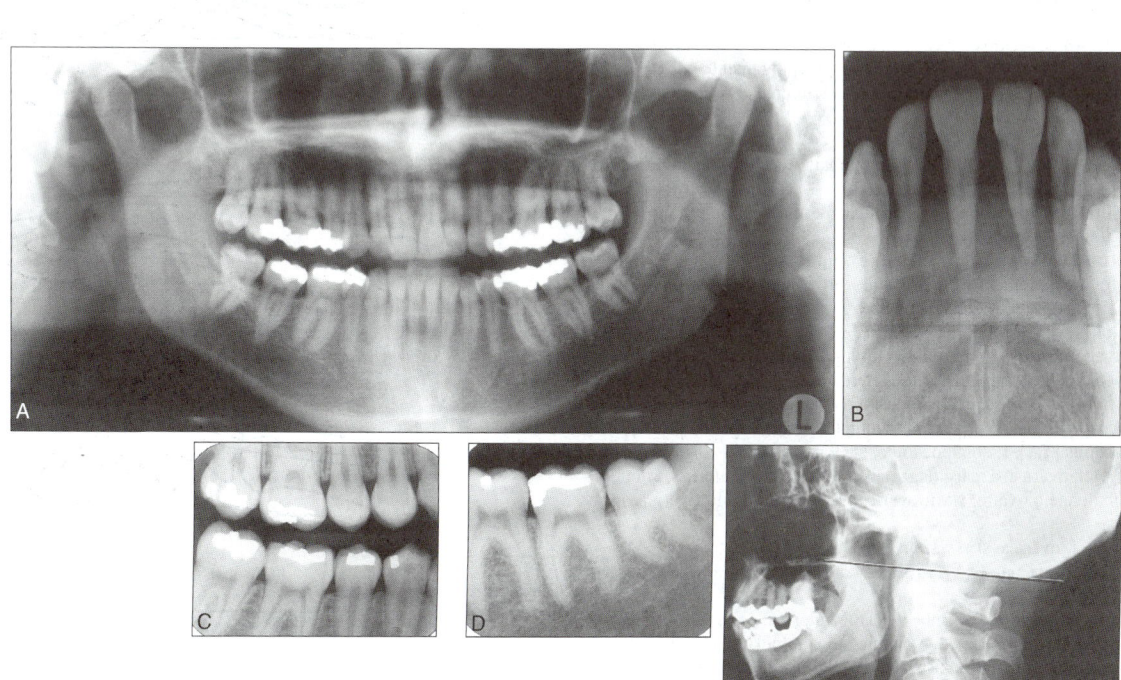

técnicas de radiografia dentária: (A) panorâmica; (B) oclusal; (C) "bite-wing"; (D) periapical; (E) cefalométrica

low-pass f., f. de baixa freqüência, f. de passagem baixa; dispositivo ou material com o efeito oposto ao do f. de alta freqüência; a maioria dos tecidos atua como filtros de baixa freqüência de sinais do ultra-som.
nitinol f., f. de nitinol; f. para a veia cava, fabricado com um metal, que adquire a forma final quando é aquecido até a temperatura corporal pelo sangue após sua inserção por meio de um cateter.
vena cava f., f. para a veia cava; f. utilizado para ocluir a veia cava inferior, a fim de impedir o embolismo pulmonar; p.ex., o f. de Greenfield. SIN venocaval f.
venocaval f., f. para a veia cava. SIN vena cava f.
fil·tra·ble, fil·ter·a·ble (fil′trā - bl, fil′ter - ā - bl). Filtrável; capaz de passar por um filtro; termo freqüentemente aplicado a vírus menores e a algumas bactérias.
fil·trate (fil′trāt). Filtrado; aquilo que passou através de um filtro.
fil·tra·tion (fil - trā′shŭn). Filtração. **1.** O processo de passar um líquido ou gás através de um filtro. **2.** Em radiologia, o processo de atenuação e têmpera de um feixe de raios X ou gama por meio da interposição de um filtro (3) entre a fonte de radiação e o objeto que está sendo irradiado; f. inerente é aquela causada pelo próprio aparelho, tal como o vidro de um tubo de raios X, sem a adição de um filtro. SIN percolation (1).
gel f., f. em gel, cromatografia em gel; separação de partículas com o tamanho de moléculas realizada pela passagem de uma mistura através de colunas de contas de dextranas entrecruzadas ou material similar e relativamente inerte de uma fileira de poros de tamanho bem definido; quanto maior a molécula, menor o tempo gasto no interior das contas, emergindo, dessa forma, mais rapidamente da coluna do que as moléculas menores.
fil·trum (fil′trŭm). Filtro. SIN filter (1). [L. mediev.]
Merkel f. ventric'uli, f. do ventrículo de Merkel. SIN f. ventriculi.
f. ventric'uli, f. do ventrículo; sulco situado entre as duas proeminências, em cada parede lateral do vestíbulo da laringe, e formado pelas cartilagens cuneiforme e aritenóidea. SIN Merkel f. ventriculi.
fi·lum, pl. **fi·la** (fī′lŭm, -lă) [TA]. Filamento; estrutura de aparência filamentosa ou semelhante a um fio. [L. fio]
f. du'rae ma'tris spina'lis, parte dural do f. terminal. SIN dural part of filum terminale.
fi'la olfacto'ria [TA], nervos olfatórios. SIN olfactory nerves [CNI], em nerve.
olfactory fila, nervos olfatórios; SIN olfactory nerves [CNI], em nerve.
radicular fi'la, filamentos radiculares; pequenos fascículos de fibras individuais dentro dos quais as raízes de todos os nervos espinais e de vários nervos cranianos (hipoglosso, vago, oculomotor) se dividem em forma de leque antes de penetrarem na medula espinal e no tronco encefálico, ou sair dos mesmos; a raiz dorsal pode dividir-se em oito a 12 radículas. SIN fila radicularia [TA], root filaments.
fi'la radicula'ria [TA], filamentos radiculares. SIN radicular fila.
f. of spinal dura mater, parte dural do f. terminal. SIN dural part of filum terminale.
terminal f., f. terminal; fio longo de tecido conectivo (pia-máter) que se estende da extremidade do cone medular até a face interna do fundo do saco dural espinal (parte pial do filamento terminal [TA], filamento terminal interno [alt TA]); fios espessos de tecido conectivo que ligam o fundo do saco dural espinal ao cóccix (parte dural do filamento terminal [TA], ligamento coccígeo [alt TA], filamento terminal externo [alt TA]). SIN f. terminale [TA], nervus impar, terminal thread.
f. termina'le [TA], f. terminal. SIN terminal f.
f. terminale externum, parte dural do f. terminal; *termo oficial alternativo para dural part of filum terminale.
f. terminale internum, parte pial do f. terminal; *termo oficial alternativo para pial part of filum terminale.
fim·bria, pl. **fim·bri·ae** (fim′brē - ă, - brē - ē). Fímbria. **1.** [TA]. Qualquer estrutura com forma semelhante a uma franja. SIN fringe. **2.** SIN pilus (2). [L. franja]
f. hippocam'pi [TA], f. do hipocampo; crista estreita e bordas pontiagudas de substância branca, contínua com o álveo do hipocampo e fixada na margem medial do hipocampo; é composta de fibras eferentes do hipocampo que formam o fórnice, de fibras da comissura do hipocampo e de fibras septo-hipocampais. SIN f. of hippocampus [TA], corpus fimbriatum (1), tenia hippocampi.
f. of hippocampus [TA], f. do hipocampo. SIN f. hippocampi.
ovarian f. [TA], f. ovárica; a mais longa das fímbrias da tuba uterina; estende-se do infundíbulo até o ovário. SIN f. ovarica [TA], infundibulo-ovarian ligament.
f. ova'rica [TA], f. ovárica. SIN ovarian f.
fim'briae tu'bae uteri'nae [TA], fímbrias da tuba uterina. SIN fimbriae of uterine tube.
fim'briae of uterine tube [TA], fímbrias da tuba uterina; processos irregularmente ramificados ou fimbriados que circundam a ampola na abertura abdominal da tuba uterina; a maioria das células epiteliais de revestimento apresenta cílios que batem em direção ao útero. SIN fimbriae tubae uterinae [TA], laciniae tubae.
fim·bri·ate, fim·bri·at·ed (fim′brē - āt, - ā - ted). Fimbriado; que possui fímbrias.

fim·bri·ec·to·my (fim′brē - ek′tō - mē). Fimbriectomia; excisão de fímbrias. [L. *fimbria,* franja, + G. *ektomē,* excisão]
fim·brin (fim′brin). Fimbrina; proteína ligadora de actina que forma ligações cruzadas firmes entre filamentos adjacentes, com formação de fibras paralelas de actina nas células dos vertebrados. Essa proteína auxilia na manutenção da polaridade e do desenvolvimento celulares. [L. *fimbriae,* fios, fibras, + -in]
fim·bri·o·cele (fim′brē - ō - sēl). Fimbriocele; hérnia do corpo fimbriado do oviduto. [L. *fimbria,* franja, + G. *kēlē,* hérnia]
fim·bri·o·plas·ty (fim′brē - ō - plas - tē). Fimbrioplastia; operação corretiva nas fímbrias da tuba uterina. [L. *fimbria,* franja, + G. *plastos,* formado]
finasteride. Finasterida; um inibidor competitivo da 5α-redutase, uma enzima intracelular que converte testosterona em 5α-diidrotestosterona, um potente andrógeno; utilizado no tratamento da hiperplasia prostática benigna; também é prescrito para calvície de padrão masculino e para promover novo crescimento de cabelo.
Finckh, Johann, psiquiatra alemão, *1873. VER F. test.
find·ing. Achado; observação clinicamente significativa; termo geralmente utilizado em relação a algo encontrado no exame físico ou em um teste laboratorial.
fine·ness (fīn′nes). Grau de pureza; indicador do teor de metal precioso de uma liga, e 1.000 pontos correspondem a 24 quilates ou ouro puro.
fin·ger (fing′ger) [TA]. Dedo da mão, quirodáctilo. SIN digitus manus [TA]. [A.S.]
baseball f., d.-de-beisebol, dedo-em-martelo; avulsão parcial ou completa de um extensor longo do dedo da base da falange distal. SIN drop f., hammer f., mallet f.
blubber f., erisipelóide. SIN erysipeloid.
clubbed f.'s, baqueteamento digital. VER clubbing.
dead f.'s, acroasfixia. SIN acroasphyxia.
drop f., dedo-de-beisebol. SIN baseball f.
fifth f., quinto dedo da mão. SIN little f.
first f., polegar, primeiro dedo da mão. SIN thumb.
fourth f., dedo anular, quarto dedo da mão. SIN ring f.
hammer f., d. em martelo, dedo-de-beisebol. SIN baseball f.
hippocratic f.'s, baqueteamento digital. VER clubbing.
index f. [TA], d. indicador; o segundo dedo (o polegar é considerado o primeiro). SIN digitus (manus) secundus [II]*, forefinger, index (1), second f.
jerk f., dedo-em-gatilho. SIN trigger f.
little f. [TA], d. mínimo; o quinto dedo da mão. SIN digitus (manus) minimus [TA], digitus auricularis, digitus (manus) quintus [V], fifth f.
lock f., dedo-em-gatilho. SIN trigger f.
mallet f., d. em martelo. SIN baseball f.

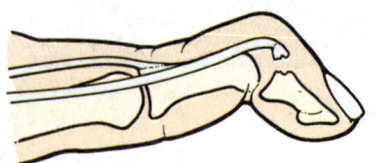

deformidade em botoeira

ruptura do tendão do músculo flexor profundo do dedo

dedo em martelo

dedo da mão: deformidades e fraturas

middle f. [TA], d. médio; terceiro dedo da mão. SIN digitus (manus), medius [TA], digitus (manus) tertius [III]*, third f.
ring f. [TA], d. anular; quarto dedo da mão. SIN digitus anularis [TA], digitus (manus) quartus IV*, fourth f.

sausage f.'s, dedos em salsicha; dedos grossos e curtos encontrados na acromegalia; dedos simétricos e difusamente inchados; alteração inicial da esclerose sistêmica.
seal f.'s, erisipelóide. SIN erysipeloid.
second f., segundo dedo da mão, dedo indicador. SIN index f.
snap f., dedo-em-gatilho. SIN trigger f.
spade f.'s, dedos em pá; os dedos curtos e grossos encontrados na acromegalia e no mixedema.
spider f., aracnodactilia. SIN arachnodactyly.
spring f., dedo-em-gatilho. SIN trigger f.
stuck f., dedo-em-gatilho. SIN trigger f.
third f., terceiro dedo da mão, dedo médio. SIN middle f.
trigger f., dedo-em-gatilho; condição na qual o movimento do d. é interrompido por um momento em flexão ou extensão e, em seguida, continua de forma abrupta; resulta de tumefação localizada no tendão que interfere no seu deslizamento através das "polias" da palma da mão. SIN jerk f., lock f., snap f., spring f., stuck f.
waxy f.'s, acroasfixia. SIN acroasphyxia.
webbed f.'s, dedos palmados; dois ou mais dedos unidos e envolvidos por uma bainha de pele comum.
whale f.'s, erisipelóide. SIN erysipeloid.
white f.'s, dedos brancos, doença dos dedos brancos; doença ocupacional encontrada em operadores de furadeiras pneumáticas que ficam expostos ao frio.
zinc f., d. de zinco; domínio de ligação do zinco em uma estrutura proteica freqüentemente observado em certas proteínas reguladoras de genes, p.ex., fatores de transcrição.
fin·ger·nail (fing′ger - nāl).Unha (dos dedos da mão). VER nail.
fin·ger·print (fing′ger-print′). Impressão digital. **1.** Impressão da polpa da falange distal de um dedo da mão previamente manchada com tinta, que exibe a configuração das linhas da superfície, utilizada como uma forma de identificação. VER TAMBÉM dermatoglyphics, Galton system of classification of f.'s. **2.** Termo, às vezes utilizado de modo informal, que se refere a qualquer método analítico capaz de detectar diferenças sutis entre compostos similares ou entre padrões de gel; p.ex., o padrão de uma curva de absorção infravermelha ou de um cromatógrafo em papel, bidimensional. **3.** Em genética, a análise de fragmentos de DNA para determinar a identidade de um indivíduo ou a paternidade de uma criança. SIN genetic f.

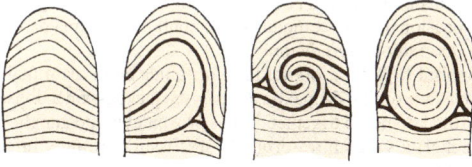

impressões digitais humanas: visão esquemática; da esquerda para a direita: arco, alça, alça dupla, verticilo

Galton system of classification of f.'s, sistema de classificação de impressões digitais de Galton; um sistema de classificação baseado nas variações dos padrões de linhas, que são agrupadas em arcos (*arches*), alças (*loops*) e verticilos (*whorls*) — *A.L.W. system* ou *arch-loop-whorl system*. Os arcos são formados quando as linhas correm de um lado para o outro da polpa do dedo, sem fazer nenhuma volta para trás; os verticilos, quando há uma volta que forma no mínimo um círculo completo; incluem-se também todas as espirais duplas. As abreviaturas utilizadas ao se fazer um registro das impressões digitais são: *a*, para arco; *l*, para alça (loop); *w*, para verticilo; *i*, para alça com uma inclinação interna (para o lado do polegar); *o*, para alça com uma inclinação externa (para o lado do dedo mínimo). Os dez dedos são agrupados em quatro grupos diferenciados por letras maiúsculas, como mostrado a seguir: *A*, para os dedos indicador, médio e anular da mão direita; *B*, para os dedos indicador, médio e anular da mão esquerda; *C*, para o polegar e dedo mínimo da mão direita; *D*, para o polegar e dedo mínimo da mão esquerda. VER TAMBÉM dermatoglyphics.
genetic f., i. d. genética. SIN fingerprint (3).
fin·ger spel·ling. Alfabeto dactilológico; sistema de comunicação por meio de palavras soletradas, utilizado com pessoas que apresentam comprometimento significativo da audição, no qual as letras do alfabeto são representadas por diferentes posições dos dedos das mãos.
Fink, R.P., anatomista norte-americano do século XX. VER F.-Heimer *stain*.
Finkeldey, Wilhelm, patologista alemão do século XX. VER Warthin-F. *cells*, em *cell*.
Finney, John M.T., cirurgião norte-americano, 1863–1942. VER F. *operation*, *pyloroplasty*.

fire (fīr).Queima; em odontologia, a mistura de água e pó que contém caulim, feldspato e outras substâncias, a fim de produzir a porcelana utilizada em restaurações e dentes artificiais.
fire·damp (fīr′damp). Grisu; metano ou outro hidrocarboneto leve que forma uma mistura explosiva, quando misturado com sete ou oito volumes de ar.
first aid. Primeiros socorros; assistência imediata administrada no caso de trauma ou doença súbita por um espectador ou outra pessoa leiga, antes da chegada de pessoal médico treinado.
Fischer, Emil, químico alemão, laureado com o prêmio Nobel, 1852–1919. VER F. projection formulas of *sugars*; Kiliani-Fischer *synthesis*; Kiliani-Fischer *reaction*.
Fischer, Louis, pediatra norte-americano, 1864–1945. VER F. *sign*, *symptom*.
Fishberg, Arthur M., médico norte-americano, *1898. VER F. concentration *test*.
fish ber·ry. As sementes da *Anamirta paniculata* que contêm o amaróide picrotoxina; estimulante do SNC e sistema respiratório, utilizado em medicina veterinária como um antídoto para barbituratos. O nome deriva da prática de amassar e atirar as bagas nos rios, a fim de intoxicar ou incapacitar os peixes.
Fisher, C. Miller, neurologista norte-americano, *1910. VER F. *syndrome*.
Fisher, Ronald A., geneticista e estatístico médico britânico, 1890–1962; criou muitos testes estatísticos.
Fishman-Lerner unit. Unidade de Fishman-Lerner. VER em unit.
fis·sion (fish′un). Fissão, divisão. **1.** O ato de dividir, p.ex., a divisão amitótica de uma célula e seu núcleo. **2.** Divisão do núcleo de um átomo. [L. *fissio*, uma fenda, de *findo*, pp. *fissus*, fender]
binary f., divisão binária; f. simples na qual as duas novas células são aproximadamente do mesmo tamanho.
bud f., divisão por brotamento. SIN gemmation.
multiple f., divisão múltipla; divisão do núcleo, simultânea ou sucessivamente, em vários núcleos-filhos, seguida pela divisão do corpo celular em um número igual de partes, cada uma contendo um núcleo.
simple f., divisão simples; divisão do núcleo e, em seguida, do corpo celular em duas partes. VER TAMBÉM binary f.
fis·si·par·i·ty (fis - i - par′i - tē). Fissiparidade. SIN schizogenesis. [L. *fissio*, fenda, de *findo*, fender, + *pario*, parir]
fis·sip·a·rous (fi - sip′a - rŭs).Fissíparo; que se reproduz ou se propaga por fissão. [L. *findo*, pp. *fissus*, fenda, + *pario*, parir]
fissula (fiz - ū - la). Diminutivo de fissura; uma pequena fissura ou fenda.
f. ante fenestram [TA], pequena passagem, semelhante a uma fenda, localizada na parede labiríntica da cavidade timpânica, que se estende obliquamente a partir da região do processo cocleariforme até o vestíbulo do labirinto ósseo, anteriormente à janela oval; é considerada uma extensão do espaço perilinfático, mas é preenchida por uma pequena faixa de tecido conectivo, contínua com a mucosa da cavidade timpânica.

FISSURA

fis·su·ra, pl. **fis·su·rae** (fi - soo′rā, - soo′re)[TA]. Fissura. **1.** SIN fissure. **2.** Em neuroanatomia, um sulco particularmente profundo da superfície do cérebro ou da medula espinal. [do L. *findo*, fender]
f. antitragohelici′na [TA], f. antitrago-helicina; fissura localizada na cartilagem da orelha, entre a cauda da hélice e o antitrago. SIN antitragohelicine fissure.
f. calcari′na, sulco calcarino. SIN calcarine *sulcus*.
fissu′rae cerebel′li [TA], fissuras do cerebelo. SIN cerebellar fissures, em *fissure*.
f. cer′ebri latera′lis, sulco lateral. SIN lateral *sulcus*.
f. choroi′dea [TA], f. corióidea. SIN optic *fissure*.
f. collatera′lis, sulco colateral. SIN collateral *sulcus*.
f. denta′ta, sulco hipocampal. SIN hippocampal *sulcus*.
f. hippocam′pi, sulco hipocampal. SIN hippocampal *sulcus*.
f. horizonta′lis [TA], f. horizontal do cerebelo. SIN horizontal *fissure* [TA] of cerebellum.
f. horizonta′lis pulmo′nis dex′tri [TA], f. horizontal do pulmão direito. SIN horizontal *fissure* of the right lung.
f. intersemilunaris [TA], f. lunográcil. SIN ansoparamedian *fissure*.
f. intraculminalis [TA], f. intraculminal. SIN intraculminate *fissure*.
f. ligamen′ti tere′tis hepatis [TA], f. do ligamento redondo. SIN *fissure* for ligamentum teres.
f. ligamen′ti veno′si [TA], f. do ligamento venoso. SIN *fissure* for ligamentum venosum.
f. longitudina′lis cer′ebri [TA], f. longitudinal do cérebro. SIN longitudinal cerebral *fissure*.
f. media′na ante′rior medul′lae oblonga′tae [TA], f. mediana anterior do bulbo. SIN anterior median *fissure* of medulla oblongata.
f. media′na ante′rior medul′lae spina′lis [TA], f. mediana anterior da medula espinal. SIN anterior median *fissure* of spinal cord.

f. obli'qua pulmon'is [TA], f. oblíqua do pulmão. SIN oblique fissure of lung.
f. orbita'lis infe'rior [TA], f. orbital inferior. SIN inferior orbital fissure.
f. orbita'lis supe'rior [TA], f. orbital superior. SIN superior orbital fissure.
f. parietooccipita'lis, f. parietooccipital; SIN parietooccipital sulcus.
f. petro-occipita'lis [TA], f. petrooccipital. SIN petrooccipital fissure.
f. petrosquamo'sa [TA], f. petroescamosa. SIN petrosquamous fissure.
f. petrotympan'ica [TA], f. petrotimpânica. SIN petrotympanic fissure.
f. posterior superior [TA], f. póstero-superior. SIN posterior superior fissure.
f. posterolatera'lis [TA], f. póstero-lateral. SIN posterolateral fissure.
f. precentralis [TA], f. pré-central. SIN precentral fissure.
f. preculminalis [TA], f. pré-culminal. SIN preculminate fissure.
f. prepyramidalis [TA], f. pré-piramidal. SIN prepyramidal fissure.
f. pri'ma cerebel'li [TA], f. primária do cerebelo. SIN primary fissure of cerebellum.
f. pterygoid'ea, incisura pterigóidea. SIN pterygoid notch.
f. pterygomaxilla'ris [TA], f. pterigomaxilar. SIN pterygomaxillary fissure.
f. pterygopalati'na, f. pterigopalatina. SIN pterygomaxillary fissure.
f. puden'di, rima do pudendo. SIN pudendal cleft.
f. secun'da cerebel'li [TA], f. secundária do cerebelo. SIN secondary fissure [TA] of cerebellum.
f. sphenopetro'sa [TA], f. esfenopetrosa. SIN petrosphenoidal fissure.
f. transver'sa cerebel'li, f. transversa do cerebelo. SIN transverse fissure of cerebellum.
f. transver'sa cer'ebri [TA], f. transversa do cérebro. SIN transverse cerebral fissure.
f. tympanomastoid'ea [TA], f. timpanomastóidea. SIN tympanomastoid fissure.
f. tympanosquamo'sa [TA], f. timpanoescamosa. SIN tympanosquamous fissure.

fis·sur·al (fish′ŭ-răl). Fissural; relativo a uma fissura.
fis·su·ra·tion (fish′ŭ-rā′shŭn). Fissuração; estado de ser fissurado.

FISSURE

fis·sure (fish′ŭr) [TA]. Fissura. **1.** Sulco, fenda ou abertura profunda. (Para a maioria das fissuras do cérebro, ver as entradas em sulcus.) **2.** Em odontologia, uma fratura ou falha do desenvolvimento localizada no esmalte do dente. SIN fissura (1) [TA]. [L. *fissura*]
abdominal f., f. abdominal; falha congênita no fechamento da parede ventral do corpo. VER TAMBÉM celosomia, gastroschisis.
Ammon f., f. de Ammon; abertura redonda na esclera observada durante o início da embriogênese.
anal f., f. anal; rachadura ou fenda localizada na mucosa do ânus, muito dolorosa e de difícil cicatrização.
ansoparamedian f. [TA], fissura lunográcil; f. que separa o lóbulo H VII A — o pilar II do lóbulo ansiforme — do lóbulo H VII B — o lóbulo paramediano —, localizados no lobo posterior do cerebelo. SIN fissura intersemilunaris [TA], intersemilunar f.
anterior median f. of medulla oblongata [TA], f. mediana anterior do bulbo; sulco longitudinal localizado na linha média da face anterior do bulbo; constitui-se no equivalente bulbar da fissura mediana anterior da medula espinal e termina no forame cego posterior; sua parte caudal é obliterada pela decussação das pirâmides. SIN fissura mediana anterior medullae oblongatae [TA], anteromedian groove (1).
anterior median f. of spinal cord [TA], f. mediana anterior da medula espinal; f. mediana profunda observada na superfície anterior da medula espinal. SIN fissura mediana anterior medullae spinalis [TA], anteromedian groove (2), sulcus ventralis.
antitragohelicine f., f. antitrago-helicina. SIN fissura antitragohelicina.
ape f., f. simiesca; termo obsoleto para o sulco semilunar (lunate *sulcus* [TA]) do lobo occipital.
auricular f., f. timpanomastóidea. SIN tympanomastoid f.
azygos f., f. ázigo; prega pleural, composta por quatro camadas, que separa o lobo ázigo do resto do lobo superior direito do pulmão, observada como uma linha oblíqua que se curva para baixo a partir do ápice direito em direção à sombra do mediastino em uma radiografia de tórax. A veia ázigo é projetada como uma sombra em forma de lágrima na extremidade inferior da f. ázigo.
Bichat f., f. de Bichat; f. quase circular que corresponde à margem medial do manto cerebral (palial), marca o hilo do hemisfério cerebral e é formada pelas fissuras calosomarginal e corióidea ao longo do hipocampo, ambas contínuas com o tronco da f. de Sylvius na extremidade anterior do lobo temporal.
branchial f., f. branquial; fenda branquial persistente.
Broca f., f. de Broca; f. que circunda o giro de Broca.

calcarine f., sulco calcarino. SIN calcarine sulcus.
callosomarginal f., sulco do cíngulo. SIN cingulate sulcus.
caudal transverse f., f. transversa caudal. SIN porta hepatis.
cerebellar f.'s, fissuras do cerebelo; sulcos profundos que dividem os lóbulos do cerebelo. VER TAMBÉM postcentral f., primary f. of cerebellum, secondary f. [TA] of cerebellum. SIN fissurae cerebelli [TA].
cerebral f.'s, fissuras do cérebro; fissuras dos hemisférios cerebrais nomeadas de modo variado. VER TAMBÉM *sulci* cerebri, em *sulcus*.
choroid f., f. corióidea. SIN optic f.
choroidal f. [TA], f. corióidea; **(1)** SIN optic f.; **(2)** fenda estreita localizada na parede medial do ventrículo lateral ao longo das margens onde se fixa o plexo corióideo; a f. está situada entre a superfície superior do tálamo e a margem lateral do fórnice na parte central do ventrículo, e entre a estria terminal e a fímbria do hipocampo no corno inferior. SIN fissura choroidea ventriculi lateralis [TA], choroid f.
Clevenger f., f. de Clevenger, sulco temporal inferior. SIN inferior temporal sulcus.
collateral f., sulco colateral. SIN collateral sulcus.
decidual f., f. da decídua; fenda localizada na decídua basal ou placenta.
dentate f., sulco hipocampal. SIN hippocampal sulcus.
Duverney f.'s, fissuras de Duverney, incisuras na cartilagem do meato acústico. SIN notch in cartilage of acoustic meatus.
Ecker f., f. de Ecker, f. petroccipital. SIN petrooccipital f.
enamel f., f. do esmalte; sulco profundo localizado entre cúspides contíguas que permite a retenção de agentes causadores de cáries.
glaserian f., f. de Glaser, f. petrotimpânico. SIN petrotympanic f.
great horizontal f., f. horizontal do cerebelo. SIN horizontal f. [TA] of cerebellum.
great longitudinal f., f. longitudinal do cérebro. SIN longitudinal cerebral f.
Henle f.'s, fissuras de Henle; pequenos espaços preenchidos com tecido conectivo e localizados entre os fascículos musculares do coração.
hippocampal f., sulco hipocampal. SIN hippocampal sulcus.
horizontal f. of right lung, f. horizontal do pulmão direito. SIN horizontal f. of the right lung.
horizontal f. [TA] of cerebellum, f. horizontal do cerebelo; f. horizontal que divide o lóbulo ansiforme em suas partes principais: o lóbulo semilunar superior (*crus I*) e o lóbulo semilunar inferior (*crus II*). SIN fissura horizontalis [TA], great horizontal f.
inferior accessory f., f. acessória inferior; f. que geralmente separa o segmento basal medial do lobo inferior do pulmão direito de outros segmentos basais, observada ocasionalmente como uma linha oblíqua próxima da borda direita do coração nas radiografias de tórax.
inferior orbital f. [TA], f. orbital inferior; fenda entre a asa maior do osso esfenóide e a face orbital da maxila, através da qual passam a divisão maxilar e o ramo orbital do nervo trigêmeo, fibras provenientes do gânglio pterigopalatino (Meckel) e vasos infra-orbitais. SIN fissura orbitalis inferior [TA], sphenomaxillary f.
intersemilunar f. [TA], f. lunográcil. SIN ansoparamedian f.
intraculminate f. [TA], f. intraculminal; f. do lobo anterior do cerebelo, localizada no interior do cúlmen, que separa os lóbulos IV e V e se estende para a margem lateral do cerebelo. SIN fissura intraculminalis [TA].
lateral cerebral f., sulco lateral do cérebro. SIN lateral sulcus.
left sagittal f., f. sagital esquerda; sulco sagital, localizado na superfície inferior do fígado, formado pela fissura do ligamento redondo, anteriormente, e pela fissura do ligamento venoso, posteriormente.
f. for ligamentum teres [TA], f. do ligamento redondo; sulco localizado na superfície inferior do fígado, estendendo-se da margem inferior até a extremidade esquerda da porta do fígado; essa f. aloja o ligamento redondo do fígado. SIN fissura ligamenti teretis hepatis [TA], f. for round ligament of liver*, fossa venae umbilicalis, umbilical f., umbilical fossa.
f. for ligamentum venosum [TA], f. do ligamento venoso; sulco profundo que se estende da porta do fígado até a veia cava inferior, entre o lobo esquerdo e o lobo caudado; essa f. aloja o ligamento venoso e é, dessa forma, um vestígio da fossa do ducto venoso. SIN fissura ligamenti venosi [TA], f. of venous ligament.
linguogingival f., f. linguogengival; f. que, às vezes, existe sobre a superfície lingual de um dos incisivos superiores e se estende para dentro do cemento.
f.'s of liver, fissuras do fígado. VER left sagittal f., right sagittal f., *porta* hepatis, f. for ligamentum teres, f. for ligamentum venosum.
longitudinal cerebral f. [TA], f. longitudinal do cérebro; fenda profunda que separa os dois hemisférios do cérebro. SIN fissura longitudinalis cerebri [TA], great longitudinal f.
lunate f. [TA], sulco semilunar. SIN lunate sulcus.
f.'s of lung, fissuras do pulmão. VER transverse f. of the right lung, oblique f. of lung.
major f., f. oblíqua do pulmão. SIN oblique f. of lung.
minor f., f. horizontal do pulmão direito. SIN horizontal f. of the right lung.
oblique f., f. oblíqua do pulmão. SIN oblique f. of lung.
oblique f. of lung [TA], f. oblíqua do pulmão; fissura profunda, presente em

cada um dos pulmões, que corre obliquamente para baixo e para a frente. Essa fissura separa o lobo superior do lobo inferior no pulmão esquerdo e separa os lobos superior e médio do lobo inferior no pulmão direito. SIN fissura obliqua pulmonis [TA], major f., oblique f.

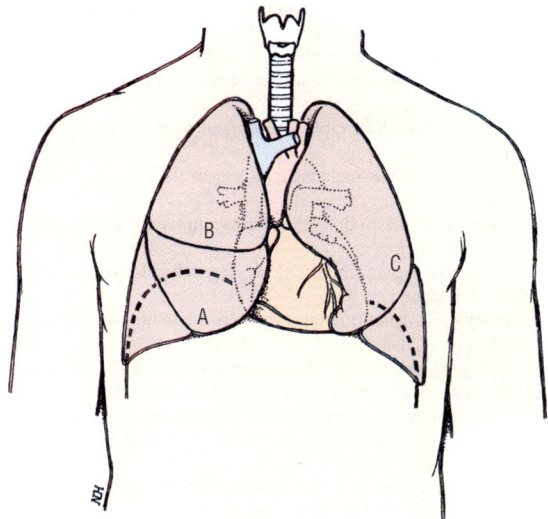

fissuras do pulmão: (A) f. oblíqua e (B) f. horizontal do pulmão direito; (C) f. oblíqua do pulmão esquerdo

optic f., f. corióidea; no embrião, a lacuna temporária localizada na margem ventral do cálice óptico em desenvolvimento. SIN choroidal f. (1) [TA], fissura choroidea [TA], choroid f.
oral f. [TA], rima da boca; a abertura da boca. SIN rima oris [TA], oral opening*.
palpebral f. [TA], rima das pálpebras; fenda da pálpebra ou fissura entre as pálpebras. SIN rima palpebrarum [TA].
Pansch f., f. de Pansch; f. do cérebro (sulco) que corre da extremidade inferior da f. central (sulco) até próximo à extremidade do lobo occipital.
paracentral f., sulco paracentral. VER paracentral *sulcus*.
parietooccipital f., sulco parietoccipital. SIN parietooccipital *sulcus*.
petrooccipital f. [TA], f. petrooccipital; fissura, localizada entre a parte petrosa do osso temporal e a parte basilar do osso occipital, que se estende anteromedialmente a partir do forame jugular; essa f. inclui o forame jugular (na sua extremidade posterior). SIN fissura petro-occipitalis [TA], Ecker f.
petrosphenoidal f. [TA], f. esfenopetrosa; abertura bastante variável localizada entre a parte medial da margem posterior da asa maior do osso esfenóide (posterior ao forame oval) e a parte medial da margem anterior da parte petrosa do osso temporal; essa f. pode ser observada como uma extensão ampla lateral do forame lacerado no crânio seco ou pode estar fechada, especialmente na parte lateral, tomando a forma de uma sutura petroesfenoidal em vez de uma fissura. SIN fissura sphenopetrosa [TA], sphenopetrosal f.
petrosquamous f. [TA], f. petroescamosa; fissura rasa que indica externamente a linha de fusão das partes petrosa e escamosa do osso temporal. SIN fissura petrosquamosa [TA].
petrotympanic f. [TA], f. petrotimpânica; fissura localizada entre as partes timpânica e petrosa do osso temporal; essa f. conduz o nervo corda do tímpano através de uma pequena parte aberta, o canalículo anterior do nervo corda do tímpano. SIN fissura petrotympanica [TA], glaserian f.
portal f., porta do fígado. SIN *porta hepatis*.
postcentral f., sulco pós-central; f. localizada na superfície superior do cerebelo e que separa o cúlmen do lóbulo central.
posterior median f. of the medulla oblongata, sulco mediano posterior do bulbo. SIN posterior median *sulcus* of medulla oblongata.
posterior median f. of spinal cord, sulco mediano posterior da medula espinal. SIN posterior median *sulcus* of spinal cord.
posterior superior f. [TA], f. posterior superior; fissura localizada entre os lóbulos VI e VII do lobo posterior do cerebelo e que se estende até a margem lateral do cerebelo. SIN fissura posterior superior [TA].
posterolateral f. [TA], f. póstero-lateral; última fissura a aparecer durante o desenvolvimento do cerebelo; essa f. separa o flóculo e o nódulo da tonsila e da úvula. SIN fissura posterolateralis [TA], prenodular f.
posthippocampal f., sulco calcarino. SIN calcarine *sulcus*.
postlingual f., f. pós-lingual; fissura transversa localizada no verme superior do cerebelo, separando a língula do lóbulo central.

postlunate f., f. pós-semilunar; fissura transversa localizada no verme superior do cerebelo, separando o lóbulo semilunar inferior, situado anteriormente, do lóbulo ansiforme, situado posteriormente.
postpyramidal f., f. pós-piramidal, fissura secundária do cerebelo; fissura localizada entre a úvula do cerebelo e a pirâmide. SIN fissura secunda cerebelli.
postrhinal f., f. pós-rinal; f. que separa o hipocampo do giro colateral.
precentral f. [TA], f. pré-central; f. localizada entre as partes anterior e posterior (lóbulos II e III) do lóbulo central do lobo anterior do cerebelo; essa f. se estende do verme até a margem do cerebelo; a f. pré-central é encontrada entre os lóbulos I e II, e este último forma a parte anterior do lóbulo central. SIN fissura precentralis [TA].
preculminate f. [TA], f. pré-culminal; f. localizada entre os lóbulos III e IV do lobo anterior do cerebelo, representando a f. entre o lóbulo central e o cúlmen; essa f. se estende do verme até a margem do cerebelo. SIN fissura preculminalis [TA].
prenodular f., f. póstero-lateral. SIN posterolateral f.
prepyramidal f. [TA], f. pré-piramidal, f. entre a pirâmide do cerebelo e o túber do cerebelo. SIN fissura prepyramidalis [TA].
primary f. of cerebellum [TA], f. primária do cerebelo; a f. mais profunda do cerebelo; demarca a divisão entre os lobos anterior e posterior do cerebelo; embriologicamente, é a segunda f. a aparecer. SIN fissura prima cerebelli [TA].
pterygoid f., incisura pterigóidea. SIN pterygoid *notch*.
pterygomaxillary f., f. pterigomaxilar; abertura estreita localizada entre a lâmina pterigóide lateral e a superfície infratemporal da maxila, através da qual a fossa infratemporal se comunica com a fossa pterigóidea; dá passagem à terceira parte da artéria maxilar e às artérias alveolares superiores posteriores, às veias e aos nervos. SIN fissura pterygomaxillaris [TA], fissura pterygopalatina.
rhinal f., sulco rinal. SIN rhinal *sulcus*.
right sagittal f., f. sagital direita; sulco sagital, localizado na superfície inferior do fígado, formado pela fossa da vesícula biliar, anteriormente, e pelo sulco da veia cava, posteriormente.
f. of Rolando, f. de Rolando, sulco central. SIN central *sulcus*.
f. for round ligament of liver, f. do ligamento redondo do fígado; *termo oficial alternativo para f. for ligamentum teres.
Santorini f.'s, fissuras de Santorini, incisura da cartilagem do meato acústico. SIN notch in cartilage of acoustic meatus.
secondary f. [TA] **of cerebellum,** f. secundária do cerebelo, f. pós-piramidal; f. localizada no cerebelo que separa a úvula, no verme inferior, da pirâmide. SIN fissura secunda cerebelli [TA], postpyramidal f.
simian f., sulco semilunar. SIN lunate *sulcus*.
sphenoidal f., f. orbital superior. SIN superior orbital f.
sphenomaxillary f., f. orbital inferior. SIN inferior orbital f.
sphenopetrosal f., f. esfenopetrosa. SIN petrosphenoidal f.
squamotympanic f., f. timpanoescamosa. SIN tympanosquamous f.
superior orbital f. [TA], f. orbital superior; fenda entre a asa maior e a asa menor do osso esfenóide que estabelece um canal de comunicação entre a fossa média do crânio e a órbita, através do qual passam os nervos oculomotor e troclear, a divisão oftálmica do nervo trigêmeo, o nervo abducente e as veias oftálmicas. SIN fissura orbitalis superior [TA], foramen lacerum anterius, sphenoidal f.
superior temporal f., sulco temporal superior. SIN superior temporal *sulcus*.
sylvian f., f. of Sylvius, sulco lateral. SIN lateral *sulcus*.
transverse f. of cerebellum, f. transversa do cerebelo; fenda provocada pela protrusão do lobo anterior do cerebelo sobre os pedúnculos cerebelares superior e médio. SIN fissura transversa cerebelli.
transverse cerebral f., f. transversa do cérebro; espaço triangular, localizado entre o corpo caloso e o fórnice, acima, e a superfície dorsal do tálamo, abaixo; é limitado lateralmente pela f. corióidea do ventrículo lateral, sendo revestido pela pia-máter, e abre-se caudalmente na cisterna da veia cerebral magna do espaço subaracnóideo. SIN fissura transversa cerebri [TA].
transverse f. of the right lung [TA], f. horizontal do pulmão direito; f. profunda que separa os lobos superior e médio do pulmão direito. SIN fissura horizontalis pulmonis dextri [TA], horizontal f. of right lung, minor f.
tympanomastoid f. [TA], f. timpanomastóidea; f. que separa a parte timpânica da parte mastóidea do osso temporal; a f. conduz o ramo auricular do nervo vago. SIN fissura tympanomastoidea [TA], auricular f., tympanomastoid suture.
tympanosquamous f. [TA], f. timpanoescamosa; f. que separa a parte timpânica da parte escamosa do osso temporal; é contínua medialmente com as fissuras petrotimpânica e petroescamosa. SIN fissura tympanosquamosa [TA], squamotympanic f.
umbilical f., f. do ligamento redondo. SIN f. for ligamentum teres.
f. of venous ligament, f. do ligamento venoso. SIN f. for ligamentum venosum.
vestibular f. of cochlea, f. vestibular da cóclea; f. delgada, localizada na parte inferior do primeiro giro da cóclea, formada por uma lâmina espiral que se projeta da parede externa da cóclea, mas não alcança completamente a lâmina espiral óssea, deixando, dessa forma, uma lacuna estreita.
zygal f., figura formada por duas fissuras cerebrais paralelas e próximas unidas por uma f. curta em ângulo reto, resultando em um H.

FISTULA

fis·tu·la, pl. **fis·tu·lae**, **fis·tu·las** (fis'tū-lă, -tū-lē, -tū-lăs). Fístula; comunicação anormal entre uma superfície epitelial e outra superfície epitelial. [L. um cano, um tubo]

abdominal f., f. abdominal; passagem fistulosa que comunica uma víscera abdominal com a superfície externa.

amphibolic f., amphibolous f., f. anfibólica; f. anal completa que se abre tanto interna como externamente.

anal f., f. anal; f. que se abre no ânus ou próximo a este; em geral, porém nem sempre, abre-se no reto, acima do esfíncter interno.

arteriovenous f., f. arteriovenosa; comunicação anormal, ou espontânea, ou criada cirurgicamente entre uma artéria e uma veia.

f. au'ris congen'ita, f. auricular congênita; f. congênita, anterior à raiz da hélice e resultante de um defeito na formação da aurícula da orelha.

biliary f., f. biliar; f. que conduz a alguma parte das vias biliares.

f. bimuco'sa, f. bimucosa; f. completa cujas extremidades se abrem em superfícies mucosas.

blind f., f. em fundo cego; f. que termina em fundo-de-saco, tendo apenas uma das extremidades aberta. SIN incomplete f.

BP f., f. broncopleural. SIN bronchopleural f.

branchial f., f. branquial; f. congênita localizada no pescoço e que resulta do fechamento incompleto de uma fenda ou bolsa branquial.

Brescia-Cimino f., f. de Brescia-Cimino; f. arteriovenosa direta, criada cirurgicamente; utilizada para facilitar a hemodiálise crônica.

bronchobiliary f., f. broncobiliar; comunicação entre um brônquio e as vias biliares; p.ex., após a ruptura de um abscesso hepático.

bronchocavitary f., f. broncocavitária; comunicação entre um brônquio e uma cavidade formada por um abscesso pulmonar.

bronchoesophageal f. f. broncoesofágica; comunicação entre um brônquio e o esôfago; pode ocorrer em associação a uma infecção ou a tumores que envolvem um brônquio ou o esôfago.

bronchopleural f., f. broncopleural; comunicação entre um brônquio e a cavidade pleural; é geralmente causada por pneumonia necrosante ou por empiema; pode também ocorrer após cirurgia ou irradiação do pulmão. SIN BP f.

bronchopleural-cutaneous f., f. broncopleurocutânea; comunicação entre a árvore traqueobrônquica e a pele, atravessando o espaço pleural.

carotid-cavernous f., f. carótico-cavernosa; comunicação fistulosa, de origem espontânea ou traumática, entre o seio cavernoso e a artéria carótida interna transversa; exoftalmia unilateral pulsátil e um sopro craniano detectável são manifestações habituais.

cholecystoduodenal f., f. colecistoduodenal; comunicação anormal entre a vesícula biliar e o duodeno, freqüentemente secundária a colecistite grave com perfuração e formação de abscesso; quando existem cálculos na vesícula biliar, eles podem provocar erosão da parede adjacente do duodeno; se grandes cálculos biliares passarem para o duodeno, eles poderão causar íleo paralítico.

chyle f., f. quilosa; extravasamento de quilo de um vaso linfático para a superfície da pele; uma complicação da dissecção radical do pescoço, quando o ducto torácico é lesado.

coccygeal f., f. coccígea; abertura fistulosa de um cisto dermóide na região coccígea.

colocutaneous f., f. colocutânea; passagem fistulosa que liga o cólon à pele.

coloileal f., f. coloileal; f. que comunica o cólon com o íleo.

colonic f., f. colônica; **(1)** interna, passagem fistulosa que comunica o cólon com uma víscera oca; **(2)** externa, passagem fistulosa que comunica o cólon com a pele.

colovaginal f., f. colovaginal; passagem fistulosa que comunica o cólon com a vagina.

colovesical f., f. colovesical; passagem fistulosa que comunica o cólon com a bexiga urinária. SIN vesicocolic f.

complete f., f. completa; f. que apresenta suas duas extremidades abertas.

congenital pulmonary arteriovenous f., f. arteriovenosa pulmonar congênita; comunicação anormal congênita entre artérias e veias pulmonares, geralmente encontrada no parênquima do pulmão.

dental f., f. dentária, f. gengival. SIN gingival f.

duodenal f., f. duodenal; comunicação que atravessa a parede do duodeno até o interior de um outro órgão revestido por epitélio, ou até a parede abdominal.

dural cavernous sinus f., f. do seio cavernoso da dura-máter; "shunt" vascular entre os ramos meníngeos das artérias carótidas interna e externa. VER internal ou external carotid *arteries* em *artery* e cavernous *sinus*.

Eck f., f. de Eck; transposição da circulação portal para a sistêmica por meio de uma anastomose entre a veia cava e a veia porta e, depois, fazendo uma ligadura desta última próximo ao fígado.

enterocutaneous f., f. enterocutânea; passagem fistulosa que comunica o intestino com a pele do abdome.

enterovaginal f., f. enterovaginal; passagem fistulosa que comunica o intestino com a vagina.

enterovesical f., f. enterovesical; passagem fistulosa que comunica o intestino com a bexiga.

ethmoidal-lacrimal f., f. lacrimoetmoidal; comunicação fistulosa entre o saco lacrimal e o seio etmoidal. SIN internal lacrimal f.

external f., f. externa; passagem fistulosa que comunica uma víscera oca com a pele.

fecal f., f. intestinal. SIN intestinal f.

gastric f., f. gástrica; passagem fistulosa que comunica o estômago com a parede abdominal.

gastrocolic f., f. gastrocólica; passagem fistulosa que comunica o estômago com o cólon.

gastrocutaneous f., f. gastrocutânea; passagem fistulosa que comunica o estômago com a pele.

gastroduodenal f., f. gastroduodenal; passagem fistulosa que comunica o estômago com o duodeno.

gastrointestinal f., f. gastrointestinal; passagem fistulosa que comunica o estômago com o intestino.

genitourinary f., f. genitourinária; abertura fistulosa no sistema urogenital. SIN urogenital f.

gingival f., f. gengival; trajeto sinuoso que se origina em um abscesso periférico e se abre para o interior da cavidade oral sobre a gengiva. SIN dental f.

hepatic f., f. hepática; passagem fistulosa que conduz ao fígado.

hepatopleural f., f. hepatopleural; passagem fistulosa que comunica o fígado com o espaço pleural.

horseshoe f., f. em ferradura; f. anal que circunda parcialmente o ânus e cujas extremidades se abrem na superfície cutânea.

H-type f., f. em H; forma rara de f. traqueoesofágica congênita, na qual não há atresia do esôfago e que se manifesta através de pneumonias aspirativas. SIN H-type tracheoesophageal f.

H-type tracheoesophageal f., f. traqueoesofágica em H. SIN H-type f.

incomplete f., f. incompleta. SIN blind f.

internal f., f. interna; passagem fistulosa que comunica vísceras ocas.

internal lacrimal f., f. lacrimal interna, f. lacrimoetmoidal. SIN ethmoidal-lacrimal f.

intestinal f., f. intestinal; trajeto que conduz da luz intestinal para o exterior. SIN fecal f.

labyrinthine f., f. labiríntica; f. entre um compartimento repleto de líquido da orelha interna e um outro compartimento repleto de líquido da orelha interna (interna), ou um espaço externo à orelha interna, p.ex., a orelha média, as células aéreas mastoideas ou o espaço subaracnóideo (externa); dependendo de sua localização, pode causar distúrbios auditivos e vestibulares.

lacrimal f., f. lacrima'lis, f. lacrimal; abertura anormal que se abre no interior do ducto lacrimal ou do saco lacrimal.

lacteal f., f. mamária, abertura fistulosa para dentro de um dos ductos lactíferos. SIN mammary f.

lymphatic f., f. linfática; f. congênita, localizada no pescoço, que se comunica com um vaso linfático e permite a saída de linfa.

mammary f., f. mamária. SIN lacteal f.

Mann-Bollman f., f. de Mann-Bollman; f. utilizada em investigações experimentais; após isolamento de uma alça do íleo, sua extremidade distal (aboral) é anastomosada lateralmente ao duodeno ou ao intestino delgado, e sua extremidade proximal (oral) aberta é suturada à parede abdominal; as ondas peristálticas avançam da extremidade oral até a aboral, sendo o extravasamento para o exterior, dessa forma, reduzido a um mínimo.

metroperitoneal f., f. uteroperitoneal. SIN uteroperitoneal f.

oroantral f., f. oroantral; comunicação patológica entre a cavidade oral e o seio maxilar, na maioria das vezes uma complicação da extração de um dente da maxila ou de um dente molar.

orofacial f., f. orofacial; comunicação patológica entre a cavidade oral e a face.

oronasal f., f. oronasal; comunicação patológica entre a cavidade oral e a cavidade nasal.

parietal f., f. parietal, f. torácica; f. em fundo cego ou completa que se abre na parede do tórax ou do abdome. SIN thoracic f.

perilymphatic f., f. perilinfática; f. entre o vestíbulo da orelha interna e a orelha média, através da qual a perilinfa pode vazar, causando distúrbios auditivos e vestibulares; os locais comuns de uma f. perilinfática são a janela do vestíbulo através ou ao redor da base do estribo, ou a janela da cóclea através da membrana da janela da cóclea.

perineovaginal f., f. perineovaginal; passagem fistulosa que comunica o períneo com a vagina.

pilonidal f., f. pilonidal, seio pilonidal. SIN pilonidal *sinus.*

pulmonary f., f. pulmonar; f. parietal que se comunica com o pulmão.

rectolabial f., f. retolabial; passagem fistulosa que comunica o reto com a superfície de um dos lábios maiores do pudendo. SIN rectovulvar f.

rectourethral f., f. retouretral; passagem fistulosa que comunica o reto com a uretra.

rectovaginal f., f. retovaginal; passagem fistulosa que comunica o reto com a vagina.
rectovesical f., f. retovesical; passagem fistulosa que comunica o reto com a bexiga.
rectovestibular f., f. retovestibular; passagem fistulosa que comunica o reto com o vestíbulo da vagina.
rectovulvar f., f. retovulvar. SIN rectolabial f.
reverse Eck f., f. de Eck inversa; anastomose látero-lateral da veia porta com a veia cava inferior e ligadura desta última acima da anastomose, porém abaixo das veias hepáticas; o sangue proveniente da parte inferior do corpo é, dessa forma, dirigido através da circulação hepática.
salivary f., f. salivar; comunicação patológica entre um ducto ou glândula salivar com a superfície cutânea.
sigmoidovesical f., f. sigmoidovesical; passagem fistulosa que comunica o cólon sigmóide com a bexiga.
spermatic f., f. espermática; f. que se comunica com o testículo ou com qualquer um dos canais seminais.
T-E f., f. traqueoesofágica. SIN tracheoesophageal f.
Thiry f., f. de Thiry; f. artificial para coletar secreções intestinais de um animal com finalidades experimentais; isolamento de uma alça do intestino com preservação das conexões vasculares e nervosas e restauração do tubo intestinal por meio de uma anastomose término-terminal; uma das extremidades do segmento isolado é fechada, e a outra é ligada à pele do abdome.
Thiry-Vella f., f. de Thiry-Vella; isolamento experimental de um segmento de intestino em um animal; isolamento de uma alça intestinal com preservação das conexões vasculares e nervosas e restauração do tubo intestinal por meio de uma anastomose término-terminal; cada extremidade do segmento isolado é conectada a uma abertura independente na parede abdominal. SIN Vella f.
thoracic f., f. torácica, f. parietal. SIN parietal f.
tracheobiliary fistula, fístula traqueobiliar; anastomose congênita rara entre um brônquio acessório e ductos biliares aberrantes.
tracheoesophageal f., f. traqueoesofágica; passagem fistulosa que comunica a traquéia com o esôfago; está freqüentemente associada à atresia de esôfago; pode também ser adquirida; no adulto, a etiologia é semelhante à da f. broncoesofágica. SIN T-E f.

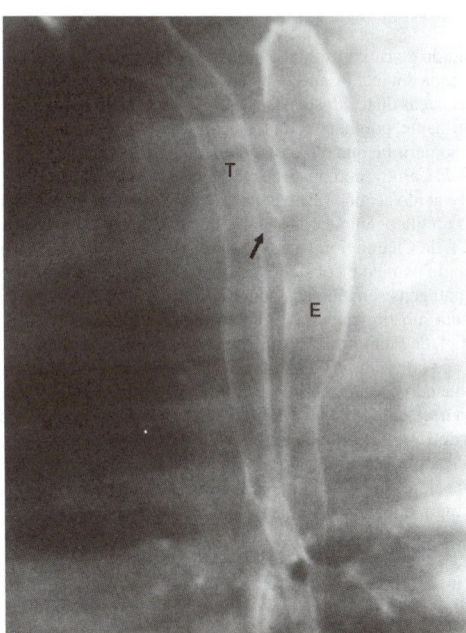

fístula traqueoesofágica: a traquéia (T) e o esôfago (E) estão ligados por uma fístula (seta)

umbilical f., f. umbilical; passagem fistulosa que comunica o intestino ou o úraco com o umbigo.
urachal f., f. do úraco; passagem fistulosa que comunica o úraco com um órgão oco.
ureterocutaneous f., f. ureterocutânea; f. entre o ureter e a pele.
ureterovaginal f., f. ureterovaginal; f. entre a parte inferior do ureter e a vagina.
urethrocutaneous f., f. uretrocutânea; f. entre a uretra e a pele do pênis; a maioria delas é provavelmente uma complicação da correção de hipospádia.
urethrovaginal f., f. uretrovaginal; f. entre a uretra e a vagina.
urinary f., f. urinária; f. que causa drenagem anormal da urina para a pele ou para um outro órgão.

urogenital f., f. urogenital, f. genitourinária. SIN genitourinary f.
uteroperitoneal f., f. uteroperitoneal; passagem fistulosa que comunica a cavidade do útero com a cavidade peritoneal. SIN metroperitoneal f.
Vella f., f. de Vella. SIN Thiry-Vella f.
vesical f., f. vesical; passagem fistulosa da bexiga.
vesicocolic f., f. vesicocólica, f. colovesical. SIN colovesical f.
vesicocutaneous f., f. vesicocutânea; f. entre a bexiga e a pele.
vesicointestinal f., f. vesicointestinal; passagem fistulosa que comunica a bexiga com o intestino delgado.
vesicouterine f., f. vesicouterina; f. entre a bexiga e o útero.

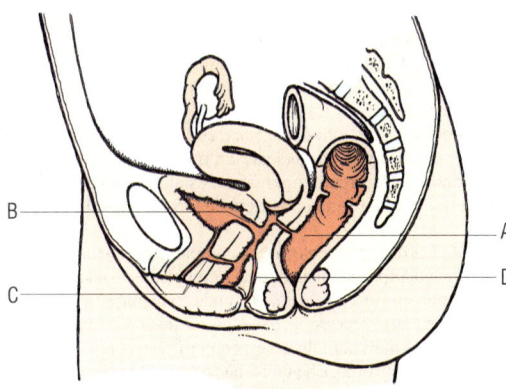

fístula: (A) retovaginal; (B) vesicovaginal; (C) uretrovaginal; (D) vaginoperineal

vesicovaginal f., f. vesicovaginal; f. entre a bexiga e a vagina.
vesicovaginorectal f., f. vesicovaginorretal; passagem fistulosa que comunica a bexiga com a vagina e esta com o reto.
vitelline f., f. vitelina; f. entre o umbigo e o íleo terminal, ao longo do trajeto de um ducto vitelino persistente. VER Meckel *diverticulum*.

fis·tu·la·tion, fis·tu·li·za·tion (fis-tū-lā′shŭn, -tū-li-zā′shŭn). Fistulização; formação de uma fístula em uma região; que se torna fistuloso.
fis·tu·la·tome (fis′tū-lă-tōm). Fistulótomo; bisturi longo com lâmina fina e uma sonda na ponta, utilizado para abrir uma fístula. SIN fistula knife, syringotome. [fistula + G. *tomē*, uma incisão]
fis·tu·lec·to·my (fis-tū-lek′tō-mē). Fistulectomia; excisão de uma fístula. SIN syringectomy. [fistula + G. *ektomē*, excisão]
fis·tu·lo·en·ter·os·to·my (fis′tū-lō-en-ter-os′tō-mē). Fistuloenterostomia; operação que comunica uma fístula com o intestino. [fistula + G. *enteron*, intestino, + *stoma*, boca]
fis·tu·lot·o·my (fis-tū-lot′ō-mē). Fistulotomia; incisão ou alargamento cirúrgico de uma fístula. SIN syringotomy. [fistula + G. *tomē*, incisão]
fis·tu·lous (fis′tū-lŭs). Fistuloso; relativo a ou que contém uma fístula.
fit. 1. Uma crise de uma doença aguda ou o aparecimento súbito de alguns sintomas, tais como a tosse. **2.** Uma convulsão. **3.** (plural) epilepsia. **4.** Em odontologia, a adaptação de uma restauração dentária, p.ex., de um bloco ao preparo cavitário feito em um dente, ou de uma dentadura ao seu suporte basal. [A.S. *fitt*]
induced f., adaptação induzida; alteração conformacional em uma macromolécula (p.ex., proteína), como resultado de múltiplas interações fracas com um ligante ou substrato.
uncinate f., epilepsia do lobo temporal. SIN temporal lobe *epilepsy*.
FITC Abreviatura de fluorescein isothiocyanate (isoticianato de fluoresceína).
fit·ness (fit′nes). **1.** Bem-estar; aptidão; adequação; **1.** Bem-estar. **2.** Conveniência. **3.** Em genética de populações, uma medida da sobrevida relativa e do sucesso reprodutivo de determinado indivíduo ou fenótipo, ou de um subgrupo da população. **4.** Condicionamento; conjunto de atributos, basicamente respiratórios e cardiovasculares, que se relacionam com a capacidade de realizar tarefas que exigem gasto de energia.
clinical f., bem-estar clínico; ausência de doença franca ou de precursores subclínicos.
evolutionary f., adequação evolucionária; a probabilidade de que a linha de descendência de um indivíduo com um traço específico não desaparecerá.
genetic f., adequação genética; o número médio de descendentes sobreviventes que um fenótipo gera durante seu tempo de vida, expresso em geral como uma fração ou porcentagem da adequação genética média da população.
physical f., bem-estar físico; estado de bem-estar no qual o desempenho é máximo.
Fitz-Hugh, T., Jr., médico norte-americano, 1894–1963. VER Fitz-Hugh and Curtis *syndrome*.

fix·a·tion (fik - sā'shŭn). Fixação. **1.** Condição de estar firmemente fixado ou imóvel. **2.** Em histologia, a morte rápida dos elementos de um tecido e a conservação e endurecimento dos mesmos, a fim de reter o mais cedo possível as mesmas relações que apresentavam no corpo vivo. SIN fixing. **3.** Em química, a conversão de um gás para a forma sólida ou líquida por meio de reações químicas, com ou sem o auxílio de tecidos vivos. **4.** Em psicanálise, a qualidade de estar firmemente ligado a uma pessoa, objeto ou período em particular durante seu desenvolvimento. **5.** Em fisiologia óptica, o posicionamento e a acomodação coordenados dos dois olhos que permitem trazer para a fóvea ou manter sobre ela uma imagem nítida de um objeto imóvel ou em movimento. [L. *figo*, pp. *fixus*, fixar, atar]
ammonia f., assimilação da amônia. SIN ammonia *assimilation*.
bifoveal f., f. binocular. SIN binocular f.
binocular f., f. binocular; condição na qual os dois olhos estão simultaneamente direcionados para o mesmo alvo. SIN bifoveal f.
circumalveolar f., f. circum-alveolar; estabilização de um segmento de fratura ou de uma tala cirúrgica por meio de um fio passado através e ao redor do processo alveolar dentário.
circummandibular f., f. circum-mandibular; estabilização de um segmento de fratura ou de uma tala cirúrgica por meio de um fio passado ao redor da mandíbula.
circumzygomatic f., f. circum-zigomática; estabilização de um segmento de fratura ou de uma tala cirúrgica por meio de um fio passado ao redor do arco zigomático.
complement f., f. do complemento; a f. do complemento em um soro pela combinação antígeno-anticorpo, por meio da qual o complemento não está mais disponível para completar uma reação em uma segunda combinação antígeno-anticorpo, na qual o complemento é necessário; o segundo sistema geralmente atua como um indicador (hemácias mais hemolisina específica); se o complemento se fixar ao complexo antígeno-anticorpo, a hemólise não ocorrerá; porém, se o complemento não for assim removido, ele causará hemólise no segundo sistema; essa técnica é a base dos testes de fixação de complemento, amplamente utilizados em laboratórios para a detecção de antígenos e anticorpos. VER TAMBÉM Bordet-Gengou *phenomenon*, Wassermann *test*. SIN CF test, complement binding assay.
craniofacial f., f. craniofacial; estabilização de fraturas faciais que se estendem até a base do crânio por meio de f. direta por fio ou f. externa esquelética por pinos.
crossed f., f. cruzada; no estrabismo convergente, o uso do olho direito virado para dentro para olhar para os objetos à esquerda, e o olho esquerdo virado para dentro para olhar para os objetos à direita, a fim de evitar a rotação ocular.
eccentric f., f. excêntrica; condição monocular na qual a linha de visão conecta um objeto a uma área extrafoveal da retina.
elastic band f., f. com bandagem elástica; estabilização dos segmentos ósseos de uma fratura do maxilar ou da mandíbula por meio de elásticos intermaxilares ligados a suportes ou aparelhos.
external f., f. externa; f. de ossos fraturados por meio de suportes, curativos plásticos ou pinos de transfixação.
external pin f., f. externa por pinos; em cirurgia oral, a estabilização de fraturas da mandíbula, da maxila ou do zigoma por meio de pinos ou parafusos introduzidos na parte óssea através da pele suprajacente e ligados por uma barra metálica.
external pin f., biphase, f. externa por pinos, bifásica; f. por pinos por meio da substituição do conector de barra metálica rígida por uma barra acrílica adaptada no momento da redução da fratura.
freudian f., f. freudiana. VER fixation (4).
genetic f., f. genética; aumento da freqüência de um gene por desvio genético até que nenhum outro alelo seja preservado em uma população finita específica.
intermaxillary f., f. intermaxilar; f. de fraturas da mandíbula ou da maxila por meio da colocação de bandagens elásticas ou fios de aço inoxidável entre as barras dos arcos maxilar e mandibular ou por outros tipos de suporte. SIN mandibulomaxillary f., maxillomandibular f.
internal f., f. interna; estabilização de uma fratura por meio de f. direta dos fragmentos ósseos entre si com fios, parafusos, pinos, talas ou placas cirúrgicas. SIN intraosseous f.
intraosseous f., f. intra-óssea, f. interna. SIN internal f.
mandibulomaxillary f., f. mandibulomaxilar, f. intermaxilar. SIN intermaxillary f.
maxillomandibular f., f. maxilomandibular, f. intermaxilar. SIN intermaxillary f.
nasomandibular f., f. nasomandibular; imobilização da mandíbula, principalmente de mandíbulas desprovidas de dentes, com o uso de suportes maxilomandibulares fixados por meio da conexão de um fio circum-mandibular com um fio interósseo e intra-oral que passa através de um orifício perfurado dentro da espinha nasal anterior das maxilas.
nitrogen f., f. do nitrogênio; processo no qual o nitrogênio atmosférico é convertido a amônia.
fix·a·tive (fik'să - tiv). Fixador. **1.** Que serve para fixar, ligar ou tornar firme ou estável. **2.** Substância utilizada na conservação de amostras histológicas e espessas de tecido ou de células individuais, em geral por desnaturação e precipitação ou ligação cruzada dos elementos proteicos. VER TAMBÉM fluid, solution.
acetone f., f. de acetona; acetona empregada em temperaturas baixas para fixar enzimas, principalmente fosfatases; remove gordura e glicogênio.

AFA f., f. AFA; combinação de álcool, formalina e ácido acético utilizada para a fixação de nematódeos, trematódeos e cestóideos.
alcohol-glycerin f., f. com álcool-glicerina; álcool (70%) e glicerina a 5%; adequado para a fixação da maioria dos nematódeos.
Altmann f., f. de Altmann; um f. de ácido ósmico-dicromato.

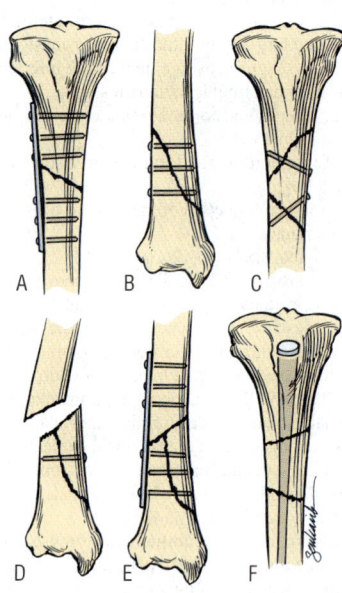

fixação interna: (A) placa e seis parafusos em uma fratura transversa ou oblíqua curta; (B) parafusos em uma fratura oblíqua longa ou em espiral; (C) parafusos em um fragmento em borboleta longo; (D), (E) placa e seis parafusos em um fragmento em borboleta curto; (F) haste medular em uma fratura segmentar

Bouin f., líquido de Bouin; solução de ácido acético glacial, formalina e ácido pícrico, utilizada em tecidos moles e delicados (como aqueles dos embriões) e em pequenas peças de tecidos; conserva o glicogênio e os núcleos e permite a coloração brilhante, porém penetra lentamente, altera o tecido renal e as mitocôndrias e não permite que o método de Feulgen core o DNA.
Carnoy f., f. de Carnoy; composto de etanol, clorofórmio e ácido acético (6:3:1) ou de etanol e ácido acético (3:1); é um f. extremamente rápido empregado na conservação do glicogênio e como um f. nuclear.
Champy f., f. de Champy; mistura composta de dicromato de potássio, ácido crômico e ácido ósmico e considerada um excelente f. citológico com vantagens e desvantagens semelhantes àquelas do f. de Flemming; difere do f. de Flemming pela substituição do dicromato por ácido acético.
Flemming f., f. de Flemming; mistura de ácido crômico, ácido ósmico e ácido acético que age como um excelente f. para citoplasma e cromossomas, principalmente quando o ácido acético é retirado; suas desvantagens são a pobre penetração, a necessidade de lavagem por longo tempo e a rápida deterioração.
formaldehyde f., f. de formaldeído; agente fixador amplamente empregado em histologia patológica; a solução comercial é composta de formaldeído a 37–40% e é conhecida como formalina ou formol a 100%; o ácido fórmico é uma impureza comum que tem de ser neutralizada ou, então, o f. deve ser preparado em solução tamponada; tecidos fixados podem apresentar um pigmento precipitado (artefato).
formol-calcium f., f. de cálcio-formol; f. para a conservação de lipídios.
formol-Müller f., f. de Müller-formol; f. de Müller que contém formalina comercial a 2%.
formol-saline f., f. de solução salina-formol; f. de uso geral empregado em preparações histológicas e histoquímicas.
formol-Zenker f., líquido de Zenker-formol; líquido de Zenker no qual o ácido acético glacial foi substituído pela formalina.
glutaraldehyde f., solução de glutaraldeído; f. empregado em tampões fosfato ou cacodilato em uso em microscopia eletrônica e como um f. de cromatina e enzimas; pode ser utilizado antes do ácido ósmico como um f. auxiliar para conservação das membranas para a microscopia eletrônica.
Golgi osmiobichromate f., f. de ácido ósmico e dicromato, de Golgi; mistura de ácido ósmico e dicromato utilizada para revelar células nervosas e seus processos.
Helly f., líquido de Helly; mistura composta de dicromato de potássio, cloreto de mercúrio, formaldeído e água destilada, empregada em anatomia microscópica como um f. para grânulos citoplasmáticos e colorações nucleares; apresenta as mesmas desvantagens do líquido de Zenker.

Hermann f., f. de Hermann; f. endurecedor composto de ácido acético glacial, ácido ósmico e cloreto de platina.

Kaiserling f., f. de Kaiserling; método de conservação de peças histológicas e patológicas, sem que ocorra alteração de cor, por meio da imersão das peças em uma solução aquosa de nitrato de potássio, acetato de potássio e formalina.

Luft potassium permanganate f., f. de permanganato de potássio de Luft; f. utilizado em microscopia eletrônica na conservação citológica de complexos de lipoproteínas em membranas e na mielina, por causa de suas propriedades oxidativas.

Marchi f., f. de Marchi; mistura composta pelo f. de Müller e por tetróxido de ósmio e na qual o dicromato de potássio do f. de Müller é substituído por clorato de potássio para a obtenção de melhores resultados; utilizado para revelar mielina em degeneração. VER TAMBÉM Marchi *stain*.

methanol f., f. de metanol; f. utilizado em esfregaços de sangue seco e freqüentemente incorporado ao corante empregado.

Müller f., f. de Müller; f. endurecedor composto de dicromato de potássio, sulfato de sódio e água destilada, similar ao f. de Regaud.

neutral buffered formalin f., f. de formalina neutra tamponada; f. histológico de uso geral que apresenta menor probabilidade de formar depósitos de formalina no tecido do que o f. de solução salina-formol.

Newcomer f., f. de Newcomer; f. que contém isopropanol, ácido propiônico e dioxano e é recomendado como substituto para o f. de Carnoy na conservação da cromatina; é também utilizado para fixar polissacarídeos; pequenas peças de tecido precisam ser fixadas, embora retração excessiva ainda possa ocorrer.

Orth f., f. de Orth; formalina adicionada ao f. de Müller; utilizado para destacar a afinidade cromafínica, estudar os processos degenerativos iniciais e a necrose e demonstrar a presença de riquétsias e bactérias.

osmic acid f., f. de ácido ósmico; f. utilizado isoladamente em tampões ou como um pós-fixador após o uso de uma solução fixadora de glutaraldeído em microscopia eletrônica; é um excelente f. de membrana, porém conserva precariamente a cromatina.

Park-Williams f., f. de Park-Williams; f. para espiroquetas, composto de uma solução de ácido ósmico a 2%; as bactérias são expostas durante alguns segundos aos vapores dessa solução.

picroformol f., f. de picroformol; f. que contém formalina e ácido pícrico.

PVA f., f. PVA (*polyvinyl alcohol*); f. de Shaudinn que utiliza uma base de cloreto de mercúrio ou de sulfato de zinco ou de sulfato de cobre; contém pó plástico de álcool polivinílico, utilizado como adesivo em amostras de fezes na preparação de esfregaços permanentes para subseqüente coloração.

Regaud f., f. de Regaud; f. que contém formaldeído e dicromato de sódio e é empregado na conservação de mitocôndrias, mas não de gordura; exige tratamento pós-cromação e lavagem abundante.

SAF f., f. SAF; mistura composta de acetato de *só*dio, ácido *a*cético e *f*ormalina utilizada para fixar amostras de fezes para subseqüente concentração e coloração de esfregaços.

Schaudinn f., f. de Schaudinn; solução de cloreto de mercúrio, cloreto de sódio, álcool e ácido acético glacial, empregada em esfregaços frescos para fixação citológica.

single vial f.'s, fixadores em frasco único; soluções patenteadas e comercialmente disponíveis utilizadas para a fixação de fezes; uma solução, um corante permanente e alguns procedimentos de imunoensaio podem ser elaborados a partir de um único frasco.

Thoma f., f. de Thoma; ácido nítrico em álcool a 95%, empregado em ossos descalcificados para a preparação de peças histológicas.

Zenker f., líquido de Zenker; f. rápido composto de cloreto de mercúrio, dicromato de potássio, sulfato de sódio, ácido acético glacial e água e utilizado em colorações tricrômicas; deve ser lavado para a remoção do dicromato de potássio e tratado com solução de iodo para a remoção do cloreto de mercúrio; os tecidos tendem a tornar-se friáveis se deixados no fixador por mais de 24 horas.

fix·a·tor (fik-sā′ter). Fixador; dispositivo que proporciona imobilização rígida por meio da fixação externa dos ossos, utilizando-se varetas (fixadores) fixadas a pinos os quais são colocados no osso (ou através dele).

fix·ing (fik′sing). Fixação. SIN fixation (2).

flac·cid (flak′sid, flas′id). Flácido; relaxado, frouxo ou sem tônus. [L. *flaccidus*]

flac·cid·i·ty (fla-sid′i-tē). Flacidez; a condição ou o estado de estar flácido.

Flack, Martin W., fisiologista britânico, 1882–1931. VER F. *node*; Keith and F. *node*.

fla·gel·la (flă-jel′ă). Flagelos; plural de flagellum.

fla·gel·lar (fla-jel′ăr). Relativo a um flagelo ou à extremidade de um protozoário.

Flag·el·la·ta (flaj′ĕ-lā′tă). Antigo nome de Mastigophora.

flag·el·late (flaj′ĕ-lāt). Flagelado. **1.** Que possui um ou mais flagelos. **2.** Nome comum dado a um membro da classe Mastigophora.
  collared f., coanomastigota. SIN choanomastigote.

flag·el·lat·ed (flaj′ĕ-lā-ted). Flagelado; que possui um ou mais flagelos.

flag·el·la·tion (flaj′ĕ-lā′shŭn). Flagelação. **1.** Chicotear a si mesmo (autoflagelação) ou outra pessoa como forma de despertar ou aumentar o prazer sexual. **2.** Padrão de formação de flagelos. [L. *flagellatus*, de *flagello*, chicotear ou açoitar]

fla·gel·lin (flaj′ĕ-lin). Flagelina; qualquer membro de uma classe de proteínas que contém o aminoácido ε-N-metillisina; essa classe representa o principal componente proteico dos flagelos das bactérias.

flag·el·lo·sis (flaj′ĕ-lō′sis). Infecção por protozoário flagelado, localizada no trato intestinal ou genital, p.ex., tricomoníase.

fla·gel·lum, pl. **fla·gel·la** (flă-jel′ŭm, -ă). Flagelo; organela de locomoção, semelhante a um chicote, com arranjo estrutural constante, que consiste em nove pares de microtúbulos periféricos e dois microtúbulos centrais; origina-se um grânulo basal intensamente corado, freqüentemente ligado ao núcleo por uma fibra, o rizoplasto. Embora o flagelo seja uma característica dos protozoários da classe Mastigophora, estruturas comparáveis são comumente encontradas em muitos outros grupos, p.ex., em espermatozóides. [L. dim. de *flagrum*, um chicote]

flam·ma·ble (flam′ă-bl). Inflamável; propriedade que consiste em queimar pronta e rapidamente. SIN inflammable. [L. *flamma*, chama]

flange (flanj). Rebordo; a parte da base da dentadura que se estende das extremidades cervicais dos dentes até a borda da dentadura.
  buccal f., rebordo bucal; parte do rebordo de uma dentadura que ocupa o vestíbulo bucal da boca.
  denture f., rebordo da dentadura; **(1)** a extensão comumente vertical do corpo da dentadura para dentro de um dos vestíbulos da cavidade oral; também, em uma dentadura inferior, a extensão comumente vertical ao longo do lado lingual do sulco alveololingual; **(2)** as extensões bucal e labial verticais da base da dentadura superior ou inferior, e a extensão lingual vertical da dentadura inferior; os rebordos bucal e labial da dentadura apresentam duas superfícies: a superfície bucal ou labial e a superfície do suporte basal; o rebordo lingual inferior também apresenta duas superfícies: a superfície do suporte basal e a superfície lingual.
  labial f., rebordo labial; parte do rebordo de uma dentadura que ocupa o vestíbulo labial da boca.
  lingual f., rebordo lingual; parte do rebordo de uma dentadura mandibular que ocupa o espaço adjacente à língua.

flank [TA]. Flanco; área do abdome situada em cada lado da região umbilical, entre o plano transpilórico e o plano intertubercular ou interespinal. SIN latus [TA], lateral abdominal region*, lateral region of abdominal region*, regio abdominis lateralis*, regio lateralis abdominis*.

flap. Retalho. **1.** Tecido para transplante, vascularizado por um pedículo. VER TAMBÉM local f., distant f. **2.** Movimento não controlado, como o que pode ocorrer com as mãos. VER asterixis. [I. m. *flappe*]
  Abbe f., r. de Abbe; parte média do lábio inferior transferida para o lábio superior e vascularizada pela artéria labial.
  advancement f., r. de avanço, r. bipediculado. SIN bipedicle f.
  arterial f., r. arterial; r. com uma artéria nutriente e veias de drenagem conhecidas. Cf. random pattern f.
  axial pattern f., r. de padrão axial; r. que inclui uma artéria específica direta dentro de seu eixo longitudinal.
  bipedicle f., r. bipediculado, r. de avanço; retalho com dois pedículos, um em cada extremidade. SIN advancement f., double pedicle f.
  bone f., r. ósseo; parte do crânio que foi removida, mas permanece ligada ao suprimento sanguíneo do revestimento musculofascial; o termo é freqüentemente utilizado de forma incorreta para uma secção do crânio completamente isolada, ou seja, um enxerto ósseo.

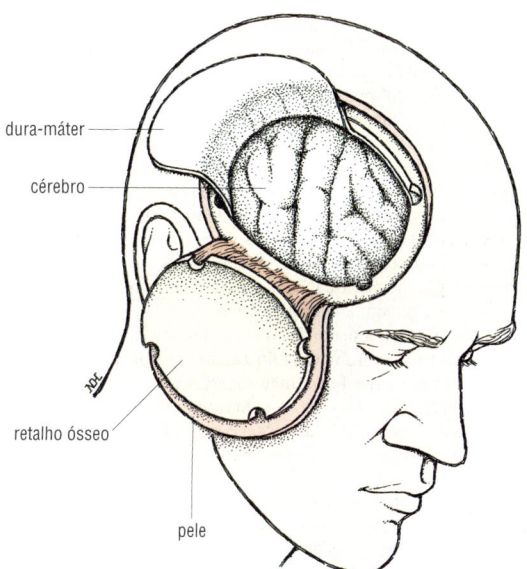

retalho ósseo

buried f., r. sepultado; r. transferido para dentro dos tecidos subcutâneos, após a retirada do epitélio da superfície e da derme superficial.
Byars f., r. de Byars; r. de pele feito de prepúcio dorsal e utilizado para cobrir a parte ventral do pênis em pacientes com corda peniana e/ou hipospádia.
composite f., compound f., r. composto; r. formado por dois ou mais tecidos, que compreendem pele, músculo subcutâneo, osso ou cartilagem.
cross f., r. cruzado; r. de pele transferido de uma parte do corpo para outra parte correspondente, p.ex., r. transferido de um braço para o outro.
delayed f., r. tardio; r. que sofre incisão e/ou é levantado de sua área doadora em duas ou mais etapas, a fim de aumentar as possibilidades de sucesso após a transferência.
deltopectoral f., r. deltopeitoral; r. de pele de padrão axial das regiões deltóidea e peitoral ligado aos vasos mamários internos.
direct f., r. direto; r. completamente levantado e transferido na mesma etapa do procedimento.
distant f., r. a distância; r. de uma área doadora que está distante da área receptora. No passado, esse procedimento exigia várias etapas; agora os retalhos a distância são transferidos por meio de anastomose microvascular da artéria e veia.
double pedicle f., r. bipediculado, r. de avanço. SIN bipedicle f.
Eloesser f., r. de Eloesser; abertura criada cirurgicamente na camada pele–revestimento para a drenagem crônica de um empiema, que freqüentemente acompanha a pneumonectomia. VER TAMBÉM Eloesser *procedure*.
envelope f., r. em envelope; r. mucoperiostal retraído a partir de uma incisão horizontal ao longo da margem gengival livre.
Estlander f., r. de Estlander; r. de espessura total do lábio, transferido do lado de um lábio para o mesmo lado do outro lábio. Variações epônimas desse princípio são os retalhos de Sabbatini, de Stein e de Abbe.
Filatov f., r. de Filatov, r. tubular. SIN tubed f.
Filatov-Gillies f., r. de Filatov-Gillies, r. tubular. SIN tubed f.
free f., r. livre; r. no qual os vasos doadores são seccionados, o tecido é transportado para outra área e o r. é revascularizado por meio de anastomoses feitas entre os vasos do leito receptor e a artéria e a(s) veia(s) do r.
free bone f., r. ósseo livre; parte do crânio removida e isolada das estruturas sobrejacentes de tecidos moles.
full-thickness f., r. de espessura total; r. de espessura total de mucosa e submucosa ou de pele e tecidos subcutâneos.
gingival f., r. gengival; parte da gengiva cuja margem coronal é cirurgicamente isolada do dente e do processo alveolar.
hinged f., r. em dobradiça; r. de rotação transferido para a área receptora levantando-o como se o pedículo fosse uma dobradiça.
Indian f., r. de uma área contígua, tal como a bochecha ou a testa, utilizado para a reconstrução do nariz.
interpolated f., r. que é rodado sobre a pele intacta para uma área adjacente.
island f., r. em ilha; r. cujo pedículo consiste somente em uma artéria nutriente e veia(s) de drenagem e, às vezes, em um nervo.
Italian f., r. proveniente de uma área distante; termo geralmente utilizado em referência a um r. do braço para reconstruir o nariz.
jump f., r. em salto; r. distante transferido em etapas através de um transportador intermediário; p.ex., um r. abdominal é fixo ao punho e, em uma etapa posterior, daí para a face.
lined f., r. revestido; r. coberto com epitélio dos dois lados; p.ex., um r. de pele dobrada.
liver f., VER asterixis.
local f., r. local; r. transferido para uma área adjacente, com o pedículo intacto.
mucoperichondrial f., r. mucopericondrial; r. composto de mucosa e pericôndrio, como o obtido do septo nasal.
mucoperiosteal f., r. mucoperiosteal; r. composto de mucosa e periósteo, como os obtidos do palato duro e da gengiva.
musculocutaneous f., r. miocutâneo. SIN myocutaneous f.
myocutaneous f., r. miocutâneo; r. de pele pediculado, freqüentemente um r. em ilha, acompanhado do músculo subjacente, de revestimentos e de suprimento sanguíneo. SIN musculocutaneous f., myodermal f.
myodermal f., r. miocutâneo. SIN myocutaneous f.
neurovascular f., r. neurovascular; r. que contém um nervo sensorial; utilizado para restaurar a sensibilidade da área receptora.
omental f., r. omental; segmento de omento, com seu suprimento de vasos sangüíneos, transplantado com um pedículo intacto, ou como tecido solto, para uma área distante e revascularizado por meio de anastomoses arteriais e venosas.
osteoplastic bone f., r. osteoplásico; tecido vascularizado que compreende osso vivo, geralmente acompanhado de fáscia e músculo, que pode ser ligado por seu pedículo ou transferido por meio de anastomose microvascular de uma área para outra.
pedicle f., r. pediculado; em cirurgia periodontal, um r. utilizado para aumentar a largura da gengiva inserida ou para cobrir a superfície de uma raiz, pelo deslocamento da gengiva inserida, que permanece presa em um dos lados, para uma posição adjacente e pela sutura da extremidade livre.
pericoronal f., r. pericoronal; r. de gengiva que cobre um dente que não sofreu erupção, principalmente o terceiro molar inferior.

pharyngeal f., r. faríngeo; r. de mucosa e músculo destacado da parede posterior da faringe e fixado ao palato mole, a fim de obturar a passagem velofaríngea e, assim, corrigir o escape de ar nasal; utilizado em pacientes com disfunção velofaríngea, em geral acompanhada de fenda palatina.
random pattern f., r. de padrão aleatório; r. no qual o suprimento sangüíneo do pedículo deriva aleatoriamente da rede de vasos da área, em vez de derivar de uma única artéria longitudinal como ocorre em um r. de padrão axial.
rotation f., r. de rotação; r. pediculado que é rodado a partir do local doador para uma área receptora adjacente.
skin f., r. de pele; r. composto de pele e de seu tecido subcutâneo subjacente.

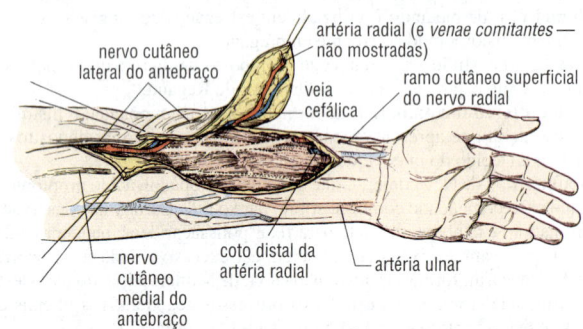

retalho radial do antebraço

subcutaneous f., r. subcutâneo; r. pediculado, desprovido de epitélio e introduzido no tecido subcutâneo da área receptora.
tubed f., r. tubular; antiga técnica de transferência de pele, na qual se retirava um r. retangular, suturava-se um dos lados com o outro e inseria-se o tubo assim formado dentro de outra área. SIN Filatov f., Filatov-Gillies f., tubed pedicle f.
tubed pedicle f., r. pediculado tubular. SIN tubed f.
V-Y f., r. em V-Y; r. no qual a incisão é feita em forma de V, e que é suturado em forma de Y, a fim de se ganhar comprimento adicional de tecido. SIN V-Y plasty.
flare (flār). **1.** Afunilamento gradual ou dilatação para fora. **2.** Rubor; vermelhidão difusa da pele que se estende para além da reação local à aplicação de um agente irritante; é causada pela dilatação de arteríolas e capilares; depende de um reflexo nervoso desencadeado pela liberação de uma substância histamina-símile na pele, quando lesada. VER TAMBÉM triple *response*.
aqueous f., o efeito Tyndall observado no líquido da câmara anterior do olho.
flash. 1. Clarão de luz ou emissão de calor súbitos e breves. **2.** Material em excesso eliminado entre os cortes de uma mufla no processo de moldagem das bases de dentaduras ou outras restaurações dentárias.
hot f., fogacho; coloquialismo para um dos sintomas vasomotores do climatério que pode envolver o corpo inteiro como uma onda de calor; também utilizado de forma intercambiável com hot *flush*.
flash·back. Flashback; relembrar involuntariamente alguns elementos de uma experiência alucinatória ou distorção da percepção que ocorre algum tempo após a ingestão de alucinógeno que produziu o efeito original e sem ingestão subseqüente da substância.
flask. Frasco, balão de vidro, mufla; pequeno recipiente, geralmente de vidro, utilizado para armazenar líquidos, pós ou gases. [I.m. keg, do Fr. *flasque*, do Alemão]
casting f., mufla refratária. SIN refractory f.
crown f., mufla para coroas. SIN denture f.
denture f., mufla para dentaduras; caixa de metal dividida em duas partes na qual é feito um molde seccional de gesso ou pedra, com o propósito de comprimir e curar dentaduras ou outras restaurações de resina. SIN crown f.
Dewar f., frasco de Dewar; recipiente de vidro, freqüentemente prateado, com duas paredes, cujo espaço interno é evacuado; utilizado para manter materiais sob temperatura constante ou, mais comumente, sob baixas temperaturas. SIN vacuum f.
Erlenmeyer f. f. de Erlenmeyer; f. com uma base larga, corpo cônico e gargalo estreito; sua forma permite que o conteúdo líquido seja agitado lateralmente sem derramamento.
Fernbach f., frasco de Fernbach; f. utilizado em fermentações microbianas nas quais uma grande superfície de substrato líquido é necessária.
Florence f., balão de Florence; garrafa de vidro fino, globular e com gargalo longo utilizada para armazenar água ou outro líquido em trabalhos laboratoriais.
hatching f., frasco para incubação; f. pintado de cor escura de forma que somente uma pequena área de água desclorada no topo seja exposta à luz, simulando assim as condições encontradas em reservatórios de água, que estimulam a incubação de ovos de esquistossomas vivos presentes em fezes e sedi-

mentos urinários frescos colocados no f.; utilizado na pesquisa de larvas — miracídeos — liberadas por certos caramujos que atuam como hospedeiros intermediários.

injection f., mufla de injeção; mufla de dentadura projetada de forma a permitir o fluxo forçado do material de base da dentadura a partir de um reservatório para dentro do molde, após a mufla ter sido fechada e durante a cura.

refractory f., mufla refratária; tubo de metal no qual é feito um molde refratário para fundir restaurações ou aparelhos dentários de metal. SIN casting f., casting ring.

vacuum f., frasco de vácuo. SIN Dewar f.

volumetric f., frasco volumétrico; f. calibrado e de gargalo estreito que armazena ou fornece uma quantidade definida de líquido.

flask·ing. Inclusão em mufla; processo de inclusão do gesso e de uma dentadura de cera em uma mufla preparatória, a fim de moldar o material de base da dentadura na forma da dentadura.

Flatau, Edward, neurologista polonês, 1869–1932. VER F. *law.*

flat·foot (flat′fut). Pé plano. SIN *pes planus.*

flat·u·lence (flat′u - lens). Flatulência; excesso de gás no estômago e nos intestinos. [L. mod. *flatulentus,* do L. *flatus,* um sopro, de *flo,* pp. *flatus,* soprar]

flat·u·lent (flat′u - lent). Flatulento; relativo a ou que sofre de flatulência.

fla·tus (flā′tus). Flato; gás ou ar dentro do sistema gastrointestinal que pode ser expelido através do ânus. [L. um sopro]

f. vagina'lis, f. vaginal; expulsão de gás proveniente da vagina.

flat·worm (flat′werm). Platelminto; membro do filo Platyhelminthes, que inclui tênias parasitas e trematódeos.

fla·ve·do (fla - vē′dō). Amarelamento; tom amarelado ou palidez da pele. [L. *flavus,* amarelo]

fla·vi·an·ic ac·id (flā - vē - an′ik) [I.C. 10316]. Ácido flaviânico; corante derivado do naftol, utilizado na precipitação e subseqüente determinação da arginina e de outras substâncias básicas.

fla·vin, fla·vine (flā′vin, - vēn, flav′in, - ēn). 1. Riboflavina. SIN riboflavin. 2. Flavina; corante amarelo de acridina encontrado em preparações utilizadas como agente anti-séptico. [L. *flavus,* amarelo]

f. adenine dinucleotide (FAD), flavina adenina dinucleotídeo; produto da condensação da riboflavina e da adenosina 5′-difosfato; a coenzima de diversas desidrogenases aeróbicas, p.ex., a ácido D-amino oxidase e a aldeído desidrogenase; estritamente falando, essa substância não é um dinucleotídeo, uma vez que contém um álcool de açúcar; a coenzima é reduzida de maneira reversível a $FADH_2$.

electron transfer f., f. transportadora de elétrons; flavoproteínas que participam da via de transporte de elétrons.

f. mononucleotide (FMN), flavina mononucleotídeo; riboflavina 5′-fosfato; a coenzima de várias enzimas de óxido-redução; p.ex., a NADH desidrogenase. Estritamente falando, essa substância não é um nucleotídeo, visto que contém um álcool de açúcar em vez de um açúcar; a coenzima é reduzida de maneira reversível a $FMNH_2$. SIN riboflavin 5′-phosphate.

Fla·vi·vi·ri·dae (flā′vī - vī′rā - dā). Família de vírus ARN de filamento único de sentido positivo e envoltos por um envelope, com 40 a 60 mm de diâmetro, antigamente classificada como "grupo B" dos arbovírus, que engloba os vírus da febre amarela e da dengue; mantido na natureza pela transmissão de vetores artrópodes a hospedeiros vertebrados.

Fla·vi·vi·rus (flā′vi - vī - rŭs). Gênero da família Flaviviridae que engloba os vírus da febre amarela, da dengue e da encefalite de St. Louis. [L. *flavus,* amarelo, + virus]

Fla·vo·bac·te·ri·um (flā - vō - bak - tēr′ē - ŭm). Gênero de bactérias aeróbicas e anaeróbicas facultativas, não-esporuladas, móveis e imóveis (família Achromobacteraceae), composto de bacilos Gram-negativos; as células móveis são peritríquias. Esses microrganismos produzem, caracteristicamente, pigmentos amarelos, laranja, vermelhos ou castanho-amarelados. São encontrados no solo e na água fresca e salgada. Algumas espécies são patogênicas. A espécie-tipo é *F. aquatile.* [L. *flavus,* amarelo]

F. aqua'tile, espécie encontrada na água que contém alta porcentagem de carbonato de cálcio; é a espécie típica do gênero *Flavobacterium.*

F. bre've, espécie encontrada nos esgotos; é patogênica para animais de laboratório.

F. meningisepticum, espécie de bactéria — encontrada na flora normal do sistema respiratório humano — que provoca ocasionalmente infecção nosocomial, que engloba a meningite neonatal.

F. piscici'da, nome antigo da *Pseudomonas piscicida.*

fla·vo·en·zyme (flā - vō - en′zim). Flavoenzima; qualquer enzima que possui uma flavina nucleotídeo como coenzima; p.ex., xantina oxidase, succinato desidrogenase. SIN yellow enzyme.

fla·vo·ki·nase (flā - vō - kī′nās). Flavocinase. SIN riboflavin kinase.

fla·vone (flā′vōn). Flavona. 1. Pigmento vegetal que constitui a base dos flavonóides; potente inibidor da biossíntese das prostaglandinas. 2. Composto que pertence a uma classe de compostos que têm como base a flavona (1).

fla·vo·noids (flā′vō - noydz). Flavonóides. 1. Substâncias de origem vegetal que contêm flavona em diversas combinações (antoxantinas, apigeninas, flavonas, quercitinas, etc.) e que apresentam atividades biológicas variadas. 2. Derivados da flavona.

fla·vo·nol (flā′ - vō - nol). Flavonol. 1. Flavona reduzida. 2. Flavona (1) hidroxilada na posição 3; um membro de uma classe de pigmentos vasculares. 3. Qualquer flavona hidroxilada.

fla·vo·pro·tein (flā′vō - prō′tēn). Flavoproteína; proteína composta que possui uma flavina como grupo prostético. Cf. flavoenzyme.

fla·vor (flā′ver). 1. Sabor; qualidade (influenciada pelo odor) que afeta o gosto de qualquer substância. 2. Aromatizante; substância terapeuticamente inerte, adicionada à fórmula de um medicamento para dar um sabor agradável ao preparado. [I.m., do Fr. ant., do L. ant. *flator,* aroma, de *flo,* soprar]

fla·vox·ate hy·dro·chlo·ride (flā - vok′sāt). Cloridrato de flavoxato; agente relaxante da musculatura lisa para o sistema urinário.

fla·vus (flā′vŭs). Flavo; amarelo, em latim. [L.]

flax·seed (flaks′sēd). Semente do linho, linhaça; SIN linseed.

f. oil, óleo de linhaça. SIN linseed oil.

flea (flē). Pulga; inseto da ordem Siphonaptera, caracterizado por achatamento bilateral, aparelho bucal sugador, capacidade extraordinária para pular e vida adulta ectoparasítica entre os pêlos e as penas de animais de sangue quente. Dentre as pulgas importantes estão: *Ctenocephalides felis* (p. do gato), *C. canis* (p. do cão), *Pulex irritans* (p. do homem), *Tunga penetrans* (bicho-de-pé, bicho-de-porco), *Echidnophaga gallinacea* (p. do picão), *Xenopsylla* (p. do rato) e *Ceratophyllus.* VER TAMBÉM Copepoda.

fle·cai·nide ac·e·tate (flē - kā′nid). Acetato de flecainida; membro do grupo de antiarrítmicos estabilizadores de membrana, com atividade anestésica local, utilizado no tratamento de arritmias ventriculares refratárias.

Flechsig, Paul E., neurologista alemão, 1847–1929. VER F. *areas,* em *area,* ground *bundles,* em *bundle; fasciculi,* em *fasciculus, tract;* oval *area* of F.; semilunar *nucleus* of F.

Flegel, H., dermatologista alemão do século XX. VER F. *disease.*

Fleisch, Alfred, médico e fisiologista suíço, 1892–1973. VER F. *pneumotachograph.*

Fleischer, Bruno, oftalmologista alemão, 1874–1965. VER F. *ring, vortex;* Kayser-F. *ring;* Fleischer-Strümpell *ring.*

Fleischmann, Friedrich Ludwig, anatomista alemão do século XIX. VER sublingual *bursa.*

Fleischner, Felix, radiologista austro-americano, 1893–1969. VER F. *lines,* em *line.*

Fleitmann, Theodore, químico alemão do século XIX. VER F. *test.*

Fleming, Sir Alexander, bacteriologista escocês, 1881–1955, co-ganhador do prêmio Nobel de 1945 pela descoberta da penicilina.

Flemming, Walther, anatomista alemão, 1843–1905. VER intermediate *body* of F.; germinal *center* of F.; *fixative,* triple *stain.*

Flesch, Rudolf F., educador austríaco, *1911. VER F. *formula.*

flesh (flĕsh). 1. A carne de animais utilizada como alimento. 2. Tecido muscular. SIN muscular *tissue.* [A.S. *flaesc*]

goose f., cutis anserina. SIN *cutis anserina.*

proud f., c. esponjosa; termo histórico para denominar as granulações exuberantes presentes no tecido de granulação encontrado na superfície de uma ferida.

flesh·flies (flesh′flīz). Moscas varejeiras; membros da ordem Diptera, cujas larvas se desenvolvem em tecidos vivos ou em putrefação. As larvas de tecidos vivos produzem miíase e incluem larvas de gasterofilídeos (tanto as invasoras primárias como as secundárias); as larvas da lã de carneiro; as moscas varejeiras ou as larvas da pele de humanos e animais domésticos (incluindo as moscas do berne); as moscas varejeiras da cabeça ou do nariz de carneiros, bodes, cavalos, camelos e veados; e as moscas varejeiras dos cavalos, cujas larvas se desenvolvem no estômago, duodeno e reto dos cavalos.

flex (fleks). Flexionar; dobrar; mover uma articulação de tal forma que ocorra a aproximação das duas partes que ela articula. [L. *flecto,* pp. *flexus,* dobrar]

flex·i·bil·i·tas ce·rea (flek - si - bil′i - tas sē′rē - ā). A rigidez da catalepsia, que pode ser vencida por força externa suave, mas que retorna imediatamente, mantendo o membro firmemente na nova posição. [L. flexibilidade cérea]

flex·im·e·ter (flek - sim′e - ter). Goniômetro. SIN goniometer (3).

flex·ion (flek′shŭn). [TA]. Flexão. 1. O ato de flexionar ou dobrar, p.ex., o dobramento de uma articulação de modo a aproximar as partes que ela articula; a flexão da coluna de forma que a concavidade da curvatura se volte para a frente. 2. A condição de estar fletido ou dobrado. [L. *flecto,* pp. *flexus,* dobrar]

palmar f., f. palmar; a flexão da mão ou dos dedos da mão em direção à superfície palmar.

plantar f., f. plantar; a flexão do pé ou dos artelhos em direção à superfície plantar.

Flexner, Simon, patologista norte-americano, 1863–1946. VER F. *bacillus.*

flex·or (flek′ser, - sōr) [TA]. Flexor; músculo cuja ação é a de flexionar uma articulação.

flex·u·ra, pl. **flex·u·'rae** (flek - shūr′ā, - shūr′ē). [TA]. Flexura. SIN flexure. [L. uma curvatura]

f. anorectalis [TA], f. anorrectal. SIN anorectal *flexure.*

f. colica splenica, f. esquerda do cólon; *termo oficial alternativo para left colic flexure.
f. co'li dex'tra [TA], f. direita do cólon. SIN right colic flexure.
f. coli hepatis, f. direita do cólon. SIN right colic flexure.
f. co'li sinis'tra [TA], f. esquerda do cólon. SIN left colic flexure.
f. duode'ni infe'rior [TA], f. inferior do duodeno. SIN inferior duodenal flexure.
f. duode'ni supe'rior [TA], f. superior do duodeno. SIN superior duodenal flexure.
f. duode'nojejuna'lis [TA], f. duodenojejunal. SIN duodenojejunal flexure.
f. perinea'lis (canalis ani), f. anorretal; *termo oficial alternativo para anorectal flexure.
f. sacra'lis rec'ti [TA], f. sacral. SIN sacral flexure of rectum.
f. sigmoid'ea, cólon sigmóide. SIN sigmoid colon.
flex·ur·al (flek′sher-ăl). Flexural; relativo a uma flexura.
flex·ure (flek′sher) [TA]. Flexura; uma curvatura, como as encontradas em órgãos ou estruturas do corpo. SIN flexura [TA]. [L. *flexura*]
  anorectal f. [TA], f. anorretal; curva ou ângulo ântero-posterior da junção anorretal, com convexidade direcionada para a frente; o tônus do músculo puborretal produz o ângulo que mantém a continência fecal; o relaxamento do músculo diminui o ângulo, permitindo a defecação. SIN flexura anorectalis [TA], flexura perinealis (canalis ani)*, perineal f. of anal canal*, anorectal angle, perineal f. of rectum.
  basicranial f., f. pontina. SIN pontine f.
  caudal f., f. sacral; curvatura localizada na região lombossacral do embrião. SIN sacral f.

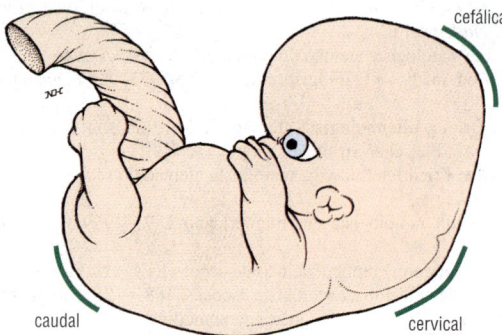

flexuras: observadas em um embrião de seis semanas

  cephalic f., f. cefálica; curva acentuada, ventralmente côncava, localizada no mesencéfalo em desenvolvimento do embrião. SIN cerebral f., cranial f., mesencephalic f.
  cerebral f., f. cefálica. SIN cephalic f.
  cervical f., f. cervical; curva ventralmente côncava localizada na junção do tronco encefálico com a medula espinal do embrião.
  cranial f., f. cefálica. SIN cephalic f.
  dorsal f., f. dorsal; f. localizada na região dorsal média do embrião.
  duodenojejunal f., [TA], f. duodenojejunal; curvatura acentuada localizada no intestino delgado na junção do duodeno com o jejuno. SIN flexura duodenojejunalis [TA], duodenojejunal angle.
  hepatic f., f. direita do cólon; *termo oficial alternativo para right colic f.
  inferior duodenal f. [TA], f. inferior do duodeno; curvatura localizada na junção das partes descendente e horizontal do duodeno. Ocasionalmente, existe uma curvatura, a flexura inferior esquerda do duodeno, na junção das partes horizontal e ascendente. SIN flexura duodeni inferior [TA].
  left colic f. [TA], f. esquerda do cólon; curvatura localizada na junção do cólon transverso com o cólon descendente. SIN flexura coli sinistra [TA], flexura colica splenica*, splenic f.*.
  lumbar f., lordose lombar. SIN lumbar lordosis.
  mesencephalic f., f. cefálica. SIN cephalic f.
  perineal f. of anal canal, f. anorretal; *termo oficial alternativo para anorectal f.
  perineal f. of rectum, f. anorretal. SIN anorectal f.
  pontine f., f. pontina; curvatura dorsalmente côncava do rombencéfalo do embrião; sua presença indica a divisão do rombencéfalo em mielencéfalo e metencéfalo. SIN basicranial f., transverse rhombencephalic f.
  right colic f. [TA], f. direita do cólon; curvatura do cólon localizada na junção das partes ascendente e transversa. SIN flexura coli dextra [TA], hepatic f.*, flexura coli hepatis.
  sacral f., f. sacral. SIN caudal f.
  sacral f. of rectum [TA], f. sacral; curva ântero-posterior, com concavidade voltada para a frente, da primeira parte do reto. SIN flexura sacralis recti [TA].
  sigmoid f., cólon sigmóide. SIN sigmoid colon.
  splenic f., f. esquerda do cólon; *termo oficial alternativo para left colic f.
  superior duodenal f. [TA], f. superior do duodeno; a flexura localizada na junção das partes superior e descendente do duodeno. SIN flexura duodeni superior [TA].
  telencephalic f., f. telencefálica; f. que aparece na região do prosencéfalo embriônico.
  transverse rhombencephalic f., f. pontina. SIN pontine f.
flick·er (flik′er). Bruxoleio; sensação visual causada pela estimulação da retina por uma série de clarões de luz intermitentes, que ocorrem em determinada freqüência. VER TAMBÉM flicker *fusion*, critical flicker fusion *frequency*.
flicks (fliks). Adejar; movimentos de fixação do olho rápidos e involuntários, que formam um arco de 5–10 minutos. SIN flick movements.
Flieringa, Henri J., oftalmologista holandês, *1891. VER F. *ring*.
flight in·to dis·ease. Fuga para a doença; ganho conseqüente de doença ou de suposta simulação de doença. VER primary *gain*, secondary *gain*.
flight in·to health. Fuga para a saúde; em psicoterapia dinâmica, o desaparecimento precoce, porém freqüentemente temporário, dos sintomas que, ostensivamente, levaram o paciente a fazer uma terapia; defesa contra a ansiedade engendrada pela perspectiva de futura exploração psicanalítica dos conflitos do paciente.
Flint, Austin, Jr., fisiologista norte-americano, 1836–1915. VER F. *arcade*.
Flint, Austin, médico norte-americano, 1812–1886. VER Austin F. *murmur*; F. *murmur*; Austin F. *phenomenon*.
flip. Uma queimadura encontrada em apenas um dos lados do local de entrada do projétil em um ferimento por projétil de arma de fogo localizado nas partes moles.
flitter. *Flutter*-fibrilação. SIN impure *flutter*.
float·er (flōt′er). Flutuante; um objeto dentro do campo de visão que se origina no corpo vítreo. VER TAMBÉM muscae volitantes.
float·ing (flōt′ing). Flutuante. 1. Livre ou não-fixado. 2. Incomumente móvel; fora da posição normal; que indica uma condição anormal e ocasional de certos órgãos, tais como os rins, o fígado, o baço, etc.
floc (flok). Floco; termo coloquial para o produto de uma floculação, isto é, a separação da fase dispersa de uma suspensão coloidal em partículas distintas, em geral visíveis, como ocorre em certos testes sorológicos de precipitação.
floc·cil·la·tion (flok-si-lā′shŭn). Carfologia, crocidismo; o ato sem propósito de um indivíduo de pegar a roupa de cama, a felpa de cobertores, como se estivesse arrancando fios ou tufos de algodão. [L. mod. *flocculus*]
floc·cose (flok′ōs). Flocose; em bacteriologia, termo aplicado a um agrupamento de filamentos ou cadeias curtos e curvos, dispostos próxima e irregularmente. [L. *floccus*, um floco de lã]
floc·cu·la·ble (flok′ū-lă-bl). Capaz de sofrer floculação.
floc·cu·lar (flok′ū-lar). Flocular; relativo a um flóculo de qualquer tipo ou, mais especificamente, ao flóculo do cerebelo.
floc·cu·late (flok′ū-lāt). Flocular; tornar-se flocoso.
floc·cu·la·tion (flok-ū-lā′shŭn). Floculação; precipitação de solução na forma de massas lanosas; o processo de tornar-se flocoso. SIN flocculence.
floc·cule (flok′ūl). Flóculo. SIN flocculus.
floc·cu·lence (flok′ū-lens). Flocosidade, floculação. SIN flocculation.
floc·cu·lent (flok′ū-lent). Flocoso. 1. Que se assemelha a tufos de algodão ou lã; que indica um líquido, tal como a urina, que contém numerosos filamentos ou partículas flocosas de muco ou outro material branco ou branco-acinzentado. 2. Em bacteriologia, indica uma cultura líquida na qual há numerosas colônias, tanto flutuando no meio líquido como depositadas de forma solta no fundo.
floc·cu·lo·nod·u·lar (flok′ū-lō-nod′ū-lar). Floculonodular. VER flocculonodular *lobe*.
floc·cu·lus, pl. **floc·cu·li** (flok′ū-lŭs, -lī). Flóculo. 1. Tufo ou retalho de algodão ou lã, ou de qualquer tecido semelhante. 2. [TA]. Pequeno lobo do cerebelo localizado na margem posterior do pedúnculo cerebelar médio, anteriormente ao lóbulo biventre; está associado ao nódulo do verme; juntas, essas duas estruturas compõem a parte vestibular do cerebelo. SIN floccule. [L. mod. dim. de L. *floccus*, um tufo de lã]
  accessory f., f. acessório; pequeno lóbulo ocasional do cerebelo, adjacente ao flóculo.
Flocks, Milton, oftalmologista norte-americano, *1914. VER Harrington-F. *test*.
Flood, Valentine, anatomista e cirurgia irlandesa, 1800–1847. VER F. *ligament*.
flood (flŭd). Hemorragia. 1. Sangramento profuso do útero após o parto ou em casos de menorragia. 2. Coloquialismo para um fluxo menstrual intenso. [A.S. *flōd*]
flood·ing (flŭd′ing). Hemorragia; imersão. 1. Sangramento profuso do útero, principalmente após o parto ou em casos graves de menorragia. 2. Hemorragia uterina intensa. 3. Tipo de terapia comportamental; estratégia em psicoterapia, utilizada logo no início, na qual os pacientes imaginam a cena que mais lhes provoca ansiedade e, em seguida, mergulham completamente ("*flood*") nela. Cf. systematic *desensitization*.
floor (flōr) [TA]. Assoalho; superfície interna inferior de um espaço aberto ou de um órgão oco.

f. of orbit [TA], parede inferior da órbita; a menor das quatro paredes da órbita que se inclinam para cima a partir da margem orbital; é formada pela maxila e pelo processo orbital do osso palatino. SIN paries inferior orbitae [TA], inferior wall of orbit.

f. of tympanic cavity, parede jugular da orelha média; *termo oficial alternativo para jugular *wall of middle ear.*

flo·ra (flō′ra). Flora. 1. Vida vegetal, em geral de certa localidade ou região. 2. A população de microrganismos que habita as superfícies interna e externa de animais considerados saudáveis. SIN microbial associates. [L. *Flora*, deusa das flores, de *flos* (*flor*-), uma flor]

flor·an·ty·rone (flor - an′ti - rōn). Florantirona; agente que aumenta o volume de bile sem aumentar a quantidade de corpos sólidos na bile ou estimular o esvaziamento da vesícula biliar.

Florence, Albert, médico francês, 1851–1927. VER F. *crystals*, em *crystal*.

Florence flask. Balão de Florence. Ver em flask.

Florey, Sir Howard W., patologista australiano-britânico laureado com o prêmio Nobel, 1898–1968. VER F. *unit*.

flor·id (flōr′id). 1. De coloração vermelho-brilhante; que indica certas lesões cutâneas. 2. Completamente desenvolvido. [L. *floridus*, florido]

Florschütz, Georg, médico alemão, *1859. VER F. *formula*.

floss. 1. Fio dental. SIN dental f. **2.** O uso do fio dental na higiene oral.

dental f., f. dental; fio não-torcido feito de seda ou fibras sintéticas finas e curtas e freqüentemente encerado; utilizado para limpar os espaços interproximais e entre as áreas de contato dos dentes. SIN floss silk, floss (1).

flo·ta·tion (flō - tā′shun). Flotação; processo para a separação de sólidos baseado na tendência que possuem para flutuar ou afundar em um líquido.

Flourens, Marie Jean Pierre, fisiologista francês, 1794–1867. VER F. *theory*.

flow (flō). Fluxo. **1.** Sangramento uterino menos intenso do que uma hemorragia. **2.** A menstruação. **3.** O movimento de um líquido ou gás; mais especificamente, o volume de líquido ou gás que passa por determinado ponto por unidade de tempo. Em fisiologia respiratória, o símbolo para o fluxo de gás é V̇ e, para o fluxo de sangue, é Q̇, seguidos por subscritos que indicam a localização e a espécie química. **4.** Em reologia, uma deformação permanente de um corpo que evolui com o tempo. [A.S. *flōwan*]

Bingham f., f. de Bingham; f. característico exibido por um plástico de Bingham.

Doppler color f., Doppler colorido; imagem colorida gerada por computador, produzida pela ultra-sonografia com Doppler, na qual direções diferentes do f. são representadas por diferentes tons. VER Doppler *ultrasonography*.

effective renal blood f. (ERBF), f. sanguíneo renal efetivo; volume de sangue que flui para as partes do rim envolvidas na produção de constituintes da urina.

effective renal plasma f. (ERPF), f. plasmático renal efetivo; volume de plasma que flui para as partes do rim que atuam na produção dos constituintes da urina; corresponde à depuração de substâncias, tais como o iodopiraceto e o ácido *p*-amino-hipúrico, partindo do pressuposto de que a razão de extração nos capilares peritubulares seja de 100%.

forced expiratory f. (FEF), f. expiratório forçado; f. expiratório obtido durante a medida da capacidade vital forçada; os valores subscritos especificam o parâmetro que está sendo avaliado, p.ex., instantâneo máximo, o f. instantâneo em algum ponto específico na curva de volume expirado *versus* tempo, ou, na curva de fluxo–volume, o f. médio entre dois volumes expirados.

gene f., f. de genes; alterações que ocorrem ao longo do tempo na composição genética de uma população em conseqüência de migração e não de mutação e seleção.

laminar f., f. laminar; o movimento relativo dos elementos de um líquido, ao longo de vias paralelas lisas, que ocorre em valores menores do número de Reynolds.

newtonian f., f. newtoniano; o tipo de f. característico de um fluido newtoniano.

peak expiratory f., f. expiratório máximo; o f. máximo presente no início da expiração forçada; encontra-se reduzido de modo proporcional à gravidade da obstrução das vias aéreas, como ocorre na asma.

shear f., f. de cisalhamento; f. de um material no qual planos paralelos imaginários se deslocam em uma direção paralela um em relação ao outro.

Flower, Sir William H., anatomista e cirurgião inglês, 1831–1899. VER F. *bone*, dental *index*.

flow·er bas·ket of Bochdalek. Parte do plexo corióideo do quarto ventrículo que se projeta através do forame de Luschka e repousa sobre a superfície dorsal do nervo glossofaríngeo.

flow·ers (flow′erz). Flores, nata; substância mineral, no estado de pó, após sublimação.

f. of antimony, trióxido de antimônio. SIN antimony trioxide.

f. of benzoin, ácido benzóico. SIN benzoic acid.

f. of sulfur, f. de enxofre. SIN sublimed sulfur.

f. of zinc, óxido de zinco. SIN zinc oxide.

flow·me·ter (flō′mē - ter). Fluxômetro; dispositivo utilizado para medir a velocidade ou o volume de fluxo de líquidos e gases.

electromagnetic f., f. eletromagnético, medidor eletromagnético; um f. no qual o fluxo sanguíneo é examinado pela aplicação de um campo magnético a um vaso sanguíneo e pela análise da voltagem resultante no vaso.

flox·a·cil·lin (flok′sa - sil′in). Floxacilina; antibiótico do grupo das penicilinas resistente à β-lactamase (penicilinase).

flox·ur·i·dine (flok - soo′ri - dēn). Floxuridina; desoxinucleosídeo da fluoruracila; agente antineoplásico. A fluoruracila é metabolizada a floxuridina que, por sua vez, é metabolizada a 5-fluoro-2′-desoxiuridina 5′-monofosfato. Esta última substância inibe a timidilato sintetase; a uridina fosfatase também é inibida.

flu (floo). Gripe, *influenza*. SIN influenza.

flu·an·i·sone (floo - an′i - sōn). Fluanisona; agente ansiolítico.

flu·cry·late (floo′kri - lāt). Flucrilato; tecido adesivo utilizado em cirurgia.

fluctuance. Flutuação, oscilação, vibração. SIN fluctuation (2).

fluc·tu·ate (flŭk′tū - āt). Flutuar; oscilar, vibrar. **1.** Mover-se em ondas. **2.** Oscilar, variar, alterar de vez em quando, no que se refere a qualquer quantidade ou qualidade, p.ex., a altura da pressão sanguínea, a concentração de uma substância na urina ou no sangue, a atividade secretória, etc. [L. *fluctuo*, pp. *-atus*, fluir em ondas]

fluc·tu·a·tion (flŭk - tū - ā′shŭn). Flutuação; oscilação, vibração. **1.** O ato de flutuar. **2.** Movimento semelhante a uma onda, sentido durante a palpação de uma cavidade com paredes não-rígidas, principalmente se cheia de líquido. SIN fluctuance.

flu·cy·to·sine (floo - si′tō - sēn). Flucitosina; agente antifúngico.

flu·dro·cor·ti·sone ac·e·tate (floo - drō - kōr′ti - sōn). Acetato de fludrocortisona; potente mineralocorticóide. SIN 9α-fluorocortisol, 9α-fluorohydrocortisone acetate.

flu·ence (H) (floo′ens). Fluxo; em radiologia diagnóstica, a medida da quantidade de radiação X em um feixe, o f. de partículas – o número de fótons que passam por uma abertura de unidade de área transversalmente seccionada –, ou o f. de energia – o somatório das energias dos fótons que passam através de uma unidade de área. Cf. flux. [L. *fluentia*, um fluxo, de *fluo*, fluir]

flu·en·cy (floo′en - sē). Fluência; o fluxo suave dos sons da fala em discurso conexo, sem interrupções ou repetições. [L. *fluentia*, um fluxo, de *fluo*, fluir]

flu·ent (floo′ent). Fluente; relativo à fluência.

flu·fen·am·ic ac·id (floo-fen-am′ik). Ácido flufenâmico; agente antiinflamatório; assemelha-se ao ácido mefenâmico.

flu·id (floo′id) [TA]. Fluido, líquido. **1.** Substância não-sólida, tal como um líquido ou um gás, que tende a fluir ou assumir a forma do recipiente. **2.** Que consiste em partículas ou entidades distintas que conseguem alterar rapidamente suas posições relativas; isto é, que tendem a se mover ou que são capazes de fluir. [L. *fluidus*, de *fluo*, fluir]

allantoic f., líquido alantóico; o l. que ocupa a cavidade da alantóide.

amnionic f., líquido amniótico; líquido presente no âmnio que circunda o feto e o protege de traumas mecânicos. SIN liquor amnii.

Brodie f., líquido de Brodie; solução salina aquosa utilizada em manômetros projetados para testar a evolução ou a captação de gás, como na respiração celular.

bronchoalveolar f., líquido broncoalveolar; líquido que contém várias enzimas líticas e serve para remover partículas inspiradas das vias aéreas inferiores.

Callison f., líquido de Callison; líquido diluente para a contagem de hemácias, composto de 1 ml de azul de metileno alcalino de Loeffler, 1 ml de formalina, 10 mL de glicerol, 1 g de oxalato de amônio neutro e 2,5 g de cloreto de sódio adicionados a 90 ml de água destilada; após ser bem misturada, a solução é deixada para descansar até que os sólidos sejam dissolvidos e o reagente se torne claro; a preparação é filtrada antes de ser utilizada.

cerebrospinal f. (CSF) [TA], líquido cerebrospinal; líquido secretado em grande parte pelos plexos corióideos dos ventrículos do cérebro, que preenche as cavidades ventriculares e o espaço subaracnóideo do cérebro e da medula espinal. SIN liquor cerebrospinalis [TA].

crevicular f., líquido gengival. SIN gingival f.

Dakin f., solução de Dakin. SIN Dakin *solution*.

dentinal f., líquido dentinal; a linfa ou o l. da dentina que aparece na superfície da dentina recém-cortada, especialmente dos dentes jovens; é um transudato do l. extracelular, principalmente do citoplasma de processos odontoblásticos, proveniente da polpa dentária e passando através dos túbulos da dentina. SIN dental lymph.

extracellular f. (ECF), líquido extracelular (LEC); **(1)** o l. intersticial e o plasma, que constituem cerca de 20% do peso do corpo; **(2)** o termo é, às vezes, utilizado para se referir a todo o líquido que está fora das células, excluindo-se geralmente o líquido transcelular.

extravascular f., líquido extravascular; todo o l. que está fora dos vasos sanguíneos, ou seja, os líquidos intracelular, intersticial e transcelular; constitui cerca de 48 a 58% do peso do corpo.

Farrant mounting f., líquido de montagem de Farrant; solução aquosa que contém goma arábica, trióxido de arsênico, glicerol e água e é utilizada na montagem de cortes histológicos diretamente a partir da água; podem ser feitas algumas modificações que envolvem a adição de acetato de potássio, para

líquido cerebrospinal humano	
(valores médios, mg/dl)	
volume	120 – 200 ml
densidade	1,006 – 1,008
reação	pH ~ 7,5
ponto de congelamento	0,55° (0,52° - 0,58°)
pressão (lombar, paciente reclinado)	70 – 220 mm H₂O
proteína	15 – 25
glicose	40 – 60 (até 80)
ácido fosfatídico	~ 1,0
colesterol	0,3 – 0,6
cloreto	730 – 740
fosfato	3 – 5

tornar o pH neutro, e a substituição de outros conservantes como o cresol ou o timol por trióxido de arsênico.

gingival f., líquido gengival; l. que contém proteínas plasmáticas e é encontrado em quantidades crescentes na inflamação gengival. SIN crevicular f., sulcular f.

infranatant f., l. claro que, após a decantação de um líquido ou sólido insolúvel pela ação da gravidade ou de força centrífuga, ocupa a parte inferior do conteúdo de um recipiente.

interstitial f., líquido intersticial; l. encontrado nos espaços entre as células dos tecidos e que constitui cerca de 16% do peso do corpo; sua composição é muito semelhante à da linfa. SIN tissue f.

intracellular f. (ICF), líquido intracelular (LIC); l. encontrado dentro das células dos tecidos e que constitui cerca de 30 a 40% do peso do corpo. SIN intracellular water.

intraocular f., humor aquoso. SIN aqueous humor.

newtonian f., líquido newtoniano; l. no qual o fluxo e a taxa de cisalhamento são sempre proporcionais à tensão aplicada; esse l. obedece precisamente à lei de Poiseuille. Cf. non-newtonian f.

non-newtonian f., líquido não-newtoniano; l. no qual o fluxo e a taxa de cisalhamento não são sempre proporcionais à tensão aplicada e que não obedecem à lei de Poiseuille. Ver anomalous *viscosity*; Fahraeus-Lindqvist *effect*; Bingham *plastic*. Cf. newtonian f.

pleural f., líquido pleural; a delgada película de l. encontrada entre as pleuras visceral e parietal. Pode aumentar de forma significativa em estados patológicos, quando é, então, denominado de derrame pleural.

prostatic f., l. prostático; *succus prostaticus*; secreção esbranquiçada que é um dos constituintes do sêmen.

pseudoplastic f., l. pseudoplástico; l. que exibe adelgaçamento por cisalhamento.

Rees-Ecker f., l. de Rees-Ecker; solução aquosa de citrato de sódio, sucrose e azul de cresil brilhante utilizada na contagem de plaquetas.

Scarpa f., l. de Scarpa, endolinfa. SIN endolymph.

seminal f., l. seminal, sêmen. SIN semen (1).

sulcular f., l. gengival. SIN gingival f.

supernatant f., sobrenadante; l. claro que, após a decantação de um líquido ou sólido insolúveis pela ação da gravidade ou de força centrífuga, ocupa a parte superior do conteúdo de um recipiente.

synovial f. [TA], l. sinovial; l. tixotrópico claro, cuja principal função é atuar como um lubrificante em uma articulação, bainha tendínea ou bolsa; é composto principalmente de mucina e um pouco de albumina, gordura, epitélio e leucócitos; o l. sinovial também auxilia na nutrição da cartilagem articular avascular. SIN synovia [TA], joint oil.

thixotropic f., l. tixotrópico; l. que tende a se transformar em um gel, quando deixado em repouso, mas que retorna à forma líquida, quando agitado, seja por vibrações, seja por adequado cisalhamento.

tissue f., l. intersticial. SIN interstitial f.

transcellular f.'s, líquidos transcelulares; líquidos que não estão dentro das células, mas encontram-se separados do plasma e do l. intersticial por barreiras celulares; p.ex., o l. cerebrospinal, o l. sinovial e o l. pleural.

ventricular f., líquido ventricular; a parte do l. cerebrospinal que está contida dentro dos ventrículos do cérebro.

flu·id·ex·tract (floo-id-eks′trakt). Extrato líquido; preparação líquida farmacológica de drogas vegetais, feita por percolação, que contém álcool como solvente e/ou conservante, sendo elaborada de tal forma que cada mililitro contém os constituintes terapêuticos de 1 g da droga-padrão que representa. SIN liquid extract.

flu·id·glyc·er·ates (floo-id-glis′er-āts). Gliceratos líquidos; formas farmacêuticas, antigamente consideradas oficiais pelo NF (*National Formulary*), que contêm aproximadamente 50% de glicerina por volume, mas nenhum álcool e a mesma potência medicamentosa dos extratos líquidos.

flu·id·ism (floo′i-dizm). Humorismo. SIN humoral doctrine.

flu·id·i·ty (floo-id′i-tē). Fluidez; o oposto de viscosidade; unidade: rhe = poise⁻¹.

flu·id·ounce (floo′id-owns′). Onça líquida; uma medida de capacidade: 8 dracmas líquidas. A o. l. imperial é uma medida que contém 1 onça avoirdupois, 437,5 grãos de água destilada a 15,6°C e é igual a 28,4 ml; a o. l. norte-americana corresponde a 1/128 galão, contém 454,6 grãos de água destilada a 25°C e é igual a 29,57 ml.

flu·i·drachm, flu·i·dram (floo′i-dram′). Dracma líquida; uma medida de capacidade: 1/8 de uma onça líquida; uma colher de chá cheia. A d. l. imperial contém 54,8 grãos de água destilada e é igual a 3,55 ml; a d. l. norte-americana contém 57,1 grãos de água destilada e é igual a 3,70 ml.

fluke (flook). Trematódeo; nome comum dado aos membros da classe Trematoda (filo Platyhelminthes). Todos os trematódeos de mamíferos (ordem Digenea) são parasitas internos na fase adulta e caracterizam-se por apresentar ciclos de vida digenéticos complexos. Os ciclos envolvem um hospedeiro inicial — um caramujo — no qual ocorrem a multiplicação larval e a liberação de larvas nadantes (cercárias), que penetram diretamente a pele do hospedeiro definitivo (como os esquistossomas), encistam-se nas plantas (como os membros do gênero *Fasciola*) ou encistam-se no interior de um hospedeiro intermediário ou sobre ele (como os parasitas do gênero *Clonorchis* e outros trematódeos transmitidos pelo peixe). Os trematódeos de vertebrados inferiores (ordem Monogenea), principalmente de peixes, são freqüentemente ectoparasitas monogenéticos ou parasitas de guelras. Os trematódeos do sangue vivem na corrente sanguínea mesentérico-portal e estão associados aos plexos venosos vesical e pélvico; incluem *Schistosoma haematobium* (t. sanguíneo vesical), *S. mansoni* (t. sanguíneo intestinal de Manson) e *S. japonicum* (t. do sangue do Oriente). Outros trematódeos importantes são *Paragonimus westermani* (t. dos brônquios e do pulmão), *Opisthorchis felineus* (t. do fígado do gato), *Clonorchis sinensis* (t. do fígado chinês ou Oriental), *Heterophyes heterophyes* (t. egípcio ou do intestino delgado), *Fasciolopsis buski* (t. do intestino grosso), *Dicrocoelium dendriticum*, *Fasciola hepatica* (t. hepática ou do fígado de carneiro) e *Paramphistomum* (t. do rúmen). [A.S. *flōc*, peixe achatado]

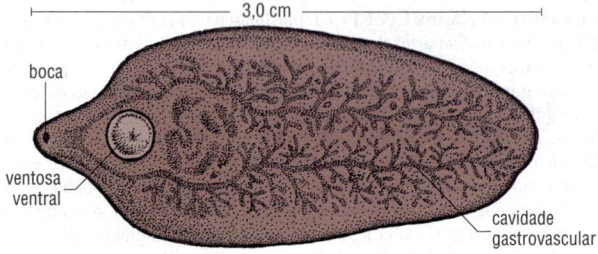

trematódeo do fígado (*Fasciola hepatica*)

flu·maz·en·il (floo′mā-zē-nil). Flumazenil; benzodiazepina com propriedades antagonistas no local de reconhecimento de benzodiazepinas do complexo benzodiazepina-GABA-canais de cloreto. Utilizada no tratamento da *overdose* de depressores do sistema nervoso central semelhantes aos benzodiazepínicos.

flu·men, pl. **flu·mi·na** (floo′men, floo′min-ā). Flúmen; fluxo ou corrente. SIN stream. [L.]

flumina pilo′rum, correntes dos pêlos. SIN hair streams, em stream.

flu·meth·a·sone (floo-meth′ā-sōn). Flumetasona; o sal 21-pivalato e o acetato também estão disponíveis.

flu·me·thi·a·zide (floo′me-thī′ā-zīd). Flumetiazida; agente diurético, efetivo por via oral, quimicamente relacionado à clorotiazida e com ações farmacológicas semelhantes. Inibe a anidrase carbônica.

flu·mi·na (floo′mi-nā). Flumens; plural de flúmen.

flu·nar·i·zine (floo-nar′ī-zēn). Flunarizina; agente bloqueador de íons cálcio com propriedades anticonvulsivantes.

flu·nis·o·lide (floo-nis′ō-līd). Flunisolida; corticosteróide antiinflamatório utilizado por via nasal ou inalação no tratamento de alergias e da asma.

flu·ni·traz·e·pam (flū′nī-trāz′ē-pam). Flunitrazepam; composto benzodiazepínico com propriedades sedativas e hipnóticas.

O flunitrazepam, conhecido como o sedativo e hipnótico mais prescrito na Europa, embora não tenha licença para ser vendido nos Estados Unidos, tem sido motivo de crescente preocupação, uma vez que a distribuição ilegal e o uso abusivo têm se espalhado dos estados do sul para outras partes desse país. O abuso é particularmente prevalente entre estudantes do curso secundário e universitário. Ingerido isoladamente, o flunitrazepam provoca leve euforia e sedação. É freqüentemente misturado a outras substâncias, a fim de, por exemplo, aumentar a euforia provocada pela heroína ou atenuar a depressão após o uso de cocaína ou *crack*. O flunitrazepam e o álcool apresentam ação sinérgica, produzindo desinibição e amnésia quando tomados juntos. Por essa razão, a droga pode ser adicionada furtivamente a bebidas alcoólicas para facilitar o estupro. Parte da popularidade da droga advém de seu baixo custo e da disponibilidade de comprimidos puros manufaturados por indústrias legítimas. O flunitrazepam é comercializado pelo Hoffman-La Roche com o nome comercial Rohypnol. Nos Estados Unidos, a droga é conhecida nas ruas como "circles", "Mexican Valium", "la rocha", "R2", "rib", "roaches", "roachies", "Roche", "roofenol", "roofies", "rope", "rophies" e "ruffies", e o estado produzido por sua ação é denominado de "roached out". Os efeitos do flunitrazepam começam 30 minutos após a ingestão, atingem seu máximo em 2 horas e podem persistir por 8 horas ou mais. As reações adversas incluem sonolência, confusão, amnésia, excitação ou agressividade paradoxais, distúrbios visuais, hipotensão, distúrbios gastrointestinais e retenção urinária. A *overdose* fatal é incomum. O uso prolongado causa dependência física. Os sinais e sintomas da síndrome de abstinência variam de cefaléia, dor muscular, inquietação e confusão a perda de identidade, alucinações, delírio, convulsões e colapso cardiovascular. As crises de abstinência podem ocorrer uma semana ou mais após a interrupção do uso. O fenobarbital é utilizado para facilitar a retirada da droga feita sob supervisão médica. Em 1997, em resposta à preocupação quanto ao uso do flunitrazepam em casos de estupro, o Hoffman-LaRoche reformulou seus comprimidos de forma que se dissolvam mais lentamente em líquidos e liberem uma cor azul-brilhante para facilitar sua detecção.

fluo-. Fluo- **1.** Forma combinante que indica fluxo. **2.** Prefixo freqüentemente utilizado para se referir ao flúor (empregado nos nomes genéricos das drogas). VER TAMBÉM fluor-. [L. *fluo*, pp. *fluxus*, fluir]

flu·o·cin·o·lone ac·e·to·nide (floo - ō - sin′ō - lōn as′e - tō - nīd). Acetonida de fluocinolona; corticosteróide fluorado para uso tópico utilizado no tratamento de algumas dermatoses.

flu·o·cin·o·nide (floo - ō - sin′ō - nīd). Fluocinonida; corticosteróide antiinflamatório utilizado em preparações tópicas.

flu·o·cor·to·lone (floo - ō - kōr′tō - lōn). Fluocortolona; um glicocorticóide.
f. caproate, caproato de f.; éster da f. utilizado topicamente no tratamento de doenças da pele. SIN f. hexanoate.
f. hexanoate, hexanoato de f. SIN f. caproate.
f. pivalate, pivalato de f.; um éster da f.

fluor-, fluoro-. Flúor.

flu·or·ap·a·tite (flōr - ap′a - tīt). Fluorapatita; fluorofosfato de cálcio de ocorrência natural.

9H-flu·o·rene (flōr′ēn). 9H-fluoreno; composto que dá origem ao 2-acetilaminofluoreno; encontrado no alcatrão de hulha.

flu·o·res·ca·mine (flōr - es′ka - mēn). Fluorescamina; reagente não-fluorescente que reage com aminas primárias a fim de formar compostos fluorescentes.

flu·o·resce (fluō - res′). Fluorescer; produzir ou exibir fluorescência.

flu·o·res·ce·in (flōr - es′ē - in) [I.C. 45350]. Fluoresceína; pó cristalino laranja-avermelhado que emite uma fluorescência verde-brilhante quando em solução e é reduzido a fluorescina; indicador não-tóxico e hidrossolúvel utilizado com fins diagnósticos para rastrear fluxo de água. SIN resorcinol phthalic anhydride, resorcinolphthalein.
f. sodium, fluoresceína sódica; corante utilizado no diagnóstico de certas doenças oculares, na diferenciação ou delineação de partes de órgãos em cirurgia e na determinação do tempo de circulação. SIN resorcinolphthalein sodium, uranin.

flu·o·res·ce·in iso·thi·o·cy·a·nate (FITC) (ī′sō - thī - ō - sī′a - nāt). Isotiocianato de fluoresceína; corante fluorocromo freqüentemente ligado a anticorpos utilizados para localizar e identificar antígenos específicos.

flu·o·res·cence (flōr - es′ens). Fluorescência; emissão de uma radiação de comprimento de onda mais longo por uma substância, como conseqüência da absorção de energia de uma radiação de comprimento de onda mais curto, que continua apenas enquanto existir o estímulo; é diferente da fosforescência, na qual a emissão persiste por um período de tempo considerável após o estímulo ter sido removido. VER photoelectric *effect*. [*fluor*spar + *-escence*, sufixo de verbos incoativos]

flu·o·res·cence·ac·ti·vat·ed cell sort·er (FACS) (flōr - es′ens). Classificador de células ativadas por fluorescência; aparelho que separa e analisa células, tais como linfócitos, marcadas com anticorpo conjugado com fluorocromo, por meio de sua fluorescência e de seus padrões de dispersão de luz.

flu·o·res·cent (flōr - es′ent). Fluorescente; que possui a qualidade da fluorescência.

flu·o·res·cin (flōr′ - es - in). Fluorescina; fluoresceína reduzida, com usos semelhantes aos da fluoresceína.

flu·o·ri·da·tion (flōr′i - dā′shŭn). Fluoração; adição de fluoretos ao suprimento de água de uma comunidade, geralmente cerca de 1 ppm, a fim de reduzir a incidência de cárie dentária.

flu·o·ride (flōr′īd). Fluoreto. **1.** Um composto de flúor com um metal, um não-metal ou um radical orgânico. **2.** O aniônte de flúor; inibe a enolase; encontrado na apatita do osso e do dente; o f. apresenta efeito cariostático; altos níveis são tóxicos.

flu·o·ride num·ber. Número do fluoreto; porcentagem de inibição da pseudocolinesterase produzida pelos fluoretos; utilizado para diferenciar as pseudocolinesterases normais das atípicas. VER TAMBÉM dibucaine number.

flu·o·ri·di·za·tion (flōr′i - di - zā′shŭn). Fluoração; uso terapêutico de fluoretos para reduzir a incidência de cáries dentárias; termo utilizado às vezes para se referir à aplicação tópica de agentes fluorados nos dentes.

flu·o·rine (F) (flōr′ēn). Flúor; elemento químico gasoso com n.° atômico 9 e massa atômica 18,9984032; o F^{18} (meia-vida de 1,83 h) é utilizado como um auxiliar diagnóstico em diversos exames de tecidos. [L. *fluere*, fluxo]

fluoro-. Fluoro-; VER fluor-.

flu·o·ro·chrome (flōr′ō - krōm). Fluorocromo; qualquer corante fluorescente utilizado para marcar ou corar.

flu·or·o·chrom·ing (flōr′ō - krōm - ing). Coloração com fluorocromo. **1.** Marcação de anticorpos com corante fluorescente para permitir que eles possam ser observados ao microscópio, utilizando-se luz ultravioleta; método para estudar a origem, a distribuição e os locais de reação com o antígeno nos tecidos. **2.** Detecção microscópica de componentes químicos celulares e tissulares (DNA, RNA, proteínas, polissacarídeos) com o auxílio de fluorocromos ligados a esses componentes.

9α-flu·o·ro·cor·ti·sol (flōr - ō - kōr′ti - sol). 9α-fluorocortisol. SIN fludrocortisone acetate.

flu·o·ro·cyte (flōr′ō - sīt). Fluorócito; termo utilizado ocasionalmente para um reticulócito que exibe fluorescência.

flu·o·ro-2,4-di·ni·tro·ben·zene (FDNB) (flōr′ō - dī - nī - trō - ben′zēn). Fluoro-2,4-dinitrobenzeno; reagente que se combina com grupamentos amino livres de resíduos aminoacil de um peptídeo, marcando, dessa forma, esses resíduos; as formas combinadas são conhecidas como proteínas-DNP, aminoacil-Dnp, etc., sendo o flúor substituído para deixar um resíduo dinitrofenil (DNP, Dnp ou N$_2$Ph–) ligado ao grupamento NH$_2$. Em conseqüência, as cadeias laterais do aminoácido *N*-terminal e da lisina sofrem modificações covalentes. SIN Sanger reagent.

flu·o·rog·ra·phy (flōr - og′ra - fē). Fluorografia. SIN photofluorography.

9α-flu·o·ro·hy·dro·cor·ti·sone ac·e·tate (flōr′ō - hī - drō - kōr′ti - sōn). Acetato de 9α-fluoro-hidrocortisona. SIN fludrocortisone acetate.

flu·o·rom·e·ter (flōr - om′e - ter). Fluorômetro; dispositivo que emprega uma fonte de luz ultravioleta, monocromadores para a escolha do comprimento de onda e um detector de luz visível; utilizado em fluorometria.

flu·o·ro·meth·o·lone (flōr - ō - meth′o - lōn). Fluorometolona; glicocorticóide para uso tópico.

flu·o·rom·e·try (flōr - om′e - trē). Fluorometria; método analítico para a detecção de compostos fluorescentes, utilizando um feixe de luz ultravioleta que excita esses compostos e faz com que emitam luz visível. [fluoro- + G. *metron*, medida]

flu·o·ro·pho·tom·e·try (flōr′ō - fō - tom′e - trē). Fluorofotometria; tubo fotomultiplicador para a medida da fluorescência emitida do interior do olho após administração intravenosa de fluoresceína; utilizada para medir a velocidade de formação de humor aquoso ou observar a integridade da vasculatura retiniana.

fluoroquinolone (flōr - ō - kwin′ō - lōn). Fluoroquinolona. SIN quinolones.

flu·o·ro·quin·o·lones (flōr′ō - kwin′ō - lōnz). Fluoroquinolonas; classe de antibióticos com um amplo espectro de atividade antimicrobiana; são bem absorvidas por via oral e apresentam boa penetração tecidual e efeito relativamente prolongado.

As fluoroquinolonas, introduzidas na década de 1980, são particularmente úteis em infecções por Gram-negativos. O ácido nalidíxico, uma quinolona não-fluorada, tem sido utilizado há várias décadas no tratamento de infecções do trato urinário, porém seu valor é limitado em virtude de sua baixa distribuição sistêmica e pelo rápido desenvolvimento de resistência bacteriana. Em contraste, as fluoroquinolonas que contêm um átomo de flúor alcançam rapidamente concentrações terapêuticas no plasma, nos tecidos e na urina após a administração oral, e a resistência desenvolve-se lentamente. O átomo de flúor também amplia o espectro desses agentes, conferindo-lhes atividade contra algumas bactérias Gram-positivas.

São úteis nas infecções dos tratos respiratório e urinário, da pele e dos ossos sensíveis às fluoroquinolonas. Vários desses agentes estão aprovados pela FDA para o tratamento oral, por dose única, da gonorréia que não apresenta complicações. Em geral, são inativos contra anaeróbios e estreptococos β-hemolíticos. As fluoroquinolonas inibem a DNA girase bacteriana, necessária para a replicação do DNA, bem como de plasmídeos envolvidos em certos tipos de resistência bacteriana. A eliminação é principalmente renal, e a dose tem de ser ajustada nos pacientes com insuficiência renal. São, em geral, bem toleradas. Os efeitos colaterais mais freqüentes são náuseas, dor abdominal e vertigem. Essas drogas acumulam-se na cartilagem articular e podem causar grave lesão durante a fase de crescimento rápido desse tecido; conseqüentemente, elas são contra-indicadas para pessoas com menos de 18 anos. O uso durante exercício físico extenuante pode ser prejudicial para as articulações e causar ruptura de tendão. Essas drogas podem interferir na biotransformação hepática da teofilina e da varfarina.

flu·o·ro·roent·gen·og·ra·phy (flōr′ō - rent - gen - og′ră - fē). Fotofluorografia. SIN photofluorography.

flu·o·ro·scope (flōr′ō - skōp). Fluoroscópio; aparelho obsoleto que torna visível ao olho adaptado ao escuro os padrões de raios X que passam através de um corpo sob exame, por meio da interposição de uma lâmina de vidro coberta com materiais fluorescentes, tais como tungstato de cálcio; atualmente, utiliza-se um intensificador de imagens e um monitor de vídeo; exame de um paciente utilizando um fluoroscópio, obsoleto ou moderno. [fluorescence + G. *skopeō*, examinar]

flu·o·ro·scop·ic (flōr - ō - skop′ik). Fluoroscópico; relativo a ou realizado por meio do fluoroscópio (isto é, biopsia percutânea).

flu·o·ros·co·py (flōr - os′kŏ - pē). Fluoroscopia; exame dos tecidos e de estruturas profundas do corpo por meio de raios X, utilizando o fluoroscópio ou seu sucessor, o videofluoroscópio. (q.v.).

video f., videofluoroscopia; f. que utiliza um amplificador de imagens e uma câmera de televisão para detectar imagens e um monitor de vídeo para a exibição de imagens.

flu·o·ro·sis (flōr - ō′sis). Fluorose. **1.** Condição causada por ingestão excessiva de fluoretos (2 ou mais p.p.m. na água potável), caracterizada principalmente por mosqueamento, coloração e hipoplasia do esmalte dos dentes, embora os ossos do esqueleto também sejam afetados. **2.** Intoxicação crônica dos animais domésticos por fluoretos que enegrece e amolece os dentes em desenvolvimento e reduz os ossos a estruturas calcárias quebradiças; mais freqüentemente causada pela ingestão de contaminantes de forragem próximo a grandes fábricas de alumínio.

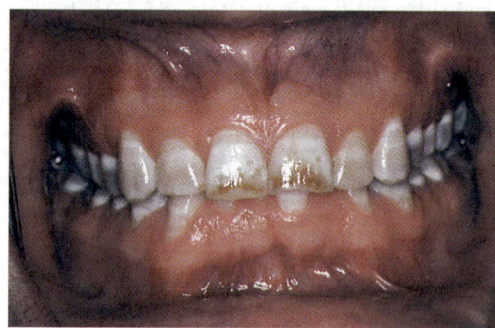

fluorose dentária: arcada dentária exibindo esmalte difusamente branco e opaco com áreas de descoloração marrom de um paciente com história de ingestão crônica excessiva de fluoreto

chronic endemic f., f. crônica endêmica; f. causada pelo excesso de flúor no suprimento natural de água, como observado em algumas partes da Índia; pode ocorrer osteoesclerose com ancilose da coluna vertebral.

flu·o·ro·u·ra·cil (flōr - ō - ū′rǎ - sil). Fluoruracil; análogo da pirimidina; antineoplásico efetivo no tratamento de alguns carcinomas; as células de certas neoplasias incorporam a uracila ao ácido ribonucleico mais rapidamente do que as células do tecido normal. VER TAMBÉM floxuridine.

flu·o·sol-DA (flu′ō - sol). Solução de perfluorocarbono experimental sob investigação para ser utilizada como um substituto artificial do sangue.

flu·ox·e·tine hy·dro·chlo·ride (floo - oks′e - tēn). Cloridrato de fluoxetina; antidepressivo oral; impede seletivamente a recaptação da serotonina.

flu·ox·y·mes·ter·one (floo - ok - sē - mes′ter - ōn). Fluoximesterona; esteróide halogenado, sintético, efetivo por via oral, que possui estrutura química e ação farmacológica semelhantes às da metiltestosterona, porém mais potentes.

flu·pen·tix·ol (floo-pen-tik′sol). Flupentixol; um neuroléptico.

flu·per·o·lone ac·e·tate (floo - per′o - lōn). Acetato de fluperolona; um corticosteróide sintético.

flu·phen·a·zine (floo - fen′ă - zēn). Flufenazina; tranqüilizante utilizado como um agente antipsicótico e neuroléptico.

f. enanthate, enantato de flufenazina; antipsicótico de ação prolongada utilizado por via parenteral.

f. hydrochloride, cloridrato de flufenazina; antipsicótico utilizado no tratamento da esquizofrenia aguda e crônica, das psicoses involutiva, senil e tóxica e na fase maníaca da psicose maníaco-depressiva.

flu·pred·nis·o·lone (floo - pred - nis′o - lōn). Fluprednisolona; glicocorticóide com ação antiinflamatória e toxicidade similares às do cortisol.

flur·an·dren·o·lide (floor - an - dren′o - līd). Flurandrenolida; glicocorticóide com ação antiinflamatória utilizado em preparações tópicas.

flur·az·e·pam hy·dro·chlo·ride (floor - az′ē - pam). Cloridrato de flurazepam; hipnótico e sedativo oral do grupo dos benzodiazepínicos.

flur·bi·pro·fen (floor - bi′prō - fen). Flurbiprofeno; agente antiinflamatório não-esteróide com ações analgésica, antiinflamatória e antipirética, semelhante ao ibuprofeno.

flur·o·ges·tone ac·e·tate (floor - ō - jes′tōn). Acetato de flurogestona; agente progestacional.

flur·oth·yl (floor′ō - thil). Flurotila; convulsionante inalatório; produz convulsões do tipo grande mal.

flur·ox·ene (floor - ok′sēn). Fluroxeno; anestésico inalatório, volátil e halogenado. SIN 2,2,2-trifluoroethyl vinyl.

flush (flŭsh). **1.** Lavagem com um jato de líquido. **2.** Rubor; eritema transitório causado por calor, exercício, estresse ou doença. **3.** Ao nível de; em linha ou nivelado com outra superfície.

carcinoid f., rubor carcinóide; hiperemia periódica (sufusão) da pele da face e de outras partes do corpo, observada em pacientes com tumor carcinóide; os tumores produzem várias monoaminas e hormônios peptídeos, porém a causa exata do rubor é incerta; o rubor pode ser provocado pelo álcool, por alimentos, pelo estresse ou pela palpação do fígado.

hectic f., r. héctico; vermelhidão da face associada a elevação da temperatura em diversos tipos de febre.

histamine f., r. causado pela histamina; vasodilatação e eritema que ocorrem como resultado da liberação de histamina; acredita-se que seja um fator na gênese do rubor da síndrome carcinóide.

hot f., fogacho; coloquialismo para um sintoma vasomotor do climatério, caracterizado por vasodilatação súbita acompanhada de uma sensação de calor que, em geral, acomete a face, o pescoço e a parte superior do tórax. Cf. hot *flash*.

malar f., r. malar; r. héctico localizado e acompanhado de calor encontrado na região das eminências malares, que ocorre com freqüência na tuberculose e é, às vezes, observado na febre reumática e no lúpus eritematoso sistêmico.

flu·tam·ide (floo′tă - mīd). Flutamida; substância sintética não-esteróide utilizada no tratamento do câncer de próstata; antineoplásico (hormonal).

flut·ter (flŭt′er). *Flutter*; agitação; tremor. [A.S. *floterian*, flutuar sobre]

atrial f., auricular f., f. atrial, f. auricular; contrações atriais rápidas e regulares que ocorrem geralmente em uma freqüência que varia entre 250 e 330 por minuto (f. atrial de tipo I) e freqüentemente produzem ondas serrilhadas no eletrocardiograma, especialmente nas derivações II, III e aVF. O f. atrial de tipo II apresenta uma freqüência de 330 a 450 por minuto. Diferentemente do tipo I, o tipo II não é interrompido pelo marcapasso.

diaphragmatic f., f. diafragmático; contrações rítmicas e rápidas (média de 150/minuto) do diafragma, simulando o f. atrial clínica e, às vezes, eletrocardiograficamente.

impure f., *flutter*-fibrilação; mistura de ondas de *flutter* atrial (FF) e ondas de fibrilação (ff) no eletrocardiograma. SIN fibrilloflutter, flitter, flutter-fibrillation.

ocular f., f. ocular; oscilação espontânea, breve, intermitente e horizontal dos olhos que ocorre durante a fixação; freqüentemente coexiste com dismetria ocular nas síndromes cerebelares.

ventricular f., f. ventricular; forma de taquicardia ventricular rápida na qual os complexos eletrocardiográficos assumem um padrão ondulante e regular sem complexos QRS e ondas T distintos.

flut·ter-fi·bril·la·tion. *Flutter*-fibrilação. SIN impure *flutter*.

flux (flŭks). **1.** Eliminação de grande volume de material líquido de uma cavidade ou superfície do corpo. VER TAMBÉM diarrhea. **2.** Material eliminado pelos intestinos. **3.** Material utilizado para remover óxidos da superfície do metal fundido e protegê-lo, quando fundido; serve a um propósito semelhante na soldagem. É, também, um dos componentes da porcelana dentária que, devido a sua baixa temperatura de fusão, auxilia na união das partículas de sílica. **4.** (*J*). Densidade de fluxo; os moles de uma substância que atravessam uma unidade de área de uma camada ou membrana limitante por unidade de tempo. SIN flux density (1). **5.** Movimento bidirecional de uma substância em uma membrana ou superfície. **6.** Em radiologia diagnóstica, o fluxo de fótons por unidade de tempo. **7.** A força de um campo de força (p.ex., magnética),

ortogonal a uma unidade de área. **8.** A velocidade de transformação ou translocação química ou física de uma substância por unidade de tempo. [L. *fluxus*, um fluxo]
   luminous f., f. luminoso; quantidade de luz emitida por uma fonte puntiforme em determinado tempo; sua unidade é o lúmen.
   net f., f. resultante; a diferença entre os dois fluxos unidirecionais.
   unidirectional f., f. unidirecional; o f. de uma substância de uma das superfícies de uma camada ou membrana limitante até a outra, independentemente de qualquer f. que contrabalance em outra direção, como medido por técnica de rastreamento.

fly (flī). Mosca; inseto com duas asas da ordem Diptera. Dentre as moscas importantes estão: *Simulium* (mosca-negra), *Calliphora, Piophila casei* (m.-do-queijo), *Chrysops, Siphona irritans, Fannia scolaris* (m. das latrinas), *Oestrus ovis* e *Gasterophilus hemorrhoidalis, Cochliomyia hominivorax* (mosca-varejeira) e *C. macellaria* (mosca-varejeira), *Stomoxys calcitrans* (mosca-dos-estábulos), *Glossina* (m. tsé-tsé) e membros da ordem Trichoptera. Para alguns tipos de moscas não arroladas como subentradas aqui (geralmente escritas com uma palavra), ver o nome completo (p.ex., blowfly, botfly, gadfly, horsefly, housefly). [A.S. *fleóge*]
   flesh f., m. -varejeira; gêneros de moscas incluindo *Wohlfahrtia, Sarcophaga* e *Parasarcophaga* que se alimentam de fezes e de carne e peixe em decomposição; podem causar doença no homem.
   heel f., m.-do-berne, mosca-de-ura, mosca-berneira. VER botfly.
   louse f.'s, hipoboscídeos; dípteros pupíparos, achatados dorsoventralmente e ectoparasitas da família Hippoboscidae. VER TAMBÉM *Hippobosca*.
   mangrove f., m.-do-mangue; espécie de *Chrysops* encontrada na África e que age como vetor da *Loa loa*; p.ex., *Chrysops silacea*.
   Russian f., Spanish f., *Lytta vesicatoria*. SIN cantharis.
   warble f., m.-do-berne. VER botfly.

Flynn, P., médico norte-americano. VER F.-Aird *syndrome*; F. *phenomenon*.
Fm Símbolo do fermium (férmio).
FMD Abreviatura de foot-and-mouth *disease* (febre aftosa).
fMet Abreviatura de *N*-formylmethionine (*N*-formilmetionina).
fMet-tRNA Abreviatura de formylmethionyl tRNA (formilmetionil RNAt).
FMLH Abreviatura de familial hemophagocytic lymphohistiocytosis (linfohistiocitose hemafagocítica familiar).
FMN Abreviatura de *flavin* mononucleotide (flavina mononucleotídeo).
FMR1. Síndrome do X frágil humano. SIN fragile X *syndrome*.
FNA Abreviatura de fine needle aspiration biopsy (biopsia por aspiração com agulha fina).
foam (fōm). **1.** Espuma; massas de pequenas bolhas sobre a superfície de um líquido. **2.** Espumar; a produção de tais bolhas. **3.** Esponja; massas de células aéreas em um sólido ou semi-sólido, como na espuma de borracha.
   human fibrin f., esponja de fibrina humana; esponja artificial e seca de fibrina humana, preparada pela coagulação da espuma de uma solução de fibrinogênio humano pela trombina; a espuma coagulada é seca a partir do estado congelado e aquecida; utilizada como um agente anticoagulante tópico.

fo·cal (fō'kal). Focal. **1.** Que se refere a um foco. **2.** Relativo a uma área localizada.
fo·cal spot size. O tamanho medido de um ponto focal de um tubo de raios X; corresponde a uma função do tamanho real do cátodo e à angulação da superfície do ânodo. VER focal *spot*.
fo·ci (fō'sī). Focos; plural de focus.
fo·cim·e·ter (fō - sim'ē - ter). Focômetro. SIN lensometer.
fo·cus, pl. **fo·ci** (fō'kŭs, fō'sī). Foco. **1.** (F). O ponto no qual os raios de luz se encontram após cruzarem uma lente convexa. **2.** O centro, ou o ponto de início, de um processo mórbido. [L. uma lareira]
   conjugate foci, focos conjugados; dois pontos relacionados a uma lente ou a um espelho côncavo de tal forma que uma imagem em um ponto é focalizada no outro, e vice-versa.
   Ghon f., f. de Ghon. SIN Ghon *tubercle*.
   natural f. of infection, f. natural de infecção; ecossistema no qual um agente infeccioso persiste normalmente na natureza; p.ex., o vírus da febre amarela em um ecossistema formado por um macaco selvagem e o mosquito do gênero *Haemagogus*.
   principal f., f. principal; o ponto de encontro real ou virtual de raios que passam por uma lente paralelamente ao seu eixo.
   real f., f. real; o ponto de encontro de raios convergentes.
   virtual f., f. virtual; o ponto a partir do qual raios divergentes parecem proceder, ou o ponto no qual os raios se encontrariam, caso fossem prolongados para trás.

fo·drin (fō'drin). Fodrina; proteína semelhante à espectrina que se liga transversalmente aos filamentos de actina adjacentes nas células dos vertebrados.
Fogarty, Thomas J., cirurgião torácico norte-americano, *1934. VER F. embolectomy *catheter*, *clamp*.
fog·ging (fog'ing). Método de refração no qual a acomodação é relaxada pela correção excessiva por uma lente esférica convexa.
fo·go sel·va·gem (fō'gŏ sel'vă - jem). Fogo selvagem, pênfigo do Brasil; forma de pênfigo foliáceo encontrada no sul do Brasil e na qual lesões bolhosas aparecem na face e na parte superior do tronco, espalham-se, tornam-se variegadas, eritrodérmicas e esfoliativas e são imunologicamente indistinguíveis das lesões do pênfigo foliáceo ou do pênfigo vulgar. SIN Brazilian pemphigus, wildfire. [Pt. fogo selvagem]
foil (foyl). Papel laminado; uma folha extremamente fina e flexível de metal.
Foix, Charles, neurologista francês, 1882–1927. VER F.-Alajouanine *myelitis*, *syndrome*; F.-Cavany-Marie *syndrome*.
fo·late (fō'lāt). Folato; um sal ou éster do ácido fólico.

FOLD

fold (fōld) [TA]. Prega. **1.** Crista ou margem aparentemente formada pela dobra de uma lâmina. SIN plica. **2.** No embrião, uma elevação transitória ou reduplicação de tecido na forma de uma lâmina.
   adipose f.'s of the pleura, pregas adiposas da pleura. SIN fatty f.'s of pleura.
   alar f.'s of intrapatellar synovial fold [TA], pregas alares da prega sinovial infrapatelar; franjas ou expansões, situadas nas partes lateral e medial da p. sinovial infrapatelar, que se assemelham a asas e são preenchidas por gordura. SIN plicae alares plicae synovialis infrapatellaris.
   amnionic f., p. amniótica; p. da membrana do âmnio que envolve o pedículo vitelino e se estende do ponto de inserção do cordão umbilical até o saco vitelino; nos répteis e nas aves, corresponde à borda refletida do âmnio, que se dobra para cobrir o embrião durante o início do seu desenvolvimento. SIN Schultze f.
   ampullary f.'s of uterine tube, pregas da ampola da tuba uterina; pregas da mucosa localizadas na extremidade fimbriada da tuba uterina. SIN plicae ampullares tubae uterinae.
   anterior axillary f., p. axilar anterior; p. que limita a axila anteriormente; formada pela pele e pela fáscia que cobre a margem inferior do músculo peitoral maior.
   aryepiglottic f. [TA], p. ariepiglótica; prega proeminente da membrana mucosa que se estende entre a margem lateral da epiglote e a cartilagem aritenóidea em ambos os lados; a p. envolve o músculo ariepiglótico. SIN plica aryepiglottica [TA], arytenoepiglottidean f.
   arytenoepiglottidean f., p. ariepiglótica. SIN aryepiglottic f.
   axillary f., p. axilar; uma das pregas de pele e de tecido muscular que limitam a axila anterior e posteriormente. SIN plica axillaris.
   caval f., p. da cava; p. próxima à base do lado direito do mesentério dorsal, na qual um segmento primordial da veia cava inferior se desenvolve entre a veia subcardinal direita e os vasos intra-hepáticos.
   cecal f.'s [TA], pregas cecais; as duas pregas peritoneais que limitam a fossa retrocecal. SIN plicae cecales [TA].
   f. of chorda tympani, p. da corda do tímpano; prega de mucosa que circunda o nervo corda do tímpano em seu curso através da cavidade timpânica. SIN plica chordae tympani.
   ciliary f.'s [TA], pregas ciliares; várias cristas baixas localizadas nos sulcos entre os processos ciliares; essas pregas, juntamente com os processos ciliares, constituem a coroa ciliar. SIN plicae ciliares [TA].
   circular f.'s of small intestine [TA], pregas circulares do intestino delgado; numerosas pregas da mucosa do intestino delgado, estendendo-se transversalmente por cerca de dois terços da circunferência do intestino. SIN plicae circulares intestini tenuis [TA], Kerckring f.'s, Kerckring valves, valvulae conniventes.
   Dennie-Morgan f., p. de Dennie-Morgan; p. ou linha localizada abaixo de ambas as pálpebras inferiores, provocada por edema na dermatite atópica. SIN Dennie line.
   dinucleotide f., domínio estrutural encontrado em certas proteínas que se ligam ao NAD^+ ou ao $NADP^+$. SIN dinucleotide domain.
   Douglas f., p. de Douglas, p. retouterina. SIN rectouterine f.
   Duncan f.'s, pregas de Duncan; pregas encontradas na face peritoneal do útero imediatamente após o parto.
   duodenojejunal f., p. duodenal superior; *termo oficial alternativo para superior duodenal f.
   duodenomesocolic f., p. duodenal inferior; *termo oficial alternativo para inferior duodenal f.
   epicanthal f., p. palpebronasal. SIN palpebronasal f.
   epigastric f., p. umbilical lateral. SIN lateral umbilical f.
   epiglottic f.'s, pregas epiglóticas; uma das três pregas de membrana mucosa encontradas entre a língua e a epiglote, a p. glossoepiglótica lateral de um dos lados e a p. glossoepiglótica mediana. SIN plicae epiglotticae.
   falciform retinal f., p. falciforme da retina; p. congênita que se estende do disco até a região ciliar, encontrada no quadrante temporal inferior da retina.
   fatty f.'s of pleura, pregas adiposas da pleura; lóbulos de gordura encapsulados situados na pleura, principalmente na vizinhança do recesso costomediastinal. SIN adipose f.'s of the pleura, plicae adiposae pleurae.

fimbriated f. of inferior surface of tongue [TA], p. franjada da superfície inferior da língua; uma de várias pregas que se dirigem para fora a partir do frênulo na face inferior da língua. SIN plica fimbriata faciei inferioris linguae [TA].
gastric f.'s [TA], pregas gástricas; pregas características da mucosa gástrica, especialmente evidentes quando o estômago está contraído. SIN plicae gastricae [TA], gastric rugae*, ruga gastrica, rugae of stomach.
gastropancreatic f.'s [TA], pregas gastropancreáticas; pregas do peritônio, localizadas na bolsa omental, que envolvem as artérias hepática e gástrica esquerda, enquanto esses vasos se dirigem aos seus destinos. SIN plicae gastropancreaticae [TA].
genital f., p. genital. SIN urogenital ridge.
giant gastric f.'s, pregas gástricas gigantes; cristas de submucosa gástrica hipertrofiada revestidas por mucosa hiperplásica, como observado na síndrome de Zollinger-Ellison, na doença de Ménétrièr e na gastropatia hipertrófica hipersecretora.
glossopalatine f., arco palatoglosso. SIN palatoglossal arch.
gluteal f. [TA], p. glútea; p. proeminente que marca o limite superior da coxa a partir do limite inferior das nádegas; a p. coincide com a margem inferior do músculo glúteo máximo; sulco entre as nádegas e a coxa. SIN sulcus gluteus [TA], gluteal furrow.
Guérin f., p. de Guérin. SIN valve of navicular fossa.
Hasner f., p. de Hasner. SIN lacrimal f.
head f., p. da cabeça; prega ventral da extremidade cefálica localizada no disco embrionário, de forma que o cérebro se posiciona rostralmente em relação à boca e ao pericárdio.
Houston f.'s, pregas de Houston. SIN transverse f.'s of rectum.
ileocecal f. [TA], p. ileocecal; prega de peritônio que limita a fossa ileocecal ou ileoapendicular. SIN plica ileocecalis [TA], Treves f.
incudal f., p. da bigorna; prega variável de mucosa que se estende do teto da cavidade timpânica até o corpo e o ramo curto da bigorna. SIN plica incudis.
inferior duodenal f. [TA], p. duodenal inferior; prega de peritônio que limita o recesso duodenal inferior. SIN plica duodenalis inferior [TA], duodenomesocolic f.*, plica duodenomesocolica*.
infrapatellar synovial f. [TA], p. sinovial infrapatelar; prega de membrana sinovial que se estende desde um ponto abaixo do nível da face articular da patela até a parte anterior da fossa intercondilar. SIN plica synovialis infrapatellaris [TA], plica synovialis patellaris.
inguinal f., p. inguinal. SIN plica inguinalis.
inguinal aponeurotic f., p. aponeurótica inguinal. SIN inguinal falx.
interarytenoid f., p. interaritenóidea; tecido frouxo localizado entre as cartilagens aritenóideas. SIN posterior commissure of the larynx.
interdigital f.'s, pregas interdigitais. SIN web of fingers/toes.
interureteric f., p. interuretérica. SIN interureteric crest.
f.'s of iris [TA], pregas da íris; numerosas pregas radiais, muito finas e quase microscópicas, localizadas na face posterior da íris, que se estendem ao redor da margem pupilar. SIN plicae iridis [TA].
Kerckring f.'s, pregas de Kerckring. SIN circular f.'s of small intestine.
Kohlrausch f.'s, pregas de Kohlrausch. SIN transverse f.'s of rectum.
labioscrotal f.'s, pregas labioescrotais; pregas laterais encontradas em ambos os lados da membrana cloacal embrionária que dão origem ou ao escroto, ou aos lábios maiores do pudendo.
lacrimal f. [TA], p. lacrimal; prega de mucosa que protege a abertura inferior do ducto lacrimonasal. SIN plica lacrimalis [TA], Hasner f., Huschke valve, Rosenmüller valve.
f. of laryngeal nerve, p. do nervo laríngeo superior. SIN f. of superior laryngeal nerve.
lateral f.'s, pregas laterais; pregas ventrais das margens laterais do disco embrionário; o desenvolvimento dessas pregas auxilia o estabelecimento da forma definitiva do corpo embrionário.
lateral glossoepiglottic f. [TA], p. glossoepiglótica lateral; prega de membrana mucosa que se estende da margem da epiglote até a parede faringeal e a base da língua bilateralmente, formando o limite lateral da valécula epiglótica. SIN plica glossoepiglottica lateralis [TA], pharyngoepiglottic f.
lateral nasal f., p. lateral do nariz. SIN lateral nasal prominence.
lateral umbilical f. [TA], p. umbilical lateral; crista formada pelos vasos epigástricos inferiores e localizada na face peritoneal da parede anterior do abdome. SIN plica umbilicalis lateralis [TA], epigastric f., plica epigastrica.
f. of left vena cava [TA], p. da veia cava esquerda; prega do pericárdio, situada entre a veia oblíqua do átrio esquerdo e a veia pulmonar esquerda superior, que contém os resquícios obliterados da veia cava superior esquerda. SIN plica venae cavae sinistrae [TA], Marshall vestigial f., vestigial f.
longitudinal f. of duodenum [TA], p. longitudinal do duodeno; prega de mucosa situada na parede medial da parte descendente do duodeno, acima da papila maior do duodeno, provavelmente formada pela relação com o ducto colédoco. SIN plica longitudinalis duodeni [TA].
malar f., p. malar; sulco mal definido na pele e que se estende para baixo e medialmente a partir do ângulo lateral do olho.
mallear f.'s [TA], pregas maleares; duas faixas ligamentosas – anterior e posterior – que formam pregas no lado timpânico da membrana timpânica e que se estendem de cada extremidade da incisura timpânica até a proeminência malear; as pregas marcam o limite entre as partes tensa e flácida da membrana timpânica. SIN plicae malleares (anterior e posterior) [TA], plica membranae tympani.
mammary f., p. mamária. SIN mammary ridge.
Marshall vestigial f., p. vestigial de Marshall. SIN f. of left vena cava.
medial canthic f., p. palpebronasal; *termo oficial alternativo para palpebronasal f.
medial nasal f., p. medial do nariz. SIN medial nasal prominence.
medial umbilical f. [TA], p. umbilical medial; prega do peritônio, localizada na parte inferior da parede anterior do abdome, que reveste a artéria umbilical obliterada em ambos os lados do úraco. SIN plica umbilicalis medialis [TA], plica hypogastrica.
median glossoepiglottic f. [TA], p. glossoepiglótica mediana; prega de membrana mucosa, localizada na linha média, que se estende do dorso da língua até a epiglote, formando o limite medial da valécula epiglótica. SIN plica glossoepiglottica mediana [TA], frenulum epiglottidis, middle glossoepiglottic f.
median umbilical f. [TA], p. umbilical mediana; prega de peritônio localizada na parede anterior do abdome e que reveste o úraco ou os resquícios do pedículo da alantóide. SIN middle umbilical f., plica urachi, urachal f.
medullary f.'s, pregas neurais. SIN neural f.'s.
mesonephric f., p. mesonéfrica. SIN mesonephric ridge.
middle glossoepiglottic f., p. glossoepiglótica mediana. SIN median glossoepiglottic f.
middle transverse rectal f., p. transversa do reto. VER transverse f.'s of rectum.
middle umbilical f., p. umbilical mediana. SIN median umbilical f.
mongolian f., p. palpebronasal. SIN palpebronasal f.
mucobuccal f., p. mucobucal; linha de flexura da membrana mucosa que se estende da mandíbula ou das maxilas até a bochecha.
mucosal f.'s of gallbladder [TA], pregas da mucosa da vesícula biliar; pregas entrelaçadas da mucosa que produzem uma aparência de favos de mel no interior da vesícula biliar. SIN plicae mucosae vesicae biliaris [TA], rugae of gallbladder*, rugae vesicae biliaris*.
nail f., p. da unha. SIN nail wall.
nasojugal f., p. nasojugal; sulco raso na pele que se estende para baixo e lateralmente a partir do ângulo medial do olho.
Nélaton f., p. de Nélaton. VER transverse f.'s of rectum.
neural f.'s, pregas neurais; as margens elevadas do sulco neural. SIN medullary f.'s.
opercular f., p. opercular; tecido que forma uma ponte ou uma aderência entre a tonsila e o pilar anterior das fauces.
palmate f.'s of cervical canal, pregas palmadas do canal cervical; duas cristas — anterior e posterior —, localizadas na mucosa que reveste o canal do colo do útero, ramificando-se em numerosas pregas ou rugas secundárias. SIN plicae palmatae canalis cervicis uteri [TA], arbor vitae uteri, lyra uterina.
palpebronasal f. [TA], p. palpebronasal; prega de pele que se estende da raiz do nariz até a terminação medial da sobrancelha, sobrepondo-se ao ângulo medial do olho; sua presença é normal durante a vida fetal e em alguns asiáticos. SIN plica palpebronasalis [TA], medial canthic f.*, epicanthal f., epicanthus, mongolian f.
paraduodenal f. [TA], p. paraduodenal; prega em forma de foice do peritônio, encontrada às vezes formando um arco entre o lado esquerdo da flexura duodenojejunal e a margem medial do rim esquerdo; sua margem direita livre contém o ramo ascendente da artéria cólica esquerda e a veia mesentérica inferior; a p. forma o limite anterior do recesso paraduodenal. VER TAMBÉM paraduodenal recess. SIN plica paraduodenalis [TA], Treitz arch.
pharyngoepiglottic f., p. glossoepiglótica. SIN lateral glossoepiglottic f.
pleuropericardial f., p. pleuropericárdica; p. de tecido que se projeta para dentro do canal pericardioperitoneal direito ou esquerdo do embrião; a p. separa o pericárdio em desenvolvimento da cavidade pleural e é formada pelo crescimento da veia cardinal comum até a linha média do corpo. SIN pericardiopleural membrane, pleuropericardial membrane.
pleuroperitoneal f., p. pleuroperitoneal; p. de tecido que faz saliência para dentro da parte caudal do canal pericardioperitoneal do embrião; a p. desenvolve-se para dentro da parte dorsal do diafragma definitivo e é formada pelos pulmões, que crescem no sentido caudal, e pelo fígado, que se expande cranialmente. SIN pleuroperitoneal membrane.
posterior axillary f., p. axilar posterior; limita a axila posteriormente; é formada por pele e fáscia revestindo os músculos latíssimo do dorso e redondo maior e os tendões de inserção.
presplenic f., p. pré-esplênica; p. em forma de leque de peritônio que se estende do ligamento gastroesplênico, próximo da extremidade inferior do baço, até o ligamento frenicocólico, com o qual se funde. Contém ramos da artéria esplênica ou da gastroepilóica esquerda.
rectal f.'s, pregas transversas do reto. SIN transverse f.'s of rectum.
rectouterine f. [TA], p. retouterina; prega de peritônio que contém o músculo retouterino e se estende do sacro até a base do ligamento largo em ambos os

lados, formando o limite lateral da escavação retouterina (Douglas). SIN plica rectouterina [TA], Douglas f., sacrouterine f.

rectovesical f., p. retovesical. SIN sacrovesical f.

retinal f., p. da retina; p. congênita ou adquirida, resultante da contração da membrana, que produz pregas em forma de estrela e meridionais ou circulares na retina.

retroauricular f., p. retroauricular; dobra de pele formada pela junção da pele da orelha externa com a pele pós-auricular.

retrotarsal f., fórnice da conjuntiva. SIN conjunctival fornix.

Rindfleisch f.'s, pregas de Rindfleisch; pregas semilunares da superfície serosa do pericárdio que envolvem o início da aorta.

sacrogenital f.'s, pregas sacrogenitais; pregas peritoneais que se estendem para trás a partir dos dois lados da bexiga, no homem, ou do útero, na mulher, passando em ambos os lados do reto, até o sacro, formando os limites laterais da escavação retovesical. VER sacrouterine f., sacrovesical f.

sacrouterine f., p. retouterina. SIN rectouterine f.

sacrovaginal f., p. sacrovaginal; parte inferior da p. sacrouterina. SIN plica rectovaginalis.

sacrovesical f., p. retovesical; p. de peritônio, presente no homem, que limita a escavação retovesical lateralmente. SIN rectovesical f.

salpingopalatine f. [TA], p. salpingopalatina; crista de membrana mucosa que se estende da margem anterior da abertura da tuba auditiva (eustaquiana) até o palato. SIN plica salpingopalatina [TA], plica tubopalatina.

salpingopharyngeal f. [TA], p. salpingofaríngea; crista de mucosa que se estende da extremidade inferior da elevação da tuba ao longo da parede da faringe, cobrindo o músculo salpingofaríngeo. SIN plica salpingopharyngea [TA].

Schultze f., p. de Schultze. SIN amnionic f.

semilunar f. [TA], p. semilunar; prega curva que une o arco palatoglosso ao arco palatofaríngeo acima da fossa supratonsilar; quando presente, a p. sempre contém tecido linfático. SIN plica semilunaris [TA].

semilunar f.'s of colon [TA], pregas semilunares do cólon; pregas encontradas da parede do cólon entre as saculações. SIN plicae semilunares coli [TA], plicae semilunares of colon.

semilunar conjunctival f., p. semilunar da conjuntiva. SIN plica semilunaris of conjunctiva.

spiral f. of cystic duct [TA], p. espiral do ducto cístico; uma série de pregas, em forma de crescente, de membrana mucosa localizada na parte superior do ducto cístico, disposta de forma levemente espiralada. SIN plica spiralis ductus cystici [TA], Amussat valve, Heister valve, spiral valve of cystic duct, valvula spiralis.

stapedial f., p. estapedial. SIN f. of stapes.

f. of stapes [TA], p. estapedial; reflexão da delicada mucosa da parede posterior da cavidade timpânica que reveste o estribo. SIN plica stapedialis, stapedial f.

sublingual f. [TA], p. sublingual; elevação localizada no assoalho da boca debaixo da língua, encontrada em ambos os lados, marcando o local da glândula sublingual. SIN plica sublingualis [TA].

superior duodenal f. [TA], p. duodenal superior; prega de peritônio que limita o recesso duodenal superior. SIN plica duodenalis superior [TA], duodenojejunal f.*, plica duodenojejunalis*.

f. of superior laryngeal nerve [TA], p. do nervo laríngeo superior; fina prega de mucosa, localizada no recesso piriforme da faringe, que envolve o nervo laríngeo superior. SIN plica nervi laryngei superioris [TA], f. of laryngeal nerve.

synovial f., p. sinovial; crista ou projeção da membrana sinovial de uma articulação que se estende em direção às duas faces articulares ou entre elas. SIN plica synovialis.

tail f., p. caudal; prega ventral da extremidade caudal do disco embrionário.

tarsal f., p. tarsal; p. que marca a união do músculo levantador da pálpebra superior na pele da pálpebra superior.

transverse palatine f. [TA], p. palatina transversa; vestígio do aparelho mastigatório encontrado no palato duro; uma de várias cristas irregulares, às vezes ramificadas, de tecido frouxo que se irradiam das regiões mais anteriores das papilas incisivas e se estendem a uma pequena distância para trás, cruzando o palato duro e atingindo lateralmente distâncias variáveis. SIN plica palatina transversa [TA], ruga palatina, transverse palatine ridge.

transverse f.'s of rectum [TA], pregas transversas do reto; três ou quatro pregas, em forma de crescente, dispostas horizontalmente na mucosa retal; a p. retal superior está situada no lado esquerdo, próxima do início do reto; a p. retal média (p. de Houston ou de Kohlrausch) é mais proeminente e consistente, projetando-se do lado direito cerca de 8 cm acima do ânus (aproximadamente ao nível do assoalho da escavação retouterina ou retovesical); a p. retal inferior está localizada no lado esquerdo, cerca de 5 cm acima do ânus. SIN plicae transversales recti [TA], Houston f.'s, Kohlrausch f.'s, plicae recti, rectal f.'s, rectal valves.

transverse vesical f., p. vesical transversa; duplicação do peritônio que passa sobre a bexiga vazia e torna-se obliterada quando a víscera está repleta. SIN plica vesicalis transversa.

Treves f., p. de Treves. SIN ileocecal f.

triangular f. [TA], p. triangular; p. inconstante de mucosa, anterior à tonsila palatina, que se origina no arco palatoglosso. SIN plica triangularis [TA].

urachal f., p. umbilical mediana. SIN median umbilical f.

ureteric f., p. uretérica. SIN interureteric crest.

urorectal f., p. urorretal. SIN urorectal septum, urorectal membrane.

f.'s of uterine tubes [TA], pregas das tubas uterinas; várias pregas longitudinais situadas na mucosa da tuba uterina (falópio). SIN plicae tubariae, tubae uterinae [TA].

uterovesical f., p. uterovesical. SIN uterovesical ligament.

vascular f. of the cecum [TA], p. cecal vascular; prega peritoneal que forma um arco sobre um ramo da artéria ileocólica e limita, em frente a um recesso estreito, o recesso ileocecal superior (ou ileocólico). SIN plica cecalis vascularis [TA].

Vater f., p. de Vater; p. de mucosa situada no duodeno, exatamente acima da papila maior do duodeno.

ventricular f., p. ventricular. SIN vestibular f.

vestibular f. [TA], p. vestibular; duas pregas de mucosa que revestem os ligamentos vestibulares e se estendem de lado a lado da cavidade da laringe, do ângulo da cartilagem tireóidea até a cartilagem aritenóidea; o par de pregas – direita e esquerda – encerra um espaço denominado de rima do vestíbulo ou falsa glote e forma o limite superior do ventrículo da laringe. SIN plica vestibularis [TA], false vocal cord, plica ventricularis, ventricular band of larynx, ventricular f.

vestigial f., p. da veia cava esquerda. SIN f. of left vena cava.

vocal f. [TA], p. vocal; prega de margem afiada que reveste o ligamento vocal e se estende pelas paredes da laringe, do ângulo entre as lâminas da cartilagem tireóidea até o processo vocal da cartilagem aritenóidea; as pregas vocais são os elementos relacionados com a produção da voz. SIN plica vocalis [TA], chorda vocalis, Ferrein cords, labium vocale, true vocal cord, vocal cord, vocal shelf.

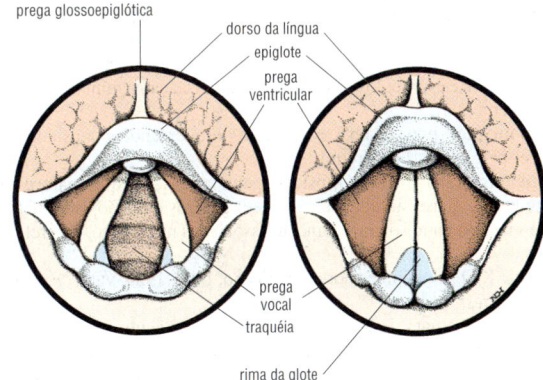

cordas vocais: interior da laringe, observado com o laringoscópio; (esquerda) rima da glote totalmente aberta, (direita) rima da glote fechada

Foley, Frederic E.B., urologista norte-americano, 1891–1966. VER F. *catheter*, Y-plasty *pyeloplasty*.

fo·lia (fō′lē-ă). Folhas; plural de folium.

fo·li·a·ceous (fō-lē-ā′shŭs). Foliáceo. SIN foliate.

fo·li·ar (fō′lē-ăr). Foliar. SIN foliate.

fo·li·ate (fō′lē-āt). Foliáceo; relativo ou que se assemelha a uma folha ou folhinha. SIN foliaceous, foliar, foliose.

---

fo·lic ac·id (fō′lik). Ácido fólico. **1.** Termo coletivo dos ácidos pteroilglutâmicos e seus ácidos oligoglutâmicos conjugados. O ácido *N*-[p-[[(2-amino-4-hidroxipteridin-6-il)metil]amino]benzoil]-L(+)-glutâmico; especificamente, o ácido pteroilmonoglutâmico; VER TAMBÉM homocysteine. **2.** O fator de crescimento do *Lactobacillus casei* e um membro do complexo da vitamina B necessário para a produção normal de hemácias; é uma vitamina hematopoética presente, com ou sem as porções L-(+) do ácido glutâmico, nas ligações peptídicas no fígado, nos vegetais verdes e nas leveduras; utilizado no tratamento da deficiência de folato e da anemia megaloblástica e para ajudar a reduzir os níveis de homocisteína. SIN *Lactobacillus casei* factor, liver *Lactobacillus casei* factor, pteroylmonoglutamic acid. [L. *folium*, folha, + -ic]

> Pesquisas recentes permitiram um melhor entendimento do papel do ácido fólico no metabolismo humano; os problemas de saúde associados à deficiência dietética de ácido fólico forneceram evidências sobre os benefícios terapêuticos da suplementação de ácido fólico e sugeriram que as doses dietéticas de ácido fólico recomendadas no passado (200 μg/dia

para homens; 180 μg/dia para mulheres) são insuficientes para certas pessoas, incluindo as gestantes. As fontes naturais de ácido fólico incluem pães integrais e cereais, suco de laranja, lentilhas, feijões, leveduras, fígado e vegetais com folhas verdes, tais como brócolis, couve e espinafre. O ácido fólico e a cobalamina (vitamina B_{12}) são componentes de coenzimas nas reações de 1 carbono, como a metilação de homocisteína a metionina. A deficiência de ácido fólico causa anemia macrocítica por prejudicar a síntese de eritrócitos e está associada à elevação dos níveis plasmáticos de homocisteína, um fator de risco para doença cardiovascular, incluindo arteriosclerose coronariana, acidente vascular cerebral e tromboembolismo. A deficiência de ácido fólico na gravidez está associada a um risco aumentado de defeitos no tubo neural, como espinha bífida e anencefalia, bem como a um risco aumentado de parto prematuro e recém-nascidos de baixo peso. As pessoas com deficiência hereditária da enzima ácido 5,10 metilenotetraidrofólico redutase possuem necessidades dietéticas aumentadas de ácido fólico. A prevalência da forma homozigota dessa deficiência pode exceder 10% da população geral. A ingestão de ácido fólico, piridoxina (vitamina B_6) e cobalamina acima da cota dietética atualmente recomendada tem sido associada a um risco substancialmente menor de doença coronariana e de defeitos do tubo neural. Os nutricionistas recomendam pelo menos 400 μg/dia de ácido fólico para todas as pessoas e 1 mg/dia ou mais para gestantes e pessoas com níveis plasmáticos de homocisteína elevados. A Food and Drug Administration exige a suplementação de grãos e cereais com ácido fólico.

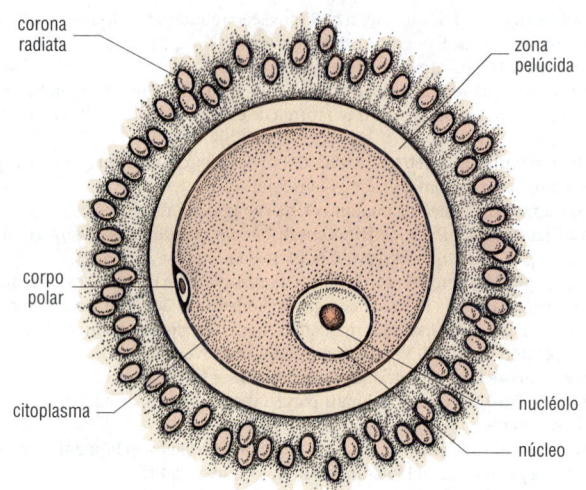

folículo ovárico: contendo um óvulo

fo·lie (fō-lē′). Demência; termo antigo para a loucura ou insanidade. [Fr. loucura]
  f. à deux (ã-du), transtorno psicótico compartilhado; distúrbios mentais idênticos ou semelhantes, tais como uma fixação paranóide, geralmente afetando dois membros da mesma família que vivem juntos. SIN shared psychotic disorder. [Fr. dois]
  f. du doute (du-doot), mania de dúvida; dúvida excessiva sobre todos os assuntos da vida e escrupulosidade mórbida com relação a minúcias. [Fr. proveniente da dúvida]
  f. du pourquoi (poor-kwah′), psicose do porquê; tendência psicopatológica de fazer perguntas. [Fr. porque]
  f. gémellaire (zha-mel-ār′), psicose gemelar; psicose que aparece simultaneamente, ou quase simultaneamente, em gêmeos que não estão necessariamente vivendo juntos ou intimamente associados na ocasião. [Fr. relativo aos gêmeos]
Folin, Otto K.O., bioquímico norte-americano, 1867–1934. VER F. *reaction*, *test*; F.-Looney *test*.
fo·li·nate (fō′li-nāt). Folinato; um sal ou éster do ácido folínico.
fo·lin·ic ac·id (fō-lin′ik). Ácido folínico. **1.** A forma ativa do ácido fólico que age como transportador do grupamento formila nas reações de transformilação; a leucovorina cálcica tem uso terapêutico. **2.** O termo é ocasionalmente aplicado a outros folatos. SIN citrovorum factor, leucovorin.
fo·li·ose (fō′lē-ōs). Foliáceo. SIN foliate.
fo·li·um, pl. **fo·lia** (fō′lē-ŭm, -lē-ă). [TA]. Folha; estrutura larga, delgada e semelhante a uma folha. [L. uma folha]
  fo′lia cerebel′li [TA], folhas do cerebelo. SIN folia of cerebellum.
  folia of cerebellum [TA], folhas do cerebelo; giros estreitos, semelhantes a folhas, do córtex cerebelar. VER TAMBÉM f. of vermis. SIN folia cerebelli [TA].
  fo′lia lin′guae, papilas folhadas. SIN foliate *papillae*, em *papilla*.
  f. ver′mis [TA], f. do verme. SIN f. of vermis.
  f. of vermis [TA], f. do verme; subdivisão pequena e posterior do verme superior do cerebelo, formada pelo lóbulo VIIA. SIN f. vermis [TA].
Folli, Folius. Cecilio (Caesilius), anatomista veneziano, 1615–1660. VER Folli *process*, follian *process*.
fol·li·cle (fol′i-kl) [TA]. Folículo. **1.** Massa mais ou menos esférica de células, contendo geralmente uma cavidade. **2.** Cripta ou fundo-de-saco minúsculo, como a depressão localizada na pele da qual o pêlo emerge. SIN folliculus [TA]. [L. *folliculus*, um pequeno saco, dim. de *follis*, um par de foles]
  aggregated lymphatic f.'s of small intestine, nódulos linfáticos agregados do intestino delgado. SIN aggregated lymphoid *nodules* of small intestine, em *nodule*.
  aggregated lymphatic f.'s of vermiform appendix, nódulos linfáticos agregados do apêndice vermiforme. SIN aggregated lymphoid *nodules*, em *nodule*.
  anovular ovarian f., f. ovárico anovular; f. que não contém um óvulo.
  antral f., f. ovárico vesiculoso. SIN vesicular ovarian f.
  atretic ovarian f., f. ovárico atrésico; f. que se degenera antes de se tornar maduro; existe um grande número de folículos atrésicos no ovário antes da puberdade; em mulheres sexualmente maduras, vários folículos atrésicos são formados a cada mês. SIN corpus atreticum.
  dental f., f. dentário, f. dental; saco dentário que contém o órgão odontogênico e o dente em desenvolvimento.
  gastric f.'s, glândulas gástricas. SIN gastric *glands*, em *gland*.
  graafian f., folículo de de Graaf. SIN vesicular ovarian f.
  growing ovarian f., f. ovárico em desenvolvimento; f. que possui várias camadas de células foliculares proliferativas circundando o óvulo, porém separadas dele por uma camada glicoproteica extracelular (zona pelúcida).
  hair f. [TA], f. piloso; invaginação da epiderme que se assemelha a um tubo, a partir da qual a haste do pêlo se desenvolve e para dentro da qual as glândulas sebáceas se abrem; o folículo é revestido por uma bainha radicular celular interna e externa de origem epidérmica e recoberto por uma bainha fibrosa derivada da derme. SIN folliculus pili [TA].
  intestinal f.'s, glândulas intestinais. SIN intestinal *glands*, em *gland*.
  Lieberkühn f.'s, folículos de Lieberkühn. SIN intestinal *glands*, em *gland*.
  lingual f.'s, folículos da língua. SIN *folliculi linguales*, em *folliculus*.
  luteinized unruptured f., f. luteinizado não-roto; f. que sofreu luteinização sem ter sofrido ruptura prévia; acreditava-se que esse f. causasse infertilidade, porém agora sabe-se que existe com a mesma freqüência, tanto em mulheres férteis como em inférteis.
  lymphatic f.'s of larynx, nódulos do anel linfático da laringe. SIN laryngeal lymphoid *nodules*, em *nodule*.
  lymphatic f.'s of rectum, folículos linfáticos do reto. SIN *folliculi lymphatici recti*, em *folliculus*.
  mature ovarian f., f. ovárico maduro; o f. pronto para a ovulação; no ovário humano, o antro desse f. atinge um diâmetro de 6 a 8 mm e apresenta uma superfície abaulada; a primeira divisão de maturação do óvulo (meiótica) geralmente ocorre imediatamente antes da ruptura do f.
  Montgomery f.'s, folículos de Montgomery. SIN areolar *glands*, em *gland*.
  multilaminar primary f., f. primário multilaminado; f. ovárico primário com duas ou mais camadas de células foliculares cubóides cobrindo o oócito.
  nabothian f., f. de Naboth. SIN nabothian *cyst*.
  ovarian follicle, folículo ovárico; um dos agregados de células esferoidais localizados no ovário, contendo um óvulo.
  polyovular ovarian f., f. ovárico poliovular; f. que contém mais de um óvulo.
  primary ovarian f., f. ovárico primário; f. ovariano antes do aparecimento de um antro; caracterizado por mudanças evolutivas no oócito e nas células foliculares, de modo que estas últimas formam uma ou mais camadas de células cubóides ou colunares; o f. torna-se circundado por um invólucro de estroma, a teca. SIN folliculus ovaricus primarius.
  primordial ovarian f., f. ovárico primordial; f. no qual o oócito primordial está rodeado por uma única camada de células foliculares achatadas.
  sebaceous f.'s, glândulas sebáceas. SIN sebaceous *glands*, em *gland*.
  secondary ovarian f., f. ovárico secundário. SIN vesicular ovarian f.
  solitary f.'s, nódulos linfáticos solitários. SIN solitary lymphatic *nodules*, em *nodule*.
  solitary lymphatic f.'s, nódulos linfáticos solitários. SIN solitary lymphatic *nodules*, em *nodule*.
  splenic lymph f.'s, nódulos linfáticos do baço; pequenas massas nodulares de tecido linfático aderidas aos lados das ramificações arteriais menores. SIN folliculi lymphatici lienales, malpighian bodies, malpighian corpuscles (2), malpighian glands, malpighian nodules, splenic corpuscles, splenic lymph nodules.
  f.'s of thyroid gland, folículos da glândula tireóide. SIN *folliculi glandulae thyroideae*, em *folliculus*.

unilaminar primary f., f. primário unilaminado; f. ovárico primário com uma única camada de células foliculares cubóides cobrindo o oócito.
vesicular f., f. ovárico vesiculoso. SIN vesicular ovarian f.
vesicular ovarian f., f. ovárico vesiculoso; f. cujo oócito atinge o tamanho máximo e é cercado por uma camada glicoproteica extracelular (zona pelúcida), que o separa de uma camada periférica de células foliculares, permeada por um ou mais antros preenchidos com líquido; a teca do f. desenvolve-se formando uma camada interna e outra externa. SIN antral f., folliculus ovaricus vesiculosus, graafian f., secondary ovarian f., vesicular f.

fol·lic·u·lar (fō-lik′ū-lar). Folicular; relativo a um folículo ou a vários folículos.
fol·lic·u·li (fō-lik′ū-lī). Folículos; plural de folliculus.
fol·lic·u·lin (fō-lik′oo-lin). Estrona. SIN estrone.
folliculin hydrate. Estriol. SIN estriol.
fol·lic·u·li·tis (fō-lik-ū-lī′tis). Foliculite; reação inflamatória que ocorre em folículos pilosos; as lesões podem ser pápulas ou pústulas.
  f. absce′dens et suffo′diens, f. dissecante do couro cabeludo; f. pustulosa progressiva crônica encontrada no couro cabeludo.
  f. bar′bae, f. da barba. SIN tinea barbae.
  f. decal′vans, f. descalvante; inflamação papulosa ou pustulosa dos folículos pilosos do couro cabeludo, de causa desconhecida, observada principalmente em homens, resultando na formação de fibrose e perda de cabelos na área afetada.
  eosinophilic pustular f., f. pustulosa eosinofílica; dermatose caracterizada por pápulas e pústulas pruriginosas e estéreis que coalescem para formar placas com bordas papulovesiculosas; exacerbações e remissões espontâneas podem ser acompanhadas de leucocitose periférica e/ou de eosinofilia e podem resultar na destruição dos folículos pilosos e formação de abscessos eosinofílicos; tem sido encontrada em pacientes com AIDS/SIDA. Uma forma possivelmente distinta da f. pustulosa eosinofílica é observada em bebês. SIN Ofuji disease.
  f. keloida′lis, f. queloidal. SIN acne keloid.
  f. na′res per′forans, f. perfurante do nariz; inflamação de um folículo piloso localizado no nariz; a infecção estende-se para a superfície cutânea, perfurando-a.
  perforating f., f. perfurante; pápulas eritematosas com uma rolha central de queratina, disseminadas pelos braços, pelas coxas e nádegas; em biopsias, fibras dérmicas são vistas estendendo-se para dentro do folículo; alterações similares são observadas principalmente em diabéticos submetidos a hemodiálise. VER TAMBÉM hyperkeratosis follicularis et parafollicularis.
  f. ulerythemato′sa reticula′ta, f. uleritematosa reticulada; cicatrizes eritematosas com forma de "furador de gelo" ou deprimidas localizadas nas bochechas; tipo de foliculite cicatricial associado a ceratose pilar e comumente herdado como um traço autossômico dominante.

fol·lic·u·lo·ma (fō-lik-ū-lō′ma). **1.** Tumor de células da granulosa. SIN granulosa cell tumor. **2.** Hipertrofia cística de um folículo de de Graaf.
fol·lic·u·lo·sis (fō-lik-ū-lō′sis). Foliculose; presença de folículos linfáticos em número anormalmente elevado.
fol·lic·u·lus, pl. **fol·lic·u·li** (fō-lik′ū-lŭs, -ū-lī) [TA]. Folículo. SIN follicle. [L. um pequeno saco, dim. de follis, foles]
follic′uli glan′dulae thyroi′deae, folículos da glândula tireóide; as pequenas estruturas esféricas vesiculosas da glândula tireóide revestidas com epitélio e contendo quantidades variáveis de colóide; o colóide serve para o armazenamento do precursor do hormônio da tireóide, a tireoglobulina. SIN follicles of thyroid gland.
follic′uli lingua′les, folículos da língua; agrupamentos de tecido linfático localizados na mucosa da parte faríngea da língua, posteriormente ao sulco terminal, que formam em conjunto a tonsila lingual. SIN lenticular papillae, lingual follicles.
follic′uli lymphat′ici aggrega′ti, nódulos linfáticos agregados. SIN aggregated lymphoid nodules of small intestine, em nodule.
follic′uli lymphat′ici aggrega′ti appen′dicis vermifor′mis, folículos linfáticos agregados do apêndice vermiforme. SIN aggregated lymphoid nodules, em nodule.
folliculi lymphat′ici gas′trici, nódulos linfáticos do estômago. SIN gastric lymphoid nodules, em nodule.
follic′uli lymphat′ici laryn′gei, folículos do anel linfático da laringe. SIN laryngeal lymphoid nodules, em nodule.
follic′uli lymphat′ici liena′les, folículos linfáticos do baço. SIN splenic lymph follicles, em follicle.
follic′uli lymphat′ici rec′ti, folículos linfáticos do reto; agrupamentos disseminados de tecido linfático localizados na parede do reto. SIN lymphatic follicles of rectum.
follic′uli lymphat′ici solita′rii, nódulos linfáticos solitários. SIN solitary lymphatic nodules, em nodule.
f. lymphat′icus, nódulo linfóide. SIN lymphoid nodule.
f. ovar′icus prima′rius, f. ovárico primário. SIN primary ovarian follicle.
f. ovar′icus vesiculo′sus, f. ovárico vesiculoso. SIN vesicular ovarian follicle.
f. pi′li [TA], f. piloso. SIN hair follicle.

Folling, Ivar A., médico norueguês, 1888–1973. VER F. disease.

fol·li·stat·in (fol-ī-stat-′n). Folistatina; peptídeo sintetizado pelas células granulosas em resposta ao FSH, que suprime a atividade do FSH, provavelmente ligando-se a ativinas. [folliclë + -stat + -in]
fol·li·tro·pin (fol-i-trō′pin). Folitropina, hormônio foliculoestimulante (FSH); hormônio glicoproteico, produzido pela hipófise anterior, que estimula os folículos de Graaf do ovário e auxilia subseqüentemente na maturação folicular e na secreção de estradiol; no homem, o hormônio estimula o epitélio dos túbulos seminíferos e é parcialmente responsável pela indução à espermatogênese. SIN follicle-stimulating hormone, follicle-stimulating principle, gametokinetic hormone. [follicle + G. tropē, uma volta, + -in]
Foltz, Jean C.E., anatomista e oftalmologista francês, 1822–1876. VER F. valvule.
fo·men·ta·tion (fō-men-tā′shŭn). Fomentação. **1.** Aplicação quente. VER TAMBÉM poultice, stupe. **2.** Aplicação de calor e umidade no tratamento de doenças. [L. fomento, pp. -atus, fomentar, de fomentum, um cataplasma, de foveo, manter aquecido]
fo·mes, pl. **fom·i·tes** (fō′mēz, fōm′i-tēz). Fomites; objetos, tais como roupas, toalhas e utensílios, que possivelmente abrigam um agente patogênico e são capazes de transmiti-lo; o termo é geralmente utilizado no plural. SIN fomite. [L. pavio, de foveo, manter aquecido]
fo·mite (fō′mīt). Fomites. SIN fomes. [L. fomitis, gen. de fomes. VER fomes]
fom·i·tes (fō′mi-tēz). Fomites; plural de fomes.
fo·na·zine mes·y·late (fō′na-zēn). Mesilato de fonazina; inibidor da serotonina com propriedades miorrelaxantes. SIN dimethothiazine mesylate.
Fonio, Anton, médico suíço, 1881–1968. VER F. solution.
Fonsecaea (fon-sē-sē′a). Gênero de fungos do qual pelo menos duas espécies, F. pedrosoi e F. compacta, causam cromoblastomicose.
Fontan, François M., cirurgião torácico francês, *1929. VER F. procedure, operation.
Fontana, Arturo, dermatologista italiano, 1873–1950. VER F. stain; F.-Masson silver stain; Masson-F. ammoniac silver stain.
Fontana, Felice, fisiologista italiano, 1730–1805. VER F. canal, spaces, em space.
fon·ta·nelle (fon′tă-nel′). [NA]. Fontículo, fontanela; uma das várias áreas membranáceas localizadas nas margens dos ossos do crânio do bebê. VER cranial f.'s. SIN fonticulus. [Fr. dim. de fontaine, fonte, nascente]
  anterior f. [NA], f. anterior; área membranácea, em forma de diamante, localizada na junção das suturas coronal, sagital e frontal (metópica), onde os ângulos dos ossos parietais encontram as duas metades separadas do osso frontal. SIN bregmatic f., fonticulus anterior, frontal f.

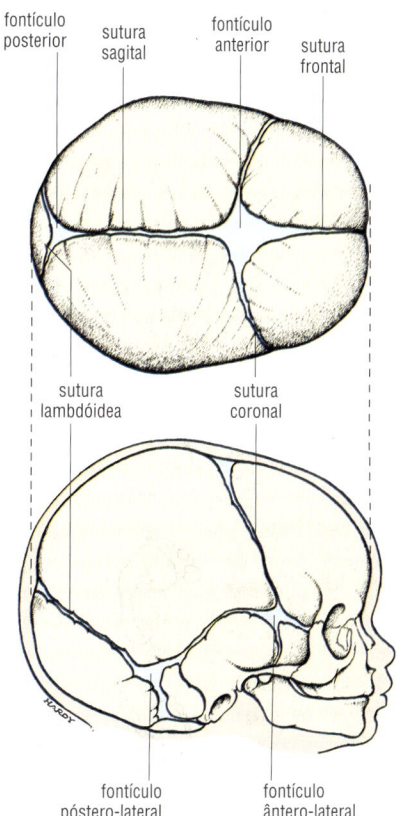

fontículos e suturas do crânio fetal: (acima) vista de cima; (abaixo) vista lateral

anterolateral f., f. ântero-lateral. SIN sphenoidal f.
bregmatic f., f. anterior. SIN anterior f.
Casser f., f. de Casser, f. póstero-lateral. SIN mastoid f.
cranial f.'s [NA], fontículos do crânio; áreas membranáceas localizadas entre os ângulos dos ossos do crânio nos lactentes; incluem a f. anterior e a f. posterior, situadas na linha média, as duas fontanelas ântero-laterais e as duas fontanelas póstero-laterais. SIN fonticuli cranii.
frontal f., f. anterior. SIN anterior f.
Gerdy f., f. de Gerdy. SIN sagittal f.
mastoid f. [NA], f. póstero-lateral; área membranácea, localizada em ambos os lados do crânio, entre o ângulo mastóideo do osso parietal, a parte petrosa do osso temporal e o osso occipital. SIN fonticulus mastoideus [NA], fonticulus posterolateralis*, Casser f., posterolateral f.
occipital f., f. occipital. SIN posterior f.
posterior f., f. posterior; área triangular, localizada na união das suturas lambdóidea e sagital, onde os ângulos occipitais dos ossos parietais encontram o osso occipital. SIN fonticulus posterior, occipital f.
posterolateral f., f. póstero-lateral. SIN mastoid f.
sagittal f. [NA], f. sagital; f. ocasional, semelhante a um defeito, localizada na sutura sagital do recém-nascido. SIN Gerdy f.
sphenoidal f. [NA], f. ântero-lateral; área com forma irregular, localizada em ambos os lados do crânio, onde o osso frontal, o ângulo esfenoidal do osso parietal, a parte escamosa do osso temporal e a asa maior do osso esfenóide se encontram. SIN fonticulus sphenoidalis [NA], fonticulus anterolateralis*, anterolateral f.
fon·tic·u·lus, pl. **fon·tic·u·li** (fon - tĭk′ū - lŭs, - lī). Fontículo, fontanela. SIN fontanelle. VER cranial *fontanelles*, em *fontanelle*. [L. dim. de *fons* (*font-*), fonte, nascente]
f. ante′rior, f. anterior. SIN anterior *fontanelle*.
f. anterolatera′lis, f. ântero-lateral; *termo oficial alternativo para sphenoidal *fontanelle*.
fontic′uli cra′nii, fontículos do crânio. SIN cranial *fontanelles*, em *fontanelle*.
f. mastoi′deus [NA], f. póstero-lateral. SIN mastoid *fontanelle*.
f. poste′rior, f. posterior. SIN posterior *fontanelle*.
f. posterolatera′lis, f. póstero-lateral; *termo oficial alternativo para mastoid *fontanelle*.
f. sphenoida′lis [NA], f. ântero-lateral. SIN sphenoidal *fontanelle*.
food (food). Alimento; o que é ingerido para fornecer elementos nutritivos necessários. [A.S. *fōda*]
Foot, N. C., patologista norte-americano do século XX. VER F. reticulin impregnation *stain*.
foot (fut) [TA]. Pé. **1.** Extremidade inferior (podálica) da perna. SIN pes (1). **2.** Unidade de comprimento contendo 12 polegadas, que corresponde a 30,48 cm. [A.S. *fōt*]
 athlete's f., pé-de-atleta, tinha do pé. SIN *tinea* pedis.
 claw f., pé em garra. VER clawfoot.
 club f., pé torto. VER *talipes* equinovarus.

contracted f., pé cavo. SIN *talipes* cavus.
drop f., pé caído. VER footdrop.
f. of hippocampus, pé do hipocampo; a extremidade espessada anterior do hipocampo. SIN pes hippocampi [TA], digitationes hippocampi.
immersion f., pé-de-trincheira; condição que resulta da exposição prolongada à umidade e ao frio; o membro permanece inicialmente frio e anestesiado, porém, ao ser aquecido novamente, torna-se hiperemiado, parestésico e hiperidrótico; a recuperação é freqüentemente lenta. SIN trench f.
Madura f., pé de Madura, micetoma. SIN mycetoma.
Morand f., pé de Morand; pé com oito artelhos.
mossy f., pé musgoso; proliferação papilomatosa, aveludada e profusa que se transforma em grandes projeções verrucosas; causada por estase e linfedema crônicos acompanhados de maceração e infecção. SIN lymphedematous keratoderma, lymphostatic verrucosis.
sandal f., pé em sandália; espaço amplo entre o primeiro e o segundo artelhos, observado em pessoas com síndrome de Down.
spastic flat f., pé plano espástico; eversão do pé acompanhada de espasmo dos músculos (fibular) do lado externo; está freqüentemente associada a faixas anormais de cartilagem óssea ou tecido fibroso entre os ossos calcâneo e navicular (escafóide), ou entre o osso navicular e o tálus, resultando numa coalizão tarsal.
trench f., pé-de-trincheira. SIN immersion f.
foot·can·dle (fut′kan-dl). Pé-vela; iluminação ou claridade equivalente a 1 lúmen por pé quadrado; substituído no sistema SI por candela.
foot·drop (fut′drop). Pé caído; incapacidade parcial ou total para realizar a dorsiflexão do pé; como conseqüência, os dedos do pé arrastam-se pelo solo durante a locomoção, a menos que o paciente adote uma marcha eqüina; é, em geral, decorrente de fraqueza dos músculos que realizam a dorsiflexão do pé (principalmente do tibial anterior), porém possui muitas causas, incluindo distúrbios do sistema nervoso central, da unidade motora, dos tendões e dos ossos.
foot·ling (foot′ling). Pé fetal, em particular o pé que desce para o canal de parto na apresentação pélvica incompleta. [foot, de A.S. *fōt*, + *-ling*, dim. sufixo]
foot·plate, foot-plate (fut′plāt). **1.** Base do estribo; *termo oficial alternativo para base of stapes. **2.** Pedicelo *termo oficial alternativo para pedicel.
foot-pound (fut′pownd). Pé-libra; energia despendida ou trabalho realizado ao erguer-se verticalmente uma massa de 1 libra (454 g aprox.) a uma altura de 1 pé (= 30,48 cm) contra a força da gravidade.
foot-pound·al (fut′pownd - ăl). Pé-poundal; energia despendida ou trabalho realizado quando uma força de 1 poundal (= 421,4 ergs ou 13,825 dinas) é aplicada a um corpo, deslocando-o 1 pé (= 30,48 cm) na direção da força; corresponde a aproximadamente 0,01 caloria.
foot·print·ing (fut′prĭnt-ing). Impressão digital genética; método utilizado para determinar a área de DNA com ligação proteica; consiste na digestão do complexo proteína-DNA pela nuclease, seguida da análise da região do DNA que ficou protegida pela interação com a proteína.
for·age (for - ahzh′). Operação que consiste em cortar um canal por meio de diatermia cirúrgica através de uma próstata hipertrofiada. [Fr. perfuração]

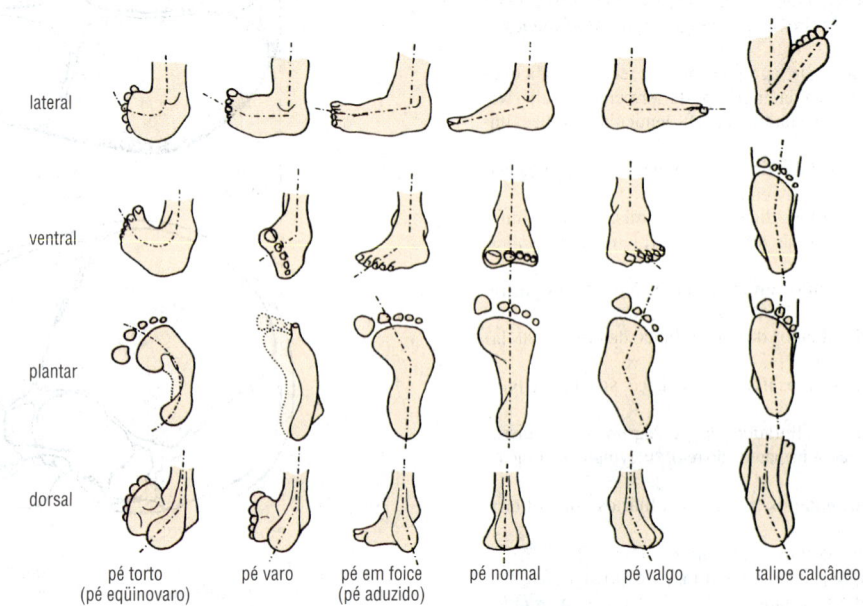

deformidades do pé

FORAMEN

fo·ra·men, pl. **fo·ram·i·na** (fō-rā′men, fō-ram′i-nă). [TA]. Forame; abertura ou perfuração que atravessa um osso ou uma estrutura membranácea. SIN trema (1). [L. uma abertura, de *foro*, furar, perfurar]

foram'ina alveola'ria corporis maxillae [TA], forames alveolares da maxila. SIN alveolar foramina of maxilla.

alveolar foramina of maxilla [TA], forames alveolares da maxila; aberturas dos canais dentários posteriores localizadas na face infratemporal da maxila. SIN foramina alveolaria corporis maxillae [TA].

anterior condyloid f., canal do nervo hipoglosso. SIN hypoglossal *canal*.

anterior palatine f., f. palatino maior. SIN greater palatine f.

aortic f., hiato aórtico. SIN aortic *hiatus*.

apical dental f., f. do ápice do dente. SIN apical f. of tooth.

apical f. of tooth [TA], f. do ápice do dente; abertura localizada no ápice da raiz de um dente que dá passagem para o nervo e vasos sanguíneos. SIN f. apicis dentis [TA], apical dental f., root f.

f. ap'icis den'tis [TA], f. do ápice do dente. SIN apical f. of tooth.

arachnoid f., abertura mediana do quarto ventrículo. SIN median *aperture* of fourth ventricle.

f. of Arnold, f. de Arnold. SIN f. petrosum.

blind f. of frontal bone, f. cego do osso frontal. SIN f. cecum of frontal bone.

blind f. of the tongue, f. cego da língua. SIN f. cecum of tongue.

Bochdalek f., f. de Bochdalek. SIN pleuroperitoneal *hiatus*.

Botallo f., f. de Botallo; orifício de comunicação entre os dois átrios do coração fetal. VER TAMBÉM f. ovale.

f. cae'cum medul'lae oblonga'tae [TA], f. cego da medula oblonga; pequena depressão triangular, localizada entre a margem inferior da ponte e a pirâmide, que marca o limite superior da fissura mediana anterior da medula oblonga. SIN f. caecum posterius, Vicq d'Azyr f.

carotid f., f. da carótida. SIN *openings* of carotid canal, em *opening*.

cecal f. of frontal bone, f. cego do frontal. SIN f. cecum of frontal bone.

cecal f. of the tongue, f. cego da língua. SIN f. cecum of tongue.

f. cecum of frontal bone [TA], f. cego do osso frontal; f. cego formado imediatamente à frente da crista etmoidal por uma depressão na extremidade inferior da crista frontal e sua articulação com o osso etmóide. É insignificante no período pós-natal, porém dá passagem a vasos durante o desenvolvimento. SIN f. cecum ossis frontalis [TA], blind f. of frontal bone, cecal f. of frontal bone.

f. ce'cum lin'guae [TA], f. cego da língua. SIN f. cecum of tongue.

f. ce'cum os'sis fronta'lis [TA], f. cego do frontal. SIN f. cecum of frontal bone.

f. cae'cum poste'rius, f. cego da medula oblonga. SIN f. caecum medullae oblongatae.

f. cecum of tongue [TA], f. cego da língua; fossa mediana localizada no dorso da parte posterior da língua, de onde partem os ramos de um sulco com forma de V, dirigindo-se para a frente e para fora; é o local de origem da glândula tireóide e do subseqüente ducto tireoglosso no embrião. SIN f. cecum linguae [TA], blind f. of the tongue, cecal f. of the tongue, Morgagni f. (1).

conjugate f., f. conjugado; f. formado pelas incisuras de dois ossos justapostos.

f. costotransversa'rium [TA], f. costotransversário. SIN costotransverse f.

costotransverse f. [TA], f. costotransversário; abertura localizada entre o colo de uma costela e o processo transverso de uma vértebra e preenchida pelo ligamento costotransversário. SIN f. costotransversarium [TA].

cribriform foramina [TA], forames da lâmina cribriforme; aberturas, localizadas na lâmina cribriforme do osso etmóide, por onde passam aproximadamente 20 feixes de fibras nervosas que, em conjunto, constituem o nervo olfatório (NC I). SIN foramina cribrosa [TA], olfactory f.

foramina cribrosa [TA], forames da lâmina cribriforme. SIN cribriform foramina.

f. diaphrag'matis sel'lae, f. do diafragma da sela. SIN f. of sellar diaphragm.

epiploic f., f. omental; *termo oficial alternativo para omental f.

f. epiplo'icum, f. omental; *termo oficial alternativo para omental f.

ethmoidal f. [TA], f. etmoidal; um dos dois forames formados na parede medial da órbita por sulcos nas duas margens da incisura etmoidal do osso frontal e completados por sulcos semelhantes no osso etmóide: f. etmoidal anterior, localizado em posição anterior, e f. etmoidal posterior, localizado em posição posterior. SIN f. ethmoidale (anterior et posterior) [TA].

f. ethmoida'le (anterior et posterior) [TA], f. etmoidal (anterior e posterior). SIN ethmoidal f.

external acoustic f., poro acústico externo. SIN external acoustic *pore*.

external auditory f., poro acústico externo. SIN external acoustic *pore*.

Ferrein f., f. de Ferrein. SIN *hiatus* for greater petrosal nerve.

frontal f., f. frontal; pequena abertura encontrada ocasionalmente na margem supra-orbital do osso frontal, medialmente ao forame supra-orbital. VER TAMBÉM frontal *notch*. SIN f. frontale.

f. fronta'le, f. frontal. SIN frontal f.

great f., f. magno. SIN f. magnum.

greater palatine f. [TA], f. palatino maior; abertura localizada no canto póstero-lateral do palato duro, em frente ao último dente molar, e que marca a extremidade inferior do canal pterigopalatino. SIN f. palatinum majus [TA], anterior palatine f.

Huschke f., f. de Huschke; abertura no assoalho da parte óssea do meato acústico externo, próxima da membrana timpânica e geralmente fechada no adulto.

Hyrtl f., f. de Hyrtl. SIN *porus* crotaphytico-buccinatorius.

incisive f. [TA], f. incisivo; uma das várias (geralmente quatro) aberturas dos canais incisivos para dentro da fossa incisiva. SIN f. incisivum [TA], incisor f., Stensen f.

f. incisi'vum [TA], f. incisivo. SIN incisive f.

incisor f., f. incisivo. SIN incisive f.

inferior dental f., f. dental inferior. SIN mandibular f.

infraorbital f. [TA], f. infra-orbital; abertura externa do canal infra-orbital, localizada na face anterior do corpo da maxila. SIN f. infraorbitale [TA].

f. infraorbita'le [TA], f. infra-orbital. SIN infraorbital f.

interatrial f. pri'mum, óstio interatrial primário; (1) no coração embrionário, a abertura temporária localizada entre os átrios direito e esquerdo, situada entre a margem inferior do septo primário e os coxins do canal atrioventricular; (2) no coração já formado, a persistência anormal da já mencionada comunicação, que é normal em embriões jovens. SIN f. subseptale, ostium primum, primary interatrial f.

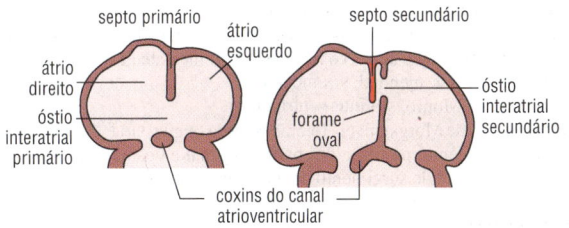

óstios interatriais primário e secundário: observados no coração embrionário; (esquerda) quinta semana de gestação; (direita) sexta semana de gestação

interatrial f. secun'dum, óstio interatrial secundário; abertura secundária que aparece na parte superior do septo primário na sexta semana de vida embrionária, antes do fechamento do f. interatrial primário. SIN ostium secundum, secondary interatrial f.

f. intermesocolica transversa, f. intermesocólico transverso.

internal acoustic f., poro acústico interno. SIN internal acoustic *pore*.

internal auditory f., poro acústico interno. SIN internal acoustic *pore*.

interventricular f. [TA], f. interventricular; passagem curta, freqüentemente semelhante a uma fenda, tanto no lado esquerdo como no direito, que comunica o terceiro ventrículo cerebral (do diencéfalo) com os ventrículos laterais (dos hemisférios cerebrais); a passagem é limitada anteromedialmente pela coluna do fórnice e posterolateralmente pelo pólo anterior e tubérculo anterior do tálamo dorsal. SIN f. interventriculare [TA], Monro f., porta (2).

f. interventricula're [TA], f. interventricular. SIN interventricular f.

intervertebral f. [TA], f. intervertebral; uma de várias aberturas localizadas no interior do canal vertebral, limitadas pelos pedículos das vértebras adjacentes, acima e abaixo, pelo corpo vertebral (geralmente da vértebra superior) e pelo disco intervertebral anteriormente, e pelos processos articulares que formam a articulação zigapofisária, posteriormente. SIN f. intervertebrale [TA].

f. intervertebra'le [TA], f. intervertebral. SIN intervertebral f.

f. ischiad'icum (anterior et posterior), f. isquiático (maior e menor). SIN sciatic f.

f. ischiadicum majus et minor [TA], f. isquiático maior e menor. SIN sciatic f.

jugular f. [TA], f. jugular; passagem localizada entre a parte petrosa do osso temporal e o processo jugular do occipital, às vezes dividida em duas passagens pelos processos intrajugulares; contém a veia jugular interna, o seio petroso inferior, o nervo glossofaríngeo, o nervo vago, o nervo acessório e ramos meníngeos das artérias faríngea ascendente e occipital. SIN f. jugulare [TA], f. lacerum posterius.

f. jugula're [TA], f. jugular. SIN jugular f.

f. of Key-Retzius, f. de Key-Retzius. SIN lateral *aperture* of fourth ventricle.

lacerated f., f. lacerado. SIN f. lacerum.

f. lac'erum [TA], f. lacerado; abertura irregular, preenchida com cartilagem (cartilagem basal) durante a vida, localizada entre o ápice da parte petrosa do osso temporal, o corpo do osso esfenóide e a parte basilar do osso occipital. Várias estruturas passam ao longo das margens do f. em sentido quase hori-

zontal, porém nenhuma estrutura passa através do f. verticalmente. SIN f. lacerum medium, lacerated f., sphenotic f.
f. lac'erum ante'rius, fissura orbital superior. SIN superior orbital *fissure*.
f. lac'erum me'dium, f. lacerado. SIN f. lacerum.
f. lac'erum poste'rius, f. jugular. SIN jugular f.
Lannelongue foramina, forames de Lannelongue. SIN *openings* of smallest cardiac veins, em *opening*.
f. latera'lis ventric'uli quar'ti, abertura lateral do quarto ventrículo. SIN lateral *aperture* of fourth ventricle.
lesser palatine foramina [TA], forames palatinos menores; aberturas, localizadas no palato duro, de canais palatinos que passam verticalmente através da tuberosidade do osso palatino e que conduzem os nervos palatinos menores e os vasos. SIN foramina palatina minora [TA], posterior palatine foramina.
f. of Luschka, f. de Luschka. SIN lateral *aperture* of fourth ventricle.
f. of Magendie, f. de Magendie. SIN median *aperture* of fourth ventricle.
f. mag'num [TA], f. magno; grande abertura localizada na parte basal do osso occipital, através da qual a medula espinal se torna contínua com o bulbo. SIN great f.
malar f., f. zigomaticofacial. SIN zygomaticofacial f.
f. mandib'ulae [TA], f. da mandíbula. SIN mandibular f.
mandibular f. [TA], f. da mandíbula; abertura localizada no canal da mandíbula, situada na face medial do ramo da mandíbula, que dá passagem para o nervo, artéria e veia alveolares inferiores. SIN f. mandibulae [TA], inferior dental f.
mastoid f. [TA], f. mastóideo; abertura localizada na parte posterior do processo mastóide, que conduz o ramo mastóideo da artéria occipital até a duramáter e uma veia emissária até o seio sigmóideo. SIN f. mastoideum [TA].
f. mastoi'deum [TA], f. mastóideo. SIN mastoid f.
mental f. [TA], f. mentual; abertura anterior do canal da mandíbula, localizada no corpo da mandíbula, lateral e superiormente ao tubérculo mentual e que dá passagem à artéria mentual e ao nervo mentual. SIN f. mentale [TA], mental canal.
f. menta'le [TA], f. mentual. SIN mental f.
Monro f., f. de Monro. SIN interventricular f.
Morgagni f., f. de Morgagni; **(1)** forame ceco da língua. SIN f. cecum of tongue; **(2)** defeito congênito na fusão das partes esternal e costal do primórdio diafragmático, o local de surgimento de uma hérnia retroesternal.
nasal f., f. nasal; f. vascular que se abre na face externa de cada osso nasal.
foram'ina nervo'sa [TA], forames nervosos; perfurações localizadas ao longo do lábio timpânico da lâmina espiral óssea que dão passagem aos nervos cocleares. SIN habenulae perforatae, zona perforata.
f. nutric'ium [TA], f. nutrício. SIN nutrient f.
nutrient f. [TA], f. nutrício; abertura externa para a entrada de vasos sanguíneos em um osso. SIN f. nutricium [TA].
obturator f. [TA], f. obturado; grande abertura oval ou irregularmente triangular, localizada no osso do quadril, cujas margens são formadas pelo púbis e ísquio; é fechada no estado natural pela membrana obturadora, exceto por uma pequena abertura para a passagem dos vasos obturatórios e do nervo obturatório. SIN f. obturatum [TA].
f. obtura'tum [TA], f. obturado. SIN obturator f.
olfactory f., forames da lâmina cribriforme. SIN cribriform foramina.
omental f. [TA], f. omental; passagem, situada abaixo e atrás da porta do fígado, que une as duas bolsas do peritônio; é limitada anteriormente pelo ligamento hepatoduodenal e posteriormente pela prega peritoneal situada sobre a veia cava inferior. SIN f. omentale [TA], epiploic f.*, f. epiploicum*, aditus ad saccum peritonei minorem, f. of Winslow.
f. omentale [TA], f. omental. SIN omental f.
optic f., canal óptico. SIN optic *canal*.
f. op'ticum, canal óptico. SIN optic *canal*.
oval f. [TA], f. oval. SIN f. ovale.
f. ova'le, f. oval; **(1)** [TA], grande abertura oval, localizada na base da asa maior do osso esfenóide, que dá passagem à divisão mandibular do gânglio trigeminal e de uma pequena artéria meníngea; **(2)** incompetência do f. oval do coração; uma condição que contrasta com a aderência fibrosa incompleta de uma valva do f. oval no fechamento pós-natal; na incompetência, a valva apresenta perfurações anormais ou é de tamanho insuficiente para permitir o movimento valvar adequado no período pré-natal ou para efetuar um fechamento completo no período pós-natal. SIN oval f. [TA].
f. ovale cordis [TA], f. oval do coração. SIN f. ovale of heart.
f. ovale of heart [TA], f. oval do coração; no coração fetal, a abertura oval na margem livre do septo secundário; a parte do septo primário que persiste atua como uma valva nessa comunicação interatrial durante a vida fetal e funde-se, no período pós-natal, ao septo secundário, a fim de fechá-lo. SIN f. ovale cordis, oval f. of heart.
oval f. of heart, f. oval do coração. SIN f. ovale of heart.
foram'ina palati'na mino'ra [TA], forames palatinos menores. SIN lesser palatine foramina.
f. palati'num ma'jus [TA], f. palatino maior. SIN greater palatine f.
foram'ina papilla'ria re'nis [TA], forames papilares do rim. SIN *openings* of papillary ducts, em *opening*.

papillary foramina of kidney, aberturas dos ductos papilares do rim. SIN *openings* of papillary ducts, em *opening*.
parietal f. [TA], f. parietal; f. inconstante localizado no osso parietal, encontrado de forma ocasional bilateralmente próximo da parte posterior da margem sagital; quando presente, o f. dá passagem a uma veia emissária para o seio sagital superior. SIN f. parietale [TA].
f. parieta'le [TA], f. parietal. SIN parietal f.
petrosal f., f. petroso. SIN f. petrosum.
f. petro'sum [TA], f. petroso; abertura ocasional localizada na asa maior do osso esfenóide, entre o f. espinhoso e o f. oval, que dá passagem ao nervo petroso menor. SIN canaliculus innominatus, f. of Arnold, petrosal f.
posterior condyloid f., canal condilar posterior. SIN condylar *canal*.
posterior palatine foramina, forames palatinos menores. SIN lesser palatine foramina.
postglenoid f., f. pós-glenoidal; pequeno forame que, às vezes, existe no osso temporal imediatamente à frente do meato acústico externo.
primary interatrial f., óstio interatrial primário. SIN interatrial f. primum.
f. proces'sus transver'si, f. transversário. SIN transverse f.
f. quadra'tum, f. quadrado. SIN caval *opening* of diaphragm.
f. recessus superioris bursae omentalis, f. do recesso superior da bolsa omental. SIN f. of superior recess of omental bursa.
f. of Retzius, f. de Retzius. SIN lateral *aperture* of fourth ventricle.
root f., f. do ápice do dente. SIN apical f. of tooth.
f. rotun'dum [TA], f. redondo; abertura localizada na base da asa maior do osso esfenóide, que dá passagem ao nervo maxilar. SIN round f.
round f., f. redondo. SIN f. rotundum.
sacral foramina [TA], forames sacrais; aberturas, localizadas entre as vértebras sacrais fundidas, que dão passagem aos nervos sacrais. Os forames sacrais anteriores conduzem os ramos primários anteriores (ventrais) dos nervos sacrais. Os forames sacrais posteriores dão passagem aos ramos primários posteriores (dorsais) dos nervos sacrais. Os termos "anterior" e "posterior" são inadequados, especialmente com referência aos forames de S1/S2, uma vez que, na posição anatômica, os forames estão dispostos verticalmente, superior e inferiormente um em relação ao outro. SIN f. sacrale, foramina sacralia anterior et posterior.
f. sacra'le, f. sacral. SIN sacral foramina.
foramina sacralia anterior et posterior, forames sacrais anterior e posterior. SIN sacral foramina.
Scarpa foramina, forames de Scarpa; duas aberturas localizadas na linha da sutura intermaxilar; o f. anterior conduz o nervo nasopalatino esquerdo, e o f. posterior, o nervo nasopalatino direito.
sciatic f. [TA], f. isquiático; um dos dois forames formados pelos ligamentos sacroespinal e sacrotuberal que cruzam as incisuras ciáticas do osso do quadril: f. isquiático maior e f. isquiático menor. SIN f. ischiadicum majus et minor [TA], f. ischiadicum (anterior et posterior).
secondary interatrial f., óstio interatrial secundário. SIN interatrial f. secundum.
f. of sellar diaphragm, f. do diafragma da sela; orifício localizado no centro do diafragma da sela turca e que dá passagem ao infundíbulo do hipotálamo. SIN f. diaphragmatis sellae.
singular f., f. singular. SIN f. singulare.
f. singula're [TA], f. singular; f. localizado no meato acústico interno, posterior à área coclear, que dá passagem aos nervos para a ampola do ducto semicircular posterior. SIN singular f.
foramina of the smallest veins of heart, forames das veias mínimas do coração. SIN *openings* of smallest cardiac veins, em *opening*.
sphenoidal emissary f. [TA], f. pequeno e inconstante localizado na asa maior do osso esfenóide, anterior e medialmente ao f. oval, que dá passagem a uma pequena veia emissária proveniente do seio cavernoso. SIN f. venosum [TA], venous f., Vesalius f.
sphenopalatine f. [TA], f. esfenopalatino; f. formado a partir da incisura esfenopalatina do osso palatino, na junção deste com o osso esfenóide; o f. dá passagem à artéria esfenopalatina e aos nervos que a acompanham. SIN f. sphenopalatinum [TA].
f. sphenopalati'num [TA], f. esfenopalatino. SIN sphenopalatine f.
sphenotic f., f. lacerado. SIN f. lacerum.
f. spino'sum [TA], f. espinhoso; abertura localizada na base da asa maior do osso esfenóide, anterior à espinha do osso esfenoidal, que dá passagem à artéria meníngea média e ao ramo meníngeo (nervo espinhoso) do nervo mandibular.
Stensen f., f. de Stensen. SIN incisive f.
stylomastoid f. [TA], f. estilomastóideo; abertura distal ou externa do canal do nervo facial, localizada na face inferior da parte petrosa do osso temporal, entre os processos estilóide e mastóide; o f. dá passagem ao nervo facial e à artéria estilomastóidea. SIN f. stylomastoideum [TA].
f. stylomastoid'eum [TA], f. estilomastóideo. SIN stylomastoid f.
f. subsepta'le, óstio interatrial primário. SIN interatrial f. primum.
f. of superior recess of omental bursa, f. do recesso superior da bolsa omen-

tal; f. produzido por duas pregas de peritônio que cobrem a artéria hepática comum/própria à direita e a artéria gástrica esquerda à esquerda e que invadem e comprimem a bolsa omental; o f. forma uma comunicação entre o recesso superior do omento menor, situado acima dele, e o restante da bolsa omental. SIN f. recessus superioris bursae omentalis.
supraorbital f. [TA], incisura supra-orbital; f. localizado na margem supraorbital do osso frontal, na junção dos terços médio e intermédio. SIN f. supraorbitale [TA].
f. supraorbita'le [TA], incisura supra-orbital. SIN supraorbital f.. VER TAMBÉM supraorbital *notch*.
thebesian foramina, forames de Tebésio. SIN openings of smallest cardiac veins, em *opening*.
thyroid f. [TA], f. tireóideo; abertura ocasional presente em uma ou em ambas as lâminas da cartilagem tireóidea. SIN f. thyroideum [TA].
f. thyroid'eum [TA], f. tireóideo. SIN thyroid f.
f. transversa'rium [TA], f. transversário. SIN transverse f.
transverse f., f. transversário. SIN f. transversarium [TA], f. of transverse process, f. processus transversi, f. vertebroarteriale, vertebroarterial f.
f. of transverse process, f. transversário. SIN transverse f.
f. of vena cava, f. da veia cava. SIN caval *opening* of diaphragm.
vena caval f., f. da veia cava. SIN caval *opening* of diaphragm.
f. ve'nae ca'vae, f. da veia cava. SIN caval *opening* of diaphragm.
foramina of the venae minimae, forames das veias mínimas. SIN openings of smallest cardiac veins, em *opening*.
foram'ina vena'rum minima'rum cordis, forames das veias mínimas do coração. SIN openings of smallest cardiac veins, em *opening*.
f. veno'sum [TA], f. venoso. SIN sphenoidal emissary f.
venous f., f. venoso. SIN sphenoidal emissary f.
vertebral f. [TA], f. vertebral; f. formado pela união do arco vertebral com o corpo vertebral; na coluna vertebral articulada, os forames vertebrais em conjunto formam a coluna vertebral. SIN f. vertebrale [TA].
f. vertebra'le [TA], f. vertebral. SIN vertebral f.
vertebroarterial f., f. transversário. SIN transverse f.
f. vertebroarteria'le, f. transversário. SIN transverse f.
Vesalius f., f. de Vesalius. SIN sphenoidal emissary f.
Vicq d'Azyr f., f. de Vicq d'Azyr. SIN f. caecum medullae oblongatae.
Vieussens foramina, forames de Vieussens. SIN openings of smallest cardiac veins, em *opening*.
Weitbrecht f., f. de Weitbrecht; abertura localizada na cápsula articular da articulação do ombro e que se comunica com a bolsa subtendínea do músculo subescapular.
f. of Winslow, f. de Winslow. SIN omental f.
zygomaticofacial f. [TA], f. zigomaticofacial; abertura localizada na face lateral do osso zigomático, abaixo da margem orbital, que dá passagem ao nervo zigomaticofacial. SIN f. zygomaticofaciale [TA], malar f.
f. zygomaticofacia'le [TA], f. zigomaticofacial. SIN zigomaticofacial f.
zygomatico-orbital f. [TA], f. zigomaticoorbital; abertura em comum, localizada na face orbital do osso zigomático, de canais que dão passagem aos nervos zigomaticofacial e zigomaticotemporal; às vezes, cada um desses canais apresenta uma abertura separada, localizada na face orbital. SIN f. zygomaticoorbitale [TA].
f. zygomat'ico-orbita'le [TA], f. zigomaticoorbital. SIN zygomatico-orbital f.
zygomaticotemporal f. [TA], f. zigomaticotemporal; abertura, localizada na face temporal do osso zigomático, de canal que dá passagem ao nervo zigomaticotemporal. SIN f. zygomaticotemporale [TA].
f. zygomat'icotempora'le [TA], f. zigomaticotemporal. SIN zygomaticotemporal f.

---

fo·ram·i·na (fō-ram′i-nă). Forames, plural de foramen.
Fo·ram·i·nif·e·ra (fō-ram-i-nif′er-ă, for′ă-mi-nif′er-ă). Ordem da classe Rhizopoda que compreende seres com pseudópodes anastomosados; estes formam uma rede ao redor da célula que, geralmente, se desenvolve em uma complexa carapaça calcária; um importante elemento do fundo do mar e de leitos rochosos que cobrem lençóis de petróleo. [L. *foramen*, abertura, + *fero*, carregar]
fo·ram·i·nif·er·ous (fō-ram-i-nif′er-ŭs, for′ă-mi-nif′er-ŭs). **1.** Foraminoso; que possui aberturas ou forames. **2.** Foraminífero; relativo à ordem Foraminifera.
for·am·i·not·o·my (for′am-i-not′ō-mē). Operação em uma abertura, geralmente para abri-la, p.ex., alargamento cirúrgico do forame intervertebral. [L. *foramen*, abertura, + G. *tome*, uma excisão]
fo·ram·in·u·lum, pl. **fo·ram·in·u·la** (fōr′ă-min′ū-lŭm, ū-lă). Um forame muito pequeno. [L. mod. dim. de *foramen*]
Forbes, A.P., médico norte-americano do século XX. VER F.-Albright *syndrome*.
Forbes, Gilbert B., pediatra norte-americano, *1915. VER F. *disease*.
force (F) (fōrs). Força; aquilo que tende a produzir movimento em um corpo. [L. *fortis*, forte]
animal f., f. animal; força muscular.
chewing f., f. da mastigação. SIN f. of mastication.
dynamic f., f. dinâmica, energia. SIN energy.
electromotive f. (EMF), f. eletromotriz; a f. (medida em volts) que produz uma corrente elétrica que se desloca de um ponto para outro.
G f., f. G; f. inercial produzida pela aceleração ou pela gravidade, expressa em unidades gravitacionais; um G é igual à força da gravidade na superfície da Terra, ao nível do mar e a 45° de latitude norte (32,1725 pés/s^2 ou 980,621 cm/s^2). VER TAMBÉM *g*.
f. of mastication, f. de mastigação; f. motriz produzida pela ação dinâmica dos músculos durante o ato fisiológico da mastigação. SIN biting strength, chewing f., masticatory f.
masticatory f., f. da mastigação. SIN f. of mastication.
occlusal f., f. oclusal; o resultado da f. muscular aplicada sobre os dentes opostos.
psychic f., energia psíquica. SIN psychic *energy*.
reciprocal f.'s, forças recíprocas; em odontologia, as forças produzidas quando a resistência de um ou mais dentes é utilizada para mover um ou mais dentes opostos.
reserve f., f. de reserva; energia existente no organismo ou em qualquer de suas partes, além da necessária para o seu funcionamento normal.
van der Waals f.'s, forças de van der Waals; postuladas pela primeira vez por van der Waals, em 1873, para explicar os desvios de comportamento observados em gases reais quando comparados com um gás ideal; correspondem às forças atrativas entre os átomos ou as moléculas diferentes da eletrostática (iônica), da covalente (compartilhamento de elétrons) ou das pontes de hidrogênio (compartilhamento de um próton); em geral, são atribuídas aos efeitos bipolares e de dispersão, a elétrons π, etc.; essas forças relativamente indefinidas contribuem para a atração mútua entre as moléculas orgânicas.
vital f., f. vital. VER vitalism.
force plat·form. Plataforma de força; dispositivo utilizado para medir a força, a simetria e a latência dos movimentos posturais compensatórios, quando estímulos visuais, vestibulares e somatossensoriais são aplicados de forma variada.
for·ceps (fōr′seps). Fórceps; pinça. **1.** Instrumento utilizado para segurar uma estrutura, por compressão ou tração. Cf. clamp. **2.** [TA]. Faixas de fibras brancas localizadas no cérebro, os fórceps maior e menor. [L. um par de pinças]
Adson f., p. de Adson; pequena p. digital com dois dentes em uma das extremidades e um dente na outra.
alligator f., p. jacaré; p. longa com um pequeno mordente articulado na extremidade.
Allis f., p. de Allis; p. de preensão reta com mordentes serrilhados utilizada para realizar, com o uso da força, a preensão ou a retração de tecidos ou estruturas.
f. anterior, fórceps anterior. SIN minor f.
Arruga f., p. de Arruga; p. para a extração intracapsular de uma catarata.
arterial f., p. arterial; p. com engate e lâminas oblíquas, utilizada para segurar a extremidade de um vaso sanguíneo até que uma ligadura seja realizada.
axis-traction f., f. de tração axial; f. obstétrico provido de um segundo cabo suficientemente fixo para que uma tração possa ser aplicada na linha onde a cabeça deve se mover no eixo da pelve.
Barton f., f. de Barton; f. obstétrico com uma colher fixa e curva e uma colher articulada anterior para aplicação a uma cabeça transversa alta.
bayonet f., pinça-baioneta; p. com lâminas deslocadas do eixo do cabo, tais como aquelas para uso através de um otoscópio.
bone f., p. óssea; p. robusta utilizada para pegar e remover fragmentos de osso.
Brown-Adson f., p. de Adson com aproximadamente 16 dentes delicados em cada ponta.
bulldog f., buldogue; p. com lâminas delicadas utilizada para ocluir um vaso sanguíneo.
bullet f., p. para balas; p. cujas lâminas finas e curvas apresentam superfícies preênseis serrilhadas para a extração de um projétil de arma de fogo dos tecidos.
capsule f., p. para cápsula; p. utilizada para remover a cápsula da lente durante a extração extracapsular de uma catarata.
Chamberlen f., f. de Chamberlen; o f. obstétrico original que não apresenta curvaturas em seus ramos.
clamp f., alicate para grampos; p. com mordentes forçados projetada para prender os mordentes de um grampo de dique de borracha, de forma que eles possam ser separados para passar por cima do contorno bucolingual mais amplo de um dente. SIN rubber dam clamp f.
clip f., p. de clipe; pequena p. com um fixador de mola utilizada para ocluir a extremidade de um vaso por onde esteja ocorrendo perda de sangue.
cup biopsy f., p. para biópsias; p. delgada e flexível com mordentes móveis e em forma de concha, utilizada para a obtenção de amostras para biópsia pela introdução de um endoscópio especialmente projetado.
cutting f., p. com lâminas cortantes. SIN labitome.
DeBakey f., p. DeBakey; p. atraumática utilizada para pegar vasos sanguíneos; também conhecida nos Estados Unidos como "magics". SIN magic f.

dental f., f. para exodontia; instrumento utilizado para luxar os dentes e removê-los dos alvéolos. SIN extracting f.
dressing f., p. para curativos; p. digital para uso geral em curativos; utilizada para remover fragmentos de tecido necrótico, pequenos corpos estranhos, etc.
extracting f., f. ou tenaz para extração dentária. SIN dental f.
frontal f., fórceps frontal; *termo oficial alternativo para minor f.
f. frontalis, fórceps frontal; *termo oficial alternativo para minor f.
Graefe f., p. de Graefe; pequena p. digital com uma fileira horizontal de seis ou oito dentes delicados em cada ponta.
hemostatic f., p. hemostática; p. com uma cremalheira para prender as lâminas, utilizada para pinçar a extremidade de um vaso sanguíneo e, assim, controlar uma hemorragia.
jeweller f., p. de joalheiro; pequena p. digital com lâminas muito finas e pontiagudas, utilizada para pegar tecidos durante uma microcirurgia.
Kjelland f., f. de Kjelland; f. obstétrico que possui uma trava deslizante e pequena curvatura pélvica.
Lahey f., p. de Lahey; p. para tireóide utilizada para liberar o útero em uma histerectomia vaginal.
Laplace f., p. de Laplace; p. utilizada para aproximar os intestinos durante uma anastomose cirúrgica.
Levret f., f. de Levret; f. de Chamberlen modificado apresentando uma curvatura que corresponde à curvatura do canal de parto.
lion-jaw bone-holding f., p. em mandíbula de leão; p. robusta com dentes fortes e pontiagudos em seus mordentes, utilizada para pegar fragmentos ósseos.
Löwenberg f., p. de Löwenberg; p. com lâminas curtas e curvas cujas extremidades prêenseis arredondadas foram projetadas para remover as adenóides da nasofaringe.
magic f., p. de DeBakey. SIN DeBakey f.
Magill f., p. de Magill; p. romba e curva utilizada para facilitar a intubação nasotraqueal.
f. ma'jor [TA], fórceps occipital. SIN major f.
major f. [TA], fórceps occipital; radiação occipital do corpo caloso; parte da radiação do corpo caloso que se curva agudamente para trás e para dentro do lobo occipital do cérebro. SIN f. major [TA], occipital f.*, f. occipitalis, f. posterior, occipital part of corpus callosum, pars occipitalis corporis callosi.
f. mi'nor [TA], fórceps frontal. SIN minor f.
minor f. [TA], fórceps frontal; radiação frontal do corpo caloso; parte da radiação do corpo caloso que se curva para a frente em direção ao pólo frontal do cérebro. SIN f. minor [TA], f. frontalis*, frontal f.*, f. anterior, frontal part of corpus callosum, pars frontalis corporis callosi.
mosquito f., p. mosquito. SIN mosquito clamp.
mouse-tooth f., p. dente-de-rato; p. com uma ou duas pontas finas, posicionadas na extremidade de cada lâmina, que se ajustam dentro das depressões entre as pontas localizadas na lâmina oposta.
needle f., porta-agulhas. SIN needle-holder.
nonfenestrated f., f. não-fenestrado; f. obstétrico que não apresenta aberturas nas colheres, facilitando, dessa forma, a rotação da cabeça.
obstetrical f., f. obstétrico; f. utilizado para realizar a preensão da cabeça do feto e tracioná-la ou rotacioná-la; as colheres são introduzidas separadamente dentro do canal genital, permitindo que a cabeça do feto seja firmemente agarrada, porém com mínima compressão e, então, são articuladas após terem sido colocadas na posição correta.

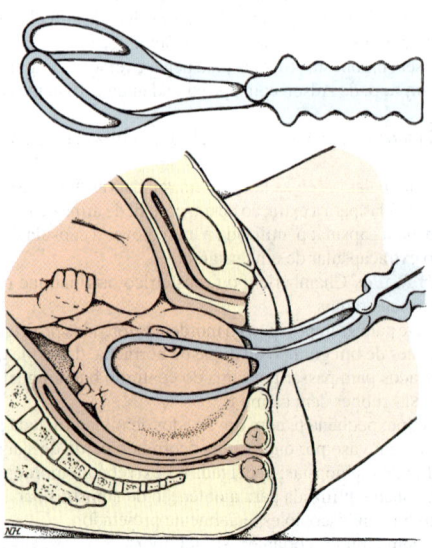

fórceps obstétrico

occipital f., fórceps occipital; *termo oficial alternativo para major f.
f. occipitalis, fórceps occipital. SIN major f.
O'Hara f., p. de O'Hara; duas pinças para grampos delgadas mantidas juntas, utilizadas no passado em anastomoses intestinais; atualmente, é um instrumento obsoleto.
Piper f., f. de Piper; f. obstétrico utilizado para facilitar a liberação da cabeça na apresentação de nádegas.
f. poste'rior, fórceps occipital. SIN major f.
Randall stone f., p. de Randall; p. com lâminas delgadas e curvas e mordentes serrilhados, utilizada para extrair cálculos da pelve ou dos cálices renais.
rubber dam clamp f., p. para grampos de dique de borracha. SIN clamp f.
Simpson f., f. de Simpson; f. obstétrico.
speculum f., p. de espéculo; p. tubular para ser utilizada através de um espéculo.
Tarnier f., f. de Tarnier; tipo de f. de tração axial.
tenaculum f., p. tenáculo, pinça de campo; p. que apresenta, na extremidade de cada um de seus ramos, um gancho reto e pontiagudo semelhante a um tenáculo.
thumb f., p. digital; p. com mola usada por compressão do polegar e do dedo indicador.
tubular f., p. tubular; p. longa e delgada para ser utilizada através de uma cânula ou de outro instrumento tubular.
Tucker-McLean f., f. de Tucker-McLean; tipo de f. de tração axial.
tying f., instrumento com pontas lisas e planas, utilizado em cirurgias oftalmológicas, especialmente para apertar suturas.
vulsella f., vulsellum f., p. vulsela; p. com ganchos na extremidade de cada lâmina. SIN volsella, vulsella, vulsellum.
Willett f., f. de Willett; termo obsoleto de um f. obstétrico para tração, utilizado na presença de placenta prévia, com o qual se traciona a cabeça fetal para baixo contra a placenta.

Forchheimer, Frederick, médico norte-americano, 1853–1913. VER F. sign.
for·ci·pate (fōr'si-pāt). Que tem a forma de uma pinça.
for·ci·pres·sure (fōr'si-presh-ūr). Forcipressão; método para sustar uma hemorragia pela compressão de um vaso sanguíneo com uma pinça.
Fordyce, John A., dermatologista norte-americano, 1858–1925. VER F. angiokeratoma, disease, granules, em granule, spots, em spot; Fox-F. disease.
fore·arm (fōr'arm) [TA]. Antebraço; o segmento do membro superior situado entre o cotovelo e o pulso. SIN antebrachium [TA].
fore·brain (fōr'brān). Prosencéfalo; *termo oficial alternativo para prosencephalon.
fore·con·scious (fōr'kon-shŭs). Pré-consciência; refere-se a lembranças, exceto as atuais, que podem ser evocadas de vez em quando, ou um processo mental inconsciente que se torna consciente somente com o cumprimento de certas condições. Cf. preconscious, foreconscious
fore·fin·ger (fōr'fing'ger). Dedo indicador. SIN index finger.
fore·gut (fōr'gŭt). Intestino anterior; parte cefálica do tubo digestivo primitivo do embrião. De seu endoderma forma-se o revestimento epitelial da faringe, da traquéia, dos pulmões, do esôfago e do estômago, a primeira parte e a metade cranial da segunda parte do duodeno e o parênquima do fígado, da vesícula biliar e do pâncreas. SIN headgut.
fore·head (fōr'ed, fōr'hed) [TA]. Fronte, testa; a parte da face situada entre as sobrancelhas e o couro cabeludo. SIN frons [TA], sinciput*, brow (2).
olympian f., fronte olímpica; testa anormalmente proeminente, alta e larga encontrada na sífilis congênita.
fore·kid·ney (fōr'kid-nē). Pronefro. SIN pronephros.
Forel, Auguste H., neurologista suíço, 1848–1931. VER F. decussation; fields of F., em field; tegmental fields of F. em field.
fore·lock (fōr'lok). Cacho, madeixa; mecha de cabelo que cresce acima da testa.
white forelock, mancha despigmentada, triangular ou em forma de diamante, com cabelos brancos, geralmente encontrada na linha média anterior do couro cabeludo; observada no piebaldismo.
fore·milk (fōr'milk). Colostro. SIN colostrum.
fo·ren·sic (fō-ren'sik). Forense; relativo ou aplicável a lesão pessoal, assassinato e outros procedimentos legais. [L. forensis, de um fórum]
fore·play (fōr'plā). Preliminares; atividade sexual excitante que precede o ato sexual.
fore·pleas·ure (fōr'plezh'er, plā'zher). Prelúdio; prazer sexual que resulta das preliminares que precedem o orgasmo genital no ato sexual.
fore·skin (fōr'skin). Prepúcio; *termo oficial alternativo para prepuce.
f. of penis [TA], prepúcio do pênis. SIN prepuce of penis.
Forestier, Jacques, reumatologista francês, 1890–1978. VER F. disease.
fore·stom·ach (fōr'stŭm'ŭk). Dilatação na porção abdominal do esôfago. SIN cardiac antrum.
fore·wa·ters (fōr'wah-terz). Bolsa-das-águas; coloquialismo para a membrana amniótica cheia de líquido e volumosa situada na frente da cabeça do feto.
for·get·ting. Esquecimento; ser incapaz de recuperar ou recordar informações que foram uma vez registradas, aprendidas e armazenadas na memória de curto prazo ou de longo prazo.
fork (fork). Forquilha. 1. Instrumento bifurcado utilizado para segurar ou levantar algo. 2. Instrumento que se assemelha a uma f. na qual há dentes.

bite f., arco facial. SIN face-bow f.
face-bow f., mordida do arco; a parte da montagem do arco facial utilizada para fixar a base de prova do maxilar ao arco facial propriamente dito. SIN bite f.
tuning f., diapasão; instrumento de aço ou liga de magnésio que se assemelha um pouco a um garfo com dois dentes, cuja vibração, quando percutido, produz um tom puro e sobretons; utilizado para testar a audição e a sensação vibratória.

form (fōrm). Forma; formato; molde. [L. *forma*]
accolé f.'s (ak-ōlā'), formas aplicadas. SIN appliqué f.'s.
appliqué f.'s (ap-li-kā'), formas aplicadas; termo aplicado à maneira pela qual a fase em anel do *Plasmodium falciparum* parasita a parte marginal dos eritrócitos. SIN accolé f.'s.
arch f., f. em arco; a forma e o contorno do arco dentário ou de um aparelho ortodôntico feito com forma desse arco.
boat f., f. de bote; a menos estável das duas conformações assumidas pelos açúcares cíclicos compostos por seis átomos de carbono (piranoses) ou pelos derivados do ciclo-hexano, em oposição à forma de cadeira. VER TAMBÉM Haworth conformational formulas of cyclic *sugars*.
cavity preparation f., f. do preparo cavitário; a configuração ou forma de um preparo cavitário.
chair f., f. de cadeira; a mais estável das duas conformações assumidas pelos açúcares cíclicos compostos por seis átomos de carbono (p.ex., as piranoses) ou pelos derivados do ciclo-hexano, em oposição à f. de bote. VER TAMBÉM Haworth conformational formulas of cyclic *sugars*.
convenience f., f. de conveniência; as alterações necessárias do lado de fora da f. de contorno básica para permitir a correta instrumentação para o preparo cavitário e a inserção de uma restauração dentária.
extension f., f. de extensão; a ampliação da f. de contorno do preparo cavitário para permitir a inclusão de áreas com cáries incipientes; essa extensão permite a criação de uma restauração dentária com margens autolimpantes ou facilmente limpáveis.
face f., f. facial; **(1)** a f. de contorno da face; **(2)** a f. de contorno da face de uma vista anterior.
half-chair f., f. de meia-cadeira. VER Haworth conformational formulas of cyclic *sugars*.
involution f., f. involutiva; célula bacteriana irregular ou atípica produzida como conseqüência da exposição a condições desfavoráveis.
L f., f. L. VER L-phase *variants*, em *variant*.
occlusal f., f. oclusal; a f. da superfície oclusal de um dente ou de uma fileira de dentes. SIN occlusal pattern.
outline f., f. de contorno; o formato da área da superfície do dente incluída dentro das margens cavossuperficiais do preparo cavitário de uma restauração dentária.
posterior tooth f., f. dos dentes posteriores; os contornos distinguíveis da superfície oclusal de diversos dentes posteriores.
replicative f. (RF), f. de replicação; **(1)** etapa intermediária da replicação, tanto do DNA viral como do RNA viral, que consiste geralmente em uma fita (filamento) dupla; **(2)** a f. de fita dupla modificada à qual o DNA de fita simples de colífago é convertido após a infecção de uma bactéria suscetível, sendo a formação da fita complementar ("minus") mediada por enzimas que existiam na bactéria antes da penetração do filamento viral de RNA ou DNA ("plus").
resistance f., f. de resistência; a forma dada a um preparo cavitário que permite que a restauração dentária resista às forças mastigatórias.
retention f., f. de retenção; a forma de um preparo cavitário que evita o deslocamento da restauração dentária pela ação de forças laterais ou diagonais, bem como de forças mastigatórias.
sickle f., f. em foice. SIN malarial *crescent*.
skew f., f. inclinada. VER Haworth conformational formulas of cyclic *sugars*.
tooth f., f. do dente; as características das curvas, das linhas, dos ângulos e dos contornos de diversos dentes que permitem sua identificação e diferenciação.
twist f., f. torcida. VER Haworth conformational formulas of cyclic *sugars*.
wave f., f. de onda. VER waveform. SIN waveshape.
wax f., f. de cera. SIN wax *pattern*.

-form. -forme; com forma de; equivalente a -oid. VER morpho-. [L. *-formis*]
Formad, Henry, médico norte-americano, 1847–1892. VER F. *kidney*.
for·mal·de·hyde (fōr-mal'dē-hīd). Formaldeído; gás irritante, cuja fórmula é HCHO; utilizado como anti-séptico, desinfetante e fixador histológico. SIN formic aldehyde, methyl aldehyde. [fórm(ico) + aldeído]
  active f., f. ativo; **(1)** derivado hidroximetil do tetraidrofolato ou do pirofosfato de tiamina; **(2)** N^5, N^{10}-metilenotetraidrofolato.
for·ma·lin (fōr'mă-lin). Formalina; solução aquosa de formaldeído a 37%. SIN formol.
for·ma·lin·ize (fōr-mă-li-nīz). Adicionar formalina, a fim de inativar vacinas sem destruir seu poder imunizante.
for·mam·i·dase (fōr-mam'i-dās). Formamidase; enzima que catalisa a hidrólise do N-formil-L-cinurenina a L-cinurenina e formiato, uma reação importante do catabolismo do L-triptofano. SIN formylase, kynurenine formamidase.
5-for·mam·i·do·im·id·a·zole-4-car·box·im·ide ri·bo·tide. Ribotídeo de 5-formamidoimidazol-4-carboximida; um produto intermediário da biossíntese da purina.
for·mant (fōr'mant). Tons e seus sobretons resultantes da produção de fonemas vocálicos.
for·mate (fōr'māt). Formiato; um sal ou éster do ácido fórmico; isto é, o radical monovalente HCOO– ou o aniônte HCOO⁻.
  active f., f. ativo; N^{10}-formiltetraidrofolato ou um produto de oxidação equivalente do tetraidrofolato.
for·ma·tio, pl. **for·ma·ti·o·nes** (fōr-mā'shē-ō, -ō'nēz) [TA]. Formação. **1.** SIN formation. **2.** Uma estrutura com forma definida ou arranjo celular. [do L. *formo*, pp. *-atus*, formar]
  f. hippocampa'lis, f. do hipocampo. VER hippocampus.
  f. reticula'ris [TA], f. reticular. SIN reticular *formation*.
for·ma·tion (fōr-mā'shŭn). [TA]. Formação. **1.** Uma formação; estrutura com formato ou arranjo celular definido. **2.** Aquilo que é formado. **3.** O ato de dar forma e contorno. SIN formatio (1) [TA].
  concept f., f. de conceito; em psicologia, o aprendizado necessário para compreender e responder por meio de idéias abstratas baseadas em uma ação ou em um objeto.
  personality f., f. da personalidade; a história da vida de uma pessoa associada ao desenvolvimento de padrões individuais e de sua individualidade.
  reaction f., f. reativa; em psicanálise, um mecanismo de defesa postulado no qual as atitudes e os comportamentos adotados por uma pessoa são o oposto daqueles esperados e de fato sentidos por essa pessoa em um nível inconsciente.
  reticular f. (RF), f. reticular; um sistema neural compacto, porém vagamente delimitado, composto de substância branca e cinzenta intimamente associadas e que se estende por toda a parte central do tronco encefálico e em direção ao diencéfalo; o termo refere-se à grande população de neurônios do tronco encefálico que não faz parte dos grupos de células neuromotoras ou dos grupos de células que formam parte dos sistemas de condução sensitiva específicos; em geral, seus neurônios apresentam dendritos longos e conexões aferentes heterogêneas, razão pela qual a f. é freqüentemente denominada de "inespecífica"; a f. reticular apresenta conexões ascendentes e descendentes complexas e com muitas sinapses que desempenham um papel importante no controle central das funções autônomas (respiração, pressão sanguínea, termorregulação, etc.) e endócrinas, bem como na postura corporal, na atividade do reflexo musculoesquelético e nos estados de comportamento gerais, tais como a vigília e o sono. SIN formatio reticularis [TA], reticular substance (2), substantia reticularis (2).
  rouleaux f., empilhamento; o arranjo das hemácias no sangue (ou em suspensões diluídas); as superfícies bicôncavas das hemácias ficam em aposição, formando, desse modo, grupos que se assemelham a pilhas de moedas. SIN pseudoagglutination (2). [Fr. pl. de *rouleau*, um rolo]
  symptom f., f. de sintoma. SIN symptom *substitution*.
for·ma·ti·o·nes (fōr-mā'shē-ō'nēz). Formações; plural de formatio.
for·ma·zan (fōr'mă-zan). Formazana; composto colorido, insolúvel em água, de estrutura geral RNH–N=CR'–N=NR'', formado pela redução de um sal de tetrazólio na demonstração histoquímica de enzimas oxidativas; cada R' corresponde, em geral, a um grupamento fenila; o neotetrazólio, o azul de tetrazólio e o nitroazul de tetrazólio são exemplos de formazanas.
form·board (fōrm'bōrd). Prancha que contém recortes de diversos formatos e dentro dos quais blocos de formato correspondente devem ser encaixados; trata-se de um teste neuropsicológico. O Tactual Performance Test, da Bateria de Halstead-Reitan, é um exemplo. VER Halstead-Reitan *battery*.
forme fruste, pl. **formes frustes** (fōrm' froost'). Forma frustra; a forma incompleta ou inaparente de uma doença. [Fr. forma incompleta]
for·mic (fōr'mik). Fórmico. **1.** Relativo ao ácido fórmico. **2.** Relativo às formigas. [L. *formica*, formiga]
for·mic ac·id. Ácido fórmico; HCOOH; o menor ácido carboxílico; um cáustico forte utilizado como adstringente e contra-irritante.
for·mic al·de·hyde. Aldeído fórmico. SIN formaldehyde.
for·mi·ca·tion (fōr-mi-kā'shŭn). Formicação, formigamento; forma de parestesia ou de alucinação tátil na qual a pessoa tem a sensação de que pequenos insetos estão andando sob a pele. [L. *formica*, formiga]
for·mim·i·no·glu·tam·ic ac·id (FIGLU) (fōr-mim'i-nō-gloo-tam'ik). Ácido formiminoglutâmico; produto intermediário do catabolismo da L-histidina na conversão da L-histidina em ácido glutâmico, com o grupamento formimino sendo transferido para o tetraidrofolato; pode aparecer na urina de pacientes com deficiência de ácido fólico ou de vitamina B_{12} ou com doença hepática.
N-for·mim·i·no·tet·ra·hy·dro·fo·late (fōr-mim'i-nō-tet'ră-hī-drō-fō'lāt). N-formiminotetraidrofolato; derivado do tetraidrofolato de um carbono formado no catabolismo da L-histidina.
formin (fōr'min). Formina; família de proteínas que participam da polarização celular, citocinese e da formação dos membros dos vertebrados. [L. *forma*, form, + -in]
for·mo·cre·sol (fōr-mō-krē'sol). Formocresol; solução aquosa que contém cresol, formaldeído e glicerina e é utilizada em dentes decíduos que necessitam de pulpotomia coronária.

for·mol (fōr′mol). Formol. SIN formalin.
for·mo·sul·fa·thi·a·zole (fōr′mō-sŭl-fă-thī′ă-zol). Formossulfatiazol; agente antimicrobiano utilizado no tratamento de infecções intestinais.

FORMULA

for·mu·la, pl. **for·mu·las, for·mu·lae** (fōr′mū-lă, -lăz, -lē). **1.** Uma receita ou prescrição médica que contém orientações sobre a composição de um preparado medicinal. **2.** Fórmula; em química, um símbolo ou conjunto de símbolos que expressa o número de átomos do elemento ou dos elementos que compõem uma molécula de uma substância, acompanhado, quando necessário, de informações relativas ao arranjo dos átomos dentro da molécula, a sua estrutura eletrônica, a sua carga, a natureza das ligações dentro da molécula, etc. **3.** Fórmula; uma expressão composta de símbolos e números da ordem ou do arranjo normal de partes ou estruturas. **4.** Fórmula; um princípio ou uma relação matemática, habitualmente representados por meio de uma equação. [L. dim. de *forma*, forma]
   Arneth f., índice de Arneth; a porcentagem normal aproximada de neutrófilos polimorfonucleares, baseada no número de segmentações existentes no núcleo: 1 segmento, 5%; 2 segmentos, 35%; 3 segmentos, 41%; 4 segmentos, 17%; 5 segmentos, 2%.
   Bazett f., f. de Bazett; f. para a correção do intervalo QT observado no eletrocardiograma em relação à freqüência cardíaca (intervalo RR): QT corrigido = $QT/\sqrt{RR}$, QT e RR em segundos.
   Bernhardt f., f. de Bernhardt; f. utilizada para calcular o peso ideal, em quilogramas, de um adulto; corresponde à altura, em centímetros, multiplicada pela circunferência do tórax, em centímetros, e dividida por 240.
   Black f., f. de Black; duração da f. de Pignet para as medidas britânicas: $F = (W + C) - H$, onde F é o fator empírico, W é o peso em libras, C circunferência do tórax em polegadas na inspiração plena e H é a altura em polegadas; um homem é classificado como "muito forte", quando F é superior a 120; "forte", entre 110 e 120; "bom", de 100 a 110; "razoável", de 90 a 100; "fraco", de 80 a 90; e "muito fraco", abaixo de 80.
   Broca f., f. de Broca; um homem completamente desenvolvido (com 30 anos de idade) deve ter um peso, em quilogramas, que corresponde ao valor, em centímetros, de sua altura acima de 1 metro.
   chemical f., f. química; expressão da estrutura de uma molécula expressa em símbolos químicos.
   Christison f., f. de Christison. SIN Häser f.
   constitutional f., f. constitucional. SIN structural f.
   Demoivre f., f. de Demoivre; f. obsoleta para calcular a expectativa de vida.
   dental f., f. dentária, f. dental; expressão na forma tabular do número de cada tipo de dente das arcadas dentárias; a f. dental para o homem é, para os dentes decíduos:

$$i. \frac{2-2}{2-2}, c. \frac{1-1}{1-1}, m. \frac{2-2}{2-2} = 20$$

para os dentes permanentes:

$$i. \frac{2-2}{2-2}, c. \frac{1-1}{1-1}, \text{pré-m.} \frac{2-2}{2-2}, m. \frac{3-3}{3-3} = 32.$$

   Dreyer f., f. de Dreyer; f. obsoleta para indicar a relação entre a capacidade vital e a área da superfície corporal.
   DuBois f., f. de DuBois; f. para predizer a área de superfície do homem a partir de seu peso e de sua altura: $A = 71,84 \cdot W^{0,425} \cdot H^{0,725}$, onde A = área da superfície, em cm², W = peso, em kg, e H = altura, em cm.
   electrical f., f. elétrica; representação gráfica por meio de símbolos da reação de um músculo a um estímulo elétrico.
   empirical f., f. empírica; em química, f. que indica o tipo e o número de átomos presentes nas moléculas de uma substância, ou sua composição, porém não indica a relação entre os átomos ou a estrutura interna da molécula. SIN molecular f.
   Fischer projection formulas, fórmulas de projeção de Fischer. VER Fischer projection formulas of *sugars*.
   Flesch f., f. de Flesch; método para determinar a dificuldade de um trecho escrito por meio de uma fórmula fornecendo uma estimativa de quantas pessoas, nos Estados Unidos, são capazes de ler e entender a passagem; utilizado para determinar a compreensão do paciente com relação aos formulários de consentimento hospitalares.
   Florschütz f., f. de Florschütz; relação exata entre a altura e a circunferência abdominal: $L : (2B - L)$, onde L representa a altura do indivíduo e B, a circunferência do abdome; o valor normal assim determinado é de 5, e qualquer valor abaixo de 5 indica obesidade.
   Gorlin f., f. de Gorlin; f. para calcular a área do orifício de uma valva cardíaca, baseada no fluxo que passa através dela e nas pressões médias do interior das câmaras situadas em ambos os lados da valva.
   graphic f., f. gráfica. SIN structural f.
   Hamilton-Stewart f., f. de Hamilton-Stewart. SIN Hamilton-Stewart *method*.
   Häser f., f. de Häser; f. para determinar o número de gramas de substâncias sólidas por litro, obtido pela multiplicação de 2,33 pelos dois últimos algarismos do valor da densidade da urina. SIN Christison f., Trapp f., Trapp-Häser f.
   Haworth perspective and conformational formulas, fórmulas de conformação e de perspectiva de Haworth. VER Haworth perspective formulas of cyclic *sugars*.
   Jellinek f., f. de Jellinek; método que estima a prevalência de alcoolismo na população de uma nação, baseado na suposição de que uma proporção previsível de pessoas viciadas em álcool morre de cirrose hepática.
   Ledermann f., f. de Ledermann; f. para calcular os níveis de dependência alcoólica. Ledermann mostrou, empiricamente, que a distribuição do consumo de álcool em uma população é log–normal; a fórmula está baseada nessa observação para estimar a prevalência de diversos graus de dependência alcoólica. Algumas perguntas têm sido levantadas sobre a validade das observações de Ledermann.
   Long f., f. de Long; f. para estimar, a partir da densidade de uma amostra de urina, a quantidade aproximada de substâncias sólidas em gramas por litro; os dois últimos algarismos do valor da densidade são multiplicados por 2,6. SIN Long coefficient.
   Mall f., f. de Mall; f. para determinar a idade (em dias) de um embrião humano, que é calculada pela raiz quadrada de seu comprimento (medido do vértice até as nádegas), em milímetros, multiplicada por 100.
   Meeh f., f. de Meeh. SIN Meeh-Dubois f.
   Meeh-Dubois f., f. de Meeh-Dubois; f. para calcular a área da superfície corporal, considerando que ela é proporcional ao peso corporal elevado à potência de 2/3. SIN Meeh f.
   molecular f., f. molecular. SIN empirical f.
   official f., f. oficial; f. contida na *Pharmacopeia* ou no *National Formulary*.
   Pignet f., f. de Pignet. VER Black f.
   Poisson-Pearson f., f. de Poisson-Pearson; f. para determinar o erro estatístico no cálculo do índice endêmico de malária: N = número total de crianças com menos de 15 anos de idade em uma localidade; n = número total de crianças que tiveram o baço examinado; x = número encontrado com o baço aumentado; $(x/n)\,100$ = proporção do baço; $e\%$ = porcentagem de erro; a porcentagem de erro será, de acordo com essa f., de:

$$e\% = \frac{200}{n} \cdot \sqrt{\frac{2x(n-x)}{n}} \cdot \sqrt{1 - \frac{n-1}{N-1}}.$$

   Ranke f., f. de Ranke; A = gramas de albumina por litro de um líquido seroso; assim, $A = (\text{densidade} - 1.000) \times 0,52 - 5,406$.
   rational f., f. racional; em química, f. que indica a constituição, bem como a composição de uma substância.
   Reuss f., f. de Reuss; um meio para estimar a quantidade aproximada de albumina em um transudato ou exsudato; a expressão 3/8 (densidade − 1.000) − 2,8 corresponde a um valor que é uma indicação previsível da porcentagem de albumina no líquido.
   Runeberg f., f. de Runeberg; f. para estimar a porcentagem de albumina em um líquido seroso; é similar à f. de Reuss, porém, em vez de 2,8, subtraem-se 2,73, no caso de um transudato, e 2,88 no caso de um exsudato inflamatório.
   spatial f., f. espacial. SIN stereochemical f.
   stereochemical f., f. estereoquímica, f. espacial; f. química na qual está indicado o arranjo espacial dos átomos ou dos grupamentos atômicos.
   structural f., f. estrutural; f. na qual estão indicadas as ligações entre os átomos e entre os grupos de átomos, bem como o tipo e o número de ligações.
   Toronto f. for pulmonary artery banding, f. de Toronto para a ligadura da artéria pulmonar; técnica que fornece um guia geral para o tamanho da ligadura em relação ao peso do paciente.
   Trapp f., f. de Trapp. SIN Häser f.
   Trapp-Häser f., f. de Trapp-Häser. SIN Häser f.
   Van Slyke f., f. de Van Slyke. SIN standard urea *clearance*.
   vertebral f., f. vertebral; f. que indica o número de vértebras em cada segmento da coluna vertebral; para os seres humanos, é: C. 7, T. 12, L. 5, S. 5, Co. 4 = 33, onde C = cervicais, T = torácicas, L = lombares, S = sacrais e Co = coccígeas.

for·mu·lary (fōr′mū-lă-rē). Formulário; conjunto de fórmulas para a composição de preparados medicinais. VER National Formulary, Pharmacopeia.
   hospital f., f. do hospital; compilação continuamente revisada de produtos farmacêuticos aprovados, além de informações adicionais importantes que refletem o julgamento clínico atual da equipe médica de uma instituição.
for·myl (f) (fōr′mil). Formila; o radical HCO–.
   active f., f. ativo; grupamento formila que participa de reações de transformilação, tendo um derivado do ácido fólico como transportador.

formyl (f)

formyl-methionyl-f., formil-metionil-formil. SIN initiation tRNA.
for·my·lase (fōr′mi-lās). Formilase. SIN formamidase.
***N*-for·myl·gly·cin·a·mide ri·bo·tide (FGAR).** Ribotídeo de *N*-formilglicinamida; um produto intermediário da biossíntese da purina.
***N*-for·myl·ky·nur·e·nine** (en-fōr′mil-ki-noor′e-nēn). *N*-formilcinurenina; o produto da clivagem oxidativa do anel indol do L-triptofano; o primeiro produto intermediário formado no catabolismo do L-triptofano.
***N*-for·myl·me·thi·o·nine (fMet)** (fōr′mil-me-thī′ō-nēn). *N*-formilmetionina; metionina acilada no grupamento NH_2 por meio de um grupamento formila (–CHO). É o resíduo inicial de aminoácido, para, virtualmente, todos os polipeptídeos bacterianos. É também observada em mitocôndrias e em cloroplastos de eucariotas. VER TAMBÉM initiating *codon*.
for·myl·me·thi·o·nyl-tRNA. Formilmetionil-RNAt; RNAt de iniciação em certos organismos.
***N*[10]-for·myl·tet·ra·hy·dro·fo·late.** *N*[10]-formiltetraidrofolato; derivado formila do tetraidrofolato que atua como uma fonte de carbono (um carbono) no metabolismo.
Forney, William R., pediatra norte-americano, *1931.
for·ni·cate (fōr′ni-kāt). **1.** Em forma de abóbada ou arqueado; que se assemelha a um fórnice. [L. *fornicatus*, arqueado, de *fornix*, abóbada, arco] **2.** Fornicar; ter relações sexuais. [ver fornication]
for·ni·ca·tion (fōr-ni-kā′shŭn). Fornicação; intercurso sexual, principalmente entre parceiros sem laços matrimoniais. [L. *fornicatio*, um subsolo da casa arqueado ou abobadado (bordel)]
for·ni·ces (fōr′ni-sēz). Fórnices; plural de fornix.
for·nix, gen. **for·ni·cis,** pl. **for·ni·ces** (fōr′niks, -ni-sis, -ni-sēz) [TA]. Fórnice. **1.** [TA]. Em geral, uma estrutura em forma de arco; freqüentemente, o teto em forma de arco (ou parte do teto) de um espaço anatômico. **2.** [TA]. O feixe compacto de fibras brancas através do qual o hipocampo de cada hemisfério cerebral se projeta para o hipocampo contralateral e também para o septo, núcleo anterior do tálamo e corpo mamilar. Partindo das células piramidais do corno de Ammon, as fibras do f. formam o álveo do hipocampo e a fímbria do hipocampo e, em seu trajeto mais adiante, compõem, em seqüência, a comissura do fórnice [TA], também denominada de comissura do hipocampo [TA] (commissura hippocampi [TA]), o pilar do fórnice [TA] (crus fornicis [TA]), o corpo do fórnice [TA] (corpus fornicis [TA]) e a coluna do fórnice [TA] (columna fornicis [TA]), que se divide em uma parte menor de fibras pré-comissurais [TA] — que passam anteriormente à comissura anterior até a área septal — e uma parte maior de fibras pós-comissurais [TA] — que passam posteriormente à comissura anterior para terminarem principalmente nos núcleos mamilares, com uma pequena extensão terminando no núcleo anterior do tálamo. SIN trigonum cerebrale. SIN cerebral trigone. [L. arco, abóbada]
f. conjuncti′vae, f. da conjuntiva. SIN conjunctival f.
conjunctival f. [TA], f. da conjuntiva; espaço formado pela junção das partes bulbar e palpebral da conjuntiva; junto à pálpebra superior, encontra-se o f. superior da conjuntiva e, junto à pálpebra inferior, o f. inferior da conjuntiva. SIN conjunctival cul-de-sac, f. conjunctivae, retrotarsal fold.
f. gastricus [TA], f. gástrico. SIN f. of stomach.
f. of lacrimal sac [TA], f. do saco lacrimal; a extremidade superior em fundo cego do saco lacrimal que se estende acima das aberturas dos canalículos lacrimais. SIN f. sacci lacrimalis [TA].
pharyngeal f., f. da faringe. SIN vault of pharynx.
f. pharyn′gis [TA], f. da faringe. SIN vault of pharynx.
f. sac′ci lacrima′lis [TA], f. do saco lacrimal. SIN f. of lacrimal sac.
f. of stomach [TA], f. gástrico; termo considerado antigamente sinônimo de "fundo do estômago" — termo registrado na *Nomina Anatomica* oficial — e utilizado mais comumente do que "fundo" em radiologia; a *Terminologia Anatomica* registra "fórnice" e "fundo" do estômago separadamente, por considerar que todos os estômagos têm um fundo, a parte mais superior do corpo do estômago, cuja mucosa apresenta a maior densidade de células fúndicas; "fórnice" é agora reservado para a parte do estômago semelhante a uma bolsa ou em forma de abóbada, situada superiormente ao orifício do cárdia e à sua esquerda, e na qual, na posição ortostática, pode ser encontrado gás. SIN f. gastricus [TA].
transverse f., comissura do hipocampo. SIN commissura fornicis.
f. u′teri, f. da vagina. SIN vaginal f.
f. vagi′nae [TA], f. da vagina. SIN vaginal f.
vaginal f. [TA], f. da vagina; recesso localizado na abóbada da vagina; é dividido em partes anterior, posterior e lateral, de acordo com sua relação com o colo do útero. A parte posterior possui importância clínica por ser o local de realização da culdocentese e da culdoscopia. Também é importante, em termos clínicos, a proximidade do ureter (abaixo) e da artéria uterina (acima), adjacentes à parte lateral do fórnice. SIN f. vaginae [TA], f. uteri.
forsk·o·lin (fōr′skō-lin). Forscolina; éster forbol que se liga à proteinoquinase C e provoca a sua ativação, imitando, dessa forma, as ações do diacilglicerol. [de *Coleus forskohlii*, nome taxonômico da fonte botânica]
Forssman, Hans, médico sueco, *1912. VER Börjeson-F.-Lehmann *syndrome*.
Forssman, John, bacteriologista e patologista sueco, 1868–1947. VER F. *antibody, antigen, reaction,* antigen-antibody *reaction*.

Förster, Richard, oftalmologista alemão, 1825–1902. VER F. *uveitis*.
fos·car·net (fos-kar′net). Foscarnet; um agente antiviral análogo ao pirofosfato.
Fosdick, Leonard S., químico norte-americano, 1903–1969. VER F.-Hansen-Epple *test*.
Foshay, Lee, bacteriologista norte-americano, 1896–1961. VER F. *test*.

FOSSA

fos·sa, gen. e pl. **fos·sae** (fos′ă, fos′ē) [TA]. Fossa; depressão com uma forma em geral mais ou menos longitudinal, localizada abaixo do nível da superfície de uma estrutura. [L. um fosso ou uma trincheira]
acetabular f. [TA], f. do acetábulo; área deprimida localizada no assoalho do acetábulo, superior à insicura do acetábulo. SIN f. acetabuli [TA].
f. acetab′uli [TA], f. do acetábulo. SIN acetabular f.
adipose fossae, fossas adiposas; espaços subcutâneos que contêm acúmulos de gordura na mama.
amygdaloid f., f. tonsilar. SIN tonsillar f.
anconal f., f. do olécrano. SIN olecranon f.
anterior cranial f. [TA], f. anterior do crânio; parte da base interna do crânio, anterior às cristas e ao limbo esfenoidais, onde os lobos frontais do cérebro se acomodam. SIN f. cranii anterior [TA], anterior cranial base.
f. anthel′icis, f. anti-hélica. SIN f. antihelica.
f. of anthelix, f. anti-hélica. SIN f. antihelica.
f. antihelica [TA], f. anti-hélica; depressão localizada na face medial da orelha e que corresponde à anti-hélice. SIN f. anthelicis, f. of anthelix, periconchal sulcus.
articular f. of temporal bone, f. mandibular. SIN mandibular f.
f. axilla′ris, f. axilar. SIN axilla.
axillary f., f. axilar. SIN axilla.
Bichat f., f. de Bichat, f. pterigopalatina. SIN pterygopalatine f.
Biesiadecki f., f. de Biesiadecki. SIN iliacosubfascial f.
Broesike f., f. de Broesike. SIN parajejunal f.
f. cani′na [TA], f. canino. SIN canine f.
canine f. [TA], f. canina; depressão localizada na face anterior da maxila, abaixo do forame infra-orbital e na parte lateral da eminência canina. SIN f. canina [TA].
f. carot′ica, trígono carótico. SIN carotid *triangle*.
cerebellar f. [TA], f. cerebelar; grandes impressões côncavas localizadas na face interna do osso occipital, em ambos os lados do forame magno e da crista occipital interna, que aloja os hemisférios cerebelares; parte da f. posterior do crânio. SIN f. cerebellaris [TA].
f. cerebellaris [TA], f. cerebelar. SIN cerebellar f.
Claudius f., f. de Claudius, f. ovárica. SIN ovarian f.
condylar f. [TA], f. condilar; depressão localizada atrás do côndilo do osso occipital, na qual repousa a margem posterior da faceta superior do atlas. SIN f. condylaris [TA].
f. condyla′ris [TA], f. condilar. SIN condylar f.
f. coronoi′dea humeri [TA], f. coronóidea do úmero. SIN coronoid f. of humerus.
coronoid f. of humerus [TA], f. coronóidea do úmero; depressão localizada na face anterior da extremidade distal do úmero, exatamente acima da tróclea, onde o processo coronóide da ulna se acomoda quando o cotovelo é fletido. SIN f. coronoidea humeri [TA].
f. cra′nii ante′rior [TA], f. anterior do crânio. SIN anterior cranial f.
f. cra′nii me′dia [TA], f. média do crânio. SIN middle cranial f.
f. cra′nii poste′rior [TA], f. posterior do crânio. SIN posterior cranial f.
crural f., f. femoral. SIN femoral f.
Cruveilhier f., f. de Cruveilhier. SIN scaphoid f. of sphenoid bone.
cubital f. [TA], f. cubital; f. localizada na frente do cotovelo e limitada, lateral e medialmente, pelas origens umerais dos músculos extensor e flexor do antebraço, respectivamente, e, superiormente, por uma linha imaginária que une os côndilos do úmero. SIN f. cubitalis [TA], antecubital space, chelidon, triangle of elbow.
f. cubita′lis [TA], f. cubital. SIN cubital f.
digastric f. [TA], f. digástrica; depressão localizada na face posterior da base da mandíbula, em ambos os lados do plano mediano; é o local da inserção do ventre anterior do músculo digástrico. SIN f. digastrica [TA].
f. digas′trica [TA], f. digástrica. SIN digastric f.
digital f., **(1)** f. trocantérica. SIN trochanteric f.; **(2)** f. do maléolo lateral. SIN f. of lateral malleolus.
f. duc′tus veno′si, f. do ducto venoso. SIN f. of ductus venosus.
f. of ductus venosus, f. do ducto venoso; sulco amplo localizado posteriormente na face inferior do fígado fetal, entre o lobo caudado e o lobo hepático esquerdo; aloja o ducto venoso e transforma-se na fissura do ligamento venoso no adulto. SIN f. ductus venosi.

fossa

duodenal fossae, recessos duodenais. VER inferior duodenal f., superior duodenal f.
duodenojejunal f., recesso duodenal superior. SIN superior duodenal f.
epigastric f. [TA], f. epigástrica; depressão suave localizada na linha média, exatamente abaixo do processo xifóide do esterno. (A TA registra esse termo como um sinônimo de epigastric *region*.) SIN f. epigastrica [TA], pit of stomach, scrobiculus cordis.
f. epigas'trica [TA], f. epigástrica. SIN epigastric f.
femoral f., f. femoral; depressão localizada na face peritoneal da parede do abdome, inferiormente ao ligamento inguinal, que corresponde à posição do anel femoral. SIN crural f., fovea femoralis.
floccular f., f. subarqueada. SIN subarcuate f.
gallbladder f., f. da vesícula biliar. SIN f. for gallbladder.
f. for gallbladder [TA], f. da vesícula biliar; depressão localizada na face visceral do fígado e anteriormente, entre o lobo quadrado e o lobo direito, que aloja a vesícula biliar. SIN f. vesicae biliaris [TA], f. vesicae felleae*, gallbladder f.
Gerdy hyoid f., f. hióide de Gerdy. SIN carotid *triangle*.
f. glan'dulae lacrima'lis [TA], f. da glândula lacrimal. SIN f. for lacrimal gland.
glenoid f., (1) cavidade glenoidal da escápula. SIN glenoid *cavity* of scapula; **(2)** f. mandibular. SIN mandibular f.
greater supraclavicular f. [TA], f. supraclavicular maior; termo antigamente considerado um sinônimo de trígono omoclavicular — "omoclavicular triangle" — (uma subdivisão do trígono posterior do pescoço); a *Terminologia Anatomica* reserva esse termo para denominar a superfície que cobre o trígono omoclavicular: uma área deprimida situada acima da parte média da clavícula, lateralmente ao músculo esternocleidomastóideo. SIN f. supraclavicularis major [TA].
Gruber-Landzert f., f. de Gruber-Landzert. SIN inferior duodenal f.
f. of helix, escafa. SIN scapha (1).
hyaloid f. [TA], f. hialóidea; depressão localizada na face anterior do corpo vítreo, na qual a lente se acomoda. SIN f. hyaloidea [TA], lenticular f., patellar f. of vitreous.
f. hyaloi'dea [TA], f. hialóidea. SIN hyaloid f.
hypophysial f. [TA], f. hipofisial; f. do osso esfenóide que aloja a hipófise. VER TAMBÉM *sella* turcica. SIN f. hypophysialis [TA], pituitary f.
f. hypophysia'lis [TA], f. hipofisial. SIN hypophysial f.
iliac f. [TA], f. ilíaca; superfície interna e lisa do osso ílio, localizada acima da linha arqueada, onde se insere o músculo ilíaco. SIN f. iliaca [TA].
f. ili'aca [TA], f. ilíaca. SIN iliac f.
iliacosubfascial f., f. iliacossubfascial; recesso peritoneal localizado entre o músculo psoas maior e a crista ilíaca. SIN Biesiadecki f., f. iliacosubfascialis.
f. iliacosubfascia'lis, f. iliacossubfascial. SIN iliacosubfascial f.
iliopectineal f., f. iliopectínea; depressão localizada entre os músculos iliopsoas e pectíneo, no centro do trígono femoral, que aloja os vasos e o nervo femorais.
f. incisi'va [TA], f. incisiva. SIN incisive f.
incisive f. [TA], f. incisiva; depressão localizada na linha média do palato duro, atrás dos incisivos centrais; é o local onde se abrem os canais incisivos. SIN f. incisiva [TA].
incudal f., f. para a bigorna. SIN f. of incus.
f. incu'dis, f. para a bigorna. SIN f. of incus.
f. of incus [TA], f. para a bigorna; pequena depressão localizada na parte inferior e posterior do recesso epitimpânico, que aloja o ramo curto da bigorna. SIN f. incudis, incudal f.
inferior duodenal f. [TA], recesso duodenal inferior; recesso peritoneal variável que está situado atrás da prega duodenal inferior e ao longo da parte ascendente do duodeno. SIN recessus duodenalis inferior [TA], Gruber-Landzert f., inferior duodenal recess.
infraclavicular f. [TA], f. infraclavicular; depressão triangular limitada pela clavícula e pelas margens adjacentes dos músculos deltóide e peitoral maior. SIN f. infraclavicularis [TA], deltoideopectoral trigone, infraclavicular triangle, Mohrenheim f., Mohrenheim space, regio infraclavicularis.
f. infraclavicula'ris [TA], f. infraclavicular. SIN infraclavicular f.
infraduodenal f., recesso retroduodenal. SIN retroduodenal *recess*.
f. infraspina'ta [TA], f. infra-espinal. SIN infraspinous f.
infraspinous f. [TA], f. infra-espinal; depressão localizada na face dorsal da escápula, inferior à sua espinha e ocupada principalmente pela inserção do músculo infra-espinal. SIN f. infraspinata [TA].
infratemporal f. [TA], f. infratemporal; cavidade localizada na parte lateral do crânio limitada: lateralmente, pelo arco zigomático e pelo ramo da mandíbula; medialmente, pela lâmina lateral do processo pterigóide; anteriormente, pelo processo zigomático da maxila e pela face infratemporal da maxila; posteriormente, pela parte timpânica e pelos processos estilóide e mastóide do osso temporal; e, superiormente, pela face infratemporal da asa maior do osso esfenóide. SIN f. infratemporalis [TA], zygomatic f.
f. infratempora'lis [TA], f. infratemporal. SIN infratemporal f.
inguinal f., f. inguinal. VER lateral inguinal f., medial inguinal f.

f. inguina'lis latera'lis [TA], f. inguinal lateral. SIN lateral inguinal f.
f. inguina'lis media'lis [TA], f. inguinal medial. SIN medial inguinal f.
f. innomina'ta, f. inominada. SIN innominate f.
innominate f., f. inominada; depressão pouco profunda localizada entre a corda vocal falsa e a prega ariepiglótica bilateralmente. SIN f. innominata.
intercondylar f. [TA], f. intercondilar; f. profunda localizada entre os côndilos femorais, na qual os ligamentos cruzados se inserem. SIN f. intercondylaris [TA], intercondyloid f. (2), intercondylic f., intercondyloid notch, popliteal notch.
f. intercondyla'ris [TA], f. intercondilar. SIN intercondylar f.
intercondyloid f., intercondylic f., (1) VER *area* intercondylaris anterior tibiae, *area* intercondylaris posterior tibiae; **(2)** f. intercondilar. SIN intercondylar f.
f. intermesocol'ica transver'sa, f. intermesocólica transversa. SIN transverse intermesocolic f.
interpeduncular f. [TA], f. interpeduncular; depressão profunda localizada na superfície inferior do mesencéfalo, entre os pilares do cérebro, cujo assoalho é formado pela substância perfurada posterior. VER interpeduncular *cistern*. SIN f. interpeduncularis [TA].
f. interpeduncula'ris [TA], f. interpeduncular. SIN interpeduncular f.
intrabulbar f., f. intrabulbar; o início dilatado da parte esponjosa da uretra masculina, localizado dentro do bulbo do pênis.
ischioanal f. [TA], f. isquioanal; espaço cuneiforme com a base voltada para o períneo, limitado, lateralmente, pela tuberosidade isquiática e pelo músculo obturador interno e, medialmente, pelo esfíncter externo do ânus e pelo músculo levantador do ânus. SIN f. ischioanalis [TA], f. ischiorectalis, ischiorectal f., Velpeau f.
f. ischioanalis [TA], f. isquioanal. SIN ischioanal f.
ischiorectal f., f. isquioanal. SIN ischioanal f.
f. ischiorecta'lis, f. isquioanal. SIN ischioanal f.
Jobert de Lamballe f., f. de Jobert de Lamballe; depressão situada exatamente acima do joelho e formada pelo músculo adutor magno e pelos músculos sartório e grácil.
Jonnesco f., f. de Jonnesco. SIN superior duodenal f.
jugular f. [TA], f. jugular; depressão oval — próxima da margem posterior da parte petrosa do osso temporal e medial ao processo estilóide — onde está situado o início da veia jugular interna (bulbo jugular). SIN f. jugularis [TA].
f. jugula'ris [TA], f. jugular. SIN jugular f.
lacrimal f., f. da glândula lacrimal; *termo oficial alternativo para f. for lacrimal gland.
f. for lacrimal gland [TA], f. da glândula lacrimal; depressão localizada na face orbital do osso frontal, formada pela margem suspensa e pelo processo zigomático e que aloja a glândula lacrimal. SIN f. glandulae lacrimalis [TA], lacrimal f.*.
f. for lacrimal sac [TA], f. do saco lacrimal; f. formada pelo osso lacrimal e pelo processo frontal da maxila, que aloja o saco lacrimal. SIN f. sacci lacrimalis [TA].
Landzert f., f. de Landzert; f. formada por duas pregas peritoneais, que envolvem a artéria cólica esquerda e a veia mesentérica inferior, respectivamente, ao lado do duodeno; é menor do que o recesso paraduodenal, às vezes encontrado na mesma região.
lateral f. of brain, f. lateral do cérebro. SIN lateral cerebral f.
lateral cerebral f. [TA], f. lateral do cérebro; depressão profunda localizada na superfície basal do cérebro anterior e cuja posição corresponde à da substância perfurada anterior. É limitada medialmente pelo trato óptico e rostralmente pela superfície orbital do lobo frontal; estende-se lateralmente ao redor do pólo suspenso do lobo temporal na fissura de Sylvius (sulco lateral). SIN f. lateralis cerebri [TA], f. of Sylvius, lateral f. of brain, vallecula sylvii.
lateral inguinal f. [TA], f. inguinal lateral; depressão localizada na superfície peritoneal da parede anterior do abdome, lateralmente à crista formada pela artéria epigástrica inferior; corresponde à posição do anel inguinal profundo e é o local de aparecimento de hérnia inguinal indireta. SIN f. inguinalis lateralis [TA].
f. latera'lis cer'ebri [TA], f. lateral do cérebro. SIN lateral cerebral f.
f. of lateral malleolus [TA], f. do maléolo lateral; depressão grande e áspera localizada na face medial da extremidade inferior da fíbula — exatamente atrás da faceta articular do tálus —, onde se inserem os ligamentos talofibular posterior e tibiofibular transverso. SIN f. malleoli lateralis [TA], digital f. (2), f. malleoli fibulae.
lenticular f., f. hialóidea. SIN hyaloid f.
lesser supraclavicular f. [TA], f. supraclavicular menor; espaço triangular localizado entre as duas cabeças de origem do músculo esternocleidomastóideo. SIN f. supraclavicularis minor [TA].
little f. of the cochlear window, fóssula da janela da cóclea. SIN f. of round window.
little f. of the oval (vestibular) window, fóssula do vestíbulo. SIN f. of oval window.
Malgaigne f., f. de Malgaigne. SIN carotid *triangle*.
f. malle'oli fib'ulae, f. do maléolo lateral. SIN f. of lateral malleolus.

f. malle'oli latera'lis [TA], f. do maléolo lateral. SIN f. of lateral malleolus.
mandibular f. [TA], f. mandibular; depressão profunda localizada na parte escamosa do osso temporal, na raiz do zigoma, na qual se acomoda o côndilo da mandíbula. SIN f. mandibularis [TA], articular f. of temporal bone, cavitas glenoidalis, glenoid cavity, glenoid f. (2), glenoid surface.
f. mandibula'ris [TA], f. mandibular. SIN mandibular f.
mastoid f., f. mastoi'dea, trígono suprameatal. SIN suprameatal *triangle*.
medial inguinal f. [TA], f. inguinal medial; depressão localizada na superfície peritoneal da parede anterior do abdome, entre as cristas formadas pela artéria epigástrica inferior e pelo ligamento umbilical medial; corresponde à posição do anel inguinal superficial e é o local de aparecimento de hérnia inguinal direta. SIN f. inguinalis medialis [TA], fovea inguinalis interna.
Merkel f., f. de Merkel; sulco localizado na parede póstero-lateral do vestíbulo da laringe, entre as cartilagens corniculada e cuneiforme.
mesentericoparietal f., f. mesentericoparietal. SIN parajejunal f.
middle cranial f. [TA], f. média do crânio; parte com forma de borboleta da base interna do crânio, situada posteriormente às cristas e ao limbo esfenoidais e anteriormente às cristas da parte petrosa dos ossos temporais e ao dorso da sela; aloja, lateralmente, os lobos temporais do cérebro e, centralmente, a hipófise. SIN f. cranii media [TA].
Mohrenheim f., f. de Mohrenheim. SIN infraclavicular f.
Morgagni f., f. de Morgagni. SIN navicular f. of urethra.
mylohyoid f., sulco milo-hióideo. SIN mylohyoid *groove*.
f. navicula'ris auric'ulae, f. triangular. SIN triangular f. of auricle.
f. navicula'ris au'ris, f. navicular da orelha; termo obsoleto para scapha (1).
f. navicula'ris Cruveil'hier, f. navicular de Cruveilhier. SIN scaphoid f. of sphenoid bone.
f. navicula'ris ure'thrae [TA], f. navicular da uretra. SIN navicular f. of urethra.
f. navicula'ris vestib'ulae vagi'nae, f. vestibular. SIN vestibular f.
navicular f. of urethra [TA], f. navicular da uretra; a parte terminal dilatada da uretra, localizada na glande do pênis. SIN f. navicularis urethrae [TA], f. terminalis urethrae, Morgagni f., Morgagni fovea.
f. olecra'ni [TA], f. do olécrano. SIN olecranon f.
olecranon f. [TA], f. do olécrano; depressão localizada no dorso da extremidade distal do úmero, acima da tróclea, na qual o processo coronóide do olécrano da ulna se acomoda quando o cotovelo é estendido. SIN f. olecrani [TA], anconal f.
oval f., f. oval; *termo oficial alternativo para f. ovalis (1).
f. ova'lis, f. oval; (1) [NA], depressão oval localizada na parte inferior do septo do átrio direito; trata-se de um vestígio do forame oval, e seu assoalho corresponde ao septo primário do coração fetal; SIN oval f.*. (2) SIN saphenous *opening*.
f. of oval window [TA], fóssula do vestíbulo; depressão situada na parede medial da orelha média, em cuja parte inferior se localiza a janela oval (fenestra vestibulae). SIN fossula fenestrae vestibuli [TA], Huguier sinus, little f. of the oval (vestibular) window.
ovarian f. [TA], f. ovárica; depressão localizada no peritônio parietal da pelve; é limitada, anteriormente, pela parte ocluída da artéria umbilical e, posteriormente, pelo ureter e pelos vasos uterinos; aloja o ovário. SIN f. ovarica [TA], Claudius f.
f. ova'rica [TA], f. ovárica. SIN ovarian f.
paraduodenal f., recesso paraduodenal. SIN paraduodenal *recess*.
parajejunal f., f. parajejunal; f. peritoneal encontrada em alguns casos nos quais o jejuno não apresenta mesentério e está fixado ao peritônio parietal posterior; a f. começa no ponto onde o mesentério termina e é observada ao se levantar as alças do intestino livre. SIN Broesike f., f. parajejunalis, mesentericoparietal f., mesentericoparietal recess.
f. parajejuna'lis, f. parajejunal. SIN parajejunal f.
pararectal f. [TA], f. pararretal; depressão peritoneal encontrada em ambos os lados do reto, formada por pregas peritoneais (sacrogenitais) que seguem da parede póstero-lateral da pelve até as vísceras localizadas no centro da pelve. Trata-se de uma extensão lateral da escavação retovesical, no homem, ou da escavação retouterina, na mulher. SIN f. pararectalis [TA], pararectal pouch.
f. pararecta'lis [TA], f. pararretal. SIN pararectal f.
paravesical f. [TA], f. paravesical; depressão peritoneal formada pela reflexão do peritônio da parede lateral da pelve sobre o teto da bexiga; na mulher, corresponde à parte lateral da escavação vesicouterina e está separada da escavação pararretal, situada posteriormente, pelo ligamento largo. SIN f. paravesicalis [TA], paracystic pouch, paravesical pouch.
f. paravesica'lis [TA], f. paravesical. SIN paravesical f.
patellar f. of vitreous, f. hialóidea. SIN hyaloid f.
peritoneal fossae, recessos peritoneais; depressões ou escavações formadas entre diversas pregas peritoneais; podem ser os locais de hérnias internas.
petrosal f., fóssula petrosa. SIN petrosal *fossula*.
piriform f. [TA], recesso piriforme; recesso localizado na parede ântero-lateral da nasofaringe, em cada lado do vestíbulo da laringe, e separado dela pelas pregas ariepiglóticas. SIN recessus piriformis [TA], piriform recess*, piriform sinus.
pituitary f., f. hipofisial. SIN hypophysial f.
f. poplit'ea [TA], f. poplítea. SIN popliteal f.

popliteal f. f. poplítea; espaço em forma de diamante, posterior à articulação do joelho e limitado, superficialmente, pela divergência formada pelos músculos bíceps femoral e semimembranáceo, acima, e pelas duas cabeças do músculo gastrocnêmio, abaixo; profundamente, a f. é limitada, superiormente, pela divergência formada entre as linhas supracondilares do fêmur e, inferiormente, pela linha para o músculo sóleo da tíbia. Conteúdo da fossa: o nervo tibial, a artéria e a veia poplíteas e gordura. SIN f. poplitea [TA], ham (1), poples, popliteal region, popliteal space, popliteus (2).
posterior cranial f. [TA], f. posterior do crânio; base interna do crânio, situada posteriormente à crista da parte petrosa dos ossos temporais e ao dorso da sela e anteriormente aos sulcos dos seios transversos, onde o cerebelo, a ponte e a medula oblonga se acomodam. SIN f. cranii posterior [TA].
f. provesica'lis, bolsa de Hartmann. SIN Hartmann *pouch*.
pterygoid f. [TA], f. pterigóidea; f. formada pela divergência posterior das lâminas do processo pterigóide do osso esfenóide; aloja a origem dos músculos pterigóideo medial e tensor do véu palatino. SIN f. pterygoidea [TA].
f. pterygoi'dea [TA], f. pterigóidea. SIN pterygoid f.
pterygomaxillary f., f. pterigopalatina. SIN pterygopalatine f.
f. pterygopalati'na [TA], f. pterigopalatina. SIN pterygopalatine f.
pterygopalatine f. [TA], f. pterigopalatina; f. esfenomaxilar, um pequeno espaço piramidal, que aloja o gânglio pterigopalatino entre o processo pterigóide, a maxila e o osso palatino. SIN f. pterygopalatina [TA], Bichat f., pterygomaxillary f., sphenomaxillary f.
radial f. of humerus [TA], f. radial do úmero; depressão rasa localizada na face anterior do úmero distal, superior ao capítulo do úmero e lateral à fossa coronóidea, na qual se acomoda, a margem da cabeça do rádio quando o cotovelo está em flexão extrema. SIN f. radialis humeri [TA].
f. radia'lis hu'meri [TA], f. radial do úmero. SIN radial f. of humerus.
retroduodenal f., recesso retroduodenal. SIN retroduodenal *recess*.
retromandibular f., f. retromandibular; depressão inferior à orelha e posterior ao ramo e ao ângulo da mandíbula. SIN f. retromandibularis.
f. retromandibula'ris, f. retromandibular. SIN retromandibular f.
retromolar f. [TA], f. retromolar; depressão triangular localizada na mandíbula, posterior ao terceiro dente molar. SIN f. retromolaris [TA].
f. retromola'ris [TA], f. retromolar. SIN retromolar f.
rhomboid f. [TA], f. rombóide; assoalho do quarto ventrículo do cérebro, formado pela superfície ventricular do rombencéfalo. SIN f. rhomboidea [TA].
f. rhomboi'dea [TA], f. rombóide. SIN rhomboid f.
Rosenmüller f., f. de Rosenmüller. SIN pharyngeal *recess*.
f. of round window [TA], fóssula da janela da cóclea; depressão situada na parede medial da orelha média, em cuja parte inferior se localiza a janela redonda (fenestra cochleae). SIN fossula fenestrae cochleae [TA], fossula rotunda, little f. of the cochlear window.
f. sac'ci lacrima'lis [TA], f. do saco lacrimal. SIN f. for lacrimal sac.
scaphoid f. [TA], f. escafóidea; depressão em forma de barco. VER TAMBÉM scaphoid f. of sphenoid bone. SIN scaphoidea [TA].
f. scaphoidea [TA], f. escafóidea. SIN scaphoid f.
f. scaphoi'dea ossis sphenoidalis, f. escafóidea do esfenóide. SIN scaphoid f. of sphenoid bone.
scaphoid f. of sphenoid bone, f. escafóidea do esfenóide; depressão longitudinal localizada na superfície posterior da parte superior (raiz) da lâmina medial do processo pterigóide; local de origem do músculo tensor do véu palatino. SIN Cruveilhier f., navicularis Cruveilhier, f. scaphoidea ossis sphenoidalis.
f. scar'pae ma'jor, trígono femoral. SIN femoral *triangle*.
sigmoid f., sulco do seio sigmóide. SIN *groove* for sigmoid sinus.
sphenomaxillary f., f. pterigopalatina. SIN pterygopalatine f.
f. subarcua'ta [TA], f. subarqueada. SIN subarcuate f.
subarcuate f. [TA], f. subarqueada; depressão irregular localizada na face posterior da parte petrosa do osso temporal, abaixo de sua crista e superior e lateralmente ao meato acústico interno. No feto, é o local onde se acomoda o flóculo do cerebelo; no adulto, é o local onde uma pequena veia penetra no osso. SIN f. subarcuata [TA], floccular f., hiatus subarcuatus.
subcecal f., f. subcecal; depressão inconstante localizada no peritônio e que se estende posteriormente ao ceco. SIN Treitz f.
subinguinal f., f. subinguinal; depressão localizada na face anterior da coxa, debaixo da virilha.
sublingual f. [TA], fóvea sublingual; depressão rasa localizada em ambos os lados da espinha mentual, na face interna do corpo da mandíbula, superior à linha milo-hióidea, que aloja a glândula sublingual. SIN fovea sublingualis [TA], sublingual pit.
submandibular f. [TA], fóvea submandibular; depressão localizada na face medial do corpo da mandíbula, inferior à linha milo-hióidea, onde a glândula submandibular está alojada. SIN fovea submandibularis [TA], f. submandibularis, fovea submaxillaris, submaxillary f.
f. submandibula'ris, fóvea submandibular. SIN submandibular f.
submaxillary f., fóvea submandibular. SIN submandibular f.
subscapular f. [TA], f. subescapular; a face ventral côncava do corpo da escápula, local de inserção do músculo subescapular. SIN f. subscapularis [TA].

f. subscapula'ris [TA], f. subescapular. SIN subscapular f.
superior duodenal f. [TA], recesso duodenal superior; recesso peritoneal que se estende para cima, atrás da prega duodenal superior. SIN recessus duodenalis superior [TA], superior duodenal recess*, duodenojejunal f., duodenojejunal recess, Jonnesco f.
f. supraclavicularis major [TA], f. supraclavicular maior. SIN greater supraclavicular f.
f. supraclavicula'ris mi'nor [TA], f. supraclavicular menor. SIN lesser supraclavicular f.
supramastoid f., fovéola suprameática. SIN suprameatal *triangle*.
f. supraspina'ta [TA], f. supra-espinal. SIN supraspinous f.
supraspinous f. [TA], f. supra-espinal; depressão localizada na face dorsal da escápula, acima de sua espinha, que aloja o músculo supra-espinal. SIN f. supraspinata [TA].
supratonsillar f. [TA], f. supratonsilar; espaço localizado entre os arcos palatoglosso e palatofaríngeo, acima da tonsila e mais visível no adulto após a regressão da tonsila. SIN supratonsillaris [TA], supratonsillar recess, Tourtual sinus.
f. supratonsilla'ris [TA], f. supratonsilar. SIN supratonsillar f.
supravesical f. [TA], f. supravesical; depressão localizada na superfície peritoneal da parede anterior do abdome, acima da bexiga e entre as pregas umbilicais mediana e média. Seu nível, em relação ao púbis, altera-se quando a bexiga está cheia. SIN f. supravesicalis [TA], fovea supravesicalis.
f. supravesica'lis [TA], f. supravesical. SIN supravesical f.
f. of Sylvius, f. de Sylvius. SIN lateral cerebral f.
temporal f. [TA], f. temporal; espaço localizado na parte lateral do crânio, limitado pelas linhas temporais e que termina abaixo no nível do arco zigomático. SIN f. temporalis [TA].
f. tempora'lis [TA], f. temporal. SIN temporal f.
f. termina'lis ure'thrae, f. navicular da uretra. SIN navicular f. of urethra.
tonsillar f. [TA], f. tonsilar; depressão localizada entre os arcos palatoglosso e palatofaríngeo e preenchida pela tonsila palatina. SIN f. tonsillaris [TA], amygdaloid f., sinus tonsillaris.
f. tonsilla'ris [TA], f. tonsilar. SIN tonsillar f.
transverse intermesocolic f., f. intermesocólica transversa; f. que ocupa a posição do recesso duodenal superior, estendendo-se, porém, transversalmente da direita para a esquerda por alguns centímetros. SIN f. intermesocolica transversa.
Treitz f., f. de Treitz. SIN subcecal f.
triangular f. of auricle [TA], f. triangular da orelha; depressão localizada na parte superior da orelha, entre os dois ramos da anti-hélice. SIN f. triangularis auriculae [TA], f. navicularis auriculae.
f. triangula'ris auriculae [TA], f. triangular da orelha. SIN triangular f. of auricle.
trochanteric f., f. trocantérica; depressão localizada na raiz do colo do fêmur, debaixo da extremidade curva do trocanter maior; é o local de inserção do tendão do músculo obturador externo. SIN digital f. (1), f. trochanterica.
f. trochanter'ica, f. trocantérica. SIN trochanteric f.
trochlear f., fóvea troclear. SIN trochlear *fovea*.
f. trochlea'ris, fóvea troclear. SIN trochlear *fovea*.
umbilical f., fissura do ligamento redondo. SIN *fissure* for ligamentum teres.
Velpeau f., f. de Velpeau. SIN ischioanal f.
f. ve'nae ca'vae, sulco da veia cava. SIN *sulcus* for vena cava.
f. ve'nae umbilica'lis, fissura do ligamento redondo. SIN *fissure* for ligamentum teres.
f. veno'sa, recesso paraduodenal. SIN paraduodenal *recess*.
vermian f., f. do verme; pequena depressão próxima da parte inferior da crista occipital interna e que aloja parte do verme inferior do cerebelo.
f. vesi'cae bilia'ris [TA], f. da vesícula biliar. SIN f. for gallbladder.
f. vesicae felleae, f. da vesícula biliar; *termo oficial alternativo para f. for gallbladder.
vestibular f. [TA], f. do vestíbulo da vagina; parte do vestíbulo da vagina situada entre o frênulo do lábio menor do pudendo e a comissura labial posterior da vulva. SIN f. vestibuli vaginae [TA], f. navicularis vestibulae vaginae, f. of vestibule of vagina.
f. of vestibule of vagina, f. do vestíbulo da vagina. SIN vestibular f.
f. vestib'uli vagi'nae [TA], f. do vestíbulo da vagina. SIN vestibular f.
Waldeyer fossae, fossas de Waldeyer. VER inferior duodenal f., superior duodenal f.
zygomatic f., f. infratemporal. SIN infratemporal f.

fos·sette (fo-set'). Fóssula. **1.** SIN fossula. **2.** Termo raramente utilizado para úlcera da córnea de pequeno diâmetro. [Fr. dim. de *fosse*, um fosso]
fos·su·la, pl. **fos·su·lae** (fos'ū-lă, -lē) [TA]. Fóssula. **1.** [NA]. Pequena fossa. **2.** Fissura diminuta ou suave depressão localizada na superfície do cérebro. SIN fossette (1). [L. dim. de *fossa*, fosso]
f. fenes'trae coch'leae [TA], f. da janela da cóclea. SIN *fossa* of round window.

f. fenes'trae vestib'uli [TA], f. da janela do vestíbulo. SIN *fossa* of oval window.
f. petro'sa [TA], f. petrosa. SIN petrosal f.
petrosal f. [TA], f. petrosa; depressão pequena e com freqüência levemente marcada, localizada na face inferior da parte petrosa do osso temporal entre a fossa jugular e a abertura do canal carótico; é o local de abertura do canalículo timpânico, que dá passagem ao nervo timpânico. SIN f. petrosa [TA], petrosal fossa, receptaculum ganglii petrosi.
f. post fenestram, pequena passagem preenchida com tecido conectivo, posterior à janela (oval) da cóclea; local onde freqüentemente ocorre otosclerose.
f. rotun'da, f. da janela da cóclea; SIN *fossa* of round window.
tonsillar fossulae [TA], fóssulas da tonsila; pequenas fossas localizadas nas aberturas das criptas tonsilares localizadas sobre a superfície externa da tonsila. São encontradas nas tonsilas palatina e faríngea. SIN fossulae tonsillarum (palatini et pharyngealis) [TA].
fos'sulae tonsilla'rum (palatini et pharyngealis) [TA], fóssulas da tonsila (palatina e faríngea). SIN tonsillar fossulae.
fos·su·late (fos'ū-lāt). Fossulado; sulcado; que contém uma fóssula ou uma pequena fossa; escavado.
Foster frame. Estrutura de Foster. VER em frame.
Foster Kennedy. VER Kennedy.
Fothergill, John, médico inglês, 1712–1780. VER F. *disease*, *neuralgia*, *sign*.
Fothergill, William E., ginecologista inglês, 1865–1926. VER F. *operation*.
Fouchet, A., médico francês, *1894. VER F. *reagent*, *stain*.
fou·lage (foo-lahzh'). Massagem e compressão dos músculos, constituindo em uma forma de massagem. [Fr. impressão]
foun·da·tion (fown-dā'shŭn). Fundação, infra-estrutura; uma base; uma estrutura de apoio.
denture f., infra-estrutura da dentadura; aquela parte das estruturas orais que está disponível para servir de apoio para uma dentadura. VER TAMBÉM denture foundation *area*, denture foundation *surface*, mean foundation *plane*.
found·er (fown'der). Fundador; uma pessoa que contribui com a estrutura genética inicial de uma população e é capaz de contribuir com uma grande proporção dos genes de seus descendentes.
four·chette (foor-shet'). Frênulo dos lábios menores do pudendo; *termo oficial alternativo para *frenulum* of labia minora. [Fr. dim. de *fourché*, de L. *furca*, forquilha]
Fou·ri·er, J.B.J., matemático e administrador francês, 1768–1830. VER Fourier *analysis*, Fourier *transform*, Fourier *transfer*.
Fourneau, Ernest F.A., químico e farmacologista francês, 1872–1949. VER F. 710, 933.
Fourneau 710. Uma quinolona sintética; um agente antimalárico. [Ernest F.A. *Fourneau*]
Fourneau 933. Cloridrato de piperoxano. SIN piperoxan hydrochloride. [Ernest F.A. *Fourneau*]
Fournier, Jean A., sifilógrafo francês, 1832–1914. VER F. *disease*, *gangrene*; *syphiloma* of F.
fo·vea, pl. **fo·ve·ae** (fō'vē-ă, fō'vē-ē) [TA]. Fóvea. Qualquer depressão natural localizada na superfície do corpo, tal como a axila, ou sobre a superfície de um osso. Cf. dimple. SIN pit (1). [L. uma cova]
f. ante'rior, f. superior. SIN superior f.
anterior f., f. superior. SIN superior f.
f. articula'ris cap'itis ra'dii [TA], f. articular (da cabeça do rádio). SIN articular *facet* of radial head.
f. articula'ris infe'rior atlan'tis, superfície articular inferior do atlas. SIN inferior articular *surface* of atlas.
f. articula'ris supe'rior atlan'tis, superfície articular superior do atlas. SIN superior articular *surface* of atlas.
f. cap'itis fem'oris [TA], f. da cabeça do fêmur. SIN f. for ligament of head of femur.
f. cardi'aca, f. do cárdia; abertura entre o intestino anterior e o intestino médio. VER TAMBÉM epigastric *fossa*. SIN anterior intestinal portal.
f. centra'lis maculae luteae [TA], f. central da retina. SIN central retinal f.
central retinal f. [TA], f. central da retina; depressão localizada no centro da retina onde há somente cones e ausência de vasos sanguíneos. SIN f. centralis maculae luteae [TA], central pit.
f. costa'lis infe'rior [TA], f. costal inferior. SIN inferior costal *facet*.
f. costa'lis proces'sus transver'si [TA], f. costal do processo transverso. SIN transverse costal *facet*.
f. costa'lis supe'rior [TA], f. costal superior. SIN superior costal *facet*.
f. den'tis atlan'tis [TA], f. do dente. SIN *facet* (of atlas) for dens.
f. ellip'tica, recesso elíptico do labirinto ósseo. SIN elliptical *recess* of bony labyrinth.
f. ethmoida'lis, f. etmoidal; o teto das células aéreas etmoidais.
f. of the femoral head, f. da cabeça do fêmur. SIN f. for ligament of head of femur.
f. femora'lis, fossa femoral. SIN femoral *fossa*.

f. hemiellip'tica, recesso elíptico do labirinto ósseo. SIN elliptical recess of bony labyrinth.
f. hemisphe'rica, recesso esférico do labirinto ósseo. SIN spherical recess of bony labyrinth.
f. infe'rior [TA], f. inferior. SIN inferior f.
inferior f. [TA], f. inferior; pequena depressão localizada no sulco limitante da fossa rombóide, abaixo das estrias medulares em ambos os lados, geralmente lateral aos trígonos do nervo hipoglosso e do nervo vago. SIN f. inferior [TA].
f. inguina'lis inter'na, fossa inguinal medial. SIN medial inguinal fossa.
f. for ligament of head of femur [TA], f. da cabeça do fêmur; depressão localizada na extremidade da cabeça do fêmur, onde se fixa o ligamento redondo do fêmur. SIN f. capitis femoris [TA], f. of the femoral head, pit of head of femur.
Morgagni f., f. de Morgagni. SIN navicular fossa of urethra.
f. oblon'ga cartilag'inis arytenoid'eae [TA], f. oblonga da cartilagem aritenóidea. SIN oblong f. of arytenoid cartilage.
oblong f. of arytenoid cartilage [TA], f. oblonga da cartilagem aritenóidea; depressão rasa e larga localizada na face ântero-lateral da cartilagem aritenóidea; é o local de inserção do músculo tireoaritenóideo. SIN f. oblonga cartilaginis arytenoideae [TA], oblong pit of arytenoid cartilage.
pterygoid f. [TA], f. pterigóidea; depressão localizada na face ântero-medial do colo do processo condilar da mandíbula; é o local de inserção do músculo pterigóideo lateral. SIN f. pterygoidea [TA], pterygoid depression, pterygoid pit.
f. pterygoid'ea [TA], f. pterigóidea. SIN pterygoid f.
f. of radial head, f. articular (da cabeça do rádio). SIN articular facet of radial head.
f. sphe'rica, recesso esférico do labirinto ósseo. SIN spherical recess of bony labyrinth.
f. sublingua'lis [TA], f. sublingual. SIN sublingual fossa.
f. submandibula'ris [TA], f. submandibular. SIN submandibular fossa.
f. submaxilla'ris, f. submaxilar. SIN submandibular fossa.
f. supe'rior [TA], f. superior. SIN superior f.
superior f. [TA], f. superior; depressão rasa, localizada no sulco limitante, em ambos os lados da fossa rombóide, acima das estrias medulares e lateralmente ao colículo facial. SIN f. superior [TA], anterior f., f. anterior.
f. supravesica'lis, fossa supravesical. SIN supravesical fossa.
triangular f. of arytenoid cartilage [TA], f. triangular da cartilagem aritenóidea; depressão profunda, localizada na parte superior da face ântero-lateral da cartilagem aritenóidea, que aloja glândulas. SIN f. triangularis cartilaginis arytenoideae [TA], triangular pit of arytenoid cartilage.
f. triangula'ris cartilag'inis arytenoid'eae [TA], f. triangular da cartilagem aritenóidea. SIN triangular f. of arytenoid cartilage.
trochlear f. [TA], f. troclear; depressão rasa, localizada no teto da órbita, próximo à margem medial, onde se fixa a polia para o tendão do músculo oblíquo superior. SIN f. trochlearis [TA], fossa trochlearis, trochlear fossa, trochlear pit.
f. trochlea'ris [TA], f. troclear. SIN trochlear f.
fo·ve·ate, fo·ve·at·ed (fō-vē-āt, -ā-ted). Foveolado; que possui fóveas ou depressões na superfície.
fo·ve·a·tion (fō-vē-ā'shŭn). Formação de cicatriz deprimida, como ocorre na varíola, na catapora (varicela) e na vacínia. [L. *fovea*, uma cova]
fo·ve·o·la, pl. **fo·ve·o·lae** (fō-vē'ō-lă, -lē) [TA]. Fovéola, fosseta, fóvea ou cova pequena. [L. mod. dim. de L. *fovea*, cova]
f. coccy'gea [TA], fosseta coccígea. SIN coccygeal f.
coccygeal f. [TA], fosseta coccígea; depressão encontrada na pele sobre o cóccix e formada pelo retináculo caudal. SIN f. coccygea [TA], coccygeal dimple, postanal dimple.
f. gas'trica [TA], f. gástrica. SIN gastric pit.
granular foveolae [TA], fovéolas granulares; covas localizadas na superfície interna do crânio, ao longo do trajeto do seio sagital superior, onde estão alojadas as granulações aracnóideas. SIN foveolae granulares [TA], granular pits, pacchionian depressions.
foveolae granula'res [TA], fovéolas granulares. SIN granular foveolae.
f. ocula'ris, f. ocular. SIN f. of retina.
f. papilla'ris, fovéola papilar; pequena depressão às vezes encontrada no ápice de uma papila renal, onde um ducto papilar se abre para o interior de um cálice.
f. of retina [TA], f. da retina; região central da fóvea central da retina, que contém apenas cones. SIN f. retinae [TA], f. ocularis.
f. retinae [TA], f. da retina. SIN f. of retina.
f. suprameatalis, f. supraméatica. SIN suprameatal triangle.
f. supramea'tica [TA], f. supraméatica. SIN suprameatal triangle.
fo·ve·o·lar (fō-vē'ō-lăr). Foveolar; relativo a uma fovéola.
fo·ve·o·late (fō've-ō-lāt, fō-vē'ō-lāt). Foveolado; que apresenta diminutas covas (fovéolas) ou pequenas depressões na superfície.
Foville, Achille L., neurologista francês, 1799–1878. VER F. *fasciculus, syndrome.*
Fowler, George R., cirurgião norte-americano, 1848–1906. VER F. *position.*
Fox, George H., dermatologista norte-americano, 1846–1937. VER F.-Fordyce *disease.*
Fox, Lewis, periodontista norte-americano, *1903. VER Goldman-F. *knives,* em *knife.*
fox·glove (foks'glŭv). Dedaleira, digital. SIN *Digitalis.*

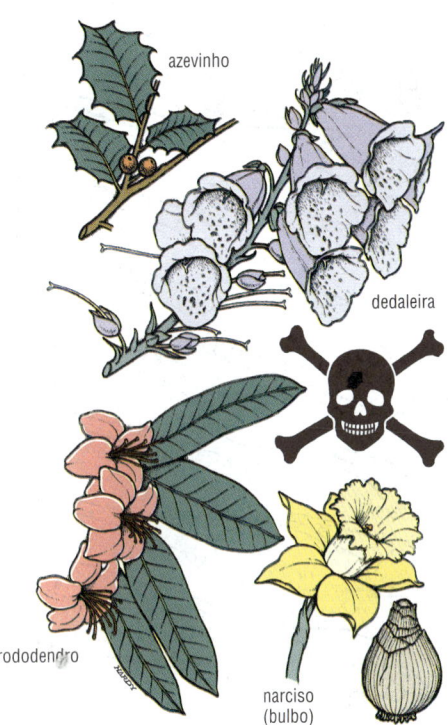

dedaleira e outras plantas tóxicas

FPLC Abreviatura de fast protein liquid chromatography (cromotografia líquida rápida de proteínas).
FPS, fps Abreviatura de foot-pound-second (pé-libra-segundo). VER foot-pound-second *system,* foot-pound-second *unit.*
Fr 1. Símbolo de Francium (frâncio).
Fraccaro, Marco, oftalmologista italiano, *1926. VER Schmid-F. *syndrome.*
Fraccaro, M., médico italiano. VER Parenti-Fraccaro *syndrome.*
F.R.A.C.P. Abreviatura de *Fellow of the Royal Australasian College of Physicians.*
fractals (frak'tălz). Fractais; padrões matemáticos desenvolvidos por Benoit Mandelbrot em 1977; segundo a teoria de Benoit, as partes pequenas apresentam a mesma forma que o todo. Os vasos sanguíneos e a árvore brônquica comportam-se como f.; algumas infecções e neoplasias também comportam-se como f. [Fr., do L. *fractus,* quebrado, pp. de *frango,* quebrar, + -al]
frac·tion (frak'shŭn). **1.** Fração; o quociente de duas quantidades. **2.** Fração; uma alíquota ou qualquer porção. **3.** Fracionar, separar em partes.
amorphous f. of adrenal cortex, f. amorfa do córtex adrenal; resíduo não-cristalino de um extrato de acetona do córtex adrenal, obtido após o isolamento de esteróides cristalinos, tais como corticosterona, desoxicorticosterona, etc.
blood plasma f.'s, frações plasmáticas do sangue; partes do plasma sanguíneo obtidas após separação por eletroforese ou outra técnica.
f. collector, coletor de fração; dispositivo utilizado para coletar o eluato de uma coluna na cromatografia em coluna.
dried human plasma protein f., f. proteica do plasma humano seco; f. proteica de plasma humano congelado e seco.
ejection f., f. de ejeção; volume de sangue contido no ventrículo no final da diástole e expelido durante a contração ventricular, isto é, o volume sistólico dividido pelo volume diastólico final, que normalmente é de 0,55 (pelo eletrocardiograma) ou maior; no início da insuficiência cardíaca congestiva, a f. de ejeção diminui, chegando às vezes a 0,10 ou menos, nos casos graves.
filtration f. (FF), f. de filtração; f. do plasma que penetra no rim e é filtrada para a luz dos túbulos renais; é determinada pela divisão da taxa de filtração glomerular pelo fluxo plasmático renal; habitualmente, é de cerca de 0,17.
human antihemophilic f., f. anti-hemofílica humana. SIN human antihemophilic *factor.*
human plasma protein f., f. proteica do plasma humano; solução estéril composta por determinadas proteínas provenientes do plasma sanguíneo de doadores humanos adultos; contém de 4,5 a 5,5 g de proteínas por 100 ml, dos

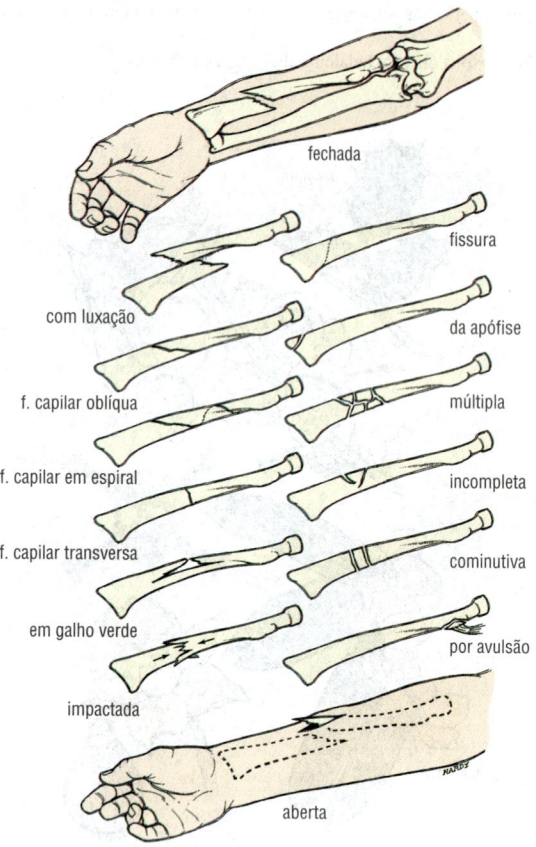

tipos de fraturas

cia; quando o tecido mole é arrancado do osso, um (ou mais) fragmento(s) ósseo(s) permanece(m) fixado(s) ao tecido mole. SIN strain f.
Barton f., f. de Barton; f. na parte distal do rádio com subluxação volar (palmar) ou luxação da articulação radiocarpal.
basal skull f., f. da base do crânio; f. que envolve a base do crânio.
bending f., f. angulada; lesão na qual um ou mais ossos longos, em geral o rádio e a ulna, estão curvados (isto é, angulados) devido a múltiplas microfraturas, e nenhuma delas pode ser observada nas radiografias.
Bennett f., f. de Bennett; f. e luxação do primeiro osso metacarpal da articulação carpometacarpal.
bimalleolar f., f. bimaleolar. SIN Pott f.
birth f., f. de nascimento; f. que ocorre durante o parto ou, ocasionalmente, antes do parto em crianças com osteogênese imperfeita.
blow-out f., f. por explosão; f. do assoalho da órbita, sem que ocorra fratura da margem orbital; é produzida por um golpe sobre o globo, sendo a força transmitida através do globo para o assoalho da órbita.

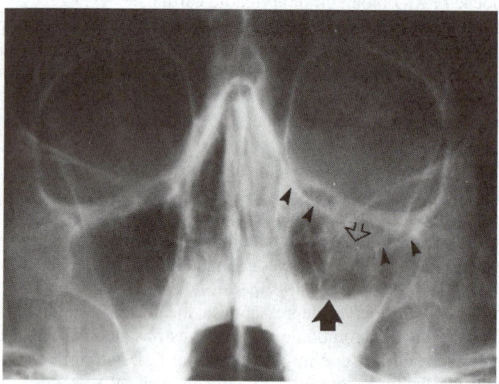

fratura por explosão do assoalho da órbita: Incidência de Waters em uma radiografia simples mostra os principais achados associados a uma lesão por explosão do assoalho da órbita: rompimento do assoalho da órbita (pontas de seta), massa de tecido frouxo na face superior do seio maxilar (seta aberta) e nível líquido no seio maxilar (seta fechada)

quais 83 a 90% correspondem a albumina, e o restante, a α- e β-globulinas; utilizada para manter o volume de sangue.
mole f., f. molar; a razão entre os moles de um composto e a soma dos moles de todos os compostos presentes em uma dada mistura.
radionuclide ejection f., f. de ejeção de radionuclídeo; exame de medicina nuclear que determina a f. de ejeção dos dois ventrículos; substitui exames de aquisição de múltiplas imagens em alguns centros médicos. VER TAMBÉM multiple-gated acquisition *scan*.
recombination f., f. recombinante; a proporção de descendentes de um casal com genótipo e fase de reprodução específicos que é recombinante; é preciso que não haja seleção diferencial entre os possíveis tipos de descendentes e a f. recombinante deve ser a mesma, independentemente dos alelos envolvidos ou da fase de reprodução.
regurgitant f., f. de regurgitação; volume de sangue regurgitado para uma câmara cardíaca dividido pelo volume sistólico; normalmente não ocorre regurgitação; em pacientes com lesões valvares graves, tais como insuficiência mitral ou aórtica, a f. de regurgitação pode aproximar-se de 80%; essa f. fornece uma medida quantitativa da gravidade da lesão valvar.
frac·tion·a·tion (frak-shŭn-ā′shŭn). Fracionamento. 1. A separação dos componentes de uma mistura. 2. A administração de radiação para tratamento de neoplasia, na qual a dose total é dividida em uma série planejada de doses, mais freqüentemente uma vez por dia por várias semanas, a fim de minimizar as lesões por radiação de tecidos normais contíguos.

FRACTURE

frac·ture (frak′choor). Fratura. 1. Quebrar. 2. Uma fratura, principalmente a fratura de um osso ou cartilagem. [L. *fractura*, uma fratura]
apophysial f., f. da apófise; separação da apófise do osso.
articular f., f. articular; uma f. que envolve a superfície articular de um osso.
avulsion f., f. por avulsão; f. que ocorre quando uma cápsula articular, um ligamento ou uma inserção muscular são arrancados do osso como resultado de um deslocamento por torção ou forte contratura do músculo contra a resistên-

boxer's f., f. do boxeador; f. do colo de um osso metacarpal, em geral do quinto metacarpal.
capillary f., f. capilar. SIN hairline f.
Chance f., f. de Chance; f. transversa, em geral na coluna torácica ou lombar, que atravessa o corpo vertebral e se estende posteriormente através dos pedículos e do processo espinhoso.
clay shoveler's f., f. dos escavadores de argila; f. por avulsão da base dos processos espinhosos de C-7, C-6 ou T-1 (em ordem de prevalência).
closed f., f. fechada, f. simples; f. na qual a pele permanece intacta no local da f. SIN simple f.
closed skull f., f. fechada de crânio, f. simples do crânio; f. na qual o couro cabeludo e/ou as membranas mucosas suprajacentes permanecem intactos. SIN simple skull f.
Colles f., f. de Colles; f. na parte distal do rádio, com deslocamento e/ou angulação dorsal do fragmento distal.
comminuted f., f. cominutiva; f. na qual o osso é quebrado em mais de dois fragmentos.
comminuted skull f., f. cominutiva do crânio; f. do crânio com fragmentação do osso.
complex f., f. complexa; f. na qual ocorre lesão significativa de tecido frouxo.
compound f., f. composta, f. exposta; f. na qual a pele é perfurada e há uma ferida aberta no local da f. SIN open f.
compound skull f., f. composta do crânio, f. exposta do crânio. SIN open skull f.
f. by contrecoup, f. por contragolpe; f. do crânio em um ponto distante do local do impacto.
cough f., f. causada pela tosse; f. de uma costela ou cartilagem, em geral a quinta ou a sétima, após tossir vigorosamente.
craniofacial dysjunction f., f. por disjunção craniofacial; f. complexa na qual os ossos da face são separados dos ossos do crânio. SIN Le Fort III craniofacial dysjunction, Le Fort III f., transverse facial f.
dentate f., f. denteada; f. na qual as superfícies opostas são ásperas, com projeções denteadas ou serrilhadas que se ajustam às partes correspondentes.
depressed f., f. de crânio com afundamento. SIN depressed skull f.
depressed skull f., f. de crânio com afundamento; f. com deslocamento para dentro de uma parte da calvária; pode ou não estar associada a rompimento da dura-máter ou do córtex cerebral subjacentes. SIN depressed f.

derby hat f., concavidade regular do crânio encontrada em lactentes; pode ou não estar associada a uma f. SIN dishpan f.
diastatic skull f., f. diastática do crânio; (**1**) separação dos ossos do crânio em uma sutura; (**2**) f. com acentuada separação dos fragmentos ósseos.
direct f., f. direta; f., principalmente do crânio, que ocorre no local do trauma.
dishpan f., f. de crânio com afundamento. SIN derby hat f.
dislocation f., f.-luxação; f. de um osso próximo a uma articulação com luxação concomitante da articulação.
double f., f. dupla. SIN segmental f.
Dupuytren f., f. de Dupuytren; f. na parte inferior da fíbula com luxação do tornozelo.
epiphysial f., epiphyseal f., f. da epífise; separação da epífise de um osso longo, causada por traumatismo. VER Salter-Harris *classification* of epiphysial plate injuries.
expressed skull f., f. exposta do crânio; f. com deslocamento para fora de uma parte do crânio.
extracapsular f., f. extracapsular; f. próxima a uma articulação, porém do lado externo da linha de inserção da cápsula da articulação.
fatigue f., f. por fadiga; f. que ocorre no osso sujeito a tensão repetitiva, mais freqüentemente sua configuração é transversa. SIN stress f.
fetal f., f. intra-uterina. SIN intrauterine f.
fissured f., f. longitudinal. SIN longitudinal f.
folding f., fratura em toro. SIN torus f.
freeze f., criofratura; procedimento, utilizado na preparação de células ou outras amostras biológicas para a microscopia eletrônica, no qual a peça é congelada rapidamente e, então, quebrada com um cortador afiado. SIN cryofracture.
Galeazzi f., f. de Galeazzi; f. da diáfise do rádio com luxação da articulação radioulnar distal.
Gosselin f., f. de Gosselin; f. em forma de V da extremidade distal da tíbia.
greenstick f., f. em galho verde; encurvamento de um osso com f. incompleta que envolve somente o lado convexo da curva.
growing f., f. de crescimento; f. linear do crânio em uma criança em fase de crescimento, em geral como resultado de laceração dural associada e formação de cisto aracnóideo na linha de fratura.
Guérin f., f. de Guérin; f. dos ossos da face na qual há uma f. horizontal na base da maxila, acima dos ápices dos dentes. SIN horizontal f., Le Fort I f.
gutter f., f. em goteira; f. com afundamento, longa e estreita, observada no crânio.
hairline f., f. capilar; f. sem separação dos fragmentos e com uma linha de fratura semelhante a um fio de cabelo; é observada às vezes no crânio. SIN capillary f.
hangman's f., f. do enforcado; f. da coluna cervical que passa pelos pedículos de C2; pode estar associada a luxação prévia entre os corpos vertebrais de C2 e C3.
horizontal f., f. horizontal. SIN Guérin f.
impacted f., f. impactada; f. na qual um dos fragmentos é cravado dentro de outro fragmento que apresenta estrutura porosa.
incomplete f., f. incompleta; f. na qual a linha de fratura não cruza completamente o osso.
indirect f., f. indireta; f., principalmente do crânio, que ocorre em um local que não corresponde à região do impacto.
intertrochanteric f., f. intertrocantérica; f. do fêmur proximal, localizada na metáfise do osso, na região entre os trocanteres maior e menor.
intraarticular f., f. intra-articular; f. que passa pela face articular para dentro da articulação.
intracapsular f., f. intracapsular; f. que ocorre próximo a uma articulação e dentro da linha de inserção da cápsula da articulação.
intrauterine f., f. intra-uterina; f. de um ou mais ossos de um feto que ocorre antes do nascimento. SIN fetal f.
Le Fort I f., f. tipo Le Fort I. SIN Guérin f.
Le Fort II f., f. tipo Le Fort II. SIN pyramidal f.
Le Fort III f., f. tipo Le Fort III. SIN craniofacial dysjunction f.
linear f., f. linear. SIN longitudinal f.
linear skull f., f. linear do crânio; f. do crânio que se assemelha a uma linha.
longitudinal f., f. longitudinal; f. que acompanha o eixo do osso. SIN fissured f., linear f.
march f., f. de marcha; f. por fadiga de um dos ossos metatarsais.
Monteggia f., f. de Monteggia; f. na parte proximal da ulna com luxação da cabeça do rádio.
multiple f., f. múltipla; (**1**) f. em dois ou mais locais de um osso; VER segmental f.; (**2**) f. em vários ossos que ocorrem simultaneamente.
neurogenic f., f. neurogênica; f. que ocorre em um osso fragilizado por doença que afeta sua inervação.
oblique f., f. oblíqua; f. cuja linha se estende obliquamente em relação ao eixo longitudinal do osso.
occult f., f. oculta; condição na qual há sinais clínicos de f., porém sem evidências radiográficas; após duas a quatro semanas, a imagem radiográfica mostra formação de osso novo; as imagens por ressonância magnética freqüentemente confirmam a fratura antes que as alterações se tornem evidentes na radiografia; é comumente observada no osso navicular do punho.
open f., f. exposta. SIN compound f.
open skull f., f. exposta do crânio; f. com laceração do couro cabeludo e/ou da mucosa suprajacentes. SIN compound skull f.
parry f., termo obsoleto para Monteggia f.
pathologic f., f. patológica; f. que ocorre em um local fragilizado por doença óssea preexistente, principalmente neoplasia ou necrose.
pertrochanteric f., f. pertrocanteriana; f. que atravessa a região intertrocantérica do fêmur; uma forma de f. extracapsular do quadril.
pilon f., f. da metáfise distal da tíbia que se estende para dentro da articulação do tornozelo.
ping-pong f., f. em pingue-pongue. VER derby hat f.
pond f., f. circular do crânio com afundamento.
Pott f., f. de Pott; f. da parte inferior da fíbula e do maléolo da tíbia com deslocamento do pé para fora. SIN bimalleolar f.
pyramidal f., f. piramidal; f. do terço médio da face na qual as linhas de fratura principais se encontram em um ponto (ápice) localizado na parte superior dos ossos nasais ou próximo a ela. SIN Le Fort II f.
segmental f., f. segmentar; f. dupla; f. em duas partes do mesmo osso. SIN double f.
Shepherd f., f. de Shepherd; f. do tubérculo lateral (processo posterior) do tálus, às vezes confundida com o deslocamento do osso trígono.
silver-fork f., f. em garfo; f. de Colles do punho na qual a deformidade provocada pela fratura apresenta a forma de um garfo de perfil.
simple f., f. simples. SIN closed f.
simple skull f., f. simples do crânio. SIN closed skull f.
Skillern f., f. de Skillern; termo obsoleto para a f. do rádio distal com f. em galho verde da parte vizinha da ulna.
skull f., f. de crânio; fratura do crânio resultante de traumatismo.
Smith f., f. de Smith; f. de Colles invertida; f. no rádio distal com deslocamento do fragmento em direção à face palmar (volar).
spiral f., f. em espiral; f. óssea que apresenta uma linha de fratura helicoidal; em geral, resulta de uma lesão por torção.
splintered f., f. estilhaçada; f. cominutiva na qual os fragmentos são longos e pontiagudos.
spontaneous f., f. espontânea; f. que ocorre sem qualquer trauma externo.
sprain f., f. por arrancamento; f. por avulsão na qual uma pequena parte de osso adjacente é arrancada.
stable f., f. estável; f. que não tende a sofrer deslocamento após ter sido reduzida e imobilizada.
stellate f., f. estrelada; f. cujas linhas de fratura irradiam de um ponto central.
stellate skull f., f. estrelada do crânio; f. do crânio com múltiplas fraturas lineares que irradiam do local do impacto.
strain f., f. por tensão. SIN avulsion f.
stress f., f. por estresse. SIN fatigue f.
subcapital f., f. subcapital; f. intracapsular do colo do fêmur, no local onde o colo do fêmur se une à cabeça do osso.
subperiosteal f., f. subperiostal; f. que ocorre debaixo do periósteo e sem luxação.
supracondylar f., f. supracondilar; f. da extremidade distal do úmero ou do fêmur, localizada acima da região condilar.
toddler's f., f. em espiral da tíbia observada freqüentemente em crianças de 1 a 2 anos de idade.
torsion f., f. por torção; f. que resulta da torção de um membro.
torus f., f. em toro; deformidade óssea encontrada em crianças na qual o osso se curva e se torce, porém não se quebra; é observada comumente no rádio ou na ulna, ou em ambos os ossos. Essa fratura ocorre somente em crianças, porque seus ossos são mais frágeis do que os dos adultos. SIN folding f.
transcervical f., f. transcervical; f. que passa pelo colo do fêmur.

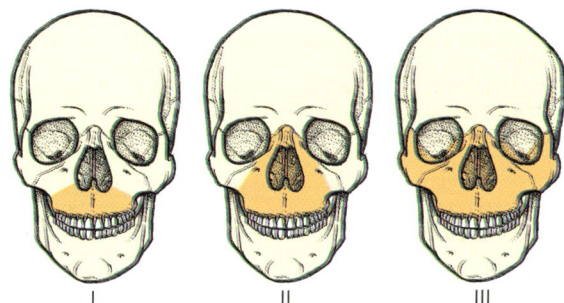

Fraturas de Le Fort

transcondylar f., f. transcondilar; f. que passa pelo côndilo do úmero ou fêmur.
transverse f., f. transversa; f. cuja linha de fratura forma um ângulo reto com o eixo longitudinal do osso.
transverse facial f., f. transversa da face. SIN craniofacial dysjunction f.
trimalleolar f., f. trimaleolar; f. do tornozelo que passa pelo maléolo lateral da fíbula e pelo maléolo medial e processo posterior da tíbia.
tripod f., f. em tripé; f. da face que envolve os três apoios da proeminência malar, ou seja, o arco do osso zigomático, o processo zigomático do osso frontal e o processo zigomático da maxila.
unstable f., f. instável; f. que apresenta uma tendência intrínseca para se deslocar após sofrer redução.
ununited f., fratura não-consolidada; f. na qual não ocorre a consolidação das extremidades do osso.

Fraenkel, Albert, médico alemão, 1848–1916. VER F. *pneumococcus*.
fra·gil·i·tas (fra-jil'i-tas). Fragilidade. SIN fragility. [L.]
  f. crin'ium, f. capilar; fragilidade do cabelo; condição na qual o cabelo ou os pêlos da face tendem a se partir ou quebrar.
  f. san'guinis, f. osmótica. SIN osmotic *fragility*.
fra·gil·i·ty (fra-jil'i-te). Fragilidade; propensão a fragmentar, romper ou desintegrar-se. SIN fragilitas. [L. *fragilitas*]
  f. of the blood, f. osmótica. SIN osmotic f.
  capillary f., f. capilar; suscetibilidade dos capilares sanguíneos a ruptura e extravasamento de hemácias sob condições de estresse elevado.
  osmotic f., f. osmótica; suscetibilidade dos eritrócitos a lise, quando expostos a soluções salinas cada vez mais hipotônicas. SIN fragilitas sanguinis, f. of the blood.
fra·gil·o·cyte (fra-jil'o-sīt). Fragilócito; hemácia que se mostra extraordinariamente frágil, quando em contato com uma solução salina hipotônica. [L. *fragilis*, frágil, + G. *kytos*, célula]
fra·gil·o·cy·to·sis (fra-jil'o-si-to'sis). Fragilocitose; condição do sangue na qual as hemácias são anormalmente frágeis.
frag·ment (frag'ment). Fragmento; uma pequena parte quebrada de uma entidade maior.
  acentric f., cromossomo(a) acêntrico. SIN acentric *chromosome*.
  Brimacombe f., f. de Brimacombe; um f. de ribonucleoproteína obtido por meio do tratamento de ribossomas com ribonuclease.
  butterfly f., f. em asa de borboleta; f. triangular largo que está habitualmente presente em fraturas cominutivas da diáfise.
  Fab f., f. Fab; f. para a ligação de um antígeno presente em uma molécula de imunoglobulina, que consiste tanto em uma cadeia leve, como de uma parte de uma cadeia pesada. SIN Fab piece.
  Fc f., f. Fc; f. cristalizável de uma molécula de imunoglobulina, composto por uma parte das moléculas pesadas e responsável pela ligação da imunoglobulina a receptores de anticorpos (receptores Fc) nas células e ao componente C1q do complemento. SIN Fc piece.
  Klenow f., f. de Klenow; fragmento terminal carboxila da DNA polimerase I, que exibe atividade de polimerase, bem como atividade de exonuclease 3' → 5' para modificar combinações incorretas.
  Okazaki f., f. de Okazaki; um fragmento relativamente curto de DNA—(100–2.000 bp na *Escherichia coli* e 100 – 200 bp em mamíferos) que, posteriormente, se une a outros fragmentos de DNA pela ação da DNA ligase, permitindo, dessa forma, o crescimento geral da cadeia 3' → 5' durante a replicação.
  one-carbon f., f. de um carbono; o grupamento formila ou o grupamento metila que participa das reações de transformilação ou transmetilação; por meio dessas reações, um grupamento com um único átomo de carbono é adicionado a um composto que está sendo biossintetizado; ocorre a adição de um grupamento metila (como na formação da timidina), a adição de um grupamento hidroximetila (como na biossíntese da serina) ou o fechamento de um anel (como na formação da purina).
  two-carbon f., f. com dois carbonos; corresponde ao grupamento acetila (CH_3CO-), que participa de reações de transacetilação, tendo a coenzima A como carreadora; é comumente denominado acetato ou ácido acético, do qual é derivado.
frag·men·ta·tion (frag-men-ta'shŭn). Fragmentação; a quebra de uma entidade em pequenas partes. SIN spallation (1).
  f. of the myocardium, f. do miocárdio; ruptura transversal das fibras musculares do coração, principalmente daquelas dos músculos papilares.
fraise (frāz). Frese; tipo de broca em forma de meia-esfera com bordas cortantes, utilizada para aumentar uma abertura no crânio, feita por um trépano, ou para cortar retalhos osteoplásticos; a suave convexidade do instrumento evita lesões na dura-máter. [Fr. morango]
Fraley, Elwin E., urologista norte-americano, *1934. VER F. *syndrome*.
fram·be·sia tro·pi·ca (fram-e'ze-ă trop'i-kă). Framboesia trópica, bouba. SIN yaws.[Fr. *framboise*, framboesa]
fram·be·si·form (fram-be'zi-form). Framboesiforme; que se assemelha à lesão da framboesia.
fram·be·si·o·ma (fram-be-ze-o'mă). Framboesoma. SIN mother *yaw*. [frambesia + *-oma*, tumor]
frame (frām). Estrutura, arcabouço; estrutura feita de partes que são ajustadas umas às outras.
  Balkan f., e. de Balkan; e. elevada, apoiada sobre pilares fixados às pernas da cama ou a um estrado separado, que permite erguer um membro imobilizado durante o tratamento de uma fratura ou doença articular. SIN Balkan beam, Balkan splint.
  Bradford f., e. de Bradford; armação retangular feita de tubos, sobre a qual são esticadas transversalmente duas faixas de lona; permite que o tronco e as extremidades inferiores de um paciente acamado se movam como uma unidade; hoje em dia, é raramente utilizada.
  Deiters terminal f.'s, estruturas terminais de Deiters; estruturas, semelhantes a lâminas, encontradas no órgão de Corti e que unem as células de Deiters às células de Hensen.
  Foster f., e. de Foster; uma cama reversível semelhante a uma e. de Stryker.
  occluding f., oclusor. SIN articulator.
  Stryker f., e. de Stryker; e. que segura o paciente e permite girá-lo em vários planos, sem que haja movimento individual de suas partes.
  trial f., e. de prova; tipo de armação de óculos com ajustes variáveis para segurar lentes de prova durante o exame oftalmológico (refração).
  Whitman f., e. de Whitman; uma e. semelhante à e. de Bradford, mas com lados curvos.
frame·shift (frām'shift). Conforme utilizado em genética: uma mutação que cria uma seqüência tal que os grupos de três bases presentes no RNAm tornam-se sem registro; a inserção ou a deleção de uma ou duas bases, por exemplo, levaria à formação de um grupo de três bases alterado que provocaria a incorporação de resíduos aminoácidos incorretos em cadeias de polipeptídeos em crescimento ou sinalizaria a terminação precoce da cadeia.
frame·work (frām'work). Estrutura. 1. VER stroma. 2. Em odontologia, o esqueleto da prótese (em geral de metal) ao redor do qual e ao qual são fixadas as partes restantes da prótese, a fim de produzir o aparelho final (dentadura parcial).
Franceschetti, Adolphe, oftalmologista suíço, 1896–1968. VER F. *syndrome*; F.-Jadassohn *syndrome*.
Francisella (fran'si-sel'lă). Gênero de bactérias aeróbias, não esporuladas e imóveis que abrange pequenos cocos e bacilos Gram-negativos. As células podem exibir coloração bipolar e raramente produzem cápsulas. São microrganismos extremamente pleomórficos; não crescem em ágar simples ou em meios líquidos sem enriquecimento especial; são patogênicas e causam a tularemia em seres humanos. A espécie típica é *F. tularensis*.
  F. tularen'sis, espécie de bactéria que causa a tularemia em seres humanos e é transmitida por insetos sugadores de sangue de animais selvagens ou por contato com animais infectados, tais como carrapatos; as principais fontes de infecção são os coelhos e os carrapatos; as bactérias conseguem penetrar na pele íntegra e causar infecção e, se inaladas, podem causar uma pneumonia rapidamente fatal; é a espécie típica do gênero *Francisella*. SIN *Pasteurella tularensis*.
fran·ci·um (Fr) (fran'se-ŭm). Frâncio; elemento radioativo da série dos metais alcalinos; o n.º atômico é 87; a meia-vida do isótopo mais estável conhecido —Fr^{223}— é de 21,8 min. [*França*, país de origem de Mlle. M. Perey (1909–1975), sua descobridora]
Francke, Karl E., médico alemão, 1859–1920. VER F. *needle*.
François, Jules, oftalmologista belga contemporâneo. VER central cloudy corneal *dystrophy* of François.
fran·gu·la (frang'goo-lă). Frângula; a casca da *Rhamnus frangula* (família Rhamnaceae); um laxante ou catártico.
fran·gu·lic ac·id (frang'ū-lik). Ácido frangúlico, emedina. SIN emodin.[VER frangula]
fran·gu·lin (frang'ū-lin). Frangulina; glicosídeo da frângula; utilizado como purgativo. SIN rhamnoxanthin.
Frank, Otto, fisiologista alemão, 1865–1944. VER F.-Starling *curve*.
frank. Franco; inconfundível; manifesto, evidente; clinicamente evidente.
Frankenhäuser, Ferdinand, ginecologista alemão, 1832–1894. VER F. *ganglion*.
Frankfort (frank'fert). VER Frankfort horizontal *plane*, Frankfort-mandibular incisor *angle*. [*Frankfurt-am-Main*, Alemanha]
frank·in·cense (frangk'in-sens). Olíbano. SIN olibanum.[L. mediev. *francum incensum*, incenso puro]
Franklin, Benjamin, físico e estadista norte-americano, 1706–1790. VER franklinic; F. *spectacles*.
Franklin, Edward C., médico e imunologista norte-americano, *1928. VER F. *disease*.
frank·lin·ic (frank'lin-ik). Frankliniano; que indica eletricidade estática ou a provocada por fricção. [B. *Franklin*]
Fräntzel (fränt'zel), Oscar Maximilian Victor, médico alemão, 1838–1894. VER Fräntzel *murmur*.

Fraser, Alexander, patologista canadense, 1869–1939. VER F.-Lendrum *stain* for fibrin.

Fraser, George R., geneticista britânico do século XX. VER F. *syndrome*.

Fraumeni, Joseph F., Jr., epidemiologista, *1933. VER Li-F. cancer *syndrome*.

Fraunhofer, Joseph von, oculista alemão, 1787–1826. VER F. *lines,* em *line*.

Frazier, Charles H., cirurgião norte-americano, 1870–1936. VER F. *needle;* F.-Spiller *operation*.

FRC Abreviatura de functional residual *capacity* (capacidade residual funcional).

F.R.C.P. Abreviatura de *Fellow of the Royal College of Physicians* (da Inglaterra).

F.R.C.P.(C) Abreviatura de *Fellow of the Royal College of Physicians* (Canadá).

F.R.C.P.(E), F.R.C.P.(Edin) Abreviatura de *Fellow of the Royal College of Physicians* (Edimburgo).

F.R.C.P.(I) Abreviatura de *Fellow of the Royal College of Physicians* (Irlanda).

F.R.C.S. Abreviatura de *Fellow of the Royal College of Surgeons* (da Inglaterra).

F.R.C.S.(C) Abreviatura de *Fellow of the Royal College of Surgeons* (Canadá).

F.R.C.S.(E), F.R.C.S.(Edin) Abreviatura de *Fellow of the Royal College of Surgeons* (Edimburgo).

F.R.C.S.(I) Abreviatura de *Fellow of the Royal College of Surgeons* (Irlanda).

freck·le (frek'l). Sarda, efélida; máculas amareladas ou acastanhadas que se desenvolvem nas partes expostas da pele, principalmente em pessoas de tez clara; o número de lesões eleva-se após exposição ao sol; a epiderme mostra-se microscopicamente normal, exceto pelo aumento de melanina. VER TAMBÉM lentigo. SIN ephelis. [I. ant. *freken*]

   Hutchinson f., s. de Hutchinson, lentigo maligno. SIN *lentigo* maligna.

   iris f.'s, sardas da íris; grupos pequenos e pigmentados de melanócitos uveais sobre a superfície da íris.

   melanotic f., s. melanótica, lentigo maligno. SIN *lentigo* maligna.

Fredet, Pierre, cirurgião francês, 1870–1946. VER F.-Ramstedt *operation*.

Freeman, Ernest A., †1975. VER F.-Sheldon *syndrome*.

freeze-dry·ing (frez'drī-ing). Congelamento-dessecação, liofilização. SIN lyophilization.

freez·ing (frē'zing). Congelamento, enrijecimento ou endurecimento pela exposição ao frio.

   gastric f., congelamento gástrico; tratamento utilizado no passado para úlcera péptica que tinha o objetivo de reduzir ou eliminar a produção de suco gástrico ácido por meio do congelamento das células secretórias com um líquido introduzido em um balão posicionado dentro do estômago.

Frei, Wilhelm S., dermatologista alemão, 1885–1943. VER F. *test;* F.-Hoffmann *reaction*.

Freiberg, Albert Henry, cirurgião norte-americano, 1869-1940. VER F. *disease*.

Frejka, Bedrich, ortopedista tcheco, 1890–1972. VER F. pillow *splint*.

fré·mis·se·ment cat·taire (frā-mēs'mon kat'air). VER fremitus.

frem·i·tus (frem'i-tŭs). Frêmito; vibração transmitida à mão que repousa sobre o tórax ou outra parte do corpo. VER TAMBÉM thrill. [L. som surdo, de *fremo,* pp. *-itus,* ressoar]

   bronchial f., f. brônquico; sons pulmonares adventícios ou sons vocais perceptíveis pela mão que repousa sobre o peito, assim como pela orelha.

   hydatid f., f. hidático. SIN hydatid *thrill*.

   pericardial f., f. pericárdico; vibração da parede do tórax produzida pela fricção das superfícies opostas e ásperas do pericárdio. VER TAMBÉM pericardial *rub*.

   pleural f., f. pleural; vibração da parede do tórax produzida pelo atrito resultante da fricção das superfícies opostas inflamadas e ásperas da pleura.

   rhonchal f., f. dos roncos; f. produzido por vibrações resultantes da passagem de ar pelos tubos brônquicos, parcialmente obstruídos por secreção mucosa.

   subjective f., f. subjetivo; vibração sentida dentro do peito pelo próprio paciente, quando cantarola com a boca fechada; ou o f. sentido quando ocorre atrito pleural ou pericárdico, em particular quando a dor é mínima.

   tactile f., f. tátil; vibração sentida com a mão sobre o tórax durante o f. vocal.

   tussive f., f. causado pela tosse; forma de f., similar ao vocal, produzido pela tosse.

   vocal f., f. vocal; vibração da parede torácica, sentida na palpação e produzida pela voz.

fre·na (frē'nă). Freios; plural de frenum.

fre·nal (frē'năl). Frenal; relativo a qualquer freio.

French. VER French *scale*.

fre·nec·to·my (frē-nek'tō-mē). Frenectomia; remoção de qualquer freio. [frenum + G. *ektomē,* excisão]

fre·no·plas·ty (frē'nō-plas-tē). Frenoplastia; correção de uma anormalidade fixada ao freio por meio do reposicionamento cirúrgico deste último. [frenum + G. *plastos,* formado]

fre·not·o·my (frē-not'ō-mē). Frenotomia; divisão de qualquer freio ou frênulo, principalmente o frênulo da língua. [frenum + G. *tomē,* um corte]

fren·u·lum, pl. **fren·u·la** (fren'ū-lŭm, -lă) [TA]. Frênulo; pequeno freio ou rédea. VER TAMBÉM frenum. SIN habenula (1) [TA]. [L. mod. dim. de L. *frenum,* freio]

   cerebellar f., f. do véu medular superior. SIN f. of superior medullary velum.

   f. cerebell'i, f. do véu medular superior. SIN f. of superior medullary velum.

   f. clitor'idis [TA], f. do clitóris. SIN f. of clitoris.

   f. of clitoris [TA], f. do clitóris; a linha de união das partes internas dos lábios menores do pudendo; na superfície inferior da glande do clitóris. SIN f. clitoridis [TA], f. preputii clitoridis.

   f. epiglot'tidis, prega glossoepiglótica mediana. SIN median glossoepiglottic *fold*.

   f. of foreskin, f. do prepúcio; [a]termo oficial alternativo para f. of prepuce.

   f. of Giacomini, f. de Giacomini. SIN uncus *band* of Giacomini.

   f. of ileal orifice [TA], f. do óstio ileal; prega, mais evidente nos cadáveres, que parte da junção das duas comissuras da válvula ileocecal em ambos os lados ao longo da parede interna da junção cecocólica. SIN f. ostii ilealis [TA], f. of ileocecal valve, f. of Morgagni, f. valvae ileocecalis, Morgagni frenum, Morgagni retinaculum.

   f. of ileocecal valve, f. do óstio ileal. SIN f. of ileal orifice.

   f. of labia minora [TA], f. dos lábios do pudendo; prega que une posteriormente os dois lábios menores do pudendo. SIN f. labiorum pudendi [TA], fourchette[a], f. labiorum minorum, f. of pudendal lips, f. pudendi.

   f. la'bii inferio'ris, f. la'bii superio'ris [TA], f. dos lábios do pudendo. SIN f. of lower lip.

   f. labio'rum mino'rum, f. dos lábios do pudendo. SIN f. of labia minora.

   f. labio'rum puden'di [TA], f. dos lábios do pudendo. SIN f. of labia minora.

   f. lin'guae [TA], f. da língua. SIN f. of tongue.

   lingual f., f. da língua. SIN f. of tongue.

   f. of lower lip, f. of upper lip [TA], f. do lábio inferior, f. do lábio superior; pregas de mucosa que se estendem da gengiva até a linha média dos lábios inferior e superior, respectivamente. SIN f. labii inferioris, f. labii superioris [TA].

   f. of M'Dowel, f. de M'Dowel; fascículos tendinosos que passam do tendão do músculo peitoral maior através do sulco bicipital.

   f. of Morgagni, f. de Morgagni. SIN f. of ileal orifice.

   f. ostii ilealis [TA], f. do óstio ileal. SIN f. of ileal orifice.

   f. of prepuce [TA], f. do prepúcio; prega de mucosa que passa da superfície inferior da glande do pênis até a superfície profunda do prepúcio. SIN f. preputii [TA], f. of foreskin[a], vinculum preputii.

   f. prepu'tii [TA], f. do prepúcio. SIN f. of prepuce.

   f. prepu'tii clitor'idis, f. do clitóris. SIN f. of clitoris.

   f. of pudendal lips, f. dos lábios do pudendo. SIN f. of labia minora.

   f. puden'di, f. dos lábios do pudendo. SIN f. of labia minora.

   f. of superior medullary velum, f. do véu medular superior; uma faixa que parte do sulco longitudinal entre os corpos geniculados até o véu medular superior. SIN f. veli medullaris superioris [TA], cerebellar f., f. cerebelli.

   synovial frenula, vínculos tendíneos dos dedos das mãos e dos pés. SIN *vincula* tendinea of digits of hand and foot, em *vinculum*.

   f. of tongue [TA], f. da língua; prega de membrana mucosa que se estende do assoalho da boca até a linha média da face inferior da língua. SIN f. linguae [TA], lingual f., vinculum linguae.

   f. val'vae ileoceca'lis, f. do óstio ileal. SIN f. of ileal orifice.

   f. ve'li medulla'ris superio'ris [TA], f. do véu medular superior. SIN f. of superior medullary velum.

fre·num, pl. **fre·na, fre·nums** (frē'nŭm, -nă, -nŭmz). Freio; **1.** Reflexão estreita ou prega de membrana mucosa que passa de uma parte mais fixa para uma parte móvel, servindo para deter um movimento indevido da última. **2.** Estrutura anatômica que se assemelha a uma prega. SIN bridle (1). [L. rédea, freio]

   Morgagni f., f. de Morgagni. SIN *frenulum* of ileal orifice.

   synovial frena, vínculos tendíneos dos dedos das mãos e dos pés. SIN *vincula* tendinea of digits of hand and foot, em *vinculum*.

fren·zy (fren'zē). Frenesi; excitação mental ou emocional extremas. [através do Fr. ant. e L. do G. *phrenēsis,* inflamação do cérebro, de *phrēn,* mente]

fre·quen·cy (v) (frē'kwen-sē). Freqüência; número de repetições regulares em determinado espaço de tempo, p.ex., batimentos cardíacos, vibrações sonoras. [L. *frequens,* repetido, freqüente, constante]

   best f., f. característica. SIN characteristic f.

   characteristic f., f. característica; f. na qual determinado neurônio responde à intensidade sonora mínima. SIN best f.

   critical flicker fusion f., f. crítica de fusão; número mínimo de clarões luminosos por segundo com o qual um estímulo luminoso intermitente não provoca mais uma sensação visual contínua.

   f. domain, domínio de f.; a expressão de uma função dada por meio de sua amplitude e fase em cada uma das freqüências componentes, conforme determina a análise de Fourier.

   dominant f., f. dominante; f. que ocorre com mais freqüência em um eletroencefalograma.

   f. encoding, codificação de f.; em ressonância magnética, um método que permite variar a força do campo magnético por local, a fim de codificar a posição de cada voxel em uma única direção.

fundamental f., f. fundamental; (1) principal componente de uma onda sonora, que apresenta o maior comprimento de onda; (2) som produzido pela vibração das pregas vocais antes de o ar alcançar quaisquer cavidades.
gene f., f. gênica; (1) a probabilidade de que um gene, escolhido ao acaso em uma população definida, seja de um tipo específico; (2) em termos epidemiológicos, a proporção de genes de um tipo específico em uma população; (3) em termos estatísticos, o cálculo estimativo de uma grandeza preceder outra grandeza.
Larmor f., f. de Larmor; em ressonância magnética, é a f. de precessão, n_0, do núcleo magnético em um plano perpendicular à direção do campo magnético externo; $v_0 = \gamma B_0/2\pi$, onde B_0 é a força do campo magnético e γ é a razão giromagnética.
f. of micturition, polaciúria; micção a intervalos curtos; pode ser resultante da formação aumentada de urina, da diminuição da capacidade da bexiga ou de inflamação do trato urinário inferior.
mutational f., f. mutacional; a proporção de mutações em uma população.
nearest neighbor f., a f. pela qual certos tipos de entidades ou estruturas estão imediatamente adjacentes a determinada estrutura.
resonant f., f. de ressonância; a f. na qual núcleos magnéticos isolados absorvem ou emitem energia de radiofreqüência em estudos de ressonância magnética. SIN resonance (6).
respiratory f. (f), f. respiratória; o número de respirações por minuto.
Frerichs, Friedrich T. von, patologista e clínico alemão, 1819–1885. VER F. *theory*.
fresh·en·ing (fresh'en - ing). Desbridamento; preparação de uma ferida aberta, parcialmente cicatrizada por segunda intenção, por meio da remoção de fibrina, granulações e tecido cicatricial inicial.
Fresnel, Augustin Jean, físico francês, 1788–1827. VER F. *lens, prism*.
fress·re·flex (fres'rē - fleks). Reflexo de alimentação; movimentos de sucção e mastigação desencadeados pela estimulação da face e dos lábios. [do Al. *fressen*, alimentar (animais)]
fret·ting (fret'ing). Corrosão; polimento abrasivo e desgaste que ocorrem na interface de duas superfícies metálicas devido a movimento repetitivo. [I.m., do I. ant. *fretan*, devorar]
fre·tum, pl. **fre·ta** (frē'tŭm, - tă). Um estreitamento; uma constrição. [L.]
Freud, Sigmund, neurologista e psiquiatra austríaco, 1856–1939, fundador da psicanálise. VER freudian; freudian *fixation*; freudian *psychoanalysis*; *freudian* slip; F. *theory*.
freud·i·an (froyd'ē - ăn). Freudiano; relativo a, ou descrito por, Sigmund Freud (1856–1939).
f. slip, ato falho; erro que ocorre durante a fala ou uma ação e que, presumivelmente, sugere algum motivo subjacente, freqüentemente de natureza sexual ou agressiva.
Freund, Jules, bacteriologista norte-americano, 1891–1960. VER F. complete *adjuvant*, incomplete *adjuvant*.
Freund, Wilhelm A., ginecologista alemão, 1833–1918. VER F. *anomaly, operation*.
Frey, Lucie, médica polonesa, 1852–1932. VER F. *syndrome*.
Frey, Max von, médico alemão, 1852–1932. VER F. *hairs*, em *hair*.
FRH Abreviatura de follitropin-releasing hormone (hormônio liberador de folitropina).
fri·a·ble (frī'ă - bl). Friável. 1. Aquilo que é facilmente reduzido a pó. 2. Em bacteriologia, denota uma cultura seca e quebradiça que se transforma em pó, quando tocada ou sacudida. [L. *friabilis*, de *frio*, esfarelar]
fric·a·tive (frik'ă - tiv). Fricativo; som da fala produzido ao se forçar o fluxo de ar através de um orifício estreito criado pela aposição dos dentes, da língua e dos lábios, a fim de emitir fonemas consonantais, tais como /f/, /v/, /s/ e /z/.
fric·tion (frik'shŭn). Fricção; atrito. 1. O ato de esfregar a superfície de um objeto contra a de outro objeto; principalmente esfregar os membros do corpo para auxiliar a circulação. 2. A força necessária para o movimento relativo de dois corpos que estão em contato. [L. *frictio*, de *frico*, friccionar]
dynamic f., atrito dinâmico; a força que precisa ser vencida para manter o movimento constante de um corpo em relação a um outro, quando ambos permanecem em contato. Cf. starting f.
starting f., atrito inicial; a força que precisa ser vencida para iniciar o movimento de um corpo em relação a outro, quando ambos repousam em contato. Cf. dynamic f. SIN static f.
static f., atrito estático. SIN starting f.
Friderichsen, Carl, médico dinamarquês, *1886. VER Waterhouse-F. *syndrome*; Friderichsen-Waterhouse *syndrome*.
Friedländer, Carl, patologista alemão, 1847–1887. VER F. *bacillus, pneumonia, stain* for capsules.
Friedman, Emanuel A., obstetra norte-americano, *1926. VER Friedman *curve*.
Friedreich, Nikolaus, neurologista alemão, 1825–1882. VER F. *ataxia, phenomenon, sign*.
Friend, Charlotte, microbiologista norte-americana, 1921–1987. VER F. *disease, virus,* leukemia *virus*.
frig·id (frij'id). Frígido. 1. SIN cold. 2. Frio ou sem resposta quanto ao temperamento, principalmente quanto ao sexo. [L. *frigidus*, frio]

fri·gid·i·ty (fri - jid'i - tē). Frigidez. 1. Impotência feminina. 2. O estado de ser frígido (2); inadequação sexual feminina que varia do conceito freudiano de incapacidade para alcançar o orgasmo a qualquer grau de resposta sexual considerada insatisfatória, tanto pela mulher quanto por seu parceiro.
frig·o·rif·ic (frig - ō - rif'ik). Frigorífico; que produz frio. [L. *frigus*, frio, + *facio*, fazer]
frig·o·rism (frig'ō - rizm). Criopatia. SIN cryopathy. [L. *frigus*, frio]
fringe (frinj). Franja, fímbria. SIN fimbria (1).
costal f., f. costal; conjunto de veias visíveis, dispostas de forma irregular, observado na pele de pessoas geralmente de meia-idade ou mais velhas; não apresenta nenhuma ligação com qualquer estrutura profunda, tal como o diafragma, nem conexão com doença visceral subjacente. SIN zona corona.
synovial f., vilosidade sinovial. SIN synovial *villi*, em *villus*.
frit (frit). Frita. 1. Material utilizado no processo de vitrificação dos dentes artificiais. 2. Pigmento em pó utilizado na coloração da porcelana de dentes artificiais. [Fr. *frit*, frito]
Fritsch, Heinrich, ginecologista alemão, 1844–1915. VER Bozeman-F. *catheter*.
Froehde, A., químico alemão do século XIX. VER F. *reagent*.
frog (frŏg). Rã; anfíbio da ordem Anura, que engloba os sapos; os gêneros mais comuns de rãs são *Rana* (rãs terrícolas) e *Hyla* (rãs arborícolas). [A.S. *frogge*]
Fröhlich, Alfred, neurologista e farmacologista austríaco, 1871–1953. VER F. *dwarfism, syndrome*.
Frohn, Damianus, médico alemão, *1843. VER F. *reagent*.
Froin, Georges, médico francês, 1874–1932. VER F. *syndrome*.
frôle·ment (frol - mon'). 1. Fricção suave ou massagem com a palma da mão. 2. Som surdo que se ouve na ausculta. [Fr.]
Froment, Jules, médico lionês, 1878–1946. VER F. *sign*.
Frommel, Richard, ginecologista alemão, 1854–1912. VER Chiari-F. *syndrome*.
frons, gen. **fron·tis** (fronz, fron'tis) [TA]. Fronte. SIN forehead. [L.]
front (frŭnt). Linha de frente; a posição da margem dianteira do solvente na cromatografia.
front·ad (frŭn'tad). Direcionado para a frente.
fron·tal (frŭn'tăl) [TA]. Frontal. 1. Na frente; relativo à parte anterior de um corpo. 2. Que se refere ao plano frontal (coronal), ao osso frontal ou à testa. SIN frontalis [TA].
fron·ta·lis (frŭn - tā'lis) [TA]. Frontal. SIN frontal. [L.]
fron·to·ma·lar (frŭn'tō - mā'lăr). Frontomalar. SIN frontozygomatic.
fron·to·max·il·lary (frŭn'tō - mak'si - lā - rē). Frontomaxilar; relativo aos ossos frontal e maxilar.
fron·to·na·sal (frŭn'tō - nā - zăl). Frontonasal; relativo aos ossos frontal e nasal.
fron·to·oc·cip·i·tal (frŭn'tō - ok - sip'i - tăl). Frontoccipital; relativo aos ossos frontal e occipital, ou à testa e ao occipício.
fron·to·pa·ri·e·tal (frŭn'tō - pa - rī'e - tăl). Frontoparietal; relativo aos ossos frontal e parietal.
fron·to·tem·po·ral (frŭn - tō - tem'pŏ - răl). Frontotemporal; relativo aos ossos frontal e temporal.
fron·to·tem·po·ra·le (frŭn'tō - tem - pō - rā'lē). Frontotemporal; ponto craniométrico localizado no ponto mais anterior da linha temporal no osso frontal.
fron·to·zy·go·mat·ic (frŭn'tō - zī'gō - mat'ik). Frontozigomático, frontomalar; relativo aos ossos frontal e zigomático. SIN frontomalar.
Froriep, August von, anatomista alemão, 1849–1917. VER F. *ganglion*.
frost. Congelamento; depósito que se assemelha àqueles produzidos pelo vapor ou orvalho congelados.
urea f., uremic f., congelamento urêmico; depósitos pulvéreos encontrados sobre a pele, principalmente da face, formados de sais de uréia e ácido úrico e resultantes da excreção de compostos nitrogenados no suor; observados na uremia grave. SIN uridrosis crystallina.
Frost, Albert D., oftalmologista norte-americano, 1889–1945. VER F. *suture*.
Frost, Wade H., epidemiologista norte-americano, 1880–1938. Ver Reed-F. *model*.
Frost, William A., oftalmologista inglês, 1853–1935.
frost·bite (frost'bit). Geladura, ulceração produzida pelo frio; destruição tecidual local resultante da exposição ao frio extremo; nos casos leves, ocorre congelamento superficial reversível acompanhado de eritema e dor fraca; nos casos graves, a lesão pode ser indolor ou parestésica e ser acompanhada de bolhas, edema persistente e gangrena. A lesão pelo frio é atualmente tratada por reaquecimento rápido.
frot·tage (frō - tahzh'). Fricção; 1. A fricção realizada nas massagens. 2. A produção de excitação sexual friccionando-se em outra pessoa. [F. uma fricção]
frot·teur (frō - tuhr'). Alguém que obtém excitação sexual por meio da fricção.
FRS Abreviatura de first rank *symptoms* (sintomas de primeira ordem de Schneider), em *symptom*.
F.R.S. Abreviatura de *Fellow of the Royal Society*.
F.R.S.C. Abreviatura de *Fellow of the Royal Society* (Canadá).
Fru Símbolo de fructose (frutose).
fruc·tan (frŭk'tan). Frutano. SIN fructosan (1).

fructo-. Fruto-; prefixo químico que indica a configuração da molécula de frutose. [L. *fructus*, fruto]

fruc·to·fu·ra·nose (frŭk - tō - foor′ă - nōs, fruk-) Frutofuranose; frutose na forma de furanose.

β-fruc·to·fu·ran·o·sid·ase (frŭk′tō - foor - ă - nō - sĭd′ās, fruk-). β-frutofuranosidase; β-*h*-frutosidase; enzima que hidrolisa os β-D-frutofuranosídeos e libera D-frutose livre; se o substrato for a sacarose, o produto será a D-glicose mais a D-frutose (açúcar invertido); o açúcar invertido é mais facilmente digerido do que a sacarose. SIN invertase, invertin, saccharase.

fruc·to·ki·nase (frŭk - tō - kī′nās, fruk-). Frutocinase; uma enzima hepática que catalisa a reação entre o ATP e a D-frutose para formar frutose 6-fosfato e ADP; indivíduos com frutosúria essencial apresentam deficiência dessa enzima (deficiência de f. hepática).

fruc·tol·y·sis (fruk - tŏl′ĭ - sis). Frutólise; conversão da frutose em lactato; reação análoga à glicólise.

fruc·to·san (frŭk′tō - san, fruk-). Frutosana. **1.** Um polissacarídeo de frutose (p.ex., inulina) que contém pequenas quantidades de outros açúcares; é encontrada em certos tubérculos. SIN fructan, levan, levulan, levulin, levulosan, polyfructose. **2.** 2,6-anidrofrutofuranose.

fruc·tose (Fru) (frŭk′tōs, fruk-). Frutose; o isômero D da frutose (também conhecido como açúcar das frutas, levoglicose, levulose e D-*arabino*-2-hexulose) é uma 2-cetoexose que, em termos fisiológicos, é considerada a mais importante das cetoexoses e é um dos dois produtos da hidrólise da sucrose; na ausência de insulina, é metabolizado ou convertido a glicogênio. [L. *fructus*, fruto, + -ose]

fruc·tose-bis·phos·pha·tase. Frutose-difosfatase; hidrolase que catalisa a conversão da frutose 1,6-difosfato em D-frutose 6-fosfato e ortofosfato na gliconeogênese; o AMP é um inibidor alostérico; a deficiência de f.-d. causa problemas relacionados com gliconeogênese defeituosa; existe uma enzima similar que age sobre a frutose 2,6-difosfato.

fruc·tose 1,6-bis·phos·phate. Frutose 1,6-difosfato; o produto intermediário mais importante da glicólise e da gliconeogênese. SIN hexosebisphosphatase, hexosediphosphatase.

fruc·tose 2,6-bis·phos·phate. Frutose 2,6-difosfato; análogo da frutose 1,6-difosfato que desempenha um papel-chave na regulação da glicólise e da gliconeogênese; ativa a fosfofrutocinase e inibe a frutose 1,6-difosfatase.

fruc·tose-bis·phos·phate al·dol·ase. Frutose-difosfato aldolase; frutose-1,6-difosfato trifosfato-liase; enzima que cliva de forma reversível a frutose 1,6-difosfato, formando diidroxiacetona fosfato e gliceraldeído 3-fosfato; age também sobre certas cetoses 1-fosfato; indivíduos com intolerância hereditária à frutose (aldolase B) apresentam deficiência dessa enzima; a deficiência de aldolase A leva à deficiência de aldolase nos eritrócitos, o que causa anemia hemolítica não-esferocítica. Cf. hereditary fructose *intolerance*. SIN 1-phosphofructaldolase, fructose-diphosphate aldolase.

fruc·tose-di·phos·phate al·dol·ase. Frutose-difosfato aldolase. SIN fructose-bisphosphate aldolase.

fruc·to·se·mia (frŭk - tō - sē′mē - ă, fruk-). Frutosemia; presença de frutose no sangue circulante. VER TAMBÉM hereditary fructose *intolerance*. SIN levulosemia.

fruc·tose 1-phos·phate. Frutose 1-fosfato; derivado da frutose que se acumula nos indivíduos com intolerância hereditária à frutose.

fruc·tose 6-phos·phate. Frutose 6-fosfato; produto intermediário da glicólise e da transcetolação da eritrose 4-fosfato. SIN Neuberg ester.

fruc·to·side (frŭk′tō - sīd, fruk′). Frutosídeo; a frutose na ligação —C—O—, na qual o grupamento —C—O— é o grupamento 2 original da frutose.

fruc·to·su·ria (frŭk - tō - soo′rē - ă, fruk-). Frutosúria; excreção de frutose na urina. SIN levulosuria. [fructose + G. *ouron*, urina]

   benign f., f. benigna, f. essencial. SIN essential f.

   essential f. f. essencial; [MIM*229800], erro inato do metabolismo, benigno e assintomático, decorrente da deficiência de frutocinase, a primeira enzima na via específica da frutose; a frutose aparece no sangue e na urina, porém é excretada inalterada; herança autossômica recessiva. Deficiência de frutocinase. VER TAMBÉM hereditary fructose *intolerance*. SIN benign f., fructokinase deficiency.

fructosyl-. Frutosil-; prefixo químico que indica a presença de frutose na ligação —C—R— (e não em —C—O—R) através de seu carbono 2 (R corresponde, em geral, a um átomo de C).

fru·se·mide (froo′se - mīd). Furosemida. SIN furosemide.

frus·tra·tion (frŭs′trā′shŭn). Frustração; termo psicológico ou psiquiátrico que indica a incapacidade de gratificar um desejo ou satisfazer um impulso ou uma necessidade. [L. *frustro*, pp. *-atus*, enganar, desapontar, de *frustra* (adv.), em vão]

FSH Abreviatura de follicle-stimulating *hormone* (hormônio folículo-estimulante).

ft. Abreviatura de L. *fiat*, faça-se; abreviatura de foot ou feet, (pé, pés).

FTA-ABS. Abreviatura de fluorescent treponemal antibody absorption (absorção de anticorpo antitreponêmico fluorescente). VER fluorescent treponemal antibody-absorption *test*.

FTI Abreviatura de free thyroxine *index* (índice de tiroxina livre).

Fuc Abreviatura de fucose (fucose).

Fuchs, Ernst, oftalmologista austríaco, 1851–1930. VER F. *adenoma*; *angle* of F.; F. heterochromic *cyclitis*, *coloboma*, endothelial *dystrophy*, black *spot*, *spur*, *stomas*, em *stoma*, *syndrome*, *uveitis*; Dalen-F. *nodules*, em *nodule*.

fuch·sin (fuk′sin). Fucsina; termo inespecífico que se refere a qualquer um dos vários corantes rosanilina vermelha utilizados em histologia e bacteriologia. [Leonhard *Fuchs*, botânico alemão, 1501–1506]

   acid f. [I.C. 42685], f. ácida; uma mistura de sais de sódio dos ácidos di e trissulfônico da rosanilina e da para-rosanilina; utilizada como corante indicador e para a coloração do citoplasma e colágeno. SIN rubin S, rubine.

   aldehyde f., f. aldeído; corante desenvolvido por Gomori e composto de f. básica para-aldeído e ácido clorídrico; cora de violeta as fibras elásticas, os grânulos dos mastócitos, as células principais do estômago, as células beta das ilhotas pancreáticas e certos grânulos beta da hipófise; outros grânulos e células da hipófise coram-se em cores diferentes. VER TAMBÉM Gomori aldehyde fuchsin *stain*.

   aniline f., f. anilina; mistura de anilina e f. básica em etanol a 30% e traços de fenol, como na coloração de Goodpasture.

   basic f. [I.C. 42500], f. básica; corante trifenilmetano, cujo componente dominante é a para-rosanilina; um corante importante em histologia, histoquímica e bacteriologia. SIN diamond f.

   carbol f., f. carbólica. VER carbol-fuchsin *paint*, Ziehl *stain*.

   diamond f., f. básica. SIN basic f.

fuch·sin·o·phil (fuk′si - nō - fil). Fucsinófilo. **1.** Que se cora facilmente com corantes à base de fucsina. SIN fuchsinophilic. **2.** Célula ou elemento histológico que se cora facilmente pela fucsina. [fuchsin + G. *philos*, amigo]

fuch·sin·o·phil·ia (fuk′si - nō - fil′ē - ă). Fucsinofilia; a propriedade de se corar rapidamente pela fucsina.

fuch·sin·o·phil·ic (fuk′si - nō - fil′ik). Fucsinófilo. SIN fuchsinophil (1).

fu·cose (Fuc) (fū′kōs). Fucose; 6-desoxigalactose; uma metilpentose cuja configuração L é encontrada nos mucopolissacarídeos das substâncias dos grupos sanguíneos, no leite humano (como um polissacarídeo) e na composição de outras substâncias encontradas na natureza. A configuração D é encontrada em certos antibióticos e em certos glicosídeos vegetais. SIN rhodeose.

α-fu·co·si·dase (fū - kōs′i - dās). α-fucosidase; enzima que catalisa a hidrólise de um α-L-fucosídeo, produzindo um álcool e L-fucose; a deficiência dessa enzima lisossômica causa fucosidose.

fu·co·si·do·sis (fū′kō - si - dō′sis). [MIM*230000]. Fucosidose; doença metabólica de armazenamento caracterizada pelo acúmulo de glicolipídios que contêm fucose e pela deficiência da enzima α-fucosidase; a deterioração neurológica progressiva começa após o primeiro ano de vida, acompanhada de espasticidade, tremor e leves alterações esqueléticas; trata-se de herança autossômica recessiva causada pela mutação no gene da α-1-fucosidase no cromossoma 1.

FUDR Abreviatura de fluorodeoxyuridine (fluorodesoxiuridina). VER floxuridine.

fu·gac·i·ty (f) (foo - gas′i - tē). Fugacidade; tendência das moléculas em um líquido, como resultado de todas as forças que agem sobre elas, de abandonar determinado local no corpo; a tendência de escape de um líquido, como ocorre na difusão, evaporação, etc. [L. *fuga*, fuga]

-fugal. Sufixo que indica afastamento da parte indicada pela raiz da palavra. [L. *fugio*, fugir]

-fuge. –fugo; fuga, sufixo que indica o local de onde a fuga acontece ou o que é posto em fuga. [L. *fuga*, uma fuga]

fu·gi·tive (fū′ji - tiv). **1.** Temporário; transitório. **2.** Fugas, fugidio; que indica certos sintomas inconstantes. [L. *fugitivus*, fugitivo, de *fugio*, pp. *fugitus*, fugir]

fugue (fūg). Fuga; condição na qual um indivíduo abandona subitamente uma atividade ou estilo de vida atuais e começa uma vida nova e diferente por certo período de tempo, freqüentemente em uma outra cidade; mais tarde, o indivíduo alega amnésia em relação aos acontecimentos que ocorreram durante o período de f., embora fatos anteriores sejam relembrados, e hábitos e habilidades não estejam em geral afetados. [Fr. do L. *fuga*, fuga]

fu·gu·tox·in (foo′goo - tok - sin). Fugutoxina; veneno potente encontrado nos ovários e na pele do baiacu do Pacífico. VER TAMBÉM tetrodotoxin.

Fukase, Masaichi. VER Crow-F. *syndrome*.

ful·crum, pl. **ful·cra, ful·crums** (ful′krŭm, - krā, - krŭmz) Fulcro; um apoio ou um ponto de apoio no qual uma alavanca gira. [L. pé de cama, de *fulcio*, apoiar]

ful·gu·rant (ful′gŭ - rănt). Fulgurante; agudo e perfurante. Cf. fulminant. SIN fulgurating (1). [L. *fulgur*, relâmpago brilhante]

ful·gu·rat·ing (ful′gŭ - rā - ting). Fulgurante. **1.** SIN fulgurant. **2.** Relativo à fulguração.

ful·gu·ra·tion (ful - gŭ - rā′shŭn). Fulguração; destruição de tecido por meio de uma corrente elétrica de alta freqüência: a **f. direta** utiliza um eletrodo isolado com um ponto de metal, conectado ao aparelho uniterminal de alta freqüência, do qual sai uma faísca de eletricidade, que invade a área a ser tratada;

a **f. indireta** envolve a conexão direta do paciente através de um cabo de metal ao uniterminal e utiliza um eletrodo ativo para completar um ciclo a partir do paciente. [L. *fulgur*, relâmpago]

ful·mi·nant (fŭl'mi-nănt). Fulminante; que ocorre subitamente, com a rapidez de um relâmpago e com alta intensidade ou gravidade; termo aplicado a certas dores, p.ex., a dor da tabes dorsal. Cf. fulgurant. [L. *fulmino*, pp. *-atus*, lançar relâmpagos, de *fulmen*, relâmpago]

ful·mi·nat·ing (fŭl'mi-nā'ting). Fulminante; que apresenta uma evolução rápida, que se agrava rapidamente.

fu·ma·rase (fū'mă-rās). Fumarase. SIN fumarate hydratase.

fu·ma·rate hy·dra·tase (fū'mă-rāt). Fumarato hidratase; enzima que catalisa a interconversão reversível do fumarato e da água a malato, uma reação importante do ciclo do ácido tricarboxílico. A deficiência dessa enzima causa retardo mental. SIN fumarase.

fu·ma·rate re·duc·tase (NADH). Fumarato redutase. SIN succinate dehydrogenase.

fu·mar·ic ac·id (fū-mar'ik). Ácido fumárico; ácido *trans*-butanodióico; ácido dicarboxílico insaturado; é um produto intermediário do ciclo do ácido tricarboxílico.

fu·mar·ic ac·i·de·mia. Acidemia fumárica; níveis elevados de fumarato no plasma sanguíneo; é decorrente da diminuição da atividade da fumarato hidratase.

fu·mar·ic am·i·nase. Aminase fumárica. SIN aspartate ammonia-lyase.

fu·mar·ic hy·dro·gen·ase. Hidrogenase fumárica. SIN succinate dehydrogenase.

fum·ar·yl·ac·e·to·ac·e·tate (fū-mă'ril-as-ē'tō-ăs-ē-tāt). Fumarilacetoacetato; intermediário no catabolismo da fenilalanina e da tirosina; está elevado na tirosinemia IA.

f. hydrolase, f. hidrolase; enzima que catalisa a hidrólise do fumarilacetoacetato a fumarato e acetoacetato; observa-se a deficiência dessa enzima na tirosinemia IA.

fu·mi·gant (fū'mi-gănt). Fumigante; substância utilizada na fumigação.

fu·mi·gate (fū'mi-gāt). Fumigar; expor à ação de fumaça ou de vapores de qualquer tipo como um meio de desinfecção ou de erradicação. [L. *fumigo* pp. *-atus*, fumigar, de *fumus*, fumaça, + *ago*, movimentar]

fu·mi·ga·tion (fū-mi-gā'shŭn). Fumigação; ato de fumigar; uso de um fumigante.

fum·ing (fūm'ing). Fumegante; que emite um vapor visível; uma propriedade dos ácidos nítrico, sulfúrico e clorídrico concentrados e de outras substâncias. [L. *fumus*, fumaça]

func·tio lae·sa (fŭngk'shē-ō lē'să). Perda da função; quinto sinal de inflamação, acrescentado por Galeno aos quatro enunciados por Celsus (calor, rubor, tumor e dor). [L.]

func·tion (fŭngk'shŭn). Função. **1.** A ação especial ou a propriedade fisiológica de um órgão ou outra parte do corpo. **2.** Diz-se do trabalho realizado por um órgão ou outra parte do corpo. **3.** As propriedades gerais de uma substância, dependentes de sua natureza química e relação com outras substâncias, que permitem agrupá-la entre os ácidos, as bases, os álcoois, os ésteres, etc. **4.** Grupamento reativo específico em uma molécula, p.ex., um grupamento funcional, como o grupamento —OH de um álcool. **5.** Uma qualidade, um traço ou um fato que está fortemente relacionado a outro, ou por meio de uma relação de dependência, ou por um deles variar de acordo com o outro. **6.** Variável ou expressão matemática. [L. *functio*, de *fungor*, pp. *functus*, realizar]

allomeric f., f. alomérica; f. associada dos vários segmentos da medula espinal e do bulbo, que se comunicam entre si por meio da substância branca.

arousal f., f. de despertar; capacidade de um estímulo sensorial de "despertar" o córtex para a vigilância ou prontidão.

atrial transport f., f. de transporte atrial; o papel dos átrios em preencher e expandir os ventrículos por meio de sua contração pré-sistólica, sem o qual a força da contração ventricular e, conseqüentemente, o débito cardíaco podem diminuir de forma significativa.

discriminant f., f. discriminante; uma combinação específica de resultados de testes variáveis e contínuos, projetados para realizar a separação de grupos; p.ex., quando um único número representa a combinação de resultados de testes laboratoriais ponderados projetados para discriminar entre classes clínicas.

isomeric f., f. isomérica; f. individual de um segmento isolado da medula espinal.

line spread f. (LSF), f. de espalhamento de linha; medida da capacidade de um sistema para formar imagens bem definidas; em radiologia, é determinada pela medida da distribuição da densidade espacial sobre o filme de imagem de raios X de uma fenda estreita em um metal pesado, tal como o urânio; a partir dessa medida, pode-se calcular a f. de transferência de modulação.

modulation transfer f. (MTF), f. de transferência de modulação; em detectores de radionuclídeos ou sistemas radiográficos, o rendimento, em cada freqüência espacial, em reproduzir a variação (contraste) na densidade do objeto ou no sinal na imagem; a f. é uma expressão da resolução espacial e é utilizada para avaliar sistemas de imagens e seus componentes; corresponde à integral da função de espalhamento de linha; também conhecida como a função de resposta de freqüência ou a função de transmissão de contraste; é geralmente dada na forma de uma tabela de porcentagem da amplitude da resposta *versus* a freqüência em ciclos por milímetro.

func·tion·al (fŭngk'shŭn-ăl). Funcional. **1.** Relativo a uma função. **2.** Que não tem origem orgânica; que indica um distúrbio no qual não se conhece ou não se detecta uma base orgânica para explicar os sintomas. VER neurosis.

func·tion·al·ism (fŭngk'shŭn-ăl-izm). Funcionalismo; ramo da psicologia relacionado com a função de processos mentais em seres humanos e em animais, principalmente o papel da mente, do intelecto, das emoções e do comportamento na adaptação do indivíduo ao ambiente. Cf. structuralism.

func·tion cor·rec·tor. Aparelho ortodôntico removível que utiliza as forças dos músculos faciais e orais para mover os dentes e, possivelmente, modificar a relação dos arcos dentários.

fun·da·ment (fŭn'dă-ment). **1.** Fundamento, fundação. **2.** O ânus. [L. *fundamentum*, fundação, de *fundus*, fundo]

fun·dec·to·my (fŭn-dek'tō-mē). Fundectomia. SIN fundusectomy. [fundus + G. *ektomē*, excisão]

fun·dic (fŭn'dik). Fúndico; relativo a um fundo.

fun·di·form (fŭn'di-fōrm). Fundiforme; em forma de alça; que tem forma de funda. [L. *funda*, uma funda, + *forma*, forma]

fun·do·pli·ca·tion (fŭn'dō-pli-kā'shŭn). Fundoplicatura; sutura do fundo do estômago parcial ou completamente ao redor da junção gastroesofágica, para tratar refluxo gastroesofágico; pode ser realizada por meio de cirurgia torácica ou abdominal a céu aberto, porém a laparoscopia tem sido o meio mais utilizado. [fundus + L. *plico*, dobrar]

Belsey f., f. de Belsey; f. parcial (270°) realizada por meio de toracotomia. SIN Belsey Mark operation, Belsey procedure.

Collis-Belsey f., f. de Collis-Belsey. SIN Collis-Nissen f.

Collis-Nissen f., f. de Collis-Nissen; f. cirúrgica para um esôfago encurtado; o esôfago é alongado por meio de grampeamento tubular do cárdia gástrico, e a f. é, então, realizada ao redor desse neo-esôfago. SIN Collis-Belsey f., Collis-Belsey procedure.

Dor f., f. de Dor; f. parcial (180°) e anterior, popular na Europa e na América do Sul, mais freqüentemente associada a miotomia para o tratamento da acalasia.

Nissen f., f. de Nissen; f. completa (360°); pode ser feita por via torácica ou abdominal; atualmente, a laparoscopia é o meio mais freqüentemente utilizado para a realização da f. SIN Nissen operation.

Toupet f., f. de Toupet; f. parcial posterior, na qual a borda do estômago é fixada ao esôfago; modificações na f. de Toupet são habitualmente adotadas na f. laparoscópica.

fun·dus, pl. **fun·di** (fŭn'dŭs, dī) [TA] Fundo; fundo ou parte inferior de um saco ou de um órgão oco; aquela parte mais distante removida a partir da abertura ou da saída; ocasionalmente, um fundo-de-saco amplo. [L. fundo]

f. albipuncta'tus [MIM*136880], distúrbio não-progressivo do epitélio pigmentado da retina caracterizado por numerosos e isolados pontos brancos; a cegueira noturna é um dos sintomas; tem sido proposta a existência de formas autossômicas dominantes e recessivas.

f. of bladder [TA], f. da bexiga; f. formado pela parede posterior do órgão, que é um pouco convexa. SIN f. vesicae urinariae [TA], bas-fond, base of bladder, f. of urinary bladder.

f. diabet'icus, retinopatia diabética. SIN diabetic retinopathy.

f. flavimacula'tus [MIM*228980], distúrbio genético que afeta o epitélio pigmentado da retina, caracterizado por um pontilhado branco-amarelado; ocorre perda parcial da visão central; é provavelmente um distúrbio autossômico recessivo.

f. of gallbladder [TA], f. da vesícula biliar; extremidade ampla e fechada da vesícula biliar situada na margem inferior do fígado. SIN f. vesicae biliaris [TA], f. vesicae felleae*.

f. gas'tricus [TA], f. gástrico. SIN f. of stomach.

f. of internal acoustic meatus [TA], f. do meato acústico interno; extremidade lateral do meato acústico interno, cuja parede é formada pela delgada placa cribriforme do osso que separa o vestíbulo do meato acústico interno; uma crista transversa divide o f. em duas regiões; na região superior, estão localizadas a área do nervo facial e a área vestibular superior; na região inferior, estão localizados a área coclear, a área vestibular inferior e o forame singular. SIN f. meatus acustici interni [TA], f. of internal auditory meatus.

f. of internal auditory meatus, f. do meato acústico interno. SIN f. of internal acoustic meatus.

leopard f., SIN tessellated f.

f. mea'tus acus'tici inter'ni [TA], f. do meato acústico interno. SIN f. of internal acoustic meatus.

mosaic f., retina tigróide. SIN tessellated f.

f. oc'uli, f. de olho; área da parte interior do globo ocular, ao redor do pólo posterior, visível por meio do oftalmoscópio. VER eyegrounds.

pepper and salt f., f. de olho "sal e pimenta"; aparência do f. de olho ao oftalmoscópio causada por atrofia coriocapilar e proliferação pigmentar.

f. polycythe'micus, f. de olho policitêmico; veias dilatadas e ingurgitadas associadas a retina cianótica, observadas na eritremia.

f. of stomach [TA], f. gástrico; parte do estômago situada acima da incisura cardíaca. SIN f. gastricus [TA], f. ventriculi, greater cul-de-sac.
tessellated f., f. de olho tigróide; f. de olho normal no qual a coróide intensamente pigmentada dá um aspecto de áreas poligonais escuras entre os vasos coroidais, principalmente na periferia. SIN f. tigré, leopard f., leopard retina, mosaic f., tigroid f., tigroid retina.
f. tigré, f. de olho tigróide. SIN tessellated f.
tigroid f., f. de olho tigróide. SIN tessellated f.
f. tym'pani, parede jugular da orelha média. SIN jugular wall of middle ear.
f. of urinary bladder, f. da bexiga. SIN f. of bladder.
f. u'teri [TA], f. do útero. SIN f. of uterus.
f. of uterus [TA], f. do útero; extremidade superior arredondada do útero, acima das aberturas das tubas uterinas (de Falópio). SIN f. uteri [TA].
f. ventric'uli, f. gástrico. SIN f. of stomach.
f. vesi'cae bilia'ris [TA], f. da vesícula biliar. SIN f. of gallbladder.
f. vesicae felleae, f. da vesícula biliar; *termo oficial alternativo para f. of gallbladder.
f. vesi'cae urina'riae [TA], f. da bexiga. SIN f. of bladder.
fun·du·scope (fŭn'dŭs-skōp). Fundoscópio, oftalmoscópio. SIN ophthalmoscope. [L. *fundus*, fundo, + G. *skopeō*, ver]
fun·dus·co·py (fŭn-dŭs'kŏ-pē). Fundoscopia, oftalmoscopia. SIN ophthalmoscopy.
fun·du·sec·to·my (fŭn-dŭ-sek'tō-mē). Fundectomia; excisão do fundo de um órgão. SIN fundectomy. [L. *fundus*, + G. *ektomē*, excisão]
fun·gal (fŭng'găl). Fungoso. SIN fungous.
fun·gate (fŭng'gāt). Crescer de forma exuberante como um fungo ou uma proliferação esponjosa.
fun·ge·mia (fŭn-jē'mē-ă). Fungiemia; infecção fúngica disseminada por meio da corrente sanguínea.
Fun·gi (fŭn'jī). Divisão de organismos eucariotas que crescem como massas irregulares, sem raízes, caules ou folhas e são desprovidos de clorofila ou outros pigmentos capazes de fotossíntese. O organismo (talo) tem uma forma que varia de unicelular a filamentosa, apresenta estruturas somáticas ramificadas (hifas), circundadas por paredes celulares compostas por glucana e/ou quitina, e contém núcleos verdadeiros. Reproduzem-se sexuada ou assexuadamente (formação de esporos) e podem obter alimento de outros organismos vivos, como parasitas, ou de matéria orgânica morta, como saprófitas. [L. *fungus*, um cogumelo]
fun·gi (fŭn'jī). Fungos; plural de fungus.
fun·gi·cid·al (fŭn-ji-sī'dăl). Fungicida; que tem uma ação mortal sobre fungos. [fungus + L. *caedo*, matar]
fun·gi·cide (fŭn'ji-sīd). Fungicida; qualquer substância que tem uma ação destrutiva mortal sobre os fungos. SIN mycocide.
fun·gi·ci·din (fŭn-ji-sī'din). Fungicidina, nistatina. SIN nystatin.
fun·gi·form (fŭn'ji-fōrm). Fungiforme; cuja forma é semelhante à de um fungo ou cogumelo; termo aplicado a qualquer estrutura que apresenta uma parte livre, larga, freqüentemente ramificada, e uma base mais estreita. SIN fungilliform.
Fun·gi Im·per·fec·ti (fŭn'jī im-per-fek'tī). Fungos imperfeitos; filo de fungos cuja reprodução sexuada é desconhecida ou do qual uma das formas de acasalamento ainda não foi descoberta. Antigamente, a maioria dos fungos causadores de doença em seres humanos era considerada assexuada e colocada nessa classe, porém estudos revelaram que muitos não são imperfeitos e que suas formas sexuadas podem ser classificadas como ascomicetos ou basidiomicetos.
fun·gil·li·form (fŭn-jil'i-fōrm). Fungiforme. SIN fungiform. [L. mod. *fungillus*, dim. de L. *fungus*]
fun·gi·stat (fŭn'ji-stat). Fungistático; agente que tem ação fungistática.
fun·gi·stat·ic (fŭn-ji-stat'ik). Fungistático; que tem uma ação inibitória sobre o crescimento de fungos. SIN mycostatic. [fungus + G. *statos*, posição]
fun·gi·tox·ic (fŭn-ji-tok'sik). Tóxico ou de algum modo deletério para o crescimento de fungos.
fun·gi·tox·ic·i·ty (fŭn'ji-tok-sis'i-tē). Propriedade de ser tóxico para os fungos.
fun·goid (fŭng'goyd). Fungóide; que se parece com um fungo; que denota um crescimento exuberante e patológico sobre a superfície do corpo.
fun·gous (fŭng'gŭs). Fungoso; relativo a um fungo. SIN fungal.
fun·gus, pl. **fun·gi** (fŭng'gŭs, fŭn'jī). Fungo; termo genérico utilizado para abranger as diversas formas morfológicas de leveduras e de fungos. Originalmente classificados como plantas primitivas sem clorofila, os fungos estão colocados no reino Fungi, e alguns no reino Protista, junto com as algas (todas, exceto as algas verde-azuladas), os protozoários e os bolores do lodo ("slime molds"). Os fungos dividem com as bactérias a importante capacidade de degradar substâncias orgânicas complexas de quase todos os tipos (celulose) e são essenciais para a reciclagem de carbono e de outros elementos no ciclo vital. Os fungos são importantes como alimentos e para o processo fermentativo no desenvolvimento de substâncias de importância industrial e médica, que incluem o álcool, os antibióticos e outras drogas e os alimentos. Relativamente poucos fungos são patogênicos para o homem, enquanto a maioria das doenças que afetam as plantas é causada por fungos. [L. *fungus*, um cogumelo]

f. cer'ebri, hérnia cerebral ulcerada com tecido de granulação projetando-se do ferimento do couro cabeludo.
dematiaceous fungi (de-māt'ē-ā-cē-ous), fungos dematiáceos; f. escuro que produz melanina. [L. mod. *Dematium* (nome do gênero), do g. *demation*, fio delgado, de *dema*, faixa, de *deō*, ligar + sufixo *-aceous*, caracterizado por]
imperfect f., f. imperfeito; f. cuja forma de reprodução sexuada ainda não é conhecida; esses fungos geralmente se reproduzem por meio de conídios.
perfect f., f. perfeito; f. que apresenta tanto a forma de reprodução sexuada, como também a assexuada, e cujas formas de acasalamento são conhecidas.
ray f., bactéria da ordem Actinomycetales.
thrush f., *Candida albicans*. SIN *Candida albicans*.
umbilical f., massa de tecido de granulação sobre o coto do cordão umbilical em um recém-nascido.
yeast f., termo obsoleto para *Saccharomyces*.
fu·nic (few'nik). Funicular; relativo ao funículo ou cordão umbilical. SIN funicular (2).
fu·ni·cle (fū'ni-kl). Funículo. SIN cord.
fu·nic·u·lar (fū-nik'ū-lăr). Funicular. **1.** Relativo a um funículo. **2.** SIN funic.
fu·nic·u·li·tis (fū-nik'ū-lī'tis). Funiculite. **1.** Inflamação de um funículo, em particular do cordão espermático. **2.** Inflamação do cordão umbilical geralmente associada a corioamnionite. [funiculus + G. *-itis*, inflamação]
endemic f., f. endêmica. SIN filarial f.
filarial f., f. filarial; celulite do cordão espermático resultante de filaríase; ocorre endemicamente no Sri Lanka e no Egito e, provavelmente, em algum outro lugar no Oriente.
fu·nic·u·lus, pl. **fu·nic·u·li** (fū-nik'ū-lŭs, -lī) [TA]. Funículo. SIN cord. [L. dim. de *funis*, cordão]
anterior f. [TA], f. anterior; coluna anterior branca da medula espinal, um feixe ou uma coluna de substância branca situada em cada lado da fissura mediana anterior, entre esta e o sulco ântero-lateral. SIN f. anterior [TA], ventral f.*.
f. ante'rior [TA], f. anterior. SIN anterior f.
cuneate f., fascículo cuneiforme. SIN cuneate *fasciculus*.
dorsal f., f. posterior; *termo oficial alternativo para posterior f.
f. dorsa'lis, f. posterior. SIN posterior f.
f. gra'cilis, fascículo grácil. SIN gracile *fasciculus*.
lateral f. [TA], f. lateral; coluna lateral branca da medula espinal situada entre as linhas de saída e entrada das raízes nervosas anteriores e posteriores. SIN f. lateralis [TA], anterolateral column of spinal cord, lateral f. of spinal cord.
f. latera'lis [TA], f. lateral. SIN lateral f.
lateral f. of spinal cord, f. lateral da medula espinal. SIN lateral f.
funic'uli medu'llae spina'lis [TA], funículos da medula espinal; as três principais colunas brancas da medula espinal.
posterior f., f. posterior; coluna posterior branca da medula espinal, o maior feixe de fibras em forma de cunha, situado entre a coluna posterior cinzenta e o septo mediano posterior e composto, em grande parte, de fibras das raízes dorsais. SIN f. posterior [TA], dorsal f.*, f. dorsalis.
f. poste'rior [TA], f. posterior. SIN posterior f.
f. sep'arans [TA], f. separativo; crista oblíqua, situada no assoalho do quarto ventrículo do cérebro, que separa a área postrema do trígono do nervo vago.
f. solita'rius, trato solitário. SIN solitary *tract*.
f. spermat'icus [TA], f. espermático. SIN spermatic *cord*.
f. te'res, eminência medial. SIN medial *eminence*.
f. umbilica'lis, cordão umbilical. SIN umbilical *cord*.
ventral f., f. anterior; *termo oficial alternativo para anterior f.
fu·ni·form (fū'ni-fōrm). Funiforme; semelhante a um cordão. [L. *funis*, cordão, + *forma*, forma]
fu·ni·punc·ture (fū-nē-pŭnk-chŭr). Cordocentese. SIN cordocentesis. [L. *funis*, cordão, + punção]
fu·nis (fū'nis). **1.** Cordão umbilical. SIN umbilical *cord*. **2.** Estrutura semelhante a um cordão. [L. um cordão]
funisitis (fū-nē-sī-tis). Funisite; inflamação do cordão umbilical. [funis + *-itis*]
fun·nel (fŭn'el). Funil. **1.** Vaso cônico e oco com um tubo de comprimento variável estendendo-se de seu ápice e utilizado para verter líquidos de um recipiente para outro, para filtrar, etc. **2.** Em anatomia, um infundíbulo.
Büchner f., f. de Büchner; f. de porcelana que possui um disco de porcelana perfurado, sobre o qual um papel de filtro pode ser colocado.
Martegiani f., f. de Martegiani; dilatação em funil localizada no disco do nervo óptico e que indica o início do canal hialóideo. SIN Martegiani area.
pial f., f. da pia-máter; canal revestido pela pia-máter que envolve cada vaso sanguíneo que penetra no cérebro; basicamente, os funis da pia-máter são extensões perivasculares do espaço subaracnóideo.
FUO Abreviatura de fever of unknown origin (febre de origem indeterminada).
fur (fer). Pêlo, pelagem. **1.** Revestimento de pêlo fino e macio de alguns mamíferos. **2.** Camada de restos epiteliais e elementos fúngicos encontrada sobre o dorso da língua. Está relacionada mais à falta de higiene oral do que a um processo patológico subjacente. [i.m. *furre*, do Fr. ant., do Al.]
fura-2 (foo'ra). Indicador fluorescente que se liga ao cálcio; é excitado por

comprimentos de onda mais longos quando não está ligado ao cálcio do que quando permanece ligado ao cálcio; a proporção da intensidade fluorescente em dois comprimentos de onda excitatórios fornece o valor da concentração de íons de cálcio livres; pode ser introduzido em células, para monitorar alterações momento a momento na concentração intracelular de íons de cálcio livres. VER TAMBÉM aequorin.

fu·ral·ta·done (fū-ral′ta-dōn). Furaltadona; agente antibacteriano.

fu·ran (fūr′an). Furano. **1.** Composto cíclico encontrado, em geral, na forma saturada, em açúcares que apresentam uma ponte de oxigênio entre os átomos de carbono 1 e 4, ou 2 e 5, ou 3 e 7, razão pela qual são conhecidos como furanoses. **2.** Oxa-2,4-ciclopentadieno.

fu·ra·nose (fūr′a-nōs). Furanose; unidade ou molécula sacarídica que contém a estrutura cíclica denominada de furano; exemplos específicos são precedidos por prefixos que indicam a configuração, p. ex., frutofuranose, ribofuranose. [furan + -ose(1)]

fu·ra·zol·i·done (fū-ră-zol′i-dōn). Furazolidona; substância que apresenta atividade antibacteriana e parasiticida contra organismos entéricos; utilizada no tratamento da enterite e da diarréia bacterianas.

fur·cal (fer′kăl). Furcado; em forma de garfo.

fur·ca·tion (fūr-kā′shūn). Bifurcação; **1.** Uma bifurcação ou um ramo, ou uma parte semelhante a um garfo. **2.** Em histologia odontológica, a região de um dente multirradicular na qual as raízes se dividem. [L. *furca*, garfo]

fur·cu·la (fer′kū-lă). Fúrcula. **1.** As clavículas fundidas que formam o osso em forma de V (osso-da-sorte) no esqueleto das aves. **2.** No embrião, elevação em forma de U invertido que aparece na parede ventral da faringe e é formada por duas cristas lineares e pela parte caudal da eminência hipobranquial; a depressão limitada pelo U é o sulco laringotraqueal. [L. dim. de *furca*, um garfo]

fur·fur, pl. **fur·fu·res** (fer′fer, fer′fū-rēz). Escama; escama epidérmica; p.ex., caspa. [L. farelo]

fur·fu·ra·ceous (fer-fū-rā′shŭs). Furfuráceo; fareláceo ou composto de pequenas escamas; que denota uma forma de descamação. SIN pityroid. [L. *furfuraceus*, de *furfur*, farelo]

fur·fu·ral (fer′fūr-ăl). Furfural; $C_4H_3O—CHO$; líquido incolor, aromático e irritante obtido na destilação de farelo com ácido sulfúrico diluído; utilizado na fabricação de agentes medicinais.

fur·fu·rol (fer′fūr-ol). Furfurol; denominação inadequada para o furfural e álcool furfurílico.

fur·fu·ryl (fer′fū-ril). Furfurila; radical monovalente derivado do álcool furfurílico pela perda do grupamento OH.
f. alcohol, álcool furfurílico; 2-furanometanol; 2-hidroximetilfurano; solvente e agente umectante.

fur·nace (fūr′năs). Forno; aparelho semelhante a um fogão e que contém uma câmara para aquecer, derreter ou fundir algo.
dental f., f. dental; **(1)** f. utilizado para eliminar a cera do molde antes da moldagem em metal; **(2)** f. utilizado para fundir e vitrificar porcelanas dentárias.
muffle f., f. de mufla; f. elétrico aquecido por transferência direta de calor de uma mufla resistente; **(2)** f. dentário aquecido por uma mufla.

fu·ro·se·mide (fū-rō′se-mid, -mīd). Furosemida; diurético utilizado nos estados edematosos e na hipertensão. SIN frusemide.

fur·row (fer′ō). Sulco, fenda; canal. [A.S. *furh*]
digital f., s. digital. SIN digital *crease*.
genital f., s. genital; sulco localizado no tubérculo genital do embrião, que aparece no final do segundo mês.
gluteal f., fenda glútea. SIN gluteal *fold*.
mentolabial f., s. mentolabial. SIN mentolabial *sulcus*.
primitive f., s. primitivo. SIN primitive *groove*.
skin f.'s, sulcos da pele. SIN skin *sulci*, em *sulcus*.

fu·run·cle (fū′rŭng-kl). Furúnculo; infecção piogênica localizada, freqüentemente causada pelo *Staphylococcus aureus* e que se origina em um folículo piloso. SIN boil, furunculus. [L. *furunculus*, um ladrão insignificante]

ℹ **fu·run·cu·lo·sis** (fū-rŭng-kū-lō′sis). Furunculose; condição caracterizada por furúnculos, sendo freqüentemente crônica e recorrente.

fu·run·cu·lus, pl. **fu·run·cu·li** (fū-rŭng′kū-lŭs, -lī). Furúnculo. SIN furuncle. [L. um ladrão insignificante, um furúnculo, dim. de *fur*, um ladrão]

Fu·sar·i·um (fū-zā′rē-ŭm). Gênero de fungos de crescimento rápido que produzem macroconídios multisseptados com forma de foice típica e que podem ser confundidos com aqueles produzidos por alguns dermatófitos. São geralmente saprófitas, porém algumas espécies, como *F. oxysporum*, *F. solani* e *F. moniliforme*, podem produzir úlceras na córnea; algumas espécies podem causar infecção disseminada. [L. *fusus*, fuso]

fu·seau (fē-zō). Fuso; macroconídio multisseptado fusiforme ou com forma de fuso. [Fr. *spindle* do L. *fusus*]

fu·si·date so·di·um (fū′si-dāt). Fusidato de sódio; o sal de sódio do ácido fusídico; possui propriedades antibacterianas. SIN sodium fusidate.

fu·sid·ic ac·id (fū-sid′ik). Ácido fusídico; produto da fermentação do *Fusidium coccineum*, um fungo parasita da planta *Veronica*; inibe a síntese proteica e a acumulação de ppGpp. VER fusidate sodium. SIN ramycin.

fu·si·form (fū′zi-fōrm, fū′si-). Fusiforme; que tem forma de fuso; que apresenta as duas extremidades afiladas. [L. *fusus*, um fuso, + *forma*, forma]

Fu·si·for·mis (fū-si-fōr′mis). Nome genérico e obsoleto às vezes utilizado para bactérias fusiformes anaeróbias encontradas na boca humana; esses microrganismos estão intimamente relacionados com os microrganismos anaeróbios encontrados no intestino humano e que pertencem ao gênero *Fusobacterium*. [ver fusiform]

fu·si·mo·tor (fū′zē-mō′ter). Fusimotor; relativo à inervação eferente das fibras musculares intrafusais por neurônios motores gama. VER TAMBÉM neuromuscular *spindle*. [L. *fusus*, fuso, + *moveo*, mover]

fusin (fū′zin). Fusina; receptor ligado à proteína G presente em certas células humanas e considerado necessário para ocorrer a fusão do HIV com uma célula-alvo. [fuse, do L. *fundo*, pp. *fusum*, fundir, + -in]

fu·sion (fū′zhŭn). Fusão. **1.** Liquefação, como o derretimento pelo calor. **2.** Consolidação, reunião de partes; p.ex., consolidação óssea. **3.** Combinação de imagens um pouco diferentes provenientes de cada olho em uma única percepção. **4.** Junção de dois ou mais dentes adjacentes durante seu desenvolvimento por meio de uma união dentária. VER TAMBÉM concrescence. **5.** Junção de dois genes, freqüentemente genes vizinhos. **6.** Junção de dois ossos em uma unidade, impedindo, dessa forma, o movimento entre eles. **7.** Processo pelo qual duas membranas são unidas. [L. *fusio*, um derramamento, de *fundo*, pp. *fusus*, derramar]
bone block f., método de fusão de dois ossos pelo qual um bloco de enxerto ósseo é colocado entre as duas superfícies, a fim de obter uma f. e corrigir uma deformidade preexistente.
cell f., f. celular; união do conteúdo de duas células por meios artificiais, sem a destruição de ambas, resultando em um heterocário que, por algumas gerações, reproduzirá sua espécie; método importante utilizado na determinação dos *loci* dos cromossomas.
centric f., f. cêntrica, translocação robertsoniana. SIN robertsonian *translocation*.
flicker f., freqüência de centelhamento. VER critical flicker fusion *frequency*.
nuclear f., f. nuclear; formação de núcleos atômicos mais complexos a partir de núcleos menos complexos com liberação de energia, como ocorre na formação dos núcleos de hélio a partir de núcleos de hidrogênio (hydrogen f.).
spinal f., spine f., f. espinal; procedimento cirúrgico para realizar uma ancilose óssea entre duas ou mais vértebras. SIN spondylosyndesis, vertebral f.
splenogonadal f., f. esplenogonadal; formação de uma massa composta de tecido do baço e tecido do testículo ou do ovário.
vertebral f., f. vertebral. SIN spinal f.

Fu·so·bac·te·ri·um (fū′zō-bak-tēr′ē-ŭm). Gênero de bactérias (família Bacteroidaceae) composto por bacilos Gram-negativos, não-esporulados, imóveis e anaeróbios obrigatórios, cujo principal produto metabólico é o ácido butírico. Esses microrganismos são encontrados nas cavidades de seres humanos e de outros animais; algumas espécies são patogênicas. A espécie típica é F. nucleatum. [L. *fusus*, um fuso, + bactéria]
F. morti′ferum, *Sphaerophorus mortiferus*; espécie de bactéria encontrada no sistema gastrointestinal e associada a infecções abdominais em seres humanos.
F. necro′phorum, *Sphaerophorus necrophorus*; espécie raramente pleomórfica que causa várias condições necróticas em animais ou está associada a estas, tais como a difteria de bezerros, a necrose labial dos coelhos, a rinite necrótica dos porcos, o apodrecimento dos pés de bovinos, ovinos e caprinos e, ocasionalmente, lesões necróticas em humanos. SIN necrosis bacillus.
F. nuclea′tum, espécie de bactéria (provavelmente o bacilo de Plaut ou de Vincent) encontrada na boca e em infecções do trato respiratório superior, da cavidade pleural e, ocasionalmente, do trato intestinal inferior; é a causa mais comum de infecção por fusobactérias em seres humanos e é a espécie típica do gênero *Fusobacterium*.

fu·so·cel·lu·lar (fū′zō-sel′ū-lar). Fusocelular; que possui células com forma de fuso.

fu·so·spi·ro·chet·al (fū-zō-spī-rō-kē′tăl). Fusoespiroquetal; que se refere a microrganismos fusiformes associados a espiroquetas, como aqueles encontrados nas lesões da angina de Vincent.

fus·tic (fŭs′tik). Conjunto de corantes naturais derivados de certas árvores da Índia Ocidental e das Américas Central e do Sul, denominadas *Rhus cotinus* e *Chlorophora tinctoria*; utilizado como corante de tecidos. Um corante importante do conjunto é a morina, que é associada ao corante maclurina.

fus·ti·ga·tion (fŭs′ti-gā′shŭn). Fustigação; forma de massagem que consiste em bater a superfície com bastões leves. [L. *fustigo*, pp. *-atus*, bater com um bastão]

Futcher, Palmer Howard, médico américo-canadense, *1910.

FVC Abreviatura de forced vital *capacity* (capacidade vital forçada).

Fy blood group. VER Duffy blood group, em Apêndice de Grupos Sanguíneos.

G

γ 1. Gama, a terceira letra do alfabeto grego. **2.** Em química, indica o terceiro carbono em uma série, o quarto carbono em um ácido alifático ou a posição 2 removida da posição α no anel benzeno. **3.** O símbolo de 10^{-4} gauss; surface *tension* (tensão superficial); activity *coefficient* (coeficiente de atividade); micrograma. **4.** O símbolo de fóton. Quanto aos termos apresentando este prefixo, ver o termo específico.

G Abreviatura ou símbolo de gravitational *units* (unidades gravitacionais), em *unit*; gap (hiato, período no ciclo celular) (3); gauss; giga-; D-glicose, como na UDPG; guanosina, como na GDP; glicina; guanina.

G Símbolo de Newtonian *constant* of gravitation (constante newtoniana de gravitação); Gibbs free *energy* (energia livre de Gibbs); G_{act} ou $G^{\ddagger}$, Gibbs *energy* of activation (energia de ativação de Gibbs).

g Abreviatura de grama; estado gasoso.

g Unidade de aceleração baseada na aceleração produzida pela atração gravitacional da Terra, onde 1 *g* = 980,621 cm/s² (cerca de 32,1725 pés/s²) ao nível do mar e a 45° de latitude. A 30° de latitude, *g* é igual a 979,329 cm/s².

G1. Símbolo de gap_1 *period* (período G1 do ciclo celular).
G2. Símbolo de *gap* 2 (período G2 do ciclo celular).
Ga Símbolo do gálio (Ga).
⁶⁷Ga Símbolo do gálio-67 (Ga⁶⁷).
⁶⁸Ga Símbolo do gálio-68 (Ga⁶⁸).
GABA Abreviatura de γ-aminobutyric acid (ácido γ-aminobutírico).
G ac·id. Ácido G; ácido 2-naftol-6,8-dissulfônico.
G-ac·tin. Actina G. VER actin.
GAD Abreviatura de *glutamate* decarboxylase (glutamato descarboxilase).
Gaddum, John H., farmacologista inglês, 1900–1965. VER G. and Schild *test*.
gad·fly (gad′flī). Mutuca, Tabanídeos. VER *Tabanus*.
gad·o·di·am·ide (gad-ō-dī′a-mid). Gadodiamida; um análogo estrutural não-iônico do gadolínio-DPTA; utilizado como contraste paramagnético em imagens por ressonância magnética.
gad·o·le·ic ac·id (gad-ō-le′ik). Ácido gadoléico; um ácido graxo cis-insaturado proveniente do óleo de fígado de bacalhau e de outras fontes. SIN 9-eicosenoic acid.
gad·o·lin·i·um (Gd) (gad-ō-lin′e-ŭm). Gadolínio; um elemento do grupo dos lantanídeos, com n.° atômico 64 e peso atômico 157,25. As propriedades paramagnéticas desse elemento são utilizadas nos contrastes para imagens por ressonância magnética. [mineral, gadolinita, de Johan *Gadolin*, químico finlandês, 1760–1852]
gad·o·pen·te·tate (gad-ō-pen′tĕ-tāt). Gadopentetato; (NMG)2, dietilenotriaminopentaacetatogadolinato de dimeglumina (III); o sal metilglucamina do gadolínio-DPTA dianiônico, um quelato cíclico; utilizado como contraste paramagnético em imagens por ressonância magnética.
gad·o·ter·i·dol (gad-ō-ter′i-dol). Gadoteridol; GdHP-DO3A; um quelato de gadolínio (III) do ácido 10-(2-hidroxipropil)-1,4,7,10-tetraazaciclododecano-1,4,7-triacético; um análogo macrocíclico não-iônico do gadolínio-DOTA; utilizado como contraste nas imagens por ressonância magnética.
Gaenslen, Frederick J., cirurgião norte-americano, 1877–1937. VER G. *sign*.
Gaffky, Georg T.A., higienista alemão, 1850–1918. VER G. *scale*, *table*.
GAG Abreviatura de glycosaminoglycan (glicosaminoglicano).
gag. 1. Ânsia de vômito. **2.** Amordaçar, silenciar. **3.** Abre-boca; um instrumento acomodado entre os dentes para impedir que a boca se feche durante cirurgias na boca ou na garganta.
  Crowe-Davis mouth g., abre-boca de Crowe-Davis; instrumento utilizado para abrir a boca, abaixar a língua, manter as vias aéreas livres e permitir a entrada de anestésicos voláteis durante uma tonsilectomia ou outra cirurgia orofaríngea.
gage (gāj). Medidor. SIN gauge.
gain (gān). Ganho; lucro; vantagem. **1.** Lucro; vantagem. **2.** A razão entre a saída e a entrada de um sistema amplificador, geralmente expresso em decibéis em ultra-som. [I.M. *gayne*, prêmio, recompensa do Fr. ant., do alemão]
  primary g., ganho primário; vantagens financeiras, sociais ou interpessoais provenientes da conversão de estresse emocional diretamente em doenças orgânicas demonstráveis (p.ex., cegueira histérica ou paralisia). Cf. secondary g.
  secondary g., vantagens sociais ou interpessoais (p.ex., assistência, atenção, compaixão) obtidas indiretamente em virtude de doença orgânica. Cf. primary g.
  time-compensated g., g. de tempo compensado. SIN time-gain *compensation*.
  time compensation g. (TCG), g. de compensação de tempo. SIN time-gain *compensation*.
  time-varied g. (TVG), g. de tempo variado. SIN time-gain *compensation*.
Gairdner, Sir William T., médico escocês, 1824–1907. VER G. *disease*.
Gaisböck, Felix, médico alemão, 1868–1955. VER G. *syndrome*.
gait (gāt). Marcha; modo de andar.
  antalgic g., m. antálgica; uma marcha característica resultante de dor, desencadeada pelo peso do próprio corpo, na qual a fase ortostática da m. é encurtada no lado afetado.
  ataxic g., m. atáxica, m. cerebelar. SIN cerebellar g.
  calcaneal g., m. calcânea; distúrbio da m. caracterizado por um andar apoiado somente sobre os calcanhares, em consequência de paralisia dos músculos da panturrilha, e observado em casos de poliomielite e em algumas outras doenças neurológicas.
  cerebellar g., m. cerebelar; marcha de base ampla com desvio lateral, instabilidade e irregularidade nos passos; freqüentemente ocorre uma tendência a cair para um ou outro lado, para a frente ou para trás. SIN ataxic g.
  Charcot g., m. de Charcot; a m. da ataxia hereditária.
  circumduction g., m. hemiplégica. SIN hemiplegic g.
  equine g., m. eqüina. SIN high-steppage g.
  festinating g., m. festinante, festinação m. na qual o tronco é fletido, ocorre a flexão dos joelhos e do quadril, porém de forma rígida, enquanto os passos são curtos e progressivamente mais rápidos; é caracteristicamente observada no parkinsonismo [ver parkinsonism (1)] e em outras doenças neurológicas. SIN festination.
  gluteus maximus g., m. do glúteo máximo; propulsão compensatória para trás do tronco para manter o centro de gravidade sobre o membro inferior de apoio.
  gluteus medius g., m. do glúteo médio; inclinação compensatória do corpo (ou arremesso do tronco) para o lado do glúteo, que se mostra enfraquecido, para colocar o centro de gravidade sobre o membro inferior de apoio.
  helicopod g., m. helicópode; m. observada em algumas reações de conversão ou em distúrbios histéricos, nos quais os pés descrevem semicírculos. SIN helicopodia.
  hemiplegic g., m. hemiplégica; m. na qual a perna permanece rígida, sem ocorrer flexão do joelho e do tornozelo, e, a cada passo, a perna sofre uma rotação para longe do corpo, voltando, em seguida, na direção deste e descrevendo, dessa forma, um semicírculo. SIN circumduction g., spastic g.
  high-steppage g., m. de passos altos, m. eqüina; uma m. na qual o pé, mais especificamente um pé caído, é erguido além do necessário, a fim de evitar que o pé fique preso no solo e é, em seguida, abaixado subitamente de forma adejante; é freqüentemente observada na paralisia do nervo fibular (isto é, no pé caído) e na tabes. SIN equine g.
  hysterical g., m. histérica; um tipo de marcha bizarra observado na reação de conversão histérica; em geral, o pé é arrastado ou arremetido para a frente, em vez de ser erguido durante o andar; o pé é freqüentemente mantido em dorsiflexão e invertido.
  scissor g., m. em tesoura; m. na qual cada perna gira medialmente, bem como para a frente, durante o andar; é geralmente resultante de espasticidade bilateral dos membros inferiores, em conseqüência de paralisia cerebral.
  spastic g., m. espástica. SIN hemiplegic g.
  steppage g., m. escarvante; uma m. na qual o pé que avança é erguido mais alto do que o normal, de modo que possa passar sobre o solo sem tocá-lo, uma vez que não pode ser dorsifletido. É observada nas neuropatias que acometem o nervo fibular, bem como em outros distúrbios nos quais ocorre dificuldade na dorsiflexão do pé. VER high-steppage g. SIN steppage.
  toppling g., m. cambaleante; uma m. na qual os passos são incertos e hesitantes, e o paciente cambaleia, às vezes caindo; é provavelmente consequência de um distúrbio do equilíbrio; pode ser observada em pacientes mais velhos após um acidente vascular cerebral.
  Trendelenburg g., m. de Trendelenburg. SIN Trendelenburg *sign*.
  waddling g., m. gingante, m. anserina; m. na qual o quadril, que suporta o peso do corpo, não está estabilizado; o quadril projeta-se para fora a cada passo, enquanto o lado oposto da pelve cai, provocando movimentos alternantes e laterais do tronco; é causada por fraqueza do músculo glúteo médio e observada na distrofia muscular entre outros distúrbios. SIN waddle.
Gal Símbolo da galactose.
galact-. VER galacto-.
ga·lac·ta·cra·sia (gă-lak′tă-krā′zē-ă). Galactocrasia; composição anormal do leite materno. [galact- + G. *akrasia*, mistura ruim, de *a-* priv. + *krasis*, uma mistura]
ga·lac·ta·gogue (gă-lak′tă-gog). Galactagogo; um agente que promove a secreção e a saída de leite. [galact- + G. *agōgos*, condutor]
ga·lac·tans (gă-lak′tanz). Galactanas; polímeros da galactose encontrados na natureza, junto com galacturonanas e arabanas, nas pectinas; p.ex., ágar. SIN galactosans.

⚠ Formas Combinantes	☆ Termo oficial alternativo para a *Terminologia Anatomica*
🛈 Indica que o termo é ilustrado, ver Índice de Ilustrações	
SIN Sinônimo	[MIM] Mendelian Inheritance in Man
Cf. Comparar, confrontar	I.C. Índice de Corantes
[NA] *Nomina Anatomica*	Termo de Alta Importância
[TA] *Terminologia Anatomica*	

ga·lac·tic (ga-lak′tik). Galáctico; relativo ao leite; que provoca a saída de leite.

ga·lac·ti·dro·sis (ga-lak-ti-dro′sis). Galactidrose; sudorese formada por um líquido leitoso. [galact- + G. *hidrōs,* suor, + *-osis,* condição]

ga·lac·ti·tol (ga-lak′ti-tol). Galactitol; um álcool de açúcar derivado da galactose; o g. acumula-se na galactosemia por deficiência de transferase.

galacto-, galact-. Leite. Cf. lact-. [G. *gala*]

ga·lac·to·blast (ga-lak′tō-blast). Galactoblasto. SIN colostrum *corpuscle.* [galacto- + *blastos,* germe]

ga·lac·to·cele (ga-lak′tō-sēl). Galactocele; cisto de retenção resultante da oclusão de um ducto lactífero. SIN lactocele. [galacto- + G. *kēlē,* tumor]

ga·lac·to·gen (ga-lak′tō-jen). Galactógeno; um polissacarídeo que contém galactose em diversas formas. [galacto- + G. *-gen,* produtor]

ga·lac·to·ki·nase (ga-lak-tō-ki′nās). Galactoquinase, galactocinase; uma enzima (fosfotransferase) que, na presença de ATP, catalisa a fosforilação da D-galactose a D-galactose L-fosfato, o primeiro passo do metabolismo da D-galactose; uma das formas de galactosemia apresenta deficiência de g.

ga·lac·tom·e·ter (gal′ak-tom′e-ter). Galactômetro; uma forma de hidrômetro utilizada na determinação da densidade do leite com indicação de seu teor de gordura. SIN lactometer. [galacto- + G. *metron,* medida]

gal·ac·toph·a·gous (gal′ak-tof′ă-gŭs). Galactófago; que subsiste de leite. [galacto- + G. *phagō,* comer]

ga·lac·to·phore (ga-lak′tō-fōr). Galactóforo; SIN lactiferous *ducts,* em *duct.* [galacto- + G. *phoros,* que transporta]

ga·lac·to·pho·ri·tis (ga-lak-tō-fō-rī′tis). Galactoforite; inflamação dos ductos lactíferos. [galacto- + G. *phoros,* que transporta, + *-itis,* inflamação]

gal·ac·toph·o·rous (gal-ak-tof′ō-rŭs). Galactóforo; que conduz o leite.

ga·lac·to·poi·e·sis (ga-lak′tō-poy-ē′sis). Galactopoese; produção de leite. [galacto- + G. *poiēsis,* que forma]

ga·lac·to·poi·et·ic (ga-lak′tō-poy-et′ik). Galactopoético; relativo à galactopoese.

ga·lac·to·pyr·a·nose (ga-lak-tō-pir′ă-nōs). Galactopiranose; galactose na forma de piranose.

ga·lac·tor·rhea (ga-lak-tō-rē′ă). Galactorréia. **1.** Qualquer secreção branca proveniente do mamilo que é persistente e se assemelha ao leite. **2.** Secreção contínua de leite das mamas que ocorre no intervalo entre cada amamentação ou após o bebê ter sido desmamado. SIN incontinence of milk, lactorrhea. [galacto- + G. *rhoia,* um fluxo]

ga·lac·tos·a·mine (ga-lak-tō-sam′ēn). Galactosamina; o derivado 2-amino-2-desoxi da galactose, no qual o NH$_2$ substitui o grupamento 2-OH; o D-isômero ocorre em diversos mucopolissacarídeos, especialmente no ácido condroitinossulfúrico e na substância do grupo sanguíneo B; é em geral encontrada na forma do derivado *N*-acetil.

ga·lac·tos·am·i·no·gly·can (ga-lak′tōs-am-i-nō-glī′kan). Galactosaminoglicana. VER mucopolysaccharide.

ga·lac·to·sans (ga-lak′tō-sanz). Galactosanas. SIN galactans.

ga·lac·to·scope (ga-lak′tō-skōp). Galactoscópio. Instrumento utilizado para avaliar a riqueza e a pureza do leite pela sua translucidez de uma camada delgada. SIN lactoscope. [galacto- + G. *skopeō,* examinar]

ga·lac·tose (Gal) (ga-lak′tōs). Galactose; uma aldoexose encontrada (na forma D) como um dos constituintes da lactose, de cerebrosídeos, de gangliosídeos, de mucoproteínas, etc., na forma de combinações galactosídeo ou galactosil; um epímero da D-glicose.

ga·lac·to·se·mia (ga-lak-tō-sē′mē-ă). Galactosemia. **1** [MIM*230400]. Um erro inato do metabolismo da galactose conseqüente à deficiência congênita da enzima galactosil-1-fosfato uridililtransferase, resultando na acumulação de galactose-1-fosfato nos tecidos; caracteriza-se por deficiência nutricional, hepatoesplenomegalia com cirrose, catarata, retardamento mental, galactosúria, aminoacidúria e albuminúria que regridem ou desaparecem, caso a galactose seja removida da dieta; herança autossômica recessiva; é causada pela mutação no gene da galactose-1-fosfato uridiltransferase (GALT) no cromossoma 9p. VER TAMBÉM galactokinase *deficiency.* **2.** Um erro inato do metabolismo, com exceção da deficiência de galactosil-1-fosfato uridiltransferase (ver as subentradas adiante). SIN galactose diabetes. [galactose + G. *haima,* sangue]

epimerase deficiency g., g. por deficiência de epimerase; um erro inato do metabolismo no qual há deficiência de uridina difosfato galactose-4-epimerase; ocorre acúmulo de galactose-1-fosfato.

galactokinase deficiency g., g. por deficiência de galactoquinase; distúrbio autossômico recessivo que acumula galactose e galactitol.

transferase deficiency g., g. por deficiência de transferase; um distúrbio autossômico recessivo no qual há uma deficiência de galactose-1-fosfato uridililtransferase (ver a entrada principal para g.).

ga·lac·tose-1-phos·phate. Galactose-1-fosfato; um derivado fosforilado da galactose; a substância-chave do metabolismo da galactose; acumula-se no organismo em certos tipos de galactosemia.

g.-1-p. uridylyltransferase, g.-1-p. uridililtransferase; uma enzima que catalisa a reação da UTP e da α-D-g.-1-p. para formar a UDP galactose e pirofosfato, o segundo e mais importante passo do metabolismo da D-galactose; a deficiência dessa enzima causa um acúmulo de galactose, de g.-1-p. e de galactitol.

ga·lac·tose-6-sul·fa·tase. Galactose-6-sulfatase; uma enzima que elimina o enxofre dos resíduos galactose-6-sulfato de certos mucopolissacarídeos, produzindo resíduos 3,6-anidrogalactose; está ausente na síndrome de Morquio de tipo A. SIN galactose-6-sulfurase.

ga·lac·tose-6-sul·fu·rase. Galactose-6-sulfurase. SIN galactose-6-sulfatase.

α-D-ga·lac·to·sid·ase (ga-lak-tō-sīd′ās). α-D-galactosidase; uma enzima que catalisa a hidrólise de α-D-galactosídeo para liberar D-galactose livre. A deficiência da α-D-galactosidase de tipo A está associada à doença de Fabry. SIN melibiase.

β-ga·lac·to·sid·ase (ga-lak′tō-si′dās). β-galactosidase; uma enzima que hidrolisa a ligação beta-galactosídea da lactose, produzindo glicose e galactose; a enzima também hidrolisa o substrato cromogênico, o isopropiltiogalactosídeo (IPTG), sendo, por isso, utilizada como um indicador de genes fundidos e da expressão gênica.

β-D-ga·lac·to·sid·ase. β-D-galactosidase; uma enzima que cinde as moléculas de açúcares; catalisa a hidrólise da lactose em D-glicose e D-galactose e a hidrólise de outros β-D-galactosídeos; a enzima também catalisa reações da galactotransferase; a deficiência de β-D-galactosidase acarreta problemas na digestão intestinal da lactose; é utilizada na produção de laticínios para adultos que não possuem a enzima intestinal; um defeito em uma das isoenzimas de β-D-galactosidase está associado à síndrome de Morquio de tipo B. Cf. lactase *persistence,* lactase *restriction.* SIN lactase.

ga·lac·to·side (ga-lak′tō-sīd). Galactosídeo; um composto no qual o H do grupamento OH do carbono-1 da galactose é substituído por um radical orgânico.

ga·lac·to·sis (gal-ak-tō′sis). Galactose; formação de leite pelas glândulas lácteas. [galacto- + G. *-osis,* condição]

ga·lac·tos·u·ria (ga-lak-tō-soo′rē-ă). Galactosúria; a excreção de galactose na urina. [galacto- + G. *ouron,* urina]

ga·lac·to·syl (ga-lak′tō-sil). Galactosil; a parte galactose de um galactosídeo.

β-ga·lac·to·syl·cer·am·i·dase. β-galactosilceramidase; uma enzima que participa do catabolismo de certas ceramidas; a deficiência de β-galactosilceramidase está associada à doença de Krabbe.

ga·lac·to·syl·cer·a·mide (ga-lak′tō-sil-ser′ă-mīd). Galactosilceramida; um esfingolipídio que se acumula no organismo de indivíduos com a doença de Krabbe.

ga·lac·to·ther·a·py (ga-lak′tō-thār′ă-pē). Galactoterapia; tratamento de doenças por meio de uma dieta láctea, exclusiva ou quase exclusiva. SIN lactotherapy.

ga·lac·tur·o·nan (ga-lak′toor-ō-nan). Galacturonana; um polissacarídeo que, ao sofrer hidrólise, produz o ácido galacturônico; um dos constituintes de algumas pectinas.

D-ga·lac·tu·ron·ic ac·id (ga-lak-toor-on′ik). Ácido D-galacturônico; o isômero D é um produto da oxidação da D-galactose, na qual o grupo 6-CH$_2$OH se transforma em um grupamento −COOH; é encontrado em muitos produtos naturais (p.ex., pectinas) e nas paredes das células. SIN pectic acid.

ga·lan·gal, ga·lan·ga (ga-lan′gal, -ga). Galanga; o rizoma da *Alpinia officinarum* (família Zingiberaceae); um estimulante e carminativo aromático. SIN Chinese ginger. [L. mediev. *galanga,* gengibre brando, do chinês]

Galant, Nikolay Fedorovich, higienista russo, *1893. VER G. *reflex.*

ga·lan·tha·mine (ga-lan′thă-mēn). Galantamina; um alcalóide derivado do *Galanthus woronowii* (família Amaryllidaceae), uma flor branca do início da primavera; do *Narcissus* spp. Um alcalóide com propriedades anticolinesterásicas; seu uso é apreciado na Europa Oriental.

ga·lea (ga′lē-ă). **1.** [NA]. Uma estrutura cuja forma se assemelha a um capacete, um elmo. **2.** Aponeurose epicraniana. SIN epicranial *aponeurosis.* **3.** Uma forma de curativo que cobre a cabeça. **4.** Coifa. SIN caul (1). [L. um elmo, um capacete]

g. aponeurot′ica [TA], g. aponeurótica. SIN epicranial *aponeurosis.*

Galeati, Domenico, médico italiano, 1686–1775. VER G. *glands,* em *gland.*

ga·le·at·o·my (ga-lē-at′ō-mē). Galeatomia; incisão da gálea aponeurótica. [galea + G. *tomē,* incisão]

Galeazzi, Riccardo, cirurgião italiano, 1886–1952. VER G. *fracture.*

Galen (Galenius, Galenos), Galeno, Claudius Galeno; médico grego e cientista médico em Roma, 130–201 d.C. VER G. *anastomosis, nerve; veins* of G., em *vein; great vein* of G.

ga·le·na (ga-lē′nă). Galena, galenita. SIN lead sulfide. [L.]

ga·len·ic (ga-len′ik). Galênico; relativo a Galeno ou a suas teorias.

ga·len·i·cals (ga-len′i-kălz). Galênicos, preparações farmacêuticas. **1.** As ervas e outras substâncias de origem vegetal; esse termo distingue-as dos medicamentos de origem mineral ou química. **2.** As drogas não processadas e as tinturas, os decoctos e outras preparações feitas a partir delas; esse termo distingue-os dos alcalóides e de outros princípios ativos. **3.** Medicamentos preparados de acordo com uma fórmula oficial. [Claudius *Galen*]

gall (gawl). Bile, bílis. **1.** SIN bile. **2.** Uma escoriação ou erosão. **3.** SIN nutgall. [A.S. *gealla*]

gal·la (gal′ă). Noz-de-galha, galha de carvalho. SIN nutgall. [L.]
gal·la·mine tri·eth·i·o·dide (gal′ă - men trī - eth - ī′o - dīd). Trietiliodeto de galamina; um composto de amônio quaternário triplo com ação comparável àquela da curarina.
Gallavardin, Louis, médico francês, 1875–1957. VER G. *phenomenon*.
gall·blad·der (gawl′blad-er) [TA]. Vesícula biliar; um receptáculo piriforme localizado na superfície inferior do fígado, em uma depressão entre o lobo direito e o lobo quadrado; serve como um reservatório para a armazenagem de bile. SIN vesica biliaris [TA], vesica fellea*, bile cyst, cholecyst, cholecystis, cystis fellea, gall bladder, vesicula fellis.
  Courvoisier g., vesícula biliar de Courvoisier; vesícula biliar aumentada, freqüentemente palpável, encontrada em pacientes com carcinoma da cabeça do pâncreas. Está associada à icterícia resultante da obstrução do ducto biliar comum (colédoco). VER Courvoisier *law*.
  porcelain g., v.b. de porcelana; calcificação intramural da v.b. comumente associada ao câncer da v.b.
  sandpaper g., v.b. em lixa; uma condição na qual a mucosa da v.b. se torna áspera; está geralmente associada a cálculos biliares.
  strawberry g., v.b. em morango; uma v.b. cuja mucosa se apresenta mosqueada, com depósitos amarelados de colesterol que contrastam com o fundo vermelho hiperêmico.

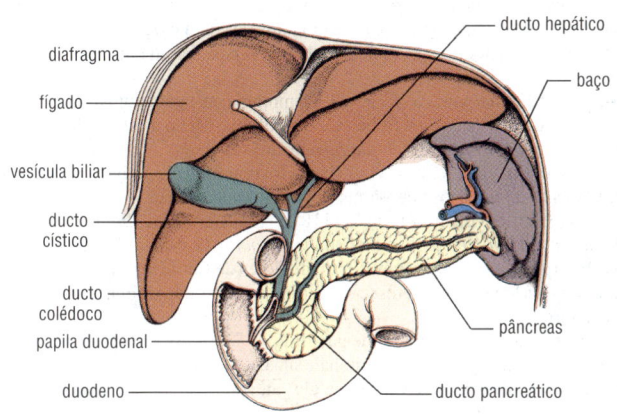

vesícula biliar, fígado e sistema biliar

Gallego dif·fer·en·ti·at·ing so·lu·tion. Solução diferenciadora de Gallego. VER solution.
gal·le·in (gal′e - in). Galeína; substância estruturalmente relacionada à fluoresceína e utilizada como indicador de tintura de anilina; torna-se rosa-avermelhado em pH > 6,6 e castanho-amarelada em pH < 4. SIN pyrogallolphthalein.
gal·lic ac·id (gal′ik). Ácido gálico; geralmente elaborado a partir de ácido tânico ou nozes-de-galha; utilizado localmente como adstringente para os mesmos propósitos que o ácido tânico.
Gallie, William E., cirurgião canadense, 1882–1959. VER G. *transplant*.
Gal·li·for·mes (gal - i - for′mez). Galiformes; uma ordem de aves que engloba o faisão, o peru e a galinha. [L. *gallus*, um galo, + *forma*, forma]
gal·li·na·ceous (gal - i - nā′shŭs). Galináceo; relativo à ordem Galliformes. [L. *gallinaceus*, de *gallina*, uma galinha]
gal·li·um (Ga) (gal′ē - ŭm). Gálio (Ga); um metal raro, com n.º atômico 31 e peso atômico 69,723. [L. *Gallia*, França]
gal·li·um-67 (^{67}Ga). Gálio-67 (Ga^{67}); um radionuclídeo produzido por cíclotron, com uma meia-vida de 3,260 dias e principais emissões de raios gama de 93, 185 e 300 keV; utilizado na forma de citrato como um radiorrastreador que localiza tumores e áreas de inflamação.
gal·li·um-68 (^{68}Ga). Gálio-68 (Ga^{68}); um emissor de positrons, com uma meia-vida radioativa de 1,130 h.
gal·lo·cy·a·nin, gal·lo·cy·a·nine (gal - o - sī′ă - nin, ă - nēn) [C.I. 51030]. Galocianina; um corante fenoxazina azul utilizado como corante de ácidos nucleicos após fervura com alúmen de cromo e empregado na determinação citofotométrica quantitativa dessas frações.
gal·lon (gal′ŭn). Galão; uma medida norte-americana de capacidade líquida que contém 4 quartos, 231 polegadas cúbicas ou 8,3293 libras de água destilada a 20°C; equivale a 3,785412 L. O galão imperial britânico contém 277,4194 polegadas cúbicas. [Fr. ant. *galon*]
gal·lop (gal′op). Galope; ritmo de galope; uma cadência tripla dos sons cardíacos; resultante da adição de uma terceira ou quarta bulha cardíaca anormal (B3, B4) às B1 e B2; é em geral indicativo de doença grave. SIN bruit de galop, cantering rhythm, gallop rhythm, Traube bruit.
  atrial g., g. atrial. SIN presystolic g.
  presystolic g., g. pré-sistólico; cadência na qual o som de galope no final da diástole é uma quarta bulha cardíaca audível devido ao enchimento ventricular vigoroso após a sístole atrial. SIN atrial g.
  protodiastolic g., g. protodiastólico; ritmo de g. no qual o som de galope ocorre no início da diástole, e trata-se de uma terceira bulha cardíaca anormal. **S$_7$ g.,** galope de somação. SIN summation g.
  summation g., g. de somação; ritmo de g. no qual o som de galope se deve à superposição de B3 e B4; é às vezes auscultado em pessoas normais com taquicardia, porém em geral é indicativo de doença do miocárdio. SIN S$_7$ g., S$_7$.
  systolic g., g. sistólico; termo obsoleto para uma cadência tripla das bulhas cardíacas na qual um batimento extra ocorre durante a sístole, em geral na forma de um "clique" sistólico.
gall·stone (gawl′stōn). Cálculo biliar; uma concreção no interior da vesícula biliar ou de um ducto biliar, composta principalmente de uma mistura de colesterol, bilirrubinato de cálcio e carbonato de cálcio e, ocasionalmente, como um cálculo puro composto apenas de uma dessas substâncias. SIN biliary calculus, cholelith.
  opacifying g.'s, cálculos biliares opacificantes; cálculos biliares que se tornam opacos nas radiografias após exposição prolongada a contrastes colecistográficos.
  silent g.'s, cálculos biliares silenciosos; cálculos biliares que não causam sintomas e são descobertos por meio de exames radiográficos ou ultra-sonográficos no momento de uma cirurgia ou necropsia.
Gal·lus (gal′ŭs). Um gênero de aves galináceas que engloba a *G. domestica*, a galinha doméstica. [L. *gallus*, um galo]
GALT Abreviatura de gut-associated lymphoid *tissue* (tecido linfóide associado ao intestino).
Galton, Sir Francis, cientista inglês, 1822–1911. VER G. *delta*, system of classification of *fingerprints*, em *fingerprint*, *law*, *whistle*.
gal·to·ni·an (gahl - tō′nē - ăn). Galtoniano; atribuído a ou descrito por Sir Francis Galton.
Gal·va·ni, Luigi, médico e anatomista italiano, 1737–1798. VER galvanism.
gal·van·ic (gal-van′ik). Galvânico; relativo ao galvanismo. SIN voltaic.
gal·va·nism (gal′vă - nizm). Galvanismo. **1.** Eletricidade por corrente contínua produzida por ação química, p.ex., por uma bateria. **2.** Manifestações orais da eletricidade por corrente contínua que ocorre quando restaurações dentárias com potenciais elétricos diferentes, tais como a prata e o ouro, são colocadas na boca; caracterizado por dor ou desenvolvimento de pequenas áreas de leucoplasia. SIN voltaism.
gal·va·ni·za·tion (gal′vă - ni - zā′shŭn). Galvanização; aplicação de eletricidade por corrente contínua (galvânica), como na galvanoplastia (eletrogalvanização).
galvano-. Prefixo que indica corrente elétrica, basicamente a corrente contínua. [ver galvanism]
gal·va·no·cau·tery (gal′vă - nō - kaw′ter - ē). Galvanocautério; um tipo de eletrocautério que utiliza um fio aquecido por uma corrente galvânica.
gal·va·no·con·trac·til·i·ty (gal′vă - nō - kon - trak - til′i - tē). Galvanocontratilidade. A capacidade de um músculo de se contrair sob o estímulo de uma corrente (contínua) galvânica.
gal·va·no·far·a·di·za·tion (gal′vă - nō - far′ă - di - sā′shŭn). Galvanofaradização. Aplicação simultânea de uma corrente galvânica e uma corrente farádica.
gal·va·nom·e·ter (gal′vă - nom′e - ter). Galvanômetro; um instrumento para medir a intensidade de uma corrente elétrica.
  d'Arsonval g., galvanômetro de d'Arsonval; um galvanômetro sensível que consiste em uma bobina móvel suspensa em um campo magnético permanente entre fios ou tiras metálicas delicadas que servem como molas de torção e condutores; um espelho colocado sobre a bobina desvia (deflexão) um feixe de luz ao longo da escala.
  Einthoven string g., g. de corda de Einthoven; o instrumento original utilizado por Einthoven para desenvolver o primeiro eletrocardiograma.
gal·va·no·mus·cu·lar (gal′vă - nō - mŭs′kū - lar). Galvanomuscular; que indica o efeito da aplicação de uma corrente (contínua) galvânica em um músculo.
gal·va·no·pal·pa·tion (gal′vă - nō - pal - pā′shŭn). Galvanopalpação. Estesiometria realizada por meio de um eletrodo pontiagudo através do qual uma corrente contínua fraca passa para o catodo aplicado sobre uma parte indiferente.
gal·va·no·scope (gal′vă - nō - skōp). Galvanoscópio. Um instrumento utilizado para detectar a presença de uma corrente galvânica. [galvano- + G. *skopeō*, ver]
gal·va·no·sur·gery (gal′vă - nō - ser′jer - ē). Galvanocirurgia; uma cirurgia na qual uma corrente elétrica contínua é utilizada.
gal·va·no·tax·is (gal′vă - nō - tak′sis). Galvanotaxia. SIN electrotaxis.
gal·va·no·ther·a·py (gal′van - ō - thār′ă - pē). Galvanoterapia. Tratamento de doenças por meio da aplicação de corrente (galvânica) contínua.

gal·va·not·o·nus (gal-vă-not'ō-nŭs). Galvanotônus. **1.** SIN electrotonus. **2.** Contração muscular tônica em resposta a um estímulo galvânico. [galvano- + G. *tonos*, tensão]

gal·va·not·ro·pism (gal-vă-not'rō-pizm). Galvanotropismo. SIN electrotaxis. [galvano- + G. *tropē*, uma volta]

gam·a·bu·fa·gin (gam-ă-boo'fă-jin). Gamabufagina. SIN gamabufotalin.

gam·a·bu·fo·gen·in (gam-ă-boo'fō-jen-in). Gamabufogenina. SIN gamabufotalin.

gam·a·bu·fo·tal·in (gam-ă-boo'fō-tal-in). Gamabufotalina; uma triidroxibufadienolida, presente no veneno de sapos (família Bufonidae), que se assemelha química e farmacologicamente aos digitálicos. SIN gamabufagin, gamabufogenin.

gam·bir (gam'bēr). Gambir; um extrato (goma-resina) proveniente das folhas da *Uncaria* (*Ourouparia*) *gambier* (família Rubiaceae); um adstringente. O g. comercial é conhecido como terra japônica.

game (gām). Jogo; uma competição, física ou mental, conduzida de acordo com um conjunto de regras e disputada por entretenimento ou em troca de um prêmio. [I.M. do I. ant. *gamen*]

language g., jogo de linguagem; em filosofia, todas as operações e todos os comportamentos contidos em símbolos (e expressos por eles), regras de linguagem e costumes sociais que dizem respeito ao uso da linguagem.

model g., jogo de modelo; o uso de jogos, principalmente de jogos de estratégia, como meio para explicar o comportamento humano (tanto o normal como o anormal).

ga·me·tan·gi·um (gam'ē-tan'jē-ŭm). Gametângio; uma estrutura onde os gametas são produzidos.

gam·ete (gam'ēt). Gameta. **1.** Uma de duas células haplóides que podem sofrer cariogamia. **2.** Qualquer célula germinativa, seja um óvulo, seja um espermatozóide. [G. *gametēs*, marido; *gametē*, mulher]

joint g., g. articular; o conjunto haplóide de genes (não-alélicos) herdados em uma única célula germinativa.

♲**gameto-.** Um gameta. [G. *gametēs*, marido, *gametē*, mulher, de *gameō*, casar]

ga·me·to·cide (gă-mē'tō-sīd). Gametocida. Um agente que destrói gametas, especialmente os gametócitos da malária. [gameto- + L. *caedo*, matar]

ga·me·to·cyst (ga-mē'tō-sist). Gametocisto. Um cisto formado ao redor de um par de gametócitos de gregarinos unidos no qual os gametas são produzidos. [gameto- + G. *kystis*, bexiga]

ga·me·to·cyte (gă-mē'tō-sīt). Gametócito. Uma célula capaz de dividir-se a fim de produzir gametas, p.ex., um espermatócito ou um oócito. SIN gamont. [gameto- + G. *kytos*, célula]

ga·me·to·gen·e·sis (gam'ē-tō-jen'ē-sis). Gametogênese. O processo de formação e desenvolvimento de gametas. [gameto- + G. *genesis*, produção]

ga·me·to·go·nia (gam'ē-tō-gō'nē-ă). Gametogonia. SIN gametogony.

gam·e·tog·o·ny (gam-ē-tog'ō-nē). Gametogonia. Uma fase do ciclo sexual de esporozoários na qual os gametas são formados, freqüentemente por esquizogonia. SIN gametogonia, gamogony. [gameto- + G. *gonē*, produção]

gam·e·toid (gam'ē-toyd). Gametóide; relativo a certas características biológicas que se assemelham às características dos gametas ou das células reprodutivas.

ga·me·to·ki·net·ic (gam'ē-tō-ki-net'ik). Gametocinético; que estimula ou causa cariogamia ou conjugação verdadeira. [gameto- + G. *kinēsis*, movimento]

gam·e·to·pha·gia (gam'ē-tō-fā'jē-ă). Gametofagia. O desaparecimento do elemento masculino ou feminino na zigose. SIN gamophagia. [gameto- + G. *phagō*, comer]

Gamgee, Joseph Sampson, cirurgião inglês, 1828–1886. VER Gamgee *tissue*.

gam·ic (gam'ik). Gâmico; relativo à, ou derivado da, união sexual; utilizado em geral como um sufixo. [G. *gamikos*, relativo ao casamento]

gam·ma (gam'ă). Gama. **1.** γ, a terceira letra do alfabeto grego. **2.** Unidade da intensidade do campo magnético que corresponde a 10^{-9} T. [G.]

gam·ma ben·zene hex·a·chlo·ride (GBH). Hexacloreto de gamabenzeno. Um dos isômeros purificados do hexaclorobenzeno utilizado como escabicida e pediculicida e aplicado topicamente na pele na forma de loções, cremes e xampus; pode ser absorvido pela pele. Suas ações são semelhantes às do DDT, mas é menos persistente. SIN hexachlorocyclohexane.

gam·ma·cism (gam'ă-sizm). Gamacismo. Má pronúncia do som da letra "g" ou dificuldade para articular esse som. [G. *gamma*, equivalente da letra g]

gam·ma·gram (gam'ă-gram). Gamagrama; termo antigo para cintigrama.

Gam·ma·her·pes·vir·i·nae (gam'ă-her'pez-vir'ī-nē). Uma subfamília de Herpesviridae que engloba o vírus Epstein-Barr e outros vírus que causam linfoproliferação.

gam·mop·a·thy (gă-mop'ă-thē). Gamopatia; um distúrbio primário da síntese de imunoglobulinas.

benign monoclonal g., g. monoclonal benigna. SIN monoclonal g. of undetermined significance.

biclonal g., uma g. na qual o soro apresenta duas imunoglobulinas monoclonais diferentes.

monoclonal g., g. monoclonal; qualquer um de um grupo de distúrbios resultantes da proliferação de um único clone de células linfóides ou plasmócitos e caracterizados pela presença de uma imunoglobulina monoclonal no soro ou na urina (visível na eletroforese como um único pico).

monoclonal g. of undetermined significance, g. monoclonal de importância indeterminada; uma paraproteinemia (uma gamaglobulina anormal, tipicamente com um componente de cadeia leve λ) de menos de 3 g/100 mL que, no momento de sua descoberta, não tem causa aparente; especificamente, não há evidências de mieloma múltiplo ou de outro distúrbio maligno. SIN benign monoclonal g.

monoclonal g. of unknown significance (MGUS), g. monoclonal de importância desconhecida; uma g. diagnosticada por eletroforese do soro de pessoas idosas assintomáticas que não apresentam outras evidências de neoplasia de plasmócitos; em 20% dos casos, evolui para um processo maligno plasmocitário.

polyclonal g., g. policlonal; uma g. na qual há um aumento heterogêneo das imunoglobulinas que envolve mais de uma linhagem de células; pode ser causada por qualquer uma de várias doenças inflamatórias, infecciosas ou neoplásicas.

Gamna, Carlos, médico italiano, 1896–1950. VER G. *disease*; G.-Favre *bodies*, em *body*; Gandy-G. *bodies*, em *body*; G.-Gandy *bodies*, em *body*, *nodules*, em *nodule*.

gam·o·gen·e·sis (gam-ō-jen'ē-sis). Gamogênese. SIN sexual reproduction. [G. *gamos*, casamento, + *genesis*, produção]

gam·og·o·ny (gam-og'ō-nē). Gamogonia. SIN gametogony.

gam·ont. Gametócito. SIN gametocyte. [G. *gamos*, casamento, + *ōn* (*ont-*), ser]

gam·o·pha·gia (gam-ō-fā'jē-ă). Gamofagia. SIN gametophagia.

gam·o·pho·bia (gam-ō-fō'bē-ă). Gamofobia. Medo mórbido de casamento. [G. *gamos*, casamento, + *phobos*, medo]

gan·ci·clo·vir (gan-sī'klō-vir). Ganciclovir; um agente antiviral utilizado no tratamento de infecções oportunistas por citomegalovírus.

Gandy, Charles, médico francês, *1872. VER Gamna-G. *bodies*, em *body*, *nodules*, em *nodule*; G.-Gamna *bodies*, em *body*; G.-Nanta *disease*.

gan·ga (gang'gă). Ganga; um extrato de flores de *Cannabis sativa* (cânhamo-indiano ou haxixe) que cresce na Índia, no Irã e na Arábia. VER TAMBÉM cannabis.

gan·glia (gang'glē-ă). Plural de ganglion.

gan·gli·al (gang'glē-ăl). Ganglionar. SIN ganglionic.

gan·gli·ate, gan·gli·at·ed (gang'glē-āt, gang'glē-ā-ted). Ganglionado; que possui gânglios. SIN ganglionated.

gan·gli·form (gang'glē-form). Gangliforme; que possui a forma ou a aparência de um gânglio. SIN ganglioform.

gan·gli·i·tis (gang-glē-ī'tis). Ganglionite. SIN ganglionitis.

gan·gli·o·blast (gang'glē-ō-blast). Ganglioblasto; uma célula embrionária a partir da qual se desenvolvem as células ganglionares. [ganglion + G. *blastos*, germe]

gan·gli·o·cyte (gang'glē-ō-sīt). Gangliócito. SIN ganglion cell.

gan·gli·o·cy·to·ma (gang'glē-ō-si-tō'mă). Gangliocitoma. Uma lesão rara formada de células neuronais (ganglionares) em um estroma glial esparso. SIN central ganglioneuroma. [ganglion + G. *kytos*, célula, + -*oma*, tumor]

gan·gli·o·form (gang'glē-ō-form). Gangliforme. SIN gangliform.

gan·gli·o·gli·o·ma (gang'glē-ō-glē-ō'mă). Glanglioglioma; um tumor raro composto por um glioma e por células neuronais (ganglionares) atípicas; em pacientes jovens, está freqüentemente associado a crises epilépticas.

gan·gli·ol·y·sis (gang-glē-ol'i-sis). Gangliólise. A dissolução ou ruptura de um gânglio.

percutaneous radiofrequency g., g. por radiofreqüência percutânea; g. produzida por correntes de radiofreqüência aplicadas a um gânglio por uma agulha que atravessa a pele.

gan·gli·o·ma (gang-glē-ō'mă). Glanglioma. SIN ganglioneuroma.

GANGLION

gan·gli·on, pl. **gan·glia, gan·gli·ons** (gang'glē-on, -glē-ă, -glē-onz). **1.** [TA]. Gânglio; originalmente, qualquer grupo de corpos de células nervosas situado no sistema nervoso central ou periférico; atualmente, um agregado de corpos de células nervosas localizado no sistema nervoso periférico. SIN nerve g., neural g., neuroganglion. **2.** Cisto sinovial; um cisto que contém líquido rico em mucopolissacarídeos dentro de tecido fibroso ou, ocasionalmente, de músculo, de osso ou de uma cartilagem semilunar; está em geral fixado a uma bainha de tendão na mão, no punho ou no pé, ou fixado à articulação subjacente. SIN myxoid cyst, peritendinitis serosa, synovial cyst. [G. uma intumescência ou um nódulo]

aberrant g., g. aberrante; um conjunto de células nervosas às vezes encontra-se sobre uma raiz nervosa espinal posterior, entre o g. espinal e a medula espinal.

acousticofacial g., g. acusticofacial; uma massa de células ganglionares primordiais, encontrada em embriões jovens, que posteriormente se diferencia no g. acústico ou espiral do nervo vestibulococlear (oitavo nervo craniano) e no g. geniculado do nervo facial (sétimo nervo craniano).

Acrel g., g. de Acrel. (1) Pseudogânglio localizado no nervo interósseo posterior situado na face dorsal da articulação do punho. (2) Um cisto encontrado em um tendão de um músculo extensor na região do punho.

Andersch g., g. de Andersch. SIN inferior g. of glossopharyngeal nerve.

aorticorenal ganglia [TA], gânglios aorticorrenais; uma parte parcialmente destacada dos gânglios celíacos, na origem de cada artéria renal; contêm os neurônios simpáticos pós-sinápticos que inervam os vasos do rim. SIN ganglia aorticorenalia [TA].

gang'lia aorticorena'lia [TA], gânglios aorticorrenais. SIN aorticorenal ganglia.

Arnold g., g. de Arnold; g. ótico. SIN otic g.

auditory g., g. auditivo; g. coclear. SIN cochlear g.

Auerbach ganglia, gânglios de Auerbach; grupos de células nervosas parassimpáticas pós-sinápticas localizados no plexo mioentérico. VER myenteric (nervous) plexus.

auricular g., g. auricular; g. ótico. SIN otic g.

autonomic ganglia, gânglios autônomos; gânglios viscerais. VER autonomic division of nervous system.

ganglia of autonomic plexuses, gânglios dos plexos autônomos; gânglios autônomos que estão situados nos plexos de fibras autônomas, p.ex., os gânglios celíacos e mesentérico inferior do simpático e os pequenos gânglios parassimpáticos do plexo mioentérico. SIN ganglia plexuum autonomicorum [TA].

basal ganglia, gânglios basais; originalmente, todas as grandes massas de substância cinzenta localizadas na base do hemisfério cerebral; atualmente, o corpo estriado (núcleos caudado e lentiforme) e os grupos de células funcionalmente associados ao corpo estriado, tais como o núcleo subtalâmico e a substância negra. VER TAMBÉM basal nuclei, em nucleus.

Bezold g., g. de Bezold; um agregado de células nervosas localizado no septo interatrial.

Bochdalek g., g. de Bochdalek; um g. do plexo do nervo dentário que está situado na maxila, acima da raiz do dente canino.

Bock g., g. de Bock. SIN carotid g.

Böttcher g., g. de Böttcher; g. situado sobre o nervo coclear no meato acústico interno.

cardiac ganglia [TA], gânglios cardíacos; gânglios parassimpáticos do plexo cardíaco que estão situados entre o arco da aorta e a bifurcação da artéria pulmonar e da extensão do plexo sobre os átrios e o sulco atrioventricular. Esses gânglios são comumente adjacentes ao ligamento arterial; os gânglios enviam fibras parassimpáticas pós-sinápticas para o tecido nodal e para os plexos periarteriais das artérias coronárias. SIN ganglia cardiaca [TA], Wrisberg ganglia.

gang'lia cardi'aca [TA], gânglios cardíacos. SIN cardiac ganglia.

carotid g., g. carotídeo; uma pequena intumescência ganglionar localizada nos filamentos oriundos do plexo carotídeo interno, que está situado na superfície inferior da artéria carótida no seio cavernoso. SIN Bock g., Laumonier g.

celiac ganglia [TA], gânglios celíacos; o maior e o mais alto grupo de gânglios simpáticos pré-vertebrais localizado na parte superior da aorta abdominal dos dois lados da origem da artéria celíaca; contêm neurônios simpáticos pós-sinápticos cujos axônios não-mielinizados pós-ganglionares inervam o estômago, o fígado, a vesícula biliar, o baço, o rim, o intestino delgado e os colos ascendente e transverso. SIN ganglia coeliaca [TA], solar ganglia, Vieussens ganglia, Willis centrum nervosum.

g. cervica'le infe'rius [TA], g. cervical inferior. SIN inferior cervical g.

g. cervica'le me'dium [TA], g. cervical médio. SIN middle cervical g.

g. cervica'le supe'rius [TA], g. cervical inferior. SIN superior cervical g.

cervicothoracic g. [TA], g. cervicotorácico; um g. do tronco simpático que está situado posteriormente à artéria subclávia, próximo à origem da artéria vertebral; é formado pela fusão do gânglio cervical inferior, na altura da sétima vértebra cervical, com o primeiro g. torácico. SIN g. cervicothoracicum [TA], g. stellatum*, stellate g. *.

g. cervicothoracicum [TA], g. cervicotorácico. SIN cervicothoracic g.

chain ganglia, gânglios do tronco simpático. SIN g. of sympathetic trunk.

g. cilia're [TA], g. ciliar. SIN ciliary g.

ciliary g. [TA], g. ciliar; um pequeno g. parassimpático situado na órbita entre o nervo óptico e o músculo reto lateral; recebe fibras pré-sinápticas do núcleo de Edinger-Westphal por meio do nervo oculomotor (III NC) e, por sua vez, dá origem a fibras pós-sinápticas que inervam o músculo ciliar e o esfíncter da íris (músculo esfíncter da pupila). SIN g. ciliare [TA], lenticular g., Schacher g.

coccygeal g., g. coccígeo. SIN g. impar.

cochlear g. [TA], g. coclear; um g. alongado formado por corpos de células nervosas sensoriais bipolares e localizado na parte coclear do nervo vestíbulo-coclear no interior do canal espiral do modíolo; cada célula do g. dá origem a um processo periférico, que passa entre as camadas da lâmina espiral óssea até o órgão de Corti, e a um axônio central, que penetra no metencéfalo como um componente da raiz inferior (coclear) do oitavo nervo craniano e conduz a sensação auditiva. SIN g. cochleare [TA], spiral g. of cochlea [TA], g. spirale cochleae*, auditory g., Corti g., spiral cochlear g.

g. cochleare [TA], g. coclear. SIN cochlear g.

gang'lia coeli'aca [TA], gânglios celíacos. SIN celiac ganglia.

Corti g., g. de Corti. SIN cochlear g.

gang'lia craniospinal'ia sensoria [TA], gânglios cranioespinais. SIN craniospinal sensory ganglia.

craniospinal sensory ganglia [TA], gânglios craniospinais sensoriais; um termo que designa de forma coletiva os gânglios sensoriais localizados nas raízes dorsais (posteriores) dos nervos espinais e nos nervos cranianos que contêm fibras sensoriais gerais e do paladar; são também denominados gânglios encefaloespinais. SIN ganglia craniospinalia sensoria [TA].

diffuse g., g. difuso; uma intumescência cística resultante de efusão inflamatória em uma ou várias bainhas de tendões adjacentes.

dorsal root g., g. da raiz dorsal; *termo oficial alternativo para spinal g.

Ehrenritter g., g. de Ehrenritter. SIN superior g. of glossopharyngeal nerve.

extracranial ganglia, gânglios extracranianos. SIN inferior g. of glossopharyngeal nerve.

g. extracrania'le, g. extracraniano. SIN inferior g. of glossopharyngeal nerve.

g. of facial nerve, g. do nervo facial. SIN geniculate g.

Frankenhäuser g., g. de Frankenhäuser. SIN uterovaginal (nervous) plexus.

Froriep g., g. de Froriep; um conjunto temporário de células nervosas localizado na face dorsal do nervo hipoglosso no embrião; corresponde a um g. sensitivo rudimentar.

gasserian g., g. de Gasser. SIN trigeminal g.

geniculate g. [TA], g. geniculado; um g. de fibras nervosas intermédias conduzidas pelo nervo facial localizado dentro do canal facial, no joelho do canal, contendo os neurônios sensitivos que inervam as papilas gustativas situadas nos dois terços anteriores da língua e uma pequena área localizada na orelha externa. SIN g. geniculi [TA], g. geniculatum*, g. of facial nerve, g. of intermediate nerve, g. of nervus intermedius, intumescentia ganglioformis.

g. geniculatum, g. geniculado; *termo oficial alternativo para geniculate g.

g. genic'uli [TA], g. geniculado. SIN geniculate g.

Gudden g., g. de Gudden. SIN interpeduncular nucleus.

g. haben'ulae, g. habenular. SIN habenular nuclei, em nucleus.

hypogastric ganglia, gânglios hipogástricos. SIN pelvic ganglia.

g. im'par [TA], g. ímpar; um g. único e na posição mais inferior do tronco simpático; sua presença é inconstante. SIN coccygeal g., Walther g.

inferior cervical g. [TA], g. cervical inferior; o g. em posição mais baixa dentre os três gânglios que compõem a parte cervical do tronco simpático e que está situado na altura da vértebra C7. Está comumente fundido ao primeiro gânglio torácico simpático, formando o gânglio cervicotorácico (estrelado). SIN g. cervicale inferius [TA].

inferior g. of glossopharyngeal nerve [TA], g. inferior do nervo glossofaríngeo; o g. inferior e mais importante do grupo de dois gânglios localizados no nervo glossofaríngeo, imediatamente inferior à sua saída do forame jugular. Os neurônios unipolares que compõem os gânglios conduzem impulsos do paladar e da sensação geral do terço posterior da língua e a sensação geral das fauces, do palato mole e da orofaringe. SIN g. inferius nervi glossopharyngei [TA], Andersch g., extracranial ganglia, g. extracraniale, petrosal g., petrous g.

inferior mesenteric g. [TA], g. mesentérico inferior; o mais inferior dos gânglios pré-vertebrais simpáticos, localizado proximo à aorta, no ponto de origem da artéria mesentérica inferior e que contém os neurônios pós-sinápticos simpáticos que inervam os colos descendente e sigmóide. SIN g. mesentericum inferius [TA].

inferior g. of vagus nerve [TA], g. inferior do nervo vago; um grande g. sensorial do nervo vago, situado anteriormente à veia jugular interna. SIN g. inferius nervi vagi [TA], g. of trunk of vagus, nodose g.

g. infe'rius ner'vi glossopharyn'gei [TA], g. inferior do nervo glossofaríngeo. SIN inferior g. of glossopharyngeal nerve.

g. infe'rius ner'vi va'gi [TA], g. inferior do nervo vago. SIN inferior g. of vagus nerve.

intercrural g., g. intercrural. SIN interpeduncular nucleus.

gang'lia interme'dia [TA], gânglios intermédios. SIN intermediate ganglia.

intermediate ganglia [TA], gânglios intermédios; pequenos gânglios simpáticos mais comumente encontrados nos ramos comunicantes na região cervical e lombar. SIN ganglia intermedia [TA].

g. of intermediate nerve, g. do nervo intermédio. SIN geniculate g.

interpeduncular g., g. interpeduncular. SIN interpeduncular nucleus.

intervertebral g., g. intervertebral. SIN spinal g.

intracranial g., g. intracraniano. SIN superior g. of glossopharyngeal nerve.

g. isth'mi, g. do istmo. SIN interpeduncular nucleus.

jugular g., g. jugular. (1) SIN superior g. of glossopharyngeal nerve; (2) SIN superior g. of vagus nerve.

Laumonier g., g. de Laumonier. SIN carotid g.

Lee g., g. de Lee. SIN uterovaginal (nervous) *plexus.*
lenticular g., g. lenticular; g. ciliar. SIN ciliary g.
Lobstein g., g. de Lobstein. SIN thoracic splanchnic g.
Ludwig g., g. de Ludwig; um pequeno grupo de células nervosas parassimpáticas localizado no septo interatrial.
gang'lia lumba'lia [TA], gânglios lombares; SIN lumbar ganglia.
lumbar ganglia [TA], gânglios lombares; quatro ou mais gânglios localizados na margem medial do músculo psoas maior em ambos os lados; formam, juntamente com os gânglios coccígeos e sacrais e suas ramificações interganglionares, a parte abdominopélvica do tronco simpático. SIN ganglia lumbalia [TA].
Meckel g., g. de Meckel. SIN pterygopalatine g.
g. mesenter'icum infe'rius [TA], g. mesentérico inferior. SIN inferior mesenteric g.
g. mesenter'icum supe'rius [TA], g. mesentérico superior. SIN superior mesenteric g.
middle cervical g. [TA], g. cervical médio; um g. simpático de tamanho pequeno e, às vezes, ausente; está localizado na altura da cartilagem cricóide. SIN g. cervicale medium [TA].
nasal g., g. nasal. SIN pterygopalatine g.
nerve g., neural g., g. nervoso. SIN ganglion (1).
g. of nervus intermedius, g. do nervo intermédio. SIN geniculate g.
nodose g., g. nodoso. SIN inferior g. of vagus nerve.
otic g. [TA], g. ótico; um g. autônomo situado inferiormente ao forame oval e medialmente ao nervo mandibular; suas fibras pós-sinápticas parassimpáticas são fibras secretomotoras distribuídas pela glândula parótida. SIN g. oticum [TA], Arnold g., auricular g., otoganglion.
g. o'ticum [TA], g. ótico. SIN otic g.
parasympathetic ganglia [TA], gânglios parassimpáticos; aqueles gânglios do sistema nervoso autônomo compostos de neurônios colinérgicos que recebem fibras pré-sinápticas provenientes de neurônios motores viscerais, tanto dos segmentos do tronco cerebral como dos segmentos espinais sacrais médios (S2 a S4); de acordo com a localização que esses gânglios parassimpáticos ocupam nos órgãos por eles inervados, a maioria deles, pelo menos dos que se situam fora da cabeça, pode ser classificada em gânglios justamurais e gânglios intramurais (isto é, localizados dentro da víscera inervada ou sobre ela). VER TAMBÉM autonomic *division* of nervous system. SIN ganglia parasympathetica [TA].
ganglia parasympathetica [TA], gânglios parassimpáticos. SIN parasympathetic ganglia.
paravertebral ganglia, gânglios paravertebrais. SIN g. of sympathetic trunk.
pelvic ganglia [TA], gânglios pélvicos; os gânglios parassimpáticos espalhados através do plexo pélvico em ambos os lados. SIN ganglia pelvica [TA], hypogastric ganglia.
gang'lia pel'vica [TA], gânglios pélvicos. SIN pelvic ganglia.
periosteal g., g. periosteal; uma cavidade subperiosteal achatada que contém um líquido claro, amarelo e viscoso, semelhante ao líquido sinovial.
petrosal g., petrous g., g. petroso. SIN inferior g. of glossopharyngeal nerve.
phrenic ganglia [TA], gânglios frênicos; vários gânglios autônomos pequenos presentes nos plexos que acompanham as artérias frênicas inferiores. SIN ganglia phrenica [TA].
gang'lia phren'ica [TA], gânglios frênicos. SIN phrenic ganglia.
gang'lia plex'uum autonomico'rum [TA], gânglios do plexo autônomo. SIN ganglia of autonomic plexuses.
prevertebral ganglia, gânglios pré-vertebrais; os gânglios simpáticos (celíaco, aorticorrenal, mesentérico superior e mesentérico inferior) que estão situados na frente da coluna vertebral; esse termo distingue-os dos gânglios do tronco simpático (gânglios paravertebrais); ocorrem principalmente ao redor da origem das ramificações da aorta abdominal mais importantes; todos estão no interior da cavidade abdominopélvica; os neurônios que compõem esses gânglios enviam fibras pós-sinápticas simpáticas até as vísceras abdominopélvicas através dos plexos periarteriais.
pterygopalatine g. [TA], g. pterigopalatino; um pequeno g. parassimpático localizado na parte superior da fossa pterigopalatina, cujas fibras pós-sinápticas secretomotoras suprem as glândulas lacrimal, nasal, palatina e faríngea. SIN g. pterygopalatinum [TA], Meckel g., nasal g., sphenopalatine g.
g. pterygopalati'num [TA], g. pterigopalatino. SIN pterygopalatine g.
Remak ganglia, gânglios de Remak. **(1)** Grupos de células nervosas localizados na parede do seio venoso, onde este se une ao átrio direito do coração. **(2)** Gânglios autônomos localizados nos nervos do estômago.
renal ganglia [TA], gânglios renais; pequenos gânglios simpáticos espalhados ao longo do plexo renal. SIN ganglia renalia [TA].
gang'lia rena'lia [TA], gânglios renais. SIN renal ganglia.
Ribes g., g. de Ribes; um pequeno g. simpático situado sobre a artéria comunicante anterior do cérebro.
sacral ganglia [TA], gânglios sacrais; três ou quatro gânglios bilaterais que constituem, juntamente com o g. ímpar e as ramificações interganglionares, a parte pélvica do tronco simpático. SIN ganglia sacralia [TA].

gang'lia sacra'lia [TA], gânglios sacrais. SIN sacral ganglia.
Scarpa g., g. de Scarpa. SIN vestibular g.
Schacher g., g. de Schacher. SIN ciliary g.
semilunar g., g. semilunar. SIN trigeminal g.
g. sensorium nervi spinalis [TA], g. sensorial do nervo espinal. SIN spinal g.
sensory g., g. sensorial; um aglomerado de neurônios sensoriais primários que formam uma intumescência geralmente visível no trajeto de um nervo periférico ou em sua raiz dorsal; essas células nervosas estabelecem a única conexão nervosa aferente entre o sistema periférico sensorial (pele, mucosas das cavidades oral e nasal, tecido muscular, tendões, cápsulas articulares, órgãos dos sentidos especiais, paredes dos vasos sanguíneos e tecidos dos órgãos internos) e o sistema nervoso central; são as células que dão origem a todas as fibras sensoriais do sistema nervoso periférico.
Soemmerring g., g. de Soemmerring. SIN *substantia* nigra.
solar ganglia, gânglios celíacos. SIN celiac ganglia.
sphenopalatine g., g. esfenopalatino. SIN pterygopalatine g.
spinal g. [TA], g. espinal; o g. da raiz posterior (dorsal) do nervo espinal de cada segmento (comumente com exceção do primeiro nervo espinal cervical); contém os corpos celulares dos neurônios sensitivos primários pseudo-unipolares, cujas ramificações periféricas (axônios) se tornam parte do nervo segmentar misto, e as ramificações centrais (axônios) penetram na medula espinal como um componente da raiz posterior sensorial. SIN g. sensorium nervi spinalis [TA], dorsal root g.*, g. spinale, intervertebral g.

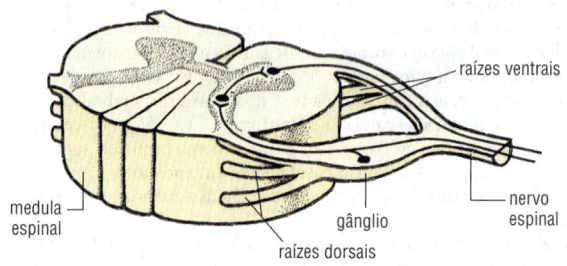

gânglio espinal (raiz dorsal)

g. spina'le, g. espinal. SIN spinal g.
spiral g. of cochlea [TA], g. coclear. SIN cochlear g.
spiral cochlear g., g. coclear. SIN cochlear g.
g. spira'le coch'leae, g. coclear; *termo oficial alternativo para cochlear g.
stellate g., g. cervicotorácico; *termo oficial alternativo para cervicothoracic g.
g. stella'tum, g. cervicotorácico; *termo oficial alternativo para cervicothoracic g.
sublingual g. [TA], g. sublingual; um minúsculo g. parassimpático encontrado ocasionalmente e situado numa posição anterior ao g. submandibular; é uma parte isolada do g. submandibular; suas fibras pós-sinápticas são secretomotoras e inervam a glândula sublingual. SIN g. sublinguale [TA].
g. sublingua'le [TA], g. sublingual. SIN sublingual g.
submandibular g. [TA], g. submandibular; um pequeno g. parassimpático pendurado no nervo lingual; suas fibras pós-sinápticas são secretomotoras e inervam as glândulas submandibulares e sublinguais; suas fibras pré-sinápticas provêm do núcleo salivatório superior através do nervo corda do tímpano. SIN g. submandibulare [TA], submaxillary g.
g. submandibula're [TA], g. submandibular. SIN submandibular g.
submaxillary g., g. submaxilar. SIN submandibular g.
superior cervical g. [TA], g. cervical superior; o g. em posição mais alta e o maior dos três gânglios do tronco simpático, situado próximo à base do crânio, entre a artéria carótida interna e a veia jugular interna. Todas as fibras póssinápticas simpáticas distribuídas para a cabeça e parte superior do pescoço são derivadas dos corpos celulares que compõem esse g. SIN g. cervicale superius [TA].
superior g. of glossopharyngeal nerve [TA], g. superior do nervo glossofaríngeo; o g. superior, menor e menos importante dos dois gânglios situados no nervo glossofaríngeo, na parte do nervo que atravessa o forame jugular; é em geral considerado uma parte isolada do g. inferior. SIN g. superius nervi glossopharyngei [TA], Ehrenritter g., intracranial g., jugular g. (1).
superior mesenteric g. [TA], g. mesentérico superior; um g. simpático, freqüentemente duplo, localizado próximo à aorta, no ponto de origem da artéria mesentérica superior. Os neurônios que compõem o g. enviam fibras pós-sinápticas para as partes dos intestinos delgado e grosso supridas pela artéria mesentérica superior. SIN g. mesentericum superius [TA].

superior g. of vagus nerve [TA], g. superior do nervo vago; um pequeno g. sensorial localizado no nervo vago, na parte do nervo que atravessa o forame jugular. SIN g. superius nervi vagi [TA], jugular g. (2).
g. supe·rius ner·vi glossopharyn·gei [TA], g. superior do nervo glossofaríngeo. SIN superior g. of glossopharyngeal nerve.
g. supe·rius ner·vi va·gi [TA], g. superior do nervo vago. SIN superior g. of vagus nerve.
sympathetic ganglia, gânglios simpáticos; os gânglios do sistema nervoso autônomo que recebem fibras eferentes originárias de neurônios pré-ganglionares motores viscerais localizados na coluna de células intermediolateral dos segmentos espinais torácicos e lombares superiores (T1–L2). De acordo com a localização dos gânglios simpáticos, eles podem ser classificados em gânglios paravertebrais (gânglios do tronco simpático) e gânglios pré-vertebrais (gânglios celíacos). VER TAMBÉM autonomic *division* of nervous system.
g. of sympathetic trunk [TA], g. do tronco simpático; os aglomerados de neurônios pós-sinápticos localizados em intervalos ao longo do tronco simpático, incluindo os gânglios cervical superior, cervical médio e cervicotorácico (estrelado), os gânglios torácicos, lombares e sacrais e o g. ímpar. SIN ganglia trunci sympathici [TA], chain ganglia, paravertebral ganglia.
terminal g. [TA], g. terminal. (1) Uma das células localizadas ao longo dos nervos terminais; SIN g. terminale [TA]. (2) Um dos neurônios pós-sinápticos autônomos espalhados pelo corpo encontrados dentro da ou próximo à parede do órgão inervado; são em geral parassimpáticos.
g. termina·le [TA], g. terminal. SIN terminal g. (1).
thoracic ganglia [TA], gânglios torácicos; gânglios simpáticos, cerca de 11 ou 12 em cada lado do corpo, situados na altura da cabeça de cada costela e que constituem, juntamente com as ramificações interganglionares, a parte torácica do tronco simpático. SIN ganglia thoracica [TA].
gang·lia thorac·ica [TA], gânglios torácicos. SIN thoracic ganglia.
thoracic splanchnic g., esplâncnico torácico; um pequeno g. simpático freqüentemente presente no trajeto do nervo esplâncnico maior. SIN g. thoracicum splanchnicum, Lobstein g.
g. thoracicum splanch·nicum, g. esplâncnico torácico. SIN thoracic splanchnic g.
trigeminal g. [TA], g. trigeminal; o grande e achatado g. sensorial do nervo trigêmeo que está adjacente ao seio cavernoso ao longo da parte medial da fossa média do crânio situada na cavidade trigeminal da dura-máter. SIN g. trigeminale [TA], gasserian g., semilunar g.
g. trigemina·le [TA], g. trigeminal. SIN trigeminal g.
Troisier g., g. de Troisier; termo histórico de um linfonodo situado imediatamente acima da clavícula, principalmente no lado esquerdo do corpo, que se apresenta aumentado à palpação como conseqüência de metástase de uma neoplasia maligna; a presença desse linfonodo indica que o local provável do acometimento neoplásico primário está em um órgão abdominal. VER TAMBÉM signal *node*. SIN Troisier node.
gang·lia trun·ci sympath·ici [TA], gânglios do tronco simpático. SIN g. of sympathetic trunk.
g. of trunk of vagus, g. do tronco do vago. SIN inferior g. of vagus nerve.
tympanic g., g. timpânico; um pequeno g. localizado na porção do nervo timpânico que passa através da parte petrosa do osso temporal. SIN g. tympanicum*.
g. tympan·icum, g. timpânico; *termo oficial alternativo para tympanic g.
Valentim g., g. de Valentim; um g. localizado no nervo alveolar superior.
vertebral g. [TA], g. vertebral; um pequeno e inconstante g. localizado ao longo da parte cervical do tronco simpático, ou uma das ramificações interganglionares que ligam o g. cervical médio ao g. cervicotorácico; em geral está situado próximo à artéria vertebral. SIN g. vertebrale [TA].
g. vertebra·le [TA], g. vertebral. SIN vertebral g.
vestibular g. [TA], g. vestibular; um conjunto de corpos de células nervosas sensoriais bipolares relacionadas com o equilíbrio e que formam uma intumescência sobre a parte vestibular do oitavo nervo craniano, no fundo do meato acústico interno; consiste em uma parte superior e em uma parte inferior unidas por um estreito istmo. SIN g. vestibulare [TA], Scarpa g.
g. vestibula·re [TA], g. vestibular. SIN vestibular g.
Vieussens ganglia, gânglios de Vieussens. SIN celiac ganglia.
Walther g., g. de Walther. SIN g. impar.
Wrisberg ganglia, gânglios de Wrisberg. SIN cardiac ganglia.

gan·gli·on·at·ed (gang'glē-o-nā'ted). Ganglionado. SIN gangliate.
gan·gli·on·ec·to·my (gang'glē-o-nek'to-mē). Gangliectomia; excisão de um gânglio. [ganglion + G. *ektomē*, excisão]
ganglioneuroblastoma (gang'lē-o-noor-o-blas-tō'ma). Ganglioneuroblastoma; um tumor de tipo celular misto, com elementos de neuroblastomas e de ganglioneuromas.
gan·gli·o·neu·ro·ma (gang'glē-o-noo-rō'ma). Ganglioneuroma; uma neoplasia benigna composta de neurônios ganglionares maduros, em número variado, espalhados isolados ou em grupos dentro de um estroma denso e relativamente abundante de neurofibrilas e fibras colágenas; é, em geral, encontrado no mediastino posterior e no retroperitônio, às vezes associado às glândulas adrenais. SIN ganglioma. [ganglion + G. *neuron*, nervo, + *-oma*, tumor]
central g., g. central; SIN gangliocytoma.
dumbbell g., g. em haltere; um g. cuja configuração macroscópica se assemelha a um haltere; p.ex., duas massas esferóides ligadas por uma porção estreita, em geral o resultado da ação de uma estrutura resistente, tal como duas costelas, sobre a massa neoplásica.
gan·gli·o·neu·ro·ma·to·sis (gang'glē-o-noo'ō-mā-tō'sis). Ganglioneuromatose; a condição de possuir muitos ganglioneuromas disseminados.
gan·gli·on·ic (gang-glē-on'ik). Ganglionar; relativo a um gânglio. SIN ganglial.
gan·gli·on·i·tis (gang'glē-o-nī'tis). Ganglionite. **1.** Inflamação de um gânglio linfático. **2.** Inflamação de um gânglio nervoso. SIN gangliitis.
gan·gli·o·nos·to·my (gang'glē-o-nos'to-mē). Ganglionostomia; fazer uma abertura em um gânglio (2). [ganglion + G. *stoma*, boca]
gan·gli·o·ple·gic (gang'glē-o-ple'jik). Ganglioplégico; um composto farmacológico que paralisa um gânglio autônomo, em geral por um período relativamente curto de tempo. [ganglion + G. *plēgē*, paralisia]
gan·gli·os·i·a·li·do·sis (gang'glē-o-si-al-ē-dō'sis). Gangliosialidose. SIN gangliosidosis.
gan·gli·o·side (gang'glē-o-sīd). Gangliosídeo; um glicoesfingolipídio quimicamente similar aos cerebrosídeos, contendo, porém, um ou mais resíduos de ácido siálico (ácido *N*-acetilneuramínico ou ácido *N*-glicolilneuramínico); encontrado principalmente no tecido nervoso, no baço e no timo; ocorre acúmulo de G_{M1} na gangliosidose generalizada e de G_{M2} na doença de Tay-Sachs. SIN sialoglycosphingolipid.
gan·gli·o·si·do·sis (gang'glē-o-si-do'sis). Gangliosidose; qualquer doença caracterizada, em parte, pelo acúmulo anormal de gangliosídeos específicos no sistema nervoso, p.ex., a gangliosidose G_{M2} e a doença de Tay-Sachs, causada pela deficiência da enzima hexosaminidase A, que leva a um acúmulo do gangliosídeo G_{M2}. SIN gangliosialidosis, ganglioside lipidosis.
G_{M1} g., g. G_{M1}; existem três formas: a infantil, generalizada, a juvenil e a forma adulta; uma g. caracterizada pelo acúmulo de um monosialogangliosídeo específico, o G_{M1}; resultante da deficiência de G_{M1}-β-galactosidase. SIN generalized g.
G_{M2} g., g. G_{M2}; uma doença metabólica hereditária; existem várias formas, dentre as quais a doença de Tay-Sachs (ver Tay-Sachs *disease*), a doença de Sandhoff (ver Sandhoff *disease*), a variante AB e o início na fase adulta; caracteriza-se pelo acúmulo de um metabólito específico, o gangliosídeo G_{M2}, que resulta da deficiência da hexosaminidase A, B ou do fator ativador de G_{M2}.
generalized g., g. generalizada. SIN G_{M1} g.
infantile G_{M2} g., g. G_{M2} infantil. SIN Tay-Sachs *disease*.
infantile, generalized G_{M1} g., g. G_{M1} infantil, generalizada; uma das doenças metabólicas hereditárias da infância; assemelha-se à doença de Tay-Sachs (ver Tay-Sachs *disease*), mas outros órgãos (ossos, fígado, rins) também são afetados. SIN familial neurovisceroipidosis, pseudo-Hurler disease, Type 1 G_{M1} g.
Type 1 G_{M1} g., g. G_{M1} de tipo 1. SIN infantile, generalized G_{M1} g.
gan·go·sa (gang-gō'sa). Gangosa; uma ulceração destrutiva que começa no palato mole e se estende para o palato duro, nasofaringe e nariz, resultando em cicatrizes mutilantes. A doença, tanto quanto se sabe, ocorre somente em certas regiões dos trópicos, principalmente nas ilhas do Pacífico e é, em geral, considerada uma seqüela da framboesia. [Esp. *gangoso*, fanhoso]
gan·grene (gang'grēn). Gangrena. **1.** Necrose resultante de obstrução, perda ou diminuição do suprimento sanguíneo; pode estar localizada em uma pequena área ou envolver toda uma extremidade ou um órgão (tal como o intestino) e pode ser úmida ou seca. SIN mortification. **2.** Necrose extensa oriunda de qualquer causa, p.ex., gangrena gasosa. [G. *gangraina*, uma ferida devoradora, de *graō*, roer]
arteriosclerotic g., g. arteriosclerótica; g. seca resultante de alterações escleróticas das artérias, com subseqüente oclusão, como observado no idoso.
cold g., g. por frio. SIN dry g.
cutaneous g., g. cutânea; g. da pele caracterizada pela formação de escaras; pode ocorrer no herpes zoster ou em qualquer infecção aguda que interfira na circulação sanguínea superficial.
decubital g., g. por decúbito. SIN decubitus *ulcer*.
diabetic g., g. diabética; g. resultante de arteriosclerose associada ao diabetes.
disseminated cutaneous g., g. cutânea disseminada. SIN dermatitis gangrenosa infantum.
dry g., g. seca; uma forma de g. na qual a parte afetada se mostra seca, bem demarcada e enrugada; é em geral resultante de doença vascular oclusiva de longa duração. SIN cold g., mummification (1).
embolic g., g. por êmbolo; g. que resulta de obstrução de uma artéria por um êmbolo.
emphysematous g., g. enfisematosa. SIN gas g.
Fournier g., g. de Fournier. SIN Fournier *disease*.
gas g., g. gasosa; g. que se desenvolve em uma ferida infectada por diversas bactérias anaeróbias esporuladas, principalmente pelo *Clostridium perfringens* e pelo *C. novyi*; causa crepitação, que se espalha rapidamente pelos tecidos

circunjacentes como resultado do gás liberado pela fermentação bacteriana, e sintomas tóxicos constitucionais e sépticos, incluindo lesão citotóxica dos rins, do fígado e de outros órgãos. SIN clostridial myonecrosis, emphysematous g., gangrenous emphysema, progressive emphysematous necrosis.

hemorrhagic g., g. hemorrágica. **(1)** SIN hemorrhagic *infarct*; **(2)** g. que ocorre raramente na septicemia meningocócica avançada.

hospital g., g. hospitalar. SIN decubitus *ulcer*.

hot g., g. quente; g. que se segue à inflamação de uma área afetada.

Meleney g., g. de Meleney. SIN Meleney *ulcer*.

moist g., g. úmida. SIN wet g.

presenile spontaneous g., g. espontânea pré-senil; g. que ocorre na meia-idade, como resultado de tromboangeíte obliterante.

pressure g., g. por pressão. SIN decubitus *ulcer*.

progressive bacterial synergistic g., g. bacteriana sinérgica progressiva. SIN Meleney *ulcer*.

senile g., g. senil; g. seca que ocorre em idosos como conseqüência de oclusão de uma artéria e que afeta particularmente os membros.

spontaneous g. of newborn, g. espontânea do recém-nascido; g. resultante de oclusão vascular de causa desconhecida e que geralmente acomete recém-nascidos marasmáticos ou desidratados.

static g., g. estática; g. úmida resultante de obstrução na circulação venosa. SIN venous g.

symmetrical g., g. simétrica; g. que afeta as extremidades do corpo bilateralmente; é observada principalmente na arteriosclerose grave, no infarto do miocárdio e no trombo esferóide.

thrombotic g., g. trombótica; g. resultante de oclusão de uma artéria por um trombo.

trophic g., g. trófica. SIN trophic *ulcer*.

venous g., g. venosa. SIN static g.

wet g., g. úmida; necrose isquêmica de um membro, acompanhada de putrefação bacteriana e que produz celulite nas áreas adjacentes à necrose. SIN moist g.

white g., g. branca; morte de uma região acompanhada da formação de escaras branco-acinzentadas. SIN leukonecrosis.

gan·gre·nous (gang'grē - nŭs). Gangrenoso; relativo a, ou afetado por, gangrena.

gan·o·blast (gan'o-blast). Ameloblasto. SIN ameloblast.

Ganong, William F., fisiologista norte-americano, *1924. VER Lown-G.-Levine *syndrome*.

Ganser, Siegbert J.M., psiquiatra alemão, 1853–1931. VER G. *commissure*, *syndrome*; *nucleus* basalis of G.

Gant, Samuel G., cirurgião norte-americano, 1869–1944. VER G. *clamp*.

gan·try (gan'trē). Uma estrutura onde se localizam o tubo de raios X, os colimadores e os detectores em uma máquina de tomografia computadorizada e que apresenta uma grande abertura, dentro da qual o paciente é colocado; um apoio mecânico para sustentar um dispositivo para que seja movido em uma trajetória circular. [I.M., do Fr. ant., do L. *cantherius*, estrutura de madeira, do G. *kanthēlia,* albarda, de *kanthos*, sela]

Gantzer, Carol F.L., anatomista alemão do século XVII. VER G. *accessory bundle*, *muscle*.

Ganz, William, cardiologista norte-americano, *1919. VER Swan-G. *catheter*.

gap. 1. Um hiato ou uma abertura em uma estrutura. **2.** Um intervalo ou uma descontinuidade em qualquer série ou seqüência. **3. (G).** Um período do ciclo celular.

g. 1 (G1), fase G1; no ciclo celular somático, o intervalo que se segue à mitose e é seguido pela síntese de DNA para a preparação do próximo ciclo.

g. 2 (G2), fase G2; no ciclo celular somático, uma pausa entre o término da síntese de DNA e o início da divisão celular.

air-bone g., diferença ar–osso; a diferença entre o limiar auditivo por condução óssea e por condução aérea.

anion g., diferença de ânions; a diferença entre a soma dos cátions e ânions quantificados no plasma ou no soro; é calculada de acordo com a fórmula a seguir: $(Na + K) - (Cl + HCO_3) = < 20$ mmol/L. Valores acima do normal podem ser encontrados na acidose diabética ou láctica; valores normais ou abaixo do normal estão presentes nas acidoses metabólicas por perda de bicarbonato. SIN cation-anion difference.

auscultatory g., hiato auscultatório; o período durante o qual os sons de Korotkoff, que indicam a pressão sistólica verdadeira, desaparecem e reaparecem em um valor pressórico mais baixo; é responsável pelo registro incorreto da pressão arterial sistólica, que se apresenta falsamente baixa em até 25 mm Hg, principalmente em pacientes hipertensivos; o erro é evitado ao se encher o manguito 30 mm Hg além da pressão sistólica palpável. SIN silent g.

Bochdalek g., intervalo de Bochdalek. SIN lumbocostal *triangle* of diaphragm.

chromosomal g., hiato cromossômico; uma área localizada de adelgaçamento encontrada em uma cromátide, que pode simular uma quebra completa.

DNA g., hiato de DNA; uma perda localizada de um dos dois filamentos na hélice dupla de DNA.

excitable g., intervalo excitável. SIN gap *phenomenon*.

interocclusal g., espaço interoclusal. SIN freeway *space*.

silent g., intervalo auscultatório. SIN auscultatory g.

Garbe, William, dermatologista canadense, *1908. VER Sulzberger-G. *disease*, *syndrome*.

Gardner, Eldon J., geneticista norte-americano, *1909. VER G. *syndrome*.

Gardner, F.H. VER G.-Diamond *syndrome*.

Gard·ner·el·la (gărd'ner - el'ă). Um gênero de bactérias (bastonetes) anaeróbias facultativas, que não formam esporos, sem cápsula, imóveis, pleomórficas, oxidase e catalase-negativas e que se coram de modo variável pelo Gram.

G. vaginalis, uma espécie que é um dos agentes etiológicos da vaginose bacteriana em seres humanos.

gar·gle (gar'gl). **1.** Gargarejar; lavar as fauces com um líquido; enquanto o líquido é mantido na cavidade oral, realiza-se expiração forçada, expelindo o ar pela própria boca e mantendo a cabeça inclinada para trás, o que produz um efeito borbulhante. **2.** Colutório; um líquido medicamentoso utilizado para gargarejar; uma lavagem da garganta. [Fr. ant. do L. *gurgulio*, fauces, traquéia]

Gariel, Maurice, médico francês, 1812–1878. VER G. *pessary*.

Garland, Hugh G., neurologista britânico, 1903–1967. VER Marinesco-Garland *syndrome*.

Garland, M., médico norte-americano, 1848–1926. VER G. *triangle*.

gar·lic (gar'lik). Alho. SIN allium.

g. oil, óleo de alho; um óleo volátil proveniente do bulbo ou da planta inteira de *Allium sativum* (família Liliaceae); contém dissulfeto de dialila e dissulfeto de alilpropila; tem sido utilizado como anti-helmíntico e rubefaciente.

Garré, Carl, cirurgião suíço, 1857–1928. VER G. *disease*; Garré *osteomyelitis*.

Gärtner, August, médico alemão, 1848–1934. VER G. *method*, vein *phenomenon*, *tonometer*.

Gartner, Herman T., anatomista e cirurgião dinamarquês, 1785–1827. VER G. *canal*, *cyst*, *duct*.

GAS Abreviatura de group A *streptococci* (estreptococos do grupo A), em *streptococcus*.

gas. Gás. **1.** Um fluido rarefeito, semelhante ao ar, capaz de expansão indefinida e conversível ao estado líquido e, por fim, ao estado sólido, quando comprimido ou exposto ao frio. **2.** Na prática clínica, um líquido que se encontra completamente em sua forma de vapor a uma atmosfera de pressão, porque a temperatura ambiente está acima de seu ponto de ebulição. [termo cunhado por J.B. van Helmont, químico e médico flamengo, 1577–1644]

alveolar g. Gás alveolar (símbolo A subscrito), o g. nos alvéolos pulmonares, onde ocorre a troca O_2-CO_2 com o sangue capilar pulmonar. SIN alveolar air.

anesthetic g., g. anestésico. VER inhalation *anesthetic*.

blood g.'s, gases sanguíneos; uma expressão clínica para a determinação das pressões parciais de oxigênio e dióxido de carbono no sangue.

carbonic acid g., ácido carbônico na forma de gás. SIN carbon dioxide.

expired g., g. expirado. **(1)** Qualquer g. que tenha sido expirado dos pulmões; **(2)** é freqüentemente utilizado como sinônimo de g. expirado misto.

hemolytic g., g. hemolítico; um gás venenoso, tal como a arsina, cuja inalação provoca hemólise com hemoglobinúria, icterícia, gastroenterite e nefrite.

ideal alveolar g., g. alveolar ideal; a composição uniforme do g. que existiria em todos os alvéolos durante uma determinada troca respiratória total, caso todos os alvéolos tivessem razões ventilação–perfusão idênticas e alcançassem equilíbrio perfeito com o sangue que deixa os capilares pulmonares.

inert g.'s, gases inertes; gases nobres. SIN noble g.'s.

inspired g. (I) (símbolo I subscrito), g. inspirado. **(1)** Qualquer g. que está sendo inalado; **(2)** especificamente, um g. após ter sido umidificado à temperatura corporal.

laughing g., g. hilariante; um termo histórico para o óxido nitroso. [assim chamado porque sua inalação às vezes desencadeia um delírio hilariante, que precede a insensibilidade]

marsh g., g. dos pântanos; metano. SIN methane.

mixed expired g., g. expirado misto; uma ou mais expirações completas de g. expirado que vem completamente misturado do espaço morto e dos alvéolos.

mustard g. (HD), g.-mostarda; um gás venenoso e vesicante, utilizado pela primeira vez na Primeira Guerra Mundial; é o precursor das chamadas mostardas nitrogenadas; foi empregado na guerra química; um conhecido carcinógeno. SIN di(2-chloroethyl)-sulfide, mustard (2), sulfur mustard.

noble g.'s, gases nobres; elementos químicos do grupo zero da tabela periódica: hélio, neônio, argônio, criptônio, xenônio e radônio. SIN inert g.'s.

sewer g., g. dos esgotos; g., provavelmente composto em sua maior parte por metano, que se origina da decomposição de matéria orgânica nos esgotos; é potencialmente explosivo e tóxico.

sneezing g., g. esternutatório. SIN sternutator.

suffocating g., g. sufocante; um g., tal como o cloro ou o fosgênio, que provoca intensa irritação nos brônquios e pulmões, acarretando edema pulmonar.

tear g., g. lacrimogêneo; um g., como acetona, brometo de benzeno e xilol, que provoca irritação da conjuntiva ocular e intenso lacrimejamento. VER TAMBÉM lacrimator.

vesicating g., g. vesicante; um g., como o g.-mostarda, que, em contato com a pele, provoca vesicação e formação de escaras; sua inalação pode causar broncopneumonia.

vomiting g., g. do vômito; um g., como a cloropicrina, que pode provocar vômito e distúrbios gastrointestinais, como cólica e diarréia.

water g., g. de água; um g. de iluminação e combustível produzido pela passagem de vapor sobre o carvão em brasa; consiste principalmente em hidrogênio, hidrocarbonetos e monóxido de carbono.

gas·e·ous (gas′ē-ŭs). Gasoso; da natureza do gás.

Gaskell, Walter H., fisiologista inglês, 1847–1914. VER G. *bridge, clamp.*

gas·om·e·ter (gas-om′ē-ter). Gasômetro; um instrumento ou vaso calibrado para medir os volumes de gases. VER TAMBÉM spirometer.

gas·o·met·ric (gas-ō-met′rik). Gasométrico; relativo à gasometria.

gas·om·e·try (gas-om′ē-trē). Gasometria; a medida de gases; a determinação da proporção relativa de gases em uma mistura.

Gass, John D.M., oftalmologista norte-americano, *1928. VER Irvine-G. *syndrome.*

Gasser (Gas·ser·i·o), Johann L., anatomista austríaco, 1723–1765. VER gasserian *ganglion.*

gas·ser·i·an (ga-ser′ē-an). Gasseriano; relativo a, ou descrito por, Johann L. Gasser.

gas·sing (gas′ing). Envenenamento por gases irrespiráveis ou de alguma forma nocivos.

Gastaut, Henri, biólogo francês, *1915. VER Lennox-G. *syndrome.*

gas·ter (gas′ter) [TA]. **1.** Estômago. SIN stomach. **2.** Gáster; parte proeminente do abdome da vespa ou da formiga, separada das outras partes do corpo por um segmento delgado. [G. *gastēr,* ventre]

Gas·ter·o·phil·i·dae (gas′ter-ō-fil′i-dē). Uma família de moscas do berne (ou varejeiras) que produzem miíase entérica nos membros da família dos cavalos (gênero *Gasterophilus*), em rinocerontes (gênero *Gyrostigma*) e em elefantes (gêneros *Cobboldia, Platycobboldia* e *Rodhainomyia*). SIN Gastrophilidae. [G. *gastēr,* ventre, estômago, + *philos,* amigo]

⚠ **gastr-.** VER gastro-.

gas·tral·gia (gas-tral′jē-ă). Gastralgia. SIN stomach ache. [gastr- + G. *algos,* dor]

gas·trec·ta·sis, gas·trec·ta·sia (gas-trek′tă-sis, gas-trek-tā′zē-ă). Gastrectasia; dilatação do estômago. [gastr- + G. *ektasis,* extensão]

gas·trec·to·my (gas-trek′tō-mē). Gastrectomia; excisão parcial ou total do estômago. [gastr- + G. *ektomē,* excisão]

Hofmeister g., g. de Hofmeister; cirurgia de Hofmeister na qual uma parte do estômago é removida e uma gastrojejunostomia retrocólica término-lateral é construída somente com a parte da curvatura maior do estômago seccionada.

Pólya g., g. de Pólya; cirurgia na qual parte do estômago é removida e uma gastrojejunostomia retrocólica é construída de forma término-lateral para se ajustar à extremidade seccionada do estômago. SIN Pólya operation.

gas·tric (gas′trik). Gástrico; relativo ao estômago. SIN gastricus.

gas·tric car·dia (gas′trik kar′dē-ă). Cárdia. SIN cardia.

gas·tric·sin (gas-trik′sin). Gastricsina; um termo alternativo para uma peptidase humana atualmente denominada pepsina C. É encontrada nos sucos gástricos da maioria dos vertebrados.

gas·tri·cus (gas′tri-kŭs). Gástrico. SIN gastric. [L.]

gas·trin·o·ma (gas-tri-nō′mă). Gastrinoma; um tumor secretor de gastrina associado à síndrome de Zollinger-Ellison.

gas·trins (gas′trinz). Gastrinas; hormônios secretados pela mucosa pilórico-antral do estômago de mamíferos que estimulam a secreção de HCl pelas células parietais das glândulas gástricas; existem três tipos principais: gastrina grande (34 resíduos aminoacil), gastrina pequena (17 resíduos) e minigastrina (14 resíduos), bem como derivados sulfatados. O pentapeptídeo C-terminal é também observado na colecistocinina e na ceruleína. [G. *gastēr,* estômago, + -in]

ℹ **gas·tri·tis** (gas-trī′tis). Gastrite; inflamação do estômago, principalmente de sua mucosa. [gastr- + G. *-itis,* inflamação]

alkaline reflux g., g. por refluxo alcalino; inflamação da mucosa gástrica que se acredita ser causada por fatores irritativos que refluem do intestino para o estômago; muito freqüente após a ressecção ou ablação do piloro. SIN bile g.

atrophic g., g. atrófica; g. crônica com atrofia da mucosa e destruição das glândulas pépticas, associada, às vezes, à anemia perniciosa ou ao carcinoma gástrico; termo também aplicado à atrofia gástrica que não apresenta alterações inflamatórias.

bile g., g. por refluxo biliar. SIN alkaline reflux g.

catarrhal g., g. catarral; g. com excessiva secreção de muco.

g. cys′tica polypo′sa, g. cística poliposa; grandes pólipos mucosos e sésseis que surgem no estômago próximo a uma antiga gastroenterostomia.

eosinophilic g., g. eosinofílica. SIN eosinophilic *gastroenteritis.*

exfoliative g., g. esfoliativa; g. com excessiva descamação de células epiteliais mucosas.

hypertrophic g., g. hipertrófica. SIN Ménétrier *disease.*

interstitial g., g. intersticial; inflamação do estômago que envolve as camadas submucosa e muscular.

polypous g., g. poliposa; uma forma de g. crônica na qual há atrofia irregular da mucosa com glândulas císticas dando uma aparência nodosa ou polipóide à superfície.

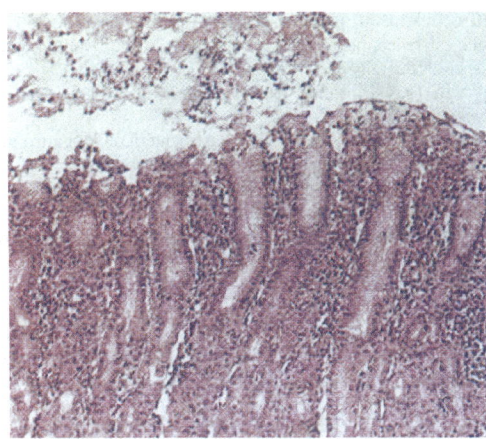

gastrite aguda: com lesão e inflamação do epitélio das glândulas gástricas

pseudomembranous g., g. pseudomembranosa; g. caracterizada pela formação de uma falsa membrana.

sclerotic g., g. esclerótica; espessamento fibroso das paredes do estômago com diminuição na capacidade do órgão.

⚠ **gastro-, gastr-.** O estômago, o abdome. [G. *gastēr,* o ventre]

gas·tro·a·ceph·a·lus (gas′trō-ă-sef′ă-lŭs). Gastroacéfalo; gêmeos desiguais e unidos, nos quais um deles é um parasita acéfalo e está ligado ao autósito. VER conjoined *twins,* em twin. [gastro- + G. *a-* priv. + *kephalē,* cabeça]

gas·tro·al·bum·or·rhea (gas′trō-al-bū-mō-rē′ă). Gastroalbuminorréia; perda de albumina para o estômago. [gastro- + albumina, + G. *rhoia,* fluxo]

gas·tro·a·mor·phus (gas′trō-ă-mōr′fŭs). Gastroamorfo; um gêmeo parasita amorfo e incluído no abdome do autósito. [gastro- + G. *amorphos,* sem forma]

gas·tro·a·nas·to·mo·sis (gas′trō-an-as-tō-mō′sis). Gastroanastomose. SIN gastrogastrostomy.

gas·tro·a·to·nia (gas′trō-ă-tō′nē-ă). Gastroatonia; termo obsoleto para a perda de tônus da musculatura do estômago. [gastro- + G. *atonia,* languidez]

gas·tro·blen·nor·rhea (gas′trō-blen-ō-rē′ă). Gastroblenorréia; excessiva produção de muco pelo estômago. [gastro- + blenorréia]

gas·tro·car·di·ac (gas′trō-kar′dē-ak). Gastrocardíaco; relativo tanto ao estômago quanto ao coração.

gas·tro·cele (gas′trō-sēl). Gastrocele; hérnia de uma parte do estômago. [gastro- + G. *kēlē,* hérnia]

gas·tro·chron·or·rhea (gas′trō-kron-ō-rē′ă). Gastrocronorréia; secreção gástrica contínua e excessiva. [gastro- + G. *chronos,* tempo, + *rhoia,* fluxo]

gas·troc·ne·mi·us (gas-trok-nē′mē-ŭs). Gastrocnêmio. SIN gastrocnemius (muscle). [G. *gastroknēmia,* a panturrilha, de *gaster* (gastr-), ventre, + *knēmē,* perna]

gas·tro·col·ic (gas′trō-kol′ik). Gastrocólico; relativo ao estômago e ao cólon.

gas·tro·co·li·tis (gas′trō-kō-lī′tis). Gastrocolite; inflamação tanto do estômago como do cólon.

gas·tro·co·lop·to·sis (gas′trō-kō-lō-tō′sis). Gastrocoloptose; deslocamento para baixo do estômago e do cólon. [gastro- + G. *kōlon,* cólon, + *ptōsis,* uma queda]

gas·tro·co·los·to·my (gas′trō-kō-los′tō-mē). Gastrocolostomia; estabelecimento de uma comunicação entre o estômago e o cólon, em geral secundária a uma úlcera gástrica ou a um processo maligno, tanto no cólon quanto no estômago. [gastro- + G. *kōlon,* cólon, + *stoma,* boca]

gas·tro·cys·to·plas·ty (gas′trō-sis′tō-plas-tē). Gastrocistoplastia; aumento da bexiga por meio de uma porção vascularizada de estômago.

gas·tro·di·al·y·sis (gas′trō-dī-al′i-sis). Gastrodiálise; diálise através da mucosa do estômago.

Gas·tro·dis·coi·des hom·i·nis (gas′trō-dis-koy′dēz hom′i-nis). Uma espécie de trematódeo às vezes encontrado nos tubos intestinais de seres humanos da Índia, do Sudeste Asiático e da China; seu hospedeiro habitual é o porco. SIN *Gastrodiscus hominis.* [gastro- + G. *diskos,* disco; L. *homo,* gen. *hominis,* homem]

Gas·tro·dis·cus hom·i·nis (gas-trō-dis′kŭs). SIN *Gastrodiscoides hominis.*

gas·tro·du·o·de·nal (gas′trō-doo′ō-dē′nal, -du-od′ē-nal). Gastroduodenal; relativo ao estômago e ao duodeno.

gas·tro·du·o·de·ni·tis (gas′trō-doo-ō-dē-nī′tis). Gastroduodenite; inflamação tanto do estômago como do duodeno.

gas·tro·du·o·de·nos·co·py (gas′trō-doo-ō-dē-nos′kō-pē). Gastroduodenoscopia; visualização do interior do estômago e do duodeno por meio de um gastroscópio. [gastro- + duodeno, + G. *skopeō,* visualizar]

gas·tro·du·o·de·nos·to·my (gas′trō-doo-ō-dĕ-nos′tō-mē). Gastroduodenostomia; estabelecimento de uma comunicação entre o estômago e o duodeno. [gastro- + duodeno + G. *stoma*, boca]

gas·tro·dyn·ia (gas-trō-din′ē-ă). Gastrodinia. SIN stomach ache. [gastro- + G. *odynē*, dor]

gas·tro·en·ter·ic (gas′trō-en-ter′ik). Gastroentérico. SIN gastrointestinal.

gas·tro·en·ter·i·tis (gas′trō-en-ter-ī′tis). Gastroenterite; inflamação da mucosa, tanto do estômago como do intestino. SIN enterogastritis. [gastro- + G. *enteron*, intestino, + *-itis*, inflamação]

  acute infectious nonbacterial g., g. infecciosa aguda não-bacteriana. SIN epidemic nonbacterial g.

  endemic nonbacterial infantile g., g. infantil endêmica não-bacteriana; g. viral endêmica que acomete crianças pequenas (6 meses a 12 anos), que se dissemina principalmente durante o inverno e é causada por cepas de rotavírus (família Reoviridae); o período de incubação é de 2 a 4 dias, e os sintomas duram de 3 a 5 dias e incluem dor abdominal, diarréia, febre e vômitos. SIN infantile g.

  eosinophilic g., g. eosinofílica; gastroenterite com dor abdominal, malabsorção e freqüentes sintomas obstrutivos associados a eosinofilia periférica e a áreas de infiltração eosinofílica no estômago, intestino delgado e/ou cólon. Pode ter uma etiologia alérgica e responde, em alguns pacientes, à eliminação do alérgeno da dieta; a terapia com corticosteróides também é efetiva. SIN eosinophilic gastritis.

  epidemic nonbacterial g., g. epidêmica não-bacteriana; doença epidêmica, de início súbito, extremamente contagiosa, porém um tanto branda e causada pelo vírus da gastroenterite epidêmica (principalmente o agente Norwalk); apresenta um período de incubação de 16 a 48 horas e uma duração de um a dois dias, afetando todos os grupos etários; a infecção está associada a febre, cólicas abdominais, náuseas, vômitos, diarréia e cefaléia, podendo um ou outro desses sintomas ser predominante. SIN acute infectious nonbacterial g.

  infantile g., g. infantil. SIN endemic nonbacterial infantile g.

  viral g., g. viral. VER endemic nonbacterial infantile g., epidemic nonbacterial g.

gas·tro·en·ter·o·a·nas·to·mo·sis (gas′trō-en-ter-ō-an-as-tō-mō′sis). Gastroenteroanastomose. SIN gastroenterostomy.

gas·tro·en·ter·o·co·li·tis (gas′trō-en′ter-ō-kō-lī′tis). Gastroenterocolite; doença inflamatória que envolve o estômago e os intestinos. [gastro- + G. *enteron*, intestino, + *kōlon*, colo, + *-itis*, inflamação]

gas·tro·en·ter·o·co·los·to·my (gas′trō-en-ter-ō-kō-los′tō-mē). Gastroenterocolostomia; formação de uma comunicação direta entre o estômago e os intestinos grosso e delgado, em geral secundária a uma úlcera gástrica ou a um processo maligno, tanto no cólon quanto no estômago. [gastro- + G. *enteron*, intestino, + *kōlon*, colo + *stoma*, boca]

gas·tro·en·ter·ol·o·gist (gas′trō-en-ter-ol′ō-jist). Gastroenterologista; um especialista em gastroenterologia.

gas·tro·en·ter·ol·o·gy (gas-trō-en-ter-ol′ō-jē). Gastroenterologia; a especialidade médica que se ocupa da função e dos distúrbios do trato gastrointestinal, incluindo o estômago, os intestinos e os órgãos associados. [gastro- + G. *enteron*, intestino, + *logos*, estudo]

gas·tro·en·ter·op·a·thy (gas′trō-en-ter-op′a-thē). Gastroenteropatia; qualquer distúrbio do canal alimentar. [gastro- + G. *enteron*, intestino, + *pathos*, sofrimento]

gas·tro·en·ter·o·plas·ty (gas′trō-en-ter-ō-plas′tē). Gastroenteroplastia; reparo cirúrgico de defeitos localizados no estômago e nos intestinos. [gastro- + G. *enteron*, intestino, + *plassō*, formar]

gas·tro·en·ter·op·to·sis (gas′trō-en-ter-ō-tō′sis). Gastroenteroptose; deslocamento para baixo do estômago e de uma porção do intestino. [gastro- + G. *enteron*, intestino, + *ptōsis*, uma queda]

gas·tro·en·ter·os·to·my (gas′trō-en-ter-os′tō-mē). Gastroenterostomia; o estabelecimento de uma nova abertura entre o estômago e o intestino, tanto anterior quanto posteriormente ao colo transverso. SIN gastroenteroanastomosis. [gastro- + G. *enteron*, intestino, + *stoma*, boca]

gas·tro·en·ter·ot·o·my (gas′trō-en-ter-ot′ō-mē). Gastroenterotomia; secção realizada tanto no estômago quanto no intestino. [gastro- + G. *enteron*, intestino, + *tomē*, incisão]

gas·tro·ep·i·plo·ic (gas′trō-ep′i-plō′ik). Gastroepiplóico; relativo ao estômago e ao omento maior (epíploo).

gas·tro·e·soph·a·ge·al (gas′trō-ē-sof′ă-jē′al). Gastroesofágico; relativo tanto ao estômago quanto ao esôfago. [gastro- + G. *oisophagos*, esôfago]

gas·tro·e·soph·a·gi·tis (gas′trō-ē-sof-ă-jī′tis). Gastroesofagite; inflamação do estômago e do esôfago.

gas·tro·e·soph·a·gos·to·my (gas′trō-ē-sof-ă-gos′tō-mē). Gastroesofagostomia. SIN esophagogastrostomy. [gastro- + G. *oisophagos*, esôfago, + *stoma*, boca]

gas·tro·gas·tros·to·my (gas′trō-gas-tros′tō-mē). Gastrogastrostomia; anastomose entre duas partes do estômago, em geral para evitar uma área de estreitamento. SIN gastroanastomosis.

gas·tro·ga·vage (gas-trō-gă-vahzh′). Gavagem. SIN gavage (1).

gas·tro·gen·ic (gas-trō-jen′ik). Gastrogênico; derivado do, ou causado pelo, estômago.

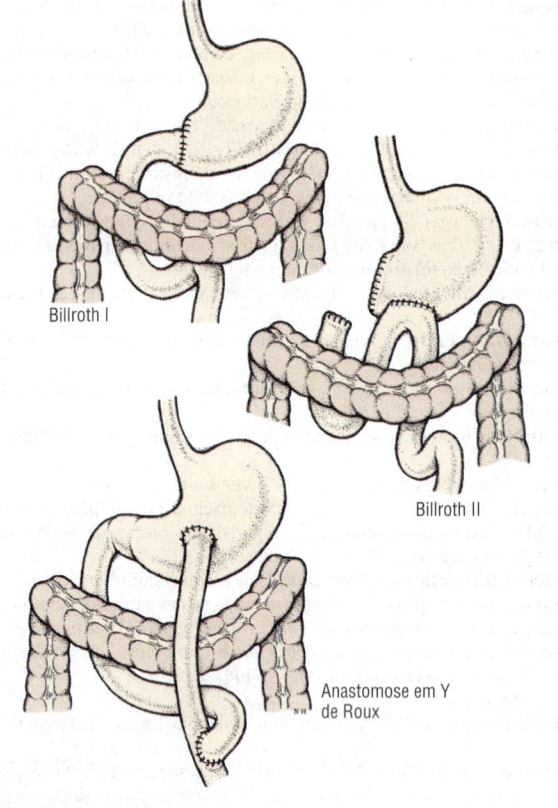

gastroenterostomia

gas·tro·graph (gas′trō-graf). Gastrógrafo; um instrumento para registrar graficamente os movimentos do estômago. SIN gastrokinesograph. [gastro- + G. *graphē*, escrever]

gas·tro·he·pat·ic (gas′trō-he-pat′ik). Gastro-hepático; relativo ao estômago e ao fígado. [gastro- + G. *hēpar* (*hēpat-*), fígado]

gas·tro·hy·dror·rhea (gas′trō-hī-drō-rē′ă). Gastro-hidrorréia; excreção para o interior do estômago de um grande volume de líquido aquoso, que não contém nem ácido clorídrico e quimosina, nem fermentos pepsina. [gastro- + G. *hydōr*, água, + *rhoia*, um fluxo]

gas·tro·il·e·i·tis (gas′trō-il-e-ī′tis). Gastroileíte; inflamação do canal alimentar na qual o estômago e o íleo são os principais órgãos acometidos.

gas·tro·il·e·os·to·my (gas′trō-il-ē-os′tō-mē). Gastroileostomia; uma ligação cirúrgica entre o estômago e o íleo; mais comumente utilizada no tratamento da obesidade grave.

gas·tro·in·tes·ti·nal (GI) (gas′trō-in-tes′tin-ăl). Gastrointestinal; relativo ao estômago e aos intestinos. SIN gastroenteric.

gas·tro·je·ju·no·col·ic (gas′trō-jē-joo′nō-kol′ik). Gastrojejunocólico; que se refere ao estômago, ao jejuno e ao cólon.

gas·tro·je·ju·nos·to·my (gas′trō-jē-joo-nos′tō-mē). Gastrojejunostomia; estabelecimento de uma comunicação entre o estômago e o jejuno. SIN gastronesteostomy. [gastro- + jejuno, G. *stoma*, boca]

gas·tro·ki·ne·so·graph (gas′trō-ki-nē′sō-graf). Gastrocinesógrafo. SIN gastrograph. [gastro- + G. *kinēsis*, movimento, + *graphē*, escrever]

gas·tro·la·vage (gas-trō-lă-vahzh′). Lavagem gástrica; lavagem do estômago.

gas·tro·li·e·nal (gas-trō-lī′ē-năl). Gastroesplênico. SIN gastrosplenic. [gastro- + L. *lien*, baço]

gas·tro·lith (gas′trō-lith). Gastrólito; uma concreção dentro do estômago. SIN gastric calculus. [gastro- + G. *lithos*, pedra]

gas·tro·li·thi·a·sis (gas′trō-li-thī′ă-sis). Gastrolitíase; presença de um ou mais cálculos dentro do estômago. [gastro- + G. *lithos*, pedra + *-iasis*, condição]

gas·trol·o·gist (gas-trol′ō-jist). Gastrologista; um especialista em gastrologia.

gas·trol·o·gy (gas-trol′ō-jē). Gastrologia; um ramo da medicina que se ocupa do estômago e de seus distúrbios. [gastro- + G. *logos*, estudo]

gas·trol·y·sis (gas-trol′i-sis). Gastrólise; secção de aderências perigástricas. [gastro- + G. *lysis*, liberação]

gas·tro·ma·la·cia (gas′trō-mă-lā′shē-ă). Gastromalacia; amolecimento das paredes do estômago. [gastro- + G. *malakia*, amolecimento]

gas·tro·meg·a·ly (gas′trō-meg′ă-lē). Gastromegalia. **1.** Aumento do estômago. **2.** Aumento do abdome. [gastro- + G. *megas* (*megal-*), grande]

gas·trom·e·lus (gas-trom′e-lŭs). Gastrômelo; uma condição na qual um indivíduo apresenta um membro supranumerário ligado ao abdome. VER conjoined *twins*, em *twin*. [gastro- + G. *melos*, um membro]

gas·tro·myx·or·rhea (gas′trō-mik-sō-rē′ă). Gastromixorréia; secreção excessiva de muco dentro do estômago. SIN myxorrhea gastrica. [gastro- + G. *myxa*, muco, + *rhoia*, um fluxo]

gas·tro·nes·te·os·to·my (gas′trō-nes-tē-os′tŏ-mē). Gastrojejunostomia. SIN gastrojejunostomy. [gastro- + G. *nēstis*, jejuno, + *stoma*, boca]

gas·trop·a·gus (gas-trop′ă-gŭs). Gastrópago; gêmeos ligados pelo abdome. VER conjoined *twins*, em *twin*. [gastro- + -*pagus*]

gas·tro·pa·ral·y·sis (gas′trō-pă-ral′i-sis). Gastroparalisia; paralisia da camada muscular do estômago.

gas·tro·par·a·si·tus (gas′trō-par-ă-sī′tŭs). Gastroparasita; gêmeos desiguais e unidos nos quais o gêmeo parasita incompleto está unido ao ou está dentro do abdome do autósito. VER conjoined *twins*, em *twin*.

gas·tro·pa·re·sis (gas-trō-pă-rē′sis, -par′e-sis). Gastroparesia; enfraquecimento da peristalse gástrica que acarreta uma demora no esvaziamento dos intestinos. [gastro- + G. *paresis*, paralisia]
  g. diabetico′rum, g. diabética; dilatação do estômago acompanhada de retenção gástrica que ocorre em diabéticos; é encontrada geralmente associada à acidose grave ou ao coma.

gas·tro·path·ic (gas-trō-path′ik). Gastropático; que se refere à gastropatia.

gas·trop·a·thy (gas-trop′ă-thē). Gastropatia; qualquer doença do estômago. [gastro- + G. *pathos*, doença]
  hypertrophic hypersecretory g., g. hipertrófica hipersecretora; espessamentos nodulares da mucosa gástrica acompanhados de hipersecreção ácida e, freqüentemente, ulceração péptica, não associada a um tumor secretor de gastrina.

gas·tro·pex·y (gas′trō-pek-sē). Gastropexia; fixação do estômago à parede abdominal ou ao diafragma. [gastro- + G. *pēxis*, fixação]

Gas·tro·phil·i·dae (gas-trō-fil′i-dē). Gasterophilidae.

gas·tro·phren·ic (gas′trō-fren′ik). Gastrofrênico; relativo ao estômago e ao diafragma. [gastro- + G. *phrēn*, diafragma]

gas·tro·plas·ty (gas′trō-plas-tē). Gastroplastia. **1.** Tratamento cirúrgico de um defeito do estômago ou a produção de um tubo gástrico na parte inferior do esôfago que utiliza a parede do estômago para a reconstrução. **2.** A colocação de uma linha de grampos através da porção superior do estômago a fim de limitar a entrada de alimentos; empregada no tratamento da obesidade grave. [gastro- + G. *plastos*, formado]
  Collis g., g. de Collis; uma técnica para alongar um esôfago "curto"; uma incisão de espessura total no cárdia, paralelamente à curvatura menor, feita em geral com uma linha de grampos, criando um tubo na parte superior do estômago a fim de alongar o esôfago.
  vertical banded g., g. com enfaixamento vertical; uma g. para tratar da obesidade mórbida, na qual uma bolsa gástrica superior é formada por uma linha vertical de grampos e uma faixa é colocada na saída para a bolsa principal a fim de impedir uma dilatação.

gas·tro·pli·ca·tion (gas′trō-pli-kā′shŭn). Gastroplicatura; uma cirurgia para reduzir o tamanho do estômago, por meio da sutura de uma prega longitudinal com as superfícies peritoneais em aposição. SIN gastroptyxis, gastrorrhaphy (2), stomach reefing. [gastro- + L. *plico*, pregar]

gas·tro·pneu·mon·ic (gas′trō-noo-mon′ik). Gastropneumônico. SIN pneumogastric. [gastro- + G. *pneumōn*, pulmão]

gas·tro·pod (gas′trō-pod). Gastrópode; nome comum dado aos membros da classe Gastropoda.

Gas·trop·o·da (gas-trop′ō-dă). Uma classe do filo Mollusca que engloba os caracóis, as conchas, as lesmas e as lapas. [gastro- + G. *pous* (*pod-*), pé]

gas·trop·to·sis, gas·trop·to·sia (gas-trō-tō′sis, -tō′sē-ă). Gastroptose; deslocamento do estômago para baixo. SIN bathygastry, descensus ventriculi, ventroptosis, ventroptosia. [gastro- + G. *ptosis*, uma queda]

gas·tro·ptyx·is (gas-trō-tik′sis). Gastroplicatura. SIN gastroplication. [gastro- + G. *ptyxis*, uma prega]

gas·tro·pul·mo·nary (gas-trō-pŭl′mo-nar-ē). Gastropulmonar. SIN pneumogastric.

gas·tro·py·lor·ic (gas′trō-pī-lōr′ik). Gastropilórico; relativo ao estômago como um todo e ao piloro.

gas·tror·rha·gia (gas-trō-rā′jē-ă). Gastrorragia; hemorragia proveniente do estômago. SIN gastric hemorrhage. [gastro- + G. *rhēgnymi*, irromper]

gas·tror·rha·phy (gas-trōr′ă-fē). **1.** Gastrorrafia; sutura de uma perfuração no estômago. **2.** Gastroplicatura. SIN gastroplication. [gastro- + G. *rhaphē*, uma costura]

gas·tror·rhea (gas-trō-rē′ă). Gastrorréia; secreção excessiva de suco gástrico ou de muco (gastromixorréia) pelo estômago. [gastro- + G. *rhoia*, um fluxo]

gas·tror·rhex·is (gas′trō-rek′sis). Gastrorrexe; uma laceração ou fenda no estômago. [gastro- + G. *rhēxis*, uma ruptura]

gas·tros·chi·sis (gas-tros′ki-sis). Gastrosquise; uma abertura congênita na parede abdominal que não envolve o cordão umbilical; é em geral acompanhada de protrusão das vísceras. [gastro- + G. *schisis*, uma fissura]

gas·tro·scope (gas′trō-skōp). Gastroscópio; um endoscópio para examinar o interior do estômago. [gastro- + G. *skopeō*, examinar]
  fiberoptic g., g. de fibra óptica; instrumento que utiliza fibras ópticas para examinar o interior do estômago.

gas·tro·scop·ic (gas-trō-skop′ik). Gastroscópico; relativo à gastroscopia.

gas·tros·co·py (gas-tros′kŏ-pē). Gastroscopia; exame do interior do estômago através de um endoscópio.

gas·tro·spasm (gas′trō-spazm). Gastroespasmo; contração espasmódica das paredes do estômago.

gas·tro·splen·ic (gas-trō-splen′ik). Gastroesplênico; relativo ao estômago e ao baço. SIN gastrolienal.

gas·tro·stax·is (gas′trō-stak′sis). Gastroestaxe; termo raramente utilizado para a exsudação de sangue a partir da mucosa do estômago. [gastro- + G. *staxis*, gotejamento]

gas·tro·ste·no·sis (gas-trō-ste-nō′sis). Gastroestenose; diminuição do tamanho da cavidade do estômago. [gastro- + G. *stenōsis*, estreitamento]

gas·tros·to·ga·vage (gas-tros′tō-gă-vahzh′). Gavagem. SIN gavage (1).

gas·tros·to·la·vage (gas-tros′tō-lă-vahzh′). Gastrostolavagem; lavagem do estômago através de uma fístula gástrica.

gas·tros·to·my (gas-tros′tō-mē). Gastrostomia; estabelecimento de uma nova abertura no estômago. [gastro- + G. *stoma*, boca]
  percutaneous endoscopic g., g. endoscópica percutânea; uma g. realizada sem a abertura da cavidade abdominal; em geral envolve gastroscopia, insuflação do estômago e perfuração da parede abdominal e do estômago seguidas da colocação de um tubo especial.

gas·tro·tho·ra·cop·a·gus (gas′trō-thōr-ă-kop′ă-gŭs). Gastrotoracópagos; gêmeos ligados, unidos pelo tórax e abdome. VER conjoined *twins*, em *twin*. [gastro- + G. *thōrax*, tórax, + *pagos*, algo fixado]

gas·tro·tome (gas′trō-tōm). Gastrótomo; uma faca para incisar o estômago.

gas·trot·o·my (gas-trot′ō-mē). Gastrotomia; incisão no estômago. [gastro- + G. *tomē*, incisão]

gas·tro·to·nom·e·ter (gas′trō-tō-nom′e-ter). Gastrotonômetro; um aparelho utilizado em gastrotonometria.

gas·tro·to·nom·e·try (gas′trō-tō-nom′e-trē). Gastrotonometria; a medida da pressão intragástrica. [gastro- + G. *tonos*, tensão, + *metron*, medida]

gas·tro·tox·ic (gas-trō-tok′sik). Gastrotóxico; venenoso para o estômago.

gas·tro·tox·in (gas-trō-tok′sin). Gastrotoxina; uma citotoxina específica para as células da mucosa do estômago.

gas·tro·tro·pic (gas-trō-trop′ik). Gastrotrópico; que afeta o estômago. [gastro- + G. *tropikos*, volta]

gas·trox·ia (gas-trok′sē-ă). Gastroxia; termo raramente utilizado para a gastroxinse. [gastro- + G. *oxys*, penetrante, ácido]

gas·trox·yn·sis (gas-trok-sin′sis). Gastroxinse; termo raramente utilizado para a secreção excessiva e intermitente de suco gástrico. [gastro- + G. *oxynō*, tornar agudo, ácido]

gas·tru·la (gas′troo-lă). Gástrula; o embrião na fase do desenvolvimento que se segue à blástula; nas formas inferiores com vitelo mínimo, é uma estrutura simples formada por uma dupla camada, consistindo em ectoderma e endoderma, que circunda o arquêntero, o qual se abre para fora através do blastóporo; nas formas com vitelo considerável, a configuração da g. é grandemente

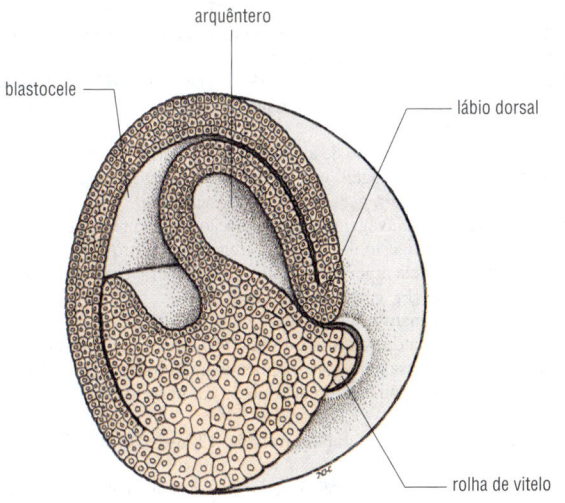

gástrula

modificada devido à persistência do vitelo durante todo o processo de gastrulação. SIN invaginate planula. [L. mod. dim. de G. *gastēr,* ventre]

gas·tru·la·tion (gas-troo-lā'shŭn). Gastrulação; transformação da blástula em gástrula; o desenvolvimento e a invaginação das camadas do broto embrionário.

Gatch, Willis D., cirurgião norte-americano, 1878–1961. VER G. *bed.*

gate (gāt). **1.** Fechar um canal iônico por meio de ação elétrica (p.ex., potencial de membrana) ou química (p.ex., neurotransmissor). **2.** Ação de uma fibra nervosa especial para bloquear a transmissão de impulsos através de uma sinapse, p.ex., barrando os impulsos dolorosos nas sinapses nos cornos dorsais. **3.** Um dispositivo que pode ser ligado e desligado eletronicamente, a fim de se controlar a passagem de um sinal. **4.** Utilizar um sinal fisiológico, tal como um ECG, para desencadear um evento, como uma exposição a raios X ou a partição de dados coletados continuamente. VER gated radionuclide *angiocardiography.* VER TAMBÉM cardiac *gating.* [I. ant. *geat*]

gate·keep·er (gāt'kēp-er). Um profissional da saúde, caracteristicamente um médico ou uma enfermeira, que tem o primeiro encontro com um paciente e que, dessa maneira, controla a entrada de pacientes no sistema de assistência médica.

gat·ing (gāt'ing). **1.** Em uma membrana biológica, a abertura e o fechamento de um canal, função que se acredita estar associada a alterações nas proteínas integrais da membrana. **2.** Um processo no qual sinais elétricos são selecionados por um portal que só deixa passar esses sinais quando existe o pulso do portal atuando como um sinal de controle, ou só deixa passar os sinais que apresentam certas características. VER gate.

cardiac gating, utilização de um sinal eletrônico, proveniente do ciclo cardíaco, a fim de desencadear um evento, tal como ocorre na criação de imagens de fases distintas da contração cardíaca.

respiratory gating, qualquer técnica que deriva um sinal proveniente da respiração para desencadear um circuito eletrônico, tal como para a coleta de dados durante a expiração. VER TAMBÉM navigator *echo.*

Gaucher, Philippe C.E., médico francês, 1854–1918. VER G. *cells,* em *cell, disease;* pseudo-G. *cell.*

Gauer, Otto Hans, fisiologista alemão, 1909–1979. VER Henry-G. *response.*

gauge (gāj). Calibrador, medidor, aferidor; um dispositivo para efetuar medições. SIN gage.

bite g., gnatodinamômetro. SIN gnathodynamometer.

Boley g., micrômetro de Boley; um instrumento de mensuração do tipo compasso, graduado em milímetros e utilizado para medir a espessura de diversos materiais dentários.

catheter g., calibrador de cateter; uma placa de metal com orifícios de diâmetro graduado utilizada para determinar o tamanho de um cateter.

strain g., calibrador de esforço; um dispositivo que emprega o princípio da ponte de Wheatstone e é utilizado para a medição acurada de forças, tais como tensão, estresse ou pressão.

undercut g., calibrador de retenção; um dispositivo, utilizado por um técnico, para localizar com precisão áreas para a colocação de componentes retentivos de grampos, ao se projetar dentaduras parciais removíveis.

gaul·the·ria oil (gawl-thēr'ē-ă). Óleo de gaultéria. SIN methyl salicylate.

gaul·the·rin (gawl'thē-rin). Gaulterina; um glicosídeo proveniente da casca de várias espécies de *Betula* (bétula); produz salicilato de metila, D-glicose e D-xilose quando submetida à hidrólise.

gaunt·let (gawnt'let). Luva. VER bandage.

Gauss, Johann K.F., físico alemão, 1777–1855. VER gauss, gaussian *curve,* gaussian *distribution.*

Gauss, Karl J., ginecologista alemão, 1875–1957. VER G. *sign.*

gauss (G) (gows). Gauss; uma unidade da intensidade de um campo magnético que equivale a 10^{-4} T. [J.K.F. *Gauss*]

Gaussel, Amans, médico francês, 1871–1937. VER Grasset-G. *phenomenon.*

gaus·si·an (gows'ē-an). Gaussiano; relativo a, ou descrito por, Johann K.F. Gauss. VER gaussian *curve.*

gauze (gawz). Gaze; um tecido de algodão branqueado de malha simples, utilizado em curativos, bandagens e esponjas absorventes; a gaze vaselinada é saturada com vaselina. [Fr. *gaze,* do Ar. *gazz,* seda crua]

ga·vage (gă-vahzh'). Gavagem. **1.** Alimentação forçada realizada através de um tubo introduzido no estômago. SIN gastrogavage, gastrostogavage. **2.** Uso terapêutico de uma dieta hipercalórica administrada através de um tubo introduzido no estômago. [Fr. *gaver,* devorar aves]

Gavard, Hyacinthe, anatomista francês, 1753–1802. VER G. *muscle.*

Gay, Alexander H., anatomista russo, 1842–1907. VER G. *glands,* em *gland.*

gay (gā). **1.** Um homossexual, principalmente um homem. **2.** Denotando um indivíduo homossexual ou o estilo de vida de um homem homossexual. VER lesbian.

Gay-Lussac, Joseph L., naturalista francês, 1778–1850. VER Gay-Lussac *equation;* Gay-Lussac *law.*

gaze (gāz). Olhar fixo; o ato de olhar de forma constante para um objeto.

conjugate g., olhar fixo conjugado; o movimento dos dois olhos com os eixos visuais paralelos.

dysconjugate g., olhar fixo não-conjugado; incapacidade de ambos os olhos de virar juntos para a mesma direção.

G-band·ing. Coloração de banda G. VER G-banding *stain.*

GBG Abreviatura de gonadal steroid-binding *globulin* (globulina ligadora de esteróide gonadal).

GBH Abreviatura de gamma benzene hexachloride (hexacloreto de gamabenzeno).

GC Abreviatura do par de bases guanina e citosina presente nos ácidos polinucleicos.

G-CSF Abreviatura de granulocyte colony-stimulatin *factor* (fator estimulante de colônias de glanulócitos).

Gd Símbolo do gadolínio.

GDP Abreviatura de guanosine 5'-diphosphate (guanosina 5'-difosfato).

GDP man·nose phos·pho·ryl·ase. GDP manose fosforilase. SIN mannose-1-phosphate guanylyltransferase (GDP).

Ge Símbolo do germânio.

Ge·doel·stia (ge-del'stē-ă). Um gênero de moscas varejeiras nasais (família Oestridae) que engloba as espécies *G. cristata* e *G. haessleri,* que parasitam gnus, caama e outros antílopes africanos e podem também causar oftalmomiíase em ovinos e seres humanos.

ge·doel·sti·o·sis (ge-del-sti-ō'sis). Gedoelstiose; infestação por larvas de moscas do gênero *Gedoelstia* que afeta herbívoros e raramente seres humanos, causando, nestes últimos, oftalmomiíase. SIN bulging eye disease.

Gehrig, Henry Louis, jogador norte-americano de beisebol; 1903–1941, vítima da doença de Lou Gehrig. VER Lou Gehrig *disease.*

Geigel, Richard, médico alemão, 1859–1930. VER G. *reflex.*

Geiger, Hans, físico alemão, 1882–1945. VER G.-Müller *counter, tube.*

gel (jel). **1.** Gel; uma gelatina ou a fase sólida ou semi-sólida de uma solução coloidal. SIN gelatum. **2.** Formar um gel ou uma gelatina; converter um sol em gel. [L. mod. *gelatum*]

colloidal g., gel coloidal; um colóide que desenvolveu resistência para fluir em conseqüência de alteração química ou térmica.

pharmacopeial g., gel farmacopeico; uma suspensão, em um meio aquoso, de uma substância insolúvel na forma hidratada na qual o tamanho das partículas se aproxima das dimensões coloidais ou as alcança.

gel·ate (jel'āt). Gelatinizar. SIN gelatinize.

gel·a·tin (jel'ă-tin). Gelatina; uma proteína derivada formada a partir do colágeno dos tecidos por meio de fervura em água; incha quando colocada em água fria e dissolve-se somente em água quente; utilizada como um hemostato, substituto do plasma e alimento proteico auxiliar na desnutrição. [L *gelo,* pp. *gelatus,* congelar, coagular]

glycerinated g., g. glicerinada; uma preparação feita com partes iguais de g. e glicerina; uma massa firme que se liquefaz sob calor brando; é utilizada como veículo para supositórios e velas uretrais. SIN glycerin jelly, glycerogelatin, glycogelatin.

Irish moss g., g. de musgo-de-irlanda; g. extraída do musgo-de-irlanda; utilizada para fazer a mucilagem do musgo-de-irlanda, empregada como um substituto da goma arábica no preparo de emulsões.

vegetable g., g. vegetal; uma substância semelhante à g. e obtida do glúten.

zinc g., g. zíncica. VER zinc gelatin.

gel·a·tin·ase (jel'ă-tin-ās). Gelatinase; pepsina B; uma metaloproteinase que hidrolisa a gelatina e vários tipos de colágeno. VER pepsin.

ge·la·ti·nif·er·ous (jel'ă-ti-nif'er-ŭs). Que produz ou contém gelatina ou apresenta uma qualidade semelhante à do gel. [gelatin + L. *fero,* conter]

ge·lat·i·ni·za·tion (jē-lat'i-ni-zā'shŭn). Gelatinização; conversão em gelatina ou em uma substância semelhante.

ge·lat·i·nize (jē-lat'i-nīz). Gelatinizar. **1.** Converter em gelatina. **2.** Tornar-se gelatinoso. SIN gelate.

ge·lat·i·noid (jē-lat'i-noyd). Gelatinóide. SIN gelatinous (2).

ge·lat·i·nous (jē-lat'i-nŭs). Gelatinoso. **1.** Relativo à, ou característico da, gelatina. **2.** Semelhante à geléia ou que se assemelha à gelatina. SIN gelatinoid.

ge·la·tion (jē-lā'shŭn). Gelação. **1.** Em química coloidal, a transformação de um sol em um gel. **2.** A solidificação de um líquido por meio de temperaturas frias.

ge·la·tum (jē-lā'tŭm). Gel. SIN gel (1). [L. mod.]

Gélineau, Jean Baptiste Edouard, médico francês, 1859–1906. VER G. *syndrome.*

Gell, Philip G.H., imunologista britânico. VER G. and Coombs *reactions,* em *reaction.*

Gellé, Marie-Ernst, otologista francês, 1834–1923. VER G. *test.*

Gellerstedt, Nils, *1896. VER Ceelen-G. *syndrome.*

ge·lo·sis (je-lō'sis). Gelose; uma massa extremamente firme encontrada em tecidos (principalmente em músculos), que apresenta uma consistência que se assemelha à do tecido congelado. [L. *gelo,* congelar, coagular, + G. *-osis,* condição]

gel·se·mine (jel'sē-mēn). Gelsemina; um alcalóide cristalizável derivado do gelsêmio (jasmim-amarelo); midriático e estimulante do sistema nervoso central. [L. mod. *gelsemium,* do Pers. *yāsmin,* jasmim]

gel·so·lin (jel-sol'in). Gelsolina; uma proteína que se liga à actina; uma proteína que separa os filamentos de actina e é ativada pelo Ca^{2+}; está relacionada, portanto, com a locomoção, secreção e endocitose.

Gély, Jules A., cirurgião francês, 1806–1861. VER G. *suture*.

gem-. Prefixo que indica substituições gêmeas em um único átomo; p.ex., a substituição *gem*-dimetil no carbono 4 do lanosterol. [L. *geminus*, gêmeo]

Ge·mel·la (jĕ - mel′a). Um gênero de bactérias cocóides, aeróbicas, anaeróbicas facultativas e móveis (família Streptococcaceae) que são observadas isoladas ou em pares, com os lados adjacentes achatados. Apresentam coloração indeterminada pelo Gram, porém possuem uma parede celular como aquela das bactérias Gram-positivas e são parasitas de mamíferos. A espécie típica é *G. haemolysans*, que é encontrada nas secreções brônquicas e no muco do trato respiratório. [L. dim. de *geminus*, gêmeo]

G. morbillorum, uma bactéria microaerófila, antigamente denominada *Streptococcus morbilorum*, incapaz de produzir β-hemólise em ágar-sangue e que não apresenta antígenos de sorogrupos distinguíveis; causa infecções graves em alguns pacientes semelhante às infecções por *Streptococcus viridans*.

ge·mel·lol·o·gy (jem - el - ol′ō - jē). O estudo de gêmeos e do fenômeno da gemelidade. [L. *gemellus*, nascido gêmeo, + G. *logos*, estudo]

ge·mel·lus (jĕ - mel′us). Gêmeo. SIN inferior gemellus (*muscle*), superior gemellus (*muscle*). [L. dim. de *geminus*, gêmeo]

gem·fi·bro·zil (jem - fī′brō - zil). Genfibrozila; um agente anti-hiperlipidêmico.

gem·i·nate (jem′i - nāt). Geminado; que está disposto aos pares. SIN geminous. [L. *gemino*, pp. *-atus*, duplicar, de *geminus*, gêmeo]

gem·i·na·tion (jem - i - nā′shŭn). Geminação; divisão embriológica parcial de um primórdio. Por exemplo, a g. de um único germe de dente resulta em duas coroas parcial ou completamente separadas sobre uma única raiz. [L. *geminatio*, uma duplicação]

gem·i·nous (jem′i - nŭs). Geminado. SIN geminate.

ge·mis·to·cyte (jĕ - mis′tō - sīt). Gemistócito. SIN gemistocytic *astrocyte*. [G. *gemistos*, carregado, de *gemizō*, encher, + cito]

ge·mis·to·cy·to·ma (jĕ - mis′tō - sī - tō′ma). Gemistocitoma. SIN gemistocytic *astrocytoma*.

gem·ma (jem′a). Gema; qualquer corpo semelhante a um botão ou bulbo, principalmente uma papila gustativa ou botão terminal. [L. botão (flor)]

gem·ma·tion (jem - ā′shŭn). Gemação, brotamento; uma forma de fissão na qual a célula-mãe não se divide, porém exterioriza um pequeno processo semelhante a um botão (célula-filha) com sua quantidade proporcional de cromatina; a célula-filha, em seguida, separa-se para começar uma existência independente. SIN bud fission, budding. [L. *gemma*, um botão]

gem·mule (jem′ūl). Gêmula. **1.** Um pequeno broto que se projeta da célula-mãe e se torna, no final, isolado, formando uma célula de uma nova origem. **2.** SIN dendritic *spines*, em *spine*. [L. *gemmula*, dim. de *gemma*, botão (de flor)]

Hoboken g.'s, gêmulas de Hoboken. SIN Hoboken *nodules*, em *nodule*.

gen-. Que nasce, que produz, que vem a ser. [G. *genos*, nascimento]

-gen. Sufixo que indica "precursor de". VER TAMBÉM pro- (2).

ge·na (jē′na). Gena; bochecha. SIN cheek. [L.]

ge·nal (jē′nal). Genal; relativo à gena ou à bochecha.

gen·der (jen′der). Gênero; categoria para a qual um indivíduo é designado por si mesmo ou por outros, de acordo com o sexo. Cf. sex, gender *role*.

gene (jēn). Gene; uma unidade funcional de hereditariedade que ocupa um lugar específico (*locus*) em um cromossoma, é capaz de auto-reproduzir-se com exatidão a cada divisão celular e controla a formação de uma enzima ou outra proteína. O g., como uma unidade funcional, consiste em um segmento bem definido de uma molécula gigante de DNA que contém as bases purínicas (adenina e guanina) e pirimidínicas (citosina e timina) na seqüência correta para codificar a seqüência de aminoácidos de um peptídeo específico. A síntese de proteínas é mediada por moléculas de RNA mensageiro formadas sobre o cromossoma, com o g. atuando como modelo. O RNA passa, em seguida, para o citoplasma e orienta-se sobre os ribossomas, onde ele, por sua vez, age como um modelo, com o propósito de organizar uma cadeia de aminoácidos a fim de formar um peptídeo. Nos organismos que se reproduzem sexuadamente, o g. encontra-se em geral disposto aos pares em todas as células, exceto nos gametas, como conseqüência do fato de que todos os cromossomas são pareados, exceto os cromossomas sexuais (X e Y) do macho. SIN factor (3). [G. *genos*, nascimento]

allelic g., g. alélico. VER allele, *dominance* of traits.

autosomal g., g. autossômico; um g. localizado em qualquer cromossoma, exceto nos cromossomas sexuais (X e Y).

BRCA1 g., g. BRCA1; um g. supressor de tumor localizado no *locus* 17q21, do cromossoma 17, e isolado em 1994; codifica a proteína p53, a qual impede que as células com DNA danificado se dividam; as portadoras de mutações na linhagem germinativa situada no g. BRCA1 são predispostas a desenvolver tanto câncer de mama como de ovário. VER TAMBÉM BRCA2 g., *carcinoma* of the breast.

BRCA2 g., g. BRCA2; um g. supressor de tumor identificado em 1995 no *locus* 13q12-q13 do cromossoma 13; um g. grande composto por 27 exons distribuídos por 70 kb e que codifica uma proteína de 3.418 aminoácidos; as portadoras de mutações de linhagem germinativa no g. BRCA2 correm um risco aumentado, semelhante ao risco apresentado pelas portadoras de mutações no g. BRCA1, de desenvolver câncer de mama e um risco moderadamente elevado de desenvolver câncer de ovário; as famílias com o g. BRCA2 também exibem uma incidência aumentada de câncer de mama masculina, de pâncreas, de próstata, de laringe e nos olhos. VER TAMBÉM BRCA1 g., *carcinoma* of the breast.

A ocorrência de câncer de mama em vários membros de uma mesma família é conhecida há muito tempo. Os cânceres de mama familiais são caracterizados por início antes dos 45 anos e pelo acometimento de três ou mais parentes próximas pertencentes a diferentes gerações. Cerca de 5% de todos os cânceres de mama resultam de herança de genes de suscetibilidade dominante, sobretudo BRCA1 e BRCA2. Enquanto as mutações espontâneas dos genes BRCA são incomuns, centenas de mutações herdadas têm sido descobertas em cada gene. A importância clínica de muitas delas é desconhecida. Como estes são cromossomas autossômicos, tanto homens como mulheres podem herdar e transmitir as mutações nos genes BRCA. A histologia do câncer de mama de mulheres com mutações nos genes BRCA1 e BRCA2 difere daquela dos casos esporádicos. A proporção de carcinomas medulares é mais alta entre os cânceres de mama associados ao g. BRCA1 do que entre todos os cânceres de mama. BRCA1 e BRCA2 são genes supressores de tumor e, quando estão funcionando normalmente, inibem o desenvolvimento de tumores. Ambos são genes grandes que codificam proteínas grandes com carga elétrica negativa. As mutações inativadoras identificadas até o momento estão distribuídas nos dois genes, com uma predominância de duas mutações distintas para BRCA1 e uma para BRCA2. Apesar da alta penetrância do gene mutante, nem todos os portadores desenvolvem câncer. Fatores hormonais, ambientais, reprodutivos e outros fatores genéticos podem influenciar a penetrância. O estradiol aumenta a proliferação e a produção celular do produto do gene BRCA1 *in vitro*, enquanto o tamoxifeno, um antagonista do estrógeno, inibe não só a proliferação celular, como também a expressão do gene BRCA1. As mutações observadas estão distribuídas por todo o gene; a maioria dessas mutações consiste em inserções, deleções ou mutações sem sentido. Duas alterações comuns (185delAG e 5382insC nos exons 2 e 20, respectivamente) são responsáveis por cerca de 19% das mutações no BRCA1. A primeira delas é encontrada em cerca de 1% dos judeus Ashkenazi e é responsável por cerca de 32% dos cânceres de mama familiais em judeus. É também encontrada em 13% das pacientes com câncer de ovário, sem história familiar de câncer de mama ou de ovário, e em 30% daquelas com história familiar, o que sugere uma doença hereditária. As mutações em BRCA1 causam um aumento de três vezes no risco de câncer de próstata em homens e um aumento de quatro vezes no risco de câncer de cólon em homens e mulheres. Estima-se que a mutação 6174delT do g. BRCA2 exista em 1,3% dos judeus Ashkenazi. As estimativas mais antigas mostravam que o risco de uma mulher com uma mutação nos genes BRCA1 ou BRCA2 desenvolver câncer de mama em algum momento em sua vida variava de 10 a 90%. Esses números foram baseados em um estudo intensivo de famílias reconhecidamente de risco. As estimativas atuais mostram que o risco de câncer de mama pode não ser maior que 30%. Além disso, 15 a 20% das mulheres com a mutação do g. BRCA1 desenvolverão câncer de ovário. Embora já existam no comércio testes para detectar as mutações genéticas em BRCA, a maioria das autoridades médicas não recomenda o rastreamento de rotina, exceto em mulheres com uma significativa história familiar de câncer. Quando se constata que a paciente tem mutações genéticas em BRCA, ela é aconselhada a começar o auto-exame da mama aos 18 anos de idade e a começar a realizar exames médicos e mamografias anuais e regulares aos 25 anos de idade. O benefício do rastreamento radiológico tem de ser avaliado em função do possível efeito da radiação sobre BRCA1 e alelo BRCA2. Além disso, as mamografias são, com freqüência, difíceis de interpretar nas mulheres jovens, por causa da densidade do tecido mamário. As portadoras de BRCA2 são também aconselhadas a iniciar uma vigilância sobre o câncer de ovário, consistindo no rastreamento anual ou semestral que utiliza a ultra-sonografia transvaginal com Doppler de fluxo colorido e o índice morfológico e da determinação dos níveis séricos de CA-125 aos 25 a 35 anos de idade. O incentivo para a realização de mastectomia e ooforectomia profiláticas está diminuindo à medida que se torna evidente que esses procedimentos drásticos não conseguem extinguir por completo o risco de câncer. Já se constatou que o tamoxifeno reduz o risco de câncer de mama em até 45% nas mulheres geneticamente predispostas.

C g., g. C; o g. que codifica as regiões constantes das cadeias de imunoglobulinas.

codominant g., g. codominante; um conjunto de dois ou mais alelos, cada um expresso fenotipicamente na presença do outro.

control g., g. de controle. VER operator g., regulator g.
dominant g., g. dominante. VER *dominance* of traits.
extrachromosomal g., g. extracromossômico; um g. localizado fora do núcleo (p.ex., os genes mitocondriais).
H g., g. H. SIN histocompatibility g.
histocompatibility g., g. de histocompatibilidade; em animais de laboratório, um g. que pode desencadear uma resposta imune e, desse modo, causar a rejeição de um homoenxerto, quando o tecido é transplantado de um indivíduo para outro; nos seres humanos, os genes de histocompatibilidade controlam os antígenos HLA. SIN H g.
holandric g., g. holândrico. SIN Y-linked g.
homeotic g.'s, genes homeóticos; um grupo de genes que regulam o desenvolvimento das partes do corpo ao definir os limites de várias regiões.
housekeeping g.'s, genes de manutenção; genes que geralmente sempre são expressos; acredita-se que esses genes estão envolvidos no metabolismo celular de rotina.
immune response g.'s, genes da resposta imune; genes localizados na região HLA-D do complexo de histocompatibilidade do cromossoma humano 6 que controla a resposta imune a antígenos específicos.
jumping g., g. saltador; um g. associado a elementos transponíveis. VER transposon.
lethal g., g. letal; um g. que produz um genótipo que leva à morte do organismo, antes que a reprodução seja possível, ou que impede a reprodução; tanto a homozigose como a heterozigose de um g. recessivo são letais.
microophthalmia transcription factor g., g. do fator de transcrição da microftalmia; g. que, quando sofre mutação, causa a síndrome de Waardenburg do tipo 2 e a síndrome de Tietz em, pelo menos, alguns subconjuntos de famílias com essas síndromes transmitidas por herança autossômica dominante.
mimic g.'s, genes mimetizantes; genes não-alelos com efeitos quase semelhantes, p.ex., a eliptocitose.
mitochondrial g., g. mitocondrial; um g. funcionante que não está localizado no núcleo de uma célula e, sim, no cromossoma da mitocôndria.
modifier g., g. modificador; um g. não-alelo que controla ou altera as manifestações de um g., ao interferir com sua transcrição.
mutant g., g. mutante; um g. que foi modificado de um tipo ancestral, não necessariamente na geração atual. VER TAMBÉM mutant, mutation.
operator g., g. operador; um g. com a função de ativar a produção de RNA mensageiro por meio de um ou mais *loci* estruturais adjacentes; parte do sistema de retroalimentação para a determinação da velocidade de produção de uma enzima.
pleiotropic g., g. pleiotrópico; um g. que apresenta manifestações fenotípicas múltiplas e aparentemente não relacionadas. SIN polyphenic g.
polyphenic g., g. pleiotrópico. SIN pleiotropic g.
regulator g., g. regulador; um g. que produz uma substância repressora, a qual se combina com um g. operador, inibindo-o. O g. impede, dessa forma, a produção de uma enzima específica. Quando a enzima se torna novamente necessária, um metabólito regulador específico inibe a substância repressora.
repressor g., g. repressor; um g. que impede que um g. não-alelo seja transcrito.
SOS g.'s, genes SOS; um grupo de genes envolvidos na reparação do DNA, com freqüência induzida por um dano grave o suficiente para causar a parada da síntese de DNA.
g. splicing, entrançamento de genes. SIN splicing (1).
split g.'s, genes fragmentados; genes nos quais as seqüências genômicas estão interrompidas por seqüências intervenientes (introns), que são retiradas do ARNm antes da tradução.
structural g., g. estrutural; um g. que codifica uma proteína ou um peptídeo específico.
transfer g.'s, genes de transferência; genes transportados por um plasmídeo conjugativo; são essenciais para a fertilidade e para o estabelecimento do estado de doador bacteriano.
transforming g., g. transformador. SIN oncogene.

tumor suppressor g., g. supressor de tumor; um gene que codifica uma proteína envolvida no controle do crescimento celular; a inativação desse tipo de gene leva à proliferação celular desordenada, como ocorre no câncer. VER TAMBÉM oncogene. SIN antioncogene.

> Em uma pessoa nascida com duas cópias normais de um gene supressor de tumor, as duas cópias têm de ser inativadas por meio de mutação pontual espontânea, deleção ou incapacidade de expressão antes que a formação do tumor ocorra. Uma mutação herdada em um gene supressor de tumor é a base da maioria das predisposições familiais ao câncer. Em uma pessoa assim predisposta, a proliferação celular maligna não acontece até que a cópia intacta restante do gene seja inativada por deleção de parte do seu cromossoma ou de todo ele. Dos muitos genes supressores de tumor, identificados até agora, o gene p53 do cromossoma 17, que codifica uma fosfoproteína que suprime a proliferação celular, parece ser o mais importante. As mutações de p53 têm sido encontradas no DNA de mais da metade de todos os cânceres humanos estudados. A síndrome de Li-Fraumeni, caracterizada por carcinomas e sarcomas de início precoce, é uma mutação herdada (autossômica dominante) no gene supressor de tumor p53. BRCA1 e BRCA2, envolvidos no câncer de mama de início precoce e no câncer de ovário, são genes supressores de tumores.

V g., g. V; o g. que codifica a parte principal da região variável de uma cadeia de imunoglobulina.
X-linked g., g. ligado ao X; um g. localizado em um cromossoma X.
Y-linked g., g. ligado ao Y; um g. localizado em um cromossoma Y. SIN holandric g.
Z g., g. Z; o g. estrutural para a β-galactosidase.
ge·ne·al·o·gy (jē-nē-awl'ō-jē). 1. Hereditariedade. 2. O agrupamento definido dos descendentes de uma pessoa ou família; pode ser de qualquer tamanho. [G. *genea*, descendência, + *logos*, estudo]
gene li·brary. Biblioteca de genes; um agrupamento aleatório de fragmentos de DNA clonado no interior de um vetor que pode conter informações genéticas sobre uma espécie.
gen·era (jen'er-a). Plural de genus (gênero).
gen·er·al·ist (jen'er-ăl-ist). Generalista; um médico generalista ou um médico de família; um médico treinado para tratar da maioria das doenças que não exigem cirurgia, incluindo, às vezes, procedimentos obstétricos.
gen·er·al·i·za·tion (jen'er-ăl-i-zā'shun). Generalização. 1. Que se torna geral, difuso ou disseminado, como quando uma doença primariamente focal se torna sistêmica. 2. O raciocínio através do qual se chega a uma conclusão básica, a qual se aplica a diferentes itens, cada um apresentando algum fator comum.
  stimulus g., g. do estímulo; no condicionamento pavloviano, a produção de uma resposta condicionada por meio de estímulos que nunca foram experimentados, mas que são similares a um determinado estímulo condicionado. VER conditioning, classical *conditioning*.
gen·er·al·ized (jen'er-ă-līzd). Generalizado; que envolve um órgão inteiro, em oposição a um processo focal ou regional.
gen·er·ate (jen'er-āt). 1. Gerar; produzir. 2. Procriar. [L. *genero*, pp. *-atus*, gerar]
gen·er·a·tion (jen-er-ā'shun). Geração; reprodução. 1. SIN reproduction (1). 2. Um estágio distinto na sucessão da descendência; p.ex., pai, filho e neto representam três gerações. [L. *generatio*, de *genero*, pp. *-atus*, gerar]
  asexual g., reprodução assexuada; reprodução por fissão, gemação, ou de qualquer outro modo, sem que ocorra a união da célula masculina com a feminina ou conjugação. VER TAMBÉM parthenogenesis. SIN heterogenesis (2), nonsexual g.
  filial g. (F), g. filial; a prole de um cruzamento (acasalamento) geneticamente especificado: primeira g. filial (símbolo F_1), a prole de pais de genótipos contrastantes; segunda g. filial (F_2), a prole de dois indivíduos F_1; terceira g. filial (F_3), quarta g. filial (F_4), etc., a prole em gerações bem-sucedidas de cruzamentos co-sanguíneos contínuos de descendentes F_1.
  nonsexual g., reprodução assexuada. SIN asexual g.
  parental g. (P_1), g. parental; os pais de um cruzamento, geralmente experimental, que envolve genótipos contrastantes; o casal original de um experimento genético; os pais da geração F_1.
  sexual g., reprodução sexuada; reprodução por conjugação ou a união de células masculina e feminina, em oposição a g. assexuada.
  skipped g., g. salteada; um fenômeno de heredogramas no qual um gene é transmitido de uma pessoa afetada para outra através de uma pessoa fenotipicamente não-afetada, por meio de recessividade (principalmente para traços ligados ao X), epistasia, expressividade variável ou ausência de um desafio ambiental, como uma toxina. A não ser em um nível fenotípico (p.ex., clínico ou comercial), esse termo torna-se progressivamente menos útil à medida que os mecanismos são elucidados.
  spontaneous g., g. espontânea; o conceito errôneo segundo o qual a matéria viva pode surgir por meio da vitalização de matéria morta. VER TAMBÉM biogenesis. SIN heterogenesis (3).
  virgin g., partenogênese. SIN parthenogenesis.
gen·er·a·tion·al. Relativo às gerações, isto é, o estagiamento bem definido na linhagem genealógica.
gen·er·a·tive (jen'er-ă-tiv). Generativo; relativo ao processo de geração.
gen·er·a·tor (jen'er-ā-ter). Gerador; um aparelho para a conversão de energia química, mecânica, atômica ou outro tipo de energia em eletricidade. [*generator*, um gerador, produtor]
  aerosol g., g. de aerosol; um dispositivo para a produção de suspensões aéreas de pequenas partículas para terapia inalatória ou trabalho experimental; p.ex., o g. La Mer, o disco de rotação ou a lâmina vibratória, cada um dos quais produz um aerosol monodisperso.
  asynchronous pulse g., g. de pulsos assíncronos; um g. no qual a freqüência de descarga é independente da atividade natural do coração. SIN fixed rate pulse g.

atrial synchronous pulse g., g. de pulsos síncronos atriais; um pulso estimulador de ventrículo cuja freqüência de descarga é determinada diretamente pela freqüência atrial. SIN atrial triggered pulse g.

atrial triggered pulse g., g. de pulsos de disparo atriais. SIN atrial synchronous pulse g.

demand pulse g., g. de pulsos de demanda. SIN ventricular inhibited pulse g.

fixed rate pulse g., g. de pulsos de freqüência fixa. SIN asynchronous pulse g.

pulse g., g. de pulsos; um dispositivo que produz uma descarga elétrica com uma onda de formato regular ou rítmico e no qual a força eletromotriz varia em um padrão específico em relação ao tempo; p.ex., em um marcapasso eletrônico, ele produz uma descarga elétrica a intervalos regulares, e esses intervalos podem ser modificados por um circuito sensor que pode reajustar o tempo de referência para a descarga subseqüente, de acordo com outra atividade elétrica, tal como aquela produzida pelo batimento cardíaco espontâneo.

radionuclide g., g. de radionuclídeos; uma coluna que contém uma grande quantidade de um determinado radionuclídeo (radionuclídeo-mãe) que se decompõe em um segundo radionuclídeo de meia-vida física mais curta; o radionuclídeo-filho é separado do radionuclídeo-mãe pelo processo da eluição e fornece um suprimento contínuo de radionuclídeos de vida relativamente curta para serem utilizados em laboratório; a eluição é vulgarmente denominada "milking" ("ordenha") e o gerador referido como uma "radioactive cow" ("vaca radioativa").

standby pulse g., g. de pulsos sobressalente. SIN ventricular inhibited pulse g.

ventricular inhibited pulse g., g. de pulsos inibidos ventriculares; um g. que suprime seu estímulo em resposta a uma atividade ventricular natural e que, na ausência dessa atividade, funciona como um g. de pulsos assíncronos. SIN demand pulse g., standby pulse g.

ventricular synchronous pulse g., g. de pulsos síncronos ventriculares; um g. que libera seu estímulo de modo síncrono com a atividade ventricular natural e que, na ausência dessa atividade, funciona como um g. de pulsos assíncronos. SIN ventricular triggered pulse g.

ventricular triggered pulse g., g. de pulsos de disparo ventriculares. SIN ventricular synchronous pulse g.

x-ray g., g. de raios X; o dispositivo eletrônico que controla a produção de raios X em uma radiografia; a função-chave é a retificação da voltagem (tensão) de linha para produzir uma voltagem de corrente contínua suave para o tubo de raios X.

ge·ner·ic (jē-nār′ik). Genérico. **1.** Relativo a, ou que indica, um gênero. **2.** Geral. **3.** Característico ou distintivo. [L. *genus* (*gener*-), nascimento]

ge·ner·ic name. Nome genérico. **1.** Em química, um substantivo que indica a classe ou o tipo de um único composto; p.ex., sal, sacarídeo (açúcar), hexose, álcool, aldeído, lactona, ácido, amina, alcano, esteróide, vitamina. O termo "classe" é mais apropriado e mais freqüentemente utilizado do que o "nome genérico". **2.** Nos campos farmacêutico e comercial, um nome impróprio para o nome não-patenteado. **3.** Em ciências biológicas, a primeira parte do nome científico (combinação binária latina ou binômio) de um organismo; escrito com uma letra maiúscula inicial e em itálico. Em bacteriologia, o nome da espécie é composto de duas partes (que formam um nome): o n. g. e o epíteto específico; em outras disciplinas da biologia, o nome da espécie é considerado como sendo composto por dois nomes: o n. g. e o nome específico.

ge·ne·si·al (je-nē′sē-ăl). Genésico; relativo à geração.

ge·ne·si·ol·o·gy (je-nē-sē-ol′ō-jē). Genesiologia; o ramo da ciência que trata da geração ou da reprodução. [G. *genesis*, geração, + *logos*, estudo]

gen·e·sis (jen′ĕ-sis). Gênese; origem ou processo inicial; também utilizado como uma forma combinante na posição de sufixo. [G.]

ge·net·ic (jē-net′ik). Genético; relativo à genética.

ge·net·i·cist (jē-net′i-sist). Geneticista; um especialista em genética.

ge·net·ics (jē-net′iks). Genética. **1.** O ramo da ciência que trata dos meios e das conseqüências da transmissão e da geração dos componentes de herança biológica. **2.** As características genéticas e a constituição de qualquer organismo isolado ou de um conjunto de organismos. [G. *genesis*, origem ou produção]

behavioral g., g. do comportamento; o estudo de fatores hereditários em padrões de comportamento por meio da análise da linhagem, de anormalidades bioquímicas ou do cariótipo.

biochemical g., g. bioquímica; o estudo da g. em função de eventos químicos (bioquímicos); estuda-se, p.ex., a maneira pela qual as moléculas de ADN se replicam e controlam a síntese de enzimas específicas por meio do código genético.

classical g., g. clássica; o método e a análise que entendem a g. como o estudo da transmissão do genótipo dos genitores para a prole; o estudo de muitos indivíduos é essencial para ela.

clinical g., g. clínica; g. aplicada ao diagnóstico, ao prognóstico, ao tratamento e à prevenção de doenças genéticas. Cf. medical g.

epidemiologic g., g. epidemiológica; o estudo da g. como um fenômeno de populações definidas pelos critérios, métodos e objetivos da epidemiologia, em vez da g. de populações.

galtonian g., g. galtoniana; o estudo dos traços pela análise dos primeiros dois momentos de dados métricos; o método de escolha para a análise dos traços que seguem a distribuição gaussiana multivariada.

Galtonian-Fisher g., g. de Galton-Fisher; a g. dos traços mensuráveis determinados pelos múltiplos *loci* que contribuem de forma independente, aditiva e aproximadamente igual. SIN multilocal g.

human g., g. humana; o estudo das características genéticas dos seres humanos considerados como uma espécie. Cf. medical g.

mathematical g., g. matemática; o estudo dos traços genéticos por meio da análise formal, p.ex., a g. quantitativa, a dinâmica das populações, a epidemiologia genética e a modelagem.

medical g., g. médica; o estudo da etiologia, da patogenia e da história natural das doenças humanas que apresentam, pelo menos, uma origem genética. Cf. clinical g., human g.

mendelian g., g. mendeliana; o estudo do padrão de segregação de fenótipos sob o controle de *loci* genéticos tomados um a um.

microbial g., g. microbiana; o estudo dos mecanismos hereditários dos micróbios.

modern g., g. moderna; o método e a análise que entendem a g. como o estudo da economia dos ácidos nucleicos e dos compostos associados.

molecular g., g. molecular; biologia molecular aplicada à g.

multilocal g., g. de Galton-Fisher. SIN Galtonian-Fisher g.

population g., g. das populações; o estudo das influências genéticas sobre os componentes de causa e efeito nas características somáticas das populações.

quantitative g., g. quantitativa; o estudo formal dos traços genéticos mensuráveis, tradicionalmente, mas não necessariamente limitados à g. galtoniana.

reverse g., g. reversa; termo que se refere à investigação de um gene responsável por uma doença por meio do aprendizado de sua posição no genoma humano. Essa abordagem não tem a pretensão de fornecer informações sobre o produto do gene. SIN positional cloning.

somatic cell g., g. das células somáticas; o estudo da estrutura, da organização e da função de um genoma por meio das técnicas de hibridização celular.

statistical g., g. estatística; o estudo das aplicações dos princípios da estatística à medicina da genética.

transplantation g., g. dos transplantes; g. aplicada ao transplante de tecidos de um animal para outro.

ge·net·o·tro·phic (jē-net-ō-trof′ik). Relativo a diferenças individuais herdadas nas necessidades nutricionais. [G. *genesis*, origem, + *trophē*, nutrição]

Ge·ne·va Con·ven·tion. Convenção de Genebra; um acordo internacional firmado em encontros em Genebra, Suíça, em 1864 e 1906, relacionado (entre questões médicas) com a salvaguarda dos feridos em batalhas, daqueles que cuidam deles e dos edifícios onde estão sendo tratados. A conseqüência direta do primeiro desses encontros foi a criação da Sociedade da Cruz Vermelha.

Ge·ne·va lens mea·sure. Medida da lente de Genebra. Ver em measure.

Gengou, Octave, bacteriologista francês, 1875–1957. VER G. *phenomenon*; Bordet-G. potato blood *agar, bacillus, phenomenon*; Bordet and G. *reaction*.

ge·ni·al, ge·ni·an (jē-nī′ăl, -nī′an). Mentoniano; mental. SIN mental (2). [G. *geneion*, queixo]

△ **-genic.** -gênico; que produz, que forma, produzido, formado por. [G. *genos*, nascimento]

ge·nic·u·la (je-nik′ū-lă). Plural de geniculum.

ge·nic·u·lar (je-nik′ū-lăr). Genicular, da região do joelho, *q.v.*

ge·nic·u·late (je-nik′ū-lāt). **1.** Geniculado; dobrado como um joelho. SIN geniculated. **2.** Que se refere ao joelho do nervo facial, que indica o gânglio que aí se encontra. **3.** Que indica o corpo geniculado medial ou lateral. [L. *geniculo*, pp. *-atus*, dobrar o joelho, de *genu*, joelho]

ge·nic·u·lat·ed (je-nik′ū-lā-ted). Geniculado. SIN geniculate (1).

ge·nic·u·lum, pl. **ge·nic·u·la** (je-nik′ū-lŭm, -lă). Joelho. **1** [TA]. Um pequeno joelho ou uma estrutura angular semelhante ao joelho. **2.** Uma estrutura semelhante a um nó. [L. dim. de *genu*, joelho]

g. cana′lis facia′lis [TA], joelho do canal do nervo facial. SIN g. of facial canal.

g. of facial canal [TA], joelho do canal do nervo facial; a dobra situada no canal do nervo facial que liga os pilares medial e lateral da parte horizontal do canal e que corresponde ao local do gânglio geniculado do nervo facial. SIN g. canalis facialis [TA], genu of facial canal.

g. of facial nerve [TA], joelho do nervo facial. **(1)** Uma dobra aguda do nervo facial no canal facial onde o nervo se curva posteriormente, a partir de seu trajeto previamente anterior, para correr dentro da parede medial da orelha média (joelho externo); **(2)** alça complexa de fibras do nervo facial situada ao redor do núcleo abducente (joelho interno). SIN g. nervus facialis [TA].

g. ner′vus facia′lis [TA], joelho do nervo facial. SIN g. of facial nerve.

△ **-genin.** -genina; sufixo utilizado para indicar a unidade esteróide básica da substância tóxica, em geral um glicosídeo esteróide (p.ex., a porção aglicona).

ge·ni·o·glos·sus (jē′nī-ō-glos′ŭs). Genioglosso. SIN genioglossus (*muscle*). [G. *geneion*, queixo, + *glōssa*, língua]

ge·ni·o·hy·oid (jē-nī′ō-hī′oyd). Genioióideo. SIN geniohyoid (*muscle*).

ge·ni·o·hy·oi·de·us (jē-nī′ō-hī-oyd′ē-ŭs). Genioióideo. SIN geniohyoid (*muscle*). [G. *geneion*, queixo, + *hyoeidēs*, com forma de Y, hióide]

ge·ni·on (jē-nī'on). Gênio; a ponta da espinha mentoniana, um ponto craniométrico. [G. *geneion*, queixo]

ge·ni·o·plas·ty (jē'nī-ō-plas-tē). Genioplastia; correção cirúrgica do contorno ósseo do queixo. [G. *geneion*, queixo, bochecha, + *plastos*, formado]

gen·i·tal (jen'i-tăl). Genital. **1.** Relativo à reprodução ou à geração. **2.** Relativo aos órgãos sexuais masculinos ou femininos primários ou genitais. **3.** Relativo a, ou caracterizado por, genitalidade. [L. *genitalis*, relativo à reprodução, de *gigno*, parir]

gen·i·ta·lia (jen'i-tā'lē-ă) [TA]. Genitália; os órgãos de reprodução ou de geração, externos e internos. SIN organa genitalia [TA], genital organs, genitals. [L. neut. pl. de *genitalis*, genital]
  ambiguous g., g. ambígua. SIN genital *ambiguity*.
  ambiguous external g., g. externa ambígua. SIN genital *ambiguity*.
  external g., g. externa; a vulva na fêmea e o pênis e o escroto no macho.
  female external g. [TA], g. feminina externa; os órgãos genitais femininos externos, a vulva e o clitóris. SIN external female genital organs, organa genitalia feminina externa.
  female internal g. [TA], g. feminina interna; os órgãos genitais femininos internos, os ovários, as tubas uterinas, o útero e a vagina. SIN internal female genital organs, organa genitalia feminina interna.
  indifferent g., g. indiferente; órgãos reprodutivos do embrião antes da formação sexual definitiva.
  male external g. [TA], g. masculina externa; os órgãos genitais masculinos externos, o pênis e o escroto. SIN external male genital organs, organa genitalia masculina externa.
  male internal g. [TA], g. masculina interna; os órgãos genitais masculinos internos, os testículos, o epidídimo, os ductos deferentes, as vesículas seminais, a próstata e as glândulas bulbouretrais. SIN internal male genital organs, organa genitalia masculina interna.

gen·i·tal·i·ty (jen-i-tal'i-tē). Genitalidade; em psicanálise, um termo que se refere aos componentes genitais da sexualidade (isto é, o pênis e a vagina), em oposição, por exemplo, à oralidade e à analidade.

gen·i·tals (jen'i-tălz). Genitália. SIN genitalia. [ver genitalia]

gen·i·to·cru·ral (jen'i-tō-kroo'răl). Genitocrural. SIN genitofemoral.

gen·i·to·fem·o·ral (jen'i-tō-fem'ō-răl). Genitofemoral; relativo à genitalia e à coxa; que indica o nervo g. SIN genitocrural.

gen·i·to·u·ri·nary (GU) (jen'i-tō-ū'ri-nar-ē). Genitourinário; relativo aos órgãos da reprodução e da micção. SIN urinogenital, urinossexual, urogenital.

ge·nius (jēn'yŭs, jēn'ē-ŭs). Gênio. **1.** Capacidade artística ou intelectual acentuadamente superior ou criatividade excepcional. **2.** Uma pessoa assim dotada. **3.** Em psicologia, um indivíduo que figura no 1% superior de todos os indivíduos em um teste de inteligência. [L.]

ge·nius ep·i·dem·i·cus (ep-i-dem'i-kŭs). A influência atmosférica, telúrica ou cósmica, ou a combinação de duas ou três delas; considerado pelos antigos como a causa das doenças endêmicas e epidêmicas. [L. mod.]

Gennari, Francesco, anatomista italiano, 1750–1795. VER G. *band, stria; line* of G.; *stripe* of G.

gen·o·blast (jen'ō-blast). Genoblasto; o núcleo do óvulo fertilizado.

gen·o·copy (jen'ō-kop-e). Genocópia; um genótipo em um *locus* que produz um fenótipo que, em alguns níveis de resolução, é indistinguível daquele produzido por um outro genótipo; p.ex., dois tipos de eliptocitose que são genocópias uma da outra, porém são diferenciadas pelo fato de que uma está ligada ao *locus* do grupo sanguíneo Rh e a outra não está.

ge·no·der·ma·tol·o·gy (jen'ō-der-mă-tol'ō-jē). Genodermatologia; o estudo das características hereditárias de distúrbios cutâneos. [G. *genos*, nascimento, descendência, + *derma*, pele, + *logos*, teoria]

ge·no·der·ma·to·sis (jen'ō-der-mă-tō'sis). Genodermatose; uma condição cutânea de origem genética.

ge·nome (je'nōm, -nom). Genoma. **1.** Um conjunto completo de cromossomas derivado de um genitor, o número haplóide de um gameta. **2.** O complemento genético total de um conjunto de cromossomas encontrado em formas de vida superiores (o conjunto haplóide dentro de uma célula eucariota) ou os arranjos lineares funcionalmente similares, porém mais simples, encontrados em bactérias e vírus. VER TAMBÉM Human Genome Project. [gene + cromossoma]

ge·nom·ic (je-nom'ik). Genômico; relativo a um genoma.

genomics (jen-ōm-'ks). Genômica; o estudo da estrutura do genoma de determinados organismos, incluindo mapeamento e seqüenciamento.
  functional g., g. funcional; o estudo de genes expressos em organismos, incluindo a identificação dos genes e os fatores que controlam a expressão diferencial.

ge·no·spe·cies (jē'nō-spē-sēz, jen'). Genoespécie; um grupo de organismos nos quais o entrecruzamento é possível, como evidenciado por transferência e recombinação genéticas.

ge·note (jē'nōt). Genoto; em genética microbiana, um elemento de recombinação no qual um dos cromossomas do par não está completo; termo geralmente utilizado como um sufixo (p.ex., endogenoto, exogenoto, genoto F). [gene + G. *-ōtēs*, sufixo toponímico]

ge·no·tox·ic (jē-nō-toks'ik). Genotóxico; que indica uma substância que danifica o DNA, podendo causar mutação ou câncer. [gene + tóxico]

gen·o·type (jen'ō-tīp). Genótipo. **1.** A constituição genética de um indivíduo. **2.** A combinação de genes em um *locus* específico ou qualquer combinação específica de *loci*. Para genótipos de grupos sanguíneos específicos, ver Apêndice sobre Grupos Sanguíneos. [G. *genos*, nascimento, descendência, + *typos*, tipo]
  ZZ g., g. ZZ; indivíduos com deficiência de α_1-antitripsina e enfisema.

gen·o·typ·ic (jēn'ō-tip-ik). Genotípico. SIN genotypical.

gen·o·typ·i·cal (jen-ō-tip'i-kăl). Genotípico; relativo ao genótipo. SIN genotypic.

gen·ta·mi·cin (jen-tă-mī'sin). Gentamicina; um antibiótico de amplo espectro da classe do aminoglicosídeos, obtido do *Micromonospora purpurea* e do *M. echinospora* e que inibe o crescimento tanto de bactérias Gram-positivas como de Gram-negativas; o sal sulfato é utilizado medicinalmente.

gen·tian, gen·tian root (jen'shŭn). Genciana, raiz de genciana; o rizoma seco e as raízes da *Gentiana lutea* (família Gentianaceae), uma erva das regiões meridional e central da Europa; um amargo simples.

gen·tian·o·phil, gen·tian·o·phile (jen'shŭn-o-fil, -fīl). Gencianófilo; que se cora prontamente com violeta de genciana. SIN gentianophilous. [gentian + G. *philos*, amigo]

gen·tian·oph·i·lous (jen-shŭn-of'i-lŭs). Gencianófilo. SIN gentianophil.

gen·tian·o·pho·bic (jen'shŭn-ō-fō'bik). Gencianofóbico; que não se cora com a violeta de genciana ou se cora mal. [gentian + G. *phobos*, medo]

gen·tian root. Raiz de genciana. VER gentian.

gen·tian vi·o·let. Violeta de genciana; uma mistura de corantes não-padronizada de rosanilinas violetas; é também utilizada topicamente como antiinfeccioso. VER crystal violet.

gen·ti·o·bi·ase (jen'shi-ō-bī'ās). Genciobiase. SIN β-D-glucosidase.

gen·ti·o·bi·o·se (jen'tē-ō-bī'ōs). Genciobiose; um dissacarídeo que contém duas moléculas de D-glicopiranose ligadas, β-1,6; um radical estrutural encontrado em muitos compostos (p.ex., amigdalina). SIN amygdalose.

gen·tis·ic ac·id (jen-tis'ik). Ácido gentísico; esse composto relaciona-se quimicamente com o salicilato e com o acetilsalicilato e compartilha com a segunda substância propriedades analgésicas e antiinflamatórias. Um metabólito da aspirina.

genu, gen. **ge·nus,** pl. **gen·ua** (jē'noo, jē'nŭs, jen'oo-ă) [TA]. Joelho. **1.** O local da articulação entre a coxa e a perna. SIN knee (1) [TA]. VER TAMBÉM knee *joint*, geniculum. **2.** Qualquer estrutura de forma angular que se assemelha a um joelho fletido. [L.]
  g. cap'sulae inter'nae [TA], j. da cápsula interna. SIN g. of internal capsule.
  g. cor'poris callo'si [TA], j. do corpo caloso. SIN g. of corpus callosum.
  g. of corpus callosum [TA], j. do corpo caloso; a extremidade anterior do corpo caloso que se dobra para baixo e para trás de si mesma, terminando no rostro. SIN g. corporis callosi [TA].
  g. of facial canal, j. do canal facial. SIN *geniculum* of facial canal.
  g. of facial nerve [TA], j. do nervo facial; a curvatura que as fibras da raiz do nervo facial descrevem ao redor do núcleo abducente no tegmento da ponte; o j. interno do nervo facial. SIN g. nervi facialis [TA].
  g. of internal capsule [TA], j. da cápsula interna; o ângulo obtuso que se abre lateralmente no plano horizontal e é formado pela união dos dois ramos (anterior e posterior) da cápsula interna. SIN g. capsulae internae [TA].
  g. ner'vi facia'lis [TA], j. do nervo facial. SIN g. of facial nerve.
  g. recurva'tum, hiperextensão do joelho que faz com que o membro inferior apresente uma curvatura para a frente. SIN back-knee.
  g. val'gum, joelho valgo; uma deformidade caracterizada por angulação lateral da perna em relação à coxa. SIN knock-knee, tibia valga.
  g. va'rum, joelho varo; uma deformidade caracterizada por angulação medial da perna em relação à coxa; arqueamento das pernas para fora. SIN bandy-leg, bowleg, bow-leg, tibia vara.

gen·u·al (jen'ū-ăl). Genicular; relativo ao joelho. [L. *genu*, joelho]

ge·nus, pl. **gen·era** (jē'nŭs, jen'er-ă). Gênero; na classificação da história natural, o nível taxonômico de divisão entre a família ou a tribo e a espécie; um grupo de espécies que se mostram iguais quanto às características gerais de sua organização, porém diferem nos detalhes, sendo incapazes de cruzamento fértil. [L. nascimento, descendência]

gen·y·an·trum (jen-ē-an'trŭm). Geniantro. SIN maxillary *sinus*. [G. *genys*, bochecha, + *antron*, caverna]

△ **geo-.** Geo-; a terra, o solo. [G. *gē*, terra]

ge·ode (jē'ōd). Geode, geodo; um espaço (ou espaços) semelhante a um cisto com ou sem um revestimento epitelial, observado radiologicamente no osso subarticular, em geral nos distúrbios artríticos. [Fr., do L. *geodes*, pedra preciosa, do G. *gē*, terra, + *-ōdēs*, aparência]

ge·o·med·i·cine (jē-ō-med'i-sin). Geomedicina; a ciência relacionada com a influência das condições climáticas e ambientais sobre a saúde e doença. SIN nosochthonography, nosogeography.

ge·o·pa·thol·o·gy (jē'ō-pă-thol'ō-jē). Geopatologia; o estudo da doença em relação às regiões, aos climas e a outras influências ambientais.

ge·o·pha·gia, ge·oph·a·gism, ge·oph·a·gy (jē - ō - fā′jē - ā, jē - of′ā - jizm, -of′ā - jē). Geofagia; a prática de comer lama ou argila. SIN dirt-eating. [geo- + G. *phago*, comer]

ge·o·phil·ic. Geófilo; terrestre, que habita o solo. [geo- + G. *philos*, amor, atração, + -ic]

Ge·oph·i·lus (jē - of′i - lūs). Um gênero de centopéias que se caracterizam por apresentar um número muito grande de pernas (47 a 67 pares); engloba *G. californius, G. rubens* e *G. umbraticus* nos Estados Unidos.

Georgi, Walter, bacteriologista alemão, 1889–1920. VER Sachs-G. *test.*

ge·o·tax·is (jē - ō - tak′sis). Geotaxia; uma forma de barotaxia positiva na qual há uma tendência a crescer ou se movimentar para a frente ou para o interior da terra. SIN geotropism. [geo- + G. *taxis*, arranjo ordenado]

ge·ot·ri·cho·sis (jē′ō - tri - kō′sis). Geotricose; uma micose sistêmica e oportunista causada pelo *Geotrichum candidum*; os sintomas atribuídos a essa doença são variados e sugestivos de infecções secundárias ou mistas. [geo- + G. *thrix*, pêlo, + -osis, condição]

Ge·ot·ri·chum (jē - ot′ri - kŭm). Um gênero de fungos, semelhantes a leveduras, que produzem artroconídeos, porém raramente blastoconídeos. Já se acreditou que o *G. candidum* fosse causador de infecções em seres humanos.

ge·ot·ro·pism (jē - ot′rō - pizm). Geotropismo. SIN geotaxis. [geo- + G. *tropē*, uma volta]

gephyrin (je-fir′in). Gefirina; uma proteína da família das proteínas relacionadas à ataxia-telangiectasia, essencial para o agrupamento dos receptores de glicina sobre as membranas dos neurônios.

geph·y·ro·pho·bia (jē - fī - rō - fō′bē - ā). Gefirofobia; medo de atravessar pontes. [G. *gephyra*, ponte, + *phobos*, medo]

gep·i·rone (je - pī′ron). Gepirona; um ansiolítico não-benzodiazepínico que se assemelha à buspirona tanto química quanto farmacologicamente. Age sobre os receptores serotoninérgicos em vez de sobre os receptores para as benzodiazepinas. Não apresenta as propriedades causadoras de dependência e a tolerância dos agentes benzodiazepínicos.

ge·ran·i·ol (jē - ra′nē - ol). Geraniol; um álcool terpênico olefínico que é o principal constituinte do óleo de rosa e do óleo de palmarosa; é também encontrado em muitos outros óleos voláteis, tais como a citronela e o capim-limão. Um isômero do linalol; um líquido oleoso com cheiro adocicado de rosa utilizado em perfumaria. É também empregado como agente que atrai insetos.

ger·a·nyl·ger·a·nyl py·ro·phos·phate (jer′a - nil - jer - a - nil pī - rō -fos′fāt). Pirofosfato de geranilgeranil; um metabólito intermediário-chave da biossíntese de muitos terpenos; o substrato-chave para a introdução do grupo geranilgeranil nas proteínas.

ger·a·nyl py·ro·phos·phate (jer′a - nil - pī - rō - fos′fāt). Pirofosfato de geranil; um metabólito intermediário-chave da biossíntese de esteróis, dolicóis, ubiquinona e proteínas preniladas.

ger·a·tol·o·gy (jār - a - tol′ō - jē). Geratologia. SIN gerontology.

Gerbich an·ti·gen. Antígeno de Gerbich. Ver em antigen.

Gerbode, Frank, cirurgião cardiotorácico norte-americano, 1907–1984. VER Gerbode *defect.*

GERD Abreviatura de gastroesophageal reflux *disease* (doença por refluxo gastroesofágico, DRGE).

Gerdy, Pierre N., cirurgião francês, 1797–1856. VER G. *fibers*, em *fiber*, *fontanelle*, hyoid *fossa, ligament*, interatrial *loop, tubercle.*

Gerhardt, Carl A.C.J., médico alemão, 1833–1902. VER G. *reaction, test* for acetoacetic acid; Gerhardt-Mitchell *disease.*

Gerhardt, Charles F., químico francês, 1816–1856. VER G. *test* for urobilin in the urine.

ger·i·at·ric (jār - ē - at′rik). Geriátrico; relativo à velhice ou à geriatria.

ger·i·at·rics (jār - ē - at′riks). Geriatria; o ramo da medicina que se ocupa dos problemas clínicos dos idosos e dos cuidados a eles dispensados. [G. *gēras*, velhice, + *iatrikos*, cura]

dental g., g. dentária; tratamento de problemas dentários próprios da idade avançada. SIN gerodontics, gerodontology.

Gerlach, Joseph, anatomista alemão, 1820–1896. VER G. annular *tendon, tonsil; valve* of vermiform appendix; G. *valvula.*

Gerlier, Felix, médico suíço, 1840–1914. VER G. *disease.*

germ (jerm). Germe. **1.** Um micróbio; um microrganismo. **2.** Um primórdio; o traço mais precoce de uma estrutura situada dentro de um embrião. [L. *germen*, grelo, broto, germe]

dental g., g. do dente, g. dentário. SIN tooth g.

enamel g., órgão do esmalte; o órgão do esmalte de um dente em desenvolvimento; uma de várias projeções semelhantes a botões e provenientes da lâmina dentária, que, posteriormente, assumem a forma de um sino e recebem em sua cavidade a papila dentária.

reserve tooth g., g. do dente reserva; o órgão e a papila do esmalte de um dente permanente.

tooth g., g. do dente, g. dentário; o órgão do esmalte e a papila da dentina, que constituem o dente em desenvolvimento. SIN dental g.

wheat g., g. do trigo; o embrião do trigo; contém tiamina, riboflavina e outras vitaminas.

ger·ma·ni·um (Ge) (jer - mān′ē - ŭm). Germânio (Ge); um elemento metálico com n.º atômico 32 e peso atômico 72,61. [L. *Germania*, Alemanha]

ger·mi·ci·dal (jer - mi - sī′dăl). Germicida. SIN germicide (1).

ger·mi·cide (jer′mi - sīd). Germicida. **1.** Destrutivo para os germes ou micróbios. SIN germicidal. **2.** Um agente com essa ação. [germ + L. *caedo*, matar]

ger·mi·nal (jer′mi - nal). Germinal; germinativo; relativo a um germe ou, em botânica, à germinação.

ger·mine (jer′mīn). Germina; um alcalóide presente nas espécies *Veratrum* e *Zygandenus*. Da mesma forma que a veratrina e a veratridina, a germina induz descargas repetitivas nas células nervosas, aparentemente por causa de distúrbios na função dos canais de sódio. É freqüentemente utilizado como derivado de acetato ou de diacetato.

ger·mi·no·ma (jer - mi - nō′mă). Germinoma; uma neoplasia do tecido germinativo das gônadas, do mediastino ou da região pineal, tal como o seminoma. [L. *germen*, broto (de flor), + -oma, tumor]

△ **gero-, geront-, geronto-.** Idade avançada, velhice. VER TAMBÉM presby-. [G. *gerōn*, homem idoso]

ger·o·der·ma (jār - ō - der′mă). Gerodermia. **1.** A pele atrófica do idoso. **2.** Qualquer condição na qual a pele se encontra adelgaçada e enrugada, assemelhando-se ao tegumento do idoso. [gero- + G. *derma*, pele]

ger·o·don·tics, ger·o·don·tol·o·gy (jār - ō - don′tiks, - don - tol′ō - jē). Gerodontia, gerodontologia. SIN dental *geriatrics*. [gero- + G. *odous*, dente]

ger·o·ma·ras·mus (jār′ō - mă - raz′mŭs). Geromarasmo. SIN senile *atrophy*. [gero- + G. *marasmos*, um desgaste]

ge·ron·tal (jār - on′tăl). Gerôntico; relativo à velhice.

ge·ron·tine (jār′on - tēn). Gerontina. SIN spermine.

△ **geronto-.** VER gero-.

ger·on·tol·o·gist (jār - on - tol′ō - jist). Gerontologista; aquele que se especializa em gerontologia.

ger·on·tol·o·gy (jār - on - tol′ō - jē). Gerontologia; o estudo científico do processo de envelhecimento e dos problemas associados à velhice. SIN geratology. [geronto- + G. *logos*, estudo]

ge·ron·to·phil·ia (jār′on - tō - fil′ē - ā). Gerontofilia; amor mórbido por pessoas idosas. [geronto- + G. *philos*, amigo]

ge·ron·to·pho·bia (jār′on - tō - fō′bē - ā). Gerontofobia; medo mórbido de pessoas idosas. [geronto- + G. *phobos*, medo]

ge·ron·to·ther·a·peu·tics (jār - on′tō - thār - ă - pū′tiks). Gerontoterapêutica; a ciência que se ocupa do tratamento do idoso.

ge·ron·to·ther·a·py (jār - on′tō - thār - ă - pē). Gerontoterapia; o tratamento de doenças encontradas nos idosos. SIN geriatric therapy.

ger·on·tox·on (jār′on - tok′son). Gerotoxo. SIN *arcus* senilis. [geronto- + G. *toxon*, arco]

Gerota, Dimitru, anatomista e cirurgião romeno, 1867–1939. VER G. *capsule, fascia, method.*

Gersh, Isidore, histologista norte-americano, *1907. VER Altmann-G. *method.*

Gerstmann, Josef, neurologista austríaco, 1887–1969. VER G. *syndrome*; G.-Sträussler-Scheinker *syndrome.*

ges·ta·gen (jes′tă - jen). Gestagênio; termo inclusivo utilizado para indicar qualquer uma das várias substâncias gestagênicas, que são em geral hormônios esteróides. SIN gestin, progestin (3).

ges·ta·gen·ic (jes - tă - jen′ik). Gestagênico; que induz efeitos progestacionais ao útero.

ge·stalt (ge-stahlt). G(u)estalt; uma entidade percebida integrada o suficiente para constituir uma unidade funcional com propriedades não-deriváveis de suas partes. VER gestaltism. [Al. forma]

ge·stalt·ism (ge-stahlt′izm). G(u)estaltismo; a teoria psicológica de que os objetos da mente surgem como formas ou configurações completas que não podem ser separadas em partes; p.ex., um quadrado é percebido como tal, e não como quatro linhas distintas. [ver gestalt]

ges·ta·tion (jes - tā′shŭn). Gestação. SIN pregnancy. [L. *gestatio*, de *gesto*, pp. *gestatus*, carregar]

ges·tin (jes′tin). Gestágeno. SIN gestagen.

ges·to·sis, pl. **ges·to·ses** (jes - tō′sis, - sēz). Gestose; qualquer distúrbio da gravidez. [L. *gesto*, carregar, + G. *-osis*, condição]

ges·ture (jes′chŭr). Gesto. **1.** Qualquer movimento expressivo de uma idéia, opinião ou emoção. **2.** Um ato. [L. *gestus*, movimento, gesto]

suicide g., g. suicida; uma tentativa aparente de suicídio praticada por alguém que deseja atrair a atenção, ganhar simpatia ou alcançar algum objetivo, exceto a autodestruição.

Gey, George O., médico e pesquisador norte-americano, 1899–1970. VER G. *solution.*

GFR Abreviatura de glomerular filtration *rate* (taxa de filtração glomerular, TFG).

GH Abreviatura de growth *hormone* (hormônio do crescimento).

GHB Abreviatura de γ-hydroxybutyrate (γ-hidroxibutirato).

ghee (gē). Uma manteiga purificada proveniente da Índia e feita a partir do leite da vaca ou da búfala que foi coagulado antes de ser desnatado; utilizada como emoliente, curativo para feridas e alimento. [Ortografia inglesa da palavra hindu *ghi*]

Ghon, Anton, patologista tcheco-eslovaco, 1866–1936. VER G. *complex, focus,* primary *lesion, tubercle.*

ghost (gōst). Um eritrócito desprovido de hemoglobina que também perdeu a maioria, se não todas, de suas proteínas internas.

GHRF, GH-RF Abreviatura de growth hormone-releasing *factor* (fator liberador do hormônio do crescimento).

GHRF, GH-RH Abreviatura de growth *hormone*-releasing *hormone* (hormônio liberador do hormônio do crescimento).

GHz Abreviatura de gigahertz; corresponde a um bilhão (10^9) de hertz; utilizada em ultra-som.

GI Abreviatura de gastrointestinal; Gingival Index.

Giacomini, Carlo, anatomista italiano, 1841–1898. VER *band* of G.; *frenulum* of G.; uncus *band* of G.

Giannuzzi, anatomista italiano, 1839–1876. VER G. *crescents,* em *crescent, demilunes,* em *demilune.*

Gianotti, F., dermatologista italiano do século XX. VER G.-Crosti *syndrome.*

gi·ar·dia (jē-ar'dē-ă). Um gênero de flagelados que parasitam o intestino delgado de muitos mamíferos, incluindo a maioria dos animais domésticos e os seres humanos; p.ex., *G. bovis* parasita o gado, *G. canis* os cães e *G. cati* os gatos. Muitas espécies já foram descritas, porém trabalhos recentes sugerem que elas devam ser reduzidas para apenas duas ou três. [Alfred *Giard*, biólogo francês, 1846–1908]

G. intestinalis, SIN *G. lamblia.*

G. lam'blia, um microrganismo achatado e em forma de coração (10 a 20 μm de comprimento) com oito flagelos; prende-se à mucosa intestinal graças a um par de órgãos sugadores; em geral não causa sintomas, exceto em infecções maciças, quando pode interferir com a absorção de gorduras e produzir flatulência, esteatorréia e desconforto agudo; é a espécie de G. mais comum no homem, porém é também encontrada em porcos. SIN *G. intestinalis.*

gi·ar·di·a·sis (jē-ar-dī'ă-sis). Giardíase; infecção pelo protozoário parasita *Giardia*; a *Giardia lamblia* pode causar diarréia, dispepsia e, ocasionalmente, má-absorção em seres humanos. SIN lambliasis.

gib·ber·el·lic ac·id (jib'er-el-ik). Ácido giberélico; uma auxina, isto é, um hormônio vegetal que estimula o crescimento; o mais importante dos metabólitos promotores do crescimento vegetal da *Gibberella fujikuroi*. Utilizada como regulador e promotor do crescimento das plantas, principalmente do crescimento das mudas. Empregada também como aditivo alimentar na maltagem da cevada.

gib·ber·el·lins. Giberelinas; uma classe de hormônios vegetais de crescimento (auxinas) da qual mais de 60 são conhecidos; foram isoladas pela primeira vez em 1938 a partir de culturas de *Gibberella fujikuroi*, o fungo que causa uma doença no arroz, a "doença das plantinhas loucas" ou "bakanae". São também encontradas nas plantas superiores; os ácidos diterpenóides estão disponíveis no comércio.

gib·bon (gib'on). Gibão; um gênero de macacos antropóides, *Hylobates*, da superfamília Hominoidea. [Fr.]

gib·bous (gib'ŭs). Giboso; corcovado, dobrado; corcunda; que indica um ângulo agudo na flexão da coluna vertebral. [L. *gibbosus*]

Gibbs, Josiah W., matemático e físico norte-americano, 1839–1903. VER G.-Donnan *equilibrium*; G.-Helmholtz *equation*; Helmholtz-G. *theory*; G. *theorem*, free *energy, energy* of activation.

gib·bus (gib'ŭs). Giba; cifose extrema, corcova ou corcunda; uma deformidade da coluna vertebral na qual há um segmento com ângulo agudo, sendo o ápice do ângulo posterior. [L. uma corcova]

Gibney, Virgil P., ortopedista norte-americano, 1847–1927. VER G. fixation *bandage, boot.*

Gibson, George A., médico escocês, 1854–1913. VER G. *murmur.*

Gibson, Kasson C., dentista norte-americano, 1849–1925. VER G. *bandage.*

Giemsa, Gustav, bacteriologista alemão, 1867–1948. VER G. *stain*, chromosome banding *stain.*

Gierke, Edgar von, patologista alemão, 1877–1945. VER G. *disease*; von G. *disease.*

Gierke, Hans P.B., anatomista alemão, 1847–1886. VER G. respiratory *bundle.*

Gifford, Harold, oftalmologista norte-americano, 1858–1929. VER G. *reflex.*

GIFT Abreviatura de gamete intrafallopian *transfer* (transferência de gametas nas tubas uterinas).

△ **giga- (G).** Prefixo utilizado nos sistemas métrico e internacional (SI) e que significa múltiplos de um bilhão (10^9). [G. *gigas*, gigante]

gi·gan·tism (jī'gan-tizm). Gigantismo; uma condição caracterizada pelo tamanho anormal ou crescimento exagerado de todo o corpo ou de qualquer uma de suas partes. SIN giantism. [G. *gigas*, gigante]

acromegalic g., g. acromegálico; uma forma de g. hipofisário na qual a altura anormal é acompanhada por sinais de acromegalia.

cerebral g., g. cerebral; uma síndrome caracterizada por peso e comprimento aumentados ao nascimento (acima do 90.º percentil), crescimento acelerado nos primeiros quatro ou cinco anos sem elevação dos níveis séricos do hormônio do crescimento e, depois, reversão para uma velocidade de crescimento normal; a fácies característica inclui prognatismo, hipertelorismo, fenda palpebral antimongolóide e dolicocefalia; também há retardo mental moderado e comprometimento da coordenação. VER Sotos *syndrome.*

eunuchoid g., g. eunucóide; g. com desenvolvimento deficiente dos órgãos sexuais; pode ser de origem hipofisária ou gonadal; é acompanhado de proporções corporais típicas do hipogonadismo durante a adolescência.

fetal g., g. fetal; feto ou recém-nascido com tamanho excessivo, p. ex., g. cerebral e bebês de mães diabéticas.

pituitary g., g. pituitário, g. hipofisário; uma forma de g. causada por hipersecreção de hormônio de crescimento hipofisário; um distúrbio raro, comumente o resultado de um adenoma de hipófise.

primordial g., g. primordial; tamanho extraordinariamente grande ao nascimento, resultante de fatores genéticos ou familiais ou do ambiente intra-uterino (p.ex., estado pré-diabético da mãe) e não de hiperpituitarismo.

△ **giganto-.** Gigante, enorme. [G. *gigas*, uma das raças de gigantes]

gi·gan·to·mas·tia (jī-gan'tō-mas'tē-ă). Gigantomastia; hipertrofia maciça das mamas. [giganto- + G. *mastos*, mama]

Gi·gan·to·rhyn·chus (ji-gan'to-ring'kŭs). Um gênero de vermes acantocéfalos muito grandes. VER TAMBÉM *Macracanthorhynchus, Moniliformis.* [giganto- + G. *rhynchos*, tromba]

Gigli, Leonardo, ginecologista italiano, 1863–1908. VER G. *saw.*

GIH Abreviatura de growth *hormone*-inhibiting *hormone* (hormônio inibidor do hormônio do crescimento).

Gi·la mon·ster (hē'lă). Monstro-de-gila; um lagarto grande e venenoso, *Heloderma suspectum*, do Novo México, Arizona e norte do México. [*Gila*, um rio do Arizona]

Gilbert, Nicholas A., médico francês, 1858–1927. VER G. *disease, syndrome.*

Gilbert, Walter, microbiologista norte-americano laureado com um Prêmio Nobel, *1932. VER Maxim-G. *sequencing.*

gil·bert. Gilbert; a unidade de força magnetomotriz ou de potencial magnético. [W. *Gilbert*, físico inglês, 1544–1603]

Gilchrist, Thomas C., médico norte-americano, 1862–1927. VER G. *disease.*

Gilford, Hastings, médico inglês, 1861–1941. VER Hutchinson-G. *disease, syndrome.*

Gilles de la Tourette, Georges, médico francês, 1857–1904. VER G. de la T. *disease, syndrome*; Tourette *disease*; Tourette *syndrome.*

Gillespie, Frank, oftalmologista norte-americano, *1927. VER G. *syndrome.*

Gillette, Eugène P., cirurgião francês, 1836–1886. VER G. suspensory *ligament.*

Gilliam, David Tod, ginecologista norte-americano, 1844–1923. VER G. *operation.*

Gillies, Sir Harold D., cirurgião plástico britânico, 1882–1960. VER G. *operation*; Filatov-G. *flap.*

Gillmore nee·dle. Agulha de Gillmore. Ver em needle.

Gilman, Alfred G., *1941, co-ganhador do Prêmio Nobel de 1994 pelo trabalho relacionado com as proteínas G, q.v.

Gilmer, Thomas L., cirurgião oral norte-americano, 1849–1931. VER G. *wiring.*

Gil-Vernet, José Maria Vila, urologista espanhol, *1922. VER Gil-Vernet *operation.*

Gimbernat, Antonio de, anatomista e cirurgião espanhol, 1734–1816. VER G. *ligament.*

gin·ger (jin'jer). Gengibre; o rizoma seco de *Zingiber officinale* (família Zingiberaceae), conhecido no comércio como g. da Jamaica, g. africano e g. da Cochinchina. As camadas corticais externas são com freqüência parcial ou completamente removidas; é utilizado como carminativo e agente aromatizante. SIN zingiber.

Chinese g., g. chinês. SIN *galangal.*

Indian g., g. indiano. SIN *Asarum canadense.*

g. oleoresin, óleo-resina de gengibre; um agente carminativo, estimulante e aromatizante.

wild g., g. selvagem. SIN *Asarum canadense.*

gin·gi·li oil (jin'ji-lē). Óleo de gergelim. SIN *sesame* oil.

gin·gi·va, gen. e pl. **gin·gi·vae** (jin'ji-vă, -vē) [TA]. Gengiva; o tecido denso e fibroso e a mucosa de revestimento que envolvem os processos alveolares das maxilas superior e inferior e circundam os colos dos dentes. SIN gum (2)*. [L.]

alveolar g., g. alveolar; o tecido gengival relacionado ao osso alveolar.

attached g., g. inserida; a parte da mucosa oral que está firmemente ligada ao dente e ao processo alveolar.

buccal g., g. vestibular; a porção da g. que cobre as superfícies vestibulares dos dentes e do processo alveolar.

free g., g. livre; a porção da g. que circunda o dente e não está diretamente fixada à superfície do dente; a parede externa do sulco gengival.

labial g., g. labial; a porção da g. que cobre as superfícies labiais (vestibulares) dos dentes e do processo alveolar.

lingual g., g. lingual; a porção da g. que cobre as superfícies linguais dos dentes e do processo alveolar.

septal g., g. septal; a porção da g. que cobre o septo interdentário.

gin·gi·val (jin'ji-văl). Gengival; relativo às gengivas.

Gin·gi·val In·dex (GI). Índice Gengival; um índice de doença periodontal baseado na gravidade e localização da lesão.

Gin·gi·val-Per·i·o·don·tal In·dex (GPI). Índice Gengivoperiodontal; um índice de gengivite, irritação gengival e de doença periodontal avançada.

gin·gi·vec·to·my (jin - ji - vek′tō - mē). Gengivectomia; ressecção cirúrgica de tecido gengival descolado. SIN gum resection. [gengiva + G. *ektomē,* excisão]

gin·gi·vi·tis (jin - ji - vī′tis). Gengivite; inflamação da gengiva em resposta à placa bacteriana localizada no dente adjacente; caracterizada por eritema, edema e hipertrofia fibrosa da gengiva, sem reabsorção do osso alveolar subjacente. [gengiva + G. *-itis,* inflamação]

   acute necrotizing ulcerative g. (ANUG), g. ulcerativa necrosante aguda. VER necrotizing ulcerative g.

   atypical g., g. atípica. SIN plasma cell g.

   chronic desquamative g., g. descamativa crônica; um termo clínico para uma condição da gengiva de etiologia desconhecida, encontrada em geral em mulheres de meia-idade e idosas, caracterizada por eritema, atrofia da mucosa e descamação, sendo freqüentemente acompanhada por sensação de queimação e dor; o diagnóstico é geralmente feito por meio de biopsia e imunofluorescência direta. SIN gingivosis.

   diabetic g., g. diabética; g. na qual a resposta do hospedeiro à placa bacteriana é modificada provavelmente pelas alterações metabólicas encontradas nos pacientes com diabetes não-controlado.

   dilantin g., g. por difenil-hidantoína. SIN diphenylhydantoin g.

   diphenylhydantoin g., g. por difenil-hidantoína; g. exacerbada por tratamento em longo prazo com difenil-hidantoína; a resposta do hospedeiro à placa bacteriana é caracterizada por hiperplasia acentuada do tecido conectivo fibroso e, em menor grau, do epitélio de superfície, levando a aumento evidente das papilas interdentárias que podem coalescer e encobrir as coroas clínicas dos dentes. SIN dilantin g.

   fusospirochetal g., g. por fusoespiroquetas. SIN necrotizing ulcerative g.

   hormonal g., g. hormonal; g. na qual a resposta do hospedeiro à placa bacteriana é provavelmente exacerbada pelas alterações hormonais que ocorrem durante a puberdade, gravidez, uso de contraceptivos orais e menopausa. SIN pregnancy g.

   hyperplastic g., g. hiperplásica; g. de duração prolongada na qual a gengiva se torna hipertrofiada e de consistência firme como conseqüência de proliferação do tecido conectivo fibroso.

   leukemic hyperplastic g., g. leucêmica hiperplásica; gengiva hipertrófica em conseqüência de infiltração por células leucêmicas e infecção proveniente de fatores locais na vigência de resposta diminuída por parte do hospedeiro.

   marginal g., g. marginal; g. cujas alterações clínicas estão confinadas à gengiva marginal e não acometem a gengiva inserida.

   necrotizing ulcerative g. (NUG), g. ulcerativa necrosante; g. aguda ou recidivante que acomete jovens e adultos de meia-idade, caracterizada clinicamente por eritema e dor gengivais, odor fétido e necrose e descamação das papilas interdentárias e da gengiva marginal que dá origem a uma pseudomembrana cinzenta; febre, linfadenopatia regional e outras manifestações sistêmicas também podem ocorrer. Um bacilo fusiforme e o *Treponema vincentii* podem ser isolados dos tecidos gengivais em grande número e acredita-se que esses microrganismos têm uma participação significativa, porém mal definida, na patogênese. SIN fusospirochetal g., trench mouth, ulceromembranous g., Vincent disease, Vincent infection.

   plasma cell g., g. plasmocitária; edema hiperêmico intenso e inflamação da gengiva resultantes de uma reação de hipersensibilidade. Um denso infiltrado de plasmócitos é observado na lâmina própria. SIN atypical g.

   pregnancy g., g. gravídica. SIN hormonal g.

   proliferative g., g. proliferativa; alterações inflamatórias localizadas na gengiva e caracterizadas por proliferação dos elementos gengivais.

   suppurative g., g. supurativa; g. na qual um exsudato purulento pode ser espremido da superfície da gengiva.

   ulceromembranous g., g. ulceromembranosa. SIN necrotizing ulcerative g.

gingivo-. Gengivo-; as gengivas da boca. [L. *gingiva*]

gin·gi·vo·ax·i·al (jin′ji - vō - ak′sē - ăl). Gengivoaxial; relativo ao ângulo formado pelas paredes gengival e axial de uma cavidade.

gin·gi·vo·glos·si·tis (jin′ji - vō - glos - sī′tis). Gengivoglossite; inflamação tanto dos tecidos gengivais como da língua. VER TAMBÉM stomatitis.

gin·gi·vo·la·bi·al (jin′ji - vō - lā′bē - ăl). Gengivolabial; que se refere ao ângulo formado pela junção das paredes gengival e labial de uma cavidade (classe III ou IV).

gin·gi·vo·lin·guo·ax·i·al (jin′ji - vō - ling′gwō - ak′sē - ăl). Gengivolinguoaxial; que se refere ao ângulo formado pelas paredes gengival, lingual e axial de uma cavidade.

gin·gi·vo-os·se·ous (jin′ji - vō - os′ē - ŭs). Gengivo-ósseo; que se refere à gengiva e ao osso subjacente a ela.

gin·gi·vo·plas·ty (jin′ji - vō - plas - tē). Gengivoplastia; um procedimento cirúrgico que dá uma nova forma e um novo contorno ao tecido gengival, com o objetivo de alcançar as formas estética, fisiológica e funcional.

gin·gi·vo·sis (jin - ji - vō′sis). Gengivite descamativa crônica. SIN chronic desquamative gingivitis.

gin·gi·vo·sto·ma·ti·tis (jin′ji - vō - stō′mă - tī′tis). Gengivoestomatite; inflamação da gengiva e de outras mucosas orais. [gengivo- + G. *stoma,* boca, + *-itis,* inflamação]

   primary herpetic g., g. herpética primária. SIN primary herpetic *stomatitis.*

gin·gly·form (jing′gli - form, ging-). Ginglimoidal. SIN ginglymoid. [G. *ginglymos,* uma articulação em dobradiça, + L. *forma,* forma]

gin·glym·o·ar·thro·di·al (jing′gli - mō - ar - thrō′dē - ăl, ging-). Ginglimoartrodial; que indica uma articulação que tem características tanto de gínglimo como de artrodia, ou seja, de articulação sinovial uniaxial e de articulação deslizante.

gin·gly·moid (jing′gli - moyd, ging-). Ginglimoidal; relativo ou que se assemelha a uma articulação sinovial uniaxial. SIN ginglyform. [G. *ginglymos,* uma articulação com movimento em um único plano, + *eidos,* que se assemelha]

gin·gly·mus (jing′gli - mŭs, ging-) [TA]. Gínglimo. SIN hinge *joint.* [G. *ginglymos*]

   helicoid g., g. helicoidal, articulação trocóidea. SIN pivot *joint.*

   lateral g., g. lateral, articulação trocóidea. SIN pivot *joint.*

Ginkgo biloba. Ginkgo biloba, nogueira-do-Japão, gincgo; uma árvore alta, decídua e ornamental da família Ginkgoaceae com folhas bilobadas, diferentes e em forma de leque; as árvores femininas carregam sementes comestíveis envoltas por uma cobertura carnuda que, quando madura, exala um forte cheiro de ácido butírico; é nativa da China, mas a árvore silvestre está extinta, sendo apenas encontrada em cultivos; os extratos das folhas contêm gincgoheterosídeos e lactonas terpênicas e são utilizados medicinalmente em doenças vasculares cerebrais e periféricas. SIN maiden-hair tree.

As folhas da árvore de gincgo têm sido utilizadas na medicina tradicional chinesa e japonesa há muitos séculos nas doenças do cérebro, do coração e dos pulmões. Vários estudos bem controlados têm mostrado que os extratos de gincgo aumentam tanto o fluxo sanguíneo cerebral como o periférico em algumas síndromes de insuficiência vascular. Aliviam os sintomas na demência, vertigem e zumbido de origem vascular, na claudicação intermitente e na síndrome pré-menstrual. Os extratos de gincgo também inibem a agregação plaquetária e eliminam os radicais livres. A dosagem habitual é de 120 a 240 mg/dia divididos em 2 a 3 doses. A administração durante várias semanas pode ser necessária antes que os efeitos benéficos sejam observados. Embora a *G. biloba* seja oferecida como uma "pílula inteligente" pelos fornecedores de medicamentos à base de ervas, ela não melhora a função mental de pessoas sem doença vascular cerebral. Os efeitos colaterais são incomuns e incluem distúrbios gastrointestinais, cefaléia e erupção cutânea. Já foram relatados alguns casos de hemorragia subaracnóidea e hifema, particularmente em pessoas que também tomam ácido acetilsalicílico. A administração do extrato de gincgo deve ser interrompida antes de cirurgias.

gin·seng (jin′seng). Ginseng; as raízes de várias espécies de *Panax* (família Araliaceae), apreciada como de grande virtude medicinal pelos chineses, amplamente utilizadas como um "alimento medicamentoso"; supõe-se que o ginseng melhore as funções físicas e mentais. [Ch.]

Giordano-Giovannetti di·et. Dieta de Giordano-Giovannetti. Ver em diet.

GIP Abreviatura de gastric inhibitory *polypeptide* (polipeptídeo inibidor gástrico); gastric inhibitory *peptide* (peptídeo inibitório gástrico).

Girard, Alfred C., cirurgião naturalizado norte-americano nascido na Suíça, 1841–1914. VER G. *reagent.*

gir·dle (ger′dl) [TA]. Cinturão, halo, couraça, cíngulo. Uma estrutura que possui a forma de um cinturão ou uma cinta. SIN cingulum (1) [TA]. [A.S. *gyrdel*]

   Hitzig g., couraça de Hitzig, couraça tabética. SIN tabetic *cuirass.*

   Neptune g., uma faixa úmida aplicada ao redor do abdome.

   pectoral g. [TA], cíngulo do membro superior; o anel ósseo incompleto formado pelas clavículas e escápulas e que sustenta os membros superiores, ligando o esqueleto apendicular ao esqueleto axial (manúbrio do esterno). SIN cingulum pectorale [TA], cingulum membri superioris*, shoulder g.*, thoracic g.

   pelvic g. [TA], cíngulo do membro inferior; os ossos direito e esquerdo do quadril unidos na sínfise púbica e por meio dos quais o esqueleto apendicular dos membros inferiores é ligado ao esqueleto axial (sacro); os ossos unem-se de tal modo que formam um anel ósseo; a pelve óssea. SIN cingulum pelvici [TA], cingulum membri inferioris*.

   shoulder g., cíngulo do membro superior; *termo oficial alternativo para pectoral g.

   thoracic g., cíngulo do membro superior. SIN pectoral g.

   white limbal g. of Vogt, halo límbico branco de Vogt; depósitos branco-amarelados, simétricos e curvos, localizados na região periférica da córnea e freqüentemente observados em pacientes com mais de 40 anos de idade.

Girdlestone, Gathorne Robert, ortopedista britânico, 1881–1950. VER G. *procedure.*

gi·tal·in (jit′ă - lin). Gitalina; um extrato de *Digitalis purpurea* (dedaleira) que contém uma mistura de glicosídeos e agliconas, com ação e usos similares aos dos digitálicos.

gith·a·gism (gith′ă - jizm). Gitagismo; uma doença semelhante ao latirismo; acredita-se que seja resultante do envenenamento por sementes de gitago ou nigela-dos-trigos, *Agrostemma githago* ou *Lychnis githago*. [L. *gith*, uma planta, coentro romano, + *ago*, conduzir]

gi·tog·e·nin (jit′ō - jen - in). Gitogenina; a genina da gitonina; um agente cardiotônico.

gi·to·nin (jit′ō - nin). Gitonina; um tetraglicosídeo gitogenina composto de duas galactoses, uma glicose e uma xilose; a gitogenina F possui uma galactose, duas glicoses e uma xilose. Ambas são agentes cardiotônicos.

gi·tox·i·gen·in (ji - toks′ē - jen - in). Gitoxigenina; a aglicona de gitoxina.

gi·tox·in (ji - tok′sin). Gitoxina; um glicosídeo cardíaco secundário proveniente da *Digitalis purpurea* e da *D. lanata*. SIN anhydrogitalin, bigitalin, pseudodigitoxin.

git·ter·zel·le (git′er - zel - e). Fagócito microglial preenchido por lipídios. SIN gitter cell. [Al. de *Gitter*, treliça, + *Zelle*, célula]

Gla Abreviatura de 4-carboxyglutamic acid (ácido 4-carboxiglutâmico).

gla·bel·la (glă - bel′ă) [TA]. Glabela. **1.** Uma proeminência lisa, muito acentuada no homem, localizada no osso frontal acima da raiz do nariz. **2.** O ponto que mais se projeta para a frente, localizado na linha média da fronte na altura das cristas supra-orbitais. SIN mesophryon. VER TAMBÉM antinion. SIN intercilium. [L. *glabellus*, calvo, liso, dim. de *glaber*]

gla·bel·lad (glă - bel′ad). Em direção à glabela.

gla·brous, gla·brate (glā′brŭs, glā′brăt). Glabro; liso ou sem pêlos; que indica as áreas do corpo onde normalmente não há pêlos, isto é, as regiões palmares ou plantares. [L. *glaber*, liso]

glad·i·ate (glad′ē - āt). Xifóide, ensiforme. SIN xiphoid. [L. *gladius*, uma espada]

glad·i·o·lus (glă - dī′ō - lŭs, glad′ē - ō′lŭs). Corpo do esterno. SIN body of sternum. [L. dim. de *gladius*, uma espada]

GLAND

gland [TA]. Glândula; um agregado organizado de células que funciona como um órgão secretório ou excretório. SIN glandula (1) [TA]. [L. *glans*, bolota, glande (fruto do carvalho)]

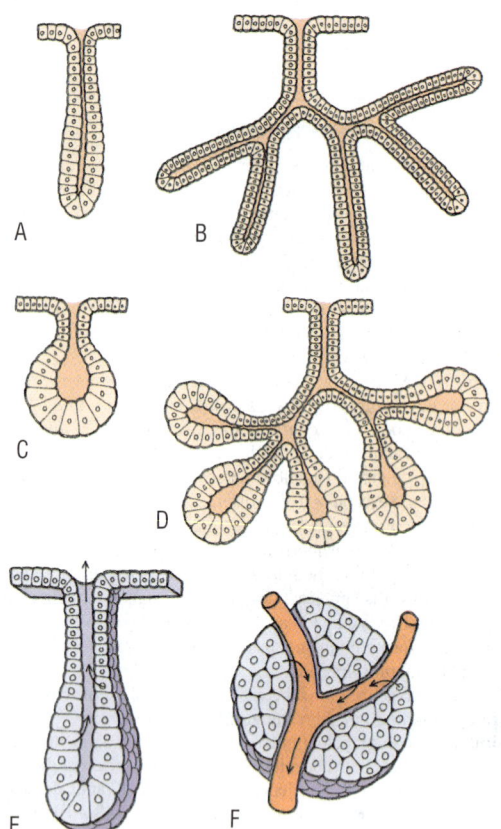

tipos de **glândulas:** (A) tubular, (B) tubular composta, (C) acinosa, (D) acinosa composta, (E) exócrina, (F) endócrina

accessory g., g. acessória; uma pequena massa de estrutura glandular, destacada porém próxima a uma outra g. maior, a qual é similar em estrutura e, provavelmente, em função.

accessory lacrimal g.'s [TA], glândulas lacrimais acessórias; glândulas pequenas, tubulares, compostas, ramificadas, localizadas às vezes na parte média da pálpebra (glândulas de Wolfring, 1872, ou glândulas de Ciaccio, 1874) ou ao longo dos fórnices superior e inferior do saco conjuntival (glândulas de Krause, 1854). Essas g. acessórias são porções ectópicas do tecido da g. lacrimal; todas elas produzem o mesmo tipo de lágrima, que é secretado sobre a superfície conjuntival. As "glândulas" de Henle e Baumgarten não são de fato glândulas, mas meras invaginações epiteliais. SIN glandulae lacrimales accessoriae [TA].

accessory parotid g. [TA], g. parótida acessória; uma ilhota ocasional de tecido da parótida separada da massa da glândula, que se situa anteriormente logo acima do início do ducto da parótida. SIN glandula parotidea accessoria [TA], admaxillary g., glandula parotis accessoria, socia parotidis.

accessory suprarenal g.'s [TA], glândulas supra-renais acessórias; massas isoladas, freqüentemente diminutas, de tecido supra-renal, às vezes encontradas próximo às glândulas principais ou no ligamento largo ou no epidídimo. SIN glandulae suprarenales accessoriae [TA].

accessory thyroid g. [TA], g. tireóide acessória; uma massa isolada, ou uma de várias massas isoladas, de tecido da tireóide, às vezes presente no lado do pescoço ou variando sua posição desde logo acima do osso hióide (glândula tireóide acessória supra-hióidea) até o arco da aorta inferiormente. SIN glandula thyroidea accessoria [TA], accessory thyroid, prehyoid g., suprahyoid g., thyroidea accessoria, thyroidea ima, Wölfler g.

acid g., g. ácida; uma das glândulas gástricas que secretam o ácido clorídrico do suco gástrico. SIN oxyntic g.

acinotubular g., g. acinotubular, g. tubuloacinar. SIN tubuloacinar g.

acinous g., g. acinosa; uma g. na qual a(s) unidade(s) secretória(s) possui(em) a forma de um cacho de uvas e um lúmen muito pequeno; p.ex., a parte exócrina do pâncreas.

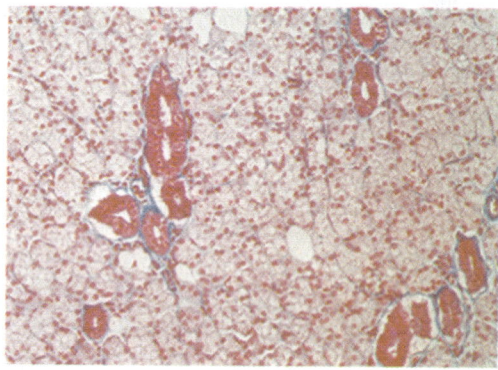

glândula acinosa: glândula parótida mostrando o sistema de ductos ramificados

admaxillary g., g. parótida acessória. SIN accessory parotid g.

adrenal g., g. supra-renal. SIN suprarenal g.

aggregate g.'s, linfonodos agregados do intestino delgado. SIN aggregated lymphoid *nodules* of small intestine, em *nodule*.

agminate g.'s, agminated g.'s, linfonodos agregados do intestino delgado. SIN aggregated lymphoid *nodules* of small intestine, em *nodule*.

Albarran g.'s, glândulas de Albarran; diminutas glândulas submucosas ou túbulos ramificados localizados na região subcervical da próstata, que se esvaziam em geral na parte posterior da uretra. SIN Albarran y Dominguez tubules.

albuminous g., g. albuminosa; uma g. que secreta um líquido aquoso.

alveolar g., g. alveolar; uma g. na qual a(s) unidade(s) secretória(s) possui(em) a forma de um saco e um lúmen evidente; p.ex., a glândula mamária ativa.

anal g., g. anal. **(1)** Uma de várias glândulas sudoríferas grandes localizadas na mucosa do ânus; **(2)** um sinônimo incorreto para o saco anal.

anterior lingual g., g. lingual anterior; uma das pequenas glândulas mistas localizadas profundamente próximo ao ápice da língua em cada lado do frênulo. SIN apical g., Bauhin g., Blandin g., glandula lingualis anterior, Nuhn g.

apical g., g. lingual anterior. SIN anterior lingual g.

apocrine g., g. apócrina; uma g. cujo produto secretado inclui uma porção apical da célula secretória, tal como ocorre na secreção de gotículas de lipídios na lactação.

apocrine sweat g.'s, glândulas sudoríferas apócrinas; glândulas sudoríferas que se desenvolvem em associação aos folículos pilosos e sofrem hipertrofia e desenvolvimento secretório na puberdade; secretam um suor viscoso e inodoro que sustenta o crescimento de bactérias produtoras de um cheiro acre; a

gland

secreção ocorre por meio de um mecanismo écrino, e não apócrino. SIN axillary sweat g.'s.

areolar g.'s [TA], glândulas areolares; várias glândulas sebáceas maiores que formam pequenas projeções arredondadas na superfície da aréola da mama; sofrem hipertrofia na gravidez e, durante a lactação, secretam uma substância que, presumivelmente, impede a formação de fissuras. SIN glandulae areolares [TA], Montgomery follicles, Montgomery g.'s.

arteriococcygeal g., glomo coccígeo. SIN coccygeal body.

arytenoid g.'s, glândulas laríngeas. SIN laryngeal g.'s.

Aselli g., g. de Aselli; um linfonodo único e grande situado ventralmente à aorta abdominal que recebe toda a linfa proveniente dos intestinos em muitos dos mamíferos menores. SIN Aselli pancreas.

g.'s of auditory tube, glândulas da tuba auditiva. SIN tubal g.'s of pharyngotympanic tube.

axillary g.'s, linfonodos axilares. SIN axillary *lymph nodes*, em *lymph node*.

axillary sweat g.'s, glândulas sudoríferas axilares. SIN apocrine sweat g.'s.

Bartholin g., g. de Bartholin; g. vestibular maior. SIN greater vestibular g.

basal g., hipófise. SIN pituitary g.

Bauhin g., g. de Bauhin, g. lingual anterior. SIN anterior lingual g.

Baumgarten g.'s, glândulas de Baumgarten. SIN Henle g.'s.

biliary g.'s, glândulas do ducto colédoco; *termo oficial alternativo para g.'s of (common) bile duct.

g.'s of biliary mucosa, glândulas da mucosa biliar; pequenas glândulas mucosas e tubuloalveolares, localizadas na mucosa dos ductos biliares maiores e principalmente no colo da vesícula biliar. SIN glandulae mucosae biliosae, Luschka cystic g.'s, Theile g.'s.

Blandin g., g. de Blandin, g. lingual anterior. SIN anterior lingual g.

Bowman g., g. de Bowman, g. olfatórias. SIN olfactory g.'s. VER olfactory g.'s.

brachial g., linfonodo braquial; um dos linfonodos do braço.

bronchial g.'s [TA], glândulas bronquiais; glândulas mucosas e seromucosas cujas unidades secretórias estão situadas fora do músculo dos brônquios. SIN glandulae bronchiales [TA].

Bruch g.'s, linfonodos localizados na conjuntiva da pálpebra. SIN trachoma g.'s.

Brunner g.'s, glândulas de Brunner, g. duodenais. SIN duodenal g.'s.

buccal g.'s [TA], glândulas das bochechas; numerosas glândulas racemosas, mucosas e serosas localizadas no tecido submucoso das bochechas. SIN glandulae buccales [TA], genal g.'s.

bulbourethral g. [TA], g. bulbouretral; uma de duas glândulas pequenas, compostas e racemosas, que produzem uma secreção mucóide e estão situadas lado a lado ao longo da uretra membranácea, acima do bulbo do pênis; secretam através de um pequeno ducto para a parte esponjosa da uretra. SIN glandula bulbourethralis [TA], Cowper g., Méry g.

cardiac g., g. do cárdia, g. cárdica; uma g. tubular, enrolada, localizada no cárdia do estômago; secreta basicamente muco.

cardiac g.'s, glândulas cárdicas, g. do cárdia. SIN cardiac g.'s of stomach.

cardiac g.'s of esophagus, glândulas cárdicas, g. do cárdia. SIN cardiac g.'s of stomach.

cardiac g.'s of stomach [TA], glândulas cárdicas, g. do cárdia; glândulas localizadas na lâmina própria da porção mais inferior do esôfago; assemelham-se às glândulas cárdicas do estômago e são constituídas de túbulos ramificados de células mucosas secretoras de um muco neutro que, presumivelmente, fornece proteção contra o refluxo de ácido. SIN cardiac g.'s of esophagus, cardiac g.'s.

ceruminous g.'s, glândulas ceruminosas; glândulas sudoríferas apócrinas localizadas no meato acústico externo. SIN glandulae ceruminosae (1).

cervical g.'s, glândulas cervicais. SIN glandulae cervicales uteri [TA]. SIN cervical g.'s of uterus.

cervical g.'s of uterus [TA], glândulas cervicais do útero; glândulas ramificadas, secretoras de muco, localizadas na mucosa do colo do útero. SIN cervical g.'s.

Ciaccio g.'s, glândulas de Ciaccio. VER accessory lacrimal g.'s.

ciliary g.'s [TA], glândulas ciliares; várias glândulas sudoríferas apócrinas modificadas localizadas nas pálpebras, com ductos que, em geral, se abrem no interior dos folículos dos cílios. SIN glandulae ciliares [TA], Moll g.'s.

circumanal g.'s, glândulas circum-anais; grandes glândulas sudoríferas apócrinas que circundam o ânus. SIN Gay g.'s, glandulae circumanales.

coccygeal g., glomo coccígeo. SIN coccygeal body.

coil g., g. convoluta; uma g. cuja parte secretória é enrolada. SIN convoluted g.

g.'s of (common) bile duct [TA], glândulas do ducto colédoco; glândulas tubuloalveolares, secretoras de mucina, dispostas em cachos ao longo das paredes do ducto colédoco. SIN glandulae ductus choledochi [TA], biliary g.'s*, glandulae ductus biliaris*.

compound g., g. composta; uma g. cujos ductos excretórios maiores se ramificam repetidas vezes em ductos menores, que, por fim, drenam as unidades secretórias.

conjunctival g.'s [TA], glândulas conjuntivais; aglomerados de células mucosas localizados no epitélio da conjuntiva e encontrados em maior número na conjuntiva do bulbo. SIN glandulae conjunctivales [TA], Terson g.'s.

convoluted g., g. convoluta. SIN coil g.

Cowper g., g. de Cowper; g. bulbouretral. SIN bulbourethral g.

cutaneous g.'s, glândulas da pele; qualquer uma das glândulas da pele. SIN glandulae cutis [TA].

ductless g.'s, glândulas endócrinas. SIN endocrine g.'s.

duodenal g.'s [TA], glândulas duodenais; pequenas glândulas tubulares convolutas e ramificadas que estão presentes principalmente na submucosa do primeiro terço do duodeno; secretam uma substância mucóide alcalina que neutraliza o suco gástrico. SIN glandulae duodenales [TA], Brunner g.'s, Wepfer g.'s.

Duverney g., g. de Duverney, g. vestibular maior. SIN greater vestibular g.

Ebner g.'s, glândulas de Ebner, g. gustativas serosas, na parte posterior da língua, próximas às papilas circunvaladas.

eccrine g., g. écrina; uma g. sudorífera tubular e convoluta (diferente das glândulas apócrinas) que é encontrada na pele em quase todas as partes do corpo.

ecdysial g.'s, glândulas ecdisiais; estruturas dos insetos que se originam do ectoderma da parte ventrocaudal da cabeça e servem como fonte de ecdisona. SIN peritracheal g.'s, prothoracic g.'s, thoracic g.'s, ventral g.'s.

Eglis g.'s, glândulas de Eglis; pequenas glândulas mucosas inconstantes do ureter e da pelve renal.

endocrine g.'s [TA], glândulas endócrinas; glândulas que não possuem ductos e cujas secreções são absorvidas diretamente para o sangue. SIN glandulae endocrinae [TA], ductless g.'s, endocrine system, g.'s of internal secretion, glandulae sine ductibus.

esophageal g.'s, glândulas esofágicas; um número variável de glândulas mucosas, compostas e pequenas, localizadas na submucosa do esôfago. SIN glandulae esophageae.

g.'s of eustachian tube, glândulas da tuba de Eustáquio, g. da tuba auditiva. SIN tubal g.'s of pharyngotympanic tube.

excretory g., g. excretora; um g. que retira material não-aproveitável do sangue.

exocrine g., g. exócrina; uma g. cujas secreções alcançam alguma superfície livre do corpo através de ductos.

external salivary g., g. salivar externa,. g. parótida. SIN parotid g.

g.'s of the female urethra, glândulas uretrais da mulher. SIN urethral g.'s of female.

follicular g., g. folicular; uma g. composta de folículos.

fundic g.'s, glândulas gástricas. SIN gastric g.'s.

Galeati g.'s, glândulas de Galeati, g. intestinais. SIN intestinal g.'s.

gastric g.'s [TA], glândulas gástricas; glândulas tubulares e ramificadas localizadas na mucosa do fundo e do corpo do estômago; essas glândulas contêm células parietais que secretam ácido clorídrico, células zimogênicas que produzem pepsina e células mucosas. SIN glandulae gastricae [TA], fundic g.'s, gastric follicles, Wasmann g.'s.

Gay g.'s, glândulas de Gay, g. circum-anais. SIN circumanal g.'s.

genal g.'s, glândulas da bochecha. SIN buccal g.'s.

genital g., (1) Testículo. SIN testis; (2) Ovário. SIN ovary.

Gley g.'s, glândulas de Gley, g. paratireóides. VER parathyroid g.

glomiform g.'s, Glomo. SIN glomus (2).

greater vestibular g. [TA], g. vestibular maior; uma de duas glândulas tubuloalveolares secretoras de muco localizadas em ambos os lados da parte inferior da vagina; equivalem às glândulas bulbouretrais no homem; são embainhadas juntamente com os bulbos vestibulares pelos músculos isquiocavernosos. Assim, a ereção e a concomitante contração muscular provocam secreção para o interior do vestíbulo da vagina. SIN glandula vestibularis major [TA], Bartholin g., Duverney g., Tiedemann g., vulvovaginal g.

Guérin g.'s, glândulas de Guérin, g. uretrais da mulher. SIN urethral g.'s of female.

hemal g., nó hemolinfático. SIN hemal node.

hematopoietic g., g. hematopoética; um órgão formador de sangue, tal como o baço.

hemolymph g., nó hemolinfático. SIN hemal node.

Henle g.'s, glândulas de Henle; antigamente consideradas glândulas lacrimais acessórias, essas invaginações epiteliais estão localizadas próximo aos fórnices na parte medial da conjuntiva da pálpebra; abrem-se na superfície da conjuntiva. VER TAMBÉM accessory lacrimal g.'s. SIN Baumgarten g.'s.

hibernating g., g. hibernante. SIN brown fat.

holocrine g., g. holócrina; uma g. cuja secreção consiste em células desintegradas da própria glândula, p.ex., uma g. sebácea, em contraste com uma g. merócrina.

internal salivary g., g. salivar interna; as glândulas sublinguais e submandibulares consideradas como uma só glândula.

g.'s of internal secretion, glândulas de secreção interna. SIN endocrine g.'s.

interscapular g., tecido adiposo multilocular. SIN brown fat.

interstitial g., células intersticiais. VER interstitial *cells*, em *cell*.

intestinal g.'s [TA], glândulas intestinais; as glândulas tubulares localizadas na mucosa dos intestinos delgado e grosso. SIN glandulae intestinales [TA], crypts of Lieberkühn, Galeati g.'s, intestinal follicles, Lieberkühn follicles, Lieberkühn g.'s.

intraepithelial g.'s, glândulas intra-epiteliais; aglomerados de células glandulares localizados dentro do epitélio, como aqueles da uretra.
jugular g., linfonodo-sentinela. SIN signal lymph node.
Knoll g.'s, glândulas de Knoll; glândulas localizadas nas pregas ventriculares da laringe (cordas vocais falsas).
Krause g.'s, glândulas de Krause. (1) VER accessory lacrimal g.'s; (2) as glândulas localizadas na mucosa da cavidade timpânica. VER accessory lacrimal g.'s.
labial g.'s [TA], glândulas labiais; glândulas mucosas localizadas no tecido submucoso dos lábios. SIN glandulae labiales [TA].
lacrimal g. [TA], g. lacrimal; a glândula que secreta lágrimas; consiste em seis a 12 glândulas serosas, tubuloalveolares, compostas e separadas, localizadas na parte látero-superior da órbita; é parcialmente dividida em uma parte palpebral menor (pars palpebralis) e uma parte orbital maior (pars orbitalis) pela aponeurose do músculo levantador da pálpebra. SIN glandula lacrimalis [TA].
lactiferous g., g. mamária. SIN mammary g.
g.'s of large intestine [TA], glândulas do intestino grosso; túbulos de epitélio mucoso, perpendiculares à superfície luminal e semelhantes a uma peneira, por causa da abundância de aberturas glandulares; as glândulas são revestidas por células epiteliais colunares curtas — principalmente células caliciformes com algumas células enteroendócrinas que absorvem água intercaladas; as glândulas do intestino grosso são mais longas (mais profundas), mais abundantes, mais intimamente apostas e apresentam uma densidade maior de células caliciformes (com exceção das células de Paneth), quando comparadas com as glândulas do intestino delgado. VER TAMBÉM g.'s of small intestine. SIN glandulae intestini crassi [TA], crypts of Lieberkühn of large intestine.
laryngeal g.'s [TA], glândulas laríngeas; um grande número de glândulas mistas localizadas na mucosa da laringe; de acordo com sua localização, são denominadas anteriores, médias e posteriores. SIN glandulae laryngeae [TA], arytenoid g.'s.
lesser vestibular g.'s [TA], glândulas vestibulares menores; várias glândulas mucosas diminutas que se abrem na superfície do vestíbulo entre os orifícios da vagina e uretra. SIN glandulae vestibulares minores [TA].
Lieberkühn g.'s, glândulas de Lieberkühn, g. intestinais. SIN intestinal g.'s.
Littré g.'s, glândulas de Littré, g. uretrais do homem. SIN urethral g.'s of male.
Luschka g., (1) Tonsila faríngea. SIN pharyngeal tonsil; (2) antigo nome para *corpus* coccygeum (glomo coccígeo).
Luschka cystic g.'s, glândulas císticas de Luschka, g. da mucosa biliar. SIN g.'s of biliary mucosa.
lymph g., gânglio linfático, linfonodo. SIN lymph node.
major salivary g.'s [TA], glândulas salivares maiores; uma categoria de glândulas salivares englobando as três maiores glândulas da cavidade oral e que também secretam a maior parte da saliva: as glândulas parótidas, submandibulares e sublinguais. SIN glandulae salivariae majores [TA].
g.'s of the male urethra, glândulas uretrais do homem. SIN urethral g.'s of male.
malpighian g.'s, corpúsculos de Malpighi, folículos linfáticos esplênicos. SIN splenic lymph follicles, em follicle.
mammary g. [TA], g. mamária; a potencial e ativa g. alveolar, composta, apócrina e secretora de leite, que está situada dentro da mama. Consiste em 15 a 24 lobos, cada um formado por muitos lóbulos, separados por septos fibrosos e tecido adiposo; o parênquima da glândula feminina pós-puberal em repouso é composto por ductos; os alvéolos desenvolvem-se apenas durante a gravidez, permanecendo ativos até a lactação. Normalmente, a glândula permanece rudimentar (indistinguível daquela da infância) nos homens. VER TAMBÉM breast. SIN glandula mammaria [TA], lactiferous g., milk g.
marrow-lymph g., um tipo de nó hemolinfático cuja estrutura e provável função assemelham-se à da medula óssea.
master g., hipófise. SIN pituitary g.
maxillary g., g. submandibular. SIN submandibular g.
meibomian g.'s, glândulas de Meibomio, g. tarsais. SIN tarsal g.'s.
merocrine g., g. merócrina; uma g. que libera apenas um produto secretório acelular, em contraste com uma g. holócrina.
Méry g., g. de Méry, g. bulbouretral. SIN bulbourethral g.
mesenteric g.'s, linfonodos mesentéricos. VER mesenteric lymph nodes, em lymph node.
milk g., g. mamária. SIN mammary g.
minor salivary g.'s [TA], glândulas salivares menores; as menores glândulas exócrinas, que secretam sobretudo muco, presentes na cavidade oral; consistem nas glândulas labiais, molares, linguais, palatinas e das bochechas. SIN glandulae salivariae minores [TA].
mixed g., g. mista. (1) Uma g. que contém tanto unidades secretórias mucosas como serosas; (2) uma g. que é tanto exócrina como endócrina, p.ex., o pâncreas.
molar g.'s [TA], glândulas molares; quatro ou cinco glândulas bucais grandes situadas na vizinhança do último dente molar. SIN glandulae molares [TA].
Moll g.'s, glândulas de Moll, g. ciliares. SIN ciliary g.'s.
Montgomery g.'s, glândulas de Montgomery, g. areolares. SIN areolar g.'s.

g.'s of mouth [TA], glândulas da boca; glândulas que se esvaziam na cavidade oral. SIN glandulae oris [TA].
mucilaginous g., g. mucilaginosas; termo obsoleto para uma das vilosidades sinoviais que, para Havers, eram as responsáveis pela secreção da sinóvia.
muciparous g., g. mucosa. SIN mucous g.
mucous g., g. mucosa; uma glândula que secreta muco. SIN glandula mucosa, muciparous g.
mucous g.'s of auditory tube, glândulas mucosas da tuba auditiva. SIN tubal g.'s of pharyngotympanic tube.
nasal g.'s [TA], glândulas nasais; glândulas seromucosas localizadas na região respiratória da membrana mucosa nasal. SIN glandulae nasales [TA].
Nuhn g., g. de Nuhn, g. lingual anterior. SIN anterior lingual g.
odoriferous g., g. odorífera. (1) Uma g., tal como a g. de Tyson (g. prepucial), cuja secreção possui um cheiro forte; (2) VER sweat g.'s.
oil g.'s, glândulas sebáceas. SIN sebaceous g.'s.
olfactory g.'s [TA], glândulas olfatórias; glândulas (de Bowman) tubuloalveolares, ramificadas e serosas localizadas na membrana mucosa da região olfatória da cavidade nasal. SIN glandulae olfactoriae [TA], Bowman g.
oxyntic g., g. oxíntica. SIN acid g.
pacchionian g.'s, granulações de Pacchioni, fovéolas granulares. SIN arachnoid granulations, em granulation.
palatine g.'s [TA], glândulas palatinas; numerosas glândulas racemosas e mucosas localizadas na metade posterior do tecido submucoso que cobre o palato duro. SIN glandulae palatinae [TA].
palpebral g.'s, glândulas tarsais. SIN tarsal g.'s.
parathyroid g. [TA], g. paratireóide; um par de duas pequenas glândulas endócrinas pareadas, superior e inferior, encontradas em geral embebidas em uma cápsula de tecido conectivo na superfície posterior da glândula tireóide; secretam paratormônio, que regula o metabolismo do cálcio e do fósforo. O parênquima é composto de células principais e oxínticas dispostas em cordões anastomosantes. A remoção inadvertida de todas as glândulas paratireóides, como ocorre durante uma tireoidectomia, provoca tetania e pode ser fatal na ausência de reposição hormonal. SIN glandula parathyroidea [TA], epithelial body, parathyroid (2).
paraurethral g.'s, glândulas uretrais da mulher. SIN urethral g.'s of female.
parotid g. [TA], g. parótida; a maior das glândulas salivares, uma das glândulas acinosas, compostas e bilaterais situadas abaixo e à frente da orelha, dos dois lados, estendendo-se do ângulo da mandíbula, inferiormente, até o arco zigomático, superiormente, posteriormente ao músculo esternocleidomastóideo, medialmente à fossa infratemporal (profundamente em relação ao ramo da mandíbula); é subdividida em uma parte superficial (pars superficialis) e em uma parte profunda (pars profunda) por ramos emergentes do nervo facial e secreta através do ducto parotídeo. SIN glandula parotidea [TA], external salivary g., glandula parotis.
pectoral g.'s, linfonodos axilares. VER axillary lymph nodes, em lymph node.
peptic g., g. péptica; uma g. que secreta pepsina. VER gastric g.'s.
peritracheal g.'s, glândulas peritraqueais, g. ecdisiais. SIN ecdysial g.'s.
perspiratory g.'s, glândulas sudoríferas. SIN sweat g.'s.
Peyer g.'s, linfonodos de Peyer. SIN aggregated lymphoid nodules of small intestine, em nodule.
pharyngeal g.'s [TA], glândulas faríngeas; glândulas mucosas e racemosas situadas sob a mucosa da faringe. SIN glandulae pharyngeales [TA].
Philip g.'s, glândulas de Philip; glândulas profundas e aumentadas, logo acima da clavícula e encontradas em crianças com tuberculose pulmonar e, ocasionalmente, em outras crianças.
pileous g., g. pilosa; uma g. sebácea que drena em um folículo piloso.
pineal g. [TA], g. pineal. SIN pineal body.
pituitary g. [TA], hipófise (pituitária); uma glândula composta e única, suspensa da base do hipotálamo por uma curta extensão do infundíbulo — o pedúnculo do infundíbulo ou da hipófise. A g. consiste em duas subdivisões principais: 1) a neuro-hipófise, que compreende o infundíbulo e sua terminação bulbosa — a parte neural ou o processo infundibular (lobo posterior) —, composta de pituitócitos semelhantes à neuróglia, vasos sanguíneos e fibras nervosas não-mielinizadas do trato hipotálamo-hipofisário, cujos corpos celulares residem nos núcleos supra-óptico e paraventricular do hipotálamo e que conduzem os hormônios neurossecretórios, oxitocina e hormônio antidiurético ao lobo para armazenamento e liberação; 2) a adeno-hipófise, que compreende a parte distal, maior — uma extensão desse lobo (parte infundibular) que se assemelha a uma manga e reveste o pedúnculo do infundíbulo —, e uma parte intermédia, delgada (pouco desenvolvida em seres humanos) e situada entre os lobos anterior e posterior; o lobo anterior é formado por cordões de células de vários tipos diferentes intercaladas por capilares do sistema porta hipotálamo-hipofisário; a secreção de somatotrofinas, prolactina, hormônio tireoestimulante, gonadotrofinas, adrenocorticotrofina e outros peptídeos pela adeno-hipófise é regulada por fatores de liberação e de inibição elaborados por neurônios localizados no hipotálamo e que são captados por um plexo primário de capilares na eminência mediana e transportados, por meio dos vasos portais da parte infundibular, e do tronco infundibular, até um plexo secundá-

rio de capilares situado na parte distal. SIN hypophysis [TA], glandula pituitaria*, basal g., glandula basilaris, hypophysis cerebri, master g.

Poirier g., um linfonodo localizado na artéria uterina, no ponto onde ela cruza com o ureter.

prehyoid g., g. tireóide acessória. SIN accessory thyroid g.

preputial g.'s [TA], glândulas prepuciais; glândulas sebáceas da coroa e do colo da glande do pênis, que produzem uma substância odorífera denominada esmegma. SIN glandulae preputiales [TA], Tyson g.'s.

prostate g., próstata; SIN prostate.

prothoracic g.'s, g. ecdisiais. SIN ecdysial g.'s.

pyloric g.'s [TA], glândulas pilóricas; as glândulas tubulares e enroladas do piloro, cujas células secretam muco. SIN glandulae pyloricae [TA].

racemose g., g. racemosa; uma g. que possui a aparência de um cacho de uvas, (reconstrução tridimensional), p.ex., uma g. alveolar ou acinosa composta.

Rivinus g., g. de Rivinus, g. sublingual. SIN sublingual g.

Rosenmüller g., linfonodo inguinal profundo proximal. SIN proximal deep inguinal lymph node.

saccular g., g. sacular; uma g. alveolar única.

salivary g. [TA], g. salivar; qualquer uma das glândulas exócrinas secretoras de saliva da cavidade oral. VER TAMBÉM major salivary g.'s, minor salivary g.'s. SIN glandula salivaria [TA].

sebaceous g.'s [TA], glândulas sebáceas; numerosas glândulas holócrinas, localizadas na derme, que se abrem em geral nos folículos pilosos e que secretam uma substância semifluida e oleosa, o sebo. SIN glandulae sebaceae [TA], oil g.'s, sebaceous follicles.

seminal g. [TA], g. seminal; uma de duas estruturas glandulares, saculadas e pregueadas, que compõem um divertículo do ducto deferente; sua secreção corresponde a um dos componentes do sêmen; de modo diferente do que historicamente se pensou, essa g. em geral não armazena espermatozóides. SIN glandula vesiculosa [TA], glandula seminalis*, seminal vesicle*, vesicula seminalis*, gonecyst, gonecystis, seminal capsule.

sentinel g., gânglio-sentinela; um linfonodo único e aumentado localizado no omento; pode ser sinal de uma úlcera oposta a ele e situada na curvatura maior ou na curvatura menor do estômago.

seromucous g., g. seromucosa. (1) Uma glândula na qual algumas das células secretoras são serosas e outras mucosas; (2) uma glândula cujas células secretam um líquido intermediário entre uma substância aquosa e uma mucóide viscosa. SIN glandula seromucosa.

serous g., g. serosa; uma glândula que secreta uma substância aquosa que pode ou não conter uma enzima. SIN glandula serosa.

Serres g.'s, glândula de Serres; restos de células epiteliais encontrados no tecido conectivo subepitelial situado no palato do recém-nascido, semelhantes àqueles encontrados nas gengivas.

sexual g., testículo ou ovário. VER testis, ovary.

Skene g.'s, glândulas de Skene, g. uretral da mulher. SIN urethral g.'s of female.

g.'s of small intestine [TA], glândulas do intestino delgado; fossas (criptas) epiteliais, tubulares e paralelas que se abrem nas bases dos vilos intestinais; suas paredes delgadas são formadas por células epiteliais colunares, principalmente por células-mãe indiferenciadas e células intermediárias e por um número crescente de células caliciformes, conforme o intestino delgado avança distalmente; todas as células migram para fora das glândulas, sobre os vilos, exceto as células de Paneth, secretoras de proteínas (enzimas), que permanecem nas glândulas. VER TAMBÉM g.'s of large intestine. SIN glandulae intestini tenuis [TA] crypts of Lieberkühn, g.'s of small intestine.

solitary g.'s, linfonodos solitários. SIN solitary lymphatic nodules, em nodule.

sublingual g. [TA], g. sublingual; uma de duas glândulas salivares localizadas no assoalho da boca, sob a língua, e que secretam através dos ductos sublinguais; a maioria das unidades secretoras da glândula dos seres humanos produz secreção mucosa e apresenta estruturas com forma de meia-lua que produzem secreção serosa. SIN glandula sublingualis [TA], Rivinus g.

submandibular g. [TA], g. submandibular; uma de duas glândulas salivares situadas no pescoço, no espaço limitado pelos dois ventres do músculo digástrico e pelo ângulo da mandíbula; as unidades secretoras são predominantemente serosas, embora existam alguns alvéolos mucosos que apresentam estruturas com forma de meia-lua que produzem secreção serosa. SIN glandula submandibularis [TA], maxillary g., submaxillary g.

submaxillary g., g. submandibular. SIN submandibular g.

sudoriferous g.'s, glândulas sudoríferas. SIN sweat g.'s.

suprahyoid g., g. tireóide acessória. SIN accessory thyroid g.

suprarenal g. [TA], g. supra-renal; um corpo achatado e quase triangular posicionado na extremidade superior de cada rim, porém primariamente fixado aos pilares do diafragma; é uma das glândulas endócrinas (sem ductos) que fornece secreções internas (epinefrina e norepinefrina provenientes da medula supra-renal e hormônios esteróides provenientes do córtex supra-renal). SIN glandula suprarenalis [TA], adrenal body, adrenal capsule, adrenal g., atrabiliary capsule, glandula atrabiliaris, paranephros, suprarenal body, suprarenal capsule.

Suzanne g., g. de Suzanne; uma pequena g. mucosa situada no assoalho da boca.

sweat g.'s [TA], glândulas sudoríferas; as glândulas enroladas da pele que secretam o suor em resposta a uma emoção ou para permitir o resfriamento por evaporação em um ambiente quente. SIN glandulae sudoriferae [TA], perspiratory g.'s, sudoriferous g.'s.

target g., g.-alvo; o órgão efetor que funciona quando estimulado pela secreção interna de uma outra glândula ou por algum outro estímulo.

tarsal g.'s [TA], glândulas tarsais; glândulas sebáceas incrustadas na placa tarsal de cada pálpebra e que se abrem na margem da pálpebra, próximo à borda posterior. Suas secreções criam uma barreira lipídica, ao longo da margem das pálpebras, que retém as secreções normais no saco conjuntival, impedindo que o líquido aquoso transborde para fora da barreira quando o olho está aberto. SIN glandulae tarsales [TA], meibomian g.'s, palpebral g.'s.

Terson g.'s, glândulas de Terson, g. conjuntivais. SIN conjunctival g.'s.

Threile g.'s, glândulas de Threile, g. da mucosa biliar. SIN g.'s of biliary mucosa.

thoracic g.'s, glândulas ecdisiais. SIN ecdysial g.'s.

thymus g., timo. SIN thymus.

thyroid g. [TA], tireóide; uma glândula endócrina (sem ductos) composta de folículos irregularmente esferoidais, situada na frente e nos lados da parte superior da traquéia e que apresenta a forma de uma ferradura, ou seja, com dois lobos laterais unidos por uma porção central estreita, o istmo; às vezes uma ramificação alongada, o lobo piramidal, passa acima do istmo, na frente da traquéia. É irrigada por ramos das artérias carótida externa e subclávia, e seus nervos são provenientes dos gânglios cervical médio e cervicotorácico do sistema simpático. Secreta hormônio tireóideo e calcitonina. SIN glandula thyroidea [TA], thyroid body, thyroidea.

Tiedemann g.'s, g. de Tiedemann, g. vestibular maior. SIN greater vestibular g.

tracheal g.'s [TA], glândulas traqueais; numerosas glândulas tubuloalveolares e mistas localizadas principalmente na submucosa da traquéia; abrem-se no interior do lúmen da traquéia através de ductos curtos. SIN glandulae tracheales [TA].

trachoma g.'s, glândulas do tracoma. SIN Bruch g.'s.

tubal g.'s of pharyngotympanic tube [TA], glândulas tubárias da tuba faringotimpânica; glândulas localizadas principalmente próximo à extremidade faríngea da tuba auditiva. SIN g.'s of auditory tube, g.'s of eustachian tube, glandulae tubariae, mucous g.'s of auditory tube.

tubular g., g. tubular; uma g. composta de um ou mais túbulos que terminam em uma extremidade sem saída.

tubuloacinar g., g. tubuloacinar; uma g. cujos elementos secretórios são compostos por ácinos alongados. SIN acinotubular g.

tubuloalveolar g., g. tubuloalveolar; uma g. que apresenta unidades secretórias compostas por túbulos curtos.

tympanic g., g. timpânica; uma das glândulas mucosas localizadas na mucosa da cavidade timpânica. SIN tympanic body.

Tyson g.'s, glândulas de Tyson, g. prepuciais. SIN preputial g.'s.

unicellular g., g. unicelular; uma única célula secretória, tal como uma célula mucosa calicial.

urethral g.'s, glândulas uretrais. VER urethral g.'s of female, urethral g.'s of male.

urethral g.'s of female [TA], glândulas uretrais da mulher; numerosas glândulas mucosas localizadas na parede da uretra da mulher. SIN glandulae urethrales femininae [TA], g.'s of the female urethra, Guérin g.'s, paraurethral g.'s, Skene g.'s.

urethral g.'s of male [TA], glândulas uretrais do homem; numerosas glândulas mucosas localizadas na parede da uretra peniana. SIN glandulae urethrales masculinae [TA], g.'s of the male urethra, Littré g.'s.

uterine g.'s [TA], glândulas uterinas; numerosas glândulas tubulares, simples, localizadas na mucosa uterina e que secretam um líquido mucoso, rico em glicogênio, durante a fase lútea do ciclo menstrual. SIN glandulae uterinae [TA].

vaginal g., g. vaginal; uma das glândulas mucosas localizadas na mucosa da vagina.

vascular g., nó hemolinfático. SIN hemal node.

ventral g.'s, glândulas ecdisiais. SIN ecdysial g.'s.

vesical g., g. vesical; um de vários folículos mucosos, e não de glândulas verdadeiras, localizados na mucosa próximo ao colo da bexiga.

vestibular g.'s, glândulas vestibulares. VER greater vestibular g., lesser vestibular g.'s.

vulvovaginal g., g. vestibular maior. SIN greater vestibular g.

Waldeyer g.'s, glândulas de Waldeyer; glândulas convolutas situadas próximo às margens das pálpebras.

Wasmann g.'s, glândulas de Wasmann, g. gástricas. SIN gastric g.'s.

Weber g.'s, glândulas de Weber; glândulas mucíparas localizadas na margem da língua em ambos os lados, posteriormente.

Wepfer g.'s, glândulas de Wepfer, g. duodenais. SIN duodenal g.'s.

Wölfler g., g. de Wölfler, g. tireóide acessória. SIN accessory thyroid g.

Wolfring g.'s, glândulas de Wolfring, g. lacrimais acessórias. VER accessory lacrimal g.'s.

Zeis g.'s, glândulas de Zeis; glândulas sebáceas que se abrem nos folículos dos cílios.

glan·ders (glan′derz). Mormo; uma doença debilitante e crônica de cavalos e de outros eqüídeos, como também de alguns membros da família dos gatos, causada por *Pseudomonas mallei* e transmissível aos homens. Ataca as mucosas das narinas do cavalo, levando à produção alterada e aumentada de secreção e eliminação de muco, bem como à hipertrofia e endurecimento das glândulas da mandíbula inferior. [Fr. ant. *glandres*, glândulas]

glan·des (glan′dēz). Plural de glans (glande).

glan·di·lem·ma (glan - di - lem′ă). Glandilema; a cápsula de uma glândula. [L. *glandula*, glândula, + G. *lemma*, bainha]

glan·du·la, pl. **glan·du·lae** (glan′doo - lă, -lē) [TA]. **1.** [NA]. Glândula. SIN gland. **2.** Pequena glândula. SIN glandule. [L. gland, dim. de *glans*, bolota (fruto do carvalho)]

glan′dulae areola′res [TA], glândulas areolares. SIN areolar *glands*, em *gland*.
g. atrabilia′ris, supra-renal. SIN suprarenal *gland*.
g. basila′ris, hipófise, pituitária. SIN pituitary *gland*.
glandulae bronchiales [TA], glândulas bronquiais. SIN bronchial *glands*, em *gland*.
glan′dulae bucca′les [TA], glândulas da bochecha. SIN buccal *glands*, em *gland*.
g. bulbourethra′lis [TA], g. bulbouretral. SIN bulbourethral *gland*.
glan′dulae cerumino′sae, glândulas ceruminosas. **(1)** SIN ceruminous *glands*, em *gland*; **(2)** glândulas tubuloalveolares do meato auditivo externo; acredita-se que sejam glândulas sudoríferas apócrinas modificadas; secretam o cerúmen, uma substância cérea.
glan′dulae cervica′les uteri [TA], glândulas do colo do útero. SIN cervical *glands*, em *gland*.
glan′dulae cilia′res [TA], glândulas ciliares. SIN ciliary *glands*, em *gland*.
glan′dulae circumana′les, glândulas circum-anais. SIN circumanal *glands*, em *gland*.
glan′dulae conjunctiva′les [TA], glândulas conjuntivais. SIN conjunctival *glands*, em *gland*.
glan′dulae cu′tis [TA], glândulas da pele. SIN cutaneous *glands*, em *gland*.
glandulae ductus biliaris, glândulas do ducto colédoco; *termo oficial alternativo para glands of (common) bile duct, em *gland*.
glandulae ductus choledochi [TA], glândulas do ducto colédoco. SIN glands of (common) bile duct, em *gland*.
glan′dulae duodena′les [TA], glândulas duodenais. SIN duodenal *glands*, em *gland*.
glan′dulae endocri′nae [TA], glândulas endócrinas. SIN endocrine *glands*, em *gland*.
glan′dulae esopha′geae, glândulas esofágicas. SIN esophageal *glands*, em *gland*.
glan′dulae gas′tricae [TA], glândulas gástricas. SIN gastric *glands*, em *gland*.
glan′dulae glomifor′mes, glomo. **(1)** SIN glomus (2); **(2)** glândulas tubulares da pele, cuja extremidade sem saída é enrolada em forma de bola ou de glomérulo; termo coletivo para as glândulas sudoríferas écrinas pequenas e apócrinas grandes.
glan′dulae intestina′les [TA], glândulas intestinais. SIN intestinal *glands*, em *gland*.
glandulae intestini crassi [TA], glândulas do intestino grosso. SIN glands of large intestine, em *gland*.
glandulae intestini tenuis [TA], glândulas do intestino delgado. SIN glands of small intestine, em *gland*.
glan′dulae labia′les [TA], glândulas labiais. SIN labial *glands*, em *gland*.
glan′dulae lacrima′les accesso′riae [TA], glândulas lacrimais acessórias. SIN accessory lacrimal *glands*, em *gland*.
g. lacrima′lis [TA], g. lacrimal. SIN lacrimal *gland*.
glan′dulae laryn′geae [TA], glândulas laríngeas. SIN laryngeal *glands*, em *gland*.
g. lingua′lis ante′rior, g. lingual anterior. SIN anterior lingual *gland*.
g. mamma′ria [TA], g. mamária. SIN mammary *gland*.
glan′dulae mola′res [TA], glândulas molares. SIN molar *glands*, em *gland*.
g. muco′sa, g. mucosa. SIN mucous *gland*.
glan′dulae muco′sae bilio′sae, glândulas da mucosa biliar. SIN glands of biliary mucosa, em *gland*.
glan′dulae nasa′les [TA], glândulas nasais. SIN nasal *glands*, em *gland*.
glan′dulae olfacto′riae [TA], glândulas olfatórias. SIN olfactory *glands*, em *gland*.
glan′dulae o′ris [TA], glândulas da boca. SIN glands of mouth, em *gland*.
glan′dulae palati′nae [TA], glândulas palatinas. SIN palatine *glands*, em *gland*.
g. parathyroi′dea [TA], paratireóide. SIN parathyroid *gland*.
g. parotid′ea [TA], g. parótida. SIN parotid *gland*.
g. parotid′ea accesso′ria [TA], g. parótida acessória. SIN accessory parotid *gland*.
g. paro′tis, g. parótida. SIN parotid *gland*.
g. paro′tis accesso′ria, g. parótida acessória. SIN accessory parotid *gland*.
glan′dulae pharyngea′les [TA], glândulas faríngeas. SIN pharyngeal *glands*, em *gland*.
g. pinealis [TA], g. pineal. SIN pineal *body*.
g. pituita′ria, hipófise (pituitária); *termo oficial alternativo para pituitary *gland*.
glan′dulae preputia′les [TA], glândulas prepuciais. SIN preputial *glands*, em *gland*.
g. prosta′tica, próstata. SIN prostate.
glan′dulae pylor′icae [TA], glândulas pilóricas. SIN pyloric *glands*, em *gland*.
g. saliva′ria [TA], g. salivar. SIN salivary *gland*.
glandulae salivariae majores [TA], glândulas salivares maiores. SIN major salivary *glands*, em *gland*.
glandulae salivariae minores [TA], glândulas salivares menores. SIN minor salivary *glands*, em *gland*.
glan′dulae seba′ceae [TA], glândulas sebáceas. SIN sebaceous *glands*, em *gland*.
g. semina′lis, g. seminal; *termo oficial alternativo para seminal *gland*, seminal *gland*.
g. seromuco′sa, g. seromucosa. SIN seromucous *gland*.
g. sero′sa, g. serosa. SIN serous *gland*.
glan′dulae sine duc′tibus, glândulas sem ductos, g. endócrinas. SIN endocrine *glands*, em *gland*.
g. sublingua′lis [TA], g. sublingual. SIN sublingual *gland*.
g. submandibula′ris [TA], g. submandibular. SIN submandibular *gland*.
glan′dulae sudorif′erae [TA], glândulas sudoríferas. SIN sweat *glands*, em *gland*.
glan′dulae suprarena′les accesso′riae [TA], glândulas supra-renais acessórias. SIN accessory suprarenal *glands*, em *gland*.
g. suprarena′lis [TA], supra-renal. SIN suprarenal *gland*.
glan′dulae tarsa′les [TA], glândulas tarsais. SIN tarsal *glands*, em *gland*.
g. thyroi′dea [TA], tireóide. SIN thyroid *gland*.
g. thyroi′dea accesso′ria, pl. **glan′dulae thyroi′deae accesso′riae** [TA], g. tireóide acessória. SIN accessory thyroid *gland*.
glan′dulae trachea′les [TA], glândulas traqueais. SIN tracheal *glands*, em *gland*.
glan′dulae tuba′riae, glândulas tubárias da tuba faringotimpânica. SIN tubal *glands* of pharyngotympanic tube, em *gland*.
glan′dulae urethra′les femini′nae [TA], glândulas uretrais da mulher. SIN urethral *glands* of female, em *gland*.
glan′dulae urethra′les masculi′nae [TA], glândulas uretrais do homem. SIN urethral *glands* of male, em *gland*.
glan′dulae uteri′nae [TA], glândulas uterinas. SIN uterine *glands*, em *gland*.
g. vesiculosa [TA], g. seminal. SIN seminal *gland*.
glan′dulae vestibula′res mino′res [TA], glândulas vestibulares menores. SIN lesser vestibular *glands*, em *gland*.
g. vestibula′ris ma′jor [TA], g. vestibular maior. SIN greater vestibular *gland*.

glan·du·lar (glan′doo - lăr). Glandular, glanduloso; relativo a uma glândula. SIN glandulous.

glan·dule (glan′dool). Uma pequena glândula. SIN glandula (2) [TA]. [L. *glandula*]

glan·du·lous (glan′doo - lŭs). Glanduloso, glandular. SIN glandular.

glans, pl. **glan·des** (glanz, glan′dēz) [TA]. Glande; uma estrutura cônica com forma de bolota (fruto do carvalho). [L. bolota (fruto do carvalho)]
g. clitor′idis [TA], g. do clitóris. SIN g. of clitoris.
g. of clitoris, g. do clitóris; uma pequena massa de tecido erétil, extremamente sensível, que cobre o corpo do clitóris. SIN g. clitoridis [TA].
g. pe′nis [TA], g. do pênis, bálano; a expansão cônica do corpo esponjoso que forma a cabeça do pênis. SIN balanus.

glan·u·lar (glan′ū - lar). Relativo à glande do pênis. [irreg. de *glans*, por analogia a *glandular*]

Glanzmann, Eduard, clínico suíço, 1887–1959. VER G. *disease*, *thrombasthenia*.

gla·phen·ine (gla - fen′ēn). Glafenina; um agente antiinflamatório com propriedades analgésicas.

glare (glār). Ofuscamento; uma sensação causada pelo brilho, dentro do campo visual, suficientemente maior do que a luminosidade à qual os olhos estão adaptados; provoca irritação, desconforto e desempenho visual diminuído.
blinding g., o. de velamento; o. resultante de iluminação excessiva. SIN veiling g.
dazzling g., o. deslumbrante; o. produzida por iluminação excessiva no campo periférico.
peripheral g., o. periférico; o. que ocorre quando a claridade circundante é maior do que o brilho do objeto focalizado.
specular g., o. especular; o. que se origina da luz refletida especularmente.
veiling g., o. de velamento. SIN blinding g.

gla·rom·e·ter (glā - rom′ĕ - ter). Glarômetro; um instrumento que mede a sensibilidade ao clarão central dos faróis dianteiros de um veículo que se aproxima.

Glaser (Glaserius), Johann H., anatomista suíço, 1629–1675. VER glaserian *artery*; glaserian *fissure*.

gla·se·ri·an (gla - ser′ē - an). Glaseriano; relativo a, ou descrito por, Johann H. Glaser.

Glasgow, William C., médico norte-americano, 1845–1907. VER G. *sign*.

Glasgow co·ma scale. Escala de coma, de Glasgow. VER coma *scale*.

glass (glas). Vidro; uma substância transparente composta de sílica e óxidos de diversas bases. [A.S. *glaes*]

  cover g., lamínula; uma lâmina ou um disco delgado de vidro que cobre um objeto examinado sob o microscópio. SIN coverslip.

  Crookes g., v. de Crookes; uma lente para óculos combinada com óxidos metálicos para absorver os raios infravermelhos ou ultravioleta.

  crown g., v. óptico; um composto de óxido de cálcio, potassa, alumina e sílica; geralmente utilizado em lentes; apresenta uma baixa dispersão (52,2) em relação ao índice de refração (1,523).

  cupping g., ventosa; um vaso de v. do qual o ar foi retirado por meio de calor ou de um aparelho de sucção especial; antigamente aplicado à pele, a fim de atrair o sangue até a superfície. VER TAMBÉM cupping, cup. SIN cup (2).

  flint g., cristal; v. que contém óxido de chumbo em vez de óxido de cálcio, com o objetivo de aumentar o índice de refração; utilizado nos segmentos para leitura de lentes bifocais fundidas.

  object g., objetiva. SIN objective (1).

  quartz g., cristal de quartzo; um cristal transparente e incolor, feito pela fusão de areia de quartzo puro, que conduz a luz ultravioleta.

  soluble g., v. solúvel; um silicato de potássio ou de sódio, solúvel em água quente, porém sólido sob temperaturas normais; utilizado em curativos fixos. SIN water g.

  vita g., um v. especialmente preparado, transparente aos raios ultravioleta do espectro.

  water g., v. líquido. SIN soluble g.

  Wood g., v. de Wood; um v. que contém óxido de níquel e é utilizado na lâmpada de Wood.

glass·es (glas′ez). **1.** Óculos. SIN spectacles. **2.** Lentes para corrigir erros de refração nos olhos.

Glauber, Johann R., químico alemão, 1604–1670. VER G. *salt*.

glau·cine (glaw′sēn). Glaucina; a forma *d*, predominante na natureza. Encontrada nas espécies *Glaucium flavum* (*G. luteum scop.*), *Papaveraceae* e *Dicentra* e *Corydalis*, da família *Fumariceae*. Um agente antitussígeno. SIN boldine dimethyl ether.

glau·co·ma (glaw - kō′mä). Glaucoma; uma doença do olho caracterizada por pressão intra-ocular aumentada, escavação e atrofia do nervo óptico; produz defeitos no campo visual. [G. *glaukōma*, opacidade da lente (cristalino), de *glaukos*, verde-azulado]

  absolute g., g. absoluto; o estágio final de cegueira no g.

  acute g., g. de ângulo agudo. SIN angle-closure g.

  angle-closure g., g. de ângulo fechado, g. de ângulo agudo; g. primário no qual o contato da íris com a periferia da córnea afasta o humor aquoso da rede de drenagem trabecular. SIN acute g., closed-angle g., narrow-angle g.

  aphakic g., g. afácico; g. que ocorre após a remoção de catarata.

  chronic g., g. crônico, g. simples. SIN open-angle g.

  α-chymotrypsin-induced g., g. induzido pela α-quimotripsina; g. secundário transitório que ocorre após o uso de α-quimotripsina na extração de catarata.

  closed-angle g., g. de ângulo fechado, g. de ângulo agudo. SIN angle-closure g.

  combined g., g. combinado; g. que apresenta os mecanismos do g. de ângulo agudo e do g. simples (ângulo aberto) no mesmo olho.

  compensated g., g. compensado, a. simples. SIN open-angle g.

  congenital g., g. congênito, buftalmia. SIN buphthalmia.

  corticosteroid-induced g., g. induzido por corticosteróide; g. causado por uma predisposição hereditária, na qual a instilação local de colírios que contém corticosteróide provoca aumento da pressão intra-ocular.

  g. ful′minans, g. fulminante; instalação rápida de g. de ângulo agudo seguida por cegueira.

  ghost cell g., g. de células fantasmas; g. que ocorre após vitrectomia e resulta do bloqueio dos canais de escoamento do humor aquoso por membranas de eritrócitos.

  hemorrhagic g., g. hemorrágico; g. secundário à formação de novos vasos sanguíneos na íris.

  hypersecretion g., g. por hipersecreção; g. causado por formação excessiva de humor aquoso.

  low-tension g., g. de baixa tensão, g. normotenso; atrofia do nervo óptico e escavação fisiológica com defeitos de campos típicos do g., porém sem aumento anormal da pressão intra-ocular. SIN normal-tension g.

  malignant g., g. maligno; g. secundário causado por deslocamento para a frente da íris e da lente, que oblitera a câmara anterior; em geral ocorre após uma operação de filtração para o glaucoma primário.

  narrow-angle g., g. de ângulo estreito, g. de ângulo agudo. SIN angle-closure g.

  neovascular g., g. neovascular; g. que ocorre na rubeose da íris.

  normal-tension g., g. normotenso. SIN low-tension g.

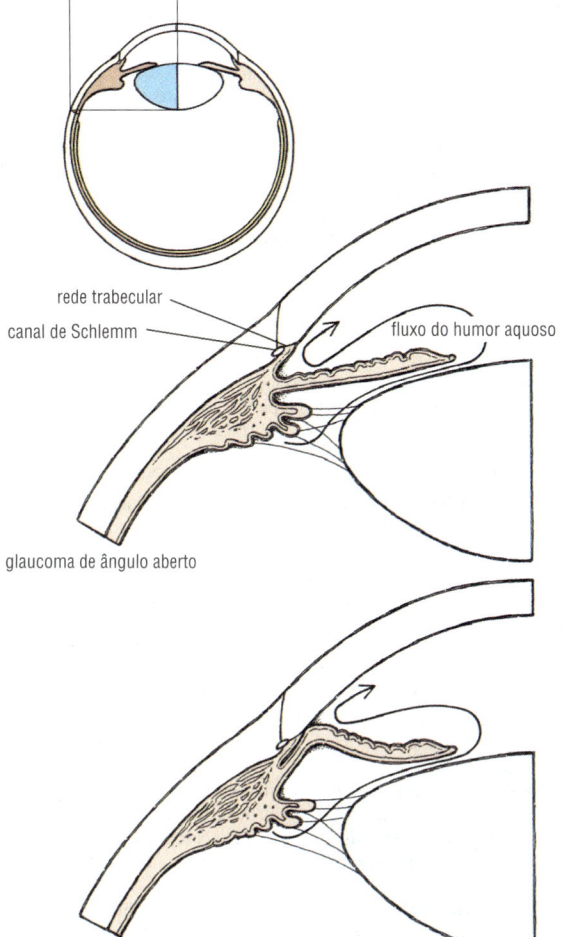

rede trabecular
canal de Schlemm
fluxo do humor aquoso
glaucoma de ângulo aberto
glaucoma de ângulo fechado

glaucoma

  open-angle g., g. de ângulo aberto, g. simples; g. primário no qual o humor aquoso possui livre acesso à rede trabecular. SIN chronic g., compensated g., simple g., g. simplex.

  phacogenic g., g. facogênico, g. facomórfico. SIN phacomorphic g.

  phacolytic g., g. facolítico; g. secundário à catarata hipermadura e à oclusão da rede de drenagem trabecular por material da lente.

  phacomorphic g., g. facomórfico; g. secundário causado tanto pelo tamanho excessivo da lente como pela sua forma esférica. SIN phacogenic g.

  pigmentary g., g. pigmentar; g. associado à erosão do pigmento da íris posterior e ao acúmulo de partículas de pigmento na rede trabecular.

  pseudoexfoliative g., g. pseudo-esfoliativo; g. que ocorre em associação à deposição disseminada de organelas celulares sobre a cápsula da lente, os vasos sanguíneos oculares, a íris e o corpo ciliar. VER TAMBÉM *pseudoexfoliation* of lens capsule.

  pupillary block g., g. por bloqueio pupilar; g. secundário à incapacidade de o humor aquoso passar através da pupila para a câmara anterior.

  secondary g., g. secundário; g. que ocorre como seqüela de uma doença ou lesão ocular preexistente.

  simple g., g. sim′plex, g. simples, g. de ângulo aberto. SIN open-angle g.

glau·co·ma·to·cy·clit·ic (glaw - kō′mä - tō - si - klit′ik). Glaucomatociclítico; que indica pressão intra-ocular aumentada associada a evidências de ciclite. VER TAMBÉM glaucomatocyclic *crisis*.

glau·co·ma·tous (glaw - kō′mä - tus). Glaucomatoso; relativo ao glaucoma.

glau·co·su·ria (glaw′kō - soo′rē - ä). Glaucosúria; termo obsoleto para indicanúria. [G. *glaukos*, verde-azulado, + *ouron*, urina]

GLC Abreviatura de gas-liquid *chromatography* (cromatografia líquido-gasosa).

Glc, GlcA, GlcN, GlcNAc, GlcUA Símbolos dos radicais de D-glicose, ácidos glicônico e glicurônico, glicosamina, *N*-acetil-glicosamina e ácido glicurônico, respectivamente.

Gleason, Donald F., patologista norte-americano, *1920. VER G. tumor *grade*, *score*.

gleet (glēt). Termo obsoleto para secreção uretral crônica que surge após a gonorréia. [I.M. *glet*, substância viscosa, do Fr. ant. *glette*, do L. *glittus*, pegajoso]

Glenn, William W., *1914. VER Glenn *shunt*.

Glenner, George B., histologista e patologista norte-americano, *1927. VER G.-Lillie *stain* for pituitary.

gle·no·hu·mer·al (glē'nō - hū'mer - ăl). Glenoumeral; relativo à cavidade glenóide e ao úmero.

gle·noid (glē'noyd, glen'oyd). Glenóide; que se assemelha a um encaixe; indica a depressão articular da escápula que entra na formação da articulação do ombro. [G. *glēnoeidēs*, de *glēnē*, pupila do olho, encaixe de articulação, favo de mel, + *eidos*, aparência]

Gley, Marcel E., fisiologista francês, 1857–1930. VER G. *glands*, em *gland*.

glia (glī'ă). Glia, neuróglia. SIN neuroglia. [G. cola]

gli·a·cyte (glī'ă - sĭt). Gliócito; uma célula da neuróglia. VER neuroglia. [G. *glia*, cola, + *kytos*, célula]

gli·a·din (glī'ă - din). Gliadina; uma classe de proteínas separáveis dos glutens do trigo e do centeio; um membro das prolaminas (proteínas ricas em prolina), insolúvel em água, álcool absoluto e em solventes neutros, porém solúvel em álcool a 50 — 90%.

gli·al (glī'ăl). Glial; relativo à glia ou neuróglia.

gli·cla·zide (glī'klă - zīd). Gliclazida; um agente antidiabético oral (sulfoniluréia) utilizado no tratamento do diabetes melito de tipo II; libera a insulina endógena das células beta das ilhotas de Langerhans localizadas no pâncreas; assemelha-se à glipizida e à tolbutamida.

glide (glīd). Deslizamento; um movimento contínuo e suave ou sem esforço.
    mandibular g., deslizamento mandibular; o movimento látero-lateral, protrátil e intermediário da mandíbula que ocorre quando os dentes ou outras superfícies oclusivas estão em contato.

glide·wire (glīd'wīr). Fio-guia; um fio-guia hidrofílico ou lubrificado, utilizado em geral no trato urinário. VER TAMBÉM guidewire.

glio-. Glio-; cola, semelhante a cola (relativo especificamente à neuróglia). [G. *glia*, cola]

gli·o·blast (glī'ō - blast). Glioblasto; uma célula neural primária em desenvolvimento, semelhante ao neuroblasto e proveniente da célula ependimária primária do tubo neural; dá origem às células neurogliais e ependimárias, aos astrócitos e aos oligodendrócitos. VER TAMBÉM spongioblast. [glio- + G. *blastos*, germe]

gli·o·blas·to·ma multiforme (glī'ō - blas - tō'mă). Glioblastoma multiforme; um glioma que consiste principalmente em células anaplásicas indiferenciadas de origem astrocítica que exibem acentuado pleomorfismo nuclear, necrose e proliferação endotelial vascular; com freqüência, as células tumorais estão dispostas de maneira radial ao redor de um foco irregular de necrose; essa neoplasia cresce rapidamente, é bastante invasiva e surge mais freqüentemente no cérebro de adultos. [G. *glia*, cola, + *blastos*, germe, + -*oma*, tumor]
    giant cell g. m., g. m. de células gigantes; uma forma histológica do glioblastoma com células tumorais grandes, freqüentemente multinucleadas e bizarras. SIN giant cell monstrocellular sarcoma of Zülch, gigantocellular glioma.

gli·o·blas·to·sis ce·re·bri. Glioblastose cerebral, gliomatose cerebral. SIN *gliomatosis* cerebri.

gli·o·ma (glī - ō'mă). Glioma; qualquer neoplasia derivada de um dos diferentes tipos de células que formam o tecido intersticial do cérebro, da medula espinal, da glândula pineal, da neuro-hipófise e da retina. [G. *glia*, cola, + -*oma*, tumor]
    brainstem g., g. do tronco cerebral; um g., em geral um astrocitoma, que surge na medula oblonga (bulbo), na ponte ou no mesencéfalo.
    gigantocellular g., g. gigantocelular, glioblastoma de células gigantes. SIN giant cell *glioblastoma multiforme*.
    mixed g., g. misto; um glioma composto de dois ou mais elementos malignos, mais freqüentemente um astrocitoma e um oligodendroglioma.
    nasal g., g. nasal; termo para uma lesão que, provavelmente, não é uma neoplasia verdadeira, mas um teratoma formado por tecido glial com astrócitos reativos, neurônios ganglionares e células ependimárias em pequenos nódulos no dorso do nariz, freqüentemente com conexões intracranianas.
    g. of optic chiasm, g. do quiasma óptico; um tumor de crescimento lento, em geral um astrocitoma, que afeta o quiasma óptico de crianças.
    optic nerve g., g. do nervo óptico; um g., em geral um astrocitoma, que envolve o nervo ou o quiasma óptico.
    g. of the spinal cord, g. da medula espinal; um tumor glial da medula espinal, geralmente um ependimoma; as neoplasias da medula espinal são relativamente raras, porém os gliomas constituem cerca de um quarto do total.
    telangiectatic g., g. telangiecto'des, g. telangiectásico; um g. no qual o estroma apresenta numerosos e evidentes capilares e vasos sanguíneos, freqüentemente dilatados, bem como grandes lagos de sangue margeados por endotélio.

gli·o·ma·to·sis (glī - ō - mă - tō'sis). Gliomatose; crescimento neoplásico de células neurogliais no cérebro ou na medula espinal; o termo é utilizado em especial com referência a uma neoplasia relativamente grande ou a múltiplos focos. SIN neurogliomatosis.
    g. cerebri (glī'ō - blas - tō'sis ser'ĕ - brī). Gliomatose cerebral; uma neoplasia intracraniana difusa de origem astrocítica. SIN astrocytosis cerebri, glioblastosis cerebri.

gli·o·ma·tous (glī - ō'mă - tŭs). Gliomatoso; relativo a, ou caracterizado por, um glioma.

gli·o·myx·o·ma (glī'ō - mik - sō'mă). Gliomixoma; um mixoma que contém uma quantidade considerável de células gliais em proliferação e fibras.

gli·o·neu·ro·ma (glī'ō - noo - rō'mă). Glioneuroma; um ganglioneuroma derivado de neurônios, com numerosas células gliais e fibras na matriz.

gli·o·sar·co·ma (glī'ō - sar - kō'mă). Gliossarcoma; um glioblastoma multiforme com um componente mesenquimal maligno associado. O termo é, às vezes, utilizado para uma neoplasia maligna derivada do tecido conectivo (p.ex., uma neoplasia associada a vasos sangüíneos no cérebro), na qual há células gliais em proliferação.

gli·o·sis (glī - ō'sis). Gliose; crescimento exagerado de astrócitos em uma área de lesão no cérebro ou na medula espinal.
    isomorphous g., g. isomorfa; gliose cujas fibras gliais estão dispostas de forma ordenada e regular.
    piloid g., g. pilóide; área de astrocitose reativa e crônica composta de células delgadas e piliformes em uma disposição vagamente paralela.
    g. u'teri, g. uterina; tecido neural fetal que persiste ou recorre localmente como uma condição benigna no endométrio ou no colo; é possivelmente derivada de um homoenxerto de estroma glial fetal.

GLIP Abreviatura de glucagonlike insulinotropic *peptide* (peptídeo insulinotrópico glucagon-símile).

glip·i·zide (glip'i - zīd). Glipizida; uma sulfoniluréia oral utilizada no tratamento do diabetes de tipo II.

Glisson, Francis, anatomista, fisiologista, patologista e médico inglês, 1597–1677. VER G. *capsule, cirrhosis, sphincter*.

glis·so·ni·tis (glis - ō - nī'tis). Glissonite; inflamação da cápsula de Glisson ou do tecido conectivo que circunda a veia porta, a artéria hepática e os ductos biliares.

glitazones (glī'ta - zonz). Glitazonas; nome comum dado aos agentes antidiabéticos que agem diminuindo a resistência periférica à insulina por meio de alterações pouco conhecidas no metabolismo dos ácidos graxos. SIN thiazolidinediones. [Proveniente dos nomes químicos genéricos das substâncias que pertencem a essa classe.]

Gln Símbolo de glutamine (glutamina) ou seu radical acila, glutaminil (glutaminyl).

glob·al (glō'băl). Global; o aspecto completo, generalizado, integral ou total.

glo·bal warm·ing (glō'bal warm'ing). Aquecimento global; um aumento generalizado nas temperaturas globais; poderia representar um risco de epidemia de malária em áreas montanhosas da África tropical ao guiar a transmissão da malária até essas áreas povoadas.

globe (glōb). Globo, bulbo. SIN globus.
    g. of eye, bulbo do olho. SIN eyeball.
    pale g., g. pálido. SIN *globus* pallidus.

glo·bi (glō'bī). Globos. 1. Plural de globus. 2. Corpos castanhos encontrados, às vezes, nas lesões granulomatosas da hanseníase, em adição aos macrófagos que contêm os bacilos álcool-ácido-resistentes (BAAR); considerados como formas degeneradas dessas células, nas quais os microrganismos não são mais viáveis e tornaram-se granulares ou amorfos.

glo·bin (glō'bin). Globina; a proteína da hemoglobina; a α-g. e a β-g. representam os dois tipos de cadeias encontradas na hemoglobina do adulto. SIN hematohiston.

Glo·bo·ceph·a·lus (glō - bō - sef'ă - lŭs). Um gênero de anciléstomos (subfamília Uncinariinae, família Ancylostomatidae) que consiste em aproximadamente cinco espécies encontradas principalmente no intestino delgado de porcos. A espécie *G. urosubalatus*, de distribuição mundial, é um anciléstomo comum de porcos domésticos e selvagens.

glo·bo·side (glō'bō - sīd). Globosídeo; um glicoesfingolipídio; especificamente, um tetrassacarídeo de ceramida (tetraglicosilceramida) isolado dos rins e eritrócitos; acumula-se em indivíduos com a doença de Sandhoff.

glo·bo·tri·a·o·syl·cer·a·mide (glō'bō - trī - ă - ō - sil - ser - a - mīd). Globotriaosilceramida; um esfingolipídio que contém três radicais de açúcar e acumula-se em indivíduos com a doença de Fabry. SIN trihexosylceramide.

glob·ule (glob'ūl). Glóbulo. 1. Um pequeno corpo esférico de qualquer tipo. 2. Uma pequena gota de gordura no leite. SIN globulus. [L. *globulus*, dim. de *globus*, uma bola]
    dentin g., g. de dentina; calcosferitas formadas por calcificação ou mineralização da dentina que ocorre em áreas globulares.
    Morgagni g.'s, glóbulos de Morgagni; vesículas situadas abaixo da cápsula e entre as fibras da lente no início da catarata. SIN Morgagni spheres.
    polar g., corpúsculo polar. SIN *polar body*.

glob·u·lif·er·ous (glob - ū - lif'er - ŭs). Globulífero; que contém glóbulos ou corpúsculos, principalmente hemácias. [L. *globulus*, glóbulo, + *fero*, carregar]

glob·u·lin (glob′ū - lin). Globulina; nome de uma família de proteínas precipitadas do plasma (ou soro) por semi-saturação com sulfato de amônio (isto é, por adição de um volume igual de sulfato de amônio saturado). As globulinas podem ser, além disso, fracionadas por solubilidade, eletroforese, ultracentrifugação e por outros métodos de separação em muitos subgrupos. Os principais grupos são α-, β- e γ-g., os quais contêm a maioria dos anticorpos. [L. *globulus*, glóbulo]

accelerator g. (AcG, ac-g), g. aceleradora; g. do soro que promove a conversão da protrombina em trombina na presença de tromboplastina e cálcio ionizado. VER *factor V₃, factor V, serum accelerator g.*

antihemophilic g. (AHG), (1) g. anti-hemofílica; SIN *factor VIII;* **(2)** fator anti-hemofílico humano. SIN human antihemophilic *factor.*

antihemophilic g. A, g. anti-hemofílica A. SIN *factor VIII.*

antihemophilic g. B, g. anti-hemofílica B. SIN *factor IX.*

antihuman g., g. anti-humana; soro de um coelho ou de outro animal previamente imunizado com g. humana purificada para preparar anticorpos contra uma imunoglobulina humana; alguns desses anticorpos podem ser utilizados nos testes de Coombs direto e indireto. SIN Coombs serum.

antilymphocyte g. (ALG), g. antilinfócitos. SIN antilymphocyte *serum.*

β₁C g., g. β₁C; fração de globulina do soro que contém o terceiro componente (C3) do complemento. VER *component* of complement.

chickenpox immune g. (human), imunoglobulina humana antivaricela; fração de g. do soro de pessoas recentemente recuperadas de infecção por herpes zoster; utilizada na prevenção de infecção em crianças de alto risco. SIN chickenpox immunoglobulin.

corticosteroid-binding g. (CBG), g. fixadora de corticosteróides. SIN transcortin.

gonadal steroid-binding g. (GBG), g. fixadora de esteróides das gônadas; uma proteína que transporta 65% da testosterona do plasma. SIN sex steroid-binding g.

human gamma g., gamaglobulina humana; um preparado de proteínas do soro humano líquido que contém os anticorpos (principalmente IgG) de adultos normais; é obtido da combinação do soro humano líquido de vários doadores e pode ser elaborado por precipitação sob condições controladas de pH, concentração iônica e temperatura. SIN human normal immunoglobulin.

immune serum g., imunoglobulina sérica; uma solução estéril de globulinas que contém muitos anticorpos normalmente presentes no sangue humano dos adultos; um agente de imunização passiva freqüentemente utilizado na profilaxia contra a hepatite A e no tratamento da doença de Kawasaki, da púrpura trombocitopênica idiopática e de algumas imunodeficiências.

measles immune g. (human), imunoglobulina humana anti-sarampo; uma solução estéril de globulinas derivadas do plasma sanguíneo de doadores humanos adultos com títulos elevados para o sarampo: é preparada a partir de imunoglobulina sérica que obedece ao padrão de referência dos anticorpos do sarampo; um agente de imunização passiva. SIN measles immunoglobulin.

pertussis immune g., imunoglobulina anticoqueluche; uma solução estéril de globulinas derivadas do plasma de doadores humanos adultos que foram imunizados com a vacina anticoqueluche; utilizada tanto profilática como terapeuticamente. SIN pertussis immunoglobulin.

plasma accelerator g., fator V. SIN *factor V.*

poliomyelitis immune g. (human), imunoglobulina humana contra a poliomielite; uma solução estéril de globulinas que contém anticorpos normalmente presentes no sangue humano do adulto com títulos elevados para a poliomielite e que confere proteção temporária, porém significativa, contra a poliomielite. SIN poliomyelitis immunoglobulin.

rabies immune g. (human), imunoglobulina humana anti-rábica; fração de globulina de plasma combinado de pessoas imunizadas com altos títulos de anticorpos anti-rábicos. SIN rabies immunoglobulin.

RH₀(D) immune g., imunoglobulina RH₀(D); uma fração de g. de anticorpo obtida de doadores humanos e específica para o antígeno mais comum do grupo Rh, o Rh₀(D); utilizada na prevenção da sensibilização ao Rh de uma mulher Rh-negativa após o parto de um feto Rh-positivo. SIN anti-D immunoglobulin, Rh₀(D) immunoglobulin.

serum accelerator g., uma substância encontrada no soro que acelera a conversão da protrombina em trombina na presença de tromboplastina e cálcio; produzida pela ação de traços de trombina sobre a g. aceleradora plasmática (fator V).

sex hormone-binding g. (SHBG), g. fixadora de hormônios sexuais; uma β-globulina plasmática produzida pelo fígado e que se liga à testosterona e, com menor afinidade, ao estrógeno; nas mulheres, os níveis séricos dessa globulina correspondem ao dobro dos níveis observados nos homens; as concentrações séricas estão aumentadas em certos tipos de doença hepática e no hipertireoidismo, e diminuem com o envelhecimento, no hipotireoidismo e durante o uso de andrógenos. SIN testosterone-estrogen-binding g.

sex steroid-binding g., g. fixadora de esteróides sexuais. SIN gonadal steroid-binding g.

specific immune g. (human), imunoglobulina humana específica; fração de g. de soros (ou plasma) combinados e selecionados que apresentem títulos altos de anticorpos específicos para um determinado antígeno ou de pessoas especificamente imunizadas.

testosterone-estrogen-binding g., g. fixadora de estrógeno e testosterona. SIN sex hormone-binding g.

tetanus immune g., imunoglobulina antitetânica; uma solução estéril de globulinas derivadas do plasma sanguíneo de doadores humanos adultos que foram imunizados com toxóide tetânico; um agente de imunização passiva. SIN tetanus immunoglobulin.

thyroxine-binding g. (TBG), g. transportadora de tiroxina; uma α-globulina do sangue com uma forte afinidade para se ligar à tiroxina; liga-se à triiodotironina de um modo muito menos firme; a deficiência ou o excesso dessa proteína podem ocorrer como um distúrbio raro e benigno ligado ao X. SIN thyroxine-binding protein (1).

zoster immune g., imunoglobulina antizoster; uma fração de g. de plasma combinado de indivíduos que se recuperaram de herpes zoster; utilizada profilaticamente em crianças imunodeprimidas expostas à varicela e terapeuticamente para obter uma melhora em uma infecção por varicela.

glob·u·li·nu·ria (glob′ū - li - noo′rē - ă). Globulinúria; a excreção de globulina na urina, em geral associada à albumina sérica.

glob·u·lus (glob′ū - lŭs). Glóbulo. SIN globule. [L.]

glo·bus, pl. **glo·bi** (glō′bŭs, - bī). Globo. **1** [TA]. Um corpo redondo; uma bola. **2.** VER globi. SIN globe. [L.]

g. hyster'icus, g. histérico; dificuldade para engolir; sensação como se houvesse uma bola na garganta, ou como se a garganta estivesse comprimida; um sintoma de transtorno de conversão (conversion *disorder*).

g. ma'jor, cabeça do epidídimo. SIN *head* of epididymis.

g. mi'nor, cauda do epidídimo. SIN *tail* of epididymis.

g. pal'lidus [TA], g. pálido; a parte cinzenta mais interna e mais clara do núcleo lentiforme; é composto de um segmento lateral (g. pallidus lateralis [TA]) e um segmento medial (g. pallidus medialis [TA]) separados por uma lâmina de fibras orientadas verticalmente, a lâmina medular medial [TA] (lamina medullaris medialis [TA]). O segmento medial pode também estar dividido de forma incompleta em uma parte lateral [TA] (pars lateralis [TA]) e uma parte medial [TA] (pars medialis [TA]) pela lâmina medular acessória [TA] (lamina medullaris accessoria [TA]). VER TAMBÉM paleostriatum. SIN pallidum [TA], pale globe.

glo·mal (glō′măl). Glômico; relativo a ou que envolve um glomo.

glo·man·gi·o·ma (glō - man - jē - ō′mă). Glomangioma; uma variante do tumor glômico, freqüentemente caracterizada por múltiplos tumores que se assemelham ao hemangioma cavernoso q.v., e revestida por células glômicas. VER TAMBÉM glomus.

glo·man·gi·o·sis (glō - man - jē - ō′sis). Glomangiose; a ocorrência de múltiplos complexos de pequenos canais vasculares, cada um assemelhando-se a um glomo.

pulmonary g., g. pulmonar; g. que ocorre dentro de pequenas artérias pulmonares na hipertensão pulmonar grave e na cardiopatia congênita.

glome (glōm). Glomo. SIN glomus.

glo·mec·to·my (glō - mek′tō - mē). Glomectomia; excisão de um tumor glômico. [L. *glomus* + G. *ektomē*, remoção]

glom·era (glom′er - ă). Plural de glomus (glomo).

glom·era aor·ti·ca. Glomos paraaórticos. *termo oficial alternativo para paraaortic *bodies*, em *body*.

glo·mer·u·lar (glō - măr′u - lăr). Glomerular; relativo a ou que afeta um glomérulo ou os glomérulos. SIN glomerulose.

glom·er·ule (glom′er - ūl). Glomérulo. SIN glomerulus.

glo·mer·u·li·tis (glō - măr′u - lī′tis). Glomerulite; inflamação de um glomérulo, especificamente dos glomérulos renais, como na glomerulonefrite.

glo·mer·u·lo·ne·phri·tis (glō - măr′u - lō - nef - rī′tis). Glomerulonefrite; doença renal caracterizada por alterações inflamatórias difusas nos glomérulos que não correspondem à resposta aguda dos rins à infecção. SIN glomerular nephritis. [glomerulus + G. *nephros*, rim, + *-itis*, inflamação]

acute g., g. aguda; g. que freqüentemente ocorre como uma complicação tardia de uma faringite ou infecção de pele, sendo causada por uma cepa nefritogênica de estreptococos β-hemolíticos e caracterizada por início abrupto de hematúria, edema de face, oligúria, azotemia variável e hipertensão; os glomérulos renais geralmente mostram proliferação celular ou infiltrado de leucócitos polimorfonucleares. SIN acute hemorrhagic g., acute nephritis, acute poststreptococcal g.

acute crescentic g., g. aguda em crescente. SIN rapidly progressive g.

acute hemorrhagic g., g. hemorrágica aguda. SIN acute g.

acute poststreptococcal g., g. pós-estreptocócica aguda. SIN acute g.

anti-basement membrane g., g. antimembrana basal; g. causada por anticorpos antimembrana basal e caracterizada por depósitos lineares e lisos de IgG e C3 ao longo das paredes dos capilares glomerulares; inclui a g. rapidamente progressiva e a g. da síndrome de Goodpasture.

Berger focal g., g. focal de Berger. SIN focal g.

chronic g., g. crônica; g. caracterizada por proteinúria persistente, insuficiência renal crônica e hipertensão; apresenta início insidioso ou ocorre como uma

seqüela tardia da g. aguda; os rins mostram-se simetricamente contraídos e granulares, com fibrose e perda de glomérulos e presença de atrofia tubular e fibrose intersticial. SIN chronic nephritis.
diffuse g., g. difusa; g. que afeta a maioria dos glomérulos renais; pode levar à azotemia.
exudative g., g. exsudativa; g. com glomérulos apresentando um infiltrado de leucócitos polimorfonucleares e que ocorre na g. aguda.
focal g., g. focal; g. que afeta uma pequena proporção de glomérulos renais e, em geral, caracterizada por hematúria; pode estar associada, em homens jovens, a infecção respiratória superior que, em geral, não é causada por estreptococos; está associada a depósitos de IgA no mesângio glomerular e pode também estar associada a doença sistêmica, como na púrpura de Henoch-Schönlein. SIN Berger disease, Berger focal g., focal nephritis, IgA nephropathy.
focal embolic g., g. embólica focal; g. associada a endocardite bacteriana subaguda, que freqüentemente provoca hematúria microscópica sem azotemia.
hypocomplementemic g., g. hipocomplementêmica. SIN membranoproliferative g.
immune complex g., g. por complexos imunes; complexos imunes são depositados nos glomérulos renais, onde se ligam ao complemento e iniciam um processo inflamatório que atrai neutrófilos e macrófagos, os quais causam uma alteração na camada basal dos rins. A doença pode levar à destruição do glomérulo e à falência renal.
lobular g., g. lobular. SIN membranoproliferative g.
local g., g. local. SIN segmental g.
membranoproliferative g., g. membranoproliferativa; g. crônica caracterizada por proliferação de células mesangiais, separação lobular aumentada dos glomérulos, espessamento das paredes dos capilares glomerulares, aumento da matriz mesangial e baixos níveis séricos de complemento; ocorre principalmente em crianças maiores, com um curso progressivo e variavelmente lento, episódios de hematúria ou edema e hipertensão. É classificada em três tipos: tipo 1, o mais comum, no qual há depósitos subendoteliais elétron-densos; tipo 2, doença de depósitos densos, no qual a lâmina densa está bastante espessada por material extremamente elétron-denso; tipo 3, no qual há tanto depósitos subendoteliais como subepiteliais. SIN hypocomplementemic g., lobular g., mesangiocapillary g.
membranous g., g. membranosa; g. caracterizada por espessamento difuso das membranas basais dos capilares glomerulares devido, em parte, a depósitos subepiteliais de imunoglobulinas, separados por espículas de material de membrana basal; caracteriza-se clinicamente por síndrome nefrótica de início insidioso e fracasso na tentativa de interromper a proteinúria; a doença é mais comumente idiopática, porém pode ser secundária a tumores malignos, a substâncias, a infecções ou ao lúpus eritematoso sistêmico.
mesangial proliferative g., g. proliferativa mesangial; g. caracterizada clinicamente por síndrome nefrótica e histologicamente por aumentos glomerulares difusos nas células endocapilares e mesangiais, bem como na matriz mesangial; em alguns casos, há depósitos mesangiais de IgM e complemento. SIN diffuse mesangial proliferation, IgM nephropathy.
mesangiocapillary g., g. mesangiocapilar. SIN membranoproliferative g.
proliferative g., g. proliferativa; g. com hipercelularidade dos glomérulos, resultante de proliferação de células endoteliais e mesangiais; ocorre na g. aguda e na g. membranoproliferativa.
rapidly progressive g., g. rapidamente progressiva; g. que geralmente se apresenta de forma insidiosa, sem infecção estreptocócica precedente, com insuficiência renal progressiva, que leva à uremia dentro de alguns meses; na necropsia, os rins exibem tamanho normal, há numerosos crescentes epiteliais nas cápsulas dos glomérulos e anticorpos antimembrana basal são freqüentemente encontrados. SIN acute crescentic g.
segmental g., g. segmentar; g. que afeta apenas parte de um glomérulo ou dos glomérulos. SIN local g.
subacute g., g. subaguda; termo indesejável para a g. com proteinúria, hematúria e azotemia que persiste durante muitas semanas; as alterações renais são variáveis, incluindo aquelas da g. rapidamente progressiva e da g. membranoproliferativa. SIN subacute nephritis.
glo·mer·u·lop·a·thy (glō - mār - ū - lop′ă - thē). Glomerulopatia; doença glomerular de qualquer tipo. [glomerulus + G. *pathos*, sofrimento]
focal sclerosing g., g. esclerosante focal; uma glomeruloesclerose focal segmentar, relatada em crianças e adultos, que apresenta complemento sérico normal e progride para glomerulonefrite crônica.
glo·mer·u·lo·scle·ro·sis (glo - mār′ū - lō - sklĕ - rō′sis). Glomeruloesclerose; depósitos hialinos ou fibrose nos glomérulos renais, um processo degenerativo que ocorre em associação à arterioesclerose renal ou ao diabetes. SIN glomerular sclerosis. [glomerulus + G. *sklērōsis*, endurecimento]
diabetic g., g. diabética; proteinúria e, por fim, insuficiência renal que ocorre no diabetes de longa duração e caracteriza-se por nódulos hialinos arredondados ou laminados localizados na periferia dos glomérulos, com espessamento da membrana basal dos capilares e aumento da matriz mesangial. SIN intercapillary g.

focal segmental g., g. focal segmentar; colapso segmentar de capilares glomerulares com espessamento das membranas basais e aumento da matriz mesangial; observada em alguns glomérulos de pacientes com síndrome nefrótica ou glomerulonefrite proliferativa mesangial.
intercapillary g., g. intercapilar, g. diabética. SIN diabetic g.
glo·mer·u·lose (glō - mār′ū - lōs). Glomerular. SIN glomerular.
glo·mer·u·lus, pl. **glo·mer·u·li** (glō - mār′ū - lŭs, - ū - lī). Glomérulo. **1.** Um plexo de capilares. **2.** Um tufo formado por alças capilares no começo de cada túbulo néfrico do rim; esse tufo com sua cápsula (cápsula de Bowman) constitui o corpúsculo renal (corpúsculo de Malpighi). SIN malpighian g., malpighian tuft. **3.** A porção secretória retorcida de uma glândula sudorífera. **4.** Um aglomerado de ramificações dendríticas e de terminais de axônios que formam uma conexão sináptica complexa circundada por uma bainha glial. SIN glomerule. [L. mod. dim. de L. *glomus*, uma bola de fio]

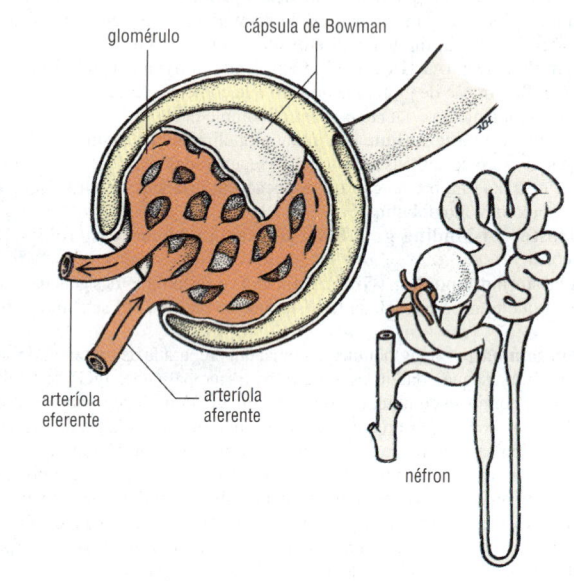

glomérulo

juxtamedullary g., g. justamedular; um g. próximo à margem medular.
malpighian g., corpúsculo de Malpighi. SIN glomerulus (2).
g. of mesonephros, g. de mesonefro; um dos tufos de vasos capilares localizados dentro do mesonefro e derivados de um ramo lateral da aorta primitiva; cada g. está ligado a um túbulo.
olfactory g., g. olfativo; uma das pequenas estruturas esféricas localizadas no bulbo olfatório nas quais os dendritos das células tufosas e mitrais fazem sinapse com os axônios das células receptoras olfatórias.
g. of pronephros, g. do pronefro; um dos tufos de vasos capilares localizados no pronefro e derivados de um ramo lateral da aorta.
glo·mus, pl. **glom·era** (glō′mŭs, glom′er - ă). Glomo. **1.** [TA]. Um pequeno corpo globular. **2.** Uma anastomose arteriolovenular bastante organizada que forma um diminuto foco nodular localizado no leito ungueal, nas polpas dos dedos das mãos e dos pés, nas orelhas, nas mãos e nos pés e em muitos outros órgãos do corpo. A arteríola aferente penetra na cápsula de tecido conectivo do g., torna-se desprovida de uma membrana elástica interna e desenvolve uma parede muscular epitelióide relativamente espessa e um pequeno lúmen; a anastomose pode ser ramificada e convoluta, ricamente inervada por nervos simpáticos e mielinizados e ligada a uma curta veia com parede fina que drena para uma veia periglômica e, então, para uma das veias da pele. O g. funciona como um mecanismo que regula o desvio ou o atalho do fluxo de sangue, da temperatura e da preservação do calor local, bem como do controle indireto da pressão sanguínea e de outras funções do sistema circulatório. SIN glandulae glomiformes (1), glomiform glands, glomus body. SIN glome. [L. *glomus*, uma bola]
aortic glomera, glomos aórticos; *termo oficial alternativo para paraaortic bodies, em body.
g. aorticum [TA], g. aórtico. SIN paraaortic bodies, em body.
g. carot'icum [TA], g. carótico. SIN carotid body.
choroid g., g. corióideo. SIN choroid enlargement.
g. choroi'deum [TA], g. corióideo. SIN choroid enlargement.
g. coccy'geum, g. coccígeo. SIN coccygeal body.
intravagal g., g. intravagal; um diminuto conjunto de células quimiorreceptoras localizadas no ramo auricular do nervo vago. Um tumor desse g. pode causar surdez e zumbido. SIN g. intravagale.

g. intravaga'le, g. intravagal. SIN intravagal g.
jugular g., g. jugular; um conjunto microscópico de tecido quimiorreceptor localizado na adventícia do bulbo jugular; um tumor desse g. pode produzir paralisia das cordas vocais, crises de vertigem, desmaios e nistagmo. SIN g. jugulare.
g. jugula're, g. jugular. SIN jugular g.
g. pulmona'le, g. pulmonar. SIN pulmonary g.
pulmonary g., g. pulmonar; uma estrutura semelhante ao corpo carótico, encontrada próximo à artéria pulmonar. SIN g. pulmonale.

gloss-. VER glosso-.
glos·sa (glos'sa). Glossa, língua. SIN tongue (1). [G.]
glos·sag·ra (glos - ag'ra). Glossagra; glossalgia de origem gotosa. [gloss- + G. *agra,* uma crise]
glos·sal (glos'al). Glóssico, lingual. SIN lingual (1).
glos·sal·gia (glos - al'jē - a). Glossalgia. SIN glossodynia. [gloss- + G. *algos,* dor]
glos·sec·to·my (glo - sek'tō - mē). Glossectomia; ressecção ou amputação da língua. SIN elinguation, glossosteresis. [gloss- + G. *ektomē,* excisão]
Glos·si·na (glo - sī'na). Um gênero de dípteros hematófagos (moscas tsé-tsé) da família dos muscídeos limitados à África; atuam como vetores de tripanosomas patogênicos que causam diversas formas de doença do sono africana em seres humanos e em animais domésticos e selvagens. [G. *glōssa,* língua]
G. mor'sitans, uma espécie originalmente considerada como a única transmissora do *Trypanosoma brucei brucei,* o causador da nagana na região central da África; essa espécie transmite a doença em algumas regiões, porém não é a única e nem sempre o principal agente transmissor; é o vetor do *T. brucei rhodesiense,* um dos agentes patogênicos da doença do sono aguda, rodesiana ou da África Oriental.
G. pallid'ipes, a principal espécie transmissora da nagana; também transmite o *Trypanosoma brucei rhodesiense.*
G. palpa'lis, uma espécie de *G.* que transmite o *Trypanosoma brucei gambiense,* um dos parasitas patogênicos da doença do sono crônica, gambiense ou da África Ocidental.
glos·si·tis (glo - sī'tis). Glossite; inflamação da língua. [gloss- + G. *-itis,* inflamação]
g. area'ta exfoliati'va, g. esfoliativa, língua geográfica. SIN geographic *tongue*.
atrophic g., g. atrófica; língua eritematosa, edemaciada e dolorosa que se apresenta lisa devido à perda de papilas filiformes e, às vezes, fungiformes, secundária a determinadas deficiências nutricionais, principalmente deficiências de vitamina B, como observado na pelagra, deficiência de tiamina e distúrbios, tais como a anemia perniciosa (g. de Hunter ou de Moeller). SIN bald tongue.
benign migratory g., g. migratória benigna, língua geográfica. SIN geographic *tongue.*
g. desic'cans, g. dessecante; uma afecção dolorosa da língua, de origem desconhecida, na qual a superfície se torna áspera e fissurada.
Hunter g., g. de Hunter, g. atrófica. VER atrophic g.
median rhomboid g., g. rombóide mediana; uma área eritematosa, macular, rombóide ou ovóide e assintomática com ausência de papilas na parte mediana do dorso da língua, anteriormente às papilas circunvaladas; considerada um tubérculo ímpar persistente.
Moeller g., g. de Moeller, g. atrófica. VER atrophic g.
glosso-, gloss-. Glosso-; linguagem; corresponde ao L. linguo-. Cf. linguo-. [G. *glōssa,* língua]
glos·so·cele (glos'ō - sēl). Glossocele; tumefação e protrusão da língua para fora da boca. VER TAMBÉM macroglossia. [glosso- + G. *kēlē,* tumor, hérnia]
glos·so·cin·es·thet·ic (glos'ō - sin - es - thet'ik). Glossocinestésico. SIN glossokinesthetic.
glos·so·don·to·tro·pism (glos - ō - don'tō - trō - pizm). Glossodontotropismo; uma manifestação de tensão ou ansiedade, na qual a língua é "atraída" para os dentes ou para as falhas dentárias. [glosso- + G. *odous (odont-),* dente, + *tropē,* uma volta]
glos·so·dy·na·mom·e·ter (glos'ō - dī - na - mom'e - ter). Glossodinamômetro; um aparelho utilizado para estimar a força contrátil dos músculos da língua. [glosso- + G. *dynamis,* força, + *metron,* medida]
glos·so·dyn·ia (glos'ō - din'ē - a). Glossodinia; uma condição caracterizada por queimação ou dor na língua. SIN burning tongue, glossalgia, glossopyrosis. [glosso- + G. *odynē,* dor]
glos·so·dyn·i·o·tro·pism (glos - ō - din'ē - o - trō - pizm). Glossodiniotropismo; satisfação aparente obtida ao se submeter a língua à sensação dolorosa produzida por uma falha dentária; considerado por alguns como um comportamento ou uma manifestação masoquista. [glosso- + G. *odynē,* dor, + *tropē,* uma volta]
glos·so·ep·i·glot·tic, glos·so·ep·i·glot·tid·e·an (glos'ō - ep - i - glot'ik, glos'ō - ep - i - glo - tid'ē - an). Glossoepiglótico; relativo à língua e à epiglote.
glos·so·graph (glos'ō - graf). Glossógrafo; um instrumento utilizado para registrar os movimentos da língua durante a fala. [glosso- + G. *graphō,* escrever]

glos·so·hy·al (glos - ō - hī'al). Glossoial. SIN hyoglossal.
glos·so·kin·es·thet·ic (glos'ō - kin - es - thet'ik). Glossocinestésico; indica a sensação subjetiva dos movimentos da língua. SIN glossocinesthetic. [glosso- + G. *kinēsis,* movimento, + *aisthētikos,* perceptivo]
glos·so·la·lia (glos - ō - lā'lē - a). Glossolalia; termo raramente utilizado para um dialeto ou balbucio ininteligível. [glosso- + G. *lalia,* conversa, bate-papo]
glos·sol·o·gy (glos - ol'ō - jē). Glossologia; o ramo da ciência médica relacionado com a língua e suas doenças. SIN glottology. [glosso- + G. *logos,* estudo]
glos·son·cus (glos - ong'kus). Glossoncose; qualquer tumefação que envolve a língua, incluindo as neoplasias. [glosso- + G. *onkos,* massa, tumor]
glos·so·pal·a·ti·nus (glos'ō - pal - a - tī'nus). Glossopalatino. SIN palatoglossus *(muscle).* [glosso- + L. mod. *palatinus,* do L. *palatum,* palato]
glos·sop·a·thy (glos - op'a - thē). Glossopatia; uma doença da língua. [glosso- + G. *pathos,* sofrimento]
glos·so·pha·ryn·ge·al (glos'ō - fa - rin'jē - al). Glossofaríngeo; relativo à língua e à faringe.
glos·so·pha·ryn·ge·us (glos'ō - fa - rin'jē - us). Glossofaríngeo. VER superior pharyngeal constrictor *(muscle).*
glos·so·plas·ty (glos'ō - plas - tē). Glossoplastia; cirurgia plástica da língua. [glosso- + G. *plastos,* formado]
glos·so·ple·gia (glos - ō - plē'jē - a). Glossoplegia; paralisia da língua. [glosso- + G. *plēgē,* paralisia]
glos·sop·to·sis, glos·sop·to·sia (glos - op - tō'sis, - op - tō'sē - a). Glossoptose; deslocamento da língua para baixo, em direção à faringe. [glosso- + G. *ptōsis,* uma queda]
glos·so·py·ro·sis (glos - ō - pī - rō'sis). Glossopirose, glossodinia. SIN glossodynia. [glosso- + G. *pyrōsis,* uma queimação]
glos·sor·rha·phy (glo - sōr'a - fē). Glossorrafia; sutura de uma ferida da língua. [glosso- + G. *rhaphē,* sutura]
glos·so·spasm (glos'ō - spazm). Glossoespasmo; contração espasmódica da língua.
glos·so·ste·re·sis (glos'ō - ste - rē'sis). Glossectomia. SIN glossectomy.
glos·sot·o·my (glo - sot'ō - mē). Glossotomia; qualquer incisão realizada na língua, em geral para obter um acesso maior à faringe. [glosso- + G. *tomē,* incisão]
glos·so·trich·ia (glos - ō - trik'ē - a). Glossotriquia; língua pilosa. SIN hairy *tongue.* [glosso- + G. *thrix,* pêlo]
glot·tal (glot'al). Glótico; relativo à glote.
glot·tal·iza·tion (glot'al - ī - zā'shun). Glotalização; fonação em uma freqüência anormalmente baixa. SIN vocal *fry.*
glot·tic (glot'ik). Glótico; relativo (1) à língua ou (2) à glote.
glot·ti·do·spasm (glot'i - dō - spazm). Glotidoespasmo. SIN laryngospasm.
glot·tis, pl. **glot·ti·des** (glot'is, glot'i - dēz) [TA]. Glote; o aparelho vocal da laringe, consistindo em pregas vocais de mucosa, que revestem o ligamento vocal e o músculo vocal em ambos os lados; nas margens livres nas pregas, que correspondem às cordas vocais; e em uma fissura mediana, a rima da glote. [G. *glōttis,* abertura da laringe]
false g., g. falsa, rima do vestíbulo. SIN rima vestibuli.
g. respirato'ria, g. respiratória. SIN intercartilaginous *part* of rima glottidis.
g. spu'ria, g. falsa, rima do vestíbulo. SIN rima vestibuli.
true g., g. verdadeira, rima da glote. SIN rima glottidis.
g. ve'ra, g. verdadeira, rima da glote. SIN rima glottidis.
g. voca'lis, g. vocal. SIN intermembranous *part* of rima glottidis.
glot·ti·tis (glo - tī'tis). Glotite; inflamação da parte glótica da laringe.
glot·tol·o·gy (glo - tol'ō - jē). Glotologia, glossologia. SIN glossology. [G. *glōssa, glōtta,* língua, + *logos,* estudo]
GLP-1 Abreviatura de glucagonlike *peptide* (peptídeo glucagon-símile).
Glp Abreviatura de 5-oxoproline (5-oxoprolina).
Glu Símbolo do glutamic acid (ácido glutâmico) ou de seu radical acila, glutamil (glutamyl).
glu·ca·gon (gloo'ka - gon). Glucagon; um hormônio que consiste em um polipeptídeo de cadeia reta, com 29 resíduos aminoacil, extraído das células alfa do pâncreas. A administração parenteral de 0,5 a 1 mg de glucagon resulta em pronta mobilização do glicogênio hepático, elevando, assim, a concentração de glicose do sangue. Ativa a fosforilase hepática, que, dessa forma, aumenta a glicogenólise, diminui a motilidade gástrica e as secreções gástrica e pancreática e aumenta a excreção urinária de nitrogênio e potássio; não apresenta efeito sobre a fosforilase muscular. Na forma de cloridrato, é utilizado no tratamento da doença do armazenamento de glicogênio (von Gierke) e da hipoglicemia, particularmente do coma hipoglicêmico resultante de insulina administrada exogenamente. SIN HG factor, hyperglycemic-glycogenolytic factor, pancreatic hyperglycemic hormone. [glucose + G. *agō,* conduzir]
gut g., g. intestinal; uma substância de origem intestinal secretada no sangue após a ingestão de glicose e atua como um potente estímulo para a secreção de insulina; sua estrutura química e os efeitos biológicos que produz são diferentes daqueles do g., e reage cruzadamente com os anticorpos antiglucagon.
glu·ca·gon·o·ma (gloo'ka - gon - ō'ma). Glucagonoma; um tumor que secreta glucagon e deriva, em geral, das células das ilhotas do pâncreas.

glu·cal (gloo′kăl). Glical. SIN glycal.
glu·can (gloo′kan). Glicana. SIN glucosan.
1,4-α-D-glu·can-branch·ing en·zyme. Enzima ramificadora da 1,4-α-D-glicana; amilo-(1,4 → 1,6)-transglicosilase ou transglicosidase; uma enzima encontrada no músculo e nas plantas (enzima Q) que cinde as ligações α-1,4 do glicogênio ou do amido, transferindo os fragmentos para as ligações α-1,6, criando ramificações nas moléculas de polissacarídeos; nas plantas, a enzima converte a amilose em amilopectina; ocorre deficiência dessa enzima nos indivíduos com a doença do armazenamento de glicogênio tipo IV. SIN α-glucan-branching glycosyltransferase, amylo-1,4: 1,6-glucantransferase, amylo-(1,4 → 1,6)-transglucosidase, amylo-(1,4 → 1,6)-transglucosylase, branching enzyme.
α-glu·can-branch·ing gly·co·syl·trans·fer·ase. Glicosiltransferase ramificadora da α-glicana. SIN 1,4-α-D-glucan-branching enzyme.
1,4-α-D-glu·can 6-α-D-glu·co·syl·trans·fer·ase. 1,4-α-D-glicano 6-α-D-glicosiltransferase; uma glicosiltransferase que transfere um resíduo α-glicosil de uma 1,4-α-glicana para o grupamento hidroxila primário da glicose de uma 1,4-α-glicana. VER TAMBÉM 1,4-α-D-glucan-branching enzyme. SIN oligoglucan-branching glycosyltransferase.
4-α-D-glu·can·o·trans·fer·ase. 4-α-D-glicanotransferase; dextrina transglicosilase ou glicosiltransferase; uma 4-glicosiltransferase que converte maltodextrinas em amilose e glicose por meio da transferência de partes de cadeias de 1,4-glicana para novas posições-4 na glicose ou em outras 1,4-glicanas. SIN amylomaltase, D enzyme, dextrin glycosyltransferase, dextrin transglycosylase, disproportionating enzyme.
α-glu·can phos·pho·ryl·ase. α-glicana fosforilase, fosforilase. SIN phosphorylase.
glu·cep·tate (gloo - sep′tat). Gliceptato; contração de glico-heptonato aprovada pelo USAN (United States Adopted Names).
glu·ci·phore (gloo′si - fōr). Glicíforo; termo cunhado para os grupamentos químicos considerados responsáveis pelo sabor doce. [G. glykys, doce, + phoros, portador]
♻ **gluco-.** Glico-; forma combinante que indica uma relação com a glicose. VER TAMBÉM glyco-. [G. gleukos, mosto, doçura]
glu·co·am·y·lase (gloo - kō - am′i - lās). Glicoamilase. SIN exo-1,4-α-D-glucosidase.
glu·co·a·scor·bic ac·id (gloo′kō - as - kōr′bik). Ácido glicoascórbico; um composto que se assemelha ao ácido ascórbico, mas com um —CHOH— adicional entre o C-5 e o C-6 do ácido ascórbico; quando adicionado à dieta, o composto exibe efeitos tóxicos que, aparentemente, não são causados por antagonismo ao ácido ascórbico.
β-glu·co·cer·e·bro·sid·ase (gloo′kō - ser′ē - brō - sīd - ās). β-glicocerebrosidase; uma enzima que hidrolisa os β-glicosídeos em cerebrosídeos; a deficiência dessa enzima causa a doença de Gaucher.
glu·co·cer·e·bro·side (gloo′kō - ser′ē - brō - sīd). Glicocerebrosídeo. SIN glucosylceramide.
glu·co·cor·ti·coid (gloo - kō - kōr′ti - koyd). Glicocorticóide. **1.** Qualquer composto semelhante a um esteróide capaz de influenciar de maneira significativa o metabolismo intermediário, promovendo a deposição de glicogênio hepático e a produção de um efeito antiinflamatório clinicamente útil. O cortisol (hidrocortisona) é o mais potente dos glicocorticóides existentes na natureza; a maioria dos glicocorticóides semi-sintéticos são derivados do cortisol. **2.** Que indica esse tipo de atividade biológica. SIN glycocorticoid.
glu·co·cor·ti·co·tro·phic (gloo′kō - kōr′ti - kō - trōf′ik). Glicocorticotrófico; indica um princípio — que se postulou existir na hipófise anterior — que estimula a produção de hormônios glicocorticóides pelo córtex da supra-renal; não foi identificado nenhum hormônio que exerça apenas esse efeito, porém o ACTH estimula a produção corticóide pela supra-renal.
glu·co·cy·a·mine (gloo - kō - sī′a - mēn). Glicociamina. SIN glycocyamine.
glu·co·fu·ra·nose (gloo - kō - foor′a - nōs). Glicofuranose; glicose na forma de furanose.
glu·co·gen·e·sis (gloo - kō - jen′ē - is). Glicogênese; formação de glicose. [gluco- + G. genesis, produção]
glu·co·gen·ic (gloo - kō - jen′ik). Glicogênico; que dá origem à ou que produz glicose. SIN glucoplastic.
glu·co·in·vert·ase (gloo - kō - in′ver - tās). Glicoinvertase. SIN α-D-glucosidase.
glu·co·ki·nase (gloo - kō - kī′nās). Glicocinase; uma fosfotransferase que catalisa a conversão da D-glicose e do ATP em D-glicose 6-fosfato e ADP; a enzima hepática possui um valor de K_m mais alto para a D-glicose do que a hexocinase e não é fortemente inibida pelo produto D-glicose 6-fosfato.
glu·co·ki·net·ic (gloo′kō - ki - net′ik). Glicocinético; que tende a mobilizar glicose; geralmente evidenciado por redução dos depósitos de glicogênio nos tecidos, a fim de produzir uma elevação na concentração da glicose que circula no sangue.
glu·co·lip·ids (gloo - kō - lip′idz). Glicolipídios; lipídios que contêm D-glicose.
glu·col·y·sis (gloo - kol′i - sis). Glicólise. SIN glycolysis.

glu·co·ne·o·gen·e·sis (gloo′kō - nē - ō - jen′ē - sis). Gliconeogênese; a formação de glicose a partir de não-carboidratos, tais como proteínas e gorduras. SIN glyconeogenesis (2).
glu·con·ic ac·id (gloo - kon′ik). Ácido glicônico; o ácido hexônico (aldônico) derivado da glicose pela oxidação do grupamento –CHO, formando o grupamento –COOH.
glu·con·o·lac·to·nase (gloo′kon - o - lak′tō - nās). Gliconolactonase; uma enzima que catalisa a hidrólise da D-glicono-δ-lactona em ácido D-glicônico. SIN lactonase.
glu·co·pe·nia (gloo - kō - pē′nē - ă). Glicopenia, hipoglicemia. SIN hypoglycemia. [gluco- + G. penia, pobreza]
glu·co·plas·tic. Glicoplástico, glicogênico. SIN glucogenic.
glu·co·pro·tein (gloo - kō - prō′tēn). Glicoproteína; uma glicoproteína na qual o açúcar é a glicose.
glu·co·pyr·a·nose (gloo - kō - pir′a - nōs). Glicopiranose; glicose na forma de piranose.
glu·co·sa·mine (gloo′kō - sā - mēn). Glicosamina; um aminoaçúcar encontrado na quitina, nas membranas celulares e nos mucopolissacarídeos em geral; utilizada como um produto auxiliar farmacêutico.
glu·cos·a·mi·no·gly·cans (gloo - kōs - ă - mē′nō - glī′kans). Glicosaminoglicanas (ou mucopolissacarídeos) nas quais todos os aminoaçúcares constituintes são glicosaminas.
glu·co·san (gloo′kō - san). Glicosana; um polissacarídeo que, ao ser hidrolisado, produz glicose; p.ex., calose, celulose, glicogênio, amido, dextrinas. SIN glucan.
D-glu·cose (G, Glc) (gloo′kōs). D-glicose; dextrose; um monossacarídeo (hexose) dextrorrotatório encontrado, na forma livre, nas frutas e em outras partes das plantas e, na forma combinada, em glicosídeos, dissacarídeos (freqüentemente com a frutose, em açúcares), oligossacarídeos e polissacarídeos; é o produto da hidrólise completa da celulose, do amido e do glicogênio. A glicose livre também está presente no sangue, onde é a principal fonte de energia utilizada pelos tecidos do corpo (concentração humana normal de 70 a 100 mg/100 mL); no diabetes melito, aparece na urina. Os epímeros da D-g. são a D-alose, a D-manose, a D-galactose e a L-idose. A dextrose não deve ser confundida com o isômero L, que é a sinistrose. SIN cellohexose.
  activated g., g. ativada; uma difosfoglicose nucleosídeo, tal como a UDPglicose.
  g. dehydrogenase, g. desidrogenase; converte a β-D-glicose em D-glicono-δ-lactona, transferindo hidrogênio para NAD^+ ou $NADP^+$. Cf. g. oxidase.
  liquid g., g. líquida; uma solução farmacêutica que consiste em dextrose, dextrinas, maltose e água e é obtida por meio da hidrólise incompleta do amido.
  g. oxidase, g. oxidase; uma enzima (flavoproteína) antibacteriana, obtida do Penicillum notatum e de outros fungos e com ação antibacteriana apenas na presença da glicose e do oxigênio, sendo seu efeito devido à oxidação da D-glicose em D-glicono-δ-lactona, com a co-conversão do O_2 em H_2O_2; utilizada na conservação de alimentos e nas análises dos níveis de glicose. SIN g. oxyhydrase, microcide.
  g. oxyhydrase, g. oxidase. SIN g. oxidase.
  g. phosphomutase, g. fosfomutase. SIN phosphoglucomutase.
D-glu·cose 1,6-bis·phos·phate. D-glicose 1,6-difosfato; um derivado difosforilado da D-glicose; trata-se de um intermediário necessário para a interconversão da D-glicose 1-fosfato em D-glicose 6-fosfato.
glu·cose-6-phos·pha·tase. Glicose-6-fosfatase; uma enzima hepática que catalisa a hidrólise da D-glicose 6-fosfato para D-glicose e ortofosfato; ocorre deficiência dessa enzima na doença do armazenamento de glicogênio de tipo Ia.
glu·cose 6-phos·phate. Glicose 6-fosfato; um éster da glicose com o ácido fosfórico; elaborado durante o metabolismo da glicose pelas células dos mamíferos e por outras células; um constituinte normal do músculo em repouso, provavelmente sempre em equilíbrio com a frutose 6-fosfato.
D-glu·cose 1-phos·phate. D-glicose 1-fosfato; um importante intermediário da glicogênese e da glicogenólise. SIN Cori ester.
D-glu·cose 6-phos·phate. D-glicose 6-fosfato; um intermediário-chave da glicólise, da glicogenólise, do desvio da via pentose fosfato etc.; níveis elevados de D-glicose 6-fosfato inibem a hexocinase cerebral e a glicólise. SIN Robison ester, Robinson-Embden ester.
glu·cose-6-phos·phate de·hy·dro·gen·ase. Glicose-6-fosfato desidrogenase; uma enzima ($NADP^+$) que catalisa a desidrogenação da D-glicose 6-fosfato a 6-fosfo-D-glicono-δ-lactona, ou seja, a reação que inicia o desvio da via pentose. A deficiência dessa enzima pode levar à anemia hemolítica grave e ao favismo. A deficiência da enzima nos leucócitos impede que ocorra a explosão respiratória nos neutrófilos. SIN Robison ester dehydrogenase, Zwischenferment.
glu·cose-phos·phate isom·er·ase. Glicose-fosfato isomerase; uma enzima que catalisa a interconversão reversível da D-frutose 6-fosfato e da D-glicose 6-fosfato; uma parte da glicólise e da gliconeogênese; a deficiência dessa enzima corresponde a um distúrbio hereditário que resulta em glicogênese hepá-

tica e em anemia hemolítica. SIN hexosephosphate isomerase, phosphohexomutase, phosphohexose isomerase.

glu·cose-1-phos·phate ki·nase. Glicose-1-fosfato cinase. SIN phosphoglucokinase.

glu·cose-1-phos·phate phos·pho·dis·mu·tase. Glicose-1-fosfato fosfodismutase; uma fosfotransferase que catalisa a transferência reversível de um resíduo fosfato de uma D-glicose 1-fosfato para uma outra, produzindo D-glicose 1,6-difosfato e D-glicose. Essa enzima fornece um intermediário crucial necessário para a glicose-fosfato isomerase.

glu·cose-6-phos·phate trans·lo·case. Glicose-6-fosfato translocase; uma proteína de transporte encontrada na membrana do retículo endoplasmático; a deficiência dessa proteína está associada à doença do armazenamento de glicogênio de tipo Ib.

glu·cose-1-phos·phate uri·dyl·yl·trans·fer·ase. Glicose-1-fosfato uridililtransferase; uma enzima que ativa D-glicose por meio da reação da D-glicose 1-fosfato com UTP, produzindo pirofosfato e UDPglicose; um passo crucial da biossíntese do glicogênio.

α-D-glu·co·si·dase (gloo′kō-si-dās). α-D-glicosidase; maltase; uma glicoidrolase que remove os resíduos terminais, não-redutíveis, da α-glicose 1,4-ligados por hidrólise, produzindo α-glicose; a deficiência da enzima lisossomial está associada à doença do armazenamento de glicogênio de tipo II. Existem, pelo menos, cinco isoenzimas da maltase. SIN glucoinvertase.

β-D-glu·co·si·dase. β-D-glicosidase; uma glicoidrolase, semelhante à α-D-glicosidase, que reage com os β-glicosídeos e libera a β-D-glicose. SIN amygdalase, cellobiase, gentiobiase.

glu·co·si·das·es (gloo′kō-sid-ās-ez). Glicosidases; enzimas que hidrolisam os glicosídeos.

glu·co·side (gloo′kō-sīd). Glicosídeo; um composto de glicose com um álcool ou com outro composto R–OH que envolve a perda do átomo de H do grupamento 1-OH (hemiacetal) da glicose, produzindo uma ligação –C–O–R a partir do C-1 da glicose; um glicosídeo da glicose.

glucosinolates. Glicosinolatos; um grupo de metabólitos vegetais secundários presentes nas plantas crucíferas, principalmente nos vegetais do gênero *Brassica* (tal como o repolho); são hidrolisados em uma ampla gama de compostos biologicamente ativos, incluindo os isotiocianatos, que exibem atividade anticarcinógena.

glu·co·sone (gloo′kō-sōn). Glicosona; um produto da 2-desidrogenação (2-ceto) da glicose; um possível intermediário da formação da glicosamina a partir da glicose. [glicose + -ona]

glu·co·sul·fone so·di·um (gloo-kō-sŭl′fōn). Glicossulfona sódica; um agente utilizado no tratamento da hanseníase; a administração parenteral é mais bem tolerada do que a administração oral.

glu·cos·u·ria (gloo-kō-soo′rē-ă). Glicosúria; a excreção urinária de glicose, em geral em quantidades aumentadas. SIN glycosuria (1), glycuresis (1). [glicose + G. *ouron*, urina]

glu·co·syl (gloo′kō-sil). Glicosil; o radical da glicose que perdeu seu hemiacetal (C-1) OH.

glu·co·syl·cer·a·mide (gloo′kō-sil-ser′ă-mīd). Glicosilceramida; um glicolipídio neutro que contém quantidades eqüimolares de ácido graxo, glicose e esfingosina (ou um derivado); acumula-se nos indivíduos com a doença de Gaucher. SIN glucocerebroside.

glu·co·syl·trans·fer·ase (gloo′kō-sil-trans′fer-ās). Glicosiltransferase; qualquer enzima que transfere grupamentos glicosila de um composto para outro; as glicosiltransferases estão na subclasse 2.4 da EC (glicosiltransferases). SIN transglucosylase.

glu·cu·ro·nate (gloo-koor′ō-nāt). Glicuronato; um sal ou um éster do ácido glicurônico.

glu·cu·rone (gloo′koo-rōn). Glicurona. SIN D-glucuronolactone.

glu·cu·ron·ic ac·id (gloo-koo-ron′ik). Ácido glicurônico; o ácido urônico da glicose no qual o C-6 é oxidado a um grupamento carboxila; o isômero D detoxifica ou inativa diversas substâncias (p.ex., o ácido benzóico, o fenol, a cânfora e os hormônios sexuais femininos), sofrendo conjugação com tais substâncias no fígado. Os glicuronídeos assim formados são excretados na urina.

β-D-glu·cu·ron·i·dase (gloo-koo-ron′i-dās). β-D-glicuronidase; uma enzima que catalisa a hidrólise de diversos β-D-glicuronídeos, liberando ácido D-glicurônico livre e um álcool; a deficiência dessa enzima está associada à síndrome de Sly. SIN glusulase, glycuronidase.

glu·cu·ro·nide (gloo-koo′rŏn-īd). Glicuronídeo. um glicosídeo do ácido glicurônico; muitos produtos químicos estranhos, como também produtos catabólicos de constituintes normais do corpo (p.ex., hormônios esteróides), são geralmente excretados na urina como D-glicuronídeos, após conjugação hepática. SIN glucuronoside.

D-glu·cu·ron·o·lac·tone (gloo′kŭ-rō′nō-lak′tōn). D-glicuronolactona; utilizada como um meio para a administração oral de ácido glicurônico para o tratamento de doenças do colágeno e das articulações. SIN glucurone.

glu·cu·ro·no·side (gloo-koo-ron′ō-sīd). Glicuronosídeo. SIN glucuronide.

glu·cu·ron·o·syl·trans·fer·ase (gloo-koo-ron′ō-sil-trans′fer-ās). Glicuronosiltransferase; uma enzima de uma família de enzimas que transferem D-glicuronato para um aceptor, formando glicuronosídeos; p.ex., a UDPglicuronato-bilirrubina glicuronosiltransferase.

glue-sniff·ing (gloo′snif-ing). Inalação de cola; inalação dos vapores provenientes de cimentos plásticos; os solventes, que induzem o tolueno, o xileno e o benzeno, induzem estimulação do sistema nervoso central, seguida por depressão. VER TAMBÉM solvent *inhalation*.

Gluge, Gottlieb, histologista alemão, 1812–1898. VER G. *corpuscles*, em *corpuscle*.

glu·sul·ase (gloo′sŭl-ās). Glusulase. SIN β-D-glucuronidase.

glu·ta·con·ic ac·id (gloo′tă-kon-ik). Ácido glutacônico; ácido dicarboxílico que se acumula nos indivíduos com acidemia glutárica de tipo I.

glu·ta·mate (gloo′tă-māt). Glutamato; um sal ou um éster do ácido glutâmico.

g. **acetyltransferase,** g. acetiltransferase. **(1)** Uma enzima que catalisa a transferência de um grupamento acetila de N^2-acetilornitina para o L-g., formando L-ornitina e *N*-acetil-L-glutamato, um ativador do ciclo da uréia; **(2)** uma enzima que catalisa a transferência de um grupamento acetila da acetil-CoA para o L-g. para formar a coenzima A e o *N*-acetil-L-g., um ativador do ciclo da uréia. SIN ornithine acetyltransferase.

g. **decarboxylase (GAD),** g. descarboxilase; uma carboxiliase que converte o L-g. em 4-aminobutirato e CO_2, bem como o L-aspartato em 3-aminopropanoato e CO_2; acredita-se que um defeito na ligação dessas coenzimas de proteínas seja a causa da dependência de piridoxina acompanhada de crises. SIN aspartate 1-decarboxylase.

g. **dehydrogenases,** g. desidrogenases; enzimas que catalisam a reação do L-g., da H_2O e do NAD^+ (ou do $NADP^+$ em alguns casos) que produz o α-cetoglutarato (2-oxoglutarato), a amônia e o NADH; em mamíferos, esse é o mais importante contribuinte para a desaminação oxidativa. SIN glutamic acid dehydrogenases.

g. **formiminotransferase,** g. formiminotransferase; uma enzima que catalisa a transferência do radical formimino do *N*-formimino-L-glutamato para o tetraidrofolato; a deficiência dessa enzima causa aumento nos níveis de formiminoglutamato.

g. **γ-semialdehyde,** g. γ-semi-aldeído; um intermediário do metabolismo da L-prolina e da L-ornitina; encontra-se elevado na hiperprolinemia de tipo II.

g. **synthase,** g. sintase; uma enzima que converte a L-glutamina, o α-cetoglutarato e o NADH (em alguns casos, o NADPH) em dois L-glutamatos e NAD^+ (ou $NADP^+$); aparentemente, essa enzima não existe nos mamíferos. Em algumas plantas, essa é uma reação dependente de ferredoxina.

γ-glu·ta·mate (glu·ta·mate γ-) car·box·y·pep·ti·dase. γ-glutamato carboxipeptidase. SIN γ-glutamyl hydrolase.

glu·tam·ic ac·id (E, Glu) (gloo-tam′ik). Ácido glutâmico; um aminoácido; o sal sódico é o glutamato monossódico. Cf. glutamate.

g. **a. dehydrogenases,** desidrogenase do ácido glutâmico. SIN *glutamate dehydrogenases.*

g. **a. hydrochloride,** cloridrato do ácido glutâmico; um acidificador gástrico que se supõe auxiliar na digestão; é também utilizado na terapia de substituição do HCl gástrico.

glu·tam·ic-as·par·tic trans·am·i·nase. Transaminase glutâmico aspártica, aspartato aminotransferase (AST). SIN *aspartate aminotransferase.*

glu·tam·ic-ox·a·lo·ace·tic trans·am·i·nase (GOT). Transaminase glutâmico oxaloacética (TGO), aspartato aminotransferase (AST). SIN aspartate aminotransferase.

glu·tam·ic-py·ru·vic trans·am·i·nase (GPT). Transaminase glutâmico pirúvica (TGP), alanina aminotransferase (ALT). SIN alanine aminotransferase.

glu·ta·min·ase (gloo-tam′in-ās). Glutaminase; uma enzima encontrada nos rins e em outros tecidos que catalisa a hidrólise da L-glutamina a amônia e ácido L-glutâmico; uma importante enzima para a formação da amônia urinária.

glu·ta·min·ate (gloo-tam′in-āt). Glutaminato; a forma aniônica da glutamina.

glu·ta·mine (Gln, Q) (gloo′tă-mēn, -tă-min, gloo-tam′in). Glutamina; a δ-amida do ácido glutâmico, derivada por oxidação da prolina, no fígado, ou pela combinação do ácido glutâmico com a amônia; o isômero L existe nas proteínas e no sangue e em outros tecidos; é uma importante fonte de amônia urinária, sendo quebrada nos rins pela ação da enzima glutaminase; é convertida a 5-oxoprolina sem a ação de enzimas.

g. **aminotransferase,** g. aminotransferase; uma enzima que promove a reação reversível da L-glutamina com o α-cetoglutarato para produzir o α-cetoglutaramato e o L-glutamato; o α-cetoglutaramato está elevado em certos casos de coma hepático. SIN g. transaminase.

g. **synthetase,** g. sintetase; uma enzima que catalisa a reação do ácido L-glutâmico, da amônia e do ATP para g., ADP e ortofosfato; uma das poucas enzimas de mamíferos conhecidas que utiliza íons de amônio como substrato em condições fisiológicas.

g. **transaminase,** g. transaminase. SIN g. aminotransferase.

glu·tam·i·nyl (Gln, Glx, Q) (gloo-tam′i-nil). Glutaminil; o radical acila da glutamina.

glu·tam·o·yl (gloo - tam′ō - il). Glutamoil; o radical do ácido glutâmico do qual tanto o grupamento α- como o δ-hidroxila foram removidos.

glu·tam·yl (E, Glu, Glx) (gloo - tam′il, gloo′tă - mil). Glutamil; o radical do ácido glutâmico do qual ou o grupamento α-, ou o δ-hidroxila foi removido.

γ-glu·tam·yl car·box·yl·ase. γ-glutamil carboxilase; uma enzima que catalisa a formação de resíduos γ-carboxiglutamil em muitas proteínas. Várias dessas proteínas são encontradas na cascata da coagulação sanguínea.

γ-glu·ta·myl·cys·teine (gloo′tă - mil - sis′te - in). γ-glutamilcisteína; um precursor necessário na biossíntese da glutationa; contém uma ligação isopeptídica em vez de eupeptídica.

   γ-g. synthetase, γ-g. sintetase; uma enzima que catalisa o primeiro passo da biossíntese da glutationa, reagindo o L-glutamato, a L-cisteína e o ATP para formar γ-g., ADP e ortofosfato; é inibida por tióis, tais como a glutationa.

γ-glu·tam·yl hy·dro·lase. γ-glutamil hidrolase; uma enzima que cliva os resíduos L-glutamil dos oligoglutamatos da pteridina; é utilizada em certos tratamentos antitumorais. SIN carboxypeptidase G, γ-glutamate (glutamate γ-) carboxypeptidase.

γ-glu·tam·yl·trans·fer·ase (gloo - tam′il - trans′fer - ās). γ-glutamil transferase; uma enzima que catalisa a transferência de um grupamento γ-glutamil de um γ-glutamilpeptídeo (em geral da glutationa) para outro peptídeo, certos aminoácidos ou para a água; a deficiência dessa enzima resulta em glutationúria. SIN γ-glutamyl transpeptidase.

γ-glu·tam·yl trans·pep·ti·dase. γ-glutamil transpeptidase, γ-glutamiltransferase (GGT). SIN γ-glutamyltransferase.

glu·ta·ral (gloo′tă - ral). Glutaral, glutaraldeído SIN glutaraldehyde.

glu·tar·al·de·hyde (gloo - tă - ral′dĕ - hīd). Glutaraldeído; um dialdeído utilizado como fixador em microscopia eletrônica, principalmente em morfologia nuclear e na localização de atividade enzimática; é também utilizado como agente germicida na desinfecção e esterilização de instrumentos ou equipamentos que não podem ser esterilizados por aquecimento. SIN glutaral.

glu·tar·ic ac·id (gloo - tar′ik). Ácido glutárico; ácido pentanodióico; um intermediário do catabolismo do triptofano; acumula-se nos indivíduos com acidemia glutárica.

glu·ta·ryl-CoA (gloo′tă - ril). Glutaril-CoA; o éster de monotiol da coenzima A e do ácido glutárico; um intermediário do catabolismo da L-lisina e do L-triptofano.

   g.-CoA dehydrogenase, g.-CoA desidrogenase; uma enzima que catalisa a reação da g.-CoA com um aceptor para formar crotonil-CoA, CO_2 e o aceptor reduzido; a deficiência dessa enzima causa acidemia glutárica de tipo I ou hiperoxalúria de tipo II.

   g.-CoA synthetase, g.-CoA sintetase; uma enzima similar à acil-CoA sintetase, mas que cliva o ATP, o GTP ou o ITP em difosfato de nucleosídeo e ortofosfato ao agir sobre o glutarato, formando, desse modo, a g.-CoA.

glu·ta·thi·one (GSH) (gloo - tă - thī′ōn). Glutationa; um tripeptídeo da glicina, da L-cisteína e do L-glutamato com o L-glutamato que possui uma ligação isopeptídica com o radical amino da L-cisteína. A g. tem numerosas funções em uma célula; é o tiol não-proteico mais prevalente. O dissulfeto de g. consiste em duas glutationas ligadas por uma ponte de dissulfeto; o termo g. oxidada para o dissulfeto de g. deve ser evitado, uma vez que esse termo (g. oxidada) inclui as sulfonas e os sulfóxidos de g. O termo g. reduzida não é necessário, uma vez que a g. está na forma de tiol. A deficiência de g. pode causar hemólise com estresse oxidativo. É também utilizada no curso do metabolismo intermediário como uma doadora de grupamentos tiol (SH) e é essencial para a detoxificação do acetoaminofeno. VER TAMBÉM oxidized g., reduced g., g. reductase.

   oxidized g., g. oxidada. (1) A g. que age nas células como um aceptor de hidrogênio; é reduzida pela g. redutase; dissulfeto de glutationa; **(2)** as sulfonas ou os sulfóxidos de glutationa ou o dissulfeto de glutationa.

   g. peroxidase, g. peroxidase; uma enzima que catalisa a reação de duas glutationas com H_2O_2, formando dissulfeto de glutationa e duas moléculas de água; uma enzima crucial na detoxificação do peróxido de hidrogênio.

   reduced g., g. reduzida; g. que atua como doadora de hidrogênio; glutationa.

   g. reductase, g. redutase; uma enzima que catalisa a reação do dissulfeto de g. com o NADH (ou com o NADPH), formando duas glutationas e NAD^+ (ou $NADP^+$); está envolvida em muitas reações do tipo redox; sua deficiência pode causar hemólise com estresse oxidativo.

   g. synthetase, g. sintetase; uma enzima que catalisa a formação de g., ADP e ortofosfato a partir da γ-glutamilcisteína, do ATP e da glicina; sua deficiência causa acidose metabólica e disfunção cerebral progressiva.

   g. S-transferase, g. S-transferase; uma classe de enzimas que catalisam a reação da g. com uma molécula aceptora (p.ex., um óxido de hidrocarboneto que contém pelo menos um anel aromático), para formar uma g. S-substituída; uma etapa fundamental na detoxificação de muitas substâncias; o início da via do ácido mercaptúrico. SIN ligandin.

glu·ta·thi·o·nu·ria (gloo - tă - thī′ō - nur - ē - ă). Glutationúria; níveis elevados de glutationa e/ou de dissulfeto de glutationa na urina.

glu·te·al (gloo′tē - ăl). Glúteo; relativo às nádegas. [G. *gloutos*, nádega]

glu·te·lins (gloo′tē - linz). Glutelinas; uma classe de proteínas simples presentes nas sementes de grãos; são solúveis em ácidos e bases diluídos, mas não em soluções neutras (p.ex., a glutenina do trigo e a oricenina no arroz). Possuem domínios ricos em glutamina e atuam como proteínas de armazenamento.

glu·ten (gloo′tĕn). Glúten; a proteína insolúvel (prolaminas) que participa da constituição do trigo e de outros grãos; uma mistura de gliadina, glutenina, prolaminas e de outras proteínas; a presença do g. permite que a farinha cresça. SIN wheat gum. [L. *gluten*, cola]

   g. casein, caseína do g.; uma proteína que existe no g. e que se assemelha à caseína.

glu·te·nin (gloo′tĕ - nin). Glutenina; qualquer glutelina encontrada no endosperma das sementes do trigo; acredita-se que a g. seja responsável pelas propriedades viscoelásticas da massa da farinha do trigo.

glu·te·o·fem·o·ral (gloo′tē - ō - fem′ō - răl). Gluteofemoral; relativo à nádega e à coxa.

glu·te·o·in·gui·nal (gloo′tē - ō - ing′gwi - năl). Gluteoinguinal; relativo à nádega e à virilha.

glu·teth·i·mide (gloo - teth′i - mīd). Glutetimida; um depressor do sistema nervoso central, empregado como hipnótico na insônia simples; antigamente era utilizado como sedativo diurno.

glu·te·us (gloo - tē′us). Glúteo. VER gluteus maximus (*muscle*), gluteus medius (*muscle*), gluteus minimus (*muscle*).

glu·ti·noid (gloo′ti - noyd). Glutinóide, albuminóide (3). SIN albuminoid (3).

glu·ti·nous (gloo′tin - us). Glutinoso; pegajoso.

glu·ti·tis (gloo - tī′tis). Glutite; inflamação dos músculos da nádega. [G. *gloutos*, nádega, + *-itis*, inflamação]

Glx Símbolo de glutamil (glutamyl) (Glu), de glutaminil (glutaminyl) (Gln) e/ou de qualquer substância que, ao sofrer hidrólise ácida de um peptídeo, produz glutamato (p.ex., 5-oxoprolina, 4-carboxiglutamato).

Gly Símbolo de glycine (glicina) ou de seu radical acila, glicila (glycyl).

gly·bu·ride (glī′bū - rīd). Gliburida; hipoglicemiante oral utilizado no tratamento do diabetes de tipo II.

gly·cal (glī′kăl). Glical; um derivado de açúcar insaturado no qual os grupamentos hidroxila adjacentes foram removidos — um deles localizado sobre o carbono 1 da aldose (ou o carbono 2 da cetose) —, produzindo um CH=CH entre essas duas posições. SIN glucal.

gly·can (glī′kan). Glicana, polissacarídeo. SIN polysaccharide. VER TAMBÉM heteroglycan, homoglycan.

gly·can·o·hy·dro·las·es (glī′kan - ō - hī′drō - lā - sez) [EC 3.2.1.x]. Glicanohidrolases; hidrolases que atuam sobre glicanas; p.ex., quitinase, hialuronoglicosidase.

gly·cate (glī′kāt). Glicato; o produto da reação não-enzimática entre um açúcar e o(s) grupamento(s) amina livre(s) de proteínas, nas quais não se sabe se o açúcar está ligado por uma ligação glicosil ou glicosídica, ou se formou uma base de Schiff.

gly·ca·tion (glī - kā′shun). Glicação; a reação não-enzimática que forma um glicato.

gly·ce·mia (glī - sē′mē - ă). Glicemia; a presença de glicose no sangue. [G. *glykys*, doce, + *haima*, sangue]

glyc·er·al·de·hyde (glis - er - al′dĕ - hīd). Gliceraldeído; uma triose e a aldose opticamente ativa mais simples; o isômero dextrorrotatório é tomado como o ponto de referência estrutural para todos os compostos D, e o isômero levorrotatório, para todos os compostos L. SIN glyceric aldehyde.

glyc·er·al·de·hyde 3-phos·phate. Gliceraldeído 3-fosfato; um intermediário do desdobramento glicolítico da D-glicose; um dos produtos da cisão da frutose 1,6-difosfato sob a influência catalítica da frutose-difosfato aldolase.

gly·cer·ic ac·id (gli - ser′ik, glīs′er - ik). Ácido glicérico; o ácido graxo análogo do glicerol; ocorre particularmente na forma de derivados fosforilados como um intermediário da glicólise.

D-gly·cer·ic ac·i·dur·i·a (gli - ser′ic as - id - oo - rē - ă). Acidúria D-glicérica. **1.** Níveis elevados de ácido D-glicérico na urina. **2.** Um erro inato do metabolismo que causa acidúria D-glicérica [D-glyceric aciduria (1)].

L-gly·cer·ic ac·i·du·ria. Acidúria L-glicérica; excreção de ácido L-glicérico na urina; um erro metabólico primário devido à deficiência da desidrogenase D-glicérica que resulta na excreção dos ácidos L-glicérico e oxálico, levando à síndrome clínica da oxalose com formação freqüente de cálculos renais de oxalato.

gly·cer·ic al·de·hyde. Aldeído glicérico, gliceraldeído. SIN glyceraldehyde.

glyc·er·i·das·es (glis′er - ī - dās - ez). Gliceridases; termo geral para as enzimas que catalisam a hidrólise de ésteres do glicerol (glicerídeos); p.ex., a triacilglicerol lipase.

glyc·er·ide (glis′er - id, - īd). Glicerídeo; um éster do glicerol. O termo é geralmente utilizado em combinação com fosfo- (fosfoglicerídeo). O uso dos termos mono-, di- e triglicerídeo está sendo substituído pelo uso de termos mais precisos, tais como mono-, di- e triacilglicerol, respectivamente.

   mixed g.'s, glicerídeos mistos; glicerídeos que, ao sofrerem hidrólise, produzem mais de um tipo de ácidos graxos.

glyc·er·in (glis′er - in). Glicerina, glicerol. SIN glycerol.

g. jelly, gelatina de g, gelatina glicerinada. SIN glycerinated gelatin.
glyc·er·ite (glis′er - īt). Glicerita. **1.** SIN glycerol. **2.** Uma preparação farmacêutica elaborada a partir da trituração da substância medicinal ativa com glicerol.
  starch g., g. de amido; uma preparação que contém 100 g de amido, 2 g de ácido benzóico, 200 mL de água purificada e 700 g de glicerina em cada 1.000 g; um emoliente tópico.
  tannic acid g., g. de ácido tânico; g. de tanino que contém ácido tânico, citrato de sódio, sulfeto de sódio não-hidratado e glicerina; um adstringente.
glyc·er·o·gel·a·tin (glis′er - ō - jel′a - tin). Glicerogelatina, gelatina glicerinada. SIN glycerinated gelatin.
glyc·er·o·ki·nase (glis′er - ō - kī′nās). Glicerocinase. SIN glycerol kinase.
glyc·er·ol (glis′er - ol). Glicerol; um líquido viscoso e doce, obtido pela saponificação de gorduras e óleos; utilizado como solvente, emoliente da pele, na forma injetável ou de supositórios para tratar a prisão de ventre e como veículo e agente adoçante. SIN 1,2,3-propanetriol, glycerin, glycerite (1), glyceryl alcohol.
  iodinated g., g. iodado; uma forma de iodo ligado organicamente que libera iodo no organismo; tem sido utilizado como fonte medicinal de iodo e como expectorante no lugar de iodetos inorgânicos como o iodeto de potássio. SIN iodopropylidene glycerol, organidin.
  g. kinase, g. cinase, glicerocinase; uma enzima que catalisa a reação entre ATP e glicerol para produzir sn-glicerol 3-fosfato e ADP; no tecido adiposo, o primeiro passo e também a etapa que regula a velocidade da síntese dos triacilgliceróis; a deficiência dessa enzima resulta em disfunção das supra-renais, dos músculos e/ou do fígado e do cérebro. SIN glycerokinase.
  g. phosphate, g. fosfato; o ânion de um éster fosfórico de g.; o derivado-3 é o componente central dos fosfatidatos (R-glicerol 3-fosfato). SIN glycerophosphate.
glyc·er·ol-3-phos·phate ac·yl·trans·fer·ase. Glicerol-3-fosfato aciltransferase; uma enzima que participa da biossíntese dos fosfolipídios e catalisa a transferência de um grupamento acila, proveniente de um acil-CoA graxo, para o sn-glicerol 3-fosfato, produzindo coenzima A e ácido lisofosfatídico.
glyc·er·ol-3-phos·phate de·hy·dro·gen·ase (NAD⁺). Glicerol-3-fosfato desidrogenase; α-glicerofosfato desidrogenase; 3-fosfoglicerol desidrogenase; uma flavoenzima que catalisa a interconversão do fosfato de diidroxiacetona e do sn-glicerol 3-fosfato, com a participação de NAD^+; sua ação fornece a fração glicerol do carboidrato durante a lipogênese.
gly·cer·one. Glicerona; o nome recomendado pela IUPAC (*International Union of Pure and Applied Chemistry*) para a diidroxiacetona.
glyc·er·o·phos·phate (glis′er - ō - fos′fāt). Glicerofosfato. SIN glycerol phosphate.
glyc·er·o·phos·pho·cho·line (glis′er - ō - fos - fō - kō′lēn). Glicerofosfocolina; um componente das fosfatidilcolinas (lecitinas), nas quais as duas OH da g. estão esterificadas com ácidos graxos. SIN glycerophosphorylcholine.
glyc·er·o·phos·phor·ic ac·id (glis′er - ō - fos - fōr′ik). Ácido glicerofosfórico; um éster fosfórico do glicerol. VER TAMBÉM glycerol phosphate.
glyc·er·o·phos·pho·ryl·cho·line (glis′er - ō - fos′fōr - il - kō′lēn). Glicerofosforilcolina. SIN glycerophosphocholine.
glyc·er·ul·ose (glis - er′ul - ōse). Glicerulose. SIN dihydroxyacetone.
glyc·er·yl (glis′er - il). Glicerila. **1.** O radical trivalente do glicerol, $C_3H_5^{3-}$; é freqüentemente utilizado de forma incorreta como glicero- ou glicerol-. **2.** Qualquer grupamento derivado do glicerol pela remoção de um ou mais grupamentos hidroxila.
  g. alcohol, glicerol, glicerina. SIN glycerol.
  g. borate, borato de g., boroglicerina. SIN boroglycerin.
  g. guaiacolate, guaiacolato de g. SIN guaifenesin.
  g. iodide, iodeto de g.; uma forma orgânica de iodo que, após administração por via oral, libera lentamente iodo no corpo. É utilizado primariamente como expectorante/mucolítico. SIN 3-iodo-1,2-propanediol, γ-iodopropyleneglycol.
  g. monostearate, monoestearato de g.; o éster do glicerol e uma molécula de ácido esteárico; é utilizado na manufatura de cremes cosméticos e preparações dermatológicas.
  g. triacetate, triacetato de g., triacetina. SIN triacetin.
  g. tributyrate, tributirato de g., tributirina. SIN tributyrin.
  g. tricaprate, tricaprato de g., tricaprilina. SIN caprin.
  g. trinitrate, trinitrato de g., nitroglicerina. SIN nitroglycerin.
glyc·in·am·ide ri·bo·nu·cle·o·tide (glī - sin′a - mīd). Glicinamida ribonucleotídeo. VER glycineamide ribonucleotide.
gly·cin·ate (glī′sin - āt). Glicinato. **1.** Um sal de glicina. **2.** O ânion de glicina.
gly·cine (G, Gly) (glī′sēn). Glicina; o aminoácido mais simples; um componente importante da gelatina e da fibrína da seda; é empregado como substância nutriente e como suplemento dietético e em soluções para irrigação; é utilizada no tratamento da síndrome dos pés suados. SIN gelatin sugar.
  g. acyltransferase, g. aciltransferase; uma enzima que catalisa a transferência reversível de um grupamento acila da acil-CoA para a g., produzindo coenzima A livre e N-acilglicina; uma etapa em uma via de detoxificação.
  g. amidinotransferase, g. amidinotransferase; uma enzima que catalisa a transferência de um grupo amidina da L-arginina para a glicina, formando guanidinoacetato e L-ornitina; uma reação importante da biossíntese da creatina; pode também atuar sobre a canavanina. SIN g. transamidinase.
  g. betaine, glicina-betaína, betaína, licina. SIN betaine.
  g. cleavage complex, complexo de clivagem da g.; um complexo de várias proteínas que catalisam a reação reversível entre a g. e o tetraidrofolato que produz CO_2, NH_3 e N^5, N^{10}-metilenotetraidrofolato; a deficiência dessa enzima (ou de uma de suas subunidades) causa hiperglicinemia não-cetótica. SIN g. synthase.
  g. dehydrogenases, g. desidrogenases; enzimas que catalisam a conversão da glicina em glioxilato e amônia, utilizando ou NAD^+ ou ferricitocromo c.
  g. synthase, g. sintase. SIN g. cleavage complex.
  g. transamidinase, g. transamidinase. SIN g. amidinotransferase.
gly·cine·a·mide ri·bo·nu·cle·o·tide, gly·cin·am·ide ri·bo·nu·cle·o·tide (glī′sin - ā - mīd, glī - sin′a - mīd). Glicinamida ribonucleotídeo; um intermediário da biossíntese da purina, no qual o nitrogênio da amida da glicinamida está ligado ao C-1 de uma porção ribosila.
gly·cin·in (glī - sen′in). Glicinina; a principal proteína da soja; uma globulina que é estruturalmente similar à araquina, à edestina e à excelsina.
gly·ci·ni·um (glī - sen - ē - um). Glicínio; o cátion da glicina.
gly·ci·nu·ria (glī - si - noo′rē - ā). Glicinúria; a excreção de glicina na urina. [glycine + G. *ouron*, urina]
  familial g. [MIM*138500], g. familial; um distúrbio metabólico; acredita-se que seja causado por defeitos na reabsorção renal de glicina; pode ou não se acompanhar de urolitíase por oxalato; seria o estado heterozigoto da iminoglicinúria; herança autossômica dominante.
♲ **glyco-.** Glico-; forma combinante que indica relação com os açúcares (p.ex., glicogênio) ou com a glicina (p.ex., glicocolato). VER TAMBÉM gluco-. [G. *glykys*, doce]
gly·co·bi·ar·sol (glī - ko - bī′ar - sol). Glicobiarsol; um arsenical pentavalente que contém bismuto; é utilizado no tratamento de formas mais brandas de amebíase intestinal ou como terapia subseqüente.
gly·co·ca·lyx (glī - ko - kā′liks). Glicocálice; um revestimento filamentoso e PAS-positivo, localizado na superfície apical de certas células epiteliais e composto de radicais de carboidratos de proteínas que se projetam da superfície livre da membrana plasmática. [glyco- + G. *kalyx*, casca, concha]
gly·co·cho·late (glī - ko - kō′lāt). Glicocolato; um sal ou éster do ácido glicocólico.
  g. sodium, g. de sódio; um constituinte normal da bile de humanos e de herbívoros; o g. de sódio dos herbívoros é purificado e utilizado como colerético e colagogo.
gly·co·cho·lic ac·id (glī - ko - kō′lik). Ácido glicocólico; N-colilglicina; um dos principais ácidos conjugados da bile, formado pela condensação do grupamento —COOH do ácido cólico com o grupamento amina da glicina; substância hidrossolúvel e um poderoso detergente.
gly·co·con·ju·gates (glī - ko - kon′joo - gātz). Glicoconjugados; uma classe geral de macromoléculas do corpo que contêm açúcares; inclui os glicolipídios, as glicoproteínas e as proteoglicanas.
gly·co·cor·ti·coid (glī′ko - kōr′ti - koyd). Glicocorticóide. SIN glucocorticoid.
gly·co·cy·a·mine (glī - ko - sī′a - mēn). Glicociamina; ácido 2-guanidinoacético; formado pela transferência do grupamento amidina da L-arginina para a glicina. SIN glucocyamine.
gly·co·gel·a·tin (glī - ko - jel′a - tin). Glicogelatina, gelatina glicerinada. SIN glycerinated gelatin.
gly·co·gen (glī′ko - jen). Glicogênio; uma glicosana de alto peso molecular e com uma estrutura semelhante à da amilopectina [com ligações α(1,4)], apresentando-se, porém, com mais ramificações [ligações α(1,6) além de um pequeno número de ligações α(1,3)]; é encontrada na maioria dos tecidos do corpo, principalmente nos tecidos hepático e muscular; como principal reserva de carboidratos, é prontamente convertida em glicose. SIN animal dextran, animal starch, hepatin, liver starch.
  g. phosphorylase, g. fosforilase, fosforilase. SIN phosphorylase.
  g. synthase, g. starch synthase, g. sintase, g. amido sintase; uma glicosiltransferase que catalisa a incorporação da D-glicose, proveniente da UDP-D-glicose, nas cadeias de 1,4-α-D-glicosil. A deficiência dessa enzima hepática pode causar um tipo de hipoglicemia.
gly·co·ge·nase (glī′ko - jĕ - nās). Glicogenase. SIN α-amylase, β-amylase.
gly·co·gen·e·sis (glī - ko - jen′e - sis). Glicogênese; formação de glicogênio a partir da D-glicose por meio da glicogênio sintase e da dextrina dextranase; a primeira enzima catalisa a formação de uma poliglicose com ligações α-1,4 a partir da UDPglicose, e a segunda enzima cliva fragmentos de uma cadeia e transfere-os para uma ligação α-1,6 em outra cadeia. [glyco- + G. *genesis*, produção]
gly·co·ge·net·ic (glī′ko - jĕ - net′ik). Glicogênico; relativo à glicogênese. SIN D-glycogenous.
gly·co·gen·ic (glī - ko - gen′ik). Glicogênico; que dá origem ao glicogênio ou que o produz.
gly·co·gen·ol·y·sis (glī′ko - jĕ - nol′i - sis). Glicogenólise; a hidrólise do glicogênio a glicose.

gly·co·ge·no·sis (glī'kō - jĕ - nō'sis). Glicogenose; qualquer uma das doenças do armazenamento de glicogênio caracterizadas por acúmulo de glicogênio de estrutura química normal ou anormal nos tecidos; pode haver aumento do fígado, do coração e do músculo estriado, incluindo a língua, com fraqueza muscular progressiva. São conhecidos sete tipos (classificação de Cori), que se diferenciam segundo a deficiência enzimática envolvida, sendo todos de herança autossômica recessiva, mas apresentando um gene diferente em cada uma das deficiências enzimáticas. [MIM: 1, *232200, *232220, *232240; 2, *232300; 3, *232400; 4, *232500; 5, *232600; 6, *232700; 7, *232800]. SIN dextrinosis, glycogen-storage disease.
brancher deficiency g., g. por deficiência de enzima ramificadora. SIN brancher glycogen storage *disease*.
generalized g., g. generalizada. SIN type 2 g.
glucose-6-phosphatase hepatorrenal g., g. hepatorrenal por deficiência de glicose-6-fosfatase. SIN type 1 g.
hepatophosphorylase deficiency g., g. por deficiência de hepatofosforilase. SIN type 6 g.
myophosphorylase deficiency g., g. por deficiência de miofosforilase. SIN type 5 g.
type 1 g., g. de tipo 1; g. devido à deficiência de glicose-6-fosfatase, que resulta no acúmulo de quantidades excessivas de glicogênio de estrutura química normal, sobretudo no fígado e nos rins. SIN Gierke disease, glucose-6-phosphatase hepatorrenal g., von Gierke disease.
type 2 g., g. de tipo 2; g. devido à deficiência de α-1,4-glicosidase lisossomial, que resulta no acúmulo de quantidades excessivas de glicogênio de estrutura química normal no coração, nos músculos, no fígado e no sistema nervoso. SIN generalized g., Pompe disease.
type 3 g., g. de tipo 3; g. devido à deficiência de amilo-1,6-glicosidase, que resulta no acúmulo de glicogênio anormal, com cadeias externas curtas, no fígado e nos músculos. SIN Cori disease, debranching deficiency limit dextrinosis, limit dextrinosis, Forbes disease.
type 4 g., g. de tipo 4; cirrose hepática familial com armazenamento de glicogênio anormal; g. resultante da deficiência da enzima ramificadora 1,4-α-glicana que resulta em acúmulo de glicogênio anormal, com cadeias internas e externas longas, no fígado, nos rins, nos músculos e em outros tecidos. SIN Andersen disease.
type 5 g., g. de tipo 5; g. devido à deficiência de glicogênio fosforilase que resulta no acúmulo de glicogênio de estrutura química normal nos músculos. SIN McArdle disease, McArdle syndrome, McArdle-Schmid-Pearson disease, myophosphorylase deficiency g.
type 6 g., g. de tipo 6; g. devido à deficiência de glicogênio fosforilase hepática que resulta no acúmulo de glicogênio de estrutura química normal no fígado e nos leucócitos. SIN hepatophosphorylase deficiency g., Hers disease.
type 7 g., g. de tipo 7; deficiência de fosfofrutocinase muscular que resulta em cãibras musculares e mioglobinúria aos esforços físicos excessivos. O quadro clínico assemelha-se ao da g. de tipo 5.
D-gly·cog·e·nous (glī - kojʹe - nŭs). D-glicogênico. SIN glycogenetic.
gly·co·geu·sia (glī - kō - gooʹsē - ă). Glicogeusia; um sabor doce subjetivo. [glyco- + G. *geusis*, sabor]
gly·co·gly·ci·nu·ria (glīʹkō - glī - si - nooʹrē - ă). [MIM*138070]. Glicoglicinúria; um distúrbio metabólico caracterizado por glicosúria e hiperglicinúria; herança autossômica dominante.
gly·co·his·to·chem·is·try (glī - kō - his - tō - kemʹis - trē). Glico-histoquímica; o estudo das frações de açúcares específicos nos tecidos.
lectin glycohistochemistry, g. da lectina; técnica para quantificar os ligantes endógenos de frações de açúcares específicos, tais como a aglutinina do amendoim e do germe do trigo, na caracterização do epitélio de superfície.
gly·col (glīʹkol). Glicol. 1. Um composto que contém dois grupamentos álcool. 2. Etilenoglicol, $HOCH_2CH_2OH$, o glicol mais simples.
gly·col·al·de·hyde (glī - kol - alʹdĕ - hīd). Glicolaldeído; $HOCH_2CHO$; o açúcar de dois carbonos mais simples; o produto da desaminação aeróbica da etanolamina. SIN diose.
active g., g. ativo; pirofosfato de 2-(1,2-diidroxietil)tiamina; um derivado formado no metabolismo dos carboidratos.
gly·col·al·de·hyde·trans·fer·ase (glī - kol - alʹdĕ - hīd - transfʹer - ās). Glicolaldeidotransferase. SIN transketolase.
gly·co·late (glī - kōʹlāt). Glicolato; um sal ou éster do ácido glicólico.
gly·co·leu·cine (glīʹkō - loo - sin). Glicoleucina. SIN norleucine.
gly·col·ic ac·id (glī - kolʹik). Ácido glicólico; um intermediário da interconversão da ácido láctico. SIN hydroxyacetic acid.
gly·col·ic ac·i·du·ria. Acidúria glicólica; excreção excessiva de ácido glicólico na urina; um defeito metabólico primário resultante da deficiência da 2-hidroxi-3-oxoadipato carboxilase e que causa a excreção dos ácidos glicólico e oxálico, levando à síndrome clínica da oxalose.
gly·co·lip·id (glī - kō - lipʹid). Glicolipídio; um lipídio com um ou mais açúcares unidos por ligações covalentes.
gly·co·lyl (glīʹkō - lil). Glicolila; $HOCH_2CO$—; o radical acila do ácido glicólico, que substitui o radical acetila em alguns ácidos siálicos; os produtos são denominados ácidos *N*-glicolilneuramínicos.
gly·co·lyl·u·rea (glīʹkō - lil - ū - rēʹa). Glicoliluréia. SIN hydantoin.
gly·col·y·sis (glī - kolʹi - sis). Glicólise; a conversão da D-glicose em ácido láctico (em vez de produtos da oxidação do piruvato), acompanhada de produção de energia, que ocorre em diversos tecidos, especialmente nos músculos, quando não existe oxigênio suficiente disponível (como ocorre em uma situação de emergência); como o oxigênio molecular não é consumido no proces-

	tipos de glicogenoses			
tipo	glicogenose	enzima deficiente	diagnóstico bioquímico	manifestações clínicas
1	g. hepatorrenal, doença de Gierke	glicose-6-fosfatase	glicogênio normal; quantidades excessivas no fígado e nos rins	hipoglicemia, hiperlipemia, cetose, hiperuricemia, hepatomegalia, nanismo
2	g. generalizada, maligna; doença de Pompe; cardiomegalia glicogênica	α-1,4-glicosidase	glicogênio normal, excessivo em todos os órgãos	hipotonia muscular, insuficiência cardíaca, sintomas neurológicos, morte no primeiro ano de vida
3	g. hepatomuscular, benigna; doença de Cori, doença de Forbes (com subvariantes 3b até f)	amilo-1,6-glicosidase	glicogênio anormal, com cadeias externas curtas, no fígado e (mais raramente) nos músculos	hepatomegalia, hipoglicemia; evolução benigna
4	g. hepática, cirrótica, reticuloendotelial; doença de Anderson; amilopectinose	α-1,4-glicana: α-1,4-glicano-6-glicosiltransferase	glicogênio anormal, com cadeias externas longas, no fígado, baço e linfonodos	cirrose do fígado; hepatoesplenomegalia
5	g. muscular, doença de McArdle-Schmid-Pearson	α-glicanofosforilase muscular	glicogênio normal, quantidades excessivas nos músculos	miastenia e mialgia generalizadas, mioglobinúria
6	g. hepática, doença de Hers	α-glicanofosforilase hepática	glicogênio normal, quantidades excessivas no fígado	hepatomegalia, relativamente benigna
7	g. muscular; doença de Tarui	fosfofrutocinase muscular	glicogênio normal, nos músculos esqueléticos	cãibras musculares, mioglobinúria
8	g. hepática; herança ligada ao cromossoma X	fosforilase-b cinase hepática	glicogênio normal, no fígado	manifestação clinicamente branda, hepatomegalia, hipoglicemia

so, a g. é freqüentemente denominada "g. anaeróbica". Cf. Embden-Meyerhof-Parnas *pathway*. SIN glucolysis. [glyco- + G. *lysis*, liberação]

gly·co·lyt·ic (glī - kō - lit′ik). Glicolítico; relativo à glicólise.

gly·co·ne·o·gen·e·sis (glī′kō - nē - ō - jen′ē - sis). Gliconeogênese. **1.** A formação de glicogênio a partir de não-carboidratos, tais como proteínas ou gorduras, pela conversão dos não-carboidratos em D-glicose. VER TAMBÉM glycogenesis. **2.** SIN gluconeogenesis. [glyco- + G. *neos*, novo, + *genesis*, produção]

gly·con·ic ac·ids (glī - kon′ik). Ácidos glicônicos. SIN aldonic acids.

gly·co·pe·nia (glī - kō - pē′nē - ā). Glicopenia; a deficiência de qualquer um ou de todos os açúcares em um órgão ou tecido. [glyco- + G. *penia*, pobreza]

gly·co·pep·tide (glī - kō - pep′tīd). Glicopeptídeo; um composto que contém açúcar(es) ligado(s) a aminoácidos (ou preponderantemente a peptídeos), como nas paredes das células bacterianas. Cf. peptidoglycan.

Gly·co·pha·gus (glī - kof′ā - gŭs). Um gênero comum de ácaros de grãos, freqüentemente implicados em dermatites que afetam manipuladores de alimentos. VER TAMBÉM *Tyrophagus putrescentiae*. [glyco- + G. *phagō*, comer]

gly·co·phil·ia (glī - kō - fil′ē - ā). Glicofilia; uma condição na qual há uma clara tendência a desenvolver hiperglicemia, mesmo após a ingestão de uma quantidade relativamente pequena de glicose. [glyko- + G. *phileō*, amar]

gly·co·pho·rins (glī - kō - fōr′ins). Glicoforinas; um grupo de glicoproteínas encontradas nas membranas dos eritrócitos; certas glicoforinas estão associadas a antígenos dos grupos sanguíneos; a glicoforina A é a mais importante; a deficiência de glicoforina C é observada na eliptocitose hereditária de tipo 4.

gly·co·pro·tein (glī - kō - prō′tēn). Glicoproteína. **1.** Uma proteína de um grupo de proteínas que contêm carboidratos unidos por ligações covalentes, dentre os quais os mais importantes são as mucinas, o mucóide e o amilóide. **2.** Termo às vezes restrito às proteínas que contêm pequenas quantidades de carboidratos, em contraste com os mucóides ou com as mucoproteínas, geralmente medidas como hexosamina; tais proteínas conjugadas são encontradas em muitos locais, especialmente nas γ-globulinas, α$_1$-globulinas, α$_2$-globulinas, transferrina, etc., e estão contidas no muco e nas mucinas. VER TAMBÉM mucoprotein.

α$_1$-**acid g.**, α$_1$-glicoproteína ácida. SIN orosomucoid.

gly·cop·ty·a·lism (glī - kō - tī′ā - lizm). Glicoptialismo. SIN glycosialia. [glyco- + G. *ptyalon*, saliva]

gly·co·pyr·ro·late (glī - kō - pī′rō - lāt). Glicopirrolato; um composto parassimpaticolítico (como a atropina), utilizado como medicação pré-anestésica antes de anestesia geral, como um antagonista aos efeitos bradicárdicos da neostigmina durante a reversão do curare e como um adjunto no tratamento da úlcera péptica.

gly·cor·rha·chia (glī - kō - rā′kē - ā, - rak - ē - ā). Glicorraquia; presença de açúcar no líquido cefalorraquidiano. [glyco- + G. *rhachis*, espinha]

gly·cor·rhea (glī - kō - rē′ā). Glicorréia; eliminação de açúcar do corpo, como ocorre na glicosúria, especialmente em quantidades extraordinariamente grandes. [glyco- + G. *rhoia*, um fluxo]

gly·cos·am·i·no·gly·can (GAG) (glī′kōs - am - i - nō - glī′kan). Glicosaminoglicana. VER TAMBÉM mucopolysaccharide.

gly·co·se·cre·to·ry (glī′kō - sē - krē′tō - rē). Glicossecretor; que causa a secreção de glicogênio ou que está envolvido nesse processo.

gly·co·si·a·lia (glī′kō - sī - al′ē - ā, - ā′lē - ā). Glicossialia; a presença de açúcar na saliva. SIN glycoptyalism. [glyco- + G. *sialon*, saliva]

gly·co·si·a·lor·rhea (glī - kō - sī′ā - lō - rē′ā). Glicossialorréia; secreção excessiva de saliva que contém glicose. [glyco- + G. *sialon*, saliva, + *rhoia*, um fluxo]

gly·cos·i·dases (glī - kō - sīd - ās′ez). Glicosidases; uma classe de enzimas hidrolíticas que atuam sobre os glicosídeos; as α-glicosidases atuam sobre as ligações α-glicosídicas (p.ex., a α-amilase), enquanto as β-glicosidases atuam sobre as ligações β-glicosídicas (p.ex., β-glicosidase). Elas podem também ser divididas em enzimas que atuam sobre os compostos O-glicosil, N-glicosil e S-glicosil.

gly·co·side (glī′kō - sīd). Glicosídeo; o produto da condensação de um açúcar com qualquer radical que envolve a perda da OH do hemiacetal ou do hemicetal do açúcar, deixando o carbono anomérico como a ligação; dessa forma, a condensação do carbono com um álcool que perde o hidrogênio de seu grupamento hidroxila, produz um álcool-glicosídeo (ou um glicosídeo-álcool); as ligações com um grupamento –NH– da purina ou da pirimidina produzem compostos glicosil (ou N-glicosil).

cardiac g.'s, glicosídeos cardíacos; termo genérico dado a um grande número de substâncias com a capacidade de aumentar a força de contração do coração em processo de falência. Os exemplos incluem os extratos digitálicos (dedaleira), bem como aqueles obtidos de outras fontes animais ou vegetais.

cyanogenic g., g. cianogênico; um g. capaz de gerar CN^- ao sofrer metabolismo (p.ex., amigdalina).

N-**gly·co·side.** *N*-glicosídeo; nome impróprio para a glicosila.

gly·co·sid·ic (glī - kō - sid′ik). Glicosídico; que se refere a ou que indica um glicosídeo ou uma ligação glicosídica.

gly·co·sphin·go·lip·id (glī′kō - sfing - gō - lip′id). Glicoesfingolipídio; uma ceramida unida a um ou mais açúcares por meio do grupamento OH terminal; entre os glicoesfingolipídios estão os cerebrosídeos, os gangliosídeos e os oligossacarídeos da ceramida (oligoglicosilceramidas). O prefixo glyc- pode ser substituído pelos prefixos gluc, galact, lact, etc. SIN ceramide saccharide.

gly·co·stat·ic (glī - kō - stat′ik). Glicostático; que indica a propriedade de certos extratos da hipófise anterior (adeno-hipófise) que permitem ao corpo manter seus depósitos de glicogênio nos músculos, no fígado e em outros tecidos.

gly·cos·ur·ia (glī - kō - soo′rē - ā). Glicosúria. **1.** SIN glucosuria. **2.** Excreção urinária de carboidratos. SIN glycuresis (2). [glyco- + G. *ouron*, urina]

alimentary g., g. alimentar; g. observada após a ingestão de uma quantidade moderada de açúcar ou de amido, que normalmente seria eliminado sem aparecer na urina; a g. ocorre porque a velocidade de absorção intestinal excede a capacidade do fígado e de outros tecidos de remover a glicose, permitindo, dessa forma, que os níveis sanguíneos desse açúcar se tornem altos o suficiente para que ocorra sua excreção renal. SIN alimentary diabetes, digestive g.

benign g., g. benigna; g. que não está associada ao diabetes melito; é resultante de um limiar renal baixo para os açúcares.

digestive g., g. digestiva, g. alimentar. SIN alimentary g.

nondiabetic g., g. não-diabética. SIN nonhyperglycemic g.

nonhyperglycemic g., g. não-hiperglicêmica; a presença de glicose na urina sem hiperglicemia e resultante de uma anormalidade na reabsorção tubular renal de glicose filtrada. SIN nondiabetic g., orthoglycemic g.

normoglycemic g., g. normoglicêmica, g. renal. SIN renal g.

orthoglycemic g. (ōr - thō - glī′cēm - ik), g. ortoglicêmica. SIN nonhyperglycemic g.

pathologic g., g. patológica; excreção crônica de quantidades relativamente grandes de açúcar na urina.

phlorizin g., phloridzin g., g. por florizina, g. por floridizina; a presença de açúcar na urina após a administração experimental de florizina, que reduz o limiar renal para a reabsorção de glicose. SIN phlorizin diabetes.

renal g., g. renal; a excreção recorrente ou persistente de glicose na urina associada a níveis normais de glicose sanguínea; é resultante da incapacidade dos túbulos renais proximais de reabsorver a glicose do filtrado glomerular a uma velocidade normal (limiar renal baixo); um defeito no transportador de glicose do nefro. SIN normoglycemic g., renal diabetes.

gly·co·syl (glī′kō - sil). Glicosila; o radical que resulta da separação da OH do hemiacetal ou do hemicetal de um sacarídeo. Cf. glycoside.

gly·co·sy·la·tion (glī′kō - si - lā′shŭn). Glicosilação; a formação de ligações com os grupamentos glicosila, como ocorre entre a D-glicose e a cadeia da hemoglobina para formar a fração hemoglobina A$_{1C}$, cujo nível aumenta de acordo com a concentração de D-glicose sanguínea aumentada no diabetes melito não-controlado ou mal controlado. VER TAMBÉM glycosylated *hemoglobin*.

gly·co·syl·trans·fer·ase (glī′kō - sil - trans′fer - ās). Glicosiltransferase; qualquer enzima (EC subclasse 2.4) que transfere grupamentos glicosila de um composto para outro. SIN transglycosylase.

gly·co·tro·pic, gly·co·tro·phic (glī - kō - tropi′k, - trof′ik). Glicotrópico, glicotrófico; relativo a um princípio encontrado nos extratos do lobo anterior da hipófise que antagoniza a ação da insulina e causa hiperglicemia. [glyco- + G. *trophē*, nutrição; *tropē*, uma volta]

glyc·u·re·sis (glī - koo - rē′sis). Glicurese, glicosúria. **1.** SIN glucosuria. **2.** SIN glycosuria (2). [glyco- + G. *ourēsis*, micção]

gly·cu·ron·ate (glī - koor′on - āt). Glicuronato; um sal ou éster de um ácido glicurônico.

gly·cu·ron·ic ac·id (glī - koor - on′ik). Ácido glicurônico; o ácido urônico de um açúcar no qual o carbono terminal é oxidado a um grupo carboxila.

gly·cu·ron·i·dase (glī - koor - on′i - dās). Glicuronidase. SIN β-D-glucuronidase.

gly·cu·ro·nide (glī - koor′on - īd). Glicuronídeo; um glicosídeo de um ácido urônico; p.ex., glucuronídeo.

gly·cu·ro·nu·ria (glī - koo - rō - noo′rē - ā). Glicuronúria; a presença de ácido glicurônico na urina.

gly·cy·cla·mide (glī - sī′klā - mīd). Gliciclamida; um agente hipoglicemiante oral. SIN cyclamide, tolcyclamide, tolhexamide.

gly·cyl (Gly) (glī′sil). Glicila; o radical acila da glicina.

glyc·yr·rhi·za (glis - ĭ - rī′zā). Glicirriza; o rizoma e a raiz secos da *Glycyrrhiza glabra* (família Leguminoseae) e espécies afins; um demulcente, laxativo suave e expectorante; é também utilizado para mascarar o sabor de outros medicamentos; sua ação parece depender do ácido glicirrízico, um glicosídeo com a propriedade de reter sal que mimetiza a ação da aldosterona. SIN licorice, liquorice. [G. de *glykys*, doce, + *rhiza*, raiz]

gly·ox·al (glī - oks′al). Glioxal; OHC—CHO; o dialdeído mais simples. SIN oxalaldehyde.

gly·ox·a·lase (glī - oks′ā - lās). Glioxalase; uma enzima, a lactoilglutationa liase (g. I) ou a hidroxiacilglutationa hidrolase (g. II), encontrada nas hemácias e em outros tecidos, que converte o glioxal e os substitutos dos glioxais ligados à glutationa nos hidroxi-ácidos livres correspondentes (g. II) ou em glioxais (g. I).

gly·ox·y·late trans·a·cet·y·lase (glī - oks'i - lāt). Glioxilato transacetilase. SIN *malate* synthase.

gly·ox·yl·di·u·reide (glī - oks - il - dī'ū - rīd). Glioxildiureída. SIN allantoin.

gly·ox·yl·ic ac·id (glī - oks - il'ik). Ácido glioxílico; OHC—COOH; é produzido pela ação das glicinas desidrogenases sobre a glicina ou sobre a sarcosina, ou a partir do ácido alantóico pela alantoicase ou pela alanina:glioxilato aminotransferase. SIN oxoacetic acid.

gm Abreviatura antiga de gram (grama).

GM-CSF Abreviatura de granulocyte-macrophage colony-stimulating *factor* (fator estimulante de colônias de granulócitos-macrófagos, FEC-GM).

Gmelin, Leopold, fisiologista e químico alemão, 1788–1853. VER G. *test;* Rosenbach-G. *test.*

GMP Abreviatura de guanylic acid (ácido guanílico).

GMP re·duc·tase Abreviatura de *guanylic acid* reductase (redutase do ácido guanílico).

GMP syn·the·tase Abreviatura de *guanylic acid* synthetase (sintetase do ácido guanílico).

GMS Abreviatura de Gomori methenamine-silver *stain* (coloração de Gomori metenamina-prata), em *stain.*

gnash·ing (nash'ing). O ato de ranger os dentes como uma função não-mastigatória; está às vezes associado à tensão emocional. VER TAMBÉM bruxism.

gnat (nat). Maruim, mosquito-pólvora, borrachudo; termo genérico aplicado a várias espécies de diminutos insetos, incluindo as espécies de *Simulium* (borrachudo do búfalo) e de *Hippelates* (borrachudo-dos-olhos). Os autores britânicos incluem às vezes os mosquitos nesse grupo, porém isso não é feito nos Estados Unidos. [A.S. *gnaet*]

gnath-. VER gnatho-.

gnath·ic (nath'ik). Gnático; relativo à mandíbula ou ao processo alveolar. [G. *gnathos,* mandíbula]

gnath·i·on (nath'ē - on). Gnátio; o ponto mais inferior da mandíbula, localizado na linha média. Em cefalometria, é o ponto médio entre o ponto mais anterior e o ponto mais inferior do queixo ósseo, medido na intersecção da linha de referência da mandíbula com a linha násio-pogônio. [G. *gnathos,* mandíbula]

gnatho-, gnath-. Gnato-; a mandíbula. [G. *gnathos*]

gnath·o·ceph·a·lus (nath - ō - sef'ā - lŭs). Gnatocéfalo; uma malformação fetal na qual toda a cabeça se apresenta pouco desenvolvida, exceto as mandíbulas. [*gnatho-* + G. *kephalē,* cabeça]

gnath·o·dy·nam·ics (nath'ō - dī - nam'iks). Gnatodinâmica; o estudo das relações de grandeza e de direção das forças desenvolvidas pelos e sobre os componentes do sistema mastigatório durante sua função. [*gnatho-* + G. *dynamis,* força]

gnath·o·dy·na·mom·e·ter (nath'ō - dī - nă - mom'ē - ter). Gnatodinamômetro; um dispositivo utilizado para medir a pressão da mordida. SIN bite gauge, occlusometer. [*gnatho-* + dinamômetro]

gnath·og·ra·phy (nă - thog'ră - fē). Gnatografia; o registro da ação do aparelho mastigatório, quando em funcionamento.

gnath·o·log·i·cal (nath - ō - loj'i - kăl). Gnatológico; relativo à gnatodinâmica.

gnath·ol·o·gy (nă - thol'ō - jē). Gnatologia; a ciência do sistema mastigatório, incluindo a fisiologia, os distúrbios funcionais e o tratamento.

gnath·os·chi·sis (nă - thos'ki - sis). Gnatosquise; fissura da mandíbula. [*gnatho-* + G. *schisis,* uma fenda]

gnath·o·stat·ics (nath - ō - stat'iks). Gnatoestática; em diagnóstico ortodôntico, um procedimento técnico para orientar a dentição a determinados pontos cranianos. [*gnatho-* + G. *statikos,* que se mantém em posição]

Gna·thos·to·ma (nă - thos'tō - mă). Um gênero de vermes nematódeos (família Gnathostomatidae), caracterizados por várias fileiras de espinhos cuticulares ao redor da cabeça e por ciclos de vida aquáticos com múltiplos hospedeiros; inclui parasitas patogênicos de gatos, bovinos e suínos. [*gnatho-* + G. *stoma,* boca]

G. doloresi, espécie de nematódeo encontrada em porcos domésticos e selvagens; infestações de seres humanos (larva migrans cutânea) já foram descritas no Japão.

G. hispidum, espécie de nematódeo encontrada em porcos domésticos e selvagens; infestações de seres humanos (larva migrans cutânea) já foram descritas no Japão.

G. nipponicum, espécie de nematódeo encontrada em doninhas; infestações de seres humanos (larva migrans cutânea) já foram descritas no Japão.

G. siamen'se, nome incorreto dado ao *G. spinigerum.*

G. spinig'erum, um parasita de gatos, cães e carnívoros selvagens; é ocasionalmente encontrado em seres humanos no Extremo Oriente; é transmitido por copépodes e peixes; a infestação humana é geralmente confinada à pele, porém vários casos de infecção ocular e cerebral com larvas migratórias dessa espécie já foram descritos.

gna·thos·to·mi·a·sis (nath - ō - stō - mī'ă - sis). Gnatostomíase; edema migratório ou uma erupção serpiginosa resultante de infestação cutânea por larvas do *Gnathostoma spinigerum.* SIN Yangtze edema.

gnos·co·pine (nos'kō - pēn). Gnoscopina; um alcalóide do ópio, $C_{22}H_{23}NO_7$, obtido a partir da racemização da noscapina; um antitussígeno. SIN *dl*-narcotine.

gno·sia (nō'sē - ă). Gnosia; a faculdade perceptiva que capacita alguém a reconhecer a forma e a natureza das pessoas e das coisas; a capacidade de perceber e reconhecer as coisas. [G. *gnōsis,* conhecimento]

gno·to·bi·ol·o·gy (nō'tō - bī - ol'ō - jē). Gnotobiologia; o estudo de animais na ausência de microrganismos contaminantes; isto é, de animais "livres de germes". [G. *gnotos,* conhecido, + *bios,* vida, + *logos,* estudo]

gno·to·bi·o·ta (nō'tō - bī - ō'tă). Gnotobiota; colônias ou espécies vivas, agrupadas a partir de amostras isoladas puras. [G. *gnotos,* conhecido, + L. mod. *biota,* do G. *bios,* vida]

gno·to·bi·ote (nō - tō - bī'ōt). Gnotobioto; um organismo único proveniente de um grupo reunido a partir de amostras isoladas puras (gnotobiota).

gno·to·bi·ot·ic (nō'tō - bī - ot'ik). Gnotobiótico; que indica algo livre de germes ou, antigamente, os organismos livres de germes nos quais a composição de qualquer flora microbiana associada, se presente, é completamente definida. [VER gnotobiota]

GnRH Abreviatura de gonadotropin-releasing *hormone* (hormônio liberador de gonadotropina).

goal (gōl). Objetivo, meta; em psicologia, qualquer objeto ou objetivo que um organismo busca atingir ou alcançar. [I.M. *gol*]

Godélier, Charles P., médico francês, 1813–1877. VER G. *law.*

Godman, John D., anatomista norte-americano, 1794–1830. VER G. *fascia.*

Godwin, John T., patologista norte-americano, *1917. VER G. *tumor.*

Goeckerman, William H., dermatologista norte-americano, 1884–1954. VER G. *treatment.*

Gofman, Moses, médico alemão, *1887. VER G. *test.*

Goggia, Carlo P., médico italiano do século XX. VER G. *sign.*

gog·gle (gog'gl). **1.** Uma tela protetora para os olhos. **2.** Óculos de proteção; um tipo de óculos com escudos auxiliares para a proteção dos olhos. [I.M. *gogelen,* olhar semicerrado]

plethysmographic g., óculos pletismográficos; óculos de proteção especialmente projetados para serem utilizados como um oftalmodinamômetro, ao mesmo tempo que permitem alterações visuais subjetivas e oculares objetivas durante um aumento transitório da pressão intra-ocular.

goi·ter (goy'ter). Bócio; aumento crônico da glândula tireóide, que não é resultante de neoplasia e que ocorre endemicamente em certas localidades, sobretudo em regiões onde ocorreu glaciação e o solo se apresenta pobre em iodo e, esporadicamente, em outros lugares. SIN struma (1). [Fr. do L. *guttur,* garganta]

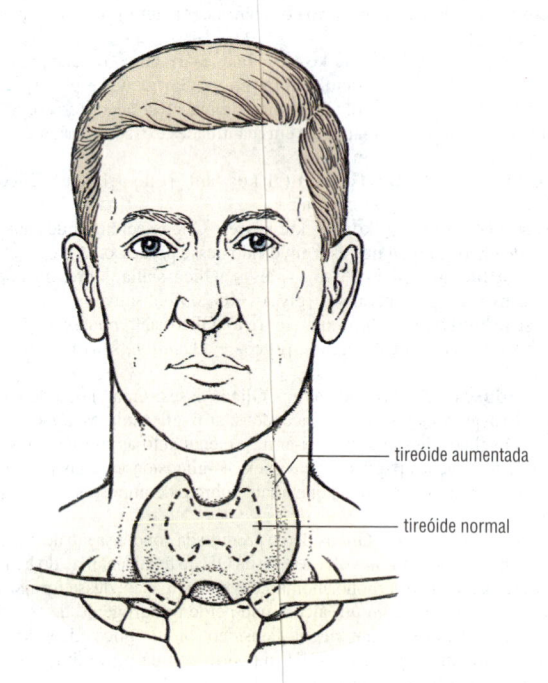

bócio

aberrant g., b. aberrante; aumento de uma glândula tireóide supranumerária. SIN struma aberrata.

acute g., b. agudo; um b. que se desenvolve muito rapidamente.

adenomatous g., b. adenomatoso; aumento da glândula tireóide resultante do crescimento de um ou mais adenomas encapsulados ou de múltiplos nódulos colóides não-encapsulados em sua substância.

Basedow g., b. de Basedow; b. colóide que se torna hiperfuncionante após a ingestão de iodo em excesso, o fenômeno de Jod-Basedow. VER Jod-Basedow *phenomenon*.

cabbage b., b. do repolho; b. resultante da ingestão de repolho ou outros alimentos bociogênicos.

colloid g., b. colóide; uma forma de b. na qual o conteúdo dos folículos aumenta muito, causando atrofia do epitélio por compressão de maneira que a substância gelatinosa predomina no tumor. SIN struma colloides.

cystic g., b. cístico; aumento da região tireoidiana resultante da presença de um ou mais cistos na glândula.

diffuse g., b. difuso; b. no qual o processo mórbido envolve toda a glândula, em oposição ao b. nodular ou ao adenoma da tireóide.

diving g., b. migratório; b. móvel que se encontra ora acima, ora abaixo da incisura esternal. SIN wandering g.

endemic g., b. endêmico; b., geralmente do tipo simples, prevalente em certas regiões onde a cota de iodo ingerida na dieta está abaixo do nível considerado ótimo.

exophthalmic g., b. exoftálmico; qualquer uma das diversas formas de hipertireoidismo nas quais a glândula tireóide está aumentada e existe exoftalmia.

familial g., b. familial; um grupo de distúrbios hereditários da tireóide nos quais o b. se torna aparente pela primeira vez durante a infância; está freqüentemente associado a retardo esquelético e/ou mental e a outros sinais de hipotireoidismo que podem desenvolver-se com a idade. Vários tipos de b. familial já foram identificados: 1) defeito no transporte de iodeto [MIM*274400]; distúrbio de herança autossômica recessiva resultante de mutação no gene do cotransportador de iodeto de sódio (SLC5A5) no 19p. A glândula mostra-se incapaz de concentrar iodeto; 2) defeito na organificação [MIM*274500 e *274600], no qual ocorre falha na iodação da tirosina; 3) síndrome de Pendred [MIM*274600]; distúrbio de herança autossômica recessiva resultante de mutação no gene da síndrome de Pendred (PDS) em 7q; 4) defeito de acoplamento, no qual um defeito no acoplamento das iodotirosinas para formar iodotironinas causa cretinismo [MIM*274700]; 5) defeito da iodotirosina desiodinase, no qual a desiodinação das iodotirosinas não é satisfatória, levando a considerável perda glandular desses precursores hormonais e a possível cretinismo [MIM*274800]; 6) distúrbio da iodoproteína plasmática [MIM*274900], no qual uma proteína sérica iodada anormal, insolúvel em butanol ácido, está presente; 7) hipertireoidismo hereditário.

fibrous g., b. fibroso; hiperplasia firme da tireóide e de sua cápsula.

follicular g., b. folicular, b. parenquimatoso. SIN parenchymatous g.

lingual g., b. lingual; um tumor do tecido da tireóide que envolve o vestígio embrionário situado na base da língua.

microfollicular g., b. microfolicular; b. no qual o tecido glandular consiste em folículos extraordinariamente pequenos e preenchidos com colóide e áreas de tecido indiferenciado com formação indistinta de folículos.

multinodular g., b. multinodular; b. adenomatoso com vários nódulos colóides.

nontoxic g., b. atóxico; b. que não é acompanhado de hipertireoidismo.

parenchymatous g., b. parenquimatoso; uma forma de b. na qual há um grande aumento dos folículos, com proliferação do epitélio. SIN follicular g.

simple g., b. simples; um aumento da tireóide que não é acompanhado de efeitos constitucionais, p.ex., de hipo ou hipertireoidismo; é freqüentemente causado por ingestão de cotas inadequadas de iodo na dieta.

substernal g., b. subesternal; aumento da glândula tireóide, principalmente da parte inferior do istmo, palpável com dificuldade ou impalpável.

suffocative g., b. sufocante; um b. que provoca compressão, acarretando dispnéia extrema.

thoracic g., b. torácico; aumento do tecido tireóide acessório situado no tórax, acompanhado ou não de hipertireoidismo.

toxic g., b. tóxico; um b. que produz secreção excessiva, desencadeando sinais e sintomas de hipertireoidismo.

wandering g., b. migratório. SIN diving g.

goi·tro·gen (goy′trō - jen). Bociogênico; qualquer substância que induz a formação de bócio, p.ex., o repolho, a colza, etc.

goi·tro·gen·ic (goy - trō - jen′ik). Bociogênico; que causa bócio.

goi·trous (goy′trus). Bocioso; denotando ou característico de um bócio.

gold (Au). Ouro (Au); um elemento metálico amarelo, de número atômico 79 e peso atômico 196,96654; o Au[198] (meia-vida de 2,694 dias) é utilizado no tratamento de certos tumores, na sinovectomia por radioisótopos e em técnica de imagens. SIN aurum.

cohesive g., o. coesivo; o. quase puro tratado de tal modo que permanece livre de gases adsorvidos pela superfície e de impurezas, fundindo-se sob pressão em temperatura ambiente; em odontologia, é utilizado para restaurações, sendo colocado diretamente na cavidade e fundido por pressão.

colloidal radioactive g., o. coloidal radioativo. SIN radiogold colloid.

mat g., o. em pó; o. formado por meio de precipitação eletrolítica, comprimido em tiras e sinterizado.

noncohesive g., o. não-coesivo; o. que não sofre fusão por causa da adsorção de gases em sua superfície; algumas formas podem ser transformadas em o. coesivo por meio de tratamento pelo calor; em odontologia, é utilizado como material de preenchimento direto.

powdered g., o. em pó; o. formado pela atomização ou pela precipitação química, levemente pré-condensado e embalado com folhas finas de o. para formar comprimidos.

g. sodium thiomalate, aurotiomalato sódico; utilizado no tratamento da artrite reumatóide. SIN sodium aurothiomalate.

g. sodium thiosulfate, aurotiossulfato sódico; utilizado no tratamento do lúpus eritematoso e em alguns casos de artrite reumatóide. SIN sodium aurothiosulfate.

g. standard, padrão ouro; termo utilizado para descrever um método ou procedimento que é amplamente reconhecido como o melhor disponível. [jargão]

g. thioglucose, aurotioglucose. SIN aurothioglucose.

Goldblatt, Harry, patologista norte-americano, 1891–1977. VER G. *hypertension, kidney, hypertension*.

Gol·den, Ross, radiologista norte-americano, 1889–1975. VER S *sign* of Golden.

Goldenhar, Maurice, médico norte-americano do século XX. VER G. *syndrome*.

gold·en seal (gōld′n sēl). Hidraste-do-canadá (*Hydrastis canadensis*). SIN hydrastis.

Goldflam, Samuel V., neurologista polonês, 1852–1932. VER G. *disease*.

gold foil. Folha de ouro; ouro puro enrolado em folhas extremamente finas; é utilizado na restauração de dentes cariados ou fraturados. VER TAMBÉM cohesive *gold*, noncohesive *gold*.

Goldie, James H., epidemiologista canadense do século XX. VER G.-Coldman *hypothesis*.

Goldman, David E., fisiologista norte-americano, *1910. VER G. *equation*; G.-Hodgkin-Katz *equation*.

Goldman, Henry M., periodontista norte-americano, 1911–1980. VER G.-Fox *knives*, em *knife*.

Goldmann, Hans, oftalmologista suíço, 1899–1991. VER G. *perimeter*, applanation *tonometer*.

Goldscheider, Johannes K.A.E., neurologista alemão, 1858–1935. VER G. *test*.

Goldstein, Hyman I., médico norte-americano, 1887–1954. VER G. toe *sign*.

Golgi, Camillo, histologista italiano, laureado com o Prêmio Nobel, 1843–1926. VER G. *apparatus, complex, corpuscle*, tendon *organ*, internal *reticulum, zone, cells*, em *cell*, osmiobichromate *fixative, stain*; G.-Mazzoni *corpuscle*; Holmgrén-G. *canals*, em *canal*.

gol·gi·o·ki·ne·sis (gol′jē - ō - ki - nē′sis). Golgiocinese; na mitose, o processo de divisão do aparelho de Golgi e sua distribuição entre as duas células-filhas.

Goll, Friedrich, anatomista suíço, 1829–1903. VER G. *column*; *nucleus* of G.; *tract* of G.

Goltz, Robert W., dermatologista norte-americano, *1923. VER G. *syndrome*.

Gombault, Albert F., patologista e neurologista francês, 1844–1904. VER G. *triangle*.

go·me·nol (gō′me - nol). Gomenol; um óleo volátil obtido de uma planta, *Melaleuca viridiflora*; seu principal constituinte é o cineol. Possui ação germicida, não apresenta propriedades irritativas e é utilizado nas inflamações crônicas das mucosas pulmonares e como vermífugo. SIN oleogomenol. [*Gomen*, uma localidade da Nova Caledônia, + L. *oleum*, óleo]

gom·i·to·li (gō - mē′tō - lē). Vasos capilares intrincadamente enovelados presentes em grande parte na haste infundibular superior do pedúnculo da hipófise; constituem uma parte da circulação portal da hipófise. [It. *gomitolo*, rolo]

gom·mel·in (gom′mē - lin). Gomelina; uma forma de dextrina.

Gomori, George, histoquímico húngaro, radicado nos Estados Unidos, 1904–1957. VER Grocott-G. methenamine-silver *stain*; G. nonspecific alkaline phosphatase *stain*, one-step trichrome *stain*, silver impregnation *stain*, chrome alum hematoxylin-phloxine *stain*. Ver as entradas em stain.

Gompertz, Benjamin, atuário inglês, 1779–1865. VER G. *hypothesis, law*.

gom·pho·sis (gom - fō′sis) [TA]. Gonfose; uma forma de articulação fibrosa na qual um processo semelhante a uma cavilha se ajusta a um orifício, como a raiz de um dente no interior da cavidade do alvéolo. SIN articulatio dentoalveolaris, dentoalveolar joint, gompholic joint, peg-and-socket articulation, peg-and-socket joint, socket. [G. *gomphos*, parafuso, prego, + *-osis*, condição]

go·nad (gō′nad). Gônada; um órgão que produz células sexuais; um testículo ou um ovário. [L. mod. do G. *gonē*, semente]

female g., g. feminina, ovário. SIN ovary.

indifferent g., g. indiferente; o órgão primordial encontrado em um embrião, antes de sua diferenciação em testículo ou ovário. VER indifferent *genitalia*.

male g., g. masculina, testículo. SIN testis.

streak g., g. vestigial, faixa gonadal. SIN gonadal *streak*.

gonad-. VER gonado-.

go·nad·al (gō - nad′al). Gonadal; relativo a uma gônada.

go·nad·ec·to·my (gō - nad - ek′tō - mē). Gonadectomia; excisão do ovário ou testículo. VER TAMBÉM castration, orchiectomy, ovariectomy. [gonado- + G. *ektomē*, excisão]

gonado-, gonad-. Gonado-, gonad-; as gônadas. [G. *gonē*, semente]

go·nad·o·blas·to·ma (gō-nad-ō-blas-tō'ma). Gonadoblastoma; neoplasia benigna composta de células germinativas, cordões sexuais, células estromais; surge em casos de disgenesia gonadal pura ou mista; em geral, o tumor é pequeno (1–3 cm) e parcialmente calcificado, porém pode dar origem a tumores malignos de células germinativas, mais freqüentemente a um seminoma/disgerminoma ou a tumores embrionários.

go·nad·o·crins (gō-nad'ō-krinz). Gonadócrinos; peptídeos que estimulam a liberação tanto do hormônio folículo-estimulante (FSH) quanto do hormônio luteinizante da hipófise; encontrados no líquido folicular dos ovários de ratas. [gonad + G. *krinō*, secretar]

go·nad·o·lib·er·in (gō-nad-ō-lib'er-in). Gonadoliberina. **1.** Uma substância hipotalâmica que promove a liberação de gonadotropina. SIN gonadotropin-releasing factor, gonadotropin-releasing hormone. **2.** Um decapeptídeo proveniente do hipotálamo de porcos que induz a liberação tanto de lutropina quanto de folitropina em proporções constantes e, dessa forma, age como a luliberina e a foliberina. SIN luteinizing hormone/follicle-stimulating hormone-releasing factor. [gonad + L. *libero*, liberar, + -in]

gon·a·dop·athy (gon-ă-dop'ă-thē). Gonadopatia; doença que afeta as gônadas. [gonado- + G. *pathos*, sofrimento]

go·nad·o·rel·in hy·dro·chlo·ride (gō-nad-ō-rel'in). Cloridrato de gonadorrelina; $C_{55}H_{75}N_{17}O_{13}·xHCl$; um hormônio liberador de gonadotropina obtido de ovinos, suínos ou de outros animais e utilizado na avaliação da capacidade funcional dos gonadotrofos da hipófise anterior. [*gonado*tropin-*rele*asing + -in]

go·nad·o·troph (gō-nad'ō-trōf, -gon'ă-dō-). Gonadotrofo; uma célula endócrina da adeno-hipófise que influencia determinadas células do ovário ou testículo.

go·nad·o·tro·phic (gō'nad-o-trōf'ik, gon'ă-dō-). Gonadotrófico. SIN gonadotropic. [gonado- + G. *trophē*, nutrição]

go·nad·o·tro·phin (gō'nad-ō-trō'fin, gon'ă-dō-). Gonadotrofina. SIN gonadotropin. [para gonadotrophin, de gonad + G. *trophē*, nutrição]

go·nad·o·tro·pic (gō'nad-ō-trōp'ik, gon'ă-dō-). Gonadotrópico. **1.** Descritivo das ou relacionado com as ações de uma gonadotropina. **2.** Que promove o crescimento e/ou a função das gônadas. SIN gonadotrophic. [gonado- + G. *tropē*, uma volta]

go·nad·o·tro·pin (gō'nad-ō-trō'pin, gon'ă-dō-). Gonadotropina. **1.** Um hormônio capaz de promover o crescimento e a função das gônadas; esses efeitos, quando exercidos por um único hormônio, estão em geral limitados a funções distintas ou a componentes histológicos de uma gônada, tais como a estimulação do crescimento folicular ou da formação de andrógenos; a maioria das gonadotropinas exerce seus efeitos em ambos os sexos, embora o efeito de uma determinada g. seja diferente em machos e fêmeas. **2.** Qualquer hormônio que estimula a função das gônadas. **3.** Qualquer substância que possui os efeitos combinados do hormônio folículo-estimulante (FSH) e do hormônio luteinizante (LH). SIN gonadotrophin, gonadotropic hormone.
anterior pituitary g., g. da hipófise anterior; qualquer g. que se origina na hipófise; termo utilizado no passado para designar um único hormônio, pois acreditava-se que a hipófise anterior secretava apenas uma única g. SIN pituitary gonadotropic hormone.
chorionic g. (CG), g. coriônica; uma glicoproteína com uma fração de carboidrato composta de D-galactose e hexosamina, extraída da urina de gestantes e produzida pelas células trofoblásticas da placenta; seu papel mais importante parece ser a estimulação, durante o primeiro trimestre, da secreção ovariana de estrógeno e progesterona necessária para a integridade do concepto; acredita-se que desempenhe um papel de menor importância nos dois últimos trimestres da gravidez, uma vez que o estrógeno e a progesterona são então formados pela placenta. SIN β-HCG, choriogonadotropin, chorionic gonadotropic hormone, chorionic gonadotrophic hormone, placenta g., placentagonadotropin.
human chorionic g. (HCG, hCG), g. coriônica humana. VER chorionic g.
β-human chorionic g., fração β da g. coriônica humana; uma subunidade com 145 aminoácidos, exclusiva da g. coriônica humana que possui uma cadeia α igual à dos hormônios folículo-estimulante, luteinizante e tireoestimulante. Os testes para detectar a gravidez específicos para a β-HCG são mais sensíveis, uma vez que não ocorre confusão com outras gonadotropinas secretadas pela hipófise.
human menopausal g. (HMG, hMG), g. menopáusica humana; um hormônio da hipófise obtido originalmente da urina de mulheres após a menopausa e, agora, produzido sinteticamente; é utilizado para induzir a ovulação. VER TAMBÉM menotropins.
placenta g. (plă-sen'tă-gō'nad-ō-trō-pin), g. placentária. SIN chorionic g.

gon·a·duct (gon'ă-dŭkt). **1.** Ducto seminal. SIN seminal duct. **2.** Tuba uterina. SIN uterine tube. [gonado- + ducto]

go·nal·gia (gō-nal'jē-ă). Gonalgia; termo obsoleto para a dor no joelho. [G. *gony*, joelho, + *algos*, dor]

gon·ane (gon'ān). Gonana; o hipotético hidrocarboneto (17-carbonos) do qual se originam os hormônios esteróides das gônadas, tais como a estrana ou a androstana, que foi concebido para atingir formas de nomenclatura sistemática.

gon·ar·thri·tis (gon-ar-thrī'tis). Gonartrite; artrite inflamatória da articulação do joelho. [G. *gony*, joelho, + *arthron*, articulação, + *-itis*, inflamação]

gon·e·cyst, gon·e·cys·tis (gon'ē-sist, gon-ē-sis'tis). Glândula seminal. SIN seminal gland. [G. *gonē*, semente, + *kystis*, bexiga]

Gon·gy·lo·ne·ma (gon'ji-lō-nē'mă). Um gênero de nematódeos que parasitam o canal alimentar de aves e mamíferos; são transmitidos por diversos insetos, principalmente por besouros, que transportam as larvas infectantes encistadas. Várias espécies apresentam importância veterinária e uma delas é também conhecida por parasitar seres humanos. [G. *gongylos*, redondo, + *nēma*, fio]
G. pul'chrum, verme que parasita o esôfago de bovinos; uma espécie que penetra na submucosa do esôfago ou do rúmen de muitos ruminantes domésticos e selvagens, porcos, ursos e humanos (os casos em humanos são principalmente causados por vermes imaturos); é transmitido por besouros coprófagos e apresenta distribuição universal.

gon·gy·lo·ne·mi·a·sis (gon'ji-lō-nē-mī'ă-sis). Gongilonemíase; infestação causada por nematódeos do gênero *Gongylonema* que afeta animais e, raramente, seres humanos.

go·nia (gō'nē-ă). Plural de gonion (gônio).

gonio-. Gonio-; ângulo. [G. *gonia*]

go·ni·o·cra·ni·om·e·try (gō'nē-ō-krā-nē-om'e-trē). Goniocraniometria; medida dos ângulos do crânio. [G. *gōnia*, ângulo, + *kranion*, crânio, + *metron*, medida]

go·ni·o·dys·gen·e·sis (gō'nē-ō-dis-jen'e-sis). Goniodisgenesia; aberração do desenvolvimento do segmento ocular anterior. [G. *gōnia*, ângulo, + disgenesia]

go·ni·om·e·ter (gō-nē-om'e-ter). Goniômetro. **1.** Um instrumento para medir ângulos. **2.** Aparelho utilizado para executar o teste estático para doenças do labirinto que consiste em uma prancha na qual uma das extremidades pode ser elevada até a altura desejada e a outra extremidade é gradualmente elevada até o ponto no qual um paciente perde o equilíbrio. **3.** Um dispositivo calibrado projetado para medir o arco ou a amplitude do movimento de uma articulação. SIN arthrometer, fleximeter, pronometer. **4.** Dispositivo utilizado para medir o desvio da cabeça no estrabismo ou no nistagmo. [G. *gōnia*, ângulo, + *metron*, medida]

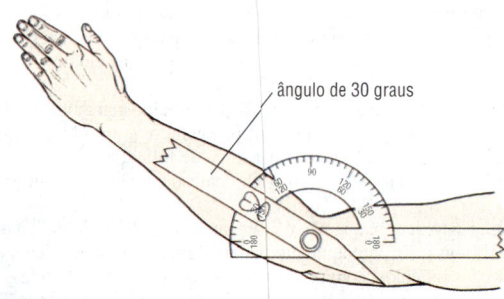

goniômetro: utilizado para medir os graus de movimento de uma articulação; este exemplo mostra 30 graus de flexão no cotovelo

go·ni·on, pl. **go·nia** (gō-nē-on, gō'nē-ă) [TA]. Gônio; o ponto posterior mais baixo e mais externo do ângulo da mandíbula. Em cefalometria, é medido pela bissecção do ângulo formado pelas tangentes das margens inferior e posterior da mandíbula; na radiografia de perfil, quando os ângulos dos dois lados da mandíbula aparecem, corresponde ao ponto médio entre os lados direito e esquerdo. [G. *gōnia*, um ângulo]

go·ni·o·punc·ture (gō'nē-ō-pŭnk'choor). Goniopunção; uma operação para o glaucoma congênito na qual se faz uma punção no ângulo de filtração da câmara anterior.

go·ni·o·scope (gō-nē-ō-skōp). Gorioscópio; uma lente projetada para estudar o ângulo da câmara anterior do olho. [G. *gōnia*, ângulo, + *skopeō*, examinar]

go·ni·os·co·py (gō-nē-os'ko-pē). Gonioscopia; exame do ângulo da câmara anterior do olho com um gonioscópio ou com uma lente prismática de contato.

go·ni·o·syn·ech·ia (gō'nē-ō-si-nek'ē-ă). Goniossinéquia; a aderência da íris à superfície posterior da córnea, no ângulo da câmara anterior; está associada ao glaucoma de ângulo fechado. SIN peripheral anterior synechia. [G. *gōnia*, ângulo, + *synechis*, ajuntar]

go·ni·ot·o·my (gō-nē-ot'ō-mē). Goniotomia; abertura cirúrgica da rede trabecular no glaucoma congênito. [G. *gōnia*, ângulo, + *tomē*, incisão]

gon·o·cho·rism, gon·o·cho·ris·mus (gon-ok'ō-rizm, -ō-riz'mŭs). Gonocorismo; diferenciação normal das gônadas, apropriada ao sexo. [G. *gonē*, semente, sexo, + *chōrizō*, separar]

gon·o·cide (gon′o-sīd). Gonococida. **1.** Destrutivo para os gonococos. **2.** Um agente que mata os gonococos. SIN gonococcicide.

gon·o·coc·cal (gon′o-kok′al). Gonocócico; relativo aos gonococos. SIN gonococcic.

gon·o·coc·ce·mia (gon′o-kok-sē′mē-a). Gonococcemia; a presença de gonococos no sangue circulante. [gonococcus + G. *haima*, sangue]

gon·o·coc·ci (gon-o-kok′sī). Plural de gonococcus (gonococo).

gon·o·coc·cic (gon′o-kok′sik). Gonocócico. SIN gonococcal.

gon·o·coc·ci·cide (gon-o-kok′si-sīd). Gonocicida. SIN gonocide. [gonococcus + L. *caedo*, matar]

gon·o·coc·cus, pl. **gon·o·coc·ci** (gon-o-kok′us, -sī). Gonococo. SIN *Neisseria gonorrhoeae*. [G. *gone*, semente, + *kokkos*, baga]

gon·o·cyte (gon′o-sit). Gonócito, célula germinativa primordial. SIN primordial germ *cell*. [G. *gone*, semente, + *kytos*, oco (célula)]

gon·o·he·mia (gon-o-hē′mē-a). Gonoemia; termo obsoleto para gonococcemia.

gon·o·op·so·nin (gon-o-op′so-nin). Gono-opsonina; uma opsonina gonocócica específica.

gon·o·phage (gon′o-fāj). Um bacteriófago gonocida.

gon·o·phore, gon·oph·o·rus (gon′o-fōr, go-nof′o-rus). Gonóforo; qualquer estrutura com a função de acumular ou conduzir as células sexuais; o oviducto, o ducto espermático, o útero ou a vesícula seminal; um órgão reprodutivo acessório. [G. *gone*, semente, + *phoros*, portador]

gon·or·rhea (gon-o-rē′a). Gonorréia; inflamação catarral e contagiosa da mucosa genital, transmitida principalmente pelo coito e causada pela *Neisseria gonorrhoeae*; pode acometer os tratos genitais superior e inferior, principalmente a uretra, a endocérvice e as tubas uterinas, ou disseminar-se pelo peritônio e, menos freqüentemente, afetar o coração, as articulações ou outras estruturas através da corrente sanguínea. [G. *gonorrhoia*, de *gone*, semente, + *rhoia*, um fluxo]

gon·or·rhe·al (gon-o-rē′al). Gonorreico; relativo à gonorréia.

gon·o·some (gon′o-sōm). Cromossomos sexuais. SIN sex *chromosomes*, em *chromosome*. [G. *gone*, semente + *soma*, corpo]

gon·o·tox·e·mia (gon′o-tok-sē′mē-a) Gonotoxemia; condição tóxica causada pela disseminação hematogênica de gonococos e pelos efeitos resultantes da absorção de sua endotoxina.

gon·o·tox·in (gon-o-tok′sin). Gonotoxina; a endotoxina elaborada pelo gonococo *Neisseria gonorrhoeae*.

gon·o·tyl (gon′o-til). Gonotil; uma estrutura semelhante a uma ventosa que envolve o poro genital dos trematódeos da família Heterophyidae. [G. *gonos*, prole, + *tyle*, botão]

Go·ny·au·lax cat·a·nel·la (gon-e-aw′laks kat-a-nel′a). Um protozoário dinoflagelado marinho produtor de uma toxina poderosa que se acumula nos tecidos do mexilhão e de outros crustáceos que se alimentam por meio da filtração da água do mar; pode causar intoxicação fatal por mexilhões em seres humanos. [G. *gony*, joelho, + *aulakos*, um sulco]

go·ny·camp·sis (gon-e-kamp′sis). Gonicampse; termo obsoleto para ancilose ou para qualquer curvatura anormal do joelho. [G. *gony*, joelho, + *kampsis*, uma inclinação ou curvatura]

Goodell, William, ginecologista norte-americano, 1829–1894. VER G. *sign*.

good·ness of fit. Adequação; o grau de concordância entre uma distribuição empiricamente observada e uma distribuição teórica ou matemática.

Goodpasture, Ernest W., patologista norte-americano, 1886–1960. VER G. *stain*, *syndrome*.

Goormaghtigh, Norbert, médico belga, 1890–1960. VER G. *cells*, em *cell*.

goose·flesh (goos′flesh). Pele anserina, cútis anserina. SIN *cutis anserina*.

Gopalan, C., bioquímico indiano do século XX. VER G. *syndrome*.

Gordius (gōr′dē-us). Antigo nome dado ao gênero *Dracunculus* — composto de vermes nematódeos — aplicado adequadamente aos membros do filo Nematomorpha, freqüentemente denominados gordiáceos ou górdios. [L., do G. *Gordios*, o rei de Górdio, na Frígia; uma alusão às protuberâncias, semelhantes a nós, que esses vermes apresentam]

Gordon, Alfred, neurologista norte-americano, 1869–1953. VER G. *reflex, sign, symptom*.

Gor·do·na (gor′dō-na). Um gênero de bactérias aeróbicas, que são actinomicetos Gram-positivos ou Gram-variáveis, encontradas no trato respiratório humano; algumas espécies estão associadas a bronquiectasia e a abscessos pulmonares de flora mista; a espécie típica é *Gordona bronchialis*.

Gordon and Sweet stain. Coloração de Gordon e Sweet. Ver em stain.

gor·get (gōr′jet). Gorjal; uma tenacânula ou um guia com um sulco amplo para ser utilizado em litotomia.

probe g., g. em sonda; um g. com uma extremidade pontiaguda.

Gorham, Lemuel W., médico norte-americano, 1885–1968. VER G. *disease*; Gorham *syndrome*.

Goriaew rule. Regra de Goriaew. Ver em rule.

Gorlin, Richard, fisiologista e cardiologista norte-americano, *1926. VER G. *formula*.

Gorlin, Robert J., patologista oral norte-americano, *1923. VER G. *sign, syndrome*; G.-Chaudhry-Moss *syndrome*.

go·ron·dou (gō-ron′doo). Gundu. SIN goundou.

goserelin (gos′er-e-lin). Goserelina; um decapeptídeo sintético agonista análogo ao LHRH (GnRH). Inibe a secreção de gonadotropina hipofisária e é utilizado no tratamento do câncer de próstata, do câncer de mama, da endometriose e no adelgaçamento prévio do endométrio antes da ablação ou ressecção do endométrio.

Gosselin, Léon Athanese, cirurgião francês, 1815–1887. VER G. *fracture*.

Gosset, William Sealy, estatístico e químico britânico, que utilizava o pseudônimo "Student" (Estudante), 1876–1937.

gos·sy·pol (gos′i-pol). Gossipol; um princípio tóxico, isolado da semente do algodoeiro (*Gossypium*), que reduz a contagem de espermatozóides; é utilizado na China como contraceptivo oral masculino.

gos·sy·pose (gos′i-pōs). Rafinose. SIN raffinose.

GOT Abreviatura de glutamic-oxaloacetic transaminase (transaminase glutâmico-oxaloacética, TGO).

Göthlin, Gustaf F., fisiologista sueco, 1874–1949. VER G. *test*.

Gottlieb, Bernard, dentista austríaco, 1885–1950. VER epithelial *attachment* of Gottlieb.

gouge (gowj). Goiva, escopro; um cinzel curvo e robusto utilizado em operações ósseas.

Gougerot, Henri, dermatologista francês, 1881–1955. VER G. and Blum *disease*; G.-Sjögren *disease*; G.-Carteaud *syndrome*.

Gould, Sir Alfred P., cirurgião inglês, 1852–1922. VER G. *suture*.

Gouley, John W.S., urologista norte-americano, 1832–1920. VER G. *catheter*.

goun·dou (goon′doo). Gundu; uma doença, endêmica na África Ocidental, caracterizada por exostose dos processos nasais dos ossos maxilares, que provoca tumefação simétrica em cada lado do nariz; acredita-se que seja uma osteíte associada à bouba. SIN anákhré, dog nose, gorondou, henpuye. [nome nativo]

gout (gowt). Gota; um distúrbio do metabolismo da purina, que afeta principalmente os homens, sendo caracterizado por um aumento variável no nível sanguíneo de ácido úrico e artrite aguda recorrente e grave de início súbito e resultante da deposição de cristais de urato de sódio nos tecidos conectivos e na cartilagem articular; a maioria dos casos de gota é hereditário e resulta de várias anormalidades no metabolismo da purina. O acometimento familial é sobretudo galtoniano, com um limiar de expressão determinado pela solubilidade do ácido úrico. Entretanto, a g. é também uma característica da síndrome de Lesch-Nyhan (Lesch-Nyhan *syndrome*), um distúrbio ligado ao X [MIM*308000]. [L. *gutta*, gota]. VER Lesch-Nyhan *syndrome*.

abarticular g., termo raramente utilizado para a g. que afeta estruturas do corpo, exceto as articulações.

articular g., g. articular; a forma comum de g. que ataca uma ou mais articulações.

calcium g., pseudogota. SIN pseudogout.

idiopathic g., g. idiopática; episódios agudos de sinovite induzida por cristais resultantes de anormalidade no metabolismo da purina; a excreção urinária de urato mais baixa do que o normal leva à hiperuricemia e a episódios agudos de inflamação nas articulações. SIN primary g.

interval g., g. intercrítica; uma fase assintomática observada entre ataques agudos de g.

latent g., g. latente; hiperuricemia sem sintomas de gota. Termo freqüentemente utilizado como sinônimo de g. intercrítica. SIN masked g.

lead g., g. induzida pelo chumbo, g. saturnina. SIN saturnine g.

masked g., g. latente. SIN latent g.

primary g., g. primária. SIN idiopathic g.

retrocedent g., g. retrocedente; termo obsoleto para a ocorrência de sintomas gástricos, cardíacos e cerebrais graves durante um ataque de g., principalmente quando os sintomas articulares e outros declinam subitamente e ao mesmo tempo.

saturnine g., g. saturnina; g. que ocorre em uma pessoa com intoxicação por chumbo. SIN lead g.

secondary g., g. secundária; g. resultante de níveis séricos aumentados de ácido úrico, como conseqüência de uma doença prévia, tal como uma doença proliferativa do sangue e da medula óssea, a intoxicação por chumbo ou a insuficiência renal crônica prolongada (sob diálise).

tophaceous g., g. tofácea; g. na qual depósitos de ácido úrico e de uratos ocorrem como tofos gotosos.

gouty (gow′tē). Gotoso; relativo à, ou característico da, gota.

Gowers, Sir William R., neurologista inglês, 1845–1915. VER G. *column, contraction, disease, syndrome, tract*.

GPI Abreviatura de Gingival-Periodontal Index (Índice Gengivo-Periodontal).

GPT Abreviatura de glutamic-pyruvic transaminase (transaminase glutâmico-pirúvica, TGP).

gr Abreviatura de grain (3) (grão).

Graaf, Reijnier de, histologista e fisiologista holandês, 1641–1673. VER graafian *follicle*.

graafian, de De Graaf; relativo a, ou descrito por, R. de Graaf.

grac·i·lis (gras′i-lis). **1.** Grácil, delgado; que indica uma estrutura fina ou delgada. **2.** Músculo grácil. SIN gracilis (*muscle*). [L.]

grad. Abreviatura do L. *gradatim*, gradualmente.

grade (grād). Grau. **1.** Uma posição, uma divisão ou um nível da escala de um sistema de valores. **2.** Em patologia oncológica, uma classificação baseada no grau de malignidade ou de diferenciação do tecido tumoral; p. ex., bem diferenciado, moderadamente diferenciado, mal diferenciado e indiferenciado ou anaplásico. **3.** Na prova de esforço, a medida de uma elevação ou queda vertical, como uma porcentagem da distância horizontal percorrida. [L. *gradus*, passo]

Gleason tumor g., g. do tumor de Gleason; uma classificação de adenocarcinomas da próstata baseada na evolução do padrão de diferenciação glandular; o g. do tumor, conhecido como índice de Gleason, corresponde à soma dos padrões dominante e secundário, cada um numerado em uma escala que varia de 1 a 5.

Heath-Edwards g.'s, graus de Heath-Edwards; um sistema que descreve a patologia da doença vascular pulmonar hipertensiva.

Gradenigo, Giuseppe, otologista italiano, 1859–1926. VER G. *syndrome*.

gra·di·ent (grā′dē-ent). Gradiente; a taxa de modificação da temperatura, da pressão, do campo magnético ou de outra variável como uma função da distância, do tempo, etc.

atrioventricular g., g. atrioventricular; a diferença da pressão diastólica entre o átrio e o ventrículo.

concentration g., g. de concentração, g. de densidade. SIN density g.

density g., g. de densidade; uma solução na qual a concentração (densidade) de um soluto aumenta de modo contínuo do topo ao fundo, ou de uma extremidade a outra de um recipiente (p.ex., o tubo para centrifugação em uma centrifugação por gradiente de densidade). SIN concentration g.

electrochemical g., g. eletroquímico; a medida da tendência de um íon a mover-se passivamente de um ponto para outro, levando em consideração as diferenças em sua concentração e nos potenciais elétricos entre os dois pontos; é comumente expresso como a voltagem adicional necessária para alcançar o equilíbrio.

g. encoding, codificação de gradiente, codificação de fase. SIN *phase* encoding.

field g., g. de campo magnético. SIN magnetic field g.

magnetic field g., g. de campo magnético; nas imagens por ressonância magnética, um campo magnético que varia com a posição e é superposto ao campo uniforme do magneto, a fim de modificar a freqüência de ressonância dos núcleos e permitir o cálculo da posição espacial dos mesmos. SIN field g.

mitral g., g. mitral; a diferença da pressão diastólica entre o átrio esquerdo e o ventrículo esquerdo.

systolic g., g. sistólico; a diferença na pressão entre duas câmaras cardiovasculares comunicantes durante a sístole, p.ex., entre o ventrículo esquerdo e a aorta na estenose aórtica.

ventricular g., g. ventricular; a soma algébrica (isto é, a diferença elétrica final entre) da área envolvida dentro do complexo QRS com aquela dentro da onda T do eletrocardiograma.

grad·u·ate (grad′ū-āt). Tubo graduado; um vaso em geral de vidro e marcado de forma apropriada, utilizado para medir o volume de líquidos; cilindro graduado. [L. mediev. *graduatus*, do L. *gradus*, passo]

grad·u·at·ed (grad′ū-āt′ed). Graduado. **1.** Marcado com linhas ou de outro modo para indicar capacidade, graus, porcentagens, etc. **2.** Dividido ou disposto em níveis, graus ou estágios sucessivos.

Graefe, Albrecht von, oftalmologista alemão, 1828–1870. VER G. *forceps*, *knife*, *operation*, *sign*; pseudo-G. *phenomenon*; G. *sign*; von G. *sign*.

Graefenberg, Ernst, ginecologista alemão, radicado na América, 1881–1957. VER G. *ring*.

Graffi, Arnold, patologista alemão, *1910. VER G. *virus*.

GRAFT

graft (graft). **1.** Enxerto; qualquer tecido ou órgão utilizado em transplantes. **2.** Enxertar; o ato de transplantar tais estruturas. VER TAMBÉM flap, implant, transplant. [A.S. *graef*]

allogeneic g., e. alogênico, aloenxerto. SIN allograft.

animal g., e. animal. SIN zoograft.

autogeneic g., e. autogênico, auto-enxerto. SIN autograft.

autologous g., e. autólogo, auto-enxerto. SIN autograft.

autoplastic g., auto-enxerto. SIN autograft.

bone g., e. ósseo; osso transplantado de uma área doadora para uma área receptora, sem anastomose de vasos nutrientes; o osso pode ser transplantado de um local para outro em um mesmo indivíduo (isto é, enxerto autogênico), ou entre indivíduos diferentes (isto é, enxerto alogênico). VER TAMBÉM osteoplasty.

chorioallantoic g., e. corioalantóico; o transplante de material vivo para a membrana corioalantóidea do embrião de pinto.

composite g., e. composto; um e. composto de vários tecidos, tais como pele e cartilagem, ou um segmento de espessura total da orelha.

corneal g., e. corneano, ceratoplastia. SIN keratoplasty.

Davis g., e. de Davis; "pitadas de enxerto", isto é, pequenos fragmentos (2–3 mm) de enxertos de pele de espessura total.

delayed g., e. tardio; adiar a aplicação de um e. de pele por vários dias até o leito da região receptora estar limpo ou ter parado de sangrar.

dermal g., e. dérmico; um e. de derme, feito a partir de pele cuja epiderme foi retirada.

dermal-fat g., e. dermogorduroso; um e. dérmico acompanhado de gordura subcutânea.

dowel g., e. em cavilha ou espiga; em cirurgia ortopédica, um tipo específico de e. ósseo que se caracteriza por apresentar uma forma circular, geralmente obtida por meio de instrumentos especiais, e utilizado como um e. ósseo estrutural para produzir uma fusão entre duas vértebras adjacentes. SIN dowel (4).

epidermic g., enxerto epidérmico. SIN Reverdin g.

fascia g., e. de fáscia; um e. de tecido fibroso, em geral da fáscia lata.

fascicular g., e. fascicular; um e. de nervo no qual cada feixe de fibras é aproximado e suturado separadamente.

fat g., e. de tecido gorduroso, um e. só de gordura.

free g., e. livre; um e. transplantado de uma área para outra, sem sua fixação normal (sem um pedículo).

full-thickness g., e. de espessura total; um e. de toda a espessura da mucosa e submucosa, ou de pele e tecido subcutâneo.

funicular g., e. funicular; um e. de nervo no qual cada funículo (composto de dois ou mais fascículos) é aproximado e suturado separadamente.

H g., e. em H. SIN H *shunt*.

heterologous g., e. heterólogo, xenoenxerto. SIN xenograft.

heteroplastic g., xenoenxerto. SIN xenograft.

heterotopic g., e. heterotópico; transplante de um tecido ou órgão para uma posição diferente daquela que normalmente ocupa.

homologous g., e. homólogo, aloenxerto. SIN allograft.

homoplastic g., aloenxerto. SIN allograft.

inlay g., e. embutido, um e. de pele envolto (com o lado cruento para fora) ao redor de um material de suporte rígido e inserido no interior de uma bolsa cirúrgica preparada. SIN epithelial *inlay*.

isogeneic g., e. isogênico, e. singênico. SIN syngraft.

isologous g., e. isólogo, e. isogênico, e. singênico. SIN syngraft.

isoplastic g., e. singênico. SIN syngraft.

Krause g., e. de Krause; um e. de pele de espessura total. SIN Krause-Wolfe g.

Krause-Wolfe g., e. de Krause-Wolfe. SIN Krause g.

mesh g., e. em malha; e. de pele de espessura parcial no qual foram feitas múltiplas incisões verticais, a fim de permitir a expansão do fragmento; é utilizado na cobertura de ferimentos complicados, ou quando há pouca pele doadora.

mucosal g., e. de mucosa; um e. de mucosa, em geral de toda a espessura do revestimento da bochecha ou do lábio inferior.

nerve g., e. de nervo; um nervo, ou parte de um nervo, utilizado como um e.

Ollier g., e. de Ollier; um e. de espessura parcial delgado. SIN Ollier-Thiersch g.

Ollier-Thiersch g., e. de Ollier-Thiersch. SIN Ollier g.

onlay g., um e. ósseo aplicado sobre o lado externo do(s) osso(s) receptor(es).

orthotopic g., e. ortotópico; transplante de um tecido ou órgão para a sua posição anatômica normal.

osteoperiosteal g., e. osteoperiosteal; um e. ósseo acompanhado de seu periósteo.

partial-thickness g., e. de espessura parcial. SIN split-thickness g.

pedicle g., e. pediculado. VER pedicle *flap*.

periosteal g., e. periosteal; um e. de periósteo.

pinch g., técnica antiga na qual pequenos fragmentos de pele, de espessura parcial ou total, são removidos de uma área saudável e aplicados sobre um ferimento aberto. SIN Davis g.

porcine g., e. de tecido de porco; um e. de espessura parcial proveniente de um porco e aplicado a uma área cruenta, em um ser humano, como um curativo temporário.

primary skin g., e. de pele primário; um e. de pele transferido imediatamente após a criação de uma área cruenta.

punch g.'s, enxertos em saca-bocado (*punch*); pequenos enxertos de espessura total do escalpo, removidos por meio de pinça em saca-bocado (*punch*) circular e transplantados para uma área calva para que produzam cabelos.

Reverdin g., e. epidérmico; um segmento de epiderme é implantado sobre uma superfície cruenta. SIN epidermic g.

skin g., e. de pele; um fragmento de pele transplantado de uma parte do corpo para outra, a fim de cobrir uma área desnuda.

sleeve g., e. em manga; um e. utilizado para reparar um nervo seccionado por meio da conexão das extremidades periférica e central com uma estrutura semelhante a uma manga, comumente um segmento de veia.

split-skin g., e. de pele de espessura parcial. SIN split-thickness g.

split-thickness g., e. de espessura parcial; um e. composto das partes superiores da pele, isto é, de epiderme e parte da derme, ou de mucosa e submucosa. SIN partial-thickness g., split-skin g.
Stent g., e. de Stent; e. de pele embutido, ou um e. de pele mantido no local por fios de sutura presos a um curativo amoldado/imobilizante.
syngeneic g., e. singênico. SIN syngraft.
tendon g., e. de tendão; um e. de tendão, como ocorre no transplante de tendão.
Thiersch g., e. de Thiersch; termo antigo dado ao e. de espessura parcial. VER Ollier-Thiersch g.
Wolfe g., e. de Wolfe; um e. de toda a espessura total da pele, sem gordura subcutânea. SIN Wolfe-Krause g.
Wolfe-Krause g., e. de Wolfe-Krause. SIN Wolfe g.
xenogeneic g., e. xenogênico, xenoenxerto. SIN xenograft.
zooplastic g., e. zooplástico. SIN zoograft.

graft·ing. Enxertar. O processo de aplicar um enxerto.
Graham, Evarts Ambrose, cirurgião norte-americano, 1883–1957. Em 1924, realizou com W.H. Cole a primeira colecistografia bem-sucedida; em 1933, realizou com J. J. Singer a primeira remoção em um estágio bem-sucedida de um pulmão com câncer. VER Graham-Cole *test*.
Graham, Thomas, químico inglês, 1805–1869. VER G. *law*.
Gra·ha·mel·la (grā-am-el′a). Um gênero antigo de bactérias aeróbicas e imóveis, que agora estão reclassificadas como membros do gênero *Bartonella*. [G.S. *Graham-Smith*]
Graham Steell, VER Steell.
grain (grān). Grão. **1.** Cereais, tais como o milho, o trigo ou o centeio, ou uma semente de um deles. **2.** Uma partícula diminuta e dura de qualquer substância, como a da areia. **3 (gr).** Uma unidade de peso, na qual 1 grão = 1/60 dracma (farmacêutica ou troy), 1/437,5 onça avoirdupois, 1/480 onça troy, 1/5.760 libra troy, 1/7.000 libra avoirdupois; o equivalente a 0,064799 g. **4.** Um grupo macroscopicamente visível de organismos que vivem nos tecidos de pacientes com actinomicose ou micetoma. [L. *granum*]
grains (grānz). Grãos; núcleos paraceratósicos situados dentro da camada córnea da epiderme, encontrados na ceratose folicular.
Gram, Hans C.J., bacteriologista dinamarquês, 1853–1938. VER G. *iodine*, *stain*; G.-chromotrope *stain*; Weigert-G. *stain*.
gram (g, gm). Grama; uma unidade de peso do sistema métrico ou centesimal; equivale a 15,432358 grãos ou 0,03527 onças avoirdupois.

⚠ **-gram.** -grama; um registro, feito em geral por um instrumento. Cf. -graph. [G. *gramma*, caractere, marca]
gram-cen·ti·me·ter. Grama-centímetro; a energia exercida, ou o trabalho realizado, quando um corpo de 1 g é elevado a uma altura de 1 cm; equivale a $9,807 \times 10^{-5}$ J ou N/m (Newton-metro).
gram·i·ci·din (gram-i-sī′din). Gramicidina; um antibiótico de um grupo de antibióticos polipeptídicos produzidos pelo *Bacillus brevis* que apresentam primariamente ação bacteriostática contra cocos e bacilos Gram-positivos. As preparações comerciais contêm várias gramicidinas conhecidas, como a g. A, B, C e D; a g. S (de "Soviet") é cíclica, e as demais são lineares.
gram·i·on. Íon-grama; o peso em gramas de um íon; corresponde à soma dos pesos atômicos dos átomos que compõem o íon.
gram-me·ter. Grama-metro; uma unidade de energia que corresponde a 100 gramas-centímetros.
gram-mol·e·cule. Molécula-grama. Ver em molecule.
Gram-neg·a·tive. Gram-negativo; refere-se à incapacidade de uma bactéria em resistir à descoloração pelo álcool, após ser tratada com violeta cristal de Gram. Contudo, após a descoloração, essas bactérias podem ser prontamente coradas com safranina, que dá uma cor rósea ou vermelha à bactéria, quando visualizada sob um microscópio óptico. Essa reação é, em geral, uma indicação de que a estrutura externa da bactéria consiste em uma membrana citoplasmática (interna), envolta por uma camada peptidioglicana relativamente delgada, que, por sua vez, é envolta por uma membrana externa. VER Gram *stain*.
Gram-pos·i·tive. Gram-positivo; refere-se à capacidade de uma bactéria de resistir à descoloração pelo álcool, após ser tratada com o corante violeta cristal de Gram, que dá uma cor violeta à bactéria quando visualizada ao microscópio óptico. Essa reação é, em geral, uma indicação de que a estrutura externa da bactéria consiste em uma membrana citoplasmática envolta por uma parede celular espessa e rígida composta de peptidioglicana. VER Gram *stain*.
gra·na (grā′nā). Grãos; corpúsculos, encontrados no interior dos cloroplastos de células vegetais, formados por camadas compostas de clorofila e fosfolipídios. [pl. do L. *granum*, grão]
gra·na·tum (gra-nā′tum). Romã. SIN pomegranate. [L. *granatus*, que possui muitas sementes]
gran·di·ose (gran′dē-ōs). Grandioso; que se refere aos sentimentos de grande importância, de efusividade ou às ilusões de grandeza. [It. *grandioso*, do L. *grandis*, grande]
Granger, Amedee, radiologista norte-americano, 1879–1939. VER G. *line*.
Granit, Ragnar A., neurofisiologista fino-sueco, laureado com o Prêmio Nobel, 1900–1991. VER G. *loop*.

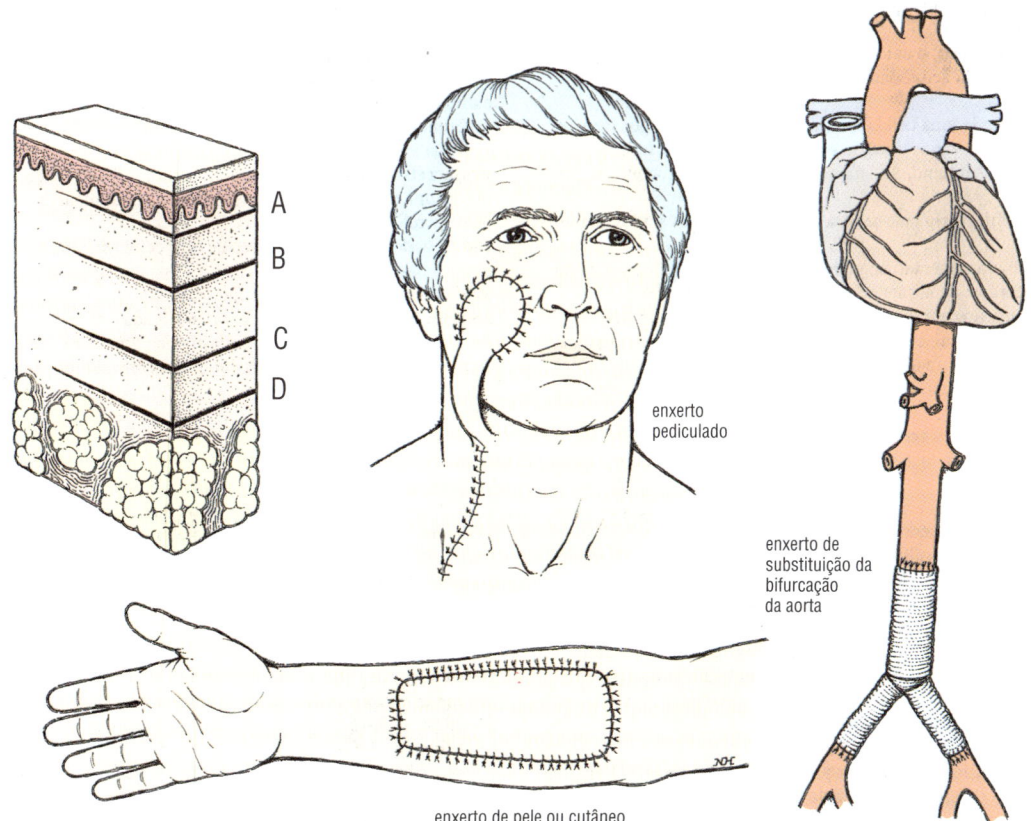

tipos de enxerto: (A, B, C) enxertos de espessura parcial, (D) enxerto de espessura total

enxerto pediculado

enxerto de substituição da bifurcação da aorta

enxerto de pele ou cutâneo

gran·u·lar (gran´u-lar). Granular. **1.** Composto de ou que se assemelha a grânulos ou granulações. **2.** Partículas com forte afinidade por corantes nucleares, observadas em muitas espécies de bactérias.

gra·nu·la·tio, pl. **gran·u·la·ti·o·nes** (gran-u-lā´shē-ō, -shē-o´nēz). Granulação. SIN granulation. [L.]

granulatio'nes arachnoideae [TA], granulações aracnóideas; SIN arachnoid granulations, em granulation. VER TAMBÉM arachnoid villi, em villus.

gran·u·la·tion (gran´u-lā´shŭn). Granulação **1.** A formação de grãos ou grânulos; o estado de ser granular. **2.** Uma massa granular na ou sobre a superfície de qualquer órgão ou membrana; ou um dos grânulos individuais que formam essa massa. **3.** A formação de diminutas projeções arredondadas e carnosas de tecido conectivo, encontradas na superfície de um ferimento, uma úlcera ou uma superfície de tecido inflamado no processo de cicatrização; um dos grânulos carnosos que compõem essa superfície. VER TAMBÉM granulation tissue. **4.** Granulagem; em farmácia, a formação de cristais por meio da agitação constante de uma solução supersaturada de um sal; o produto utilizado na fabricação de comprimidos para uso oral. SIN granulatio. [L. *granulatio*]

arachnoid g.'s [TA], granulações aracnóideas; prolongamentos tufosos da piaaracnóide, compostos de numerosos vilos aracnóideos que penetram nos seios venosos durais e efetuam a transferência de líquido cerebrospinal para o sistema venoso. Na idade avançada, as granulações são mais numerosas e tendem a calcificar-se. SIN arachnoidal g.'s [TA], granulationes arachnoideae [TA], pacchionian bodies, pacchionian corpuscles, pacchionian glands, pacchionian g.'s.

arachnoidal g.'s [TA], granulações aracnóideas. SIN arachnoid g.'s.

pacchionian g.'s, granulações de Pacchioni. SIN arachnoid g.'s.

gran·u·la·ti·o·nes (gran-u-lā-shē-o´nēz). Plural de granulatio.

gran·ule (gran´ūl). Grânulo. **1.** Uma partícula semelhante a um grão; uma granulação; uma massa diminuta e isolada. **2.** Uma pílula muito pequena, em geral revestida de gelatina ou açúcar, que contém uma substância a ser administrada em uma dose pequena. **3.** Uma colônia de bactérias ou fungos que causam uma doença ou que simplesmente colonizam os tecidos do paciente. Em pacientes imunocomprometidos, a diferenciação é difícil. **4.** Uma pequena partícula que pode ser observada ao microscópio eletrônico; contém material armazenado. [L. *granulum,* dim. de *granum,* grão]

α **g.'s,** grânulos α; grânulos grandes, semelhantes a bastões ou filamentosos, encontrados em vários tipos de células, principalmente nas plaquetas, nas quais são o tipo mais numeroso de g.; contêm proteínas secretoras, que incluem o fibrinogênio, a fibronectina, a trombospondina, o fator de von Willebrand (coletivamente conhecidas como proteínas adesivas) e outras proteínas (o fator plaquetário 4, o fator de crescimento derivado das plaquetas, o fator V da coagulação, etc.).

acidophil g., g. acidófilo; um g. que se cora com um corante ácido como a eosina. SIN oxyphil g.

acrosomal g., g. acrossômico; o único g., rico em glicoproteínas, encontrado no interior de uma vesícula acrossômica e resultante da coalescência de grânulos pró-acrossômicos.

alpha g., g. alfa; um g. de uma célula alfa; denominado alfa ou por ter sido considerado o primeiro de vários tipos de grânulos, ou por ser acidófilo.

Altmann g., (1) g. de Altmann. SIN fuchsinophil g.; (2) mitocôndria. SIN mitochondrion.

amphophil g., g. anfófilo; um g. que se cora tanto com corantes ácidos quanto com básicos.

argentaffin g.'s, grânulos argentafins; grânulos que reduzem os íons de prata de uma solução de corante de nitrato de prata amoniacal.

azurophil g., g. azurófilo; um g. que se cora de uma cor púrpura-avermelhada com um corante azul-celeste; tais grânulos são observados em esfregaços secos de determinadas células sanguíneas maduras e em desenvolvimento; são lisossomas primários ligados à membrana que contêm enzimas. SIN kappa g.

basal g., corpúsculo basal. SIN basal *body.*

basophil g., g. basófilo; um g. que se cora prontamente com um corante básico.

Bensley specific g.'s, grânulos específicos de Bensley; grânulos encontrados nas células das ilhotas de Langerhans do pâncreas.

beta g., g. beta; um g. de uma célula beta.

Birbeck g., g. de Birbeck, g. de Langerhans. SIN Langerhans g.

Bollinger g.'s, grânulos de Bollinger. (1) Grânulos branco-amarelados ou amarelo-pálidos relativamente pequenos, mas freqüentemente visíveis ao microscópio, observados na lesão granulomatosa ou no exsudato da botriomicose; os grânulos consistem em agregados irregulares ou colônias de cocos Grampositivos, em geral de estafilococos; (2) termo às vezes utilizado de modo incorreto como sinônimo de corpúsculos de Bollinger.

chromatic g., g. cromático. g. cromófilo. SIN chromophil g. (2).

chromophil g., g. cromófilo; (1) Qualquer g. prontamente corável; (2) um g. de substância cromófila (Nissl). SIN chromatic g.

chromophobe g.'s, grânulos cromófobos; grânulos que não se coram ou que se coram fracamente com os corantes comuns; esses grânulos são encontrados em algumas células do lobo anterior da hipófise.

cone g., g. do cone; o núcleo de uma célula da retina, que se comunica com um dos cones.

Crooke g.'s, grânulos de Crooke; massas grumosas de material basofílico encontradas nas células basófilas do lobo anterior da hipófise; estão associados à doença de Cushing ou surgem após a administração de ACTH.

delta g., g. delta; um g. de uma célula delta.

elementary g., g. elementar; uma partícula de poeira de sangue ou de hemocônia.

eosinophil g., g. eosinófilo; um g. que se cora com eosina.

Fordyce g.'s, grânulos de Fordyce, manchas de Fordyce. SIN Fordyce *spots,* em *spot.*

fuchsinophil g., g. fucsinófilo; um g. que possui afinidade pela fucsina. SIN Altmann g. (1).

glycogen g., g. de glicogênio; glicogênio presente nas células como grânulos beta, que apresentam um diâmetro médio de cerca de 300 Å, ou como grânulos alfa, que são agregados de partículas menores, com 900 Å.

iodophil g., g. iodófilo; um g. que se cora de castanho com o iodo; é encontrado em muitos dos leucócitos polimorfonucleares na pneumonia, erisipela, escarlatina e em outras doenças agudas.

juxtaglomerular g.'s, grânulos justaglomerulares; grânulos secretores osmofílicos presentes nas células justaglomerulares; acredita-se que contenham renina.

kappa g., g. capa, g. azurófilos. SIN azurophil g.

keratohyalin g.'s, grânulos cerato-hialinos; grânulos basofílicos com forma irregular encontrados nas células do estrato granuloso da epiderme.

lamellar g., g. lamelar. SIN keratinosome.

Langerhans g., g. de Langerhans; um pequeno g. envolto por uma membrana e com forma de raquete de tênis que apresenta uma ultra-estrutura interna característica; foi registrado pela primeira vez nas células de Langerhans da epiderme. SIN Birbeck g.

Langley g.'s, grânulos de Langley; grânulos encontrados nas células secretoras serosas.

membrane-coating g., g. lamelar, queratinossoma. SIN keratinosome.

metachromatic g.'s, grânulos metacromáticos. (1) Grânulos que se coram de uma cor diferente daquela do corante utilizado; VER TAMBÉM metachromasia; (2) termo às vezes empregado como sinônimo de volutin (volutina).

mucinogen g.'s, grânulos mucinógenos; grânulos que produzem mucina, como nas células das glândulas salivares e nas mucosas gástrica e intestinal.

Neusser g.'s, grânulos de Neusser; minúsculos grânulos basofílicos às vezes observados em uma zona indistinta ao redor do núcleo de um leucócito.

neutrophil g., g. neutrófilo; o corado pelo componente neutro dos corantes, p.ex., pelos corantes de sangue do tipo Romanovsky.

Nissl g.'s, grânulos de Nissl. SIN Nissl *substance.*

oxyphil g., g. oxífilo. SIN acidophil g.

Palade g., g. de Palade, ribossoma. SIN ribosome.

proacrosomal g.'s, grânulos pró-acrossômicos; pequenos grânulos ricos em carboidratos que aparecem no interior de vesículas do aparelho de Golgi das espermátides; coalescem formando um único g. acrossômico contido em uma vesícula acrossômica.

prosecretion g.'s, grânulos pró-secreção; grânulos encontrados no citoplasma de uma célula indicativos de uma etapa preliminar da formação de um produto secretório.

rod g., g. do bastonete; o núcleo de uma célula da retina que se comunica com um dos bastonetes.

Schüffner g.'s, grânulos de Schüffner. SIN Schüffner *dots,* em *dot.*

secretory g., g. secretor; uma partícula ligada à membrana, em geral uma proteína, formada no retículo endoplasmático granular e no complexo de Golgi.

seminal g., g. seminal; um dos diminutos corpúsculos granulares presentes no sêmen.

specific g.'s, grânulos específicos; os característicos grânulos dos leucócitos basófilos, eosinófilos e neutrófilos, em oposição aos grânulos azurófilos não-específicos.

volutin g.'s, grânulos de volutina. SIN volutin.

Zimmermann g., g. de Zimmermann; termo obsoleto dado às plaquetas.

zymogen g., g. de zimogênio; g. secretor encontrado nas células acinares do pâncreas.

granulo-. Granulo-; granular, grânulos. [L. *granulum,* um pequeno grão-]

gran·u·lo·blast (gran´u-lō-blast). Granuloblasto; termo raramente utilizado para uma célula hematopoética imatura capaz de dar origem aos granulócitos. [granulo- + G. *blastos,* germe]

gran·u·lo·cyte (gran´u-lō-sit) Granulócito; um leucócito granular maduro, que inclui os tipos neutrofílico, acidofílico e basofílico de leucócitos polimorfonucleares, isto é, respectivamente, os neutrófilos, os eosinófilos e os basófilos. [granulo- + G. *kytos,* célula]

immature g., g. imaturo; um neutrófilo imaturo; pode ser de caráter neutrofílico, acidofílico ou basofílico.

gran·u·lo·cy·to·pe·nia (gran´u-lō-si-tō-pē´nē-a). Granulocitopenia; número menor do que o normal de leucócitos granulares no sangue. SIN granulopenia, hypogranulocytosis. [granulocyte + G. *penia,* pobreza]

gran·u·lo·cy·to·poi·e·sis (gran′ū-lō-sī′tō-poy-ē′sis). Granulocitopoese. SIN granulopoiesis.

gran·u·lo·cy·to·poi·et·ic (gran′ū-lō-sī′tō-poy-et′ik). Granulocitopoético. SIN granulopoietic. [granulocyte + G. *poieō,* fazer]

gran·u·lo·cy·to·sis (gran′ū-lō-si-tō′sis). Granulocitose; uma condição caracterizada por um número maior do que o normal de granulócitos no sangue circulante ou nos tecidos.

GRANULOMA

gran·u·lo·ma (gran-ū-lō′mă). Granuloma; termo aplicado às lesões inflamatórias nodulares, em geral pequenas ou granulares, firmes, persistentes e que contêm fagócitos modificados agrupados de modo compacto, tais como células epitelióides, células gigantes e outros macrófagos. VER TAMBÉM granulomatosis. [granulo- + G. *-oma,* tumor]

actinic g., g. actínico; erupção anular, encontrada na pele exposta ao sol; ao exame microscópico, há fagocitose das fibras elásticas da derme por células gigantes e histiócitos. SIN Miescher g.

amebic g., g. amebiano. SIN ameboma.

g. annula′re, g. anular; erupção cutânea papular crônica ou recorrente, em geral autolimitada, que tende a desenvolver-se nas partes distais dos membros e sobre as proeminências, embora a condição possa ser generalizada; as pápulas céreas tendem a formar lesões anulares caracterizadas ao microscópio por focos de necrose dérmica com depósitos de mucina, circundados por histiócitos com núcleos em paliçada.

apical g., g. apical, g. periapical. SIN periapical g.

beryllium g., g. de berílio; uma reação granulomatosa, semelhante ao sarcóide, resultante da exposição ao berílio, seja por inalação, seja por cortes cutâneos por fragmentos de vidro de lâmpadas fluorescentes.

bilharzial g., g. da bilharziose. SIN schistosome g.

Capillaria **g.**, g. de *Capillaria*; lesões granulomatosas encontradas no fígado e nos pulmões; são uma resposta tecidual local ao parasita e a seus ovos.

cholesterol g., g. de colesterol; g. com fendas proeminentes de colesterol circundados por células gigantes de corpo estranho e encontrados na otite média crônica e na sinusite.

coccidioidal g., g. da coccidioidomicose. SIN secondary *coccidioidomycosis*.

cutaneous leishmaniasis g., g. da leishmaniose cutânea; granulomas linfocíticos com centros necróticos encontrados durante o processo de cicatrização.

dental g., g. dentário, g. periapical. SIN periapical g.

Enterobius **g.**, g. de *Enterobius*; lesões que contêm vermes e ovos mortos desse nematódeo; são encontrados na vagina, no colo uterino, nas tubas uterinas, no omento, no peritônio, no fígado, nos rins e nos pulmões.

eosinophilic g., g. eosinofílico; uma forma de histiocitose de Langerhans que acomete predominantemente os ossos de pessoas jovens; pode ser único ou múltiplo; composto histologicamente de células de Langerhans e eosinófilos.

g. facia′le, g. facial; nódulos castanho-avermelhados bem demarcados, persistentes e de causa desconhecida que, em geral, aparecem sobre a face de pessoas de meia-idade e consistem em um infiltrado dérmico denso de eosinófilos e neutrófilos, separado da epiderme e dos folículos pilosos e acompanhado de vasculite fibrinóide de origem desconhecida.

fish-tank g., g. de piscina. SIN swimming pool g.

foreign body g., g. de corpo estranho; um g. resultante da presença de material particulado estranho nos tecidos e caracterizado por uma reação histiocítica com células gigantes de corpo estranho.

g. gangrenes′cens, g. letal da linha média. SIN lethal midline g.

giant cell g., g. de células gigantes; uma lesão não-neoplásica caracterizada por proliferação de tecido de granulação contendo numerosas células gigantes multinucleadas; ocorre na gengiva e na mucosa alveolar (ocasionalmente, em outros tecidos moles), nas quais se apresenta como uma tumefação nodular hemorrágica vermelho-clara e azulada; também ocorre na mandíbula ou na maxila como uma imagem radiotransparente uni ou multilocular; lesões microscopicamente semelhantes ocorrem nos ossos tubulares das mãos e dos pés e acredita-se que sejam neoplásicas, podendo apresentar uma evolução maligna. Lesões ósseas idênticas podem ser observadas no hiperparatireoidismo e no querubismo. VER TAMBÉM giant cell *tumor* of bone. SIN giant cell epulis, reparative giant cell g.

g. gravida′rum, g. gravídico; um g. piogênico que se desenvolve na gengiva durante a gravidez; acredita-se que esteja relacionado à resposta hormonalmente alterada das mucosas da boca a irritantes locais, tais como placas bacterianas sobre os dentes adjacentes. SIN pregnancy tumor.

infectious g., g. infeccioso; qualquer lesão granulomatosa que se sabe ser causada por um agente vivo; p.ex., por bactérias, fungos, helmintos.

g. inguina′le, g. inguinal; um g. específico classificado como doença venérea e causado pelo *Calymmatobacterium granulomatis*, microrganismo observa-do no interior de macrófagos como corpúsculos de Donovan; as lesões granulomatosas ulcerantes ocorrem na região inguinal e na genitália; a disseminação periférica das lesões produz destruição extensa. SIN g. venereum.

laryngeal g., g. laríngeo; uma projeção polipóide de tecido granulomatoso para a luz da laringe, que freqüentemente ocorre após uma intubação traqueal traumática.

lethal midline g., g. letal de linha média. **(1)** Destruição do septo nasal, do palato duro, das paredes nasais laterais, dos seios paranasais, da pele da face, da órbita e da nasofaringe causada por um infiltrado inflamatório com células histiocíticas e linfocíticas atípicas; na maioria dos casos, uma forma de linfoma. **(2)** Termo obsoleto para polymorphic *reticulosis* (reticulose polimórfica). SIN g. gangrenescens, malignant g., midline malignant reticulosis granuloma.

lipoid g., g. lipóide; g. caracterizado por agregados ou acúmulos de fagócitos mononucleares razoavelmente grandes que contêm lipídios.

lipophagic g., g. lipofágico; uma lesão formada como resultado da reação inflamatória desencadeada por focos de necrose na gordura subcutânea, como ocorre em determinados tipos de ferimento traumático; a região central do material necrótico é circundada por uma zona irregular de numerosos macrófagos, muitos dos quais preenchidos por minúsculos glóbulos de lipídios.

lymphatic filariasis g., g. da filaríase linfática; lesão granulomatosa freqüentemente encontrada ao redor de microfilárias mortas.

Majocchi g.'s, granulomas de Majocchi; tinha inflamatória da pele glabra. SIN tinea profunda.

malignant g., g. maligno. SIN lethal midline g.

Miescher g., g. de Miescher. SIN actinic g.

g. multifor′me, g. multiforme; uma erupção anular granulomatosa crônica da pele da parte superior do corpo encontrada em idosos da África central; de causa desconhecida.

ocular larva migrans g., g. de larva migrans ocular; granuloma eosinofílico encontrado ao redor de vermes mortos (em geral, *Toxocara* spp.), no olho; pode mimetizar o retinoblastoma.

oily g., g. oleoso; reação à inclusão de um grande volume de líquido insolúvel (freqüentemente de uma substância oleosa) que perdura vários meses, às vezes anos, após a injeção do material.

paracoccidioidal g., g. da paracoccidioidomicose. SIN paracoccidioidomycosis.

Paragonimus **g.**, g. de *Paragonimus*; lesões causadas pelos ovos e vermes adultos do trematódeo pulmonar aprisionado no parênquima pulmonar.

periapical g., g. periapical; proliferação de tecido de granulação que circunda o ápice de um dente morto e surge em resposta à necrose pulpar. SIN apical g., dental g., root end g.

pulse g., angiopatia hialina de células gigantes. SIN giant cell hyaline angiopathy.

pyogenic g., g. pyogen′icum, g. piogênico; uma pequena massa arredondada adquirida de tecido de granulação bastante vascularizado, freqüentemente com uma superfície ulcerada, que se projeta da pele, principalmente da face, ou da mucosa oral; histologicamente, a massa é um hemangioma capilar lobular. SIN lobular capillary hemangioma.

reparative g., g. reparador; complicação de estapedectomia na qual um g. se forma na janela oval ao redor da prótese; resulta em perda auditiva sensorial.

reparative giant cell g., g. reparador de células gigantes. SIN giant cell g.

root end g., g. periapical. SIN periapical g.

sarcoidal g., g. sarcóide; um g. de células epitelióides não-necrosante semelhante ao observado na sarcoidose.

schistosome g., g. esquistossomótico; uma lesão granulomatosa que se forma ao redor dos ovos de esquistossoma embebidos nos tecidos nos casos de esquistossomose (bilharziose); tipicamente, esses granulomas são encontrados nos tecidos intestinais (infestação por *Schistosoma japonicum* ou por *S. mansoni*), no tecido vesical (*S. haematobium*) e no tecido hepático (todos os esquistossomos humanos). SIN bilharzial g.

sea urchin g., g. de ouriço-do-mar; nódulos granulomatosos, do tipo corpo estranho ou compostos de células epitelióides, resultantes da retenção de espinhos de ouriço-do-mar, que ocorrem vários meses após a lesão da pele.

silica g., g. de sílica; erupção de lesões granulomatosas resultante da inoculação traumática da pele com areia ou materiais que contenham sílica; essa condição pode seguir-se à dermoabrasão feita com lixa.

silicotic g., g. de sílica; nódulo granulomatoso resultante da deposição de partículas de sílica, que em geral ocorre nos pulmões.

swimming pool g., g. de piscina; uma lesão verrucosa crônica, mais comumente observada nos joelhos e resultante de infecção por *Mycobacterium marinum*. SIN fish-tank g.

trichinosis g., g. da triquinose; lesões causadas pela morte de células após a penetração de larvas migratórias de nematódeos recém-nascidos.

g. trop′icum, Bouba. SIN yaws.

umbilical g., g. umbilical; tecido de granulação úmido encontrado no centro do umbigo de neonatos.

g. vene′reum, g. venéreo, g. inguinal. SIN g. inguinale.

zirconium g., g. de zircônio; g. geralmente encontrado nas axilas e composto de sais de zircônio provenientes de antiperspirantes que contêm esse material ou da aplicação de solução de óxido de zircônio nas lesões de hera venenosa.

gran·u·lo·ma·to·sis (gran'ū-lō-mă-tō'sis). Granulomatose; qualquer condição caracterizada por granulomas múltiplos.
  allergic g., g. alérgica. SIN Churg-Strauss *syndrome.*
  lipid g., lipoid g., g. lipídica, g. lipóide. SIN xanthomatosis.
  lymphomatoid g., g. linfomatóide; linfoma angiocêntrico maligno de pulmão; pode afetar o trato respiratório superior e outras partes do corpo. VER TAMBÉM polymorphic *reticulosis*.
  g. siderot'ica, g. siderótica; uma forma de g. na qual focos marrons de consistência firme, contendo pigmento de ferro (corpúsculos de Gamna), são encontrados em um baço aumentado.
  Wegener g., g. de Wegener; uma doença, que ocorre principalmente na quarta e quinta décadas de vida, caracterizada por granulomas e ulcerações necrosantes do trato respiratório superior, acompanhadas de rinorréia purulenta, obstrução nasal e, às vezes, otorréia, hemoptise, infiltração e cavitação pulmonares e febre; podem ocorrer exoftalmia, acometimento da laringe e faringe e glomerulonefrite; a condição subjacente é uma vasculite que afeta os pequenos vasos e é, possivelmente, resultante de distúrbio imunológico. VER TAMBÉM lymphomatoid g.

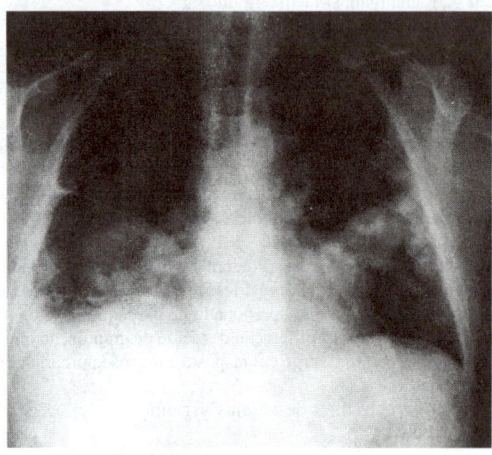

granulomatose de Wegener (radiografia): granulomas nos dois pulmões

gran·u·lom·a·tous (gran-ū-lom'ă-tŭs). Granulomatoso; que possui as características de um granuloma.
gran·u·lo·mere (gran'ū-lō-mēr). Granulômero; a parte interna de uma plaqueta do sangue. SIN chromomere (2). [granulo- + G. *meros*, uma parte]
gran·u·lo·pe·nia (gran'ū-lō-pē'nē-ă). Granulopenia, granulocitopenia. SIN granulocytopenia.
gran·u·lo·plasm (gran'ū-lō-plazm). Granuloplasma; a substância interna de uma ameba ou de outro microrganismo unicelular, situada no ectoplasma e ao redor do núcleo.
gran·u·lo·plas·tic (gran'ū-lō-plas'tik). Granuloplásico; que forma grânulos.
gran·u·lo·poi·e·sis (gran'ū-lō-poy-ē'sis). Granulopoese; a produção de granulócitos. Nos adultos, os granulócitos são produzidos principalmente na medula óssea vermelha dos ossos planos. SIN granulocytopoiesis. [granulo(cyte) + G. *poiēsis*, produção]
gran·u·lo·poi·et·ic (gran'ū-lō-poy-et'ik). Granulopoético; relativo à granulopoese. SIN granulocytopoietic.
gran·u·lo·sa (gran-ū-lō'să). Granulosa. SIN *stratum* granulosum folliculi ovarici vesiculosi.
gran·u·lo·sis (gran-ū-lō'sis). Granulose; uma massa de diminutos grânulos de qualquer natureza.
  g. ru'bra na'si, g. rubra do nariz; eritema, pápulas e ocasionais vesículas, encontrados na ponta do nariz, que se estendem para cima e para os lados, em direção às bochechas; é resultante da oclusão e inflamação crônica dos ductos sudoríferos.
gra·num (grā'nŭm). Singular de grana (grana).
gran·zymes (gran'zimz). Proteases com atividade serina esterase que representam a maior parte do conteúdo dos grânulos das células T citotóxicas. Não se sabe se a célula T citotóxica necessita dessas enzimas para matar. [granule + -zyme]

graph (graf). Gráfico. **1.** Uma linha ou um traçado que indica os valores variáveis de bens e serviços, temperatura, débito urinário, etc.; mais genericamente, qualquer representação geométrica ou ilustrada de medidas que poderiam de outro modo ser expressas de forma tabular. **2.** A apresentação visual da relação entre duas variáveis, na qual os valores de uma são colocados no eixo horizontal, e os valores da outra, no eixo vertical; os gráficos tridimensionais, que mostram as relações entre três variáveis, podem ser descritos e visualmente compreendidos em duas dimensões. [G. *graphō*, escrever]
-graph. -grafo. **1.** Algo escrito, como em monografia, radiografia. **2.** O instrumento utilizado para fazer um registro, como em cimógrafo. Cf. -gram. [G. *graphō*, escrever]
graph·an·es·the·sia (graf'an-es-thē'zē-ă). Grafanestesia; incapacidade tátil para reconhecer números ou letras escritos sobre a pele; pode ser resultante de doença da medula espinal ou do cérebro. [G. *graphē*, escrita + *anaisthēsia*, de *an-* priv. + *aisthēsis*, percepção]
graph·es·the·sia (graf-es-thē'zē-ă). Grafestesia; capacidade tátil para reconhecer a escrita sobre a pele. [G. *graphē*, escrita, + *aisthēsis*, percepção]
graph·ite (graf'īt). Grafite, grafita; forma cristalizável, preta e macia de carbono. SIN black lead, plumbago.
grapho-. Grafo-; uma escrita, descrição. [G. *graphō*, escrever]
gra·phol·o·gy (gră-fol'ō-jē). Grafologia; o estudo da caligrafia como um meio que indica o temperamento, o caráter ou a personalidade de alguém. [grapho- + G. *logos*, estudo]
graph·o·ma·nia (graf-ō-mā'ne-ă). Grafomania; impulso mórbido e excessivo para escrever. [grapho- + G. *mania*, insanidade]
graph·o·mo·tor (graf-ō-mō'ter). Grafomotor; relativo aos movimentos utilizados na escrita. [grapho- + L. *motus*, de *movere*, mover]
graph·o·pa·thol·o·gy (graf'ō-path-ol'ō-jē). Grafopatologia; interpretação dos distúrbios da personalidade a partir de um estudo da caligrafia. VER graphology. [grapho- + pathology]
graph·o·pho·bia (graf-ō-fō'be-ă). Grafofobia; medo mórbido de escrever. [grapho- + G. *phobos*, medo]
graph·o·spasm (graf'ō-spazm). Grafospasmo. SIN writer's *cramp*.
-graphy. -grafia; uma composição literária ou musical, uma descrição. [G. *graphō*, escrever]
grasp. Pega, empunhadura; o ato de pegar algo de modo seguro e segurar firmemente.
  palm g., pega ou empunhadura palmar; segurar um objeto envolvendo-o com a palma da mão e dedos.
  pen g., pega ou empunhadura digital; método de agarrar um instrumento semelhante àquele para segurar uma caneta durante a escrita.
GRASS Abreviatura de gradient-recalled *acquisition* in the steady state (aquisição rápida de imagens em equilíbrio dinâmico).
Grasset, Joseph, médico francês, 1849–1918. VER G. *law, phenomenon, sign*; G.-Gaussel *phenomenon*; Landouzy-G. *law*.
Gratiolet, Louis P., anatomista, fisiologista e médico francês, 1815–1865. VER G. *fibers*, em *fiber, radiation*.
grat·tage (gră-tazh'). Palavra francesa que significa raspadura ou escovadela de uma úlcera ou superfície com granulações pequenas a fim de estimular o processo de cicatrização. [Fr. raspagem]
grave (grāv). Sério, grave; que indica sintomas de caráter sério ou perigoso. [L. *gravis*, pesado, grave]
grav·el (grav'l). Gravela; pequenas concreções, em geral de ácido úrico, oxalato de cálcio ou fosfatos, formadas nos rins e que passam pelos ureteres, pela bexiga e pela uretra. SIN urocheras (1), uropsammus (1). [I.M., do Fr. ant.]
Graves, Robert James, médico irlandês, relembrado por sua descrição do bócio exoftálmico em 1835, 1796–1853. VER G. *disease, ophthalmopathy, orbitopathy*.
grav·id. Grávida. SIN pregnant.
grav·i·da (grav'i-dă). Grávida; gestante. Em inglês, a palavra *gravida* (para), quando seguida de um algarismo romano ou precedida por um prefixo latino (primi-, secundi-, etc.), designa a mulher grávida pelo número de gravidezes; p.ex., **gravida I** (gesta I) primigesta, uma mulher em sua primeira gravidez; **gravida II** (gesta II) secundigesta, uma mulher em sua segunda gravidez. Cf. para. [L. *gravidus* (adj.), fem. *gravida*, de *gravis*, pesado]
grav·id·ic (grav-id'ik). Gravídico; relativo à gravidez ou a uma gestante.
grav·id·ism (grav'id-izm). Gravidez, gestação. SIN pregnancy.
gra·vid·i·tas (grav-vid'i-tas). Gravidez, gestação. SIN pregnancy. [L.]
  g. examnia'lis, g. extra-amniótica. SIN extraamniotic *pregnancy*.
  g. exochoria'lis, g. extracorial. SIN extrachorial *pregnancy*.
gra·vid·i·ty (gră-vid'i-tē). O número de gravidezes (completas ou incompletas) de uma mulher. [L. *graviditas*, gravidez]
gra·vim·e·ter (gră-vim'ē-ter). Gravímetro. SIN hydrometer. [L. *gravis*, pesado, + G. *metron*, medida]
grav·i·met·ric (grav-i-met'rik). Gravimétrico; relativo ao ou determinado pelo peso.
grav·i·re·cep·tors (grav'i-rē-sep'terz). Gravirreceptores; órgãos receptores e terminações nervosas muito especializadas localizados na orelha inter-

na, nas articulações, nos tendões e nos músculos que fornecem ao cérebro informações sobre a posição do corpo, equilíbrio, direção das forças gravitacionais e sensação de "para baixo" e "para cima". [L. *gravis*, pesado, + receptor]

grav·i·ta·tion (grav-i-tā'shŭn). Gravitação; a força de atração entre dois corpos no universo; varia diretamente com o produto de suas massas e inversamente com o quadrado da distância entre seus centros; é expressa pela fórmula $F = Gm_1m_2l^{-2}$, onde G (constante de gravitação de Newton) = 6,67259 × 10^{-11} m³ kg⁻¹ s⁻², m_1 e m_2 correspondem às massas dos dois corpos (em kg) e l é a distância que os separa (em metros). [L. *gravitas*, peso]

grav·i·ty (grav'i-tē). Gravidade; a atração em direção à Terra que faz com que qualquer massa exerça uma força para baixo ou tenha peso. Estritamente falando, a g. é a soma algébrica da atração gravitacional da Terra com a força centrífuga, oposta e resultante da rotação da massa ao redor da Terra. Assim, a atração gravitacional nos pólos norte e sul é maior do que no equador. Um satélite em uma órbita estável apresenta gravidade zero, porque a força centrífuga do movimento orbital corresponde exatamente à força de atração gravitacional da Terra. [L. *gravitas*]
  specific g. (sp. gr.), peso específico; o peso de um corpo comparado com o peso de um outro corpo de igual volume, considerado como unidade; em geral, o peso de um líquido comparado com o peso da água destilada.
  zero g., g. zero. VER zero gravity.

Grawitz, Paul, patologista alemão, 1850–1932. VER G. *basophilia, tumor*.

gray (Gy) (grā). A unidade do SI de dose absorvida de radiação ionizante; equivale a 1 J/kg de tecido; 1 Gy = 100 rad. SIN griseus. [Louis H. *Gray*, radiologista britânico, 1905–1965]

Greeff, Richard, oftalmologista alemão, 1862–1938. VER Prowazek-G. *bodies*, em *body*.

green (grēn). Verde; uma cor do espectro situada entre o azul e o amarelo. Para corantes verdes individuais, ver os nomes específicos.
  Scheele g., verde-de-scheele, arsenito cúprico. SIN cupric arsenite.

Greenfield, L., cirurgião americano que projetou o filtro de Greenfield. VER Greenfield *filter*.

greg·a·loid (greg'a-loyd). Gregalóide; que indica uma colônia de protozoários formada pela união casual de células independentes, principalmente de sarcodinos com aderência de pseudópodes. [L. *grex* (*greg-*), um grupo]

Greg·a·ri·na (greg-ă-rī'nă). Um gênero de protozoários (esporozoários) do filo Apicomplexa, subclasse Gregarinia, parasitas de anelídeos e artrópodes; não ocorre esquizogonia nem endodiogenia no ciclo de vida. [L. *gregarius*, gregário, de *grex* (*greg-*), um grupo]

greg·a·rine (greg'a-rēn). Gregarino; um membro da subclasse Gregarinia.

Greg·a·ri·nia (greg'a-rin'i-ă). Uma subclasse de esporozoários que consiste em vários parasitas da cavidade do corpo e do trato intestinal de invertebrados, principalmente de anelídeos e artrópodes; os gêneros típicos englobam *Gregarina*, nos insetos, e *Monocystis*, nas minhocas.

greg·a·ri·no·sis (greg'a-ri-nō'sis). Gregarinose; uma doença resultante da presença de gregarinos.

Greig, David M., médico escocês; 1864–1936. VER G. *syndrome*.

gres·sion (gres'shŭn). Deslocamento de um dente para trás. [L. *grador*, pp. *gressus*, andar, de *gradus*, um passo]

grey mat·ter. Substância cinzenta. VER gray *matter*.

Grey Turner, VER Turner.

GRH Abreviatura de gonadotropin-releasing *hormone* (hormônio liberador de gonadotropina).

grid (grid). Grade. **1.** Um gráfico com linhas horizontais e perpendiculares utilizado para assinalar curvas. **2.** Nas imagens por raios X, um dispositivo formado de tiras de chumbo ou alumínio utilizado para impedir que a radiação dispersa alcance o filme de raios X. [I.M. *gridel*, do L. *craticula*, treliça]
  Amsler g., tela de Amsler. SIN Amsler *chart*.
  focused g., g. antidifusora; uma g. (2), composta por tiras de chumbo, que torna paralelo o feixe divergente de raios X, de uma distância particular, que por ela passa.
  Wetzel g., grade de Wetzel; gráfico de crescimento que assinala a altura, o peso, a adaptação física e os aspectos correlatos de crianças pequenas e adolescentes durante a fase de crescimento.

Gridley, Mary F., tecnóloga médica norte-americana, 1908–1954. VER G. *stain, stain* for fungi.

grief (grēf). Pesar, tristeza; uma resposta emocional normal a uma perda externa; diferencia-se de um distúrbio depressivo, uma vez que, em geral, melhora após um período de tempo razoável.

Griesinger, Wilhelm, neurologista alemão, 1817–1868. VER G. *disease*; bilious *typhoid* of G.; G. *sign*.

grin·de·lia (grin-dē'lē-ă). Grindélia; as folhas secas e os topos florescentes de *G. camporum*, *G. humilius* e *G. squarrosa* (família Compositae); utilizada como expectorante; um extrato líquido tem sido utilizado externamente no tratamento da intoxicação por plantas do gênero *Rhus*. [David H. *Grindel*, botânico alemão, 1776–1836]

grind·ing (grīnd'ing). Desgaste, desbastamento. SIN abrasion (3).
  selective g., desgaste seletivo; a modificação das formas oclusais dos dentes por desgaste de acordo com um plano ou por desgaste em locais selecionados marcados com fita ou papel de articulação.

grind·ing-in. Desgaste corretivo intrabucal; termo utilizado para indicar o ato de corrigir os problemas oclusais por meio do desgaste dos dentes naturais ou artificiais.

grip. 1. Gripe. SIN influenza. **2.** Preensão, fixação; pega; empunhadura. VER grasp.
  devil g., Pleurodinia epidêmica. SIN epidemic *pleurodynia*.

grippe (grip). Gripe. SIN influenza. [Fr. *gripper*, pegar]

gris·e·o·ful·vin (gris'ē-ō-ful'vin). Griseofulvina; um antibiótico fungistático produzido por *Penicillium griseofulvin*, *P. patulum* e *P. janczewskii*; utilizado no tratamento sistêmico de micoses superficiais causadas pelos dermatófitos *Microsporum*, *Trichophyton* e *Epidermophyton*; inibe a organização dos microtúbulos.

gris·e·us (gris'ē-ŭs). Cinzento. SIN gray. [L.]

Gri·so·nel·la ra·tel·li·na (gri-so-nel'a ra-te-lī'nă). Uma doninha da América do Sul, um hospedeiro-reservatório para o *Trypanosoma cruzi*.

gris·tle (gris'l). Cartilagem. SIN cartilage. [A.S.]

Gritti, Rocco, cirurgião italiano, 1828–1920. VER G. *operation*; G.-Stokes *amputation*.

Grocco, Pietro, médico italiano, 1857–1916. VER G. *sign, triangle*; Orsi-G. *method*.

Grocott-Gomori meth·en·a·mine-sil·ver stain. Corante prata-metenamina de Grocott-Gomori. Ver em stain.

Groenouw, Arthur, oftalmologista alemão, 1862–1945. VER G. corneal *dystrophy*.

groin (groyn) [TA]. Virilha. **1.** Área topográfica do abdome inferior relacionada com o canal inguinal e situada ao lado da região púbica. SIN inguen [TA], inguinal region*, regio inguinalis*, iliac region. **2.** Termo às vezes utilizado para indicar apenas a dobra localizada na junção da coxa com o tronco.

Grönblad, Ester E., oftalmologista sueca, *1898. VER G.-Strandberg *syndrome*.

GROOVE

groove (groov) [TA]. Sulco, incisura; uma depressão ou fenda alongada e estreita, localizada em qualquer superfície. VER TAMBÉM sulcus.
  alveolobuccal g., s. alveolobucal; a metade superior e inferior do vestíbulo bucal de cada lado. SIN alveolobuccal sulcus, gingivobuccal g., gingivobuccal sulcus.
  alveololabial g., s. alveololabial. **(1)** A metade superior e inferior do vestíbulo labial; **(2)** no embrião, o s. formado pelo aprofundamento do sulco labial; sua parede interna torna-se incorporada ao processo alveolar da mandíbula ou da maxila, e sua parede externa, aos lábios e às bochechas. SIN alveololabial sulcus, gingivolabial g., gingivolabial sulcus.
  alveololingual g., s. alveololingual. **(1)** A parte da cavidade oral, em cada lado do frênulo da língua, entre a língua e o processo ou a crista alveolar mandibular; **(2)** no embrião, o s. em cada lado entre o primórdio lingual e as elevações alveolares da mandíbula. SIN alveololingual sulcus, gingivolingual g., gingivolingual sulcus.
  ampullary g. [TA], s. ampular; o sulco localizado sobre a superfície externa da ampola de cada ducto semicircular, onde o nervo penetra na crista ampular. SIN sulcus ampullaris [TA], ampullary sulcus.
  anterior auricular g., incisura anterior da orelha. SIN anterior *notch* of auricle.
  anterior intermediate g., s. intermédio anterior. SIN anterior intermediate *sulcus*.
  anterior interventricular g., s. interventricular anterior. SIN anterior interventricular *sulcus*.
  anterolateral g., s. ântero-lateral. SIN anterolateral *sulcus*.
  anteromedian g., **(1)** Fissura mediana anterior do bulbo. SIN anterior median *fissure* of medulla oblongata; **(2)** fissura mediana anterior da medula espinal. SIN anterior median *fissure* of spinal cord.
  g. for arch of aorta, s. do arco da aorta; um sulco largo e profundo que se arqueia sobre o hilo na superfície mediastinal do pulmão esquerdo, formado no cadáver como resultado da impressão do arco da aorta sobre o pulmão.
  arterial g.'s [TA], sulcos arteriais; sulcos ramificados, localizados sobre a superfície interior da abóbada craniana, nos quais passam as artérias meníngeas; os sulcos mais proeminentes estão relacionados aos ramos da artéria meníngea média. SIN sulci arteriosi [TA].
  atrioventricular g., s. coronário; SIN coronary *sulcus*.
  g. for auditory tube, s. da tuba auditiva. SIN *sulcus* for pharyngotympanic tube.
  auriculoventricular g., s. coronário; SIN coronary *sulcus*.
  bicipital g., s. intertubercular; *termo oficial alternativo para intertubercular *sulcus*.

branchial g., s. branquial; um s. embrionário externo situado entre arcos branquiais contíguos. VER TAMBÉM branchial clefts, em cleft.
carotid g., s. carótico do esfenóide. SIN cavernous g.
carpal g. [TA], s. do carpo; a concavidade localizada na superfície anterior do arco formado pelos ossos carpais. SIN sulcus carpi [TA], carpal canal (2).
cavernous g. [TA], s. carótico do esfenóide; o sulco no corpo do osso esfenóide sobre o qual a artéria carótida interna atravessa o seio cavernoso. SIN sulcus caroticus [TA], carotid g., carotid sulcus.
chiasmatic g., s. pré-quiasmático. SIN prechiasmatic sulcus.
coronary g., s. coronário. SIN coronary sulcus.
costal g. [TA], s. da costela; um sulco, localizado na margem interna inferior da costela, que aloja os vasos e o nervo intercostais. SIN sulcus costae [TA], subcostal g.
g. of crus of helix [TA], s. do ramo da hélice; uma fissura transversa, localizada na superfície craniana da orelha, que corresponde ao ramo da hélice. SIN sulcus cruris helicis [TA].
dental g., s. dentário; uma depressão transitória localizada na superfície gengival da mandíbula embrionária ao longo da linha de crescimento interno da lâmina dentária.
g. for the descending aorta, s. para a aorta descendente; um sulco largo, profundo e vertical localizado posteriormente ao hilo, na superfície mediastinal do pulmão esquerdo do cadáver e formado como resultado da impressão da aorta descendente sobre o pulmão.
developmental g.'s, sulcos de desenvolvimento; linhas finas encontradas no esmalte de um dente que marcam a junção dos lobos da coroa durante o seu desenvolvimento. SIN developmental lines.
digastric g., incisura mastóidea. SIN mastoid notch.
ethmoidal g. [TA], s. etmoidal; um sulco localizado na superfície interna de cada osso nasal e que aloja o ramo nasal externo do nervo etmoidal anterior. SIN sulcus ethmoidalis [TA].
g. of first rib for subclavian artery [TA], s. da artéria subclávia da primeira costela; um sulco localizado posteriormente ao tubérculo do músculo escaleno, na superfície superior da primeira costela e ao longo do qual passa a artéria subclávia. SIN sulcus arteriae subclaviae costae primae [TA], sulcus costae arteriae subclaviae.
frontal g.'s, sulcos frontais. VER inferior frontal sulcus, middle frontal sulcus, superior frontal sulcus.
gingival g., s. gengival. SIN gingival sulcus.
gingivobuccal g., s. gengivobucal. SIN alveolobuccal g.
gingivolabial g., s. gengivolabial. SIN alveololabial g.
gingivolingual g., s. gengivolingual. SIN alveololingual g.
greater palatine g. [TA], s. palatino maior; um sulco localizado tanto no corpo da maxila como na lâmina perpendicular do osso palatino; quando os ossos se articulam, os sulcos formam o canal palatino maior. SIN sulcus palatinus major [TA], pterygopalatine g., sulcus for greater palatine nerve, sulcus pterygopalatinus.
g. for greater petrosal nerve [TA], s. do nervo petroso maior no temporal; o sulco, localizado na superfície anterior da parte petrosa do osso temporal, que aloja o nervo petroso maior. SIN sulcus nervi petrosi majoris [TA].
Harrison g., s. de Harrison; uma deformidade das costelas resultante da tração exercida pelo diafragma sobre as costelas enfraquecidas pelo raquitismo ou por outra condição que cause amolecimento ósseo.
inferior petrosal g., s. do seio petroso inferior. SIN g. for inferior petrosal sinus.
g. for inferior petrosal sinus [TA], s. do seio petroso inferior; um sulco que aloja o seio petroso inferior e é formado pela união de sulcos que apresentam nomes semelhantes e estão localizados na parte petrosa do osso temporal e na parte basilar do osso occipital. SIN sulcus sinus petrosi inferioris [TA], inferior petrosal g., inferior petrosal sulcus.
g. for inferior venae cava, s. da veia cava inferior. SIN sulcus for vena cava.
infraorbital g. [TA], s. infra-orbital; um sulco localizado na face orbital da maxila, que se aprofunda gradualmente e se dirige ao canal infra-orbital. SIN sulcus infraorbitalis [TA].
interosseous g., (1) Sulco do calcâneo. SIN calcaneal sulcus; (2) sulco do tálus. SIN sulcus tali.
interosseous g. of calcaneus, s. do calcâneo. SIN calcaneal sulcus.
interosseous g. of talus, s. do tálus. SIN sulcus tali.
intertubercular g. [TA], s. intertubercular. SIN intertubercular sulcus.
interventricular g.'s, sulcos interventriculares. VER anterior interventricular sulcus, posterior interventricular sulcus.
lacrimal g. [TA], s. lacrimal; o sulco localizado na face nasal da maxila que, juntamente com o osso lacrimal, forma a fossa do saco lacrimal. SIN sulcus lacrimalis [TA].
laryngotracheal g., s. laringotraqueal; a depressão localizada no assoalho da extremidade caudal da faringe embrionária, que se continua para trás sobre a parede ventral do intestino anterior; a partir desse s., desenvolvem-se a parte inferior da laringe, a traquéia, os brônquios e os pulmões. SIN tracheobronchial g.

lateral bicipital g. [TA], s. bicipital lateral da região braquial; o sulco situado ao longo da face lateral do braço que separa o músculo bíceps braquial dos músculos braquiais. SIN sulcus bicipitalis lateralis [TA], sulcus bicipitalis radialis*.
g. of lesser petrosal nerve [TA], s. do nervo petroso menor; o sulco situado na face anterior da parte petrosa do osso temporal que acomoda o nervo petroso menor em seu trajeto até o gânglio ótico. SIN sulcus nervi petrosi minoris [TA].
linguogingival g., s. linguogengival; um s. que separa a parte mandibular embrionária da língua do restante do processo mandibular.
Lucas g., s. de Lucas. SIN stria spinosa.
g. of lung for subclavian artery, s. da artéria subclávia no pulmão; um sulco localizado na superfície do pulmão do cadáver, abaixo do ápice, que corresponde ao trajeto da artéria subclávia. SIN sulcus subclavius.
major g., s. maior; em uma análise detalhada da estrutura do DNA, é possível observar dois tipos de sulcos: o s. maior tem os átomos de nitrogênio e oxigênio dos pares de bases apontando para dentro e para a frente do eixo helicoidal, enquanto, no s. menor, os átomos de nitrogênio e oxigênio apontam para fora; é importante por ser mais dependente da composição das bases e, também, pela possibilidade de ser o local para o reconhecimento proteico de regiões ou de seqüências específicas do DNA.
malleolar g. [TA], s. maleolar; um sulco largo localizado na face posterior do maléolo medial, através do qual corre o tendão do músculo tibial posterior. SIN sulcus malleolaris [TA], g. for tibialis posterior tendon, malleolar sulcus.
mastoid g., incisura, mastóidea. SIN mastoid notch.
medial bicipital g. [TA], s. bicipital medial da região braquial; o sulco localizado ao longo da face medial do braço e que separa o músculo bíceps braquial dos músculos braquiais. SIN sulcus bicipitalis medialis [TA], sulcus bicipitalis ulnaris*.
median g. of tongue, s. mediano da língua. SIN median sulcus of tongue.
medullary g., s. neural; SIN neural g.
middle meningeal artery g., s. da artéria meníngea média; um s. estreito localizado sobre a lâmina interna da calvária e observado nas radiografias de perfil como uma linha fina e escura, que pode ser confundida com uma fratura de crânio. VER sulci arteriosi, em sulcus.
g. for middle temporal artery [TA], s. da artéria temporal média; um sulco vertical localizado acima do meato acústico externo, na face externa da parte escamosa do osso temporal. SIN sulcus arteriae temporalis mediae [TA], sulcus for middle temporal artery.
minor g., s. menor. VER major g.
musculospiral g., s. do nervo radial. SIN radial g.
mylohyoid g. [TA], s. milo-hióideo; um sulco localizado na face medial do ramo da mandíbula, começando na língula; aloja a artéria e o nervo milo-hióideos. SIN sulcus mylohyoideus [TA], mylohyoid fossa.
g. of nail matrix, s. da matriz da unha. SIN sulcus matricis unguis.
nasolabial g., s. nasolabial. SIN nasolabial sulcus.
nasopalatine g., s. nasopalatino; um s. localizado sobre o vômer, que aloja o nervo nasopalatino.
nasopharyngeal g., s. nasofaríngeo; uma linha indistinta que marca o limite entre as cavidades nasais e a nasofaringe.
neural g., s. neural; o s. semelhante a uma calha, formado na linha média da superfície dorsal do embrião pela elevação progressiva das margens laterais da placa neural; a fusão dorsal definitiva das margens resulta na formação do tubo neural. SIN medullary g.
obturator g. [TA], s. obturatório; um sulco profundo localizado na face interna do ramo superior do púbis. SIN sulcus obturatorius [TA].
occipital g. [TA], s. occipital; um sulco estreito, medial à incisura mastóidea do osso temporal, que aloja a artéria occipital. SIN sulcus arteriae occipitalis [TA], sulcus of occipital artery.
olfactory g., s. olfatório. SIN olfactory sulcus.
olfactory g. of nasal cavity [TA], s. olfatório da cavidade nasal; sulco estreito, localizado na cavidade nasal, acima da crista do nariz, que se estende desde o átrio do meato médio até a área olfatória. SIN sulcus olfactorius cavi nasi [TA], olfactory sulcus of nasal cavity.
optic g., s. pré-quiasmático. SIN prechiasmatic sulcus.
palatine g.'s [TA], sulcos palatinos; vários sulcos localizados na face inferior do processo palatino da maxila nos quais repousam os vasos e nervos palatinos. SIN sulci palatini [TA].
palatovaginal g. [TA], s. palatovaginal; uma fenda localizada sobre a face inferior do processo vaginal do osso esfenóide que se comunica abaixo com o processo esfenóide do osso palatino para formar o canal palatovaginal. SIN sulcus palatovaginalis [TA].
paraglenoid g., s. paraglenóide, s. pré-auricular. SIN preauricular g.
pharyngeal g.'s, sulcos faríngeos; sulcos embrionários endodérmicos ou ectodérmicos situados entre arcos faríngeos sucessivos.
pharyngotympanic g., s. da tuba auditiva. SIN sulcus for pharyngotympanic tube.
pontomedullary g., s. bulbopontino. SIN medullopontine sulcus [TA].

popliteal g., s. poplíteo. SIN g. for popliteus.
g. for popliteus [TA], s. poplíteo; um s. localizado no côndilo lateral do fêmur, entre o epicôndilo e a margem articular. Sua extremidade anterior dá origem ao músculo poplíteo, e a posterior aloja o tendão do músculo, quando o joelho está completamente fletido. SIN sulcus popliteus [TA], popliteal g.
posterior auricular g. [TA], s. posterior da orelha; o s. situado entre o antitrago e a cauda da hélice, cobrindo a fissura antitrago-helicina. SIN sulcus posterior auriculae [TA].
posterior intermediate g., s. intermédio posterior. SIN posterior intermediate sulcus.
posterior interventricular g., s. interventricular posterior. SIN posterior interventricular sulcus.
posterolateral g., s. póstero-lateral. SIN posterolateral sulcus.
preauricular g., s. pré-auricular; um s. na face pélvica do ílio, lateralmente à face auricular; é mais pronunciado na mulher. SIN paraglenoid g., paraglenoid sulcus, preauricular sulcus, sulcus paraglenoidalis.
primary labial g., s. labial no embrião. SIN labial sulcus.
primitive g., s. primitivo; a depressão mediana localizada na linha primitiva, ladeada pelas cristas primitivas. SIN primitive furrow.
g. of promontory of labyrinthine wall of tympanic cavity [TA], s. do promontório na parede labiríntica da cavidade timpânica; um sulco estreito e ramificado que corre verticalmente na superfície do promontório da orelha média e aloja o plexo timpânico. SIN sulcus promontorii cavitatis tympanicae [TA], sulcus of promontory of tympanic cavity.
g. for pterygoid hamulus [TA], s. do hâmulo pterigóideo; um sulco situado na base do hâmulo pterigóideo que forma uma polia para o tendão do músculo tensor do véu palatino. SIN sulcus hamuli pterygoidei [TA], sulcus of pterygoid hamulus.
g. of pterygoid hamulus [TA], incisura pterigomaxilar; a incisura ou fissura situada entre a tuberosidade da maxila e o hâmulo pterigóideo do osso esfenóide. SIN hamular notch, pterygomaxillary notch.
pterygopalatine g., s. palatino maior. SIN greater palatine g.
pulmonary g., s. pulmonar; o recesso profundo situado em cada lado da coluna vertebral formado pela extensão posterior da curvatura das costelas. SIN sulcus pulmonalis [TA], paravertebral gutter, pulmonary sulcus.
radial g. [TA], s. radial; o sulco raso que passa ao redor da diáfise do úmero; aloja o nervo radial e a artéria braquial profunda. SIN sulcus nervi radialis [TA], g. for radial nerve*, musculospiral g., spiral g.
g. for radial nerve, s. do nervo radial no úmero; *termo oficial alternativo para radial g.
retention g., s. retentivo; um dos sulcos que formam as constrições verticais opostas em um dente para auxiliar na retenção de uma restauração dentária.
rhombic g.'s, sulcos rômbicos; sete pares de fendas transversas localizadas no assoalho do cérebro posterior embrionário.
sagittal g., s. do seio sagital superior. SIN g. for superior sagittal sinus.
Sibson g., s. de Sibson; um s. ocasionalmente observado no lado externo do tórax e formado pela margem inferior proeminente do músculo peitoral maior.
sigmoid g., s. do seio sigmóide. SIN g. for sigmoid sinus.
g. for sigmoid sinus [TA], s. do seio sigmóide; um sulco largo encontrado na fossa craniana posterior; começa na parte lateral do osso occipital e, a seguir, curva-se ao redor do processo jugular sobre a parte mastóidea do osso temporal e que, por fim, gira agudamente sobre o ângulo inferior posterior do osso parietal, tornando-se contínuo com o sulco transverso; aloja o seio transverso. SIN sulcus sinus sigmoidei [TA], sigmoid fossa, sigmoid g., sigmoid sulcus.
skin g.'s, sulcos da pele. SIN skin sulci, em sulcus.
g. for spinal nerve [TA], s. do nervo espinal na vértebra; o sulco direcionado lateralmente e situado sobre a face superior dos processos transversos das vértebras cervicais típicas, entre os tubérculos anterior e posterior, ao longo do qual passa o nervo espinal emergente. SIN sulcus nervi spinalis [TA].
spiral g., s. do nervo radial. SIN radial g.
subclavian g. [TA], s. do músculo subclávio; um sulco, localizado na face inferior do corpo da clavícula, no qual se fixa o músculo subclávio. SIN sulcus musculi subclavii [TA], g. for subclavius*, subclavian sulcus, sulcus subclavianus.
g. for subclavian vein [TA], s. da veia subclávia na primeira costela; um sulco, situado anteriormente ao tubérculo do escaleno da primeira costela, que marca o trajeto da veia subclávia através da costela. SIN sulcus venae subclaviae [TA].
g. for subclavius, s. do músculo subclávio na clavícula; *termo oficial alternativo para subclavian g.
subcostal g., s. da costela. SIN costal g.
g. for superior petrosal sinus [TA], s. do seio petroso superior; um sulco, localizado sobre a crista da parte petrosa do osso temporal, no qual repousa o seio petroso superior. SIN sulcus sinus petrosi superioris [TA], superior petrosal sulcus.
g. for superior sagittal sinus, s. do seio sagital superior; o sulco localizado na linha média da lâmina interna da calvária, que aloja o seio sagital superior. SIN sagittal g., sagittal sulcus, sulcus sinus sagittalis superioris, superior longitudinal sulcus.
g. for superior vena cava, s. da veia cava superior; um s., localizado na superfície do pulmão direito do pulmão, acima do hilo, no qual corre a veia cava superior. SIN sulcus venae cavae cranialis.
supplemental g., s. suplementar; uma depressão curvilínea normalmente encontrada em cada lado de uma crista triangular (crista triangularis).
supra-acetabular g. [TA], s. supra-acetabular; um sulco, póstero-superior ao acetábulo, onde se fixa a cabeça refletida do músculo reto femoral. SIN sulcus supraacetabularis [TA], supraacetabular sulcus.
g. for tendon of fibularis longus [TA], s. do tendão do músculo fibular longo. (1) O s. situado abaixo da tróclea fibular do calcâneo; (2) o s. localizado distalmente à tuberosidade do osso cubóide. SIN sulcus tendinis musculi fibularis longi [TA], g. for tendon of peroneus longus*, sulcus tendinis musculi peronei longi (1)*.
g. for tendon of flexor hallucis longus [TA], s. do tendão do músculo flexor longo do hálux; um s. vertical localizado no processo posterior do tálus, contínuo com um outro sulco (de mesmo nome), situado na face inferior do sustentáculo do tálus do calcâneo. SIN sulcus tendinis musculi flexoris hallucis longi [TA].
g. for tendon of peroneus longus, s. do tendão do músculo fibular longo; *termo oficial alternativo para g. for tendon of fibularis longus.
g. for tibialis posterior tendon, s. maleolar. SIN malleolar g.
tracheobronchial g., s. traqueobrônquico. SIN laryngotracheal g.
transverse anthelicine g., s. transverso da antélice; um sulco profundo, localizado sobre a face craniana da orelha, que separa as eminências da fossa triangular da concha. SIN sulcus anthelicis transversus.
transverse nasal g., s. nasal transverso. SIN stria nasi transversa.
g. for transverse sinus [TA], s. do seio transverso; o sulco localizado sobre a face interna do osso occipital e que marca o trajeto do seio transverso; o tentório está fixo às suas margens. SIN sulcus sinus transversi [TA], sulcus for transverse sinus.
tympanic g., s. timpânico. SIN tympanic sulcus.
g. for ulnar nerve [TA], s. do nervo ulnar no úmero; uma fenda na face posterior do epicôndilo medial do úmero e que aloja o nervo ulnar. SIN sulcus nervi ulnaris [TA].
urethral g., s. uretral; o s. situado na superfície ventral do pênis embrionário e que, no final, fecha-se para formar a parte peniana da uretra.
venous g.'s [TA], sulcos venosos; sulcos ocasionalmente encontrados na face interna do osso parietal e nos quais estão situadas as veias. SIN sulci venosi [TA].
vertebral g., s. vertebral; a depressão, limitada pelos processos espinhosos e pelas lâminas das vértebras, na qual repousam os músculos profundos das costas.
g. for vertebral artery [TA], s. da artéria vertebral; o s., localizado na face superior do arco posterior do atlas, que conduz a artéria vertebral medialmente em direção ao forame magno. SIN sulcus arteriae vertebralis [TA], sulcus for vertebral artery.
vomeral g., s. do vômer. SIN vomerine g.
vomerine g. [TA], s. do vômer; o sulco localizado na margem anterior do vômer e que recebe a cartilagem septal. SIN sulcus vomeris [TA], sulcus vomeralis, vomeral g., vomeral sulcus.
vomerovaginal g. [TA], s. vomerovaginal; um s. localizado na face inferior do processo vaginal do osso esfenóide e que, juntamente com a asa do vômer, forma o canal vomerovaginal. SIN sulcus vomerovaginalis [TA].

Gross, Ludwik, oncologista norte-americano, *1904. VER G. virus, leukemia virus.
gross (gros). Macroscópico; grosseiro ou grande; grande bastante para ser visível a olho nu. [L. *grossus*, espesso]
group (groop). Grupo, grupamento. **1.** Vários objetos semelhantes ou correlatos. **2.** Em química, um radical. Para grupamentos químicos individuais, ver o nome específico.
blood g., g. sanguíneo. VER blood group.
characterizing g., g. caracterizador; um g. de átomos de uma molécula que distingue de todas as outras classes a classe de substâncias no qual está presente; assim, a carbonila (CO) é o g. característico das cetonas; COOH, dos ácidos orgânicos, etc.
connective tissue g., g. de tecidos conectivos; um nome coletivo dado ao tecido mucoso, à dentina, ao osso, à cartilagem e ao tecido conectivo comum, todos derivados do mesênquima.
control g., g.-controle; um g. de indivíduos que participa de um experimento como um outro g. de indivíduos que também participa, mas que não é exposto à variável sob investigação. VER TAMBÉM experimental g.
cytophil g., g. citófilo; a parte de um anticorpo que o liga a uma célula.
determinant g., g. determinante. SIN antigenic *determinant.*
diagnosis-related g. (DRG), g. de diagnóstico homogêneo; um esquema criado para possibilitar a cobrança pelos serviços médicos prestados, principal-

mente hospitalares, no qual as doenças estão reunidas em grupos de acordo com os recursos exigidos pela atenção médica dispensada, que está disposta em categorias diagnósticas. Um valor em dólares é atribuído a cada grupo como a base para o pagamento de todos os casos desse grupo, sem relação com o custo real da assistência médica ou com a duração da hospitalização de qualquer caso em particular, como mecanismo para motivar os provedores de assistência de saúde a economizar.

encounter g., g. de encontro; uma forma de treinamento da sensibilidade psicológica que enfatiza a experiência dos relacionamentos individuais dentro do g. e minimiza o aporte de dados intelectuais e didáticos; o g. enfoca o presente em vez de ocupar-se com o passado ou com os problemas externos de seus membros. VER TAMBÉM sensitivity training g.

experimental g., g. experimental; um g. de indivíduos expostos à variável de um experimento, em oposição ao g.-controle.

functional g., g. funcional. VER function (4).

HACEK g., g. HACEK; um grupo de bactérias Gram-negativas que engloba *Haemophilus* spp., *Actinobacillus actinomycetemcomitans*, *Cardiobacterium hominis*, *Eikenella corrodens* e *Kingella kingae*. As bactérias desse grupo têm em comum a necessidade de que os meios de culturas apresentem uma atmosfera enriquecida com dióxido de carbono e apresentam a capacidade de infectar as valvas cardíacas humanas.

linkage g., g. de ligação; um conjunto de dois ou mais *loci* que, como demonstrado por meio de análise de ligação, encontram-se fisicamente próximos no genoma, mas que ainda não foram associados a cromossomas específicos. Está se tornando um termo antiquado.

matched g.'s, grupos pareados; um método de controle experimental no qual os indivíduos de um g. são combinados com os indivíduos de outros grupos em uma relação de um para um, levando em consideração todas as variáveis do organismo (p. ex., a idade, o sexo, a altura, o peso) que o experimentador acredita poderiam influenciar a variável sob investigação.

prosthetic g., g. prostético; um composto — que não é um aminoácido — ligado a uma proteína, em geral de modo reversível, que confere novas propriedades à proteína conjugada assim produzida. VER TAMBÉM coenzyme.

sensitivity training g., g. de treinamento da sensibilidade; um g., mais popular durante as décadas de 60 e 70, no qual os membros buscam desenvolver o autoconhecimento e uma compreensão dos processos grupais, em vez de obter tratamento para um distúrbio emocional. VER TAMBÉM encounter g., personal growth *laboratory*.

symptom g., g. de sintomas. VER syndrome, complex (1).

T g., g. T; abreviatura de training g. (g. de treinamento).

therapeutic g., g. terapêutico; qualquer g. de pacientes que se reúnem para buscar mutuamente um desenvolvimento pessoal e psicoterapêutico, assim como planos de mudança de vida.

training g. (T g.), g. de treinamento; qualquer g. que enfatiza o treinamento do autoconhecimento e a dinâmica de grupo. VER sensitivity training g.

Grover, Ralph W., dermatologista norte-americano, *1920. VER G. *disease*.

growth (grōth). Crescimento; o aumento no tamanho de um ser vivo, ou de qualquer uma de suas partes, que ocorre durante o processo de desenvolvimento.

accretionary g., c. por acreção; c. por um aumento de material intercelular.

appositional g., c. por aposição; c. realizado pela adição de novas camadas sobre aquelas previamente formadas; p.ex., a adição de lamelas na formação do osso; é o método característico de c., quando materiais rígidos estão envolvidos.

auxetic g., c. por auxese; c. por aumento no tamanho das células componentes. SIN intussusceptive g.

bacterial g., c. bacteriano; c. de uma cultura bacteriana por aumento do material celular ou do número de células.

differential g., c. diferencial; diferentes velocidades de c. em tecidos ou estruturas associados; utilizado principalmente em embriologia, quando as diferenças nas velocidades de c. resultam em alterações nas proporções ou relações originais.

exponential g., c. exponencial. VER logarithmic *phase*.

interstitial g., c. intersticial; c. de vários centros diferentes dentro de uma área; em contraste com o c. por aposição, ele pode ocorrer apenas quando os materiais envolvidos não são rígidos.

intussusceptive g., c. por auxese. SIN auxetic g.

multiplicative g., c. multiplicativo; c. por aumento do número de células.

new g., neoformação. SIN neoplasm.

grub (grŭb). Larva, lagarta ou berne semelhante a um verme de certos insetos, sobretudo das ordens Coleoptera, Diptera e Hymenoptera e do gênero *Hypoderma*.

Gruber, George B., médico alemão, 1884–1977. VER Meckel-G. *syndrome*; Martin-G. *anastomosis*.

Gruber, Josef, otologista austríaco, 1827–1900. VER G. *method*.

Gruber, Max von, higienista alemão, 1853–1927. VER G. *reaction*; G.-Widal *reaction*.

Gruber, Wenzel (Wenaslaus) L., anatomista russo, 1814–1890. VER G. *cul-de-sac*; G.-Landzert *fossa*.

gru·el (groo′el). Mingau, papa; um alimento semilíquido de farinha de aveia ou outro cereal fervido em água; mingau ralo. [atr. do Fr. ant., do L. mediev. *grutum*, refeição]

gru·mous (groo′mŭs). Grumoso; espesso e grumoso, como o coágulo sanguíneo. [L. *grumus*, um pequeno monte]

Grunert spur. Esporão de Grunert. Ver em spur.

Grunstein-Hogness as·say. Análise de Grunstein-Hogness. Ver em assay.

Grünwald. VER May-Grünwald *stain*.

Grütz, O., dermatologista alemão, *1886. VER Bürger-G. *syndrome*.

Grynfeltt, Joseph C., cirurgião francês, 1840–1913. VER G. *triangle*.

gry·o·chrome (grī′ō-krōm). Griocroma; termo aplicado por Nissl às células nervosas nas quais a parte corável existe na forma de diminutos grânulos, sem um arranjo definido. [G. *gry*, algo insignificante, + *chrōma*, cor]

gry·po·sis (gri-pō′sis). Gripose; uma curvatura anormal. [G. *grypos*, recurvado, em forma de gancho, + *-osis*, condição]

GSH Abreviatura de glutathione (glutationa).

GSR Abreviatura de galvanic skin *response* (resposta cutânea galvânica).

GSSG Abreviatura de glutathione disulfide (dissulfeto de glutationa).

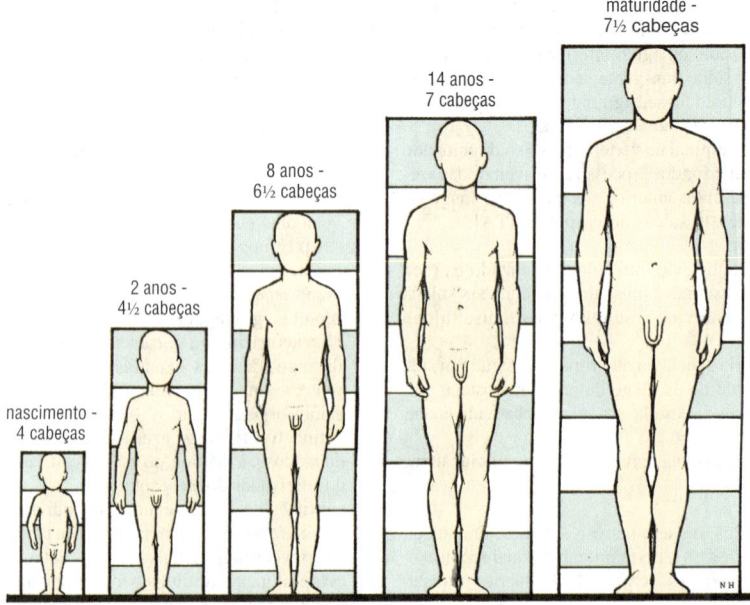

crescimento: proporções em diversas idades

G-stro·phan·thin. Estrofantina G. VER ouabain.
gt. Abreviatura de gutta (gota).
g-tol·er·ance. Tolerância G; a tolerância de uma pessoa ou uma peça de um equipamento às forças que se desenvolvem como resultado da aceleração ou desaceleração.
GTP Abreviatura de guanosine 5′-triphosphate (5′-trifosfato de guanosina).
gtt. Abreviatura de guttae (gotas).
GU Abreviatura de genitourinary (genitourinário).
Gua Abreviatura de guanine (guanina).
guai·ac (gwī′ak). Guaiaco; a resina do *Guaiacum officinale* ou do *G. sanctum* (família Zygophyllaceae); um agente nauseante, diaforético e estimulante e um reagente utilizado na detecção de sangue oculto. SIN guaiac gum. [Esp. *guayaco*, imitação do nome nativo caribenho]
guai·a·cin (gwī′ă-sin). Guaiacina; a saponina do guaiaco, um dos constituintes do guaiaco, utilizado como reagente em reações com oxidases, nas quais se colore de azul.
guai·a·col (gwī′ă-kol). Guaiacol; tem sido utilizado como expectorante e desinfetante intestinal; está também disponível como carbonato de g.
  g. glyceryl ether, éter gliceril guaiacol. SIN guaifenesin.
  g. phosphate, fosfato de guaiacol; éter guaiacil fosfórico, um pó branco cristalino, insolúvel em água; é utilizado como anti-séptico intestinal e nos estados febris.
guai·fen·e·sin (gwī-fen′ĕ-sin). Guaifenesina; um expectorante que, supostamente, reduz a viscosidade do escarro, facilitando, dessa forma, sua eliminação. SIN glyceryl guaiacolate, guaiacol glyceryl ether.
guan·a·benz ac·e·tate (gwahn-ă-benz′). Acetato de guanabenzo; um anti-hipertensivo antiadrenérgico com ação central, que age de modo semelhante à clonidina.
gua·na·cline sul·fate (gwahn′ă-klēn). Sulfato de guanaclina; um anti-hipertensivo.
gua·na·drel sul·fate (gwahn′ă-drel). Sulfato de guanadrel; uma droga anti-hipertensiva cuja ação é semelhante à da guanetidina.
gua·nase (gwahn′ās). Guanase. SIN *guanine deaminase.*
guanazolo (gwahn-ă-zōl′ō). Guanazol. SIN 8-azaguanine.
gua·neth·i·dine sul·fate (gwahn-eth′i-dēn). Sulfato de guanetidina; um potente agente anti-hipertensivo. Parece interferir na liberação do mediador químico (norepinefrina) na junção neuroefetora simpática; tomado nas doses recomendadas, não produz bloqueio ganglionar ou parassimpático. Em oftalmologia, é utilizado topicamente no tratamento do glaucoma e na neutralização da retração das pálpebras da doença de Graves.
guan·fa·cine (gwan′fă-sēn). Guanfacina; um agente anti-hipertensivo; um agonista α_2-adrenérgico que age no sistema nervoso central, reduzindo a ação do sistema nervoso simpático; seu perfil farmacológico é semelhante ao da clonidina.
gua·ni·dine (gwahn′i-dēn, -din). Guanidina; um composto fortemente alcalino geralmente encontrado (em algumas plantas e animais inferiores) na forma de cloridrato; um dos constituintes da creatina e da arginina; administrado como estimulante colinérgico da musculatura estriada.
guan·id·i·ni·um (gwahn′i-din-ē-um). Guanidínio; que se refere à porção guanidina em uma molécula (p.ex., na arginina).
gua·ni·di·no·ac·e·tate (gwahn′i-din-ō-ăs-ĕ-tāt). Guanidinoacetato; um intermediário da biossíntese da creatina.
gua·ni·di·no·ac·e·tate *N*-meth·yl·trans·fer·ase. Guanidinoacetato *N*-metiltransferase; a enzima que catalisa a transferência de um grupamento metila da *S*-adenosil-L-metionina ("metionina ativa") para o guanidinoacetato (glicociamina), formando creatina e *S*-adenosil-L-homocisteína.
gua·nine (Gua, G) (gwahn′ēn, -in). Guanina; 2-amino-6-oxipurina; uma das duas principais purinas (a outra é a adenina) que está presente em todos os ácidos nucleicos.
  g. aminase, g. aminase. SIN g. deaminase.
  g. deaminase, g. desaminase; uma desaminase do fígado que catalisa a hidrólise da guanina em xantina e amônia; o primeiro passo da degradação da purina. SIN guanase, g. aminase.
  g. deoxyribonucleotide, desoxirribonucleotídeo de g. SIN deoxyguanylic acid.
  g. ribonucleotide, ribonucleotídeo de g. SIN guanylic acid.
gua·no·chlor sul·fate (gwahn′ō-klor). Sulfato de guanocloro; utilizado como agente bloqueador α-adrenérgico no tratamento da hipertensão essencial.
gua·no·sine (G, Guo) (gwahn′ō-sēn, -sin). Guanosina; 9-β-D-ribosilguanina (a combinação do N-9 da guanina com o C-1 da β-D-ribose); um dos principais constituintes do RNA e dos nucleotídeos de guanina. SIN 9-β-D-ribofuranosylguanine.
  cyclic g. 3′,5′-monophosphate (cGMP), 3′,5′-monofosfato cíclico de g.; um análogo do AMPc; um segundo mensageiro para o fator natriurético atrial. SIN cyclic GMP.
gua·no·sine 5′-di·phos·phate (GDP). 5′-difosfato de guanosina; guanosina esterificada na sua posição 5′ com o ácido difosfórico; apresenta-se fortemente ligada nos microtúbulos.
gua·no·sine 5′-monophos·phate. 5′-monofosfato de guanosina. SIN guanylic acid.

gua·no·sine 5′-tri·phos·phate (GTP). 5′-trifosfato de guanosina; um precursor imediato dos nucleotídeos de guanina do ARN; semelhante ao ATP; é crucial na formação dos microtúbulos.
  GTP cyclohydrolase, ciclo-hidrolase de 5′-trifosfato de guanosina; uma enzima que catalisa a reação entre 5′-trifosfato de guanosina e H_2O, que forma formato e um precursor da tetraidrobiopterina; a deficiência dessa enzima resulta em uma forma de hiperfenilalaninemia maligna.
guan·ox·an sul·fate (gwahn-ok′san). Sulfato de guanoxano; um agente anti-hipertensivo.
gua·nyl (gwahn′il). Guanila; o radical da guanina.
  g. cyclase, g. ciclase. SIN guanylate cyclase.
guan·y·late cy·clase (gwahn′i-lāt). Guanilato ciclase; substância análoga à adenilato (adenilil) ciclase, que promove a transformação cíclica de 5′-trifosfato de guanosina em 3′:5′-monofosfato cíclico de guanosina e também produz pirofosfato; é ativada pelo óxido nítrico. SIN guanyl cyclase, guanylyl cyclase.
gua·nyl·ic ac·id (GMP) (gwă-nil′ik). Ácido guanílico; um componente importante dos ácidos ribonucleicos. SIN guanine ribonucleotide, guanosine 5′-monophosphate.
  g. a. reductase (GMP reductase), a. g. redutase; uma enzima que catalisa a reação do ácido guanílico com o NADPH, que produz IMP, NH_3 e $NADP^+$; uma parte da via de recuperação da purina.
  g. a. synthetase (GMP synthetase), a. g. sintetase; uma enzima que catalisa a reação entre L-glutamina, XMP e ATP para produzir GMP, L-glutamato, AMP e pirofosfato; uma etapa-chave da biossíntese da purina.
gua·nyl·o·ri·bo·nu·cle·ase (gwahn′i-lō-rī-bō-noo′klē-ās). Guanilorribonuclease. SIN RNase T_1. Ver as entradas em ribonuclease.
gua·nyl·yl (gwahn′i-lil). Guanilila; o radical do ácido guanílico.
  g. cyclase, g. ciclase. SIN guanylate cyclase.
gua·ra·na (gwah-rah-nah′). Guaraná; uma pasta seca de sementes esmagadas de *Paullinia cupana* (família Sapindaceae), uma planta trepadeira cultivada de forma extensiva no Brasil. Contém guaranina (cafeína), saponina, um óleo volátil e ácido paulinitânico. Tem sido utilizado no alívio da cefaléia. [palavra nativa brasileira]
gua·ra·nine (gwahr′ă-nēn). Guaranina. SIN caffeine.
guard·ing (gard′ing). Defesa muscular; espasmo muscular que visa minimizar o movimento ou a agitação dos locais afetados por um ferimento ou por uma doença.
  abdominal g., d. m. abdominal; espasmo dos músculos da parede abdominal, detectado durante a palpação, que visa proteger as vísceras abdominais inflamadas da compressão; é, em geral, resultante de inflamação da superfície parietal do peritônio, como ocorre na apendicite, diverticulite ou peritonite generalizada.
  involuntary g., d. m. involuntária; espasmo dos músculos abdominais causado por inflamação do retroperitônio e que não pode ser intencionalmente suprimido.
  voluntary g., d.m. voluntária; espasmo dos músculos abdominais que pode ser intencionalmente suprimido.
Guarnieri, Giuseppi, médico italiano, 1856–1918. VER G. *bodies*, em *body*.
gu·ber·nac·u·lum (goo′ber-nak′ū-lŭm) [TA]. Gubernáculo; um cordão fibroso que liga duas estruturas. Uma coluna mesenquimatosa de tecido que liga o testículo fetal ao escroto em desenvolvimento; parece participar na descida dos testículos. SIN g. testis. [L. um timão, um leme]
  g. den′tis, g. do dente; uma faixa de tecido conectivo que une o saco dentário à gengiva.
  Hunter g., g. de Hunter; termo obsoleto para g. testis.
  g. tes′tis, g. do testículo. SIN gubernaculum.
Gubler, Adolphe, médico francês, 1821–1879. VER G. *line, paralysis, syndrome*; Millard-G. *syndrome*.
Gudden, Bernhard A. von, neurologista alemão, 1824–1886. VER G. *commissure, ganglion,* tegmental *nuclei*, em *nucleus*.
Guedel, Arthur Ernest, anestesiologista norte-americano, 1883–1956. VER G. *airway*.
Guéneau de Mussy, Noël F.O., médico francês, 1813–1885. VER G. de M. *point*.
Guérin, Alphonse F.M. cirurgião francês, 1816–1895. VER G. *fold fracture, glands,* em *gland, sinus, valve*.
Guérin, Camille, bacteriologista francesa, 1872–1961. VER bacille Calmette-Guérin; bacillus Calmette-Guérin *vaccine*; Calmette *test*; Calmette-Guérin *bacillus*; Calmette-Guérin *vaccine*.
guid·ance (gī′dăns). Guia, orientação, direção. **1.** O ato de guiar. **2.** Uma guia.
  condylar g., guia condilar; o dispositivo mecânico que é colocado sobre um articulador e tem por objetivo guiar o movimento do articulador, de modo semelhante à orientação produzida pelas trajetórias dos côndilos nas articulações temporomandibulares. VER TAMBÉM condylar guidance *inclination*. SIN condylar guide.
  incisal g., guia incisal; a influência produzida pelas superfícies de contato dos dentes anteriores da maxila e mandíbula sobre os movimentos da mandíbula durante incursões excêntricas. SIN incisal path.
guide (gīd). Guia, fio-guia. **1.** Guiar por um trajeto fixo. **2.** Qualquer dispositivo ou instrumento que guia um segundo dispositivo em sua trajetória adequada, p.ex., uma tentacânula, um fio-guia de cateter. [I.M., do Fr. ant. *guier*, mostrar o caminho, do alemão]

anterior g., g. anterior. SIN incisal g.
catheter g., fio-guia de cateter; um fio metálico e flexível ou uma sonda delgada sobre os quais um cateter é colocado e que permitem que o cateter avance pelo interior de uma estrutura, como um vaso sanguíneo ou a uretra, até alcançar sua posição final. VER TAMBÉM stylet.
condylar g., g. condilar. SIN condylar *guidance.*
incisal g., g. incisal; em odontologia, a parte de um articulador sobre a qual o pino da g. anterior repousa para manter a dimensão vertical da oclusão e do ângulo da g. incisal, conforme estabelecido pela guia incisal; pode ser ajustável, apresentando uma superfície superior que pode ser modificada, a fim de fornecer variações no ângulo da g. incisal, ou feita sob medida, sendo moldada individualmente em plástico para permitir outra orientação, além da guia incisal de linha reta, nos movimentos excêntricos. SIN anterior g.
mold g., g. de molde; uma g. utilizada para pormenorizar a forma dos dentes artificiais ou de um dente artificial.
guide·line (gīd′līn). Diretriz; protocolo; uma marca na forma de uma linha que serve como guia ou referência.
clasp g., Linha de nivelamento. SIN survey line.
clinical practice g.'s, protocolos da prática clínica; uma conduta formal sobre uma determinada tarefa ou função da prática clínica, como os testes diagnósticos desejáveis ou o regime de tratamento ótimo para um diagnóstico específico; em geral, são baseados na melhor evidência disponível, p.ex., estudos controlados randomizados avaliados por um grupo colaborador Cochrane. VER TAMBÉM Cochrane *collaboration.*
Cummer g., linha de nivelamento de Cummer. SIN survey line.
practice g.'s, protocolos clínicos; recomendações sobre o atendimento médico elaboradas por grupos de médicos clínicos e baseadas em várias evidências. SIN practice parameters.
guide·wire (gīd′wīr). Fio-guia; fio ou mola utilizada como guia para a colocação de um dispositivo ou prótese maior, tal como um cateter ou um pino intramedular.
Guillain, Georges, neurologista francês, 1876–1961. VER G.-Barré *reflex, syndrome;* Landry-G.-Barré *syndrome.*
guil·lo·tine (gīl′ō-tēn, gē′ō-tēn). Guilhotina; um instrumento com a forma de um anel de metal através do qual corre uma lâmina deslizante de bisturi; é utilizado na excisão de uma tonsila. [Fr. um instrumento para execução por decapitação]
guin·ea green B (gin′ē) [C.I. 42085]. Verde-guiné B; um corante de diaminotrifenilmetano ácido, utilizado como indicador nas determinações do íon H (muda de magenta para verde em pH 6,0) e como corante de fibras citoplasmáticas em determinados procedimentos de coloração de tricrômio de Masson.
guin·ea pig (gin′ē). Porquinho-da-índia, cobaia. SIN *Cavia porcellus.*
Guldberg, C., químico norueguês, 1862–1902. VER G.-Waage *law.*
gul·let (gŭl′et). Garganta. SIN throat (1). [L. *gula*, garganta]
Gull·strand, Allvar, oftalmologista sueco laureado com o Prêmio Nobel, 1862–1930. VER biomicroscope.
L-gu·lon·ic ac·id (goo-lon′ik). Ácido L-gulônico; o produto da redução do ácido glicurônico (–CHO → –CH$_2$OH); o produto da oxidação da L-gulose (–CHO → –COOH); um precursor (exceto em determinados primatas, nos porquinhos-da-índia, em certos peixes e no morcego das frutas indiano) do ácido ascórbico por meio da L-gulonolactona.
L-gu·lon·o·lac·tone (goo-lon′ō-lak-tōn). L-gulonolactona; o precursor imediato do ácido ascórbico nos animais capazes de realizar a biossíntese do ácido ascórbico. SIN dihydroascorbic acid, L-gulono-γ-lactone.
L-g. oxidase, L-g. oxidase; a enzima que catalisa a conversão de L-g. e O$_2$ em H$_2$O$_2$ e L-*xilo*-hexulonolactona, um precursor do ácido ascórbico; está ausente nos seres humanos.
L-gul·o·no·γ·lac·tone. L-gulono-γ-lactona. SIN L-gulonolactone.
gu·lose (goo′lōs). Gulose; um dos oito pares (D e L) de aldoses; a D-g. é um epímero da D-galactose.
gum (gŭm). **1.** Goma, resina; a seiva exsudada e seca de várias árvores e arbustos que forma uma massa amorfa e friável; em geral forma uma solução mucilaginosa na água e é freqüentemente utilizada como um agente de suspensão em preparações líquidas de drogas insolúveis. [L. *gummi*] **2.** Gengiva; *termo oficial alternativo para gingiva. [A.S. *goma*, mandíbula] **3.** Glicanas solúveis em água que, freqüentemente, contêm ácidos urônicos e são encontradas em muitas plantas.
g. arabic, goma-arábica. SIN acacia. VER TAMBÉM arabin.
Bassora g., goma de Bassora; uma g. proveniente do Irã e da Turquia que se assemelha ao tragacanto, à acácia e ao exsudato gomoso da cerejeira e ameixeira; é utilizada para fazer o estoraque.
g. benjamin, g. benzoin, benjoim. SIN benzoin.
British g., goma inglesa; uma forma de dextrina.
eucalyptus g., goma de eucalipto; um exsudato gomoso seco proveniente do *Eucalyptus rostrata* e de outras espécies de *Eucalyptus* (família Myrtaceae); é utilizado como adstringente (em colutórios e pastilhas) e como agente antidiarreico. SIN red g.
ghatti g., goma *ghatti.* SIN Indian g.
guaiac g., guaiaco. SIN guaiac.
guar g., guar; os endospermas moídos de *Cyamopsis tetragonolobus*; utilizados em formulações farmacêuticas gelatinosas.
Indian g., goma indiana; exsudação da *Anogeisus latifolia* (família Combrettaceae); sua mucilagem é utilizada como um substituto para a mucilagem da acácia. SIN ghatti g.
karaya g., goma caraia, estercúlia. SIN sterculia g.
locust g., algaroba. SIN algaroba.
g. opium, ópio. SIN opium.
red g., g. de eucalipto. SIN eucalyptus g.
senegal g., goma-do-senegal; a g. da *Acacia senegal.* VER acacia.
starch g., dextrina, goma de amido. SIN dextrin.
sterculia g., estercúlia; exsudação gomosa seca de *Sterculia urens, S. villosa, S. tragacantha* ou de outra espécie de *Sterculia*, ou de *Cochlospermum gossypium* ou outra espécie de *Cochlospermum* (família Bixaceae); é utilizada como laxativo hidrofílico e na fabricação de loções e pastas. SIN karaya g.
wheat g., glúten. SIN gluten.
gum·boil (gŭm′boyl). Abscesso gengival. SIN gingival *abscess.*
gum·ma, pl. **gum·ma·ta, gum·mas** (gŭm′a̧, a̧-ta, -z̆). Goma; um granuloma infeccioso característico da sífilis terciária, mas que nem sempre se desenvolve; pode ser solitário (atingindo até 8–10 cm de diâmetro) ou múltiplo e difusamente disseminado (com 1 mm ou menos de diâmetro). As gomas caracterizam-se por apresentar uma parte central irregular e firme, às vezes parcialmente hialinizada, que consiste em necrose de coagulação, na qual o arcabouço das estruturas pode ser reconhecido; uma zona média mal definida de células epitelióides, com eventuais células gigantes multinucleadas; e uma zona periférica composta de fibroblastos e numerosos capilares, com um infiltrado de linfócitos e plasmócitos. À medida que as gomas envelhecem, persiste uma cicatriz irregular ou um nódulo fibroso arredondado. SIN syphiloma. [L. *gummi*, gengiva, do G. *kommi*]
Gumprecht, Ferdinand A., médico alemão, 1864–1941. VER Klein-Gumprecht shadow *nuclei*, em *nucleus*; G. *shadows*, em *shadow.*
Gunn, Robert Marcus, oftalmologista britânico, 1850–1909. VER G. *phenomenon, dots*, em *dot, sign, syndrome*; Marcus G. *pupil.*
Günning, Jan W., químico holandês, 1827–1901. VER G. *reaction.*
Gunning, Thomas B., dentista norte-americano, 1813–1889. VER G. *splint.*
Günz, Justus W., anatomista alemão, 1714–1815. VER G. *ligament.*
Günzberg, Alfred, médico alemão, *1861. VER G. *reagent, test.*
Guo Símbolo de guanosine (guanosina).
gur·ney (gŭr′nē). Uma maca ou cama de lona com rodas, utilizada no transporte de pacientes. [Sir Goldsworthy *Gurney*, médico e inventor britânico, 1793–1875]
gush·er (gŭsh′er). Jato; um fluxo abundante de líquido.
perilymphatic g., j. de perilinfa; fluxo anormal de perilinfa que ocorre quando a base do estribo é perfurada; ocorre na surdez mista ligada ao X (DFN 3), resultante de uma mutação no gene POU3F4, e em outras condições.
Gussenbauer, Carl, cirurgião alemão, 1842–1903. VER G. *suture.*
gus·ta·tion (gŭs-tā′shŭn). Gustação, paladar. **1.** O ato de provar. **2.** O sentido do gosto. [L. *gustatio*, de *gusto*, pp. -*atus*, provar]

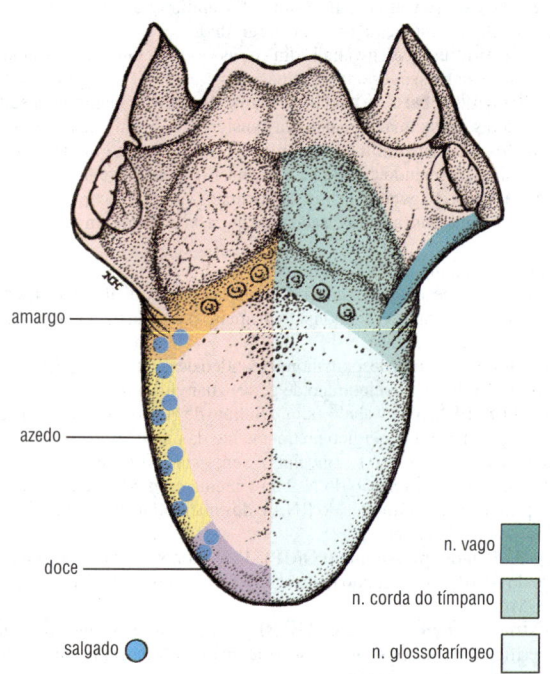

gustação: regiões de percepção do paladar e seus nervos gustativos

gus·ta·to·ry (gŭsʹtă-tōr-ē). Gustatório, gustativo; relativo à gustação ou ao paladar.

gust·duc·in (gŭst-dus-in). Gustoducina; uma proteína mensageira encontrada nas papilas gustativas e ativada em resposta às substâncias doces; é uma subunidade α da proteína G. [L. *gustus*, gosto, + *duco*, induzir, provocar, + -in]

gut (gŭt). **1.** Intestino. SIN intestine. **2.** Tubo digestivo embrionário. **3.** Forma abreviada de catgut. VER TAMBÉM suture. [A.S.]

   blind g., ceco. SIN cecum (1).

   postanal g., i. pós-anal; uma extensão do intestino posterior, caudalmente ao ponto onde se forma a abertura anal. SIN postcloacal g., tailgut.

   postcloacal g., i. pós-cloacal. SIN postanal g.

   preoral g., bolsa de Seessel. SIN Seessel *pocket.*

   primitive g., intestino primitivo; uma lâmina plana de endoderma intra-embrionário que se transforma em um intestino tubular, devido às flexões do corpo embrionário — cabeça, cauda e pregas corporais laterais. SIN archenteron, celenteron, endodermal canal, subgerminal cavity.

Guthrie, George J., oftalmologista inglês, 1785–1856. VER G. *muscle.*

Guthrie, Robert, pediatra norte-americano, 1916–1995. VER G. *test.*

Gutmann, Carl, médico alemão, *1872. VER Michaelis-G. *body.*

gut·ta (gt.), pl. **gut·tae (gtt.)** (gŭtʹă, -ē). **1.** Gota; um pingo. **2.** Um politerpeno semelhante à borracha e encontrado na guta-percha. Cf. chicle, gutta-percha. [L.]

   g. sere·na, g.-serena; antigo termo para a cegueira de etiologia desconhecida; o termo "serena" sugeria que o segmento anterior do olho estava claro e tranqüilo e que não havia nenhuma causa visível para a cegueira, ou seja, nenhuma cicatriz na córnea, nem inflamação ou catarata. Assim, g.-serena tornou-se o termo utilizado para se referir à cegueira resultante de alguma causa posterior insondável, alguma lesão na retina, no nervo óptico ou no cérebro. Esse foi o nome dado à cegueira de John Milton. Com a criação do oftalmoscópio, em 1851, o diagnóstico da g.-serena tornou-se, em pouco tempo, antiquado e inadequado.

gut·tae. Plural de gutta (gota). [L.]

gut·ta-per·cha (gŭtʹă-perʹchă). Guta-percha; o suco leitoso, coagulado, purificado e seco das árvores dos gêneros *Palaguium* e *Payena* (família Sapotaceae); é empregado como material para obturações em odontologia e na fabricação de talas e isolantes elétricos; uma solução de g.-p. é utilizada como substituto do colódio, um protetor, e para fechar feridas feitas por incisão. Cf. chicle, gutta. [Malaio *gatah*, goma, + *percha*, o nome de uma árvore]

guttat. Abreviatura do L. *guttatim*, gota a gota.

gut·tate (gŭtʹtāt). Com a forma de, ou que se assemelha a, uma gota, que caracteriza certas lesões cutâneas.

gut·ter [TA]. Goteira, canal, calha; recesso ou sulcos profundos.

   paracolic gutters [TA], goteiras paracólicas; os sulcos localizados entre a face lateral do cólon ascendente ou descendente e a parede abdominal. SIN sulci paracolici [TA], paracolic recesses.

   paravertebral gutter, sulco pulmonar. SIN pulmonary *groove.*

Guttman, L.L., epidemiologista norte-americano do século XX. VER G. *scale.*

gut·tur·al (gŭtʹer-ăl). Gutural; relativo à garganta.

gut·tur·o·tet·a·ny (gŭtʹer-ō-tetʹă-nē). Guturotetania; espasmo laríngeo que provoca gaguez temporária. [L. *guttur*, garganta, + G. *tetanos*, tensão convulsiva]

Gutzeit, Max A.G., químico alemão, 1847–1915. VER G. *test.*

Guyon, Jean C.F., cirurgião francês, 1831–1920. VER G. *amputation, isthmus, sign;* Guyon tunnel *syndrome.*

GVH Abreviatura de graft versus host (enxerto-versus-hospedeiro).

GVHR Abreviatura de graft versus host *reaction* (reação enxerto-versus-hospedeiro).

Gy Abreviatura de gray.

gym-di·ol. VER gym-*diol.*

Gym·na·moe·bi·da (jim-nă-mēʹbi-dă). Uma ordem de amebas desprovidas de um envoltório quitinoso (*testa*), embora possa haver uma camada envoltória de ectoplasma condensado; engloba o gênero *Amoeba*. [G. *gymnos*, nu, + *amoibē*, mudança (ameba)]

gym·nas·tics (jim-nasʹtiks). Ginástica; exercícios musculares realizados em recinto fechado (em contraste com o atletismo, praticado a céu aberto) e, em geral, por meio de aparelhos especiais. [G. *gymnos*, nu]

   Swedish g., g. sueca. SIN Swedish *movements*, em *movement.*

Gym·no·as·ca·ce·ae (jimʹnō-as-kāʹsē-ē). Uma família de fungos que engloba o estado ascomiceto de muitos dos dermatófitos e alguns dos patógenos sistêmicos de seres humanos (*Histoplasma capsulatum, Blastomyces dermatitidis*, etc.). Até as formas sexuais serem identificadas, esses patógenos eram classificados como Fungos Imperfeitos.

Gymnodinium (jim-nō-dinʹē-um). Gênero de dinoflagelados marinhos englobando o organismo unicelular que causa a maré vermelha.

   G. breve, uma espécie de alga microscópica que causa a maré vermelha; produz uma toxina que afeta o sistema nervoso central dos peixes, paralisando-os e matando-os.

Gym·no·phal·loi·des (jim-nōfal-oyʹdēz). Pequeno trematódeo (família Gymnophallidae) normalmente encontrado nas aves; na Coréia, há freqüentes relatos sobre o encontro desse trematódeo no intestino humano; supõe-se que o hospedeiro intermediário seja uma ostra ou um molusco bivalve marinhos.

   g. seoi, trematódeo encontrado nos habitantes de uma ilha a sudoeste da península da Coréia; a infestação por esse trematódeo provoca sintomas intestinais vagos; é um parasita de seres humanos sob condições naturais, não ocorrendo infecções acidentais, e os moluscos bivalves são os hospedeiros intermediários.

gym·no·pho·bia (jim-nō-fōʹbē-ă). Gimnofobia; temor mórbido de ver uma pessoa nua ou uma parte descoberta do corpo. [G. *gymnos*, nu, + *phobos*, medo]

gym·no·the·ci·um (jimʹnō-theʹsē-um). Gimnotécio; um corpo produtor de ascomicetos composto por hifas frouxamente entremeadas. [G. *gymnos*, nu, + *thēkion*, bolsa, invólucro, dim. de *thēkē*, caixa]

GYN Abreviatura de gynecology (ginecologia).

♻ **gyn-, gyne-, gyneco-, gyno-.** Mulher, fêmea. [G. *gynē*, mulher]

gy·nan·drism (ji-nanʹdrizm, gīʹnan-drizm). Ginandrismo, ginandria; uma anormalidade do desenvolvimento caracterizada por hipertrofia do clitóris e união dos lábios maiores do pudendo, que simulam o aspecto do pênis e do escroto. VER hermaphroditism, female *pseudohermaphroditism.* [gyn- + G. *anēr* (*andr-*), homem]

gy·nan·dro·blas·to·ma (ji-nanʹdrō-blas-tōʹmă, gī-). Ginandroblastoma. **1.** Tumor de células Sertoli-Leydig. SIN Sertoli-Leydig cell *tumor.* **2.** Uma rara variedade de arrenoblastoma de ovário, que contém elementos das células da granulosa ou da teca e produz efeitos androgênicos e estrogênicos simultâneos.

gy·nan·droid (gī-nanʹdroyd, jī-). Ginandróide; um indivíduo que exibe ginandrismo. [gyn- + G. *anēr* (*andr-*), homem, + *eidos*, semelhança]

gy·nan·dro·mor·phism (gī-nan-drō-mōrʹfizm, jī-). Ginandromorfismo. **1.** Uma combinação anormal de características masculinas e femininas. **2.** A presença de cromossomas sexuais masculinos e femininos em diferentes tecidos; mosaicismo de cromossomas sexuais. [gyn- + G. *anēr* (*andr-*), um humano do sexo masculino, + *morphē*, forma]

gy·nan·dro·mor·phous (gī-nan-drō-mōrʹfŭs, jī-). Ginandromorfo; que apresenta tanto características masculinas como femininas.

gy·na·tre·sia (gī-nă-trēʹzē-ă, jī-). Ginatresia; a oclusão de alguma parte do trato genital feminino, principalmente a oclusão da vagina por uma membrana espessa. [gyn- + G. *a-* priv. + *trēsis*, um orifício]

♻ **gyne-.** Gine-; VER gyn-.

gy·ne·cic (gī-nēʹsik, jī-) Pertinente a ou associado às mulheres.

gy·ne·co·gen·ic (gīʹne-kō-jenʹik, jinʹē-). **1.** Que dá à luz predominantemente mulheres. **2.** Termo obsoleto que significa algo que produz características femininas.

gy·ne·coid (gī-ne-koyd, jinʹē-). Ginecóide; que possui forma e estrutura semelhantes às de uma mulher. [gyneco- + G. *eidos*, semelhança]

gy·ne·co·log·ic, gy·ne·co·log·i·cal (gīʹne-kō-lojʹik, jinʹē-; -lojʹi-kăl). Ginecológico; relativo à ginecologia.

gy·ne·col·o·gist (gī-ne-kolʹo-jist, jī-nē-). Ginecologista; um médico que se especializa em ginecologia.

gy·ne·col·o·gy (GYN) (gī-ne-kolʹō-jē, jin-ē-). Ginecologia; a especialidade médica que se ocupa das doenças do trato genital feminino, bem como da endocrinologia e da fisiologia reprodutiva da mulher. [gyneco- + G. *logos*, estudo]

gy·ne·co·ma·nia (gīʹne-kō-māʹnē-ă, jinʹē-). Ginecomania; desejo mórbido ou excessivo por mulheres. [gyneco- + G. *mania*, frenesi]

gy·ne·co·ma·stia, gy·ne·co·mas·ty (gīʹne-kō-masʹtē-ă, jinʹē-; -masʹtē). Ginecomastia; desenvolvimento excessivo das glândulas mamárias masculinas, resultante principalmente de proliferação ductal acompanhada de edema periductal; é freqüentemente secundária a níveis elevados de estrógenos, contudo, g. discreta pode ocorrer na adolescência normal. [gyneco- + G. *mastos*, mama]

   refeeding g., g. por realimentação; aumento temporário das mamas quando suporte nutricional é oferecido a mulheres que passaram fome durante certo período de tempo. É provável que represente um desequilíbrio da função endócrina, no qual alguns sistemas aumentam a função antes que outros; observada de forma mais notável quando as prisioneiras dos campos de concentração e das forças aliadas foram libertadas no final da Segunda Guerra Mundial.

gy·ne·pho·bia (gī-ne-fōʹbē-ă, jin-ē-). Ginofobia, ginecofobia; medo mórbido de mulheres ou do sexo feminino. [gyne- + G. *phobos*, medo]

gy·ni·at·rics (gī-ne-atʹriks, jin-ē-). Giniatria; o tratamento das doenças das mulheres. SIN gyniatry. [gyn- + G. *iatrikos*, de medicamento ou cirurgia]

gy·ni·at·ry (gī-ne-atʹrē, jin-ē). Giniatria. SIN gyniatrics.

♻ **gyno-.** Gino-; VER gyn-.

gy·no·car·dia oil (gī-nō-karʹdē-ă). Óleo de ginocárdia, óleo de chaulmogra. SIN chaulmoogra oil.

gy·no·gen·e·sis (gī-nō-jenʹe-sis, jin-ō-). Ginogênese; o desenvolvimento do ovo ativado por um espermatozóide, sem que haja contribuição de material genético do gameta masculino. [gyno- + G. *genesis*, produção]

gy·nop·a·thy (gī-nopʹă-thē, jī-). Ginopatia; qualquer doença própria de mulheres. [gyno- + G. *pathos*, sofrimento]

gynoplasty (gi′nō-plas-tiks). Ginoplastia; cirurgia reparativa ou plástica dos órgãos genitais femininos. [gyno- + G. *plassō*, formar]

gyp·sum (jip′sŭm). Gipso, gipsita, gesso; a forma hidratada natural do sulfato de cálcio; um dos componentes do gesso de moldar, do gesso de Paris e de revestimentos utilizados em odontologia. [L. do G. *gypsos*]

gy·rase (gi′rās). Girase; a topoisomerase II procariótica que utiliza ATP para produzir superespirais negativas de DNA. [L. *gyro*, girar em círculos, de *gyrus*, G. *gyros*]

gy·rate (ji′rāt). **1.** Com forma de anel ou convoluta. **2.** Girar, revolver. [L. *gyro*, pp. *gyratus*, girar ao redor de um círculo, *gyrus*]

gy·ra·tion (ji-rā′shŭn). **1.** Giro; um movimento circular ou uma revolução. **2.** A disposição das circunvoluções ou dos giros do córtex cerebral.

gy·rec·to·my (ji-rek′tō-mē). Girectomia; excisão de um giro cerebral. [G. *gyros*, anel, + *ektomē*, excisão]

gyr·en·ce·phal·ic (ji′ren-se-fal′ik). Girencefálico; que indica cérebros, como os humanos, nos quais o córtex cerebral apresenta circunvoluções, em contraste com os cérebros lissencefálicos (lisos) de pequenos mamíferos, como os roedores. [G. *gyros*, anel (giro), + *enkaphalē*, cérebro]

gy·ri (ji′ri). Plural de *gyrus*. [L.]

gy·ro·chrome (ji′rō-krōm). Girocromo; que indica uma célula nervosa na qual a substância cromófila está disposta de forma quase anular. [G. *gyros*, um anel, um círculo, + *chrōma*, uma cor]

Gy·ro·mi·tra es·cu·len·ta (gi-rō-mē′tra es-kū-len′ta). Uma espécie de cogumelo que pode produzir uma toxina monometil-hidrazina, que provoca náuseas, diarréia e outros sintomas; em casos graves, pode levar à morte. SIN *Helvella esculenta*.

gy·rose (ji′rōs). Girose; caracterizado por linhas curvas irregulares, como a superfície de um hemisfério cerebral. [G. *gyros*, círculo]

gy·ro·spasm (ji′rō-spazm). Girospasmo; movimentos rotatórios espasmódicos da cabeça. [G. *gyros*, círculo, + *spasmos*, espasmo]

GYRUS

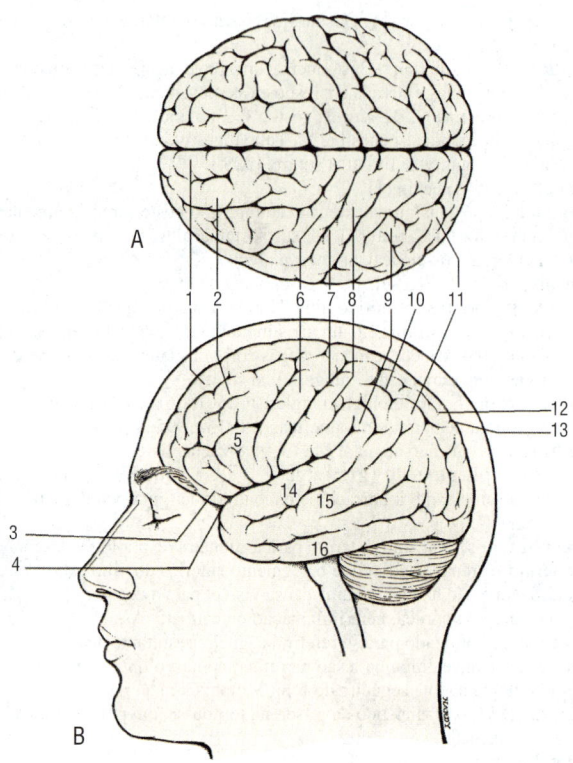

giros: (A) vista superior e (B) vista lateral do cérebro. (1) giro frontal superior; (2) giro frontal médio; (3) giros orbitais; (4) fossa cerebral lateral; (5) giro frontal inferior; (6) giro pré-central; (7) sulco central; (8) giro pós-central; (9) giro supramarginal; (10) sulco intraparietal; (11) lóbulo parietal inferior; (12) sulco intraparietal; (13) lóbulo parietal superior; (14) giro temporal superior; (15) giro temporal médio; (16) giro temporal inferior

gy·rus, gen. e pl. **gy·′ri** (ji′rŭs, -ri) [TA]. Giro; uma das elevações arredondadas e proeminentes que formam os hemisférios cerebrais, cada uma consistindo em uma parte superficial exposta e uma parte oculta da visão localizada na parede e no assoalho do sulco. [L. do G. *gyros*, círculo]

angular g. [TA], g. angular; uma circunvolução preguenda encontrada no lóbulo parietal inferior e formada pela união das extremidades posteriores dos giros temporais superior e médio; um g. localizado ao redor da terminação caudal do sulco temporal superior. SIN g. angularis [TA], angular convolution.

g. angula′ris [TA], g. angular. SIN angular g.

annectent g., g. transicional. SIN transitional g.

anterior central g., g. pré-central. SIN precentral g.

anterior paracentral g. [TA], g. paracentral anterior; a parte anterior do lóbulo paracentral; a continuação medial do córtex somatomotor primário (giro pré-central), na qual a coxa, a perna e o pé estão representados. SIN g. paracentràlis anterior [TA].

anterior piriform g., g. piriforme anterior. SIN prepiriform g.

anterior transverse temporal g. [TA], g. temporal transverso anterior. VER transverse temporal gyri. SIN g. temporalis transversus anterior [TA].

ascending frontal g., g. pré-central. SIN precentral g.

ascending parietal g., g. pós-central. SIN postcentral g.

gy′ri bre′ves in′sulae [TA], giros curtos da ínsula. SIN short gyri of insula.

callosal g., g. do cíngulo. SIN cingulate g.

central gyri, giros centrais; os giros pré-central e pós-central.

cerebral gyri [TA], giros do cérebro. SIN gyri cerebri.

gy′ri cer′ebri [TA], giros do cérebro; os giros ou as circunvoluções do córtex cerebral. SIN cerebral gyri [TA].

cingulate g., g. do cíngulo; uma circunvolução curva e longa localizada na superfície medial do hemisfério cortical e que se arqueia sobre o corpo caloso, do qual está separada pelo sulco profundo do corpo caloso; juntamente com o g. para-hipocampal, com o qual se continua atrás do corpo caloso, forma o g. fornicatus. SIN g. cinguli [TA], callosal convolution, callosal g., cingulate convolution, falciform lobe, lobus falciformis.

g. cin′guli [TA], g. do cíngulo. SIN cingulate g.

deep transitional g., g. transicional profundo; o g. transverso do embrião que, durante o desenvolvimento, assume nova posição no fundo do sulco central do hemisfério cerebral.

dentate g. [TA], g. dentado; um dos dois giros conectados que compõem o hipocampo; o outro giro é o corno de Ammon. SIN g. dentatus [TA], dentate fascia, fascia dentata hippocampi.

g. denta′tus [TA], g. dentado. SIN dentate g.

fasciolar g. [TA], g. fasciolar; uma pequena faixa dupla que passa ao redor do esplênio do corpo caloso, a partir da estria longitudinal lateral até o g. denteado. SIN g. fasciolaris [TA], fascia cinerea, fasciola cinerea.

g. fascio′laris [TA], g. fasciolar. SIN fasciolar g.

fornicate g., g. do fórnice; a circunvolução cortical em forma de ferradura que circunda o hilo do hemisfério cerebral; seu ramo superior é formado pelo g. do cíngulo, e o inferior, pelo g. para-hipocampal. SIN g. fornicatus (1).

g. fornica′tus, (1) Giro do fórnice. SIN fornicate g.; **(2)** termo utilizado no passado para se referir a todo o sistema límbico.

g. fronta′lis infe′rior [TA], g. frontal inferior. SIN inferior frontal g.

g. frontalis medialis [TA], g. frontal medial. SIN medial frontal g.

g. fronta′lis me′dius [TA], g. frontal médio. SIN middle frontal g.

g. fronta′lis supe′rior [TA], g. frontal superior. SIN superior frontal g.

fusiform g., g. occipitotemporal lateral; uma circunvolução extremamente longa que se estende longitudinalmente sobre a face inferior dos lobos temporal e occipital; é limitada medialmente pelo sulco colateral, a partir do g. lingual, e pela parte anterior do g. para-hipocampal e, lateralmente, pelo sulco temporal inferior, a partir do g. temporal inferior. SIN g. occipitotemporalis lateralis [TA], lateral occipitotemporal g. [TA], g. fusiformis, lobulus fusiformis.

g. fusifor′mis, g. occipitotemporal lateral. SIN fusiform g.

Heschl gyri, giros de Heschl, giros temporais transversos. SIN transverse temporal gyri.

hippocampal g., g. para-hipocampal. SIN parahippocampal g.

inferior frontal g. [TA], g. frontal inferior; uma circunvolução larga, localizada na convexidade do lobo frontal do cérebro, entre o sulco frontal inferior e a fissura de Sylvius; é dividida pelas ramificações da fissura de Sylvius em três partes: a parte opercular [TA] (pars opercularis [TA]), a parte triangular [TA] (pars triangularis [TA]) e a parte orbital [TA] (pars orbitalis [TA]); as duas primeiras partes constituem uma porção do opérculo frontal. SIN g. frontalis inferior [TA], inferior frontal convolution.

inferior occipital g. [TA], g. occipital inferior; um g. situado abaixo do sulco occipital lateral, na parte inferior da face lateral do lobo occipital.

inferior parietal g., g. parietal inferior. SIN inferior parietal *lobule*.

inferior temporal g. [TA], g. temporal inferior; uma circunvolução sagital localizada na margem ínfero-lateral do lobo temporal do cérebro e separada do g. temporal médio pelo sulco temporal inferior. Na superfície inferior do lobo temporal, é separada do g. occipitotemporal medial pelo sulco occipitotemporal. Engloba o g. occipitotemporal lateral. SIN g. temporalis inferior [TA], inferior temporal convolution, third temporal convolution.

gy'ri in'sulae [TA], giros da ínsula. SIN insular gyri.

insular gyri [TA], giros da ínsula; os giros curtos e o giro longo da ínsula. SIN gyri insulae [TA].

interlocking gyri, giros conectados; vários giros pequenos que se localizam nas paredes do sulco central do hemisfério; os giros opostos encaixam-se uns nos outros.

lateral occipitotemporal g. [TA], g. occipitotemporal lateral; SIN fusiform g.

lateral olfactory g. [TA], g. olfatório lateral; camadas superficiais de células localizadas próximo à estria olfatória lateral; pouco desenvolvidas em animais microsmáticos, mas bem desenvolvidas em macrosmáticos. SIN g. olfactorius lateralis [TA].

lingual g. [TA], g. lingual; uma circunvolução horizontal relativamente curta, localizada sobre a face ínfero-medial dos lobos occipital e temporal e separada do g. occipitotemporal lateral ou fusiforme pelo sulco colateral profundo e do cúneo pelo sulco calcarino; sua extremidade anterior está em contato com o istmo do g. para-hipocampal; a faixa medial ou superior do g., que forma a margem inferior do sulco calcarino, corresponde à metade inferior da área estriada ou do córtex visual primário e representa o quadrante superior contralateral do campo binocular da visão. SIN g. lingualis [TA], g. occipitotemporalis medialis [TA], medial occipitotemporal g. [TA].

g. lingua'lis [TA], g. lingual. SIN lingual g.

long g. of insula [TA], g. longo da ínsula; o mais posterior e mais longo dos giros delgados e retos que compõem a ínsula. SIN g. longus insulae [TA].

g. lon'gus in'sulae [TA], g. longo da ínsula. SIN long g. of insula.

marginal g., g. frontal superior. SIN superior frontal g.

medial frontal g. [TA], g. frontal medial; termo às vezes utilizado para designar a parte do giro frontal superior que envolve e se localiza sobre a face medial do lobo frontal. SIN g. frontalis medialis [TA].

medial occipitotemporal g. [TA], g. occipitotemporal medial. SIN g. occipitotemporalis medialis.

medial olfactory g. [TA], g. olfatório medial; camadas de células localizadas próximo à estria olfatória medial; apresentam-se bem desenvolvidas nos animais macrosmáticos, mas pouco desenvolvidas nos microsmáticos. SIN g. olfactorius medialis [TA].

middle frontal g., g. frontal médio; uma circunvolução localizada sobre a convexidade de cada lobo frontal do cérebro e que corre na direção ântero-posterior, entre os sulcos frontais superior e inferior. SIN g. frontalis medius [TA], middle frontal convolution.

middle temporal g. [TA], g. temporal médio; um g. longitudinal localizado sobre a superfície lateral do lobo temporal, entre os sulcos temporais superior e inferior. SIN g. temporalis medius [TA], middle temporal convolution, second temporal convolution.

occipital gyri, giros occipitais. VER inferior occipital g., superior occipital g.

g. occip'itotempora'lis latera'lis [TA], g. occipitotemporal lateral. SIN fusiform g.

g. occip'itotempora'lis media'lis [TA], g. occipitotemporal medial; a porção medial do g. occipitotemporal, na superfície inferior do hemisfério cerebral, separada da porção lateral pelo sulco occipitotemporal e do giro para-hipocampal pelo sulco colateral.

g. olfactorius lateralis [TA], g. olfatório lateral. SIN lateral olfactory g.

g. olfactorius medialis [TA], g. olfatório medial. SIN medial olfactory g.

orbital gyri [TA], giros orbitais; várias circunvoluções pequenas e irregulares que ocupam a superfície inferior côncava de cada lobo frontal do cérebro. SIN gyri orbitales [TA].

gy'ri orbita'les [TA], giros orbitais. SIN orbital gyri.

g. paracentralis anterior [TA], g. paracentral anterior. SIN anterior paracentral g.

g. paracentralis posterior [TA], g. paracentral posterior. SIN posterior paracentral g.

parahippocampal g. [TA], g. para-hipocampal; uma circunvolução longa, localizada na superfície medial do lobo temporal, que forma a parte inferior do g. do fórnice e se estende da parte posterior do esplênio do corpo caloso para a frente, ao longo do g. dentado do hipocampo, do qual é separada pela fissura do hipocampo. O extremo anterior do g. curva-se para trás sobre si mesmo, formando o unco, a principal parte do córtex olfatório. VER TAMBÉM entorhinal *area*. SIN g. parahippocampalis [TA], hippocampal convolution, hippocampal g.

g. par'ahippocampa'lis [TA], g. para-hipocampal. SIN parahippocampal g.

paraterminal g. [TA], g. paraterminal. SIN subcallosal g.

g. paratermina'lis [TA], g. paraterminal. SIN subcallosal g.

postcentral g. [TA], g. pós-central; a circunvolução anterior do lobo parietal, limitada anteriormente pelo sulco central (fissura de Rolando) e, posteriormente, pelo sulco interparietal. SIN g. postcentralis [TA], ascending parietal convolution, ascending parietal g., posterior central convolution, posterior central g.

g. postcentra'lis [TA], g. pós-central. SIN postcentral g.

posterior central g., g. central posterior. SIN postcentral g.

posterior paracentral g. [TA], g. paracentral posterior; a parte posterior do lóbulo paracentral; a continuação medial do córtex somatossensorial primário (giro pós-central), no qual os impulsos sensitivos provenientes da coxa, da perna e do pé estão representados. SIN g. paracentralis posterior [TA].

posterior transverse temporal g. [TA], g. temporal transverso posterior; a parte posterior do córtex auditivo primário, onde existem dois giros. VER TAMBÉM transverse temporal gyri. SIN g. temporalis transversus posterior [TA].

precentral g. [TA], g. pré-central; é limitado posteriormente pelo sulco central e, anteriormente, pelo sulco pré-central. SIN g. precentralis [TA], anterior central convolution, anterior central g., ascending frontal convolution, ascending frontal g.

g. precentra'lis [TA], g. pré-central. SIN precentral g.

prepiriform g., g. pré-piriforme; um g. que cobre o corpo amigdalóide, localizado mais profundamente; está relacionado com a função olfatória. SIN anterior piriform g.

g. rec'tus [TA], g. reto. SIN straight g.

Retzius g., g. de Retzius; o g. intralímbico localizado na parte cortical do rinencéfalo.

short gyri of insula [TA], giros curtos da ínsula; vários giros curtos e radiados que convergem em direção à base da ínsula, compondo aproximadamente os dois terços anteriores do córtex da ínsula. SIN gyri breves insulae [TA].

splenial g., g. do esplênio; uma faixa do córtex, localizada na superfície medial do hemisfério cerebral, que passa ao redor do esplênio do corpo caloso, estreita-se anteriormente e, por fim, funde-se com o indúsio cinzento.

straight g. [TA], g. reto; um g. que corre ao longo da parte medial da superfície orbital do lobo frontal do hemisfério cerebral. É limitado lateralmente pelo sulco olfatório. SIN g. rectus [TA].

subcallosal g., área subcalosa; uma faixa esbranquiçada vertical e delgada imediatamente anterior à lâmina terminal e à comissura anterior; ao contrário do que seu nome indica, não se trata de uma circunvolução cortical e, sim, da continuação ventral do septo pelúcido. A pequena crista de tecido, rostral à lâmina terminal, é às vezes considerada uma parte separada da área subcalosa e denominada giro paraterminal [TA] (gyrus paraterminalis [TA]). SIN area subcallosa [TA], g. paraterminalis [TA], g. subcallosus [TA], paraterminal g. [TA], subcallosal area [TA], corpus paraterminale, paraterminal body, peduncle of corpus callosum, pedunculus corporis callosi, precommissural septal area, Zuckerkandl convolution.

g. subcallo'sus [TA], área subcalosa. SIN subcallosal g.

superior frontal g. [TA], g. frontal superior; uma circunvolução larga que corre em uma direção ântero-posterior na margem medial da superfície convexa e que envolve a superfície medial de cada lobo frontal. SIN g. frontalis superior [TA], marginal g., superior frontal convolution.

superior occipital g., g. occipital superior; um g. situado acima do sulco occipital lateral na superfície lateral do lobo occipital.

superior parietal g., lóbulo parietal superior. SIN superior parietal *lobule*.

superior temporal g. [TA], g. temporal superior; um g. longitudinal localizado na superfície lateral do lobo temporal, entre a fissura lateral (de Sylvius) e o sulco temporal superior. SIN g. temporalis superior [TA], first temporal convolution, superior temporal convolution.

supracallosal g., Indúsio cinzento. SIN *indusium* griseum.

supramarginal g. [TA], g. supramarginal; uma circunvolução preguada que ultrapassa a extremidade posterior do sulco lateral (de Sylvius); juntamente com o g. angular, forma o lóbulo parietal inferior. SIN g. supramarginalis [TA], supramarginal convolution.

g. supramargina'lis [TA], g. supramarginal. SIN supramarginal g.

gy'ri tempora'les transver'si [TA], giros temporais transversos. SIN transverse temporal gyri.

g. tempora'lis infe'rior [TA], g. temporal inferior. SIN inferior temporal g.

g. tempora'lis me'dius [TA], g. temporal médio. SIN middle temporal g.

g. tempora'lis supe'rior [TA], g. temporal superior. SIN superior temporal g.

g. temporalis transversus anterior [TA], g. temporal transverso anterior. SIN anterior transverse temporal g. VER transverse temporal gyri.

g. temporalis transversus posterior [TA], g. temporal transverso posterior. SIN posterior transverse temporal g.

transitional g., g. transicional; uma pequena circunvolução que liga dois lobos ou dois giros importantes na profundidade de um sulco. SIN annectent g., transitional convolution.

transverse temporal gyri [TA], giros temporais transversos; duas ou três circunvoluções que correm transversalmente na superfície superior do lobo temporal, margeando a fissura lateral (de Sylvius), e separados uns dos outros pelos sulcos temporais transversos. SIN gyri temporales transversi [TA], Heschl gyri, transverse temporal convolutions.

uncinate g., unco. SIN uncus (2).

H

H Abreviatura ou símbolo para hydrogen (hidrogênio); hyperopia (hiperopia); hyperopic (hiperópico); horizontal, Hauch, unidade *unit* Holzknecht; henry; *unit* of electrical inductance (unidade de indutância elétrica); a linha Fraunhofer em λ 3968, devido ao cálcio; histidina; magnetic field strength (força do campo magnético); heroin (heroína), histone (histona); histamine (histamina).
H⁺ Símbolo do íon hidrogênio (hidrogen *ion*), o próton.
¹H Símbolo de hidrogênio-1 (H¹).
²H Símbolo do hidrogênio-2 (H²).
³H Símbolo do hidrogênio-3 (H³).
H Símbolo de enthalpy (entalpia), heat content (conteúdo de calor), na equação para free energy (energia livre); fluence (fluência); magnetic field strength (força do campo magnético).
h Símbolo de hecto-; height (altura); hour (hora).
hν. Símbolo de *photon* (fóton), representa a energia do fóton, onde h = constante de Planck e ν = freqüência da onda eletromagnética.
h Símbolo da constante de Planck; $h = h/2\pi$.
HAA Abreviatura de hepatitis-associated *antigen* (antígeno associado à hepatite).
Haab, Otto, oftalmologista suíço, 1850–1931.
Haase rule. Ver em rule.
ha·be·na, pl. **ha·be·nae** (hă-bē′nă, -bē′nē). Habena. **1.** Um freio ou faixa fibrosa restritora. **2.** Faixa restritora. **3.** Habênula. SIN habenula (2). [L. tira]
hab·e·nal, ha·be·nar (habʹe-nal, ha-bēʹnar). Habenal; relativo a habena.
ha·ben·u·la, pl. **ha·ben·u·lae** (ha-benʹū-lă, -lē)[TA]. Habênula. **1.** Frênulo. SIN frenulum. **2.** [TA] Em neuroanatomia, o termo indicava, originalmente, o pedúnculo da glândula pineal (habênula pineal; pedúnculo do corpo pineal); entretanto, passou gradualmente a referir-se a um grupo vizinho de células nervosas com as quais se acreditava que a glândula pineal estivesse associada, o núcleo habenular. Hoje em dia, o termo TA refere-se, exclusivamente, a essa massa de células circunscritas nas faces caudal e dorsal do tálamo dorsal, embebida na extremidade posterior da estria bulbar, da qual recebe a maioria de suas fibras aferentes. Através do fascículo retroflexo (trato habenulointerpeduncular), projeta-se para o núcleo interpeduncular e outros grupos de células paramedianas do tegumento do mesencéfalo. Apesar de sua proximidade com o pedúnculo pineal, não se conhece a existência de qualquer conexão com fibras habenulopineais. Trata-se de uma parte do epitálamo. SIN habena (3). [L.]
 h. of cecum, h. do ceco; extensão da tênia mesocólica do cólon, dorsal ou ventralmente ao íleo terminal.
 Haller h. h. de Haller; termo raramente utilizado para referir-se ao remanescente em forma de cordão do processo vaginal do peritônio. SIN Scarpa h.
 habenʹulae perforaʹtae, forames nervosos. SIN *foramina* nervosa, under *foramen*.
 pineal h., h. pineal; o pedúnculo da glândula pineal. VER habenula (2).
 Scarpa h. h. de Scarpa. SIN Haller h.
 h. urethraʹlis, h. da uretra; uma das duas linhas esbranquiçadas e finas que seguem um percurso desde o meato uretral até o clitóris em meninas e mulheres jovens; vestígios da parte anterior do corpo esponjoso.
ha·ben·u·lar (ha-benʹū-lar). Habenular; relativo a uma habênula, especialmente o pedúnculo do corpo pineal.
Haber, Henry, dermatologista inglês, 1900–1962. VER H. *syndrome*.
Habermann, R., dermatologista alemão, 1884–1941. VER Mucha-H. *disease*.
hab·it. Hábito. **1.** Ato, resposta comportamental, prática ou costume estabelecido no repertório do indivíduo através de repetição freqüente do mesmo ato. VER TAMBÉM addiction. **2.** Uma variável básica no estudo do condicionamento e da aprendizagem, utilizada para designar uma nova resposta aprendida, seja por associação ou seguida de um evento de recompensa ou reforço. VER conditioning, learning. [L. habeo, pp. habitus, ter]
ha·bit·u·a·tion (ha-bit-choo-āʹshun). Habituação. **1.** O processo de formação de um hábito, referindo-se, em geral, à dependência psicológica no uso contínuo de uma substância para manter uma sensação de bem-estar, podendo levar a dependência química. **2.** Método pelo qual o sistema nervoso reduz ou inibe a responsividade durante um estímulo repetido.
habʹi·tus (habʹi-tŭs). Constituição; as características físicas de uma pessoa. [L. constituição]
 fetal h., c. fetal; relação de uma parte fetal com outra. SIN fetal attitude.
 gracile h., constituição esguia; estatura baixa, aparência frágil com peso inferior ao normal.
Hab·ro·ne·ma (ha-brō-nēʹmă). Gênero de nematódeos espiruróides que habitam o estômago de cavalos; as larvas desses nematódeos se desenvolvem em larvas de moscas-domésticas e moscas-dos-estábulos, que vivem no esterco, tornando-se infecciosas quando as larvas das moscas se transformam em ninfas e são transportadas pelas moscas adultas para feridas abertas nos cavalos, onde são deixadas, causando habronemíase cutânea; a reinfecção do estômago do cavalo por *H.* ocorre por ingestão acidental de moscas infectadas ou ao lamber feridas nas quais se encontram larvas infectantes. [G. habros, delicado, gracioso + nēma, filamento]
 H.maʹjus, uma de duas espécies (sendo a outra *H. microstoma*) semelhantes, quanto ao aspecto, hospedeiro, distribuição e ciclo de vida, a *H. muscae*; o hospedeiro intermediário é a mosca-dos-estábulos, *Stomoxys calcitrans*.
 H. megasʹtoma, espécie que causa tumores na mucosa gástrica contendo numerosos nematódeos pequenos; as larvas causam habronemíase cutânea; o hospedeiro intermediário é a mosca-doméstica comum, *Musca domestica*.
 H. microsʹtoma, VER *H. majus*.
 H. musʹcae, espécie que ocorre no estômago do cavalo, da mula, do asno ou da zebra; o hospedeiro intermediário é a mosca-doméstica comum, *Musca domestica*, ou moscas relacionadas.
hack·ing (hakʹing). Golpes aplicados de forma cadenciada com a borda da mão em massagem.
Hadfield, Geoffrey, médico inglês, 1889–1968. VER Clarke-H. *syndrome*.
Ha·dru·rus (hă-drooʹrŭs). Gênero de escorpiões encontrados no sudoeste dos Estados Unidos, caracterizados por numerosas cerdas no ferrão; a espécie mais comum é *H. arizonensis*. VER TAMBÉM Scorpionida. [G. *hadros*, espesso, forte + *ouro*, cauda]
Haeckel, Ernst H.P.A., naturalista alemão, 1834–1919. VER H. gastrea *theory, law*.
⌬ **haem-.** VER hem-.
Hae·ma·dip·sa cey·lon·i·ca (hē-mă-dipʹsă să-lonʹi-kă). Espécie de sanguessuga do solo encontrada em Sri Lanka; fixa-se à pele de animais ou do ser humano. Sua picada é dolorosa, e numerosas picadas podem provocar anemia. [G. *haima*, sangue, + *dipsa*, sede]
Hae·ma·moe·ba (hē-mă-mēʹbă). Termo antigo para referir-se a protozoários amebóides atualmente classificados na subordem Haemosporina, hemoparasitas que incluem o gênero *Plasmodium*. [G. *haima*, sangue, + *amoibē*, mudança]
Hae·ma·phy·sa·lis (hē-mă-fīʹsă-lis). Gênero de pequenos carrapatos sem olhos e sem marcas características. As larvas e as ninfas são encontradas principalmente em pequenos mamíferos e aves; os adultos são encontrados em mamíferos maiores e em algumas aves. São importantes como vetores de protozoários e vírus (p. ex., o vírus da doença da floresta de Kyasanur. [G. *haima*, sangue, + *physaleos*, cheio de vento]
 H. cinnabariʹna, carrapato que ocorre principalmente no distrito seco da Colúmbia Britânica; essa espécie pode causar paralisia do carrapato tanto em seres humanos quanto em animais. [G. *kinnabarinos*, semelhante ao cinabre, vermelhão]
 H. concinʹna, espécie de carrapato comum de roedores da região antes conhecida como União Soviética, vetor e reservatório da febre maculosa do Mediterrâneo.
 H. leachʹi, espécie da África, da Ásia e da Austrália, que ocorre em carnívoros domésticos e selvagens, em pequenos roedores e, às vezes, no gado bovino; transmite a babesiose canina e a febre botonosa.
 H. spinigeʹra, espécie da floresta tropical da Índia, que é um vetor da doença de Floresta de Kyasanur; vários roedores e insetívoros servem como hospedeiros dos carrapatos imaturos dessa espécie, que transmitem um arbovírus do complexo do grupo B de doença de primavera-verão da Rússia; os macacos atuam como reservatórios da infecção humana.
Hae·ma·to·pi·nus (hēʹmă-tō-piʹnŭs). Gênero importante de piolhos sugadores (família Haematopinidae), que afeta suínos e outros animais domésticos e selvagens; normalmente, não é patogênico. O *H. asini* afeta cavalos, mulas e asnos; o *H. eurysternus* e o *H. quadripertusus*, bovinos; e o *H. suis*, suínos. [G. *haima*, sangue, + L. *pinus*, pinheiro]
Hae·mo·coc·cid·i·um (hēʹmō-kok-sidʹē-ŭm). Termo antigo para referir-se às espécies de *Plasmodium*. [G. *haima*, sangue, + *kokkos*, baga]
Hae·mo·dip·sus ven·tri·co·sus (hē-mō-dipʹsŭs ven-tri-kōʹsŭs). O piolho do coelho, transmissor de *Francisella tularensis*. [G. *haima*, sangue, + *dipsos*, sede; L. *venter* (*ventr-*), ventre]
Hae·mo·greg·a·ri·na (hēʹmō-greg-ă-rīʹnă). Gênero de esporozoário coccídeo (ordem Euroccidiida, família Haemogregarinidae) que parasita as células sanguíneas de animais de sangue frio e o sistema digestivo de hospedeiros

---

⌬ Formas Combinantes	☆ Termo oficial alternativo para a *Terminologia Anatomica*
🔲 Indica que o termo é ilustrado, ver Índice de Ilustrações	
	[MIM] Mendelian Inheritance in Man
SIN Sinônimo	
Cf. Comparar, confrontar	I.C. Índice de Corantes
[NA] *Nomina Anatomica*	
[TA] *Terminologia Anatomica*	Termo de Alta Importância

primários invertebrados, num ciclo obrigatório de dois hospedeiros. [G. *haima,* sangue, + L. *grex,* rebanho]

Hae·mon·chus (hē-mong′kŭs). Gênero economicamente importante de parasitas nematódeos (família Trichostrongylidae), que ocorre no abomaso de ruminantes e causa anemia grave, especialmente em animais jovens ou anteriormente não-expostos; algumas espécies significativas incluem *H. placei* (em bovinos, ovinos e caprinos), *H. similis* (em bovinos e ovinos) e *H. contortus,* o verme do estômago, espiralado ou enrolado de bovinos, ovinos, caprinos e outros ruminantes, com poucos casos relatados em seres humanos; parasita acidental do homem. [G. *haima,* sangue, + *onchos,* lança]

Hae·moph·i·lus (hē-mof′i-lŭs). Gênero de bactérias imóveis, aeróbicas a anaeróbicas facultativas (família Brucellaceae), constituídas por diminutas células Gram-negativas, em forma de bastonete, que, algumas vezes, formam filamentos e são pleomórficas; esses microrganismos são estritamente parasitas e crescem melhor ou apenas em meios de cultura contendo sangue. Podem ou não ser patogênicas. Ocorrem em várias lesões e secreções, bem como nas vias respiratórias normais de vertebrados. A espécie típica é *H. influenzae.* [G. *haima,* sangue, + *philos,* amigo]

H. actinomycetemcomi′tans, SIN *Actinobacillus actinomycetemcomitans.*
H. aegyp′tius, espécie que causa conjuntivite infecciosa aguda ou subaguda em climas quentes. SIN Koch-Weeks bacillus.
H. aphroph′ilus, espécie encontrada no sangue e, raramente, na válvula cardíaca como causa de endocardite.
H. ducrey′i, espécie que causa o cancro mole (cancróide) sexualmente transmitido. SIN Ducrey bacillus.
H. haemolyt′icus, espécie habitualmente não-patogênica, mas que, em raras ocasiões, provoca endocardite subaguda.
H. influen′zae, espécie encontrada nas vias respiratórias, causando infecções respiratórias agudas, incluindo pneumonia, conjuntivite aguda, otite e meningite purulenta em crianças (raramente em adultos, nos quais contribui para a sinusite e para a bronquite crônica); originalmente considerada como causa da influenza, é a espécie típica do gênero *H.* SIN influenza bacillus, Weeks bacillus.
H. influenzae Type b, *H. influenzae* Tipo b; o sorotipo mais virulento (existem seis sorotipos, a-f, com base na tipagem antigênica da cápsula de polissacarídeo); espécie responsável pela meningite e por infecções respiratórias em crianças pequenas.
nontypeable *H. influenzae, H. influenzae* não-tipável; espécie que é um importante patógeno na otite média aguda.
H. parahaemoly′ticus, espécie encontrada nas vias respiratórias inferiores e associada freqüentemente à faringite; em certas ocasiões, provoca endocardite subaguda.
H. parainfluen′zae, espécie que, habitualmente, não é patogênica mas causa, por vezes, endocardite subaguda.
H. paratropicalis, espécie relativamente não-patogênica que tem sido associada a infecção nos seres humanos, incluindo casos de endocardite.
H. segnis, espécie habitualmente saprofítica que, algumas vezes, causa meningite, endocardite e outras infecções nos seres humanos.

Hae·mo·pro·te·us (hē′mō-prō′tē-ŭs). Gênero de esporozoários (subordem Haemosporina), parasitas de aves e répteis associado a *Leucocytozoon, Hepatocystis* e a outros gêneros da família Haemoproteidae; a esquizogonia ocorre em células endoteliais dos vasos sanguíneos, especialmente nos pulmões do hospedeiro, enquanto os gametócitos em forma de halteres são encontrados nas hemácias. A infecção é transmitida por dípteros pupíparos, como moscas dos piolhos (Hippoboscidae) e por mosquitos-pólvora hematófagos (*Culicoides*). [G. *haima,* sangue, + *Proteus,* deus marinho que tinha o poder de assumir diferentes formas]

Hae·mo·spo·ri·na (hē′mō-spo-rī′nă). Subordem de coccídeos (classe Sporozoea) que não apresentam sigígia, com desenvolvimento separado de macrogametas e microgamontes, produzindo estes últimos oito microgametas flagelados; heteróxenos com merogania em vertebrados e esporogonia em insetos hematófagos; inclui os gêneros *Haemoproteus, Leucocytozoon* e *Plasmodium.* [G. *haima,* sangue, + *sporos,* semente]

Haens·zel, William M., epidemiologista/estatístico norte-americano, 1910–1998. VER Mantel-Haenszel *test.*
Haffkine, Waldemar M.W., médico russo, 1860–1930. VER H. *vaccine.*
Haf·nia (haf′nē-ah). Gênero pertencente à família Enterobacteriaceae; encontrada em fezes humanas, constitui uma rara causa de infecções hospitalares; associada a doença diarreica de mecanismo indefinido. Existe uma única espécie, *Hafnia alvei.*
haf·ni·um (Hf) (haf′nē-ŭm). Elemento químico raro, número atômico 72, peso atômico 178,49. [L. *Hafnia,* Copenhague]
Hagedorn, Hans Christian, médico dinamarquês, *1888. VER NPH *insulin.*
Hagedorn, Werner, cirurgião alemão, 1831–1894. VER H. *needle.*
Hageman. Sobrenome de pessoa na qual foi observada pela primeira vez a deficiência do fator Hageman (Hageman *factor*).
hag·i·o·ther·a·py (hag′ē-ō-thār′a-pē). Hagioterapia; tratamento da doença por meio de contato com relíquias de santos, visitas a santuários e outras práticas religiosas. [G. *hagios,* sagrado]

Haglund, S.E. Patrik, ortopedista sueco, 1870–1937. VER H. *deformity, disease.*
Hahnemann, Christian F.S., médico alemão e fundador da homeopatia, 1755–1843. VER hahnemannian.
hah·ne·man·ni·an (hah-nē-mahn′ē-an). Hahnemanniano; relativo à homeopatia, ensinada por Christian F. Samuel Hahnemann.
Hahn ox·ine re·a·gent. Ver em reagent.
Haidinger, Wilhelm von, mineralogista austríaco, 1795–1871. VER H. *brushes,* em *brush.*
Hailey, Hugh E., dermatologista norte-americano, *1909. VER H.-H. *disease.*
Hailey, W. Howard, dermatologista norte-americano, 1898–1967. VER H.-H. *disease.*

hair (hār). [TA]. Pêlo, cabelo. **1.** Crescimento epidérmico filamentoso fino e queratinizado que surge na pele do corpo dos mamíferos, exceto nas regiões palmares e plantares e superfícies flexoras das articulações; o comprimento total e a textura dos pêlos variam acentuadamente em diferentes partes do corpo. SIN pilus (1) [TA]. **2.** Um dos delicados processos piliformes das células auditivas do labirinto e de outras células sensoriais, denominados pêlos auditivos, pêlos sensoriais, etc. SIN thrix [TA]. [A.S. *haer*]
auditory h.'s, pêlos auditivos; cílios encontrados na superfície livre das células auditivas.
axillary h.'s [TA]; pêlo axilar; pêlo das axilas. SIN hircus (2).
bamboo h., p. em bambu; pêlos com nódulos regularmente espaçados ao longo da haste, produzidos por quebras intermitentes com invaginação do pêlo distal na porção proximal, com segmentos intercalados de pêlo normal, dando a aparência de bambu; observado na síndrome de Netherton; caráter autossômico recessivo. SIN trichorrhexis invaginata.
bayonet h., p. em baioneta; defeito de desenvolvimento em forma de fuso, que ocorre na ponta afunilada do pêlo.
beaded h., p. em contas de rosário. SIN monilethrix.
burrowing h.'s, pêlo encravado. SIN ingrown h.'s.
club h., p. em clava; p. em estado de repouso antes de cair, em que o bulbo se transformou numa massa claviforme.
downy h. [TA], p. de lanugem; pêlo fetal fino e macio, ligeiramente pigmentado, com hastes diminutas e grandes papilas; aparece aproximadamente no final do terceiro mês de gestação. SIN lanugo [TA], primary h.*, lanugo h.
exclamation point h., p. em ponto de exclamação; o tipo de pêlo anágeno distrófico encontrado nas margens de placas de alopecia areata; o bulbo está ausente.
Frey h.'s, pêlos de Frey; pêlos curtos de vários graus de rigidez, colocados em ângulo reto na extremidade de um cabo de madeira; utilizados para avaliar a presença de sensação.
h.'s of head [TA], cabelos; pêlos do couro cabeludo. SIN scalp h.
ingrown h.'s, pêlos encravados; pêlos que crescem em ângulos mais agudos do que o normal e em todas as direções; saem incompletamente do folículo, voltam-se para trás e provocam pseudofoliculite. SIN burrowing h.'s.
kinky h., p. retorcido; p. encarapinhado ou crespo. VER kinky-hair *disease.*
lanugo h., p. de lanugem. SIN downy h.

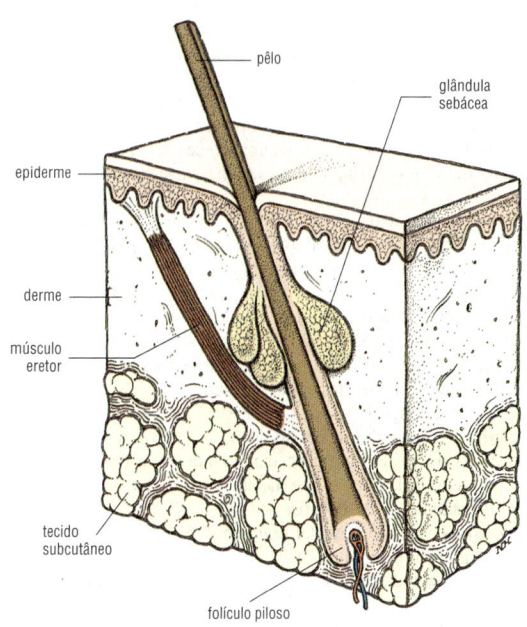

pêlo: com estruturas anatômicas associadas

moniliform h., p. moniliforme. SIN monilethrix.
nettling h.'s, pêlos irritantes; pêlos pontiagudos de certas lagartas que causam dermatite quando entram em contato com a pele.
primary h., p. primário;* termo oficial alternativo para downy h.
pubic h. [TA], pêlo pubiano; um dos pêlos pubianos; o pêlo da região pubiana imediatamente acima dos órgãos genitais externos. SIN pubes (1) [TA].
ringed h., pêlo anular; condição rara em que o pêlo exibe segmentos pigmentados e translúcidos alternados, sendo estes últimos devido a cavidades de ar no interior do córtex. SIN pili annulati.
scalp h., pêlo do couro cabeludo. SIN h.'s of head.
Schridde cancer h.'s, pêlos de câncer de Schridde; pêlos espessos e foscos, dispersos na região da barba e na região temporal; afirma-se que ocorrem em pacientes cancerosos, mas são também encontrados em indivíduos com outras condições caquéticas.
spun glass h., p. em vidro puxado. SIN uncombable hair *syndrome*.
stellate h., p. estrelado; pêlos divididos em diversos fios na extremidade livre.
taste h.'s, pêlos gustativos; projeções piliformes das células gustativas dos botões gustativos; as micrografias eletrônicas mostram que esses pêlos consistem em aglomerados de microvilosidades.
terminal h., p. terminal; pêlo maduro, pigmentado e grosseiro.
h.'s of tragus [TA], pêlos do trago; pêlos que crescem no trago da orelha.
twisted h.'s, pêlos retorcidos. SIN pili torti, under pilus.
vellus h., penugem; pêlo incolor, fino e macio encontrado desde o período pós-natal até a vida adulta.
h.'s of vestibule of nose [TA], vibrissa; um dos pêlos que crescem na narina ou vestíbulo do nariz. SIN vibrissa [TA].
woolly h., p. lanoso; p. fortemente espiralado, oval em corte transversal, com a textura de lã.
hair·pin [TA] (hār'pin). Grampo. **1.** Estrutura formada por um ácido polinucleico através do emparelhamento de bases entre seqüências complementares vizinhas de um único filamento de DNA ou de RNA. **2.** Estrutura observada numa prostaglandina e em que dois segmentos da molécula dobram-se para trás um sobre o outro.
hair·worm (hār'werm). VER *Trichostrongylus, Gordius*.
hairy (hār'ē). Cabeludo, piloso. **1.** Semelhante ao cabelo. **2.** Coberto com pêlos. VER TAMBÉM hirsutism. SIN pilar, pilary, pilose.
ha·la·tion (hā - lā'shŭn). Halo; turvação da imagem visual por luz forte.
hal·a·zone (hal'ă - zōn). Halazona; cloramina utilizada para a esterilização da água potável.
Halbeisen, William A., médico norte-americano, *1915. VER Stryker-H. *syndrome*.
Halberstaedter, Ludwig, médico alemão, 1876–1949. VER Halberstaedter-Prowazek *bodies*, em *body*.
Haldane, John B.S., bioquímico e geneticista inglês, 1892–1964. VER H. *relationship*.
Haldane, John S., fisiologista escocês em Oxford, 1860–1936. VER H. *apparatus, effect, transformation, tube;* H.-Priestley *sample*.
Hale col·loi·dal iron stain. Corante de ferro coloidal de Hale. Ver em stain.
Hales, Stephen, fisiologista inglês, 1677–1761. VER H. *piesimeter*.
half-hap·ten (haf - hap'ten). Meio-hapteno; substância que desencadeia uma reação antígeno-anticorpo, porém sem precipitação.
half-life (haf'līf). Meia-vida; período durante o qual a radioatividade ou o número de átomos de substância radioativa se reduz à metade; termo igualmente aplicado a qualquer substância, como uma droga no soro, cuja quantidade diminui de modo exponencial com o tempo. Cf. half-time.
biologic h.-l., meia-vida biológica; tempo necessário para que ocorra perda da metade de determinada quantidade de uma substância através de processos biológicos.
effective h.-l., meia-vida efetiva; tempo necessário para que a carga corporal de uma dose administrada de radioatividade sofra redução à metade através de uma combinação de desintegração radioativa e eliminação biológica.
physical h.-l., meia-vida física; tempo necessário para que metade dos átomos de um radionuclídeo sofra desintegração.
half-moon (haf'moon). Meia-lua. SIN lunule of nail.
red h.-m., meia-lua vermelha; pigmentação vermelha irregular da meia-lua, geralmente pálida na base das unhas dos dedos das mãos; pode ser observada na insuficiência congestiva, em doenças malignas ou na hepatopatia, porém não é específica de nenhuma dessas doenças.
half-time (haf'tīm). Meio-tempo; o tempo, numa reação química (ou enzimática) de primeira ordem, para que metade da substância (substrato) seja convertida ou desapareça. Cf. half-life.
half·way house (haf'wā hows). Clínica de tratamento parcial; instalação para indivíduos que não necessitam mais de todos os recursos de um hospital ou clínica, mas que ainda não estão preparados para voltar a ter uma vida independente.
hal·i·but liv·er oil (hal'i - bŭt). Óleo de fígado de hipoglosso; o óleo fixo obtido da carne ou do fígado adequado conservado de espécies do gênero *Hippoglossus* (família Pleuronectidae); fonte suplementar de vitaminas A e D.

hal·ide (hal'īd). Halóide; sal de um halogênio.
hal·i·pha·gia (hal - i - fā'jē - ă). Halifagia; ingestão de uma quantidade excessiva de sal ou sais, especialmente cloreto de sódio, sais de cálcio, magnésio ou potássio, ou de bicarbonato de sódio. [G. *hals*, sal, + *phagō*, comer]
hal·i·ste·re·sis (hă - lis - ter - ē'sis). Halisterese; deficiência de sais de cálcio nos ossos. SIN halosteresis. [G. *hals*, sal, + *sterēsis*, privação, de *stereō*, privar]
hal·i·ste·ret·ic (hă - lis - ter - et'ik). Halisterético; relativo a, ou caracterizado por, halisterese.
hal·i·to·sis (hal - i - tō'sis). Halitose; hálito com cheiro desagradável. SIN fetor oris, ozostomia, stomatodysodia. [L. *halitus*, respiração, + G. *-osis*, condição]
hal·i·tus (hal'i - tŭs). Hálito; qualquer exalação, como de uma respiração ou vapor. [L., de *halo*, respirar]
hal·la·chrome (hal'ă - krōm). Halacromo; intermediário de quinona, derivado da L-dopa, na formação da melanina a partir da L-tirosina.
Hallé, Adrien H.M.N., médico francês, 1859–1947. VER H. *point*.
Haller, Albrecht von, fisiologista suíço, 1708–1777. VER H. *ansa, anulus, arches,* em *arch, circle, cones,* under *cone, habenula, insula, line, plexus, rete*, vascular *tissue, tripod, tunica* vasculosa, *unguis, vas* aberrans.
Hallermann, Wilhelm, oftalmologista alemão, 1901–1976. VER H.-Streiff *syndrome*; Hallermann-Streiff-François *syndrome*.
Hallervorden, Julius, neurologista alemão, 1882–1965. VER H. *syndrome*; H.-Spatz *disease, syndrome*.
hal·lex, pl. **hal·li·ces** (hal'eks, hal'i - sēz). Hálux. SIN great toe I. [L.]
Hallgren, Bertil, geneticista sueco do século XX. VER H. *syndrome*.
Hallopeau, François H., dermatologista francês, 1842–1919. VER H. *disease*.
Hallpike, C.S., otologista inglês do século XX. VER Dix-H. *maneuver*.
hal·lu·cal (hal'oo - kăl). Halucal; relativo ao hálux.
hal·lu·ci·na·tion (ha - loo'si - nā'shŭn). Alucinação; a aparente percepção subjetiva, freqüentemente intensa, de um objeto ou acontecimento quando não há esse estímulo ou situação; pode ser visual, auditiva, olfativa, gustativa ou tátil. [L. *alucinor*, vaguear com o pensamento]
auditory h., a. auditiva; um sintoma freqüentemente observado num distúrbio esquizofrênico que consiste, na ausência de uma fonte externa, em ouvir uma voz ou outro estímulo auditivo que outros indivíduos não percebem.
command h., a. de comando; um sintoma, habitualmente auditivo, mas algumas vezes visual, que consiste numa mensagem, sem nenhuma fonte externa, para fazer algo.
formed visual h., a. visual figurada; alucinação composta de cenas, freqüentemente de paisagens.
gustatory h., a. gustativa; a sensação de paladar na ausência de estímulo gustativo; pode ser observada na epilepsia do lobo temporal.
haptic h., a. háptica; a sensação de toque na ausência de estímulos; pode ser observada no *delirium tremens* do alcoolismo.
hypnagogic h., a. hipnagógica; alucinação que ocorre ao deitar, no período entre a vigília e o sono; um dos componentes da narcolepsia.
hypnopompic h., a. hipnopômpica; alucinações vívidas que ocorrem ao despertar do sono; ocorre na narcolepsia, porém associada a alucinação hipnagógica.
kinesthesia h., a. de cinestesia; sensação de movimento de um ou mais músculos, quando não ocorre nenhum movimento.
lilliputian h., a. liliputiana; alucinação de tamanho reduzido de objetos ou pessoas.
mood-congruent h., a. com humor congruente; alucinação em que o conteúdo é apropriado para o humor.
mood-incongruent h., a. com humor não-congruente; alucinação que não é condizente com os estímulos externos; o conteúdo não é congruente com o humor maníaco ou deprimido.
olfactory h., a. olfativa; falsa percepção do olfato.
stump h., dor do membro fantasma. SIN phantom limb *pain*.
tactile h., a. tátil; percepção falsa de movimento ou de sensação, como de um membro amputado, ou sensação rastejante na pele.
unformed visual h., a. visual não-formada; alucinação composta de faíscas, luzes ou esferas de luz explodindo.
hal·lu·ci·no·gen (ha - loo'si - nō - jen). Alucinógeno; substância química, droga ou agente que tem a propriedade de alterar a mente, especificamente uma substância química cuja ação farmacológica mais proeminente é exercida no sistema nervoso central (p. ex., mescalina); em indivíduos normais, desencadeia alucinações ópticas ou auditivas, despersonalização, distúrbios de percepção e distúrbios dos processos do pensamento. SIN psychedelic drug, psychodysleptic drug, psycholytic drug, psychotomimetic drug. [L. *alucinor*, vaguear com pensamento, + G. *-gen*, produzindo]
hal·lu·ci·no·gen·e·sis (ha - loo'si - nō - jen'ĕ - sis). Alucinogênese; o processo de produzir uma alucinação.
hal·lu·ci·no·gen·ic (ha - loo'si - nō - jen'ik). Alucinogênico. SIN psychedelic.
hal·lu·ci·no·sis (ha - loo - si - nō'sis). Alucinose; uma síndrome, habitualmente de origem orgânica, caracterizada por alucinações mais ou menos persistentes, como, p. ex., alucinação alcoólica.
organic h., a. orgânica; o estado de experimentar uma falsa percepção sensorial na ausência de estímulo externo, observado em indivíduos com um dos

hallucinosis

distúrbios mentais orgânicos (p. ex., as sensações assustadoras que ocorrem na alucinose alcoólica ou apresentadas por uma pessoa que ingeriu LSD ou outra droga com a propriedade de alterar a mente). VER hallucination.

hal·lus (hal′ŭs). Hálux. SIN great toe I.

hal·lux, pl. **hal·lu·ces** (hal′ŭks, hal′ū - sēz)[TA]. Hálux. SIN great toe I. [forma L. Mod. para *hallex (hallic-)*, grande artelho]

  h. doloro'sus, h. doloroso; condição habitualmente associada a pé plano, em que a marcha provoca dor intensa na articulação metatarsofalangiana do dedo grande do pé. SIN painful toe.

  h. exten'sus, h. esticado; deformidade em que o primeiro artelho é mantido rigidamente em extensão.

  h. flex'us, h. em martelo. SIN h. malleus.

  h. mal'leus, h. em martelo; primeiro artelho em martelo. SIN h. flexus.

  h. rig'idus, h. rígido; condição em que ocorre rigidez na primeira articulação metatarsofalângica; geralmente associada ao desenvolvimento de esporões ósseos na superfície dorsal. SIN stiff toe.

  h. val'gus, h. valgo; desvio da ponta do hálux ou de seu eixo principal para a face lateral do pé.

  h. va'rus, h. varo; desvio do eixo principal do hálux para o lado interno do pé, afastando-o do segundo dedo.

ha·lo (hā′lo). Halo. **1.** Anel amarelo avermelhado que circunda o disco óptico, devido a um alargamento do anel da esclerótica, tornando as estruturas mais profundas visíveis. **2.** Fulguração anular de luz em torno de um corpo luminoso ou anel despigmentado ao redor de uma mola. VER halo *nevus*. **3.** SIN areola (4). **4.** Faixa metálica circular usada em molde ou suporte, fixada ao crânio com pinos. [G. *halōs,* eira na qual andavam os bois em círculo; halo em redor do sol ou da lua]

  anemic h., h. anêmico; áreas pálidas e relativamente avasculares na pele, observadas ao redor de aranhas vasculares, angiomas vermelho-cereja e, algumas vezes, erupções maculares agudas.

  glaucomatous h., h. glaucomatoso; **(1)** anel branco amarelado em torno do disco óptico, indicando atrofia da coróide no glaucoma. SIN glaucomatous ring. **(2)** h. circundando luzes, produzido por edema da córnea no glaucoma. SIN rainbow symptom.

  senile h., h. senil; halo circumpapilar observado na atrofia coróide do idoso.

hal·o·al·kyl·a·mines (hal - ō - al - kil′ā - mēnz). Haloalquilaminas; classe de drogas, incluindo a fenoxibenzamina e a diabenamina, que se ligam aos receptores α-adrenérgicos e os alquilam, tornando-os irreversivelmente ativados.

hal·o·gen (hal′ō - jen). Alógeno, alogênio; um dos elementos do grupo do cloro (flúor, cloro, bromo, iodo, astatínio); os alogênios formam ácidos monobásicos com o hidrogênio, e seus hidróxidos (o flúor não forma nenhum) também são ácidos monobásicos. [G, *hals,* sal, + *-gen,* produzindo]

hal·o·gen·a·tion (hal′ō - jĕ - nā′shŭn). Alogenação; incorporação de um ou mais átomos de alogênio numa molécula.

hal·o·gen·o·der·ma (hal - ō - gen′ō - der - mă). Alogenoderma; dermatose causada pela ingestão ou injeção de alogênios, mais notavelmente brometos e iodetos. [halogen + G. *derma,* pele]

Hal·o·ge·ton (hal - ō - jē′ton). Gênero de plantas (família Chenopodiaceae) encontradas em regiões de pastagem natural no oeste dos Estados Unidos e em outras regiões áridas do mundo; provoca envenenamento no gado e nas ovelhas, devido à presença de oxalatos solúveis.

ha·lom·e·ter (hal - om′ĕ - ter). Alômetro; instrumento utilizado para medir o halo de difração de uma hemácia; baseado na premissa de que o halo dos grandes eritrócitos da anemia perniciosa é menor do que o da célula normal; o halo nebuloso e incolor de tamanho normal é característico da anemia secundária.

hal·o·phil, hal·o·phile (hal′ō - fil, - fil). Alópilo; microrganismo cujo crescimento é intensificado por uma elevada concentração de sal ou depende dela. [G. *hals,* sal, + *philos,* amigo]

hal·o·phil·ic (hal - ō - fil′ik). Alópilo; que exige uma alta concentração de sal para seu crescimento.

hal·o·ste·re·sis (hā - los - tĕ - rē′sis). Alosterese. SIN halisteresis.

hal·o·thane (hal′ō - thān). Halotano; potente anestésico inalatório, não-inflamável e não-explosivo, amplamente utilizado, com rápido início e reversão; os efeitos colaterais consistem em depressão respiratória e cardiovascular e sensibilização a arritmias induzidas por epinefrina. Freqüentemente utilizado em crianças, visto ser o seu odor menos pungente do que aquele de alguns outros agentes anestésicos.

Halstead, Ward C., psicólogo norte-americano, 1908–1968. VER H.-Reitan *battery.*

Halsted, William Stewart, cirurgião norte-americano, 1852–1922. VER H. *law, operation, suture.*

Hal·te·rid·i·um (hawl - tĕ - rid′ē - ŭm). Nome antigo de *Haemoproteus.* [G. *haltēres,* peso mantido nas mãos ao saltar]

hal·zoun (hal′zŭn). Nome local de uma infecção bucofaríngea que ocorre no Líbano, provavelmente causada por larvas pentastomídeas de *Linguatula serrata,* que migram para a garganta do hospedeiro humano após a ingestão de carne crua de ovinos ou de fígado ou linfonodos de caprinos. [Ar., snail]

Ham, Thomas Hale, médico norte-americano, 1905–1987. VER H. *test.*

ham. 1. Fossa poplítea. SIN popliteal *fossa.* **2.** As nádegas e a parte posterior da coxa. [A.S.]

HAMA Abreviatura para anticorpo anticamundongo humano (human antimouse antibody).

ham·a·me·lis (ham′ă - mē′lis). Hamamélis; um arbusto ou pequena árvore, *Hamamelis virginiana* (família Harmarmelidaceae), cuja casca e folhas secas têm sido aplicadas externamente a contusões e outras lesões, na cefaléia e para a cura de hemorróidas não-inflamatórias; a água de hamamélis, popularmente conhecida como "extrato de aveleira-de-bruxa", é feita com a casca e contém álcool a 14%. SIN witch hazel. [L. Mod. fr. G. *hama- mēlis,*fr. *hama,* junto + *mēlon,*maçã]

ha·mar·tia (ham - ar′shē - ă). Hamartia; distúrbio localizado de desenvolvimento, caracterizado por um arranjo e/ou combinações anormais dos tecidos normalmente presentes na área. [G. *hamartion,* defeito corporal]

ham·ar·to·blas·to·ma (hă - mar′tō - blas - tō′mă). Hamartoblastoma; neoplasia maligna de células anaplásicas indiferenciadas que se acredita seja derivada de um hamartoma. [hamartoma + blastoma]

ham·ar·to·chon·dro·ma·to·sis (ham - ar′tō - kon′drō - mă - tō′sis). Hamartocondromatose; focos de tecido cartilaginoso de aspecto neoplásico em locais onde a cartilagem é um constituinte normal, mas em que o crescimento das células cartilaginosas é desproporcional ao de outros elementos do órgão. [G. *hamartion,* defeito corporal, + *chondros,* cartilagem, + *-osis,* condição]

ham·ar·to·ma (ham - ar - tō′mă). Hamartoma; malformação focal que se assemelha a uma neoplasia, macroscópica e até microscopicamente, mas que resulta do desenvolvimento defeituoso em determinado órgão; composto de uma mistura anormal de elementos teciduais ou de proporção anormal de um único elemento, normalmente presente nesse local, que se desenvolve e cresce praticamente na mesma velocidade que os componentes normais; não tende a causar compressão dos tecidos adjacentes (ao contrário de uma neoplasia). [G. *hamartion,* defeito corporal, + *-oma,* tumor]

  fibrous h. of infancy, h. fibroso do lactente; tumor que aparece habitualmente no braço ou no ombro nos dois primeiros anos de vida, consistindo em tecido fibroso celular que se infiltra no tecido subcutâneo.

  pulmonary h., h. pulmonar; produz uma lesão numular composta primariamente de cartilagem e epitélio brônquico.

ham·ar·tom·a·tous (ham - ar - tō′mă - tŭs). Hamartomatoso; relativo a hamartoma.

ham·ar·to·pho·bia (ham′ar - tō - fō′bē - ă). Hamartofobia; temor mórbido de erro ou pecado. [G. *hamartia,* erro, + *phobos,* medo]

ha·mate. Hamato. VER hamate (*bone*).

ha·ma·tum (ha - mā′tŭm). Hamato. SIN hamate (*bone).* [L. neut. De *hamatus,* em gancho, fr. *hamus,* gancho]

Hamburger, Hartog J., fisiologista holandês, 1859–1924. VER H. *phenomenon.*

Hamman, Louis, médico norte-americano, 1877–1946. VER H. *disease, murmur, sign, syndrome;* Hamman-Rich *syndrome.*

Hammarsten, Olof, químico fisiologista sueco, 1841–1932. VER H. *reagent.*

ham·mer (ham′er). Martelo. SIN malleus.

Hammerschlag, Albert, médico austríaco, 1863–1935. VER H. *method.*

Hammond, William A., neurologista norte-americano, 1828–1900. VER H. *disease.*

Hampton, Aubrey Otis, radiologista norte-americano, 1900–1955. VER H. *line, maneuver, technique, hump.*

ham·ster. *Hamster,* criceto; qualquer um dos quatro gêneros (subfamília Cricetinae, família Muridae) de pequenos roedores amplamente utilizados em pesquisa e como animais de estimação: *Cricetus, Cricetulus, Mesocricetus* e *Phodopus.* Todos os *hamsters* alimentam-se de sementes e plantas, armazenam o alimento, hibernam no inverno e procriam o ano todo em condições de laboratório.

ham·string. Tendões do jarrete. **1.** Um dos tendões que ladeiam a fossa poplítea; a **porção medial** compreende os tendões dos músculos semimembranoso e semitendinoso; a **porção lateral** é o tendão do músculo bíceps femoral. Os músculos posteriores da coxa (a) originam-se da tuberosidade isquiática, (b) atuam através de ambas as articulações do quadril e do joelho (produzindo extensão e flexão, respectivamente) e (c) são inervados pela porção tibial do nervo isquiático. A porção medial do tendão contribui para a rotação medial da perna na articulação do joelho flexionado, enquanto a porção lateral contribui para a rotação lateral. **2.** Em animais domésticos, a combinação de tendões do flexor digital superficial, tríceps sural, bíceps femoral e músculos semitendinosos, que são designados como tendão calcâneo comum (tendo calcaneus communis); está fixado à tuberosidade do calcanhar.

ham·u·lar (ham′ū - lăr). Hamular; em forma de gancho; unciforme. [L. *hamulus, q.v.*]

ham·u·lus, gen. e pl. **ham·u·li** (ham′ū - lŭs, - lī) [TA]. Hâmulo; qualquer estrutura semelhante a um gancho (unciforme). SIN hook (2)*. [L. dim. de *hamus,* gancho]

  h. coch'leae, h. da lâmina espiral. SIN h. of spiral lamina.

lacrimal h. [ITA], h. lacrimal; extremidade inferior unciforme da crista lacrimal, que se curva entre o processo frontal e a superfície orbital da maxila, formando a abertura superior da porção óssea do canal nasolacrimal. SIN h. lacrimalis [TA], hamular process of lacrimal bone.
h. lacrima'lis [TA], h. lacrimal. SIN lacrimal h.
h. lam'inae spira'lis [TA], h. da lâmina espiral. SIN h. of spiral lamina.
h. os'sis hama'ti [TA], h. do osso hamato. SIN hook of hamate.
pterygoid h. [TA], h. pterigóideo; a extremidade inferior unciforme da placa medial do processo pterigóideo, que atua como roldana (tróclea) para o tendão do músculo tensor do palato mole. SIN hamular process of sphenoid bone, h. pterygoideus.
h. pterygoid'eus, h. pterigóideo. SIN pterygoid h.
h. of spiral lamina [TA], h. da lâmina espiral; a terminação superior unciforme da lâmina espiral óssea do ápice da cóclea. SIN h. laminae spiralis [TA], h. cochleae, hook of spiral lamina.
Hancock, Henry, cirurgião inglês, 1809–1880. VER H. *amputation.*
Hand, Alfred, pediatra norte-americano, 1868–1949. VER H.-Schüller-Christian *disease.*
hand [TA]. Mão; parte do membro superior distalmente à articulação radiocárpica, constituída pelo punho, palma e dedos. SIN manus [TA], main. [A.S.]
accoucheur h., m. de parteiro, m. obstétrica; posição da mão na tetania ou na distrofia muscular; os dedos são flexionados nas articulações metacarpofalângicas e estendidos nas articulações falângicas, com o polegar em flexão e adução em direção à face palmar da mão; semelhante à posição da mão do médico ao fazer um exame vaginal. SIN obstetric h.
ape h., m. de macaco; deformidade caracterizada pela extensão do polegar no mesmo plano da palma e dos dedos da mão. SIN monkey h., monkey-paw.
claw h., m. em garra. VER clawhand.
cleft h., m. fendida; deformidade congênita em que a divisão entre os dedos, especialmente entre o terceiro e o quarto, estende-se até a região metacarpal. VER TAMBÉM lobster-claw *deformity.* SIN split h.
club h., m. em clava; deformidade de angulação congênita ou adquirida da mão, associada à ausência parcial ou completa do rádio ou da ulna; geralmente associada a deformidades intrínsecas da mão em variantes congênitas.
crab h., erisipelóide. SIN erysipeloid.
dorsum of h. [TA], dorso da mão. SIN dorsum manus [TA].
drop h., queda do punho. SIN *wrist*-drop.
ghoul h., m. de *ghoul*, condição observada em negros africanos, provavelmente uma manifestação de bouba terciária, caracterizada por despigmentação das regiões palmares e contração da pele, conferindo à mão um aspecto semelhante a uma garra e a um cadáver.
Marinesco succulent h., m. suculenta de Marinesco; edema da mão com frieza e lividez da pele, observada na siringomielia. SIN main succulente.
monkey h., m. simiesca. SIN ape h.
obstetric h., m. obstétrica. SIN accoucheur h.
opera-glass h., m. em binóculo; deformidade observada na artrite absortiva crônica, em que os dedos e os punhos estão encurtados e cobertos com pele enrugada nas pregas transversas; as falanges parecem estar retraídas uma dentro da outra, como um binóculo ou um telescópio em miniatura.
simian h., h. símia; deformidade caracterizada por retificação da eminência tenar, com o polegar em adução e extensão; geralmente causada por lesão de nervo mediano.
skeleton h., m.-de-esqueleto; extensão dos dedos das mãos com atrofia dos tecidos; ocorre na atrofia muscular progressiva.
spade h., m. em pá; mão grosseira, espessa e quadrada da acromegalia ou do mixedema.
split h., m. fendida. SIN cleft h.
trident h., m. em tridente; mão em que os dedos são de comprimento quase igual e defletidos na primeira articulação interfalângica, conferindo um aspecto de garfo; encontrada na acondroplasia.
writing h., m.-de-escritor; contração dos músculos da mão no parkinsonismo, com os dedos colocados aproximadamente na posição de segurar uma caneta.
hand·ed·ness (hand'ed - nes). Destreza no uso da mão; preferência pelo uso de uma das mãos, mais comumente a direita, associada à dominância do hemisfério cerebral oposto; pode resultar também de treinamento ou hábito.
hand·i·cap (hand'i - kap). Desvantagem. **1.** Condição física, mental ou emocional que interfere no funcionamento normal do indivíduo. **2.** Redução na capacidade de um indivíduo de desempenhar um papel social em conseqüência de comprometimento, treinamento inadequado para o papel ou outras circunstâncias. VER TAMBÉM disability. [fr. *hand in cap,* (jogo)]
hand·piece (hand'pēs). Instrumento dentário motorizado mantido na mão, utilizado para segurar instrumentos rotatórios de corte, esmerilhamento ou polimento enquanto estão sendo acionados.
hand·shapes (hand'shāps). Alfabeto manual; símbolos manuais de sons falados utilizados para comunicação de surdos-mudos.
HANE Acrônimo de hereditary angioneurotic *edema* (edema angioneurótico hereditário).

hang·nail (hang'nāl). Cutícula; retalho frouxo triangular de pele fixado proximalmente na dobra ungueal medial ou lateral.
Hanhart, Ernst, internista suíço, 1891–1973. VER H. *syndrome.*
Hanks, Horace Tracy, cirurgião norte-americano, 1837–1900. VER H. *dilators.*
Hanks so·lu·tion. Solução de Hanks. Ver em solution.
Hanlon, C. Rollins, cirurgião cardiovascular e torácico norte-americano, *1915. VER Blalock-H. *operation.*
Hannover, Adolph, anatomista dinamarquês, 1814–1894. VER H. *canal.*
Hanot, Victor C., médico francês, 1844–1896. VER H. *cirrhosis.*
Hansen, Gerhard A., médico norueguês, 1841–1912. VER H. *bacillus, disease.*
Han·ta·vi·rus (han'tă - vă - rŭs). Gênero de Bunyaviridae responsável pela pneumonia e por febres hemorrágicas; até o momento, já foram reconhecidos pelo menos 7 membros do gênero: vírus Hantaan, Puumala, Seoul, Prospect Hill, Thailand, Thottapalayam e Sin Nombre. Várias outras espécies ainda não foram classificadas. O vírus Hantaan causa a febre hemorrágica da Coréia. Diversas espécies de roedores são portadores assintomáticos desses vírus, que são eliminados na saliva, na urina e nas fezes. A infecção humana é direta ou ocorre por via respiratória a partir de espécies contaminadas; a transmissão interpessoal é considerada rara. No oeste dos Estados Unidos, numa região onde se encontram as fronteiras dos estados do Arizona, Utah, Colorado e New Mexico, foi identificado, em 1993, um surto de infecção por hantavírus, a síndrome pulmonar por Hantavírus (SPH), e o agente responsável foi subseqüentemente denominado vírus Sin Nombre.
hap·a·lo·nych·ia (hap'ă - lō - nik'ē - ă). Hapaloníquia; adelgaçamento das unhas resultando em encurvamento e ruptura da extremidade livre, com fissuras longitudinais. SIN egg shell nail. [G. *hapalos,* mole, + G. *onyx (onych-),* unha]
haph·al·ge·sia (haf - al - jē'zē - ă). Afalgesia; dor ou sensação extremamente desagradável causada pelo mais simples toque. SIN Pitres sign (1). [G. *haphē,* toque, + *algēsis,* sensação de dor]
hap·haz·ard. Ao acaso; que carece de qualquer sistema, organização ou objetivo coerente; não confundir com randômico ou caótico.
haph·e·pho·bia (haf - ē - fō'bē - ă). Hafefobia; desgosto mórbido ou medo de ser tocado. [G. *haphē,* toque, + *phobos,* medo]
haplo-. Haplo-. Simples, único. [G. *haplous*]
hap·lo·dont (hap'lō - dont). Haplodonte; que tem dentes molares com coroas simples, isto é, dentes cônicos simples sem sulcos ou tubérculos. [haplos- + G. *odous,* dente]
hap·loid (hap'loyd). Haplóide; indica o número de cromossomas, no espermatozóide ou no óvulo, que é metade do número das células somáticas (diplóide); o número h. nos seres humanos normais é 23. SIN monoploid. [G. *haplos,* único, + *eidos,* aspecto]
hap·lol·o·gy (hap - lol'ō - jē). Haplologia; omissão de sílabas devido à velocidade excessiva da fala. [haplo- + G. *logos,* estudo]
hap·lo·pro·tein (hap - lō - prō'tēn). Haploproteína; o complexo funcional entre uma apoproteína e o grupo prostético que, em conjunto, é responsável pela atividade biológica.
hap·lo·scope (hap'lō - skōp). Haploscópio; instrumento para mostrar imagens separadas a cada olho, de modo que possam ser vistas como uma só imagem. [haplo- + G. *skopeō,* ver]
mirror h., h. de espelho; haploscópio que utiliza espelhos para deslocar o campo de visão dos dois olhos, como no amblioscópio de Worth e no sinoptóforo.
hap·lo·scop·ic (hap - lō - skop'ik). Haploscópico; relativo a um haploscópio.
Hap·lo·spo·rid·ia (hap'lō - spō - rid'ē - ă). Ordem de esporozoários, atualmente colocada no filo dos protozoários Ascetospora, da classe Stellatosporea, que se reproduzem assexuadamente por esquizogonia e produzem esporos, mas não flagelos, embora possa haver pseudópodes. [haplo- + G. *sporos,* semente]
hap·lo·type (hap'lō - tīp). Haplótipo. **1.** Constituição genética de um indivíduo em relação a um membro de um par de genes alelos; os indivíduos são do mesmo h. (mas de genótipos diferentes) quando semelhantes em relação a um alelo de um par, porém diferentes em relação ao outro alelo de um par. **2.** Em imunogenética, a porção do fenótipo determinada por um conjunto de genes estreitamente ligados e herdados de um dos genitores (isto é, genes localizados em um dos pares de cromossomas). [haplo- + G. *typos,* impressão, modelo]
hap·ten (hap' - ten). Hapteno; molécula que é incapaz, isoladamente, de causar a produção de anticorpos, mas que, entretanto, tem a capacidade de se combinar com uma molécula antigênica maior, denominada transportador. O complexo hapteno-transportador pode estimular a produção de anticorpos, dos quais alguns se combinam com a porção h. do complexo. VER TAMBÉM hapten *inhibition* of precipitation. SIN incomplete antigen, partial antigen. [G. *haptō,* fixar, ligar]
conjugated h., h. conjugado; hapteno capaz de induzir a produção de anticorpos após a sua ligação covalente a proteínas. SIN conjugated antigen.
Forssman h., h. de Forssman; glicolipídios de órgãos de mamíferos; trata-se de um pentassacarídeo ceramida. Cf. Forssman *antibody,* Forssman *antigen.*
half. h., meio-hapteno. VER half-hapten.

hap·to·dys·pho·ria (hap'tō - dis - fō'rē - ā). Haptodisforia; sensação desagradável em conseqüência do toque de certos objetos. [G. *haptō*, tocar, + disforia]

hap·to·glo·bin (HP) (hap - tō - glō'bin) [MIM*140100 & MIM* 140210]. Haptoglobina (HP); grupo de α_2-globulinas no soro humano, assim denominada em virtude de sua capacidade de se combinar com a hemoglobina, impedindo a sua perda na urina. Os tipos variantes formam um sistema polimórfico, sendo as cadeias polipeptídicas α e β controladas por *loci* genéticos separados. Os níveis de haptoglobina estão diminuídos nos distúrbios hemolíticos e elevados em condições inflamatórias ou em caso de lesão tecidual. [G. *haptō*, segurar + hemoglobina]

hap·tom·e·ter (hap - tom'e - ter). Haptômetro; instrumento para medir a sensibilidade ao tato. [G. *haptō*, tocar, + *metron*, medida]

Har Abreviatura de homoarginine (homoarginina).

Harada, Einosuke, cirurgião japonês, 1892–1947. VER H. *disease, syndrome;* Harada-Ito *procedure.*

Harada, T., patologista japonês do século XX. VER H.-Mori filter paper strip *culture.*

Harden, Sir Arthur, bioquímico inglês e ganhador do Prêmio Nobel, 1865–1940. VER H.-Young *ester.*

hardening (har'den - ing). **1.** Condição de redução das reações a alérgenos em decorrência de exposição não-terapêutica repetida ou prolongada, semelhante à hipossensibilização. **2.** Qualquer método na preparação de tecidos para exame, como corte para microscopia, capaz de tornar o tecido mais rígido.

har·di·ness (har'di - nes). Resistência; traço de comportamento que fortalece a saúde e que se acredita aumente a resistência do indivíduo à doença; caracteriza-se por alto nível de controle pessoal, compromisso e ação ao responder a eventos da vida diária. [I.M., do Fr. ant. *hardi*, através do germânico]

Harding, Harold E., patologista inglês do século XX. VER H.-Passey *melanoma.*

hard·ness (hard'nes). **1.** Dureza; grau de firmeza de um sólido, determinado pela sua resistência à deformação, arranhadura ou abrasão. VER TAMBÉM hardness *scale*, *number*. **2.** Dureza; poder relativo de penetração de um feixe de raios X, utilizado dentro da faixa de energia para diagnóstico e em radioterapia; expresso em termos da espessura de camada de meio-valor.

indentation h., d. de indentação; número relacionado ao tamanho da impressão feita por um indentador (ou instrumento) de tamanho e forma específicos, sob uma carga conhecida.

hard·ware. Hardware; componente eletrônico de um computador.

Hardy, George. H., matemático inglês, 1877–1947. VER H.-Weinberg *equilibrium, law.*

Hardy, LeGrand H., oftalmologista norte-americano, 1894–1954. VER H.-Rand-Ritter *test.*

hare·lip (hār'lip). Lábio leporino, fenda labial. SIN cleft *lip.*

har·ma·line (har'mā - līn). Harmalina; inibidor da amina oxidase e estimulante do sistema nervoso central; obtida das sementes de *Peganum harmala* (família Zygophyllaceae) e de *Banisteria caapi* (família de Malpighiaceae); tem sido utilizada no parkinsonismo. SIN harmidine.

har·mi·dine (har'mi - dēn). Harmidina. SIN harmalina.

har·mine (har'mēn). Harmina; estimulante do sistema nervoso central e potente inibidor da monoamina oxidase obtido de *Peganum harmala* (família Zygophyllaceae) e de *Banisteria caapi* (família Malpighiaceae); os efeitos psíquicos assemelham-se aos produzidos pelo LSD, porém as qualidades sedativas e depressivas podem predominar sobre as manifestações alucinatórias. SIN banisterine, leucoharmine, telepathine. [G. *harmala*, harmal, fr. Ar. *harmalah*, + ine]

har·mo·nia (har - mō'nē - ā). Sutura plana. SIN plane *suture*. [L. e G. uma união]

har·mon·ic (har - mon'ik). Harmônico; componente de um som complexo, cuja freqüência é um múltiplo da freqüência fundamental. A freqüência fundamental é denominada a primeira harmônica; a segunda harmônica tem duas vezes a freqüência da fundamental, e assim por diante.

har·mo·ny (har'mō - nē). Harmonia; num som complexo, refere-se a uma relação matemática entre as freqüências do som fundamental e seus sons harmônicos, de modo que as freqüências desses últimos são múltiplos inteiros ou parciais da freqüência do som fundamental; o efeito auditivo resultante tem uma qualidade musical ou agradável, em oposição ao ruído. [G., L. *harmonia*, acordo, articulação, fr. *harmos*, união]

functional occlusal h., oclusiva funcional; relação oclusiva de dentes opostos em todas as faixas e movimentos funcionais, proporcionando a máxima eficiência de mastigação, sem produzir esforço ou traumatismo indevido sobre os tecidos de sustentação, dentes e músculos.

occlusal h., oclusiva; oclusão sem contatos oclusivos defletivos ou interceptivos em relação à mandíbula cêntrica, bem como em movimentos excêntricos.

har·pax·o·pho·bia (har'paks - ō - fō'bē - ā). Harpaxofobia; temor mórbido de ladrões. [G. *harpax*, ladrão, + *phobos*, medo]

har·poon (har - poon'). Arpão; pequeno instrumento pontiagudo com uma cabeça farpada, utilizado para extrair pedaços de tecido para exame microscópico.

Harrington, David O., oftalmologista norte-americano, *1904. VER H.-Flocks *test.*

Harris, Henry A., anatomista inglês, 1886–1968. VER H. *lines*, em *line*.

Harris, Henry F., médico norte-americano, 1867–1926. VER H. *hematoxylin*.

Harris, R.I., ortopedista canadense do século XX. VER Salter-H. *classification* of epiphysial plate injuries.

Harris, Seale, médico norte-americano, 1870–1957, que investigou as condições alimentares e doenças nutricionais. VER Harris *syndrome*.

Harris, Wilfred, neurologista inglês, 1869–1960. VER H. *migraine*.

Harris and Ray test. Teste de Harris e Ray. Ver em *test*.

Harrison, Edward, médico inglês. 1766–1838. VER H. *groove*.

Hartel, Fritz, cirurgião alemão. VER H. *technique*.

Hartman, LeRoy L., dentista norte-americano, 1893–1951. VER H. *solution*.

Hartmann, Alexis F., pediatra norte-americano, 1898–1964. VER H. *solution;* Shaffer-H. *method*.

Hartmann, Arthur, laringologista alemão, 1849–1931. VER H. *curette*.

Hartmann, Henri A.C.A., cirurgião francês, 1860–1952. VER H. *operation*, *pouch*.

Hart·man·nel·la (hart - mă - nel'ă). Ameba comum de vida livre, encontrada no solo, em esgotos e na água; invade invertebrados (lesmas, gafanhotos, ostras); suspeita mas não confirmada como agente da meningoencefalite amebiana primária humana.

Hartnup. Sobrenome da família inglesa na qual a doença foi descrita pela primeira vez. VER Hartnup *disease,* Hartnup *syndrome*.

harts·horn (harts'hōrn). Carbonato de amônio; mistura de bicarbonato de amônia e carbamato de amônio obtido do sulfato de amônio e carbonato de cálcio por sublimação; utilizado como expectorante e em sais aromáticos; assim denominado por ter sido originalmente obtido dos chifres do cervo.

har·vest bug. Micuim; a larva de espécies de *Trombicula*.

Harvey, William, 1578–1657. Anatomista, fisiologista e médico inglês que descreveu pela primeira vez a circulação do sangue, em 1628. Ele percebeu que o septo interventricular não é poroso, de modo que o sangue não consegue atravessá-lo. Demonstrou que o volume de sangue que flui de modo unidirecional através de um segmento de uma veia periférica excede o volume de sangue no corpo, razão pela qual o sangue deve recircular. Descreveu a organização da circulação fetal e a transição da organização pós-natal.

has·a·mi·ya·mi (has'ă - mē - yah'mē). Hasamiyami; febre que ocorre no outono no Japão; assemelha-se à doença de Weil, porém é mais branda e causada pelo sorotipo *autumnalis* de *Leptospira interrogans*. SIN akiyami, autumn fever (2), sakushu fever, seven-day fever (2).

Häser, Heinrich, médico alemão, 1811–1884. VER H. *formula;* Trapp-H. *formula*.

Hashimoto, cirurgião japonês, 1881–1934. VER H. *disease, struma, thyroiditis*.

hash·ish (hash'ish). Haxixe; forma de maconha que consiste, em grande parte, em resina das sumidades floridas e brotos de plantas femininas cultivadas; contém a maior concentração de canabinóis entre as preparações derivadas da maconha. [Ar. feno]

Hasner, Joseph Ritter von, oftalmologista tchecoslovaco, 1819–1892. VER H. *fold*.

Hassall, Arthur, médico inglês, 1817–1894. VER H. *bodies*, em *body;* concentric *corpuscle*, em *corpuscle;* H.-Henle *bodies*, em *body;* Virchow-H. *bodies*, em *body*.

Hasselbalch, Karl, bioquímico e médico dinamarquês, 1874–1962. VER Henderson-H. *equation*.

hatch·et. Machadinha; instrumento dentário com lâmina cortante na extremidade, colocada em ângulo com o eixo do cabo e possuindo um ou dois biséis; no primeiro caso, feito como pares direito e esquerdo, denominados machadinhas de esmalte; utilizada para remover o esmalte e a dentina dos dentes.

Haubenfelder (how'ben - fel'der). VER *fields* of Forel, em *field*. [Ger.]

Hauch (H) (howkh). Hauch (H); termo utilizado para designar o antígeno flagelar de bactérias. VER TAMBÉM H *antigen*. [Ger. respiração]

Haudek, Martin, radiologista austríaco, 1880–1931. VER H. *niche*.

Hauser, G.A., ginecologista alemão do século XX. VER Mayer-Rokitansky-Küster-H. *syndrome,* Rokitansky-Küster-H. *syndrome*.

haus·to·ri·um, pl. **haus·to·ria** (haw - stō'rē - ŭm, - stō'rē - ă). Haustório; órgão para absorção de nutrientes. [Mod. L. fr. L. *hautus*, bebida]

haus·tra (haw'stră). Haustros; plural de haustrum. [L.]

haus·tral (hos'trăl). Haustral; relativo a um haustro.

haus·tra·tion (hos'trā'shŭn). Haustração. **1.** Processo de formação de um haustro. **2.** Aumento na proeminência dos haustros.

h.'s of colon, h. do cólon. SIN *haustra* of colon, em *haustrum*.

haus·trum, pl. **haus·tra** (hos'trŭm, haw'stră) [TA]. Haustro; um dentre uma série de sáculos ou bolsas, assim denominado em virtude de uma semelhança imaginária a baldes numa roda hidráulica. [L. uma máquina para retirar água, fr. *haurio*, pp. *haustus*, puxar para cima, beber]

haus'tra co'li [TA], Haustros do cólon. SIN haustra of colon.

haustra of colon [TA], Haustros do cólon; as saculações do cólon produzidas pelas tênias ou faixas longitudinais, que são um pouco mais curtas do que o intestino, de modo que este apresenta pregas ou bolsas. SIN haustra coli [TA], cellulae coli, haustrations of colon, sacculation of colon.

haus·tus (haws'tŭs). Hausto; poção ou bebida medicinal. [L. bebida, gole]
HAV Abreviatura de hepatitis A *virus* (vírus da hepatite A).
Ha·ver·hil·lia mul·ti·for·mis (ha - ver - hĭl'ē - ă mŭl - ti - fōr'mis). VER *Streptobacillus moniliformis*.
Havers, Clopton, anatomista inglês, 1650–1702. VER haversian *canals*, em *canal;* haversian *lamella;* haversian *spaces;* haversian *system*.
ha·ver·si·an (ha - ver'shan). Haversiano; relativo a Clopton Havers e às várias estruturas ósseas por ele descritas.
Hawley, C.A., ortodontista norte-americano. VER H. *appliance, retainer*.
Haworth, Sir Walter Norman, químico inglês e ganhador do Prêmio Nobel, 1883–1950. VER H. *conformational formulas of cyclic sugars, perspective formulas of cyclic sugars*.
Hayem, Georges, médico francês, 1841–1933. VER H. *hematoblast, solution;* H.-Widal *syndrome*.
Hayflick, Leonard, microbiologista norte-americano, *1928. VER H. *limit*.
Haygarth, John, médico inglês, 1740–1827. VER H. *nodes,* em *node*.
ha·zel·wort (hā'zel - wort). Aveleira. SIN *Asarum europaeum*.
Hb Abreviatura de hemoglobin (hemoglobina).
Hb$_{Chesapeake}$ Abreviatura de *hemoglobin* Chesapeake (hemoglobina Chesapeake).
HB$_e$Ab Abreviatura de antibody to the hepatitis B e *antigen* (anticorpo contra o antígeno e da hepatite B).
HB$_c$Ab Abreviatura de antibody to the hepatitis B core *antigen* (anticorpo contra o antígeno do cerne da hepatite B).
HB$_s$Ab Abreviatura de antibody to the hepatitis B surface *antigen* (anticorpo contra o antígeno de superfície da hepatite B).
HB$_c$Ag Abreviatura de hepatitis B core *antigen* (antígeno do cerne da hepatite B).
HB$_s$Ag Abreviatura de hepatitis B surface *antigen* (antígeno de superfície da hepatite B).
HbCO Abreviatura de carboxyhemoglobin (carboxiemoglobina).
HBE Abreviatura de His bundle *electrogram* (eletrograma do feixe de His).
Hbe, HB$_e$Ag Abreviatura de hepatitis B e *antigen* (antígeno e da hepatite B).
HbO$_2$ Abreviatura de oxyhemoglobin (oxiemoglobina).
Hb S Abreviatura de sickle cell *hemoglobin* (hemoglobina falciforme).
HBV Abreviatura de hepatitis B *virus* (vírus da hepatite B).
HCC Abreviatura de 25-hydroxycholecalciferol (25-hidroxicolecalciferol).
HCFA Abreviatura de *Health Care Financing Administration*.
HCG, hCG Abreviatura de human chorionic *gonadotropin* (gonadotropina coriônica humana).
β-HCG. Gonadotropina coriônica humana. SIN *chorionic gonadotropin*.
H chain. Cadeia H. SIN *heavy chain*.
HCS Abreviatura de human chorionic somatomammotropic *hormone* (hormônio somatomamotrópico humano); human chorionic *somatomammotropin* (somatomamotropina coriônica humana).
Hct Abreviatura de hematocrit (hematócrito).
HCV Abreviatura de hepatitis C *virus* (vírus da hepatite C).
Hcy Abreviatura de homocysteine (homocisteína).
HD Abreviatura de mustard *gas* (gás mostarda).
h.d. Abreviatura do L. *hora decubitus,* ao deitar.
HDCV Abreviatura de human diploid cell *vaccine* (vacina de células diplóides humanas); human diploid cell rabies *vaccine* (vacina anti-rábica de células diplóides humanas).
HDL Abreviatura de high density lipoprotein (lipoproteína de alta densidade). VER lipoprotein.
HDV Abreviatura de hepatitis delta *virus* (vírus delta da hepatite).
He Símbolo do hélio.
³He, ⁴He Símbolos de hélio-3 (He^3) e hélio-4 (He^4), respectivamente.
Head, Sir Henry, neurologista inglês, 1861–1940. VER H. *areas,* em *area; lines,* em *line; zones,* em *zone*.
🛈 **head** (hed) [TA]. Cabeça. **1.** [TA]. Extremidade superior ou anterior do corpo de um animal, contendo cérebro e os órgãos da visão, audição, paladar e olfato. **2.** [TA]. A extremidade superior, anterior ou maior, expandida ou arredondada, de qualquer corpo, órgão ou outra estrutura anatômica. **3.** Extremidade arredondada de um osso. **4.** Extremidade de um músculo fixada à parte menos móvel do esqueleto. SIN caput [TA]. [A.S. *heāfod*]
bulldog h., c. de buldogue; a cabeça larga com abóbada alta observada na acondroplasia.
h. of caudate nucleus [TA], c. do núcleo caudado; cabeça ou extremidade anterior do núcleo caudado, que se projeta para dentro do corno anterior do ventrículo lateral. SIN caput nuclei caudati [TA], anterior extremity of caudate nucleus.
clavicular h. of pectoralis major muscle [TA], c. clavicular do músculo grande peitoral. VER pectoralis major (*muscle*). SIN pars clavicularis musculi pectoralis majoris [TA], clavicular part of pectoralis major (muscle).
deep h. of flexor pollicis brevis [TA], c. profunda do flexor curto do polegar; cabeça do flexor curto do polegar que se origina nos ossos trapezóide e capitato e ligamentos cárpicos transversos. É inervada pelo nervo ulnar profundo e considerada por muitas autoridades no assunto como o primeiro músculo interósseo palmar. SIN caput profundum musculi flexoris pollicis brevis [TA].

h. of epididymis [TA], c. do epidídimo; a extremidade superior e maior do epidídimo. SIN caput epididymidis [TA], caput epididymis, globus major.
h. of femur [TA], c. do fêmur; a superfície articular hemisférica na extremidade superior do osso da coxa. SIN caput femoris [TA], caput ossis femoris, h. of thigh bone.
h. of fibula [TA], c. da fíbula; extremidade superior da fíbula, que se articula por uma faceta com a superfície interior do côndilo lateral da tíbia. SIN caput fibulae [TA], upper extremity of fibula.
hourglass h., c. em ampulheta; na sífilis congênita, crânio com sutura coronária deprimida.
humeral h. [TA], c. do úmero; termo aplicado às cabeças dos músculos do antebraço que se fixam ao úmero. A *Terminologia Anatomica* relaciona os seguintes músculos com cabeças umerais (caput humerale ...): 1) m. flexor ulnar do punho (... musculi flexoris carpi ulnaris [TA]); 2) m. pronador redondo (... musculi pronatoris teretis [TA]); e 3) m. extensor ulnar do punho (... musculi extensoris carpi ulnaris [TA]). SIN caput humerale [TA].
humeroulnar h. of flexor digitorum superficialis muscle [TA], c. umeroulnar do músculo flexor superficial dos dedos; a cabeça do flexor superficial dos dedos, que se insere tanto no úmero quanto na ulna. SIN caput humeroulnare musculi flexoris digitorum superficialis [TA].
h. of humerus [TA], c. do úmero; extremidade arredondada superior que se encaixa na cavidade glenóide da escápula. SIN caput humeri [TA].
lateral h. [TA], c. lateral; cabeça que se origina mais longe da linha média. A *Terminologia Anatomica* relaciona os seguintes músculos com c. lateral (caput laterale ...): 1) m. tríceps braquial (... musculi tricipitis brachii [TA]); 2) m. gastrocnêmio (... musculi gastrocnemii [TA]); e 3) m. flexor curto do hálux (... musculi flexoris hallucis brevis [TA]). SIN caput laterale [TA].
little h. of humerus, capítulo do úmero. SIN *capitulum* of humerus.
long h. [TA], c. longa; cabeça que tem a origem mais proximal. A *Terminologia Anatomica* relaciona os seguintes músculos com c. longa (caput longum ...): 1) m. bíceps braquial (... musculi bicipitis brachii [TA]); 2) m. bíceps femoral (... musculi bicipitis femoris [TA]); e 3) m. tríceps braquial (... musculi tricipitis brachii [TA]). SIN caput longum [TA].
h. of malleus [TA], c. do martelo; porção arredondada do martelo, que se articula com o corpo da bigorna. SIN caput mallei [TA].
h. of mandible [TA], c. da mandíbula; porção articular expandida do processo condilar da mandíbula. SIN caput mandibulae [TA].
medial h. [TA], c. medial; a cabeça de origem mais próxima da linha média. A *Terminologia Anatomica* relaciona os seguintes músculos com c. medial (caput mediale ...): 1) m. tríceps braquial (... musculi tricipitis brachii [TA]); 2) m. gastrocnêmio (... musculi gastrocnemii [TA]); e 3) flexor curto do hálux (... musculi flexoris hallucis brevis [TA]). SIN caput mediale [TA].
Medusa h., c. de medusa. SIN *caput medusae*.
h. of metacarpal [TA], c. de osso metacarpal; extremidade distal expandida de um metacarpo que se articula com a falange proximal do mesmo dedo. SIN caput ossis metacarpalis [TA].
h. of metatarsal [TA], c. de osso metatarsal; extremidade distal expandida de um osso metatarso, que se articula com a falange proximal do mesmo artelho. SIN caput ossis metatarsalis [TA].
oblique h. [TA], c. oblíqua; cabeça de origem diagonalmente situada. A *Terminologia Anatomica* relaciona os seguintes músculos com cabeça oblíqua (caput obliquum ...): 1) m. adutor do hálux (... musculi adductoris hallucis [TA]); e 2) m. adutor do polegar (... musculi adductoris pollicis [TA]). SIN caput obliquum [TA].
optic nerve h., disco óptico. SIN *optic disk*.
h. of pancreas [TA], c. do pâncreas; porção do pâncreas localizada na concavidade do duodeno. SIN caput pancreatis [TA].
h. of phalanx (of hand or foot) [TA], c. da falange (da mão ou do pé); superfície articular arredondada na extremidade distal das falanges proximal e média de cada dedo da mão e do pé. SIN caput phalangis (manus et pedis) [TA].
h. of radius [TA], c. do rádio; extremidade superior em forma de disco, que se articula com capítulo do úmero. SIN caput radii [TA].
h. of rib [TA], c. da costela; extremidade medial arredondada de uma costela que, à exceção das costelas 1, 10, 11 e 12, articula-se, por meio de duas facetas, com os corpos de duas vértebras contíguas. SIN caput costae [TA].
saddle h., clinocefalia. SIN *clinocephaly*.
short h. [TA], c. curta; para um músculo com duas cabeças de origem (um músculo "bíceps"), refere-se à cabeça que se origina mais próximo da inserção. VER short h. of biceps brachii, short h. of biceps femoris. SIN caput breve [TA].
short h. of biceps brachii [TA], c. curta do bíceps braquial, que se origina do processo coracóide da escápula. SIN caput breve musculii bicipitis brachii [TA].
short h. of biceps femoris [TA], c. curta do bíceps femoral; parte do bíceps femoral que se origina da linha áspera da metade distal do fêmur. SIN caput breve musculi bicipitis femoris [TA].
h. of stapes [TA], c. do estribo; porção do estribo que se articula com o processo lenticular da bigorna. SIN caput stapedis [TA].
sternocostal h. of pectoralis major (muscle) [TA], c. esternocostal do grande peitoral (músculo); porção do m. grande peitoral que se origina do esterno

e das costelas; atuando isoladamente, a parte esternocostal estende o braço na articulação do ombro; atuando com a cabeça clavicular, aduz o braço. VER pectoralis major (*muscle*). SIN pars sternocostalis musculi pectoralis majoris [TA], sternocostal part of pectoralis major muscle.

superficial h. of flexor pollicis brevis [TA], c. superficial do flexor curto do polegar; cabeça do flexor curto do polegar que se origina do ligamento carpal transverso (retináculo flexor) e trapézio. É inervada pelo ramo recorrente do nervo mediano. SIN caput superficiale musculi flexoris pollicis brevis [TA].

h. of talus [TA], c. do tálus; porção anterior arredondada que se articula com o osso navicular. SIN caput tali [TA].

h. of thigh bone, c. do fêmur. SIN h. of femur.

transverse h. [TA], c. transversa; cabeça de origem de um músculo transversalmente situada. A *Terminologia Anatomica* relaciona os seguintes músculos com c. transversa (caput transversum ...): 1) m. adutor do hálux (... musculi adductoris hallucis [TA]); e 2) m. adutor do polegar (... musculi adductoris pollicis [TA]). SIN caput transversum [TA].

h. of ulna [TA], c. da ulna; pequena extremidade distal arredondada da ulna que se articula com a incisura ulnar do rádio e com o disco articular. SIN caput ulnae [TA].

ulnar h. [TA], c. da ulna; termo aplicado a uma cabeça de origem de um músculo do antebraço que tem a sua origem na ulna. A *Terminologia Anatomica* relaciona os seguintes músculos com c. ulnar (caput ulnare ...): 1) m. flexor ulnar do punho (... musculi flexoris carpi ulnaris [TA]); 2) m. pronador redondo (... musculi pronatoris teritis [TA]); e 3) m. extensor ulnar do punho (... musculi extensoris carpi ulnaris [TA]). SIN caput ulnare [TA].

head·ache (hed′āk). Cefaléia; dor em diversas partes da cabeça, não limitada à área de distribuição de qualquer nervo. VER TAMBÉM cephalodynia. SIN cephalalgia, encephalalgia, encephalodynia.

benign exertional h., c. de esforço benigna; cefaléia que ocorre com o esforço na ausência de qualquer doença intracraniana.

bilious h., enxaqueca. SIN migraine.

blind h., enxaqueca. SIN migraine.

cluster h., c. em salvas; possivelmente devido a hipersensibilidade à histamina; caracterizada por cefaléia orbitotemporal unilateral, grave e recorrente, associada a fotofobia, lacrimejamento e congestão nasal ipsolaterais. SIN histaminic cephalalgia, histaminic h., Horton cephalalgia, Horton h.

coital h., c. do coito; forma de cefaléia de esforço benigna que ocorre durante a atividade sexual. SIN benign coital cephalalgia.

fibrositic h., c. fibrosítica; cefaléia localizada na região occipital, devido à fibrosite dos músculos occipitais; existem áreas hipersensíveis, e, comumente, são encontrados nódulos hipersensíveis no couro cabeludo, na região occipital inferior.

histaminic h., histamínica. SIN cluster h.

Horton h., c. de Horton. SIN cluster h.

ice pick h., c. em punhalada idiopática. SIN idiopathic stabbing h.

idiopathic stabbing h., c. em punhalada idiopática; dores agudas repetitivas e de breve duração na área têmporo-parietal da cabeça. SIN ice pick h.

migraine h., enxaqueca. VER migraine.

muscle contraction h., c. por contração muscular. SIN tension h.

nodular h., c. nodular; dor que se irradia na cabeça, acompanhada de tumefações nodulares nos músculos esplênio, frontal e trapézio e em outros músculos.

organic h., c. orgânica; cefaléia devida a doença intracraniana.

posttraumatic h., c. pós-traumática; cefaléia que ocorre após traumatismo da cabeça ou pescoço.

reflex h., c. reflexa. SIN symptomatic h.

sick h., hemicrania. SIN migraine.

spinal h., c. espinal; habitualmente frontal ou occipital, após punção lombar, precipitada pela postura sentada ou ortostática do paciente e aliviada pelo decúbito; causada por extravasamento de líquido cefalorraquidiano (LCR) através do local de punção, com conseqüente redução da pressão do LCR e tração sobre os vasos da dura-máter e do cérebro. SIN postlumbar puncture syndrome.

symptomatic h., c. sintomática; cefaléia secundária a outra condição orgânica. SIN reflex h.

tension h., c. tensional; cefaléia associada a tensão nervosa, ansiedade, etc., freqüentemente relacionada com a contração crônica dos músculos do couro cabeludo. VER TAMBÉM posttraumatic neck *syndrome*. SIN muscle contraction h., tension-type h.

tension-type h., c. tensional. SIN tension h.

thunderclap h., c. "em trovoada"; dor de cabeça não-localizada súbita e intensa, que não está associada a nenhum achado neurológico anormal; de etiologia variada, incluindo hemorragia subaracnóide, enxaqueca, dissecção da artéria carótida ou da artéria vertebral, trombose do seio cavernoso e idiopática.

vacuum h., c. em vácuo; cefaléia devida ao fechamento do seio frontal.

vascular h., c. vascular. SIN migraine.

head·gear (hed′gēr). Touca; dispositivo extra-oral removível, utilizado como fonte de tração para aplicar uma força aos dentes e à mandíbula.

head·gut (hed′gut). Intestino anterior. SIN foregut.

head-nod·ding (hed′nod-ing). Tremores da cabeça; movimentos da cabeça associados a nistagmo congênito, espasmo nutante e nistagmo de mineiros. SIN head tremors.

head-tilt (hed′tilt). Inclinação da cabeça; posição anormal da cabeça adotada para evitar a visão dupla resultante da subatividade dos músculos oculares verticais.

heal (hēl). Curar. **1.** Restabelecer a saúde, especialmente promovendo a cicatrização de úlcera ou ferida. **2.** Sentir-se bem, curado; cicatrizado ou fechado, quando se fala de uma úlcera ou ferida. [A.S. *healan*]

heal·er (hē′ler). **1.** Médico; alguém que cura. **2.** Curandeiro; aquele que declara curar por meio de preces, misticismo, novas idéias ou outras formas de sugestão.

heal·ing (hēl′ing). Cura. **1.** Restabelecimento da saúde; que promove o fechamento de feridas e úlceras. **2.** O processo de retorno à saúde. **3.** Cicatrização; fechamento de uma ferida. VER TAMBÉM union.

faith h., cura pela fé; tratamento utilizado desde a antigüidade, baseado em preces e numa profunda crença na intervenção divina nos acontecimentos dos seres humanos.

h. by first intention, cicatrização por primeira intenção; cicatrização por aderência fibrosa, sem supuração ou formação de tecido de granulação. SIN primary adhesion, primary union.

h. by second intention, cicatrização por segunda intenção; fechamento tardio de duas superfícies de granulação. SIN secondary adhesion, secondary union.

h. by third intention, cicatrização por terceira intenção; enchimento lento de uma cavidade de ferimento ou úlcera por granulação, com cicatrização subseqüente.

health (helth). Saúde. **1.** O estado do organismo quando funciona de modo ideal, sem qualquer evidência de doença ou anormalidade. **2.** Estado de equilíbrio dinâmico em que a capacidade de um indivíduo ou de um grupo de lidar com todas as circunstâncias de vida encontra-se num nível ótimo. **3.** Estado caracterizado por integridade anatômica, fisiológica e psicológica, capacidade de desempenhar pessoalmente um papel na família, no trabalho e na comunidade; capacidade de lidar com estresses físicos, biológicos, psicológicos e sociais; sensação de bem-estar; e ausência de risco de doença e morte prematura. [A.S. *haelth*]

behavioral h., saúde comportamental; área interdisciplinar dedicada a promover uma filosofia de saúde que destaca a responsabilidade do indivíduo na aplicação do conhecimento e das técnicas da ciência comportamental e biomédica à manutenção da saúde e prevenção da doença e disfunção por meio de inúmeras atividades individuais e compartilhadas.

h. education, educação sanitária; processo pelo qual indivíduos e grupos de indivíduos aprendem a se comportar de modo proveitoso na promoção, manutenção ou restauração da saúde.

mental h., s. mental; maturidade ou normalidade emocional, comportamental e social; ausência de distúrbio mental ou comportamental; um estado de bem-estar psicológico em que o indivíduo alcança uma integração satisfatória de seus impulsos instintivos aceitáveis tanto para ele próprio como para o meio social; um equilíbrio apropriado de procura de amor, trabalho e lazer.

public h., s. pública; a arte e a ciência da saúde comunitária, relacionada com estatística, epidemiologia, higiene e prevenção e erradicação de doenças epidêmicas; esforço organizado pela sociedade para promover, proteger e restaurar a saúde das pessoas; a s. pública é uma instituição social, um serviço e uma prática.

Health Care Fi·nanc·ing Ad·min·is·tra·tion (HCFA). Organização federal dos Estados Unidos que determina o reembolso para programas federais.

health cen·ter. Centro de saúde; instituição ou grupo de instituições que oferecem todos os tipos de assistência médica e serviços profiláticos para uma população.

Health Resources and Services Administration (HRSA). Organização federal dos Estados Unidos responsável pelo manejo dos bancos de dados nacionais, como o *National Practitioner Data Bank*, bem como por outros programas de assistência à saúde.

healthy (helth′ē). Sadio; bem; num estado de funcionamento normal; livre de doença.

Heaney, Noble Sproat, cirurgião ginecológico e obstetra norte-americano, 1880–1955. VER H. *operation*.

hear (hēr). Ouvir; perceber sons; refere-se à função da orelha. [A.S. *hēran*]

hear·ing (hēr′ing). Audição; a capacidade de perceber sons; a sensação de sons em oposição à vibração. SIN audition.

color h., a. colorida; percepção subjetiva de cor produzida por certos sons. VER TAMBÉM pseudochromesthesia. SIN chromatic audition.

normal h., a. normal. SIN acusia.

hear·ing aid (hēr′ing ād). Aparelho auditivo; aparelho amplificador eletrônico destinado a levar o som para dentro da orelha; consiste num microfone, amplificador e receptor. SIN hearing instrument.

behind-the-ear h. a., aparelho auditivo atrás da orelha; aparelho auditivo colocado na face medial da aurícula.

completely in the canal h. a. (CIC), a. auditivo totalmente no canal; aparelho auditivo que se encaixa totalmente no canal auditivo externo, não sendo visível na superfície do corpo.
digital h. a., a. auditivo digital; aparelho auditivo programável que pode ser feito sob medida, de acordo com o grau de perda de audição do usuário.
in-the-canal h. a., a. auditivo no canal; aparelho auditivo colocado no canal auditivo externo, porém ainda visível.
in-the-ear h. a., a. auditivo na orelha; aparelho auditivo que se encaixa dentro da concha da orelha.

HEARING IMPAIRMENT

hear·ing im·pair·ment, hear·ing loss. Comprometimento da audição, perda de audição; surdez; redução na capacidade de perceber sons; pode variar desde uma leve incapacidade até uma surdez completa. VER TAMBÉM deafness, threshold *shift*.
acoustic trauma hearing loss, surdez por traumatismo agudo; perda de audição sensorial, devido à exposição a ruídos de alta intensidade.
Alexander h. i. [MIM*203500], redução da audição de Alexander; redução da audição de alta freqüência devido à displasia coclear membranosa.
boilermaker's hearing loss, surdez dos caldeireiros. SIN noise-induced h. i.
conductive h. i., diminuição da audição condutiva; forma de comprometimento da audição devido a uma lesão no canal auditivo externo ou orelha média.
functional h. i., diminuição de audição funcional. SIN psychogenic h. i.
hereditary h. i., diminuição hereditária da audição; comprometimento da audição que ocorre em formas sindrômicas (nas quais são observadas outras anomalias além do comprometimento da audição) e formas não-sindrômicas (em que o comprometimento da audição constitui o único achado anormal), com modos de herança autossômico dominante e recessivo, ligado ao X e mitocondrial; pode ser congênita, de início precoce na infância ou de início tardio na meia-vida e na velhice.
high-frequency h. i., diminuição da audição de alta freqüência; perda seletiva da audição para altas freqüências, geralmente associada a lesão sensorial; comum na surdez por traumatismo acústico e surdez induzida por ruídos.
hysterical h. i., diminuição histérica da audição. SIN psychogenic h. i.
industrial hearing loss, surdez industrial. SIN noise-induced h. i.
low-tone hearing loss, surdez para tons graves; incapacidade de ouvir notas graves ou de baixa freqüência.
mixed h. i., diminuição de audição mista; combinação de surdez condutiva e surdez sensorineural.
Mondini h. i., surdez de Mondini; comprometimento da audição devido à aberração estrutural da displasia de Mondini.
neural h. i., surdez neural; forma de surdez sensorineural devido a uma lesão na divisão auditiva do oitavo par craniano.
noise-induced h. i., diminuição da audição induzida por ruídos; surdez sensorial devido a exposição a sons intensos ou contínuos. SIN boilermaker's hearing loss, industrial hearing loss, occupational hearing loss.
occupational hearing loss, surdez ocupacional. SIN noise-induced h. i.
organic h. i., diminuição orgânica da audição; comprometimento da audição devido a um processo patológico ou causa orgânica, em contraste com a surdez psicogênica.
perceptive h. i., surdez perceptiva; termo mais antigo para referir-se à surdez sensorineural.
psychogenic h. i., surdez psicogênica; comprometimento da audição sem qualquer evidência de causa orgânica; com freqüência, ocorre após choque psíquico grave. SIN functional h. i., hysterical h. i.
retrocochlear h. i., surdez retrococlear; termo utilizado para referir-se à surdez sensorineural; sugere uma lesão proximal à cóclea.
Scheibe h. i., surdez de Scheibe; comprometimento da audição devido a displasia cocleossacular; em geral, de herança autossômica recessiva.
sensorineural h. i., surdez sensorineural; forma de perda da audição em decorrência de uma lesão da divisão auditiva do 8.º par craniano ou do ouvido interno.
sensory h. i., surdez sensorial; forma de surdez sensorineural causada por lesão do ouvido interno.

heart (hart) [TA]. Coração; órgão muscular oco que recebe o sangue das veias e o impele para as artérias. Nos mamíferos, é dividido por um septo musculo-

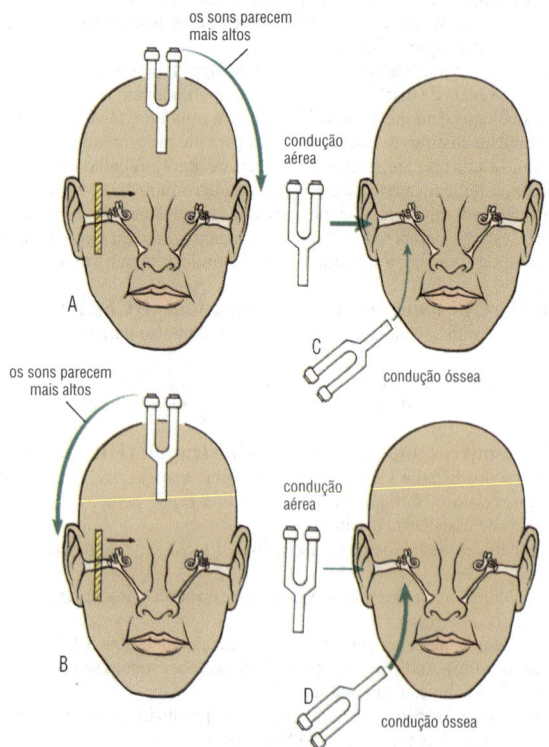

perda de audição: (A) surdez sensorineural demonstrada pelo teste de Weber; (B) surdez condutiva demonstrada pelo teste de Weber; (C) teste de Rinne: com audição normal ou surdez sensorineural, os sons parecem mais altos pela condução do ar do que pela condução óssea; (D) teste de Rinne: com surdez condutiva, os sons parecem mais altos por condução óssea

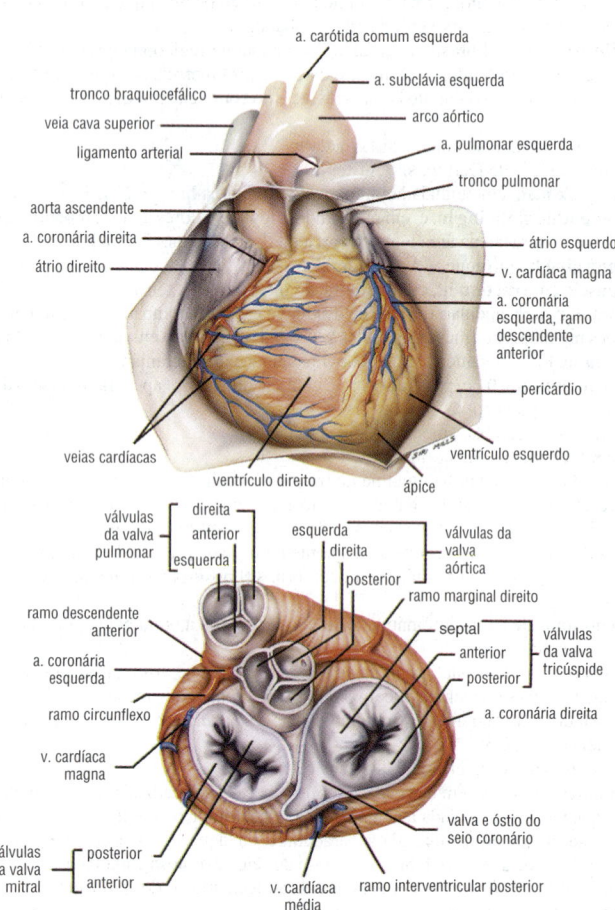

coração humano (em cima) vista ventral com pericárdio aberto, (embaixo) corte transversal ao nível das valvas

membranoso em duas metades — direita ou venosa e esquerda ou arterial —, cada uma das quais consiste numa câmara receptora (átrio) e numa câmara ejetora (ventrículo). SIN cor [TA], coeur. [A.S. *heorte*]

armor h., c. em couraça; calcificação extensa ou completa (raramente ossificação) do pericárdio, produzindo geralmente pericardite constritiva.

armored h., c. blindado; depósitos calcários no pericárdio devido a pericardite subaguda ou crônica. SIN panzerherz.

artificial h., c. artificial; bomba mecânica utilizada para substituir a função de um coração lesado, seja temporariamente ou como prótese permanente.

athlete's h., c. de atleta; designação mais ou menos indefinida para referir-se aos achados cardíacos em atletas sadios que seriam ou poderiam ser anormais em pacientes com doença, incluindo bloqueio atrioventricular, hipertrofia ventricular esquerda e, algumas vezes, arritmias benignas e bloqueios atrioventriculares.

athletic h., c. atlético; hipertrofia do coração supostamente devida a um condicionamento atlético sistemático.

beer h., c. dos bebedores de cerveja. SIN alcoholic *cardiomyopathy*.

beriberi h., c. do beribéri; doença cardíaca causada por deficiência de tiamina, que pode ser epidêmica ou esporádica, caracterizada por lesão metabólica cardíaca e insuficiência do miocárdio, freqüentemente do tipo de "alto débito", com edema (exceto no beribéri seco) e polineurite. O termo deriva do cingalês, "Sou incapaz".

bony h., c. ósseo; presença de placas calcárias extensas no pericárdio e nas paredes do coração, algumas das quais desenvolvem cronicamente alterações ósseas.

chaotic h., c. caótico; ação ou ritmo cardíaco com incoordenação aparentemente total.

crisscross h., c. entrecruzado; anomalia em que as relações ventriculares não são aquelas esperadas para a determinada conexão atrioventricular.

drop h., cardioptose. SIN cardioptosia.

fatty h., c. adiposo; **(1)** degeneração gordurosa do miocárdio; **(2)** acúmulo de tecido adiposo na superfície externa do coração, com infiltração ocasional de gordura entre os feixes musculares da parede cardíaca. SIN cor adiposum.

frosted h., c. congelado; hialoserosite que acomete o pericárdio. SIN icing h.

globular h., c. globular. SIN round h.

hairy h., pericardite fibrinosa. SIN fibrinous *pericarditis*.

Holmes h., c. de Holmes; variante de ventrículo esquerdo de entrada dupla em que a conexão ventrículo-arterial está em conformidade, enquanto o ventrículo direito é rudimentar.

horizontal h., c. horizontal; descrição da posição elétrica do coração; reconhecido no eletrocardiograma quando o QRS na derivação aVL assemelha-se àquele em V_6, e o QRS na derivação aVF assemelha-se àquele em V_1; refere-se também, de forma imprecisa, ao eixo elétrico situado entre $-30°$ e $+30°$.

hyperthyroid h., c. hipertireóideo; resposta do coração ao hipertireoidismo, essencialmente a conseqüência da estimulação simpática, produzindo uma freqüência cardíaca rápida e, em última análise, insuficiência cardíaca e fibrilação se o distúrbio não for tratado.

hypoplastic h., c. hipoplásico; coração pequeno, como aquele observado na doença de Addison.

icing h., c. gelado. SIN frosted h.

intermediate h., c. intermediário; descrição geral do eixo elétrico do coração quando dirigido aproximadamente entre $+30°$ e $+60°$. Quanto à posição cardíaca, reconhecido no eletrocardiograma quando os complexos QRS tanto na derivação aVL quanto na derivação aVF assemelham-se àqueles em V_6.

Jarvik artificial h., c. artificial de Jarvik; coração artificial pneumático.

left h., c. esquerdo; o átrio e o ventrículo esquerdos.

mechanical h., c. mecânico; termo aplicado de modo generalizado a qualquer aparelho de assistência circulatória mecânica.

movable h., c. móvel. SIN cor mobile.

myxedema h., c. mixedematoso; coração de volume aumentado, associado ao hipotireoidismo grave não-tratado, muitas vezes acompanhado de derrame pericárdico; raro na medicina moderna.

ox h., c. bovino; coração muito grande devido a hipertensão crônica ou, com mais freqüência, a valvulopatia aórtica, especialmente regurgitação. SIN bucardia, cor bovinum.

parchment h., c. em pergaminho; condição congênita ou adquirida em que ocorre adelgaçamento do miocárdio ventricular direito. VER Uhl *anomaly*. SIN right ventricular hypoplasia.

pendulous h., c. em pêndulo. SIN cor pendulum.

pulmonary h., c. pulmonar; o átrio e o ventrículo direitos, recebendo sangue venoso e propelindo-o para os pulmões. VER TAMBÉM cor pulmonale.

right h., c. direito; o átrio e o ventrículo direitos.

round h., c. redondo; contornos arqueados anormalmente lisos do coração no imageamento, devido à presença de doença dos ventrículos ou a um falso aspecto do coração, produzido por líquido pericárdico excessivo. SIN globular h.

sabot h., c. em tamanco. SIN coeur en sabot.

semihorizontal h., c. semi-horizontal; refere-se, de modo geral, ao eixo elétrico do coração quando dirigido em aproximadamente $0°$. Como posição elétrica cardíaca, reconhecido no eletrocardiograma quando o complexo QRS na derivação aVL assemelha-se a V_6, enquanto aquele na derivação aVF é pequeno em termos algébricos ou absolutos.

semivertical h., c. semivertical; descreve de forma indeterminada o eixo elétrico do coração quando este está dirigido em aproximadamente $+60°$. Como posição elétrica cardíaca, reconhecido no eletrocardiograma quando o complexo QRS na derivação aVF assemelha-se à V_6, ao passo que, na derivação aVL, é pequeno em termos algébricos ou absolutos.

stone h., c. de pedra. SIN ischemic *contracture* of the left ventricle.

systemic h., c. sistêmico; o átrio e o ventrículo esquerdos, recebendo o sangue arejado dos pulmões e propelindo-o através do corpo.

three-chambered h., c. de três câmaras; anormalidade congênita caracterizada por um único átrio com dois ventrículos ou um único ventrículo com dois átrios. Pode haver partes rudimentares dos septos interatrial e interventricular, porém estes são incompetentes para impedir uma câmara única virtual em ambos os casos.

tiger h., c. de tigre; coração adiposo degenerado em que a gordura se deposita na forma de listras interpostas no miocárdio subendocárdico.

tobacco h., c. do fumante; irritabilidade cardíaca caracterizada por ação irregular, palpitação e, algumas vezes, dor; acredita-se que ocorre em consequência do uso maciço de tabaco.

univentricular h., c. univentricular; anomalia em que todo o sangue flui através de um ventrículo ou em que as válvulas atrioventriculares deságuam apenas numa câmara na massa ventricular.

venous h., c. venoso; o lado direito do coração, incluindo tanto o átrio quanto o ventrículo.

vertical h., c. vertical; descrição geral do eixo elétrico do coração quando este é dirigido em aproximadamente $+90°$. Como posição elétrica cardíaca, reconhecido no eletrocardiograma quando o complexo QRS na derivação aVL assemelha-se a V_1, enquanto aquele na derivação aVF assemelha-se a V_6.

wooden-shoe h., c. em tamanco. SIN coeur en sabot.

heart·beat (hart′bēt). Batimento cardíaco; um único ciclo completo de contração e dilatação do músculo cardíaco.

heart·burn (hart′bern). Pirose. SIN pyrosis.

heart·worm. Dirofilária. SIN *Dirofilaria immitis*.

heat (q) (hēt). Calor. **1.** Temperatura elevada; a sensação produzida pela proximidade do fogo ou de um objeto incandescente, em oposição ao frio. **2.** A energia cinética dos átomos e das moléculas, bem como a rotação e vibração. **3.** Estro. SIN estrus. **4.** Entalpia. SIN enthalpy. [A.S. *haete*]

atomic h., atômico; o calor necessário para elevar a temperatura de um átomo de 0 a 1°C; aproximadamente o mesmo para todos os elementos (cerca de 25 kJ/átomo-grama).

h. of combustion, c. de combustão; o calor liberado por molécula-grama quando uma substância sofre oxidação completa.

h. of compression, c. de compressão; calor produzido quando um gás é comprimido.

conductive h., c. por condução; calor transmitido por contato direto, como por uma almofada elétrica ou uma garrafa de água quente.

convective h., c. por convecção; calor transferido por um meio quente, como ar ou água, em movimento a partir de sua fonte.

conversive h., c. de conversão; calor produzido num corpo pela absorção de ondas que não são, em si, quentes, como raios solares ou irradiação infravermelha.

h. of crystallization, c. de cristalização; o calor liberado ou absorvido por mol quando uma substância passa para o estado cristalino.

h. of dissociation, c. de dissociação; o calor (expresso em calorias ou joules) consumido na dissociação de 1 mol de uma substância em produtos específicos.

h. of evaporation, c. de evaporação; o calor absorvido na evaporação da água, do suor ou de outro líquido; para a água, é de 540 cal/g a 100°C. SIN h. of vaporization.

h. of formation, c. de formação, o calor (expresso em calorias ou joules) absorvido ou liberado durante a reação (hipotética) em que um mol de determinado composto é formado a partir dos elementos necessários, na forma elementar.

initial h., c. inicial; a primeira salva de calor produzida após o início de uma contração muscular; descrita por A.V. Hill.

innate h., c. inato; na antiga medicina grega, o calor do coração sustentado pelo pneuma e distribuído pelas artérias através do corpo.

latent h., c. latente; o calor que uma substância absorveria sem aumento da temperatura, como na conversão do estado sólido em líquido (gelo em água a 0°C) ou do estado líquido para o gasoso (água para o vapor a 100°C). Cf. sensible h.

molecular h., c. molecular; o produto do calor específico de um corpo multiplicado pelo seu peso molecular.

prickly h., miliária rubra. SIN *miliaria* rubra.

radiant h., c. radiante; calor emitido de qualquer corpo na forma de ondas infravermelhas.

sensible h., c. sensível; o calor que, quando absorvido pela substância, causa elevação da temperatura. Cf. latent h.

h. of solution, c. de solução; o calor absorvido ou emitido quando um sólido é dissolvido em líquido.

specific h., c. específico; o calor necessário para elevar a temperatura de qualquer substância em 1°C, em comparação com a elevação do mesmo volume de água em 1°C.

h. of vaporization, c. de vaporização. SIN h. of evaporation.

heat·la·bile (hēt'lā'bl). Termolábil; destruído ou alterado pelo calor.

heat·sta·ble (hēt'stā'bl). Termoestável. SIN thermostabile.

heat·stroke (hēt'strōk). Termoplegia; doença grave, freqüentemente fatal, produzida pela exposição a temperaturas excessivamente elevadas, sobretudo quando acompanhada de esforço acentuado; caracterizada por cefaléia, vertigem, confusão, pele seca e quente e discreta elevação da temperatura corporal; nos casos graves, ocorrem febre muito alta, colapso vascular e coma. SIN heat apoplexy. (1), heat hyperpyrexia, malignant hyperpyrexia, thermic fever.

Heb·e·lo·ma (heb-ē-lō'mā). Gênero de cogumelos, fonte de toxinas gastrointestinais.

he·be·phre·nia (hē-bē-frē'nē-ā, hebʹē-). Hebefrenia; síndrome caracterizada por afeto superficial e inapropriado, riso afetado e comportamento regressivo tolo e maneirismos; subtipo de esquizofrenia que, hoje em dia, recebeu a nova denominação de esquizofrenia desorganizada (disorganized *schizophrenia*). [G. *hēbē*, puberdade, + *phrēn*, mente]

he·be·phren·ic (hē-bē-frēn'ik, heb-ē-). Hebefrênico; relativo a, ou caracterizado por, hebefrenia.

Heberden, William, médico inglês, 1710–1801. VER H. *angina; nodes,* em *node;* Rougnon-H. *disease.*

he·bet·ic (hē-bet'ik). Hebético; pertinente à juventude. [G. *hēbētikos,* juventude, fr. *hēbē,* jovem]

heb·e·tude (heb'ē-tood). Hebetude. SIN moria (1). [L. *hebetudo,* fr. *hebeo,* ser estúpido]

he·bi·at·rics (hē-bē-at'riks). Hebiatria; medicina do adolescente. SIN adolescent *medicine.* [G. *hēbē,* juventude, + *iatrikos,* relativo à medicina]

Hebra, Ferdinand von, dermatologista austríaco, 1816–1880. VER H. *prurigo.*

hec·a·ter·o·mer·ic (hekʹa-ter-ō-mer'ik). Hecatomérico; indica um neurônio espinal cujo axônio se divide e dá origem a processos em ambos os lados da medula espinal; em geral, o mesmo que neurônio heteromérico. SIN hecatomeral, hecatomeric. [G. *hekateros,* cada um de dois, + *meros,* parte]

hec·a·tom·er·al, hec·a·to·mer·ic (hekʹa-tom'er-āl, hekʹa-tō-mer'ik). Hecatomérico. SIN hecateromeric.

Hecht, Victor, patologista austríaco do início do século XX. VER H. *pneumonia.*

Heck, John W., dentista norte-americano, *1923. VER H. *disease.*

hec·tic (hek'tik). Héctico; refere-se a uma elevação vespertina e diária da temperatura, acompanhada de ruborização das bochechas, que ocorre na tuberculose ativa e em outras infecções; o uso do termo baseia-se no aspecto do gráfico da temperatura. [G. *hektikos,* habitual, ético, consuntivo, fr. *hexis,* hábito]

♻ **hecto- (h).** Hecto; prefixo utilizado no sistema SI e sistema métrico indicando múltiplos de uma centena (10^2). [G. *hekaton,* uma centena]

hec·to·gram (hek'tō-gram). Hectograma; uma centena de gramas, o equivalente a 1543,7 grãos.

hec·to·li·ter (hek'tō-lē-ter). Hectolitro; uma centena de litros, o equivalente a 105,7 quartos ou 26,4 galões americanos (22 imperiais).

hed·e·o·ma (he-dē-ō-ma). Hedeoma. VER pennyroyal.

hed·er·i·form (hed'er-i-fōrm). Hederiforme; que apresenta a forma de hera; termo utilizado para referir-se a certas terminações sensoriais na pele. [L. *hedera,* hera, + *forma,* forma]

he·do·no·pho·bia (hē-dō-nō-fō'bē-ā). Hedenofobia; medo mórbido do prazer. [G. *hēdonē,* de leite, + *phobos,* medo]

Hedström, Gustav, endodontista sueco. VER H. *file.*

heel (hēl) [TA]. Calcanhar. 1. Porção proximal da superfície plantar do pé. 2. SIN calx (2). 3. SIN distal *end.* [A.S. *hēla*]

black h., petéquias no calcâneo. SIN calcaneal *petechiae.*

cracked h., ceratoderma plantar sulcado. SIN keratoderma *plantare sulcatum.*

painful h., calcaneodinia; condição em que a sustentação do peso sobre o calcanhar provoca dor de intensidade variável. SIN calcaneodynia.

prominent h., c. proeminente; condição caracterizada por tumefação dolorosa à palpação do calcanhar devido a espessamento do periósteo ou tecido fibroso que recobre a parte posterior do osso do calcanhar.

Heerfordt, Christian Frederick, oftalmologista dinamarquês, *1871. VER H. *disease.*

Hegar, Alfred, ginecologista alemão, 1830–1914. VER H. *dilators,* em *dilator, sign.*

Hegglin, Robert M.P., médico suíço, 1907–1970. VER H. *anomaly, syndrome;* May-H. *anomaly.*

Hehner, Otto, químico inglês, 1853–1924. VER H. *number.*

Heidenhain, Rudolph P.H., histologista e fisiologista alemão, 1834–1897. VER H. *crescents,* em *crescent, demilunes,* em *demilune, law, azan stain, iron hematoxylin stain, pouch;* Biondi-H. *stain.*

height (h) (hīt). Altura; medida vertical.

anterior facial h. (AFH), a. facial anterior; em cefalometria, medida linear do násio até o queixo.

h. of contour, a. de contorno; linha que circunda um dente ou outra estrutura em sua proeminência ou diâmetro maior. Relaciona-se a uma via selecionada de inserção de um aparelho dentário.

cusp h., a. de cúspide; (1) a distância mais curta entre a ponta de uma cúspide e seu plano basal; (2) a distância mais curta entre a parte mais profunda da fossa central de um dente posterior e uma linha que une os pontos das cúspides do dente.

facial h., a. facial; dimensão linear na linha média, desde a linha de implantação dos cabelos até o queixo.

nasal h., a. nasal; distância entre o násio e a borda inferior da abertura nasal.

orbital h., a. orbital; distância entre os pontos médios das margens superior e inferior da órbita.

Heilbronner, Karl, médico holandês, 1869–1914. VER H. *thigh.*

Heim, Ernst L., médico alemão, 1747–1834. VER H.-Kreysig *sign.*

Heimlich, Henry J., cirurgião torácico norte-americano, *1920. VER H. *maneuver.*

Heine, Leopold, oftalmologista alemão, 1870–1940.

Heineke, Walter, cirurgião alemão, 1834–1901. VER H.-Mikulicz *pyloroplasty.*

Heinz, Robert, patologista alemão, 1865–1924. VER H. body *anemia, bodies,* em *body, body test;* H.-Ehrlich *body;* H. body *anemia.*

Heister, Lorenz, anatomista alemão, 1683–1758. VER H. *diverticulum, valve.*

HeLa (hē'la). Hela; refere-se a células da primeira cepa de carcinoma (cervical humano) continuamente cultivada. [*H*enrietta *La*cks (d. 1951), cujo carcinoma cervical foi a fonte da linhagem celular]

hel·co·me·nia (hel-kō-mē'nē-ā). Helcomenia; ocorrência de úlceras por ocasião da menstruação. [G. *helkos,* úlcera, + *emmēnos,* mensalmente]

Held, Hans, anatomista alemão, 1866–1942. VER H. *bundle, decussation.*

he·li·an·thine (hē-li-an'thin). Heliantina. SIN methyl orange.

hel·i·cal (hel'i-kăl). 1. Helicoidal; relativo a uma hélice. SIN helicine (2). 2. Helicóide. SIN helicoid. [G. *helix,* espiral]

hel·i·ces (hel'i-sēz). Hélices; plural de helix.

hel·i·cine (hel'i-sēn). Helicino. 1. Espiralado. 2. Helicoidal. SIN helical (1). [G. *helix,* espiral]

Hel·i·co·bac·ter (hel'ī-kō-bakʹter). Gênero de bactérias microaerofílicas helicoidais, espiraladas ou lineares, com extremidades arredondadas e múltiplos flagelos com bainha (unipolares ou bipolares e laterais), com bulbos terminais. Formam colônias não-pigmentadas e transparentes de 1–2 mm de diâmetro, catalase e oxidase-positivas. Encontrado na mucosa gástrica de primatas, incluindo seres humanos e doninhas. Algumas espécies de *Helicobacter* estão associadas a úlceras gástricas e pépticas e predispõem ao desenvolvimento de carcinoma gástrico. A espécie típica é *Helicobacter pylori.*

H. cinaedi, espécie associada a casos de proctite e colite em homens homossexuais.

H. fennelliae, espécie associada a proctite e colite em homens homossexuais.

H. heilmannii, espécie observada na mucosa gástrica. Esse agente apresenta baixa prevalência (menos de 1% dos pacientes), não foi cultivado *in vitro,* e sua importância patogênica permanece desconhecida.

H. pylo'ri, espécie que produz urease e provoca gastrite; envolvido na maioria dos casos de úlcera péptica do estômago e duodeno. A infecção por esse microrganismo também desempenha um papel etiológico (provavelmente em associação a co-fatores dietéticos) na displasia e metaplasia da mucosa gástrica, adenocarcinoma gástrico distal e linfoma não-Hodgkin do estômago. SIN *Campylobacter pylori.*

O microrganismo foi observado pela primeira vez em 1982, por Robin Warren e Barry J. Marshall, no Royal Perth Hospital, na Austrália Ocidental, em amostras de biópsia de pacientes com gastrite crônica. Originalmente considerado como espécie de *Campylobacter,* o microrganismo foi reclassificado como *Helicobacter pylori* em 1989. O *Helicobacter pylori,* um bacilo Gram-negativo flagelado curvo ou espiralado, coloniza a mucosa gástrica, fixando-se à superfície das células colunares secretoras de muco. A capacidade do microrganismo de sobreviver em meio ácido é devida à sua capacidade de produzir urease, que converte a uréia em amônia e alcaliniza a película de muco onde reside. A infecção por *Helicobacter pylori* é comum no mundo inteiro, e a sua incidência aumenta com a idade, atingindo cerca de 50% entre indivíduos com 60 anos de idade. Acredita-se que a transmissão seja interpessoal, por via orofecal. A ocorrência da infecção em vários membros de uma família e a sua maior incidência entre negros e hispânicos foram atribuídas a fatores mais sociais do que genéticos. Uma vez instalada a infecção, ela tipicamente dura por toda a vida, a não ser que seja tratada com antibióticos. A infecção recém-adquirida resulta em extensa lesão das células parietais, com gastrite aguda acompanhada de comprometimento na produção de ácido, que pode ser transitório. Os indivíduos infectados são, em sua maioria, assintomáticos (possivelmente pelo fato de algumas cepas de *Helicobacter pylori* não produzirem citotoxinas); todavia, verifica-se o desenvolvimento de úlcera péptica em cerca de 1% dos adultos infectados por *Helicobacter pylori* anualmente. O risco de progressão para úlcera péptica aumenta com o tabagismo e com o uso prolongado de agentes antiinflamatórios não-esteróides. Cerca de 70% de todos os indivíduos com úlceras gástricas e 90% daqueles com úlceras duodenais estão infectados por *Helicobacter pylori*. Nos Estados Unidos, ocorrem cerca de 500.000 novos casos de úlcera péptica por ano. A doença é responsável por 3–4 milhões de consultas médicas e por aproximadamente 16.000 mortes a cada ano. A infecção por *Helicobacter pylori* não tem sido associada a dispepsia sem úlcera nem a distúrbios inflamatórios do trato digestivo, a não ser a ulceração péptica. Todavia, a incidência de adenocarcinoma e de linfoma gástricos é maior em indivíduos infectados por esse microrganismo. Além disso, essa bactéria foi implicada em alguns casos de colecistite e tireoidite auto-imune, e alguns estudos sugeriram que a infecção gástrica por *Helicobacter pylori* pode constituir um fator, através de algum mecanismo desconhecido, em alguns casos de síndrome de morte súbita do lactente (SMSL). O diagnóstico de infecção por *Helicobacter pylori* pode ser confirmado pela identificação do microrganismo em cortes corados de material obtido por biópsia gástrica, por cultura do material de biópsia, avaliação do material de biópsia quanto à sua atividade de urease, identificação do antígeno bacteriano nas fezes, detecção de anticorpos IgG no soro (constituindo o método de escolha para confirmar a presença de infecção num paciente previamente não-tratado) ou detecção da atividade de urease através de vários testes bioquímicos. O teste de depuração respiratória da uréia é mais útil do que o teste sorológico para confirmar a erradicação de *Helicobacter pylori* após um curso de tratamento, visto que os níveis de anticorpos IgG podem permanecer elevados por mais de 1 ano após a erradicação. A erradicação do microrganismo com antibióticos não proporciona uma cicatrização mais rápida da úlcera péptica do que o tratamento com agentes anti-secretores; todavia, reduz acentuadamente a probabilidade de recidiva da úlcera. Os esquemas recomendados para a erradicação do *Helicobacter pylori* consistem em combinações de subsalicilato de bismuto com dois antibióticos (metronidazol ou claritromicina e tetraciclina ou amoxicilina). A resistência adquirida do *Helicobacter pylori* aos antibióticos macrolídeos e imidazólicos representa um problema crescente. Nos Estados Unidos, calcula-se que cerca de 30% das cepas desse microrganismo sejam resistentes ao metronidazol, enquanto quase 10% exibem resistência aos macrolídeos. Um importante fator no desenvolvimento de cepas resistentes parece consistir no fracasso do primeiro tratamento ou na administração de um primeiro curso de tratamento inadequado. A vacinação ativa, com administração oral de uma subunidade recombinante enzimaticamente inativa de urease de *Helicobacter pylori* combinada com adjuvante mucoso (toxina lábil de *Escherichia coli*), já produziu cura microbiológica e clínica da infecção por *Helicobacter pylori* em estudos de animais e em estudos clínicos limitados realizados em seres humanos.

hel·i·coid (hel′i - koyd). Helicóide; semelhante a uma hélice. SIN helical (2). [G. *helix*, uma espiral, + *eidos*, semelhante]

hel·i·co·po·dia (hel′i - kō - pō′dē - ǎ). Helicopodia; marcha helicópode. SIN helicopod gait. [G. *helix*, uma espiral, + *pous*, pé]

hel·i·co·tre·ma (hel′i - kō - trē′mǎ) [TA]. Helicotrema; abertura semilunar no ápice da cóclea, através da qual a rampa vestibular e a rampa timpânica da cóclea comunicam-se entre si. SIN Breschet hiatus, Scarpa hiatus. [G. *helix*, espiral, + *trēma*, orifício]

Helie, Louis T., ginecologista francês, 1804–1867. VER H. bundle.

he·li·en·ceph·a·li·tis (hē - lē - en - sef - ǎ - lī′tis). Heliencefalite; inflamação do cérebro após insolação. [G. *helios*, sol, + *enkephalos*, cérebro, + -*itis*, inflamação]

△ **helio-.** Hélio-. O sol. [G. *hēlios*]

he·li·o·aer·o·ther·a·py (hē′lē - ō - ār - ō - thār′ǎ - pē). Helioaeroterapia; tratamento da doença pela exposição à luz solar e ao ar fresco.

he·li·op·a·thy (hē - lē - op′ǎ - thē). Heliopatia; lesão por exposição à luz solar. [helio- + G. *pathos*, sofrimento]

he·li·o·pho·bi·a (hē′lē - ō - fō′bē - ǎ). Heliofobia; temor mórbido de exposição aos raios solares. [helio- + G. *phobos*, medo]

he·li·o·sis (hē - lē - ō′sis). Heliose. SIN sunstroke. [helio- + G. -*osis*, condição]

he·li·o·tax·is (hē - lē - ō - tak′sis). Heliotaxia; forma de fototaxia e, talvez, de termotaxia em que ocorre tendência ao crescimento ou movimento em direção (h. positiva) ou afastando-se (h. negativa) do sol ou da luz solar. SIN heliotropism. [helio- + G. *taxis*, distribuição ordenada]

he·li·o·tro·pism (hē - lē - ot′rō - pizm). Heliotropismo, heliotaxia. SIN heliotaxis. [helio- + G. *tropē*, uma tropa]

He·li·o·zo·ea (hē′lē - ō - zō′ē - ǎ). Classe de protozoários (subfilo Sarcodina) caracterizados por axópodes rígidos que se irradiam em todos os lados, geralmente nus, embora alguns possuam um esqueleto de escamas e espinhas silicosas, porém sem cápsula central. São, em sua maioria, formas dulcícolas, sendo comum a formação de colônias. [helio- + G. *zōon*, animal]

he·li·um (He) (hē′lē - ŭm). Hélio; elemento gasoso presente em diminutas quantidades na atmosfera (0,000524% de volume seco); número atômico 2, peso atômico 4,002602; utilizado como diluente de gases medicinais; utilizado como diluente do oxigênio principalmente em aplicações não-médicas e, em sua forma líquida, como refrigerante para ímãs supercondutores (como nas imagens por ressonância magnética). [G. *hēlios*, sol]

he·li·um-3. Hélio-3; o raro isótopo estável do hélio (1,37 partes por milhão de h. comum); produzido pela decomposição beta do trício.

he·li·um-4. Hélio-4; o isótopo comum do hélio, constituindo 99,999% do hélio natural; é emitido na forma de raios alfa (que são núcleos de hélio), a partir de vários radionuclídeos.

he·lix, pl. **hel·i·ces** (hē′liks, hel′i - sēz) [TA]. Hélice. **1** [NA]. A margem da orelha; borda preguada da cartilagem que forma a parte superior da parte anterior, superior e maior das margens posteriores da aurícula. **2.** Linha em forma de espiral (ou de mola, ou os sulcos de um parafuso), sendo cada ponto eqüidistante de uma linha reta que é o eixo do cilindro no qual cada ponto da hélice se localiza; com freqüência, o termo é incorretamente aplicado a uma espiral. [L. fr. G. *helix*, uma espiral]

3_{10} h., h. 3_{10}, um tipo de hélice orientada para a direita, encontrada em pequenos fragmentos em diversas proteínas; possui três resíduos de aminoácidos por giro.

3.6_{13} h., h. $3,6_{13}$; h. α. SIN α h.

α h., h. α; forma helicoidal (comumente orientada para a direita) observada em muitas proteínas, deduzida por Pauling e Corey através de estudos de difração por raios X de proteínas, como a α-ceratina; a hélice é estabilizada por pontes de hidrogênio entre grupos, como, p.ex., $R_2C=O$ e HNR_2' (simbolizados pelo ponto central em $R_2CO·HNR_2'$) de diferentes ligações eupeptídicas. Numa verdadeira h. α, existem 3,6 resíduos de aminoácidos por giro da hélice e uma elevação de 1,5 Å por resíduo. SIN $3,6_{13}$ h., Pauling-Corey h.

collagen h., h. do colágeno, uma hélice extensa orientada para a esquerda, resultante dos níveis elevados de glicina, L-prolina e L-hidroxiprolina presentes nos colágenos. Existem 3,3 aminoácidos por giro da hélice. Três dessas hélices orientadas para a esquerda formam uma super-hélice tripla orientada para a direita.

DNA h., h. do DNA. SIN Watson-Crick h.

double h., h. dupla. SIN Watson-Crick h.

π h., h. π; uma hélice rara orientada para a direita, encontrada apenas em pequenas porções de certas proteínas. Estabilizada por pontes de hidrogênio semelhantes, como aquelas na hélice α; existem 4,3 resíduos de aminoácidos por giro.

Pauling-Corey h., h. de Pauling-Corey. SIN α h.

triple h., h. tríplice; a super-hélice formada (orientada para a direita) a partir de três hélices individuais de colágeno (sendo cada uma delas orientada para a esquerda).

twin h., h. gêmea. SIN Watson-Crick h.

Watson-Crick h., h. de Watson-Crick; estrutura helicoidal assumida por dois filamentos de ácido desoxirribonucleico, mantidos unidos em toda a sua extensão por pontes de hidrogênio entre bases nos filamentos opostos, uma disposição conhecida como emparelhamento de bases de Watson-Crick. VER base *pair*. SIN DNA h., double h., twin h.

hel·le·bore (hel′ē - bōr). Helébore; planta do gênero *Helleborus*, especialmente *H. niger* (h. negro). VER TAMBÉM *Veratrum album*, *Veratrum viride*. [G. *helleboros*]

false h., h. -falso. SIN adonis.

hel·le·bo·rin (hē - leb′o - rin, hel - ē - bō′rin). Heleborina; glicosídeo tóxico do *Veratrum viride* (helébore verde); narcótico.

hel·le·bor·ism (hel′ē - bōr - izm). Heleborismo; condição resultante do envenenamento por *Veratrum helleborus*.

hel·leb·o·rus (hel - leb′o - rŭs). Helébore-preto; o rizoma e raízes secos do *Helleborus niger* (família Ranunculaceae); utilizado como tônico cardíaco e arterial, diurético e catártico. [G. *helleboros*]

Heller, Arnold L. G., patologista alemão, 1840–1913. VER H. plexus.

Heller, Ernst, cirurgião alemão, 1877–1964. VER H. operation.

Hellin, Dyonizy (Dionys), patologista polonês, 1867–1935. VER H. law.

Helly, Konrad, patologista suíço, *1875. VER H. fixative.

Helmholtz, Hermann L.F., von, médico, físico e fisiologista alemão, 1821–1894. VER H. axis *ligament*, *energy*, *theory* of accommodation, *theory* of color vision, *theory* of hearing; H.-Gibbs *theory*; Gibbs-H. *equation*; Young-H. *theory* of color vision.

hel·minth (hel′minth). Helminto; parasita intestinal vermiforme, primariamente nematódeos, cestódeos, trematódeos e acantocéfalos. [G. *helmins*, verme]

hel·min·tha·gogue (hel - min th′ǎ - gog). Helmintagogo. SIN anthelmintic (1). [G. *helmins*, verme, + *agōgos*, que conduz]

hel·min·them·e·sis (hel - min - them′ē - sis). Helmintêmese; vômito ou expulsão de vermes intestinais pela boca. [G. *helmins*, verme + *emesis*, vômito]

hel·min·thi·a·sis (hel - min - thī′ā - sis). Helmintíase; condição de albergar parasitas vermiformes intestinais. SIN helminthism, invermination.

hel·min·thic (hel - min′thik). **1.** Helmíntico. **2.** SIN anthelmintic (1).

hel·min·thism (hel′min - thizm). Helmintismo. SIN helminthiasis.

hel·min·thoid (hel - min′thoyd). Helmintóide; vermiforme. [G. *helminthōdes*, semelhante a verme, fr. *helmins*, verme, + *eidos*, semelhança]

hel·min·thol·o·gy (hel - min - thol′ō - jē). Helmintologia; o ramo da ciência relacionado aos parasitas; especialmente o ramo da zoologia e medicina relacionado com parasitas vermiformes intestinais. SIN scolecology. [G. *helmins*, verme, + *logos*, estudo]

hel·min·tho·ma (hel - min - thō′mā). Helmintoma; nódulo isolado de inflamação granulomatosa (incluindo o estágio cicatrizado), causado por um helminto ou seus produtos, assim denominado em virtude de certas semelhanças macroscópicas com uma neoplasia. [G. *helmins*, verme, + *-oma*, tumor]

hel·min·tho·pho·bia (hel′min - thō - fō′bē - ā). Helmintofobia; temor mórbido de vermes. [G. *helmins*, verme, + *phobos*, medo]

Hel·min·tho·spo·ri·um (hel - min - thō - spor′ē - ŭm). Fungo saprófico habitualmente isolado em laboratórios clínicos; possui conidióforos determinantes de paredes paralelas; termo que costuma ser aplicado incorretamente para referir-se a *Drechslera* isolados.

hel·min·tic (hel - min′tik). Helmíntico. **1.** Relativo a vermes parasitários ou infectado por eles. **2.** SIN anthelmintic (1).

He·lo·der·ma (he - lō - der′mā). O único gênero de lagartos venenosos, como o monstro-de-Gila, assim denominado devido às escamas tuberculares que lhe recobrem o corpo. São nativos do México e sudoeste dos Estados Unidos. [G. *hēlos*, unha, + *derma*, pele]

Hel·vel·la es·cu·len·ta (hel - vel′ā es - kū - len′tā). SIN *Gyromitra esculenta*.

Helweg, Hans K.S., médico dinamarquês, 1847–1901. VER H. *bundle*.

Helweg-Larssen, Helweg-Larssen, Hans F., dermatologista dinamarquês do século XX. VER Helweg-Larssen *syndrome*.

♻ **hem-, hema-.** hem-, hema-. Sangue. VER TAMBÉM hemat-, hemato-, hemo-. [G. *haima*]

he·ma·chrome (hē′mā - krōm, hem′ā-). Hemacromo; a matéria corante do sangue, hemoglobina ou hematina. [hema- + G. *chrōma*, cor]

he·ma·cy·tom·e·ter (hē′mā - sī - tom′e - ter, hem′ā-). Hemocitômetro. SIN hemocytometer.

he·ma·cy·to·zo·on (hē′mā - sī - tō - zō′on, hem′ā). Hemocitozoário. SIN hemocytozoon.

he·ma·do·ste·no·sis (hē′mā - dō - ste - nō′sis, hem′ad - ō). Hemadostenose; contração das artérias. [G. *haimas, (haimad-)*, corrente de sangue, + *stenōsis*, estreitamento]

he·mad·sorp·tion (hē′mad - sōrp - shŭn, hem′ad-). Hemadsorção; fenômeno que se manifesta por um agente ou substância que está aderindo ou sendo adsorvido à superfície de um eritrócito.

he·ma·fa·ci·ent (hē - mā - fā′shē - ent, hem - ā-). Hemopoético. SIN hemopoietic.

he·mag·glu·ti·na·tion (hē - mā - gloo′ti - nā′shŭn). Hemaglutinação; a aglutinação de eritrócitos; pode ser imune, em consequência de anticorpo específico dirigido contra antígenos eritrocitários em si ou contra outros antígenos que recobrem os eritrócitos, ou pode ser não-imune, como na hemaglutinação causada por vírus ou outros micróbios. SIN hemoagglutination.

passive h., h. passiva; tipo de aglutinação passiva em que são utilizados eritrócitos, habitualmente modificados por tratamento leve com ácido tânico ou outras substâncias químicas, para a adsorção de antígeno solúvel em sua superfície; a seguir, esses eritrócitos sofrem aglutinação na presença de anti-soro específico para o antígeno adsorvido. SIN indirect hemagglutination test.

reverse passive h., h. passiva invertida; técnica diagnóstica para infecção viral que utiliza a aglutinação de eritrócitos por vírus previamente recobertos por anticorpos específicos contra o vírus.

viral h., h. viral; aglutinação não-imune de eritrócitos suspensos por alguns dentre uma ampla gama de vírus não relacionados nos demais aspectos, habitualmente pelo próprio virion, mas, em alguns casos, por produtos de crescimento viral (p. ex., subunidades), em que as espécies de eritrócitos aglutinados diferem com o vírus diferente. VER TAMBÉM hemagglutination *inhibition*.

he·mag·glu·ti·nin (hē′mā - gloo′ti - nin, hem-). Hemaglutinina; substância, anticorpo ou outro produto que produz hemaglutinação. SIN hemoagglutinin.

he·ma·gog·ic (hē - mā - goj′ik, hem - ā-). Hemagógico; que promove um fluxo de sangue.

he·mal (hē - māl). Hemal. **1.** Relativo ao sangue ou vasos sanguíneos. **2.** Refere-se ao lado ventral dos corpos vertebrais ou seus precursores, onde o coração e os grandes vasos estão localizados, em oposição a neural (2). [G. *haima*, sangue]

he·mal·um (hē - mal′ŭm, hem-). Hemalume; solução de hematoxilina e alume utilizada como corante nuclear em histologia, especialmente com eosina como contracorante.

he·mam·e·bi·a·sis (hē′mā - me - bī′ā - sis, hem′ā-). Hemamebíase; qualquer infecção por formas amebóides de parasitas nos eritrócitos, como na malária.

he·ma·nal·y·sis (hē - mā - nal′ī - sis, hem-). Hemanálise; análise do sangue; um exame de sangue, especialmente com referência a métodos químicos. [G. *haima*, sangue, + *análise*]

he·man·gi·ec·ta·sis, he·man·gi·ec·ta·sia (hē - man - jē - ek′tāsis, hem - an-; - ek - tā′zē - ā). Hemangiectasia; dilatação de vasos sanguíneos. [G. *haima*, sangue, + *angeion*, vaso, + *ektasis*, distensão]

♻ **hemangio-.** Hemangio-. Refere-se a vasos sanguíneos. [G. *haima*, sangue, + *angeion*, vaso]

he·man·gi·o·blast (he - man′jē - ō - blast). Hemangioblasto; célula embrionária primitiva, de origem mesodérmica, que produz células das quais derivam o endotélio vascular, elementos reticuloendoteliais e células hematopoéticas de todos os tipos. [hemangio- + G. *blastos*, germe]

he·man·gi·o·blas·to·ma (he - man′jē - ō - blas - tō′mā). Hemangioblastoma; neoplasia benigna que, freqüentemente, surge no cerebelo, constituída por células endoteliais formadoras de vasos capilares e por células do estroma; tumor de crescimento lento que afeta primariamente indivíduos de meia-idade; incidência aumentada na doença de von Hippel-Lindau. SIN angioblastoma, Lindau tumor.

he·man·gi·o·en·do·the·li·o·blas·to·ma (he - man′jē - ō - en - dō - thē′ - lē - ō - blastō′mā). Hemangioendotelioblastoma; hemangioendotelioma em que as células endoteliais parecem ser formas especialmente imaturas. [hemangio- + endotélio + G. *blastos*, germe, + *-oma*, tumor]

he·man·gi·o·en·do·the·li·o·ma (he - man′jē - ō - en - dō - thē - lē - ō′mā). Hemangioendotelioma; neoplasia derivada de vasos sanguíneos, caracterizada por numerosas células endoteliais proeminentes que ocorrem isoladamente, em agregados e como revestimento de congéries de tubos ou canais vasculares; no indivíduo idoso pode ser maligno (angiossarcoma ou hemangiossarcoma); entretanto, em crianças, essas neoplasias são benignas e, provavelmente, representam um estágio de crescimento do hemangioma capilar. [hemangio- + endotélio + G. *-oma*, tumor]

h. tubero′sum mul′tiplex, h. tuberoso múltiplo; erupção de pápulas rosadas, causada por hiperplasia do endotélio dos vasos sanguíneos superficiais.

he·man·gi·o·fi·bro·ma (he - man′jē - ō - fi - brō′mā). Hemangiofibroma; hemangioma com estrutura abundante de tecido fibroso.

juvenile h., h. juvenil. SIN juvenile *angiofibroma*.

he·man·gi·o·ma (he - man′jē - ō′mā). Hemangioma; anomalia congênita em que a proliferação de vasos sanguíneos leva à formação de uma massa que se assemelha a uma neoplasia; pode ocorrer em qualquer parte do corpo; entretanto, é mais freqüentemente observado na pele e nos tecidos subcutâneos; a maioria dos hemangiomas sofre regressão. VER TAMBÉM nevus. [hemangio- + G. *-oma*, tumor]

capillary h., h. capilar; crescimento excessivo de vasos sanguíneos capilares, observado mais comumente na pele, por ocasião do nascimento ou pouco depois, na forma de nódulo ou placa vermelho-viva a púrpura, de consistência mole, habitualmente desaparecendo no quinto ano de vida. Trata-se do tipo mais comum de hemangioma. SIN capillary angioma, capillary h. of infancy, nevus vascularis, nevus vasculosus, superficial angioma.

capillary h. of infancy, h. capilar do lactente. SIN capillary h.

ℹ **cavernous h.,** h. cavernoso; termo antigo para referir-se ao hemangioma cutâneo profundo que manifesta involução espontânea. Termo também utilizado incorretamente para referir-se a uma malformação venosa.

lobular capillary h., h. capilar lobular. SIN pyogenic *granuloma*.

racemose h., h. racemoso. SIN cirsoid *aneurysm*.

sclerosing h., h. esclerosante; **(1)** lesão pulmonar ou brônquica benigna; freqüentemente subpleural, algumas vezes múltipla, que forma tecido conjuntivo hialinizado. **(2)** SIN dermatofibroma.

senile h., h. senil; pápulas vermelhas, produzidas por enfraquecimento das paredes capilares da derme, que não empalidecem ao serem pressionadas; observado principalmente em indivíduos com mais de 30 anos de idade. SIN cherry angioma, De Morgan spots.

spider h., angioma aracniforme. SIN spider *angioma*.

strawberry h., h. em morango; hiperproliferação de vasos capilares imaturos, habitualmente na cabeça e no pescoço, presente ao nascimento ou nos primeiros 2–3 meses do período pós-natal, que costuma regredir sem formação de cicatriz.

verrucous h., h. verrucoso; termo incorreto para referir-se a uma malformação vascular cutânea constituída por capilares e linfáticos anormais.

he·man·gi·o·ma·to·sis (he - man′jē - ō - mā - tō′sis). Hemangiomatose; condição em que existem numerosos hemangiomas.

he·man·gi·o·per·i·cy·to·ma (he - man′jē - ō - per′i - sī - tō′mā). Hemangiopericitoma; neoplasia vascular incomum, habitualmente benigna, constituída por células arredondadas e fusiformes derivadas dos pericitos e que circundam vasos revestidos de endotélio; é difícil distinguir microscopicamente o h. maligno da forma benigna. [hemangio- + pericito + G. *-oma*, tumor]

he·man·gi·o·sar·co·ma (he - man′jē - ō - sar - kō′mā). Hemangiossarcoma; neoplasia maligna rara, caracterizada por células anaplásicas de rápida proliferação, que se infiltram extensamente, derivadas de vasos sanguíneos e que revestem espaços irregulares cheios de sangue ou nodulares.

he·ma·phe·ic (hē - mă - fē′ik, hem - ă-). Hemafeico; relativo à hemafeína ou que contém esse pigmento.

he·ma·phe·in (hē - mă - fē′in, hem - ă-). Hemafeína; pigmento patológico castanho derivado da hemoglobina; considerada uma combinação de indican e urobilina. [G. *haima,* sangue, + *phaios,* pardo]

he·ma·phe·ism (hē - mă - fē′izm, hem - ă-). Hemafeísmo; presença de hemafeína no plasma sanguíneo e na urina.

he·mar·thro·sis (hē′mar - thrō′sis, hem′ar-). Hemartrose; presença de sangue numa articulação. [G. *haima,* sangue, + *arthron,* articulação]

he·ma·stron·ti·um (hē - mă - stron′shē - ŭm, hem - ă-). Hemastrôncio; corante feito pela adição de cloreto de estrôncio e uma solução de hemateína e cloreto de alumínio em ácido cítrico e álcool; utilizado em histologia.

△ **hemat-.** hemat-. Sangue. VER TAMBÉM hem-, hemato-, hemo-. [G. *haima (haimat-)*]

he·ma·ta·chom·e·ter (hē′mă - tă - kom′e - ter, hem′ă-). Hematacômetro. SIN hemotachometer.

he·mat·ap·os·te·ma (hē′mat - ă - pos - tē′mă, hem′at-). Hematapostema; abscesso em que houve derrame de sangue. [hemat- + G. *apostēma,* abscesso]

he·ma·te·in (hē - mă - tē′in, hem - ă). Hemateína; produto de oxidação da hematoxilina.
   Baker acid h., h. ácida de Baker; solução ácida de hematoxilina oxidada, utilizada em cortes congelados para a coloração de fosfolipídios.

he·ma·tem·e·sis (hē - mă - tem′e - sis, hem - ă-). Hematêmese; vômito de sangue. SIN *vomitus cruentes.* [hemat- + G. *emesis,* vômito]

he·mat·en·ceph·a·lon (hē′mat - en - sef′ă - lon, hem′at-). Hematencéfalo. SIN cerebral *hemorrhage.* [hemat- + G. *enkephalos,* cérebro]

he·ma·ther·a·py (hē - mă - thăr′ă - pē, hem′ă-). Hematoterapia. SIN hemotherapy.

he·ma·therm (hē′mă - therm, hem′ă-). Homeotérmico. SIN homeotherm. [G. *haima,* sangue, + *thermos,* calor]

he·ma·ther·mal (hē - mă - ther′măl, hem′ă-). Homeotérmico. SIN homeothermic. [G. *haima,* sangue, + *thermos,* calor]

he·ma·ther·mous (hē - mă - ther′mŭs, hem - ă-). Homeotérmico. SIN homeothermic.

he·ma·tho·rax (hē - mă - thŏr′aks, hem - ă-). Hemotórax. SIN hemothorax.

he·mat·ic (hē - mat′ik). Hemático. **1.** Relativo ao sangue. SIN hemic. **2.** Hematínico. SIN hematinic (2).

he·ma·tid (hē′mă - tid, hem′ă-). Hemátide. **1.** Termo obsoleto para eritrócito. **2.** Termo obsoleto para referir-se a uma erupção cutânea presumivelmente causada por uma substância no sangue circulante. [hemat- + *-id*]

he·ma·ti·dro·sis (hē′mat - i - drō′sis, hem′at-). Hematidrose; excreção de sangue ou pigmento sanguíneo no suor; distúrbio extremamente raro. [hemat- + G. *hidrōs,* suor]

he·ma·tim·e·ter (hē - mă - tim′e - ter, hem - ă-). Hematímetro. SIN hemocytometer.

hem·a·tin (hē′mă - tin, hem′ă-). Hematina; heme em que o ferro encontra-se na forma Fe(III) (Fe^{3+}); o grupo prostético da metemoglobina. SIN ferriheme, hematosin, hydroxyhemin, oxyheme, oxyhemochromogen, phenodin.
   h. chloride, cloreto de h. SIN hemin.
   reduced h., h. reduzida. SIN heme.

he·ma·ti·ne·mia (hē′mă - ti - nē′mē - ă, hem′ă-). Hematinemia; presença de heme no sangue circulante. [hematina + G. *haima,* sangue]

hem·a·tin·ic (hē - mă - tin′ik, hem - ă-). Hematínico. **1.** Que melhora a condição do sangue. **2.** Agente que melhora a qualidade do sangue ao aumentar o número de eritrócitos e/ou a concentração de hemoglobina. SIN hematic (2). SIN hematonic.

△ **hemato-.** hemato-. Forma combinante que se refere ao sangue. VER TAMBÉM hem-, hemat-, hemo-. [G. *haima (haimat-)*]

he·ma·to·bil·ia (hē′mă - tō - bil′ē - ă). Hematobilia. SIN hemobilia.

he·ma·to·bi·um (hē - mă - tō′bē - ŭm, hem - ă-). Hematóbio; qualquer microrganismo parasita no sangue, especialmente numa forma animal ou hemozoário. [hemato- + G. *bios,* vida]

he·ma·to·blast (hē′mă - tō - blast, hem′ă-). Hematoblasto; forma primitiva e não-diferenciada de célula sanguínea a partir da qual se originam os eritroblastos, linfoblastos, mieloblastos e outras células sanguíneas imaturas; provavelmente idêntica ou muito semelhante ao hemocitoblasto e hemoistioblasto; na medula óssea normal, é encontrado apenas em pequeno número, sendo a sua identificação difícil em esfregaços, visto que os hematoblastos são frágeis e sofrem fácil desintegração; quando a medula óssea é hiperplásica, podem ser observados em pequenos grupos. [hemato- + G. *blastos,* germe]
   Hayem h., h. de Hayem; termo obsoleto para referir-se a uma plaqueta.

he·ma·to·cele (hē′mă - tō - sēl, hem′ă-). Hematocele. **1.** SIN hemorrhagic *cyst.* **2.** Derrame de sangue num canal ou numa cavidade do corpo. **3.** Aumento de volume devido ao derrame de sangue na túnica vaginal do testículo. [hemato- + G. *kēlē,* tumor]
   pelvic h., h. pélvica; derrame intraperitoneal de sangue na pelve.
   pudendal h., h. pudenda; derrame de sangue no grande lábio.

hem·a·to·ceph·a·ly (hē′mă - tō - sef′ă - lē, hem′ă-). Hematocefalia; derrame intracraniano de sangue, comumente em um feto. [hemato- + G. *kephalē,* cabeça]

he·ma·to·che·zia (hē′mă - tō - kē′zē - ă, hem′ă-). Hematoquezia; eliminação de fezes sanguinolentas, em contraposição a melena ou fezes alcatroadas. [hemato- + G. *chezō,* eliminar com fezes]

he·ma·to·chlo·rin (hē′mă - tō - klō′rin, hem′ă-). Hematoclorina; substância corante verde derivada da hemoglobina obtida da placenta. [hemato- + G. *chlōros,* luz verde + *-in*]

he·ma·to·chy·lu·ria (hē′mă - tō - kī - loo′rē - ă, hem′ă-). Hematoquilúria; presença de sangue, bem como de quilo, na urina. [hemato- + G. *chylos,* suco, + *ouron,* urina]

he·ma·to·col·po·me·tra (hē′mă - tō - kol′pō - mē′tră). Hematocolpometria; acúmulo de sangue no útero e na vagina, resultante de hímen imperfurado ou outra obstrução vaginal inferior. [hemato- + G. *kolpos,* vagina, + *mētra,* útero]

he·ma·to·col·pos (hē′mă - tō - kol′pos, hem′ă-). Hematocolpia; acúmulo de sangue menstrual na vagina, em conseqüência de hímen imperfurado ou outra obstrução. SIN retained menstruation. [hemato- + G. *kolpos,* vagina]

he·mat·o·crit (Hct) (hē′mă - tō - krit, hem′ă-). Hematócrito. **1.** Percentagem do volume de uma amostra de sangue ocupada por células. Cf. plasmacrit. **2.** Termo obsoleto para referir-se a uma centrífuga ou aparelho para separar as células e outros elementos particulados do sangue do plasma. [hemato- + G. *krinō,* separar]

he·ma·toc·ry·al (hē - mă - tok′rē - ăl, hem - ă-). Pecilotérmico. SIN poikilothermic. [hemato- + G. *kryos,* frio]

he·ma·to·cyst (hē′mă - tō - sist, hem′ă-). Hematocisto. SIN hemorrhagic *cyst.*

he·ma·to·cys·tis (hē′mă - tō - sis′tis, hem′ă-). Hematocistia; presença de sangue na bexiga. [hemato- + G. *kystis,* bexiga]

he·ma·to·cyte (hē′mă - tō - sīt, hem′ă-). Hematócito. SIN hemocyte.

he·ma·to·cy·to·blast (hē′mă - tō - sī′tō - blast, hem′ă-). Hematocitoblasto. SIN hemocytoblast.

he·ma·to·cy·tol·y·sis (hē′mă - tō - sī′ - tol′e - sis, hem′ă-). Hematocitólise. SIN hemocytolysis.

he·ma·to·cy·tom·e·ter (hē′mă - tō - sī - tom′e - ter, hem′ă-). Hematocitômetro. SIN hemocytometer.

he·ma·to·cy·to·zo·on (hē′mă - tō - sī′tō - zō′on, hem′ă-). Hemotocitozoário. SIN hemocytozoon.

he·ma·to·dys·cra·sia (hē′mă - tō - dis - krā′zē - ă, hem′ă-). Hematodiscrasia. SIN hemodyscrasia.

he·ma·to·dys·tro·phy (hē′mă - tō - dis′trō - fē, hem′ă-). Hematodistrofia. SIN hemodystrophy.

he·ma·to·gen·e·sis (hē′mă - tō - jen′e - sis, hem′ă-). Hematogênese. SIN hemopoiesis. [hemato- + G. *genesis,* produção]

he·ma·to·gen·ic, he·ma·tog·e·nous (hē′mă - tō - jen′ik, hem′ă-; hem - ă - toj′en - ŭs). Hematogênico. **1.** SIN hemopoietic. **2.** Relativo a qualquer coisa produzida, derivada ou transportada pelo sangue.

he·ma·to·his·ti·o·blast (hē′mă - tō - his′tē - ō - blast, hem′ă-). Hemato-histioblasto. SIN hemohistioblast.

he·ma·to·his·ton (hē′mă - tō - his′ton, hem′ă-). Hemato-histona, globina. SIN globin.

he·ma·toi·din (hē - mă - toy′din). Hematoidina; pigmento derivado da hemoglobina que não contém ferro, mas que está estreitamente relacionado ou é idêntico à bilirrubina. A hematoidina é formada no interior da célula, presumivelmente em células reticuloendoteliais; todavia, é muitas vezes encontrada extracelularmente depois de 5–7 dias em focos de hemorragia anterior. Ocorre na forma de grânulos refratários, castanho-amarelados e vermelho-alaranjados, porém, mais tipicamente, como placas rombóides dispostas em padrão radial, a chamada h. crenada. SIN blood crystals, hematoidin crystals. [hemato- + G. *eidos,* semelhança, + *-in*]

he·ma·tol·o·gist (hē - mă - tol′ō - jist, hem - ă-). Hematologista; médico treinado e especializado em hematologia, isto é, proficiente na realização de exames diagnósticos de sangue e medula óssea ou no tratamento dessas doenças ou em ambas as áreas.

he·ma·tol·o·gy (hē - mă - tol′ō - jē, hem - ă-). Hematologia; a especialidade médica relativa à anatomia, fisiologia, patologia, sintomatologia e terapêutica do sangue e tecidos hematopoéticos. SIN hemology. [hemato- + G. *logos,* estudo]

he·ma·to·lymph·an·gi·o·ma (hē′mă - tō - limf′an - jē - ō′ - mă). Hematolinfangioma; anomalia congênita que consiste em numerosos vasos linfáticos de tamanho variável, estreitamente aglomerados e em canais maiores, associados a um número moderado de vasos sanguíneos de um tipo semelhante.

he·ma·tol·y·sis (hē - mă - tol′ĭ - sis, hem - ă-). Hematólise. SIN hemolysis.

he·ma·to·lyt·ic (hē - mă - tō - lit′ik, hem′ă-). Hematolítico. SIN hemolytic.

he·ma·to·ma (hē - mă - tō′mă, hem - ă-). Hematoma; massa localizada de sangue extravasado, relativa ou completamente limitada dentro de um órgão ou tecido, espaço ou espaço potencial; o sangue geralmente está coagulado (ou parcialmente coagulado) e, dependendo do tempo de seu confinamento, pode

manifestar vários graus de organização e pigmentação. [hemato- + G. -oma, tumor]
communicating h., h. comunicante, pseudo-aneurisma. SIN pseudoaneurysm.
corpus luteum h., h. do corpo lúteo. SIN *corpus* hemorrhagicum.
epidural h., h. epidural. SIN extradural *hemorrhage.*
intracranial h., h. intracraniano. VER intracranial *hemorrhage.*
intramural h., h. intramural; hematoma na parede de uma estrutura, como intestino ou bexiga, que habitualmente resulta de traumatismo ou de anticoagulação excessiva.
pulsatile h., h. pulsátil. SIN pseudoaneurysm.
subdural h., h. subdural. SIN subdural *hemorrhage.*
he·ma·to·me·tra (hē′mă-tō-mē′tră, hem′ă-). Hematometra; acúmulo ou retenção de sangue na cavidade uterina. SIN hemometra. [hemato- + G. *mētra,* útero]
he·ma·tom·e·try (hē-mă-tom′e-trē, hem-ă). Hematometria; exame do sangue para determinar os seguintes dados: 1) número total, tipos e proporções relativas das diversas células sanguíneas; 2) número e proporção de outros elementos figurados; 3) percentagem de hemoglobina. Em alguns casos, a h. é utilizada para incluir a determinação da pressão arterial. SIN hemometry. [hemato- + G. *metron,* medida]
he·mat·om·pha·lo·cele (hē′mat-om-făl′ō-sēl, hem′at-). Hematonfalocele; hérnia umbilical em que ocorreu derrame de sangue. [hemato- + G. *omphalos,* umbigo, + *kēlē,* hérnia]
he·ma·to·my·e·lia (hē′mă-tō-mē′ē-lē-ă). Hematomielia; hemorragia na substância da medula espinal; em geral, trata-se de uma lesão pós-traumática, mas também pode ser encontrada em casos de telangiectasia da medula espinal. SIN hematorrachis interna, myelapoplexy, myelorrhagia. [hemato- + G. *myelos,* medula]
he·ma·to·my·e·lo·pore (hē′mă-tō-mī′e-lō-pōr). Hematomieloporo; formação de porosidades na medula espinal em consequência de hemorragias. [hemato- + G. *myelos,* medula, + *poros,* poro]
he·ma·ton·ic (hē-mă-ton′ik, hem-ă-). Hematônico. SIN hematinic.
he·ma·to·pa·thol·o·gy (hē′mă-tō-păth-ol′ō-jē, hem′ă-). Hematopatologia; a divisão da patologia relacionada a doenças do sangue e dos tecidos hemopoético e linfóide. SIN hemopathology. [hemato- + G. *pathos,* sofrimento + *logos,* estudo]
he·ma·top·a·thy (hē-mă-top′ă-thē, hem-ă-). Hematopatia. SIN hemopathy.
he·ma·to·pe·nia (hē′mă-tō-pē′nē-ă, hem′ă-). Hematopenia; deficiência de sangue, incluindo hipocitose ou citopenia. [hemato- + G. *penia,* pobreza]
he·ma·to·pha·gia (hē′mă-tō-fā′jē-ă, hem′ă-). Hematofagia; que se alimenta do sangue de outro animal, como faz o morcego vampiro ou a sanguessuga. SIN hemophagia. [hemato- + G. *phagō,* comer]
he·ma·toph·a·gous (hē′mă-tof′ă-gŭs, hem′ă-). Hematófago; que se alimenta de sangue. [hemato- + G. *phagō,* comer]
he·ma·toph·a·gus (hē′mă-tof′ă-gŭs, hem′ă-). Hematófago; que se alimenta de sangue, especialmente insetos sugadores de sangue. [hemato- + G. *phagō,* comer]
he·ma·to·plas·tic (hē′mă-tō-plăs′tik, hem′ă-). Hematoplásico. SIN hemopoietic. [hemato- + G. *plassō,* formar]
he·ma·to·poi·e·sis (hē′mă-tō-poy-ē′sis, hem′ă-). Hematopoese. SIN hemopoiesis.
he·ma·to·poi·et·ic (hē′mă-tō-poy-et′ik). Hematopoético. SIN hemopoietic.
he·ma·to·poi·e·tin (hē′mă-tō-poy′ĕ-tin, hem′ă-). Hematopoetina. SIN erythropoietin.

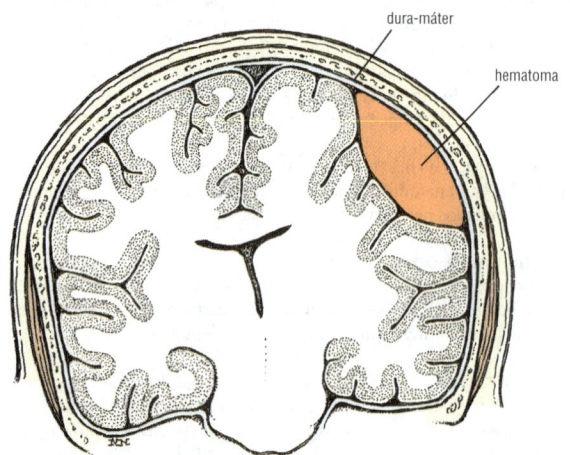

hematoma subdural: corte frontal do cérebro

he·ma·to·por·phyr·ia (hē′mă-tō-pōr-fir′ē-ă, hem′ă-). Hematoporfiria; termo obsoleto para referir-se a qualquer distúrbio do metabolismo da porfirina, independentemente da causa. [hemato- + G. *porphyra,* púrpura]
he·ma·to·por·phy·rin (hē′mă-tō-pōr′fi-rin, hem′ă-). Hematoporfirina; porfirina vermelho-escura, quase púrpura, resultante da decomposição da hemoglobina; a composição química é a do heme com o ferro removido e dois grupos vinil ($-CH=CH_2$) hidratados a hidroxietil ($-CH(OH)-CH_3$). SIN hemoporphyrin.
he·ma·to·por·phy·ri·ne·mia (hē′mă-tō-pōr′fi-ri-nē′mē-ă, hem′ă-). Hematoporfirinemia; termo antigo utilizado para designar a ocorrência de hematoporfirina no sangue circulante.
he·ma·to·por·phy·rin·u·ria (hē′mă-tō-pōr′fi-ri-noo′rē-ă, hem′ă-). Hematoporfirinúria; termo antigo utilizado para designar a excreção urinária aumentada de porfirinas.
he·ma·top·sia (hē-mă-top′sē-ă, hem-ă-). Hematopsia. SIN hemophthalmia. [hemato- + G. *opsis,* visão]
he·ma·tor·rha·chis (hē-mă-tōr′ă-kis, hem-ă-). Hematorraquia; hemorragia espinal. [hemato- + G. *rhachis,* espinha]
h.exter′na, h. externa; hemorragia no canal espinal externo à coluna vertebral, no interior ou fora da dura-máter. SIN extradural h., subdural h.
  extradural h., h. extradural. SIN h. externa.
  h. inter′na, h. interna. SIN hematomyelia.
  subdural h., h. subdural. SIN h. externa.
he·ma·to·sal·pinx (hē′mă-tō-săl′pinks, hem′ă-). Hematossalpinge; coleção de sangue numa trompa, frequentemente associada a gravidez tubária. SIN hemosalpinx. [hemato- + G. *salpinx,* trompa]
he·ma·to·sep·sis (hē′mă-tō-sep′sis, hem′ă-). Hematossepse; termo obsoleto para referir-se à septicemia.
he·ma·to·sin (hē-mă-tō′sin, hem-ă-). Hematosina. SIN hematin.
he·ma·to·sis (hē-mă-tō′sis, hem-ă-). Hematose. **1.** SIN hemopoiesis. **2.** Oxigenação do sangue venoso nos pulmões.
he·ma·to·spec·tro·scope (hē′mă-tō-spek′trō-skōp, hem′ă-). Hematospectroscópio; espectroscópio especialmente adaptado para exame do sangue.
he·ma·to·spec·tros·co·py (hē′mă-tō-spek-tros′kō-pē, hem′ă-). Hematospectroscopia; exame do sangue por meio de um espectroscópio.
he·ma·to·sper·mat·o·cele (hē′mă-tō-sper′mă-tō-sēl, hem′ă-). Hematospermatocele; uma espermatocele que contém sangue.
he·ma·to·sper·mia (hē′mă-tō-sper′mē-ă, hem′ă-). Hematospermia. SIN hemospermia.
he·ma·to·stat·ic (hē′mă-tō-stat′ik, hem′ă-). Hematostático. **1.** Variante de hemostático. **2.** Devido à estagnação ou parada de sangue nos vasos da região.
he·ma·to·stax·is (hē′mă-tō-stak′sis, hem′ă-). Hematostaxia; sangramento espontâneo devido a uma doença do sangue. [hemato- + G. *staxis,* gotejamento]
he·ma·tos·te·on (hē-mă-tos′tē-on, hem-ă). Hematósteo; sangramento na cavidade medular de um osso. [hemato- + G. *osteon,* osso]
he·ma·to·ther·mal (hē′mă-tō-ther′măl, hem′ă-). Homeotérmico. SIN homeothermic.
he·ma·to·tox·in (hē′mă-tō-toks′in, hem′ă-). Hematotoxina. SIN hemotoxin.
he·ma·to·tro·pic (hē′mă-tō-trop′ik, hem′ă-). Hematotrópico. SIN hemotropic.
he·ma·to·tym·pa·num (hē′mă-tō-tim′păn-ŭm, hem′ă-). Hematotímpano. SIN hemotympanum.
he·ma·tox·in (hē-mă-toks′in, hem-ă). Hematoxina. SIN hemotoxin.
he·ma·tox·y·lin (hē-mă-toks′i-lin, hem-ă-) [C.I. 75290]. Hematoxilina; composto cristalino contendo a substância corante de *Haematoxylon campechianum* (pau de campeche), a partir do qual é obtido por extração com éter. A hematoxilina é utilizada como corante em histologia, sobretudo para os núcleos celulares e cromossomas, estrias musculares transversais e células enterocromafins; suas propriedades tintoriais dependem da oxidação da hemateína e mordente com alumes de cromo e ferro. É também utilizada como indicador (vermelho a amarelo em pH 0,0 a 1,0, amarelo a violeta em pH 5,0 a 6,0).
Boehmer h., h. de Boehmer; tipo de alume de hematoxilina cujo amadurecimento natural ocorre em cerca de 8 a 10 dias, permanecendo a solução boa durante muitos meses.
Delafield h., h. de Delafield; tipo de alume de hematoxilina utilizado em histologia; o amadurecimento natural leva cerca de 2 meses, e a solução permanece boa durante anos.
Harris h., h. de Harris; tipo de alume de hematoxilina semelhante à h. de Delafield, mas que utiliza o amadurecimento químico para produzir oxidação da hematoxilina para uso imediato.
iron h., h. férrica; lagos férricos peculiares de hemateína que produzem colorações azul-escuras profundas; útil para o estudo de detalhes citológicos, como cromossomas, fibras fusiformes, aparelho de Golgi, miofibrilas e mitocôndrias; é também útil para demonstrar *Entamoeba histolytica.* VER TAMBÉM Heidenhain iron hematoxylin *stain,* Weigert iron hematoxylin *stain.*
phosphotungstic acid h. (PTAH), h. de ácido fosfotúngstico; corante com ampla aplicação em citologia e histologia; os núcleos, as mitocôndrias, a fibrina,

as fibrilas neurogliais e as estrias cruzadas de músculo esquelético e músculo cardíaco coram-se de azul; a substância fundamental da cartilagem, o retículo ósseo e a elastina aparecem em tonalidades de amarelo-alaranjado e vermelho-acastanhado; também útil para demonstração de astrócitos anormais ou enfermos, freqüentemente em combinação com a coloração com ácido periódico Schiff e azul resistente de Luxol. SIN Mallory phosphotungstic acid hematoxylin stain.

he·ma·to·zo·ic (hē'ma-tō-zō'ik, hem'ă). Hematozóico. SIN hemozoic.

he·ma·to·zo·on (hē'ma-tō-zō'on, hem'ă-). Hematozoário. SIN hemozoon.

he·ma·tu·ria (hē-mă-too'-rē-ă, hem-ă-). Hematúria; presença de sangue ou de eritrócitos na urina. [hemato- + G. *ouron*, urina]

    Egyptian h., h. egípcia. SIN *schistosomiasis* haematobium.

    endemic h., h. endêmica. SIN *schistosomiasis* haematobium.

    false h., h. falsa, pseudo-hematúria. SIN pseudohematuria.

    gross h., h. macroscópica; presença de sangue na urina em quantidade suficiente para ser visível a olho nu.

    initial h., h. inicial; presença de sangue apenas na primeira fração da urina eliminada, indicando, em geral, uma fonte uretral ou prostática de sangramento.

    microscopic h., h. microscópica; presença de células sanguíneas na urina, visíveis apenas ao microscópio.

    painful h., h. dolorosa; hematúria associada a disúria, indicando habitualmente a coexistência de infecção, traumatismo, cálculos ou corpos estranhos nas vias urinárias inferiores.

    painless h., h. indolor; hematúria não associada a disúria, indicando freqüentemente uma etiologia vascular ou neoplásica.

    renal h., h. renal; hematúria resultante do extravasamento de sangue para os espaços glomerulares, túbulos ou pelve renal.

    terminal h., h. terminal; presença de sangue apenas na última fração de urina eliminada, indicando habitualmente uma fonte prostática de sangramento.

    total h., h. total; presença de sangue em todas as frações de urina eliminada, indicando comumente uma fonte de sangramento na via urinária superior ou média.

    urethral h., h. uretral; hematúria em que a uretra constitui o local de sangramento.

    vesical h., h. vesical; hematúria em que a bexiga constitui o local de sangramento.

heme (hēm). Heme. **1.** O quelato porfirina de ferro em que o ferro encontra-se na forma Fe(II) (ou Fe^{2+}); o grupo prostético transportador de oxigênio e responsável pela cor da hemoglobina. **2.** O ferro ligado a não-porfirinas, mas a estruturas tetrapirrólicas relacionadas (p. ex., heme biliverdina). **3.** Ferro quelado com qualquer porfirina, independentemente do estado de valência do átomo de ferro. SIN ferroheme, ferroprotoporphyrin, reduced hematin. [G. *haima*, sangue]

    h. a., h. a; derivado do heme encontrado no citocromo aa_3.

    h. c., h. c; derivado do heme encontrado nos citocromos c, b_4 e f.

hem·er·a·lo·pia (hem'er-al-ō'pē-ă). Hemeralopia; incapacidade de ver distintamente na luz clara, bem como na iluminação reduzida; observada em pacientes com comprometimento da função dos cones. SIN day blindness, hemeranopia, night sight. [G. *hēmera*, dia, + *alaos*, obscuro, + *ōps*, olho]

hem·er·a·no·pia (hem'er-ă-nō'pē-ă). Hemeranopia. SIN hemeralopia. [G. *hemera*, dia, + *an-*, priv., + *ōps*, olho]

he·me·ryth·rins (hē-mē-rith'rinz, hem-ē-). Hemeritrinas; proteínas contendo ferro, que se ligam ao oxigênio, encontradas em certos invertebrados, cujo peso molecular é aproximadamente igual ao da hemoglobina, mas que difere desta pela ausência de grupos porfirina na molécula. A h. oxigenada é a oxiemeritrina. [G. *haima*, sangue, + G. *erythros*, vermelho, + -in]

hemi-. Hemi-. Refere-se a uma metade. Cf. semi-. [G.]

hem·i·car·di·us (hem'ē-ă-kar'dē-ŭs). Hemicárdio; um dos fetos gêmeos em que apenas uma parte da circulação é realizada pelo próprio coração, sendo o restante pelo coração do outro gêmeo. [hemi- + G. *a-* priv. + *kardia*, coração]

hem·i·ac·e·tal (hem'ē-as'e-tal). Hemiacetal; RCH(OH)OR', um produto da adição de um álcool a um aldeído (o acetal é formado pela adição de um álcool a um hemiacetal). Nos açúcares aldoses, a formação de hemiacetal é interna e lábil, produzida pelo ataque de 4-OH ou 5-OH na carbonila O, produzindo as estruturas furanose ou piranose; as formas hemiacetal dos açúcares estão envolvidas em todos os polissacarídeos, como glicosilas ou glicosídeos. VER TAMBÉM hemiketal, acetal.

hem·i·ac·ro·so·mia (hem'ē-ak-rō-sō'mē-ă). Hemiacrossomia; forma congênita de hemi-hipertrofia de um membro. [hemi- + G. *akron*, extremidade, + *sōma*, corpo]

hem·i·a·geu·sia (hem'ē-ă-goo'sē-ă). Hemiageusia; perda do paladar de um lado da língua. SIN hemiageustia, hemigeusia. [hemi- + G. *a-* priv. + *geusis*, paladar]

hem·i·a·geus·tia (hem'ē-ă-goos'tē-ă). Hemiageusia. SIN hemiageusia.

hem·i·al·gia (hem-ē-al'jē-ă). Hemialgia; dor que afeta a metade do corpo. [hemi- + G. *algos*, dor]

hem·i·an·al·ge·sia (hem'ē-an'al-jē'zē-ă). Hemianalgesia; analgesia que afeta uma metade do corpo.

hem·i·an·en·ceph·a·ly (hem'ē-an-en-sef'ă-lē). Hemianencefalia; anencefalia de um lado apenas ou afetando mais um lado do que outro.

hem·i·an·es·the·sia (hem'ē-an-es-thē'-zē-ă). Hemianestesia; anestesia de um lado do corpo. SIN unilateral anesthesia.

    alternate h., h. alternada; hemianestesia que afeta a cabeça de um lado e o corpo e membros do outro lado. SIN crossed h.

    crossed h., h. cruzada. SIN alternate h.

hem·i·a·no·pia (hem'ē-ă-nō'pē-ă). Hemianopia; perda da visão para metade do campo visual de um ou de ambos os olhos. SIN hemianopsia.

    absolute h., h. absoluta; hemianopia em que o campo afetado é totalmente insensível a todos os estímulos visuais. SIN complete h.

    altitudinal h., h. altitudinal; defeito no campo visual em que a metade superior ou inferior é perdida; pode ser unilateral ou bilateral.

    binasal h., h. binasal; cegueira no campo nasal de visão dos dois olhos.

    bitemporal h., h. bitemporal; cegueira no campo temporal de visão dos dois olhos.

    complete h., h. completa. SIN absolute h.

    congruous, h., h. congruente; hemianopia em que os defeitos dos campos visuais em ambos os olhos são completamente simétricos na sua extensão e intensidade.

    crossed h., h. cruzada. SIN heteronymous h.

    heteronymous h., h. heterônima; hemianopia altitudinal envolvendo o campo superior de um olho e o campo inferior do outro; ou h. binasal ou bitemporal. SIN crossed h.

    homonymous h., h. homônima; cegueira no campo correspondente (direito ou esquerdo) da visão de cada olho.

    incomplete h., h. incompleta; hemianopia afetando menos da metade do campo visual de cada olho.

    incongruous h., h. incongruente; h. incompleta ou homônima assimétrica.

    pseudo-h., pseudo-h.; condição em que os estímulos individuais são vistos corretamente; entretanto, quando o campo visual nasal de um olho e o campo visual temporal do outro são estimulados simultaneamente, um campo é cego. SIN visual extinction.

    quadrantic h., quadrantanopia. SIN quadrantanopia.

    unilateral h., h. unilateral; perda da visão em metade do campo visual de apenas um olho. SIN unilocular h.

    unilocular h., h. unilocular. SIN unilateral h.

hem·i·a·nop·ic (hem'ē-an-op'ik). Hemianópico; relativo à hemianopia.

hem·i·a·nop·sia (hem'ē-an-op'sē-ă). Hemianopsia. SIN hemianopia. [hemi- + G. *an-* priv. + *opsis*, visão]

hem·i·an·os·mia (hem'ē-an-oz'mē-ă). Hemianosmia; perda do sentido do odor em um dos lados. [hemi- + G. *an-* priv. + *osmē*, odor]

hem·i·a·pla·sia (hem'ē-ă-plā'zē-ă). Hemiaplasia; ausência de um lobo de um órgão bilobado. Termo utilizado especialmente para referir-se à glândula tireóide. [hemi- + aplasia]

hem·i·a·prax·ia (hem'ē-ă-prak'sē-ă). Hemiapraxia; apraxia que afeta um lado do corpo.

hem·i·arthro·plas·ty (hem-ē-ar'thrō-plas-tē). Hemiartroplastia; artroplastia em que uma superfície articular é substituída por material artificial, geralmente metal.

hem·i·a·syn·er·gia (hem'ē-ă-sin-er'jē-ă). Hemiassinergia; assinergia que afeta um lado do corpo.

hem·i·a·tax·ia (hem'ē-ă-tak'sē-ă). Hemiataxia; ataxia que afeta um lado do corpo.

hem·i·ath·e·to·sis (hem'ē-ath'ē-tō'sis). Hemiatetose; atetose que afeta apenas uma mão ou uma mão e um pé.

hem·i·at·ro·phy (hem-ē-at'rō-fē). Hemiatrofia; atrofia de uma metade lateral de uma parte ou de um órgão, como a face ou a língua.

    facial h., h. facial; atrofia habitualmente progressiva, que afeta os tecidos de um lado da face. SIN facial h. of Romberg, Romberg disease, Romberg syndrome.

    facial h. of Romberg, h. facial de Romberg. SIN facial h.

    lingual h., h. da língua; atrofia de uma metade lateral da língua.

hem·i·bal·lism (hem-ē-bal'izm). Hemibalismo. SIN hemiballismus. [hemi- + G. *ballismos*, saltar]

hem·i·bal·lis·mus (hem-ē-bal-iz'mŭs). Hemibalismo; balismo afetando um lado do corpo. SIN hemiballism. [hemi- + G. *ballismos*, saltar]

hem·i·block (hem'ē-blok). Hemibloqueio. SIN divisional block.

he·mic (hē-mik). Hêmico. SIN hematic (1).

hem·i·car·dia (hem-ē-kar'dē-ă). Hemicardia. **1.** Qualquer metade lateral do coração, incluindo o átrio e o ventrículo. **2.** Malformação congênita do coração em que são formadas apenas duas das quatro câmaras habituais. [hemi- + G. *kardia*, coração]

    h. dex'tra, h. direita; lado direito do coração.

    h. sinis'tra, h. esquerda; lado esquerdo do coração.

hem·i·cel·lu·lose (hem-ē-sel'ū-lōs). Hemicelulose; polissacarídeos da parede celular de vegetais estreitamente associados à celulose, como xilanos, mananos e galactanos. SIN cellulosan.

hem·i·cen·trum (hem′ē - sen′trŭm). Hemicentro; uma das duas metades laterais do corpo das vértebras. [hemi- + G. *kentron*, centro]

hem·i·ceph·a·lal·gia (hem′ē - sef′ă - lal′jē - ă). Hemicefalalgia; cefaléia unilateral característica da enxaqueca típica. SIN hemicrania (2). [hemi- + G. *kephalē*, cabeça, + *algos*, dor]

hem·i·ce·pha·lia (hem - ē - se - fā′lē - ă). Hemicefalia; falha congênita no desenvolvimento normal do cérebro; em geral, o cerebelo e os gânglios da base são representados pelo menos em forma rudimentar. SIN partial anencephaly. [hemi- + G. *kephalē*, cabeça]

hem·i·cer·e·brum (hem′ē - ser′ē - brŭm). Hemicérebro; um hemisfério cerebral.

hem·i·cho·lin·i·um (hem′ē - kō - lin′ē - ŭm). Hemicolínio; substância química que interfere na síntese da acetilcolina nas terminações nervosas colinérgicas.

Hem·i·chor·da (hem - ē - kor′dă). Hemicordado. SIN Hemichordata.

Hem·i·chor·da·ta (hem′ē - kōr - dā′tă). Filo composto de animais marinhos vermiformes bilateralmente simétricos, de corpo mole, com fendas branquiais até a faringe e probóscida cônica; estágio larvário ciliado que se assemelha ao dos equinodermas. SIN Hemichorda. [hemi- + L. Mod. *chordata*, que possui um notocórdio, fr. G. *chordē*, cordão]

hem·i·cho·rea (hem′ē - kōr - ē′ă). Hemicoréia; coréia afetando os músculos em apenas um lado. SIN hemilateral chorea.

hem·i·col·ec·to·my (hem′ē - kō - lek′tō - mē). Hemicolectomia; remoção do lado direito ou esquerdo do cólon. [hemi- + G. *kolon*, cólon, + *ektomē*, excisão]

hem·i·cor·po·rec·to·my (hem′ē - kōr - pō - rek′tō - mē). Hemicorporectomia; remoção cirúrgica da metade inferior do corpo, incluindo os membros inferiores, a pelve óssea, a genitália e vários dos conteúdos pélvicos, incluindo a parte inferior do reto e ânus. [hemi- + L. *corpus*, corpo, + G. *ektomē*, excisão]

hem·i·cra·nia (hem - ē - krā′nē - ă). Hemicrânia. **1.** Enxaqueca. SIN migraine. **2.** Hemicefalalgia. SIN hemicephalalgia. [hemi- + G. *kranion*, crânio]

hem·i·cra·ni·ec·to·my (hem′ē - krā - nē - ek′tōmē). Hemicraniectomia. SIN hemicraniotomy. [hemi- + G. *kranion*, crânio, + *ektomē*, excisão]

hem·i·cra·ni·o·sis (hem′ē - krā - nē - ō′sis). Hemicraniose; aumento de volume de um lado do crânio.

hem·i·cra·ni·ot·o·my (hem′ē - krā - nē - ot′ō - mē). Hemicraniotomia; separação e reflexão da maior parte ou de toda a metade do crânio, como preliminar para uma operação no cérebro. SIN hemicraniectomy. [hemi- + G. *kranion*, crânio, + *tomē*, corte]

hem·i·des·mo·somes (hem - ē - desmō - sōmz). Hemidesmossomas; metade de desmossomas que ocorrem na superfície basal do extrato basal do epitélio escamoso estratificado.

hem·i·di·a·pho·re·sis (hem′ē - dī - ă - fō - rē′sis). Hemidiaforese; diaforese ou sudorese na metade do corpo. SIN hemidrosis, hemihidrosis.

hem·i·dro·sis (hem - i - drō′sis). Hemidrose. SIN hemidiaphoresis.

hem·i·dys·es·the·sia (hem′ē - dis - es - thē′ - zē - ă). Hemidisestesia; disestesia que afeta um lado do corpo.

hem·i·dys·tro·phy (hem - ē - dis′trō - fē). Hemidistrofia; subdesenvolvimento da metade lateral do corpo. [hemi- + G. *dys-*, doente + *trophē*, nutrição, crescimento]

hem·i·ec·tro·me·lia (hem′ē - ek - trō - mē′lē - ă). Hemiectromelia; desenvolvimento defeituoso dos membros de um lado do corpo. [hemi- + ectromelia]

hem·i·fa·cial (hem - ē - fā′shăl). Hemifacial; relativo a um lado da face.

hem·i·gas·trec·to·my (hem′ē - gas - trek - tō - mē). Hemigastrectomia; excisão da metade distal do estômago.

hem·i·geu·sia (hem′ē - goo′sē - ă). Hemigeusia. SIN hemiageusia.

hem·i·glos·sal (hem′ē - glos′ăl). Hemilingual. SIN hemilingual. [hemi- + G. *glōssa*, língua]

hem·i·glos·sec·to·my (hem′ē - glos - ek′tō - mē). Hemiglossectomia; remoção cirúrgica de metade da língua. [hemi- + G. *glōssa*, língua, + *ektomē*, excisão]

hem·i·glos·si·tis (hem′ē - glos - ī′tis). Hemiglossite; erupção vesicular em um dos lados da língua e superfície interna correspondente da bochecha, provavelmente herpética. [hemi- + G. *glōssa*, língua, + *-itis*, inflamação]

hem·i·gna·thia (hem - ē - nath′ē - ă). Hemignatia; desenvolvimento defeituoso de um lado da mandíbula. [hemi- + G. *gnathos*, manbídula]

hem·i·hep·a·tec·to·my (hem′ē - hep - ă - tek′tō - mē). Hemi-hepatectomia; remoção cirúrgica de metade ou de um lobo do fígado.

hem·i·hi·dro·sis (hem′ē - hī - drō′sis). Hemi-hidrose. SIN hemidiaphoresis.

hem·i·hy·dran·en·ceph·a·ly (hem - ē - hī′dran - en - sef′ă - lē). Hemi-hidrancencefalia; forma unilateral de hidrancencefalia.

hem·i·hyp·al·ge·sia (hem′ē - hī - pal - je′zē - ă). Hemi-hipalgesia; hipalgesia que afeta um lado do corpo.

hem·i·hy·per·es·the·sia (hem′ē - hī′per - es - thē′zē - ă). Hemi-hiperestesia; hiperestesia ou sensibilidade tátil ou dolorosa aumentada, que afeta um lado do corpo.

hem·i·hy·per·hi·dro·sis (hem′ē - hī - per - hī - drō′sis). Hemi-hiper-hidrose; sudorese excessiva limitada a um lado do corpo. [hemi- + G. *hyper*, sobre + *hidrōsis*, sudorese]

hem·i·hy·per·to·nia (hem′ē - hī - per - tō′nē - ă). Hemi-hipertonia; tonicidade muscular exagerada em um lado do corpo. [hemi- + G. *hyper*, sobre + *tonos*, tônus]

hem·i·hy·per·tro·phy (hem′ē - hī - per′trō - fē). Hemi-hipertrofia; hipertrofia muscular ou óssea de um lado da face ou do corpo.

hem·i·hyp·es·the·sia (hem′ē - hī - pes - thē′zē - ă). Hemi-hipestesia; sensibilidade diminuída de um lado do corpo. SIN hemihypoesthesia. [hemi- + G. *hypo*, abaixo + *aesthēses*, sensação]

hem·i·hy·po·es·the·sia (hem′ē - hī - pō - es - thē′zē - ă). Hemi-hipoestesia. SIN hemihypesthesia. [hemi- + G. *hypo*, abaixo + *aisthēses*, sensação]

hem·i·hy·po·to·nia (hem′ē - hī - pō - tō′nē - ă). Hemi-hipotonia; perda parcial da tonicidade muscular de um lado do corpo. [hemi- + G. *hypo*, abaixo + *tonos*, tônus]

hem·i·kar·y·on (hem - i - kar′i - on). Hemicario; núcleo celular contendo um número haplóide de cromossomas. [hemi- + G. *karyon*, nós (núcleo)]

hem·i·ke·tal (hem′ē - kē - tăl). Hemicetal; RC(R′)(OH)OR″, um produto da adição de um álcool a uma cetona. Nos açúcares cetose, a formação de hemicetal provém de ataque da carbonila da cetona por um OH interno, resultando em ciclização intramolecular (furanose ou piranose); as formas hemicetais dos açúcares estão envolvidas na formação de polissacarídeos, como glicosilas ou glicosídeos. VER TAMBÉM hemiacetal, ketal.

hem·i·lam·i·nec·to·my (hem′ē - lam - i - nek′tō - mē). Hemilaminectomia; remoção de uma parte de uma lâmina vertebral, habitualmente efetuada para exploração ou descompressão do conteúdo intra-espinhal ou para acesso a esse conteúdo. [hemi- + L. *lamina*, camada + G. *ektomē*, excisão]

hem·i·lar·yn·gec·to·my (hem′ē - lar - in - jek′tō - mē). Hemilaringectomia; excisão de uma metade lateral da laringe. [hemi- + G. *larynx (laryng-)*, laringe + *ektomē*, excisão]

hem·i·lat·er·al (hem - ē - lat′er - ăl). Hemilateral; relativo a uma metade lateral.

hem·i·le·sion (hem - ē - lē′zhŭn). Hemilesão; lesão unilateral.

hem·i·lin·gual (hem - ē - ling′gwăl). Hemilingual; relativo a uma metade lateral da língua. SIN hemiglossal. [hemi- + L. *lingua*, língua]

hem·i·mac·ro·glos·sia (hem′ē - mak′rō - glos′ē - ă). Hemimacroglossia; aumento de volume da metade da língua. [hemi- + G. *makros*, grande + *glōssa*, língua]

hem·i·man·dib·u·lec·to·my (hem′ē - man - dib′ū - lek′tō - mē). Hemimandibulectomia; ressecção de metade da mandíbula.

hemimelia (hem - ē - mēl′ē - ă). Hemimelia; ausência parcial congênita de parte de um membro, p. ex., ausência da fíbula e presença da tíbia. [hemi- + G. *melos*, membro + *-ia*]

hem·i·me·tab·o·lous (hem′ē - me - tab′ō - lŭs). Hemimetábolo; termo que se refere a um membro da série da ordem dos insetos Hemimetabola, em que ocorre metamorfose simples ou incompleta. [hemi- + G. *metabolē*, mudança]

he·min (hēm′in). Hemina. **1.** Cloreto do heme em que o Fe^{2+} transformou-se em Fe^{3+}. Os cristais de hemina são denominados cristais de Teichmann (Teichmann *crystals*), em *crystal*. **2.** Qualquer complexo de coordenação de cloro (porfirinato) ferro (III). SIN chlorohemin, factor X for *Haemophilus*, ferriheme chloride, ferriporphyrin chloride, ferriprotoporphyrin, hematin chloride.

hem·i·o·pal·gia (hem′ē - ō - pal′jē - ă). Hemiopalgia; dor em um olho, geralmente acompanhada de hemicrania. [hemi- + G. *ōps*, olho + *algos*, dor]

hem·ip·a·gus (hem - ip′ă - gŭs). Hemípago; gêmeos unidos lateralmente no tórax; a zona de união também pode incluir o pescoço e as mandíbulas. VER conjoined *twins*, em *twin*. [hemi- + G. *pagos*, algo fixo]

hem·i·pan·cre·at·ec·to·my (hem′ē - pan′ - krē - ă - tek′tō - mē). Hemipancreatectomia; ressecção cirúrgica de metade do pâncreas.

hem·i·pa·re·sis (hem - ē - pa - rē′sis, - par′ē - sis). Hemiparesia; fraqueza que afeta um lado do corpo.

hem·i·pel·vec·to·my (hem′ē - pel - vek′tō - mē). Hemipelvectomia; amputação de um membro inferior, juntamente com parte da pelve ipsolateral. SIN hindquarter amputation, Jaboulay amputation. [hemi- + L. *pelvis*, bacia (pelve), + G. *ektomē*, excisão]

hem·i·ple·gia (hem - ē - plē′jē - ă). Hemiplegia; paralisia de um lado do corpo. [hemi- + G. *plēgē*, golpe]

alternating h., h. alternante; hemiplegia em um lado, com paralisia contralateral de nervos cranianos. SIN crossed h., crossed paralysis.

contralateral h., h. contralateral; paralisia que ocorre no lado oposto à lesão central causal.

crossed h., h. cruzada. SIN alternating h.

double h., h. dupla. SIN diplegia.

facial h., h. facial; paralisia de um lado da face, sem comprometimento dos músculos dos membros.

infantile h., h. infantil; hemiparesia aguda que ocorre no lactente, habitualmente causada por acidente vascular, como infarto cerebral ou trombose; freqüentemente associada a convulsões.

spastic h., h. espástica; hemiplegia com tônus aumentado nos músculos antigravitacionais do lado afetado.

hem·i·ple·gic (hem - ē - ple'jik). Hemiplégico; relativo à hemiplegia.
He·mip·tera (hem - ip'ter - ă). Ordem de artrópodes da classe Insecta que inclui muitos piolhos de vegetais e outros percevejos verdadeiros; os da subfamília Triatominae são hematófagos e de importância médica. A espécie mais bem conhecida é *Cimex lectularius*, o percevejo comum. [hemi- + G. *pteron*, asa]
hem·i·sec·tion (hem - ē - sek'shŭn). Hemissecção; remoção cirúrgica de uma raiz de um dente multirradicular e sua porção coronária relacionada.
hem·i·sen·so·ry (hem'ē - sen'sōr - ē). Hemissensorial; perda da sensação de um lado do corpo. Cf. hemianesthesia.
hem·i·sep·tum (hem - ē - sep'tŭm). Hemissepto; metade lateral de qualquer septo.
hem·i·spasm (hem'ē - spazm). Hemiespasmo; espasmo que afeta um ou mais músculos de um lado da face ou do corpo.
hem·i·sphere (hem'i - sfēr) [TA]. Hemisfério; metade de uma estrutura esférica. SIN cerebral h. (1) [TA]. (hemi- + G. *sphaira*, bola, globo)
  h. of bulb of penis, h. do bulbo do pênis; uma das metades laterais do bulbo do pênis separadas por um sulco mediano na parte posterior da superfície. SIN hemispherium bulbi urethrae.
  h. of cerebellum, h. do cerebelo. SIN h. of cerebellum HII-HX.
  h. of cerebellum HII-HX, h. do cerebelo HII-HX; a grande parte do cerebelo lateralmente ao verme do cerebelo. SIN hemispherium cerebelli [HII-HX] [TA], hemispherium (2) [TA], h. of cerebellum, hemispericum cerebelli HII-HX, hemisphericum.
  cerebral h. [TA], h. cerebral; **(1)** SIN hemisphere; **(2)** a grande massa do telencéfalo, de cada lado da linha média, consistindo no córtex cerebral e seus sistemas de fibras associados, juntamente com os núcleos telencefálicos subcorticais de localização mais profunda (isto é, gânglios da base [núcleos]). SIN hemispherium cerebri [TA], hemispherium (1) [TA].
  dominant h., h. dominante; o hemisfério cerebral que contém a representação da fala e controla o braço e a perna utilizados preferencialmente em movimentos delicados; em geral, o hemisfério esquerdo.
hem·i·spher·ec·to·my (hem'ē - sfēr - ek'tō - mē). Hemiesferectomia; excisão de um hemisfério cerebral; realizada para tumores malignos, epilepsia intratável geralmente associada a hemiplegia infantil causada por traumatismo do nascimento e outras condições cerebrais.
hem·i·spher·i·cum. Hemisfério. SIN *hemisphere* of cerebellum HII-HX.
  hemispericum cerebelli HII-HX, hemisfério cerebelar HII-HX. SIN *hemisphere* of cerebellum HII-HX.
hem·i·sphe·ri·um (hem'i - sfēr'ē - ŭm). [TA]. Hemisfério. **1.** SIN cerebral *hemisphere*. **2.** SIN *hemisphere* of cerebellum HII-HX. [G. *hemisphairion*]
  h. bul'bi ure'thrae, h. do bulbo uretral. SIN *hemisphere* of bulb of penis.
  h. cerebel'li [HII-HX] [TA], h. cerebelar [HII-HX]. SIN *hemisphere* of cerebellum HII-HX.
  h. cer'ebri [TA], h. cerebral. SIN cerebral *hemisphere*.
Hem·i·spo·ra (hem'ē - spō'ră). Nome genérico de certas espécies de *Fungi Imperfecti* (Fungos Imperfeitos), nos quais se desenvolvem cadeias de conídeos a partir de estruturas tubulares que se formam em conseqüência de uma constrição na extremidade de cada uma das séries de curtos ramos de hifas; existem septações estreitas que dividem o conteúdo do tubo em segmentos relativamente quadrados, de paredes espessas e intensamente corados, que acabam se separando, transformando-se em esporos arredondados, de paredes espessas e superfície rugosa. Os *H.* aparecem com razoável freqüência como contaminantes em culturas para outros fungos; em geral, são considerados formas não-patogênicas; entretanto, existem alguns casos relatados em que foram aparentemente os agentes causais de doença. [hemi- + G. *sporos*, semente]
hem·i·stru·mec·to·my (hem'ē - stroo - mek'tō - mē). Heminstrumectomia; termo raramente utilizado para referir-se à excisão de quase metade de um bócio. [hemi- + L. *struma* + G. *ektomē*, excisão]
hem·i·sub·stance (hem'ē - sŭb'stan s). Hemissubstância; substância amorfa encontrada em paredes celulares.
hem·i·syn·drome (hem'ē - sin - drōm). Hemissíndrome. **1.** Condição em que metade do corpo está atrofiada ou com hipertrofia. **2.** Lesão unilateral da medula espinal.
hem·i·ter·pene (hem - ē - ter'pēn). Hemiterpeno; isopreno ou derivado de um isopreno.
hem·i·ther·mo·an·es·the·sia (hem'ē - ther'mō - an - es - thē'zē - ă). Hemitermoanestesia; perda da sensibilidade ao calor e ao frio, afetando um lado do corpo.
hem·i·tho·rax (hem - ē - thō'raks). Hemitórax; um lado do tórax.
hem·i·trem·or (hem'ē - trem'er, - trē'mer). Hemitremor; tremor que afeta os músculos de um lado do corpo.
hem·i·trun·cus (hem'ē - trunk'ŭs). Hemitronco; tronco arterial variante em que apenas uma artéria pulmonar origina-se do tronco arterial.
hem·i·ver·te·bra (hem - ē - ver'tĕ - bră). Hemivértebra; defeito congênito da coluna em que um lado de uma vértebra não se desenvolve por completo.
hem·i·zy·gos·i·ty (hem'i - zī - gos'i - tē). Hemizigosidade; o estado de ser hemizigoto.
hem·i·zy·gote (hem - i - zī'gōt). Hemizigoto; indivíduo hemizigoto em relação a um ou mais *loci* específicos; p. ex., um macho normal é hemizigoto em relação a todos os genes ligados ao cromossoma X ou aos genes ligados ao cromossoma Y em seu genoma. [hemi- + G. *zygōtos*, emparelhado]
hem·i·zy·got·ic (hem'i - zī - got'ik). Hemizigótico. SIN hemizygous.
hem·i·zy·gous (hem - i - zī'gŭs). Hemizigótico; que possui genes não-emparelhados numa célula diplóide sob os demais aspectos. Os machos são normalmente hemizigotos para genes existentes nos dois cromossomas sexuais. SIN hemizygotic.
hem·lock (hem'lok). Cicuta. SIN conium.
hemo-. Hemo-; forma combinante que significa sangue. VER TAMBÉM hem-, hemat-, hemato-. [G. *haima*]
he·mo·ag·glu·ti·na·tion (hē'mō - ă - gloo'ti - nā'shŭn). Hemoaglutinação. SIN hemagglutination.
he·mo·ag·glu·ti·nin (hē'mō - ă - gloo'ti - nin). Hemaglutinina. SIN hemagglutinin.
he·mo·an·ti·tox·in (hē'mō - an - ti - tok'sin). Hemantitoxina; anticorpo que neutraliza os efeitos de uma hemotoxina, como o material hemolítico existente no veneno de serpentes *Naja*.
he·mo·bil·ia (hē - mō - bil'ē - ă). Hemobilia; sangramento nas vias biliares, geralmente em conseqüência de traumatismo hepático ou de neoplasia no fígado ou nas vias biliares. SIN hematobilia.
he·mo·blast (hēm'ō - blast). Hemoblasto. SIN hemocytoblast.
  lymphoid h. of Pappenheim, h. linfóide de Pappenheim; termo obsoleto para referir-se ao pronormoblasto. VER TAMBÉM erythroblast.
he·mo·blas·to·sis (hē'mō - blas - tō'sis). Hemoblastose; condição proliferativa dos tecidos hematopoéticos em geral.
he·mo·ca·thar·sis (hē'mō - ka - thar'sis). Hemocatarse; limpeza de sangue. [hemo- + G. *katharsis*, limpeza]
he·mo·cath·e·re·sis (hē'mō - kath - e - rē'sis). Hemocaterese; destruição das células sanguíneas, especialmente dos eritrócitos (hemocitocaterese). [hemo- + G. *kathairesis*, destruição]
he·mo·cath·e·ret·ic (hē'mō - kath - e - ret'ik). Hemocaterético; relativo a, ou que se caracteriza por, hemocaterese.
he·mo·cele (hē'mō - sēl). Hemocele; o sistema de espaços contendo sangue por todo o corpo dos artrópodes. [hemo- + G. *koilōma*, cavidade]
he·mo·cho·le·cys·ti·tis (hē'mō - kō'lē - sis - tī'tis). Hemocolecistite; colecistite hemorrágica.
he·mo·chro·ma·to·sis (hē'mō - krō - mă - tō'sis). Hemocromatose; distúrbio do metabolismo do ferro caracterizado por absorção excessiva de ferro ingerido, saturação da proteína de ligação do ferro e deposição de hemossiderina nos tecidos, particularmente no fígado, no pâncreas e na pele; podem ocorrer cirrose hepática, diabetes (diabetes bronzeado), pigmentação bronzeada da pele e, por fim, insuficiência cardíaca; além disso, pode resultar da administração de grandes quantidades de ferro por via oral, por injeção ou na forma de transfusão sanguínea. [hemo- + G. *chrōma*, cor + *-osis*, condição]
  exogenous h., h. exógena; hemossiderose devida a transfusões sanguíneas repetidas; pode evoluir para a cirrose pigmentar.
  primary h. [MIM*235200], h. primária; defeito metabólico hereditário específico, com absorção aumentada e acúmulo de ferro com dieta normal; herança autossômica recessiva causada por uma mutação no gene da hemocromatose (HFE) em 6p, menos florida no sexo feminino; a h. juvenil pode representar um estado homozigoto do mesmo gene.
  secondary h., h. secundária; ingestão aumentada e acúmulo de ferro secundariamente a uma causa conhecida, como terapia com ferro oral ou múltiplas transfusões.
he·mo·chrome (hē'mō - krōm). Hemocromo. SIN hemochromogen.
he·mo·chro·mo·gen (hē - mō - krō'mō - jen). Hemocromogênio; termo originalmente utilizado para referir-se a combinações de ferro- ou ferriporfirinas com dois moles de uma base nitrogenada ou proteína, como, p. ex., piridina ferroporfirina. SIN hemochrome. [hemo- + G. *chrōma*, cor + *-gen*, produzindo]
he·moc·la·sis, he·mo·cla·sia (hē - mok'lă - sis, hē'mō - klā'zē - ă). Hemoclasia; ruptura, dissolução (hemólise) ou outro tipo de destruição dos eritrócitos. [hemo- + G. *klasis*, ruptura]
he·mo·clas·tic (hē'mō - klas'tik). Hemoclástico; relativo à hemoclasia.
he·mo·con·cen·tra·tion (hē'mō - kon - sen - trā'shŭn). Hemoconcentração; diminuição do volume de plasma em relação ao número de eritrócitos; aumento na concentração de eritrócitos no sangue circulante.
he·mo·co·nia (hē - mō - kō'nē - ă). Hemocônia; termo obsoleto para descrever pequenas partículas refratárias no sangue circulante, consistindo, provavelmente, em material lipídico associado a estroma fragmentado de eritrócitos. SIN blood dust, blood motes, dust corpuscles. [hemo- + G. *konis*, poeira]
he·mo·co·ni·o·sis (hē'mō - kō - nē - ō'sis). Hemoconiose; condição em que existe uma quantidade anormal de hemocônia no sangue.
he·mo·cry·os·co·py (hē'mō - krī - os'kō - pē). Hemocrioscopia; determinação do ponto de congelamento do sangue. [hemo- + G. *kryos*, frio + *skopeō*, examinar]
he·mo·cu·pre·in (hē - mō - koo'prē - in). Hemocupreína. SIN cytocuprein.
he·mo·cy·a·nin (hē - mō - sī'ă - nin). Hemocianina; pigmento transportador de oxigênio (pesos moleculares entre 0,45 e 13×10^6) de animais marinhos infe-

riores (incluindo moluscos e crustáceos) e artrópodes; o cobre é um componente essencial, mas não contém heme; utilizada como antígeno experimental.

he·mo·cyte (hē′mō-sīt). Hemócito; qualquer célula ou elemento figurado do sangue. SIN hematocyte. [hemo- + G. *kytos*, cavidade (célula)]

he·mo·cy·to·blast (hē′mō-sī′tō-blast). Hemocitoblasto; célula sanguínea derivada do mesênquima embrionário, caracterizada por citoplasma basófilo e núcleo relativamente grande, com uma rede esponjosa e frouxa de cromatina e vários nucléolos; as mitocôndrias são extremamente finas e delicadas. Os hemocitoblastos representam as células-tronco (células primordiais) primitivas da teoria monofilética da origem do sangue e têm o potencial de desenvolver-se em eritroblastos, formas jovens da série granulocítica, megacariócitos, etc. SIN hematocytoblast, hemoblast. [hemo- + G. *kytos*, célula + *blastos*, germe]

he·mo·cy·to·cath·er·e·sis (hē′mō-sī′tō-kă-therē-sis). Hemocitocaterese; hemólise ou outro tipo de destruição dos eritrócitos. [hemo- + G. *kytos*, uma cavidade (célula) + *kathairesis*, destruição]

he·mo·cy·tol·y·sis (hē′mō-sī-tol′i-sis). Hemocitólise; dissolução das células sanguíneas, incluindo hemólise. SIN hematocytolysis. [hemo- + G. *kytos*, célula + *lysis*, dissolução]

he·mo·cy·tom·e·ter (hē′mō-sī-tom′ē-ter). Hemocitômetro; aparelho para avaliar o número de células sanguíneas num volume de sangue quantitativamente medido; consiste numa pipeta de vidro com ampola para a colheita e diluição do sangue e numa câmara de contagem quadriculada. SIN hemacytometer, hematimeter, hematocytometer. [hemo- + G. *kytos*, célula + *metron*, medida]

he·mo·cy·tom·e·try (hē′mō-sī-tom′ē-trē). Hemocitometria; a contagem de eritrócitos.

he·mo·cy·to·trip·sis (hē′mō-sī-tō-trip′sis). Hemocitotripsia; fragmentação ou desintegração de células sanguíneas por meio de traumatismo mecânico, como, p. ex., compressão entre superfícies duras. [hemo- + G. *kytos* + *tripsis*, trituração]

he·mo·cy·to·zo·on (hē′mō-sī-tō-zō′on). Hemocitozoário; protozoário parasita de células sanguíneas. SIN hemacytozoon, hematocytozoon. [hemo- + G. *kytos*, célula + *zōon*, animal]

he·mo·di·ag·no·sis (hē′mō-dī-ag-nō′sis). Hemodiagnóstico; diagnóstico através do exame de sangue.

he·mo·di·al·y·sis (hē′mō-dī-al′i-sis). Hemodiálise; diálise de substâncias solúveis e água do sangue por meio de difusão através de uma membrana semipermeável; a separação de elementos celulares e colóides de substâncias solúveis é obtida pelas dimensões dos poros na membrana e pelas velocidades de difusão.

he·mo·di·a·lyz·er (hē-mō-dī′ă-lī-zer). Hemodialisador; máquina para hemodiálise na insuficiência renal aguda ou crônica; as substâncias tóxicas no sangue são removidas pela exposição ao líquido dialisador através de uma membrana semipermeável. SIN artificial kidney.
  ultrafiltration h., h. por ultrafiltração; hemodiálise que utiliza diferenças de pressão do líquido para produzir a perda (geralmente) de líquido desprovido de proteínas do sangue para a solução.

he·mo·di·a·stase (hē-mō-dī′as-tās). Hemodiastase; amilase sanguínea.

he·mo·di·lu·tion (hē-mō-di-loo′shŭn). Hemodiluição; aumento do volume de plasma em relação aos eritrócitos; concentração reduzida de eritrócitos na circulação.

he·mo·dy·nam·ic (hē′mō-dī-nam′ik). Hemodinâmico; relativo aos aspectos físicos da circulação sanguínea.

he·mo·dy·nam·ics (hē′mō-dī-nam′iks). Hemodinâmica; o estudo da dinâmica da circulação sanguínea. [hemo- + G. *dynamis*, poder, força]

he·mo·dys·cra·sia (hē′mō-dis-krā′zē-ă). Hemodiscrasia; qualquer condição anormal ou distúrbio do sangue e do tecido hematopoético; termo utilizado especialmente para referir-se aos distúrbios que resultam em alterações nos elementos figurados do sangue. SIN hematodyscrasia. [hemo- + G. *dyscrasia*, temperamento ruim]

he·mo·dys·tro·phy (hē-mō-dis′trō-fē). Hemodistrofia; qualquer doença ou condição anormal do sangue e dos tecidos hematopoéticos, exceto alterações transitórias simples. SIN hematodystrophy.

he·mo·fil·tra·tion (hē′mō-fil-trā′shŭn). Hemofiltração; processo semelhante à hemodiálise através do qual o sangue é dialisado utilizando-se a ultrafiltração, geralmente para remover um produto específico do volume de líquido.

he·mo·flag·el·lates (hē-mō-flaj′e-lāts). Hemoflagelados; protozoários flagelados da família Trypanosomatidae, que são parasitas do sangue de muitas espécies de animais e aves domésticos e selvagens, bem como do ser humano; incluem os gêneros *Leishmania* e *Trypanosoma*, dos quais várias espécies são patógenos importantes. [hemo- + L. *flagellum*, dim. de *flagrum*, chicote]

he·mo·fus·cin (hē-mō-fŭs′in). Hemofuscina; pigmento castanho, derivado da hemoglobina, que ocorre na urina ocasionalmente com a hemossiderina; em geral, indica aumento da destruição dos eritrócitos; ocorre também no fígado com hemossiderina em casos de hemocromatose.

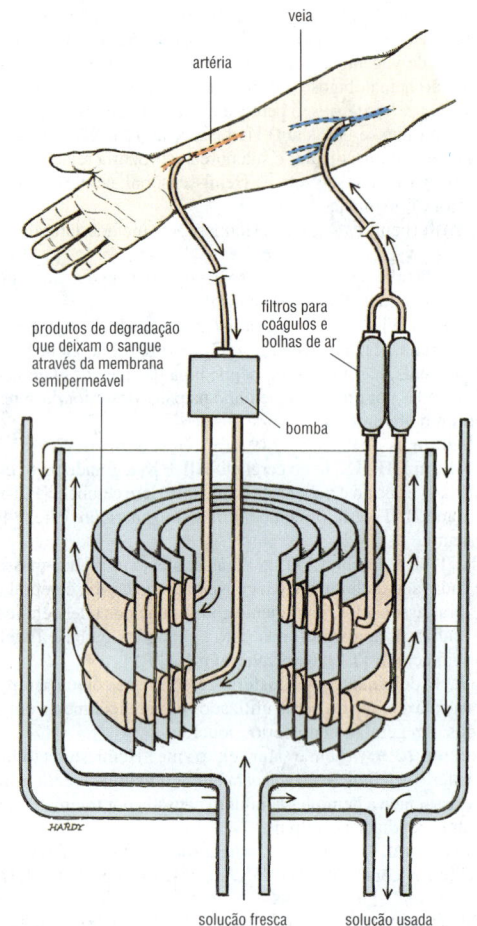

hemodiálise

he·mo·gen·e·sis (hē-mō-jen′ē-sis). Hemogênese. SIN hemopoiesis.
he·mo·gen·ic (hē-mō-jen′ik). Hemogênico. SIN hemopoietic.

HEMOGLOBIN

he·mo·glo·bin (Hb) (hē-mō-glō′bin). [MIM*141800–142310]. Hemoglobina (Hb); a proteína respiratória vermelha dos eritrócitos, que consiste em cerca de 3,8% de heme e 96,2% de globina, com peso molecular de 64.450, que, na forma de oxiemoglobina (HbO$_2$), transporta o oxigênio dos pulmões para os tecidos, onde o oxigênio é prontamente liberado e a HbO$_2$ transforma-se em Hb. Quando a Hb é exposta a determinadas substâncias químicas, sua função respiratória normal é bloqueada; assim, p. ex., o oxigênio na HbO$_2$ é facilmente deslocado pelo monóxido de carbono, levando, assim, à formação de carboxiemoglobina (HbCO) bastante estável, como na asfixia decorrente da inalação de gases expelidos por motores a gasolina. Quando o ferro na Hb é oxidado do estado ferroso ao estado férrico, como na intoxicação por nitratos e alguns outros produtos químicos, forma-se um composto não-respiratório, a metemoglobina (MetHb).

Nos seres humanos, existem pelo menos cinco tipos de Hb normal: duas Hb embrionárias (Hb Gower-1, Hb Gower-2), a Hb fetal (Hb F) e dois tipos adultos (Hb A, Hb A$_2$). Existem duas cadeias de globina α contendo 141 resíduos aminoácidos e dois outros tipos (β, γ, δ, ε ou ζ), contendo, cada uma, 146 resíduos aminoácidos em quatro das Hb. A Hb Gower-1 possui duas cadeias ζ e duas cadeias ε. A produção de cada tipo de cadeia de globina é controlada por um gene estrutural de designação semelhante em letra grega; os indivíduos normais são homozigotos para o alelo normal em cada *locus*. Pode ocorrer substituição de um aminoácido por outro na cadeia polipeptídica em qualquer códon de qualquer um dos cinco *loci*, resultando na produção de muitas centenas de tipos de Hb anormais, a maioria sem importância clínica conhecida. Além

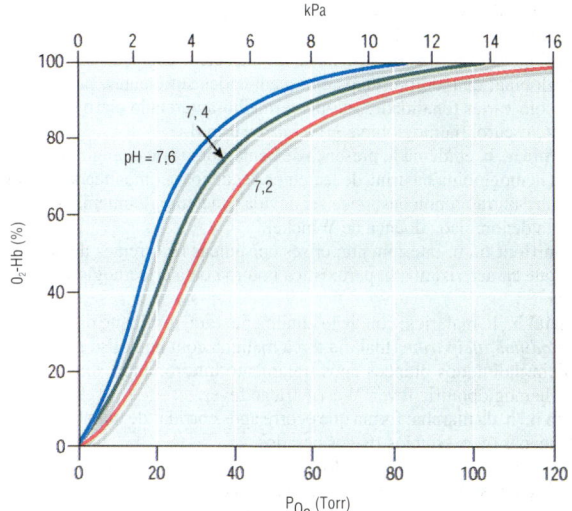

curvas de dissociação do oxigênio da hemoglobina: *ordenada*, saturação de oxigênio; *abscissa*, pressão de oxigênio do ar alveolar

disso, foram identificadas deleções de um ou mais resíduos aminoácidos, bem como rearranjos gênicos, devido a um *crossing-over* desigual entre cromossomas homólogos. Os tipos de Hb relacionados a seguir incluem os principais tipos anormais que, reconhecidamente, têm importância clínica.

Os tipos de Hb normais recém-descobertos recebem primeiro um nome, geralmente do lugar onde foram descobertos, sendo acrescentada uma fórmula molecular, quando esta é determinada. A fórmula consiste em letras gregas para designar as cadeias básicas, com o subscrito 2 nos casos em que existem duas cadeias idênticas; adiciona-se uma letra sobrescrita (^{A} quando normal para a Hb do adulto, etc.), ou o sobrescrito pode designar o local da substituição do aminoácido (numeração dos resíduos de aminoácidos a partir da extremidade N-terminal do polipeptídeo), com especificação da mudança, utilizando abreviaturas padrões para os aminoácidos. Existe uma lista exaustiva de hemoglobinas variantes na MIM, em que se utiliza um sistema de números compostos.

h. A [MIM*141800], h. A; Hb normal do adulto (Hb A), com fórmula $\alpha_2^A \beta_2^A$ ou $\alpha_2 \beta_2$.

h. A$_2$ [MIM*141850], h. A$_2$; Hb normal (Hb A$_2$) da fórmula $\alpha_2^A \delta_2$ ou $\alpha_2 \delta_2$, que compõe cerca de 2,5% da concentração total de hemoglobina do adulto. Já foram descritas pelo menos 18 variantes mutantes da cadeia δ.

h. A$_{Ic}$, h. A$_{Ic}$; a principal fração da hemoglobina glicosilada.

aberrant h., h. aberrante; Hb mutante que funciona normalmente. Cf. variant h.

h. anti-Lepore, h. anti-Lepore; um grupo de hemoglobinas anormais semelhantes à h. Lepore. Essas hemoglobinas possuem cadeias α normais, porém a cadeia não-α consiste na porção N-terminal da cadeia β unida à porção C-terminal da cadeia δ. Trata-se do padrão de *crossing-over* oposto observado na h. Lepore. Os exemplos de h. anti-Lepore incluem: Hb$_{Miyada}$, Hb P$_{Congo}$, Hb P$_{Nilotic}$ e Hb $_{Lincoln\ Park}$. Existe também uma variante que consiste tanto em h. Lepore quanto em h. anti-Lepore (Hb$_{Parchman}$). Cf. h. Lepore.

h. Bart [MIM*142309], h. de Bart; homotetrâmero de Hb (todos os quatro polipeptídeos idênticos) de fórmula γ_4, encontrado no início da vida embrionária e na α-talassemia 2; não é efetiva no transporte de oxigênio; não exibe o efeito Bohr.

bile pigment h., coleglobina. SIN choleglobin.

h. C [MIM*141900.0038], h. C; Hb anormal com substituição do resíduo glutamil pelo resíduo lisil na sexta posição da cadeia β, de fórmula $\alpha_2^A \beta_2^{6Glu \rightarrow Lys}$; esse tipo de Hb reduz a plasticidade normal dos eritrócitos. Heterozigotos: traço Hb C, cerca de 28–44% da Hb total consistem em Hb C, sem anemia. Homozigotos: quase toda a Hb consiste em Hb C, anemia hemolítica normocítica moderada. São conhecidos indivíduos heterozigotos tanto para Hb C e Hb S (doença da Hb SC) quanto para Hb C e talassemia, com anemias hemolíticas atípicas; o afoiçamento está aumentado na doença da Hb SC.

h. C$_{Georgetown}$, h. C$_{Harlem}$ [MIM*141900.0039], h. C$_{Georgetown}$, h. C$_{Harlem}$; duas Hb anormais, ambas com a substituição do resíduo glutamil pelo resíduo valil na sexta posição da cadeia β, como na Hb S; além disso, cada uma exibe uma segunda substituição de um resíduo aspartil por um resíduo asparaginil na posição 73 da cadeia β; ambos os tipos causam afoiçamento dos eritrócitos, semelhante ao produzido pela Hb S.

carbon monoxide h., h. de monóxido de carbono. SIN carboxihemoglobin.

h. Chesapeake (Hb$_{Chesapeake}$) [MIM*141800.0018], h. Chesapeake (Hb$_{Chesapeake}$); hemoglobina anormal com uma única substituição da cadeia α, com fórmula molecular $\alpha_2^{92Arg \rightarrow Leu} \beta_2^A$; os heterozigotos apresentam policitemia, aparentemente para compensar o aumento de afinidade do oxigênio por essa Hb, resultando em menor liberação de oxigênio nos tecidos.

h. Constant Spring, h. Constant Spring; hemoglobina anormal com cadeia polipeptídica ampliada (31 resíduos aminoacil adicionais) na cadeia α (por conseguinte, a cadeia α tem 172 aminoácidos de comprimento); cerca de 20% dos indivíduos com doença Hb H também apresentam esse defeito.

h. D$_{Punjab}$ [MIM*141900.0065], h. D$_{Punjab}$; Hb anormal com uma única substituição na cadeia β, com fórmula molecular $\alpha_2^A \beta_2^{121Glu \rightarrow Gln}$; os heterozigotos são assintomáticos, enquanto os homozigotos exibem anemia hemolítica leve; ocorre aumento na afinidade do O$_2$; idêntica às h. D$_{Los\ Angeles}$, h. D$_{North\ Carolina}$, h. D$_{Portugal}$, h. D$_{Chicago}$ e h. Oak Ridge.

h. E [MIM*141900.0071], h. E; Hb anormal com uma única substituição na cadeia β, com fórmula molecular $\alpha_2^A \beta_2^{26Glu \rightarrow Lys}$, comum no Sudeste Asiático, especialmente na Tailândia; os heterozigotos são assintomáticos, com 35–45% da Hb E, enquanto os homozigotos apresentam anemia hemolítica leve a moderada, com 90–100% de Hb E e o restante de Hb F.

embryonic h., h. embrionária. VER h. Gower-1, h. Gower-2.

h. F [MIM*142200], h. F; Hb fetal normal (Hb F) com fórmula molecular $\alpha_2^A \gamma_2^F$; trata-se do principal componente de Hb durante a vida intra-uterina, diminuindo rapidamente durante o primeiro ano de vida para atingir uma concentração de menos de 0,5% em crianças e adultos normais; a concentração de Hb F aumenta em algumas hemoglobinopatias e em alguns casos de anemia hipoplásica, anemia perniciosa e leucemia; a Hb F tem afinidade mais fraca do que a Hb A pelo 2,3-difosfoglicerato. Já foram descritas mais de 50 variantes mutantes da cadeia γ. SIN fetal h.

fetal h., h. fetal. SIN h. F.

h. F (hereditary persistence of) [MIM*142200.0026], h. F (persistência hereditária da); condição devida a um alelo que deprime a síntese de cadeias β e δ (como na talassemia), porém totalmente compensada por um aumento na síntese de cadeia γ; não ocorre anemia. Existem três tipos: 1) tipo africano, nenhuma síntese de cadeia β ou δ pelo cromossoma com gene anormal, os heterozigotos apresentam 20–30% de Hb F e ligeira redução da Hb A$_2$, enquanto os homozigotos não formam nenhuma Hb A ou Hb A$_2$; 2) tipo grego, redução da síntese de cadeias β e δ, os heterozigotos apresentam 10–20% de Hb F e Hb A$_2$ normal; 3) tipo suíço, os heterozigotos apresentam apenas 1–3% de Hb F e Hb A$_2$ normal.

glycosylated h., h. glicosilada; qualquer uma das quatro frações de Hb A (A$_{Ia1}$, A$_{Ia2}$, A$_{Ib}$ ou A$_{Ic}$) às quais se ligam a D-glicose e monossacarídeos relacionados de forma covalente; as concentrações estão aumentadas nos eritrócitos de pacientes com diabetes melito e podem ser utilizadas como índice retrospectivo de controle da glicose nesses pacientes.

h. Gower-1, h. Gower-1; Hb de fórmula molecular $\zeta_2 \epsilon_2$, encontrada como Hb de componente menor na fase embrionária inicial; desaparece no terceiro mês de gravidez, sendo substituída pela h. Gower-2 e h. Portland e, a seguir, pela Hb F; a cadeia ζ possui 141 resíduos de aminoácidos. A síntese da cadeia ζ está deficiente em casos de hidropsia fetal. Cf. h. Gower-2, h. Portland.

h. Gower-2, h. Gower-2; Hb normal de fórmula molecular $\alpha_2^A \epsilon_2$, que é um componente principal da Hb da fase embrionária inicial; a produção de cadeias ϵ cessa normalmente por volta do terceiro mês de desenvolvimento fetal, sendo substituída pela Hb F. Cf. h. Gower-1, h. Portland.

green h., coleglobina. SIN choleglobin.

h. H [MIM*142309], h. H; homotetrâmero de Hb (todos os quatro polipeptídeos são idênticos) de forma molecular β_4, encontrado apenas quando a síntese de cadeia α está deprimida e não é efetiva no transporte de oxigênio. A doença da Hb H (α-talassemia intermediária) é uma síndrome semelhante à talassemia em indivíduos heterozigotos para os genes tanto graves quanto leves da α-talassemia; presença de anemia moderada e anormalidades dos eritrócitos com 25–35% de Hb Bart ao nascimento, porém com substituição posterior da Hb Bart pela Hb H e diminuição da Hb A$_2$. A Hb H não exibe nenhuma cooperatividade com a ligação do O$_2$, nem efeito Bohr.

h. I [MIM*141800.0055], h. I; Hb anormal com uma única substituição na cadeia α, com fórmula molecular $\alpha_2^{16Lys \rightarrow Glu} \beta_2^A$; síndrome semelhante à talassemia encontrada em indivíduos heterozigotos para os genes da Hb I e da α-talassemia, com formação de cerca de 70% de Hb I.

h. J$_{Capetown}$ [MIM*141800.0063], h. J$_{Capetown}$; Hb anormal com uma única substituição na cadeia α, fórmula molecular $\alpha_2^{92Arg \rightarrow Gln} \beta_2^A$; os heterozigotos apresentam policitemia, devido a aumento da afinidade dessa Hb pelo oxigênio.

h. Kansas [MIM*141900.0145], h. Kansas; Hb anormal com fórmula molecular $\alpha_2^A \beta_2^{102Asn \rightarrow Thr}$; encontrada em associação à cianose familiar, devido a diminuição da afinidade dessa Hb pelo oxigênio.

h. Lepore [MIM 142000-various], h. Lepore; grupo de hemoglobinas anormais com cadeias α normais, cujas cadeias não-α consistem na porção N-terminal da cadeia δ unida à porção C-terminal da cadeia β, aparentemente em consequência do emparelhamento e *crossing-over* não-homólogo entre os genes para as cadeias β e δ. Os principais tipos incluem: Hb Lepore$_{Boston}$ (idênti-

hemoglobin (Hb)

ca à Hb Lepore$_{Washington}$), Hb Lepore$_{Hollandia}$ e Hb Lepore$_{Baltimore}$, que diferem na região do *crossing-over* (δ87–β116, δ22–β50 e δ50–β86, respectivamente). Os heterozigotos formam cerca de 10% de Hb Lepore, quantidades normais de Hb A$_2$ e quantidades moderadamente aumentadas de Hb F e, em geral, apresentam anemia leve, microcitose e hipocromia; os homozigotos formam apenas Hb Lepore e Hb F e apresentam anemia grave. Cf. h. anti-Lepore.

h. M [MIM*142310 & various], h. M; grupo de hemoglobinas anormais em que uma única substituição de aminoácido favorece a formação de metemoglobina, a despeito de quantidades normais da metemoglobina redutase. Estritamente falando, as Hb M são hemoglobinas com mutações nos resíduos histidil proximais ou distais. Outras Hb M tendem a favorecer o estado Fe(III). Os heterozigotos apresentam metemoglobinemia congênita; o estado homozigoto desses genes é desconhecido e presumivelmente fatal. Os tipos específicos incluem: Hb M$_{Iwate}$, α$_2^{87His \to Tyr}$ (cadeia α, posição 87, histidina substituída pela tirosina); Hb M$_{Hyde Park}$, β$^{92His \to Tyr}$; Hb M$_{Boston}$, α$^{58His \to Tyr}$; Hb M$_{Saskatoon}$, β$^{63His \to Tyr}$; Hb M$_{Milwaukee-1}$, β$^{67Val \to Glu}$.

mean corpuscular h. (MCH), h. corpuscular média (HCM); o conteúdo de hemoglobina do eritrócito médio, calculado a partir da concentração de hemoglobina e contagem de eritrócitos, nos índices eritrocitários.

muscle h., mioglobina. SIN myoglobin.

oxygenated h., oxiemoglobina. SIN oxyhemoglobin.

h. Portland, h. Portland; uma forma de Hb embrionária contendo as cadeias ζ da Hb Gower-1 e as cadeias γ da Hb F, apresentando, assim, a fórmula ζ$_2$γ$_2$; essencialmente, desaparece no terceiro mês de gravidez. Cf. h. Gower-1, h. Gower-2.

h. Rainier [MIM*141900-0232]; h. de Rainier; Hb anormal com fórmula molecular α$_2^A$β$_2^{145Tyr \to Cys}$; os heterozigotos apresentam policitemia, devido a aumento da afinidade dessa Hb pelo oxigênio.

reduced h., h. reduzida; a forma de Hb nos eritrócitos após a liberação do oxigênio da oxiemoglobina nos tecidos.

h. S [MIM*141900], h. S; Hb anormal com substituição do ácido glutâmico pela valina na sexta posição da cadeia β; a fórmula é α$_2^A$β$_2^S$ ou, mais especificamente, α$_2^A$β$_2^{6Glu \to Val}$. Estado heterozigoto: traço falciforme, ausência de anemia, Hb S 20–45% do total, sendo o restante constituído de Hb A. Estado homozigoto: anemia falciforme, Hb S 75–100% do total, sendo o restante constituído de Hb F ou Hb A$_2$. SIN sickle cell h.

sickle cell h. (Hb S), h. falciforme (Hb S). SIN h. S.

unstable h.'s, hemoglobinas instáveis; grupo de hemoglobinas raras com substituições de aminoácidos (ou deleções de aminoácidos em três tipos), que alteram a forma tridimensional da globina de modo a tornar a molécula instável; essas hemoglobinas exibem tendência aumentada, porém variável, à auto-oxidação e formação de corpúsculos de Heinz, e estão associadas à anemia hemolítica não-esferocítica congênita. As anormalidades da cadeia β instáveis incluem: hemoglobinas de Genova, Gun Hill, Hammersmith, Köln, Philly, Sabine, Santa Ana, Sydney, Wien e Zürich; as anormalidades da cadeia α instáveis incluem as hemoglobinas Bibba, Sinai e Torino.

variant h., h. variante; forma mutante inócua de Hb.

h. Yakima [MIM*141900-0301], h. Yakima; Hb anormal de fórmula molecular α$_2^A$β$_2^{99Asp \to His}$; os heterozigotos apresentam policitemia, devido a aumento da afinidade dessa Hb pelo oxigênio.

---

he·mo·glo·bi·ne·mia (hē'mō - glo - bi - nē'mē - ā). Hemoglobinemia; presença de hemoglobina livre no plasma sanguíneo, como ocorre na hemólise intravascular.

paroxysmal nocturnal h., h. paroxística noturna; distúrbio adquirido das células-tronco (células primordiais) hematopoéticas, que se caracteriza pela formação de plaquetas, granulócitos, eritrócitos e, possivelmente, linfócitos defeituosos. A anormalidade dos eritrócitos provoca lise intravascular mediada pelo complemento, que pode manifestar-se de maneira irregular ou, até mesmo, oculta.

puerperal h., h. puerperal. SIN postparturient *hemoglobinuria.*

he·mo·glo·bi·no·cho·lia (hē'mō - glō'bi - nō - kō'lē - ā). Hemoglobinocolia; presença de hemoglobina na bile. [hemoglobina + G. *cholē,* bile]

he·mo·glo·bi·nol·y·sis (hē'mō - glō - bi - nol'i - sis). Hemoglobinólise; destruição ou clivagem química da hemoglobina. SIN hemoglobinopepsia. [hemoglobina + G. *lysis,* dissolução]

he·mo·glo·bi·nop·a·thy (hē'mō - glō - bi - nop'ă - thē). Hemoglobinopatia; distúrbio ou doença causada pela, ou associada à, presença de hemoglobinas anormais no sangue, como, p. ex., anemia falciforme, distúrbios das hemoglobinas C, D, E, H ou I. Em certas ocasiões, são observadas combinações de hemoglobinas anormais nas hemoglobinopatias. [hemoglobina + G. *pathos,* doença]

he·mo·glo·bi·no·pep·sia (hē - mō - glō'bi - nō - pep'sē - ā). Hemoglobinopepsia. SIN hemoglobinolysis. [hemoglobina + G. *pepsis,* digestão]

he·mo·glo·bi·no·phil·ic (hē'mō - glō'bi - nō - fil'ik). Hemoglobinofílico; refere-se a certos microrganismos que não podem ser cultivados, exceto na presença de hemoglobina. [hemoglobina + G. *phileō,* amar]

hemolysin

he·mo·glo·bi·nu·ria (hē'mō - glō - bi - noo'rē - ā). Hemoglobinúria; presença de hemoglobina na urina, incluindo certos pigmentos estreitamente relacionados, que são formados a partir de uma discreta alteração da molécula de hemoglobina; quando presentes em quantidades suficientes, produzem uma urina com várias tonalidades, desde vermelho-amarelado claro até vermelho bastante escuro. [hemoglobina + G. *ouron,* urina]

epidemic h., h. epidêmica; presença de hemoglobina ou de pigmentos derivados da hemoglobina na urina de lactentes pequenos acompanhada de cianose, icterícia e outras condições; pode ser devida à metemoglobinemia secundária; também denominada doença de Winckel.

intermittent h., h. intermitente; crises episódicas recorrentes de hemoglobinúria que caracterizam a h. paroxística noturna ou a crioemoglobinúria paroxística.

malarial h., h. malárica; condição atualmente rara, resultante da infecção por *Plasmodium falciparum* (malária terçã maligna com hemólise grave); observada em indivíduos brancos após tratamento interrompido. SIN black-water fever, hemoglobinuric fever, West African fever.

march h., h. da marcha; forma que ocorre após corridas de maratona, marchas prolongadas ou exercícios físicos pesados.

paroxysmal cold h., crioemoglobinúria paroxística; distúrbio raro em que ocorre hemólise aguda grave após exposição ao frio.

paroxysmal nocturnal h., h. paroxística noturna; distúrbio raro com início insidioso (habitualmente na terceira ou na quarta década de vida) e evolução crônica, que se caracteriza por episódios de anemia hemolítica, hemoglobinúria (principalmente à noite), palidez, icterícia ou bronzeamento da pele, grau moderado de esplenomegalia e, algumas vezes, de hepatomegalia; em geral, os eritrócitos são macrocíticos e variam consideravelmente de tamanho, porém não há evidências de esferocitose, eritrofagocitose ou leucócitos anormais. O distúrbio resulta de uma anormalidade da membrana dos eritrócitos, que torna essas células extremamente sensíveis à lise pelo complemento. SIN Marchiafava-Micheli anemia, Marchiafava-Micheli syndrome.

postparturient h., h. pós-parto; doença hemolítica súbita e grave que aparece esporadicamente em vacas leiteiras bem nutridas, 2–4 semanas após o parto; em geral, ocorre nos animais de estábulo no inverno e no início da primavera; a causa não é conhecida, embora a doença esteja freqüentemente associada a hipofosfatemia. SIN puerperal hemoglobinemia.

toxic h., h. tóxica; hemoglobinúria que ocorre após a ingestão de vários venenos, em certas doenças sanguíneas e em determinadas infecções.

he·mo·glo·bi·nu·ric (hē'mō - glō - bi - noo'rik). Hemoglobinúrico; relativo a, ou caracterizado por, hemoglobinúria.

he·mo·gram (hē'mō - gram). Hemograma; registro detalhado e completo dos achados num exame total do sangue, especialmente com referência ao número, às proporções e às características morfológicas dos elementos figurados. [hemo- + G. *gramma,* desenho]

he·mo·his·ti·o·blast (hē'mō - his'tē - ō - blast). Hemo-histioblasto; célula mesenquimatosa primitiva que se acredita seja capaz de se desenvolver em todos os tipos de células sanguíneas, incluindo monócitos, e em histiócitos. SIN Ferrata cell, hematohistioblast. [hemo- + G. *histion,* tecido + *blastos,* germe]

he·mo·la·mel·la (hē'mō - lā - mel'ă). Hemolamela; termo obsoleto para plaqueta.

he·mo·li·pase (hē - mō - lip'ās). Hemolipase; lipase sanguínea.

he·mo·lith (hē'mō - lith). Hemólito; concreção na parede de um vaso sanguíneo. [hemo- + G. *lithos,* pedra]

he·mol·o·gy (hē - mol'ō - jē). Hematologia. SIN hematology.

he·mo·lymph (hē'mō - limf). Hemolinfa. 1. O sangue e a linfa, no sentido de um "tecido circulante". 2. O líquido nutriente de certos invertebrados. [hemo- + L. *lympha,* água clara]

he·mol·y·sate (hē - mol'i - sāt). Hemolisado; preparação resultante da lise dos eritrócitos.

he·mo·ly·sin (hē - mol'i - sin). Hemolisina. 1. Qualquer substância elaborada por um agente vivo, capaz de provocar lise dos eritrócitos e liberação de sua hemoglobina. SIN erythrocytolysin, erythrolysin. 2. Anticorpo sensibilizante (fixador de complemento) que se combina com eritrócitos do tipo antigênico que estimulou a formação da hemolisina, complemento fixador, em que a união anticorpo—célula resulta em lise das células.

α' h., h. α. VER α' *hemolysis.*

β h., h. β. VER β *hemolysis.*

bacterial h., h. bacteriana; qualquer agente hemolítico elaborado por diversas espécies de bactérias ou por determinadas cepas de uma espécie.

cold h., crioemolisina. SIN Donath-Landsteiner cold *autoantibody.*

heterophil h., h. heterófila; anticorpo sensibilizante que pode combinar-se com eritrócitos de diversas espécies (além daquelas utilizadas como antígeno para estimular a formação da hemolisina), resultando em hemólise na presença da quantidade apropriada de complemento.

immune h., h. imune; anticorpo hemolítico fixador do complemento e sensibilizante, formado em um animal em conseqüência da administração parenteral de eritrócitos ou de sangue total de outra espécie; a hemolisina imune também pode ser formada em seres humanos aos quais se administram transfusões de sangue humano que é antigênico no receptor, como, p. ex., a formação de anticorpo anti-Rh num indivíduo Rh-negativo tratado com eritrócitos Rh-positivos.

natural h., h. natural; hemolisina que ocorre no plasma de um animal de determinada espécie, como, p. ex., cão, que fixa o complemento com os eritrócitos de alguma outra espécie, p. ex., coelho, causando, assim, lise de células sanguíneas do coelho, apesar de o cão não ter sido anteriormente exposto a estímulo antigênico com essas células.

specific h., h. específica; anticorpo hemolítico, fixador de complemento e sensibilizante, que reage, total ou completamente, com eritrócitos do tipo antigênico utilizados para estimular a formação da hemolisina.

warm-cold h., h. quente-fria; hemolisina que se combina com os eritrócitos em temperaturas < 20°C e que são eluídos em temperaturas mais altas, como, p. ex., 30–37%. VER Donath-Landsteiner cold *autoantibody,* hemagglutinating cold *autoantibody.*

he·mo·ly·sin·o·gen (hē′mō-lī-sin′ō-jen). Hemolisinogênio; material antigênico nos eritrócitos que estimula a formação de hemolisina.

he·mol·y·sis (hē-mol′i-sis). Hemólise; alteração, dissolução ou destruição dos eritrócitos, de tal modo que a hemoglobina é liberada no meio em que as células estão suspensas, como, p. ex., por anticorpos específicos fixadores de complemento, toxinas, vários agentes químicos, tonicidade, alteração da temperatura. SIN erythrocytolysis, erythrolysis, hematolysis. [hemo- + G. *lysis,* destruição]

α′ h., h. α; hemólise observada em culturas de cepas ocasionais de pneumococos ou estreptococos em ágar-sangue; a zona de hemólise próxima à colônia é esverdeada, devido à decomposição parcial da hemoglobina.

β h., h. β; hemólise completa ou verdadeira observada em culturas de diversas bactérias em ágar-sangue, especialmente estreptococos hemolíticos e estafilococos; praticamente todos os eritrócitos são destruídos numa zona circular relativamente ampla e regularmente circunscrita próxima à colônia, produzindo, assim, um "halo" claro de ágar transparente; a zona de hemólise é freqüentemente muito mais larga do que o diâmetro da colônia; o grau de mudança varia de acordo com a espécie de eritrócitos.

biologic h., h. biológica; hemólise causada por materiais elaborados por diversos organismos vivos.

conditioned h., h. condicionada. SIN immune h.

γ h., h. γ; termo algumas vezes utilizado para indicar que não há hemólise em relação a colônias bacterianas em ágar-sangue; assim, os microrganismos não-hemolíticos podem ser designados como produtores de h. γ.

immune h., h. imune; hemólise causada pelo complemento quando os eritrócitos foram sensibilizados por anticorpo específico fixador de complemento. SIN conditioned h.

phenylhydrazine h. (fen′il-hī′-drā-zin), h. por fenilidrazina; teste *in vitro* para a deficiência de glicose-6-fosfato-desidrogenase (G6PD); hemólise decorrente da adição *in vitro* de fenilidrazina ao sangue com eritrócitos deficientes em G6PD, com aparecimento de corpúsculos de Heinz-Ehrlich.

venom h., h. por veneno; causada por material hemolítico existente no veneno de diversas espécies de cobras ou outros animais peçonhentos.

viridans h., h. viridans. VER α′ h.

he·mo·lyt·ic (hē-mō-lit′ik). Hemolítico; destrutivo para as células sanguíneas, resultando em liberação de hemoglobina. SIN hematolytic, hemotoxic (2), hematotoxic, hemotaxic.

he·mo·ly·za·tion (hē′mol-i-zā′shŭn). Hemolização; produção ou ocorrência de hemólise.

he·mo·lyze (hē′mō-līz). Hemolisar; produzir hemólise ou liberação de hemoglobina dos eritrócitos.

he·mo·me·di·as·ti·num (hē′mō-mē-dē-ā-stī′nŭm). Hemomediastino; presença de sangue no mediastino.

he·mo·me·tra (hē-mō-mē′tră). Hemometra. SIN hematometra.

he·mom·e·try (hē-mom′ĕ-trē). Hemometria. SIN hematometry.

he·mo·pa·thol·o·gy (hē′mō-pa-thol′ō-jē). Hemopatologia. SIN hematopathology.

he·mop·a·thy (hē′mop′á-thē). Hemopatia; qualquer condição anormal ou doença do sangue ou dos tecidos hematopoéticos. SIN hematopathy. [hemo- + G. *pathos,* sofrimento]

he·mo·per·fu·sion (hē′mō-per-fū′zhŭn). Hemoperfusão; passagem de sangue através de colunas de material adsortivo, como carvão ativado, para remover as substâncias tóxicas do sangue. [hemo- + L. *perfusio,* passar através de]

he·mo·per·i·car·di·um (hē′mō-pār′-i-kar′dē-ŭm). Hemopericárdio; presença de sangue no saco pericárdico.

he·mo·per·i·to·ne·um (hē′mō-pār-i-tō-nē′ŭm). Hemoperitônio; presença de sangue na cavidade peritoneal.

he·mo·pex·in (hēm-ō-peks′in). Hemopexina; glicoproteína sérica relacionada às β-globulinas, com peso molecular de cerca de 57.000, contendo 22% de carboidrato; importante na ligação do heme e das porfirinas, impedindo a excreção e, talvez, regulando o heme no metabolismo de drogas. [hemo- + G. *pēxis,* fixação, + -in]

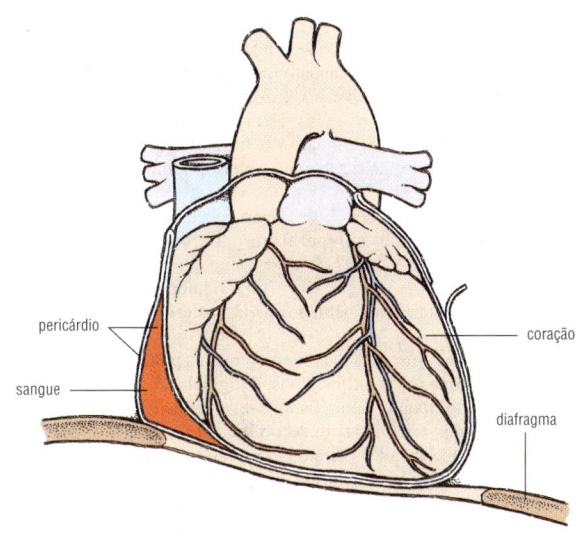

hemopericárdio

he·mo·pha·gia (hē-mō-fā′jē-ā). Hemofagia. SIN hematophagia. [hemo- + G. *phagein,* comer]

he·mo·phag·o·cy·to·sis (hē′mō-fag′ō-sī-tō′sis). Hemofagocitose; o processo de ingestão (e, habitualmente, destruição) das células sanguíneas pelos diversos tipos de células fagocíticas; termo utilizado especialmente para referir-se à fagocitose de eritrócitos e outras células da série eritróide.

he·mo·phil, he·mo·phile (hē-mō-fil, -fīl). Hemófilo; microrganismo que cresce preferencialmente em meios de cultura contendo sangue. [hemo- + G. *philos,* amigo]

he·mo·phil·ia (hē-mō-fil′ē-ā). Hemofilia; distúrbio hereditário da coagulação sanguínea caracterizado por tendência permanente a hemorragias, espontâneas ou traumáticas, devido a um defeito no mecanismo da coagulação sanguínea. [hemo- + G. *philos,* amigo]

h. A [MIM*306700-various], h. A; hemofilia devido à deficiência do fator VIII; condição recessiva ligada ao X que ocorre quase exclusivamente no sexo masculino em seres humanos, mas que também afeta várias raças de cães, caracterizada por prolongamento do tempo de coagulação, formação diminuída de tromboplastina e diminuição da conversão de protrombina. SIN classic h.

h. B [MIM*306900-various], h. B; distúrbio da coagulação que se assemelha à h. A, causado pela deficiência hereditária do fator IX; também observado como condição recessiva ligada ao X na raça terrier Cairn de cães. SIN Christmas disease.

h. C, h. C; hemofilia devida à deficiência de fator XI; do ponto de vista clínico, assemelha-se às hemofilias A e B, porém é transmitida como herança autossômica dominante; ocorre primariamente em indivíduos de ancestralidade judia.

classic h., h. clássica. SIN h. A.

he·mo·phil·i·ac (hē-mō-fil′ē-ak). Hemofílico; indivíduo que sofre de hemofilia.

he·mo·phil·ic (hē-mō-fil′ik). Hemofílico; relativo à hemofilia.

he·mo·phil·o·sis (hē-mō-fil-ō′sis). Hemofilose; qualquer doença causada por bactérias do gênero *Haemophilus.*

he·mo·pho·bia (hē-mō-fō′bē-ā). Hemofobia; temor mórbido de sangue ou de hemorragia. [hemo- + G. *phobos,* medo]

he·mo·pho·re·sis (hē′mō-fō-rē′sis). Hemoforese; convecção ou irrigação dos tecidos por sangue. [hemo- + G. *phoreō,* levar]

he·moph·thal·mia, he·moph·thal·mus (hē-mof-thal′mē-ah, -mof′-thal′mŭs). Hemoftalmia; derrame de sangue no olho. SIN hematopsia. [hemo- + G. *ophthalmos,* olho]

he·moph·thi·sis (hē-mof′thi-sis, hē-mof-thī′sis). Hemotísica; termo obsoleto para a anemia causada por degeneração anormal ou destruição de eritrócitos, ou por deficiência na formação destes. [hemo- + G. *phthisis,* consunção]

he·mo·plas·tic (hē-mō-plas′tik). Hemoplásico. SIN hemopoietic.

he·mo·plas·ty (hē′mō-plas-tē). Hemoplastia; formação ou elaboração de sangue pelos tecidos hematopoéticos. [hemo- + G. *plasso,* formar]

he·mo·pneu·mo·per·i·car·di·um (hē′mō-noo′mō-pār-i-kar′dē-ŭm). Hemopneumopericárdio; presença concomitante de sangue e de ar no pericárdio. SIN pneumohemopericardium. [hemo- + G. *pneuma,* ar + pericárdio]

he·mo·pneu·mo·tho·rax (hē′mō-noo-mō-thō′raks). Hemopneumotórax; acúmulo de ar e de sangue na cavidade pleural. SIN pneumohemothorax. [hemo- + G. *pneuma,* ar + tórax]

he·mo·poi·e·sis (hē′mō-poy-ē′sis). Hemopoese; o processo de formação e desenvolvimento dos vários tipos de células sanguíneas e outros elementos figurados. SIN hematogenesis, hematopoiesis, hematosis (1), hemogenesis, sanguification. [hemo- + G. *poiēsis,* fazer]

he·mo·poi·et·ic (hē′mō-poy-et′ik). Hemopoético; relativo ou relacionado à formação de células sanguíneas. SIN hemafacient, hematogenic (1), hematogenous, hematoplastic, hematopoietic, hemogenic, hemoplastic, sanguifacient.

he·mo·poi·e·tin (hē-mō-poy′ē-tin). Hemopoetina. SIN erythropoietin.

he·mo·por·phy·rin (hē-mō-pōr′fi-rin). Hemoporfirina. SIN hematoporphyrin.

he·mo·pre·cip·i·tin (hē′mō-prē-sip′i-tin). Hemoprecipitina; anticorpo que se combina com material antigênico solúvel dos eritrócitos causando a sua precipitação.

he·mo·pro·tein (hē-mō-prō′tēn). Hemoproteína; proteína ligada a um composto metal-porfirina (p. ex., citocromos, mioglobina, catalase).

he·mop·ty·sis (hē-mop′ti-sis). Hemoptise; emissão de sangue proveniente dos pulmões ou dos brônquios em decorrência de hemorragia pulmonar ou brônquica. SIN bronchostaxis. [hemo- + G. *ptysis,* emissão]
  endemic h., h. endêmica. SIN parasitic h.
  parasitic h., h. parasitária; a expressão clínica da paragonimíase, caracterizada por tosse e emissão de sangue proveniente dos pulmões. SIN endemic h.

he·mo·py·el·ec·ta·sis, he·mo·py·el·ec·ta·sia (hē′mō-pī′e-lek′tă-sis, -lek-tā′zē-ă). Hemopielectasia; termo obsoleto para descrever a dilatação da pelve renal com sangue e urina. [hemo- + pielectasia]

he·mo·re·pel·lant (hē′mō-rē-pel′ant). Hemorrepelente. **1.** Substância ou superfície que dificulta a aderência de sangue. **2.** Que possui essa ação.

he·mo·rhe·ol·o·gy (hē′mō-rē-ol′ō-jē). Hemorreologia; a ciência do fluxo de sangue em relação à pressão, ao fluxo, volume e resistência nos vasos sanguíneos, especialmente em termos de viscosidade sanguínea e deformação dos eritrócitos na microcirculação. [hemo- + G. *rheos,* corrente, fluxo + *logos,* estudo]

hem·or·rhage (hem′ō-rij). Hemorragia. **1.** Escape de sangue do espaço intravascular. **2.** Sangrar. [G. *haimorrhagia,* fr. *haima,* sangue + *rhēgnymi* irromper]
  brainstem h., hemorragia do tronco cerebral; sangramento para a ponte ou para o mesencéfalo, freqüentemente secundária à deformação do tronco cerebral por hérnia transtentorial, devido a lesões intracranianas rapidamente expansivas.
  cerebral h., h. cerebral; hemorragia na substância do cérebro, habitualmente na região da cápsula interna em conseqüência da ruptura da artéria lenticuloestriada. SIN hematencephalon, intracerebral h.
  concealed h., h. oculta. SIN internal h.
  Duret h., h. de Duret; pequena hemorragia do tronco cerebral em decorrência da deformação do tronco cerebral secundária a hérnia transtentorial.
  extradural h., h. extradural; acúmulo de sangue entre o crânio e a dura-máter. SIN epidural hematoma.
  gastric h., h. gástrica. SIN gastrorrhagia.
  intermediate h., h. intermediária; hemorragia recidivante.
  internal h., h. interna; sangramento para órgãos ou cavidades do corpo. SIN concealed h.
  intracerebral h., h. intracerebral. SIN h. cerebral.
  intracranial h., h. intracraniana; sangramento na abóbada craniana; inclui a h. cerebral e a h. subaracnóide.
  intrapartum h., h. intraparto; hemorragia que ocorre durante o trabalho de parto e o parto normais.
  intraventricular h., h. intraventricular; extravasamento de sangue para o sistema ventricular do cérebro.
  nasal h., h. nasal. SIN epistaxis.
  parenchymatous h., h. parenquimatosa; sangramento na substância de um órgão.
  h. per rhex'is. hemorragia causada por ruptura de um vaso sanguíneo.
  petechial h., h. petequial; hemorragia capilar para a pele, formando petéquias. SIN punctate h.
  pontine h., h. pontina; hemorragia que ocorre na substância da ponte, tipicamente em pacientes hipertensos.
  postpartum h., h. pós-parto; hemorragia do canal do parto superior a 500 ml, após parto vaginal, ou de 1.000 ml após cesárea, nas primeiras 24 horas após o parto.
  primary h., h. primária; hemorragia que ocorre imediatamente após uma lesão ou cirurgia, diferente da h. intermediária ou secundária.
  punctate h., h. puntiforme. SIN petechial h.
  renal h., h. renal; hematúria cuja origem é o rim.
  secondary h., h. secundária; hemorragia que ocorre em certo intervalo após uma lesão ou cirurgia.
  serous h., h. serosa; termo obsoleto para referir-se a uma transudação profusa de plasma através das paredes dos capilares.
  splinter h.'s, h. subungueal; diminutas hemorragias subungueais longitudinais, tipicamente observadas na endocardite bacteriana, triquinose, etc, embora não sejam diagnósticas.
  subarachnoid h., h. subaracnóide; extravasamento de sangue para o espaço subaracnóide, freqüentemente devido a ruptura de aneurisma e que se dissemina, em geral, através das vias do líquido cefalorraquidiano.
  subdural h., h. subdural; extravasamento de sangue entre as membranas da dura-máter e da aracnóide; ocorrem formas agudas e crônicas; os hematomas crônicos podem tornar-se encapsulados por neomembranas. SIN subdural hematoma.
  subgaleal h., h. subgaleal; coleção de sangue sob a aponeurose epicrânica.
  syringomyelic h., h. siringomiélica; sangramento para uma cavidade siringomiélica.

hem·or·rhag·ic (hem-ō-raj′ik). Hemorrágico; relativo a, ou caracterizado por, hemorragia.

hem·or·rhag·ins (hem-ō-raj′inz,-rā′jins). Hemorraginas; citolisinas encontradas em certos venenos e materiais verminosos de algumas plantas, como, p. ex., veneno de cascavel e ricina; as hemorraginas causam degeneração e lise das células endoteliais nos capilares e pequenos vasos, resultando, desse modo, em numerosas pequenas hemorragias nos tecidos. [hemorragia + in]

hem·or·rhoid (hem′ō-royd). Hemorróida; refere-se a um dos tumores ou varizes que constituem as hemorróidas.

hem·or·rhoi·dal (hem-ō-roy′dăl). Hemorroidário. **1.** Relativo a hemorróidas. **2.** Termo antigamente aplicado a certas artérias e veias que suprem a região do reto e do ânus, atualmente descritas como "anais" ou "retais".

hem·or·rhoid·ec·to·my (hem′ō-roy-dek′tō-mē). Hemorroidectomia; remoção cirúrgica de hemorróidas; em geral, realizada por excisão dos tecidos hemorroidários através de dissecção ou pela aplicação de ligadura elástica na base dos feixes hemorroidários, produzindo necrose isquêmica e, por fim, ablação das hemorróidas. [hemorróidas + G. *ektomē,* excisão]

hem·or·rhoids (hem′ō-roydz). Hemorróidas; condição varicosa das veias hemorroidárias externas, causando intumescimento doloroso no ânus. SIN piles. [G. *haimorrhois,* pl. *haimorrhoides,* veias que provavelmente sangrarão, fr. *haima,* sangue + *rhoia,* fluxo]
  cutaneous h., h. cutâneas; hiperplasia do tecido conjuntivo em uma ou mais das pregas irradiantes normais da pele que circunda imediatamente o ânus.
  external h., h. externas; veias dilatadas que formam tumores no lado externo do esfíncter anal.
  internal h., h. internas; veias dilatadas sob a membrana mucosa, no interior do esfíncter.

he·mo·sal·pinx (hē′mō-sal′pinks). Hemossalpinge. SIN hematosalpinx.

he·mo·si·al·em·e·sis (hē′mō-sī-ăl-em′ē-sis). Hemossialêmese; vômito de sangue e saliva. [hemo- + G. *sialon,* saliva + *emesis,* vômito]

he·mo·sid·er·in (hē-mō-sid′er-in). Hemossiderina; proteína insolúvel amarelo-ouro ou amarelo-acastanhada produzida pela digestão fagocítica da hematina; encontrada na maioria dos tecidos, especialmente no fígado, baço e medula óssea, sob a forma de grânulos muito maiores do que as moléculas de ferritina (das quais se acredita sejam agregados), porém com teor mais elevado de ferro, de até 37%; cora-se de azul pelo azul-da-Prússia de Perl. [hemo- + G. *sidēros,* ferro + -in]

he·mo·sid·er·o·sis (hē′mō-sid-er-ō′sis). Hemossiderose; acúmulo de hemossiderina nos tecidos, particularmente no fígado e no baço. VER hemochromatosis. [hemosiderina + *osis,* condição]
  idiopathic pulmonary h., h. pulmonar idiopática; ataques súbitos e repetidos de dispnéia e hemoptise, resultando em hemossiderose pulmonar difusa, observada mais comumente em crianças; de causa desconhecida; entretanto, alguns casos podem estar associados à síndrome de Goodpasture. SIN Ceelen-Gellerstedt syndrome.
  nutritional h., h. nutricional; doença que resulta da ingestão de ferro em alimentos preparados em vasilhames de ferro.

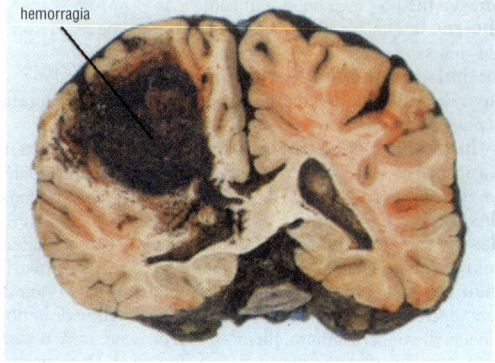

hemorragia: espécime de necropsia mostrando hemorragia maciça no hemisfério cerebral

he·mo·sper·mia (hē'mō-sper'mē-ă). Hemospermia; presença de sangue no líquido seminal. SIN hematospermia. [hemo- + G. *sperma*, semente]
  h. spu'ria, h. espúria; h. que ocorre na uretra prostática.
  h. ve'ra, h. verdadeira; h. proveniente das vesículas seminais.
he·mo·spo·rid·i·um (hē'mō-spō-rid'ē-ŭm). Hemosporídio; parasita sanguíneo da ordem Haemosporidia. [hemo- + L. Mod. dim. do G. *sporos*, semente]
he·mo·spo·rines (hē'mō-spō-rēnz). Hemosporinas; termo comum para referir-se a membros da ordem Haemosporidia.
he·mo·sta·sia (hē-mō-stā'zē-ă). Hemostasia. SIN *hemostasis.*
he·mo·sta·sis (hē'mō-stā-sis, hē-mos'tă-sis). Hemostasia. **1.** Cessação do sangramento. **2.** Parada da circulação em alguma parte. **3.** Estagnação do sangue. SIN hemostasia. [hemo- + G. *stasis*, parada]
he·mo·stat (hē'mō-stat). Hemostato. **1.** Qualquer agente que interrompe, química ou mecanicamente, o fluxo de sangue de um vaso aberto. **2.** Instrumento que faz cessar a hemorragia por compressão do vaso hemorrágico.
he·mo·stat·ic (hē-mō-stat'ik). Hemostático. **1.** Que interrompe o fluxo de sangue no interior dos vasos. **2.** SIN *antihemorrhagic.*
he·mo·styp·tic (hē-mo-stip'tik). Hemostíptico. SIN *styptic (2).* [hemo- + G. *styptikos*, adstringente]
he·mo·suc·cus pan·cre·a·ti·cus. Sangramento para o ducto pancreático, geralmente em conseqüência de traumatismo, tumor, inflamação ou pseudoaneurisma associado a pseudocisto.
he·mo·ta·cho·gram (hē-mō-ta'chō-gram). Hematograma; registro obtido pelo hematocômetro. [hemo + tachos + G. *gramma*, algo escrito]
he·mo·ta·chom·e·ter (hē'mō-tā-kom'ĕ-ter). Hematocômetro; instrumento para medir a velocidade do fluxo nas artérias. SIN hematachometer. [hemo- + G. *tachos*, rapidez + *metron*, medida]
he·mo·ther·a·py, he·mo·ther·a·peu·tics (hē'mō-thār'ă-pē, thār-ă-pū'tiks). Hemoterapia, hemoterapêutica; tratamento da doença pelo uso de sangue ou hemoderivados, como na transfusão. SIN hematherapy.
he·mo·tho·rax (hē-mō-thōr'aks). Hemotórax; presença de sangue na cavidade pleural. SIN hemathorax.
he·mo·tox·ic, he·ma·to·tox·ic, he·ma·tox·ic (hē-mō-tok'sik; hē'mă-tō-toks'ik, hem'ă; hē-mă-toks'ik, hem-ă-). Hemotóxico, hematotóxico, hematóxico. **1.** Que causa intoxicação do sangue. **2.** Hemolítico. SIN *hemolytic.*
he·mo·tox·in (hē-mō-tok'sin). Hemotoxina; qualquer substância que provoca destruição dos eritrócitos, incluindo várias hemolisinas; em geral, termo utilizado para referir-se a substâncias de origem biológica, em contraste com produtos químicos. SIN hematotoxin, hematoxin.
  cobra h., h. de *Naja*; o constituinte do veneno de serpentes *Naja* (Elapidae) que hemolisa os eritrócitos de várias espécies.
he·mo·troph, he·mot·ro·phe (hēm'ō-trof). Hemotrofo; materiais nutritivos fornecidos aos embriões de mamíferos com placenta através da corrente sanguínea materna. Cf. embryotroph, histotroph. [hemo- + G. *trophē*, alimento]
he·mo·tro·pic (hē-mō-trop'ik). Hemotrópico; relativo ao mecanismo pelo qual uma substância nas células sanguíneas, especialmente nos eritrócitos, atrai células fagocíticas; estas últimas mudam a sua direção e migram para as células hemotrópicas. SIN hematotropic. [hemo- + G. *tropos*, direção (ou *tropē*, uma volta)]
he·mo·tym·pa·num (hē'mō-tim'pă-nŭm). Hemotímpano; presença de sangue no ouvido médio. SIN hematotympanum.

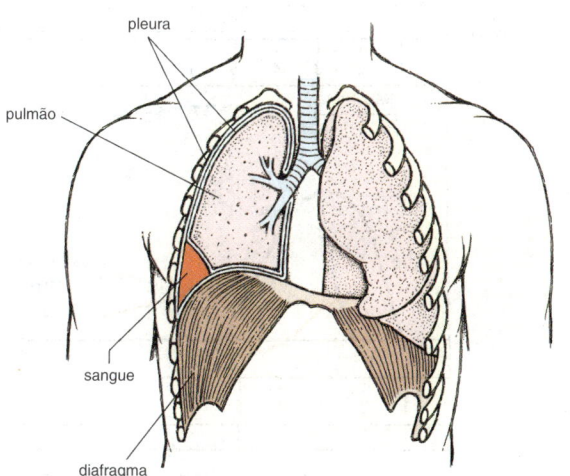

hemotórax: na cavidade pulmonar direita

he·mo·zo·ic (hē-mō-zō'ik). Hemozóico; parasita no sangue de vertebrados; refere-se a determinados protozoários. SIN hematozoic.
he·mo·zo·on (hē-mō-zō'on). Hemozoário; animal parasita que vive no sangue, como os tripanossomas ou as microfilárias de *Wuchereria* ou *Brugia*. SIN hematozoon. [hemo- + G. *zōon*, animal]
HEMPAS Abreviatura de *h*ereditary *e*rythroblastic *m*ultinuclearity associated with *p*ositive *a*cidified *s*erum (multinuclearidade eritroblástica hereditária associada a soro acidificado positivo). VER HEMPAS *cells*, em *cell.*
hen·bane (hen'bān). Meimendro. SIN *hyoscyamus.*
Henderson, Lawrence J., bioquímico norte-americano, 1878–1942. VER H.-Hasselbalch *equation.*
Hendersonula toruloidea. SIN *Nattrassia mangiferae.*
Henke, Wilhelm, anatomista alemão, 1834–1896. VER H. *space.*
Henle, Friedrich G.J., anatomista, patologista e histologista alemão, 1809–1885. VER *crypts* of H. em *crypt;* H. *ampulla, ansa, glands,* em *gland, fissures,* em *fissure, layer, fiber layer, nervous layer, loop, membrane,* fenestrated elastic *membrane, reaction, sheath, spine, tubules,* em *tubule, warts,* em *wart;* Hassal-H. *bodies,* em *body.*
hen·na (hen'ă). Hena; as folhas da hena egípcia, *Lawsonia inermis;* usada como cosmético e corante de cabelos. [Ar. *hennā*]
Hen·ne·bert. Camille, otologista belga, 1867–1958. VER Hennebert *sign.*
Henoch, Eduard H., pediatra alemão, 1820–1910. VER H. *chorea, purpura;* H.-Schönlein *purpura, syndrome;* Schönlein-H. *syndrome.*
hen·pu·ye (hen-poo'yē). Henpuye. SIN *goundou.* [termo nativo da Costa do Ouro (Gana) que significa "nariz de cachorro"]
Hen·ri, Victor, bioquímico francês do século XX. VER Michaelis-Menten *equation;* H.-Michaelis-Menten *equation.*
Henry, James Paget, fisiologista norte-americano.*1914. VER H.-Gauer *response.*
Henry, Joseph, físico norte-americano, 1797–1878. VER Dalton-H. *law.*
Henry, William, químico inglês, 1774–1836. VER H. *law.*
hen·ry (H) (hen'rē). Henry (H); a unidade de indutância elétrica quando 1 V é induzido por uma mudança na corrente de 1 A/s. [Joseph *Henry*]
Henseleit, K., internista alemão, *1907. VER Krebs-H. *cycle.*
Hensen, Victor, anatomista e fisiologista alemão, 1835–1924. VER H. *canal, cell, disk, duct, knot, line, node, stripe.*
Hensing, Friedrich W., anatomista alemão, 1719–1745. VER H. *ligament.*
He·pad·na·vi·ri·dae (hē-pa'd'nă-vī'rā-dā). Família de vírus de DNA icosaédricos contendo lipídios, de 42 nm de diâmetro, cujo genoma consiste numa única molécula de DNA circular fechado de forma não-covalente, de filamento parcialmente simples e parcialmente duplo; associados à hepatite em várias espécies de animais. O principal gênero, ortho Hepadnavirus, está associado à hepatite B em mamíferos, enquanto o gênero Avihepadnavirus provoca doença em aves; a infecção persistente é comum e está associada a doença crônica e câncer hepático. [*hep*atite + *DNA* + *v*írus]
he·par, gen. **hep·a·tis** (hē'par, hē'pah-tis). [TA]. Fígado. SIN *liver.* [L. emprestado do G. *hēpar,* gen. *hēpatos,* fígado]
  h. loba'tum, fígado lobado; fígado fissurado devido a fibrose de gomas sifilíticas cicatrizadas.
hep·a·ran N-sul·fa·tase (hep'ă-ran). Heparana N-sulfatase; enzima que participa na degradação por etapas do sulfato de heparana; a heparana N-sulfatase hidrolisa o componente sulfato fixado ao grupamento amino do resíduo glicosamina do sulfato de heparana; a deficiência dessa enzima está associada à mucopolissacaridose IIIA (síndrome de Sanfilippo A).
hep·a·ran sul·fate. Sulfato de heparana. SIN *heparitin sulfate.*
hep·a·rin (hep'ă-rin). Heparina; princípio anticoagulante que é um componente de vários tecidos (especialmente o fígado e o pulmão) e mastócitos nos seres humanos e em várias espécies de mamíferos; seu constituinte principal e ativo é um glicosaminoglicano composto de ácido D-glicurônico e D-glicosamina, ambos sulfatados, em ligação 1,4-α, de peso molecular de 6.000 a 20.000. Em conjunção com um co-fator de proteína sérica (o denominado co-fator da heparina), a heparina atua como antitrombina e antiprotrombina. São freqüentemente utilizadas preparações sintéticas na anticoagulação terapêutica. Além disso, potencializa a atividade dos "fatores de limpeza" (lipoproteína lipases). SIN heparinic acid.
  h. eliminase, h. eliminase. SIN *h. lypase.*
  h. lyase, h. liase; enzima que elimina os resíduos Δ-4,5-D-glicuronato da heparina e poliglicuronatos de ligação 1,4 semelhantes. SIN h. eliminase, heparinase.
  h. sodium, h. sódica; uma mistura de princípios ativos (habitualmente obtidos de vários tecidos de animais domésticos) com a propriedade de prolongar o tempo de coagulação do sangue humano.
hep·a·rin·ase (hep'ă-rin-ās). Heparinase. SIN *heparin lyase.*
hep·a·ri·ne·mia (hep'ă-ri-nē'mē-ă). Heparinemia; presença de níveis demonstráveis de heparina no sangue circulante.
hep·a·rin·ic ac·id (hep-ă-rin'ik). Ácido heparínico. SIN *heparin.*
hep·a·rin·ize (hep'ă-rin-īz). Heparinizar; proceder à administração terapêutica de heparina.

hep·a·rit·in sul·fate (hep′ă - rit - in). Sulfato de heparitina; heteropolissacarídeo que possui o mesmo dissacarídeo repetido da heparina, porém com menos grupamentos sulfato e mais grupamentos acetila. Acumula-se em indivíduos com certos tipos de mucopolissacaridoses. SIN heparan sulfate.

♻ **hepat-, hepato-**. Hepat-, hepato-. O fígado. [G. hēpar (hēpat−)]
hep·a·ta·tro·phia, hep·a·tat·ro·phy (hep′ă - tă - trō′fē - ă, hep - ă - tat′rō - fē). Hepatatrofia; atrofia do fígado.
hep·a·tec·to·my (hep - ă - tek′tō - mē). Hepatectomia; remoção do fígado, completa ou parcial. [hepat- + G. ektomē, excisão]
he·pa·tic (he-pat′ik). Hepático; relativo ao fígado. [G. hēpatikos]
he·pat·i·co·do·chot·o·my (he - pat′i - kō - dō - kot′ō - mē). Hepatodocotomia; hepatotomia e coledocotomia combinadas.
he·pat·i·co·du·o·de·nos·to·my (he - pat′i - kō - doo′ō - de - nos′tō - mē). Hepatoduodenostomia; estabelecimento de uma comunicação entre os ductos hepáticos e o duodeno. SIN hepatoduodenostomy. [hepatico- + duodenostomia]
he·pat·i·co·en·ter·os·to·my (he - pat′i - kō - en - ter - os′tō - mē). Hepatoenterostomia; estabelecimento de uma comunicação entre os ductos hepáticos e o intestino. SIN hepatocholangioenterostomy. [hepatico- + enterostomia]
he·pat·i·co·gas·tros·to·my (he - pat′i - kō - gas - tros′tō - mē). Hepatogastrostomia; estabelecimento de uma comunicação entre o ducto hepático e o estômago. [hepatico- + gastrostomia]
he·pat·i·co·li·thot·o·my (he - pat′i - kō - li - thot′ō - mē). Hepatolitotomia; remoção de um cálculo de um ducto hepático. [hepatico- + G. lithos, pedra + tomē, corte]
he·pat·i·co·lith·o·trip·sy (he - pat′i - kō - lith′ō - trip - sē). Hepatolitotripsia; esmagamento ou fragmento de um cálculo biliar no ducto hepático. [hepatico- + G. lithos, pedra + tripsis, fricção]
he·pat·i·co·pul·mo·nary (he - pat′i - kō - pul′mō - năr - ē). Hepatopulmonar. SIN hepatopneumonic.
he·pat·i·cos·to·my (he - pat - i - kŏs′tō - mē). Hepatostomia; estabelecimento de uma abertura para o ducto hepático. [hepatico- + G. stoma, boca]
he·pat·i·cot·o·my (he - pat - i - kot′ō - mē). Hepatotomia; incisão no ducto hepático. [hepatico- + G. tomē, incisão]
hep·a·tin (hep′ă - tin). Hepatina. SIN glycogen.
hep·a·tit·ic (hep - ă - tit′ik). Hepatítico; relativo à hepatite.

hep·a·ti·tis (hep - ă - tī′tis). Hepatite; inflamação do fígado, geralmente devido a infecção viral, porém algumas vezes devido a agentes tóxicos. [hepat- + -itis]

> Anteriormente endêmica na maioria dos países em desenvolvimento, a hepatite viral representa, hoje em dia, um importante problema de saúde pública nas nações industrializadas. Os três tipos mais comuns de hepatite viral (A, B e C) acometem milhões de pessoas no mundo inteiro. A hepatite viral aguda caracteriza-se por graus variáveis de febre, mal-estar, fraqueza, anorexia, náuseas e distúrbio abdominal. A lesão hepatocelular causa retenção de bilirrubina, muitas vezes com icterícia, e elevação dos níveis séricos de certas enzimas (particularmente transaminases). A hepatite A, causada por um enterovírus, é transmitida por via orofecal, mais freqüentemente através da ingestão de água ou alimentos contaminados. A taxa de casos fatais é de menos de 1%, e a recuperação é completa. A presença de anticorpo contra o vírus da hepatite A indica infecção prévia, não-infectividade e imunidade a ataques futuros. A hepatite B, causada por um pequeno DNA vírus, é transmitida através de contato sexual, agulhas compartilhadas por usuários de drogas IV, lesões por picadas de agulha em profissionais de saúde e da mãe para o feto. A incidência anual nos Estados Unidos é de 300.000 casos. O período de incubação é de 6–24 semanas. Alguns pacientes tornam-se portadores, e, em alguns, o desenvolvimento de uma resposta imune ao vírus induz uma fase crônica, que leva ao desenvolvimento de cirrose, insuficiência hepática e risco de carcinoma hepatocelular. O antígeno de superfície da hepatite B (HBsAg) pode ser detectado no soro no estágio inicial; sua persistência correlaciona-se com infecção crônica e infectividade. O antígeno do cerne (HBcAg) aparece num estágio mais tardio e também indica infectividade. A hepatite C constitui a principal forma de hepatite transmitida por transfusões; com freqüência, verifica-se o desenvolvimento de uma forma crônica ativa. A infecção aguda pelos vírus da hepatite B ou C apresenta maior taxa de mortalidade do que a hepatite A. Já existem vacinas efetivas para imunização ativa contra as hepatites A e B. O interferon-alfa produz remissão clínica em alguns casos de hepatites B e C. A hepatite D é causada por um RNA vírus que só pode produzir doença em indivíduos previamente infectados pelo vírus da hepatite B. A hepatite E, que ocorre principalmente nas regiões tropicais, assemelha-se à hepatite A pelo fato de ser transmitida por via orofecal e a infecção não se tornar crônica ou resultar em estado de portador; todavia, está associada a uma taxa de mortalidade muito mais elevada.

h. A, h. A. SIN viral h. type A.
acute parenchymatous h., h. parenquimatosa aguda. SIN acute massive liver necrosis.
anicteric h., h. anictérica; hepatite sem icterícia.
anicteric virus h., h. viral anictérica; hepatite relativamente leve, sem icterícia, causada por vírus; os sinais e sintomas físicos principais consistem em aumento de tamanho do fígado, dos linfonodos e, freqüentemente, do baço, juntamente com cefaléia, fadiga contínua, náuseas, anorexia, súbita aversão ao fumo, dores abdominais e, algumas vezes, febre baixa; os exames laboratoriais revelam evidências de hepatite.
h. B, h. B. SIN viral h. type B.
h. C, h. C. SIN viral h. type C.
cholangiolitic h., h. colangiolítica; hepatite com alterações inflamatórias ao redor dos pequenos ductos biliares, produzindo icterícia principalmente obstrutiva; pode ser devido a infecção viral ou bacteriana que ascende pela árvore biliar em virtude da obstrução.
cholestatic h., h. colestática; icterícia com estase biliar nos ductos biliares intra-hepáticos inflamados; em geral, causada pelos efeitos tóxicos de uma droga.
chronic h., h. crônica; qualquer um dos vários tipos de hepatite que persistem por mais de seis meses, evoluindo freqüentemente para cirrose. SIN chronic active liver disease.
chronic active h., h. crônica ativa; hepatite com inflamação porta crônica estendendo-se ao parênquima, com necrose em saca-bocado e fibrose que habitualmente evolui para cirrose pós-necrótica grosseiramente nodular. SIN juvenile cirrhosis, posthepatitic cirrhosis, subacute h.
chronic interstitial h., h. intersticial crônica; termo obsoleto para referir-se à cirrose do fígado.
chronic persistent h., h. persistente crônica. SIN chronic persisting h.
chronic persisting h., h. persistente crônica; forma de hepatite habitualmente benigna, que não evolui para a cirrose; em geral, assintomática sem qualquer achado físico, porém com anormalidades contínuas nas provas de função hepática. SIN chronic persistent h.
h. D, h. D. SIN viral h. type D.
delta h., h. delta. SIN viral h. type D.
drug-induced h., h. fármaco-induzida; lesão hepatocelular causada por uma droga.
h. E, h. E. SIN viral h. type E.
epidemic h., h. epidêmica. SIN viral h. type A.
h. exter'na, periepatite. SIN perihepatitis.
h. F, h. F; doença causada por um DNA vírus ainda pouco caracterizado.
fulminant h., h. fulminante; perda grave e rapidamente progressiva da função hepática, devido a infecção viral ou outra causa de destruição inflamatória do tecido hepático.
h. G, h. G; doença causada por um RNA vírus semelhante ao vírus da hepatite.
giant cell h., h. de células gigantes. SIN neonatal h.
halothane h., h. por halotano; lesão hepatocelular considerada resultante da administração de anestesia por halotano.
infectious h. (IH), h. infecciosa (IH). SIN viral h. type A.
long incubation h., h. de incubação prolongada; termo obsoleto para a hepatite B, com base no seu período de incubação mais longo (faixa de 30–180 dias,

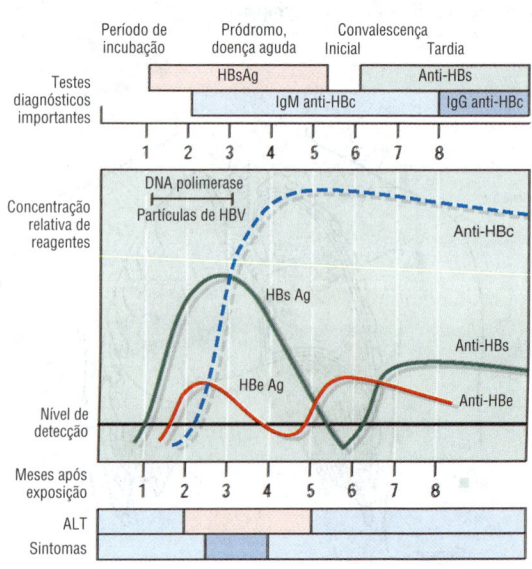

infecção pelo vírus da hepatite B: eventos clínicos e sorológicos

nomenclatura dos antígenos da hepatite e anticorpos correspondentes		
doença	componente do sistema	definição
Hepatite A	HAV	Vírus da hepatite A. Agente etiológico da hepatite infecciosa. Um picornavírus, o protótipo de um novo gênero, *Hepatovirus*.
	Anti-HAV	Anticorpo anti-HAV. Detectável no início dos sintomas; persistência durante toda a vida.
	IgM anti-HAV	Anticorpo da classe IgM dirigido contra o HAV. Indica infecção recente pela hepatite A; positivo dentro de até 4–6 meses após a infecção.
Hepatite B	HBV	Vírus da hepatite B. Agente etiológico da hepatite sérica (hepatite de incubação longa). Hepadnavírus.
	HBsAG	Antígeno de superfície da hepatite B. Os antígenos de superfície do HBV são detectáveis em grandes quantidades no soro; já foram identificados vários subtipos.
	HBcAG	Antígeno do cerne do vírus da hepatite B.
	Anti-HBs	Anticorpo contra o HBsAg. Indica infecção passada por HBV e imunidade ao vírus, presença de anticorpo passivo proveniente de HBIG ou resposta imune à vacina contra HBV.
	Anti-HBe	Anticorpo dirigido contra o HBeAg. A sua presença no soro de portadores de HBsAg sugere títulos mais baixos de HBV.
	Anti-HBc	Anticorpo contra o HBcAg. Indica infecção por HBV em algum momento não-definido do passado.
	IgM anti-HBc	Anticorpo da classe IgM contra o HBcAg. Indica infecção recente por HBV; positivo durante 4-8 meses após a infecção.
Hepatite C	HCV	Vírus da hepatite C, agente etiológico comum da hepatite pós-transfusional. Flavivírus.
	Anti-HCV	Anticorpo contra o HCV.
Hepatite D	HDV	Vírus da hepatite D. Agente etiológico da hepatite D; provoca infecção apenas na presença de HBV.
	HDAg	Antígeno delta (Ag-delta). Detectável na fase inicial da infecção aguda por HDV.
	Anti-HDV	Anticorpo contra o Ag-delta (antidelta). Indica infecção passada ou atual por HDV.
Hepatite E	HEV	Vírus da hepatite E. Vírus da hepatite transmitida por via entérica. Provoca grandes epidemias na Ásia e no Norte da África; transmissão orofecal ou através da água. Talvez um calicivírus.
Imunoglobulinas	IG	Imunoglobulina USP. Contém anticorpos contra o HAV; nenhum anticorpo contra HBsAg, HCV ou HIV.
	HBIG	Imunoglobulina da hepatite B. Contém títulos elevados de anticorpos contra o HBV.

em geral 60–90 dias) em comparação com a hepatite A (15–45 dias, média de 30 dias).
lupoid h., h. lupóide; icterícia com evidências de lesão dos hepatócitos e provas positivas para anticorpo antinuclear e célula LE, porém sem qualquer evidência de lúpus eritematoso sistêmico; em geral, as biópsias hepáticas revelam h. crônica ativa, com infiltração por plasmócitos, ou cirrose pós-necrótica; o soro é negativo para o antígeno da hepatite B. SIN plasmacell h.
MS-1 h., h. MS-1. SIN viral h. type A.
NANB h., h. NANB. SIN non-A, non-B h.
NANBNC h., h. NANBNC; abreviatura para hepatite não-A, não-B, não-C.
neonatal h., h. neonatal; hepatite no período neonatal atribuída a várias causas, principalmente vírus; caracterizada por bilirrubinemia direta e indireta, degeneração hepatocelular e aparecimento de células gigantes multinucleadas; pode ser difícil diferenciá-la da atresia biliar, porém é mais provável que termine com recuperação, embora possa haver desenvolvimento de cirrose. SIN giant cell h.
non-A-E h., h. não-A-E; hepatite aguda não causada por qualquer um dos agentes virais identificados de A até E.
non-A, non-B h., h. não-A não-B; hepatite causada por qualquer número de agentes infecciosos não-detectáveis pelos métodos que revelam a presença dos vírus da hepatite A e B. SIN NANB h.
non-A, non-B, non-C h. (NANBNC h.), h. não-A, não-B, não-C (h. NANBNC); hepatite causada por outros microrganismos virais diferentes dos vírus da hepatite A, B ou C.
peliosis h., h. da peliose; condição rara em que o fígado contém pequenos espaços muito numerosos, repletos de sangue, algumas vezes revestidos por endotélio; pode ser encontrada incidentalmente, ou a ruptura pode causar hemorragia intraperitoneal.
plasma cell h., h. lupóide. SIN lupoid h.
serum h. (SH), h. B. SIN viral h. type B.
short incubation h., h. A. SIN viral h. type A.
subacute h., h. crônica ativa. SIN chronic active h.
suppurative h., h. supurativa; hepatite com formação de abscesso; freqüentemente de origem amebiana.
transfusion h., h. B. SIN viral h. type B.
viral h., h. viral; **(1)** hepatite causada por qualquer um de, pelo menos, 7 vírus imunologicamente não-relacionados: vírus da hepatite A, vírus da hepatite B, vírus da hepatite C, vírus da hepatite D, vírus da hepatite E, vírus da hepatite F, vírus da hepatite G; **(2)** hepatite causada por infecção viral, incluindo o vírus Epstein-Barr e citomegalovírus. SIN virus h.
viral h. type A, h. viral tipo A; doença viral com período de incubação curto (em geral, 15–50 dias), causada pelo vírus da hepatite A, um membro da família Picornaviridae, freqüentemente transmitido por via orofecal; pode ser inaparente, leve, grave ou, em certas ocasiões, fatal, ocorrendo de modo esporádico ou em epidemias, comumente em crianças em idade escolar e adultos jovens; a necrose dos hepatócitos periporta com infiltração de linfócitos e plasmócitos é característica, e a icterícia é um sintoma comum. SIN epidemic h., h. A, infectious h., MS-1 h., short incubation h., virus A h.
viral h. type B, h. viral do tipo B; doença viral com período de incubação longo (em geral, 50–160 dias), causada pelo vírus da hepatite B, um DNA vírus, membro da família Hepadnaviridae, habitualmente transmitido pela injeção de sangue ou hemoderivados infectados ou pelo uso de agulhas, lancetas ou outros instrumentos contaminados; assemelha-se, clínica e patologicamente, à hepatite viral do tipo A; todavia, não há imunidade protetora cruzada; o HB_sAg é encontrado no soro, e o vírus da hepatite delta ocorre em alguns pacientes. SIN h. B, serum h., transfusion h., virus B h.
viral h. type C, h. viral do tipo C (NANB); principal causa de h. pós-transfusional não-A, não-B; causada por um RNA vírus classificado na família Flaviviridae. O período de incubação é de 6–8 semanas, com 75% das infecções subclínicas evoluindo para a infecção persistente crônica. Uma alta percentagem desses casos desenvolve hepatopatia crônica, resultando em cirrose e possível carcinoma hepatocelular. SIN h. C, virus C h.
viral h. type D, h. viral do tipo D; hepatite aguda ou crônica causada por vírus satélite, o delta vírus da hepatite, um RNA vírus defeituoso que necessita da presença do HBV para a sua replicação, visto que ele utiliza o HB_sAg como seu próprio revestimento. O tipo agudo ocorre em duas formas: 1) coinfecção, ocorrência simultânea de infecções pelo vírus da hepatite e vírus da hepatite delta, que é habitualmente autolimitada. 2) superinfecção, o aparecimento de infecção pelo vírus da hepatite delta em portador do vírus da hepatite B, que freqüentemente resulta em h. crônica. O tipo crônico parece ser mais grave do que os outros tipos de hepatite viral. SIN delta h., h. D.
viral h. type E, h. viral do tipo E; hepatite causada por um vírus de RNA de sentido positivo, filamento simples, sem envoltório, de 27–34 nm de diâmetro, não relacionado a outros vírus da hepatite e pertencente à família Caliciviridae; constitui a principal causa de hepatite NANB epidêmica trans-

mitida por via entérica e pela água, que ocorre primariamente na Ásia, África e América do Sul. SIN h. E.
  virus h., hepatite viral. SIN viral h.
  virus A h., h. por vírus A. SIN viral h. type A.
  virus B h., h. por vírus B. SIN viral h. type B.
  virus C h., h. por vírus C. SIN viral h. type C.
hep·a·ti·za·tion (hep′ă - ti - zā - shŭn). Hepatização; conversão de um tecido frouxo numa massa firme como a substância do fígado macroscopicamente, indicando, em particular, uma alteração nos pulmões na consolidação da pneumonia.
  gray h., h. cinzenta; o segundo estágio da hepatização da pneumonia, quando o exsudato começa a degenerar antes de se decompor; a cor é cinza-amarelado ou mosqueado.
  red h., h. vermelha; o primeiro estágio da hepatização, em que o exsudato é cor de sangue.
  yellow h., h. amarela; o estágio final de hepatização, em que o exsudato está se tornando purulento.
△ **hepato-.** Hepato. VER hepat-.
he·pa·to·blas·to·ma (hep′ă - tō - blas - tō′mă). Hepatoblastoma; neoplasia maligna que ocorre em crianças pequenas, primariamente no fígado, composta de tecido semelhante ao epitélio hepático embrionário ou fetal ou de tecidos epiteliais e mesenquimatosos mistos.
he·pa·to·car·ci·no·ma (hep′ă - tō - kar - si - nō′mă). Hepatocarcinoma. SIN hepatocellular carcinoma.
he·pa·to·cele (hep′ă - tō - sēl, he - pat′ō - sēl). Hepatocele; protrusão de parte do fígado através da parede abdominal ou do diafragma. [hepato- + G. kēlē, hérnia]
he·pa·to·chol·an·gi·o·en·ter·os·to·my (hep′ă - tō - kō - lan′jē - ō - en - ter - os′tō - mē). Hepatocolangioenterostomia. SIN hepaticoenterostomy. [hepato- + G. cholē, bile + angeion, vaso + enteron, intestino + stoma, boca]
he·pa·to·chol·an·gi·o·je·ju·nos·to·my (hep′ă - tō - kō - lan′jē - ō - jē - joo - nos′tō - mē). Hepatocolangiojejunostomia; união do ducto hepático ao jejuno. [hepato- + G. cholē, bile + angeion, vaso + jejunostomia]
he·pa·to·chol·an·gi·os·to·my (hep′ă - tō - kō - lan - jē - os′tō - mē). Hepatocolangiostomia; criação de uma abertura para o colédoco para estabelecer uma drenagem.
he·pa·to·chol·an·gi·tis (hep′ă - tō - kō - lan - jī′tis). Hepatocolangite; inflamação do fígado e da árvore biliar.
he·pa·to·cu·pre·in (hep′ă - tō - koo′prē - in). Hepatocupreína. SIN cytocuprein.
he·pa·to·cys·tic (hep′ă - tō - sis′tik). Hepatocístico; relativo à vesícula biliar ou ao fígado e à vesícula biliar. [hepato- + G. kystis, bexiga]
He·pa·to·cys·tis (hep′ă - tō - sis′tis). Gênero de hemosporinas que parasitam o sangue (família Plasmodiidae), com gametócitos nos eritrócitos e esquizontes exoeritrocitários semelhantes a cistos no parênquima hepático; parasitas de primatas do Velho Mundo, morcegos e esquilos, mas não de animais domésticos ou no hemisfério ocidental. A espécie *H. kochi*, um parasita comum de babuínos africanos e outros macacos, é transmitida pelo mosquito-pólvora, *Culicoides*. [hepato- + G. kystis, bexiga]
he·pa·to·cyte (hep′ă - tō - sīt). Hepatócito; célula do parênquima hepático.
he·pa·to·du·o·de·nos·to·my (hep′ă - tō - doo - ō - de - nos′tō - mē). Hepatoduodenostomia. SIN hepaticoduodenostomy.
he·pa·to·dys·en·tery (hep′ă - tō - dis′en - ter - ē). Hepatodisenteria; disenteria associada a hepatopatia.
he·pa·to·en·ter·ic (hep′ă - tō - en - těr′ik). Hepatoentérico; relativo ao fígado e ao intestino. [hepato- + G. enteron, intestino]
hep·a·to·fu·gal (hep′ă - tō - fū′gal). Hepatófugo; que se afasta do fígado, referindo-se, em geral, ao fluxo sanguíneo porta.
he·pa·to·gas·tric (hep′ă - tō - gas′trik). Hepatogástrico; relativo ao fígado e ao estômago.
he·pa·to·gen·ic, he·pa·tog·e·nous (hep - ă - tō - jen′ik, - toj′en - ŭs). Hepatogênico; de origem hepática; formado no fígado.
he·pa·tog·raphy (hep - ă - tog′ră - fē). Hepatografia; radiografia do fígado. [hepato- + G. graphē, escrita]
he·pa·to·he·mia (hep′ă - tō - hē′mē - ă). Hepatoemia; termo raramente utilizado para referir-se à congestão do fígado. [hepato- + G. haima, sangue]
he·pa·toid (hep′ă - toyd). Hepatóide; semelhante ao fígado. [hepato- + G. eidos, semelhança]
he·pa·to·jug·u·la·rom·e·ter (hep′ă - tō - jŭg′ū - lă - rom′e - ter). Hepatojugularômetro; aparelho utilizado para o controle quantitativo e medida da pressão e força aplicadas sobre o fígado para analisar o refluxo hepatojugular. [hepato- + L. jugulum, garganta + G. metron, medida]
he·pa·to·li·en·og·ra·phy (hep′ă - tō - lī - en - og′ră - fē). Hepatolienografia. SIN hepatosplenography. [hepato- + L. lien, baço + G. graphē, escrita]
he·pa·to·li·en·o·meg·a·ly (hep′ă - tō - lī′ē - nō - meg′ă - lē). Hepatolienomegalia. SIN hepatosplenomegaly.
he·pa·to·lith (hep′ă - tō - lith). Hepatólito; concreção no fígado. [hepato- + G. lithos, pedra]

he·pa·to·li·thec·to·my (hep′ă - tō - li - thek′tō - mē). Hepatolitectomia; remoção de um cálculo do fígado. [hepato- + G. lithos, pedra + ektomē, excisão]
he·pa·to·li·thi·a·sis (hep′ă - tō - li - thī′ă - sis). Hepatolitíase; presença de cálculos no fígado. [hepato- + G. lithiasis, presença de cálculo]
he·pa·tol·o·gist (hep - ă - tol′ō - jist). Hepatologista; especialista em hepatologia.
he·pa·tol·o·gy (hep - ă - tol′ō - jē). Hepatologia; o ramo da medicina relacionado com as doenças do fígado. [hepato- + G. logos, estudo]
he·pa·tol·y·sin (hep - ă - tol′ĭ - sin). Hepatolisina; uma citolisina que destrói células parenquimatosas do fígado.
he·pa·to·ma (hep - ă - tō′mă). Hepatoma. VER malignant h. [hepato- + G. –oma, tumor]
  malignant h., h. maligno. SIN hepatocellular carcinoma.
he·pa·to·ma·la·cia (hep′ă - tō - mă - lā′shē - ă). Hepatomalacia; amolecimento do fígado. [hepato- + G. malakia, amolecimento]
he·pa·to·meg·a·ly, he·pa·to·me·ga·lia (hep′ă - tō - meg′ă - lē, - mē - gā′lē - ă). Hepatomegalia; aumento de tamanho do fígado. [hepato- + G. megas, grande]
he·pa·to·mel·a·no·sis (hep′ă - tō - mel′ă - nō′sis). Hepatomelanose; pigmentação densa do fígado. [hepato- + G. melas, negro + -osis, condição]
he·pa·tom·pha·lo·cele (hep′ă - tom - fal′ō - sēl, hep - ă - tom′fă - lō - sēl). Hepatonfalocele; hérnia umbilical com comprometimento do fígado. SIN hepatomphalos. [hepato- + onfalocele]
he·pa·tom·pha·los (hep - ă - tom′fă - lōs). Hepatônfalo. SIN hepatomphalocele.
he·pa·to·ne·cro·sis (hep′ă - tō - ne - krō - sis). Hepatonecrose; morte de células hepáticas.
he·pa·to·neph·ric (hep′ă - tō - nef′rik). Hepatonéfrico. SIN hepatorenal.
he·pa·to·neph·ro·meg·a·ly (hep′ă - tō - nef′rō - meg′ă - lē). Hepatonefromegalia; aumento de tamanho do fígado e do rim ou de ambos os rins. [hepato- + G. nephros, rim + megas, grande]
he·pa·to·path·ic (hep′ă - tō - path′ik). Hepatopático; que lesiona o fígado.
he·pa·top·a·thy (hep - ă - top′ă - thē). Hepatopatia; doença do fígado. [hepato- + G. pathos, sofrimento]
he·pa·to·per·i·to·ni·tis (hep′ă - tō - păr′i - tō - nī′tis). Hepatoperitonite. SIN perihepatitis.
hep·a·to·pet·al (hep′ă - tō - pet′al). Hepátopeto; em direção ao fígado, referindo-se, em geral, à direção normal do fluxo sanguíneo porta.
he·pa·to·pex·y (hep′ă - tō - pek - sē). Hepatopexia; ancoramento do fígado à parede abdominal. [hepato- + G. pēxis, fixação]
he·pa·to·phy·ma (hep′ă - tō - fī′mă). Hepatofima; tumor arredondado ou nodular do fígado. [hepato- + G. phyma, tumor]
he·pa·to·pneu·mon·ic (hep′ă - tō - noo - mon′ik). Hepatopneumônico; relativo ao fígado e aos pulmões. SIN hepaticopulmonary, hepatopulmonary. [hepato- + G. pneumonikos, pulmonar]
he·pa·to·por·tal (hep′ă - tō - pōr′tal). Hepatoporta; relativo ao sistema porta do fígado.
he·pa·top·to·sis (hep′ă - top - tō′sis, tō - tō′sis). Hepatoptose; deslocamento do fígado para baixo. SIN wandering liver. [hepato- + G. ptōsis, queda]
he·pa·to·pul·mo·nary (hep′ă - tō - pŭl′mō - năr′ē). Hepatopulmonar. SIN hepatopneumonic.
he·pa·to·re·nal (hep - ă - tō - rē′năl). Hepatorrenal; relativo ao fígado e ao rim. SIN hepatonephric. [hepato- + L. renalis, renal, fr. renes, rins]
he·pa·tor·rha·gia (hep′ă - tō - rā′jē - ă). Hepatorragia; sangramento para o fígado ou oriundo deste. [hepato- + G. rhēgnymi, irromper]
he·pa·tor·rha·phy (hep - ă - tōr′ă - fē). Hepatorrafia; sutura de uma ferida do fígado. [hepato- + G. rhaphē, sutura]
he·pa·tor·rhex·is (hep′ă - tō - rek′sis). Hepatorrexe; ruptura do fígado. [hepato- + G. rhēxis, ruptura]
he·pa·tos·co·py (hep - ă - tos′kō - pē). Hepatoscopia; exame do fígado. [hepato- + G. skopeō, examinar]
he·pa·to·sple·ni·tis (hep′ă - tō - splē - nī′tis). Hepatoesplenite; inflamação do fígado e do baço.
he·pa·to·sple·nog·ra·phy (hep′ă - tō - splē - nog′ră - fē). Hepatoesplenografia; uso de contraste para delinear ou desenhar o fígado e o baço radiograficamente. SIN hepatolienography.
he·pa·to·splen·o·meg·a·ly (hep′ă - tō - splē - nō - meg′ă - lē). Hepatoesplenomegalia; aumento de tamanho do fígado e do baço. SIN hepatolienomegaly. [hepato- + G. splēn, baço + megas, grande]
he·pa·to·sple·nop·a·thy (hep′ă - tō - splē - nop′ă - thē). Hepatoesplenopatia; doença do fígado e do baço.
he·pa·tos·to·my (hep - ă - tos′tō - mē). Hepatostomia; estabelecimento de uma fissura para o fígado. [hepato- + G. stoma, boca]
he·pa·to·ther·a·py (hep′ă - tō - thăr′ă - pē). Hepatoterapia; termo raramente utilizado para: **1.** Tratamento de doença do fígado. **2.** Uso terapêutico de extrato hepático ou da substância natural do fígado.
he·pa·tot·o·my (hep - ă - tot′ō - mē). Hepatotomia; incisão no fígado. [hepato- + G. tomē, incisão]

he·pa·to·tox·e·mia (hep′a-tō-tok-sē′mē-ă). Hepatoxemia; auto-intoxicação atribuída ao funcionamento inadequado do fígado. [hepato- + G. *toxikon*, veneno + *haima*, sangue]

he·pa·to·tox·ic (hep′a-tō-tok′sik). Hepatotóxico; relativo a um agente que causa lesão do fígado ou relativo a essa ação.

he·pa·to·tox·ic·i·ty. Hepatotoxicidade; a capacidade de uma droga, substância química ou outra exposição de produzir lesão do fígado. Os agentes com hepatotoxicidade reconhecida incluem: tetracloreto de carbono, álcool, dantroleno sódico, ácido valpróico, hidrazida do ácido isonicotínico (isoniazida).

he·pa·to·tox·in (hep′a-tō-tok′sin). Hepatotoxina; toxina destrutiva para as células parenquimatosas do fígado.

He·pa·to·zo·on (hep′a-tō-zō′on). Gênero de parasitas coccidianos (família Haemogregarinidae), cuja esquizogonia ocorre nas vísceras, enquanto a gametogonia ocorre nos leucócitos ou eritrócitos de animais vertebrados, e a esporogonia, em certos carrapatos e outros invertebrados hematófagos; *H. canis* ocorre em cães, gatos, chacais e hienas, porém é mais patogênico em cães, nos quais pode causar doença grave e morte; foram descritas outras espécies em ratos, camundongos, coelhos e esquilos. [hepato- + G. *zōon*, animal]

HEPES. Um composto sem efeito farmacológico, amplamente utilizado como tampão biológico em experimentos *in vitro*.

hepta-. Hepta-. Prefixo que indica sete. Cf. septi-, sept-. [G. *hepta*]

hep·ta·chlor (hep′ta-klōr). Heptoclor; inseticida hidrocarboneto clorado para controle da broca do casulo de algodão. Trata-se de um veneno que pode penetrar no corpo por contaminação da pele, inalação ou ingestão. Devido ao problema de toxicidade humana, esse composto químico possui aplicação apenas limitada.

hep·tad (hep′tad). Heptavalente; radical ou elemento químico septivalente.

hep·ta·nal (hep′tă-nal). Heptanal; obtido do ácido ricinoleico do óleo de rícino por meios químicos, utilizado na fabricação de etil enantato, um constituinte de muitas essências (aromas) artificiais. SIN enanthal, oenanthal.

hep·ta·pep·tide (hep-ta-pep′tĭd). Heptapeptídeo; peptídeo contendo sete aminoácidos.

hep·tose (hep′tōs). Heptose; açúcar com sete átomos de carbono em sua molécula; p. ex., sedoeptulose.

hep·tu·lose (hep′too-lōs). Heptulose. SIN ketoheptose.

D-*altro*-2-hep·tu·lose. D-*altro*-2-heptulose. SIN sedoheptulose.

D-*manno*-hep·tu·lose. D-*mano*-heptulose. Uma cetoeptose da configuração da manose presente na urina de indivíduos que ingeriram grandes quantidades de abacate.

***n*-hep·tyl·pen·i·cil·lin** (hep′til-pen-ĭ-sil′in). *n*-heptilpenicilina; penicilina K.

Herbert, Herbert, cirurgião oftalmologista inglês, 1865–1942.

her·biv·o·rous (her-biv′ō-rŭs). Herbívoro; que se alimenta de vegetais. [L. *herba*, herva + *voro*, devorar]

herd (hĕrd). Bando, rebanho; grupo de pessoas ou animais em determinada área. [O.E. *heord*]

he·red·i·tary (hĕ-red′i-ter-ē). Hereditário; transmissível de um genitor para seus descendentes através das informações codificadas na célula germinativa parental. [L. *hereditarius*; fr. *heres* (*hered-*), herdeiro]

he·red·i·ty (hĕ-red′i-tē). Hereditariedade. **1.** Transmissão de caracteres dos genitores para os descendentes através das informações codificadas nas células germinativas parentais. **2.** Genealogia. [L. *hereditas*, herança, fr. *heres* (*hered-*), herdeiro]

heredo-. Heredo-. Hereditariedade. [L. *heres*, herdeiro]

her·e·do·path·ia atac·ti·ca pol·y·neu·ri·ti·for·mis (her′ē-dō-path′ē-ă ă-tak′ti-kă pol′ē-noo-ri-ti-fōr′mis). Heredopatia atáxica polineuritiforme. SIN Refsum disease.

her·e·do·tax·ia. Heredotaxia. SIN Friedreich ataxia.

Herelle, Felix H. VER d'Herelle.

He·rel·lea (hĕ-rel′ē-ă). Nome genérico bacteriano que foi oficialmente rejeitado em virtude de sua espécie típica, *H. vaginicola*, ser um membro do gênero *Acinetobacter*.

Hering, Heinrich Ewald, fisiologista alemão, 1866–1948. VER sinus *nerve* of H.; H.-Breuer *reflex*; Traube-H. *curves*, em *curve*.

Hering, Karl E.K., fisiologista alemão, 1834–1918. VER H. *test*, *theory* of color vision; *canal* of H.; Traube-H. *curves*, em *curve*; *waves*, em *wave*; Semon-Hering *theory*.

her·i·ta·bil·i·ty (her′i-tă-bil′i-tē). Hereditariedade. **1.** Em psicometria, termo estatístico utilizado para referir-se ao grau de variação de um índice total ou de uma resposta do indivíduo atribuível a um suposto componente genético, em contraste com um componente adquirido. **2.** Em genética, um termo estatístico utilizado para referir-se à proporção de variação fenotípica, devido à variância nos genótipos, que é geneticamente determinada, indicada pelo símbolo tradicional h^2. [ver heredity]

h. in the broad sense, h. em sentido amplo: a proporção da variação fenotípica total que pode ser atribuída a qualquer tipo de fatores genéticos (aditivos, aqueles decorrentes de efeitos de dominância, epístase e hipóstase e interações de todos os tipos).

h. in the narrow sense, h. em sentido estrito; a proporção da variação fenotípica total que pode ser atribuída apenas à variação genética aditiva. Reflete a semelhança entre genitores e descendentes e está relacionada ao valor comercial da reprodução.

her·i·tage (her′i-tij). Herança; a totalidade dos caracteres herdados. [O. Fr.]

Herlitz, Gillis, pediatra sueco, *1902. VER H. *syndrome*.

Herman, E., histologista norte-americano do século XX. VER Padykula-Herman *stain* for myosin ATPase.

Hermann, Friedrich, anatomista alemão, 1859–1920. VER H. *fixative*.

Hermansky, Frantisek, médico tcheco do século XX. VER H.-Pudlak *syndrome*.

her·maph·ro·dism (her-maf′rō-dizm). Hermafrodismo. SIN hermaphroditism.

her·maph·ro·dite (her-maf′rō-dīt). Hermafrodita; indivíduo com hermafroditismo. [G. *Hermaphroditos*, o filho de *Hermēs*, Mercúrio + *Aphroditē*, Vênus]

her·maph·ro·dit·ism (her-maf′rō-dīt-izm). Hermafroditismo; presença em um indivíduo de tecido tanto ovariano quanto testicular, isto é, h. verdadeiro. SIN hermaphrodism.

adrenal h., h. supra-renal; aspecto alterado da genitália devido a distúrbios da função adrenocortical, mais freqüentemente virilização feminina; não é um exemplo de h. verdadeiro.

bilateral h., h. bilateral; hermafroditismo verdadeiro com ovotestículo em ambos os lados.

dimidiate h., h. lateral. SIN lateral h.

false h., pseudo-hermafroditismo. SIN pseudohermaphroditism.

female h., h. feminino; ambigüidade dos órgãos reprodutores, de modo que o sexo do indivíduo não é exclusivamente masculino nem feminino, porém h. predominantemente feminino, em que existem apenas ovários.

lateral h., h. lateral; forma em que existe um testículo em um lado e um ovário no outro. SIN dimidiate h.

male h., h. masculino; mais corretamente designado como pseudo-hermafroditismo masculino, como é comumente utilizado; entretanto, pode referir-se a um caso de h. verdadeiro em que as características corporais visíveis são de h. predominantemente masculino, existindo apenas testículos.

transverse h., h. transverso; pseudo-hermafroditismo em que os órgãos genitais externos são característicos de um sexo, enquanto as gônadas são características do outro sexo.

true h., h. verdadeiro; hermafroditismo em que ambos os tecidos, ovariano e testicular, estão presentes. Presença das características somáticas de ambos os sexos; também denominado intersexo verdadeiro.

unilateral h., h. unilateral, hermafroditismo em que a duplicação das características sexuais ocorre apenas em um lado: ovotestículo em um lado e ovário ou testículo no outro.

her·met·ic (her-met′ik). Hermético; impermeável; refere-se a um recipiente fechado ou selado, de modo que o ar não pode penetrar nem sair dele.

HERNIA

her·nia (her′nē-ă). Hérnia; protrusão de uma parte ou estrutura através do tecido que normalmente a contém. SIN rupture (1). [L. *rupture*]

abdominal h., h. abdominal; hérnia que se projeta através ou para dentro de qualquer parte da parede abdominal. SIN laparocele.

Barth h., h. de Barth; uma alça do intestino entre um ducto vitelino persistente e a parede abdominal.

Béclard h., h. de Béclard; hérnia através da abertura para a veia safena.

bilocular femoral h., h. femoral bilocular. SIN Cooper h.

h. of the broad ligament of the uterus, h. do ligamento largo do útero; alça do intestino contida numa bolsa que se projeta para dentro da substância do ligamento largo.

cecal h., h. cecal; hérnia que contém o ceco.

cerebral h., h. cerebral; protrusão da substância cerebral através de um defeito no crânio.

Cloquet h., h. de Cloquet; hérnia femoral que perfura a aponeurose do pectíneo e insinua-se entre essa aponeurose e o músculo, localizando-se, portanto, atrás dos vasos femorais.

complete h., h. completa; hérnia inguinal indireta, cujo conteúdo se estende para a túnica vaginal.

concealed h., h. oculta; hérnia não encontrada à inspeção ou palpação.

congenital diaphragmatic h., h. diafragmática congênita; **(1)** ausência da membrana pleuroperitoneal esquerda; **(2)** SIN Morgagni foramen h.

Cooper h., h. de Cooper; hérnia femoral com dois sacos, estando o primeiro no canal femoral, enquanto o segundo passa através de um defeito na fáscia superficial, aparecendo imediatamente abaixo da pele. SIN bilocular femoral h., Hey h.

crural h., h. crural. SIN femoral h.
diaphragmatic h., h. diafragmática; protrusão do conteúdo abdominal no tórax através de um enfraquecimento no diafragma respiratório; tipo comum de hérnia de hiato.
direct inguinal h., h. inguinal direta. VER inguinal h.
double loop h., h. de alça dupla. SIN "w" h.
dry h., h. seca; hérnia com saco e conteúdo aderentes.
duodenojejunal h., h. duodenojejunal; hérnia nos tecidos subperitoneais. SIN retroperitoneal h., Treitz h.
h. en bissac, h. em alforje. SIN properitoneal inguinal h.
epigastric h., h. epigástrica; hérnia através da linha alba acima do umbigo.
extrasaccular h., h. extra-sacular. SIN sliding h.
fascial h., h. fascial; protuberância do músculo através de um defeito em sua fáscia.
fat h., h. de gordura; hérnia em que o tecido que faz protrusão de sua localização normal é constituído apenas de gordura.
fatty h., h. de gordura. SIN pannicular h.
femoral h., h. femoral; hérnia através do anel femoral. SIN crural h., femorocele.
foramen of Bochdalek h., h. do forame de Bochdalek. SIN Morgagni foramen h.
gastroesophageal h., h. gastroesofágica; hérnia hiatal no tórax.
gluteal h., h. ciática. SIN sciatic h.
Hesselbach h., h. de Hesselbach; hérnia com divertículos através da fáscia cribriforme, exibindo um contorno lobular.
Hey h., h. de Hey. SIN Cooper h.
hiatal h., hiatus h., h. hiatal, h. de hiato; hérnia de uma parte do estômago através do hiato esofágico do diafragma; essas hérnias são classificadas em hérnia por deslizamento (junção esofagogástrica acima do diafragma) ou paraesofágica (junção esofagogástrica abaixo do diafragma).
Holthouse h., h. de Holthouse; hérnia inguinal com extensão da alça do intestino ao longo do ligamento de Poupart.
iliacosubfascial h., h. ilíaco-subfascial; hérnia cujo saco passa através da fáscia ilíaca e localiza-se na fossa ilíaca, em contato com o músculo ilíaco.
incarcerated h., h. encarcerada. SIN irreducible h.
incisional h., h. incisional, hérnia que ocorre através de uma incisão ou cicatriz cirúrgica.
indirect inguinal h., h. inguinal indireta. VER inguinal h.
infantile h., h. infantil; hérnia na qual uma alça intestinal desce por trás da túnica vaginal, apresentando, portanto, três camadas peritoneais na sua frente.
inguinal h., h. inguinal; hérnia na região inguinal: a hérnia inguinal direta envolve a parede abdominal entre a artéria epigástrica profunda e a borda do músculo reto; a hérnia inguinal indireta envolve o anel inguinal interno e passa para dentro do canal inguinal.
inguinocrural h., inguinofemoral h., h. inguinofemoral; hérnia bilocular ou dupla, tanto inguinal quanto femoral.
inguinolabial h., h. inguinolabial; h. inguinal que desce para o lábio.
inguinoscrotal h., h. inguinoscrotal; hérnia inguinal que desce para o escroto.
inguinosuperficial h., h. inguinossuperficial; hérnia inguinal que se virou em direção cefálica, afastando-se do escroto e assumindo uma localização subcutânea na parede abdominal.
internal h., h. interna; protrusão de uma víscera intraperitoneal num compartimento ou sob uma faixa constritora no interior da cavidade abdominal.

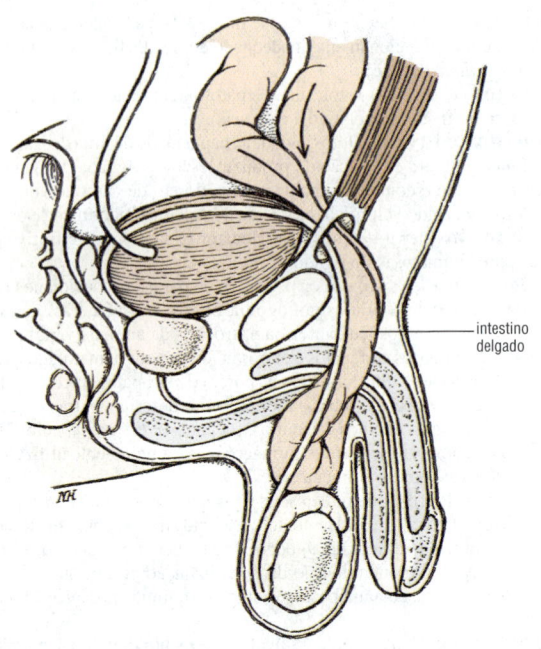

hérnia inguinal indireta

intersigmoid h., h. intersigmóide; hérnia na fossa intersigmóide na superfície inferior da raiz do mesossigmóide, próximo à borda interna do músculo grande psoas.
interstitial h., h. intersticial; hérnia cuja protrusão encontra-se entre qualquer das camadas da parede abdominal.
intraepiploic h., h. intra-epiplóica; alça intestinal encarcerada num saco omental.
intrailiac h., h. intra-ilíaca; hérnia intersticial que se projeta a partir do anel inguinal interno.
intrapelvic h., h. intrapélvica; hérnia intersticial que se projeta para dentro da pelve a partir do anel inguinal interno.
irreducible h., h. irredutível, h. encarcerada; hérnia que não pode ser reduzida sem cirurgia. SIN incarcerated h.
ischiatic h., h. isquiática; hérnia através do forame sacroisquiático.
Krönlein h., h. de Krönlein. SIN properitoneal inguinal h.
labial h., h. labial; hérnia através do canal de Nuck.
lateral ventral h., h. ventrolateral. SIN spigelian h.
Laugier h., h. de Laugier; hérnia que passa através de uma abertura no ligamento lacunar.
levator h., h. perineal. SIN perineal h.
Littré h., h. de Littré; (1) SIN parietal h; (2) hérnia do divertículo de Meckel.
lumbar h., h. lombar; hérnia entre a última costela e a crista ilíaca, onde a aponeurose do músculo transverso é coberta apenas pelo m. latíssimo do dorso.
Malgaigne h., h. de Malgaigne; hérnia inguinal infantil que ocorre antes da descida dos testículos.
meningeal h., h. meníngea; herniação das meninges através de uma espinha bífida ou craniosquise.
mesenteric h., h. mesentérica; hérnia através de uma abertura no mesentério.
Morgagni foramen h., h. do forame de Morgagni; hérnia anterior retrosternal congênita do conteúdo abdominal, mais freqüentemente apenas do omento, mas, em certas ocasiões, do estômago, geralmente através do forame de Morgagni retrosternal direito, através do qual passa a artéria mamária interna, que se transforma em artéria epigástrica superior; com freqüência, assintomática. SIN congenital diaphragmatic h. (2), foramen of Bochdalek h., parasternal h., retrosternal h.
obturator h., h. obturadora; hérnia através do forame obturado.
orbital h., h. orbital; deslocamento da gordura orbitária, através de um defeito no septo orbitário ou na cápsula de Tenon, para dentro dos tecidos subcutâneos da pálpebra, ou subconjuntivamente.
pannicular h., h. panicular; escape de gordura subcutânea através de uma lacuna em uma fáscia ou aponeurose. SIN fatty h.
pantaloon h., h. em pantalão; hérnia inguinal que envolve um componente tanto indireto quanto direto.
paraduodenal h., h. paraduodenal; tipo de hérnia interna resultante da rotação anormal ou incompleta do intestino médio, envolvendo um dos vários espaços paraduodenais.

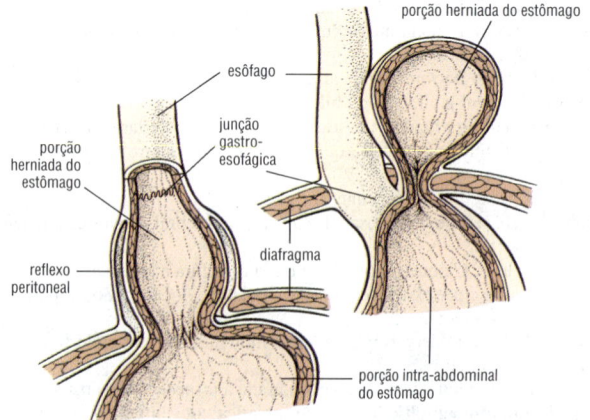

hérnias do hiato esofágico por deslizamento e paraesofágica: nas hérnias do hiato esofágico por deslizamento (à esquerda), a parte superior do estômago e a junção cardioesofágica deslizam para dentro e para fora do tórax; nas hérnias paraesofágicas (à direita), todo o estômago, ou parte dele, passa através do diafragma, próximo à junção gastroesofágica

paraesophageal h., h. paraesofágica; hérnia através do hiato esofágico do diafragma, ou adjacente a ele, em que a junção esofagogástrica permanece abaixo do diafragma, com rolamento do estômago no tórax.

parahiatal h., h. para-hiatal; hérnia através do diafragma que ocorre num ponto distinto do hiato esofágico.

paraperitoneal h., h. paraperitoneal; hérnia vesical em que apenas uma parte do órgão que faz protrusão é coberta pelo peritônio do saco.

parasaccular h., h. por deslizamento. SIN sliding h.

parasternal h., h. paraesternal. SIN Morgagni foramen h.

parietal h., h. parietal; hérnia em que apenas uma porção da parede do intestino está envolvida. SIN Littré h. (1), partial enterocele, Richter h.

perineal h., hérnia que se projeta através do diafragma pélvico. SIN levator h., pudendal h.

Petit h., h. de Petit; hérnia lombar que ocorre no triângulo de Petit.

posterior vaginal h., h. vaginal posterior; deslocamento da bolsa de Douglas para baixo.

properitoneal inguinal h., h. inguinal properitoneal; hérnia complicada que possui um saco duplo, uma parte do canal inguinal e a outra projetando-se a partir do anel inguinal interno para os tecidos subperitoneais. SIN h. em bissac, Krönlein h.

pudendal h., h. pudenda. SIN perineal h.

reducible h., h. redutível; hérnia em que o conteúdo do saco pode ser devolvido à sua localização normal.

retrograde h., h. retrógrada; hérnia de alça dupla, cuja alça central se localiza na cavidade abdominal.

retroperitoneal h., h. retroperitoneal. SIN duodenojejunal h.

retropubic h., h. retropubiana; hérnia que se projeta para baixo, nos tecidos subperitoneais, a partir do anel inguinal interno.

retrosternal h., h. retroesternal. SIN Morgagni foramen h.

Richter h., h. de Richter. SIN parietal h.

Rokitansky h., h. de Rokitansky; separação das fibras musculares do intestino, permitindo a protrusão de um saco da membrana mucosa.

sciatic h., h. isquiática; protrusão do intestino através do grande forame sacro isquiático. SIN gluteal h., ischiocele.

scrotal h., h. escrotal; hérnia inguinal completa, localizada no escroto.

sliding h., h. por deslizamento; hérnia em que uma víscera abdominal forma parte do saco. SIN extrasaccular h., parasaccular h., slipped h.

sliding esophageal hiatal h., h. do hiato esofágico por deslizamento; deslocamento da junção cardioesofágica e do estômago através do hiato esofágico no mediastino. SIN sliding hiatal h.

sliding hiatal h., h. de hiato por deslizamento. SIN sliding esophageal hiatal h.

slipped h., h. por deslizamento. SIN sliding h.

spigelian h., h. de Spigel; hérnia abdominal através da linha semilunar. SIN lateral ventral h.

strangulated h., h. estrangulada; hérnia irredutível em que a circulação está interrompida; ocorre gangrena, a não ser que o alívio seja imediato.

synovial h., h. sinovial; protrusão de uma dobra do estrato sinovial através de uma laceração no estrato fibroso de uma cápsula articular.

Treitz h., h. de Treitz. SIN duodenojejunal h.

umbilical h., h. umbilical; hérnia em que o intestino ou o omento faz protrusão através da parede abdominal sob a pele, ao nível do umbigo. VER TAMBÉM onphalocele. SIN exomphalos (2), exumbilication (2).

h. uteri inguinale, h. inguinal uterina. SIN persistent müllerian duct syndrome.

Velpeau h., h. de Velpeau; hérnia femoral em que o intestino está em frente dos vasos sanguíneos.

ventral h., h. ventral; hérnia incisional abdominal.

vesicle h., h. vesical; protrusão de um segmento da bexiga através da parede abdominal ou no interior do canal inguinal e escroto.

vitreous h., h. vítrea; prolapso do humor vítreo para dentro da câmara anterior; pode ocorrer após remoção ou deslocamento do cristalino do espaço lenticular.

"w" h., h. em "w"; presença de duas alças do intestino num saco herniário. SIN double loop h.

---

her·nial (her'nē-ăl). Herniário; relativo a uma hérnia.

her·ni·at·ed (her'nē-ā-ted). Herniado; refere-se a qualquer estrutura que faz protrusão através de uma abertura herniária.

her·ni·a·tion (her-nē-ā'shŭn). Herniação; protrusão de uma estrutura anatômica (p. ex., disco intervertebral) a partir de sua posição anatômica normal.

caudal transtentorial h., h. transtentorial caudal; deslocamento de estruturas temporais mediais através da incisura, com ou sem desvio do tronco cerebral rostrocaudal. SIN uncal h.

cingulate h., h. cingulada; deslocamento do giro cingulado sob a foice.

contained disk h., h. de disco contida; material herniado do disco que permanece recoberto por uma fina camada do anel fibroso posterior ou ligamento longitudinal posterior; a protrusão de um disco é um exemplo de h. discal contida.

disk h., h. de disco; extensão de material discal além do anel fibroso posterior e ligamento longitudinal posterior para o canal espinal.

foraminal h., h. do forame; deslocamento das amígdalas cerebelares através do forame magno.

noncontained disk h., h. de disco não-contida; material discal herniado que entra diretamente em contato com o espaço epidural anterior através de um defeito completo no anel fibroso posterior e ligamento longitudinal posterior; existem dois tipos principais: (1) extrusão do material herniado que está em continuidade com o espaço discal, mas que se estende completamente ao espaço epidural, e (2) material seqüestrado que perdeu qualquer continuidade com o espaço discal, tornando-se um fragmento livre no espaço epidural.

rostral transtentorial h., h. transtentorial rostral; deslocamento das estruturas cerebelares anteriores através da incisura, com ou sem desvio do tronco cerebral caudorrostral.

sphenoidal h., h. esfenóidea; deslocamento do tecido lobar frontal ventral sobre a crista esfenóidea.

subfalcial h., h. subfalcial; herniação abaixo da foice do cérebro; geralmente do giro cingulado.

tonsillar h., h. amigdaliana; h. das amígdalas cerebelares através do forame magno.

transtentorial h., h. transtentorial; herniação na incisura, por cima (h. transtentorial rostral) ou por baixo (h. transtentorial caudal).

uncal h., h. uncal. SIN caudal transtentorial h.

hernio-. Hernio. Uma hérnia. [L. hernia, ruptura]

her·ni·o·en·ter·ot·o·my (her'nē-ō-en-ter-ot'ō-mē). Hernioenterotomia; incisão do intestino após redução de uma hérnia.

her·ni·og·ra·phy (her-nē-og'ră-fē). Herniografia; exame radiográfico de uma hérnia após injeção de contraste no saco herniário. [hernia + G. graphō, escrever]

her·ni·oid (her'nē-oyd). Hernióide; semelhante a uma hérnia. [hernio- + G. eidos, semelhança]

her·ni·o·lap·a·rot·o·my (her'nē-ō-lap-ă-rot'ō-mē). Herniolaparotomia; laparotomia para correção de hérnia.

her·ni·o·punc·ture (her'nē-ō-pŭnk'choor). Herniopunção; inserção de uma agulha oca numa hérnia para reduzir o tamanho do tumor através da retirada de gás ou de líquido.

her·ni·or·rha·phy (her'nē-ōr'ă-fē). Herniorrafia; reparo cirúrgico de uma hérnia. [hernio- + G. rhaphē, sutura]

Bassini h., h. de Bassini; herniorrafia para reparo de hérnia inguinal indireta; após a redução da hérnia, o saco é torcido, ligado e seccionado; a seguir, efetua-se um novo assoalho inguinal através da união da borda do músculo oblíquo interno ao ligamento inguinal, colocando-se o cordão sobre este e cobrindo o último com o músculo oblíquo externo. SIN Bassini operation.

her·ni·o·tome (her'nē-ō-tōm). Herniótomo. SIN hernia knife.

Cooper h., h. de Cooper; bisturi fino, com borda cortante curta para dividir os tecidos constritores no colo de um saco herniário.

her·ni·ot·o·my (her-nē-ot'ō-mē). Herniotomia; divisão cirúrgica da constrição ou do estrangulamento de uma hérnia, freqüentemente seguida de herniorrafia. [hernio- + G. tomē, corte]

Petit h., h. de Petit; herniotomia sem incisão no saco.

he·ro·ic (hē-rō'ik). Heróico; indica um procedimento agressivo e ousado, em um paciente em estado grave, e que, por si só, pode ser perigoso para o paciente, mas que também tem a possibilidade de ser bem-sucedido, enquanto uma ação menos agressiva resultaria em fracasso. [G. hērōikos, próprio de um herói]

her·o·in (H) (her'ō-in). Heroína; alcalóide, $C_{17}H_{17}(OC_2H_3O)_2ON$, preparado a partir da morfina por acetilação; rapidamente metabolizada a morfina no corpo; antigamente utilizada para alívio da tosse. Exceto para pesquisa, seu uso nos Estados Unidos é proibido por lei federal, devido a seu potencial de causar dependência. SIN diacetylmorphine. [nome comercial (foi comercializada como "heroína" de agentes analgésicos)]

He·roph·i·lus. Médico e anatomista grego da Escola de Alexandria, cerca de 300 a.C. VER torcular herophili.

her·pan·gi·na (her-pan'ji-nă, herp-an-jī'nă). Herpangina; doença causada por tipos de vírus Coxsackie e caracterizada por lesões vesiculopapulares com cerca de 1–2 mm de diâmetro, encontradas ao redor das fauces, sofrendo rápida decomposição para formar úlceras amarelo-acinzentadas; acompanhada de febre de início súbito, perda do apetite, disfagia, faringite e, algumas vezes, dor abdominal, náuseas e vômitos. [G. herpēs, erupção vesicular + L. angina, quinsy, fr. ango, estrangular]

her·pes (her'pēz). Herpes; doença cutânea inflamatória causada pelo vírus herpes simples (herpes simplex virus) ou vírus varicela-zoster (varicella-zoster virus); erupção de grupos de vesículas de localização profunda sobre bases eritematosas. SIN serpigo (2). [G. herpēs, erupção cutânea disseminada, cobreiro, fr. herpō, serpentear]

h. catarrh'alis, h. simples. SIN h. simplex.

h. cor'neae, ceratite herpética. SIN herpetic keratitis.

h. digita'lis, h. digital; infecção do dedo pelo vírus herpes simples.

h. facia'lis, h. simples. SIN h. simplex.
h. febri'lis, h. simples. SIN h. simplex.
h. generalisa'tus, h. generalizado; infecção generalizada pelo vírus herpes simples.
h. genita'lis, genital h., h. genital; infecção dos órgãos genitais pelo vírus herpes simples, mais comumente pelo vírus herpes simples tipo 2.
h. gestatio'nis, h. gestacional; erupção polimorfa e bolhosa, mais comum nos membros e no abdome do que na parte superior do tronco, com aspecto de penfigóide ou dermatite herpetiforme; começa no segundo ou terceiro trimestre, com exacerbação próxima à época do parto e regressão subseqüente; geralmente recidivante durante a gravidez seguinte. Demonstração de C3 linear na membrana basal epidérmica por imunofluorescência direta. Não é causado por infecção viral.
h. gladiato'rum, h. do gladiador; infecção pelo vírus herpes simples associada a traumatismo do tecido cutâneo.
h. labia'lis, h. simples. SIN h. simplex.
neonatal h., h. neonatal; infecção pelo vírus herpes simples tipo 1 ou 2, transmitida pela mãe ao recém-nascido, freqüentemente durante a passagem através do canal de parto infectado; a gravidade varia desde leve até uma infecção generalizada fatal; esta última é observada particularmente no herpes genital materno primário.
h. progenita'lis, h. progenital; infecção herpética genital causada pelo vírus herpes simples.
h. sim'plex, h. simples; várias infecções causadas por herpesvírus dos tipos 1 e 2; as infecções pelo vírus tipo 1 caracterizam-se mais comumente pela erupção de um ou mais grupos de vesículas na borda dos lábios ou na porção externa das narinas, enquanto a infecção pelo vírus tipo 2 caracteriza-se por essas lesões na genitália; os dois tipos são freqüentemente recrudescentes e reaparecem durante outras doenças febris ou, até mesmo, em estados fisiológicos, como a menstruação. Com freqüência, os vírus tornam-se latentes e podem não se manifestar durante anos. SIN h. catarrhalis, h. facialis, h. febrilis, h. labialis, Simplexvirus.
traumatic h., h. traumático; infecção pelo vírus herpes simples no local de traumatismo ou de queimadura, algumas vezes acompanhada de elevação da temperatura e mal-estar.
h. whitlow, inflamação da base das unhas das mãos pelo vírus herpes simples.
h. zos'ter, h. zoster; infecção causada por herpesvírus (vírus varicela-zoster), caracterizada por erupção de grupos de vesículas no lado do corpo seguindo o trajeto de um nervo, devido à inflamação de gânglios e raízes nervosas dorsais em decorrência da ativação do vírus que, em muitos casos, permaneceu latente durante anos após varicela primária; a condição é autolimitada, mas pode ser acompanhada ou seguida de intensa dor pós-herpética. VER TAMBÉM varicela. SIN zona (2) [TA], shingles, zoster.
h. zos'ter ophthal'micus, h. zoster oftálmico; comprometimento herpético do ramo oftálmico do nervo trigêmeo, que pode resultar em ulceração da córnea.
h. zos'ter o'ticus, h. zoster ótico; infecção dolorosa pelo vírus da varicela, que se manifesta na forma de erupção vesicular da aurícula, com ou sem paralisia do nervo facial. SIN geniculate zoster, Ramsay Hunt syndrome (2).
h. zos'ter varicello'sus, h. zoster variceloso; herpes zoster associado a lesões variceliformes disseminadas.
Her·pes·vir·i·dae (her'pēs-vir'i-dē). Família heterogênea de vírus morfologicamente semelhantes, contendo todos eles DNA de filamento duplo; infectam o homem e uma ampla variedade de outros vertebrados. As infecções produzem corpúsculos de inclusão do tipo A; em muitos casos, a infecção pode permanecer latente durante muitos anos, mesmo na presença de anticorpos circulantes específicos. Os vírions possuem envoltório, são sensíveis ao éter e seu diâmetro varia até 200 nm; os nucleocapsídeos têm 100 nm de diâmetro e simetria icosaédrica, com 162 capsômeros. A família é subdividida em três subfamílias: Alphaherpesvirinae, Betaherpesvirinae e Gammaherpesvirinae, incluindo o vírus herpes simples, o vírus varicela-zoster, o citomegalovírus e o vírus EB (todos os quais infectam o homem), o vírus da pseudo-raiva de suínos, o vírus da rinopneumonia eqüina, o vírus da rinotraqueíte bovina infecciosa, o herpes vírus canino, o vírus B de macacos do Velho Mundo, diversos vírus de macacos do Novo Mundo, o vírus III de coelhos, o vírus da laringotraqueíte infecciosa de aves domésticas, o vírus da doença de Marek de galinhas, o vírus do tumor de Lucké de rãs e muitos outros.

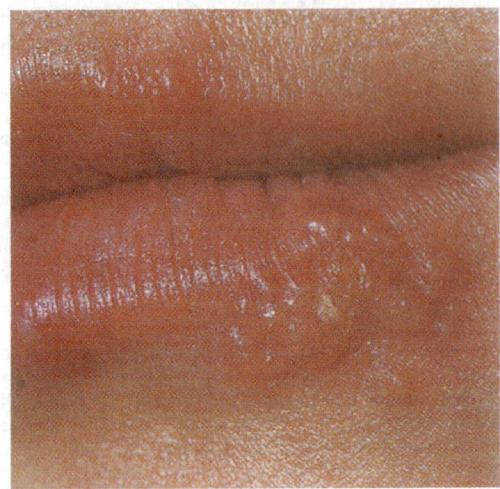

herpes simples: do lábio

her·pes·vi·rus (her'pēz-vī'rŭs). Herpesvírus; qualquer vírus pertencente à família Herpesviridae.
cercopithecrine h., h. cercopitecrino; herpesvírus da família Herpesviridae que afeta macacos do Velho Mundo, muito semelhante morfologicamente ao vírus herpes simples; pode ocorrer infecção fatal em seres humanos após a mordida de um macaco infectado, embora também tenham sido documentados outros modos de transmissão. SIN B virus.
human h. 1, h. humano 1; vírus herpes simples tipo 1. VER *herpes* simplex.
human h. 2, h. humano 2; vírus herpes simples tipo 2. VER *herpes* simplex.
human h. 3, h. humano 3. SIN varicella-zoster *virus.*
human h. 4, h. humano 4. SIN Epstein-Barr *virus.*
human h. 5, h. humano 5; um herpesvírus extremamente espécie-específico (citomegalovírus), com afinidade particular pelo tecido glandular salivar. SIN salivary gland virus, salivary virus.
human h. 6, h. humano 6; herpesvírus humano encontrado em certos distúrbios linfoproliferativos; replica-se em vários tipos diferentes de leucócitos e está associado à doença infantil roséola (exantema súbito).

classificação dos herpesvírus humanos

subfamília	gênero	exemplos		propriedades biológicas	
		nome oficial	nome comum	citopatologia	infecções latentes
Alfaherpesvirinae	*Simplexvirus*	herpesvírus humano 1 herpesvírus humano 2	vírus herpes simples tipo 1 vírus herpes simples tipo 2	citolítico	neurônios
	Varicellovirus	herpesvírus humano 3	vírus varicela-zoster		
Betaherpesvirinae	*Cytomegalovirus*	herpesvírus humano 5	citomegalovírus	citomegálico	glândulas, rins
	Roseolovirus	herpesvírus humano 6 herpesvírus humano 7	herpesvírus humano 6 herpesvírus humano 7	linfoproliferativo	tecido linfóide
Gamaherpesvirinae	*Lymphocryptovirus*	herpesvírus humano 4	vírus de Epstein-Barr	linfoproliferativo	tecido linfóide
	Rhadinovirus	herpesvírus humano 8	herpesvírus associado ao sarcoma de Kaposi		

human h. 7, h. humano 7; vírus encontrado em associação a linfócitos T de seres humanos, liberado na saliva da maioria dos adultos; todavia, não foi estabelecida nenhuma relação causal com qualquer doença conhecida.

human h. 8, h. humano 8; vírus de DNA de filamento duplo linear, que induz o sarcoma de Kaposi (SK) em indivíduos imunodeficientes. Seqüências de DNA exclusivas desse vírus são encontradas regularmente em amostras de SK de indivíduos HIV-negativos. O vírus também está associado a várias síndromes linfoproliferativas raras em pacientes com AIDS/SIDA, incluindo doença de Castleman multicêntrica e linfoma de derrame primário (linfoma em cavidades corporais).

Entre os indivíduos com AIDS/SIDA, o sarcoma de Kaposi é observado em 15–25% dos homens homossexuais, porém apenas em 1–3% dos indivíduos que contraíram AIDS/SIDA por vias não-sexuais (p. ex., hemofílicos e outros receptores de transfusões). Esses achados apóiam a hipótese de que o vírus é sexualmente transmitido. O SK caracteriza-se, histologicamente, por vascularização anormal e presença de células endoteliais proliferativas, fibroblastos, leucócitos infiltrantes e células tumorais fusiformes. Ocorre replicação do HHV8 apenas num pequeno subgrupo de células fusiformes, porém a maioria dessas células apresenta infecção latente. A proliferação de células fusiformes é aparentemente desencadeada por fatores de crescimento liberados pelas células infectadas pelo HIV. Por sua vez, as células fusiformes produzem fatores que promovem a angiogênese. O DNA do HHV8 também pode ser encontrado nos linfócitos B CD19 circulantes de 40–50% dos pacientes aidéticos com SK. Existem provas sorológicas para anticorpos anti-HHV8, cuja maioria utiliza antígeno viral de linhagens celulares derivadas de linfomas em cavidades corporais. A replicação viral é insensível ao aciclovir, porém é inibida por ganciclovir, foscarnet, cidofovir e interferon alfa.

h. saimiri, h. saimiri; infecção ubíqua de saguis, que é extremamente oncogênica quando injetada em outras espécies de macacos.
suid h., h. de suínos; agente causador da pseudo-raiva.
her·pet·ic (her-pet′ik). Herpético. **1.** Relativo a, ou caracterizado por, herpes. **2.** Relativo a, ou causado por, herpesvírus.
her·pet·i·form (her-pet′i-form). Herpetiforme; semelhante ao herpes.
her·pe·tol·o·gist (her-pet-ol′ō-jist). Herpetologista; especializado em herpetologia.
her·pe·tol·o·gy (her-pet-ol′ō-jē). Herpetologia; o ramo da zoologia relacionado ao estudo dos répteis e anfíbios.
Her·pe·to·mo·nas (her-pē-tom′ō-nas). Gênero de flagelados monogenéticos assexuados (família Trypanosomatidae) que são estritamente parasitas de insetos, com várias formas corporais, incluindo promastigotas (leptomonas), epimastigotas (critídeos), amastigotas (leishmânias) e tripomastigotas (semelhantes a tripanossomas); as formas infecciosas são eliminadas nas fezes do hospedeiro. *H. muscae domesticae,* a espécie típica, é encontrada na mosca-doméstica comum. [G. *herpeton,* réptil (fr. *herpō,* rastejar) + *monas,* unidade (uma das *Monodidae*)]
Her·pet·o·vir·i·dae. Termo obsoleto para referir-se a Herpesviridae.
her·pe·to·vi·rus (her′pē-tō-vī′rus). Herpetovírus; termo obsoleto para referir-se a um vírus pertencente à família Herpesviridae. VER TAMBÉM herpesvírus.
Herring, Percy T., fisiologista inglês, 1872–1967. VER H. *bodies,* em *body.*
Herrmann, C., Jr., século XX. VER H. *syndrome.*
Hers, G., bioquímico francês. VER H. *disease.*
her·sage (ār-sahzh′). Separação, divisor; que separa as fibras individuais de um tronco nervoso. [Fr. (de L. *hirpex,* um grande ancinho), uma grade]
Hertwig, Richard, zoologista alemão, 1850–1937. VER Magendie-H. *sign, syndrome.*
Hertwig, Wilhelm A.O., embriologista alemão, 1849–1922. VER H. *sheath.*
Hertz, Heinrich R., físico alemão, 1857–1894. VER hertz; hertzian *experiments,* em *experiment.*
hertz (Hz) (herts). Hertz; unidade de freqüência equivalente a 1 ciclo/s; esse termo não deve ser utilizado para a freqüência radial (circular) ou velocidade angular, casos em que se deve utilizar o termo s^{-1}. [H.R. *Hertz*]
hertz·i·an (hert′zē-an). Hertziano; atribuído a, ou descrito por, Heinrich R. Hertz.
Herxheimer, Karl, dermatologista alemão, 1861–1944. VER H. *reaction;* Jarisch-H. *reaction.*
herz·stoss (hārz′stos). Sístole cardíaca que produz um esforço pré-cordial difuso, com ou sem qualquer ponto definindo o impulso máximo. [Ger. *heart thrust*]
Heschl, Richard L., patologista austríaco, 1824–1881. VER H. *gyri,* em *gyrus.*
hes·i·tan·cy (hez′i-tan-sē). Hesitação; atraso involuntário ou incapacidade de iniciar o jato urinário.

hes·i·tant (hez′i-tant). Hesitante; termo utilizado para descrever o estado da RNA polimerase quando suscetível a sinais de pausa, interrupção ou terminação. VER TAMBÉM overdrive, antitermination.
hes·per·i·din (hes-per′i-din). Hesperidina; diglicosídeo de flavona obtido de fruta cítrica verde, ao qual se atribui uma atividade de vitamina P. SIN cirantin.
Hess, Carl von, oftalmologista alemão, 1860–1923. VER H. *screen.*
Hess, Walter R., fisiologista suíço e ganhador do Prêmio Nobel, 1881–1973. VER trophotropic *zone* of H.
Hesselbach, Franz K., anatomista e cirurgião alemão, 1759–1816. VER H. *fascia, hernia, ligament, triangle.*
het·a·starch (het′ā-starch). Hetamido; derivado do amido utilizado como agente crioprotetor para os eritrócitos. Também utilizado como expansor do volume plasmático sanguíneo.
△ **heter-.** Heter-. VER hetero-.
het·er·a·del·phus (het-er-ā-del′fŭs). Heteradelfo; gêmeos conjugados desiguais em que o parasita incompleto menor está ligado ao autósito maior, de tamanho quase normal. VER conjoined *twins,* em *twin.* [heter- + G. *adelphos,* irmão]
het·er·a·li·us (het-er-ā′lē-ŭs). Heterálio; gêmeos conjugados desiguais em que o parasita parece ser pouco mais do que uma excrescência ao autósito. VER conjoined *twins,* em *twin.* [heter- + G. *halios,* sem uso]
het·er·ax·i·al (het-er-ak′sē-ăl). Heteraxial; que possui eixos mutuamente perpendiculares de comprimento desigual.
het·er·e·cious (het-er-ē′shŭs). Heterécio; que possui mais de um hospedeiro; diz-se de um parasita que passa diferentes estágios de seu ciclo de vida em diferentes animais. SIN metoxenous. [heter- + G. *oikion,* lar]
het·er·e·cism (het-er-ē-sizm). Heterecismo; a ocorrência, num parasita, de dois ciclos de desenvolvimento que se passam em dois hospedeiros diferentes. SIN metoxeny (1). [heter- + G. *oikion,* lar]
het·er·es·the·sia (het-er-es-thē′zē-ă). Heterestesia; mudança que ocorre no grau (seja para mais ou para menos) da resposta sensorial a um estímulo cutâneo quando este cruza certa linha na superfície. [heter- + G. *aisthēsis,* sensação]
△ **hetero-, heter-.** Hetero-, heter-. O outro, diferente; oposto de homo-. [G. *heteros,* outro]
het·er·o·ag·glu·ti·nin (het′er-ō-ă-gloo′ti-nin). Heteroaglutinina; uma forma de hemaglutinina que aglutina os eritrócitos de espécies diferentes daquela em que ocorre. VER TAMBÉM hemagglutinin.
het·er·o·al·leles (het′er-ō-ă-lēlz′). Heteroalelos; genes que sofreram mutação em diferentes posições do nucleotídeo, resultando, portanto, de eventos mutacionais diferentes. Cf. eualleles.
het·er·o·an·ti·body (het′er-ō-an′ti-bod-ē). Heteroanticorpo; anticorpo que é heterólogo em relação ao antígeno, em contraposição ao isoanticorpo.
het·er·o·an·ti·se·rum (het′er-ō-an′ti-sē-rŭm). Heteroanti-soro; anti-soro desenvolvido numa espécie animal contra antígenos ou células de outra espécie.
het·er·o·at·om (het′er-ō-at′om). Heteroátomo; um átomo diferente do carbono, localizado na estrutura em anel de um composto orgânico, como o N nas piridinas ou pirimidinas (compostos heterocíclicos).
het·er·o·blas·tic (het-er-ō-blas′tik). Heteroblástico; que se desenvolve a partir de mais de um único tipo de tecido. [hetero- + G. *blastos,* germe]
het·er·o·cel·lu·lar (het′er-ō-sel′ū-lăr). Heterocelular; formado de células de diferentes tipos.
het·er·o·cen·tric (het′er-ō-sen′trik). Heterocêntrico. **1.** Que possui centros diferentes; diz-se de raios que não se encontram num foco comum. Cf. homocentric. **2.** SIN allocentric. [hetero- + G. *kentron,* centro]
het·er·o·ceph·a·lus (het′er-ō-sef′ă-lŭs). Heterocéfalo; gêmeos conjugados com cabeças de tamanho desigual. VER conjoined *twins,* em *twin.* [hetero- + G. *kephalē,* cabeça]
het·er·o·chei·ral, het·er·o·chi·ral (het-er-ō-kī′răl). Heteroquiro; relativo ou referente à outra mão. [hetero- + G. *cheir,* mão]
het·er·o·chro·mat·ic (het′er-ō-krō-mat′ik). Heterocromático; característico de heterocromatina.
het·er·o·chro·ma·tin (het′er-ō-krō′mă-tin). Heterocromatina; parte do cromonema que permanece bem espiralada e condensada durante a interfase e, assim, cora-se prontamente. SIN heterophyknotic chromatin.
constitutive h., h. constitutiva; h. repetitiva localizada em constrições secundárias nos organizadores nucleares.
facultative h., h. facultativa; h. não-repetitiva que compreende seqüências de DNA passíveis de tradução.
satellite-rich h., h. rica em satélites; heterocromatina que codifica os componentes 18 S e 28 S do RNA ribossomal e está localizada próximo aos centrômeros de certos cromossomas.
het·er·o·chro·mia (het′er-ō-krō′mē-ă). Heterocromia; diferença na coloração de duas estruturas que, normalmente, têm a mesma cor. [hetero- + G. *chrōma,* cor]
atrophic h., h. atrófica; h. da íris após traumatismo ou inflamação ou na velhice.
binocular h., h. binocular; aumento ou diminuição na pigmentação de um olho, com ou sem defeitos pigmentares extra-oculares.

h. i'ridis, h. of iris, h. da íris; diferença na coloração das íris. VER binocular h. **monocular h.,** h. monocular. SIN *iris* bicolor.
simple h., h. simples; h. da íris que aparece como defeito de desenvolvimento, sem qualquer defeito de inervação.
sympathetic h., h. simpática; h. da íris que ocorre após lesões dos nervos simpáticos cervicais.

het·er·o·chro·mous (het′er-ō-krō′mŭs). Heterocrômico; que possui uma diferença anormal na coloração.

het·er·o·chron (het′er-ō-kron). Heterócrono; que tem ritmos variáveis. [hetero- + G. *chronos*, tempo]

het·er·o·chro·nia (het-er-ō-krō′nē-ă). Heterocronia; origem ou desenvolvimento de tecidos ou órgãos em tempo incomum ou fora da seqüência regular. Cf. synchronia. [hetero- + G. *chronos*, tempo]

het·er·o·chron·ic (het-er-ō-kron′ik). Heterocrônico. SIN heterochronous.

het·er·och·ro·nous (het-er-ok′rō-nŭs). Heterocrônico; relativo à heterocronia. SIN heterochronic.

het·er·o·clad·ic (het′er-ō-klad′ik). Heteroclárico; refere-se a uma anastomose entre ramos de diferentes troncos arteriais, distinguindo-se do homoclárico. [hetero- + G. *klados*, ramo]

het·er·o·crine (het′er-ō-krin). Heterócrino; refere-se à secreção de dois ou mais tipos de materiais. [hetero- + G. *krinō*, separar]

het·er·o·cri·sis (het′er-ō-krī′sis). Heterocrise; termo raramente utilizado para referir-se a uma crise irregular, que ocorre num tempo anormal ou com sintomas incomuns.

het·er·o·cy·to·tro·pic (het′er-ō-sī′tō-trop′ik). Heterocitotrópico; que possui afinidade por células de uma espécie diferente. [hetero- + G. *kytos*, célula + *tropē*, uma volta]

het·er·o·dis·perse (het′er-ō-dis-pers′). Heterodisperso; de tamanho variável; descreve aerossóis cujas partículas não são de tamanho uniforme.

het·er·o·dont (het′er-ō-dont). Heterodonte; que possui dentes de formas variáveis, como os dos seres humanos e da maioria dos mamíferos, em contraste com os homodontes. [hetero- + G. *odous*, dente]

Het·er·o·dox·us spi·ni·ger (het-er-ō-dok′sŭs spī′ni-ger). Piolho do cão, algumas vezes denominado piolho canguru.

het·er·od·ro·mous (het-er-od′rō-mŭs). Heterodrômico; que se move em direção oposta. [hetero- + G. *dromos*, corrida]

het·er·o·du·plex (het′er-ō-doo′pleks). Heteroduplex. **1.** Uma molécula de DNA cujos dois filamentos constitutivos derivam de fontes distintas e, portanto, tendem a ser um tanto incompatíveis. **2.** Híbrido de DNA-RNA. [hetero- + L. *duplex*, duas vezes]

het·er·od·y·mus (het-er-od′i-mŭs). Heteródimo; gêmeos conjugados desiguais em que o parasita incompleto, consistindo em cabeça e pescoço e, até certo grau, tórax, está fixado à superfície anterior do autósito. VER conjoined *twins*, em *twin*. [hetero- + G. *didymos*, gêmeo]

het·er·o·e·rot·i·cism (het′er-ō-ē-rot′i-sism). Heteroerotismo; condição de excitação sexual produzida por contato com uma pessoa do sexo oposto.

het·er·o·ga·met·ic (het′er-ō-gă-met′ik). Heterogamético; que possui gametas sexuais de tipos contrastantes; o sexo masculino humano é heterogamético. SIN digametic. [hetero- + G. *gametikos*, conubial]

het·er·og·a·mous (het-er-og′ă-mŭs). Heterogâmico; relativo à heterogamia.

het·er·og·a·my (het-er-og′ă-mē). Heterogamia. **1.** Conjugação de gametas diferentes. **2.** Que possui diferentes tipos de flores. **3.** Reprodução por métodos indiretos de polinização. [hetero- + G. *gamos*, casamento]

het·er·o·ge·ne·i·ty (het′er-ō-jē-nē′i-tē). Heterogeneidade; estado ou qualidade heterogênica.

genetic h., h. genética; o caráter de um fenótipo produzido por mutação de mais de um gene ou por mais de um mecanismo genético. VER genocopy.

het·er·o·ge·neous (het′er-ō-jē′nē-ŭs). Heterogêneo; constituído por elementos com propriedades diversas e diferentes.

het·er·o·gen·e·sis (het′er-ō-jen′e-sis). Heterogênese. **1.** Alternação de gerações. **2.** Geração assexuada. SIN asexual *generation*. **3.** Geração espontânea. SIN spontaneous *generation*. [hetero- + G. *genesis*, produção]

het·er·o·ge·net·ic (het′er-ō-jē-net′ik). Heterogenético; relativo à heterogênese.

het·er·o·gen·ic, het·er·o·ge·ne·ic (het′er-ō-jen′ik, -jĕ-nē′ik). Heterogênico; que possui diferentes constituições gênicas, sobretudo em espécies diversas.

het·er·o·ge·note (het′er-ō-jē′nōt). Heterogenota; em genética microbiana, um microrganismo que contém material genético exógeno que difere um pouco da região correspondente de seu próprio genoma original, mas, de um modo muito limitado, assemelha-se a um heterozigoto.

het·er·og·e·nous (het-er-oj′e-nŭs). Heterogêneo; de origem estranha.

het·er·o·gly·can (het′er-ō-glī′kan). Heteroglicana. SIN heteropolysaccharide.

het·er·o·graft (het′er-ō-graft). Heteroenxerto. SIN xenograft.

het·er·o·kar·y·on (het′er-ō-kar′ē-on). Heterocárion; célula contendo diversos núcleos no interior de um citoplasma comum, geralmente resultante da fusão artificial de duas células de espécies diferentes. [hetero- + G. *karyon*, grão, noz]

het·er·o·kar·y·ot·ic (het′er-ō-kar-ē-ot′ik). Heterocariótico; que tem as propriedades de um heterocárion.

het·er·o·ker·a·to·plas·ty (het′er-ō-ker′ă-tō-plas-tē). Heteroceratoplastia; ceratoplastia em que a córnea de uma espécie de animal é enxertada no olho de um animal de outra espécie.

het·er·o·ki·ne·sia (het′er-ō-ki-nē′zē-ă). Heterocinesia; que executa movimentos inversos aos que se pede que faça. SIN heterokinesis (2). [hetero- + G. *kinēsis*, movimento]

het·er·o·ki·ne·sis (het′er-ō-ki-nē′sis). Heterocinese. **1.** Distribuição diferencial dos cromossomas X e Y durante a divisão meiótica da célula. **2.** SIN heterokinesia.

het·er·o·lat·er·al (het′er-ō-lat′er-ăl). Heterolateral. SIN contralateral. [hetero- + L. *latus*, lado]

het·er·o·lip·ids (het′er-ō-lip′idz). Heterolipídios. **1.** Lipídios contendo átomos N e P além dos átomos habituais C, H e O. **2.** Qualquer lipídio complexo. Cf. homolipids.

het·er·o·lit·er·al (het′er-ō-lit′er-ăl). Heteroliteral; substituição de uma letra por outra na pronúncia de certas palavras. [hetero- + L. *littera*, letra]

het·er·ol·o·gous (het-er-ol′ō-gŭs). Heterólogo. **1.** Relativo a elementos citológicos ou histológicos que ocorrem onde normalmente não são encontrados. VER TAMBÉM xenogeneic. **2.** Derivado de um animal de espécie diferente, como o soro de um cavalo, que é heterólogo para um coelho. [hetero- + G. *logos*, proporção, relação]

het·er·ol·o·gy (het-er-ol′ō-jē). Heterologia; afastamento do normal quanto à estrutura, arranjo ou modo ou tempo de desenvolvimento.

het·er·o·ly·sin (het-er-ol′i-sin). Heterolisina; lisina formada numa espécie animal que manifesta atividade lítica nas células de uma espécie diferente.

het·er·ol·y·sis (het-er-ol′i-sis). Heterólise; dissolução ou digestão de células ou componentes proteicos de uma espécie por um agente lítico de uma espécie diferente. [hetero- + G. *lysis*, afrouxamento]

het·er·o·lyt·ic (het′er-ō-lit′ik). Heterolítico; relativo à heterólise ou ao efeito de uma heterolisina.

het·er·o·mas·ti·gote (het-er-ō-mas′ti-gōt). Heteromastigota; flagelado que possui dois flagelos, um anterior e outro posterior. [hetero- + G. *mastix*, chicote]

het·er·om·er·al (het′er-om′er-ăl). Heteromérico. SIN heteromeric (2).

het·er·o·mer·ic (het′er-ō-mār′ik). Heteromérico. **1.** Que possui composição química diferente. **2.** Refere-se a neurônios espinais que possuem prolongamentos que passam para o lado oposto da medula. SIN heteromeral, heteromerous. [hetero- + G. *meros*, parte]

het·er·om·er·ous (het′er-om′er-ŭs). Heteromérico. SIN heteromeric (2).

het·er·o·me·tab·o·lous (het′er-ō-me-tab′ō-lŭs). Heterometábolo; relativo a um membro da Heterometabola, uma superordem algumas vezes utilizada para referir-se a uma série de ordens de insetos nos quais ocorre metamorfose incompleta. [hetero- + G. *metabolē*, mudança]

het·er·o·met·a·pla·sia (het′er-ō-met-ă-plā′zē-ă). Heterometaplasia; transformação tecidual que resulta na produção de um tecido estranho à área onde é produzido.

het·er·o·met·ric (het′er-ō-met′rik). Heterométrico; que envolve ou depende de uma mudança no tamanho. [hetero- + G. *metron*, medida]

het·er·o·me·tro·pia (het′er-ō-me-trō′pē-ă). Heterometropia; condição em que a refração é diferente nos dois olhos. [hetero- + G. *metron*, medida + *ōps*, olho]

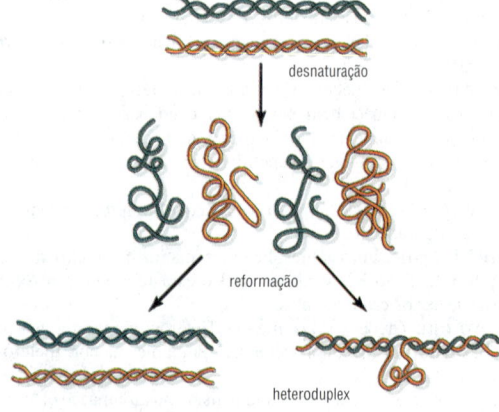

formação de heteroduplex: esquemático

het·er·o·mor·phism (het′er-ō-mōrf′izm). Heteromorfismo; em citogenética, uma diferença na forma ou no tamanho na metáfase entre os dois cromossomas homólogos. [hetero- + G. *morphē*, forma]

het·er·o·mor·pho·sis (het′er-ō-mor-fō′sis). Heteromorfose. **1.** Desenvolvimento de um tecido a partir de outro tipo de tecido. **2.** Desenvolvimento embrionário de tecido ou de um órgão inapropriado para seu local. [hetero- + G. *morphōsis*, moldagem]

het·er·o·mor·phous (het′er-ō-mōr′fŭs). Heteromorfo; que difere da forma normal.

het·er·on·o·mous (het-er-on′ō-mŭs). Heterônomo. **1.** Diferente do tipo; anormal. **2.** Sujeito à direção ou ao controle de outro, que não se autogoverna. Cf. autonomous. [hetero- + G. *nomos*, lei]

het·er·on·o·my (het-er-on′ō-mē). Heteronomia; a condição ou estado de ser heterônomo. [hetero- + G. *nomos*, lei]

het·er·o·nu·cle·ar (het′er-ō-noo′klē-er). Heteronuclear; indica um heterocárion que perdeu parte do material nuclear do qual a linhagem celular era originalmente constituída.

het·er·on·y·mous (het-er-on′i-mŭs). Heterônimo; que possui nomes diferentes ou expresso em termos diferentes. [G. *heterōnymos*, que tem um nome diferente, *onyma* ou *onoma*, nome]

het·er·op·a·gus (het-er-op′a-gŭs). Heterópago; gêmeos conjugados desiguais em que o parasita imperfeitamente desenvolvido está fixado à porção ventral do autósito. VER conjoined *twins*, em *twin*. VER TAMBÉM epigastrius. [hetero- + G. *pagos*, fixado]

het·er·op·a·thy (het′er-op′a-thē). Heteropatia. **1.** Sensibilidade anormal a estímulos. **2.** Alopatia. SIN allopathy. [hetero- + G. *pathos*, sofrimento]

het·er·oph·a·gy (het-er-of′a-jē). Heterofagia; digestão, no interior de uma célula, de uma substância exógena fagocitada do ambiente da célula. [hetero- + G. *phagō*, comer]

het·er·o·phil, het·er·o·phile (het′er-ō-fil, -fīl). Heterófilo. **1.** Relativo a antígenos heterogenéticos ou de reação cruzada que ocorre em diferentes espécies ou a anticorpos dirigidos contra esses antígenos. **2.** O leucócito neutrófilo no homem; em alguns animais, os grânulos variam de tamanho e reação a corantes. [hetero- + G. *philos*, amigo]

het·er·o·pho·nia (het′er-ō-fō′nē-ă). Heterofonia. **1.** A mudança da voz na puberdade. **2.** Qualquer anormalidade nos sons vocais. SIN heterophthongia. [hetero- + G. *phōnē*, voz]

het·er·o·pho·ria (het′er-ō-fō′rē-ă). Heteroforia; tendência a desvio dos olhos do paralelismo, evitada pela visão binocular. [hetero- + G. *phora*, movimento]

het·er·oph·thal·mus (het′er-of-thal′mŭs). Heteroftalmia; termo raramente utilizado para referir-se a uma diferença no aspecto dos dois olhos, geralmente devido a heterocromia da íris. SIN allophthalmia. [hetero- + G. *ophthalmos*, olho]

het·er·oph·thon·gia (het-er-of-thon′jē-ă). Heeroftongia. SIN heterophonia. [G. *heterophthongos*, fr. *heteros*, diferente + *phthongos*, som, voz]

Het·er·o·phy·es (het-er-of′i-ēz). Gênero de vermes digenéticos (família Heterophyidae) parasitas de aves e mamíferos que se alimentam de peixes, incluindo o homem; as cercárias de caramujos infectados penetram nos peixes, onde se encistam; os peixes são consumidos pelos hospedeiros finais. [hetero- + G. *phyē*, estatura, forma]

H. brevicae'ca, espécie relatada em seres humanos nas Filipinas e responsável por lesões cardíacas causadas pelos ovos desse minúsculo verme, transportado da mucosa intestinal para obstruir os capilares coronários.

H. heteroph'yes, o verme intestinal egípcio ou verme do intestino delgado, uma espécie que infecta o intestino delgado e o ceco dos seres humanos e de outros mamíferos que se alimentam de peixes no Egito e no Extremo Oriente.

H. katsura'dai, uma espécie, um pouco menor do que *H. heterophyes,* encontrada no Japão.

het·er·o·phy·i·a·sis (het′er-ō-fī-ī′ă-sis). Heterofíase; infecção por um trematódeo heterofiídeo, particularmente *Heterophyes heterophyes*. SIN heterophyidiasis.

het·er·o·phy·id (het′er-o-fī′id). Heterofiídeo; nome comum para um membro da família Heterophyidae.

Het·er·o·phy·i·dae (het-er-o-fī′i-dē). Família de minúsculos trematódeos transportados por peixes, incluindo o gênero *Heterophyes* e seu parasita humano comum, *H. heterophyes.*

het·er·o·phy·id·i·a·sis (het′er-ō-fī-id-ī′ă-sis). Heterofiidíase. SIN heterophyiasis.

het·er·o·pla·sia (het′er-ō-plā′zē-ă). Heteroplasia. **1.** Desenvolvimento de elementos citológicos e histológicos que não são normais para o órgão ou para a parte em questão, como crescimento de osso num local onde normalmente existe tecido conjuntivo fibroso. **2.** Posição incorreta de tecido ou de uma parte normal sob os demais aspectos, como um ureter que se desenvolve no pólo inferior de um rim. SIN alloplasia. [hetero- + G. *plasis*, formação]

het·er·o·plas·tic (het′er-ō-plas′tik). Heteroplásico. **1.** Relativo a ou que manifesta heteroplasia. **2.** Relacionado à heteroplasia.

het·er·o·plas·tid (het′er-ō-plas′tid). Heteroplastídeo; o enxerto na heteroplasia.

het·er·o·ploid (het′er-ō-ployd). Heteroplóide; relativo à heteroploidia.

het·er·o·ploi·dy (het′er-ō-ploy′dē). Heteroploidia; estado de uma célula que possui algum número de conjuntos haplóides completos diferentes do normal. [hetero- + G. *ploides*, em forma]

het·er·o·pol·y·sac·cha·ride (het′er-ō-pol-ē-sak′ă-rīd). Heteropolissacarídeo; polissacarídeo composto de dois ou mais tipos diferentes de monossacarídeos. Cf. glycan, homoglycan. SIN heteroglycan.

het·er·o·pro·te·ose (het′er-ō-prō′tē-ōs). Heteroproteose. VER primary *proteose.*

het·er·o·pyk·no·sis (het′er-ō-pik-nō′sis). Heteropicnose; qualquer estado de densidade ou condensação variável, geralmente em diferentes cromossomas ou entre regiões diferentes do mesmo cromossoma, uma região pode ser atenuada (**h. negativa**) ou acentuada (**h. positiva**). [hetero- + G. *pyknos*, denso]

het·er·o·pyk·not·ic (het′er-ō-pik-not′ik). Heteropicnótico; relativo a, ou caracterizado por, heteropicnose.

het·er·o·re·cep·tor (het′er-ō-rē-sep′ter). Heterorreceptor; local, em um neurônio, que se liga a um neuro-regulador modulador diferente daquele liberado pelo neurônio. [hetero- + receptor]

het·er·o·sac·cha·ride (het′er-ō-sak′ă-rīd). Heterossacarídeo; glicosídeo em que um grupamento açúcar liga-se a um grupamento não-açúcar; p. ex., amigdalina.

het·er·o·sced·as·tic·i·ty (het′er-ō-skĕd-as-tis′ī-tē). Heteroscedasticidade; não-constância da variação de uma medida acima dos níveis do fator estudado. [hetero- + G. *skedastikos*, relativo à dispersão, fr. *skedannumi*, dispersar]

het·er·o·sex·u·al (het′er-ō-sek′shoo-al). Heterossexual. **1.** Indivíduo cuja orientação sexual é dirigida para pessoas do sexo oposto. **2.** Relativo a, ou caracterizado por, heterossexualidade. **3.** Indivíduo cujos interesses e comportamentos são característicos de heterossexualidade.

het·er·o·sex·u·al·i·ty (het′er-ō-sek-shoo-al′i-tē). Heterossexualidade; atração, predisposição ou atividade eróticas, incluindo relação sexual entre indivíduos do sexo oposto.

het·er·o·side (het′er-ō-sīd). Heterosídeo; composto contendo dois ou mais resíduos de carboidratos diferentes, ligados de modo covalente a um componente não-carboidrato.

het·er·o·sis (het-er-ō′sis). Heterose; o efeito benéfico, ao nível do fenótipo, do cruzamento (hibridização) sobre o crescimento, vigor e qualidades físicas ou mentais numa cepa de plantas ou numa raça animal, medido pela diferença entre o fenótipo médio dos pais e aquele da geração F_1; também denominado vigor híbrido. [hetero- + *-osis*, condição]

het·er·os·mia (het-er-os′mē-ă). Heterosmia. SIN allotriosmia.

het·er·o·some (het′er-ō-sōm). Heterossoma; em genética, o par de cromossomas que é diferente nos dois sexos. VER sex *chromosomes*, em *chromosome*. [hetero- + G. *sōma*, corpo]

het·er·o·spe·cif·ic (het′er-ō-spe-sif′ik). Heteroespecífico; heterólogo; referente a exertos.

het·er·o·sug·ges·tion (het′er-ō-sŭg-jes′chŭn). Heterossugestão; termo raramente utilizado para sugestão hipnótica recebida de outra pessoa; oposto a auto-sugestão.

het·er·o·tax·ia (het′er-ō-taks′ē-ă). Heterotaxia; distribuição anormal de órgãos ou partes do corpo um em relação ao outro. SIN heterotaxis, heterotaxy. [hetero- + G. *taxis*, disposição, distribuição]

cardiac h., h. cardíaca. VER dextrocardia.

het·er·o·tax·ic (het′er-ō-taks′ik). Heterotáxico; anormalmente colocado ou distribuído.

het·er·o·tax·is, het·er·o·taxy (het-er-ō-taks′is, het′er-ō-taks-ē). Heterotaxia. SIN heterotaxia.

het·er·o·thal·lic (het′er-ō-thal′ik). Heterotálico; nos fungos, refere-se a um tipo de reprodução sexuada em que um esporo sexual é produzido apenas pela fusão com o núcleo de outro tipo de par. Cf. homothallic. [hetero- + G. *thallos*, broto novo]

het·er·o·therm (het′er-ō-therm). Heterotermo; animal heterotérmico.

het·er·o·ther·mic (het′er-ō-ther′mik). Heterotérmico; que possui regulação parcial da temperatura corporal; entre poicilotérmico e homeotérmico.

het·er·ot·ic (het-er-ot′ik). Heterótico; relativo à heterose.

het·er·o·to·nia (het′er-ō-tō′nē-ă). Heterotonia; anormalidade ou variação na tensão ou no tônus. [hetero- + G. *tonos*, tensão]

het·er·o·to·pia (het′er-ō-tō′pē-ă). Heterotopia. **1.** SIN ectopia. **2.** Em neuropatologia, deslocamento da substância cinzenta, tipicamente para a substância branca cerebral profunda. [hetero- + G. *topos*, local]

h. mac'ulae, h. da mácula. SIN *ectopia* maculae.

het·er·o·top·ic (het-er-ō-top′ik). Heterotópico. **1.** SIN ectopic (1). **2.** Relativo à heteropia (2). [hetero- + *topos*, local + sufixo *-ic*, relativo a]

het·er·ot·o·pous (het-er-ot′ō-pŭs). Heterótopo; heterotópico, particularmente no que concerne a teratomas compostos de tecidos que estão fora do local na região em que se encontram.

het·er·o·trans·plan·ta·tion (het′er-ō-tranz-plan-tā′shŭn). Heterotransplante; transferência de um heteroenxerto (xenoenxerto).

het·er·o·tri·cho·sis (het′er-ō-tri-kō′sis). Heterotricose; condição caracterizada pelo crescimento de pêlos de cor variegada. [hetero- + G. *trichōsis*, crescimento de pêlos]

het·er·o·troph (het′er-ō-trof, -trōf). Heterótrofo; microrganismo que obtém seu carbono, bem como sua energia, de compostos orgânicos. VER TAMBÉM autotroph. [hetero- + G. *trophē*, nutrição]

het·er·o·tro·phic (het′er-ō-tro-fik). Heterotrófico. **1.** Relativo à ou que exibe as propriedades da heterotrofia. **2.** Relativo a um heterótrofo.

het·er·ot·ro·phy (het′er-ō-trō-fē). Heterotrofia; a capacidade ou a necessidade de sintetizar todos os metabólitos a partir de compostos orgânicos.

het·er·o·tro·pia, het·er·ot·ro·py (het′er-ō-trō′pē-a, het-er-ot′rō-pē). Heterotropia. SIN strabismus. [hetero- + G. *tropē*, uma volta]

het·er·o·typ·ic (het′er-ō-tip′ik). Heterotípico; de um tipo ou forma diferente ou incomum.

het·er·o·xan·thine (het′er-ō-zan′thin). Heteroxantina; 7-metilxantina; uma das bases aloxúricas na urina, representando os produtos terminais do metabolismo das purinas.

het·er·ox·e·nous (het-er-oks′e-nŭs). Heteroxeno. SIN digenetic (1). [hetero- + G. *xenos*, estranho]

het·er·o·zo·ic (het-er-ō-zō′ik). Heterozóico; relativo a outro animal ou espécie de animal. [hetero- + G. *zōikos*, relativo a um animal]

het·er·o·zy·gos·i·ty, het·er·o·zy·go·sis (het′er-ō-zī-gos′i-tē, -zī-gō′sis). Heterozigosidade; o estado de ser heterozigoto. [hetero- + G. *zygon*, união]

het·er·o·zy·gote (het′er-ō-zī′gōt). Heterozigoto; indivíduo heterozigoto. [hetero- + G. *zygotos*, unido]

   compound h., h. composto; em genética médica, a presença de dois alelos mutantes diferentes nos mesmos *loci*. SIN genetic compound.

   manifesting h., h. manifesto; organismo heterozigoto para o qual existe habitualmente uma condição recessiva que, em decorrência de mecanismos especiais (como lionização, exclusão alélica ou deleção no cromossoma homólogo), apresenta manifestações fenotípicas. SIN manifesting carrier.

het·er·o·zy·gous (het′er-ō-zī′gŭs). Heterozigoto; que possui diferentes alelos em um *locus* no que concerne a um caráter específico; heterótico.

   doubly h., h. duplo; na análise da ligação entre dois *loci*, refere-se ao genótipo em que um genitor é heterozigoto em ambos os *loci*, o estado em que, em média, contém a informação máxima relativa à ligação.

Heubner, Johann O.L., pediatra alemão, 1843–1926. VER *artery* of H.; H. *arteritis.*

Heurenius, Johannes. VER van Horne.

Heuser, Chester H., embriologista norte-americano, 1885–1965. VER H. *membrane.*

HEV HEV. Abreviatura para hepatitis E *virus* (vírus da hepatite E).

♻ **hexa-, hex-.** hex(a); prefixo que significa seis. [G. *hex*]

hex·a·canth (hek′sa-kanth). Hexacanto; a larva móvel de primeiro estágio dos cestóides ciclofilídeos, dotada de seis ganchos ou espinhos; eclode do ovo e abre ativamente seu caminho através do intestino do hospedeiro intermediário antes de se desenvolver no próximo estágio larvário; p. ex., o hexacanto da *Taenia saginata*, que penetra no intestino de uma vaca que ingeriu o ovo, formando, em seguida, um cisticerco nos músculos do hospedeiro intermediário. SIN oncosphere. [hetero- + G. *akantha*, gancho ou espinho]

hex·a·chlo·ro·cy·clo·hex·ane (hek-sa-klō′rō-sī-klō-hek′san). Hexaclorociclo-hexano. SIN gamma benzene hexachloride.

hex·a·chlo·ro·phane (hek-sa-klō′rō-fān). Hexaclorofano. SIN hexachlorophene.

hex·a·chlo·ro·phene (hek-sa-klō′rō-fēn). Hexaclorofeno; antibacteriano; muito utilizado, no passado, em sabões e detergentes para inibir o crescimento bacteriano; o uso excessivo provoca lesões neurológicas; hoje em dia, tem uso limitado. SIN hexachlorophane.

hex·a·co·sa·no·ic ac·id (heks′a-kō′san-ō-ik). Ácido hexacosanóico; nome sistêmico para o ácido cerotínico.

hex·a·co·sa·nol (heks-a-kō′sa-nol). Hexacosanol. VER ceryl.

hex·a·co·syl (heks-a-kō′sil). Hexacosil. SIN ceryl.

hex·ad (heks′ad). Elemento ou radical com seis valências.

hex·a·dac·ty·ly, hex·a·dac·tyl·ism (hek′sa-dak′ti-lē, -lizm). Hexadactilia; presença de seis dedos em uma ou ambas as mãos ou pés. [hexa- + G. *daktylos*, dedo]

hex·a·dec·a·no·ic ac·id (heks′a-dek-a-nō′ik). Ácido hexadecanóico, ácido palmítico. SIN palmitic acid.

1-hex·a·dec·a·nol (hek-sa-dek′a-nol). 1-hexadecanol, álcool cetílico. SIN cetyl alcohol.

hex·a·flu·o·ren·i·um bro·mide (hek′sa-floo-rēn′ē-ŭm). Brometo de hexafluorênio; potencializador para a succinilcolina em anestesiologia, devido à produção de leve bloqueio neuromuscular não-despolarizante; inibe também a colinesterase plasmática.

hex·a·mer (hek′sa-mer). Hexâmero. **1.** Grupo de seis subunidades proteicas que formam um capsômero na superfície de um vírus icosaédrico. **2.** Complexo ou composto contendo seis subunidades ou componentes (p. ex., um complexo proteico com seis cadeias polipeptídicas ou um oligopeptídeo com seis resíduos aminoácidos). [hexa- + G. *meros*, parte]

hex·a·mer·ic (heks′a-mer-ik). Hexamérico; que contém seis subunidades ou componentes.

hex·a·met·a·zime (HMPAO). Hexametazima [HMPAO]; substância lipofílica que atravessa facilmente a barreira hematoencefálica; combinada com Tc^{99m} para produzir um radiofármaco para obtenção de imagens por SPECT ou para avaliação do fluxo sanguíneo cerebral. SIN hexamethylpropyleneamine oxime.

hex·a·meth·yl·prop·yl·ene·a·mine ox·ime (heks-ã-meth′il-prō′pi-lēn-ã-mēn oks′em). Hexametilpropilenamina oxima. SIN hexametazime.

hex·am·i·dine is·e·thi·o·nate (hek-sam′i-dēn). Isetionato de hexamidina; anti-séptico tópico.

hex·a·mine (hek′sa-mēn). Hexamina. SIN methenamine.

hex·ane (hek′san). Hexano; hidrocarboneto saturado, C_6H_{14}, da série das parafinas (tipicamente *n*-h., $CH_3-(CH_2)_4-CH_3$).

hex·a·no·ate (hek′sa-nō-āt). Hexanoato. SIN caproylate.

n-hex·a·no·ic ac·id (hek-sa-nō′ik). Ácido *n*-hexanóico. SIN *n-caproic acid*.

hex·a·no·yl (hek′sa-nō-il). Hexanoil. SIN caproyl.

hex·a·pep·tide (heks′a-pep′tīd). Hexapeptídeo; peptídeo constituído por seis resíduos aminoácidos.

hex·a·ploid·y (heks′a-ploy-dē). Hexaploidia. VER polyploidy.

Hex·a·po·da (hek-sap′ō-da). Classe dos Arthropoda. SIN Insecta. [hexa- + G. *pous*, pé]

hex·es·trol (hek-ses′trol). Hexestrol; composto *meso* sintético com atividade estrogênica.

hex·i·tol (heks′i-tol). Hexitol; o poliol (álcool açúcar) obtido com a redução de uma hexose (p. ex., D-sorbitol).

hex·o·ki·nase (heks-ō-kī′nās). Hexocinase; fosfotransferase presente na levedura, no músculo, no cérebro e em outros tecidos que catalisam a fosforilação ATP-dependente da D-glicose e de outras hexoses para formar D-glicose-6-fosfato (ou outras hexoses-6-fosfato); a primeira etapa da glicólise; a deficiência de h. pode resultar em anemia hemolítica e comprometimento da glicólise.

hex·on (heks′on). Hexon; grupo de seis unidades proteicas (unidade hexamérica) na face triangular de um capsômero icosaédrico em certos vírus. [hex- + -on]

hex·on·ic ac·id (heks-on′ik). Ácido hexônico; o ácido aldônico obtido na oxidação do grupamento aldeído de uma aldo-hexose a ácido carboxílico (p. ex., ácido glicônico a partir da glicose).

hex·os·a·mine (hek′sō-sam′ēn). Hexosamina; derivado amina (com substituição do OH por NH_2) de uma hexose; p. ex., glicosamina.

hex·os·a·min·i·dase (hek′sō-sa-min′i-dās). Hexosaminidase; termo genérico para referir-se a enzimas que clivam resíduos *N*-acetil-hexose (p. ex., *N*-acetilglicosamina) a partir de oligossacarídeos semelhantes a glicosídeos. São conhecidas pelo menos quatro enzimas específicas que efetuam esse tipo de reação: α-*N*-acetil-D-galactosaminidase, α-*N*-acetil-D-glicosaminidase, β-*N*-acetil-D-hexosaminidase e β-*N*-acetil-D-galactosaminidase, sendo cada uma específica para a configuração e o tipo de açúcar incluído no nome.

   h. A, h. A; enzima hidrolítica que atua sobre o gangliosídeo G_{M2}, produzindo *N*-acetil-D-galactosamina e gangliosídeo G_{M3}; a deficiência dessa enzima está associada à doença de Tay-Sachs.

   h. B, h. B; enzima hidrolítica que atua sobre o gangliosídeo G_{M1}, produzindo gangliosídeo G_{M1} e galactose, bem como no globosídeo, produzindo *N*-acetil galactosamina e triexosilceramida; a deficiência dessa enzima está associada à doença de Sandhoff.

hex·o·sans (hek′sō-sanz). Hexosanos; polissacarídeos com a fórmula geral $(C_6H_{10}O_5)_x$ que, na hidrólise, liberam hexoses; estão incluídos glicosanos (glicanos), mananos, galactanos e frutosanos (frutanos). SIN polyhexoses.

hex·ose (hek′sōs). Hexose; monossacarídeo contendo seis átomos carbono na molécula ($C_6H_{12}O_6$); a D-glicose é a principal hexose na natureza.

hex·ose·bis·phos·pha·tase, hex·ose·di·phos·pha·tase (hek′sōs-bis-fos′fa-tās, -dī-). Hexose difosfatase. SIN fructose 1,6-bisphosphate.

hex·ose phos·pha·tase (hek′sōs fos′fa-tāz). Hexose fosfatase; enzima que catalisa a hidrólise de um fosfato de hexose em hexose (p. ex., glicose-6-fosfatase).

hex·ose·phos·phate isom·er·ase (hek-sōs-fos′fāt). Hexose fosfato isomerase. SIN glucose-phosphate isomerase.

hex·ose-1-phos·phate uri·dyl·yl·trans·fer·ase. Hexose-1-fosfato uridililtransferase. SIN UDPglucose-hexose-1-phosphate uridylyltransferase.

hex·u·lose (hek′sū-lōs). Hexulose. SIN ketohexose.

hex·u·ron·ic ac·id (hek-sūr-on′ik). Ácido hexurônico; o ácido urônico de uma hexose.

hex·yl (hek′sil). Hexil; o radical do hexano, $CH_3(CH_2)_4CH_2-$.

hex·yl·res·or·cin·ol (hek′sil-re-sōr′si-nol). Hexilresorcinol; anti-helmíntico de largo espectro e anti-séptico.

Hey, William, cirurgião inglês, 1736–1819. VER H. *amputation, hernia*, ligamento.

Heyer, W.T., cientista norte-americano, *1902. VER H.-Pudenz *valve.*
Hf Hf. Símbolo de hafnium (háfnio).
Hg Símbolo do *mercury* (mercúrio). O nome antigo era hydrargyrum (hidrargírio).
HGE Abreviatura de human granulocytic *ehrlichiosis* (erliquiose granulocítica humana).
HGF Abreviatura do hyperglycemic-glycogenolytic *factor* (fator hiperglicêmico-glicogenolítico).
HGH Abreviatura do human growth hormone (hormônio do crescimento humano). VER somatotropin.
HGPRT Abreviatura de *hypoxanthine* guanine phosphoribosyl-transferase (hipoxantina guanina fosforribosil transferase).
HGSIL Abreviatura de high-grade squamous intraepithelial *lesion* (lesão intra-epitelial escamosa de alto grau).
HGV Abreviatura de hepatitis G *virus* (vírus da hepatite G).
HHV Abreviatura de human herpesvirus (herpesvírus humano).
hi·a·tal (hī-āʹtăl). Hiatal; relativo a um hiato.
hi·a·tus (hī-āʹtŭs) [TA]. Hiato; uma abertura, orifício ou forame. [L. uma abertura, fr. *hio,* p. *hiatus,* abrir-se]
  adductor h. [TA], h. dos adutores; a abertura na inserção aponeurótica do músculo adutor magno, que transmite a artéria e a veia femorais do canal adutor para o espaço poplíteo. SIN h. adductorius [TA], femoral opening, h. tendineus, tendinous opening.
  h. adductoʹrius [TA], h. dos adutores. SIN adductor h.
  aortic h. [TA], h. aórtico; abertura no diafragma limitada pelos dois pilares, pela coluna vertebral e ligamento arqueado mediano, através da qual passa a aorta e o ducto torácico. SIN h. aorticus [TA], aortic foramen, aortic opening.
  h. aorʹticus [TA], h. aórtico. SIN aortic h.
  Breschet h., h. de Breschet. SIN helicotrema.
  h. canaʹlis faciaʹlis, h. do canal do nervo petroso maior. SIN h. for greater petrosal nerve.
  h. canaʹlis nerʹvi petroʹsi majoʹris [TA], h. do canal do nervo petroso maior. SIN h. for greater petrosal nerve.
  h. canaʹlis nerʹvi petroʹsi minoʹris [TA], h. do canal do nervo petroso menor. SIN h. for lesser petrosal nerve.
  esophageal h. [TA], h. esofágico; abertura no pilar direito do diafragma, entre o tendão central e o hiato aórtico, através da qual passa o esôfago e os dois nervos vagos. SIN h. esophageus [TA], esophageal opening.
  h. esophaʹgeus [TA], h. semilunar. SIN esophageal h.
  h. ethmoidaʹlis, h. semilunar. SIN semilunar h.
  h. of facial canal, h. do canal do nervo petroso maior. SIN h. for greater petrosal nerve.
  fallopian h., h. do canal do nervo petroso maior. SIN h. for greater petrosal nerve.
  h. for greater petrosal nerve [TA], h. do canal do nervo petroso maior; a abertura na face anterior da parte petrosa do osso temporal que leva ao canal facial e dá passagem ao nervo petroso maior. SIN h. canalis nervi petrosi majoris [TA], fallopian h., Ferrein foramen, h. canalis facialis, h. of facial canal.
  h. for lesser petrosal nerve [TA], h. do canal do nervo petroso menor; a pequena abertura no poço petroso lateral ao hiato para o nervo petroso maior, que dá passagem ao nervo petroso menor. SIN h. canalis nervi petrosi minoris [TA], Arnold canal, canalis nervi petrosi superficialis minoris.
  h. maxillaʹris [TA], h. maxilar. SIN maxillary h.
  maxillary h. [TA], h. maxilar; a grande abertura no seio maxilar na superfície nasal da maxila. SIN h. maxillaris [TA].
  pleuropericardial h., h. pleuropericárdico; abertura que conecta as cavidades pleural e pericárdica; em geral, o resultado do desenvolvimento incompleto da prega pleuropericárdica do embrião.
  pleuroperitoneal h., h. pleuroperitoneal; abertura, através do diafragma, conectando as cavidades pleural e peritoneal, geralmente o resultado do desenvolvimento defeituoso da membrana pleuroperitoneal no embrião; se o defeito for extenso, pode haver herniação dos órgãos digestivos para a cavidade pleural. VER TAMBÉM diaphragmatic *hernia.* SIN Bochdalek foramen.
  sacral h. [TA], h. sacral; lacuna de ocorrência natural na extremidade inferior do sacro, expondo o canal vertebral devido à não-coalescência das lâminas do último segmento sacral. É fechado pelo ligamento sacrococcígeo e fornece acesso canular ao espaço epidural sacral para a administração de anestésicos (bloqueio nervoso caudal). SIN h. sacralis [TA].
  h. sacraʹlis [TA], h. sacral. SIN sacral h.
  saphenous h., h. safeno. SIN saphenous *opening.*
  h. sapheʹnus [TA], h. safeno. SIN saphenous *opening.*
  scalene h., triângulo interescalênico; hiato triangular delimitado pelos músculos escaleno anterior e escaleno médio e pela primeira costela à qual se inserem os músculos; o hiato fornece a passagem para a artéria subclávia e para as raízes do plexo braquial. A compressão das estruturas que passam através do hiato por qualquer causa manifesta-se na forma da "síndrome do desfiladeiro torácico". SIN interscalene triangle.
  Scarpa h., h. de Scarpa, helicotrema. SIN helicotrema.
  semilunar h. [TA], h. semilunar; sulco profundo e estreito na parede lateral do meato médio da cavidade nasal, no qual se abrem o seio maxilar, o ducto frontonasal e as células etmóides médias. SIN h. semilunaris [TA], h. ethmoidalis.
  h. semilunaʹris [TA], h. semilunar. SIN semilunar h.
  h. subarcuaʹtus, fossa subarqueada. SIN subarcuate *fossa.*
  h. tendinʹeus, h. dos adutores. SIN adductor h.
  h. totaʹlis sacraʹlis, h. sacral total; fenda de desenvolvimento observado em todas as vértebras sacrais; pode envolver também vértebras lombares adjacentes.
hi·ber·na·tion (hī-ber-nāʹshŭn). Hibernação; condição de entorpecimento em que certos animais passam os meses de frio. Os hibernantes verdadeiros, como as marmotas, os esquilos terrestres, os arganazes e alguns outros animais, têm temperaturas corporais reduzidas até quase o ponto de congelamento, com freqüência cardíaca muito lenta, metabolismo baixo e incursões respiratórias infreqüentes. Os hibernantes parciais, como os ursos, as doninhas e os guaxinins, possuem atividade fisiológica reduzida durante os meses frios, mas não se encontram num estado comatoso. Cf. estivation. SIN winter sleep. [L. *hibernus,* relativo ao inverno]
hi·ber·no·ma (hīʹber-nōʹmă). Hibernoma; um tipo raro de neoplasia benigna em seres humanos, constituída por gordura castanha que se assemelha à gordura em certos animais hibernantes; as células tumorais individuais contêm múltiplas gotículas de lipídios. VER TAMBÉM brown *fat.* [L. *hibernus,* relativo ao inverno + G. -*ōma,* tumor]
  interscapular h., h. interescapular. SIN brown *fat.*
hic·cup, hic·cough (hikʹŭp). Soluço, singulto; espasmo diafragmático que provoca uma súbita inalação, interrompida pelo fechamento espasmódico da glote e produzindo um ruído. SIN singultus.
  epidemic h., s. epidêmico; s. persistente que ocorre como complicação da *influenza* (gripe).
Hickman, Robert O., cirurgião pediatra norte-americano do século XX. VER H. *catheter.*
Hicks, Hicks, VER Braxton Hicks.
HIDA Abreviatura de dimethyl iminodiacetic acid (ácido dimetil iminodiacético).
△ **hidr-.** VER hidro-.
hi·drad·e·ni·tis (hī-dradʹē-nīʹtis). Hidradenite; inflamação das glândulas sudoríparas. SIN hydradenitis. [G. *hidrōs,* suor + *adēn,* glândula + -*itis,* inflamação]
  h. suppuratiʹva, h. supurativa; foliculite supurativa crônica da pele contendo glândulas sudoríparas apócrinas das áreas perianal, axilar e genital ou inframamária, que surge após a puberdade e produz abscessos ou fístulas com fibrose.
  neutrophilic eccrine h., h. écrina neutrofílica; condição inflamatória que ocorre em pacientes submetidos a quimioterapia, com infiltração profunda das glândulas écrinas por neutrófilos.
hi·drad·e·no·ma (hī-dradʹ-ē-nōʹmă). Hidradenoma; neoplasia benigna derivada de células epiteliais das glândulas sudoríparas. SIN hydradenoma. [G. *hidrōs,* suor + *adēn,* glândula + -*oma,* tumor]
  clear cell h., h. de células claras; tumor derivado das glândulas sudoríparas écrinas, composto de células claras ricas em glicogênio. SIN eccrine acrospiroma, nodular h.
  nodular h., h. nodular. SIN clear cell h.
  papillary h., h. papilar; tumor benigno solitário, cístico e papilar, que ocorre em mulheres, geralmente nos lábios maiores do pudendo, composto de epitélio que se assemelha ao das glândulas apócrinas. SIN apocrine adenoma, h. papilliferum.
  h. papillifeʹrum, h. papilar. SIN papillary h.
△ **hidro-, hidr-.** hidro-., hidr-. Refere-se a suor, glândulas sudoríparas. Cf. sudor-. [G. *hidrōs*]
hi·droa (hī-drōʹă). Hidroa. SIN hydroa.
hi·dro·cys·to·ma (hīʹdrō-sis-tōʹmă). Hidrocistoma; forma cística de hidradenoma, geralmente apócrina. SIN hydrocystoma (2), syringocystoma. [hidro- + G. *kystis,* bexiga + -*ōma,* tumor]
  apocrine h., cisto sudorífero. SIN sudoriferous *cyst.*
hi·dro·mei·o·sis (hīʹdrō-mī-ōʹsis). Hidromeiose; declínio na taxa de sudorese durante a exposição ao calor, especialmente durante banhos quentes. [hidro- + G. *meiōsis,* redução]
hi·dro·poi·e·sis (hīʹdrō-poy-ēʹsis, hidʹrō-). Hidropoese; formação do suor. [hidro- + G. *poiēsis,* formação]
hi·dros·che·sis (hī-drosʹkē-sis, hid-rosʹ). Hidroquese; supressão do suor. [hidro- + G. *schesis,* interrupção]
hi·dro·sis (hi-drōʹsis, hī-). Hidrose; a produção e a excreção de suor. [G. *hidrōs,* suor + -*osis,* condição]
hi·drot·ic (hi-drotʹik, hī-). Hidrótico; relativo a ou que provoca hidrose.
hi·er·ar·chy (hīʹer-ar-kē, hīʹ-i-rarʹkē). Hierarquia. **1.** Qualquer sistema de pessoas ou coisas ordenadas segundo uma ordem de prioridade. **2.** Em psicologia e psiquiatria, uma organização de hábitos ou conceitos nos quais os componentes mais simples são combinados para formar integrações cada vez mais complexas. [G. *hierarchia,* regra ou poder do sacerdote superior]

dominance h., h. de dominância; situação social em que um organismo domina todos os outros abaixo dele, o seguinte todos abaixo, e assim por diante até chegar ao organismo dominado por todos os demais; p. ex., a hierarquia social observada em macacos, focas, galinhas de terreiro e outras espécies.

Maslow h., h. de Maslow; classificação de necessidades que os seres humanos presumivelmente preenchem de modo sucessivo da ordem mais inferior para a mais elevada: necessidades fisiológicas, amor e afiliação, auto-estima e auto-realização.

response h., h. de resposta; reações ou modos alternativos de adaptação a determinada situação dispostos na ordem provável de efetividade anterior; p. ex., a mãe que tenta disciplinar um filho rebelde pode inicialmente pedir, adular, em seguida suplicar, ralhar e, por fim, castigar; seus comportamentos podem ser ordenados ao longo de uma h. de respostas para monitoração adicional da efetividade.

h. of terms, h. de termos; em radiologia, o conceito semântico de utilizar diferentes termos para descrever estruturas anatômicas ou patológicas confrontadas com as imagens diagnósticas resultantes.

hi·er·o·pho·bia (hī″er-ō-fō′bē-ə). Hierofobia; temor mórbido de objetos religiosos ou sagrados. [G. *hieros*, sagrado + *phobos*, medo]

hi·er·o·ther·a·py (hī″er-ō-thār′ă-pē). Hieroterapia; tratamento de doenças por orações e práticas religiosas. [G. *hieros*, sagrado + *therapeia*, terapia]

Higashi, Ototaka, médico japonês. VER Chédiak-H. *disease;* Chédiak-Steinbrinck-H. *anomaly, syndrome.*

Highmore, Nathaniel, anatomista inglês, 1613–1685. VER *antrum* of H.; H. *body.*

Higoumenakia sign. Sinal de Higoumenakia. Ver em *sign.*

hi·la (hī′lă). Hilos; plural de hilum.

hi·lar (hī′lăr). Hilar; relativo a um hilo.

hi·li·tis (hī-lī′tis). Hilite; inflamação da membrana de revestimento de qualquer hilo.

Hill, Archibald V., biofísico inglês e ganhador do Prêmio Nobel, 1886–1977. VER H. *equation, plot;* initial *heat.*

Hill, Austin Bradford, médico estatístico inglês, 1897–1991. VER H.'s criteria of evidence, em *criterion.*

Hill, Harold A., radiologista norte-americano do século XX. VER H.-Sachs *lesion.*

Hill, Sir Leonard Erskine, fisiologista inglês, 1866–1952. VER H. *sign, phenomenon.*

Hill, Lucius D., cirurgião torácico norte-americano, *1921. VER H. *operation.*

Hill, Robert, fisiologista botânico inglês, *1899. VER H. *reaction.*

Hillis, David S., obstetra-ginecologista norte-americano, 1873–1942. VER H.-Müller *maneuver.*

hil·lock (hil′lok). Proeminência; em anatomia, qualquer elevação ou proeminência pequena.

axon h., p. axônica; cone de implantação; a área cônica de origem do axônio a partir do corpo da célula nervosa; contém séries paralelas de microtúbulos e é desprovido de substância de Nissl. SIN implantation cone.

facial h., colículo facial. SIN facial *colliculus.*

seminal h., colículo seminal. SIN seminal *colliculus.*

Hilton, John, cirurgião inglês, 1804–1878. VER H. *law;* white *line, method, sac.*

hi·lum, pl. **hi·la** (hī′lŭm, hī′lă). [TA]. Hilo. **1.** Parte de um órgão onde os nervos e os vasos penetram e de onde saem. SIN porta (1). **2.** Depressão ou fenda semelhante ao hilo no núcleo olivar do cérebro. [L. um pedacinho ou ninharia]

h. of dentate nucleus [TA], h. do núcleo denteado; a boca do núcleo denteado, em forma de frasco, do cerebelo, orientada para dentro e que propicia a saída de muitas das fibras que compõem o pedúnculo cerebelar superior. SIN h. nuclei dentati [TA].

h. of inferior olivary nucleus [TA], h. do núcleo olivar inferior; a abertura orientada medialmente, na camada celular preguada que compõe o núcleo olivar inferior, através da qual saem as fibras eferentes do núcleo. SIN h. nuclei olivaris inferioris [TA].

h. of kidney [TA], h. do rim; a depressão na borda medial do rim através da qual passam os vasos renais segmentares e nervos renais e onde se encontra o ápice da pelve renal. SIN h. renalis [TA], porta renis.

h. li′enis, h. do baço; *termo oficial alternativo para splenic h.

h. of lung [TA], h. do pulmão; uma depressão cuneiforme na superfície mediastinal de cada pulmão, onde os brônquios, vasos sanguíneos, nervos e linfáticos penetram na víscera ou dela saem. SIN h. pulmonis [TA], porta pulmonis.

h. of lymph node [TA], h. do linfonodo; a área deprimida da superfície de um linfonodo através da qual os linfáticos eferentes saem da medula e os vasos sanguíneos nela penetram e deixam o linfonodo. SIN h. nodi lymphatici [TA].

h. no′di lympha′tici [TA], h. do linfonodo. SIN h. of lymph node.

h. nu′clei denta′ti [TA], h. do núcleo denteado. SIN h. of dentate nucleus.

h. nu′clei oliva′ris inferioris [TA], h. do núcleo olivar inferior. SIN h. of inferior olivary nucleus.

h. ova′rii, h. do ovário. SIN h. of ovary.

h. of ovary, h. do ovário; a depressão ao longo da margem mesovariana, na inserção do mesovário, onde os vasos sanguíneos e nervos penetram no ovário ou dele saem. SIN h. ovarii.

h. pulmo′nis [TA], h. do pulmão. SIN h. of lung.

h. rena′lis [TA], h. do rim. SIN h. of kidney.

h. of spleen, h. do baço. SIN splenic h.

splenic h. [TA], h. do baço; fissura na superfície gástrica do baço que dá passagem aos vasos e nervos esplênicos. SIN h. splenicum [TA], h. lienis*, h. of spleen, porta lienis.

h. sple′nicum [TA], h. do baço. SIN splenic h.

hi·lus (hī′lŭs) [TA], hilo; designação antiga e incorreta para referir-se ao hilum. [uma variante inglesa de L. *hilum*]

hi·man·to·sis (hī-man-tō′sis). Himantose; úvula inusitadamente longa. [G. *himas*, correia + *-osis*, condição]

hind·brain (hīnd′brān) [TA]. Rombencéfalo. SIN rhombencephalon.

hind·gut (hīnd′gut). Intestino posterior. **1.** Parte caudal ou terminal do intestino embrionário. **2.** Cólon descendente e sigmóide, reto e canal anal; alguns incluem todo o intestino grosso. SIN endgut.

hind·wa·ter (hīnd′wah-ter). Coloquialismo para referir-se ao líquido amniótico *in utero* atrás da parte de apresentação do feto.

hinge-bow (hinj′bō). Arco em dobradiça, charneira. SIN face-bow.

Hinman, Frank, Jr., urologista norte-americano, *1915. VER H. *syndrome.*

Hinton, William A., médico norte-americano, 1883–1959. VER H. *test;* Mueller-H. *agar.*

hip. Quadril. **1.** Proeminência lateral da pelve da cintura até a coxa. SIN coxa (1) [TA]. **2.** Cabeça, colo e trocanter maior e trocanter menor do fêmur. Este é o sentido do termo nas expressões comuns "fratura de quadril" ou "artroplastia femoral". **3.** Mais estritamente, refere-se à articulação coxofemoral. [A.S. *hype*]

snapping h., q. estalante; condição em que a fáscia lata ou o músculo glúteo máximo sob tensão, movendo-se sobre o trocanter maior na extremidade proximal do fêmur, ou o tendão do iliopsoas move-se sobre o trocanter menor, causando um estalido.

hip·ber·ries. Frutos de rosas silvestres. SIN rose hips.

Hippel, Eugen von. VER von H.

Hip·pe·la·tes (hip-ē-lā′tēz). Moscas-dos-olhos; um gênero de moscas da família Chloropidae (moscas-das-frutas), que são atraídas pelas secreções de líquidos corporais de animais e seres humanos, particularmente dos olhos. Acredita-se que *H.* transmite certos tipos de conjuntivite (como a conjuntivite aguda contagiosa), mastite bovina e bomba (framboesia tropical). [G. *hippelatēs*, condutor de cavalos]

Hip·po·bos·ca (hip-ō-bos′kă). Gênero de moscas pupíparas (família Hippoboscidae) relacionadas à mosca tsé-tsé; são ectoparasitas de aves e mamíferos. [G. *hippos*, cavalo + *boskein*, alimentar]

hip·po·cam·pal (hip-ō-kam′păl). Hipocampal; relativo ao hipocampo.

hip·po·cam·pus (hip-ō-kam′pŭs) [TA]. Hipocampo; a estrutura complexa e internamente convoluta que forma a margem medial ("bainha") do manto cortical do hemisfério cerebral, margeando a fissura coróide do ventrículo lateral; constituída de dois giros (corno de Ammon e giro denteado), juntamente com sua substância branca, o álveo e a fímbria do hipocampo. Nos macacos e nos seres humanos, o hipocampo é limitado ao lobo temporal pelo desenvolvimento maciço do corpo caloso. O hipocampo, que, citoarquiteturalmente, é uma forma singular de alocórtex (arquicórtex), faz parte do sistema límbico (antigamente rinencéfalo). Suas principais conexões aferentes são com a área entorrinal do giro para-hipocampal e com o septo transparente; através do fórnice, projeta-se para o septo, núcleo anterior do tálamo e corpo mamilar. SIN h. major, major h. [G. *hippocampos*, cavalo-marinho]

h. ma′jor, hipocampo. SIN hippocampus.

major h., hipocampo. SIN hippocampus.

h. mi′nor, *calcar avis.* SIN calcarine *spur.*

minor h., *calcar avis.* SIN calcarine *spur.*

Hippocrates of Cos. Hipócrates da ilha Cos; médico grego, considerado o "Pai da Medicina", cerca de 460–377 a.C. VER hippocratic *facies*, hippocratic *fingers*, em *finger*, hippocratic *nails*, em *nail*, hippocratic *school*, hippocratic *succussion*.

hip·po·crat·ic (hip-ō-krat′ik). Hipocrático; relativo a, descrito por ou atribuído a Hipócrates.

Hip·po·crat·ic Oath. Juramento de Hipócrates; juramento habitualmente feito por médicos ao iniciar a prática de sua profissão, que, apesar de ser habitualmente atribuído a Hipócrates de Cos, é provavelmente um juramento antigo dos asclepitanos. Sua forma original, hoje em dia freqüentemente revisada, aparece num livro da coleção de Hipócrates da seguinte maneira:

"Juro por Apolo, o médico, por Aesculapius, Hygeia e Panacea, e tomo como testemunha todos os deuses e todas as deusas para, de acordo com a minha capacidade e meu conhecimento, cumprir o seguinte juramento:

Considerar tão estimado quanto meus pais aquele que me ensinou essa arte; viver em comum com ele e, se necessário, compartilhar com ele meus bens; encarar seus filhos como meus próprios irmãos, ensinar-lhes essa arte se assim o desejarem, sem pagamento ou promessas escritas; deixar que compartilhem dos preceitos e da instrução meus filhos e os filhos do mestre que me ensinou, bem como os discípulos que concordaram com as regras da profissão, porém apenas a eles. Prescreverei dietas para o bem dos meus pacientes, de acordo com a minha capacidade e meu julgamento, e nunca para prejudicar alguém. Jamais, para agradar alguém, prescreverei uma droga mortal, nem darei conselho que possa causar a morte. Nunca darei a uma mulher um pessário para causar aborto. Preservarei a pureza da minha vida e da minha arte. Não farei nenhuma operação para cálculos, mesmo em pacientes nos quais a doença é manifesta; deixarei essa operação para os especialistas nessa arte. Em toda casa, entrarei somente para o bem dos meus pacientes, mantendo-me afastado de toda ação má e sedução intencionais, especialmente dos prazeres do amor, com mulheres ou com homens, sejam eles livres ou escravos. Tudo que possa chegar ao meu conhecimento, no exercício de minha profissão ou fora dela ou no contato diário com homens, que não deva ser divulgado, manterei em segredo e jamais revelarei. Se eu mantiver esse juramento fielmente, que eu possa viver a minha vida e praticar a minha arte, sendo respeitado por todos os homens e em todos os momentos; mas, se eu faltar ao juramento ou violá-lo, que meu destino seja o contrário."

hip·poc·ra·tism (hi-pok′rǎ-tizm). Hipocratismo; sistema de medicina, atribuído a Hipócrates e seus discípulos, baseado na imitação dos processos da natureza na conduta terapêutica da doença.

hip·pu·rate (hip′ū-rāt). Hipurato; sal ou éster do ácido hipúrico.

hip·pu·ria (hi-pū′rē-ǎ). Hipúria; excreção de uma quantidade anormalmente grande de ácido hipúrico na urina.

hip·pu·ric ac·id (hi-pūr′ik). Ácido hipúrico; produto de desintoxicação e excreção do benzoato encontrado na urina de seres humanos e de muitos animais herbívoros; utilizado terapeuticamente na forma de seus sais (hipuratos de cálcio e de amônio). [G. *hippos,* cavalo + *ouron,* urina]

hip·pu·ri·case (hi-pūr′i-cās). Hipuricase. SIN aminoacylase.

hip·pus (hip′ŭs). Atetose pupilar; dilatação e constrição pupilares intermitentes, independentes da iluminação, convergência ou estímulos psíquicos. [G. *hippos,* cavalo, de uma sugestão imaginária de movimentos de galope]

  respiratory h., dilatação das pupilas que ocorre durante a inspiração voluntária forçada e contração pupilar durante a expiração.

hir·ci. Hircos. Plural de hircus.

hir·cis·mus (her-siz′mŭs). Hircismo; odor desagradável das axilas. [L. *hircus,* bode]

hir·cus, gen. e pl. **hir·ci** (her′kŭs, her′sī). **1.** Hirco; o cheiro das axilas. **2.** [TA]. Pêlos axilares. SIN axillary hairs, em hair. **3.** Trago. SIN tragus (1). [L. bode]

Hirschberg, Julius, oftalmologista alemão, 1843–1925. VER H. *method.*

Hirschfeld, Isador, dentista norte-americano, 1881–1965. VER H. *canals,* em *canal.*

Hirsch-Peiffer stain. Coloração de Hirsch-Peiffer. Ver em stain.

Hirschsprung, Harald, médico dinamarquês, 1830–1916. VER H. *disease.*

hir·sute (her-soot′). Hirsuto; relativo a, ou caracterizado por, hirsutismo. [L. *hirsutus,* peludo]

hir·su·ti·es (her-su′tē-ēz). Hirsutismo. SIN hirsutism. [L. Mod. fr. L. *hirsutus,* peludo]

hir·sut·ism (her′soo-tizm). Hirsutismo; presença excessiva de pêlos corporais e faciais, geralmente num padrão masculino, especialmente nas mulheres; pode ocorrer em adultos normais como expressão de uma característica étnica, ou desenvolver-se em crianças ou adultos em consequência de excesso de andrôgenios, devido a tumores, drogas ou a drogas não-androgênicas. SIN hirsuties, pilosis. [L. *hirsutus,* peludo]

  constitutional h., h. constitucional; grau leve a moderado de hirsutismo presente num indivíduo cujas funções endócrinas e reprodutoras são normais sob os demais aspectos.

  idiopathic h., h. idiopático; hirsutismo de origem incerta em mulheres, que, além disso, exibiriam anormalidades menstruais e infertilidade.

hir·tel·lous (hīr′te-lŭs). Hirteloso; que possui ou que se assemelha a pêlos finos; termo utilizado para descrever o polissacarídeo proteico filamentoso que recobre as microvilosidades. VER glycocalyx. [L. *hirtus,* cabeludo, peludo]

hir·u·di·cide (hi-roo′di-sīd). Hirudicida; agente que mata sanguessugas. [L. *hirudo,* sanguessuga + *caedo,* matar]

hir·u·din (hir′ū-din). Hirudina; substância antitrombínica extraída das glândulas salivares da sanguessuga e que tem a propriedade de impedir a coagulação do sangue. [L. *hirudo,* sanguessuga]

Hir·u·din·ea (hir′oo-din′ē-ǎ). As sanguessugas, uma classe de vermes (filo Annelida) com corpo segmentado achatado, uma ventosa na extremidade posterior e, com frequência, uma ventosa menor na extremidade anterior; são predadoras de tecidos de invertebrados ou alimentam-se do sangue e dos exsudatos teciduais de vertebrados. [L. *hirudo,* sanguessuga]

hir·u·di·ni·a·sis (hi-roo-di-nī′ǎ-sis). Hirudiníase; condição resultante da fixação de sanguessugas à pele ou de sua entrada pela boca ou nariz durante a ingestão de líquido. [L. *hirudo,* sanguessuga + G. *-iasis,* condição]

hir·u·din·i·za·tion (hi-roo′di-ni-zā′shun). Hirudinização. **1.** Processo de tornar o sangue incoagulável pela injeção de hirudina. **2.** A aplicação de sanguessugas.

Hir·u·do (hi-roo′dō). Gênero de sanguessugas (classe Hirudinea, família Gnathobdellidae). As espécies antigamente utilizadas em medicina são: *H. australis,* a sanguessuga australiana; *H. decora,* a sanguessuga americana; *H. interrupta* ou *H. troctina,* uma sanguessuga do norte da África; *H. medicinalis,* a sanguessuga mosqueada sueca ou alemã, a espécie anteriormente de uso mais generalizado; *H. m. officinalis,* uma variedade da precedente; *H. provincialis,* a sanguessuga verde ou húngara; *H. quinquestriata,* a sanguessuga com cinco estrias. [L. sanguessuga]

His, Wilhelm, Jr., médico alemão, 1863–1934. VER H. *band, bundle,* bundle *electrogram, spindle;* Kent-H. *bundle;* H.-Tawara *system.*

His, Wilhelm, Sr., anatomista e embriologista suíço na Alemanha, 1831–1904. VER H. *copula, line,* perivascular *space; isthmus* of H.

His–, –His– His. Símbolo de histidyl (histidil).

–His His. Símbolo de histidino (histidino).

His His. Símbolo de histidine (histidina).

Hiss, Philip, bacteriologista norte-americano, 1868–1913. VER H. *stain.*

his·ta·mi·nase (his-tam′i-nās). Histaminase. SIN amine oxidase (copper-containing).

his·ta·mine (H) (his′tǎ-mēn). Histamina; amina vasodepressora derivada da histidina pela ação da histidina descarboxilase, encontrada no esporão do centeio e em tecidos de animais. Trata-se de um poderoso estimulante da secreção gástrica, de um constritor da musculatura lisa brônquica e de um vasodilatador (capilares e arteríolas) que provoca queda da pressão arterial. A h., ou uma substância de ação indistinguível, é liberada na pele em consequência de lesão. Quando injetada por via intradérmica em alta diluição, provoca a resposta tríplice.

  h. phosphate, fosfato de h.; utilizado no tratamento de certas alergias, cefalgia e esclerose múltipla aguda, com resultados variáveis; também utilizado para avaliar a função secretora gástrica, no diagnóstico de feocromocitoma e no tratamento da doença de Ménière; também disponível na forma de fosfato ácido de h.

his·ta·mine-fast. Histamina-resistente; indica ausência de resposta normal à histamina, especialmente no que concerne à verdadeira falta de acidez gástrica.

his·ta·mi·ne·mia (his′tǎ-mi-nē′mē-ǎ). Histaminemia; presença de histamina no sangue circulante. [histamina + G. *haima,* sangue]

his·ta·mi·nu·ria (his′tǎ-mi-noo′rē-ǎ). Histaminúria; excreção de histamina na urina. [histamina + G. *ouron,* urina]

his·tan·gic (his-tan′jik). Histângico. SIN histoangic.

his·ti·dase (his′ti-dās). Histidase. SIN histidine ammonia-lyase.

his·ti·din·al (his′ti-din-āl). Histidinal; análogo aldeído da histidina (−CHO substituindo −COOH).

his·ti·di·nase (his′ti-di-nās). Histidinase. SIN histidine ammonia-lyase.

his·ti·dine (H, His) (his′ti-dēn). Histidina; ácido α-amino-β-(4-imidazolil)-propiônico; o L-isômero de um aminoácido básico encontrado na maioria das

histamina	
receptores H₁	receptores H₂
pulmão	
contração dos músculos brônquicos (seres humanos)	relaxamento dos músculos brônquicos (ovelhas)
coração/sistema circulatório	
efeito batmotrópico positivo efeito dromotrópico positivo vasoconstrição (vasos < 80 μm)	efeito inotrópico positivo efeito cronotrópico positivo
vasodilatação (vasos > 80 μm)	
distribuição da adrenalina contração endotelial e, portanto, aumento da permeabilidade (edema tecidual)	
útero	
contração (cobaia)	relaxamento (rato)
intestino	
contração	
estômago	
	aumento da secreção de ácido

proteínas. Trata-se de um aminoácido nutricionalmente essencial nos mamíferos.
  h. ammonia-lyase, h. amônia-liase; enzima que catalisa a desaminação da L-histidina a urocanato e amônia; essa enzima está ausente ou deficiente em indivíduos com histidinemia. SIN histidase, histidinase, h. deaminase.
  h. deaminase, h. desaminase. SIN h. ammonia-lyase.
  h. decarboxylase, h. descarboxilase; enzima que catalisa a descarboxilação piridoxal fosfato-dependente da L-histidina em histamina e CO_2; por conseguinte, participa na constrição do músculo liso brônquico.
his·ti·di·ne·mia (his′ti-di-nē′mē-a). [MIM*235800]. Histidinemia; distúrbio metabólico caracterizado por defeitos da fala, deficiência de crescimento e leve retardo mental em alguns pacientes; associado a elevação dos níveis sanguíneos de histidina e excreção de histidina e metabólitos imidazólicos relacionados na urina, devido à deficiência de histidina amônia-liase ou histidinase; herança autossômica recessiva causada por uma mutação no gene da histidinase (HIS) no cromossoma 12q. [histidina + G. *haima,* sangue + -ia]
his·ti·dino (–His) (his′ti-din-ō). Histidino; o radical da histidina produzido pela remoção de um hidrogênio do átomo de nitrogênio; com prefixo $N^α$, $N^τ$ ou $N^π$.
his·ti·di·nol (his′ti-di-nol). Histidinol; o álcool análogo da histidina (−COOH transforma-se em −CH_2OH)
his·ti·di·nu·ria (his′ti-di-noo′rē-a). Histidinúria; excreção de quantidades consideráveis de histidina na urina; freqüentemente observada nos últimos meses de gravidez, bem como na histidinemia.
his·ti·dyl (His–) (his′ti-dil). Histidil; o radical acil da histidina.
△ **histio-.** Histio-; tecido; especialmente o tecido conjuntivo. [G. *histion,* tecido]
his·ti·o·blast (his′tē-ō-blast). Histioblasto; célula formadora de tecido. SIN histoblast. [histio- + G. *blastos,* germe]
his·ti·o·cyte (his′tē-ō-sīt). Histiócito; macrófago tecidual; a classe inclui células de Kupffer hepáticas, macrófagos alveolares, células gigantes de granulomas, osteoclastos e células de Langerhans da derme. Essas células originam-se de precursores que, normalmente, residem na medula óssea, mas que migram através da corrente sanguínea para penetrarem nos tecidos, para diferenciação final. SIN histocyte. [histio- + G. *kytos,* célula]
  cardiac h., h. cardíaco; grande célula mononuclear encontrada no tecido conjuntivo da parede cardíaca em condições inflamatórias, especialmente no corpúsculo de Aschoff. O núcleo ovóide contém uma massa de cromatina central que aparece como uma barra ondulada em corte longitudinal. SIN Anitschkow cell, Anitschkow myocyte, caterpillar cell.
  sea-blue h., h. azul-marinho; um histiócito contendo grânulos citoplasmáticos que se coram de azul brilhante com corantes hematológicos, como o Wright-Giemsa; encontrado na medula óssea e no baço, associado a hepatoesplenomegalia e púrpura trombocitopênica, bem como em outras doenças hematológicas.
his·ti·o·cy·to·ma (his′tē-ō-sī-tō′mā). Histiocitoma; tumor composto de histiócitos. [histio- + G. *kytos,* célula + *-ōma,* tumor]
  fibrous h., h. fibroso. SIN dermatofibroma; VER dermatofibroma.
  generalized eruptive h., h. eruptivo generalizado; erupção generalizada recorrente rara em adultos, de pápulas eritematosas ou cor da carne, que permanecem localizadas na pele e consistem em nódulos dérmicos de histiócitos mononucleares que não se coram para lipídios. SIN nodular non-X histiocytosis.
  malignant fibrous h., h. fibroso maligno; sarcoma de potencial maligno variável, que ocorre mais freqüentemente nos membros e no retroperitônio; com freqüência, sofre recidiva local após ressecção e, menos comumente, metastatiza; exibe diferenciação histiocítica e fibroblástica parcial, com padrão em roda de carroça variável, áreas mixóides e células gigantes.
his·ti·o·cy·to·sis (his′tē-ō-sī-tō′sis). Histiocitose; proliferação generalizada de histiócitos. SIN histocytosis.
  Langerhans cell h., h. de células de Langerhans; um conjunto de distúrbios estreitamente unificados por um elemento proliferante comum, a célula de Langerhans. São reconhecidas três síndromes clínicas superpostas: uma doença afetando um único local (granuloma eosinofílico), um processo unissistêmico multifocal (síndrome de Hand-Schüller-Christian) e uma histiocitose multissistêmica multifocal (síndrome de Letter-Siwe). Antigamente, esse processo era conhecido como histiocitose X. SIN h. X.
  lipid h., h. lipídica; histiocitose com acúmulo citoplasmático de lipídios, consistindo em fosfolipídios (doença de Niemann-Pick) ou glicocerebrosídeos (doença de Gaucher).
  malignant h., h. maligna; forma rapidamente fatal de linfoma, caracterizada por febre, icterícia, pancitopenia e aumento de tamanho do fígado, do baço e dos linfonodos; os órgãos acometidos exibem necrose focal e hemorragia, com proliferação de histiócitos e fagocitose de eritrócitos.
  nodular non-X h., h. nodular não-X. SIN generalized eruptive *histiocytoma.*
  nonlipid h., h. não-lipídica. SIN Letterer–Siwe *disease.*
  sinus h. with massive lymphadenopathy, h. sinusal com linfadenopatia maciça; doença crônica que ocorre em crianças, caracterizada por linfadenopatia cervical maciça indolor, devido à distensão dos seios linfáticos por macrófagos contendo linfócitos ingeridos e por fibrose capsular e pericapsular. SIN Rosai-Dorfman disease.
  h. X, h. X. SIN Langerhans cell h.
  h. Y, h. Y. SIN verrucous *xanthoma.*
his·ti·o·gen·ic (his′tē-ō-jen′ik). Histiogênico. SIN histogenous.
his·ti·oid (his′tē-oyd). Histióide. SIN histoid.
his·ti·o·ma (his-tē-ō′mā). Histioma. SIN histoma.
his·ti·on·ic (his-tē-on′ik). Histiônico; relativo a qualquer tecido.
△ **histo-.** Histo-. Tecido. [G. *histos,* web (tecido)]
his·to·an·gic (his-tō-an′jik). Histoângico; relativo à estrutura dos vasos sanguíneos, especialmente em termos de sua função. SIN histangic. [histo- + G. *angeion,* vaso]
his·to·blast (his′tō-blast). Histoblasto. SIN histioblast.
his·to·chem·is·try (his′tō-kem′is-trē). Histoquímica. SIN cytochemistry.
his·to·com·pat·i·bil·i·ty (his′tō-kom-pat-i-bil′i-tē). Histocompatibilidade; um estado de semelhança (ou identidade) imunológica que permite a realização bem-sucedida de transplante de homoenxerto.
his·to·cyte (his′tō-sīt). Histiócito. SIN histiocyte.
his·to·cy·to·sis (his′tō-sī-tō′sis). Histiocitose. SIN histiocytosis.
his·to·dif·fer·en·ti·a·tion (his′tō-dif-er-en-shē-ā′shŭn). Histodiferenciação; o aparecimento morfológico de características teciduais durante o desenvolvimento.
his·to·flu·o·res·cence (his-tō-flōr-es′ens). Histofluorescência; fluorescência dos tecidos com exposição aos raios ultravioleta após a injeção de uma substância fluorescente ou em conseqüência de uma substância fluorescente natural.
his·to·gen·e·sis (his-tō-jen′e-sis). Histogênese; a origem de tecido; a formação e o desenvolvimento dos tecidos do organismo. SIN histogeny. [histo- + G. *genesis,* origem]
his·to·ge·net·ic (his-tō-jĕ-net′ik). Histogenético; relativo à histogênese.
his·tog·e·nous (his-toj′e-nŭs). Histogênico; formado pelos tecidos; p. ex., as células histogênicas, num exsudato, que se originam da proliferação das células teciduais fixas. SIN histiogenic. [histo- + G. *-gen,* produzindo]
his·tog·e·ny (his-toj′ĕ-nē). Histogenia. SIN histogenesis.
his·to·gram (his′tō-gram). Histograma. **1.** Representação gráfica em colunas ou barras para comparar magnitudes de freqüências ou número de itens. **2.** Representação gráfica da distribuição da freqüência de uma variável em que os retângulos são traçados com as suas bases numa escala linear uniforme, representando intervalos, sendo as suas alturas proporcionais aos valores em cada um dos intervalos. [histo- + G. *gramma,* escrita]
his·toid (his′toyd). Históide. **1.** Semelhante, em termos de estrutura, a um dos tecidos do organismo. **2.** Termo algumas vezes utilizado para referir-se à estrutura histológica de uma neoplasia derivada de um único tipo relativamente simples de tecido neoplásico, que se assemelha estreitamente ao tecido normal, como em certos fibromas e leiomiomas. SIN histioid. [histo- + G. *eidos,* semelhança]
his·to·in·com·pat·i·bil·i·ty (his′tō-in′kom-pat-i-bil′i-tē). Histoincompatibilidade; um estado de falta de semelhança imunológica de tecidos suficiente para causar a rejeição de um homoenxerto quando o tecido é transplantado de um indivíduo para outro; implica uma diferença nos genes de histocompatibilidade entre doador e receptor.
his·to·log·ic, his·to·log·i·cal (his-tō-log′ik, i-kăl). Histológico; relativo à histologia.
his·tol·o·gist (his-tol′ō-jist). Histologista; indivíduo especializado na ciência da histologia. SIN microanatomist.
his·tol·o·gy (his-tol′o-jē). Histologia; a ciência relacionada com a ultra-estrutura das células, dos tecidos e dos órgãos em relação à sua função. VER microscopic *anatomy.* SIN microanatomy. [histo- + G. *logos,* estudo]
  pathologic h., histopatologia. SIN histopathology.
his·tol·y·sis (his-tol′i-sis). Histólise; desintegração de tecidos. [histo- + G. *lysis,* dissolução]
his·to·ma (his-tō′mā). Histoma; neoplasia benigna cujos elementos citológicos e histológicos assemelham-se muito àqueles do tecido normal do qual derivam as células neoplásicas. SIN histioma. [histo- + G. *-oma,* tumor]
his·to·met·a·plas·tic (his′tō-met-ā-plas′tik). Histometaplásico; que estimula a metaplasia tecidual.
his·to·mor·phom·e·try (his′tō-mōr-fom′e-trē). Histomorfometria; a medida quantitativa e a caracterização de imagens microscópicas utilizando um computador; a análise da imagem digital, manual ou automatizada, envolve tipicamente medidas e comparações de áreas geométricas selecionadas, perímetros, comprimento, ângulo de orientação, fatores morfológicos, centro de gravidade, coordenadas, bem como ampliação da imagem. [histo- + G. *morphē,* forma + *metron,* medida]
his·tone (H) (his′tōn). Histona; uma de várias proteínas simples (freqüentemente encontradas no núcleo celular) contendo uma alta proporção de aminoácidos básicos; são solúveis em água, ácidos diluídos e álcalis e não são coaguláveis pelo calor; p. ex., as proteínas associadas aos ácidos nucleicos nos núcleos de tecidos vegetais e animais. Constituem cerca da metade da massa dos cromossomas das células eucarióticas.
his·to·nec·to·my (his-tō-nek′tō-mē). Histonectomia. SIN periarterial *sympathectomy.* [histo- + G. *ektomē,* excisão]

his·to·neu·rol·o·gy (his-tō-noo-rol′ō-jē). Histoneurologia. SIN neurohistology.

his·ton·o·my (his-ton′ō-mē). Histonomia; uma lei do desenvolvimento e da estrutura dos tecidos do organismo. [histo- + G. *nomos*, lei]

his·to·nu·ria (his-tō-noo′rē-ā). Histonúria; excreção de histona na urina, como a que ocorre em certos casos de leucemia, doenças febris e doenças debilitantes. [histona + G. *ouron*, urina]

his·to·path·o·gen·e·sis (his′tō-path-ō-jen′e-sis). Histopatogênese; desenvolvimento embrionário ou crescimento anormais de tecido. [histogênese + patogênese]

his·to·pa·thol·o·gy (his′tō-pa-thol′ō-jē). Histopatologia; a ciência ou o estudo que trata da estrutura citológica e histológica do tecido anormal ou doente. SIN pathologic histology.

his·to·phys·i·ol·o·gy (his′tō-fiz-ē-ol′ō-jē). Histofisiologia; o estudo microscópico dos tecidos em relação às suas funções.

His·to·plas·ma cap·su·la·tum (his-tō-plaz′mā kap-soo-lā′tŭm). Espécie de fungo dimórfico, de distribuição mundial, que provoca histoplasmose nos seres humanos e em outros mamíferos; no seu estado de ascomiceto, é denominado *Ajellomyces capsulatum*. O habitat natural desse microrganismo é o solo fertilizado com dejetos de aves e morcegos, onde cresce na forma de bolor, cujos fragmentos, após inalação, produzem infecção pulmonar primária; nos tecidos do hospedeiro mamífero, os fragmentos inalados de micélios crescem como leveduras uninucleares, que se reproduzem por brotamento. Essa forma parasitária também pode ser induzida em laboratório mediante cultura da fase de micélio a 37°C em meio enriquecido com sangue; o crescimento reverte à forma de micélio quando a temperatura se torna inferior a 37°C. *H. c.* var. *duboisii* causa uma doença clinicamente distinta, a histoplasmose africana, na qual são encontradas grandes células leveduriformes com paredes mais espessas nos tecidos, em contraste com as pequenas células leveduriformes de *H. c.* var. *farciminosum*, que causam linfangite epizoótica. [histo- + G. *plasma*, algo formado]

his·to·plas·min (his′tō-plas′min). Histoplasmina; extrato antigênico de *Histoplasma capsulatum*, utilizado em testes imunológicos para o diagnóstico da histoplasmose; também utilizado em testes cutâneos na análise de populações para determinar a distribuição geográfica do fungo e prever aqueles que são endêmicos para a histoplasmose.

his·to·plas·mo·ma (his′tō-plaz-mō-mā). Histoplasmoma; granuloma infeccioso causado por *Histoplasma capsulatum*.

his·to·plas·mo·sis (his′tō-plaz-mō′sis). Histoplasmose; doença infecciosa amplamente distribuída, causada por *Histoplasma capsulatum*, que ocorre algumas vezes em surtos; geralmente adquirida por inalação de esporos do fungo na poeira do solo e manifestada por pneumonia autolimitada. Em pacientes com enfisema, a infecção pode ser crônica e causar doença fibrocavitária pulmonar, assemelhando-se à tuberculose; em pacientes imunossuprimidos e, raramente, em pacientes normais, a histoplasmose pode causar doença disseminada do sistema reticuloendotelial, que se manifesta por febre, emagrecimento, esplenomegalia e leucopenia. SIN Darling disease.
  acute h., h. aguda; causada pela inalação de microconídeos, resultando em doença que varia desde uma doença gripal até pneumonite difusa aguda observada com exposição maciça. Com freqüência, após doença as lesões cicatrizam, deixando nódulos calcificados.
  African h., h. africana; uma forma de histoplasmose causada pelo fungo *Histoplasma capsulatum* var. *duboisii*, observada apenas na África tropical; a infecção manifesta-se como lesões granulomatosas crônicas no osso, na pele e em outros órgãos.
  chronic h., h. crônica; doença habitualmente observada em pacientes com anormalidade subjacente do parênquima pulmonar, particularmente enfisema e doença pulmonar bolhosa. A doença é de evolução indolente, caracterizada por tosse e produção de escarro e, radiograficamente, por perda gradual do volume pulmonar.
  chronic mediastinal h., h. mediastinal crônica; fibrose mediastinal causada pelo comprometimento de linfonodos por histoplasmose. Pode produzir uma enorme massa fibrótica afetando muitas estruturas importantes no mediastino.
  disseminated h., h. disseminada; infecção disseminada que acomete muitos órgãos; ocorre em lactentes e em pacientes imunocomprometidos, como indivíduos com AIDS/SIDA.
  presumed ocular h., h. ocular presumida; neovascularização sub-retiniana na região macular, associada a atrofia coriorretiniana e proliferação de pigmento adjacente ao disco óptico, com atrofia coriorretiniana periférica.

his·to·ra·di·og·ra·phy (his′tō-rā-dē-og′rā-fē). Historradiografia; radiografia de tecido, particularmente de cortes microscópicos; em geral, microrradiografia.

his·tor·rhex·is (his-tō-rek′sis). Historrexe; ruptura de tecido por algum agente diferente de infecção. [histo- + G. *rhexis*, ruptura]

his·to·tome (his′tō-tōm). Histótomo. SIN microtome. [histo- + G. *tomē*, corte]

his·tot·o·my (his-tot′ō-mē). Histotomia. SIN microtomy.

his·to·tope (his′tō-tōp). Histótopo; parte da molécula de histocompatibilidade principal da Classe II que interage com o receptor de células T. [histo- + -topo]

his·to·tox·ic (his-tō-tok′sik). Histotóxico; relativo à intoxicação do sistema enzimático respiratório dos tecidos.

his·to·troph (his′tō-trof). Histotrofo; a parte da nutrição do embrião derivada de fontes celulares diferentes do sangue. Cf. embryotroph, hemotroph.

his·to·tro·phic (his-tō-trof′ik). Histotrófico; que fornece nutrição ou que favorece a formação de tecido. [histo- + G. *trophē*, nutrição]

his·to·tro·pic (his-tō-trop′ik). Histotrópico; atraído para os tecidos, refere-se a certos parasitas, corantes e compostos químicos. [histo- + G. *tropikos*, uma volta]

his·to·zo·ic (his-tō-zō′ik). Histozóico; que vive nos tecidos, fora de um corpo celular; refere-se a certos protozoários parasitas. [histo- + G. *zōikos*, relativo a um animal]

his·to·zyme (his′tō-zīm). Histozima. SIN aminoacylase.

hitch·hik·er (hitch′hik-er). "Carona"; um gene que não possui nenhuma vantagem seletiva ou que pode ser até mesmo prejudicial, mas que se torna temporariamente disseminado em virtude de estar muito ligado e acoplado a um gene bastante vantajoso, que é fortemente selecionado.

Hitzig, Eduard, psiquiatra alemão, 1838–1907. VER H. *girdle*.

HIV. Abreviatura de human immunodeficiency *virus* (vírus da imunodeficiência humana).

HIV-1. Abreviatura de human immunodeficiency virus-1 (vírus da imunodeficiência humana 1).

HIV-2. Abreviatura de human immunodeficiency virus-2 (vírus da imunodeficiência humana 2). VER human immunodeficiency *virus*.

hives (hīvz). **1.** Urticária. SIN urticaria. **2.** Pápula. SIN wheal.
  giant h., u. gigante. SIN angioedema.

hK3. Abreviatura de human glandular *kallikrein* 3 (calicreína glandular humana 3).

HL-7. Abreviatura de Health Level 7 (Nível de Saúde 7), um padrão de informática médica que facilita a comunicação entre diferentes sistemas digitais.

HLA Abreviatura de human leukocyte *antigens* (antígenos leucocitários humanos), em *antigen*.

HMB-45. Anticorpo contra uma glicoproteína pré-melanossoma encontrada em melanomas e em outros tumores derivados de melanócitos.

HME Abreviatura de human monocytic *ehrlichiosis* (ehrliquiose monocítica humana).

HMG, hMG Abreviatura de human menopausal *gonadotropin* (gonadotropina menopáusica humana).

HMG-CoA Abreviatura de β-hydroxy-β-methylglutaryl-CoA (β-hidroxi-β-metilglutaril-CoA).

HMO. Abreviatura de hypothetical mean *organism* (organismo médio hipotético); health maintenance *organization* (organização de manutenção de saúde).

HMPAO Abreviatura de hexametazime ou hexamethylpropyleneamine oxime (hexametazima ou hexametilpropilenoneamina oxima).

HMS Abreviatura de hypothetical mean *strain* (cepa média hipotética).

HN2 Símbolo de nitrogen mustard (mostarda nitrogenada). VER nitrogen *mustards*, em *mustard*.

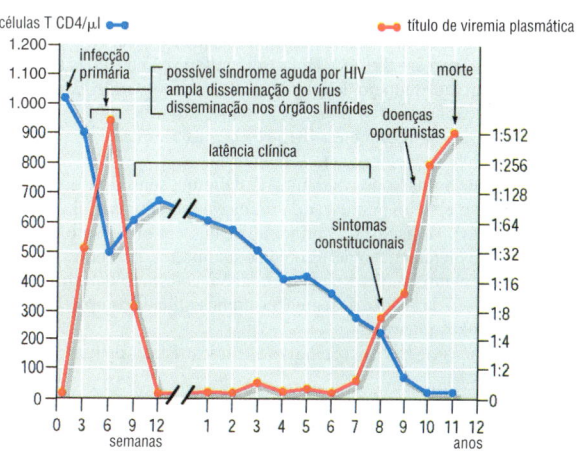

infecção por HIV: evolução típica: durante o período inicial, após infecção primária, ocorre ampla disseminação do vírus, e verifica-se redução acentuada no número de células T CD4 no sangue periférico; surge uma resposta imune ao HIV, com diminuição da viremia detectável, seguida de um período prolongado de latência clínica; os ensaios sensíveis para o RNA viral detectam o vírus no plasma em todas essas fases; a contagem de células T CD4 continua diminuindo durante os anos seguintes até atingir um nível crítico abaixo do qual surge um risco significativo de doenças oportunistas

hnRNA Abreviatura de heterogeneous nuclear RNA (RNA nuclear heterogêneo).
Ho Símbolo do holmium (hólmio).
Hoagland sign. Sinal de Hoagland. Ver em sign.
hoarse (hōrs). Rouco; que possui voz rouca. [A.S. *hās*]
hoarse·ness (hōrs′nes). Rouquidão, traquifonia; alteração do timbre, da tonalidade ou da altura da voz, que se torna mais grave.
Hoboken, Nicholaus van, anatomista e médico holandês, 1632–1678. VER H. *gemmules,* em *gemmule, nodules,* em *nodule, valves,* em *valve.*
HOCA Abreviatura de high osmolar contrast agent (agente de contraste com alta osmolaridade). SIN HOCM.
Hoche, Alfred E., psiquiatra alemão, 1865–1943. VER H. *bundle, tract.*
HOCM Abreviatura de high osmolar contrast medium (meio de contraste com alta osmolaridade). SIN HOCA.
Hodge, Hugh L., ginecologista norte-americano, 1796–1873. VER H. *pessary.*
Hodgkin, Alan L., fisiologista inglês e ganhador do Prêmio Nobel, *1914. VER Goldman-H. –Katz *equation.*
Hodgkin, Thomas, médico inglês, 1798–1866. VER H. *disease;* H.-Key *murmur;* non-H. *lymphoma.*
Hodgson, Joseph, médico inglês, 1788–1869. VER H. *disease.*
ho·do·neu·ro·mere (hō - dō - noo′rō - mēr). Hodoneurômero; em embriologia, termo obsoleto para referir-se a um segmento metamérico do tubo neural, com seu par de nervos e seus ramos. [G. *hodos,* via + *neuron,* nervo + *meros,* parte]
ho·do·pho·bia (hō - dō - fō′bē - ǎ). Hodofobia; temor mórbido de viajar. [G. *hodos,* via + *phobos,* medo]
HOECHST 33258. Corante dibenzimidazólico empregado em citoquímica e microscopia de fluorescência como um indicador sensível de DNA nos cromossomas, especificamente heterocromatina constitutiva.
Hoeppli, Reinhard J.C., parasitologista alemão, 1893–1973. VER Splendore-H. *phenomenon.*
hof (hōf). A cavidade no citoplasma de uma célula que aloja o núcleo. [Al. pátio]
Hofbauer, J. Isfred I., ginecologista norte-americano, 1878–1961. VER H. *cell.*
Hoffa, Albert, cirurgião alemão, 1859–1907. VER H. *operation.*
Hoffman, August Wilhelm, químico alemão, 1818–1892. VER Frei-Hoffmann *reaction,* Hoffman *violet.*
Hoffmann, Friedrich (Fredericus), médico alemão, 1660–1742. Professor de Anatomia e Cirurgia em Halle, reputado pelas suas observações clínicas sobre várias doenças infecciosas.
Hoffmann, Johann, neurologista alemão, 1857–1919. VER H. muscular *atrophy, phenomenon, reflex, sign;* Werdnig-H. *disease;* Werdnig-Hoffmann muscular *atrophy.*
Hoffmann, Moritz, anatomista alemão, 1622–1698. VER H. *duct.*
Hofmann (Hofmann-Wellenhof), Georg von, bacteriologista austríaco, 1843–1890. VER H. *bacillus.*
Hofmeister, Franz, bioquímico alemão, 1850–1922. VER H. *series, gastrectomy.*
Hofmeister, Franz von, cirurgião alemão, 1867–1926. VER H. *operation;* H.-Pólya *anastomosis.*
Hog·ben, Lawrence, matemático inglês, *1895. VER H. *number.*
Hogness, D.S., biologista molecular norte-americano, *1925. VER Grunstein-H. *assay;* H. *box.*
hol·an·dric (hol - an′drik). Holândrico; relativo a genes localizados no cromossoma Y. [G. *holos,* inteiro + *aner,* homem]
hol·ar·thrit·ic (hol-ar-thrit′ik). Holartrítico; relativo à holartrite.
hol·ar·thri·tis (hol - ar - thrī′tis). Holartrite; inflamação de todas as articulações ou de um grande número delas. [G. *holos,* inteiro + *arthron,* articulação + *-itis,* inflamação]
Holden, Luther, anatomista inglês, 1815–1905. VER H. *line.*
Holder. VER Virchow-Holder *angle.*
hole in ret·i·na. Solução de continuidade da retina sensorial, permitindo a separação entre o epitélio pigmentar da retina e a retina sensorial.
ho·lism (hō′lizm). Holismo. **1.** O princípio de que um organismo ou uma de suas ações não é meramente igual à soma de suas partes, devendo ser percebido ou estudado como um todo. **2.** A abordagem ao estudo de um fenômeno psicológico através da análise de fenômeno como entidade completa em si. Cf. atomism. [G. *holos,* inteiro]
ho·lis·tic (hō - lis′tik). Holístico; relativo às características do holismo ou psicologias holísticas.
Holl, Mortiz, cirurgião austríaco, 1852–1920. VER H. *ligament.*
Hollander, Franklin, fisiologista norte-americano, 1899–1966. VER H. *test.*
Hollenhorst, Robert W., oftalmologista norte-americano, *1913. VER H. *plaques,* em *plaque.*
Hol·li·day, R. VER H. *junction, structure.*
hol·low (hol′ō). Oco; uma concavidade ou depressão.
Sebileau h., oco de Sebileau; depressão entre a face inferior da língua e as glândulas sublinguais.
Holmes, Sir Gordon M., neurologista inglês, 1876–1965. VER H.-Adie *pupil, syndrome;* Stewart-H. *sign.*

Holmes, Oliver Wendell, médico norte-americano, 1809–1894, que identificou o modo de disseminação e o controle da febre puerperal.
Holmes, Thomas, psiquiatra norte-americano, *1918. VER H.-Rahe *questionnaire.*
Holmes, Walter Chapin, 1884–1932. VER H. *stain.*
Holmgren, Alarik Frithiof, fisiologista sueco, 1831–1897. VER H. wool *test.*
Holmgren, Emil A., histologista sueco, 1866–1922. VER Holmgren-Golgi *canals,* em *canal.*
hol·mi·um (Ho) (hol′mē - ŭm). Hólmio; elemento do grupo dos lantanídeos de número atômico 67, peso atômico 164,93032. [L. *Holmia,* de Stockholm]
△ **holo-.** Holo-; inteiro, completo. [G. *holos*]
hol·o·a·car·di·us (hol′ō - ǎ - kar′dē - ŭs). Holoacárdia; gêmeo separado, macroscopicamente defeituoso, que carece de coração, sendo seu suprimento sanguíneo dependente de uma derivação da circulação placentária de um gêmeo quase normal; gêmeo parasita placentário ou onfalósito. Cf. acardius. [holo- + G. *a-* priv. + *kardia,* coração]
  h. aceph′alus, h. acéfalo; holoacárdia que também não possui cabeça.
  h. amor′phus, h. amorfo; holoacárdia em que o corpo do parasita é representado apenas por uma massa informe. VER TAMBÉM anideus.
ho·lo-ACP syn·thase. Holo-ACP sintase; enzima que catalisa a transferência do resíduo 4′-fosfopanteteinil da coenzima A para uma serina de apo-ACP (proteína transportadora de acil) para formar holo-ACP, liberando 3′,5′-difosfato de adenosina; etapa necessária à biossíntese de ácidos graxos.
hol·o·a·cra·nia (hol′ō - ǎ - krā′nē - ǎ). Holoacrania; defeito congênito do crânio em que os ossos da abóbada estão ausentes. [holo- + G. *a-* priv. + *kranion,* crânio]
hol·o·an·en·ceph·a·ly (hol′ō - an - en - sef′ǎ - lē). Holoanencefalia; ausência completa do crânio e do cérebro. [holo- + G. *an-* priv. + *enkephalos,* cérebro]
hol·o·blas·tic (hol - ō - blas′tik). Holoblástico; refere-se à participação de todo o óvulo (isolécito ou moderadamente telolécito) na clivagem. [holo- + G. *blastos,* germe]
hol·o·car·box·y·lase syn·the·tase (hōl - ō - kar - boks′il - ās sen′thē - tās). Holocarboxilase sintetase; uma de várias enzimas que fazem a biotinilação de outras proteínas (p. ex., carboxilases); a deficiência de h. s. resulta em acidemia orgânica.
hol·o·ce·phal·ic (hol′ō - sē - fal′ik). Holocefálico; refere-se a um feto com uma cabeça completa, porém com deficiências em outras partes do corpo. [holo- + G. *kephale* cabeça]
hol·o·cord (hol′ō - kōrd). Holocorda; relativo a toda a medula espinal, estendendo-se desde a junção cervicobulbar até o cone medular.
hol·o·crine (hol′ō - krin). Holócrino. VER holocrine *gland.* [holo- + G. *krino,* separar]
hol·o·di·a·stol·ic (hol′ō - dī - ǎ - stol′ik). Holodiastólico; relativo a ou que ocupa todo o período diastólico.
hol·o·en·dem·ic (hol′ō - en - dem′ik). Holoendêmico; endêmico em toda população, como o tracoma nas aldeias da Arábia Saudita.
hol·o·en·zyme (hol - ō - en′zīm). Holoenzima; enzima completa, isto é, apoenzima mais coenzima, co-fator, íon metálico e/ou grupamento prostético.
hol·o·gas·tros·chi·sis (hol′ō - gas - tros′ki - sis). Hologastrosquise; malformação congênita em que uma fenda se estende por toda a extensão do abdome. [holo- + G. *gaster,* ventre + *schisis,* clivagem]
hol·o·gram (hol′ō - gram). Holograma; imagem tridimensional produzida por reconstrução da frente de onda e registrada numa chapa fotográfica. [holo- + G. *gramma,* algo escrito]
hol·og·ra·phy (hō - log′rǎ - fē). Holografia; processo de produzir um holograma.
hol·o·gyn·ic (hol - ō - jin′ik). Hologínico; relativo aos caracteres manifestados apenas em fêmeas. [holo- + G. *gyne,* mulher]
hol·o·mas·ti·gote (hol - ō - mas′ti - gōt). Holomastigota; que possui flagelos em toda a superfície. [holo- + G. *mastix,* chicote]
hol·o·me·tab·o·lous (hol′ō - me - tab′ō - lŭs). Holometábolo; pertencente a um membro dos Holometabola, várias ordens de insetos em que ocorre metamorfose complexa ou completa. [holo- + G. *metabole,* mudança]
hol·o·mi·ant·ic (in·fec·tion) (hol′ōm - ī - an - tik). Holomiântica (infecção); surto infeccioso devido à exposição de um grupo de indivíduos a determinado agente que afeta ou é comum a todos os membros do grupo. [holo + C. *miantos,* poluído, fr. *miaino,* poluir + *-ic*]
hol·o·mor·pho·sis (hol′ō - mōr - fō′sis). Holomorfose; termo raramente utilizado para referir-se ao que atinge ou restabelece a integridade física. [holo- + G. *morphosis,* forma]
hol·o·phyt·ic (hol - ō - fit′ik). Holofítico; semelhante a um vegetal no modo de obter nutrientes, denotando certos protozoários fotossintéticos, como, p. ex., *Euglena.* [holo- + G. *phyton,* planta]
hol·o·pros·en·ceph·a·ly (hol′ō - pros - en - sef′ǎ - lē). Holoprosencefalia; presença de um único hemisfério ou lobo no prosencéfalo; ocorre cicloplia na forma mais grave. Com freqüência, é acompanhada de déficit no desenvolvimento facial mediano. [holo- + G. *proso,* para frente + *enkephalos,* cérebro]
hol·o·pro·tein (hō - lō - prō - tēn). Holoproteína; proteína completa; isto é, apoproteína mais íon metálico e/ou grupamento prostético.

hol·o·ra·chis·chi·sis (hol'ō-ră-kis'ki-sis). Holorraquísquise; espinha bífida em toda a coluna vertebral. SIN araphia, rachischisis totalis. [holo- + G. *rhachis*, espinha + *schisis*, fissura]

hol·o·side (hŏl'ō-sīd). Holosídio; composto contendo um ou mais carboidratos idênticos ligados glicosidicamente.

hol·o·sys·tol·ic (hol'ō-sis-tol'ik). Holossistólico. SIN pansystolic.

hol·o·tel·en·ceph·a·ly (hol'ō-tel-en-sef'ă-lē). Holotelencefalia; holoprosencefalia associada a arrinencefalia. [holo- + telencéfalo]

hol·o·thur·ins (hōl-ō-thu'rins). Holoturinas; classe de glicosídeos esteróides sulfatados muito tóxicos, secretados por holotúrias (*Holothurioidea*).

ho·lot·ri·chous (ho-lot'ri-kŭs). Holotríquio; que possui cílios em toda a superfície. [holo- + G. *thrix*, pêlo]

hol·o·zo·ic (hol-ō-zō'ik). Holozóico; semelhante a um animal no modo de obter a sua nutrição, carecendo da capacidade de fotossíntese; refere-se a certos protozoários para diferenciá-los de outros que são holofíticos. [holo- + G. *zōon*, animal]

Holt, Mary, cardiologista inglesa do século XX. VER H.-Oram *syndrome*.

Holter, Norman, biofísico norte-americano, 1914–1983. VER H. *monitor*.

Holthouse, Carsten, cirurgião inglês, 1810–1901. VER H. *hernia*.

Holzknecht, Guido, radiologista austríaco, 1872–1931. VER H. *unit*.

hom·a·lo·ceph·a·lous (hom'ă-lō-sef'ă-lŭs). Homalocéfalo; que tem a cabeça achatada. [G. *homalos*, plano + *kephalē*, cabeça]

Ho·ma·lo·my·ia (hom'ă-lō-mī'yă). Gênero de moscas cujas larvas algumas vezes infestam o intestino dos seres humanos ou de animais. [G. *homalos*, plano + *myia*, mosca]

hom·a·lu·ria (hom-ă-loo'rē-ă). Homalúria; termo raramente utilizado para referir-se ao fluxo normal de urina. [G. *homalos*, nível + *ouron*, urina]

Homans, John, cirurgião norte-americano, 1877–1954. VER H. *sign*.

ho·mat·ro·pine (hō-mat'rō-pēn). Homatropina; agente anticolinérgico, midriático e ciclopégico; disponível na forma de bromidrato e metil bromide. SIN mandelytropine, tropine mandelate.

hom·ax·i·al (hō-mak'sē-ăl). Homoaxial; que possui todos os eixos iguais, como uma esfera. [G. *homos*, igual + *axis*]

Home, Sir Everard, cirurgião inglês, 1756–1832. VER H. *lobe*.

homeo-. Homeo-; o mesmo, semelhante. VER TAMBÉM homo- (1). [G. *homoios*, semelhante]

ho·me·o·box. *Homeoboxe!* seqüência de DNA bastante conservada de cerca de 180 pares de bases próximo à extremidade 3' de genes homeóticos específicos; codifica um domínio de ligação de DNA, permitindo que as proteínas do homeoboxe se liguem à expressão gênica no desenvolvimento e a regulem. SIN homeodomain.

ho·me·o·do·main (hō'mē-ō-dō-mān'). Homeodomain. SIN homeobox.

ho·me·o·met·ric (hō'mē-ō-met'rik). Homeométrico; sem alteração no tamanho. [homeo- + G. *metron*, medida]

ho·me·o·mor·phous (hō'mē-ō-mōr'fŭs). Homeomorfo; de forma semelhante, mas não necessariamente com a mesma composição. [homeo- + G. *morphē*, forma]

ho·me·o·path (hō'mē-ō-path). Homeopata. SIN homeopathist.

ho·me·o·path·ic (hō'mē-ō-path'ik). Homeopático. **1.** Relacionado à homeopatia. SIN homeotherapeutic (1). **2.** Refere-se a uma dose extremamente pequena de um agente farmacológico que, teoricamente, imita os sintomas produzidos pela condição que está sendo tratada, como a que pode ser utilizada em homeopatia; mais genericamente, uma dose supostamente muito pequena para produzir o efeito habitualmente esperado do agente. Forma alternativa de medicina em relação à alopatia, em que as drogas utilizadas antagonizam os efeitos da doença. Cf. pharmacologic (2), physiologic (4), supraphysiologic. [homeo- + G. *pathos*, doença]

ho·me·op·a·thist (hō-mē-op'ă-thist). Homeopata; médico que exerce a homeopatia. SIN homeopath.

ho·me·op·a·thy (hō-mē-op'ă-thē). Homeopatia; sistema de tratamento desenvolvido por Samuel Hahnemann, baseado na "lei da semelhança", do aforismo *similia similibus curantur* (os semelhantes são curados por semelhantes), que afirma que uma substância medicinal capaz de desencadear certos sintomas em indivíduos sadios seria efetiva no tratamento de doenças com sintomas semelhantes, se administrada em doses muito pequenas. [homeo- + G. *pathos*, sofrimento]

ho·me·o·pla·sia (hō'mē-ō-plā'zē-ă). Homeoplasia; formação de novo tecido do mesmo caráter daquele já existente na parte. SIN homoioplasia. [homeo- + G. *plasis*, moldagem]

ho·me·o·plas·tic (hō'mē-ō-plas'tik). Homeoplásico; relativo a, ou caracterizado por, homeoplasia.

ho·me·or·rhe·sis (hō'mē-ō-rē'sis). Homeorrese; o conjunto de processos pelos quais os desequilíbrios e outros defeitos em ontogenia são corrigidos antes que o desenvolvimento esteja completo. SIN ontogenic homeostasis, waddingtonian homeostasis. [homeo- + G. *rheos*, corrente]

ho·me·o·sis (hō-mē-ō'sis). Homeose; formação de uma parte do corpo com características normalmente encontradas numa parte correlata ou homóloga em outra localização no corpo. [homeo- + G. *-osis*, condição]

ho·me·o·sta·sis (hō'mē-ō-stā'sis, -os'tā-sis). Homeostasia. **1.** O estado de equilíbrio (equilíbrio entre pressões opostas) no corpo no que concerne a diversas funções e à composição química dos líquidos e tecidos. **2.** Os processos através dos quais é mantido esse equilíbrio corporal. [homeo- + G. *stasis*, parada]
Bernard-Cannon h., h. de Bernard-Cannon; o conjunto de mecanismos responsáveis pelo ajuste cibernético de estados fisiológicos e bioquímicos na vida pós-natal. SIN physiologic h.
genetic h., h. genética. SIN Lerner h.
Lerner h., h. de Lerner; os mecanismos restauradores que tendem a corrigir perturbações na composição genética de uma população. SIN genetic h.
ontogenic h., h. ontogênica. SIN homeorrhesis.
physiologic h., h. fisiológica. SIN Bernard-Cannon h.
waddingtonian h., h. de Waddington. SIN homeorrhesis.

ho·me·o·stat·ic (hō'mē-ō-stat'ik). Homeostático; relativo à homeostasia.

ho·me·o·ther·a·peu·tic (hō'mē-ō-thār-ă-pū'tik). Homeoterapêutico. **1.** SIN Homeopathic (1). **2.** Relativo à homeoterapia.

ho·me·o·ther·a·py, ho·me·o·ther·a·peu·tics (hō'mē-ō-thār'ă-pē, -thār-ă-pū'tiks). Homeoterapia; tratamento ou prevenção de uma doença utilizando os princípios da homeopatia.

ho·me·o·therm (hō'mē-ō-therm). Homeotermo; animais, incluindo mamíferos e aves, que tendem a manter uma temperatura corporal constante. SIN hematherm, warm-blooded animal. [homeo- + G. *thermos*, calor]

ho·me·o·ther·mal (hō'mē-ō-ther'mal). Homeotérmico. SIN homeothermic.

ho·me·o·ther·mic (hō'mē-ō-ther'mik). Homeotérmico; relativo a ou que possui a característica essencial de homeotermos. Cf. poikilothermic heterothermic. SIN hemathermal, hemathermous, hematothermal, homeothermal, homoiothermal, homothermal, warm-blooded.

ho·me·ot·ic (hō-mē-ot'ik). Homeótico; relativo a, ou caracterizado por, homeose.

ho·me·o·typ·i·cal (hō'mē-ō-tip'i-kăl). Homeotípico; que se assemelha ao tipo usual.

hom·er·gy (hom'er-jē). Homergia; termo obsoleto para referir-se ao metabolismo normal e seus resultados. [G. *homos*, igual + *ergon*, trabalho]

hom·i·cid·al (hom-i-sī'dăl). Homicida; que tem tendência a homicídio.

hom·i·cide (hom'i-sīd). Homicídio; a morte de um ser humano praticada por outro. [L. *homo*, homem + *caedo*, matar]

ho·mid·i·um bro·mide (hō-mid'ē-ŭm). Brometo de homídio; tripanocida utilizado em medicina veterinária. SIN ethidium.

Hom·in·i·dae (hō-min'i-dē). A família de primatas que inclui o homem moderno (*Homo sapiens*) e vários grupos fósseis.

Ho·mi·noi·dea (hō-mi-noy'dē-ă). Uma superfamília de primatas que inclui os macacos antropóides e o homem. Dividida nas famílias Pongidae (macacos antropóides) e Hominidae (seres humanos). [L. *homo* (*homin-*), homem + G. *eidos*, forma]

Ho·mo (hō'mō). Gênero de primatas que inclui os seres humanos. [L. homem]
H. sa'piens, o homem moderno. [L. homem inteligente]

homo-. Homo-. **1.** Forma combinante que significa igual, semelhante; oposto de hetero-. VER TAMBÉM homeo-. **2.** Em química, prefixo utilizado para indicar a inserção de mais um átomo de carbono numa cadeia (isto é, a inserção de um componente metileno). [G. *homos*, o mesmo]

ho·mo·ar·gi·nine (Har) (hō-mō-ar'ji-nēn). Homoarginina; homólogo da arginina que apresenta um grupamento metileno adicional.

ho·mo·bi·o·tin (hō-mō-bī'ō-tin). Homobiotina; composto que se assemelha à biotina, exceto pela substituição do enxofre por um átomo de oxigênio e presença de um grupamento CH_2 adicional na cadeia lateral; um antagonista ativo da biotina.

ho·mo·blas·tic (hō-mō-blas'tik). Homoblástico; que se desenvolve a partir de um único tipo de tecido. [homo- + G. *blastos*, germe]

ho·mo·car·no·sine (hō-mō-kar'nō-sēn). Homocarnosina; N^2-(4-aminobutiril)-L-histidina; constituinte do cérebro formado de L-histidina e ácido γ-aminobutírico.

ho·mo·car·no·sin·o·sis (hō-mō-kar'nō-sēn-ō-sis). Homocarnosinose; erro inato do metabolismo em que os níveis de homocarnosina estão elevados, sobretudo no líquido cefalorraquidiano.

ho·mo·cen·tric (hō'mō-sen'trik). Homocêntrico; que tem o mesmo centro; indica raios que se encontram num foco comum. Cf. heterocentric (1).

ho·moch·ro·nous (hō-mōk'rō-nŭs). Homócrono, homocrônico. **1.** SIN synchronous. **2.** Que ocorre na mesma idade em cada geração. [homo- + G. *chronos*, tempo]

ho·mo·cit·rul·li·nu·ria (hō-mō-sit'ru-lēn-oor'ē-ă). Homocitrulinúria; distúrbio herdado associado a níveis urinários elevados de homocitrulina.

ho·mo·clad·ic (hō-mō-klad'ik). Homocládico; refere-se à anastomose entre ramos do mesmo tronco arterial, em contraposição a heterocládico. [homo- + G. *klados*, um ramo]

ho·mo·cys·te·ine (Hcy) (hō-mō-sis'tē-ēn, -sis'tīn). Homocisteína; $HSCH_2CH_2CH(NH_3)+COO-$; um homólogo da cisteína, produzido pela desmetilação da metionina e intermediário na biossíntese de L-cisteína a partir da L-metionina através da L-cistationina. Níveis elevados de h. têm sido associados a certas formas de cardiopatia. VER TAMBÉM folic acid.

A elevação do nível de homocisteína no plasma constitui um fator de risco independente de doença cardiovascular (incluindo infarto do miocárdio, acidente vascular cerebral, doença tromboembólica e claudicação intermitente) e (em gestantes) de defeitos do tubo neural no feto, como espina bífida e anencefalia. Já foi relatado que o aumento nos níveis plasmáticos totais de homocisteína está associado a um risco independente de doença vascular, semelhante àquele do tabagismo ou da hiperlipidemia, complicando o risco associado ao tabagismo e hipertensão. Em cerca de 25% dos indivíduos com aterosclerose, observa-se uma elevação dos níveis plasmáticos de homocisteína acima de 15 mmol/L. Como os níveis de homocisteína aumentam após infarto do miocárdio e permanecem elevados por vários meses, algumas autoridades no assunto questionaram o papel causal atribuído a esse aumento na doença vascular. Diversos estudos prospectivos não conseguiram estabelecer qualquer conexão entre os níveis de homocisteína e o risco de coronariopatia. A homocisteína parece exercer um efeito tóxico direto sobre a íntima das artérias, além de induzir a oxidação das lipoproteínas de baixa densidade (LDL) e predispor à formação de trombos ao ativar as plaquetas e os fatores da coagulação. Em estudos de reprodução animal, promove defeitos do tubo neural, anomalias cardíacas e falha de fechamento ventral. Ocorre elevação dos níveis plasmáticos de homocisteína em diversas condições, incluindo distúrbios genéticos, deficiências nutricionais e doenças crônicas. Os níveis apresentam-se mais elevados nos homens e tendem a aumentar com o avançar da idade. A doença cardiovascular prematura foi associada pela primeira vez a elevação da homocisteína em indivíduos com homocistinúria, um raro distúrbio genético em que a deficiência da enzima cistationina β-sintase resulta em elevação dos níveis de homocisteína no plasma e de seu produto de oxidação, a homocistina, na urina. Um distúrbio genético mais comum associado a níveis anormalmente elevados de homocisteína resulta da mutação do gene que codifica a enzima metileno tetraidrofolato redutase. A acentuada elevação dos níveis de homocisteína que ocorre após a menopausa participaria na incidência aumentada de doença vascular, câncer e osteoporose nas mulheres pós-menopáusicas. A deficiência dietética de ácido fólico, vitamina B_6 (piridoxina) e vitamina B_{12} também está associada a elevação da homocisteína, da mesma forma que a insuficiência renal crônica, o hipotireoidismo e alguns processos malignos. Foi constatado que a redução da concentração sérica de homocisteína com a administração de ácido fólico diminui o risco de eventos cardiovasculares adversos em indivíduos com homocistinúria. Em estudos de animais, a administração de ácido fólico impede o efeito teratogênico da homocisteína. Aconselha-se a triagem dos níveis elevados de homocisteína em indivíduos com coronariopatia desproporcional aos fatores de risco conhecidos, bem como para aqueles com história familiar de doença aterosclerótica prematura. A administração de ácido fólico, numa dose de 1 mg/dia ou mais, reduz os níveis de homocisteína a valores quase normais e protege contra a doença vascular assim como contra os defeitos congênitos.

ho·mo·cys·tine (hō-mō-sis′tēn). Homocistina; o dissulfeto resultante da oxidação leve da homocisteína; um análogo da cistina.
ho·mo·cys·ti·ne·mia (hō′mō-sis-ti-nē′mē-ă). Homocistinemia; excesso de homocistina no plasma, como na homocistinúria.
ho·mo·cys·ti·nu·ria (hō′mō-sis-ti-noo′rē-ă) [MIM*236200]. Homocistinúria; distúrbio metabólico caracterizado por cabelos louros escassos, membros longos, peito escavado, ectopia da lente do olho, deficiência no desenvolvimento, retardo mental, distúrbios psiquiátricos e episódios tromboembólicos; em alguns pacientes, os sintomas são aliviados com piridoxina, enquanto outros não respondem a esse tratamento; associada a excreção urinária aumentada de homocistina e metionina. Herança autossômica recessiva; todavia, os portadores correm risco aumentado de doença vascular oclusiva; a doença é causada por mutação do gene da cistationa beta-sintase (CBS) no cromossoma 21q. Além disso, existem sete outras causas de homocistinúria: (1) defeito no metabolismo da vitamina B_{12} [MIM*277400], (2) deficiência de N-metileno tetraidrofolato redutase [MIM*236250], (3) malabsorção intestinal seletiva de vitamina B_{12} [MIM*261100], (4) h. responsiva à vitamina B_{12}, tipo cb1E [MIM*236270], (5) deficiência de metilcobalamina, tipo cb1G [MIM*250940], (6) defeito metabólico da vitamina B_{12}, tipo 2 [MIM*277410] e (7) deficiência de transcobalamina 2 [MIM*275350].
ho·mo·cy·to·tro·pic (hō′mō-sī′tō-trop′ik). Homocitotrópico; que possui afinidade por células da mesma espécie ou de uma espécie estreitamente relacionada. [homo- + G. kytos, célula + tropē, uma volta]
ho·mo·dont (hō′mō-dont). Homodonte; que tem todos os dentes de forma igual, como os dos vertebrados inferiores, em contraste com heterodonte. [homo- + G. odous, dente]
ho·mod·ro·mous (hō-mod′rō-mŭs). Homódromo; que se move na mesma direção. [homo- + G. dromos, que corre]
△**homoeo-**. Homoeo-. VER homeo-.
ho·mo·er·ot·ism, ho·mo·e·rot·i·cism (hō-mō-er′ō-tizm, -ĕ-rot′i-sizm). Homoerotismo. SIN homosexuality. [homo- + G. erōs, amor]
ho·mo·ga·met·ic (hō′mō-gă-met′ik). Homogamético; que produz apenas um tipo de gameta em relação aos cromossomas sexuais; nos seres humanos e na maioria dos animais, a fêmea é homogamética. SIN monogametic. [homo- + gametikos, conjugal]
ho·mog·a·my (hō-mog′ă-mē). Homogamia; semelhança entre marido e mulher num traço específico. [homo- + G. gamos, casamento]
ho·mog·e·nate (hō-moj′ĕ-nāt). Homogeneizado; tecido triturado até obter uma consistência cremosa na qual a estrutura celular está desintegrada (denominada "livre de célula"). Cf. brei.
ho·mo·ge·neous (hō-mō-jē′nē-ŭs). Homogêneo; de estrutura ou composição totalmente uniforme. [homo- + G. genos, raça]
ho·mo·gen·e·sis (hō-mō-jen′ĕ-sis). Homogênese; produção de descendentes semelhantes aos genitores, em contraste com heterogênese. SIN homogeny. [homo- + G. genesis, produção]
ho·mog·e·ni·za·tion (hō-moj′ĕ-ni-zā′shŭn). Homogeinização; processo pelo qual um material é tornado homogêneo.
ho·mog·e·nize (hō-moj′ĕ-nīz). Homogeinizar; tornar homogêneo.
ho·mog·e·nous (hō-moj′ĕ-nŭs). Homogênico; que possui semelhança estrutural por descender de um ancestral comum. Termo comumente confundido com homogêneo (homogeneous). [homo- + G. genos, família, espécie]
ho·mo·gen·tis·ate 1,2-di·ox·y·gen·ase (hō-mō-jen′tis-āt). Homogentisato 1,2-dioxigenase; enzima contendo ferro e que catalisa a clivagem oxidativa do anel benzeno no ácido homogentísico pelo O_2, formando 4-maleilacetoacetato; a ausência/deficiência dessa enzima resulta em alcaptonúria. SIN homogentisic acid oxidase.
ho·mo·gen·tis·ic ac·id (hō′mō-jen-tis′ik). Ácido homogentísico; ácido glicosúrico; ácido (2,5-diidroxifenil) acético; intermediário no catabolismo da L-fenilalanina e L-tirosina; ao se tornar alcalino, sofre rápida oxidação no ar a uma quinona, que se polimeriza num material semelhante à melanina; são observados níveis elevados em indivíduos com alcaptonúria. SIN alcapton, alkapton.
h. a. oxidase, a. h. oxidase. SIN homogentisate 1,2-dioxygenase.
ho·mog·e·ny (hō-moj′ĕ-ne). Homogenia. SIN homogenesis.
ho·mo·gly·can (hō-mō-glī′kan). Homoglicana; polissacarídeo constituído apenas por um tipo de subunidade de monossacarídeo (p. ex., glicano). Cf. heteroglycan, glycan.
ho·mo·graft (hō′mō-graft). Homoenxerto. SIN allograft.
ho·moi·o·pla·sia (hō′moy-ō-plā′zē-ă). Homeoplasia. SIN homeoplasia.
ho·moi·o·ther·mal (hō-moy-ō-ther′mal). Homeotérmico. SIN homeothermic.
ho·mo·kar·y·on (hō-mō-kar′ē-on). Homocárion; núcleos múltiplos e geneticamente idênticos num citoplasma comum, geralmente decorrentes da fusão de duas células da mesma espécie. [homo- + G. karyon, núcleo]
ho·mo·kar·y·o·tic (hō′mō-kar-ē-ot′ik). Homocariótico; que exibe as propriedades de um homocárion.
ho·mo·ker·a·to·plas·ty (hō′mō-ker′ă-tō-plas-tē). Homoceratoplastia; transplante de córnea entre membros da mesma espécie.
ho·mo·lat·er·al (hō-mō-lat′er-ăl). Homolateral. SIN ipsilateral. [homo- + L. latus, lado]
ho·mo·lip·ids (hō-mō-lip′idz). Homolipídios; lipídios que contêm apenas C, H e O. Cf. heterolipids. SIN simple lipids.
ho·mo·log, ho·mo·logue (hom′ō-log). Homólogo; membro de um par homólogo de uma série. [homo- + G. logos, palavra, proporção, relação]
ho·mol·o·gous (hō-mol′ō-gŭs). Homólogo; correspondente ou semelhante em certos atributos essenciais. **1.** Em biologia ou zoologia, refere-se a órgãos ou partes correspondentes na sua origem evolutiva e semelhantes, até certo ponto, na sua estrutura, porém não necessariamente na sua função. **2.** Em química, indica uma única série química, que difere por incrementos fixos. **3.** Em genética, refere-se a cromossomas ou partes de cromossomas idênticos em relação à sua construção e conteúdo genético. **4.** Em imunologia, refere-se ao soro ou tecido derivados de membros de uma única espécie, ou a um anticorpo em relação ao antígeno que induziu a sua produção. **5.** Proteínas que possuem funções idênticas ou semelhantes (sobretudo no que concerne a proteínas de espécies diferentes). [ver homolog]
ho·mol·o·gy (hō-mol′ō-jē). Homologia; o estado de ser homólogo.
h. of chains, h. de cadeias; o grau de semelhança entre as seqüências de bases de filamentos de dois DNA. SIN h. of strands.
DNA h., h. do DNA; o grau (ou percentagem) de hibridização possível entre o DNA de diferentes microrganismos.
h. of strands, h. de filamentos. SIN h. of chains.

ho·mol·y·sin (hō-mol′i-sin). Homolisina; anticorpo hemolítico sensibilizante (hemolisina) formado em decorrência da estimulação por um antígeno proveniente de um animal da mesma espécie. [homo- + hemolisina]

ho·mol·y·sis (hō-mol′i-sis). Homólise; lise de eritrócitos por uma hemolisina e complemento.

ho·mo·mor·phic (hō-mō-mōr′fik). Homomórfico; indica duas ou mais estruturas de forma e tamanho semelhantes. [homo- + G. *morphē*, forma, aspecto]

ho·mon·o·mous (hō-mon′o-mŭs). Homônomo; refere-se a partes, com forma e estrutura semelhantes, dispostas numa série, como os dedos das mãos e dos pés. [G. *homonomos*, sob as mesmas leis, *homos*, o mesmo + *nomos*, lei]

ho·mon·o·my (hō-mon′o-mē). Homonomia; a condição de ser homônomo.

ho·mo·nu·cle·ar (hō′mō-noo′klē-er) Homonuclear; refere-se a uma linhagem celular que conserva o complemento cromossômico original.

ho·mon·y·mous (hō-mon′i-mŭs). Homônimo; que possui o mesmo nome ou expresso nos mesmos termos, como, p. ex., as metades correspondentes (direita ou esquerda, inferior ou superior) das retinas. [G. *homōnymous*, do mesmo nome, *onyma*, nome]

ho·mo·phenes (hō′mō-fēnz). Homófonos; vocábulos em que os órgãos visíveis da fala comportam-se da mesma maneira, como, p. ex., paço e passo.

ho·mo·phil (hō′mō-fil). Homófilo; refere-se a um anticorpo que só reage contra o antígeno específico indutor de sua formação. [homo- + G. *philos*, amar]

homophobia (hō-mō-fō′bē-ă). Homofobia; medo irracional de sentimentos, pensamentos, comportamentos ou indivíduos homossexuais.
  internalized h., h. internalizada; homofobia que ocorre num indivíduo homossexual, freqüentemente associada a aversão de si próprio, autocensura e autocrítica.

ho·mo·plas·tic (hō-mō-plas′tik). Homoplásico; semelhante quanto à forma e estrutura, mas não quanto à origem. [homo- + G. *plastos*, formado]

ho·mo·pol·y·mer (hō-mō-pol′i-mer). Homopolímero; polímero composto por uma série de radicais idênticos; p. ex., polilisina, ácido poli(adenílico), poliglicose.

ho·mo·pro·line (hō-mō-prō′lēn). Homoprolina. SIN pipecolic acid.

ho·mo·pro·to·cat·e·chu·ic ac·id (hō′mō-prō′tō-kat-ē-choo′ik). Ácido homoprotocatequínico; ácido (3,4-diidroxifenil) acético; isômero do ácido homogentísico encontrado na urina; produto de degradação da L-tirosina, L-dopa e hidroxitiramina.

hom·or·gan·ic (hom-ōr-gan′ik). Homorgânico; produzido pelos mesmos órgãos ou por órgãos homólogos.

ho·mo·sal·ate (hō-mō-sal′āt). Homossalato; agente protetor contra raios ultravioleta para aplicação tópica à pele.

ho·mo·sced·as·tic·i·ty (hō′mō-skē-das-tis′i-tē). Homoscedasticidade; constância da variação de uma medida sobre os níveis do fator em estudo.

ho·mo·ser·ine (hō-mō-ser′ēn). Homosserina; ácido amino-4-hidroxibutírico; um ácido hidroxiamino que difere da serina pela presença de um grupamento CH₂ adicional. Intermediário na biossíntese da cistationina, treonina e metionina.
  h. deaminase, h. desaminase. SIN cystathionine γ-lyase.
  h. dehydratase, h. desidratase. SIN cystathionine γ-lyase.
  h. lactone, h. lactona; o éster cíclico (isto é, a δ-lactona) da homosserina; formado pela reação do brometo de cianogênio em resíduos metionil em peptídeos e proteínas.

ho·mo·sex·u·al (hō-mō-sek′shoo-ăl). Homossexual. **1.** Relativo a, ou característico de, homossexualidade. **2.** Indivíduo cujos interesses e comportamentos são característicos da homossexualidade. VER gay, lesbian.

ho·mo·sex·u·al·i·ty (hō′mō-sek-shoo-al′i-tē). Homossexualidade; atração ou atividade erótica, incluindo relação sexual, entre indivíduos do mesmo sexo, especialmente após a puberdade. SIN homoerotism, homoeroticism.
  ego-dystonic h., h. ego distônica; distúrbio psicológico ou psiquiátrico em que um indivíduo apresenta incômodo persistente associado à preferência pelo mesmo sexo e uma forte necessidade de mudar o comportamento ou, pelo menos, aliviar o desconforto associado à homossexualidade; não é mais um diagnóstico reconhecido como DSM; hoje em dia, é incluído entre os distúrbios sexuais ainda não-especificados.
  female h., h. feminina; predisposição ou atividade erótica, incluindo relação sexual, entre duas mulheres após a idade da puberdade.
  latent h., h. latente; inclinação erótica por pessoas do mesmo sexo não conscientemente experimentada nem expressa de forma liberal, em oposição à homossexualidade aberta. Esse termo vem sendo pouco usado tanto pelo seu efeito potencialmente iatrogênico quanto pela sua incapacidade de validar o fenômeno por meio de técnicas fora da teoria psicanalítica. SIN unconscious h.
  male h., h. masculina; predisposição ou atividade erótica, incluindo relação sexual, entre dois homens após a idade da puberdade.
  overt h., h. franca; inclinações homossexuais conscientemente experimentadas e expressas em comportamento homossexual real.
  unconscious h., h. inconsciente. SIN latent h.

D-ho·mo·ster·oid (hō-mō-ster′oyd). D-homosteróide; esteróide em que o anel D é composto de seis átomos de carbono, em lugar dos cinco habituais.

ho·mo·ster·oid. Homosteróide; esteróide que teve pelo menos um dos anéis expandido em sua estrutura.

4-ho·mo·sul·fa·nil·a·mide (hō′mō-sŭl-fă-nil′ă-mīd). 4-homossulfanilamida. SIN mafenide.

ho·mo·thal·lic (hō-mō-thal′ik). Homotálico; nos fungos, refere-se a uma forma de reprodução sexual em que o núcleo de um talo é capaz de se fundir com outro núcleo do mesmo talo ou de tipo correspondente. Cf. heterothallic. [homo- + G. *thallos*, broto novo]

ho·mo·ther·mal (hō-mō-ther′măl). Homotérmico. SIN homeothermic. [homo- + G. *thermē*, calor]

ho·mo·ton·ic (hō-mō-ton′ik). Homotônico; de tensão ou tônus uniforme.

ho·mo·top·ic (hō-mō-top′ik). Homotópico; relativo a ou que ocorre no mesmo local ou parte do corpo. [homo- + G. *topos*, lugar]

ho·mo·trans·plan·ta·tion (hō′mō-tranz-plan-tā′shŭn). Homotransplante. SIN allotransplantation.

ho·mo·trop·ic (hō-mō-trō-pik). Homotrópico; refere-se à ligação do mesmo ligante a uma macromolécula; p. ex., a ligação de quatro O₂ à hemoglobina é uma cooperatividade homotrópica.

ho·mo·type (hō′mō-tīp). Homótipo; qualquer parte ou órgão de estrutura ou função iguais a outro, especialmente ao do lado oposto do corpo. [homo- + G. *typos*, tipo]

ho·mo·typ·ic, ho·mo·typ·i·cal (hō-mō-tip′ik, i-kăl). Homotípico; do mesmo tipo ou forma; correspondente a um entre dois órgãos ou partes pareadas.

ho·mo·va·nil·lic ac·id (HVA) (hō′mō-vă-nil′ik). Ácido homovanílico; ácido 4-hidroxi-3-metoxifenilacético; um fenol encontrado na urina humana; produzido através da metilação do ácido homoprotocatequínico sobre o grupamento *meta*-OH. Trata-se do principal metabólito urinário da dopa e dopamina.

ho·mo·zo·ic (hō-mō-zō′ik). Homozóico; relativo ao mesmo animal ou à mesma espécie de animal. [homo- + G. *zōikos*, relativo a um animal]

ho·mo·zy·gos·i·ty, ho·mo·zy·go·sis (hō′mō-zī-gos′i-tē, -zī-gō′sis). Homozigosidade; o estado de ser homozigoto. [homo- + G. *zygon*, união]

ho·mo·zy·gote (hō-mō-zī′gōt). Homozigoto; indivíduo homozigoto. [homo- + G. *zygōtos*, união]

ho·mo·zy·gous (hō-mō-zī′gŭs). Homozigoto; que possui alelos idênticos em um ou mais *loci*.

ho·mo·zy·gous by de·scent. Homozigoto por descendência; que possui dois alelos idênticos, em um determinado *locus*, que são descendentes de uma única fonte, como pode ocorrer no casamento consangüíneo.

ho·mun·cu·lus (hō-mŭngk′u-lŭs). Homúnculo. **1.** Corpo excessivamente pequeno que, de acordo com os pontos de vista de desenvolvimento defendidos por alguns cientistas médicos dos séculos XVI e XVII, estava contido numa célula sexual. Acreditava-se que o corpo humano se desenvolvia a partir dessa estrutura pré-formada, porém infinitamente pequena. VER TAMBÉM preformation *theory*, animalcule. **2.** A figura de um ser humano algumas vezes superposta em desenhos da superfície do cérebro para representar regiões motoras e sensitivas ali representadas. [L. dim. de *homo*, homem]

Hon·du·ras bark (hon-doo′răs). Casca-de-honduras, cáscara-amara. SIN cascara amara.

hon·ey (hŭn′ē). Mel; mel puro; substância sacarínica depositada na colméia pela abelha doméstica, *Apis mellifera*; utilizado como excipiente, aromatizante em gargarejos e antitussígeno, e como alimento. SIN mel (1). [A.S. *hunig*]

honk (hawnk). Grasnada. **1.** Em termos médicos, som que pode ser comparado ao grito de um ganso. **2.** Algumas vezes, esse termo é especificamente utilizado para referir-se a um som de origem laríngea emitido pelas cordas vocais vibrando numa expiração forçada e devido a um anel vascular congênito comprimindo a traquéia. [echoic]
  systolic h., g. sistólico; sopro sistólico um tanto musical, semelhante ao grasnar de um ganso; algumas vezes de origem inocente, porém inexplicada; outras vezes, constituindo um sinal de insuficiência mitral. SIN systolic whoop.

hood (hud). Capuz, capela. **1.** Parte anterior do tegumento dos carrapatos moles (família Argasidae) que se estende sobre o capítulo e forma o teto do cameróstomo. **2.** Estrutura expandida de revestimento, que se assemelha ao capelo de uma capa ou manto na sua forma ou função, como as expansões digitais extensoras que se superpõem à face dorsal das cabeças dos metacarpos. [O.E. *hōd*, chapéu]
  dorsal h., aponeurose palmar. SIN extensor digital *expansion*.

hook (huk). Gancho. **1.** Instrumento curvo ou dobrado próximo à sua extremidade, utilizado para fixação de uma parte ou para tração. **2.** Hâmulo, *termo oficial alternativo para hamulus. [A.S. *hōk*]
  calvarial h., gancho da calvária; instrumento utilizado para retirada do topo do crânio após ter sido serrado em volta em necrópsias e dissecções.
  h. of hamate, hâmulo do hamato; processo unciforme na parte distal ou medial da superfície palmar do osso hamato. SIN hamulus ossis hamati [TA].
  palate h., g. do palato; instrumento para tracionar o palato mole para a frente, a fim de facilitar a rinoscopia posterior.
  sliding h., g. deslizante; fixação móvel utilizada em aparelho ortodôntico para a aplicação de tração elástica ou força de arreios.

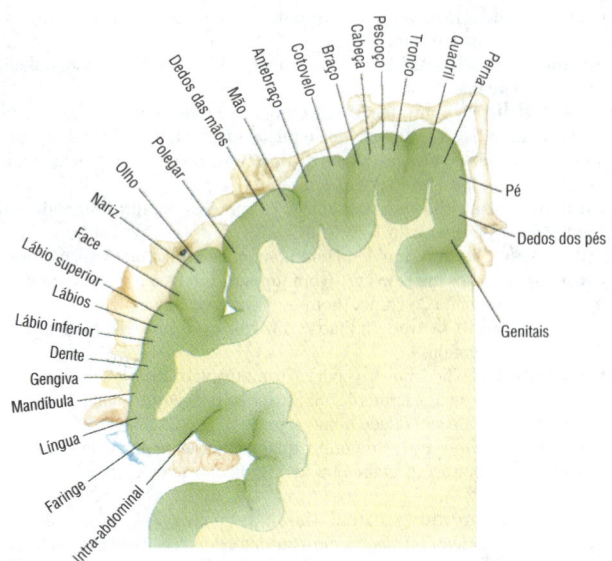

projeção somatotrópica da superfície corporal no córtex somatossensorial primário (homúnculo): o mapa é um corte transversal através do giro pós-central; os neurônios em cada área são mais responsivos às partes do corpo ilustradas acima de cada um deles

h. of spiral lamina, hâmulo da lâmina espiral. SIN hamulus of spiral lamina.
squint h., g. do estrabismo; instrumento cirúrgico utilizado para levantar os músculos oculares.
tracheotomy h., g. de traqueotomia; gancho de ângulo reto utilizado para manter a traquéia na posição desejada durante uma traqueotomia.
Hooke, Robert, físico experimental inglês, 1635–1703. VER hookean *behavior*; H. *law*.
hook·lets (huk′letz) Ganchos. **1.** Ganchos quitinosos e retráteis, em forma de pinças, que rodeiam ou alinham-se no rostelo do escólex de certas tênias para a sua fixação à mucosa intestinal, com o auxílio adicional de ventosas; os ganchos podem ser retirados e o rostelo invertido quando a tênia se move. As diversas distribuições e formas dos ganchos caracterizam as famílias de cestóides tenióides. **2.** Ganchos dos escóleces degenerados de espécies *Echinococcus* nos líquidos do cisto hidático. **3.** Os ganchos da oncosfera, pelos quais ela se fixa à bainha de sua membrana após eclodir e penetrar na parede intestinal do hospedeiro; esses ganchos podem ser posteriormente encontrados no cercômero do procercóide e cisticercóide.
hook·worm (huk′werm). Ancilostomatídeo; nome comum de nematódeos hematófagos da família Ancylostomatidae, principalmente membros dos gêneros *Ancylostoma* (ancilostomatídeo do Velho Mundo), *Necator* e *Uncinaria*, incluindo a espécie *A. caninum* (ancilóstomo do cão) e *N. americanus* (ancilóstomo do Novo Mundo).
Hoover, Charles F., médico norte-americano, 1865–1927. VER H. *signs*, em *sign*.
Hopkins, H.H., físico óptico inglês do século XX. VER H. *rod-lens telescope*.
Hopkins, Sir Frederick G., bioquímico inglês e ganhador do Prêmio Nobel, 1861–1947. VER Benedict-H.-Cole *reagent*.
Hop·lop·syl·lus anom·a·lus (hop-lō-sil′us ā-nom′a-lŭs). Espécie de pulga parasita de tâmias no oeste dos Estados Unidos, vetor da peste. [G. *hoplo*, ferramenta, lança + *psyll*, pulga]
Hopmann, Carl M., rinologista alemão, 1849–1925. VER H. *papilloma, polyp*.
hops. Lúpulo. SIN humulus.
hor. decub. Abreviatura do L. *hora decubitus*, ao deitar.
hor·de·nine (hōr′den-ēn). Hordenina; amina biogênica isolada pela primeira vez da cevada; aumenta a pressão arterial. [L. *hordeum*, cevada + -*in*]
hor·de·o·lum (hōr-dē′o-lŭm). Hordéolo; inflamação supurativa de uma glândula da pálpebra. [L. Mod., *hordeolus*, terçol no olho, dim. de *hordeum*, cevada]
h. exter′num, h. externo; inflamação da glândula sebácea de uma pálpebra. SIN sty, stye.
h. inter′num, h. interno; infecção purulenta aguda de uma glândula tarsal (de meibomio). SIN acute chalazion, h. meibomianum, meibomian sty.
h. meibomia′num, h. de meibomio, h. tarsal. SIN h. internum.
Horecker, Bernard L., bioquímico norte-americano, *1914. VER Warburg-Dickens-Horecker *shunt*.
hore·hound, hoar·hound (hōr-hound). Marroio-branco, marroio-comum; *Marrubium vulgare* (família Labitae); o componente amargo é o marrúbio, um óleo volátil. Composto ao qual se atribuem propriedades expectorantes, freqüentemente encontrado em pastilhas para tosse e outros remédios patenteados. [O.E. *hār*, esbranquiçado + *hūne*, erva]
hor·i·zon·ta·lis (hōr-i-zon-tā′lis). Horizontal; refere-se ao plano do corpo, perpendicular ao plano vertical, em ângulos retos com os planos mediano e coronal, que separa o corpo em partes superior e inferior. [L.]
hor·me·sis (hōr-mē′sis). Hórmese; o efeito estimulante de concentrações subinibitórias de qualquer substância tóxica sobre qualquer organismo. [G. *hormēsis*, movimento rápido]
hor·mi·on (hōr′mē-on). Hórmio; craniométrico na junção da borda posterior do vômer com o osso esfenóide. [G. *hormos*, cordão, cadeia, corrente]
hor·mo·gon·al (hōr-mō′gō-nal). Hormogonal; referente a uma classe de cianobactérias cujas células crescem em filamentos.
hor·mo·nal (hōr-mōn′ăl). Hormonal; relativo a hormônios.

HORMONE

hor·mone (hōr′mōn). Hormônio; substância química formada em determinado órgão ou parte do corpo e transportada pelo sangue para outro órgão ou parte; dependendo da especificidade de seus efeitos, os hormônios conseguem alterar a atividade funcional e, algumas vezes, a estrutura de apenas um órgão ou tecido ou de vários deles. Numerosos hormônios são formados por glândulas sem ductos, porém a secretina, a colecistocinina e a pancreozimina, que são formadas no trato gastrointestinal, também são, por definição, hormônios. Para os hormônios não relacionados a seguir, ver os nomes específicos. [G. *hormōn*, particípio presente de *hormaō*, estimular ou colocar em movimento]
adipokinetic h., adipocinina. SIN adipokinin.
adrenal androgen-stimulating h. (AASH), h. estimulante dos androgênios supra-renais (AASH); um suposto hormônio hipofisário que seria responsável pelo aumento da secreção dos androgênios supra-renais na época da puberdade.
adrenocortical h.'s, h. adrenocorticais; hormônios secretados pelo córtex supra-renal humano; p. ex., cortisol, aldosterona, corticosterona.
adrenocorticotropic h. (ACTH), h. adrenocorticotrópico (ACTH); o hormônio do lobo anterior da hipófise que governa a nutrição e o crescimento do córtex supra-renal, estimula-o a exercer sua atividade funcional e também possui atividade adipocinética extra-supra-renal; trata-se de um polipeptídeo contendo 39 aminoácidos, apesar de a sua estrutura exata variar de uma espécie para outra;

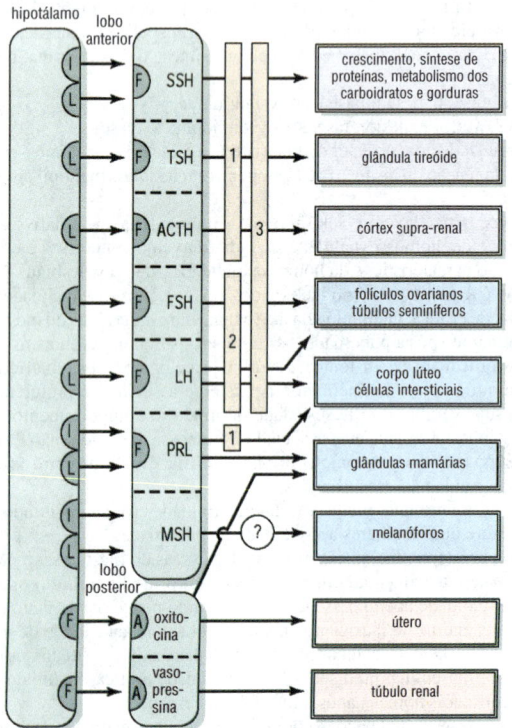

hormônios hipofisários: (I) hormônios de inibição, (L) hormônios de liberação, (F) formação, (A) armazenamento, (1) hormônios metabólicos, (2) gonadotropinas, (3) hormônios glandulotrópicos

algumas vezes, o termo é precedido pelo prefixo α para distingui-lo da β-corticotropina. Os primeiros 13 aminoácidos na região N-terminal são idênticos à α-melanotropina. SIN adrenocorticotropin; adrenotropic h., adrenotropin, corticotropic h., corticotropin (1).

adrenomedullary h.'s, h. adrenomedulares; hormônios produzidos pela medula supra-renal, sobretudo as catecolaminas epinefrina e norepinefrina.

adrenotropic h., h. adrenocorticotrópico. SIN adrenocorticotropic h.

androgenic h., h. androgênico; qualquer hormônio capaz de produzir um efeito masculinizante; dentre os hormônios androgênicos de ocorrência natural, a testosterona é o mais potente.

antidiuretic h. (ADH), h. antidiurético (HAD). SIN vasopressin.

anti-müllerian h., h. antimülleriano. SIN müllerian inhibiting substance.

cardiac h., h. cardíaco. SIN herz h.

chorionic gonadotropic h., chorionic gonadotrophic h., h. gonadotrópico coriônico, h. gonadotrófico coriônico. SIN chorionic gonadotropin.

chorionic "growth h.-prolactin" (CGP), "prolactina-hormônio do crescimento" coriônico (CGP). SIN human placental lactogen.

cortical h.'s, h. corticais; hormônios esteróides produzidos pelo córtex supra-renal.

corticotropic h., h. adrenocorticotrópico. SIN adrenocorticotropic h.

corticotropin-releasing h. (CRH), hormônio liberador da corticotropina (CRH); fator secretado pelo hipotálamo, que estimula a liberação de hormônio adrenocorticotrópico pela hipófise. SIN corticotropin-releasing factor.

ectopic h., h. ectópico; hormônio formado por um tecido fora do local endócrino normal de produção; p. ex., produção de h. adrenocorticotrópico por um carcinoma broncogênico. SIN inappropriate h.

endocrine h.'s, h. endócrinos; hormônios produzidos pelo sistema endócrino. Cf. tissue h.'s.

erythropoietic h., h. eritropoético; (1) genericamente, qualquer hormônio capaz de promover a formação dos eritrócitos, p. ex., testosterona; (2) eritropoetina. SIN erythropoietin.

estrogenic h., estradiol. SIN estradiol.

follicle-stimulating h. (FSH), h. folículo-estimulante (FSH). SIN follitropin.

follicular h., estrona. SIN estrone.

galactopoietic h., prolactina. SIN prolactin.

gametokinetic h., folitropina. SIN follitropin.

gastrointestinal h., h. gastrointestinal; qualquer secreção da mucosa gastrointestinal que afeta o ritmo e o volume das várias secreções digestivas (p. ex., secretina) ou que causa aumento da motilidade do órgão-alvo (p. ex., colecistocinina).

gonadal h.'s, h. gonadais. SIN sex h.'s.

gonadotropic h., gonadotropina. SIN gonadotropin.

gonadotropin-releasing h. (GnRH, GRH), h. liberador das gonadotropinas (GnRH, GRH). SIN gonadoliberin (1).

growth h. (GH), h. do crescimento (GH). SIN somatotropin.

growth h.-inhibiting h. (GIH), h. inibidor do hormônio do crescimento (GIH). SIN somatostatin.

growth h.-releasing h. (GHRH, GH-RH), h. liberador do hormônio do crescimento (GHRH, GH-RH). SIN somatoliberin.

heart h., h. do coração. SIN herz h.

herz h., h. cardíaco; substância presente em extratos de tecido cardíaco que aumenta a contração cardíaca; possivelmente adenosina, uma catecolamina ou algum estimulante inespecífico geralmente encontrado nos tecidos. SIN cardiac h., heart h.

human chorionic somatomammotropic h. (HCS), h. somatomamotrópico coriônico humano (HCS). SIN human placental lactogen.

hypophysiotropic h., h. hipofisiotrópico; hormônio que estimula a taxa de secreção dos hormônios hipofisários; p. ex., fator de liberação; fator hipotalâmico (regulador).

inappropriate h., h. ectópico. SIN ectopic h.

interstitial cell-stimulating h. (ICSH), h. estimulante das células intersticiais (ICSH), lutropina. SIN lutropin.

lactation h., prolactina. SIN prolactin.

lactogenic h., prolactina. SIN prolactin.

lipid-mobilizing h., lipotropina. SIN lipotropin.

lipotropic h. (LPH), lipotropic pituitary h., h. lipotrópico (LPH), h. hipofisário lipotrópico, lipotropina. SIN lipotropin.

local h., h. local; produto metabólico secretado por um conjunto de células que afeta a função de células adjacentes; altacóide; p. ex., prostaglandinas e neurotransmissores.

luteinizing h. (LH), h. luteinizante (LH), lutropina. SIN lutropin.

luteinizing hormone-releasing h. (LH-RH, LRH), h. liberador do hormônio luteinizante (LH-RH, LRH). SIN luliberin.

mammotropic h., h. mamotrópico. SIN prolactin.

melanocyte-stimulating h. (MSH), h. melanócito-estimulante (MSH). SIN melanotropin.

melanotropin release-inhibiting h. (MIH), h. inibidor da liberação de melanotropina (MIH). SIN melanostatin.

melanotropin-releasing h. (MRH), h. liberador da melanotropina. SIN melanoliberin.

neurohypophysial h.'s, h. neuro-hipofisários; hormônios produzidos no hipotálamo; p. ex., oxitocina, vasopressina.

ovarian hormone, hormônio ovariano. SIN relaxin.

pancreatic hyperglycemic h., glucagon. SIN glucagon.

parathyroid h. (PTH), paratormônio (PTH); hormônio peptídico formado pelas glândulas paratireóides; produz elevação dos níveis séricos de cálcio quando administrado por via parenteral, causando reabsorção óssea, reduzindo a depuração renal de cálcio e aumentando a eficiência da absorção de cálcio no intestino. Atua em conjunção com a calcitonina e outros hormônios. SIN parathormone, parathyrin.

pituitary gonadotropic h., h. gonadotrópico hipofisário. SIN anterior pituitary gonadotropin.

pituitary growth h., somatotropina. SIN somatotropin.

placental growth h., lactogênio placentário humano. SIN human placental lactogen.

pregnancy h., progesterona. SIN progesterone.

progestational h., progesterona. SIN progesterone.

proparathyroid h., h. pró-paratormônio; precursor imediato do paratormônio; o h. pró-paratormônio difere do paratormônio por uma extensão hexapeptídica N-terminal.

releasing h. (RH), fatores liberadores. SIN releasing factors.

salivary gland h., parotina. SIN parotin.

sex h.'s, h. sexuais; termo genérico abrangendo os hormônios esteróides que são formados pelos tecidos testicular, ovariano e adrenocortical, consistindo em androgênios ou estrogênios. SIN gonadal h.'s.

somatotropic h. (STH), somatotropina. SIN somatotropin.

somatotropin release-inhibiting h. (SIH), hormônio inibidor da liberação de somatotropina (SIH). SIN somatostatin.

somatotropin-releasing h. (SRH), h. liberador da somatotropina (SRH). SIN somatoliberin.

steroid h.'s, h. esteróides; hormônios que possuem o sistema em anel esteróide; p. ex., androgênios, estrogênios, hormônios adrenocorticais.

sympathetic h., h. simpático. SIN sympathin.

thyroid-stimulating h. (TSH), h. tireoestimulante (TSH). SIN thyrotropin.

thyrotropic h., h. tireotrópico, tirotropina. SIN thyrotropin.

thyrotropin-releasing h. (TRH), h. liberador da tireotropina (TRH). SIN thyroliberin.

tissue h.'s, h. teciduais; hormônios sintetizados por células diferentes daquelas do sistema endócrino. Cf. endocrine h.'s.

tropic h.'s, trophic h.'s, h. trópicos, h. tróficos; hormônios do lobo anterior da hipófise que afetam o crescimento, a nutrição ou a função de outras glândulas endócrinas (p. ex., TRH, ACTH).

vertebrate h.'s, h. de vertebrados; hormônios sintetizados em vertebrados.

---

hor·mo·no·gen·e·sis (hōr'mō-nō-jen'ĕ-sis). Hormonogênese; formação dos hormônios. SIN hormonopoiesis.

hor·mo·no·gen·ic (hōr'mō-nō-jen'ik). Hormonogênico; relativo à formação de um hormônio. SIN hormonopoietic.

hor·mo·no·poi·e·sis (hōr'mō-nō-poy'ē'sis). Hormonopoese. SIN hormonogenesis. [hormone + G. poiēsis, produção]

hor·mo·no·poi·et·ic (hōr'mō-nō-poy-et'ik). Hormonopoético. SIN hormonogenic.

hor·mo·no·priv·ia (hōr'mō-nō-priv'ē-ă). Hormonoprivo; termo obsoleto que significa privação parcial ou total de hormônios. [hormônio + G. privus, privado de]

hor·mo·no·ther·a·py (hōr'mō-nō-thār'ă-pē). Hormonoterapia; tratamento com hormônios.

horn (hōrn) [TA]. Corno; qualquer estrutura semelhante cuja forma lembra um corno. SIN cornu (1). [A.S.]

Ammon h. [TA], corno de Ammon; um dos dois giros entrelaçados que compõem o hipocampo, sendo o outro o giro denteado. Com base em características citoarquitetônicas, o c. de Ammon pode ser dividido em: região I [TA] (regio I cornus ammonis [TA]), região II [TA] (regio II cornus ammonis [TA]), região III [TA] (regio III cornus ammonis [TA]) e região IV [TA] (regio IV cornus ammonis [TA]). SIN cornu ammonis. [G. Ammōn, divindade egípcia Amūn]

anterior h. [TA], c. anterior; (1) a divisão frontal ou anterior do ventrículo lateral do cérebro, estendendo-se adiante do forame interventricular de Monro; VER lateral ventricle; (2) o c. anterior ou coluna cinzenta ventral da medula espinal, como aparece em corte transversal. O c. anterior é composto pela lâmina espinal VIII-IV [TA] de Rexed, com porções de VII estendendo-se também para seus limites geográficos nos níveis lombossacro e cervical. Os núcleos do c. anterior são: o núcleo ântero-lateral [TA] ou núcleo ventrolateral [TAalt] (nucleus anterolateralis [TA]), o núcleo anterior [TA] (nucleus anterior [TA]), o núcleo ântero-medial [TA] ou núcleo ventromedial [TAalt] (nucleus anteromedialis [TA]), o núcleo póstero-lateral [TA] ou núcleo dorsola-

teral [TAalt] (nucleus posterolateralis [TA]), o núcleo lateral retroposterior [TA] ou núcleo lateral retrodorsal [TAalt] (nucleus retroposterolateralis [TA]), o núcleo póstero-medial [TA] ou núcleo dorsomedial [TAalt] (nucleus posteromedialis [TA]), o núcleo central [TA], (nucleus centralis [TA]) e o núcleo acessório e núcleo frênico, ambos encontrados apenas em níveis cervicais. VER TAMBÉM anterior *column*, gray *columns*, em *column*. SIN cornu anterius [TA], ventral h.
cicatricial h., corno cicatricial; corno ceratinoso que se projeta para fora de uma cicatriz.
coccygeal h., c. coccígeo. SIN coccygeal *cornu*.
cutaneous h., c. cutâneo; proliferação ceratótica que se projeta da pele; a base pode exibir alterações de ceratose actínica ou carcinoma. SIN cornu cutaneum, warty h.
frontal h. [TA], c. frontal. VER inferior h. of lateral ventricle, inferior h.
greater h. of hyoid bone [TA], c. maior do hióide; o maior e mais lateral dos dois processos de cada lado do osso hióide. SIN cornu majus ossis hyoidei [TA].
h.'s of hyoid bone, cornos do hióide. VER greater h. of hyoid bone, lesser h. of hyoid.
iliac h., c. ilíaco; esporão ósseo da parte posterior do ílio, freqüentemente encontrado na síndrome de unha–patela.
inferior h., c. inferior; prolongamento inferior ou descendente de uma parte ou estrutura do corpo. SIN cornu inferius [TA].
inferior h. of falciform margin of saphenous opening [TA], c. inferior da margem falciforme da abertura safena; parte inferior da margem falciforme da abertura na fáscia lata através da qual passa a veia grande safena. SIN cornu inferius marginis falciformis hiatus sapheni [TA], crus inferius marginis falciformis hiatus sapheni*.
inferior h. of lateral ventricle, c. inferior do ventrículo lateral; parte do ventrículo lateral que se estende para baixo e para frente na parte medial do lobo temporal. VER lateral *ventricle*. SIN cornu inferius ventriculi lateralis [TA], cornu temporale ventriculi lateralis [TA], temporal h. [TA].
inferior h. of thyroid cartilage [TA], c. inferior da cartilagem tireóidea; um dos dois prolongamentos descendentes situados na parte posterior da cartilagem tireóide; articula-se de cada lado com a cartilagem cricóide. SIN cornu inferius cartilaginis thyroideae [TA].
lateral h. [TA], c. lateral; a pequena coluna cinzenta lateral da medula espinal; aparece em corte transversal, contendo a coluna de células interomediais. VER TAMBÉM gray *columns* em *column*. SIN cornu laterale [TA].
lesser h. of hyoid [TA], c. menor do hióide; o menor e mais medial dos dois processos de cada lado do osso hióide. SIN cornu minus ossis hyoidei [TA], styloid cornu.
occipital h. [TA], c. occipital. SIN posterior h.
posterior h., c. posterior; (1) divisão occipital ou posterior do ventrículo lateral do cérebro, estendendo-se para trás no lobo occipital; VER TAMBÉM posterior *column*; (2) [TA], o c. posterior ou coluna cinzenta da medula espinal, como aparece em corte transversal. O corno posterior [TA] ou corno dorsal [TAalt] contém as lâminas espinais I-VI [TA] de Rexed. Os núcleos do c. posterior são: o núcleo marginal [TA] (nucleus marginalis [TA]), a substância gelatinosa [TA] (substantia gelatinosa [TA]), o núcleo próprio [TA], a substância cinzenta visceral secundária [TA] (substantia visceralis secundaria [TA]), o núcleo basilar interno [TA] (nucleus basilar internus [TA]), o núcleo cervical medial [TA] (nucleus cervicalis medialis [TA]), o núcleo posterior do funículo lateral [TA] (nucleus posterior funiculi lateralis [TA]) e o núcleo cervical lateral. SIN cornu posterius ventriculi lateralis [TA], cornu posterius [TA], occipital h. [TA], cornu of spinal cord.
pulp h., c. da polpa; prolongamento da polpa que se estende em direção à cúspide de um dente.
sacral h., c. sacral;* termo oficial alternativo de sacral *cornu*.
h.'s of saphenous opening, cornos da abertura safena. VER inferior h. of falciform margin of saphenous opening, superior h. of falciform margin of saphenous opening.
sebaceous h., c. sebáceo; proliferação sólida de um cisto sebáceo.
superior h. of falciform margin of saphenous opening [TA], c. superior da margem falciforme da abertura safena; parte superior da margem falciforme da abertura na fáscia lata através da qual passa a veia grande safena. SIN cornu superius marginalis falciformis [TA], Burns falciform process, Burns ligament, crus superius marginis falciformis hiatus sapheni, Hey ligament.
superior h. of thyroid cartilage [TA], c. superior da cartilagem tireóidea; um dos dois prolongamentos ascendentes da cartilagem tireóidea, ao qual se fixa o ligamento hiotireóideo lateral. SIN cornu superius cartilaginis thyroideae [TA].
temporal h. [TA], c. temporal. SIN inferior h. of lateral ventricle.
h.'s of thyroid cartilage, cornos da cartilagem tireóidea. VER inferior h. of thyroid cartilage, superior h. of thyroid cartilage.
uterine h., h. of uterus [TA], c. uterino, c. do útero; parte do útero em que a parte intramural da trompa uterina penetra na direita ou na esquerda. SIN cornu uteri [TA].

ventral h., c. ventral. SIN anterior h.
warty h., c. verrucoso. SIN cutaneous h.
Horner, Johann F., oftalmologista suíço, 1831–1886. VER H. *syndrome*, *pupil*; Bernard-H. *syndrome*; H.-Trantas *dots* em *dot*.
Horner, William E., anatomista norte-americano, 1793–1853. VER H. *muscle*, *teeth*, em *tooth*.
horny (hōrn'e) . Córneo; da natureza ou estrutura de um corno. SIN keratinous (2).
ho·rop·ter (hō - rop'ter). Horóptero; a soma dos pontos no espaço, cujas imagens para determinado ponto de fixação caem nos pontos correspondentes da retina. Se o ponto de fixação estiver a 2 m, o horóptero é uma linha reta; se estiver a uma distância menor, o horóptero é uma curva côncava para a face; se for mais distante, uma curva convexa. [G. *horos*, limite + *optēr*, espião, observador, fr. *oraō*, fut. *opsomai*, ver]
empirical h., h. empírico; elipse experimentalmente determinada que passa através dos centros ópticos dos dois olhos através dos quais pontos adjacentes ao ponto de fixação, ambos situados na elipse, são percebidos estimulando pontos correspondentes na retina.
hor·rip·i·la·tion (ho - rip - i - la'shun). Horripilação; ereção dos pêlos finos à contração dos eretores dos pêlos. [L. *horreo*, arrepiar + *pilus*, pêlo]
hor·ror (hor'er). Horror; pavor; medo. [L.]
h. autotox'icus, h. autotóxico; termo introduzido por Ehrlich, significando que a imunidade é dirigida contra materiais estranhos, mas não contra os constituintes do próprio corpo; as exceções a esse conceito são as reações e as doenças auto-alérgicas. SIN self-tolerance. [L., pavor de auto-intoxicação]
h. fusio'nis, projeção simultânea na consciência de imagens retinianas tão diferentes que a fusão é impossível. SIN macular evasion. [L., pavor de fusão]
horse-fly (hōrs'flī). Mutuca. VER *Tabanus*, *Anthomyia canicularis*.
horse·pow·er (hōrs'pow - er). Cavalo-vapor; unidade de potência equivalente a 550 pés-libras/s ou 745,7 W.
Horsfall, Frank L., Jr., médico norte-americano, 1906–1971. VER Tamm-H. *mucoprotein*, *protein*.
Horsley, Sir Victor A.H., cirurgião inglês, 1857–1916. VER H. bone *wax*.
hor. som. Abreviatura do L. *hora somni*, antes de dormir, ao deitar.
Hortega, Pio del Rio, neuro-histologista espanhol na América do Sul, 1882–1945. VER H. *cells*, em *cell*, neuroglia *stain*.
Horton, Bayard T., médico norte-americano, *1895. VER H. *arteritis*, *cephalalgia*, *headache*.
hos·pice (hos'pis). Asilo; instituição que oferece um programa centralizado de serviços paliativos e de suporte a indivíduos moribundos e suas famílias, na forma de assistência física, psicológica, social e espiritual; esses serviços são fornecidos por uma equipe interdisciplinar de profissionais e voluntários, disponíveis para atendimento domiciliar ou em unidades especializadas para pacientes internados. [L. *hospitium*, hospitalidade, alojamento, fr. *hospes*, hóspede]
hospi·tal (hos'pi - tăl). Hospital; instituição para tratamento, assistência e cura de um indivíduo doente ou ferido, para o estudo de doenças e para o treinamento de médicos, enfermeiras e outros profissionais de saúde. [L. *hospitalis*, para um hóspede, fr. *hospes (hospit-)*, hóspede, hospedeiro]

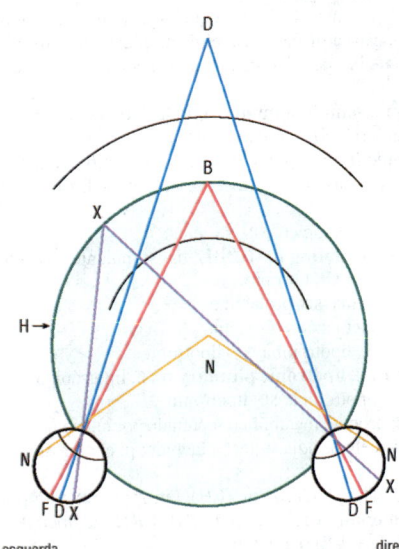

plano do horóptero: um ponto de fixação (B) é representado na fóvea (F) enquanto outro ponto de fixação (X) é representado na mesma distância, a partir da fóvea, em ambos os olhos; os objetos fora do plano do horóptero (D) exibem disparidade nasal, enquanto aqueles no seu interior (N) exibem disparidade temporal

base h., h. de base; unidade hospitalar localizada em acampamento militar ou recreativo; em geral, de pequeno tamanho e recursos limitados, para assistência imediata de doenças e lesões. SIN camp h.

camp h., h. de campo. SIN base h.

closed h., h. fechado; hospital que limita os membros de sua equipe de atendimento ou consulta, algumas vezes a médicos empregados ou médicos de uma lista seletiva, limitando, assim, os que podem internar e tratar pacientes.

day h., h. diurno; instituição especial, ou área dentro de um ambiente hospitalar, que permite ao paciente ir ao hospital para tratamento durante o dia e retornar a casa ou a outro estabelecimento à noite. Cf. night h.

general h., h. geral; qualquer grande hospital civil, equipado para tratar de casos clínicos, cirúrgicos, obstétricos e psiquiátricos, que, em geral, possui uma equipe médica residente.

government h., h. público; hospital administrado por funcionários municipais, estaduais ou federais. SIN public h.

group h., h. de grupo; hospital particular organizado e controlado por um grupo de médicos e restrito à recepção e à assistência de seus próprios pacientes.

maternity h., h.-maternidade; hospital especial para o atendimento de mulheres em trabalho de parto.

mental h., h. psiquiátrico; instituição médica para atendimento e tratamento de pessoas com distúrbios psiquiátricos e psicológicos.

municipal h., h. municipal; hospital público administrado por funcionários municipais.

night h., h. noturno; instituição especial, ou área dentro de um ambiente hospitalar, que fornece tratamento e alojamento noturno para pacientes capazes de trabalhar na comunidade durante o dia. Cf. day h.

open h., h. aberto; hospital para onde todos os médicos, e não apenas os membros da equipe regular, ou aqueles numa lista seletiva, podem enviar seus pacientes e controlar seu tratamento; extremamente raro, visto que a maioria dos hospitais limita, em certo grau, o acesso a médicos.

philanthropic h., h. filantrópico. SIN voluntary h.

private h., h. particular; **(1)** hospital semelhante a um hospital de grupo, exceto por ser controlado por um único médico ou por ele e seus associados no consultório; **(2)** hospital que visa obter lucros. SIN proprietary h.

proprietary h., h. particular. SIN private h.

public h., h. público. SIN government h.

special h., h. especializado; hospital para assistência médica e cirúrgica de pacientes com tipos específicos de doenças, como para ouvido, nariz e garganta, olhos ou doenças mentais.

state h., h. estadual; hospital sustentado, em parte, por contribuintes de imposto de renda e administrado por funcionários estaduais.

teaching h., h.-escola; hospital que também funciona como centro formal de ensino para o treinamento de médicos, enfermeiros e outros profissionais de saúde.

Veterans Administration h., hospital que funciona à custa do governo federal norte-americano, administrado pela Veterans Administration para assistência de veteranos de guerras e militares reformados dos Estados Unidos.

voluntary h., h. voluntário; hospital sustentado, em parte, por contribuições voluntárias e sob o controle de um conselho local de administradores, geralmente autonomeados; hospital sem fins lucrativos. SIN philanthropic h.

weekend h., h. de fim de semana; instituição especial, ou instalação dentro de um ambiente hospitalar, que permite ao paciente trabalhar na comunidade durante os dias úteis da semana e receber tratamento hospitalar nos fins de semana.

hos·pi·tal·ist (hos′pit - al - ist). Hospitalista. **1.** Médico cujas atividades profissionais são realizadas, em grande parte, num hospital, como, p. ex., anestesiologistas, médicos de emergência, intensivistas (especialistas em cuidados intensivos), patologistas e radiologistas. SIN hospital-based physician. **2.** Médico de atendimento primário (não-residente) que assume a responsabilidade de pela observação e tratamento de pacientes hospitalizados, devolvendo-os aos cuidados de seus médicos particulares ao receberem alta. [hospital + -ist]

Os hospitalistas podem ser funcionários de um hospital ou HMO, contratantes ou médicos particulares. Os médicos de atendimento primário que atuam nos hospitais dispensam os clínicos gerais da necessidade de efetuar visitas diárias aos pacientes hospitalizados. Embora a disponibilidade de médicos orientados para o atendimento de pacientes internados melhore a eficiência da assistência e reduza a permanência do paciente no hospital, alguns profissionais consideraram-na uma ameaça à integridade da relação médico-paciente tradicional. A medicina organizada possui relações contratuais opostas, incluindo cláusulas de atendimento gerenciado (*managed care*), em que os médicos particulares devem passar a um hospitalista a responsabilidade pela assistência a todos os pacientes internados no hospital. Embora esse acordo tenha muitas semelhanças com o sistema inglês de consultoria e clínicos gerais, alguns assinalaram que a restrição dos médicos de cuidados primários à prática em consultório pode levar a uma redução das habilidades diagnósticas e terapêuticas essenciais e a um declínio de prestígio entre colegas e o próprio público. O impacto do sistema de hospitalistas sobre a educação médica e sobre o sistema de equipe hospitalar, através do qual médicos e consultores mantêm "privilégios" ao fornecerem assistência hospitalar a seus próprios pacientes de acordo com regulamentos ou estatutos, também tem causado certa preocupação.

hos·pi·tal·i·za·tion (hos′pi - tăl - i - zā′shŭn). Hospitalização; internação para estudo diagnóstico e tratamento.

host. Hospedeiro; organismo no qual vive um parasita, obtendo sua substância ou energia corporal desse hospedeiro. [L. *hospes*, hóspede, hospedeiro]

accidental h., h. acidental; hospedeiro que abriga um organismo que, habitualmente, não o infecta.

amplifier h., h. amplificador; hospedeiro em que os agentes infecciosos multiplicam-se rapidamente em níveis elevados, proporcionando uma importante fonte de infecção para vetores em doenças transmitidas por vetores.

dead-end h., h. final; hospedeiro em que os agentes infecciosos não são transmitidos a outros hospedeiros suscetíveis.

definitive h., h. definitivo; hospedeiro em que um parasita alcança o estágio adulto ou estágio sexualmente maduro. SIN final h.

final h., h. final, h. definitivo. SIN definitive h.

intermediate h., intermediary h., h. intermediário; **(1)** hospedeiro em que ocorrem os estágios larvário ou de desenvolvimento; **(2)** hospedeiro através do qual pode passar o microrganismo ou que contém um estágio assexuado de um parasita. SIN secondary h.

paratenic h., h. paratênico; hospedeiro intermediário em que não ocorre desenvolvimento do parasita, embora sua presença possa ser necessária como elo essencial para completar o ciclo de vida do parasita; p. ex., os sucessivos peixes hospedeiros que transportam o plerocercóide do *Diphyllobothrium latum*, a grande tênia do peixe, até peixes maiores que acabam sendo consumidos por seres humanos ou outros hospedeiros finais. SIN transport h.

reservoir h., h. reservatório; o hospedeiro de uma infecção cujo agente infeccioso multiplica-se e/ou desenvolve-se e do qual o agente depende para a sua sobrevida na natureza; o h. essencial para a manutenção da infecção durante os períodos em que não ocorre transmissão ativa.

secondary h., h. secundário. SIN intermediate h.

transport h., h. de transporte. SIN paratenic h.

Hounsfield, Godfrey N., engenheiro eletrônico inglês, *1919. Desenvolveu o primeiro aparelho prático de tomografia computadorizada, o *scanner* EMI; recebeu o Prêmio Nobel de Medicina em 1979, juntamente com o físico A. M. Cormack. VER H. *unit*, *number*.

house·fly (hows′flī). Mosca-doméstica. VER *Musca*, *Fannia*.

house of·fi·cer. Residente; pessoa com grau médico empregada por um hospital para fornecer assistência a pacientes enquanto recebe treinamento numa especialidade médica.

Houssay, Bernardo A., fisiologista argentino e ganhador do Prêmio Nobel, 1887–1971. VER H. *animal*, *phenomenon*, *syndrome*.

Houston, John, médico irlandês, 1802–1845. VER H. *folds*, em *fold*, *muscle*.

Hovius, Jacob, oftalmologista holandês, 1710–1786. VER *canal* of H.

Howard, John Eager, internista e endocrinologista norte-americano, 1902–1985. VER H. *test*; Ellsworth-H. *test*.

Howell, William H., fisiologista norte-americano, 1860–1945. VER H. *unit*; H.-Jolly *bodies*, em *body*.

Howship, John, cirurgião inglês, 1781–1841. VER H. *lacunae*, em *lacuna*.

Hoyer, Heinrich F., anatomista e histologista polonês, 1834–1907. VER H. *anastomoses*, em *anastomosis*, *canals*, em *canal*; Sucquet-H. *canals*, em *canal*.

HP Abreviatura de haptoglobin (haptoglobina).

HPL Abreviatura de human placental *lactogen* (lactogênio placentário humano).

HPLC Abreviatura de high-pressure liquid chromatography (cromatografia líquida de alta pressão); high-performance liquid *chromatography* (cromatografia líquida de alto desempenho).

HPV Abreviatura de human papillomavirus (papilomavírus humano).

H₂Q Símbolo de ubiquinol (ubiquinol).

h.r.a. Abreviatura de health risk *assessment* (avaliação de risco de saúde).

HRCT Abreviatura de high-resolution computed *tomography* (tomografia computadorizada de alta resolução).

HRSA Abreviatura de *Health Resources and Services Administration*.

HRT Abreviatura de hormone replacement *therapy* (terapia de reposição hormonal).

h.s. Abreviatura de L. *hora somni*, antes de dormir, ao deitar.

HSIL Abreviatura de high-grade squamous intraepithelial *lesion* (lesão intraepitelial escamosa de alto grau).

hsp Abreviatura de heat shock *proteins* (proteínas de choque térmico), em *protein*.

HSV Abreviatura de herpes simplex *virus* (vírus herpes simples).

5-HT Abreviatura de 5-hydroxytryptamine (5-hidroxitriptamina).
Ht Abreviatura de total *hyperopia* (hiperopia total).
HTLV Abreviatura de human T-cell lymphoma/leukemia *virus* (vírus de linfoma/leucemia de células T humano).
HTLV-I Abreviatura de T-cell lymphotrophic virus type I (vírus linfotrópico de células T tipo I); human lymphotropic virus, type 1 (vírus linfotrópico humano tipo 1).
HTLV-II Abreviatura de T-cell lymphotrophic virus type II (vírus linfotrópico de células T tipo II); human lymphotropic virus, type 2 (vírus linfotrópico humano tipo 2).
HTLV-III Abreviatura antiga de human T-cell lymphotropic virus type III (vírus linfotrópico de células T tipo III). VER human immunodeficiency *virus*.
hU, hu Abreviatura de dihydrouridine (diidrouridina).
Hubrecht, Ambrosius A.W., zoologista e anatomista comparativo holandês, 1853–1915. VER H. protochordal *knot*.
Hucker-Conn stain. Corante de Hucker-Conn. VER em stain.
Hudson, Arthur Cyril, oftalmologista inglês, 1875–1962. VER H.-Stähli *line*.
hue (hū) . Tonalidade; uma das três qualidades da cor; propriedade pela qual as cores do espectro são distinguidas umas das outras e dos cinzas de brilho semelhante; determinada pelo comprimento de onda ou por uma combinação de comprimentos de onda de luz.
Hueck, Alexander F., anatomista alemão, 1802–1842. VER H. *ligament*.
Huët, G.J., médico holandês, *1879. VER Pelger-Huët nuclear *anomaly*.
Hueter, Karl, cirurgião alemão, 1838–1882. VER H. *maneuver*.
Hüfner, Carl Gustav von, médico alemão, 1840–1908. VER H. *equation*.
Huguier, Pierre C., cirurgião francês, 1804–1873. VER H. *canal, circle, sinus*.
Huhner, Max, urologista norte-americano, 1873–1947. VER H. *test*.
Hull, Edgar, cardiologista norte-americano, *1904.
hum (hum) . Zumbido, sopro; sopro contínuo baixo. [echoic]
  venous h., s. venoso; ruído breve ou contínuo que se origina nas veias do pescoço e pode ser confundido com sopros cardíacos, em particular com o sopro contínuo do canal arterial persistente. SIN bruit de diable, nun's murmur.
Human Genome Initiative. Projeto Genoma Humano. SIN Human Genome Project.

Human Genome Project. Projeto Genoma Humano; empreendimento abrangente por biologistas moleculares do mundo inteiro com a finalidade de mapear o genoma humano, que consiste em cerca de 100.000 genes ou 3 bilhões de pares de bases de nucleotídeos. SIN Human Genome Initiative.

> Iniciado pelo Congresso, em 1990, o *U.S. Human Genome Project (Projeto Genoma Humano dos Estados Unidos)* é um empreendimento multidisciplinar de 15 anos de duração, conjuntamente administrado pelo *Department of Energy* e pelos *National Institutes of Health*, para mapear o genoma humano e estabelecer a sua seqüência. Empreendimentos semelhantes foram iniciados na Grã-Bretanha, no Japão e em outros países, bem como por organizações financiadas pelo setor privado. Se fosse impresso, o genoma humano, em sua totalidade, preencheria 1.000 listas telefônicas de cidades grandes, cada uma com 1.000 páginas. Segundo estimativas, a determinação da seqüência do DNA em todos os 46 cromossomos deverá levar 15 anos, com um custo de $3 bilhões de dólares, mesmo com a ajuda das reações da cadeia de polimerase, hibridização *in situ* com fluorescência, clonagem de segmentos de DNA e tecnologia de determinação automática de seqüências. O mapa resultante será uma representação bastante idealizada, como uma ilustração num atlas de anatomia, visto que não existem duas pessoas, exceto (talvez) os gêmeos idênticos, que tenham exatamente a mesma constituição genética. O estabelecimento do mapa genômico ampliará nossos conhecimentos de biologia humana e deverá facilitar a detecção e o tratamento de doenças genéticas. Existem também projetos em andamento para estudar os genomas de bactérias, leveduras, plantas de cultivo, animais de fazenda e outros organismos, que deverão promover avanços na agricultura, na ciência do meio ambiente e nos processos industriais. Cerca de 5% do orçamento do *Human Genome Project* foram reservados antecipadamente para a resolução de questões éticas, legais e sociais que poderão surgir com essa pesquisa.

---

hu·man pap·il·lo·ma·vi·rus (HPV). Papilomavírus humano; DNA vírus icosaédrico de 55 nm de diâmetro, do gênero *Papillomavirus*, família Papovaviridae; certos tipos causam verrugas cutâneas e genitais, enquanto outros tipos estão associados a neoplasia intra-epitelial cervical grave e carcinomas anogenital e laríngeo. Mais de 70 tipos já foram caracterizados com base na sua relação do DNA. SIN infectious papilloma virus.

> A infecção pelo papilomavírus humano constitui a doença viral sexualmente transmissível mais comum. O intervalo entre a exposição e a manifestação clínica da doença varia de 3 semanas a 8 meses. Um único contato com um indivíduo infectado sem proteção está associado a um risco de infecção de 60%. Pelo menos 80% dos casos de câncer de colo uterino são atribuídos à infecção por HPV, e acredita-se que 25% de todos os resultados irregulares nos esfregaços de Papanicolaou resultem da presença do vírus, que é freqüentemente assintomático nos demais aspectos. A tipagem do HPV em mulheres com células escamosas atípicas de importância indeterminada (ASCUS, *atypical squamous cells of undetermined significance*) no esfregaço de colo uterino de Papanicolaou ajuda a identificar aquelas nas quais é necessária uma vigilância mais intensiva à procura de qualquer alteração pré-maligna. O câncer cervical invasivo está associado aos tipos 16, 18, 31, 33 e outros tipos. Em cerca de 40% das mulheres HIV-positivas, verifica-se o desenvolvimento de displasia cervical grave causada por HPV, que, em muitos casos, evolui para um câncer fatal com agressividade não comumente observada em mulheres HIV-positivas. As verrugas genitais externas (condiloma acuminado) são habitualmente causadas por HPV tipo 6 ou 11. As mulheres com verrugas genitais externas não correm risco aumentado de câncer cervical e não precisam ser submetidas a colposcopia ou outros procedimentos especiais de vigilância se o esfregaço de Papanicolaou de rotina for negativo. Cerca de 20–30% das infecções por HPV sofrem regressão espontânea. O diagnóstico de infecção por HPV baseia-se na inspeção visual (incluindo colposcopia com aplicação de ácido acético ao colo uterino), esfregaço de Papanicolaou e biopsia, com detecção do DNA viral no tecido. As opções de tratamento incluem excisão cirúrgica, criocirurgia, ablação com laser, excisão eletrocirúrgica com alça e injeção intralesional de interferon. As verrugas genitais externas respondem habitualmente ao tratamento tópico com gel podofilox ou ao imiquimod (agente indutor de citocinas), que pode ser aplicado pela própria paciente. Pode não ser possível erradicar a infecção subclínica por HPV, detectável apenas pelo esfregaço de Papanicolaou ou outros métodos laboratoriais. O vírus não pode ser cultivado, e não existe nenhum teste para confirmar a cura.

---

hu·mec·tant (hū - mek'tănt) . Umectante. **1.** Umectante. **2.** Substância utilizada para obter um efeito umectante (p. ex., solução de glicerina).
hu·mec·ta·tion (hū - mek - tā'shŭn) . Umectação. **1.** Aplicação terapêutica de umidade. **2.** Infiltração serosa dos tecidos. **3.** Maceração de uma droga no seu estado integral em água na preparação de um extrato. [L. *humecto*, pp. *-mectus*, umedecer, fr. *humeo*, molhar]
hu·mer·al (hū'mer - ăl) . Umeral; relativo ao úmero.
hu·mer·o·ra·di·al (hū'mer - ō - rā'dē - ăl) . Umerorradial; relativo tanto ao úmero quanto ao rádio; indica especialmente a relação de comprimento entre ambos.
hu·mer·o·scap·u·lar (hū'mer - ō - skap'ū - lăr) . Umeroescapular; relativo ao úmero e à escápula.
hu·mer·o·ul·nar (hū'mer - ō - ŭl'năr) . Umeroulnar; relativo tanto ao úmero quanto à ulna; indica especialmente a relação de comprimento entre ambos.
hu·mer·us, gen. e pl. **hu·mer·i** (hū'mer - ŭs, - ī) [TA]. Úmero; o osso do braço, que se articula com a escápula em cima e com o rádio e a ulna embaixo. SIN arm bone. [L. ombro]
hu·mid·i·ty (hū - mid'i - tē) . Umidade; umidade, como a do ar. [L. *humiditas*, umidade]
  absolute h., u. absoluta; a massa de vapor d'água realmente presente por unidade de volume de gás ou ar.
  relative h., u. relativa; a quantidade real de vapor d'água presente no ar ou num gás, dividida pela quantidade necessária para a saturação na mesma temperatura e pressão; expressa como percentagem.
hu·min (hū'min) . Humina; resíduo acastanhado ou preto insolúvel, obtido da hidrólise ácida de glicoproteínas.
Hummelsheim, Eduard K.M.J., oftalmologista alemão, 1868–1952. VER H. *operation*; Hummelsheim *procedure*.
hu·mor, gen. **hu·mor·is** (hū'mer, hū - mōr'is) [TA]. Humor. **1.** [NA]. Qualquer líquido claro ou substância anatômica hialina semilíquida. **2.** Um dos líquidos corporais elementares que eram a base dos ensinamentos fisiológicos e patológicos da escola hipocrática: sangue, bile amarela, bile preta e flegma. VER TAMBÉM humoral *doctrine*. [L. corretamente, *humor*, líquido]
  aqueous h. [TA], h. aquoso; líquido aquoso que preenche as câmaras anterior e posterior do olho. É secretado por processos ciliares para as câmaras posteriores e passa através da pupila para a câmara anterior, onde é filtrado através da rede trabecular, sendo reabsorvido no sistema venoso, no ângulo iridocorneano, por meio do seio venoso da esclerótica. SIN h. aquosus [TA], intraocular fluid.
  h. aquo'sus [TA], h. aquoso. SIN aqueous h.
  Morgagni h., h. de Morgagni. SIN Morgagni *liquor*.

ocular h., ocular h; um dos humores do olho: aquoso e vítreo.
peccant humors, humores mórbidos; com base na teoria humoral histórica da doença, esses humores ou líquidos anormais no corpo eram considerados como as causas diretas de várias doenças.
vitreous h. [TA], h. vítreo; o líquido componente do corpo vítreo, com o qual é quase sempre erroneamente igualado. SIN h. vitreus [TA].
h. vit'reus [TA] h. vítreo. SIN vitreous h.
hu·mor·al (hū'mŏr-ăl). Humoral; relativo a um humor em qualquer sentido.
hu·mor·al·ism, hu·mor·ism (hū'mŏr-ăl-izm, -mŏr-izm). Humoralismo. SIN humoral *doctrine.* [L. *umor, humor,* umidade]
hump (hŭmp). Corcunda, giba; protuberância ou saliência arredondada.
buffalo h., giba de búfalo. SIN buffalo *type.*
dowager h., c. de viúva; cifose cervical pós-menopáusica de mulheres idosas, devido à osteoporose e fraturas de vértebras por compressão.
Hampton h., c. de Hampton; densidade de tecido mole pulmonar justapleural em radiografia de tórax, convexa em direção ao hilo, geralmente no ângulo costofrênico; descrita como manifestação de infarto pulmonar devido a embolia pulmonar.
hump·back (hŭmp'back). Corcunda; termo não-científico para referir-se a cifose ou giba.
Humphry, Sir George M., cirurgião inglês, 1820–1896. VER H. *ligament.*
hu·mu·lin (hū'moo-lin). Humulina. SIN lupulin.
hu·mu·lus (hū'moo-lŭs). Lúpulo; os frutos secos (estróbilos) de *Humulus lupulus* (família Moraceae), uma erva trepadeira da Ásia Central e do Norte, Europa e América do Norte; amargo aromático, levemente sedativo e diurético; primariamente utilizado na fermentação industrial para dar aroma e sabor à cerveja. SIN hops. [L. Medieval]
hunch·back (hŭnch'bak). Corcunda; termo não-científico para referir-se a cifose ou giba.
Hünermann, Carl, médico alemão. VER Conradi-Hünermann *disease.*
hun·ger (hŭn'ger). Fome. **1.** Desejo ou necessidade de alimentação. **2.** Qualquer apetite, desejo forte ou desejo mórbido. [A.S.]
affect h., f. de afeto; fome emocional pelo amor materno e sentimento de proteção e cuidados implícitos na relação mãe–filho.
narcotic h., f. de narcóticos; desejo fisiológico mórbido por narcóticos.
Hunner, Guy L., cirurgião norte-americano, 1868–1957. VER H. *ulcer;* Fenwick-H. *ulcer.*
Hunt, James Ramsay, neurologista norte-americano, 1872–1937. VER H. *neuralgia,* paradoxic *phenomenon, syndrome;* Ramsay H. *syndrome.*
Hunt, William E., neurocirurgião norte-americano, *1921. VER Tolosa-H. *syndrome.*
Hunter, Charles, médico canadense, 1872–1955. VER H. *syndrome.*
Hunter, John, cirurgião escocês, anatomista, fisiologista e patologista, 1728–1793. VER H. *canal, gubernaculum, operation;* H.-Schreger *bands* em *band; lines,* em *line.*
Hunter, William, anatomista e obstetra escocês, 1718–1783. VER H. *ligament, line, membrane.*
Hunter, William, patologista inglês, 1861–1937. VER H. *glossitis.*
hunt·ing (hŭnt'ing). Busca; a oscilação de uma variável controlada, como a temperatura de um termostato, em torno de seu ponto de ajuste. VER hunting *reaction.*
Huntington, George, médico norte-americano, 1850–1916. VER H. *chorea, disease.*
Hurler, Gertrud, pediatra austríaco, 1889–1965. VER H. *disease, syndrome;* Pfaundler-H. *syndrome.*
Hurst, Edward Weston, médico australiano do século XX. VER H. *disease.*
Hurst, Sir Arthur Frederick (nascido Hertz), médico inglês, 1879–1944.
Hürthle, Karl W., histologista alemão, 1860–1945. VER H. *cell, cell adenoma, cell carcinoma.*
Huschke, Emil, anatomista alemão, 1797–1858. VER H. *cartilages,* em *cartilage, foramen,* em *teeth,* em *tooth valve.*
Hutchinson, Sir Jonathan, cirurgião inglês, 1828–1913. VER H. *facies, freckle, mask,* crescentic *notch, patch, pupil, teeth,* em *tooth, triad;* H.-Gilford *disease, syndrome.*
Hutchison, Sir Robert, pediatra inglês, 1871–1960. VER H. *syndrome.*
Huxley, Thomas H., biologista, fisiologista e anatomista comparativo inglês, 1825–1895. VER H. *layer, membrane, sheath.*
Huygens, Christian, físico holandês, 1629–1695. VER H. *ocular, principle.*
HV Abreviatura de half-value (meio-valor).
HVA Abreviatura de homovanillic acid (ácido homovanílico).
HVL Abreviatura de half-value *layer* (camada de meio-valor).
△ **hyal-.** Hial-. SIN hyalo-.
hy·a·lin (hī'ă-lin). Hialina; substância homogênea clara e eosinofílica que ocorre na degeneração celular; p. ex., nas paredes arteriolares na esclerose arteriolar e nos tufos glomerulares na glomerulosclerose diabética. [G. *hyalos,* vidro]
alcoholic h., h. alcoólica. SIN Mallory *bodies,* em *body.*
hy·a·line (hī'ă-lin, -lēn). Hialino; relativo a hifas ou outras estruturas fúngicas incolores. SIN hyaloid. [G. *hyalos,* vidro]

hy·a·lin·i·za·tion (hī'ă-lin-i-zā'shŭn). Hialinização; formação de hialina.
hy·a·li·no·sis (hī'ă-li-nō'sis). Hialinose; degeneração hialina (hyaline *degeneration*), especialmente aquela de grau relativamente extenso.
h. cutis et mucosae, h. cutânea e mucosa. SIN lipoid *proteinosis.*
systemic h., h. sistêmica. SIN juvenile hyalin *fibromatosis.*
hy·a·li·nu·ria (hī-ă-li-noo'rē-ă). Hialinúria; excreção de hialina ou de cilindros de material hialino na urina. [hialina + G. *ouron,* urina]
hy·a·li·tis (hī-ă-lī'tis). Hialite. SIN vitreitis.
suppurative h., h. supurativa; humor vítreo purulento, devido à exsudação de estruturas adjacentes, como na panoftalmite.
△ **hyalo-, hyal-.** Hialo-, Hial-; vítreo, hialino. Cf. vitreo-. [G. *hyalos,* vidro]
hy·a·lo·bi·u·ron·ic ac·id (hī'ă-lō-bī-ūr-on'ik). Ácido hialobiurônico; dissacarídeo composto de ácido D-glicurônico e *N*-acetil-D-glicosamina numa ligação β1,3; ocorre no ácido hialurônico como unidade repetitiva.
hy·a·lo·cyte (hī'ă-lō-sīt). Hialócito. SIN vitreous *cell.* [hialo- + G. *kytos,* célula]
hy·al·o·gens (hī-al'ō-jenz). Hialogênios; substâncias semelhantes a mucóides que são encontradas em muitas estruturas animais (p. ex., cartilagem, humor vítreo, cistos hidáticos) e liberam açúcares com a sua hidrólise.
hy·a·lo·hy·pho·my·co·sis (hī'ă-lō-hī'fō-mī-kō'sis). Hialo-hifomicose; termo geral para referir-se à infecção tecidual causada por um fungo com micélio hialino (incolor). Se for possível identificar o fungo, a doença deve receber um nome específico, como aspergilose ou fusariose. [hialo- + G. *hyphē,* tecido + *mykēs,* fungo + *-osis,* condição]
hy·a·loid (hī'ă-loyd). Hialóide. SIN hyaline. [hyalo- + G. *eidos,* semelhança]
hy·al·o·mere (hī'ă-lō-mēr). Hialômero; a periferia clara de uma plaqueta sanguínea. [hialo- + G. *meros,* parte]
Hy·a·lom·ma (hī-ă-lom'ă). Gênero do Velho Mundo (cerca de 21 espécies) de grandes carrapatos ixodídeos com olhos submarginais, festão coalescente e escudo ornado, com rostro longo. Os adultos parasitam todos os animais domésticos, bem como uma ampla variedade de animais selvagens; as larvas ou ninfas podem parasitar pequenos mamíferos, aves e répteis. As espécies abrigam uma grande variedade de patógenos de seres humanos e animais, e também causam considerável lesão mecânica. [hialo- + G. *omma,* olho]
H. anato'licum, nome antigo para *H. anatolicum anatolicum.*
H. anato'licum anato'licum, uma subespécie que infesta gado, camelos e cavalos na Ásia, Oriente Próximo e Oriente Médio, sudeste da Europa e África do Norte; trata-se de um vetor da teileriose tropical bovina, da babesiose eqüina e da febre hemorrágica humana da Criméia–Congo.
H. margina'tum, uma espécie particularmente comum de carrapatos transportados por aves que migram entre a Europa e a Ásia e África, constituindo o provável vetor do vírus da febre hemorrágica da Criméia.
H. variega'tum, espécie de carrapato, vetor do agente viral da coriomeningite linfocítica na Etiópia.
hy·a·lo·pha·gia, hy·a·loph·a·gy (hī'ă-lō-fā'jē-ă, hī-ă-lof'ă-jē). Hialofagia; ato de ingerir ou mastigar vidro. [hyalo- + G. *phagō,* comer]
hy·a·lo·pho·bia (hī'ă-lō-fō'bē-ă). Hialofobia; medo mórbido de objetos de vidro. SIN crystallophobia. [hyalo- + G. *phobos,* medo]
hy·al·o·plasm, hy·a·lo·plas·ma (hī'ă-lō-plazm, -plaz'mă). Hialoplasma; substância líquida protoplasmática de uma célula. [hyalo- + G. *plasma,* coisa formada]
nuclear h., h. nuclear. SIN karyolymph.
hy·a·lo·se·ro·si·tis (hī'ă-lō-ser-ō-sī'tis). Hialosserosite; inflamação de uma membrana serosa com exsudato fibrinoso que acaba por se tornar hialinizada, produzindo um revestimento relativamente espesso, denso, opaco, brilhante, branco ou branco-acinzentado; quando o processo envolve as membranas serosas viscerais de vários órgãos, a condição macroscopicamente aparente recebe algumas vezes a denominação coloquial de fígado com glacê, baço recoberto de açúcar, coração congelado, e assim por diante, dependendo do local acometido. [hyalo- + L. Mod. *serosa,* membrana serosa + *-itis,* inflamação]
hy·a·lo·sis (hī-ă-lō'sis). Hialose; alterações degenerativas no corpo vítreo. [hyalo- + G. *-osis,* condição]
asteroid h., h. asteróide; presença de numerosos corpúsculos esféricos pequenos (opacidades em "bola de neve") no corpo vítreo, visíveis à oftalmoscopia; uma alteração relacionada à idade, habitualmente unilateral, que não afeta a visão.
punctate h., h. pontilhada; condição caracterizada por minúsculas opacidades no vítreo.
hy·a·lo·some (hī-al'ō-sōm). Hialossoma; estrutura oval ou redonda no interior de um núcleo celular, que se cora fracamente, mas que se assemelha a um nucléolo nos demais aspectos. [hyalo- + G. *sōma,* corpo]
hy·a·lu·rate (hī-ă-loo'răt). Hialurato. SIN hyaluronate.
hy·a·lu·ro·nate (hī-ă-loo'ron-āt). Hialuronato; sal ou éster do ácido hialurônico. SIN hyalurate.
h. lyase, h. liase; uma liase que catalisa a clivagem dos ácidos hialurônicos, produzindo diversas 3-(4-desoxi-β-D-glic-4-enuronosil)-*N*-acetil-D-glicosaminas (ácido hialobiurônico). VER TAMBÉM hyaluronidase (1), hyaluronoglucosaminidase. SIN hyaluronic lyase.

hy·al·u·ron·ic ac·id (hī'ă - loo - ron'ik). Ácido hialurônico; mucopolissacarídeo constituído por resíduos de ligação β1,4 alternados de ácido hialobiurônico, formando um material gelatinoso nos espaços teciduais e atuando como lubrificante e absorvente de choque geralmente por todo o corpo; é hidrolisado a unidade de dissacarídeos ou tetrassacarídeos pela hialuronidase.

hy·al·u·ron·ic ly·ase. Liase hialurônica. SIN *hyaluronate lyase.*

hy·al·u·ron·i·dase (hī'ă - loo - ron'i - dās). Hialuronidase. **1.** Termo utilizado livremente para referir-se à hialuronato liase, hialuronoglicosaminidase e hialuronoglicuronidase, das quais uma ou mais estão presentes nos testículos, espermatozóides, outros órgãos, venenos de abelhas e cobras, pneumococos do tipo II, certos estreptococos hemolíticos etc. SIN diffusing factor, Duran-Reynals permeability factor, Duran-Reynals spreading factor, invasin, spreading factor. **2.** Produto enzimático solúvel preparado a partir de testículos de mamíferos; utilizado para aumentar o efeito de anestésicos locais e permitir uma infiltração mais ampla de líquidos administrados por via subcutânea, sendo sugerido no tratamento de certas formas de artrite para promover a regressão do tecido redundante; utilizado para acelerar a reabsorção de edema e hematoma traumáticos ou pós-operatórios, em combinação com a colagenase para dissociar órgãos, como fígado e coração, em suspensões de células viáveis, e, em histoquímica, empregado em secreções teciduais para verificar a presença de ácido hialurônico ou de sulfatos de condroitina.

hy·al·u·ron·o·glu·cos·a·min·i·dase (hī - ă - loo'ron - ō - gloo'kō - să - min'i - dās). Hialuronoglicosaminidase; enzima que hidrolisa ligações β1,4- nos hialuronatos. VER TAMBÉM hyaluronidase (1), *hyaluronate* lyase.

hy·al·u·ron·o·glu·cu·ron·i·dase (hī - ă - loo'ron - ō - gloo - kur - on'i - dās). Hialuronoglicuronidase; enzima que hidrolisa ligações β1,3-nos hialuronatos. VER TAMBÉM hyaluronidase (1).

hy·bar·ox·ia (hī - bă - rok'sē - ă). Hibaroxia; oxigenoterapia com pressões superiores a uma atmosfera ou pressão de oxigênio ambiente aplicada a todo o corpo numa câmara ou quarto. [G. *hyper*, acima + *baros*, pressão, + *oxys*, aguda]

hy·ben·zate (hī - ben'zāt). Hibenzato; contração aprovada pela USAN para *o*-(4-hidroxibenzoil) benzoato.

hy·brid (hī'brid). Híbrido. **1.** Indivíduo (planta ou animal) cujos genitores consistem em variedades diferentes da mesma espécie ou que pertencem a espécies diferentes, porém estreitamente relacionadas. **2.** Fusão de células de cultura de tecido, como ocorre no hibridoma. **3.** Ligação ou valência orbital obtida pela combinação linear de dois ou mais orbitais atômicos diferentes. SIN cross-breed (1). [L. *hybrida*, descendente de uma porca doméstica e de um javali, fr. G. *hybris*, violação, libertinagem]

DNA-RNA h., h. DNA-RNA; ácidos polinucleicos de filamento duplo em que um dos filamentos consiste em DNA, enquanto o outro consiste no RNA complementar; formado durante a transcrição e a multiplicação de RNA vírus oncogênicos.

SV40-adenovirus h., h. SV40-adenovírus; virion que consiste em material genético SV40 contido num capsídeo de adenovírus.

hy·brid·ism (hī'brid - izm). Hibridismo; estado de ser híbrido.

hy·brid·i·za·tion (hī'brid - i - zā'shŭn). Hibridização. **1.** Processo de procriação de um híbrido. **2.** *Crossover* entre genes relacionados, porém não-alélicos. **3.** Reassociação específica de filamentos complementares de ácidos polinucleicos; p. ex., formação de um híbrido DNA-RNA. **4.** O processo ou ato de formar um híbrido macromolecular em que as subunidades são obtidas de diferentes fontes. SIN crossbreeding.

cell h., h. celular; fusão de duas ou mais células desiguais, levando à formação de um sincárion.

cross h., h. cruzada; união de uma sonda de DNA a uma molécula de DNA de complementaridade imperfeita.

DNA h., h. de DNA; técnica utilizada para determinar as relações de microrganismos através da velocidade e eficiência da reassociação de DNA de filamento simples para formar DNA de filamento duplo, quando um dos filamentos se origina de um organismo, e o outro filamento, do outro organismo; ocorre quando as seqüências de bases são complementares ou quase.

fluorescence in situ h., h. *in situ* com fluorescência. SIN *fluorescent in situ h.*

fluorescent in situ h., h. *in situ* com fluorescência; método empregado para determinar a localização de cromossomas ou o padrão de expressão de fragmentos de cDNA ou DNA genômico. A porção do DNA a ser mapeada (a "sonda") é marcada com corante fluorescente e hibridizada a uma preparação de cromossomas ou a um corte tecidual. A sonda une-se a seqüências complementares de DNA ou de RNA. O exame dos cromossomas ou do corte tecidual ao microscópio de fluorescência revela o número, o tamanho e a localização das seqüências-alvo. SIN fluorescence in situ h.

nucleic acid h., h. de ácidos nucleicos. SIN *anneal (5).*

overlap h., h. de superposição. SIN *chromosome* walking.

in situ h., h. *in situ*; técnica desenvolvida em 1969 para a união de sondas de ácido nucleico ao DNA celular para detecção por auto-radiografia. Em condições laboratoriais apropriadas, o processo de ligação ocorre espontaneamente. A h. *in situ* constitui uma etapa-chave na impressão do DNA (DNA *fingerprinting*). SIN in situ nucleic acid h.

in situ nucleic acid h., h. de ácidos nucleicos *in situ*. SIN *in situ h.*

somatic cell h., h. de células somáticas; produção de um heterocárion.

hy·brid·o·ma (hī - brid - ō'mă). Hibridoma; tumor de células híbridas utilizado na produção *in vitro* de anticorpos monoclonais específicos; produzido pela fusão de uma linhagem de cultura tecidual estabelecida de células tumorais linfocitárias (p. ex., células do plasmocitoma de camundongos) e células produtoras de anticorpos específicos (p. ex., esplenócitos de camundongos especificamente imunizados); as fusões são obtidas pelo uso de polietilenoglicol ou outros métodos. [G. *hybris*, violação, libertinagem + -*ōma*, tumor]

hy·clate (hī'klāt). Hiclato; contração aprovada pela USAN para o monocloridrato de hemietanolato hemiidratado, HCl.1/2C₂H₅OH.1/2H₂O.

hy·dan·to·in (hī - dan'tō - in). Hidantoína; 2,4-imidazolidinediona; derivada da uréia ou da alantoína; o grupamento NH—CH₂—CO é protótipo dos α-aminoácidos. Os derivados de hidantoína são formados pela reação do fenilisotiocianato e um polipeptídeo. SIN glycolylurea.

hy·dan·to·in·ate (hī - dan - tō'in - āt). Hidantoinato; sal de hidantoína.

hy·da·tid (hī'da - tid). **1.** Hidátide, cisto hidático. SIN *hydatid cyst.* **2.** Estrutura vesicular que se assemelha a um cisto de *Echinococcus*. [G. *hydatis*, gota de água, hidátide]

Morgagni h., h. de Morgagni, apêndices vesiculosos do epoóforo. SIN vesicular *appendages* of epoophoron, em *appendage.*

nonpedunculated h., apêndice do testículo. SIN *appendix* of testis.

pedunculated h., apêndice do epidídimo. SIN *appendix* of epididymidis.

sessile h., apêndice do testículo. SIN *appendix* of testis.

stalked h., apêndices vesiculosos do epoóforo. SIN vesicular *appendages* of epoophoron, em *appendage.*

hy·da·tid·i·form (hī - da - tid'i - form). Hidatiforme; que possui a forma ou o aspecto de hidátide.

hy·da·tid·o·cele (hī - da - tid'ō - sēl). Hidatidocele; massa cística composta por uma ou mais hidátides formadas no escroto. [hydatid + G. *kē - lē*, tumor]

hy·da·tid·o·sis (hī'da - ti - dō'sis). Hidatidose; estado mórbido causado pela presença de cistos hidáticos.

hy·da·ti·dos·to·my (hī'da - ti - dos'tō - mē). Hidatidostomia; evacuação cirúrgica de um cisto hidático. [hydatid + G. *stoma*, boca]

Hy·da·tig·e·ra tae·ni·ae·for·mis (hī - da - tij'er - ă tē - ni - ē - fōr'mis). SIN *Taenia taeniaeformis.*

hy·da·toid (hī'da - toyd). Hidatóide. **1.** Humor aquoso. **2.** Membrana hialóide. **3.** Relativo a humor aquoso. **4.** Aquoso ou semelhante à água. [G. *hydōr* (*hydat*-), água + *eidos*, semelhança]

hyd·no·car·pus oil (hid - nō - kar'pŭs). Óleo de hidnocarpo, óleo de chaulmogra. SIN *chaulmoogra oil.*

△ **hydr-.** Hidr-. VER hidro-.

hy·drac·e·tin (hī - drasʹē - tin). Hidracetina; forma pura de acetilfenilidrazina.

hy·drad·e·ni·tis (hī'drad - ē - nī'tis). Hidradenite. SIN *hidradenitis.*

hy·drad·e·no·ma (hī'drad - ē - nō'mă). Hidradenoma. SIN *hidradenoma.*

hy·dra·gogue (hī'drā - gog). Hidragogo; que produz uma descarga de líquido aquoso; refere-se a uma classe de catárticos que retêm líquido no intestino e ajudam na remoção de líquidos de edema, como, p. ex., catárticos salinos. [hydr- + G. *agōgos*, fazer sair]

hy·dral·a·zine hy·dro·chlo·ride (hī - dralʹă - zēn). Cloridrato de hidralazina; agente anti-hipertensivo vasodilatador.

hy·dral·lo·stane (hī - drallʹō - stān). Hidralostano; 11β,17α,21-triidroxi-5β-pregnano-3,20-diona; metabólito do cortisol, reduzido na ligação dupla 4,5. SIN 4,5α-dihydrocortisol.

hy·dra·mi·tra·zine tar·trate (hī - dră - mīʹtră - zēn). Tartarato de hidramitrazina; antiespasmódico intestinal.

hy·dram·ni·os, hy·dram·ni·on (hī - dram'nē - os, - nē - on). Hidrâmnio; presença de volume excessivo de líquido amniótico, geralmente mais de 2.000 mL. SIN polyhydramnios. [G. *hidōr*, água + âmnio]

hy·dran·en·ceph·a·ly (hī'dran - en - sefʹă - lē). Hidranencefalia; ausência de hemisférios cerebrais, que foram substituídos por sacos cheios de líquido, revestidos por leptomeninges. O crânio e as cavidades cerebrais estão normais. [hydr- + G. *an-* priv. + *enkephalos*, cérebro]

hy·drar·gyr·ia, hy·drar·gy·rism (hī - drar - jirʹē - ă, hī - drar'jir - izm). Hidrargiria. SIN mercury *poisoning.* [L. *hydrargyrum*, mercúrio]

hy·drar·gy·rum (hī - drarʹji - rŭm). Hidrargírio. SIN *mercury.* [G. *hydrargyros*, azougue, fr. *hydōr*, água + *argyros*, prata]

hy·drar·thro·di·al (hī - drar - thrōʹdē - ăl). Hidrartrodial; relativo a hidrartrose.

hy·drar·thro·sis (hī - drar - thrō'sis). Hidrartrose; derrame de líquido seroso para uma cavidade articular. [hydr- + G. *arthron*, articulação]

intermittent h., h. intermitente; distúrbio caracterizado por derrame seroso periodicamente recidivante na cavidade de uma articulação; a articulação pode ser a sede de artrite crônica ou pode estar aparentemente normal nos intervalos dos ataques.

hy·drase (hī'drās). Hidrase; nome antigo de hydratase (hidratase).

hy·dras·tine (hī - drasʹtēn). Hidrastina; alcalóide do hidraste; isoquinolina quimicamente relacionada à narcotina. Como cloridrato, era utilizado localmente no tratamento da inflamação catarral das mucosas e internamente no tratamento da inflamação gástrica, como estimulante uterino e para deter a hemorragia uterina.

hy·dras·ti·nine (hī-dras′ti-nēn). Hidrastinina; alcalóide semi-sintético preparado a partir da hidrastina; o cloridrato tem sido utilizado na hemorragia uterina e como oxitóxico; em altas doses, trata-se de um poderoso depressor de todo o sistema motor (córtex motor, nervo e músculo).

hy·dras·tis (hī-dras′tis). Hidraste; rizoma seco de *Hydrastis canadensis* (família Ranunculaceae), nativo do leste dos Estados Unidos; utilizado antigamente no tratamento de estados catarrais crônicos das mucosas e na metrorragia. SIN golden seal, jaundice root, yellow root. [L. Mod. fr. G. *hydōr* (*hydro-*), água + *draō*, realizar]

hy·dra·tase (hī′drā-tās). Hidratase; nome comum aplicado, juntamente com desidratase, a certas hidroliases (EC 4.2.1.x) que catalisam a hidratação–desidratação; p. ex., interconversão de fumarato-malato pela fumarato hidratase.

hy·drate (hī′drāt). Hidrato; solvato aquoso (em terminologia antiga, hidróxido); composto que se cristaliza com uma ou mais moléculas de água; p. ex., $CuSO_4 \cdot 5H_2O$.

hy·drat·ed (hī-drāt-ed). Hidratado; combinado com água, formando um hidrato. SIN hydrous.

hy·dra·tion (hī-drā′shŭn). Hidratação. **1.** Quimicamente, adição de água; deve ser diferenciada da hidrólise, na qual a união com a água é acompanhada de clivagem da molécula original e da molécula de água. VER TAMBÉM solvation. **2.** Clinicamente, captação de água; termo utilizado comumente no sentido de h. reduzida ou desidratação. **3.** Formação de uma camada de moléculas de água ao redor de uma entidade molecular.
  absolute h., h. absoluta; excesso real de água, medido por uma diferença do normal ou a partir de determinado conteúdo de água.

hy·dra·zide (hī′drā-zīd). Hidrazida; composto orgânico de fórmula geral $RCO–NHNH_2$; derivado acil da hidrazina.

hy·dra·zine (hī′drā-zēn). Hidrazina; $H_2N–NH_2$, líquido oleoso do qual derivam a fenilidrazina e produtos semelhantes. É muito tóxica e, possivelmente, trata-se de um carcinógeno.

hy·dra·zine yel·low. Amarelo de hidrazina, tartrazina. SIN tartrazine.

hy·dra·zi·nol·y·sis (hī-drā-zi-nol′i-sis). Hidrazinólise; clivagem de ligações químicas pela hidrazina; aplicada em degradações de proteínas e ácidos nucleicos.

hy·dra·zone (hī′drā-zōn). Hidrazona; substância derivada de aldeídos e cetonas pela reação com a hidrazina, ou derivado da hidrazina, formando o grupamento $R'R''C=N–NHR$.

hy·dre·mia (hī-drē′mē-ă). Hidremia; condição em que ocorre aumento do volume sanguíneo em conseqüência de aumento no conteúdo de água do plasma, com ou sem redução na concentração de proteínas; há um excesso de plasma em proporção aos elementos figurados, com redução correspondente do hematócrito. SIN dilution anemia, polyplasmia. [hydr- + G. *haima*, sangue]

hy·dren·ceph·a·lo·cele (hī-dren-sef′ă-lō-sēl). Hidrencefalocele; protrusão, através de uma fenda no crânio, de substância cerebral expandida num saco contendo líquido. SIN encephalocystocele, hydrocephalocele, hydroencephalocele. [hydr- + G. *enkephalos*, cérebro + *kēlē*, tumor]

hy·dren·ceph·a·lo·me·nin·go·cele (hī-dren-sef′ă-lō-me-ning′gō-sēl). Hidrencefalomeningocele; protrusão, através de um defeito no crânio, de um saco contendo meninges, substância cerebral e líquido cefalorraquidiano.

hy·dren·ceph·a·lus (hī-dren-sef′ă-lŭs). Hidrencefalia; termo raramente utilizado para referir-se à hidrocefalia interna (internal *hydrocephalus*). [hydr- + G. *enkephalos*, cérebro]

hy·dri·at·ric, hy·dri·a·tic (hī-drē-at′rik, -at′ik). Hidriático; relativo ao uso obsoleto de água para tratamento ou cura de doença. SIN hydrotherapeutic. [hydr- + G. *iatrikos*, relativo a remédio, tratamento]

hy·dric (hī′drik). Hídrico; relativo ao hidrogênio em combinação química.

hy·dride (hī′drīd). Hidreto; hidrogênio com carga elétrica negativa (isto é, $H:^-$) ou composto de hidrogênio em que ele assume uma carga elétrica negativa formal, p. ex., boroidreto de sódio ($NaBH_4$).

hy·drin·dan·tin (hī-drin-dan′tin). Hidrindantina; forma reduzida de ninidrina. Freqüentemente utilizada em conjunção com a ninidrina na detecção de grupos amino ou imino.

♻ **hydro-, hydr-.** Hidro-, hidro-. **1.** Água, aquoso. **2.** Que contém ou que se combina com hidrogênio. **3.** Hidátide. [G. *hydōr*, água]

hy·droa (hī-drō′ă). Hidroa; qualquer erupção vesicular ou bolhosa. SIN hidroa. [hydro + G. *ōon*, ovo]
  h. aesti·va′le, h. estival. SIN h. vacciniforme.
  h. puero′rum, h. vaciniforme. SIN h. vacciniforme.
  h. vacciniforme, h. vaciniforme; erupção recidivante de eritema que evolui para a formação de bolhas umbilicadas; ocorre após exposição ao sol e afeta principalmente crianças do sexo masculino, com regressão antes da vida adulta. Nos casos graves, pode haver desenvolvimento de deformidades nas mãos e na face e opacidade da córnea. SIN h. aestivale, h. puerorum.

hy·dro·a·dip·si·a (hī′drō-ă-dip′sē-ă). Hidroadipsia, hidradipsia; ausência de sede de água. [hydro- + G. *a-* priv. + *dipsa*, sede]

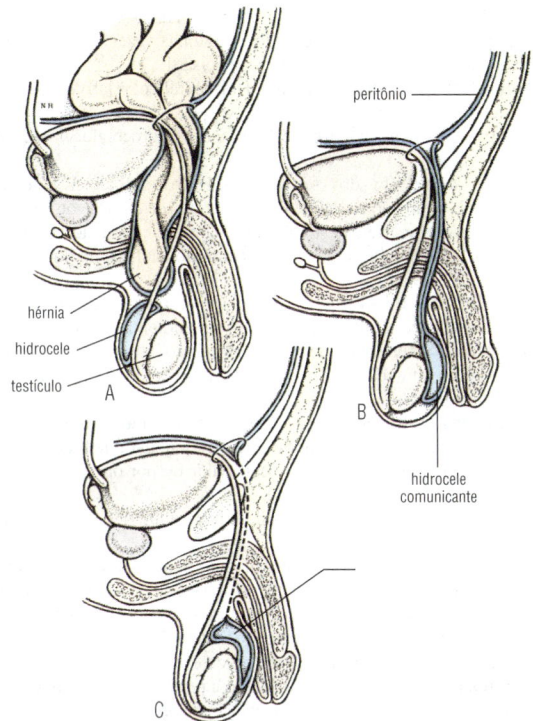

tipos de hidrocele: peritônio mostrado em azul, hidrocele em azul-claro

hy·dro·ap·pen·dix (hī′drō-ă-pen′diks). Hidroapêndice; distensão do apêndice vermiforme com líquido seroso.

hy·dro·bil·i·ru·bin (hī′drō-bil-i-roo′bin). Hidrobilirrubina; pigmento castanho-avermelhado escuro, que seria formado quando a bilirrubina é reduzida.

hy·dro·bro·mate (hī-drō-brō′māt). Bromidrato; sal do ácido hidrobrômico.

hy·dro·bro·mic ac·id (hī-drō-brō′mik). Ácido hidrobrômico; solução aquosa de brometo de hidrogênio (HBr); seus sais são brometos.

hy·dro·cal·y·co·sis (hī′drō-kal-i-kō′sis). Hidrocalicose; anomalia habitualmente assintomática do cálice renal, que está dilatado em conseqüência da obstrução do infundíbulo; em geral, descoberta casualmente na pielografia ou necropsia; pode tornar-se infectada. [hydro- + G. *kalyx*, cálice de uma flor]

hy·dro·car·bon (hī-drō-kar′bŏn). Hidrocarboneto; composto contendo apenas hidrogênio e carbono.
  Diels h., h. de Diels; derivado de fenantreno obtido pela desidrogenação de vários esteróides.
  saturated h., h. saturado; hidrocarboneto que contém o maior número possível de átomos de hidrogênio, de modo que a molécula não contém anéis nem ligações múltiplas.

ℹ **hy·dro·cele** (hī′drō-sēl). Hidrocele; coleção de líquido seroso numa cavidade saculada; especificamente, coleção no espaço da túnica vaginal do testículo ou numa bolsa separada, ao longo do cordão espermático. [hydro- + G. *kēlē*, hérnia]
  cervical h., h. cervical; cisto formado por secreção para um ducto persistente ou fissura do pescoço; quando envolve canais linfáticos, trata-se habitualmente de um linfangioma. SIN h. colli.
  h. col′li, h. do pescoço. SIN cervical h.
  communicating h., h. comunicante; associada a um processo vaginal persistente.
  congenital h., h. congênita; coleção de líquido no processo vaginal persistente, que se estende da cavidade abdominal até o envoltório do testículo.
  cord h., h. do cordão; hidrocele isolada do cordão espermático. SIN funicular h.
  Dupuytren h., h. de Dupuytren; hidrocele bilocular em que o saco enche o escroto e também se estende para a cavidade abdominal, abaixo do peritônio.
  h. fem′inae, h. da mulher; acúmulo de líquido seroso no lábio maior do pudendo ou no canal de Nuck. SIN Nuck h.
  filarial h., h. por filárias; hidrocele devida a microfilárias (principalmente de *Wuchereria bancrofti*) na túnica vaginal.
  funicular h., h. funicular. SIN cord h.
  noncommunicating h., h. não-comunicante; hidrocele do cordão espermático ou do escroto sem comunicação com a cavidade peritoneal, devido à obliteração do processo vaginal.
  Nuck h., h. de Nuck. SIN h. feminae.
  h. spina′lis, h. espinal. SIN *spina* bifida.

hy·dro·ce·lec·to·my (hi′drō-sē-lek′tō-mē). Hidrocelectomia; excisão de hidrocele por drenagem de seu líquido e, algumas vezes, excisão parcial da túnica vaginal. [hydrocele + G. *ektomē*, excisão]

hy·dro·ce·phal·ic (hi′drō-se-fal′ik). Hidrocefálico; relativo a ou que sofre de hidrocefalia.

hy·dro·ceph·a·lo·cele (hī-drō-sef′a-lō-sēl). Hidrocefalocele. SIN hydrencephalocele.

hy·dro·ceph·a·loid (hī-drō-sef′a-loyd). Hidrocefalóide. **1.** Semelhante à hidrocefalia. **2.** Condição em lactentes acometidos de diarréia ou outra doença debilitante, em que ocorrem desidratação e manifestações generalizadas semelhantes às da hidrocefalia, sem qualquer acúmulo anormal de líquido cefalorraquidiano.

hy·dro·ceph·a·lus (hī-drō-sef′a-lūs). Hidrocefalia; condição caracterizada pelo acúmulo excessivo de líquido cefalorraquidiano, resultando em dilatação dos ventrículos cerebrais e elevação da pressão intracraniana. Além disso, pode resultar em aumento do crânio e atrofia do cérebro. SIN hydrocephaly. [hydro- + G. *kephalē*, cabeça]

communicating h., h. comunicante; tipo de hidrocefalia em que existe uma anormalidade na absorção do líquido cefalorraquidiano; não há obstrução ao fluxo cefalorraquidiano no sistema ventricular ou por onde passa o líquido cefalorraquidiano para o canal espinal.

congenital h., h. congênita; hidrocefalia devido a um defeito de desenvolvimento do cérebro. SIN primary h.

double compartment h., h. de compartimento duplo; hidrocefalia supra e infratentorial independente, devido a uma oclusão oculta do aqueduto de Sylvius.

external h., h. externa; **(1)** acúmulo de líquido nos espaços subaracnóides do cérebro; **(2)** acúmulo de líquido no espaço subdural, devido a uma comunicação persistente entre os espaços subaracnóide e subdural.

h. ex vac′uo, h. *ex vacuo*; hidrofilia devido à perda ou atrofia do tecido cerebral; menos comumente associada a elevação da pressão intracraniana.

internal h., h. interna; hidrocefalia em que o acúmulo de líquido limita-se aos ventrículos.

noncommunicating h., h. não-comunicante. SIN obstructive h.

normal pressure h., h. com pressão normal; tipo de hidrocefalia que se desenvolve habitualmente em indivíduos idosos, devido à falta de absorção do líquido cefalorraquidiano pelas granulações de Pacchioni; clinicamente, caracteriza-se por demência progressiva, marcha instável, incontinência urinária e, em geral, pressão normal do líquido cefalorraquidiano. SIN occult h.

obstructive h., h. obstrutiva; hidrocefalia secundária ao bloqueio do fluxo de líquido cefalorraquidiano no sistema ventricular ou entre o sistema ventricular e o canal espinal. SIN noncommunicating h.

occult h., h. oculta. SIN normal pressure h.

otitic h., h. otítica; forma de hidrocefalia associada a otite média e trombose de um ou de ambos os seios sigmóides da dura-máter; caracterizada por elevação acentuada da pressão do líquido cefalorraquidiano.

postmeningitic h., h. pós-meningítica; dilatação ventricular após a meningite e secundária à obstrução das vias do líquido cefalorraquidiano.

posttraumatic h., h. pós-traumática; dilatação ventricular após lesão, devido ao comprometimento da circulação e/ou absorção de líquido cefalorraquidiano ou devido à perda de substância cerebral (h. *ex vacuo*).

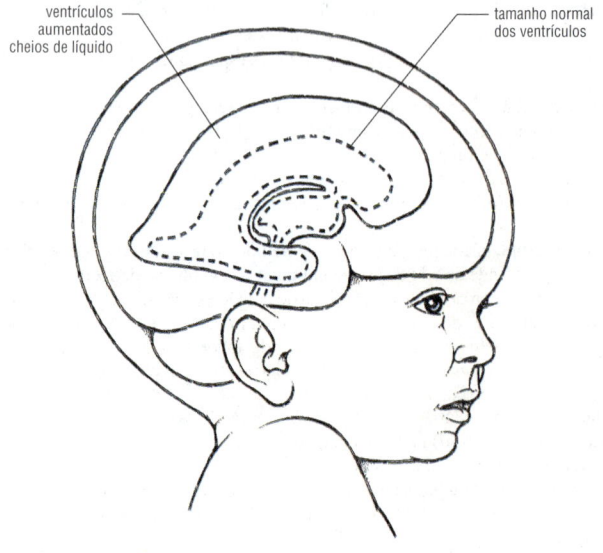

hidrocefalia

primary h., h. primária. SIN congenital h.

secondary h., h. secundária; acúmulo de líquido na cavidade craniana devido a meningite ou obstrução ao fluxo venoso.

thrombotic h., h. trombótica; aumento do líquido cefalorraquidiano e da pressão intracraniana após trombose das veias ou seios cerebrais; causada por infecção séptica, desidratação, tuberculose, tifóide, leucemia e outras doenças.

toxic h., h. tóxica; hidrocefalia trombótica associada a alguma infecção geral ou estado tóxico.

hy·dro·ceph·a·ly (hī-drō-sef′a-lē). Hidrocefalia. SIN hydrocephalus.

hy·dro·chlo·ric ac·id (hī-drō-klōr′ik). Ácido clorídrico; HCl; o ácido do suco gástrico. O produto comercial é utilizado como escarótico; o gás e a solução concentrada são irritantes fortes. SIN muriatic acid.

diluted h., a. c. diluído; preparação que contém, em cada 100 mL, 10 g de HCl; utilizado internamente para a acloridria.

hy·dro·chlo·ride (hī-drō-klōr′īd). Cloridrato; composto formado pela adição de uma molécula de ácido clorídrico a um radical básico na substância; p. ex., cloridrato de guanina, cloridrato de glicina.

hy·dro·chlo·ro·thi·a·zide (hi′drō-klōr-ō-thī′a-zīd). Hidroclorotiazida (HCTZ); poderoso agente diurético e anti-hipertensivo efetivo por via oral, relacionado com a clorotiazida; pode causar hipopotassemia e hiperglicemia.

hy·dro·cho·le·cys·tis (hi′drō-kō-lē-sis′tis). Hidrocolecisto; termo raramente utilizado para referir-se a um derrame de líquido seroso na vesícula biliar. [hydro- + G. *cholē*, bile + *kystis*, bexiga]

hy·dro·cho·le·re·sis (hi′drō-kō-ler-ē′sis, -kol-er-). Hidrocolerese; aumento do débito de bile aquosa de baixa densidade, viscosidade e conteúdo sólido. [hydro- G. *cholē*, bile + *hairesis*, tomada]

hy·dro·cho·le·ret·ic (hi′drō-kō-ler-et′ik). Hidrocolerético; relativo à hidrocolerese.

hy·dro·co·done (hī-drō-kō′dōn). Hidrocodona; potente analgésico derivado da codeína, utilizado como antitussígeno e analgésico. Freqüentemente associada ao ácido acetilsalicílico ou acetaminofeno. SIN dihydrocodeinone.

hy·dro·col·loid (hī-drō-kol′oyd). Hidrocolóide; colóide gelatinoso em equilíbrio instável com seu conteúdo de água, útil em odontologia para impressões, em virtude de sua estabilidade dimensional em condições controladas.

irreversible h., h. irreversível; hidrocolóide cujo estado físico é alterado por uma reação química irreversível, quando se adiciona água a um pó e forma-se uma substância insolúvel.

reversible h., h. reversível; hidrocolóide composto de uma substância básica cujo estado físico pode ser alterado de um sólido ou semi-sólido para um líquido através da aplicação de calor e, em seguida, modificado em gel elástico por esfriamento.

hy·dro·col·po·cele, hy·dro·col·pos (hī-drō-kol′pō-sēl, -kōl′pos). Hidrocolpocele; acúmulo de muco ou outro líquido não-sanguinolento na vagina. [hydro- + G. *kolpos*, vagina]

hy·dro·cor·ta·mate hy·dro·chlo·ride (hī-drō-kōr′ta-māt). Cloridrato de hidrocortamato; sal éster de hidrocortisona utilizado topicamente no tratamento de dermatoses agudas e crônicas.

hy·dro·cor·ti·sone (hī-drō-kōr′ti-sōn). Hidrocortisona; produto de redução (em C-11) da cortisona; hormônio esteróide secretado pelo córtex suprarenal (o hormônio ativo secretado na maior quantidade pelas glândulas adrenais) e o mais potente dos glicocorticóides de ocorrência natural nos seres humanos; agente antiinflamatório. SIN cortisol.

h. acetate, acetato de h.; éster de hidrocortisona com ações e usos semelhantes à hidrocortisona. SIN cortisol acetate.

h. cyclopentylpropionate, ciclopentilpropionato de h.; éster de hidrocortisona.

h. cypionate, cipionato de h.; éster ciclopentanopropiônico da cortisona, para administração oral.

h. hydrogen succinate, succinato de hidrogênio de h.; forma de hidrocortisona administrada por via intravenosa.

h. sodium phosphate, fosfato sódico de h.; agente antiinflamatório para administração intravenosa ou intramuscular.

h. sodium succinate, succinato sódico de h.; sal éster muito solúvel de hidrocortisona (cortisol), utilizado por via parenteral no tratamento de emergências resultantes de insuficiência supra-renal aguda.

hy·dro·co·tar·nine (hī-drō-kō-tar′nēn). Hidrocotarnina; princípio alcalóide derivado da cotarnina; trata-se do produto hidrolítico básico da narcotina; também obtida do líquido-mãe da tebaína.

hy·dro·cy·an·ic ac·id (hi′drō-sī-an′ik). Ácido hidrociânico; HCN; líquido muito tóxico, com odor de amêndoas amargas, presente em amêndoas amargas (amigdalina), caroços de pêssegos, ameixas e outros frutos, bem como nas folhas do louro; a inalação de 300 p.p.m. causa morte. SIN hydrogen cyanide, prussic acid.

hy·dro·cy·an·ism (hī-drō-sī′an-izm). Hidrocianismo; envenenamento com ácido hidrociânico.

hy·dro·cyst (hī′drō-sist). Hidrocisto; cisto com conteúdo claro e aquoso. [hydro- + G. *kystis*, vesícula]

hy·dro·cys·to·ma (hi′drō-sis′tō′mā). Hidrocistoma. **1.** Erupção de vesículas situadas profundamente, devido à retenção de líquido nos folículos sudoríparos. 2. SIN hidrocystoma. [hydro- + G. *kystis*, vesícula, + *-oma*, tumor]

hy·dro·dip·sia (hī-dro-dip′sē-a). Hidrodipsia; sede de água, uma característica de animais que habitualmente bebem água. [hydro- + G. *dipsa*, sede]

hy·dro·dip·so·ma·nia (hī′dro-dip′so-mā′nē-a). Hidrodipsomania; episódios periódicos de sede incontrolável, ocasionalmente observados em pacientes epilépticos. [hydro- + G. *dipsa*, sede + *mania*, frenesi, mania]

hy·dro·di·u·re·sis (hī′dro-dī-u-rē′sis). Hidrodiurese; diurese efetuada pela água.

hy·dro·dy·nam·ics (hī′dro-dī-nam′iks). Hidrodinâmica; ramo da física relacionado com o fluxo de líquidos. [hydro- + G. *dynamis*, força]

hy·dro·en·ceph·a·lo·cele (hī′dro-en-sef′a-lō-sēl). Hidroencefalocele. SIN hydrencephalocele.

hy·dro·flu·o·ric ac·id (hī-dro-flōr′ik). Ácido fluorídrico; solução de gás de fluoreto de hidrogênio em água; líquido espumoso cáustico e tóxico utilizado na limpeza de metais e na gravação do vidro; extremamente irritante para a pele e para os pulmões.

hy·dro·gel (hī′dro-jel). Hidrogel; colóide cujas partículas estão na fase externa ou de dispersão, e a água, na fase interna ou dispersa. Cf. hydrosol.

hy·dro·gen (H) (hī′dro-jen). Hidrogênio. 1. Elemento gasoso, de número atômico 1 e peso atômico 1,00794. 2. Forma molecular (H_2) do elemento. SIN dihydrogen. [hydro- + G. *-gen*, produzindo]

  activated h., h. ativado; hidrogênio removido por uma desidrogenase, p. ex., através de uma flavoproteína, de um metabólito para transferência a outra substância com a qual se combina.

  arseniureted h., h. arseniado. SIN arsine.

  h. bromide, brometo de h.; HBr; gás incolor que possui cheiro muito irritante e que emite vapores no ar úmido; em solução aquosa, é o ácido hidrobrômico.

  h. chloride, cloreto de h.; HCl; gás muito solúvel que, em solução, forma ácido clorídrico.

  h. cyanide, ácido hidrociânico. SIN hydrocyanic acid.

  h. dehydrogenase, h. desidrogenase; flavoproteína que catalisa a conversão do NAD^+ em NADH pelo hidrogênio molecular (H_2); isto é, $H_2 + NAD^+ \rightarrow H^+ + NADH$.

  h. dioxide, dióxido de h. SIN peroxide.

  heavy h., h. pesado. SIN hydrogen-2.

  h. peroxide, peróxido de h.; composto instável facilmente decomposto a água e oxigênio, uma reação catalisada por diversos metais em pó e pela enzima catalase; utiliza-se uma solução a 3% como anti-séptico leve para a pele e mucosas. SIN h. dioxide, hydroperoxide.

  h. phosphide, fosfeto de h. SIN phosphine.

  phosphureted h., h. fosforado. SIN phosphine.

  h. sulfide, sulfeto de h.; H_2S; gás tóxico inflamável e incolor, com cheiro familiar de "ovos podres", formado na decomposição de matéria orgânica contendo enxofre; utilizado como reagente e na fabricação de produtos químicos. SIN sulfureted h.

  sulfureted h., h. sulfurado. SIN h. sulfide.

hy·dro·gen-1 (^1H). Hidrogênio-1; isótopo comum de hidrogênio compondo 99,985% dos átomos de hidrogênio que ocorrem na natureza. SIN protium.

hy·dro·gen-2 (^2H). Hidrogênio-2; isótopo de hidrogênio de peso atômico 2; o isótopo estável de hidrogênio menos comum, representando até 0,015% dos átomos de hidrogênio que ocorrem na natureza; o núcleo é constituído por um próton e por nêutron. SIN deuterium, heavy hydrogen.

hy·dro·gen-3 (^3H). Hidrogênio-3; isótopo de hidrogênio de peso atômico 3; fracamente radioativo, emite partículas beta, transformando-se no hélio-3 estável; meia-vida de 12,32 anos. SIN tritium.

hy·dro·gen·ase (hī′dro-je-nās, hī-drj′e-nās). Hidrogenase. 1. Qualquer enzima capaz de remover um íon hidreto (ou $H:^-$) do NADH (ou do NADPH). SIN hydrogenlyase. 2. Enzima que catalisa a reação do $2H^+$ com ferro e citocromo ou ferredoxina, gerando H_2.

hy·dro·gen·a·tion (hī′dro-je-nā′shŭn, hī-drj′e-nā-shŭn). Hidrogenação; adição de hidrogênio a um composto, especialmente a uma gordura insaturada ou ácido graxo; assim, as gorduras moles ou os óleos são solidificados ou "endurecidos".

hy·dro·gen ex·po·nent. Expoente de hidrogênio; logaritmo decádico da concentração de íons hidrogênio no sangue ou em outro líquido; seu negativo é o pH desse líquido.

hy·dro·gen·ly·ase (hī′dro-gen-lī′ās). Hidrogenliase. SIN hydrogenase (1).

hy·dro·ki·net·ic (hī′dro-ki-net′ik). Hidrocinético; relativo ao movimento de líquidos e às forças que dão origem a esse movimento.

hy·dro·ki·net·ics (hī′dro-ki-net′iks). Hidrocinética; ramo da cinética relacionado com os líquidos em movimento.

hy·dro·la·bile (hī-dro-lā′bil). Hidrolábil; instável na presença de água.

hy·dro·la·bil·i·ty (hī-dro-la-bil′i-tē). Hidrolabilidade; estado em que a quantidade de líquido nos tecidos modifica-se facilmente.

hy·dro·las·es (hī′dro-lās-ez). Hidrolases; enzimas (EC classe 3) que clivam substratos com a adição de H_2O no ponto de clivagem; p. ex., esterases, fosfatases, nucleases, peptidases. SIN hydrolyzing enzymes.

  cysteine h., cisteína h.; hidrolases que utilizam um local ativo de resíduo cisteinil para o evento catalítico.

  serine h., serina h.; hidrolases que utilizam um local ativo de resíduo seril para o evento catalítico.

hy·dro·ly·as·es (hī-dro-lī′as-ez). Hidroliases; classe de liases (EC 4.2.1.x) constituída por enzimas que removem H e OH na forma de água, levando à formação de ligações duplas novas no interior da molécula afetada; os nomes triviais geralmente contêm desidratase ou hidratase.

hy·dro·lymph (hī′dro-limf). Hidrolinfa; líquido circulante em muitos invertebrados.

hy·drol·y·sate (hī-drol′i-sāt). Hidrolisado; solução contendo os produtos de hidrólise.

hy·drol·y·sis (hī-drol′i-sis). Hidrólise; processo químico pelo qual um composto é clivado em dois ou mais compostos mais simples, com captação das partes H e OH da molécula de água em cada lado da ligação química clivada; a hemólise é efetuada pela ação de ácidos, álcalis ou enzimas. Cf. hydration. SIN hydrolytic cleavage. [hydro- + G. *lysis*, dissolução]

hy·dro·lyt·ic (hī-dro-lit′ik). Hidrolítico; que se refere a ou que produz hidrólise.

hy·dro·lyze (hī′dro-līz). Hidrolisar; submeter a hidrólise.

hy·dro·ma (hī-dro′ma). Hidroma. SIN hygroma.

hy·dro·mas·sage (hī′dro-mā-sahzh). Hidromassagem; massagem produzida por correntes de água.

hy·dro·me·nin·go·cele (hī′dro-men-ing′go-sēl). Hidromeningocele; protrusão das meninges do cérebro ou da medula espinal através de um defeito na parede óssea; o saco assim formado contém líquido cefalorraquidiano. [hydro- + G. *mēninx*, membrana + *kēlē*, hérnia]

hy·drom·e·ter (hī-drom′e-ter). Hidrômetro; instrumento para determinar a densidade de um líquido. SIN areometer, gravimeter. [hydro- + G. *mēron*, medida]

hy·dro·me·tra (hī-dro-mē′tra). Hidrometria; acúmulo de muco fino ou outro líquido aquoso na cavidade do útero. [hydro- + G. *metra*, útero]

hy·dro·met·ric (hī-dro-met′rik). Hidrométrico; relativo a hidrometria ou a hidrômetro.

hy·dro·me·tro·col·pos (hī′dro-mē-tro-kol′pos). Hidrometrocolpo; distensão do útero e da vagina por outro líquido que não sangue ou pus. [hydro- + G. *metra*, útero + *kolpos*, vagina]

hy·drom·e·try (hī-drom′e-trē). Hidrometria; determinação da gravidade específica de um líquido por meio de um hidrômetro.

hy·dro·mi·cro·ceph·a·ly (hī′dro-mī-krō-sef′a-lē). Hidromicrocefalia; microcefalia associada a um volume aumentado de líquido cefalorraquidiano.

hy·dro·mor·phone hy·dro·chlo·ride (hī-dro-mōr′fon). Cloridrato de hidromorfona; derivado sintético da morfina, com potência analgésica cerca de 10 vezes a da morfina. SIN dihydromorphinone hydrochloride.

hy·drom·pha·lus (hī-drom′fa-lŭs). Hidrônfalo; tumor cístico no umbigo, mais comumente um cisto vitelointestinal. [hydro- + G. *omphalos*, umbigo]

hy·dro·my·e·lia (hī-dro-mī-ē′lē-a). Hidromielia; aumento de líquido no canal central dilatado da medula espinal ou em cavidades congênitas em outra parte na substância da medula espinal. [hydro- + G. *myelos*, medula]

hy·dro·my·e·lo·cele (hī-dro-mī′e-lō-sēl). Hidromielocele; protrusão de uma porção da medula espinal, adelgaçada num saco distendido com líquido cefalorraquidiano, através de uma espina bífida. [hydro- + G. *myelos*, medula + *kēlē*, tumor, hérnia]

hy·dro·ne·phro·sis (hī′dro-ne-frō′sis). Hidronefrose; dilatação da pelve e dos cálices de um ou de ambos os rins. Pode resultar de obstrução ao fluxo de urina, refluxo vesicoureteral ou pode constituir uma deformidade congênita primária sem causa aparente. SIN pelvocaliectasis, pyeloureterectasis. [hydro- + G. *nephros*, rim + *-osis*, condição]

hy·dro·ne·phrot·ic (hī′dro-ne-frot′ik). Hidronefrótico; relativo à hidronefrose.

hy·dro·ni·um (hī-dro′nē-um). Hidrônio. VER hydronium ion.

hy·dro·par·a·sal·pinx (hī′dro-par-ā-sal′pinks). Hidroparassalpinge; acúmulo de líquido seroso nas trompas acessórias do oviduto. [hydro- + G. *para*, além + *salpinx*, trompa]

hy·dro·path·ic (hī-dro-path′ik). Hidropático; relativo à hidropatia.

hy·drop·a·thy (hī-drop′a-thē). Hidropatia; uso obsoleto de água para o tratamento e cura de doenças.

hy·dro·pe·nia (hī-dro-pē′nē-a). Hidropenia; redução ou privação de água. [hydro- + G. *penia*, pobreza]

hy·dro·pe·nic (hī-dro-pē′nik). Hidropênico; relativo a, ou caracterizado por, hidropenia.

hy·dro·per·i·car·di·um (hī′dro-par-i-kar′dē-um). Hidropericárdio; acúmulo não-inflamatório de líquido no saco pericárdico.

hy·dro·per·i·to·ne·um, hy·dro·per·i·to·nia (hī′dro-par-i-tō-nē′um, -tō′nē-a). Hidroperitônio. SIN ascites. [hydro- + G. peritônio]

hy·dro·per·ox·i·das·es (hī′dro-per-oks′i-dā-sez). Hidroperoxidases; aquelas oxidorredutases que necessitam de H_2O_2 como aceptores de hidrogênio; p. ex., peroxidase, catalase.

hidronefrose (causas)

I. obstrução mecânica do trato urinário
  a) alterações no interior do trato urinário
     1. hiperplasia e carcinoma da próstata
     2. tumores das vias urinárias eferentes
     3. cicatriz no ureter ou na uretra
     4. formação de cálculos
     5. deformidades congênitas ou outras deformidades (nefroptose)
  b) alterações fora do trato urinário
     1. tumores da pelve (carcinoma cervical)
     2. tumores e processos proliferativos do retroperitônio
     3. fibrose retroperitoneal
     4. pressão de artérias renais aberrantes ou aneurismas das artérias renais
     5. pressão de aderências
II. problemas neuromusculares
    espina bífida, paraplegia, tabes dorsal, esclerose múltipla
III. gravidez
IV. causas desconhecidas
    estreitamento funcional do ureter na passagem da pelve renal: síndrome de megaloureter-megacisto

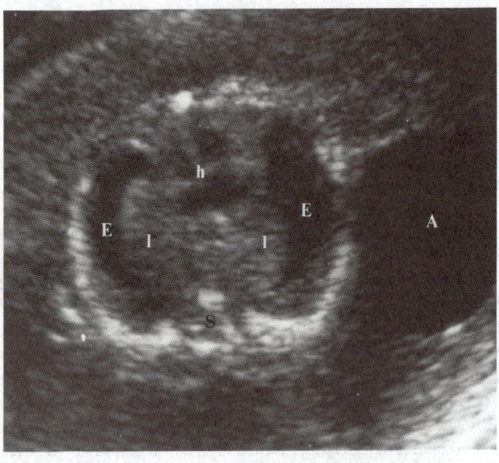

hidropisia fetal: imagem transversal através do tórax do feto, ao nível do coração (h), mostrando derrames pleurais bilaterais (E) contornando os pulmões (l); o tórax fetal é visto de cima, com a coluna (S) posterior; esse feto também tinha ascite; presença de uma bolsa de líquido amniótico (A) adjacente ao lado direito do feto

hy·dro·per·ox·ide (hi′drō - per - ok′sīd). Hidroperóxido. SIN *hydrogen* peroxide.
hy·dro·phil, hy·dro·phile (hi′drō - fil, - fīl). Hidrófilo; substância hidrofílica.
hy·dro·phil·ia (hi - drō - fīl′ē - ă). Hidrofilia; tendência do sangue e dos tecidos a absorver líquidos. [hydro- + G. *philos,* amigo]
hy·dro·phil·ic (hi - drō - fil′ik). Hidrofílico. **1.** Que se refere à propriedade de atrair moléculas de água ou de associar-se a elas, possuído por radicais ou íons polares, em oposição a hidrofóbico (2). **2.** Tendência a dissolver-se em água. **3.** Polar. SIN hydrophilous.
hy·droph·i·lous (hi - drof′i - lŭs). Hidrófilo. SIN *hydrophilic.*
hy·dro·pho·bia (hi - drō - fō′bē - ă). Hidrofobia. SIN *rabies.* [hydro- + G. *phobos,* medo; decorrente de relatórios sobre a incapacidade de deglutir e conseqüente resistência a líquidos orais na raiva humana e animal]
hy·dro·pho·bic (hi - drō - fōb′ik). Hidrofóbico. **1.** Relativo a, ou que sofre de, hidrofobia. **2.** Que carece de afinidade por moléculas de água, em oposição a hidrofílico. SIN apolar (2). **3.** Que tende a não se dissolver em água. **4.** Não-polar.
hy·droph·thal·mia, hy·droph·thal·mos, hy·droph·thal·mus (hi′drof - thal′mē - ă, - thal′mos). Hidroftalmia. SIN *buphthalmia.* [hydro- + G. *ophthalmos,* olho]
Hy·dro·phy·i·dae (hi - drō - fī′i - dē). Família de cobras, as serpentes marinhas verdadeiras, caracterizadas por cauda verticalmente comprimida, conferindo-lhe um aspecto de remo; suas presas, como as das cobras, são pequenas, sulcadas e permanentemente eretas. São comuns em águas rasas costeiras em muitas regiões da bacia do Pacífico e têm importância clínica na Malásia Ocidental e na costa do Vietnã. Existem numerosas espécies, todas venenosas, porém poucas picam seres humanos.
hy·drop·ic (hi - drop′ik). Hidrópico; que contém um excesso de água ou de líquido aquoso. SIN dropsical.
hy·dro·pneu·ma·to·sis (hi - drō - noo - mă - tō′sis). Hidropneumatose; enfisema e edema combinados; presença de líquido e de gás nos tecidos. [hydro- + G. *pneuma,* respiração, espírito]
hy·dro·pneu·mo·per·i·car·di·um (hi - drō - noo′mō - per - i - kar′dē - ŭm). Hidropneumopericárdio; presença de derrame seroso e de gás no saco pericárdico. SIN pneumohydropericardium. [hydro- + G. *pneuma,* ar + pericárdio]
hy·dro·pneu·mo·per·i·to·ne·um (hi - drō - noo′mō - par - i - tō - nē′ŭm). Hidropneumoperitônio; presença de gás e de líquido seroso na cavidade peritoneal. SIN pneumohydroperitoneum. [hydro- + G. *pneuma,* ar + peritônio]
hy·dro·pneu·mo·tho·rax (hi - drō - noo - mō - thōr′aks). Hidropneumotórax; presença de gás e de líquidos na cavidade pleural. SIN pneumohydrothorax, pneumoserothorax. [hydro- + G. *pneuma,* ar + tórax]
hy·dro·po·sia (hi - drō - pō′zē - ă). Hidroposia; ingestão de água, uma característica de animais que habitualmente bebem água. [hydro- + G. *posis,* bebendo]
hy·drops (hi′drops). Hidropisia; acúmulo excessivo de líquido aquoso e claro em qualquer um dos tecidos ou cavidades do corpo; sinônimo, de acordo com o seu caráter e sua localização, de ascite, anasarca, edema, etc. [G. *hydrōps*]
endolymphatic h., h. endolinfática. SIN *Ménière disease.*
fetal h., h. fetal'is, h. fetal; acúmulo anormal de líquido seroso nos tecidos fetais, como na eritroblastose fetal.
h. follic'uli, h. folicular; acúmulo de líquido num folículo de Graaf (folículo ovárico vesiculoso).
h. of gallbladder, h. da vesícula biliar; acúmulo de líquido aquoso e claro na vesícula biliar, em conseqüência de obstrução prolongada do ducto cístico.
immune fetal h., h. fetal imune; edema e ascite fetais, secundários à incompatibilidade materno-fetal de grupo sanguíneo.
nonimmune fetal h., h. fetal não-imune; edema e ascite fetais não relacionados a incompatibilidade materno-fetal de grupo sanguíneo; múltiplas etiologias, incluindo cardiopatia fetal, doença viral no feto e anomalias estruturais fetais.
h. ova'rii, h. do ovário. SIN *hydrovarium.*
h. pericardii, h. drops per - i - kar′dē - i), h. do pericárdio; termo obsoleto para derrame pericárdico (pericardial *effusion*).
h. tu'bae, h. da trompa. SIN *hydrosalpinx.*
h. tu'bae pro'fluens, h. intermitente da trompa. SIN intermitent *hydrosalpinx.*
hy·dro·py·o·ne·phro·sis (hi′drō - pī′ō - ne - frō′sis). Hidropionefrose; presença de urina purulenta na pelve e nos cálices renais após obstrução do ureter. [hydro- + G. *pyon,* pus + nefrose]
hy·dro·quin·ol (hi - drō - kwin′ol). Hidroquinol. SIN *hydroquinone.*
hy·dro·qui·none (hi - drō - kwin′ōn). Hidroquinona; antioxidante utilizado em pomadas. SIN hydroquinol, quinol.
hy·dror·chis (hi - drōr′kis). Hidrorquia; coleção de líquido (hidrocele) ao redor do testículo, como na túnica vaginal ou ao longo do cordão espermático. [hydro- + G. *orchis,* testículo]
hy·dro·rhe·o·stat (hi - drō - rē′ō - stat). Hidrorreostato; reostato em que a resistência ao fluxo da corrente elétrica é fornecida pela água.
hy·dror·rhea (hi - drō - rē′ă). Hidrorréia; secreção profusa de líquido aquoso de qualquer parte do corpo. [hydro- + G. *rhoia,* fluxo]
h. grav'idae, h. gravida'rum, h. da gravidez; secreção de líquido aquoso da vagina durante a gravidez.
hy·dro·sal·pinx (hi - drō - sal′pinks). Hidrossalpinge; acúmulo de líquido seroso na trompa de Falópio, freqüentemente um resultado final de piossalpinge. SIN hydrops tubae. [hydro- + G. *salpinx,* trompa]
intermittent h., h. intermitente; secreção intermitente de líquido aquoso do oviduto. SIN hydrops tubae profluens.
hy·dro·sar·ca (hi - drō - sar′kă). Hidrossarca. SIN *anasarca.* [hydro- + G. *sarx,* carne]
hy·dro·sar·co·cele (hi - drō - sar′kō - sēl). Hidrossarcocele; intumescimento crônico do testículo complicado com hidrocele. [hydro- + G. *sarx,* carne + *kēlē,* tumor]
hy·dro·sol (hi′drō - sol). Hidrossol; colóide em solução aquosa, estando as partículas na fase dispersa ou interna, e a água, na fase externa ou de dispersão. Cf. hydrogel.
hy·dro·sphyg·mo·graph (hi - drō - sfig′mō - graf). Hidroesfigmógrafo; esfigmógrafo em que o batimento do pulso é transmitido ao registrador através de uma coluna de água.
hy·dro·stat (hi′drō - stat). Hidrostato; dispositivo para regular o nível de água. [hydro- + G. *statikos,* produzindo uma parada]
hy·dro·stat·ic (hi - drō - stat′ik). Hidrostático; relativo à pressão de líquidos ou às suas propriedades quando em equilíbrio.

hy·dro·su·dop·a·thy (hī′drō-soo-dop′ă-thē). Hidrossudopatia. SIN hydrosudotherapy. [hydro- + L. *sudor*, suor + G. *pathos*, sofrimento]

hy·dro·su·do·ther·a·py (hī′drō-soo′dō-thăr′ă-pē). Hidrossudoterapia; hidroterapia combinada com sudorese induzida, como no banho turco. SIN hydrosudopathy.

hy·dro·sy·rin·go·my·e·lia (hī′drō-sī-rin′gō-mī-ē′lē-ă). Hidrossiringomielia. SIN syringomyelia. [hydro- + G. *hydōr*, água + *syrinx*, tubo + *myelos*, medula]

hy·dro·tax·is (hī-drō-tak′sis). Hidrotaxia; movimento de células ou organismos em relação à água. [hydro- + G. *taxis*, arranjo, disposição]

hy·dro·ther·a·peu·tic (hī′drō-thăr′ă-pū′tik). Hidroterapêutico. SIN hydriatic.

hy·dro·ther·a·peu·tics (hī′drō-thăr′ă-pū′tiks). Hidroterapêutica. SIN hydrotherapy.

hy·dro·ther·a·py (hī-drō-thăr′ă-pē). Hidroterapia; uso terapêutico da água por aplicação externa, seja pelo seu efeito de pressão ou como meio de aplicar uma energia física aos tecidos. SIN hydrotherapeutics. [hydro- + G. *therapeia*, terapia]

hy·dro·ther·mal (hī-drō-ther′măl). Hidrotérmico; relativo à água quente. [hydro- + G. *thermē*, calor]

hy·dro·thi·o·ne·mia (hī′drō-thī-ō-nē′mē-ă). Hidrotionemia; presença de sulfeto de hidrogênio no sangue circulante. [hydro- + G. *theion*, enxofre + *haima*, sangue]

hy·dro·thi·o·nu·ria (hī-drō-thī-ō-noo′rē-ă). Hidrotionúria; excreção de sulfeto de hidrogênio na urina. [hydro- + G. *theion*, enxofre, + *ouron*, urina]

hy·dro·tho·rax (hī-drō-thōr′aks). Hidrotórax. SIN pleural *effusion*.
chylous h., quilotórax. SIN chylothorax.

hy·drot·o·my (hī-drot′ō-mē). Hidrotomia; em histologia, separação de elementos teciduais por injeção de água. [hydro- + G. *tomē*, corte]

hy·dro·tro·pism (hī-drō-trō′pizm, hī-drot′rō-pizm). Hidrotropismo; propriedade dos organismos em crescimento de voltar-se para uma superfície úmida (**h. positivo**) ou afastar-se dela (**h. negativo**). [hydro- + G. *tropos*, uma volta]

hy·dro·tu·ba·tion (hī′drō-too-bā′shŭn). Hidrotubação; injeção de um medicamento líquido ou solução salina através do colo uterino para a cavidade uterina e das tubas uterinas para dilatação e/ou tratamento das trompas.

hy·dro·u·re·ter (hī′drō-ū-rē′ter, -ūr′ē-ter). Hidroureter. SIN ureterectasia.

hy·dro·ure·ter·o·ne·phro·sis (hī-drō-ū-rē′ter-ō-nef-rō′sis). Hidroureteronefrose. SIN ureterohydronephrosis.

hy·drous (hī′drŭs). Hidratado. SIN hydrated.

hy·dro·va·ri·um (hī-drō-vā′rē-um). Hidrovário; coleção de líquido no ovário. SIN hydrops ovarii.

hy·drox·am·ic ac·ids (hī-drok-sam′ik). Ácidos hidroxâmicos; R–CO–NH–OH ↔ RC(OH)=N–OH; derivados hidroxilamina de ácidos carboxílicos, incluindo aminoácidos, formados pela ação da hidroxilamina.

hy·drox·ide (hī-drok′sīd). Hidróxido. **1.** Composto contendo um grupamento hidroxila potencialmente ionizável, principalmente um composto que libera OH− com dissolução em água. **2.** O ânion hidróxido, OH−.

hy·drox·o·co·bal·a·min (hī-drok′sō-kō-bal′ă-min). Hidroxocobalamina; vitamina B$_{12b}$, que difere da cianocobalamina (vitamina B$_{12}$) pela presença de íon hidroxila no lugar do íon cianeto na sexta posição coordenada do átomo de cobalto. VER TAMBÉM *vitamina* B$_{12}$. SIN hydroxocobemine.

hy·drox·o·co·be·mine (hī-drok′sō-kō-bē-mēn). Hidroxocobemina. SIN hydroxocobalamin.

♲ **hydroxy-**. Hidroxi-; prefixo indicando adição ou substituição do grupamento –OH ao ou no composto cujo nome se segue. VER TAMBÉM oxa-, oxo-, oxy-.

hy·drox·y·ace·tic ac·id (hī-drok′sē-a-sē′tik). Ácido hidroxiacético. SIN glycolic acid.

hy·drox·y ac·id (hī′drok′sē). Hidroxiácido; ácido orgânico contendo grupamentos OH e COOH; p. ex., ácido láctico.

3-hy·drox·y·ac·yl-CoA de·hy·dro·gen·ase (hī-drok′sē-as′il). 3-hidroxiacil-CoA desidrogenase; β-hidroxiacil desidrogenase; enzima que catalisa a oxidação de L-3-hidroxiacil-CoA a 3-cetoacil-CoA, com redução concomitante do NAD$^+$; uma das enzimas da β-oxidação de ácidos graxos. SIN β-ketohydrogenase, β-ketoreductase.

hy·drox·y·a·cyl·glu·ta·thi·one hy·dro·lase (hī-drok′sē-as′il-gloo-tă-thī′ōn). Hidroxiacilglutationa hidrolase; enzima com atividade catalítica semelhante à da lactoilglutationa liase, porém mais generalizada; catalisa a hidrólise de uma *S*-2-hidroxiacilglutationa, produzindo glutationa e um ânion 2-hidroxiácido. VER TAMBÉM glyoxalase.

3-hy·drox·y·anth·ran·il·ic ac·id (hī-drok′sē-anth-ra-nil′ik). Ácido 3-hidroxiantranílico; metabólito da degradação do triptofano, podendo servir como precursor na biossíntese de NAD$^+$.

hy·drox·y·ap·a·tite (hī-drok′sē-ap-ă-tīt). Hidroxiapatita; estrutura mineral natural que se assemelha muito à rede cristalina dos ossos e dos dentes (isto é, h. amorfa); utilizada em cromatografia dos ácidos nucleicos; também encontrada em calcificações patológicas (p. ex., aorta aterosclerótica). SIN hydroxylapatite.

amorphous h., h. amorfa; que contém contaminantes iônicos (p. ex., 6–8% de CO$_3^{2-}$, 3-5% de Mg^{2+}, F$^-$, Cl$^-$, etc.); encontrada em tecido conjuntivo mineralizado (p. ex., osso, dentina, cimento). SIN poorly crystalline h.
poorly crystalline h., h. amorfa. SIN amorphous h.

3-hy·drox·y·bu·ta·no·ic ac·id. Ácido 3-hidroxibutanóico. SIN 3-hydroxybutyric acid.

γ-hydroxybutyrate (GHB) (gam′ă-hī-drok′sē-byu′tir-āt). γ-hidroxibutirato; ácido graxo de cadeia curta de ocorrência natural, um metabólito do ácido γ-aminobutírico (GABA) encontrado em todos os tecidos do corpo, com as maiores concentrações no cérebro; afeta os níveis de GABA, dopamina, 5-hidroxitriptamina e acetilcolina e pode atuar ele próprio como neurotransmissor. O acúmulo de GHB em indivíduos com distúrbio hereditário no metabolismo do GABA provoca ataxia e retardo mental. O GHB sintético, antigamente utilizado em anestesia e no tratamento da narcolepsia e abstinência de álcool, foi proibido pela *Food and Drug Administration*, devido aos efeitos colaterais neurológicos, cardiovasculares, respiratórios e gastrointestinais graves. SIN 4-hydroxybutyrate.

> O uso ilícito do GHB tornou-se cada vez mais popular, particularmente entre fisiculturistas, visto que é fabricado facilmente e com baixo custo em casa e supostamente suprime o apetite, alivia a depressão, aumenta a massa muscular, ao estimular a liberação de hormônio do crescimento, e melhora o sono. Além disso, tem sido utilizado como euforizante e (por ser inodoro e quase sem sabor e induzir rapidamente sedação com amnésia retrógrada) para facilitar o estupro. Os nomes populares comuns do GHB incluem "grievous bodily harm", "liquid ecstasy", "liquid E", "liquid X," e "scoop". A droga sofre rápida absorção, após administração oral, e atravessa facilmente a barreira hematoencefálica. Trata-se primariamente de um depressor do SNC; entretanto, o GHB também diminui a temperatura corporal, a freqüência cardíaca e o débito cardíaco. A intoxicação aguda pode manifestar-se como sonolência, confusão, comportamento agressivo e autolesivo, náuseas, tremores, tonteira e coma. O GHB atua de modo sinérgico com o álcool, os benzodiazepínicos e os narcóticos, produzindo depressão respiratória e do SNC profunda. Os episódios tóxicos ocorrem, em sua maioria, em homens de 18–25 anos de idade e também envolvem o consumo de álcool. Já foi relatada a ocorrência de dependência e de sintomas intensos de abstinência. O tratamento dos efeitos tóxicos é puramente de suporte; não existe nenhum antídoto. Como o solvente γ-butirolactona industrial e utilizado como produto doméstico é metabolizado a GHB, foi comercializado ilicitamente como suplemento nutricional, atribuindo-lhe os mesmos efeitos terapêuticos do GHB. Seu uso tem sido associado a inúmeros relatos de eventos adversos, incluindo morte.

4-hydroxybutyrate. 4-Hidroxibutirato. SIN γ-hydroxybutyrate.

β-hy·drox·y·bu·tyr·ic ac·id. Ácido β-hidroxibutírico. SIN 3-hydroxybutyric acid.

3-hy·drox·y·bu·tyr·ic ac·id (hī-drōk′sē-bū-tir′ik). Ácido 3-hidroxibutírico; o D-estereoisômero é um dos corpos cetônicos e é formado na cetogênese; trata-se de uma importante fonte de energia para os tecidos extra-hepáticos; como derivado acil, é também um intermediário na biossíntese de ácidos graxos. O L-isômero é encontrado como derivado da coenzima A na β-oxidação de ácidos graxos. SIN 3-hydroxybutanoic acid, β-hydroxybutyric acid.
D-3-h. a. dehydrogenase, a. D-3-hidroxibutírico desidrogenase; enzima que catalisa irreversivelmente a interconversão dos dois corpos cetônicos principais, catalisando a reação acetoacetato + NADH + H$^+$ ↔ D-3-hidroxibutirato + NAD$^+$.

4-hy·drox·y·bu·ty·ric ac·i·du·ria (hī-drok′sē-bū-tir′ik). 4-hidroxibutiricacidúria; refere-se a níveis elevados de 4-hidroxibutirato na urina. Distúrbio hereditário que também pode resultar em hipotonia e retardo mental.

hy·drox·y·car·bam·ide (hī-drok′sē-kar′bă-mīd). Hidroxicarbamida. SIN hydroxyurea.

hy·drox·y·chlo·ro·quine sul·fate (hī-drok′sē-klōr′ō-kwīn). Sulfato de hidroxicloroquina; derivado da quinolina; agente antimalárico cujas ações e usos assemelham-se aos do fosfato de cloroquina; também utilizado no tratamento do lúpus eritematoso e da artrite reumatóide.

25-hy·drox·y·cho·le·cal·cif·er·ol (HCC) (hī-drok′sē-kō′lē-kal-sif′er-ol) 25-hidroxicolecalciferol. SIN calcidiol.

7α-hy·drox·y·cho·les·ter·ol (hī-droks′ē-kol-es-ter-ol). 7α-hidroxicolesterol; primeiro intermediário na conversão do colesterol em ácidos biliares; formado na principal etapa de limitação da taxa de biossíntese de ácidos biliares.

hy·drox·y·chro·man (hī-drok-sē-krō′man). Hidroxicromano. SIN chromanol.

hy·drox·y·chro·mene (hī-drok-sē-krō′mēn). Hidroxicromeno. SIN chromenol.

hy·drox·y·eph·ed·rine (hī-drok'sē-ĕ-fed'rēn). Hidroxiefedrina; agente simpaticomimético utilizado no tratamento do choque.

25-hy·drox·y·er·go·cal·cif·er·ol (hī-drok'sēr'go-kal-sif'er-ol). 25-hidroxiergocalciferol; metabólito circulante importante e biologicamente ativo da vitamina D_2. SIN ercalcidiol.

α-hy·drox·y·eth·yl·thi·a·min py·ro·phos·phate. α-hidroxietiltiamina pirofosfato. SIN activated acetaldehyde.

hy·drox·y·fat·ty ac·id (hī-drok'sē-fat'te). Ácido hidroxigraxo; um ácido graxo que possui um grupamento hidroxila ligado de forma covalente (p. ex., na hidroxinervona).

3-hy·drox·y·glu·tar·ic ac·id (hī-drok'sē-gloo-tar'ik). Ácido 3-hidroxiglutárico; ácido dicarboxílico que se acumula em indivíduos com acidemia glutárica tipo I.

hy·drox·y·he·min (hī-drok-sē-hē'min). Hidroxiemina. SIN hematin.

β-hy·drox·y·i·so·bu·tyr·ic ac·id (hī-droks'ē-ī-sō-byu-ter-ik). Ácido β-hidroxiisobutírico; intermediário na degradação da L-valina.

3-L-hy·drox·y·ky·nu·ren·ine (hī-drok'sē-ki-noo-rĕ-nēn). 3-L-hidroxicinurenina; intermediário no catabolismo do L-triptofano e precursor do xanturenato; elevado em casos de deficiência de vitamina B_6.

hy·drox·y·ky·nu·re·ni·nu·ria (hī-drok'sē-kī-noo'rĕ-ni-noo'rē-ă) [MIM*236800]. Hidroxicinureninúria; anormalidade no metabolismo do triptofano, provavelmente devido a um defeito na cinureninase; caracterizada por retardo mental leve, cefaléias semelhantes a enxaqueca e excreção urinária de grandes quantidades de cinurenina, 3-hidroxicinurenina e ácido xanturênico; herança autossômica recessiva.

hy·drox·yl (hī-drok'sil). Hidroxila; radical –OH.

hy·drox·yl·a·mine (hī-drok'sil-ā'mēn). Hidroxilamina. **1.** NH_2OH; um derivado parcialmente oxidado da amônia; reage com grupos carbonila para produzir oximas; forma sais ácidos, como, p. ex., cloridrato de hidroxilamina. Trata-se de um mutágeno químico que causa desaminação de resíduos de citosina no DNA. **2.** Qualquer composto contendo RNH–OH.

h. reductase, h. redutase; enzima que catalisa a redução reversível da hidroxilamina a amônia com uma variedade de doadores (p. ex., azul-de-metileno, flavina). VER TAMBÉM NADH-hydroxylamine reductase.

hy·drox·yl·a·mi·no (hī-drok'sil-am-i-nō). Hidroxilamino; grupo monovalente –NH–OH.

hy·drox·yl·ap·a·tite (hī-drok'sil-ap-ă-tīt). Hidroxilapatita. SIN hydroxyapatite.

hy·drox·y·las·es (hī-drok'si-lā-sez). Hidroxilases; enzimas que catalisam a formação de grupamentos hidroxila por adição de um átomo de oxigênio, oxidando portanto o substrato; a maioria é encontrada na subclasse EC 1.14.

hy·drox·yl·a·tion (hī-drok-si-lā'shŭn). Hidroxilação; colocação de um grupo hidroxila num composto, numa posição onde não se encontrava antes.

δ-hy·drox·y·ly·sine. δ-Hidroxilisina. SIN 5-hydroxylysine.

5-hy·drox·y·ly·sine (5Hyl). 5-Hidroxilisina; aminoácido hidroxilado encontrado em certos colágenos. A capacidade reduzida de formar 5-hidroxilisina está associada à síndrome de Ehlers-Danlos tipo VI. SIN δ-hydroxylysine.

p-hy·drox·y·mer·cur·i·ben·zo·ate (hī-drok'sē-mer'kū-rē-ben'zō-āt). Benzoato de p-hidroxi mercúrio; mercurial orgânico formado espontaneamente pela hidrólise do benzoato de p-cloromercúrio. VER TAMBÉM p-mercuribenzoate.

β-hy·drox·y-β-meth·yl·glu·tar·yl-CoA (HMG-CoA). β-hidroxi-β-metilglutaril-CoA (HMG-CoA); intermediário-chave na síntese de corpos cetônicos, esteróides e derivados farnesil e geranil. SIN 3-hydroxy-3-methylglutaryl-CoA.

β-h.-β-m.-CoA lyase, β-h.-β-m.-CoA liase; enzima encontrada primariamente no fígado e no epitélio do rume, que catalisa a formação de acetil-CoA e acetoacetato a partir de β-h.-β-m.-CoA; etapa-chave na cetogênese; a deficiência dessa enzima resulta em episódios de acidose metabólica grave sem cetose.

β-h.-β-m.-CoA reductase, β-h.-β-m.-CoA redutase; enzima que catalisa a etapa que limita a velocidade de biossíntese do colesterol: β-h.-β-m.-CoA + 2NADPH + $2H^+$ → (R)-mevalonato + 2NADP$^+$ + CoA.

β-h.-β-m.-CoA synthase, β-h.-β-m.-CoA sintase; enzima encontrada nas mitocôndrias que catalisa a reação da acetil-CoA com acetoacetil-CoA e água para formar (S)-β-h.-β-m.-CoA e coenzima A, uma etapa necessária tanto para a cetogênese quanto para a esteroidogênese.

3-hy·droxy-3-meth·yl·glu·tar·yl-CoA. 3-hidroxi-3-metilglutaril-CoA. SIN β-hydroxy-β-methylglutaryl-CoA.

hy·drox·y·ner·vone (hī-drok-sē-ner'vōn). Hidroxinervona; cerebrosídeo contendo ácido α-hidroxinervônico. SIN oxynervone.

hy·drox·y·ner·von·ic ac·id (hī-drok'sē-ner-von'ik). Ácido hidroxinervônico; importante constituinte de certos cerebrosídeos.

p-hy·drox·y·phe·nyl·ac·e·tate (hī-droks'ē-fen'il-as'e-tāt). p-hidroxifenilacetato; produto de menor importância da degradação da L-tirosina, cuja concentração está elevada na urina em casos de tirosinemia neonatal e síndrome de Richner-Hanhart.

p-hy·drox·y·phe·nyl·lac·tate (hī-droks'ē-fen'il-lak'tāt). p-hidroxifenilactato; metabólito na degração da tirosina, elevado em indivíduos com síndrome de Richner-Hanhart.

p-hy·drox·y·phe·nyl·py·ru·vate (hī-droks'ē-fen'il-pī'roo-vāt). p-hidroxifenilpiruvato; metabólito formado pela transaminação da tirosina; elevado na urina de indivíduos com tirosinemia.

hy·drox·y·phen·yl·u·ria (hī-drok'sē-fen-il-oo'rē-ă). Hidroxifenilúria; excreção urinária de tirosina e fenilalanina, em consequência da deficiência de ácido ascórbico; ocorre notavelmente em prematuros que carecem dessa vitamina.

3α-hy·drox·y-5α-preg·nan-20-one. 3α-hidroxi-5α-pregnan-20-ona; catabólito da progesterona; encontrado na urina de gestantes.

17α-hy·drox·y·pro·ges·ter·one (hī-drok'sē-prō-jes'ter-ōn). 17α-hidroxiprogesterona; hormônio esteróide cuja aplicação clínica assemelha-se à da progesterona. O acetato é um derivado efetivo por via oral, útil em condições nas quais se indica a administração parenteral de progesterona ou caproato; possui alguma potência androgênica, podendo causar alterações virilizantes no feto feminino. O caproato ou hexanoato tem essencialmente as mesmas ações e usos que a progesterona, porém é mais potente e tem maior duração de ação. Precursor dos androgênios, estrogênios e hormônios córtico-supra-renais.

21-hy·drox·y·pro·ges·ter·one. 21-Hidroxiprogesterona. SIN deoxycorticosterone.

3-hy·drox·y·pro·line (3Hyp) (hī-drok'sē-prō'lēn). 3-Hidroxiprolina; derivado da prolina encontrado em certos colágenos, particularmente no colágeno da membrana basal. SIN 3-hydroxy-2-pyrrolidinecarboxylic acid.

4-hy·drox·y·pro·line (4Hyp, Hyp). 4-Hidroxiprolina; ácido-4-hidroxi-2-pirrolidinocarboxílico; o trans-L-isômero é uma pirrolidina encontrada entre os produtos de hidrólise do colágeno; não encontrado em outras proteínas que não as do tecido conjuntivo. A deficiência de vitamina C resulta em comprometimento da formação de h.

h. oxidase, h. oxidase; (**1**) flavoenzima que catalisa a conversão da h. em Δ'-pirrolina-3-hidroxi-5-carboxilato, utilizando FAD; essa enzima parece estar deficiente em indivíduos com hiperidroxiprolinemia; (**2**) enzima que catalisa a reação da h. com NAD$^+$ para formar NADH e 4-oxoprolina. SIN 4-oxoproline reductase.

hy·drox·y·pro·li·ne·mia (hī-drok'sē-prō-li-nē'mē-ă) [MIM*237000]. Hidroxiprolinemia; distúrbio metabólico caracterizado por retardo mental e hematúria microscópica em alguns pacientes; associado à elevação das concentrações plasmáticas e excreção urinária de hidroxiprolina livre devido à deficiência de hidroxiprolina oxidase; herança autossômica recessiva.

β-hy·drox·y·pro·pi·o·nic ac·id (hī-drok'sē-prō'pē-on'ik). Ácido β-hidroxipropiônico; intermediário de menor importância no metabolismo do propionato e do metilmalonato. SIN β-hydroxypropionic aciduria.

β-hy·drox·y·pro·pi·o·nic ac·i·du·ria. Acidúria β-hidroxipropiônica; níveis elevados de ácido β-propiônico na urina; observada em defeitos do metabolismo do ácido metilmalônico e propionato, bem como na síndrome de hiperglicinemia cetótica.

15-hy·drox·y·pros·ta·glan·din de·hy·dro·gen·ase (hī-drok'sē-pros-tă-glan'din). 15-Hidroxiprostaglandina desidrogenase; enzima que catalisa a oxidação das prostaglandinas inativas, através da conversão do grupamento 15-hidroxila em grupamento ceto utilizando o NAD$^+$.

6-hy·drox·y·pu·rine. 6-Hidroxipurina. SIN hypoxanthine.

3-hy·droxy-2-pyr·ro·li·di·ne·car·box·yl·ic ac·id. Ácido 3-hidroxi-2-pirrolidinocarboxílico. SIN 3-hydroxyproline.

8-hy·drox·y·quin·o·line (hī-drok-sē-kwin'ō-lin). 8-Hidroxiquinolina; fungistático e agente quelante. SIN quinolinol.

3β-hy·drox·y·ste·roid sul·fa·tase (hī-drok'sē-stēr'ōid). 3β-Hidroxiesteróide sulfatase; enzima encontrada na maioria dos tecidos de mamíferos que tem a capacidade de hidrolisar ligações de éster de sulfato de vários esteróis sulfatados; a deficiência dessa enzima resulta em ictiose ligada ao X.

hy·drox·y·stil·bam·i·dine is·e·thi·o·nate (hī-drok'sē-stil-bam'i-dēn). Isetionato de hidroxiestilbamidina; agente antifúngico e antiprotozoário utilizado no tratamento da forma cutânea não-progressiva da blastomicose.

hy·drox·y·to·lu·ic ac·id (hī-drok'sē-tō-loo'ik). Ácido hidroxituico. SIN mandelic acid.

5-hy·drox·y·tryp·ta·mine (5-HT) (hī-drok-sē-trip'tă-mēn). 5-Hidroxitriptamina. SIN serotonin.

hy·drox·y·tryp·to·phan de·car·box·yl·ase (hī-drok-sē-trip'tō-fan). Hidroxitriptofano descarboxilase. SIN aromatic D-amino acid decarboxylase.

3-hy·drox·y·ty·ra·mine (hī-drok-sē-tī'ră-mēn). 3-Hidroxitiramina. SIN dopamine.

hy·drox·y·u·rea (hī-drok'sē-ū-rē'ă). Hidroxiuréia; agente antineoplásico oral que inibe a síntese de DNA; utilizado no tratamento de uma variedade de processos malignos, incluindo melanoma, leucemia mielocítica crônica e carcinoma de ovário. SIN hydroxycarbamide.

hy·drox·y·zine (hī-drok'si-zēn). Hidroxizina; sedativo leve e tranqüilizante menor utilizado em neuroses; disponível como cloridrato e pamoato. Utilizado com freqüência na prevenção de náuseas e para intensificar os efeitos dos narcóticos.

Hy·dro·zoa (hī-drō-zō'ă). Classe de celenterados ou águas vivas, incluindo *Hydra*, um pólipo de água doce; *Physalia*, a caravela; a *Millepora*, um coral urticante, e *Chironex heckeri* e *Chiropsalmus quadrigatus*, cujas células urticantes podem causar urticária intensa, dor e necrose cutânea e, em certas ocasiões, morte rápida por depressão respiratória e cardíaca. [hydro- + G. *zōon*, animal]

hy·giei·ol·o·gy (hī-jē-yol'ō-jē). Higiologia; a ciência da higiene e do saneamento e sua prática. [G. *hygieia*, saúde + *-logia*]

hy·gie·ist (hī'jē-ist). Higienista. SIN hygienist. [G. *hygieia*, saúde]

hy·giene (hī'jēn). Higiene. 1. A ciência da saúde e sua manutenção. 2. Limpeza que promove a saúde e o bem-estar, especialmente de natureza pessoal. [G. *hygieinos*, sadio, fr. *hygiēs*, saudável]

  criminal h., h. criminal; termo obsoleto para referir-se ao ramo da h. mental ou penologia dedicada ao estudo das causas e profilaxia da criminalidade e tratamento de criminosos.

  industrial h., h. industrial; práticas adotadas por uma empresa industrial para minimizar as doenças e/ou lesões ocupacionais.

  mental h., h. mental; a ciência e a prática da manutenção e restauração da saúde mental; um ramo da psiquiatria do início do século XX, que se tornou um campo interdisciplinar, incluindo subespecialidades em psicologia, enfermagem, assistência social, lei e outras profissões.

  oral h., h. oral; a limpeza da boca por meio de escova, fio dental, irrigação, massagem ou uso de outros dispositivos. VER TAMBÉM oral *physiotherapy*.

hy·gien·ic (hī-jen'ik, hī-jē-en'ik). Higiênico, sadio; relativo à higiene; que tende a manter a saúde.

hy·gien·ist (hī-jē'nist, hī'jē-en-ist). Higienista; indivíduo especializado na ciência da saúde e sua manutenção. SIN hygieist.

  dental h., h. dentário; auxiliar profissional em odontologia, que é tanto um clínico quanto educador da saúde oral, que utiliza métodos profiláticos, terapêuticos e educacionais para o controle das doenças orais.

hygr-. Higr-. VER hygro-.

hy·gric (hī'grik). Hígrico. Relativo à umidade. [G. *hygros*, úmido]

hy·gric ac·id. Ácido hígrico. *N*-metilprolina, cuja metilbetaína é a estaquidrina.

hygro-, hygr-. Higro-, higr-; umidade; oposto de xero-. [G. *hygros*, úmido]

hy·gro·ma (hī-grō'mǎ). Higroma; intumescimento cístico contendo líquido seroso, como o joelho da doméstica, etc. SIN hydroma. [hygro- + G. *-oma*, tumor]

  h. axilla're, higroma da região axilar.

  cervical h., h. cervical; proliferação cística benigna de linfáticos do pescoço, ocorrendo por ocasião do nascimento, que pode formar uma grande massa tumoral. SIN h. colli cysticum.

  h. col'li cys'ticum, h. cístico do pescoço. SIN cervical h.

  cystic h., h. cístico; malformação fetal de acúmulo de líquido, geralmente na região do pescoço e do ombro; pode ser simples ou complexo; freqüentemente associado à síndrome de Turner.

  subdural h., h. subdural; acúmulo, no espaço subdural, de líquido proteináceo, habitualmente derivado do soro ou do líquido cefalorraquidiano, devido a uma laceração na membrana aracnóide.

hy·grom·e·ter (hī-grom'ē-ter). Higrômetro; qualquer aparelho para medir o vapor d'água na atmosfera, em geral indicando diretamente a umidade relativa. [hygro- + G. *metron*, medida]

hy·grom·e·try (hī-grom'ē-trē). Higrometria. SIN psychrometry.

hy·gro·pho·bia (hī-grō-fō'bē-ǎ). Higrofobia; medo mórbido de umidade. [hygro- + G. *phobos*, medo]

hy·gro·scop·ic (hī-grō-skop'ik). Higroscópico; indica uma substância capaz de absorver e reter facilmente a umidade; p. ex., NaOH, CaCl₂.

hy·gro·sto·mia (hī'grō-stō'mē-ǎ). Higrostomia. SIN sialorrhea. [hygro- + G. *stoma*, boca]

Hyl Símbolo de hydroxylysine (hidroxilisina) ou hydroxylysyl (hidroxilisil) (5Hyl refere-se, especificamente, à 5-hidroxilisina).

5Hyl Abreviatura de 5-hydroxylysine (5-hidroxilisina).

hy·la (hī'lǎ). Hilos; extensão lateral do aqueduto cerebral (ou de Sylvius). [G. *hylē*, floresta]

hy·le·pho·bia (hī-lē-fō'bē-ǎ). Hilefobia; medo mórbido de florestas. [G. *hylē*, floresta + *phobos*, medo]

hy·men (hī'men) [TA]. Hímen; dobra membranosa delgada, de aspecto bastante variável, que oclui parcialmente o orifício da vagina antes de sua ruptura (que pode ocorrer por várias razões). Está freqüentemente ausente (mesmo em virgens), embora seja comum a presença de remanescentes na forma de carúnculas himenais. [G. *hymēn*, membrana]

  h. bifenestra'tus, h. bifo'ris, h. bifenestrado; hímen em que existem duas aberturas separadas por um septo largo. Cf. septate h.

  cribriform h., h. cribriforme; hímen com diversas perfurações pequenas.

  denticulate h., h. denticulado; hímen com bordas acentuadamente serrilhadas.

  imperforate h., h. imperfurado; hímen em que não existe abertura, com oclusão completa da vagina pela membrana.

  infundibuliform h., h. infundibuliforme; hímen em forma de funil, com uma abertura central e bordas inclinadas.

  h. sculpta'tus, h. esculpido; hímen com bordas acentuadamente irregulares.

  septate h., h. septado; hímen em que existem duas aberturas separadas por uma estreita faixa de tecido. Cf. h. bifenestratus.

  h. subsep'tus, h. subseptado; hímen em que a abertura é parcialmente fechada por um septo.

  vertical h., h. vertical; hímen em que a abertura é perpendicular.

hy·men·al (hī'men-ǎl). Himenal; relativo ao hímen.

hy·me·nec·to·my (hī-me-nek'tō-mē). Himenectomia; excisão do hímen. (G. *hymēn*, membrana + *ektomē*, excisão]

hy·me·ni·tis (hī-me-nī'tis). Himenite; inflamação do hímen.

hy·men·oid (hī'men-oyd). Himenóide. 1. SIN membranous. 2. Semelhante ao hímen.

hy·me·no·le·pi·a·sis (hī'me-nō-lē-pī'ǎ-sis). Himenolepíase; doença causada pela infestação por tênias do gênero *Hymenolepis*.

hy·me·no·lep·i·did (hī'men-ō-lep'i-did). Himenolepidídeo; nome comum das tênias da família Hymenolepididae.

Hy·men·o·lep·i·di·dae (hī'men-ō-lep'i-did-ē). Família de tênias (ordem Cyclophyllidea) que inclui o gênero clinicamente importante *Hymenolepis*. [G. *hymēn*, membrana + *lepis*, casca]

Hy·me·nol·e·pis (hī-me-nol'e-pis). O maior gênero (família Hymenolepididae) de cestóides da ordem Cyclophyllidea; parasitas especialmente comuns de roedores, musaranhos e aves aquáticas. [G. *hymēn*, membrana + *lepis*, casca]

  ***H. diminu'ta**, h. diminuta; espécie de tênia de ratos e camundongos, raramente encontrada no homem; suas larvas cisticercóides são albergadas por besouros, pulgas, lagartas e outros insetos.

  ***H. lanceola'ta**, tênia de aves aquáticas, raramente encontrada nos seres humanos.

  ***H. na'na**, a tênia anã do camundongo; uma pequena tênia do homem, algumas vezes encontrada em grande número no intestino; os cisticercóides podem desenvolver-se por duas vias: no hospedeiro final, em que o ovo proveniente de um ser humano é diretamente infectante para outro hospedeiro humano, no qual ocorrem os estágios tanto larvário quanto do adulto; ou através de dois hospedeiros, um inseto (ou crustáceo) intermediário e um hospedeiro final vertebrado, o ciclo obrigatório de dois hospedeiros da maioria dos cestódeos ciclofilídeos; além disso, *H. nana* pode reinfectar internamente o mesmo ser humano ou hospedeiro roedor, produzindo reinfecção maciça.

  ***H. na'na**, var. *frater'na*, uma raça, cepa ou subespécie de *H. nana* adaptada a camundongos, embora possa permanecer a infectividade para os seres humanos; a forma humana, *H. nana*, deriva presumivelmente da cepa de roedores.

hy·me·nol·o·gy (hī-mē-nol'ō-jē). Himenologia; o ramo da anatomia e da fisiologia relacionado às membranas do corpo. [G. *hymēn*, membrana + *logos*, estudo]

Hy·me·nop·tera (hī-me-nop'ter-ǎ). Ordem de insetos, incluindo as abelhas, vespas e formigas, caracterizada por pares fechados de asas membranosas e alto desenvolvimento em termos de comportamento social ou em colônias. [G. *hymēn*, membrana + *pteron*, asa]

hy·me·nor·rha·phy (hī-me-nōr'ǎ-fē). Himenorrafia; procedimento obsoleto de sutura do hímen para fechar a vagina. [G. *hymēn*, membrana + *raphē*, sutura]

hy·men·ot·o·my (hī-me-not'ō-mē). Himenotomia; divisão cirúrgica de um hímen. [G. *hymēn*, membrana + *tomē*, incisão]

Hynes, Wilfred, cirurgião plástico inglês, *1903.

hyo-. Hio-. Em forma de U, hióide. [G. *hyoeides*, em forma da letra ipsilon, υ]

hy·o·ep·i·glot·tic (hī'ō-ep-i-glot'ik). Hioepiglótico; relativo ao osso hióide e à epiglote; refere-se ao ligamento h. elástico que une as duas estruturas. SIN hyoepiglottidean.

hy·o·ep·i·glot·tid·e·an (hī'ō-ep-i-glo-tid'ē-an). Hioepiglótico. SIN hyoepiglottic.

hy·o·glos·sal (hī'ō-glos'ǎl). Hioglosso; relativo ao osso hióide e à língua. SIN glossohyal.

hy·o·glos·sus (hī'ō-glos'ǔs). Hioglosso. SIN hyoglossus (*muscle*).

hy·oid (hī'oyd). Hióide; em forma de U ou em forma de V; refere-se ao *osso* hióide e ao *aparelho* hióide. [G. *hyoeidēs*, com forma semelhante à letra ipsilon, υ]

hy·o·pha·ryn·ge·us (hī'ō-far'in-jē'us). Hiofaríngeo. VER middle constrictor (*muscle*) of pharynx.

hy·o·scine (hī'ō-sēn). Hioscina. SIN scopolamine.

  h. hydrobromide, de escopolamina. SIN *scopolamine* hydrobromide.

hy·o·scy·a·mine (hī-ō-sī'ǎ-mēn). Hiosciamina; alcalóide encontrado no hioscíamo, na beladona, na duboisina e no estramônio; o componente levorotatório da mistura racêmica, atropina; utilizada como antiespasmódico, analgésico e sedativo; o bromidrato de hiosciamina é utilizado para os mesmos propósitos. SIN daturine.

  h. sulfate, sulfato de h; antiespasmódico, hipnótico e sedativo, também utilizado no parquinsonismo para aliviar o tremor, a rigidez e a salivação excessiva.

***dl*-hy·o·scy·a·mine**. *dl*-hiosciamina. SIN atropine.

hy·o·scy·a·mus (hī-ō-sī'ǎ-mǔs). Hioscíamo; as folhas e sumidades floridas de *Hyoscyamus niger* (família Solanaceae); contém hiosciamina e hioscina (escopolamina); anticolinérgico e antiespasmódico. SIN henbane. [G. *hyoskyamos*, meimendro negro ou fava de porco, fr. *hys*, gen. *hyos*, porco + *kyamos*, fava]

hy·o·thy·roid (hī′ō-thī′royd). Hiotireóideo. VER thyrohyoid *membrane*.

Hyp Abreviatura de hypoxanthine (hipoxantina); hidroxoprolina (a 3Hyp e a 4Hyp referem-se especialmente à 3-hidroxiprolina e 4-hidroxiprolina, respectivamente].

3Hyp Abreviatura de 3-hydroxyproline (3-hidroxiprolina).

4Hyp Abreviatura de 4-hydroxyproline (4-hidroxiprolina).

♻ **hyp-.** Hip-. Variação do prefixo hipo-, freqüentemente utilizado antes de uma vogal. Cf. sub-.

hyp·a·cu·sia (hī′pă-koo′zē-ă, hipʹă-). Hipoacusia, hipacusia. SIN hypacusis.

hyp·a·cu·sis (hī′pă-koo′sis, hipʹă-). Hipoacusia, hipacusia; diminuição da audição de natureza condutora ou neurossensorial. SIN hypacusia, hypoacusis. [hypo- + G. *akousis*, audição]

hyp·al·bu·mi·ne·mia (hī′pal-bū-mi-nē′mē-ă, hipʹal-). Hipoalbuminemia. SIN hypoalbuminemia. [G. *hypo*, abaixo + albuminemia]

hyp·al·ge·sia (hī′pal-jē′zē-ă, hipʹal-). Hipalgesia, hipoalgesia; diminuição da sensibilidade à dor. SIN hypoalgesia. [G. *hypo*, abaixo + *algēsis*, sensação de dor]

hyp·al·ge·sic, hyp·al·get·ic (hī′pal-jē′sik, hipʹal-; -jetʹik). Hipalgésico; relativo à hipalgesia; que apresenta diminuição da sensibilidade à dor.

hyp·am·ni·on, hyp·am·ni·os (hī-pamʹnē-on, -nē-os). Hipâmnio. SIN oligo-hydramnios.

hyp·an·a·ki·ne·sia, hyp·an·a·ki·ne·sis (hī-panʹă-ki-nēʹsē-ă, -kin-ēʹsis). Hipanacinesia; diminuição dos movimentos gástricos ou intestinais normais. [G. *hypo*, abaixo + *anakinēsis*, movimento de vai-e-vem]

hyp·ar·te·rial (hīpar-tērʹē-ăl, hipʹar-). Hiparterial; abaixo de ou sob uma artéria. [G. *hypo*, abaixo + *artēria*, artéria]

hyp·ax·i·al (hī-pakʹsē-ăl, hip-akʹ). Hipaxial; abaixo de qualquer eixo, como o eixo da coluna vertebral ou o eixo de um membro. VER hypomere. [G. *hypo*, abaixo + eixo]

hyp·az·o·tu·ria (hī′paz-ō-tooʹrē-ă). Hipazotúria. SIN hypoazoturia.

hyp·en·ceph·a·lon (hī′pen-sefʹă-lon). Hipencéfalo; o mesencéfalo, a ponte e o bulbo. [G. *hypo*, abaixo + *enkephalos*, cérebro]

hyp·en·gy·o·pho·bia (hī-penʹgi-ō-fōʹbē-ă). Hipengiofobia; medo mórbido de responsabilidade. [G. *hypengyos*, responsável + *phobos*, medo]

♻ **hyper-.** Hiper-. Excessivo, acima do normal; oposto de hipo-. [G. *hyper*, acima, sobre]

hy·per·ab·duc·tion. Hiperabdução. SIN superabduction.

hy·per·a·cid·i·ty (hī′per-a-sidʹi-tē). Hiperacidez; grau anormalmente alto de acidez, como suco gástrico.

hy·per·ac·tiv·i·ty (hī′per-ak-tivʹi-tē). Hiperatividade. **1.** SIN superactivity. **2.** Inquietude geral ou movimento excessivo, como o que caracteriza crianças com transtorno de déficit de atenção ou hipercinesia.

hy·per·a·cu·sis, hy·per·a·cu·sia (hī′per-a-kooʹsis, -kooʹsē-ă). Sensibilidade auditiva anormal. SIN auditory hyperesthesia. [hyper- + G. *akousis*, audição]

hy·per·ad·e·no·sis (hī′per-ad-ē-nōʹsis). Hiperadenose; aumento de volume glandular, especialmente das glândulas linfáticas. [hyper- + G. *adēn*, glândula + -*ōsis*, condição]

hy·per·ad·i·po·sis, hy·per·ad·i·pos·i·ty (hī′per-ad-i-pōʹsis, -posʹi-tē). Hiperadiposidade; grau extremo de adipose ou gordura.

hy·per·ad·re·nal·cor·ti·cal·ism (hī′per-ă-drēʹnal-kōrʹti-kăl-izm). Hiperadrenocorticismo. SIN hypercorticoidism.

hy·per·a·dre·no·cor·ti·cal·ism (hī′per-ă-drēʹnō-kōrʹti-kăl-izm). Hiperadrenocorticalismo. SIN hypercorticoidism.

hy·per·al·a·nine·mia (hī′per-alʹă-nēn-ēʹmē-ă). Hiperalaninemia; níveis séricos elevados de alanina.

hy·per-β-al·a·nine·mia (hī′per-bāʹta-alʹă-nen-ēʹmē-a). Hiper-β-alaninemia; níveis elevados de β-alanina no soro; acredita-se que seja devido a uma deficiência de β-alanina: piruvato aminotransferase; resulta em comprometimento da função do SNC.

hy·per·al·dos·te·ron·ism (hī′per-al-dosʹter-on-izm). Hiperaldosteronismo. SIN aldosteronism.

hy·per·al·ge·sia (hī-per-al-jēʹzē-ă). Hiperalgesia; sensibilidade extrema a estímulos dolorosos. [hyper- + G. *algos*, dor]

hy·per·al·ge·sic, hy·per·al·get·ic (hī′per-al-jēʹsik, -jetʹik). Hiperalgésico; relativo à hiperalgesia.

hy·per·al·i·men·ta·tion (hī′per-alʹi-men-tāʹshŭn). Hiperalimentação; administração ou consumo de nutrientes além das necessidades normais mínimas, numa tentativa de repor deficiências nutricionais. SIN superalimentation, suralimentation.

enteral h., h. enteral; hiperalimentação através da administração de nutrientes elementares por um cateter colocado no tubo digestivo; habitualmente utilizada em pacientes com pelo menos uma parte do intestino delgado funcional.

parenteral h., h. parenteral; hiperalimentação de nutrientes através de cateter venoso central em pacientes que não podem consumir alimentos adequados pela via enteral.

hy·per·al·lan·to·in·u·ria (hī′per-ă-lanʹtō-i-nooʹrē-ă). Hiperalantoinúria; excreção aumentada de alantoína na urina.

hy·per·al·pha·lip·o·pro·tei·ne·mia (hī′per-alʹfa-lip-ō-prōʹtēn-ēʹmē-ă). Hiperalfalipoproteinemia; defeito herdado que resulta em níveis elevados de lipoproteínas de alta densidade no soro.

hy·per·a·mi·no·ac·i·du·ria (hī′per-amʹi-nō-as-i-dooʹrē-ă). Hiperaminoacidúria. SIN aminoaciduria.

hy·per-β-ami·no·iso·bu·ty·ric ac·i·du·ria. Hiperacidúria β-aminoisobutírica; níveis elevados de ácido β-aminoisobutírico na urina; acredita-se que o distúrbio se deva a uma deficiência da β-aminoisobutirato: piruvato aminotransferase hepática.

hy·per·am·mo·ne·mia (hī′per-am-ō-nēʹmē-ă) Hiperamonemia. SIN ammonemia.

hy·per·am·y·la·se·mia (hī′per-amʹi-lā-sēʹmē-ă). Hiperamilasemia; níveis séricos elevados de amilase, geralmente observada como uma das manifestações da pancreatite aguda. [hyper- + amilase, G. *haima*, sangue]

hy·per·an·a·ci·ne·sia, hy·per·an·a·ci·ne·sis (hī′per-an-ă-si-nēʹzē-ă, -nēʹsis). Hiperanacinesia. SIN hyperanakinesia.

hy·per·an·a·ki·ne·sia, hy·per·an·a·ki·ne·sis (hī′per-an-ă-ki-nēʹzē-ă, -ki-nēʹsis). Hiperanacinesia; movimento de vai-e-vem excessivo, como, p. ex., do estômago ou do intestino. SIN hyperanacinesia, hyperanacinesis. [hyper- + G. *anakinēsis*, movimento de vai-e-vem]

hy·per·a·phia (hī′per-āʹfē-ă). Hiperafia; sensibilidade extrema ao tato. SIN oxyaphia, tactile hyperesthesia. [hyper- + G. *haphē*, toque, tato]

hy·per·aph·ic (hī-per-afʹik). Hiperáfico; caracterizado por hiperafia.

hy·per·ar·gi·ni·ne·mia (hī′per-ar-jen-in-ē-mē-a). Hiperargininemia; níveis elevados de arginina no plasma sanguíneo; condição habitualmente associada a deficiência de arginase.

hy·per·bar·ic (hī-per-barʹik). Hiperbárico. **1.** Refere-se à pressão de gases ambientes acima de uma atmosfera. **2.** Relativo a soluções mais densas do que o diluente ou meio; p. ex., na anestesia raquiana, uma solução hiperbárica tem uma densidade maior que a do líquido cefalorraquidiano. [hyper- + G. *baros*, peso]

hy·per·bar·ism (hī-per-barʹizm). Hiperbarismo; distúrbios corporais resultantes da pressão de gases ambientes acima de uma atmosfera; p. ex., narcose por nitrogênio, intoxicação por oxigênio, mal-dos-caixões. [hyper- + G. *baros*, pesos]

hy·per·be·ta·lip·o·pro·tein·e·mia (hī′per-bet-ă-lipʹō-prō-tē-nēʹmē-ă). Hiperbetalipoproteinemia; aumento da concentração sanguínea de β-lipoproteínas.

familial h., h. familiar. VER type II familial *hyperlipoproteinemia*.

familial h. and hyperprebetalipoproteinemia, h. familiar e hiper pré-β-lipoproteinemia. SIN type III familial *hyperlipoproteinemia*.

hy·per·bil·i·ru·bi·ne·mia (hī′per-bilʹi-roo-bi-nēʹmē-ă). Hiperbilirrubinemia; níveis anormalmente elevados de bilirrubina no sangue circulante, resultando em icterícia clinicamente aparente quando a concentração é suficiente.

neonatal h., h. neonatal; nível sérico de bilirrubina > 12,9 mg/dl (220 μmol/L) ou aumentando numa taxa de mais de 5 mg/dl por dia; termo também aplicado a um padrão não-fisiológico de hiperbilirrubinemia, isto é, a ocorrência de icterícia nas primeiras 24 horas de vida ou estendendo-se além da primeira semana de vida em recém-nascidos a termo.

hy·per·brach·y·ceph·a·ly (hī′per-brak-ē-sefʹă-lē). Hiperbraquicefalia; grau extremo de braquicefalia, com índice cefálico > 85. [hyper- + G. *brachys*, curto + *kephalē*, cabeça]

ℹ **hy·per·cal·ce·mia** (hī′per-kal-sēʹmē-ă). Hipercalcemia; concentração anormalmente elevada de compostos contendo cálcio no sangue circulante; termo comumente utilizado para indicar uma concentração elevada de íons cálcio no sangue.

humoral h. of benignancy, h. humoral de processos benignos; h. induzida por proteína paratormônio-símile de tumor benigno.

idiopathic h. of infants, h. idiopática de lactentes; hipercalcemia persistente de causa desconhecida em crianças muito pequenas, associada a osteosclerose, insuficiência renal e, algumas vezes, hipertensão; além disso, pode estar associada a estenose aórtica supravalvar, fácies de elfo e retardo mental.

hy·per·cal·ci·nu·ria (hī′per-kal-si-nooʹrē-ă). Hipercalcinúria. SIN hypercalciuria.

hy·per·cal·ci·u·ria (hī′per-kal-sē-yuʹrē-ă). Hipercalciúria; excreção de quantidades anormalmente grandes de cálcio na urina, como no hiperparatireoidismo e em tipos de raquitismo hipofosfatêmico hereditário. SIN calcinuric diabetes, hypercalcinuria, hypercalcuria.

hy·per·cal·cu·ria (hī′per-kal-kūʹrē-ă). Hipercalcúria. SIN hypercalciuria.

hy·per·cap·nia (hī-per-kapʹnē-ă). Hipercapnia; aumento anormal da tensão arterial de dióxido de carbono. SIN hypercarbia. [hyper- + G. *kapnos*, fumaça, vapor]

hy·per·car·bia (hī-per-karʹbē-ă). Hipercarbia. SIN hypercapnia.

hy·per·car·dia (hī-per-karʹdē-ă). Hipercardia; hipertrofia do coração. [hyper- + G. *kardia*, coração]

diagnóstico diferencial da hipercalcemia	
processos malignos	hipercalcemia hipocalciúrica familiar
com comprometimento esquelético	hipercalcemia idiopática do lactente
erosão tumoral direta do osso	superdosagem de vitaminas
produção tumoral local de agentes de reabsorção óssea	vitamina D
(isto é, prostaglandina E_2)	vitamina A
ausência de comprometimento esquelético (hipercalcemia	doença granulomatosa
humoral de processos malignos)	sarcoidose
proteína relacionada ao paratormônio	tuberculose
fator(es) de crescimento (fator de crescimento tumoral,	beriliose
fator de crescimento epidérmico, fator de crescimento	coccidioidomicose
derivado das plaquetas)	insuficiência renal
neoplasia hematológica	insuficiência renal crônica
citocinase (interleucina-1, fator de necrose tumoral, linfotoxina)	insuficiência renal aguda—fase diurética
1,25-diidroxivitamina D (linfoma)	após transplante renal
hiperparatireoidismo primário coexistente	diuréticos clorotiazídicos
hiperparatireoidismo primário	terapia com lítio
adenoma, hiperplasia, carcinoma	síndrome leite-álcali
familiar	imobilização
neoplasia endócrina múltipla tipo I com tumores hipofisários	aumento das proteínas séricas
e pancreáticos	hemoconcentração
neoplasia endócrina múltipla tipo II com carcinoma medular	hiperglobulinemia devido ao mieloma múltiplo
da tireóide e feocromocitoma	
outros distúrbios endócrinos	
hipertireoidismo	
hipotireoidismo	
acromegalia	
insuficiência supra-renal aguda	
feocromocitoma	

hy·per·cat·a·bol·ic (hī′per - kat - ă - bol′ik). Hipercatabólico; relativo ao hipercatabolismo.

hy·per·cat·ab·o·lism (hī′per - kă - tab′ŏ - lizm). Hipercatabolismo; degradação metabólica excessiva de uma substância específica ou tecido corporal em geral, resultando em perda de peso e consunção.

hy·per·ca·thar·sis (hī′per - kă - thar′sis). Hipercatarse; defecação excessiva e freqüente. [hyper- + G. *katharsis*, limpeza]

hy·per·ca·thex·is (hī′per - kă - thek′sis). Hipercatexe; em psicanálise, investimento excessivo da libido ou do interesse de um indivíduo num objeto, numa pessoa ou numa idéia. [hyper- + G. *kathexis*, contenção, retenção]

hy·per·ce·men·to·sis (hī′per - sē - men - tō′sis). Hipercementose; deposição excessiva de cemento secundário na raiz de um dente, que pode ser causada por traumatismo localizado ou inflamação, erupção dentária excessiva ou osteíte deformante, podendo ocorrer de forma idiopática. SIN cementum hyperplasia. [hyper- + L. *caementum*, pedra áspera + *-osis*, condição]

hy·per·chlor·e·mia (hī′per - klō - rē′mē - ă). Hipercloremia; níveis anormalmente elevados de íons cloreto no sangue circulante. SIN chloremia (2).

hy·per·chlor·hy·dria (hī′per - klōr - hī′drē - ă). Hipercloridria; presença de quantidade excessiva de ácido clorídrico no estômago. SIN chlorhydria, hyperhydrochloria. [hyper- + (ácido) clorídrico]

hy·per·chlor·u·ria (hī′per - klōr - ū′rē - ă). Hiperclorúria; excreção aumentada de íons cloreto na urina.

hy·per·cho·les·ter·e·mia (hī′per - kō - les′ter - ē′mē - ă). Hipercolesterolemia. SIN hypercholesterolemia.

hy·per·cho·les·ter·in·e·mia (hī′per - kō - les′ter - i - nē′mē - ă). Hipercolesterinemia. SIN hypercholesterolemia.

hy·per·cho·les·ter·ol·e·mia (hī′per - kō - les′ter - ol - ē′mē - ă). Hipercolesterolemia; presença de níveis anormalmente elevados de colesterol no sangue. SIN hypercholesteremia, hypercholesterinemia.
  familial h., h. familiar. VER type II familial *hyperlipoproteinemia*.
  familial h. with hyperlipemia, h. familiar com hiperlipemia. SIN type III familial *hyperlipoproteinemia*.

hy·per·cho·les·ter·o·lia (hī′per - kō - les′ter - ō′lē - ă). Hipercolesterolia; presença de quantidade anormalmente grande de colesterol na bile.

hy·per·cho·lia (hī - per - kō′lē - ă). Hipercolia; condição em que ocorre formação de uma quantidade anormalmente grande de bile no fígado. [hyper- + G. *cholē*, bile]

hy·per·chro·maf·fin·ism (hī′per - krō′maf - in - izm). Hipercromafinismo; presença de feocromocitoma funcionante.

hy·per·chro·ma·sia (hī′per - krō - mā′zē - ă). Hipercromasia. SIN hyperchromatism.

hy·per·chro·mat·ic (hī′per - krō - mat′ik). Hipercromático. **1.** Coloração anormalmente intensa, excessivamente corado ou hiperpigmentado. SIN hyperchromic (1). **2.** Que apresenta aumento da cromatina. [hyper- + G. *chrōma*, cor]

hy·per·chro·ma·tism (hī′per - krō′mă - tizm). Hipercromatismo. **1.** Pigmentação excessiva. **2.** Capacidade de coloração aumentada, especialmente dos núcleos celulares pela hematoxilina. **3.** Aumento da cromatina nos núcleos celulares. SIN hyperchromasia, hyperchromia. [hyper- + G. *chrōma*, cor]

hy·per·chro·mia (hī - per - krō′mē - ă). Hipercromia. SIN hyperchromatism.
  macrocytic h., h. macrocítica; macrocitemia hipercromática; termo incorreto, visto que os eritrócitos são maiores do que o normal, a quantidade total de hemoglobina por célula está aumentada, porém a percentagem de hemoglobina por célula está habitualmente na faixa normocrômica.

hy·per·chro·mic (hī - per - krōm′ik). Hipercrômico. **1.** SIN hyperchromatic (1). **2.** Indica aumento da absorção de luz. **3.** Indica uma coloração mais intensa do que o normal. **4.** Descreve eritrócitos que contêm ou parecem conter mais hemoglobina do que o normal.

hy·per·chy·lia (hī - per - kī′lē - ă). Hiperquilia; secreção excessiva de suco gástrico. [hyper- + G. *chylos*, suco]

hy·per·chy·lo·mi·cro·ne·mia (hī′per - kī′lō - mī - krō - nē′mē - ă). Hiperquilomicronemia; concentrações plasmáticas aumentadas de quilomícrons.
  familial h., h. familiar. SIN type I familial *hyperlipoproteinemia*.
  familial h. with hyperprebetalipoproteinemia, h. familiar com hiper pré-β-lipoproteinemia. SIN type V familial *hyperlipoproteinemia*.

hy·per·ci·ne·sis, hy·per·ci·ne·sia (hī′per - si - nē′sis, - si - nē′zē - ă). Hipercinese, hipercinesia. SIN hyperkinesis.

hy·per·co·ag·u·la·bil·i·ty (hī′per - kō - ag′oo - lă - bil - i - tē). Hipercoagulabilidade; aumento anormal da coagulabilidade.

hy·per·co·ag·u·la·ble (hī′ - per - kō - ag′oo - lă - bl). Hipercoagulável; caracterizado por aumento anormal da coagulação.

hy·per·cor·ti·coid·ism (hī′per - kōr′ti - koyd - izm). Hipercorticoidismo; secreção excessiva de um ou mais hormônios esteróides do córtex supra-renal; algumas vezes, o termo é também utilizado para designar o estado produzido pela administração terapêutica de grandes quantidades de esteróides com atividade glicocorticóide, como, p. ex., hidrocortisona. VER TAMBÉM Cushing *syndrome*. SIN adrenalism, hyperadrenalcorticalism, hyperadrenocorticalism.

hy·per·cor·ti·sol·ism (hī′per-kōr′ti-sol-izm). Hipercortisolismo. VER hyperadrenocorticalism.

hy·per·cry·al·ge·sia (hī′per-krī-al-jē′zē-ă) Hipercrialgesia. SIN hypercryesthesia. [hyper- + G. *kryos*, frio + *algēsis*, sentido da dor]

hy·per·cry·es·the·sia (hī′per-krī-es-thē′zē-ă). Hipercriestesia; sensibilidade extrema ao frio. SIN hypercryalgesia. [hyper- + G. *kryos*, frio + *aisthēsis*, sensação]

hy·per·cu·pre·mia (hī′per-koo-prē′mē-ă). Hipercupremia; nível plasmático anormalmente elevado de cobre. [hyper- + G. *cuprum*, cobre + *haima*, sangue]

hy·per·cy·a·not·ic (hī′per-sī-ă-not′ik). Hipercianótico; caracterizado por cianose extrema.

hy·per·cy·e·sis, hy·per·cy·e·sia (hī′per-sī-ē′sis, -ē′zē-ă). Hiperciese. SIN superfetation. [hyper- + G. *kyēsis*, gravidez]

hy·per·cy·the·mia (hī′per-sī-thē′mē-ă). Hipercitemia; presença de número anormalmente elevado de eritrócitos no sangue circulante. SIN hypererythrocytemia. [hyper- + G. *kytos*, célula + *haima*, sangue]

hy·per·cy·to·chro·mia (hī′per-sī-tō-krō′mē-ă). Hipercitocromia; intensidade aumentada de coloração de uma célula, especialmente células sanguíneas. [hyper- + G. *kytos*, célula + *chrōma*, cor]

hy·per·cy·to·sis (hī′per-sī-tō′sis). Hipercitose; termo obsoleto para referir-se a qualquer condição caracterizada por um aumento anormal no número de células no sangue circulante ou nos tecidos; freqüentemente utilizado como sinônimo de leucocitose.

hy·per·di·crot·ic (hī′per-dī-krot′ik). Hiperdicrótico; acentuadamente dicrótico. SIN superdicrotic.

hy·per·di·cro·tism (hī-per-dik′rō-tizm, -dī′krō-tizm). Hiperdicrotismo; dicrotismo extremo.

hy·per·dip·loid (hī′per-dip′loid). Hiperdiplóide; que possui um número de cromossomas maior do que o número diplóide.

hy·per·dip·sia (hī-per-dip′sē-ă). Hiperdipsia; sede intensa e relativamente temporária. [hyper- + G. *dipsa*, sede]

hy·per·dis·ten·tion (hī′per-dis-ten′shŭn). Hiperdistensão; distensão extrema. SIN superdistention.

hy·per·ech·o·ic (hī′per-ĕ-kō′ik). Hiperecóico. 1. Em ultra-sonografia, relativo a material que produz ecos de maior amplitude ou densidade do que o meio circundante. 2. Refere-se a uma região numa imagem ultra-sonográfica em que os ecos são mais fortes do que o normal ou do que as estruturas circundantes.

hyperekplexia (hī′per-ek-pleks′ē-ă). [MIM#149400]. Hiperecplexia; distúrbio hereditário caracterizado por respostas de sobressalto patológicas, isto é, reações protetoras a qualquer tipo de estímulo inesperado e potencialmente ameaçador, particularmente auditivo; os estímulos quase sempre induzem contrações súbitas disseminadas e violentas da musculatura da cabeça, pescoço, coluna e, por vezes, membros, resultando em gritos, movimentos bruscos, estremecimento e queda involuntários; formas de herança autossômica dominante e recessiva, estando o gene responsável localizado no cromossoma 5q; resulta provavelmente da ausência de neurotransmissores inibitórios, glicina ou GABA. SIN kok disease, startle disease. [hyper- + G. *ekplēxia*, choque súbito, fr. *ekplēssō*, sobressaltar]

hy·per·em·e·sis (hī-per-em′ĕ-sis). Hiperêmese; vômitos excessivos. [hyper- + G. *emesis*, vômitos]

 h. gravida'rum, h. da gravidez; vômitos perniciosos durante a gravidez.

 h. lacten'tium, h. do lactente; vômitos de lactentes com estenose pilórica.

hy·per·e·met·ic (hī′per-ĕ-met′ik). Hiperemético; caracterizado por vômitos excessivos.

hy·per·e·mia (hī-per-ē′mē-ă). Hiperemia; fluxo sanguíneo aumentado numa parte ou órgão. VER TAMBÉM congestion. [hyper- + G. *haima*, sangue]

 active h., h. ativa; hiperemia devido a um afluxo aumentado de sangue arterial para capilares dilatados. SIN arterial h., fluxionary h.

 arterial h., h. arterial. SIN active h.

 Bier h., h. de Bier; termo obsoleto para referir-se à hiperemia causada pelo método de Bier (2). [Bier *method* (2)].

 collateral h., h. colateral; aumento do fluxo sanguíneo através de canais colaterais abundantes, quando a circulação pela artéria principal para uma parte está interrompida.

 fluxionary h., h. de fluxo. SIN active h.

 passive h., h. passiva; hiperemia devido a uma obstrução do fluxo de sangue da parte afetada, com distensão das radículas venosas. SIN venous h.

 peristatic h., h. peristática. SIN peristasis.

 reactive h., h. reativa; hiperemia que ocorre após parada e restabelecimento subseqüente do suprimento sanguíneo para uma parte.

 venous h., h. venosa. SIN passive h.

hy·per·e·mic (hī-per-ē′mik). Hiperêmico; indica hiperemia.

hy·per·en·ceph·a·ly (hī′per-en-sef′ă-lē). Hiperencefalia; deficiência de desenvolvimento fetal da abóbada craniana, expondo o cérebro precariamente formado. [hyper- + G. *enkephalos*, cérebro]

hy·per·e·o·sin·o·phil·ia (hī′per-ē-ō-sin-ō-fil′ē-ă). Hipereosinofilia; grau maior de aumento anormal no número de granulócitos eosinofílicos no sangue circulante ou nos tecidos; p. ex., nas doenças em que o grau de eosinofilia geralmente varia de 10–30%, a ocorrência de um aumento de 50 ou 60% (ou mais) poderia ser considerada como hipereosinofilia.

hy·per·er·gia (hī′per-er′jē-ă). Hiperergia; hipersensibilidade alérgica. SIN hypergia.

hy·per·er·gic (hī-per-er′jik). Hiperérgico; relativo à hiperergia. SIN hypergic.

hy·per·e·ryth·ro·cy·the·mia (hī′per-ē-rith′rō-sī-thē′mē-ă). Hipereritrocitemia. SIN hypercythemia.

hy·per·es·o·pho·ria (hī′per-es-ō-fō′rē-ă). Hiperesoforia; tendência de um olho a desviar-se para cima e para dentro, impedida pela visão binocular. [hyper- + G. *esō*, para dentro + *phora*, movimento]

hy·per·es·the·sia (hī′per-es-thē′zē-ă). Hiperestesia; acuidade anormal da sensibilidade tátil, dolorosa ou a outros estímulos sensoriais. [hyper- + G. *aisthēsis*, sensação]

 auditory h., h. auditiva. SIN hyperacusis.

 cervical h., h. cervical; hipersensibilidade dos dentes, na área cervical, devido à exposição da dentina.

 gustatory h., h. gustativa. SIN hypergeusia.

 muscular h., h. muscular; sensibilidade dos músculos à pressão.

 olfactory h., h. olfacto'ria, h. olfatória. SIN hyperosmia.

 h. op'tica, h. óptica; sensibilidade extrema dos olhos à luz. VER photophobia, photosensitivity.

 tactile h., h. tátil. SIN hyperaphia.

hy·per·es·thet·ic (hī′per-es-thet′ik). Hiperestésico; caracterizado por hiperestesia.

hy·per·eu·ry·pro·so·pic (hī′per-ū′ri-prō-sop′ik). Hipereuriprosópico; relativo a, ou que se caracteriza por, uma face muito baixa e larga. [hyper- + G. *eurys*, largo + *prosōpon*, face]

hy·per·ex·o·pho·ria (hī′per-ek-sō-fō′rē-ă). Hiperexoforia; tendência de um olho a desviar-se para cima e para fora, impedida pela visão binocular. [hyper- + G. *exō*, para fora + *phora*, movimento]

hy·per·ex·ten·sion (hī′per-eks-ten′shŭn). Hiperextensão; extensão de um membro ou parte além do limite normal. SIN overextension, superextension.

hy·per·fer·re·mia (hī′per-fer-ē′mē-ă). Hiperferremia; níveis séricos elevados de ferro; observada na hemocromatose.

hy·per·fi·bri·no·ge·ne·mia (hī′per-fī-brin′ō-jĕ-nē′ē-ă). Hiperfibrinogenemia; aumento dos níveis de fibrinogênio no sangue. SIN fibrinogenemia.

hy·per·fi·bri·nol·y·sis (hī′per-fī-brin-ol′i-sis). Hiperfibrinólise; fibrinólise acentuadamente aumentada, como nos hematomas subdurais.

hy·per·flex·ion (hī-per-flek′shŭn). Hiperflexão; flexão de um membro ou parte além do limite normal. SIN superflexion.

hy·per·fruc·to·se·mia (hī′per-frŭk-tō-sē-mē-ă). Hiperfrutosemia; níveis séricos elevados de frutose.

hy·per·gal·ac·to·sis (hī′per-ga-lak-tō′sis). Hipergalactose; secreção excessiva de leite. [hyper- + G. *gala*, leite + *-ōsis*, condição]

hy·per·gam·ma·glob·u·lin·e·mia (hī′per-gam-ă-glob′ū-li-nē′mē-ă). Hipergamaglobulinemia; nível aumentado das γ-globulinas no plasma, como ocorre freqüentemente em doenças infecciosas crônicas.

hy·per·gan·gli·on·o·sis (hī-per-gang-glē-ō-nō′sis). Hiperganglionose. SIN neuronal *hyperplasia*.

hy·per·gen·e·sis (hī-per-jen′ĕ-sis). Hipergênese; desenvolvimento excessivo ou produção redundante de partes ou órgãos do corpo. [hyper- + G. *genesis*, produção]

hy·per·ge·net·ic (hī-per-jĕ-net′ik). Hipergenético; relativo à hipergênese.

hy·per·gen·i·tal·ism (hī-per-jen′i-tăl-izm). Hipergenitalismo; desenvolvimento excessivo e anormal da genitália.

hy·per·geu·sia (hī-per-goo′sē-ă,-joo′sē-ă). Hipergeusia; acuidade anormal do sentido do paladar. SIN gustatory hyperesthesia. [hyper- + G. *geusis*, paladar]

hy·per·gia (hī-per′jē-ă). Hipergia. SIN hyperergia.

hy·per·gic (hī-per′jik). Hipérgico. SIN hyperergic.

hy·per·glan·du·lar (hī-per-glan′dyŭ-lăr). Hiperglandular; que se caracteriza por superatividade ou aumento de tamanho de uma glândula.

hy·per·glob·u·lia, hy·per·glob·u·lism (hī′per-glob-ū′lē-ă, -glob′ū-lizm). Hiperglobulia, hiperglobulismo; termo antigo para referir-se à policitemia. [hyper- + G. *globulus*, glóbulo]

hy·per·glob·u·lin·e·mia (hī′per-glob′ū-lin-ē′mē-ă). Hiperglobulinemia; concentração anormalmente elevada de globulinas no plasma sanguíneo circulante.

hy·per·gly·ce·mia (hī′per-glī-sē′mē-ă). Hiperglicemia; concentração anormalmente elevada de glicose no sangue circulante, observada especialmente em pacientes com diabetes melito. SIN hyperglycosemia. [hyper- + G. *glykys*, doce + *haima*, sangue]

 ketotic h., h. cetótica; erro inato do metabolismo da glicina caracterizado por letargia, vômitos, convulsões, hipertonia e dificuldade da respiração; a proteína do leite e a caseína induzem ataques; herança autossômica recessiva.

nonketotic h., h. não-cetótica. SIN hyperosmolar (hyperglycemic) nonketotic coma.

posthypoglycemic h., h. pós-hipoglicêmica. SIN Somogyi *phenomenon.*

hy·per·glyc·er·i·de·mia (hī′per - glis′er - i - dē′mē - ă). Hipergliceridemia; concentração plasmática elevada de glicerídeos.

endogenous h., h. endógena; hiperlipoproteinemia familiar tipo IV ou, mais comumente, uma variedade esporádica não-familiar.

exogenous h., h. exógena; hipergliceridemia persistente devido à remoção tardia do plasma dos quilomícrons de origem dietética; ocorre no alcoolismo, no hipotireoidismo, no diabetes melito insulinopênico, na hiperlipoproteinemia tipos I e V e durante a pancreatite aguda.

hy·per·gly·ci·ne·mia (hī′per - glī - si - nē′mē - ă). Hiperglicinemia; concentração plasmática elevada de glicina.

ketotic h., h. cetótica; defeito metabólico hereditário decorrente de uma deficiência de propionil coenzima A carboxilase, a enzima que converte o propionato em metilmalonato; a enzima exige biotina como co-fator; clinicamente, os lactentes afetados apresentam doença devastadora, com letargia, acidose metabólica com cetose, hipotonia; tipicamente, ocorrem coma e convulsões com morte precoce; o ácido propiônico está acentuadamente elevado no plasma e na urina; além disso, há hiperamonemia, bem como níveis elevados de outros metabólitos, incluindo glicina, daí o nome original da síndrome. SIN methylmalonic acidemia, propionic acidemia.

nonketotic h. [MIM*238300], h. não-cetótica; erro inato do metabolismo da glicina devido à deficiência da proteína P glicina dicarboxilase (GCSP), um componente do sistema de clivagem da glicina; doença tipicamente devastadora no período neonatal, com coma, convulsões e morte ou, com menos freqüência, início gradual com ausência de desenvolvimento, convulsões focais e retardo mental; elevação maciça dos níveis plasmáticos de glicina, com níveis elevados no líquido cefalorraquidiano e na urina; ocorrem hiperosmolalidade plasmática e desidratação intensa sem cetoacidose; herança autossômica recessiva; causada por uma mutação no gene GCSP no cromossoma 9p.

hy·per·gly·ci·nu·ri·a (hī′per - glī - si - noo′rē - ă). Hiperglicinúria; aumento da excreção urinária de glicina.

hy·per·gly·co·gen·ol·y·sis (hī′per - glī′kō - jĕ - nol′i - sis). Hiperglicogenólise; glicogenólise excessiva. [hyper- + glicogênio + G. *lysis,* dissolução]

hy·per·gly·cor·rha·chia (hī′per - glī - kō - rak′ē - ă). Hiperglicorraquia; excesso de açúcar no líquido cefalorraquidiano. [hyper- + G. *glykys,* doce + *rhachis,* espinha]

hy·per·gly·co·se·mia (hī′per - glī - kō - sē′mē - ă). Hiperglicosemia. SIN hyperglycemia.

hy·per·gly·co·su·ri·a (hī′per - glī - kō - soo′rē - ă). Hiperglicosúria; excreção persistente de quantidades inusitadamente elevadas de glicose na urina; isto é, grau extremo de glicosúria.

hy·per·gly·ox·yl·e·mia (hī′per - glī - ok′si - lē′mē - ă). Hiperglioxilemia; aumento das concentrações plasmáticas (e, possivelmente, teciduais) de glioxilato; pode surgir durante a deficiência de tiamina.

hy·per·gno·sis (hī - per - nō′sis). Hipergnose. **1.** Projeção de conflitos internos no meio ambiente. **2.** Percepção exagerada, como a expansão de um pensamento isolado. [hyper- + G. *gnōsis,* conhecimento]

hy·per·go·nad·ism (hī - per - gō′nad - izm). Hipergonadismo; estado clínico resultante da secreção aumentada de hormônios gonadais.

hy·per·go·nad·o·tro·pic (hī - per - gō′nă - dō - trop′ik). Hipergonadotrópico; indica a produção ou a excreção aumentada de hormônios gonadotrópicos.

hy·per·gran·u·lo·sis (hī′per - gran - ū - lō′sis). Hipergranulose; aumento da espessura da camada granular da epiderme, em associação com hiperceratose. [hyper- + (stratum) granulosum + -osis, condição]

hy·per·guan·i·di·ne·mia (hī′per - gwan′i - di - nē′mē - ă). Hiperguanidinemia; condição caracterizada por níveis anormalmente elevados de guanidina no sangue circulante.

hy·per·gy·ne·cos·mia (hī′per - gī - nē - koz′mē - ă). Hiperginecosmia; superdesenvolvimento dos caracteres sexuais secundários da mulher madura ou seu desenvolvimento precoce numa menina pequena. [hyper- + G. *gyne,* mulher + *kosmeō,* decorar]

hy·per·he·do·nia, hi·per·he·do·nism (hī′per - hē - dō′nē - ă, - hē′don - izm). Hiperedonia, hiperedonismo; sentimento de um prazer anormalmente grande em qualquer ato ou em decorrência de qualquer acontecimento. [hyper- + G. *hēdonē,* prazer]

hy·per·he·mo·glo·bi·ne·mia (hī′per - hē′mō - glō - bi - nē′mmē - ă). Hiperhemoglobinemia; níveis anormalmente elevados de hemoglobina no plasma sanguíneo circulante; isto é, muito mais do que o habitualmente observado na maioria dos exemplos de hemoglobinemia.

hy·per·hep·a·ri·ne·mia (hī′per - hep′ar - in - ē′mē - ă). [MIM*144050]. Hiper-heparinemia; concentrações plasmáticas elevadas de heparina; acredita-se que seja a causa de uma tendência hemorrágica hereditária; provavelmente de herança autossômica dominante.

hy·per·hi·dro·sis (hī′per - hī - drō′sis). Hiperidrose; sudorese excessiva ou profusa. SIN polyhidrosis, sudorrhea. [hyper- + hidrose]

gustatory h., h. gustatória; sudorese excessiva dos lábios, nariz e testa após a ingestão de certos alimentos; é fisiológica em muitas pessoas; entretanto, ocorre algumas vezes após cirurgia da parótida ou em consequência de lesão dos nervos parassimpáticos ou simpáticos da cabeça e do pescoço.

hy·per·hy·dra·tion (hī′per - hī - drā′shŭn). Hiperidratação; teor excessivo de água no corpo, podendo resultar da administração intravenosa de quantidades indevidamente grandes de solução de glicose. SIN overhydration.

hy·per·hy·dro·chlo·ria (hī′per - hī - drō - klōr′ē - ă). Hiperidrocloria. SIN hyperchlorhydria.

hy·per·hy·dro·chlo·rid·i·a (hī′ - per - hī′drō - chlōr - id - ē - ă). Hiperidrocloridia; secreção excessiva de ácido pelo estômago; associada à úlcera péptica. [hyper- + ácido *clorídrico,* + -ia]

hy·per·hy·dro·pexy, hy·per·hy·dro·pex·is (hī - per - hī′drō - pek - sē, hī′per - hī - drō - pek′sis). Hiperidropexia; fixação aumentada de água nos tecidos. [hyper- + G. *hydōr,* água + *pēgnymi,* jejuar]

hy·per·hy·drox·y·pro·line·mia (hī′per - hī - drok′sē - prō - lēn - ē - mē - ă). Hiperidroxiprolinemia. VER hydroxyprolinemia.

hy·per·i·mi·do·di·pep·ti·du·ri·a (hī′per - im′i - dō - dī - pep′tid - oor - ē - ă). Hiperimidodipeptidúria; níveis elevados de imidodipeptídeos (p. ex., Xaa–Pro) na urina, devido à deficiência de prolidase.

hy·per·im·mune (hī′per - im - mum′). Hiperimune; que apresenta níveis elevados de anticorpos específicos no soro em decorrência de imunizações ou infecções repetidas.

hy·per·im·mu·ni·ty (hī′per - i - mu′ - ni - tē). Hiperimunidade; elevado grau de imunidade.

hy·per·im·mu·ni·za·tion (hī′per - im - oo - nī - zā′shŭn). Hiperimunização. **1.** Indução de um estado de alta imunidade mediante administração de doses repetidas de antígeno, freqüentemente utilizada na dessensibilização da energia. **2.** Imunidade passivamente adquirida pela injeção de gamaglobulina hiperimune.

hy·per·in·di·can·e·mia (hī′per - in′di - kan - ē′mē - ă). Hiperindicanemia; nível inusitadamente elevado de indicana no sangue circulante; isto é, maior do que o observado na maioria dos casos de indicanemia.

hy·per·in·fec·tion (hī′per - in - fek′shŭn). Hiperinfecção; infecção por um número muito grande de organismos em consequência de deficiência imunológica. Cf. superinfection.

hyperinflation (hī - per - in - flā′shŭn). Hiperinflação; superdistensão das vias aéreas e alvéolos, resultando algumas vezes em enfisema, causada por doença pulmonar obstrutiva; ocorre reversivelmente com asma e pode ocorrer localmente com aspiração de um corpo estranho, com fenômeno subsequente de válvula esférica. [hyper- + inflação]

hy·per·i·no·se·mia (hī′per - i′nō - sē′mē - ă, -hī′per - in′ō-). Hiperinosemia; nível acentuadamente aumentado de fibrinogênio no sangue circulante; em certas condições, pode haver formação de quantidades anormalmente grandes de fibrina, levando, assim, a um maior grau de coagulabilidade do sangue. SIN hyperinosis. [hyper- + G. *is (in-),* fibra + *haima,* sangue]

hy·per·i·no·sis (hī - per - i - nō′sis). Hiperinose. SIN hyperinosemia.

hy·per·in·su·li·ne·mia (hī′per - in′soo - lin - ē′ - mē - ă). Hiperinsulinemia. SIN hyperinsulinism.

hy·per·in·su·lin·ism (hī′per - in′soo - lin - izm). Hiperinsulinismo; níveis aumentados de insulina no plasma, devido a um aumento da secreção de insulina pelas células beta das ilhotas pancreáticas; a remoção hepática diminuída de insulina constitui uma causa em alguns pacientes, embora o hiperinsulinismo esteja habitualmente associado a uma resistência à insulina, sendo comumente encontrado na obesidade em associação a graus variáveis de hiperglicemia. SIN hyperinsulinemia.

alimentary h., h. alimentar; níveis elevados de insulina no plasma após a ingestão de refeições por indivíduos com esvaziamento gástrico anormalmente rápido (p. ex., após gastroenterostomia ou vagotomia); a absorção rápida de glicose resulta em liberação excessiva de insulina que, por sua vez, pode levar a uma acentuada queda da glicemia para níveis hipoglicêmicos.

hy·per·in·vo·lu·tion (hī′per - in′vō - loo′shŭn). Hiperinvolução. SIN superinvolution.

hy·per·i·so·ton·ic (hī′per - ī - sō - ton′ik). Hiperisotônico. SIN hypertonic.

hy·per·ka·le·mia (hī′per - kă - lē′mē - ă). Hiperpotassemia; concentração de íons potássio no sangue circulante maior do que o normal. SIN hyperkaliemia, hyperpotassemia. [hyper- + L. Mod. *kalium,* potássio + G. *haima,* sangue]

hy·per·kal·i·e·mia (hī′per - kal - i - ē′mē - ă). Hipercaliemia, hiperpotassemia. SIN hyperkalemia.

hy·per·kal·u·re·sis (hī′per - kal - ū - rē′sis). Hipercaliurese; excreção urinária excessiva de potássio. [hyper- + L. Mod. *kalium,* potássio + G. *oureō,* urinar]

hy·per·ker·a·tin·i·za·tion (hī′per - ker′at - i - ni - zā′shŭn). Hiperceratinização. SIN hyperkeratosis.

hy·per·ker·a·to·sis (hī′per - ker - ă - tō′sis). Hiperceratose; espessamento da camada córnea da epiderme ou mucosa. VER TAMBÉM keratoderma, keratosis. SIN hyperkeratinization.

h. congen′ita, h. congênita. SIN *ichthyosis* vulgaris.

diffuse h. of palms and soles, h. difusa das regiões palmares e plantares; distúrbio autossômico dominante com início na lactância; caracterizado por placas hiperceratóticas descamativas e, com freqüência, hiperidrose das regiões palmares e plantares. SIN Unna-Thost syndrome.
epidermolytic h. [MIM*144200]. h. epidermolítica; caracterizada por lesões localizadas, ceratose palmar e plantar e níveis elevados de IgE, associada a hiperceratose, hipergranulose e degeneração reticular na parte superior da epiderme; herança autossômica dominante, causada pela mutação do gene do ceratoderma palmoplantar epidermolítico (CPPE) no cromossoma 17q. Ocorre h. epidermolítica generalizada no eritroderma ictiosiforme congênito bolhoso. SIN porcupine skin.
h. follicula'ris et parafollicula'ris, h. folicular e parafolicular; tampões foliculares córneos isolados e confluentes numa base crateriforme, ocorrendo freqüentemente nos braços e nas pernas de pacientes diabéticos com insuficiência renal; possivelmente, trata-se de uma forma grave de foliculite perfurante. VER TAMBÉM perforating *folliculitis.* SIN Kyrle disease.
generalized epidermolytic h., h. epidermolítica generalizada. SIN bullous congenital ichthyosiform *erythroderma.*
h. lenticula'ris per'stans [MIM*144150], h. lenticular persistente; pequenas pápulas hiperceratóticas no dorso dos pés e pernas e, em certas ocasiões, em outras partes, com pápulas ceratóticas puntiformes nas regiões palmares e plantares; início na terceira e quarta décadas de vida; caráter autossômico dominante. SIN Flegel disease.
hy·per·ke·to·ne·mia (hī'per-kē'tō-nē'mē-ă). Hipercetonemia; concentrações elevadas de corpos cetônicos no sangue.
hy·per·ke·ton·u·ria (hī'per-kē'tō-noo'rē-ă). Hipercetonúria; excreção urinária aumentada de corpos cetônicos.
hy·per·ki·ne·mia (hī'per-ki-nē'mē-ă). Hipercinemia; aumento da velocidade da circulação; aumento do volume de fluxo através da circulação; débito cardíaco supernormal. [hyper- + G. *kineō,* mover + *haima,* sangue]
hy·per·ki·ne·sis, hy·per·ki·ne·sia (hī'per-ki-nē'sis, -nē'zē-ă). Hipercinese, hipercinesia. **1.** Motilidade excessiva. **2.** Atividade muscular excessiva. SIN hypercinesis, hypercinesia, supermotility. [hyper- + G. *kinēsis,* movimento]
hy·per·ki·net·ic (hī'per-ki-net'ik). Hipercinético; relativo a, ou que se caracteriza por, hipercinesia.
hy·per·lac·ta·tion (hī'per-lak-tā'shŭn). Hiperlactação. SIN superlactation.
hy·per·leu·ko·cy·to·sis (hī'per-loo'kō-sī-tō'sis). Hiperleucocitose; aumento inusitadamente grande do número e da proporção de leucócitos no sangue circulante ou nos tecidos; isto é, muito mais do que o habitualmente observado na maioria dos casos de leucocitose.
hy·per·lex·ia (hī-per-lek'sē-ă). Hiperlexia; em crianças com retardo mental, presença de capacidade de leitura relativamente avançada. [hyper- + G. *lexis,* palavra, frase]
hy·per·li·pe·mia (hī'per-li-pē'mē-ă). Hiperlipemia; níveis elevados de lipídios no plasma sangüíneo. Existem vários tipos de hiperlipemia. Uma delas está associada à deficiência de δ-aminoadípico semialdeído sintetase. VER TAMBÉM lipemia.
carbohydrate-induced h., h. induzida por carboidratos. SIN type III familial *hyperlipoproteinemia,* type IV familial *hyperlipoproteinemia.*
combined fat- and carbohydrate-induced h., h. induzida por gordura e carboidratos combinados. SIN type V familial *hyperlipoproteinemia.*
familial combined h., h. combinada familiar. VER familial *hyperlipoproteinemia.*
familial fat-induced h., h. familiar induzida por gordura. SIN type I familial *hyperlipoproteinemia.*
idiopathic h., h. idiopática. SIN type I familial *hyperlipoproteinemia.*
mixed h., h. mista. SIN type V familial *hyperlipoproteinemia.*
hy·per·lip·id·e·mia (hī'per-lip-i-dē'mē-ă).Hiperlipidemia. SIN lipemia.
mixed h., h. mista. SIN mixed hyperlipoproteinemia familial type 5 h.
mixed hyperlipoproteinemia familial, type 5 h., h. hiperlipoproteinemia familiar mista, h. tipo 5; elevações das VLDL e dos quilomícrons no plasma. SIN mixed h.
hy·per·lip·oi·de·mia (hī'per-lip-oy-dē'mē-ă). Hiperlipoidemia. SIN lipemia.
hy·per·lip·o·pro·tein·e·mia (hī'per-lip'ō-prō'tē-in-ē'mē-ă, -prō'tēn-). Hiperlipoproteinemia; aumento das concentrações sangüíneas de lipoproteínas.
acquired h., h. adquirida; h. não-familiar que se desenvolve em decorrência de alguma doença primária, como deficiência da tireóide.
familial h., h. familiar; grupo de doenças caracterizadas por alterações na concentração de β-lipoproteínas e pré-β-lipoproteínas e dos lipídios a elas associados. VER type I familial h., type II familial h., type III familial h., type IV familial h., type V familial h.
lipoprotein(a) h., h. de lipoproteína (a); níveis elevados de lipoproteína (a) no soro; associada a um risco aumentado de coronariopatia.
type I familial h. [MIM*238600], h. familiar do tipo I; hiperlipoproteinemia caracterizada por níveis elevados de quilomícrons e triglicerídeos no plasma quando o paciente segue uma dieta normal e seu desaparecimento com dieta desprovida de gordura; baixos níveis de α e β-lipoproteínas com dieta normal, verificando-se uma elevação com dieta desprovida de gordura; atividade lipolítica diminuída pós-heparina plasmática e baixa atividade da lipoproteína lipase tecidual. É acompanhada de episódios de dor abdominal, hepatoesplenomegalia, pancreatite e xantomas eruptivos; herança autossômica recessiva; causada por uma mutação do gene da lipoproteína lipase (LPL) no cromossoma 8p. VER TAMBÉM familial lipoprotein lipase *inhibitor.* SIN Bürger-Grütz syndrome, familial fat-induced hyperlipemia, familial hyperchylomicronemia, familial hypertriglyceridemia (1), idiopathic hyperlipemia.
type II familial h. [MIM*143890 e MIM*144400], h. familiar do tipo II; hiperlipoproteinemia caracterizada por níveis plasmáticos elevados de β-lipoproteínas e colesterol, níveis normais ou elevados de triglicerídeos; os heterozigotos apresentam alterações lipídicas leves e são suscetíveis à aterosclerose na meia-idade, enquanto os homozigotos exibem alterações pronunciadas — freqüentemente com xantomatose generalizada, xantelasma, arco corneano e aterosclerose clínica franca quando adultos jovens. Esse distúrbio é dividido em duas classes, ambas herdadas como caráter autossômico dominante, em que os homozigotos estão mais gravemente afetados do que os heterozigotos: 1) tipo IIA, que se caracteriza por níveis elevados de LDL, porém com níveis normais de triglicerídeos, devido à deficiência do receptor de LDL, um defeito do receptor ou uma LDL-apolipoproteína B-100 modificada, causado por uma mutação no gene do receptor de LDL (LDLR) no cromossoma 19p. SIN familial hypercholesterolemia; 2) tipo IIB, caracterizado por níveis elevados de LDL, colesterol e triglicerídeos, devido à desregulação da 3-hidroxi-3-metilglutaril coenzima A redutase (HMG CoA redutase), a enzima que controla a velocidade no processo de biossíntese do colesterol. SIN familial hyperbetalipoproteinemia, familial hypercholesterolemic xanthomatosis.
type III familial h. [MIM*107741], h. familiar tipo III; hiperlipoproteinemia caracterizada por níveis plasmáticos elevados de LDL, β-lipoproteínas, pré-β-lipoproteínas, colesterol, fosfolipídios e triglicerídeos; hipertrigliceridemia induzida por dieta rica em carboidratos, com tolerância anormal à glicose; xantomas eruptivos e ateromatose freqüentes, particularmente coronariopatia; o defeito bioquímico é observado nas apolipoproteínas; existem muitas variedades; uma delas é causada pela mutação do gene APOE no cromossoma 19q. SIN carbohydrate-induced hyperlipemia, dysbetalipoproteinemia, familial hyperbetalipoproteinemia and hyperprebetalipoproteinemia, familial hypercholesterolemia with hyperlipemia.
type IV familial h. [MIM*144600], h. familiar tipo IV; os níveis plasmáticos de VLDL, pré-β-lipoproteínas e triglicerídeos estão aumentados com uma dieta normal, porém as β-lipoproteínas, o colesterol e os fosfolipídios estão normais; hipertrigliceridemia induzida por dieta rica em carboidratos; pode ser acompanhada de tolerância anormal à glicose e suscetibilidade à cardiopatia isquêmica; provavelmente de herança autossômica dominante, embora haja a possibilidade de heterogeneidade genética. SIN carbohydrate-induced hyperlipemia, familial hyperprebetalipoproteinemia, familial hypertriglyceridemia (2).
type V familial h. [MIM*144650], h. familiar tipo V; hiperlipoproteinemia caracterizada por níveis plasmáticos aumentados de quilomícrons, VLDL, pré-β-lipoproteínas e triglicerídeos e discreto aumento do colesterol com uma dieta normal, com níveis normais de β-lipoproteínas; pode ser acompanhada de crises de dor abdominal, hepatoesplenomegalia, suscetibilidade à aterosclerose e tolerância à glicose anormal; provavelmente de herança autossômica recessiva. SIN combined fat- and carbohydrate-induced hyperlipemia, familial hyperchylomicronemia with hyperprebetalipoproteinemia, mixed hyperlipemia.
hy·per·li·po·sis (hī'per-li-pō'sis). Hiperlipose. **1.** Adiposidade excessiva. **2.** Grau extremo de degeneração gordurosa. [hyper- + G. *lipos,* gordura]
hy·per·li·thu·ria (hī'per-li-thu'rē-ă). Hiperlitúria; excreção excessiva de ácido úrico (lítico) na urina.
hy·per·lo·gia (hī-per-lō'jē-ă). Hiperlogia; verbosidade ou loquacidade mórbida. VER logorrhea. [hyper- + G. *logios,* eloqüente]
hy·per·lor·do·sis (hī'per-lōr-dō'sis). Hiperlordose; lordose extrema.
hy·per·lu·cent (hī'-per-loo'sent). Hipertransparente; região, numa radiografia de tórax, em que o filme está mais escuro do que o normal em virtude da maior transmissão dos raios X. VER unilateral hyperlucent *lung.* [hyper- + L. *lucens,* brilhante, fr. *luceo,* brilhar]
hy·per·ly·ne·mia (hī'per-lī-si-nē'mē-ă) [MIM*238700]. Hiperlisinemia; distúrbio metabólico caracterizado por retardo mental, convulsões, anemia e astenia; associada a elevação anormal dos níveis do aminoácido lisina no sangue circulante devido a deficiência de lisina-cetoglutarato redutase. Uma variante [MIM*268700] está associada a deficiência de semialdeído α-aminoadípico sintase, resultando em hiperlisinemia e sacaropinemia.
hy·per·ly·si·nu·ria (hī'per-lī-si-noo'rē-ă). Hiperlisinúria; presença de concentrações anormalmente elevadas de lisina na urina; forma de aminoacidúria que ocorre na cistinúria, na degeneração hepatolenticular e na síndrome de Fanconi.
hy·per·mag·ne·se·mia (hī'per-mag-nē-sē'mē-ă). Hipermagnesemia; concentração anormalmente elevada de magnésio no soro sangüíneo.

hy·per·mas·tia (hī-per-mas′tē-ă). Hipermastia. **1.** SIN polymastia. **2.** Glândulas mamárias excessivamente grandes. [hyper- + G. *mastos*, mama]

hy·per·men·or·rhea (hī′per-men-ō-rē′ă). Hipermenorréia; menstruação excessivamente prolongada ou profusa. SIN menorrhagia. [hyper- + G. *mēn*, mês + *rhoia*, fluxo]

hy·per·me·tab·o·lism (hī′per-me-tab′ō-lizm). Hipermetabolismo; produção acima do normal de calor pelo corpo, como na tireotoxicose.
   extrathyroidal h., h. extratireóideo; estado de metabolismo aumentado com níveis normais de produção de hormônio tireóideo.

hy·per·met·a·mor·pho·sis (hī′per-met-ă-mōr′fō-sis). Hipermetamorfose; mudança excessiva e rápida de idéias que ocorre num distúrbio mental. VER mania, manic-depressive, manic *excitement*. [hyper- + G. *metamorphōsis*, transformação]

hy·per·me·thi·o·nine·mia (hī-per-meth-ī-ō-mēn-ē-mē-ă). Hipermetioninemia; níveis séricos elevados de metionina.

hy·per·me·tria (hī-per-mē′trē-ă). Hipermetria; ataxia caracterizada por exceder-se no desejo de um objeto ou meta; habitualmente observada na presença de distúrbios cerebelares. Cf. hypometria. [hyper- + G. *metron*, medida]

hy·per·met·rope (hī-per-met′rōp). Hipermétrope. SIN hyperope.

hy·per·me·tro·pia (hī′per-me-trō′pē-ă). Hipermetropia. SIN hyperopia. [hyper- + G. *metron*, medida + *ōps*, olho]
   index h., h. índice; hipermetropia que se origina de uma refratariedade diminuída da lente do olho.

hy·perm·ne·sia (hī-perm-nē′zē-ă). Hipermnésia. **1.** Extrema capacidade de memória. **2.** Capacidade, sob hipnose, de registro imediato e lembrança exata de muito mais itens individuais do que se considera possível em circunstâncias normais. Cf. hypomnesia. [hyper- + G. *mnēmē*, memória]

hy·per·mo·bil·i·ty (hī′per-mō-bil′i-tē). Hipermobilidade; aumento do arco de movimento das articulações e frouxidão articular, ocorrendo normalmente em crianças e adolescentes ou em decorrência de doença, como, p. ex., síndrome de Marfan ou de Ehlers-Danlos.

hy·per·morph (hī′per-mōrf). Hipermorfo. **1.** Pessoa cuja altura sentada é baixa em proporção à altura em pé, devido ao comprimento excessivo dos membros. Cf. hypomorph, ectomorph. **2.** Gene mutante que provoca aumento na atividade controlada pelo gene. Cf. hypomorph. [hyper- + G. *morphē*, forma]

hy·per·my·ot·ro·phy (hī′per-mī-ot′rō-fē). Hipermiotrofia; hipertrofia muscular. [hyper- + G. *mys*, músculo + *trophē*, nutrição]

hy·per·na·tre·mia (hī′per-nă-trē′mē-ă). Hipernatremia; concentração plasmática anormalmente elevada de íons sódio. [hyper- + L. *natrium*, sódio + G. *haima*, sangue]

hy·per·ne·o·cy·to·sis (hī′per-nē′ō-sī-tō′sis). Hiperneocitose; hiperleucocitose caracterizada por um número considerável de células imaturas e jovens (especialmente na série granulocítica), isto é, "desvio para a esquerda" no hemograma. SIN hyperskeocytosis. [hyper- + G. *neos*, novo + *kytos*, célula + *-osis*, condição]

hy·per·neph·roid (hī-per-nef′royd). Hipernefróide; semelhante a ou do tipo da glândula supra-renal. [hyper- + G. *nephros*, rim + *eidos*, aspecto]

hy·per·noia (hī-per-noy′ă). Hipernóia. **1.** Grande rapidez de pensamento. **2.** Atividade mental ou imaginação excessiva do tipo observado na fase maníaca da depressão maníaca. VER depression. [hyper- + G. *noeō*, pensar]

hy·per·nom·ic (hī-per-nom′ik). Hipernômico; controlado ao excesso. [hyper- + G. *nomos*, lei]

hy·per·nu·tri·tion (hī′per-noo-trish′ŭn). Hipernutrição. SIN supernutrition.

hy·per·on·cot·ic (hī′per-on-kot′ik). Hiperoncótico; indica uma pressão oncótica acima do normal, como, p. ex., a do plasma sanguíneo.

hy·per·o·nych·ia (hī′per-ō-nik′ē-ă). Hiperoníquia; hipertrofia das unhas. [hyper- + G. *onyx*, (*onych-*), unha]

hy·per·ope (hī′per-ōp). Hiperope; que sofre de hiperopia. SIN hypermetrope (hipermetrope).

hy·per·o·pia (H) (hī-per-ō′pē-ă). Hiperopia; presbiopia; condição óptica em que apenas os pares convergentes podem ser focalizados na retina. SIN far sight, farsightedness, hypermetropia, long sight. [hyper- + G. *ōps*, olho]
   absolute h., h. absoluta; hiperopia manifesta, que não pode ser superada por um esforço de acomodação.
   axial h., h. axial; hiperopia devido ao encurtamento do diâmetro ântero-posterior do globo ocular.
   curvature h., h. por curvatura; hiperopia causada por refração diminuída do segmento ocular anterior.
   facultative h., h. facultativa. SIN manifest h.
   latent h., h. latente; a diferença entre a hiperopia total e a manifesta.
   manifest h., h. manifesta; hiperopia que pode ser compensada por acomodação. SIN facultative h.
   total h. (Ht), h. total; a que pode ser determinada após paralisia completa da acomodação por meio de um agente cicloplégico.

hy·per·o·pic (H) (hī-per-ō′pik). Hiperópico; relativo à hiperopia.

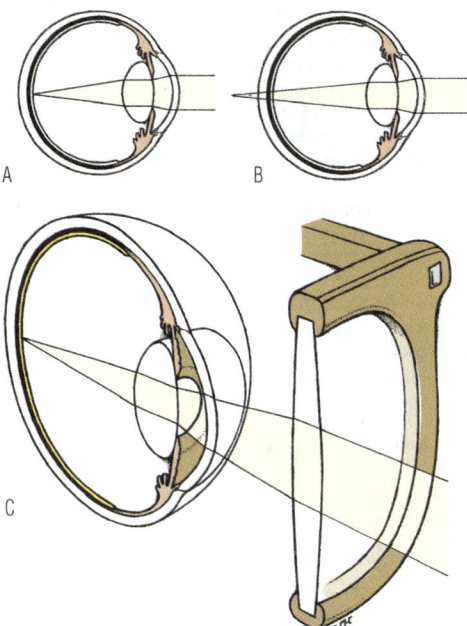

hiperopia: (A) visão normal (20/20), com foco preciso dos raios luminosos na retina; (B) visão hiperópica (hiperopia), em que os raios luminosos de objetos próximos entram em foco preciso atrás da retina; (C) hiperopia corrigida com lente convexa

hy·per·o·ral·i·ty (hī′per-ō-ral′i-tē). Hiperoralidade; condição em que objetos inapropriados são colocados na boca. [hyper- + L. *os* (*or-*), boca]

hy·per·o·rex·ia (hī′per-ō-rek′sē-ă). Hiperorexia. SIN bulimia nervosa. [hyper- + G. *orexis*, apetite]

hy·per·or·ni·thi·ne·mia (hī′per-ōrn′ă-thēn-ē-mē-ă). Hiperornitinemia; níveis séricos elevados de ornitina; algumas vezes associada a hiperamonemia e homocitrulinúria.

hy·per·or·tho·cy·to·sis (hī′per-ōr′thō-sī-tō′sis). Hiperortocitose; hiperleucocitose em que a percentagem relativa dos vários tipos de leucócitos encontra-se dentro da faixa normal e não se observam formas imaturas. [hyper- + G. *orthos*, correto + *kytos*, célula + *osis*, condição]

hy·per·os·mia (hī-per-oz′mē-ă). Hiperosmia. Sentido do olfato exagerado ou anormalmente agudo. SIN olfactory hyperesthesia, hyperesthesia olfactoria. [hyper- + G. *osmē*, sentido do olfato]

hy·per·os·mo·lal·i·ty (hī′per-oz-mō-lal′i-tē). Hiperosmolalidade; concentração osmótica aumentada de uma solução expressa em osmoles de soluto por quilograma de soro.

hy·per·os·mo·lar·i·ty (hī′per-oz-mō-lar′i-tē). Hiperosmolaridade; aumento na concentração osmótica de uma solução expressa como osmoles de soluto por litro da solução.

hy·per·os·mot·ic (hī′per-oz-mot′ik). Hiperosmótico. **1.** Que possui osmolalidade superior à de outro líquido, habitualmente considerado plasma ou líquido extracelular. **2.** Relativo a aumento da osmose.

hy·per·os·te·oi·do·sis (hī′per-os-tē-oy-dō′sis). Hiperosteoidose; formação excessiva de osteóide, conforme observado no raquitismo e na osteomalacia.

hy·per·os·to·sis (hī′per-os-tō′sis). Hiperostose. **1.** Hipertrofia do osso. **2.** Exostose. SIN exostosis. [hyper- + G. *osteon*, osso + *-ōsis*, condição]
   ankylosing h., h. anquilosante. SIN diffuse idiopathic skeletal h.
   h. cortica′lis defor′mans [MIM*239000], h. cortical deformante; espessamento irregular e acentuado do crânio e do córtex ósseo, com espessamento e alargamento das diáfises dos ossos longos e níveis séricos elevados de fosfatase alcalina; herança autossômica recessiva.
   diffuse idiopathic skeletal h. (DISH), h. esquelética idiopática difusa (HEID); distúrbio articular espinal e extra-espinal generalizado, caracterizado por calcificação e ossificação de ligamentos, particularmente do ligamento longitudinal anterior; distinta da espondilite anquilosante ou doença articular degenerativa. SIN ankylosing h., Forestier disease, hyperostotic spondylosis.
   flowing h., h. de fluxo. SIN rheostosis.
   h. fronta′lis inter′na, h. frontal interna; deposição anormal de osso na face interna do osso frontal, visível aos raios X; pode constituir parte da síndrome de Morgagni.
   generalized cortical h., h. cortical generalizada. SIN van Buchem *syndrome*.
   infantile cortical h., [MIM*114000], h. cortical infantil; formação óssea subperióstea neonatal sobre muitos ossos, especialmente a mandíbula, as clavículas

e as diáfises dos ossos longos; surge após a ocorrência de febre, habitualmente antes dos 6 meses de idade, desaparecendo durante a infância; os casos familiares são herdados como caráter autossômico dominante. SIN Caffey disease, Caffey syndrome, Caffey-Silverman syndrome.
streak h., h. estriada. SIN rheostosis.
hy·per·o·var·i·an·ism (hī′per-ō-vā′rē-an-izm). Hiperovarianismo; precocidade sexual em meninas jovens devido à maturação prematura do eixo hipotálamo–hipófise e desenvolvimento dos ovários acompanhado de secreção de hormônios ovarianos. SIN true precocious puberty.
hy·per·ox·al·u·ria (hī′per-ok-sā-loo′rē-ā). Hiperoxalúria; presença de quantidade inusitadamente grande de ácido oxálico ou oxalatos na urina; podem ocorrer cálculos renais. SIN oxaluria.
primary h. and oxalosis [MIM*259900 & MIM*260000], h. primária e oxalose; distúrbio metabólico, que geralmente se torna clinicamente evidente na primeira década de vida, caracterizado por nefrocalcinose e nefrolitíase de oxalato de cálcio, oxalose extra-renal e aumento do débito urinário de ácidos oxálico e glicólico, resultando em insuficiência renal progressiva e uremia. O tipo I é devido a deficiência de alanina-glioxilato aminotransferase, e o tipo II, a deficiência de D-glicerato desidrogenase; esta última forma é uma doença mais leve, com prognóstico em longo prazo mais favorável em termos de função renal. Os dois tipos são herdados como caráter autossômico recessivo, causados por uma mutação no gene da alanina-glioxilato aminotransferase (AGXT) no cromossoma 2q.
hy·per·ox·ia (hī-per-ok′sē-ā). Hiperoxia. **1.** Quantidade aumentada de oxigênio nos tecidos e órgãos. **2.** Tensão de oxigênio maior do que o normal, como a produzida pela respiração de ar ou oxigênio em pressões acima de uma atmosfera.
hy·per·ox·i·da·tion (hī′per-oks-i-dā′shŭn). Hiperoxidação; oxidação excessiva.
hy·per·pan·cre·a·tism (hī′per-pan′krē-ā-tizm). Hiperpancreatismo; condição de atividade aumentada do pâncreas, havendo um excesso de tripsina entre as enzimas.
hy·per·par·a·site (hī-per-par′ā-sīt). Hiperparasita; parasita secundário capaz de se desenvolver no interior de um parasita previamente existente.
hy·per·par·a·sit·ism (hī-per-par′ā-sit-izm). Hiperparasitismo; condição em que um parasita secundário desenvolve-se no interior de um parasita previamente existente. SIN biparasitism.
hy·per·par·a·thy·roid·ism (hī′per-par-ā-thī′royd-izm). Hiperparatireoidismo; condição decorrente de um aumento na secreção das paratireóides, produzindo elevação dos níveis séricos de cálcio, níveis séricos diminuídos de fósforo e excreção aumentada de cálcio e fósforo, formação de cálculos de cálcio e, algumas vezes, osteíte fibrosa cística generalizada.
primary h., h. primário; hiperparatireoidismo devido a neoplasias ou hiperplasia idiopática das glândulas paratireóides.
secondary h., h. secundário; hiperparatireoidismo que surge em consequência de distúrbio do metabolismo, produzindo hipocalcemia, como na uremia crônica devido a doença renal, malabsorção, raquitismo ou osteomalacia; associado a hiperplasia das glândulas paratireóides.
hy·per·pa·rot·i·dism (hī′per-pa-rot′i-dizm). Hiperparotidismo; aumento da atividade das glândulas parótidas.
hy·per·path·ia (hī-per-path′ē-ā). Hiperpatia; resposta subjetiva exagerada a estímulos dolorosos, com sensação contínua de dor após ter cessado o estímulo. [hyper- + G. *pathos,* sofrimento]
hy·per·pep·sia (hī-per-pep′sē-ā). Hiperpepsia. **1.** Digestão anormalmente rápida. **2.** Digestão prejudicada com hipercloridria. [hyper- + G. *pepsis,* digestão]
hy·per·pep·sin·ia (hī′per-pep-sin′ē-ā). Hiperpepsinia; excesso de pepsina no suco gástrico.
hy·per·per·i·stal·sis (hī′per-per-i-stal′sis). Hiperperistaltismo; rapidez excessiva da passagem do alimento através do estômago e do intestino.
hy·per·pha·gia (hī-per-fā′jē-ā). Hiperfagia; glutonaria; hiperalimentação. [hyper- + G. *phagein,* comer]
hy·per·pha·lan·gism (hī′per-fā-lan′jizm). Hiperfalangismo; presença de falange supranumerária num dedo da mão ou do pé. SIN polyphalangism.
hy·per·phen·yl·a·ni·ne·mia (hī′per-fen′il-al-ā-ni-nē′mē-ā). Hiperfenilalaninemia. Presença de níveis sanguíneos anormalmente elevados de fenilalanina, que podem ou não estar associados a níveis elevados de tirosina em recém-nascidos (prematuros e a termo), em associação ao estado heterozigoto da fenilcetonúria, fenilcetonúria materna ou deficiência transitória de fenilalanina hidroxilase ou ácido *p*-hidroxifenilpirúvico oxidase.
malignant h., h. maligna; **(1)** forma com deficiência de dHPR; distúrbio hereditário caracterizado pela ausência ou deficiência da diidropteridina redutase (DHPR); resulta em comprometimento da regeneração de tetraidrobiopterina, causando elevação dos níveis de fenilalanina; **(2)** forma gTP-CH; distúrbio hereditário caracterizado por deficiência de guanosina trifosfato ciclo-hidrolase, uma enzima envolvida na biossíntese da tetraidrobiopterina; **(3)** forma 6-PTS; distúrbio hereditário caracterizado pela deficiência da 6-piruvoil tetraidropterina sintetase, uma enzima que participa na biossíntese da tetraidrobiopterina. SIN nonclassical phenylketonuria.
non-PKU h., h. não-PKU; fenótipo benigno em que a fenilalanina monooxigenase está deficiente, porém acima de 1% dos níveis normais.
hy·per·pho·ne·sis (hī′per-fō-nē′sis). Hiperfonese; aumento do som de percussão ou do som vocal à ausculta. [hyper- + G. *phonēsis,* som]
hy·per·pho·nia (hī′per-fō′nē-ā). Hiperfonia; esforço excessivo na produção da voz, caracterizado por intensidade ou tensão indevida dos músculos vocais. [hyper- + G. *phonē,* som, voz]
hy·per·pho·ria (hī-per-fō′rē-ā). Hiperforia; tendência do eixo visual de um olho a sofrer desvio para cima, evitada pela visão binocular. [hyper- + G. *phora,* movimento]
hy·per·phos·pha·ta·se·mia (hī′per-fos′fā-tā-sē′mē-ā). Hiperfosfatasemia; teor anormalmente elevado de fosfatase alcalina no sangue circulante. VER TAMBÉM hyperphosphatasia.
hy·per·phos·pha·ta·sia (hī′per-fos-fā-tā′zē-ā). [MIM*239000 e MIM*239300]. Hiperfosfatasia; displasia esquelética caracterizada por nanismo, macrocrânio, expansão das diáfises dos ossos tubulares com múltiplas fraturas, osteosclerose difusa, arqueamento das pernas e, em certas ocasiões, retardo mental; níveis séricos elevados de fosfatase alcalina; herança autossômica recessiva.
hy·per·phos·pha·te·mia (hī′per-fos-fā-tē′mē-ā). Hiperfosfatemia; concentração anormalmente elevada de fosfatos no sangue circulante.
hy·per·phos·pha·tu·ria (hī′per-fos-fā-too′rē-ā). Hiperfosfatúria; excreção aumentada de fosfatos na urina.
hy·per·phre·nia (hī-per-frē′nē-ā). Hiperfrenia; termo raramente utilizado para referir-se a um grau excessivo de atividade intelectual; uma forma de mania. [hyper- + G. *phrēn* mente]
hy·per·pi·e·sis, hy·per·pi·e·sia (hī′per-pī-ē′sis, -pī-ē′zē-ā). Hiperpiese. SIN hypertension. [hyper- + G. *piesis,* pressão]
hy·per·pi·et·ic (hī-per-pī-et′ik). Hiperpiético; relativo a, ou caracterizado por, pressão arterial elevada.
hy·per·pig·men·ta·tion (hī′per-pig-men-tā′shŭn). Hiperpigmentação; excesso de pigmento num tecido ou parte.
hy·per·pip·e·co·la·te·mia (hī-per-pip′e-kō-lā-tē′mē-ā). Hiperpipecolatemia; distúrbio metabólico em que as concentrações séricas de ácido pipecólico estão acentuadamente elevadas; caracterizada por hepatomegalia e desmielinização generalizada e progressiva do sistema nervoso. SIN hyperpipecolic acidemia.
hy·per·pip·e·co·lic ac·i·de·mia (hī′per-pī′pē-ko-lik). Hiperacidemia pipecólica. SIN hyperpipecolatemia.
hy·per·pi·tu·i·ta·rism (hī′per-pi-too′i-tā-rizm). Hiperpituitarismo; produção excessiva de hormônios da hipófise anterior, especialmente hormônio do crescimento; pode resultar em gigantismo ou acromegalia.
hy·per·pla·sia (hī-per-plā′zhē-ā). Hiperplasia; aumento no número de células normais de um tecido ou órgão, excluindo a formação tumoral, em que a maior parte do órgão pode estar aumentada. VER TAMBÉM hypertrophy. SIN numerical hypertrophy, quantitative hypertrophy. [hyper- + G. *phasis,* moldagem]
adenomatous h., h. adenomatosa. SIN complex endometrial h.
angiofollicular mediastinal lymph node h., h. dos linfonodos mediastinais angiofolicular. SIN benign giant lymph node h.
angiolymphoid h. with eosinophilia, h. angiolinfóide com eosinofilia; pequenos nódulos eritematosos cutâneos benignos, solitários ou múltiplos, que ocorrem principalmente na cabeça e pescoço de adultos jovens, caracterizados pela proliferação dérmica de vasos sanguíneos com células endoteliais histiocitóides vacuoladas e com infiltrado variado de eosinófilos, linfócitos que podem formar folículos e histiócitos. SIN Kimura disease.
atypical endometrial h., h. endometrial atípica; aumento no número de giândulas que apresentam pouco ou nenhum estroma para separá-las, mas que conservam uma arquitetura organizada, diferenciando-as do adenocarcinoma.
atypical melanocytic h., h. melanocítica atípica; proliferação de melanócitos mostrando atipicidade nuclear, especialmente como células isoladas espalhadas na parte superior da epiderme; interpretada por alguns patologistas como melanoma maligno *in situ.*
basal cell h., h. de células basais; aumento no número de células num epitélio, assemelhando-se a células basais.
benign giant lymph node h., h. de linfonodos gigantes benigna; massas solitárias de tecido linfóide contendo agregados perivasculares concêntricos de linfócitos, ocorrendo, em geral, no mediastino ou na região hilar de adultos jovens; já foram relatadas alterações semelhantes fora do mediastino, e, quando associadas a camadas interfoliculares de plasmócitos, podem progredir para o linfoma ou plasmocitoma. SIN angiofollicular mediastinal lymph node h., Castleman disease.
benign prostatic h., h. prostática benigna; aumento progressivo da próstata devido à hiperplasia dos componentes tanto glandulares quanto do estroma; tipicamente, começa na quinta década de vida e, algumas vezes, produz sintomas obstrutivos e/ou irritativos; não evolui para câncer.
cementum h., h. do cimento. SIN hypercementosis.
complex endometrial h., h. endometrial complexa; agregação estreita das glândulas endometriais, com uma única camada de células exibindo núcleos

ligeiramente aumentados que, em geral, estão localizados na base. SIN adenomatous h.

congenital adrenal h., h. congênita da supra-renal; grupo de distúrbios herdados como caráter autossômico recessivo, associados a uma deficiência de uma das enzimas envolvidas na biossíntese do cortisol, resultando em elevação dos níveis de ACTH e superprodução e acúmulo de precursores do cortisol proximalmente ao bloqueio; ocorre produção de androgênios em excesso, causando virilização. O distúrbio mais comum é a deficiência de 21-hidroxilase, causada por mutação do gene da 21-hidroxilase do citocromo P450 (CYP21) no cromossoma 6p. Existem quatro tipos principais com algumas semelhanças clínicas, porém com diferenças genéticas e bioquímicas notáveis: 1) forma perdedora de sal [MIM*201710, MIM*201810 e MIM*201910], 2) a forma hipertensiva [MIM*202010 e MIM*202110], 3) a forma virilizante simples [MIM*201910] e 4) a forma pseudo-hermafrodita [MIM*201810 e MIM*202110].

congenital virilizing adrenal h., h. supra-renal virilizante congênita; um grupo de erros inatos do metabolismo com hiperplasia do córtex supra-renal e superprodução de hormônios virilizantes. As formas mais comuns são causadas pela deficiência parcial ou completa da 21-hidroxilase, resultando em aumento da produção de ACTH pela hipófise, estimulando o crescimento e a função das glândulas supra-renais. A forma grave caracteriza-se por um estado perdedor de sal.

cystic h., h. cística; formação de múltiplos cistos de retenção devido à obstrução dos ductos ou glândulas por hiperplasia do epitélio de revestimento, como na doença fibrocística da mama e na metropatia hemorrágica.

cystic h. of the breast, h. cística da mama. SIN fibrocystic condition of the breast.

denture h., h. fibrosa inflamatória. SIN inflammatory fibrous h.

ductal h., h. ductal; hiperplasia caracterizada pela proliferação intraductal das células epiteliais, como, p. ex., na mama.

endometrial h., h. endometrial; aumento no número de glândulas endometriais, geralmente secundário a hiperestrinismo; classificada em h. simples, h. complexa ou h. complexa com atipia; esta última pode evoluir para o adenocarcinoma.

fibromuscular h., h. fibromuscular; espessamento da média arterial por fibrose e hiperplasia muscular, afetando habitualmente as artérias renais e produzindo estenose multifocal e hipertensão; uma variedade de displasia fibromuscular.

focal epithelial h., h. epitelial focal; múltiplas lesões nodulares moles dos lábios, da mucosa bucal, da língua e de outros locais orais em crianças e adolescentes; as lesões sofrem regressão espontânea depois de um período de vários meses e foram atribuídas a papovavírus. SIN Heck disease.

gingival h., h. gengival; aumento da gengiva devido à proliferação de tecido conjuntivo fibroso. SIN gingival proliferation.

inflammatory fibrous h., h. fibrose inflamatória; proliferação de tecido na prega mucobucal ou labial, induzida por traumatismo crônico de dentaduras mal adaptadas. SIN denture h., epulis fissuratum.

inflammatory papillary h., h. papilar inflamatório; pápulas estreitamente distribuídas da mucosa palatina subjacentes a uma dentadura mal ajustada. SIN palatal papillomatosis.

intravascular papillary endothelial h., h. endotelial papilar intravascular; proliferação endotelial papilar florida benigna no interior das veias da pele ou subcútis, menos freqüentemente em vasos sanguíneos viscerais.

neuronal h., h. neuronal; aumento no número de células ganglionares com hiperplasia do plexo mientérico e atividade aumentada da acetilcolinesterase nos nervos da mucosa e submucosa. Clinicamente, a h. neuronal imita a doença de Hirschsprung. São observados achados semelhantes em pacientes com síndrome de neoplasia endócrina múltipla, tipo IIB, e na neurofibromatose. SIN hyperganglionosis, neuronal intestinal dysplasia.

nodular h. of prostate, h. nodular da próstata; hiperplasia glandular e do estroma que ocorre com muita freqüência na zona de transição e no estroma fibromuscular anterior de homens idosos, formando nódulos que podem obstruir cada vez mais a uretra.

nodular regenerative h., h. regenerativa nodular. SIN nodular transformation of the liver.

pseudoepitheliomatous h., pseudocarcinomatous h., h. pseudo-epiteliomatosa, h. pseudocarcinomatosa; aumento pronunciado e benigno e crescimento das células epidérmicas para baixo; observada nas dermatoses inflamatórias crônicas e em algumas neoplasias dérmicas e nevos; ao exame microscópico, assemelha-se ao carcinoma de células escamosas bem diferenciado.

senile sebaceous h., h. sebácea senil; hiperplasia de glândulas sebáceas maduras, formando um nódulo na pele da face ou da testa em indivíduos idosos.

simple endometrial h., h. endometrial simples; aumento na quantidade de tecido endometrial, com glândulas separadas por estroma abundante. SIN Swiss cheese endometrium.

squamous cell h., h. de células escamosas; aumento no número de células num epitélio escamoso. SIN hypertrophic dystrophy.

verrucous h., h. verrucosa; hiperplasia da mucosa oral que ocorre no indivíduo idoso; caracterizada por projeções papilares ascendentes afiladas ou rombas do epitélio escamoso.

hy·per·plas·tic (hī-per-plas'tik). Hiperplásico; relativo à hiperplasia.

hy·per·pnea (hī-per-nē'a, hī-perp'nē-a). Hiperpnéia; respiração mais profunda e mais rápida do que o normal em repouso. [hyper- + G. pnoē, respiração]

hy·per·po·lar·i·za·tion (hī'per-pō'lăr-i-zā'shŭn). Hiperpolarização; aumento na polarização de membranas de células nervosas ou musculares; alteração inversa daquela associada à ação excitatória.

hy·per·po·tas·se·mia (hī'per-pō-tas-ē'mē-a). Hiperpotassemia. SIN hyperkalemia.

hy·per·pre·be·ta·lip·o·pro·tein·e·mia (hī'per-prē-bā'ta-lip-ō-prō'tē-in-ē'mē-a,-prō'tēn-). Hiperpré-β-lipoproteinemia; concentrações aumentadas de pré-β-lipoproteínas no sangue.

familial h., h. familiar. SIN type IV familial hyperlipoproteinemia.

hy·per·pro·chor·e·sis (hī'per-prō-kōr-ē'sis). Hiperprocorese; termo raramente utilizado para referir-se ao hiperperistaltismo. [hyper- + G. pro-choreō, ir para diante]

hy·per·pro·in·su·lin·e·mia (hī'per-prō-in'sŭl-i-nē'mē-a). Hiperpróinsulinemia; níveis plasmáticos elevados de pró-insulina ou de material pró-insulina-símile.

hy·per·pro·lac·ti·ne·mia (hī'per-prō-lak-ti-nē'mē-a). Hiperprolactinemia; níveis elevados de prolactina no sangue, constituindo uma reação fisiológica normal durante a lactação, porém patológica nas demais situações; a prolactina também pode estar elevada nos casos de certos tumores hipofisários, freqüentemente ocorrendo amenorréia.

hy·per·pro·li·ne·mia (hī'per-prō-li-nē'mē-a). [MIM*239500 & MIM*239510]. Hiperprolinemia; distúrbio metabólico caracterizado por aumento das concentrações plasmáticas de prolina e da excreção urinária de prolina, hidroxiprolina e glicina; herança autossômica recessiva. A h. do tipo I está associada a deficiência de prolina oxidase e doença renal. A h. do tipo II está associada a deficiência de Δ-pirrolina-5-carboxilato desidrogenase, retardo mental e convulsões, sendo causada pela mutação do gene do δ-pirrolina-5-carboxilato (P5CD) no cromossoma 1p.

hy·per·pro·tein·e·mia (hī'per-prō'tē'in-ē'mē-a, -prō'tēn-). Hiperproteinemia; concentração anormalmente elevada de proteína no plasma.

hy·per·pro·te·o·sis (hī'per-prō-tē-ō'sis). Hiperproteose; condição causada por excesso de proteínas na dieta.

hy·per·py·ret·ic (hī'per-pī-ret'ik). Hiperpirético; relativo à hiperpirexia. SIN hyperpyrexial.

hy·per·py·rex·ia (hī'per-pī-rek'sē-a). Hiperpirexia; febre extremamente alta. [hyper- + G. pyrexis, estado febril]

fulminant h., h. fulminante. SIN malignant hyperthermia.

heat h., h. por calor. SIN heatstroke.

malignant h., h. maligna. SIN heatstroke.

hy·per·py·rex·i·al (hī'per-pī-rek'sē-ăl). Hiperpirético. SIN hyperpyretic.

hy·per·re·flex·ia (hī'per-rē-flek'sē-a). Hiper-reflexia; condição em que os reflexos tendinosos profundos estão exagerados.

detrusor h., h. do detrusor. SIN detrusor instability.

hy·per·res·o·nance (hī-per-rez'ō-nans). Hiper-ressonância. **1.** Grau extremo de ressonância. **2.** Ressonância aumentada acima do normal e, com freqüência, de baixo grau à percussão de uma área do corpo; ocorre no tórax devido à hiperinsuflação do pulmão, como no enfisema ou pneumotórax, bem como no abdome sobre o intestino distendido.

hy·per·sal·e·mia (hī'per-sal-ē'mē-a). Hipersaliemia; termo obsoleto para referir-se ao aumento no teor de sal do sangue circulante.

hy·per·sa·line (hī-per-sā'lēn,-sā'līn). Hipersalino; caracterizado por concentrações aumentadas de sal numa solução salina.

hy·per·sal·i·va·tion (hī'per-sal-i-vā'shŭn). Hipersalivação; aumento da salivação.

hy·per·sar·co·si·ne·mia (hī'per-sar-kō-si-nē'mē-a). Hipersarcosinemia. SIN sarcosinemia.

hy·per·se·cre·tion. Hipersecreção; secreção excessiva de qualquer tecido ou glândula.

gastric h., h. gástrica; formação excessiva de suco gástrico, especialmente o componente ácido.

hy·per·seg·men·ta·tion. Hipersegmentação; divisão excessiva de um tecido ou parte em segmentos.

hereditary hypersegmentation of neutrophils, hipersegmentação hereditária dos neutrófilos; distúrbio autossômico dominante caracterizado pela hipersegmentação dos neutrófilos; os indivíduos afetados são assintomáticos.

hy·per·sen·si·tiv·i·ty (hī'per-sen-si-tiv'i-tē). Hipersensibilidade; sensibilidade anormal, uma condição em que ocorre uma resposta exagerada do corpo ao estímulo de um agente estranho. VER allergy.

contact h., h. de contato; (1) SIN contact dermatitis; (2) SIN delayed reaction.

delayed h., h. tardia; (1) SIN cell-mediated immunity; (2) SIN delayed reaction; (3) resposta mediada por células que ocorre em indivíduos imunes, com pico

24–48 horas após estímulo com o mesmo antígeno utilizado no estímulo inicial. A resposta é iniciada pela interação de linfócitos T auxiliares I com células apresentadoras de antígeno positivas para MHC da classe II. Essa interação induz as células T auxiliares 1 e os macrófagos no local a secretarem citocinas, que desempenham o principal papel na reação. Denominada h. de tipo tuberculínico.

immediate h., h. imediata; resposta imune exagerada mediada por anticorpos produzidos dentro de poucos minutos após exposição de um indivíduo sensibilizado ao antígeno; também denominada h. Tipo I. As manifestações clínicas consistem em alergia tópica e anafilaxia sistêmica. O antígeno induz anticorpos IgE, que se ligam à maioria das células e basófilos. A exposição subseqüente ao antígeno determina a ligação à IgE citofílica, resultando na liberação de mediadores. VER allergy.

tuberculin-type h., h. do tipo tuberculínico. SIN delayed reaction.

hy·per·sen·si·ti·za·tion (hī′per-sen′si-ti-zā′shŭn). Hipersensibilização; processo imunológico pelo qual a hipersensibilidade é induzida.

hy·per·se·ro·to·ne·mia (hī′per-sēr′ō-tō-nē′mē-ă). Hiperserotonemia; níveis inusitadamente elevados de serotonina no sangue circulante; provável causa de alguns dos sinais e sintomas da síndrome carcinoide.

hy·per·ske·o·cy·to·sis (hī′per-skē′ō-si-tō′sis). Hiperesqueocitose. SIN hyperneocytosis. [G. *skaios*, esquerda + *kytos*, célula + *-osis*, condição]

hy·per·so·ma·to·tro·pism (hī′per-sō′mă-tō-trō′pizm). Hipersomatotropismo; estado caracterizado pela secreção anormalmente aumentada de hormônio do crescimento (somatotropina) pela hipófise.

hy·per·som·nia (hī-per-som′nē-ă). Hipersonia; condição em que os períodos de sono são excessivamente longos, porém o indivíduo responde normalmente nos intervalos; distingue-se da sonolência. [hyper- + L. *somnus*, sono]

hy·per·son·ic (hī-per-son′ik). Hipersônico; relativo a, ou caracterizado por, velocidades supersônicas ≥ 5 Mach. Embora qualquer velocidade acima da velocidade do som possa ser considerada como supersônica, as velocidades ≥ 5 Mach são especificamente designadas como hipersônicas. [hyper- + L. *sonus*, som]

hy·per·sphyx·ia (hī-per-sfik′sē-ă). Condição de pressão arterial elevada e aumento da atividade circulatória. [hyper- + G. *sphyxis*, pulso]

hy·per·splen·ism (hī-per-splēn′izm). Hiperesplenismo; grupo de condições em que os componentes celulares do sangue ou plaquetas são removidos de forma anormalmente rápida pelo baço, resultando em baixos níveis circulantes.

hy·per·ste·a·to·sis (hī′per-stē-ă-tō′sis). Hiperesteatose; secreção sebácea excessiva.

hy·per·sthe·nia (hī-per-sthē′nē-ă). Hiperestenia; tensão ou força excessiva. [hyper- + G. *sthenos*, força]

hy·per·sthen·ic (hī-per-sthen′ik). Hiperestênico; relativo a, ou caracterizado por, hiperestenia.

hy·per·sthen·u·ria (hī′per-sthen-ū′rē-ă). Hiperestenúria; excreção de urina de densidade e concentração de solutos inusitadamente altas, devido, em geral, à perda ou privação de água. [hyper- + G. *sthenos*, força + *ouron*, urina]

hy·per·sus·cep·ti·bil·i·ty (hī′per-sŭ-sep-ti-bil′i-tē). Hipersuscetibilidade; aumento da suscetibilidade ou da resposta a um agente infeccioso, químico ou outro tipo de agente.

hy·per·sys·to·le (hī-per-sis′tō-lē). Hipersístole; força ou duração anormal da sístole cardíaca.

hy·per·sys·tol·ic (hī′per-sis-tol′ik). Hipersistólico; relativo a, ou caracterizado por, hipersístole.

hy·per·tel·or·ism (hī-per-tel′or-izm). Hipertelorismo; distância anormal entre dois órgãos pares. [hyper- + G. *tēle*, longe + *horizō* + separar, fr. *horos*, limite]

Bixler type h., h. tipo Bixler; as características associadas incluem microtia e fenda do lábio, palato e nariz, deficiência mental, atresia dos canais auditivos, rins ectópicos e hipoplasia tenar; herança autossômica recessiva.

canthal h., h. cantal. SIN telecanthus.

ocular h. [MIM*145400], h. ocular; aumento da distância entre os olhos devido à parada de desenvolvimento das asas maiores do osso esfenóide, fixando as órbitas na posição fetal amplamente separada; herança autossômica dominante. O hipertelorismo ocular é uma característica de muitas síndromes. Uma forma distinta [MIM*145410] apresenta outros defeitos congênitos, com hipospadias e anomalias esofágicas. VER TAMBÉM faciodigitogenital *dysplasia*. SIN Greig syndrome, Opitz BBB syndrome, Opitz G syndrome.

hy·per·ten·sin (hī-per-ten′-sin). Hipertensina; nome antigo da angiotensina.

hy·per·ten·sin·o·gen (hī′per-ten-sin′ō-jen). Hipertensinogênio; nome antigo para referir-se ao angiotensinogênio.

---

hy·per·ten·sion (hī′per-ten′shŭn). Hipertensão; pressão arterial elevada; elevação transitória ou persistente da pressão arterial sistêmica para um nível passível de induzir lesão cardiovascular ou outras conseqüências adversas. A hipertensão foi arbitrariamente definida por uma pressão arterial (PA) sistólica acima de 140 mm Hg e PA diastólica superior a 90 mm Hg. As conseqüências da hipertensão descontrolada incluem: lesão vascular retiniana (alterações de Keith-Wagener-Barker), doença e acidente vasculares cerebrais, hipertrofia e insuficiência ventricular esquerda, infarto do miocárdio, aneurisma dissecante e doença vascular renal. Pode-se identificar um distúrbio subjacente (p. ex., doença renal, síndrome de Cushing, feocromocitoma) em menos de 10% de todos os casos de hipertensão. Os demais casos, tradicionalmente designados como hipertensão "essencial", derivam provavelmente de uma variedade de distúrbios nos mecanismos de regulação da pressão normal (que envolvem barorreceptores, influências autônomas sobre a freqüência e força de contração cardíaca e tônus vascular, retenção renal de sal e de água, formação de angiotensina II sob a influência da renina e da enzima conversora de angiotensina e outros fatores, tanto conhecidos quanto desconhecidos), sendo a maioria provavelmente determinada geneticamente. SIN hyperpiesis, hyperpiesia. [hyper- + L. *tensio*, tensão]

Devido à sua ampla prevalência e a seu impacto sobre a saúde cardiovascular, a hipertensão constitui uma importante causa de doença e morte nas sociedades industrializadas. Estima-se que 50–70 milhões de norte-americanos, incluindo cerca de 50% de todos os indivíduos com mais de 60 anos de idade, tenham hipertensão, porém apenas cerca de um terço tem conhecimento de sua condição e recebe tratamento apropriado. Nos Estados Unidos, a hipertensão é responsável por 35.000 mortes anualmente, sendo um fator contribuinte em mais 180.000 mortes. A hipertensão está associada a um aumento de três vezes no risco de infarto do miocárdio e aumento de 7 a 10 vezes no risco de acidente vascular cerebral. A prevalência da hipertensão e a incidência de conseqüências não-fatais e fatais são significativamente maiores em afro-americanos. Embora os indivíduos com pressão diastólica extremamente elevada possam apresentar cefaléia, tonteira e até mesmo encefalopatia, a hipertensão não-complicada raramente produz sintomas. Por conseguinte, o diagnóstico de hipertensão é habitualmente estabelecido em decorrência da triagem de indivíduos aparentemente sadios ou que estão sob tratamento para outra condição. Os fatores de risco da hipertensão incluem história familiar de hipertensão, ser afro-americano, idade avançada, estado pós-menopáusico, ingestão excessiva de sódio na dieta, obesidade, consumo excessivo de álcool, estilo de vida sedentário e estresse emocional crônico. As opções de tratamento incluem mudança do estilo de vida (manutenção de um peso saudável; pelo menos 30 minutos de exercício aeróbico várias vezes por semana; limitação da ingestão de sódio a 2,4 g por dia e do consumo diário de etanol a 31 g; consumo de quantidades adequadas de potássio, cálcio e magnésio; e evitar qualquer estresse emocional excessivo) e uma ampla variedade de drogas, incluindo diuréticos, beta-bloqueadores, bloqueadores dos canais de cálcio, inibidores da enzima conversora de angiotensina, antagonistas do receptor de angiotensina II, antagonistas α₁-adrenérgicos, agonistas alfa de ação central e outros agentes. Nestas últimas décadas, a detecção precoce e o tratamento agressivo da hipertensão reduziram as taxas de morbidade e mortalidade associadas. Os atuais padrões de prática exigem uma conduta ainda mais diligente, incluindo profilaxia ao evitar os fatores de risco conhecidos, bem como controle dos co-fatores que, reconhecidamente, aumentam o risco de lesão cardiovascular em indivíduos com hipertensão (tabagismo, hipercolesterolemia, diabetes melito). Alguns estudos sugerem que a meta do tratamento deve consistir numa pressão diastólica de 80 ou menos.

---

accelerated h., h. acelerada; hipertensão que progride rapidamente com elevação progressiva dos níveis tensionais, associada a sinais e sintomas agudos que se agravam rapidamente.

adrenal h., h. supra-renal; hipertensão produzida por feocromocitoma da medula supra-renal ou devido à hiperatividade ou tumor funcionante do córtex supra-renal.

benign h., h. benigna; hipertensão que segue uma evolução relativamente longa e assintomática.

borderline h., h. limítrofe, por consenso, zona de pressão arterial entre a pressão arterial "normal" mais elevada aceitável e valores hipertensivos. O *Framingham Heart Study* define essa zona como a de pressões situadas entre 140 e 160 mm Hg para a pressão sistólica e 90 e 95 mm Hg para a diastólica.

episodic h., h. episódica; hipertensão que se manifesta de modo intermitente, desencadeada por ansiedade ou por fatores emocionais. SIN paroxysmal h.

essential h., h. essencial; hipertensão sem causa conhecida. SIN idiopathic h., primary h.

gestational h., h. gestacional; hipertensão que ocorre durante a gravidez numa mulher previamente normotensa, ou agravamento da hipertensão durante a gravidez numa mulher hipertensa. SIN pregnancy-induced h.

Goldblatt h., h. de Goldblatt; aumento da pressão arterial após obstrução do fluxo sanguíneo de um rim.

idiopathic h., h. idiopática. SIN essential h.

labile h., h. lábil; alteração freqüente dos níveis de pressão arterial elevada.

malignant h., h. maligna; hipertensão grave que segue uma evolução rápida, causando necrose das paredes arteriolares no rim, na retina, etc.; ocorrem he-

morragias, e a morte é mais freqüentemente causada por uremia ou ruptura de um vaso cerebral.
pale h., h. pálida; hipertensão com palidez da pele, uma forma grave com constrição pronunciada dos vasos periféricos.
paroxysmal h., h. paroxística. SIN episodic h.
portal h., h. porta; hipertensão no sistema porta, como a que se observa na cirrose hepática e em outras condições que causam obstrução da veia porta.
postpartum h., h. pós-parto; elevação da pressão arterial imediatamente após o trabalho de parto.
pregnancy-induced h., h. induzida por gravidez. SIN gestational h.
primary h., h. primária. SIN essential h.
pulmonary h., h. pulmonar; hipertensão no circuito pulmonar; pode ser primária ou secundária a doença pulmonar ou cardíaca, como, p. ex., fibrose do pulmão ou estenose mitral.
renal h., h. renal; hipertensão secundária a doença renal.
renovascular h., h. renovascular; hipertensão produzida por obstrução da artéria renal.
secondary h., h. secundária; hipertensão arterial produzida por uma causa conhecida, como, p. ex., hipertireoidismo, doença renal, etc., em contraste com a hipertensão primária, que é de causa desconhecida.
systemic venous h., h. venosa sistêmica; aumento da pressão nas veias, levando, em última análise, ao átrio direito, quase sempre devido a doença do coração direito ou do pericárdio; todavia, ocasionalmente devido ao bloqueio de uma ou de ambas as veias cavas.
hy·per·ten·sive (hī - per - ten′siv). Hipertensivo. **1.** Caracterizado por pressão arterial elevada. **2.** Refere-se a um indivíduo que sofre de pressão arterial elevada.
hy·per·ten·sor (hī - per - ten′ser, - sōr). Hipertensor. SIN pressor.
hy·per·tes·toid·ism (hī - per - tes′toyd - izm). Hipertestoidismo; hipergonadismo no sexo masculino, caracterizado pela proliferação das células de Leydig, com produção excessiva de testosterona.
hy·per·the·co·sis (hī′per - thē - kō′sis). Hipertecose; hiperplasia difusa das células da teca dos folículos de Graaf.
stromal h., h. do estroma; condição em que as células luteinizadas estão presentes no estroma ovariano, a certa distância das estruturas foliculares.
hy·per·the·lia (hī - per - thē′lē - ă). Hipertelia. SIN polythelia. [hyper- + G. thēlē, mamilo]
hy·per·ther·mal·ge·sia (hī′per - ther - măl - jē′zē - ă). Hipertermalgesia; sensibilidade extrema ao calor. [hyper- + G. thermē, calor + algēsis, dor]
hy·per·ther·mia (hī - per - ther′mē - ă). Hipertermia; hiperpirexia induzida terapeuticamente. [hyper- + G. thermē, calor]
malignant h., h. maligna; início rápido de febre extremamente elevada, com rigidez muscular, precipitada em indivíduos geneticamente suscetíveis por agentes exógenos, especialmente por halotano ou succinilcolina. Cf. futile cycle. SIN fulminant hyperpyrexia.
hy·per·ther·moes·the·sia (hī - per - ther′mō - es - thē′zē - ă). Hipertermoestesia; sensibilidade extrema ao calor. [hyper- + G. thermē, calor + aisthēsis, sensação]
hy·per·throm·bi·ne·mia (hī′per - throm - bi - nē′mē - ă). Hipertrombinemia; aumento anormal da trombina no sangue, freqüentemente resultando em tendência à coagulação intravascular.
hy·per·thy·mia (hī - per - thī′mē - ă). Hipertimia; estado de hiperatividade, maior do que a média e menor do que a hiperatividade do estado maníaco do distúrbio maníaco depressivo. [hyper- + G. thymos, alma, pensamento]
hy·per·thy·mic (hī - per - thī′mik). Hipertímico. **1.** Relativo à hipertimia. **2.** Relativo ao hipertimismo.
hy·per·thy·mism (hī - per - thī′mizm). Hipertimismo; atividade excessiva da glândula timo; antigamente considerado como fator causal em certos casos de morte inesperada e súbita, como o estado tímico linfático. SIN hyperthymization.
hy·per·thy·mi·za·tion (hī′per - thī - mi - zā′shŭn). Hipertimização. SIN hyperthymism.
hy·per·thy·rea (hī′per - thī - rē - ă). Hipertireose. SIN hyperthyroidism.
hy·per·thy·roid·ism (hī - per - thī′royd - izm). Hipertireoidismo; anormalidade da glândula tireóide cuja secreção de hormônio tireóideo está habitualmente aumentada e não se encontra mais sob o controle regulador dos centros hipotalâmico-hipofisários; caracteriza-se por um estado hipermetabólico, geralmente com perda de peso, tremores, níveis plasmáticos elevados de tiroxina e/ou triiodotironina e, algumas vezes, exoftalmia; pode progredir para fraqueza intensa, consunção, hiperpirexia e outras manifestações da tempestade tireóidea; freqüentemente associado a exoftalmia. VER TAMBÉM thyrotoxicosis. SIN hyperthyrea, thyroidism (1), thyrointoxication.
hereditary h., h. hereditário; distúrbio hereditário (autossômico dominante) raro com estimulação constitutiva dos tireócitos.
iodine-induced h., h. induzido por iodo. SIN Jod-Basedow phenomenon.
masked h., h. mascarado, hipertireoidismo que ocorre das manifestações habituais, particularmente ausência de hiperatividade e dos achados oculares, freqüentemente com hipoatividade e, até mesmo, sonolência. A manifestação pode limitar-se à insuficiência cardíaca.

ophthalmic h., h. oftálmico. SIN Graves disease.
primary h., h. primário; hipertireoidismo devido a um distúrbio da glândula tireóide, em contraste com aquele de origem hipofisária; pode ser devido a uma hiperatividade generalizada da glândula, a um nódulo hiperativo localizado ou a anticorpos circulantes, que estimulam a glândula (estimulador tireóideo de ação prolongada [long-acting thyroid stimulator]).
secondary h., h. secundário; hipertireoidismo devido ao estímulo da glândula tireóide por um excesso de tireotropina secretada pela hipófise.
hy·per·thy·rox·i·ne·mia (hī′per - thī - rok - si - nē′mē - ă). Hipertiroxinemia; concentração elevada de tiroxina no sangue.
hy·per·to·nia (hī - per - tō′nē - ă). Hipertonia; tensão extrema dos músculos ou das artérias. SIN hypertonicity (1). [hyper- + G. tonos, tensão]
h. polycythe′mica, h. policitêmica; forma de policitemia sem esplenomegalia proeminente, mas com pressão arterial elevada.
simpathetic h., h. simpática; hiperfunção do sistema nervoso simpático, freqüentemente manifestada como ansiedade.
hy·per·ton·ic (hī - per - ton′ik). Hipertônico. **1.** Que apresenta maior grau de tensão. SIN spastic (1). **2.** Que possui pressão osmótica maior do que uma solução de referência, que é habitualmente considerada como sendo o plasma sanguíneo ou líquido intersticial; mais especificamente, refere-se a um líquido no qual as células se retraem. SIN hyperisotonic.
hy·per·to·nic·i·ty (hī′per - tō - nis′i - tē). Hipertonicidade. **1.** Hipertonia. SIN hypertonia. **2.** Aumento da pressão osmótica efetiva dos líquidos corporais.
hy·per·tri·chi·a·sis (hī′per - tri - kī′ă - sis). Hipertriquíase. SIN hypertrichosis.
hy·per·trich·o·phry·dia (hī′per - trik - ō - fri′dē - ă). Hipertricofridia; sobrancelhas excessivamente espessas. [hyper- + G. thrix, pêlo + ophrys, sobrancelha]
hy·per·tri·cho·sis (hī′per - tri - kō′sis). Hipertricose; crescimento de pêlos acima do normal. VER TAMBÉM hirsutism. SIN hypertrichiasis. [hyper- + G. trichōsis, cabeludo]
h. lanugino′sa, h. lanuginosa; crescimento excessivo de lanugem associado a neoplasia maligna interna.
nevoid h., h. nevóide; crescimento congênito de pêlos anormais quanto à sua localização, textura, cor ou comprimento; freqüentemente associado a outros nevos melanocíticos congênitos.
h. partia′lis, h. parcial; crescimento piloso anormalmente excessivo, em placas, em áreas incomuns.
h. universa′lis, h. universal; crescimento piloso excessivo generalizado.
hy·per·tri·glyc·er·i·de·mia (hī′per - tri - glis′er - i - dē′mē - ă). Hipertrigliceridemia; concentração elevada de triglicerídeos no sangue.
familial h., h. familiar; **(1)** SIN type I familial hyperlipoproteinemia; **(2)** SIN type IV familial hyperlipoproteinemia.
hy·per·troph (hī′per - trof). Hipertrofo; microrganismo que necessita de células vivas para suprir os sistemas enzimáticos necessários para seu crescimento e sua reprodução.
hy·per·tro·phia (hī - per - trō′fē - ă). Hipertrofia. SIN hypertrophy.
hy·per·tro·phic (hī - per - trof′ik). Hipertrófico; relativo a, ou caracterizado por, hipertrofia.
hy·per·tro·phy (hī - per′trō - fē). Hipertrofia; aumento generalizado no volume de uma parte ou de um órgão, não devido à formação de tumor. O uso do termo pode ser restrito para indicar um maior volume através de aumento no tamanho de células ou outros elementos teciduais individuais, mas não de seu número. SIN hypertrophia. [hyper- + G. trophē, nutrição]
adaptive h., h. adaptativa; espessamento das paredes de um órgão oco, como a bexiga, quando existe obstrução ao fluxo.
benign prostatic h., h. prostática benigna; termo incorreto, freqüentemente considerado como sinônimo de hiperplasia nodular da próstata (nodular hyperplasia of prostate).
compensatory h., h. compensatória; aumento no tamanho de um órgão, ou de parte de um órgão ou tecido, quando surge a necessidade de executar um trabalho adicional ou efetuar o trabalho de tecido destruído ou de um órgão par.
compensatory h. of the heart, h. compensatória do coração; espessamento das paredes do coração em resposta a doença vascular, valvar ou a outra cardiopatia ou condicionamento atlético.
complementary h., h. complementar; aumento no tamanho ou expansão de parte de um órgão ou tecido para preencher o espaço deixado pela destruição de outra porção do mesmo órgão ou tecido.
concentric h., h. concêntrica; espessamento das paredes do coração ou de qualquer cavidade com aparente diminuição da capacidade da cavidade.
eccentric h., h. excêntrica; espessamento da parede do coração ou de outra cavidade, com dilatação.
endemic h., h. endêmica; aumento do calcâneo, precedido de febre e dor no calcanhar, relatada na Costa do Ouro (atualmente Gana) e Tailândia, entre a população nativa.
false h., h. falsa. SIN pseudohypertrophy.
functional h., h. funcional. SIN physiologic h.
giant h. of gastric mucosa, h. gigante da mucosa gástrica. SIN Ménétrier disease.
hemangiectatic h., h. hemangiectásica. SIN Klippel-Trenaunay-Weber syndrome.

lipomatous h., h. lipomatosa. SIN lipomatous *infiltration.*
numerical h., h. numérica. SIN hyperplasia.
physiologic h., h. fisiológica; aumento temporário no tamanho de um órgão ou parte para proporcionar um aumento natural de função, como a do tipo que ocorre nas paredes do útero e da mama durante a gravidez. SIN functional h.
quantitative h., h. quantitativa. SIN hyperplasia.
simple h., h. simples; aumento no tamanho das células.
simulated h., h. simulada; aumento no tamanho de uma parte, devido ao crescimento contínuo irrestrito por atrito, conforme observado no caso dos dentes de certos animais, quando os dentes opostos foram destruídos.
true h., h. verdadeira; aumento de tamanho envolvendo todos os tecidos diferentes que compõem a parte considerada.
vicarious h., h. vicariante; hipertrofia de um órgão após falência de outro devido a uma relação funcional entre eles; p. ex., aumento de tamanho da hipófise após destruição da tireóide.
hy·per·tro·pia (hī′per-trō′pē-ā). Hipertropia; desvio ocular em que um olho é mais alto do que outro. [hyper- + G. *tropē,* uma volta]
hy·per·ty·ro·si·ne·mia (hī′per-tī′rō-si-nē′mē-ā). Hipertirosinemia. SIN tyrosinemia.
hy·per·ura·cil thy·mi·nu·ria (hī′per-oor′a-sil). Hiperuracil timinúria; distúrbio hereditário caracterizado por níveis elevados de uracila e timina na urina; associada a deficiência de diidropirimidina desidrogenase, com conseqüente comprometimento da função do SNC.
hy·per·u·ri·ce·mia (hī′per-ū-rē-sē′mē-ā). Hiperuricemia; concentração sanguínea aumentada de ácido úrico.
hy·per·u·ri·ce·mic (hī′per-ū-ri-sē′mik). Hiperuricêmico; relativo a, ou caracterizado por, hiperuricemia.
hy·per·u·ri·cu·ria (hī′per-ū-ri-kū′rē-ā). Hiperuricúria; aumento da excreção urinária de ácido úrico.
hy·per·vac·ci·na·tion (hī′per-vak-si-nā′shŭn). Hipervacinação; inoculação repetida num indivíduo já imunizado; utilizada como meio de preparar um anti-soro hiperpotente.
hy·per·val·i·ne·mia (hī′per-val-i-nē′mē-ā). Hipervalinemia; concentrações plasmáticas anormalmente elevadas de valina, um achado comum na doença da urina em xarope de bordo.
hy·per·vas·cu·lar (hī′per-vas′kū-ler). Hipervascular; anormalmente vascular; que contém um número excessivo de vasos sanguíneos. [hyper- + L. *vas,* vaso]
hy·per·ven·ti·la·tion (hī′per-ven-ti-lā′shŭn). Hiperventilação; aumento da ventilação alveolar em relação à produção metabólica de dióxido de carbono, de modo que a pressão de dióxido de carbono alveolar cai abaixo do normal. SIN overventilation.
hy·per·vi·ta·min·o·sis (hī′per-vī′tă-mi-nō′sis). Hipervitaminose; condição produzida pela ingestão excessiva de determinado preparado vitamínico, em que os sintomas variam de acordo com a vitamina particular; podem-se observar efeitos graves causados pela superdosagem de vitaminas lipossolúveis, especialmente A ou D, e, raramente, com vitaminas hidrossolúveis.
hy·per·vo·le·mia (hī′per-vō-lē′mē-ā). Hipervolemia; volume anormalmente aumentado de sangue. SIN plethora (1), repletion. [hyper- + L. *volumen,* volume + G. *haima,* sangue]
hy·per·vo·le·mic (hī′per-vō-lē′mik). Hipervolêmico; relativo a, ou caracterizado por, hipervolemia.
hy·per·vo·lia (hī-per-vō′lē-ā). Hipervolia; aumento no conteúdo de água ou no volume de determinado compartimento; p. ex., hipervolia celular.
hyp·es·the·sia (hī-pes-thē′zē-ā). Hipestesia; sensibilidade diminuída a estímulos. SIN hypoesthesia. [G. *hypo,* abaixo + *aisthēsis,* sensação]
olfactory h., h. olfatória. SIN hyposmia.
hy·pha, pl. **hy·phae** (hī′fă, hī′fē). Hifa; célula tubular ramificada característica dos fungos filamentosos (bolores). Na maioria das espécies, as hifas são divididas por paredes cruzadas (septos) em hifas multicelulares; as hifas intercomunicantes constituem um micélio, a colônia visível em substratos naturais ou meios artificiais de laboratório. Os termos hifa e micélio são freqüentemente utilizados como sinônimos. [G. *hyphē,* teia, tecido]
racquet h., h. em raquete; hifa vegetativa com extremidades distais de células sucessivas infladas, assemelhando-se a um cordão de raquetes de neve alongadas; observada em muitos fungos com micélios, como, p. ex., muitas espécies de dermatófitos em cultura.
spiral hyphae, hifas espiraladas; hifas que terminam numa espiral plana ou helicoidal, como nas colônias de *Trichophyton mentagrophytes* em laboratório.
hyp·he·do·nia (hĭp-hē-dō′nē-ā). Hipo-hedonismo; grau habitualmente diminuído ou atenuado de prazer por algo que normalmente produziria muito prazer. [G. *hypo,* sob + *hēdonē,* prazer]
hy·phe·ma (hī-fē′mă). Hifema; sangue na câmara anterior do olho. [G. *hyphaimos,* sufusão de sangue]
hy·phe·mia (hī-fē′mē-ā). Hifemia. SIN hypovolemia. [hypo- + G. *haima,* sangue]
intertropical h., tropical h., h. intertropical, h. tropical. SIN ancylostomiasis.
Hy·pho·my·ces des·tru·ens (hī-fō-mī′sēs des′troo-enz). Nome antigo de *Pythium insidiosum.*

Hy·pho·my·ce·tes (hī′fō-mī-sē′tēs). Classe de fungos que inclui todos os membros filamentosos dos Fungos Imperfeitos que não formam acérvulos nem picnídios. Não ocorre reprodução sexuada; a maioria dos membros desse grupo produz esporos assexuados. [G. *hyphe,* teia, tecido + *mykēs,* fungo]
hy·pho·my·co·sis (hī′fō-mī-kō′sis). Hifomicose; doença de cavalos e mulas (raramente de seres humanos) causada pelo fungo *Pythium insidiosum (Hyphomyces destruens),* caracterizada por lesões granulomatosas e necróticas que aparecem na cabeça e na parte inferior das pernas, ulceram e aumentam por extensão subcutânea.
hypn-. VER hipno-.
hyp·na·gog·ic (hip-nă-goj′ik). Hipnagógico; refere-se a um estado de transição, relacionado ao hipnóide, que precede o sono; aplica-se também a várias alucinações que podem manifestar-se nessa ocasião. VER hypnoidal. [hypno- + G. *agōgos,* que leva]
hypno-, hypn-. Hipno-, hipn-. Sono, hipnose. [G. *hypnos*]
hyp·no·a·nal·y·sis (hip′nō-ă-nal′i-sis). Hipnoanálise; psicanálise ou outra psicoterapia que emprega a hipnose como técnica auxiliar.
hyp·no·an·a·lyt·ic (hip′nō-an-ă-lit′ik). Hipnoanalítico; relativo à hipnoanálise.
hyp·no·ca·thar·sis (hip′nō-kă-thar′sis). Hipnocatarse; ventilação da tensão emocional suprimida ou reprimida, conflitos e ansiedade sob hipnose. [hypno- + G. *katharsis,* purificação]
hyp·no·cyst (hip′nō-sist). Hipnocisto; cisto quiescente ou "adormecido", protozoário encistado, cuja atividade reprodutora está suspensa. [hypno- + G. *kystis,* bexiga (cisto)]
hyp·no·gen·e·sis (hip-nō-jen′ĕ-sis). Hipnogênese; indução do sono ou do estado hipnótico. [hypno- + G. *genesis,* produção]
hyp·no·gen·ic, hyp·nog·e·nous (hip-nō-jen′ik, -noj′ĕ-nŭs). Hipnogênico. **1.** Relativo à hipnogênese. **2.** Agente capaz de induzir um estado hipnótico. VER hypnosis.
hypnoid. Hipnóide. SIN hypnoidal.
hyp·noi·dal (hip-noy′dal). Hipnoidal; semelhante à hipnose; refere-se ao estado de subvigília, uma condição mental intermediária entre o sono e a vigília. VER hypnagogic. SIN hypnoid. [hypno- + G. *eidos,* semelhança]
hyp·no·pho·bia (hip-nō-fō′bē-ā). Hipnofobia; medo mórbido de dormir. [hypno- + G. *phobos,* medo]
hyp·no·pom·pic (hip-nō-pom′pik). Hipnopômpico; indica a ocorrência de visões ou sonhos durante o estado de sonolência após o sono. [hypno- + G. *pompē,* procissão]
hyp·no·sis (hip-nō′sis). Hipnose; estado semelhante ao transe induzido artificialmente, semelhante ao sonambulismo, em que o indivíduo é altamente suscetível a sugestões, esquecido de tudo e facilmente responsivo a comandos do hipnotizador; sua validade científica foi aceita e rejeitada em vários momentos no decorrer dos últimos dois séculos. VER mesmerism. SIN hypnotic sleep, hypnotic state. [G. *hypnos,* sono + *-osis,* condição]

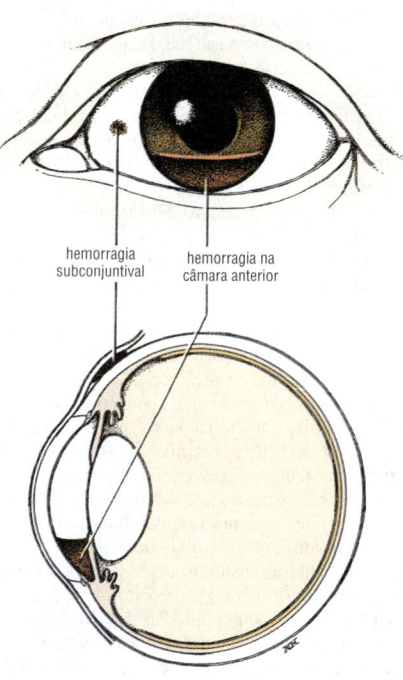

hifema (hemorragia na câmara anterior) e hemorragia subconjuntival

lethargic h., h. letárgica; sono profundo que se segue à hipnose maior. SIN trance coma.

major h., h. maior; estado de extrema sugestibilidade na hipnose, em que o indivíduo torna-se insensível a todas as impressões externas, exceto aos comandos do hipnotizador.

minor h., h. menor; estado induzido, semelhante ao sono normal, em que o indivíduo é suscetível a sugestões, embora não até o ponto de catalepsia ou sonambulismo.

hyp·no·ther·a·py (hip - no - thãr′ã - pē). Hipnoterapia. **1.** Tratamento psicoterapêutico por meio do hipnotismo. **2.** Tratamento de doença pela indução de um sono semelhante ao transe.

hyp·not·ic (hip - not′ik). Hipnótico. **1.** Que causa sono. **2.** Agente que promove o sono. SIN soporific (2). **3.** Relativo ao hipnotismo. [G. *hypnōtikos,* que produz sono]

hyp·no·tism (hip′no - tizm). Hipnotismo. **1.** Processo ou ato de induzir hipnose. SIN somnolism. **2.** A prática ou o estudo da hipnose. VER mesmerism. [G. *hypnos,* sono]

hyp·no·tist (hip′nō - tist). Hipnotizador; aquele que pratica o hipnotismo.

hyp·no·tize (hip′nō - tīz). Hipnotizar; induzir alguém à hipnose.

hyp·no·zo·ite (hip - no - zō′īt). Hipnozoíta; esquizozoíta exoeritrocitário de *Plasmodium vivax* ou *P. ovale* no fígado humano, caracterizado por desenvolvimento primário tardio; considerado responsável pela recidiva da malária.

hypo-. Hipo-. **1.** Prefixo que indica deficiente, abaixo do normal. VER TAMBÉM hyp-. Cf. sub-. **2.** Em química, indica o mais baixo ou menos rico em oxigênio de uma série de compostos químicos. [G. *hypo,* sob]

hy·po·ac·id·i·ty (hī′pō - a - sid′i - tē). Hipoacidez; grau de acidez menor do que o normal, como o do suco gástrico.

hy·po·a·cu·sis (hī′pō - ã - koo′sis). Hipoacusia, hipacusia. SIN hypacusis.

hy·po·a·de·nia (hī - po - ã - dē′nē - ã). Hipoadenia; qualquer deficiência na função de um órgão ou tecido glandular. [hypo- + G. *adēn,* glândula]

hy·po·a·dre·nal·ism (hī′pō - ã - drē′nal - izm). Hipoadrenalismo; redução da função adrenocortical.

hy·po·al·bu·mi·ne·mia (hī′pō - al - boo - mi - nē′mē - ã). Hipoalbuminemia; concentração anormalmente baixa de albumina no sangue. SIN hypalbuminemia.

hy·po·al·dos·ter·on·ism (hī′pō - al - dos′ter - on - izm). Hipoaldosteronismo; condição causada pela secreção deficiente de aldosterona; pode ocorrer em duas formas: 1) como parte de insuficiência adrenocortical generalizada; 2) como deficiência seletiva causada por um defeito primário da glândula supra-renal ou defeito no controle da secreção de aldosterona.

hyporeninemic h., h. hiporreninêmico; deficiência seletiva de aldosterona em decorrência da baixa produção de renina.

isolated h., h. isolado. SIN selective h.

selective h., h. seletivo; deficiência de aldosterona sem deficiência concomitante de hormônios glicocorticóides. SIN isolated h.

hy·po·al·dos·ter·on·u·ria (hī′pō - al - dos′ter - on - oo′rē - ã). Hipoaldosteronúria; níveis anormalmente baixos de aldosterona na urina.

hy·po·al·ge·sia (hī - pō - al - jē′zē - ã). Hipoalgesia. SIN hypalgesia. [hypo- + G. *algēsis,* sensação de dor]

hy·po·al·i·men·ta·tion (hī′pō - al - i - men - tā′shŭn). Hipoalimentação. SIN subalimentation.

hy·po·az·o·tu·ria (hī′pō - az - ō - too′rē - ã). Hipoazotúria; excreção de quantidades anormalmente pequenas de material nitrogenado não-proteico (especialmente uréia) na urina. SIN hypazoturia. [hypo- + Fr. *azote,* nitrogênio + G. *ouron,* urina]

hy·po·bar·ia (hī - pō - bar′ē - ã). Hipobaria. SIN hypobarism.

hy·po·bar·ic (hī - pō - bar′ik). Hipobárico. **1.** Relativo à pressão de gases ambientais abaixo de uma atmosfera. **2.** Em relação a soluções, menos denso do que o diluente ou meio; p. ex., na anestesia raquiana, uma solução hipobárica tem uma densidade mais baixa que a do líquido cefalorraquidiano. [hypo- + G. *baros,* peso]

hy·po·bar·ism (hī - pō - bar′izm). Hipobarismo; disbarismo resultante da pressão barométrica diminuída sobre o corpo sem hipoxia; os gases nas cavidades corporais tendem a se expandir, e os gases dissolvidos nos líquidos orgânicos tendem a abandonar a solução na forma de bolhas. Cf. decompression *sickness.* SIN hypobaria.

hy·po·ba·rop·a·thy (hī′pō - ba - rop′ã - thē). Hipobaropatia; doença produzida por redução da pressão barométrica; nem sempre diferenciada do hipobarismo e da doença de altitude. [hypo- + G. *baros,* peso + *pathos,* sofrimento]

hy·po·be·ta·lip·o·pro·tein·e·mia (hī′pō - bā′tã - lip′ō - prō′tēn - ē′mē - ã) [MIM*107730]. Hipobetalipoproteinemia; níveis anormalmente baixos de β-lipoproteínas no plasma, ocasionalmente com acantocitose e sinais neurológicos; herança autossômica dominante; causada pela mutação do gene da apolipoproteína B (APOB) no cromossoma 2p. VER TAMBÉM abetalipoproteinemia.

familial h., h. familiar; distúrbio semelhante à abetalipoproteinemia; ainda ocorre formação de quilomícrons, porém os níveis de LDL estão tipicamente baixos.

h. with apo B-37, h. com apo B-37; distúrbio caracterizado por níveis muito baixos de LDL, má absorção leve de gordura e formação de apolipoproteína B-37 truncada.

hy·po·blast (hī′pō - blast). Hipoblasto; camada celular adjacente à cavidade do saco vitelino e subjacente ao epiblasto de um embrião com dupla camada. [hypo- + G. *blastos,* germe]

hy·po·blas·tic (hī - pō - blas′tik). Hipoblástico; relativo a, ou derivado do, hipoblasto.

y·po·bran·chi·al (hī - pō - brang′kē - ãl). Hipobranquial; localizado abaixo do aparelho branquial.

hy·po·bro·mite (hī - pō - brō′mīt). Hipobrometo; sal do ácido hipobromoso.

hy·po·bro·mous ac·id (hī - pō - brō′mŭs). Ácido hipobromoso; um ácido, HOBr, cuja solução aquosa possui propriedades oxidantes e descorantes.

hy·po·cal·ce·mia (hī′pō - kal - sē′mē - ã). Hipocalcemia; níveis anormalmente baixos de cálcio no sangue circulante; indica comumente concentrações subnormais de íons cálcio.

hy·po·cal·ci·fi·ca·tion (hī′pō - kal - si - fi - kā′shŭn). Hipocalcificação; calcificação deficiente de ossos ou dentes.

enamel h. [MIM*104500]. h. do esmalte; defeito de maturação do esmalte caracterizado por esmalte mole opaco ou branco-amarelado, sem brilho. Variedade de amelogênese imperfeita. Existem formas autossômica dominante, autossômica recessiva e recessiva ligada ao X.

hy·po·cap·nia (hī - pō - kap′nē - ã). Hipocapnia; tensão arterial de dióxido de carbono anormalmente diminuída. SIN hypocarbia. [hypo- + G. *kapnos,* fumaça, vapor]

hy·po·car·bia (hī - pō - kar′bē - ã). Hipocarbia. SIN hypocapnia.

hy·po·ce·lom (hī - pō - sē′lom). Hipoceloma; termo raramente utilizado para referir-se à porção ventral do celoma ou cavidade corporal do embrião. [hypo- + G. *koilos,* oco]

hy·po·chlor·e·mia (hī′pō - klō - rē′mē - ã). Hipocloremia; nível anormalmente baixo de íons cloreto no sangue circulante.

hy·po·chlor·e·mic (hī′pō - klō - rē′mik). Hipoclorêmico; relativo a, ou caracterizado por, hipocloremia.

hy·po·chlor·hy·dria (hī′pō - klōr - hī′drē - ã, - hī′drī - ah). Hipocloridria; quantidade anormalmente pequena de ácido clorídrico no estômago. SIN hypohydrochloria.

hy·po·chlo·rite (hī - pō - klō′rīt). Hipocloreto; sal do ácido hipocloroso.

hy·po·chlo·rous ac·id (hī - pō - klōr′ŭs). Ácido hipocloroso; um ácido, HOCl, com propriedades oxidantes e descorantes.

hy·po·chlo·ru·ria (hī - pō - klōr - u′rē - ã). Hipoclorúria; excreção de quantidades anormalmente pequenas de íons cloreto na urina.

hy·po·cho·les·ter·e·mia (hī′pō - kō - les - tē - rē′mē - ã). Hipocolesteremia. SIN hypocholesterolemia.

hy·po·cho·les·ter·in·e·mia (hī′pō - kō - les′tē - ri - nē′mē - ã). Hipocolesterinemia. SIN hypocholesterolemia.

hy·po·cho·les·ter·ol·e·mia (hī′pō - kō - les′ter - ol - ē′mē - ã). Hipocolesterolemia; níveis anormalmente baixos de colesterol no sangue circulante. SIN hypocholesteremia, hypocholesterinemia.

hy·po·cho·lia (hī - pō - kō′lē - ã). Hipocolia; termo raramente utilizado para referir-se a oligocolia.

hy·po·chon·dria (hī - pō - kon′drē - ã). Hipocondria. SIN hypochondriasis.

hy·po·chon·dri·ac (hī - pō - kon′drē - ak). Hipocondríaco. **1.** Pessoa com excessiva preocupação somática, incluindo atenção mórbida para os detalhes do funcionamento do corpo e exageração de qualquer sintoma, independentemente do quanto sejam insignificantes. **2.** Pessoa que manifesta hipocondríase. **3.** Abaixo das costelas; relacionado ao hipocôndrio.

hy·po·chon·dri·a·cal (hī′pō - kon - drī′ã - kãl). Hipocondríaco; relativo a, ou que sofre de, hipocondríase.

diagnóstico diferencial da hipocalcemia

hipoalbuminemia

insuficiência renal crônica

deficiência de magnésio

hipoparatireoidismo

pseudo-hipoparatireoidismo

osteomalacia e raquitismo por deficiência de vitamina D ou resistência à vitamina D

pancreatite hemorrágica e edematosa aguda

fase de cicatrização de doença óssea do hiperparatireoidismo tratado, hipertireoidismo e neoplasias hematológicas (síndrome do osso ávido)

hy·po·chon·dri·a·sis (hī'pō-kon-drī'ă-sis). Hipocondria; preocupação mórbida a respeito da própria saúde e atenção exagerada para qualquer sensação corporal ou mental incomum; delírio de que está sofrendo de alguma doença para a qual não existe nenhuma base física evidente. SIN hypochondria, hypochondriacal neurosis. [fr. hypochondrium, considerado como o local do hipocôndrio + G. -iasis, condição]

hy·po·chon·dri·um, pl. **hy·po·chon·dria** (hī-pō-kon'drē-ŭm,-ă) [TA]. Hipocôndrio. SIN hypochondriac region. [L. fr. G. hypochondrion, abdome, ventre, de hypo, sob + chondros, cartilagem (de costelas)]

hy·po·chon·dro·pla·sia (hī'pō-kon-drō-plā'zē-ă). [MIM*146000]. Hipocondroplasia; displasia esquelética caracterizada por nanismo com manifestações semelhantes àquelas da acondroplasia, porém muito mais brandas; crânio e fácies normais; as manifestações não são clinicamente evidentes até metade da infância. Herança autossômica dominante, causada, em alguns casos, por mutação do gene do receptor do fator de crescimento dos fibroblastos 3 (FGFR3) no cromossoma 4p. [hypo- + G. chondros, cartilagem + plasis, moldagem]

hy·po·chord·al (hī-pō-kōr'dăl). Hipocordal; no lado ventral da medula espinal. [hypo- + G. chordē, cordão]

hy·po·chro·ma·sia (hī'pō-krō-mā'zē-ă). Hipocromasia. SIN hypochromia.

hy·po·chro·mat·ic (hī'-pō-krō-mat'ik). Hipocromático; que contém uma pequena quantidade de pigmento ou menos do que a quantidade normal para o tecido individual. SIN hypochromic (1). [hypo- + G. chrōma, cor]

hy·po·chro·ma·tism (hī-pō-krō'mă-tizm). Hipocromatismo. **1.** Condição de ser hipocromático. **2.** SIN hypochromia.

hy·po·chro·mia (hī-pō-krō'mē-ă). Hipocromia; condição anêmica em que a percentagem de hemoglobina nos eritrócitos é inferior à faixa normal. SIN hypochromasia, hypochromatism (2), hypochrosis. [hypo- + G. chrōma, cor]

hy·po·chro·mic (hī-pō-krō'mik). Hipocrômico. **1.** SIN hypochromatic. **2.** Indica uma diminuição na absorção de luz, com desvio do comprimento de onda para um comprimento menor.

hy·po·chro·sis (hī-pō-krō'sis). Hipocrose. SIN hypochromia. [hypo- + G. chrōsis, tintura]

hy·po·chy·lia (hī-pō-kī'lē-ă). Hipoquilia; termo raramente utilizado para referir-se à oligoquilia. [hypo- + G. chylos, suco]

hy·po·ci·ne·sis, hy·po·ci·ne·sia (hī'pō-si-nē'sis, -nē'zē-ă). Hipocinese. SIN hypokinesis.

hy·po·cit·ra·tur·ia (hī'pō-si-tră-toor'ē-ă). Hipocitratúria; concentração anormalmente baixa de citrato na urina.

hy·po·com·ple·men·te·mia (hī'pō-kom'plĕ-men-tē'mē-ă). Hipocomplementemia; condição em que um ou outro componente do complemento está faltando ou está quantitativamente diminuído; associada a doenças por imunocomplexos e casos de glomerulonefrite membranoproliferativa em que existe o fator nefrítico. São conhecidas várias formas autossômicas, tanto dominantes [MIM*120550 e MIM*120980] quanto recessivas [MIM*216950 e MIM*217070].

hy·po·cone (hī'pō-kōn). Hipocone; cúspide distolingual de um dente molar superior. [hypo- + G. kōnos, pinha]

hy·po·con·id (hī-pō-kon'id). Hipoconide; cúspide distobucal de um dente molar inferior.

hy·po·con·ule (hī-pō-kon'ūl). Hipocônule; quinta cúspide ou cúspide distal de um dente molar superior. [hypo- + L. Mod. dim. do L. conus, cone]

hy·po·con·u·lid (hī-pō-kon'ū-lid). Hipoconulídeo; quinta cúspide ou cúspide distal de um dente molar inferior. [hypo- + L. Mod. dim. do L. conus, cone]

hy·po·cor·ti·coid·ism (hī-pō-kōr'ti-koyd-izm). Hipocorticoidismo. SIN adrenocortical insufficiency.

hy·po·cu·pre·mia (hī'pō-koo-prē'mē-ă). Hipocupremia; conteúdo reduzido de cobre no sangue; observada na doença de Wilson, devido aos níveis diminuídos de ceruloplasmina, embora o nível sérico de cobre ligado à albumina esteja aumentado. [hypo- +L. cuprum, cobre + G. haima, sangue]

hy·po·cy·cloi·dal (hī'-pō-sī-kloy'dăl). Hipocicloidal; movimento tricíclico utilizado por unidades de tomografia mecânica para melhorar o embaçamento e reduzir os artefatos. [hypo- + G. kuklos, círculo + -oeidēs, aparência]

hy·po·cys·tot·o·my (hī'pō-sis-tot'ō-mē). Hipocistotomia; cistotomia perineal.

hy·po·cy·the·mia (hī'pō-sī-thē'mē-ă). Hipocitemia; hipocitose do sangue circulante, como a observada na anemia aplásica. [hypo- + G. kytos, célula + haima, sangue]

hy·po·cy·to·sis (hī'pō-sī-tō'sis). Hipocitose; graus variáveis de número anormalmente baixo de eritrócitos, leucócitos e outros elementos figurados do sangue; em alguns casos, o termo também é utilizado para indicar escassez de células componentes de qualquer tecido. VER TAMBÉM cytopenia, pancytopenia. [hypo- + G. kytos, célula + -osis, condição]

hy·po·dac·ty·ly, hy·po·dac·tyl·ia, hy·po·dac·tyl·ism (hī'pō-dak'ti-lē, -dak-til'ē-ă, -dak'til-izm). Hipodactilia; menos do que o número total normal de dedos. [hypo- + G. daktylos, dedo]

hy·po·derm (hī'pō-derm). Hipoderme. SIN subcutaneous tissue. [hypo- + G. derma, pele]

Hy·po·der·ma (hī-pō-der'mă). Gênero de mosca cujas larvas são a causa de uma forma tropical de miíase linear (larva migrans cutânea) do homem; em certas ocasiões, invadem o interior do olho. Duas espécies, *H. bovis* e *H. lineatum*, são moscas de gado. Os ovos de *H. bovis* são depositados nos pêlos das pernas, e as larvas penetram na pele e migram através dos tecidos até a pele do dorso do animal, onde aparecem no final do inverno como tumores de berne comuns; esses tumores ulceram até a superfície, e as larvas maduras escapam no início do verão, caem ao solo, transformam-se em pupas e dão origem a uma nova geração de moscas. [hypo- + G. derma, pele]

hy·po·der·mat·oc·ly·sis (hī'pō-der-mă-tok'li-sis). Hipodermatóclise; termo raramente utilizado para hipodermóclise.

hy·po·der·mat·o·my (hī'pō-der-mat'ō-mē). Hipodermatomia; divisão subcutânea de uma estrutura. [hypo- + G. derma, pele + tomē, incisão]

hy·po·der·ma·to·sis (hī'pō-der-mă-tō'sis). Hipodermatose; infecção de herbívoros e seres humanos com larvas de moscas do gênero *Hypoderma*.

hy·po·der·mic (hī'pō-der'mik). Hipodérmico. **1.** Subcutâneo. SIN subcutaneous. **2.** Injeção hipodérmica. SIN hypodermic injection. **3.** Seringa hipodérmica. SIN hypodermic syringe.

hy·po·der·mis (hī-pō-der'mis). Hipoderme; ★termo oficial alternativo para subcutaneous tissue.

hy·po·der·moc·ly·sis (hī'pō-der-mok'li-sis). Hipodermóclise; injeção subcutânea de soro fisiológico ou outra solução. [hypo- + G. derma, pele + klysis, lavagem] (hī'-pō-dip'loid). Hipodiplóide; que apresenta um número de cromossomas inferior ao número diplóide.

hy·po·dip·sia (hī-pō-dip'sē-ă). Hipodipisia; condição fisiológica, talvez causada pela hipertonicidade dos líquidos corporais, insuficiente para iniciar a ingestão de líquidos, porém algumas vezes insuficiente para mantê-la quando iniciada; de forma imprecisa, oligodipisia. SIN insensible thirst, subliminal thirst. [hypo- + G. dipsa, sede]

hy·po·don·tia (hī-pō-don'shē-ă). Hipodontia; condição de apresentar um conjunto de dentes menor do que o normal, na forma congênita ou adquirida. SIN oligodontia, partial anodontia. [hypo- + G. odous, dente]

hy·po·dy·nam·ia (hī'pō-dī-nā'mē-ă, -dī-nam'ē-ă). Hipodinamia; força diminuída. [hypo- + G. dynamis, força]
  h. cor'dis, h. do coração; força diminuída da contração cardíaca.

hy·po·dy·nam·ic (hī'pō-dī-nam'ik). Hipodinâmico; que possui ou exibe força subnormal.

hy·po·ec·cri·sis (hī'pō-ek'ri-sis). Hipoecrisia; excreção reduzida de produtos de degradação. [hypo- + G. eccrisis, separação]

hy·po·ec·crit·ic (hī'pō-ĕ-krit'ik). Hipoecrítico; caracterizado por hipoecrisia.

hy·po·ech·o·ic (hī'pō-e-kō'ik). Hipoecóico; região na imagem de ultrasonografia em que os ecos são mais fracos ou menores do que o normal ou nas regiões circundantes. [hypo- + echo + -ic]

hy·po·e·o·sin·o·phil·ia (hī'pō-ē'ō-sin-ō-fil'ē-ă). Hipoeosinofilia. SIN eosinopenia.

hy·po·es·o·pho·ria (hī'pō-es-ō-fō'rē-ă). Hipoesoforia; tendência do eixo visual de um olho a desviar-se para baixo e para dentro, evitada pela visão binocular. [hypo- + G. esō, dentro + phoros, transportando]

hy·po·es·the·sia (hī'pō-es-thē'zē-ă). Hipoestesia. SIN hypesthesia.

hy·po·ex·o·pho·ria (hī'pō-ek-sō-fō'rē-ă). Hipoexoforia; tendência do eixo visual de um olho a desviar-se para baixo e para fora, evitada pela visão binocular. [hypo- + G. exō, sem + phoros, transportando]

hy·po·fer·re·mia (hī'pō-fer-ē'mē-ă). Hipoferremia; deficiência de ferro no sangue circulante.

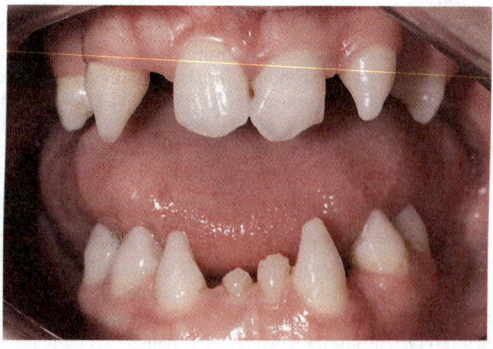

hipodontia: dentição mostrando dentes decíduos retidos e ausência de numerosos dentes permanentes que nunca se desenvolveram

hy·po·fi·brin·o·ge·ne·mia (hī′pō - fī - brin′ō - jĕ - nē′mē - ă). Hipofibrinogenemia; concentração anormalmente baixa de fibrinogênio no plasma sanguíneo circulante.

hypofrontality (hī′pō - fron - tal′i - tē). Hipofrontalidade; diminuição da atividade neuronal de várias áreas dos lobos frontais, de várias etiologias e associada a diversos sintomas clínicos ou distúrbios.

hy·po·func·tion (hī′pō - fŭnk - shŭn). Hipofunção; função reduzida, baixa ou inadequada.

hy·po·ga·lac·tia (hī′pō - ga - lak′shē - ă). Hipogalactia; secreção de leite menor do que o normal. [hypo- + G. *gala*, leite]

hy·po·ga·lac·tous (hī′pō - ga - lak′tŭs). Hipogalácteo; que produz ou secreta menos leite do que o normal.

hy·po·gam·ma·glo·bi·ne·mia (hī′pō - gam′ă - glō′bi - nē′mē - ă). Hipogamaglobinemia. SIN hypogammaglobulinemia.

hy·po·gam·ma·glob·u·lin·e·mia (hī′pō - gam′ă - glob′ū - li - nē′mē - ă). Hipogamaglobulinemia; quantidade diminuída da fração gama das globulinas séricas; algumas vezes, termo utilizado de modo impreciso para referir-se a uma quantidade diminuída de imunoglobulinas em geral, associada a aumento da suscetibilidade a infecções piogênicas. SIN hypogammaglobinemia.
  acquired h., h. adquirida. SIN common variable *immunodeficiency.*
  primary h., h. primária; hipogamaglobulinemia devida a uma imunodeficiência primária de células formadoras de imunoglobulinas (linfócitos B).
  secondary h., h. secundária. SIN secondary *immunodeficiency.*
  transient h. of infancy, h. transitória do lactente; tipo de imunodeficiência primária que ocorre em lactentes de ambos os sexos, habitualmente antes do sexto mês de vida, provavelmente em decorrência de imaturidade do tecido linfóide. SIN transient agammaglobulinemia.
  X-linked h., X-linked infantile h., h. ligada ao X, h. infantil ligada ao X; imunodeficiência primária congênita, caracterizada por número diminuído (ou ausência) de linfócitos B circulantes, com redução correspondente nas imunoglobulinas das cinco classes; associada a uma suscetibilidade acentuada a infecções por bactérias piogênicas (notavelmente pneumococos e *Haemophilus influenzae*), começando após a perda dos anticorpos maternos; herança recessiva ligada ao X, causada por mutação no gene da tirosina-cinase de Bruton (BTK) no cromossoma Xq.
  X-linked h. with growth hormone deficiency, h. ligada ao X com deficiência de hormônio do crescimento; hipogamaglobulinemia combinada a um número reduzido de células B; caracterizada por estatura baixa, puberdade tardia e infecções recorrentes.

hy·po·gan·gli·o·no·sis (hī′pō - gang - lē - on - ō′sis). Hipoganglionose; redução no número de células nervosas ganglionares.

hy·po·gas·tric (hī - pō - gas′trik). Hipogástrico; relativo ao hipogástrio.

hy·po·gas·tri·um (hī′pō - gas′trē - ŭm) [TA]. Hipogástrio. SIN pubic *region.* [G. *hypogastrion*, parte inferior do ventre, fr. *hypo*, sob + *gaster*, ventre, barriga]

hy·po·gas·tro·cele (hī′pō - gas′trō - sēl). Hipogastrocele; hérnia da parte inferior do abdome. [hypogastrium + G. *kēlē*, hérnia]

hy·po·gas·trop·a·gus (hī′pō - gas - trop′a - gŭs). Hipogastrópago; gêmeos unidos no hipogástrio. VER conjoined *twins*, em *twin*. [hypogastrium + G. *pagos*, fr. *pēgnynai*, jejuar]

hy·po·gas·tros·chi·sis (hī′pō - gas - tros′ki - sis). Hipogastrosquise; fenda congênita na parede abdominal, na região hipogástrica. [hypogastrium + G. *schisis*, clivagem]

hy·po·gen·e·sis (hī′pō - jen′ĕ - sis). Hipogênese; defeito congênito de crescimento com subdesenvolvimento de partes ou órgãos do corpo. [hypo- + G. *genesis*, origem]
  polar h., h. polar; grau de desenvolvimento abaixo do normal na extremidade cefálica ou caudal do embrião.

hy·po·ge·net·ic (hī′pō - jĕ - net′ik). Hipogenético; relativo à hipogênese.

hy·po·gen·i·tal·ism (hī - pō - jen′i - tāl - izm). Hipogenitalismo; falha parcial ou completa de maturação da genitália; em geral, representa uma conseqüência do hipogonadismo.

hy·po·geu·sia (hī - pō - gū′sē - ă). Hipogeusia; diminuição do sentido do paladar. Pode ser: 1) geral a todas as substâncias experimentadas, parcial a algumas delas ou específica a uma ou mais delas; 2) devido a distúrbios de transporte (acesso à parte inferior dos botões gustativos) ou a distúrbios sensorioneurais (que afetam as células sensoriais ou nervos gustativos ou as vias neurais gustativas centrais); e 3) hereditária ou adquirida. [hypo- + G. *geusis*, paladar]

hy·po·glob·u·lia (hī′pō - glo - bū′lē - ă). Hipoglobulia; termo obsoleto para referir-se a um número anormalmente baixo de eritrócitos no sangue circulante; também utilizado raramente para referir-se a proporções anormalmente diminuídas de elementos eritróides na medula óssea. [hypo- + G. *globulus*, glóbulo]

hypo·glos·sal (hī - pō - glos′ăl). Hipoglosso. **1.** Abaixo da língua. **2.** Relativo ao décimo segundo nervo craniano, o nervo hipoglosso. SIN hypoglossus. [L. *hypoglossus* fr. hypo- + *glossus*, língua]

hy·po·glos·sis (hī - pō - glos′is). Hipoglosse. SIN hypoglottis.

hy·po·glos·sus (hī′pō - glos′ŭs). Hipoglosso. SIN hypoglossal. [L.]

hy·po·glot·tis (hī′pō - glot′is). Hipoglote; superfície inferior da língua. SIN hypoglossis. [G. *hypoglossis*, ou *-glottis*, superfície inferior da língua, fr. *hypo*, sob + *glossa*, língua]

hy·po·gly·ce·mia (hī′pō - glī - sē′mē - ă). Hipoglicemia. **1.** Sintomas produzidos por baixos níveis de glicemia (faixa normal da glicose: 60–100 mg/dL [3,3 a 5,6 mmol/L]), que são autônomos ou neuroglicopênicos. Os sintomas autônomos consistem em sudorese, tremor, sensação de calor, ansiedade e náuseas. Os sintomas neuroglicopênicos incluem sensação de tonteira, confusão, cansaço, dificuldade em falar, cefaléia e incapacidade de concentração. **2.** Doença orgânica que, mais freqüentemente, resulta em sintomas neuroglicopênicos, distúrbios funcionais e sintomas autônomos. A hipoglicemia funcional é de existência duvidosa; a denominada síndrome de hipoglicemia pós-prandial não foi confirmada por determinações da glicemia. Não foram encontradas provas convincentes sobre a existência de hipoglicemia do diabetes precoce ou hipoglicemia alimentar. SIN glucopenia.
  fasting h., h. de jejum; glicemia excessivamente baixa em associação ao jejum; pode ser observada em pacientes com hiperinsulinismo, mas também ocorre na ausência de doença definível.
  ketotic h., h. cetótica; forma mais comum de hipoglicemia infantil depois do período neonatal; em geral, surge entre 18 meses e 5 anos de idade e desaparece espontaneamente no final da infância; manifesta-se por episódios hipoglicêmicos que, habitualmente, ocorrem durante doenças de menor gravidade que causam diminuição do apetite; provavelmente devida a um defeito na gliconeogênese e reservas limitadas de glicogênio.
  leucine h., h. por leucina; redução da concentração de glicose no sangue produzida pela administração de leucina; acredita-se que reflita a capacidade desse aminoácido de estimular a secreção de insulina.
  leucine-induced h., h. induzida por leucina; causa rara de hipoglicemia que ocorre após a ingestão de leucina. Observada particularmente em lactentes. SIN leucine-sensitive h.
  leucine-sensitive h., h. sensível à leucina. SIN leucine-induced h.
  mixed h., h. mista; hipoglicemia devido a mais de uma causa.
  neonatal h. [MIM*240900], h. neonatal; início familiar de hipoglicemia sintomática durante a lactância, com nível de glicemia persistentemente baixo; uma forma variante [MIM*240800] é induzida por leucina, com hiperinsulinismo e retardo mental variável.

hy·po·gly·ce·mic (hī′pō - glī - sē′mik). Hipoglicêmico; relativo a, ou caracterizado por, hipoglicemia.

hy·po·gly·co·gen·ol·y·sis (hī′pō - glī′kō - jĕ - nol′i - sis). Hipoglicogenólise; glicogenólise deficiente.

hy·po·gly·cor·rha·chia (hī′pō - glī - kō - rak′ē - ă). Hipoglicorraquia; concentração diminuída de glicose no líquido cefalorraquidiano; característica de meningite bacteriana, fúngica e tuberculosa. [hypo- + G. *glykys*, doce + *rhachis*, espinha]

hy·pog·na·thous (hī′pō - nath′ŭs, hī - pog′na - thŭs). Hipognato; que apresenta maxilar inferior pequeno, de desenvolvimento congenitamente defeituoso. [hypo- + G. *gnathos*, mandíbula]

hy·pog·na·thus (hī′pō - nath′ŭs, hī - pog′na - thŭs). Hipognato; gêmeos unidos desiguais, em que o parasita rudimentar está fixado à mandíbula do autósito. VER conjoined *twins*, em *twin*. [hypo- + G. *gnathos*, mandíbula]

hy·po·gon·ad·ism (hī′pō - gō′nad - izm). Hipogonadismo; função gonadal inadequada, manifestada por deficiências na gametogênese e/ou secreção de hormônios gonadais; resulta em atrofia ou desenvolvimento deficiente dos caracteres sexuais secundários e, quando ocorre em indivíduos pré-puberais do sexo masculino, em alteração do biotipo caracterizada por tronco curto e membros longos.
  familial hypogonadotropic h. [MIM*312100 & MIM*307300], h. hipogonadotrópico familiar; grupo de distúrbios caracterizados pela falta de desenvolvimento sexual, devido à secreção inadequada de gonadotropinas hipofisárias; talvez ligado ao X, embora existam provavelmente formas de herança autossômica dominante e recessiva.
  hypergonadotropic h., h. hipergonadotrópico; deficiência no desenvolvimento gonadal ou na função das gônadas, em decorrência de níveis elevados de gonadotropinas.
  hypogonadotropic h., h. hipogonadotrópico; deficiência no desenvolvimento e/ou função gonadal em decorrência da secreção inadequada de gonadotropinas hipofisárias. SIN hypogonadotropic eunuchoidism, secondary h.
  male h., h. masculino. SIN eunuchoidism.
  primary h., h. primário; deficiência no desenvolvimento e/ou função gonadal devido a uma anormalidade ou perda da própria gônada.
  secondary h., h. secundário. SIN hypogonadotropic h.
  h. with anosmia, h. com anosmia; falta de desenvolvimento sexual secundariamente à secreção inadequada de gonadotropinas hipofisárias, associada a anosmia devido à agenesia dos lobos olfativos do cérebro. Existem formas de herança autossômica dominante [MIM*147950], autossômica recessiva [MIM*244200] e recessiva ligada ao X [MIM*308700]; a forma ligada ao X

é causada pela mutação do gene Kallmann (KAL1) no cromossoma Xp. SIN Kallmann syndrome.

hy·po·go·nad·o·tro·pic (hī'pō - gon'a - dō - trop'ik). Hipogonadotrópico; indica uma secreção inadequada de gonadotropinas e suas conseqüências.

hy·po·gran·u·lo·cy·to·sis (hī'pō - gran'u - lō - si - tō'sis). Hipogranulocitose. SIN granulocytopenia.

hy·po·he·pat·ia (hī'pō - hē - pat'ē - a). Hipoepatia; termo raramente utilizado para referir-se à deficiência de função hepática. [hypo- + G. hēpar, fígado]

hy·po·hi·dro·sis (hī'pō - hī - drō'sis). Hipoidrose; perspiração diminuída.

hy·po·hy·dre·mia (hī'pō - hī - drē'mē - a). Hipoidremia; qualquer deficiência na quantidade de líquido no sangue. [hypo- + G. hydōr, água + haima, sangue]

hy·po·hy·dro·chlo·ria (hī'pō - hī - drō - klōr'ē - a). Hipoidrocloria. SIN hypochorhydria.

hy·po·i·so·ton·ic (hī'pō - ī - sō - ton'ik). Hipoisotônico. SIN hypotonic.

hy·po·ka·le·mia (hī'pō - ka - lē'mē - a). Hipocaliemia, hipopotassemia; concentração anormalmente baixa de íons potássio no sangue circulante; ocorre na paralisia periódica familiar e na depleção de potássio devido à perda excessiva pelo trato gastrointestinal ou pelos rins. As alterações na hipocaliemia podem incluir vacuolização do citoplasma das células epiteliais tubulares renais, com comprometimento da capacidade de concentração urinária e acidificação, achatamento da onda T no eletrocardiograma e fraqueza muscular. SIN hypopotassemia. [hypo- + L. Mod. kalium, potássio + G. haima, sangue]

hy·po·ki·ne·mia (hī'pō - ki - nē'mē - a). Hipocinemia; redução da velocidade de circulação; redução do fluxo de volume através da circulação; débito cardíaco subnormal. [hypo- + G. kineo, mover + haima, sangue]

hy·po·ki·ne·sis, hy·po·ki·ne·sia (hī'pō - ki - nē'sis, - nē'zē - a). Hipocinese, hipocinesia; movimento diminuído ou lento. SIN hypocinesis, hypocinesia, hypomotility. [hypo- + G. kinēsis, movimento]

hy·po·ki·net·ic (hī'pō - ki - net'ik). Hipocinético; relativo a, ou caracterizado por, hipocinesia.

hy·po·leu·ke·mia (hī'pō - loo - kē'mē - a). Hipoleucemia. SIN subleukemic leukemia.

hy·po·ley·dig·ism (hī - pō - lī'dig - izm). Hipoleidigismo; secreção subnormal de androgênios pelas células intersticiais (de Leydig) dos testículos.

hy·po·lip·o·pro·teine·mia (hī'pō - lip'ō - prō - tēn - ē - mē - a). Hipolipoproteinemia; níveis diminuídos de lipoproteína no soro.

hy·po·li·po·sis (hī'pō - li - pō'sis). Hipolipose; quantidade anormalmente pequena de gordura nos tecidos.

hy·po·lo·gia (hī'pō - lō'jē - a). Hipologia; redução da capacidade de falar. [hypo- + G. logos, palavra]

hy·po·lym·phe·mia (hī'pō - lim - fē'mē - a). Hipolinfemia; número anormalmente pequeno de linfócitos no sangue circulante.

hy·po·mag·ne·se·mia (hī'pō - mag - nē - sē'mē - a). Hipomagnesemia; concentração sérica subnormal de magnésio; pode causar convulsões e hipocalcemia concomitante.

hy·po·ma·nia (hī'pō - mā'nē - a). Hipomania; grau leve de mania.

hy·po·mas·tia (hī'pō - mas'tē - a). Hipomastia; atrofia ou pequenez congênita das mamas. [hypo- + G. mastos, mama]

hy·po·mel·an·cho·lia (hī'pō - mel - an - kō'lē - a). Hipomelancolia; grau leve de depressão mental.

hy·po·mel·a·no·sis (hī'pō - mel - a - nō'sis). Hipomelanose. SIN leukoderma.
h. of Ito [MIM*146150 e MIM*308300], h. de Ito; não se trata de uma entidade específica, mas representa manifestações de muitas formas diferentes de mosaicismo; caracterizada por máculas hipopigmentadas unilaterais ou bilaterais em espirais, estrias e placas num padrão em "bolo de mármore", variavelmente associada a nevos epidérmicos, alopecia e anormalidades oculares, esqueléticas e neurais. VER TAMBÉM incontinentia pigmenti. SIN incontinentia pigmenti achromians.

hy·po·me·lia (hī - pō - mē'lē - a). Hipomelia; termo geral para referir-se à hipoplasia de alguma ou de todas as partes de um ou mais membros. [hypo- + G. melos, membro]

hy·po·men·or·rhea (hī'pō - men - ō - rē'a). Hipomenorréia; redução do fluxo ou da duração da menstruação. [hypo- + G. mēn, mês + rhoia, fluxo]

hy·po·mere (hī'pō - mēr). Hipômero. **1.** Porção do miótono que se estende ventrolateralmente para formar o músculo da parede corporal e do membro, inervada pelo ramo ventral primário de um nervo espinal. VER hypaxial. **2.** Menos comumente, as camadas somática e esplâncnica do mesoderma lateral que dão origem ao revestimento do celoma. [hypo- + G. meros, parte]

hy·po·me·tab·o·lism (hī'pō - me - tab'ō - lizm). Hipometabolismo; metabolismo reduzido. VER TAMBÉM hypometabolic state.
euthyroid h., h. eutireóideo; condição incomum semelhante ao mixedema, porém com glândula tireóide aparentemente normal.

hy·po·met·ria (hī - pō - mē'trē - a). Hipometria; ataxia caracterizada pela incapacidade de atingir um objeto ou meta; observada na doença cerebelar. Cf. hypermetria. [hypo- + G. metron, medida]

hy·pom·ne·sia (hī - pō - nē'zē - a). Hipomnésia; comprometimento da memória. Cf. hypermnesia. [hypo- + G. mnēmē, memória]

hy·po·morph (hī'pō - mōrf). Hipomorfo. **1.** Indivíduo cuja altura de pé é menor do que a altura sentada, devido ao encurtamento dos membros. Cf. hypermorph, endomorph. **2.** Gene mutante que provoca uma redução parcial na atividade controlada por ele. Cf. hypermorph. [hypo- + G. morphē, forma]

hy·po·mo·til·i·ty (hī'pō - mō - til'i - tē). Hipomotilidade. SIN hypokinesis.

hy·po·my·e·li·na·tion, hy·po·my·e·lin·o·gen·e·sis (hī'pō - mī'ē - lin - ā - shun, - ō - jen'ē - sis). Hipomielinização; formação deficiente de mielina na medula espinal e no cérebro; base de diversas doenças desmielinizantes.

hy·po·my·o·to·nia (hī'pō - mī - ō - tō'nē - a). Hipomiotonia; condição de diminuição do tônus muscular. [hypo- + G. mys (myo-) músculo + tonos, tensão]

hy·po·myx·ia (hī'pō - mik'sē - a). Hipomixia; condição caracterizada por redução na secreção de muco. [hypo- + G. myxa, muco]

hy·po·na·tre·mia (hī'pō - na - trē'mē - a). Hiponatremia; concentrações anormalmente baixas de íons sódio no sangue circulante. [hypo- + sódio + G. haima, sangue]
depletional h., h. por depleção; concentrações séricas diminuídas de sódio associadas à perda de sódio do sangue circulante através do trato GI, dos rins, da pele ou no "terceiro espaço". Acompanhada de estado hipovolêmico e hipotônico.

hy·po·ne·o·cy·to·sis (hī'pō - nē'ō - sī - tō'sis). Hiponeocitose; leucemia associada à presença de leucócitos imaturos e jovens (especialmente da série granulocítica), isto é, "desvio para a esquerda" no hemograma. SIN hyposkeocytosis. [hypo + G. neos, novo + kytos, célula + -osis, condição]

hy·po·noia (hī'pō - noy' - a). Hiponóia; atividade mental ou imaginação deficiente ou lenta. [hypo- + G. noeō, pensar]

hy·po·nych·i·al (hī'pō - nik'ē - al). Hiponiquial. **1.** SIN subungual. **2.** Relativo ao hiponíquio.

hy·po·nych·i·um (hī'pō - nik'ē - um) [TA]. Hiponíquio; epitélio do leito ungueal, particularmente sua parte proximal na região da raiz da unha e lúnula, formando a matriz ungueal. [hypo- + G. onyx, unha]

hy·pon·y·chon (hī - pon'i - kon). Hiponíquio; hemorragia subungueal. [hypo- + G. onyx, unha]

hy·po·on·cot·ic (hī'pō - on - kot'ik). Hipooncótico; indica uma pressão oncótica abaixo da normal, como, p. ex., do plasma sanguíneo.

hy·po·or·tho·cy·to·sis (hī'pō - ōr'thō - sī - tō'sis). Hiportocitose; leucopenia em que o número relativo dos vários tipos de leucócitos situa-se dentro da faixa normal, não havendo nenhuma célula imatura no sangue circulante. [hypo- + G. orthos, correto + kytos, célula, + -osis, condição]

hy·po·var·i·an·ism (hī'pō - ō - vā'rē - an - izm). Hipovarianismo; função ovariana inadequada, referindo-se comumente à secreção diminuída de hormônios ovarianos. SIN hypovarianism.

hy·po·pan·cre·a·tism (hī'pō - pan'krē - a - tizm). Hipopancreatismo; condição de atividade diminuída da secreção de enzimas digestivas pelo pâncreas.

hy·po·pan·cre·or·rhea (hī'pō - pan'krē - ō - rē - a). Hipopancreorréia; liberação reduzida de secreções enzimáticas digestivas do pâncreas. [hypo- + pâncreas + G. rhoia, fluxo]

hy·po·par·a·thy·roid·ism (hī'pō - par - a - thī'royd - izm). Hipoparatireoidismo; condição causada pela redução ou ausência da secreção de hormônios paratireóideos, com baixos níveis séricos de cálcio e tetania e, algumas vezes, com aumento da densidade óssea. VER TAMBÉM pseudohypoparathyroidism. SIN parathyroid insufficiency.
familial h., h. familiar; hipoparatireoidismo isolado hereditário, caracterizado por hipocalcemia, hiperfosfatemia, cataratas, calcificações intracerebrais e tetania; são conhecidas todas as três formas mendelianas de herança (ligada ao sexo, autossômica dominante e autossômica recessiva) [MIM*146200, MIM*241400 e MIM*307700]. A forma autossômica dominante é causada por mutação no gene do hormônio paratireóideo (PTH) no cromossoma 11p, ou do gene do receptor sensor de cálcio (CASR) no cromossoma 3q.

hy·po·pep·sia (hī - pō - pep'sē - a). Hipopesia; comprometimento da digestão, especialmente devido a uma deficiência de pepsina. SIN oligopepsia. [hypo- + G. pepsis, digestão]

hy·po·per·i·stal·sis (hī'pō - per - i - stal'sis). Hipoperistaltismo; peristaltismo reduzido ou inadequado.

hy·po·pha·lan·gism (hī'pō - fa - lan'jizm). Hipofalangismo; ausência congênita de uma ou mais das falanges de um dedo da mão ou do pé.

hy·po·phar·ynx (hī'pō - fa'rinks). Hipofaringe; *termo oficial alternativo para laryngopharynx.

hy·po·pho·ne·sis (hī'pō - fō - nē'sis). Hipofonese; à percussão ou ausculta, som diminuído ou mais fraco do que o habitual. [hypo- + G. phōnēsis, som]

hy·po·pho·nia (hī'pō - fō'nē - a). Hipofonia; voz anormalmente fraca, devido à incoordenação dos músculos relacionados à vocalização. SIN leptophonia, microphonia, microphony. [hypo- + G. phōnē, voz]

hy·po·pho·ria (hī'pō - fō'rē - a). Hipoforia; tendência do eixo visual de um olho a desviar-se para baixo, evitada pela visão binocular. [hypo- + G. phora, movimento]

hy·po·phos·pha·ta·se·mia (hī'pō - fos'fa - tā - sē'mē - a). Hipofosfatasemia. SIN hypophosphatasia.

hy·po·phos·pha·ta·sia (hī′pō-fos′fă-tā′zē-ă). Hipofosfatasia; concentração anormalmente baixa de fosfatase alcalina no sangue circulante. SIN hypophosphatasemia.
   adult h., h. do adulto; caráter autossômico dominante com perda precoce dos dentes, arqueamento e crânio em cobre batido; há evidências de que o defeito básico esteja na fosfatase alcalina hepática.
   childhood h., h. infantil; forma autossômica recessiva relativamente leve de hipofosfatasia; pode ser alélica com a h. congênita.
   congenital h. [MIM*241500]; h. congênita; distúrbio raro associado a baixos níveis de fosfatase alcalina no soro, hiperfosfatúria, hipercalcemia, anormalidades esqueléticas, fraturas patológicas, craniostenose, perda prematura dos dentes e, com freqüência, morte prematura; os olhos podem apresentar esclerótica azul, retração palpebral, ceratopatia em faixa, cataratas, papiledema e atrofia óptica; herança autossômica recessiva, causada pela mutação do gene da fosfatase alcalina hepática (ALPL) no cromossoma 1p.

hy·po·phos·pha·te·mia (hī′pō-fos-fā-tē′mē-ă). Hipofosfatemia; concentrações anormalmente baixas de fosfatos no sangue circulante. Ver também as entradas em *rickets*.

hy·po·phos·pha·tu·ria (hī′pō-fos′fă-too′rē-ă). Hipofosfatúria; excreção urinária diminuída de fosfatos.

hy·po·phos·pho·rous ac·id (hī-pō-fos′fō-rŭs). Ácido hipofosforoso; solução aquosa contendo 31% de HPH_2O_2. Utilizado como agente redutor estabilizante em preparações farmacêuticas.

hy·po·phra·sia (hī′pō-frā′zē-ă). Hipofrasia; lentidão ou deficiência da fala associada a psicose ou lesão cerebral. [hypo- + G. *phrasis,* fala]

hy·po·phy·se·al (hī′pō-fiz′ē-ăl). Hipofisário. SIN hypophysial.

hy·po·phy·sec·to·mize (hī′pof-i-sek′tō-mīz). Hipofisectomizar; remover a hipófise.

hy·poph·y·sec·to·my (hī′pof-i-sek′tō-mē). Hipofisectomia; remoção cirúrgica da hipófise ou glândula pituitária.

hy·po·phys·e·o·priv·ic (hī′pō-fiz′ē-ō-priv′ik). Hipofisoprivo. SIN hypophysiopriv ic.

hy·po·phys·e·o·trop·ic (hī′pō-fiz′ē-ō-trop′ik). Hipofisotrópico. SIN hypophysiotropic.

hy·po·phy·si·al (hī′pō-fiz′ē-ăl). Hipofisário; relativo à hipófise. SIN hypophyseal.

hy·poph·y·sin (hī-pof′i-sin). Hipofisina; extrato aquoso do lobo posterior da hipófise fresca de bovino; contém oxitocina e vasopressina.

hy·po·phys·i·o·priv·ic (hī′pō-fiz′ē-ō-priv′ik). Hipofisoprivo; indica a condição em que a hipófise pode estar funcionalmente inativa ou ausente, como, p. ex., após hipofisectomia. SIN hypophyseoprivic. [hypophysis + G. *privus,* privado de]

hy·po·phys·i·o·trop·ic (hī′pō-fiz′ē-ō-trop′ik). Hipofisiotrópico; refere-se a um hormônio estimulador que atua sobre a hipófise (glândula pituitária). SIN hypophyseotropic.

hy·poph·y·sis (hī-pof′i-sis). Hipófise. SIN pituitary gland. VER TAMBÉM hypothalamus. [G. subcrescimento]
   h. cere'bri, hipófise cerebral. SIN pituitary gland.
   pharyngeal h., h. faríngea; tecido residual, derivado do divertículo hipofisário, que se situa na lâmina própria da nasofaringe; suas células e distribuição são idênticas àquelas da parte distal. SIN pars pharyngea hypophyseos.
   h. sic'ca, h. seca. SIN posterior pituitary.

hy·poph·y·si·tis (hī-pof-i-sī′tis). Hipofisite, inflamação da hipófise.
   lymphocytic h., h. linfocítica; reação linfocítica aguda da hipófise anterior, caracterizada, clinicamente, por sinais e sintomas de insuficiência da hipófise anterior; trata-se, provavelmente, de um distúrbio auto-imune, devido à presença de anticorpos anti-hipofisários no soro. SIN lymphoid h.
   lymphoid h., h. linfóide. SIN lymphocytic h.

hy·po·pi·e·sis (hī′pō-pī-ē′sis). Hipopiese. SIN hypotension (1). [hypo- + G. *piesis,* pressão]
   orthostatic h., h. ortostática. SIN orthostatic hypotension.

hypopigmentation (hī-pō-pig-men-tā′shun). Hipopigmentação; deficiência de melanina cutânea em relação à pele circundante. VER albinism. [hypo- + pigmentação]

hy·po·pi·tu·i·ta·rism (hī′pō-pi-too′i-tă-rizm). Hipopituitarismo; condição devido à atividade diminuída do lobo anterior da hipófise, com secreção inadequada, em graus variáveis, de um ou mais dos hormônios da hipófise anterior.

hy·po·pla·sia (hī′pō-plā′zē-ă). Hipoplasia. **1.** Subdesenvolvimento de um tecido ou órgão, em geral por deficiência no número de células. **2.** Atrofia devido à destruição de alguns dos elementos, e não apenas à redução geral de tamanho. [hypo- + G. *plasis,* modelagem]
   cartilage-hair h. [MIM*250250 & MIM*250460], h. da cartilagem-cabelo; displasia esquelética prevalente entre os Amish, caracterizada por nanismo com membros curtos, cabelos esparsos e de cor clara, defeito imunológico das células T responsável pela suscetibilidade a infecções e achados radiográficos de displasia metafisária. Herança autossômica recessiva, com o gene situado no cromossoma 9p. SIN McKusick metaphyseal dysplasia.
   enamel h., h. do esmalte; distúrbio do desenvolvimento dos dentes caracterizado pela formação deficiente ou defeituosa da matriz do esmalte; pode ser hereditária, como na amelogênese imperfeita, ou adquirida, como a encontrada na fluorose dentária, em infecções localizadas, febres infantis e sífilis congênita.
   focal dermal h. [MIM*305600], h. dérmica focal; herdada como caráter dominante ligado ao X, com letalidade *in utero* para fetos do sexo masculino; caracteriza-se por áreas lineares de atrofia ou hipoplasia dérmica, herniação da gordura devido a defeitos dérmicos e papilomas da mucosa ou da pele; pode estar associada a anomalias digitais, oculares e orais; retardo mental; estriações ósseas. SIN Goltz syndrome.
   optic nerve h., h. do nervo óptico; disco óptico congenitamente pequeno devido a reduzido número de células dos gânglios da retina e, portanto, a reduzido número de axônios; o distúrbio visual pode ser pronunciado. VER de Morsier *syndrome.*
   renal h., h. renal; rim anormalmente pequeno, de morfologia normal, porém com reduzido número de néfrons ou néfrons menores.
   h. of right ventricle, h. do ventrículo direito; falha de desenvolvimento do ventrículo direito, resultando em pouco músculo e muito tecido conjuntivo, em vez do inverso.
   right ventricular h., h. ventricular direita. SIN parchment heart.
   thymic h., h. do timo. SIN DiGeorge *syndrome.*

hy·po·plas·tic (hī′pō-plas′tik). Hipoplásico; relativo a, ou caracterizado por, hipoplasia.

hy·po·pnea (hī-pop′nē-ă). Hiponpéia; respiração mais superficial e/ou mais lenta do que o normal. SIN oligopnea. [hypo- + G. *pnoē,* respiração]

hy·po·po·sia (hī′pō-pō′sē-ă). Hiposia; hipodipsia, primariamente devido à tendência reduzida a ingerir líquido e não à sensação reduzida de sede. [hypo- + G. *posis,* bebida]

hy·po·po·tas·se·mia (hī′pō-pō-ta-sē′mē-ă). Hipopotassemia. SIN hypokalemia.

hy·po·pro·ac·cel·er·i·ne·mia (hī′pō-prō-ak-sel′er-i-nē′mē-ă). Hipoproacelerinemia; concentração anormalmente baixa do fator V da coagulação sanguínea, isto é, pró-acelerina, no sangue circulante.

hy·po·pro·con·ver·ti·ne·mia (hī′pō-prō-kon-ver′ti-nē′mē-ă). Hipoproconvertinemia; concentração anormalmente baixa do fator VII da coagulação sanguínea, isto é, pró-convertina no sangue circulante; deficiência que causa prolongamento quantitativo do tempo de protrombina.

hy·po·pro·tein·e·mia (hī′pō-prō′tē-in-ē′mē-ă, -prō-tēn-). Hipoproteinemia; níveis anormalmente baixos de proteínas totais no plasma sanguíneo circulante.

hy·po·pro·tein·o·sis (hī′pō-prō′tē-in-ō′sis, -prō′tēn-). Hipoproteinose; condição devida a deficiência dietética de proteínas, observada sobretudo em crianças; caracterizada por anorexia, vômitos, retardo do crescimento, anemia e maior suscetibilidade a infecções.

hy·po·pro·throm·bin·e·mia (hī′pō-prō-throm′bin-ē′mē-ă). Hipoprotrombinemia; níveis anormalmente baixos de protrombina no sangue circulante. SIN prothrombinopenia.

hy·pop·ty·a·lism (hī′pō-tī′ă-lizm). Hipoptialismo. SIN hyposalivation. [hypo- + G. *ptyalon,* saliva]

hy·po·py·on (hī-pō′pi-on). Hipópio; presença de leucócitos na câmara anterior do olho. [hypo- + G. *pyon,* pus]
   recurrent h., h. recorrente. SIN Behçet-*syndrome.*

hy·po·re·flex·ia (hī′pō-rē-flek′sē-ă). Hiporreflexia; condição em que os reflexos estão enfraquecidos.

hy·po·ren·i·ne·mia (hī′pō-ren-i-nē′mē-ă). Hiporreninemia; baixos níveis de renina no sangue circulante.

hy·po·ren·i·nem·ic (hī′pō-ren-i-nē′mik). Hiporreninêmico; relativo a, ou caracterizado por, hiporreninemia.

hy·po·ri·bo·fla·vin·o·sis (hī′pō-rī′bō-flā-vi-nō′sis). Hiporriboflavinose; termo mais correto do que o mais comumente utilizado de arriboflavinose, *q.v.*

hy·po·sal·i·va·tion (hī′pō-sal′i-vā′shun). Hipossalivação; salivação reduzida. SIN hypoptyalism.

hy·pos·che·ot·o·my (hī-pos-kē-ot′ō-mē). Hiposqueotomia; incisão ou função numa hidrocele, no seu ponto mais dependente. [hypo- + G. *oscheon,* escroto + *tomē,* incisão]

hy·po·scle·ral (hī-pō-sklēr′ăl). Hipoesclerótico; abaixo da camada esclerótica do globo ocular.

hy·po·sen·si·tiv·i·ty (hī′pō-sen-si-tiv′i-tē). Hipossensibilidade; condição de sensibilidade subnormal, em que a resposta a um estímulo é inusitadamente tardia ou de grau reduzido.

hy·po·sen·si·ti·za·tion. Hipossensibilização. SIN desensitization.

hy·po·ske·o·cy·to·sis (hī′pō-skē′ō-sī-tō′sis). Hipoesqueocitose. SIN hyponeocytosis. [hypo- + *skaios,* esquerda + *kytos,* célula + *-osis,* condição]

hy·pos·mia (hī-poz′mē-ă). Hiposmia; diminuição do sentido do olfato. Pode ser: 1) geral a todos os odorantes, parcial a alguns odorantes ou específica a um ou mais odorantes; 2) devida a distúrbios de transporte (na obstrução nasal) ou sensorineurais (que afetam o neuroepitélio olfatório ou as vias neurais olfatórias centrais); e 3) hereditária ou adquirida. SIN olfactory hypesthesia. [hypo- + G. *osmē,* odor]

hy·pos·mo·sis (hī-pos-mō'sis). Hiposmose; redução na rapidez da osmose.

hy·pos·mot·ic (hī-pos-mot'ik). Hiposmótico; que tem uma osmolalidade menor que a de outro líquido, habitualmente considerado como plasma ou líquido extracelular.

hy·po·so·ma·to·tro·pism (hī'pō-sō'mă-tō-trō'pizm). Hipossomatotropismo; estado caracterizado pela secreção deficiente de hormônio do crescimento (somatotropina) pela hipófise.

hy·po·so·mi·a (hī'pō-sō'mē-ă). Hipossomia; desenvolvimento inadequado do corpo. [hypo- + G. *sōma,* corpo]

hy·po·som·ni·ac (hī'pō-som'nē-ak). Hipossoníaco; indivíduo com redução do tempo de sono. [hypo- + L. *somnus,* sono]

hy·po·spa·di·ac (hī'pō-spā'dē-ak). Hipospadíaco; relativo a hipospádias.

hy·po·spa·di·as (hī'pō-spā'dē-ăs). Hipospádia; anomalia de desenvolvimento caracterizada por um defeito na superfície ventral do pênis, de modo que o meato uretral se situa proximalmente à sua localização normal; pode estar associada a cordas; refere-se também a um defeito semelhante na mulher em que a uretra se abre na vagina. Cf. epispadias. SIN urogenital sinus anomaly. [hypo- + G. *spaō,* rasgar ou abrir canal]

  balanic h., h. balânica. SIN glandular h.
  coronal h., h. coronal; posição ventral e proximal incorreta do meato no sulco coronal.
  glanular h., h. glanular; posição glanular ventral e proximal incorreta do meato uretral no sexo masculino. SIN balanic h.
  penile h., h. peniana; posição incorreta do meato uretral no corpo peniano ventral.
  penoscrotal h., h. peniana escrotal; posição incorreta do orifício uretral na junção do pênis com o escroto.
  perineal h., h. perineal; hipospádia em que o meato uretral se abre no períneo, próximo ao ânus; o escroto habitualmente está fendido.
  scrotal h., h. escrotal; hipospádia com orifício uretral na superfície do escroto.
  subcoronal h., h. subcoronal; posição incorreta do meato no sulco coronal.

hy·po·sphyg·mia (hī'pō-sfig'mē-ă). Hiposfigmia; pressão arterial anormalmente baixa, com lentidão da circulação. [hypo- + G. *sphyxis,* pulso]

hy·po·splen·ism (hī'pō-splen'izm). Hipoesplenismo; ausência ou redução da função esplênica, geralmente devido a remoção cirúrgica, aplasia congênita, substituição por tumor ou acidente vascular esplênico. É comum a existência de anormalidades eritrocitárias, como inclusões, eritrócitos nucleados e células em alvo. Os pacientes com hipoesplenismo correm risco aumentado de sépsis bacteriana, especialmente por pneumococos.

hy·pos·ta·sis (hi-pos'tă-sis). Hipóstase. **1.** Formação de sedimento no fundo de um líquido. **2.** SIN hypostatic *congestion.* **3.** Fenômeno pelo qual o fenótipo que normalmente se manifestaria em um *locus* é obscurecido pelo genótipo em outro *locus* epistático; p. ex., nos seres humanos, o fenótipo para o *locus* do grupo sanguíneo ABO só pode ser expresso na presença de seu precursor, a substância H. O fator Bombay no estado homozigoto bloqueia a formação da substância H e obscurece o fenótipo ABO. [G. *hypo-stasis,* permanecer sob, sedimento]

  postmortem h., h. *post-mortem.* SIN postmortem *livedo.*
  pulmonary h., h. pulmonar; congestão hidrostática do pulmão.

hy·po·stat·ic (hī-pō-stat'ik). Hipostático. **1.** Sedimentar; resultante de posição em declive. **2.** Relativo a hipóstase.

hy·pos·the·nu·ri·a (hī'pos-the-noo're-ă). Hipostenúria; excreção de urina de baixa densidade; devido à incapacidade dos túbulos renais de produzir uma urina concentrada; ocorre também após a ingestão excessiva de água no diabetes insípido. [hypo- + G. *sthenos,* força + *ouron,* urina]

hy·po·stome (hī'pō-stōm). Hipóstomo; órgão central ímpar, em forma de gancho, do capítulo do carrapato; o hipóstomo é coberto por espinhos recurvados que o tornam capaz de servir de gancho de ancoragem enquanto o carrapato se alimenta. [hypo- + G. *stoma,* boca]

hy·po·sto·mia (hī'pō-stō'mē-ă). Hipostomia; forma de microstomia em que a abertura oral consiste numa pequena fenda vertical. [hypo- + G. *stoma,* boca]

hyp·os·to·sis (hīp-os-tō'sis). Hipostose; desenvolvimento deficiente do osso. [hypo- + G. *osteon,* osso + *-osis,* condição]

hy·po·supra·dren·al·ism (hī'pō-soo'pra-ă-drē'nal-izm). Hipossuprarenalismo. SIN chronic adrenocortical *insufficiency.*

hy·po·sys·to·le (hī'pō-sis'tō-lē). Hipossístole; sístole cardíaca fraca ou incompleta.

hy·po·tel·or·ism (hī-pō-tel'or-izm). Hipotelorismo; aproximação anormal dos olhos. [hypo- + G. *tēle,* longe + *horizō,* separar, fr. *horos,* limite]

hy·po·ten·sion (hī'pō-ten'shun). Hipotensão. **1.** Pressão arterial subnormal. SIN hypopiesis. **2.** Redução da pressão ou tensão de qualquer tipo. [hypo- + L. *tensio,* estiramento]

  arterial h., h. arterial. VER hypotension (1).
  idiopathic orthostatic h., h. ortostática idiopática; tendência da pressão arterial a cair, por razões desconhecidas, ao assumir a posição ortostática.
  induced h., controlled h., h. induzida, h. controlada; redução aguda deliberada da pressão arterial, a fim de reduzir a perda sanguínea operatória, por meios farmacológicos, durante a anestesia e a cirurgia.
  intracranial h., h. intracraniana; pressão subnormal do líquido cefalorraquidiano; ocorre, mais comumente, após punção lombar e está associada a cefaléia, náuseas, vômitos, rigidez de nuca e, algumas vezes, febre; pode resultar também de desidratação.
  orthostatic h., h. ortostática; forma de pressão arterial baixa que ocorre na posição ortostática. SIN orthostatic hypopiesis, postural h.
  postural h., h. postural. SIN orthostatic h.

hy·po·ten·sive (hī'pō-ten'siv). Hipotensivo; caracterizado por pressão arterial baixa ou que provoca redução da pressão arterial.

hy·po·ten·sor (hī-pō-ten'ser, -sōr). Hipotensor. SIN depressor (4).

hy·po·thal·a·mo·hy·po·phy·si·al (hī'pō-thal'ă-mō-hī'pō-fiz'ē-ăl). Hipotálamo-hipofisário; relativo ao hipotálamo e à hipófise.

hy·po·thal·a·mus (hī'pō-thal'ă-mŭs). Hipotálamo; a região ventral e medial do diencéfalo que forma as paredes da metade ventral do terceiro ventrículo; delineado a partir do tálamo do sulco hipotalâmico, situado medialmente à cápsula interna e subtálamo, em continuidade com o septo pré-comissural, na parte anterior, e com o tegmento mesencefálico da substância cinzenta central, na parte posterior. Sua superfície ventral caracteriza-se, de diante para trás, pelo quiasma óptico, pelo infundíbulo ímpar, que se estende, por meio do pedículo infundibular, até o lobo posterior da hipófise, e pelos corpos mamilares pares. O hipotálamo consiste na área hipotalâmica anterior [TA], área hipotalâmica dorsal [TA], área hipotalâmica intermediária [TA], área hipotalâmica lateral [TA] e área hipotalâmica posterior [TA], contendo, cada uma delas, núcleos específicos. Possui conexões de fibras aferentes com o mesencéfalo, sistema límbico, cerebelo, e conexões de fibras eferentes com as mesmas estruturas e com o lobo posterior da hipófise; sua conexão funcional com o lobo anterior da hipófise é estabelecida pelo sistema porta hipotálamo-hipofisário. O hipotálamo está proeminentemente envolvido nas funções do sistema nervoso autônomo (motor visceral) e, através de sua ligação vascular, com o lobo anterior da hipófise, nos mecanismos endócrinos; além disso, parece participar nos mecanismos neurais subjacentes aos estados de humor e motivação. VER TAMBÉM pituitary *gland.* [hypo- + thalamus]

hy·po·the·nar (hī'pō-thē'nar, hī-poth'ē-nar) [TA]. Hipotenar. **1.** [NA]. SIN hypothenar *eminence.* **2.** Indica qualquer estrutura em relação à eminência hipotenar ou seus componentes coletivos subjacentes. [hypo- + G. *thenar,* palma]

hy·po·ther·mal (hī-pō-ther'măl). Hipotérmico; relativo a hipotermia.

hy·po·ther·mia (hī'pō-ther'mē-ă). Hipotermia; temperatura corporal significativamente abaixo de 37°C. [hypo- + G. *thermē,* calor]

  accidental h., h. acidental; diminuição não-intencional da temperatura corporal, especialmente no recém-nascido, em lactentes e indivíduos idosos, sobretudo durante operações.

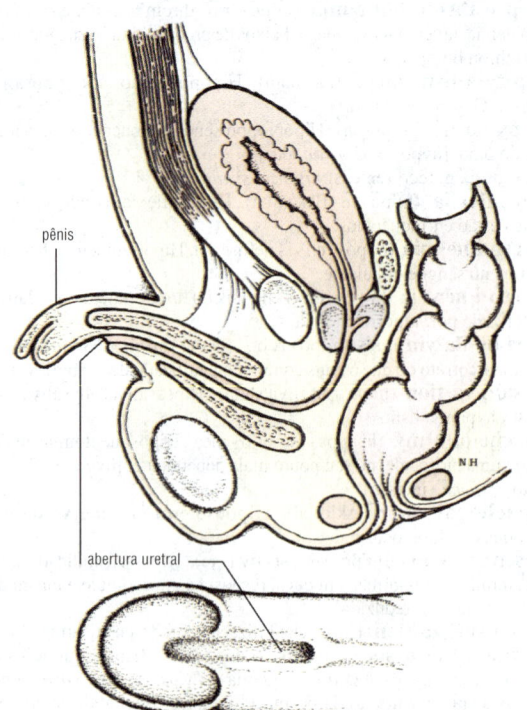

hipospádia: (em cima) vista mediossagital, (embaixo) vista ventral do pênis

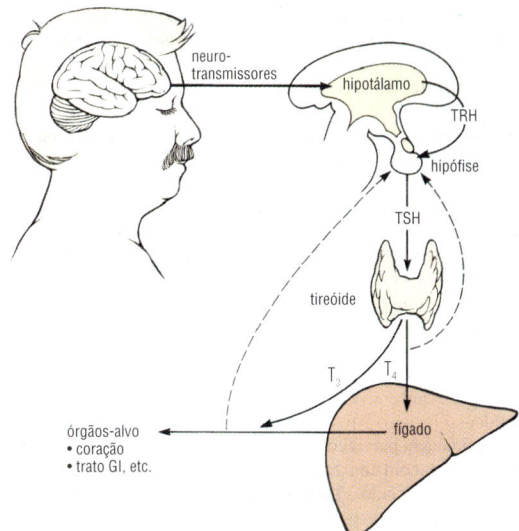

eixo hipotálamo–hipófise–tireóide: o hormônio liberador do hormônio tireóideo (TRH) do hipotálamo estimula a hipófise a secretar o hormônio tireoestimulante (TSH). O TSH atua na produção de hormônio tireóideo (T_3 e T_4). Os níveis circulantes elevados de T_3 e T_4 inibem a secreção adicional de TSH e a produção de hormônios tireóideos através de um mecanismo de retroalimentação negativa (linhas tracejadas).

moderate h., h. moderada; temperatura corporal de 23–32°C, induzida por resfriamento superficial.
profound h., h. profunda; temperatura corporal de 12–20°C.
regional h., h. regional; redução da temperatura de uma extremidade ou órgão pelo frio externo ou por perfusão com sangue ou soluções frios.
total body h., h. corporal total; redução deliberada da temperatura corporal total, a fim de reduzir o metabolismo tecidual.
hy·poth·e·sis (hī-poth′ē-sis). Hipótese; suposição emitida para fins heurísticos, expressa numa forma acessível a confirmação ou refutação através da realização de experimentos definíveis e organização crítica de dados empíricos; não deve ser confundida com suposição, postulação ou especulação não focada. VER TAMBÉM postulate, theory. [G. fundação, pressuposição fr. *hypotithenai,* formular]
adaptor h., h. do adaptador; hipótese proposta por F.H.C. Crick, segundo a qual deve existir uma molécula adaptadora entre o DNA contendo a informação e a proteína que está sendo sintetizada.
alternative h., h. alternativa; no teste de Neyman-Pearson de uma hipótese, refere-se à hipótese ou conjunto de hipóteses acerca do valor numérico de um parâmetro se, e apenas se, a hipótese nula for rejeitada como insustentável.
autocrine h., h. autócrina; hipótese de que as células tumorais que contêm oncogenes virais podem ter codificado um fator de crescimento, normalmente produzido por outros tipos celulares e, dessa maneira, produzir o fator de modo autônomo, resultando em proliferação descontrolada.
Avogadro h., h. de Avogadro. SIN Avogadro *law.*
Bayesian h., conjunto de supostos valores de um parâmetro a serem explorados individualmente à luz de um conjunto atual de dados, sendo preservada simetria lógica acima de tudo. Os méritos de cada hipótese aventada baseiam-se em quantidade, a probabilidade prévia. A probabilidade dos dados condicionais sobre a hipótese é computada como probabilidade condicionada para cada uma; o produto das duas para cada hipótese é a probabilidade conjunta, e a relação de cada probabilidade conjunta com a soma de todas as probabilidades conjuntas é a probabilidade posterior dessa hipótese. Ao contrário do teste de Neyman-Pearson para hipóteses, a resposta é uma declaração sobre a hipótese, não sobre a mesma condicional sobre a hipótese. Nenhuma hipótese é preferida ou prevalece à revelia. O procedimento pode ser aplicado repetidamente por qualquer número de vezes, à medida que forem surgindo dados disponíveis.
frustration-aggression h., h. de frustração-agressão; teoria de que a frustração pode levar à agressão, mas que a agressão é sempre o resultado de alguma forma de frustração.
gate-control h., h. de controle do portão. SIN gate-control *theory.*
Goldie-Coldman h., h. de Goldie-Coldman; modelo matemático que prevê a mutação de células tumorais num fenótipo resistente, cuja taxa depende de sua instabilidade genética intrínseca. A probabilidade de que um câncer contenha clones resistentes a drogas depende da taxa de mutação e do tamanho do tumor. De acordo com essa hipótese, até mesmo os menores cânceres detectá-

veis devem conter pelo menos um clone fármaco-resistente; por conseguinte, a melhor chance de cura seria utilizar todos os agentes quimioterápicos efetivos; na prática, isso significa utilizar dois esquemas diferentes de quimioterapia sem resistência cruzada em ciclos alternados.
Gompertz h., h. de Gompertz; teoria segundo a qual a força de mortalidade aumenta em progressão geométrica, baseando-se na suposição de que a exaustão média da capacidade de um indivíduo de evitar a morte é tal que, no final de intervalos de tempo iguais e infinitamente pequenos, as perdas individuais são iguais às proporções da capacidade de opor-se à destruição disponível no início de cada um desses intervalos.
insular h., h. insular; teoria obsoleta da origem do diabetes melito a partir da destruição ou perda de função das ilhotas de Langerhans no pâncreas.
Knudsen h., h. de Knudsen; explicação para a ocorrência bilateral (e mais precoce) do retinoblastoma hereditário; se houver mutação de um gene supressor tumoral por herança, é necessária apenas uma mutação somática para inativar o outro alelo. Na forma esporádica, são necessárias duas mutações que inativam cada alelo.
Lyon h., h. de Lyon. SIN lyonization.
Makeham h., h. de Makeham; desenvolvimento da hipótese de Gompertz quanto à força da mortalidade seguindo alguma lei matemática. Makeham propôs que a morte é a conseqüência de duas causas geralmente coexistentes: 1) chance; 2) deterioração ou maior incapacidade de enfrentar a destruição. A primeira delas é constante, a segunda, uma progressão geométrica crescente.
Michaelis-Menten h., h. de Michaelis-Menten; hipótese de que um complexo se forma entre uma enzima e seu substrato (também conhecida como h. de O'Sullivan-Tompson), com decomposição subseqüente do complexo, produzindo a enzima livre e produtos da reação (também descrita como h. de Brown), sendo esta última etapa a que determina a velocidade para a taxa global de conversão do substrato em produto. VER TAMBÉM Michaelis-Menten *constant,* Michaelis-Menten *equation.*
mnemic h., h. mnemônica; a teoria segundo a qual os estímulos ou irritantes deixam traços definidos (em gramas) no protoplasma do animal; quando esses estímulos são regularmente repetidos, induzem um hábito que persiste mesmo após a cessação dos estímulos. SIN mnemic theory, mnemism, Semon-Hering theory.
monoamine h., h. da monoamina; a teoria clássica da base neuroquímica da depressão, ligando-a a uma deficiência de, pelo menos, um dos três neurotransmissores monoamínicos: noradrenalina, serotonina ou dopamina.
Neyman-Pearson statistical h., h. estatística de Neyman-Pearson; conjectura formal acerca do valor numérico de um parâmetro a ser testado exclusivamente à luz de um conjunto imediato de dados, sem qualquer atenção para conhecimentos ou convicções anteriores e ignorando outros conjuntos de evidências tratados de forma semelhante. A resposta é uma afirmativa não sobre a veracidade da hipótese, mas se esta fornece uma explicação aceitável dos dados ou deve ser rejeitada a favor de outra hipótese.
Norton-Simon h., h. de Norton-Simon; hipótese de que um tumor é constituído de populações de células de crescimento mais rápido, que são sensíveis à terapia, e de células mais resistentes e de crescimento mais lento. Como apenas a terapia que erradica por completo todas as células tumorais é curativa, isso tem mais probabilidade de ser alcançado com esquemas seqüenciais sem resistência cruzada. O esquema inicial tem de ser efetivo o suficiente para resultar numa baixa carga tumoral residual, sendo seguido de um ou mais tratamentos sem resistência cruzada para erradicar o restante do câncer.
null h., h. nula; hipótese estatística de que uma variável não tem nenhuma associação com outra variável ou conjunto de variáveis ou de que duas ou mais populações não diferem entre si; a afirmativa de que os resultados não diferem daqueles esperados pela atuação exclusiva da casualidade; se for rejeitada, aumenta a confiabilidade da hipótese.
sequence h., h. da seqüência; hipótese segundo a qual a seqüência de aminoácidos de uma proteína é determinada por uma seqüência particular de nucleotídeos (o cistron) no DNA do organismo que está produzindo a proteína.
sliding filament h., h. do filamento deslizante; teoria de que a contração muscular encurta o músculo devido ao deslizamento de dois conjuntos de filamentos um sobre o outro.
Starling h., h. de Starling; o princípio de que a filtração efetiva através das membranas capilares é proporcional à diferença da pressão hidrostática transmembrana menos a diferença da pressão oncótica transmembrana; apesar de bem estabelecida, é denominada h. de Starling para distingui-la da lei de Starling do coração.
upregulation/downregulation h., h. da regulação de incremento/regulação de decremento; teoria da base neuroquímica da depressão (uma elaboração da h. da monoamina) associando-a a um aumento no número (regulação de incremento) de receptores pós-sinápticos de monoamina, cujo número é então efetivamente diminuído (regulação de decremento) em decorrência da atividade antidepressora. VER TAMBÉM monoamine h.
wobble h., h. da oscilação. VER wobble *base,* oscilação.
zwitter h., h. do *zwitter;* hipótese segundo a qual uma molécula anfotérica (p. ex., um aminoácido) tem, em seu ponto isoelétrico, número igual de cargas elétricas positivas e negativas, tornando-se, assim, um *zwitterion.*

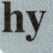

hy·po·throm·bi·ne·mia (hī′pō - throm - bin - ē′mē - ā). Hipotrombinemia; níveis anormalmente baixos de trombina no sangue circulante, resultando em tendência hemorrágica.

hy·po·throm·bo·plas·ti·ne·mia (hī′pō - throm′bō - plas - ti - nē′mē - ā). Hipotromboplastinemia; níveis anormalmente baixos de tromboplastina no sangue, em consequência da liberação de quantidades deficientes dos tecidos.

hy·po·thy·mia (hī′pō - thī′mē - ā). Hipotimia; depressão de ânimo; tristeza, melancolia. [hypo- + G. *thymos*, mente, alma]

hy·po·thy·mic (hī - pō - thē′mik). Hipotímico; relativo a, ou caracterizado por, hipotimia.

hy·po·thy·mism (hī′pō - thī′mizm). Hipotimismo; termo obsoleto para referir-se à função inadequada do timo.

hy·po·thy·roid (hī′pō - thī′royd). Hipotireóideo; caracterizado por redução da função da tireóide.

hy·po·thy·roid·ism (hī′pō - thī′royd - izm). Hipotireoidismo; produção diminuída de hormônio tireóideo; resulta em manifestações clínicas de insuficiência da tireóide, incluindo baixa taxa metabólica, tendência a ganhar peso, sonolência e, algumas vezes, mixedema. SIN athyrea (1). [hypo- + G. *thyreoeidés*, tireóide]
  congenital h., h. congênito; ausência de secreção da tireóide. VER infantile h.
  infantile h., h. infantil; pode ser devido a bócio congênito endêmico; os casos não-endêmicos são habitualmente devidos a embriogênese defeituosa da tireóide, função hipotálamo-hipofisária deficiente, defeitos congênitos na síntese ou na ação dos hormônios tireóideos ou exposição intra-uterina a agentes bociogênicos. SIN Brissaud infantilism, congenital myxedema, dysthyroidal infantilism, hypothyroid dwarfism, hypothyroid infantilism, infantile myxedema, myxedematous infantilism.
  secondary h., h. secundário; hipotireoidismo que surge em decorrência da secreção inadequada de tireotropina pela hipófise anterior.

hy·po·thy·rox·i·ne·mia (hī′pō - thī - rok - sin - ē′mē - ā). Hipotiroxinemia; concentração subnormal de tiroxina no sangue.

hy·po·to·nia (hī′pō - tō′nē - ā). Hipotonia. **1.** Tensão reduzida em qualquer parte, como no globo ocular. **2.** Relaxamento das artérias. **3.** Condição em que existe diminuição ou perda da tonicidade muscular. SIN hypotonicity (1), hypotonus, hypotony. [hypo- + G. *tonos*, tônus]
  benign congenital h., h. congênita benigna; hipotonia não-progressiva de etiologia desconhecida em lactentes e crianças; devem ser excluídas outras causas conhecidas de hipotonia.

hy·po·ton·ic (hī - pō - ton′ik). Hipotônico. **1.** Que apresenta grau menor de tensão. **2.** Que possui pressão osmótica menor do que uma solução de referência, que habitualmente é considerada o plasma sanguíneo ou líquido intersticial; mais especificamente, refere-se a um líquido no qual as células devem inchar. SIN hypoisotonic.

hy·po·to·nic·i·ty (hī′pō - tō - nis′i - tē). Hipotonicidade. **1.** SIN hypotonia. **2.** Diminuição da pressão osmótica efetiva.

hy·po·to·nus, hy·pot·o·ny (hī′pō - tō′nŭs, hī - pot′ō - nē). Hipotonia. SIN hypotonia.

hy·po·tri·chi·a·sis (hī′pō - tri - kī′a - sis). Hipotriquíase. **1.** Hypotrichosis. **2.** SIN *alopecia* congenitalis. [hypo- + G. *trichiasis*, pilosidade]

hy·po·tri·cho·sis (hī′pō - tri - kō′sis). Hipotricose; quantidade de cabelos ou pêlos menor do que o normal na cabeça e/ou corpo. SIN hypotrichiasis (1), oligotrichia, oligotrichosis. [hypo- + G. *trichōsis*, pilosidade]

hy·po·tro·pia (hī - pō - trōp′pē - ā). Hipotropia; desvio ocular em que um olho é mais baixo do que o outro. [hypo- + G. *tropē*, volta]

hy·po·tym·pa·not·o·my (hī′pō - tim - pā - not′ō - mē). Hipotimpanotomia; procedimento cirúrgico para excisão, sem sacrifício da audição, de pequenos tumores limitados à porção inferior da cavidade timpânica. [hypo- + G. *tympanon*, tímpano + *tomē*, incisão]

hy·po·tym·pa·num (hī′pō - tim′pā - nŭm). Hipotímpano; parte inferior da cavidade timpânica. É separada do bulbo jugular por uma parede óssea.

hy·po·u·re·sis (hī′pō - ū - rē′sis). Hipourese; redução do fluxo de urina.

hy·po·u·ri·ce·mia (hī′pō - ū - ri - sē′mē - ā). Hipouricemia; concentração sanguínea reduzida de ácido úrico.

hy·po·u·ri·cu·ria (hī′pō - ū′ri - kū′rē - ā). Hipouricúria; excreção reduzida de ácido úrico na urina.
  hereditary renal h., h. renal hereditária; distúrbio autossômico recessivo causado por reabsorção deficiente de urato no túbulo proximal renal.

hy·po·var·i·an·ism (hī′pō - vā′rē - an - izm). Hipovarianismo. SIN hypoovarianism.

hy·po·ven·ti·la·tion (hī′pō - ven - ti - lā′shŭn). Hipoventilação; redução da ventilação alveolar em relação à produção metabólica de dióxido de carbono, de modo que a pressão alveolar de dióxido de carbono se eleva acima do normal. SIN underventilation.

hy·po·vi·ta·min·o·sis (hī′pō - vī′ta - min - ō′sis). Hipovitaminose; estado de deficiência nutricional caracterizado pela insuficiência relativa de uma ou mais vitaminas na dieta; manifesta-se inicialmente por depleção dos níveis teciduais, a seguir, por alterações funcionais e, por fim, pelo aparecimento de lesões morfológicas. Cf. avitaminosis.

hy·po·vo·le·mia (hī′pō - vō - lē′mē - ā). Hipovolemia; volume diminuído de sangue no corpo. SIN hyphemia. [hypo- + L. *volumen*, volume + G. *haima*, sangue]

hy·po·vo·le·mic (hī′pō - vō - lē′mik). Hipovolêmico; relativo a, ou caracterizado por, hipovolemia.

hy·po·vo·lia (hī - pō - vō′lē - ā). Hipovolia; conteúdo de água ou volume diminuído de determinado compartimento; p. ex., hipovolia extracelular. [hypo- + L. *volumen*, volume]

hy·po·xan·thine (Hyp) (hī - pō - zan′thin). Hipoxantina; 6-oxipurina; purina-6(1*H*)-ona; purina existente nos músculos e em outros tecidos, formada durante o catabolismo da purina por desaminação da adenina; elevada na deficiência do co-fator molibdênio. SIN 6-hydroxypurine.
  h. guanine phosphoribosyltransferase (HGPRT), h. guanina fosforribosiltransferase (HGPRT). SIN *h. phosphoribosyltransferase.*
  h. oxidase, h. oxidase. SIN *xanthine* oxidase.
  h. phosphoribosyltransferase, h. fosforribosiltransferase; enzima presente no tecido humano e que converte a hipoxantina e a guanina em seus respectivos 5′nucleotídeos, em que o 5-fosforribose 1-difosfato atua como doador de ribose-fosfato; a deficiência parcial dessa enzima pode resultar em aumento da biossíntese de purinas, com consequente desenvolvimento de gota; outro nível de deficiência está associado à síndrome de Lesch-Nyhan. SIN h. guanine phosphoribosyltransferase.

hy·po·xan·thin·o·sine (hī′pō - zan - thēn′ō - sēn). Hipoxantinosina. SIN *inosine.*

hy·pox·e·mia (hī - pok - sē′mē - ā). Hipoxemia; oxigenação subnormal do sangue arterial, à exceção da anoxia. [hypo- + oxigênio + G. *haima*, sangue]

hy·pox·ia (hī - pok′sē - ā). Hipoxia; diminuição do oxigênio abaixo dos níveis normais nos gases inspirados, no sangue arterial ou no tecido, à exceção da anoxia. [hypo- + oxigênio]
  anemic h., h. anêmica; hipoxia resultante de concentração diminuída de hemoglobina funcional ou de um número reduzido de eritrócitos; é causada por hemorragia ou anemia de vários tipos ou por intoxicação com monóxido de carbono, nitritos ou cloratos.
  diffusion h., h. de difusão; diminuição transitória abrupta na tensão de oxigênio alveolar quando o ar ambiente é inalado na conclusão de uma anestesia com óxido nitroso, visto que o óxido nitroso que se difunde do sangue dilui o oxigênio alveolar.
  hypoxic h., h. hipóxica; hipoxia resultante de um mecanismo defeituoso de oxigenação nos pulmões; pode ser causada por baixa tensão de oxigênio, função pulmonar anormal ou obstrução respiratória ou por derivação da direita para a esquerda do coração.
  ischemic h., h. isquêmica; hipoxia tecidual caracterizada por oligoemia dos tecidos e causada por obstrução ou vasoconstrição arterial ou arteriolar.
  oxygen affinity h., h. por afinidade de oxigênio; hipoxia devido a uma capacidade reduzida da hemoglobina de liberar oxigênio.
  stagnant h., h. estagnante; hipoxia tecidual caracterizada não por oligoemia do tecido (estando o volume de sangue decidual normal ou até mesmo aumentado), mas pela estase intravascular em consequência de comprometimento do fluxo venoso ou (em alguns casos) diminuição do fluxo arterial.

hy·pox·ic (hī - pok′sik). Hipóxico; relativo a, ou caracterizado por, hipoxia.

hyp·sa·rhyth·mia, hyp·sar·rhyth·mia (hip′sā - rith′mē - ā). Hipsarritmia; eletroencefalograma anormal e tipicamente caótico que costuma ser encontrado em pacientes com espasmos infantis. [G. *hypsi*, alto + *a*- priv. + *rhythmos*, ritmo]

hypsi-, hypso-. Hipsi-, hipso-. Alto, altura. [G. *hypsos*, altura]

hyp·si·brach·y·ce·phal·ic (hip - sē - brak′ē - sē - fal′ik). Hipsobraquicefálico; que possui uma cabeça alta e larga. [hypsi- + G. *brachys*, largo + *kephalē*, cabeça]

hyp·si·ceph·a·ly (hip - si - sef′a - lē). Hipsocefalia. SIN *oxycephaly.* [hypsi- + G. *kephalē*, cabeça]

hyp·si·con·chous (hip - si - kon′kŭs). Hipsoconcho; que possui uma órbita alta, com índice orbitário > 85. [hypsi- + G. *konchos*, concha, parte superior do crânio]

hyp·si·loid (hip′si - loyd). Hipsilóide, ipsilóide; em forma de Y; em forma de U. SIN upsiloid, ypsiliform. [G. *upsilon (ypsilon)*]

hyp·si·sta·phyl·ia (hip′si - stā - fil′ē - ā). Hipsistafilia; condição em que o palato é alto e estreito. [hypsi- + G. *staphylē*, úvula]

hyp·si·sten·o·ce·phal·ic (hip - si - sten′ō - sē - fal′ik). Hipsistenocefálico; que tem a cabeça alta e estreita. [hypsi- + G. *stenos*, estreito + *kephalē*, cabeça]

hypso-. Hipso-. VER hypsi-.

hyp·so·ceph·a·ly (hip - sō - sef′a - lē). Hipsocefalia. SIN *oxycephaly.* [hypso- + G. *kephalē*, cabeça]

hyp·so·chro·mic (hip - sō - krōm′ik). Hipsocrômico; refere-se ao desvio de um espectro de absorção máximo para um comprimento de onda mais curto (maior energia). [hypso- + G. *chroma*, cor]

hyp·so·dont (hip′sō - dont). Hipsodonte; que possui dentes longos. [hypso- + G. *odous*, dente]

hy·pur·gia (hī - per′jē - ā). Hipurgia; termo raramente utilizado para qualquer fator menor capaz de modificar a evolução de uma doença para uma melhora

sinais e sintomas de hipoxia sistêmica			
órgão/função	leve	moderada	grave
mental	euforia, desorientação	distúrbios visuais, ansiedade	tonteira, delírio, coma
trato gastrointestinal	náusea	ânsia de vômito	vômito
sintomas subjetivos	cefaléia	dor precordial	
respiração	aumento da freqüência e profundidade	apnéia após a administração de O_2	deprimida, irregular, respiração de Cheyne-Stokes, apnéia
pressão arterial	discreta elevação (sistólica e diastólica)	elevação	queda abrupta
pulso	rápido, tornando-se irregular	lento, alternante, irregular	muito fraco, irregular, falhando
sistema muscular	incoordenação	espasmos, rigidez, convulsões	fraqueza, paralisia
pele			
com Hb normal	cianótica (dependendo da Hb) quente, úmida	intensamente cianótica, quente, úmida	intensamente cianótica, fria e úmida
na anemia	azulada, seca	cinza-ardósia, úmida a diaforética	cinzenta, fria e úmida
pupilas	irregulares	dilatadas	dilatadas ao máximo e fixas
pressão venosa central	discreta elevação	acentuada elevação	queda

ou piora, especialmente a primeira. [G. *hypourgia*, ajuda, serviço, fr. *hypo*, + *ergon*, trabalho]

Hyrtl, Joseph, anatomista austríaco, 1811–1894. VER H. *anastomosis, foramen, loop,* epitympanic *recess, sphincter.*

hyster-. Hister-. VER hystero-.

hys·ter·al·gia (his′ter-al′jē-ă). Histeralgia; dor no útero. SIN hysterodynia, metrodynia. [hystero- + G. *algos,* dor]

hys·ter·a·tre·sia (his′ter-ă-trē′zē-ă). Histeratresia; atresia da cavidade uterina, geralmente em decorrência de aderências endocervicais inflamatórias.

hys·ter·ec·to·my (his-ter-ek′tō-mē). Histerectomia; remoção do útero; salvo especificação em contrário, indica habitualmente a remoção do útero (corpo e colo). [hystero- + G. *ektomē,* excisão]
   abdominal h., h. abdominal; remoção do útero através de uma incisão na parede abdominal. SIN abdominohysterectomy.
   abdominovaginal h., h. abdominovaginal; abordagem cirúrgica vaginal e abdominal combinada que permite a remoção parcial ou completa da vagina, vulva, reto e períneo (via de acesso abdominoperineal), bem como dos órgãos pélvicos; em geral, efetuada em casos de câncer pélvico avançado.
   cesarean h., h. com cesariana; cesariana seguida de histerectomia. SIN Porro h.
   laparoscopic-assisted vaginal h., h. vaginal assistida por laparoscopia; histerectomia vaginal em que o pedículo ovariano, o ligamento largo e os ligamentos uterossacrais são cirurgicamente excisados utilizando instrumentos laparoscópicos, sendo o procedimento concluído através de colpotomia efetuada de modo habitual.
   modified radical h., h. radical modificada; histerectomia ampla em que uma porção da vagina superior é removida; os ureteres são expostos e puxados para baixo lateralmente, sem dissecção do leito ureteral. SIN TeLinde operation.
   Porro h., h. de Porro. SIN cesarean h.
   radical h., h. radical; remoção completa do útero, da porção superior da vagina e paramétrio.
   subtotal h., h. subtotal. SIN supracervical h.
   supracervical h., h. supracervical; remoção do fundo do útero, deixando o colo *in situ.* SIN subtotal h.
   vaginal h., h. vaginal; remoção do útero através da vagina, sem qualquer incisão da parede do abdome. SIN colpohysterectomy, vaginohysterectomy.

hys·ter·e·sis (his-ter-ē′sis). Histerese. **1.** Incapacidade de um de dois fenômenos relacionados de acompanhar o ritmo do outro, ou qualquer situação em que o valor de um depende do aumento ou da redução do outro. **2.** Atraso de um efeito magnético em relação à sua causa. SIN magnetic inertia. **3.** Temperatura diferencial que existe quando uma substância, como hidrocolóide reversível, funde-se numa temperatura e solidifica-se em outra. **4.** Base de um tipo de cooperatividade observada em muitas reações catalisadas por enzimas, em que o grau de cooperatividade está associado a uma alteração lenta da configuração da enzima. Cf. allosterism, cooperativity. [G. *hysterēsis,* que chega mais tarde]
   static h., h. estática; diferença do valor atingido por uma variável dependente num valor constante particular da variável independente, dependendo da aproximação deste último valor para cima ou para baixo; p. ex., na medida das relações de pressão–volume dos pulmões, se o indivíduo expirar por completo e, a seguir, inspirar um determinado volume, mantendo-o constante, a pressão transpulmonar necessária para manter esse volume pulmonar será maior do que se tivesse inspirado por completo e, a seguir, expirado o mesmo volume, mantendo-o constante.

hys·te·ria (his-ter′ē-ă, his′tēr′). Histeria; transtorno somatoforme (psiconeurótico ou psicossomático), caracterizado por uma alteração ou perda da função física sugerindo um distúrbio físico, como paralisia de um braço ou distúrbio da visão, mas que, na verdade, constitui aparentemente a expressão de um conflito ou necessidade psicológicos; termo diagnóstico que se refere a uma ampla variedade de sintomas psicogênicos envolvendo distúrbios da função, que podem ser mentais, sensoriais, motores ou viscerais. VER somatoform *disorder.* [G. *histera,* útero, com base na noção original de distúrbios relacionados ao útero em mulheres]
   anxiety h., h. de ansiedade; histeria caracterizada por ansiedade manifesta.
   conversion h., h. de conversão; histeria caracterizada pela substituição, através de transformação psíquica, da ansiedade em sinais ou sintomas físicos; em geral, restrita a sintomas importantes, como cegueira, surdez e paralisia, ou sinais menores, como visão embaçada e dormência. SIN conversion hysteria neurosis, conversion neurosis, conversion reaction.
   dissociative h., h. dissociativa; processo inconsciente algumas vezes observado em pacientes com múltiplas personalidades ou na histeria, em que um grupo de processos mentais é separado do resto dos processos de pensamento, resultando em funcionamento independente desses processos e perda das relações habituais entre eles.
   epidemic h., h. epidêmica. SIN mass h.
   mass h., h. de massa; **(1)** desenvolvimento *en masse* espontâneo de sintomas físicos e/ou emocionais idênticos entre um grupo de indivíduos, conforme observado numa sala de aula de crianças; **(2)** frenesi socialmente contagioso de comportamento irracional num grupo de pessoas como reação a um acontecimento. SIN epidemic h., mass sociogenic illness.

hys·ter·i·cal, hys·ter·ic (his-ter′ē-kăl, -ter′ik). Histérico; relativo a, ou caracterizado por, histeria.

hys·ter·ics (his-ter′iks). Histérico; expressão de emoção freqüentemente acompanhada de choro, riso e gritos.

hystero-, hyster-. Histero-, hister-. **1.** Útero. VER TAMBÉM metr-, utero-. [G. *hystera,* útero] **2.** Histeria [G. *hystera,* útero] **3.** Mais tarde, depois de [G. *hysteros,* mais tarde]

hys·ter·o·cat·a·lep·sy (his′ter-ō-kat′ă-lep-sē). Histerocatalepsia; histeria com manifestações catalépticas.

hys·ter·o·cele (hist′ter-ō-sēl). Histerocele. **1.** Hérnia abdominal ou perineal contendo parte do útero ou todo ele. **2.** Protrusão do conteúdo uterino numa área enfraquecida e abaulada da parede uterina. [hystero- + G. *kēlē,* hérnia]

hys·ter·o·clei·sis (his′ter-ō-klī′sis). Histeroclise; oclusão cirúrgica do útero. [hystero- + G. *kleisis,* fechamento]

hys·ter·o·col·po·scope (his′ter-ō-kol′pō-skōp). Histerocolposcópio; instrumento para inspeção da cavidade uterina e vagina. [hystero- + G. *kolpos,* vagina + *skopeō,* ver]

hys·ter·o·cys·to·pexy (his′ter-ō-sis′tō-pek-sē). Histerocistopexia; fixação do útero e da bexiga à parede abdominal para corrigir um prolapso. [hystero- + G. *kystis*, bexiga + *pēxis*, fixação]

hys·ter·o·dyn·ia (his′ter-ō-din′ē-ă). Histerodinia. SIN hysteralgia. [hystero- + G. *odynē*, dor]

hys·ter·o·gen·ic, hys·ter·og·en·ous (his-ter-ō-jen′ik, his-ter-oj′ē-nŭs). Histerogênico; que produz sintomas ou reações histéricas. [hysteria + G. *-gen*, produzindo]

hys·ter·o·gram (his′ter-ō-gram). Histerograma. **1.** Exame radiológico do útero, utilizando habitualmente contraste. **2.** Registro da força das contrações uterinas.

hys·ter·o·graph (his′ter-ō-graf). Histerógrafo; aparelho para registrar a força das contrações uterinas.

hys·ter·og·ra·phy (his′ter-og′ra-fē). Histerografia. **1.** Exame radiográfico da cavidade uterina cheia de contraste. **2.** Procedimento gráfico utilizado para registrar as contrações uterinas. [hystero- + G. *graphō*, escrever]

hys·ter·oid (his′ter-oyd). Histeróide; semelhante a ou que simula histeria. [hystero- + G. *eidos*, semelhança]

hys·ter·ol·y·sis (his-ter-ol′i-sis). Histerólise; ruptura de aderências entre o útero e as partes vizinhas. [hystero- + G. *lysis*, dissolução]

hys·ter·om·e·ter (his-ter-om′ē-ter). Histerômetro; sonda graduada para medir a profundidade da cavidade uterina. SIN uterometer. [hystero- + G. *metron*, medida]

hys·ter·o·my·o·mec·to·my (his′ter-ō-mī-ō-mek′tō-mē). Histeromiomectomia. SIN myomectomy. [hysteromyoma + G. *ektomē*, excisão]

hys·ter·o·my·ot·o·my (his′ter-ō-mī-ot′ō-mē). Histeromiotomia; incisão nos músculos do útero. [hystero- + G. *mys*, músculo + *tomē*, incisão]

hys·ter·o·oph·o·rec·to·my (his′ter-ō-ō′of-ō-rek′tō-mē). Histerooforectomia; remoção cirúrgica do útero e dos ovários. [hystero- + G. *ōon*, ovo + *phoros*, que transporta + *ektomē*, excisão]

hys·ter·op·a·thy (his-ter-op′a-thē). Histeropatia; qualquer doença do útero. [hystero- + G. *pathos*, sofrimento]

hys·ter·o·pex·y (his′ter-ō-pek-sē). Histeropexia; fixação de útero deslocado ou anormalmente móvel. SIN uterofixation, uteropexy. [hystero- + G. *pēxis*, fixação]

abdominal h., h. abdominal; fixação do útero à parede anterior do abdome.

hys·ter·o·plas·ty (his′ter-ō-plas-tē). Histeroplastia. SIN uteroplasty.

hys·ter·or·rha·phy (his-ter-ōr′a-fē). Histerorrafia; reparo por sutura de útero lacerado. [hystero- + G. *rhaphē*, sutura]

hys·ter·o·sal·pin·gec·to·my (his′ter-ō-sal-pin-jek′tō-mē). Histerossalpingectomia; cirurgia para remoção do útero e de uma ou de ambas as tubas uterinas. [hystero- + G. *salpinx*, trompa + *ektomē*, excisão]

hys·ter·o·sal·pin·gog·ra·phy (his′ter-ō-sal-ping-gog′ra-fē). Histerossalpingografia; radiografia do útero e das trompas de Falópio após injeção de material radiopaco. SIN hysterotubography, uterosalpingography, uterotubography. [hystero- + G. *salpinx*, trompa + *graphō*, escrever]

hys·ter·o·sal·pin·go-o·oph·o·rec·to·my (his′ter-ō-sal-ping′gō-ō-of-ō-rek′tō-mē). Histerossalpingoforectomia; excisão do útero, das trompas e dos ovários. [hystero- + G. *salpinx*, trompa + *ōon*, ovo + *phoros*, transportar + *ektomē*, excisão]

hys·ter·o·sal·pin·gos·to·my (his′ter-ō-sal-ping-gos′tō-mē). Histerossalpingostomia; operação para estabelecer a perviedade da trompa uterina. [hystero- + G. *salpinx*, trompa + *stoma*, boca]

hys·ter·o·scope (his′ter-ō-skōp). Histeroscópio; endoscópio utilizado no exame visual direto da cavidade uterina. SIN uteroscope. [hystero- + G. *skopeō*, ver]

contact h., h. de contato; histeroscópio com lente de índice de refração graduado; não exige distensão para visualização e permite vistas com comprimento focal muito curto; aparelho apropriado para localizar hemorragias.

flexible h., h. flexível; histeroscópio flexível de pequeno diâmetro, para procedimentos diagnósticos ou cirúrgicos, que não necessita de uma bainha externa, possui fibra óptica para visualização e tem de ser utilizado com gás para distensão da cavidade.

hys·ter·os·co·py (his-ter-os′kō-pē). Histeroscopia; inspeção instrumental visual da cavidade uterina. SIN uteroscopy.

hys·ter·o·spasm (his′ter-ō-spazm). Histerospasmo; espasmo do útero.

hys·ter·o·sys·to·le (his-ter-ō-sis′tō-lē). Histerossístole; contração tardia do coração; oposta à contração prematura ou extra-sístole. [G. *hysteros*, depois de + *systolē*, contração]

hys·ter·o·ther·mom·e·try (his′ter-ō-ther-mom′ē-trē). Histerotermometria; medida da temperatura uterina.

hys·ter·ot·o·my (his-ter-ot′ō-mē). Histerotomia; incisão do útero. SIN metrotomy, uterotomy. [hystero- + G. *tomē*, incisão]

abdominal h., h. abdominal; incisão transabdominal no útero. SIN abdominohysterotomy.

vaginal h., h. vaginal; incisão no útero através da vagina. SIN colpohysterotomy.

hys·ter·o·trach·e·lec·to·my (his′ter-ō-trak-el-ek′tō-mē). Histerotraquelectomia; remoção do colo uterino. [hystero- + G. *trachēlos*, pescoço + *ektomē*, excisão]

hys·ter·o·trach·e·lo·plas·ty (his′ter-ō-trak′e-lō-plas-tē). Histerotraqueloplastia; cirurgia plástica do colo uterino. [hystero- + G. *trachēlos*, pescoço + *plastos*, formado]

hys·ter·o·tra·che·lor·rha·phy (his′ter-ō-trak′e-lōr′a-fē). Histerotraquelorrafia; reparo do colo uterino lacerado por sutura. [hystero- + G. *trachēlos*, pescoço + *rhaphē*, sutura]

hys·ter·o·trach·e·lot·o·my (his′ter-ō-trak-e-lot′ō-mē). Histerotraquelotomia; incisão do colo uterino. [hystero- + G. *trachēlos*, pescoço + *tomē*, incisão]

hys·ter·o·tu·bog·ra·phy (his′ter-ō-too-bog′ra-fē). Histerotubografia. SIN hysterosalpingography.

Hz Abreviatura de hertz.

I

ι A nona letra do alfabeto grego, iota.

I 1. símbolo do iodo; intensidade (*intensity*) luminosa ou intensidade radiante; intensidade (*strength*) iônica (em mol/L); isoleucina, inosina. **2.** Abreviatura (em itálico) da intensidade de corrente elétrica, expressa em ampères. **3.** Como subscrito, símbolo de gás (*gas*) inspirado. **4.** Designação do grupo sanguíneo I (ver apêndice sobre Grupos Sanguíneos).

^{123}**I** Símbolo do iodo-123 (I^{123}).

^{125}**I** Símbolo do iodo-125 (I^{125}).

^{127}**I** Símbolo do iodo-127 (I^{127}).

^{131}**I** Símbolo do iodo-131 (I^{131}).

^{132}**I** Símbolo do iodo-132 (I^{132}).

♲ **-ia.** -ia. Sufixo utilizado para formar termos referentes a estados ou condições freqüentemente anormais. Cf. -ism. [G. *-ia*, um antigo sufixo formador de substantivos]

IAHS IAHS. Abreviatura de infection-associated hemophagocytic syndrome (síndrome hemofagocítica associada a infecção).

IANC IANC. Abreviatura de *International Anatomical Nomenclature Committee*. VER *Nomina Anatomica*.

IAP Abreviatura de intermittent acute *porphyria* (porfiria intermitente aguda).

♲ **-iasis.** -íase. Condição ou estado especialmente mórbido; em neologismos médicos, tem o mesmo valor que -ose, sendo às vezes utilizado como sinônimo. [G. sufixo formador de substantivos a partir de verbos]

ia·tra·lip·tic (ī′a - trā - lip′tik). Iatralíptico; termo obsoleto para referir-se a tratamento por meio de unção. [G. *iatros*, médico + *aleiptēs*, aquele que efetua a unção]

ia·tra·lip·tics (ī′a - trā - lip′tiks). Iatralíptica; tratamento por meio de medicamentos externos, como unturas e fricções.

iat·ric (ī - at′rik). Iátrico; relativo à medicina ou a um médico ou curandeiro. [G. *iatros*, médico]

♲ **iatro-.** Iatro-. Médico, medicina, tratamento. Cf. medico-. [G. *iatros*, médico]

iat·ro·chem·i·cal (ī - at - rō - kem′i - kǎl). Iatroquímico; referente a uma escola de medicina que pratica a iatroquímica.

iat·ro·chem·ist (ī - at - rō - kem′ist). Iatroquímico; membro da escola de iatroquímica.

iat·ro·chem·is·try (ī - at - rō - kem′is - trē). Iatroquímica; estudo da química em relação aos processos fisiológicos e patológicos e tratamento da doença por substâncias químicas, conforme praticado por uma escola de pensamento médico no século XVII.

iat·ro·gen·ic (ī - at - rō - jen′ik). Iatrogênico; referente a uma resposta a tratamento clínico ou cirúrgico induzida pelo próprio tratamento; termo habitualmente utilizado para indicar respostas desfavoráveis. [iatro- + G. *-gen*, produzindo]

ia·trol·o·gy (ī - a - trol′ō - jē). Iatrologia; termo raramente utilizado para a ciência médica. [iatro- + G. *logos*, estudo]

iat·ro·math·e·mat·i·cal (ī - at′rō - math - ē - mat′i - kǎl). Iatromatemático; relativo a iatromatemática ou seguidor de seus princípios. SIN iatrophysical.

iat·ro·me·chan·i·cal (ī - at′rō - mē - kan′i - kǎl). Iatromecânico. SIN iatrophysical.

iat·ro·phys·i·cal (ī - at′rō - fiz′i - kǎl). Iatrofísico; escola de pensamento médico do século XVII que explicava todos os fenômenos fisiológicos e patológicos pelas leis da física. SIN iatromathematical, iatromechanical.

iat·ro·phys·i·cist (ī - at′rō - fiz′ - i - sist). Iatrofísico; membro da escola de iatrofísica.

iat·ro·phys·ics (ī - at′rō - fiz′iks). Iatrofísica; física aplicada à medicina.

iat·ro·tech·nique (ī - at′rō - tek - nēk′). Iatrotécnica; termo raramente utilizado para referir-se à arte da medicina e da cirurgia; a técnica ou modo de aplicação da ciência médica. [iatro- + G. *techne*, arte]

IBC Abreviatura de iron-binding *capacity* (capacidade de ligação do ferro).

ibo·ga·ine (ī′bō - gān). Ibogaína; alcalóide indólico do grupo *iboga*. Obtida de várias partes do arbusto africano *Tabernanthe iboga* (família Apocynaceae). Utilizada por caçadores africanos para paralisar os movimentos do caçador; alucinogênico, antidepressivo e euforizante.

ibo·ten·ic ac·id (ī′bō - ten - ik). Ácido ibotênico; substância química semelhante ao ácido caínico extraído de cogumelos venenosos das espécies *Amanita muscaria* e *A. pantherina* (família Agaricaceae). Possui importantes propriedades neuroexcitatórias. Utilizado em pesquisa neurofarmacológica.

ibu·pro·fen (ī - boo′prō - fen). Ibuprofeno; analgésico e antiinflamatório não-esteróide derivado do ácido propiônico.

♲ **-ic.** -Ic. **1.** Sufixo indicando de ou relativo a. **2.** Sufixo químico indicando um elemento em determinado composto em uma de suas maiores valências. Cf. -ous (1). **3.** Sufixo indicador de ácido. [L. *-icus*, fr. G. *-ikos*]

ICAM-1 ICAM-1. Abreviatura de intercellular adhesion *molecule*-1 (molécula de adesão intercelular 1).

ic·co·somes (ī′kō - sōmz). Icossomas; estrutura citoplasmática em forma de contas encontrada em células dendríticas foliculares; acredita-se que seja um local de depósito de antígenos. [*immune complex coated* (recoberto por imunocomplexo) + some]

ICD CID. Abreviatura de *International Classification of Diseases of the World Health Organization* (Classificação Internacional de Doenças da Organização Mundial de Saúde).

ICDA Abreviatura de *International Classification of Diseases Adapted for Use in the United States* (Classificação Internacional de Doenças Adaptada para Uso nos EUA); inclui uma classificação de intervenções cirúrgicas e outros procedimentos diagnósticos e terapêuticos.

ice pack. Compressa de gelo; aplicação local de frio para limitar ou reduzir a inchação de tecidos recém-traumatizados; geralmente na forma de uma bolsa impermeável contendo gelo. Com freqüência, são utilizados meios improvisados de colocação do gelo (bolsas de plástico, toalhas, etc.), bem como sacos químicos que, quando comprimidos, permitem a mistura de substâncias químicas que reagem de modo endotérmico.

ICF LIC. Abreviatura de intracellular *fluid* (líquido intracelular).

ichor (ī′kōr). Icor; termo raramente utilizado para referir-se a uma secreção aquosa rala de uma úlcera ou ferida não-cicatrizada. [G. *ichōr*, soro]

icho·re·mia (ī - kō - rē′mē - ǎ). Icoremia. SIN ichorrhemia.

icho·roid (ī′kō - royd). Icoróide; refere-se a secreção purulenta rala. [G. *ichōr*, soro + *eidos*, semelhança]

ichor·ous (ī′kōr - ŭs). Icoroso; relativo ou semelhante ao icor.

ichor·rhea (ī′kō - rē′ǎ). Icorréia; secreção icorosa profusa. [G. *ichōr*, soro + *rhoia*, fluxo]

ichor·rhe·mia (ī - kō - rē′mē - ǎ). Icorremia; sepse resultante de infecção acompanhada de secreção icorosa. SIN ichoremia. [G. *ichōr*, soro + *rhoia*, fluxo + *haima*, sangue]

ICHPPC Abreviatura de *International Classification of Health Problems in Primary Care* (Classificação Internacional de Problemas de Saúde em Assistência Primária).

ich·tham·mol (ik′tham - mol). Ictamol; líquido viscoso, de coloração castanho-avermelhada a preto-acastanhada, com forte odor empireumático (acre) característico, solúvel em água e em glicerina; obtido da destilação destrutiva de certos xistos betuminosos, sulfonatando o destilado e neutralizando o produto com amônia. É utilizado em distúrbios cutâneos; seu efeito benéfico se deve à sua discreta ação irritante, estimulante, anti-séptica e analgésica; tem sido utilizado em concentração de 10 e 20% na forma de pomada ("ungüento de drenagem"). SIN ammonium ichthosulfonate.

ich·thy·ism (ik′thi - izm). Ictiosismo; intoxicação por ingestão de carne de peixe deteriorada ou de peixe impróprio por outra causa. SIN ichthyismus. [G. *ichthys*, peixe]

ich·thy·is·mus (ik - thi - iz′mŭs). Ictiosismo. SIN ichthyism. [G. *ichthys*, peixe]
i. exanthemat'icus, i. exantemático; erupção eritematosa tóxica devido à ingestão de peixe estragado.
i. hys'trix, i. histrix. SIN bullous congenital ichthyosiform *erythroderma*.

♲ **ichthyo-.** Ictio-. Peixe. [G. *ichthys*]

ich·thy·o·a·can·tho·tox·ism (ik′thi - ō - ǎ - kan′thō - tok′sizm). Ictioacantotoxismo; intoxicação por ferrões ou espinhos de peixes venenosos. [ichthyo- + G. *akantha*, espinho + *toxikon*, veneno]

ich·thy·o·col·la (ik - thē - ō - kol′ǎ). Itiocola; gelatina de peixe obtida de bexigas natatórias de peixes como a merluza, o bacalhau e o esturjão; utilizada como cola, como substituto alimentar e agente clarificador. SIN isinglass. [ichthyo- + G. *kolla*, cola]

ich·thy·o·he·mo·tox·in (ik′thē - ō - hē′mō - tok′sin). Ictio-hemotoxina; substância tóxica presente no sangue de certos peixes. [ichthyo- + G. *haima*, sangue + *toxikon*, veneno]

ich·thy·o·he·mo·tox·ism (ik′thē - ō - hē′mō - tok′sizm). Ictio-hemotoxismo; intoxicação decorrente da ingestão de carne de peixe contendo a substância tóxica ictio-hemotoxina.

♲ Formas Combinantes	★ Termo oficial alternativo para a *Terminologia Anatomica*
🛈 Indica que o termo é ilustrado, ver Índice de Ilustrações	
SIN Sinônimo	[MIM] Mendelian Inheritance in Man
Cf. Comparar, confrontar	I.C. Índice de Corantes
[NA] *Nomina Anatomica*	
[TA] *Terminologia Anatomica*	**Termo de Alta Importância**

ich·thy·oid (ik′thē-oyd). Ictióide; que tem a forma de peixe. [ichthyo- + G. *eidos*, semelhança]

ich·thy·o·o·tox·in (ik′thē-ō-ō-tok′sin). Ictiotoxina; substância tóxica restrita à ova dos peixes. [ichthyo- + G. *ōon*, ovo + *toxikon*, veneno]

ich·thy·oph·a·gous (ik-thē-of′ă-gŭs). Ictiófago; que se alimenta de peixe. [ichthyo- + G. *phagō*, comer]

ich·thy·o·pho·bia (ik′thē-ō-fō′bē-ă). Ictiofobia; medo mórbido de peixes. [ichthyo- + G. *phobos*, medo]

ich·thy·o·sar·co·tox·in (ik′thē-ō-sar′kō-tok′sin). Ictiossarcotoxina; substância tóxica encontrada na carne ou nos órgãos de peixes. [ichthyo- + G. *sarx*, carne + *toxikon*, veneno]

ich·thy·o·sar·co·tox·ism (ik′thē-ō-sar′kō-tok′sizm). Ictiossarcotoxismo; intoxicação causada pela substância tóxica (ictiossarcotoxina) presente na carne ou nos órgãos de peixes. [ichthyo- + G. *sarx*, carne + *toxikon*, veneno]

ich·thy·o·sis (ik-thē-ō′sis). Ictiose; distúrbio congênito de ceratinização, caracterizado por ressecamento não-inflamatório e descamação da pele, freqüentemente em associação a outros defeitos e a anormalidades do metabolismo dos lipídios; distinguível genética, clínica e microscopicamente e pela cinética das células epidérmicas. SIN alligator skin, fish skin, sauriasis. [ichthyo- + G. *-osis*, condição]
   acquired i., i. adquirida; espessamento e descamação da pele associados a algumas doenças malignas (p. ex., linfoma de Hodgkin), lepra e deficiências nutricionais graves.
   i. congenita, i. congênita. SIN lamellar i.
   i. congen′ita neonato′rum, i. congênita do recém-nascido; ictiose generalizada com pele semelhante a pergaminho, observada em prematuros.
   i. cor′neae, i. da córnea; complicação ocular de uma anormalidade congênita da pele, com ceratinização, ressecamento e descamação da córnea.
   i. feta′lis, i. fetal. **(1)** SIN harlequin *fetus;* **(2)** condição recessiva em gado bovino Holstein e norueguês, semelhante ao feto arlequim nos seres humanos.
   i. follicula′ris, i. folicular; forma de ictiose de tipo autossômico dominante, com tampões (rolhas) foliculares córneos nas superfícies extensoras dos membros; início nos primeiros anos de vida.
   harlequin i. [MIM*242500]; i. arlequim; forma fetal de ictiose, considerada distinta da i. lamelar, em que as placas têm forma semelhante a um losango, lembrando o traje de um arlequim; os ceratinócitos contêm quantidades aumentadas de tonofibrilas, que são proteínas estruturais fibrilares; herança autossômica recessiva.
   i. hys′trix, i. histrix. SIN bullous congenital ichthyosiform *erythroderma*. [G. *hystrix*, porco-espinho]
   lamellar i. [MIM*242300], i. lamelar; forma seca de eritrodermia ictiosiforme congênita, caracterizada por ectrópio e grandes escamas de textura grosseira na maior parte do corpo, com espessamento das regiões palmares e plantares; pode ser fatal, com complicações de sépsis, perda de proteínas e eletrólitos no primeiro ano de vida; a histologia revela hiperceratose, camada granular proeminente na epiderme, acantose discreta, numerosas figuras mitóticas e renovação normal ou reduzida das células epidérmicas. Herança autossômica recessiva, causada por uma mutação no gene que codifica a ceratinócito transglutaminase (TGM1) no cromossoma 14q. VER TAMBÉM collodion *baby*, harlequin *fetus*. SIN i. congenita.
   i. linea′ris circumflex′a, i. linear circunflexa; eritema policíclico migratório infantil e descamação que exibe uma margem dupla periférica; persiste por toda a vida e pode estar associada a tricorrexe invaginata na síndrome de Netherton [MIM*256500]; herança autossômica recessiva.
   nacreous i., i. nacarada; variante de ictiose caracterizada por escamas secas aperoladas.
   i. palma′ris et planta′ris, i. palmar e plantar. SIN palmoplantar *keratoderma*.
   i. scutula′ta, i. escutular; ictiose caracterizada por lesões em forma de diamante ou em forma de escudo.
   i. sim′plex, i. simples. SIN i. vulgaris.
   i. vulga′ris [MIM*146700], i. vulgar; caráter autossômico dominante, de início na infância, com escamas no tronco e nos membros, mas não nas áreas de flexão, em associação a atopia e marcas palmares e plantares proeminentes; histologicamente, há hiperceratose, ausência de camada granular na epiderme e renovação normal das células epidérmicas. SIN hyperkeratosis congenita, i. simplex.
   X-linked i. [MIM*308100], i. ligada ao X; forma de ictiose com início ao nascimento ou nos primeiros meses de vida, que afeta os homens; caracterizada por descamação predominantemente no couro cabeludo, pescoço e tronco, com progressão centrípeta; as regiões palmares e plantares são poupadas; as manifestações histológicas consistem em hiperceratose, camada granular na epiderme e renovação normal das células epidérmicas. Herança recessiva ligada ao X, causada por uma mutação no gene da esteróide sulfatase (STS) no cromossoma Xp. SIN steroid sulfatase deficiency.

ich·thy·ot·ic (ik-thē-ot′ik). Ictiótico; relativo à ictiose.

ich·thy·o·tox·i·col·o·gy (ik′thē-ō-tok-si-kol′ō-jē). Ictiotoxicologia; o estudo dos venenos produzidos por peixes e seu reconhecimento, efeitos e antídotos. [ichthyo- + G. *toxikon*, veneno + *logos*, estudo]

ich·thy·o·tox·i·con (ik-thē-ō-tok′si-kon). Ictiotóxico; princípio tóxico presente em certos peixes. SIN fish poison (1). [ichthyo- + G. *toxicon*, veneno]

ich·thy·o·tox·in (ik′thē-ō-tok′sin). Ictiotoxina; princípio hemolítico ativo do soro da enguia. [ichthyo- + G. *toxicon*, veneno]

ich·thy·o·tox·ism (ik′thē-ō-tok′sizm). Ictiotoxismo; intoxicação por peixes. [ichthyo- + G. *toxikon*, veneno]

ICIDH Abreviatura de *International Classification of Impairments, Disabilities and Handicaps* (Classificação Internacional de Diminuição da Capacidade Funcional, Incapacidade e Deficiência Física).

ico·sa·he·dral (ī′kō-să-hē′dral). Icosaédrico; que possui 20 superfícies triangulares eqüilaterais e 12 vértices, conforme observado na maioria dos vírus com simetria cúbica. [G. *eikosi*, vinte + *-edros*, que possui lados ou bases]

n·ico·sa·no·ic ac·id (ī′kō-să-nō′ik). Ácido *n*-icosanóico. SIN arachidic acid.

ICP PIC. Abreviatura de intracranial *pressure* (pressão intracraniana).

ICRP Abreviatura de *International Commission on Radiological Protection* (Comissão Internacional sobre Proteção Radiológica).

-ics. -ica; conhecimento organizado, prático, tratamento. [-ic + -s]

ICSH Abreviatura de interstitial cell-stimulating *hormone* (hormônio estimulante das células intersticiais).

ic·tal (ik′tal). Ictal, comicial; relativo a, ou causado por, *ictus* ou convulsão. [L. *ictus*, golpe]

ic·ter·ic (ik-ter′ik). Ictérico; relativo a, ou caracterizado por, icterícia. [G. *ikterikos*, ictérico]

ictero-. Ictero-. Icterícia. [G. *ikteros*, icterícia]

ic·ter·o·a·ne·mia (ik′ter-ō-ă-nē′mē-ă). Icteroanemia. SIN acquired hemolytic *icterus.*

ic·ter·o·gen·ic (ik′ter-ō-jen′ik). Icterogênico; que provoca icterícia. [ictero- + G. *-gen*, produzindo]

ic·ter·o·he·ma·tu·ric (ik′ter-ō-hē′mă-too′rik). Íctero-hematúrico; indica icterícia, com eliminação de sangue na urina. [ictero- + G. *haima*, sangue + *ouron*, urina]

ic·ter·o·he·mo·glo·bi·nu·ria (ik′ter-ō-hē′mō-glō-bi-noo′rē-ă). Ícterohemoglobinúria; icterícia com presença de hemoglobina na urina.

ic·ter·oid (ik′ter-oyd). Icteróide; de tonalidade amarela ou aparentemente ictérico. [ictero- + G. *eidos*, semelhança]

ic·ter·us (ik′ter-ŭs). Icterícia. SIN jaundice. [G. *ikteros*]
   acquired hemolytic i., i. hemolítica adquirida; icterícia e anemia que ocorrem em associação a esplenomegalia moderada, fragilidade aumentada dos eritrócitos e quantidade aumentada de urobilina na urina. SIN icteroanemia.
   benign familial i., i. familiar benigna. SIN familial nonhemolytic *jaundice*.
   cholestatic hepatosis i. gravidarum, i. hepática colestática da gravidez. SIN intrahepatic *cholestasis of pregnancy*.
   chronic familial i., i. familiar crônica. SIN hereditary *spherocytosis*.
   congenital hemolytic i., i. hemolítica congênita. SIN hereditary *spherocytosis*.
   cythemolytic i., i. cito-hemolítica; icterícia causada pela absorção de bile produzida em excesso através de estimulação pela hemoglobina livre decorrente da destruição de eritrócitos.
   i. gra′vis, i. grave; icterícia associada a febre alta e delírio; observada na hepatite grave e em outras doenças do fígado com insuficiência funcional grave. SIN malignant jaundice.
   infectious i., i. infecciosa. SIN Weil *disease*.
   i. mel′as, i. negra; forma em que a pele torna-se castanho-escura.
   i. neonato′rum, icterícia do recém-nascido. SIN physiologic i. SIN physiologic *jaundice*.
   physiologic i., i. fisiológica. SIN i. neonatorum.
   i. prae′cox, i. precoce; tipo relativamente inócuo, porém rapidamente progressivo, de icterícia com anemia leve no recém-nascido, mais freqüentemente causada por incompatibilidade ABO entre a mãe e o feto.

ic·tom·e·ter (ik-tom′ē-ter). Ictômetro; aparelho para determinar a força do batimento do ápice cardíaco. [L. *ictus*, golpe + G. *metron*, medida]

ic·tus (ik′tŭs). Ictus, icto. **1.** Golpe ou ataque. **2.** Batimento. [L.]
   i. cor′dis, i. cardíaco, batimento cardíaco. SIN heart *beat*.
   i. epilep′ticus, i. epiléptico; convulsão epiléptica.
   i. paralyt′icus, i. paralítico; crise de paralisia.
   i. so′lis, i. solar. SIN sunstroke.

ICU UTI. Abreviatura de intensive care *unit* (unidade de tratamento intensivo).

I.D. I.D. Abreviatura de infecting dose (dose infectante). VER minimal infecting *dose*.

id. id. **1.** Em psicanálise, um dos três componentes do aparelho psíquico no modelo estrutural froidiano, sendo os outros dois o ego e o superego. O id encontra-se totalmente no plano inconsciente, é desorganizado e constitui o reservatório de energia psíquica ou libido, estando sob a influência dos processos primários. **2.** A totalidade da energia psíquica disponível nas necessidades biológicas inatas, apetites, necessidades corporais e impulsos no recémnascido; através da socialização, essa energia difusa e sem direção torna-se canalizada em direções mais egocêntricas e mais sociáveis (desenvolvimento do ego a partir do id). [L. *id*, esse]

-id., -ide. 1. Estado de sensibilidade da pele em que uma parte remota da lesão primária reage ("reação -ide") a substâncias do patógeno, dando origem a uma lesão inflamatória secundária; a lesão que manifesta reação é designada pelo uso de -ide como sufixo. [G. *-eidēs*, semelhante, através do Fr. *-ide*]. **2.** Espécime pequeno e jovem. [G. *-idion*, sufixo diminutivo]

IDA IDA. Abreviatura de imunodiacetoato (imunodiacetato), cujos derivados são utilizados em radiofarmacêutica com marcador Tc^{99m}. VER HIDA. VER TAMBÉM DISIDA.

IDDM DMID. Abreviatura de insulin-dependent *diabetes* mellitus (diabetes melito insulino-dependente).

-ide. -Eto, -ídio. 1. Sufixo que indica o elemento mais eletronegativo num composto químico binário; antigamente designado pela qualificação -ureted (-uretado); p. ex., sulfeto de hidrogênio, antigamente hidrogênio sulfuretado. **2.** Sufixo (num nome de açúcar) indica a substituição do hemiacetal OH pelo H; p. ex., glicosídeo.

idea (ī-dē′ă). Idéia; qualquer imagem ou conceito mental. [G. forma, aparência, fr. *idein*, ter visto, fr. obs. *eidō*, ver]

autochthonous i.'s, idéias autóctones; pensamentos que irrompem subitamente no plano da consciência como se fossem vitalmente importantes, freqüentemente como se proviessem de uma fonte externa.

compulsive i., i. compulsiva; idéia fixa e repetidamente recorrente.

dominant i., i. dominante; idéia que governa todas as ações e todos os pensamentos do indivíduo.

fixed i., i. fixa. **(1) N**oção, crença ou ilusão exagerada que persiste, a despeito de provas em contrário, controlando a mente; **(2)** convicção obstinada de uma pessoa psicótica acerca da validade de um delírio. SIN idée fixe, overvalued i.

flight of i.'s, fuga de idéias; sintoma incontrolável da fase maníaca de um distúrbio depressivo bipolar, em que ocorrem sucessões de palavras e idéias não-relacionadas numa velocidade impossível de vocalizar, a despeito de um acentuado aumento no débito global de palavras do indivíduo. VER TAMBÉM mania.

overvalued i., i. superestimada. SIN fixed i.

i. of reference, i. de referência; interpretação incorreta de que as afirmações ou os atos de outra pessoa ou objetos neutros no ambiente estão dirigidos para si, quando, de fato, não estão.

ide·al (ī-dēl′). Ideal; padrão de perfeição.

ego i., ideal do ego. Parte da personalidade que compreende os objetivos, as aspirações e metas do indivíduo, que habitualmente tem a sua origem na emulação de uma pessoa importante com a qual se identificou.

ide·a·tion (ī-dē-ā′shŭn). Ideação; formação de idéias ou pensamentos.

ide·a·tion·al (ī-dē-ā′shŭn-ăl). Ideacional; relativo à ideação.

idée fixe (ē-dā′feks′). Idéia fixa. SIN fixed *idea*. [Fr. obsessão]

iden·ti·fi·ca·tion (ī-den′ti-fī-kā′shŭn). Identificação. **1.** Ato ou processo de determinar a classificação ou natureza de. **2.** Sensação de unidade ou continuidade psíquica com outra pessoa ou grupo; um dos mecanismos de defesa freudianos comuns a todas as pessoas, em que a ansiedade relativa à identidade ou valor pessoal dissipa-se através do mecanismo de percepção de que possui características em comum com uma pessoa reconhecida publicamente ou na identificação infantil com uma pessoa mais poderosa, como um genitor. SIN incorporation. [Mediev. L. *identicus*, fr. L. *idem*, o mesmo + *facio*, fazer]

projective i., i. projetiva; ato de atribuir, de modo defensivo, seus próprios processos psíquicos a outra pessoa.

synthetic sentence i., i. de sentença sintética; teste de integridade da via auditiva central em que um conjunto fechado de 10 sentenças de sintaxe incompleta é apresentado com uma mensagem apropriada para identificação.

iden·ti·ty (ī-den′ti-tē). Identidade; o papel social da pessoa e sua percepção do mesmo.

ego i., i. do ego; o sentido de que o ego tem a sua própria identidade.

gender i., i. sexual; consistência e persistência da individualidade como masculina, feminina ou andrógena. Particularmente experimentada na autopercepção; representação internalizada do papel sexual. Cf. gender *role*, sex *role*.

sense of i., senso de i.; sentido de que a pessoa tem sua própria identidade ou individualidade psicológica.

ideo-. Idéias; ideação Cf. idio-. [G. *idea*, forma, noção]

ide·o·ki·net·ic (ī′dē-ō-ki-net′ik). Ideocinético. SIN ideomotor.

ide·ol·o·gy (ī-dē-ol′ō-jē, id-ē-). Ideologia; o sistema composto de idéias, crenças e atitudes que constituem a visão organizada do indivíduo ou de um grupo em relação aos outros. [ideo- + G. *logos*, estudo]

ide·o·mo·tion (ī-dē-ō-mō′shŭn). Ideomoção; movimento muscular executado sob a influência de uma idéia dominante, sendo praticamente automático e não-volicional.

ide·o·mo·tor (ī′dē-ō-mō′ter). Ideomotor; relativo à ideomoção. SIN ideokinetic.

ide·o·pho·bia (ī′dē-ō-fō′bē-ă). Ideofobia; medo mórbido de ter idéias novas ou diferentes.

idio-. Idio-. Privado, distinto, peculiar. Cf. ideo-. [G. *idios*, o próprio]

id·i·o·ag·glu·ti·nin (id′ē-ō-ă-gloo′tin-in). Idioaglutinina; aglutinina que ocorre naturalmente no sangue de uma pessoa ou de um animal, sem a injeção de antígeno estimulante ou transferência passiva de anticorpo.

id·i·o·dy·nam·ic (id′ē-ō-dī-nam′ik). Idiodinâmico; independentemente ativo.

id·i·o·gen·e·sis (id′ē-ō-jen′ē-sis). Idiogênese; origem sem causa evidente; refere-se especialmente à origem de uma doença idiopática. [idio- + G. *genesis*, produção]

id·i·o·glos·sia (id′ē-ō-glos′ē-ă). Idioglossia; forma extrema de lalia ou substituição de vogais ou consoantes, em que a fala de uma criança pode tornar-se ininteligível e parecer outro idioma a alguém que não possui a "chave" das alterações literais. [idio- + G. *glōssa*, língua, fala]

id·i·o·glot·tic (id′ē-ō-glot′ik). Idioglótico; relativo à idioglossia.

id·i·o·gram (id′ē-ō-gram). Idiograma. **1.** SIN karyotype. **2.** Representação diagramática da morfologia cromossômica característica de uma espécie ou população. [idio- + G. *gramma*, algo escrito]

id·i·o·graph·ic (id′ē-ō-graf′ik). Idiográfico; relativo às características ou comportamento de um indivíduo específico como indivíduo, em oposição a nomotético. [idio- + G. *graphō*, escrever]

id·i·o·het·er·o·ag·glu·ti·nin (id′ē-ō-het′er-ō-ă-gloo′tin-in). Idio-heteroaglutinina; idioaglutinina que ocorre no sangue de um animal, mas que tem a capacidade de se combinar com o material antigênico de outra espécie. [idio- + G. *heteros*, outro + aglutinina]

id·i·o·het·er·o·ly·sin (id′ē-ō-het-er-ol′i-sin). Idio-heterolisina; idiolisina que ocorre no sangue de um animal de uma espécie, mas que tem a capacidade de se combinar com os eritrócitos de outra espécie, causando, assim, hemólise na presença do complemento.

id·i·o·hyp·no·tism (id′ē-ō-hip′nō-tizm). Idio-hipnotismo. SIN autohypnosis.

id·i·o·i·so·ag·glu·ti·nin (id′ē-ō-ī′sō-ă-gloo′tin-in). Idioisoaglutinina; idioaglutinina presente no sangue de um animal de determinada espécie e que tem a capacidade de aglutinar as células de animais da mesma espécie. [idio- + G. *isos*, igual + aglutinina]

id·i·o·i·sol·y·sin (id′ē-ō-ī-sol′i-sin). Idioisolisina; idiolisina presente no sangue de um animal de determinada espécie e que tem a capacidade de se combinar com os eritrócitos de animais da mesma espécie, causando, assim, hemólise na presença do complemento.

id·i·o·la·lia (id′ē-ō-lā′lē-ă). Idiolalia; uso de uma linguagem inventada pela própria pessoa. [idio- + G. *lalia*, fala]

id·i·ol·y·sin (id-ē-ol′i-sin). Idiolisina; lisina que ocorre naturalmente no sangue de uma pessoa ou de um animal, sem injeção de um antígeno estimulante ou transferência passiva de anticorpo.

id·i·o·mus·cu·lar (id′ē-ō-mŭs′kū-lăr). Idiomuscular; relativo apenas aos músculos, independentemente do controle nervoso.

id·i·o·nod·al (id′ē-ō-nō′dăl). Idionodal; que se origina do próprio nó AV; aplica-se ao ritmo ventricular no bloqueio sinoatrial (SA) ou atrioventricular (AV) completo ou em outras formas de dissociação AV, quando o nó AV, mais do que um foco ventricular ectópico, controla os ventrículos. Mais precisamente, idiojunção, visto ser habitualmente impossível localizar com uma precisão um ritmo "nodal AV"; o nó AV faz parte da junção AV. VER TAMBÉM idioventricular.

id·i·o·pa·thet·ic (id′ē-ō-pă-thet′ik). Idiopatético; termo raramente utilizado para idiopático.

id·i·o·path·ic (id′ē-ō-path′ik). Idiopático; refere-se a uma doença de causa desconhecida. SIN agnogenic. [idio- + G. *pathos*, sofrimento]

id·i·op·a·thy (id-ē-op′ă-thē). Idiopatia; doença idiopática. [idio- + G. *pathos*, sofrimento]

id·i·o·phren·ic (id′ē-ō-fren′ik). Idiofrênico; relativo a ou que se origina apenas nas mentes ou no cérebro, não reflexo nem secundário. [idio- + G. *phrēn*, mente]

id·i·o·psy·cho·log·ic (id′ē-ō-sī-kō-loj′ik). Idiopsicológico; relativo a idéias desenvolvidas na própria mente, independentemente de qualquer sugestão do exterior.

id·i·o·re·flex (id-ē-ō-rē′fleks). Idiorreflexo; reflexo devido a um estímulo ou irritação que se origina no órgão ou na parte onde ocorre o reflexo.

id·i·o·some (id′ē-ō-sōm). Idiossoma; centrossoma de uma espermátide ou de um ovócito. [idio- + G. *sōma*, corpo]

id·i·o·syn·cra·sy (id′ē-ō-sin′krā-sē). Idiossincrasia. **1.** Característica ou peculiaridade mental, comportamental ou física do indivíduo. **2.** Em farmacologia, uma reação anormal a uma substância, algumas vezes especificada como geneticamente determinada. [G. *idiosynkrasia*, de *idios*, o próprio + *synkrasis*, mistura]

id·i·o·syn·crat·ic (id′ē-ō-sin-krat′ik). Idiossincrásico, idiossincrático; relativo a, ou caracterizado por, idiossincrasia.

id·i·o·tope (id′ē-ōtōp). Idiótopo; determinante antigênico único, de um idiótipo. VER TAMBÉM idiotypic antigenic *determinant*. SIN idiotypic antigenic determinant. [idio- + -tope]

set of idiotopes, conjunto de idiótopos (determinantes antigênicos) das regiões variáveis da imunoglobulina ou do receptor de células T.

id·i·ot-prod·i·gy (id′ē-ŏt prŏd′i-jē). Idiota-prodígio. SIN idiot-savant.

id·i·o·tro·phic (id′ē-ō-trŏf′ik). Idiotrófico; capaz de escolher seu próprio alimento. [idio- + G. *trophē*, alimento]

id·i·o·tro·pic (id′ē-ō-trŏp′ik). Idiotrópico; que está voltado para dentro de si próprio. [idio- + G. *tropē*, uma volta]

id·i·ot-sa·vant (ē-dē-ō′ sah-vahn′). Idiota-prodígio; indivíduo de baixo nível de inteligência geral que possui uma faculdade incomum para executar certas tarefas mentais que a maioria dos indivíduos normais é incapaz de realizar. SIN idiot-prodigy. [Fr.]

id·i·o·type (id′ē-ō-tīp). Idiotipo; conjunto de idiotopos, na região variável, que confere à molécula de imunoglobulina uma "individualidade" antigênica e que constitui freqüentemente um atributo exclusivo de determinado anticorpo em um animal específico. Trata-se do produto de um número limitado de clones de linfócitos B; também encontrado no receptor de células T. VER idiotope. [idio- + G. *typos*, modelo].

id·i·o·ven·tric·u·lar (id-ē-ō-ven-trik′ū-lăr). Idioventricular; relativo a ou associado apenas aos ventrículos cardíacos.

id·i·tol (ī′di-tŏl). Iditol; produto de redução da hexose idose.

IDL IDL. Abreviatura de intermediate density *lipoprotein* (lipoproteína de densidade intermediária).

id·ose (ī′dōs). Uma das aldoexoses, isomérica da galactose; a L-idose é epimérica com a D-glicose. VER sugar.

idox·ur·i·dine (IDU) (ī-dŏks-ū′ri-dēn). Idoxuridina; análogo da pirimidina que produz efeitos tanto antivirais quanto anticancerosos através de interferência na síntese de DNA; utilizada localmente no olho para tratamento da ceratite produzida por herpes simples ou vacínia.

IDP IDP. Abreviatura de inosine 5′-diphosphate (inosina 5′-difosfato).

IDU IDU. Abreviatura de idoxuridine (idoxuridina).

id·ur·o·nate (ī-door-ŏn′āt). Iduronato; sal ou éster do ácido idurônico.
 i. sulfatase, i. sulfatase; enzima necessária para dessulfatação de resíduos de 2-sulfato iduronato no sulfato de heparan. É também necessária na degradação do sulfato de dermatan; a síndrome de Hunter está associada à deficiência dessa enzima.

idur·on·ic ac·id (ī-door-ŏn′ik). Ácido idurônico; ácido urônico da idose; constituinte do sulfato de dermatan.

α·L·id·ur·on·id·ase (ī-door-ŏn′i-dās). α-L-iduronidase; enzima que hidrolisa resíduos de ácido α-L-idurônico dessulfatados terminais do sulfato de dermatan e do sulfato de heparan; a deficiência dessa enzima está associada à síndrome de Hurler e à síndrome de Scheie.

IEP Abreviatura de isoelectric *point* (ponto isoelétrico).

IF Abreviatura de initiation *factor* (fator de iniciação); intrinsic *factor* (fator intrínseco).

IFN IFN. Abreviatura de *interferon* (interferon).

IFN-α IFN-α. Abreviatura de *interferon* alfa (α-interferon).

IFN-β IFN-β. Abreviatura de *interferon* beta (β-interferon).

IFN-γ IFN-γ. Abreviatura de *interferon* gama (γ-interferon).

Ig Ig. Abreviatura de immunoglobulin (imunoglobulina).

IgA Abreviatura de immunoglobulin A (imunoglobulina A).

IgD Abreviatura de immunoglobulin D (imunoglobulina D).

IgE Abreviatura de immunoglobulin E (imunoglobulina E).

IGF Abreviatura de insulinlike growth *factor* (fator de crescimento insulino-símile).

IgG Abreviatura de immunoglobulin G (imunoglobulina G).

IgM Abreviatura de immunoglobulin M (imunoglobulina M).

ig·na·tia (ig-nā′shē-ă). Inácia; semente madura seca de *Strychnos ignatii* (família Loganiaceae). Suas propriedades assemelham-se às da noz vômica e constitui uma fonte de estriquinina. [*St. Ignatius*]

ig·ni·pe·di·tes (ig′ni-pe-dī′tēz). Pé ígneo; dor em queimação nas plantas dos pés na neurite múltipla. [L. *ignis*, fogo + *pes (ped-)*, pé + G. *itēs*]

ig·ni·punc·ture (ig′ni-pŭngk-choor). Ignipuntura; procedimento original de fechar uma ruptura da retina no descolamento da retina por transfixação da ruptura com cautério. [L. *ignis*, fogo + puntura]

ig·no·tine (ig′nō-tēn). Ignotina. SIN carnosine.

IH HI. Abreviatura de infectious *hepatitis* (hepatite infecciosa).

IJP IJP. Abreviatura de inhibitory junction *potential* (potencial de junção inibitório).

iko·ta (ī-kō′tă). Ikota; neurose semelhante a *latah*, que afeta mulheres casadas entre os samoiedos da Sibéria.

IL-1 Abreviatura de interleukin-1 (interleucina-1).
IL-2 Abreviatura de interleukin-2 (interleucina-2).
IL-3 Abreviatura de interleukin-3 (interleucina-3).
IL-4 Abreviatura de interleukin-4 (interleucina-4).
IL-5 Abreviatura de interleukin-5 (interleucina-5).
IL-6 Abreviatura de interleukin-6 (interleucina-6).
IL-7 Abreviatura de interleukin-7 (interleucina-7).
IL-8 Abreviatura de interleukin-8 (interleucina-8).
IL-9 Abreviatura de interleukin-9 (interleucina-9).
IL-10 Abreviatura de interleukin-10 (interleucina-10).
IL-11 Abreviatura de interleukin-11 (interleucina-11).
IL-12 Abreviatura de interleukin-12 (interleucina-12).
IL-13 Abreviatura de interleukin-13 (interleucina-13).
IL-14 Abreviatura de interleukin-14 (interleucina-14).
IL-15 Abreviatura de interleukin-15 (interleucina-15).
IL-16 Abreviatura de interleukin-16 (interleucina-16).
IL-17 Abreviatura de interleukin-17 (interleucina-17).
IL-18 Abreviatura de interleukin-18 (interleucina-18).

ILA ILA. Abreviatura de insulinlike *activity* (atividade insulina-símile).

il·e·ac (il′ē-ak). Ileal. **1.** Relativo ao íleo paralítico. **2.** Relacionado ao íleo.

il·e·a·del·phus (il′ē-ă-del′fŭs). Ileadelfo. SIN *duplicitas* posterior.

il·e·al (il′ē-ăl). Ileal; do ou relativo ao íleo.

il·e·ec·to·my (il-ē-ek′tō-mē). Ilectomia; remoção do íleo. [ileum + G. *ektomē*, excisão]

il·e·i·tis (il-ē-ī′tis). Ileíte; inflamação do íleo.
 backwash i., ileíte por contracorrente; comprometimento do íleo terminal por alterações inflamatórias e ulcerativas, observado na colite ulcerativa crônica; diferencia-se do comprometimento do íleo e cólon proximal por enterite regional (granulomatosa) (p. ex., doença de Crohn do íleo terminal e do cólon proximal]
 distal i., regional i., terminal i., i. distal, i. regional, i. terminal. SIN regional enteritis.

ileo-. Íleo-. O íleo [L. Novo *ileum*, virilha]

il·e·o·ce·cal (il′ē-ō-sē′kăl). Ileocecal; relativo tanto ao íleo quanto ao ceco.

il·e·o·ce·co·cys·to·plas·ty (il′ē-ō-sē′kō-sis′tō-plas-tē). Ileocecocistoplastia; reconstrução da bexiga e aumento com um segmento vascularizado isolado do ileoceco. [ileo- + ceco- + G. *kystis*, bexiga + *plastos*, formado]

il·e·o·ce·cos·to·my (il′ē-ō-sē-kos′tō′mē). Ileocecostomia; anastomose do íleo ao ceco. SIN cecoileostomy.

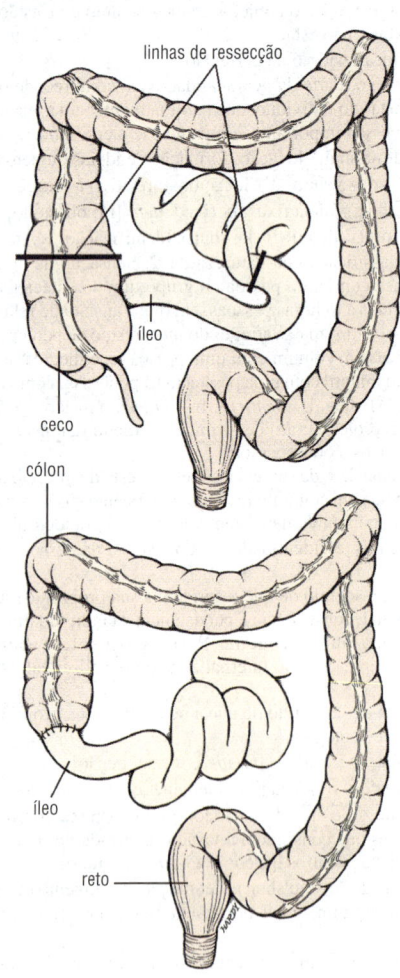

ileocolostomia: ressecção das porções acometidas do íleo e ceco (A) e anastomose das extremidades ressecadas (B).

il·e·o·ce·cum (il - ē - ō - sē´kŭm). Ileoceco; íleo e ceco combinados.
il·e·o·co·lic (il´ē - ō - kol´ik). Ileocólico; relativo ao íleo e ao cólon. SIN ileocolonic.
il·e·o·co·li·tis (il´ē - ō - kō - lī´tis). Ileocolite; inflamação, em grau variável, da mucosa do íleo e do cólon.
il·e·o·co·lon·ic (il´ē - ō - kō - lon´ik). Ileocolônico. SIN ileocolic.
il·e·o·co·los·to·my (il´ē - ō - kō - los´tō - mē). Ileocolostomia; anastomose do íleo ao cólon. [ileo- + colostomia]
il·e·o·cys·to·plas·ty (il´ē - ō - sis´tō - plas - tē). Ileocistoplastia; reconstrução da bexiga com um segmento vascularizado isolado do íleo para aumentar a capacidade vesical. [ileo- + G. *kystis*, bexiga + *plastos*, formado]
il·e·o·en·tec·tro·py (il´ē - ō - en - tek´trō - pē). Ileoentropia; termo raramente utilizado para referir-se à eversão de um segmento do íleo. [ileo- + G. *entos*, dentro + *ek*, fora + *tropē*, uma volta]
il·e·o·il·e·os·to·my (il´ē - ō - il - ē - os´tō - mē). Ileoileostomia. **1.** Anastomose entre segmentos do íleo. **2.** A abertura assim estabelecida. [ileum + ileum + G. *stoma*, boca]
il·e·o·je·ju·ni·tis (il´ē - ō - je - joo - nī´tis). Ileojejunite; condição inflamatória crônica afetando o jejuno e partes ou a maioria do íleo; ocorre em diferentes formas: um estado granulomatoso semelhante à ileíte regional, pseudodivertículos ou estenose cicatricial do intestino.
il·e·o·pexy (il´ē - ō - pek´sē). Ileopexia; fixação cirúrgica do íleo. [ileo- + G. *pēxis*, fixação]
il·e·o·proc·tos·to·my (il´ē - ō - prok - tos´tō - mē). Ileoproctostomia; anastomose entre o íleo e o reto. SIN ileorectostomy. [ileo- + G. *prōktos*, ânus (reto) + *stoma*, boca]
il·e·o·rec·tos·to·my (il´ē - ō - rek - tos´tō - mē). Ileorretostomia. SIN ileoproctostomy. [ileum + reto + G. *stoma*, boca]
il·e·or·rha·phy (il´ē - ōr´a - fē). Ileorrafia; sutura do íleo. [ileo- + G. *rhaphē*, sutura]
il·e·o·sig·moid·os·to·my (il´ē - ō - sig´moyd - os´tō - mē). Ileossigmoidostomia; anastomose entre o íleo e o cólon sigmóide. [ileo- + G. sigmóide + G. *stoma*, boca]
il·e·os·to·my (il´ē - os´tō - mē). Ileostomia; estabelecimento de uma fístula através da qual o íleo elimina diretamente seu conteúdo para fora do corpo. [ileo- + G. *stoma*, boca]

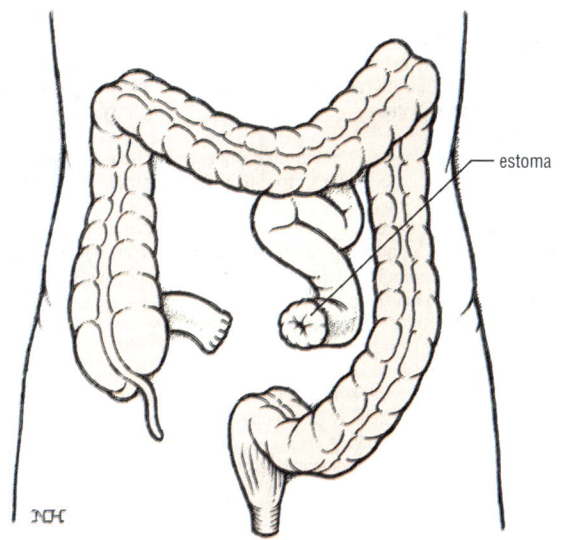

ileostomia

Brooke i., i. de Brooke; ileostomia em que o íleo proximal seccionado, levado através da parede abdominal, é evaginado e sua borda é suturada à derme; o resultado desejado do procedimento consiste numa protrusão de 2 cm.
Kock i., i. de Kock. SIN Kock pouch.
il·e·ot·o·my (il´ē - ot´ō - mē). Ileotomia; incisão no íleo. [ileo- + G. *tomē*, incisão]
il·e·o·trans·ver·sos·to·my (il´ē - ō - tranz - vers - os´tō - me). Ileotransversostomia; anastomose do íleo ao cólon transverso. [íleo + cólon transverso + G. *stoma*, boca]
il·e·um (il´ē - ŭm) [TA]. Íleo; a terceira porção mais longa do intestino delgado, com cerca de 30 cm de comprimento nos seres humanos, que se estende desde uma junção indistinta com o jejuno até a abertura ileocecal. Em geral, é distinto do jejuno pelo seu diâmetro tipicamente menor com paredes mais finas, pregas circulares menores e menos complexas (pregas circulares), maior quantidade de gordura no mesentério e artérias (artérias ileais) que formam mais fileiras de arcadas arteriais com vasos retos mais curtos. [L. do G. *eileo*, enrolar, torcer]
i. du´plex, i. duplo; duplicações segmentares tubulares e císticas do trato alimentar.
il·e·us (il´ē - ŭs). Íleo paralítico ou adinâmico; obstrução mecânica, dinâmica ou adinâmica, do intestino; pode ser acompanhado de dor em cólica intensa, distensão abdominal, vômitos, ausência de evacuações e, com freqüência, febre e desidratação. [G. *eileos*, cólica intestinal, de *eilō*, enrolar de modo apertado]
adynamic i., i. adinâmico; obstrução do intestino devido à paralisia da parede intestinal, habitualmente em decorrência de peritonite localizada ou generalizada ou de choque. SIN paralytic i.
dynamic i., i. dinâmico; obstrução intestinal devido à contração espástica de um segmento do intestino. SIN spastic i.
gallstone i., i. por cálculos biliares; obstrução do intestino delgado produzida pela eliminação de um cálculo pelas vias biliares (em geral, a vesícula biliar em consequência de colecistite) no tubo intestinal (em geral, através de uma conexão fistulosa entre a vesícula biliar e o intestino delgado); a ocorrência e o local da obstrução dependem do tamanho do cálculo, porém a localização habitual é na junção ileocecal ou próximo a ela.
mechanical i., i. mecânico; obstrução do intestino, devido a alguma causa mecânica, como, p. ex., vôlvulo, cálculo biliar, aderências.
meconium i., i. meconial; obstrução intestinal no feto e no recém-nascido após espessamento do mecônio, causada pela ausência de tripsina; associado a fibrose cística.
occlusive i., i. oclusivo; bloqueio mecânico completo da luz intestinal.
paralytic i., i. paralítico. SIN adynamic i.
spastic i., i. espástico. SIN dynamic i.
i. subpar´ta, obstrução do intestino grosso por compressão do útero grávido.
terminal i., i. terminal; obstrução da parte inferior do intestino delgado. SIN pars terminalis ilei [TA].
verminous i., i. por vermes; obstrução devido a massas de parasitas intestinais.
il·i·ac (il´ē - ak). Ilíaco; relativo ao ílio.
il·i·a·cus (il - ī´ă - kŭs). Ilíaco. VER iliacus (*muscle*).
il·i·a·del·phus (il - ē - a - del´fŭs). Iliadelfo. SIN *duplicitas* posterior. [L. *ilium* + G. *adelphos*, irmão]
ilio-. O ílio. [L. *ilium*]
il·i·o·coc·cyg·e·al (il´ē - ō - kok - sij´ē - ăl). Iliococcígeo; relativo ao ílio e ao cóccix.
il·i·o·co·lot·o·my (il´ē - ō - kō - lot´ō - mē). Iliocolotomia; operação de abertura do cólon na região inguinal (ilíaca). [ilio- + G. *kolon*, cólon + *tomē*, incisão]
il·i·o·cos·tal (il´ē - ō - kos´tăl). Iliocostal; relativo ao ílio e às costelas; refere-se aos músculos que passam entre as duas partes.
il·i·o·cos·ta·lis (il´ē - ō - kos - tā´lis). Iliocostal. VER iliocostalis (*muscle*).
il·i·o·fem·o·ral (il´ē - ō - fem´ō - răl). Iliofemoral; relativo ao ílio e ao fêmur.
il·i·o·fem·o·ro·plas·ty (il - ē - o - fem´ōr - ō - plas - tē). Iliofemoroplastia; método obsoleto para garantir uma fusão do quadril por uma técnica extra-articular (procedimento de derivação articular), em que um retalho ósseo dobrado para baixo do ílio é colocado numa fenda do grande trocanter.
il·i·o·hy·po·gas·tric (il´ē - ō - hī - pō - gas´trik). Ílio-hipogástrico; relativo ao ílio e à região hipogástrica.
il·i·o·in·gui·nal (il´ē - ō - ing´gwi - năl). Ilioinguinal; relativo à região ilíaca e à virilha.
il·i·o·lum·bar (il - ē - ō - lŭm´băr). Iliolombar; relativo ao ilíaco e às regiões ilíaca e lombar.
il·i·op·a·gus (il - ē - op´a - gŭs). Iliópago; gêmeos conjuntos em que a fusão se restringe à região ilíaca. VER conjoined *twins*, em *twin*. [ilio- + G. *pagos*, algo fixo]
il·i·o·pec·tin·e·al (il´ē - ō - pek - tin´ē - ăl). Iliopectíneo; relativo ao ílio e ao púbis.
il·i·o·pel·vic (il´ē - ō - pel´vik). Iliopélvico; relativo à região ilíaca e à cavidade pélvica.
il·i·o·sa·cral (il´ē - ō - sā´krăl). Iliossacro; relativo ao ílio e ao sacro.
il·i·o·sci·at·ic (il´ē - ō - sī - at´ik). Ilioisquiático; relativo ao ílio e ao ísquio.
il·i·o·spi·nal (il´ē - ō - spī´năl). Iliospinhal; relativo ao ílio e à coluna vertebral.
il·i·o·tho·ra·cop·a·gus (il´ē - ō - thōr - ă - kop´a - gŭs). Iliotoracopago; gêmeos conjuntos em que a união ocorre através dos ílios e estende-se envolvendo o tórax. VER conjoined *twins*, em *twin*. SIN ischiothoracopagus. [ilio- + G. *thorax*, tórax + *pagos*, fixado]
il·i·o·tib·i·al (il´ē - ō - tib´ē - ăl). Iliotibial; relativo ao ílio e à tíbia.
il·i·o·tro·chan·ter·ic (il´ē - ō - trō - kan - ter´ik). Iliotrocantérico; relativo ao ílio e ao grande trocanter do fêmur.

il·i·o·xi·phop·a·gus (il′ē-ō-zī-fop′ă-gŭs). Ilioxifópago; gêmeos conjuntos em que a fusão se estende desde o xifóide até a região ilíaca. VER conjoined *twins* em *twin*. [ilio- + xifóide + G. *pagos*, fixado]

il·i·um, pl. **il·ia** (il′ē-ŭm, il′ē-ă) [TA]. Ílio; porção larga do osso do quadril, distinta ao nascimento mas que, posteriormente, se funde com o ísquio e púbis; consiste num corpo que se une ao púbis e ao ísquio para formar o acetábulo e em uma porção larga e delgada, denominada asa, ladeada, superiormente, por uma crista mais espessa. O corpo transmite o peso do tronco ao fêmur, enquanto a asa e a crista recebem a inserção muscular e protegem as vísceras abdominopélvicas. SIN os ilium [TA], flank bone, iliac bone, os iliacum. [L. virilha, flanco]

il·lic·i·um (il-lis′ē-ŭm). Anis estrelado ou anis chinês. Fruto seco de *Illhicium verum* (família Magnoliaceae), um arbusto de folhas persistentes ou uma pequena árvore do sul da China; utilizado como carminativo estimulante. [L. sedução, de *il-licio*, seduzir]

il·lin·i·tion (il-in-ish′ŭn). Ilinição; fricção de uma superfície para facilitar a absorção de uma pomada. [L. *il-lino*, pp. *-litus*, esfregar sobre (*in* + *lino*)]

ill·ness (il′nes). Doença. SIN disease (1).
   environmental i., d. ambiental. SIN multiple chemical sensitivity.
   factitious i. by proxy, d. factícia por proximidade. SIN Munchausen syndrome by proxy.
   functional i., d. funcional. SIN functional disorder.
   manic-depressive i., d. maníaco-depressiva; termo antigo para referir-se ao transtorno maníaco-depressivo (maniac-depressive *disorder*), que é atualmente denominado distúrbio bipolar (bipolar *disorder*) no atual DSM (*Diagnostic and Statistical Manual of Mental Disorders*).
   mass sociogenic i., d. sociogênica de massa. SIN mass hysteria.
   mental i., d. mental. **(1)** Termo bastante abrangente, indicando, em geral, uma ou todas as seguintes doenças: 1) doença do cérebro, com sintomas comportamentais predominantes, como na paresia ou no alcoolismo agudo; 2) doença da "mente" ou da personalidade, evidenciada por comportamento anormal, como na histeria ou na esquizofrenia; também denominada doença, distúrbio ou desordem mental ou emocional ou distúrbio de comportamento; **(2)** qualquer doença psiquiátrica relacionada na *Current Medical Information and Terminology* da Associação Americana de Medicina ou no *Diagnostic and Statistical Manual of Mental Disorders* (DSM) da Associação Psiquiátrica Americana. VER TAMBÉM behavior *disorder*.
   nonspecific building-related i.'s, doenças inespecíficas relacionadas a construções; grupo heterogêneo de sintomas relacionados ao trabalho ou ao domicílio, sem achados físicos ou laboratoriais objetivos e claros. Cf. specific building-related i.'s.
   severity of i., gravidade da d.; grau de doença e risco de doença manifestados por pacientes, baseando-se em dados clínicos obtidos de registros médicos ou em dados provenientes de alta/faturas hospitalares. As comparações finais são habitualmente interpretadas em termos de gravidade de doença para garantir a interpretação de dados significativos.
   specific building-related i.'s, doenças específicas relacionadas a construções; grupo de doenças infecciosas, alérgicas e imunológicas, com sinais clínicos bastante homogêneos, cujas causas podem ser atribuídas a fatores existentes em construções onde os pacientes acometidos trabalham ou residem. Cf. nonspecific building-related i.'s.

il·lu·mi·na·tion (i-loo′mi-nā′shŭn). Iluminação. **1.** Emissão de luz sobre o corpo ou uma parte ou no interior de uma cavidade para fins diagnósticos. **2.** Iluminação de um objeto sob um microscópio. [L. *il-lumino*, pp. *-atus*, iluminar]
   axial i., i. axial; transmissão ou reflexo de luz na direção do eixo de um sistema óptico. SIN central i.
   central i., i. central. SIN axial i.
   contact i., i. de contato; iluminação do olho por meio de um instrumento em contato com a córnea ou com a conjuntiva bulbar.
   critical i., i. crítica; focalização precisa da fonte luminosa diretamente sobre o objeto a ser examinado.
   dark-field i., i. em campo escuro; método em que se utiliza um escudo negro circular para bloquear a maior parte dos raios luminosos de direção vertical (p. ex., o campo é escuro), e utiliza-se uma superfície espelhada circunferencial, em ângulo apropriado, para dirigir os raios periféricos horizontalmente contra o objeto, refletindo, assim, a luz verticalmente através da objetiva e ao longo do eixo óptico; assim, o objeto fica bem iluminado contra um fundo escuro contrastante. SIN dark-ground i.
   dark-ground i., i. de fundo escuro. SIN dark-field i.
   direct i., i. direta; iluminação em que os raios luminosos são dirigidos para baixo, quase perpendicularmente à superfície superior do objeto, que reflete os raios para cima no sistema óptico. SIN erect i., vertical i.
   erect i., i. ereta. SIN direct i.
   focal i., i. focal; iluminação em que um feixe de luz é dirigido diagonalmente para um objeto, de modo que este fica brilhantemente iluminado, enquanto a área circundante se encontra na sombra. SIN lateral i., oblique i.
   Köhler i., i. de Köhler; método de iluminação de objetos microscópicos em que a imagem da fonte luminosa é focalizada na subplatina do diafragma do condensador e o diafragma da fonte luminosa é focado no mesmo plano com o objeto a ser examinado; aumenta ao máximo tanto o brilho quanto a uniformidade do campo iluminado.
   lateral i., i. lateral. SIN focal i.
   oblique i., i. oblíqua. SIN focal i.
   vertical i., i. vertical. SIN direct i.

il·lu·mi·nism (i-loo′mi-nizm). Iluminismo; estado psicótico de exaltação em que o indivíduo apresenta delírios e alucinações de comunhão com seres sobrenaturais ou exaltados.

il·lu·sion (i-loo′zhŭn). Ilusão; percepção falsa; ato de confundir algo por aquilo que não é. [L. *illusio*, de *il-ludo*, pp. *-lusus*, brincar, zombar]
   i. of doubles, i. de duplos. SIN Capgras syndrome.
   i. of movement, i. de movimento; estimulação sucessiva de pontos vizinhos da retina, causando a sensação de movimento.
   oculogravic i., i. oculogravítica; movimento aparente do campo visual quando o corpo é submetido a aceleração; devido à gravidade.
   oculogyral i., i. oculógira; ilusão que ocorre na aceleração angular, em que a posição da luz fixa parece deslocar-se.
   optical i., i. óptica; falsa interpretação da cor, forma, tamanho ou movimento de uma sensação visual.

il·lu·sion·al (i-loo′zhŭn-ăl). Ilusório; relativo a, ou da natureza de, uma ilusão.

Ilosvay, Lajos de, químico húngaro, 1851–1936. VER I. *reagent*.

IM Abreviatura de internal *medicine* (medicina interna).

I.M., i.m. Abreviatura de intramuscular.

ima (ī′mă). O mais inferior. VER TAMBÉM imus. [L.]

im·age (im′ij). Imagem. **1.** Representação de um objeto feita pelos raios luminosos que emanam dele ou que nele se refletem. **2.** Representação produzida por raios X, ultra-som, tomografia, termografia, radioisótopos, etc. **3.** Produzir essas representações. [L. *imago*, semelhança]
   accidental i., i. acidental. SIN afterimage.
   body i., i corporal; **(1)** Representação cerebral de toda a sensação corporal organizada no córtex parietal; **(2)** concepção pessoal do próprio corpo em contraste com o corpo anatômico real ou a concepção de outras pessoas sobre o próprio corpo. SIN body schema.
   catatropic i., i. catatrópica. SIN Purkinje-Sanson i.'s.
   direct i., i. direta. SIN virtual i.
   eidetic i., i. eidética; imagem mental vívida na forma de um sonho, fantasia ou capacidade incomum de memória ou visualização de objetos previamente vistos ou imaginados.
   false i., i. falsa; imagem formada no olho desviado no estrabismo.
   heteronymous i., imagem heterônima; imagem dupla na diplopia fisiológica, quando a fixação é dirigida além do objeto; a imagem direita origina-se do olho esquerdo, enquanto a imagem esquerda origina-se do olho direito; isto é, existe diplopia cruzada.
   homonymous i.'s, imagens homônimas; imagens duplas produzidas por estímulo, que se originam de pontos proximais do horóptero. SIN homonymous diplopia, simple diplopia, uncrossed diplopia.
   hypnagogic i., i. hipnagógica; imagem que ocorre entre a vigília e o sono.
   hypnopompic i., i. hipnopômpica; imagem que ocorre após o estado de sono e antes do despertar completo; semelhante à imagem hipnagógica, exceto quanto ao momento de sua ocorrência.
   inverted i., i. invertida. SIN real i.
   magnitude i., i. de magnitude; nas imagens (*imaging*) obtidas por ressonância magnética, imagem formada a partir da amplitude do sinal, distinta das informações de fase. VER TAMBÉM magnetic resonance *imaging*.
   mental i., i. mental; visualização de um objeto não presente, produzida na mente pela memória ou imaginação.
   mirror i., i. -espelho; representação de um objeto, ou parte dele, como se fosse a sua imagem refletida num espelho.
   motor i., i. motora; imagem dos movimentos corporais.
   negative i., i. negativa. SIN afterimage.
   optical i., i. óptica; imagem formada pela refração ou reflexão da luz.
   phase i., i. de fase; imagem de ressonância magnética mostrando apenas a informação de desvio de fase para detectar o movimento.
   Purkinje i.'s, imagens de Purkinje. SIN Purkinje-Sanson i.'s.
   Purkinje-Sanson i.'s, imagens de Purkinje-Sanson, as duas imagens formadas pelas superfícies anterior e posterior da córnea e as duas imagens formadas pelas superfícies anterior e posterior do cristalino. SIN catatropic i., Purkinje i.'s, Sanson i.'s.
   real i., i. real; imagem formada pela convergência dos raios luminosos provenientes de um objeto. SIN inverted i.
   retinal i., i. da retina; imagem real formada na retina.
   Sanson i.'s, imagens de Sanson. SIN Purkinje-Sanson i.'s.
   sensory i., i. sensorial; imagem baseada em um ou mais tipos de sensação.
   specular i., i. especular; imagem de uma fonte de luz que se torna visível pela reflexão de um espelho.
   tactile i., i. tátil; imagem de um objeto percebido pelo sentido do tato.

unequal retinal i., i. retiniana desigual. SIN aniseikonia.
virtual i., i. virtual; imagem ereta formada pela projeção de raios divergentes de um sistema óptico. SIN direct i.
visual i., i. visual; coleção de focos que correspondem a todos os pontos luminosos de um objeto.

im·age in·ten·si·fi·er. Intensificador de imagem. SIN image amplifier.

im·ag·e·ry (im′ij-rē). Imaginação; técnica, em terapia comportamental, pela qual o cliente ou o paciente é condicionado a substituir os sentimentos desagradáveis associados a ansiedade por fantasias agradáveis.

imag·i·nal (ī-maj′i-nāl). Imaginário; relativo a uma imagem ou ao processo de imaginação.

imag·ing (im′ā-jing). Imagens clínicas obtidas através de raios X, ultra-som, tomografia computadorizada, ressonância magnética, cintilografia e termografia; especialmente, imagens transversais, como ultra-sonografia, TC ou RM. VER image.
blood pool i., i. do reservatório sanguíneo; estudo de medicina nuclear utilizando um radionuclídeo confinado ao compartimento vascular.
exercise i., prova de esforço. VER stress test.
magnetic resonance i. (MRI), imagens por ressonância magnética; modalidade radiológica diagnóstica que utiliza a tecnologia da ressonância magnética nuclear, em que os núcleos magnéticos (especialmente prótons) de um paciente são alinhados num campo magnético forte e uniforme, absorvem energia de pulsos de radiofreqüência e emitem sinais de radiofreqüência à medida que a sua excitação declina. Esses sinais, cuja intensidade varia de acordo com a abundância nuclear e com o ambiente químico molecular, são convertidos em conjuntos de imagens tomográficas ao utilizar gradientes de campo no campo magnético, permitindo uma localização tridimensional das fontes puntiformes dos sinais. SIN nuclear magnetic resonance i., NMR i., nuclear magnetic resonance tomography.
nuclear magnetic resonance i., NMR i., ressonância magnética nuclear. SIN magnetic resonance i.
pharmacologic stress i., prova de esforço farmacológico. VER stress test.
through transfer i., i. de transferência. SIN transfer i.
transfer i., i. de transferência; produção de uma imagem de ultra-som por detecção e análise do som no lado oposto do corpo a partir do transdutor emissor. SIN through transfer i.

imag·ing de·part·ment. Departamento de radiologia diagnóstica. VER imaging, radiology.

ima·go, pl. **imag·ines** (i-mā′gō, i-maj′i-nēz). Imago. **1.** Último estágio de um inseto após ter completado toda a sua metamorfose através de ovo, larva e pupa; a forma adulta do inseto. **2.** Arquétipo. SIN archetype (2). [L. imagem]

im·bal·ance (im-bal′ans). Desequilíbrio. **1.** Falta de igualdade entre forças oponentes. **2.** Falta de igualdade em algum aspecto da visão binocular, como equilíbrio muscular, tamanho da imagem e/ou forma da imagem. [L. *in-* neg. + *bi-lanx (-lanc-)*, que possui dois pratos, de *bis*, duplo + *lanx*, prato de balança]
autonomic i., d. autônomo; falta de equilíbrio entre os sistemas nervosos simpático e parassimpático, especialmente em relação aos distúrbios vasomotores. SIN vasomotor i.
occlusal i., d. oclusal; relação desarmônica entre os dentes do maxilar e da mandíbula durante o fechamento ou os fechamentos funcionais da mandíbula.
sex chromosome i., d. dos cromossomas sexuais; qualquer padrão anormal dos cromossomas sexuais; p. ex., XXY em homens com disgenesia dos túbulos seminíferos, XO em mulheres com síndrome de Turner; os padrões mais raros de desequilíbrio incluem XXX, XXXY e XYY. VER TAMBÉM isochromosome.
sympathetic i., d. simpático. SIN vagotonia.
vasomotor i., d. vasomotor. SIN autonomic i.

im·be·cile (im′bē-sil). Imbecil; termo obsoleto para referir-se a uma subclasse de *retardo* mental ou ao indivíduo assim classificado. [L. *imbecillus*, fraco, tolo]

im·bed. Incluído, incrustado. SIN embed.

im·bi·bi·tion (im-bi-bish′ŭn). Embebição. **1.** Absorção de líquido por um corpo sólido sem alteração química resultante em ambos. **2.** Captação de água por um gel, aumentando assim o seu tamanho. [L. *im-bibo*, beber (*in* + *bibo*)]

im·bri·cate, im·bri·cat·ed (im′bri-kāt, im′bri-kā-ted). Imbricar, imbricado; superposto como telhas. [L. *imbricatus*, coberto com telhas]

im·bri·ca·tion (im′bri-kā′shŭn), Imbricação; superposição cirúrgica de camadas de tecido no fechamento de feridas ou reparo de defeitos. [ver imbricar]
eyelid i., i. palpebral; anormalidade da posição das pálpebras em que a pálpebra superior superpõe-se à pálpebra inferior estando o olho fechado, resultando em irritação ocular crônica.

im·id·a·zole (im-id-az′ōl). Imidazol; composto heterocíclico com cinco elementos que ocorre na L-histidina e em outros compostos biologicamente importantes.
i. alkaloids, alcalóides de i.; alcalóides contendo um ou mais radicais de imidazol como parte de sua estrutura (p. ex., pilocarpina).

4-im·id·a·zo·lone-5-pro·pi·on·ate (im-id-a-zō′lōn). 4-imidazolona-5-propionato; intermediário na degradação da histidina; presente em níveis reduzidos na acidúria urocânica.

im·id·az·o·lyl (im-id-az′ō-lil). Imidazolil; radical do imidazol. SIN iminazolyl.

im·ide (im′id). Imida. Radical, grupo ou componente, =NH, fixado a dois grupamentos –CO–.

imido-. Imido-. Prefixo indicando radical de uma imida, formado pela perda do H do grupamento =NH.

im·i·do·di·pep·ti·dase (im′i-dō-dī-pep′ti-dās). Imidodipeptidase. SIN *proline* dipeptidase.

im·id·o·di·pep·ti·du·ria (im-idō-dī-pep′tid-oor-ē-ā). Imidodipeptidúria; níveis elevados de dipeptídeos contendo prolina na urina; associada a deficiência de prolidase (peptidase D); resultando em comprometimento do desenvolvimento.

im·i·dole (im′i-dōl). Imidol. SIN pyrrole.

im·in·az·o·lyl (im-in-az′ō-lil). Iminazolil. SIN imidazolyl.

-imine. -Imina. Sufixo indicando o grupamento =NH.

imino-. Imino-. Prefixo indicando o grupamento =NH.

im·i·no ac·ids (im′i-nō, i-mē′nō). Iminoácidos; compostos com moléculas contendo tanto um grupamento ácido (em geral, a carboxila –COOH) e um grupamento imino (=NH).

im·i·no·car·bon·yl (im′i-nō-kar′bon-il). Iminocarbonil. VER carboxamide.

im·i·no·di·pep·ti·dase (im′i-nō-dī-pep′ti-dās). Iminodipeptidase. SIN *prolyl* dipeptidase.

im·i·no·gly·ci·nu·ria (im′i-nō-glī-si-noo′rē-ā). [MIM*242600]. Iminoglicinúria; erro inato benigno do transporte de aminoácidos nos túbulos renais e no intestino; a glicina, a prolina e a hidroxiprolina são excretadas na urina; provavelmente de herança autossômica recessiva; foi sugerida uma heterogeneidade genética.

im·i·no·hy·dro·las·es (im′i-nō-hī′drō-lās-ez) [EC class 3.5.3]. Iminohidrolases; enzimas que hidrolisam grupamentos imino; p. ex., arginina desiminase. SIN deiminases.

im·in·os·til·benes (im′i-nō-stil′benz). Iminostilbenos; classe química de agentes dos quais o mais proeminente é a carbamazepina, um agente antiepiléptico.

im·i·pen·em (im-i-pen′em). Imipenem; antibiótico tienamicina com amplo espectro de atividade, associado à cilastina no tratamento de várias infecções.

imip·ra·mine hy·dro·chlo·ride (im-ip′ra-mēn). Cloridrato de imipramina; antidepressivo tricíclico. Metabolizado para formar desipramina, outro antidepressivo tricíclico.

imiquimod. Modificador da resposta imune utilizado na pele no tratamento de verrugas genitais e perianais externas.

IML Abreviatura de intermediolateral cell column (coluna de células intermediolaterais) da substância cinzenta da medula espinal.

Imlach, Francis, anatomista e cirurgião escocês, 1819–1891. VER I. *fat-pad*.

im·me·di·ca·ble (im-med′i-kā-bl). Imedicável; termo obsoleto significando não-curável por medicamentos. [L. *in-* neg. + *medicabilis*, curável]

im·mer·sion (i-mer′zhŭn). Imersão. **1.** Colocação de um corpo debaixo de água ou de outro líquido. **2.** Em microscopia, preenchimento do espaço entre a objetiva e a parte superior da lamínula com um líquido, como água ou óleo, para reduzir a aberração esférica e aumentar a abertura numérica efetiva por eliminação dos efeitos refratários que resultam da interface ar-vidro; obtém-se a melhor resolução quando o espaço entre o condensador e a lâmina também está cheio de líquido. [L. *immergo*, pp. *-mersus*, mergulhar (*in* + *mergo*)]
homogeneous i., i. homogênea; em microscopia de imersão, uso de um líquido, como óleo, que tem um índice de refração praticamente idêntico ao do vidro, fornecendo a máxima abertura numérica possível.
oil i., water i., i. em óleo, i. em água. VER immersion (2).

im·mis·ci·ble (i-mis′i-bl). Imiscível; incapaz de solução mútua; p. ex., óleo e água. [L. *im. misceo*, misturar (*in* + *misceo*)]

immission (im-ish′in). Imissão; concentração ambiental de um poluente, resultante de uma combinação de imissões e dispersões; utilizado freqüentemente como sinônimo de exposição. [L. *immissio*, introdução, de *im- mitto*, introduzir]

im·mit·tance (i-mit′ans). Imitância; medida da impedância e complacência do ouvido médio. SIN admittance [L. *immitto*, enviar]

im·mo·bi·li·za·tion (i-mo′bi-li-zā′shŭn). Imobilização; o ato de tornar imóvel. [ver imobilizar]

im·mo·bi·lize (i-mō′bi-līz). Imobilizar; tornar fixo ou incapaz de se mover. [L. *in-* neg. + *mobilis*, móvel]

im·mor·tal·i·za·tion (i-mōr′tāl-i-zā′shŭn). Imortalização; que confere a células normais cultivadas *in vitro* a propriedade de uma sobrevida infinita, em decorrência de mutação espontânea, exposição a carcinógenos químicos ou por infecção viral. A imortalização de células primárias em cultura constitui a primeira de várias etapas na expressão de genes de transformação de vírus tumorais de DNA, oncogenes retrovirais e oncogenes celulares derivados de células cancerosas humanas.

im·mune (i-mūn′). Imune. **1.** Livre da possibilidade de adquirir determinada doença infecciosa; resistente a uma doença infecciosa. **2.** Relativo ao meca-

immune

nismo de sensibilização em que a reatividade é tão alterada por contato prévio com um antígeno que os tecidos capazes de responder o fazem rapidamente com um contato subseqüente, ou a reações *in vitro* com soro contendo anticorpos desses indivíduos sensibilizados. [L. *immunis*, livre de serviço, de *in*, neg., + *munus* (*muner-*), serviço]

im·mu·ni·fa·cient (im'ū - ni - fā'shent). Imunifaciente; que torna imune após uma doença específica. [L. *immunis*, isento + *faciens*, fazendo, pr. part. de *facio*]

im·mu·ni·ty (i - mū'ni - tē). Imunidade. **1.** Estado ou qualidade de ser imune (1). **2.** Proteção contra doenças infecciosas. SIN insusceptibility. [L. *immunitas* (ver immune)]

acquired i., i. adquirida; resistência resultante de exposição prévia do indivíduo a um agente infeccioso ou antígeno; pode ser *ativa* e *específica*, em conseqüência de infecção adquirida naturalmente (evidente ou inaparente) ou vacinação intencional (i. ativa artificial); ou pode ser *passiva*, sendo adquirida por transferência de anticorpos de outra pessoa ou de animal, seja naturalmente, como da mãe para o feto, ou por inoculação intencional (i. passiva artificial) e, em relação aos anticorpos particulares transferidos, *específica*. A imunidade passiva mediada por células, produzida pela transferência de células linfóides vivas de um animal imune (alérgico ou sensível) para um animal normal, às vezes é denominada i. adotiva.

active i., i. ativa. VER acquired i.
adoptive i., i. adotiva. VER acquired i.
antiviral i., i. antiviral; imunidade resultante de infecção por vírus, seja adquirida naturalmente ou produzida por vacinação intencional; comparada com algumas imunidades bacterianas, tem duração relativamente longa, mas isso pode ser o resultado de uma imunidade à infecção em vez de ser peculiar à infecção viral em si, visto que ocorre também na imunidade bacteriana após infecções como a febre tifóide.

resumo das defesas inespecíficas do hospedeiro

tipo	mecanismo
barreiras anatômicas	
pele	barreira mecânica que retarda a penetração de micróbios
	meio ácido (pH = 3–5) retarda o crescimento de micróbios
mucosas	a flora normal compete com os micróbios por nutrientes e locais de ligação
	o muco retém os microrganismos estranhos
	os cílios impelem os microrganismos para fora do organismo
barreiras fisiológicas	
temperatura	a temperatura corporal inibe o crescimento de alguns patógenos
	a resposta febril inibe o crescimento de alguns patógenos
pH baixo	o pH ácido do estômago destrói a maioria dos microrganismos ingeridos
mediadores químicos	a lisozima fragmenta a parede celular das bactérias
	o interferon induz o estado antiviral em células não-infectadas
	o complemento lisa os microrganismos ou facilita a fagocitose dos mesmos
barreiras fagocíticas/endocíticas	
	várias células internalizam (endocitose) e fragmentam macrocélulas
	células especializadas (monócitos sanguíneos, neutrófilos, macrófagos teciduais) fagocitam, destroem e digerem microrganismos inteiros
barreiras inflamatórias	
	lesão tecidual e infecção induzem extravasamento de líquido vascular, contendo proteínas séricas com atividade antibacteriana, e influxo de células fagocíticas para a área afetada

immunoassay

artificial active i., i. ativa artificial. VER acquired i.
artificial passive i., i. passiva artificial. VER acquired i.
bacteriophage i., i. por bacteriófagos; estado induzido numa bactéria por lisogenização, sendo a bactéria lisogênica insensível a nova lisogenização ou a um ciclo lítico por um bacteriófago superinfectante, em contraposição com resistência a bacteriófagos.
cell-mediated i. (CMI), cellular i., i. mediada por células (IMC), i. celular; respostas imunes que são desencadeadas por uma célula apresentadora de antígeno que interage com linfócitos T (p. ex., rejeição de enxerto, hipersensibilidade de tipo tardio). SIN delayed hypersensitivity (1).
concomitant i., i. concomitante. SIN infection i.
general i., i. generalizada; imunidade associada a mecanismos amplamente difusos, que tende a proteger o corpo como um todo, em comparação com a i. local.
group i., i. de grupo. SIN herd i.
herd i., i. de grupo; resistência a invasão e disseminação de um agente infeccioso num grupo ou comunidade, baseando-se na resistência de uma alta proporção de membros do grupo à infecção; a resistência é um produto do número de indivíduos suscetíveis e da probabilidade de que esses indivíduos entraram em contato com uma pessoa infectada. SIN group i.
humoral i., i. humoral; imunidade associada a anticorpos circulantes, em contraposição com a i. celular.
infection i., i. à infecção; estado imune paradoxal em que a resistência à reinfecção coincide com a persistência da infecção original. SIN concomitant i.
innate i., i. inata; resistência manifestada por uma espécie (ou por raças, famílias e indivíduos numa espécie) que não foi imunizada (sensibilizada, alergizada) por infecção ou vacinação prévia; grande parte da imunidade inata resulta de mecanismos corporais que ainda não estão bem elucidados, mas que diferem daqueles responsáveis pela reatividade alterada associada à natureza específica da imunidade adquirida; em geral, a imunidade inata não é específica nem é estimulada por antígenos específicos. VER TAMBÉM self. SIN natural i., nonspecific i.
local i., i. local; imunidade natural ou adquirida a certos agentes infecciosos, manifestada por um órgão ou por tecido, como um todo ou em parte.
maternal i., i. materna; imunidade adquirida pelo feto devido à presença de IgG materna que atravessa a placenta.
natural i., nonspecific i., i. natural, i. inespecífica. SIN innate i.
passive i., i. passiva. VER acquired i.
relative i., i. relativa; resistência modificada, não totalmente efetiva, que surge quando existe um tipo de "equilíbrio flutuante" entre os mecanismos de defesa do hospedeiro e o agente infeccioso.
specific i., i. específica; o estado imune em que existe uma reatividade alterada dirigida apenas contra os determinantes antigênicos (agente infeccioso ou outro) que a estimularam. VER acquired i.
specific active i., i. ativa específica. VER acquired i.
specific passive i., i. passiva específica. VER acquired i.
stress i., i. ao estresse; resistência ou ausência de suscetibilidade aos efeitos de tensão emocional.

im·mu·ni·za·tion (im - mū'ni - zā'shŭn). Imunização; proteção de indivíduos suscetíveis contra doenças contagiosas por meio da administração de um agente modificado vivo (p. ex., vacina contra febre amarela), de uma suspensão de microrganismos mortos (p. ex., vacina contra coqueluche) ou de uma toxina inativada (p. ex., tétano). VER TAMBÉM vaccination, allergization.
active i., i. ativa; produção de imunidade ativa.
passive i., i. passiva; produção de imunidade passiva.

im·mu·nize (im'ū - nīz). Imunizar. **1.** Tornar imune. **2.** Administrar uma imunização.

immuno-. Imuno-. Imune, imunidade. [L. *immunis*, imune]

im·mu·no·ad·ju·vant (im'ū - nō - ad'joo - vant). Imunoadjuvante. VER adjuvant (2).

im·mu·no·ag·glu·ti·na·tion (im'ū - nō - ă - gloo - ti - nā'shŭn). Imunoaglutinação; aglutinação específica efetuada por anticorpos.

im·mu·no·as·say (im'ū - nō - ăs'ā, im - ū'nō). Imunoensaio; detecção e ensaio de substâncias por métodos sorológicos (imunológicos); na maioria das aplicações, a substância em questão serve como antígeno, tanto na produção de anticorpos quanto na medida do anticorpo pela substância do teste. VER TAMBÉM enzyme-linked immunosorbent *assay*, radio-immunoassay, radioimmunoelectrophoresis, immunologic pregnancy *test*. SIN immunochemical assay.
double antibody i., i. de anticorpo duplo. SIN double antibody *precipitation*.
enzyme i., i. enzimático; inclui vários métodos de imunoensaio que utilizam uma enzima ligada de modo covalente a um antígeno ou anticorpo como marcador; os tipos mais comuns são o ensaio imunossorvente ligado a enzima (ELISA) e a técnica de imunoensaio multiplicado por enzima (EMIT). VER TAMBÉM enzyme-linked immunosorbent *assay*, enzyme-multiplied i. technique.
enzyme-multiplied i. technique (EMIT), técnica de i. multiplicado por enzima; tipo de imunoensaio em que o ligante é marcado com uma enzima e o complexo enzima–ligante–anticorpo é enzimaticamente inativo, permitindo a quantificação do ligante não-marcado. VER TAMBÉM competitive binding *assay*, enzyme-linked immunosorbent *assay*.

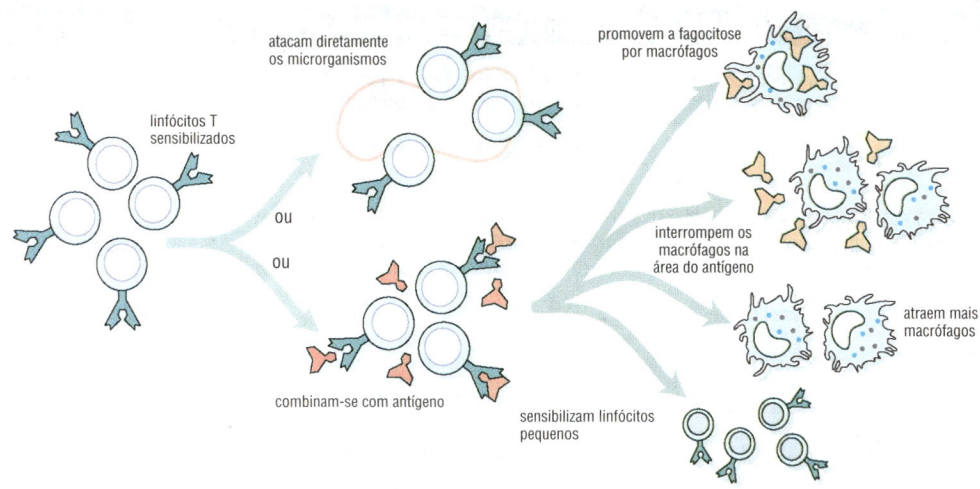

imunidade mediada por células

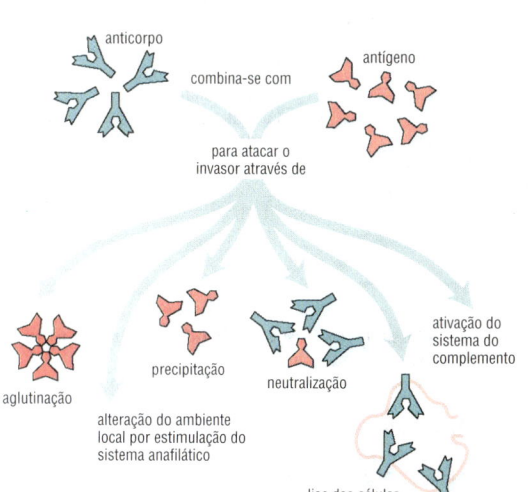

imunidade humoral

solid phase i., i. de fase sólida; imunoensaio em que o antígeno ou soro é ligado a uma superfície sólida, como uma parede de microplaca ou os lados de um tubo, estando os outros reagentes livres na solução.

thin-layer i., i. de camada fina; método de detecção de reações antígeno-anticorpo, aplicável à detecção do antígeno ou do anticorpo, baseando-se no fato de que qualquer reagente, quando adicionado a uma superfície de polistireno (como um orifício numa placa de polistireno), é absorvido como uma delgada camada e atua como imunossorvente capaz de ligar-se ao segundo reagente.

im·mun·o·bi·ol·o·gy (im′ū-nō-bī-ol′-ō-ijē, im-oo′nō). Imunobiologia; estudo dos fatores imunes que afetam o crescimento, o desenvolvimento e a saúde dos organismos biológicos.

im·mu·no·blast (im′ū-nō-blast). Imunoblasto; linfócito estimulado antigenicamente; grande célula com citoplasma basófilo bem definido, núcleo grande com membrana nuclear proeminente, nucléolos distintos e cromatina agregada. VER TAMBÉM lymphoblast, lymphocyte *transformation*. [immuno- + G. *blastos*, germe]

im·mu·no·blot, im·mu·no·blot·ting (i′mū-nō-blot′). Immunoblot, immunoblotting. Processo que permite a separação de antígenos por eletroforese, que aderem a camadas de nitrocelulose, onde se ligam de modo inespecífico e, a seguir, são identificados por coloração com anticorpos apropriadamente marcados. VER TAMBÉM Western blot *analysis*.

im·mu·no·blot·ting. Immunoblotting. VER immunoblot.

im·mu·no·chem·is·try (im′ū-nō-kem′is-trē). Imunoquímica; campo da química relacionado aos aspectos químicos dos fenômenos imunológicos, como, p. ex., as reações químicas relacionadas à estimulação antigênica dos tecidos, estudos químicos dos antígenos e anticorpos.

im·mu·no·com·pe·tence (im′ū-nō-kom′pĕ-tens). Imunocompetência; capacidade de produzir uma resposta imune normal.

im·mu·no·com·pe·tent (im′ū-nō-kom′pĕ-tent). Imunocompetente; que tem a capacidade de desenvolver uma resposta imune normal.

im·mu·no·com·plex. Imunocomplexo; complexo de anticorpo e antígeno. VER immune *complex*.

im·mu·no·com·pro·mised (im′ū-nō-kom′pro-mīzd). Imunocomprometido; refere-se a um indivíduo cujo mecanismo imunológico é deficiente devido a um distúrbio de imunodeficiência ou à indução desse estado por agentes imunossupressores.

im·mu·no·con·glu·ti·nin (im′ū-nō-kon-gloo′ti-nin). Imunoconglutinina; imunoglobulina (IgM) semelhante a um auto-anticorpo, formado em animais (ou no homem) contra seu próprio complemento após injeção de complexos contendo complemento ou bactérias sensibilizadas.

im·mu·no·cyte (im′ū-nō-sit, im-oo′nō). Imunócito; leucócito imunologicamente competente, que tem a capacidade, ativa ou potencial, de produzir anticorpos ou de reagir em reações de imunidade celular. VER TAMBÉM I *cell*. [immuno- + G. *kytos*, célula]

im·mu·no·cy·to·ad·her·ence (im′ū-nō-sī′tō-ad-her′ens). Imunocitoaderência; método para determinar as propriedades das superfícies celulares, em que uma imunoglobulina ou receptores sobre a superfície de uma população de células induz a aderência das células com configurações moleculares correspondentes em sua superfície, formando rosetas em torno das células.

im·mu·no·cy·to·chem·is·try (im′ū-nō-si-tō-kem′is-trē). Imunocitoquímica; o estudo dos constituintes celulares por métodos imunológicos, como o uso de anticorpos fluorescentes ou da coloração com imunoperoxidase.

im·mu·no·de·fi·cien·cy (im′ū-nō-dē-fish′en-sē, im-ū′). Imunodeficiência; condição resultante de deficiência do mecanismo imunológico; pode ser *primária* (devido a um defeito no próprio mecanismo imunológico) ou *secundária* (dependente de outro processo mórbido), *específica* (devido a um defeito no sistema de linfócitos B ou de linfócitos T ou ambos) ou *inespecífica* (devido a um defeito em um ou outro componente do mecanismo imunológico inespecífico: o sistema do complemento, da properdina ou fagocítico). SIN immune deficiency, immunity deficiency, immunologic deficiency.

cellular i. with abnormal immunoglobulin synthesis, i. celular com síntese anormal de imunoglobulinas; grupo mal definido de distúrbios esporádicos, de causa desconhecida, que ocorrem em homens e mulheres e estão associados a infecções por bactérias, fungos, protozoários e vírus recorrentes; ocorre hipoplasia do timo com depressão da imunidade celular (linfócitos T) associada a imunidade humoral defeituosa (linfócitos B), embora os níveis de imunoglobulinas possam ser normais. SIN Nezelof syndrome.

combined i., i. combinada; imunodeficiência tanto dos linfócitos B quanto dos linfócitos T.

common variable i., i. comum variável; imunodeficiência de causa desconhecida e, em geral, não-classificável; o início ocorre habitualmente depois dos 15 anos de idade, mas pode ser observado em qualquer idade em ambos os sexos; a quantidade total de imunoglobulina costuma ser inferior a 300 mg/dL; a contagem de linfócitos B situa-se freqüentemente dentro dos limites normais, porém há uma falta de plasmócitos no tecido linfóide; a imunidade celular (linfócitos T) está habitualmente intacta; ocorre susceptibilidade aumentada a infecção piogênica e, com freqüência, a doença auto-imune. SIN acquired agammaglobulinemia, acquired hypogammaglobulinemia.

classificação dos distúrbios de imunodeficiência primária			
imunodeficiências humorais (células B)	**imunodeficiências celulares (células T)**	**deficiências combinadas de células B (humoral) e de células T (celular)**	**doenças de disfunção fagocítica**
agamaglobulinemia ligada ao X	anomalia de DiGeorge	imunodeficiência combinada grave (incluindo SCID ligada ao X, síndrome de Nezelof, etc.)	síndromes neutropênicas
hipogamaglobulinemia transitória do lactente	candidíase mucocutânea crônica	imunodeficiência combinada com defeitos de sinalização ou da membrana das células T	doença granulomatosa crônica
imunodeficiência comum variável	deficiência múltipla de co-carboxilase biotina-dependente	síndrome de Wiskott-Aldrich	deficiência de glicose-6-fosfato-desidrogenase leucocitária
síndrome da hiper-IgM	deficiência de células *natural killer*	ataxia–telangiectasia	síndrome de Chediak-Higashi
deficiência de IgA	linfopenia idiopática de células CD4	síndrome de ruptura de Nijmegen	deficiência de mieloperoxidase
deficiência de IgM		imunodeficiência com nanismo de membros curtos, hipoplasia da cartilagem e cabelo	deficiência de grânulos específicos
deficiências de subclasses de IgG		imunodeficiência com deficiência enzimática: adenosina desaminase ou nucleosídeo fosforilase	doença de armazenamento do glicogênio tipo 1b
falta de responsividade a polissacarídeos		doença de enxerto-*versus*-hospedeiro	síndrome de Job/hiper-IgE
deficiência de transcobalamina		síndrome do linfócito nu	defeito na adesão leucocitária
imunodeficiência com timoma		síndrome de Omenn	síndrome de Schwachman
		disgenesia reticular	deficiência de tuftsina
		síndrome linfoproliferativa ligada ao X	síndromes de periodontite

SCID, doença por imunodeficiência combinada grave

phagocytic dysfunction i., i. por disfunção fagocítica; supressão do número ou da função das células fagocíticas, como na doença granulomatosa crônica. SIN phagocytic dysfunction disorders i.
phagocytic dysfunction disorders i., i. dos distúrbios de disfunção fagocítica. SIN phagocytic dysfunction i.
secondary i., i. secundária; imunodeficiência em que não há defeito evidente nos tecidos linfóides, mas há sinais de hipercatabolismo ou perda de imunoglobulinas; conforme observado na hipoproteinemia hipercatabólica idiopática familiar ou em defeitos associados à síndrome nefrótica. SIN secondary agammaglobulinemia, secondary antibody deficiency, secondary hypogammaglobulinemia.
severe combined i. (SCID) [MIM*202500, MIM*300400 e MIM*312863], i. combinada grave (IDCG); imunodeficiência caracterizada pela ausência de imunidade tanto humoral quanto celular com linfopenia (tanto de linfócitos do tipo B quanto do tipo T); caracterizada por atrofia do timo, ausência de hipersensibilidade tardia e acentuada suscetibilidade a infecções por bactérias, vírus, fungos, protozoários e vacinas vivas; embora o transplante de medula óssea tenha sido efetivo, pode ocorrer morte no primeiro ano de vida. Ocorrem formas tanto autossômicas recessivas quanto ligadas ao X; cerca da metade dos indivíduos com SCID autossômica recessiva apresenta deficiência de adenosina desaminase. A forma ligada ao X é causada por mutação no gene do receptor da interleucina-2 gama (IL2RG) no cromossoma Xq. SIN Swiss type agammaglobulinemia.
i. with elevated IgM, i. com IgM elevada; imunodeficiência com redução das células que transportam IgG e IgA; ocorre infecção piogênica recorrente; forma ligada ao cromossoma X em algumas famílias.
i. with hypoparathyroidism, i. com hipoparatireoidismo. SIN DiGeorge *syndrome.*
im·mu·no·de·fi·cient (im′ū-nō-dē-fish′ent). Imunodeficiente; falta de alguma função essencial no sistema imune.
im·mu·no·de·pres·sant (im′ū-nō-dē-pres′ănt). Imunodepressor. SIN immunosuppressant.
im·mu·no·de·pres·sor (im′ū-nō-dē-pres′ŏr, -ōr). Imunodepressor. SIN immunosuppressant.
im·mu·no·di·ag·no·sis (im′ū-nō-dī-ag-nō′sis). Imunodiagnóstico; processo de determinação das características imunológicas específicas de indivíduos ou de células, soro ou outras amostras biológicas.
im·mu·no·dif·fu·sion (im′ū-nō-di-fū′zhŭn, im-ū′nō-). Imunodifusão; técnica de estudo das reações antígeno-anticorpo (Ag-Ac) pela observação de precipitados formados por complexos Ag-Ac, que são formados pela combinação de antígeno e anticorpos específicos que se difundiram em um gel no qual foram colocados separadamente.
double i., i. dupla. VER gel diffusion precipitin *tests* in two dimensions, em *test.*
radial i. (RID), i. radial. VER gel diffusion precipitin *tests* in one dimension, em *test.*
single i., i. simples. VER gel diffusion precipitin *tests* in one dimension, em *test,* gel diffusion precipitin *tests* in two dimensions, em *test.*
im·mu·no·e·lec·tro·pho·re·sis (im′ū-nō-ē-lek′trō-fō-rē′sis). Imunoeletroforese; tipo de teste de precipitina em que os componentes de um grupo de reagentes imunológicos (em geral, uma mistura de antígenos) são inicialmente separados com base na sua mobilidade eletroforética em ágar ou outro meio; a seguir, os componentes separados são identificados por meio da técnica de dupla difusão, com base nos precipitados formados pela reação com componentes do outro grupo de reagentes (anticorpos).
crossed i., i. cruzada. SIN two-dimensional i.
rocket i., i. em foguete; método quantitativo para proteínas séricas que envolve a eletroforese de antígenos em gel contendo anticorpos; essa técnica restringe-se à detecção de antígenos que se movem para o pólo positivo na eletroforese. VER electroimmunodiffusion.
two-dimensional i., i. bidimensional; combinação da separação eletroforética convencional e eletroimunodifusão; efetua-se em primeiro lugar a eletroforese; a seguir, a tira eletroforética é colocada numa segunda lâmina, e deixa-se uma solução de agarose contendo anticorpo solidificar em sua adjacência; a seguir, efetua-se a eletroforese em ângulo reto com a separação original. SIN crossed i.
im·mu·no·en·hance·ment (im′ū-nō-en-hans′ment). Intensificação imune; aumento da resposta imune; além do anticorpo, substâncias inespecíficas também podem atuar para intensificar a resposta imune. SIN immunologic enhancement.
im·mu·no·en·hanc·er (im′ū-nō-en-hans′er). Imunointensificador; qualquer substância específica ou inespecífica capaz de aumentar o grau da resposta imune.
im·mu·no·fer·ri·tin (im′ū-nō-fer′i-tin). Imunoferritina; conjugado de anticorpo–ferritina utilizado para identificar antígenos específicos por microscopia eletrônica.
im·mu·no·flu·o·res·cence (im′ū-nō-flōr-es′ens, i-mū′nō-). Imunofluorescência; técnica imuno-histoquímica que utiliza marcação de anticorpos por corante fluorescente para identificar o material antigênico específico para o anticorpo marcado; a ligação específica do anticorpo pode ser determinada microscopi-

camente através da produção de uma luz visível característica pela aplicação de raios ultravioleta à preparação. VER TAMBÉM fluorescent antibody *technique*.
direct i., i. direta; microscopia de fluorescência de tecido de lesões após a aplicação de anticorpos marcados. VER TAMBÉM fluorescent antibody *technique*.
indirect i., i. indireta; microscopia de fluorescência de tecido normal após a aplicação do soro do paciente para detectar anticorpos dirigidos contra componentes normais do tecido (auto-anticorpos). VER TAMBÉM fluorescent antibody *technique*.
im·mu·no·gen (i - mū′nō - jen). Imunógeno. SIN antigen.
im·mu·no·ge·net·ics (im′ū - nō - jĕ - net′iks, im - ū′nō-). Imunogenética; estudo da genética da rejeição de transplantes e tecidos, *loci* histoquímicos, resposta imunológica, estrutura das imunoglobulinas e imunossupressão.

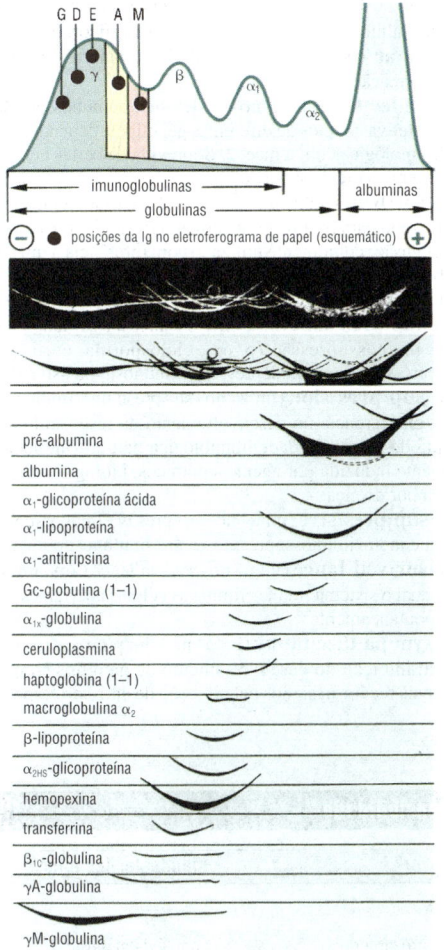

imunoeletroforese: distribuição das proteínas plasmáticas

im·mu·no·gen·ic (im′ū - nō - jen′ik). Imunogênico. SIN antigenic.
im·mu·no·ge·nic·i·ty (im′ū - nō - jĕ - nis′i - tē). Imunogenicidade. SIN antigenicity.

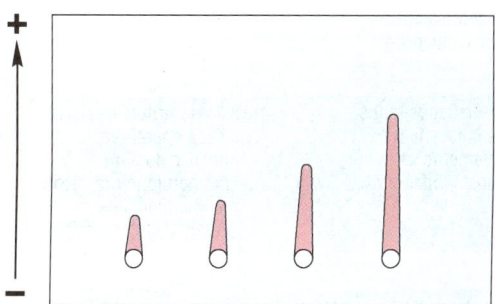

imunoeletroforese em foguete: vista esquemática da eletroforese de antígeno em gel contendo anticorpo; quanto maior a concentração de antígeno, mais longa e mais densa a zona de precipitação

im·mu·no·glob·u·lin (Ig) (im′ū - nō - glob′ū - lin). Imunoglobulina; uma classe de proteínas estruturalmente relacionadas, consistindo, cada uma, em dois pares de cadeias polipeptídicas, um par de cadeias leves (L) [de baixo peso molecular] (κ ou λ) e um par de cadeias pesadas (H) (γ, α, μ, δ e ε), estando todas as quatro habitualmente ligadas por pontes de dissulfeto. Com base nas propriedades estruturais e antigênicas das cadeias H, as Ig são classificadas (por ordem de quantidades relativas presentes no soro humano normal) em IgG (7S de tamanho, 80%), IgA (10–15%), IgM (19S, um pentâmero da unidade básica, 5–10%), IgD (menos de 0,1%) e IgE (menos de 0,01%). Todas essas classes são homogêneas e suscetíveis à análise da seqüência de aminoácidos. Cada classe de cadeia H pode associar-se a cadeias L κ ou λ. As subclasses de Ig, com base em diferenças nas cadeias H, são designadas como IgG1, etc.

Quando clivada pela papaína, a IgG dá origem a três fragmentos: o fragmento Fc, que consiste na porção C-terminal das cadeias H, sem qualquer atividade de anticorpo, porém com a capacidade de fixar o complemento e cristalizável; e dois fragmentos Fab idênticos, que possuem os sítios de ligação do antígeno, consistindo, cada um deles, numa cadeia L ligada ao remanescente de uma cadeia H.

Os anticorpos são Ig, e todas as imunoglobulinas provavelmente funcionam como anticorpos. Entretanto, a Ig refere-se não apenas aos anticorpos habituais, mas também a grande número de proteínas patológicas, classificadas como proteínas do mieloma, que aparecem no mieloma múltiplo, juntamente com proteínas de Bence-Jones, globulinas de mieloma e fragmentos Ig.

A partir das seqüências de aminoácidos das proteínas de Bence-Jones, sabe-se que todas as cadeias L são divididas numa região de seqüência variável (V_L) e uma região de seqüência constante (C_L), cada uma compreendendo cerca da metade do comprimento da cadeia L. As regiões constantes de todas as cadeias L humanas do mesmo tipo (κ ou λ) são idênticas, exceto por uma substituição de único aminoácido, que está sob controle genético. As cadeias H são igualmente divididas, embora a região V_H, se bem que semelhante à região V_L no seu comprimento, tem apenas um terço ou um quarto do comprimento da região C_H. Os locais de ligação constituem uma combinação de regiões de proteína V_L e V_H. O grande número de combinações possíveis das cadeias L e H compõe as "bibliotecas" de anticorpos de cada indivíduo.

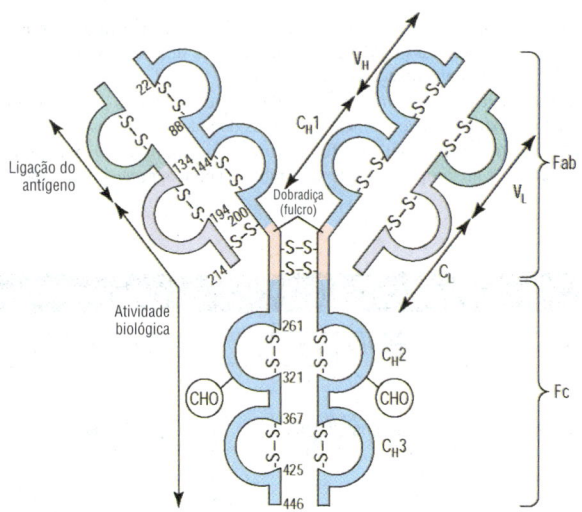

imunoglobulina (estrutura esquemática)

anti-D i., i. anti-D. SIN $RH_0(D)$ immune *globulin*.
chickenpox i., i. da varicela. SIN chickenpox immune *globulin* (human).
i. domains, domínios da imunoglobulina; unidades estruturais das cadeias pesadas ou leves de imunoglobulina, compostas de aproximadamente 110 aminoácidos. As cadeias leves de uma imunoglobulina são compostas de um domínio constante e um domínio variável. As cadeias pesadas são constituídas de três ou quatro domínios constantes e um domínio variável.
i. G subclass deficiency, deficiência de subclasses da i. G; distúrbio hereditário raro caracterizado por níveis reduzidos de uma ou mais subclasses de IgG, devido a genes defeituosos das cadeias pesadas ou anormalidade na regulação da mudança de isotipo.
human normal i., i. normal humana. SIN human gamma *globulin*.
measles i., i. do sarampo. SIN measles immune *globulin* (human).
monoclonal i., imunoglobulina homogênea resultante da proliferação de um único clone de plasmócitos e que, durante a eletroforese do soro, aparece como uma banda estreita ou "espícula"; caracteriza-se por cadeias pesadas de uma única classe e subclasse e cadeias leves de um único tipo. SIN M protein (2), monoclonal protein, paraprotein (2).

pertussis i., i. da coqueluche. SIN pertussis immune *globulin.*
poliomyelitis i., i. da poliomielite. SIN poliomyelitis immune *globulin* (human).
rabies i., i. anti-rábica. SIN rabies immune *globulin* (human).
Rh₀D i., i. de Rh₀(D). SIN RH₀(D) immune *globulin.*
secretory i., i. secretora; habitualmente IgA, podendo ser IgM ligada a um componente secretor e encontrada em secreções mucosas.
secretory i. A, i.A secretora; subclasse de IgA encontrada primariamente em secreções, como lágrimas e colostro. Essa forma de IgA é protegida da degradação proteolítica pela presença de um componente secretor.
selective i. A deficiency, deficiência de i. A seletiva; distúrbio hereditário caracterizado por acentuada redução ou ausência de IgA, resultando em células B transportadoras de IgA imaturas.
tetanus i., i. antitetânica. SIN tetanus immune *globulin.*
thyroid-stimulating i.'s (TSI), imunoglobulinas tireoestimulantes; na doença de Graves, anticorpos dirigidos contra os receptores de TSH na glândula tireóide. Esses anticorpos são produzidos pelos linfócitos B e estimulam os receptores, causando hipertireoidismo. Antigamente denominada LATS (*long-acting* thyroid *stimulator,* estimulador tireóideo de ação prolongada).
im·mu·no·he·ma·tol·o·gy (im′ū - nō - hē - mă - tol′ō - jē, im - ū′nō-). Imunoematologia; divisão da hematologia relacionada com as reações imunes ou antígeno-anticorpo, bem como com as alterações relacionadas no sangue.
im·mu·no·his·to·chem·is·try (im′ū - nō - his′tō - kem′is - trē). Imunoistoquímica; demonstração de antígenos específicos em tecidos através do uso de marcadores, que consistem em corantes fluorescentes ou enzimas, como a peroxidase do rábano-bastardo.
im·mu·no·lo·cal·i·za·tion (im′ū - nō - lō′cal - ī - zā - shŭn). Imunolocalização; refere-se ao uso de técnicas imunológicas, incluindo anticorpos específicos, para identificar a localização de moléculas ou estruturas no interior das células ou tecidos.
im·mu·nol·o·gist (im - ū - nol′ō - jist). Imunologista; especialista na ciência da imunologia.
im·mu·nol·o·gy (im′ū - nol′ō - jē). Imunologia. **1.** Ciência relacionada com os diversos fenômenos da imunidade, sensibilidade induzida e alergia. **2.** Estudo da estrutura e função do sistema imune. [immuno- + G. *logos,* estudo]
im·mu·no·mod·u·la·to·ry (im′ū - nō - mod′ū - la - to - rē). Imunomodulador. **1.** Capaz de modificar ou de regular uma ou mais funções imunes. **2.** Ajuste, regulação ou potencialização imunológica.
im·mu·no·pa·thol·o·gy (im′ū - nō - pă - thol′ō - jē, i - moo′nō-). Imunopatologia; estudo de doenças ou condições resultantes de reações imunes.
im·mu·no·phil·ins (im′ū - nō - fil′inz). Imunofilinas; proteínas receptoras de alta afinidade no citoplasma, que se combinam com agentes imunossupressores, resultando em inibição da rotamase e, nas células T, em interrupção da ativação celular. [*immune* + G. *philos,* amigo + in]
im·mu·no·po·ten·ti·a·tion (im′ū - nō - pō - ten - shē - ā′shŭn). Imunopotenciação; intensificação da resposta imune através do aumento de sua velocidade ou prolongamento de sua duração.
im·mu·no·po·ten·ti·a·tor (im′ū - nō - pō - ten′shē - ā - tōr). Imunopotencializador; qualquer uma de uma ampla variedade de substâncias específicas ou inespecíficas que, ao serem inoculadas, intensificam ou aumentam uma resposta imune.
im·mu·no·pre·cip·i·ta·tion (im′ū - nō - prē - sip - i - tā′shŭn). Imunoprecipitação; fenômeno de agregação de antígenos sensibilizados após a adição de anticorpo específico (precipitina) ao antígeno em solução. SIN immune precipitation.
im·mu·no·re·ac·tion (im′ū - nō - rē - ak′shŭn). Imunorreação; reação imunológica, especialmente *in vitro* entre antígeno e anticorpo.
im·mu·no·re·ac·tive (im′ū - nō - rē - ak′tiv). Imunorreativo; relativo a ou que exibe imunorreação.
im·mu·no·se·lec·tion (im′ū - nō - se - lek′shŭn). Imunosseleção. **1.** Morte ou sobrevida seletiva de fetos de diferentes genótipos, dependendo da incompatibilidade imunológica com a mãe. **2.** Sobrevida de certas células, dependendo de sua antigenicidade de superfície.
im·mu·no·sor·bent (im′ū - nō - sōr′bent). Imunossorvente; anticorpo (ou antígeno) utilizado para remover um antígeno (ou anticorpo) específico da solução ou suspensão; comumente utilizado com referência a um anticorpo ligado a uma substância particulada, como polímero de dextrana empregado para remover antígenos solúveis (p. ex., insulina) da solução.
im·mu·no·sup·pres·sant (im′ū - nō - sŭ - pres′ant). Imunossupressor; agente que induz imunossupressão (p. ex., ciclosporina, corticosteróides). SIN immunodepressant, immunodepressor, immunosuppressive (2).
im·mu·no·sup·pres·sion (im′ū - nō - sŭ - presh′ŭn). Imunossupressão; prevenção ou interferência no desenvolvimento da resposta imunológica; pode refletir falta de responsividade imunológica natural (intolerância), pode ser artificialmente induzida por agentes químicos, biológicos ou físicos ou pode ser causada por doença.
im·mu·no·sup·pres·sive (im′ū - nō - sŭ - pres′iv). Imunossupressivo. **1.** Relativo a ou que induz imunossupressão. **2.** SIN immunosuppressant.
im·mu·no·sur·veil·lance (im′ū - nō - ser - vā′lance). Imunovigilância; teoria segundo a qual o sistema imune elimina as células aberrantes ou tumorais que surgem espontaneamente.
im·mu·no·sym·pa·thec·to·my (im′ū - nō - sim′pă - thek′tō - mē). Imunossimpatectomia; inibição do desenvolvimento de gânglios simpáticos, induzida em animais recém-nascidos pela injeção de anti-soro específico para pro-

classificação das reações de hipersensibilidade

tipo	nome descritivo	tempo de início	mecanismo	manifestações típicas
			reações imediatas	

tipo I	hipersensibilidade mediada por IgE	2–30 min	o Ag induz ligação cruzada da IgE ligada aos mastócitos e basófilos, com liberação de mediadores vasoativos	anafilaxia sistêmica
				anafilaxia localizada:
				    febre do feno, asma,
				    urticária, alergias
				    alimentares, eczema

tipo II	hipersensibilidade citotóxica mediada por anticorpo	5–8 h	o Ac contra antígenos da superfície celular medeia a destruição das células através da ativação do complemento ou citotoxicidade mediada por células anticorpo-dependente	reações transfusionais eritroblastose fetal anemia hemolítica auto-imune

tipo III	hipersensibilidade mediada por imunocomplexos	2–8 h	os complexos Ag-Ac depositados em vários tecidos induzem ativação do complemento e conseqüente resposta inflamatória	reação de Arthus localizada
				reações generalizadas:
				    doença do soro,
				    glomerulonefrite, artrite
				    reumatóide, lúpus
				    eritematoso sistêmico

			reações tardias	
tipo IV	hipersensibilidade mediada por células	24–72 h	as células T_{DTH} sensibilizadas liberam citocinas que ativam os macrófagos ou as células T_C, que medeiam a lesão celular direta	dermatite de contato lesões tuberculosas rejeição de enxerto

teína que intensifica seletivamente o crescimento dos neurônios simpáticos.

im·mu·no·ther·a·py (im'ū-nō-thār'ā-pē). Imunoterapia; originalmente, administração terapêutica de soro ou de imunoglobulina contendo anticorpos préformados, produzidos por outro indivíduo; hoje em dia, a imunoterapia inclui estimulação sistêmica inespecífica, adjuvante, imunoterapia específica ativa e imunoterapia adotiva. As novas formas de imunoterapia incluem o uso de anticorpos monoclonais. SIN biologic i.

> Esse método foi amplamente adotado em oncologia, particularmente para os casos que não respondem a outro tratamento. A imunoterapia procura reforçar a função do sistema imune, através da administração de interferons e interleucina-2, ou atacar diretamente as células cancerosas, através da injeção de anticorpos monoclonais. Já foram também utilizadas diversas técnicas de imunoterapia na AIDS/SIDA. Além disso, afirma-se que várias práticas de medicina alternativa intensificam a função imune, e várias substâncias adquiridas sem receita médica ganharam popularidade em virtude dessa suposta propriedade.

adoptive i., i. adotiva; transferência passiva de imunidade de um doador imune, através da inoculação de linfócitos sensibilizados ou anticorpos no soro ou gamaglobulina. A vacinação com DNA de plasmídio está sendo atualmente objeto de pesquisa.
biologic i., i. biológica. SIN immunotherapy.
im·mu·no·tol·er·ance (im'ū-nō-tol'er-ăns). Imunotolerância. SIN immunologic *tolerance*.
im·mu·no·trans·fu·sion (im'ū-nō-trans-fū'zhŭn, i-moo'nō-). Imunotransfusão; transfusão indireta, em que o doador é inicialmente imunizado por meio de injeções de um antígeno preparado a partir dos microrganismos isolados do receptor; posteriormente, colhe-se sangue do doador, que é desfibrinado e, em seguida, administrado ao paciente; presume-se que este último seja, então, passivamente imunizado por meio de anticorpos produzidos no doador, como, p. ex., anticorpos que reagem contra os microrganismos existentes no paciente.
IMP Abreviatura de inosine 5'-monophosphate (inosina 5'-monofosfato).
im·pact. Impacto **1.** (im'pakt). Choque de um corpo contra outro. **2.** (im-pakt'). Pressionar dois corpos, duas partes ou fragmentos estreitamente, de tal modo que as duas partes se movam como uma única entidade. [L. *impingo,* pp. *-pactus,* bater em (*in* + *pango*), fixar, entrar]
im·pact·ed (im-pak'ted). Impactado; encravado ou comprimido fortemente, de modo a mover-se como uma unidade.
im·pac·tion (im-pak'shŭn). Impacção; processo ou condição de impactado.
dental i., i. dentária; confinamento de um dente no alvéolo e impedimento de sua erupção na posição normal. VER TAMBÉM impacted *tooth*.
fecal i., i. fecal; coleção imóvel de fezes comprimidas ou endurecidas no cólon ou no reto.
food i., i. alimentar; encravamento forçado de alimento entre dentes adjacentes durante a mastigação, produzindo recessão gengival e formação de bolsas.
mucus i., de muco; enchimento dos brônquios proximais e também dos bronquíolos com muco.
im·pair·ment (im-pār'ment). Comprometimento; defeito físico ou mental a nível de um sistema corporal ou órgão. A definição oficial da OMS (*Organização Mundial de Saúde*) é a seguinte: qualquer perda ou anormalidade de estrutura ou função psicológica, fisiológica ou anatômica.
mental i., c. mental; distúrbio caracterizado por um defeito intelectual, manifestado na forma de redução da eficiência cognitiva, interpessoal, social e vocacional, quantitativamente avaliado por exame e avaliação psicológica.
IMP-as·par·tate li·gase. IMP-aspartato ligase. SIN adenylosuccinate synthase.
im·pat·ent (im-pat'ent, im-pā'tent). Não-pérvio; fechado.
im·ped·ance (im-pē'dăns). Impedância. **1.** Oposição total ao fluxo. Em eletricidade, quando o fluxo é constante, a impedância consiste simplesmente na resistência, como, p. ex., a pressão impulsora por unidade de fluxo; quando o fluxo é variável, a impedância também inclui os fatores que se opõem a alterações do fluxo. Assim, os desvios da impedância a partir de resistência ôhmica simples, devido aos defeitos de capacitância e indutância, tornam-se mais importantes na corrente alternada à medida que aumenta a freqüência das oscilações. Nas analogias dos líquidos (p. ex., fluxo pulsátil de sangue, fluxo de vaivém dos gases respiratórios), a impedância depende não apenas da resistência viscosa, como também da compressibilidade, complacência, inertância e freqüência das oscilações impostas. **2.** Resistência de um sistema acústico a ser colocado em movimento.
acoustic i., i. acústica; a resistência que determinado material oferece à passagem de uma onda sonora (coloquial); propriedade de um meio calculada como produto da densidade pela velocidade de propagação do som (i. acústica característica). As descontinuidades na impedância acústica são responsáveis pelos ecos nos quais se baseia a ultra-sonografia. Unidade: o rayl.

im·per·cep·tion (im-per-sep'shŭn). Impercepção; incapacidade de formar uma imagem mental de um objeto pela associação dos dados sensoriais recolhidos. [L. *in-,* não + *per-cipio,* pp. *-ceptus,* perceber]
im·per·fo·rate (im-per'fŏr-āt). Imperfurado. SIN atretic.
im·per·fo·ra·tion (im-per-fŏr-ā'shŭn). Imperfuração; condição de ser atrésico, ocluído ou fechado; indicada em palavras compostas pelo prefixo *atreto-* ou *-atresia*. [L. *im-* neg. + *per-foro,* pp. *-atus,* perfurar]
im·per·me·a·ble (im-per'mē-ă-bl). Impermeável; não-permeável; que não permite a passagem de substâncias (p. ex., líquidos, gases) ou de calor através de uma membrana ou outra estrutura. SIN impervious. [L. *impermeabilis,* que não é atravessado]
im·per·me·ant (im-per'mē-ant). Impermeante; incapaz de passar através de uma membrana semipermeável em particular. [L. *im-,* neg, + *permano,* penetrar]
im·per·sis·tence (im-per-sis'tens). Impersistência; existência ou ocorrência transitória, de pouca duração. [L. *im-,* neg. + *persisto,* persistir]
motor i., i. motora; incapacidade de manter um movimento.
im·per·vi·ous (im-per'vē-ŭs). Impérvio. SIN impermeable.
im·pe·tig·i·ni·za·tion (im'pe-tij'i-ni-zā'shŭn). Impetiginização; ocorrência de impetigo em uma área de dermatose preexistente.
im·pe·tig·i·nous (im-pe-tij'i-nŭs). Impetiginoso; relativo ao impetigo.
ℹ️ **im·pe·ti·go** (im-pe-tī'gō). Impetigo; piodermia superficial contagiosa, causada por *Staphylococcus aureus* e/ou estreptococos do grupo A, começando com uma vesícula flácida superficial que sofre ruptura e forma uma crosta amarelada espessa, ocorrendo mais comumente em crianças. SIN i. contagiosa, i. vulgaris. [L. erupção crostosa, de *im-peto (inp-),* acometer, atacar]
Bockhart i., i. de Bockhart. SIN follicular i.
i. bullo'sa, i. bolhosa; impetigo com lesões de grande tamanho, formando bolhas.
bullous i. of newborn, i. bolhosa do recém-nascido; em geral, lesões bolhosas, amplamente disseminadas, que aparecem pouco depois do nascimento, causadas pela infecção por *Staphylococcus aureus*. SIN i. neonatorum (2), pemphigus gangrenosus (2).
i. circina'ta, i. circinada; configuração anelar de lesões bolhosas de impetigo formada pela confluência de diversas bolhas ou pela ruptura de uma única lesão, com formação de crosta na periferia.
i. contagio'sa, i. contagiosa. SIN impetigo.
i. contagio'sa bullo'sa, i. contagiosa bolhosa; lesões cutâneas purulentas distintas, observadas ocasionalmente com piodermia estreptocócica.
follicular i., i. folicular; erupção pustular folicular superficial que acomete o couro cabeludo ou outra área pilosa. SIN Bockhart i.
i. herpetifor'mis, i. herpetiforme; piodermia rara, que pode estar relacionada à psoríase pustular, ocorrendo mais comumente em gestantes no terceiro trimestre na forma de erupção de pequenas pústulas estreitamente agregadas, que se desenvolvem numa base inflamatória e são acompanhadas de sintomas constitucionais graves e morte fetal; sofre recidiva com gestações subseqüentes.
i. neonato'rum, i. do recém-nascido. **(1)** SIN *dermatitis* exfoliativa infantum; **(2)** SIN bullous i. of newborn.
i. vulga'ris, i. vulgar. SIN impetigo.
im·pe·tus (im'pe-tŭs). Ímpeto; em psicanálise, o elemento motor de um instinto; quantidade de força da energia do indivíduo exigida pelo impulso instintivo. [L. início, de *im-peto,* atacar]
im·plant. Implante. **1** (im-plant'). Enxertar ou inserir. **2.** Material inserido em tecidos não-vivos. VER TAMBÉM graft, transplant. **3.** (im'plant). Em cirurgia genitourinária, dispositivo inserido para restaurar a continência ou a potência. Refere-se também a um material injetável para criar uma competência valvular da junção ureterovesical ou orifício vesical. VER TAMBÉM prosthesis. [L. *im-,* in, + *planto,* pp. *-atus,* plantar, de *planta,* broto, rebento]
carcinomatous i.'s, implantes carcinomatosos; transferência de células de carcinoma de um tumor primário para tecidos adjacentes, onde continua o crescimento.
ℹ️ **cochlear i.**, i. coclear; dispositivo eletrônico consistindo em um microfone, processador da fala e eletrodos que são implantados no ouvido médio para estimular as fibras nervosas remanescentes da parte auditiva do oitavo nervo craniano em adultos e crianças com acentuado comprometimento auditivo e surdez. Muitos receptores de implantes cocleares conseguem um amplo reconhecimento de um conjunto aberto de palavras, podendo até mesmo entender as palavras por telefone. VER TAMBÉM auditory *prosthesis*. SIN cochlear prosthesis.
ℹ️ **dental i.'s,** implantes dentários; coroas, pontes ou dentaduras fixadas permanentemente à mandíbula por meio de âncoras de metal, mais freqüentemente suportes de titânio.

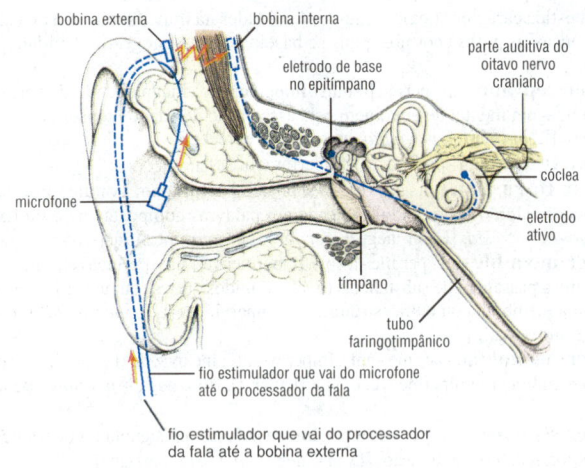

implante coclear

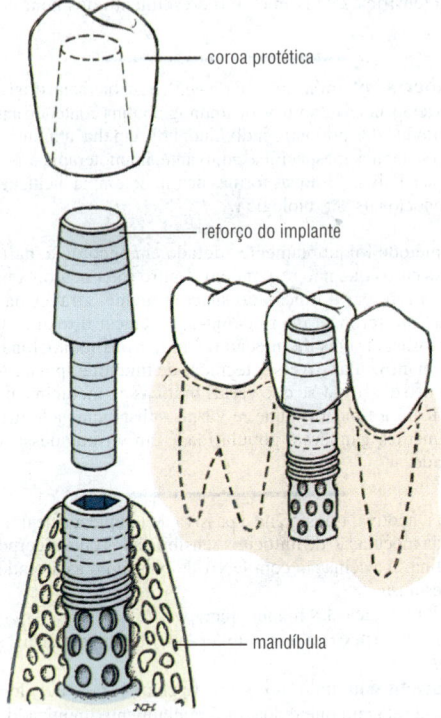

implante dental

endometrial i.'s, implantes endometriais; fragmentos de mucosa endometrial implantados na estrutura pélvica após transferência retrógrada através dos ovidutos. SIN endometriosis.
endo-osseous i., i. endósseo; implante no osso alveolar, inserido através do canal preparado da raiz de um dente, a fim de aumentar o comprimento efetivo da raiz.
endosseous i., i. endósseo. SIN endosteal i.
endosteal i., i. endósteo; implante inserido no osso alveolar, e/ou basal que faz protrusão através do muco periósteo. SIN endosseous i.
inflatable i., i. inflável; bolsa de borracha de silicone vazia com um tubo de entrada e uma válvula, inserida na mama ou atrás dela, que é então inflada com líquido até o tamanho desejado; utilizado na mamoplastia de aumento e na reconstrução de mama.
intracorneal i.'s, implantes intracorneanos; implantes colocados no interior de bolsas corneanas para alterar o poder de refração do olho.
intraocular i., i. intra-ocular; lente de plástico colocada na câmara anterior ou posterior do olho para substituir a lente removida na extração de catarata.
magnetic i., i. magnético; metal magnetizado tolerado por tecidos, que é colocado dentro do osso para ajudar na retenção da dentadura; coloca-se um magneto semelhante na dentadura suprajacente para completar o campo.
orbital i., i. orbitário; dispositivo de vidro, plástico ou metal colocado no cone muscular após enucleação de um olho.
penile i., i. peniano; dispositivo rígido, flexível ou inflável, que é colocado cirurgicamente nos corpos cavernosos para produzir ereção.
pin i., i. de pino; tipo de implante dentário, geralmente em forma de bastonete, utilizado na área dos seios maxilares.
post i., implante de suporte; porção de uma subestrutura de implante dentário, que faz protrusão através da mucosa para unir-se à restauração.
root-form i., i. em forma de raiz; implante cuja forma é semelhante à raiz de um dente.
silicone i., i. de silicone; implante composto de silicone; forma comum de implante mamário para aumento.
submucosal i., i. submucoso; implante dentário que repousa abaixo da mucosa. VER TAMBÉM implant *denture*.
subperiosteal i., i. subperiósteo; dispositivo metálico artificial para adaptar-se à forma de um osso, colocado sobre a sua superfície, por baixo do periósteo. VER implant denture *substructure*.
supraperiosteal i., i. supraperiósteo; enxerto aloplástico inserido superficialmente ao periósteo para modificar o contorno de uma área.
testicular i., i. testicular; dispositivo colocado cirurgicamente na bolsa escrotal de homens com ausência ou hipoplasia pronunciada do testículo. SIN testicular prosthesis.
threaded i., i. em parafuso; implante com fios semelhantes a parafuso, que é parafusado no osso previamente aparafusado por um tampão ou por autotamponamento, os fios de corte do implante no osso quando inserido num orifício perfurado.
triplant i., i. de três implantes; combinação de três implantes de pinos para formar um único reforço para sustentar ou reter uma prótese dentária.
im·plan·ta·tion (im - plan - tā′shŭn). Implantação. **1.** Fixação do óvulo fertilizado (blastocisto) ao endométrio e sua penetração subseqüente na camada compacta, que ocorre 6 ou 7 dias após a fertilização do óvulo nos seres humanos. **2.** Processo de colocar um dispositivo ou uma substância no corpo, como, p. ex., colocação de um dispositivo repleto de solução salina por debaixo da mama. **3.** Inserção de um dente natural num alvéolo construído artificialmente. **4.** Enxerto de tecido. VER TAMBÉM transplantation.

central i., i. central; implantação em que o blastocisto permanece na cavidade uterina, como nos carnívoros, macacos *rhesus* e coelhos. SIN circumferential i., superficial i.
circumferential i., i. circumferencial. SIN central i.
collagen i., i. de colágeno. SIN collagen *injection*.
cortical i., i. cortical; implantação do blastocisto no córtex ovariano, resultando em gravidez ovariana. VER ectopic *pregnancy*.
eccentric i., i. excêntrica; implantação em que o blastocisto se localiza numa cripta uterina, como no camundongo, rato e *hamster*.
interstitial i., i. intersticial; implante em que o blastocisto se localiza dentro da substância do endométrio, como nos seres humanos e nas cobaias.
nerve i., i. de nervo; implante de um nervo na bainha de outro.
pellet i., i. de grânulo; inserção intramuscular ou subcutânea de agente terapêutico ativo na forma de grânulos, a fim de obter uma absorção prolongada numa velocidade mais lenta do que a injeção subcutânea ou intramuscular e como meio de proporcionar um efeito terapêutico contínuo sem administração repetida.
periosteal i., i. periostea; inserção de um tendão normal no periósteo como parte de uma operação de transplante de tendão.
subcutaneous i., i. subcutânea; inserção de material sob a pele.
superficial i., i. superficial. SIN central i.
im·plo·sion (im - plō′shŭn). Implosão. **1.** Colapso súbito, como de um vaso esvaziado, em que ocorre uma explosão para dentro, mais do que para fora, como numa explosão. **2.** Tipo de terapia comportamental, semelhante ao *flooding*, durante a qual o paciente é submetido a exposição maciça de estímulos que despertam extrema ansiedade, pedindo-lhe que descreva e, assim, volte a viver em sua imaginação os eventos ou situações da vida que tipicamente produziram essas reações emocionais esmagadoras. À medida que o paciente prossegue, o terapeuta procura extinguir a influência futura desse material inconsciente sobre a conduta e os sentimentos do paciente, sendo as respostas prévias de evitar esses estímulos substituídas por respostas mais apropriadas.
im·po·tence, im·po·ten·cy (im′pŏ - tens, - ten - sē). Impotência. **1.** Fraqueza; falta de força. **2.** Especificamente, incapacidade de o macho conseguir e/ou manter a ereção do pênis e, assim, praticar a cópula; manifestação de disfunção neurológica, vascular ou psicológica. [L. *impotentia*, incapacidade, de *in*- neg. + *potencia*, força]
psychic i., i. psíquica; impotência causada por fatores psicológicos.
vasculogenic i., i. vasculogênica; impotência causada por alterações no fluxo de sangue do pênis.
im·preg·nate (im - preg′nāt). Impregnar. **1.** Fecundar; produzir gravidez. **2.** Difundir-se ou permear com outra substância. VER TAMBÉM saturate. [L. *im*-, in, + *praegnans*, grávida]
im·preg·na·tion (im - preg - nā′shŭn). Impregnação. **1.** Ato de engravidar. **2.** Processo de difundir-se ou permear com outra substância, como na impregna-

ção metálica de componentes teciduais com nitrato de prata ou prata amoniacal. VER TAMBÉM saturation.

im·pres·sio, pl. **im·pres·si·o·nes** (im‑prĕs′ē‑ō, im‑prĕs‑ē‑ō′nēz)[TA]. Impressão. SIN impression. [L.]
  i. aortica pulmonis sinistri, i. da aorta pulmonar esquerda. SIN aortic impression of left lung.
  i. cardi'aca faciei diaphragmaticae hep'atis [TA], i. cardíaca da superfície diafragmática do fígado. SIN cardiac impression of diaphragmatic surface of liver.
  i. cardi'aca pulmo'nis, i. cardíaca do pulmão. SIN cardiac impression on lung.
  i. col'ica hepatis [TA], i. cólica hepática. SIN colic impression on liver.
  impressio'nes digita'tae, impressões digitais; *termo oficial alternativo para impressions of cerebral gyri.
  i. duodena'lis hepatis [TA], i. duodenal hepática. SIN duodenal impression on liver.
  i. espha'gea hepatis [TA], i. esofágica hepática. SIN esophageal impression on liver.
  i. gas'trica hepatis [TA], i. gástrica hepática. SIN gastric impression on liver.
  impressiones gyrorum [TA], i. impressões dos giros. SIN impressions of cerebral gyri.
  i. ligamen'ti costoclavicula'ris [TA], i. do ligamento costoclavicular. SIN impression for costoclavicular ligament.
  i. petro'sa pal'lii, i. petrosa do pálio. SIN petrosal impression of the pallium.
  i. rena'lis hepatis [TA], i. renal do fígado. SIN renal impression on liver.
  i. suprarena'lis hepatis [TA], i. supra-renal do fígado. SIN suprarenal impression on liver.
  i. trigemina'lis [TA], i. do trigêmeo. SIN trigeminal impression.

im·pres·sion (im‑presh′ŭn).Impressão. **1.** Marca feita aparentemente pela compressão de uma estrutura ou órgão sobre outro, observada especialmente em dissecções de cadáveres. VER TAMBÉM *groove* para as várias impressões dos pulmões, como, p. ex., a aorta descendente, artéria subclávia e veia cava. **2.** Efeito produzido sobre a mente por algum objeto externo que atua através dos órgãos dos sentidos. SIN mental i. **3.** Impressão ou imagem negativa; especialmente a forma negativa dos dentes e/ou de outros tecidos da cavidade oral, feita em material plástico que se torna relativamente duro enquanto em contato com esses tecidos, feita para reproduzir uma forma positiva ou molde dos tecidos registrados; classificada, de acordo com os materiais empregados, em i. hidrocolóide reversível e irreversível, i. de plástico de modelagem, i. de gesso e i. de cera. SIN impressio [TA]. [L. *impressio*, de *im- primo*, pp. *-pressus*, exercer pressão sobre]
  aortic i. of left lung, i. aórtica do pulmão esquerdo; sulco profundo e largo na face medial do pulmão esquerdo, acima e atrás do íleo, que recebe o arco da aorta e aorta torácica. SIN aortic sulcus, impressio aortica pulmonis sinistri, sulcus aorticus.
  basilar i., i. basilar; invaginação da base do crânio no interior da fossa posterior, com compressão do tronco cerebral e estruturas cerebelares no forame magno. Cf. platybasia.
  cardiac i. of diaphragmatic surface of liver [TA], i. cardíaca da superfície diafragmática do fígado; depressão na área superior da superfície diafragmática do fígado, que corresponde à posição do coração. SIN impressio cardiaca faciei diaphragmaticae hepatis [TA].
  cardiac i. on lung [TA], i. cardíaca do pulmão; depressão na superfície medial de cada pulmão, produzida pela presença do coração. É mais pronunciada no pulmão esquerdo. SIN impressio cardiaca pulmonis.
  i. of cerebral gyri [TA], i. dos giros cerebrais; depressões na superfície interna do crânio que correspondem às circunvoluções do cérebro. SIN impressiones gyrorum [TA], impressiones digitatae*, juga cerebralia*, digitate i.'s.
  colic i. on liver [TA], i. cólica do fígado; depressão na superfície visceral do lobo direito do fígado, na parte anterior, que corresponde à localização da flexura direita e início do cólon transverso. SIN impressio colica hepatis [TA].
  colic i. of spleen [TA], i. cólica do baço; parte da superfície visceral do baço em contato com o cólon. SIN facies colica splenis [TA], colic surface of spleen.
  complete denture i., i. de dentadura completa. **(1)** Impressão de uma arcada desdentada com o objetivo de construir uma dentadura completa; **(2)** registro negativo de toda a área estabilizadora de suporte da dentadura do maxilar ou da mandíbula; **(3)** registro negativo de toda a base da dentadura e áreas limítrofes presentes na boca desdentada.
  i. for costoclavicular ligament [TA], i. para o ligamento costoclavicular; área deprimida irregular na superfície inferior da clavícula, na sua extremidade externa, permitindo a fixação ao ligamento costoclavicular. SIN impressio ligamenti costoclavicularis [TA], costal tuberosity, rhomboid i., tuberositas costalis.
  deltoid i., i. deltóide. SIN deltoid tuberosity (of humerus).
  digitate i., impressões digitais. SIN i. of cerebral gyri.
  direct bone i., i. direta de osso; impressão de osso desnudado, utilizada na construção de implantes subperiósteos de dentadura.
  duodenal i. on liver [TA], i. duodenal do fígado; depressão na superfície visceral do lobo direito do fígado, ao longo da vesícula biliar, marcando a localização do duodeno. SIN impressio duodenalis hepatis [TA].
  esophageal i. on liver [TA], i. esofágica do fígado; marca do esôfago sobre a parte posterior do lobo esquerdo do fígado. SIN impressio esophagea hepatis [TA].
  i.'s of esophagus, impressões do esôfago. SIN esophageal constrictions, em constriction.
  final i., i. final; em odontologia, a impressão utilizada para fazer o molde-mestre.
  gastric i. on liver [TA], i. gástrica do fígado; depressão na superfície visceral do lobo esquerdo do fígado que corresponde à localização do estômago. SIN impressio gastrica hepatis [TA].
  gastric i. on spleen [TA], i. gástrica do baço; superfície do baço em contato com o estômago. SIN facies gastrica splenis [TA], gastric surface of spleen.
  mental i., i. mental. SIN impression (2).
  partial denture i., i. de dentadura parcial; impressão ou cópia negativa de toda a área ou arcada dentária parcialmente desdentada, ou de parte dela, efetuada com o propósito de projetar ou construir uma dentadura parcial.
  petrosal i. of the pallium, i. petrosa do pálio; impressão superficial na superfície inferior do hemisfério cerebral, efetuada pela margem superior da parte petrosa do osso temporal. SIN impressio petrosa pallii.
  preliminary i., i. preliminar; em odontologia, impressão feita com o objetivo de diagnosticar ou construir uma bandeja. SIN primary i.
  primary i., i. primária. SIN preliminary i.
  renal i. on liver [TA], i. renal do fígado; depressão na superfície visceral do lobo direito do fígado, na qual se localiza o rim direito. SIN impressio renalis hepatis [TA].
  renal i. of spleen [TA], i. renal do baço; porção da superfície visceral do baço que faz contato com o rim esquerdo. SIN facies renalis splenis [TA], facies renalis lienis*, renal surface of spleen.
  rhomboid i., i. rombóide. SIN i. for costoclavicular ligament.
  sectional i., i. seccional; impressão feita em seções.
  suprarenal i. on liver [TA], i. supra-renal do fígado; depressão na superfície visceral do lobo direito do fígado, adjacente ao sulco da veia cava inferior, onde se localiza a glândula supra-renal direita. SIN impressio suprarenalis hepatis [TA].
  trigeminal i. [TA], i. do trigêmeo; depressão na superfície anterior da porção petrosa do osso temporal, próxima ao ápice, formada em relação ao gânglio trigêmeo. SIN impressio trigeminalis [TA].

im·print·ing. *Imprinting.* Impressão; forma particular de aprendizagem, caracterizada pela sua ocorrência nas primeiras horas de vida e que determina o comportamento de reconhecimento da espécie.
  genomic i., i. genômica; processo epigenético que leva à inativação do alelo paterno ou materno de certos genes suscetíveis a regulação epigenética; responsável, entre outras, pelas síndromes de Angelman e de Prader-Willi.

im·pro·mi·dine (im′prō‑mī‑dēn). Impromidina; agente que atua como agonista nos receptores de histamina tipo H₂. Provoca a secreção de ácido gástrico e taquicardia. As ações podem ser bloqueadas com agentes como a cimetidina e a ranitidina.

im·pulse (im′pŭls).Impulso. **1.** Súbito empurrão ou força impulsora. **2.** Determinação súbita, freqüentemente irracional, para executar algum ato. **3.** Potencial de ação de uma fibra nervosa. [L. *im-pello*, pp. *-pulsus*, empurrar, impelir (*inp-*)]
  apex i., i. apical; por convenção, a área mais baixa e mais à esquerda de pulsação cardíaca habitualmente palpável.
  cardiac i., i. cardíaco; movimento da parede torácica produzido pela contração cardíaca.
  ectopic i., i. ectópico; impulso elétrico de uma área cardíaca diferente do nodo sinusal.
  escape i., i. de escape; um ou mais impulsos (atriais, juncionais ou ventriculares) que se originam em conseqüência do atraso na formação ou na chegada de impulsos de marcapasso predominante.
  irresistible i., i. irresistível; compulsão para atuar que o indivíduo sente ou à qual afirma não poder resistir.
  morbid i., i. mórbido; impulso que impele uma pessoa a cometer algum ato, habitualmente de natureza proibida, a despeito dos esforços para se conter.
  right parasternal i., impulso paraesternal direito; atividade cardíaca palpável ou passível de registro à direita do esterno.

im·pul·sion (im‑pŭl′shŭn). Impulsão, necessidade anormal de executar determinada atividade.

im·pul·sive (im‑pŭl′siv). Impulsivo; relativo a, ou que atua por, impulso, em vez de controlado pela razão ou deliberação cuidadosa.

imus (ī′mŭs). Imo; o mais baixo; a mais inferior ou caudal de várias estruturas semelhantes. [L.]

IMV Abreviatura de intermittent mandatory *ventilation* (ventilação mandatória intermitente).

IMViC Acrônimo de *i*ndole production, *m*ethyl red, *V*oges-Proskauer reaction, and ability to use *c*itrate as a sole source of carbon (o segundo *i* é inserido por eufonia); utilizado primariamente para diferenciar *Escherichia coli* de *Enterobacter aerogenes* e microrganismos relacionados.

In Símbolo de índio; inulina.

[113m]**In** Abreviatura de índio-113m (In[113m]).
[111]**In** Símbolo do índio-111 (In[111]).

in-. In-. **1.** Negação, semelhante ao G. a-, an- ou ao inglês un-. **2.** Em, no interior de, dentro de. **3.** Muito; aparece como im-, antes de b, p ou m. [L.]

-in. -Ina. Sufixo amplamente utilizado para formar nomes de substâncias bioquímicas, incluindo proteínas (p. ex., *globulina*), lipídios (*lecitina*), hormônios (*insulina*), princípios botânicos (*digoxina*), antibióticos (*estreptomicina*), drogas sintéticas (*aspirina*), corantes (*eosina*) e outras; inicialmente, uma variante de *-ine*. [G. *-inos*, L. *-inus*, adj. Sufixos]

in·ac·tion (in - ak'shŭn). Inação; inatividade, repouso ou ausência de resposta a um estímulo.

in·ac·ti·vate (in - ak'ti - vāt). Inativar; destruir a atividade ou os efeitos biológicos de determinado agente ou substância, como, p. ex., a destruição da atividade do complemento quando se aquece o soro.

in·ac·ti·va·tion (in - ak - ti - vā'shŭn). Inativação; processo de destruir ou remover a atividade ou os efeitos de determinado agente ou substância; p. ex., pode-se destruir o efeito complementar de um soro através de inativação a 56°C durante 30 min.
  insertional i., i. de inserção; método da tecnologia do DNA recombinante utilizado para selecionar bactérias que transportam plasmídios recombinantes; um fragmento de DNA estranho é inserido num sítio de restrição dentro de um gene para resistência antibiótica, tornando conseqüentemente o gene não-funcional.
  X i., i. do X. VER lyonization.

in·an·i·mate (in - na'i - māt). Inanimado; sem vida. [L. *in-* neg. + *anima*, respiração, alma]

in·a·ni·tion (in'a - nish'ŭn). Inanição; fraqueza e consunção intensas, como as que ocorrem em conseqüência da falta de alimentos, defeitos na assimilação ou doença neoplásica. [L. *inanis*, vazio]

in·ap·par·ent (in'ă - par'ent). Inaparente; não-aparente; abaixo do limiar do reconhecimento clínico, como infecção inaparente.

in·ap·pe·tence (in - ap'ē - tens). Inapetência; falta de desejo ou de anseio. [L. *in-* neg. + *ap-peto*, pp. *-petitus*, procurar, desejar ardentemente (*adp-*)]

in·ar·tic·u·late (in - ar - tik'ū - lit). Inarticulado. **1.** Não articulado em fala inteligível. **2.** Incapaz de se expressar satisfatoriamente com palavras.

in·as·sim·i·la·ble (in - ă - sim'il - ă - bl). Não-assimilável; incapaz de sofrer assimilação. VER assimilation.

in·at·ten·tion (in - ă - ten'shŭn). Inatenção; falta de atenção; negligência.
  selective i., i. seletiva; aspecto da atenção em que uma pessoa procura ignorar ou evitar perceber aquilo que gera ansiedade.
  sensory i., i. sensorial; incapacidade de sentir um estímulo tátil quando um estímulo semelhante, apresentado simultaneamente numa área homóloga do corpo, é percebido.
  visual i., i. visual; incapacidade de perceber um estímulo fótico num campo visual quando um estímulo semelhante, porém percebido, é apresentado simultaneamente no campo homólogo.

in·born (in'bōrn). Inato; que começa durante o desenvolvimento *in utero*. No contexto específico de erro inato do metabolismo, refere-se a um distúrbio genético de uma enzima. VER inborn *errors* of metabolism, under *error*. SIN innate.

in·bred. Endógamo; refere-se a populações (grupos, linhagens genéticas, etc.) que provêm, ao longo de várias gerações, quase exclusivamente de um pequeno grupo de ancestrais, exibindo, portanto, uma elevada taxa de consangüinidade, que é freqüentemente oculta.

in·breed·ing (in'brēd - ing). Endogamia. **1.** Acasalamento entre organismos que são geneticamente mais relacionados do que aqueles selecionados ao acaso na população. **2.** Prática de acasalamento de animais estreitamente relacionados. O termo está claramente relacionado ao tipo de definição da população; quanto maior a endogamia na população, menor o número de relações sexuais no acasalamento individual.

in·car·cer·at·ed (in - kar'ser - ā - ted). Encarcerado; confinado; aprisionado; capturado. [L. *in*, em + *carcero*, pp. *-atus*, aprisionar, de *carcer*, prisão]

in·car·nant (in - kar'nant). Encarnante; que promove ou acelera a granulação de uma ferida. SIN incarnative. [L. *incarno*, de *in* + *caro* (*carn-*), carne]

in·car·na·tive (in - kar'nă - tiv). Encarnativo. SIN incarnant.

in·cen·di·a·rism (in - sen'di - ă - rizm). Incendiarismo. SIN pyromania. [L. *incendiarius*, que causa conflagração]

in·cen·tive (in - sen'tiv). Incentivo; em psicologia experimental, um objeto ou objetivo de comportamento motivado. [LL. *incentivus*, provocativo]

in·cer·tae se·dis (in - ser'tē sē'dis). *Incertae sedis.* De afiliação duvidosa ou incerta ou deposição duvidosa, referindo-se a organismos nas classificações taxonômicas. [L.]

in·cest (in'sest). Incesto. **1.** Relações sexuais entre pessoas intimamente relacionadas pelo sangue, sobretudo entre genitores e seus filhos, irmão e irmã. **2.** Crime de praticar relações sexuais entre pessoas relacionadas pelo sangue, em que essa coabitação é proibida por lei. [*incestus*, não-casto, de *in-*, não + *castus*, casto]

in·ces·tu·ous (in - ses'choo - ŭs). Incestuoso. **1.** Relativo a incesto. **2.** Culpado de incesto.

in·ci·dence (in'si - dens). Incidência. **1.** O número de novos eventos especificados, como, p. ex., pessoas que adoecem com doença específica, durante determinado período, numa população específica. **2.** Em óptica, intersecção de um raio luminoso com uma superfície. [L. *incido*, atingir, acontecer]

in·ci·dent (in'si - dent). Incidente; dirigir-se a; incidir em, como os raios incidentes. [L. *incido*, pp. *-casus*, atingir, encontrar-se com]

in·ci·dent·a·lo·ma (in'si - den - tă - lō'mă). Incidentaloma; lesão expansiva, habitualmente da glândula supra-renal, detectada casualmente durante uma tomografia computadorizada efetuados por outras razões. [incidental + *-oma*, tumor]

in·ci·sal (in - sī'zăl). Incisal; cortante; relativo às bordas cortantes dos dentes incisivos e caninos. [L. *incido*, pp. *-cisus*, cortar]

in·cise (in - sīz'). Incisar; cortar com faca.

in·ci·sion (in - sizh'ŭn). Incisão; corte; ferida cirúrgica; divisão das partes moles, habitualmente feita com bisturi. [L. *inciso*]

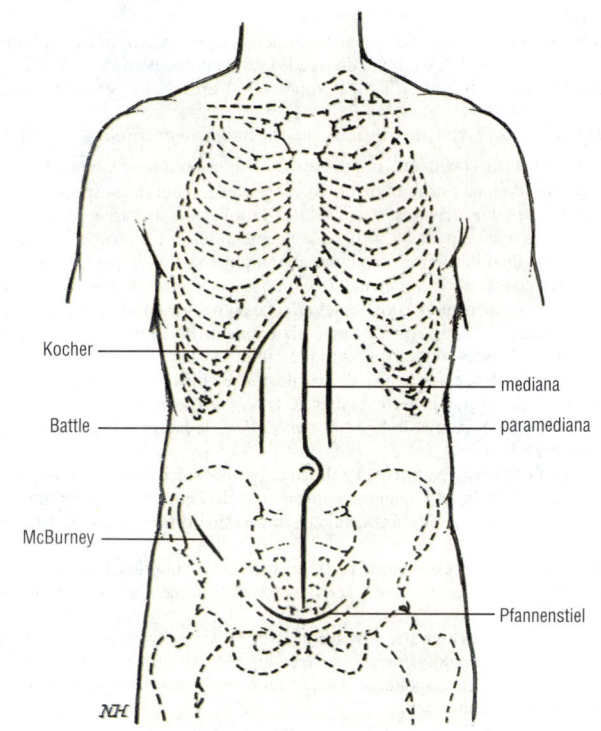

incisões cirúrgicas

bucket-handle i., i. em alça de balde; incisão abdominal subcostal bilateral.
celiotomy i., i. de celiotomia; incisão através da parede abdominal.
chevron i., em chevron; incisão subcostal bilateral no abdome, na forma de "V" invertido; utilizada em procedimentos abdominais superiores.
clamshell i., i. em concha de molusco; incisão efetuada de toracotomias anteriores submamárias bilaterais conectadas por uma esternotomia transversa e proporcionando acesso semelhante ao de uma esternotomia padrão. VER TAMBÉM transverse *thoracosternotomy*. SIN clamshell thoracotomy.
collar i., i. em colar; incisão cervical, efetuada poucos centímetros acima da incisura esternal, freqüentemente utilizada em procedimentos da glândula tireóide ou das paratireóides.
Deaver i., i. de Deaver; incisão no quadrante inferior direito do abdome, com deslocamento medial do músculo reto.
Dührssen i.'s, incisões de Dührssen; três incisões cirúrgicas de um colo uterino incompletamente dilatado, correspondendo, aproximadamente, a 2, 6 e 10 horas, efetuadas como meio de conseguir a expulsão imediata do feto quando a sua cabeça fica retida durante uma apresentação de nádegas.
endaural i., i. endaural; incisão através do canal auditivo externo, evitando a cartilagem, para permitir a cirurgia do mastóide.
Fergusson i., i. de Fergusson; incisão utilizada na maxilectomia, ao longo da junção do nariz com a bochecha, com bissecção do lábio superior.
flank i., i. de flanco; incisão habitualmente feita próximo e paralelamente à décima segunda costela, entre a crista ilíaca e a costela.

Kocher i., i. de Kocher; incisão feita várias polegadas abaixo da margem costal direita e paralelamente a ela.
lumbotomy i., i. de lombotomia. SIN posterior nephrectomy.
McBurney i., i. de McBurney; incisão paralela ao trajeto do músculo oblíquo externo, a uma ou duas polegadas em sentido cefálico da espinha ântero-superior do ílio.
midline i., incisão abdominal vertical efetuada na aponeurose da linha mediana, entre as duas bainhas dos músculos retos do abdome.
paramedian i., i. paramediana; incisão lateral à linha mediana.
Pfannenstiel i., i. de Panestil; incisão efetuada transversalmente e através da bainha externa dos músculos retos, aproximadamente a uma polegada acima do púbis, sendo os músculos separados na linha mediana, na direção de suas fibras.
postauricular i., i. pós-auricular; incisão feita paralelamente e a poucos milímetros posteriormente à dobra retroauricular para ter acesso ao córtex do mastóide.
transmeatal i., i. transmeatal; incisão na pele do canal auditivo externo posterior, que se estende logo acima da dobra maleolar posterior até uma posição de 6 horas, inferiormente; feita para ter acesso à parte posterior do ouvido médio.
transverse abdominal i., i. abdominal transversa; incisão abdominal feita perpendicularmente ao eixo dos músculos retos do abdome.

in·ci·sive (in - sī′siv). Incisivo. **1.** Cortante; que tem a capacidade de cortar. **2.** Relativo aos dentes incisivos.

in·ci·sor (in - sī′zor). Incisivo. SIN incisor tooth. [L. incido, cortar]
central i., i. central; o primeiro dente no maxilar e na mandíbula de cada lado do plano médio sagital da cabeça.
Hutchinson i.'s, incisivos de Hutchinson. SIN Hutchinson teeth, em tooth.
lateral i., i. lateral. SIN second i.
second i., segundo i.; segundo dente decíduo ou permanente do maxilar ou da mandíbula de cada lado do plano médio sagital da cabeça. SIN lateral i.

INCISURA

in·ci·su·ra, pl. **in·ci·su·rae** (in′sī - soo′ră, in′si - soo′rē) [TA]. Incisura. SIN notch. [L. um corte]
i. acetab′uli [TA], i. acetabular. SIN acetabular notch.
i. angula′ris [TA], i. angular. SIN angular incisure.
i. anterior auriculae [TA], **i. ante′rior au′ris,** i. anterior da orelha. SIN anterior notch of auricle.
i. ap′icis cor′dis [TA], i. do ápice do coração. SIN notch of cardiac apex.
i. cardi′aca, i. cardíaca. SIN cardial notch.
i. cardi′aca pulmo′nis sinis′tri [TA], i. cardíaca do pulmão esquerdo. SIN cardiac notch of left lung.
i. cardialis [TA], i. da cárdia. SIN i. cardialis. SIN i. cardialis [TA].
i. cartilag′inis mea′tus acus′tici [TA], i. na cartilagem do meato acústico. SIN notch in cartilage of acoustic meatus.
i. cerebel′li ante′rior, i. anterior do cerebelo. SIN anterior cerebellar notch.
i. cerebel′li poste′rior, i. posterior do cerebelo. SIN posterior cerebellar notch.
i. clavicula′ris [TA], i. clavicular. SIN clavicular notch of sternum.
incisurae costa′les [TA], incisuras costais. SIN costal notches, em notch.
i. ethmoida′lis [TA], i. etmoidal. SIN ethmoidal notch.
i. fibula′ris [TA], i. fibular. SIN fibular notch.
i. fronta′lis [TA], i. frontal. SIN frontal notch.
i. interarytenoi′dea [TA], i. interaritenóide. SIN interarytenoide notch.
i. intertrag′ica [TA], i. intertrágica. SIN intertragic notch.
i. ischiad′ica ma′jor [TA], i. isquiática maior. SIN greater sciatic notch.
i. ischiad′ica mi′nor [TA], i. isquiática menor. SIN lesser sciatic notch.
i. jugula′ris os′sis occipita′lis [TA], i. jugular do osso occipital. SIN jugular notch of occipital bone.
i. jugula′ris os′sis tempora′lis [TA], i. jugular do osso temporal. SIN jugular notch of petrous part of temporal bone.
i. jugula′ris sterna′lis [TA], i. jugular do esterno. SIN jugular notch of sternum.
i. lacrima′lis [TA], i. lacrimal. SIN lacrimal notch.
i. ligamen′ti tere′tis hep′atis [TA], i. para o ligamento redondo do fígado. SIN notch for ligamentum teres.
i. mandib′ulae [TA], i. da mandíbula. SIN mandibular notch.
i. mastoi′dea [TA], i. da mastóide. SIN mastoid notch.
i. nasa′lis [TA], i. nasal. SIN nasal notch.
i. pancrea′tis [TA], i. do pâncreas. SIN pancreatic notch.
i. parieta′lis [TA], i. parietal. SIN parietal notch.
i. preoccipita′lis [TA], i. pré-occipital. SIN preoccipital notch.
i. pterygoi′dea, i. pterigóide. SIN pterygoid notch.
i. radia′lis [TA], i. radial. SIN radial notch.
i. rivi′ni, i. timpânica. SIN tympanic notch.
i. santori′ni, i. na cartilagem do meato acústico. SIN notch in cartilage of acoustic meatus.
i. scap′ulae, i. escapular. SIN suprascapular notch.
i. semiluna′ris ul′nae, i. semilunar da ulna. SIN trochlear notch.
i. sphenopalati′na [TA], i. esfenopalatina. SIN sphenopalatine notch.
i. supraorbita′lis [TA], i. supra-orbitária. SIN supraorbital notch; VER TAMBÉM supraorbital foramen.
i. tento′rii [TA], i. tentorial. SIN tentorial notch.
i. of tentorium, i. do tentório; *termo oficial alternativo para tentorial notch.
i. terminalis auricularis [TA], i. terminal da aurícula. SIN terminal notch of auricle.
i. termina′lis au′ris, i. terminal da aurícula. SIN terminal notch of auricle.
i. thyroi′dea infe′rior [TA], i. tireóidea inferior. SIN inferior thyroid notch.
i. thyroi′dea supe′rior [TA], i. tireóidea superior. SIN superior thyroid notch.
i. trag′ica, i. trágica. SIN intertragic notch.
i. trochlea′ris [TA], i. da tróclea. SIN trochlear notch.
i. tympan′ica [TA], i. timpânica. SIN tympanic notch.
i. ulna′ris [TA], i. da ulna. SIN ulnar notch.
i. umbilica′lis, i. umbilical. SIN notch for ligamentum teres.
i. vertebra′lis [TA], i. vertebral. SIN vertebral notch.

in·ci·sure (in - sī′zhoor). Incisura. SIN notch. [L. incisura]
angular i. [TA], i. angular; acentuada depressão angular na curvatura menor do estômago, na junção do corpo com o canal pilórico. SIN incisura angularis [TA], angular notch, sulcus angularis.
Lanterman i.'s, incisuras de Lanterman. SIN Schmidt-Lanterman i.'s.
Rivinus i., i. de Rivinus. SIN tympanic notch.
Santorini i.'s, incisuras de Santorini. SIN notch in cartilage of acoustic meatus.
Schmidt-Lanterman i.'s, i. incisuras de Schmidt-Lanterman, interrupções afuniladas na estrutura regular da bainha de mielina das fibras nervosas, antigamente interpretadas como verdadeiras rupturas na bainha, mas que, à microscopia eletrônica, correspondem a uma faixa de citoplasma que separa localmente as duas membranas oligodendrogliais fundidas (ou, nos nervos periféricos, células de Schwann) que compõem a bainha de mielina. SIN Lanterman i.'s, Schmidt-Lanterman clefts.
tympanic i., i. timpânica. SIN tympanic notch.

in·cli·na·tio, pl. **in·cli·na·ti·o·nes** (in′kli - nā′shē - ō, - nā - shē - ō′nēz) [TA]. Inclinação. SIN inclination. [L.]
i. pel′vis [TA], i. da pelve. SIN pelvic inclination.

in·cli·na·tion (in - kli - nā′shŭn) [TA]. Inclinação. **1.** Inclinação ou declive. **2.** Em odontologia, desvio do eixo longitudinal de um dente da perpendicular. SIN inclinatio [TA], version (3). [L. inclinatio, inclinação]
condylar guidance i., i. da guia condilar; ângulo de inclinação da guia condilar para um plano horizontal convencionado.
enamed rod i., i. dos bastonetes de esmalte; direção dos bastonetes de esmalte em relação à superfície externa do esmalte de um dente.
lateral condylar i., i. lateral do côndilo; a direção da via lateral do côndilo.
pelvic i. [TA], i. da pelve; ângulo que o plano da abertura superior da pelve faz com o plano horizontal. SIN inclinatio pelvis [TA], i. of pelvis.
i. of pelvis, i. da pelve. SIN pelvic i.

in·cli·nom·e·ter (in′kli - nom′ē - ter). Inclinômetro; instrumento obsoleto para determinar a direção dos eixos oculares no astigmatismo. [L. inclino, inclinar + G. metron, medida]

in·clu·sion (in - kloo′zhŭn). Inclusão. **1.** Qualquer substância estranha ou heterogênea contida numa célula ou em qualquer tecido ou órgão, não introduzida em conseqüência de traumatismo. **2.** Processo pelo qual uma estrutura estranha ou heterogênea é colocada erroneamente em outro tecido. [L. inclusio, resguardar, encerrar, de includo, pp. -clusis, fechar]
cell i.'s, i. inclusões celulares. **(1)** Elementos residuais do citoplasma que são produtos metabólicos da célula, como, p. ex., grânulos de pigmento ou cristais; **(2)** materiais de armazenamento, como glicogênio ou gordura; **(3)** material englobado, como carvão ou outras substâncias estranhas. VER TAMBÉM inclusion bodies em body.
Döhle i.'s, inclusões de Döhle. SIN Döhle bodies, em body.
fetal i., i. fetal; gêmeos conjugados desiguais em que o parasita incompletamente desenvolvido está totalmente incluído no autósito.
leukocyte i.'s, i. inclusões leucocitárias. SIN Döhle bodies em body.

in·co·her·ent (in - kō - her′ent). Incoerente; sem coerência; desintegrado; confuso; indica uma falta de conexão ou organização de partes durante a expressão verbal. [L. in-, neg. + co-haereo, pp. -haesus, aderir, unir, de haereo, aderir, grudar]

in·com·pat·i·bil·i·ty (in′kom - pat - i - bil′i - tē). Incompatibilidade. **1.** A qualidade de ser incompatível. **2.** Maneira de classificar os plasmídios bacterianos; dois plasmídios são incompatíveis quando não podem coexistir numa célula hospedeira.
physiologic i., i. fisiológica; forma de incompatibilidade em que as substâncias numa mistura exercem ações fisiológicas opostas. SIN therapeutic i.
Rh antigen i., i. de antígeno Rh. SIN erythroblastosis fetalis.
therapeutic i., i. terapêutica. SIN physiologic i.

in·com·pat·i·ble (in - kom - pat′i - bl). Incompatível. **1.** Sem composição apropriada para ser combinada ou misturada com outro agente ou substância, sem produzir uma reação indesejável (incluindo alteração química ou destruição ou efeito farmacológico). **2.** Refere-se a indivíduos que são incapazes de se associar entre si sem que isso resulte em ansiedade e conflitos. **3.** Que tem genótipos que colocam a progênie em alto risco de distúrbios recessivos graves ou que promovem uma reação materno-fetal prejudicial (p. ex., a eritroblastose fetal é causada por Rh incompatível). **4.** Falta de identidade antigênica entre um doador e um receptor. [L. *in-* neg., + *con-*, com + *patior*, pp. *passus*, sofrer, tolerar]

in·com·pe·tence, in·com·pe·ten·cy (in - kom'pe - tens, in - kom'pĕ - ten - sē). Incompetência. **1.** Qualidade de ser incompetente ou incapaz de executar determinada função, especialmente a incapacidade de fechamento completo das valvas cardíacas ou venosas. **2.** Em psiquiatria forense, a incapacidade de distinguir o certo do errado ou de administrar os próprios negócios. [L. *in-*, neg. + *com-peto*, empenhar-se]
  aortic i., i. aórtica; fechamento defeituoso da valva aórtica, permitindo a regurgitação no ventrículo esquerdo durante a diástole.
  cardiac i., i. cardíaca; incapacidade dos ventrículos de bombear o sangue de volta para os átrios com rapidez suficiente para impedir uma elevação anormal da pressão atrial ou bombear sangue suficiente para manter a função circulatória normal.
  cardiac valvular i., i. valvar cardíaca; incapacidade de uma válvula de executar a sua função: manutenção de um fluxo unidirecional; manifesta-se por regurgitação de sangue na direção oposta quando a valva deveria estar fechada.
  mitral i., i. mitral; fechamento defeituoso da valva mitral, permitindo a regurgitação de sangue no átrio esquerdo durante a sístole.
  muscular i., i. muscular; fechamento imperfeito de uma valva cardíaca anatomicamente normal, em conseqüência da ação defeituosa dos músculos papilares.
  pulmonary i., pulmonic i., i. pulmonar; fechamento defeituoso da valva pulmonar, permitindo a regurgitação no ventrículo direito durante a diástole.
  pyloric i., i. pilórica; estado dilatado ou falta de tônus do piloro, permitindo a passagem de alimento para o intestino antes que a digestão gástrica esteja completa.
  relative i., i. relativa; fechamento imperfeito de uma valva cardíaca em conseqüência da dilatação excessiva da cavidade correspondente do coração.
  tricuspid i., i. tricúspide; fechamento defeituoso da valva tricúspide, permitindo a regurgitação para o átrio direito durante a sístole.
  valvular i., i. valvar. SIN valvular *regurgitation.*

in·con·stant (in - kon'stant). Inconstante. **1.** Irregular. **2.** Em anatomia, refere-se a uma estrutura, como uma artéria, nervo, etc., que pode ou não estar presente.

in·con·ti·nence (in - kon'ti - nens). Incontinência. **1.** Incapacidade de impedir a expulsão de uma excreção, especialmente urina ou fezes. **2.** Falta de restrição do apetite, especialmente sexual. Cf. intemperance. SIN incontinencia. [L. *in-continentia*, de *in-*. neg. + *con-tineo*, manter junto, de *teneo*, segurar]
  fecal i., i. fecal. SIN i. of feces.
  i. of feces, i. de fezes; evacuação involuntária de fezes na roupa ou nos lençóis, geralmente em decorrência de patologia que afeta o controle esfincteriano ou de perda das funções cognitivas. SIN fecal i.
  i. of milk, i. de leite. SIN galactorrhea.
  overflow i., i. de fluxo constante; perda involuntária de urina associada a hiperdistensão da bexiga, com ou sem contração do músculo detrusor. SIN paradoxical i., passive i.
  paradoxical i., i. paradoxal. SIN overflow i.
  passive i., i. passiva. SIN overflow i.
  i. of pigment, i. de pigmento; perda de melanina da epiderme e seu acúmulo em melanófagos na derme superior; observada em diversas doenças inflamatórias da pele e na incontinência pigmentar.
  reflex i., i. reflexa; perda de urina devido à hiper-reflexia involuntária do detrusor.
  stress urinary i. (SUI), i. urinária de estresse; vazamento de urina em conseqüência de tosse, esforço ou qualquer movimento voluntário súbito, devido à incompetência dos mecanismos esfincterianos. SIN urinary exertional i.
  urge i., urgency i., i. de urgência; extravasamento de urina por contração involuntária do detrusor na vigência de forte desejo de urinar.
  urinary exertional i., i. urinária de esforço. SIN stress urinary i.
  i. of urine, i. de urina; eliminação involuntária de urina nas roupas ou lençóis. Problema comum em indivíduos idosos, sobretudo aqueles que se encontram em asilos; pode ser devido a anormalidades neurológicas, perda da função esfincteriana (especialmente comum em mulheres multíparas), obstrução crônica do orifício vesical ou perda das funções cognitivas.

in·con·ti·nent (in - kon'ti - nent). Incontinente; relativo à incontinência.

in·con·ti·nen·tia (in - kon'ti - nen'shē - ā). Incontinência. SIN incontinence. [L.]
  i. pigmen'ti [MIM*146150, MIM*308300 e MIM*308310], i. pigmentar; genodermatose rara caracterizada por lesões hiperpigmentadas em configuração linear, zebrada e outras configurações bizarras, seguindo as linhas de Blaschko; algumas vezes acompanhada de outras anormalidades de desenvolvimento dos olhos, dentes, unhas, esqueleto, coração. As manifestações dermatológicas podem ser divididas em quatro estágios: o estágio I caracteriza-se por eritema, vesículas e pústulas; o estágio II, por pápulas, lesões verrucosas e hiperceratose; o estágio III, por hiperpigmentação; e o estágio IV, por palidez, atrofia e cicatrizes. Historicamente, acreditava-se que existiam duas formas: 1) a forma esporádica de i. pigmentar (IP1), que atualmente é conhecida como *hipomelanose* de Ito, e 2) o tipo familiar (IP2), que é dominante ligado ao X e genético letal nos homens. VER TAMBÉM *hypomelanosis* of Ito. SIN Bloch-Sulzberger disease, Bloch-Sulzberger syndrome.
  i. pigmen'ti achro'mians [MIM*146150], i. pigmentar do acrômio. SIN *hypomelanosis* of Ito.

in·co·or·di·na·tion (in - kō - ōr - di - nā'shŭn). Incoordenação. SIN ataxia. [L. *in-* neg. + coordenação]

in·cor·po·ra·tion (in - kōr - pŏ - rā'shŭn). Incorporação. SIN identification. [L. *in-*, em + *corporare*, pp. *corporatus*, transformar-se num corpo]

in·crease (in'krēs). Aumento; qualquer aumento de quantidade.
  absolute cell i., a. absoluto de células; aumento verdadeiro em um dos tipos de leucócitos, sendo o número absoluto de leucócitos por mm^3 de sangue obtido multiplicando-se a contagem total de leucócitos pela percentagem dos tipos celulares em questão.
  base i. at low levels, a. base de baixos níveis; estratégia de processamento de sinais de auxílio da audição para aumentar gradualmente a amplificação de baixas freqüências em níveis de baixa densidade.
  treble i. at low levels, a. agudo em baixos níveis; estratégia de processamento de sinais de auxílio auditivo para aumentar gradualmente a amplificação de sons de alta freqüência em baixos níveis.

in·cre·ment (in'kre - ment). Incremento; mudança no valor de uma variável; em geral, aumento, sendo o termo "decremento" aplicado para referir-se a diminuição, embora o termo "incremento" também possa ser corretamente aplicado às duas situações. [L. *incrementum*, aumento]

incretin. Incretina; termo genérico para referir-se a todas as substâncias insulinotrópicas que se originam no trato gastrointestinal, liberadas na circulação por refeições contendo glicose. Uma delas é o polipeptídeo insulinotrópico glicose-dependente, que é liberado na circulação pelas células crípticas no duodeno proximal e jejuno após refeições contendo glicose ou ácidos graxos de cadeia longa. Outra incretina é o polipeptídeo derivado do pró-glucagon, produto de clivagem do glucagon, que é posteriormente processado em peptídeo-1 glucagon-símile e, a seguir, em peptídeo insulinotrópico glucagon-símile.

in·cre·tion (in - krē'shŭn). Increção; atividade funcional de uma glândula endócrina. [in- + secreção]

in·crus·ta·tion (in'krŭs - tā'shŭn). Incrustação. **1.** Formação de crosta ou casca de ferida. **2.** Revestimento de algum material advertício ou de exsudato; crosta. [L. *in-crusto*, pp. *-atus*, incrustar, de *crusta*, crosta]

in·cu·ba·tion (in'kū - bā'shŭn). Incubação. **1.** Ato de manter condições ambientais controladas, com o objetivo de favorecer o crescimento ou desenvolvimento de culturas microbianas ou teciduais ou manter condições ideais para uma reação química ou imunológica. **2.** Manutenção de um ambiente artificial para um recém-nascido, geralmente prematuro ou hipóxico, fornecendo-lhe temperatura apropriada, umidade e, em geral, oxigênio. **3.** Desenvolvimento, na ausência de sinais ou sintomas, de uma infecção desde o momento de entrada do agente infeccioso até o aparecimento dos primeiros sinais ou sintomas. [L. *incubo*, depender de]

in·cu·ba·tor (in'kū - bā'tōr). Incubadora. **1.** Recipiente no qual podem ser mantidas condições ambientais controladas; p. ex., para a cultura de microrganismos. **2.** Aparelho para manter um recém-nascido (habitualmente prematuro) num ambiente de oxigenação, umidade e temperatura apropriadas.

in·cu·bus (in'koo - bŭs). Incubo; originalmente, espírito demoniacal que se deitava em cima e oprimia pessoas dormindo; especialmente um espírito masculino que copulava com mulheres dormindo. Cf. succubus. [L. de *incubo*, deitar sobre]

in·cu·dal (in'koo - dăl). Incudal; relativo à bigorna.

in·cu·dec·to·my (in - koo - dek'tō - mē). Incudectomia; remoção da bigorna do tímpano. [incus + G. *ektomē*, excisão]

in·cu·des (in - koo'dēz). Plural de incus (bigorna). [L.]

in·cu·di·form (in - koo'di - fōrm). Incudiforme; com forma de bigorna. [L. *incus (incud-)*, bigorna]

in·cu·do·mal·le·al (in - koo'dō - mal'lē - ăl). Incudomaleal; relativo à bigorna e ao martelo; indica articulação entre a bigorna e o martelo no ouvido médio. SIN ambomalleal.

in·cu·do·sta·pe·di·al (in - koo'dō - stā - pē'dē - ăl). Incudoestapedial; relativo à bigorna e ao estribo; indica a articulação entre a bigorna e o estribo no ouvido médio.

in·cur·a·ble (in - kūr'ă - bl). Incurável; refere-se a uma doença ou processo mórbido que não responde ao tratamento clínico ou cirúrgico.

in·cur·va·tion (in'ker - vā'shŭn). Encurvamento; curvatura para dentro. Flexão para dentro.

in·cus, gen. **in·cu·dis,** pl. **in·cu·des** (ing'kŭs, in - koo'dis, in - koo'dēz) [TA]. Bigorna; o ossículo médio dos três ossículos no ouvido médio; possui um corpo e duas ramificações ou processos (ramo longo da bigorna e ramo curto da bigorna); na extremidade do ramo longo, existe um pequeno nódulo, o processo lenticular, que se articula com a cabeça do estribo. SIN anvil. [L. anvil]

in·cy·clo·duc·tion (in - sī - klō - dŭk'shŭn). Inciclodução; ciclodução em que o pólo superior da córnea sofre rotação interna (medialmente). [in- + cyclo- + L. *duco,* pp. *ductus,* levar a]

in·cy·clo·pho·ria (in - sī'klō - fō'rē - ă). Incicloforia; cicloforia em que a posição da íris em 12 horas tende a desviar-se medialmente. [L. in- + cyclo- + G. *phora,* transportar]

in·cy·clo·tro·pia (in - sī - klō - trō'pē - ă). Inciclotropia; ciclotropia em que os pólos superiores das córneas sofrem rotação interna (medialmente) um em relação ao outro. [in- + cyclo- + G. *tropē,* uma volta]

in d. Abreviatura do L. *in dies,* diariamente.

in·dan·e·di·one de·riv·a·tives. Derivados da indanediona; anticoagulantes semelhantes à warfarina na sua ação. A anisindiona e a fenindiona são utilizadas clinicamente; a difenadiona possui ação muito longa e é utilizada como raticida.

in·dan·e·di·ones (in'dăn - dī - ōnz). Indanedionas; classe de anticoagulantes de ação indireta, eficazes por via oral, cujo representante é a fenindiona.

in·de·cid·u·ate (in - dē - sid'ū - āt). Indecíduo; relativo a mamíferos (indecidual) que não eliminam nenhum tecido uterino materno quando a placenta é expelida no parto (p. ex., égua, porca), em contraste com os mamíferos decíduos (p. ex., seres humanos, cão, roedores).

in·den·i·za·tion (in - den - i - zā'shŭn). Indenização. SIN innidiation. [*in-* + denizen]

in·den·ta·tion (in - den - tā'shŭn). Indentação. **1.** Ato de sulcar ou escavar. **2.** Chanfradura. **3.** Estado de estar sulcado. [Mediev. L. *indento,* pp. *-atus,* fazer sulcos semelhantes a dentes, de L. *dens (dent-),* dente]

in·de·pen·dence. Independência. **1.** Relação entre dois ou mais eventos em que nenhuma informação acerca de qualquer combinação de alguns deles contém qualquer informação acerca de qualquer combinação dos outros. **2.** Estado de desligamento mútuo entre unidades autônomas.

causal i., i. causal; estado de sistemas que não compartilham nenhuma causa ou efeito.

stochastic i., i. estocástica; independência de dois ou mais eventos ou variáveis; estado em que sua probabilidade conjunta ou distribuição é igual ao produto de suas probabilidades ou distribuições marginais.

INDEX

in·dex, gen. **in·di·cis,** pl. **in·di·ces, in·dex·es** (in'deks, - di - sis, - di - sēz, - dek - sēz) **1.** Dedo indicador [NA]. SIN index *finger.* **2.** Índice; guia, padrão, indicador, símbolo ou número que indica a relação quanto ao tamanho, capacidade ou função de uma parte ou coisa com outra. VER TAMBÉM quotient, ratio. **3.** Molde utilizado para registrar ou manter a posição relativa de um dente ou dentes entre si e/ou com um molde. **4.** Guia, habitualmente feito de gesso, utilizado para recolocar dentes, moldes ou partes. **5.** Em epidemiologia, escala, escala de graduação. [L. aquele que indica, informante, indicador, índice, de *in-dico,* pp. *-atus,* declarar]

absorbancy i., i. de absorbância. **(1)** SIN specific absorption *coefficient;* **(2)** SIN molar absorption *coefficient.*

alveolar i., i. alveolar; **(1)** SIN gnathic i; **(2)** SIN basilar i.

amnionic fluid i., i. de líquido amniótico; soma dos diâmetros da bolsa vertical maior de líquido amniótico em cada um dos quatro quadrantes do útero, obtidos por ultra-som; medida do volume de líquido durante a gravidez.

anesthetic i., i. anestésico; relação entre o número de unidades de anestésico necessárias para anestesia e o número de unidades de anestésico necessárias para produzir insuficiência respiratória ou cardiovascular.

antitryptic i., i. antitríptico; termo obsoleto para referir-se ao retardo relativo na perda de viscosidade de uma solução de caseína incubada com tripsina, à qual foi adicionada uma gota de soro sanguíneo anormal (p. ex., de paciente canceroso), em comparação com uma solução semelhante à qual foi adicionado soro normal; se a primeira gotejar através do tubo do viscosímetro em 100 segundos e a segunda em 104 segundos, o i. antitríptico é de 4.

apnea-hypopnea i., i. de apnéia-hipopnéia; número de episódios de apnéia e hipopnéia combinados por hora de sono.

Arneth i., i. de Arneth; expressão baseada na soma das percentagens de neutrófilos polimorfonucleares com núcleos de 1 ou 2 lobos com metade da percentagem dos que apresentam núcleos com três lobos; o valor normal é de 60%. VER TAMBÉM Arneth *formula,* Arneth *count.*

auricular i., i. auricular; relação da largura com a altura da orelha externa: (largura da orelha externa × 100)/comprimento da orelha externa.

Ayala i., i. de Ayala; i. cerebroespinal quando são removidos 10 ml de líquido cefalorraquidiano. SIN Ayala quotient, spinal quotient.

basilar i., i. basilar; relação entre a linha basialveolar e o comprimento máximo do crânio, de acordo com a fórmula: (linha basialveolar × 100)/comprimento do crânio. SIN alveolar i. (2).

Bödecker i., i. de Bödecker; modificação do i. de cárie DMF.

body mass i., i. de massa corporal; medida antropométrica da massa corporal, definida como o peso em quilogramas dividido pela altura em metros quadrados; método de determinar o estado nutricional calórico.

buffer i., i. tampão. SIN buffer *value.*

cardiac i., i. cardíaco; volume de sangue ejetado pelo coração numa unidade de tempo, dividido pela área de superfície corporal; em geral, expresso em litros por minuto por metro quadrado.

centromeric i., i. centromérico; a relação entre o comprimento do braço curto do cromossoma e o do cromossoma total; habitualmente expresso em percentagem.

cephalic i., i. cefálico; a relação entre largura máxima e o comprimento máximo da cabeça, obtida pela fórmula: (largura × 100)/comprimento. SIN length-breadth i.

cephalo-orbital i., i. céfalo-orbitário; a relação do conteúdo cúbico das duas órbitas com o da cavidade craniana multiplicada por 100.

cerebral i., i. cerebral; a relação do diâmetro transverso com o ântero-posterior da cavidade craniana multiplicada por 100.

cerebrospinal i., i. cefalorraquidiano; o valor obtido ao multiplicar a pressão do líquido cefalorraquidiano, após retirada do mesmo por punção espinal, pelo volume de líquido retirado e, em seguida, dividido pela pressão original.

chemotherapeutic i., i. quimioterápico; a relação entre a dose efetiva mínima de um agente quimioterápico e a dose máxima tolerada. Originalmente utilizado por Ehrlich para expressar a toxicidade relativa de um agente quimioterápico sobre um parasita e seu hospedeiro.

chest i., i. torácico. SIN thoracic i.

cranial i., i. craniano; a relação entre a largura máxima e o comprimento máximo do crânio, obtida pela fórmula: (largura × 100)/comprimento.

Cumulative I. Medicus, coleção de literatura médica, publicada anualmente, que começou no consultório do *Army Surgeon General* dos Estados Unidos, no final da Guerra Civil. A *National Library of Medicine* assumiu a sua continuidade, transformando-se numa base de dados denominada MEDLINE.

Dean fluorosis i., i. de fluorose de Dean; índice que mede o grau de esmalte mosqueado (fluorose) nos dentes; utilizado mais freqüentemente em estudos epidemiológicos de campo.

def caries i., DEF caries i., i. de cáries DEF ou DEF; um índice de cáries já ocorridas, com base no número de dentes decíduos (indicados por letras minúsculas) ou permanentes (indicados por letras maiúsculas) cariados, extraídos e obturados (*d*ecayed *e*xtracted, and *f*illed).

degenerative i., i. degenerativo; a percentagem de granulócitos que contêm grânulos tóxicos no citoplasma, em comparação com a percentagem total de granulócitos.

dental i. (DI), i. dentário (ID). **(1)** Relação entre o comprimento do dente (distância da superfície mesial do primeiro pré-molar até a superfície distal do terceiro molar) e o comprimento basinasal (do básio ao násio): (comprimento do dente × 100)/comprimento basinasal; **(2)** sistema de números para indicar o tamanho comparativo dos dentes. SIN Flower dental i.

df caries i., DF caries i., i. de cáries df ou DF; índice de cáries já ocorridas, com base no número de dentes decíduos (indicados por letras minúsculas) ou permanentes (indicados por letras maiúsculas) cariados e obturados (*d*ecayed and *f*illed). SIN df. DF.

diet quality i., i. de qualidade dietética; medida da qualidade da dieta utilizando um conjunto de oito recomendações relativas ao consumo de alimentos e nutrientes da *National Academy of Sciences* (NAS). Atribui-se um valor 0 quando se seguem todos os critérios do padrão; um valor 1 quando se alcançam 30% do padrão; e um valor 2 quando a diferença é de mais de 30%. O índice obtido pode ser um valor situado entre 0–16, sendo o menor valor o melhor. As recomendações da NAS incluem: redução da ingestão total de gordura a 30% ou menos da energia total; redução da ingestão de ácidos graxos saturados a menos de 10% da energia; diminuição da ingestão de colesterol a menos de 300 mg/dia; ingestão de 5 ou mais porções de vegetais e frutas diariamente; aumento da ingestão de amidos e outros carboidratos complexos através da ingestão de seis ou mais porções de pão, cereais e legumes diariamente; manutenção da ingestão de proteínas em níveis moderados (níveis inferiores a duas vezes a cota dietética recomendada [CDR]); limitar a ingestão diária total de sódio a 2.400 mg ou menos; e manutenção de uma ingestão adequada de cálcio (aproximadamente a CDR).

dmfs caries i., DMFS caries i., i. de cáries dmfs ou DMFS; índice de cáries já ocorridas, com base no número de dentes decíduos (indicados por letras minúsculas) ou permanentes (indicados por letras maiúsculas) cariados, ausentes ou obturados (*d*ecayed, *m*issing and *f*illed).

effective temperature i., i. de temperatura efetiva; índice composto de conforto ambiental que é comparado após exposição a diferentes combinações de temperatura, umidade e movimento do ar.

empathic i., i. empático; grau de empatia ou compreensão emocional experimentado por um profissional de saúde ou outra pessoa em relação a outro indivíduo, mais particularmente a uma pessoa que esteja sofrendo de alguma condição emocional ou somática.

endemic i., i. endêmico; percentagem de crianças infectadas com malária ou outra doença endêmica, em determinada localidade.

erythrocyte indices, índices eritrocitários; cálculos para determinar o tamanho médio, o conteúdo de hemoglobina e a concentração de hemoglobina dos eritrócitos, especificamente o volume corpuscular médio (VCM), a hemoglobina corpuscular média (HCM) e a concentração de hemoglobina corpuscular média (CHCM); os resultados costumam ser utilizados na classificação e no diagnóstico dos distúrbios eritrocitários.

facial i., i. facial; relação entre o comprimento da face e a sua largura máxima entre as proeminências zigomáticas; para obter o **i. facial superior,** o comprimento da face é medida do násio até o ponto alveolar: (comprimento nasialveolar × 100)/largura bizigomática; para o **i. facial total,** o comprimento é medido do násio até o tubérculo mentoniano: (comprimento nasimentoniano × 100)/largura bizigomática.

Flower dental i., i. dentário de Flower. SIN dental i.

free thyroxine i. (FTI), i. de tiroxina livre (FTI); um valor arbitrário obtido ao multiplicar a captação da triiodotironina (T_3) pela concentração sérica de tiroxina (T_4); corrige, em grande parte, as variações da concentração de globina ligada ao hormônio tireóideo ao fornecer uma estimativa clinicamente válida da tiroxina livre fisiologicamente ativa; o ensaio direto ou a medida laboratorial da tiroxina sérica livre fornecem um valor mais acurado.

glycemic i., i. glicêmico; grau de elevação da glicose sérica a partir do consumo de vários produtos alimentares.

gnathic i., i. gnático; relação entre os comprimentos basialveolar (do básio até o ponto alveolar) e basinasal (do básio ao násio): (comprimento basialveolar × 100)/comprimento basinasal; o resultado indica o grau de projeção do maxilar superior. SIN alveolar i. (1).

health status i., i. do estado de saúde; conjunto de medidas destinadas a detectar flutuações em curtos prazos na saúde dos membros de uma população; em geral, as medidas incluem função física, bem-estar emocional, atividades diárias, sentimentos, etc.

height-length i., i. altura-comprimento. SIN vertical i.

international sensitivity i. (ISI), i. de sensibilidade internacional; a inclinação da linha de melhor adaptação relacionando o log do tempo de protrombina obtido com reagente padrão com o log do tempo de protrombina obtido com o reagente de trabalho para indivíduos normais e pacientes em uso de terapia anticoagulante oral estável; os reagentes padrões utilizados para obter esse valor são preparações de referência calibradas contra o reagente padrão da *Organização Mundial de Saúde*. VER TAMBÉM international normalized *ratio*.

iron i., índice de ferro, índice obsoleto de ferro obtido ao dividir o valor do conteúdo médio de ferro no sangue normal (42,74 mg) pela contagem de eritrócitos em milhões; normalmente, varia entre 8 e 9; na anemia perniciosa, o índice é habitualmente superior a 10, mas tende a ser normal na anemia secundária crônica.

karyopyknotic i., i. cariopicnótico; índice utilizado para monitorizar o estado hormonal da paciente, refletido pelas células vaginais esfoliadas e sua morfologia; expressão da percentagem de células intermediárias e superficiais de células escamosas do epitélio vaginal que possuem núcleos picnóticos.

length-breadth i., i. de comprimento–largura. SIN cephalic i.

length-height i., i. de comprimento–largura. SIN vertical i.

leukopenic i., i. leucopênico; diminuição significativa da contagem dos leucócitos após a ingestão de alimentos aos quais o paciente é hipersensível, utilizando-se uma contagem efetuada durante o estado de jejum normal como base para avaliação da contagem pós-prandial.

maturation i., i. de maturação; índice que indica o grau de maturação alcançado pelo epitélio vaginal, a julgar pelos tipos de células esfoliadas; serve como meio objetivo para avaliar a secreção ou a resposta hormonal; representa a percentagem de células parabasais/intermediárias/superficiais, nessa ordem; a ocorrência de "desvio para a esquerda" indica a presença de células mais imaturas na superfície (atrofia), enquanto um "desvio para a direita" indica um epitélio mais maduro.

metacarpal i., i. metacarpal; a relação média entre o comprimento e a largura dos metacarpos II a V; essa relação está aumentada na síndrome de Marfan.

mitotic i., i. mitótico; a proporção de células, em determinado tecido que está sofrendo mitose, freqüentemente expressa como o número de células numa área específica de corte tecidual ou como percentagem da amostra total de células.

molar absorbancy i., i. de absorbância molar. SIN molar absorption *coefficient*.

nasal i., i. nasal; relação da maior largura da abertura nasal com o comprimento de uma linha traçada do násio até a borda inferior da abertura nasal: (largura nasal × 100)/altura nasal.

nucleoplasmic i., i. nucleoplasmático; o quociente do volume nuclear dividido pelo volume citoplasmático.

obesity i., i. de obesidade; peso corporal dividido pelo volume corporal.

opsonic i., i. opsônico; valor que indica o conteúdo relativo de opsonina no sangue de um indivíduo com doença infecciosa, avaliado *in vitro* em comparação com uma amostra de sangue presumivelmente normal; o i. opsônico é calculado a partir da seguinte equação: i. fagocítica do soro normal ÷ i. fagocítico do soro do teste = 1 ÷ x, onde x representa o i. opsônico.

orbital i., i. orbitário; relação da altura da órbita com a sua largura: (altura orbitária × 100)/largura da órbita.

orbitonasal i., i. orbitonasal; relação da largura entre os ângulos laterais dos olhos, medida com uma fita métrica passando sobre a raiz do nariz vezes 100, com a largura entre os ângulos laterais dos olhos, medidos com calibrador.

palatal i., palatine i., i. do palato, i. palatino. SIN palatomaxillary i.

palatomaxillary i., i. palatomaxilar; relação da largura palatomaxilar, medida entre as bordas externas do arco alveolar, imediatamente acima do meio do segundo dente molar, com o comprimento palatomaxilar, medido a partir do ponto alveolar até o meio de linha transversa, tocando as bordas posteriores dos dois maxilares: (largura palatomaxilar × 100)/comprimento palatomaxilar; indica as formas variáveis da arcada dentária do palato. SIN palatal i., palatine i.

Pearl i., i. de Pearl; o número de falhas de um método contraceptivo por 100 mulheres-anos de exposição.

pelvic i., i. pélvico; a relação entre os diâmetros conjugado do estreito pélvico e transverso da pelve: (diâmetro conjugado do estreito pélvico × 100)/diâmetro transverso.

phagocytic i., i. fagocítico; o número médio de bactérias ou outras partículas observadas no citoplasma de leucócitos polimorfonucleares ou de outras células fagocíticas após mistura e incubação a 37°C. Refletirá o número médio de partículas ingeridas ou a taxa de depuração de partículas do sangue ou de uma cultura.

Pirquet i., i. de Pirquet; um método obsoleto para estabelecer a presença de desnutrição ao dividir o peso corporal (gramas/10) pela altura na posição sentada (em cm); a raiz cúbica do quociente, quando < 0,945, era considerada como indicadora de desnutrição.

PMA i., índice que mede a presença ou ausência de inflamação gengival que ocorre nas papilas ou gengivas marginais ou fixas.

ponderal i., i. ponderal; raiz cúbica do peso corporal vezes 100 dividida pela altura em cm.

pressure-volume i., i. de pressão-volume, método de avaliação da hidrodinâmica do líquido cefalorraquidiano.

pulsatility i., i. de pulsatilidade; cálculo de medidas Doppler das velocidades sistólica e diastólica nas circulações uterina, umbilical ou fetal.

refractive i., (n), i. de refração; velocidade relativa da luz em outro meio, quando comparada com a velocidade no ar; p. ex., no caso do ar para o vidro, $n = 1,52$; no caso do ar para a água, $n = 1,33$. VER TAMBÉM *law* of refraction.

Robinson i., i. de Robinson; índice utilizado para calcular a carga de trabalho cardíaco. VER double *product*.

Röhrer i., i. de Röhrer; peso corporal em gramas vezes 100 dividido pelo cubo da altura em centímetros.

root caries i., i. de cáries de raiz; relação entre o número de dentes com lesões de cáries da raiz e/ou restaurações da raiz e o número de dentes com superfícies expostas das raízes.

sacral i., i. sacral; relação obtida ao multiplicar a maior largura do sacro por 100, dividindo-se pelo comprimento.

saturation i., i. de saturação; indicação da concentração relativa de hemoglobina nos eritrócitos, calculada da seguinte maneira: gramas de hemoglobina por 100 ml (expressos em percentagem do normal) ÷ valor do hematócrito (expresso como percentagem do normal) = i. de saturação. O índice normal para adultos e lactentes é de 0,97 a 1,02; na anemia primária e secundária, o índice é, em geral, consideravelmente inferior a 0,97.

Schilling i., i. de Schilling. SIN Schilling *blood count*.

shock i., i. de choque; o quociente da freqüência cardíaca dividido pela pressão arterial sistólica; normalmente, é de cerca de 0,5, mas, no choque (p. ex., freqüência crescente do pulso com queda da pressão arterial), o índice pode atingir 1,0.

short increment sensitivity i., i. de sensibilidade a incrementos curtos; medida da capacidade de detectar pequenos incrementos (1dB) na intensidade; quando há lesões cocleares, essa capacidade ultrapassa o normal.

small increment sensitivity i., i. de sensibilidade a pequenos incrementos. VER SISI *test*.

spiro-i., i. espiro. VER spiro-index.

splenic i., i. esplênico; indicação aproximada de salubridade ou o reverso em relação à malária numa determinada localidade particular, a julgar pela ausência relativa ou prevalência de baços aumentados na população.

staphyloopsonic i., i. estafilopsônico; índice opsônico calculado em relação a uma infecção estafilocócica, com cultura jovem de *Staphylococcus aureus* ou da cepa de estafilococo do paciente submetido ao teste.

stroke work i., i. do impulso apical; medida do trabalho realizado pelo coração em cada contração, ajustada para a área de superfície corporal; igual ao volume sistólico do coração multiplicado pela pressão arterial e dividido pela área de superfície corporal; o i. do impulso apical normal não ultrapassa 40 g-m/m².

therapeutic i., i. terapêutico; a relação entre LD_{50} e ED_{50}, utilizada na comparação quantitativa de substâncias.

thoracic i., i. torácico; diâmetro ântero-posterior do tórax vezes 100 dividido pelo diâmetro transverso do tórax. SIN chest i.
tibiofemoral i., i. tibiofemoral; a relação obtida ao multiplicar o comprimento da tíbia por 100, dividindo-se pelo comprimento do fêmur.
transversovertical i., i. transverso vertical. SIN vertical i.
tuberculoopsonic i., i. tuberculopsônico; índice opsônico calculado em relação à infecção tuberculosa, sendo utilizada no teste uma cultura em crescimento ativo de *Mycobacterium tuberculosis* ou da cepa do bacilo da tuberculose do paciente.
ultraviolet i., i. ultravioleta; índice diário publicado pelo *U.S. National Weather Service* para muitas cidades, prevendo a quantidade de luz ultravioleta perigosa que deverá chegar à superfície da terra no dia seguinte, aproximadamente ao meio-dia.
uricolytic i., i. uricolítico; percentagem de ácido úrico oxidado a alantoína antes de ser secretado.
vertical i., i. vertical; a relação entre altura e comprimento do crânio: (altura × 100)/comprimento. SIN height-length i., length-height i., transversovertical i.
vital i., i. vital; relação entre nascimentos e mortes dentro de uma população durante determinado período de tempo.
Volpe-Manhold i. (V-MI), i. de Volpe-Manhold (V-MI); índice para comparar a quantidade de cálculo dentário nos indivíduos.
volume i., i. de volume; indicação do tamanho relativo (p. ex., volume) dos eritrócitos, calculado da seguinte maneira: valor do hematócrito expresso em percentagem do normal ÷ contagem dos eritrócitos expressa em percentagem do normal = i. de volume
zygomaticoauricular i., i. zigomático auricular; relação entre os diâmetros zigomático e auricular do crânio ou da cabeça.

---

in·di·can (in′di-kan). Indicana. **1.** Indoxil β-D-glicosídeo da espécie *Indigofera* e *Polygonium tinctorium;* fonte de índigo. SIN plant i. **2.** Ácido 3-indoxilsulfúrico; uma substância encontrada (na forma de seus sais) no suor e em quantidades variáveis na urina; quando presente em quantidade significativa, indica putrefação proteica no intestino (indicanúria). SIN metabolic i., uroxanthin.
metabolic i., i. metabólica. SIN indican (2).
plant i., i. vegetal. SIN indican (1).
in·di·can·i·dro·sis (in′di-kan-i-drō′sis). Indicanidrose; excreção de indicana no suor. [indican + G. *hidrōs,* suor]
in·di·cant (in′di-kant). Indicador. **1.** Que assinala; indica. **2.** Indicação; especialmente um sintoma indicando a linha adequada de tratamento. [L. *in-dico,* pres. P. *-ans* (*-ant*), apontar]
in·di·can·u·ria (in′di-kan-ū′rē-ă). Indicanúria; excreção urinária aumentada de indicana, um derivado do indol formado principalmente no intestino quando ocorre putrefação das proteínas; o indol também é formado durante a putrefação de proteínas em outros locais.
in·di·ca·tion (in-di-kā′shŭn). Indicação; a base para início do tratamento de uma doença ou de teste diagnóstico; pode ser fornecida por um conhecimento da causa (**i. causal**), pelos sintomas presentes (**i. sintomática**) ou pela natureza da doença (**i. específica**). [L. de *in-dico,* p. *-atus,* apontar, de *dico,* proclamar]
off label i., uso de medicação para uma finalidade diferente daquela aprovada pela FDA.
in·di·ca·tor (in′di-kā-ter, -tōr). Indicador. **1.** Em análise química, uma substância que muda de cor dentro de certa faixa definida de pH ou potencial de oxidação ou que, de alguma forma, torna visível o término de uma reação química; p. ex., litmo, fenolsulfaftaleína. **2.** Isótopo utilizado como traçador. **3.** Sustância marcada cuja distribuição entre reagentes de um sistema é utilizada para determinar a quantidade de analisado presente. [L. aquele que indica]
alizarin i., i. alizarina; solução consistindo em 1 g de sulfonato sódico de alizarina dissolvido em 100 ml de água destilada; utilizada como indicador para acidez livre no conteúdo gástrico.
clinical i., i. clínico; medida, processo ou resultado utilizado para avaliar uma determinada situação clínica e indicar se o tratamento administrado foi apropriado.
health i., i. de saúde; variável, passível de medida direta, que reflete o estado de saúde das pessoas numa comunidade.
oxidation-reduction i., i. de oxirredução; substância que sofre uma mudança de coloração definida num potencial de oxidação específico. SIN redox i.
redox i., i. redox. SIN oxidation-reduction i.
in·di·ces (in′di-sēz). Índices. Plural alternativo de *index.*
In·di·el·la (in-dē-el′ă). Denominação antiga de *Madurella.*
in·dig·e·nous (in-dij′e-nŭs). Indígena; nativo; nascido no país ou na região onde foi encontrado. [L. *indigenus,* nascido de *indu,* dentro (antiga forma de *in*), + G. *-gen,* produzindo]
in·di·ges·tion (in-di-jes′chŭn). Indigestão; termo inespecífico para referir-se a vários sintomas resultantes de uma deficiência de digestão e absorção adequadas do alimento no trato alimentar.
acid i., i. ácida; indigestão resultante de hipercloridria; termo freqüentemente utilizado por leigos como sinônimo de pirose.
fat i., i. de gordura. SIN steatorrhea.
gastric i., i. gástrica. SIN dyspepsia.
nervous i., i. nervosa; indigestão causada por problemas ou estresse emocionais.
in·di·go (in′dī-gō) [C.I. 73000]. Índigo; corante azul obtido de *Indigofera tinctoria* e de outras espécies de *Indigofera* (família Leguminosae); também produzido sinteticamente. SIN indigo blue, indigotin. [L. *indicum,* do G. *indikon,* índigo, ntr. de *Indikos,* indu]
in·di·go blue. Índigo-azul. SIN indigo.
in·di·go car·mine [C.I. 73015]. Índigo-carmim, indigotindissulfonato de sódio; corante azul utilizado para medir a função renal e como corante especial para corpúsculos de Negri. SIN sodium indigotin disulfonate.
in·di·go·tin (in-dig′ō-tin, in-di-gō′tin). Indigotina. SIN indigo.
in·di·go·u·ria, in·di·gu·ria (in′dī-gō-ū′rē-ă, in-di-goo′rē-ă). Indigoúria, indigúria; excreção de índigo na urina.
in·dis·po·si·tion (in-dis-pō-zish′ŭn). Indisposição; doença geralmente branda; mal-estar. [L. *in* neg. + *dispositio,* arranjo, de *dis-pono,* pp. *-positus,* colocar de lado]
in·di·um (In) (in′dē-ŭm). Índio; elemento metálico, de número atômico 49, peso atômico 114,82. [*indigo,* em virtude de sua linha azul no espectro]
in·di·um-111 (^{111}**In**). Índio-111 (In^{111}). Radionuclídeo produzido no ciclotron com meia-vida de 2,8049 dias e com emissão de raios gama de 171,2 e 245,3 quiloeletronvolts. Numa forma cloreto, é utilizado como marcador da medula óssea e de localização de tumor; numa forma quelato, como marcador do líquido cefalorraquidiano. É também utilizado como agente marcador de eritrócitos e como marcador de anticorpos.
i. chloride, i. trichloride, cloreto de índio, tricloreto de índio, Cl$_3$In; utilizado em microscopia eletrônica para corar ácidos nucleicos em cortes teciduais finos.
in·di·um-113m (^{113m}**In**). Índio-113m (In^{113m}). Isômero radiativo do In^{113}; possui meia-vida de 1,658 hora, tem sido utilizado na cisternografia e como auxiliar diagnóstico na determinação do débito cardíaco.
in·di·vid·u·a·tion (in′di-vid-ū-ā′shŭn). Individuação. **1.** Desenvolvimento do indivíduo a partir do específico. **2.** Em psicologia jungiana. O processo pelo qual a personalidade do indivíduo diferencia-se, desenvolve-se e se expressa. **3.** Atividade regional num embrião em resposta a um organizador.
in·do·cy·a·nine green (in-dō-sī′ă-nēn). Verde de indocianina; corante tricarbocianina que se liga à albumina sérica; utilizado na determinação do volume sanguíneo e em provas de função hepática.
in·do·cy·bin (in-dō-sī′bin). Indocibina. SIN psilocybin.
in·dol·ac·e·tu·ria (in′dōl-as-ĕ-too′rē-ă). Indolacetúria; excreção de quantidade apreciável de ácido indolacético na urina; manifestação da doença de Hartnup, também observada em pacientes com tumores carcinoides.
in·dol·a·mine (in-dol′ă-mēn). Indolamina; termo genérico para um indol ou seu derivado contendo um grupamento amina primário, secundário ou terciário (p. ex., serotonina).
in·dole (in′dōl). Indol. **1.** 2,3-Benzopirrol; base de muitas substâncias biologicamente ativas (p. ex., serotonina, triptofano); formado na degradação do triptofano. SIN ketole. **2.** Qualquer um de muitos alcalóides contendo a estrutura indol (1).
in·do·lent (in′dō-lent). Indolente; inativo; preguiçoso; indolor ou quase, referindo-se a um processo mórbido. [L. *in-.* neg. + *doleo,* pr. p. *dolens* (*-ent-*), sentir dor]
in·dol·ic ac·ids (in-dōl′ik). Ácidos indólicos; metabólitos do L-triptofano formados no interior do corpo ou por microrganismos intestinais; os principais ácidos indólicos encontrados na urina são o ácido indolacético, a indolacetilglutamina, o ácido 5-hidroxindolacético e o ácido indoleláctico.
in·do·log·e·nous (in′dō-loj′ĕ-nŭs). Indológeno; que produz ou leva à produção de indol.
in·do·lu·ria (in-dō-loo′rē-ă). Indolúria; excreção de indol na urina; refere-se comumente aos ácidos indólicos e indoxil, visto que o indol propriamente dito raramente aparece na urina.
in·do·lyl (in′dō-lil). Indolil; radical do indol.
in·do·meth·a·cin (in-dō-meth′ă-sin). Indometacina; agente analgésico, antipirético e antiinflamatório não-esteróide utilizado para tratamento da artrite reumatóide, osteoartrite, espondilite anquilosante e gota. É também utilizada para induzir o fechamento do canal arterial persistente em lactentes.
in·do·phe·nol·ase (in-dō-fē′nol-ās). Indofenolase. SIN cytochrome *c* oxidase.
in·do·phe·nol ox·i·dase (in-dō-fē′nol). Indofenol oxidase. SIN cytochrome *c* oxidase.
in·dor·a·min (in-dor′ă-min). Indoramina; antagonista α$_1$-competitivo seletivo que tem sido utilizado no tratamento da hipertensão; atua também como antagonista nos receptores histamínicos H$_1$ e receptores 5-HT.
in·dox·yl (in-dok′sil). Indoxil; radical do 3-hidroxindol; produto da degradação bacteriana intestinal do ácido indolacético, excretado na urina como ácido

indoxyl 794 **infant**

indolacetúrico (conjugado com glicina) como sulfato (indicana urinária) ou como glicuronídeo (glicosiduronato); são excretadas quantidades aumentadas na fenilcetonúria.

in·dox·yl·u·ria (in-dok-sil-ū′rē-ă). Indoxilúria; excreção de indoxil, especialmente sulfato de indoxil, na urina; a indoxilúria pode estar associada a indicanúria, visto que a hidrólise da indicana resulta na formação de indoxil.

in·duce (in-doos′). Induzir; causar ou provocar. VER induction.

in·duc·er (in-doos′er). Indutor; molécula, geralmente um substrato de uma via enzimática específica, que se combina com um repressor ativo (produzido por um gene regulador) e o desativa; isso permite a um gene operador previamente reprimido ativar os genes estruturais por ele controlados, resultando em produção enzimática; mecanismo homeostático para regular a produção enzimática num sistema enzimático indutível.
  embryonal i., i. embrionário; qualquer composto que efetuará a diferenciação nos estágios iniciais do desenvolvimento.
  gratuitous i., i. gratuito; análogo de um indutor natural, capaz de induzir um operon, apesar de não servir de substrato para a enzima que está sendo induzida.

in·duc·tance (L) (in-dŭk′tans). Indutância; coeficiente de indução eletromagnética; a unidade de indutância é o henry. [ver induction]

in·duc·tion (in-dŭk′shŭn). Indução. **1.** Produção ou causa. **2.** Produção de uma corrente elétrica ou estado magnético num corpo pela eletricidade ou magnetismo em outro corpo próximo ao primeiro. **3.** O período a partir do início da anestesia até o estabelecimento de uma profundidade anestésica adequada para uma intervenção cirúrgica. **4.** Em embriologia, a influência exercida por um organizador ou evocador sobre a diferenciação de células adjacentes ou o desenvolvimento de uma estrutura embrionária. **5.** Modificação imposta sobre a progênie pela ação do ambiente sobre as células germinativas de um ou de ambos os genitores. **6.** Em microbiologia, mudança do pró-bacteriófago em fago vegetativo, que pode ocorrer espontaneamente ou após estimulação por certos agentes físicos e químicos. **7.** Em enzimologia, o processo de aumentar a quantidade ou a atividade de uma proteína. VER TAMBÉM inducer. **8.** Estágio no processo de hipnose. **9.** Análise causal; método de raciocínio no qual uma inferência é feita a partir de uma ou mais observações específicas para uma declaração mais geral. Cf. deduction. [L. *inductio,* levar para dentro]
  electromagnetic i., i. eletromagnética; ondas eletromagnéticas propagadas por indução num campo eletromagnético.
  lysogenic i., i. lisogênica; indução que ocorre quando o profago é transferido para uma bactéria não-lisogênica por conjugação ou transdução.
  spinal i., i. espinal; modo pelo qual um estímulo sensorial reduz o limiar de outro.

in·duc·tor (in-dŭk′ter, -tōr). Indutor. **1.** Que produz indução. **2.** Em embriologia, um evocador ou organizador.

in·duc·to·ri·um (in-dŭk-tō′rē-ŭm). Indutório; instrumento antigamente utilizado em experimentos fisiológicos para gerar pulsos de eletricidade induzida para estimular um nervo ou músculo.

in·duc·to·therm (in-dŭk′tō-therm). Indutotermo; aparelho utilizado na indutotermia.

in·duc·to·ther·my (in-dŭk′tō-ther-mē). Indutotermia; produção artificial de febre por meio de indução eletromagnética. [induction + G. *thermē,* calor]

in·du·lin (in′doo-lin) [C.I. 50400-50415]. Indulina; um corante quinona-imina azul relacionado com a nigrosina; algumas vezes utilizada como corante em histologia e bacteriologia.

in·du·lin·o·phil, in·du·lin·o·phile (in-doo-lin′ō-fil, -fīl). Indulinófilo; que tem a propriedade de captar facilmente um corante de indulina. [indulin + G. *philos,* amigo]

in·du·rat·ed (in′doo-rāt-ed). Indurado, endurecido; termo habitualmente utilizado para referir-se a tecidos moles cuja consistência se tornou extremamente firme, porém não tão dura quanto a do osso. [L. *in-duro, pp. -duratus,* endurecer, de *durus,* duro]

in·du·ra·tion (in-doo-rā′shŭn). Induração, endurecimento. **1.** Processo de se tornar extremamente firme ou duro ou que apresenta essas características físicas. **2.** Foco ou região de tecido endurecido. SIN sclerosis (1). [L. *induratio* (ver indurated)]
  brown i. of the lung, i. castanha do pulmão; condição caracterizada por pulmões de consistência firme e coloração castanha associada a macrófagos pigmentados com hemossiderina nos alvéolos, em conseqüência de congestão prolongada devido a cardiopatia. SIN pigment i. of the lung.
  cyanotic i., i. cianótica; endurecimento relacionado à congestão venosa crônica e persistente num órgão ou tecido, resultando freqüentemente em espessamento fibroso das paredes das veias e fibrose final do tecido adjacente; a consistência do tecido afetado torna-se mais firme do que o normal e tende a exibir uma coloração vermelho-azulada incomum.
  gray i., i. cinza; condição que ocorre nos pulmões durante e após processos pneumônicos, em que não ocorre resolução; verifica-se um aumento perceptível de tecido conjuntivo fibroso nas paredes dos alvéolos, bem como no seu interior (p. ex., organização fibrosa de exsudato); em contraste com a induração castanha, não há habitualmente nenhum grau proeminente de pigmentação, a não ser que ocorra também congestão passiva crônica.
  pigment i. of the lung, i. pigmentar do pulmão. SIN brown i. of the lung.
  plastic i., i. plástica; esclerose do corpo cavernoso do pênis.
  red i., i. vermelha; condição observada nos pulmões, caracterizada por grau avançado de congestão passiva aguda, pneumonite aguda ou processo patológico semelhante.

in·du·ra·tive (in′doo-rā-tiv). Indurado; relativo a, causado por ou caracterizado por, induração.

in·du·si·um, pl. **in·du·sia** (in-doo′zē-ŭm, -zē-ă). Indúsio. **1.** Camada ou revestimento membranoso. **2.** O âmnio. [L. roupa íntima feminina, de *induo,* colocar]
  i. gris′eum [TA], i. cinzento; camada delgada de substância cinzenta na superfície dorsal do corpo caloso, na qual estão mergulhadas as estrias longitudinais mediais e laterais. O indúsio cinzento é um componente rudimentar do hipocampo, caudalmente contínuo em torno do esplênio do corpo caloso com o giro fasciolar, uma fina convolução que, por sua vez, é contínua com o giro denteado do hipocampo; rostralmente, o i. cinzento curva-se ao redor do joelho e rostro do corpo caloso e estende-se ventralmente para o trígono olfatório como *tenia tecta* ou hipocampo rudimentar, oculto na profundidade do sulco parolfatório posterior, que marca a borda anterior do giro subcaloso ou septo pré-comissural. SIN supracallosal gyrus.

♻ **-ine.** -Ina, -ino, -ina. **1.** Sufixo utilizado para formar nomes de substâncias químicas (p. ex., *clorina*), incluindo bases orgânicas (*guanina*), aminoácidos (*glicina*), princípios botânicos (*cafeína*), produtos farmacêuticos (*meperidina*) e outros. **2.** Sufixo de adjetivo geral (p. ex., *eqüino, uterino*). **3.** Sufixo diminutivo (p. ex., *colerina*). [G. *-inos,* L. *-inus,* sufixos adj.]

in·e·bri·ant (in-ē′brē-ant). Inebriante. **1.** Que torna bêbado; que intoxica. **2.** Intoxicante, como álcool. [ver inebriety]

in·e·bri·a·tion (in-ē-brē-ā′shŭn). Inebriamento; intoxicação, especialmente por álcool. [ver inebriety]

in·e·bri·e·ty (in-ē-brī′e-tē). Embriaguez; indulgência habitual com bebidas alcoólicas em quantidades excessivas. [L. *in-* intensivo + *ebrietas,* embriaguez]

In·er·mi·cap·si·fer (in-er-mi-cap′si-fer). Gênero de tênia (ordem Cyclophyllidae) reconhecido pela primeira vez em seres humanos, em 1935; acredita-se que um artrópode esteja envolvido na transmissão (de roedores para seres humanos, seres humanos para seres humanos).
  I. madagascariensis, cestóide freqüentemente responsável por infestações humanas em Cuba, acometendo crianças de 1–3 anos de idade e causando sintomas intestinais vagos; suspeita-se de um vetor artrópode; a proglote, os ovos e as suas cápsulas assemelham-se aos de *Raillietina* spp.

in·ert (in-ert′). Inerte. **1.** De ação lenta; indolente; inativo. **2.** Desprovido de propriedades químicas ativas, como os gases inertes. **3.** Refere-se a uma droga ou agente que não possui ação farmacológica ou terapêutica. [L. *iners,* inábil, preguiço, de *in,* neg. + *ars,* arte]

in·er·tia (in-er′shē-ă, in-er′shah). Inércia. **1.** Tendência de um corpo físico a opor-se a qualquer força que tenda a movê-lo de uma posição de repouso ou a modificar seu movimento uniforme. **2.** Indica inatividade ou falta de força, falta de vigor físico ou mental ou lentidão de pensamento ou ação. [L. falta de habilidade, indolência]
  magnetic i., i. magnética. SIN hysteresis (2).
  psychic i., i. psíquica; termo psiquiátrico que indica resistência a qualquer mudança de idéias ou progresso; fixação de uma idéia.
  uterine i., i. uterina; ausência de contrações uterinas efetivas durante o trabalho de parto.
  primary uterine i., true uterine i., i. uterina primária, i. uterina verdadeira; inércia uterina que ocorre quando o útero deixa de se contrair com força suficiente para efetuar uma dilatação contínua ou apagamento do colo uterino ou descida ou rotação da cabeça do feto e quando o útero é facilmente indentável no acme da contração; **secondary uterine i.,** i. uterina secundária; inércia uterina que ocorre quando as contrações uterinas são inicialmente vigorosas, porém diminuem em seguida, cessando a evolução do trabalho de parto.

in ex·tre·mis (in eks-trē′mis). *In extremis;* no ponto de morte. [L. *extremus,* último]

in·fan·cy (in′fan-sē). Lactância; primeira infância; o período inicial de vida extra-uterina; aproximadamente o primeiro ano de vida.

in·fant. Lactente. Criança com menos de 1 ano de idade. [L. *infans,* não-falante]
  i. Hercules, termo aplicado para descrever crianças pequenas com desenvolvimento sexual e muscular precoce, devido a um distúrbio adrenocortical virilizante.
  liveborn i., nascido vivo; o produto de um nascimento; recém-nascido que apresenta sinais de vida; considera-se que existe vida após o nascimento quando se observa qualquer um dos seguintes sinais: 1) respiração; 2) batimentos cardíacos; 3) ocorrência de pulsação do cordão umbilical; ou 4) movimento definido dos músculos voluntários.

postmature i., recém-nascido pós-maduro; aquele nascido depois de mais de 42 semanas de gestação e correndo risco devido à função inadequada da placenta. Em geral, o recém-nascido apresenta pele enrugada e, algumas vezes, anormalidades mais graves.
postterm i., recém-nascido pós-termo; aquele com idade gestacional de 42 semanas completas ou mais (294 dias ou mais).
preterm i., prematuro ou pré-termo; aquele com idade gestacional de mais de 20 semanas e menos de 37 semanas completas (259 dias completos).
stillborn i., natimorto; aquele que atingiu 20 semanas de gestação e não exibe nenhum sinal de vida após o nascimento. Cf. liveborn i.
term i., recém-nascido a termo; aquele com idade gestacional entre 37 semanas completas (259 dias completos) e 42 semanas completas (294 dias completos).

in·fan·ti·cide (in - fan'ti - sīd). Infanticida. **1.** O homicídio de lactente. **2.** Aquele que assassina um lactente. [lactente + L. *caedo,* matar]
in·fan·tile (in'fǎn - tīl). **1.** Relativo a, ou característico de, lactentes ou do primeiro ano de vida. **2.** Infantil; refere-se a um comportamento característico da criança.
in·fan·ti·lism (in-fan'ti-lizm). Infantilismo. **1.** Estado caracterizado pelo desenvolvimento lento da mente e do corpo. SIN infantile dwarfism. **2.** Infantilidade, como, p. ex., caracterizada por acesso de fúria ou raiva de adolescente ou adulto. **3.** Subdesenvolvimento dos órgãos sexuais.
Brissaud i., i. de Brissaud. SIN infantile *hypothyroidism.*
dysthyroidal i., i. distireóideo. SIN infantile *hypothyroidism.*
hepatic i., i. hepático; desenvolvimento retardado em consequência de hepatopatia.
hypophysial i., i. hipofisário; deficiência do hormônio do crescimento, devido à insuficiência de hormônio de liberação do hormônio do crescimento (também conhecido como somatocrinina) hipotalâmico.
hypothyroid i., i. hipotireóideo. SIN infantile *hypothyroidism.*
idiopathic i., i. idiopático; nanismo geralmente associado a hipogonadismo; pode ser causado pela secreção deficiente de hormônios da hipófise anterior. SIN Lorain disease, proportionate i., universal i.
Lorain-Lévi i., i. de Lorain-Lévi. SIN pituitary *dwarfism.*
myxedematous i., i. mixedematoso. SIN infantile *hypothyroidism.*
pancreatic i., i. pancreático; infantilismo associado a deficiência ou ausência de secreção pancreática.
pituitary i., i. hipofisário. SIN pituitary *dwarfism.*
proportionate i., i. proporcional. SIN idiopathic i.
renal i., i. renal. SIN renal *rickets.*
sexual i., i. sexual; falta de desenvolvimento das características sexuais secundárias após a época normal da puberdade.
static i., i. estático; condição observada em crianças pequenas que se assemelha à paralisia espinal espástica; caracterizado por hipotonia dos músculos do tronco e hipertonia dos músculos dos membros.
tubal i., i. tubário; termo descritivo de uma trompa de Falópio semelhante a um saca-rolha, conforme observado durante a vida fetal.
universal i., i. universal. SIN idiopathic i.

in·farct (in'farkt). Infarto; área de necrose resultante de uma súbita insuficiência de suprimento sanguíneo arterial ou venoso. SIN infarction (2). [L. *in-farcio,* pp. *-fartus (-ctus,* uma forma incorreta), encher, obstruir]
anemic i., i. anêmico; infarto em que ocorre pouco ou nenhum sangramento para os espaços teciduais quando o suprimento sanguíneo é obstruído. SIN pale i., white i. (1).
bland i., infarto não-infectado.
bone i., i. ósseo; área de tecido ósseo que se tornou necrótica em consequência da perda de seu suprimento sanguíneo arterial.
Brewer i.'s, infartos de Brewer; áreas cuneiformes vermelho-escuras que se assemelham aos infartos observados em cortes de um rim na pielonefrite.
embolic i., i. embólico; infarto causado por êmbolo.
hemorrhagic i., i. hemorrágico; infarto de cor vermelha devido à infiltração de sangue dos vasos colaterais na área necrótica. SIN hemorrhagic gangrene (1), red i.
pale i., i. anêmico. SIN anemic i.
red i., i. hemorrágico SIN hemorrhagic i.
Roesler-Dressler i., i. de Roesler-Dressler; infarto do miocárdio em forma de halteres, afetando as porções anterior e posterior do ventrículo esquerdo e o lado esquerdo do septo interventricular.
septic i., i. séptico; área de necrose resultante de obstrução vascular por êmbolos compostos de aglomerados de bactérias ou material infectado.
thrombotic i., i. trombótico; infarto causado por trombo.
uric acid i., i. de ácido úrico; precipitados de ácido úrico distendendo os túbulos coletores renais no recém-nascido; como não há necrose, o uso do termo infarto é incorreto.
white i., (1) i. anêmico. SIN anemic; i; **(2)** i. branco; na placenta, fibrina intervilosa com necrose isquêmica das vilosidades.
Zahn i., i. de Zahn; pseudo-infarto do fígado, consistindo numa área de congestão com atrofia parenquimatosa, porém sem necrose; devido à obstrução de um ramo da veia porta.

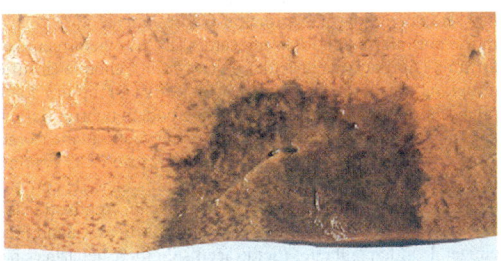

infarto de Zahn: corte de fígado

in·farc·tion (in - fark'shŭn). **1.** Infartação; insuficiência súbita de suprimento sanguíneo arterial ou venoso, devido a êmbolos, trombos, fatores mecânicos ou pressão que produz uma área macroscópica de necrose; qualquer órgão pode ser afetado. **2.** Infarto. SIN infarct.
anterior myocardial i., i. miocárdico anterior; infarto afetando a parede anterior do ventrículo esquerdo e produzindo alterações eletrocardiográficas indicativas nas derivações torácicas anteriores e, com freqüência, nas derivações dos membros, DI e aVL.
anteroinferior myocardial i., i. miocárdico ântero-inferior; infarto acometendo ambas as paredes anterior e inferior do coração simultaneamente.
anterolateral myocardial i., i. miocárdico ântero-lateral; infarto anterior extenso, produzindo alterações indicativas através do precórdio, freqüentemente também em DI e aVL.
anteroseptal myocardial i., i. miocárdico ântero-septal; infarto anterior cujas alterações eletrocardiográficas indicadoras limitam-se às derivações torácicas mediais ($V_1 - V_4$).
apical i., i. apical. SIN inferolateral myocardial i.
cardiac i., i. cardíaco. SIN myocardial i.
diaphragmatic myocardial i., i. miocárdico diafragmático. SIN inferior myocardial i.
Freiberg i., i. de Freiberg. SIN Freiberg *disease.*
inferior myocardial i., i. miocárdico inferior; infarto em que a parede inferior ou diafragmática do coração está afetada, produzindo alterações indicadoras em DII, DIII e aVF do eletrocardiograma. SIN diaphragmatic myocardial i.
inferolateral myocardial i., i. miocárdico ínfero-lateral; infarto que afeta as superfícies inferior e lateral do coração, produzindo alterações indicadoras no eletrocardiograma, nas derivações II, III, aVF, V_5 e V_6. SIN apical i.
lateral myocardial i., i. miocárdico lateral; infarto que afeta apenas a parede lateral do coração, produzindo alterações eletrocardiográficas indicadoras, limitadas a DI, aVL ou V_5 e V_6.

myocardial i. (MI), i. do miocárdio (IM); infarto de uma área do músculo cardíaco, habitualmente em decorrência da oclusão de uma artéria coronária. SIN cardiac i., heart attack.

O infarto do miocárdio constitui a causa mais comum de morte nos Estados Unidos. Cerca de 800.000 pessoas sofrem anualmente infartos do miocárdo pela primeira vez, com taxa de mortalidade de 30%, enquanto 450.000 sofrem infartos do miocárdio recorrentes, com taxa de mortalidade de 50%. A causa mais comum de IM consiste em trombose de uma artéria coronária aterosclerótica. As causas menos comuns incluem anomalias das artérias coronárias, vasculite ou espasmo induzido por cocaína, derivados do esporão do centeio ou outros agentes. Os fatores de risco do IM incluem: sexo masculino, história familiar de IM, obesidade, hipertensão, tabagismo e elevação dos níveis de colesterol total, LDL-colesterol, homocisteína, lipoproteína (a) ou proteína C-reativa. Pelo menos 80% dos casos de IM ocorrem em indivíduos com história pregressa de angina de peito, e 20% dos casos não são reconhecidos, uma vez que não provocam nenhum sintoma (infarto silencioso) ou porque os sintomas presentes são atribuídos a outras causas. Cerca de 20% dos indivíduos que sofrem IM morrem antes de chegarem ao hospital. O sintoma clássico do IM consiste em dor torácica anterior constritiva ou esmagadora, que se irradia para o pescoço, ombro ou braço, com mais de 30 minutos de duração e não aliviada pela nitroglicerina. Tipicamente, a dor é acompanhada de dispnéia, diaforese, fraqueza e náuseas. Os achados físicos significativos, que muitas vezes estão ausentes, incluem ritmo de galope atrial (quarta bulha cardíaca) e atrito pericárdico. O eletrocardiograma revela elevação do segmento ST (que, posteriormente, muda para depressão) e inversão da onda T em derivações que refletem a área de infarto. As ondas Q indicam lesão transmural e prognóstico mais sombrio. O diagnóstico é corroborado por uma elevação aguda nos níveis séricos de CK-MB (isoenzima de mioglobina da creatina cinase), desidrogenase láctica e troponinas. As evidências inequívocas de IM podem não ser encontradas nas primeiras 6 horas em até 50% dos pacientes. A morte por infarto agudo do miocárdio (IAM) é geralmente causada por arritmia (fibrilação ventricular ou assistolia), choque (insuficiência anterógrada), insuficiência cardíaca congestiva ou ruptura do músculo papilar. Outras complicações graves, que podem ocorrer durante a convalescença, incluem cardiorrexia, aneurisma ventricular e trombomural. O IAM é tratado (idealmente com monitorização ECG contínua em uma unidade de tratamento intensivo ou em uma unidade coronariana) com analgésicos narcóticos, oxigênio por inalação, administração intravenosa de agente trombolítico, agentes antiarrítmicos, quando indicados, e, em geral, anticoagulantes (ácido acetilsalicílico, heparina), beta-bloqueadores e inibidores da ECA. Os pacientes com sinais de isquemia persistente devem ser submetidos a angiografia e podem ser candidatos a angioplastia com balão. Os dados do *Framingham Heart Study* mostram que uma maior percentagem de IAM é silenciosa ou não reconhecida em mulheres e idosos. Diversos estudos constataram que as mulheres e os idosos tendem a aguardar mais tempo antes de procurar assistência médica, após o aparecimento de sintomas coronarianos agudos, do que os homens e indivíduos mais jovens. Além disso, as mulheres que procuram tratamento de emergência para sintomas sugestivos de coronariopatia aguda têm menos probabilidade de serem admitidas para avaliação do que homens que apresentam sintomas semelhantes, e as mulheres são encaminhadas menos freqüentemente do que os homens para exames diagnósticos, como cineangiocoronariografia. Outros estudos revelaram importantes diferenças nos sintomas iniciais e no reconhecimento clínico do IM em ambos os sexos. A dor torácica constitui o sintoma mais comum relatado por ambos os sexos, porém os homens tendem mais a se queixar de diaforese, enquanto as mulheres têm mais probabilidade de apresentar dor no pescoço, na mandíbula ou nas costas, náuseas, vômitos, dispnéia ou insuficiência cardíaca, além da dor torácica. As taxas de incidência de edema pulmonar agudo e choque cardiogênico no IM são maiores em mulheres, e as taxas de mortalidade em 28 dias e 6 meses também são maiores.

through-and-through myocardial i., i. miocárdico transmural. SIN transmural myocardial i.
transmural myocardial i., i. miocárdico transmural; infarto que afeta toda a espessura do músculo cardíaco, desde o endocárdio até o epicárdio. SIN through-and-through myocardial i.
watershed i., i. divisório; infarto numa área em que a distribuição das principais artérias cerebrais se encontram ou se superpõem.

in·fect (in-fekt′). Infectar. 1. Penetração, invasão ou estabelecimento de um microrganismo em outro organismo, produzindo infecção ou contaminação. 2. Instalar-se internamente, de forma endoparasítica, em oposição a externamente (infestação). [L. *in-ficio*, pp. *-fectus*, mergulhar, corromper, infectar, de *in + facio*, fazer]

in·fec·tion (in-fek′shŭn). Infecção; invasão do corpo por organismos que têm o potencial de causar doença.
agonal i., i. agônica. SIN terminal i.

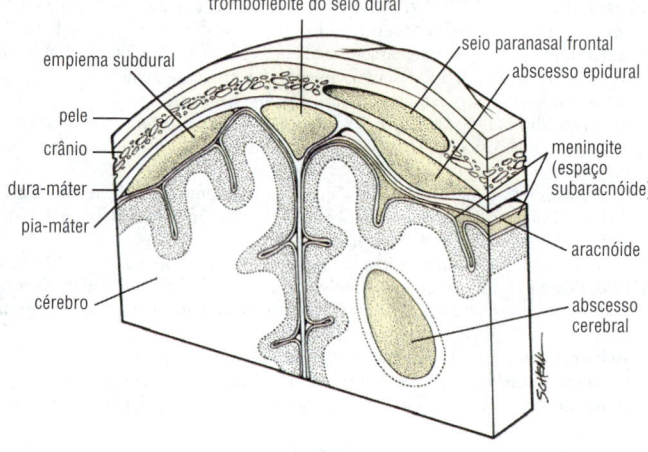

infecções intracranianas secundárias a sinusite

airborne i., i. transportada pelo ar; mecanismo de transmissão de um agente infeccioso por partículas, poeira ou perdigotos suspensos no ar.
apical i., i. apical; implantação de microrganismos no ápice de um dente, geralmente em consequência da migração de microrganismos do canal da polpa através do forame apical.
cross i., i. cruzada; infecção disseminada de uma fonte para outra, interpessoal, de um animal para uma pessoa, de uma pessoa para um animal, de um animal para outro animal.
cryptogenic i., i. criptogênica; infecção bacteriana, viral ou por outro agente, cuja fonte é desconhecida.
disseminated gonococcal i., i. gonocócica disseminada; infecção causada por *Neisseria gonorrheae*, que se dissemina para partes distantes do corpo além da porta original de entrada (habitualmente, o trato genital inferior). Em geral, manifesta-se por erupção cutânea e artrite.
droplet i., i. por perdigotos; infecção adquirida através da inalação de gotículas ou aerossóis de saliva ou de escarro contendo vírus ou outros microrganismos expelidos por outra pessoa durante espirros, tosse, riso ou conversa.
endogenous i., i. endógena; infecção causada por um agente infeccioso já presente no corpo, cuja infecção prévia foi inaparente.
focal i., i. focal; termo antigo que diferencia as infecções locais (focais) das infecções generalizadas (sépsis).
inapparent i., i. inaparente; infecção num hospedeiro sem a ocorrência de sinais ou sintomas reconhecíveis.
latent i., i. latente; infecção assintomática capaz de manifestar sintomas em circunstâncias particulares ou quando ativada.
mass i., i. maciça; infecção resultante da entrada de grande número de patógenos na circulação ou nos tecidos.
mixed i., i. mista; infecção por mais de um tipo de microrganismos patogênicos.
pyogenic i., i. piogênica; infecção caracterizada por intensa inflamação local, habitualmente com formação de pus, causada, em geral, por uma das bactérias piogênicas.
Salinem i., i. de Salinem. SIN Salinem *fever*.
scalp i., i. do couro cabeludo; infecção externa à gálea; p. ex., foliculite ou celulite.
secondary i., i. secundária; infecção, habitualmente séptica, que ocorre numa pessoa ou animal que está sofrendo de infecção de outra natureza.

infarto do miocárdio

nontransmural myocardial i. (NTMI), i. miocárdico não-transmural; necrose do músculo cardíaco que não se estende completamente do endocárdio para o epicárdio, muitas vezes considerado de modo errôneo como relativamente benigno.
posterior myocardial i., i. miocárdico posterior; infarto que acomete a parede posterior do coração; termo também utilizado de maneira errônea para infartos afetando a superfície inferior ou diafragmática do coração.
silent myocardial i., i. miocárdico silencioso; aquele que não provoca nenhum dos sintomas e sinais característicos de infarto do miocárdio.
subendocardial myocardial i., i. miocárdico subendocárdico; infarto que afeta apenas a camada de músculo subjacente ao endocárdio.

terminal i., i. terminal; infecção aguda, comumente pneumônica ou séptica, que ocorre no final de qualquer doença e constitui freqüentemente a causa de morte. SIN agonal i.

urinary tract i. (UTI), i. do trato urinário (ITU); infecção microbiana, geralmente bacteriana, de qualquer parte do trato urinário; pode acometer o parênquima do rim, a pelve renal, o ureter, a bexiga, a uretra ou combinações desses órgãos; com freqüência, ocorre comprometimento de todo o trato urinário; o microrganismo mais comum responsável por essa infecção é *Escherichia coli.*

vector-borne i., i. transmitida por vetores; classe de infecções transmitidas por inseto ou animal vetor. O vetor pode simplesmente ser um transportador passivo do agente infeccioso, porém muitos tipos de agentes infecciosos passam por um estágio de desenvolvimento biológico no vetor, isto é, tanto o vetor quanto o hospedeiro humano são essenciais à sobrevida do agente infeccioso.

Vincent i., i. de Vincent. SIN necrotizing ulcerative *gingivitis.*

zoonotic i., i. zoonótica; infecção compartilhada na natureza pelos seres humanos e outras espécies de animais.

in·fec·tion-im·mu·ni·ty. Imunidade por infecção. VER infection *immunity.*

in·fec·ti·os·i·ty (in-fek-shē-os′i-tē). Infecciosidade. SIN infectiousness.

in·fec·tious (in-fek′shŭs). 1. Infecciosa; doença capaz de ser transmitida de pessoa para pessoa, com ou sem contato real. 2. Infectante. SIN infective. 3. Infecciosa; refere-se a uma doença causada pela ação de um microrganismo.

in·fec·tious·ness (in-fek′shŭs-nes). Infecciosidade; estado ou qualidade de ser infeccioso. SIN infectiosity.

in·fec·tive (in-fek′tiv). Infectante; capaz de transmitir uma infecção. SIN infectious (2).

in·fec·tiv·i·ty (in-fek-tiv′i-tē). Infectividade. 1. Característica de um agente patológico que possui a capacidade de penetrar, sobreviver e multiplicar-se num hospedeiro suscetível, causando doença. 2. Proporção de exposições em circunstâncias definidas que resultam em infecção.

in·fe·cun·di·ty (in-fē-kŭn′di-tē). Infecundidade. SIN female *sterility.* [L. *infecunditas,* esterilidade]

in·fer·ence (in′fer-ens). Inferência; processo lógico de passar de observações e axiomas para generalizações; em estatística, desenvolvimento de generalizações a partir de dados de amostras, geralmente com graus calculados de incerteza.

in·fe·ri·or (in-fē′rē-ōr). Inferior. 1. Situado abaixo ou dirigido para baixo. 2. [TA]. Em anatomia humana, situado mais próximo das plantas dos pés em relação a um ponto de referência específico; oposto a superior. 3. Menos útil ou de menor qualidade. SIN Lower. [L. inferior]

in·fe·ri·or·i·ty (in-fēr-ē-ōr′i-tē). Inferioridade; condição ou estado de ser ou sentir-se inadequado ou inferior, especialmente em relação a semelhantes ou a outras pessoas igualmente situadas.

in·fer·til·i·ty (in-fer-til′i-tē). Infertilidade; capacidade diminuída ou ausente de produzir uma prole; tanto no homem quanto na mulher, não é tão irreversível quanto a esterilidade. [L. *in-* neg. + *fertilis,* fértil]

in·fest (in-fest′). Infestar; ocupar um local e instalar-se de forma ectoparasitária no tecido superficial externo, em oposição a internamente (infectar). [L. *infesto,* pp. *-atus,* atacar]

in·fes·ta·tion. Infestação; desenvolvimento de um agente patogênico sobre o corpo (mais do que no seu interior), como, p. ex., piolhos do corpo. SIN ectoparasitism.

in·fib·u·la·tion (in-fib-oo-la′shun). Infibulação; fechamento do vestíbulo da vagina através de fusão dos lábios maiores do pudendo; tipicamente efetuada após excisão dos pequenos lábios e do clitóris e incisão dos grandes lábios para criar superfícies rugosas que podem ser cirurgicamente unidas por meio de grampos, de modo que possam crescer juntas; efetuada por motivos culturais, e não médicos. VER TAMBÉM female *circumcision.* [L. *infibulo,* pregar ou prender, unir cirurgicamente (Celsus), de *in-* + *fibula,* grampo, gancho]

in·fil·trate (in′-fil-trāt, in-fil′trāt). 1. Infiltrar; realizar ou sofrer infiltração. 2. Infiltrado. SIN Infiltration (2). 3. Infiltração celular (1) no pulmão, deduzida pelo aspecto de uma imagem hipotransparente localizada e maldefinida na radiografia de tórax; termo comumente utilizado para descrever uma sombra numa radiografia. [L. *in* + Mediev. L. *filtro,* pp. *-atus,* coar através de um feltro, de *filtrum,* feltro]

Assmann tuberculous i., i. tuberculoso de Assmann. SIN infraclavicular i.

infraclavicular i., i. infraclavicular; lesão incipiente de infecção tuberculosa. SIN Assmann tuberculous i.

in·fil·tra·tion (in′fil-tra′shŭn). Infiltração. 1. Ato de permear ou de penetrar numa substância, célula ou tecido; refere-se a gases, líquidos ou matéria em solução. 2. O gás, líquido ou matéria dissolvida que penetrou em qualquer substância, célula ou tecido. SIN infiltrate (2). 3. Injeção de solução em tecidos, como na anestesia por infiltração. 4. Extravasamento de soluções destinadas à injeção intravascular.

adipose i., i. adiposa; crescimento de células adiposas adultas normais em locais onde não estão habitualmente presentes.

calcareous i., i. calcárea. SIN calcification.

cellular i., i. celular; migração de células de suas fontes de origem ou extensão direta de células em conseqüência de crescimento e multiplicação incomuns, resultando em focos bem definidos, acúmulos irregulares ou células individuais difusamente distribuídas no tecido conjuntivo e nos interstícios de vários órgãos ou tecidos; termo utilizado especialmente para referir-se a alterações associadas a inflamações e a certos tipos de neoplasias malignas.

epituberculous i., i. epituberculosa; infiltração superposta a uma lesão tuberculosa.

fatty i., i. gordurosa; acúmulo anormal de gotículas de gordura no citoplasma das células, particularmente de gordura proveniente do exterior das células. VER TAMBÉM fatty *degeneration.*

gelatinous i., i. gelatinosa. SIN gray i.

gray i., i. cinzenta; termo algumas vezes empregado para referir-se ao exsudato cinzento ou cinzento-esbranquiçado semi-sólido de formação relativamente rápida (constituído principalmente por células necróticas e remanescentes de tecidos e macrófagos), resultante de infecção tuberculosa difusa, maciça e inusitadamente aguda nos pulmões. SIN gelatinous i.

lipomatous i., i. lipomatosa; tecido adiposo não-encapsulado formando uma massa semelhante a um lipoma, habitualmente no septo interatrial cardíaco, onde pode causar arritmia e morte súbita. SIN lipomatous hypertrophy.

paraneural i., i. paraneural. SIN perineural i.

perineural i., i. perineural; infiltração adjacente a, ou ao longo de, um nervo. SIN paraneural i.

in·fin·i·ty (in-fin′i-tē). Infinito. SIN infinite *distance.*

in·firm (in-ferm′). Enfermo; fraco ou débil devido à idade avançada ou doença. [L. *in-firmus,* de *in-* neg. + *firmus,* forte]

in·fir·ma·ry (in-fer′ma-rē). Clínica ou pequeno hospital, especialmente numa escola ou instituição. [L. *infirmarium;* ver infirm]

in·fir·mi·ty (in-fer′mi-tē). Enfermidade; fraqueza; condição anormal, mais ou menos incapacitante, da mente ou do corpo. [ver infirm]

in·flam·ma·ble (in-flam′a-bl). Inflamável. SIN flammable. [L. *in-,* intensivo + *flamma,* chama]

in·flam·ma·tion (in-flă-mā′shŭn). Inflamação; processo patológico fundamental que consiste num complexo dinâmico de reações citológicas e químicas, ocorrendo nos vasos sanguíneos e tecidos adjacentes afetados, em resposta a uma lesão ou estímulo anormal produzidos por um agente físico, químico ou biológico, incluindo: 1) as reações locais e alterações morfológicas resultantes; 2) a destruição ou remoção do material lesado; 3) as respostas que levam ao reparo e à cura. Os denominados "sinais cardinais" da inflamação são: *rubor,* vermelhidão; *calor,* calor; *tumor,* intumescimento; e *dolor,* dor; algumas vezes, acrescenta-se um quinto sinal, *functio laesa,* inibição ou perda da função. Todos os sinais podem ser observados em certas circunstâncias, porém nenhum deles está necessariamente sempre presente. [L. *inflammo,* pp. *-atus,* de *in,* in, + *flamma,* chama]

active i., i. ativa. SIN acute i.

acute i., i. aguda; qualquer inflamação que possui início bastante rápido, torna-se rapidamente intensa e, em geral, manifesta-se durante apenas alguns dias, mas que pode persistir por algumas semanas; caracterizada, histologicamente, por edema, hiperemia e infiltrados de leucócitos polimorfonucleares. SIN active i.

adhesive i., i. adesiva; inflamação em que a quantidade de fibrina no exsudato é suficiente para resultar em aderência leve ou moderada dos tecidos adjacentes, como na cicatrização por primeira intenção.

allergic i., i. alérgica. VER allergic *reaction.*

alterative i., i. alterativa; reação local à lesão, algumas vezes observada nas paredes de vasos sanguíneos e em células parenquimatosas de diversos órgãos em reação a certos agentes químicos, vírus e outros agentes intracelulares; a resposta caracteriza-se por alterações degenerativas no citoplasma e no núcleo, resultando freqüentemente em necrose; todavia, a exsudação (quando presente) só costuma ser observada na parede do vaso afetado ou nos interstícios, imediatamente adjacentes ao vaso acometido ou às células parenquimatosas. SIN degenerative.

atrophic i., i. atrófica; forma de inflamação crônica, ou de episódios repetidos de inflamação aguda, em que a proliferação contínua ou recorrente de fibroblastos leva à formação de tecido fibroso que, finalmente, se retrai, resultando em compressão e atrofia do tecido parenquimatoso. SIN fibroid i.

catarrhal i., i. catarral; termo obsoleto para referir-se a um processo inflamatório situado mais freqüentemente no trato respiratório, mas que pode ocorrer em qualquer membrana mucosa; caracteriza-se por hiperemia dos vasos da mucosa, edema do tecido intersticial, aumento das células epiteliais secretoras (que proliferam e formam glóbulos evidentes de muco) e camada irregular de material viscoso e mucinoso na superfície; à medida que progride a exsudação, ocorre migração de um número variável de neutrófilos para o tecido afetado, que são incluídos no exsudato, juntamente com fragmentos de células epiteliais degeneradas e necróticas; essa inflamação pode tornar-se freqüentemente mucopurulenta.

chronic i., i. crônica; inflamação que pode começar de forma relativamente rápida ou de maneira lenta, insidiosa e até mesmo despercebida, tendendo a persistir por várias semanas, meses ou anos, com término vago e indefinido; ocorre quando o agente lesivo (ou produtos resultantes de sua presença) persiste na lesão, e os tecidos do hospedeiro respondem de modo (ou em grau) insuficiente para superar por completo os efeitos contínuos do agente lesivo;

caracterizada, do ponto de vista histopatológico, por infiltrados de linfócitos, plasmócitos e histiócitos, fibrose e formação de granulomas.

chronic active i., i. ativa crônica; coexistência de inflamação crônica e inflamação aguda superposta.

degenerative i., i. degenerativa. SIN alterative i.

exudative i., i. exsudativa; inflamação em que a característica manifesta ou diferencial consiste em exsudato, que pode ser principalmente seroso, serofibrinoso, fibrinoso ou mucoso (p. ex., com presença de relativamente poucas células) ou que pode caracterizar-se por um número relativamente grande de neutrófilos, eosinófilos, linfócitos, monócitos ou plasmócitos, muitas vezes com um ou dois tipos predominantes; ocorre não apenas como processo patológico separado e distinto, mas também, freqüentemente, como parte de certas inflamações granulomatosas.

fibrinopurulent i., i. fibrinopurulenta; inflamação purulenta, cujo exsudato contém uma quantidade inusitadamente grande de fibrina; além disso, inflamação fibrinosa ou serofibrinosa, em que o acúmulo de grande número de leucócitos polimorfonucleares resulta em necrose liquefativa do tecido e na formação de pus, com quantidade relativamente grande de fibrina.

fibrinous i., i. fibrinosa; inflamação exsudativa caracterizada por uma quantidade desproporcionalmente grande de fibrina.

fibroid i., i. fibróide. SIN atrophic i.

granulomatous i., i. granulomatosa; forma de inflamação proliferativa. VER TAMBÉM granuloma.

hyperplastic i., i. hiperplásica. SIN proliferative i.

immune i., i. imune. VER allergic *reaction*.

intersticial i., i. intersticial; inflamação em que a reação inflamatória é observada principalmente no tecido conjuntivo fibroso de suporte ou no estroma de um órgão.

necrotic i., necrotizing i., i. necrótica, i. necrozante; em geral, reação inflamatória aguda em que a alteração histológica predominante consiste em necrose bastante rápida, que ocorre de forma difusa ou extensa em focos relativamente grandes por todo o tecido afetado, freqüentemente com apenas pouca ou nenhuma evidência de células no exsudato.

productive i., i. produtiva; termo vago habitualmente empregado para referir-se a inflamação proliferativa, com ou sem exsudato; termo também utilizado algumas vezes para indicar inflamação em que se forma um exsudato macroscopicamente visível.

proliferative i., i. proliferativa; reação inflamatória em que a característica diferencial consiste em aumento real no número de células teciduais, especialmente macrófagos reticuloendoteliais, em contraste com as células exsudadas dos vasos sanguíneos; além disso, vários tipos de exsudatos tendem a ser observados em granulomas e em outras formas de inflamação proliferativa; todavia, estas últimas podem ocorrer sem a formação de exsudato (como em certas infecções causadas por vírus). SIN hyperplastic i.

pseudomembranous i., i. pseudomembranosa; forma de inflamação exsudativa que acomete as membranas mucosas e serosas; a presença de quantidades relativamente grandes de fibrina no exsudato resulta em um revestimento semelhante a uma membrana, bastante tenaz, que adere bastante ao tecido subjacente agudamente inflamado; em geral, a pseudomembrana contém (além da densa rede de fibrina) quantidades variáveis de proteínas plasmáticas, elementos degenerados e necróticos do tecido acometido, leucócitos polimorfonucleares, bactérias etc.

purulent i., i. purulenta; inflamação exsudativa aguda em que o acúmulo de leucócitos polimorfonucleares é suficientemente grande para que suas enzimas produzam liquefação dos tecidos afetados, seja de modo focal ou difuso; o exsudato purulento é freqüentemente denominado pus e consiste em plasma e seus constituintes, produtos finais da digestão enzimática do tecido, células degeneradas e necróticas e seus detritos, leucócitos polimorfonucleares e outros leucócitos, o agente causal da inflamação, etc. SIN suppurative i.

sclerosing i., i. esclerosante; inflamação que leva à formação extensa de tecido fibroso e cicatricial.

serofibrinous i., i. serofibrinosa; inflamação cujo exsudato consiste principalmente em líquido seroso, com proporção inusitadamente grande de fibrina.

serous i., i. serosa; inflamação exsudativa em que o exsudato é predominantemente líquido (p. ex., exsudato de vasos sanguíneos), contendo proteína, eletrólitos e outros materiais; observa-se um número relativamente pequeno (ou ausente) de células.

subacute i., i. subaguda; inflamação de duração intermediária entre a inflamação aguda e a inflamação crônica, que persiste geralmente por mais de 3 ou 4 semanas.

suppurative i., i. supurativa. SIN purulent i.

in·flam·ma·to·ry (in - flam′ă - tōr - ē). Inflamatório; relativo a, caracterizado por, que causa, resulta de ou torna-se afetado por inflamação.

in·fla·tion (in - flā′shŭn). Inflação, insuflação; distensão por líquido ou gás. [L. *inflatio*, de *in-flo*, pp. *-flatus*, soprar para dentro, inflar]

in·fla·tor (in - flā′ter, - tōr). Inflator; instrumento para injetar ar.

in·flec·tion, in·flex·ion (in - flek′shŭn). Inflexão. **1.** Flexão para dentro. **2.** Termo obsoleto para difração. [L. *in-flecto*, pp. *-flexus*, dobrar]

in·flu·en·za (in - floo - en′ză). *Influenza*, gripe; doença respiratória infecciosa aguda, causada por vírus da influenza pertencentes à família Orthomyxoviridae, que, quando inalados, atacam as células epiteliais respiratórias de pessoas suscetíveis, produzindo inflamação catarral; caracteriza-se por início súbito, calafrios, febre de curta duração (3–4 dias), prostração intensa, cefaléia, dores musculares e tosse, habitualmente seca e podendo ser seguida de infecção bacteriana secundária que pode persistir por 10 dias. A doença ocorre comumente em epidemias, algumas vezes em pandemias, que se desenvolvem e disseminam rapidamente; em geral, a taxa de mortalidade é baixa, mas pode ser alta nos casos com pneumonia bacteriana secundária, particularmente no idoso e naqueles com doenças debilitantes subjacentes; o indivíduo desenvolve imunidade cepa-específica, porém as mutações no vírus são freqüentes, e a imunidade geralmente não afeta as cepas antigenicamente diferentes. SIN flu, grip (1), grippe. [It. influência (de planetas ou estrelas), do L. *influentia*, do *in-fluo*, fluir]

i. A, i. A; tipo mais comum de *influenza*. Essas cepas têm alta propensão a mudança antigênica em conseqüência de mutações, em parte porque podem infectar diversos animais onde podem ocorrer infecções duplas, dando origem a novas cepas híbridas. As infecções ocorrem em epidemias, que podem surgir a cada 2–3 anos, variando conforme sua extensão e gravidade; talvez o mais importante dos três tipos de *influenza* (A, B e C).

Asian i., i. asiática; *influenza* mundial que teve aparentemente a sua origem na China, no verão de 1957; provoca uma doença mais branda do que a da pandemia de 1917–1919.

i. B, i. B; *influenza* causada por cepas do vírus influenza do tipo B; em geral, os surtos são mais limitados do que os do vírus influenza do tipo A, embora as infecções pelos dois tipos sejam clinicamente indistinguíveis; em certas ocasiões, associada à síndrome de Reye.

i. C, i. C; *influenza* causada por cepas do vírus influenza do tipo C; a doença é mais branda do que a causada pelos tipos A e B e, nestes últimos anos, tornou-se incomum.

endemic i., i. endêmica; em geral, trata-se de um tipo menos grave, que ocorre com algum grau de regularidade durante o inverno, especialmente nas maiores cidades do mundo. SIN i. nostras.

Hong Kong i., i. de Hong Kong; *influenza* causada por um sorotipo do vírus influenza tipo A, identificado pela primeira vez em Hong-Kong, em 1968.

i. nos'tras, i. endêmica. SIN endemic i.

Russian i., i. russa; pandemia de uma cepa do vírus influenza A que se acredita tenha se originado na Rússia; ocorreu em 1978.

Spanish i., i. espanhola; *influenza* que causou várias ondas de pandemia em 1918–1919, resultando em mais de 20 milhões de mortes em todo o mundo; foi particularmente grave na Espanha (daí o seu nome), mas, atualmente, acredita-se que tenha se originado nos Estados Unidos, como uma forma de *influenza* suína.

swine i., i. suína; doença respiratória aguda de suínos, causada por cepas do vírus influenza do tipo A; acredita-se que se adaptou a suínos nos Estados Unidos durante a grande pandemia humana, em 1918; casos fatais, como os da *influenza* pandêmica no homem, estão comumente associados a pneumonia bacteriana secundária.

in·flu·en·zal (in - floo - en′zăl). Gripal; relativo a, caracterizado por ou resultante de gripe ou *influenza*.

In·flu·en·za vi·rus (in - floo - en′ză - vī - rŭs). Vírus influenza; a família Orthomyxoviridae contém 3 gêneros: vírus influenza A, B; vírus influenza C e "vírus Thogoto-símiles". Cada tipo de vírus tem um antígeno de grupo de nucleoproteínas estável, comum a todas as cepas do tipo, porém distinto do antígeno de outro tipo; o genoma consiste em RNA monofilamentar, de sentido negativo, em 6–8 segmentos; cada um também possui um mosaico de antígenos de superfície (hemaglutinina e neuraminidase), que caracterizam as cepas e que estão sujeitos a variações de dois tipos: 1) um desvio algo contínuo, que ocorre independentemente nos antígenos hemaglutinina e neuraminidase; 2) depois de um período de anos, um súbito desvio (notavelmente no vírus do tipo A de origem humana) para um antígeno hemaglutinina e neuraminidase diferente. Os desvios principais súbitos constituem a base das subdivisões do vírus tipo A de origem humana, que ocorrem após a infecção do hospedeiro animal por duas cepas diferentes ao mesmo tempo, resultando em vírus híbrido. As notações da cepa indicam o tipo, a origem geográfica, o ano de isolamento e, no caso das cepas do tipo A, os subtipos que caracterizam os antígenos hemaglutinina e neuraminidase (p. ex., A/Hong Kong/1/68 (H_3N_2); B/Hong Kong/5/72).

in·fold (in - fōld′). Envolver; incluir dentro de uma dobra, como se faz ao "envolver" uma úlcera do estômago, em que as paredes de ambos os lados da lesão são unidas e suturadas.

informatics (in-for-mat′iks). Informática. **1.** Estudo da informação e meios de processá-la, especialmente através da tecnologia da informação, isto é, computadores e outros aparelhos eletrônicos para rápida transferência, processamento e análise de grandes quantidades de dados. **2.** A ciência do arranjo e da organização do produto de estudos genômicos e genômicos funcionais, visando obter informações úteis. VER TAMBÉM bioinformatics. [*informa*tion + *-ics*]

in·formed con·sent. Formulário de consentimento. Consentimento voluntário fornecido por uma pessoa ou responsável legal (p. ex., um dos pais) para participação em um estudo, programa de imunização, esquema de tratamento, procedimento invasivo, etc., após ter sido informado do propósito, dos métodos, procedimentos, benefícios e riscos. Os critérios essenciais do formulário de consentimento são que o indivíduo tenha conhecimento e compreensão, que o consentimento seja voluntariamente fornecido, sem nenhuma forma de coerção ou influência indevida, e que o direito de abandono a qualquer momento seja claramente comunicado ao indivíduo. Outros aspectos do formulário de consentimento no contexto das pesquisas epidemiológicas e biomédicas e os critérios a serem preenchidos na sua obtenção são especificados nos *International Guidelines for Ethical Review of Epidemiologic Studies* (Geneva: CIOMS/WHO 1991) e *International Ethical Guidelines for Biomedical Research Involving Human Subjects* (Geneva: CIOMS/WHO 1993).

in·for·mo·fers (in-fōr′mō-fers). Informoferos; nome sugerido para as partículas proteicas que aparecem quando o RNA é removido de partículas de nucleoproteína. [*inform*ation + -fer]

in·for·mo·somes (in-fōr′mō-sōmz). Informossomas; nome sugerido para os corpúsculos constituídos de RNA mensageiro (informativo) e proteína, que são encontrados no citoplasma de células animais. [*inform*ation + G. *sōma*, corpo]

infra-. Infra-. Posição abaixo da parte descrita pela palavra à qual se junta. [L. *abaixo*]

in·fra·ax·il·lary (in′frā-ak′si-lār-ē). Infra-axilar. SIN subaxillary.

in·fra·bulge (in′frā-būlj). Infraprotrusão. **1.** Porção da coroa de um dente gengival em relação à altura do contorno. **2.** Área de um dente onde a parte de retenção de um gancho de uma dentadura parcial removível é colocada.

in·fra·car·di·ac (in′frā-kar′dē-ak). Infracardíaco; abaixo do coração; abaixo do nível do coração.

in·fra·ce·re·bral (in′frā-ser′e-brăl). Infracerebral; relativo à porção do sistema nervoso abaixo do nível do cérebro.

in·fra·cla·vic·u·lar (in′frā-klā-vik′ū-lăr). Infraclavicular. SIN subclavian (1).

in·fra·clu·sion (in-frā-kloo′zhŭn). Infra-oclusão; estado em que um dente não sofreu erupção no plano maxilomandibular de interdigitação. SIN infraocclusion, infraversion (3).

in·fra·cor·ti·cal (in-frā-kōr′ti-kăl). Infracortical; abaixo do córtex de um órgão, referindo-se principalmente ao cérebro ou ao rim. VER subcortical.

in·fra·cos·tal (in-frā-kos′tăl). Infracostal. SIN subcostal (1).

in·fra·cot·y·loid (in-frā-kot′i-loyd). Infracotilóide; abaixo do acetábulo ou cavidade cotilóide.

in·fra·cris·tal (in-frā-kris′tăl). Infracrista; abaixo da crista supraventricular do ventrículo direito; termo habitualmente utilizado para referir-se a um defeito no septo interventricular [infra- + L. *crista*, crista]

in·frac·tion (in-frak′shŭn). Termo obsoleto para fratura; especialmente sem luxação. [L. *infractio*, ruptura, de *infringere*, romper]

in·fra·den·ta·le (in′frā-den-tā′lē). Infradental; em craniometria, o ápice do septo entre os incisivos centrais mandibulares. SIN lower alveolar point.

in·fra·di·an (in-frā′dē-ăn). Relativo a variações ou ritmos biológicos que ocorrem em ciclos com menos de 24 horas. [infra- + L. *dies*, dia]

in·fra·di·a·phrag·mat·ic (in′frā-dī′ă-frag-mat′ik). Infradiafragmático. SIN subdiaphragmatic.

in·fra·duc·tion (in-frā-dŭk′shŭn). Infradução. SIN deorsumduction.

in·fra·gle·noid (in′frā-glē′noyd). Infraglenóide; abaixo da cavidade glenóide da escápula. SIN subglenoid.

in·fra·glot·tic (in-frā-glot′ik). Infraglótico; abaixo da glote. SIN subglottic.

in·fra·he·pa·tic (in-frā-he-pat′ik). Infra-hepático. SIN subhepatic.

in·fra·hy·oid (in′frā-hī′oyd). Infra-hióide; abaixo do osso hióide; refere-se particularmente a um grupo de músculos: o esterno-hióideo, esternotireóideo, tireo-hióideo e homo-hióideo. SIN subhyoid, subhyoidean.

in·fra·mam·il·lary (in-frā-mam′i-lār-ē). Inframamilar; relativo ao que se encontra situado abaixo do mamilo.

in·fra·mam·ma·ry (in-frā-mam′ă-rē). Inframamário; abaixo da glândula mamária. SIN submammary (2).

in·fra·man·dib·u·lar (in-frā-man-dib′ū-lăr). Inframandibular. SIN submandibular.

in·fra·mar·gin·al (in-frā-mar′ji-năl). Inframarginal; abaixo de qualquer margem ou borda.

in·fra·max·il·lary (in-frā-mak′si-lā-rē). Inframaxilar. SIN mandibular.

in·fra·na·tant (in′frā-nā′tănt). Infranadante. **1.** VER infranatant *fluid*. **2.** Estendendo-se abaixo de. [infra- + L. *natare*, nadar]

in·fra·oc·clu·sion (in′frā-ŏ-kloo′zhŭn). Infra-oclusão. SIN infraclusion.

in·fra·or·bit·al (in′frā-ōr′bi-tăl). Infra-orbitário; abaixo ou por baixo da órbita. SIN suborbital.

in·fra·pa·tel·lar (in-frā-pa-tel′ăr). Infrapatelar; inferiormente à patela; indica especialmente uma bolsa, coxim de gordura ou dobra sinovial. SIN subpatellar (2).

in·fra·psy·chic (in-frā-sī′kik). Infrapsíquico; indica idéias ou ações que se originam abaixo do nível da consciência.

in·fra·red (IR, ir) (in′frā-red). Infravermelho; parte do espectro eletromagnético com comprimento de onda entre 730 e 1.000 nm.

in·fra·scap·u·lar (in-frā-skap′ū-lăr). Infra-escapular; abaixo da escápula. SIN subscapular (2).

in·fra·son·ic (in′frā-son′ik). Infra-sônico; refere-se às freqüências situadas abaixo da faixa da audição humana. [infra- + L. *sonus*, som]

in·fra·spi·na·tus (in-frā-spī-nā′tŭs). Infra-espinal. VER infraspinatus (*muscle*).

in·fra·spi·nous (in-frā-spī′nŭs). Infra-espinal; abaixo da espinha ou processo espinhoso; especificamente, a fossa infra-espinal. SIN subspinous (1).

in·fra·splen·ic (in′frā-splen′ik, -sple′nik). Infra-esplênico; abaixo ou por baixo do baço.

in·fra·ster·nal (in-frā-ster′năl). Infra-esternal; abaixo do esterno. SIN substernal (2).

in·fra·sub·spe·cif·ic (in′frā-sŭb-spe-si′fik). Infra-subespecífico; indica uma categoria de organismos de situação inferior à subespécie.

in·fra·tem·po·ral (in-frā-tem′pō-răl). Infratemporal; abaixo da fossa temporal.

in·fra·tho·rac·ic (in′frā-thō-ras′ik). Infratorácico; abaixo ou na porção inferior do tórax.

in·fra·ton·sil·lar (in-frā-ton′si-lăr). Infratonsilar; abaixo das tonsilas palatina ou cerebelar.

in·fra·troch·le·ar (in′frā-trok′lē-ăr). Infratroclear; abaixo da tróclea ou polia do músculo oblíquo superior do olho.

in·fra·um·bil·i·cal (in′frā-ŭm-bil′i-kăl). Infra-umbilical; abaixo do umbigo. SIN subumbilical.

in·fra·ver·sion (in′frā-ver′shŭn). Infraversão. **1.** Giro (versão) para baixo. **2.** Em óptica fisiológica, rotação de ambos os olhos para baixo. **3.** SIN infraclusion.

in·fric·tion (in-frik′shŭn). Aplicação de linimentos ou pomadas combinada com fricção. [L. *in*, sobre + *frictio*, fricção]

in·fun·dib·u·la (in-fŭn-dib′ū-lă). Infundíbulos; plural de infundibulum.

in·fun·dib·u·lar (in-fŭn-dib′ū-lăr). Infundibular; relativo a um infundíbulo.

in·fun·dib·u·lec·to·my (in′fŭn-dib′ū-lek′tō-mē). Infundibulectomia; excisão do infundíbulo, especialmente do septo ventricular do miocárdio hipertrofiado, comprimindo o efluxo ventricular na tetralogia de Fallot. [infundibulum + G. *ektomē*, excisão]

in·fun·dib·u·li·form (in-fŭn-dib′ū-li-fōrm). Infundibuliforme. SIN choanoid. [L. *infundibulum*, funil + *forma*, forma]

in·fun·dib·u·lin (in-fŭn-dib′ū-lin). Infundibulina; solução a 20% de um extrato do lobo posterior da hipófise cerebral.

in·fun·dib·u·lo·ma (in-fŭn-dib′ū-lō-mă). Infunduloma; astrocitoma pilocítico que surge na neuro-hipófise. [infundibulum + G. *-oma*, tumor]

in·fun·dib·u·lo·ovar·i·an (in-fŭn-dib′ū-lō-ō-vā′rē-an). Infundibulovariano; relacionado à extremidade fimbriada de uma tuba uterina e ovário.

in·fun·dib·u·lo·pel·vic (in-fŭn-dib′ū-lō-pel′vik). Infundibulopélvico; relativo a qualquer uma das duas estruturas denominadas infundíbulo e pelve, como a porção expandida de um cálice e a pelve do rim ou a extremidade fimbriada da tuba uterina e a pelve.

in·fun·dib·u·lum, pl. **in·fun·dib·u·la** (in-fŭn-dib′ū-lŭm, -ū-lă). Infundíbulo. **1.** [TA]. Funil ou estrutura ou passagem em forma de funil. **2.** Infundíbulo da tuba uterina. SIN i. of uterine tube. **3.** A porção alargada de um cálice quando se abre na pelve renal. **4.** [TA]. Cone arterial SIN conus arteriosus. **5.** Terminação de um bronquíolo no alvéolo. **6.** Terminação do canal coclear abaixo da cúpula. **7.** [TA]. Proeminência ímpar, em forma de funil, da base do hipotálamo, atrás do quiasma óptico, encerrando o recesso infundibular do terceiro ventrículo e contínuo com o pedículo da hipófise. [L. um funil]
ethmoid i., i. etmóide. SIN ethmoidal i.
ethmoidal i. [TA], i. etmóide; passagem do meato médio do nariz, que se comunica com as células etmoidais anteriores e com o seio frontal. SIN i. ethmoidale [TA], ethmoid i.
i. ethmoida′le [TA], i. etmóide. SIN ethmoidal i.
i. of gallbladder [TA], i. da vesícula biliar; porção afunilada da vesícula biliar, oposta ao fundo, à medida que o corpo da vesícula se estreita até o colo (a partir do qual segue o ducto cístico). SIN i. vesicae biliaris [TA], i. vesicae felleae*.
i. hypophysis [TA], i. da hipófise. SIN i. of pituitary gland.
i. hypothal′ami [TA], i. da hipófise. SIN i. of pituitary gland.
hypothalamic i., i. da hipófise. SIN i. of pituitary gland.
i. of lungs, i. dos pulmões; no embrião, uma das extremidades expandidas das subdivisões dos brotos pulmonares; no desenvolvimento posterior, aparecem minúsculas bolsas (os sacos aéreos) em sua parede.
i. of pituitary gland [TA], i. da hipófise; porção apical do tuber cinéreo que se estende para dentro do pedículo hipofisário. SIN i. hypothalami [TA], hypothalamic i.
i. of right ventricle [TA], cone arterial do ventrículo direito. SIN conus arteriosus.

i. tu'bae uteri'nae [TA], i. da tuba uterina. SIN i. of uterine tube.
i. of uterine tube [TA], i. da tuba uterina; expansão afunilada da extremidade abdominal da tuba uterina (de Falópio). SIN i. tubae uterinae [TA], infundibulum (2).
i. vesicae biliaris [TA], i. da vesícula biliar. SIN i. of gallbladder.
i. vesicae felleae, i. da vesícula biliar; *termo oficial alternativo para i. of gallbladder.
in·fu·si·ble (in-foo′zi-bl). **1.** Infusível; incapaz de ser fundido ou derretido. **2.** Capaz de ser transformado em infusão.
in·fu·sion (in-fū′zhŭn). Infusão. **1.** Processo de macerar uma substância em água, seja fria ou quente (abaixo do ponto de ebulição), a fim de extrair seus princípios solúveis. **2.** Preparado medicinal obtido ao macerar a substância original em água. **3.** A introdução de líquido que não seja sangue, como, p. ex., soro fisiológico, numa veia. [L. *infusio*, de *in-fundo*, pp. *-fusus*, despejar]
In·fu·so·ria (in-foo-sō′rē-ă). Infusórios (ramo taxonômico); termo arcaico para os Ciliophora. [L. Mod., relativo a ou encontrado em infusão, de *in-fundo*, pp. *in-fusus*, despejar]
in·fu·so·ri·an (in-fū-sō′rē-an). Infusório; termo arcaico para referir-se a um membro da classe dos infusórios, atualmente o filo Ciliophora.
Ingelfinger, Franz, nefrologista e editor norte-americano, 1910–1980. VER I. *rule*.
in·ges·ta (in-jes′tă). Ingestão; nutrientes sólidos ou líquidos introduzidos no corpo. [pl. do L. *ingestum*, ntr. pp. of *in-gero, -gestus*, carregar]
in·ges·tion (in-jes′chŭn). Ingestão. **1.** Introdução de alimentos e líquidos no estômago. **2.** Incorporação de partículas no citoplasma de uma célula fagocítica através de invaginação de parte da membrana celular que serve de vacúolo. [L. *in-gero*, transportar]
in·ges·tive (in-jes′tiv). Ingestivo; relativo a ingestão.
Ingrassia, Giovanni F., anatomista italiano, 1510–1580. VER I. *process*.
in·gra·ves·cent (in-gră-ves′ent). Ingravescente; que aumenta de gravidade. [L. *in-gravesco*, tornar mais pesado, de *gravis*, pesado]
in·guen (ing′gwen) [TA]. Virilha. SIN groin (1). [L.]
in·gui·nal (ing′gwi-năl). Inguinal; relativo à virilha.
in·gui·no·cru·ral (ing′gwi-nō-krool′răl). Inguinocrural; relativo à virilha e à coxa.
in·gui·no·dyn·ia (ing′gwi-nō-din′ē-ă). Inguinodinia; termo raramente utilizado para referir-se à dor na virilha. [L. *inguen (inguin-)*, virilha + G. *odynē*, dor]
in·gui·no·la·bi·al (ing′gwi-nō-lā′bē-ăl). Inguinolabial; relativo à virilha e ao lábio maior do pudendo.
in·gui·no·per·i·to·ne·al (ing′gwi-nō-per′i-tō-nē′ăl). Inguinoperitoneal; relativo à virilha e ao peritônio.
in·gui·no·scro·tal (ing′gwi-nō-skrō′tăl). Inguinoscrotal; relativo à virilha e ao escroto.
INH INH. Abreviatura de isonicotinic acid hydrazide (hidrazida do ácido isonicotínico).
in·hal·ant (in-hā′lant). Inalante. **1.** Aquilo que é inalado; medicamento administrado por inalação. **2.** Droga (ou combinação de drogas) com alta pressão de vapor, transportada por uma corrente de ar nas vias nasais, onde produz seus efeitos. **3.** Grupo de produtos consistindo em drogas finamente pulverizadas ou na forma líquida, que são transportados nas vias respiratórias pelo uso de dispositivos especiais, como recipientes de aerossol de baixa pressão. SIN insufflation (2). VER TAMBÉM inhalation, aerosol. [ver inhalation]
in·ha·la·tion (in-hă-lā′shŭn). Inalação. **1.** Ato de inalar na respiração. SIN inspiration. **2.** Aspirar um vapor medicamentoso na respiração. **3.** Solução de uma droga ou combinação de drogas para administração na forma de névoa nebulizada para alcançar a árvore respiratória. [L. *in-halo*, pp. *-halatus*, respirar em]
solvent i., i. de solvente; inalação de solventes orgânicos voláteis utilizados na cola, removedor de esmalte de unhas, solventes de vernizes, líquido para limpeza, fluido de isqueiro e gasolina, com o propósito de auto-intoxicação. VER TAMBÉM glue-sniffing.
in·hale (in-hāl′). Inalar; aspirar na respiração. SIN inspire.
in·hal·er (in-hāl′er). Inalador. **1.** SIN respirator (2). **2.** Aparelho para a administração de agentes farmacologicamente ativos por inalação.
metered-dose i., i. com dosímetro; aparelho utilizado para administrar uma dose definida de medicamento por inalação; utilizado freqüentemente no tratamento da asma e outras condições respiratórias.
in·her·ent (in-her′ent). Inerente; que ocorre como parte natural ou conseqüência; iminente; latente; intrínseco. [L. *inhaerens*, aderindo a]
in·her·i·tance (in-her′i-tans). Herança. **1.** Características ou qualidades que são transmitidas de um genitor para sua descendência através de dados citológicos codificados; que é herdado. **2.** Herança cultural ou legal. **3.** Ato de herdar. [L. *heredito*, herdar, de *heres (hered-)*, herdeiro]
alternative i., h. alternativa. **(1)** SIN mendelian i; **(2)** termo galtoniano para uma forma pressuposta em que todos os caracteres derivam de um dos genitores.
blending i., i. combinada; termo galtoniano para uma herança em que nenhum componente é evidente ou imposto.
codominant i., h. co-dominante; herança em que dois alelos se expressam individualmente na presença do outro; pode haver outros alelos disponíveis no *locus*, que podem ou não exibir co-dominância.
collateral i., h. colateral; aparecimento de caracteres em membros colaterais de um grupo familiar, como, p. ex., quando um tio e uma sobrinha apresentam o mesmo caráter herdado de um ancestral comum; em caracteres recessivos, pode aparecer irregularmente, em contraste com caracteres dominantes, que são transmitidos diretamente de uma geração para a próxima.
cytoplasmic i., h. citoplasmática; transmissão de caracteres dependentes de elementos autoperpetuantes de origem não-nuclear (p. ex., DNA mitocondrial). SIN extranuclear i.
dominant i., h. dominante. VER *dominance* of traits.
extrachromosomal i., h. extracromossômica; transmissão de caracteres dependentes de algum fator não ligado aos cromossomas.
extranuclear i., h. extranuclear. SIN cytoplasmic i.

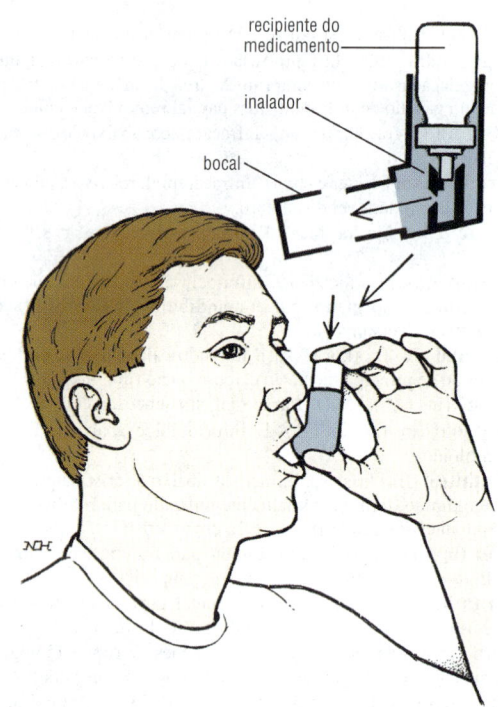

inalador com dosímetro

galtonian i., h. galtoniana; herança em que um fenótipo mensurável é produzido por muitos *loci*, cujas contribuições são estatisticamente independentes, aditivas e de valor quase igual. (Estas últimas estão de acordo com o limite central clássico e justificam o uso da distribuição normal multivariada na genética galtoniana). SIN polygenic i.
holandric i., h. holândrica. SIN Y-linked i.
hologynic i., h. hologínica; transmissão de um caráter da mãe para todas as filhas, mas para nenhum dos filhos, atribuída a cromossomas X fixados (parcialmente fundidos), a herança citoplasmática ou a limitação sexual com segregação anormal, como, p. ex., hematocolpia.
maternal i., h. materna; transmissão de caracteres que dependem das propriedades do citoplasma do ovo produzidas por genes nucleares e/ou mitocondriais.
mendelian i., h. mendeliana; herança em que caracteres estáveis e não-desintegráveis, controlados por completo ou maciçamente por um único *locus* genético, são transmitidos durante muitas gerações. VER Mendel first *law, law of segregation, law of independent assortment*. SIN alternative i. (1).
mosaic i., h. em mosaico; herança em que a influência materna é dominante em um grupo de células, e a materna, em outro. Cf. lyonization.
multifactorial i., h. multifatorial; herança envolvendo muitos fatores, dos quais pelo menos um é genético, porém nenhum de importância fundamental, como na produção de uma doença por múltiplos fatores genéticos e ambientais. Cf. galtonian i.
polygenic i., h. poligênica. SIN galtonian i.
recessive i., h. recessiva. VER *dominance* of traits.

sex-influenced i., h. influenciada pelo sexo; herança autossômica, mas que apresenta intensidade de expressão diferente nos dois sexos, como, p. ex., calvície de padrão masculino.
sex-limited i., h. limitada ao sexo; herança de um traço que só pode ser expresso em um sexo, como, p. ex., feminização testicular.
sex-linked i., h. ligada ao sexo; padrão de herança que pode resultar de um gene mutante localizado no cromossoma X ou Y.
X-linked i., h. ligada ao X; padrão de herança que pode resultar de um gene mutante localizado num cromossoma X.
Y-linked i., h. ligada ao Y; padrão de herança que pode resultar de um gene mutante localizado num cromossoma Y. SIN holandric i.
in·her·it·ed (in-her′it-ed). Hereditário; derivado de um código genético pré-formado existente nos genitores. Em contraste com adquirido.
in·hib·in (in-hib′in). Inibina; uma das várias proteínas que participam na diferenciação e crescimento. Duas glicoproteínas, a inibina A e a inibina B, são secretadas pelas células de Sertoli nos testículos e nas células granulosas do ovário, inibindo a secreção de FSH através de sua ação direta sobre a hipófise. [inibir + -in]
in·hib·it (in-hib′it). Inibir; reprimir ou restringir.
in·hib·i·tine (in - hib′i - tēn). Inibitina. SIN carnosine.
in·hi·bi·tion (in - hi - bish′ŭn). Inibição. **1.** Depressão ou parada de uma função. VER TAMBÉM inhibitor. **2.** Em psicanálise, a restrição de impulsos ou tendências instintuais ou inconscientes, especialmente se estiverem em conflito com a consciência do indivíduo ou com as exigências sociais. **3.** Em psicologia, termo genérico para referir-se a uma variedade de processos associados à atenuação gradual, mascaramento e extinção de uma resposta previamente condicionada. **4.** Redução na velocidade de uma reação ou processo. [L. *inhibeo*, pp. *-hibitus*, deter, reter, de *habeo*, ter]
allogeneic i., i. alogênica; inibição ou lesão de células alogênicas que ocorre quando linfócitos são misturados e cultivados com outras células de diferentes genótipos *in vitro*.
central i., i. central; supressão ou diminuição de impulsos provenientes de um centro reflexo.
competitive i., i. competitiva; bloqueio da ação de uma enzima por um composto que se liga à enzima livre, impedindo a ligação do substrato e, portanto, a ação da enzima sobre ele. O inibidor competitivo é freqüentemente um análogo do substrato, que se liga ao sítio ativo; entretanto, esse requisito não é absolutamente necessário para a inibição competitiva. A inibição pode ser removida por concentrações saturadas de substrato. Cf. isostery. SIN selective i.
contact i., i. de contato; interrupção da replicação das células em divisão que entram em contato, como no centro de uma ferida em cicatrização.
end product i., i. pelo produto final. SIN feedback i.
feedback i., i. por retroalimentação; inibição da atividade por um produto final da via da qual faz parte essa atividade; p. ex., a tireoliberina estimula a produção de tireoglobulina, e esta última diminui a formação de tireotropina. SIN end product i., retroinhibition.
hapten i. of precipitation, i. de precipitação por hapteno; inibição da precipitação que ocorre quando o anticorpo se combinou com o hapteno da mesma especificidade do antígeno subseqüentemente adicionado.
hemagglutination i., i. da hemaglutinação; inibição da hemaglutinação não-imune por anticorpo específico contra a hemaglutinina; p. ex., não ocorre hemaglutinação por vírus se anticorpo antiviral específico for adicionado antes da adição dos eritrócitos. A inibição é específica e amplamente utilizada na identificação de vírus e determinação dos anticorpos.
noncompetitive i., i. não-competitiva; tipo de inibição enzimática, em que o composto inibidor não compete com o substrato natural pelo sítio ativo da enzima, porém inibe a reação ao combinar-se com o complexo enzima–substrato ou com a enzima livre.
potassium i., i. por potássio; parada cardíaca no estado totalmente relaxado, em conseqüência de intoxicação por potássio.
proactive i., i. proativa; tipo de interferência ou transferência negativa, observado em experiências de memória e outras situações de aprendizagem, quando algo aprendido previamente interfere com o aprendizado atual ou com a recordação. Cf. retroactive i.

product i., i. pelo produto; inibição de uma atividade enzimática por um produto da reação catalisada por essa enzima.
reciprocal i., i. recíproca. **(1)** SIN reciprocal *innervation;* **(2)** SIN systematic *desensitization.*
reflex i., i. reflexa; situação em que os estímulos sensoriais diminuem a atividade reflexa.
residual i., i. residual; inibição ou supressão do zumbido pelo uso de um dispositivo gerador de som (inibidor residual) que mascara o zumbido e produz um efeito residual inibidor de som quando o aparelho é desligado.
retroactive i., i. retroativa; obliteração parcial ou completa da memória por um acontecimento mais recente, particularmente um novo aprendizado. Cf. proactive i.
selective i., i. seletiva. SIN competitive i.
substrate i., i. pelo substrato; inibição de uma atividade enzimática por um substrato da reação catalisada por essa enzima; com freqüência, esse tipo de inibição ocorre com concentrações elevadas de substrato, em que este se liga a um segundo sítio não-ativo da enzima.
uncompetitive i., i. não-competitiva; efeito inibitório sobre uma função metabólica, como uma enzima, que não se baseia na competição pelo sítio de ligação do substrato de ocorrência natural, porém num efeito diferente sobre a molécula cuja função está sendo inibida.
Wedensky i., i. de Wedensky; inibição da resposta muscular resultante da aplicação de uma série de estímulos rapidamente repetidos ao nervo motor, em que uma freqüência mais lenta de estimulação leva a uma resposta muscular.
in·hib·i·tor (in - hib′i - ter, -tōr). Inibidor. **1.** Agente que restringe ou retarda uma ação fisiológica, química ou enzimática. **2.** Nervo cujo estímulo reprime a atividade. VER TAMBÉM inhibition.

α-glucosidase i., i. da α-glicosidase; agente oral que ajuda a controlar o diabetes melito ao retardar a absorção de glicose do trato digestivo.

> Os inibidores da α-glicosidase, como a acarbose, bloqueiam a função de enzimas produzidas pelas células mucosas da porção proximal do intestino delgado, que normalmente decompõem os carboidratos complexos da dieta em açúcares simples, incluindo glicose. Em conseqüência, a elevação pós-prandial da glicemia ocorre de modo muito mais gradual. Quando administrada antes das refeições, a acarbose pode reduzir os níveis pós-prandiais máximos de glicose em até 75 mg/dL. Por conseguinte, permite a redução na dose dos agentes hipoglicemiantes orais ou da insulina. A droga não é absorvida na circulação e atua apenas topicamente sobre as células de revestimento intestinais. A acarbose em si não consegue induzir hipoglicemia; entretanto, ao reduzir a necessidade de insulina, pode aumentar o risco de hipoglicemia para uma determinada dose de sulfoniluréia ou insulina. Pode causar flatulência, distensão abdominal e diarréia quando os carboidratos complexos atingem o cólon em lugar de serem digeridos e absorvidos.

angiotensin-converting enzyme i.'s (ACEI), inibidores da enzima conversora de angiotensina (IECA); classe de drogas utilizadas no tratamento da hipertensão e da insuficiência cardíaca congestiva; produzem redução da resistência arterial periférica, embora o mecanismo exato de ação não esteja totalmente determinado; bloqueiam a conversão da angiotensina I em angiotensina II, um poderoso vasoconstritor.
aromatase i.'s, inibidores da aromatase; drogas como a aminoglutetimida, que inibem a aromatase, uma enzima utilizada na síntese de estrogênios.
Bowman-Birk i., i. de Bowman-Birk; polipeptídeo que inibe tanto a tripsina quanto a quimotripsina.
carbonate-dehydratase i., i. da carbonato desidratase; agente, em geral quimicamente relacionado com as sulfonamidas, que inibe a atividade da carbonato desidratase, produzindo diminuição geral na formação de H_2CO_3 nos tecidos. VER TAMBÉM acetazolamide, dichlorphenamide. SIN carbonic anhydrase i.
carbonic anhydrase i., i. da anidrase carbônica. SIN carbonate dehydratase i.

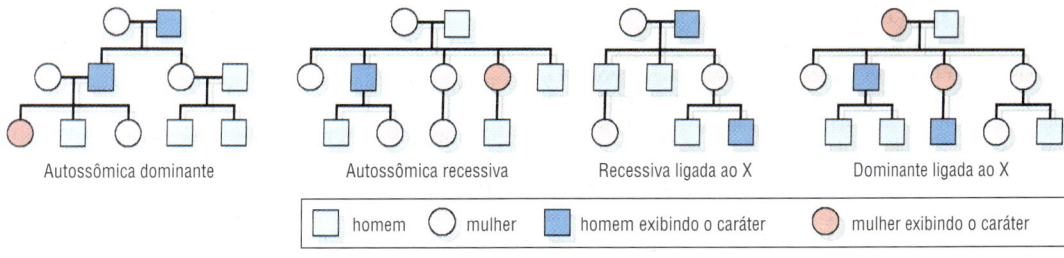

herança mendeliana: principais modos

C1 esterase i., i. da C1 esterase; α₂-neuraminoglicoproteína que inibe a atividade enzimática da C1 esterase, o primeiro componente ativado do complemento. A deficiência desse inibidor resulta em falta de inibição de C1r e C1s, resultando em ativação descontrolada da cascata do complemento e edema.

cholinesterase i., i. da colinesterase; droga, como a neostigmina, que, ao inibir a biodegradação da acetilcolina, restabelece a função mioneural na miastenia grave ou após a administração de relaxantes neuromusculares não-despolarizantes.

familial lipoprotein lipase i., i. da lipoproteína lipase familiar; inibidor, encontrado em certos indivíduos, que inibe a lipoproteína lipase, resultando em acúmulo de quilomícrons, VLDL e triacilgliceróis; os sintomas assemelham-se aos da deficiência familiar de lipoproteína lipase.

glucosidase i., inibidores da glicosidase; agentes, como a acarbose, que reduzem a absorção gastrointestinal de carboidratos. Esses fármacos, como grupo, são conhecidos popularmente como "bloqueadores de amido". Reduzem os níveis plasmáticos de glicose e tendem a causar perda de peso. Um efeito colateral limitante consiste na ocorrência de flatulência.

HMG CoA-reductase i.'s, inibidores da HMG CoA-redutase; drogas que interferem na biossíntese do colesterol; utilizados no tratamento da hiperlipidemia.

Os inibidores da HMG-CoA redutase, genericamente denominados estatinas, reduzem os níveis de colesterol total e LDH-colesterol em indivíduos com hiperlipidemia, retardam a progressão da aterosclerose e diminuem o risco de morbidade e mortalidade cardiovasculares. Na síntese de colesterol no fígado, a 3-hidroxi-3-metilglutaril coenzima A (HMG-CoA) é convertida em ácido mevalônico pela enzima HMG-CoA redutase. Normalmente, essa enzima é inibida pela ingestão significativa de colesterol, e, por outro lado, a redução do colesterol da dieta pode aumentar a atividade da HMG-CoA redutase. As drogas que bloqueiam a ação da HMG-CoA redutase são análogos estruturais da HMG-CoA e inibem competitivamente a enzima, impedindo a síntese de colesterol. A ocorrência de um declínio nos níveis intracelulares de colesterol promove um aumento na expressão de receptores de LDL na superfície celular e captação das LDL circulantes. Estudos controlados mostraram que, em indivíduos com história de angina de peito ou IAM, a lovastatina, a pravastatina e a sinvastatina reduzem significativamente a mortalidade cardiovascular, conferindo proteção contra a angina instável e reduzindo o risco de infarto do miocárdio fatal e não-fatal, o número e a duração das internações, a necessidade de procedimentos de revascularização e a incidência de ataques isquêmicos transitórios (AIT) e acidentes vasculares cerebrais (AVC). Estudos prospectivos sobre o uso desses agentes por indivíduos com níveis normais de colesterol mostraram uma redução significativa no risco de um evento coronariano importante em mulheres pós-menopáusicas e em pessoas de ambos os sexos com mais de 65 anos de idade. Em contraste, os estudos nos quais o colesterol foi reduzido apenas com dieta ou com o uso de outros fármacos (p. ex., colestiramina, genfibrozil) não demonstraram nenhum efeito consistente sobre a taxa de infartos do miocárdio ou AVC. Os efeitos benéficos da redução dos níveis de colesterol com as estatinas são independentes do uso de medicamentos concomitantes, como ácido acetilsalicílico, β-bloqueadores e bloqueadores dos canais de cálcio. Por conseguinte, a regressão física do ateroma pode não representar o principal mecanismo pelo qual a redução do colesterol modifica o risco cardíaco. Há evidências experimentais de que as estatinas afetam a função imune e a proliferação e o metabolismo dos macrófagos e das células endoteliais, independentemente de alterações nas concentrações plasmáticas de LDL. Estudos realizados em animais sugerem que as estatinas podem reduzir o risco de trombose, após ruptura da placa, ao inibirem a agregação plaquetária e ao manterem um equilíbrio favorável entre os mecanismos pró-trombótico e fibrinolítico. Nem todas as estatinas exercem efeito protetor igual. Os benefícios só foram claramente demonstrados com as estatinas "naturais" produzidas por fermentação (lovastatina, pravastatina e sinvastatina). As estatinas sintéticas possuem estruturas químicas diferentes e são metabolizadas diferentemente; apesar de reduzirem os níveis de LDL-colesterol, não há dados mostrando que elas prolongam a vida ou diminuem o risco de IAM.

human α₁-protease i. (α₁PI), i. da α₁-protease humana. SIN α₁-antitrypsin.

β-lactamase i.'s, inibidores da β-lactamase; drogas, como ácido clavulânico, que são utilizadas para inibir as β-lactamases bacterianas; freqüentemente associadas a uma penicilina ou cefalosporina para superar a resistência medicamentosa.

lipoprotein-associated coagulation i. (LACI), i. da coagulação associada à lipoproteína (ICAL); antigamente conhecida como anticonvertina; proteína que inibe a via extrínseca da coagulação ao ligar-se ao complexo fator III tecidual-fator VII-Ca²⁺-fator Xa.

mechanism-based i., i. baseado no mecanismo. SIN suicide substrate.

monoamine oxidase i. (MAOI), i. da monoamina oxidase (IMAO); classe de compostos químicos que exercem efeito antidepressivo através da inibição reversível ou irreversível da monoamina oxidase A.

ovulation i., i. da ovulação; composto que inibe a ovulação; freqüentemente presente em anticoncepcionais orais.

protease i., i. da protease (IP); classe de fármacos sintéticos recém-desenvolvidos, utilizados no tratamento da infecção por HIV, cujo modo de ação difere daquele dos agentes anti-retrovirais anteriormente empregados, incluindo análogos de nucleosídeo.

A atividade protease do HIV-1 é fundamental para a maturação final dos virions infecciosos. Os IP específicos para o HIV-1 inibem competitivamente essa enzima, impedindo, assim, a maturação dos virions capazes de infectar outras células. Esses agentes podem reduzir a carga viral (nível sérico de RNA do HIV) abaixo dos níveis mensuráveis no paciente com AIDS/SIDA. Foi constatado que seu uso diminui o risco de progressão da doença e reduz a mortalidade em pacientes com infecção por HIV. Além disso, verificou-se que esses agentes aumentam as contagens de células CD4 e revertem a demência da AIDS/SIDA em alguns pacientes. Os IP são associados a análogos de nucleosídeos (inibidores nucleosídeos da transcriptase reversa) para explorar os diferentes modos de ação dessas duas classes de agentes antivirais. Como o aparecimento de resistência aos inibidores da protease já constitui um problema, os esquemas de combinação, incluindo três agentes, representam o tratamento. Algumas cepas de HIV exibem resistência a todos os inibidores da protease disponíveis. Os efeitos colaterais significativos dos IP incluem elevação dos níveis de colesterol e triglicerídeos, resistência à insulina e desenvolvimento de diabetes melito franco e lipodistrofia esteticamente problemática (acúmulo excessivo de gordura no abdome e nas mamas, acompanhado de perda de gordura na face, nos membros e nas nádegas). Os IP usados atualmente incluem indinavir, nelfinavir, ritonavir e saquinavir. Vários outros encontram-se em diferentes estágios de desenvolvimento e testes.

proton pump i., i. da bomba de prótons; agentes que bloqueiam o transporte de íons hidrogênio no estômago e, portanto, mostram-se úteis no tratamento da hiperacidez gástrica, conforme observado na úlcera.

5α-reductase i.'s, inibidores da 5α-redutase; drogas que inibem a ação da 5α-redutase, resultando em níveis mais baixos de diidrotestosterona prostática, produzida pela enzima a partir da testosterona como principal androgênio na próstata.

residual i., i. residual; dispositivo gerador de sons, utilizado na orelha, que inibe ou suprime o zumbido (tinido) por meio de mascaramento, com efeito inibitório residual quando o aparelho é desligado.

respiratory i., i. respiratório; composto que inibe a cadeia respiratória. SIN respiratory poison.

selective norepinephrine reuptake i., i. seletivo da recaptação de norepinefrina; classe de compostos químicos que inibem seletivamente, em graus variáveis, a recaptação de norepinefrina pelos neurônios pré-sinápticos; supõe-se que exerçam seu efeito antidepressivo através desse mecanismo.

selective serotonin-reuptake i., i. seletivo da recaptação de serotonina; classe de compostos químicos que inibem seletivamente, em graus variáveis, a recaptação de serotonina pelos neurônios pré-sinápticos; supõe-se que exerçam seu efeito antidepressivo através desse mecanismo.

serine protease i.'s, inibidores da serina protease; classe de inibidores altamente polimórficos da tripsina, elastase e algumas outras proteases sintetizadas pelos hepatócitos e macrófagos. VER TAMBÉM α₁-antitrypsin. SIN serpins.

serotonin norepinephrine reuptake i., i. da recaptação de serotonina e noradrenalina; classe de agentes antidepressivos cuja ação é atribuída à inibição da recaptação pré-sináptica de serotonina e norepinefrina.

suicide i., i. i. suicida. SIN suicide substrate.

trypsin i., i. da tripsina. (1) Peptídeo formado a partir do tripsinogênio através de hidrólise, sob a influência catalítica da enteropeptidase, resultando também na produção de tripsina; assim denominado pelo fato de o peptídio mascarar ou inibir o sítio ativo da molécula da tripsina; (2) um dos peptídeos, de várias fontes (p. ex., colostro humano e bovino, soja, clara do ovo), que inibe a ação da tripsina. Cf. Bowman-Birk i.

α₁-trypsin i., i. da α₁-tripsina. SIN α₁-antitrypsin.

uncompetitive i., i. não-competitivo; tipo de inibidor enzimático em que o composto inibitório só se liga ao complexo enzima-substrato.

in·hib·i·to·ry (in-hib'i-tōr-ē). Inibitório, inibidor; que restringe; que tende a inibir.

in·i·ac (in'ē-ak). Iníaco; relativo ao ínio. SIN inial (inial).

in·i·ad (in'ē-ad). Inial; em direção ao ínio. [L. ad, para]

in·i·al (in'ē-ăl). Ineal. SIN iniac.

in·i·en·ceph·a·ly (in'ē-en-sef'ă-lē). Iniencefalia; malformação que consiste num defeito craniano no occipúcio, com exposição do cérebro; com freqüência, ocorre em associação a raquísquise cervical e retroflexão. [G. inion, parte posterior da cabeça + enkephalos, cérebro]

in·i·on (in′ē-on) [TA]. Ínio; ponto localizado na protuberância occipital externa, na interseção da linha média com uma linha tangente à convexidade superior das linhas nucais superiores direita e esquerda. [G. nuca]

in·i·op·a·gus (in′ē-op′ă-gŭs). Iniópago. SIN *craniopagus occipitalis*. [inion + G. *pagos*, fixo]

in·i·ops (in′ē-ops). Iniopsia. SIN *janiceps asymmetrus*. [inion + G. *ōps*, olho, face]

in·i·ti·a·tion (i-ni-shē-ā′shŭn). Início, iniciação. **1.** Primeiro estágio de indução tumoral por um carcinógeno; alteração sutil de células por exposição a um agente carcinogênico, de modo que tendem a formar um tumor com exposição subseqüente a um agente promotor (promoção). **2.** Ponto inicial de replicação ou tradução na biossíntese de macromoléculas. **3.** Início de uma reação química ou enzimática. **4.** Primeira etapa numa reação em cadeia.

in·i·tis (in-ī′tis). Inite. **1.** Inflamação de tecido fibroso. **2.** SIN myositis. [G. *is* (*in-*), fibra + *-itis*, inflamação]

in·ject (in-jekt′). Injetar; introduzir no corpo; refere-se a um líquido forçado abaixo da pele ou num vaso sanguíneo. VER TAMBÉM injection. [L. *injicio*, introduzir]

in·ject·a·ble (in-jek′tă-bl). Injetável. **1.** Capaz de ser injetado em algo. **2.** Capaz de receber uma injeção.

in·ject·ed (in-jek′ted). Injetado. **1.** Indica um líquido introduzido no corpo. **2.** Refere-se a vasos sanguíneos visíveis distendidos por sangue.

in·jec·tion (in-jek′shŭn). Injeção. **1.** Introdução de uma substância medicinal ou material nutritivo no tecido subcutâneo (i. subcutânea ou hipodérmica), no tecido muscular (i. intramuscular), numa veia (i. intravenosa), numa artéria (i. intra-arterial), no reto (i. retal ou enema), na vagina (ducha vaginal), na uretra ou em outros canais ou cavidades do corpo. **2.** Preparação farmacêutica injetável. **3.** Congestão ou hiperemia. [L. *injectio*, introduzir em, de *in-jicio*, introduzir]
   adrenal cortex i., i. de córtex supra-renal; tratamento obsoleto envolvendo a administração parenteral de extrato do córtex supra-renal; antigamente utilizada no tratamento da *doença* de Addison.
   collagen i., i. de colágeno; correção de deformidades superficiais de tecidos moles, cicatrizes de acne ou alterações cutâneas relacionadas com a idade por injeção (implantação) de colágeno; são utilizadas comumente preparações de colágeno bovino. É necessário um teste intradérmico prévio para excluir a possibilidade de hipersensibilidade. SIN collagen implantation.
   depot i., i. de depósito; injeção de uma substância em veículo que tende a mantê-la no local de injeção, de modo que a absorção ocorre durante um período prolongado.
   hypodermic i., i. hipodérmica; administração de um medicamento na forma líquida por injeção nos tecidos subcutâneos. SIN hypodermic (2).
   insulin i., .de insulina; preparação que, habitualmente, contém 100 unidades de insulina USP por ml; é administrada por via subcutânea, algumas vezes por via intravenosa, com rápido início de ação e duração breve (5 a 7 horas); é compatível para misturar com preparações de insulina de ação longa; utilizada no tratamento da acidose diabética e do coma insulínico. SIN regular insulin i.
   intracytoplasmic sperm i., i. intracitoplasmática de espermatozóide; procedimento em que um único espermatozóide é injetado no ovócito durante a fertilização *in vitro*.
   intrathecal i., i. intratecal; introdução de material para difusão através do espaço subaracnóide por meio de punção lombar.
   intraventricular i., i. intraventricular; introdução de materiais para difusão através do espaço ventricular e subaracnóide por meio de punção ventricular.
   jet i., i. a jato; injeção hipodérmica de medicamentos por injetor a jato.
   lactated Ringer i., i. de lactato de Ringer; solução estéril de cloreto de cálcio, cloreto de potássio, cloreto de sódio e lactato de sódio em água para injeção; utilizada por via intravenosa como alcalinizante sistêmico e na reposição de líquidos e eletrólitos.
   regular insulin i., i. de insulina regular. SIN insulin i.
   Ringer i., i. de Ringer; solução estéril de cloreto de sódio, cloreto de potássio e cloreto de cálcio contendo, em cada 100 ml, 820 a 900 mg de cloreto de sódio, 25 a 35 mg de cloreto de potássio e 30 a 37 mg de cloreto de cálcio; utilizada por via intravenosa na reposição de líquidos e eletrólitos.
   selective i., i. seletiva; injeção de contraste após cateterismo seletivo de uma artéria ou veia para angiografia.
   sensitizing i., i. sensibilizante; injeção que sensibiliza um indivíduo, de tal modo que a exposição subseqüente ao antígeno (alérgeno) desencadeia uma resposta alérgica.
   test i., i. de teste; injeção intravenosa de alguns mililitros de meio de contraste radiográfico para triagem de respostas alérgicas ou idiossincrásicas.
   Z-tract i., i. em forma de Z; técnica em que a pele e o tecido subcutâneo são colocados lateralmente antes de inserir a agulha por via intramuscular; utilizada para evitar o vazamento ao longo do trajeto da agulha e a conseqüente irritação do tecido.

in·jec·tor (in-jek′ter). Injetor; aparelho para aplicar injeções.
   jet i., i. a jato; injetor que utiliza uma alta pressão para forçar um líquido através de um pequeno orifício, numa velocidade suficiente para penetrar na pele ou na mucosa sem o uso de agulha.
   power i., i. de potência; injetor para injeção rápida de meio de contraste na angiografia ou na tomografia computadorizada.

in·jure (in′jer). Lesar; ferir, prejudicar ou danificar.

in·ju·ry (in′jer-ē). Lesão; dano ou ferida de traumatismo. [L. *injuria*, de *in-* neg. + *jus* (*jur-*), reto]
   blast i., l. por explosão; laceração do tecido pulmonar ou ruptura de qualquer tecido ou órgão sem lesão externa, como, p. ex., pela força de uma explosão.
   brachial plexus i., l. do plexo braquial; lesão do plexo braquial relacionada ao parto; associada a estiramento lateral excessivo da cabeça, tipicamente em casos de distocia do ombro ou apresentação de nádegas. VER TAMBÉM brachial birth *palsy*.

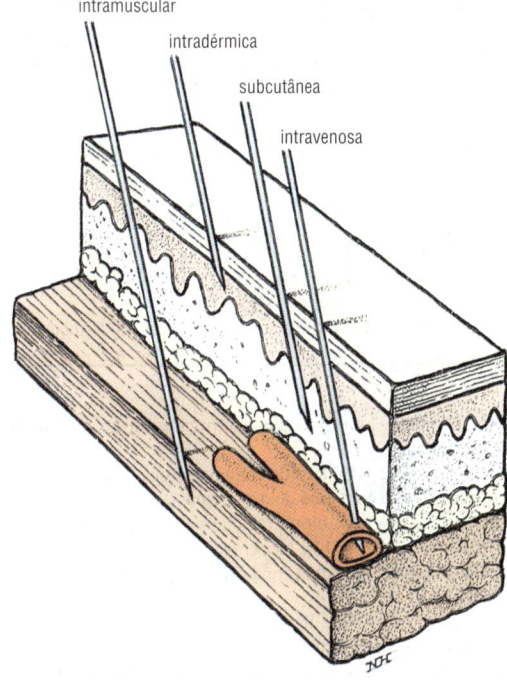

injeção

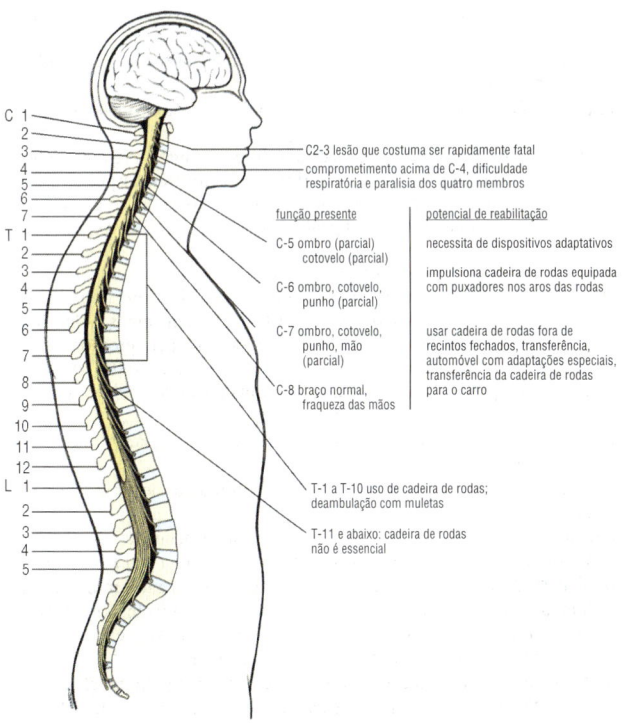

lesão da medula espinal: seqüelas em vários níveis

   closed head i., l. fechada da cabeça; lesão cefálica em que é mantida a continuidade do couro cabeludo e das mucosas.
   contrecoup i. of brain, l. cerebral por contragolpe; lesão que ocorre por baixo do crânio, em posição oposta à área de impacto.

coup i. of brain, l. cerebral por golpe; lesão que ocorre diretamente abaixo do crânio, na área de impacto.
current of i., corrente de l. VER *current* of injury.
degloving i., l. de desluvamento; avulsão da pele de parte do corpo (mais comumente nos membros), em que a parte é descarnada pela remoção da maior parte ou de toda a pele e tecido subcutâneo.
egg-white i., l. em clara de ovo. SIN *egg-white syndrome.*
flexion-extension i., l. por flexão-extensão; movimento vigoroso para frente e para trás da cabeça sem apoio que pode lesionar a coluna cervical ou o cérebro.
hyperextension-hyperflexion i., l. por hiperextensão-hiperflexão; violência corporal levando a cabeça sem apoio a mover-se rapidamente para trás e para frente, resultando em hiperextensão e hiperflexão do pescoço; não indica qualquer patologia ou traumatismo resultante específico.
i. of intervertebral disk, l. de disco intervertebral. VER *traumatic cervical discopathy.*
open head i., l. aberta da cabeça; lesão cefálica em que ocorre perda de continuidade do couro cabeludo ou das mucosas; o termo é algumas vezes empregado para indicar uma comunicação entre o exterior e a cavidade intracraniana. VER TAMBÉM *penetrating wound.*
pneumatic tire i., l. por pneumáticos; separação da pele e do tecido subcutâneo da fáscia subjacente, que ocorre classicamente quando o pneu de um veículo esmaga um membro e rola por cima dele; entretanto, pode ocorrer através de outros mecanismos que produzem forças de cisalhamento; semelhante a uma lesão de desluvamento, porém a pele e as camadas de tecido subcutâneo permanecem em continuidade.
reperfusion i., l. de reperfusão; comprometimento do miocárdio, habitualmente com arritmia, após abertura de bloqueio arterial; acredita-se que seja causada por radicais livres derivados do oxigênio.
sterring wheel i., i. causada por volante; traumatismo da parede torácica anterior causada por impacto com o volante durante um acidente automobilístico; pode consistir em fratura de esterno e costelas, contusão cardíaca, laceração da aorta e de outros grandes vasos, bem como lesões pulmonares.
whiplash i., l. em chicotada; termo popular para a lesão por flexão–extensão.
in·lay (in′lā). Incrustação, bloco. **1.** Em odontologia, restauração pré-fabricada, fixada na cavidade com cimento. **2.** Enxerto de osso numa cavidade óssea. **3.** Enxerto de pele numa cavidade de ferida para epitelialização. **4.** Em ortopedia, dispositivo ortomecânico inserido num sapato; comumente denominado "suporte de arco".
epithelial i., enxerto epitelial. SIN *inlay graft.*
gold i., b. de ouro; restauração de ouro fabricada por fusão em molde feito a partir de um padrão de cera; a restauração é fixada na cavidade preparada com cimento dentário.
porcelain i., b. de porcelana; restauração de porcelana fundida colocada na cavidade preparada de um dente.
in·let [TA]. Entrada, estreito, ádito; passagem que leva a uma cavidade. SIN *aditus* [TA].
laryngeal i. [TA], ádito da laringe; abertura entre a faringe e a laringe, delimitada pelas bordas superiores da epiglote (anteriormente) pelas pregas ariepiglóticas (lateralmente) e pela mucosa entre as aritenóides (posteriormente). SIN *aditus laryngis* [TA], *laryngeal aditus* [TA], *i. of larynx, laryngeal aperture.*
i. of larynx, ádito da laringe. SIN *laryngeal i.*
pelvic i. [TA], abertura pélvica; abertura superior da pelve verdadeira, limitada, anteriormente, pela sínfise pubiana e crista púbica em ambos os lados, lateralmente pelas linhas iliopectíneas e, posteriormente, pelo promontório do sacro. SIN *apertura pelvis superior* [TA], *aditus pelvis, first parallel pelvic plane, pelvic brim, pelvic plane of inlet, plane of inlet, superior pelvic aperture.*
thoracic i., a. torácica. SIN *superior thoracic aperture.*
in·nate (i′nāt, i - nāt′). Inato. SIN *inborn.* [L. *in-nascor,* pp. *-natus,* nascer em, pp. adjetivado, inato]
in·ner·va·tion (in′er - vā′shŭn). Inervação; suprimento de fibras nervosas funcionalmente ligadas a uma parte. [L. *in,* em + *nervus,* nervo]
reciprocal i., i. recíproca; a contração num músculo é acompanhada de perda de tônus ou relaxamento do músculo antagonista. SIN *reciprocal inhibition* (1).
in·nid·i·a·tion (i - nid - ē - ā′shŭn). Colonização; crescimento e multiplicação de células anormais em outra localização para a qual foram transportadas através da linfa e/ou da corrente sanguínea. VER TAMBÉM *metastasis.* SIN *colonization* (1), *indenization.* [L. *in,* em + *nidus,* ninho]
in·no·cent (in′ō - sent). Inocente. **1.** Aparentemente não-prejudicial. **2.** Livre de erro legal ou moral. [L. *innocens* (-*ent-*), de *in,* neg. + *noceo,* lesar]
in·noc·u·ous (i - nok′ū - ŭs). Inócuo; inofensivo. SIN *innoxious.* [L. *in-nocuus*]
in·nom·i·nal (i - nom′i - nā - tăl). Inominado; relativo ao osso ilíaco.
in·nom·i·nate (i - nom′i - nāt). Inominado; sem nome; termo antigamente aplicado aos grandes vasos no tórax (atualmente denominados tronco e veia braquiocefálicos) e ao osso do quadril. SIN *anonyma.* [L. *innominatus,* de *in-* neg. + *nomen* (*nomin-*), nome]
in·nox·ious (i - nok′shŭs). Inócuo. SIN *innocuous.* [L. *in-noxius,* de *in,* neg. + *noceo,* lesão]

INO Acrônimo de *internuclear ophthalmoplegia* (oftalmoplegia internuclear).
Ino Símbolo de inosine (inosina).
ino-, in-. Ino-, in-. Fibra, fibroso. VER TAMBÉM *fibro-.* [G. *is* (*in-*), fibra]
in·oc·u·la·bil·i·ty (i - nok′ū - lă - bil′i - tē). Inoculabilidade; qualidade de ser inoculável.
in·oc·u·la·ble (i - nok′ū - lă - bl). Inoculável. **1.** Passível de ser transmitido por inoculação. **2.** Suscetível a uma doença transmissível por inoculação.
in·oc·u·late (i - nok′ū - lāt). Inocular. **1.** Introduzir o agente de uma doença ou outro material antigênico no tecido subcutâneo, em vaso sanguíneo ou através de uma superfície escoriada ou absorvente para fins profiláticos, curativos ou experimentais. **2.** Implantar microrganismos ou material infeccioso em meios de cultura. **3.** Transmitir uma doença através da transferência de seu vírus. [L. *inoculo,* pp. *-atus,* introduzir]
in·oc·u·la·tion (i - nok - ū - lā′shŭn). Inoculação; introdução, no corpo, do organismo causal de uma doença. O termo também é algumas vezes empregado, de modo incorreto, para referir-se à imunização com qualquer tipo de vacina.
stress i., i. de estresse; em psicologia clínica, abordagem destinada a fornecer ao paciente habilidades cognitivas e de atitudes que poderão ser utilizadas para enfrentar o estresse.

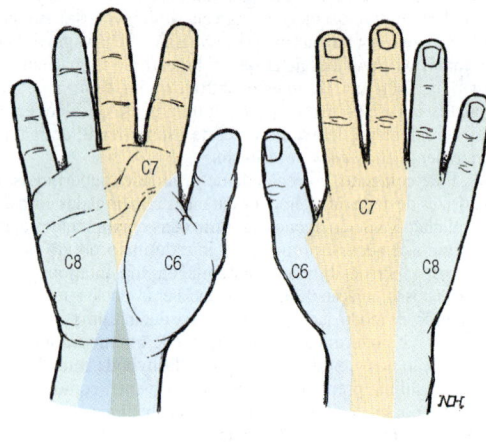
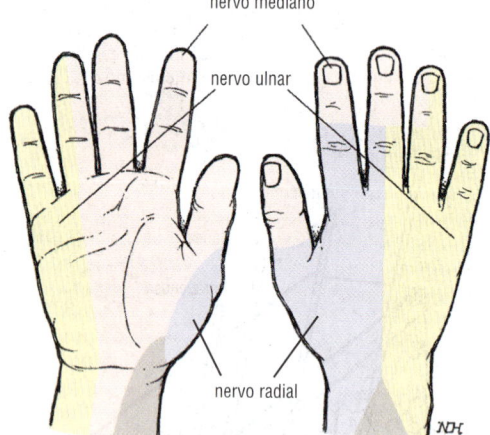

inervação da mão e do punho: (A) dermátomos segmentares, (B) distribuição dos nervos cutâneos

in·oc·u·lum (i - nok′ū - lŭm). Inóculo; microrganismo ou outro material introduzido por inoculação.
In·o·cy·be (i - nō′si - bē). Gênero de cogumelos que inclui diversas espécies possuidoras de elevado conteúdo de muscarina.
in·o·pec·tic (in - ō - pek′tik). Inopéctico, inopéxico; relativo à inopexia.
in·op·er·a·ble (in - op′er - ă - bl). Inoperável; indica que não pode ser submetido a operação ou refere-se a uma condição que, provavelmente, não pode ser curada por cirurgia.
in·o·pex·ia (in - ō - pek′sē - ă). Inopexia; tendência à coagulação espontânea do sangue. [ino + G. *pexis,* fixação + *-ia*]
in·or·gan·ic (in - ōr - gan′ik). Inorgânico. **1.** Não-orgânico, que não é formado por organismos vivos. **2.** VER *inorganic compound.* **3.** Que não contém carbono.

in·os·a·mine (in-ōs'à-mēn). Inosamina; inositol em que um grupo −OH é substituído por um grupamento −NH₂.

in·os·co·py (in-os'ko-pē). Inoscopia; exame microscópico de materiais biológicos (p. ex., tecido, escarro, sangue coagulado) após dissecção ou digestão química dos elementos fibrilares e feixes de fibrina. [ino- + G. *skopeō*, olhar]

in·ose (in'ōs). Inose. SIN inositol.

in·o·se·mia (in-ō-sē'mē-à). Inosemia. **1.** Presença de inositol no sangue circulante. **2.** SIN fibremia. [inose + G. *haima*, sangue]

in·o·si·nate (in-ō'si-nāt). Inosinato; sal ou éster do ácido inosínico.

in·o·sine (I, Ino) (in'ō-sēn). Inosina; 9-β-D-ribosil-hipoxantina; nucleosídeo formado pela desaminação da adenosina. SIN hypoxanthinosine.

in·o·sine 5'-di·phos·phate (IDP). Inosina 5'-difosfato (IDP). Inosina esterificada em sua posição 5' com ácido difosfórico.

in·o·sine 5'-mon·o·phos·phate (IMP). Inosina 5'-monofosfato (IMP). SIN inosinic acid.

    IMP dehydrogenase, IMP desidrogenase; enzima que catalisa a reação de IMP, água e NAD⁺ para formar NADH e xantosina 5'-monofosfato (XMP), o precursor imediato do GMP.

in·o·sine pran·o·bex (in'ō-sēn pran'ō-beks). Inosina pranobex; complexo molar 1:3 de 1-dimetilaminopropano-2-ol-4-acetamidobenzoato e inosina, utilizado como agente antiviral.

in·o·sine 5'-tri·phos·phate (ITP) (in'ō-sēn). Inosina 5'-trifosfato (ITP); inosina com ácido trifosfórico esterificado em sua posição 5'; participa em diversas reações catalisadas por enzimas.

in·o·sin·ic ac·id (in-ō-sin'ik). Ácido inosínico; mononucleotídeo encontrado no músculo e em outros tecidos; intermediário-chave na biossíntese de purinas; também produzido em níveis relativamente altos no músculo. SIN inosine 5'-monophosphate.

in·o·sin·i·case (in-o-sin'-a-kās). Inosinicase; enzima que atua na biossíntese de purinas e catalisa a reação de fechamento do anel que produz ácido inosínico a partir de 5'-fosforribosil 5-formamidoimidazol-4-carboxamida.

in·o·sin·yl (in-ō'si-nil). Inosinil; radical do ácido inosínico.

in·o·site (in'ō-sīt). Inosita. SIN inositol.

in·o·si·tide (in-ō'si-tīd). Inositídeo; termo utilizado para referir-se ao fosfatidilinositol ou a qualquer fosfolipídio contendo inositol.

in·o·si·tol (in-ō'si-tōl, -tol). Inositol; 1,2,3,4,5,6-hexaidroxicicloexano; membro do complexo da vitamina B necessário para o crescimento de leveduras e de camundongos; a sua ausência na dieta produz alopecia e dermatite em camundongos, e "olhos de óculos" em ratos. Ocorre em diversas formas estereoisoméricas: *cis-, epi-, alo-, neo-, mio-, muco-, quiro-* e *cilo*-inositóis; a forma de ocorrência natural mais abundante é o *mio*-inositol (geralmente subentendido quando aparece o termo "inositol" sem prefixo). SIN antialopecia factor, inose, inosite, lipositol, mouse antialopecia factor.

    i. niacinate, niacinato de i.; vasodilatador periférico.

    i. 1,3,4,5-tetraphosphate, i. 1,3,4,5-tetrafosfato; derivado fosforilado do inositol, formado a partir do inositol 1,4,5-trifosfato, que induz a entrada de Ca²⁺ do citosol a partir do meio extracelular; inativado por hidrólise, formando inositol 1,3,4-trifosfato.

    i. 1,4,5-triphosphate (IP₃), i. 1,4,5-trifosfato (IP₃); segundo mensageiro formado a partir do fosfatidilinositol 4,5-difosfato; deflagra a liberação de íons cálcio de vesículas especiais do retículo endoplasmático; participa na ativação dos neutrófilos.

    meso-**in·o·si·tol.** *Meso*-inositol. **1.** Termo genérico para qualquer isômero do *meso*-inositol, em que os grupamentos hidroxila estão distribuídos de tal modo que a molécula, como um todo, possui um plano de simetria e é opticamente inativa. **2.** Termo antigo para referir-se ao *mio*-inositol.

    myo-**in·o·si·tol.** Mio-inositol; 1,2,3,5/4,6-inositol; constituinte de diversos fosfatidilinositóis, representando a forma mais amplamente distribuída de inositol encontrada em microrganismos, vegetais e animais superiores. Nos vegetais, é encontrado como ácido fítico e fitina; ocorrem formas parcialmente fosforiladas e livres em toda a natureza e em muitos tecidos.

in·o·si·tu·ria (in'ō-si-too'rē-à). Inositúria; excreção de inositol na urina. SIN inosuria (1). [inositol + G. *ouron*, urina]

in·o·su·ria (in-ō-soo'rē-a). Inosúria. **1.** SIN inosituria. **2.** Ocorrência de fibrina na urina.

in·o·tro·pic (in-ō-trop'ik). Inotrópico; que influencia a contratilidade do tecido muscular. [in + G. *tropos*, uma volta]

    negatively i., negativamente i.; enfraquecimento da ação muscular.

    positively i., positivamente i.; reforço da ação muscular.

Ino·vir·i·dae (i-nō-vir'i-dē). Família de vírus filamentosos que infectam bactérias Grã-negativas com genoma de DNA monofilamentar (PM 1,9–2,7 × 10⁶). O colífago fd, a espécie-tipo do gênero do grupo de fagos fd, adsorve as pontas das fímbrias de enterobactérias masculinas, e, após multiplicação, as partículas são liberadas sem produzir lise da bactéria hospedeiro. [ino + vírus]

in phase. Em fase; que se move na mesma direção ao mesmo tempo; possível característica de duas oscilações simultâneas de freqüência semelhante.

in·quest (in'kwest). Inquérito; investigação legal sobre a causa de morte súbita, violenta ou misteriosa. [L. *in*, em + *quaero*, pp. *quaesitus*, procurar]

in·qui·line (in'kwi-līn, -lin). Inquilino; animal que vive habitualmente na moradia de outra espécie (um caranguejo no interior da concha de uma ostra), causando pouco ou nenhum inconveniente ao hospedeiro. VER TAMBÉM commensal. [L. *inquilinus*, habitante de um lugar que não lhe pertence, de *in*, em + *colo*, habitar]

INR RNI. Abreviatura de international normalized *ratio* (relação normalizada internacional).

in·sa·lu·bri·ous (in-sā-loo'brē-ŭs). Insalubre; prejudicial; não-saudável; referindo-se habitualmente ao clima. [L. *in-salubris*, insalubre]

in·sane (in-sān'). Insano. **1.** Que tem mente doente; com grave comprometimento mental; demente; louco. **2.** Relativo à insanidade. [L. *in-* neg. + *sanus*, são]

in·san·i·tary (in-san'i-tār-ē). Anti-higiênico; lesivo à saúde, referindo-se habitualmente a um ambiente sujo ou contaminado. SIN unsanitary. [L. *in-* neg. + *sanus*, sadio]

in·san·i·ty (in-san'i-tē). Insanidade. **1.** Termo obsoleto que se refere a grave doença mental ou psicose. **2.** Juridicamente, refere-se ao grau de doença mental que nega a responsabilidade legal de um indivíduo ou a sua capacidade. [L. *in-* neg. + *sanus*, saudável]

    criminal i., i. criminal; em psiquiatria forense, termo utilizado para descrever o grau de competência mental, definido por precedentes legais comumente aplicáveis, como a *American Law Institute rule*, a *Durham rule*, a *M'Naghten rule* e a *New Hampshire rule*.

    i. defense, i. de defesa; em psiquiatria forense; uso, no tribunal, de insanidade como fator lenitivo na defesa de um indivíduo julgado por grave delito criminoso. VER criminal i.

in·scrip·tio (in-skrip'shē-ō). Inscrição. SIN inscription. [L. de *in-scribo*, pp. -*scriptus*, escrever]

    i. tendin'ea, i. tendínea. SIN tendinous *intersection*.

in·scrip·tion (in-skrip'shŭn). Inscrição. **1.** Parte principal de uma prescrição; a que indica os medicamentos e a quantidade de cada um deles a ser usada na mistura. **2.** Marca, faixa ou linha. SIN inscriptio. [L. *inscriptio*]

    tendinous i., i. tendinosa. SIN tendinous *intersection*.

In·sec·ta (in-sek'tà). Insetos; a maior classe do filo Arthropoda e o maior e principal grupo de seres vivos, caracterizados, principalmente, por asas, grande adaptabilidade, vasto número de espécies em ambientes terrestres e dulcícolas, apresentando três pares de patas articuladas e, em geral, dois pares de asas. Alguns são parasitas, enquanto outros servem como hospedeiros intermediários para parasitas, incluindo os que causam muitas doenças humanas. Alguns não têm asas; outros, como os Diptera, têm apenas um par de asas. A respiração é feita por traquéias, que consistem em tubos de ar revestidos de cutícula através dos quais o ar chega diretamente aos tecidos. Nas formas superiores, o desenvolvimento é holometabólico e passa pelos estágios característicos de ovo, larva, pupa e adulto. SIN Hexapoda. [L. pl. of *insectus*, inseto, de *in-seco*, pp. -*sectus*, cortar]

in·sec·tar·i·um (in-sek-tā'rē-ŭm). Insectário; local próprio para manter e reproduzir insetos para finalidades científicas. [L.]

in·sec·ti·cide (in-sek'ti-sīd). Inseticida; agente que mata insetos. [inseto + L. *caedo*, matar]

in·sec·ti·fuge (in-sek'ti-fooj). Insetífugo; substância que repele insetos. [inseto + L. *fugos*, pôr em fuga]

In·sec·tiv·o·ra (in-sek-tiv'ō-rà). Ordem de pequenos mamíferos plantígrados e placentários, que são extremamente ativos e, com freqüência, extremamente predadores; alimentam-se principalmente de insetos e pequenos roedores, embora os *jes* ou potomogales da África se alimentem de peixes. Oito famílias vivas incluem os solenodontes de Cuba e do Haiti, os tanreques de Madagascar, porcos espinhos da Europa e Ásia e musaranhos e toupeiras dos Estados Unidos, África e Ásia. [inseto + L. *voro*, devorar]

in·sec·tiv·o·rous (in-sek-tiv'ō-rŭs). Insetívoro; que se alimenta de insetos. [inseto + L. *voro*, devorar]

in·se·cu·ri·ty (in-sē-kūr'i-tē). Insegurança; sentimento de falta de proteção e desamparo.

in·sem·i·na·tion (in-sem-i-nā'shŭm). Inseminação; deposição de líquido seminal no interior da vagina, normalmente durante o coito. SIN semination. [L. *in-semino*, pp. -*atus*, semear ou plantar, de *semen*, semente]

    artificial i., i. artificial; introdução de sêmen na vagina sem coito.

    donor i., i. de doador. SIN heterologous i.

    heterologous i., i. heteróloga; inseminação artificial com sêmen de um doador que não é o marido da paciente. SIN donor i.

    homologous i., i. homóloga; inseminação artificial com sêmen do marido.

    intrauterine i. (IUI), i. intra-uterina; colocação de esperma do qual foi removido o líquido seminal diretamente no útero, sem passar pelo colo uterino.

in·se·nes·cence (in-sē-nes'ens). Senescência; processo de envelhecer. [L. *insenesco*, começar a envelhecer]

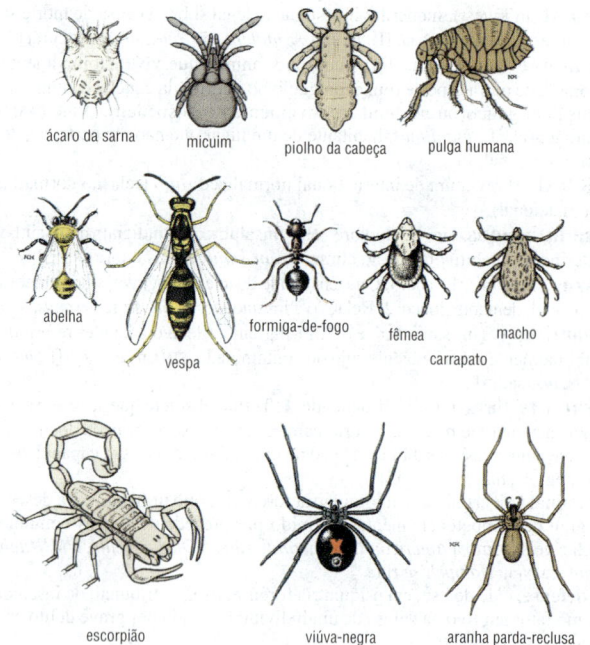

insetos e aracnídeos que picam e ferroam: (em cima) inócuos, (no meio) potencialmente perigosos, (embaixo) potencialmente fatais; os insetos não estão desenhados na escala

in·sen·si·ble (in-sen'si-bl). Insensível. **1.** SIN unconscious. **2.** Não apreciável pelos sentidos. [L. *in-sensibilis*, de *in*, neg. + *sentio*, pp. *sensus*, sentir]

in·sert (in'sert). Inserção, suplemento inserido. **1.** Extensão adicional de pares de bases introduzida no DNA. **2.** Extensão adicional de bases que foi introduzida no RNA. **3.** Extensão adicional de resíduos de aminoácidos que foi introduzida numa proteína.

in·ser·tion (in-ser'shŭn). Inserção. **1.** Colocação em. **2.** A inserção habitualmente mais distal de um músculo à parte mais móvel do esqueleto, distinguindo-a da origem. **3.** Em odontologia, colocação intra-oral de uma prótese dentária. **4.** Introdução de fragmentos de qualquer tamanho, desde moleculares até citogenéticos, no genoma normal. [L. *insertio*, plantar em, de *insero*, *-sertus*, plantar]
 parasol i., i. em guarda-chuva. SIN velamentous i.
 velamentous i., i. velamentosa; forma de inserção dos vasos sanguíneos fetais na placenta em que os vasos se separam antes de alcançá-la e desenvolvem-se em sua direção numa dobra do âmnio, assemelhando-se discretamente às varetas de um guarda-chuva aberto. SIN parasol i.

in·sheathed (in-shēthd'). Embainhado; encerrado numa bainha ou cápsula.

in·sid·i·ous (in-sid'ē-ŭs). Insidioso; traiçoeiro; furtivamente; indica uma doença que evolui gradualmente com sintomas inaparentes. [L. *insidiosus*, astúcia, de *insidiae* (pl.). emboscada]

in·sight (in'sīt). Insight, introvisão, autopercepção; compreensão dos motivos e das razões por detrás de suas próprias ações ou das ações de outra pessoa.

in si·tu (in sī'too). *In situ*; na posição, que não se estende além do foco ou nível de origem. [L. *in*, em + *situs*, local]

in·so·la·tion (in-sō-lā'shŭn). **1.** Exposição aos raios solares. **2.** Insolação, febre térmica. SIN sunstroke. [L. *insolare*, colocar no sol]

in·sol·u·ble (in-sol'ū-bl). Insolúvel, não-solúvel.

in·som·nia (in-som'nē-ă). Insônia; incapacidade de dormir, na ausência de impedimentos externos, como ruídos, luz brilhante, etc., durante o período em que o sono deveria normalmente ocorrer; pode variar de intensidade, desde inquietação ou cochilo perturbado até encurtamento da duração normal do sono ou vigília total. SIN sleeplessness. [L. de *in-* priv. + *somnus*, sono]
 conditioned i., i. condicionada; forma de insônia que resulta de comportamentos condicionados incompatíveis com o sono, como, p. ex., toda vez que a pessoa se dirige ao quarto, seu primeiro pensamento é de que ela não será capaz de dormir.
 subjective i., i. subjetiva; condição caracterizada pela experiência subjetiva de uma acentuada redução do sono dentro do contexto de uma medida fisiológica relativamente normal de sono.

in·som·ni·ac (in-som'nē-ak). Insone. **1.** Que sofre de insônia. **2.** Que apresenta, tende a ter ou produz insônia.

in·sorp·tion (in-sōrp-shŭn). Absorção; movimento de substâncias da luz do intestino para o sangue. [L. *in*, em + *sorbeo*, sugar]

inspection. Inspeção.

visual i. with acetic acid, i. visual com ácido acético. SIN acetowhitening, cervicoscopy.

in·sper·sion (in-sper'shŭn, -zhŭn). Insperção; borrifar com líquido ou com pó. [L. *inspersio*, espalhar, de *in-spergo*, pp. *-spersus*, espalhar, fr. *spargo*, espalhar]

in·spi·ra·tion (in-spi-rā'shŭn). Inspiração. SIN inhalation (1). [L. *inspiratio*, de *in-spiro*, pp. *-atus*, inspirar]
 crowing i., i. ruidosa; respiração ruidosa associada a obstrução respiratória, geralmente na laringe.

in·spi·ra·to·ry (in-spī'ră-tō-rē). Inspiratório; relativo a ou regulado durante a inspiração.

in·spire (in-spīr). Inspirar. SIN inhale.

in·spi·rom·e·ter (in-spī-rom'ē-ter). Inspirômetro; instrumento para medir a força, a freqüência ou o volume das inspirações. [L. *in-spiro*, inspirar + G. *metron*, medida]

in·spis·sate (in-spis'āt). Inspissar, tornar espesso; realizar ou sofrer inspissação.

in·spis·sa·tion (in-spi-sā'shŭn). Inspissação. **1.** Ato de espessar ou de condensar, como, p. ex., por evaporação ou absorção de líquido. **2.** Aumento da espessura ou diminuição da fluidez. [L. *in*, intensivo + *spisso*, pp. *-atus*, espessar]

in·spis·sa·tor (in-spis'ă-tor). Inspissador; aparelho para evaporar líquidos.

in·sta·bil·i·ty (in-stă-bil'i-tē). Instabilidade; estado de ser instável ou falta de estabilidade.
 detrusor i., i. do detrusor; contrações involuntárias do detrusor que podem ocorrer com volumes vesicais abaixo da capacidade. SIN detrusor hyperreflexia.
 spinal i., instabilidade da coluna; incapacidade da coluna vertebral, com cargas fisiológicas, em manter a sua configuração normal; pode resultar em lesão da medula espinal ou de raízes nervosas ou levar ao desenvolvimento de deformidade espinal dolorosa.

in·star (in'stahr). Instar; qualquer uma das etapas sucessivas de linfa na metamorfose de insetos hemimetabólicos (metamorfose simples ou incompleta) ou dos estágios de mudança larvária por mudas sucessivas, que caracterizam os insetos holometabólicos (metamorfose complexa ou completa). [L. forma]

in·step. Dorso do pé; arco ou parte mais elevada do dorso do pé. VER TAMBÉM tarsus.

in·stil·la·tion (in-sti-lā'shŭn). Instilação; gotejamento de um líquido sobre ou numa parte do corpo. [L. *instillatio*, de *in-stillo*, pp. *-atus*, despejar em gotas, de *stilla*, uma gota]

in·stil·la·tor (in'sti-lā-ter). Instilador; aparelho ou dispositivo para efetuar a instilação. SIN dropper.

in·stinct (in'stinkt). Instinto. **1.** Disposição ou tendência permanente de um organismo a atuar de maneira organizada ou biologicamente adaptada, característica de sua espécie. **2.** Impulso irracional para executar alguma ação proposital sem a consciência imediata do resultado ao qual pode levar essa ação. **3.** Em teoria psicanalítica, as forças ou impulsos que, supostamente, existem por trás da tensão causada pelas necessidades do id. [L. *instinctus*, impulso]
 aggressive i., i. agressivo. SIN death i.
 death i., i. de morte; instinto das criaturas vivas para a autodestruição, morte ou retorno ao estado inorgânico sem vida do qual se originaram. SIN aggressive i.
 ego i.'s, instintos do ego; necessidades de autopreservação e auto-estima, em oposição ao amor por objetos; impulsos que são primariamente eróticos.
 herd i., i. de grupo; tendência ou inclinação a unir-se e compartilhar os costumes de outros seres de um grupo, conformando-se com as opiniões e adotando os pontos de vista do grupo. SIN social i.
 life i., i. de vida; instinto de autopreservação e procriação sexual; necessidade básica de preservação da espécie. SIN sexual i.
 sexual i., i. sexual. SIN life i.
 social i., i. social. SIN herd i.

in·stinc·tive, in·stinc·tu·al (in-stink'tiv, -stink'choo-ăl). Instintivo; relativo ao instinto.

in·stru·ment (in'stroo-ment). Ferramenta, utensílio, aparelho, prótese. [L. *instrumentum*]
 diamond cutting i.'s, instrumentos de corte em losangos; em odontologia, cilindros, discos e outros instrumentos de corte aos quais são fixadas numerosas e pequenas pirâmides em losango por meio de uma chapa de metal.
 hearing i., prótese auditiva. SIN hearing aid.
 Krueger i. stop, i. de limitação de Krueger; dispositivo mecânico que limita a inserção de um instrumento para tratamento de canal dentro de um canal.
 plugging i., i. de encaixe. SIN plugger.
 purse-string i., i. em bolsa de tabaco; pinça intestinal com mordentes em ângulo com o cabo; quando fechada no intestino, grandes serrilhas interdigitadas e sulcadas permitem a passagem de uma agulha e sutura através de cada lado para formar uma sutura em bolsa de tabaco, seguida de remoção da pinça.
 Sabouraud-Noiré i., i. de Sabouraud-Noiré; dispositivo obsoleto para medir a quantidade de raios X por meio da mudança de cor de um disco de platinocianeto de bário produzida pela exposição aos raios; a unidade utilizada nesse método é denominada tonalidade B (tint B). VER erythema dose.

stereotactic i., stereotaxic i., i. estereotático, i. estereotáxico; aparelho fixado à cabeça, utilizado para localizar com precisão uma área do cérebro através de coordenadas relacionadas com as estruturas intracerebrais.

test handle i., i. de cabo de teste; i. de canal de raiz cujo cabo assemelha-se a um mandril e que pode ser mantido em posição sobre o i. do canal para ajustar seu comprimento eficaz.

in·stru·men·tar·i·um (in'stroo-men-tār'ē-ŭm). Instrumentário; coleção de instrumentos e outros equipamentos para uma operação cirúrgica ou procedimento clínico.

in·stru·men·ta·tion (in'stroo-men-tā'shŭn). Instrumentação. **1.** Uso de instrumentos. **2.** Em odontologia, aplicação do armamentário num procedimento de restauração.

in·suc·ca·tion (in'sŭ-kā'shŭn). Maceração ou infiltração, especialmente de uma droga no seu estado integral, a fim de prepará-la para posterior operação farmacêutica. [L. *insuco,* pp. *-atus,* infiltrar, de *in,* em + sucus, suco, seiva (improp. *succ-*)]

in·su·date (in'soo-dāt). Insudato; acúmulo de líquido no interior de uma parede arterial (habitualmente seroso), diferindo do exsudato por não se localizar extramuralmente. [L. *in,* em + *sudo,* pp. *-atus,* suar]

in·suf·fi·cien·cy (in-sŭ-fish'en-sē). Insuficiência; impossibilidade de completar a função ou poder. VER TAMBÉM incompetence. [L. *in-,* neg. + *sufficientia,* de *sufficio,* ser suficiente]
  accommodative i., i. acomodativa; falta de acomodação apropriada para um foco próximo.
  acute adrenocortical i., i. córtico-supra-renal aguda; grave insuficiência córtico-supra-renal quando uma doença intercorrente ou traumatismo provoca um aumento na demanda de hormônios adrenocorticais num paciente com insuficiência supra-renal devido a doença ou ao uso de doses relativamente grandes de hormônios semelhantes como terapia; caracteriza-se por náuseas, vômitos, hipotensão e, com freqüência, hipertermia, hiponatremia, hipercalemia e hipoglicemia; pode ser fatal se não for tratada. SIN addisonian crisis, adrenal crisis, Bernard-Sergent syndrome.
  adrenocortical i., i. adrenocortical; perda, em graus variáveis, da função adrenocortical. SIN hypocorticoidism.
  aortic i., i. aórtica. VER valvular *regurgitation.*
  cardiac i., i. cardíaca. SIN heart *failure* (1).
  chronic adrenocortical i., i. córtico-supra-renal crônica; insuficiência córtico-supra-renal que, habitualmente, resulta de atrofia idiopática ou destruição de ambas as glândulas supra-renais por tuberculose, processo auto-imune ou outras doenças; caracteriza-se por fadiga, diminuição da pressão arterial, perda de peso, aumento de peso, aumento da pigmentação de melanina da pele e das mucosas, anorexia e náuseas ou vômito; na ausência de terapia de reposição apropriada, pode evoluir para a insuficiência córtico-supra-renal aguda. SIN Addison disease, addisonian syndrome, hyposupradrenalism, morbus Addisonii.
  convergence i., i. de convergência; condição em que uma exoforia ou exotropia é mais pronunciada para a visão próxima do que para a visão a distância.
  coronary i., i. coronária; circulação coronária inadequada, resultando em dor anginosa. SIN coronarism (1).
  divergence i., i. de divergência; condição em que uma exoforia ou exotropia é mais pronunciada para a visão a distância do que para a visão próxima.
  exocrine pancreatic i., i. pancreática exócrina; falta de secreção exócrina do pâncreas devido à destruição dos ácinos, geralmente em decorrência de pancreatite crônica; ausência de enzimas digestivas do pâncreas resulta em diarréia, habitualmente com excesso de gordura (esteatorréia), devido à falta de enzimas pancreáticas.
  hepatic i., i. hepática; atividade funcional deficiente dos hepatócitos.
  latent adrenocortical i., i. córtico-supra-renal latente; insuficiência córtico-supra-renal não clinicamente evidente, mas que pode tornar-se grave se aparecer um estresse súbito, como uma doença aguda intercorrente.
  mitral i., i. mitral. VER valvular *regurgitation.*
  muscular i., i. muscular; incapacidade de qualquer músculo de contrair-se com sua força normal, referindo-se, especialmente, a qualquer dos músculos oculares.
  myocardial i., i. miocárdica. SIN heart *failure* (1).
  parathyroid i., i. das paratireóides. SIN hypoparathyroidism.
  partial adrenocortical i., i. córtico-supra-renal parcial; função adrenocortical basal normal, com ausência de resposta da reserva córtico-supra-renal à estimulação do ACTH.
  primary adrenocortical i., i. córtico-supra-renal primária; insuficiência córtico-supra-renal causada por doença, destruição ou remoção cirúrgica do córtex supra-renal.
  pulmonary i., i. pulmonar. VER valvular *regurgitation.*
  pyloric i., i. pilórica; incompetência do piloro, permitindo a regurgitação do conteúdo duodenal para o estômago.
  renal i., i. renal; função deficiente dos rins, com acúmulo de produtos de degradação (sobretudo escórias nitrogenadas no sangue).
  respiratory i., i. respiratória; incapacidade de fornecer oxigênio adequadamente às células do organismo e de remover delas o excesso de dióxido de carbono.
  secondary adrenocortical i., i. córtico-supra-renal secundária; insuficiência córtico-supra-renal causada pela deficiência de secreção de ACTH devido a doença da hipófise anterior ou inibição da produção de ACTH em conseqüência de terapia com esteróides exógenos.
  thyroid i., i. da tireóide; secreção subnormal de hormônios pela glândula tireóide. VER TAMBÉM hypothyroidism.
  tricuspid i., i. tricúspide. VER valvular *regurgitation.*
  uterine i., i. uterina; atonia da musculatura uterina.
  valvular i., i. valvar. SIN valvular *regurgitation.*
  velopharyngeal i., i. velofaríngea; deficiência anatômica ou funcional no palato mole ou no músculo constritor superior da faringe, resultando em incapacidade de obter o fechamento velofaríngeo.
  venous i., i. venosa; drenagem inadequada do sangue venoso de uma parte, resultando em edema ou dermatose.

in·suf·flate (in-sŭf'lāt). Insuflar; introduzir ar ou gás sob pressão numa cavidade ou câmara do corpo, como, p. ex., injeção de dióxido de carbono no peritônio para produzir pneumoperitônio durante a laparoscopia e cirurgia laparoscópica. [L. *in-sufflo,* soprar sobre ou para dentro]

in·suf·fla·tion (in-sŭf-lā'shŭn). Insuflação. **1.** Ato ou processo de insuflar. **2.** SIN inhalant (3).
  perirenal i., i. perirrenal; técnica obsoleta que consiste na injeção de ar ou de dióxido de carbono em torno dos rins para radiografia das glândulas supra-renais.
  peritoneal i., i. peritoneal; introdução de um gás, geralmente dióxido de carbono, na cavidade peritoneal para facilitar procedimentos laparoendoscópicos.

in·suf·fla·tor (in'sŭf-lā-ter). Insuflador; instrumento utilizado na insuflação.

in·su·la, gen. e pl. **in·su·lae** (in'soo-lă, -lē) [TA]. Ínsula, ilha. **1** [TA]. Região oval do córtex cerebral que recobre a cápsula externa, lateralmente ao núcleo lenticular, mergulhada na profundidade da fissura lateral do cérebro (fissura de Sylvius), separada dos opérculos adjacentes pelo sulco circular da ínsula. SIN insular area, insular cortex, island of Reil. **2.** SIN island. **3.** Qualquer corpo circunscrito ou placa na pele. [L. ilha]
  Haller i., i. de Haller; duplicação do ducto torácico durante parte de seu trajeto através do tórax. SIN Haller anulus.

in·su·lar (in'soo-lăr). Insular; relativo a qualquer ínsula, especialmente a ínsula de Reil.

in·su·late (in'sŭ-lāt). Isolar; impedir a passagem de energia elétrica ou radiante pela interposição de uma substância não-condutora. [L. *insulatus,* feito como uma ilha]

in·su·la·tion (in-sŭ-lā'shŭn). Isolamento. **1.** Ato de isolar. **2.** A substância não-condutora utilizada para essa finalidade. **3.** Estado de ser isolado.

in·su·la·tor (in'sŭ-lā-ter). Isolador; substância não-condutora utilizada para insulação ou isolamento.

in·su·lin (in'sŭ-lin). Insulina; hormônio polipeptídico, secretado pelas células beta das ilhotas de Langerhans, que promove a utilização da glicose, a síntese de proteínas e a formação e o armazenamento de lipídios neutros; disponível em várias apresentações, incluindo insulina humana obtida por engenharia genética, que atualmente é a forma preferida; utilizada por via parenteral no tratamento do diabetes melito. [L. *insula,* ilha + -in]
  biphasic i., i. bifásica; o princípio antidiabético específico do pâncreas do boi numa solução daquele do pâncreas do corpo.
  globin i., i. globina. SIN regular i.
  globin zinc i., i. globina zinco; solução estéril de insulina modificada pela adição de cloreto de zinco e globina; contém 100 unidades por ml; a duração de ação é de cerca de 18 horas.
  human i., i. humana; proteína que tem a estrutura normal da insulina produzida pelo pâncreas humano, preparada por técnicas de DNA recombinante e por processos semi-sintéticos.
  immunoreactive i., i. imunorreativa; porção da insulina no sangue medida por métodos imunoquímicos para o hormônio; pressupõe-se que representa a fração livre (não-ligada) e biologicamente ativa da insulina sanguínea total.
  isophane i., i. isófana; forma modificada de insulina composta de insulina, protamina e zinco; preparação de ação intermediária utilizada para o tratamento do diabetes melito. SIN NPH i.
  lente i., i. lenta. SIN insulin zinc *suspension.*

  lispro i., i. lispro; versão modificada da insulina humana natural, sintetizada por uma cepa geneticamente programada de *Escherichia coli* não-patogênica, em que são transpostos os aminoácidos lisina (Lys) e prolina (Pro) próximo à extremidade da cadeia B. Essa alteração química produz uma insulina com início de ação muito mais rápido, que atinge seu efeito máximo antes da insulina regular. [Lys + Pro]

  A insulina lispro, introduzida em 1996, tem o mesmo peso molecular e as mesmas funções bioquímicas do hormônio natural; quando adminis-

insulina (efeitos metabólicos)			
alteração metabólica	efeito	mecanismo	principal órgão
1. transporte de glicose	+	desconhecido	músculos, tecido adiposo
2. transporte de aminoácidos	+	desconhecido	músculos, tecido adiposo
3. transporte de potássio	+	desconhecido; algumas vezes em conjunção com o transporte de glicose	fígado, músculos
4. oxidação da glicose	+	aumento do transporte da glicose para as células	músculos, tecido adiposo
5. síntese de glicogênio	+	aumento do transporte de glicose para as células; ativação da glicogênio sintetase através de desfosforilação da enzima	músculos, fígado
6. síntese de ácidos graxos	+	como em 4; além disso, redução da acil-CoA, aumento da acetil-CoA a partir da glicose, resultante da ativação da piruvato desidrogenase, liberação de acetil-CoA carboxilase	tecido adiposo, fígado
7. síntese de lipídios	+	como em 4; além disso, produção de α-glicerofosfato a partir da glicose	tecido adiposo, fígado, músculos
8. síntese de proteínas	+	ativação dos ribossomas (tradução do RNA mensageiro)	músculos, fibroblastos
9. lipólise	−	antagonista dos hormônios lipolíticos; inibição da adenilato ciclase	tecido adiposo, fígado
10. cetogênese	−	inibição da produção de ácidos graxos através de antilipólise (ver 9)	fígado
11. gliconeogênese e glicogenólise	−	inibição da liberação de glicose estimulada pelo glucagon; inibição da adenilato ciclase	fígado
12. proteólise	−	desconhecido; inibição da produção de uréia no fígado através da produção diminuída de aminoácidos	fígado, músculo

trada por via intravenosa, seus efeitos são praticamente indistinguíveis daqueles da insulina regular. Entretanto, quando injetada por via subcutânea, atinge seu nível sérico máximo em 30–90 minutos, em comparação com 50–120 minutos para a insulina regular; além disso, possui meia-vida mais curta. Apesar de a indicação original da insulina lispro ter sido o seu uso como insulina pré-prandial de ação rápida, a experiência clínica mostrou que ela melhora os níveis pós-prandiais de glicose, diminui a incidência de hipoglicemia grave e hipoglicemia noturna e melhora o controle da glicose quando medida pela hemoglobina glicosilada, ao se efetuarem ajustes apropriados para o nível de insulina basal, prandial e durante o exercício físico. Em contraste com outras insulinas, nos EUA a insulina lispro não é disponível sem prescrição médica. Não é recomendada para uso durante a gravidez, visto que seus efeitos sobre o feto ainda não foram avaliados.

NPH i., i. NPH. SIN isophane i. [*Neutral Protamine Hagedorn*]
protamine zinc i., i. protamina-zinco; insulina modificada pela adição de protamina e cloreto de zinco; contém 100 unidades por ml.
regular i., i. regular; forma de insulina de ação rápida, consistindo numa solução clara que pode ser administrada por via intravenosa ou subcutânea; pode ser misturada com formas de insulina de ação mais prolongada para maior duração de seus efeitos. O início dos efeitos é observado em 1/2 a 1 hora; os efeitos máximos ocorrem em 2 a 3 horas, e a duração dos efeitos é de cerca de 5 a 7 horas. SIN globin i.
semilente i., i. semilenta. SIN prompt insulin zinc *suspension.*
ultralente i., i. ultralenta; forma de insulina zíncica precipitada em suspensão, cujo tamanho das partículas é grande, tornando lenta a sua liberação na corrente sanguínea após injeção subcutânea; pode ser misturada com outras insulinas apresentando partículas de diferentes tamanhos para obter diferentes durações de atividade. Pode derivar de insulina suína, bovina ou humana obtida por engenharia genética.
in·su·li·ne·mia (in′sū-li-nē′mē-ă). Insulinemia; literalmente, insulina no sangue circulante; em geral, indica concentrações anormalmente grandes de insulina no sangue circulante. [insulina + G *haima,* sangue]
in·su·lin·o·gen·e·sis (in′sū-lin-ō-jen′ĕ-sis). Insulinogênese; produção de insulina. [insulina + G. *genesis,* produção]
in·su·lin·o·gen·ic, in·su·lo·gen·ic (in′sū-lin-ō-jen′ik, in′sū-lō-jen′ik). Insulinogênico; relativo à insulinogênese.
in·su·li·no·ma (in′sū-li-nō′mă). Insulinoma; adenoma de células das ilhotas que secreta insulina.
in·su·li·tis (in′sū-lī′tis). Insulite; inflamação das ilhotas de Langerhans, com infiltração linfocítica, que pode resultar de infecção viral e constituir a lesão inicial do diabetes melito insulino-dependente. [L. *insula,* ilha + *-itis,* inflamação]
in·sult (in′sŭlt). Insulto; agressão, lesão, ataque ou traumatismo. [LL. *insultus,* de L. *insulto,* saltar sobre]
insurance. Seguro.
fee-for-service i., seguro de honorários; cobertura que reembolsa participantes e profissionais após apreciação de um pedido. Os participantes têm poucas restrições ou nenhuma no que concerne aos hospitais ou médicos escolhidos.
in·sus·cep·ti·bil·i·ty (in′sŭ-sep′ti-bil′i-tē). Insuscetibilidade. SIN immunity. [L. *suscipio,* pp. *-ceptus,* tomar sobre si, de *sub,* sob + *capio,* tomar]
int. cib. Abreviatura do L. *inter cibos,* entre as refeições.
in·te·gral (int′ĕ-gral). Integral. **1.** Constituinte. **2.** Integrado. **3.** VER integration (3).
in·te·gra·tion (in-tĕ-grā′shŭn). Integração. **1.** Estado de estar combinado ou o processo de combinação em um todo completo e harmonioso. **2.** Em fisiologia, processo de construir, como, p. ex., por acreção, anabolismo, etc. **3.** Em matemática, processo de avaliar uma função a partir de seu diferencial. **4.** Em biologia molecular, evento de recombinação no qual é inserido um elemento genético. [L. *integro,* pp. *-atus,* tornar completo, de *integer,* completo, um todo]
personality i., i. da personalidade; organização efetiva de experiências, dados e capacidades emocionais antigas e recentes na personalidade; a organização harmoniosa da personalidade.
in·te·grins (in-te′grinz). Integrinas; família de glicoproteínas da membrana celular que consistem em heterodímeros constituídos de subunidades de cadeias α e β. Atuam como receptores glicoproteicos da matriz extracelular, envolvidos na adesão celular, como, p. ex., a mediação da adesão dos neutrófilos às células endoteliais. [L. *integer,* integral, intacto, de *in-* + *tango,* tocar + *-in*]
in·teg·ri·ty (in-teg′ri-tē). Integridade; perfeição ou inteireza de uma estrutura; condição perfeita ou intacta.
marginal i. of amalgam, i. marginal de amálgama; capacidade de uma restauração de amálgama dentário de manter a sua forma marginal original nas margens da superfície da cavidade.
in·teg·u·ment (in-teg′ū-ment) [TA]. Integumento, tegumento. **1.** A membrana que envolve o corpo; inclui, além da epiderme e da derme, todos os de-

rivados da epiderme, como, p. ex., pêlos, unhas, glândulas sudoríparas e sebáceas e glândulas mamárias. **2.** Revestimento externo, cápsula ou cobertura de qualquer corpo ou parte. SIN tegument (2). SIN integumentum commune [TA], integumentary system, tegument (1). [L. *integumentum*, revestimento, cobertura, de *intego*, cobrir]

in·teg·u·men·ta·ry (in-teg-ū-men′tă-rē). Integumentar, tegumentar; relativo ao integumento. VER TAMBÉM cutaneous, dermal.

in·teg·u·men·tum com·mune (in-teg-ū-men′tŭm kō-moo′nē) [TA]. Integumento comum. SIN integument.

in·tel·lec·tu·al·i·za·tion (in-te-lek′choo-ăl-i-zā′shŭn). Intelectualização; mecanismo de defesa inconsciente pelo qual o indivíduo utiliza o raciocínio, a lógica, a atenção e a verbalização de minúcias intelectuais numa tentativa de evitar o confronto com um impulso, afeto ou situação interpessoal objetável ou desagradável. [L. *intellectus*, percepção, discernimento]

in·tel·li·gence (in-tel′i-jens). Inteligência. **1.** Capacidade conjunta de um indivíduo para agir propositadamente, pensar racionalmente e lidar efetivamente com o ambiente, sobretudo com relação à extensão de sua efetividade percebida em enfrentar desafios. **2.** Em psicologia, uma posição relativa do indivíduo em dois índices quantitativos, a inteligência medida e a efetividade do comportamento adaptativo; um índice quantitativo ou índice semelhante em ambos constitui a definição operacional de inteligência. [L. *intelligentia*]
abstract i., i. abstrata; capacidade de compreender e manejar idéias abstratas e símbolos.
artificial i., i. artificial. **(1)** Ramo da ciência da computação em que são feitas tentativas de reproduzir funções intelectuais humanas. Uma aplicação consiste no desenvolvimento de programas computadorizados para diagnóstico. Esses programas baseiam-se, com freqüência, na análise epidemiológica dos dados em grande número de prontuários; **(2)** máquina que reproduz as funções intelectuais humanas, embora até agora nenhuma máquina (isto é, computador) tenha a capacidade de preencher essa função.
measured i., i. medida; inteligência que pode ser classificada em relação a uma idade ou índice quantitativo de grupo de indivíduos semelhantes pelo uso de escores em provas de inteligência.
mechanical i., i. mecânica; capacidade de compreender e manejar mecanismos técnicos.
social i., i. social; capacidade de compreender e manejar relações humanas e questões sociais.

in·tem·per·ance (in-tem′per-ăns). Intemperança; falta de autocontrole adequado, referindo-se, em geral, ao uso de bebidas alcoólicas. Cf. incontinence (2). [L. *intemperantia*, de *in-*, neg. + *temperantia*, moderação]

in·ten·si·ty (in-ten′si-tē). Intensidade. **1.** Tensão pronunciada; grande atividade; termo utilizado com freqüência para indicar simplesmente uma medida do grau ou quantidade de alguma qualidade. **2.** Magnitude do fluxo de energia, força de campo ou força. [L. *in-tendo*, pp. *-tensus*, distender]
luminous i. (I), i. luminosa; fluxo luminoso por unidade de ângulo sólido em determinada direção. SIN candle-power, radiant i.
performance i., i. de desempenho; melhora no reconhecimento de palavras faladas que ocorre com o aumento da intensidade do som.
radiant i. (I), i. radiante. SIN luminous i.
i. of sound, i. do som; medida objetiva da amplitude de vibração de uma onda sonora.

in·ten·sive (in-ten′siv). Intensivo; relativo a, ou caracterizado por, intensidade; indica uma forma de tratamento por meio de doses muito grandes ou de substâncias que possuem grande força ou atividade.

in·ten·tion (in-ten′shŭn). Intenção. **1.** Objetivo. **2.** Em cirurgia, processo ou operação. [L. *intentio*, distensão; intenção]

△ **inter-**. Inter-. Entre, no meio de. [L. *inter*, entre]

in·ter·ac·i·nar (in-ter-as′i-nar). Interacinar. SIN interacinous.

in·ter·ac·i·nous (in-ter-as′i-nŭs). Interacinar; entre os ácinos de uma glândula. SIN interacinar.

in·ter·ac·tion (int′er-ak′shŭn). Interação. **1.** Ação recíproca entre duas entidades no ambiente comum, como, p. ex., i. química, i. ecológica, i. social, etc. **2.** Efeitos resultantes da cooperação de duas entidades que não seriam observados com ambas as entidades isoladas. **3.** Em estatística, farmacologia e genética quantitativa, fenômeno segundo o qual os efeitos combinados de duas causas diferem da soma dos efeitos separados (como no sinergismo e no antagonismo). **4.** Operação independente de duas ou mais causas para produzir ou impedir um efeito. **5.** Em estatística, necessidade de um termo de produtos num modelo linear. **6.** Transferência de energia entre partículas elementares ou entre campos de energia.
apolar i., i. apolar. SIN hydrophobic i.
hydrophobic i., i. hidrofóbica; interação entre substituintes sem carga em diferentes moléculas sem compartilhar elétrons ou prótons; i. impulsionada por entropia. SIN apolar i.

in·ter·al·ve·o·lar (in′ter-al-vē′ō-lăr). Interalveolar; entre quaisquer alvéolos, referindo-se especialmente aos alvéolos dos pulmões.

in·ter·an·nu·lar (in-ter-an′ū-lăr). Interanular; entre qualquer de duas estruturas ou constrições anulares. [inter- + L. *anulus*, anel]

in·ter·arch (in′ter-arch). Distância interarco. VER interarch *distance*.

in·ter·ar·tic·u·lar (in-ter-ar-tik′ū-lăr). Interarticular. **1.** Entre duas articulações. Cf. intra-articular. **2.** Entre duas superfícies articulares. [inter- + L. *articulus*, articulação]

in·ter·ar·y·te·noid (in′ter-ăr′i-tē′noyd). Interaritenóide; entre as cartilagens aritenóides.

in·ter·as·ter·ic (in-ter-ă-stē′rik). Interastérico; entre dois astérios. VER asterion.

in·ter·a·tri·al (in-ter-ā′trē-ăl). Interatrial; entre os átrios do coração. SIN interauricular (1).

in·ter·au·ral (in-ter-aw′ral). Interaural; relativo a diferenças entre as orelhas, particularmente eventos temporais que ocorrem nas orelhas ou delas surgem.

in·ter·au·ric·u·lar (in′ter-aw-rik′ū-lăr). Interauricular. **1.** SIN interatrial. **2.** Entre as aurículas ou pavilhões das orelhas.

in·ter·body (in′ter-bod′ē). Intercorporal; entre os corpos de duas vértebras adjacentes.

in·ter·ca·dence (in-ter-kā′dens). Intercadência; ocorrência de batimento cardíaco suplementar entre dois batimentos regulares. [inter- + L. *cado*, pr. p. *cadens* (*-ent-*), cair]

in·ter·ca·dent (in-ter-kā′dent). Intercadente; que apresenta ritmo irregular, caracterizado por intercadência.

in·ter·ca·lary (in-ter′kă-ler-ē, in-ter-kal′er-ē). Intercalar. **1.** Que ocorre entre dois outros; como no traçado do pulso, traço ascendente interposto entre dois batimentos normais. **2.** Nos fungos, localizado numa hifa ou entre segmentos de hifa, e não em sua terminação. [L. *intercalarius*, relativo a uma inserção]

in·ter·ca·lat·ed (in-ter′kă-lā-ted). Intercalado; interposto; inserido entre dois outros. [L. *intercalatus*]

in·ter·ca·la·tion (in′ter-kă′lā-shun). Intercalação; processo de inserção entre duas outras entidades; p. ex., inserção de um corante ou droga entre bases "empilhadas" no DNA.

in·ter·can·a·lic·u·lar (in-ter-kan-ă-lik′ū-lăr). Intercanalicular; entre canalículos.

in·ter·cap·il·lary (in′ter-kap′i-lā-rē). Intercapilar; entre, ou no meio de, vasos capilares.

in·ter·ca·rot·ic, in·ter·ca·rot·id (in-ter-ka-rot′ik, -id). Intercarotídeo; entre as artérias carótidas interna e externa.

in·ter·car·pal (in-ter-kar′păl). Intercarpal; entre os carpos.

in·ter·car·ti·lag·i·nous (in′ter-kar-ti-laj′i-nŭs). Intercartilaginoso; entre cartilagens ou conectando-as. SIN interchondral.

in·ter·cav·ern·ous (in′ter-kav′er-nŭs). Intercavernoso; entre duas cavidades.

in·ter·cel·lu·lar (in-ter-sel′ū-lăr). Intercelular; situado entre células ou no meio delas.

in·ter·cen·tral (in-ter-sen′trăl). Intercentral; que conecta ou está localizado entre dois ou mais centros.

in·ter·ce·re·bral (in′ter-ser′ē-brăl). Intercerebral; entre os hemisférios cerebrais.

in·ter·chon·dral (in-ter-kon′drăl). Intercondral. SIN intercartilaginous. [inter- + L. *chondros*, cartilagem]

in·ter·cil·i·um (in-ter-sil′ē-ŭm). Intercílio. SIN glabella. [inter- + L. *cilium*, pálpebra]

in·ter·cla·vic·u·lar (in-ter-kla-vik′ū-lăr). Interclavicular; entre ou conectando as clavículas.

in·ter·coc·cyg·e·al (in′ter-kok-sij′ē-ăl). Intercoccígeo; situado entre segmentos não-fundidos do cóccix.

in·ter·co·lum·nar (in-ter-kō-lŭm′nar). Intercolunar; entre quaisquer duas colunas, como as colunas do anel inguinal superficial.

in·ter·con·dy·lar, (in·ter·con·dyl·ic, in·ter·con·dy·loid) (in-ter-kon′di-lăr, -kon-dil′ik, -kon′di-loyd). Intercondilar; entre dois côndilos.

in·ter·con·ver·sion (in-ter-kon-ver′shun). Interconversão; alteração mútua da natureza física ou química de uma substância ou entidade; p. ex., interconversão de compostos químicos ou produtos alimentares.
enzyme i., i. enzimática; transformação reversível de uma forma enzimática em outra, tipicamente com alteração na atividade ou regulação enzimática, como, p. ex., fosforilação de uma glicogênio fosforilase.

in·ter·cos·tal (in-ter-kos′tăl). Intercostal; entre as costelas. [inter- + L. *costa*, costela]

in·ter·cos·to·hu·mer·al (in′ter-kos′tō-hū′mer-ăl). Intercostoumeral; relativo a um espaço intercostal e ao braço. VER intercostobrachial *nerves*, em *nerve*.

in·ter·cos·to·hu·mer·a·lis (in-ter-kos′tō-hū-mer-ā′lis). Intercostoumeral. VER intercostobrachial *nerves*, em *nerve*.

in·ter·course (in′ter-kōrs). Intercurso; comunicação ou relação entre pessoas. [L. *intercursus*, corrida entre]

sexual i., i. sexual. SIN coitus.

in·ter·cri·co·thy·rot·o·my (in-ter-krī′kō-thī-rot′ō-mē). Intercricotireotomia. SIN cricothyrotomy.

in·ter·crines (in′ter-krīnz). Intercrinas. SIN chemokines. [inter- + G. *krinō*, separar, secretar]

in·ter·cris·tal (in-ter-kris′tăl). Intercristal; entre duas cristas, como entre as cristas do ílio, aplicado a uma das medidas pélvicas.

in·ter·cross (in′ter-kros). Cruzamento; acasalamento entre dois indivíduos heterozigotos em um *locus* ou *loci* específicos.

in·ter·cru·ral (in-ter-kroo′răl). Intercrural; entre dois ramos; p. ex., os pedículos cerebrais do cérebro, etc.

in·ter·cur·rent (in-ter-ker′ent). Intercorrente; interveniente; refere-se a uma doença que acomete um indivíduo já afetado por outra doença. [inter- + L. *curro,* pr. p. *currens* (-*ent*-), correr]

in·ter·cus·pa·tion (in′ter-kŭs-pā′shŭn). Intercuspidiano. **1.** Relação entre cúspide e fossa dos dentes posteriores maxilares e mandibulares entre si. **2.** Encaixe das cúspides de dentes opostos. SIN interdigitation (4). SIN intercusping.

in·ter·cusp·ing (in-ter-kŭs′ping). Intercúspide. SIN intercuspation. [L. *inter*, entre, mutuamente + cúspide]

in·ter·cu·ta·ne·o·mu·cous (in′ter-kū-tā′nē-ō-mū′kŭs). Intercutaneomucoso; entre a pele e a mucosa, como na bochecha, lábio ou na borda mucocutânea dos lábios ou do ânus.

in·ter·de·fer·en·tial (in-ter-def-er-en′shăl). Interdeferencial; entre os ductos deferentes.

in·ter·den·tal (in-ter-den′tăl). Interdental. **1.** Entre os dentes. **2.** Indica a relação entre as superfícies proximais dentes da mesma arcada. [inter- + L. *dens,* dente]

in·ter·den·ti·um (in-ter-den′shē-ŭm). Interdentário; intervalo entre dois dentes contíguos.

in·ter·dig·it (in-ter-dij′it). Interdígito; parte da mão ou do pé localizada entre dois dedos adjacentes.

in·ter·dig·i·tal (in-ter-dij′i-tăl). Interdigital; entre os dedos das mãos ou dos pés.

in·ter·dig·i·ta·tion (in′ter-dij-i-tā′shŭn). Interdigitação. **1.** Encaixe mútuo de processos denteados ou lingüiformes. **2.** Os processos assim engatados. **3.** Dobras ou pregas de membranas celulares ou plasmáticas adjacentes. **4.** SIN intercuspation (2). [inter- + L. *digitus,* dedo]

in·ter·dis·ci·pli·nary (in-ter-dis′i-pli-năr-ē). Interdisciplinar; refere-se a uma superposição de interesses de diferentes campos da medicina e da ciência. [inter- + L. *disciplina,* instrução, ensino]

in·ter·face (in′ter-fās). Interface. **1.** Superfície que forma um limite comum entre dois corpos. **2.** Limite entre regiões que diferem quanto à radiopacidade e a suas propriedades acústicas ou de ressonância magnética; projeção da interface entre tecidos com diferentes propriedades numa imagem.
 crystalline i., i. cristalina; em odontologia, limite entre cristais adjacentes.
 dermoepidermal i., i. dermoepidérmica; linha de encontro da derme com a epiderme.
 metal i., i. metálica; em odontologia, limite entre o metal e a solda não-solvente, ou entre o metal e o óxido da superfície.
 structural i., i. estrutural; em odontologia, limite entre o dente e o material de restauração.

in·ter·fa·cial (in-ter-fā′shăl). Interfacial; relativo a uma interface.

in·ter·fas·cic·u·lar (in′ter-fă-sik′ū-lăr). Interfascicular; entre fascículos.

in·ter·fem·o·ral (in-ter-fem′ō-răl). Interfemoral; entre as coxas.

in·ter·fer·ence (in-ter-fēr′ens). Interferência. **1.** Chegada simultânea de ondas em vários meios, de modo que as cristas de uma correspondem às depressões da outra, resultando em neutralização mútua, ou de modo que as cristas das duas ondas correspondem, aumentando, assim, as excursões de ambas as ondas. **2.** Colisão no miocárdio de duas ondas de excitação na junção dos territórios controlados por cada uma, conforme observado na dissociação AV. **3.** Também na dissociação AV, o distúrbio do ritmo regular dos ventrículos por um impulso conduzido a partir dos átrios, como, p. ex., por uma captura ventricular (batimento de interferência). **4.** Condição em que a infecção de uma célula por um vírus impede a superinfecção por outro vírus, ou que a superinfecção impede os efeitos resultantes da infecção por qualquer vírus isoladamente, embora ambos os vírus persistam. [inter- + L. *ferio,* bater]
 bacterial i., i. bacteriana; condição em que a colonização por uma cepa bacteriana impede a colonização por outra cepa.
 cuspal i., i. das cúspides. SIN deflective occlusal *contact.*

in·ter·fer·om·e·ter (in′ter-fe-rom′ē-ter). Interferômetro; instrumento para medir distâncias ou movimentos diminutos através da interferência de ondas luminosas assim produzidas. [interfere + G. *metron,* medida]
 electron i., i. eletrônico; interferômetro que emprega um feixe de elétrons em lugar de um feixe luminoso.

in·ter·fer·o·me·try (in′ter-fe-rom′e-trē). Interferometria; medida de distâncias ou movimentos diminutos pela interação de ondas de energia eletromagnética.
 electron i., i. eletrônica; interferometria em que se utiliza um feixe de elétrons em lugar de um feixe luminoso.

in·ter·fer·on (IFN) (in-ter-fēr′on). Interferon; classe de pequenas citocinas proteicas e glicoproteicas (15–28 kD), produzidas pelas células T, pelos fibroblastos e por outras células em resposta a infecções virais e outros estímulos biológicos e sintéticos. Os interferons ligam-se a receptores específicos nas membranas celulares; seus efeitos consistem em indução de enzimas, supressão da proliferação celular, inibição da proliferação viral, intensificação da atividade fagocítica dos macrófagos e aumento da atividade citotóxica dos linfócitos T. Os interferons são divididos em cinco grandes classes (alfa, beta, gama, tau e ômega) e várias subclasses (indicadas por algarismos arábicos e letras) com base nas propriedades físico-químicas, células de origem, modo de indução e reações humorais. [interfere + -on]

 A descoberta, em 1957, de que a infecção viral de células humanas induz a formação de agentes antivirais naturais fez surgir uma esperança de que essas substâncias pudessem ter potencial terapêutico. Os estudos preliminares mostraram que, ao contrário dos anticorpos, os interferons mostram-se ativos contra uma ampla variedade de vírus; entretanto, os progressos na aplicação desse conhecimento à medicina humana foram retardados devido à dificuldade em produzir interferons em quantidades suficientes. Na década de 80, o desenvolvimento da tecnologia do DNA recombinante superou esse obstáculo, e, hoje em dia, os interferons são importantes no tratamento não apenas das infecções virais, como também de certos processos malignos. Os interferons comercialmente disponíveis são produzidos por colônias geneticamente alteradas de *Escherichia coli* ou de células do ovário de *hamsters* chineses, ou são induzidos por infecção viral controlada em misturas de leucócitos humanos. Os interferons alfa têm mostrado aplicação mais ampla em medicina. (A designação alfa é utilizada para referir-se a interferons de ocorrência natural; de acordo com as convenções internacionais para nomes genéricos de drogas, a designação alfa aparece em nomes de formulações farmacêuticas.) Os interferons alfa são utilizados no tratamento das hepatites B e C crônicas, leucemia de células pilosas, leucemia mielógena crônica, sarcoma de Kaposi relacionado à AIDS/SIDA, melanoma maligno, condiloma acuminado e papilomatose respiratória recorrente por papilomavírus humano e hemangiomatose infantil. Em cerca de 50% dos pacientes com hepatite B crônica tratados com interferon-alfa, ocorre desaparecimento do antígeno B_e da hepatite (HB$_e$Ag), bem como normalização da alanina aminotransferase. O índice de resposta na hepatite C crônica é menor (15–25%), porém são obtidos melhores resultados com o uso de terapia mais agressiva (administração diária, em lugar de duas vezes por semana) e sua manutenção por mais tempo (12 meses no mínimo). As formulações modificadas de interferon-alfa conjugado com polietilenoglicol (PEG), que produziram resultados promissores na hepatite C com administração de uma dose uma vez por semana, encontram-se em estudos de fase III. Os interferons beta reduzem as recidivas clínicas e a progressão da lesão da mielina na esclerose múltipla. O interferon gama mostra-se eficaz para retardar as alterações teciduais na osteopetrose e na esclerodemia sistêmica, bem como na redução da freqüência e gravidade de infecções na doença granulomatosa crônica. Os interferons são administrados por via parenteral (intravenosa, intramuscular, subcutânea, intranasal, intratecal ou intralesional), podendo ser necessárias várias semanas de tratamento para que se possa observar uma resposta clínica. Mais de 50% dos pacientes apresentam uma síndrome gripal de fadiga, mialgia e artralgia. Os efeitos colaterais gastrointestinais e do SNC também são comuns, e pode ocorrer mielossupressão com tratamento prolongado.

usos clínicos de interferons aprovados pela FDA	
alfa	
leucemia de células pilosas	hepatite B
condiloma acuminado	hepatite C
sarcoma de Kaposi	melanoma maligno (pós-cirúrgico)
beta	**gama**
esclerose múltipla	doença granulomatosa crônica

 i. alfa 2b, i. alfa 2b; proteína hidrossolúvel (PM de 19.271) secretada por células infectadas por vírus; utilizado no tratamento de leucemia de células pilosas, melanoma maligno, condiloma acuminado, sarcoma de Kaposi relacionado à AIDS/SIDA e hepatite C crônica.

i. alpha (IFN-α), i. alfa (IFN-α); o principal interferon produzido por leucócitos induzidos por vírus; existem diferentes subtipos que são elaborados por leucócitos em resposta à infecção viral ou estimulação com RNA de duplo filamento. Existem 14 genes no braço curto do cromossoma 9 que codificam essas substâncias nos seres humanos. O IFN-α-2A e -2B são produtos proteicos produzidos por técnicas de DNA recombinante; utilizados como agentes antineoplásicos. SIN leukocyte i.
antigen i., i. antigênico. SIN i. gamma.
i. beta (IFN-β), i. beta (IFN-β); interferon elaborado por fibroblastos e micrófagos em resposta aos mesmos estímulos que induzem o i. alfa; apenas um gene codifica esse interferon. SIN fibroblast i.
i. beta 1b, i. beta 1b; proteína purificada contendo 165 aminoácidos (PM de aproximadamente 18.500), com efeitos antivirais e imunomoduladores, utilizada no tratamento da esclerose múltipla em recidiva-remissão para diminuir a freqüência de exacerbações clínicas.
fibroblast i., i. de fibroblastos. SIN i. beta.
i. gamma (IFN-γ), i. gama (IFN-γ); interferon elaborado por linfócitos T em resposta a um antígeno específico ou estimulação mitogênica; apenas um gene codifica o interferon γ. O interferon γ comporta-se como um modificador da resposta biológica e é altamente imunorregulador. SIN antigen i., immune i.
immune i., i. imune. SIN i. gamma.
leukocyte i., i. leucocitário. SIN i. alpha.
i. -omega, i. ômega; forma de interferon conhecido como interferon-alfa-2.
i. -tau, i. tau; interferon secretado por conceptos bovinos, com potente atividade anti-retroviral; em uso experimental. SIN trophoblast i., trophoblastin.
trophoblast i., i. trofoblástico. SIN i.-tau.
type I i., i. tipo I; interferons antivirais, incluindo o interferon-alfa e o interferon-beta.
type II i., i. tipo II; interferon imune, interferon-gama.
in·ter·fer·on-β2. Interferon-β2. SIN interleukin-6.
in·ter·fi·bril·lar, in·ter·fi·bril·lary (in′ter-fī′bri-lăr, -fī′bri-lār-ē; -fi-bril′ăr) Interfibrilar; entre as fibrilas.
in·ter·fi·brous (in-ter-fī′brŭs). Interfibroso; entre fibras.
in·ter·fil·a·men·tous (in′ter-fil-ă-men′tŭs). Interfilamentoso; entre filamentos.
in·ter·fron·tal (in-ter-fron′tăl). Interfrontal; entre as metades não-fundidas do osso frontal; indica uma sutura persistente presente nesse local (anormal).
in·ter·gan·gli·on·ic (in′ter-gang′lē-on′ik). Interganglionar; entre gânglios ou unindo-os.
in·ter·gem·mal (in′ter-jem′ăl). Interpapilar, interbulbar; entre dois ou mais corpos semelhantes a botões ou bulbos, como os botões ou papilas gustativas; refere-se, especialmente, a uma terminação nervosa entre dois bulbos terminais. [inter- + L. *gemma*, botão]
in·ter·ge·nal (in-ter-jēn′al). Intergênico; entre dois genes.
in·ter·glob·u·lar (in-ter-glob′u-lăr). Interglobular; entre glóbulos.
in·ter·glu·te·al (in-ter-gloo′tē-ăl). Interglúteo; entre as nádegas. [inter- + G. *gloutos*, nádega]
in·ter·go·ni·al (in-ter-gō′nē-ăl). Intergonial; entre dois gônios VER gonion. [inter- + G. *gōnia*, ângulo]
in·ter·gy·ral (in-ter-jī′răl). Intergiral; entre os giros ou circunvoluções do cérebro.
in·ter·hem·i·ce·re·bral (in′ter-hem′ē-ser′ē-brăl). Inter-hemisférico; entre os hemisférios cerebrais.
in·ter·ic·tal (in-ter-ik′tăl). Interictal; refere-se ao período entre convulsões. [inter- + L. *ictus*, choque]
in·te·ri·or (in-tēr′ē-ŏr). Interior; relativo ao lado interno; situado dentro.
in·ter·is·chi·ad·ic (in-ter-is-kē-ad′ik). Interisquiático; entre os dois ísquios; refere-se, especialmente, à posição entre as duas tuberosidades dos ísquios. SIN interisciatic.
in·ter·ki·ne·sis (in′ter-ki-nē′sis). Intercinese; período entre a primeira e a segunda divisão da meiose; comparável à interfase da mitose. [inter- + G. *kinēsis*, movimento]
in·ter·la·mel·lar (in′ter-lă-mel′ăr, -lam′ē-lăr). Interlamelar; entre lamelas.
in·ter·leukin. Interleucina; nome dado a um grupo de citocinas multifuncionais uma vez conhecida a sua estrutura de aminoácidos. São sintetizadas por linfócitos, monócitos, macrófagos e por algumas outras células. VER lymphokine, cytokine. [inter- + *leukocyte* + -in]
recombinant human i. 11, i. humana recombinante 11, droga que aumenta o número de plaquetas sanguíneas; útil para melhorar a trombocitopenia grave resultante de quimioterapia do câncer. SIN rhIL-11.
in·ter·leu·kin-1 (IL-1) (in-ter-loo′kin). Interleucina-1 (IL-1); citocina derivada primariamente de fagócitos mononucleares, que intensifica a proliferação de células T auxiliares e o crescimento e a diferenciação de células B. Quando em quantidades maiores, atua como mediador da inflamação, penetrando na corrente sanguínea e causando febre, induzindo à síntese de proteínas de fase aguda e iniciando a degradação metabólica. Existem duas formas distintas de IL-1: α e β, ambas as quais desempenham as mesmas funções, porém representam proteínas diferentes.
in·ter·leu·kin-2 (IL-2). Interleucina-2 (IL-2); citocina derivada de linfócitos T auxiliares que causa proliferação dos linfócitos T e linfócitos B ativados.
in·ter·leu·kin-3 (IL-3). Interleucina-3 (IL-3); citocina derivada de linfócitos CD4+ ativados, fibroblastos e células endoteliais que aumenta a produção de monócitos. Atua na hematopoese controlando a produção e a diferenciação dos granulócitos. SIN multicolony-stimulating factor.
in·ter·leu·kin-4 (IL-4). Interleucina-4 (IL-4); citocina derivada de linfócitos T4 que induz a diferenciação de linfócitos B. Promove a mudança de classe das Ig. Estimula a biossíntese de DNA. SIN B cell differentiating factor.
in·ter·leu·kin-5 (IL-5). Interleucina-5 (IL-5); citocina derivada de linfócitos T que induz a ativação dos linfócitos B e a diferenciação dos eosinófilos.
in·ter·leu·kin-6 (IL-6). Interleucina-6 (IL-6); citocina derivada de macrófagos e de células endoteliais que aumenta a síntese e a secreção de imunoglobulinas por linfócitos B; além disso, induz a formação de proteínas de fase aguda. Nos hepatócitos, induz reagentes de fase aguda. SIN B cell stimulatory factor 2, interferon-β2.
in·ter·leu·kin-7 (IL-7). Interleucina-7 (IL-7); citocina derivada de células da medula óssea que causa a proliferação de linfócitos B e T.
in·ter·leu·kin-8 (IL-8). Interleucina-8 (IL-8); citocina (quimiocina) derivada de células endoteliais, fibroblastos, ceratinócitos, macrófagos e monócitos que induz a quimiotaxia de neutrófilos e linfócitos T. SIN anionic neutrophil-activating peptide, monocyte-derived neutrophil chemotactic factor, neutrophil chemotactant factor, neutrophil-activating factor.
in·ter·leu·kin-9 (IL-9). Interleucina-9 (IL-9); citocina derivada de células T que induz o crescimento e a proliferação de células T IL-2/IL-4-independentes.
in·ter·leu·kin-10 (IL-10). Interleucina-10 (IL-10); citocina derivada de linfócitos T auxiliares (TH$_2$) que inibe a secreção de γ-interferon (IFNγ) e IL-2 por linfócitos T (TH$_1$), bem como a inflamação por células mononucleares.
in·ter·leu·kin-11 (IL-11). Interleucina-11 (IL-11); citocina e fator de crescimento derivado de células do estroma da medula óssea (células endoteliais, macrófagos e pré-adipócitos) que estimula concentrações plasmáticas aumentadas de proteínas de fase aguda e atua como fator de crescimento com múltiplos efeitos hematopoéticos.
in·ter·leu·kin-12 (IL-12). Interleucina-12 (IL-12); citocina derivada de linfócitos B e macrófagos que induz a expressão do gene do γ-interferon (IFNγ) e a IL-2 nos linfócitos T e células NK, além de infra-regular citocinas derivadas de linfócitos TH$_2$.
in·ter·leu·kin-13 (IL-13). Interleucina-13 (IL-13); citocina derivada de linfócitos T auxiliares que inibe a inflamação por células mononucleares e é considerada como modulador das respostas das células B.
in·ter·leu·kin-14 (IL-14). Interleucina-14 (IL-14); citocina derivada de células T que estimula a proliferação de células B e inibe a secreção de Ig.
in·ter·leu·kin-15 (IL-15). Interleucina-15 (IL-15); citocina derivada de células T que estimula a proliferação de células T e a ativação de células NK.
in·ter·leu·kin-16 (IL-16). Interleucina-16 (IL-16); citocina produzida por células T que atua como potente quimioatraente para células T CD4+.
in·ter·leu·kin-17 (IL-17). Interleucina-17 (IL-17); citocina pró-inflamatória produzida por células T.
in·ter·leu·kin-18 (IL-18). Interleucina-18 (IL-18); citocina produzida por macrófagos; potente indutor do interferon-γ por células T e células NK.
in·ter·lo·bar (in-ter-lō′bar). Interlobar; entre os lobos de um órgão ou de outra estrutura.
in·ter·lo·bi·tis (in′ter-lō-bī′tis). Interlobite; inflamação da pleura que separa dois lobos pulmonares.
in·ter·lob·u·lar (in-ter-lob′u-lăr). Interlobular; entre os lóbulos de um órgão.
in·ter·mal·le·o·lar (in-ter-mal-ē′ō-lăr). Intermaleolar; entre os maléolos.
in·ter·mam·ma·ry (in-ter-mam′ă-rē). Intermamário; entre as mamas. [inter- + L. *mamma*, mama]
in·ter·mam·mil·lary (in-ter-mam′i-lā-rē). Intermamilar; entre as mamas; entre os mamilos; indica uma linha traçada entre os dois mamilos. [inter- + L. *mammilla*, mama, mamilo]
in·ter·mar·riage (in-ter-mar′ij). **1.** Casamento entre parentes. **2.** Casamento de pessoas de raças ou culturas diferentes.
in·ter·max·il·la (in-ter-maks-il′ă). Intermaxilar. SIN incisive bone.
in·ter·max·il·lary (in-ter-mak′si-lā-rē). Intermaxilar; entre os maxilares ou ossos do maxilar superior.
in·ter·me·di·ary (in′ter-mē′dē-ăr-ē). Intermediário; que ocorre entre. [L. *in-termedius*, situado entre, de *medius*, meio]
in·ter·me·di·ate (in′ter-mē′dē-it) [TA]. Intermediário. **1.** Entre dois extremos, interposto; interveniente. **2.** Substância formada no decorrer de reações químicas que, em seguida, participa em reações posteriores; essas substâncias, quando aparecem durante as reações envolvidas no metabolismo, são intermediários metabólicos. **3.** Em odontologia, base de cimento. **4.** Elemento ou órgão entre estruturas direita e esquerda (ou lateral e medial). SIN intermedius [TA].

replicative i., i. replicativo; durante a cópia do RNA de um vírus de RNA, o filamento de sentido oposto que serve de modelo para produção do filamento positivo.

in·ter·me·din (in-ter-mē′din). Intermedina. SIN melanotropin.

in·ter·me·di·o·lat·er·al (in-ter-mē′dē-ō-lat′er-ăl). Intermediolateral; intermediário e para um lado, não-central. Termo utilizado especialmente para referir-se à coluna de células intermediolaterais da substância cinzenta da medula espinal, abreviado por IML, a localização de todos os corpos celulares dos nervos simpáticos pré-sinápticos. VER intermediolateral *nucleus*.

in·ter·me·di·us (in-ter-mē′dē-ŭs) [TA]. Intermédio. SIN intermediate (4). [L.]

in·ter·mem·bra·nous (in-ter-mem′brā-nŭs). Intermembranoso; entre membranas.

in·ter·me·nin·ge·al (in′ter-me-nin′jē-ăl). Intermeníngeo; entre as meninges.

in·ter·men·stru·al (in-ter-men′stroo-ăl). Intermenstrual; entre dois períodos menstruais consecutivos.

in·ter·met·a·car·pal (in-ter-met′ă-kar′păl). Intermetacarpal; entre os ossos metacárpicos.

in·ter·met·a·mer·ic (in′ter-met′ă-mer′ik). Intermetamérico; entre dois metâmeros; refere-se especialmente aos discos intervertebrais.

in·ter·met·a·tar·sal (in-ter-met′ă-tar′săl). Intermetatarsal; entre os ossos metatársicos.

in·ter·met·a·tar·se·um (in-ter-met′ă-tar′sē-ŭm). Intermetatarso. SIN *os intermetatarseum.*

in·ter·mis·sion (in-ter-mish′ŭn). Intermissão. **1.** Interrupção temporária dos sintomas ou de qualquer ação. **2.** Intervalo entre dois paroxismos de uma doença, como a malária. [L. *intermissio,* de *intermitto,* deixar, interromper, de *mitto,* enviar]

in·ter·mit. Interromper; cessar por algum tempo.

in·ter·mit·tence, in·ter·mit·ten·cy (in-ter-mit′ens, -en-sē). Intermitência. **1.** Condição caracterizada por intermissões ou interrupções na evolução de uma doença ou de outro processo ou estado ou em qualquer ação contínua; indica especialmente a perda de um ou mais batimentos do pulso. **2.** Cessação completa dos sintomas entre dois períodos de atividade de uma doença.

in·ter·mit·tent (in-ter-mit′ent). Intermitente; caracterizado por intervalos de quietude completa entre dois períodos de atividade.

in·ter·mus·cu·lar (in-ter-mŭs′kŭ-lăr). Intermuscular; entre os músculos.

in·tern (in′tern). Residente; estudante de nível superior ou recém-formado prosseguindo a sua educação posterior (em geral, primeiro ano de pós-graduação) ao participar nos cuidados clínicos ou cirúrgicos de pacientes hospitalizados, com supervisão e instrução; antigamente, aquele que residia na instituição. [F. *interne,* dentro]

in·ter·nal (in-ter′năl). Interno; afastado da superfície; com freqüência, termo utilizado incorretamente para significar medial. SIN internus [TA]. [l. *internus*]

in·ter·nal·i·za·tion (in-ter′năl-i-zā′shŭn). Internalização; adoção de padrões e valores de outra pessoa ou sociedade como se fossem seus.

in·ter·na·ri·al (in-ter-nā′rē-ăl). Internasal; situado entre as narinas. SIN internasal.

in·ter·na·sal (in-ter-nā′săl). Internasal. SIN internarial.

In·ter·na·tion·al Clas·si·fi·ca·tion of Dis·eas·es (ICD, ICDA). *Classificação Internacional de Doenças* (CID); a classificação de condições específicas e grupos de condições, determinada por um comitê especializado e internacionalmente representativo da *Organização Mundial de Saúde,* instituição que publica a lista completa num livro periodicamente revisado, o *Manual of the International Statistical Classification of Diseases, Injuries and Causes of Death.* A Décima Revisão (ICD-10) foi publicada em 1992; contém 20 capítulos, cada um com uma distribuição hierárquica de subdivisões (rubricas); há capítulos etiológicos, outros relacionados a sistemas orgânicos, alguns a classes de condições e outros a procedimentos.

In·ter·na·tion·al Clas·si·fi·ca·tion of Health Prob·lems in Pri·ma·ry Care (ICHPPC); *classificação Internacional dos Problemas Sanitários nos Cuidados Primários*; classificação de doenças, condições e problemas para uso nos cuidados primários, onde a precisão diagnóstica é raramente possível.

In·ter·na·tion·al Clas·si·fi·ca·tion of Im·pair·ments, Dis·a·bil·i·ties and Hand·i·caps (ICIDH). *Classificação Internacional de Danos, Incapacidades e Dificuldades*; taxonomia numérica patrocinada pela OMS dos danos, incapacidades e dificuldades decorrentes de lesão e doença.

In·ter·na·tion·al Com·mit·tee of the Red Cross. *Comitê Internacional da Cruz Vermelha;* organização suíça politicamente neutra que serve como intermediária entre tropas lutando em conflitos armados, na guerra civil ou em lutas internas para ajudar as vítimas a receberem proteção e outra assistência humanitária sob a Convenção de Genebra, de acordo com os princípios fundamentais da Cruz Vermelha.

In·ter·na·tion·al Sys·tem of Units (SI). *Sistema Internacional de Unidades;* sistema de medidas, baseado no sistema métrico, adotado na *11th General Conference on Weights and Measures* (*11.ª Conferência Geral de Pesos e Medidas*) da *International Organization for Standardization* (*Organização Internacional de Padronização,* 1960), para abranger tanto as unidades coerentes (unidades básicas, suplementares e derivadas) como os decimais múltiplos e submúltiplos dessas unidades formados pelo uso de prefixos propostos para uso técnico e científico internacional geral. O SI propõe sete unidades básicas: metro (m), quilograma (kg), segundo (s), ampère (A), Kelvin (K), candela (cd) e mole (mol) para as quantidades básicas de comprimento, massa, tempo, corrente elétrica, temperatura, intensidade luminosa e quantidade de substância, respectivamente; as unidades suplementares propostas incluem: radiano (rad) para o ângulo plano e esteradiano (sr) para o ângulo sólido; as unidades derivadas (p. ex., força, potência, freqüência) são expressas em termos das unidades básicas (p. ex., velocidade em metros por segundo, m s^{-1}). Os múltiplos (prefixos) em ordem descendente são: exa- (E, 10^{18}), peta- (P, 10^{15}), tera- (T, 10^{12}), giga- (G, 10^{9}), mega- (M, 10^{6}), quilo- (k, 10^{3}), hecto- (h, 10^{2}), deca- (da, 10^{1}), deci- (d, 10^{-1}), centi- (c, 10^{-2}), mili- (m, 10^{-3}), micro- (μ, 10^{-6}), nano- (n, 10^{-9}), pico- (p, 10^{-12}), fento- (f, 10^{-15}), ato- (a, 10^{-18}). Os prefixos propostos são zeta- (z, 10^{21}), yota (y, 10^{24}), zepto- (z, 10^{-21}) e yocto- (y, 10^{-24}). São recomendados os que envolvem um múltiplo de 10^{3}, enquanto não se recomendam os compostos destes últimos (p. ex., mμ para n). [Fr. *Système International d'Unités*]

in·terne. Interno.

in·ter·neu·ro·mer·ic (in′ter-noor-ō-mer′ik). Interneuromérico; entre os neurômeros.

in·ter·neu·rons (in′ter-noo′ronz). Interneurônios; combinações ou grupos de neurônios entre neurônios sensoriais e motores que governam a atividade coordenada.

in·tern·ist (in-ter′nist, in′ter-nist). Internista; médico treinado em medicina interna.

in·ter·nod·al (in-ter-nō′dăl). Internodal; situado entre dois nodos; relacionado a um internodo.

in·ter·node (in′ter-nōd). Internodo. SIN internodal *segment.*

in·ter·nu·cle·ar (in-ter-noo′klē-ăr). Internuclear; entre grupos de células nervosas no cérebro ou na retina.

in·ter·nun·ci·al (in′ter-nun′sē-ăl). Internuncial. **1.** Indica um neurônio funcionalmente interposto entre dois ou mais neurônios. **2.** Que atua como meio de comunicação entre dois órgãos. [L. *inernuntius* ou *-nuncius*), um mensageiro entre duas partes, de *inter,* entre + *nuncius,* um mensageiro]

in·ter·nus (in-ter′nŭs) [TA]. Interno. SIN internal. [L.]

in·ter·oc·clu·sal (in′ter-ō-kloo′săl). Interoclusal; entre as superfícies de oclusão de dentes opostos.

in·ter·o·cep·tive (in′ter-ō-sep′tiv). Interoceptivo; relativo às células nervosas sensoriais que inervam as vísceras (órgãos torácicos, abdominais e pélvicos e o sistema cardiovascular), a seus órgãos terminais sensoriais ou às informações que transmitem à medula espinal e ao cérebro. [inter- + L. *capio,* captar]

in·ter·o·cep·tor (in′ter-ō-sep′ter). Interoceptor; uma das várias formas de pequenos órgãos terminais sensoriais (receptores), situados no interior das paredes das vias respiratórias, do trato gastrointestinal ou de outras vísceras. [inter- + L. *capio,* tomar]

in·ter·ol·i·vary (in-ter-ol′i-vār-ē). Interolivar; entre as olivas inferiores esquerda e direita do bulbo.

in·ter·or·bit·al (in-ter-ōr′bi-tăl). Interorbitário; situado entre as órbitas.

in·ter·os·se·al (in-ter-os′ē-ăl). Interósseo. SIN interosseous.

in·ter·os·sei (in-ter-os′ē-ī). Interósseos; plural de interosseus.

in·ter·os·se·ous (in′ter-os′ē-ŭs). Interósseo; situado entre ossos ou unindo-os; refere-se a certos músculos e ligamentos. SIN interosseal. [inter- + L. *os,* osso]

in·ter·os·se·us, pl. **in·ter·os·sei** (in′ter-os′ē-ŭs, -os′e-ī). Interósseo. VER muscle.

in·ter·pal·pe·bral (in-ter-pal′pe-brăl). Interpalpebral; situado entre as pálpebras.

in·ter·pa·ri·e·tal (in′ter-pă-rī′e-tăl). Interparietal; situado entre as paredes de uma parte ou entre os ossos parietais. [inter- + L. *paries,* parede]

in·ter·par·ox·ys·mal (in′ter-par-ok-siz′măl). Interparoxístico; que ocorre entre paroxismos sucessivos de uma doença.

in·ter·pe·dic·u·late (in-ter-pe-dik′ū-lăt). Interpedicular; entre pedículos vertebrais.

in·ter·pe·dun·cu·lar (in-ter-pe-dŭnk′ū-lăr). Interpeduncular; situado entre dois pedúnculos.

in·ter·per·son·al (in-ter-per′son-ăl). Interpessoal; relativo a relações e intercâmbios sociais entre pessoas.

in·ter·pha·lan·ge·al (in′ter-fă-lan′jē-ăl). Interfalângico; situado entre duas falanges; refere-se às articulações dos dedos das mãos ou dos pés.

in·ter·phase (in′ter-fāz). Interfase; estágio entre duas divisões sucessivas de um núcleo celular em que ocorrem as funções bioquímicas e fisiológicas das células, bem como a replicação da cromatina. SIN karyostasis.

in·ter·phy·let·ic (in′ter - fī - let′ik). Interfilético; indica as formas de transição entre dois tipos de células durante a evolução da metaplasia. [inter- + G. *phylē*, tribo]

in·ter·plant. Interimplante; material transferido do doador para o hospedeiro na interimplantação.

in·ter·plant·ing. Interimplantação; em embriologia experimental, a transferência de uma massa celular primordial de um embrião para um meio indiferente em outro embrião, como nos enxertos corioalantóicos ou nos transplantes intra-oculares.

in·ter·pre·ta·tion (in - ter - pre - tā′shŭn). Interpretação. **1.** Em psicanálise, a intervenção terapêutica característica do analista. **2.** Em psicologia clínica, a elaboração de inferências e a formulação do significado em termos da dinâmica psicológica inerente às respostas de um indivíduo a testes psicológicos ou durante a psicoterapia.

in·ter·prox·i·mal (in - ter - prok′si - măl). Interproximal; entre superfícies adjacentes.

in·ter·pu·bic (in - ter - pū′bik). Interpúbico; situado entre os dois ossos púbicos.

in·ter·pu·pil·lary (in - ter - pū′pi - lār - ē). Interpupilar; situado entre as pupilas.

in·ter·ra·di·al (in - ter - rā′dē - ăl). Inter-radial; situado entre os rádios ou raios.

in·ter·re·nal (in - ter - rē′năl). Inter-renal; situado entre os dois rins.

in·ter·scap·u·lar (in - ter - skap′ū - lār). Interescapular; situado entre as escápulas.

in·ter·scap·u·lum (in - ter - skap′ū - lŭm). Interescápulo; parte do dorso entre os ombros ou entre as escápulas.

in·ter·sci·at·ic (in - ter - sī - at′ik). Interisquiático. SIN interischiadic.

in·ter·sec·tio, pl. **in·ter·sec·ti·o·nes** (in′ter - sek′shē - ō, - sek - shē - ō′nēz) [TA]. Interseção. SIN intersection. [L.]

intersectiones tendineae musculi recti abdominis [TA]. Interseções tendinosas dos músculos retos abdominais. SIN tendinous *intersections* of rectus abdominis, under *intersection.*

i. tendin'ea [TA], i. tendinosa. SIN tendinous *intersection.*

in·ter·sec·tion (in′ter - sek - shŭn) [TA]. Intersecção; local de cruzamento de duas estruturas. SIN intersectio [TA].

tendinous i. [TA], i. tendinosa; faixa ou parte tendinosa que cruza um músculo. SIN intersectio tendinea [TA], inscriptio tendinea, tendinous inscription.

tendinous i.'s of rectus abdominis [TA], interseções tendinosas do músculo retoabdominal; em geral, três e, algumas vezes, quatro faixas fibrosas transversas ou faixas parciais que ocorrem a intervalos como interrupções das porções contráteis e carnosas do músculo retoabdominal; ocorrem habitualmente no umbigo e acima dele. SIN intersectiones tendineae musculi recti abdominis [TA].

in·ter·sec·ti·o·nes (in - ter - sek - shē - ō′nēz). Interseções; plural de intersectio.

in·ter·seg·men·tal (in - ter - seg - men′tăl). Intersegmentar; entre dois segmentos, como metâmeros ou miótomos.

in·ter·sep·tal (in - ter - sep′tăl). Interseptal; situado entre dois septos.

in·ter·sep·to·val·vu·lar (in′ter - sep - tō - val′vū - lār). Interseptovalvular; entre o septo embrionário primum e o septo espúrio.

in·ter·sep·tum (in - ter - sep′tŭm). Intersepto. SIN diaphragm (1). [L.]

in·ter·sex·u·al (in - ter - seks′ū - ăl). Intersexual; relativo a, ou caracterizado por, intersexualidade.

in·ter·sex·u·al·i·ty (in′ter - seks - ū - al′i - tē). Intersexualidade; condição de apresentar características tanto masculinas quanto femininas; intermediário entre os dois sexos.

in·ter·space (in′ter - spās). Interespaço; qualquer espaço existente entre dois objetos semelhantes, como o interespaço costal ou intervalo entre duas costelas.

in·ter·spi·nal (in - ter - spī′năl). Interespinal; entre duas espinas, como os processos espinosos das vértebras. SIN interspinous.

in·ter·spi·na·lis (in - ter - spī - nā′lis). Interespinal. VER interspinales (*muscles*), em *muscle.*

in·ter·spi·nous (in - ter - spī′nŭs). Interespinal. SIN interspinal.

in·ter·stice, pl. **in·ter·stic·es** (in - ter′stis, - sti - siz). Interstício. SIN interstitium. [L. *interstitium,* de *sisto,* permanecer]

in·ter·sti·tial (in - ter - stish′ăl). Intersticial. **1.** Relativo a espaços ou interstícios em qualquer estrutura. **2.** Relativo a espaços no interior de um tecido ou órgão, porém excluindo os espaços como as cavidades corporais ou espaço potencial. Cf. intracavitary.

in·ter·sti·ti·um (in - ter - stish′ē - ŭm). Interstício; pequena área, espaço ou lacuna na substância de um órgão ou tecido. VER TAMBÉM connective *tissue.* SIN interstice. [L.]

in·ter·tar·sal (in - ter - tar′săl). Intertarsal; refere-se às articulações dos ossos társicos entre si. SIN tarsotarsal.

in·ter·tha·lam·ic (in - ter - thal′ă - mik). Intertalâmico; situado entre os tálamos.

in·ter·trans·ver·sa·lis (in - ter - trans - ver - sā′lis). Intertransversal, intertransversários. VER muscle.

in·ter·trans·verse (in′ter - trans′vers). Intertransverso; situado entre os processos transversos das vértebras.

in·ter·trig·i·nous (in - ter - trij′i - nŭs). Intertriginoso; caracterizado por, ou relacionado a, intertrigo.

in·ter·tri·go (in - ter - trī′gō). Intertrigo; dermatite irritante que ocorre entre dobras ou superfícies justapostas de pele, como entre as nádegas, entre o escroto e as coxas, no sulco inframamário (mamas pêndulas), etc.; causada por fricção, retenção de suor, umidade, calor e proliferação concomitante de microrganismos residentes; ocorre em crianças pequenas (ver diaper *dermatitis*) e adultos obesos. [L. uma irritação, escoriação da pele, de *inter,* entre + *tero,* esfregar, friccionar]

in·ter·tro·chan·ter·ic (in′ter - trō - kan - tār′ik). Intertrocantérico; situado entre os dois trocânteres do fêmur.

in·ter·tu·bu·lar (in - ter - too′bū - lār). Intertubular; situado entre, ou no meio de, túbulos.

in·ter·u·re·ter·al (in′ter - ū - rē′ter - ăl). Interureteral; situado entre os dois ureteres. SIN interureteric.

in·ter·u·re·ter·ic (in - ter - ū - rē - tār′ik). Interuretérico. SIN interureteral.

in·ter·val (in′ter - văl). Intervalo; tempo ou espaço entre dois períodos ou objetos; solução de continuidade. [L. *inter-vallum,* espaço entre defesas num acampamento, intervalo, de *vallum,* parapeito, parede]

a-c i., i. a-c; intervalo entre o início de uma onda a e aquele da onda c do pulso jugular.

AH i., i. AH; intervalo entre a rápida deflexão inicial da onda atrial e a rápida deflexão inicial do potencial do feixe de His (H); corresponde, aproximadamente, ao tempo de condução através do nodo AV (normalmente, 50–120 ms).

AN i., i. AN; intervalo entre o início da deflexão atrial e potencial nodal (normalmente, 40–100 ms).

atrioventricular i., i. atrioventricular. SIN auriculoventricular i.

auriculoventricular i., i. auriculoventricular; espaço entre a despolarização dos átrios e do ventrículo. SIN atrioventricular i.

AV i., i. AV; intervalo entre o início da sístole atrial e o começo da sístole ventricular, medido pelos pulsos de pressão ou pelas curvas de volume cardíaco em animais ou a partir do eletrocardiograma nos seres humanos.

BH i., i. BH; duração das deflexões do feixe de His (normalmente, 15–20 ms).

calibration i., i. de calibração; período de tempo ou série de medidas durante os quais se pode esperar que a calibração permaneça estável dentro de limites especificados e documentados.

cardioarterial i., c-a i., i. cardioarterial, i. c-a; intervalo entre o batimento apical do coração e o batimento do pulso radial.

confidence i., i. de confiança; faixa de valores de determinada variável, construída de tal modo que ela possui uma probabilidade específica de incluir o verdadeiro valor da variável.

coupling i., i. de acoplamento; intervalo expresso em milissegundos entre um batimento sinusal normal e o batimento prematuro seguinte.

escape i., i. de escape; intervalo entre o último batimento do ritmo básico do paciente (batimento ectópico ou sinusal) e um batimento de um foco de escape espontâneo ou o impulso do marcapasso eletrônico inicial (intervalo preestabelecido no circuito); pode ser um período mais curto ou mais longo do que o i. do pulso.

focal i., i. focal; distância entre os pontos focais anterior e posterior do olho.

HV i., i. HV; intervalo entre a deflexão inicial do potencial do feixe de His (H) e o início da atividade ventricular (normalmente 35–45 ms).

interectopic i., i. interectópico; distância entre complexos ectópicos consecutivos no eletrocardiograma.

isovolumic i., i. isovolumétrico; tempo durante o qual estão fechadas uma valva AV e uma valva semilunar.

lucid i., i. lúcido; em psicoses ou no delírio, período racional que aparece no decurso do distúrbio mental.

PA i., i. PA; intervalo entre o início da onda P e a rápida deflexão inicial da onda A no eletrograma do feixe de His (normalmente 25–45 ms); representa o tempo de condução intra-atrial.

PJ i., i. PJ; intervalo decorrido desde o início da onda P até o final do complexo QRS (J para junção entre o QRS e a onda T) no eletrocardiograma.

P-P i., i. P-P; distância entre ondas P consecutivas no eletrocardiograma.

PQ i., i. PQ. SIN PR i.

PR i., i. PR; no eletrocardiograma, o tempo que decorre entre o início da onda P e o início do complexo QRS seguinte; corresponde ao intervalo a-c do pulso venoso e, normalmente, é de 0,12–0,20 s. SIN PQ i.

QR i., i. QR; tempo decorrido desde o início do complexo QRS até o pico da onda R ou onda R final; mede o tempo de início da deflexão intrinsecóide quando determinado num traçado de derivação unipolar apropriado.

QRB i., i. QRB; intervalo entre o início da onda Q do complexo QRS e o potencial de ramo do feixe direito (normalmente, 15–20 ms).

QRS i., i. QRS; duração do complexo QRS no eletrocardiograma.
QS₂ i., i. QS₂. SIN electromechanical *systole*.
QT i., i. QT; no eletrocardiograma, tempo decorrido desde a onda Q até o final da onda T correspondendo à sístole elétrica.
R-R i., i. R-R; tempo decorrido entre duas ondas R consecutivas no eletrocardiograma.
serial i., i. seriado; intervalo entre fases análogas de uma doença infecciosa em casos sucessivos de uma cadeia de infecção de transmissão interpessoal. VER TAMBÉM mass action *principle,* infection transmission *parameter.*
sphygmic i., i. esfígmico; período, no ciclo cardíaco, em que as valvas semilunares estão abertas e o sangue está sendo ejetado dos ventrículos para o sistema arterial. SIN ejection period .
Sturm i., i. de Sturm; distância entre as linhas focais anterior e posterior numa combinação de lentes esferocilíndricas.
systolic time i.'s, intervalos de tempo sistólico. VER electromechanical *systole,* left ventricular ejection *time,* preejection *period.*
in·ter·vas·cu·lar (in - ter - vas′kŭ - lăr). Intervascular; entre os vasos sanguíneos ou linfáticos.
in·ter·ven·tion (in - ter - ven′shŭn). Intervenção; ação ou administração que produz um efeito ou que pretende alterar a evolução de um processo patológico. [L. *inter-ventio,* intromissão, de *intervenio,* intrometer-se]
crisis i., i. na crise; técnica psicoterápica visando o aconselhamento por ocasião de uma crise existencial aguda e limitada, com o objetivo de ajudar a resolver a crise.
in·ter·ven·tric·u·lar (in - ter - ven - trik′ū - lăr). Interventricular; entre os ventrículos.
in·ter·ver·te·bral (in - ter - ver′te - brăl). Intervertebral; situado entre duas vértebras.
interview. Entrevista.
Zarit burden i., e. de carga de Zarit; interação verbal estruturada utilizada para avaliar os níveis de estresse em membros da família ou pessoas que cuidam de pacientes com doença de Alzheimer.
in·ter·vil·lous (in - ter - vil′ŭs). Interviloso; situado entre, ou no meio de, vilosidades.
in·tes·ti·nal (in - tes′ti - năl). Intestinal; relativo ao intestino.
i. pseudo-obstruction, pseudo-obstrução i.; manifestações clínicas que sugerem falsamente uma obstrução do intestino delgado, ocorrendo habitualmente em pacientes com múltiplos divertículos jejunais.
in·tes·tine (in - tes′tin). [TA]. Intestino; o tubo digestivo que se estende do estômago até o ânus. É dividido primariamente em intestino delgado e intestino grosso. SIN bowel, gut (1), intestinum (1). [L. *intestinum*]

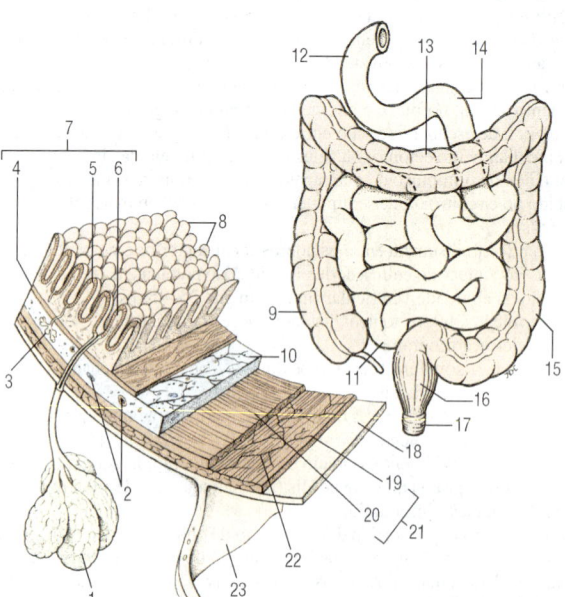

Intestinos: (embaixo) diagrama das quatro camadas principais da parede do tubo digestivo: mucosa, submucosa, muscular e serosa (abaixo do diafragma); (acima) visão anterior do intestino na cavidade abdominal; (1) glândula extra-intestinal, mas que se desenvolve a partir do intestino (fígado), (2) vasos sanguíneos, (3) glândula na submucosa, (4) muscular da mucosa, (5) epitélio, (6) lâmina própria, (7) mucosa, (8) vilosidades, (9) cólon ascendente, (10) submucosa, (11) íleo, (12) duodeno, (13) cólon transverso, (14) jejuno, (15) cólon descendente, (16) reto, (17) ânus, (18) serosa, (19) músculo circular, (20) músculo longitudinal, (21) muscular, (22) plexo mioentérico, (23) mesentério

large i., i. grosso; parte do tubo digestivo que se estende desde a válvula ileocecal até o ânus; compreende o ceco, o cólon, o reto e o canal anal. SIN intestinum crassum [TA].
small i. [TA], i. delgado; parte do tubo digestivo entre o estômago e o ceco ou início do intestino grosso; consiste em três porções: duodeno, jejuno e íleo. SIN intestinum tenue [TA].
in·tes·ti·no·tox·in (in - tes′ti - nō - tok′sin). Intestinotoxina; termo obsoleto para enterotoxina.
in·tes·ti·num, pl. **in·tes·ti·na** (in - tes - tī′nŭm, - nă). Intestino. 1. [TA]. SIN intestine. 2. Interior; interno. [neutro de *intestinus*] [L. *intestinus,* como substantivo, as entranhas, de *intus,* dentro]
i. ce'cum, i. cego. SIN cecum (1).
i. cras'sum [TA], i. grosso. SIN large *intestine.*
i. il'eum, i. íleo; VER ileum.
i. jeju'num, i. jejuno. VER jejunum.
i. rec'tum, i. reto. VER rectum.
i. ten'ue [TA], i. delgado. SIN small *intestine.*
i. ten'ue mesenteria'le, i. delgado mesentérico. SIN mesenteric *portion* of small intestine.
in·ti·ma (in′ti - mă). Íntima; mais interna. VER *tunica* intima. [L. fem. de *intimus,* a parte mais interna]
in·ti·mal (in′ti - măl). Íntima; relativo à íntima ou ao revestimento interno de um vaso.
in·ti·mi·tis (in - ti - mī′tis). Intimite; inflamação de uma íntima, como na endangiite. [íntima + G. *-itis,* inflamação]
proliferative i., i. proliferativa; erupção caracterizada por eritema escuro e pequenas úlceras, devido a alterações proliferativas no leito capilar.
in·toe (in′tō). Hálux valgo. SIN *metatarsus* adductus.
in·tol·er·ance (in - tol′er - ăns). Intolerância; anormalidade no metabolismo, na excreção ou em outro processamento de determinada substância; termo freqüentemente utilizado para referir-se a um comprometimento na utilização ou processamento de constituintes alimentares.
hereditary fructose i. [MIM*229600], i. hereditária a frutose; erro metabólico devido à deficiência de frutose-1,6-difosfato aldolase B hepática (que também atua sobre a frutose-1-fosfato), a segunda enzima na via específica da frutose. A ingestão de frutose é acompanhada de vômitos e hipoglicemia; a ingestão prolongada de frutose em crianças pequenas resulta em retardo do crescimento, icterícia, hepatomegalia, albuminúria, aminoacidúria e, algumas vezes, caquexia e morte; herança autossômica recessiva causada por uma mutação no gene da aldolase B (ALDOB) no cromossoma 9q.
lactose i., i. a lactose; distúrbio caracterizado por cólicas abdominais e diarréia após consumo de alimentos contendo lactose (p. ex., leite, sorvete); acredita-se que reflita uma deficiência de lactase intestinal; pode aparecer pela primeira vez em adultos jovens que toleravam bem o leite quando lactentes.
lysinuric protein i., i. à proteína lisinúrica; distúrbio autossômico recessivo, caracterizado por níveis elevados de aminoácidos dibásicos (p. ex., L-lisina, L-arginina e L-ornitina) na urina; aparentemente devido a um defeito no transporte de aminoácidos dibásicos.
in·tor·sion (in - tōr′shŭn). Intorção; rotação conjugada dos pólos superiores de cada córnea para dentro. [L. *in-torqueo,* pp. *tortus,* torção]
in·tor·tor (in - tōr′tŏr). Rotador medial. SIN medial *rotator.*
in·tox·a·tion (in - tok - sā′shŭn). Intoxicação; envenenamento, especialmente produtos tóxicos de bactérias ou animais peçonhentos, diferente da intoxicação por álcool. [ver intoxication]
in·tox·i·cant (in - tok′si - kant). Intoxicante. **1.** Que tem a capacidade de intoxicar. **2.** Agente intoxicante, como o álcool.
in·tox·i·ca·tion (in - tok - si - kā′shŭn). Intoxicação. **1.** SIN poisoning (2). **2.** SIN acute *alcoholism.* [L. *in,* em + G. *toxikon,* veneno]
acid i., i. ácida; envenenamento por produtos ácidos (ácido β-oxibutírico, ácido diacético ou acetona) formados em conseqüência de metabolismo defeituoso (p. ex., diabetes melito não-controlado) ou por ácidos introduzidos do exterior; caracterizada por dor epigástrica, cefaléia, perda de apetite, constipação, inquietação e odor de acetona na respiração, seguido de dispnéia, coma e colapso.
anaphylactic i., i. anafilática; intoxicação após uma reação anafilática.
citrate i., i. por citrato; condição tóxica que pode desenvolver-se durante a terapia de reposição maciça com sangue transfundido contendo citrato como anticoagulante; o citrato combina-se com íons cálcio e pode resultar em tetania.
intestinal i., i. intestinal. SIN autointoxication.
septic i., i. séptica. SIN septicemia.
water i., i. hídrica; encefalopatia metabólica decorrente de hiperidratação grave.
intra-. Intra-. No interior, dentro; oposto a extra-. VER TAMBÉM endo-, ento-. [L. dentro]
in·tra·ab·dom·i·nal (in′tră - ab - dom′i - năl). Intra-abdominal; dentro do abdome.
in·tra·ac·i·nous (in - tră - as′i - nŭs). Intra-acinoso; dentro de um ácino.

in·tra·ad·e·noi·dal (in′trā - ad - ē - noy′dăl). Intra-adenóide; dentro das adenóides.

in·tra·ar·te·ri·al (in′trā - ar - tēr′ē - ăl). Intra-arterial; dentro de uma artéria ou das artérias.

in·tra·ar·tic·u·lar (in′trā - ar - tik′ūlăr). Intra-articular; dentro da cavidade de uma articulação. [intra- + L. *articulus*, articulação]

in·tra·a·tri·al (in′trā - ā - trē - ăl). Intra-atrial; dentro de um ou de ambos os átrios do coração.

in·tra·au·ral (in′trā - aw′răl). Intra-aural; dentro do ouvido. [intra- + L. *auris*, ouvido]

in·tra·au·ric·u·lar (in′trā - aw - rik′ū - lăr). Intra-auricular; dentro de uma aurícula (p. ex., do ouvido).

in·tra·bron·chi·al (in - trā - brong′kē - ăl). Intrabrônquico; dentro dos brônquios ou tubos brônquicos. SIN endobronchial.

in·tra·buc·cal (in - trā - buk′ăl). Intrabucal. 1. Dentro da boca. 2. Dentro da substância da bochecha. [intra- + L. *bucca*, bochecha]

in·tra·can·a·lic·u·lar (in′trā - kan - ā - lik′ū - lăr). Intracanalicular; dentro de um canalículo ou canalículos.

in·tra·cap·su·lar (in′trā - kap′soo - lăr). Intracapsular; dentro de uma cápsula, especialmente a cápsula de uma articulação.

in·tra·car·di·ac (in′trā - kar′dē - ak). Intracardíaco; dentro de uma das câmaras do coração. SIN endocardiac (1), endocardial, intracordal. [intra- + G. *kardia*, coração]

in·tra·car·pal (in - trā - kar′păl). Intracárpico; dentro do carpo; entre os ossos cárpicos.

in·tra·car·ti·lag·i·nous (in′trā - kar - ti - laj′i - nŭs). Intracartilaginoso; dentro de uma cartilagem ou tecido cartilaginoso. SIN enchondral, endochondral.

in·tra·cath·e·ter (in′trā - kath′e - ter). Intracateter; tubo de plástico, habitualmente fixado à agulha de punção, introduzido num vaso sanguíneo para infusão, injeção ou monitorização da pressão.

in·tra·cav·i·tary (in′trā - cav′i - tār - ē). Intracavitário; dentro de um órgão ou cavidade corporal.

in·tra·ce·li·al (in′trā - sē′lē - ăl). Intracelíaco, dentro de qualquer uma das cavidades corporais, especialmente dentro de um dos ventrículos cerebrais. [intra- + G. *koilia*, cavidade]

in·tra·cel·lu·lar (in - trā - sel′ū - lăr). Intracelular; dentro de uma célula ou células.

in·tra·cer·e·bel·lar (in′trā - ser - ē - bel′ăr). Intracerebelar; dentro do cerebelo.

in·tra·ce·re·bral (in′trā - ser′ē - brăl). Intracerebral; dentro do cérebro.

in·tra·cer·e·bro·ven·tric·u·lar (in - tra - ser - ē′ - brō - ven - trik′ - ū - lar). Intracerebroventricular; local de administração de fármacos ou substâncias químicas no sistema ventricular do cérebro. Freqüentemente utilizado em estudos de animais e, algumas vezes, para a introdução de agentes antiinfecciosos que não penetram na barreira hematoencefálica no cérebro humano.

in·tra·cer·vi·cal (in′trā - ser′vi - kăl). Intracervical. SIN endocervical (1).

in·tra·cis·ter·nal (in′trā - sis - ter′năl). Intracisternal; dentro de uma das cisternas subaracnóides; em geral, refere-se à introdução de uma cânula na cisterna cerebelobulbar para aspiração de líquido cefalorraquidiano ou injeção de ar nos ventrículos cerebrais.

in·tra·co·lic (in′trā - kol′ik). Intracólico; dentro do cólon.

in·tra·cor·dal (in′trā - kōr′dăl). Intracardíaco, intracordial. SIN intracardiac. [intra- + L. *cor*, coração]

in·tra·cor·o·nal (in′trā - kōr′o - năl). Intracoronal; dentro da porção da coroa de um dente.

in·tra·cor·po·re·al (in′trā - kōr - po′rē - ăl). Intracorporal. 1. Dentro do corpo. 2. Dentro de qualquer estrutura anatomicamente semelhante a um corpo. [intra- + L. *corpus*, corpo]

in·tra·cor·pus·cu·lar (in′trā - kōr - pŭs′kū - lăr). Intracorpuscular; dentro de um corpúsculo, especialmente um eritrócito. SIN intraglobular (2).

in·tra·cos·tal (in′trā - kos′tăl). Intracostal; na superfície interna das costelas.

in·tra·cra·ni·al (in′trā - krā′nē - ăl). Intracraniano; dentro do crânio.

intracrine (in′trā - krin). Intrácrino; indica auto-estimulação através da produção celular de um fator que atua no interior da célula. [intra- + G. *krino*, separar, secretar]

in·trac·ta·ble (in′trak′tă - bl). Intratável. 1. SIN refractory (1). 2. SIN obstinate (1). [L. *in-tractabilis*, de *in-* neg. + *tracto*, levar, transportar]

in·tra·cu·ta·ne·ous (in′trā - koo - tā′nē - ŭs). Intracutâneo; dentro da substância da pele, particularmente a derme. SIN intradermal, intradermic. [intra- + L. *cutis*, pele]

in·tra·cys·tic (in′trā - sis′tik). Intracístico; dentro de um cisto ou dentro da bexiga.

in·trad (in′trăd). Em direção à parte interna.

in·tra·der·mal, in·tra·der·mic (in′trā - der′măl, - der′mik). Intradérmico. SIN intracutaneous. [intra- + G. *derma*, pele]

in·tra·duct (in′trā - dŭkt). Intraducto; dentro do ducto ou dos ductos de uma glândula.

in·tra·du·ral (in′trā - doo′răl). Intradural; dentro de, ou encerrado pela, dura-máter.

in·tra·em·bry·on·ic (in′trā - em - brē - on′ik). Intra-embrionário; dentro do corpo embrionário, p. ex., a porção da veia umbilical dentro do embrião (em contraste com a porção do cordão umbilical que é descartada por ocasião do nascimento). Cf. extraembryonic.

in·tra·ep·i·der·mal (in′trā - ep - i - der′măl). Intra-epidérmico; dentro da epiderme.

in·tra·ep·i·phys·i·al (in′trā - ep - i - fiz′ē - ăl). Intra-epifisário; dentro da epífise de um osso longo.

in·tra·ep·i·the·li·al (in′trā - ep - i - thē′lē - ăl). Intra-epitelial; dentro ou no meio das células epiteliais.

in·tra·far·a·di·za·tion (in′trā - fa - rā - di - zā′shŭn). Intrafaradização; aplicação de uma corrente cauterizadora farádica à superfície interna de uma cavidade ou órgão oco.

in·tra·fas·cic·u·lar (in′trā - fă - sik′ū - lăr). Intrafascicular; dentro dos fascículos de um tecido ou de uma estrutura (p. ex., fascículo intrafascicular).

in·tra·fe·brile (in′trā - fē′bril, - feb′ril). Intrafebril; que ocorre durante o estágio febril de uma doença. SIN intrapyretic.

in·tra·fi·lar (*in′trā - fī′lăr*). Intrafilamentar; situado dentro da malha de uma rede. [intra- + L. *filum*, filamento]

in·tra·fu·sal (in′trā - fū′săl). Intrafusal; aplica-se às estruturas existentes dentro do fuso muscular.

in·tra·gal·va·ni·za·tion (in′trā - gal - van - i - zā′shŭn). Intragalvanização; aplicação de uma corrente cauterizante galvânica ao interior de uma cavidade ou órgão oco.

in·tra·gas·tric (in′trā - gas′trik). Intragástrico; dentro do estômago.

in·tra·gem·mal (in′trā - jem′ăl). Intrapapilar, intrabulbar; dentro de qualquer corpo semelhante a um botão ou bulbo; indica especialmente uma terminação nervosa dentro de um bulbo terminal ou papila gustativa. [intra- + L. *gemma*, broto, botão]

in·tra·ge·nal (in′trā - jēn′ăl). Intragênico; dentro de um gene.

in·tra·glan·du·lar (in′trā - glan′doo - lăr). Intraglandular; dentro de uma glândula ou tecido glandular.

in·tra·glob·u·lar (in′trā - glob′ū - lăr). 1. Intraglobular; dentro de um glóbulo em qualquer sentido. 2. Intracorpuscular. SIN intracorpuscular.

in·tra·gy·ral (in′trā - ji′răl). Intragiral; dentro de um giro ou circunvolução cerebral.

in·tra·he·pat·ic (in′trā - he - pat′ik). Intra-hepático; dentro do fígado.

in·tra·hy·oid (in′trā - hī′oyd). Intra-hióide; dentro do osso hióide. Indica certas glândulas acessórias da tireóide situadas na cavidade ou dentro da substância do osso hióide.

in·tra·la·ryn·ge·al (in′trā - lā - rin′jē - ăl). Intralaríngeo; no interior da laringe.

in·tra·lig·a·men·tous (in′trā - lig - ă - men′tŭs). Intraligamentoso; dentro de um ligamento, referindo-se especialmente ao ligamento largo do útero.

in·tra·lo·bar (in′trā - lō′bar). Intralobar; dentro de um lobo de qualquer órgão ou estrutura.

in·tra·lob·u·lar (in′trā - lob′ū - lăr). Intralobular; dentro de um lóbulo.

in·tra·loc·u·lar (in - trā - lok′ū - lăr). Intralocular; dentro dos lóculos de qualquer parte.

in·tra·lu·mi·nal (in - trā - loo′mi - năl). Intraluminal. SIN intratubal.

in·tra·med·ul·lary (in′trā - med′u - lăr - ē). 1. Intramedular; dentro da medula óssea. 2. Intramedular; dentro da medula espinal. 3. Intrabulbar; dentro do bulbo.

in·tra·mem·bra·nous (in′trā - mem′brā - nŭs). Intramembranoso. 1. Dentro das camadas de uma membrana ou entre elas. 2. Indica o método de formação óssea diretamente a partir de células mesenquimatosas sem uma fase cartilaginosa intermediária (que ocorre, p. ex., na calvária), distinguindo-se da formação óssea intracartilaginosa.

in·tra·me·nin·ge·al (in′trā - mē - nin′jē - ăl). Intrameníngeo; no interior das, ou encerrado pelas, meninges do cérebro ou da medula espinal.

in·tra·mi·to·chon·dri·al (in′trā - mī - tō - kon′drē - ăl). Intramitocondrial; no interior das mitocôndrias.

in·tra·mo·lec·u·lar (in′trā - mō - lek′ū - lăr). Intramolecular; refere-se a situações e eventos dentro de uma molécula.

in·tra·mu·ral (in′trā - mū′răl). Intramural; dentro da substância da parede de qualquer cavidade ou órgão oco. SIN intraparietal (1).

in·tra·mus·cu·lar (I.M., i.m.) (in′trā - mŭs′kū - lăr). Intramuscular; dentro da substância de um músculo.

in·tra·my·o·car·di·al (in′trā - mī′ō - kard′ē - ăl). Intramiocárdico; dentro do miocárdio.

in·tra·my·o·me·tri·al (in′trā - mī′ō - mē′trē - ăl). Intramiométrico; dentro da camada muscular do útero.

in·tra·na·sal (in′tră - nā′săl). Intranasal; dentro da cavidade nasal.

in·tra·na·tal (in′tră - nā′tăl). Intranatal; durante o, ou por ocasião do, nascimento. [intra- + L. *natalis*, relacionado ao nascimento]

in·tra·neu·ral (in′tră - noo′răl). Intraneural; dentro de um nervo. [intra- + G. *neuron*, nervo]

in·tra·nu·cle·ar (in′tră - noo′klē - ăr). Intranuclear; dentro do núcleo de uma célula.

in·tra·oc·u·lar (in′tră - okū - lăr). Intra-ocular; dentro do globo ocular.

in·tra·o·ral (in′tră - ō′răl). Intra-oral; dentro da boca. [intra- + L. *os*, boca]

in·tra·or·bit·al (in′tră - ōr′bi - tăl). Intra-orbitário; dentro da órbita.

in·tra·os·se·ous (in′tră - os′ē - ŭs). Intra-ósseo; dentro do osso. SIN intraosteal. [intra- + L. *os*, osso]

in·tra·os·te·al (in′tră - os′tē - ăl). Intra-ósseo. SIN intraosseous.

in·tra·o·var·i·an (in′tră - ō - vā′rē - an). Intra-ovariano; dentro do ovário.

in·tra·ov·u·lar (in′tră - ov′ū - lăr). Intra-ovular; dentro do óvulo.

in·tra·pa·ri·e·tal (in′tră - pă - ri′ē - tăl). Intraparietal. **1.** SIN intramural. **2.** Indica o sulco intraparietal. VER intraparietal *sulcus*.

in·tra·par·tum (in′tră - par′tŭm). Intraparto; durante o trabalho de parto e o parto ao nascimento. Cf. antepartum, postpartum. [intra- + L. *partus*, parto]

in·tra·pel·vic (in′tră - pel′vik). Intrapélvico; dentro da cavidade pélvica.

in·tra·per·i·car·di·ac, in·tra·per·i·car·di·al (in′tră - per′ē - kar′dē - ak, - kar′dē - ăl). Intrapericárdico; dentro da cavidade pericárdica. SIN endopericardiac.

in·tra·per·i·to·ne·al (I.P., i.p.) (in′tră - per′i - tō - nē′ăl). Intraperitoneal; dentro da cavidade peritoneal.

in·tra·per·son·al (in′tră - per′sŏn - ăl). Intrapessoal. SIN intrapsychic.

in·tra·pi·al (in′tră - pī′ăl). Intrapial; dentro da pia-máter.

in·tra·pleu·ral (in′tră - ploo′răl). Intrapleural; dentro da pleura ou da cavidade pleural.

in·tra·pon·tine (in′tră - pon′tīn). Intrapontino; dentro da ponte do tronco cerebral.

in·tra·pros·tat·ic (in′tră - pros - tat′ik). Intraprostático; dentro da próstata.

in·tra·pro·to·plas·mic (in′tră - prō - tō - plas′mik). Intraprotoplasmático; dentro do protoplasma de uma célula.

in·tra·psy·chic (in′tră - sī′kik). Intrapsíquico; indica a dinâmica psicológica que ocorre dentro da mente, sem referir-se a trocas individuais com outras pessoas ou eventos. SIN intrapersonal.

in·tra·pul·mo·nary (in′tră - pul′mo - năr - ē). Intrapulmonar; dentro dos pulmões.

in·tra·py·ret·ic (in′tră - pī - ret′ik). Intrapirético. SIN intrafebrile. [intra- + L. *pyretos*, febre]

in·tra·rec·tal (in′tră - rek′tăl). Intra-retal; dentro do reto.

in·tra·re·nal (in′tră - rē′năl). Intra-renal; dentro do rim. [intra- + L. *ren*, rim]

in·tra·ret·i·nal (in′tră - ret′i - năl). Intra-retiniano; dentro da retina.

in·trar·rha·chid·i·an, in·tra·ra·chid·i·an (in′tră - ră - kid′ē - an). Intra-raquidiano. SIN intraspinal. [intra- + G. *rachis*, raque, espinha]

in·tra·scro·tal (in′tră - skrō′tăl). Intra-escrotal; dentro do escroto.

in·tra·spi·nal (in′tră - spī′năl). Intra-espinal; dentro do canal vertebral ou da medula espinal. SIN intrarrhachidian, intrarachidian.

in·tra·splen·ic (in′tră - splen′ik). Intra-esplênico; dentro do baço.

in·tra·stro·mal (in′tră - strō′măl). Intra-estromal; dentro do estroma ou da substância fundamental de qualquer órgão ou parte.

in·tra·syn·ov·i·al (in′tră - si - nō′vē - ăl). Intra-sinovial; dentro do saco sinovial de uma articulação ou de uma bainha sinovial de tendão.

in·tra·tar·sal (in′tră - tar′săl). Intratarsal; dentro do tarso; entre os ossos tarsais.

in·tra·the·cal (in′tră - thē′kăl). Intratecal. **1.** Dentro de uma bainha. **2.** No espaço subaracnóide ou subdural.

in·tra·tho·rac·ic (in′tră - thō - ras′ik). Intratorácico; dentro da cavidade do tórax.

in·tra·ton·sil·lar (in′tră - ton - si - lăr). Intratonsilar; dentro da substância de uma tonsila.

in·tra·tub·al (in′tră - too′băl). Intratubário; dentro de qualquer tubo. SIN intraluminal.

in·tra·tu·bu·lar (in′tră - too′bū - lăr). Intratubular; dentro de qualquer túbulo.

in·tra·tym·pan·ic (in′tră - tim - pan′ik). Intratimpânico; dentro do ouvido médio ou da cavidade timpânica.

in·tra·u·ter·ine (in′tră - ū′ter - in). Intra-uterino; dentro do útero.

in·tra·vas·cu·lar (in′tră - vas′kū - lăr). Intravascular; dentro dos vasos sanguíneos ou linfáticos.

in·tra·ve·nous (I.V., i.v.) (in′tră - vē′nŭs). Intravenoso; dentro de uma veia ou veias. SIN endovenous.

in·tra·ven·tric·u·lar (I-V) (in′tră - ven - trik′ū - lăr). Intraventricular; dentro de um ventrículo do cérebro ou coração.

in·tra·ves·i·cal (in′tră - ves′i - kăl). Intravesical; dentro de uma vesícula, referindo-se especialmente à bexiga.

in·tra vi·tam (in′tră vī′tăm). *Intra vitam*; durante a vida. [L. *vita*, vida]

in·tra·vi·tel·line (in′tră - vi - tel′in, - ēn). Intravitelino; dentro do vitelo.

in·tra·vit·re·ous (in′tră - vit′rē - ŭs). Intravítreo; dentro do corpo vítreo.

in·trin·sic (in - trin′sik). Intrínseco. **1.** Que pertence inteiramente a uma parte. **2.** Em anatomia, indica os músculos cuja origem e inserção encontram-se na estrutura em consideração, diferentemente dos músculos extrínsecos, que têm a sua origem fora da estrutura em consideração; termo aplicado especialmente aos membros, mas também ao músculo ciliar para distingui-lo dos músculos retos e outros músculos orbitários que estão fora do globo ocular. SIN essential (6). [L. *intrinsecus*, no lado de dentro, no interior]

intro-. Intro-. No interior, dentro de; oposto de extra-. Cf. intra-. [L. *intro*, dentro de]

in·tro·duc·er (in - trō - doos′er). Intubador; instrumento, como cateter, agulha ou tubo endotraqueal, para a introdução de um dispositivo flexível. SIN intubator. [L. *intro-duco*, levar para dentro, introduzir]

in·tro·flec·tion, in·tro·flex·ion (in′trō - flek′shŭn). Introflexão; inclinação para dentro. [intro- + L. *flecto*, pp. *flectus*, inclinar, flexionar]

in·tro·gas·tric (in - trō - gas′trik). Intragástrico; que leva para o estômago ou que é nele introduzido. [intro- + G. *gastēr*, ventre, estômago]

in·tro·i·tus (in - trō′i - tŭs). Intróito; entrada num canal ou órgão oco, como a vagina. [L. entrada, de *intro-eo*, entrar]
   i. cana′lis, i. do canal facial. SIN i. of facial canal.
   i. of facial canal, i. do canal facial; entrada para o canal facial, através do qual passa o nervo facial, no final do meato acústico interno. SIN i. canalis.
   vaginal i., i. vaginal. SIN *vestibule* of vagina.

introject (in′trō - jekt). Introjetado; representação interna dinamicamente fixa e permanente de um objeto.

in·tro·jec·tion (in - trō - jek′shŭn). Introjeção; mecanismo de defesa psicológica que envolve a apropriação de um acontecimento externo e sua assimilação pela personalidade, tornando-o parte do *self*. [intro- + L. *jacto*, arremessar]

in·tro·mis·sion (in - trō - mish′ŭn). Intromissão; inserção ou introdução de uma parte em outra. [intro- + L. *mitto*, enviar]

in·tro·mit·tent (in - trō - mit′ent). Intromitente; que transporta ou envia para dentro de um corpo ou cavidade.

in·tron (in′tron). Intron; porção do DNA situada entre dois exons, transcrita em RNA, mas que não aparece nesse mRNA após maturação, visto que o intron é removido e os exons reunidos, de modo que não é expresso (como proteína) na síntese de proteínas. Por costume, o termo aplica-se também às regiões correspondentes na transcrição primária do mRNA, antes da maturação. SIN intervening sequence. [inter- + -on]

in·tro·spec·tion (in - trō - spek′shŭn). Introspecção; que olha para dentro; auto-análise; contemplação dos próprios processos mentais. [intro- + L. *specto*, olhar, inspecionar]

in·tro·spec·tive (in - trō - spek′tiv). Introspectivo; relativo à introspecção.

in·tro·sus·cep·tion (in′trō - sŭs - sep′shŭn). Introssuscepção. SIN intussusception.

in·tro·ver·sion (in - trō - ver′zhŭn). Introversão. **1.** Giro de uma estrutura sobre si própria. VER TAMBÉM intussusception, invagination. **2.** Preocupação para consigo próprio, praticada por uma pessoa introvertida. Cf. extraversion. [intro- + L. *verto*, p. *versus*, virar, girar]

in·tro·vert. 1. (in′trō - vert). Introvertido; indivíduo que tende a ser inusitadamente tímido, introspectivo, autocentrado e que evita ter qualquer interesse ou envolvimento nos assuntos de outros. Cf. extrovert. **2.** (in - trō - vert′). Introverter; girar uma estrutura sobre si mesma, inverter.

in·tu·bate (in′too - bāt). Intubar; introduzir um tubo.

in·tu·ba·tion (in - too - bā′shŭn). Intubação; inserção de um dispositivo tubular num canal, órgão oco ou cavidade; especificamente, a passagem de um tubo oro- ou nasotraqueal para anestesia ou para controlar a ventilação pulmonar. [L. *in*, em + *tuba*, tubo]
   altercursive i., i. altercursiva; termo raramente utilizado para referir-se ao desvio de secreção intermitentemente para o exterior a partir de seu destino normal, como, p. ex., da bile do intestino.
   aqueductal i., i. aquedutal; inserção de um tubo no aqueduto de Sylvius para alívio da atresia ou estreitamento do aqueduto.
   blind nasotracheal i., i. nasotraqueal às cegas; passagem de um tubo através do nariz para a traquéia sem utilizar um laringoscópio.
   endotracheal i., i. endotraqueal; passagem de um tubo através do nariz ou da boca para o interior da traquéia para manutenção das vias aéreas durante a anestesia, ou para suporte ventilatório ou manutenção de uma via aérea em risco. SIN intratracheal i.
   intratracheal i., i. intratraqueal. SIN endotracheal i.
   nasotracheal i., i. nasotraqueal; intubação traqueal através do nariz.
   orotracheal i., i. orotraqueal; intubação traqueal através da boca.
   tracheal i., i. traqueal; passagem de um tubo através do nariz, da boca ou de traqueotomia para dentro da traquéia para manutenção da perviedade das vias aéreas.

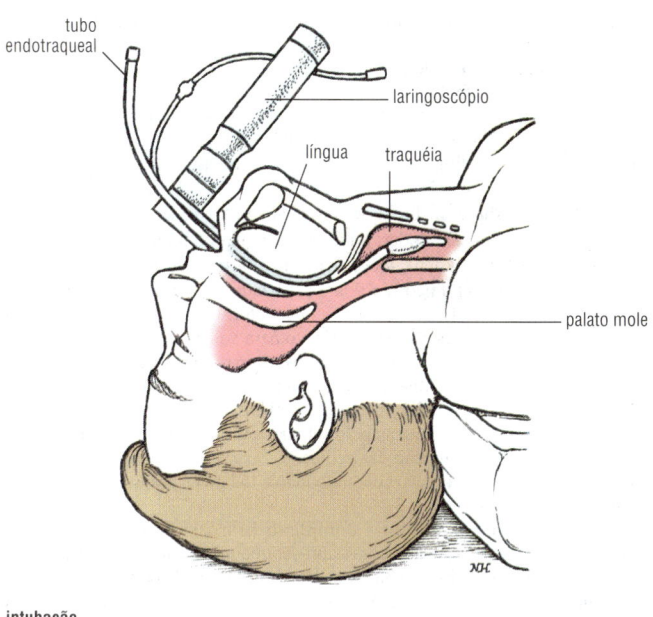
intubação

in·tu·ba·tor (in′too - bā - tor). Intubador. SIN introducer.
in·tu·mesce (in - too - mes′). Intumescer; inchar; aumentar de volume. [L. *intumesco,* intumescer, inchar, de *tumeo,* inchar]
in·tu·mes·cence (in - too - mes′ens). Intumescimento. **1.** SIN enlargement. **2.** Processo de aumento de volume ou inchação; termo utilizado para descrever aumentos espinais.
  tympanic i., i. timpânico. SIN tympanic *enlargement.*
in·tu·mes·cent (in - too - mes′ent). Intumescente; que aumenta de volume; tornando-se aumentado ou intumescido.
in·tu·mes·cen·tia (in - too - mes - sen′shē - ä) [TA]. Intumescência. SIN enlargement. [L. Mod.]
  i. cervica'lis [TA], i. cervical. SIN cervical *enlargement.*
  i. gangliofor'mis, i. gangliforme. SIN geniculate *ganglion.*
  i. lumbosacra'lis [TA], i. lombossacra. SIN lumbosacral *enlargement.*
  i. tympan'ica [TA], i. timpânica. SIN tympanic *enlargement.*
in·tus·sus·cep·tion (in′tŭs - sŭ - sep′shŭn). Intussuscepção. **1.** Captação ou introdução de uma parte dentro de outra, referindo-se, especialmente, à invaginação de um segmento do intestino dentro de outro. VER TAMBÉM introversion, invagination. **2.** Com freqüência, refere-se, especificamente, ao processo de incorporação de novo material no crescimento da parede celular. SIN introsusception. [L. *intus,* dentro + *sus-cipio,* captar, de *sub* + *capio,* tomar]
  colic i., i. cólica; embainhamento de uma porção do cólon em outra.
  double i., i. dupla; segunda intussuscepção que envolve o intestino acima da primeira; a primeira intussuscepção é seguida de contração da parede intestinal ao seu redor, e a massa sólida assim formada é envolvida pela porção proximal do intestino, produzindo, desse modo, a segunda intussuscepção.
  ileal i., i. ileal; intussuscepção em que uma porção do íleo é embainhada em outra porção da mesma divisão do intestino.
  ileocecal i., i. ileocecal; intussuscepção em que o segmento inferior do íleo passa através da válvula do cólon para dentro do ceco.
  ileocolic i., i. ileocólica; intussuscepção em que a porção inferior do íleo com a válvula do ceco passa para dentro do cólon ascendente.
  jejunogastric i., i. jejunogástrica; complicação rara, após gastrojejunostomia, em que a alça aferente ou eferente do intestino invagina-se dentro do estômago.
  retrograde i., i. retrógrada; invaginação de um segmento inferior do intestino dentro de um segmento imediatamente acima.
in·tus·sus·cep·tive (in′tŭs - sŭ - sep′tiv). Intussusceptivo; relativo a, ou caracterizado por, intussuscepção.
in·tus·sus·cep·tum (in′tŭs - sŭ - sep′tŭm). Intussuscepto; o segmento interno numa intussuscepção; a parte do intestino que é invaginada dentro da outra parte.
in·tus·sus·cip·i·ens (in′tŭ - sŭ - sip′ē - enz). Intussuscipiente; a porção do intestino, na intussuscepção, que recebe a outra porção. [L. *intus,* dentro + *suspiciens,* pr. p. de *suscipio,* captar]
in·u·lase (in′ū - lās). Inulase. SIN inulinase.
in·u·lin (In) (in′ū - lin). Inulina; polissacarídeo de frutose do rizoma de *Inula helenium* ou *elecampane* (família Compositae) e de outros vegetais; utilizada por injeção intravenosa, sendo filtrada pelos glomérulos renais, mas não reabsorvida; por conseguinte, pode ser utilizada para determinar a taxa de filtração glomerular; também utilizada no pão para diabéticos. Cf. inulin *clearance.* SIN alant starch, alantin, dahlin.
in·u·lin·ase (in′ū - lin - ās). Inulinase; enzima que atua sobre as ligações 2,1, -β-D-frutose na inulina, liberando a D-frutose. SIN inulase.
in·u·lol (in′ū - lol). Inulol. SIN alantol.
in·unc·tion (in′ - ŭngk′shŭn). Inunção; administração de um medicamento na forma de pomada friccionada para causar a absorção do ingrediente ativo. [L. *inunctio,* ungüento, de *inunguo,* pp. *-unctus,* esfregar sobre]
in·vac·ci·na·tion (in - vak - si - nā′shŭn). Termo obsoleto para referir-se à inoculação acidental de alguma doença, como, p. ex., sífilis, durante a vacinação.
in·vac·uo (in vak′ū - ō). A vácuo; no vácuo, como, p. ex., sob pressão reduzida. [L.]
in·vag·i·nate (in - va′ji - nāt). Invaginar; embainhar, envolver ou inserir uma estrutura dentro dela própria ou de outra. [L. *in,* em + *vagina,* bainha]
in·vag·i·na·tion (in - vaj′i - nā′shŭn). Invaginação. **1.** Embainhamento, penetração ou inserção de uma estrutura dentro de si própria ou de outra. **2.** Estado de ser invaginado. VER TAMBÉM introversion, intussusception.
  basilar i., i. basilar. SIN platybasia.
in·vag·i·na·tor (in - vag′i - nā - ter, - tōr). Invaginador; instrumento para introduzir qualquer tecido.
in·va·lid (in′vă - lid). Inválido. **1.** Fraco; enfermo. **2.** Indivíduo parcial ou totalmente incapacitado. [L. *in-* neg. + *validus,* forte]
in·va·lid·ism (in′vă - lid - izm). Invalidez; condição de ser inválido.
in·va·sin (in - vā′sin). Invasina. SIN hyaluronidase (1).
in·va·sion (in - vā′zhŭn). Invasão. **1.** Início ou incursão de uma doença. **2.** Disseminação local de uma neoplasia maligna por infiltração ou destruição do tecido adjacente; no caso de neoplasias epiteliais, a invasão significa infiltração abaixo da membrana basal epitelial. **3.** Entrada de células estranhas num tecido, como os leucócitos polimorfonucleares na inflamação. [L. *invasio,* de *in-vado,* pp. *–vasus,* entrar, atacar]
in·va·sive (in - vā′siv). Invasivo. **1.** Indica ou caracteriza-se por invasão. **2.** Indica um procedimento que exige a introdução de um instrumento ou dispositivo no corpo através da pele ou de um orifício corporal para diagnóstico ou tratamento.
in·ven·to·ry (in′ven - tōr - ē). Inventário; lista detalhada e freqüentemente descritiva de itens.
  Millon clinical multiaxial i. (MCMI), i. multiaxial clínico de Millon. SIN Millon Clinical Multiaxial Inventory *test.*
  Minnesota Multiphasic Personality I., i. de personalidade multifásico de Minnesota. SIN Minnesota Multiphasic Personality Inventory *test.*
  personality i., i. de personalidade; teste psicológico para avaliação dos modos habituais de comportamento, pensamento e sentimentos baseando-se nas características comparáveis de indivíduos dentro de um grupo homogêneo.
in·ver·mi·na·tion (in - ver - mi - nā′shŭn). Verminose, helmintíase; SIN helminthiasis. [L. *in,* em + *vermis* (*vermin-*), verme]
in·ver·sion (in - ver′zhŭn). Inversão. **1.** Ato de virar para dentro, ao contrário ou em qualquer direção contrária à existente. **2.** Conversão por hidrólise de um dissacarídeo ou polissacarídeo em monossacarídeo; especificamente, a hidrólise da sacarose em D-glicose e D-frutose; assim denominada em virtude da mudança de rotação óptica. **3.** Alteração de uma molécula de DNA efetuada ao remover um fragmento, ao reverter a sua orientação e ao colocá-lo de novo no local. **4.** Transição da sílica induzida por calor em que o quartzo tridimita ou cristobalita altera suas propriedades físicas quanto à expansão térmica. **5.** Conversão de um centro quiral em sua imagem especular. [L. *inverto,* pp. *-versus,* virar ao contrário, inverter]
  i. of chromosomes, i. de cromossomas; aberração cromossômica resultante de uma dupla ruptura num segmento do cromossoma, com rotação término-terminal do fragmento entre as linhas de fratura e refusão dos fragmentos; esse processo resulta em inversão da ordem dos genes no segmento.
  paracentric i., i. paracêntrica; inversão, num cromossoma, de um único segmento em que o centrômero não é incluído.
  pericentric i., i. pericêntrica; inversão, num cromossoma, de um único segmento que inclui o centrômero.
  i. of the uterus, i. do útero; inversão do útero, habitualmente após o parto.
  visceral i., i. visceral. SIN *situs inversus viscerum.*
in·vert (in′vert). Invertido. **1.** Em química, submetido a inversão, como, p. ex., açúcar invertido. **2.** Inverter a direção, seqüência ou efeito. **3.** Termo raramente utilizado para referir-se a um indivíduo homossexual. VER inversion.
in·vert·ase (in′ver - tās). Invertase. SIN β-fructofuranosidase.
In·ver·te·bra·ta (in - ver - tĕ - brā′tă). Invertebrados; categoria geral do reino Animalia (animais multicelulares), incluindo os filos cujos membros não têm notocorda; isto é, todos os animais, à exceção dos vertebrados no filo Chordata.
in·ver·te·brate (in - ver′tĕ - brăt). Invertebrado. **1.** Que não possui uma coluna vertebral. **2.** Qualquer animal que carece de coluna vertebral.

in·vert·ed re·peat. Repetição invertida; seqüência de nucleotídeos que é repetida quase sem nenhuma alteração, exceto na direção oposta, geralmente em algum ponto distante da seqüência original; freqüentemente associada a inserção gênica.

in·ver·tin (in′ver - tin). Invertina. SIN β-fructofuranosidase.

in·ver·tor (in - ver′ter, - tōr). Inversor; músculo que inverte, causa inversão ou vira uma parte, como o pé, para dentro. [ver inversion]

in·vest·ing. Revestimento, investimento. **1.** Em odontologia, ato de cobrir ou envolver algo totalmente ou em parte, como dentadura, dente, molde de cera, coroa, etc., com material refratário antes de tratá-lo, soldá-lo ou fundi-lo. **2.** Em psicanálise, ato de carregar um objeto com energia psíquica ou catexia.
  vacuum i., r. a vácuo; revestimento de um padrão utilizando um vácuo para remover o ar aprisionado do material de revestimento.

in·vest·ment. Revestimento, investimento. **1.** Em odontologia, qualquer material utilizado no revestimento. **2.** Em psicanálise, a carga psíquica ou catexia investida num objeto.
  refractory i., r. refratário; material de revestimento que pode suportar as elevadas temperaturas utilizadas na solda ou fusão.

in·vet·er·ate (in - vet′er - āt). Inveterado; instalado há muito tempo; firmemente estabelecido; refere-se a uma doença ou a hábitos crônicos. [L. *in-vetero,* pp. *-atus,* envelhecer, de *vetus,* velho]

in·vis·ca·tion (in - vis - kā′shŭn). Inviscação. **1.** Untar com matéria mucilaginosa. **2.** Mistura do alimento, durante a mastigação, com a saliva. [L. *in,* em, sobre + *viscum,* visgo]

in vit·ro (in vē′trō). *In vitro;* em ambiente artificial, referindo-se a um processo ou reação que ocorre nesse ambiente, como em um tubo de ensaio ou meio de cultura. Cf. *in vivo.* [L. em vidro]

in vi·vo (in vē′vō). *In vivo;* no organismo vivo, referindo-se a um processo ou reação que ocorre em seres vivos. Cf. *in vitro.* [L. no ser vivo]

in·vo·lu·cre (in′vō - loo - ker). Invólucro. SIN involucrum.

in·vo·lu·crin (in - vō - loo′krin). Involucrina; precursor não-solúvel em ceratina da proteína de ligação altamente cruzada, conhecida como envoltório do corneócito. [do L. *involucrum,* envoltório]

in·vo·lu·crum, pl. **in·vo·lu·cra** (in - vō - loo′krŭm, - loo′krä). Invólucro. **1.** Membrana envolvente, como, p. ex., bainha ou saco. **2.** A bainha de novo osso que se forma ao redor de um seqüestro. SIN involucre. [L. um envoltório, de *in-volvo,* enrolar]

in·vol·un·tary (in - vol′ŭn - tār - ē). Involuntário. **1.** Independente da vontade; não-volicional. **2.** Contrário à vontade. [L. *in-* neg. + *voluntarius,* querer, de *volo,* querer, desejar]

in·vo·lu·tion (in - vō - loo′shŭn). Involução. **1.** Retorno de um órgão aumentado a seu tamanho normal. **2.** Ato de enrolar as bordas de uma parte para a face ventral. **3.** Em psiquiatria, declínio mental associado ao envelhecimento. SIN catagenesis. [L. *in-volvo,* pp. *-volutus,* enrolar]
  senile i., i. senil; regressão de órgãos vitais e processos psicológicos com o envelhecimento.
  i. of the uterus, i. do útero; processo de redução do útero a seu tamanho e estado normais antes da gravidez e do parto.

in·vo·lu·tion·al (in - vō - loo′shŭn - ăl). Involutivo; relativo à involução.

io·ben·zam·ic ac·id (ī - ō - ben - zam′ik). Ácido iobenzâmico; contraste radiográfico utilizado antigamente para colecistografia oral.

io·ce·tam·ic ac·id (ī′ō - sē - tam′ik). Ácido iocetâmico; contraste radiográfico utilizado antigamente para colecistografia oral.

io·da·mide (ī - ō′dă - mīd). Iodamida; contraste radiográfico utilizado antigamente para colecistografia oral. SIN ametriodinic acid.

Iod·a·moe·ba (ī - od - ă - mē′bă). Gênero de amebas parasitas da superclasse Rhizopoda, ordem Amoebida.
  I. bütsch′lii, ameba parasita do intestino grosso dos seres humanos; os trofozoítas têm habitualmente 9–14 μm de diâmetro; os cistos têm, em geral, 8–10 μm de diâmetro, são uninucleados e discretamente irregulares quanto à sua forma, com parede espessa e grande massa compacta de glicogênio que se cora intensamente com solução de iodo; a amebíase clinicamente reconhecível causada por esse microrganismo é rara, e os sintomas assemelham-se aos da doença crônica causada por *Entamoeba histolytica.* Também encontrada em outros primatas, constituindo a ameba mais comum nos suínos.

io·date (ī′ō - dāt). Iodato; sal do ácido iódico.

iod·ic (ī - od′ik). Iódico. **1.** Relativo a, ou causado por, iodo ou iodeto. **2.** Indica um composto de iodo em seu estado pentavalente.

iod·ic ac·id. Ácido iódico; pó cristalino, hidrossolúvel; utilizado como adstringente, cáustico, desinfetante, desodorante e, antigamente, como anti-séptico.

io·dide (ī′ō - dīd). Iodeto. **1.** O íon negativo do iodo, I$^-$. **2.** Qualquer sal do ácido hidroiódico. **3.** Qualquer composto contendo um átomo de iodo ligado a um carbono.
  i. peroxidase, i. peroxidase; óxido redutase que catalisa reações entre o iodo e a água, produzindo iodeto e H_2O_2; também catalisa a iodação e a desiodação de compostos de tirosina; a deficiência dessa enzima resulta em perda dos derivados de iodo tirosina e iodo da tireóide, com desenvolvimento de bócio. SIN iodinase, iodotyrosine deiodase.
  sodium i. iodine-131, i. de sódio iodo-131; preparado a partir do iodo radioativo (I^{131}); nominalmente sem transportador, com meia-vida de 8,1 dias; utilizado como agente diagnóstico nos casos de suspeita de doença da tireóide e no tratamento de doenças tireóideas selecionadas.

io·dim·e·try (ī - ō - dim′ē - trē). Iodimetria. SIN iodometry.[iodo + G. *metron,* medida]

io·di·nase (ī′ō - din - ās). Iodinase. SIN *iodide* peroxidase.

io·di·nate (ī′ō - di - nāt). Iodar; tratar ou combinar com iodo.

io·dine (I) (ī′ō - dīn, - dēn). Iodo; elemento químico não-metálico, de número atômico 53, peso atômico 126,90447; utilizado na fabricação de compostos de iodo e como catalisador, reagente, marcador, componente de contrastes radiográficos, anti-séptico tópico, antídoto para venenos alcalóides e em certos corantes e soluções; antigamente utilizado para profilaxia da deficiência de iodo. [G. *īodēs,* semelhante a uma violeta, de *ion,* violeta, + *eidos,* forma]
  butanol-extractable i. (BEI), i. extraível em butanol; iodo que pode ser separado das proteínas plasmáticas pelo butanol ou outros solventes extraíveis; utilizado para medir a função da tireóide.
  Gram i., i. de Gram; solução contendo iodo e iodato de potássio, utilizado na coloração de Gram.
  povidone i., iodo-povidona; complexo hidrossolúvel de iodo com polivinilpirrolidina. Aplicado como anti-séptico na forma de soluções ou pomadas, libera iodo. Utilizado na limpeza e desinfecção da pele, preparação da pele no pré-operatório e tratamento de infecções suscetíveis ao iodo. SIN polyvinylpyrrolidone-iodine complex, povidone-iodine.
  protein-bound i. (PBI), i. ligado à proteína; hormônio tireóideo em sua forma circulante, consistindo em uma ou mais iodotironinas ligadas a uma ou mais das proteínas séricas.
  radioactive i., i. radioativo; os radioisótopos do iodo, I^{131}, I^{125} ou I^{123}, utilizados como marcadores em biologia e medicina.
  tamed i., i. suavizado. SIN iodophor.
  i. tincture, tintura de i; solução hidroalcoólica contendo 2% de i. elementar e 2,4% de iodeto de potássio para facilitar a dissolução e 47% de álcool; utilizada como anti-séptico/germicida na superfície da pele para cortes e arranhaduras. Tem sido utilizada como desinfetante da pele antes da cirurgia, mas, hoje em dia, é substituída, em grande parte, por formas orgânicas de iodo.

io·dine-123 (^{123}I). Iodo-123 (I^{123}); radioisótopo do iodo com emissão gama de 159 keV e meia-vida física de 13,2 h; utilizado para estudos de doença da tireóide e da função renal.

io·dine-125 (^{125}I). Iodo-125 (I^{125}); isótopo de iodo radioativo que se desintegra pela captação de K (conversão interna), com meia-vida de 59,4 dias; utilizado como marcador em imunoensaio e técnicas de imagem; antigamente utilizado em estudos da tireóide e como marcador em técnicas de imagem.

io·dine-127 (^{127}I). Iodo-127 (I^{127}); iodo estável não-radioativo; trata-se do isótopo de iodo mais abundante na natureza; a deficiência dietética provoca bócio simples; utilizado para bloquear a captação tireóidea de iodo radioativo liberado de acidentes nucleares.

io·dine-131 (^{131}I). Iodo-131 (I^{131}); isótopo radioativo de iodo; emissor beta e gama, com meia-vida de 8,1 dias; utilizado como marcador em estudos da tireóide, como tratamento no hipertireoidismo e câncer da tireóide e como marcador em imunoensaios e estudos de imagem; utilizado outrora como terapia na doença cardíaca.

io·dine-132 (^{132}I). Iodo-132 (I^{132}); radioisótopo de iodo emissor beta e gama, com meia-vida de 2,28 h, habitualmente obtido de gerador de radionuclídeos de telúrio-132; seu uso clínico foi suplantado pelo I^{131} e I^{123}.

io·dine·fast. Resistente ao iodo; indica o hipertireoidismo que não responde à terapia com iodo, que se desenvolve freqüentemente na maioria dos casos assim tratados.

io·din·o·phil, io·din·o·phile (ī - ō - din′ō - fil, - fīl). Iodófilo. **1.** Que se cora facilmente pelo iodo. SIN iodinophilous. **2.** Qualquer elemento histológico que se cora facilmente pelo iodo. [iodo + G. *philos,* amigo]

io·din·oph·i·lous (ī - ō - din - of′i - lŭs). Iodófilo. SIN iodinophil (1).

io·dip·a·mide (ī - ō - dip′a - mīd). Iodipamida; contraste radiográfico iônico, dimérico e hidrossolúvel para colangiografia intravenosa; utilizada como sal sódico ou de metilglucamina. SIN Adipiodone.
  methylglucamine i., i. de metilglucamina; composto de iodo orgânico hidrossolúvel, utilizado para colangiografia intravenosa e colecistografia.

io·dism (ī′ō - dizm). Iodismo; intoxicação pelo iodo, uma condição caracterizada por coriza intensa, erupção cutânea acneiforme, fraqueza, salivação e mau hálito; causado pela administração contínua de iodo ou de um dos iodetos.

io·dix·an·ol (ī - ō - diks′a - nol). Iodixanol; 5,5′-[(2-hidroxi-1,3-propano)bis(acetilamino)]bis[*N,N′*-bis(2,3-diidroxipropil)-2,4,6-triiodo-1,3-benzenodicarboxamida]; contraste radiográfico dimérico, não-iônico, de baixa osmolaridade e hidrossolúvel para uso intravascular.

io·dize (ī′ō - dīz). Iodizar; tratar ou impregnar com iodo.

i·o·dized oil (ī'ō - dīzd). Óleo iodado; produto de adição de iodo de óleos vegetais, contendo não menos de 38 e não mais de 42% de iodo combinado organicamente; meio radiopaco.

io·do·a·cet·a·mide (ī - ō'dō - ă - sē'tă - mĭd). Iodoacetamida; ICH_2-CONH_2; substância química que reage facilmente com grupos sulfidrila, constituindo, portanto, um forte inibidor de muitas enzimas.

io·do·al·phi·on·ic ac·id (ī - ō'dō - al - fē - on'ik). Ácido iodoalfiônico; contraste radiográfico utilizado antigamente para colecistografia.

io·do·ca·sein (ī - ō - dō - kā'sēn). Iodocaseína; composto de iodo com caseína em que o iodo está fixado a moléculas de tirosina; possui atividade de tiroxina.

io·do·chlor·hy·drox·y·quin, io·do·chlo·ro·hy·drox·y·quin·o·line (ī·o - dō - klōr'hī - drok'si - kwin, - klōr'ō - hī - drok'si - kwin'ō - lēn). Iodocloroidroxiquina, iodocloroidroxiquinolina. Antiinfeccioso tópico. SIN chloriodoquin, clioquinol.

io·do·chlo·rol (ī'ō - dō - klōr'ol). Iodoclorol. SIN chloriodized oil.

io·do·der·ma (ī - ō'dō - der'mă). Iododermia; erupção de pápulas foliculares e pústulas ou paniculite, causada por intoxicação ou sensibilidade ao iodo.

io·do·form (ī - ō'dō - fōrm). Iodofórmio; anti-séptico tópico. SIN triiodomethane.

io·do·glob·u·lin (ī - ō'dō - glob'u - lin). Iodoglobulina. SIN thyroglobulin (1).

io·do·gor·go·ic ac·id (ī - ō'dō - gōr - gō'ik). Ácido iodogorgóico; 3,5-diiodotirosina; precursor da tiroxina.

io·do·hip·pu·rate so·di·um (ī - ō'dō - hip'poo - rāt). Iodoipurato sódico; composto radiopaco antigamente utilizado por via intravenosa, por via oral ou para urografia retrógrada. Quando marcado com iodo-131, é utilizado para medir o fluxo plasmático renal efetivo e para obter imagens dos rins na renografia radioisotópica.

io·do·meth·a·mate so·di·um (ī - ō'dō - meth'ă - māt). Iodometamato sódico; contraste radiográfico bastante osmolar, iônico e hidrossolúvel, antigamente utilizado na forma de sal dissódico para urografia intravenosa.

io·do·met·ric (ī - ō'dō - met'rik). Iodométrico; relativo à iodometria.

io·dom·e·try (ī - ō - dom'ē - trē). Iodometria; técnicas analíticas que envolvem titulações, em que são formadas ou consumidas formas visíveis de iodo, sendo o ponto final marcado pelo súbito aparecimento ou desaparecimento do iodo. SIN iodimetry. [iodo + G. *metron*, medida]

io·do·pa·no·ic ac·id (ī - ō'dō - pa - nō'ik). Ácido iodopanóico. SIN iopanoic acid.

io·do·phen·dyl·ate (ī - ō'dō - fen'dil - āt). Iodofendilato. SIN iophendylate.

io·do·phil·ia (ī - ō'dō - fil'ē - ă). Iodofilia; afinidade pelo iodo, manifestada por alguns leucócitos em certas condições. Quando tratados com uma solução de iodo e iodeto de potássio, os leucócitos polimorfonucleares (PMN) normais coram-se de amarelo brilhante; em certas condições patológicas, os leucócitos polimorfonucleares muitas vezes coram-se difusamente de castanho ou castanho-amarelado; a reação pode ser intracelular (conforme descrito) ou extracelular, afetando as partículas nas vizinhanças imediatas dos leucócitos. [iodo + G. *phileō*, amar]

io·do·phor (ī - ō'dō - fōr). Iodóforo; combinação de iodo com um transportador surfactante, geralmente polivinilpirrolidona. As preparações comerciais geralmente contêm 1% de iodo "disponível", que é lentamente liberado para exercer seu efeito contra microrganismos; utilizado como desinfetante da pele, particularmente para limpezas cirúrgicas. SIN tamed iodine. [iodo + G. *phora*, transportador]

io·do·phtha·lein (ī - ō'dō - thal'ēn, - dof - thal'ē - in). Iodoftaleína; contraste radiográfico. O sal dissódico já foi utilizado para radiografia da vesícula biliar. SIN tetraiodophenolphthalein sodium.

3-io·do-1,2-pro·pane·di·ol. 3-iodo-1,2-propanediol. SIN *glyceryl* iodide.

γ-io·do·pro·py·lene·gly·col. γ-iodopropilenoglicol. SIN *glyceryl* iodide.

io·do·pro·pyl·i·dene·glyc·er·ol. Iodopropilidenoglicerol. SIN iodinated glycerol.

io·do·pro·teins (ī - ō'dō - prō'tēnz). Iodoproteínas; proteínas contendo iodo ligado a grupamentos tirosil.

io·dop·sin (ī - ō - dop'sin). Iodopsina; qualquer um de três pigmentos visuais compostos de 11-*cis*-retinal ligado a opsina, encontrados nos cones da retina. SIN visual violet. [G. *ion*, violeta, + *ōps*, olho + -in]

io·do·py·ra·cet (ī - ō'dō - pī'ră - set). Iodopiraceto; contraste radiográfico antigamente utilizado para urografia intravenosa; também utilizado para determinar o fluxo plasmático renal e a massa excretora tubular renal. SIN diodone.

io·do·qui·nol (ī - ō'dō - kwin'ol). Iodoquinol; fármaco utilizado como amebicida, preparado pela ação do monocloreto de iodo sobre a 8-hidroxiquinolina.

io·do·ther·a·py (ī'ō - dō - thăr'ă - pē). Iodoterapia; tratamento com iodo.

io·do·thy·ro·nines (ī - ō'dō - thī'rō - nēnz). Iodotironinas; derivados iodados da tironina.

io·do·ty·ro·sine (ī - ō'dō - tī'rō - sēn). Iodotirosina; tirosina iodada.
 i. deiodase, i. desiodase. SIN *iodide* peroxidase.

io·dox·a·mate meg·lu·mine (ī - ō - doks'ă - māt). Iodoxamato de meglumina; o sal metilglucamina de um contraste iônico, hidrossolúvel e dimérico; outrora utilizado principalmente para colangiografia intravenosa.

io·du·ria (ī - ō - doo'rē - ă). Iodúria; excreção urinária de iodo.

io·gly·cam·ic ac·id (ī'ō - glī - kam'ik). Ácido ioglicâmico; ácido 3,3'-[oxibis(metileno carbonilimino)]bis[2,4,6,-trioidobenzóico]; contraste radiográfico iônico, hidrossolúvel e dimérico, utilizado outrora para colangiografia intravenosa.

io·hex·ol (ī'ō - heks'ol). Ioexol; contraste radiográfico monomérico, não-iônico, hidrossolúvel e de baixa osmolaridade para urografia e angiografia. Utilizado por via intratecal e intravascular.

iom·e·ter (ī - om'ē - ter). Iômetro; aparelho para medir a ionização. [ion + G. *metron*, medida]

ion (ī'on). Íon; átomo ou grupamento de átomos que transportam uma carga elétrica em conseqüência do ganho ou da perda de um ou mais elétrons. Os íons carregados com eletricidade negativa (ânions) dirigem-se para um pólo positivo (anodo); aqueles carregados com eletricidade positiva (cátions) dirigem-se para um pólo negativo (catodo). Os íons podem existir em ambientes sólidos, líquidos ou gasosos, embora aqueles em meio líquido (eletrólitos) sejam mais comuns e familiares. [G. *iōn*, que vai]
 aquo-i., aquo ion. VER aquo-ion.
 dipolar i.'s, íons dipolares; íons que possuem tanto uma carga elétrica negativa quanto uma positiva, cada uma localizada em um ponto diferente na molécula que, assim, possui "pólos" positivo e negativo; os aminoácidos são os íons dipolares mais notáveis, contendo um grupamento NH_3^+ de carga elétrica positiva e um grupamento COO^- de carga elétrica negativa em pH neutro. SIN amphions, zwitterions.
 gram-i., i.-grama. VER gram-ion.
 hydride i., i. hidreto; o íon H^-, transferido para moléculas aceptoras em algumas oxidações biológicas.
 hydrogen i. (H^+), íon hidrogênio; um átomo de hidrogênio menos seu elétron e, portanto, transportando uma carga elétrica positiva unitária (isto é, um próton); na água, combina-se com uma molécula de água para formar o íon hidrônio, H_3O^+.
 hydronium i., i. hidrônio; o próton hidratado, H_3O^+, uma forma em que o íon hidrogênio existe em soluções aquosas; além disso, $H_3O^+ \cdot H_2O$, $H_3O^+ \cdot 2H_2O$, etc. SIN oxonium i.
 oxonium i., i. oxônio. SIN hydronium i.
 sulfonium i., i. sulfônio; composto em que um átomo de enxofre possui três ligações covalentes simples e, portanto, uma carga positiva análoga à do hidrogênio de um composto de amônio; p. ex., *S*-adenosil-L-metionina.

Ionescu. VER Jonnesco.

ion ex·change (ī'on eks - chanj'). Troca iônica. VER anion exchange, cation exchange, ion exchange *chromatography*.

ion ex·chang·er (ī'on eks - chanj'er). Trocador de íons. VER anion exchanger, cation exchanger.

ion·ic (ī - on'ik). Iônico; relativo a um íon.

i·o·ni·um (ī - ō'nē - ŭm). Iônio; termo antigo para o tório-230. [G. *iōn*, que vai]

ion·i·za·tion (ī'on - i - zā'shŭn). Ionização. **1.** Dissociação em íons que ocorre quando um eletrólito é dissolvido em água ou em certos líquidos, ou quando moléculas são submetidas a descarga elétrica ou radiação ionizante. **2.** Produção de íons em conseqüência da interação da irradiação com a matéria. **3.** SIN iontophoresis.

ion·ize (ī'on - īz). Ionizar; separar em íons; dissociar átomos ou moléculas em átomos ou radicais com carga elétrica.

ion·o·gram (ī'on - ō - gram). Ionograma. SIN electropherogram.

io·none (ī'ō - nōn). Ionona; uma de duas cetonas terpênicas cíclicas com odor de violeta ou de cedro, cujas variedades α e β diferem na localização da dupla ligação no anel: as pró-vitaminas A e a vitamina A possuem configuração ionona na porção do anel; o α-caroteno contém uma α e uma β-ionona; o β-caroteno contém duas β-iononas; e o γ-caroteno contém uma β-ionona.

ion·o·pher·o·gram (ī'on - ō - fer'ō - gram). Ionoferograma. SIN electropherogram.

ion·o·phore (ī - on'ō - fōr). Ionóforo; composto ou substância que forma um complexo com um íon e o transporta através da membrana. [ion + G. *phore*, transportador]

ion·o·pho·re·sis (ī - on'ō - fōr - ē'sis). Ionoforese. SIN electrophoresis. [ion + G. *phorēsis*, transportando]

ion·o·pho·ret·ic (ī - on'ō - fōr - et'ik). Ionoforético. SIN electrophoretic.

ion·to·pho·re·sis (ī - on'tō - fōr - ē'sis). Iontoforese; introdução nos tecidos, por meio de uma corrente elétrica, de íons de um medicamento escolhido. SIN ionic medication, ionization (3), iontotherapy. [ion + G. *phorēsis*, transportador]

ion·to·pho·ret·ic (ī - on'tō - fōr - et'ik). Iontoforético; relativo à iontoforese.

ion·to·ther·a·py (ī - on'tō - thăr'ă - pē). Iontoterapia. SIN iontophoresis.

io·pam·i·dol (ī'ō - pam'i - dol). Iopamidol; contraste radiográfico monomérico, não-iônico, hidrossolúvel e de baixa osmolaridade para urografia ou angiografia.

io·pa·no·ic ac·id (ī′ō - pa - nō′ik). Ácido iopanóico; contraste radiográfico insolúvel em água; já foi muito utilizado para colecistografia oral. SIN iodopanoic acid.

io·pen·tol (ī′ō - pen′tol). Iopentol; N,N′-Bis(2,3-diidroxipropil)-5-[N-(2-hidroxi-3-metoxipropil) acetamido]-2,4,6-triiodoisoftalamida; contraste radiográfico não-iônico, monomérico e de baixa osmolaridade para urografia intravenosa ou angiografia.

io·phen·dyl·ate (ī - ō - fen′dil - āt). Iofendilato; mistura de isômeros de etil iodofenilundecilato, um ácido graxo iodado de baixa viscosidade; utilizado para radiografia da medula espinal. SIN iodophendylate.

io·phe·no·ic ac·id (ī′ō - fen - ō - ik). Ácido iofenóico. SIN iophenoxic acid.

io·phen·ox·ic ac·id (ī′ō - fen - oks′ik). Ácido iofenóxico; contraste radiográfico; utilizado antigamente para colecistografia oral. SIN iophenoic acid.

io·pho·bia (ī - ō - fō′bē - ā). Iofobia; medo mórbido de venenos. [G. *ios*, veneno + *phobos*, medo]

io·pro·mide (ī - ō′prō - mid). Iopromida; N,N′ Bis(2,3,-diidroxi propil)-2,4-6-triiodo-5-(2-metoxiacetamido)-N-metil isoftalamida; um contraste radiográfico monomérico, não-iônico, hidrossolúvel e de baixa osmolaridade para urografia intravenosa ou angiografia.

i·o·ta (ι) (ī - ōt′a). Iota. **1.** A nona letra do alfabeto grego. **2.** Em química, indica o nome de uma série ou o nono átomo de um grupo carboxila ou outro grupo funcional. **3.** Uma quantidade minúscula ou diminuta.

io·ta·cism (ī - ō′ta - sizm). Iotacismo; defeito da fala caracterizado pela substituição freqüente de vogais por um som *e* longo (confusão do i com o j). [G. *iōta*, a letra ι]

io·tha·lam·ic ac·id (ī′ō - thā - lam′ik). Ácido iotalâmico; contraste radiográfico iônico, monomérico e hidrossolúvel, amplamente utilizado na forma de sal sódico ou de metilglucamina (iotalamato) para urografia intravenosa e angiografia.

io·thi·o·u·ra·cil so·di·um (ī′ō - thī - ō - ūr′a - sil). Iotiouracil sódico; o sal sódico do 5-iodo-2-tiouracil; derivado de iodo orgânico do tiouracil com ação involutiva do iodo sobre a tireóide e capacidade de inibir a produção de tiroxina.

io·trol (ī′ō - trol). Iotrol. SIN iotrolan.

io·tro·lan (ī - ō′trō - lan). Iotrolan; 5,5′-[malonilbis(metilimino)]bis[N,N′-bis[2,3-diidroxi-1-(hidroximetil)propil]-2,4,6-triiodoisoftalamida; contraste radiográfico dimérico, não-iônico, hidrossolúvel e de baixa osmolaridade, utilizado para mielografia e outras aplicações não-vasculares. SIN iotrol.

io·ver·sol (ī - ō - ver′sol). Ioversol; N,N′-bis(2,3-diidroxipropil)-5-[N-(2-hidroxietil)glicolamido]-2,4,6-triiodoisoftalamida; contraste radiográfico hidrossolúvel, não-iônico, de baixa osmolaridade.

iox·ag·late (ī - oks - ag′lāt). Ioxaglato; meio radiopaco diagnóstico que consiste, habitualmente, numa combinação de ioxaglato meglumina ($C_{24}H_{21}I_3N_5O_8 \cdot C_7H_{17}NO_5$) e ioxaglato sódico ($C_{24}H_{20}I_6N_5NaO_8$); utilizado em angiografia, aortografia, arteriografia, venografia e urografia.

iox·i·lan (ī - oks′ī - lan). Ioxilan. N-(2,3-diidroxipropil)-5-[N (2,3-diidroxipropil)acetamido]-N′-(2-hidroxietil)-2,4,6-triiodoisoftalamida; contraste radiográfico monomérico, não-iônico, hidrossolúvel, de baixa osmolaridade para urografia ou angiografia.

iox·i·thal·a·mate (ī - oks - ī - thal′ā - māt). Ioxitalamato; ácido 5-acetamido-2,4,6-triiodo-N-(2-hidroxietil)isoftálmico; contraste radiográfico iônico, monomérico e hidrossolúvel para urografia e angiografia.

I.P., i.p. Abreviatura de intraperitoneal (intraperitoneal) ou intraperitoneally (intraperitonealmente); isoelectric *point* (ponto isoelétrico).

IP$_3$ Abreviatura de *inositol* 1,4,5-trisphosphate (inositol 1,4,5-trifosfato).

IPA Abreviatura de independent practice *association* (associação de prática independente), isopropyl alcohol (álcool isopropílico).

ip·e·cac (ip′ē - kak). Ipeca. SIN ipecacuanha.
  powdered i., i. em pó; forma de ipeca utilizada na preparação do xarope de ipeca.

ip·e·cac·u·a·nha (ip - ē - kak - ū - an′ā). Ipecacuanha; a raiz seca de *Uragoga (Cephaelis) ipecacuanha* (família Rubiaceae), um arbusto do Brasil e de outras partes da América do Sul; contém emetina, cefalina, emetamina, ácido ipecacuânico, psicotrina e metilpsicotrina; possui propriedades expectorantes, eméticas e antidisentéricas. SIN ipecac. [palavra brasileira nativa]
  de-emetinized i., i. desemetinizada; ipecacuanha da qual foi extraído o princípio emético; tem sido utilizada como agente antidisentérico.
  prepared i., i. preparada; pó fino contendo 2% dos alcalóides totais da ipecacuanha, calculados como emetina.

IPF Abreviatura de idiopathic pulmonary *fibrosis* (fibrose pulmonar idiopática) ou interstitial pulmonary *fibrosis* (fibrose pulmonar intersticial).

ipo·date (ī′pō - dāt). Ipodato; contraste radiográfico, administrado por via oral na forma de sal sódico ou, mais freqüentemente, sal de cálcio para opacificação da vesícula biliar e da árvore biliar central.

ip·o·mea (ī - pō - mē′a). Ipoméia; raiz seca de *Ipomea orizabensis* (família Convolvulaceae). VER TAMBÉM ipomea resin SIN orizaba jalap root. [G. *ips (ip-)*, verme + *homoios*, semelhante]

Ip·o·moea (ī - pō - mē′a). Ipomoea; gênero de planta da família Convolvulaceae, incluindo a ipoméia. [L. ipomea]
  I. rubrocoeru′lea var. *prae′cox*, as sementes contêm amida do ácido lisérgico, amida do ácido isolérgico, chanoclavina, elimoclavina e outros alcalóides do esporão do centeio (indol); a ingestão das sementes produz efeitos alucinatórios e eufóricos. SIN morning glory (1).
  I. versico′lor, uma espécie cujas sementes contêm alcalóides alucinogênicos do esporão do centeio (indol).

IPPB Abreviatura de intermittent positive pressure *breathing* (ventilação com pressão positiva intermitente).

IPPV Abreviatura de intermittent positive pressure *ventilation* (ventilação por pressão positiva intermitente).

ipra·tro·pi·um (i - prā - trō′pē - ŭm). Ipratrópio; composto de amônio quaternário sintético, quimicamente relacionado com a atropina, que possui atividade anticolinérgica e é utilizado por via inalatória como broncodilatador.

ipro·ni·a·zid (i - prō - nī′ā - zid). Iproniazida; agente antituberculoso e antidepressivo semelhante à isoniazida, porém mais tóxico e raramente utilizado; inibe a monoamina oxidase (MAO). O primeiro agente antidepressivo.

ipro·ver·a·tril (ī - prō - ver′ā - tril). Iproveratril. SIN verapamil.

iPrSGal Abreviatura de isopropylthiogalactoside (isopropiltiogalactosídeo).

Ips Abreviatura de pipsyl (pipsil).

Ip·se·fact (ip′se - fakt). Todas as partes ou aspectos do ambiente que o indivíduo, a colônia, a população ou a espécie de animal tenha modificado, química ou fisicamente, por seu próprio comportamento (p. ex., ninho ou lar, rastros de roedores ou cervos, excremento, feromonas). [L. *ipse*, o próprio + *factum*, coisa feita]

ip·si·lat·er·al (ip - si - lat′er - āl). Ipsolateral; do mesmo lado, referindo-se a determinado ponto, como, p. ex., pupila dilatada no mesmo lado que um hematoma extradural com membros contralaterais paréticos. SIN homolateral. [L. *ipse*, mesmo + *latus (later-)*, lado]

IPSP Abreviatura de inhibitory postsynaptic *potential* (potencial pós-sináptico inibitório, PPSI).

IPTG Abreviatura de isopropylthiogalactoside (isopropiltiogalactosídeo).

IPV Abreviatura de inactivated poliovirus *vaccine* (vacina de poliovírus inativado). VER poliovirus *vaccines,* em *vaccine*.

IQ Abreviatura de intelligence *quotient* (quociente de inteligência, QI).

IR, ir Abreviatura de infrared (infravermelho).

Ir Símbolo de irídio.

IRB Abreviatura de institutional review *board* (comissão de revisão institucional).

△**irid-. Irid-** VER irido-.

ir·i·dal (ī′ri - dāl, ir′i - dāl). Irial; relativo à íris. SIN iridial, iridian, iridic.

ir·i·dec·to·my (ir′i - dek′tō - mē). Iridectomia. **1.** Excisão de parte da íris. **2.** O orifício, na íris, produzido por uma iridectomia cirúrgica. [irido- + G. *ektomē*, excisão]
  buttonhole i., i. em casa de botão. SIN peripheral i.
  optical i., i. óptica; iridectomia efetuada com o objetivo de melhorar a visão, fazendo uma pupila artificial.
  peripheral i., i. periférica; no glaucoma de ângulo agudo, remoção cirúrgica de uma diminuta porção da íris em sua raiz; na extração intracapsular de catarata, remoção de uma ou mais seções diminutas, próximo à borda periférica, deixando a margem pupilar intacta. SIN button-hole i., stenopeic i..
  sector i., i. de setor; iridectomia em que parte da margem pupilar é excisada.
  stenopeic i., i. estenopéica. SIN peripheral i.
  therapeutic i., i. terapêutica; iridectomia realizada para profilaxia ou cura de doença, como, p. ex., glaucoma de ângulo fechado.

ir·i·den·clei·sis (ir′i - den′klī′sis). Iridênclise; o encarceramento de porção da íris por incisão corneoescleral no glaucoma para efetuar a filtração entre a câmara anterior e o espaço subconjuntival. [irido- + G. *enkleiō*, fechar]

ir·i·der·e·mia (ir′i - der - ē′mē′ā, ī′rid-). Irideremia; condição em que a íris é tão rudimentar a ponto de parecer ausente. Cf. aniridia. [irido- + G. *erēmia*, ausência]

ir·i·des (ir′i - dēz). Íris; plural de iris. [G.]

ir·i·des·cent (ir - i - des′ent). Iridescente; que apresenta múltiplas cores refringentes brilhantes, tipicamente em conseqüência de interferência óptica quando a luz branca incidente é decomposta em seus componentes espectrais ao ser refletida de volta através de várias películas de camada fina. [G. *iris*, arco-íris]

irid·e·sis (i - rid′ē - sis, ī - ri - dē′sis). Iridese; ligadura de porção da íris efetuada através de uma incisão na córnea. [irido- + G. *desis*, união, junção]

irid·i·al, irid·i·an, irid·ic (ī - ridē - al; ī - ridē - an; ī - rid′ik, i - rid′-). Irial, iridiano. SIN iridal.

ir·i·din (ir′i - din). Iridina. **1.** Irigenina 7-glicosídeo do rizoma do lírio-florentino, *Iris florentina*. **2.** Resinóide do lírio-azul, *Iris versicolor*; utilizado como colagogo e catártico. SIN irisin.

irid·i·um (Ir) (i - rid′ē - ŭm). Irídio; elemento metálico branco prateado, de número atômico 77, peso atômico 192,22; o Ir^{192} é um radioisótopo (meia-vida de 77,83 dias) que tem sido utilizado no tratamento intersticial de certos tumores. [L. *iris*, arco-íris]

irido-, irid-. Irido-, irid-. A íris. [G. *ris (irid-)*, arco-íris]

ir·i·do·a·vul·sion (ir′i - dō - ā - vŭl′shŭn). Iridoavulsão; avulsão ou dilaceração da íris.

ir·i·do·cele (ir′i - dō - sēl). Iridocele; herniação de uma porção da íris através de um defeito da córnea. [irido- + G. *kēlē*, hérnia]

ir·i·do·cho·roid·i·tis (ir′i - dō - kō - roy - dī′tis). Iridocoroidite; inflamação da íris e da coróide.

ir·i·do·col·o·bo·ma (ir′i - dō - ko - lō - bō′mă). Iridocoloboma; coloboma ou defeito congênito da íris. [irido- + G. *kolobōma*, coloboma]

ir·i·do·cor·ne·al (ir′i - dō - kōr′nē - ăl). Iridocorneano; relativo à íris e à córnea.

ir·i·do·cy·clec·to·my (ir′i - dō - sī - klek′tō - mē). Iridociclectomia; remoção da íris e do corpo ciliar para excisão de um tumor. [irido- + G. *kyklos*, círculo (corpo ciliar) + *ektomē*, excisão]

ir·i·do·cy·cli·tis (ir′i - dō - sī - klī′tis). Iridociclite; inflamação da íris e do corpo ciliar. VER TAMBÉM iritis, uveitis. [irido- + G. *kyklos*, círculo (corpo ciliar) + *-itis*, inflamação]
  i. sep't·ica, i. séptica. SIN Behçet *syndrome.*

ir·i·do·cy·clo·cho·roid·i·tis (ir′i - dō - sī′klō - kō - royd - ī′tis). Iridociclocoroidite; inflamação da íris envolvendo o corpo ciliar e a coróide.

ir·i·do·cys·tec·to·my (ir′i - dō - sis - tek′tō - mē). Iridocistectomia; operação para produzir uma pupila artificial quando a extração extracapsular de catarata é acompanhada de sinéquias posteriores; a borda da íris e uma porção da cápsula do cristalino são puxadas através de uma incisão na córnea e seccionadas. [irido- + G. *kystis*, bexiga (cápsula) + *ektomē*, excisão]

ir·i·do·di·ag·no·sis (ir′i - dō - dī - ag - nō′sis). Iridodiagnóstico; diagnóstico de doenças sistêmicas através da observação de alterações na forma e na cor da íris.

ir·i·do·di·al·y·sis (ir′i - dō - dī - al′i - sis). Iridodiálise; defeito colobomatoso da íris causado pela sua separação do esporão da esclerótica. [irido- + G. *dialysis*, afrouxamento]

ir·i·do·di·la·tor (ir′i - dō - dī - lā′ter). Iridodilatador; que causa dilatação da pupila; aplica-se ao músculo dilatador da pupila.

ir·i·do·do·ne·sis (ir′i - dō - dō - nē′sis). Iridodonese; movimento agitado da íris. SIN tremulous iris. [irido- + G. *doneō*, agitar]

ir·i·do·ki·net·ic (ir′i - dō - ki - net′ik). Iridocinético; relativo aos movimentos da íris.

ir·i·dol·o·gy (ir - i - dol′ō - jē). Iridologia; sistema de medicina hipotético, não baseado em evidências, que recorre ao exame da íris utilizando um gráfico em que certas áreas da íris são consideradas diagnosticamente específicas para determinados órgãos, sistemas e estruturas. [irido- + G. *logos*, estudo]

ir·i·do·ma·la·cia (ir′i - dō - mă - lā′shē - ă). Iridomalacia; amolecimento degenerativo da íris. [irido- + G. *malakia*, amolecimento]

ir·i·do·mes·o·di·al·y·sis (ir′i - dō - mes′ō - di - al′i - sis). Iridomesodiálise; separação de aderências ao redor da margem interna da íris. [irido- + G. *mesos*, meio + *dialysis*, afrouxamento]

ir·i·do·mo·tor (ir′i - dō - mō′tor). Iridomotor. SIN pupillomotor.

ir·i·do·par·al·y·sis (ir′i - dō - pă - ral′i - sis). Iridoparalisia. SIN iridoplegia.

ir·i·dop·a·thy (ir′i - dop′ă - thē). Iridopatia; lesões patológicas da íris.

ir·i·do·ple·gia (ir′i - dō - plē′jē - ă). Iridoplegia; paralisia do esfíncter muscular da íris. SIN iridoparalysis. [irido- + G. *plēgē*, golpe]
  complete i., i. completa; paralisia dos músculos dilatador e esfincteriano da íris.
  reflex i., i. reflexa; ausência do reflexo pupilar à luz, como na pupila de Argyll Robertson.
  sympathetic i., i. simpática; iridoplegia devido à paralisia do músculo dilatador da pupila de inervação simpática.

ir·i·dop·to·sis (ir′i - dop - tō′sis). Iridoptose; prolapso da íris. [irido- + G. *ptōsis*, queda]

ir·i·dor·rhex·is (ir′i - dō - rek′sis). Iridorrexia; ruptura cirúrgica deliberada da íris do esporão da esclerótica para aumentar a largura de um coloboma. [irido- + G. *rhēxis*, ruptura]

ir·i·dos·chi·sis (ir - i - dos′ki - sis). Iridosquise; separação da camada anterior da íris da camada posterior; as fibras anteriores rotas flutuam no humor aquoso. [irido- + G. *schisma*, fenda]

ir·i·do·scle·rot·o·my (ir′i - dō - skle - rot′ō - mē). Iridoesclerotomia; incisão envolvendo tanto a esclerótica quanto a íris. [irido- + esclerótica + G. *tomē*, incisão]

ir·i·dot·o·my (ir - i - dot′ō - mē). Iridotomia; divisão transversa de algumas das fibras da íris, formando uma pupila artificial. [irido- + G. *tomē*, incisão]
  laser i., i. a laser; iridectomia periférica efetuada por laser.

Ir·i·do·vir·i·dae (i - do - vir′i - dē). Família de vírus incluindo os vírus iridescentes de insetos (Iridovírus) e os vírus que infectam rãs e peixes. Esses vírus são grandes, icosaédricos (120–170 nm de diâmetro) e contêm lipídios. O genoma consiste numa única molécula de DNA de filamento duplo, com peso molecular de $130–160 \times 10^6$.

Ir·i·do·vi·rus (ir′i - dō - vī′rŭs). Iridovírus; gênero de vírus (família Iridoviridae) constituído por vírus iridescentes de insetos, cuja espécie-tipo é o vírus iridescentes tipula.

iri·gen·in (ī - ri - jen′in). Irigenina; componente triiodoxi trimetoxi isoflavona da iridina.

iris, pl. **ir·i·des** (ī′ris, iri - dēz). Íris; a divisão anterior da túnica vascular do olho, um diafragma, perfurado no centro (a pupila), fixada perifericamente ao esporão da esclerótica; composta por estroma e por uma dupla camada de epitélio retiniano pigmentado, do qual derivam os músculos esfincteriano e dilatador da pupila. SIN orris. [G. rainbow, a íris do olho]
  i. bicolor, i. bicolor; íris variegada ou de duas cores. SIN monocular heterochromia.
  i. bombé, i. arqueada; condição que ocorre na sinéquia anular posterior, em que o aumento de líquido na câmara posterior provoca um abaulamento da íris periférica para frente.
  plateau i., i. em platô; no glaucoma de ângulo fechado, aspecto achatado da íris, em lugar de uma convexidade para frente.
  tremulous i., i. trêmula. SIN iridodonesis.

iris frill. Beira enrugada da íris. SIN collarette.

iri·sin (ī′ri - sin). Irisina. SIN iridin (2).

irit·ic (ī - rit′ik). Irítico; relativo à irite.

iri·tis (ī - rī′tis). Irite; inflamação da íris. VER TAMBÉM iridocyclitis, uveitis.
  fibrinous i., i. fibrinosa; inflamação aguda da íris, com exsudato profuso; ocorre na uveíte da sífilis terciária.
  follicular i., i. folicular; termo raramente utilizado para referir-se à irite crônica com nódulos vítreos situados profundamente entre as camadas anterior e posterior da íris.
  i. glaucomato'sa, i. glaucomatosa; derramamento de exsudato e células após controle do glaucoma de ângulo fechado.
  hemorrhagic i., i. hemorrágica; irite com hiperemia tão intensa a ponto de ocorrer hifema.
  nodular i., i. nodular; irite com agregações de células redondas na íris.
  plastic i., i. plástica; irite com exsudação fibrinosa.
  quiet i., i. silenciosa; irite sem sinais inflamatórios, como vermelhidão ou edema da córnea.
  serous i., i. serosa; inflamação da íris com exsudato seroso na câmara anterior.
  sympathetic i., i. simpática; irite consecutiva a uma condição semelhante no outro olho.

iron (Fe) (ī′ern, ī′rŭn). Ferro; elemento metálico, de número atômico 26, peso atômico 55,847, que ocorre no heme da hemoglobina, na mioglobina, na transferrina, na ferritina e nas porfirinas contendo ferro, além de ser um componente essencial de enzimas como catalase, peroxidase e os vários citocromos; seus sais são utilizados medicinalmente. Para os sais individuais não relacionados adiante, ver as subentradas ferric e ferrous. [A.S. *iren*]
  albuminized i., i. albuminate, f. albuminizado; composto de óxido de ferro e albumina, solubilizado pela presença de citrato de sódio; ocorre na forma de grânulos castanho-avermelhados brilhantes, inodoros ou quase; utilizado na anemia.
  i. alum, alúmen férrico. SIN *ferric* ammonium sulfate.
  i. filings, limalha de ferro; pequenos aglomerados de ovos de *Paragonimus* spp. que podem ser observados no escarro; os aglomerados de ovos tendem a ser castanho-amarelados.
  i. protoporphyrin, ferro protoporfirina; protoporfirina ligada a um átomo de ferro; p. ex., heme.
  i. pyri'tes, pirita férrica; sulfeto nativo de ferro.

iron-52 (^{52}Fe). Ferro-52 (Fe^{52}); isótopo radioativo de ferro; emissor de positrons produzido por cicloton, com meia-vida de 8,28 horas, utilizado para o estudo do metabolismo do ferro.

iron-55 (^{55}Fe). Ferro-55 (Fe^{55}); isótopo do ferro; emissor de positrons com meia-vida de 2,73 anos; utilizado (com menos freqüência do que o Fe^{59}) como marcador no estudo do metabolismo do ferro e da perfusão do sangue.

iron-59 (^{59}Fe). Ferro-59 (Fe^{59}); isótopo do ferro; emissor gama e beta com meia-vida de 44,51 dias; utilizado como marcador no estudo do metabolismo do ferro, determinação do volume sanguíneo e em estudo de transfusão sanguínea.

ir·ra·di·ate (i - rā′dē - āt). Irradiar; aplicar radiação de determinada fonte a uma estrutura ou organismo. [ver irradiation]

ir·ra·di·a·tion (i - rā - dē - ā′shŭn). Irradiação. **1.** Aumento subjetivo de um objeto brilhante observado contra um fundo escuro. **2.** Exposição à ação da irradiação eletromagnética (p. ex., calor, luz, raios X). **3.** A disseminação de impulsos nervosos de uma área no cérebro ou na medula espinal ou de um trato para outro trato. VER TAMBÉM radiation. [L. *irradio, (in-r)*, pp. *-radi-atus*, irradiar]

ir·ra·tion·al (i - rash′ŭn - ăl). Irracional; não-racional; não-razoável (contrário à razão) ou ilógico (que não exerce a razão). [L. *irrationalis*, sem razão]

ir·re·duc·i·ble (ir - rē - doo'si - bl, i - rē-). Irredutível. **1.** Não-redutível; incapaz de se tornar menor. **2.** Em química, incapaz de se tornar mais simples ou ser substituído, hidrogenado ou reduzido na sua carga elétrica positiva.

ir·re·spir·a·ble (ir - rē - spir'a - bl). Irrespirável. **1.** Incapaz de ser inalado devido à irritação das vias aéreas, resultando em suspensão da respiração. **2.** Indica um gás ou vapor venenoso ou contendo oxigênio em quantidade insuficiente. **3.** Indica um aerossol composto de partículas com tamanho aerodinâmico > 10 μ.

ir·re·spon·si·bil·i·ty (ir're - spons - i - bil'i - tē). Irresponsabilidade; estado de não atuar de modo responsável, por motivos conscientes ou inconscientes.
  criminal i., criminal; o estado, habitualmente atribuído a algum defeito ou doença mental, que torna uma pessoa não-responsável por sua conduta criminosa.

ir·re·sus·ci·ta·ble (ir'rē - sŭs'i - tā - bl). Incapaz de ser reanimado.

ir·re·vers·i·ble (ir - rē - ver'si - bl). Irreversível; incapaz de ser revertido; permanente. [L. *in-* (*ir-*) neg. + *re-verto,* pp. *-versus,* retornar]

ir·ri·gate (ir'i - gāt). Irrigar; efetuar uma irrigação. [L. *ir-rigo,* pp. *-atus,* irrigar, de *in,* sobre + *rigo,* regar]

ir·ri·ga·tion (ir - i - gā'shŭn). Irrigação; lavagem de uma cavidade corporal, espaço ou ferida com líquido. [ver irrigate]

ir·ri·ga·tor (ir'i - gā - ter). Irrigador; dispositivo utilizado na irrigação.

ir·ri·ta·bil·i·ty (ir'i - tā - bil'i - tē). Irritabilidade; propriedade inerente do protoplasma de reagir a um estímulo. [L. *irritabilitas,* de *irrito,* pp. *-atus,* excitar]
  electric i., i. elétrica; a resposta de um nervo ou músculo à passagem de uma corrente elétrica; em casos de degeneração no nervo ou no músculo, essa irritabilidade encontra-se alterada ou perdida. VER modal *alteration,* qualitative *alteration,* quantitative *alteration.*
  myotatic i., i. miotática; capacidade de um músculo de se contrair em resposta ao estímulo produzido por estiramento abrupto.

ir·ri·ta·ble (ir'i - tā - bl). Irritável. **1.** Capaz de reagir a um estímulo. **2.** Que tende a reagir imoderadamente a um estímulo. Cf. excitable.

ir·ri·tant (ir'i - tant). Irritante. **1.** Excitante; que produz irritação. **2.** Qualquer agente com essa ação.
  primary i., i. primário; substância que causa inflamação e outras evidências de irritação, particularmente da pele, ao primeiro contato ou exposição, ou como reação a contatos cumulativos, independentemente do mecanismo de sensibilização.

ir·ri·ta·tion (ir - i - tā'shŭn). Irritação. **1.** Reação inflamatória incipiente extrema dos tecidos a uma lesão. **2.** A resposta normal do nervo ou do músculo a um estímulo. **3.** Evocação de uma resposta normal ou exagerada nos tecidos pela aplicação de um estímulo. [L. *irritatio*]

ir·ri·ta·tive (ir - i - tā'tiv). Irritativo; que causa irritação.

ir·ru·ma·tion (ir'oo - mā'shŭn). Felação, coito bucal. SIN fellatio. [L. *irrumo,* pp. *-atus,* amamentar]

ir·rup·tion (i - rŭp'shŭn). Irrupção; ato ou processo de irromper através de uma superfície. [L. *irruptio,* de *irrumpo,* romper]

ir·rup·tive (i - rŭp'tiv). Irruptivo; relativo a, ou caracterizado por, irrupção.

IRS-1 Abreviatura de insulin receptor *substrate-1* (substrato do receptor de insulina 1).

IRV Abreviatura de inspiratory reserve *volume* (volume de reserva inspiratório, VRI).

Irvine, A. Ray, Jr., oftalmologista norte-americano, *1917. VER I.-Gass *syndrome.*

ISA Abreviatura de intrinsic sympathomimetic *activity* (atividade simpaticomimética intrínseca).

Is·a·mine blue (is'ā - mēn, ī'sā-). Azul de isamina. SIN pyrrol blue.

is·aux·e·sis (ī - sawk - zē'sis). Isauxese; crescimento de partes na mesma velocidade do que o crescimento do todo. [G. *isos,* igual + *auxēsis,* aumento]

is·che·mia (is - kē'mē - ā). Isquemia; anemia localizada devido a obstrução mecânica (principalmente por estenose ou ruptura arterial) do suprimento sanguíneo. [G. *ischō,* reter + *haima,* sangue]
  myocardial i., i. do miocárdio; circulação inadequada do sangue para o miocárdio, geralmente em conseqüência de coronariopatia. VER TAMBÉM *angina* pectoris, myocardial *infarction.*
  postural i., i. postural; redução da pressão arterial e do fluxo sanguíneo induzida em uma parte, como, p. ex., a perna ou o pé, elevando-a acima do nível do coração; utilizada para reduzir o sangramento durante intervenções cirúrgicas nos membros.
  i. ret'inae, i. da retina; diminuição do suprimento sanguíneo na retina, devido à insuficiência da circulação arterial; pode ocorrer em conseqüência de embolia ou espasmo arterial; intoxicação, como, p. ex., pela quinina; ou exsanguinação de hemorragias profusas recidivantes; pode ocorrer cegueira bilateral transitória ou permanente.
  silent i., i. silenciosa; i. do miocárdio sem sinais ou sintomas associados de angina de peito; pode ser detectada por ECG e outras técnicas laboratoriais. VER TAMBÉM silent myocardial *infarction.*

is·che·mic (is - kē'mik). Isquêmico; relativo a, ou afetado por, isquemia.

is·che·sis (is - kē'sis). Isquese; supressão de qualquer secreção, especialmente uma secreção normal. [G. *ischō,* reter]

is·chia (is'kē - ā). Ísquios; plural de ischium.

is·chi·ad·ic (is - kē - ad'ik). Isquiático. SIN sciatic (1).

is·chi·a·di·cus (is - kē - ad'i - kŭs). Isquiático. SIN sciatic. [L.]

is·chi·al (is'kē - ăl). Isquiático. SIN sciatic (1).

is·chi·al·gia (is - kē - al'jē - ā). Isquialgia. **1.** Termo obsoleto para referir-se à dor no quadril; especificamente, o ísquio. SIN ischiodynia. **2.** Termo obsoleto para ciática. [G. *ischion,* quadril + *algos,* dor]

is·chi·at·ic (is - kē - at'ik). Isquiático. SIN sciatic (1).

△ **ischio-.** Ísquio-. O ísquio. [G. *ischion,* articulação do quadril, anca (ísquio)]

is·chi·o·a·nal (is - kē - ō - ā'năl). Isquioanal; relativo ao ísquio e ao ânus.

is·chi·o·bul·bar (is - kē - ō - bŭl'bar). Isquiobulbar; relativo ao ísquio e ao bulbo do pênis.

is·chi·o·cap·su·lar (is - kē - ō - kap'soo - lăr). Isquiocapsular; relativo ao ísquio e à cápsula da articulação do quadril; indica a parte da cápsula fixada ao ísquio.

is·chi·o·cav·er·no·sus. Isquiocavernoso. VER ischiocavernous (*muscle*).

is·chi·o·cav·ern·ous (is - kē - ō - kav'er - nŭs). Isquiocavernoso; relativo ao ísquio e ao corpo cavernoso.

is·chi·o·cele (is'kē - ō - sēl). Isquiocele. SIN sciatic *hernia.* [ischio- + G. *kēlē,* hérnia]

is·chi·o·coc·cyg·e·al (is - kē - ō - kok - sij'ē - ăl). Isquiococcígeo; relativo ao ísquio e ao cóccix.

is·chi·o·coc·cyg·e·us (is - kē - ō - kok - sij'ē - ŭs). Isquiococcígeo. SIN coccygeus *muscle.* VER muscle.

is·chi·o·dyn·ia (is'kē - ō - din'ē - ā). Isquiodinia. SIN ischialgia (1). [ischio- + G. *odynē,* dor]

is·chi·o·fem·o·ral (is - kē - ō - fem'ō - răl). Isquiofemoral; relativo ao ísquio ou osso do quadril e ao fêmur ou osso da coxa.

is·chi·o·fib·u·lar (is'kē - ō - fib'u - lăr). Isquiofibular; relativo a ou que une o ísquio e a fíbula.

is·chi·o·me·lus (is - ki - om'ē - lŭs). Isquiômelo; gêmeos conjugados desiguais em que o parasita, freqüentemente representado apenas por um braço ou uma perna, origina-se da região pélvica do autósito. VER conjoined *twins,* em *twin.* [ischio- + G. *melos,* membro]

is·chi·o·ni·tis (is'kē - ō - nī'tis). Isquionite; inflamação do ísquio.

is·chi·op·a·gus (is - kē - op'ă - gŭs). Isquiópago; gêmeos conjugados unidos pela região isquiática. VER conjoined *twins,* em *twin.* [ischio- + G. *pagos,* fixo]

is·chi·o·per·i·ne·al (is'kē - ō - per - i - nē'ăl). Isquioperineal; relativo ao ísquio e ao períneo.

is·chi·o·pu·bic (is'kē - ō - poo'bik). Isquiopúbico; relativo ao ísquio e ao púbis.

is·chi·o·rec·tal (is'kē - ō - rek'tăl). Isquiorretal; relativo ao ísquio e ao reto.

is·chi·o·sa·cral (is - kē - ō - sā'krăl). Isquiossacral; relativo ao ísquio e ao sacro.

is·chi·o·tho·ra·cop·a·gus (is'kē - ō - thōr - ă - kop'ă - gŭs). Isquiotoracópago. SIN iliothoracopagus.

is·chi·o·tib·i·al (is - kē - ō - tib'ē - ăl). Isquiotibial; relativo ao ísquio e à tíbia ou ao que os une.

is·chi·o·vag·i·nal (is - kē - ō - vaj'i - năl). Isquiovaginal; relativo ao ísquio e à vagina.

is·chi·o·ver·te·bral (is - kē - ō - ver'tē - brăl). Isquiovertebral; relativo ao ísquio e à coluna vertebral.

is·chi·um, gen. **is·chii,** pl. **is·chia** (is'kē - ŭm, is'kē - ī, is'kē - ā). [TA]. Ísquio; a parte inferior e posterior do osso do quadril, distinta ao nascimento, mas que, posteriormente, se funde com o íleo e o púbis; consiste em um corpo, onde se une ao íleo e ramo superior do púbis para formar o acetábulo, e num ramo que se une ao ramo inferior do púbis. SIN os ischii [TA], ischial bone. [L. Mod. do G. *ischion,* quadril]

is·cho·chy·mia (is - kō - kī'mē - ā). Iscoquimia; retenção de alimento no estômago devido à dilatação desse órgão. [G. *ischō,* reter + *chymos,* suco]

is·chu·ret·ic (is - koo - ret'ik). Iscurético. **1.** Relativo a ou que alivia a iscúria. **2.** Agente que alivia a retenção ou a supressão de urina.

is·chu·ria (is - koo'rē - ā). Iscúria; retenção ou supressão da urina. [G. *ischō,* reter + *ouron,* urina]

is·e·thi·o·nate (ī - se - thī'ō - nāt). Isetionato; sal ou éster do ácido isetiônico.

is·e·thi·on·ic ac·id (ī'se - thī - on'ik). Ácido isetiônico; ácido 2-hidroxietanossulfônico; líquido viscoso incolor, miscível com água e álcoois, que forma sais cristalinos com ácidos orgânicos.

Ishak, VER Luna-Ishak *stain.*

Ishihara, Shinobu, oftalmologista japonês, 1879-1963. VER I. *test.*

ISI Abreviatura de international sensitivity *index* (índice de sensibilidade internacional).

isin·glass (ī'zing-glas). Cola de peixe. SIN ichthyocolla. [Alemão antigo *huysenblas*, bexiga de esturjão]

is·land (ī'land). Ilha; em anatomia, qualquer parte isolada, separada dos tecidos circundantes por um sulco, ou caracterizada por uma diferença na estrutura. SIN insula (2) [TA]. [A.S. *īgland*]
  blood i., ilhota sanguínea; agregação de células mesodérmicas esplâncnicas no saco vitelino embrionário, com a potencialidade de formar endotélio vascular e células sanguíneas primitivas. SIN blood islet.
  bone i., ilhota óssea; foco macroscópico de osso cortical dentro do osso medular, comumente observado como imagens densas redondas ou ovais em radiografias da pelve, da cabeça do fêmur, do úmero ou das costelas.
  i.'s of Calleja, ilhotas de Calleja; aglomerados densos de células nervosas muito pequenas (células granulosas), características do tubérculo olfatório na base do prosencéfalo.
  epimyoepithelial i.'s (ep'ē-mī-ō-ep'ē-thē'lī-al). Ilhotas epimioepiteliais; proliferação de epitélio ductal e mioepitélio das glândulas salivares. Características de lesões linfoepiteliais benignas e da síndrome de Sjögren.
  Langerhans i.'s, ilhotas de Langerhans. SIN *islets* of Langerhans, em *islet*.
  pancreatic i.'s, ilhotas pancreáticas. SIN *islets* of Langerhans, em *islet*.
  i. of Reil, i. de Reil. SIN insula (1).

is·let (ī'let). Ilhota; uma pequena ilha.
  blood i., i. sanguínea. SIN blood *island*.
  i.'s of Langerhans, ilhotas de Langerhans; massas celulares que variam desde algumas a centenas de células localizadas no tecido intersticial do pâncreas; são constituídas por diferentes tipos celulares, que compreendem a porção endócrina do pâncreas e constituem a fonte de insulina e glucagon. SIN islet tissue, Langerhans islands, pancreatic islands, pancreatic i.'s.

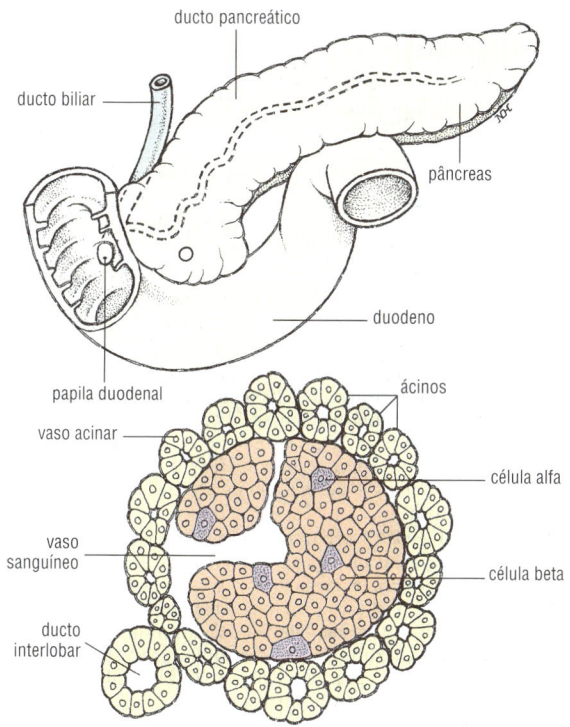

ilhotas de Langerhans

  pancreatic i.'s, ilhotas pancreáticas. SIN i.'s of Langerhans.

-ism. -Ismo. **1.** Condição, doença ou intoxicação. **2.** Indica uma prática ou doutrina. Cf. -ia, -ismus. [G. *-isma, -ismos,* sufixo formador de substantivo]

-ismus. -Ismo. L. para -ism; habitualmente utilizado para indicar espasmo, contração. [L. do G. *-ismos,* sufixo formador de substantivos de ação]

iso-. Iso-. **1.** Prefixo que significa igual, semelhante. **2.** Em química, prefixo que indica "isômero de" (isomerismo); p. ex., isocianato *vs.* cianato. **3.** Em imunologia, prefixo que designa igualdade em relação a espécies; nestes últimos anos, o significado mudou para igualdade em relação à constituição genética de indivíduos. [G. *isos,* igual]

iso·ac·cept·or tRNA (ī'sō-ak'sep-tor). tRNA isoaceptor; diferentes espécies de tRNA que se ligam a códons alternados para o mesmo resíduo de aminoácido; pode ser um tRNA que reconhece os vários códons que representam aqueles para o resíduo de aminoácido específico.

iso·ag·glu·ti·na·tion (ī'sō-ă-gloo-ti-nā'shŭn). Isoaglutinação; aglutinação de eritrócitos em consequência da reação entre uma isoaglutinina e um antígeno específico nas células. SIN isohemagglutination. [iso- + L. *ad,* para + *gluten,* cola]

iso·ag·glu·ti·nin (ī'sō-ă-gloo'ti-nin). Isoaglutinina; isoanticorpo que provoca aglutinação de células de membros geneticamente diferentes da mesma espécie. SIN isohemagglutinin.

iso·ag·glu·tin·o·gen (ī'sō-ă-gloo-tin'ō-jen). Isoaglutinógeno; isoantígeno que induz a aglutinação das células às quais está ligado após exposição a seu isoanticorpo específico.

iso·al·lele (ī'sō-ă-lēl'). Isoalelo; um de vários dos alelos que podem ser distinguidos apenas por análises especiais.

iso·al·lox·a·zine (ī'sō-ă-loks'ă-zēn). Isoaloxazina; composto heterocíclico que forma a base estrutural da riboflavina e de outras flavinas.

iso·am·i·nile (ī-sō-am'i-nīl). Isoaminila; agente antitussígeno.

iso·am·yl (ī-sō-am'il). Isoamila. VER amyl.

iso·am·y·lase (ī-sō-am'il-ās). Isoamilase; hidrolase que cliva as ligações de ramificação 1,6-α-D-glicosídicas no glicogênio, na amilopectina e suas dextrinas β-limites; parte do complexo conhecido como enzima desramificante; semelhante à α-dextrina 1,6-α-glicosidase, porém incapaz de atuar sobre o pululano.

iso·an·dros·ter·one (ī'sō-an-dros'ter-ōn). Isoandrosterona. SIN epiandrosterone.

iso·an·ti·body (ī'sō-an'ti-bod-ē). Isoanticorpo. **1.** Anticorpo que ocorre em alguns indivíduos de uma espécie e reage especificamente com um isoantígeno estranho específico. Para os isoanticorpos específicos de grupos sanguíneos, ver apêndice de Grupos Sanguíneos. **2.** Termo algumas vezes utilizado como sinônimo de aloanticorpo. [G. *isos,* igual]

iso·an·ti·gen (ī'sō-an'ti-jen). Antiantígeno. **1.** Substância antigênica que só ocorre em alguns indivíduos de uma espécie, como os antígenos de grupos sanguíneos dos seres humanos. Para isoantígenos específicos de grupos sanguíneos, ver o apêndice de Grupos Sanguíneos. **2.** Termo algumas vezes utilizado como sinônimo de aloantígeno.

iso·bar (ī'sō-bar). Isóbaro. **1.** Um de dois ou mais nuclídios que possui o mesmo número total de prótons mais nêutrons, porém com distribuição diferente; p. ex., argônio-40 com 18 prótons e 22 nêutrons, potássio-40 com 19 prótons e 21 nêutrons, cálcio-40 com 20 prótons e 20 nêutrons. O produto de uma β-desintegração é um isóbaro de seu original. **2.** Em um mapa, linha que liga pontos de pressão barométrica igual. **3.** Qualquer curva ou equação relacionando quantidades medidas na mesma pressão. [iso- + G. *baros,* peso]

iso·bar·ic (ī-sō-bar'ik). Isobárico. **1.** Que apresenta peso ou pressão igual. **2.** Com relação a soluções, que tem a mesma densidade do que o diluente ou meio; p. ex., na anestesia raquiana, uma solução isobárica tem a mesma densidade do líquido cefalorraquidiano.

iso·bor·nyl·thi·o·cy·a·no·ac·e·tate (ī-sō-bōr'nil thī-ō-sī'ă-nō-as'ē-tāt). Isobornil tiocianoacetato; $C_{13}H_{19}NO_2S$; pediculicida.

iso·bu·tane (ī'sō-bū'tān). Isobutano. VER butane.

iso·bu·te·ine (ī-sō-bū'tē-ēn). Isobuteína. S-(2-carboxipropil)cisteína; composto contendo enxofre encontrado na urina.

iso·bu·tyl ni·trite. Nitrato de isobutila; líquido presente no nitrito de amila comercial, com propriedades antiespasmódicas e vasodilatadoras semelhantes.

iso·bu·tyr·ic ac·id (ī'sō-bū-tir'ik). Ácido isobutírico. VER butyric acid.

iso·cap·nia (ī-sō-kap'nē-ă). Isocapnia; estado em que a pressão arterial de dióxido de carbono permanece constante ou inalterada. [iso- + G. *kapnos,* vapor]

iso·cel·lu·lar (ī'sō-sel'ū-lăr). Isocelular; composto de células de tamanho igual ou caráter semelhante. [iso- + L. *cellula,* dim. de *cella,* uma sela, depósito]

iso·chor·ic (ī'sō-kōr'ik). Isocórico. SIN isovolumic. [iso- + G. *chōra,* espaço]

iso·chro·mat·ic (ī-sō-krō-mat'ik). Isocromático. **1.** De cor uniforme. SIN isochroous. **2.** Indica dois objetos da mesma cor. [iso- + G. *chrōma,* cor]

iso·chro·mat·o·phil, iso·chro·mat·o·phile (ī'sō-krō-mat'ō-fil, fīl). Isocromatófilo; que tem afinidade igual para o mesmo corante; refere-se a células ou tecidos. [iso- + G. *chrōma,* cor + *philos,* amigo]

iso·chro·mo·some (ī'sō-krō'mō-sōm). Isocromossoma; aberração cromossômica que surge em consequência da divisão transversal, e não longitudinal, do centrômero durante a meiose; formam-se dois cromossomas, faltando, em cada um, um braço cromossômico, porém com o outro duplicado.

iso·chro·nia (ī-sō-krō'nē-ă). Isocronismo. **1.** Estado de ter a mesma cronaxia. **2.** Concordância entre dois processos quanto ao tempo, velocidade ou freqüência. [iso- + G. *chronos,* tempo]

isoch·ro·nous (ī-sok'rō-nŭs). Isócrono; que ocorre durante o mesmo tempo.

isoch·ro·ous (ī-sok'rō-ŭs). Isocromático. SIN isochromatic (1).

iso·cit·rase, iso·cit·ra·tase (ī - sō - sit′rās,   - sit′rā - tās). Isocitrase, isocitratase. SIN *isocitrate* lyase.
iso·ci·trate (ī - sō - sit′rāt),   (ī - sit′rāt). Isocitrato; sal ou éster do ácido isocítrico.
   i. dehydrogenase, i. desidrogenase; uma de duas enzimas que catalisa a conversão do *treo*-D$_s$-isocitrato, o produto da ação da aconitase e da isocitrato-liase, em α-cetoglutarato (2-oxoglutarato) e CO_2; uma das isozimas utiliza NAD+ (que participa no ciclo do ácido tricarboxílico), enquanto a outra utiliza $NADP^+$. SIN isocitric acid dehydrogenase, oxalosuccinic carboxylase.
   i. lyase, i. liase; enzima que catalisa a condensação aldol reversível do glioxilato e succinato, formando *treo*-D$_2$-isocitrato; participa no ciclo do glioxilato. SIN isocitrase, isocitratase, isocitritase.
iso·cit·ric ac·id (ī - sō - sit′rik). Ácido isocítrico; intermediário no ciclo dos ácidos tricarboxílicos.
   i. a. dehydrogenase, desidrogenase do ácido isocítrico. SIN *isocitrate* dehydrogenase.
iso·cit·ri·tase (ī - sō - sit′ri - tās). Isocitritase. SIN *isocitrate* lyase.
iso·cline (ī′sō - klīn). Isóclina; numa região geográfica, linha que liga todos os pontos em que, numa população, existe a mesma freqüência média para os diversos alelos em determinado *locus* genético. VER TAMBÉM cline. [iso- + G. *klino,* inclinar]
iso·con·a·zole (ī′sō - kō′nă - zōl). Isoconazol; agente antibacteriano e antifúngico relacionado ao cetoconazol e oxiconazol.
iso·co·ria (ī - sō - kō′rē - ă). Isocoria; dimensão igual das duas pupilas. [iso- + G. *korē,* pupila]
iso·cor·tex (ī - sō - kōr′teks) [TA]. Isocórtex; termo criado por O. e C. Vogt para referir-se à parte maior do córtex cerebral de mamíferos, que difere do alocórtex por ser composto de maior número de células nervosas dispostas em seis camadas. VER TAMBÉM cerebral *cortex.* SIN neocortex [TA], homotypic cortex, neopallium.
iso·cy·a·nate (ī - sō - sī′ă - nāt). Isocianato; o radical —N=C=O do ácido isociânico.
iso·cy·an·ic ac·id (ī - sō - sī′ă - nik). Ácido isociânico; substância química altamente reativa, HNCO.
iso·cy·a·nide (ī - sō - sī′ă - nīd). Isocianeto; o radical —NC; os isocianetos orgânicos são denominados isonitrilas.
iso·cy·tol·y·sin (ī′sō - sī - tol′i - sin). Isocitolisina; citolisina que reage com as células de alguns outros animais da mesma espécie, mas não com as células do indivíduo que a formou.
iso·dac·tyl·ism (ī - sō - dak′ti - lizm). Isodactilia; condição em que os dedos das mãos ou dos pés têm, todos eles, aproximadamente o mesmo comprimento. [iso- + G. *daktylos,* dedo]
iso·dense (ī′sō - dens). Isodenso; indica um tecido que possui radiopacidade (radiodensidade) semelhante à do outro tecido ou tecido adjacente.
iso·des·mo·sine (ī - sō - des′mō - sēn). Isodesmosina; aminoácido de ligação cruzada formado a partir de resíduos lisil; encontrada na elastina.
isodose. Isodose; área de dose de irradiação equivalente. [iso- + dose]
iso·dul·cit (ī - sō - dŭl′sit). Isodulcita. SIN L-rhamnose.
iso·dy·nam·ic (ī′sō - dī - nam′ik). Isodinâmico. **1.** De força igual. **2.** Relativo a alimentos ou a outros materiais que liberam a mesma quantidade de energia na combustão. [iso- + G. *dynamis,* força]
iso·dy·na·mo·gen·ic (ī′sō - dī - nă - mō - jen′ik,   - dī - nam′ō-). Isodinamogênico. **1.** SIN isoenergetic. **2.** Que produz força nervosa igual. [iso- + G. *dynamis,* força + *-gen,* produzindo]
iso·e·lec·tric (īsō - ē - lek′trik). Isoelétrico; de potencial elétrico igual. Cf. isoelectric *point.* SIN isopotential.
   i. focusing, focalização isoelétrica; eletroforese de pequenas moléculas ou macromoléculas em gradiente de pH.
iso·en·er·get·ic (ī′sō - en - er - jet′ik). Isoenergético; que exerce força igual; igualmente ativo. SIN isodynamogenic (1).
iso·en·zyme (ī - sō - en′zīm). Isoenzima; uma de um grupo de enzimas que catalisam a mesma reação, mas que podem ser diferenciadas por variações nas suas propriedades físicas, como ponto isoelétrico, mobilidade eletroforética, parâmetros cinéticos ou modos de regulação; p. ex., lactato desidrogenase, um tetrâmero composto de quantidades variáveis de subunidades α e β (isto é, 4α, 3α + 1β, 2α + 2β, 1α + 3β e 4β). SIN isozyme.
   creatine kinase i.'s, isoenzimas da creatinocinase; a creatinocinase (CK) é um dímero com subunidades M (músculo) e/ou B (cérebro); existe em três formas de isoenzimas: CK-MM, a forma predominante, encontrada primariamente no músculo esquelético; CK-MB, encontrada no músculo cardíaco, na língua, no diafragma e, em pequenas quantidades, no músculo esquelético; e CK-BB, encontrada no cérebro, no músculo liso, na tireóide, nos pulmões e na próstata. As elevações detectadas por eletroforese ou outras metodologias podem ser utilizadas para ajudar no diagnóstico diferencial de uma variedade de estados mórbidos, sendo a elevação da CK-MB um importante marcador após infartos do miocárdio, enquanto as elevações da CK-MM constituem um indicador de doença muscular, e os aumentos da CK-BB, um achado ocasional após infartos cerebrais, infartos intestinais ou na presença de certos processos malignos.

iso·e·ryth·rol·y·sis (ī′sō - ĕ - rith - rol′i - sis). Isoeritrólise; destruição de eritrócitos por isoanticorpos. [isso- + eritrócito + G. *lysis,* dissolução]
   neonatal i., i. neonatal. **(1)** Isoeritrólise no animal recém-nascido; **(2)** icterícia hemolítica do recém-nascido.
iso·flu·or·phate (ī - sō - flōr′fāt). Isofluorofato; agente colinérgico tóxico que atua através da inibição irreversível da colinesterase; agente colinérgico oftálmico utilizado no tratamento do glaucoma; também utilizado na pesquisa bioquímica como inibidor enzimático. SIN diisopropyl fluorophosphate.
iso·flu·rane (ī - sō - floor′ān). Isoflurano; éter alogenado não-inflamável, não-explosivo, com poderosa ação anestésica; isômero do enflurano.
iso·ga·mete (ī - sō - gam′ēt). Isogameta. **1.** Uma de duas ou mais células semelhantes que sofrem conjugação ou fusão e, subseqüentemente, dividem-se, resultando em reprodução. **2.** Gameta do mesmo tamanho do gameta com o qual se une. [iso- + G. *gametēs* ou *gametē,* marido ou esposa]
isog·a·my (ī - sog′ă - mē). Isogamia; conjugação entre dois gametas iguais ou duas células individuais semelhantes em todos os aspectos. [iso- + G. *gamos,* casamento]
iso·ge·ne·ic, iso·gen·ic (ī′sō - jĕ - nē′ik,   - jen′ik). Isogênico. SIN syngeneic.
isog·e·nous (ī - soj′ĕ - nŭs). Isogênico; da mesma origem, como no desenvolvimento do mesmo tecido ou célula. [iso- + G. *genos,* família, tipo, espécie]
iso·gen·ti·o·bi·ose (ī′sō - jen - shi - ō - bī′ōs). Isogentibiose. SIN isomaltose.
iso·glu·ta·mine (ī - sō - gloo′tă - mēn). Isoglutamina; amida glutâmica.
iso·gna·thous (ī - sog′nă - thŭs). Isognato; que possui mandíbulas com, aproximadamente, a mesma largura. [iso- + G. *gnathos,* mandíbula]
iso·graft (ī′sō - graft). Isoenxerto. SIN syngraft.
iso·he·mag·glu·ti·na·tion (ī′sō - hē′mă - gloo′ti - nā′shŭn). Isoemaglutinação. SIN isoagglutination. [iso- + G. *haima,* sangue, + L. *ad,* para + *gluten,* cola]
iso·he·mag·glu·ti·nin (ī′sō - hē′mă - gloo′ti - nin). Isoemaglutinina. SIN isoagglutinin.
iso·he·mo·ly·sin (ī′sō - hē - mol′i - sin). Isoemolisina; isolisina que reage com eritrócitos.
iso·he·mol·y·sis (ī′sō - hē - mol′i - sis). Isoemólise; forma de isólise em que ocorre dissolução dos eritrócitos em conseqüência da reação entre uma isolisina (isoemolisina) e o antígeno específico presente nas células ou sobre elas. [iso- + G. *haima,* sangue + *lysis,* dissolução]
iso·hy·dric (ī - sō - hī′drik). Isoídrico; indica duas substâncias que possuem o mesmo pH.
iso·hy·dru·ria (ī′sō - hī - droo′rē - ă). . Isoidrúria; fixação do pH da urina sem variação habitual. [iso- + G. *hydor,* água, + *ouron,* urina + -ia]
iso·im·mu·ni·za·tion (ī′sō - im′ū - ni - zā′shŭn). Isoimunização; desenvolvimento de um título significativo de anticorpo específico em decorrência de estimulação antigênica com material contido nos eritrócitos de outro indivíduo da mesma espécie; p. ex., é provável ocorrer imunização quando uma pessoa Rh-negativa recebe uma transfusão de sangue Rh-positivo de outro ser humano, ou uma mulher Rh-negativa tem uma gravidez em que o feto tem eritrócitos Rh-positivos.
iso·late (ī′sō - lāt). **1.** Isolar, separar, colocar de lado; aquele que é assim tratado. **2.** Isolar; livrar-se de contaminantes químicos. **3.** Isolar; em psicanálise, separar idéias, experiências ou lembranças dos afetos a elas relacionados. **4.** Isolado; em psicoterapia de grupo, um indivíduo que não é considerado por outros no grupo. **5.** Microorganismos viáveis isolados em uma única ocasião de uma amostra obtida de um hospedeiro ou sistema de cultura. **6.** População que, por motivos geográficos, lingüísticos, culturais, sociais, religiosos ou outros motivos, está sujeita a pouco ou nenhum fluxo gênico. SIN genetic i. [It. *isolare;* L. Mediev. *insulo,* pp. *-atus,* isolar, de L. *insula,* ilha]
   genetic i., i. genético. SIN isolate (6).
   mating i., i. de acasalamento; população separada de seus vizinhos por qualquer meio, de modo que todos ou a maioria dos acasalamentos ocorrem dentro do grupo populacional.
iso·la·tion. Isolamento. **1.** Em microbiologia, separação de um microrganismo de outros, geralmente através de culturas seriadas. **2.** Separação, durante o período de contagiosidade, de indivíduos ou animais infectados uns dos outros, de modo a impedir ou limitar a transmissão direta ou indireta do agente infeccioso dos indivíduos infectados para aqueles que são suscetíveis.
iso·lec·i·thal (ī - sō - les′i - thăl). Isolécito; indica um ovo em que existe uma quantidade moderada de vitelo uniformemente distribuído.
iso·leu·cine (I) (ī - sō - loo′sēn). Isoleucina; ácido 2-amino-3-metilvalérico; o L-aminoácido encontrado em quase todas as proteínas; isômero da leucina e, como ela, um aminoácido essencial da dieta.
iso·leu·cyl (ī - sō - loo′sil). Isoleucila; radical acila da isoleucina.
iso·leu·ko·ag·glu·ti·nin (ī′sō - loo′kō - ă - gloo′ti - nin). Isoleucoaglutinina; anticorpo anormal no sangue de alguns indivíduos, capaz de aglutinar leucócitos humanos.

isol·o·gous (ī - sol'o - gŭs). Isólogo. SIN syngeneic. [iso- + G. *logos*, relação, proporção]

isol·y·sin (ī - sol'i - sin). Isolisina; anticorpo que se combina com células que contêm o isoantígeno específico, sensibiliza-as e resulta em fixação do complemento e dissolução dessas células; as isolisinas ocorrem no sangue de alguns membros de uma espécie e reagem com as células dessa espécie, mas não com as do indivíduo (ou do mesmo tipo) em que são naturalmente formadas.

isol·y·sis (ī - sol'i - sis). Isólise; lise ou dissolução de células em conseqüência da reação entre uma isolisina e um antígeno específico nas células. VER TAMBÉM isohemolysis. [iso- + G. *lysis*, dissolução]

iso·lyt·ic (ī - sō - lit'ik). Isolítico; relativo a, caracterizado por ou que causa isólise.

iso·malt·ase (ī - sō - mal'tās). Isomaltase. SIN oligo-α-1,6-glucosidase. VER TAMBÉM sucrose α-D-glucohydrolase.

iso·malt·ose (ī - sō - mal'tōs). Dissacarídeo em que duas moléculas de glicose estão unidas por uma ligação α-1,6 em lugar de uma ligação α-1,4, como na maltose. SIN isogentiobiose.

iso·mas·ti·gote (ī - sō - mas'ti - gōt). Isomastigota; indica um protozoário que possui dois ou quatro flagelos de comprimento igual em uma extremidade. [iso- + G. *mastix*, chicote]

iso·mer (ī'sō - mer). Isômero. **1.** Uma de duas ou mais substâncias que exibem isomerismo (q.v.); p. ex., L-glicose e D-glicose ou citrato e isocitrato. Cf. stereoisomer. **2.** Um de dois ou mais nuclídeos que possuem o mesmo número atômico e número de massa, mas que diferem nos estados de energia por determinado período de tempo; p. ex., Tc^{99m} e Tc^{99}. [iso- + G. *meros*, parte] **geometric i.**, i. geométrico. VER geometric *isomerism*.

isom·er·ase (ī - som'er - ās). Isomerase; classe de enzimas (EC classe 5) que catalisam a conversão de uma substância numa forma isomérica; p. ex., glicose fosfato isomerase.

iso·mer·ic (ī - sō - mār'ik). Isomérico; relativo a, ou caracterizado por, isomerismo. SIN isomerous.

isom·er·ism (ī - som'er - izm). Isomerismo; a existência de um composto químico em duas ou mais formas que são idênticas quanto à composição percentual, mas que diferem em relação à posição de um ou mais átomos dentro das moléculas, bem como quanto às suas propriedades físicas e químicas.
geometric i., i. geométrico; forma de isomerismo, apresentada por compostos insaturados ou em um anel, em que está restrita a rotação livre em torno de uma ligação (em geral, uma ligação carbono-carbono); p. ex., o isomerismo de um composto *cis-* ou *trans-*, como no ácido oleico e ácido elaídico. Cf. cis-, entgegen, trans-, zusammen.
optic i., i. óptico; estereoisomerismo envolvendo o arranjo de substituintes em torno de um átomo ou átomos assimétricos (habitualmente carbono), de tal modo que existe uma diferença no comportamento dos vários isômeros no tocante à extensão de sua rotação no plano da luz polarizada. Cf. stereoisomerism.
stereochemical i., i. estereoquímico. SIN stereoisomerism.
structural i., i. estrutural; isomerismo envolvendo os mesmos átomos em arranjos diferentes; p. ex., os ácidos butíricos, a leucina e isoleucina, a glicose e a frutose.

isom·er·i·za·tion (ī - som'er - ī - zā'shŭn). Isomerização; processo em que um isômero é formado a partir de outro, como na ação das isomerases.
enzyme i., i. enzimática; alterações reversíveis na conformação enzimática.

isom·er·ous (ī - som'er - ŭs). Isômero. SIN isomeric.

iso·meth·a·done (ī - sō - meth'a - dōn). Isometadona; analgésico narcótico.

iso·meth·ep·tene (ī'sō - meth - ep'ten). Isometepteno; amina simpaticomimética alifática insaturada, com ações antiespasmódica e vasoconstritora.

iso·met·ric (ī - sō - met'rik). Isométrico. **1.** De dimensões iguais. **2.** Em fisiologia, indica a condição em que as extremidades de um músculo em contração são mantidas fixas, de modo que a contração produz aumento de tensão num comprimento global constante. Cf. auxotonic, isotonic (3), isovolumic. [iso- + G. *metron*, medida]

iso·me·tro·pia (ī'sō - me - trō'pē - ă). Isometropia; igualdade na refração dos dois olhos. [iso- + G. *metron*, medida + ōps (ŏp-) olho]

iso·mor·phic (ī - sō - mōr'fik). Isomórfico. SIN isomorphous.

iso·mor·phism (ī - sō - mōr'fizm). Isomorfismo; semelhança de forma entre dois ou mais organismos ou entre partes do corpo. [iso- + G. *morphē*, forma]

iso·mor·phous (ī - sō - mōr'fŭs). Isomorfo; que tem a mesma forma ou que é morfologicamente igual. SIN isomorphic.

iso·naph·thol (ī - sō - naf'thol). Isonaftol. VER naphthol.

ison·cot·ic (ī - son - kot'ik). Isoncótico; que possui pressão oncótica igual.

iso·ni·a·zid (ī - sō - nī'a - zid). Isoniazida (INH); hidrazida do ácido isonicotínico; fármaco antituberculoso de primeira linha e, provavelmente, utilizado mais comumente. Os microrganismos desenvolvem rapidamente resistência a essa droga quando utilizada isoladamente no tratamento da doença ativa. O principal efeito colateral consiste em hepatotoxicidade.

iso·nic·o·tin·ic ac·id (ī - sō - nik - ō - tin'ik). Ácido isonicotínico; a substância cuja hidrazida é a isoniazida.

iso·ni·trile (ī - sō - nī'tril). Isonitrila; iocianeto orgânico.

iso·ni·tro·so·ac·e·tone (ī'sō - nī - trō - sō - as'ē - tōn). Isonitrosoacetona; reativador da colinesterase que pode penetrar facilmente na barreira hematoencefálica e produzir reativação significativa da acetilcolinesterase fosforilada no sistema nervoso central; utilizada para proteger seres humanos e animais contra uma intoxicação por agentes anticolinesterásicos organofosforados que, de outro modo, seria letal. SIN monoisonitrosoacetone, pyruvaldoxine.

iso·os·mot·ic (ī'sō - os - mot'ik). Isosmótico. SIN isosmotic.

isop·a·thy (ī - sop'ă - thē). Isopatia; tratamento de doença por meio do agente causal ou por um produto da mesma doença; ou tratamento de um órgão enfermo por um extrato de um órgão semelhante de um animal sadio. VER TAMBÉM homeopathy. [iso- + G. *pathos*, sofrimento]

iso·pen·ten·yl·py·ro·phos·phate (ī - sō - pen - tēn - il'pī - rō - fos'fāt). Isopentenilpirofosfato; intermediário na biossíntese de esteróides, terpenos, dolicol e proteínas preniladas.

iso·pen·tyl (ī - sō - pen'til). Isopentila. SIN amyl.

iso·pep·tide (ī - sō - pep'tīd). Isopeptídeo. VER isopeptide *bond*.

isoph·a·gy (ī - sof'ă - jē). Isofagia. SIN autolysis. [iso- + G. *phagō*, comer]

iso·plas·sonts (ī - sō - plas'onts). Isoplassontes; entidades de formação semelhante que exibem certos aspectos em comum. [iso- + G. *plassō*, formar]

iso·plas·tic (ī - sō - plas'tik). Isoplástico. SIN syngeneic. [iso- + G. *plassō*, formar]

iso·pleth (ī - sō - pleth). Isopleta; linha sobre um nomograma cartesiano consistindo em todos os pontos que representam determinado valor de uma variável; p. ex., uma isóbara é uma isopleta para uma pressão particular.

iso·po·ten·tial (ī'sō - pō - ten'chŭl). Isopotencial. SIN isoelectric.

iso·pre·cip·i·tin (ī'sō - prē - sip'i - tin). Isoprecipitina; anticorpo que se combina com material antigênico solúvel e o precipita no plasma ou no soro ou num extrato de células de outro membro, mas não de todos os membros da mesma espécie. [iso- + precipitina]

iso·pren·a·line hy·dro·chlo·ride (ī - sō - pren'ă - lēn). Cloridrato de isoprenalina. SIN isoproterenol hydrochloride.

iso·pren·a·line sul·fate. Sulfato de isoprenalina. SIN isoproterenol sulfate.

iso·prene (ī'sō - prēn). Isopreno; 2-metil-1,3-butadieno; hidrocarboneto de cinco carbonos insaturado com cadeia ramificada que, no reino vegetal e animal, é utilizado como base para a formação de isoprotenóides; p. ex., terpenos, carotenóides e pigmentos relacionados, borracha. As vitaminas lipossolúveis são isoprenóides ou possuem cadeias laterais isoprenóides; os esteróides são sintetizados através de intermediários isoprenóides, assim como a ubiqüinona, o dolicol e as proteínas preniladas.

iso·pre·noids (ī - sō - prēn'oydz). Isoprenóides; polímeros cujos esqueletos de carbono consistem, na sua totalidade ou em grande parte, em unidades de isopreno ligadas de modo término-terminal; p. ex., caroteno, licopeno, vitamina A. As vitaminas K e E e as coenzimas Q possuem cadeias laterais isoprenóides.

iso·pre·nyl·a·tion (ī - sō - pren'il - ā'shun). Isoprenilação. VER prenylation.

iso·pro·pa·nol (ī - sō - prō'pă - nol). Isopropanol. SIN isopropyl alcohol.

iso·pro·phen·a·mine hy·dro·chlo·ride (ī'sō - prō - fen'ă - mēn). Cloridrato de isoprofenamina. SIN clorprenaline hydrochloride.

iso·pro·pyl al·co·hol (ī - sō - prō'pil). Álcool isopropílico; isômero do álcool propílico e homólogo do álcool etílico, com propriedades semelhantes às deste último quando utilizado externamente, porém mais tóxico quando ingerido; utilizado como ingrediente de várias preparações cosméticas e medicinais para uso externo; também disponível como álcool de fricção isopropílico, que contém 68 a 72% de álcool isopropílico (por volume) em água; utilizado como rubefaciente. SIN dimethylcarbinol, isopropanol.

iso·pro·pyl·ar·te·re·nol hy·dro·chlo·ride (ī - sō - prō'pil - ar - ter'ē - nol). Cloridrato de isopropilarterenol. SIN isoproterenol hydrochloride.

iso·pro·pyl·car·bi·nol (ī'sō - prō - pil - kar'bin - ol). Isopropilcarbinol. VER *butyl* alcohol.

iso·pro·pyl myr·is·tate (ī - sō - prō'pil). Miristato de isopropila; auxiliar farmacêutico utilizado em preparações medicinais tópicas para promover a absorção através da pele.

iso·pro·pyl·thi·o·ga·lac·to·side (iPrSGal, IPTG) (ī - sō - prō'pil - thī'ō - gă - lak'tō - sīd). Isopropiltiogalactosídeo; galactosídeo artificial capaz de induzir a β-galactosidase em *Escherichia coli* sem ser clivado, como o são os substratos naturais, como a lactose.

iso·pro·te·re·nol hy·dro·chlo·ride (ī'sō - prō - ter'ē - nol). Cloridrato de isoproterenol; estimulante dos receptores β-simpaticomiméticos que possui as ações excitatórias cardíacas, mas não vasoconstritoras da epinefrina. Quimicamente, difere da epinefrina por apresentar um grupamento isopropila substituindo o grupamento metila fixado ao átomo de nitrogênio; utilizado no tratamento da asma brônquica e do bloqueio atrioventricular, incluindo crises de Adams-Stokes. SIN isoprenaline hydrochloride, isopropylarterenol hydrochloride.

iso·pro·te·re·nol sul·fate. Sulfato de isoproterenol; utilizado como aerossol no tratamento das crises asmáticas agudas e do enfisema pulmonar crônico;

hoje em dia, é raramente empregado, uma vez que são preferidos agentes menos tóxicos e mais específicos. SIN isoprenaline sulfate.

isop·ter (ī - sop′ter). Isóptero; linha de sensibilidade retiniana igual no campo visual. [iso- + G. *optēr*, observador]

iso·pyk·nic (ī - sō - pik′nik). Isopícnico; que tem a mesma densidade. [iso- + G. *phknos*, espesso, denso + -ic]

iso·py·ro·cal·cif·er·ol (ī - sō - pī′rō - cal - sif′er - ol). Isopirocalciferol; 9β-ergosterol; produto da decomposição térmica do calciferol; estereoisômero do pirocalciferol e ergosterol.

iso·quin·o·line (ī - sō - kwin′ō - lēn). Isoquinolina. **1.** Estrutura em anel característica do grupo dos alcalóides do ópio, representado pela papaverina. **2.** Classe de alcalóides contendo a estrutura em anel da isoquinolina (1).

iso·ri·bo·fla·vin (ī′sō - rī′bō - flā - vin). Isorriboflavina; 8-desmetil-6-metilrriboflavina; antimetabólito da riboflavina, que difere desta última pela localização dos grupamentos metila no núcleo isoaloxazina nas posições 6,7 em lugar de 7,8.

isor·rhea (ī - sō - rē′a). Isorréia; igualdade na ingestão e excreção de água; manutenção do equilíbrio hídrico. [iso- + G. *rhoia*, fluxo]

isos·best·ic (ī - sos - bes′tik). Isosbéstico; indica o comprimento de onda da luz em que dois compostos relacionados exibem coeficientes idênticos de extinção; p. ex., o comprimento de onda em que os espectros de absorção da hemoglobina e da oxiemoglobina se cruzam em seu ponto isosbéstico. A espectrofotometria, nesse comprimento de onda, mede a concentração total de hemoglobina, independentemente do grau em que possa estar oxigenada. [Ger. *isosbestisch*, de G. *isos*, igual + *sbestos*, extinto]

iso·schiz·o·mer (ī - sō - skiz′ō - mer). Isosquisômero; endonuclease de restrição de diferentes organismos, que reconhece e hidrolisa a mesma seqüência de DNA. [Jiso- + G. *schizō*, clivar, dividir + -mer]

iso·sen·si·tize (ī - sō - sen′si - tīz). Isossensibilizar. SIN autosensitize.

iso·sex·u·al (ī - sō - sek′shoo - ăl). Isossexual; que descreve as características somáticas de um indivíduo ou dos processos que nele ocorrem, que estão de acordo com o sexo desse indivíduo.

is·os·mot·ic (ī′sos - mot′ik). Isosmótico; que tem a mesma pressão osmótica total ou osmolalidade de outro líquido (habitualmente, o líquido intracelular); esse líquido não é isotônico quando inclui solutos que permeiam livremente as membranas celulares. SIN iso-osmotic.

iso·sor·bide. Isossorbida; composto com propriedades diuréticas preparado por desidratação ácida do D-glucitol.

iso·sor·bide di·ni·trate (ī - sō - sōr′bĭd dī - nī′trāt). Dinitrato de isossaorbida; dilatador coronariano que atua através da formação de óxido nítrico.

Isos·po·ra (ī - sos′pō - ră). Gênero de coccídios (família Eimeriidae, classe Sporozoea), com espécies principalmente em mamíferos; os oocistos maduros contêm dois esporocistos, contendo, cada um, quatro esporozoítas. Atualmente, sabe-se que esse gênero está estreitamente relacionado a *Toxoplasma* e *Sarcocystis*, com uma fase sexuada semelhante no ciclo de vida e um complexo apical semelhante. [iso- + G. *sporos*, semente]

I. bel′li, Espécie relativamente rara que ocorre no intestino delgado do homem, mais comum nos trópicos, porém, provavelmente, de distribuição mundial; as infecções são, em sua maioria, subclínicas, mas podem algumas vezes causar diarréia mucosa.

I. bigem′ina, espécie que ocorre no intestino delgado de cães, gatos, raposas, visão e, possivelmente, outros carnívoros; trata-se do coccídio mais patogênico em cães e gatos, causando enterite e diarréia; os oocistos são habitualmente esporulados, quando eliminados nas fezes, porém indistintos daqueles de *Toxoplasma gondii*, permanecendo, assim, uma considerável dúvida quanto ao estado desses parasitas.

I. ca′nis, espécie de distribuição mundial, que é discretamente patogênica em cães, mas não é infecciosa em gatos.

I. fe′lis, espécie encontrada no intestino delgado e, algumas vezes, no ceco e no cólon de gatos, leões e outros felinos; é apenas um pouco patogênica em gatos, não sendo infecciosa em cães.

I. rivol′ta, espécie que ocorre no intestino delgado de cães, gatos, dingos e, provavelmente, outros carnívoros selvagens; as possibilidades patogênicas assemelham-se às de *I. bigemina*.

I. su′is, espécie que parasita o intestino delgado de suínos, produzindo diarréia leve.

isos·po·ri·a·sis (ī - sos - pō - rī′ă - sis). Isosporíase; doença causada por infecção por uma espécie de *Isospora*, como *I. belli* nos seres humanos; em geral, a doença humana é leve, exceto em casos de imunossupressão, como na AIDS/SIDA, em que pode causar diarréia refratária.

isos·stere (ī′sō - stēr). Isóstero; um de dois ou mais átomos ou moléculas que possuem a mesma distribuição de elétrons; p. ex., N_2 e CO. [iso- + G. *stereos*, sólido]

isos·stery (ī - sō - stēr′ē). Isosterismo; regulação enzimática ou metabólica fisiológica através de inibição competitiva por análogos estruturais dos substratos naturais.

isos·the·nu·ria (ī - sos′thē - noo′rē - ă, ī′sō - sthē-). Isostenúria; estado, numa doença renal crônica, em que o rim é incapaz de formar urina com densidade superior ou inferior à do plasma livre de proteínas; a densidade da urina torna-se fixa em torno de 1,010, independentemente da ingestão de líquido. [iso- + G. *sthenos*, força + *ouron*, urina]

iso·suc·cin·ic ac·id (ī′sō - sŭk - sin′ik). Ácido isossuccínico. SIN methylmalonic acid.

iso·sul·fan blue (ī - sō - sŭl′fan). Azul de isossulfano; corante utilizado como auxiliar radiográfico para marcar os vasos linfáticos durante a linfografia.

iso·ther·mal (ī - sō - ther′măl). Isotérmico; que possui a mesma temperatura. [iso- + G. *thermē*, calor]

iso·thi·o·cy·a·nate (ī′sō - thī - ō - sī′ă - nāt). Isotiocianato; o radical do ácido isotiociânico, —N=C=S.

iso·thi·pen·dyl (ī′sō - thī - pen′dil). Isotipendil; anti-histamínico H_1.

iso·tone (ī′sō - tōn). Isotono; um de vários nuclídeos apresentando o mesmo número de nêutrons em seus núcleos; p. ex., K_{19}^{39} e Ca_{20}^{40}, cada um com 20, Fe_{26}^{56} e Ni_{28}^{58} cada um com 30. [iso- + G. *tonos*, estiramento, tensão]

iso·to·nia (ī - sō - tō′nē - ă). Isotonia; condição de igualdade tônica em que a tensão ou pressão osmótica em duas substâncias ou soluções é a mesma. [iso- + G. *tonos*, tensão]

iso·ton·ic (ī - sō - ton′ik). Isotônico. **1.** Relativo à isotonicidade ou isotonia. **2.** Que possui tensão igual; indica soluções que apresentam a mesma pressão osmótica; mais especificamente, limita-se a soluções nas quais as células não estão aumentadas nem diminuídas de volume. Assim, uma solução que é isosmótica com o líquido intracelular não será isotônica se incluir um soluto que, como a uréia, atravessa facilmente as membranas celulares. **3.** Em fisiologia, indica a condição em que um músculo em contração se encurta com uma carga constante, como ao levantar um peso. Cf. auxotonic, isometric (2).

iso·to·nic·i·ty (ī - sō - tō - nis′i - tē). Isotonicidade. **1.** A qualidade de possuir e de manter um tônus ou tensão uniforme. **2.** A propriedade que uma solução apresenta de ser isotônica.

iso·tope (ī′sō - tōp). Isótopo; um de dois ou mais nuclídeos que são quimicamente idênticos, exibindo o mesmo número de prótons, mas que diferem no número de massa, visto que seus núcleos contêm números diferentes de nêutrons; os isótopos individuais são denominados com a inclusão de seu número de massa na posição superior (C^{12}) e o número atômico (prótons nucleares) na posição inferior (C_6). No primeiro uso, os números de massa seguem o símbolo químico (C-12). [iso- + G. *topos*, parte, local]

daughter i., i.-filho; elemento produzido por decomposição radioativa de outro. VER radionuclide *generator*, cow.

radioactive i., i. radioativo; isótopo com composição nuclear instável; esses núcleos sofrem decomposição espontânea pela emissão de um elétron nuclear (partícula β) ou núcleo de hélio (partícula α) e irradiação (raios γ), alcançando, assim, uma composição nuclear estável; utilizado como traçador e como fonte de irradiação e energia. VER half-life.

stable i., i. estável; nuclídeo não-radioativo; isótopo que não exibe tendência a sofrer decomposição radioativa.

iso·to·pic (ī - sō - top′ik). Isotópico; de composição química idêntica, porém diferindo em alguma propriedade física, como o peso atômico.

iso·trans·plan·ta·tion (ī′sō - tranz - plan - tā - shŭn). Isotransplante; transferência de isoenxerto (syngraft).

iso·tret·i·noin (ī - sō - tret′i - noyn). Isotretinoína; retinóide utilizado no tratamento da acne cística recalcitrante intensa; teratógeno humano conhecido.

iso·tro·pic, isot·ro·pous (ī - sō - trop′ik, ī - sot′rō - pŭs). Isotrópico; que possui propriedades que são as mesmas em todas as direções. [iso- + G. *tropē*, uma volta]

iso·type (ī′sō - tīp). Isotipo; determinante antigênico (marcador) que ocorre em todos os membros de uma classe ou subclasse nas cadeias pesadas de uma imunoglobulina ou no tipo e subtipo de cadeias leves de uma molécula de imunoglobulina. Enquanto se acredita que determinado marcador ou determinante alotípico só ocorre numa subclasse, um marcador antigênico isotípico numa subclasse também pode ocorrer como marcador alotípico em outra subclasse. [iso- + G. *typos*, modelo]

iso·typ·ic (ī - sō - tip′ik). Isotípico; relativo a um isotipo.

iso·va·ler·ic ac·id (ī′sō - vă - lăr′ik, - lēr′ik). Ácido isovalérico; ácido 3-metilbutírico; intermediário metabólico nos processos oxidativos; elevado em casos de acidemia isovalérica.

iso·va·ler·ic ac·i·de·mia [MIM*243500]. Acidemia isovalérica; erro inato do metabolismo da leucina, caracterizado por retardo psicomotor, odor específico que lembra pés suados, vômitos, acidose e coma; associada à produção excessiva de ácido isovalérico após ingestão de proteína ou durante episódios infecciosos; resulta da deficiência de isovaleril-CoA desidrogenase; a acidose metabólica grave resulta das grandes quantidades de ácido formado. Herança autossômica recessiva; são conhecidas duas formas: 1) a forma neonatal aguda, com acidose metabólica fulminante e morte rápida, e 2) a forma carateriza, caracterizada por episódios intermitentes de cetoacidose grave. SIN sweaty feet syndrome.

iso·va·ler·yl-CoA (ī - sō - vă′ler - il). Isovaleril-CoA; produto de condensação do ácido valérico e da coenzima A; intermediário no catabolismo da L-leucina. SIN isovalerylcoenzyme A.

isovaleryl-CoA

i.-CoA dehydrogenase, isovaleril-CoA desidrogenase; enzima que participa no catabolismo da L-leucina; converte a isovaleril-CoA em 3-metilcrotonil-CoA, utilizando FAD; a deficiência dessa enzima resulta em acidemia isovalérica.

iso·va·ler·yl·co·en·zyme A. Isovaleril coenzima A. SIN isovaleryl-CoA.

iso·val·thine (ī - sō - val′thēn). Isovaltina; composto contendo enxofre encontrado na urina.

iso·vol·ume (ī - sō - vol′ūm). Isovolume; que possui o mesmo volume. VER TAMBÉM isovolumic.

iso·vol·u·met·ric (ī′sō - vol - ū - met′rik). Isovolumétrico. SIN isovolumic.

iso·vol·u·mic (ī′sō - vol - ū′mik). Isovolumétrico; que ocorre sem alteração associada no volume, como, p. ex., quando as fibras musculares aumentam inicialmente a sua tensão sem encurtamento no início da sístole ventricular, de modo que o volume ventricular permanece inalterado. VER TAMBÉM isometric. SIN isochoric, isovolumetric.

isox·su·prine hy·dro·chlo·ride (ī - soks′soo - prēn). Cloridrato de isoxuprina; amina simpaticomimética com poderosos efeitos inibitórios sobre os músculos lisos vasculares, uterinos e outros músculos lisos; utilizado como vasodilatador em diversas doenças vasculares e como relaxante uterino.

iso·zyme (ī′sō - zīm). Isozima. SIN isoenzyme.

is·sue (ish′ū). Vazão, saída; termo arcaico para a eliminação de pus, sangue ou outro material. [Fr. saída]
  nature-nurture i., controvérsia sobre a importância relativa da hereditariedade (natureza) e do ambiente (educação) em vários aspectos do desenvolvimento individual, como inteligência, personalidade ou doença mental.

isth·mec·to·my (is - mek′tō - mē). Istmectomia; excisão da porção média da tireóide. [G. *isthmos*, istmo + *ektomē*, excisão]

isth·mic, isth·mi·an (is′mik, is′mē - an). Ístmico; relativo a um istmo anatômico.

isth·mo·pa·ral·y·sis (is′mō - pă - ra′li - sis). Istmoparalisia; paralisia do véu do pêndulo do palato e dos músculos que formam os pilares anteriores das fauces. SIN faucial paralysis, isthmoplegia. [G. *isthmos*, istmo + paralisia]

isth·mo·ple·gia (is′mō - plē′jē - ă). Istmoplegia. SIN isthmoparalysis. [G. *isthmos*, istmo + *plēgē*, golpe]

isth·mus, pl. **isth·mi, isth·mus·es** (is′mŭs, - mī, - mŭs - ez) [TA]. Istmo. **1.** Constrição no tubo neural embrionário delineando a porção anterior do robencéfalo, o futuro metencéfalo, formando o mesencéfalo de localização mais rostral. **2.** SIN rhombencephalici. [G. *isthmos*]
  i. of aorta, i. da aorta. SIN aortic i.
  i. aor′tae [TA], i. da aorta. SIN aortic i.
  aortic i. [TA], i. da aorta; discreta constrição da aorta, imediatamente distal à artéria subclávia esquerda, no ponto de fixação do canal arterial. SIN i. aortae [TA], i. de aorta.
  i. of auditory tube, i. da tuba auditiva. SIN i. of pharyngotympanic tube.
  i. of cartilage of ear, i. da cartilagem da orelha. SIN i. of cartilaginous auricle.
  i. of cartilaginous auricle [TA], i. da cartilagem da orelha; ponte estreita unindo a cartilagem do meato acústico externo e a lâmina do trago com a porção principal da cartilagem da auricula. SIN i. cartilaginis auris, i. of cartilage of ear.
  i. cartilaginis auricularis [TA], **i. cartilag′inis au′ris** [TA], i. da cartilagem da orelha externa. SIN i. of cartilaginous auricle.
  i. of cingulate gyrus [TA], i. do giro cingulado; estreitamento do giro cingulado, em sua transição com o giro hipocampo, atrás e abaixo do esplênio do corpo caloso, produzido pela extensão anterior dos sulcos parieto-occipital e calcarino em conjunto. SIN i. gyri cinguli [TA], i. of gyrus fornicatus, i. of limbic lobe.
  i. of eustachian tube, i. da trompa de Eustáquio. SIN i. of pharyngotympanic tube.
  i. of external acoustic meatus, i. do meato acústico externo; a porção mais estreita desse canal na parte óssea, próximo à sua terminação profunda. SIN i. meatus acustici externi.
  i. of fauces [TA], i. das fauces; espaço constrito e curto que estabelece a conexão entre a cavidade da boca e a orofaringe, delimitado, anteriormente, pelas pregas palatolinguais e, posteriormente, pelas pregas palatofaríngeas; o orifício lateral é a fossa tonsilar. SIN i. faucium [TA], oropharyngeal i.
  i. fau′cium [TA], i. das fauces. SIN i. of fauces.
  i. glan′dulae thyroid′eae [TA], i. da glândula tireóide. SIN i. of thyroid gland.
  Guyon i., i. de Guyon. SIN i. of uterus.
  i. gy′ri cin′guli [TA], i. do giro cingulado. SIN i. of cingulate gyrus.
  i. of gy′rus fornica′tus, i. do giro cingulado. SIN i. of cingulate gyrus.
  i. of His, i. de His. SIN rhombencephalic i.
  Krönig i., i. de Krönig; porção estreita semelhante a uma fita do campo ressonante que se estende sobre o ombro, ligando as áreas maiores de ressonância sobre o ápice pulmonar, na frente e atrás.
  i. of limbic lobe, i. do lobo límbico. SIN i. of cingulate gyrus.
  i. mea′tus acus′tici exter′ni, i. do meato acústico externo. SIN i. of external acoustic meatus.
  oropharyngeal i., i. orofaríngeo. SIN i. of fauces.
  pharyngeal i., i. da faringe. SIN i. of pharynx.
  i. pharyngis, i. da faringe. SIN i. of pharynx.
  i. pharyngonasa′lis, i. faringonasal. SIN choanae.
  i. of pharyngotympanic tube [TA], i. da tuba faringotimpânica. A porção mais estreita da tuba auditiva, na junção das porções cartilaginosa e óssea. SIN i. tubae auditivae [TA], i. tubae auditoriae*, i. of auditory tube, i. of eustachian tube.
  i. of pharynx [TA], i. da faringe; passagem posterior para o palato mole através da qual se comunicam a nasofaringe e a orofaringe (isto é, a junção da naso- e orofaringe), fechada durante a deglutição pela elevação do palato mole e contração do fascículo posterior do palato faríngeo (músculo), formando o coxim de Passavant. SIN i. pharyngis, pharyngeal i.
  pleural i., i. pleural. SIN mesopneumonium.
  i. pros′tatae [TA], i. da próstata. SIN i. of prostate.
  i. of prostate [TA], i. da próstata; parte média estreita da próstata, anteriormente à uretra. SIN i. prostatae [TA].
  i. rhombenceph′ali, i. do rombencéfalo. SIN rhombencephalic i.
  rhombencephalic i., i. do rombencéfalo. **(1)** Constrição do tubo neural embrionário, delineando o mesencéfalo do rombencéfalo, **(2)** porção anterior do rombencéfalo unida ao mesencéfalo. SIN isthmus (2) [TA], i. of His, i. rhombencephali.
  i. of thyroid gland [TA], i. da glândula tireóide; parte central da glândula tireóide que une os dois lobos laterais. SIN i. glandulae thyroideae [TA].
  i. tu′bae auditi′vae [TA], i. da tuba auditiva. SIN i. of pharyngotympanic tube.
  i. tubae auditoriae, i. da tuba auditiva; *termo oficial alternativo para i. of pharyngotympanic tube.
  i. tu′bae uteri′nae [TA], i. da trompa uterina. SIN i. of uterine tube.
  i. u′teri [TA], i. do útero. SIN i. of uterus.
  i. of uterine tube [TA], i. da trompa uterina; a porção estreita da trompa uterina que se une ao útero. SIN i. tubae uterinae [TA].
  i. of uterus [TA], i. do útero; constrição alongada na junção do corpo e do colo do útero. SIN i. uteri [TA], Guyon i., orificium internum uteri, os uteri internum, ostium uteri internum.
  Vieussens i., i. de Vieussens. SIN limbus fossae ovalis.

it·a·con·ic ac·id (it′ă - kon′ik). Ácido itacônico; produto de descarboxilação do ácido *cis*-acotínico. SIN methylenesuccinic acid.

itch. Prurido. **1.** Sensação irritante na pele que desperta o desejo de coçar. SIN pruritus (2). **2.** Nome comum para sarna. [A. S. *gikkan*]
  azo i., p. por azo; prurido que ocorre entre pessoas que trabalham com corantes azo.
  baker i., p. do padeiro; erupção cutânea que aparece nas mãos e nos braços de padeiros, devido a reação alérgica à farinha ou a outras substâncias manipuladas ou ao ácaro de cereais.
  barber i., p. do barbeiro. SIN tinea barbae.
  bath i., p. do banho. SIN bath pruritus.
  copra i., p. da copra; dermatite que ocorre em trabalhadores em moinhos de copra, causada pela presença de um ácaro, *Tyrophagus putrescentiae*.
  Cuban i., alastrim. SIN alastrim.
  frost i., p. do inverno. SIN winter i.
  grain i., p. causado por cereais; erupção cutânea observada ocasionalmente em fazendeiros e manipuladores de cereais, causada pela ação do ácaro *Pyemotes ventricosus*.
  grocer i., p. dos merceeiros; dermatite vesicular observada em merceeiros e padeiros que manuseiam açúcar ou farinha; causado por um ácaro do gênero *Glycophagus*.
  ground i., p. da larva migrans cutânea. SIN cutaneous larva migrans.
  kabure i., p. de kabure, esquistossomose japônica. SIN schistosomiasis japonica.
  Norway i., p. da escabiose norueguesa. SIN Norwegian scabies.
  poultryman's i., p. dos manuseadores de aves domésticas; erupção causada por infestação pelo ácaro *Dermanyssus gallinae*.
  rice i., p. do arroz; esquistossomose japônica. SIN schistosomiasis japonica.
  Saint Ignatius i., p. de Santo Inácio; pelagra. SIN pellagra.
  straw i., straw-bed i., p. da palha; erupção urticariforme causada pelo ácaro *Pyemotes ventricosus*, que pode infestar a palha utilizada em colchões. SIN dermatitis pediculoides ventricosus.
  summer i., p. do verão. SIN pruritus aestivalis.
  swimmer's i., p. do nadador. SIN schistosomal dermatitis.
  water i., p. da água. **(1)** SIN cutaneous larva migrans; **(2)** SIN schistosomal dermatitis.
  winter i., p. do inverno; eczema recorrente que aparece com o início da temperatura fria. SIN dermatitis hiemalis, frost i., pruritus hiemalis.

itch·ing. Prurido; sensação desagradável de irritação da pele ou das mucosas que leva à coçadura ou fricção das partes afetadas. SIN pruritus (1).

-ite. -Ite. **1.** Da natureza de, semelhante a. **2.** Sal de um ácido que tem a terminação -ous. **3.** Em anatomia comparada, sufixo que indica uma porção essencial da parte a cujo nome se liga. VER TAMBÉM -ites. [G. *-itēs*, fem. *-itis*]

iter (ī′ter). Iter; passagem de uma parte anatômica para outra. VER TAMBÉM canaliculus. [L. *iter (itiner-)* via, caminho]
  i. chor′dae ante′rius, i. da corda anterior. SIN anterior *canaliculus* of chorda tympani.
  i. chor′dae poste′rius, i. da corda posterior. SIN posterior *canaliculus* of chorda tympani.

i. den'tis, i. dos dentes; via ou vias pelas quais um ou mais dentes irrompem. SIN i. dentium

i. den'tium, i. dos dentes. SIN i. dentis.

i. a ter'tio ad quar'tum ventric'ulum. SIN cerebral *aqueduct*. [L. via do terceiro para o quarto ventrículo]

iter·al (i'ter-ăl). Iteral; relativo a um iter.

-ites. -Ites. sufixo adjetival grego ligado a substantivos, correspondendo a L. *-alis* ou *-inus* ao inglês -y ou -like. O adjetivo formado com esse sufixo é algumas vezes utilizado isoladamente, representando uma frase a partir da qual foi removido um substantivo (p. ex., tympanites para *tympanitēs hydrōps*, aumento de volume do abdome que se distende como um tambor. VER TAMBÉM -ite, -itis. [G. *itēs*]

-itides. Plural de -itis.

-itis. -Ite; forma feminina do sufixo adjetival grego -ites. Um adjetivo formado com esse sufixo algumas vezes é utilizado isoladamente, representando uma frase a partir da qual foi retirado um substantivo, como, p. ex., nephritis (nefrite) para *nephritis nosos,* doença dos rins. Assim, transforma-se, de fato, num sufixo de substantivo. Além disso, sua ocorrência freqüente em termos que se referem a distúrbios inflamatórios levou-o a adquirir o significado de inflamação. VER TAMBÉM -ites. [G. *-ites*]

Ito, Minor, dermatologista japonês do século XX. VER Ito *nevus; hypomelanosis* of *I.*

Ito, Toshio, médico japonês do século XX. VER I. *cells,* em *cell.*

ITP Abreviatura de idiopathic thrombocytopenic *purpura* (púrpura trombocitopênica idiopática, PTI); inosine 5'-triphosphate (inosina 5'-trifosfato)

itra·min tos·yl·ate (i'tră-min). Tosilato de itramina; vasodilatador.

IU Abreviatura de *International Unit* (Unidade Internacional, UI).

IUB Abreviatura de *International Union of Biochemistry* (*União Internacional de Bioquímica*).

IUCD Abreviatura de intrauterine contraceptive *device* (dispositivo contraceptivo intra-uterino), em *device.*

IUD Abreviatura de intrauterine *device* (dispositivo intra-uterino, DIU), em *device.*

IUI Abreviatura de intrauterine *insemination* (inseminação intra-uterina, IIU).

IUPAC Abreviatura de *International Union of Pure and Applied Chemistry* (*União Internacional de Química Pura e Aplicada*).

I-V Abreviatura de intraventricular.

I.V., i.v. Abreviatura de intravenous ou intravenously (intravenoso ou por via intravenosa).

IVB Abreviatura de intraventricular *block* (bloqueio intraventricular).

IVC Abreviatura de inferior *vena* cava (veia cava inferior, VCI).

Ivemark, Björn, patologista sueco, *1925. VER I. *syndrome.*

iver·mec·tin (i-ver-mek'tin). Ivermectina; antibiótico macrolídio semi-sintético efetivo no tratamento da filaríase; destrói *Onchocerca microfilaria* e *Filaria bancrofti*. Também aprovada pela FDA para o tratamento da escabiose através de administração tópica.

IVF Abreviatura de *in vitro fertilization* (fertilização *in vitro*, FIV).

IVF-ET Abreviatura de in vitro fertilization and in vivo transfer of the embryo to the uterus, Fallopian tube, or the peritoneal cavity (fertilização *in vitro* e transferência *in vivo* do embrião para o útero, tuba uterina ou cavidade peritoneal).

IVP Abreviatura de intravenous *pyelography* ou pyelogram (pielografia intravenosa, PIV).

IVU Abreviatura de intravenous urogram (urografia intravenosa); preferida em vez de IVP. VER intravenous *urography.*

Ivy, Robert H., cirurgião oral e plástico norte-americano, 1881-1974. VER I. loop *wiring,* bleeding time *test.*

Ix·o·des (ik-so'dēz). Gênero de carrapatos duros (família Ixodidae), do qual muitas espécies são parasitas de seres humanos e animais; caracterizam-se por um sulco que circunda o ânus anteriormente, ausência de olhos e festões e dimorfismo sexual acentuado; já foram descritas cerca de 40 espécies na América do Norte. [G. *ixōdēs,* viscoso, como visgo, de *ixos,* visgo + *eidos,* forma]

I. cook'ei, espécie que é um vetor do vírus Powassan no Canadá.

I. damm'ini, espécie que é um vetor da doença de Lyme (*Borrelia burgdorferi*) e da babesiose humana (*Babesia microti*) nos Estados Unidos. As picadas que causam a doença de Lyme em seres humanos são feitas por ninfas de carrapatos que têm aproximadamente o tamanho de uma ponta de lápis, infectados por *B. burgdorferi* de camundongos do campo. Os carrapatos adultos completam o seu ciclo de vida de dois anos alimentando-se em cervos.

I. pacif'icus, espécie de carrapato que é o vetor da doença de Lyme no oeste dos Estados Unidos.

I. persulca'tus, uma espécie de carrapato eurasiana que é um vetor da encefalite de primavera-verão da Rússia e doença de Lyme.

I. redikorzevi, espécie eurasiana de carrapato que causou toxicose humana em Israel.

I. rici'nus, uma espécie eurasiana de carrapato que infesta bovinos, ovinos e animais selvagens e transmite o piroplasma *Babesia divergens,* o vírus da encefalite transmitida por carrapato, e a doença de Lyme.

I. scapula'ris, uma espécie de carrapato encontrada em animais no sul e leste dos Estados Unidos; trata-se do vetor primário da doença de Lyme nos Estados Unidos.

I. spinipal'pis, uma espécie de carrapato parasita de roedores selvagens na Colúmbia Britânica e vetor do vírus Powassan em camundongos do gênero *Peromyscus.*

ix·o·di·a·sis (ik-so-di'ă-sis). Ixodíase; lesões cutâneas causadas por picadas de carrapatos ixodídeos.

ix·od·ic (ik-sod'ik). Ixódico; relativo a, ou causado por, carrapatos.

ix·o·did (ik'sō-did). Ixodídeo; nome comum para membros da família Ixodidae.

Ix·od·i·dae (ik-sod'i-dē). Família de carrapatos (ordem Acarina, subordem Ixodidea), os denominados carrapatos "duros", caracterizados por uma forma corporal rígida, presença de escudo dorsal e capítulo que se projeta anteriormente; inclui os gêneros *Ixodes, Hyalomma, Amblyomma, Boophilus, Margaropus, Dermacentor, Haemaphysalis* e *Rhipicephalus,* cujas espécies transmitem muitas doenças humanas a animais importantes e causam a paralisia do carrapato; em certas ocasiões, atacam os seres humanos, porém alguns o fazem habitualmente. [G. *ixōdes,* viscoso]

Ix·o·doi·dea (ik'sō-dō-id'ē-ă). Superfamília da ordem Acarina, incluindo as famílias Ixodidae e Argasidae. [G. *ixōdēs,* viscoso]

J

J Símbolo de Joule; *equivalente* de Joule; densidade de corrente elétrica.
J Símbolo de fluxo (4); constante de acoplamento; coeficiente de acoplamento.
Ja·bo·ran·di. Jaborandi. SIN pilocarpus.
Jaboulay, Mathieu, cirurgião francês, 1860–1913. VER J. *pyloroplasty, amputation.*
Jaccoud, François Sigismond, médico francês, 1830–1913. VER J. *arthritis, arthropathy.*
jack·et (jak'et). Colete, jaqueta. **1.** Uma atadura fixa aplicada ao redor do corpo a fim de imobilizar a coluna vertebral. **2.** Em Odontologia, termo comumente usado para designar uma coroa artificial constituída por porcelana vitrificada ou resina acrílica. [I.M., do Fr. Ant. *jaquet,* dim. de *jaque,* túnica, de *Jacques,* apelido dos camponeses franceses.]
  Minerva j., c. de minerva, aparelho gessado que imobiliza a cabeça e o tronco, geralmente usado em casos de fratura da coluna cervical.
jack·screw (jak'skroo). Macaco-de-rosca, macaco-de-parafuso; dispositivo usado em aparelhos para separar dentes ou mandíbulas aproximados.
Jackson, Jabez N., cirurgião norte-americano, 1868–1935. VER J. *membrane, veil.*
Jackson, John Hughlings, neurologista inglês, 1835–1911. VER jacksonian *epilepsy;* J. *law, rule, sign.*
jack·so·ni·an (jak - sō'nē - an). Jacksoniano. Descrito por John Hughlings Jackson. VER jacksonian *epilepsy,* jacksonian *seizure.*
Jacobaeus, Hans C., cirurgião sueco, 1879–1937. VER J. *operation.*
Jacobson, Ludwig L., anatomista dinamarquês, 1783–1843. VER J. *anastomosis, canal, cartilage, nerve, organ, plexus, reflex.*
Jacquart, Henri, médico francês do século XIX. VER J. *facial angle.*
Jacquemet, Marcel, anatomista francês, 1872–1908. VER J. *recess.*
Jacquemin, Emile, químico francês do século XIX. VER Jacquemin *test.*
Jacques, Paul, médico francês do século XIX. VER J. *plexus.*
Jadassohn, Josef, dermatologista alemão na Suíça, 1863–1936; introduziu o teste cutâneo para dermatite de contato. VER J. *nevus;* Borst-J. *type intraepidermal epithelioma;* J.-Pellizzari *anetoderma;* Franceschetti-J. *syndrome;* J.-Lewandowski *syndrome.*
Jaeger, Eduard, Ritter von Jaxthal, oftalmologista austríaco, 1818–1884. VER J. *test types.*
Jaffe, Max, bioquímico alemão, 1841–1911. VER J. *reaction, test.*
Jaffe, Henry L., patologista norte-americano, 1896–1979. VER J.-Lichtenstein *disease.*
Jakob, Alfons M., neuropsiquiatra alemão, 1884–1931. VER Creutzfeldt-Jakob *disease.*
jal·ap. Jalapa. A raiz tuberosa seca de *Exogonium purga, E. jalapa* ou *Ipomoea purga* (família Convolvulaceae); usada como catártico. [*Jalapa* ou *Xalapa,* uma cidade mexicana de onde a substância era exportada.]
James, George C.W., radiologista norte-americano, 1915–1972. VER Swyer-J. *syndrome;* Swyer-J.-MacLeod *syndrome.*
James, Thomas N., cardiologista e fisiologista norte-americano, *1925. VER J. *fibers,* em *fiber, tracts* em *tract.*
James·town weed. Estramônio; figueira-brava. SIN *Datura stramonium.*
Janet, Pierre M.F., neurologista francês, 1859–1947. VER J. *test.*
Janeway, Edward G., médico norte-americano, 1841–1911. VER J. *lesion.*
jan·i·ceps (jan'i-seps). Janícipite, janicéfalo; gêmeos monozigóticos que possuem as cabeças fundidas, com as faces voltadas em direções opostas. VER conjoined *twins,* em *twin.* VER TAMBÉM craniopagus, syncephalus. [L. *Janus,* divindade romana que possuía duas faces, + *caput,* cabeça.]
  j. asym'metrus, j. assimétrico; iníope, sincéfalo assimétrico; j. com uma face muito pequena e mal desenvolvida. SIN iniops, syncephalus asymmetros.
  j. parasit'icus, j. parasita; j. no qual um dos gêmeos é um parasita pequeno e incompletamente formado fixado ao autósito mais bem formado.
Jansen, Albert, otorrinolaringologista alemão, 1859–1933. VER J. *operation.*
Jansky, Jan, médico tcheco, 1873–1921. VER J.-Bielschowsky *disease;* J. *classification.*
Janus green B [C.I. 11050]. Verde B de Janus. Um corante básico usado em histologia e na coloração supravital de mitocôndrias.
jar. 1. Agitar ou sacudir. **2.** Agitação, sacudidela, sobressalto ou choque.
  heel j., o paciente de pé, na ponta dos pés, sente dor ao apoiar subitamente os calcanhares no chão: **(1)** na coluna vertebral na doença de Pott ou na infecção do disco intervertebral; **(2)** em uma região lombar no caso de litíase renal.
jar·gon (jar'gŏn). Jargão. Linguagem ou terminologia peculiar a um campo, profissão ou grupo específico. VER TAMBÉM paraphasia. [Fr. gibberish]
Jarisch, Adolf, dermatologista austríaco, 1850–1902. VER J.-Herxheimer *reaction;* Bezold-J. *reflex.*
Jarman, Brian, um clínico-geral inglês do século XX. VER J. *score.*
Jar·vik, Robert Koffler, cardiologista norte-americano. VER Jarvik artificial *heart.*

Ja·tro·pha (jat'rōfa). Jatrofa. Gênero de plantas da família Euphorbiaceae; uma planta venenosa encontrada no leste da África e nas Antilhas. [G. *iatros,* médico, + *trophē,* nutrição]
  J. cur'cas, pinhão de purga ou pinhão-do-paraguai, cuja semente contém um óleo purgante semelhante ao óleo de Cróton. SIN *J. glandulifera.*
  J. glandulife'ra, SIN *J. curcas.*
  J. u'rens, cansanção-de-leite, urtiga-cansanção; uma espécie da América do Sul; as folhas frescas maceradas são usadas como rubefaciante e cataplasma estimulante; as sementes fornecem um óleo purgante.
jaun·dice (jawn'dis). Icterícia; uma coloração amarelada do tegumento, das escleróticas, dos tecidos mais profundos e das excreções por pigmentos biliares, resultante de níveis aumentados no plasma. SIN icterus. [Fr. *jaune,* amarelo]
  acholuric j., i. acolúrica; icterícia com concentrações plasmáticas excessivas de bilirrubina não-conjugada e sem pigmentos biliares na urina.
  anhepatic j., i. não-hepática; icterícia devida a hemólise, com função normal do fígado e das vias biliares. SIN anhepatogenous j.
  anhepatogenous j., i. não-hepatogênica; SIN anhepatic j.
  choleric j., i. colérica; icterícia associada a derivados biliares na urina; ocorre na hiperbilirrubinemia por regurgitação.
  cholestatic j., i. colestática; icterícia produzida por bile espessada ou rolhas de bile nas pequenas vias biliares no fígado.
  chronic acholuric j., i. acolúrica crônica; SIN hereditary *spherocytosis.*
  chronic familial j., i. familiar crônica; SIN hereditary *spherocytosis.*
  chronic idiopathic j., i. idiopática crônica; SIN Dubin-Johnson *syndrome.*
  congenital hemolytic j., i. hemolítica congênita; SIN hereditary *spherocytosis.*
  familial nonhemolytic j. [MIM*143500], i. não-hemolítica familiar; icterícia leve devida a aumento das concentrações plasmáticas de bilirrubina não-conjugada sem evidências de lesão hepática, obstrução biliar ou hemólise; atribuída a um erro congênito do metabolismo no qual a excreção de bilirrubina pelo fígado é deficiente, atribuída à diminuição da conjugação de bilirrubina como um glucuronídio ou comprometimento da captação de bilirrubina hepática; herança autossômica dominante. SIN benign familial icterus, constitutional hepatic dysfunction, Gilbert disease, Gilbert syndrome.
  hematogenous j., i. hematogênica; SIN hemolytic j.
  hemolytic j., i. hemolítica; icterícia resultante do aumento da produção de bilirrubina a partir da hemoglobina em virtude de qualquer processo (tóxico, genético ou imune) que cause aumento da destruição das hemácias. SIN hematogenous j., toxemic j.
  hepatocellular j., i. hepatocelular; icterícia resultante de lesão ou inflamação difusa ou de falha da função dos hepatócitos, geralmente referindo-se à hepatite viral ou tóxica.
  hepatogenous j., i. hepatogênica; icterícia resultante de doença hepática, diferente daquela devida a alterações do sangue.
  homologous serum j., i. por soro homólogo; designação obsoleta de hepatite viral tipo B; viral *hepatitis* type B.
  human serum j., i. por soro humano; designação obsoleta da hepatite transmitida por via parenteral, geralmente por sangue ou hemoderivados; geralmente é causada pelo vírus da hepatite B.
  infectious j., i. infecciosa; **(1)** SIN Weil *disease;* **(2)** designação obsoleta de hepatite viral tipo A; viral *hepatitis* type A.
  infective j., i. infecciosa; início agudo de mal-estar, febre, mialgia, náuseas, anorexia, dor abdominal e icterícia causados por membros do gênero *Leptospira.*
  leptospiral j., i. por *Leptospira;* icterícia associada a infecção por várias espécies de *Leptospira.*
  malignant j., i. maligna; SIN icterus *gravis.*
  mechanical j., i. mecânica; SIN obstructive j.
  neonatal j., i. neonatal; SIN physiologic j.
  j. of the newborn, i. do recém-nascido. SIN physiologic j.
  nonobstructive j., i. não-obstrutiva; qualquer icterícia na qual as vias biliares principais não estejam obstruídas, p. ex., i. hemolítica ou i. causada por hepatite.
  nuclear j., i. nuclear; SIN kernicterus.
  obstructive j., i. obstrutiva; icterícia resultante da obstrução do fluxo de bile para o duodeno, seja intra- ou extra-hepática. SIN mechanical j.

△ Formas Combinantes	☆ Termo oficial alternativo para a *Terminologia Anatomica*
🛈 Indica que o termo é ilustrado, ver Índice de Ilustrações	
SIN Sinônimo	[MIM] Mendelian Inheritance in Man
Cf. Comparar, confrontar	I.C. Índice de Corantes
[NA] *Nomina Anatomica*	
[TA] *Terminologia Anatomica*	Termo de Alta Importância

painless j., i. indolor; icterícia não associada a dor abdominal; termo geralmente usado para descrever a i. obstrutiva resultante de obstrução do colédoco na cabeça do pâncreas por um tumor ou impactação de um cálculo.
physiologic j., i. fisiológica; uma forma de i. observada freqüentemente em recém-nascidos nas primeiras 1–2 semanas de vida. É causada por vários fatores, incluindo uma massa eritrocitária ao nascimento relativamente alta em comparação à dos adultos, menor período de vida das hemácias, comprometimento transitório da conjugação da bilirrubina no fígado e ausência de flora intestinal (úteis no metabolismo intestinal e na excreção de bilirrubina); está relacionada à bilirrubinemia indireta (não-conjugada) que atinge seu nível máximo em 2–3 dias de idade em lactentes a termo, normais e, mais tarde, com maiores níveis em prematuros, sendo acentuada em lactentes que recebem leite materno. SIN icterus neonatorum, j. of the newborn, neonatal j.
postarsphenamine j., i. pós-arsfenamina; intoxicação hepática, causando i. em um paciente que receber arsfenamina.
recurrent j. of pregnancy, i. recorrente da gravidez. SIN intrahepatic *cholestasis of pregnancy.*
regurgitation j., i. por regurgitação; i. devida à obstrução biliar, tendo o pigmento biliar sido conjugado e secretado pelas células hepáticas e depois reabsorvido para a corrente sanguínea.
retention j., i. por retenção; i. devida à insuficiência da função hepática ou a excesso da produção de pigmento biliar; a bilirrubina não é conjugada porque não atravessou os hepatócitos.
Schmorl j., i. de Schmorl; kernicterus.
spherocytic i., i. esferocítica; i. hemolítica associada à esferocitose.
spirochetal j., i. por espiroqueta; i. causada por infecção por espécies de *Leptospira,* geralmente *Leptospira icterohemorrhagica.*
toxemic j., i. toxêmica. SIN hemolytic j.
jaun·dice root. *Hydrastis canadensis, raiz-amarela;* hidraste. SIN hydrastis.
jaw. Mandíbula ou maxilar. **1.** Uma das duas estruturas ósseas nas quais os dentes estão implantados e que formam o arcabouço da boca. **2.** Denominação comum da maxila ou da mandíbula. [A.S. *ceōwan,* mastigar]
crackling j., crepitação mandibular; subluxação crônica com estalido ao movimento.
Hapsburg j., m. dos Hapsburg; prognatismo e protrusão do lábio inferior, característicos da dinastia imperial hispano-austríaca.
jaw winking, movimento paradoxal das pálpebras associado a movimentos da mandíbula.
lock-j., trismo; SIN trismus.
lower j., mandíbula ou maxilar inferior. SIN mandible.
lumpy j., actinomicose em gado. SIN actinomycosis.
parrot j., mandíbula de papagaio; distúrbio causado por protrusão dos dentes incisivos.
upper j., maxilar superior. SIN maxilla.
Jaworski, Walery, médico polonês, 1849–1924. VER J. *bodies,* em *body.*
Jeanselme, Edouard, dermatologista francês, 1858–1935. VER J. *nodules,* em *nodule.*
Jeghers, Harold, médico norte-americano. *1904. VER Peutz-J. *syndrome;* J.-Peutz *syndrome.*
△ **jejun-.** VER jejuno-.
je·ju·nal (je - joo′ - nāl). Jejunal; relativo ao jejuno.
je·ju·nec·to·my (je - joo - nek′tō - mē). Jejunectomia; excisão de todo o jejuno ou de parte do mesmo. [jejunum + G. *ektomē,* excisão]
je·ju·ni·tis (je - joo - nī′tis). Jejunite; inflamação do jejuno.
△ **jejuno-, jejun-.** O jejuno, jejunal. [L. *jejunus,* vazio]
je·ju·no·co·los·to·my (je - joo - nō - kō - los′tō - mē). Jejunocolostomia; uma anastomose entre o jejuno e o cólon. [jejuno- + cólon + G. *stoma,* boca]
je·ju·no·il·e·al (je - joo′nō - il′ē - āl). Jejunoileal; relativo ao jejuno e ao íleo.
je·ju·no·il·e·i·tis (je - joo′nō - il - ē - ī′tis). Jejunoileíte; inflamação do jejuno e íleo.
je·ju·no·il·e·os·to·my (je - joo′ - nō - il - ē - os′tō - mē). Jejunoileostomia; uma anastomose entre o jejuno e o íleo. [jejuno- + íleo + G. *stoma,* boca]
je·ju·no·je·ju·nos·to·my (je - joo′nō - je - ju - nos′tō - mē). Jejunojejunostomia; uma anastomose entre duas partes do jejuno. [jejuno- + jejuno- + G. *stoma,* boca]
je·ju·no·plas·ty (je - joo′nō - plas - tē). Jejunoplastia. Um procedimento cirúrgico corretivo no jejuno. [jejuno- + G. *plastos,* moldado]
je·ju·nos·to·my (je - joo - nos′tō - mē). Jejunostomia. Estabelecimento cirúrgico de uma fístula do jejuno até a parede abdominal, geralmente com criação de um estoma. [jejuno- + G. *stoma,* boca]
je·ju·not·o·my (je - joo - not′ō - mē). Jejunotomia. Incisão do jejuno. [jejuno- + G. *tomē,* incisão]
je·ju·num (jē - joo′nŭm) [TA]. Jejuno. A porção do intestino delgado, com cerca de 240 cm de comprimento, situada entre o duodeno e o íleo. O jejuno é distinto do íleo por ser mais proximal, ter maior diâmetro com uma parede mais espessa, ter pregas circulares mais desenvolvidas, ser mais vascularizado (aspecto mais vermelho), com as artérias jejunais formando menos fileiras de arcadas arteriais e vasos retos mais longos. [L. *jejunus,* vazio]
Jellinek, Edward J., médico inglês especializado em distúrbios relacionados ao álcool, 1890–1963. VER Jellinek *formula.*
jel·ly (jel′ē). Geléia. **1.** Composto semi-sólido trêmulo, geralmente contendo alguma forma de gelatina em solução aquosa. **2.** SIN jellyfish. [L. *gelo,* congelar]
box j., SIN *Chiropsalmus quadrumanus.*
cardiac j., geléia cardíaca; termo introduzido por C.L. Davis para designar o material acelular e gelatinoso entre o revestimento endotelial e a camada miocárdica do coração em embriões muito pequenos; em uma fase mais avançada do desenvolvimento, serve como substrato para o mesênquima cardíaco.
interlaminar j., geléia interlaminar; termo introduzido por B.M. Patten para designar o material gelatinoso entre o ectoderma e o endoderma que serve como substrato para o qual as células mesenquimais migram.
Wharton j., geléia de Wharton; o tecido conjuntivo mucoso do cordão umbilical.
jel·ly·fish (jel′ē - fish). Medusa; água-viva; celenterados marinhos (classe Hydrozoa), incluindo algumas espécies venenosas, sobretudo *Physalia,* a caravela; a toxina é injetada na pele por nematocistos presentes nos tentáculos, produzindo vergões lineares. SIN jelly (2).
Jendrassik, Ernö, médico húngaro, 1858–1921. VER J. *maneuver.*
Jenner, Edward, 1749–1823; médico e naturalista inglês que descobriu o método de vacinação contra varíola mediante a inoculação de vacínia em pessoas susceptíveis; o método de Jenner levou diretamente à erradicação da varíola em todo o mundo em 1977, a maior conquista já obtida pela saúde pública.
Jenner, Harley D., médico canadense, *1907. VER J.-Kay *unit.*
Jenner, Louis, médico inglês, 1866–1904. VER J. *stain.*
Jennings, E.R., estatístico norte-americano do século XX. VER Levey-J. *chart.*
Jensen, Edmund Z., oftalmologista dinamarquês, 1861–1950. VER J. *disease.*
Jensen, Carl O., cirurgião veterinário e patologista dinamarquês, 1864–1934. VER J. *sarcoma.*
jerk. Reflexo; abalo. **1.** Uma tração súbita. **2.** SIN deep *reflex.*
ankle j., reflexo aquileu. SIN Achilles *reflex.*
chin j., reflexo mandibular. SIN jaw *reflex.*
crossed j., reflexo cruzado. SIN crossed *reflex.*
crossed adductor j., reflexo adutor cruzado. SIN crossed adductor *reflex.*
crossed knee j., reflexo patelar cruzado. SIN crossed knee *reflex.*
elbow j., reflexo tricipital. SIN triceps *reflex.*
jaw j., reflexo mandibular. SIN jaw *reflex.*
knee j., reflexo patelar. SIN patellar *reflex.*
supinator j., reflexo braquiorradial. SIN brachioradial *reflex.*
jerks (pl.). Coréia ou qualquer forma de tique.
Jervell, Anton, cardiologista norueguês do século XX. VER J. and Lange-Nielsen *syndrome.*
Jes·u·its bark. Chinchona; cinchona. SIN cinchona.
jet. Jato; uma região de velocidade muito alta do sangue logo após a estenose de um vaso.
jet lag. Dessincronose; desequilíbrio do ritmo circadiano normal resultante de viagem em velocidade subsônica ou supersônica através de um número variado de fusos horários, que leva à fadiga, irritabilidade e a vários distúrbios funcionais.
Jeune, M., pediatra francês do século XX. VER J. *syndrome.*
Jewett, Hugh J., urologista norte-americano, 1903–1990. VER J. *sound* e Strong *staging.*
Jewett, Eugene Lyon, cirurgião ortopédico norte-americano e inventor de muitos instrumentos ortopédicos, *1900.
jig·ger. Bicho-do-pé; nome comum da *Tunga penetrans.* VER TAMBÉM chigoe.
jim·son weed. Estramônio. SIN *Datura stramonium.*
Jk blood group. Grupo sanguíneo Jk. Ver grupo sanguíneo de Kidd no apêndice de Grupos Sanguíneos.
JNA Abreviação de *Jena Nomina Anatomica,* 1935. VER *Terminologia Anatomica.*
Jobert de Lamballe, Antoine J., cirurgião francês, 1799–1867. VER J. de L. *fossa, suture.*
Jod-Basedow, jod·bas·e·dow (yod - bas′ē - dō). Hipertireoidismo induzido por iodo. VER Jod-Basedow *phenomenon.* [Al. *Jod,* iodo, + K.A. von *Basedow*]
Joffroy, Alexis C., médico francês, 1844–1908. VER J. *reflex, sign.*
Johne, H. Albert, médico alemão, 1839–1910. VER johnin.
joh·nin (yō′nin). Jonina, ionina; produto utilizado como agente diagnóstico, análogo à tuberculina, mas produzido pelo *Mycobacterium paratuberculosis* (o microrganismo causador da doença de Johne) cultivado em caldo de cultura contendo *Mycobacterium phlei* (bacilo do capim rabo-de-rato); usada como alérgeno para provocar reações em animais infectados. [H.A. *Johne*]

Johnson, Frank B., patologista norte-americano, *1919. VER Dubin-J. *syndrome*.
Johnson, Frank C., pediatra norte-americano, 1894–1934. VER Stevens-J. *syndrome*.
Johnson, Harry B., dentista norte-americano. VER J. *method*.
Johnson, Treat Baldwin, químico norte-americano, 1875–1947. VER Wheeler-J. *test*.

JOINT

joint (joynt) [TA]. Articulação. Em anatomia, o local de união, em geral mais ou menos móvel, entre dois ou mais ossos. Articulações entre elementos ósseos exibem uma grande variedade de formas e funções, e são classificadas em três tipos morfológicos gerais: articulações fibrosas; articulações cartilaginosas; e articulações sinoviais. SIN junctura (1) [TA], arthrosis (1), articulation (1), articulus. [L. *junctura*; de *jungo*, pp. *junctus*, unir]
acromioclavicular j. [TA], a. acromioclavicular; uma articulação sinovial plana (artrodial) entre a extremidade acromial da clavícula e a margem medial do acrômio. SIN articulatio acromioclavicularis [TA].
ankle j. [TA], a. talocrural; uma articulação sinovial tipo gínglimo entre a tíbia e a fíbula, acima, e o tálus, abaixo. SIN articulatio talocruralis [TA], ankle (1), mortise j., talocrural articulation, talocrural j.
anterior intraoccipital j., sincondrose intra-occipital anterior. SIN anterior intraoccipital *synchondrosis*.
arthrodial j., a. artrodial. SIN plane j.
atlantoaxial j., a. atlantoaxial; a. composta entre a primeira e a segunda vértebras cervicais.
atlanto-occipital j. [TA], a. atlanto-occipital; uma articulação sinovial condilar entre as facetas articulares superiores do atlas e os côndilos do osso occipital. SIN articulatio atlanto-occipitalis [TA], atlanto-occipital articulation.
j.'s of auditory ossicles [TA], articulações dos ossículos da audição; as articulações da cadeia de ossículos, que consistem nas incudomaleolar, a. incudoestapedial e a sindesmose timpanoestapedial. SIN articulationes ossiculorum auditus [TA], articulationes ossiculorum auditoriorum*, j.'s of ear bones.
ball and socket j., a. esferóidea; uma articulação sinovial multiaxial na qual uma esfera mais ou menos extensa na cabeça de um osso encaixa-se em uma cavidade arredondada no outro osso, como na articulação do quadril. SIN articulatio spheroidea [TA], enarthrosis*, spheroidal j.*, articulatio cotylica, cotyloid j., enarthrodial j., socket j., spheroid articulation.
biaxial j., a. biaxial, ovóide; a. na qual há dois eixos principais de movimento formando ângulos retos entre si; p. ex., a. selar.
bicondylar j., [TA], a. bicondilar; uma articulação sinovial na qual duas superfícies arredondadas de um osso, mais ou menos distintas, articulam-se com depressões rasas em outro osso. SIN articulatio bicondylaris [TA], bicondylar articulation.
bilocular j., a. bilocular; articulação na qual o disco intra-articular está completo, dividindo a a. em duas cavidades distintas.
Budin obstetrical j., a. obstétrica de Budin. SIN posterior intraoccipital *synchondrosis*.
calcaneocuboid j. [TA], a. calcaneocubóidea; uma articulação sinovial em formato de sela entre a superfície anterior do calcâneo e a superfície posterior do cubóide. Este é o elemento lateral da articulação transversa composta do tarso. SIN articulatio calcaneocuboidea [TA].
capitular j., a. da cabeça da costela. SIN j. of head of rib.
carpal j.'s [TA], a. do carpo; as articulações sinoviais entre os ossos do carpo. SIN articulatio carpi [TA], articulationes carpi [TA], articulationes intercarpales*, intercarpal j.'s *.
carpometacarpal j.'s [TA], a. carpometacarpais; as articulações sinoviais entre os ossos do carpo e do metacarpo; estas são todas articulações planas, exceto a do polegar, que tem forma de sela. SIN articulationes carpometacarpales [TA].
carpometacarpal j. of thumb [TA], a. carpometacarpal do polegar; a articulação sinovial em forma de sela entre o trapézio e a base do primeiro osso metacarpal. SIN articulatio carpometacarpalis pollicis.
cartilaginous j. [TA], a. cartilagínea; uma articulação na qual as superfícies ósseas apostas são unidas por cartilagem; são divididas em sincondroses e sínfises; nas sincondroses, a cartilagem que une as superfícies apostas é, como regra geral, finalmente convertida em osso, como entre as epífises e diáfises dos ossos longos; são exceções as sincondroses esternais e a união cartilaginosa da primeira costela e o manúbrio do esterno; nas sínfises, os ossos são unidos por um disco plano de fibrocartilagem que permanece não-ossificado por toda a vida; p. ex., o disco intervertebral e a sínfise púbica. SIN junctura cartilaginea [TA], articulatio cartilaginis, cartilaginous articulation, synarthrodial j. (2).
Charcot j., a. de Charcot. SIN neuropathic j.
Chopart j., a. de Chopart. SIN transverse tarsal j.
Clutton j.'s, articulações de Clutton; artrose simétrica, principalmente das articulações do joelho, em casos de sífilis congênita.
coccygeal j., a. sacrococcígea. SIN sacrococcygeal j.
cochlear j., a. coclear; um tipo de a. em gínglimo na qual a elevação e a depressão, respectivamente, nas superfícies articulares opostas formam parte de uma espiral, sendo a flexão então acompanhada por certo desvio lateral. SIN screw j., spiral j.
complex j. [TA], a. composta; uma articulação composta de três ou mais elementos ósseos, ou na qual duas articulações anatomicamente distintas funcionam como uma unidade. Por exemplo, as articulações talonavicular e calcaneocubóidea atuam juntas como a articulação transversa composta do tarso. SIN articulatio composita [TA], articulatio complexa, composite j., compound articulation, compound j.
composite j., a. composta. SIN complex j.
compound j., a. composta. SIN complex j.

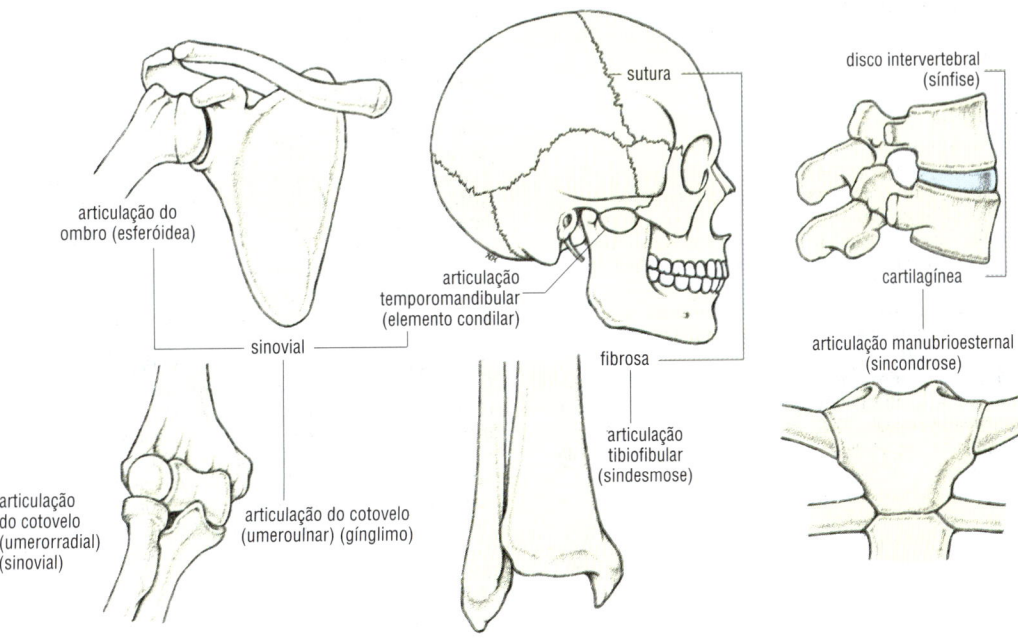

articulações

condylar j. [TA], a. condilar, a. elipsóidea; uma articulação sinovial esferoidal modificada na qual as superfícies articulares são alongadas ou elipsóides; é uma articulação biaxial, isto é, dois eixos de movimento formando ângulos retos entre si, sendo a articulação radiocarpal um exemplo. SIN articulatio ellipsoidea [TA], ellipsoidal j. *, articulatio condylaris, condylar articulation.

costochondral j.'s [TA], a. costocondrais; as articulações cartilaginosas entre a extremidade esternal das costelas e as extremidades laterais das cartilagens costais. SIN articulationes costochondrales [TA], costochondral junctions.

costotransverse j., a. costotransversa; a articulação sinovial entre o colo e o tubérculo de uma costela e o processo transverso de uma vértebra. SIN articulatio costotransversaria.

costovertebral j.'s [TA], a. costovertebrais; as articulações sinoviais que unem costelas e vértebras; consistem na a. da cabeça da costela e na a. costotransversa. SIN articulationes costovertebrales [TA].

cotyloid j., a. cotilóidea, a. esferoidal. SIN ball and socket j.

cranial synovial j.'s [TA], a. sinoviais do crânio; a. sinoviais da cabeça, compostas pela a. temporomandibular (ATM) e a. atlanto-occipital. SIN articulationes cranii [TA].

cricoarytenoid j. [TA], a. cricoaritenóidea; a articulação sinovial entre o corno inferior da cartilagem tireóide e o lado da cartilagem cricóide. SIN articulatio cricoarytenoidea [TA], cricoarytenoid articulation.

cricothyroid j. [TA], a. cricotireóidea; a articulação sinovial entre a base de cada cartilagem aritenóide e a borda superior da lâmina da cartilagem cricóide. SIN articulatio cricothyroidea [TA], cricothyroid articulation.

Cruveilhier j., a. de Cruveilhier. SIN median atlantoaxial j.

cubital j., a. do cotovelo. SIN elbow j.

cuboideonavicular j., a. cuboideonavicular; a. fibrosa entre partes adjacentes dos ossos cubóide e navicular; ocasionalmente é encontrada uma cavidade sinovial aqui como extensão da a. cuneonavicular.

cuneocuboid j., a. cuneocubóidea; a. sinovial entre a superfície lateral do cuneiforme lateral e os dois terços anteriores da superfície medial do cubóide.

cuneometatarsal j.'s, a. cuneometatarsais. SIN tarsometatarsal j.'s.

cuneonavicular j., a. cuneonavicular; a a. sinovial entre a superfície anterior do navicular e as superfícies posteriores dos três ossos cuneiformes. SIN articulatio cuneonavicularis [TA], cuneonavicular articulation.

cylindrical j., a. cilíndrica; uma classe de articulações livremente móveis que giram em torno de um eixo longitudinal único, incluindo articulações em pivô e gínglimo. SIN articulatio cylindrica [TA].

dentoalveolar j., a. dentoalveolar; gonfose. SIN gomphosis.

diarthrodial j., a. diartrodial. SIN synovial j.

digital j.'s, a. digitais. SIN interphalangeal j.'s of hand.

DIP j.'s, a. interfalângicas distais. SIN distal interphalangeal j.'s.

distal interphalangeal j.'s, a. interfalângicas distais; as articulações sinoviais entre as falanges média e distal dos dedos das mãos e dos pés. SIN DIP j.'s.

distal radioulnar j. [TA], a. radioulnar distal; a articulação sinovial em pivô entre a cabeça da ulna e a incisura ulnar no rádio; um disco articular atravessa a parte distal da articulação. SIN articulatio radioulnaris distalis [TA], distal radioulnar articulation, inferior radioulnar j.

distal tibiofibular j., a. tibiofibular distal. SIN tibiofibular syndesmosis.

j.'s of ear bones, a. dos ossículos da audição. SIN j.'s of auditory ossicles.

elbow j. [TA], a. do cotovelo; uma articulação sinovial tipo gínglimo composta entre o úmero e os ossos do antebraço; consiste na a. umerorradial e na a. umeroulnar. SIN articulatio cubiti [TA], cubital j.

ellipsoidal j., a. elipsóidea; * termo alternativo oficial para condylar j.

enarthrodial j., a. esferóidea. SIN ball and socket j.

facet j.'s, a. dos processos articulares. SIN zygapophysial j.'s.

false j., a. falsa. SIN pseudarthrosis.

femoropatellar j., a. femoropatelar; a articulação das facetas na superfície articular da patela com as superfícies correspondentes nos côndilos femorais.

fibrous j. [TA], a. fibrosa; união de dois ossos por tecido fibroso de forma que não haja cavidade articular e quase nenhum movimento é possível; os tipos de articulações fibrosas são suturas, sindesmoses e gonfoses. SIN junctura fibrosa [TA], articulatio fibrosa, immovable j., synarthrodia, synarthrodial j. (1).

flail j., a. instável; uma a. com perda da função causada por perda da capacidade de estabilizar a a. em qualquer plano dentro de sua amplitude de movimento normal.

j.'s of foot [TA], articulações do pé; incluem as articulações talocrurais, intertarsais, tarsometatarsais, intermetatarsais, metatarsofalângicas e interfalângicas. SIN articulationes pedis [TA], articulations of foot.

j.'s of free inferior limb, articulações da parte livre do membro inferior. SIN synovial j.'s of free lower limb.

j.'s of free superior limb, articulações da parte livre do membro superior. SIN synovial j.'s of free upper limb.

ginglymoid j., a. ginglimóide. SIN hinge j.

glenohumeral j. [TA], a. glenoumeral; uma articulação sinovial esferoidal entre a cabeça do úmero e a cavidade glenóide da escápula. SIN articulatio humeri [TA], articulatio glenohumeralis*, shoulder j.*, glenohumeral articulation, humeral articulation.

gliding j., a. deslizante. SIN plane j.

gompholic j., gonfose. SIN gomphosis.

j.'s of hand [TA], articulações da mão; incluem a articulação radiocarpal ou do punho; articulações intercarpais, carpometacarpais, intermetacarpais; metacarpofalângicas e interfalângicas. SIN articulationes manus [TA], articulations of hand.

j. of head of rib [TA], a. da cabeça da costela; a. sinovial entre uma costela e os corpos de duas vértebras adjacentes; a cavidade articular é dividida por um ligamento intra-articular que se fixa ao disco intervertebral; a primeira, a décima, a décima primeira e a décima segunda costelas articulam-se apenas com uma vértebra. SIN articulatio capitis costae [TA], capitular j.

hemophilic j., a. hemofílica; artropatia crônica devida à hemartrose repetida em um hemofílico.

hinge j. [TA], gínglimo; uma articulação uniaxial na qual uma convexidade transversalmente cilíndrica e larga em um osso encaixa-se em uma concavidade correspondente no outro, permitindo movimento apenas em um plano, como no cotovelo. SIN ginglymus [TA], ginglymoid j.

hip j. [TA], a. do quadril; a a. sinovial esferoidal entre a cabeça do fêmur e o acetábulo. SIN articulatio coxae [TA], coxa (2) [TA], articulatio coxofemoralis*, thigh j.

humeroradial j. [TA], a. umerorradial; a porção da articulação do cotovelo entre o capítulo do úmero e a cabeça do rádio. SIN articulatio humeroradialis [TA], humeroradial articulation.

humeroulnar j. [TA], a. umeroulnar; a porção da articulação do cotovelo entre a tróclea do úmero e a incisura troclear da ulna. SIN articulatio humeroulnaris [TA].

hysterical j., a. histérica; simulação de doença articular, com sintomas de dor, com possível edema e comprometimento do movimento.

immovable j., a. imóvel. SIN fibrous j.

incudomalleolar j. [TA], a. incudomaleolar; a articulação sinovial selar entre a bigorna e o martelo. SIN articulatio incudomallearis [TA], incudomalleolar articulation.

incudostapedial j. [TA], a. incudoestapedial; a a. sinovial entre o processo lenticular no ramo longo da bigorna e a cabeça do estribo. SIN articulatio incudostapedia [TA], incudostapedial articulation.

j.'s of inferior limb girdle, articulações do cíngulo do membro inferior. SIN j.'s of pelvic girdle.

inferior radioulnar j., a. radioulnar inferior. SIN distal radioulnar j.

inferior tibiofibular j., a. tibiofibular inferior. SIN tibiofibular syndesmosis.

interarticular j.'s, articulações interarticulares. SIN zygapophysial j.'s.

intercarpal j.'s, *articulações intercarpais; termo alternativo oficial para carpal j.'s.

interchondral j.'s [TA], articulações intercondrais; as articulações sinoviais entre as superfícies contíguas da quinta, sexta, sétima, oitava, nona e décima cartilagens costais, formando o arco costal. SIN articulationes interchondrales [TA], interchondral articulations.

intercuneiform j.'s [TA], articulações intercuneiformes; as articulações entre superfícies contíguas dos ossos cuneiformes. VER TAMBÉM intertarsal j.'s. SIN articulationes intercuneiformes [TA].

intermetacarpal j.'s [TA], articulações intermetacarpais; as articulações sinoviais entre as bases do segundo, terceiro, quarto e quinto ossos metacarpais. SIN articulationes intermetacarpales [TA].

intermetatarsal j.'s [TA], articulações intermetatarsais; as articulações sinoviais entre as bases dos cinco ossos metatarsianos. SIN articulationes intermetatarsales [TA], intermetatarsal articulations.

interphalangeal j.'s of foot [TA], articulações interfalângicas do pé; as articulações sinoviais tipo gínglimo entre as falanges dos dedos dos pés. SIN articulationes interphalangeae pedis [TA].

interphalangeal j.'s of hand [TA], articulações interfalângicas da mão; as articulações sinoviais tipo gínglimo entre as falanges dos dedos das mãos. SIN articulationes interphalangeae manus [TA], digital j.'s, interphalangeal articulations, phalangeal j.'s.

intersternebral j.'s, articulações interesternebrais. SIN synchondroses intersternebrales, em synchondrosis.

intertarsal j.'s, articulações intertarsianas; as articulações sinoviais que unem os ossos do tarso. SIN articulationes intertarseae, intertarsal articulations, tarsal j.'s.

jaw j., a. mandibular. SIN temporomandibular j.

knee j. [TA], a. do joelho; uma articulação sinovial condilar composta que consiste na articulação entre os côndilos do fêmur e os côndilos da tíbia, meniscos articulares (cartilagens semilunares) interpostos e articulação entre fêmur e patela. SIN articulatio genus [TA].

lateral atlantoaxial j. [TA], a. atlantoaxial lateral; uma articulação sinovial condilar entre as facetas articulares inferiores do atlas e as facetas articulares superiores do áxis. SIN articulatio atlantoaxialis lateralis [TA], lateral atlantoepistrophic j.

lateral atlantoepistrophic j., a. atlantoaxial lateral. SIN lateral atlantoaxial j.

Lisfranc j.'s, articulações de Lisfranc. SIN tarsometatarsal j.'s.

lumbosacral j. [TA], a. lombossacral; a articulação da quinta vértebra lombar com o sacro. SIN articulatio lumbosacralis [TA], junctura lumbosacralis.

Luschka j.'s, articulações de Luschka. SIN uncovertebral j.'s.

mandibular j., a. temporomandibular. SIN temporomandibular j.

manubriosternal j. [TA], a. manubrioesternal; a união precoce, por cartilagem hialina, do manúbrio ao corpo do esterno, que mais tarde torna-se uma articulação do tipo sínfise. SIN synchondrosis manubriosternalis [TA].

median atlantoaxial j. [TA], a. atlantoaxial mediana; uma articulação sinovial em pivô entre o dente do áxis e o anel formado pelo arco anterior e o ligamento transverso do atlas. SIN articulatio atlantoaxialis mediana [TA], Cruveilhier j., middle atlantoepistrophic j.

metacarpophalangeal j.'s [TA], a. metacarpofalângicas; as articulações sinoviais condilares ou elipsóideas entre as cabeças dos ossos metacarpais e as bases das falanges proximais. As faces palmares das cabeças dos ossos metacarpais são parcialmente divididas, de forma que a articulação é quase bicondilar. SIN articulationes metacarpophalangeae [TA], metacarpophalangeal articulations, MP j.'s (1).

metatarsophalangeal j.'s [TA], a. metatarsofalângicas; as articulações sinoviais condilares ou elipsóideas entre as cabeças dos ossos metatarsais e as bases das falanges proximais dos artelhos. SIN articulationes metatarsophalangeae [TA], metatarsophalangeal articulations, MP j.'s (2).

midcarpal j. [TA], a. mediocarpal; a articulação sinovial entre as fileiras proximal e distal dos ossos do carpo. SIN articulatio mediocarpalis [TA], middle carpal j.

middle atlantoepistrophic j., a. atlantoaxial média. SIN median atlantoaxial j.

middle carpal j., a. mediocarpal. SIN midcarpal j.

middle radioulnar j., a. radioulnar média. SIN radioulnar syndesmosis.

midtarsal j., a. mediotarsal. SIN transverse tarsal j.

mortise j., a. talocrural. SIN ankle j.

movable j., a. móvel. SIN synovial j.

MP j.'s, articulações metacarpofalângicas. (1) SIN metacarpophalangeal j.'s; (2) SIN metatarsophalangeal j.'s.

multiaxial j., a. multiaxial; a. na qual há movimento em vários eixos. VER ball and socket j. SIN polyaxial j.

neurocentral j., a. neurocentral. SIN neurocentral synchondrosis.

neuropathic j., a. neuropática; doença articular destrutiva causada por diminuição da propriocepção, com destruição gradual da articulação por lesão subliminar repetida, comumente associada à tabes dorsal ou neuropatia diabética. SIN Charcot j., neuropathic arthropathy.

j.'s of pectoral girdle [TA], articulações do cíngulo do membro superior; as articulações que unem as escápulas e as clavículas entre si, e estas últimas ao esterno, formando a cintura escapular; estas são as articulações acromioclavicular e esternoclavicular. SIN articulationes cinguli pectoralis*, articulationes cinguli membri superioris, j.'s of superior limb girdle, juncturae membri superioris.

peg-and-socket j., gonfose. SIN gomphosis.

j.'s of pelvic girdle [TA], articulações do cíngulo do membro inferior; as articulações que unem o sacro e os dois ossos do quadril para formar a cintura pélvica; estas são as articulações sacroilíacas, a sínfise púbica, os ligamentos sacrotuberal e sacroespinhal, e a membrana obturadora. SIN articulationes cinguli pelvici [TA], articulationes cinguli membri inferioris, j.'s of inferior limb girdle.

petrooccipital j., a. petrooccipital. SIN petrooccipital synchondrosis.

phalangeal j.'s, articulações interfalângicas. SIN interphalangeal j.'s of hand.

PIP j.'s, articulações interfalângicas proximais. SIN proximal interphalangeal j.'s.

pisiform j. [TA], a. do pisiforme; a a. sinovial entre os ossos pisiforme e piramidal; é separada das outras articulações intercarpais. SIN articulatio ossis pisiformis [TA], articulation of pisiform bone, pisotriquetral j.

pisotriquetral j., a. pisopiramidal. SIN pisiform j.

pivot j. [TA], a. em pivô, articulação trocóidea; uma a. sinovial na qual uma secção de um cilindro de um osso encaixa-se em uma cavidade correspondente no outro, como na articulação radioulnar proximal. SIN articulatio trochoidea [TA], helicoid ginglymus, lateral ginglymus, rotary j., rotatory j., trochoid articulation, trochoid j.

plane j. [TA], a. plana, uma a. sinovial na qual as superfícies oponentes são quase planas e na qual há apenas um discreto movimento de deslizamento, como as articulações intermetacarpais. SIN articulatio plana [TA], arthrodia, arthrodial articulation, arthrodial j., gliding j.

polyaxial j., a. poliaxial. SIN multiaxial j.

posterior intraoccipital j., sincondrose intra-occipital posterior. SIN posterior intraoccipital synchondrosis.

proximal interphalangeal j.'s, articulações interfalângicas proximais; as articulações sinoviais entre as falanges proximais e médias dos dedos das mãos e artelhos. SIN PIP j.'s.

proximal radioulnar j. [TA], a. radioulnar proximal; a articulação sinovial em pivô entre a cabeça do rádio e o anel formado pela incisura radial da ulna e o ligamento anular. SIN articulatio radioulnaris proximalis [TA], proximal radioulnar articulation, superior radioulnar j.

proximal tibiofibular j., a. tibiofibular proximal. SIN tibiofibular j.

radiocarpal j. a. radiocarpal. SIN wrist j.

rotary j., rotatory j., a. trocóidea. SIN pivot j.

sacrococcygeal j. [TA], a. sacrococcígea; a a. cartilaginosa do cóccix com o sacro. SIN articulatio sacrococcygea [TA], coccygeal j., junctura sacrococcygea, sacrococcygeal junction, symphysis sacrococcygea.

sacroiliac j. [TA], a. sacroilíaca; a a. sinovial de cada lado entre a superfície auricular do sacro e a do ílio. SIN articulatio sacroiliaca [TA], sacroiliac articulation.

saddle j. [TA], a. selar; uma a. sinovial biaxial na qual o movimento duplo é efetuado pela oposição de duas superfícies, cada uma côncava em uma direção e convexa na outra; como na articulação carpometacarpal do polegar. SIN articulatio sellaris [TA], articulatio ovoidalis.

schindyletic j., a. esquindilese. SIN schindylesis.

screw j., a. em espiral. SIN cochlear j.

secondary cartilaginous j. [TA], a. cartilagínea secundária. SIN symphysis.

shoulder j., a. do ombro; *termo oficial alternativo para glenohumeral j.

simple j. [TA], a. simples; a. composta apenas por dois ossos. SIN articulatio simplex [TA].

socket j., a. esferóidea. SIN ball and socket j.

sphenooccipital j., sincondrose esfenooccipital. SIN sphenooccipital synchondrosis.

spheroidal j., a. esferóidea; *termo oficial alternativo para ball and socket j.

spiral j., a. espiral. SIN cochlear j.

sternal j.'s, sincondroses esternais. SIN sternal synchondroses, em synchondrosis.

sternoclavicular j. [TA], a. esternoclavicular; a articulação sinovial entre a extremidade medial da clavícula e o manúbrio do esterno e a cartilagem da primeira costela; um disco articular subdivide a articulação em duas cavidades. SIN articulatio sternoclavicularis [TA].

sternocostal j.'s [TA], articulações esternocostais; as articulações entre as cartilagens das sete primeiras costelas e o esterno; as cavidades sinoviais têm ocorrência variável nessas articulações. SIN articulationes sternocostales [TA], sternocostal articulations.

stress-broken j., conector flexível. SIN nonrigid connector.

subtalar j. [TA], a. talocalcânea; uma articulação sinovial plana entre a superfície inferior do astrágalo e a superfície articular posterior do calcâneo. O termo também é usado clinicamente para se referir à articulação composta formada pelas articulações talocalcânea e talocalcaneonavicular. SIN articulatio subtalaris [TA], articulatio talocalcanea*, talocalcaneal j.*.

j.'s of superior limb girdle, articulações do cíngulo do membro superior. SIN j.'s of pectoral girdle.

superior radioulnar j., a. radioulnar superior. SIN proximal radioulnar j.

superior tibiofibular j., a. tibiofibular superior; *termo oficial alternativo para tibiofibular j.

suture j., sutura. SIN suture (1).

synarthrodial j., sinartrose. (1) SIN fibrous j; (2) SIN cartilaginous j.

synchondrodial j. [TA], sincondrose. SIN synchondrosis.

syndesmodial j., syndesmotic j., sindesmose. SIN syndesmosis.

synovial j. [TA], a. sinovial; uma a. na qual as superfícies ósseas oponentes são recobertas por uma camada de cartilagem hialina ou fibrocartilagem; há uma cavidade articular contendo líquido sinovial, revestida por membrana sinovial e reforçada por uma cápsula fibrosa e ligamentos; e há algum grau de movimento possível. SIN junctura synovialis [TA], articulatio*, diarthrosis*, articulatio synovialis, diarthrodial j., movable j., perarticulation.

synovial j.'s of free lower limb [TA], articulações sinoviais da parte livre do membro inferior; as articulações que unem os ossos da parte livre do membro inferior entre si e à cintura pélvica; elas são as articulações do quadril, joelho, tibiofibulares e do tornozelo e pé. SIN articulationes membri inferioris liberi [TA], j.'s of free inferior limb, juncturae membri inferioris liberi.

synovial j.'s of free upper limb [TA], articulações sinoviais da parte livre do membro superior; as articulações que unem os ossos dos membros superiores livres; estas são as articulações do ombro, cotovelo, radioulnares e do punho e da mão. SIN articulationes membri superioris liberi [TA], j.'s of free superior limb, juncturae membri superioris liberi.

synovial j.'s of thorax [TA], articulações sinoviais do tórax; articulações sinoviais do esqueleto torácico, incluindo as articulações costovertebrais, esternocostais, costocondrais e intercondrais. SIN articulationes thoracis [TA].

talocalcaneal j., a. talocalcânea; *termo oficial alternativo para subtalar j.

talocalcaneonavicular j. [TA], a. talocalcaneonavicular; uma articulação sinovial esferoidal, parte da qual participa da articulação transversa do tarso, formada pela cabeça do astrágalo que se articula com o osso navicular e com a parte anterior do calcâneo. SIN articulatio talocalcaneonavicularis [TA].

talocrural j., a. talocrural. SIN ankle j.

talonavicular j., a. talonavicular; a parte da a. talocalcaneonavicular que forma o elemento medial da a. transversa do tarso composta.

tarsal j.'s, articulações tarsais. SIN intertarsal j.'s.

tarsometatarsal j.'s [TA], articulações tarsometatarsais; as três articulações sinoviais entre os ossos tarsais e metatarsais, que consistem em uma articulação medial entre o primeiro cuneiforme e o primeiro osso metatarsal, uma articulação intermediária entre o segundo e terceiro cuneiformes e os ossos metatarsais correspondentes, e uma articulação lateral entre o cubóide e o quarto e quinto ossos metatarsais. SIN articulationes tarsometatarsales [TA], cuneometatarsal j.'s, Lisfranc j.'s.

temporomandibular j. [TA], a. temporomandibular (ATM); a articulação sinovial entre a cabeça da mandíbula e a fossa mandibular e o tubérculo articular do osso temporal; um disco articular fibrocartilaginoso divide a articulação em duas cavidades. SIN articulatio temporomandibularis [TA], articulatio mandibularis, jaw j., mandibular j., temporomandibular articulation.

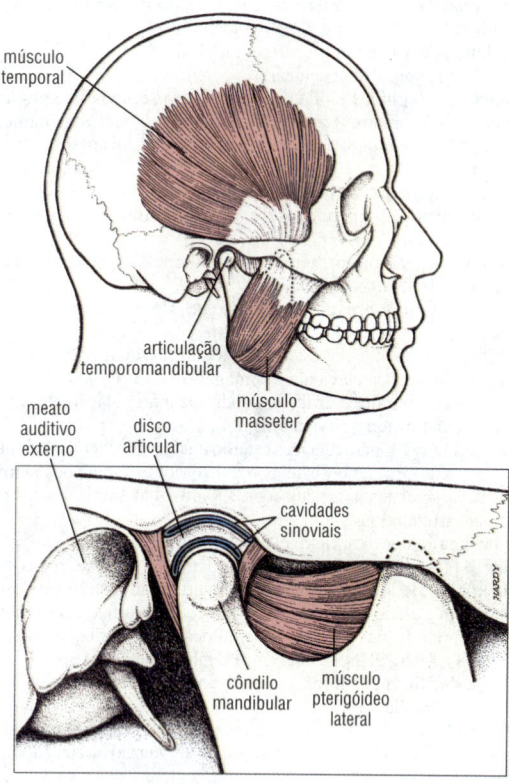

articulação temporomandibular

thigh j., a. do quadril. SIN hip j.
tibiofibular j. [TA], a. tibiofibular; a articulação sinovial plana entre o côndilo lateral da tíbia e a cabeça da fíbula. SIN articulatio tibiofibularis [TA], superior tibiofibular j.*, proximal tibiofibular j., superior tibial articulation, tibiofibular articulation (1).
transverse tarsal j. [TA], a. tarsal transversa; as articulações sinoviais entre o astrágalo e o osso navicular, medialmente, e o calcâneo e o osso navicular, lateralmente, que atuam como uma unidade, permitindo que a frente do pé gire em relação à parte posterior do pé em torno do eixo longitudinal deste, contribuindo para os movimentos de inversão e eversão total. SIN articulatio tarsi transversa [TA], Chopart j., midtarsal j., transverse tarsal articulation.
trochoid j., a. trocóidea. SIN pivot j.
uncovertebral j.'s, articulações uncovertebrais; pequenas articulações sinoviais entre os lábios laterais adjacentes dos corpos das vértebras cervicais inferiores. SIN Luschka j.'s.
uniaxial j., a. uniaxial; a. na qual o movimento se faz ao redor apenas de um eixo.
unilocular j., a. unilocular; aquela na qual um disco intra-articular é incompleto ou ausente, com a a. possuindo apenas uma cavidade.
wedge-and-groove j., esquindilese. SIN schindylesis.
wrist j. [TA], a. radiocarpal; a articulação sinovial entre a extremidade distal do rádio e seu disco articular e a fileira proximal de ossos do carpo, à exceção do osso pisiforme. SIN articulatio radiocarpalis [TA], radiocarpal articulation, radiocarpal j.
xiphisternal j. [TA], sínfise xifosternal; a união cartilaginosa entre o processo xifóide e o corpo do esterno. SIN symphysis xiphosternalis [TA], synchondrosis xiphosternalis.
zygapophysial j.'s [TA], articulações dos processos articulares; as articulações sinoviais entre zigapófises ou processos articulares das vértebras. SIN articulationes zygapophysiales [TA], facet j.'s, interarticular j.'s, juncturae zygapophysiales.

Joint Commission on Accreditation of Healthcare Organizations. Uma organização privada, sem fins lucrativos, que avalia e aprova organizações de assistência à saúde nos Estados Unidos, incluindo hospitais e outras organizações que prestam assistência domiciliar (*home care*), assistência em longo prazo, assistência à saúde mental e serviços ambulatoriais.

Jolles, Adolf, químico austríaco, 1863–1944. VER J. *test*.
Jolly, Friedrich, neurologista alemão, 1844–1904. VER J. *reaction*.
Jolly, Justin, histologista francês, 1870–1953. VER J. *bodies*, em *body*; Howell-J. *bodies*, em *body*.
Jones, Ernest, psiquiatra britânico, 1879–1958. VER Ross-J. *test*.
Jones, Henry Bence. VER Bence J.
Jones, T. Duckett, cardiologista norte-americano do século XX, 1899–1954. VER J. *criteria*, em *criterion*.
Jonesia dentrificans. Uma espécie de bactérias móveis, Gram-positivas, antes classificadas como *Listeria dendrificans;* o único membro do gênero *Jonesia.*
Jonnesco (Ionescu), Thomas, cirurgião romeno, 1860–1926. VER J. *fossa*.
Joseph, Jacques, cirurgião alemão, 1865–1934.
Joubert, Marie, neurologista canadense do século XX. VER J. *syndrome*.
Joule, James P., físico britânico, 1818–1889. VER joule; J. *equivalent*.
joule (J) (jool, jowl). Joule. Uma unidade de energia; o calor gerado, ou a energia gasta, por um ampère fluindo através de 1 ohm por 1 segundo; igual a 10^7 ergs e a 1 newton-metro. É um múltiplo aprovado da unidade fundamental do SI de energia, o erg, e tem por objetivo substituir a caloria (4,184 J). SIN unit of heat (3). [J.P. *Joule*]
Judkins, Melvin P., radiologista norte-americano, 1922–1985; pioneiro em cineangiocoronariografia e angioplastia. VER J. *technique*.
ju·ga (joo′gă). Plural de jugum.
ju·gal (joo′găl). Jugal. **1.** Ligado, emparelhado. **2.** Relacionado ao osso zigomático. [L. *jugalis*, ligado, de *jugum*, uma conexão]
ju·ga·le (joo - gā′lē). Ponto jugal; um ponto craniométrico na união dos processos temporal e frontal do osso zigomático. SIN jugal point.
ju·go·max·il·lary (joo′gō - mak′si - lār - ē). Jugomaxilar; relativo aos ossos zigomático e maxilar.
jug·u·lar (jŭg′u - lar). Jugular. **1.** Relativo à garganta ou ao pescoço. **2.** Relativo às veias jugulares. **3.** Uma veia j. [L. *jugulum*, garganta]
jug·u·lum (jŭg′u - lŭm). Garganta. SIN throat (2).
ju·gum, pl. **ju·ga** (joo′gŭm, -gă) [TA]. Jugo. **1.** Uma crista ou sulco ligando dois pontos. SIN yoke [TA]. **2.** Um tipo de pinça. [L. um jugo]
juga alveola'ria [TA], jugos alveolares. SIN alveolar *yokes*, em *yoke*.
juga cerebralia, *termo oficial alternativo para *impressions* of cerebral gyri.
j. sphenoida'le [TA], jugo esfenoidal; uma superfície plana no osso esfenóide, na frente da sela túrcica, ligando as duas asas menores e formando parte da fossa anterior do crânio, e particularmente, mais tarde, o teto da porção mais anterior do seio esfenoidal. SIN planum sphenoidale [TA], sphenoidal yoke*.
juice (joos). Suco, seiva. **1.** O líquido intersticial de uma planta ou animal. **2.** Uma secreção digestiva. [L. *jus*, caldo]
appetite j., s. do apetite; s. gástrico secretado quando a pessoa vê ou sente o aroma do alimento e por ocasião das refeições, influenciado pelo aspecto dos alimentos e pelo prazer no alimento ingerido; um reflexo condicionado.
gastric j., s. gástrico; o líquido digestivo secretado pelas glândulas gástricas; um líquido incolor, ralo, de reação ácida, contendo basicamente ácido clorídrico, quimosina, pepsinogênio e fator intrínseco mais muco.
intestinal j., s. intestinal; um líquido alcalino, cor de palha, secretado pelas glândulas intestinais; suas enzimas (peptidases, sacarases, nucleases, lecitinases, fosfatases, lipases) completam a hidrólise dos carboidratos, proteínas e lipídios.
pancreatic j., s. pancreático; a secreção externa do pâncreas; um líquido alcalino transparente que contém várias enzimas: α-amilase, nucleases, tripsinogênio, quimiotripsinogênio e triacilglicerol lipase.
Jukes (jooks). O pseudônimo de uma família famosa, cuja maioria dos membros eram desajustados sociais, débeis mentais e degenerados. O tema de argumentos sobre teorias de superioridade genética, agora desacreditadas. VER TAMBÉM Kallikak.
junctio. Junção. * Termo oficial alternativo para junction.
junctio anorectalis [TA], junção anorretal. SIN anorectal *junction.*
junc·tion (jŭngk′shŭn) [TA]. Junção; o ponto, a linha ou a superfície de união de duas partes, principalmente ossos ou cartilagens. SIN juncture. SIN junctura (2) [TA], junctio*.
adhering j.'s, junções de adesão, junções intermediárias; junções intercelulares, incluindo zônulas de aderência, hemidesmossomas e desmossomas, cuja função básica é unir células fisicamente.
amelodental j., amelodentinal j., j. amelodentária; j. amelodentinária; termos raramente usados para designar a j. da dentina com o esmalte.
amnioembryonic j., j. amnioembrionária; a linha de fixação amniótica na periferia do disco embrionário.
anorectal j. [TA], j. anorretal; transição do reto para o canal anal; corresponde à flexura perineal, ou o nível no qual o intestino perfura o diafragma pélvico;

aqui a ampola retal se estreita abruptamente em uma fenda estreita. SIN junctio anorectalis [TA].

AV j., j. AV; zona mal definida circundando e incluindo o nodo AV e o miocárdio atrial e ventricular adjacente.

cardioesophageal j., j. cardioesofágica. SIN esophagogastric j.

cementodentinal j., j. cementodentinária; a superfície na qual o cimento e a dentina da raiz de um dente se unem. SIN dentinocemental j.

cementoenamel j., j. esmaltodentinária; a superfície na qual o esmalte da coroa e o cemento da raiz de um dente se unem. VER TAMBÉM cervical *line*.

choledochoduodenal j., j. coledocoduodenal; a parte da parede duodenal atravessada pelo colédoco, ducto pancreático e ampola.

communicating j., j. comunicante. SIN gap j.

corneoscleral j., j. corneoescleral. SIN corneal *limbus*.

costochondral j.'s, junções costocondrais. SIN costochondral *joints*, em *joint*.

dentinocemental j., j. dentinocementária. SIN cementodentinal j.

dentinoenamel j., j. amelodentária; a superfície na qual o esmalte e a dentina da coroa de um dente se unem.

duodenojejunal j., j. duodenojejunal; ponto ao longo do trajeto do trato gastrointestinal onde termina o duodeno e começa o jejuno; ocorre aproximadamente ao nível da vértebra L2, 2–3 cm à esquerda da linha média; geralmente toma a forma de um ângulo agudo, a flexura duodenojejunal, e é sustentada pela fixação do músculo (ligamento) suspensor do duodeno. VER TAMBÉM duodenojejunal *flexure*.

electrotonic j., j. eletrotônica. SIN gap j.

esophagogastric j., j. esofagogástrica; extremidade terminal do esôfago e início do estômago no cárdia; local do esfíncter esofágico inferior fisiológico. SIN cardioesophageal j.

gap j., sinapse, mácula comunicante, nexo. **(1)** uma j. intercelular antes considerada uma j. intermembrana impermeável (*macula occludens*), sabendo-se agora que existe uma fenda de 2 nm entre membranas celulares apostas; a fenda não é vazia, mas contém subunidades na forma de gelosia poligonal; é encontrada em epitélios, entre determinadas células nervosas e na musculatura lisa e cardíaca; acredita-se que medeie o acoplamento eletrotônico que permite a passagem de correntes iônicas de uma célula para outra. VER TAMBÉM synapse; **(2)** áreas de comunicação eletroquímica aumentada entre células miometriais que ajudam na propagação das contrações do trabalho de parto. SIN communicating j., electrotonic j., electrotonic synapse, macula communicans, nexus.

Holliday j., j. de Holliday; a estrutura de filamentos cruzados formada quando duas duplas de ADN se cruzam em um evento de recombinação. SIN Holliday structure.

ileocecal j., j. ileocecal; ponto ao longo do trajeto do trato gastrointestinal onde o intestino delgado (íleo) termina abrindo-se na porção cecal do intestino grosso; ocorre geralmente na fossa ilíaca, demarcada internamente como orifício ileocecal.

impermeable j., j. impermeável. SIN zonula occludens.

intercellular j.'s, junções intercelulares; especializações das margens celulares que contribuem para a adesão ou permitem a comunicação entre células; incluem a *macula adherens* (desmossoma), a *zonula adherens*, a *zonula occludens* e o nexo (gap junction).

intermediate j., j. intermediária. SIN zonula adherens.

j. of lips, j. dos lábios. SIN commissure of lips.

manubriosternal j., j. manubrioesternal. SIN sternal *angle*.

mucocutaneous j., j. cutâneo-mucosa; o local de transição da epiderme para o epitélio de uma mucosa.

muscle-tendon j., inserção musculotendinosa. SIN muscle-tendon *attachment*.

myoneural j., j. mioneural; a conexão sináptica do axônio do neurônio motor com uma fibra muscular. VER motor *endplate*. SIN neuromuscular j.

neuroectodermal j., j. neuroectodérmica; j. neurossomática; a margem da placa neural embrionária que a separa do ectoderma da superfície embrionária; as células dessa região formam a crista neural. SIN neurosomatic j.

neuromuscular j., j. neuromuscular. SIN myoneural j.

neurosomatic j., j. neurossomática. SIN neuroectodermal j.

rectosigmoid j., j. retossigmóide; o local no qual o cólon sigmóide torna-se o reto; geralmente tem a forma de um ângulo agudo, demarcado externamente por uma interrupção dos apêndices epiplóicos, um afastamento das tênias do cólon para circundar completamente o reto e, conseqüentemente, interrupção das saculações (haustrações) entre as tênias.

right splicing j., j. direita; limite entre a extremidade direita de um intron e a extremidade esquerda do exon adjacente. SIN acceptor splicing site.

sacrococcygeal j., j. sacrococcígea. SIN sacrococcygeal *joint*.

sclerocorneal j., j. esclerocorneana. SIN corneal *limbus*.

squamocolumnar j., j. escamocolunar; o local de transição do epitélio escamoso estratificado para o epitélio colunar, geralmente caracterizado por epitélio cubóide estratificado.

ST j., j. ST. SIN J *point*.

sternomanubrial j., j. esternomanubrial. SIN manubriosternal *symphysis*.

tight j., j. impermeável. SIN zonula occludens.

tympanostapedial j., j. timpanoestapédica. SIN tympanostapedial *syndesmosis*.

ureteropelvic j. (UPJ), j. ureteropélvica; local de origem do ureter na pelve renal, uma localização comum de obstrução congênita ou adquirida.

ureterovesical j., j. ureterovesical; o local de entrada do ureter na bexiga, com uma angulação oblíqua através do detrusor para evitar refluxo. VER TAMBÉM vesicoureteral *reflux*.

junc·tu·ra, pl. **junc·tu·rae** (jŭngk - too′ră, - rē) [TA]. **1.** Articulação. SIN joint. **2.** Junção; junta. SIN junction. [L. uma junção]

j. cartilagi′nea [TA], a. cartilagínea. SIN cartilaginous *joint*.

j. fibro′sa [TA], a. fibrosa. SIN fibrous *joint*.

j. lumbosacra′lis, a. lombossacra. SIN lumbosacral *joint*.

junctu′rae mem′bri inferio′ris li′beri, articulações da parte livre dos membros inferiores. SIN synovial *joints* of free lower limb, em *joint*.

junctu′rae mem′bri superio′ris, articulações da parte livre dos membros superiores. SIN joints of pectoral girdle, em *joint*.

junctu′rae mem′bri superio′ris li′beri, articulações da parte livre dos membros superiores. SIN synovial *joints* of free upper limb, em *joint*.

junctu′rae os′sium, junções ósseas, designação alternativa de articulações. VER articulatio.

j. sacrococcy′gea, a. sacrococcígea. SIN sacrococcygeal *joint*.

j. synovia′lis [TA], a. sinovial. SIN synovial *joint*.

junctu′rae ten′dinum, junções tendinosas. SIN intertendinous *connections* of extensor digitorum, em *connection*.

junctu′rae zygapophysia′les, a. dos processos articulares. SIN zygapophysial *joints*, em *joint*.

junc·ture (jŭngk′choor). Junção. SIN junction.

Jung, Carl Gustav, psiquiatra e psicólogo suíço, 1875–1961. VER jungian *psychoanalysis*.

Jung, Karl G., anatomista suíço, 1793–1864. VER J. *muscle*.

jung·i·an (yung′ē - an). Junguiano; o sistema psicológico ou a forma de tratamento psicanalítico derivada dele; desenvolvido por Carl Gustav Jung.

Jüngling, Adolph O., cirurgião alemão, 1884–1944. VER J. *disease*.

ju·ni·per (joo′ni-per). Zimbro; juníparo; o fruto maduro e seco de *Juniperus communis* (família Pinaceae). [L. a árvore do zimbro]

j. berry oil, óleo de baga de juníparo. SIN oil of juniper.

j. tar, alcatrão de zimbro; óleo de cade ou oxicedro; o óleo volátil de odor acre obtido da porção lenhosa do *Juniperus oxycedrus*; usado externamente para doenças cutâneas. SIN cade oil.

jur·is·pru·dence (joor-is-proo′dens). Jurisprudência. A ciência da lei, seus princípios e conceitos. [L. *juris prudentia*, conhecimento da lei]

dental j., odontologia forense ou odontologia legal. SIN forensic *dentistry*.

medical j., medicina legal, medicina forense. SIN forensic *medicine*.

jus·tice. Justiça; o princípio ético de que as pessoas, em circunstâncias e condições semelhantes, devem ser tratadas da mesma forma; algumas vezes conhecida como justiça de distribuição. [L. *justitia*, de *jus*, direito, lei]

jus·to ma·jor (jus′tō mā′jer). Pelve maior. VER *pelvis* justo major.

jus·to mi·nor (jus′tō mī′ner). Pelve menor. VER *pelvis* justo minor.

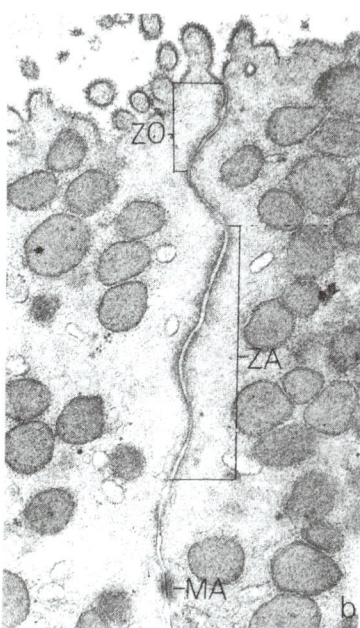

junção intercelular: micrografia eletrônica das porções apicais de duas células epiteliais adjacentes da mucosa gástrica, mostrando o complexo juncional; MA, *macula adherens*; ZA, *zonula adherens*; e ZO, *zonula occludens*; 30.000×

ju·ve·nile de·lin·quent. Delinqüente juvenil; um menor que não pode ser controlado pela autoridade paterna e comete atos anti-sociais ou criminosos, como vandalismo, violência ou roubo.

jux·ta·crine (juks'tă - krin). Justácrina; forma de ação hormonal que exige que a célula que produz o efetor esteja em contato direto com a célula que contém o receptor apropriado. [L. *juxta*, próximo a, + G. *krinō*, separar]

jux·ta·ep·i·phys·i·al (jŭks'tă - ep - i - fiz'ē - ăl). Justaepifisário. Próximo ou adjacente a uma epífise.

jux·ta·glo·mer·u·lar (jŭks'tă - glō - mer'ū - lăr). Justaglomerular. Próximo ou adjacente a um glomérulo renal.

jux·tal·lo·cor·tex (jŭks'tă - lō - kōr'teks). Justalocórtex; termo coletivo criado por O. Vogt para designar várias regiões do córtex cerebral que ocupam uma posição intermediária entre o isocórtex e o alocórtex.

jux·ta·med·ul·lary (jŭks'tă - med'ū - lār - ē). Justamedular; próximo ou adjacente à borda medular.

jux·ta·po·si·tion (jŭks - tă - pō - zish'ŭn). Justaposição; posição lado a lado. VER TAMBÉM apposition, contiguity. [L. *juxta*, próximo a, + *positio*, uma localização, de *pono*, pp. *positus*, colocar]

K

κ Símbolo de kappa, a décima letra do alfabeto grego.

K **1.** Símbolo de potássio (L. *kalium*); filoquinona; kelvin; lisina; lisil. **2.** Em óptica, o coeficiente de rigidez da esclerótica. **3.** Na adaptação de lentes de contato, o raio da curvatura do meridiano mais plano da córnea apical.

^{39}**K** Símbolo de potássio-39 (K^{39}).

^{40}**K** Símbolo de potássio-40 (K^{40}).

^{42}**K** Símbolo de potássio-42 (K^{42}).

^{43}**K** Símbolo de potássio-43 (K^{43}).

K Símbolo da *constante* de dissociação; *energia* cinética; eficiência luminosa (dissociation *constant*; kinetic *energy*; luminous efficiency). VER K_d.

K_a Símbolo da *constante* de dissociação de um ácido (dissociation *constant* of an acid); constante de associação (association *constant*) (2) (freqüentemente usada com gases).

K_b Símbolo da *constante* de dissociação de uma base (dissociation *constant* of base).

K_d Símbolo da *constante* de dissociação (dissociation *constant*).

K_{eq} Símbolo da *constante* de equilíbrio (equilibrium *constant*).

K_i Símbolo da constante de dissociação de um inibidor; na cinética das enzimas, K_{ii} reflete os valores de K_i que afetam o intercepto de uma representação duplo-recíproca, enquanto K_{is} reflete os valores de K_i que afetam a inclinação da mesma representação.

K_m Símbolo da *constante* de Michaelis (Michaelis *constant*); constante de Michaelis-Menten (Michaelis-Menten *constant*).

K_w Símbolo da constante de autoprotólise da água.

k Símbolo de quilo-.

k Símbolo das *constantes* de velocidade; rate *constants*, em *constant* ou velocity *constants* em *constant*; Boltzmann constant.

k_{cat} A taxa catalítica global de uma enzima; símbolo do *número* de renovação (turnover *number*); V_{max} dividido pela concentração total de enzimas.

ka·bu·re (kah - boo′rē). SIN schistosomiasis japonica.

Kaes, Theodor, neurologista alemão, 1852–1913. VER *line* of K.; *band* of K.-Bechterew.

ka·fin·do (kā - fin′dō). Cafindo. SIN onyalai.

kai·nic ac·id (kā′in - ik). Ácido caínico; um análogo glutamato que exibe atividade excitatória e tóxica potente e prolongada sobre os neurônios; usado como ferramenta de pesquisa em neurobiologia para destruir neurônios e como ativador dos receptores de glutamato. Tem sido usado como anti-helmíntico contra nematódeos.

kai·ro·mones (kī′rō - mōn). Cairomônios; mensageiros químicos emitidos por organismos de uma espécie, mas que beneficiam ou afetam organismos de outra espécie; por exemplo, um perfume de flores usado para atrair ou repelir outras espécies. Cf. pheromones, allomones.

Kaiserling, Karl, patologista alemão, 1869–1942. VER K. *fixative*.

⚠ **kak-, kako-.** VER caco-.

⚠ **kal-, kali-.** Cali-, calio-; potássio; algumas vezes impropriamente escritas como kalio-. [L. *kalium*, potássio]

ka·la azar (kah′lah ah - zahr′). Calazar. SIN visceral leishmaniasis. [Hind. *kala*, preto, + *azar*, veneno]

ka·le·mia (kā - lē′mē - ā). Calemia. A presença de potássio no sangue.

ka·li·o·pe·nia (kā′lē - ō - pē′nē - ā). Caliopenia; insuficiência de potássio no corpo. VER TAMBÉM hypokalemia. [L. Mod. *kalium*, potássio, + G. *penia*, escassez]

ka·li·o·pe·nic (kā′lē - ō - pē′nik). Caliopênico; relativo à caliopenia.

Kalischer, Siegfried, médico alemão, *1862. VER Sturge-K.-Weber *syndrome*.

ka·li·um (K) (kā′lē - ŭm). Potássio. SIN potassium. [L. Mod. do Ar. *quali*, potash]

ka·li·u·re·sis (kā′lē - ū - rē′sis). Caliurese. SIN kaluresis.

ka·li·u·ret·ic (kā′lē - ū - ret′ik). Caliurético. SIN kaluretic.

kal·li·din (kal′i - din). Calidina. Bradicinina com um grupamento lisil ligado à terminação amino; esse grupamento pode ser removido por uma aminopeptidase no sangue para produzir bradicinina; um vasodilatador decapeptídio. SIN bradykininogen, k. 10, k. II, lysyl-bradykinin.

  k. 9, bradicinina. SIN bradykinin.

  k. 10, calidina. SIN kallidin.

  k. I, bradicinina. SIN bradykinin.

  k. II, calidina. SIN kallidin.

Kal·li·kak (kal′ī - kak). Nome fictício de uma família de Nova Jérsei, descrita pelo sociólogo norte-americano H.H. Goddard com duas linhas de descendentes, uma de cidadãos respeitáveis, a outra de desajustados sociais e criminosos. VER TAMBÉM Jukes.

kal·li·kre·in (kal - i - krē′in). Calicreína; um grupo de enzimas (p. ex., c. plasmática, tecidual, pancreática, urinária, submandibular) que conseguem converter o cininogênio, por proteólise, em bradicinina ou calidina; a tripsina e a plasmina também conseguem realizar a conversão; a c. plasmática ativa o fator de Hageman e atua sobre o cininogênio. A c. tecidual é uma endopeptidase sérica que consegue gerar calidina a partir do cininogênio. SIN kininogenase, kininogenin.

  human glandular k. 3 (hK3), c. glandular humana; antígeno prostático específico. SIN prostate-specific antigen.

Kallmann, Franz Josef, geneticista médico e psiquiatra norte-americano, 1897–1965. VER K. *syndrome*.

kal·u·re·sis (kal - ū - rē′sis). Caliurese; o aumento da excreção urinária de potássio. SIN kaliuresis. [L. Mod. *kalium*, potássio, + G. *ourēsis*, micção]

kal·u·ret·ic (kal - ū - rēt′ik). Caliurético. Relativo a, ou que causa ou se caracteriza por caliurese. SIN kaliuretic.

Kandori, Fumio, oftalmologista japonês, *1904. VER fleck *retina* of Kandori.

Kanner, Leo, psiquiatra austríaco nos EUA, 1894–1981. VER K. *syndrome*.

kan·yem·ba (kan - yem′bă). Caniemba. SIN chiufa.

ka·od·ze·ra (kah′od - ze′ră). Tripanossomíase rodesiense; uma doença prevalente no Zimbabwe (antiga Rodésia), semelhante à doença do sono, causada pelo *Trypanosoma rhodesiense*. VER TAMBÉM Rhodesian *trypanosomiasis*.

ka·o·lin (kā′ō - lin). Caolim; silicato de alumínio hidratado; quando pulverizado e isento de partículas arenosas por eluição, o c. é usado como emoliente e adsorvente; em odontologia, é usado para aumentar a rigidez e a opacidade dos dentes de porcelana. SIN aluminum silicate. [Ch. *kao lin*, Crista Alta, nome de uma localidade na China onde a substância é encontrada em abundância]

ka·o·lin·o·sis (kā′ō - lin - ō′sis). Caolinose; pneumoconiose causada pela inalação da poeira de argila.

Kaposi, Moritz, (nascido Moritz Kohn), dermatologista húngaro na Áustria, 1837–1902. VER K. varicelliform *eruption, sarcoma*.

kap·pa (κ) (kap′a). **1.** A décima letra do alfabeto grego. **2.** Em química, designa a posição de um substituto localizado no décimo átomo do grupamento carboxila ou outro grupamento funcional. **3.** Uma medida do grau de consenso não-aleatório entre observadores ou medidas da mesma variável categórica.

kap·pa·cism (kap′ă - sizm). Capacismo; pronúncia errada do som da letra "k". [G. *kappa*, a letra κ]

Karman can·nu·la. Cânula de Karman; VER cannula.

Karmen, Albert, clínico e patologista norte-americano. *1930. VER K. *unit*.

Karnofsky, David A., médico norte-americano do século XX, † 1970. VER K. *scale*.

Kartagener, Manes, médico suíço, 1897–1975. VER K. *syndrome, triad*.

⚠ **karyo-.** Cario-; núcleo. Cf. nucleo-. [G. *karyon*, núcleo]

kar·y·o·chrome (kar′ē - ō - krōm). Cariocroma; o corpo de uma célula nervosa contendo pouca ou nenhuma substância de Nissl visível, mas um núcleo que se cora intensamente. [karyo- + G. *chroma*, cor]

kar·y·oc·la·sis (kar - ē - ok′lă - sis). Carioclase. SIN karyorrhexis. [karyo- + G. *klasis*, uma ruptura]

kar·y·o·cyte (kar′ē - ō - sīt). Cariócito; um normoblasto jovem, imaturo. [karyo- + G. *kytos*, célula]

kar·y·o·gam·ic (kar - ē - ō - gam′ik). Cariogâmico; relativo a ou caracterizado por cariogamia.

kar·y·og·a·my (kar - ē - og′ă - mē). Cariogamia; fusão dos núcleos de duas células, como ocorre na fertilização ou na conjugação verdadeira. [karyo- + G. *gamos*, casamento]

kar·y·o·gen·e·sis (kar - ē - ō - jen′ē - sis). Cariogênese; formação do núcleo de uma célula. [karyo- + G. *genesis*, produção]

kar·y·o·gen·ic (kar - ē - ō - jen′ik). Cariogênico; relativo à cariogênese; formando o núcleo.

kar·y·o·go·nad (kar′ē - ō - gō′nad). Cariogônada. SIN micronucleus (2). [karyo- + G. *gonē*, geração, descendência]

kar·y·o·gram (kar′ē - ō - gram). Cariograma. SIN karyotipe.

kar·y·ol·o·gy (kar′ē - ol′o - jē). Cariologia; o ramo da citologia que estuda o núcleo celular, suas organelas, estruturas e funções. [karyo + -logy]

kar·y·o·lymph (kar′ē - ō - limf). Cariolinfa; a substância presumivelmente líquida ou gel do núcleo na qual se acreditava haver elementos coráveis suspensos; grande parte do que antes era considerado cariolinfa agora se sabe ser eucromatina. SIN nuclear hyaloplasma, nuclear sap, nucleochylema, nucleochyme. [karyo- + L. *lympha*, água clara]

kar·y·ol·y·sis (kar - ē - ol′i - sis). Cariólise; destruição aparente do núcleo de uma célula por tumefação e perda da afinidade de sua cromatina por corantes básicos. [karyo- + G. *lysis*, dissolução]

⚠ Formas Combinantes	★ Termo oficial alternativo para a *Terminologia Anatomica*
📖 Indica que o termo é ilustrado, ver Índice de Ilustrações	[MIM] Mendelian Inheritance in Man
SIN Sinônimo	
Cf. Comparar, confrontar	I.C. Índice de Corantes
[NA] *Nomina Anatomica*	
[TA] *Terminologia Anatomica*	__Termo de Alta Importância__

kar·y·o·lyt·ic (kar′ē-ō-lit′ik). Cariolítico; relativo à cariólise.

kar·y·o·mere (kar′ē-ō-mer′). Cariômero; uma vesícula contendo apenas uma pequena parte do núcleo típico, geralmente após uma mitose anormal. [karyo- + G. *meros*, parte]

kar·y·o·mi·cro·some (kar-ē-ō-mī′krō-sōm). Cariomicrossoma; umas das diminutas partículas ou grânulos que formam a substância do núcleo celular. SIN nucleomicrosome. [karyo- + G. *mikros*, pequeno, + *soma*, corpo]

kar·y·o·mi·to·me (kar′-ē-ōm-i-tom). Cariomitoma; a rede de cromatina nuclear. [karyo- + mitosis + -ome]

kar·y·o·mor·phism (kar′ē-ō-mōr′fizm). Cariomorfismo. **1.** Desenvolvimento do núcleo de uma célula. **2.** Designa os formatos nucleares das células, principalmente leucócitos. [karyo- + G. *morphē*, forma]

kar·y·on (kar′ē-on). Cárion. SIN nucleus (1). [G. *karyon*, uma noz, castanha]

kar·y·o·phage (kar′ē-ō-fāj). Cariófago; um parasita intracelular que se alimenta do núcleo do hospedeiro. [karyo- + G. *phagō*, devorar]

kar·y·o·plasm (kar′ē-ō-plazm). Carioplasma; termo raramente usado para nucleoplasma.

kar·y·o·plas·mol·y·sis (kar′ē-ō-plaz-mol′i-sis). Carioplasmólise. SIN achromatolysis.

kar·y·o·plast (kar′ē-ō-plast). Carioplasto; um núcleo celular circundado por uma faixa estreita de citoplasma e uma membrana plasmática. [karyo- + G. *plastos*, formado]

kar·y·o·plas·tin (kar′ē-ō-plas′tin). Carioplastina; o material nuclear acromático que forma o fuso mitótico.

kar·y·o·pyk·no·sis (kar′ē-ō-pik-nō′sis). Cariopicnose; características citológicas das células superficiais ou cornificadas de epitélio escamoso estratificado no qual há retração dos núcleos e condensação da cromatina em massas sem estrutura. [karyo- + G. *pyknos*, espesso, reunido, + *-osis*, condição]

kar·y·o·pyk·not·ic (kar′ē-ō-pik-not′ik). Cariopicnótico; relativo ou causador de cariopicnose.

kar·y·or·rhex·is (kar-ē-ō-rak′sis). Cariorrexe, carioclase; fragmentação do núcleo na qual sua cromatina é distribuída irregularmente por todo o citoplasma; um estágio de necrose geralmente seguido por cariólise. SIN karyoclasis. [karyo- + G. *rhexis*, ruptura]

kar·y·o·some (kar′ē-ō-sōm). Cariossoma; uma massa de cromatina freqüentemente encontrada no núcleo celular em interfase representando uma zona mais condensada de filamentos de cromatina. SIN chromatin nucleolus, chromocenter, false nucleolus, net knot. [karyo- + G. *sōma*, corpo]

kar·y·os·ta·sis (kar-ē-os′tā-sis). Cariostase. SIN interphase. [karyo- + G. *stasis*, parada]

kar·y·o·the·ca (kar′ē-ō-thē′kă). Carioteca. SIN nuclear envelope. [karyo- + G. *thēkē*, caixa, bainha]

kar·y·o·type (kar′ē-ō-tīp). Cariótipo; as características cromossomiais de uma célula individual ou de uma linhagem celular, geralmente apresentadas como um arranjo sistematizado de cromossomas em metáfase em uma fotomicrografia de um núcleo celular em pares em ordem decrescente de tamanho e de acordo com a posição do centrômero. SIN idiogram (1), karyogram. [karyo- + G. *typos*, modelo]

kar·y·o·zo·ic (kar′ē-ō-zō′ik). Cariozóico; designa um parasita que habita o núcleo celular de seu hospedeiro. [karyo- + G. *zōon*, animal]

Kasabach, Haig H., médico norte-americano, 1898–1943. VER K.-Merritt *syndrome.*

Kasai, Morio, cirurgião japonês. VER K. *operation.*

ka·sai (kă-sī′). Anemia do Congo Belga; uma forma de anemia que ocorre na região do rio Congo, com edema associado dos tecidos subcutâneos, regiões despigmentadas na pele e vários distúrbios gastrointestinais; atribuída a deficiências nutricionais. SIN Belgian Congo anemia.

Kashin, Nikolai I., ortopedista russo, 1825–1872. VER K.-Bek *disease.*

Kasten, Frederick H., histoquímico e biólogo celular norte-americano, *1927. VER K. fluorescente Schiff *reagents,* em *reagent,* fluorescent Feulgen *stain,* fluorescent PAS *stain.*

kat Abreviatura de katal.

kata-. Cata; grafia alternativa de cata-; embaixo. [G. *kata*, embaixo]

kat·al (kat) (kat′ăl). Catal; unidade de atividade catalítica igual a 1 mol de produto formado (ou substrato consumido) por segundo, como a quantidade de enzima que catalisa a transformação de 1 mol de substrato por segundo.

kat·a·ther·mom·e·ter (kat′ă-ther-mom′e-ter). Catatermômetro; um termômetro cheio de álcool, de desenho específico, que é aquecido acima da temperatura ambiente e depois deixado esfriar; o tempo que leva para esfriar entre temperaturas específicas é uma medida do conteúdo de calor do ambiente, que leva em conta o movimento e a temperatura do ar. O bulbo pode ser prateado, para minimizar os efeitos da radiação, ou preto para maximizá-los.

Katayama, Kunika, médico japonês, 1856–1931. VER K. *fever, test.*

kathexis. Catexia; um distúrbio raro caracterizado por retenção na medula óssea de elementos mielóides que levam à neutropenia periférica grave; os neutrófilos têm um aspecto distintamente anormal; os níveis de FEC-Gm (fator estimulante de colônias de granulócitos e macrófagos) são indetectáveis, e a administração dessa substância é terapeuticamente efetiva. SIN myelokathexis.

Katz, Sir Bernard, neurofisiologista alemão-britânico, laureado com o Prêmio Nobel, *1911. VER Goldman-Hodgkin-K. *equation.*

ka·va (kah′vah). Cava-cava. **1.** SIN methysticum. **2.** SIN yaqona. [Tongan and Marquesan, Litter]

Kawasaki, Tomisaku, pediatra japonês do século XX. VER K. *disease, syndrome.*

Kay, Herbert D., bioquímico britânico, *1893. VER Jenner-K. *unit.*

Kayser, Bernhard, médico alemão, 1869–1954. VER K.-Fleischer *ring.*

Kazanjian, Varaztad H., otorrinolaringologista armênio nos EUA, 1879–1974. VER K. *operation.*

kb Abreviatura de quilobase.

K blood group, k blood group. Grupo sanguíneo K. VER Kell blood group, no apêndice de Grupos Sanguíneos.

kc Abreviatura de quilociclo.

kcal Abreviatura de quilograma de caloria (kilogram *calorie*); quilocaloria.

Kearns, Thomas P., oftalmologista norte-americano, *1922. VER K.-Sayre *syndrome.*

Keating-Hart, Walter V., médico francês, 1870–1922. VER Keating-Hart *method.*

keel (kēl). Febre paratifóide ou salmonelose de filhotes de pato.

Keen, William W., cirurgião norte-americano, 1837–1932. VER K. *operation.*

Kegel, A.H., ginecologista norte-americano do século XX. VER K. *exercises,* em *exercise.*

Kehr, Hans, cirurgião alemão, 1862–1916. VER K. *sign.*

Keith, Sir Arthur, anatomista escocês, 1866–1955. VER K. *bundle, node* e Flack *node.*

ke·lec·tome (kē′lek-tōm). Queléctomo; instrumento usado, como um arpão, para retirar uma amostra de substância tumoral para exame. [G. *kēlē*, tumor, + *ektomē*, excisão]

Kell blood group. Grupo sanguíneo de Kell. Ver apêndice Grupos Sanguíneos.

Keller, William Lordan, cirurgião norte-americano, 1874–1959. VER K. *bunionectomy.*

Kellie, George, anatomista escocês do século XVIII. VER Monro-K. *doctrine.*

Kelly, Howard A., ginecologista norte-americano, 1858–1943. VER K. *clamp, operation,* rectal *speculum.*

Kelly, Adam B., otolaringologista britânico, 1865–1941. VER Paterson-K. *syndrome;* Paterson-Brown-K. *syndrome.*

ke·loid (kē′loyd). Quelóide; uma massa nodular, de consistência firme, móvel, não-encapsulada, freqüentemente linear de tecido cicatricial hiperplásico, sensível e freqüentemente dolorosa, que consiste em faixas largas de colágeno

cariótipo de uma célula humana normal

distribuídas irregularmente; ocorre no derma e no tecido subcutâneo adjacente, geralmente após traumatismo, cirurgia, queimadura ou doença cutânea grave como acne cística, sendo mais comum em negros. SIN cheloid. [G. *kēlē*, um tumor (ou *Kēlis*, uma mancha), + *eidos*, aspecto]

acne k., quelóide acneico; uma erupção crônica de pápulas fibrosas que se desenvolvem no local de foliculite profunda, geralmente na nuca (na linha de implantação do cabelo). SIN folliculitis keloidalis.

ke·loi·do·sis (kē'loy-dō'sis). Queloidose; quelóides múltiplos.

ke·lo·so·mia (kē-lō-sō'mē-ā). Quelossomia. SIN celosomia.

Kelvin, Lord William Thomson, físico escocês, 1824–1907. VER kelvin; K. *scale*.

kel·vin (K). Uma unidade de temperatura termodinâmica igual a 273,16⁻¹ da temperatura termodinâmica do ponto triplo da água. VER Kelvin *scale*. [Lord *Kelvin*]

Kendall, J., patologista norte-americano do século XX. VER Abell-Kendall *method*.

Kendall. VER Abell-Kendall *method*.

Kennedy, Edward, dentista norte-americano, *1883. VER K. *classification*.

Kennedy, Robert Foster, neurologista norte-americano, 1884–1952. VER K. *syndrome*; Foster K. *syndrome*.

Kennedy, William, neurologista norte-americano. VER Kennedy *disease*.

Kenny, Elizabeth, enfermeira australiana, 1880–1952. VER K. *treatment*.

keno-. VER ceno- (3). [G. *kenos*, vazio]

Kent, Albert F.S., fisiologista inglês, 1863–1958. VER K. *bundle*; K.-His *bundle*.

keph·a·lin (kef'ă-lin). Cefalina. SIN cephalin.

Kerandel, Jean F., médico francês, 1873–1934. VER Kerandel *sign*.

ker·a·sin (ker'ă-sin). Cerasina; designação obsoleta de glicocerebrosídeo. SIN cerasin.

kerat-. Cerat-. VER kerato-.

ker·a·tan sul·fate (ker'ă-tan). Sulfato de queratano; um tipo de mucopolissacarídeo sulfatado contendo D-galactose no lugar do ácido urônico, do ácido hialurônico ou condroitina; também contendo *N*-acetil-D-glucosamina não-sulfatada e 6-sulfatada; encontrado em cartilagem, osso, tecido conjuntivo, córnea, aorta e discos intervertebrais; acumula-se na síndrome de Morquio; o s.q. I é abundante na córnea e é fixado a uma proteína através de um resíduo asparaginil; o s.q. II é encontrado no tecido conjuntivo frouxo e no osso e está ligado a um resíduo seril ou treonil. SIN keratosulfate.

ker·a·tec·ta·sia (ker-ă-tek-tā'zē-ă). Ceratoectasia. SIN keratoectasia. [kerato- + G. *ektasis*, extrusão]

ker·a·tec·to·my (ker-ă-tek'tō-mē). Ceratectomia; uma cirurgia realizada para modificar a refração da córnea; é removido um pedaço do estroma corneano em formato de crescente e a ferida resultante na córnea é suturada. Isso aprofunda a córnea e aumenta sua eficácia nesse eixo. VER TAMBÉM keratotomy. [kerato- + G. *ektome*, excisão]

automated lamellar k., c. lamelar automatizada; ressecção de um disco de tecido corneano utilizando um aparelho preciso para alterar o poder de refração do olho.

photorefractive k. (PRK), c. fotorrefrativa; remoção de parte da córnea com um *laser* para modificar seu formato e, assim, também o erro de refração do olho (reduzir sua miopia, por exemplo).

phototherapeutic k. (PTK), c. fototerapêutica; ablação do tecido corneano doente utilizando um *laser* excimer.

ker·a·te·in (ker'-ă-tē-in). Ceratína; o produto de redução da queratina, facilmente digerido, no qual as ligações dissulfeto são reduzidas a grupamentos SH, sendo as cadeias peptídicas individuais separadas.

ker·a·tin (ker'ă-tin). Queratina; nome coletivo para um grupo de proteínas que formam os filamentos intermediários nas células epiteliais. As queratinas possuem um peso molecular entre 40 e 68 kD, e são separadas entre si por eletroforese e focalização isoelétrica; assim separados, são numerados seqüencialmente de 1–20, e também subdivididos em proteínas de peso molecular baixo, intermediário e alto. De acordo com sua mobilidade isoelétrica são ácidas ou básicas. Em geral, cada proteína queratina ácida tem seu equivalente básico ao qual se une para formar os filamentos intermediários; entretanto, algumas proteínas queratinas existem sem par. Várias células epiteliais contêm diferentes proteínas queratinas, em uma forma tecido-específica. Os anticorpos contra as proteínas queratinas são amplamente usados para tipagem histológica dos tumores, e são úteis sobretudo para distinguir entre carcinomas e sarcomas, linfomas e melanomas. SIN ceratin, cytokeratin. [G. *keras (kerat-)*, corno, + -in]

ker·a·tin·as·es (ker'ă-tin-ās-ez). Queratinases; hidrolases que catalisam a hidrólise da queratina; cada uma possuindo especificidades um pouco diferentes.

ker·a·tin·i·za·tion (ker'ă-tin-i-zā'shŭn). Queratinização; formação de queratina ou desenvolvimento de uma camada córnea; também pode ser aplicado à formação prematura de queratina. SIN cornification.

ker·a·tin·ized (ker'ă-ti-nīzd). Queratinizado; que se tornou córneo. SIN cornified.

ke·rat·i·no·cyte (ke-rat'i-nō-sīt). Ceratinócito; queratinócito; célula da epiderme viva e determinado epitélio oral que produz queratina no processo de diferenciação em células mortas e totalmente queratinizadas do estrato córneo.

ke·rat·i·no·phil·ic (ke-rat'i-nō-fil'ik). Ceratinofílico; queratinofílico; designa fungos que usam queratina como substrato, p. ex., dermatófitos. [keratin + Gr. *philos*, amor, atração, + -ic]

ke·rat·i·no·some (ke-rat'i-nō-sōm). Ceratinossoma; queratinossoma; um grânulo ligado à membrana, com 100 a 500 nm de diâmetro, localizado nas camadas superiores do estrato espinhoso de determinados epitélios escamosos estratificados. SIN lamellar granule, membrane-coating granule, Odland body.

ke·rat·i·nous (ke-rat'i-nŭs). Ceratinoso; queratinoso. **1.** Relativo à queratina. **2.** SIN horny.

ker·a·ti·tis (ker-ă-tī'tis). Ceratite; inflamação da córnea. VER TAMBÉM keratopathy. [kerato- + G. *-itis*, inflamação]

actinic k., c. actínica; uma reação da córnea à luz ultravioleta.

deep punctate k., c. pontilhada profunda; opacidades bem definidas em uma córnea sem outros problemas, ocorrendo na irite sifilítica.

dendriform k., dendritic k., c. dendriforme; c. dendrítica; uma forma de c. herpética.

diffuse deep k., c. profunda difusa. SIN k. profunda.

Dimmer k., c. de Dimmer. SIN k. nummularis.

disciform k., c. disciforme; grande infiltração em forma de disco do estroma corneano central ou paracentral. Essa lesão é profunda e não-supurativa, sendo observada em infecções virais, sobretudo herpéticas. SIN k. disciformis.

k. discifor'mis, c. disciforme. SIN disciform k.

exposure k., c. por exposição; inflamação da córnea resultante de irritação causada por incapacidade de fechar as pálpebras. SIN lagophthalmic k.

fascicular k., c. fascicular; uma c. flictenular seguida pela formação de uma faixa ou fascículo de vasos sanguíneos que se estendem da margem para o centro.

filamentary k., c. filamentar; condição caracterizada pela formação de filamentos epiteliais de vários tamanhos e comprimentos na superfície da córnea. SIN k. filamentosa.

k. filamento'sa, c. filamentosa. SIN filamentary k.

geographic k., c. geográfica; c. com coalescência de lesões superficiais na ceratite herpética.

herpetic k., c. herpética; inflamação da córnea (ou córnea e conjuntiva) causada pelo vírus herpes simples. SIN herpes corneae, herpetic keratoconjunctivitis.

interstitial k., c. intersticial; inflamação do estroma corneano, freqüentemente com neovascularização.

lagophthalmic k., c. lagoftálmica. SIN exposure k.

k. linea'ris mi'grans, c. linear migratória; opacidade corneana linear profunda, que se estende de um limbo a outro; associada à sífilis congênita.

marginal k., c. marginal; inflamação corneana no limbo.

metaherpetic k., c. metaerpética; uma inflamação corneana pós-infecciosa, na c. herpética, levando a erosão epitelial; não se deve à replicação viral.

mycotic k., c. micótica; infecção da córnea do olho causada por um fungo.

necrotizing k., c. necrotizante; inflamação e destruição grave do tecido corneano, podendo observar-se em resposta à infecção herpética.

neuroparalytic k., c. neuroparalítica. SIN neurotrophic k.

neurotrophic k., c. neurotrófica; inflamação da córnea após anestesia. SIN neuroparalytic k.

k. nummula'ris, c. numular; c. de Dimmer; áreas acinzentadas em forma de moeda ou redondas, distintas, medindo 0,5 a 1,5 mm de diâmetro, dispersas pelas várias camadas da córnea. SIN Dimmer k.

phlyctenular k., c. flictenular; c. escrofulosa; inflamação da conjuntiva corneana com a formação de pequenos nódulos vermelhos de tecido linfóide (flictênulas) próximo do limbo corneoescleral. SIN scrofulous k.

pneumococcal/suppurative k., c. pneumocócica/supurativa. SIN serpiginous k.

polymorphic superficial k., c. superficial polimórfica; degeneração epitelial que ocorre na inanição.

k. profun'da, c. profunda; inflamação do estroma corneano posterior. SIN diffuse deep k.

punctate k., k. puncta'ta, c. pontilhada. SIN keratic precipitates, em precipitate.

sclerosing k., c. esclerosante; inflamação da córnea que complica a esclerite; caracterizada por opacificação do estroma corneano.

scrofulous k., c. escrofulosa. SIN phlyctenular k.

serpiginous k., c. serpiginosa; uma úlcera supurativa, central, de evolução lenta, grave, freqüentemente causada por pneumococos. SIN pneumococcal/suppurative k., serpent ulcer of cornea.

k. sic'ca, c. seca. SIN keratoconjunctivitis sicca.

superficial linear k., c. linear superficial; c. dolorosa, espontânea com erosão epitelial e pregas na membrana de Bowman.

superficial punctate k., c. pontilhada superficial; c. pontilhada epitelial associada à conjuntivite viral. SIN Thygeson disease.

trachomatous k., c. tracomatosa. VER pannus, corneal *pannus*.

vascular k., c. vascular; infiltração celular superficial da córnea e neovascularização entre a membrana de Bowman e o epitélio.

vesicular k., c. vesicular; c. com coalescência de áreas de edema corneano epitelial.

xerotic k., c. xerótica. SIN keratomalacia.
△ **kerato-, kerat-.** Cerato-, cerat-; querato-, querat-. **1.** A córnea. **2.** Tecido ou células córneas. VER TAMBÉM cerat-, cerato-. [G. *keras,* corno]
ℹ **ker·a·to·ac·an·tho·ma** (ker'ă-tō-ak'an-thō'-mă). Ceratoacantoma; um tumor de crescimento rápido, por vezes umbilicado, que costuma ocorrer nas áreas expostas da pele em homens brancos idosos, invadindo a derme, mas permanecendo localizado, e geralmente desaparece espontaneamente se não tratado; microscopicamente, o nódulo é composto de epitélio pavimentoso bem diferenciado, com uma massa de queratina central que se abre na superfície cutânea. [kerato- + G. *akantha,* espinho, + *-oma,* tumor]
ker·a·to·an·gi·o·ma (ker'ă-tō-an-jē-ō'mă). Ceratoangioma. SIN angiokeratoma.
ker·a·to·cele (ker'ă-tō-sēl). Ceratocele; hérnia da membrana de Descemet através de um defeito nas camadas externas da córnea. [kerato- + G. *kēlē,* hérnia]
ker·a·to·con·junc·ti·vi·tis (ker'ă-tō-kon-jŭngk'ti-vī'tis). Ceratoconjuntivite; inflamação da conjuntiva e da córnea.
 atopic k., c. atópica; inflamação papilar crônica da conjuntiva mostrando pontos de Trantas em um paciente com história pregressa de atopia.
 epidemic k., c. epidêmica; conjuntivite folicular seguida por infiltrados corneanos subepiteliais; freqüentemente causada por adenovírus tipo 8, menos comumente por outros tipos. SIN virus k.
 flash k., c. luminosa. SIN ultraviolet k.
 herpetic k., c. herpética. SIN herpetic *keratitis.*
 microsporidian k., c. por microsporídios; uma forma de c. freqüentemente associada a pessoas imunodeprimidas, como aquelas que sofrem de AIDS/SIDA.
 k. sic'ca, c. seca; c. associada a diminuição das lágrimas. VER TAMBÉM Sjögren *syndrome.* SIN dry eye syndrome, keratitis sicca.
 superior limbic k., c. límbica superior; edema inflamatório do limbo corneoescleral superior.
 ultraviolet k., c. por ultravioleta; c. aguda resultante da exposição à radiação ultravioleta intensa. SIN actinic conjunctivitis, arc-flash conjunctivitis, flash k., ophthalmia nivalis, snow conjunctivitis, welder's conjunctivitis.
 vernal k., c. primaveral. SIN vernal *conjunctivitis.*
 virus k., c. viral. SIN epidemic k.
ℹ **ker·a·to·co·nus** (ker'ă-tō-cō'nŭs). Ceratocone; protrusão cônica da córnea causada por adelgaçamento do estroma; geralmente bilateral. VER TAMBÉM Fleischer *ring,* Munson *sign.* SIN conical cornea. [kerato- + G. *kōnos,* cone]

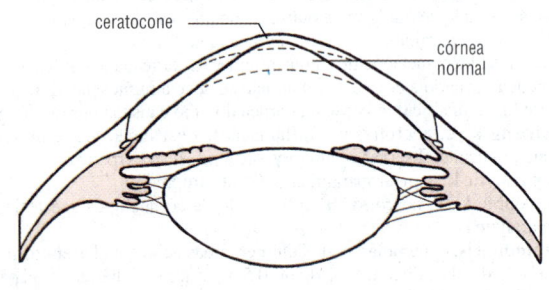

ceratocone

circumscribed posterior k., c. posterior circunscrito; defeito congênito da córnea caracterizado por um defeito semelhante a uma cratera na superfície posterior da córnea.
ker·a·to·cri·coid (ker'ă-tō-krī'koyd). Ceratocricóide. SIN ceratocricoid.
ker·a·to·cyst (ker'ă-tō-sist). Ceratocisto; cisto odontogênico derivado de remanescentes da lâmina dentária e apresentando-se como uma radiotransparência unilocular ou multilocular que pode produzir expansão da mandíbula; o revestimento epitelial é caracterizado microscopicamente por espessura uniforme, uma camada superficial corrugada de paraqueratina e uma camada basal proeminente composta de células cilíndricas em paliçada; associado à síndrome do nevo de células basais com arcos costais bífidos.
 odontogenic k. (ke-rā'tō-sist), c. odontogênico; cisto com origem na lâmina dentária com elevada taxa de recorrência e critérios histológicos bem definidos de uma superfície de paraqueratina corrugada, epitélio uniformemente fino e uma camada basal em paliçada. Uma manifestação da síndrome do nevo basocelular.
ker·a·to·cyte (ker'ă-tō-sīt). Ceratócito; célula fibroblástica do estroma da córnea.
ker·a·to·der·ma (ker'ă-tō-der'mă). Ceratoderma. **1.** Qualquer crescimento superficial córneo. **2.** Espessamento generalizado da camada córnea da epiderme. [kerato- + G. *derma,* pele]

 k. blennorrhag'ica, c. blenorrágico. SIN *keratosis* blennorhagica.
 k. blennorrhagicum (blen-ō-raji-kŭm). c. blenorrágico; as lesões cutâneas hiperceratóticas, espessadas, dispersas, observadas na síndrome de Reiter.
 lymphedematous k., c. linfedematoso. SIN mossy *foot.*
 mutilating k. [MIM*124500], c. mutilante; c. difuso dos membros, com o desenvolvimento, durante a infância, de faixas fibrosas constrictivas ao redor da falange média dos dedos das mãos ou dos pés que podem levar a amputação espontânea; pode haver surdez congênita; herança autossômica dominante, causada por mutação no gene para loricrina (LOR), um componente do complexo de diferenciação epidérmico em 1q. SIN keratoma hereditarium mutilans, Vohwinkel syndrome.
 k. palma'ris et planta'ris, c. palmar e plantar. SIN palmoplantar k.
 palmoplantar k. [MIM*148600 & MIM*244850], c. plantar; a ocorrência de áreas difusas ou segmentares simétricas de hipertrofia da camada córnea da epiderme nas regiões palmares e plantares; um grupo de displasias ectodérmicas de variedade considerável e herança autossômica dominante ou recessiva. SIN ichthyosis palmaris et plantaris, k. palmaris et plantaris, k. symmetrica, keratoma plantare sulcatum, keratosis palmaris et plantaris, tylosis palmaris et plantaris.
 k. planta're sulca'tum, c. plantar sulcado; hiperceratose e formação de fissuras na região plantar. SIN cracked heel.
 punctate k. [MIM*175860], c. pontilhado; pápulas córneas sobre as palmas das mãos, plantas dos pés e dedos que desenvolvem crateras centrais; comumente observadas em negros; herança autossômica dominante. SIN keratoma disseminatum, keratosis punctata.
 senile k., c. senil. SIN actinic *keratosis.*
 k. symmet'rica, c. simétrico. SIN palmoplantar k.
 type III punctate palmoplantar k., c. palmoplantar pontilhado tipo III. SIN acrokeratoelastoidosis.
ker·a·to·der·ma·ti·tis (ker'ă-tō-der-mă-tī'tis). Ceratodermatite; inflamação com proliferação da camada córnea da pele. [kerato- + G. *derma,* skin, + *-itis,* inflamação]
ker·a·to·ec·ta·sia (ker'ă-tō-ek-tā'zē-ă). Ceratoectasia; uma saliência anterior da córnea. SIN corneal ectasia, keratectasia.
ker·a·to·elas·toid·o·sis (ker'ă-tō-ă-las'toy-dō-sis). Ceratoelastoidose; hiperceratose e degeneração do tecido elástico dérmico. VER TAMBÉM acrokeratoelastoidosis. [kerato- + L. Mod. *elasticus,* elástico, do G. *elastikos,* propulsivo, de *elaunō,* guiar + *eidos,* semelhança, + sufixo *-ōsis,* condição]
 k. marginalis (mar-gin-āl'is), c. marginal; hiperceratose e elastose solar que se apresentam como pápulas lineares ao longo da junção da região palmar com a superfície dorsal das mãos em idosos. [L. marginal]
ker·a·to·ep·i·the·li·o·plas·ty (ker'ă-tō-ep-i-thē'lē-ō-plas-tē). Ceratoepitelioplastia; um procedimento cirúrgico para o reparo de defeitos epiteliais corneanos persistentes. Todo o epitélio corneano é removido da córnea do receptor, e pequenos pedaços de córnea do doador, com epitélio fixado, são colocados no limbo corneoescleral. O epitélio corneano do doador cresce e espalha-se para cobrir a córnea do receptor. [kerato- + epithelio- + G. *plastos,* formado]
ker·a·to·gen·e·sis (ker'ă-tō-jen'ĕ-sis). Ceratogênese; produção ou origem de tecido ou células córneas. [kerato- + G. *genesis,* produção]
ker·a·to·ge·net·ic (ker'ă-tō-jĕ-net'ik). Ceratogenético; relativo à ceratogênese.
ker·a·tog·e·nous (keră-toj'ĕ-nŭs). Ceratógeno; que causa crescimento de células produtoras de queratina, resultando na formação de tecido córneo, como unhas, escamas, penas, etc.
ker·a·to·glo·bus (keră-tō-glō'bŭs). Ceratoglobo; anomalia congênita que consiste em um segmento anterior do olho aumentado. SIN anterior megalophthalmos, megalocornea. [kerato- + L. *globus,* bola]
ker·a·tog·ra·phy (ker'ah-tog'ra-fē). Ceratografia; registro ou retrato da córnea. VER photokeratoscope, videokeratoscope. [kerato- + G. *graphō,* escrever]
ker·a·to·hy·al (ker'ă-tō-hī'al). Ceratoióide. SIN ceratohyal.
ker·a·to·hy·a·lin (ker'ă-tō-hī'ă-lin). Ceratoialino; substância presente nos grânulos basófilos grandes do estrato granuloso da epiderme rica em prolina e grupamentos sulfidrila. [kerato- + hyalin]
ker·a·toid (ker'ă-toyd). Ceratóide; semelhante ao tecido corneano. [kerato- + G. *eidos,* semelhança]
ker·a·to·lep·tyn·sis (ker'ă-tō-lep-tin'sis). Ceratoleptinse. **1.** SIN gutter *dystrophy* of cornea. **2.** Uma cirurgia para remoção da superfície da córnea e substituição por conjuntiva bulbar para fins cosméticos. [kerato- + G. *leptynsis,* adelgaçamento]
ker·a·to·leu·ko·ma (ker'ă-tō-loo-kō'mă). Ceratoleucoma; uma opacidade de corneana branca. [kerato- + G. *leukos,* branco, + *-ōma,* crescimento]
ker·a·tol·y·sis (ker-ă-tol'i-sis). Ceratólise. **1.** Separação ou afrouxamento da camada córnea da epiderme. **2.** Especificamente, uma doença caracterizada por desprendimento da epiderme que recorre a intervalos mais ou menos regulares. SIN deciduous skin. [kerato- + G. *lysis,* afrouxamento]

k. exfoliati'va [MIM*270300], ceratólise esfoliativa; desprendimento contínuo da pele, de origem familiar, caracterizado por separação do estrato córneo em flocos foliáceos em todo o corpo, exceto nas regiões palmares e plantares; herança autossômica recessiva. SIN erythema exfoliativa.
pitted k., c. sulcada; infecção bacteriana por microrganismos Gram-positivos não-inflamatória das superfícies plantares que produz pequenas depressões no estrato córneo, associadas freqüentemente a umidade e hiperidrose. SIN k. plantare sulcatum.
k. planta're sulca'tum, c. plantar sulcada. SIN pitted k.
ker·a·to·lyt·ic (ker′a - to - lit′ik). Ceratolítico; relativo à ceratólise.
ker·a·to·ma (ker - a - to′ma). Ceratoma. 1. SIN callosity. 2. Um tumor córneo. [kerato- + G. -oma, tumor]
k. dissemina'tum, c. disseminado. SIN punctate keratoderma.
k. heredita'rium mu'tilans, c. hereditário mutilante. SIN mutilating keratoderma.
k. planta're sulca'tum, c. plantar sulcado. SIN palmoplantar keratoderma.
senile k., c. senil. SIN actinic keratosis.
ker·a·to·ma·la·cia (ker′a - to - ma - la′she - a). Ceratomalacia; ressecamento com ulceração e perfuração da córnea, com ausência de reações inflamatórias, que ocorre em crianças caquéticas; resulta de deficiência acentuada de vitamina A. SIN xerotic keratitis. [kerato- + G. malakia, maciez]
ker·a·tome (ker′a - tom). Ceratótomo; um bisturi usado para incisão da córnea. SIN keratotome.
ker·a·tom·e·ter (ker - a - tom′e - ter). Ceratômetro; instrumento para medir a curvatura da superfície anterior da córnea. SIN ophthalmometer. [kerato- + G. metron, medida]
ker·a·tom·e·try (ker - a - tom′e - tre). Ceratometria; medida dos raios de curvatura da córnea.
ker·a·to·mi·leu·sis (ker′a - to - mi - loo′sis). Ceratomileuse; alteração cirúrgica de erro de refração (ceratoplastia) pela modificação do formato de uma camada profunda da córnea: a lamela anterior é removida, congelada e reesculpida em sua superfície posterior em um torno mecânico; ou parte do estroma da córnea pode ser removida do leito com um laser ou bisturi. [cunhagem, prov. do G. keras (kerat-), corno, + smileusis, gravadura]
laser-assisted in situ k. (LASIK), c. in situ assistida por laser; procedimento de refração para correção de miopia no qual é retirado um retalho da córnea, realizada ablação do estroma da córnea com laser excimer e o retalho é devolvido à sua posição original.
ker·a·to·my·co·sis (ker - a - to - mi - ko′sis). Ceratomicose; infecção fúngica da córnea.
ker·a·to·no·sis (ker′a - to - no′sis). Ceratonose; qualquer afecção anormal não-inflamatória, geralmente hipertrófica, da camada córnea da pele. [kerato- + G. -osis, condição]
ker·a·to·pach·y·der·ma (ker′a - to - pak - i - der′ma). Ceratopaquidermia; uma síndrome de surdez congênita com desenvolvimento de hiperceratose da pele das regiões palmares e plantares, cotovelos e joelhos na infância, e com constrições dos dedos das mãos em forma de faixas. [kerato- + G. pachys, espesso, + derma, pele]
ker·a·to·path·i·a (ker′a - to - path′e - a). Ceratopatia. SIN keratopathy.
k. guttata, c. em gota; crescimento endotelial semelhante a uma verruga na superfície posterior da córnea.
ker·a·top·a·thy (ker - a - top′a - the). Ceratopatia; qualquer doença, lesão, disfunção ou anormalidade da córnea. SIN keratopathia. [kerato- + G. pathos, sofrimento, doença]
band-shaped k., c. em faixa; uma opacidade interpalpebral cinza, horizontal da córnea que começa na periferia e progride centralmente; ocorre na hipercalcemia, iridociclite crônica e doença de Still.
bullous k., c. bolhosa; edema do estroma e do epitélio da córnea; ocorre na distrofia endotelial de Fuchs, glaucoma avançado, iridociclite e, algumas vezes, após implante de lente intra-ocular.
chronic actinic k., c. actínica crônica. SIN climatic k.
climatic k., c. climática; distrofia simétrica e bilateral da córnea, causada por exposição prolongada a extremos de calor ou frio; as opacidades nodulares são limitadas à área interpalpebral e a visão é apenas um pouco afetada. SIN chronic actinic k., climatic droplike k., Labrador k., spheroidal degeneration.
climatic droplike k., c. climática semelhante a uma gota. SIN climatic k.
filamentary k., c. filamentar; formação de prolongamentos delgados de epitélio corneano em estados inflamatórios, edematosos e degenerativos.
infectious crystalline k., c. cristalina infecciosa; depósitos em forma de agulha, semelhantes a samambaias, que podem ser observados na ceratite bacteriana, sobretudo aquela causada por estreptococos α-hemolíticos. VER α-hemolytic streptococci, em streptococcus.
Labrador k., c. de Labrador. SIN climatic k.
lipid k., c. lipídica; ocorrência de gorduras em uma área de vascularização corneana.
neuroparalytic k., c. neuroparalítica; inflamação ou ulceração da córnea associada à disfunção do ramo oftálmico do nervo trigêmeo.

striate k., c. estriada; edema do estroma corneano com formação de feixes entrecruzados.
vesicular k., c. vesicular; edema epitelial corneano com formação de vacúolos.
ker·a·to·pha·kia (ker′a - to - fak′e - a). Ceratofaquia; implantação de uma córnea de doador ou lente de plástico no estroma corneano para modificar erro de refração. SIN keratophakic keratoplasty. [kerato- + G. phakos, lente]
ker·a·to·plas·ia (ker′a - to - pla′ze - a). Ceratoplasia; a formação ou renovação de uma camada córnea. [kerato- + G. plasso, modelar]
ker·a·to·plas·ty (ker′ato - plas - te). Ceratoplastia; qualquer modificação cirúrgica da córnea; a remoção de uma parte da córnea contendo uma opacidade e a inserção, em seu lugar, de um pedaço de córnea do mesmo tamanho e formato removido de outra parte. SIN corneal graft, corneal transplantation, corneal trepanation, trepanation of cornea, transplantation of cornea. [kerato- + G. plasso, formar]
allopathic k., c. alopática; transplante de córnea de vidro, plástico ou outro material inerte.
autogenous k., c. autógena; transplante de córnea com material do mesmo indivíduo.
epikeratophakic k., c. epiceratofáquica. SIN epikeratophakia.
heterogenous k., c. heterogênea; transplante de córnea com material de outra espécie.
homogenous k., c. homogênea; transplante de córnea com material de outro indivíduo da mesma espécie.
keratophakic k., c. ceratofáquica. SIN keratophakia.
lamellar k., layered k., c. lamelar, c. em camada. SIN nonpenetrating k.
nonpenetrating k., c. não-penetrante; c. na qual apenas a camada anterior da córnea é usada (não uma c. tectônica). SIN lamellar k., layered k.
optical k., c. óptica; transplante de tecido corneano transparente para substituir um leucoma ou cicatriz que comprometa a visão.
penetrating k., c. penetrante; transplante de córnea com substituição de todas as camadas da córnea, mas preservando a córnea periférica. SIN perforating k.
perforating k., c. perfurante. SIN penetrating k.
refractive k., c. refrativa; qualquer procedimento no qual o formato da córnea é modificado, com o objetivo de modificar o erro de refração do olho; por exemplo, se a córnea for achatada, o olho torna-se menos míope. VER photorefractive keratectomy, keratophakia, lamellar k., thermokeratoplasty, keratomileusis, radial keratotomy. SIN keratorefractive surgery.
tectonic k., c. tectônica; enxerto para substituir tecido corneano perdido.
total k., c. total; transplante de córnea no qual toda a córnea é removida e substituída.
ker·a·to·pros·the·sis (ker′a - to - pros - the′sis). Ceratoprótese; substituição da área central de uma córnea opacificada por plástico. [kerato- + G. prosthesis, adição]
ker·a·to·rhex·is, ker·a·tor·rhex·is (ker′a - to - rek′sis). Ceratorrexe; ruptura da córnea devida a traumatismo ou úlcera perfurante. [kerato- + G. rhexis, ruptura]
ker·a·to·rus (ker - a - to′rus). Ceratoro; herniação abobadada da córnea com astigmatismo miópico regular grave. [kera- + L. torus, tumefação, protuberância, saliência]

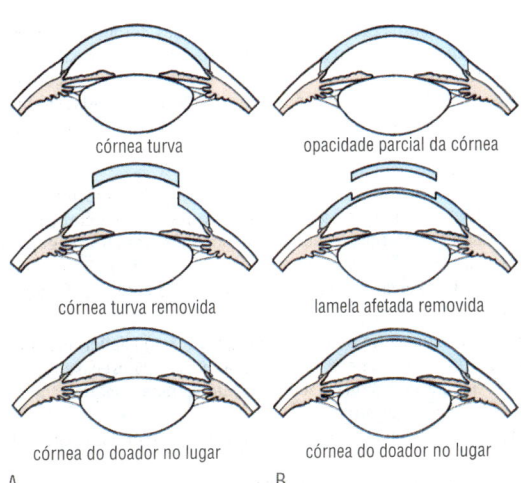

transplante de córnea total e parcial: (A) ceratoplastia penetrante: é removido um disco de espessura total (7 a 8 mm) do receptor e substituído por um botão de espessura total compatível do doador; (B) ceratoplastia lamelar; uma fina camada de tecido corneano é excisada do olho do receptor, preservando o estroma e todo o endotélio

ker·a·to·scle·ri·tis (ker'ă-tō-skle-rī'tis). Ceratoesclerite; inflamação da córnea e da esclerótica.

ker·a·to·scope (ker'ă-tō-skōp). Ceratoscópio; instrumento marcado com linhas ou círculos por meio do qual pode ser observado o reflexo corneano. SIN Placido da Costa disk. [kerato- + G. *skopeō,* examinar]

ker·a·tos·co·py (ker-ă-tos'kŏ-pē). Ceratoscopia. **1.** Exame dos reflexos da superfície anterior da córnea a fim de determinar o caráter e o grau de astigmatismo da córnea. **2.** Um termo aplicado pela primeira vez por Cuignet a seu método de retinoscopia. [kerato- + G. *skopeō,* examinar]

ker·a·to·sis, pl. **ker·a·to·ses** (ker-ă-tō'sis,-sēz). Ceratose; ceratíase; qualquer lesão da epiderme caracterizada por proliferações circunscritas da camada da córnea. [kerato- + G. *-osis,* distúrbio]

actinic k., c. actínica; uma lesão verrucosa pré-maligna que ocorre na pele exposta ao sol da face ou das mãos em pessoas idosas de pele clara; a hiperceratose pode formar um corno cutâneo, e pode haver desenvolvimento de carcinoma de células pavimentosas de baixo grau de malignidade em uma pequena proporção de pacientes não-tratados. SIN senile keratoderma, senile keratoma, senile k., k. senilis, senile wart, solar k., verruca plana senilis, verruca senilis.

arsenical k., c. arsenical; múltiplas ceratoses pontilhadas, mais comumente nas regiões palmares e plantares, mas também nos dedos das mãos e porções proximais dos membros, resultantes da ingestão prolongada de arsênico; assemelham-se à doença de Bowen microscopicamente e podem tornar-se carcinoma basocelular ou epidermóide.

k. blennorrhag'ica, c. blennorrágica; pústulas e crostas associadas com síndrome de Reiter. SIN keratoderma blennorrhagica.

k. follicula'ris [MIM*124200], c. folicular; um distúrbio autossômico dominante caracterizado por erupção, que começa geralmente no final da segunda infância, no qual pápulas ceratóticas originadas tanto dos folículos como da epiderme interfolicular do tronco, face, couro cabeludo e axilas tornam-se crostosas e verrucosas; quase sempre, as pápulas são muito pruriginosas. Microscopicamente, são observadas células disceratóticas denominadas corpos redondos (*corps ronds*) na epiderme. Faixas ungueais longitudinais são freqüentes. SIN Darier disease.

inverted follicular k., c. folicular invertida; um tumor epitelial benigno solitário, com origem nos folículos pilosos infundibulares, encontrado na face e consistindo em uma proliferação epidérmica lobulada voltada para a parte interna do folículo, composta por células escamosas queratinizadas com um padrão de redemoinhos ou espirais.

k. labia'lis, c. labial; espessamento do estrato córneo labial.

lichenoid k., c. liquenóide; pápula ou placa benigna solitária, com aspectos microscópicos semelhantes ao líquen plano, em pele exposta ao sol ou não. SIN lichen planus-like k.

lichen planus-like k., c. semelhante ao líquen plano. SIN lichenoid k.

k. obtu'rans, c. obliterante; uma acreção de epitélios no canal auditivo externo. SIN laminated epithelial plug.

k. palma'ris et planta'ris, c. palmar e plantar. SIN palmoplantar *keratoderma*.

k. pilaris, c. pilosa; uma erupção benigna comum que consiste em pápulas descamativas dos folículos; afeta basicamente as superfícies extensoras dos braços e coxas.

k. pila'ris atroph'icans facie'i, c. pilosa atrófica da face; eritema e tampões córneos das porções externas das sobrancelhas com destruição dos folículos; início nos primeiros meses de vida.

k. puncta'ta, c. pontilhada. SIN punctate *keratoderma*.

seborrheic k., k. seborrhe'ica, c. seborreica; lesões gordurosas superficiais, benignas, verrucosas, freqüentemente pigmentadas, que consistem em proliferação de células epidérmicas, semelhantes a células basais, encerrando cistos córneos; geralmente ocorrem após a terceira década de vida. SIN basal cell papilloma, seborrheic verruca.

senile k., k. seni'lis, c. senil. SIN actinic k.

solar k., c. solar. SIN actinic k.

tar k., c. do alcatrão; lesões verrucosas na face e nas mãos resultantes de exposição repetida e prolongada ao alcatrão e ao piche; também ocorre como lesões semelhantes ao ceratoacantoma que podem se tornar malignas, sobretudo no escroto.

ker·a·to·sul·fate (ker'ă-tō-sŭl-fāt). Ceratossulfato. SIN keratan sulfate.

ker·a·to·tome (ker'ă-tō-tōm). Ceratótomo. SIN keratome.

ker·a·tot·o·my (ker'ă-tot'ō-mē). Ceratotomia. **1.** Qualquer incisão através da córnea. **2.** Uma cirurgia que realiza uma incisão da espessura parcial da córnea para achatá-la e reduzir seu poder de refração naquele meridiano. [kerato- + G. *tomē,* incisão]

delimiting k., c. delimitante; incisão na córnea ao longo da margem de uma úlcera progressiva.

radial k., c. radial; uma c. com incisões radiais ao redor de uma zona central clara. Uma forma de ceratoplastia refrativa usada no tratamento da miopia.

refractive k., c. refrativa; modificação da curvatura córnea por meio de incisões na córnea para minimizar hiperopia, miopia ou astigmatismo.

ke·rau·no·pho·bia (kē-raw'nō-fō'bē-ă). Ceraunofobia; temor mórbido de trovões e relâmpagos. [G. *keraunos,* raio, + *phobos,* medo]

Kerckring (Kerckringius), Theodor, anatomista dinamarquês, 1640–1693. VER K. *center, folds,* em *fold*; ossicle; K. *valves,* em *valve*.

ke·ri·on (kē'rē-on). Quérion; uma lesão granulomatosa secundariamente infectada complicando a infecção fúngica dos pêlos; tipicamente, uma lesão elevada de consistência mole. [G. *kērion,* favo de mel; uma doença cutânea, de *kēros,* cera de abelha]

Kerley, Peter J., radiologista inglês, 1900–1979. VER K. B *lines,* em *line*.

ker·nel (ker'nĕl). Cerne, âmago; a porção central da expressão do *software* de um algoritmo matemático, como na tomografia computadorizada. [O.E. *cyrnel,* um pequeno corno]

ker·nic·ter·us (ker-nik'ter-ŭs). Kernicterus, icterícia nuclear; icterícia associada a altos níveis de bilirrubina não-conjugada, ou em prematuros pequenos com graus mais modestos de bilirrubinemia; coloração amarela e lesões degenerativas são encontradas principalmente nos gânglios da base, incluindo o núcleo lenticular, subtálamo, corno de Ammon e outras áreas; pode ocorrer em distúrbios hemolíticos como eritroblastose Rh ou ABO ou deficiência de G6PD, bem como na sépsis neonatal ou na síndrome de Crigler-Najjar; as características clínicas iniciais são opistótono, choro agudo, letargia e má sucção, bem como reflexo de Moro anormal ou ausente e perda do movimento ocular para cima; as conseqüências posteriores incluem surdez, paralisia cerebral, outros déficits neurossensoriais e retardo mental. SIN bilirubin encephalopathy, nuclear jaundice. [Al. *Kern,* cerne (núcleo), + *Ikterus,* icterícia]

Kernig, Vladimir, médico russo, 1840–1917. VER K. *sign*.

Kernohan, James W., patologista norte-americano, 1896–1981. VER K. *notch*.

ker·o·sene (ker'ō-sēn). Querosene; mistura de hidrocarbonetos do petróleo, principalmente da série metano; a quinta fração na destilação do petróleo, usada como combustível para lamparinas e fogões, como desengordurante e para limpeza, e em inseticidas. O contato com a pele humana pode causar irritação e infecção; a inalação pode causar cefaléia, sonolência, coma; a ingestão causa irritação, vômito e diarréia. O vômito não deve ser induzido, pois a aspiração de vômito causa pneumonite. [G. *kēros,* cera, + *-ene*]

Kerr, Harry Hyland, cirurgião norte-americano, 1881–1963. VER Parker-K. *suture*.

Kestenbaum, Alfred, oftalmologista norte-americano, 1890–1961. VER Kestenbaum *sign,* Kestenbaum *number,* Kestenbaum *procedure*.

ke·tal (kē'tal). Cetal; RC(OR')(R'')OR'''; uma cetona hidratada na qual ambos os grupamentos hidroxila são esterificados com álcoois.

ket·a·mine (kēt'ă-mēn). Cetamina; um anestésico administrado por via parenteral que produz catatonia, analgesia profunda, aumento da atividade simpática e pouco relaxamento dos músculos esqueléticos; os efeitos colaterais incluem sialorréia e disforia acentuada ocasional, principalmente em adultos; quimicamente relacionado à fenciclidina (PCP), pode produzir alucinações.

ke·tan·ser·in (kēt-an'ser-in). Cetanserina; antagonista específico do receptor $5HT_2$ da serotonina com propriedades anti-hipertensivas; a droga também reduz a agregação plaquetária produzida pela serotonina.

ke·tene (kē'tēn). Ceteno. **1.** $CH_2=C=O$; um agente acetilante muito reativo, usado em sínteses químicas. **2.** Qualquer c. substituto.

ket·i·mine (kē'ta-mēn). Cetimina; R—N=C(R')(R''); um tautômero de uma aldimina, formado em muitas reações de catálise enzimática; p. ex., aminotransferases.

keto-. Ceto-; forma combinante que indica um composto contendo um grupamento cetona; substituído por oxo- na nomenclatura sistemática. [Al.]

ke·to ac·id (kē'tō). Cetoácido; um ácido contendo um grupamento cetona (—CO—) além do(s) grupamento(s) ácido; α-c. a. refere-se a um 2-oxoácido (p. ex., ácido pirúvico); β-c. a. refere-se a um 3-oxoácido (p. ex., ácido acetoacético), etc. SIN oxo acid.

α-k. a. dehydrogenase, α-c. a. desidrogenase; um dos vários complexos multienzimáticos distintos que catalisam a formação de um derivado acil-CoA, CO_2 e NADH a partir de um α-cetoácido, NAD^+ e coenzima A; a doença da urina em xarope de bordo resulta de vários defeitos hereditários diferentes no complexo mitocondrial de desidrogenase do α-cetoácido de cadeia ramificada.

3-ke·to·ac·id-CoA trans·fer·ase. 3-cetoácido-CoA transferase. SIN 3-oxoacid-CoA transferase.

ke·to·ac·i·de·mia (kē'tō-as-id-ē'mē-ă). Cetoacidemia. SIN maple syrup urine *disease*.

ke·to·ac·i·do·sis (kē'tō-as-i-dō'sis). Cetoacidose; acidose, como no diabetes ou na inanição, causada pelo aumento da produção de corpos cetônicos.

ke·to·ac·i·du·ria (kē'tō-as-i-doo'rē-ă). Cetoacidúria; excreção de urina com elevado conteúdo de cetoácidos.

branched chain k., c. de cadeia ramificada. SIN maple syrup urine *disease*.

β-ke·to·ac·yl-ACP re·duc·tase (kē-tō-as'il). β-cetoacil-ACP redutase. SIN 3-oxoacyl-ACP reductase.

β-ke·to·ac·yl-ACP syn·thase. β-cetoacil-ACP sintase. SIN 3-oxoacyl-ACP synthase.

3-ke·to·ac·yl-CoA thi·o·lase. 3-cetoacil-CoA tiolase. SIN acetyl-CoA acyl-transferase.

2-ke·to·a·dip·ic ac·id (kē'tō-a-dip'ik). Ácido 2-cetoadípico; um intermediário no catabolismo do L-triptofano e L-lisina; o a. 2-c. acumula-se em determinados distúrbios hereditários, provavelmente devido à deficiência de uma das proteínas no complexo α-cetoadipato desidrogenase; ácido 2-oxoadípico; ácido 2-oxo-hexadióico.

2-k. a. dehydrogenase complex, complexo a. 2-c. desidrogenase; o complexo multienzimático pelo qual o a. 2-c. reage com a coenzima A e com o NAD$^+$ para produzir glutaril-CoA, CO_2 e NADH + H$^+$ no catabolismo da L-lisina e do L-triptofano; a deficiência de uma das proteínas nesse complexo resulta em 2-cetoadípico acidemia.

2-ke·to·a·dip·ic ac·i·de·mi·a (kē′tō - a - dip′ik). 2-cetoadípico acidemia; níveis séricos elevados de ácido 2-cetoadípico.

ke·to·con·a·zole (kē - tō - kō′na - zōl). Cetoconazol; um agente antifúngico de amplo espectro usado no tratamento de infecções fúngicas sistêmicas e tópicas.

α-ke·to·de·car·box·y·lase (kē′tō - dē - kar - boks′i - lās). α-cetodescarboxilase; outrora, o sistema enzimático que convertia piruvato (um 2-oxoácido) em acetil-CoA e CO_2, com redução de NAD$^+$ para NADH e a participação de lipoamida e tiamina pirofosfato; agora se sabe que envolve pelo menos três enzimas em sucessão: piruvato desidrogenase, diidrolipoamida aceltransferase e diidrolipoamida desidrogenase. Cf. *pyruvate* dehydrogenase (lipoamide).

ke·to·gen·e·sis (kē - tō - jen′e - sis). Cetogênese; produção metabólica de cetonas ou corpos cetônicos.

ke·to·gen·ic (kē - tō - jen′ik). Cetogênico; que dá origem a corpos cetônicos no metabolismo.

α-ke·to·glu·tar·am·ic ac·id (kē′tō - gloo - tar - ik). Ácido α-cetoglutarâmico; um metabólito da glutamina formado pela ação da glutamina aminotransferase; elevado em determinados casos de coma hepático. SIN 2-oxoglutaric acid.

α-ke·to·glu·tar·ate. α-cetoglutarato; um sal ou éster do ácido α-cetoglutárico.

α-k. dehydrogenase, α-c. desidrogenase; uma enzima que catalisa a descarboxilação oxidativa do ácido 2-cetoglutárico em succinildiidrolipoato; o grupamento succinil é posteriormente transferido para CoA e o lipoato reduzido é oxidado por NAD$^+$; um complexo que é uma parte do ciclo do ácido tricarboxílico. SIN 2-oxoglutarate dehydrogenase, α-ketoglutarate dehydrogenase complex.

ke·to·hep·tose (kē - tō - hep′tōs). Cetoeptose; heptulose; um açúcar de sete carbonos que possui um grupamento cetona. SIN heptulose.

ke·to·hex·ose (kē - tō - heks′ōs). Cetoexose; hexulose; um açúcar de seis carbonos que possui um grupamento cetona; p. ex., frutose. SIN hexulose.

β-ke·to·hy·dro·gen·ase (kē - tō - hī′drō - jen - ās). β-cetoidrogenase. SIN 3-hydroxyacyl-CoA dehydrogenase.

ke·to·hy·drox·y·es·trin (kē - tō - hī - drok - sē - es′trin). Cetoidroxiestrina. SIN estrone.

ke·tol (kē′tol). Cetol; uma cetona que tem um grupamento OH próximo ao grupamento CO. Em um α-c., o OH está fixado a um átomo de carbono que está fixado ao átomo de carbono CO; em um β-c., há um átomo de carbono interposto.

ke·tole (kē′tōl). Cetol. SIN indole (1).

ke·tole group. Grupamento cetol; carbonos 1 e 2 de uma 2-cetose (HOCH$_2$CO-); a *trans*-cetolação de D-xilose 5-fosfato para C-1 de aldoses é importante em várias vias metabólicas envolvendo carboidratos (p. ex., fotossíntese, *shunt* de Dickens); a unidade de dois carbonos é transferida como α,β-diidroxietiltiamina pirofosfato.

ke·to·lyt·ic (kē - tō - lit′ik). Cetolítico; que causa a dissolução de substâncias à base de cetona ou acetona, referindo-se geralmente a produtos de oxidação da glicose e substâncias correlatas.

ke·tone (kē′tōn). Cetona; uma substância com o grupamento carbonila ligando dois átomos de carbono; a c. mais importante na medicina e mais simples é a dimetil c. (acetona).

$$\begin{array}{c} O \\ \| \\ - CO - \end{array}$$

ke·tone al·co·hol. Álcool cetônico; uma substância contendo um grupamento carbonila ou cetona, bem como um grupamento hidroxila; p. ex., diidroxiacetona.

ke·tone-al·de·hyde mu·tase. Cetona-aldeído mutase. SIN lactoylglutathione lyase.

ke·to·ne·mia (kē - tō - nē′mē - ā). Cetonemia; a presença de concentrações reconhecíveis de corpos cetônicos no plasma. [ketone + G. *haima*, sangue]

ke·ton·ic (kē - tōn′ik). Cetônico; relativo a, ou que possui as características de, uma cetona.

ke·to·ni·za·tion (kē - tō - ni - zā′shŭn). Cetonização; conversão em uma cetona.

ke·ton·u·ria (kē - tō - noo′rē - ā). Cetonúria; aumento da excreção urinária de corpos cetônicos.

branched chain k., c. de cadeia ramificada. SIN maple syrup urine *disease*.

ke·to·pan·to·ic ac·id (kē′tō - pan - tō′ik). Ácido cetopantóico; precursor oxidado do ácido pantóico, intermediário na via de síntese entre o ácido α-cetoisovalérico e o ácido pantotênico.

ke·to·pen·tose (kē - tō - pen′tōs). Cetopentose; um açúcar de cinco carbonos no qual os carbonos 2, 3 ou 4 fazem parte de um grupamento carbonil; p. ex., ribulose.

β-ke·to·re·duc·tase (kē′tō - rē - dŭk′tās). β-Cetorredutase. SIN 3-hydroxyacyl-CoA dehydrogenase.

ket·or·o·lac. Cetorolaco; um antiinflamatório não-esteróide pirrolo-pirrólico com propriedades antipiréticas e analgésicas; tem ações semelhantes às do ibuprofeno, mas é significativamente mais potente e capaz de aliviar dores fortes. Freqüentemente usado na forma injetável.

ke·tose (kē′tōs). Cetose; um carboidrato contendo o grupamento carbonil característico das cetonas; isto é, uma poliidroxicetona; p. ex., frutose, ribulose, sedoeptulose; a maioria das cetoses de ocorrência natural possuem o grupamento carbonil no segundo átomo de carbono.

ke·tose-1-phos·phate al·dol·ase. Cetose-1-fosfato aldolase; frutose bifosfato aldolase.

ke·tose re·duc·tase. Cetose redutase. SIN D-sorbitol-6-phosphate dehydrogenase.

ke·to·sis (kē - tō′sis). Cetose; um distúrbio caracterizado pelo aumento da produção de corpos cetônicos, como no diabetes melito ou inanição. [ketone + -*osis*, distúrbio]

bovine k., c. bovina; uma doença metabólica comum de vacas que costuma surgir algumas semanas após o parto; caracterizada por hipoglicemia, cetonúria, perda do apetite, letargia, queda da produção de leite e emaciação rápida.

17-ke·to·ste·roids (17-KS) (kē - tō - stēr′oydz). 17-Cetosteróides; nominalmente, qualquer esteróide com um grupamento carbonila em C-17; comumente usado para designar metabólitos esteróides C_{19} urinários de hormônios androgênios e adrenocorticais que possuem essa característica estrutural. SIN 17-oxosteroids.

α-ke·to·suc·ci·nam·ic ac·id (kē′tō - sŭk - si - nam′ik). Ácido α-cetossuccinâmico; o produto da transaminação da asparagina; transformado pela ω-amidase.

ke·to·suc·ci·nic ac·id (kē - tō - sŭk′si - nik). Ácido cetossuccínico. SIN oxaloacetic acid.

ke·to·su·ria (kē′tō - su′rē - ā′). Cetosúria; a presença de cetonas na urina.

ke·to·tet·rose (kē′tō - tet′rōs). Cetotetrose; um açúcar de quatro carbonos que possui um grupamento cetona; p. ex., eritrulose.

β-ke·to·thi·o·lase (kē - tō - thī′ō - lās). β-Cetotiolase. SIN *acetyl-CoA* acyltransferase.

ke·to·tic (kē′tot - ik). Cetótico; relativo aos corpos cetônicos; acidose devida à produção excessiva de corpos cetônicos como ocorre no diabetes insulinodependente não-controlado.

ke·to·tri·ose (kē′tō - trī′ōs). Cetotriose; um açúcar de três carbonos que possui um grupamento cetona; isto é, diidroxiacetona.

keV. Abreviação de quiloelétron volts, uma unidade de energia usada em radiografia diagnóstica e medicina nuclear, equivalente à energia cinética ganha por um elétron que cai através de um potencial de 1 volt.

Key, Charles Alston, médico inglês, 1793–1849.

Key, Ernst, A.H., anatomista e médico sueco, 1832–1901. VER *foramen* of K.-Retzius; *sheath* of K. and Retzius.

key·way (kē′wā). A porção fêmea de uma conexão.

kg Abreviação de quilograma.

khat (kot). Qat; khat; partes macias frescas de *Catha edulis*.

khel·lin (kel′in). Quelina; o princípio ativo em extratos de *Ammi visnaga*, vegetal umbelífero que cresce no Oriente Próximo; usada na angina do peito e na asma. [Ar. *khella*]

KHN Abreviação de Knoop hardness *number*.

kick (kik). Estímulo mecânico vigoroso.

atrial k., estímulo atrial; a contribuição de força impulsora da contração atrial imediatamente antes da sístole ventricular para aumentar a eficiência da ejeção ventricular devido a um aumento agudo da pré-carga.

idioventricular k., estímulo idioventricular; aumento da contratilidade das fibras ventriculares em contração que, por estiramento das fibras que se contraem mais tarde, aumenta sua força por contração.

Kidd blood group. Grupo sanguíneo de Kidd. Ver apêndice Grupos Sanguíneos.

kid·ney (kid′nē). Rim; um dos dois órgãos que excretam urina. Os rins são órgãos em forma de feijão (cerca de 11 cm de comprimento, 5 cm de largura e 3 cm de espessura) situados de cada lado da coluna vertebral, posteriores ao peritônio, aproximadamente opostos à décima segunda vértebra torácica e às primeiras três vértebras lombares. SIN nephros, ren. [A.S. *cwith*, ventre, abdome, + *neere*, rim (L. *ren*, G. *nephros*)]

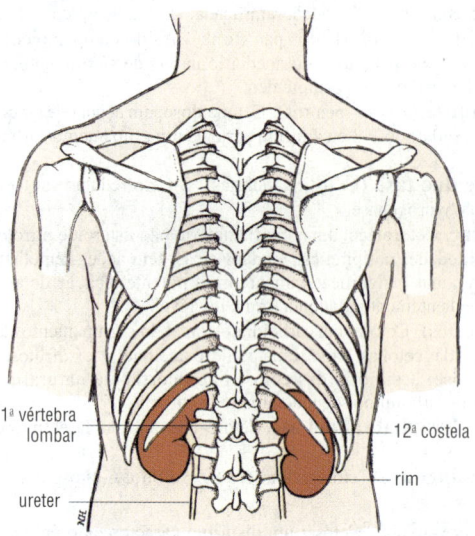

rim: localização

amyloid k., r. amilóide; um r. que sofreu amiloidose, geralmente em associação com alguma doença crônica, como mieloma múltiplo, tuberculose, osteomielite ou outra inflamação supurativa crônica; esses rins apresentam aumento moderado e seu aspecto macroscópico é céreo, com amilóide depositado sob o endotélio nas alças glomerulares e nas arteríolas, aparentemente começando como focos de espessamento das membranas basais. SIN waxy k.
Armanni-Ebstein k., r. de Armanni-Ebstein; vacuolização glicogênica das alças de Henle, observada em diabéticos antes da introdução da insulina. SIN Armanni-Ebstein change.
arteriolosclerotic k., r. arteriolosclerótico; um r. no qual há esclerose das arteríolas, isto é, nefrosclerose arteriolar resultante de hipertensão benigna crônica. Esses rins tendem a ser castanho-avermelhados pálidos ou relativamente cinza, de tamanho moderadamente reduzido, e mais firmes que os órgãos normais; as superfícies capsulares apresentam granularidade fina uniforme. A maioria das arteríolas apresentam-se espessadas e hialinizadas, assim resultando em graus variáveis de estreitamento das luzes, isquemia e fibrose no tecido intersticial, levando à contração uniforme da cortical.
arteriosclerotic k., r. arteriosclerótico; um rim no qual há esclerose dos vasos arteriais maiores que as arteríolas. Esses rins geralmente não sofrem redução significativa do tamanho, mas tendem a ser mais pálidos que o habitual; a superfície capsular pode ser caracterizada por algumas, possivelmente várias, cicatrizes cônicas, em forma de V, relativamente profundas, que resultam de fibrose e atrofia isquêmica da região suprida pelo vaso afetado.
artificial k., r. artificial. SIN hemodialyzer.
Ask-Upmark k., r. de Ask-Upmark; hipoplasia renal verdadeira com diminuição dos lóbulos e sulcos transversais profundos nas superfícies corticais do rim.
atrophic k., r. atrófico; um rim cujo tamanho está diminuído devido à circulação inadequada e/ou perda de néfrons.
cake k., r. em bolo; um órgão sólido, irregularmente lobulado, de formato bizarro, geralmente situado na pelve em direção à linha média, produzido por fusão do primórdio renal.
contracted k., r. contraído; um rim difusamente fibrosado no qual a quantidade de relativamente grande de tecido fibroso anormal e a atrofia isquêmica levam a redução moderada ou grande do tamanho do órgão, como na nefrosclerose arteriolar e na glomerulonefrite crônica.
cow k., r. de vaca; um rim contendo um número anormalmente grande de pequenos cálices, semelhantes à anatomia renal bovina normal.
crush k., r. do esmagamento; insuficiência renal oligúrica aguda após lesões musculares por esmagamento; os rins mostram alterações de lesão tubular hipóxica, mais cilindros de pigmentos nos túbulos renais que contêm mioglobina.
cystic k., r. cístico; um termo geral usado para indicar um rim que contém um ou mais cistos, incluindo doença policística, cisto solitário, múltiplos cistos simples e cistos de retenção (associados à fibrose do parênquima).
disk k., r. discóide. SIN pancake k.
duplex k., r. duplo; um rim no qual há dois sistemas pelvicaliceais.
fatty k., r. gorduroso; um rim no qual há metamorfose gordurosa das células do parênquima, principalmente degeneração gordurosa.
flea-bitten k., r. picado por pulga; o rim observado à necropsia em alguns casos de endocardite bacteriana, sendo causado por hemorragias petequiais difusas resultantes de glomerulonefrite focal.

floating k., r. flutuante; o rim anormalmente móvel que, freqüentemente, desce até a borda da pelve quando o paciente fica de pé; nefroptose. SIN movable k., wandering k.
Formad k., r. de Formad; um rim aumentado e deformado algumas vezes observado no alcoolismo crônico.
fused k., r. fundido; um órgão único, anômalo, produzido por fusão do primórdio renal.
Goldblatt k., r. de Goldblatt; um rim cujo suprimento sanguíneo arterial foi comprometido; uma conseqüência é a hipertensão arterial (renovascular).
granular k., r. granular; um rim no qual focos de cicatrização bastante uniformes, situados de forma difusa e uniforme, do tecido intersticial da cortical (e algumas vezes cicatrização dos glomérulos) e o pequeno grau associado de saliência de grupos de túbulos dilatados levam ao desenvolvimento de uma superfície com mínimos relevos; esses rins são observados na nefrosclerose arteriolar ou glomerulonefrite crônica. SIN sclerotic k.
head k., cabeça renal. SIN pronephros (1).
hind k., r. posterior. SIN metanephros.
horseshoe k., r. em ferradura; união das extremidades inferiores ou, algumas vezes, das extremidades superiores dos dois rins por uma faixa de tecido que se estende através da coluna vertebral.
medullary sponge k., r. esponjoso medular; doença cística das pirâmides renais associada à formação de cálculos e hematúria; difere da doença cística da medula renal porque não costuma haver desenvolvimento de insuficiência renal.
middle k., r. médio. SIN mesonephros.
mortar k., r. em argamassa. SIN putty k.
movable k., r. móvel. SIN floating k.
pancake k., r. em panqueca; r. discóide; um órgão em forma de disco produzido por fusão de ambos os pólos do primórdio renal contralateral. SIN disk k.
pelvic k., r. pélvico; uma anormalidade congênita na qual o rim está na pelve; geralmente o suprimento sanguíneo arterial provém da bifurcação da aorta ou da artéria ilíaca.

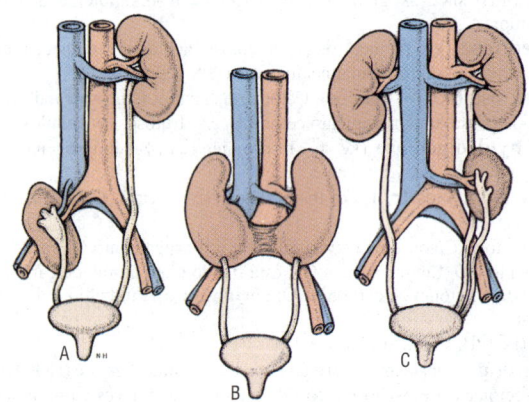

anomalias renais: (A) rim pélvico, (B) rim em ferradura, (C) rim supranumerário

polycystic k., r. policístico; uma doença progressiva caracterizada pela formação de múltiplos cistos de tamanhos variáveis, dispersos difusamente nos dois rins, resultando em compressão e destruição do parênquima renal, geralmente com hipertensão, hematúria macroscópica e uremia levando à insuficiência renal progressiva. Há dois tipos principais: 1) com início no lactante ou na criança pequena, geralmente com herança autossômica recessiva [MIM*263200]; 2) com início na vida adulta, de herança autossômica dominante com heterogeneidade genética [MIM*173900, 173910 e 600666]; pode ser causado por mutação no gene policistina-1 do cromossoma 16p, gene da policistina-2 em 4q, ou gene(s) ainda não identificados. SIN polycystic disease of kidneys.
primordial k., r. primordial. SIN pronephros.
putty k., r. em massa de vidraceiro; um rim contendo material caseoso aprisionado por estreitamento do ureter devido a granulações tuberculosas na tuberculose renal. SIN mortar k.
pyelonephritic k., r. pielonefrítico; um rim deformado por múltiplas cicatrizes causadas por infecção renal crônica ou recorrente.
Rose-Bradford k., r. de Rose-Bradford; uma forma de rim fibrótico, de origem inflamatória, encontrado em pessoas jovens.
sclerotic k., r. esclerótico. SIN granular k.
sigmoid k., r. sigmóide; pólo superior de um rim fundido ao pólo inferior do outro.
supernumerary k., r. supranumerário; um rim, além dos dois geralmente presentes, desenvolvido pela divisão do blastema nefrogênico ou por um blaste-

ma metanéfrico separado, no qual uma duplicação parcial ou completa da haste ureteral entra para formar um rim separado, capsulado; em alguns casos, a separação do órgão duplicado é incompleta.
  thoracic k., r. torácico; rim ectópico situado parcialmente acima do diafragma no mediastino posterior.
  wandering k., r. móvel. SIN floating k.
  waxy k., r. céreo. SIN amyloid k.

Kiel clas·si·fi·ca·tion. Classificação de Kiel. Ver em classification.

Kielland. VER Kjelland.

Kien, Alphonse M.J., médico alemão do século XIX. VER Kussmaul-K. *respiration.*

Kienböck, Robert, radiologista austríaco, 1871–1953. VER K. *disease, dislocation, unit.*

Kiernan, Francis, médico inglês, 1800–1874. VER K. *space.*

Kiesselbach, Wilhelm, laringologista alemão, 1839–1902. VER K. *area.*

Kikuchi, M, hematologista japonês do século XX. VER K. *disease.*

Kilian, Hermann F., ginecologista alemão, 1800–1863. VER K. *line.*

Kiliani, H., químico, 1855–1945. VER Kiliani-Fischer *synthesis;* Kiliani-Fischer *reaction.*

Killian, Gustav J., laringologista alemão, 1860–1921. VER K. *bundle, operation, triangle.*

♻ **kilo- (k).** Quilo-; prefixo usado no SI e no sistema métrico significando mil (10^3). [G. *chilioi,* mil]

kil·o·base (kb) (kĭl'ō-bās). Quilobase; unidade usada para designar o comprimento de uma seqüência de ácidos nucleicos; 1 kb é igual a uma seqüência de 1.000 bases purina ou pirimidina.

kil·o·cal·o·rie (kcal) (kil'ō-kal-ō-rē). Quilocaloria. SIN large *calorie.*

kil·o·cy·cle (kc) (kil'ō-sī-kl). Quilociclos; mil ciclos por segundo.

kil·o·gram (kg) (kil'ō-gram). Quilograma; a unidade de massa do SI, 1.000 g; equivalente a 15.432,358 grãos, 2,2046226 libras avoirdupois ou 2,6792289 libras troy.

kil·o·gram-me·ter. Quilograma-metro; a energia despendida, ou trabalho realizado, quando uma massa de 1 kg é levantada a uma altura de 1 m; igual a 9,80665 J no sistema SI.

kil·o·hertz. Quilohertz; uma unidade de freqüência igual a 10^3 hertz.

kil·ohm. Quiloohm; uma unidade de resistência elétrica igual a 10^3 ohms. [kilo + ohm]

kil·o·joule. Quilojoule; uma unidade de energia, trabalho ou quantidade de calor igual a 10^3 joules. [kilo + joule]

kil·o·volt (kv) (kil'ō-vōlt). Quilovolt; uma unidade de potencial elétrico, diferença de potencial ou força eletromotriz igual a 10^3 volts. [kilo + volt]

kil·o·volt-me·ter (kil'ō-vōlt-mē'ter). Quilovoltímetro; instrumento designado para medir a força eletromotriz em quilovolts.

Kimmelstiel, Paul, patologista alemão nos EUA, 1900–1970. VER K.-Wilson *disease, syndrome.*

Kimura, T., patologista japonês do século XX. VER K. *disease.*

♻ **kin-, kine-.** Cin-; cine-; movimento. VER TAMBÉM cine-. [G. *kineō,* mover, colocar em movimento]

kin·an·es·the·sia (kin-an-es-thē'zē-ă). Cinanestesia; distúrbio da sensibilidade profunda na qual há incapacidade de perceber a direção ou a extensão do movimento, sendo o resultado da ataxia. SIN cinanesthesia. [G. *kinēsis,* movimento, + *an-* neg. + *aisthēsis,* sensação]

ki·nase (kī'nās). Cinase; quinase. **1.** Uma enzima que catalisa a conversão de uma proenzima em uma enzima ativa; p. ex., enteropeptidase (enterocinase). **2.** Uma enzima que catalisa a transferência de grupamentos fosfato. Quanto a cinases individuais, ver o nome específico.

ki·nase II. Cinase II. SIN peptidyl dipeptidase A.

kind·ling. Alterações epileptogênicas de longa duração induzidas por estimulação cerebral elétrica subliminar diária sem lesão neuronal aparente.

kin·dred. Parentes; parentesco; um conjunto de pessoas geneticamente relacionadas; diferente do heredograma, que é uma representação estilizada de um parentesco. [I. ant. *kynrēde,* de *cyn,* parente, + *rēde,* condição]
  degree of k., grau de parentesco; grau de parentesco entre dois membros de um heredograma, o número mínimo de etapas entre um e outro. Parentes em primeiro grau são irmãos, pais e filhos; parentes em segundo grau são tios, tias, sobrinhos e sobrinhas, e assim por diante. O termo é definido para fins legais, p. ex., casamentos consangüíneos, e pode induzir erros em genética. O uso de grupos formados por reunião de "parentes em primeiro grau", independentemente do sexo ou do modo de herança em questão, deve ser evitado, pois não distingue entre filhos e irmãos.

kin·e·mat·ics (kin-ē-mat'iks). Cinemática; em fisiologia, a ciência que trata dos movimentos das partes do corpo. SIN cinematics. [G. *kinēmatica,* coisas que se movem]

kin·e·mom·e·ter (kin-ē-mom'ē-ter). Cinemômetro; aparelho eletromagnético, semelhante, em princípio, ao balistocardiógrafo de velocidade, usado para medir a contração e o relaxamento produzidos em um reflexo tendíneo. [G. *kinēsis,* movimento, + *metron,* medida]

♻ **kinesi-, kinesio-, kineso-.** Cinese-, cinesio-, cineso-; movimento. [G. *kinēsis*]

ki·ne·si·a (ki-nē'sē-ă,-nē'zē-). Doença do movimento. SIN motion *sickness.* [G. *kinēsis,* movimento]

ki·ne·si·at·rics (ki-nē'sē-at'riks). Cinesiatria. SIN kinesitherapy. [G. *kinēsis,* movimento, + *iatrikos,* relativo à medicina]

ki·ne·sics (ki-nē'siks). Cinesia; estudo do movimento corporal não-verbal na comunicação. VER body *language.*

kin·e·sim·e·ter (kin-ē-sim'ē-ter). Cinesímetro; cinesiômetro; um instrumento para medir a extensão de um movimento. SIN kinesiometer. [G. *kinēsis,* movimento, + *metron,* medida]

ki·ne·sin (ki-nē'sin). Cinesina; uma proteína motora associada a microtúbulos; participa do transporte ATP-dependente de vesículas e outros; orienta o transporte axonal anterógrado.

♻ **kinesio-.** Cinesio-. VER kinesi-.

ki·ne·si·ol·o·gy (ki-nē-sē-ol'ō-jē). Cinesiologia; a ciência ou o estudo do movimento e das estruturas ativas e passivas envolvidas. [G. *kinēsis,* movimento, + *-logos,* estudo]

ki·ne·si·om·e·ter (ki-nē-sē-om'ē-ter). Cinesiômetro. SIN kinesimeter.

kin·e·sip·a·thist (kin-ē-sip'ă-thist). Cinesiopatista; indivíduo que não é médico e trata doenças por movimentos de vários tipos.

ki·ne·sis (ki-nē'sis). Cinese; movimento. Como terminação, usada para designar movimento ou ativação, particularmente o tipo induzido por um estímulo. [G.]

ki·ne·si·ther·a·py (ki-nē-si-thār'ă-pē). Cinesioterapia; fisioterapia envolvendo exercícios de movimento e amplitude de movimento. VER movement. SIN kinesiatrics.

♻ **kineso-.** Cineso-. VER kinesi-.

ki·ne·so·pho·bia (ki-nē-so-fō'bē-ă). Cinesiofobia; medo mórbido de movimento. [G. *kinēsis,* movimento, + *phobos,* medo]

kin·es·the·sia (kin'es-thē'zē-ă). Cinestesia. **1.** A percepção do movimento; percepção muscular. **2.** Uma ilusão de movimento no espaço. [G. *kinēsis,* movimento, *aisthēsis,* sensação]

kin·es·the·si·om·e·ter (kin'es-thē'zē-om'ē-ter). Cinestesiômetro; instrumento para determinar o grau de percepção muscular. [kinesthesia, + G. *metron,* medida]

kin·es·the·sis (kin'es-thē-sēz). Cinestesia. VER kinesthesia.

kin·es·thet·ic (kin-es-thet'ik). Cinestésico. **1.** Relativo à cinestesia. **2.** Usado para descrever uma pessoa que utiliza preferencialmente a fantasia mental do que sentiu. VER TAMBÉM internal *representation.*

ki·net·ic (ki-net'ik). Cinético; relativo ao movimento. [G. *kinētikos,* e movimento, de *kinētos,* em movimento]

ki·net·ics (ki-net'iks). Cinética; o estudo do movimento, aceleração ou velocidade de mudança.
  chemical k., c. química; o estudo das velocidades das reações químicas.
  enzyme k., c. das enzimas; o estudo das velocidades, bem como das alterações dessas velocidades, de reações catalisadas por enzimas; inclui as reações catalisadas por sinzimas, abzimas e ribozimas.

♻ **kineto-.** Cineto-; movimento. [G. *kinētos,* em movimento, móvel]

ki·ne·to·car·di·o·gram (ki-nē'tō-kar'dē-ō-gram, ki-net'ō-). Cinetocardiograma; um tipo de registro gráfico das vibrações da parede torácica produzidas pela atividade cardíaca.

ki·ne·to·car·di·o·graph (ki-nē'tō-kar'dē-ō-graf, ki-net'ō-). Cinetocardiógrafo; aparelho para registrar impulsos precordiais causados pelo movimento cardíaco; o deslocamento absoluto de um ponto na parede torácica é registrado em relação a um ponto de referência fixo acima do paciente em decúbito.

ki·ne·to·chore (ki-nē'tō-kōr, ki-net'ō-). Cinetócoro; a porção estrutural do cromossoma à qual se fixam os microtúbulos. Cf. centromere. [kineto- + G. *chōra,* espaço]

ki·ne·to·chores (ki-nē'tō-korz). Cinetócoros; a região do centrômero ligada a proteínas.

ki·ne·to·gen·ic (ki-nē-tō-jen'ik, ki-net-ō-). Cinetogênico; que causa ou produz movimento.

ki·ne·to·plasm (ki-nē'tō-plazm). Cinetoplasma. **1.** A parte mais contrátil de uma célula. **2.** O citoplasma da gotícula que cobre a cabeça do espermatozóide durante a maturação. SIN cinetoplasm, cinetoplasma, kinoplasm. [kineto- + G. *plasma,* uma coisa formada]

ki·ne·to·plast (ki-nē'tō-plast, ki-net'ō-). Cinetoplasto; uma estrutura de DNA extranuclear, baciliforme, discóide ou esférica, encontrada em flagelados parasitas (família Trypanosomatidae), próxima da base do flagelo, posterior ao blefaroplasto e, freqüentemente, formando ângulos retos com o núcleo. As micrografias eletrônicas mostram que é parte de uma mitocôndria gigante única, que ocupa a maior parte do citoplasma de flagelados amastigotas, sendo a porção cinetoplasto visível à microscopia óptica. O DNA do cinetoplasto é denominado kDNA (DNAc) para distinguir-se do DNA nuclear, ou nDNA

(DNAn). O cinetoplasto divide-se independentemente, juntamente com o corpúsculo basal, antes da divisão nuclear. O termo cinetoplasto anteriormente incluía o corpúsculo parabasal e o blefaroplasto em um aparelho locomotor, mas agora é reconhecido como uma organela distinta da maioria dos tripanossomatídeos. VER TAMBÉM parabasal *body*. [kineto- + G. *plastos*, formado]

ki·ne·to·scope (kī - ne'to - skōp). Cinetoscópio; aparelho para obter fotografias seriadas para registrar o movimento. [kineto- + G. *skopeō*, examinar]

ki·net·o·some (ki - nē'tō - sōm, ki - net'ō-). Cinetossoma. SIN basal *body*. [kineto- + G. *sōma*, corpo]

King, Earl J., bioquímico canadense, 1901–1962. VER K. *unit;* K.-Armstrong *unit*.

king·dom (king'dum). Reino; uma das quatro categorias nas quais geralmente são classificados os objetos naturais: o reino animal, incluindo todos os animais; o reino vegetal, incluindo todos os vegetais; o reino mineral, incluindo todos os objetos e substâncias sem vida; e o protista, incluindo todos os microrganismos unicelulares. [A.S. *cyningdōm*, de *cyning*, rei, + *-dom*, estado, condição]

Kin·gel·la (kin - jel'ah). Gênero da família Neisseriaceae; os membros são cocos e cocobacilos imóveis, aeróbios e anaeróbios facultativos, Gram-negativos, de tamanho médio, em pares ou cadeias curtas, que não são bem descorados por acetona-álcool; são oxidase-positivos e fermentam a glicose com ácido, mas não com gás. A espécie modelo é a *K. kingae*.
K. indolog'enes, designação antiga de *Suttonella indologenes*, uma espécie de bactéria que é o agente causador de infecções oculares e endocardite em válvulas cardíacas lesadas (principalmente próteses).
K. kin'gae, uma espécie de bactéria β-hemolítica que causa endocardite, osteomielite e artrite séptica em seres humanos; antigamente *Moraxella kingae*. VER HACEK *group*. SIN *Moraxella kingae*.

king's evil. Mal do rei; designação histórica da linfadenite tuberculosa cervical (escrófula), que se acreditava antigamente ser curada pelo toque de um rei.

Kingsley, Norman W., dentista norte-americano, 1829–1913. VER K. *splint*.

kin·ic ac·id (kin'ik). Ácido quínico. SIN quinic acid.

ki·nin (kī'nin). Cinina; uma dentre várias substâncias muito diferentes, apresentando efeitos fisiológicos acentuados e dramáticos. Algumas (p. ex., calidina e bradicinina) são polipeptídios, formados no sangue por proteólise secundária a algum processo patológico, que estimulam o músculo liso visceral, mas relaxam o músculo liso vascular, assim produzindo vasodilatação; outras (p. ex., cinetina) são reguladores do crescimento vegetal. [G. *kineō*, movimentar, + *-in*]
k. 9, cinina 9. SIN bradykinin.

ki·nin·o·gen (ki - nin'ō - jen). Cininogênio; a globulina precursora de uma cinina (plasmática).
high molecular weight k., c. de alto peso molecular; uma proteína plasmática de peso molecular 110.000 que existe normalmente no plasma em um complexo 1:1 com pré-calicreína. O complexo é um co-fator na ativação do fator da coagulação XII. O produto dessa reação, XIIa, por sua vez, ativa a pré-calicreína em calicreína. SIN Fitzgerald factor, Flaujeac factor, Williams factor.
low molecular weight k., c. de baixo peso molecular; uma proteína de peso molecular 50.000 presente em vários tecidos normais e que, após clivagem pela calicreína ou outros cininogênios, forma a calidina. A calidina, por sua vez, é convertida em bradicinina.

ki·nin·o·ge·nase (ki - nin'ō - jĕ - nās). Cininogenase. SIN kallikrein.

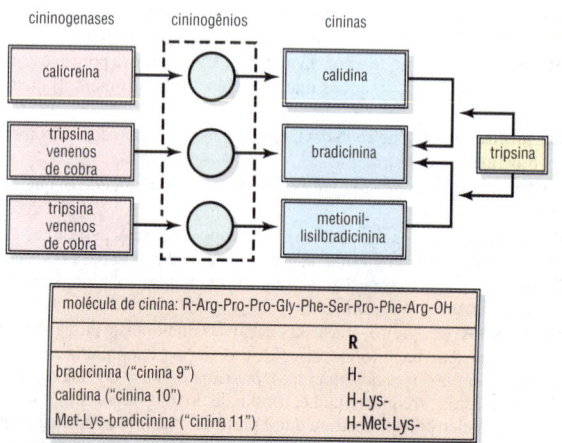

cininas

ki·nin·o·gen·in (ki - nin'ō - jen - in). Cininogenina. SIN kallikrein.

kink. Torcedura; uma angulação, torção ou giro.
Lane k., torcedura de Lane. SIN Lane *band*.

kino-. Cino-; movimento. [G. *kineō*, movimentar]

kin·o·cen·trum (kin - ō - sen'trŭm). Cinocentro; citocentro. SIN cytocentrum. [kino- + G. *kentron*, centro]

ki·no·cil·i·um (kī - nō - sil'ē - ŭm). Cinocílio; um cílio, geralmente móvel, que possui nove microtúbulos duplos periféricos e dois centrais. [kino- + cilium]

kin·o·mom·e·ter (kin - ō - mom'ĕ - ter). Cinomômetro; um instrumento para medir o grau de movimento. [kino- + G. *metron*, medida]

kin·o·plasm (kin'ō - plazm, kī'nō). Cinoplasma; cinetoplasma. SIN kinetoplasm.

kin·o·plas·mic (kin - ō - plas'mik, kī - nō-). Cinoplásmico; relativo ao cinoplasma (cinetoplasma).

kin·ship. Parentesco; a condição de ser geneticamente relacionado.

Kinyoun, Joseph J., médico norte-americano, 1860–1919. VER K. *stain*.

ki·on (kī'on). Quion; designação obsoleta de úvula. Ver entradas em cion- como uma forma combinante de úvula. [G. *kiōn*, pilar, a úvula]

kion-, kiono-. Quion-, quiono-; a úvula. VER uvulo-, uvul-. [G. *kiōn*, úvula]

Kirk, Norman Thomas, cirurgião do exército norte-americano, 1888–1960. VER K. *amputation*.

Kirkland, Olin, periodontista norte-americano, 1876–1969. VER K. *knife*.

Kirschner, Martin, cirurgião alemão, 1879–1942. VER K. *apparatus, wire*.

Kisch, Bruno, fisiologista alemão, 1890–1966. VER K. *reflex*.

Kitasato, Shibasaburo, Barão, bacteriologista japonês, 1853–1931. VER K. *bacillus*.

Kjeldahl, Johan G.C., químico dinamarquês, 1849–1900. VER K. *apparatus, method;* macro-K. *method;* micro-K. *method*.

Kjelland (Kielland), Christian, obstetra norueguês, 1871–1941. VER K. *forceps*.

Klatskin, Gerald, clínico norte-americano (falecido em 1988). VER K. *tumor*.

Klebs, Theodor Albrecht Edwin, médico alemão, 1834–1913. VER *Klebsiella;* K.-Loeffler *bacillus*.

Kleb·si·el·la (kleb - sē - el'ă). Gênero de bactérias aeróbicas, facultativamente anaeróbicas, imóveis e não-formadoras de esporos (família Enterobacteriaceae) contendo bastões Gram-negativos, encapsulados que ocorrem isoladamente, em pares ou em cadeias curtas. Esses microrganismos produzem acetilmetilcarbinol e lisina descarboxilase ou ornitina descarboxilase. Geralmente não liquefazem a gelatina. O citrato e a glicose são comumente usados como fontes de carbono únicas. Esses microrganismos podem ou não ser patogênicos. Ocorrem nos tratos respiratório, intestinal e urogenital dos seres humanos, bem como no solo, na água e em grãos. A espécie típica é a *K. pneumoniae*. [E. *Klebs*]
K. mo'bilis, SIN *Enterobacter aerogenes*.
K. oxytoca, uma espécie caracterizada por sua capacidade de produzir indol. Clinicamente assemelha-se a *K. pneumoniae;* entretanto, cepas hospitalares tendem a exibir uma maior propensão a desenvolver resistência a antibióticos.
K. ozae'nae, uma espécie bacteriana que ocorre em casos de ozena e outras doenças crônicas das vias respiratórias. SIN *K. pneumoniae* subesp. *ozaenae*.
K. pneumo'niae, uma espécie bacteriana encontrada no solo e na água, em grãos, e no trato intestinal de seres humanos e outros animais; também pode ser associada a vários distúrbios patológicos, infecções urinárias, escarro, fezes e metrite em éguas; os tipos capsulares 1, 2 e 3 desse microrganismo podem ser os agentes causadores da pneumonia; microrganismos previamente identificados como cepas imóveis de *Aerobacter aerogenes* agora são colocados nessa espécie; é a espécie típica de *K*. SIN Friedländer bacillus, pneumobacillus.
K. pneumo'niae subesp. *ozae'nae,* SIN *K. ozaenae*.
K. rhinosclero'matis, uma espécie bacteriana encontrada em casos de rinoscleroma.

klee-blatt·schä·del (klā - blat - she'dl). Crânio em folha de trevo. VER cloverleaf skull *syndrome*. [Al. crânio em folha de trevo]

Kleffner, Frank, neurologista norte-americano do século XX. VER Landau-Kleffner *syndrome*.

Kleihauer. VER Kleihauer *stain*, Betke-Kleihauer *test*.

Klein, Edward E., histologista húngaro, 1844–1925. VER K.-Gumprecht shadow *nuclei*, em *nucleus*.

Kleine, Willi, neuropsiquiatra alemão do século XX. VER K.-Levin *syndrome*.

klep·to·ma·nia (klep - tō - mā'nē - ă). Cleptomania; distúrbio do controle de impulsos caracterizado por uma tendência mórbida a furtar. [G. *kleptō*, furtar, + *mania*, insanidade]

klep·to·ma·ni·ac (klep - tō - mā'nē - ak). Cleptomaníaco; pessoa portadora de cleptomania.

klep·to·pho·bia (klep - tō - fō'bē - ă). Cleptofobia; medo mórbido de furtar ou de se tornar um ladrão. [G. *kleptō*, furtar, + *phobos*, medo]

Klinefelter, Harry F., Jr., médico norte-americano, *1912. VER K. *syndrome*.

Klippel, Maurice, neurologista francês, 1858–1942. VER K.-Feil *syndrome;* K.-Trenaunay-Weber *syndrome*.

Klumpke, VER Dejerine-K.
Klüver, Heinrich, neurologista alemão, naturalizado americano, 1897–1975. VER K.-Barrera Luxol fast blue *stain*; K.-Bucy *syndrome*.
Kluy·ve·ra (klooy - ver'ah). Gênero da família Enterobacteriaceae; os microrganismos são móveis, fermentam lactose e são diferenciados dos outros gêneros por perfis fenotípicos específicos e por parâmetros de hibridização DNA-DNA; algumas espécies foram associadas à infecção humana; a espécie típica é *K. ascorbata.*
Knapp, Herman J., oftalmologista norte-americano, 1832–1911. VER K. *streaks,* em *streak, striae,* em *stria.*
knee (nē) [TA]. Joelho. **1.** SIN genu (1). **2.** Qualquer estrutura de formato angular semelhante a um joelho fletido. [A.S. *cnēōw*]
 Brodie k., j. de Brodie; sinovite hipertrófica crônica do joelho. SIN Brodie disease (1).
 housemaid's k., j. da dona-de-casa; uma bursite ocupacional adventícia que ocorre sobre a área de contato quando a pessoa está ajoelhada; não deve ser confundida com bursite infrapatelar. SIN prepatellar bursitis.
 locked k., j. travado; um distúrbio no qual não há extensão nem flexão completa do joelho devido a um distúrbio interno, geralmente resultante de uma laceração do menisco.
 runner's k., j. do corredor; uma síndrome de uso excessivo da face anterior do joelho, dor associada a movimento lateral excessivo da patela durante a atividade. SIN patellofemoral stress syndrome.
 Wilbrand k., j. de Wilbrand; feixe de fibras nasais inferiores do nervo óptico que servem ao campo visual temporal superior e cruzam no quiasma óptico anterior (anterior optic *chiasm*), entrando por um breve espaço no nervo óptico posterior (posterior optic *nerve*) contralateral [NC II] antes de seguirem para o trato óptico (optic *tract*) contralateral. Pesquisas recentes indicam que este pode ser um artefato de degeneração da retina e não existir na anatomia normal.
knee·cap (nē'kap). Patela. SIN patella.
Kne·mi·do·kop·tes (nē'mi - dō - kop'tēz). Um gênero de ácaros sarcoptídeos escavadores microscópicos, que infestam aves domésticas e pássaros cativos; as espécies incluem *K. laevis* var. *gallinae,* o ácaro da desplumação, e *K. mutans,* o ácaro da descamação da perna. [G. *knēmē,* perna, + *koptō,* cortar]

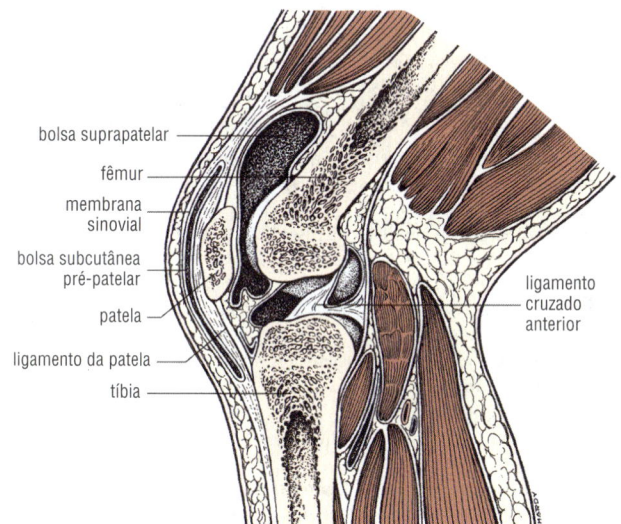

articulação do joelho: corte sagital mostrando as bolsas subcutâneas pré-patelar e suprapatelar

KNF mod·el Modelo KNF; abreviação de Koshland-Némethy-Filmer *model.*
Kniest, Wilhelm, pediatra alemão do século XX. VER K. *syndrome.*
knife, pl. **knives** (nīf, nīvz). Bisturi; instrumento cortante usado em cirurgia e dissecção. [I.M. *knif,* de A.S. *cnif,* do O. Norse *knīfr*]
 amputation k., b. de amputação; um b. de lâmina larga usado basicamente para transecção de músculos grandes durante grandes amputações.
 Beer k., b. de Beer; um b. triangular com extremidade e borda agudas, usado antigamente para incisão de catarata.
 cartilage k., b. de cartilagem; condrótomo. SIN chondrotome.
 cautery k., b.-cautério; um b. que cauteriza ao cortar, diminuindo o sangramento.
 chemical k., b. químico; termo usado algumas vezes para a endonuclease de restrição (restriction *endonuclease*).
 electrode k., b. elétrico; instrumento elétrico em forma de lâmina usado para cortar tecidos por meio de uma corrente elétrica de alta freqüência.
 fistula k., b. para fístulas; fistulótomo. SIN fistulatome.
 free-hand k., b. manual; um b. ou lâmina operado manualmente geralmente usado para obter enxertos cutâneos de espessura parcial; p. ex., b. de Blair-Brown, b. de Humby.
 gamma k., b. gama; um sistema radiocirúrgico de invasividade mínima usado no tratamento de neoplasias intracranianas benignas e malignas e malformações arteriovenosas. VER TAMBÉM radiosurgery.

> Como etapa preliminar ao uso do bisturi gama, a lesão a ser retirada é localizada precisamente por técnicas de imagem como a RM, TC, PET e angiografia. Feixes de raios gama de 200 fontes de cobalto-60 são dirigidos por um computador de forma a convergirem sobre a lesão. É feita uma série de exposições durante um período de aproximadamente 1 hora. Lesões com mais de 3 cm não podem ser tratadas. O mecanismo é volumoso e dispendioso, mas o procedimento mostrou uma taxa de sucesso de aproximadamente 85% no tratamento de malformações arteriovenosas e 50–95% em neoplasias. Além de evitar os riscos e complicações da cirurgia a céu aberto, o bisturi gama permite o tratamento de lesões cuja localização proíbe qualquer tentativa de remoção cirúrgica. Além disso, o desconforto do paciente é mínimo, e a maioria dos pacientes permanecem no hospital por apenas 1 noite; muitos retornam para casa, ou mesmo para o trabalho, no dia do tratamento. Espera-se que o bisturi gama mostre-se útil no tratamento de outros distúrbios, como tumores do olho e da hipófise, neuralgia do trigêmeo, epilepsia, parkinsonismo e outros distúrbios do movimento.

 Goldman-Fox knives, bisturis de Goldman-Fox; um conjunto de bisturis usados em cirurgia periodontal.
 Graefe k., b. de Graefe; um b. de lâmina estreita usado para fazer um corte na córnea.
 hernia k., herniótomo; b. de lâmina fina com borda cortante curta, para dividir os tecidos constritores na boca do saco herniário. SIN herniotome.
 Kirkland k., b. de Kirkland; um b. em forma de coração usado em cirurgias da gengiva.
 lenticular k., b. lenticular; cureta que se assemelha a uma colher afiada.
 Liston knives, bisturis de Liston; bisturis de lâminas longas de vários tamanhos usados em amputações.
 Merrifield k., b. de Merrifield; um b. longo, estreito, triangular, usado em cirurgias da gengiva.
 valvotomy k., b. para valvulotomia; um b. usado em cirurgia mitral ou valvular venosa; também denominado valvulótomo.
knis·mo·gen·ic (nis'mō - jen'ik). Cnismogênico; que causa sensação de cócegas. [G. *knismos,* cócegas, + *-gen,* produção]
knit·ting (nit'ing). Coaptação; termo não-médico que designa o processo de união dos fragmentos de um osso fraturado ou das bordas de uma ferida. [I.M., *knitten,* amarrar, do A.S. *cnyttan*]
knob (nob). Nó; nódulo; botão; uma protuberância; uma massa.
 aortic k., botão aórtico; a sombra proeminente do arco aórtico em uma radiografia do tórax frontal.
 Engelmann basal k.'s, nódulos basais de Engelmann; epônimo obsoleto para blefaroplasto.
 malarial k.'s, nódulos maláricos; protrusões arredondadas de uma hemácia infestada pelo *Plasmodium falciparum,* responsável pela adesão das hemácias infestadas entre si e ao endotélio dos vasos sangüíneos que contêm essas células infestadas; resulta em bloqueio capilar responsável por grande parte das alterações histopatológicas da malária terçã maligna.
knock (nok). Batimento; golpe; batida. **1.** Coloquialismo para uma pancada, especialmente na cabeça. **2.** Um som semelhante ao de uma batida ou pancada.
 pericardial k., batimento pericárdico; um som no início da diástole que é uma variante da terceira bulha, mas que ocorre distintamente antes, devido à interrupção abrupta do enchimento ventricular rápido pelo pericárdio restritivo; uma qualidade realmente de "pancada" é rara.
knock-knee (nok'nē). Joelho valgo. SIN *genu valgum.*
knock-out (nok'out). Nocaute; um organismo modificado por engenharia genética no qual o genoma foi alterado por recombinação direcionada para o local de forma que um gene é deletado.
Knoll, Philipp, fisiologista da Boêmia, 1841–1900. VER K. *glands,* em *gland.*
Knoop, Hedwig, médico alemão, *1908. VER K. *theory.*
Knoop hard·ness num·ber (KHN). Ver em number.
knot (not). Nó. **1.** Um entrelaçamento das extremidades de dois cordões, fitas ou fios de sutura, de tal forma que não possam ser facilmente separados; ou um entrelaçamento ou dobramento semelhante de um cordão em sua continuidade. **2.** Em anatomia ou patologia, um linfonodo, gânglio ou tumefação circunscrita sugestiva de um nó. [A.S. *cnotta*]

false k.'s, false k.'s of umbilical cord, nós falsos, nós falsos do cordão umbilical; aumentos locais no comprimento ou na varicosidade da veia umbilical, causando torção do cordão bastante aparente.

granny k., nó da vovó; um nó duplo no qual as extremidades livres da segunda alça são assimétricas e não estão no mesmo plano que as extremidades livres da primeira alça.

Hensen k., nó de Hensen. SIN primitive *node*.

Hubrecht protochordal k., nó do protocórdio de Hubrecht. SIN primitive *node*.

laparoscopic k., nó laparoscópico; um nó feito dentro do corpo através de um instrumento laparoscópico. O nó em si pode ser dado fora do corpo e introduzido no corpo através de uma cânula, ou pode ser feito e amarrado dentro do corpo.

net k., cariossoma. SIN karyosome.

primitive k., nó primitivo. SIN primitive *node*.

protochordal k., nó do protocórdio. SIN primitive *node*.

square k., nó direito ou quadrado; um nó duplo no qual as pontas livres da segunda alça são assimétricas e estão no mesmo plano que as extremidades livres da primeira alça.

surgeon's k., nó de cirurgião, a primeira alça do nó tem 2 fios trançados em vez de um. A segunda alça tem apenas 1 fio trançado, que é colocado em um nó direito, deixando as pontas livres no mesmo plano da primeira alça.

syncytial k., nó sincicial; uma agregação localizada de núcleos de sinciciotrofoblastos nas vilosidades da placenta no início da gravidez. SIN syncytial bud, syncytial sprout.

true k., true k. of umbilical cord, nó verdadeiro, nó verdadeiro do cordão umbilical; entrelaçamento real de um segmento do cordão umbilical; a circulação geralmente não é obstruída.

vital k., nó vital. SIN noued vital.

knuck·le (nŭk′l). Nó dos dedos; articulação. **1.** Uma articulação de um dedo quando o punho é fechado, principalmente uma articulação metacarpofalangiana. **2.** Uma torção ou alça de intestino, como em uma hérnia. [I.M. *knokel*]

aortic k., botão aórtico; o contorno do arco aórtico saliantando-se em relação à silhueta do mediastino em uma radiografia ântero-posterior (AP) do tórax.

cervical aortic k., botão aórtico cervical; um arco aórtico anômalo, no qual a aorta estende-se até o pescoço e forma um arco ântero-posterior, que pode alcançar a altura do osso hióide; a artéria carótida comum de um lado emerge do pico do arco, e a carótida comum do outro lado emerge da parte mais proximal da aorta; o arco pulsátil pode ser confundido com um aneurisma, mas os pulsos radiais são iguais.

Kobelt, Georg L., médico alemão, 1804–1857. VER K. *tubules,* em *tubule*.

Kober, Philip A., químico norte-americano, *1884, ver K. *test*.

Köbner, Heinrich, dermatologista alemão, 1838–1904. VER K. *phenomenon*.

Koch, Robert, bacteriologista alemão premiado com o Nobel, 1843–1910. VER K. *bacillus, law,* old *tuberculin, phenomenon, postulates* em *postulate*; K.-Weeks *bacillus*.

Koch, Walter, cirurgião alemão, *1880. VER K. *node, triangle*.

Kocher, Emil Theodor, cirurgião suíço premiado com o Nobel, 1841–1917. VER K. *clamp, incision, sign*; K.-Debré-Sémélaigne *syndrome*.

Kock, Nils G., cirurgião sueco do século XX. VER K. *pouch*.

Koenig, Franz, cirurgião alemão, 1832–1910. VER K. *syndrome*.

Koerber, H., oftalmologista alemão do século XX. VER Koerber-Salus-Elschnig *syndrome*.

Koerte, Werner, cirurgião alemão, 1853–1937. VER K.-Ballance *operation*.

Koettstorfer, J., químico alemão do século XIX. VER K. *number*.

Kogoj, Franjo, médico iugoslavo, 1894–1983. VER spongiform *pustule* de K.

Köhler, Alban, radiologista alemão, 1874–1947. VER K. *disease*.

Köhler, August, microscopista alemão, 1866–1948. VER K. *illumination*.

Kohlrausch, Otto L.B., médico alemão, 1811–1854. VER K. *muscle, folds,* em *fold*.

Kohn, Hans N., patologista alemão, *1866. VER K. *pores,* em *pore*.

Kohnstamm, Oskar, médico alemão, 1871–1917. VER K. *phenomenon*.

koi·lo·cyte (koy′lō-sĭt). Coilócito; uma célula escamosa, freqüentemente binucleada, mostrando um halo perinuclear; característica da infecção por papilomavírus humano. [G. *koilos,* oco, + *kytos,* célula]

koi·lo·cy·to·sis (koy′lō-sī-tō′sis). Coilocitose; vacuolação perinuclear. VER TAMBÉM koilocyte. [G. *koilos,* oco, + *kytos,* célula, + *-osis,* condição]

koi·lo·nych·ia (koy-lō-nĭk′ē-ă). Coiloníquia; uma malformação das unhas na qual a superfície externa é côncava; freqüentemente associada à deficiência de ferro ou amolecimento por contato ocupacional com óleos. SIN spoon nail. [G. *koilos,* oco, + *onyx, (onych-),* unha]

koil·o·ster·nia (koy-lō-ster′nē-ă). Coilosternia. SIN *pectus* excavatum. [G. *koilos,* oco, + *sternon,* tórax (esterno)]

Kojewnikoff (Kozhevnikov), Aleksei Y., neurologista russo, 1836–1902. VER K. *epilepsy*.

ko·jic ac·id (kō′jik). Ácido cójico; um antibiótico, produto do catabolismo da D-glicose em alguns fungos; pode ser convertido em aromatizantes.

Kokoskin, Evelyn, patologista canadense do século XX. VER K. *stain*.

ko·la (kō′lă). Cola; os cotilédones secos de *Cola nitida* ou outra espécie de *Cola* (família Sterculiaceae); contém cafeína, teobromina e um princípio solúvel, colatina; usada como estimulante cardíaco e do sistema nervoso central. SIN cola (1).

Kölliker, Rudolph A. von, histologista suíço, 1817–1905. VER K. *layer, reticulum*.

Kollmann, Arthur, urologista alemão do século XIX. VER K. *dilator*.

Kolmer, John A., patologista norte-americano, 1886–1962. VER K. *test*.

Kolopp, P., dermatologista francês do século XX. VER Woringer-K. *disease*.

♻ **kolp-.** Colp-. VER colpo-.

ko·lyt·ic (kō-lit′ik). Colítico; indica uma ação inibidora. [G. *kolyō,* impedir]

Kondoleon, Emmanuel, cirurgião grego, 1879–1939. VER K. *operation*.

ko·ni·o·cor·tex (kō′nē-ō-kor′teks). Coniocórtex; regiões do córtex cerebral caracterizadas por uma camada granular interna particularmente bem desenvolvida (camada 4); esse tipo de córtex cerebral é representado pela área sensorial primária 17 do córtex visual, áreas 1 a 3 do córtex sensorial somático e área 41 do córtex auditivo. VER TAMBÉM cerebral *cortex*. [G. *konis,* poeira, + L. *cortex,* casca]

konzo (kon′zō). Konzo; uma doença do neurônio motor superior causada por cianeto, que se manifesta principalmente como paraplegia espástica, observada na África e resultante do consumo de raízes de mandioca impropriamente preparadas, que contêm altas concentrações de glicosídios cianogênicos. [Yaka, pernas cansadas]

Koplik, Henry, médico norte-americano, 1858–1927. VER K. *spots,* em *spot*.

kop·o·pho·bia (kop-ō-fō′bē-ă). Copofobia; medo mórbido de fadiga. [G. *kopos,* fadiga, + *phobos,* medo]

♻ **kopro-.** VER copro-.

Korff, Karl von, anatomista e histologista alemão do século XX. VER K. *fibers,* em *fiber*.

Kornberg, Arthur, bioquímico norte-americano premiado com o Nobel, *1918. VER K. *enzyme*.

Kornzweig, Abraham L., médico norte-americano, *1900. VER Bassen-K. *syndrome*.

ko·ro (kō′rō). Koro; um estado de delírio agudo, que ocorre nos Macassars, nativos das Celebes (Indonésia) e de outras partes do Oriente, no qual o indivíduo tem a sensação de que o pênis está encolhendo ou entrando no abdome. SIN shook jong.

ko·ro·ni·on (kō-rō′nē-on). Corônio. SIN coronion.

Korotkoff, Nikolai S., médico russo, 1874–1920. VER K. *sounds,* em *sound, test*.

Korsakoff, Sergei S., neurologista russo, 1853–1900. VER K. *psychosis, syndrome;* Wernicke-k. *encephalopathy, syndrome*.

Koshland, Daniel E., bioquímico norte-americano, *1920. VER Adair-K.-Némethy-Filmer *model*; K.-Némethy-Filmer *model*.

Kossa, VER von Kossa.

Koyanagi, Yosizo, oftalmologista japonês, 1880–1954. VER Vogt-K. *syndrome*.

Koyter, VER Coiter.

Kr Símbolo de criptônio.

Krabbe, Knud H., neurologista dinamarquês, 1885–1961. VER K. *disease;* Christensen-K. *disease*.

krait (krīt). Cobra elapídea do gênero *Bungarus,* encontrada no norte da Índia, cuja picada está associada a efeitos anestésicos e paralíticos generalizados, em oposição à dor local, alteração da cor ou edema local; os sintomas neurotóxicos são semelhantes àqueles induzidos por veneno de naja. [Hindi *karait*]

Krantz, Kermit E., ginecologista-obstetra norte-americano, *1923. VER Marshall-Marchetti-K. *operation*.

Kraske, Paul, cirurgião alemão, 1851–1930. VER K. *operation*.

krau·ro·sis vul·vae (kraw-rō′sis vŭl′vē). Craurose vulvar; atrofia e retração do epitélio da vagina e vulva, freqüentemente acompanhada por reação inflamatória crônica nos tecidos mais profundos; um termo antigo para líquen escleroso e atrófico da vulva. SIN leukokraurosis. [G. *krauros,* seco, quebradiço]

Krause, Fedor, cirurgião alemão, 1857–1937. VER K. *graft;* Wolfe-K. *graft*.

Krause, Karl F.T., anatomista alemão, 1797–1868. VER K. *glands,* em *gland, ligament*.

Krause, Wilhelm J.F., anatomista alemão, 1833–1910. VER K. *bone,* end *bulbs,* em *bulb,* respiratory *bundle, valve*.

kreb·i·o·zen (krē′bē-oz′en). Um extrato de sementes de pêssego, cuja composição não foi totalmente descrita, mas que ganhou notoriedade nas décadas de 1960 e 1970 como um remédio duvidoso, mas explorado para tratamento do câncer; atualmente não é considerado efetivo. [Al. *Krebs,* caranguejo, câncer]

Krebs, Edwin G., bioquímico norte-americano, *1918, ganhador associado do Prêmio Nobel de 1992 pela descoberta da fosforilação proteica reversível como um mecanismo regulador biológico.

Krebs, Sir Hans Adolph, bioquímico alemão na Inglaterra e premiado com o Nobel, 1900–1981. VER K. *cycle;* K.-Henseleit *cycle;* K.-Ringer *solution.*

Kretschmann, Friederich, otologista alemão, 1858–1934. VER K. *space.*

Kreysig, Friedrich L., médico alemão, 1770–1839. VER K. *sign;* Heim-K. *sign.*

kriging (krī′jing). Um método usado pela primeira vez nas ciências da terra para uniformizar dados de medidas de pontos dispersos espacialmente, usado em epidemiologia geográfica. [D. G. *Krige,* engenheiro sul-africano]

krin·gle (krin′gle). Um elemento (motivo) ou domínio estrutural observado em determinadas proteínas nas quais uma prega de grandes alças é estabilizada por ligações dissulfeto; uma característica estrutural importante em fatores da coagulação sanguínea. [Al. *Kringel,* espiral]

Krogh, August, fisiologista dinamarquês e premiado com o Nobel, 1874–1949. VER K. *spirometer.*

Kronecker, Karl H., fisiologista suíço, 1839–1914. VER K. *stain.*

Krönig, Georg, médico alemão, 1856–1911. VER K. *isthmus, steps,* em *step.*

Krönlein, Rudolf U., cirurgião suíço, 1847–1910. VER K. *operation, hernia.*

Krueger in·stru·ment stop. Ver em instrument.

Krukenberg, Adolph, anatomista alemão, 1816–1877. VER K. *veins,* em *vein.*

Krukenberg, Friedrich, patologista alemão, 1871–1946. VER K. *amputation, spindle, tumor.*

Kruse, Walther, bacteriologista alemão, 1864–1943. VER K. *brush;* Shiga-Kruse *bacillus.*

krymo-, kryo-. VER crymo-, cryo-.

kryp·ton (Kr) (krip′ton). Criptônio. Um dos gases nobres, presente em pequenas quantidades na atmosfera (1,14 ppm por volume seco); número atômico 36, peso atômico 83,80; Kr^{85} (meia-vida de 10,73 anos) foi usado em estudos de anormalidades cardíacas. [G. *kryptos,* oculto]

17-KS Abreviatura de 17-cetosteróides (17-ketosteroids).

KUB Abreviatura de rins, ureteres, bexiga (kidneys, ureters, bladder); designação arcaica de radiografia simples frontal do abdome em decúbito dorsal.

ku·bi·sa·ga·ri, ku·bi·sa·ga·ru (koo - bi - sah - gah′rē, koo - bi - sah - gah′roo). Neuronite vestibular. SIN vestibular *neuronitis.* (Jap. *kubi,* cabeça, pescoço, + *sagaru,* pendurar]

Kufs, Hugo, psiquiatra alemão, 1871–1955. VER K. *disease.*

Kugel anastomotic ar·tery. Artéria anastomótica de Kugel. Ver em *artery.*

Kugelberg, Eric, neurologista sueco, 1913–1983. VER K.-Welander *disease;* Wohlfart-K.-Welander *disease.*

Kühne, Wilhelm (Willy) F., fisiologista e histologista alemão, 1837–1900. VER K. *fiber, methylene blue, phenomenon, plate, spindle.*

Kuhnt, Hermann, oftalmologista alemão, 1850–1925. VER K. *spaces,* em *space.*

Kulchitsky, Nicholas, histologista russo, 1856–1925. VER K. *cells,* em *cell.*

Külz, Rudolph E., médico alemão, 1845–1895. VER K. *cylinder.*

Küntscher, Gerhard, cirurgião alemão, 1902–1972. VER K. *nail.*

Kupffer, Karl W. von, anatomista alemão, 1829–1902. VER K. *cells,* em *cell.*

kur·chi bark (ker′chē). Casca de kurchi. SIN conessi.

Kürsteiner (Kuersteiner), W., anatomista alemão do século XIX. VER K. *canals,* em *canal.*

kur·to·sis (kur - tō′sis). Curtose; a extensão com que uma distribuição unimodal atinge o máximo. [G., uma curva]

ku·ru (koo′roo). Kuru; uma forma progressiva fatal de encefalopatia espongiforme, endêmica no povo Fore nas regiões montanhosas da Nova Guiné, inicialmente atribuída a infecção por um "vírus lento", mas agora se sabe que é causada por prions. Acredita-se que a transmissão se dê por contaminação e ingestão durante rituais de canibalismo. É caracterizada por ataxia, tremores, ausência de coordenação e morte; as lesões histopatológicas no cérebro incluem perda neuronal, ostrocitose e estado esponjoso. VER prion. [dialeto nativo, tremer de medo ou frio]

Kurzrok-Ratner test. Teste de Kurzrok-Ratner. Ver em *test.*

Kussmaul, Adolph, médico alemão, 1822–1902. VER K. *respiration, coma, disease, sign;* K.-Kien *respiration.*

Küster, Herman, ginecologista alemão do início do século XX. VER Mayer-Rokitansky-K.-Hauser *syndrome;* Rokitansky-K.-Hauser *syndrome.*

Küstner, Heinz, ginecologista alemão, *1897. VER Prausnitz-K. *antibody, reaction;* reversed K. *reaction.*

kv Abreviação de quilovolt.

Kveim, Morton A., médico norueguês, *1892. VER K. *antigen, test;* K.-Siltzbach *antigen, test;* Nickerson-K. *test.*

kVp Abreviação de pico em quilovolts, a maior voltagem instantânea através de um tubo de raios X, correspondente aos raios X de máxima energia emitidos.

kwa·shi·or·kor (kwah - shē - ōr′kor). Kwashiorkor; pelagra infantil; uma doença observada originalmente em africanos, sobretudo em crianças entre 1 e 3 anos, devida à deficiência alimentar, particularmente de proteínas; caracterizada por hipoalbuminemia acentuada, anemia, edema, abdome protuberante, despigmentação cutânea, perda de pêlos ou alteração da cor dos mesmos para vermelho, e fezes volumosas contendo alimento não-digerido; alterações gordurosas nas células hepáticas, atrofia das células acinares do pâncreas e hialinização dos glomérulos renais são encontradas *postmortem.* SIN infantile pellagra, malignant malnutrition. [Ga, uma linguagem de Gana, menino vermelho ou criança deslocada]

  marasmic k., k. marasmático; desnutrição proteico-calórica grave, caracterizada por emagrecimento extremo, fraqueza e manifestações de k.

△ **ky-.** Quanto às palavras que começam assim e não são encontradas a seguir, ver cy-.

ky·mo·gram (kī′mō - gram). Quimograma; cimograma; curva gráfica feita por um quimógrafo.

ky·mo·graph (kī′mō - graf). Quimógrafo, cimógrafo, osciloscópio; instrumento obsoleto para registrar movimentos em forma de onda ou modulação, principalmente para registrar variações da pressão arterial; consiste em um tambor, geralmente girado por um mecanismo de relógio e coberto com papel enfumaçado no qual um estilete ou outro tipo de objeto pontiagudo inscreve a curva. [G. *kyma,* onda, + *graphō,* registrar]

ky·mog·ra·phy (kī - mog′ră - fē). Quimografia; cimografia; uso do quimógrafo.

ky·mo·scope (kī′mō - skōp). Quimoscópio; cimoscópio; aparelho usado antigamente para medir as ondas de pulso ou a variação na pressão arterial. [G. *kyma,* onda, + *skopeō,* olhar]

kyn·u·ren·ic ac·id (kin - ū - rē′nik, - ren′ik). Ácido quinurênico; um produto do metabolismo do L-triptofano; aparece na urina humana em estados de acentuada deficiência de piridoxina.

kyn·u·ren·i·nase (kī - noo - ren′i - nās). Quinurreninase; enzima hepática que catalisa a hidrólise da cadeia lateral da L-cinurrenina, com a formação de ácido antranílico e L-alanina, no metabolismo do L-triptofano.

kyn·u·ren·ine (kī - noo′rē - nēn, - nin). Quinurrenina; um produto do metabolismo do L-triptofano, excretada em pequenas quantidades na urina; elevada em casos de deficiência de vitamina B_6.

  k. formamidase, q. formamidase. SIN formamidase.
  k. 3-hydroxylase, q. 3-hidroxilase. SIN k. 3-monooxygenase.
  k. 3-monooxygenase, q. 3-monoxigenase; uma enzima que catalisa a adição de um grupamento hidroxila à L-quinurrenina, com o auxílio do NADPH e O_2, produzindo 3-hidroxi-L-quinurrenina, $NADP^+$ e água; uma etapa no catabolismo do L-triptofano. SIN k. 3-hydroxylase.

ky·phos (kī′fos). Cifo, corcunda, corcova, a proeminência convexa na cifose. [G.]

ky·pho·sco·li·o·sis (kī - fō - skō′lē - ō - sis). Cifoescoliose; curvatura lateral e posterior da coluna vertebral; a insuficiência cardíaca congestiva grave pode ser uma complicação tardia. SIN scoliokyphosis. [G. *kyphōsis,* cifose, + *scoliosis,* curvo]

ky·pho·sis (kī - fō′sis). Cifose. **1.** Uma curvatura côncava anteriormente da coluna vertebral; as cifoses normais das regiões torácica e sacral são porções preservadas da curvatura primária (cifose) da coluna vertebral. **2.** Uma curvatura anterior (flexão) da coluna vertebral; a coluna torácica normalmente tem uma leve cifose; a curvatura anterior excessiva da coluna torácica pode representar uma condição anormal. [G. *kyphōsis,* corcova, de *kyphos,* curvo, corcova]

  juvenile k., c. juvenil. SIN Scheuermann *disease.*
  sacral k. [TA], c. sacral; a curvatura anteriormente côncava normal do sacro (segmento sacral da coluna vertebral), na qual a curvatura primária do embrião fetal é mantida até a maturidade. SIN k. sacralis [TA].
  k. sacralis [TA], c. sacral. SIN sacral k.
  thoracic k. [TA], c. torácica; a curvatura anteriormente côncava normal do segmento torácico da coluna vertebral, na qual a curvatura primária do embrião fetal é mantida até a maturidade. SIN k. thoracica [TA].
  k. thoracica [TA], c. torácica. SIN thoracic k.

ky·phot·ic (kī - fot′ik). Cifótico; relativo a, ou que sofre de, cifose.

Kyrle, Josef, dermatologista alemão, 1880–1926. VER K. *disease.*

△ **kyto-.** VER cyto-.

L

Λ 1. A 11.ª letra do alfabeto grego, lambda. **2.** Símbolo (λ) do Avogadro *number* (número de Avogadro); wavelength (comprimento de onda); radioactive *constant* (constante radioativa); Ostwald solubility *coefficient* (coeficiente de solubilidade de Ostwald); molar conductivity (condutividade molar) de um eletrólito (Λ). **3.** Em química, indica a posição de um substituto localizado no 11.º átomo de um grupamento carboxila ou de outro grupamento funcional (λ).

L 1. Abreviatura de left (esquerda, p.ex., olho esquerdo); lombar vertebrae (vértebras lombares, L1 a L5). **2.** Símbolo para inductance (indutância); liter (litro); leucine (leucina); leucyl (leucil). **3.** Abreviatura para limes; usado como uma letra minúscula, mais sinal, letra subscrita ou subscrita mais sinal como um símbolo para várias doses de toxina. VER dose.

L Símbolo para linking *number* (número de encadeamento).

l Símbolo de liter (litro); liquid (líquido); length (comprimento) (em itálico).

⚠ *l-.* Levorrotatório. Cf. *d-*. [L. *laevus*, no lado esquerdo]

⚠ **L-.** Prefixo indicando um composto químico que é estruturalmente (estearicamente) relacionado ao L-gliceraldeído. Cf. D-.

La Símbolo do lanthanum (lantânio).

Laband, Peter F., odontólogo norte-americano, *1900. VER L. *syndrome*.

Labbé, Ernest M., médico francês, 1870–1939.

Labbé, Leon, cirurgião francês, 1832–1916. VER L. *triangle, vein*.

la·bel. 1. Marcar; incorporar uma substância que seja facilmente detectada, como um radionuclídeo, em um composto, por meio do qual seu metabolismo possa ser seguido ou sua distribuição física seja detectada. **2.** Marcador; a substância incorporada dessa maneira.

la belle in·dif·fér·ence (lah bel an-dif-er-ahns′). A bela indiferença; a carência ingênua e imprópria de emoção ou preocupação com as percepções pelos outros da incapacidade da pessoa, tipicamente observada na pessoa com histeria de conversão. [Fr.]

la·bet·a·lol hy·dro·chlo·ride (la - bet′ă - lol). Cloridrato de labetalol; um agente bloqueador α-adrenérgico e β-adrenérgico empregado no tratamento da hipertensão arterial.

la·bia (lā′bē - ă). Lábios; plural de labium.

la·bi·al (lā′bē - ăl). Labial. **1.** Relativo aos lábios ou a qualquer lábio. **2.** Em direção a um lábio. **3.** Uma das letras formadas por meio dos lábios. [L. *labium*, lábio]

la·bi·al·ism (lā′bē - ăl - izm). Labialismo; uma forma de balbucio em que existe confusão no uso das consoantes labiais.

la·bi·al·ly (lā′bē - ăl - ē). Labialmente; em direção aos lábios.

la·bile (lā′bīl, - bil). Lábil; instável; não-fixo; indicando: **1.** Uma adaptabilidade à alteração ou modificação, ou seja, com relativa facilidade de ser alterado ou redistribuído. **2.** Determinados constituintes do soro afetados por aumentos da temperatura. **3.** Um eletrodo que é mantido em movimento sobre a superfície durante a passagem de uma corrente elétrica. **4.** Em psicologia ou psiquiatria, indica o humor ou a expressão comportamental livre e descontrolada das emoções. **5.** Facilmente removível; p.ex., um átomo de hidrogênio l. [L. *labilis*, capaz de se partir, de *labor*, pp. *lapsus*, deslocar]

la·bil·i·ty (lă - bil′i - tē). Labilidade; o estado de ser lábil.

⚠ **labio-.** Lábio-; os lábios. VER TAMBÉM cheilo-. [L. *labium*, lábio]

la·bi·o·cer·vi·cal (lā - bē - ō - ser′vi - kăl). Labiocervical; relativo a um lábio e um colo; especificamente, à superfície labial ou bucal de um dente. [labio- + L. *cervix*, pescoço]

la·bi·o·cli·na·tion (lā′bē - ō - kli - nā′shŭn). Labioclinação; inclinação da posição mais no sentido dos lábios que o normal; diz-se de um dente.

la·bi·o·den·tal (lā - bē - ō - den′tăl). Labiodental; relativo aos lábios e aos dentes; indica determinadas letras cujo som é formado pelos lábios e dentes. [labio- + L. *dens*, dente]

la·bi·o·gin·gi·val (lā′bē - ō - jin′ji - văl). Labiogengival; relativo ao ponto de junção da borda labial à linha gengival na superfície distal ou mesial de um dente incisivo.

la·bi·o·glos·so·la·ryn·ge·al (lā′bē - ō - glos′ō - lă - rin′jē - ăl). Labioglossolaríngeo; relativo aos lábios, língua e laringe; descreve a paralisia bulbar em que essas partes estão envolvidas. [labio- + G. *glōssa*, língua, + larynx]

la·bi·o·glos·so·pha·ryn·ge·al (lā′bē - ō - glos′ō - fă - rin′jē - ăl). Labioglossofaríngeo; relativo aos lábios, língua e faringe; descreve a paralisia bulbar que envolve essas partes. [labio- + G. *glōssa*, língua, + pharynx]

la·bi·o·graph (lā′bē - ō - graf). Um instrumento para registrar os movimentos dos lábios na fala. [labio- + G. *graphō*, registrar]

la·bi·o·men·tal (lā′bē - ō - men′tăl). Labiomentual; relativo ao lábio inferior e ao queixo. [labio- + L. *mentum*, queixo]

la·bi·o·na·sal (lā′bē - ō - nā′săl). Labionasal. **1.** Relativo ao lábio superior e ao nariz, ou a ambos os lábios e o nariz. **2.** Indica uma letra que é labial e nasal na produção de seu som.

la·bi·o·pal·a·tine (lā′bē - ō - pal′ă - tīn). Labiopalatino; relativo aos lábios e ao palato.

la·bi·o·place·ment (lā′bē - ō - plās′ment). Labiocolocação; posicionamento (p.ex., de um dente) mais no sentido dos lábios que o normal.

la·bi·o·plas·ty (lā′bē - ō - plas - tē). Labioplastia; cirurgia plástica de um lábio. [labio- + G. *plastos*, formado]

la·bi·o·ver·sion (lā′bē - ō - ver - zhŭn). Labioversão; posição incorreta de um dente anterior em relação à linha normal de oclusão, ou seja, mais próximo dos lábios.

lab·i·tome (lab′i - tōm). Labítomo; uma pinça com lâminas cortantes. SIN cutting forceps. [G. *labis*, pinças, + *tomē*, uma incisão]

la·bi·um, gen. **la·bii,** pl. **la·bia** (lā′bē - ŭm, - bē - ē, - bē - ă) [TA]. Lábio, lábios. **1.** SIN lip. **2.** Qualquer estrutura com formato de lábio. [L.]

l. ante′rius os′tii u′teri [TA], l. anterior do óstio do útero. SIN anterior lip of external os of uterus.

l. exter′num cris′tae ili′acae [TA], l. externo da crista ilíaca. SIN outer lip of iliac crest.

l. infe′rius o′ris [TA], l. inferior do vestíbulo da boca. SIN lower lip.

l. inter′num cris′tae ili′acae [TA], l. interno da crista ilíaca. SIN inner lip of iliac crest.

l. latera′le lin′eae as′perae [TA], l. lateral da linha áspera. SIN lateral lip of linea aspera.

l. lim′bi tympan′icum la′minae spira′lis ossei [TA], l. do limbo timpânico da lâmina espiral óssea. SIN tympanic lip of spiral limbus.

l. limbi tympanicum limbi spiralis ossei [TA], l. timpânico do limbo da espiral óssea. SIN tympanic lip of spiral limbus.

l. lim′bi vistibula′re la′minae spi′ralis ossei [TA], l. do limbo vestibular da lâmina espiral óssea. SIN vestibular lip of spiral limbus.

l. limbi vestibulare limbi spiralis ossei [TA], l. do limbo vestibular da espiral óssea. SIN vestibular lip of spiral limbus.

l. ma′jus [TA], l. maior do pudendo; uma das duas pregas arredondadas do tegumento que formam os limites laterais da fenda interglútea. Os lábios maiores do pudendo são o homólogo feminino da bolsa escrotal. SIN l. majus pudendi [TA], large pudendal lip.

l. ma′jus puden′di, pl. **la′bia majo′ra** [TA], l. maior do pudendo. SIN l. majus.

l. media′le lin′eae as′perae [TA], l. medial da linha áspera. SIN medial lip of linea aspera.

l. mi′nus [TA], l. menor do pudendo; uma das duas pregas longitudinais estreitas de mucosa que fecham a fenda pudenda nos lábios maiores do pudendo; posteriormente, fundem-se com os lábios maiores do pudendo, unindo-se para formar o frênulo dos lábios do pudendo (fércula); anteriormente, cada l. divide-se em duas porções que se unem com aquelas do lado oposto em frente à glande do clitóris, de modo a formar o prepúcio. SIN l. minus pudendi, small pudendal lip.

l. mi′nus puden′di, pl. **la′bia mino′ra,** l. menor do pudendo. SIN l. minus.

la′bia o′ris [TA], lábios do vestíbulo da boca. SIN lips of mouth, em lip. VER lip (1).

l. poste′rius os′tii u′teri [TA], l. posterior do óstio do útero. SIN posterior lip of external os of uterus.

l. supe′rius o′ris [TA], l. superior do vestíbulo da boca. SIN upper lip.

tympanic l. of limbus of spiral lamina, l. timpânico do limbo da espiral óssea. SIN tympanic lip of spiral limbus.

l. ure′thrae, l. da uretra; uma das duas margens laterais do óstio uretral externo no sexo feminino.

la′bia u′teri, lábios do óstio do útero. VER anterior lip of external os of uterus, posterior lip of external os of uterus.

vestibular l. of limbus of spiral lamina, l. do limbo vestibular da lâmina espiral. SIN vestibular lip of spiral limbus.

l. voca′le, pl. **la′bia voca′lia,** l. vocal. SIN vocal fold.

la·bor (lā′bor). Trabalho de parto; o processo de expulsão do feto e da placenta a partir do útero. Os **estágios do trabalho de parto** incluem: **primeiro estágio,** começando com o estabelecimento das contrações uterinas através do período de dilatação do óstio uterino; **segundo estágio,** o período do esforço expulsivo, começando com a dilatação completa do colo e terminando com a expulsão do concepto; **terceiro estágio** ou **estágio placentário,** o período que começa com a expulsão do concepto e termina com a expulsão completa da placenta e das membranas. [L. trabalho, sofrimento]

active l., trabalho de parto ativo; as contrações que resultam no apagamento e dilatação progressivos do colo.

dry l., trabalho de parto seco; termo obsoleto para indicar o trabalho de parto após a perda espontânea do líquido amniótico.

⚠ Formas Combinantes

🔲 Indica que o termo é ilustrado, ver Índice de Ilustrações

SIN Sinônimo

Cf. Comparar, confrontar

[NA] *Nomina Anatomica*

[TA] *Terminologia Anatomica*

☆ Termo oficial alternativo para a *Terminologia Anatomica*

[MIM] Mendelian Inheritance in Man

I.C. Índice de Corantes

Termo de Alta Importância

false l., trabalho de parto falso; contrações que não produzem a dilatação ou apagamento cervical.
missed l., trabalho de parto ausente; contrações uterinas breves que não levam ao trabalho de parto e à expulsão do concepto, mas que cessam, resultando na retenção indefinida do concepto (usualmente morto) quer *in utero*, quer na cavidade abdominal.
precipitate l., trabalho de parto precipitado; trabalho de parto muito rápido que termina na expulsão do feto.
premature l., trabalho de parto prematuro; o estabelecimento do trabalho de parto depois de 20 semanas e antes da 37.ª semana completa de gestação, contada a partir do último período menstrual normal.
trial of l. after cesarean section, tentativa de trabalho de parto depois de cesariana; a tentativa de expulsão por via vaginal depois de uma cesariana; comporta algum risco de ruptura da cicatriz uterina.

lab·o·ra·to·ri·an (lab′o - ra - tōr′e - an). Laboratorista; aquele que trabalha em laboratório; na área de saúde, aquele que examina ou realiza os exames (ou supervisiona esses procedimentos) com tipos variados de materiais químicos e biológicos, principalmente como complemento do diagnóstico, tratamento e controle da doença, ou como uma base para práticas de saúde e sanitária.

lab·o·ra·tory (lab′o - ra - tō - re, lab′ra-). Laboratório; um local equipado para a realização de exames, experiências e procedimentos investigativos, bem como para a preparação de reagentes, materiais químicos farmacêuticos e assim por diante. [L. M. *laboratorium*, um local de trabalho, do L. *laboro*, pp. *-atus*, trabalhar]
  personal growth l., laboratório de desenvolvimento pessoal; um ambiente de treinamento sensorial em que a ênfase primária se faz sobre as potencialidades de cada participante para a criatividade, empatia e liderança. VER TAMBÉM sensitivity training *group*.

la·bra (la′brä). Lábios; plural de labrum. [L.]
la·bra·le in·fe·ri·us (lä - brä′lē in - fē′rē - ŭs). Um ponto onde o limite da borda do vermelhão do lábio inferior e a pele é cruzado pelo plano mediano.
la·bra·le su·pe·ri·us (lä - brä′lē soo - pē′rē - ŭs). O ponto no lábio superior que se situa no plano mediossagital em uma linha desenhada no limite da borda do vermelhão e a pele.

lab·ro·cyte (lab′rō - sīt). Mastócito. SIN mast *cell.*

la·brum, pl. **la·bra** (la′brŭm, la′brä) [TA]. Lábio. **1.** Um lábio. **2.** Uma estrutura em formato de lábio. **3.** Um lábio fibrocartilaginoso ao redor da borda da porção côncava de algumas articulações. SIN articular l., articular lip, l. articulare. [L.]
  acetabular l. [TA], l. acetabular; uma borda fibrocartilaginosa presa à margem do acetábulo do osso do quadril. SIN l. acetabulare [TA], acetabular lip, circumferential cartilage (1), cotyloid ligament, ligamentum cotyloideum.
  l. acetabula′re [TA], l. acetabular. SIN acetabular l.
  articular l., l. articular. SIN labrum (3).
  l. articula′re, l. articular. SIN labrum (3).
  l. glenoida′le scapulae [TA], l. glenóide da escápula. SIN glenoid l. of scapula.
  glenoid l. of scapula [TA], l. glenóide da escápula; um anel de fibrocartilagem preso à margem da cavidade glenóide da escápula para aumentar sua profundidade. SIN l. glenoidale scapulae [TA], articular margin, circumferential cartilage (2), glenoid ligament (1), glenoidal lip, ligamentum glenoidale.

lab·y·rinth (lab′i-rinth) [TA]. Labirinto; qualquer uma das várias estruturas anatômicas com inúmeros canais ou células intercomunicantes. **1.** O ouvido interno, composto de canais semicirculares, vestíbulo e cóclea. **2.** Qualquer grupo de cavidades comunicantes, como em cada massa lateral do osso etmóide. **3.** Um grupo de tubos de ensaio em posição vertical que termina, abaixo, em uma base de tubos comunicantes alternados, em forma de U, invertidos e voltados para cima, usados para isolar os organismos móveis dos imóveis na cultura, ou de um organismo móvel de um menos móvel (como o bacilo tifóide em relação ao bacilo colônico), onde o primeiro se movimenta mais rápido e por uma distância maior, através dos tubos, que o último.
  bony l. [TA], l. ósseo; uma série de cavidades (cóclea, vestíbulo e canais semicirculares) contida na cápsula ótica da porção petrosa do osso temporal; o labirinto ósseo é cheio de perilinfa, na qual fica suspenso o delicado labirinto membranoso cheio de endolinfa. SIN labyrinthus osseus [TA], osseous l.
  cochlear l. [TA], l. coclear; a porção do labirinto membranoso relacionada à sensação da audição (cf. o labirinto vestibular, que está relacionado à sensação de equilíbrio) e inervada pelo nervo coclear; localiza-se dentro da cóclea do labirinto ósseo e consiste no canal coclear, que contém o órgão espiral. SIN labyrinthus cochlearis [TA], organ of hearing.
  ethmoidal l. [TA], l. etmoidal; uma massa de células aéreas com finas paredes ósseas que formam parte da parede lateral da cavidade nasal; as células estão dispostas em três grupos, anterior, médio e posterior, e são fechadas lateralmente pela placa orbitária que forma a parte da parede da órbita. SIN labyrinthus ethmoidalis [TA], ectethmoid, ectoethmoid, lateral mass of ethmoid bone.
  Ludwig l., l. de Ludwig. SIN convoluted *part* of kidney lobule.
  membranous l. [TA], l. membranáceo; um arranjo complexo de sacos e canalículos membranosos comunicantes, cheios de endolinfa e circundados por perilinfa, suspensos dentro da cavidade do labirinto ósseo; suas divisões principais são o ducto coclear e o labirinto vestibular. SIN labyrinthus membranaceus [TA].
  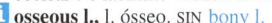 **osseous l.,** l. ósseo. SIN bony l.

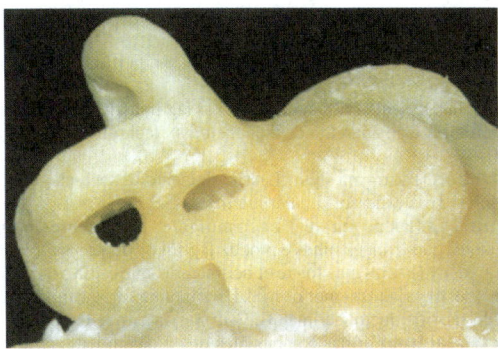
labirinto ósseo: removido da porção petrosa do osso temporal

  renal l., parte convoluta do lóbulo renal. SIN convoluted *part* of kidney lobule.
  Santorini l., l. de Santorini. SIN prostatic venous *plexus.*
  vestibular l. [TA], l. vestibular; a porção do labirinto membranáceo relacionada ao equilíbrio (cf. o labirinto coclear, que está relacionado à audição) e inervada pelo nervo vestibular; localiza-se nos canais semicirculares e do vestíbulo do labirinto ósseo, e consiste no utrículo, sáculo e ductos semicircular, utriculossacular e endolinfático. SIN labyrinthus vestibularis [TA], vestibular organ.

lab·y·rin·thec·to·my (lab - ĭ - rin - thek′tō - me). Labirintectomia; a excisão do labirinto; uma cirurgia destrutiva para extinguir a função labiríntica. [labyrinth + G. *ektome*, excisão]
lab·y·rin·thine (lab - ĭ - rin′thin). Labiríntico; relativo a qualquer labirinto.
lab·y·rin·thi·tis (lab′ĭ - rin - thī′tis). Labirintite; inflamação do labirinto (o ouvido interno), por vezes acompanhada por vertigem e surdez. SIN otitis interna.
lab·y·rin·thot·o·my (lab - ĭ - rin - thot′o - me). Labirintotomia; incisão dentro do labirinto. [labyrinth + G. *tome*, incisão]
lab·y·rin·thus (lab - i - rin′thŭs). Labirinto. SIN convoluted *part* of kidney lobule. [L. do G. *labyrinthos*, labirinto]
  l. cochlea′ris [TA], l. coclear. SIN cochlear *labyrinth.*
  l. ethmoida′lis [TA], l. etmoidal. SIN ethmoidal *labyrinth.*
  l. membrana′ceus [TA], l. membranáceo. SIN membranous *labyrinth*
  l. os′seus [TA], l. ósseo. SIN bony *labyrinth.*
  l. vestibula′ris [TA], l. vestibular. SIN vestibular *labyrinth.*

lac, gen. **lac·tis** (lak, lak′tis). Leite. **1.** SIN milk (1). **2.** Qualquer líquido esbranquiçado, semelhante ao leite. [L. leite]
  l. sul′furis, l. sulfúrico. SIN precipitated *sulfur.*
  l. vacci′num, leite de vaca.

lac·ca (lak′ä). Laca. SIN shellac.

lac·case (lak′ās). Lacase; uma enzima que oxida benzenodióis em semiquinonas com O_2. SIN monophenol monooxygenase (2), phenol oxidase, phenolase, polyphenol oxidase, uroshiol oxidase.

lac·er·a·ble (las′er - ă - bl). Lacerável; capaz de ser lacerado ou estar sujeito a laceração. [L. *lacero*, cortar em pedaços, de *lacer*, dilacerado]

lac·er·at·ed (las′er - ā - ted). Lacerado; roto; rasgado; que possui uma borda lacerada. [L. *lacero*, pp. *-atus*, rasgar em pedaços]

lac·er·a·tion (las - er - ā′shŭn). Laceração. **1.** Uma ferida lacerada ou rota, ou uma ferida cortada acidentalmente. **2.** O processo ou ato de lacerar os tecidos. [L. *lacero*, pp. *-atus*, cortar em pedaços]
  brain l., l. cerebral; laceração macroscópica do tecido nervoso.
  scalp l., l. do couro cabeludo; laceração da derme ou dos tecidos subjacentes e da gálea aponeurótica do couro cabeludo.
  through-and-through laceration, laceração transfixiante; uma l. que penetra as duas superfícies de uma estrutura, geralmente restrita às superfícies da pele ou mucosa, como a bochecha, lábio, asas do nariz, orelha, etc.
  vaginal l., l. vaginal; laceração da parede vaginal. SIN colporrhexis.

la·cer·tus (lä - ser′tŭs) [TA]. Lacerto. **1** [TA]. Uma faixa, feixe ou tira fibrosa relacionada a um músculo. **2.** Originalmente, a parte muscular do membro superior, desde o ombro até o cotovelo. [L.]
  l. cor′dis, l. do coração; uma das trabéculas carnosas.
  l. fibro′sus, aponeurose bicipital; *termo oficial alternativo para bicipital *aponeurosis.*
  l. of lateral rectus muscle, l. do músculo reto lateral; a parte do tendão de origem do músculo reto lateral que se insere na asa maior do osso esfenóide, lateralmente ao anel tendinoso comum; com freqüência, erroneamente igualado ao ligamento controlador lateral do globo ocular. SIN l. musculi recti lateralis.
  l. me′dius, ligamento longitudinal anterior. SIN anterior longitudinal *ligament.*
  l. mus′culi rec′ti latera′lis, l. do músculo reto lateral. SIN l. of lateral rectus *muscle.*

lach·ry·mal (lak′ri - măl). Lacrimal. SIN lacrimal.

LACI Abreviatura de lipoprotein-associated coagulation *inhibitor* (inibidor da coagulação associada a lipoproteína).

la·cin·i·ae tu·bae (la - sin′ē - ē too′bē). Lacíneas da trompa. SIN *fimbriae of uterine tube*, em *fimbria*. [L. *lacinia*, orla]

lac·ri·mal (lak′ri - mǎl). Lacrimal; relativo às lágrimas, à sua secreção, às glândulas secretoras e ao aparelho de drenagem. SIN lachrymal. [L. *lacrima*, uma lágrima]

lac·ri·ma·tion (lak′ri - mā′shŭn). Lacrimejamento; a secreção das lágrimas, especialmente em excesso. [L. *lacrimatio*]

lac·ri·ma·tor (lak′ri - mā - ter). Lacrimejante; um agente (como o gás lacrimejante) que irrita os olhos e produz lágrimas. [L. *lacrima*, lágrima]

lac·ri·ma·to·ry (lak′ri - mā - tō - rē). Lacrimatório; que causa o lacrimejamento.

lac·ri·mot·o·my (lak - ri - mot′ō - mē). Lacrimotomia; a cirurgia de fazer uma incisão do saco ou ducto lacrimal. [L. *lacrima*, lágrima, + G. *tomē*, incisão]

△ **lact-, lacti-, lacto-.** Formas combinantes que indicam leite; leite. VER TAMBÉM galacto-. [L. *lac, lactis*]

lac·tac·i·de·mia (lak - tas - i - dē′mē′ǎ). Lactacidemia. SIN *lactic acidemia.*

lac·tac·i·do·sis (lak - tas - i - dō′sis). Lactacidose; acidose decorrente do ácido lático aumentado.

lac·tal·bu·min (lak - tal - bū′min). Lactalbumina; a fração albumina do leite. Contém duas proteínas: α- e β-l.; a primeira, l. minor, interage com a galactosil transferase para formar a lactose sintase, que sintetiza a lactose a partir da D-glicose e UDP-galactose na produção do leite; a β-l. é a principal proteína do soro no leite bovino; a α-l. é a mais termoestável das proteínas do soro.

lac·tam, lac·tim (lak′tam, -tim). Contrações de "lactoneamina" e "lactoneimina" e aplicadas às formas tautoméricas –NH–CO– e –N=C(OH)–, respectivamente, observadas em muitas purinas, pirimidinas e outras substâncias; a última forma contribui para as propriedades ácidas do ácido úrico.

β-lac·tam. β-Lactâmico; uma classe de antibióticos de largo espectro que estão relacionados, do ponto de vista estrutural e farmacológico, às penicilinas e cefalosporinas.

lactamase (lak′ta - māz). Lactamase. SIN *β-lactamase.*

β-lac·ta·mase (lak′ta - mās). β-lactamase; uma enzima produzida por muitas espécies de bactérias que rompem o anel β-lactâmico de quatro componentes dos grupos da penicilina e cefalosporina dos antibióticos, destruindo suas atividades antimicrobianas. A capacidade de um microrganismo de produzir uma β-lactamase pode ser cromossomial e constitutiva ou uma propriedade adquirida associada a um plasmídeo. SIN cephalosporinase, lactamase, penicillinase (1).

lac·tase (lak′tās). Lactase. SIN *β-D-galactosidase.*

lac·tate (lak′tāt). Lactato. **1.** Um sal ou éster do ácido lático. **2.** Para produzir leite nas glândulas mamárias.

l. dehydrogenase (LDH), l. desidrogenase, desidrogenase láctica; nome para inúmeras enzimas, incluindo: L-l. desidrogenase (citocromo), D-l. desidrogenase (citocromo), L-l. desidrogenase e D-l. desidrogenase. As duas primeiras enzimas transferem hidrogênio para o ferricitocromo *c* ou para o citocromo b_2; as duas últimas enzimas transferem-no para o NAD$^+$, ao catalisar a oxidação do lactato em piruvato; a distribuição da isoenzima da l. desidrogenase cardíaca e muscular é de uso significante nos casos de infarto do miocárdio; uma deficiência de uma subunidade resultará em mioglobinúria depois do exercício intenso. SIN lactic acid dehydrogenase.

excess l., l. em excesso; o aumento na concentração de l. além daquele que seria esperado a partir do aumento na concentração de piruvato, resultante de uma modificação no potencial redox; usado como índice do metabolismo anaeróbico dos carboidratos.

Ringer l., l. de Ringer, solução de Ringer lactato. SIN *Ringer solution.*

lac·tate 2-mon·o·ox·y·gen·ase. Lactato 2-monoxigenase; uma oxirredutase da flavoproteína que catalisa a oxidação (com O_2) do L-lactato em acetato mais CO_2 e água. SIN lactic acid oxidative decarboxylase.

lac·ta·tion (lak - tā′shŭn). Lactação. **1.** Produção de leite. **2.** Período após o parto durante o qual o leite é secretado pelas mamas. [L. *lactatio*, sugar]

lac·ta·tion·al (lak - tā′shŭn - ǎl). Lactacional; relativo à lactação.

lac·te·al (lak′tē - ǎl). Lácteo. **1.** Relativo ou semelhante ao leite. **2.** Um vaso linfático que conduz o quilo. SIN chyle vessel, lacteal vessel.

central l., l. central; um capilar linfático de extremidade cega no centro de uma vilosidade intestinal.

lac·te·nin (lak′tē - nin). Lactenina; um agente antibacteriano ativo contra os estreptococos isolados do leite de vaca.

lac·tes·cent (lak-tes′ent). Lactescente; que se assemelha ao leite; leitoso.

△ **lacti-.** Lacti-; VER lact-.

lac·tic (lak′tik). Lático; relativo ao leite. [L. *lac (lact-)*, leite]

lac·tic ac·id. Ácido lático, ácido láctico; um intermediário normal na fermentação (oxidação, metabolismo) do açúcar. Na forma pura, um líquido xaroposo, inodoro e incolor obtido pela ação do bacilo do ácido lático sobre o leite ou lactose; na forma concentrada, um cáustico usado internamente para evitar a fermentação gastrointestinal. Uma cultura do bacilo, ou o leite que o contém, em geral é administrado em lugar do ácido. O L-a. lático também é conhecido como ácido sarcolático.

lac·tic ac·id de·hy·dro·gen·ase. Lactato desidrogenase, desidrogenase láctica. SIN *lactate* dehydrogenase.

lac·tic ac·i·de·mia (lak′tik - as - i - dē′mē - ǎ). Laticacidemia; a presença do ácido lático dextrorrotatório no sangue circulante. SIN lactacidemia. [lactic acid + G. *haima*, sangue]

lac·tic ac·id ox·i·da·tive de·car·box·yl·ase. Descarboxilase oxidativa do ácido lático. SIN *lactate 2-mono-oxygenase.*

lac·tif·er·ous (lak - tif′er - ŭs). Lactífero; que fornece leite. [lacti- + L. *fero*, conduzir]

lac·tif·u·gal (lak′ - tif′ū - gǎl). Lactífugo. SIN *lactifuge (1).*

lac·ti·fuge (lak′ti - fūj). Lactífugo. **1.** Que causa a parada da secreção do leite. SIN lactifugal. **2.** Um agente que possui esse efeito. [lacti- + L. *fugo*, ir para longe]

lac·tig·e·nous (lak - tij′ē - nŭs). Lactígeno; que produz leite. [lacti- + -*gen*, que produz]

lac·tim (-tim). VER lactam.

lac·ti·mor·bus (lak - ti - mōr′bŭs). Lactimorbo; SIN *milk sickness.* [lacti- + L. *morbus*, doença]

lac·ti·nat·ed (lak′ti - nā - ted). Lactinado; preparado com ou que contém lactose.

△ **lacto-.** Lacto-; VER lact-.

Lac·to·bac·il·la·ce·ae (lak′tō - bas′i - lā′sē - ē). Uma família de bactérias aeróbicas a anaeróbicas facultativas, em geral imóveis (ordem Eubacteriales), contendo bastonetes Gram-positivos retos ou curvos, que geralmente ocorrem de forma isolada ou em cadeias; as células móveis são peritricosas. Esses microrganismos têm exigências nutricionais orgânicas complexas; eles produzem ácido lático a partir de carboidratos. Eles são encontrados em produtos de fermentação animal e vegetal onde há disponibilidade de carboidratos; também são encontrados na boca, vagina e trato intestinal de vários animais de sangue quente, inclusive em seres humanos. Apenas algumas espécies são patogênicas. O gênero típico é o *Lactobacillus*, que contém 56 espécies.

lac·to·ba·cil·li (lak - tō - ba - sil′ī). Lactobacilos; plural de lactobacillus.

lac·to·ba·cil·lic ac·id (lak′tō - bǎ - sil′ik). Ácido lactobacílico; um importante constituinte dos lipídios dos lactobacilos; notável pela presença de um anel ciclopropano na molécula.

Lac·to·ba·cil·lus (lak′tō - bǎ - sil′ŭs). Lactobacilo; um gênero de bactérias microaerofílicas ou anaeróbicas, não-formadoras de esporos, comumente imóveis (família Lactobacillaceae), contendo bastonetes Gram-positivos curvos ou retos, que variam de células longas e finas a cocobacilos curtos; as cadeias são comumente produzidas, em especial na parte tardia da fase logarítmica do crescimento. Esses microrganismos possuem requisitos nutricionais complexos, geralmente característicos para cada espécie; o metabolismo é fermentativo, e pelo menos metade do produto final é formado por ácido lático. Elas são encontradas em laticínios, efluentes de derivados de grãos e carne de vaca, água, esgoto, cerveja, vinho, frutas e sucos de fruta, vegetais em conserva e massas azedas, assim como fazem parte da flora normal da boca, trato intestinal e vagina de muitos animais de sangue quente, inclusive seres humanos; como flora normal, elas produzem bacterocidinas protetoras contra as bactérias patogênicas; raramente são patogênicas. A espécie típica é *L. delbrueckii*. [lacto- + bacillus]

L. acidoph'ilus, uma espécie de bactéria encontrada nas fezes de lactentes e, também, nas fezes de pessoas idosas com uma dieta rica em leite, lactose ou dextrina.

L. bre'vis, uma espécie de bactéria amplamente distribuída na natureza, especialmente nos produtos vegetais e animais; também é encontrada na boca e no trato intestinal de seres humanos e ratos.

L. buch'neri, uma espécie de bactéria amplamente distribuída nas substâncias em fermentação.

L. bulgar'icus, uma espécie bacteriana usada na produção de iogurte.

L. ca'sei, uma espécie de bactéria encontrada no leite e no queijo.

L. catenafor'mis, uma espécie bacteriana anaeróbica encontrada nos intestinos e cavidades pulmonares de seres humanos.

L. crispa'tus, uma espécie bacteriana encontrada no pus oriundo de um abscesso dentário.

L. curva'tus, uma espécie bacteriana encontrada no esterco bovino, na atmosfera dos estábulos, no leite e em um caso de endocardite.

L. delbrueck'ii, uma espécie de bactéria encontrada nos vegetais e cereais em fermentação; é a espécie típica do gênero *L.*

L. fermen'tum, uma espécie bacteriana amplamente distribuída na natureza, principalmente nos produtos vegetais e animais em fermentação. Também encontrado na boca de seres humanos.

L. jensen'ii, uma espécie bacteriana isolada de fontes humanas, como secreção vaginal e coágulo sanguíneo.

L. planta'rum, uma espécie bacteriana encontrada em laticínios e no ambiente, plantas fermentadoras, silagem, chucrute, picles, derivados de tomate deteriorados, polvilho azedo, esterco de vaca e na boca, trato intestinal e fezes de seres humanos.

L. saliva'rius, uma espécie bacteriana encontrada na boca e no trato intestinal do *hamster*, na boca de seres humanos e no trato intestinal da galinha.

L. tricho'des, uma espécie bacteriana encontrada em vinhos que contêm etanol a 20% e em sedimentos na Califórnia, Austrália, França e Espanha; na Califórnia, esse microrganismo é comumente referido como o bacilo do pêlo, bacilo algodoado, mofo algodoado ou mofo de Fresno.

lac·to·ba·cil·lus (lak - tō - ba - sil′ŭs). Lactobacilo; um termo vernacular usado para descrever qualquer membro do gênero *Lactobacillus*.
lactobezoar (lak′tō - bē′zor). Lactobezoar; um bezoar atribuído ao conteúdo enriquecido de cálcio ou caseína em alguns leites artificiais preparados para neonatos prematuros. [lacto- + bezoar]
lac·to·bu·ty·rom·e·ter (lak′tō - bū - ti - rom′e - ter). Lactobutirômetro; um tipo de lactócrito. [lacto- + G. *boutyron*, manteiga, + *metron*, medida]
lac·to·cele (lak′tō - sēl). Lactocele. SIN galactocele. [lacto- + G. *kēlē*, tumor]
lac·to·chrome (lak′tō - krōm). Lactocromo. SIN lactoflavin (1).
lac·to·crit (lak′tō - krit). Lactócrito; um instrumento usado para estimar o teor de gordura da manteiga no leite. [lacto- + G. *krinō*, separar]
lac·to·den·sim·e·ter (lak′tō - den - sim′e - ter). Lactodensímetro; um tipo de galactômetro; [lacto- + L. *densus*, espesso, + G. *metron*, medida]
lac·to·fer·rin (lak′tō - far - in). Lactoferrina; transferrina encontrada no leite de várias espécies de mamíferos e que se acredita estar envolvida no transporte de ferro para eritrócitos; concentrações relativamente altas são encontradas no leite humano.
lac·to·fla·vin (lak′tō - flā - vin). Lactoflavina. **1.** A flavina no leite. SIN lactochrome. **2.** Riboflavina. SIN riboflavin.
lac·to·gen (lak′tō - jen). Lactogênio; um agente que estimula a produção ou secreção de leite. [lacto- + G. -*gen*, produzindo]
 human placental l. (HPL), l. placentário humano; l. isolado das placentas humanas e estruturalmente similar à somatotropina; sua atividade biológica mimetiza fracamente aquela da somatotropina e prolactina; secretado na circulação materna; a deficiência de HPL durante a gestação leva à concepção de crianças com crescimento pós-natal e intra-uterino anormal. SIN choriomammotropin, chorionic "growth hormone-prolactin", human chorionic somatomammotropic hormone, human chorionic somatomammotropin, placenta protein, placental growth hormone, purified placental protein.
lac·to·gen·e·sis (lak - tō - jen′e - sis). Lactogênese; produção de leite. [lacto- + G. *genesis*, produção]
lac·to·gen·ic (lak - tō - jen′ik). Lactogênico; pertinente à lactogênese.
lac·to·glob·u·lin (lak - tō - glob′u - lin). Lactoglobulina; a globulina presente no leite, constituindo 50–60% da proteína do soro bovino.
lac·tom·e·ter (lak - tom′e - ter). Lactômetro. SIN galactometer. [lacto- + G. *metron*, medida]
lac·to·nase (lak′tō - nās). Lactonase. SIN gluconolactonase.
lac·tone (lak′tōn). Lactona; um anidrido orgânico intramolecular formado a partir de um hidroxiácido pela perda de água entre uma hidroxila e um grupamento –COOH; um éster cíclico.
lac·to·per·ox·i·dase (lak′tō - per - oks′i - dās). Lactoperoxidase; uma peroxidase obtida a partir do leite. Também catalisa a oxidação do iodeto em iodo.
lac·to·pro·tein (lak - tō - prō′tēn). Lactoproteína; qualquer proteína normalmente presente no leite.
lac·tor·rhea (lak - tō - rē′ă). Lactorréia, galactorréia. SIN galactorrhea. [lacto- + G. *rhoia*, um fluxo]
lac·to·scope (lak′tō - skōp). Lactoscópio. SIN galactoscope. [lacto- + G. *skopeō*, visualizar]
lac·tose (lak′tōs). Lactose; dissacarídeo presente no leite de mamíferos, que ocorre naturalmente como α- e β-l.; obtida do leite de vaca e usada na preparação de leite modificado, no alimento para os neonatos e convalescentes, e nas preparações farmacêuticas; as doses grandes atuam como diurético osmótico e laxativo. O leite humano contém l. a 6,7%. SIN milk sugar, saccharum lactis.
 l. synthase, l. sintase; a enzima responsável pela síntese da l., que catalisa a reação entre UDP-galactose e D-glicose em l. e UDP.
lac·tos·u·ria (lak′tō - soo′rē - ă). Lactosúria; a excreção de lactose (açúcar do leite) na urina; um achado comum durante a gestação e lactação, bem como em neonatos, principalmente nos lactentes prematuros. [lactose + G. *ouron*, urina, + -ia]
lac·to·ther·a·py (lak - tō - thăr′ă - pē). Lactoterapia. SIN galactotherapy.
lactotrophic. Lactotrófico; termo obsoleto para produtor de prolactina.
lac·to·tro·pin (lak - tō - trō′pin). Lactotropina, prolactina. SIN prolactin.
lac·to·veg·e·tar·i·an (lak′tō - vej - ē - tā′rē - ăn). Lactovegetariano. **1.** Alguém que vive sob uma dieta mista de leite e laticínios, ovos e vegetais, mas recusa a carne. **2.** Um vegetariano que consome leite e laticínios, mas não ingere ovos ou carnes nem frutos-do-mar.
lac·to·yl·glu·ta·thi·one ly·ase (lak′tō - il - gloo - tă - thī′ōn). Lactoilglutationa liase; glioxilase I; uma liase que cliva a S-D-lactoilglutationa em glutationa e metilglioxal. SIN aldoketomutase, ketone-aldehyde mutase, methylglyoxalase.
lac·tu·lose (lak′too - lōs). Lactulose; um dissacarídeo sintético usado para tratar a encefalopatia hepática e constipação crônica.
α-lac·tyl·thi·am·in py·ro·phos·phate. α-Lactil-tiamina pirofosfato. SIN active *pyruvate*.
la·cu·na, pl. **la·cu·nae** (lă - koo′nă, - koo′nē). Lacuna, lacunas. **1** [TA]. Um pequeno espaço, cavidade ou depressão. **2.** Um intervalo ou defeito. **3.** Um espaço anormal entre extratos ou entre os elementos celulares da epiderme. **4.** SIN corneal *space*. [L. uma depressão, dim. de *lacus*, uma cavidade, um lago]
 cartilage l., l. cartilaginosa; uma cavidade na matriz cartilaginosa, ocupada por um condrócito. SIN cartilage space.

 cerebral l., l. cerebral; pequena perda circunscrita de tecido cerebral causada pela oclusão de uma das pequenas artérias penetrantes. SIN l. cerebri.
 l. cer′ebri, l. cerebral. SIN cerebral l.
 Howship lacunae, lacunas de Howship; pequenas depressões, fóveas ou sulcos irregulares no osso que está sendo reabsorvido pelos osteoclastos. SIN resorption lacunae.
 intervillous l., l. intervilosas; um dos espaços sanguíneos na placenta em que se projetam as vilosidades coriônicas.
 lateral lacunae [TA], lacunas laterais do seio sagital superior. SIN lateral lacunae of superior sagittal sinus.
 lacunae laterales [TA], lacunas laterais do seio sagital superior. SIN lateral lacunae of superior sagittal sinus.
 lateral lacunae of superior sagittal sinus [TA], lacunas laterais do seio sagital superior; expansões laterais do seio sagital superior da dura-máter, cuja largura comumente aumenta com a idade até que, no muito idoso, elas podem estender-se por 2 cm lateralmente à linha média; as luzes das lacunas revestidas por endotélio geralmente são reduzidas a um labirinto semelhante a uma esponja por numerosas granulações aracnóides e trabéculas durais. SIN lacunae laterales [TA], lateral lacunae [TA], lateral lakes, lateral venous lacunae, parasinoidal sinuses.
 lateral venous lacunae, lacunas laterais do seio sagital superior. SIN lateral lacunae of superior sagittal sinus.
 l. mag′na, l. magna; um recesso no teto da fossa navicular do pênis, formada por uma prega da mucosa, a válvula da fossa navicular.
 Morgagni l., l. de Morgagni. SIN urethral l.
 muscular l., espaço muscular. SIN muscular *space* of retroinguinal *compartment*.
 l. musculo′rum, l. muscular. SIN muscular *space* of retroinguinal compartment.
 l. musculorum retroinguinalis, l. muscular do compartimento retroinguinal. SIN muscular *space* of retroinguinal compartment.
 osseous l., l. óssea; uma cavidade no tecido ósseo ocupada por um osteócito.
 pharyngeal l., l. da faringe; uma depressão próxima à abertura faríngea da tuba auditiva. SIN l. pharyngis.
 l. pharyn′gis, l. da faringe. SIN pharyngeal l.
 resorption lacunae, lacunas de reabsorção. SIN Howship lacunae.
 trophoblastic l., l. trofoblástica; um dos espaços na camada sinciciotrofoblástica inicial do cório antes da formação das vilosidades; nos embriões humanos, o sangue materno entra nesses espaços no 10.º dia; com a diferenciação das vilosidades coriônicas, transformam-se em espaços intervilosos, por vezes chamados de lacunas intervilosas.
 urethral l. [TA], l. uretral; um dos inúmeros pequenos recessos na mucosa da uretra esponjosa, nos quais desembocam os canais das glândulas uretrais. SIN l. urethralis [TA], Morgagni l.
 l. urethra′lis, pl. **lacu′nae urethra′les** [TA], lacuna uretral. SIN urethral l.
 vascular l., espaço vascular do compartimento retroinguinal. SIN vascular *space* of retroinguinal compartment.
 l. vasorum, espaço vascular do espaço retroinguinal. SIN vascular *space* of retroinguinal compartment.
 l. vasorum retroinguinalis [TA], espaço vascular do compartimento retroinguinal. SIN vascular *space* of retroinguinal compartment.
la·cu·nar (lă - koo′năr). Lacunar; relativo a uma lacuna.
la·cu·nule (lă - koo′nool). Lacúnula; uma lacuna muito pequena. [L. mod. *lacunula*, dim. do L. *lacuna*]
la·cus, pl. **la·cus** (lā′kŭs) [TA]. Lago. SIN lake (1). [L. lago]
 l. lacrima′lis [TA], l. lacrimal. SIN lacrimal *lake*.
 l. semina′lis, l. seminal. SIN seminal *lake*.
LAD Abreviatura de leukocyte adhesion *deficiency* (deficiência de adesão leucocitária).
Ladd, William E., cirurgião pediátrico norte-americano, 1880–1967. VER L. *band, operation*.
Ladd-Franklin, Christine, psicóloga norte-americana, 1847–1930. VER Ladd-Franklin *theory*.
Lae·laps echid·ni·nus (lē′laps ē - kid - nī′nŭs). Ácaro espinhoso do rato, um ectoparasita mundialmente comum do rato selvagem da Noruega e ocasionalmente encontrado no camundongo domiciliar, rato algodoado e outros roedores; é o vetor natural do *Hepatozoon muris* e pode transmitir experimentalmente o agente da tularemia. O vírus Junin foi isolado a partir dessa espécie na América do Sul.
Laënnec, René T. H., médico francês, 1781–1826. VER L. *cirrhosis, pearls,* em *pearl*.
la·e·trile (lā′ē - tril). Laetrila; um medicamento supostamente antineoplásico que consiste principalmente em amigdalina derivada de fibras de damasco; seu efeito antitumoral ainda não foi comprovado.
△ **laev-.** VER levo-.
Lafora, Gonzalo Rodriguez, neurologista espanhol, 1887–1971. VER L. *body, body disease, disease*.
lag. Demora. **1.** Mover-se ou progredir mais lentamente que o normal; atrasar-se. **2.** O ato ou condição de se atrasar. **3.** O intervalo de tempo entre uma modificação em uma variável e a consequente alteração em outra variável.

anaphase l., atraso de anáfase; a diminuição da velocidade ou parada na migração normal dos cromossomas durante a anáfase, resultando na exclusão desses cromossomas de uma das células-filhas.

homeostatic l., atraso homeostático; o intervalo em um processo homeostático entre uma modificação do traço controlado e a resposta apropriada, devido aos componentes aferentes, eferentes e centrais. O atraso pode ser uma variável ocasional pura, p.ex., o tempo de espera de um processo exponencial ou o somatório de vários desses processos alcançando qualquer valor maior que zero, mas com uma média consideravelmente maior que zero; por vezes, pode ser determinante, ou quase isso, e com um mínimo bem definido e maior que zero por motivos anatômicos. Por exemplo, as pressões parciais de oxigênio e de dióxido de carbono são controladas nos pulmões, mas baseadas nas informações aferentes oriundas do corpo carotídeo, que já estão ultrapassadas, por causa do tempo de circulação de 10 segundos ou mais entre os dois locais.

la·ge·na, pl. **la·ge·nae** (lā - jē′nä, - jē - nē). **1.** Ceco cupular do ducto coclear. SIN cupular *cecum* of the cochlear duct. **2.** Uma das três partes do labirinto membranoso do ouvido interno dos vertebrados inferiores; nos mamíferos, transforma-se na cóclea. [L. frasco]

lag·ging. Retardo; movimento ventilatório retardado ou diminuído do lado afetado do tórax devido a doença pleural com imobilização muscular ou colapso de um pulmão.

lag·o·morph (lā′gō - morf).Lagomorfo; um membro da ordem Lagomorpha.

Lag·o·mor·pha (lā - gō - mor′fä). Uma ordem de mamíferos herbívoros (classe Eutheria) que se assemelham aos roedores (ordem Rodentia), mas que possuem dois pares de incisivos superiores, um atrás do outro; inclui os coelhos, lebres e lagômios. [G. *lagōs*, lebre, + *morphē*, forma]

lag·oph·thal·mia (lag - of - thal′mē - ä). Lagoftalmia. VER lagophthalmos.

lag·oph·thal·mos, lag·oph·thal·mia (lag - of - thal′mōs, lag - of - thal′mē - ä). Lagoftalmia; uma condição em que o fechamento completo das pálpebras sobre o bulbo do olho é difícil ou impossível. [G. *lagōs*, lebre, + *ophthalmos*, olho]

Lagrange, Pierre F., oftalmologista francês, 1857–1928.

Lahey, Frank H., cirurgião norte-americano, 1880–1935. VER L. forceps.

LAK Abreviatura de limphokine activated killer cells (células destruidoras ativadoras).

lake (lāk) [TA]. Lago. **1.** Uma pequena coleção de líquido. SIN lacus [TA]. **2.** Fazer o plasma sanguíneo ficar avermelhado em consequência da liberação de hemoglobina dos eritrócitos, como ocorre quando os últimos estão suspensos em água. VER TAMBÉM lacuna. [A.S. *lacu*, do L. *lacus*, lago]

capillary l., l. capilar; a massa total de sangue contida nos vasos capilares.

lacrimal l. [TA], a pequena área semelhante a uma cisterna na conjuntiva no ângulo medial do olho, em que as lágrimas se coletam depois de banhar a superfície anterior do globo ocular e o saco conjuntival. SIN lacus lacrimalis [TA], lacrimal bay.

lateral l.'s, lacunas laterais do seio sagital superior. SIN lateral *lacunae* of superior sagittal sinus, em *lacuna*.

seminal l., l. seminal; a cúpula da vagina depois da inseminação. SIN lacus seminalis.

subchorial l., espaço subcorial. SIN subchorial *space*.

venous l.'s, lagos venosos; **(1)** vasos sanguíneos dilatados, azulados e com paredes finas, que esmaecem sob pressão, comumente encontrados nos ouvidos e, menos amiúde, nos lábios e na face e pescoço de homens idosos com a pele lesionada pelo sol; **(2)** cavidades ou canais venosos descontínuos cf. marginal *sinuses* of placenta, em *sinus*; **(3)** na radiografia de crânio, focos arredondados ou ovais, radiotransparentes, nos ossos frontais ou parietais, causados por canais venosos diplóicos dilatados.

Laki-Lorand fac·tor. Fator de Laki-Lorand. Ver em factor.

laky (lā′kē).Pertinente ao aspecto vermelho-vivo transparente do plasma ou soro sanguíneo, desenvolvendo-se em consequência da liberação da hemoglobina por eritrócitos destruídos.

la·li·a·try (lā - lī′ä - trē).Laliatria; o estudo e o tratamento dos distúrbios da fala. [G. *lalia*, fala, balbucio, + *iatria*, medo]

lal·i·o·pho·bia (lal′ē - o - fō′bē - ä). Liofofobia; medo mórbido de falar ou balbuciar. [G. *lalia*, fala, + *phobos*, medo]

Lallemand, Claude F., cirurgião francês, 1790–1853. VER L. *bodies*, em *body*; Trousseau-L. *bodies*, em *body*.

lal·ling (lal′ing). Uma forma de tartamudez em que a fala é quase ininteligível. [G. *laleō*, balbuciar]

Lallouette, Pierre, médico francês. 1711–1792. VER L. *pyramid*.

lal·o·che·zia (lal - ō - kē′zē - ä).Laloquezia; descarga emocional obtida pela pronúncia de palavras indecentes ou obscenas. [G. *lalia*, fala, + *chezo*, aliviar-se]

lal·og·no·sis (lal′og - nō′sis).Lalognose; compreensão e conhecimento da fala. [G. *lalia*, fala, + *gnosis*, conhecimento]

la·lo·ple·gia (la - lō - plē′jē - ä).Laloplegia; paralisia dos músculos ligados ao mecanismo da fala. [G. *lalia*, fala, + *plēgē*, um golpe]

Lamarck, Jean-Baptiste P.A., botânico, zoólogo e filósofo biólogo francês, 1744–1829. VER lamarckian *theory*.

Lamaze, Fernand, obstetra francês, 1890–1957. VER L. *method*.

LAMB Acrônimo de *l*entigines, *a*trial mixoma, *m*ucocutaneous myxomas, e *b*lue nevi (lentigo, mixoma atrial, mixomas mucocutâneos e nevos azuis). VER LAMB *syndrome*.

Lam B. Proteína da membrana externa de bactérias Gram-negativas.

lamb·da (lam′dä).Lambda. **1.** A 11.ª letra do alfabeto grego, λ. **2.** O ponto craniométrico na junção das suturas sagital e lambdóide.

lamb·da·cism (lam′dä - sizm).Lambdacismo. **1.** Pronúncia errônea ou desarticulação da letra *l*. **2.** Substituição da letra *l* pela letra *r*. [G. *lambda*, a letra L]

lamb·doid (lam′doyd). Lambdóide; que se assemelha à letra grega lambda (λ), como a sutura lambdóidea. [lambda + G. *eidos*, semelhança]

Lambert, Edward H., médico norte-americano, *1915. VER L.-Eaton *syndrome*; Eaton-L. *syndrome*.

lam·bert (lam′bert). Uma unidade de brilho; o brilho de uma superfície difusora perfeita que emite ou reflete um fluxo luminoso total de 1 lúmen/cm² de superfície. [J.H. *Lambert*, físico e matemático alemão, 1728–1777]

Lamblia intestinalis (lam′blē - ä in - tes - ti - nā′lis). Denominação obsoleta da *Giardia lamblia*, ainda frequentemente usado, em especial por protozoólogos na antiga União Soviética.

lam·bli·a·sis (lam - blī′ä - sis). Lamblíase, giardíase. SIN giardiasis.

lam·bo lam·bo (lam′bō - lam′bō). Piomiosite tropical. SIN tropical *pyomyositis*.

Lambrinudi, Constantine, cirurgião ortopédico britânico, 1890–1943. VER Lambrinudi *operation*.

la·mel·la, pl. **la·mel·lae** (lä - mel′ä, - mel′ē) [TA]. Lamela. **1** [TA]. Uma lâmina ou camada fina (como a que ocorre no osso compacto) ou subcamada. **2.** Uma preparação na forma de um disco gelatinoso de medicamento, usado como um meio de fazer aplicações locais na conjuntiva em lugar das soluções. SIN discus [TA], disk (2) [TA]. [L. dim. de *lamina*, placa, folha]

annulate lamellae, lamelas anulares; vários pares de membranas lisas e paralelas, com cada par contendo poros regularmente espaçados que se assemelham aos do envelope nuclear; elas ocorrem nas células germinativas, células embrionárias e células neoplásicas.

articular l., l. articular; a camada compacta de osso, em sua superfície articular, que está firmemente presa à cartilagem articular suprajacente.

l. of bone, l. óssea; uma l. concêntrica, circunferencial ou intersticial.

circumferential l., l. circunferencial; uma l. óssea que envolve a superfície externa ou interna de um osso.

concentric l., l. concêntrica; uma das camadas tubulares concêntricas de osso que circundam o canal central em um ósteon. SIN haversian l.

cornoid l., l. cornóide; uma estreita coluna vertical de paraceratose no estrato córneo epidérmico; característica da poroceratose.

elastic l., l. elástica; uma lâmina fina ou membrana composta de fibras elásticas; diferenciada da membrana elástica, que, em geral, se refere a uma massa condensada de fibras, como em uma artéria, enquanto uma l. elástica pode ser uma camada elástica mais frouxa, como a encontrada em uma veia ou no trato respiratório.

enamel l., l. do esmalte; defeito orgânico no esmalte; uma estrutura fina, semelhante a uma folha, que se estende desde a superfície do esmalte no sentido da junção dentinoesmalte.

glandulopreputial l., l. glandulopreputial; uma camada de tecido epitelial embrionário que origina o prepúcio.

ground l., l. fundamental. SIN interstitial l.

haversian l., l. de Havers. SIN concentric l.

intermediate l., l. intermediária. SIN interstitial l.

interstitial l., l. intersticial; uma das lamelas dos ósteons parcialmente reabsorvidos que ocorrem entre os ósteons completos mais novos. SIN ground l., intermediary system, intermediate l.

triangular l., l. triangular. SIN tela *choroidea* of third ventricle.

l. tympanica (laminae spiralis ossei) [TA], l. timpânica (das lâminas ósseas espirais) da cóclea. SIN tympanic l. (of osseous spiral lamina).

tympanic l. (of osseous spiral lamina) [TA], l. timpânica (da lâmina óssea espiral) da cóclea; a mais fina das duas placas de osso, separadas de forma incompleta entre si por canais para fibras periféricas derivadas do gânglio espiral (coclear), que compreendem, em conjunto, a lâmina espiral óssea; essa placa situa-se no lado da rampa do tímpano, que forma uma parte de sua parede. SIN l. tympanica (laminae spiralis ossei) [TA].

l. vestibularis (laminae spiralis ossei) [TA], l. vestibular (das lâminas espirais ósseas) da cóclea. SIN vestibular l. (of osseous spiral lamina).

vestibular l. (of osseous spiral lamina) [TA], lamela vestibular (da lâmina espiral óssea) da cóclea; a camada mais espessa de duas placas ósseas, separadas de forma incompleta por canais para as fibras periféricas originárias do gânglio espiral da cóclea, que compreendem, em conjunto, a lâmina espiral óssea; essa placa situa-se no lado da rampa do vestíbulo; espessamento do periósteo, o limbo espiral, insere-se na lamela vestibular no canal coclear. SIN l. vestibularis (laminae spiralis ossei) [TA].

vitreous l., l. basilar da corióide. SIN lamina basalis choroideae.

lam·el·lar (lam′e - lär, lä - mel′är). Lamelar, lamelado **1.** Disposto em finas placas ou escamas. SIN lamelate, lamellated. **2.** Relativo às lamelas.

lam·el·late, lam·el·lat·ed (lam′e - lāt, - ed). Lamelado; SIN lamellar (1).

la·mel·li·po·di·um, pl. **la·mel·li·po·dia** (lä - mel - i - pō′dē - ŭm, - ä). Lamelipódio; um véu citoplasmático produzido em todos os lados dos leucócitos polimorfonucleares migratórios.

LAMINA

lam·i·na, pl. **lam·i·nae** (lam′i-nă, lam′i-nē)[TA]. Lâmina. SIN plate (1). VER TAMBÉM layer, stratum. [L.]
l. affix′a [TA], l. afixa; a parte da parede ependimária medial do ventrículo lateral do cérebro embrionário que, no desenvolvimento posterior, adere à superfície superior do tálamo e, dessa maneira, forma o assoalho da parte central do ventrículo lateral; cobre as veias tálamo-estriada e coróides.
l. ala′ris, l. alar. SIN alar l. of neural tube.
alar l. of neural tube, l. alar do tubo neural; a divisão dorsal das paredes laterais do tubo neural no embrião; dá origem aos neurônios que retransmitem os impulsos aferentes para os centros superiores; no adulto, esses neurônios compõem os núcleos sensoriais da medula espinal e do tronco cerebral. SIN alar plate of neural tube, dorsolateral plate of neural tube, l. alaris, l. dorsalis, wing plate.
lam′inae al′bae cerebel′li, lâminas medulares do cerebelo; camadas de substância branca observadas no corte do cerebelo. SIN laminae medullares cerebelli.
l. anterior fasciae thoracolumbalis [TA], l. anterior da aponeurose toracolombar. SIN anterior layer of thoracolumbar fascia.
anterior limiting l. [TA], l. limitante anterior; a periferia da córnea que determina o término da membrana de Descemet e a borda anterior da rede trabecular; um marco importante na gonioscopia. SIN l. limitans anterior [TA], anterior limiting ring, Schwalbe ring.
l. ante′rior vagi′nae mus′culi rec′ti abdo′minis, l. anterior da bainha do músculo reto do abdome. SIN anterior layer of rectus sheath.
l. ar′cus ver′tebrae [TA], l. do arco vertebral. SIN l. of vertebral arch.
basal l., l. basal; **(1)** uma camada extracelular amorfa aplicada à superfície basal do epitélio e que também reveste as células musculares, células adiposas e células de Schwann; acredita-se que seja um filtro seletivo e tenha funções estrutural e morfogenética. É composta de uma rede de 20–100 nm de filamentos chamados de l. densa, que parece densa no microscópio eletrônico, e, em ambos ao lado dessa camada, está uma camada menos densa, a l. rara. VER TAMBÉM basement membrane, l. densa; **(2)** l. densa. SIN l. densa.
basal l. of choroid [TA], l. basilar da coróide. SIN l. basalis choroideae.
basal l. of ciliary body [TA], l. basilar do corpo ciliar; a camada interna do corpo ciliar, contínua com a camada basal da coróide e que sustenta o epitélio pigmentar da retina ciliar. SIN l. basilaris corporis ciliaris [TA], basal layer of ciliary body, l. basalis corporis ciliaris.
basal l. of cochlear duct [TA], l. basilar da parede timpânica do ducto coclear; a l. que se estende da lâmina espiral óssea até a crista basilar da cóclea; forma a maior parte do assoalho do canal coclear, separando o último da rampa do tímpano, e sustenta o órgão de Corti. SIN l. basilaris ductus cochlearis [TA], basilar l., basilar membrane of cochlear duct, l. basilaris cochleae, membrana basilaris.

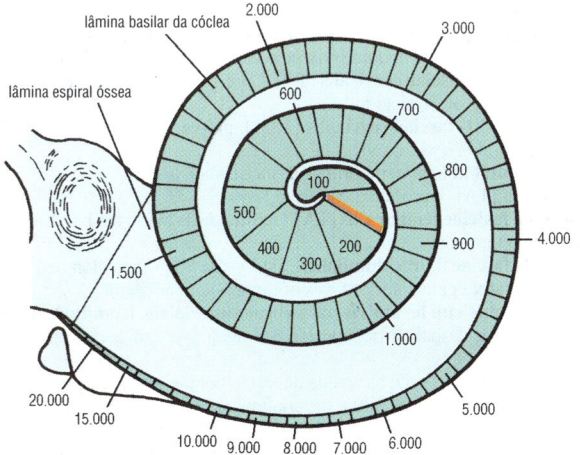

membrana basilar: a figura indica as freqüências sonoras em Hz pertinentes a cada local

l. basalis, l. basal. SIN basal l. of neural tube.
l. basa′lis choroi′deae [TA], lâmina basilar da coróide, a camada interna transparente, quase sem estrutura, da coróide em contato com a camada pigmentada da retina. SIN basal l. of choroid [TA], basal layer of choroid [TA], Bruch membrane, Henle membrane, l. vitrea, vitreous lamella, vitreous membrane (3).
l. basalis corporis ciliaris, l. basilar do corpo ciliar. SIN basal l. of ciliary body.
basal l. of neural tube, l. basal do tubo neural; a divisão central das paredes laterais do tubo neural no embrião; contém neuroblastos que originam os neurônios motores somáticos e viscerais. SIN basal plate of neural tube, l. basalis, l. ventralis, ventral plate of neural tube.
basal l. of semicircular duct, l. basilar dos canais semicirculares. SIN basal membrane of semicircular duct.
basement l., l. basilar da parede timpânica do ducto coclear. SIN basement membrane.
basilar l., l. basilar da parede timpânica do ducto coclear. SIN basal l. of cochlear duct.
l. basilaris cochleae, l. basilar da parede timpânica do ducto coclear. SIN basal l. of cochlear duct.
l. basilaris corporis ciliaris [TA], l. basilar do corpo ciliar. SIN basal l. of ciliary body.
l. basilaris ductus cochlearis [TA], l. basilar da parede timpânica do ducto coclear. SIN basal l. of cochlear duct.
boundary l., l. limitante; uma estrutura semelhante à membrana basal que reveste as células musculares, células adiposas e células de Schwann. VER TAMBÉM basement membrane, basal l.
capillary l. of choroid [TA], l. corioideocapilar; a porção interna ou profunda da coróide do olho, composta de uma rede capilar muito próxima. SIN l. choroidocapillaris [TA], choriocapillaris, choriocapillary layer, entochoroidea, l. chorocapillaris, membrana choriocapillaris, Ruysch membrane.
l. cartilag′inis cricoi′deae [TA], l. da cartilagem cricóidea. SIN l. of cricoid cartilage.
l. cartilag′inis thyroi′deae [TA], l. da cartilagem tireóidea. SIN l. of thyroid cartilage.
l. choriocapilla′ris, l. corioideocapilar. SIN capillary l. of choroid.
l. choroi′dea, l. epitelial. SIN epithelial l.
l. choroi′dea epithelia′lis, l. epitelial. SIN epithelial l.
l. choroidocapilla′ris [TA], l. corioideocapilar. SIN capillary l. of choroid.
l. cine′rea, l. terminal do cérebro. SIN l. terminalis of cerebrum.
l. cribro′sa os′sis ethmoida′lis [TA], l. cribriforme do osso etmóide. SIN cribriform plate of ethmoid bone.
l. cribrosa of sclera [TA], l. cribriforme da esclera; a porção da esclerótica através da qual passam as fibras do nervo óptico. SIN l. cribrosa sclerae [TA], cribrous l., perforated layer of sclera.
l. cribro′sa scle′rae [TA], l. cribriforme da esclera. SIN l. cribrosa of sclera.
cribrous l., l. cribriforme da esclera. SIN l. cribrosa of sclera.
l. of cricoid cartilage [TA], l. da cartilagem cricóidea; uma placa quadrada que forma a parte posterior da cartilagem cricóidea. Ela assemelha-se ao escudo de um anel de sinete, com o arco da cricóide representando o restante do anel. SIN l. cartilaginis cricoideae [TA].
deep l., l. profunda. SIN deep layer.
l. den′sa, l. densa; **(1)** a camada elétron-densa da l. basal, conforme observada no microscópio eletrônico. VER TAMBÉM basement membrane; **(2)** a l. basal extraordinariamente espessa do glomérulo renal. SIN basal l. (2).
dental l., l. dentária. SIN dental ledge.
l. denta′ta, lábio do limbo vestibular do limbo espiral. SIN vestibular lip of spiral limbus.
dentogingival l., l. dentogengival. SIN dental ledge.
l. dorsa′lis, l. dorsal. SIN alar l. of neural tube.
l. du′ra, l. dura; a camada dura que reveste os alvéolos dentários.
l. elas′tica ante′rior, l. limitante anterior da córnea. SIN anterior limiting layer of cornea.
l. elas′tica poste′rior, l. limitante posterior da córnea. SIN posterior limiting l. of cornea.
elastic laminae of arteries, lâminas elásticas das artérias; 1) externa: a camada de tecido conjuntivo elástico que se localiza imediatamente externo à musculatura lisa da túnica média; 2) interna: uma camada fenestrada de tecido elástico da túnica íntima. SIN elastic layers of arteries, Henle fenestrated elastic membrane.
l. epiphysialis [TA], placa epifisária. SIN epiphysial plate.
episcleral l., l. episcleral. SIN episcleral layer of fibrous layer of eyeball.
l. episclera′lis [TA], l. episcleral da túnica fibrosa do bulbo. SIN episcleral layer of fibrous layer of eyeball.
epithelial l., l. epitelial; a camada de células ependimárias modificadas que formam a camada interna da tela corióidea, de frente para o ventrículo. SIN epithelial choroid layer, l. choroidea epithelialis, l. choroidea, l. epithelialis.
l. epithelialis, l. epitelial. SIN epithelial l.
l. externa calvaria [TA], l. externa da calvária. SIN external table of calvaria.
l. exter′na cra′nii, l. externa da calvária. SIN external table of calvaria.
external medullary l. [TA], l. medular externa. VER medullary laminae of thalamus.
l. fibrocartilagin′ea interpu′bica, disco interpúbico. SIN interpubic disk.
l. fibroreticula′ris, l. fibrorreticular; uma camada da membrana basal em continuidade com o tecido conjuntivo associado; com freqüência, é descontínua e, em alguns casos, pode estar totalmente ausente.
l. fusca of sclera, l. supracoróide da esclera. SIN suprachoroid l. of sclera.

l. fusca sclerae [TA], l. supracorióide da esclera. SIN suprachoroid l. of sclera.
hepatic laminae, lâminas hepáticas; as placas de células hepáticas que se irradiam do centro do lóbulo do fígado.
l. horizonta'lis os'sis palati'ni [TA], l. horizontal do palatino; SIN horizontal plate of palatine bone.
l. interna calvariae [TA], l. interna da calvária. SIN internal table of calvaria.
l. inter'na cra'nii, l. interna da calvária. SIN internal table of calvaria.
internal medullary l. [TA], l. medular interna. VER medullary laminae of thalamus.
l. interna ossium cranii, l. interna dos ossos do crânio. SIN vitreous table.
iridopupillary l., l. iridopupilar; precursor embrionário do estroma anterior da íris que forma a parede interna (posterior ou profunda) da câmara anterior primária do olho. Sua porção central torna-se atenuada como a membrana pupilar (membrana pupillaris [NA]).
labiogingival l., l. labiogengival; uma faixa de células epiteliais ectodérmicas que se desenvolve no mesênquima da mandíbula embrionária, entre o lábio em desenvolvimento e a elevação gengival em crescimento; mais adiante, abre-se para formar o sulco labiogengival.
lateral l. of cartilage of pharyngotympanic (auditory) tube [TA], l. lateral da cartilagem da tuba auditiva. SIN l. lateralis cartilaginis tubae auditivae [TA], l. lateralis cartilaginis tubae auditoriae*, lateral cartilaginous plate, lateral plate of cartilaginous auditory tube.
l. latera'lis cartila'ginis tu'bae auditi'vae [TA], l. lateral da cartilagem da tuba auditiva. SIN lateral l. of cartilage of pharyngotympanic (auditory) tube.
l. latera'lis cartilag'inis tubae auditoriae, l. lateral da cartilagem da tuba auditiva; *termo oficial alternativo para lateral l. of cartilage of pharyngotympanic (auditory) tube.
l. latera'lis proces'sus pterygoid'ei [TA], l. lateral do processo pterigóide. SIN lateral pterygoid plate.
lateral medullary l. [TA] **of lentiform nucleus**, l. medular lateral do núcleo lentiforme; uma camada fina e bem definida de fibras que separam o putame do globo pálido. SIN l. medullaris lateralis nuclei lentiformis [TA].
l. of lens, l. da lente; uma da série de camadas concêntricas compostas de fibras da lente que constituem a substância da lente.
l. limitans anterior [TA], l. limitante anterior. SIN anterior limiting l.
l. lim'itans ante'rior cor'neae, l. limitante anterior da córnea. SIN anterior limiting layer of cornea.
l. lim'itans poste'rior cor'neae, l. limitante posterior da córnea. SIN posterior limiting l. of cornea.
l. lu'cida, l. lúcida; a camada levemente corável da membrana basal em contato com o plasmalema das células epiteliais ou de outras células que possuem um revestimento de membrana basal.
medial l. of cartilage of pharyngotympanic (auditory) tube [TA], l. medial da cartilagem da tuba auditiva; a ampla porção medial da parte cartilaginosa da tuba auditiva. SIN l. medialis cartilaginis tubae auditivae [TA], l. medialis cartilaginis tubae auditoriae*, medial cartilaginous plate, medial plate of cartilaginous auditory tube.
l. media'lis cartila'ginis tu'bae auditi'vae [TA], l. medial da cartilagem da tuba auditiva. SIN medial l. of cartilage of pharyngotympanic (auditory) tube.
l. media'lis cartilag'inis tubae auditoriae, l. medial da cartilagem da tuba auditiva; *termo oficial alternativo para medial l. of cartilage of pharyngotympanic (auditory) tube.
l. media'lis proces'sus pterygoi'dei [TA], l. medial do processo pterigóide. SIN medial pterygoid plate.
medial medullary l. [TA] **of lentiform nucleus**, l. medular medial do núcleo lentiforme; uma camada de fibras que separa os segmentos lateral e medial do globo pálido. SIN l. medullaris medialis nuclei lentiformis [TA].
lam'inae medulla'res cerebel'li, lâminas medulares do cerebelo. SIN laminae albae cerebelli.
lam'inae medulla'res thal'ami, lâminas medulares do tálamo. SIN medullary laminae of thalamus.
l. medullaris lateralis [TA], l. medular lateral. VER medullary laminae of thalamus.
l. medulla'ris latera'lis nuclei lentiformis [TA], l. medular lateral do núcleo lentiforme. SIN lateral medullary l. [TA] of lentiform nucleus.
l. medullaris medialis [TA], l. medular medial. VER medullary laminae of thalamus.
l. medulla'ris media'lis nuclei lentiformis [TA], l. medular medial do núcleo lentiforme. SIN medial medullary l. [TA] of lentiform nucleus.
medullary laminae of thalamus, lâminas medulares do tálamo; camadas de fibras mielinizadas que aparecem nos cortes transversais do tálamo; a l. medular lateral [TA] (external medullary lamina [TA]) marca as bordas ventral e lateral do tálamo e o delimitam do subtálamo e núcleo reticular do tálamo; a l. medular medial [TA] (internal medullary lamina [TA]) fica interposta entre os núcleos mediodorsal e ventral do tálamo e engloba os núcleos intralaminares (núcleos centromediano, paracentral e lateral central). SIN laminae medullares thalami, medullary layers of thalamus.
l. membrana'cea cartila'ginis tu'bae auditi'vae [TA], l. membranácea da cartilagem da tuba auditiva. SIN membranous l. of cartilage of pharyngotympanic (auditory) plate.

l. membranacea cartilaginis tubae auditoriae, l. membranácea da cartilagem da tuba auditiva; *termo oficial alternativo para membranous l. of cartilage of pharyngotympanic (auditory) plate.
membranous l. of cartilage of pharyngotympanic (auditory) plate [TA], l. membranácea da cartilagem da tuba auditiva; a membrana de tecido conjuntivo que, com as lâminas lateral e medial, completa as paredes lateral e inferior da parte cartilaginosa da tuba auditiva. SIN l. membranacea cartilaginis tubae auditivae [TA], l. membranacea cartilaginis tubae auditoriae*, membranous layer.
l. of mesencephalic tectum, l. do teto do mesencéfalo; a lâmina do teto do mesencéfalo formado pelos corpos quadrigêmeos. SIN l. tecti [TA], tectal plate [TA], tectum mesencephali [TA], l. quadrigemina, quadrigeminal l., quadrigeminal plate, tectum of midbrain.
l. modi'oli cochleae [TA], l. do modíolo da cóclea. SIN l. of modiolus of cochlea.
l. of modiolus of cochlea [TA], l. do modíolo da cóclea; uma placa óssea, a continuação do modíolo e do septo entre as convoluções do canal espiral da cóclea, que se estende para cima, em direção à cúpula, formando, com o hâmulo, o helicotrema. SIN l. modioli cochleae [TA], plate of modiolus.
l. molecularis corticis cerebri [TA], l. molecular do córtex cerebral. SIN molecular layer of cerebral cortex.
l. muscula'ris muco'sae, l. muscular da mucosa. SIN muscularis mucosae.
nuclear l., l. nuclear; uma camada rica em proteína que reveste a superfície interna da membrana nuclear nas células em interfase.
orbital l. of ethmoid bone, l. orbital do osso etmóide. SIN orbital plate of ethmoid bone.
l. orbita'lis os'sis ethmoida'lis [TA], l. orbital do osso etmóide; SIN orbital plate of ethmoid bone.
osseous spiral l. [TA], l. espiral óssea; uma placa dupla de osso que se espirala ao redor do modíolo, dividindo de maneira incompleta o canal espiral da cóclea em dois, ou seja, a rampa do tímpano e a rampa do vestíbulo; entre as duas placas dessa lâmina, as fibras do nervo coclear alcançam o órgão espiral (de Corti). SIN l. spiralis ossea [TA], spiral plate.
l. papyra'cea, l. orbital do osso etmóide. SIN orbital plate of ethmoid bone.
l. parieta'lis [TA], l. parietal. SIN parietal layer.
l. parietalis pericar'dii serosi [TA], l. parietal do pericárdio seroso. SIN parietal layer of serous pericardium.
l. parietalis tu'nicae vagina'lis tes'tis [TA], l. parietal da túnica vaginal do testículo. SIN parietal layer of tunica vaginalis of testis.
periclaustral l., l. periclaustral. SIN external capsule.
l. perpendicula'ris [TA], l. perpendicular. SIN perpendicular plate.
l. perpendicula'ris os'sis ethmoida'lis [TA], l. perpendicular do etmóide. SIN perpendicular plate of ethmoid bone.
l. perpendicula'ris os'sis palati'ni [TA], l. perpendicular do palatino. SIN perpendicular plate of palatine bone.
posterior limiting l. of cornea [TA], l. limitante posterior da córnea; uma camada acelular homogênea transparente entre a substância própria e a camada endotelial da córnea; considerado como sendo uma membrana basal muito desenvolvida. SIN Descemet membrane, Duddell membrane, entocornea, hyaloid membrane, l. elastica posterior, l. limitans posterior corneae, membrana hyaloidea, membrana vitrea, posterior elastic layer, posterior limiting layer of cornea, tunica vitrea, vitreous membrane (1).
l. poste'rior vagi'nae mus'culi rec'ti abdo'minis [TA], l. posterior da bainha do músculo reto do abdome. SIN posterior layer of rectus sheath.
l. pretrachea'lis fasciae cervicalis [TA], l. pré-traqueal da fáscia cervical. SIN pretracheal layer of cervical fascia.
l. prevertebra'lis fasciae cervicalis [TA], l. pré-vertebral da fáscia cervical. SIN prevertebral layer of cervical fascia.
primary dental l., l. dentária primária. SIN dental ledge.
l. profun'da [TA], l. profunda. SIN deep layer.
l. profunda fas'ciae tempora'lis [TA], l. profunda da fáscia temporal. SIN deep layer of temporal fascia.
l. profunda fasciae thoracolumbalis, l. anterior da fáscia toracolombar; *termo oficial alternativo para anterior layer of thoracolumbar fascia.
l. profunda mus'culi levato'ris pal'pebrae superio'ris, l. profunda do músculo levantador da pálpebra superior. SIN deep layer of levator palpebrae superioris.
l. propria [TA], l. própria; a camada de tecido conjuntivo que fica subjacente ao epitélio de uma mucosa. SIN l. propria mucosae.
l. pro'pria muco'sae, l. própria da mucosa. SIN l. propria.
pterygoid laminae, lâminas pterigóides. VER lateral pterygoid plate, medial pterygoid plate.
l. quadrigem'ina, l. do teto do mesencéfalo. SIN l. of mesencephalic tectum.
quadrigeminal l., l. do teto do mesencéfalo. SIN l. of mesencephalic tectum.
l. ra'ra, l. rara; a camada relativamente elétron-transparente em ambos os lados da l. densa da membrana basal.
reticular l., l. reticular; **(1)** um componente importante da membrana basal, conforme observado à microscopia óptica; consiste, em grande parte, em fibras reticulares e substância fundamental; **(2)** a placa de tecido conjuntivo em que estão embebidas as terminações que sustentam os cílios das células sensoriais auditivas do órgão de Corti.

retrorectal l. of endopelvic fascia, fáscia pré-sacral. SIN presacral *fascia*.
retrorectal l. of hypogastric sheath, fáscia pré-sacral. SIN presacral *fascia*.
l. retrorectalis fasciae endopelvicae, fáscia pré-sacral. SIN presacral *fascia*.
l. of Rexed, l. de Rexed; uma divisão da substância cinzenta da medula espinal dentro de nove lâminas (I–IX) e uma área cinzenta ao redor do canal central (área X) baseada nos aspectos da citoarquitetura; o corno dorsal (posterior) é composto pelas lâminas I–VI, zona intermediária da lâmina VII e corno ventral das lâminas VIII e IX; a correlação geral das lâminas com alguns dos núcleos principais: I, núcleo posteromarginal; II, substância gelatinosa; III e IV, núcleo próprio do corno dorsal; V e VI, por vezes descrito como contendo a formação reticular espinal; VII, núcleo de Clarke, coluna celular intermediolateral; VIII, núcleo comissural, interneurônios; IX, núcleos motores do corno ventral.
rostral l., l. rostral; uma linha esbranquiçada observada nos cortes perfeitamente medianos do cérebro como uma fina ponte que une o rostro do corpo caloso com a lâmina terminal; a l. rostral não contém fibras comissurais; em lugar disso, ela corresponde à linha ao longo da qual a pia-máter reflete da superfície medial de um hemisfério para a do outro. SIN l. rostralis, rostral layer, taeniola corporis callosi.
l. rostra'lis, l. rostral. SIN rostral l.
secondary spiral l. [TA], l. espiral secundária; uma crista na parede externa da primeira volta da cóclea oposta à l. espiral. SIN l. spiralis secundaria [TA], secondary spiral plate.
l. sep'ti pellu'cidi, l. do septo pelúcido. SIN l. of septum pellucidum.
l. of septum pellucidum, l. do septo pelúcido; uma das duas camadas finas do septo pelúcido que se estendem desde o corpo caloso até o fórnice; freqüentemente separadas entre si por um espaço, a cavidade do septo pelúcido. SIN l. septi pellucidi.
spinal l. II, l. espinal II, substância gelatinosa; *termo oficial alternativo para gelatinous *substance*.
l. spinalis II, l. espinal II, substância gelatinosa; *termo oficial alternativo para gelatinous *substance*.
l. spira'lis os'sea [TA], l. espiral óssea. SIN osseous spiral l.
l. spira'lis secunda'ria [TA], l. espiral secundária. SIN secondary spiral l.
successional l., l. de sucessão; um brotamento ectodérmico no lado labial da l. dental que se desenvolve em um dente permanente.
superficial l., l. superficial. SIN superficial *layer*.
l. superficia'lis [TA], l. superficial. SIN superficial *layer*.
l. superficia'lis fas'ciae cervica'lis [TA], l. superficial da fáscia cervical. SIN investing *layer* of cervical fascia.
l. superficia'lis fas'ciae tempora'lis [TA], l. superficial da fáscia temporal. SIN superficial *layer* of temporal fascia.
l. superficia'lis mus'culi levato'ris pal'pebrae superio'ris, l. superficial do músculo levantador da pálpebra superior. SIN superficial *layer* of the levator palpebrae superioris.
suprachoroid l. of sclera [TA], l. fosca da esclera; uma camada excessivamente delicada de tecido conjuntivo pigmentado frouxo, entre a superfície interna da esclera e a superfície externa da corióide, unindo-as; originalmente, a l. fusca e a l. supracorióide eram consideradas duas camadas adjacentes. SIN l. fusca sclerae [TA], brown layer, ectochoroidea, l. fusca os sclera, membrana fusca, suprachoroidea.
l. supraneuropor'ica, aquela parte da membrana corióide do terceiro ventrículo que forma o teto do forame de Monro.
l. tec'ti [TA], l. do teto do mesencéfalo. SIN l. of mesencephalic tectum.
l. termina'lis [TA], l. terminal. SIN l. terminalis of cerebrum.
l. terminalis of cerebrum [TA], l. terminal; uma fina placa que se dirige para cima, a partir do quiasma óptico, e que forma o limite rostral do terceiro ventrículo; a membrana que fecha o neuroporo rostral. SIN l. terminalis [TA], l. cinerea, terminal plate, velum terminale.
l. of thyroid cartilage [TA], l. da cartilagem tireóidea; uma das placas quadrilaterais finas pareadas (esquerda e direita) que são unidas anteriormente e formam um ângulo aberto, posteriormente. SIN l. cartilaginis thyroideae [TA].
tragal l. [TA], l. do trago; uma placa curva longitudinal da cartilagem, o início da porção cartilaginosa do meato acústico externo. SIN l. tragi [TA], l. of tragus.
l. tra'gi [TA], l. do trago. SIN tragal l.
l. of tragus, l. do trago. SIN tragal l.
vascular l. of choroid [TA], l. vascular da corióide; a porção externa ou superficial da corióide do olho, que contém os vasos sanguíneos mais calibrosos. SIN l. vasculosa choroideae [TA], Haller vascular tissue, uvaeformis, vascular layer of choroid coat of eye, vascular layer.
l. vasculo'sa choroi'deae [TA], l. vascular da corióide. SIN vascular l. of choroid.
l. ventra'lis, l. basilar do tubo neural. SIN basal l. of neural tube.
l. of vertebral arch [TA], l. do arco vertebral; a porção posterior achatada do arco vertebral que se estende entre os pedículos e a linha média, formando a parede dorsal do forame vertebral, e de cuja junção na linha média se estende o processo espinhoso. SIN l. arcus vertebrae [TA], neurapophysis.
l. viscera'lis [TA], camada visceral. SIN visceral *layer*.
l. viscera'lis pericar'dii, l. visceral do pericárdio. SIN visceral *layer* of serous pericardium.
l. viscera'lis tu'nicae vagina'lis tes'tis [TA], l. visceral da túnica vaginal do testículo. SIN visceral *layer* of tunica vaginalis of testis.
l. vit'rea, l. basilar da corióide. SIN l. basalis choroideae.

lam·i·na·gram (lam'i-nă-gram). Laminograma; uma imagem feita por laminografia (q.v.). VER TAMBÉM tomography.
lam·i·na·graph (lam'i-nă-graf). Laminógrafo; um aparelho para a laminografia; um laminograma.
lam·i·nag·ra·phy, lam·i·nog·ra·phy (lami-nahg'ră-fē, lam-i-nog'-ră-fē). Laminografia; a técnica radiográfica em que as imagens dos tecidos acima e abaixo do plano de interesse são borradas pelo movimento recíproco do tubo de raios X e do chassi, para mostrar com maior nitidez uma área específica. VER TAMBÉM tomography. [lamina + G. *graphē*, uma escrita]
lam·i·nar (lam'i-nar). Laminar. **1.** Disposto em placas ou lâminas. SIN laminated. **2.** Relativo a qualquer lâmina.
lam·i·nar·ia (lam-i-nā'rē-ă). Lamináría; bastão estéril feito de algas (gênero *Laminaria*) que é hidrofílico e, quando colocado no canal cervical, absorve a umidade, intumesce e dilata gradualmente o colo. [L. *lamina*, uma lâmina]
lam·i·na·rin (lam-i-nar'in). Laminarina; um polissacarídeo de algas, constituído principalmente de resíduos β-D-glicose, obtidos de espécies de *Laminaria* (família Laminariaceae); proporções variáveis de cadeias de glicose contêm, na extremidade redutora potencial, uma molécula de manitol que pode ser sulfatada.
l. sulfate, sulfato de laminária; l. sulfatada em graus variados; dois grupamentos sulfato por unidade de glicose resultam na estabilidade máxima e na atividade anticoagulante similar à da heparina; a l. com menos grupamentos sulfato possui apenas atividade antilipêmica.
lam·i·nat·ed (lam'i-nāt-ed). Laminado. SIN laminar (1).
lam·i·na·tion (lam-i-nā'shŭn). Laminação. **1.** Disposição na forma de placas ou lâminas. **2.** Embriotomia por retirada da cabeça fetal em fatias.
lam·i·nec·to·my (lam'i-nek'tō-mē). Laminectomia; a excisão de uma lâmina vertebral; termo comumente empregado para indicar a retirada do arco posterior. [L. *lamina*, camada, + G. *ektomē*, excisão]
lam·i·nin (lam'i-nin). Laminina; um grande componente glicoproteico multimérico da membrana basal; principalmente de suas lâminas não-coradas; um importante componente proteico das lâminas do glomérulo renal.
lam·i·ni·tis (lam-i-nī'tis). Laminite; a inflamação de qualquer lâmina.
lam·i·nog·ra·phy (lam-i-nog'-ră-fē). Laminografia. VER laminagraphy.
lam·i·not·o·my (lam-'i-not'ō-mē). Laminotomia; a excisão de uma parte de uma lâmina vertebral, na qual o forame intervertebral é aumentado pela remoção de uma parte da lâmina. SIN rachiotomy. [L. *lamina*, camada, + G. *tomē*, incisão]
lam·ins (lam'inz). Rede fibrosa associada às membranas internas dos núcleos das células, composta de polipeptídeos de pesos moleculares variados (60.000 a 80.000) e classificados como A, B, C, etc., com base nas propriedades físicas; a fosforilação da l. está associada à mitose.
lam·o·tri·gine (lă-mō'trī-jen). Lamotrigina; uma nova classe estrutural de antiepilépticos; um anticonvulsivante que parece, nos estudos pré-clínicos, assemelhar-se à fenitoína.
lamp (lamp). Lâmpada; dispositivo de iluminação; fonte de luz. VER TAMBÉM light.
annealing l., uma l. de álcool com uma chama livre empregada em odontologia para retirar a camada de gás protetora NH_3 da superfície da folha de ouro coesiva.
Edridge-Green l., l. de Edridge-Green; uma lanterna utilizada para testar a identificação de sinais coloridos; emite uma luz única com filtros coloridos em discos rotatórios, que podem ser modificados para simular as condições do tempo e atmosfera. Esse teste para a cegueira para cores foi oficialmente adotado na Grã-Bretanha em 1915, em lugar do teste de Holmgren, mas é raramente utilizado hoje em dia.
heat l., l. de calor; uma lâmpada que emite luz infravermelha e produz calor; empregada para aplicação de calor tópico na pele.
mercury vapor l., l. de vapor de mercúrio; uma lâmpada em que o arco elétrico está em uma atmosfera de vapor de mercúrio ionizado; produz luz ultravioleta que pode ser usada de forma terapêutica ou em fotometria diagnóstica.
mignon l., lâmpada elétrica diminuta utilizada em diversos instrumentos endoscópicos.
slit l., de fenda; uma combinação de microscópio e um feixe estreito de luz colimada, empregada para examinar os olhos.
spirit l., l. usada principalmente para aquecimento no trabalho laboratorial, na qual álcool é queimado.
tungsten arc l., l. de arco de tungstênio; uma l. que possui elementos de tungstênio bastante comprimidos.
ultraviolet l., l. ultravioleta; uma l. que emite raios na faixa ultravioleta do espectro. VER TAMBÉM ultraviolet.
Wood l., l. de Wood; uma l. ultravioleta com um filtro de óxido de níquel que permite a passagem apenas da luz com um comprimento de onda máximo de cerca de 3.660 Å; usada para detectar, através de fluorescência, os pêlos infectados por *Microsporum audouinii*, *M. canis*, var. *distortum*, ou *M. ferrugineum*, produzindo fluorescência amarelo-esverdeada.

Lamy, Maurice, médico francês, 1895–1975. VER Maroteaux-L. *syndrome.*

la·na, gen. e pl. **la·nae** (lan'ă, lan'ē).Lã. SIN wool. [L.]

la·nat·o·side D (lā - nat'ō - sīd).Lanatosídeo D; um glicosídeo digitálico obtido das folhas da *Digitalis lanata,* que fornece a genina diginatigenina (12-hidroxigitoxigenina; 16-hidroxidigoxigenina).

la·nat·o·sides A, B e C (lā - nat'ō - sīdz).Lanatosídeos A, B e C; digilanídeos A, B e C; os glicosídeos precursores cardioativos obtidos da *Digitalis lanata.* A retirada do grupamento acetil fornece os desacetilanatosídeos A, B e C (glicosídeos purpúreos A, B e C, respectivamente); a retirada da glicose dos lanatosídeos A, B e C fornece acetildigitoxina, acetilgitoxina e acetildigoxina, respectivamente; a retirada da glicose e do grupamento acetil fornece digitoxina, gitoxina e digoxina, respectivamente. VER TAMBÉM purpurea glycosides A.

lance (lans). **1.** Lancetar; incisar uma parte, como um abscesso ou bolha. **2.** Uma lanceta. [L. *lancea,* uma lança fina]

Lancefield, Rebecca Craighill, bacteriologista norte-americana, 1895–1981. VER L. *classification.*

lan·cet (lan'set). Lanceta; um bisturi cirúrgico com uma lâmina curta, larga, apontada, e duas bordas cortantes. [Fr. *lancette*]

  gum l., l. para gengiva; uma l. usada para fazer incisão na gengiva sobre a coroa de um dente em erupção.

  spring l., l. de mola; uma lanceta com um cabo que contém uma lâmina, a qual é ativada por uma mola.

  thumb l., l. de polegar; uma l. com lâmina curta e achatada, que se dobra para trás, quando fechada, entre duas placas do manúbrio.

lan·ci·nat·ing (lan'si - nāt'ing).Lancinante; indica uma dor dilacerante ou cortante aguda. [L. *lancino,* pp. *-atus,* lacerar]

Lancisi, Giovanni M., médico italiano, 1654–1720. VER L. *sign; striae* lancisi, em *stria.*

Landau-Kleffner syn·drome. Síndrome de Landau-Kleffner. Ver em syndrome.

Landouzy, Louis T. J., neurologista francês, 1845–1917. VER L.-Dejerine *dystrophy;* L.-Grasset *law.*

Landry, Jean B. O., médico francês, 1826–1865. VER L. *paralysis, syndrome;* L.-Guillain-Barré *syndrome.*

Landschutz tu·mor. Tumor de Landschutz. Ver em tumor.

Landsteiner, Karl, patologista austríaco-norte-americano e laureado com Nobel, 1868–1943. VER L.-Donath *test;* Donath-L. cold *autoantibody, phenomenon.*

Landström, John, cirurgião sueco, 1869–1910. VER L. *muscle.*

Landzert, T., anatomista alemão do século XIX. VER L. *fossa;* Gruber-L. *fossa.*

Lane, Sir William Arbuthnot, cirurgião inglês, 1856–1943. VER L. *band, disease.*

Lang, Basil T., oftalmologista inglês, 1880–1928.

Lange, Carl F. A., bioquímico alemão, *1883. VER L. *solution, test.*

Lange, Cornelia de. Ver em de Lange.

Langenbeck, Bernhard R. K. von, cirurgião alemão, 1810–1887. VER L. *triangle.*

Langendorff, Oscar, fisiologista alemão, 1853–1908. VER L. *method.*

Lange-Nielsen, F., cardiologista norueguês do século XX. VER Jervell and Lange-Nielsen *syndrome.*

Langer, Carl (Ritter von Edenberg), anatomista austríaco, 1819–1887. VER L. *arch, lines,* em *line, muscle.*

Langer, Leonard O., médico norte-americano. VER Langer-Saldino *syndrome.*

Langerhans, Paul, anatomista alemão, 1847–1888. VER L. *cells,* em *cell, granule, islands,* em *island; islets* of L., em *islet.*

Langhans, Theodor, patologista alemão, 1839–1915. VER L. *cells,* em *cell;* L.-type giant *cells,* em *cell;* L. *layer, stria.*

Langley, John N., fisiologista inglês, 1852–1925. VER L. *granules,* em *granule.*

Langmuir, Irving, químico norte-americano e laureado com Nobel, 1881–1957. VER L. *trough.*

lan·guage (lang'gwij). Linguagem; o uso de símbolos falados, manuais, escritos e outros símbolos para expressar, representar ou receber comunicação. [L. *lingua*]

  American Sign L. (ASL), a linguagem manual por sinais e gestos utilizada pela comunidade surda nos Estados Unidos. É uma l. distinta do inglês, com sua própria gramática e sintaxe, mas não na forma escrita.

  body l., l. corporal; **(1)** a expressão dos pensamentos e sentimentos por meio de movimentos corporais não-verbais, p.ex., gestos, ou através dos sintomas da conversão histérica. VER kinesics; **(2)** comunicação por meio dos sinais corporais.

lan·i·ary (lan'i - ār - ē). Adaptado para dilacerar; em anatomia, por vezes aplicado aos dentes caninos. [L. *lanio,* rasgar em pedaços]

lan·ka·my·cin (lan'kā - mi - sin). Lancamicina; antibiótico macrolídeo produzido por *Streptomyces violaceoniger* a partir do solo do Sri Lanka.

Lannelongue, Odilon M., cirurgião e patologista francês, 1840–1911. VER L. *foramina,* em *foramen, ligaments,* em *ligament.*

lan·o·lin (lan'ō - lin). Lanolina. SIN *adeps* lanae. [L. *lana,* lã, + *oleum,* óleo]

  anhydrous l., l. anidra; l. que contém não mais que 0,25% de água; usado como base de pomada hidroadsorvível.

la·nos·ter·ol (lan - ō'stēr - ol).Lanosterol; um zoosterol sintetizado do esqualeno e um precursor para o colesterol.

Lanterman, A. J., anatomista norte-americano no século XIX em Strasbourg. VER L. *incisures,* em *incisure, segments,* em *segment;* Schmidt-L. *clefts,* em *cleft, incisures,* em *incisure.*

lan·tha·nic (lan'thă - nik). Lantânico; termo raramente utilizado que indica um processo patológico que não produz sintomas nem evidências clínicas de doença. [G. *lanthanō,* permanecer escondido]

lan·tha·nides (lan'thă - nīdz).Lantanídeos; os elementos de número atômico 57 a 71 muito semelhantes entre si do ponto de vista químico e, outrora, difíceis de separar uns dos outros. SIN rare earth elements. [*lanthanum,* primeiro elemento da série]

lan·tha·num (La) (lan'thă - nŭm).Lantânio; elemento metálico, símbolo La, número atômico 57, peso atômico 138,91, primeiro dos elementos terrosos raros (lantanídeos). [G. *lanthanō,* ficar oculto]

  l. nitrate, nitrato de lantânio; La(NO$_3$)$_3$; usado na microscopia eletrônica como corante para mucopolissacarídeos extracelulares.

lan·thi·o·nine (lan - thi'ō - nēn).Lantionina; 3,3'-tiodialanina; um aminoácido obtido da madeira que se assemelha à cistina, mas possui apenas um átomo de enxofre na molécula, em vez de dois; ou seja, um sulfeto em vez de um dissulfeto.

la·nu·go (lă - noo'gō) [TA]. Lanugo. SIN downy *hair.* [L. *lanuginoso,* de *lana,* lã]

Lanz, Otto, cirurgião suíço em Amsterdam, 1865–1935. VER L. *line.*

LAO. Abreviatura de left anterior oblique projection (incidência oblíqua anterior esquerda [OAE]), usada na radiografia de tórax, especialmente para avaliar o tamanho do ventrículo e átrio esquerdos.

LAP Abreviatura de leukocyte alkaline phosphatase (fosfatase alcalina leucocitária). VER alkaline *phosphatase.*

laparo-. Laparo-; os flancos (menos corretamente, o abdome em geral). [G. *lapara,* flanco]

lap·a·ro·cele (lap'ă - rō - sēl).Hérnia abdominal. SIN abdominal *hernia.* [laparo- + G. *kēlē,* hérnia]

laparoendoscopic (lap'ă - rō - en - dō - skop'ik).Laparoendoscópico; referente à introdução de um laparoscópio na cavidade abdominal para diversos procedimentos intracavitários.

lap·a·ro·gas·tros·co·py (lap'ă - rō - gas - tros'kŏ - pē). Laparogastroscopia; inspeção do interior do estômago após uma gastrotomia. [laparo- + G. *gastēr,* estômago, + *skopeō,* visualizar]

lap·a·ro·my·o·si·tis (lap'ă - rō - mī'ō - sī'tis).Laparomiosite; inflamação dos músculos abdominais laterais. [laparo- + G. *mys,* músculo, + *-itis,* inflamação]

lap·a·ror·rha·phy (lap'ă - rōr'ă - fē).Laparorrafia. SIN celiorrhaphy.

lap·a·ro·sal·pin·go-o·o·pho·rec·to·my (lap'ă - rō - sal'ping - gō - ō - of'ō - rek'tŏ - mē). Salpingo-ooforectomia; remoção da tuba uterina e ovário através de uma incisão abdominal.

lap·a·ro·scope (lap'ă - rō - skōp).Laparoscópio; um endoscópio para examinar a cavidade peritoneal. SIN peritoneoscope. [laparo- + G. *skopeō,* visualizar]

lap·a·ros·co·py (lap - ă - ros'kŏ - pē). Laparoscopia; exame da cavidade abdominopélvica com um laparoscópio introduzido através da parede abdominal. VER TAMBÉM peritoneoscopy. SIN abdominoscopy.

A laparoscopia tornou-se clinicamente exequível com o desenvolvimento da fibra óptica na década de 60 e de bulbos de halogênio de alta intensidade e baixo calor nos anos 70. A técnica foi padronizada, em casos selecionados, para muitos procedimentos cirúrgicos de rotina que antes exigiam laparotomia, como apendicectomia, colecistectomia, herniorrafia inguinal, ooforectomia, revisão após excisão de um tumor de ovário e avaliação diagnóstica de endometriose e infertilidade feminina. Em primeiro lugar, a cavidade peritoneal é insuflada com gás CO_2, sendo o laparoscópio introduzido por uma pequena incisão na parede abdominal. Em geral, é feita uma segunda incisão para proporcionar o acesso cirúrgico até a área de interesse. Um arsenal elaborado de instrumentos cirúrgicos foi desenvolvido para incisão, drenagem, excisão, cautério, laqueadura, sutura e outros procedimentos com o laparoscópio. O risco de complicações intra-operatórias e pós-operatórias, o custo do tratamento e o tempo de hospitalização são, em geral, menores com a cirurgia laparoscópica do que com os procedimentos a céu aberto tradicionais.

  closed l., l. fechada; l. realizada após insuflação da cavidade abdominal, usando uma agulha inserida por via percutânea.

  open l., l. aberta; l. realizada após insuflação do abdome usando um trocarte colocado sob visualização direta depois de realizar uma pequena incisão de celiotomia.

lap·a·rot·o·my (lap'ă - rot'ŏ - mē). Laparotomia. **1.** Incisão no flanco. **2.** Celiotomia. SIN celiotomy. [laparo- + G. *tomē,* incisão]

Lapicque, Louis, fisiologista francês, 1866–1952. VER L. *law.*

lap·i·ni·za·tion (lap'i - ni - zā'shŭn). Passagem seriada de um vírus ou vacina em coelhos. [Fr. *lapin,* coelho]

lap·i·nized (lap'ĭ-nīzd). Indica vírus que foram adaptados para se desenvolver em coelhos por transferências seriadas nessa espécie. [Fr. *lapin*, coelho]

Laplace, Ernest, cirurgião norte-americano, 1861–1924. VER L. *forceps*.

Laplace, Pierre S. de, fisiologista francês, 1749–1827. VER L. *law*.

Laquer, Ernst, fisiologista alemão, *1910. VER L. *stain* for alcoholic hyalin.

lard. Banha, lardo. SIN adeps (2). [L. *lardum*]
  benzoinated l., banha benzoinada; usada como lubrificante, na manufatura do sabão, para impermeabilizar lã e como fonte luminosa. Originalmente utilizada como base para pomadas.

lark·spur (lark'sper). Esporinha. SIN *Delphinium ajacis.*

Laron, Zvi, endocrinologista pediátrico israelense, *1927. VER L. type dwarfism.

Laroyenne, Lucien, cirurgião francês, 1831–1902. VER L. *operation*.

Larrey, Barão Dominique Jean de, cirurgião francês, 1766–1842. VER L. *cleft*.

Larsen, Loren J., cirurgião ortopédico, *1914. VER L. *syndrome*.

Larsson, Tage Konrad Leopold, cientista sueco, *1905. VER Sjögren-L. *syndrome*.

lar·va, pl. **lar·vae** (lar'vă, lar'vē). Larva. **1.** O estágio de desenvolvimento semelhante a um verme ou estágios de um inseto ou helminto que são muito diferentes do adulto e que sofrem subseqüente metamorfose; gusano, vareja ou lagarta. **2.** O segundo estágio no ciclo de vida de um carrapato; o estágio que se desenvolve do ovo e, depois de se ingurgitar, transforma em ninfa. **3.** Filhotes de peixes ou anfíbios que, com freqüência, diferem do adulto na aparência. [L. uma máscara]
  filariform l., l. filariforme; o terceiro estágio infeccioso da l. do *Ascaris* e de outros nematódeos com larvas penetrantes ou com larvas que migram através do corpo para alcançar o intestino.
  rhabditiform l., l. rabditiforme; os estágios iniciais (primeiro e segundo) de desenvolvimento larvar de nematódeos transmitidos pelo solo, como *Necator*, *Ancylostoma* e *Strongyloides*, que precedem o terceiro estágio infeccioso de larva filariforme.

lar·va·ceous (lar-vā'shŭs). Larvado. SIN larvate.

lar·va cur·rens (lar'vă kŭr'enz). Larva migrans cutânea causada por larvas rapidamente móveis do *Strongyloides stercoralis* (até 10 cm por hora), que se estendem tipicamente da área anal para baixo, passando pela parte superior das coxas e observadas como um trajeto urticariforme linear progressivo; também pode ser causada por espécies zoonóticas do *Strongyloides*. [L. *larva*, máscara + *currens*, corrida]

lar·val (lar'văl). **1.** Larvário; larvar; relativo à larva. **2.** Larvado. SIN larvate.

lar·va mi·grans (lar'vă mī'granz). Um verme larvário, tipicamente um nematódeo, que vagueia durante certo período nos tecidos do hospedeiro, mas que não se desenvolve no estágio adulto; geralmente, isso ocorre em hospedeiros incomuns que inibem o desenvolvimento normal do parasita. [L. *larva*, máscara, + *migro*, transferir, migrar]
  cutaneous l. m., l. migrans cutânea; escavações em forma de túnel, serpiginosas migratórias ou semelhante a uma rede, com prurido acentuado, causada por larvas de nematódeos migratórias não adaptadas para a maturação intestinal em seres humanos; especialmente comum nas costas leste e sul dos Estados Unidos e em outras áreas costeiras tropicais e subtropicais; vários nematódeos de cães e gatos têm sido implicados, principalmente *Ancylostoma braziliense* das fezes de cães e gatos em praias e caixas de areia nos Estados Unidos, mas também *Ancylostoma caninum* dos cães, *Uncinaria stenocephala*, o nematódeo de cães europeus, e *Bunostomum phlebotomum*, o nematódeo do gado; a espécie *Strongyloides* de origem animal também pode contribuir para a l. m. cutânea humana. SIN ancylostoma dermatitis, creeping eruption, cutaneous ancylostomiasis, ground itch, water itch (1).
  ocular l. m., l. m. ocular; l. m. visceral que afeta os olhos, basicamente de crianças maiores; as manifestações clínicas incluem acuidade visual diminuída e estrabismo.
  spiruroid l. m., l. m. espirurôide; a migração extra-intestinal por larvas de nematódeos da ordem Spiruroidea, não adaptadas para maturação no intestino humano; causada principalmente por espécies de *Gnathostoma spinigerum* e *G. hispidum* no Japão e Tailândia, após a ingestão de peixe cru infectado pela larva infecciosa encapsulada de terceiro estágio e, possivelmente, pela ingestão de copépodos infectados (o primeiro hospedeiro intermediário) em água potável contaminada; as larvas com espinhos anteriores escavam túneis serpiginosos na pele ou podem provocar abscesso subcutâneo ou pulmonar, ou podem invadir os olhos ou o cérebro.
  visceral l. m., l. m. visceral; uma doença, principalmente de crianças, causada pela ingestão de ovos infecciosos de *Toxocara canis*, menos comumente por outros nematódeos ascarídios não adaptados em seres humanos, cujas larvas amadurecem no intestino, penetram na parede intestinal e vagueiam pelas vísceras (principalmente no fígado) por até 18 a 24 meses; pode ser assintomática ou pode ser caracterizada por hepatomegalia (com lesões granulomatosas causadas por larvas encapsuladas no fígado dilatado), infiltração pulmonar, febre, tosse, hiperglobulinemia e eosinofilia significativa e persistente.

lar·vate (lar'vāt). Larvado; mascarado ou oculto; aplicado a uma doença com sintomas não-desenvolvidos, ausentes ou atípicos. SIN larvaceous, larval (2). [L. *larva*, máscara]

lar·vi·cid·al (lar-vi-sī'dăl). Larvicida; destrutivo para as larvas.

lar·vi·cide (lar'vi-sīd). Larvicida; um agente que mata as larvas. [larva + L. *caedo*, matar]

lar·vip·a·rous (lar-vip'ă-rŭs). Larvíparo; portador de larvas; indica a eliminação de larvas, em vez de ovos, do corpo da fêmea, como em determinados nematódeos e insetos. [larva + L. *pario*, levar]

lar·vi·phag·ic (lar'vi-fā'jik). Larvifágico; que consome larvas; determinados peixes l. são empregados no controle de mosquitos. [larva + G. *phagō*, comer]

laryng-. VER laryngo-.

la·ryn·ge·al (lă-rin'jē-ăl). Laríngeo; relativo, de qualquer modo, à laringe.

lar·yn·gec·to·mee (lar-in-jek'tō-mē). Laringectomizado; a pessoa que sofreu uma laringectomia.

la·ryn·gec·to·my (lar'in-jek'tō-mē). Laringectomia; excisão da laringe. [laringo- + G. *ektomē*, excisão]
  horizontal l., l. parcial. SIN partial l.
  partial l., l. parcial; ressecção incompleta da laringe em que a porção supraglótica é removida, preservando-se as cordas vocais. SIN horizontal l., supraglottic l.
  supraglottic l., l. supraglótica, l. parcial. SIN partial l.

la·ryn·ges (lă-rin'jēz). Laringes; plural de larynx. [L.]

lar·yn·gis·mus (lar-in-jiz'mŭs). Laringismo; estreitamento ou fechamento espasmódico da rima da glote. [L. de G. *larynx*, + *-ismos*, -ismo]
  l. strid'ulus, l. estriduloso; fechamento espasmódico da glote, causando inspiração ruidosa. Cf. *laryngitis* stridulosa. SIN pseudocroup, spasmus glottidis.

lar·yn·git·ic (lar-in-jit'ik). Laringítico; relativo a ou causado por laringite.

lar·yn·gi·tis (lar-in-jī'tis). Laringite; inflamação da mucosa da laringe. [laryngo- + G. *-itis*, inflamação]
  chronic posterior l., l. posterior crônica; uma forma de l. que envolve principalmente a área interaritenóidea; acredita-se que seja causada por regurgitação do conteúdo gástrico.
  chronic subglottic l., l. subglótica crônica. SIN chorditis vocalis inferior.
  croupous l., l. espasmódica; inflamação da porção subglótica da laringe associada a infecção respiratória e respiração ruidosa.
  membranous l., l. membranosa; uma forma de laringite em que existe um exsudato pseudomembranoso sobre as cordas vocais.
  l. sicca, l. seca; l. caracterizada por ressecamento e formação de crostas na mucosa da laringe.
  spasmodic l., l. espasmódica. SIN l. stridulosa.
  l. stridulo'sa, l. estridulosa; inflamação infecciosa da laringe em crianças, acompanhada por crises noturnas de fechamento espasmódico da glote, causando estridor inspiratório. SIN spasmodic l.

laryngo-, laryng-. Laringo-; laring-; formas combinantes relacionadas à laringe. [G. *larynx*]

la·ryn·go·cele (lă-ring'gō-sēl). Laringocele; um saco aéreo que se comunica com a laringe através do ventrículo, freqüentemente abaulando-se para fora, para os tecidos do pescoço, principalmente durante a tosse e ao se tocar um instrumento de sopro. [laryngo- + G. *kēlē*, hérnia]

la·ryn·go·fis·sure (lă-ring'gō-fish'er). Laringofissura; abertura cirúrgica na laringe, geralmente através da linha média, comumente feita para a excisão de carcinoma inicial ou correção da laringoestenose. SIN median laryngotomy, thyrofissure, thyroidotomy, thyrotomy (2).

la·ryn·go·graph (lă-ring'gō-graf). Laringógrafo; instrumento para fazer um traçado dos movimentos das cordas vocais. [laryngo- + G. *graphō*, escrever]

la·ryn·gog·ra·phy (lă-rin-gog'ră-fē). Laringografia; radiografia da laringe depois de revestir as superfícies de mucosa com contraste.

lar·yn·gol·o·gy (lar'ing-gol'ō-jē). Laringologia; o ramo da ciência médica relacionado à laringe e à voz; a especialidade das doenças da laringe. [laryngo- + G. *logos*, estudo]

la·ryn·go·ma·la·cia (lă-ring'gō-mă-lā'shē-ă). Laringomalacia. SIN chondromalacia of larynx. [laryngo- + G. *malakia*, um amolecimento]

la·ryn·go·pa·ral·y·sis (lă-ring'gō-pă-ral'i-sis). Laringoparalisia; paralisia dos músculos da laringe. SIN laryngoplegia.

la·ryn·go·pha·ryn·ge·al (lă-ring'gō-fă-rin'jē-ăl). Laringofaríngeo; relativo à laringe e à faringe ou à parte laríngea da faringe.

la·ryn·go·phar·yn·gec·to·my (lă-ring'gō-far'in-jek'tō-mē). Laringofaringectomia; ressecção ou excisão da laringe e faringe.

la·ryn·go·pha·ryn·ge·us (lă-ring'gō-far'in-jē'ŭs). Músculo constritor inferior da faringe. SIN inferior constrictor (*muscle*) of pharynx. [L.]

la·ryn·go·phar·yn·gi·tis (lă-ring'gō-far-in-jī'tis). Laringofaringite; inflamação da laringe e faringe.

la·ryn·go·phar·ynx (lă-ring'gō-far-ingks) [TA]. Parte laríngea da faringe; a parte da faringe que se situa abaixo da abertura da laringe e atrás da laringe; estende-se desde o vestíbulo da laringe até o esôfago no nível da borda inferior da cartilagem cricóidea. SIN pars laryngea pharyngis [TA], hypopharynx*, laryngeal part of pharynx, laryngeal pharynx.

la·ryn·go·phthi·sis (lă-ring'gō-thī'sis). Laringoftise; tuberculose da laringe. [laringo- + G. *phthisis*, um desgaste]

la·ryn·go·plas·ty (lă-ring'gō-plas-tē). Laringoplastia; cirurgia reparadora ou plástica da laringe. [laryngo- + G. *plassō*, formar]

la·ryn·go·ple·gia (lă-ring'gō-plē'jē-ă). Laringoplegia. SIN laryngoparalysis. [laryngo- + G. *plēgē*, golpe]

la·ryn·gop·to·sis (lă-ring-gō-tō'sis). Laringoptose; posição anormalmente baixa da laringe, que pode ser congênita ou adquirida; não compromete a saúde do neonato. Algum grau de l. ocorre com o envelhecimento. [laryngo- + G. *ptōsis*, uma queda]

la·ryn·go·scope (lă-ring'gō-skōp). Laringoscópio; qualquer um dos vários tipos de tubos, com iluminação elétrica, usados no exame ou operação da laringe através da boca. [laryngo- + G. *skopeō*, inspecionar]

la·ryn·go·scop·ic (lă-ring'gō-skop'ik). Laringoscópico; relativo à laringoscopia.

lar·yn·gos·co·pist (lar'ing-gos'kŏ-pist). Laringoscopista; uma pessoa habilitada no uso do laringoscópio.

lar·yn·gos·co·py (lar'ing-gos'kŏ-pē). Laringoscopia; inspeção da laringe por meio do laringoscópio.

  direct l., l. direta; inspeção da laringe por meio de um instrumento oco ou um cabo de fibras ópticas.

  indirect l., l. indireta; a inspeção da laringe por meio de uma imagem refletida em um espelho.

  suspension l., l. de suspensão; o suporte do laringoscópio por meio de alavancas a partir da estrutura de sustentação para proporcionar a exposição máxima da cavidade faríngea e laringe.

  transnasal fiberoptic l., l. transnasal com fibra óptica; l. realizada com um endoscópio de fibra óptica introduzido através do nariz.

la·ryn·go·spasm (lă-ring'gō-spazm). Laringospasmo; o fechamento espasmódico da abertura glótica. SIN glottidospasm, laryngospastic reflex.

la·ryn·go·ste·no·sis (lă-ring'gō-stĕ-nō'sis). Laringostenose; estenose ou estreitamento da luz da laringe. [laryngo- + G. *stenōsis*, um estreitamento]

lar·yn·gos·to·my (lar'ing-gos'tō-mē). Laringostomia; o estabelecimento de uma abertura permanente no pescoço até a laringe. [laryngo- + G. *stoma*, boca]

la·ryn·go·stro·bo·scope (lă-ring'gō-strō'bō-skōp, -strob'ō-skōp). Laringostroboscópio; aparelho para observar a movimentação das cordas vocais durante a fonação com iluminação intermitente. À medida que a freqüência da iluminação se aproxima da freqüência da abertura e fechamento das cordas vocais, elas parecem ficar paradas.

lar·yn·got·o·my (lar-ing-got'ō-mē). Laringotomia; incisão cirúrgica da laringe. [laringo- + G. *tomē*, incisão]

  inferior l., cricotirotomia. SIN cricothyrotomy.
  median l., l. mediana. SIN laryngofissure.
  superior l., l. superior; incisão através da membrana tireo-hióidea.

la·ryn·go·tra·che·al (lă-ring'gō-trā'kē-ăl). Laringotraqueal; relativo à laringe e à traquéia.

la·ryn·go·tra·che·i·tis (lă-ring'gō-trā-kē-ī'tis). Laringotraqueíte; inflamação da laringe e traquéia.

la·ryn·go·tra·che·o·bron·chi·tis (lă-ring'gō-trā'kē-ō-brong-kī'tis). Laringotraqueobronquite; uma infecção respiratória aguda que envolve a laringe, a traquéia e os brônquios. VER croup.

lar·yn·go·tra·che·o·plas·ty (lar-ing'gō-trā'kē-ō-plas'tē). Laringotraqueoplastia; cirurgia para reparar estenose subglótica.

lar·ynx, pl. **la·ryn·ges** (lar'ingks, lă-rin'jēz). Laringe, laringes; o órgão da produção da voz; a parte do trato respiratório entre a faringe e a traquéia; consiste em um arcabouço de cartilagens e membranas elásticas que alojam as cordas vocais e os músculos que controlam a posição e a tensão desses elementos. [L. mod. do G.]

  Cooper-Rand artificial l., l. artificial de Cooper-Rand; um dispositivo eletrônico para reabilitação depois da laringectomia, que produz um som intraoral articulado na forma de fala com a faringe, o palato, a língua, os lábios e os dentes.

lase (lāz). Cortar, dividir ou dissolver uma substância, ou tratar uma estrutura anatômica com laser.

Lasègue, Ernest C., médico francês, 1816-1883. VER L. *sign, syndrome.*

la·ser (lā'zer). Laser. **1.** (substantivo) Um dispositivo que concentra altas energias em um feixe estreito e intenso de radiação eletromagnética monocromática não-divergente; usado em microcirurgia, cauterização e para diversos fins diagnósticos. Os lasers podem ser baseados em numerosas fontes químicas, gás, líquido e sólido, alguns dos quais estão arrolados no quadro. Os lasers são muito utilizados em impressoras de texto ou imagens radiográficas. **2.** (verbo) Tratar uma estrutura com um feixe de laser. [acrônimo de *l*ight *a*mplification by *s*timulated *e*mission of *r*adiation, amplificação de luz por emissão estimulada de radiação]

  argon l., l. de argônio; l. usado para procedimentos oftálmicos, inclusive fotocoagulação retiniana e trabeculoplastia, consistindo em fótons no espectro azul (488 nm) ou verde (514 nm).

  continuous wave l., l. de onda contínua; um l. em que o débito de energia é constante.

  excimer l., l. de excímero; l. usado principalmente para procedimentos de refração, consistindo em fótons no espectro ultravioleta emitido por dímeros instáveis de argônio e flúor. [*exci*ted d*imer*]

  krypton l., l. de criptônio; l. usado por procedimentos oftálmicos, principalmente na fotocoagulação retiniana para hemorragia vítrea, que consiste em fótons no espectro vermelho (647 nm).

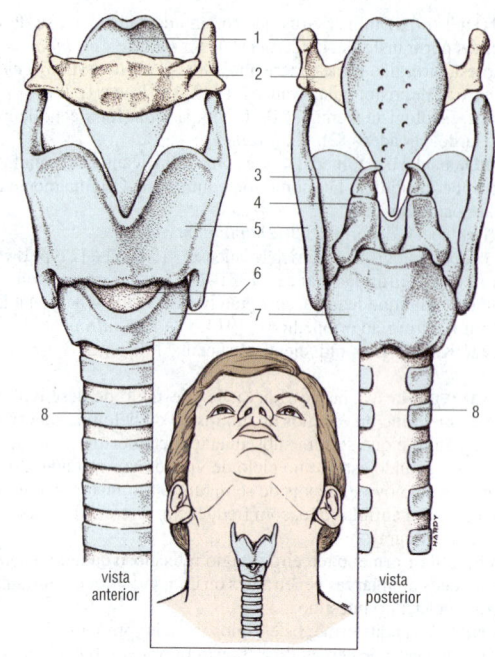

as cartilagens da laringe: (1) epiglote, (2) osso hióide, (3) cartilagem corniculada, (4) cartilagem aritenóidea, (5) cartilagem tireóidea, (6) ligamento cricotireóideo, (7) cartilagem cricóidea, (8) traquéia

  KTP l., l. na faixa do espectro azul-verde (532 nm), usado para hemostasia; produzido pela duplicação da freqüência de um l. de Nd:YAG ao passar o feixe através de um cristal KTP. [*K* (potassium) *T*itanyl *P*hosphate]

  Nd:YAG l., l. de Nd:YAG; o l. no espectro infravermelho (1.064 nm), com maior penetração que outros lasers. [*Nd* (neodymium) + *Y*ttrium-*A*luminum-*G*arnet]

  pulsed l., l. pulsado; um l. em que o débito de energia é pulsado, permitindo salvas curtas de alta energia.

  pulsed dye l., l. de corante pulsado; surtos extremamente curtos de luz amarela focalizada absorvidos pela hemoglobina; usado para tratar hemangiomas sem anestesia em crianças jovens.

  pumped l., um l. cujo nível de energia é aumentado pela aplicação de fontes separadas de elétrons ou fótons, que podem, por si mesmos, ser lasers primários.

  Q-switched l., l. mudado em Q (qualidade trocada); um l. em que a qualidade, ou capacidade de armazenamento de energia, é alterada entre um valor muito alto e um baixo.

  quasi-continuous wave l., l. de onda quase contínua; um l. cujo débito pode ser controlado em milissegundos ou por aumentos igualmente pequenos por controle eletrônico.

la·ser·ing (lā'zer-ing). O uso de um feixe de laser para cortar, dividir ou dissolver uma substância, ou para tratar uma estrutura anatômica.

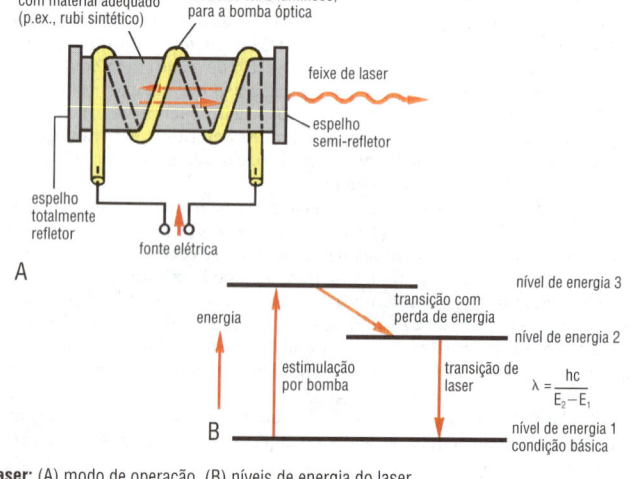

laser: (A) modo de operação, (B) níveis de energia do laser

alguns lasers comuns usados em medicina

lasers de onda contínua	comprimento de onda (nm)	algumas utilizações comuns
argônio	488/514	trabeculoplastia; preparação da superfície dentária
CO_2	10.600	dermatologia; cirurgia otológica
He-Ne*	632,8	nefelometria; guia para lasers invisíveis
criptônio	647	fotocoagulação oftálmica

lasers quase contínuos		
vapor de cobre/ bromo	510/578	lesões cutâneas pigmentadas ou vasculares
corante de argônio	577/585	lesões cutâneas vascularizadas
KTP†	532	lesões cutâneas vascularizadas; cirurgia otológica
XeCl°	308	facoablação

lasers de pulso		
érbio: YAG‡	2.940	ressuperficialização da pele; procedimentos oftálmicos
corante pulsado por bomba de lâmpada	585	lesões cutâneas vasculares
hólmio: YAG	2.100	cirurgia urológica
HF•	2.900	preparação da superfície dentária

lasers q-permutados		
alexandrita	755	lesões cutâneas pigmentadas
Nd: YAG	1.064	dermatologia; cirurgia endotraqueal
rubi	694	lesões cutâneas pigmentadas

*hélio, neon
† potássio, titanil, fosfato
‡ ítrio, alumínio, granada
• fluoreto de hidrogênio
° xenônio, cloro

laser plume. A produção de fumaça com a ablação por laser; pode provocar dificuldade respiratória para a equipe cirúrgica. [L. *pluma*, plumagem]

Lash, Abraham Fae, ginecologista-obstetra norte-americano, *1898. VER L. *operation*.

lash. Cílio.

LASIK Acrônimo de laser-assisted *in situ keratomileusis* (ceratomileuse *in situ* laser-assistida).

La·si·o·he·lea (las′ē-ō-hē′lē-ă). Um gênero de pequenos mosquitos hematófagos.

las·si·tude (las′i-tood). Lassitude, lassidão; sensação de esgotamento ou cansaço. [L. *lassitudo*, de *lassus*, cansado]

la·tah (lah′tah). Uma das síndromes de sobressalto patológico. Um transtorno ligado à cultura caracterizado por resposta física exagerada a um susto ou a uma sugestão inesperada; as pessoas involuntariamente gritam ou executam movimentos em resposta ao comando, ou imitam o que eles ouviram ou viram nos outros. VER TAMBÉM jumping *disease*. [Malaio, sensível]

Latarget, André, anatomista francês, 1877–1947. VER L. *nerve*, *vein*.

lat·e·bra (lat′ē-bră). Uma região em forma de frasco, em ovos com grandes gemas, que se estende desde o pólo animal até uma porção terminal dilatada próxima ao centro da gema; contém a massa principal da gema. [L. local oculto]

la·ten·cy (lā′ten-sē). Latência. **1.** O estado de ser latente. **2.** No condicionamento ou em outras experiências comportamentais, o período de inatividade aparente entre o momento em que o estímulo é apresentado e o momento em que acontece a resposta. **3.** Em psicanálise, o intervalo de tempo desde quase cinco anos até a puberdade.

la·tent (lā′tent). Latente; não-manifesto, oculto, quiescente, mas potencialmente discernível. [L. *lateo*, p. pres. *latens* (-*ent-*), ficar oculto]

lat·er·ad (lat′er-ad). Em direção ao lado. [L. *latus*, lado, + *ad*, para]

🅘 **lat·er·al** (lat′er-ăl) [TA]. Lateral. **1.** Do lado. SIN lateralis [TA]. **2.** Além do plano mediano ou mediossagital. SIN lateralis [TA]. **3.** Em odontologia, uma posição à direita ou esquerda do plano mediossagital. **4.** Uma incidência radiográfica feita com o filme no plano sagital; especialmente, a segunda incidência de uma série torácica. SIN lateralis [TA]. [L. *lateralis*, lateral, de *latus*, lado]

la·te·ra·lis (lat-er-ā′lis) [TA]. Lateral. SIN lateral (1), lateral (2). [L.]

lat·er·al·i·ty (lat-er-al′i-tē). Lateralidade; que se refere a um lado do corpo ou de uma estrutura; especificamente, a dominância de um lado do cérebro ou do corpo.

  crossed l., l. cruzada; a dominância direita de alguns membros, p.ex., braço ou perna, e a dominância esquerda de outros membros.

lat·er·al·i·za·tion (lat′er-al-ī′zā′shŭn). Lateralização; o processo por meio do qual determinadas assimetrias embriológicas da estrutura (como a localização do fígado no lado direito e a estrutura dos grandes vasos) e função (destreza) são ordenadas por meios filogenéticos, codificados geneticamente e percebidas ontogeneticamente.

lat·er·i·flex·ion, lat·er·i·flec·tion (lat-er-i-flek′shŭn). Lateroflexão. SIN lateroflexion.

♻ **latero-.** Lateral, para um lado. [L. *lateralis*, lateral, de *latus*, lado]

lat·er·o·ab·dom·i·nal (lat′er-ō-ab-dom′i-năl). Lateroabdominal; relativo aos lados do abdome, aos flancos ou à região lombar.

lat·er·o·de·vi·a·tion (lat′er-ō-dē-vē-ā′shŭn). Laterodesvio; uma curvatura ou deslocamento para um lado. [latero- + L. *devio*, virar para o lado, de *via*, um caminho]

lat·er·o·duc·tion (lat′er-ō-dŭk′shŭn). Lateroducção; movimento para um lado; indica a virada do bulbo do olho para fora da linha média. SIN exduction. [latero- + L. *duco*, pp. *ductus*, conduzir]

lat·er·o·flex·ion, lat·er·o·flec·tion (lat′er-ō-flek′shŭn). Lateroflexão; inclinação ou curvatura para um lado. SIN lateriflexion, lateriflection. [latero- + L. *flecto*, pp. *flexus*, inclinar]

lat·er·o·po·si·tion (lat′er-ō-pō-zish′ŭn). Lateroposição; deslocamento para um lado.

lat·er·o·pul·sion (lat′er-ō-pŭl′shŭn). Lateropulsão; movimento lateral involuntário que ocorre em determinadas afecções neurológicas. [latero- + L. *pello*, pp. *pulsus*, empurrar, dirigir]

lat·er·o·tor·sion (lat′er-ō-tōr′shŭn). Laterotorção; torção para um lado; indica a rotação do bulbo do olho ao redor de seu eixo anteroposterior, de modo que a parte superior da córnea afasta-se do plano sagital. [latero- + L. *torsio*, uma torção]

lat·er·o·tru·sion (lat′er-ō-troo′zhŭn). Laterotrusão; impulso para fora feito pelos músculos da mastigação para a rotação do côndilo mandibular durante o movimento da mandíbula. [latero- + L. *trudo*, pp. *trusus*, empurrar]

lat·er·o·ver·sion (lat′er-ō-ver′shŭn). Lateroversão; versão para um lado ou para outro, indicando principalmente uma posição errônea do útero. [latero- + L. *verto*, pp. *versus*, virar]

la·tex (lā′teks). Látex. **1.** Uma emulsão ou suspensão produzida pela seiva de alguns vegetais; contém glóbulos microscópicos suspensos de borracha natural. **2.** Materiais sintéticos similares, como poliestireno, cloreto de polivinila, etc. [L. líquido]

lathe (lādh). Torno mecânico; máquina motorizada com uma haste giratória que pode ser adaptada a vários tipos de instrumentos de corte, pedras de amolar e lâminas de polimento; usada no acabamento e polimento de próteses dentárias.

lath·y·rism (lath′i-rizm). Latirismo; uma doença que ocorre na Etiópia, Algéria e Índia, caracterizada por diversas manifestações nervosas, tremores, paraplegia espástica e parestesias; prevalente nos distritos onde favas de *Lathyrus sativus* e espécies correlatas formam o principal alimento. Experimentalmente, é uma forma de doença óssea induzida em cobaias através da alimentação com favas de *L. sativus* ou com um princípio derivado delas, especialmente β-aminoproprionitrila. SIN lupinosis. [L. *lathyrus*, ervilhaca]

lath·y·ro·gen (lath′i-rō-jen). Latirógeno; um agente ou medicamento, que ocorre naturalmente ou é usado experimentalmente e que induz o latirismo.

La·tin square. Quadrado latino; um cálculo estatístico para experiências que remove do erro experimental a variação oriunda de duas fontes, podendo ser identificado com fileiras e colunas de um quadrado. A alocação dos tratamentos experimentais é tal que cada tratamento ocorre exatamente uma vez em cada fileira e coluna. Por exemplo, um cálculo para um quadrado de 5 × 5 é o seguinte:

```
A B C D E
B A E C D
C D A E B
D E B A C
E C D B A
```

lat·i·tude (la'ti-tood). Escala cinza; a faixa de exposição à luz ou aos raios x aceitável para determinada emulsão fotográfica. VER latitude *film*. SIN digital gray scale, gray scale. [L. *latitudo*, largura, de *latus*, amplo]

La·tro·dec·tus (lat-rō-dek'tŭs). Um gênero de aranhas relativamente pequenas, as aranhas-viúvas, capazes de infligir picadas muito venenosas, neurotóxicas e dolorosas; são responsáveis, juntamente com as espécies de *Loxosceles* (as aranhas-marrons), pela maioria das reações graves do envenenamento por aranha. Espécies com importância clínica são conhecidas na Austrália, nas Américas do Norte e do Sul, na África do Sul e na Nova Zelândia. Algumas espécies venenosas, além de *L. mactans* (a aranha viúva-negra), são *L. bishopi* (a aranha viúva-negra de pernas vermelhas), *L. euracaviensis, L. geometricus* e *L. tredecimguttatus*. [L. *latro*, serviçal, ladrão, + G, *dēktēs*, um mordedor]

L. mac'tans, a aranha viúva-negra; uma aranha venenosa, de coloração preto-azeviche, encontrada em locais escuros protegidos; é especialmente comum no sul dos Estados Unidos; a fêmea adulta (com pouco mais de 1 cm de comprimento) apresenta uma marca vermelho-brilhante, em forma de haltere ou ampulheta, na face ventral do abdome; sua picada pode ser extremamente dolorosa, provocando uma síndrome semelhante a uma crise abdominal aguda; algumas mortes, embora raras, já foram relatadas, principalmente de crianças pequenas; o macho não tem a marca em ampulheta e não é venenoso.

LATS Abreviatura de long-acting thyroid *stimulator* (estimulador tireóideo de ação prolongada).

lat·tice (lat'is). Treliça, gelosia, adufa; uma disposição regular de unidades, de tal modo que um plano que passa através de duas unidades de determinado tipo, ou em determinada inter-relação, atravessará um número indefinido dessas unidades; p.ex., o arranjo de um átomo em um cristal.

la·tus, gen. **la·te·ris**, pl. **la·te·ra** (lā'tŭs, lat'er-is, lat'er-ā) [TA]. Lado, flanco. SIN flank. [L. lado]

Latzko, Wilhelm, obstetra austríaco, 1863–1945. VER L. cesarean *section*.

laud·a·ble (law'dă-bl). Louvável, saudável; um termo antigo usado para descrever o pus (espesso e cremoso) que sugeria que a lesão finalmente curaria através do processo de granulação e não levaria a sepse e morte. [L. *laudabilis*, louvável]

lau·da·nine (law'dă-nēn). Laudanina; um alcalóide isoquinolínico derivado da morfina; provoca convulsões tetanóides, com ação similar à da estricnina.

lau·da·no·sine (law'dă-nō-sēn). Laudanosina; um alcalóide isoquinolínico obtido da solução-mãe da morfina; provoca convulsões tetânicas.

lau·da·num (law'dă-nŭm). Láudano; tintura que contém ópio. [G. *lēdanon*, uma goma resinosa]

Laugier, Stanislas, cirurgião francês, 1799–1872. VER L. *hernia*.

Laumonier, Jean B. P. N. R., cirurgião francês, 1749–1818. VER L. *ganglion*.

Launois, Pierre E., médico francês, 1856–1914. VER L.-Cléret *syndrome*; L.-Bensaude *syndrome*.

Laurence, John Zachariah, oftalmologista britânico, 1830-1874. VER L.-Moon *syndrome*.

Laurer, Johann F., farmacologista alemão, 1798–1873. VER L. *canal*.

lau·ric ac·id (law'rik). Ácido láurico; um ácido graxo que ocorre no espermacete, no leite e nos óleos de louro, coco e palma, bem como em ceras e gorduras marinhas. SIN *n*-dodecanoic acid.

Lauth, Charles, químico inglês, 1836–1913. VER L. *violet*.

Lauth, Ernst A., médico alemão, 1803–1837. VER L. *canal*.

Lauth, Thomas, anatomista e cirurgião alemão, 1758–1826. VER L. *ligament*.

Lauth vi·o·let. Violeta de Lauth. SIN thionine.

LAV Abreviatura de lymphadenopathy-associated *virus* (vírus associado a linfadenopatia).

la·vage (lă-vahzh'). Lavado; a lavagem de uma cavidade ou órgão oco por injeções copiosas e retirada de líquido. [Fr. do L. *lavo*, lavar]

antral l., l. antral; irrigação do seio maxilar através de seu óstio natural ou através de punção do meato inferior.

bronchoalveolar l. (BAL), l. broncoalveolar; procedimento para analisar o meio celular dos alvéolos (inclusive microbiologia, tipos de células inflamatórias) pelo uso de um broncoscópio, ou de outro tubo oco, através do qual é instilado e, em seguida, retirado soro fisiológico dos brônquios distais.

Lavdovsky, Michail D., histologista russo, 1846–1902. VER L. *nucleoid*.

La·ver·an·ia (lav-er-ā'nē-ă). Antigo nome genérico para os protozoários causadores da malária e outros hematozoários. *L. falciparum* é um nome genérico distinto para o *Plasmodium falciparum*, sendo preferido por alguns que acreditam que os gametócitos em crescente devem ser a base para classificar o agente causal da malária falcípara em um gênero separado. VER *Plasmodium, Haemoproteus*. [C. *Laveran*, protozoologista francês e laureado com o Nobel, 1845–1922]

la·veur (lă-vūr'). Instrumento para irrigação ou lavagem. [Fr.]

LAW

law (law). Lei. **1.** Um princípio ou regra. **2.** Uma afirmação que detalha uma seqüência ou relação de fenômenos invariável em determinadas condições. VER TAMBÉM principle, rule, theorem. [A.S. *lagu*]

Alexander l., l. de Alexander; afirma que um *nistagmo* rítmico se agrava quando se olha na direção do componente rápido.

all or none l., l. do tudo-ou-nada. SIN Bowditch l.

Ångström l., l. de Ångström; uma substância absorve luz do mesmo comprimento de onda que ela emite, quando luminosa.

Arndt l., l. de Arndt; lei obsoleta que afirma que estímulos fracos excitam a atividade fisiológica, estímulos moderadamente fortes a favorecem, estímulos fortes a retardam e os muito fortes a paralisam.

Arrhenius l., l. de Arrhenius. SIN Arrhenius *doctrine*.

l.'s of association, leis de associação; os princípios formulados por Aristóteles para explicar as relações funcionais entre as idéias; a l. da contigüidade (associação) mostrou-se muito útil para psicólogos experimentais, culminando em modernos estudos de condicionamento da resposta.

l. of average localization, lei da localização média; a dor visceral é localizada com maior acurácia nas vísceras menos móveis e com menor acurácia naquelas mais móveis.

Avogadro l., l. de Avogadro; volumes iguais de gases contêm números iguais de moléculas, se forem idênticas as condições de pressão e temperatura. SIN Ampère postulate, Avogadro hypothesis, Avogadro postulate.

Baer l., l. de Baer; as características orgânicas gerais encontradas em todos os membros de um grupo aparecem mais precocemente na embriogênese que as características orgânicas especiais que diferenciam membros específicos do grupo; essa lei é a predecessora da teoria da recapitulação.

Baruch l., l. de Baruch; o efeito de qualquer procedimento hidriático é diretamente proporcional à diferença entre a temperatura da água e a da pele; quando a temperatura da água está acima ou abaixo da temperatura da pele, o efeito é estimulador; quando as duas temperaturas são idênticas, o efeito é sedativo.

Beer l., l de Beer; a intensidade de uma cor ou de um raio luminoso é inversamente proporcional à profundidade do líquido através do qual ele é transmitido; conclui-se que a absorção é dependente do número de moléculas na trajetória do raio luminoso. Cf. Beer-Lambert l.

Beer-Lambert l., l. de Beer-Lambert; a absorvância da luz é diretamente proporcional à espessura dos meios através dos quais a luz está sendo transmitida, multiplicada pela concentração de cromóforo absorvente, ou seja, $A = \varepsilon bc$, onde A é a absorvância, ε é o coeficiente de extinção molar, b é a espessura dos meios e c é a concentração.

Behring l., l. de Behring; a administração parenteral de soro de uma pessoa imunizada fornece uma imunidade passiva relativa para essa doença (ou seja, impede a doença ou modifica favoravelmente seu curso) em uma pessoa previamente susceptível.

Bell l., l. de Bell; as raízes espinais ventrais são motoras, e as dorsais, sensoriais. SIN Bell-Magendie l., Magendie l.

Bell-Magendie l., l. de Bell-Magendie. SIN Bell l.

Bernoulli l., l. de Bernoulli; quando o atrito é desprezível, a velocidade do fluxo de um gás ou líquido através de um tubo está inversamente relacionada à sua pressão contra o lado do tubo; ou seja, a velocidade é maior e a pressão é menor em um ponto de constrição. SIN Bernoulli principle, Bernoulli theorem.

Berthollet l., l. de Bertollet; os sais em solução sempre reagirão entre si, de modo a formar um sal menos solúvel, se possível.

biogenetic l., l. of biogenesis, l. biogenética. SIN recapitulation *theory*.

Blagden l., l. de Blagden; a depressão do ponto de congelamento de soluções diluídas é proporcional à quantidade da substância dissolvida.

Bowditch l., l. de Bowditch; resposta consistentemente total a qualquer estímulo efetivo. SIN all or none l.

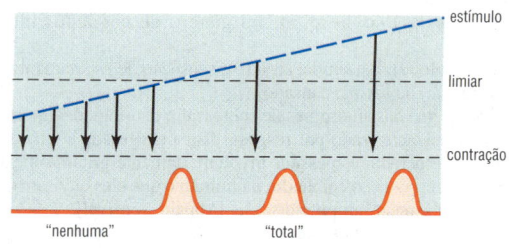

lei de Bowditch

Boyle l., l. de Boyle; em temperatura constante, o volume de determinada quantidade de gás varia inversamente com sua pressão absoluta. SIN Mariotte l.

Broadbent l., l. de Broadbent; as lesões do segmento superior do trato motor causam paralisia menos acentuada dos músculos que, habitualmente, produzem movimentos bilaterais em comparação àquelas que comumente agem de forma independente do lado oposto.

Bunsen-Roscoe l., l. de Bunsen-Roscoe; em duas reações fotoquímicas, p.ex., o escurecimento de uma placa ou filme fotográfico, se os produtos da intensidade da iluminação e o tempo de exposição são iguais, as quantidades de material químico que sofrem alteração serão iguais; a retina para curtos períodos de exposição obedece a essa l. SIN reciprocity l., Roscoe-Bunsen l.

Charles l., l. de Charles; todos os gases expandem-se de forma igual no aquecimento, isto é, 1/273,16 de seu volume a 0°C para cada grau Celsius adicional. SIN Gay-Lussac l.

l. of constant numbers in ovulation, lei do número constante na ovulação; o número de ovos liberados a cada ovulação é quase constante para determinada espécie.

l. of contiguity, l. da contigüidade; quando duas idéias ou eventos psicologicamente percebidos já ocorreram em íntima associação, é provável que eles ocorram dessa forma novamente, a ocorrência subseqüente de uma tendendo a incitar a outra; essa l. figura proeminentemente nas modernas teorias de condicionamento e aprendizado.

l. of contrary innervation, l. de Meltzer. SIN Meltzer l.

Coppet l., l. de Coppet; soluções que apresentam o mesmo ponto de congelamento possuem iguais concentrações de substâncias dissolvidas.

Courvoisier l., l. de Courvoisier; é provável que o aumento indolor da vesícula biliar associado à icterícia resulte de carcinoma da cabeça do pâncreas e não de um cálculo no colédoco, porque, no segundo caso, a vesícula biliar sofre, em geral, fibrose e não se distende. SIN Courvoisier sign.

Dale-Feldberg l., l. de Dale-Feldberg; um transmissor químico idêntico é liberado em todas as terminações funcionais de um único neurônio.

Dalton l., l. de Dalton; cada gás em uma mistura de gases exerce uma pressão proporcional à porcentagem do mesmo e independente da pressão dos outros gases presentes. SIN l. of partial pressures.

Dalton-Henry l., l. de Dalton-Henry; ao ser dissolvido em uma mistura de gases, um líquido absorverá cada gás na mistura como se esse fosse o único gás dissolvido.

l. of definite proportions, l. de proporções definidas; os pesos relativos dos vários elementos que formam um composto químico são invariáveis. SIN Proust l.

l. of denervation, l. da desnervação; quando uma estrutura é desnervada, aumenta sua sensibilidade a determinados agentes químicos; p.ex., a maior sensibilidade da pupila à acetilcolina após a secção e a degeneração do terceiro nervo, e da membrana nictitante à epinefrina (adrenalina) após a excisão do gânglio cervical superior.

Descartes l., l. de Descartes. SIN l. of refraction.

Donders l., l. de Donders; a rotação do bulbo do olho é determinada pela distância do objeto do plano mediano e da linha do horizonte.

Draper l., l. de Draper; uma alteração química é produzida em uma substância fotoquímica apenas pelos raios luminosos que são absorvidos por essa substância.

Du Bois-Reymond l., l. de Du Bois-Reymond. SIN l. of excitation.

Dulong-Petit l., l. de Dulong-Petit; o calor específico de muitos elementos sólidos é inversamente proporcional a seus pesos atômicos.

Einthoven l., l. de Einthoven; no eletrocardiograma, o potencial de qualquer onda ou complexo na derivação II (DII) é igual ao somatório de seus potenciais nas derivações I (DI) e III (DIII). SIN Einthoven equation.

Elliott l., l. de Elliott; a epinefrina (adrenalina) atua sobre as estruturas inervadas por fibras nervosas simpáticas.

l. of excitation, l. de excitação; um nervo motor responde, não ao valor absoluto, mas à alteração do valor de um momento para outro, da corrente elétrica; ou seja, a taxa de alteração da intensidade da corrente é um fator na determinação de sua efetividade. SIN Du Bois-Reymond l.

Faraday l.'s, leis de Faraday; (**1**) a quantidade de um eletrólito decomposto por uma corrente elétrica é proporcional à quantidade da corrente; (**2**) quando a mesma corrente é passada através de vários eletrólitos, as quantidades das diferentes substâncias decompostas são proporcionais a seus equivalentes químicos.

Farr l.'s, leis de Farr; um conjunto de fórmulas matemáticas, axiomas e leis enunciadas pela primeira vez nos relatos anuais submetidos por William Farr ao *Registrar General of England and Wales* de 1839 a 1883. As leis tratam da correlação entre incidência e prevalência, da história natural da epidemia e dos aspectos matemáticos de tipos comuns de epidemia. [Derivados dos escritos de William Farr, estatístico médico britânico]

Fechner-Weber l., l. de Fechner-Weber. SIN Weber-Fechner l.

Ferry-Porter l., l. de Ferry-Porter; a fusão crítica é diretamente proporcional ao logaritmo da intensidade luminosa.

Fick l.'s of diffusion, leis de difusão de Fick; (**1**) a direção do movimento dos solutos por difusão sempre se faz da concentração maior para a menor, e o fluxo de difusão J_A do soluto A através de um plano em x é proporcional ao gradiente de concentração de A em x; ou seja, $J_A = -D(C_A/x)$; (**2**) o aumento da concentração do soluto A com o tempo, C_A/t, é diretamente proporcional à alteração no gradiente de concentração, ou seja, $C_A/t = D(fl^2/x^2)$.

Flatau l., l. de Flatau; uma lei que se refere à posição excêntrica dos tratos espinais longos; quanto maior for a distância que as fibras nervosas percorrem no sentido longitudinal na medula, mais elas tendem a se situar em direção à sua periferia.

Galton l., l. de Galton; em uma população cruzada ao acaso, a progênie de um genitor com um valor extremo para um fenótipo mensurável tenderá, na média, a ter valores mais próximos à média da população do que nos ancestrais extremos. VER TAMBÉM l. of regression to mean. SIN l. of regression to mean.

Gay-Lussac l., l. de Gay-Lussac. SIN Charles l.

Godélier l., l. de Godélier; a tuberculose do peritônio está sempre associada à tuberculose da pleura em um ou em ambos os lados.

Gompertz l., l. de Gompertz; a relação proporcional entre mortalidade e idade; após 35–40 anos de idade, o aumento da taxa de mortalidade com a idade tende a ser logarítmico.

Graham l., l. de Graham; a relativa rapidez da difusão de dois gases varia inversamente à raiz quadrada de suas densidades, ou seja, seus pesos moleculares.

Grasset l., l. de Grasset. SIN Landouzy-Grasset l.

l. of gravitation, l. de Newton. SIN Newton l.

Guldberg-Waage l., l. de Guldberg-Waage. SIN l. of mass action.

Haeckel l., l. de Haeckel. SIN recapitulation *theory*.

Halsted l., l. de Halsted; o tecido transplantado crescerá apenas se não houver esse tecido no hospedeiro.

Hardy-Weinberg l., l. de Hardy-Weinberg; se o cruzamento ocorre ao acaso em relação a qualquer *locus* autossômico em uma população na qual as freqüências do gene são iguais nos dois sexos e os fatores que tendem a modificar as freqüências genéticas (mutação, seleção diferencial, migração) não existem ou são desprezíveis, então, em uma geração, as probabilidades de todos os genótipos possíveis serão iguais, na média, às mesmas proporções que ocorreriam se os genes fossem reunidos ao acaso. A lei não se aplica a dois ou mais *loci* em conjunto, nem a traços ligados ao X, nos quaias as freqüências genéticas iniciais diferem em ambos os sexos.

l. of the heart, l. de Starling; a energia liberada pelo coração quando ele contrai é uma função do comprimento de suas fibras musculares no final da diástole. SIN Starling l.

Heidenhain l., l. de Heidenhain; a secreção glandular sempre é acompanhada por uma alteração na estrutura da glândula.

Hellin l., l. de Hellin; gêmeos ocorrem uma vez a cada 89 nascimentos, trigêmeos uma vez a cada 89^2 e quadrigêmeos uma vez a cada 89^3. Se a freqüência de gêmeos em uma população é p, a freqüência de trigêmeos é p^2 e a freqüência de quadrigêmeos é p^3.

Henry l., l. de Henry; em equilíbrio, a determinada temperatura, o volume de gás dissolvido em determinado volume de líquido é diretamente proporcional à pressão parcial desse gás na fase gasosa (isso é verdadeiro apenas para os gases que não reagem quimicamente com o solvente).

Herring l., l. de Herring; afirma que músculos agonistas pareados em cada olho que operam no mesmo campo visual recebem igual inervação, enquanto músculos antagonistas pareados recebem igual inibição.

Hess l., l. de Hess; o calor gerado por uma reação é o mesmo, quer a reação aconteça em uma etapa ou em várias etapas; ou seja, os valores de ΔH (e, portanto, os valores de ΔG) são aditivos.

Hilton l., l. de Hilton; o nervo que supre uma articulação também supre os músculos que movimentam essa articulação e a pele que reveste a inserção articular desses músculos.

Hooke l., l. de Hooke; o estresse aplicado para estirar ou comprimir um corpo é proporcional à deformação ou alteração no comprimento produzidos dessa maneira, desde que o limite de elasticidade do corpo não seja excedido.

l. of independent assortment, l. da segregação independente; os genes que não são alelos são distribuídos de forma independente durante a formação dos gametas; os traços em *loci* ligados constituem uma exceção. SIN Mendel second l.

l. of intestine, reflexo mioentérico. SIN myenteric *reflex*.

inverse square l., l. do quadrado inverso; quando aplicado às fontes pontuais, a intensidade da radiação diminui em proporção ao quadrado da distância dessa fonte.

isodynamic l., l. isodinâmica; para fins energéticos, os diferentes alimentos podem substituir-se entre si, de acordo com seus valores calóricos, quando queimados em um calorímetro.

Jackson l., l. de Jackson; a perda das funções mentais devido à doença ocorre em ordem inversa ao seu desenvolvimento evolucionário.

Koch l., l. de Koch. SIN Koch *postulates*, em *postulate*.

Lambert l., l. de Lambert; (**1**) cada camada de igual espessura absorve uma fração igual da luz que a atravessa. Cf. Beer-Lambert l.; (**2**) a iluminação de uma superfície, sobre a qual a luz incide normalmente a partir de uma fonte pontual, é inversamente proporcional ao quadrado da distância dessa fonte de luz.

Landouzy-Grasset l., l. de Landouzy-Grasset; nas lesões de um hemisfério, a cabeça do paciente é virada para o lado dos músculos afetados se houver espasticidade e para o lado da lesão cerebral se houver paralisia. SIN Grasset l.

Lapicque l., l. de Lapicque; a cronaxia é inversamente proporcional ao diâmetro de um axônio.

Laplace l., l. de Laplace; a relação de equilíbrio entre a diferença de pressão transmural (ΔP), tensão da parede (T) e o raio da curvatura (R) em uma superfície côncava; para uma esfera: $\Delta P = 2T/R$; para um cilindro: $\Delta P = T/R$.

Le Chatelier l., l. de Le Chatelier; se fatores externos, como temperatura e pressão, perturbam um sistema em equilíbrio, o ajuste ocorre de tal modo que o efeito dos fatores conturbadores é reduzido a um mínimo. SIN Le Chatelier principle.

Listing l., l. de Listing; quando os olhos deixam um objeto e se fixam em outro, eles giram em torno de um eixo perpendicular a um plano que corta tanto as linhas iniciais como as novas linhas de visão.

Louis l., l. de Louis; a tuberculose em qualquer órgão está associada à tuberculose no pulmão.

Magendie l., l. de Magendie. SIN Bell l.

Marey l., l. de Marey; a freqüência de pulso varia inversamente com a pressão arterial; ou seja, o pulso é lento quando a pressão está alta; uma expressão das influências do reflexo barorreceptor sobre a freqüência cardíaca.

Marfan l., l. de Marfan; a cura da tuberculose localizada protege contra o desenvolvimento subseqüente de tuberculose pulmonar.

Mariotte l., l. de Mariotte. SIN Boyle l.

mass l., l. da ação das massas. SIN l. of mass action.

l. of mass action, l. de ação das massas; a velocidade de uma reação química é proporcional às concentrações das substâncias reagentes; quando a velocidade de reação anterógrada se iguala à velocidade da reação inversa (ou seja, em equilíbrio), então, em temperatura constante, o produto das concentrações de todos os produtos dividido pelo produto das concentrações de todos os reagentes é, por si, uma constante (K_{eq}). SIN Guldberg-Waage l., mass l.

Meltzer l., l. de Meltzer; todas as funções vitais são continuamente controladas por duas forças opostas: por um lado, o aumento ou ação e, por outro, a inibição. SIN l. of contrary innervation.

Mendeléeff l., l. de Mendeléeff; as propriedades dos elementos são funções periódicas de seus pesos atômicos; ou seja, os elementos são dispostos na ordem de seus pesos atômicos, cada elemento na série estará relacionado, segundo suas propriedades, ao oitavo elemento antes ou depois dele. SIN periodic l.

Mendel first l., primeira l. de Mendel. SIN l. of segregation.

Mendel second l., segunda l. de Mendel. SIN l. of independent assortment.

l. of the minimum, l. do mínimo; crescimento e desenvolvimento de vegetais e animais são determinados pela disponibilidade do nutriente essencial que está presente em menor quantidade.

Müller l., l. de Müller; cada tipo de terminação nervosa sensorial, desde que estimulado (por meios elétricos, mecânicos, etc.), dá origem à sua própria sensação específica; ademais, cada tipo de sensação não depende de características especiais dos diferentes nervos, mas da parte do cérebro em que terminam suas fibras. SIN l. of specific nerve energies.

l. of multiple proportions, l. de múltiplas proporções. SIN l. of reciprocal proportions.

Nasse l., l. de Nasse; uma afirmação antiga sobre o padrão da herança recessiva ligada ao X: a hemofilia afeta apenas os meninos, porém é transmitida através das mães e irmãs.

Neumann l., l. de Neumann; em compostos de constituição química análoga, o calor molecular, ou o produto do calor específico pelo peso atômico, sempre é o mesmo.

Newton l., l. de Newton; a força de atração entre dois corpos quaisquer é proporcional ao produto de suas massas e inversamente proporcional ao quadrado da distância entre seus centros. SIN l. of gravitation.

Nysten l., l. de Nysten; o *rigor mortis* afeta primeiro os músculos da cabeça e se espalha em direção aos pés.

Ochoa l., l. de Ochoa; o conteúdo do cromossoma X tende a ser conservado filogeneticamente.

Ohm l., l. de Ohm; em uma corrente elétrica que passa por um fio, a intensidade da corrente (I) em ampères é igual à força eletromotora (E) em volts dividida pela resistência (R) em ohms: $I = E/R$.

l. of partial pressures, l. das pressões parciais. SIN Dalton l.

Pascal l., l. de Pascal; os líquidos em repouso transmitem pressão igualmente em todas as direções.

periodic l., l. de Mendeléeff. SIN Mendeléeff l.

Pflüger l., l. de Pflüger. SIN l. of polar excitation.

Plateau-Talbot l., l. de Plateau-Talbot; quando estímulos luminosos sucessivos se sucedem de forma suficientemente rápida para se fundir, seu brilho aparente é diminuído.

Poiseuille l., l. de Poiseuille; no fluxo laminar, o volume de um líquido homogêneo que passa por unidade de tempo através de um tubo capilar é diretamente proporcional à diferença de pressão entre suas extremidades e à quarta potência de seu raio interno, e inversamente proporcional a seu comprimento e à viscosidade do líquido.

l. of polar excitation, l. da excitação polar; determinado segmento de um nervo é irritado pelo desenvolvimento do cateletrotônus e pelo desaparecimento do aneletrotônus, mas o inverso não se sustenta; ou seja, a excitação ocorre no catódio, quando o circuito é fechado, e no anódio, quando aberto. SIN Pflüger l.

l. of priority, l. da prioridade; o uso do nome publicado primeiro (sinônimo sênior) entre dois ou mais nomes de um organismo como o nome correto.

Profeta l., l. de Profeta; o indivíduo com sífilis congênita é imune à doença adquirida.

Proust l., l. de Proust. SIN l. of definite proportions.

Raoult l., l. de Raoult; a pressão de vapor de uma solução de um não-eletrólito não-volátil é a pressão do solvente puro multiplicada pela fração molar do solvente na solução.

l. of recapitulation, l. da recapitulação. SIN recapitulation *theory*.

l. of reciprocal proportions, l. das proporções recíprocas; os pesos relativos em que duas substâncias formam uma união química isoladamente com uma terceira são idênticos a ou múltiplos simples, daqueles a que elas se unem; um corolário da lei de proporções definidas. SIN l. of multiple proportions.

reciprocity l., l. da reciprocidade. SIN Bunsen-Roscoe l.

l. of referred pain, l. da dor referida; a dor origina-se apenas da irritação dos nervos sensíveis aos estímulos que produzem a dor quando aplicados à superfície do corpo.

l. of refraction, l. da refração; para dois determinados meios, o seno do ângulo de incidência mantém uma relação constante com o seno do ângulo de refração. SIN Descartes l., Snell l.

l. of regression to mean, l. de Galton. SIN Galton l.

Ribot l. of memory, l. da memória de Ribot; nas demências progressivas, a memória remota tende a ser preservada, enquanto a memória recente é perdida.

Ricco l., l. de Ricco; para pequenas imagens, intensidade luminosa × área = constante para o limiar.

Roscoe-Bunsen l., l. de Roscoe-Bunsen. SIN Bunsen-Roscoe l.

Rosenbach l., l. de Rosenbach; (1) nas afecções dos troncos nervosos ou centros nervosos, a paralisia dos músculos flexores surge depois da paralisia dos extensores; (2) nos casos de estimulação anormal dos órgãos com periodicidade funcional rítmica, existe, com freqüência, um agrupamento de atos individuais com aumento correspondente das pausas, de tal forma que a proporção entre repouso e atividade totais permanece quase idêntica.

Rubner l.'s of growth, leis do crescimento de Rubner; (1) a l. do consumo constante de energia: a rapidez do crescimento é proporcional à intensidade dos processos metabólicos; (2) a l. do quociente de crescimento constante: na maioria dos mamíferos jovens, 24% de toda a energia alimentar, ou calorias, são usados para o crescimento; nos seres humanos, apenas 5% são empregados dessa maneira.

Schütz l., l. de Schütz. SIN Schütz *rule*.

second l. of thermodynamics, segunda lei da termodinâmica; a entropia do universo move-se para um máximo; de modo similar, a entropia de qualquer microcosmo isolado (p.ex., uma reação química) prossegue espontaneamente apenas na direção que aumenta a entropia, sendo a entropia máxima no equilíbrio. Para citar G. N. Lewis, "Todo processo que ocorre espontaneamente é capaz de realizar trabalho; a reversão de qualquer processo deste exige o gasto de trabalho do exterior".

l. of segregation, l. da segregação; os fatores que afetam o desenvolvimento retêm sua individualidade de uma geração para outra, não se tornam contaminados quando misturados a um híbrido e, quando é formada a nova geração de gametas, separam-se uns dos outros. SIN Mendel first l.

Sherrington l., l. de Sherrington; toda raiz nervosa espinal dorsal supre determinada área da pele, o dermátomo (3), que, no entanto, é invadido, acima e abaixo, por fibras dos segmentos espinais adjacentes.

l. of similars, l. dos semelhantes. VER similia similibus curantur.

Snell l., l. de Snell. SIN l. of refraction.

Spallanzani l., l. de Spallanzani; quanto mais jovem for o indivíduo, maior será o poder de regeneração de suas células.

l. of specific nerve energies, l. de Müller. SIN Müller l.

Starling l., l. de Starling. SIN l. of the heart.

Stokes l., l. de Stokes; (1) um músculo localizado acima de uma mucosa ou serosa inflamada é, com freqüência, o local da paralisia; (2) uma relação da velocidade da queda de uma pequena esfera em um líquido viscoso; aplicável à centrifugação das macromoléculas; (3) o comprimento de onda da luz emitida por um material fluorescente é maior que a da radiação usada para excitar a fluorescência.

Tait l., l. de Tait; uma máxima obsoleta de que uma laparotomia exploradora deve ser realizada em todo caso de doença pélvica ou abdominal obscura que ameace a saúde ou a vida.

Thoma l.'s, leis de Thoma; o desenvolvimento dos vasos sanguíneos é governado por forças dinâmicas que atuam sobre suas paredes da seguinte maneira: um aumento na velocidade do fluxo sanguíneo provoca dilatação da luz vascular; um aumento na pressão lateral sobre a parede vascular faz com que ela se espesse; um aumento na pressão terminal gera a formação de novos capilares.

van't Hoff l., l. de van't Hoff; (1) em estereoquímica, todas as substâncias opticamente ativas possuem um ou mais átomos multivalentes unidos a quatro átomos ou a radicais diferentes, de modo a formar, no espaço, uma disposição assimétrica; (2) a pressão osmótica exercida por qualquer substância em uma solução muito diluída é idêntica àquela que seria exercida se houvesse gás no mesmo volume da solução; ou, em temperatura constante, a pressão osmótica de soluções diluídas é proporcional à concentração (número de moléculas) da substância dissolvida, ou seja, a pressão osmótica, Π, em soluções diluídas é $\Pi = RT\Sigma c_i$, onde R é a constante universal do gás, T é a temperatura absoluta e c_i é a concentração molar do soluto i; **(3)** a velocidade das reações químicas aumenta entre duas a três vezes para cada aumento de 10°C na temperatura.

Vogel l., l. de Vogel; quando um fenótipo pode ser transmitido por várias modalidades de herança mendeliana, a dominante terá o fenótipo menos deletério, a recessiva o mais deletério e a ligada ao X é intermediária entre os dois extremos.

wallerian l., l. de Waller; após a secção da raiz posterior de um nervo espinal entre o gânglio da raiz e a medula espinal, a porção central degenera; após a divisão da raiz anterior, a porção periférica degenera; o centro trófico da raiz posterior é, portanto, o gânglio, e o da raiz anterior, da medula espinal.

Weber l., l. de Weber. SIN Weber-Fechner l.

Weber-Fechner l., l. de Weber-Fechner; a intensidade de uma sensação varia segundo uma série de aumentos iguais (aritméticos), enquanto a potência do estímulo aumenta geometricamente; quando uma série de estímulos é aplicada e ajustada de forma que a potência de cada estímulo provoque uma alteração apenas perceptível na intensidade da sensação, então a potência de cada estímulo difere da anterior por uma fração constante; dessa maneira, se uma alteração apenas perceptível em uma sensação visual é produzida pela adição de 1 vela a uma iluminação original de 100 velas, serão necessárias 10 velas para produzir qualquer alteração na sensação quando a iluminação original era de 1.000 velas. SIN Fechner-Weber l., Weber l.

Weigert l., l. de Weigert; a perda ou destruição de uma parte ou elemento no mundo orgânico provavelmente resulta em reposição compensatória e produção excessiva de tecido durante o processo de regeneração ou reparo (ou ambos), como na formação de calo ósseo quando ocorre a consolidação de um osso fraturado. SIN overproduction theory.

Williston l., l. de Williston; à medida que se ascende a escala de vertebrados, o número de ossos do crânio diminui.

Wolff l., l. de Wolff; toda alteração na forma e na função de um osso, ou apenas em sua função, é seguida por determinadas alterações definidas em sua arquitetura interna e por alterações secundárias em sua conformação externa; essas alterações geralmente representam respostas às alterações nas forças que sustentam o peso.

Lawrence, Robert D., médico inglês, 1892–1968. VER L.-Seip *syndrome*.

law·ren·ci·um (Lr, Lw) (law-ren′sē-ŭm). Laurêncio; um elemento transplutônico artificial; número atômico 103; peso atômico 262,11. [E. O. *Lawrence*, físico norte-americano e laureado com o Nobel, 1901–1958]

lax·a·tion (lak-sā′shŭn). Laxação; defecação, com ou sem laxativos. [ver laxative]

lax·a·tive (lak′să-tiv). Laxativo, laxante. **1.** Discretamente catártico; que possui a ação de aumentar a evacuação intestinal. **2.** Um catártico discreto; um remédio que provoca defecação sem dor ou ação violenta. [L. *laxativus*, de *laxo*, pp. *-atus*, relaxar]

diphenylmethane l. 's, laxativos do tipo difenilmetano; membros de uma classe química dos agentes laxativos, incluindo a fenolftaleína e o bisacodil.

LAYER

lay·er (lā′er) [TA]. Estrato, lâmina, camada; uma lâmina de uma substância que se situa sobre a outra e diferencia-se dela por uma diferença na textura ou coloração, ou por não ser contínua com ela. VER TAMBÉM stratum, lamina. SIN panniculus.

ameloblastic l., c. ameloblástica; a c. do órgão do esmalte. SIN enamel l.

anterior elastic l., lâmina limitante anterior. SIN anterior limiting l. of cornea.

anterior limiting l. of cornea, c. limitante anterior da córnea; uma camada acelular homogênea transparente, com 6 a 9 μm de espessura, que se situa entre a c. basal da camada externa do epitélio estratificado e a substância própria da córnea; considerada uma membrana basal. SIN anterior elastic l. Bowman l., Bowman membrane, lamina elastica anterior, lamina limitans anterior corneae.

anterior l. of rectus sheath [TA], lâmina anterior da bainha do músculo reto do abdome; a porção da bainha do reto anterior ao músculo, consistindo, em seus dois terços superiores, em contribuições das aponeuroses dos músculos oblíquos externo e interno e, em seu terço inferior (abaixo da linha arqueada), de contribuições das aponeuroses de todos os três músculos da parede abdominal anterolateral. SIN lamina anterior vaginae musculi recti abdominis.

anterior l. of thoracolumbar fascia [TA], lâmina anterior da aponeurose toracolombar; membrana fascial que se estende a partir dos processos transversos das vértebras lombares. SIN lamina anterior fasciae thoracolumbalis [TA], fascia musculi quadrati lumborum*, lamina profunda fasciae thoracolumbalis*, quadratus lumborum fascia*.

bacillary l., c. parte óptica da retina. SIN l. of rods and cones.

basal l., estrato basal. SIN *stratum* basale (1).

basal cell l., estrato basal da epiderme. SIN *stratum* basale epidermidis.

basal l. of choroid [TA], lâmina basilar da corióide. SIN *lamina* basalis choroideae.

basal l. of ciliary body, lâmina basilar do corpo ciliar. SIN basal *lamina* of ciliary body.

l. of Bechterew, c. de Bechterew. SIN *band* of Kaes-Bechterew.

blastodermic l.'s, camadas blastodérmicas; as camadas de células primordiais na superfície vitelina de um ovo telolícito; nos estágios iniciais, consistem no protoderma e, em seguida, mais adiante, diferenciam-se em ectoderma, endoderma e mesoderma.

Bowman l., c. de Bowman. SIN anterior limiting l. of cornea.

brown l., lâmina supracorióide. SIN suprachoroid *lamina* of sclera.

cambium l., (1) a c. osteogênica interna do periósteo; **(2)** uma zona extremamente celular logo abaixo do epitélio, cobrindo um sarcoma botrioide.

l.'s of cerebellar cortex, estratos do córtex cerebelar. VER cerebellar *cortex*.

l.'s of cerebral cortex, lâminas do córtex cerebral. VER cerebral *cortex*.

cerebral l. of retina, parte óptica da retina; a camada interna da retina que contém os elementos neurais, conforme diferenciado do folheto externo da retina, ou a camada pigmentada. SIN pars optica retinae [TA], neural l. of retina, stratum cerebrale retinae.

Chievitz l., c. de Chievitz; na retina de um embrião em desenvolvimento, uma zona de transição entre as camadas neuroblásticas interna e externa que é desprovida dos núcleos.

choriocapillary l., lâmina corioideocapilar. SIN capillary *lamina* of choroid.

circular l. of detrusor (muscle) of urinary bladder [TA], c. circular do músculo detrusor da bexiga urinária; a camada média substancial de três camadas mal definidas, entrelaçadas (as camadas interna e externa com orientação predominantemente longitudinal) das fibras musculares lisas (involuntárias) que constituem a camada muscular da parede da bexiga. SIN stratum circulare musculi detrusoris vesicae [TA].

circular l. of muscle coat of small intestine [TA], c. helicoidal da túnica muscular do intestino delgado; a camada interna dos músculos lisos (involuntários) da túnica muscular (muscular externa) do intestino delgado, em que as fibras musculares envolvem a luz; alguns pesquisadores defendem que a orientação das fibras musculares é uma espiral ou hélice apertada em vez de ser realmente circular. SIN stratum circulare tunicae muscularis intestini tenuis [TA], short pitch helicoidal l.*, stratum helicoidale brevis gradus*.

circular l. of muscular coat [TA], c. circular da túnica muscular; a camada circular interna da musculatura lisa da túnica muscular. A *Terminologia Anatomica* relaciona as camadas circulares das túnicas musculares (stratum circulare tunicae muscularis...) das seguintes regiões: 1) do colo (...coli [TA]); 2) da parte prostática da uretra (...urethrae prostaticae [TA]); 3) do reto (...recti [TA]); 4) do intestino delgado (...intestini tenuis [TA]); 5) do estômago (...gastricae [TA]); 6) da uretra (...urethrae [TA]). SIN stratum circulare tunicae muscularis [TA].

circular l.'s of muscular tunics, camadas circulares das túnicas musculares. VER circular l. of muscular coat.

circular l. of tympanic membrane, estrato circular da membrana timpânica. SIN *stratum* circulare membranae tympani.

claustral l., claustro; a c. da substância cinzenta subcortical entre a cápsula externa e a substância branca da ínsula ou da cápsula extrema.

clear l. of epidermis, estrato lúcido. SIN *stratum* lucidum.

columnar l., estrato basal da epiderme. SIN *stratum* basale epidermidis.

conjunctival l. of bulb, conjuntiva bulbar. SIN bulbar *conjunctiva*.

conjunctival l. of eyelids, conjuntiva palpebral. SIN palpebral *conjunctiva*.

corneal l. of epidermis, estrato córneo da epiderme. SIN *stratum* corneum epidermidis.

cornified l. of nail, estrato córneo da unha. SIN *stratum* corneum unguis.

cutaneous l. of tympanic membrane, estrato cutâneo da membrana timpânica. SIN *stratum* cutaneum membranae tympani.

deep l. [TA], lâmina profunda; em uma estrutura estratificada, o estrato que se situa abaixo de todos os outros, além da superfície. VER deep l. of levator palpebrae superioris, deep l. of temporal fascia. SIN lamina profunda [TA], deep lamina.

deep gray l. of superior colliculus [TA], estrato cinzento profundo do colículo superior; uma l. de corpos celulares no colículo superior localizada entre o estrato medular intermédio e o estrato medular profundo. SIN stratum griseum profundum colliculus superioris [TA].

deep l. of levator palpebrae superioris, lâmina profunda do músculo levantador superior da pálpebra superior; as fibras mais profundas do músculo levantador da pálpebra superior que se inserem no tarso superior. SIN lamina profunda musculi levatoris palpebrae superioris.

deep l. of temporal fascia, lâmina profunda da fáscia temporal; a parte profunda da fáscia temporal que se insere na superfície medial do arco zigomático. SIN lamina profunda fasciae temporalis [TA].

deep white l. of superior colliculus [TA], estrato medular profundo do colículo superior; a camada mais interna do colículo superior; uma camada de corpos

la

celulares neuronais localizada entre o estrato medular profundo e a substância branca intermédia. SIN stratum medullare profundum [TA].
l.'s of dentate gyrus [TA], estratos do giro denteado; a partir da superfície do giro denteado, essas camadas são: o estrato molecular [TA] (stratum moleculare [TA]), que contém dendritos de células granulares e alguns axônios da via perfurante; estrato granular [TA] (stratum granulare [TA]), que contém a camada de pequenas células granulares; e o estrato multiforme [TA] (stratum multiforme [TA]), também por vezes chamado de camada polimórfica, que contém os axônios de células granulares e alguns axônios aferentes que penetram através do fórnice. SIN strata gyri dentati [TA].
elastic l.'s of arteries, lâminas elásticas das artérias. SIN elastic *laminae* of arteries, em *lamina*.
elastic l.'s of cornea, lâminas limitantes da córnea. VER anterior limiting l. of cornea, posterior limiting l. of cornea.
enamel l., c. do esmalte. SIN ameloblastic l.
ependymal l., c. ependimária; uma c. epitelial interna de células que limitam a luz do tubo neural e do cérebro embrionários, formada durante a estratificação da última e persistindo na forma modificada por toda a vida. SIN ependymal zone, ventricular l.
episcleral l. of fibrous layer of eyeball [TA], lâmina episcleral; a camada móvel delicada de tecido conjuntivo frouxo entre a superfície externa da esclera e a bainha fascial do bulbo do olho. SIN lamina episcleralis [TA], episcleral lamina.
epithelial l.'s, camadas epiteliais. VER epithelium.
epithelial choroid l., lâmina epitelial. SIN epithelial *lamina*.
epitrichial l., c. epitriquial; a camada de células superficiais achatadas da epiderme de um jovem embrião antes que ocorra a estratificação definitiva.
external nuclear l. of retina, estrato dos segmentos interno e externo da retina. SIN neuroepithelial l. of retina.
fatty l. of subcutaneous tissue [TA], panículo adiposo da tela subcutânea; porção superficial do tecido subcutâneo de determinadas áreas do corpo (p.ex., porção inferior da parede abdominal anterior) que é especializada no armazenamento adiposo e, dessa maneira, possui, com freqüência, bastante gordura, especialmente no indivíduo com sobrepeso, comparado à porção fibrosa mais profunda de tecido subcutâneo; na obesidade mórbida, esse panículo forma o núcleo de uma grande prega pendente (abdome em avental). VER TAMBÉM fatty l. of subcutaneous tissue of abdomen. SIN panniculus adiposus [TA].
fatty l. of subcutaneous tissue of abdomen [TA], panículo adiposo da tela subcutânea do abdome; a porção mais superficial e gordurosa da fáscia superficial da parede abdominal ântero-inferior. SIN panniculus adiposus telae subcutaneae abdominis [TA], Camper fascia, fatty l. of superficial fascia.
fatty l. of superficial fascia, panículo adiposo da tela subcutânea do abdome. SIN fatty l. of subcutaneous tissue of abdomen.
fibromusculocartilagenous l. of bronchi [TA], túnica fibromusculocartilagínea dos brônquios; a c. entre a submucosa e a adventícia dos brônquios, incluindo as cartilagens envolvidas no pericôndrio, contínua entre as cartilagens com uma membrana densa e fibrosa, que inclui o músculo liso e as fibras elásticas; essa camada fornece rigidez para a parede, enquanto permite a redução ativa e o aumento passivo no diâmetro dos brônquios. SIN tunica fibromusculocartilaginea bronchi [TA].
fibrous l., c. fibrosa; a c. de tecido conjuntivo denso externa do periósteo.
fibrous l. of eyeball [TA], túnica fibrosa do bulbo do olho; a camada externa do bulbo do olho composta da esclera e córnea. SIN tunica fibrosa bulbi [TA], fibrous tunic of eye, tunica externa oculi.
fibrous l. of joint capsule [TA], estrato fibroso da cápsula articular; a parte fibrosa externa da cápsula de uma articulação sinovial, que pode, em determinados locais, ser espessada para formar os ligamentos capsulares. SIN membrana fibrosa capsulae articularis [TA], fibrous layer of articular capsule*, fibrous membrane of joint capsule*, fibrous articular capsule, stratum fibrosum capsulae articularis.
fibrous l. in or on deep aspect of fatty layer of subcutaneous tissue [TA], estrato fibroso do panículo adiposo da tela subcutânea; o tecido fibroso interposto ou concentrado nas porções mais profundas do panículo adiposo da tela subcutânea em determinada região, tornando-a mais substancial, mas não organizada em uma camada membranácea uniforme. SIN stratum fibrosum panniculi adiposi telae subcutaneae [TA].
fillet l., estrato do lemnisco. SIN *stratum* lemnisci.
fusiform l., lâmina multiforme do córtex cerebral. SIN multiform l. [TA] of cerebral cortex.
ganglionic l. [TA], estrato ganglionar; a c. da retina que contém principalmente os corpos celulares de células ganglionares, embora alguns corpos celulares de células amácrinas também sejam encontrados. VER TAMBÉM ganglion *cells* of retina, em *cell*. SIN stratum ganglionicum [TA], ganglionic cell l. of retina.
ganglionic cell l. of retina, estrato ganglionar da retina. SIN ganglionic l.
ganglionic l. of cerebellar cortex, estrato purkinjense do córtex cerebelar. SIN Purkinje cell l.
ganglionic l. of cerebral cortex, lâmina piramidal interna do córtex cerebral; c. 5 do córtex cerebral.

ganglionic l. of optic nerve, c. ganglionar do nervo óptico; termo obsoleto usado para descrever os neurônios multipolares na retina que se originam nas fibras do nervo óptico. SIN stratum ganglionare nervi optici.
germ l., c. germinativa; uma das três camadas de células primordiais (ectoderma, endoderma, mesoderma) estabelecidas em um embrião durante a gastrulação.

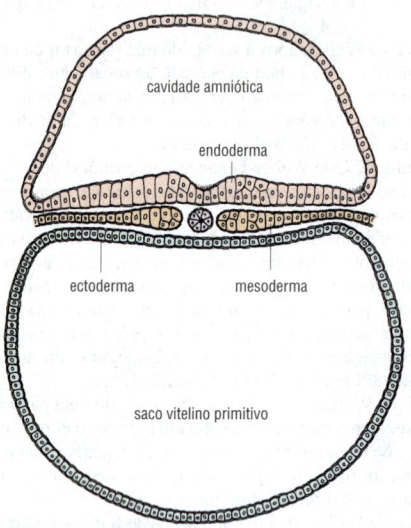

camadas germinativas do embrião

germinative l., estrato basal da epiderme. SIN *stratum* basale epidermidis.
germinative l. of nail, estrato germinativo da unha. SIN *stratum* germinativum unguis.
glomerular l. of olfactory bulb, c. glomerular do bulbo olfativo; uma c. composta de corpos esféricos, chamados glomérulos, formada pelas sinapses das células mitrais com as fibras do nervo olfatório derivadas das células do epitélio olfatório.
granular l. [TA], estrato granular do giro denteado. VER l.'s of dentate gyrus. SIN stratum granulare [TA].
granular l. of cerebellar cortex, estrato granuloso do córtex cerebelar. SIN granular l. of cerebellum.
granular l. of cerebellum [TA], estrato granuloso do córtex cerebelar; a mais profunda das três camadas do córtex; contém numerosas células com grânulos, cujos dendritos fazem sinapse com as fibras musgosas aferentes nos glomérulos cerebelares. Os axônios finos e desmielinizados das células granulosas ascendem perpendicularmente para o estrato molecular, na qual se bifurcam nas fibras que avançam em paralelo ao eixo longitudinal das folhas do verme cerebelar. As fibras em paralelo formam numerosas sinapses com os dendritos das células de Purkinje, células em cesta e células estrelares. SIN granular l. of cerebellar cortex [TA], stratum granulosum corticis cerebelli [TA].
granular l.'s of cerebral cortex, camadas granulares do córtex cerebral; as 2 camadas (externas) e 4 (internas) do córtex cerebral.
granular l. of epidermis, estrato granular da epiderme; uma c. de células algo achatadas, contendo grânulos basofílicos de cerato-hialina e situada logo acima do estrato espinhoso e profundamente ao estrato córneo. SIN stratum granulosum epidermidis.
granular l. of a vesicular ovarian follicle, estrato granuloso dos folículos ováricos vesiculosos. SIN *stratum* granulosum folliculi ovarici vesiculosi.
gray l.'s of superior colliculus, estratos cinzentos do colículo superior; termo aplicado a qualquer uma das três camadas principais da substância cinzenta do colículo superior que se alternam com as camadas compostas principalmente de fibras nervosas: 1) o estrato cinzento superficial do colículo superior, externo à camada em grande parte branca de fibras que se originam do trato óptico (lâmina óptica); 2) o estrato cinzento intermédio do colículo superior, colocado entre a lâmina óptica e uma lâmina localizada mais profundamente de fibras, a lâmina do lemnisco; 3) o estrato cinzento profundo do colículo superior, entre a lâmina do lemnisco e a substância cinzenta central que circunda o aqueduto do mesencéfalo, contendo as grandes células nervosas, a partir da qual se origina a maioria das conexões descendentes do colículo (tratos tetobulbar, tetopontino e tetospinal). SIN stratum cinereum colliculi superioris, stratum griseum colliculi superioris.
half-value l. (HVL), camada da metade do valor, camada de meio-valor; a espessura de um material absorvente específico (p.ex., alumínio) que reduzirá a intensidade de um feixe de radiação à metade de seu valor inicial.

Henle l., c. de Henle; a c. externa de células da bainha da raiz interna do folículo piloso.

Henle fiber l., c. fibrosa de Henle; a c. de fibras cônicas internas na área central da retina.

Henle nervous l., c. nervosa de Henle. SIN entoretina.

l.'s of hippocampus [TA], estratos do hipocampo; quatro camadas formadas por células e prolongamentos celulares; são, começando na superfície ventricular e álvea: estrato de orientação [TA] (stratum oriens [TA]), que contém os dendritos basais e os colaterais axônicos das células piramidais; o estrato piramidal [TA] (stratum pyramidale [TA]), que contém os corpos das grandes células piramidais do hipocampo; o estrato radiado [TA] (stratum radiatum [TA]), que contém os dendritos ramificantes das células piramidais e os colaterais axônicos recorrentes das células piramidais; e o estrato molecular e substrato lacunar [TA] (stratum moleculare et substratum lacunosum [TA]), que contêm os dendritos distais e parte dos axônios aferentes da via perfurante. SIN strata hippocampi [TA].

horny l. of epidermis, estrato córneo da epiderme. SIN *stratum* corneum epidermidis.

horny l. of nail, estrato córneo da unha. SIN *stratum* corneum unguis.

Huxley l., c. de Huxley; uma c. de células interpostas entre a c. de Henle e a cutícula da bainha da raiz interna do folículo piloso. SIN Huxley membrane, Huxley sheath.

infragranular l., c. infragranular; a faixa celular profunda à lâmina granular interna do córtex cerebral humano em desenvolvimento, que se diferencia no estrato ganglionar e na lâmina multiforme em torno do sexto mês de desenvolvimento fetal.

inner l. of eyeball [TA], túnica interna do bulbo do olho; a terceira e mais profunda das três camadas do bulbo do olho, composta da retina, parte intraocular do nervo óptico e vasos sanguíneos retinianos. SIN tunica interna bulbi [TA], nervous tunic of eyeball.

inner limiting layer [TA], estrato limitante interno; a estrutura semelhante a membrana localizada imediatamente interna à camada de fibras nervosas; composta dos prolongamentos das células da neuróglia (células de Müller) da retina. SIN stratum limitans internum [TA].

inner nuclear l. [TA], estrato nuclear interno; a c. da retina composta dos corpos celulares das células bipolares, células horizontais e parte dos corpos celulares das células amácrinas. SIN stratum nucleare internum [TA].

l. of inner and outer segments [TA], estrato dos segmentos interno e externo; a c. da retina localizada externamente à lâmina limitante externa e composta dos segmentos interno e externo dos bastonetes e cones; as extremidades externas dos segmentos de bastonetes e cones são apostas ao estrato pigmentoso. SIN stratum segmentorum externorum et internorum [TA].

inner plexiform l. [TA], estrato plexiforme interno; a c. da retina composta dos prolongamentos das células bipolares, células ganglionares e células amácrinas; uma camada que contém os contatos sinápticos. SIN stratum plexiforme internum [TA].

intermediate l., lâminas do córtex cerebral. SIN mantle l.

intermediate white l. of superior colliculus, estrato medular intermédio; uma c. de fibras mielinizadas localizada entre os estratos cinzentos intermédio e profundo do colículo superior. SIN stratum medullare intermedium [TA].

investing l. [TA], c. de revestimento; uma c. fascial que embainha ou envolve intimamente um grupo específico de músculos. SIN fascia investiens [TA].

investing l. of cervical fascia [TA], lâmina superficial da fáscia cervical; a parte da fáscia cervical que reveste os músculos esternocleidomastóideo e trapézio e que envolve por completo o pescoço. SIN lamina superficialis fasciae cervicalis [TA], superficial l. of deep cervical fascia*, investing fascia.

Kölliker l., c. de Kölliker; a c. de tecido conjuntivo na íris.

lacunar-molecular l., estrato molecular e substrato lacunar. VER l.'s of hippocampus. SIN stratum moleculare et substratum lacunosum [TA].

Langhans l., c. de Langhans. SIN cytotrophoblast.

latticed l., c. reticulada; uma c. de células corticais no hipocampo.

limiting l.'s of cornea, lâminas limitantes da córnea. VER anterior limiting l. of cornea, posterior limiting *lamina* of cornea.

longitudinal l. of muscle coat of small intestine [TA], c. longitudinal da túnica muscular do intestino delgado [TA]. SIN stratum longitudinale tunicae muscularis intestini tenuis [TA], stratum helicoidale longi gradus*.

longitudinal l. of muscular coat [TA], camada longitudinal da túnica muscular; a c. longitudinal externa da musculatura lisa da túnica muscular. A *Terminologia Anatomica* arrola as seguintes camadas longitudinais das túnicas musculares (stratum longitudinale tunicae muscularis...): 1) da parte membranácea da uretra (...urethrae intermediae [TA]); 2) do colo (...coli [TA]); 3) da parte prostática da uretra (...urethrae prostaticae [TA]); 4) do reto (...recti [TA]); 5) do intestino delgado (...intestini tenuis [TA]); 6) da parte esponjosa da uretra (...urethrae spongiosae [TA]); 7) do estômago (...gastricae [TA]). SIN stratum longitudinale tunicae muscularis [TA].

longitudinal l.'s of muscular tunics, camadas longitudinais da túnica muscular. VER longitudinal l. of muscular coat.

long pitch helicoidal l., camada helicoidal de passo longo. SIN *stratum* helicoidale longi gradus [TA].

malpighian l., estrato de Malpighi. SIN malpighian *stratum.*

mantle l., c. do manto; a zona nuclear do tubo neural em desenvolvimento entre a c. marginal e a c. ependimária; forma a substância cinzenta do sistema nervoso central. SIN intermediate l., mantle zone (1).

marginal l., zona marginal; a c. externa anuclear do tubo neural embrionário; em sua rede fibrosa crescem as fibras nervosas longitudinais que, mais adiante, transformam-se na substância branca da medula espinal e do tronco cerebral. SIN marginal zone (2).

medullary l.'s of thalamus, lâminas medulares do tálamo. SIN medullary *laminae* of thalamus, em *lamina.*

membranous l., lâmina membranácea da parte cartilagínea da tuba auditiva. SIN membranous *lamina* of cartilage of pharyngotympanic (auditory) plate.

membranous l. of subcutaneous tissue of abdomen [TA], camada membranácea da tela subcutânea do períneo; a camada mais profunda, membranosa ou lamelar, do tecido subcutâneo da parede abdominal inferior; é contínua com a camada superficial do períneo (Colles). SIN membranous l. of superficial fascia of perineum (2), membranous l. of superficial fascia (2), Scarpa fascia.

membranous l. of superficial fascia, (1) tela subcutânea do períneo. SIN subcutaneous *tissue* of perineum; **(2)** camada membranácea da tela subcutânea do períneo. SIN membranous l. of subcutaneous tissue of abdomen.

membranous l. of superficial fascia of perineum, (1) tela subcutânea do períneo. SIN subcutaneous *tissue* of perineum; **(2)** camada membranácea da tela subcutânea do períneo. SIN membranous l. of subcutaneous tissue of abdomen.

meningeal l. of dura mater, parte encefálica da dura-máter. VER cranial *dura mater.*

Meynert l., c. de Meynert. SIN pyramidal cell l.

middle gray l. of superior colliculus, c. cinzenta intermediária do colículo superior. VER gray l.'s of superior colliculus.

molecular l., estrato ou lâmina molecular; termo aplicado a qualquer lâmina do tecido cerebral que contenha poucos corpos de células nervosas e que seja composta, em grande parte, de arborizações terminais dos dendritos e axônios; os exemplos notáveis são o estrato superficial (primeira c.) do córtex cerebral e o estrato molecular do cerebelo. SIN plexiform l., stratum moleculare.

molecular l. of cerebellar cortex [TA], estrato molecular do córtex cerebelar; a lâmina externa do córtex, contendo os corpos celulares (a menos que a camada de células de Purkinje seja designada como uma camada separada) e os dendritos das células de Purkinje, os axônios das células granulares e os corpos celulares, dendritos e axônios das células em cesta. SIN stratum moleculare corticis cerebelli [TA], molecular l. of cerebellum.

molecular l. of cerebellum, estrato molecular do córtex cerebelar. SIN molecular l. of cerebellar cortex.

molecular l. of cerebral cortex [TA], lâmina molecular do córtex cerebral; camada 1 do córtex cerebral. SIN lamina molecularis corticis cerebri [TA], plexiform l. of cerebral cortex.

molecular l.'s of olfactory bulb, estratos moleculares do bulbo olfatório; as camadas compostas principalmente das fibras nervosas, nos lados externo e interno da c. de células mitrais do bulbo.

molecular l. of retina, estrato molecular da retina; nome aplicado a cada uma das camadas plexiformes da retina. SIN stratum moleculare retinae.

multiform l. [TA], estrato multiforme do giro denteado. VER l.'s of dentate gyrus. SIN stratum multiforme [TA].

multiform l. [TA] of cerebral cortex, lâmina multiforme [TA] do córtex cerebral; a camada mais interna do córtex cerebral, camada VI. SIN fusiform l., polymorphous l., spindle-celled l.

muscle l. in fatty layer of subcutaneous tissue [TA], estrato muscular do panículo adiposo da tela subcutânea; a c. de músculo liso ou estriado embebida no tecido adiposo subcutâneo para a contração ou para produzir o movimento da pele, p.ex., os músculos faciais no tecido subcutâneo da face e do pescoço, o músculo dartos na túnica darta da bolsa escrotal. SIN stratum musculorum panniculi adiposi telae subcutaneae [TA].

muscular l., túnica muscular; a camada muscular, usualmente média, de uma estrutura tubular; para a maior parte do trato gastrointestinal, consiste em uma camada longitudinal externa de músculo e uma camada interna circular. SIN tunica muscularis [TA], muscular coat*.

muscular l. of bronchi, c. muscular dos brônquios; a camada muscular da parede brônquica. SIN tunica muscularis bronchiorum [TA], muscular coat of bronchi*.

muscular l. of colon [TA], túnica muscular do colo; a camada muscular da parede do colo. SIN tunica muscularis coli [TA], muscular coat of colon*.

muscular l. of ductus deferens [TA], túnica muscular do ducto deferente; a camada muscular da parede do ducto deferente. SIN tunica muscularis ductus deferentis [TA], muscular coat of ductus deferens*.

muscular l. of esophagus [TA], túnica muscular do esôfago; a camada muscular da parede esofágica. SIN tunica muscularis esophagi [TA], muscular coat of esophagus*.

muscular l. of female urethra [TA], túnica muscular da uretra feminina; a camada muscular da parede da uretra feminina. SIN tunica muscularis urethrae femininae [TA], muscular coat of female urethra*.

muscular l. of gallbladder, túnica muscular da vesícula biliar; túnica muscular da vesícula biliar, consistindo nas camadas de fibras musculares lisas que

avançam em várias direções imediatamente externas à mucosa da vesícula biliar. SIN tunica muscularis vesicae biliaris [TA], muscular coat of gallbladder*, tunica muscularis vesicae fellae*, muscular tunic of gallbladder.
muscular l. of intermediate part of (male) urethra [TA], túnica muscular da parte membranácea da uretra (masculina); a camada interna relativamente fina de feixes de músculos lisos (involuntários), em sua maioria dispostos longitudinalmente e separados do epitélio por um fino estroma vascular de tecido conjuntivo fibroelástico, que são contínuos, superiormente, com os da parte prostática da uretra e, perifericamente, com uma c. externa, muito mais proeminente, de fibras de músculos esqueléticos (voluntários) de orientação circular que formam a parte principal, semelhante a um tubo, do esfíncter externo da uretra. VER TAMBÉM external urethral *sphincter* of male. SIN tunica muscularis partis intermediae urethrae masculinae [TA], muscular coat of intermediate part of male urethra*.
muscular l. of large intestine [TA], túnica muscular do intestino grosso; coletivamente, a c. muscular da parede de todas as partes do intestino grosso (ceco, colo, reto e canal anal). SIN tunica muscularis intestini crassi [TA], muscular coat of large intestine*.
muscular l. of male urethra [TA], túnica muscular da uretra masculina; a c. muscular das partes prostática, membranácea e esponjosa da uretra masculina. VER TAMBÉM muscular l. of intermediate part of (male) urethra. SIN tunica muscularis urethrae masculinae [TA], muscular coat of male urethra.
muscular l. of mucosa, lâmina muscular da mucosa. SIN *muscularis mucosae*.
muscular l. of pharynx [TA], túnica muscular da faringe; a camada muscular da parede faríngea. Em contraste com as camadas musculares do restante do trato gastrointestinal (excetuando-se o canal anal), a da faringe possui uma camada circular externa e uma camada longitudinal interna. SIN tunica muscularis pharyngis [TA], muscular coat of pharynx*.
muscular l. of prostatic urethra [TA], túnica muscular da parte prostática da uretra masculina; a camada interna relativamente fina de feixes de músculos lisos (involuntários), dispostos de forma circular e longitudinal e separados do epitélio por um fino estroma vascular de tecido conjuntivo fibroelástico; esses feixes são contínuos inferiormente com os da parte membranácea da uretra e perifericamente com o tecido fibromuscular da próstata, incluindo uma camada relativamente espessa, semelhante a uma calha, de músculo esquelético (voluntário) que ascende na face anterior da uretra prostática até o colo da bexiga como parte do esfíncter externo da uretra; proximal (superior) ao colículo seminal, que comporta as aberturas dos canais ejaculatórios, a camada circular de músculo liso é particularmente proeminente como uma continuação do esfíncter interno da parte intramural ou pré-prostática da uretra. VER TAMBÉM external urethral *sphincter* of male, internal urethral *sphincter*. SIN tunica muscularis partis prostaticae urethrae masculinae [TA], muscular coat of intermediate part of male urethra*, muscular coat of prostatic urethra.
muscular l. of rectum [TA], túnica muscular do reto; camada muscular da parede do reto. SIN tunica muscularis recti [TA], muscular coat of rectum*.
muscular l. of renal pelvis [TA], túnica muscular da pelve renal; a c. média (entre a adventícia externa e a mucosa interna) composta de dois tipos diferentes de músculo liso, do ponto de vista morfológico e bioquímico, dos quais um é idêntico e contínuo com o dos ureteres, enquanto o outro é único para os cálices e pelve. SIN tunica muscularis pelvis renalis [TA].
muscular l. of seminal gland [TA], túnica muscular da glândula seminal; a c. média (entre o tecido conjuntivo externo e a mucosa interna) da parede da glândula seminal, composta das camadas longitudinal externa e circular interna de músculos lisos. SIN tunica muscularis glandulae vesiculosae [TA].
muscular l. of small intestine [TA], túnica muscular do intestino delgado; a camada muscular da parede do intestino delgado. SIN tunica muscularis intestini tenuis [TA], muscular coat of small intestine*.
muscular l. of spongy (male) urethra [TA], túnica muscular da uretra esponjosa (masculina); a c. relativamente escassa de fibras musculares lisas (involuntárias) dispostas, em sua maioria, longitudinalmente entre a mucosa e o tecido erétil circunvizinho do corpo esponjoso do pênis. SIN tunica muscularis partis spongiosae urethrae masculinae [TA], muscular coat of spongy part od male urethra*.
muscular l. of stomach [TA], túnica muscular do estômago; a camada muscular do estômago, consistindo em músculos lisos em três camadas muito bem definidas; uma *camada longitudinal externa*, contínua com a do esôfago, mas que se divide na cárdia em duas faixas que correm ao longo das curvaturas maior e menor, deixando as áreas médias das paredes anterior e posterior desprovidas de fibras longitudinais; em seguida, coalescem na região pilórica em uma camada completa, que é contínua com a c. longitudinal do duodeno. A *camada circular média* é mais completa e mais forte, contínua com a camada circular do esôfago na cárdia; espessa-se progressivamente em direção ao piloro, formando, por fim, o anel muscular do esfíncter pilórico. A *camada oblíqua interna* é única para o estômago e é mais fortemente desenvolvida na região fúndica, estando ausente ao longo da curvatura menor. Essa ausência contribui para a formação do "canal gástrico". SIN tunica muscularis gastrica [TA], muscular coat of stomach*, tunica muscularis ventriculi.
muscular l. of trachea [TA], túnica muscular da traquéia; a camada muscular da parede traqueal. SIN tunica muscularis tracheae [TA], muscular coat of trachea*.
muscular l. of ureter [TA], túnica muscular do ureter; a camada muscular da parede do ureter. SIN tunica muscularis ureteris [TA], muscular coat of ureter*.
muscular l. of urinary bladder [TA], túnica muscular da bexiga; a camada muscular da parede da bexiga urinária. SIN tunica muscularis vesicae urinariae [TA], muscular coat of urinary bladder*.
muscular l. of uterine tube [TA], túnica muscular da tuba uterina; a camada muscular da parede da tuba uterina. SIN tunica muscularis tubae uterinae [TA], muscular coat of uterine tube*.
muscular l. of vagina [TA], túnica muscular da vagina; a camada muscular da parede vaginal. SIN tunica muscularis vaginae [TA], muscular coat of vagina*.
l. of nerve fibers [TA], estrato das neurofibras; a c. da retina composta dos prolongamentos axônicos das células ganglionares; esses prolongamentos convergem para formar o nervo óptico. SIN stratum neurofibrarum [TA].
neural l. of optic part of retina, c. neural da parte óptica da retina. VER retina.
neural l. of retina, parte óptica da retina. SIN cerebral l. of retina.
neuroepithelial l. of retina, estrato dos segmentos externo e interno da retina; a c. mais externa do estrato nervoso da retina, composta das células receptoras primárias da retina; essa área consiste em duas camadas: 1) uma camada dos segmentos externo e interno [TA] constituída de bastonetes e cones, os prolongamentos fotossensíveis das células receptoras; e 2) a c. nuclear externa [TA], que contém os corpos celulares dessas células; a lâmina limitante externa [TA] forma uma placa de sustentação perfurada entre as duas subcamadas; o nome refere-se ao fato de que as células receptoras retinianas são uma forma especializada de célula ependimária (epitelial) e, dessa forma, em um sentido, são comparáveis às células neuroepiteliais (p.ex., células ciliadas) de outros órgãos dos sentidos. SIN external nuclear l. of retina, stratum neuroepitheliale retinae.
Nitabuch l., membrana de Nitabuch. SIN Nitabuch *membrane*.
nuclear l.'s of retina, estratos nucleares da retina; o estrato do segmento externo, o e. 4 da retina, a c. neuroepitelial da retina, e o estrato do segmento interno, o e. 6 da retina, a camada ganglionar da retina. SIN strata nuclearia externa et interna retinae.
odontoblastic l., c. odontoblástica; uma c. de células mesenquimais na periferia da polpa dentária.
optic l., estrato óptico; **(1)** uma camada de substância branca interespaçada por corpos de células nervosas, logo abaixo da c. cinzenta superficial do colículo superior, composta de fibras mielinizadas que se originam na retina e no córtex estriado; **(2)** um termo raramente empregado para descrever o estrato interno da retina, consistindo em fibras que se originam das células do e. ganglionar da retina; em seus trajetos posteriores, essas fibras combinam-se para formar o nervo óptico. SIN stratum opticum [TA].
orbital l. of ethmoid bone, lâmina orbital do osso etmóide. SIN orbital *plate* of ethmoid bone.
oriens l. [TA], estrato de orientação. VER l.´s of hippocampus. SIN stratum oriens [TA].
osteogenetic l., c. osteogênica; a c. interna do periósteo formadora de osso.
outer limiting l. [TA], estrato limitante externo; a estrutura semelhante a membrana localizada imediatamente interna ao estrato dos segmentos externo e interno; constituída por prolongamentos das células neurogliais da retina (células de Müller); penetrada pela porção dos bastonetes e cones localizada entre os segmentos interno e externo e o corpo celular. SIN stratum limitans externum [TA].
outer nuclear l. [TA], estrato nuclear externo; a c. da retina que contém os corpos celulares dos bastonetes e cones. SIN stratum nucleare externum [TA].
outer plexiform l. [TA], estrato plexiforme externo; a c. da retina composta por prolongamentos de bastonetes e cones, células horizontais e células bipolares; uma camada que contém os contatos sinápticos. SIN stratum plexiforme externum [TA].
palisade l., estrato basal da epiderme. SIN *stratum* basale epidermidis.
papillary l., estrato papilar do cório. SIN *stratum* papillare corii.
parietal l. [TA], lâmina parietal; a c. externa de uma bolsa ou saco que envolve uma estrutura, geralmente revestindo as paredes da cavidade ou espaço ocupado pela estrutura envelopada, com a própria estrutura sendo coberta pela camada interna ou visceral do saco acondicionador; um espaço real ou potencial é envolto pelas duas camadas contínuas, interpondo-se entre as camadas parietal e visceral. A lâmina parietal é usualmente a mais substancial. SIN lamina parietalis [TA].
parietal l. of leptomeninges, aracnóide-máter. SIN arachnoid mater.
parietal l. of serous pericardium [TA], lâmina parietal do pericárdio seroso; a parte externa do pericárdio seroso sustentada pelo pericárdio fibroso. SIN lamina parietalis pericardii serosi [TA].
parietal l. of tunica vaginalis of testis [TA], lâmina parietal da túnica vaginal do testículo; a parte externa da túnica vaginal do testículo sustentada pela fáscia espermática interna. SIN lamina parietalis tunicae vaginalis testis [TA].
perforated l. of sclera, c. cribriforme da esclera. SIN *lamina* cribrosa of sclera.
periosteal l. of dura mater, c. periosteal da dura-máter. VER cranial *dura* mater.
pigmented l. of ciliary body, estrato pigmentoso do corpo ciliar. SIN *stratum* pigmenti corporis ciliaris.
pigmented l. of iris, epitélio pigmentado da íris. SIN *stratum* pigmenti iridis.

pigmented l. of retina [TA], estrato pigmentoso da retina; a c. externa da retina, consistindo em epitélio pigmentado. SIN ectoretina, stratum pigmenti bulbi, stratum pigmenti retinae, tapetum nigrum, tapetum oculi.

piriform neuron l., c. neuronal piriforme; um termo obsoleto para estrato purkinjense.

l. of piriform neurons, estrato purkinjense. SIN Purkinje cell l.

plasma l., espaço de Poiseuille. SIN still l.

plexiform l., estrato molecular. SIN molecular l.

plexiform l. of cerebral cortex, estrato molecular do giro denteado. SIN molecular l. of cerebral cortex.

plexiform l.'s of retina, estratos plexiformes da retina onde ocorrem as sinapses; no estrato externo, os prolongamentos dos bastonetes e cones fazem sinapse com os dendritos dos neurônios bipolares; no estrato interno, as terminações axônicas das células bipolares fazem sinapse com os dendritos das células ganglionares. VER retina. SIN stratum plexiforme internum [TA], stratum plexiforme externum.

polymorphous l., estrato multiforme do giro denteado. SIN multiform l. [TA] of cerebral cortex.

posterior elastic l., lâmina limitante posterior da córnea. SIN posterior limiting lamina of cornea.

posterior limiting l. of cornea, lâmina limitante posterior da córnea. SIN posterior limiting lamina of cornea.

posterior l. of rectus sheath [TA], lâmina posterior da bainha do músculo reto do abdome; a porção da bainha dos músculos reto do abdome que se situa posteriormente ao músculo e cobre apenas seus dois terços superiores é formada por contribuições das aponeuroses dos músculos oblíquo interno e transverso do abdome; sua margem inferior livre forma a linha arqueada; é deficiente abaixo desta, com a face posterior do músculo sendo coberta apenas pela fáscia transversal e peritônio. SIN lamina posterior vaginae musculi recti abdominis [TA].

pretracheal l. of cervical fascia [TA], lâmina pré-traqueal da fáscia cervical; a camada da fáscia de revestimento dos músculos infra-hióideos e que contribui para a formação da bainha carótica. SIN lamina pretrachealis fasciae cervicalis [TA], middle cervical fascia, Porter fascia, pretracheal fascia.

prevertebral l. of cervical fascia [TA], lâmina pré-vertebral da fáscia cervical, a parte da fáscia cervical que recobre os corpos das vértebras cervicais e os músculos que se inserem nessas vértebras e nas porções anteriores de seus processos transversos. SIN lamina prevertebralis fasciae cervicalis [TA] prevertebral fascia.

prickle cell l., estrato espinhoso da epiderme. SIN stratum spinosum epidermidis.

Purkinje cell l., estrato purkinjense; a c. de corpos celulares neuronais grandes localizada na interface dos estratos molecular e granular no córtex cerebelar; os dendritos dessas células espalham-se para fora, para o estrato molecular, em um plano transverso à folha do cerebelo. SIN stratum purkinjense corticis cerebelli [TA], ganglionic l. of cerebellar cortex, l. of piriform neurons, Purkinje cells, Purkinje corpuscles.

pyramidal l. [TA], estrato piramidal. VER l.'s of hippocampus. SIN stratum pyramidale [TA].

pyramidal cell l., lâminas piramidais; as camadas 3 e 5 do córtex cerebral. SIN Meynert l.

radiant l. [TA], estrato radiado. VER l.'s of hippocampus. SIN stratum radiatum [TA].

radiate l. of tympanic membrane, c. radiada da membrana timpânica. SIN stratum radiatum membranae tympani.

Rauber l., c. de Rauber; **(1)** uma membrana trofoblástica afilada sobre o disco embrionário nos carnívoros e ungulados em desenvolvimento; **(2)** a camada celular mais externa que ajuda a formar o blastodisco; chamada de blastoderma ou ectoderma primitivo.

reticular l. of corium, estrato reticular do cório. SIN stratum reticulare corii.

l.'s of retina, estratos da retina. VER retina.

l. of rods and cones, estrato dos segmentos externo e interno; a c. da retina próxima ao estrato pigmentoso e que contém os receptores visuais. VER TAMBÉM retina, neuroepithelial l. of retina. SIN bacillary l.

rostral l., lâmina rostral. SIN rostral lamina.

Sattler elastic l., c. elástica de Sattler; a c. média da corióide.

serous l. of peritoneum, túnica serosa do peritônio. SIN serosa of peritoneum.

short pitch helicoidal l., c. helicoidal de passo curto da túnica muscular do intestino delgado; *termo oficial alternativo para circular l. of muscle coat of small intestine.

l.'s of skin, camadas da pele. VER epidermis, dermis.

sluggish l., espaço de Poiseuille. SIN still l.

somatic l., c. somática; a c. externa do mesoderma lateral do embrião situada adjacente ao ectoderma e que, juntamente com este, constitui a somatopleura.

spindle-celled l., lâmina multiforme do córtex cerebral. SIN multiform l. [TA] of cerebral cortex.

spinous l., estrato espinhoso da epiderme. SIN stratum spinosum epidermidis.

splanchnic l., c. esplâncnica; a c. interna do mesoderma lateral situada adjacente ao endoderma e que, juntamente com este, forma a esplancnopleura.

spongy l. of female urethra [TA], túnica esponjosa da uretra feminina; referência imprópria à lâmina própria da mucosa da uretra feminina, caracterizada por numerosas veias, de paredes finas, outrora erroneamente comparadas ao tecido erétil. SIN tunica spongiosa urethrae femininae [TA].

spongy l. of vagina [TA], túnica esponjosa da vagina; referência coletiva imprópria aos plexos venosos abundantes da vagina, ocorrendo nas camadas mucosa e muscular (dando às rugas algo do caráter do tecido erétil), bem como na adventícia (os plexos venosos vaginais lateralmente dispostos), sugerindo falsamente uma camada bem definida de tecido erétil. SIN tunica spongiosa vaginae [TA].

still l., espaço de Poiseuille; a c. da corrente sanguínea nos vasos capilares, situada próximo à parede do vaso, que flui lentamente e transporta os leucócitos ao longo da camada da parede, enquanto, no centro, o fluxo é rápido e transporta os eritrócitos. SIN plasma l., Poiseuille space, sluggish l.

subendocardial l., c. subendocárdica; a camada de tecido conjuntivo frouxo que une o endocárdio e o miocárdio; nos ventrículos, contém ramos do sistema de condução do coração.

subendothelial l., c. subendotelial; a c. fina do tecido conjuntivo que se situa entre o endotélio e a lâmina elástica na camada íntima dos vasos sanguíneos.

subpapillary l., c. subpapilar; a c. vascular do cório.

subserous l., subserosa; *termo oficial alternativo para subserosa.

superficial l. [TA], lâmina superficial; em uma estrutura estratificada, a mais externa ou superior das camadas; a camada mais próxima da superfície. VER superficial l. of deep cervical fascia; superficial l. of levator palpebrae superioris, superficial l. of temporal fascia. SIN lamina superficialis [TA], superficial lamina.

superficial l. of deep cervical fascia, lâmina superficial da fáscia cervical; *termo oficial alternativo para investing l. of cervical fascia.

superficial gray l. [TA] of superior colliculus, estrato cinzento superficial do colículo superior. VER gray l.'s of superior colliculus.

superficial l. of the levator palpebrae superioris [TA], lâmina superficial do músculo levantador da pálpebra superior; as fibras superficiais do músculo levantador da pálpebra superior que estão inseridas na pele da pálpebra superior. SIN lamina superficialis musculi levatoris palpebrae superioris.

superficial l. of temporal fascia [TA], lâmina superficial da fáscia temporal; a parte superficial da fáscia temporal que se insere na superfície lateral do arco zigomático. SIN lamina superficialis fasciae temporalis [TA].

suprachoroid l., lâmina supracorióide. SIN suprachoroid lamina of sclera.

Tomes granular l., c. granular de Tomes; uma c. fina de dentina, adjacente ao cemento, que se mostra granular nos cortes; os grânulos são pequenos espaços não-calcificados.

vascular l., lâmina vascular da corióide. SIN vascular lamina of choroid.

vascular l. of choroid coat of eye, lâmina vascular da corióide. SIN vascular lamina of choroid.

vascular l. of eyeball [TA], túnica vascular do bulbo do olho; a camada vascular, pigmentar ou média do olho, compreendendo corióide, corpo ciliar e íris. SIN tunica vasculosa bulbi [TA], Haller tunica vasculosa, tunica vasculosa oculi, uvea, uveal tract, vascular tunic of eye.

vascular l. of testis [TA], túnica vascular do testículo; a mais interna das três camadas (com as túnicas vaginal e albugínea) que revestem os testículos, consistindo em um plexo vascular em uma delicada matriz de tecido conjuntivo frouxo que cobre a face interna da túnica albugínea e se estende profundamente, cobrindo os septos e, portanto, circundando os lóbulos do testículo. SIN tunica vasculosa testis [TA].

ventricular l., lâmina ependimária. SIN ependymal l.

visceral l. [TA], lâmina visceral; a c. interna de um saco ou bolsa envolvente que reveste a superfície externa da estrutura envolvida, em oposição à lâmina parietal que cobre as paredes do espaço ou cavidade ocupada. A lâmina visceral é geralmente fina, delicada e não evidente quando está sendo separada, assemelhando-se à superfície externa da própria estrutura. VER TAMBÉM serosa. SIN lamina visceralis [TA].

visceral l. of serous pericardium [TA], lâmina visceral do pericárdio seroso; a parte interna do pericárdio seroso aplicada diretamente sobre o coração. SIN epicardium*, lamina visceralis pericardii.

visceral l. of tunica vaginalis of testis [TA], lâmina visceral da túnica vaginal do testículo; a parte interna da túnica vaginal do testículo aplicada diretamente ao testículo e ao epidídimo. SIN lamina visceralis tunicae vaginalis testis [TA].

Waldeyer zonal l., trato póstero-lateral do funículo lateral. SIN dorsolateral fasciculus.

Weil basal l., zona basal de Weil; a c. abaixo dos odontoblastos do dente; ela contém as fibras reticulares, porém com poucas ou nenhuma célula. SIN Weil basal zone.

zonular l., estrato zonal; **(1)** uma camada fina da substância branca que cobre a superfície superior do tálamo e que forma parte do assoalho do corpo do ventrículo lateral; **(2)** uma c. de substância branca na superfície do colículo superior. SIN stratum zonale [TA].

---

laz·a·ret, laz·a·ret·to (laz'ā - ret, - ret'ō). Lazareto; termo obsoleto para: **1.** Um hospital para o tratamento de doenças contagiosas. **2.** Um local de detenção para as pessoas em quarentena. [It. *lazzaretto*, de *lazzaro*, uma lepra]

lb. Abreviatura de pound (libra).
LBF Abreviatura de *Lactobacillus bulgaricus factor* (fator do *Lactobacillus bulgaricus*).
LCAT Abreviatura de lecithin-cholesterol acyltransferase (lecitina-colesterol aciltransferase).
l-cone. Cone l; cone sensível a comprimento de onda longo (cone vermelho).
LD Abreviatura de lethal *dose* (dose letal).
LDH Abreviatura de *lactate* dehydrogenase (desidrogenase láctica).
LDL Abreviatura de low density lipoprotein (lipoproteína de baixa densidade). Ver lipoprotein.
LE, L.E. Abreviatura de left eye (olho esquerdo); *lupus* erythematosus (lúpus eritematoso).
leach·ing (lēch′ing). Lixiviação. **1.** Remoção dos constituintes solúveis de uma substância fazendo com que a água corra através dela. **2.** Solubilização dos metais, tipicamente de minérios mistos, usando bactérias litotróficas. [A. S. *leccan*, umedecer]
lead (Pb) (led). Chumbo; um elemento metálico, número atômico 82, peso atômico 207,2. SIN plumbum.
  l. acetate, acetato de chumbo; tem sido empregado como adstringente na diarréia e, em solução aquosa, como um curativo úmido em determinadas dermatoses. SIN sugar of lead.
  black l., grafite. SIN graphite.
  l. carbonate, carbonato de c. cerusa; um pó branco pesado que é insolúvel em água; ocasionalmente, é usado para aliviar a irritação na dermatite, mas é usado sobretudo na manufatura de tinta e nas artes, sendo por isso produtora de intoxicação por c. SIN ceruse, white l.
  l. chromate, cromato de c., amarelo de cromo. SIN chrome yellow.
  l. monoxide, monóxido de c., massicote, litargírio; tem sido utilizado como um ingrediente em aplicações externas, como emplastros. SIN l. oxide (yellow), litharge, massicot.
  l. oxide (yellow), óxido de c. (amarelo). SIN l. monoxide.
  red l., c. vermelho. SIN l. tetroxide.
  red oxide of l., óxido vermelho de c. SIN l. tetroxide.
  l. sulfide, sulfeto de chumbo, galena. PbS; a forma original em que o c. é principalmente encontrado. SIN galena.
  l. tetraethyl, chumbo tetraetila. SIN tetraethyllead.
  l. tetroxide, tetróxido de c.; um pó vermelho-alaranjado brilhoso que fica negro quando aquecido; usado em pomadas e emplastros. SIN red l., red oxide of l.
  white l., c. branco, carbonato de c. SIN l. carbonate.
lead (lēd). Derivação; um cabo eletrocardiográfico com conexões nos componentes eletrônicos do aparelho designados para um eletrodo colocado em determinado ponto sobre a superfície corporal.
  ABC l.'s, derivações ABC; as derivações para registrar um tipo de vetorcardiograma que utiliza o triângulo de Arrighi; suplantado pelas derivações XYZ (XYZ l.'s).
  augmented l., d. aumentada; eletrocardiograma registrado entre uma derivação e duas outras derivações. As derivações aumentadas são designadas como aVF, aVL e aVR para os registros feitos entre o pé (esquerdo), braço esquerdo e braço direito, respectivamente, e as outras duas derivações.
  bipolar l., d. bipolar; um registro obtido com dois eletrodos colocados em diferentes regiões do corpo, cada um contribuindo de modo significativo para o registro; p.ex., uma d. de membro padronizada.
  CB l., d. CB: uma d. torácica bipolar com o eletrodo negativo colocado nas costas da pessoa.
  CF l., d. CF; uma d. torácica bipolar com o eletrodo negativo colocado na perna esquerda da pessoa.
  chest l.'s, derivações torácicas ou precordiais; aquelas em que o eletrodo explorador fica sobre o tórax, sobrepondo-se ao coração ou às suas vizinhanças. SIN precordial l.'s, semidirect l.'s.
  CL l., d. CL; uma derivação torácica bipolar com o eletrodo negativo colocado no braço esquerdo da pessoa.
  CR l., d. CR; uma d. torácica bipolar com o eletrodo negativo colocado no braço direito da pessoa.
  direct l., d. direta; em eletrocardiografia, uma d. unipolar registrada com o eletrodo explorador diretamente sobre a superfície do coração exposto.
  esophageal l., d. esofágica; uma d. eletrocardiográfica introduzida no esôfago, através da garganta, para registrar o eletrocardiograma em vários níveis do esôfago; útil sobretudo para certos tipos de arritmias. De maneira similar, um transdutor para ecocardiografia pode ser introduzido no esôfago.
  indirect l., d. indireta. SIN standard limb l.
  intracardiac l., d. intracardíaca; o registro obtido quando o eletrodo explorador é colocado dentro de uma das câmaras cardíacas, geralmente por meio do cateterismo cardíaco.
  limb l., d. de membro; uma das três derivações padronizadas (derivações I, II, III) ou uma das derivações de membro unipolares (aVR, aVL, aVF).
  precordial l.'s, derivações precordiais. SIN chest l.'s.
  semidirect l.'s, derivações semidiretas. SIN chest l.'s.
  standard limb l., d. de membro padronizada; uma das três derivações de membro bipolares originais do eletrocardiograma clínico, designadas I, II e III; DI registra a diferença de potencial entre os braços direito e esquerdo; DII, a diferença entre o braço direito e o eletrodo da perna; e DIII, a diferença entre o braço esquerdo e o eletrodo da perna. SIN indirect l.
  unipolar l.'s, derivações unipolares; aquelas em que o eletrodo explorador está no tórax, nas proximidades do coração, ou em um dos membros, enquanto o outro eletrodo ou eletrodo indiferente é o terminal central.
  V l., d. V; uma d. unipolar com o terminal central como eletrodo indiferente; V é o símbolo para unipolar ("U" latino).
leaf·let (lēf′let). Folheto. **1.** Uma camada de fosfolipídios; dessa maneira, uma camada dupla possui dois folhetos. **2.** Uma estrutura ou objeto fino e achatado.
League of Red Cross So·ci·e·ties. Liga das Sociedades da Cruz Vermelha; a federação internacional da *Cruz Vermelha* nacional e sociedades similares.
learned help·less·ness. Desamparo aprendido; um modelo laboratorial de depressão que envolve técnicas de condicionamento clássicas (reatoras) e instrumentais (atuantes); a aplicação do choque inevitável é seguido por falha em lidar com situações nas quais a adequação poderia ser, de outra forma, possível.
learn·ing (lern′ing). Aprendizado; termo genérico para a alteração relativamente permanente no comportamento que acontece em conseqüência da prática. VER TAMBÉM conditioning, forgetting, memory.
  incidental l., a. incidental; a. sem uma tentativa direta. SIN passive l.
  insight l., *insight;* a obtenção da solução para um problema sem a série interveniente das etapas de tentativa e erro que estão associadas à maioria dos tipos de aprendizado (p.ex., um macaco alojado atrás das grades de uma jaula que, sem passar por inúmeras horas de tentativas fúteis com um bastão ou outra coisa, encaixa dois bastões para recuperar uma banana fora do alcance de cada bastão isoladamente).
  latent l., a. latente; aquele a. que não é evidente para o observador no momento em que ocorre, mas que é deduzido a partir do desempenho posterior, no qual o a. é mais rápido que o que seria esperado sem a experiência prévia.
  passive l., a. passivo. SIN incidental l.
  rote l., a. mecânico; o a. de relações arbitrárias, usualmente por repetição do procedimento de a. através da memorização e sem compreensão das relações.
  state-dependent l., a. dependente do estado; o a. durante um estado específico de sono ou vigília, ou durante um estado quimicamente alterado no qual a recuperação da informação aprendida (p.ex., conforme a medida do desempenho de uma resposta aprendida) não pode ser demonstrada, a menos que a pessoa retorne ao estado que originalmente existiu durante o a.
least squares. Quadrados mínimos; um princípio de estimativa, inventado por Gauss, no qual as estimativas de um conjunto de parâmetros em um modelo estatístico são as quantidades que minimizam o somatório das diferenças quadradas entre os valores observados da variável dependente e os valores previstos pelo modelo.
Le Bel, Joseph Achille, químico francês, 1847–1930. VER Le B.-van't Hoff *rule.*
Leber, Theodor, oftalmologista alemão, 1840–1917. VER L. idiopathic stellate *neuroretinitis,* hereditary optic *atrophy, plexus; amaurosis* congenita of L.
Le Chatelier, Henri, físico-químico francês, 1850–1936. VER Le C. *law, principle.*
lec·i·thal (les′i - thăl). Lecítico; que possui uma gema ou pertinente à gema de qualquer ovo; usado especificamente como sufixo. [G. *lekithos*, gema de ovo]
lec·i·thin (les′i-thin). Lecitina; termo tradicional para as 1,2-diacil-*sn*-glicero-3-fosfocolinas ou 3-*sn*-fosfatidilcolinas, os fosfolipídios que, na hidrólise, fornecem duas moléculas de ácidos graxos e uma molécula de ácido glicerofosfórico e outra de colina. Em algumas variedades de lecitina, os dois ácidos graxos são saturados, outras contêm apenas ácidos insaturados (p.ex., ácido oleico, linoleico ou araquidônico); em outros mais, um ácido graxo é saturado e o outro, insaturado. As lecitinas são substâncias céreas amareladas ou acastanhadas, prontamente miscíveis em água, na qual aparecem como partículas alongadas irregulares ao microscópio, conhecidas como "formas de mielina", e são encontradas no tecido nervoso, especialmente nas bainhas de mielina, na gema de ovo e como constituintes essenciais das células animais e vegetais. [G. *lekithos*, gema de ovo]
  l. acyltransferase, l. aciltransferase. SIN lecithin-cholesterol acyltransferase.
lec·i·thi·nase (les′i - thi - nās). Lecitinase. SIN phospholipase.
  l. A, l. A. SIN *phospholipase A*.
  l. B, l. B. SIN lysophospholipase.
  l. C, l. C. SIN *phospholipase* C.
  l. D, l. D. SIN *phospholipase* D.
lec·i·thin-cho·les·ter·ol ac·yl·trans·fer·ase (LCAT). Lecitina-colesterol aciltransferase; uma enzima que transfere de maneira reversível um resíduo acil de uma lecitina para o colesterol, formando uma 1-acilglicerofosfocolina (uma lisolecitina) e um éster de colesterol; a deficiência dessa enzima leva ao acúmulo de colesterol não-esterificado no plasma, resultando em anemia, proteinúria, insuficiência renal e opacificações da córnea; a LCAT também está baixa nos indivíduos com doença do olho de peixe. SIN lecithin acyltransferase.
lec·i·tho·blast (les′i - thō - blast). Lecitoblasto; uma das células que proliferam para formar o endoderma do saco vitelino. [G. *lekithos*, gema de ovo, + *blastos*, germe]

lec·i·tho·pro·tein (les'i - thō - prō'tēn). Lecitoproteína; uma proteína conjugada, com a lecitina como grupo prostético.
Leclef. VER Denys-Leclef *phenomenon*.
Le·cler·cia (le - clãr'cē - a). Um gênero na família Enterobacteriaceae que se assemelha ao gênero *Escherichia*, mas é separável por classificação metabólica e genética; isoladas das fezes de seres humanos e animais, foram isoladas clinicamente em amostras de sangue, fezes, escarro, urina e feridas; seu grau de patogenicidade é incerto.
lec·tin (lek'tin). Lectina; qualquer uma de um grupo de glicoproteínas de origem basicamente vegetal (em geral de sementes) que se ligam às glicoproteínas na superfície das células, causando aglutinação, precipitação ou outros fenômenos semelhantes à ação de anticorpos específicos; as lectinas incluem aglutininas vegetais (fitoaglutininas, fito-hemaglutininas), precipitinas vegetais e, talvez, determinadas proteínas animais; algumas possuem propriedades mitogênicas e induzem a transformação dos linfócitos. [L. *lego*, pp. *lectum*, selecionar, + -in]
  mitogenic l., l. mitogênica; uma l. que induz a replicação de ácidos polinucleicos e a proliferação de linfócitos.
Ledermann, Sully, psiquiatra francês. VER Ledermann *formula*.
ledge (lej). Prateleira, lâmina; em anatomia, uma estrutura que se assemelha a uma prateleira. VER TAMBÉM shelf, lamina.
  dental l., lâmina dentária; uma faixa de células ectodérmicas que cresce a partir do epitélio das mandíbulas embrionárias para dentro do mesênquima subjacente; os brotos locais oriundos de uma lâmina dentária originam os primórdios dos órgãos do esmalte dos dentes. SIN dental lamina, dental shelf, dentogingival lamina, enamel l., primary dental lamina.
  enamel l., lâmina do esmalte. SIN dental l.
Lee, Robert, médico inglês, 1793–1877. VER L. *ganglion*.
Lee, Roger I., médico norte-americano, 1881–1967. VER L.-White *method*.
leech (lēch). Sanguessuga. **1.** Um verme anelídio aquático hematófago (gênero *Hirudo*, classe Hirudinea) por vezes usado em medicina para a retirada local de sangue. Para várias espécies de s., ver *Hirudo*. **2.** Tratar medicamente pela aplicação de sanguessugas. [A.S., *laece*, um médico; uma sanguessuga, por causa de seu uso terapêutico]

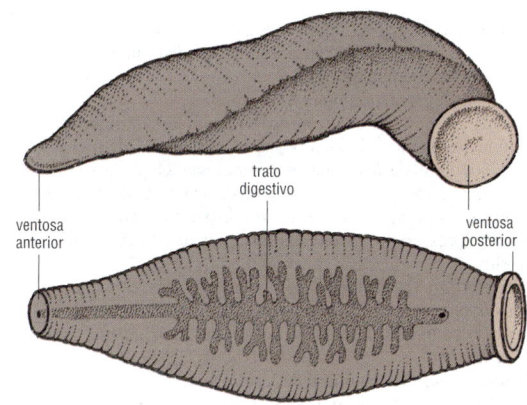

sanguessuga (*Hirudo medicinalis*)

leech·ing (lēch'ing). Sangrar; a prática antiga de aplicar sanguessugas no corpo para retirar o sangue para fins terapêuticos.
Leede, Carl S., médico norte-americano, * 1882. VER Rumpel-L. *sign, test*; L.-Rumpel *phenomenon*.
LEEP Abreviatura para loop eletrocautery excision *procedure* (procedimento de excisão por eletrocautério); loop electrosurgical excision *procedure* (procedimento de excisão eletrocirúrgica).
Leeuwenhoek, Anton van, microscopista holandês, 1632–1723. VER L. *canals*, em *canal*.
Lefèvre, Paul, dermatologista francês do século XX. VER Papillon-L. *syndrome*.
Le Fort, Léon C., cirurgião e ginecologista francês, 1829–1893. VER Le F. I *fracture*, II *fracture*, III *fracture*, *sound*, *amputation*.
left-foot·ed. Sinistropedal. SIN sinistropedal.
left-hand·ed. Sinistromanual, canhoto; indicando o uso habitual ou mais habilidoso da mão esquerda para escrever e para a maioria das operações manuais. SIN sinistromanual.
left-sid·ed·ness. A localização normal à esquerda de determinados órgãos ímpares, como o baço e a maior parte do estômago.
  bilateral l.'-s., síndrome da polisplenia; uma síndrome em que os órgãos normalmente ímpares desenvolvem-se mais simetricamente, como uma imagem em espelho; dois baços, um em cada lado, estão usualmente presentes, sendo comuns as anomalias cardiovasculares. SIN polysplenia syndrome.
leg. Perna. **1** [TA]. Anatomicamente, o segmento do membro inferior entre o joelho e o tornozelo; comumente utilizado para significar todo o membro inferior. **2.** Uma estrutura que se assemelha a uma perna. SIN crus (1) [TA].
  l. of antihelix, ramos da antélice. SIN *crura* of antihelix, em *crus*.
  bow-l., joelho varo. VER *genu* varum.
  elephant l., elefantíase. SIN elephantiasis.
  restless l.'s, síndrome das pernas inquietas. SIN restless legs *syndrome*.
  rider's l., p. de cavaleiro; distensão dos músculos adutores da coxa.
  tennis l., p. de tenista; ruptura do músculo gastrocnêmio na junção musculotendinosa, resultante de contrações forçadas dos músculos da panturrilha; comum em jogadores de tênis.
Legal, Emmo, médico alemão, 1859–1922. VER L. *test*.
Legendre, Gaston J., médico francês, *1887. VER L. *sign*.
Legg, Arthur T., cirurgião norte-americano, 1874–1939. VER L.-Calvé-Perthes *disease*.
-legia. –Legia; sufixo relacionado à leitura, diferente dos derivados gregos, -lexis e -lexy, que significam fala. [L. *lego*, ler]
Le·gion·el·la (lē - jŭ - nel'lă). Um gênero de bacilos Gram-negativos, aeróbicos, móveis, não-álcool-ácido-resistentes e não-encapsulados (família Legionellaceae) que apresentam metabolismo não-fermentativo e que exigem L-cisteína-HCl e sais de ferro para o crescimento; são aquáticos, disseminam-se por via aérea e são patogênicas para os seres humanos. Cerca de 40 espécies já foram identificadas; a espécie típica é *L. pneumophila*.
  L. bozeman'ii, espécie bacteriana que causa pneumonia em seres humanos.
  L. dumoffii, espécie bacteriana implicada na pneumonia.
  L. feeleii, espécie bacteriana implicada na pneumonia.
  L. gormanii, espécie bacteriana implicada na pneumonia.
  L. longbeachae, espécie bacteriana implicada na pneumonia.
  L. micda'dei, uma espécie bacteriana que pode ser álcool-ácido-resistente, e que causa a pneumonia de Pittsburgh, uma variante da doença dos Legionários. Representa aproximadamente 60% das pneumonias por *Legionella* diferentes daquelas causadas por *L. pneumophila*. SIN Pittsburgh pneumonia agent.
  L. pneumo'phila, espécie bacteriana que é o agente etiológico primário da doença dos Legionários; acredita-se que cresça em sistemas de encanamentos ou na água estagnada em sistemas de ventilação. A espécie típica do gênero *L.*
  L. wadsworthii, espécie bacteriana implicada na pneumonia.
le·gi·o·nel·lo·sis (lē - jŭ - nel - ō'sis). Legionelose, doença dos Legionários. SIN Legionnaires *disease*.
le·gu·min (lē - goo'min, leg'oo - min). Legumina. SIN avenin.
le·gu·mi·niv·o·rous (le - goo - mi - niv'ō - rŭs). Leguminívoro; que se alimenta de feijões, ervilhas e outros legumes.
Lehmann, J. O. Orla, médico sueco, *1927. VER Börjeson-Forssman-L. *syndrome*.
Leigh, Denis, psiquiatra britânico, *1915. VER L. *disease*.
Leiner, Karl, pediatra austríaco, 1871–1930. VER L. *disease*.
leio-. Leio-; forma combinante que significa liso. [G. *leios*]
lei·o·my·o·fi·bro·ma (lī - ō - mī'ō - fī - brō'mă). Leiomiofibroma; SIN fibroleiomyoma.
lei·o·my·o·ma (lī'ō - mī - ō'mă). Leiomioma, liomioma; neoplasia benigna derivada do músculo liso (não-estriado). [leio- + G. *mys*, músculo, + -oma, tumor]
  l. cu'tis, dermatomioma; erupção cutânea de pequenos nódulos dolorosos múltiplos, compostos de fibras musculares lisas; derivado dos músculos eretores dos pêlos. O dermatomioma solitário indolor pode originar-se de vasos sanguíneos cutâneos e da pele genital. SIN dermatomyoma.
  parasitic l., l. parasita; um l. uterino que se desprendeu do útero e aderiu a outra superfície peritoneal, da qual retira seu suprimento sanguíneo.
  vascular l., l. vascular; l. acentuadamente vascular que se origina aparentemente do músculo liso dos vasos sanguíneos. SIN angioleiomyoma, angiomyofibroma, angiomyoma.
lei·o·my·o·ma·to·sis (lī'ō - mī'ō - mă - tō'sis). Leiomiomatose, liomiomatose; o estado de ter múltiplos leiomiomas por todo o corpo.
  l. peritonealis disseminata, l. peritoneal disseminada; uma condição benigna caracterizada por nódulos pequenos e múltiplos no peritônio abdominal e pélvico que mimetiza macroscopicamente o câncer ovariano disseminado, mas com características histológicas de mioma benigno; freqüentemente associado à gestação recente.
lei·o·my·o·mec·to·my (lī'ō - mī - ō - mek'tō - mē). Leiomiomectomia, liomiomectomia; ressecção cirúrgica de um leiomioma, geralmente do útero.
lei·o·my·o·sar·co·ma (lī'ō - mī'ō - sar - kō'mă). Leiomiossarcoma, liomiossarcoma; neoplasia maligna derivada do músculo liso (não-estriado). [leio- + myosarcoma]
lei·ot·ri·chous (lī - ot'ri - kŭs). Liótrico; cujos cabelos são lisos e macios. [leio- + G. *thrix*, cabelo]
leipo-. Leipo-. VER lipo-.
Leipzig yel·low [C.I. 77600]. Amarelo de Leipzig. SIN chrome yellow.
Leishman, Sir William B., cirurgião escocês, 1865-1926. VER *Leishmania*; L. chrome *cells*, em *cell, stain*; L.-Donovan *body*.

Leish·man·ia (lēsh-man′ē-ă). Um gênero de protozoários flagelados, digenéticos, assexuados (família Trypanosomatidae) que ocorre como amastigotas nos macrófagos de hospedeiros vertebrados e como promastigotas em hospedeiros invertebrados e nas culturas. As espécies são, em grande parte, indistinguíveis do ponto de vista morfológico, mas podem ser separadas por manifestações clínicas, distribuição geográfica e epidemiologia, padrões de desenvolvimento dos promastigotas em seus hospedeiros flebótomos, testes de virulência de clones *in vivo*, efeito dos soros de teste sobre o crescimento em cultura, provas de imunidade cruzada e sorotipagem com os fatores excretados dos promastigotas; as cepas também podem ser diferenciadas por várias análises bioquímicas. Esses procedimentos identificaram todos os grupos reconhecidos e confirmaram a separação dos agentes da leishmaniose do Novo Mundo em dois complexos de espécies, *L. mexicana* e *L. braziliensis* [W. B. Leishman]

L. aethio'pica, espécie africana de *L.* responsável pela leishmaniose cutânea humana na Etiópia, com um reservatório da infecção humana em hiraces das rochas, *Procavia capensis* e *Heterohyrax brucei*, e no Quênia, com reservatórios em hiraces das árvores, *Dendrohyrax arboreus*, e no rato gigante, *Cricetomys gambianus*; os vetores são os mosquitos *Phlebotomus longipes* e *P. pedifer*. Causa leishmaniose cutânea de três tipos: a úlcera oriental clássica, a leishmaniose cutânea e a leishmaniose cutânea difusa; a ulceração é tardia ou ausente, e a cura leva de um a três ano.

L. brazilien'sis, espécie que é o agente causal da leishmaniose mucocutânea, endêmica no sul do México e nas Américas Central e do Sul, transmitida por várias espécies de *Lutzomyia* (mosquitos do Novo Mundo); roedores selvagens e outros animais arborícolas neotropicais servem como reservatórios. *L. braziliensis* é atualmente dividida em três cepas ou subespécies clínica, epidemiológica e bioquimicamente distintas: *L. b. braziliensis*, *L. b. guyanensis* e *L. b. panamensis*.

L. brazilien'sis brazilien'sis, a subespécie típica da *l. braziliensis* e o agente da leishmaniose mucocutânea. Um reservatório natural da infecção permanece desconhecido, mas o vetor comprovado no Brasil é *Lutzomyia (Psychodopygus) wellcomei*; outros mosquitos também podem transmitir a infecção.

L. brazilien'sis guyanen'sis, subespécie do complexo da *L. braziliensis*, originária do Brasil e Guiana, e a causa da leishmaniose cutânea localmente conhecida como "pian bois"; o hospedeiro reservatório é a preguiça *Choloepus hoffmani*, e o vetor é o mosquito *Lutzomyia umbratilis*.

L. brazilien'sis panamen'sis, subespécie de *L. braziliensis* encontrada no Panamá, na Colômbia e em regiões vizinhas; causa lesões ulcerantes da leishmaniose cutânea que não curam de forma espontânea e que, com freqüência, afetam os tecidos linfáticos próximos; mas o envolvimento da nasofaringe é raro. A preguiça *Choloepus hoffmani* é o reservatório no Panamá e na Costa Rica; o mosquito *Lutzomyia trapidoi* mostrou ser um vetor.

L. donova'ni, uma espécie que é o agente causal da leishmaniose visceral no Mediterrâneo e nos países adjacentes, na parte centro-sul da antiga União Soviética, leste da Índia, norte da China, Quênia, Etiópia e Sudão; também encontrado no Brasil, Argentina, Colômbia e Venezuela; no Velho Mundo, é transmitido por várias espécies de *Phlebotomus*; os vetores no Novo Mundo são as espécies de *Lutzomyia*, sendo os cães e outros carnívoros conhecidos como hospedeiros reservatórios em algumas áreas. A forma amastigota intracelular multiplica-se nos macrófagos e provoca hiperplasia reticuloendotelial, que afeta macroscopicamente o baço e o fígado, com outros tecidos linfóides também sendo envolvidos, resultando em hepatoesplenomegalia grave, a qual, em geral, é fatal, quando não-tratada.

L. donova'ni archibal'di, VER *L. donovani donovani*.

L. donova'ni chaga'si, subespécie de *L.* encontrada na América do Sul, principalmente no Brasil, que provoca a leishmaniose visceral; infecções foram encontradas em cães domésticos e em raposas, embora o hospedeiro reservatório primário não seja conhecido. O vetor permanece desconhecido, e o estado taxonômico dessa subespécie é incerto.

L. donova'ni donova'ni, subespécie típica e agente da leishmaniose visceral na Ásia, África e subcontinente indiano; alguns casos ocorrem na parte centro-sul da antiga União Soviética, bem como no Irã, Iraque e, possivelmente, Iêmen; o cão e o chacal são os reservatórios animais. A forma na África pode ser essa subespécie, embora o nome *L. donovani archibaldi* também seja empregado.

L. donova'ni infan'tum, cepa ou subespécie da *L. donovani* que provoca leishmaniose visceral em crianças pequenas nos países do Mediterrâneo; o reservatório é o cão doméstico.

L. furunculo'sa, nome antigo da *L. tropica*.

L. ma'jor, espécie responsável pela leishmaniose cutânea zoonótica em uma grande área da região mediterrânea e na Ásia Menor. Os reservatórios animais são, em geral, esquilos terrestres, como *Rhombomys opimus* na antiga União Soviética e em outros pontos na região centro-sul da Ásia, e outros roedores no noroeste da Índia, Oriente Médio e norte da África; os mosquitos vetores comprovados incluem *Phlebotomus papatasi*, *P. duboscqi* e *P. salehi*. SIN *L. tropica major*.

L. mexica'na, o agente de muitas formas de leishmaniose cutânea, atualmente considerada um complexo de várias subespécies ou, possivelmente, espécies, cada uma com características de enzimas e DNA distintas, distribuição e associação hospedeiro reservatório-vetor próprias, resultando em manifestações distintas da leishmaniose humana; os hospedeiros-reservatórios são extremamente diversos e incluem uma ampla gama de roedores arborícolas, bem como marsupiais, primatas e pequenos carnívoros. As formas de doença típica causadas por essa espécie são a úlcera de chicleiro e a leishmaniose cutânea difusa, em contraste com a leishmaniose mucocutânea, mais característica da infecção por *L. braziliensis*. SIN *L. tropica mexicana*.

L. mexica'na amazonen'sis, uma forma particularmente disseminada de *L. mexicana* na bacia do Amazonas (Bolívia, Brasil, Colômbia, Equador e sul da Venezuela), onde infecta vários roedores das florestas, os reservatórios da infecção humana. A doença é rara nos seres humanos, mas as lesões únicas ou múltiplas, quando induzidas, raramente curam de maneira espontânea; a forma disseminada é comum, mas não há envolvimento nasofaríngeo. O vetor é o mosquito *Lutzomyia flaviscutellata*.

L. mexica'na garnha'mi, uma subespécie da *L. mexicana*, encontrada no oeste da Venezuela, que causa lesões únicas ou múltiplas em seres humanos; essas lesões curam espontaneamente em cerca de 6 meses; o provável mosquito vetor é *Lutzomyia townsendi*.

L. mexica'na mexica'na, uma espécie oriunda do México, Guatemala e Belize; o agente de uma forma de leishmaniose cutânea do Novo Mundo chamada de úlcera de chicleiro, associada à goma de mascar e aos trabalhadores florestais que lidam com o mogno. O mosquito do Novo Mundo *Lutzomyia olmeca* é um vetor comprovado dessa subespécie.

L. mexica'na pifa'noi, uma cepa de *L. mexicana* que recebeu o *status* de espécie por aqueles que a consideram responsável pela forma difusa ou disseminada de leishmaniose cutânea. É responsável por essa condição na Venezuela, onde foi descrita, mas atualmente sabe-se que várias espécies e subespécies de *L.* causam formas disseminadas similares de leishmaniose em regiões muito afastadas (*L. mexicana amazonensis, L. aethiopica*); a ausência ou a supressão da resposta imune celular no hospedeiro também é um fator importante na indução da leishmaniose cutânea difusa. SIN *L. pifanoi*.

L. mexica'na venezuelen'sis, uma subespécie recentemente descrita de *L. mexicana* oriunda da Venezuela que causa o desenvolvimento de lesões únicas, indolores e nodulares de leishmaniose cutânea, por vezes associadas à leishmaniose cutânea disseminada curável; a infecção também foi encontrada em eqüinos.

L. peruvia'na, espécie de *L.* que infecta seres humanos nos elevados vales andinos do Peru e da Bolívia; causa uma forma distinta de leishmaniose cutânea do Novo Mundo chamada uta.

L. pifa'noi, SIN *L. mexicana pifanoi*.

L. trop'ica, espécie que é o agente causal da leishmaniose cutânea antroponótica; outrora endêmica por toda a bacia do Mediterrâneo, Oriente Médio, regiões do sul da área antes conhecida como União Soviética e em outros pontos na Ásia, tendo sido também reportada no oeste da África; é transmitida por *Phlebotomus papatasi*, *P. sergenti* e espécies correlatas de mosquitos; pequenos roedores, como vários esquilos terrestres, servem como hospedeiros reservatórios.

L. trop'ica ma'jor, SIN *L. major*.

L. trop'ica mexica'na. SIN *L. mexicana*.

leishmania, pl. **leishmaniae** (lēsh-man′ē-ă). Leishmânia; um membro do gênero *Leishmania*.

leishmaniae. Leishmânias; plural de *leishmania*.

leish·man·i·a·sis (lēsh′mă-nī′ă-sis). Leishmaniose; infecção por uma espécie de *Leishmania* resultando em um grupo clinicamente mal definido de doenças tradicionalmente divididas em quatro tipos principais: 1) l. visceral (calazar); 2) l. cutânea do Velho Mundo; 3) l. cutânea do Novo Mundo; 4) l. mucocutânea. Cada tipo é distinto, do ponto de vista clínico e geográfico, e cada um foi subdividido, nos últimos anos, em categorias clínicas e epidemiológicas adicionais. A transmissão é feita por várias espécies de mosquitos dos gêneros *Phlebotomus* ou *Lutzomyia*. VER tropical *diseases*, em *disease*. SIN leishmaniosis.

acute cutaneous l., l. cutânea aguda. SIN zoonotic cutaneous l.

American l., l. america'na, l. mucocutânea. SIN mucocutaneous l.

anergic l., l. cutânea difusa. SIN diffuse cutaneous l.

anthroponotic cutaneous l., l. cutânea antroponótica; uma forma de l. cutânea do Velho Mundo usualmente com um período de incubação prolongado e confinada às áreas urbanas. SIN chronic cutaneous l., dry cutaneous l., urban cutaneous l.

canine l., l. canina; uma infecção branda dos cães, geralmente confinada ao focinho ou orelhas, produzida por espécies de *Leishmania* causadoras de doença em seres humanos; os cães, portanto, são importantes reservatórios da infecção humana, como na l. visceral na região do Mediterrâneo.

chronic cutaneous l., l. cutânea crônica. SIN anthroponotic cutaneous l.

cutaneous l., l. cutânea; a infecção por promastigotos (leptomonas) da *Leishmania tropica* e da *L. major* inoculados na pele pela picada de um mosquito infectado, *Phlebotomus* (comumente *P. papatasi*); é endêmica em regiões da Ásia Menor, África setentrional e Índia; é conhecida por inúmeros nomes, incluindo úlceras tropicais e outras indicações da localidade (p.ex., úlcera de Aleppo, Bagdá, Delhi ou Jericó; úlcera de Aden; botão de Biskra); a úlcera começa como uma pápula que evolui para um nódulo e, em seguida, rompe-se em uma úlcera. As células de *leishmania* são observadas dentro dos histiócitos em cortes teciduais corados por hematoxilina-eosina. São reconhecidas duas doenças clínica e epidemiologicamente distintas: a doença rural zoonótica, mais comum e disseminada, com uma forma aguda úmida, causada pela *L. major*, com os roedores sendo os hospedeiros reservatórios, e uma forma de l. urbana, crônica, seca e antroponótica, causada pela *L. tropica*, sem um hospedeiro reservatório e, atualmente, quase controlada. VER zoonotic cutaneous l., anthroponotic cutaneous l. SIN Old World l.

diffuse l., l. cutânea difusa. SIN diffuse cutaneous l.

diffuse cutaneous l., l. cutânea difusa; l. causada por várias espécies e cepas de *Leishmania* do Novo Mundo e do Velho Mundo (*L. mexicana amazonensis, L. m. pifanoi*, possivelmente *L. m. garnhami* e *L. m. venezuelensis*; na Etiópia, *L. aethiopica*, e agentes *leishmania* não-identificados na Namíbia e Tanzânia). A condição é associada à supressão da resposta imune celular, de modo que as lesões cutâneas não-ulcerativas e não-necrotizantes podem espalhar-se amplamente pelo corpo; numerosos macrófagos repletos de parasitas são encontrados nas lesões dérmicas. A cura não parece ocorrer, a menos que possa desenvolver-se hipersensibilidade celular adquirida. SIN anergic l., diffuse l., disseminated cutaneous l., l. tegumentaria diffusa, pseudolepromatous l.

disseminated cutaneous l., l. cutânea disseminada. SIN diffuse cutaneous l.

dry cutaneous l., l. cutânea seca. SIN anthroponotic cutaneous l.

infantile l., l. do lactente; l. visceral em lactentes, causada por *Leishmania donovani infantum*.

lupoid l., l. lupóide. SIN l. recidivans.

mucocutaneous l., l. mucocutânea; doença grave causada pela *Leishmania braziliensis braziliensis*, endêmica no sul do México e nas Américas Central e do Sul, à exceção da região equatorial do Chile; o microrganismo não invade as vísceras, e a doença limita-se à pele e às mucosas, com as lesões assemelhando-se às úlceras da l. cutânea provocadas pela *L. mexicana* ou *L. tropica*; as úlceras cancróides curam após algum tempo, mas, alguns meses ou anos depois, podem aparecer formas fungosas ou erosivas de ulceração na língua e na mucosa bucal ou nasal; existem muitas variantes da doença, caracterizadas por diferenças na distribuição, vetor, epidemiologia e patologia, sugerindo que ela seria, na verdade, causada por inúmeros agentes etiológicos intimamente relacionados. VER TAMBÉM espundia. SIN American l., l. americana, bubas, nasopharyngeal l., New World l.

nasopharyngeal l., l. nasofaríngea. SIN mucocutaneous l.

New World l., l. do Novo Mundo. SIN mucocutaneous l.

Old World l., l. do Velho Mundo. SIN cutaneous l.

pseudolepromatous l., l. pseudolepromatosa. SIN diffuse cutaneous l.

l. recid'ivans, l. recidivante; uma lesão de leishmaniose parcialmente cicatrizada provocada por *Leishmania tropica* e caracterizada por uma forma extrema de resposta imune celular, produção intensa de granuloma, necrose fibrinóide sem caseação e freqüente desenvolvimento de lesões satélites que continuam a produção de tecido granulomatoso sem cicatrização, por vezes durante muitos anos; os microrganismos são difíceis de demonstrar, mas podem ser cultivados. SIN lupoid l.

rural cutaneous l., l. cutânea rural. SIN zoonotic cutaneous l.

l. tegumenta'ria diffu'sa, l. tegumentar difusa. SIN diffuse cutaneous l.

urban cutaneous l., l. cutânea urbana. SIN anthroponotic cutaneous l.

visceral l., l. visceral; **(1)** uma doença crônica, que ocorre na Índia, China, Paquistão, litoral do Mediterrâneo, Oriente Médio, Américas do Sul e Central, Ásia e África causada pela *Leishmania donovani* e transmitida pela picada de uma espécie apropriada de mosquito do gênero *Phlebotomus* ou *Lutzomyia*; os microrganismos crescem e multiplicam-se nos macrófagos, provocando, mais tarde, a rotura dos mesmos e a liberação de parasitas amastigotas, os quais, em seguida, invadem outros macrófagos; a proliferação dos macrófagos na medula óssea interfere nos elementos eritróides e mielóides, resultando em leucopenia, anemia, esplenomegalia e hepatomegalia, que são características, juntamente com o aumento dos linfonodos; febre, fadiga, indisposição e infecções secundárias também ocorrem; existem diferentes cepas de *L. donovani*: *L. infantum*, na Eurásia, *L. chagasi*, na América Latina. **(2)** l. visceral causada por *Leishmania tropica*, cultivada a partir de aspirados de medula óssea de alguns pacientes militares após a Guerra do Golfo. SIN Assam fever, black sickness, Burdwan fever, cachectic fever, Dumdum fever, kala azar, tropical splenomegaly.

wet cutaneous l., l. cutânea úmida. SIN zoonotic cutaneous l.

zoonotic cutaneous l., l. cutânea zoonótica; uma forma de l. cutânea caracterizada pela distribuição rural dos casos em seres humanos próximo a roedores infectados, principalmente esquilos terrestres comuns; caracterizada pelo desenvolvimento agudo e rápido de lesões dérmicas que se tornam muito inflamadas, com úlceras necrotizantes úmidas ou úlceras que curam em 2 a 8 meses depois de um período de incubação de 2 a 4 meses; em imigrantes não-imunes, lesões múltiplas podem desenvolver-se, as quais cicatrizam de forma mais lenta e deixam cicatrizes incapacitantes ou desfigurantes. Uma forte hipersensibilidade retardada e o envolvimento de imunocomplexos participam na necrose, que faz parte do processo de cicatrização e da forte imunidade específica que se segue. SIN acute cutaneous l. rural cutaneous l., wet cutaneous l.

leish·man·i·o·sis (lēsh'man-ē-ō'sis). Leishmaniose. SIN leishmaniasis.

leish·man·oid (lēsh'mă-noyd). Leishmanóide; que se assemelha à leishmaniose.

dermal l., l. dérmica pós-calazar. SIN post-kala azar dermal l.

post-kala azar dermal l., l. dérmica pós-calazar; erupção cutânea nodular crônica, progressiva, granulomatosa, não-ulcerante e hipopigmentada que pode surgir 6 meses a 5 anos depois da cura espontânea ou medicamentosa da leishmaniose visceral (calazar); essa condição foi descrita pela primeira vez na Índia e é mais característica do calazar nesse país. SIN dermal l.

Leiter, Russell G., psicólogo norte-americano, *1901. VER L. International Performance *Scale*.

Lejeune, Jerôme J. L. M., citogeneticista francês, 1926–1994. VER L. *syndrome*.

Lembert, Antoine, cirurgião francês, 1802–1851. VER L. *suture*; Czerny-L. *suture*.

le·mic (lē'mik), lem (o); relativo à peste ou a qualquer doença epidêmica. [G. *loimos*, peste]

Le·min·or·ella (lem'in-ō-rel'ă). Um gênero na família Enterobacteriaceae que contém duas espécies, *Leminorella grimontii* e *Leminorella richardii*, que foram isoladas em material clínico, basicamente de amostras fecais; sua importância clínica é incerta atualmente.

Lemli, Luc, pediatra norte-americano do século XX. VER Smith-L.-Opitz *syndrome*.

lem·mo·blast (lem'ō-blast). Lemoblasto; em um embrião, uma célula oriunda da crista neural capaz de formar uma célula da bainha do neurilema. [G. *lemma*, farelo, + *blastos*, germe]

lem·mo·cyte (lem'ō-sīt), lemócito. Uma das células do neurolema. [G. *lemma*, casca, + *kytos*, germe, semente]

lem·nis·cus, pl. **lem·nis·ci** (lem-nis'kŭs, -nis'ī) [TA]. Lemnisco; um feixe de fibras nervosas que ascende desde os núcleos de retransmissão sensorial até o tálamo. SIN fillet (1). [L. do G. *lēmniskos*, fita ou filete]

acoustic l., l. lateral. sin lateral l.

auditory l., lateral. sin lateral l.

gustatory l., l. gustativo; o sistema de fibras sensoriais secundárias não-cruzadas que ascende do núcleo gustativo rombencefálico até os núcleos parabraquiais (nível pontino rostral) e diretamente para o núcleo gustativo talâmico (núcleo póstero-medial ventral, parte parvocelular)

lateral l. [TA], l. lateral; um feixe de fibras ascendentes que se originam dos núcleos de retransmissão coclear e auditivo do rombencéfalo, entram no corpo trapezóide, um estrato de fibras transversas no qual cerca de metade de suas fibras decussam e, a partir daí, viram-se rostralmente ao longo do lado lateral do trato espinotalâmico; no mesencéfalo, o feixe arqueia-se dorsalmente e penetra no colículo inferior, no qual todas as suas fibras terminam; daí, a via auditiva é estendida, de forma transináptica, por meio do braço do colículo inferior, até o corpo geniculado medial do tálamo, a partir do qual, por sua vez, as radiações auditivas levam ao córtex auditivo; intercalados no corpo trapezóide e ao longo da trajetória ascendente da l. estão vários grupos celulares, nos quais parte das fibras fazem sinapse. sin l. lateralis [TA], acoustic l., auditory l., auditory tract, lateral fillet.

l. latera'lis [TA], l. lateral. sin lateral l.

medial l. [TA], l. medial; um feixe de fibras brancas que se originam dos núcleos grácil e cuneiforme e decussam na porção inferior do bulbo; daí, ele ascende através do centro da medula oblonga, próximo à rafe mediana; ao entrar na ponte, espalha-se lateralmente para formar uma faixa achatada, ascendendo sobre a borda dorsal dos núcleos pontinos; no mesencéfalo, passa sobre a borda dorsal da substância negra, sendo deslocado lateralmente pelo núcleo rubro; passando medialmente ao corpo geniculado medial, o feixe penetra e termina no núcleo ventro-posterior do tálamo. Durante todo esse trajeto, as fibras retêm uma ordem somatotópica, de tal modo que aquelas que se originam do núcleo grácil e que representam o membro inferior se situam lateralmente àquelas que se originam no núcleo cuneiforme e representam o braço. O l. medial conduz as informações somatossensoriais envolvidas na discriminação tátil (discriminação de dois pontos), propriocepção e percepção vibratória. sin l. medialis [TA], medial fillet, Reil band (2), Reil ribbon.

l. media'lis [TA], l. medial. sin medial l.

spinal l. [TA], trato espinotalâmico. sin spinothalamic *tract*.

l. spina'lis [TA], trato espinotalâmico. sin spinothalamic *tract*.

trigeminal l. [TA], l. trigeminal; termo coletivo que indica as fibras que ascendem dos núcleos sensoriais do nervo trigêmeo; um desses sistemas de fibras origina-se do núcleo espinal do nervo trigêmeo e do núcleo principal do nervo trigêmeo (sensorial), decussa e ascende como o trato trigeminotalâmico anterior [TA] em íntima associação com o l. medial, com o qual penetra no complexo ventrobasal para terminar no núcleo ventral póstero-medial; um segundo grupo de fibras, não-cruzadas, que se originam do núcleo principal do nervo trigêmeo, cujo trajeto é ascendente através das partes centrais do tegmento do mesencéfalo como o trato trigeminotalâmico posterior [TA], também termina no núcleo ventral póstero-medial. O l. trigeminal conduz impulsos táteis, dolorosos e térmicos oriundos da pele da face, mucosas das cavidades oral e nasal, e do olho, bem como informações proprioceptivas dos músculos faciais e mastigatórios. sin l. trigeminalis [TA].

l. trigemina'lis [TA], l. trigeminal. sin trigeminal l.

lem·on (lem'ŏn). Limão; o fruto do *Citrus limon* (família Rutaceae); uma fonte de ácidos cítrico e ascórbico; o suco recentemente expresso do fruto maduro é usado como diurético refrigerante na febre, na forma de limonada. sin limon. [L. *limon*]

lem·on yel·low. Amarelo de cromo, cromato de chumbo. sin chrome yellow.

Lendrum, A. C., patologista escocês do século XX. ver L. phloxine-tartrazine *stain*; Fraser-L. *stain* for fibrin.

Lenègre, Jean, cardiologista francês do século XX. ver L. *disease, syndrome*.

length(l). Comprimento; distância linear entre dois pontos.

arch l., c. de arco; o espaço necessário para os dentes permanentes, medido desde a face mesial do primeiro molar, em um lado, até a face mesial do primeiro molar, no lado oposto, medido através dos pontos de contato ao longo de uma linha imaginária na arcada dentária.

available arch l., c. de arco disponível; o espaço disponível para os dentes permanentes na arcada dentária, desde o primeiro molar permanente até o primeiro molar permanente oposto.

crown-heel l. (CH, CHL), c. vértice–tornozelo; o c. de um embrião ou feto esticado, desde o vértice do crânio até o tornozelo. ver Streeter developmental horizon(s).

crown-hump l. (CR, CRL), c. vértice–nádegas; uma medida, desde o vértice do crânio até o ponto médio entre os ápices das nádegas de um embrião ou feto, que permite a estimativa da idade embrionária ou fetal.

greatest l., c. máximo; a medida desde a extremidade craniana até a caudal do embrião antes que ele se curve.

required arch l., c. de arco necessário; o somatório das larguras mesiodistais dos dentes permanentes, desde o primeiro molar permanente até o primeiro molar do lado oposto.

resting l., c. em repouso; o comprimento em repouso a partir do qual um músculo desenvolve tensão isométrica máxima.

spinal l. (SL), c. espinal; medida desde a superfície distal do embrião, onde passa o plano através dos olhos em desenvolvimento (este é o limite craniano da medula espinal) até as nádegas.

Lenhossék, Michael (Mihály) von, anatomista húngaro, 1863–1937. ver L. *processes*, em *process*.

len·i·tive (len'i-tiv). Lenitivo. **1.** Que suaviza; que alivia o desconforto ou a dor. **2.** Termo raramente empregado para um demulcente. [L. *lenio*, pp. *lenitus*, amolecer, de *lenis*, brando]

Lennert, Karl, *1921. ver L. *lymphoma, classification*.

Lennox, William G., neurologista norte-americano, 1884–1960. ver L. *syndrome*; L.-Gastaut *syndrome*.

Lenoir, Camille A. H., anatomista francês, *1867. ver L. *facet*.

lens (lenz) [TA]. Lente. **1.** Um material transparente com uma ou ambas as superfícies apresentando uma curvatura côncava ou convexa; sob energia eletromagnética, provoca a convergência ou a divergência dos raios luminosos. **2** [TA]. A estrutura refratária celular biconvexa transparente que se situa entre a íris e o humor vítreo, consistindo em uma parte externa macia (córtex) e uma parte mais densa (núcleo), sendo circundada por uma membrana basal (cápsula); a superfície anterior apresenta epitélio cubóide, e, no equador, as células se alongam para se transformarem em fibras da lente. sin crystaline. [L. uma lentilha]

achromatic l., l. acromática; l. composta constituída de duas ou mais lentes com diferentes índices de refração, correlacionadas de forma a minimizar a aberração cromática.

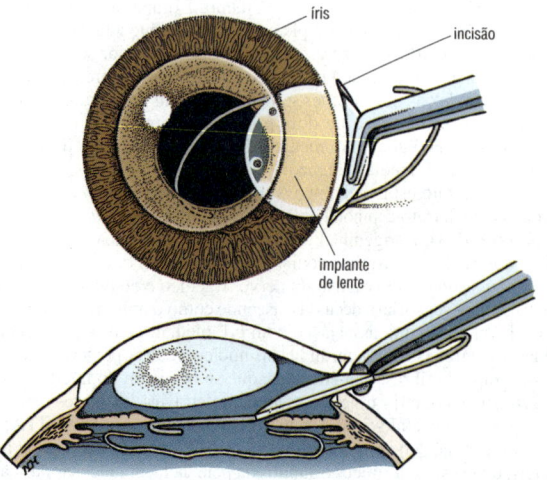

implante intra-ocular de lente: lente sendo inserida na câmara anterior do olho

acoustic l., l. acústica; em ultra-sonografia, l. utilizada para focalizar ou divergir um feixe sonoro; pode ser simulada pela manipulação eletrônica dos sinais.

aplanatic l., l. aplanática; l. destinada a corrigir a aberração simétrica e o coma (*q.v.*). sin periscopic meniscus.

apochromatic l., l. apocromática; l. composta destinada a corrigir as aberrações cromáticas e esféricas.

aspheric l., l. asférica; l. com uma superfície em parábola que elimina a aberração esférica.

astigmatic l., l. astigmática. sin cylindrical l.

bandage contact l., l. de contato de cobertura; l. de contato colocada sobre a córnea para cobrir um defeito.

biconcave l., l. bicôncava; l. que é côncava nas duas superfícies opostas. sin concavoconcave l., double concave l.

biconvex l., l. biconvexa; l. com ambas as superfícies convexas. sin convexoconvex l., double convex l.

bifocal l., l. bifocal; l. usada em casos de presbiopia, na qual uma parte é adaptada para a visão a distância, a outra para leitura e trabalhos próximos em geral; a lente para leitura acrescentada pode ser cimentada à l., fundida à superfície frontal ou preparada como uma peça única; as outras lentes bifocais são do tipo de Franklin de ápice achatado ou de mistura invisível.

cataract l., l. para catarata; qualquer l. prescrita para a afaquia.

l. clock, l. de relógio. sin Geneva lens *measure*.

compound l., l. composta; sistema óptico de duas ou mais lentes.

concave l., l. côncava; lente divergente com capacidade de aumento negativo. sin minus l.

concavoconcave l., l. bicôncava. sin biconcave l.

concavoconvex l., l. côncavo-convexa; l. com menisco convergente que é côncava em uma superfície e convexa na superfície oposta.

contact l., l. de contato; lente que se adapta sobre a córnea e a esclera ou apenas sobre a córnea; usada para corrigir erros de refração.

convex l., l. convexa; l. convergente. sin plus l.

convexoconcave l., l. convexo-côncava; lente de aumento negativo que possui uma superfície convexa e a superfície oposta côncava, com a última tendo a maior curvatura.

convexoconvex l., l. biconvexa; sin biconvex l.

corneal l., l. córnea; l. de contato de plástico sem as porções em contato com a esclera.

crystalline l., lente. sin lens (2).

cylindrical l. (cyl., C), l. cilíndrica; l. em que uma das superfícies é curvada em um meridiano e menos curvada no meridiano oposto; p.ex., uma colher de chá ou uma bola de futebol americano. sin astigmatic l.

decentered l., l. descentralizada; uma l. montada de modo que o eixo visual não passe através do eixo da l.

dislocation of l., luxação da lente. sin *ectopia* lentis.

double concave l., l. bicôncava. sin biconcave l.

double convex l., l. biconvexa. sin biconvex l.

eye l., lente ocular; a parte superior das duas lentes planoconvexas da ocular de Huygens. sin ocular l.

field l., l. de campo; a parte inferior das duas lentes planoconvexas da ocular de Huygens.

foldable intraocular l., l. intra-ocular dobrável; l. freqüentemente feita de silicone ou de um polímero acrílico que pode ser dobrada sobre si mesma para o implante intra-ocular. após a remoção da catarata.

Fresnel l., l. de Fresnel; l. com uma superfície que consiste em uma série concêntrica de zonas que duplicam o poder de uma l. ou prisma, porém com menor espessura. sin lighthouse l.

Hruby l., l. de Hruby; uma lente não de contato montada sobre uma lâmpada de fenda usada para avaliar a retina.

immersion l., l. de imersão; uma objetiva (para um microscópio) construída de tal modo que a l. inferior possa ser movida para baixo, em contato direto com um líquido, o qual é colocado no objeto a ser examinado; através do uso de um líquido com um índice de refração muito similar ao do vidro, a perda de luminosidade é minimizada.

lighthouse l., l. de Fresnel. sin Fresnel l.

meniscus l., menisco; l. que possui uma curvatura côncava esférica em um lado e uma curvatura convexa esférica no outro. sin articular crescent, articular meniscus, intraarticular cartilage (2), meniscus articularis, meniscus (1).

minus l., l. negativa, l. côncava. sin concave l.

multifocal l., l. multifocal; l. com segmentos que proporcionam duas ou mais forças de aumento; comumente, uma l. trifocal.

ocular l., l. ocular. sin eye l.

omnifocal l., l. omnifocal; l. para a visão próxima e distante em que uma parte da leitura é uma curvatura continuamente variável.

orthoscopic l., l. ortoscópica; l. de óculos corrigida para a distorção e curvatura da periferia.

periscopic l., l. periscópica; l. com uma curvatura de base de 1,25 D.

photochromic l., l. fotocrômica, l. fotocromática; l. de óculos sensível à luz que diminui a transmissão luminosa na luz solar e aumenta a transmissão na luminosidade reduzida.

planoconcave l., l. planocôncava; l. que é achatada em um lado e côncava no outro.
planoconvex l., l. planoconvexa; lente que é achatada em um lado e convexa no outro.
plus l., l. positiva, l. convexa. SIN convex l.
safety l., l. de segurança; l. que satisfaz as especificações do governo para a resistência ao impacto; a resistência aumentada ao impacto necessária para as lentes de segurança é obtida temperando-as por um processo de troca iônica ou pelo uso de lentes laminadas ou de plástico.
slab-off l., lente com um fragmento prismático retirado da parte inferior; usada na miopia desigual, para igualar o deslocamento da imagem durante a leitura.
spherical l. (S, sph.), l. esférica; l. em que todas as superfícies refratárias são esféricas.
spherocylindrical l., l. esferocilíndrica; l. esférica e cilíndrica combinada, uma superfície sendo esférica e a outra cilíndrica. SIN spherocylinder.
toric l., l. tórica; uma lente em que os dois meridianos são curvos, mas não no mesmo grau.
trial l.'s, lentes de prova; uma série de lentes cilíndricas e esféricas usadas para examinar a visão.
trifocal l., l. trifocal; l. com segmentos de três potências focais: distante, intermediária e próxima.
lens clock. Ver em lens.
lens·ec·to·my (len-sek′to-me). Lensectomia; remoção da lente do olho por um cortador de infusão–aspiração; freqüentemente feita através de incisão (punção) da parte plana durante a vitrectomia. [lens + G. *ektome*, excisão]
lens·om·e·ter (len-zom′e-ter). Lensômetro; um instrumento para medir a potência e o eixo cilíndrico de uma lente de óculos. SIN focimeter, vertometer. [lens + G. *metron*, medida]
lens·op·a·thy (lenz-op′a-the). Lensopatia; o processo pelo qual as proteínas da lágrima são depositadas em uma lente de contato. [lens + G. *pathos*, sofrimento]
len·ti·co·nus (len-ti-ko′nŭs). Lenticone; a projeção cônica da superfície anterior ou posterior da lente do olho, ocorrendo como uma anomalia do desenvolvimento. [lens + L. *conus*, cone]
len·tic·u·la (len-tik′u-lă). Núcleo lentiforme. SIN lentiform nucleus. [L. dim de *lens*]
len·tic·u·lar (len-tik′u-lar). Lenticular. 1. Que se relaciona ou se assemelha a uma lente de qualquer tipo. 2. Do formato de uma lentilha. [L. *lenticula*, uma lentilha]
len·tic·u·lo-op·tic (len-tik′u-lo-op′tik). Lentículo-óptico; relativo ao núcleo lentiforme e trato óptico; refere-se especificamente aos ramos da artéria cerebral média que parece irrigarem essas estruturas.
len·tic·u·lo·pap·u·lar (len-tik′u-lo-pap′u-lar). Lenticulopapular; indica uma erupção com pápulas em forma de cúpula ou lente.
len·tic·u·lo·stri·ate (len-tik′u-lo-stri′at). Lentículo-estriado; relativo ao núcleo lentiforme e ao núcleo caudado; refere-se especificamente aos ramos da artéria cerebral média que irrigam essas massas cinzentas.
len·tic·u·lo·tha·lam·ic (len-tik′u-lo-tha-lam′ik). Lenticulotalâmico; pertinente ao núcleo lentiforme e ao tálamo.
len·tic·u·lus, pl. **len·tic·u·li** (len-tik′u-lŭs, -li). Lentículo; termo raramente utilizado para uma prótese intra-ocular da lente colocada na câmara anterior ou posterior do olho, ou fixada à lente após a extração da catarata. SIN prosthetophacos, pseudophacos. [L. dim de *lens, lentis*, uma pequena lente]
len·ti·form (len′ti-form). Lentiforme; com a forma de lente.
len·tig·i·nes (len-tij′i-nez). Lentigos; plural de lentigo. [L.]
len·tig·i·no·sis (len-tij-i-no′sis). Lentiginose; presença de lentigos em número muito grande ou em uma configuração distinta.
  centrofacial l. [MIM*151000 & MIM*151001], l. centrofacial; síndrome autossômica dominante rara com pequenas máculas hiperpigmentadas em uma faixa horizontal através do centro da face com um ano de idade, aumentando em número até os 10 anos de idade e associada a defeitos esqueléticos e neurais.
  generalized l., l. generalizada; lentigos que ocorrem isoladamente ou em grupos a partir do primeiro ano de vida.
len·ti·glo·bus (len-ti-glo′bŭs). Lentiglobo; anomalia congênita rara com uma elevação esferóide na superfície posterior da lente do olho. [lens + L. *globus*, esfera]
len·ti·go, pl. **len·tig·i·nes** (len-ti′go, len-tij′i-nez). Lentigo; uma mácula acastanhada adquirida, benigna, assemelhando-se a uma sarda, mas tendo a borda geralmente regular e alongamento microscópico das cristas intrapapilares, com aumento do número de melanócitos e pigmento de melanina na camada de células basais. VER TAMBÉM junction nevus. SIN l. simplex. [L. de *lens (lent-)*, uma lentilha]
  l. maligna, l. maligno; uma lesão acastanhada ou negra, mosqueada, com contornos irregulares e de crescimento lento, que se assemelha a um lentigo, na qual existem um número aumentado de melanócitos atípicos espalhados na epiderme, ocorrendo, em geral, na face das pessoas idosas; depois de muitos anos, a derme pode ser invadida, sendo a lesão, então, denominada melanoma lentiginoso maligno. SIN Hutchinson freckle, melanotic freckle.
  senile l., l. senil; l. benigno variadamente pigmentado que ocorre na pele exposta de pessoas idosas da raça branca. SIN liver spot, solar l.
  l. simplex, l. simples. SIN lentigo.
  solar l., l. solar. SIN senile l.
Len·ti·vir·i·nae (len′ti-vir′i-ne). Termo utilizado outrora para descrever uma subfamília de vírus não-oncogênicos (família Retroviridae) que inclui os vírus lentos do carneiro (vírus visna e vírus maedi) e os vírus linfotrópicos da célula T humana, inclusive os vírus da imunodeficiência humana 1 e 2 (HIV-1, HIV-2). Os vírus assemelham-se aos vírus tumorais RNA do tipo C (Oncovirinae) em muitos aspectos, incluindo a produção de transcriptase reversa. [L. *lentus*, lento, preguiçoso]
len·ti·vi·rus (len′ti-vi-rŭs). Um gênero na família Retroviridae contendo 5 sorogrupos, os quais refletem o hospedeiro com o qual eles estão associados. Entre os lentivírus de primatas estão os vírus da imunodeficiência humana 1 e 2.
len·to·gen·ic (len-to-jen′ik). Lentogênico; refere à virulência de um vírus capaz de induzir infecção letal nos hospedeiros embrionários após um longo período de incubação e infecção inaparente nos hospedeiros imaturos e adultos; o termo é usado na caracterização do vírus da doença de Newcastle, principalmente das cepas usadas como vacinas administradas em água ou como aerossóis, isto é, cepas brandas ou avirulentas. [L. *lentus*, preguiçoso, inativo, + G. *-gen*, que produz]
len·tu·la, len·tu·lo (len′tu-lă, -lo). Lentual; um instrumento de fio espiralado, flexível, motorizado, empregado em odontologia para aplicar o material de enchimento pastoso no canal da raiz de um dente. [L. *lentus*, maleável, flexível]
le·on·ti·a·sis (le-on-ti′a-sis). Leontíase; as cristas e sulcos na fronte e nas bochechas de pacientes com lepra lepromatosa avançada, gerando uma aparência leonina. SIN leonine facies. [G. *leon (leont-)*, leão]
  l. os′sea, l. óssea. SIN megacephaly.
LEOPARD [MIM*151100]. Acrônimo para *l*entigos (múltiplos), anormalidades *e*letrocardiográficas, hipertelorismo *o*cular, estenose *p*ulmonar, *a*normalidades da genitália, *r*etardo do crescimento e *s*urdez (*deafness*) (sensioroneural); de herança autossômica dominante.
leop·ard's bane. Arnica. SIN arnica.
Leopold, Christian Gerhard, médico alemão, 1846–1911. VER L. maneuvers, em *maneuver*.
Lepehne, Georg, médico alemão, *1887. VER L.-Pickworth *stain*.
lep·er (lep′er). Leproso; uma pessoa que possui lepra. [G. *lepra*]
le·pid·ic (le-pid′ik). Lepídico; que contém escamas ou uma camada de revestimento escamoso. [G. *lepis (lepid-)*, escama, casca]
Lep·i·dop·tera (lep-i-dop′ter-ă). Lepidópteros; uma ordem de insetos composta de mariposas e borboletas, caracterizada por asas cobertas por escamas delicadas. [G. *lepis*, escama, + *pteron*, asa]
Lep·or·i·pox·vi·rus (lep′o-ri-poks′vi-rŭs). O gênero de vírus (família Poxviridae) que compreende os vírus do fibroma e mixoma dos coelhos; diferente dos ortopoxvírus, eles são éter-sensíveis. [L. *leporis*, gen. de *lepus*, lebre, + vírus]
lep·o·thrix (lep′o-thriks). Lepotrix. SIN trichomycosis axillaris. [G. *lepos*, casca, palha, + *thrix*, cabelo]
lep·re·chaun·ism (lep′re-kawn-izm) [MIM*246200]. Leprechaunismo; uma forma congênita de nanismo caracterizada por extremo retardo do crescimento, distúrbios endócrinos e face de elfo e orelhas grandes, com implantação baixa; herança autossômica recessiva; causado por mutação no gene do receptor de insulina (INSR) em 19p. SIN Donohue disease, Donohue syndrome. [Irlandês *leprechaun*, elfo]
lep·rid. Lépride; lesão cutânea inicial da lepra. [G. *lepra*, lepra, + *-id (1)*]
le·pro·ma (le-pro′mă). Leproma; um foco definido e razoavelmente bem circunscrito de inflamação granulomatosa, causada por *Mycobacterium leprae*, que consiste principalmente em acúmulo de grandes células fagocitárias mononucleares, nas quais o citoplasma parece finamente vacuolizado (ou seja, células espumosas); o caráter espumoso dos macrófagos está relacionado à fagocitose de numerosos microrganismos álcool-ácido-resistentes. [G. *lepros*, escamoso, + *-oma*, tumor]
lep·rom·a·tous (lep-ro′mă-tŭs). Lepromatoso; pertinente a ou caracterizado por sinais de um leproma.
lep·ro·min (lep′ro-min). Lepromina; um extrato de tecido infectado por *Mycobacterium leprae* usado nos testes cutâneos para classificar o estágio da lepra. VER TAMBÉM lepromin *reaction, test*.
lep·ro·sar·i·um (lep′ro-sar′e-ŭm). Leprosário; um hospital especialmente destinado ao tratamento daqueles que sofrem de lepra, em particular aqueles que precisam de cuidado especializado.
lep·ro·sery (lep′ro-ser-e). Leprosário; uma casa ou colônia de leprosos.
lep·ro·stat·ic (lep-ro-stat′ik). Leprostático. 1. Que inibe o crescimento do *Mycobacterium leprae*. 2. Um agente que apresenta essa ação.
lep·ro·sy (lep′ro-se). Lepra, hanseníase. 1. Uma infecção granulomatosa crônica, causada pelo *Mycobacterium leprae*, que afeta as partes corporais mais frias, especialmente a pele, os nervos periféricos e os testículos. A l. é classificada em dois tipos principais, lepromatosa e tuberculóide, representando os extremos da resposta imunológica. 2. Um nome usado na Bíblia para descrever várias doenças cutâneas, especialmente aquelas de natureza crônica ou contagiosa, que provavelmente incluía a psoríase e o leucoderma. SIN Hansen disease. [G. *lepra*, de *lepros*, escamoso]

anesthetic l., l. anestésica; uma forma de l. que afeta principalmente os nervos, caracterizada por hiperestesia seguida por anestesia e por paralisia, ulceração e vários distúrbios tróficos, terminando em gangrena e mutilação. SIN Danielssen disease, Danielssen-Boeck disease, dry l., trophoneurotic l.

borderline l., l. limítrofe; uma forma de l. que é muito instável do ponto de vista imunológico; os nervos cutâneos geralmente contêm bacilos, mas o teste da lepromina é, em geral, negativo; as lesões cutâneas são compostas de placas ou faixas achatadas. SIN dimorphous l.

dimorphous l., l. dimórfica. SIN borderline l.

dry l., l. seca. SIN anesthetic l.

histoid l., l. históide; uma forma de l. lepromatosa com lesões que se assemelham microscopicamente ao dermatofibroma ou a outros tumores de células fusiformes.

indeterminate l., l. indeterminada; forma transitória de l. em que o estado imunológico ainda não está constituído e os aspectos histológicos e clínicos ainda não são característicos de qualquer um dos tipos principais de l.

lepromatous l., l. lepromatosa; uma forma de l. em que as lesões cutâneas nodulares estão infiltradas, possuem bordas mal-definidas e são bacteriologicamente positivas; o teste da lepromina é negativo, ou seja, o sistema imunológico do paciente não responde à infecção por *Mycobacterium leprae*.

Lucio l., fenômeno de Lucio; uma forma aguda que acontece na l. lepromatosa difusa pura apresentando placas com formato irregular, intensamente eritematosas, dolorosas, especialmente nas pernas, com tendência para ulceração e fibrose. SIN Lucio leprosy phenomenon.

macular l., l. macular; uma forma de l. tuberculóide em que as lesões são pequenas, glabras e secas, mostrando-se eritematosas na pele clara e hipopigmentadas ou com coloração acobreada na pele escura.

mutilating l., l. mutilante; um estágio tardio da l. anestésica.

nodular l., l. nodular. SIN tuberculoid l.

smooth l., l. lisa. SIN tuberculoid l.

trophoneurotic l., l. trofoneurótica. SIN anesthetic l.

tuberculoid l., l. tuberculóide; uma forma benigna, estável e resistente da doença, na qual a reação à lepromina é fortemente positiva e na qual as lesões são placas eritematosas, insensíveis e infiltradas, com bordas bem delimitadas. SIN nodular l., smooth l.

lep·rot·ic (lep-rot′ik). Leproso; SIN leprous.

lep·rous (lep′rŭs). Leproso; relativo a ou que sofre de lepra. SIN leprotic.

-lepsis, -lepsy. Formas combinantes que indicam uma convulsão. [G. lēpsis]

lep·tan·dra (lep-tan′dră). Leptandra; o rizoma seco e as raízes da *Veronicastrum virginicum* (família Serophulariaceae). Nativa da América do Norte. Originalmente utilizada como catártico. SIN black root, Culver root.

lep·tin (lep′tin). Leptina; uma proteína helicoidal secretada pelo tecido adiposo e que age sobre um receptor no núcleo ventro-medial do hipotálamo para refrear o apetite e aumentar o dispêndio de energia à medida que as reservas lipídicas corporais aumentam. Os níveis de l. são 40% mais elevados nas mulheres e exibem um aumento adicional de 50% pouco antes da menarca, retornando posteriormente aos níveis basais; os níveis são diminuídos pelo jejum e aumentados pela inflamação. [G. leptos, magro, 1 -in]

Já foram identificados os genes humanos que codificam a leptina (*locus* 7q31.3) e o receptor de leptina (1p31). Os camundongos de laboratório que apresentam mutações no gene ob, que codifica a leptina, tornam-se obesos mórbidos, diabéticos e inférteis; a administração de leptina a esses camundongos melhora a tolerância à glicose, aumenta a atividade física, reduz o peso corporal em 30% e restaura a fertilidade. Os camundongos com mutações do gene db, que codifica o receptor de leptina, também se tornam obesos e diabéticos, porém não melhoram com a administração de leptina. Embora mutações nos genes da leptina e do receptor de leptina tenham sido encontradas em um pequeno número de seres humanos com obesidade mórbida e comportamento alimentar anormal, a maioria das pessoas obesas não apresentam essas mutações e têm níveis circulantes normais ou elevados de leptina. A leptina estimula o transporte de glicose mediado por insulina para dentro das células adiposas *in vitro*. Nos estudos preliminares, tanto as pessoas magras quanto as pessoas com peso excessivo mostraram discreta redução do peso com injeções subcutâneas diárias de leptina humana metionil recombinante durante vários meses. Todas as pessoas seguiram dietas de redução de peso durante o período de estudo. A perda de peso, em algumas pessoas que receberam leptina, não superou aquela conseguida pelas pessoas que receberam placebo, mas, quando ocorreu significativa redução de peso, ela foi proporcional à dosagem. A imunodeficiência observada na inanição pode resultar da secreção diminuída de leptina. Os camundongos que não têm gene para a leptina ou para seu receptor mostram comprometimento da função da célula T, e, em estudos de laboratório, a leptina induziu uma resposta proliferativa nos linfócitos CD4 humanos.

lepto-. Forma combinante que indica leve, magro, frágil. [G. *leptos*, delicado, magro, fraco]

lep·to·ceph·a·lous (lep-tō-sef′ă-lŭs). Leptocéfalo; que possui um crânio estreito e anormalmente alto. [lepto- + G. *Kephalé*, cabeça]

lep·to·ceph·a·ly (lep-tō-sef′ă-lē). Leptocefalia; uma malformação caracterizada por um crânio estreito e anormalmente alto. [lepto- + G. *kephalé*, cabeça]

lep·to·chro·mat·ic (lep′tō-krō-mat′ik). Leptocromático; que possui uma rede de cromatina muito fina.

lep·to·cyte (lep′tō-sīt). Leptócito; uma célula-alvo ou em chapéu de mexicano, ou seja, um eritrócito incomumente fino ou achatado em que existe uma área central arredondada de material pigmentado, uma zona média clara que não contém pigmento e um aro externo pigmentado na borda da célula. Acredita-se que os leptócitos sejam eritrócitos cujo envoltório ou membrana celular seja incomumente grande em relação a seu conteúdo. [lepto- + G. *kytos*, célula]

lep·to·cy·to·sis (lep′tō-sī-tō′sis). Leptocitose; a presença de leptócitos no sangue circulante, como na talassemia, em alguns casos de icterícia (mesmo na ausência de anemia), em exemplos ocasionais de doença hepática (na ausência de icterícia) e em alguns pacientes que tiveram o baço removido.

lep·to·dac·ty·lous (lep-tō-dak′ti-lŭs). Leptodactiloso; que possui dedos das mãos finos. [lepto- + G. *daktylos*, dedo]

lep·to·me·nin·ge·al (lep′tō-me-nin′jē-ăl). Leptomeníngeo; pertinente às leptomeninges.

lep·to·me·nin·ges, lep·to·me·ninx, sing. **lep·to·me·ninx** (lep-tō-me-nin′jēz, lep′tō-mē′ninks, lep′tō-mē′ninks) [TA]. Leptomeninges. SIN leptomeninx. [lepto- + G. *mēninx*, pl. mēninges, membranas]

lep·to·men·in·gi·tis (lep′tō-men-in-jī′tis). Leptomeningite; inflamação das leptomeninges. VER TAMBÉM arachnoiditis. SIN pia-arachnitis.

basilar l., l. basilar; inflamação da aracnóide na base do cérebro; freqüentemente encontrada na meningite crônica de origem tuberculosa, sifilítica ou micótica.

lep·to·mere (lep′tō-mēr). Leptômero; uma partícula muito pequena de matéria viva; Asclepíades acreditava que o corpo era composto de uma agregação de numerosos leptômeros. [lepto- + G. *meros*, parte]

lep·to·mo·nad (lep′tō-mō′nad, lep-tom′ō-nad). Leptomônada. 1. Nome comum para um membro do gênero *Leptomonas*. 2. ver promastigote.

Lep·tom·o·nas (lep′tō-mō′nas, lep-tom′ō-nŭs). Um gênero de parasitas flagelados, assexuados, monogenéticos (família Trypanosomatidae) comumente encontrados no intestino posterior de insetos. [lepto- + G. *monas*, unidade]

lep·to·ne·ma (lep-tō-nē′mă). Leptonema. SIN leptotene. [lepto- + G. *nēma*, filamento]

lep·to·pho·nia (lep′tō-fō′nē-ă). Leptofonia. SIN hypophonia. [lepto- + G. *phōnē*, som, voz]

lep·to·phon·ic (lep′tō-fon′ik). Leptofônico; com a voz enfraquecida.

lep·to·po·dia (lep-tō-pō′dē-ă). Leptopodia; a condição de apresentar pés delgados. [lepto- + G. *pous*, pé]

lep·to·pro·so·pia (lep′tō-prō-sō′pē-ă). Leptoprosopia; estreitamento da face. [kepto- + G. *prosōpon*, face]

lep·to·pro·so·pic (lep′tō-prō-sō′pik). Leptoprosópico; que possui uma face fina e estreita. Cf. leptosomatic.

lep·tor·rhine (lep′tō-rīn). Leptorrino; que possui um nariz delgado. Aplicado a um crânio com um índice nasal abaixo de 47 (concordância de Frankfort) ou 48 (Broca). [lepto- + G. *rhis*, nariz]

lep·to·scope (lep′tō-skōp). Leptoscópio; um aparelho para medir as membranas celulares.

lep·to·so·mat·ic, lep·to·som·ic (lep′tō-sō-mat′ik, -tō-sō′mik). Leptossômico; que possui um corpo delgado, leve ou magro. [lepto- + G. *sōma*, corpo]

Lep·to·spi·ra (lep′tō-spī′ră). Um gênero de bactérias aeróbicas móveis (ordem Spirochaetales) que contém microrganismos finos, firmemente espiralados, com 6 a 20 μm de comprimento. Possuem um filamento axial e uma ou as duas extremidades podem ser encurvadas em um gancho semicircular. Coram-se com dificuldade, exceto com o corante de Giemsa ou pela impregnação por prata; associados à febre íctero-hemorrágica; incluem 7 espécies patogênicas e 3 não-patogênicas; a espécie típica é *L. interrogans*. [lepto- + G. *speira*, uma mola]

L. interrogans, uma espécie que contém múltiplas sorovariantes patogênicas. Agente causal da leptospirose. É a espécie típica do gênero *L.*

lep·to·spire (lep′tō-spīr). Leptospira; nome comum para qualquer microrganismo que pertença ao gênero *Leptospira*.

lep·to·spi·ro·sis (lep′tō-spī-rō′sis). Leptospirose; infecção por *Leptospira interrogans*.

anicteric l., l. anictérica; infecção por uma das espécies do grupo *Leptospira*, usualmente branda, com envolvimento hepático e renal limitado, ao contrário da doença de Weil.

l. icterohemorrhagica (ik′ter-ō-hem-ōr-aj′ī-kă), l. íctero-hemorrágica. SIN icterohemorrhagic *fever*.

lep·to·spi·ru·ria (lep′tō-spī-roo′rē-ă). Leptospirúria; presença de espécie do gênero *Leptospira* na urina, em conseqüência da leptospirose nos túbulos renais.

lep·to·tene (lep′tō-tēn). Leptóteno; o estágio inicial da prófase na meiose, na qual os cromossomas contraem-se e tornam-se visíveis como filamentos longos bem separados entre si. [lepto- + G. *tainia*, faixa, fita]

lep·to·thri·co·sis (lep′tō-thri-kō′sis). Leptotricose; termo obsoleto para qualquer doença causada pelo gênero atualmente inválido *Leptothrix*.

Lep·to·thrix (lep′tō - thriks). Um gênero atualmente inválido de microrganismos embainhados, intimamente relacionados ao gênero *Sphaerotilus*, encontrados na água fresca.

Lep·to·trich·ia (lep - tō - trik′ē - ă). Um gênero de bactérias anaeróbicas imóveis, contendo bastonetes Gram-negativos, retos ou discretamente curvos, com 5–15 μm de comprimento, com uma ou ambas as extremidades arredondadas, freqüentemente afiladas. Os grânulos estão uniformemente distribuídos ao longo do eixo longitudinal, e um ou mais grânulos grandes podem localizar-se próximo à extremidade da célula. Não há formas ramificadas ou baqueteadas. Duas ou mais células unem-se e formam filamentos septados de comprimento variável; nas culturas mais antigas, podem formar-se filamentos de até 200 μm e que se enrolam uns nos outros; corpúsculos cocóides grandes podem ser encontrados dentro de um filamento à medida que uma célula sofre lise. O dióxido de carbono é essencial para o crescimento ótimo. Ácido lático é produzido a partir da glicose. Esses microrganismos ocorrem na cavidade oral de seres humanos. A espécie típica é *L. buccalis*. [lepto- + G. *thrix*, cabelo]

L. bucca′lis, uma espécie bacteriana encontrada na boca dos seres humanos, raramente encontrada no sangue de pacientes imunocomprometidos; é a espécie típica do gênero *L.*

Lep·to·trom·bid·i·um (lep′tō - trom - bid′ē - ŭm). Um gênero importante de ácaros trombiculídeos, antes considerado um subgênero do gênero *Trombicula*, que inclui todos os vetores do tifo rural (doença tsutsugamushi). Os membros do *L.* que servem como vetores do tifo rural pertencem ao grupo *L. deliense*: *L. akamushi* é o vetor clássico no Japão; *L. deliense* é o vetor primário, sendo encontrado desde a Nova Guiné, Austrália, Filipinas, China e Sudeste Asiático até o oeste do Paquistão; *L. fletcheri* é encontrado na Malásia, Nova Guiné e Filipinas. Cerca de oito outras espécies também foram implicadas na transmissão do tifo rural em áreas mais limitadas.

L. akamu′shi, uma de duas espécies, sendo a outra *L. deliensis* (*T. deliensis*), implicadas na transmissão de *Rickettsia tsutsugamushi*, o agente da doença tsutsugamushi no Japão e em outros pontos no Oriente; as larvas dessa espécie são parasitas característicos de roedores, que, portanto, são reservatórios das infecções humanas, embora os próprios ácaros também sejam reservatórios, visto que suas riquétsias parasitas são transmitidas por via transovariana de uma geração para outra (um requisito para a transmissão para os seres humanos, visto que apenas as larvas do ácaro se alimentam de forma parasitária e apenas uma vez em seu ciclo de vida). SIN *Trombicula akamushi*.

ler·go·trile (ler′gō - trīl). Lergotrila; um derivado do esporão do centeio que exerce propriedades agonistas sobre os receptores da dopamina; semelhantes à bromocriptina e à lisurida.

Leri, André, cirurgião ortopédico francês, 1875–1930. VER L. *pleonosteosis, sign*; L.-Weill *disease, syndrome*.

Leriche, René, cirurgião francês, 1879–1955. VER L. *operation, syndrome*.

Lermoyez, Marcel, otorrinolaringologista francês, 1858–1929. VER L. *syndrome*.

Lerner, I.M., geneticista populacional norte-americano, 1910–1967. VER L. *homeostasis*.

Leroy, Edgar August, médico francês, *1883. VER Fiessinger-L.-Reiter *syndrome*.

LES Acrônimo de *lower esophageal sphincter* (esfíncter esofágico inferior); Lambert–Eaton *syndrome* (síndrome de Lambert-Eaton).

les·bi·an (lez′bē - ăn). Lésbica. **1.** Uma mulher homossexual. **2.** Pertinente à homossexualidade entre mulheres. VER gay.

les·bi·an·ism (lez′bē - ăn - izm). Lesbianismo; homossexualidade entre mulheres. SIN sapphism. [G. *lesbios*, relativo à ilha de Lesbos]

Lesch, Michael, pediatra norte-americano, *1939. VER L.-Nyhan *syndrome*.

Leser, Edmund, cirurgião alemão, 1828–1916. VER L.-Trélat *sign*.

le·sion (lē′zhŭn). Lesão. **1.** Uma ferida ou lesão. **2.** Uma alteração patológica nos tecidos. **3.** Um dos pontos individuais ou manchas de uma doença multifocal. [L. *laedo*, pp. *laesus*, lesionar]

Baehr-Lohlein, l. de Baehr-Lohlein. SIN Lohlein-Baehr l.

Bankart l., l. de Bankart; uma laceração do lábio glenóide anterior que acompanha o descolamento do ligamento gleno-umeral inferior.

benign lymphoepithelial l., l. linfoepitelial benigna; massas de tecido linfóide semelhantes a um tumor benigno na glândula parótida, contendo pequenas ilhas de células epiteliais espalhadas, principalmente sólidas. SIN Godwin tumor.

Bracht-Wächter l., l. de Bracht-Wächter; uma coleção focal de linfócitos e células mononucleares no miocárdio na endocardite bacteriana.

caviar l., l. em caviar; uma veia dilatada ou varícola existente no sistema coletor venoso sob a língua.

coin l. of lungs, l. nodulares dos pulmões. SIN nodular *opacity*.

Dieulafoy l., l. de Dieulafoy; uma artéria submucosa anormalmente grande localizada na parte proximal do estômago que seria o local de episódios agudos e recorrentes de hemorragia maciça.

Duret l., l. de Duret; pequena hemorragia no assoalho do quarto ventrículo ou sob o aqueduto de Sylvius.

Ghon primary l., l. primária de Ghon. SIN Ghon *tubercle*.

gross l., l. macroscópica; uma l. facilmente visível a olho nu.

high-grade squamous intraepithelial l. (HSIL, HGSIL), l. intra-epitelial escamosa de alto grau (HSIL, HGSIL); termo utilizado no sistema Bethesda para relatar o diagnóstico citológico cervical/vaginal e, assim, descrever um espectro de anormalidades epiteliais cervicais não-invasivas, incluindo displasia moderada e grave, carcinoma *in situ* e graus 2 e 3 de neoplasia intra-epitelial

lesões primárias

alterações planas, impalpáveis na coloração da pele

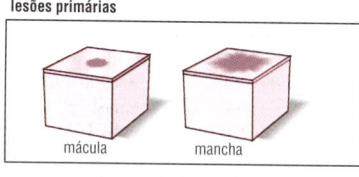

elevação formada por líquido em uma cavidade

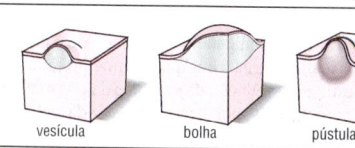

massas sólidas, palpáveis e elevadas

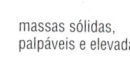
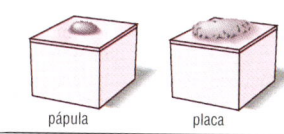
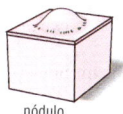
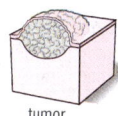
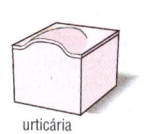

lesões secundárias

material na superfície cutânea

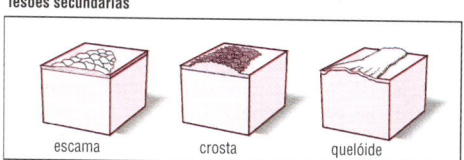

perda da superfície cutânea

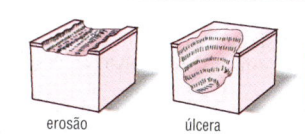
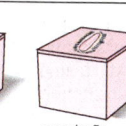
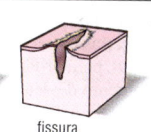

lesões vasculares

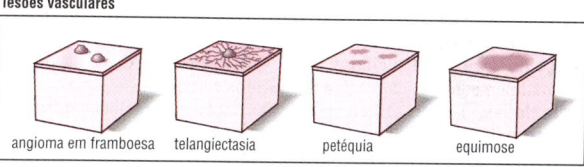

lesões: tipos de lesões primárias, secundárias e vasculares

cervical. VER TAMBÉM Bethesda *system*, ASCUS, atypical glandular *cells* of undetermined significance, em *cell*, low-grade squamous intraepithelial l.

Hill-Sachs l., l. de Hill-Sachs; uma irregularidade observada na cabeça do úmero após a luxação anterior do ombro; causada pela impacção da porção póstero-lateral da cabeça do úmero contra a borda anterior da glenóide.

Janeway l., l. de Janeway; um dos estigmas da endocardite infecciosa; máculas irregulares, eritematosas, planas e indolores nas regiões palmares, plantares, eminências tenares e hipotenares das mãos, pontas dos dedos das mãos e superfícies plantares dos artelhos; raramente uma erupção cutânea difusa. Na endocardite aguda, as lesões podem ser hemorrágicas ou purpúricas.

Lohlein-Baehr l., l. de Lohlein-Baehr; glomerulonefrite embólica focal que ocorre na endocardite bacteriana. SIN Baehr-Lohlein l.

lower motor neuron l., l. do neurônio motor inferior; a lesão das células motoras no tronco cerebral ou medula espinal, ou dos axônios delas derivados.

low-grade squamous intraepithelial l. (LGSIL, LSIL), l. intra-epitelial escamosa de baixo grau; termo utilizado no sistema Bethesda para relatar o diagnóstico citológico cervical/vaginal para descrever um espectro das anormalidades epiteliais cervicais não-invasivas; essas lesões incluem as alterações celulares associadas ao efeito citopatológico do papilomavírus humano (HPV) e displasia cervical (neoplasia intra-epitelial cervical de grau 1). VER TAMBÉM Bethesda *system*, reactive *changes*, em *change*, ASCUS, atypical glandular *cells* of undetermined significance, em *cell*.

Mallory-Weiss l., l. de Mallory-Weiss. SIN Mallory-Weiss *syndrome*.

precancerous l., l. pré-cancerosa; uma l. não-invasiva com uma probabilidade de previsível de se tornar maligna; p.ex., ceratose actínica.

radial sclerosing l., l. esclerosante radial; uma variante da adenose esclerosante da mama com formação de cicatriz central e ductos hiperplásicos que se irradiam. SIN radial scar.

ring-wall l., l. em parede anelar; um pequeno anel hemorrágico no cérebro que estimula a proliferação de um anel glial.

supranuclear l., l. supranuclear; lesão das fibras descendentes cerebrais (corticonucleares) acima do tronco cerebral ou do núcleo do nervo motor espinal. SIN upper motor neuron l.

upper motor neuron l., l. do neurônio motor superior. SIN supranuclear l.

wire-loop l., l. em alça; o espessamento da membrana basal, com coloração fibrinóide, de capilares periféricos espalhados nos glomérulos renais; característica do envolvimento renal no lúpus eritematoso sistêmico; o aspecto de uma parede capilar afetada assemelha-se a uma alça empregada em microbiologia.

Lesser, Ladislaus Leo, cirurgião naturalizado alemão nascido na Polônia, 1846–1925. VER Lesser *triangle*.

Lesshaft, Pjotr F., médico russo, 1836–1909. VER L. *triangle*.

LET Abreviatura de linear energy *transfer* (transferência linear de energia).

le·thal (lē'thǎl).Letal; pertinente a ou que causa a morte; indicando especialmente o agente causal. [L. *letalis*, de *letum*, morte]
  clinical l., um distúrbio que culmina em morte prematura.
  genetic l., um distúrbio que evita a reprodução efetiva dos indivíduos afetados; p.ex., síndrome de Klinefelter.

le·thal·i·ty (lē - thal'i - tē). Letalidade; a qualidade ou estado de ser letal.

leth·ar·gy (leth'ar - jē). Letargia; o comprometimento relativamente brando da consciência que resulta em redução da vigília e da consciência; essa condição apresenta muitas causas, mas, por fim, é provocada pela disfunção cerebral generalizada. [G. *lēthargia*, sonolência]

LETS Acrônimo de *l*arge, *e*xternal *t*ransformation-*s*ensitive fibronectin (fibronectina grande e sensível a transformação externa). VER fibronectins.

Letterer, Erich, patologista alemão, *1895. VER L.-Siwe *disease*.

Leu Símbolo de leucine (leucina); leucyl (leucil).

leuc-, leuco-. Formas combinantes que significam branco, leucócitos. VER leuko-, leuk-. [G. *leukos*, branco]

leu·cin (loo'sin). Leucina. SIN leukin.

leu·cine (L, Leu) (loo'sēn).Leucina; ácido 2-amino-4-metilvalérico; o L-isômero é um dos aminoácidos encontrados nas proteínas; um aminoácido essencial à nutrição.
  l. aminopeptidase, l. aminopeptidase; aminopeptidase (citosol).
  l. dehydrogenase, l.-desidrogenase; uma enzima que catalisa a reação da L-l., água e NAD$^+$ para produzir NADH, amônia e 4-metil-2-oxopentanoato; usada no tratamento de determinados tumores.
  l. zipper, fechamento de leucina; um motivo (*motif*) estrutural encontrado em inúmeras proteínas (p.ex., algumas das proteínas reguladoras que ligam o DNA) em que os resíduos leucil se alinham ao longo de uma borda da hélice e podem interdigitar-se com uma estrutura similar em outra molécula de proteína. [Zipper, original de uma marca comercial para um fecho com duas fileiras de dentes que se entremeiam e travam]

leu·ci·no·sis (loo'si - nō'sis). Leucinose; uma condição em que existe uma proporção anormalmente grande de leucina nos tecidos e líquidos corporais.

leu·cin·u·ri·a (loo - si - noo'rē - ǎ).Leucinúria; a excreção de leucina na urina.

leu·co·har·mine (loo - kō - har'mēn).Leucoarmina. SIN harmine.

leu·co·line (loo'kō - lēn).Leucolina. SIN quinolline (1).

leu·co·meth·yl·ene blue (lu'kō - meth'i - lēn). Leucometileno azul; a forma reduzida e incolor do azul de metileno. SIN methylene white.

Leu·co·nos·toc (loo - kō - nos'tok).Um gênero de bactérias microaerofílicas a anaeróbicas facultativas (família Lactobacillaceae) contendo células esféricas Gram-positivas, que podem, em determinadas condições, alongar-se e tornar-se afiladas e, até mesmo, formar bastonetes. Ácidos lático e acético são produzidos por esses microrganismos. Eles são encontrados nos sucos vegetais e no leite. A espécie típica é *L. mesenteroides*. [G. *leukos*, branco, + *nostoc*, um gênero de algas (uma palavra cunhada por Paracelso]
  L. mesenteroi'des, uma espécie encontrada em vegetais em fermentação e em outros materiais vegetais e nos derivados de carne preparada; é um produtor ativo de uma dextrana comumente utilizada como expansor plasmático; é a espécie típica do gênero *L*.

leu·co pa·tent blue (loo'kō pat'ent)[C.I. 42051]. Patente azul V; um corante trifenilmetano sulfonado reduzido e descolorado com zinco e ácido acético para produzir uma solução estável; usado para demonstrar a hemoglobina peroxidase. SIN patent blue V.

leu·co·vo·rin (loo'kō - vōr - in).Leucovorina. SIN folinic acid.
  l. calcium, l. cálcica; o sal de cálcio da leucovorina (ácido folínico); usada para se contrapor aos efeitos tóxicos dos antagonistas do ácido fólico, para o tratamento das anemias megaloblásticas e como adjunto para a cianocobalamina na anemia perniciosa. SIN calcium folinate.

Leudet, Théodor E., médico francês, 1825–1887. VER L. *tinnitus*.

leu·en·keph·a·lin (loo - en - kef'ǎ - lin). Leuencefalina. VER enkephalins.

leuk-. VER leuko-.

leuk·a·ne·mia (loo - kǎ - nē'mē - ǎ). Leucanemia; termo obsoleto para a eritroleucemia. [leukemia + anemia]

leuk·a·phe·re·sis (look'ǎ - fē - rē'sis).Leucaférese; um procedimento, análogo à plasmaférese, em que os leucócitos são removidos do sangue coletado e o restante do sangue é retransfundido para o doador. [leuko- + G. *aphairesis*, uma retirada]

leu·ke·mia (loo - kē'mē - ǎ). Leucemia; a proliferação progressiva de leucócitos anormais encontrados nos tecidos hematopoéticos, em outros órgãos e, em geral, no sangue em grande número. A l. é classificada pelo tipo celular dominante e pela duração desde o início até a morte. A morte ocorre na *l. aguda* em alguns meses, na maioria dos casos, estando associada a sintomas agudos, incluindo anemia grave, hemorragias e aumento discreto dos linfonodos ou do baço. A duração da *l. crônica* excede um ano, com instalação gradual dos sintomas de anemia ou do aumento acentuado do baço, fígado ou linfonodos. SIN leukocytic sarcoma. [leuko- + G. *haima*, sangue]
  acute lymphocytic leukemia (ALL), l. linfocítica aguda. VER lymphocytic l.
  acute promyelocytic l., l. promielocítica aguda; a l. que se apresenta como um distúrbio hemorrágico grave, com infiltração da medula óssea por promielócitos e mielócitos anormais, fibrinogênio plasmático baixo e coagulação defeituosa.
  adult T-cell l. (ATL), l. de células T adultas. SIN adult T-cell *lymphoma*.
  aleukemic l., l. aleucêmica; l. em que não há células anormais (ou leucêmicas) no sangue periférico.
  basophilic l., basophilocytic l., l. basófila, l. mastocitária; uma forma de l. granulocítica em que há um número incomumente grande de granulócitos basofílicos nos tecidos e no sangue circulante; em alguns casos, as formas basofílicas imaturas e maduras podem representar 40 a 80% do número total de leucócitos. SIN mast cell l.
  chronic granulocytic l., l. granulocítica crônica. SIN chronic myelocytic l.
  chronic myelocytic l., l. mielocítica crônica; um grupo heterogêneo de distúrbios mieloproliferativos que pode evoluir para l. aguda nos estágios tardios (ou seja, crise blástica). SIN chronic granulocytic l., chronic myelogenous l., chronic myeloid l.
  chronic myelogenous l. (CML), l. mielogênica crônica. SIN chronic myelocytic l.
  chronic myeloid l., l. mielóide crônica. SIN chronic myelocytic l.
  l. cu'tis, l. cutânea; lesões amarelo-cutâneas, avermelhadas, azul-avermelhadas ou purpúreas, por vezes nodulares, associadas à infiltração difusa da pele por células leucêmicas; o envolvimento pode ser difuso e generalizado, ou seja, a chamada l. cutânea universal, ou ela pode ser localizada.
  embryonal l., l. embrionária. SIN stem cell l.
  eosinophilic l., eosinophilocytic l., l. eosinofílica; uma f. de l. granulocítica em que há um número notável de granulócitos eosinofílicos nos tecidos e no sangue circulante, em um em que essas células são predominantes, na doença crônica desse tipo, a contagem de leucócitos totais pode chegar a 200.000–250.000/mm^3, com até 80 a 90% sendo eosinófilos, principalmente nas formas adultas.
  granulocytic l., l. granulocítica; uma forma de l. caracterizada por uma proliferação descontrolada de células mielopoéticas na medula óssea e em locais extramedulares, bem como pela presença de numerosas formas granulocíticas imaturas e maduras em vários tecidos (e órgãos) e no sangue circulante; a contagem total pode variar desde 1.000 (variedade aleucêmica) até várias centenas de milhares por mm^3. A célula predominante geralmente é da série neutrofílica, mas, em alguns casos, os granulócitos eosinofílicos ou basofílicos, ou mesmo os megacariócitos, podem representar a forma principal; no início da l. granulocítica, o sangue circulante pode conter um número excessivo de todas as formas granulocíticas. SIN leukemic myelosis (1), myelocytic l., myelogenic l., myelogenous l., myeloid l.

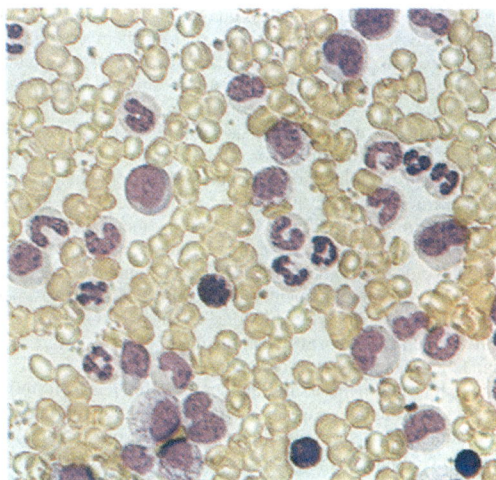

leucemia granulocítica (esfregaço sanguíneo): contagem de leucócitos alta, com mieloblastos

hairy cell l., l. de células pilosas; um distúrbio raro, usualmente crônico, caracterizado por proliferação de células pilosas no sangue e nos órgãos reticuloendoteliais.
leukemic l., l. leucêmica; um termo obsoleto redundante por vezes empregado para enfatizar a ocorrência de numerosas células leucêmicas no sangue circulante; essa forma clássica de l. é usualmente denominada apenas *leukemia* (leucemia).
leukopenic l., l. leucopênica; uma forma de l. linfocítica, granulocítica ou monocítica em que o número total de leucócitos no sangue circulante está dentro dos limites de normalidade ou pode estar diminuído em vários níveis, os quais se situam muito abaixo do normal.
lymphatic l., l. linfocítica. SIN lymphocytic l.
lymphoblastic l., l. linfocítica; l. linfocítica aguda em que as células anormais são formas principalmente (ou quase totalmente) blásticas da série linfocítica ou em que um número incomumente grande de formas imaturas ocorre em associação com os linfócitos adultos.
lymphocytic l., l. linfocítica; uma variedade de l. caracterizada por proliferação descontrolada e aumento notável do tecido linfóide em vários locais (p.ex., linfonodos, baço, medula óssea, pulmões), bem como pela ocorrência de um número aumentado de células da série linfocítica no sangue circulante e em vários tecidos e órgãos; na doença crônica, as células são linfócitos adultos, enquanto um número notável de linfoblastos é observado nas síndromes mais agudas. SIN lymphatic l., lymphoid l.
lymphoid l., l. linfocítica. SIN lymphocytic l.
mast cell l., l. de mastócitos. SIN basophilic l.
mature cell l., l. granulocítica crônica.
megakaryocytic l., l. megacariocítica; uma forma incomum da doença mielopoética que se caracteriza por proliferação aparentemente descontrolada de megacariócitos na medula óssea e, por vezes, pela presença de um número considerável de megacariócitos no sangue circulante. Quando se examina a medula óssea em vários intervalos em alguns casos de l. mielocítica crônica, a proliferação de megacariócitos é mais proeminente que a de granulócitos; nesses períodos, o sangue circulante pode conter megacariócitos e/ou fragmentos dos núcleos e citoplasmas megacariocíticos, perfazendo até 5 ou 6% do número total de leucócitos.
meningeal l., l. meníngea; infiltração das meninges por células leucêmicas, uma ocorrência comum na recidiva após a administração sistêmica de agentes quimioterápicos para pacientes leucêmicos.
micromyeloblastic l., l. micromieloblástica; uma forma de l. mielocítica em que proporções relativamente grandes de micromieloblásticos são encontradas no sangue circulante e na medula óssea e outros tecidos.
mixed l., mixed cell l., l. de células mistas; termo raramente utilizado para descrever l. granulocítica, enfatizando, assim, a ocorrência de diferentes tipos de células na série mielóide (ou seja, granulócitos neutrofílicos, eosinofílicos e basófilos), em contraste com o padrão comparativamente monótono observado na l. linfocítica e monocítica.
monocytic l., l. monocítica; uma forma de l. caracterizada por numerosas células que podem ser definitivamente identificadas como monócitos, além de células maiores, aparentemente correlatas, formadas a partir da proliferação descontrolada do tecido reticuloendotelial; a l. em que esses dois tipos de células parecem "inundar" os locais usuais do sistema reticuloendotelial, ocorrendo em número notável no sangue circulante, sendo freqüentemente referida como o tipo Schilling da l. monocítica ou, por vezes, como l. monocítica verdadeira. A doença exibe uma evolução aguda ou subaguda nas pessoas idosas, caracterizando-se por edema das gengivas, ulceração oral, sangramento na pele ou mucosas, infecção secundária e esplenomegalia.
murine l., l. murina; um distúrbio leucêmico do camundongo causado por inúmeros retrovírus do tipo C diferentes.
myeloblastic l., l. mieloblástica; uma forma de l. granulocítica em que existem numerosos mieloblastos em vários tecidos (e órgãos) e no sangue circulante; as formas imaturas podem perfazer 30 a 60% (ou mesmo uma proporção maior) do número total aumentado de leucócitos. Utilizado como sinônimo de l. granulocítica aguda. SIN leukemic myelosis (2).
myelocytic l., myelogenic l., myelogenous l., myeloid l., l. mielocítica, mielogênica, mielógena, mielóide. SIN granulocytic l.
myelomonocytic l., l. mielomonocítica; uma variante da l. granulocítica com monocitose no sangue periférico. SIN Naegeli type of monocytic l.
Naegeli type of monocytic l., l. monocítica do tipo Naegeli. SIN myelomonocytic l.
natural killer cell l., l. de células destruidoras naturais (*natural killer*); uma l. que se origina nas células *natural killer*; freqüentemente associada à presença de vírus Epstein-Barr monoclonal que infecta células tumorais; geralmente indica um subtipo leucêmico com prognóstico ruim.
neutrophilic l., l. neutrofílica; uma forma incomum de l. granulocítica crônica em que o número muito aumentado de leucócitos no sangue circulante é formado por neutrófilos polimorfonucleares maduros, com quase nenhum granulócito jovem ou imaturo sendo observado.
plasma cell l., l. de plasmócitos; uma doença incomum caracterizada por leucocitose e outros sinais e sintomas sugestivos de l., em associação com as infiltrações difusas e agregados de plasmócitos no baço, fígado, medula óssea e linfonodos, e com a presença de um número considerável de plasmócitos no sangue circulante; o número total de leucócitos no sangue pode variar desde os níveis normais até 80.000 a 90.000/mm^3, podendo 5 a 90% ser constituídos de plasmócitos; mielomas múltiplos observados em alguns exemplos de l. de plasmócitos, porém nódulos bem definidos não são formados no osso. Embora existam outras diferenças clinicopatológicas nas duas condições, elas podem ser fases do mesmo processo básico.
polymorphocytic l., l. polimorfocítica; l. granulocítica, principalmente qualquer variedade em que as células predominantes sejam granulócitos maduros e segmentados.
Rieder cell l., l. de células de Rieder; uma forma especial de l. granulocítica aguda em que os tecidos afetados e o sangue circulante contêm um número relativamente grande de mieloblastos atípicos (ou seja, células de Rieder) que apresentam o tipo de citoplasma imaturo, usual e discretamente granular, bem como um núcleo bizarro e comparativamente maduro, com várias indentações amplas e bizarras (sugestivas de lobulação).
Schilling type of monocytic l., l. monocítica do tipo Schilling. VER monocytic l.
splenic l., l. esplênica; uma forma de l. em que existe um aumento incomum do baço, conforme observado com freqüência na l. granulocítica crônica.
stem cell l., l. de células primordiais, l. de células-tronco; uma forma de l. em que se acredita que as células anormais são precursoras de linfoblastos, mieloblastos ou monoblastos. SIN embryonal l.
subleukemic l., l. subleucêmica; uma forma de l. em que existem células anormais no sangue periférico, mas a contagem total de leucócitos não está elevada. SIN hypoleukemia, leukopenic myelosis, subleukemic myelosis, subleukemia.

leu·ke·mic (loo - kē′mik). Leucêmico; pertinente a ou que possui as características de qualquer forma de leucemia.
leu·ke·mid (loo-kem′id). Leucêmide; qualquer tipo inespecífico de lesão cutânea que está freqüentemente associado à leucemia, mas não é um acúmulo localizado de células leucêmicas; p.ex., petéquias, vesículas, vergões, bolhas, hematomas e lesões de dermatite esfoliativa e herpes zoster. [leuko- + G. *haima*, sangue, + *id* (1)]
leu·ke·mo·gen (loo - kē′mō - jen). Leucemógeno; qualquer substância ou entidade (p.ex., benzeno, radiação ionizante) que seja considerado um fator causal na ocorrência da leucemia.
leu·ke·mo·gen·e·sis (loo - kē - mō - jen′ē - sis). Leucemogênese; a causa (ou indução), desenvolvimento e progressão de uma doença leucêmica. [leukemia + G. *genesis*, produção]
leu·ke·mo·gen·ic (loo - kē - mō - jen′ik). Leucemogênico; relativo à causa, indução e desenvolvimento da leucemia; que manifesta a capacidade de provocar leucemia.
leu·ke·moid (loo - kē′moyd). Leucemóide; que se assemelha a leucemia em vários sinais e sintomas, especialmente com relação às alterações no sangue circulante. VER TAMBÉM leukemoid reaction. [leukemia + G. *eidos*, semelhança]
leu·ke·moid re·ac·tion. Reação leucemóide; um grau moderado, avançado e, por vezes, extremo de leucocitose no sangue circulante, similar ao que ocorre em várias formas de leucemia, mas que não é resultado de doença leucêmica; geralmente, existe um aumento desproporcional no número de formas (incluindo estágios imaturos) em uma série de leucócitos, com vários exemplos de r. l. mielocítica, linfocítica, monocítica ou plasmocítica podendo também ser

indistinguíveis da leucocitose que está associada a determinadas formas de leucemia. As reações leucemóides são, por vezes, observadas como um sinal de: 1) doença infecciosa causada por determinadas bactérias e outros agentes biológicos, p.ex., tuberculose, difteria e varicela; 2) intoxicação de vários tipos, p.ex., eclâmpsia, queimaduras graves e intoxicação por gás mostarda; 3) neoplasias malignas, p.ex., carcinoma do colo, do pulmão, do rim ou de outros órgãos; 4) hemorragia aguda ou hemólise.

lymphocytic l. r., reação leucemóide linfocítica; leucocitose de grau variável, com os linfócitos adultos e formas imaturas alcançando até 40% (ou mais) do número total de leucócitos no sangue circulante; pode ser observada em associação a coqueluche, mononucleose infecciosa, gonorréia, varicela e sarcoidose.

monocytic l. r., reação leucemóide monocítica; leucocitose de grau variável, p.ex., 30.000 a 40.000/mm^3, com monócitos adultos e formas imaturas alcançando até 30% (ou mais) do número total de leucócitos no sangue circulante; pode ser observada em associação a tuberculose, especialmente a primeira infecção, tipo miliar.

myelocytic l. r., reação leucemóide mielocítica; leucocitose de grau pelo menos moderado, p.ex., 50.000 ou mais por mm^3, com algumas formas imaturas, p.ex., 1 ou 2% de mielócitos, mas principalmente de leucócitos polimorfonucleares maduros no sangue circulante; pode ser observada em associação a tuberculose, osteomielite crônica, vários tipos de empiema, malária, pneumonia pneumocócica, meningite meningocócica, doença de Hodgkin e metástases de carcinoma na medula óssea.

plasmocytic l. r., reação leucemóide plasmocítica; a presença de um número incomum de plasmócitos, ou seja, plasmocitose, na medula óssea; pode ser observada em associação a sarcoidose, artrite reumatóide, cirrose, doença de Hodgkin e a algumas das chamadas doenças do colágeno.

leu·kin (loo′kin). Leucina; uma substância bactericida termoestável extraída dos leucócitos. SIN leucin. [*leuko*cyte + -in]

leuko-, leuk-. Formas combinantes que indicam branco, leucócitos. Para algumas palavras assim iniciadas, ver leuc- e leuco-. [G. *leukos*, branco]

leu·ko·ag·glu·ti·nin (loo′kō-ă-gloo′ti-nin). Leucoaglutinina; um anticorpo que aglutina leucócitos.

leu·ko·bil·in (loo-kō-bil′in). Leucobilina. SIN white *bile*. [leuko- + L. *bilis*, bile]

leu·ko·blast (loo′kō-blast). Leucoblasto; um leucócito granular imaturo. SIN proleukocyte. [leuko- + G. *blastos*, germe]

leu·ko·blas·to·sis (loo′kō-blas-tō′sis). Leucoblastose; um termo geral para a proliferação anormal de leucócitos, especialmente aquela que ocorre nas leucemias mielocítica e linfocítica.

leu·ko·chlo·ro·ma (loo′kō-klō-rō′mă). Leucocloroma; termo obsoleto para mielocitomatose. [leuko- + G. *chlōros*, verde, + -*oma*, tumor]

leu·ko·ci·din (loo-kos′i-din, loo-kō-sī′din). Leucocidina; uma substância termolábil que é produzida por muitas cepas de *Staphylococcus aureus*, *Streptococcus pyogenes* e pneumococos e manifesta uma ação destrutiva sobre os leucócitos, com ou sem lise das células. [leukocyte + L. *caedo*, matar]

leu·ko·co·ria, leu·ko·ko·ria (loo-kō-kō′rē-ă, loo-kō′rē-ă). Leucocoria; reflexo a partir de uma massa esbranquiçada no olho fornecendo o aspecto de uma pupila branca. SIN leukokoria, white pupillary *reflex*. [leuko-, branco, + G. *korē*, pupila]

leu·ko·cy·tac·tic (loo′kō-sī-tak′tik). Leucocitotático. SIN leukocytotactic.

leu·ko·cy·tal (loo-kō-sī′tăl). Leucocítico; SIN leukocytic.

leu·ko·cy·tax·ia, leu·ko·cy·tax·is (loo′kō-si-tak′sē-ă, -tak′sis). Leucocitaxia. SIN leukocytotaxia.

leu·ko·cyte (loo′kō-sīt). Leucócito; um tipo de célula formada nas porções mielopoética, linfóide e reticular do sistema reticuloendotelial em várias partes do corpo, e normalmente presente nesses locais e no sangue circulante (raramente em outros tecidos). Em várias condições anormais, o número total e/ou relativo pode estar caracteristicamente aumentado, diminuído ou inalterado, podendo os leucócitos ser encontrados em outros tecidos e órgãos. Os leucócitos representam três linhas de desenvolvimento a partir dos elementos primitivos: séries mielóide, linfóide e monocítica. Com base nos aspectos observados com diversos métodos de coloração com corantes policromáticos (p.ex., corante de Wright), as células da série mielóide são freqüentemente denominadas leucócitos granulares ou granulócitos; as células das séries linfóide e monocítica também apresentam grânulos no citoplasma, porém, devido aos seus tamanhos diminutos e indistinguíveis e propriedades diferentes (freqüentemente não visualizados claramente com os métodos rotineiros), os linfócitos e monócitos são por vezes denominados leucócitos não-granulares ou agranulares. Os granulócitos são comumente conhecidos como leucócitos polimorfonucleares (também leucócitos polinucleares ou multinucleares), visto que o núcleo maduro é dividido em dois a cinco lobos arredondados ou ovóides que estão conectados com filamentos finos ou pequenas faixas de cromatina; eles consistem em três tipos distintos: neutrófilos, eosinófilos e basófilos, denominados com base nas reações de coloração dos grânulos citoplasmáticos. As células da série linfocítica ocorrem como duas variedades normais, um pouco arbitrárias: linfócitos pequenos e grandes; os primeiros representam as formas comuns e são, nitidamente, mais numerosos no sangue circulante e nos tecidos linfóides normais; os últimos podem ser encontrados no sangue circulante normal, mas são mais facilmente observados nos tecidos linfóides. Os pequenos linfócitos apresentam núcleos que se coram de forma intensa ou densa (a cromatina é grosseira e volumosa) e quase preenchem as células, com uma borda apenas discreta de citoplasma ao redor dos núcleos; os grandes linfócitos apresentam núcleos que possuem quase o mesmo tamanho, ou são apenas um pouco maiores que os das formas pequenas, mas existe uma faixa mais larga, facilmente visualizada, de citoplasma ao redor dos núcleos. As células da série monocítica são usualmente maiores que os outros leucócitos e caracterizam-se por citoplasma relativamente abundante, discretamente opaco, azul-pálido ou azul-acinzentado, que contém uma miríade de grânulos azul-avermelhados extremamente finos. Em geral, os monócitos são indentados, reniformes ou com formato similar a uma ferradura, mas, por vezes, são arredondados ou ovóides; seus núcleos são, em geral, grandes e centrais e, quando são excêntricos, são completamente circundados por uma faixa pelo menos pequena de citoplasma. SIN white blood cell. [leuko- + G. *kytos*, célula]

acidophilic l., l. eosinofílico. SIN eosinophilic l.

agranular l., l. agranular. SIN nongranular l.

basophilic l., l. basófilo, mastócito; um l. polimorfonuclear (PMN) caracterizado por grânulos grandes, grosseiros e metacromáticos (púrpura intenso ou azul-escuro, quando tratados com corante de Wright ou similares) que geralmente enchem o citoplasma e podem quase mascarar o núcleo; esses leucócitos são singulares porque geralmente seu número não aumenta como conseqüência de doença infecciosa aguda e suas qualidades fagocíticas não são provavelmente significantes; os grânulos, que contêm heparina e histamina, podem desgranular em resposta a reações de hipersensibilidade e podem ser significantes em inflamação geral. SIN basocyte, basophilocyte, mast l.

cystinotic l., l. cistinótico; um l. que possui um conteúdo aumentado de cistina, encontrado em pacientes com distúrbios caracterizados pelo armazenamento da cistina; dentro do l., a cistina, em grande parte na forma não-cristalina, está associada a partículas lisossomiais densas.

endothelial l., l. endotelial; termo obsoleto para um monócito, um tipo de l. tido como derivado do tecido reticuloendotelial.

eosinophilic l., l. eosinófilo; um l. polimorfonuclear (PMN) caracterizado por muitos grânulos citoplasmáticos grandes ou proeminentes e refráteis, bastante uniformes em tamanho e com uma coloração alaranjada ou vermelho-amarelada intensa, quando tratados com corante de Wright ou similares; os núcleos são usualmente maiores que os dos neutrófilos, não se coram com tanta intensidade e, de modo característico, possuem dois lobos (um terceiro lobo está por vezes interposto sobre o filamento de conexão da cromatina); esses leucócitos são fagócitos móveis com funções antiparasitárias distintas. SIN acidophilic l., eosinocyte, eosinophil, eosinophile, oxyphil (2), oxyphile, oxyphilic l.

filament polymorphonuclear l., l. polimorfonuclear filamentar; qualquer l. polimorfonuclear maduro, especialmente um l. neutrófilo, no qual os lobos do núcleo estão interconectados por um filamento ou faixa fina de cromatina.

globular l., l. globular; um tipo de célula migratória com um núcleo pequeno e arredondado, encontrada no epitélio e na lâmina própria da mucosa intestinal de muitos animais; seu citoplasma contém grandes glóbulos ou gotículas eosinofílicas.

granular l., l. granular; qualquer um dos leucócitos polimorfonucleares, especialmente um l. neutrófilo. VER TAMBÉM granulocyte, basophilic l., eosinophilic l.

hyaline l., l. hialino; termo obsoleto para um monócito e para um macrófago mononuclear em várias lesões.

mast l., mastócito. SIN basophilic l.

motile l., l. móvel; qualquer l. que exibe movimento amebóide ativo, especialmente um l. granulócito maduro (os eosinófilos são menos móveis que os neutrófilos ou basófilos); os monócitos exibem um movimento lento, mas persistente e semelhante a uma onda.

multinuclear l., l. multinuclear. SIN polymorphonuclear l.

neutrophilic l., l. neutrófilo; um granulócito neutrófilo, o mais freqüente dos leucócitos polimorfonucleares, e também o fagócito mais ativo entre os vários tipos de leucócitos; quando tratados com o corante de Wright (ou preparações similares), o citoplasma bastante abundante é levemente róseo, sendo reconhecidos no seu citoplasma inúmeros grânulos diminutos, discretamente refráteis, relativamente róseos brilhosos ou róseo-violeta, difusamente espalhados; o núcleo azul ou azul-purpúreo profundamente corado é bem diferenciado do citoplasma e é nitidamente lobulado, com finos filamentos de cromatina conectando os três a cinco lobos.

nonfilament polymorphonuclear l., l. polimorfonuclear não-filamentar; um eosinófilo, basófilo ou neutrófilo que não está completamente maduro, ou seja, os lobos dos núcleos permanecem conectados por faixas de cromatina, em contraste com os filamentos finos observados nas células maduras.

nongranular l., l. não-granular; um termo genérico, inespecífico, freqüentemente utilizado com referência aos linfócitos, monócitos e plasmócitos; embora o citoplasma de um linfócito ou monócito contenha grânulos diminutos, ele é "agranular" em comparação com o de um neutrófilo, basófilo ou eosinófilo. VER TAMBÉM leukocyte. SIN agranular l.

nonmotile l., l. imóvel; um termo por vezes usado em relação a linfócitos, monócitos e plasmócitos; embora essas formas realmente apresentem algum grau de motilidade, são "imóveis" em comparação com os leucócitos neutrófilos, basofílicos e eosinofílicos ativamente amebóides.

leukocyte 881 **leukodystrophy**

oxyphilic l., l. oxifílico, l. eosinofílico. SIN eosinophilic l.
polymorphonuclear l., polynuclear l., l. polimorfonuclear; termo comum para o granulócito ou l. granulocítico; o termo inclui os leucócitos basófilos, eosinófilos e neutrófilos, mas é comumente empregado com relação aos leucócitos neutrófilos. SIN multinuclear l.
segmented l., l. segmentado; qualquer l. polimorfonuclear maduro, especialmente um l. neutrófilo.
transitional l., l. transicional; termo obsoleto para monócito.
Türk l., l. de Türk. SIN Türk cell.
leu·ko·cy·the·mia (loo′kō-sī-thē′mē-ă). Leucocitemia; termo obsoleto para a leucemia. [leucocyte + G. *haima*, sangue]
leu·ko·cyt·ic (loo′kō-sit′ik). Leucocítico; pertinente a ou caracterizado por leucócitos. SIN leukocytal.
leu·ko·cy·to·blast (loo-kō-sī′tō-blast). Leucocitoblasto; um termo inespecífico para qualquer célula imatura a partir da qual se desenvolve um leucócito, incluindo linfoblasto, mieloblasto e os similares. [leukocyte + G. *blastos*, germe]
leu·ko·cy·toc·la·sis (loo′kō-sī-tok′lă-sis). Leucocitoclasia; cariorrexe dos leucócitos. [leuko- + G. *kytos*, célula, + *klasia*, uma ruptura]
leu·ko·cy·to·gen·e·sis (loo′kō-sī-tō-jen′ĕ-sis). Leucocitogênese; a formação e o desenvolvimento dos leucócitos. [leukocyte + G. *genesis*, produção]
leu·ko·cy·toid (loo′kō-sī-toyd). Leucocitóide; que se assemelha a um leucócito. [leukocyte + G. *eidos*, semelhança]
leu·ko·cy·tol·y·sin (loo′kō-sī-tol′ĭ-sin). Leucocitolisina; qualquer substância (inclusive o anticorpo lítico) que causa a dissolução dos leucócitos. SIN leukolysin.
leu·ko·cy·tol·y·sis (loo′kō-sī-tol′ĭ-sis). Leucocitólise; dissolução ou lise dos leucócitos. SIN leukolysis. [leukocyte + G. *lysis*, dissolução]
leu·ko·cy·to·lyt·ic (loo′kō-sī-tō-lit′ik). Leucocitolítico; pertinente a, que causa ou que manifesta leucocitólise. SIN leukolytic.
leu·ko·cy·to·ma (loo′kō-sī-tō′mă). Leucocitoma; termo obsoleto para um acúmulo denso, nodular e muito bem circunscrito de leucócitos. [leukocyte + G. *-oma*, tumor]
leu·ko·cy·tom·e·ter (loo′kō-sī-tom′ĕ-ter). Leucocitômetro; uma lâmina de vidro padronizada que é adequada para a contagem de leucócitos em um volume medido de sangue (ou de outras amostras) exatamente diluído. [leukocyte + G. *metron*, medida]
leu·ko·cy·to·pe·ni·a (loo′kō-sī-tō-pē′nē-ă). Leucocitopenia. SIN leukopenia.
leu·ko·cy·to·pla·ni·a (loo′kō-sī-tō-plā′nē-ă). Leucocitoplania; o movimento dos leucócitos a partir das luzes dos vasos sanguíneos, através de membranas serosas ou nos tecidos. [leukocyte + G. *planē*, um movimento errático]
leu·ko·cy·to·poi·e·sis (loo′kō-sī-tō-poy-ē′sis). Leucocitopoese. SIN leukopoiesis. [leukocyte + G. *poiēsis*, uma produção]
leu·ko·cy·to·sis (loo′kō-sī-tō′sis). Leucocitose; um número anormalmente grande de leucócitos, conforme observado nas infecções agudas, inflamação, hemorragia e outras condições. Uma contagem de leucócitos de 10.000 ou mais por mm³ geralmente indica l. Muitos exemplos de l. representam um aumento desproporcional no número de células na série neutrofílica, sendo o termo usado, com freqüência, como sinônimo de neutrofilia. A l. de 15.000 a 25.000/mm³ é freqüentemente observada em diversas condições patológicas, e os valores de até 40.000 não são incomuns; ocasionalmente, como em alguns exemplos de reações leucemóides, as contagens de leucócitos podem chegar a 100.000/mm³. [leukocyte + G. *-osis*, condição]
absolute l., l. absoluta; um aumento real no número total de leucócitos no sangue circulante, conforme distinguido de um aumento relativo (como aquele observado na desidratação).
agonal l., l. agônica. SIN terminal l.
basophilic l., l. basofílica; a presença de um número anormalmente grande de granulócitos basófilos no sangue. SIN basocytosis.
digestive l., l. digestiva; l. que ocorre normalmente após a ingestão de alimento.
distribuition l., l. de distribuição; uma proporção anormalmente grande de um ou mais tipos de leucócitos.
emotional l., l. emocional; uma contagem de leucócitos anormalmente alta possivelmente relacionada apenas a um distúrbio emocional.
eosinophilic l., l. eosinofílica; uma forma de l. relativa em que o aumento proporcional máximo é de eosinófilos. SIN eosinophilia.
lymphocytic l., linfocitose. SIN lymphocytosis.
monocytic l., monocitose. SIN monocytosis.
neutrophilic l., neutrofilia; SIN neutrophilia.
l. of the newborn, l. do recém-nascido; uma l. aparentemente "fisiológica", observada, em geral, nos recém-nascidos, nos quais as contagens de leucócitos são, amiúde, superiores a 10.000/mm³ e, por vezes, variam até 45.000/mm³, resultando principalmente do número aumentado de neutrófilos (em especial das formas únicas e bilobuladas). No terceiro ou quarto dia de vida, a contagem em geral diminui rapidamente e, em seguida, flutua por vários dias; em torno da quarta semana de vida, observa-se uma linfocitose relativa, persistindo esta, normalmente, por alguns anos.
physiologic l., l. fisiológica; qualquer forma de l. que está associada a situações aparentemente normais e que não está diretamente relacionada a uma condição patológica; p.ex., o aumento temporário do número total de leucócitos que pode acontecer durante um único dia, ou de um dia para o outro, bem como no período neonatal, durante a infância, depois do exercício extenuante, durante crises de taquicardia paroxística e em associação a várias outras situações.
relative l., l. relativa; uma proporção aumentada de um ou mais tipos de leucócitos no sangue circulante, sem um aumento real do número total de leucócitos.
terminal l., l. relativa; aquela que ocorre em uma pessoa pouco antes da morte, em especial nos casos de uma "morte lenta". SIN agonal l.
leu·ko·cy·to·tac·tic (loo′kō-sī-tō-tak′tik). Leucocitotático; pertinente a, caracterizado por ou que causa leucocitotaxia. SIN leukocytactic, leukotactic.
leu·ko·cy·to·tax·ia (loo-kō-sī-tō-tak′sē-ă). Leucocitotaxia. **1.** O movimento amebóide ativo dos leucócitos, especialmente dos granulócitos neutrófilos, em direção a (**l. positiva**) ou para longe (**l. negativa**) de determinados microrganismos, bem como várias substâncias freqüentemente formadas no tecido inflamado. **2.** A propriedade de atrair ou repelir leucócitos. SIN leukocytaxia, leukotaxia, leukocytaxis, leukotaxis. [leukocyte + *taxis*, disposição]
leu·ko·cy·to·tox·in (loo′kō-sī-tō-tok′sin). Leucocitotoxina; qualquer substância que causa degeneração e necrose dos leucócitos, incluindo leucolisina e leucocidina. SIN leukotoxin. [leukocyte + G. *toxikon*, veneno]
leu·ko·cy·tu·ri·a (loo′kō-sī-too′rē-ă). Leucocitúria; a presença de leucócitos na urina que é recentemente eliminada ou coletada por meio de um cateter. [leukocyte + G. *ouron*, urina]
leu·ko·der·ma (loo-kō-der′mă). Leucoderma; ausência de pigmento, parcial ou total, na pele. SIN hypomelanosis, leukopathia, leukopathy. [leuko- + G. *derma*, pele]
acquired l., l. adquirida, vitiligo. SIN vitiligo.
l. acquisi′tum centrifu′gum, l. adquirida centrífuga. SIN halo nevus.
l. col′li, l. sifilítica. SIN syphilitic l.
syphilitic l., l. sifilítica; um esmaecimento da roséola da sífilis secundária, deixando áreas reticuladas, despigmentadas e hiperpigmentadas, localizadas principalmente nos lados do pescoço. SIN l. colli, melanoleukoderma colli.
leu·ko·der·ma·tous (loo-kō-der′mă-tŭs). Leucodermatoso; que se relaciona ou se assemelha à leucodermia.
leu·ko·don·tia (loo-kō-don′shē-ă). Leucodontia; a condição de ter dentes brancos. [leuko- + G. *odous*, dente]
leu·ko·dys·tro·phia (loo-kō-dis-trō′fē-ă). Leucodistrofia. SIN leukodystrophy.
l. cer′ebri progressi′va, l. cerebral progressiva. SIN leukodystrophy.
leu·ko·dys·tro·phy (loo-kō-dis′trō-fē). Leucodistrofia; termo para um grupo de doenças da substância branca, algumas familiares, caracterizadas por deterioração cerebral progressiva, geralmente no início da vida e, ao exame histopatológico, por ausência primária ou degeneração da mielina nos sistemas nervosos central e periférico, com reação glial; provavelmente relacionada a um defeito no metabolismo lipídico; muitas leucodistrofias são autossômicas recessivas, várias são recessivas ligadas ao X e algumas são autossômicas dominantes. VER TAMBÉM Canavan *disease*. SIN leukodystrophia cerebri progressiva, leukodystrophy, sclerosis of white matter. [leuko- + G. *dys*, mal, + *trophe*, nutrição]
adrenal l., l. adrenal ou supra-renal; leucodistrofia sudanofílica com bronzeamento da pele e atrofia adrenal. Um distúrbio metabólico de homens jovens, caracterizado por degeneração ampla da mielina e insuficiência associada da supra-renal. A degeneração da mielina é maciça em várias porções do cérebro e, por vezes, da medula espinal, com acúmulo de produtos de degradação da mielina nos macrófagos: desmielinização sudanofílica; há atrofia das glândulas supra-renais e testículos, ocorrendo aumento acentuado de ácidos graxos de cadeia longa no cérebro e nas glândulas supra-renais. Os sinais e sintomas incluem bronzeamento da pele, disartria, cegueira cortical, hemiplegia bilateral, paralisia pseudobulbar e demência progressiva. Herança recessiva provavelmente ligada ao sexo.
globoid cell l. [MIM*245200], l. de células globóides; um distúrbio metabólico do lactente e da criança pequena caracterizado por espasticidade, convulsões e degeneração cerebral rapidamente progressiva, perda maciça de mielina, gliose astrocítica grave e infiltração da substância branca pelas características células globóides multinucleadas; metabolicamente, existe deficiência evidente de cerebrosidase lisossomal (galactosilceramida β-galactosidase); herança autossômica recessiva, causada por mutação no gene que codifica a glicosilceramida (GALC) em 14q. SIN diffuse infantile familial sclerosis, galactosylceramide lipoidosis, Krabbe disease.
metachromatic l. [MIM*250100], l. metacromática; um distúrbio metabólico, com início ocorrendo em geral no segundo ano de vida e com a morte sobrevindo, com freqüência, antes de 5 anos, com perda da mielina e acúmulo de lipídios metacromáticos (galactosil sulfatídeos) na substância branca dos sistemas nervoso central e periférico, levando a sinais e sintomas motores, paralisia, convulsões e deterioração cerebral progressiva. Herança autossômica recessiva [MIM*249900 e MIM*250100], causada por mutação no gene da aril-sulfatase A (ARSA) em 22q ou no gene da prosaposina (PSAP) em 10q. Existe uma forma dominante que ocorre em adultos [MIM*156310]. SIN arylsulfatase A deficiency, sulfatide lipidosis.

l. with diffuse Rosenthal fiber formation, l. com formação difusa de fibras de Rosenthal; um distúrbio metabólico cujo início pode se dar no lactente, no adolescente ou no adulto; caracterizada histopatologicamente por desmielinização cerebral disseminada, com proliferação de astrócitos e células primitivas da oligodendróglia; as fibras de Rosenthal refratárias resultam da degeneração dessas células proliferantes; a etiologia não é conhecida, mas, possivelmente, decorre de um defeito metabólico dos astrócitos; distúrbio recessivo ligado ao sexo.

leu·ko·en·ceph·a·li·tis (loo′kō-en-sef-ă-lī′tis). Leucoencefalite; a encefalite restrita à substância branca.

acute epidemic l., l. epidêmica aguda; doença caracterizada pelo estabelecimento agudo da febre, seguido por convulsões, delírio e coma, e associado a desmielinização perivascular e focos hemorrágicos no sistema nervoso central. SIN acute primary hemorrhagic meningoencephalitis, Strümpell disease (2).

acute hemorrhagic l., l. hemorrágica aguda. SIN acute necrotizing hemorrhagic encephalomyelitis.

acute necrotizing hemorrhagic l., l. hemorrágica necrotizante aguda. SIN acute necrotizing hemorrhagic encephalomyelitis.

sclerosing l., l. esclerosante. SIN subacute sclerosing panencephalitis.

subacute sclerosing l., l. esclerosante subaguda. SIN subacute sclerosing panencephalitis.

leu·ko·en·ceph·a·lop·a·thy (loo′kō-en-sef-ă-lop′ă-thē). Leucoencefalopatia; alterações da substância branca descritas pela primeira vez em crianças com leucemia, associada a lesão por radiação e quimioterápicos, freqüentemente associada ao metotrexato; histopatologicamente caracterizada por astrocitose reativa difusa com múltiplas áreas de focos necróticos sem inflamação. [leuko- + G. *enkephalos,* cérebro, + *pathos,* doença]

progressive multifocal l. (PML), l. multifocal progressiva; rara doença subaguda e afebril, caracterizada por áreas de desmielinização circundadas por neuróglia muito alterada, incluindo corpúsculos de inclusão nas células gliais; ocorre comumente em pessoas com AIDS/SIDA, leucemia, linfoma ou outras doenças debilitantes, ou naquelas que estão recebendo tratamento imunossupressor. Causada pelo vírus JC, um poliomavírus humano. SIN progressive subcortical encephalopathy.

leu·ko·e·ryth·ro·blas·to·sis (loo′kō-ē-rith′rō-blas-tō′sis). Leucoeritroblastose; qualquer condição anêmica que resulte de lesões expansivas na medula óssea; o sangue circulante contém células imaturas da série granulocítica e eritrócitos nucleados, freqüentemente em número desproporcional (aumentado) ao grau da anemia. SIN leukoerythroblastic anemia, myelophthisic anemia, myelopathic anemia.

leu·ko·ki·net·ic (loo′kō-ki-net′ik). Leucocinético; pertinente à leucocinética. [leukocyte + G. *kinētikos,* de movimento, de *kineō,* mover]

leu·ko·ki·net·ics (loo′kō-ki-net′iks). Leucocinética; o estudo da formação, circulação e destino dos leucócitos, usualmente pelo uso de um marcador radioativo. [leukocyte + G. *kinetikos,* de ou para colocar em movimento]

leu·ko·ko·ria (loo-kō-kō′rē-ă). Leucocoria. VER leukocoria.

leu·ko·krau·ro·sis (loo′kō-kraw-rō′sis). Leucocraurose. SIN kraurosis vulvae.

leu·kol·y·sin (loo-kol′i-sin). Leucolisina. SIN leukocytolisin.

leu·kol·y·sis (loo-kol′i-sis). Leucólise. SIN leukocytolysis.

leu·ko·lyt·ic (loo-kō-lit′ik). Leucolítico. SIN leukocytolytic.

leu·ko·ma (loo-kō′mă). Leucoma; uma opacificação esbranquiçada densa da córnea. [G. brancura, uma mancha branca no olho, de *leukos,* branco]

adherent l., l. aderente; uma cicatriz da córnea à qual se fixa uma porção da íris.

leu·ko·ma·tous (loo-kō-mă-tŭs). Leucomatoso; pertinente ao leucoma.

leu·ko·mye·li·tis (loo′kō-mī-e-lī′tis). Leucomielite; um processo inflamatório que envolve a substância branca da medula espinal.

necrotizing hemorrhage l., l. hemorrágica necrotizante; um substrato patológico responsável pelo distúrbio clínico da *mielite* necrotizante aguda.

leu·ko·my·e·lop·a·thy (loo′kō-mī′e-lop′ă-thē). Leucomielopatia; qualquer doença sistêmica que envolve a substância branca ou os tratos condutores da medula espinal. [leuko- + G. *myelos,* medula, + *pathos,* sofrimento]

leu·kon (loo′kon). Leucon; a massa total dos leucócitos circulantes, bem como das células e células leucopoéticas, a partir das quais elas se originam.

leu·ko·ne·cro·sis (loo-ko-ne-krō′sis). Leuconecrose. SIN white gangrene. [leuko- + G. *nekrōsis,* morte]

leu·ko·nych·ia (loo-kō-nik′ē-ă). Leuconíquia; a ocorrência de manchas ou placas brancas sob as unhas, de causa desconhecida; a descoloração pode ser total ou na forma de linhas (l. estriada ou transversa) ou pontos (l. pontilhada). [leuko- + G. *onyx* (onych-), unha]

leu·ko·path·ia, leu·ko·pa·thy (loo-kō-path′ē-ă, loo-kop′ă-thē). Leucoderma. SIN leukoderma. [leuko- + G. *pathos,* doença]

leu·ko·pe·de·sis (loo-kō-pē-dē′sis). Leucopedese; o movimento de leucócitos (especialmente leucócitos polimorfonucleares) através das paredes dos capilares e para os tecidos. [leuko- + G. *pēdēsis,* um salto]

leu·ko·pe·nia (loo-kō-pē′nē-ă). Leucopenia; a antítese da leucocitose; qualquer situação em que o número total de leucócitos no sangue circulante é menor que o normal, cujo limite inferior é geralmente considerado como 4.000-5.000/mm³. SIN leukocytopenia. [leuko(cyte) + G. *penia,* pobreza]

basophilic l., l. basofílica; diminuição do número de granulócitos basofílicos no sangue circulante (difícil de avaliar, devido ao número pequeno e variável normalmente existente). SIN basocytopenia, basopenia.

eosinophilic l., l. eosinofílica; diminuição no número de granulócitos eosinofílicos normalmente no sangue circulante.

lymphocytic l., linfopenia. SIN lymphopenia.

monocytic l., monocitopenia. SIN monocytopenia.

neutrophilic l., neutropenia. SIN neutropenia.

leu·ko·pe·nic (loo-kō-pē′nik). Leucopênico; pertinente à leucopenia.

leu·ko·pla·kia (loo-kō-plā′kē-ă). Leucoplaquia; uma placa branca da mucosa oral ou genital feminina que não pode ser removida e não pode ser diagnosticada clinicamente como qualquer entidade mórbida específica; no uso corrente, um termo clínico sem conotação histológica. SIN smoker's patches. [leuko- G. *plax,* prato]

hairy l., l. pilosa; uma lesão esbranquiçada que aparece na língua, ocasionalmente na mucosa bucal, de pacientes com AIDS/SIDA; uma manifestação da infecção por vírus Epstein-Barr em um hospedeiro imunocomprometido; a lesão mostra-se elevada, com uma superfície corrugada ou "pilosa" devido às projeções de queratina.

A leucoplaquia pilosa foi reconhecida pela primeira vez em 1981 como um marcador de imunossupressão em homens homossexuais com AIDS/SIDA. A incidência nas pessoas com AIDS/SIDA fica em torno de 20%. A leucoplaquia pilosa oral consiste em cristas ou pregas verticais esbranquiçadas, geralmente ao longo das bordas laterais da língua, mas, por vezes, em sua superfície inferior ou na mucosa bucal. Diferente das lesões da candidíase oral ("sapinho"), as placas não podem ser descoladas. A condição é usualmente assintomática, não provocando dor nem alteração do paladar. O estudo histológico mostra paraceratose e cilocitose com pouca inflamação. Ocasionalmente, a lesão progride para o carcinoma de células escamosas. O tratamento com a podofilina tópica ou aciclovir sistêmico geralmente induz a regressão imediata das lesões.

l. vul'vae, l. vulvar; termo clínico para placas esbranquiçadas e hiperceratóticas do epitélio vulvar; a biopsia é necessária para o diagnóstico específico.

leu·ko·poi·e·sis (loo′kō-poy-ē′sis). Leucopoese; a formação e o desenvolvimento de vários tipos de leucócitos. SIN leukocytopoiesis. [leuko- + G. *poiēsis,* uma produção]

leu·ko·poi·et·ic (loo′kō-poy-et′ik). Leucopoético; pertinente a ou caracterizado por leucopoese, conforme manifestado por porções da medula óssea e tecidos reticuloendotelial e linfóide, que formam, respectivamente, os granulócitos, monócitos e linfócitos.

leu·ko·pro·te·ase (loo-kō-prō′tē-ās). Leucoprotease; uma enzima proteolítica mal definida dos leucócitos polimorfonucleares, formada em uma área de inflamação, que provoca liquefação do tecido morto.

leu·ko·ri·bo·fla·vin (loo-kō-rī′bō-flā-vin). Leucorriboflavina; o composto diidro incolor não-fluorescente formado pela redução da riboflavina.

leu·kor·rha·gia (loo-kō-rā′jē-ă). Leucorragia, leucorréia. SIN leukorrhea. [leuko- + G. *rhēgnymi,* jorrar]

leu·kor·rhea (loo-kō-rē′ă). Leucorréia; secreção, a partir da vagina, de um líquido viscoso esbranquiçado ou amarelado que contém muco e piócitos. SIN leukorrhagia. [leuko- + G. *rhoia,* fluxo]

menstrual l., l. menstrual; l. intermitente que reincide a cada período menstrual ou exatamente antes dele.

leu·kor·rhe·al (loo-kō-rē′al). Leucorreico; relativo ou caracterizado por leucorréia.

leu·ko·tac·tic (loo-kō-tak′tik). Leucotático. SIN leukocytotactic.

leu·ko·tax·ia (loo-kō-tak′sē-ă). Leucotaxia. SIN leukocytotaxia.

leu·ko·tax·ine (loo-kō-tak′sēn). Leucotaxina; um material nitrogenado acelular preparado a partir do tecido lesionado em degeneração aguda e a partir de exsudatos inflamatórios.

leu·ko·tax·is (loo-kō-tak′sis). Leucotaxia. SIN leukocytotaxia.

leu·ko·tome (loo′kō-tōm). Leucótomo; um instrumento para realizar a leucotomia.

leu·kot·o·my (loo-kot′ō-mē). Leucotomia, lobotomia; incisão na substância branca do lobo frontal do cérebro. [leuko- + G. *tomē,* um corte]

prefrontal l., l. pré-frontal. SIN prefrontal lobotomy.

transorbital l., l. transorbital. SIN transorbital lobotomy.

leu·ko·tox·in (loo-kō-tok′sin). Leucotoxina. SIN leukocytotoxin.

leu·ko·trich·ia (loo-kō-trik′ē-ă). Leucotríquia; brancura do cabelo. [leuko- + G. *thrix,* cabelo]

leu·ko·tri·enes (LT) (loo-kō-trī′enz). Leucotrienos; produtos do metabolismo dos eicosanóides (usualmente, ácido araquidônico) com suposta atividade fisiológica, como mediadores da inflamação e nas reações alérgicas; diferem das prostaglandinas e tromboxanos correlatos por não terem um anel central; assim chamados porque foram originalmente descobertos em associação com os leucócitos e devido às suas três ligações duplas conjugadas; as letras A a F identificam os seis primeiros metabólitos isolados, com os números subscritos para indicar o número de duplas ligações (p.ex., leucotrieno C_4).

peptidyl l., peptidil leucotrieno; l. que tem um ou mais aminoácidos presentes; p.ex., LTC_4 é uma glutationa *S*-substituída, LTD_4 é uma cisteinil-glicina *S*-substituída, LTE_4 é uma cisteína *S*-substituída e LTF_4 (também conhecido como γ-glutamil-LTE_4) é uma γ-glutamilcisteína *S*-substituída.

Leu·ko·vi·rus (loo′ko - vī′rus). Termo obsoleto para um gênero original composto de vírus tumoral RNA agora incluído na família Retroviridae.

LEU M1. O epítopo para um anticorpo monoclonal gerado para a linhagem celular histiocítica humana que localiza neutrófilos, monócitos aderentes e um subgrupo de células T ativadas.

leu·pep·tin (loo-pep′tin). Leupeptina; um dos inúmeros inibidores da tripeptídeo protease modificados, a partir de espécies de *Streptomyces*, que inibem catepsina B, papaína, tripsina e catepsina D. A leupeptina mais comumente utilizada é a *N*-acetil-leucil-leucil-arginal.

leu·pro·lide ac·e·tate (loo′pro - līd). Acetato de leuprolida; um análogo nonapeptídico sintético do hormônio liberador de gonadotropina de ocorrência natural; usado no tratamento paliativo do câncer de próstata avançado.

leu·ro·cris·tine (loo′rō - kris′tin). Sulfato de vincristina. SIN *vincristine sulfate.*

Lev, Maurice, patologista norte-americano, 1908–1994. VER L. *disease, syndrome.*

Levaditi, Constantin, bacteriologista romeno em Paris, 1879–1928. VER L. *stain.*

lev·al·lor·phan tar·trate (lev - ā - lōr′fan). Tartarato de levalorfano; o análogo *N*-alil do levorfanol, antagonista das ações dos analgésicos narcóticos; usado no tratamento da depressão respiratória decorrente de *overdose* de narcóticos.

lev·am·i·so·le (lē - vam′ī - sōl). Levamisol; originalmente empregado como anti-helmíntico; aumenta as respostas imunes e é usado de forma adjuvante aos agentes antineoplásicos para melhorar a resposta e suprimir a recorrência.

lev·an (le′van). Levano. SIN *fructosan (1).*

lev·an·su·crase (lev - an - soo′krās). Levanossacarase; uma enzima que catalisa a transferência da molécula de frutose para a polifrutose (um levano), liberando D-glicose.

lev·ar·te·re·nol (lev - ar - tēr′e - nol). Levarterenol, norepinefrina. SIN *norepinephrine.*
 l. bitartrate, bitartarato de l. SIN *norepinephrine bitartrate.*

le·va·tor (le - vā′ter, tōr)[TA]. Levantador, elevador. **1.** Um instrumento cirúrgico para elevar a parte deprimida em uma fratura de crânio. **2.** Um dos vários músculos cuja ação é elevar a parte na qual se insere. [L. um levantador, de *levo*, pp. *-atus*, levantar, de *levis*, leve]

LeVeen, Harry H., cirurgião norte-americano, *1914. VER LeV. *shunt.*

lev·el (le′vel). Nível. **1.** Qualquer classificação, posição ou estado em uma escala graduada de valores. **2.** Um teste para determinar essa classificação ou posição.
 acoustic reference l., nível de referência acústica; o nível de referência biológica para medidas sonoras. Quando o termo decibel é empregado para indicar o nível de ruído, está implícita uma referência de quantidade; esse valor de referência é usualmente expresso como uma pressão sonora de 20 micronewtons por metro quadrado. O nível de referência é referido como 0 decibéis, a linha de base da escala de níveis de ruído; essa linha basal é considerada como o som mais fraco que pode ser ouvido por uma pessoa com audição muito boa em um local extremamente quieto. Outros níveis de referência equivalentes ainda em uso incluem 0,0002 microbar e 0,0002 dinas por centímetro quadrado. VER TAMBÉM *sound pressure l.*
 l. of aspiration, n. de aspiração; em psicologia clínica, o grau ou qualidade de desempenho (exibido em uma situação de teste) que uma pessoa deseja atingir ou sente que pode ser alcançado.
 background l., n. fundamental; a concentração (usualmente baixa) em que uma substância ou agente está presente ou ocorre em um determinado momento e local, sem perigo específico sob investigação; um exemplo é o nível fundamental de radiação ionizante.
 Clark l., n. de Clark; o n. de invasão do melanoma maligno primário da pele; limitado à epiderme, I; na derme papilar subjacente, II; até a junção das camadas papilar e reticular da derme, III; na derme reticular, IV; no tecido adiposo subcutâneo, V. O prognóstico é cada vez pior a cada camada sucessiva mais profunda de invasão.
 hearing l., n. de audição; a medida da audição segundo a leitura direta na escala de perda da audição de um audiômetro; descrito em decibéis como um desvio de um valor padronizado para zero no audiômetro.
 loudness discomfort l., n. de desconforto de intensidade; a intensidade em que o som, principalmente à fala, provoca desconforto.
 most comfortable l., n. mais confortável; a intensidade sonora máxima que é confortável.
 saturation sound pressure l. (SSPL), n. de saturação da pressão sonora; uma medida do débito máximo de um aparelho de audição.
 sensation l., n. de sensibilidade; o número de decibéis acima do limiar de audição de um estímulo.
 sensory acuity l., n. de acuidade sensorial; uma técnica para determinar os limiares de condução aérea sem obliteração ou com a obliteração imposta pela condução óssea na fronte; a alteração nos limiares indica a perda condutiva da audição.
 sound pressure l. (SPL), n. de pressão sonora; uma medida da energia sonora relativa a 0,002 dinas/cm^2, expressa em decibéis.
 uncomfortable l., n. desconfortável; a intensidade de som que provoca desconforto.
 window l., n. de janela; o número de TC que estabelece, em unidades Hounsfield, o ponto médio da largura da janela, correspondente à escala cinza de imagem; um n. de janela típico para obter imagens dos pulmões é de −500; para o abdome, 0.

Leventhal, Michael L., ginecologista-obstetra norte-americano, 1901–1971. VER Stein-L. *syndrome.*

le·ver (lev′er, lē′ver). Alavanca; um instrumento usado para levantar ou erguer. [Fr. *lever*, levantar]
 dental l., a. dentária. SIN *elevator (2).*

le·ver·age (lē′ver - ij). **1.** O levantamento real ou a direção da elevação de um nível ou elevador. **2.** A vantagem mecânica obtida dessa forma.

Levey, S., estatístico norte-americano do século XX. VER L.-Jenings *chart.*

Lévi, E. Leopold, endocrinologista francês, 1868–1933. VER dominantly inherited L. *disease*; Lorain-L. *dwarfism, infantilism, syndrome.*

Levin, Abraham, médico norte-americano, 1880–1940. VER L. *tube.*

Levin, Max, neurologista norte-americano, *1901. VER Kleine-L. *syndrome.*

Levine, Samuel A., cardiologista norte-americano, 1891–1966. VER Lown-Ganong-L. *syndrome.*

Le·vin·ea (lē - vin′e - ā). Um antigo gênero de bactérias (família Enterobacteriaceae) cujas espécies são atualmente designadas para o gênero *Citrobacter*. [Max *Levine*, bacteriologista norte-americano, *1889]
 L. amalona′tica. SIN *Citrobacter amalonatica.*
 L. diversus. SIN *Citrobacter diversus.*
 L. malona′tica. SIN *Citrobacter diversus.*

lev·i·ta·tion (lev - i - tā′shun). Colocação do paciente sobre um colchão de ar. [L. *levitas*, leveza]

Le·vi·vir·i·dae (lē - vi - vir′i - dē). Nome provisório para uma família de pequenos vírus bacterianos isométricos, não-envelopados, com genomas de RNA monofilamentar, de sentido positivo (peso molecular de 1×10^6). Os vírions são adsorvidos aos lados dos pêlos bacterianos e os grupos cristalinos são formados nas bactérias infectadas. A espécie típica é o fago de enterobactérias M52. [L. *levis*, leve (não pesado)]

△ **levo-.** Forma combinante que indica esquerda, em direção ao lado esquerdo. [L. *laevus*]

le·vo·bu·no·lol hy·dro·chlo·ride (lē′vō - bū′nō - lol). Cloridrato de levobunolol; um agente bloqueador β-adrenérgico usado principalmente como colírio no tratamento do glaucoma crônico de ângulo aberto e hipertensão ocular.

le·vo·car·dia (lē - vō - kar′dē - ā). Levocardia; *situs inversus* de outras vísceras, mas com o coração normalmente situado à esquerda; lesões cardíacas congênitas estão comumente associadas. [levo- + G. *kardia*, coração]

le·vo·car·di·o·gram (lē - vō - kar′dē - ō - gram). Levocardiograma; a parte do eletrocardiograma que é o efeito do ventrículo esquerdo.

levo·car·ni·tine (lē′vō - kar′nī - tēn). Levocarnitina; usada como suplemento para a deficiência de carnitina.

le·vo·cli·na·tion (lē′vō - kli - nā′shun). Levoclinação. SIN *levotorsion (2).* [levo- + L. *clino*, pp. *-atus*, inclinar]

levocycloduction. Levociclodução. SIN *sinistrotorsion.*

le·vo·cy·clo·duc·tion (lē′vō - sī - klō - dŭk′shun). Levociclodução; levotorção de um olho. [levo- + cyclo- + L. *duco*, pp. *ductus*, levar]

le·vo·do·pa (lē - vō - dō′pā). Levodopa; uma forma biologicamente ativa da dopa; um agente antiparkinsoniano que é convertido em dopamina. SIN L-dopa.

le·vo·duc·tion (lē - vō - dŭk′shun). Levodução; virar um olho para a esquerda; abdução do olho esquerdo ou adução do olho direito. [levo- + L. *duco*, pp. *ductus*, conduzir]

le·vo·form (lē′vō - fōrm). Levoforme; que indica a estrutura de uma substância que roda o plano da luz polarizada no sentido horário (para a esquerda); isto é, conforme visualizado pelo observador que olha para a fonte luminosa.

le·vo·glu·cose (lē - vō - gloo′kōs). Levoglicose; D-frutose. VER *fructose.*

le·vo·gram (lē′vō - gram). Levograma; registro eletrocardiográfico em um animal de laboratório que representa a disseminação do impulso apenas através do ventrículo esquerdo.

le·vo·gy·rate, le·vo·gy·rous (lē - vō - jī′rāt, - jī′rus). Levógiro. SIN *levorotatory.* [levo- + L. *gyro*, virar em círculos]

le·vo·nor·def·rin (lē′vō - nōr - def′rin). Levonordefrina; usado como descongestionante nasal e vasoconstritor fornecido com anestésicos de infiltração.

le·vo·fa·ce·top·er·ane (lē′vō - fa - sē - top′er′an). Levofacetoperano; um antidepressivo com propriedades anorexígenas.

le·vo·pho·bia (lev - ō - fō′bē - ā). Levofobia; o medo de objetos à esquerda.

le·vo·pro·pox·y·phene nap·syl·ate (lē′vō - prō - pok′si - fēn). Napsilato de levopropoxifeno; um antitussígeno.

le·vo·ro·ta·tion (lē - vō - rō - tā′shun). Levorrotação. **1.** Virada ou torção para a esquerda; em particular, a torção anti-horária dada ao plano da luz polarizada plana por soluções de determinadas substâncias opticamente ativas. Cf. *dextrorotation.* **2.** Sinistrotorção. SIN *sinistrotorsion.* [levo- + L. *roto*, virar]

le·vo·ro·ta·to·ry (lē-vō-rō′tă-tōr-ē). Levorrotatório. **1.** Indica a levorrotação ou determinados cristais ou soluções capazes de provocá-la; como um prefixo químico, usualmente é abreviado para *l-* ou (–). Cf. dextrorotatory. **2.** Que descreve qualquer rotação para a esquerda ou anti-horária. SIN levogyrate, levogyrous.

lev·or·pha·nol tar·trate (lev-ōrf′ă-nol). Tartarato de levorfanol; um analgésico com ação similar à morfina.

le·vo·tor·sion (lē-vō-tōr′shŭn). Levotorção. **1.** SIN sinistrotorsion. **2.** Rotação do pólo superior da córnea de um ou ambos os olhos para a esquerda. SIN levoclination. [levo- + L. *torsio*, uma torção]

le·vo·ver·sion (lē′vō-ver′zhŭn). Levoversão. **1.** Versão para a esquerda. **2.** Giro conjugado dos olhos para a esquerda. [levo- + L. *verto*, pp. *versus*, virar]

Levret, André, obstetra francês, 1703–1780. VER L. *forceps;* Mauriceau-L. *maneuver.*

lev·u·lan (lev′ū-lan). Levulano. SIN fructosan (1).

lev·u·lic ac·id (lev′ū-lik). Ácido levúlico. SIN levulinic acid.

lev·u·lin (lev′ū-lin). Levulina. SIN fructosan (1).

lev·u·li·nate (lev′ū-lin-āt). Levulinato; um sal ou éster do ácido levulínico.

lev·u·lin·ic ac·id (lev-ū-lin′ik). Ácido levulínico; ácido 4-oxopentanóico; formado pela ação de ácidos fortes e quentes sobre as hexoses. VER TAMBÉM δ-aminolevulinic acid. SIN levulic acid.

lev·u·lo·san (lev′ū-lō-san). Levulosano. SIN fructosan (1).

lev·u·lose (lev′ū-lōs). Levulose; D-frutose. SIN fructose.

lev·u·lo·se·mia (lev′ū-lō-sē′mē-ă). Levulosemia. SIN fructosemia.

lev·u·lo·su·ria (lev′ū-lō-soo′rē-ă). Levulosúria. SIN fructosuria.

Lévy, Gabrielle, neurologista francesa, 1886–1935. VER Roussy-L. *disease, syndrome.*

Lewandowski, Felix, dermatologista alemão, 1879–1921. VER Jadassohn-L. *syndrome.*

Lewis, Gilbert N., químico norte-americano, 1875–1946. VER TAMBÉM L. *acid, base;* second *law* of thermodynamics.

Lewis, Ivor, cirurgião sueco que, em 1946, reportou ao *Royal College of Surgeons* uma esofagectomia em duas etapas por laparotomia e toracotomia direita, realizada atualmente como um único procedimento. VER Ivor L. *esophagectomy.*

Lewis Blood Group, Le Blood Group. Grupo sanguíneo Lewis; ver Apêndice de Grupos Sanguíneos.

lew·is·ite (loo′i-sīt). Lewisita; um gás utilizado na guerra, um veneno sistêmico que penetra na circulação através dos pulmões ou da pele, e um veneno mitótico que paralisa a mitose na metáfase; o dimercaprol é o antídoto. SIN β-chlorovinyldichloroarsine. [W. Lee *Lewis*, químico norte-americano, 1898–1943]

Lewy (Lewey), Frederic H., neurologista alemão nos Estados Unidos, 1885–1950. VER L. *bodies,* em *body;* Lewy body *dementia;* diffuse Lewy body *disease.*

lex·i·cal (leks′ī-kal). Léxico; que indica o vocabulário da fala ou linguagem.

▷ **-lexis, -lexy.** Sufixos que se relacionam adequadamente à fala, embora freqüentemente confundidos com -legia (L. *lego*, ler) e, assim, erroneamente empregados para se ligar à leitura. [G. *lexis*, palavra, fala, de *lego*, dizer]

Leyden, Ernst V. von, médico alemão, 1832–1910. VER L. *ataxia, crystals,* em *crystal, neuritis;* L.-Möbius muscular *dystrophy.*

Leydig, Franz von, anatomista alemão, 1821–1908. VER L. *cells,* em *cell;* Leydig cell *tumor;* Sertoli-Leydig cell *tumor.*

ley·dig·ar·che (lī′dig-ar-kē). Leidigarca; termo obsoleto para o início da função gonadal no homem, p.ex., puberdade masculina. [Leydig (ver Leydig cells), + G. *archē*, início]

Lf, L_f. VER dose.

LFA Abreviatura de left frontoanterior position (posição fronto-anterior esquerda); lymphocyte function associated *antigen* (antígeno associado a linfócitos).

LFP Abreviatura de left frontoposterior position (posição fronto-posterior esquerda).

LFT Abreviatura de left frontotransverse position (posição fronto-transversa esquerda).

LGSIL Abreviatura de low-grade squamous intraepithelial *lesion* (lesão intra-epitelial escamosa de baixo grau).

LH Abreviatura de luteinizing *hormone* (hormônio luteinizante).

Lhermitte, Jean, neurologista francês, 1877–1959. VER L. *sign.*

LH/FSH-RF Abreviatura de luteinizing hormone/follicle-stimulating hormone-releasing *factor* (fator liberador de hormônio luteinizante/hormônio folículo-estimulante).

LH-RF Abreviatura de luteinizing hormone-releasing *factor* (fator liberador de hormônio luteinizante).

LH-RH Abreviatura de luteinizing hormone-releasing *hormone* (hormônio liberador de hormônio luteinizante).

Li, Frederick P., epidemiologista do século XX. VER L.-Fraumeni cancer *syndrome.*

Li Símbolo de lithium (lítio).

lib·er·a·tor (lib′er-ā-ter, -tōr). Liberador; um agente que estimula ou ativa uma ação fisiológica de uma substância química ou enzimática.

histamine l.'s, liberadores de histamina; substâncias que provocam a liberação da histamina por mastócitos ou basófilos.

li·ber·ins (lib′er-ins). Liberinas. SIN realising *factors.* [L. *libero*, liberar, + -in]

lib·er·o·mo·tor (lib′er-ō-mō′ter). Liberomotor; que se relaciona aos movimentos voluntários. [L. *liber*, livre, + *motor*, mover]

li·bid·i·ni·za·tion (li-bid′i-ni-zā′shŭn). Libidinização. SIN erotization.

li·bid·i·nous (li-bid′i-nŭs). Libidinoso; lascivo; caracterizado por ou que provoca o desejo ou energia sexual. [L. *libidinosus*, de *libido* (*libidin-*), prazer, desejo]

li·bi·do (li-bē′dō, -bī′dō). Libido. **1.** Desejo sexual consciente ou inconsciente. **2.** Qualquer interesse passional ou forma de força de vida. **3.** Na psicologia junguiana, sinônimo de energia psíquica (psychic *energy*). [L. prazer]

object l., l. de objeto; a l. investida no objeto, em contradição com a libido investida no ego.

Libman, Emanuel, médico norte-americano, 1872–1946. VER L.-Sacks *endocarditis, syndrome.*

Liborius, Paul, bacteriologista do século XIX. VER L. *method.*

li·brary (lī′brar-ē). Biblioteca; uma coleção de fragmentos clonados que representam todo o genoma.

cDNA l., b. de DNAc; uma coleção de cópias de fragmentos (DNAc) que foram produzidas pela transcriptase reversa a partir do RNAm de determinada célula, órgão ou organismo.

genomic l., b. genômica; b. em que os introns e exons estão representados; uma b. preparada a partir do DNA genômico.

l. screening, rastreamento de b.; o processo de seleção de um clone desejado a partir da coleta.

lice (līs). Piolhos; plural de louse.

li·chen (lī′ken). Líquen; uma pápula plana bem definida ou um agregado de pápulas com uma configuração ordenada semelhante ao líquen que cresce em rochas. [G. *leichēn*, líquen; uma erupção semelhante ao líquen]

l. myxedemato′sus, l. mixedematoso; erupção liquenóide de pápulas na parte superior do edema mucinoso decorrente do depósito de glicosaminoglicanas na pele e proliferação de fibroblastos, na ausência de doença endócrina. Gamopatia monoclonal é comum. VER TAMBÉM scleromyxedema. SIN papular mucinosis.

l. ni′tidus, l. nítido; pequenas pápulas esbranquiçadas ou róseas assintomáticas; as lesões, que exibem o ápice achatado, raramente coexistem com o l. plano e podem envolver a genitália masculina.

l. nu′chae, l. da nuca; l. simples do pescoço, geralmente nas mulheres.

l. obtu′sus, l. obtuso; uma forma em que as pápulas são grandes e arredondadas, em lugar de achatadas.

oral (erosive) l. planus, l. plano oral (erosivo); manifestações orais do l. plano caracterizadas por estrias esbranquiçadas (estrias de Wickham) da mucosa oral e, por vezes, associadas a ulceração; os pacientes podem ter ou não história pregressa de l. plano cutâneo.

l. planopila′ris, l. planopiloso; uma rara alopecia em área com hiperceratose folicular do couro cabeludo e perifoliculite linfocítica com l. plano em outros pontos.

l. pla′nus, l. plano; erupção de pápulas violáceas brilhosas, com o ápice achatado, nas superfícies flexoras, genitália masculina e mucosa bucal, de etiologia desconhecida; podem formar grupos lineares; caracterizadas microscopicamente por um infiltrado linfocítico subepidérmico em faixa. A resolução espontânea é comum após meses a anos.

l. pla′nus annula′ris, l. plano anular; uma forma em que as pápulas são agrupadas em figuras anelares.

l. pla′nus follicula′ris, l. plano folicular; o l. plano dos folículos pilosos, usualmente do couro cabeludo.

l. pla′nus hypertro′phicus, l. plano hipertrófico; lesões verrucóides ou verrucosas que ocorrem nas pernas e coxas em associação com o l. plano em outro local. SIN l. planus verrucosus.

l. pla′nus verruco′sus, l. plano verrucoso. SIN l. planus hypertrophicus.

l. ru′ber monilifor′mis, l. rubro moniliforme; uma rara dermatose que consiste em pequenas pápulas avermelhadas dispostas em estreitas faixas peroladas e que cobrem grandes áreas do corpo.

l. sclero′sus et atro′phicus, l. escleroso e atrófico; erupção que consiste em pápulas atróficas esbranquiçadas e pruriginosas e placas que podem ser distintas ou confluentes, podendo conter uma depressão central ou um tampão ceratótico negro evidenciando microscopicamente a hiperceratose epidérmica e atrofia, edema dérmico superficial e homogeneização, e inflamação da camada média da derme; ocorre mais amiúde nas mulheres antes da puberdade e após a menopausa; o envolvimento vulvar foi outrora denominado craurose vulvar.

l. scrofuloso′rum, l. escrofuloso; pequenas pápulas liquenosas assintomáticas no tronco de crianças com tuberculose; bacilos álcool-ácido-resistentes (BAAR) não são observados nos granulomas dérmicos. SIN papular tuberculid.

l. sim′plex chronicus, l. simples crônico; uma área espessada de pele pruriginosa que resulta de atrito e arranhadura.

l. spinulo′sus, l. espinhoso; erupção de pápulas cônicas, de etiologia desconhecida, que possuem uma superfície escamosa aderente; pode estar relacionado ao l. plano.

l. stria'tus, l. estriado; uma erupção papular autolimitada que ocorre principalmente em crianças (mais amiúde em meninas); as lesões estão dispostas em grupos lineares e, em geral, ocorrem em um membro.

li·chen·i·fi·ca·tion (lī′ken-i-fi-kā′shŭn). Liquenificação; o endurecimento coriáceo e o espessamento da pele com hiperceratose, causada por coçadura, como na dermatite de contato atópica ou crônica. [lichen + L. *facio*, fazer]

li·chen·in (lī′ken-in). Liquenina; uma variedade de polissacarídeo obtida a partir do musgo da Islândia; usada como demulcente. SIN moss starch.

li·chen·oid (lī′ke-noyd). Liquenóide. **1.** Que se assemelha ao líquen. **2.** Acentuação das marcas cutâneas normais observadas nos casos de eczema crônico. **3.** Que se assemelha microscopicamente ao líquen plano.

Lichtenstein, Louis, médico norte-americano, 1906–1977. VER Jaffe-L. *disease*.

lic·o·rice (lik′o-ris). Alcaçuz. SIN glycyrrhiza.

lid. Pálpebra. SIN eyelid. [A.S. *hlid*]
  granular l.'s, tracoma. SIN trachoma.
  lower l., p. inferior. SIN inferior eyelid.
  upper l., p. superior. SIN superior eyelid.

Liddell, Edward G.T., neurofisiologista inglês, 1895–1981. VER L.-Sherrington *reflex*.

li·do·caine hy·dro·chlo·ride (lī′dō-kān). Cloridrato de lidocaína; anestésico local com propriedades antiarrítmicas e anticonvulsivantes.

li·do·fla·zine (lī-dō-flā′zēn). Lidoflazina; vasodilatador coronariano.

lie (lī). Posição, situação; relação do eixo longitudinal do feto com o da mãe.
  longitudinal l., p. longitudinal; a relação em que o eixo longitudinal do feto é longitudinal e quase paralelo ao eixo longitudinal da mãe; a parte apresentada pode ser a cabeça ou as nádegas.
  oblique l., p. oblíqua; a relação em que o eixo longitudinal do feto atravessa o eixo materno em um ângulo diferente de um ângulo reto.
  transverse l., p. transversa; a relação em que o eixo longitudinal do feto é transverso ou está em ângulo reto ao da mãe.
  unstable l., p. instável; a orientação oblíqua do feto que não é transversa nem longitudinal, mas que se converte em uma ou outra antes ou no decorrer do trabalho de parto.

Lieberkühn, Johann N., anatomista alemão, 1711–1756. VER *crypts* of L., em *crypt*; L. *follicles*, em *follicle, gland*, em *gland*.

lie·ber·kühn (lē′ber-koon). Um refletor côncavo ao redor da objetiva de um microscópio, com a finalidade de direcionar um feixe concentrado de luz sobre o material que está sendo examinado. [J. N. *Lieberkühn*]

Liebermann, Leo von S., médico húngaro, 1852–1926. VER Burchard–L. *reaction*; L. –Burchard *test*.

Liebermeister, Carl von, médico alemão, 1833–1901. VER L. *rule*.

Liebig, Baron Justus von, químico alemão, 1803–1873. VER L. *theory*.

Liebow (lē′-bō), Averill A., patologista pulmonar austríaco-norte-americano, 1911–1978. VER usual interstitial *pneumonia* of Liebow.

lie de·tec·tor. Detetor de mentira. SIN polygraph (2).

li·en (lī′-en). Baço; *termo oficial alternativo para spleen. [L.]
  l. acces so'rius, b. acessório; *termo oficial alternativo para accessory spleen.
  l. mo'bilis, b. móvel. SIN floating spleen.
  l. succenturia'tus, b. acessório. SIN accessory spleen.

lien-, lieno-. Formas combinantes relacionadas ao baço; a maioria dos termos que começam assim são, dessa maneira, obsoletos ou em obsolescência. VER spleno-. [L. *lien*]

li·e·nal (lī′e-nāl). Esplênico. SIN splenic.

li·en·cu·lus (lī-en′kū-lŭs). Baço acessório. SIN accessory spleen. [L. mod. dim. do L. *lien*, baço]

li·e·nec·to·my (lī′e-nek′tō-mē). Lienectomia; termo obsoleto para esplenectomia.

li·e·no·med·ul·lary (lī′e-nō-med′u-lār-ē). Lienomedular. SIN splenomyelogenous. [lieno- + G. *medulla*, medula]

li·e·no·my·e·log·e·nous (lī′e-nō-mī-e-loj′e-nŭs). Lienomielógeno. SIN splenomyelogenous.

li·e·no·pan·cre·at·ic (lī′e-nō-pan′krē-at′ik). Lienopancreático. SIN splenopancreatic.

li·e·no·re·nal (lī′e-nō-rē′nal). Lienorrenal. SIN splenorenal. [lieno- + L. *ren*, rim]

li·en·ter·ic (lī-en-ter′ik). Lientérico; relativo ou marcado por lienteria.

li·en·tery (lī′en-ter-ē). Lienteria; eliminação de alimento não-digerido nas fezes. [G. *leienteria*, de *leios*, liso, + *enteron*, intestino]

li·e·nun·cu·lus (lī′e-nun′kū-lŭs). Baço acessório. SIN accessory spleen. [L. mod. dim de L. *lien*, baço]

Liesegang, Ralph E., químico alemão, 1869–1947. VER L. *rings*, em *ring*.

Lieutaud, Joseph, anatomista e patologista francês, 1703–1780. VER L. *body, triangle, trigone, uvula*.

life (līf). Vida. **1.** Vitalidade, a condição essencial de estar vivo; o estado da existência, caracterizado por certas funções como metabolismo, crescimento, reprodução, adaptação e resposta aos estímulos. **2.** Organismos vivos, como plantas e animais. [A. S. *lif*]
  half-l., meia-vida. VER half-life.

postnatal l., v. pós-natal; o intervalo da v. após o nascimento; nos seres humanos, geralmente dividido em períodos: neonatal, lactente, infância, adolescência e adulto.

prenatal l., v. pré-natal; o intervalo da vida entre a concepção e o nascimento; nos seres humanos, geralmente dividido em períodos embrionário e fetal.

quality of l., qualidade de v.; o bem-estar geral do paciente, incluindo estado mental, nível de estresse, função sexual e estado de saúde autopercebido.

sexual l., v. sexual; em psiquiatria e psicanálise, os interesses, fantasias, inclinações e condutas especificamente eróticas ou sexuais do paciente.

vegetative l., v. vegetativa; a simples atividade metabólica e reprodutiva de seres humanos ou animais, independentemente do exercício dos processos psíquicos ou mentais conscientes.

life e·vents. Eventos da vida; as ocorrências na vida diária da pessoa, algumas das quais atuam como estressores.

life·span. Espectro de vida. **1.** A duração da vida de um indivíduo. **2.** A duração normal ou média da vida dos membros de uma determinada espécie. VER TAMBÉM longevity.

life-style. Estilo de vida; o conjunto de hábitos e costumes que é influenciado pelo processo de socialização durante a vida, incluindo o uso social de substâncias, como álcool e fumo, hábitos alimentares, exercício, etc., os quais têm importantes implicações para a saúde.

LIGAMENT

lig·a·ment (lig′ă-ment)[TA]. Ligamento. **1.** Uma faixa ou bainha de tecido fibroso que conecta dois ou mais ossos, cartilagens ou outras estruturas, ou que serve como suporte para fáscias ou músculos. **2.** Uma dobra do peritônio que sustenta qualquer uma das vísceras abdominais. **3.** Qualquer estrutura que se assemelha a um l., embora não realizando a função de um. **4.** Os resquícios em forma de cordão de um vaso fetal ou de outra estrutura que perdeu sua luz original. SIN ligamentum [TA]. [L. *ligamentum*, uma faixa, atadura]

accessory l.'s, ligamentos acessórios; os ligamentos em torno de uma articulação que se somam à cápsula articular. Eles podem situar-se dentro (ligamentos intracapsulares) ou fora (ligamentos extracapsulares) da cápsula articular.

accessory plantar l.'s, ligamentos plantares. SIN plantar l.'s.

accessory volar l.'s, ligamentos palmares. SIN palmar l.'s.

acromioclavicular l. [TA], l. acromioclavicular; uma faixa fibrosa que se estende desde o acrômio da escápula até a clavícula. SIN ligamentum acromioclaviculare [TA].

alar l.'s, ligamentos alares; uma de um par de pequenas faixas curtas e retesadas que se estendem desde o lado do dente do áxis até o tubérculo na face medial do côndilo occipital. SIN check l.'s of odontoid.

alveolodental l., periodonto. SIN periodontium.

anococcygeal l., l. anococcígeo; uma faixa musculofibrosa que passa entre o ânus e o cóccix. SIN anococcygeal body, ligamentum anococcygeum, raphe anococcygea, Symington anococcygeal body.

anterior costotransverse l., l. costotransversário superior. SIN superior costotransverse l.

anterior cruciate l. [TA], l. cruzado anterior; o l. que se estende desde a área intercondilar anterior da tíbia até a parte posterior da superfície medial do côndilo lateral do fêmur. SIN ligamentum cruciatum anterius.

anterior l. of fibular head [TA], l. anterior da cabeça da fíbula; um l. que une a parte anterior da cabeça da fíbula à tíbia. SIN ligamentum capitis fibulae anterius [TA].

anterior l. of Helmholtz, l. anterior de Helmholtz. VER anterior l. of malleus.

anterior longitudinal l. [TA], l. longitudinal anterior; a ampla faixa fibrosa que interliga as superfícies anterolaterais dos corpos vertebrais, misturando-se às lamelas externas dos discos intervertebrais à medida que passam entre as vértebras. SIN ligamentum longitudinale anterius [TA], lacertus medius.

anterior l. of malleus [TA], l. anterior do martelo; consiste em duas porções: a faixa de Meckel, que vai da base do processo anterior até a espinha do esfenóide, através da fissura petrotimpânica; e o l. anterior de Helmholtz, que se estende desde a face anterior do colo do martelo até o limite posterior da incisura timpânica. SIN ligamentum mallei anterius [TA].

anterior meniscofemoral l. [TA], l. meniscofemoral anterior; a faixa ligamentosa que passa anteriormente ao l. cruzado posterior, estendendo-se entre a porção posterior do menisco lateral e a extremidade superior do l. cruzado anterior. SIN ligamentum meniscofemorale anterius [TA], Humphry l.

anterior sacrococcygeal l. [TA], l. sacrococcígeo anterior; a continuação do l. longitudinal anterior que une o sacro e o cóccix. SIN ligamentum sacrococcygeum anterius [TA], ventral sacrococcygeal l.

anterior sacroiliac l.'s [TA], ligamentos sacroilíacos anteriores; as fortes faixas fibrosas que reforçam anteriormente a articulação sacroilíaca. SIN ligamenta sacroiliaca anteriora [TA], ventral sacroiliac l.'s.

anterior sacrosciatic l., l. sacroespinal. SIN sacrospinous l.

anterior sternoclavicular l. [TA], l. esternoclavicular anterior; uma faixa fibrosa que reforça anteriormente a articulação esternoclavicular. SIN ligamentum sternoclaviculare anterius [TA].
anterior talofibular l. [TA], l. talofibular anterior; a faixa de fibras que se estende desde o maléolo lateral até o colo do talo. SIN ligamentum talofibulare anterius [TA].
anterior talotibial l., parte talotibial anterior do ligamento colateral medial. SIN anterior tibiotalar *part* of medial ligament of ankle joint. VER TAMBÉM medial l. of ankle joint.
anterior tibiofibular l. [TA], l. tibiofibular anterior; o l. que une a face anterior da sindesmose tibiofibular. SIN ligamentum tibiofibulare anterius [TA].
anterior tibiotalar l., parte tibiotalar anterior do ligamento colateral medial. SIN anterior tibiotalar *part* of medial ligament of ankle joint.
anular l. [TA], l. anular; um dos inúmeros ligamentos que envolvem várias regiões; os principais ligamentos anulares são aqueles do estribo, rádio e traquéia. VER anular l. of radius, anular l. of stapes, anular l.'s of trachea. SIN ligamentum anulare [TA], orbicular l.
anular l. of radius [TA], l. anular do rádio; o l. que envolve e sustenta a cabeça do rádio na incisura radial da ulna, formando a articulação radioulnar proximal e que possibilita a pronação/supinação do antebraço; recebe o l. colateral radial da articulação do cotovelo. SIN ligamentum anulare radii [TA], ligamentum orbiculare radii, orbicular l. of radius.
anular l. of stapes [TA], l. estapedial anular; um anel de fibras elásticas que se insere na base do estribo até a margem das fenestrações vestibulares. SIN ligamentum anulare stapedis [TA].
anular l.'s of trachea [TA], ligamentos anulares da traquéia; as membranas fibrosas que conectam as cartilagens traqueais adjacentes. SIN ligamenta anularia trachealia [TA], ligamenta trachealia.
apical l. of dens [TA], l. do ápice do dente; um l. que se estende desde o ápice do dente até a margem anterior do forame magno; inclui os vestígios do notocórdio. SIN ligamentum apicis dentis.
Arantius l., l. de Arantius. SIN *ligamentum* venosum.
arcuate popliteal l. [TA], l. poplíteo arqueado; uma faixa fibrosa larga que se insere acima do côndilo lateral do fêmur e que passa medialmente e para baixo, misturando-se à parte posterior da cápsula fibrosa da articulação do joelho, arqueando-se sobre o tendão do músculo poplíteo. SIN ligamentum popliteum arcuatum [TA], popliteal arch, posterior l. of knee.
arcuate pubic l., l. púbico inferior. SIN inferior pubic l.
arterial l., l. arterial (ducto arterial). SIN *ligamentum* arteriosum.
l.'s of auditory ossicles [TA], ligamentos dos ossículos da audição; os ligamentos que unem os ossos da orelha entre si e com as paredes da cavidade timpânica. SIN ligamenta ossiculorum auditus [TA], ligamenta ossiculorum auditorium*.
l.'s of auricle [TA], ligamentos auriculares; os três ligamentos que fixam a orelha ao lado da cabeça: l. auricular anterior (*ligamentum* auriculare anterius), que se estende desde a raiz do processo zigomático à espinha da hélice; o l. auricular posterior (*ligamentum* auriculare posterius), que se estende desde o processo mastóideo até a proeminência da concha; o l. auricular superior (*ligamentum* auriculare superius), que se estende desde a margem superior do meato acústico externo ósseo até a espinha da hélice. SIN ligamenta auricularia [TA], auricular l.'s, Valsalva l.'s
auricular l.'s, ligamentos auriculares. SIN l.'s of auricle.
axis l. of malleus, l. do eixo do martelo. SIN Helmholtz axis l.
Bardinet l., l. de Bardinet; a faixa posterior do l. colateral ulnar do cotovelo.
Barkow l.'s, ligamentos de Barkow; as porções anterior e posterior da cápsula fibrosa da articulação do cotovelo.
Bellini l., l. de Bellini; um fascículo da porção isquiofemoral da cápsula fibrosa articular maior do quadril que se estende até o trocanter maior.
Berry l.'s, ligamentos de Berry. SIN lateral thyrohyoid l.
Bertin l., l. de Bertin. SIN iliofemoral l.
Bichat l., l. de Bichat; o fascículo inferior do l. sacroilíaco posterior.
bifurcate l. [TA], l. bifurcado; um forte l. dorsal do tarso em forma de V no dorso do pé que passa desde o calcâneo, distal ao seio társico, inserindo-se nos ossos cubóide e navicular; divide-se no l. calcaneocubóideo e no l. calcaneonavicular. SIN ligamentum bifurcatum [TA], bifurcated l.
bifurcated l., l. bifurcado. SIN bifurcate l.
Bigelow l., l. de Bigelow. SIN iliofemoral l.
Botallo l., l. de Botallo. SIN *ligamentum* arteriosum.
Bourgery l., l. de Bourgery. SIN oblique popliteal l.
broad l. of the uterus [TA], l. largo do útero; uma dobra peritoneal que passa desde a margem lateral do útero até a parede da pelve em ambos os lados, e, ao fazer isso, também embainha os ovários e as trompas uterinas. SIN ligamentum latum uteri [TA].
Brodie l., l. de Brodie. SIN transverse humeral l.
Burns l., l. de Burns. SIN superior *horn* of falciform margin of saphenous opening.
calcaneocuboid l., l. calcaneocubóideo; a parte lateral do l. bifurcado. SIN ligamentum calcaneocuboideum [TA].
calcaneofibular l. [TA], l. calcaneofibular; o fascículo médio dos três fascículos que formam o l. lateral da articulação do tornozelo, reforçando o lado lateral dessa articulação e resistindo à inversão excessiva do pé; os dois ligamentos remanescentes são os ligamentos talofibulares anterior e posterior. SIN ligamentum calcaneofibulare [TA].
calcaneonavicular l. [TA], l. calcaneonavicular; a parte medial do ligamento bifurcado. SIN ligamentum calcaneonaviculare [TA].
calcaneotibial l., parte tibiocalcânea do ligamento colateral medial da articulação talocrural. SIN tibiocalcaneal *part* of medial ligament of ankle joint. VER TAMBÉM medial l. of ankle joint.
Caldani l., l. de Caldani. SIN coracoclavicular l.
Campbell l., l. de Campbell. SIN suspensory l. of axilla.
Camper l., l. de Camper. SIN perineal *membrane*.
capsular l. [TA], l. capsular; porções espessadas da membrana fibrosa de uma cápsula articular. SIN ligamentum capsulare [TA].
cardinal l. [TA], l. transverso do colo do útero; uma faixa fibrosa inserida no colo do útero e na cúpula do fórnice lateral da vagina; contínuo com o tecido que embainha os vasos pélvicos. SIN ligamentum cardinale [TA], transverse cervical l.*, cervical l. of uterus, ligamentum transversale cervicis, Mackenrodt l.
caroticoclinoid l., l. caroticoclinóide; o l. que une o processo clinóide anterior do esfenóide ao processo clinóide médio.
carpometacarpal l.'s (dorsal and palmar) [TA], ligamentos carpometacarpais (dorsal e palmar); os ligamentos que unem os ossos metacarpais e carpais. SIN ligamenta carpometacarpalia (dorsalia/palmaria) [TA]
caudal l., retináculo caudal. SIN retinaculum caudale.
ceratocricoid l. [TA], l. ceratocricóideo; um dos três ligamentos (anterior, posterior e lateral) reforçando a cápsula da articulação cricotireóidea em ambos os lados. SIN ligamentum ceratocricoideum [TA].
cervical l. of uterus, l. transverso do colo do útero; SIN cardinal l.
check l.'s of eyeball, medial and lateral, ligamentos controladores do bulbo do olho, mediais e laterais; SIN check l.'s of medial and lateral rectus muscles.
check l.'s of medial and lateral rectus muscles [TA], ligamentos controladores dos músculos retos mediais e laterais; expansões das bainhas dos músculos retos mediais e laterais do bulbo do olho que se inserem, respectivamente, no osso lacrimal e no tubérculo superficial do osso zigomático; eles servem para evitar a ação excessiva desses músculos. A *Terminologia Anatomica* reconhece apenas o l. controlador do músculo reto lateral. SIN check l.'s of eyeball, medial and lateral.
check l.'s of odontoid, ligamentos alares. SIN alar l.'s.
chondroxiphoid l., l. costoxifóideo. SIN costoxiphoid l.
ciliary l., músculo ciliar. SIN ciliary *muscle*.
Civinini l., l. de Civinini. SIN pterygospinous l.
Clado l., l. de Clado; uma prega mesentérica que corre desde o l. largo do útero, à direita, até o apêndice.
coccygeal l., l. parte dural do filamento terminal; *termo oficial alternativo para dural *part* of filum terminale.
collateral l. [TA], l. colateral; um dos inúmeros ligamentos em ambos os lados de uma articulação com movimento de dobradiça, servindo como um raio de movimento dessa articulação; ocorrem nas seguintes articulações: cotovelo, joelho, punho e articulações metacarpo- ou metatarsofalângicas, interfalângicas proximais e interfalângicas distais das mãos e dos pés. SIN ligamentum collaterale [TA].
Colles l., l. de Colles. SIN reflected inguinal l.
conoid l. [TA], l. conóide; a parte medial do l. coracoclavicular que se insere no tubérculo conóide da clavícula. O ligamento conóide e seu ligamento parceiro coracoclavicular, o ligamento trapezóide, suspendem passivamente o membro superior livre a partir do suporte formado pela clavícula. SIN ligamentum conoideum [TA].
Cooper l.'s, ligamentos de Cooper; (1) ligamentos suspensores da mama. SIN suspensory l.'s of breast; (2) ligamento pectíneo. SIN pectineal l; (3) ligamento transverso do cotovelo. SIN transverse l. of elbow.
coracoacromial l. [TA], l. coracoacromial; a forte faixa fibrosa arqueada que passa entre o processo coracóide e o acrômio acima da articulação do ombro; o arco osteofibroso assim formado impede a luxação para cima da articulação do ombro (glenoumeral). SIN ligamentum coracoacromiale [TA].
coracoclavicular l. [TA], l. coracoclavicular; o forte l. composto que une a clavícula ao processo coracóide; é subdividido no ligamento conóide e no ligamento trapezóide. O membro superior livre é passivamente suspenso, a partir da sustentação clavicular, pelo l. coracoclavicular; o l. também é importante na prevenção da luxação da articulação acromioclavicular. SIN ligamentum coracoclaviculare [TA], Caldani l.
coracohumeral l. [TA], l. coracoumeral; o l. que passa da base do processo coracóide até o tubérculo maior do úmero. SIN ligamentum coracohumerale [TA].
corniculopharyngeal l., l. cricofaríngeo. SIN cricopharyngeal l.
coronary l. of knee, l. coronário do joelho; porções da cápsula articular da articulação do joelho que ligam a circunferência dos meniscos com as margens dos côndilos da tíbia.
coronary l. of liver, l. coronário do fígado; reflexões peritoneais desde o fígado até o diafragma nas margens da área nua do fígado. SIN ligamentum coronarium hepatis [TA].

costoclavicular l. [TA], l. costoclavicular; o l. que une a primeira costela e a clavícula próximo à sua extremidade esternal; limita a elevação do ombro (na articulação esternoclavicular). SIN ligamentum costoclaviculare [TA], rhomboid l.
costocolic l., l. frenocólico. SIN phrenicocolic l.
costotransverse l. [TA], l. costotransversário; o l. que une a face dorsal do colo de uma costela à face ventral do processo transverso correspondente. VER TAMBÉM costotransverse l., superior costotransverse l. SIN ligamentum costotransversarium [TA], ligamentum colli costae, middle costotransverse l.
costoxiphoid l. [TA], l. costoxifóideo; l. que une o processo xifóide à sétima e, com freqüência, à sexta cartilagem costal. SIN ligamentum costoxiphoideum [TA], chondroxiphoid l.
cotyloid l., lábio do acetábulo. SIN acetabular *labrum*.
Cowper l., l. de Cowper; a parte da fáscia lata que fica anterior e que origina as fibras do músculo pectíneo.
cricoarytenoid l. [TA], l. cricoaritenóideo; o l. que passa para baixo a partir da borda posterior da cartilagem aritenóidea até a lâmina da cartilagem cricóidea. SIN ligamentum cricoarytenoideum posterius, posterior crycoarytenoid l.
crycopharyngeal l. [TA], l. cricofaríngeo; uma faixa elástica que une a extremidade da cartilagem corniculada (Santorini) e a lâmina da cartilagem cricóidea e que continua para a mucosa faríngea, revestindo a lâmina da cartilagem cricóidea. SIN ligamentum cricopharyngeum [TA], corniculopharyngeal l., cricosantorinian l., jugal l., ligamentum corniculopharyngeum, ligamentum jugale.
cricosantorinian l., l. cricofaríngeo. SIN cricopharyngeal l.
cricotracheal l. [TA], l. cricotraqueal; uma faixa fibrosa, na linha média, que une a cartilagem cricóidea ao primeiro anel da traquéia. SIN ligamentum cricotracheale [TA], cricotracheal membrane.
crucial l., (1) VER inferior extensor *retinaculum*, superior extensor *retinaculum*; (2) ligamentos cruzados do joelho. SIN cruciate l.'s of knee; (3) l. cruciforme do atlas. SIN cruciate l. of the atlas; (4) parte cruciforme das bainhas fibrosas dos dedos. SIN cruciform *part of fibrous digital sheath*.
cruciate l. of the atlas [TA], l. cruciforme do atlas; o forte l. que se situa posteriormente ao dente do áxis, fixando-o contra o arco anterior do atlas; consiste principalmente no l. transverso do atlas, que forma a barra da cruz e é mais importante do ponto de vista funcional, e nas faixas longitudinais do l. cruciforme, formando os feixes eretos ou verticais da cruz. SIN ligamentum cruciforme atlantis [TA], crucial l. (3), cruciform l. of atlas, ligamentum cruciatum atlantis.
cruciate l.'s of knee, ligamentos cruzados do joelho; os dois ligamentos que se originam da área intercondilar da tíbia até a fossa intercondilar do fêmur. VER anterior cruciate l., posterior cruciate l.; VER TAMBÉM anterior cruciate l., posterior cruciate l. SIN crucial l. (2), ligamenta cruciata genus.
cruciate l. of leg, retináculo inferior dos músculos extensores. SIN inferior extensor *retinaculum*.
cruciform l. of atlas, l. cruciforme do atlas. SIN cruciate l. of the atlas.
Cruveilhier l.'s, ligamentos de Cruveilhier. SIN plantar l.'s
cuboideonavicular l.'s [TA], ligamentos cuboideonaviculares; o l. que une o osso cubóide ao osso navicular. VER dorsal cuboideonavicular l., plantar cuboideonavicular l.'s. SIN ligamenta cuboideonaviculare [TA].
cuneocuboid l.'s [TA], ligamentos cuneocubóideos; os ligamentos que unem o osso cuneiforme lateral ao osso cubóide. VER dorsal cuneocuboid l., cuneocuboid interosseous l., plantar cuneocuboid l. SIN ligamentum cuneocuboideum [TA].
cuneocuboid interosseous l. [TA], l. cuneocubóideo interósseo; a faixa fibrosa que une as margens adjacentes da extremidade distal dos ossos cuneiforme lateral e cubóide. SIN interosseus cuneocuboid l., ligamentum cuneocuboideum interosseum.
cuneometatarsal interosseus l.'s [TA], ligamentos cuneometatarsais interósseos; os ligamentos que se originam dos ossos cuneiformes até os metatarsais, com aquele do primeiro cuneiforme para o segundo metatarsal sendo o mais forte. SIN ligamenta cuneometatarsalia interossea [TA], interosseous cuneometatarsal l.'s, Lisfranc l.'s.
cuneonavicular l.'s, ligamentos cuneonaviculares; os ligamentos que unem o osso cuneiforme medial com o navicular. VER TAMBÉM dorsal cuneonavicular l.'s, plantar cuneonavicular l.'s.
cystoduodenal l., l. cistoduodenal; uma prega peritoneal que por vezes se origina da vesícula biliar até a primeira parte do duodeno.
deep dorsal sacrococcygeal l., l. sacrococcígeo dorsal profundo. SIN deep posterior sacrococcygeal l.
deep posterior sacrococcygeal l., l. sacrococcígeo posterior profundo; a continuação do l. longitudinal posterior que une o sacro e o cóccix. SIN deep dorsal sacrococcygeal l., ligamentum sacrococcygeum posterius profundum.
deep transverse metacarpal l. [TA], l. metacarpal transverso profundo; o l. que interliga a superfície palmar das cabeças do segundo ao quinto metacarpais, sendo contínuo com os ligamentos palmares ou placas palmares; situa-se no plano da fáscia interóssea palmar. SIN ligamentum metacarpale transversum profundum [TA], transverse metacarpal l.
deep transverse metatarsal l. [TA], l. metatarsal transverso profundo; o l. que interliga a superfície plantar das cabeças dos metatarsais, sendo contínuo com os ligamentos plantares. SIN ligamentum metatarsale transversum profundum [TA], transverse metatarsal l.
deltoid l., l. colateral medial; *termo oficial alternativo para medial l. of ankle joint.
Denonvilliers l., l. de Denonvilliers. SIN puboprostatic l.
dentate l. of spinal cord, l. denticulado; variação raramente utilizada do l. denticulado.
denticulate l. [TA], l. denticulado; uma extensão serrilhada, semelhante a uma prateleira, da pia-máter espinal, projetando-se em um plano frontal a partir de cada lado das porções cervical e torácica da medula espinal; seus 21 processos pontiagudos se fundem lateralmente com a aracnóide-máter e dura-máter, aproximadamente a meio caminho entre as saídas das raízes dos nervos espinais adjacentes, com o processo mais elevado inserindo-se logo acima do forame magno. SIN ligamentum denticulatum [TA].
Denucé l., l. de Denucé. SIN quadrate l.
diaphragmatic l. of the mesonephros, l. diafragmático do mesonefro, mesentério urogenital; o segmento da crista urogenital que se estende desde o mesonefro até o diafragma; transforma-se no l. suspensor do ovário. SIN urogenital mesentery.
dorsal calcaneocuboid l., l. calcaneocubóideo dorsal. VER bifurcate l.
dorsal carpal l., retináculo dos músculos extensores. SIN extensor *retinaculum*.
dorsal carpometacarpal l.'s [TA], ligamentos carpometacarpais dorsais; faixas fibrosas que ligam as superfícies dorsais do carpo e ossos metacarpais. SIN ligamenta carpometacarpalia dorsalia [TA].
dorsal cuboideonavicular l. [TA], l. cuboideonavicular dorsal; o l. dorsal do tarso que une as superfícies dorsais dos ossos cubóide e navicular do tarso. SIN ligamentum cuboideonaviculare dorsale [TA].
dorsal cuneocuboid l. [TA], l. cuneocubóideo dorsal; um dos ligamentos dorsais do tarso que aparecem como uma faixa fibrosa que une as margens dorsais dos ossos cuneiforme lateral e cubóide. SIN ligamentum cuneocuboideum dorsale [TA].
dorsal cuneonavicular l.'s [TA], ligamentos cuneonaviculares dorsais; vários ligamentos que unem a superfície dorsal do navicular com os três ossos cuneiformes. SIN ligamenta cuneonavicularia dorsalia [TA].
dorsal intercuneiform l.'s [TA], ligamentos intercuneiformes dorsais; o ligamento dorsal do tarso que se estende entre os ossos cuneiformes adjacentes.
dorsal metacarpal l.'s [TA], ligamentos metacarpais dorsais; faixas fibrosas que unem as faces dorsais das bases do segundo ao quinto metacarpais. SIN ligamenta metacarpalia dorsalia [TA].
dorsal metatarsal l.'s [TA], ligamentos metatarsais dorsais; faixas fibrosas que unem as faces dorsais das bases dos metatarsais. SIN ligamenta metatarsalia dorsalia [TA].
dorsal radiocarpal l. [TA], l. radiocarpal dorsal; o l. que se estende da extremidade distal do rádio, posteriormente, à fileira proximal dos ossos do carpo. SIN ligamentum radiocarpale dorsale [TA].
dorsal sacroiliac l.'s, ligamentos sacroilíacos posteriores. SIN posterior sacroiliac l.'s.
dorsal tarsal l.'s [TA], ligamentos dorsais do tarso; os ligamentos que unem as faces dorsais dos ossos tarsais como um grupo; incluídos no grupo estão o: l. talonavicular [TA] (ligamentum talonaviculare [TA]), l. bifurcado [TA]

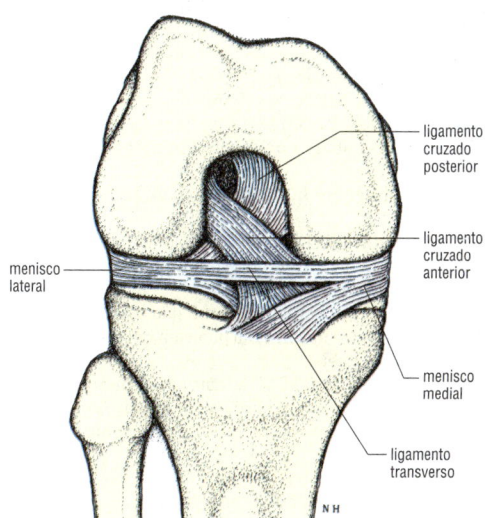

ligamentos cruzados do joelho

(ligamentum bifurcatum [TA]) e os seguintes ligamentos dorsais (ligamentum/a ... dorsalia/e): intercuneiforme [TA] (intercuneiformia [TA]), cuneocubóideo [TA] (cuneocuboideum [TA]), cuboideonavicular [TA] (cuboideonaviculare [TA]), cuneonavicular [TA] (cuneonavicularia [TA]) e calcaneocubóideo [TA] (calcaneocuboideum [TA]). sin ligamenta tarsi dorsalia [TA].

dorsal tarsometatarsal l.'s [TA], ligamentos tarsometatarsais dorsais; faixas robustas, achatadas, longitudinais e oblíquas que reforçam as faces dorsais das articulações tarsometatarsais (articulações entre os metatarsos e os ossos cubóide e cuneiforme); o primeiro metatarsal e o cuneiforme medial compartilham uma cápsula articular exclusiva, e os ligamentos tarsometatarsais dorsais mediais unem apenas esses ossos; os metatarsais remanescentes possuem inserções para múltiplos ossos, com os ligamentos reforçando a face dorsal de suas cápsulas articulares comuns. sin ligamenta tarsometatarsalia dorsalia [TA].

duodenorenal l., l. duodenorrenal; uma prega do peritônio que, ocasionalmente, se origina da terminação do l. hepatoduodenal até a parte frontal do rim direito. sin ligamentum duodenorenale.

l.'s of epididymis (inferior and superior), ligamentos do epidídimo (inferior e superior); uma das duas pregas (superior e inferior) da túnica vaginal entre o epidídimo e o testículo. sin ligamenta epididymidis (inferius et superius) [TA].

epihyal l., l. estilo-hióideo. sin stylohyoid l.

external collateral l. of wrist, l. colateral radial do carpo. sin radial collateral l. of wrist joint.

extracapsular l.'s [TA], ligamentos extracapsulares; os ligamentos associados de uma articulação sinovial, mas separados e externos à sua cápsula articular. sin ligamenta extracapsularia [TA].

falciform l., processo falciforme do l. sacrotuberal. sin falciform process of sacrotuberous ligament.

falciform l. of liver [TA], l. falciforme do fígado; uma prega em crescente do peritônio que se estende até a superfície do fígado a partir do diafragma e da parede abdominal anterior; o ligamento redondo situa-se em sua borda livre, derivado do mesogástrio ventral embrionário. sin ligamentum falciforme hepatis [TA].

fallopian l., ligamento de Falópio. sin inguinal l.

Ferrein l., l. de Ferrein. sin lateral l. of temporomandibular joint.

fibular collateral l. [TA], l. colateral fibular; o l. semelhante a um cordão que passa do epicôndilo lateral do fêmur até a cabeça da fíbula. sin ligamentum collaterale fibulare [TA], lateral l. of knee, Winslow l.

fibular collateral l. of ankle, l. colateral lateral da articulação talocrural. sin lateral l. of ankle.

Flood l., l. de Flood; uma faixa do ligamento coracoumeral, inserida na parte inferior da tuberosidade menor do úmero.

fundiform l. of clitoris [TA], l. fundiforme do clitóris; a condensação fibrosa do tecido subcutâneo que desce a partir da linha alba, acima da sínfise púbica, para se desdobrar e circundar a raiz do corpo do clitóris, antes de se fundir com a fáscia do clitóris. sin ligamentum fundiforme clitoridis [TA].

fundiform l. of foot, l. de Retzius. sin Retzius l.

fundiform l. of penis [TA], l. fundiforme do pênis; uma faixa de fibras elásticas da camada superficial da fáscia a partir da linha alba, acima da sínfise pubiana, desdobrando-se para circundar o pênis antes de se ligar à fáscia do pênis. sin ligamentum fundiforme penis [TA].

gastrocolic l. [TA], l. gastrocólico; a porção principal do omento maior, semelhante a um aventu, que se estende entre o estômago e o colo transverso. sin ligamentum gastrocolicum [TA].

gastrodiaphragmatic l., l. gastrofrênico. sin gastrophrenic l.

gastrolienal l., l. gastroesplênico. sin gastrosplenic l.

gastrophrenic l. [TA], l. gastrofrênico; a porção do omento maior que se estende desde a curvatura maior do estômago até a superfície inferior do diafragma. sin ligamentum gastrophrenicum [TA], gastrodiaphragmatic l., phrenogastric l.

gastrosplenic l. [TA], l. gastroesplênico; a porção do omento maior que se situa entre a curvatura maior do estômago e o hilo do baço. sin ligamentum gastrosplenicum [TA], ligamentum gastrolienale*, gastrolienal l., gastrosplenic omentum.

genital l., l. suspensor das gônadas; uma faixa mesenquimatosa embrionária que fornece a sustentação para a genitália interna. sin suspensory l. of gonad.

genitoinguinal l., l. genito-inguinal; no feto, uma prega do mesocórdio que contém o gubernáculo do testículo. sin ligamentum genitoinguinale, plica gubernatrix.

Gerdy l., l. de Gerdy. sin suspensory l. of axilla.

Gillette suspensory l., l. suspensor de Gillette. sin cricoesophageal tendon.

Gimbernat l., l. de Gimbernat. sin lacunar l.

gingivodental l., periodonto. sin periodontium.

glenohumeral l.'s [TA], ligamentos glenoumerais; três faixas fibrosas (ligamentos capsulares) que reforçam a parte anterior da cápsula articular do ombro; estão em continuidade com o lábio glenóide no tubérculo supraglenóide da escápula e misturam-se com a cápsula fibrosa quando se insere no colo anatômico do úmero; são perceptíveis como pregas ou cristas na face interna da cápsula articular. sin ligamenta glenohumeralia [TA].

glenoid l., (1) labioglenoidal. sin glenoid labrum of scapula; (2) ligamentos plantares. sin plantar l.'s.

glossoepiglottic l., l. glossoepiglótico; uma faixa ligamentosa elástica que se origina da base da língua até a epiglote na prega glossoepiglótica média.

Günz l., l. de Günz; uma porção da camada superficial da membrana obturadora.

hammock l., l. de rede; a parte do l. periodontal abaixo da extremidade crescente da raiz do dente.

l. of head of femur [TA], l. da cabeça do fêmur; um l. achatado que se origina da fóvea na cabeça do fêmur até as bordas da incisura do acetábulo (l. transverso do acetábulo); durante o desenvolvimento, uma artéria dirige-se para a cabeça do fêmur com o l., que pode ou não persistir na vida adulta; o l. não contribui para a integridade da articulação nem controla os movimentos nesse local. sin ligamentum capitis femoris [TA], ligamentum teres femoris, round l. of femur.

Helmholtz axis l., l. do eixo de Helmholtz; um l. que forma o eixo sobre o qual roda o martelo; consiste em duas porções que se estendem desde a borda anterior e posterior, respectivamente, da incisura timpânica até o martelo. sin axis l. of malleus.

Hensing l., l. de Hensing; o l. cólico superior esquerdo; uma pequena prega horizontal ou oblíqua serosa por vezes encontrada entre a extremidade superior do colo descendente e a parede abdominal. ver phrenicocolic l.

hepatocolic l. [TA], l. hepatocólico; uma extensão inconstante do l. hepatoduodenal até o colo transverso. sin ligamentum hepatocolicum [TA].

hepatoduodenal l. [TA], l. hepatoduodenal; a porção do omento menor que une o fígado e o duodeno. sin ligamentum hepatoduodenale [TA].

hepatoesophageal l. [TA], l. hepatoesofágico; a parte do omento menor que se estende entre o fígado e a parte abdominal do esôfago. sin ligamentum hepatoesophageum [TA].

hepatogastric l. [TA], l. hepatogástrico; a parte do omento menor que se estende entre o fígado e a curvatura menor do estômago. sin ligamentum hepatogastricum [TA].

hepatorenal l. [TA], l. hepatorrenal; um prolongamento do l. coronário para baixo, sobre o rim direito. sin ligamentum hepatorenale [TA].

Hesselbach l., l. de Hesselbach. sin interfoveolar l.

Hey ligament, ligamento de Hey. sin superior horn of falciform margin of saphenous opening.

Holl l., l. de Holl; l. que une o corpo cavernoso do clitóris na frente do meato urinário.

Hueck l., l. de Hueck. sin trabecular tissue of sclera.

Humphry l., l. de Humphry. sin anterior meniscofemoral l.

Hunter l., l. de Hunter. sin round l. of uterus.

hyalocapsular l., l. hialoideocapsular; inserção do corpo vítreo na superfície posterior da lente do olho. sin ligamentum hyaloideo-capsulare.

hyoepiglottic l. [TA], l. hioepiglótico; uma curta faixa elástica que une a epiglote à borda superior do osso hióide. sin ligamentum hyoepiglotticum [TA].

hypsiloid l., l. iliofemoral. sin iliofemoral l.

iliofemoral l. [TA], l. iliofemoral; um l. triangular preso por seu ápice na espinha ântero-inferior do ílio e na borda do acetábulo, e, por sua base, à linha intertrocantérica anterior do fêmur; a faixa medial forte está presa à parte inferior da linha intertrocantérica; a forte parte lateral fixa-se ao tubérculo na parte superior dessa linha; a faixa diverge, formando uma figura semelhante a um Y com uma área fraca entre os ramos; entre o mais forte dos ligamentos do corpo, limita a extensão na articulação do quadril. sin ligamentum iliofemorale [TA], Bertin l., Bigelow l., hypsiloid l., Y-shaped l.

iliolumbar l. [TA], l. iliolombar; o forte l. que une a quarta e a quinta vértebras lombares ao ílio, cobrindo a "incisura" entre a coluna vertebral e a asa do ílio. sin ligamentum iliolumbale [TA].

iliopectineal l., arco iliopectíneo. sin iliopectineal arch.

iliotrochanteric l., l. iliotrocantérico; a forte faixa lateral do l. iliofemoral em forma de Y; está presa abaixo do tubérculo, na parte superior da linha intertrocantérica.

inferior calcaneonavicular l., l. calcaneonavicular plantar. sin plantar calcaneonavicular l.

inferior l. of epididymis [TA], l. inferior do epidídimo; a mais inferior das pregas da túnica vaginal entre o corpo do epidídimo e o testículo. sin ligamentum epididymidis inferius [TA].

inferior pubic l. [TA], l. púbico inferior; o l. que se arqueia através da face inferior da sínfise púbica. sin ligamentum pubicum inferius [TA], arcuate pubic l., ligamentum arcuatum pubis.

inferior transverse scapular l. [TA], l. transverso inferior da escápula; uma faixa fibrosa inconstante que se origina da borda lateral da coluna vertebral da escápula até a margem posterior da cavidade glenóide. sin ligamentum transversum scapulae inferius [TA], spinoglenoid l.

infundibulo-ovarian l., l. fímbrias ovarianas. sin ovarian fimbria.

infundibulopelvic l., l. suspensor do ovário. sin suspensory l. of ovary.

inguinal l. [TA], l. inguinal; uma faixa fibrosa formada pela borda inferior espessada da aponeurose do músculo oblíquo externo que se estende desde a espinha ântero-superior do ílio até o tubérculo púbico, cobrindo as lacunas muscular e vascular; forma o assoalho do canal inguinal, dá origem às fibras mais inferiores dos músculos oblíquo interno e transverso do abdome. VER TAMBÉM *aponeurosis* of external oblique muscle. SIN ligamentum inguinale [TA], arcus inguinalis*, crural arch, fallopian arch, fallopian l., femoral arch, Poupart l.

inguinal l. of the kidney, l. inguinal do rim; o segmento do mesonefro que se estende até a região inguinal.

intercarpal l.'s [TA], ligamentos intercarpais; três grupos de feixes fibrosos curtos que se ligam, em conjunto, com as duas fileiras de ossos carpais; de acordo com suas localizações, são denominados ligamentos intercarpais dorsais (ligamenta intercarpalia dorsalia), ligamentos intercarpais interósseos (ligamenta intercarpalia interossea) e ligamentos intercarpais palmares (ligamenta intercarpalia palmaria). SIN ligamenta intercarpalia [TA].

interclavicular l. [TA], l. interclavicular; um l. forte que une as duas articulações esternoclaviculares através da borda superior do manúbrio. SIN ligamentum interclaviculare [TA].

interclinoid l., l. interclinóide; uma faixa de dura-máter que une os processos clinóides anterior e posterior do osso esfenóide; pode tornar-se ossificado.

intercornual l., l. sacrococcígeo lateral. SIN lateral sacrococcygeal l.

intercostal l.'s, membranas intercostais. SIN intercostal *membranes*, em *membrane*.

intercuneiform l.'s [TA], ligamentos intercuneiformes; as faixas fibrosas que unem os ossos cuneiformes; estão dispostos em três grupos: ligamentos intercuneiformes dorsais (ligamenta intercuneiformia dorsalia), ligamentos intercuneiformes interósseos (ligamenta intercuneiformia interossea) e ligamentos intercuneiformes plantares (ligamenta intercuneiformia plantaria). SIN ligamenta intercuneiformia [TA].

interfoveolar l. [TA], l. interfoveolar; filamentos fibrosos ou musculares que se situam medialmente ao anel inguinal profundo, estendendo-se desde a borda inferior do músculo transverso até o l. lacunar e a fáscia pectínea. SIN ligamentum interfoveolare [TA], Hesselbach l.

internal collateral l. of the wrist, l. colateral ulnar do punho. SIN ulnar collateral l. of wrist joint.

interosseous cuneocuboid l., l. cuneocubóideo interósseo. SIN cuneocuboid interosseous l.

interosseous cuneometatarsal l.'s, ligamentos cuneometatarsais interósseos. SIN cuneometatarsal interosseous l.'s.

interosseous metacarpal l.'s [TA], ligamentos metacarpais interósseos; faixas fibrosas que unem as bases do segundo ao quinto metacarpais; estendem-se entre os ligamentos metacarpais dorsais e palmares. SIN ligamenta metacarpalia interossea [TA].

interosseous metatarsal l.'s, ligamentos metatarsais interósseos. SIN metatarsal interosseous l.'s.

interosseous sacroiliac l.'s [TA], ligamentos sacroilíacos interósseos; faixas fibrosas curtas, dirigidas obliquamente, que passam entre o sacro e o ílio na estreita fenda atrás das superfícies auriculares desses ossos. SIN ligamenta sacroiliaca interossea [TA].

interosseous talocalcaneal l., l. talocalcâneo interósseo. SIN talocalcaneal interosseous l.

interosseous tibiofibular l., l. tibiofibular interósseo; a continuação distal da membrana interóssea, formando um l. forte, que une a extremidade distal da tíbia e fíbula; localiza-se profundamente ao l. tibiofibular posterior. SIN transverse tibiofibular l.

interspinous l., l. interespinal; faixas de tecido fibroso que unem os processos espinhosos das vértebras adjacentes. SIN ligamentum interspinale [TA].

intertransverse l., l. intertransversário; um dos ligamentos que unem os processos transversos das vértebras adjacentes. SIN ligamentum intertransversarium [TA].

intraarticular l. of costal head, l. intra-articular da cabeça da costela. SIN intraarticular l. of head of rib.

intraarticular l. of head of rib [TA], l. intra-articular da cabeça da costela; fibras transversas que se estendem dentro da cápsula, desde a crista entre as duas facetas na cabeça da costela até o disco intervertebral. SIN intraarticular l. of costal head, ligamentum capitis costae intraarticulare.

intraarticular sternocostal l. [TA], l. esternocostal intra-articular; um l. dentro da cápsula articular entre uma cartilagem costal e o esterno; especialmente bem desenvolvido na segunda cartilagem costal. SIN ligamentum sternocostale intraarticulare [TA].

intracapsular l.'s [TA], ligamentos intracapsulares; ligamentos localizados dentro e separados da cápsula articular de uma articulação sinovial. SIN ligamenta intracapsularia [TA].

ischiocapsular l., l. isquiofemoral. SIN ischiofemoral.

ischiofemoral l. [TA], l. isquiofemoral; a parte espessada da cápsula da articulação do quadril que se origina do ísquio, dirigindo-se para cima e lateralmente por sobre o colo do fêmur; parte de suas fibras continuam para dentro da zona orbicular. SIN ligamentum ischiofemorale [TA], ischiocapsular l., ligamentum ischiocapsulare.

jugal l., l. cricofaríngeo. SIN cricopharyngeal l.

Krause l., l. de Krause. SIN transverse perineal l.

laciniate l., retináculo dos músculos flexores dos membros inferiores. SIN flexor *retinaculum* of lower limb.

lacunar l. [TA], l. lacunar; uma faixa fibrosa curva que passa horizontalmente para trás da extremidade medial do l. inguinal até a linha pectínea; forma o limite medial do anel femoral. VER TAMBÉM *aponeurosis* of external oblique muscle. SIN ligamentum lacunare [TA], Gimbernat l.

Lannelongue l.'s, ligamentos de Lannelongue. SIN sternopericardial l.'s.

lateral l. of ankle [TA], l. colateral lateral; o l. calcaneofibular, l. talofibular anterior e l. talofibular posterior que mantêm, em conjunto, a integridade da face lateral da articulação talocrural. SIN ligamentum collaterale laterale [TA], fibular collateral l. of ankle, lateral collateral l. of ankle.

lateral arcuate l. [TA], l. arqueado lateral; espessamento da fáscia do músculo quadrado do lombo entre o processo transverso da primeira vértebra lombar e a décima segunda costela de cada lado que fornece a inserção de uma porção do diafragma (um dos arcos de Haller). SIN ligamentum arcuatum laterale [TA], arcus lumbocostalis lateralis, lateral lumbocostal arch.

lateral l. of bladder, l. lateral vesical; condensações do tecido fibroareolar que se originam de cada lado da bexiga para uni-la com a fáscia pélvica; usualmente existe músculo liso nesse tecido e é referido como retovesical (músculo retovesical). SIN ligamentum laterale vesicae [TA].

lateral collateral l. of ankle, l. colateral lateral da articulação talocrural. SIN lateral l. of ankle.

lateral costotransverse l. [TA], l. costotransversário lateral; um l. quadrangular curto, na realidade um espessamento da face posterior da articulação costotransversária, que se estende desde a extremidade do processo transverso até a superfície posterior do colo da costela. SIN ligamentum costotransversarium laterale [TA], ligamentum costotransversarium posterius, ligamentum tuberculi costae, posterior costotransverse l.

lateral l. of elbow, l. colateral lateral do cotovelo. SIN radial collateral l. of elbow joint.

lateral l. of knee, l. lateral fibular. SIN fibular collateral l.

lateral malleolar l., l. tibiofibular. VER anterior tibiofibular l., posterior tibiofibular l.

lateral l. of malleus [TA], l. lateral do martelo; um l. curto, em formato de leque, que converge da metade posterior da incisura timpânica para o colo do martelo. SIN ligamentum mallei laterale [TA].

lateral palpebral l. [TA], l. palpebral lateral; a faixa que liga as placas tarsais à eminência orbitária do osso zigomático. SIN ligamentum palpebrale laterale [TA], ligamentum palpebrale externum, ligamentum tarsale externum.

lateral puboprostatic l., l. lateral puboprostático; *termo oficial alternativo para puboprostatic l. VER puboprostatic l.

lateral sacrococcygeal l. [TA], l. sacrococcígeo lateral; um l. que se estende desde a margem inferior lateral do sacro até o processo transverso da primeira vértebra coccígea. SIN ligamentum sacrococcygeum laterale [TA], intercornual l.

lateral talocalcaneal l. [TA], l. talocalcâneo lateral; um l. que se estende desde a tróclea do tálus até a superfície lateral do calcâneo. SIN ligamentum talocalcaneum laterale [TA].

lateral temporomandibular l., l. lateral da articulação temporomandibular. SIN lateral l. of temporomandibular joint.

lateral l. of temporomandibular joint [TA], l. lateral da articulação temporomandibular; o l. capsular que avança obliquamente para baixo e para trás através da superfície lateral da articulação temporomandibular. SIN ligamentum laterale articulationis temporomandibularis [TA], Ferrein l., lateral temporomandibular l., ligamentum temporomandibulare, temporomandibular l.

lateral thyrohyoid l. [TA], l. tireo-hióideo lateral; o feixe elástico espessado que une o corno superior da cartilagem tireóidea à ponta do corno maior do osso hióide; forma a borda posterior da membrana tireóidea. SIN ligamentum thyrohyoideum laterale [TA], Berry l.'s, ligamentum hyothyroideum laterale.

lateral umbilical l., l. umbilical mediano. SIN *ligamentum* umbilicale laterale.

lateral l. of wrist, l. colateral lateral do carpo. SIN radial collateral l. of wrist joint.

Lauth l., l. de Lauth. SIN transverse l. of the atlas.

l. of left superior vena cava, l. da veia cava superior esquerda; a veia cava comum esquerda obliterada que se estende desde a veia braquiocefálica esquerda até a veia oblíqua do átrio esquerdo.

left triangular l. of liver [TA], l. triangular esquerdo do fígado; uma prega triangular de tecido conjuntivo fibroso e peritônio que se estende desde o lobo esquerdo do fígado até o diafragma. SIN ligamentum triangulare sinistrum hepatis [TA].

l. of left vena cava [TA], l. da veia cava esquerda; a veia cava comum esquerda obliterada; estende-se desde a veia braquiocefálica esquerda até a veia oblíqua do átrio esquerdo. SIN ligamentum venae cavae sinistrae [TA].

lienophrenic l., l. frenoesplênico. SIN phrenicosplenic l.

lienorenal l., l. esplenorrenal; *termo oficial alternativo para splenorenal l.

Lisfranc l.'s, ligamentos de Lisfranc. SIN cuneometatarsal interosseous l.'s.

Lockwood l., l. de Lockwood. SIN suspensory l. of eyeball.

longitudinal l.'s, ligamentos longitudinais; uma das duas extensas faixas fibrosas que acompanham o comprimento da coluna vertebral: o l. longitudinal anterior e o l. longitudinal posterior. VER TAMBÉM anterior longitudinal l., posterior longitudinal l. SIN ligamenta longitudinalia.

long plantar l. [TA], l. plantar longo; um forte l. que se estende desde o calcâneo até o cubóide e os metatarsais laterais na face plantar do pé; parte do sistema de sustentação passiva para a manutenção do arco longitudinal do pé. SIN ligamentum plantare longum [TA].

lumbocostal l. [TA], l. lombocostal; uma faixa forte que une a décima segunda costela com as extremidades dos processos transversos da primeira e segunda vértebras lombares. SIN ligamentum lumbocostale [TA].

Luschka l.'s, ligamentos de Luschka. SIN sternopericardial l.'s.

Mackenrodt l., l. de Mackenrodt. SIN cardinal l.

l.'s of malleus, ligamentos do martelo. VER anterior l. of malleus, lateral l. of malleus, superior l. of malleus.

Mauchart l.'s, ligamentos de Mauchart. VER alar l.'s.

Meckel l., l. de Meckel. SIN Meckel band.

medial l. of ankle joint [TA], l. colateral medial da articulação talocrural; l. composto que consiste em quatro ligamentos componentes, os quais passam para baixo, desde o maléolo medial da tíbia até os ossos do tarso: 1) parte tibionavicular (pars tibionavicularis [NA]), 2) parte tibiocalcânea (pars tibiocalcanea [NA]), 3) parte tibiotalar anterior (pars tibiotalaris anterior [NA]) e 4) parte tibiotalar posterior (pars tibiotalaris posterior [NA]). SIN ligamentum collaterale mediale [TA], deltoid l.*, ligamentum deltoideum*, ligamentum mediale articulationis talocruralis, medial l. of talocrural joint, tibial collateral l. of ankle joint.

medial arcuate l. [TA], l. arqueado medial; um dos arcos de Haller; um espessamento tendinoso da fáscia do psoas que se estende desde o corpo da primeira vértebra lombar até seu processo transverso de cada lado. Uma parte do diafragma origina-se dele. SIN ligamentum arcuatum mediale [TA], arcus lumbocostalis medialis, medial lumbocostal arch.

medial canthal l., l. palpebral medial. SIN medial palpebral l.

medial collateral l. of elbow, l. colateral ulnar do cotovelo. SIN ulnar collateral l. of elbow joint.

medial l. of knee, l. colateral tibial. SIN tibial collateral l.

medial palpebral l. [TA], l. palpebral medial; a faixa fibrosa que une as extremidades mediais das placas tarsais até a maxila na margem orbital medial. SIN ligamentum palpebrale mediale [TA], ligamentum tarsale internum, medial canthal l., tendo oculi, tendo palpebrarum.

medial puboprostatic l., l. pubovesical (masculino); *termo oficial alternativo para pubovesical l. (of male).

medial talocalcaneal l. [TA], l. talocalcâneo medial; um l. que se estende da tuberosidade medial do processo posterior do tálus e o sustentáculo do tálus. SIN ligamentum talocalcaneum mediale [TA].

medial l. of talocrural joint, l. colateral do pé medial. SIN medial l. of ankle joint.

medial l. of temporomandibular joint [TA], l. medial da articulação temporomandibular; o feixe intracapsular de fibras que fortalecem a parte medial da cápsula articular da articulação temporomandibular; não tão evidente quanto o ligamento lateral. SIN ligamentum mediale articulationis temporomandibularis [TA].

medial umbilical l., l. umbilical mediano. SIN cord of umbilical àrtery.

medial l. of wrist, l. colateral ulnar do punho. SIN ulnar collateral l. of wrist joint.

median arcuate l. [TA], l. arqueado mediano; uma conexão tendinosa entre o pilar do diafragma que se arqueia sobre a aorta, formando a margem ânterosuperior do hiato aórtico. SIN ligamentum arcuatum medianum [TA].

median cricothyroid l. [TA], l. cricotireóideo mediano; uma forte faixa que une as cartilagens cricóidea e tireóidea na linha média, anteriormente; continua posteriormente com o cone elástico.

median thyrohyoid l. [TA], l. tireo-hióideo mediano; a porção central espessada da membrana tireoióidea. SIN ligamentum thyrohyoideum medianum [TA], ligamentum hyothyroideum medium.

median umbilical l. [TA], l. umbilical mediano; o resquício do úraco, contido na prega umbilicai mediana; persiste como um cordão fibroso na linha média, entre o ápice da bexiga e o umbigo. SIN ligamentum umbilicale medianum [TA], middle umbilical l., urachal l.

meniscofemoral l.'s [TA], ligamentos meniscofemorais; um dos dois ligamentos que se estendem desde a parte posterior do menisco lateral até a superfície lateral do menisco medial: l. meniscofemoral anterior e l. meniscofemoral posterior. VER TAMBÉM anterior meniscofemoral l., posterior meniscofemoral l. SIN ligamenta meniscofemoralia [TA].

metatarsal interosseous l.'s [TA], ligamentos metatarsais interósseos; faixas fibrosas que unem as bases dos metatarsais; estendem-se entre os ligamentos metatarsais dorsal e plantar. SIN ligamenta metatarsalia interossea [TA], interosseou metatarsal l.'s.

middle costotransverse l., l. costotransversário. SIN costotransverse l.

middle umbilical l., l. umbilical mediano. SIN median umbilical l.

nuchal l., l. nucal; *termo oficial alternativo para *ligamentum* nuchae.

oblique l. of elbow joint, corda oblíqua da sindesmose radioulnar. SIN oblique cord of interosseous membrane of forearm.

oblique popliteal l. [TA], l. poplíteo oblíquo; tendão refletido da inserção do músculo semimembranoso; uma faixa fibrosa que se estende através da parte posterior do joelho, desde sua separação do tendão direto da inserção no côndilo medial da tíbia até o côndilo lateral do fêmur. SIN ligamentum popliteum obliquum [TA], Bourgery l.

occipitoaxial l.'s, ligamentos occipitoaxiais; os ligamentos que unem o áxis ao osso occipital. VER alar l.'s, apical l. of dens.

orbicular l., l. anular. SIN anular l.

orbicular l. of radius, l. anular do rádio. SIN anular l. of radius.

ovarian l., l. útero-ovárico. SIN l. of ovary.

l. of ovary [TA], l. útero-ovárico; um feixe de fibras, semelhante a um cordão, que passa até o lado do útero, a partir da extremidade inferior do ovário, entre as pregas do l. largo (mesovário). SIN ligamentum ovarii proprium [TA], ligamentum uteroovaricum*, ovarian l., proper l. of ovary.

palmar l.'s [TA], ligamentos palmares; as placas fibrocartilaginosas, uma localizada na face anterior de cada articulação metacarpofalângica e interfalângica, que são firmemente presas às bases das falanges e às cabeças dos ossos proximais a seguir; essas placas são sulcadas para acomodar os tendões dos flexores longos. VER TAMBÉM palmar l.'s of interphalangeal joints of hand, palmar l.'s of metacarpophalangeal joints. SIN ligamenta palmaria [TA], accessory volar l.'s.

palmar carpal l., retináculo dos músculos flexores do membro superior. SIN antebrachial flexor *retinaculum*.

palmar carpometacarpal l.'s [TA], ligamentos carpometacarpais palmares; as faixas fibrosas que unem as superfícies palmares dos ossos do carpo e os metacarpais. SIN ligamenta carpometacarpalia palmaria [TA].

palmar l.'s of interphalangeal joints of hand [TA], ligamentos palmares das articulações interfalângicas da mão; os ligamentos localizados na face anterior (palmar) das articulações interfalângicas dos dedos, flanqueados por e unidos aos ligamentos colaterais, formando a porção anterior da cápsula articular; mais leves, porém similares em estrutura e função aos ligamentos palmares das articulações metacarpofalângicas. VER TAMBÉM palmar l.'s of metacarpophalangeal joints. SIN ligamenta palmaria articulationis interphalangeae manus [TA].

palmar metacarpal l.'s [TA], ligamentos metacarpais palmares; faixas fibrosas que unem as faces palmares das bases do segundo ao quinto metacarpos. SIN ligamenta metacarpalia palmaria [TA].

palmar l.'s of metacarpophalangeal joints [TA], ligamentos palmares das articulações metacarpofalângicas; ligamentos espessos, densos, fibrocartilaginosos, localizados na face anterior (palmar) das articulações metacarpofalângicas, flanqueados por e unidos aos ligamentos colaterais, formando a porção anterior da cápsula articular; os ligamentos são sulcados longitudinalmente (em relação ao dedo) para acomodar os tendões do flexor longo dos dedos; em cada lado do sulco, eles são inseridos aos ligamentos metacarpais transversos profundos e às bainhas fibrosas dos dedos; inserem-se firmemente à base das falanges proximais, aprofundando o "encaixe" das bases das falanges para acomodar as cabeças dos metacarpos, aos quais se prendem frouxamente, permitindo a livre movimentação. SIN ligamenta palmaria articulationis metacarpophalangeae [TA], palmar plates.

palmar radiocarpal l. [TA], l. radiocarpal palmar; um forte l. que passa da extremidade distal do rádio até a fileira proximal dos ossos do carpo na superfície anterior da articulação do punho. SIN ligamentum radiocarpale palmare [TA].

palmar ulnocarpal l. [TA], l. ulnocarpal palmar; a faixa fibrosa que passa do processo estilóide da ulna até os ossos do carpo. SIN ligamentum ulnocarpale palmare [TA].

patellar l. [TA], l. da patela; uma forte faixa fibrosa achatada que passa desde o ápice e das bordas adjacentes da patela até a tuberosidade da tíbia; considerado por alguns como sendo parte do tendão do músculo quadríceps femoral, no qual a patela está embebida como um osso sesamóide. SIN ligamentum patellae [TA].

pectinate l.'s of iridocorneal angle, tecido trabecular da esclera. SIN trabecular *tissue* of sclera.

pectinate l.'s of iris, tecido trabecular da esclera. VER trabecular *tissue* of sclera.

pectineal l. [TA], l. pectíneo; uma forte e espessa faixa fibrosa que passa lateralmente, desde o l. lacunar, ao longo da linha pectínea do púbis. Esse tecido fibroso sobre a superfície óssea permite o ponto de apoio de suturas em diversos procedimentos para a reparação de hérnias inguinais. VER TAMBÉM *aponeurosis* of external oblique muscle. SIN ligamentum pectineale [TA], Cooper l.'s (2).

peridental l., periodonto. SIN periodontium.

periodontal l. [TA], periodonto. SIN periodontium.

phrenicocolic l. [TA], l. frenocólico; uma prega triangular do peritônio presa à flexura esquerda do colo e ao diafragma, sobre a qual repousa o pólo inferior ou extremidade do baço. SIN ligamentum phrenicocolicum [TA], costocolic l.

phrenicolienal l., l. frenoesplênico. SIN phrenicosplenic l.

phrenicosplenic l. [TA], l. frenoesplênico; a prega dupla do peritônio (mesentério) que se estende entre o diafragma e o baço; esta é uma porção do omento maior, sendo as distinções entre o ligamento frenoesplênico e os ligamentos adjacentes — todos fazendo parte da mesma lâmina mesentérica — freqüentemente nebulosas. SIN ligamentum phrenicosplenicum [TA], liephrenic l., ligamentum phrenicolienale, phrenicolienal l., phrenosplenic l., sustentaculum lienis.

phrenogastric l., l. gastrofrênico. SIN gastrophrenic l.
phrenosplenic l., l. frenoesplênico. SIN phrenicosplenic l.
pisohamate l. [TA], l. piso-hamato; uma forte faixa fibrosa que se estende desde o osso pisiforme até o hâmulo do osso hamato. SIN ligamentum pisohamatum [TA], pisounciform l., pisouncinate l.
pisometacarpal l. [TA], pisometacarpal; uma forte faixa fibrosa que se estende desde o osso pisiforme até a base do quinto osso metacarpal; esse l., em conjunto com o l. piso-hamato, forma o tendão de inserção do flexor ulnar do carpo, no qual o osso pisiforme é semelhante a um osso sesamóide. SIN ligamentum pisometacarpeum [TA].
pisounciform l., l. piso-hamato. SIN pisohamate l.
pisouncinate l., l. piso-hamato. SIN pisohamate l.
plantar l.'s [TA], ligamentos plantares; placas fibrocartilaginosas localizadas na face plantar de cada articulação metatarsofalângica e interfalângica do pé; os similares no pé dos ligamentos palmares na mão. VER TAMBÉM plantar l.'s of interphalangeal joints of foot, plantar l.'s of metatarsophalangeal joints. SIN ligamenta plantaria [TA], accessory plantar l.'s, Cruveilhier l.'s, glenoid l. (2).
plantar calcaneocuboid l. [TA], l. calcaneocubóideo plantar; uma forte faixa que passa para diante e medialmente, desde a superfície plantar do calcâneo até o osso cubóide, formando, na realidade, uma parte da cápsula articular da articulação calcaneocubóidea; a porção mais curta e mais profunda do ligamento plantar longo. SIN ligamentum calcaneocuboideum plantare [TA].
plantar calcaneonavicular l. [TA], l. calcaneonavicular plantar; um l. fibroelástico denso que se estende desde o sustentáculo do tálus até a superfície plantar do osso navicular; sustenta a cabeça do tálus, fazendo, na realidade, parte do "encaixe" articular para a cabeça do tálus. SIN ligamentum calcaneonaviculare plantare [TA], spring l.*, inferior calcaneonavicular l.
plantar cuboideonavicular l.'s [TA], ligamentos cuboideonaviculares plantares; os ligamentos que unem as superfícies plantares dos ossos cubóide e navicular do tarso. SIN ligamenta cuboideonavicularia plantaria [TA].
plantar cuneocuboid l. [TA], l. cuneocubóideo plantar; a faixa fibrosa que une o ápice do cuneiforme lateral com a margem medial da superfície plantar do cubóide. SIN ligamentum cuneocuboideum plantare [TA].
plantar cuneonavicular l.'s [TA], ligamentos cuneonaviculares plantares; os ligamentos que unem a superfície plantar do navicular com os três ossos cuneiformes. SIN ligamenta cuneonavicularia plantaria [TA].
plantar l.'s of interphalangeal joints of foot [TA], ligamentos plantares das articulações interfalângicas do pé; os ligamentos localizados na face inferior das articulações interfalângicas dos artelhos, flanqueados pelos ligamentos colaterais e unidos a estes, formando a porção plantar da cápsula articular; mais leves, porém semelhantes, em estrutura e função, aos ligamentos palmares das articulações metacarpofalângicas. VER TAMBÉM plantar l.'s of metatarsophalangeal joints. SIN ligamenta plantaria articulationis interphalangeae pedis [TA].
plantar l.'s of metatarsophalangeal joints [TA], ligamentos plantares das articulações metatarsofalângicas; ligamentos espessos e densos na face inferior das articulações metatarsofalângicas, flanqueados pelos ligamentos colaterais e unidos a estes, formando a porção plantar da cápsula articular; os ligamentos são sulcados longitudinalmente (em relação ao dedo) para acomodar os tendões do flexor longo dos dedos; em cada lado do sulco, são presos aos ligamentos metatarsais transversos profundos e às bainhas fibrosas dos artelhos; estão firmemente presos à base das falanges proximais, aprofundando o "encaixe" das bases das falanges para acomodar as cabeças dos metatarsais, nas quais estão frouxamente inseridos, permitindo a livre movimentação. SIN ligamenta plantaria articulationis metatarsophalangeae [TA].
plantar metatarsal l.'s [TA], ligamentos metatarsais plantares; faixas fibrosas que unem as faces plantares dos metatarsos. SIN ligamenta metatarsalia plantaria.
plantar tarsal l.'s [TA], ligamentos plantares dos ligamentos que unem as faces plantares dos ossos do tarso como um grupo; incluídos no grupo estão: o ligamento plantar longo [TA] (ligamentum plantare longum [TA]) e os seguintes ligamentos plantares (ligamentum/a ... plantare/ia): calcaneocubóideo [TA] (calcaneocuboideum [TA]), calcaneonavicular [TA] (calcaneonaviculare [TA]), cuneonavicular [TA] (cuneonavicularia [TA]), cuboideonavicular (cuboideonaviculare [TA], intercuneiforme [TA] (intercuneiformia [TA]) e cuneocubóideo [TA] (cuneocuboideum [TA]). SIN ligamenta tarsi plantaria [TA].
plantar tarsometatarsal l.'s [TA], ligamentos tarsometatarsais plantares; faixas longitudinais e oblíquas que reforçam as faces plantares das articulações tarsometatarsais (articulações entre os metatarsos e os ossos cubóide e cuneiforme); as faixas mediais são mais fortes; elas se tornam cada vez mais fracas lateralmente. SIN ligamenta tarsometatarsalia plantaria [TA].
posterior costotransverse l., l. costotransversário lateral. SIN lateral costotransverse l.
posterior cricoarytenoid l., l. cricoaritenóideo. SIN cricoarythenoid l.

posterior cruciate l. [TA], l. cruzado posterior; o forte cordão fibroso que se estende desde a área intercondilar posterior da tíbia até a parte anterior da superfície lateral do côndilo medial do fêmur. SIN ligamentum cruciatum posterius [TA].
posterior l. of fibular head [TA], l. posterior da cabeça da fíbula; um l. que une a parte posterior da cabeça da fíbula à tíbia. SIN ligamentum capitis fibulae posterius [TA], posterior l. of head of fibula.
posterior l. of head of fibula, l. posterior da cabeça da fíbula. SIN posterior l. of fibular head.
posterior l. of incus [TA], l. posterior da bigorna; faixa ligamentosa que se estende a partir da cruz posterior do estribo. SIN ligamentum incudis posterius [TA].
posterior l. of knee, l. poplíteo arqueado. SIN arcuate popliteal l.
posterior longitudinal l. [TA], l. longitudinal posterior; a faixa fibrosa que interliga as superfícies posteriores dos corpos vertebrais; estreita-se para passar entre os pedículos e abre-se para misturar-se às lamelas externas da face posterior do ânulo fibroso dos discos intervertebrais; forma a parede anterior do canal vertebral. SIN ligamentum longitudinale posterius [TA].
posterior meniscofemoral l. [TA], l. meniscofemoral posterior; a faixa que passa posteriormente até o l. cruzado posterior, estendendo-se entre o côndilo medial do fêmur e o ramo posterior do menisco lateral. SIN ligamentum meniscofemorale posterius [TA], ligamentum cruciatum tertium genus, ligamentum menisci lateralis, Wrisberg l.
posterior occipitoaxial l., membrana tectória (da articulação atlantoaxial mediana). SIN tectorial membrane (of median atlantoaxial joint).
posterior sacroiliac l.'s [TA], ligamentos sacroilíacos posteriores; as fortes faixas fibrosas que passam do ílio até o sacro, posteriores à articulação sacroilíaca. SIN ligamenta sacroiliaca posteriora [TA], dorsal sacroiliac l.'s, ligamentum sacroiliacum posterius.
posterior sacrosciatic l., l. sacrotuberal. SIN sacrotuberous l.
posterior sternoclavicular l. [TA], l. esternoclavicular posterior; uma faixa fibrosa que reforça posteriormente a articulação esternoclavicular. SIN ligamentum sternoclaviculare posterius [TA].
posterior talocalcaneal l. [TA], l. talocalcâneo posterior; o robusto l. localizado imediatamente posterior à porção lateral do l. talocalcâneo interósseo e medial ao l. talocalcâneo lateral na parte mais ampla do seio do tarso. SIN ligamentum talocalcaneum posterius [TA].
posterior talofibular l. [TA], l. talofibular posterior; a faixa fibrosa quase horizontal que se estende desde a borda posterior do tálus até a fossa maleolar. SIN ligamentum talofibulare posterius [TA].
posterior talotibial l., parte talotibial posterior do ligamento colateral medial do pé. SIN tibiotalar part of medial ligament of ankle joint. VER TAMBÉM medial l. of ankle joint.
posterior tibiofibular l. [TA], l. tibiofibular posterior; a faixa fibrosa que cruza horizontalmente a face posterior da sindesmose tibiofibular, contribuindo para a "parede" posterior do "encaixe", que recebe a tróclea do tálus. SIN ligamentum tibiofibulare posterius [TA].
posterior tibiotalar l., parte tibiotalar posterior do ligamento colateral medial do pé. SIN tibiotalar part of medial ligament of ankle joint.
Poupart l., l. de Poupart. SIN inguinal l.
proper l. of ovary, l. útero-ovárico. SIN l. of ovary.
pterygomandibular l., rafe pterigomandibular. SIN pterygomandibular raphe.
pterygospinal l., l. pterigoespinal. SIN pterygospinous l.
pterygospinous l. [TA], l. pterigoespinal; um l. membranoso que se estende a partir da espinha do esfenóide até a parte superior da borda posterior da placa lateral do esfenóide (placa pterigóidea lateral). SIN ligamentum pterygospinale [TA], Civinini l., pterygospinal l.
pubocapsular l., l. pubofemoral. SIN pubofemoral l.
pubofemoral l. [TA], l. pubofemoral; uma parte espessada da cápsula da articulação do quadril que se estende desde o ramo superior do púbis até a linha intertrocantérica do fêmur. SIN ligamentum pubofemorale [TA], ligamentum pubocapsulare, pubocapsular l.
puboprostatic l. [TA], l. puboprostático; o espessamento localizado da fáscia superior do diafragma pélvico, anteriormente, que ancora a próstata e o colo da bexiga ao púbis, em cada lado. Geralmente contém músculo liso. SIN ligamentum puboprostaticum [TA], lateral puboprostatic l.*, Denonvilliers l.
pubovesical l. (of female) [TA], l. pubovesical (do sexo feminino); na mulher, o espessamento fascial compatível com o l. puboprostático, composto dos ligamentos pubovesicais medial e lateral. SIN ligamentum pubovesicale (femininum) [TA].
pubovesical l. (of male) [TA], l. pubovesical (do sexo masculino); a parte mais anterior do arco tendinoso da fáscia pélvica (uma condensação da fáscia superior do diafragma pélvico) que se estende entre a parte inferior da sínfise pubiana e a próstata e bexiga; forma o limite inferior do espaço retropúbico potencial. SIN ligamentum pubovesicale (masculinum) [TA], ligamentum mediale puboprostaticum*, medial puboprostatic l.*.
pulmonary l. [TA], l. pulmonar; prega de duas camadas formada à medida que a pleura mediastinal se reflete por sobre o pulmão, inferior ao hilo pulmonar. SIN ligamentum pulmonale [TA], ligamentum latum pulmonis, Teutleben l.

quadrate l. [TA], l. quadrado; as fibras que passam da margem distal da incisura radial da ulna até o colo do rádio. SIN ligamentum quadratum [TA], Denucé l.

radial collateral l., l. colateral radial do cotovelo. SIN radial collateral l. of elbow joint.

radial collateral l. of elbow joint [TA], l. colateral radial da articulação do cotovelo; o l. que une o epicôndilo lateral do úmero com o l. anular do rádio. SIN ligamentum collaterale radiale articulationis cubiti [TA], lateral l. of elbow, radial collateral l.

radial collateral l. of wrist joint [TA], l. colateral radial da articulação do punho; o l. que se estende distalmente desde o processo estilóide do rádio até os ossos do carpo. SIN ligamentum collaterale carpi radiale articulationis radiocarpalis [TA], external collateral l. of wrist, lateral l. of wrist.

radiate l., l. radiado da cabeça da costela. SIN radiate l. of head of rib.

radiate carpal l. [TA], l. radiado do carpo; o ligamento que se estende desde o osso capitato até o escafóide, lunar e piramidal no lado palmar do punho. SIN ligamentum carpi radiatum [TA], radiate l. of wrist.

radiate l. of head of rib [TA], l. radiado da cabeça da costela; o l. radiado, estrelado ou costovertebral anterior que une a cabeça de cada costela aos corpos das duas vértebras com as quais ela se articula. SIN ligamentum capitis costae radiatum [TA], ligamentum radiatum, radiate l., stellate l.

radiate sternocostal l.'s [TA], ligamentos esternocostais radiados; as fibras da cápsula articular que se irradiam desde as cartilagens costais até a superfície anterior do esterno. SIN ligamenta esternocostalia radiata [TA].

radiate l. of wrist, l. radiado do carpo. SIN radiate carpal l.

reflected inguinal l. [TA], l. reflexo; a porção discretamente reforçada da aponeurose do músculo oblíquo externo, do abdome, formada por fibras derivadas da porção medial do ligamento inguinal de um lado que corre medial e discretamente no sentido superior, definindo a margem inferior do anel inguinal superficial; em seguida, as fibras dirigem-se para a face profunda do ramo medial ipsolateral, cruzando a linha alba e correndo dentro da aponeurose contralateral, em um trajeto paralelo e superior ao ligamento inguinal contralateral. VER TAMBÉM *aponeurosis* of external oblique muscle. SIN ligamentum reflexum [TA], Colles l., fascia triangularis abdominis, reflex l., triangular fascia.

reflex l., l. reflexo. SIN reflected inguinal l.

Retzius l., l. de Retzius; a inserção profunda do retináculo dos músculos extensores no seio tarsal, onde age como uma tipóia para os tendões extensores dos artelhos. SIN fundiform l. of foot.

rhomboid l., l. costoclavicular. SIN costoclavicular l.

right triangular l. of liver [TA], l. triangular direito do fígado; uma prega triangular do peritônio que passa desde o lobo inferior do fígado até o diafragma; é uma formação do l. coronário, formado à medida que o l. coronário faz um ângulo agudo após alcançar seu ponto mais lateral no lado direito, quando circunda a área desnuda do fígado. SIN ligamentum triangulare dextrum hepatis [TA].

ring l., zona orbicular (da articulação do quadril). SIN zona orbicularis (articulationis coxae).

round l. of elbow joint, corda oblíqua da membrana interóssea do antebraço. SIN oblique cord of interosseous membrane of forearm.

round l. of femur, l. da cabeça do fêmur. SIN l. of head of femur.

round l. of liver [TA], l. redondo do fígado; os resquícios da veia umbilical que correm dentro da borda livre do l. falciforme, desde o umbigo até o fígado, onde continua dentro da fissura para o l. redondo até a origem da veia porta esquerda dentro da porta hepática. SIN ligamentum teres hepatis [TA].

round l. of uterus [TA], l. redondo do útero; uma faixa fibromuscular que se insere no útero de cada lado, por diante e por baixo da abertura da tuba uterina; ele passa através do canal inguinal até o lábio maior do pudendo; corresponde ao cordão espermático do homem, no qual passa através do canal inguinal e ganha revestimentos similares, mas não é homólogo, sendo um homólogo do gubernáculo do testículo. SIN ligamentum teres uteri [TA], Hunter l.

sacrodural l., l. sacrodural; um feixe longitudinal de filamentos fibrosos que corre desde a linha média da parte inferior do saco dural até o ligamento longitudinal posterior do sacro. SIN ligamentum sacrodurale.

sacrospinous l. [TA], l. sacroespinal; a faixa fibrosa que passa desde a espinha isquiática até o sacro e o cóccix. SIN ligamentum sacrospinale [TA], anterior sacrosciatic l., ligamentum sacrospinosum.

sacrotuberous l. [TA], l. sacrotuberal; o l. que passa desde a tuberosidade isquiática até o ílio, o sacro e o cóccix, transformando a incisura isquiática no forame isquiático maior, que, então, é subdividido pelo l. sacroespinal. SIN ligamentum sacrotuberale [TA], ligamentum sacrotuberosum, posterior sacrosciatic l.

serous l., l. seroso; uma das inúmeras pregas peritoneais que fixam determinadas vísceras à parede abdominal ou entre si. SIN ligamentum serosum.

sheath l.'s, bainhas fibrosas. VER fibrous *sheaths* of digits of hand, em *sheath*, fibrous digital *sheaths* of toes, em *sheath*, fibrous tendon *sheath*.

Simonart l.'s, ligamentos de Simonart. SIN amnionic band.

skin l.'s [TA], ligamentos cutâneos; um dos inúmeros filamentos fibrosos pequenos que se estendem através da fáscia superficial, ligando a superfície profunda da derme à fáscia profunda subjacente, determinando a mobilidade da pele sobre as estruturas profundas; são especialmente bem desenvolvidos sobre a mama, onde são conhecidos como ligamentos suspensores da mama; também são bem desenvolvidos, porém curtos, nas regiões palmares e plantares. SIN retinaculum cutis [TA], retinaculum of skin.

Soemmerring l., l. de Soemmerring; pequenas fibras que prendem a glândula lacrimal à periórbita.

sphenomandibular l. [TA], l. esfenomandibular; a faixa fibrosa que passa da coluna vertebral do osso esfenóide até a língula da mandíbula; é um suporte passivo primário da mandíbula, servindo como um "eixo de oscilação", permitindo a depressão e a elevação ao redor de um eixo transverso que passa através das duas línguias, enquanto, ao mesmo tempo, permite a protração e a retração. SIN ligamentum sphenomandibulare [TA].

spinoglenoid l., l. transverso inferior da escápula. SIN inferior transverse scapular l.

spiral l. of cochlea, l. espiral do ducto coclear. SIN spiral l. of cochlear duct.

spiral l. of cochlear duct [TA], l. espiral do ducto coclear; o revestimento periósteo espessado da cóclea óssea que forma a parede externa do ducto coclear, na qual se insere a lâmina basilar. SIN ligamentum spirale ductus cochlearis [TA], crista spiralis, ligamentum spirale cochleae, spiral crest, spiral l. of cochlea.

splenorenal l. [TA], l. esplenorrenal; uma prega peritoneal (porção do omento maior) que se estende desde a face anterior do rim esquerdo até o hilo esplênico, conduzindo os vasos esplênicos a partir da parede posterior do corpo até o baço. SIN ligamentum splenorenale [TA], lienorenal l.*, ligamentum lienorenale*.

spring l., l. calcaneonavicular plantar; *termo oficial alternativo para plantar calcaneonavicular l.

Stanley cervical l.'s, ligamentos cervicais de Stanley; fibras da cápsula da articulação do quadril refletidas para o colo do fêmur.

stellate l., l. radiado da cabeça da costela. SIN radiate l. of head of rib.

sternoclavicular l.'s, ligamentos esternoclaviculares; l. que une a clavícula ao manúbrio do esterno. VER anterior sternoclavicular l., posterior sternoclavicular l. SIN ligamenta sternoclavicularia.

sternopericardial l.'s, ligamentos esternopericárdicos; feixes fibrosos que se estendem do pericárdio até o esterno. SIN ligamenta sternopericardiaca [TA], Lannelongue l.'s, Luschka l.'s.

stylohyoid l. [TA], l. estilo-hióideo; um cordão fibroso que passa da extremidade do processo estilóide até o corno menor do osso hióide; ocasionalmente está calcificado. SIN ligamentum stylohyoideum [TA], epihyal l.

stylomandibular l. [TA], l. estilomandibular; uma condensação da fáscia cervical profunda que se estende desde a extremidade do processo estilóide do osso temporal até a borda posterior do ângulo da mandíbula; mistura-se com a bainha parotídea (como um espessamento desta). SIN ligamentum stylomandibulare [TA], stylomaxillary l.

stylomaxillary l., l. estilomandibular. SIN stylomandibular l.

superficial dorsal sacrococcygeal l., l. sacrococcígeo posterior superficial. SIN superficial posterior sacrococcygeal l.

superficial posterior sacrococcygeal l. [TA], l. sacrococcígeo posterior superficial; a continuação do l. supra-espinal, desde o sacro até o cóccix. SIN ligamentum sacrococcygeum posterius superficiale [TA], ligamentum sacrococcygeum dorsale superficiale*, superficial dorsal sacrococcygeal l.

superficial transverse metacarpal l. [TA], l. metacarpal transverso superficial; espessamento da fáscia profunda na parte mais distal da base da aponeurose palmar triangular. SIN ligamentum metacarpale transversum superficiale [TA], Gerdy fibers, ligamentum natatorium.

superficial transverse metatarsal l. [TA], l. metatarsal transverso superficial; um espessamento da parte distal (base) da aponeurose plantar, ao nível das cabeças dos ossos metatarsais. SIN ligamentum metatarsale transversum superficiale [TA].

superior costotransverse l. [TA], l. costotransversário superior; a faixa fibrosa que se estende para cima desde o colo de uma costela até o processo transverso da vértebra superior seguinte. SIN ligamentum costotransversarium superius [TA], anterior costotransverse l., ligamentum costotransversarium anterius.

superior l. of epididymis [TA], l. superior do epidídimo; a mais superior das duas pregas da túnica vaginal entre a cabeça do epidídimo e o testículo. SIN ligamentum epididymidis superius [TA].

superior l. of incus [TA], l. superior da bigorna; conecta o corpo da bigorna com o teto do processo timpânico. SIN ligamentum incudis superius [TA].

superior l. of malleus [TA], l. superior do martelo; um l. que se estende desde a cabeça do martelo até o teto do recesso epitimpânico. SIN ligamentum mallei superius [TA].

superior pubic l. [TA], l. púbico superior; as fibras que passam transversalmente acima da sínfise pubiana. SIN ligamentum pubicum superius [TA].

superior transverse scapular l. [TA], l. transverso superior da escápula; o forte feixe fibroso que cruza a incisura da escápula, criando um forame que dá passagem ao nervo supra-escapular, enquanto os vasos supra-escapulares passam sobre o l. superiormente. SIN ligamentum transversum scapulae superius [TA], suprascapular l.

suprascapular l., l. transverso superior da escápula. SIN superior transverse scapular l.

supraspinous l. [TA], l. supra-espinal; o feixe fibroso longitudinal inserido às extremidades dos processos espinhosos das vértebras; na região cervical, é alterado para formar o ligamento nucal. SIN ligamentum supraspinale [TA].

suspensory l. of axilla [TA], l. suspensor da axila; a continuação da fáscia clavipeitoral para baixo, até se inserir na fáscia axilar; mantém a característica concavidade da axila. SIN ligamentum suspensorium axillae [TA], Campbell l., Gerdy l.

suspensory l.'s of breast [TA], ligamentos suspensores da mama; o retináculo cutâneo bem desenvolvido que se estende desde o estroma fibroso da glândula mamária até a pele sobrejacente. SIN retinaculum cutis mammae*, suspensory retinaculum of breast*, Cooper l.'s (1), ligamenta suspensoria mammaria, suspensory l.'s of Cooper.

suspensory l. of clitoris [TA], uma faixa fibrosa no nível fascial profundo que se estende desde a sínfise púbica até a fáscia profunda do clitóris, ancorando o clitóris à sínfise pubiana. SIN ligamentum suspensorium clitoridis [TA].

suspensory l.'s of Cooper, ligamentos suspensores de Cooper. SIN suspensory l.'s of breast.

suspensory l. of duodenum, músculo suspensor do duodeno; *termo oficial alternativo para suspensory muscle of duodenum.

suspensory l. of esophagus, tendão cricoesofágico. SIN cricoesophageal tendon.

suspensory l. of eyeball [TA], l. suspensor do bulbo do olho; um espessamento da parte inferior da bainha bulbar que suporta o bulbo do olho dentro da órbita; estende-se entre as margens orbitais lateral e medial e inclui os ligamentos controladores medial e lateral. SIN ligamentum suspensorium bulbi [TA], Lockwood l.

suspensory l. of gonad, l. suspensor das gônadas; SIN genital l.

suspensory l. of lens, zônula ciliar. SIN ciliary zonule.

suspensory l. of ovary [TA], l. suspensor do ovário; uma faixa do peritônio que se estende para cima desde o pólo superior do ovário; contém os vasos ovarianos e o plexo ovariano dos nervos. SIN ligamentum suspensorium ovarii [TA], Clado band, infundibulopelvic l.

suspensory l. of penis [TA], l. suspensor do pênis; uma faixa fibrosa na camada fascial profunda, a partir da sínfise púbica até a fáscia profunda do pênis que ancora a raiz do pênis. SIN ligamentum suspensorium penis [TA].

suspensory l. of testis, l. suspensor do testículo; a porção cranial atrófica da crista urogenital presa ao pólo cranial do testículo embrionário intra-abdominal.

suspensory l. of thyroid gland [TA], l. suspensor da glândula tireóide; uma das várias faixas fibrosas que passam desde a bainha da glândula tireóide até as cartilagens cricóidea e tireóidea. SIN ligamentum suspensorium glandulae thyroideae [TA].

sutural l., l. sutural; uma membrana delicada que liga os ossos nas suturas cranianas.

synovial l., sinovial; uma das grandes pregas sinoviais em uma articulação.

talocalcaneal l. [TA], l. talocalcâneo; qualquer um dos três ligamentos que unem o tálus ao calcâneo: l. talocalcâneo interósseo, l. talocalcâneo lateral e l. talocalcâneo medial. SIN ligamentum talocalcaneum [TA].

talocalcaneal interosseous l. [TA], l. talocalcâneo interósseo; uma forte faixa fibrosa que ocupa o seio tarsal; um dos três ligamentos interósseos do tarso. SIN interosseous talocalcaneal l., ligamentum talocalcaneare interosseum.

talonavicular l. [TA], l. talonavicular; um dos ligamentos dorsais do tarso, os quais ocorrem como um amplo hiato que passa desde o lado dorsal do colo do tálus até a superfície dorsal do osso navicular. SIN ligamentum talonaviculare [TA].

tarsal l.'s [TA], ligamentos do tarso; os ligamentos que interligam os ossos do tarso; eles são reunidos em três grupos: ligamentos dorsais do tarso, ligamentos interósseos do tarso e ligamentos plantares do tarso, sendo nomeados individualmente de acordo com suas inserções. SIN ligamenta tarsi [TA].

tarsal interosseous l.'s, ligamentos interósseos do tarso; os ligamentos mais profundos, localizados entre os ossos do tarso, interligando-os entre si; o grupo inclui os ligamentos interósseos talocalcâneo, cuneocubóideo e intercuneiforme. SIN ligamenta tarsi interossea [TA].

tarsometatarsal l.'s [TA], ligamentos tarsometatarsais; os ligamentos que unem os ossos tarsais e metatarsais; estão dispostos nos grupos interósseos dorsal, plantar e cuneometatarsais. SIN ligamenta tarsometatarsalia [TA].

temporomandibular l., l. lateral da articulação temporomandibular. SIN lateral l. of temporomandibular joint.

Teutleben l., l. de Teutleben. SIN pulmonary l.

Thompson l., l. de Thompson. SIN iliopubic tract.

thyroepiglottic l. [TA], l. tireoepiglótico; uma faixa elástica que une o pecíolo epiglótico ao interior da cartilagem tireóidea próximo à incisura tireóidea superior. SIN ligamentum thyroepiglotticum [TA].

tibial collateral l. [TA], l. colateral tibial; a larga faixa fibrosa que passa desde o epicôndilo medial do fêmur até a margem medial e superfície medial da tíbia; o menisco medial está inserido à sua superfície profunda; é contínuo com cápsula fibrosa da articulação do joelho (como um espessamento desta). SIN ligamentum collaterale tibiale [TA], medial l. of knee.

tibial collateral l. of ankle joint, l. colateral medial. SIN medial l. of ankle joint.

tibiocalcaneal l., parte tibiocalcânea do ligamento colateral medial. SIN tibiocalcaneal part of medial ligament of ankle joint.

tibiofibular l., l. tibiofibular. VER anterior tibiofibular l., interosseous *membrane* of leg, posterior tibiofibular l. VER TAMBÉM tibiofibular *syndesmosis*.

tibionavicular l., parte tibionavicular do l. colateral medial da articulação talocrural. SIN tibionavicular *part* of medial ligament of ankle joint.

transverse acetabular l. [TA], l. transverso do acetábulo; porção do lábio acetabular que passa através da incisura acetabular. SIN ligamentum transversum acetabuli [TA], transverse l. of acetabulum.

transverse l. of acetabulum, l. transverso do acetábulo. SIN transverse acetabular l.

transverse atlantal l., l. transverso do atlas. SIN transverse l. of the atlas.

transverse l. of the atlas [TA], l. transverso do atlas; faixa espessa e forte, com achatamento central, sobre o forame vertebral do atlas, à medida que se estende desde a face medial de uma massa lateral até a outra, passando dorsalmente ao dente do áxis com o qual se articula; forma a porção dorsal da abertura para o dente do áxis, envolvendo firmemente seu colo. Forma uma parte da "barra transversal" do ligamento cruciforme do atlas. VER TAMBÉM cruciate l. of the atlas. SIN ligamentum transversum atlantis [TA], Lauth l., transverse atlantal l.

transverse carpal l., retináculo dos músculos flexores. SIN flexor *retinaculum*.

transverse cervical l., l. transverso do colo do útero; *termo oficial alternativo para cardinal l.

transverse crural l., retináculo dos músculos extensores. SIN superior extensor *retinaculum*.

transverse l. of elbow, l. transverso do cotovelo; um feixe de fibras que corre desde o olécrano até o processo coronóide em associação com o l. colateral ulnar. SIN Cooper l.'s (3).

transverse genicular l., l. transverso do joelho. SIN transverse l. of knee.

transverse humeral l. [TA], l. transverso do úmero; uma faixa fibrosa que corre mais ou menos obliquamente desde o tubérculo maior até o tubérculo menor do úmero, sobre o sulco bicipital. SIN ligamentum transversum humeri [TA], Brodie l.

transverse l. of knee [TA], l. transverso do joelho; uma faixa transversa que passa entre os meniscos medial e lateral na parte anterior da articulação do joelho. SIN ligamentum transversum genus [TA], transverse genicular l.

transverse l. of leg, retináculo dos músculos extensores. SIN superior extensor *retinaculum*.

transverse metacarpal l., l. metacarpal transverso profundo. SIN deep transverse metacarpal l.

transverse metatarsal l., l. metatarsal transverso profundo. SIN deep transverse metatarsal l.

transverse l. of pelvis, l. transverso do períneo. SIN transverse perineal l.

transverse perineal l. [TA], l. transverso do períneo; a borda anterior espessada da membrana perineal. SIN ligamentum transversum perinei [TA], Krause l., ligamentum transversum pelvis, transverse l. of pelvis, transverse l. of perineum.

transverse l. of perineum, l. transverso do períneo. SIN transverse perineal l.

transverse tibiofibular l., l. tibiofibular interósseo. SIN interosseous tibiofibular l.

trapezoid l. [TA], l. trapezóide; a parte lateral do l. coracoclavicular que se insere na linha trapezóide da clavícula. SIN ligamentum trapezoideum [TA].

Treitz l., l. de Treitz. SIN suspensory *muscle* of duodenum.

triangular l., membrana do períneo. SIN perineal *membrane*.

triangular l.'s of liver, ligamentos triangulares do fígado. VER right triangular l. of liver, left triangular l. of liver.

ulnar collateral l., l. colateral ulnar da articulação do cotovelo. SIN ulnar collateral l. of elbow joint.

ulnar collateral l. of elbow joint [TA], l. colateral ulnar da articulação do cotovelo; o l. triangular que se estende desde o epicôndilo medial do úmero para o lado medial do processo coronóide e olécrano da ulna. SIN ligamentum collaterale ulnare articulationis cubiti [TA], medial collateral l. of elbow, ulnar collateral l.

ulnar collateral l. of wrist joint [TA], l. colateral ulnar do carpo; um l. que passa do processo estilóide da ulna até o pisiforme e tríquetro. SIN internal collateral l. of wrist, ligamentum collaterale carpi ulnare articulationis radiocarpalis, medial l. of wrist.

urachal l., umbilical mediano. SIN median umbilical l.

uterovesical l., prega uterovesical; uma prega peritoneal que se estende desde o útero até a porção posterior da bexiga. SIN plica uterovesicalis, plica vesicouterina, uterovesical fold, vesicouterine l.

Valsalva l.'s, ligamentos de Valsalva. SIN l.'s of auricle.

venous l., l. venoso. SIN *ligamentum* venosum.

ventral sacrococcygeal l., l. sacrococcígeo anterior. SIN anterior sacrococcygeal l.

ventral sacroiliac l.'s, ligamentos sacroilíacos anteriores. SIN anterior sacroiliac l.'s.

ventricular l., l. vestibular. SIN vestibular l.

vertebropelvic l.'s, ligamentos vertebropélvicos. VER iliolumbar l., sacrospinous l., sacrotuberous l.
vesicoumbilical l., um dos ligamentos entre a bexiga urinária e o umbigo. VER median umbilical l., *cord* of umbilical artery.
vesicouterine l., prega uterovesical. SIN uterovesical l.
vestibular l. [TA], l. vestibular; a borda inferior da membrana quadrangular que fica por baixo da prega ventricular da laringe. SIN ligamentum vestibulare [TA], ligamentum ventriculare, ventricular l.
vocal l. [TA], l. vocal; a faixa que se estende, em ambos os lados, desde a cartilagem tireóidea até o processo vocal da cartilagem aritenóidea; é a borda superior livre e espessada do cone elástico da laringe. SIN ligamentum vocale [TA].
volar carpal l., retináculo dos músculos flexores. SIN flexor *retinaculum*.
Weitbrecht l., l. de Weitbrecht. SIN oblique *cord* of interosseous membrane of forearm.
Winslow l., l. de Winslow. SIN fibular collateral l.
Wrisberg l., l. de Wrisberg. SIN posterior meniscofemoral l.
yellow l., l. amarelo. SIN ligamenta flava, em *ligamentum*.
Y-shaped l., l. iliofemoral. SIN iliofemoral l.
Zaglas l., l. de Zaglas; uma faixa fibrosa curta e espessa desde a espinha póstero-superior do ílio até o segundo tubérculo transverso do sacro.
Zinn l., l. de Zinn. SIN common tendinous *ring* of extraocular muscles.

lig·a·men·ta (ligʹă-menʹtă). Ligamentos; plural de ligamentum. [L.]
lig·a·men·to·pex·is, lig·a·men·to·pexy (ligʹă-men-tōʹpekʹsis, -pekʹse). Ligamentopexia; encurtamento de qualquer ligamento do útero. [ligament + G. *pēxis*, fixação]
lig·a·men·tous (ligʹă-menʹtŭs). Ligamentoso; relativo a ou que tem a forma ou estrutura de um ligamento.

LIGAMENTUM

lig·a·men·tum, pl. **lig·a·men·ta** (ligʹă-menʹtŭm, -menʹtă) [TA]. Ligamento, ligamentos. SIN ligament. [L. uma faixa, amarração, de *ligo*, ligar]
l. acromioclavicula're [TA], l. acromioclavicular. SIN acromioclavicular *ligament*.
l. annococcy'geum, l. anococcígeo. SIN anococcygeal *ligament*.
l. anula're [TA], l. anular. SIN anular *ligament*.
l. anula're bul'bi, tecido trabecular da esclera. SIN trabecular *tissue* of sclera.
l. anula're digito'rum, parte anular das bainhas fibrosas dos dedos das mãos e dos pés. SIN anular *part* of fibrous digital sheath of digits of hand and foot.
l. anula're ra'dii [TA], l. anular do rádio. SIN anular *ligament* of radius.
l. anula're stape'dis [TA], l. estapedial anular. SIN anular *ligament* of stapes.
ligamen'ta anula'ria trachea'lia [TA], ligamentos anulares da traquéia. SIN anular *ligaments* of trachea, em *ligament*.
l. ap'icis den'tis, l. do ápice do dente. SIN apical *ligament* of dens.
l. arcua'tum latera'le [TA], l. arqueado lateral. SIN lateral arcuate *ligament*.
l. arcua'tum media'le [TA], l. arqueado medial. SIN medial arcuate *ligament*.
l. arcua'tum media'num [TA], l. arqueado mediano. SIN median arcuate *ligament*.
l. arcua'tum pu'bis, l. púbico inferior. SIN inferior pubic *ligament*.
l. arterio'sum [TA], l. arterial; resquício fibroso do canal arterial que se estende entre o arco aórtico e o tronco pulmonar. SIN arterial ligament, Botallo ligament.
ligamen'ta auricula'ria [TA], ligamentos auriculares. SIN *ligaments* of auricle, em *ligament*.
l. bifurca'tum [TA], l. bifurcado. SIN bifurcate *ligament*.
l. calcaneocuboi'deum [TA], l. calcaneocubóideo. SIN calcaneocuboid *ligament*.
l. calcaneocuboi'deum planta're [TA], l. calcaneocubóideo plantar. SIN plantar calcaneocuboid *ligament*.
l. calcaneofibula're [TA], l. calcaneofibular. SIN calcaneofibular *ligament*.
l. calcaneonavicula're [TA], l. calcaneonavicular. SIN calcaneonavicular *ligament*.
l. calcaneonavicula're planta're [TA], l. calcaneonavicular plantar. SIN plantar calcaneonavicular *ligament*.
l. calcaneotibia'le, parte tibiocalcânea do ligamento colateral medial. SIN tibiocalcaneal *part* of medial ligament of ankle joint. VER TAMBÉM medial *ligament* of ankle joint.
l. cap'itis cos'tae intraarticula're, l. intra-articular da cabeça da costela. SIN intraarticular *ligament* of head of rib.
l. cap'itis cos'tae radia'tum [TA], l. radiado da cabeça da costela. SIN radiate *ligament* of head of rib.
l. cap'itis fem'oris [TA], l. da cabeça do fêmur. SIN *ligament* of head of femur.
l. cap'itis fib'ulae ante'rius [TA], l. anterior da cabeça da fíbula. SIN anterior *ligament* of fibular head.
l. cap'itis fib'ulae poste'rius [TA], l. posterior da cabeça da fíbula. SIN posterior *ligament* of fibular head.
ligamen'ta capitulo'rum transver'sa, ligamentos transversos profundos. VER deep transverse metacarpal *ligament*, deep transverse metatarsal *ligament*.
l. capsula're [TA], l. capsular. SIN capsular *ligament*.
l. cardinale [TA], l. transverso do colo do útero. SIN cardinal *ligament*.
l. car'pi dorsa'le, retináculo dos músculos extensores. SIN extensor *retinaculum*.
l. car'pi radia'tum [TA], l. radiado do carpo. SIN radiate carpal *ligament*.
l. car'pi transver'sum, retináculo dos músculos flexores. SIN flexor *retinaculum*.
l. car'pi vola're, retináculo dos músculos flexores. SIN flexor *retinaculum*.
ligamenta carpometacarpa'lia dorsa'lia [TA], ligamentos carpometacarpais dorsais. SIN dorsal carpometacarpal *ligaments*, em *ligament*.
ligamen'ta carpometacarpa'lia (dorsalia/palmaria) [TA], ligamentos carpometacarpais (dorsal/palmar). SIN carpometacarpal *ligaments* (dorsal and palmar), em *ligament*.
ligamenta carpometacarpa'lia palma'ria [TA], ligamentos carpometacarpais palmares. SIN palmar carpometacarpal *ligaments*, em *ligament*.
l. cauda'le, retináculo caudal. SIN *retinaculum* caudale.
l. ceratocricoi'deum [TA], l. ceratocricóideo. SIN ceratocricoid *ligament*.
l. collatera'le, pl. **ligamen'ta collatera'lia** [TA], l. colateral. SIN collateral *ligament*.
l. collatera'le car'pi radia'le articulationis radiocarpalis [TA], l. colateral radial do carpo. SIN radial collateral *ligament* of wrist joint.
l. collaterale carpi ulnare [TA], **l. collatera'le car'pi ulna're articulationis radiocarpalis,** l. colateral ulnar do carpo. SIN ulnar collateral *ligament* of wrist joint.
l. collatera'le fibula're [TA], l. colateral fibular. SIN fibular collateral *ligament*.
l. collaterale laterale [TA], l. colateral lateral da articulação talocrural. SIN lateral *ligament* of ankle.
l. collaterale mediale [TA], l. colateral medial da articulação talocrural. SIN medial *ligament* of ankle joint.
l. collatera'le radia'le articulationis cubiti [TA], l. colateral radial do cotovelo. SIN radial collateral *ligament* of elbow joint.
l. collatera'le tibia'le [TA], l. colateral tibial. SIN tibial collateral *ligament*.
l. collaterale ulnare articulationis cubiti [TA], l. colateral ulnar do cotovelo. SIN ulnar collateral *ligament* of elbow joint.
l. col'li cos'tae, l. costotransversário. SIN costotransverse *ligament*.
l. conoid'eum [TA], l. conóide. SIN conoid *ligament*.
l. coracoacromia'le [TA], l. coracoacromial. SIN coracoacromial *ligament*.
l. coracoclavicula're [TA], l. coracoclavicular. SIN coracoclavicular *ligament*.
l. coracohumera'le [TA], l. coracoumeral. SIN coracohumeral *ligament*.
l. corniculopharyn'geum, l. cricofaríngeo. SIN cricopharyngeal *ligament*.
l. corona'rium hep'atis [TA], l. coronário do fígado. SIN coronary *ligament* of liver.
l. costoclavicula're [TA], l. costoclavicular. SIN costoclavicular *ligament*.
l. costotransversa'rium [TA], l. costotransversário. SIN costotransverse *ligament*.
l. costotransversa'rium ante'rius, l. costotransversário superior. SIN superior costotransverse *ligament*.
l. costotransversa'rium latera'le [TA], l. costotransversário lateral. SIN lateral costotransverse *ligament*.
l. costotransversa'rium poste'rius [TA], l. costotransversário lateral. SIN lateral costotransverse *ligament*.
l. costotransversa'rium supe'rius [TA], l. costotransversário superior. SIN superior costotransverse *ligament*.
l. costoxiphoi'deum [TA], l. costoxifóideo. SIN costoxiphoid *ligament*.
l. cotyloid'eum [TA], lábio do acetábulo. SIN acetabular *labrum*.
l. cricoarytenoi'deum poste'rius, l. cricoaritenóideo. SIN cricoarytenoid *ligament*.
l. cricopharyn'geum [TA], l. cricofaríngeo. SIN cricopharyngeal *ligament*.
l. cricotrachea'le [TA], l. cricotraqueal. SIN cricotracheal *ligament*.
ligamen'ta crucia'ta digito'rum, parte cruciforme das bainhas fibrosas dos dedos. SIN cruciform *part* of fibrous digital sheath.
ligamen'ta crucia'ta ge'nus, ligamentos cruzados do joelho. SIN cruciate *ligaments* of knee, em *ligament*.
l. crucia'tum ante'rius, l. cruzado anterior. SIN anterior cruciate *ligament*.
l. crucia'tum atlan'tis, l. cruciforme do atlas. SIN cruciate *ligament* of the atlas.
l. crucia'tum cru'ris, retináculo inferior dos músculos extensores. SIN inferior extensor *retinaculum*.
l. crucia'tum poste'rius [TA], l. cruzado posterior. SIN posterior cruciate *ligament*.
l. crucia'tum ter'tium ge'nus, l. meniscofemoral posterior. SIN posterior meniscofemoral *ligament*.
l. crucifor'me atlan'tis [TA], l. cruciforme do atlas. SIN cruciate *ligament* of the atlas.
ligamenta cuboideonaviculare [TA], ligamentos cuboideonaviculares. SIN cuboideonavicular *ligaments*, em *ligament*.

l. cuboideonavicula're dorsa'le [TA], l. cuboideonavicular dorsal. SIN dorsal cuboideonavicular *ligament*.
ligamenta cuboideonavicula'ria planta'ria [TA], ligamentos cuboideonaviculares plantares. SIN plantar cuboideonavicular *ligaments*, em *ligament*.
l. cuneocuboideum [TA], l. cuneocubóideo. SIN cuneocuboid *ligaments*, em *ligament*.
l. cuneocuboideum dorsa'le [TA], l. cuneocubóideo dorsal. SIN dorsal cuneocuboid *ligament*.
l. cuneocuboideum interos'seum, l. cuneocubóideo interósseo. SIN cuneocuboid interosseous *ligament*.
l. cuneocuboideum planta're [TA], l. cuneocubóideo plantar. SIN plantar cuneocuboid *ligament*.
ligamen'ta cuneometatarsa'lia interos'sea [TA], ligamentos cuneometatarsais interósseos. SIN cuneometatarsal interosseous *ligament*, em *ligament*.
ligamen'ta cuneonavicula'ria dorsa'lia [TA], ligamentos cuneonaviculares dorsais. SIN dorsal cuneonavicular *ligaments*, em *ligament*.
l. cuneonavicula'ria planta'ria [TA], ligamentos cuneonaviculares plantares. SIN plantar cuneonavicular *ligaments*, em *ligament*.
l. deltoi'deum, l. colateral medial da articulação talocrural.; *termo oficial alternativo para medial *ligament* of ankle joint.
l. denticula'tum [TA], l. denticulado. SIN denticulate *ligament*.
l. duc'tus veno'si, l. venoso. SIN l. venosum.
l. duodenorena'le, l. duodenorrenal. SIN duodenorenal *ligament*.
ligamenta epididym'idis (inferius et superius) [TA], ligamentos do epidídimo (inferior e superior). SIN ligaments of epididymis (inferior and superior), em *ligament*.
l. epididym'idis infe'rius [TA], l. inferior do epidídimo. SIN inferior *ligament* of epididymis.
l. epididym'idis supe'rius [TA], l. superior do epidídimo. SIN superior *ligament* of epididymis.
ligamen'ta extracapsula'ria [TA], ligamentos extracapsulares. SIN extracapsular *ligaments*, em *ligament*.
l. falcifor'me, processo falciforme do l. sacrotuberal. SIN falciform *process* of sacrotuberous *ligament*.
l. falcifor'me hep'atis [TA], l. falciforme do fígado. SIN falciform *ligament* of liver.
ligamenta fla'va [TA], ligamentos amarelos; ligamentos pareados de tecido fibroso elástico amarelo, que ligam as lâminas de vértebras adjacentes, formando a parede dorsal do canal vertebral entre as vértebras ou lâminas; a penetração do ligamento amarelo com um trocarte durante a punção epidural ou espinal produz uma sensação distinta ("pop"), levando o profissional a saber que a ponta do trocarte penetrou no espaço epidural. SIN yellow ligament.
l. fundiforme clitoridis [TA], l. fundiforme do clitóris. SIN fundiform *ligament* of clitoris.
l. fundifor'me pe'nis [TA], l. fundiforme do pênis. SIN fundiform *ligament* of penis.
l. gastrocol'icum [TA], l. gastrocólico. SIN gastrocolic *ligament*.
l. gastroliena'le, l. gastroesplênico; *termo oficial alternativo para gastrosplenic *ligament*.
l. gastrophren'icum [TA], l. gastrofrênico. SIN gastrophrenic *ligament*.
l. gastrosple'nicum [TA], l. gastroesplênico. SIN gastrosplenic *ligament*.
l. genitoinguina'le, l. genito-inguinal. SIN genitoinguinal *ligament*.
ligamen'ta glenohumera'lia [TA], ligamentos glenoumerais. SIN glenohumeral *ligaments*, em *ligament*.
l. glenoida'le, lábio glenoidal. SIN glenoid *labrum* of scapula.
l. hepatocol'icum [TA], l. hepatocólico. SIN hepatocolic *ligament*.
l. hepatoduodena'le [TA], l. hepatoduodenal. SIN hepatoduodenal *ligament*.
l. hepatoesopha'geum [TA], l. hepatoesofágico. SIN hepatoesophageal *ligament*.
l. hepatogas'tricum [TA], l. hepatogástrico. SIN hepatogastric *ligament*.
l. hepatorena'le [TA], l. hepatorrenal. SIN hepatorenal *ligament*.
l. hyaloi'deo-capsula're, l. hialoideocapsular. SIN hyalocapsular *ligament*.
l. hyoepiglot'ticum [TA], l. hioepiglótico. SIN hyoepiglottic *ligament*.
l. hyothyroi'deum latera'le, l. tireo-hióideo lateral. SIN lateral thyrohyoid *ligament*.
l. hyothyroi'deum me'dium, l. tireo-hióideo mediano. SIN median thyrohyoid *ligament*.
l. iliofemora'le [TA], l. iliofemoral. SIN iliofemoral *ligament*.
l. iliolumba'le [TA], l. iliolumbar. SIN iliolumbar *ligament*.
l. iliopectinea'le, arco iliopectíneo. SIN iliopectineal *arch*.
l. incu'dis poste'rius [TA], l. posterior da bigorna. SIN posterior *ligament* of incus.
l. incu'dis supe'rius [TA], l. superior da bigorna. SIN superior *ligament* of incus.
l. inguina'le [TA], l. inguinal. SIN inguinal *ligament*.
ligamen'ta intercarpa'lia [TA], ligamentos intercarpais. SIN intercarpal *ligaments*, em *ligament*.
l. intercarpalia dorsalia, l. intercarpais dorsais. VER intercarpal *ligaments*, em *ligament*.
l. intercarpalia interossea, l. intercarpais interósseos. VER intercarpal *ligaments*, em *ligament*.
l. intercarpalia palmaria, l. intercarpais palmares. VER intercarpal *ligaments*, em *ligament*.
l. interclavicula're [TA], l. interclavicular. SIN interclavicular *ligament*.
ligamen'ta intercosta'lia, membranas intercostais. SIN intercostal *membranes*, em *membrane*.
ligamen'ta intercuneifor'mia [TA], ligamentos intercuneiformes. SIN intercuneiform *ligaments*, em *ligament*.
ligamenta intercuneiformia dorsalia, ligamentos intercuneiformes dorsais. VER intercuneiform *ligaments*, em *ligament*.
ligamenta intercuneiformia interossea, ligamentos intercuniformes interósseos. VER intercuneiform *ligaments*, em *ligament*.
ligamenta intercuneiformia plantaria, ligamentos intercuneiformes plantares. VER intercuneiform *ligaments*, em *ligament*.
l. interfoveola're [TA], l. interfoveolar. SIN interfoveolar *ligament*.
l. interspina'le [TA], l. interespinal. SIN interspinous *ligament*.
l. intertransversa'rium [TA], l, intertransversário. SIN intertransverse *ligament*.
ligamen'ta intracapsula'ria [TA], ligamentos intracapsulares. SIN intracapsular *ligaments*, em *ligament*.
l. ischiocapsula're, l. isquiofemoral. SIN ischiofemoral *ligament*.
l. ischiofemora'le [TA], l. isquiofemoral. SIN ischiofemoral *ligament*.
l. juga'le, l. cricofaríngeo. SIN cricopharyngeal *ligament*.
l. lacinia'tum, retináculo dos músculos flexores dos membros inferiores. SIN flexor *retinaculum* of lower limb.
l. lacuna're [TA], l. lacunar. SIN lacunar *ligament*.
l. latera'le articulatio'nis temporomandibula'ris [TA], l. lateral da articulação temporomandibular. SIN lateral *ligament* of temporomandibular joint.
l. laterale vesicae [TA], l. lateral vesical. SIN lateral *ligament* of bladder.
l. la'tum pulmo'nis, l. pulmonar. SIN pulmonary *ligament*.
l. la'tum u'teri [TA], l. largo do útero. SIN broad *ligament* of the uterus.
l. lienorena'le, l. esplenorrenal; *termo oficial alternativo para splenorenal *ligament*.
l. longitudina'le ante'rius [TA], l. longitudinal anterior. SIN anterior longitudinal *ligament*.
l. longitudina'le poste'rius [TA], l. longitudinal posterior. SIN posterior longitudinal *ligament*.
ligamenta longitudina'lia, ligamentos longitudinais. SIN longitudinal *ligaments*, em *ligament*.
l. lumbocosta'le [TA], l. lombocostal. SIN lumbocostal *ligament*.
l. mal'lei ante'rius [TA], l. anterior do martelo. SIN anterior *ligament* of malleus.
l. mal'lei latera'le [TA], l. lateral do martelo. SIN lateral *ligament* of malleus.
l. mal'lei supe'rius [TA], l. superior do martelo. SIN superior *ligament* of malleus.
l. malle'oli latera'lis, l. lateral do martelo. VER anterior tibiofibular *ligament*, posterior tibiofibular *ligament*.
l. media'le, parte tibiofibular anterior do ligamento colateral medial da articulação talocrural. SIN anterior tibiotalar *part* of medial ligament of ankle joint.
l. media'le articulatio'nis talocrura'lis, l. colateral medial da articulação talocrural. SIN medial *ligament* of ankle joint.
l. media'le articulatio'nis temporomandibula'ris [TA], l. medial da articulação temporomandibular. SIN medial *ligament* of temporomandibular joint.
l. mediale puboprostaticum, l. pubovesical (do homem); *termo oficial alternativo para pubovesical *ligament* (of male).
l. menis'ci latera'lis, l. meniscofemoral posterior. SIN posterior meniscofemoral *ligament*.
ligamen'ta meniscofemora'lia [TA], ligamentos meniscofemorais. SIN meniscofemoral *ligaments*, em *ligament*.
l. meniscofemora'le ante'rius [TA], l. meniscofemoral anterior. SIN anterior meniscofemoral *ligament*.
l. meniscofemora'le poste'rius [TA], l. meniscofemoral posterior. SIN posterior meniscofemoral *ligament*.
l. metacarpa'le transver'sum profun'dum [TA], l. metacarpal transverso profundo. SIN deep transverse metacarpal *ligament*.
l. metacarpa'le transver'sum superficia'le [TA], l. metacarpal transverso superficial. SIN superficial transverse metacarpal *ligament*.
ligamen'ta metacarpa'lia dorsa'lia [TA], ligamentos metacarpais dorsais. SIN dorsal metacarpal *ligaments*, em *ligament*.
ligamen'ta metacarpa'lia interos'sea [TA], ligamentos metacarpais interósseos. SIN interosseous metacarpal *ligaments*, em *ligament*.
ligamen'ta metacarpa'lia palma'ria [TA], ligamentos metacarpais palmares. SIN palmar metacarpal *ligaments*, em *ligament*.
l. metatarsa'le transver'sum profun'dum [TA], l. metatarsal transverso profundo. SIN deep transverse metatarsal *ligament*.
l. metatarsa'le transver'sum superficia'le [TA], l. metatarsal transverso superficial. SIN superficial transverse metatarsal *ligament*.

ligamen'ta metatarsa'lia dorsa'lia [TA], ligamentos metatarsais dorsais. SIN dorsal metatarsal ligaments, em ligament.

ligamen'ta metatarsa'lia interos'sea [TA], ligamentos metatarsais interósseos. SIN metatarsal interosseous ligaments, em ligament.

ligamen'ta metatarsa'lia planta'ria [TA], ligamentos metatarsais plantares. SIN plantar metatarsal ligaments, em ligament.

l. natato'rium, l. metacarpal transverso superficial. SIN superficial transverse metacarpal ligament.

ligamen'ta navicularicuneifor'mia, ligamentos cuneonaviculares. VER dorsal cuneonavicular ligaments, em ligament, plantar cuneonavicular ligaments, em ligament.

l. nu'chae [TA], l. nucal; uma faixa ligamentosa sagital na parte posterior do pescoço, formada por ligamentos supra-espinhosos espessados; estende-se desde a protuberância occipital externa à borda posterior do forame magno, cranialmente, e ao sétimo processo espinhoso cervical, caudalmente. SIN nuchal ligament*, apparatus ligamentosus colli.

l. orbicula're ra'dii, l. anular do rádio. SIN anular ligament of radius.

ligamenta ossiculorum auditorium, ligamentos dos ossículos da audição; *termo oficial alternativo para ligaments of auditory ossicles, em ligament.

ligamen'ta ossiculo'rum audi'tus [TA], ligamentos dos ossículos da audição. SIN ligaments of auditory ossicles, em ligament.

l. ova'rii pro'prium [TA], l. útero-ovárico. SIN ligament of ovary.

ligamen'ta palma'ria [TA], ligamentos palmares. SIN palmar ligaments, em ligament.

ligamenta palmaria articulationis interphalangeae manus [TA], ligamentos palmares das articulações interfalângicas da mão. SIN palmar ligaments of interphalangeal joints of hand, em ligament.

ligamenta palmaria articulationis metacarpophalangeae [TA], ligamentos palmares das articulações metacarpofalângicas. SIN palmar ligaments of metacarpophalangeal joints, em ligament.

l. palpebra'le exter'num, l. palpebral lateral. SIN lateral palpebral ligament.

l. palpebra'le latera'le [TA], l. palpebral lateral. SIN lateral palpebral ligament.

l. palpebra'le media'le [TA], l. palpebral medial. SIN medial palpebral ligament.

l. patel'lae [TA], l. da patela. SIN patellar ligament.

l. pectina'tum, tecido trabecular da esclera; ligamentos pectíneos do ângulo iridocorneano. VER trabecular tissue of sclera.

l. pectina'tum an'guli iridocornea'lis, tecido trabecular da esclera; ligamentos pectíneos do ângulo iridocorneano. VER trabecular tissue of sclera.

l. pectina'tum ir'idis, tecido trabecular da esclera; ligamentos pectíneos do ângulo iridocorneano. VER trabecular tissue of sclera.

l. pectinea'le [TA], l. pectíneo. SIN pectineal ligament.

l. phrenicocol'icum [TA], l. frenocólico. SIN phrenicocolic ligament.

l. phrenicolienale, l. frenoesplênico. SIN phrenicosplenic ligament.

l. phrenicosplenicum [TA], l. frenoesplênico. SIN phrenicosplenic ligament.

l. pisohama'tum [TA], l. piso-hamato. SIN pisohamate ligament.

l. pisometacarp'eum [TA], l. pisometacarpal. SIN pisometacarpal ligament.

l. planta're lon'gum [TA], l. plantar longo. SIN long plantar ligament.

ligamen'ta planta'ria [TA], ligamentos plantares. SIN plantar ligaments, em ligament.

ligamenta plantaria articulationis interphalangeae pedis [TA], ligamentos plantares das articulações interfalângicas do pé. SIN plantar ligaments of interphalangeal joints of foot, em ligament.

ligamenta plantaria articulationis metatarsophalangeae [TA], ligamentos plantares das articulações metatarsofalângicas. SIN plantar ligaments of metatarsophalangeal joints, em ligament.

l. poplit'eum arcua'tum [TA], l. poplíteo arqueado. SIN arcuate popliteal ligament.

l. poplit'eum obli'quum [TA], l. poplíteo oblíquo. SIN oblique popliteal ligament.

l. pterygospina'le [TA], l. pterigoespinal. SIN pterygospinous ligament.

l. pubicum inferius [TA], l. púbico inferior. SIN inferior pubic ligament.

l. pu'bicum supe'rius [TA], l. púbico superior. SIN superior pubic ligament.

l. pubocapsula're, l. pubocapsular. SIN pubofemoral ligament.

l. pubofemora'le [TA], l. pubofemoral. SIN pubofemoral ligament.

l. puboprostat'icum [TA], l. puboprostático. SIN puboprostatic ligament.

l. puboprostat'icum latera'le, l. puboprostático. VER puboprostatic ligament.

l. puboprostat'icum media'le, l. puboprostático. VER puboprostatic ligament.

l. pubovesica'le (femininum) [TA], l. pubovesical (feminino). SIN pubovesical ligament (of female).

l. pubovesicale (masculinum) [TA], l. pubovesical (masculino). SIN pubovesical ligament (of male).

l. pulmona'le [TA], l. pulmonar. SIN pulmonary ligament.

l. quadra'tum [TA], l. quadrado. SIN quadrate ligament.

l. radia'tum, l. radiado da cabeça da costela. SIN radiate ligament of head of rib.

l. radiocarpa'le dorsa'le [TA], l. radiocarpal dorsal. SIN dorsal radiocarpal ligament.

l. radiocarpa'le palma're [TA], l. radiocarpal palmar. SIN palmar radiocarpal ligament.

l. reflex'um [TA], l. reflexo. SIN reflected inguinal ligament.

l. sacrococcyg'eum ante'rius [TA], l. sacrococcígeo anterior. SIN anterior sacrococcygeal ligament.

l. sacrococcygeum dorsale superficiale, l. sacrococcígeo posterior superficial; *termo oficial alternativo para superficial posterior sacrococcygeal ligament.

l. sacrococcyg'eum latera'le [TA], l. sacrococcígeo lateral. SIN lateral sacrococcygeal ligament.

l. sacrococcyg'eum poste'rius profun'dum, l. sacrococcígeo posterior profundo. SIN deep posterior sacrococcygeal ligament.

l. sacrococcyg'eum poste'rius superficia'le [TA], l. sacrococcígeo posterior superficial. SIN superficial posterior sacrococcygeal ligament.

l. sacrodura'le, l. sacrodural. SIN sacrodural ligament.

ligamen'ta sacroili'aca anterio'ra [TA], ligamentos sacroilíacos anteriores. SIN anterior sacroiliac ligaments, em ligament.

ligamen'ta sacroili'aca interos'sea [TA], ligamentos sacroilíacos interósseos. SIN interosseous sacroiliac ligaments, em ligament.

ligamen'ta sacroili'aca posterio'ra [TA], ligamentos sacroilíacos posteriores. SIN posterior sacroiliac ligaments, em ligament.

l. sacroili'acum poste'rius, l. sacroilíaco posterior. SIN posterior sacroiliac ligaments, em ligament.

l. sacrospina'le [TA], l. sacroespinal. SIN sacrospinous ligament.

l. sacrospino'sum, l. sacroespinal. SIN sacrospinous ligament.

l. sacrotubera'le [TA], l. sacrotuberal. SIN sacrotuberous ligament.

l. sacrotubero'sum, l. sacrotuberoso. SIN sacrotuberous ligament.

l. sero'sum, l. seroso. SIN serous ligament.

l. sphenomandibula're [TA], l. esfenomandibular. SIN sphenomandibular ligament.

l. spira'le coch'leae, l. espiral do ducto coclear. SIN spiral ligament of cochlear duct.

l. spirale ductus cochlearis [TA], l. espiral do canal coclear. SIN spiral ligament of cochlear duct.

l. splenorena'le [TA], l. esplenorrenal. SIN splenorenal ligament.

ligamenta sternoclavicularia, ligamentos esternoclaviculares. SIN sternoclavicular ligaments, em ligament.

l. sternoclavicula're ante'rius [TA], l. esternoclavicular anterior. SIN anterior sternoclavicular ligament.

l. sternoclavicula're poste'rius [TA], l. esternoclavicular posterior. SIN posterior sternoclavicular ligament.

l. sternocosta'le intraarticula're [TA], l. esternocostal intra-articular. SIN intraarticular sternocostal ligament.

ligamen'ta sternocosta'lia radia'ta [TA], ligamentos esternocostais radiados. SIN radiate sternocostal ligaments, em ligament.

ligamen'ta sternoper'icardi'aca [TA], ligamentos esternopericárdicos. SIN sternopericardial ligaments, em ligament.

l. stylohyoi'deum [TA], l. estilo-hióideo. SIN stylohyoid ligament.

l. stylomandibula're [TA], l. estilomandibular. SIN stylomandibular ligament.

l. supraspina'le [TA], l. supra-espinal. SIN supraspinous ligament.

ligamen'ta suspenso'ria mammaria, ligamentos suspensores da mama. SIN suspensory ligaments of breast, em ligament.

l. suspensorium axillae [TA], l. suspensor da axila. SIN suspensory ligament of axilla.

l. suspensorium bulbi [TA], l., suspensor do bulbo do olho. SIN suspensory ligament of eyeball.

l. suspenso'rium clitor'idis [TA], l. suspensor do clitóris. SIN suspensory ligament of clitoris.

l. suspensorium duodeni, músculo suspensor do duodeno; *termo oficial alternativo para suspensory muscle of duodenum.

l. suspensorium glandulae thyroideae [TA], l. suspensor da glândula tireóide. SIN suspensory ligament of thyroid gland.

l. suspenso'rium ova'rii [TA], l. suspensor do ovário. SIN suspensory ligament of ovary.

l. suspenso'rium pe'nis [TA], l. suspensor do pênis. SIN suspensory ligament of penis.

l. talocalcaneum [TA], l. talocalcâneo. SIN talocalcaneal ligament.

l. talocalcanea're interos'seum, l. talocalcâneo interósseo. SIN talocalcaneal interosseous ligament.

l. talocalcaneum latera'le [TA], l. talocalcâneo lateral. SIN lateral talocalcaneal ligament.

l. talocalcaneum media'le [TA], l. talocalcâneo medial. SIN medial talocalcaneal ligament.

l. talocalcaneum posterius [TA], l. talocalcâneo posterior. SIN posterior talocalcaneal ligament.

l. talofibula're ante'rius [TA], l. talofibular anterior. SIN anterior talofibular ligament.

l. talofibula're poste'rius [TA], l. talofibular posterior. SIN posterior talofibular ligament.

l. talonavicula're [TA], l. talonavicular. SIN talonavicular ligament.

l. talotibia'le ante'rius, parte talotibial anterior do ligamento colateral medial. SIN anterior tibiotalar part of medial ligament of ankle joint. VER TAMBÉM medial ligament of ankle joint.
l. talotibia'le poste'rius, parte talotibial posterior do l. colateral medial. SIN posterior tibiotalar part of medial ligament of ankle joint. VER TAMBÉM medial ligament of ankle joint.
l. tarsa'le exter'num, l. palpebral lateral. SIN lateral palpebral ligament.
l. tarsa'le inter'num, l. palpebral medial. SIN medial palpebral ligament.
ligamen'ta tar'si [TA], ligamentos do tarso. SIN tarsal ligaments, em ligament.
ligamenta tarsi dorsalia [TA], ligamentos dorsais do tarso. SIN dorsal tarsal ligaments, em ligament.
ligamenta tarsi interossea [TA], ligamentos interósseos do tarso. SIN tarsal interosseous ligaments, em ligament.
ligamenta tarsi plantaria [TA], ligamentos plantares do tarso. SIN plantar tarsal ligaments, em ligament.
ligamen'ta tarsometatarsa'lia [TA], ligamentos tarsometatarsais. SIN tarsometatarsal ligaments, em ligament.
ligamenta tarsometatarsalia dorsalia [TA], ligamentos tarsometatarsais dorsais. SIN dorsal tarsometatarsal ligaments, em ligament.
ligamenta tarsometatarsalia plantaria [TA], ligamentos tarsometatarsais plantares. SIN plantar tarsometatarsal ligaments, em ligament.
l. temporomandibula're, l. lateral da articulação temporomandibular. SIN lateral ligament of temporomandibular joint.
l. te'res fem'oris, l. da cabeça do fêmur. SIN ligament of head of femur.
l. te'res hep'atis [TA], l. redondo do fígado. SIN round ligament of liver.
l. te'res u'teri [TA], l. redondo do útero. SIN round ligament of uterus.
l. tes'tis, l. do testículo; a porção caudal da crista urogenital embrionária; o terço superior do gubernáculo do testículo.
l. thyroepiglot'ticum [TA], l. tireoepiglótico. SIN thyroepiglottic ligament.
l. thyrohyoi'deum latera'le [TA], l. tireo-hióideo lateral. SIN lateral thyrohyoid ligament.
l. thyrohyoi'deum media'num [TA], l. tireo-hióideo mediano. SIN median thyrohyoid ligament.
l. tibiofibula're ante'rius [TA], l. tibiofibular anterior. SIN anterior tibiofibular ligament.
l. tibiofibula're me'dium, membrana interóssea da perna. SIN interosseous membrane of leg.
l. tibiofibula're poste'rius [TA], l. tibiofibular posterior. SIN posterior tibiofibular ligament.
l. tibionavicula're, parte tibionavicular do l. colateral medial da articulação talocrural. SIN tibionavicular part of medial ligament of ankle joint.
ligamen'ta trachea'lia, ligamentos anulares da traquéia. SIN anular ligaments of trachea, em ligament.
l. transversa'le cervicis, l. transverso do colo do útero. SIN cardinal ligament.
l. transver'sum acetab'uli [TA], l. transverso do acetábulo. SIN transverse acetabular ligament.
l. transver'sum atlan'tis [TA], l. transverso do atlas. SIN transverse ligament of atlas.
l. transver'sum cru'ris, retináculo superior dos músculos extensores. SIN superior extensor retinaculum.
l. transver'sum ge'nus [TA], l. transverso do joelho. SIN transverse ligament of knee.
l. transversum humeri [TA], l. transverso do úmero. SIN transverse humeral ligament.
l. transver'sum pel'vis, l. transverso do períneo. SIN transverse perineal ligament.
l. transver'sum perine'i [TA], l. transverso do períneo. SIN transverse perineal ligament.
l. transver'sum scap'ulae infe'rius [TA], l. transverso inferior da escápula. SIN inferior transverse scapular ligament.
l. transver'sum scap'ulae supe'rius [TA], l. transverso superior da escápula. SIN superior transverse scapular ligament.
l. trapezoi'deum [TA], l. trapezóide. SIN trapezoid ligament.
l. triangula're, membrana perineal. SIN perineal membrane.
l. triangula're dex'trum hepatis [TA], l. triangular direito do fígado. SIN right triangular ligament of liver.
l. triangula're sinis'trum hepatis [TA], l. triangular esquerdo do fígado. SIN left triangular ligament of liver.
l. tuber'culi cos'tae, l. costotransversário lateral. SIN lateral costotransverse ligament.
l. ulnocarpa'le palma're [TA], l. ulnocarpal palmar. SIN palmar ulnocarpal ligament.
l. umbilica'le latera'le, l. umbilical mediano; denominação antiga do l. umbicale mediale. SIN lateral umbilical ligament.
l. umbilica'le media'le, corda da artéria umbilical. SIN cord of umbilical artery.
l. umbilica'le media'num [TA], l. umbilical mediano. SIN median umbilical ligament.
l. uteroovaricum, l. útero-ovárico; *termo oficial alternativo para ligament of ovary.
l. ve'nae ca'vae sinis'trae [TA], l. da veia cava esquerda. SIN ligament of left vena cava.
l. veno'sum [TA], l. venoso; um fino cordão fibroso que se situa na fissura do ligamento venoso, os resquícios do canal venoso do feto. SIN Arantius ligament, l. ductus venosi, venous ligament.
l. ventricula're, l. vestibular. SIN vestibular ligament.
l. vestibula're [NA], l. vestibular. SIN vestibular ligament.
l. voca'le [TA], l. vocal. SIN vocal ligament

lig·and (lig'and, li'gand). Ligante. **1.** Qualquer átomo, grupo ou molécula individual ligada a um íon metálico central por múltiplas ligações coordenadas; p.ex., a porção da porfirina do heme, o núcleo corrínico das vitaminas B_{12}. **2.** Uma molécula orgânica ligada a um elemento traçador, p.ex., um radioisótopo. **3.** Uma molécula que se liga a uma macromolécula, p.ex., um l. que se acopla a um receptor. **4.** O analisado em ensaios de ligação competitiva, como o radioimunoensaio. **5.** Um átomo ou grupo que se liga por meio covalente a um átomo de carbono específico em uma molécula orgânica. [L. *ligo,* ligar].
addressin l.'s, ligantes da adressina; ligantes nas células para receptores de acoplamento específico nos linfócitos.
Fas l., l. Fas; uma molécula na superfície das células T citotóxicas que se liga a seu receptor, Fas, na superfície de outras células, iniciando a apoptose na célula-alvo.
lig·an·din (li-gan'din). Ligandina. SIN glutathione S-transferase.
li·gase (li'gās). Ligase; termo genérico para enzimas (classe 6 EC) que catalisam a ligação de duas moléculas acopladas com a clivagem de uma ligação pirofosfato no ATP ou em um composto similar. VER TAMBÉM synthetase.
li·gate (li'gāt). Ligar; aplicar uma ligadura. [L. *ligo,* pp. *-atus,* ligar]
li·ga·tion (li-gā'shun). Ligação. **1.** A aplicação de uma ligadura ou conexão. **2.** O ato de ligar, unir ou conectar. [L. *ligatio,* de *ligo,* ligar]
blunt-end l., l. em fundo cego; uma reação que une duas duplas de DNA diretamente por suas extremidades cegas.
enzyme-catalyzed l., l. catalisada por enzima; uma união da ligação fosfodiéster de dois segmentos de DNA ou RNA mediada por enzima, ou da ligação peptídica de dois polipeptídeos.
pole l., l. do pólo; uma l. na raiz de um órgão para cortar ou diminuir o suprimento sanguíneo.
surgical l., l. cirúrgica; em odontologia, a exposição cirúrgica de um dente não-eclodido, de modo que uma ligadura metálica possa ser colocada ao redor de seu colo e ajustada em um aparelho ortodôntico para facilitar a erupção.
tooth l., l. dentária; a ligação dos dentes com fios para a estabilização e imobilização após a lesão traumática ou cirurgia ortognática, ou durante a terapia periodontal.
tubal l., l. tubária; interrupção da continuidade dos ovidutos por corte, cautério ou por um dispositivo de plástico ou metal para evitar futuras concepções.
li·ga·tor (li'gā-ter, -tōr). Um instrumento utilizado na ligadura dos vasos nas partes profundas e quase inacessíveis.
lig·a·ture (lig'a-choor). Ligadura. **1.** Passar um arame, fio, filamento ou objeto semelhante apertado em torno de um vaso sanguíneo, pedículo de um tumor ou outra estrutura de modo a comprimi-la. **2.** Em ortodontia, um fio ou outro material empregado para fixar uma inserção ortodôntica ou dente em aparelho ortodôntico. [L. *ligatura,* uma faixa ou laço, de *ligo,* atar]
elastic l., l. elástica; **(1)** l. de borracha que constringe lentamente; **(2)** em ortodontia, material filiforme expansível que pode ser fixado, a partir de um dente, a um aparelho ortodôntico ou a outro dente para ganhar o movimento dessas unidades.
intravascular l., l. intravascular; oclusão por balão dos vasos nutrícios de uma malformação arteriovenosa cerebral.
nonabsorbable l., l. não-absorvível; l. permanente de material inerte, como seda, arame ou fibra sintética, que não sofre dissolução nos tecidos humanos.
occluding l., l. oclusiva; l. para cortar completamente o suprimento sanguíneo distal.
provisional l., l. provisória; l. aplicada a uma artéria em continuidade no início de uma cirurgia para evitar a hemorragia, mas removida quando se completa a cirurgia.
soluble l., l. solúvel; l. temporária de material que pode ser absorvido pelos tecidos humanos.
Stannius l., l. de Stannius; l. colocada ao redor de uma junção entre o seio venoso e o átrio do coração de uma rã ou tartaruga (primeira l. de Stannius) ou ao redor da junção atrioventricular (segunda l. de Stannius); mostra que o impulso cardíaco é conduzido do seio venoso para os átrios e ventrículos, mas que as câmaras sucessivas possuem automaticidade, visto que cada uma pode continuar a se contrair, mas os átrios passam a ter uma freqüência mais lenta que o seio venoso; o ventrículo não se contrai ou bate a uma freqüência menor que a dos átrios.
subocclusing l., l. suboclusiva; l. para diminuir o aporte sanguíneo e encorajar a circulação colateral.
suture l., l. por sutura; l. aplicada ao se passar uma agulha com o fio acoplado através ou ao redor de uma estrutura, de modo a fixar a l. com maior firmeza.

light (līt). Luz; aquela porção da radiação eletromagnética (entre 390 e 770 nm) à qual a retina é sensível (variação de comprimento de onda de 380–780 nm). VER TAMBÉM lamp. [A. S. *leōht*]
  cold l., l. fria; **(1)** SIN bioluminescence (1); **(2)** l. fluorescente em oposição à l. incandescente.
  infrared l., l. infravermelha. VER infrared.
  invisible l., l. invisível; termo histórico para X-rays (raios X).
  minimum l., limiar visual. VER visual *threshold*.
  polarized l. l. polarizada; l. em que, como resultado da reflexão ou transmissão através de determinados meios, as vibrações estão todas em um plano, transverso ao raio, e não em todos os planos.
  reflected l., l. refletida; l. que retorna após incidir em um espelho.
  refracted l., l. refratada; raios de l. curvos modificados na passagem de um meio transparente para outro de densidade desigual. VER TAMBÉM refraction.
  transmitted l., l. transmitida; l. passada através de um meio transparente.
  Wood l., l. de Wood; l. ultravioleta produzida pela lâmpada de Wood.
light·en·ing (līt′en - ing). Sensação de distensão abdominal diminuída nas últimas semanas de gestação depois da descida da cabeça do feto para a entrada pélvica.
light green SF yel·low·ish [C.I. 42095]. Verde-claro SF amarelado; um corante arilmetano ácido, usado como corante citoplasmático em histologia vegetal e animal; esmaece muito na luz brilhante.
lig·ne·ous (lig′nē - us). Lígneo, lenhoso; que tem aspecto ou consistência de madeira. [L. *ligneus*, arborizado, de *lignum*, madeira]
lig·nin (lig′nin). Lignina; um polímero ocasional do álcool coniferílico que acompanha a celulose e está presente na fibra vegetal e nas células da madeira; uma fonte de vanilina (por oxidação da l.); a composição da l. varia com espécies vegetais. É um dos biopolímeros mais abundantes na natureza. [L. *lignum*, madeira]
lig·no·cer·ic ac·id (lig - nō - sar′ik, -sēr′ik). Ácido lignocérico; um ácido presente em um tipo de esfingolipídio e, em pequenas quantidades, em triacilgliceróis. SIN *n*-tetracosanoic acid.
like·li·hood. Probabilidade; uma afirmação da chance de que uma quantidade desconhecida tem, na verdade, determinado valor com base na presteza com que contribuiria para determinado grupo de dados; dessa maneira, os méritos das diversas interpretações fornecidas podem ser comparadas.
Likert, Rensis, psicólogo social, *1903. VER Likert *scale*.
Lillie, Ralph D., patologista norte-americano, 1896–1979. VER Glenner-L. *stain* for pituitary. Ver entradas em stain.
Lilly, John C., fisiologista norte-americano, *1915. VER Silverman-L. *pneumotachograph*.
limb (lim) [TA]. **1.** Um membro; um braço ou perna. SIN member. **2.** Ramo; um segmento de qualquer estrutura articulada. VER TAMBÉM leg, crus. [A. S. *lim*]
  ampullary membranous l.'s of semicircular ducts [TA], pilares membranáceos ampulares dos ductos semicirculares; as extremidades dilatadas dos três ductos semicirculares, cada qual contendo um espessamento especializado do epitélio conhecido como crista ampular. SIN crura membranacea ampullaria ductuum semicircularium [TA], ampullary crura of semicircular ducts.
  anacrotic l., ramo anacrótico; a parte ascendente de um traçado de pulso arterial.
  anterior l. of internal capsule [TA], ramo anterior da cápsula interna entre a cabeça do núcleo caudado e o putame; situa-se anteriormente ao joelho da cápsula interna. SIN crus anterius capsulae internae [TA].
  anterior l. of stapes [TA], ramo anterior do estribo; o ramo anterior dos dois ramos curvos delicados que passam a partir da cabeça do osso até a base ou pedal. SIN crus anterius stapedis [TA], anterior crus of stapes.
  l.'s of bony semicircular canals, pilares ósseos ampulares dos canais semicirculares. SIN bony l.'s of semicircular canals.
  bony l.'s of semicircular canals [TA], pilares ósseos dos canais semicirculares; as extremidades dos canais semicirculares ósseos nos quais estão localizados os pilares membranáceos correspondentes dos ductos semicirculares; eles são os pilares ósseos comuns (crus osseum commune), pilares ósseos simples (crus osseum simplex) e polares ósseos ampulares (crus ossea ampullaria). SIN crura of bony semicircular canals, crura ossea canalium semicircularium, l.'s of bony semicircular canals.
  common membranous l. of membranous semicircular ducts, pilares membranáceos comuns dos ductos semicirculares. SIN common membranous l. of semicircular ducts.
  common membranous l. of semicircular ducts [TA], p. membranáceo comum dos ductos semicirculares; as extremidades não-ampulares unidas dos ductos semicirculares superior e posterior. SIN crus membranaceum commune ductuum semicircularium [TA], common crus of semicircular ducts, common membranous l. of membranous semicircular ducts.
  l. of helix, ramo da hélice. SIN crus of helix.
  inferior l., membro inferior. SIN lower l.
  inferior l. of ansa cervicalis, raiz inferior da alça cervical; *termo oficial alternativo para inferior *root* of ansa cervicalis.
  lateral l., pilar lateral. SIN lateral *crus*,
  long l. of incus [TA], ramo longo da bigorna; o processo da bigorna que se articula com o estribo. SIN crus longum incudis [TA], long crus of incus.
  lower l. [TA], membro inferior; o quadril, a coxa, a perna, o tornozelo e o pé. SIN inferior member [TA], membrum inferius [TA], inferior l., lower extremity, pelvic l.
  medial l., ramo medial. SIN medial *crus*.
  pelvic l., membro inferior. SIN lower l.
  phantom l., dor no membro fantasma. SIN phantom limb *pain*.
  posterior l. of internal capsule [TA], ramo posterior da cápsula interna; a subdivisão da cápsula interna caudal ao joelho e localizada entre o tálamo e o núcleo lentiforme. SIN crus posterius capsulae internae [TA].
  posterior l. of stapes [TA], pilar posterior do estribo, o ramo posterior dos dois ramos delicados do estribo que unem a cabeça e a base do osso. SIN crus posterius stapedis [TA], posterior crus of stapes.
  retrolenticular l. of internal capsule, parte retrolentiforme da cápsula interna; *termo oficial alternativo para retrolentiform l. of internal capsule.
  retrolentiform l. of internal capsule [TA], parte retrolentiforme da cápsula interna; a porção da cápsula interna caudal ao ramo posterior da cápsula interna e do núcleo lentiforme. VER TAMBÉM retrolenticular *part* of internal capsule. SIN pars retrolentiformis cruris posterior [TA], retrolenticular l. of internal capsule*.
  short l. of incus [TA], ramo curto da bigorna; o pilar curto da bigorna; o processo da bigorna que se encaixa em uma depressão (fossa da bigorna) no recesso epitimpânico. SIN crus breve incudis [TA], short crus of incus.
  simple membranous l. of semicircular duct [TA], pilar membranáceo simples do ducto semicircular; a extremidade não-ampular do ducto semicircular lateral que se abre independentemente para o utrículo. SIN crus membranaceum simplex ductus semicircularis [TA], simple crus of semicircular duct.
  sublenticular l. of internal capsule, parte sublentiforme da cápsula interna; *termo oficial alternativo para sublentiform l. of internal capsule.
  sublentiform l. of internal capsule [TA], parte sublentiforme da cápsula interna; a porção da cápsula interna localizada ventralmente às porções caudais do núcleo lentiforme. VER TAMBÉM sublenticular *part* of internal capsule. SIN pars sublentiformis cruris posterioris [TA], sublenticular l. of internal capsule*.
  superior l., membro superior. SIN upper l.
  superior l. of ansa cervicalis, raiz superior da alça cervical; *termo oficial alternativo para superior *root* of ansa cervicalis.
  thoracic l., membro superior. SIN upper l.
  upper l. [TA], membro superior; o ombro, o braço, o antebraço, o punho e a mão. SIN membrum superius [TA], superior member [TA], superior l., thoracic l., upper extremity.
lim·bic (lim′bik). Límbico. **1.** Relativo a um limbo. **2.** Relativo ao *sistema* límbico.
lim·bus, pl. **lim·bi** (lim′bŭs, lim′bī). Limbo; a borda, margem ou orla de uma parte. [L. uma borda]
  l. acetab′uli [TA], l. do acetábulo. SIN acetabular *margin*.
  l. alveola′ris, **(1)** arco alveolar da mandíbula. SIN alveolar *arch* of mandible; **(2)** arco alveolar da maxila. SIN alveolar *arch* of maxilla.
  l. anterior palpebrae [TA], l. anterior da pálpebra. SIN anterior palpebral *margin*.
  l. of cornea, l. da córnea. SIN corneal l.
  l. cor′neae, l. da córnea. SIN corneal l.
  corneal l. [TA], l. da córnea; a margem da córnea superposta pela esclera. SIN corneal margin, corneoscleral junction, l. corneae, l. of cornea, sclerocorneal junction.
  l. fos′sae ova′lis [TA], l. da fossa oval; um anel muscular que circunda a fossa oval na parede do átrio direito do coração. SIN anulus ovalis, margin of fossa ovalis, Vieussens anulus, Vieussens isthmus, Vieussens l., Vieussens ring.
  l. lam′inae spira′lis os′seae [TA], limbo espiral ósseo. SIN l. of osseous spiral lamina.
  l. membra′nae tym′pani, limbo da membrana timpânica. SIN l. of tympanic membrane.
  l. of osseous spiral lamina [TA], limbo espiral; o periósteo espessado que reveste a placa superior da lâmina espiral óssea da cóclea. SIN l. laminae spiralis osseae [TA].
  lim′bi palpebra′les [TA], limbos da pálpebra. SIN palpebral *margins*, em *margin*.
  l. penicilla′tus, borda em escova. SIN brush border.
  l. posterior palpebrae, l. posterior da pálpebra.
  l. sphenoidalis [TA], l. esfenoidal. SIN l. of sphenoid (bone).
  l. of sphenoid (bone), l. esfenoidal; crista variadamente proeminente no corpo do esfenóide (osso) que forma a borda posterior do jugo esfenoidal e a borda anterior do sulco pré-quiasmático. SIN l. sphenoidalis [TA].
  l. stria′tus, borda estriada. SIN striated *border*.
  l. of tympanic membrane, limbo da membrana timpânica; margem da membrana timpânica que se insere no sulco timpânico. SIN l. membranae tympani.
  Vieussens l., ânulo de Vieussens. SIN l. fossae ovalis.
lime (līm). **1.** Cal; CaO; um óxido de terras alcalinas que ocorre na forma de massas branco-acinzentadas (cal virgem); a exposição à atmosfera faz com que

lime

se transforme em hidrato de cálcio e carbonato de cálcio (cal extinta ao ar); a adição direta da água ao óxido de cálcio produz o hidrato de cálcio (cal extinta). SIN calcium oxide, calx (1). **2.** Limão-galego; fruto do limoeiro-galego, *Citrus medica* (família Rutaceae), que é uma fonte de ácido ascórbico e atua como agente antiescorbútico. [l. ant. *līm*, visgo]

air-slaked l., cal extinta ao ar. VER lime (1).

chlorinated l., cal clorada; uma mistura de proporções variadas dos complexos do cloro com óxido de cálcio e hidróxido de cálcio. Contém cerca de 24–37% de cloro livre. Decompõe-se nas condições úmidas para liberar o cloro. Forte irritante devido aos vapores de cloro. Usado para desinfetar água potável, esgotos, etc.; no esbranquiçamento da polpa de madeira, roupas, algodão, palha, óleos, saponáceos e lavanderia; como oxidante; na destruição de larvas; e como descontaminante para o gás mostarda e substâncias similares. SIN bleaching powder.

slaked l., cal extinta. VER lime (1).

sulfurated l., cal sulfurada. SIN crude *calcium* sulfide.

li·men, pl. **li·mi·na** (lī'men, lim'i-nă) [TA]. **1.** Límen; entrada; a abertura externa de um canal ou espaço, como l. insulae [TA]. **2.** Limiar. SIN threshold. [L.]

difference l., l. de diferença; uma mudança que mal é percebida na intensidade ou na freqüência de um estímulo.

l. insulae [TA], límen da ínsula; uma faixa de transição entre a porção anterior da substância cinzenta da ínsula e a substância perfurada anterior; é formada por uma estreita faixa do córtex olfativo ao longo do lado lateral da estria olfatória lateral. SIN threshold of island of Reil.

l. na'si [TA], limiar do nariz; uma crista que marca o limite entre a própria cavidade nasal e o vestíbulo. SIN threshold of nose.

lim·er·ence (lim'er-ens). A excitação emocional de estar apaixonado.

limes (L) (lī'mēz). Limiar; um limite, demarcação ou limiar. VER TAMBÉM L *doses*, em *dose*. [L.]

lim·i·nal (lim'i-năl). Limiar. **1.** Pertinente a um limiar. **2.** Pertinente a um estímulo suficientemente forte para excitar um tecido, p.ex., nervo ou músculo. [L. *limen* (*limin-*), um limiar]

lim·i·nom·e·ter (lim-i-nom'e-ter). Liminômetro; um instrumento para medir a força de um estímulo, o qual é apenas suficiente para produzir uma resposta reflexa. [L. *limen*, limiar, + G. *metron*, medida]

lim·it. Limite; uma demarcação ou final. [L. *limes*, limite]

critical l., l. crítico; o limite superior ou inferior de um resultado de exame laboratorial que indica um valor potencialmente fatal.

elastic l., l. elástico; a tensão máxima à qual um material pode ser sujeitado e ainda ser capaz de retornar às suas dimensões originais quando cessadas as forças.

Hayflick l., l. de Hayflick; o l. da divisão celular humana em subculturas; essas células dividem-se tipicamente apenas cerca de 50 vezes antes de morrer.

permissible exposure l., l. de exposição permissível; um padrão de saúde ocupacional para salvaguardar os trabalhadores contra contaminantes perigosos no local de trabalho.

proportional l., l. proporcional; o estresse máximo que um material consegue suportar sem qualquer desvio da proporcionalidade entre o estresse e a deformidade (lei de Hooke).

quantum l., l. quântico; o comprimento de onda mais curto encontrado no espectro de raios X.

short-term exposure l. (STEL), l. de exposição de curto prazo; a concentração máxima de uma substância química à qual os trabalhadores podem ser expostos continuamente, por até 15 minutos, sem risco para a saúde, ou trabalhar de forma segura e eficiente.

tolerance l.'s, limites de tolerância; os limites de desempenho especificados para o erro permissível para um teste; os limites selecionados devem depender do efeito do erro na significância clínica de um teste e sobre o que é tecnicamente possível de conseguir.

Lim·na·tis ni·lot·i·ca (lim-nā'tis nī-lot'i-kă). A sanguessuga eqüina; uma espécie de sanguessuga do sul da Europa e do norte da África, que pode infestar as narinas ou garganta e, prendendo-se à mucosa, provocar hemorragias e anemia em eqüinos e outros animais que bebem água infestada por sanguessuga. [G. *limnē*, lago]

lim·ne·mia (lim-nē'mē-ă). Malária crônica. SIN chronic *malaria.* [G. *limnē*, lago, + *haima*, sangue]

lim·ne·mic (lim-nē'mik). Que sofre de malária crônica.

lim·nol·o·gy (lim-nol'ō-jē). Limnologia; o estudo das condições físicas, químicas, meteorológicas e biológicas na água doce; um ramo da ecologia. [G. *limnē*, lago, + *logos*, estudo]

li·mon, gen. **li·mo·nis** (lī'mon, li-mō'nis). Limão. SIN lemon. [L.]

li·moph·thi·sis (lī-mof'thi-sis). Termo raramente utilizado para emagrecimento decorrente da falta de nutrição suficiente. [G. *limos*, fome, + *phthisis*, consunção]

limp. Claudicação; marcha claudicante com passadas incertas; marcha assimétrica. VER TAMBÉM claudication.

LINAC Acrônimo para linear *accelerator* (acelerador linear).

lin·co·my·cin (lin-kō-mī'sin). Lincomicina; substância antibacteriana, composta de pirrolidina e octapiranose substituídas, produzida por *Streptomyces lincolnensis*; ativa contra microrganismos Gram-positivos; usada medicinalmente como cloridrato de l.

linc·ture, linc·tus (link'choor, link'tŭs). Um eletuário ou uma confecção; originalmente uma preparação medicinal destinada a ser lambida. [L. *lingo*, pp. *linctus*, lamber]

lin·dane (lin'dān). Lindano; usado como escabicida, pediculicida e inseticida (10 vezes mais tóxico para moscas domésticas que o DDT).

Lindau, Arvid, patologista sueco, 1892–1958. VER L. *disease, tumor*; von Hippel-L. *syndrome*.

Lindbergh, Charles A., aviador norte-americano, 1902–1974. VER Carrel-L. *pump*.

Lindner, Karl D., oftalmologista austríaco, 1883–1961. VER L. *bodies*, em *body*.

Lindqvist, Johan Torsten, médico sueco, *1906. VER Fahraeus-L. *effect*.

LINE

line (līn) [TA]. **1.** Linha; uma marca, faixa ou limite. Em anatomia, uma longa e estreita faixa, tira ou estria diferenciada dos tecidos adjacentes por coloração, textura ou realce. VER TAMBÉM linea. **2.** Uma unidade de medida usada por histologistas no século XIX; variava em diferentes países de 1/10 – 1/12 de uma polegada inglesa. **3.** Um derivado laboratorial de uma série de organismos mantidos sob condições físicas definidas. **4.** Um corte do equipo que fornece líquidos ou que conduz impulsos para o equipamento de monitoração; p.ex., l. intravenosa, l. arterial. SIN linea [TA]. [L. *linea*, um fio de linha, uma corrente, linha, de *linum*, fibra de linho]

absorption l.'s, linhas de absorção; as linhas escuras no espectro solar decorrentes da absorção pela atmosfera solar e terrestre; o fenômeno ocorre porque os raios que emanam de um corpo incandescente através de um meio mais frio são absorvidos por elementos nesse meio.

accretion l.'s, linhas de acreção; as linhas observadas em cortes microscópicos do esmalte, marcando as sucessivas camadas do material acrescido.

alveolonasal l., l. alveolonasal; a l. que une o ponto alveolar ao násion.

Amberg lateral sinus l., l. do seio lateral de Amberg; uma l. que divide o ângulo formado pela borda anterior do processo mastóide e a l. temporal.

anocutaneous l. [TA], l. anocutânea; a borda inferior do pécten anal, onde o epitélio escamoso estratificado muda da derme anal glabra para a pele típica (pilosa); coincide comumente com a borda inferior do esfíncter anal interno. SIN linea anorectalis [TA].

anterior axillary l. [TA], l. axilar anterior; uma linha vertical que se estende para baixo a partir da prega axilar anterior. SIN linea axillaris anterior [TA], linea preaxillaris, preaxillary l.

anterior junction l., l. juncional anterior; projeção radiográfica do septo tecidual mediastinal entre os lobos superiores por trás do esterno.

anterior median l. [TA], l. mediana anterior; uma linha de interseção do plano mediossagital com a superfície anterior do corpo. SIN linea mediana anterior [TA].

arcuate l. [TA], l. arqueada; arqueamento ou linha em forma de arco. VER arcuate l. of ilium, arcuate l. of rectus sheath. SIN linea arcuata [TA].

arcuate l. of ilium [TA], l. arqueada do ílio; a porção ilíaca da linha terminal da pelve óssea. SIN linea arcuata ossis ilii [TA].

arcuate l. of rectus sheath [TA], l. arqueada da bainha dos retos; uma linha em crescente, nem sempre bem definida, que marca o limite inferior da camada posterior da bainha do músculo reto abdominal. SIN linea arcuata vaginae musculi recti abdominis [TA], Douglas l., linea semicircularis, semicircular l.

arterial l., l. arterial; um cateter intra-arterial.

axillary l., l. axilar. VER anterior axillary l., midaxillary l., posterior axillary l.

Baillarger l.'s, linhas de Baillarger; duas lâminas de fibras brancas paralelas à superfície do córtex cerebral e visíveis como as estrias da camada piramidal interna [TA] na V camada cortical (l. externa), e como as estrias da camada granular interna [TA] na IV camada cortical (l. interna), aparecendo nos cortes corados de mielina seccionados perpendicularmente à superfície; a l. de Gennari no córtex calcarino representa a mais externa dessas linhas. SIN stria laminae granularis internae [TA], stria laminae pyramidalis internae [TA], Baillarger bands.

base l., l. plano orbitomeatal. VER orbitomeatal *plane* (1).

basinasal l., l. nasobasilar; uma l. que une o básion e o násion. SIN nasobasilar l.

Beau l.'s, linhas de Beau; sulcos transversos nas unhas dos dedos das mãos após doença febril grave, desnutrição, trauma, infarto do miocárdio, etc.

l. of Bechterew, l. de Bechterew. SIN band of Kaes-Bechterew.

bismuth l., l. de bismuto; uma zona negra na borda gengival livre, freqüentemente o primeiro sinal de intoxicação a partir da administração parenteral de bismuto prolongada.

black l., l. negra. SIN *linea nigra.*

l.'s of Blaschko, linhas de Blaschko; um padrão de distribuição das lesões cutâneas ou anomalias pigmentares; lineares nos membros, curvas em forma de S no abdome e em forma de V nas costas, atribuídas a mosaicismo genético (q.v.) e à relação entre a proliferação clonal transversa e o crescimento longitudinal e flexão do embrião.

blue l., l. azul; uma l. azulada ao longo da borda livre da gengiva, ocorrendo na intoxicação crônica por metal pesado.

Brödel bloodless l., l. de Brödel; a l. que corre algo posterior à borda convexa lateral do rim entre os segmentos renais anterior e posterior, demarcando as áreas de distribuição dos ramos anterior e posterior da artéria renal; é, de fato, apenas relativamente avascular.

Burton l., l. de Burton; uma l. azulada na borda livre da gengiva, ocorrendo na intoxicação por chumbo.

calcification l.'s of Retzius, linhas de calcificação de Retzius; linhas de aumento da deposição rítmica de camadas sucessivas da matriz do esmalte durante o desenvolvimento. SIN l.'s of Retzius.

Camper l., l. de Camper; a l. que corre desde a borda inferior da asa do nariz até a borda superior do trago do ouvido.

cell l., (1) linhagem celular; em cultura de tecido, as células que crescem na primeira ou última subcultura de uma cultura primária. VER TAMBÉM established cell 1; **(2)** um clone de células cultivadas derivadas de um tipo de células parentais identificadas.

cement l., l. de cemento; o limite refratário de um ósteon ou sistema lamelar intersticial no osso compacto.

cervical l., l. cervical; uma l. curva irregular, anatômica e contínua, que marca a extremidade cervical da coroa de um dente e a junção cemento–esmalte.

Chamberlain l., l. de Chamberlain; uma l. traçada a partir da margem posterior do palato duro até o dorso do forame magno; na impressão basilar, o processo odontóide eleva-se acima dessa l.

Chaussier l., l. ântero-posterior do corpo caloso, como é vista no corte mediano do cérebro.

choroid l. [TA], tênia corióidea. SIN *tenia* choroidea.

Clapton l., l. de Clapton; coloração esverdeada da margem da gengiva nos casos de intoxicação crônica por cobre.

cleavage l.'s, linhas de clivagem. SIN tension l.'s.

Conradi l., l. de Conradi; l. que se estende desde a base do processo xifóide até a ponta do coração, correspondendo aproximadamente à borda inferior da área cardíaca.

contour l.'s of Owen, linhas de contorno de Owen. SIN Owen l.'s.

Correra l., l. de Correra. SIN pleural l.'s.

costal l. of pleural reflection, l. costal do reflexo pleural; projeção superficial da l. aguda ao longo da qual a parte costal da pleura parietal se torna contínua com a parte diafragmática, inferiormente; essa l. faz interseção com a linha hemiclavicular ao nível da 8.ª costela, com a l. axilar média ao nível da 10.ª costela e com a l. paravertebral ao nível da 12.ª costela; a toracocentese é realizada uma costela acima nessas linhas.

costoclavicular l., l. paraesternal. SIN parasternal l.

costophrenic septal l.'s, linhas septais costofrênicas. SIN Kerley B l.'s.

Crampton l., l. de Crampton; l. traçada desde o ápice da cartilagem da última costela para baixo e para diante quase até a crista ilíaca, em seguida para diante, em paralelo com ela até um pouco abaixo da espinha ântero-superior; uma guia para a artéria ilíaca comum.

Daubenton l., l. de Daubenton; a l. que passa entre o opístio e o básion. VER TAMBÉM Daubenton *angle*, Daubenton *plane*.

l. of demarcation, l. de demarcação; uma zona de reação inflamatória que separa uma área gangrenosa do tecido saudável.

demarcation l. of retina, l. de demarcação da retina; a junção da retina avascular e vascular na retinopatia da prematuridade; a linha que marca os limites de um antigo descolamento de retina.

Dennie l., l. de Dennie. SIN Dennie-Morgan *fold*.

dentate l., l. pectinada. SIN pectinate l.

developmental l.'s, linhas de desenvolvimento. SIN developmental *grooves*, em *groove*.

Douglas l., l. de Douglas. SIN arcuate l. of rectus sheath.

Eberth l.'s, linhas de Eberth; as linhas que aparecem entre as células do miocárdio, quando coradas com nitrato de prata.

Egger l., l. de Egger; termo raramente empregado para a l. circular de adesão entre o humor vítreo e a porção posterior da lente.

Ehrlich-Türk l., l. de Ehrlich-Türk; termo raramente utilizado para a deposição vertical e fina de material na superfície posterior da córnea na uveíte.

epiphysial l. [TA], l. epifisária; a linha de junção da epífise e a diáfise de um osso longo, onde o crescimento ocorre no comprimento. SIN linea epiphysialis [TA], synchondrosis epiphyseos.

established cell l., l. celular estabelecida; as células que demonstram o potencial para subcultura indefinida *in vitro*.

Farre l., l. de Farre; l. esbranquiçada que marca a inserção do mesovário no hilo do ovário.

Feiss l., l. de Feiss; l. que corre desde o maléolo medial até a face plantar da primeira articulação metacarpofalângica.

Ferry l., l. de Ferry; l. férrica que corre no epitélio corneal anterior a uma bolha (bleb).

l. of fixation, l. de fixação; uma l. que une o objeto (ou ponto de fixação) com a fóvea.

Fleischner l.'s, l. de Fleischner; imagens lineares rudes em uma radiografia de tórax, indicando as faixas de atelectasia subsegmentar.

Fraunhofer l.'s, linhas de Fraunhofer; algumas das mais proeminentes das linhas de absorção do espectro solar.

fulcrum l., l. de fulcro; uma l. imaginária ao redor da qual uma dentadura parcial removível tende a rodar. SIN rotational axis.

l. of Gennari, l. de Gennari; uma linha branca proeminente que aparece em cortes perpendiculares do córtex visual (área 17 de Brodmann) em cerca da metade da espessura da substância cinzenta cortical, correspondendo à linha externa de Baillarger particularmente bem desenvolvida nessa área cortical, sendo composta, em grande parte, de fibras de associação intracorticais tangencialmente dispostas. SIN occipital stripe [TA], stria occipitalis [TA], occipital l.*, Gennari band, Gennari stria, stripe of Gennari.

germ l., linhagem germinativa; uma coleção de células haplóides derivadas das células especializadas da gônada primitiva.

gluteal l.'s [TA], linhas glúteas; uma das três linhas curvas ásperas na superfície externa da asa do ílio: l. glútea anterior, l. glútea inferior e l. glútea posterior; as duas áreas limitadas por estas fornece a inserção para o músculo glúteo mínimo, abaixo, e glúteo médio, acima. SIN lineae gluteae [TA].

Granger l., l. de Granger; nas radiografias laterais de crânio, a l. produzida pelo sulco do quiasma óptico ou sulco pré-quiasmático (*sulcus* prechiasmaticus).

growth arrest l.'s, linhas de parada de crescimento; as linhas densas em paralelo com as placas de crescimento dos ossos longos nas radiografias, representando a lentificação temporária ou cessação do crescimento longitudinal. SIN Harris l.'s.

Gubler l., l. de Gubler; o nível da origem superficial do trigêmeo na ponte, abaixo da qual uma lesão causa a paralisia de Gubler.

gum l., l. da gengiva; a posição da margem da gengiva em relação aos dentes no arco dentário.

Haller l., l. de Haller. SIN *linea* splendens.

Hampton l., l. de Hampton; uma faixa radiotransparente fina através do colo de uma úlcera gástrica benigna cheia de contraste, indicando edema de mucosa. Cf. Carman *sign*.

Harris l.'s, linhas de Harris. SIN growth arrest l.'s.

Head l.'s, linhas de Head; faixas de hiperestesia cutânea associadas a inflamação aguda ou crônica das vísceras. SIN Head zones, tender l.'s, tender zones.

Hensen l., l. de Hensen. SIN H *band*.

highest nuchal l. [TA], l. nucal suprema; uma linha acima e em paralelo com a linha nucal superior na superfície externa do osso occipital; fornece inserção para a aponeurose epicraniana e músculo occipital. SIN linea nuchae suprema [TA].

Linhas cranianas		
órgão	**área do dermátomo**	**lado do corpo**
coração	C3–4–T1–5	frontal direito
aorta torácica	C3–4–T1–7	ambos os lados
costelas	T2–12	ipsolateral
pulmões	C3–4	ipsolateral
esôfago	T1–8	ambos os lados
estômago	T (5) 6–9	esquerdo
fígado e vesícula biliar	T (5) 6–9 (10)	direito
pâncreas	T6–9	frontal esquerdo
duodeno	T6–10	direito
jejuno	T8–11	esquerdo
íleo	T9–11	ambos os lados
ceco, colo proximal	T9–10–L1	direito
colo distal	T9–L1	esquerdo
reto	T9–L1	esquerdo
rim e ureter	T9–L1 (2)	ipsolateral
útero e ovários	T12–L1	ipsolateral
peritônio	T5–12	ambos os lados
baço	T6–10	esquerdo

C = segmentos cervicais, T = segmentos torácicos, L = segmentos lombares

high lip l., l. labial elevada; a altura mais alta a que o lábio é elevado na função normal ou durante o ato de sorrir largamente.

Hilton white l., l. branca de Hilton. SIN white l. of anal canal.

His l., l. de His; uma linha que se estende desde a ponta da espinha nasal anterior (acântio) até o ponto mais posterior na margem posterior do forame magno (opístio), dividindo a face em uma parte superior e uma inferior ou dentária.

Holden l., l. de Holden; a prega ou sulco da pele da virilha causado pela flexão da coxa.

Hudson-Stähli l., l. de Hudson-Stähli; uma l. horizontal acastanhada através do terço inferior da córnea, ocasionalmente observada no idoso e também em associação a opacificações da córnea.

Hunter l., l. de Hunter. SIN linea alba.

Hunter-Schreger l.'s, linhas de Hunter-Schreger. SIN Hunter-Shreger bands, em band.

iliopectineal l., linha terminal da pelve. SIN linea terminalis of pelvis.

imbrication l.'s of von Ebner, linhas de imbricação na dentina que refletem as variações na mineralização durante a formação da dentina; a distância entre as linhas corresponde à velocidade diária de formação da dentina. SIN incremental l.'s of von Ebner.

incremental l.'s, linhas de aumento; (1) no esmalte, as linhas de calcificação de Retzius; (2) na dentina, as linhas de imbricação ou de aumento de von Ebner e as linhas de Owen.

incremental l.'s of von Ebner, linhas de aumento de von Ebner. SIN imbrication l.'s of von Ebner.

inferior nuchal l. [TA], l. nucal inferior; uma crista que se estende lateralmente, desde a crista occipital, em direção ao processo jugular do osso occipital. SIN linea nuchae inferior [TA].

inferior temporal l. of parietal bone [TA], l. temporal inferior do osso parietal; a mais baixa das duas linhas curvas no osso parietal; marca o limite externo da inserção do músculo temporal. SIN linea temporalis inferior ossis parietalis [TA], temporal ridge.

infracostal l., plano subcostal. SIN subcostal plane.

intercondylar l. of femur [TA], l. intercondilar do fêmur; uma tênue crista transversal que separa o assoalho da fossa intercondilar da superfície poplítea do fêmur; permite a inserção da porção posterior da cápsula articular do joelho. SIN linea intercondylaris femoris [TA].

intermediate l. of iliac crest, l. intermédia da crista ilíaca. SIN intermediate zone of iliac crest.

interspinal l., l. interespinhal; a l. que passa através de ambas as espinhas ilíacas ântero-superiores, indicando o plano interespinal (interspinal *plane*). SIN linea interspinalis.

intertrochanteric l. [TA], l. intertrocantérica; uma linha áspera que separa anteriormente o colo e a diáfise do fêmur; ela passa para baixo e medialmente, desde o trocanter maior até o trocanter menor, e continua para o lábio medial da linha áspera. SIN linea intertrochanterica [TA], linea spiralis, spiral l.

intertubercular l., l. intertubercular; l. horizontal que passa através dos tubérculos de ambas as cristas ilíacas, indicando o plano intertubercular (intertubercular *plane*). SIN linea intertubercularis.

iron l., l. férrica; a l. de deposição no epitélio da córnea.

isoelectric l., l. isoelétrica; a linha basal do eletrocardiograma, registrada no intervalo TP durante os ritmos com ondas P.

l. of Kaes, l. de Kaes. SIN band of Kaes-Bechterew.

Kerley A l.'s, linhas A de Kerley; imagens dos septos interlobulares profundos; mais longas, espessas e centrais que as linhas B de Kerley; usualmente nos lobos superiores.

Kerley B l.'s, linhas B de Kerley; linhas septais periféricas finas. SIN costophrenic septal l.'s

Kerley C l.'s, linhas C de Kerley; um padrão reticular fino inespecífico nas radiografias de tórax.

Kilian l., l. de Kilian; uma l. transversa que marca o promontório da pelve.

Langer l.'s, linhas de Langer. SIN tension l.'s.

Lanz l., l. de Lanz. SIN interspinous plane.

lead l., l. plúmbica; depósitos de sulfeto de chumbo na gengiva nas áreas de inflamação crônica.

Looser l.'s, linhas de Looser; faixas radiotransparentes no córtex de um osso; geralmente indicam osteomalacia. SIN Looser zones.

low lip l., l. do lábio inferior; (1) a posição mais inferior do lábio inferior durante o ato de sorrir ou de retração voluntária; (2) a posição mais baixa do lábio superior em repouso.

M l., linha M; uma l. fina no centro da faixa A do sarcômero das miofibrilas do músculo estriado. SIN M band, mesophragma.

Mach l., l. de Mach; a l. evidente de contraste de densidade que limita a imagem de tecidos moles em uma radiografia; é uma ilusão de óptica construída pela retina do observador.

mammary l., l. mamária; l. transversa desenhada entre os dois mamilos.

mammillary l. [TA], l. mamilar; uma linha vertical que passa através do mamilo em ambos os lados. SIN linea mammilaris [TA], nipple l.

McKee l., l. de McKee; uma l. traçada a partir da ponta da cartilagem da décima primeira costela até um ponto 3,5 cm medial à espinha ântero-superior; em seguida é curvada para baixo, para diante e para dentro, até exatamente acima do anel inguinal profundo; um guia para a artéria ilíaca comum.

median l., l. mediana. VER anterior median l., posterior median l.

Mees l.'s, l. de Mees; faixas brancas horizontais nas unhas observadas na intoxicação crônica por arsênico e, ocasionalmente, na lepra. SIN Mees stripes.

mercurial l., l. mercurial; pigmentação marrom-azulada percebida na margem gengival e associada à intoxicação por mercúrio (estomatite mercurial).

Meyer l., l. de Meyer; uma l. através do eixo do primeiro pododáctilo e que passa no ponto médio do calcanhar em um pé normal.

midaxillary l. [TA], l. axilar média; uma linha vertical que faz interseção com um ponto a meio caminho entre as dobras ou linhas axilares anterior e posterior. SIN linea axillaris media [TA], linea medio-axillaris, middle axillary l.

midclavicular l. [TA], l. medioclavicular; uma linha vertical que passa através do ponto médio da clavícula. SIN linea medioclavicularis [TA].

middle axillary l., l. axilar média. SIN midaxillary l.

milk l., crista mamária. SIN mammary ridge.

Monro l., l. de Monro. SIN Monro-Richter l.

Monro-Richter l., l. de Monro-Richter; uma l. que vai do umbigo até a espinha ilíaca ântero-superior. O ponto de McBurney ocorre nessa linha. SIN Monro l., Richter-Monro l.

Muehrcke l.'s, linhas de Muehrcke; linhas brancas paralelas à lúnula e separadas entre si por áreas róseas normais; associadas a hipoalbuminemia; as linhas não se deslocam para fora com o crescimento da unha, mas desaparecem quando a albumina sérica retorna ao normal.

mylohyoid l. [TA], l. milo-hióidea; uma crista na superfície interna da mandíbula que corre desde um ponto inferior à espinha mentual, para cima e para trás, até o ramo atrás do último dente molar; fornece a inserção para o músculo milo-hióideo e parte mais inferior do músculo constritor superior da faringe. SIN linea mylohyoidea [TA], mylohyoid ridge.

nasobasilar l., l. nasobasilar. SIN basinasal l.

Nélaton l., l. de Nélaton; uma l. traçada da espinha ilíaca ântero-superior até a tuberosidade do ísquio; normalmente, o trocanter maior se localiza nessa linha, mas, nos casos de luxação de quadril ou de fratura do colo do fêmur, o trocanter é palpado acima da l. SIN Roser-Nélaton l.

neonatal l., l. neonatal; nos dentes decíduos, é uma l. de demarcação entre o esmalte pré-natal e o pós-natal. SIN neonatal ring.

nipple l., l. mamilar. SIN mammillary l.

Obersteiner-Redlich l., l. de Obersteiner-Redlich. SIN Obersteiner-Redlich zone.

oblique l. [TA], l. oblíqua; uma l. diagonal, em declive ou aclive; uma l. que não está em paralelo, nem é perpendicular, nem horizontal, nem vertical. VER oblique l. of mandible, oblique l. of thyroid cartilage. SIN linea obliqua [TA].

oblique l. of mandible [TA], l. oblíqua da mandíbula; a l. na superfície externa da mandíbula e que se estende desde o tubérculo mentual até o ramo, separando as partes alveolar e basilar do osso. SIN linea obliqua mandibulae [TA], external oblique ridge.

oblique l. of thyroid cartilage [TA], l. oblíqua da cartilagem tireóidea; uma crista na superfície externa da cartilagem tireóidea que fornece inserção para os músculos esternotireóideo e tireo-hióideo. SIN linea obliqua cartilaginis thyroideae [TA].

occipital l., estria occipital do isocórtex; *termo oficial alternativo para l. of Gennari.

l. of occlusion, l. de oclusão; o alinhamento das superfícies de oclusão dos dentes no plano horizontal. VER TAMBÉM occlusal *plane*.

Ogston l., l. de Ogston; uma l. traçada desde o tubérculo do adutor do fêmur até a incisura intercondilar; um guia para a ressecção do côndilo medial para o joelho valgo.

Ohngren l., l. de Ohngren; um plano teórico que passa entre o canto medial do olho e o ângulo da mandíbula; usado como uma l. divisória arbitrária na classificação de tumores localizados do seio maxilar; os tumores acima da l. invadem estruturas vitais precocemente seu prognóstico é pior, enquanto aqueles abaixo da l. possuem um prognóstico mais favorável.

orbitomeatal l., l. orbitomeatal. VER orbitomeatal *plane*.

Owen l.'s, linhas de Owen; as linhas de aumento acentuadas na dentina atribuídas a distúrbios no processo de mineralização. SIN contour l.'s of Owen.

paraspinal l., imagem radiográfica da interface entre o pulmão e os tecidos moles paravertebrais.

parasternal l. [TA], l. paraesternal; uma linha vertical eqüidistante entre as linhas esternal e hemiclavicular. SIN linea parasternalis [TA], costoclavicular l.

paravertebral l., l. paravertebral; uma linha vertical que corresponde às extremidades dos processos transversos das vértebras. SIN linea paravertebralis [TA].

Paris l., l. de Paris; uma unidade de medida microscópica como a usada na *Mikroskopische Anatomie* de Kölliker; era igual a 0,0888138 de uma polegada.

Paton l.'s, linhas de Paton. SIN striae retinae, em stria.

pectinate l. [TA], l. pectinada; a l. entre o epitélio colunar simples do reto e o epitélio estratificado do canal anal, usualmente definida como estando no nível das válvulas anais nas bases das colunas anais. SIN linea pectinata canalis analis [TA], dentate l.

pectineal l. of femur [TA], l. pectínea do fêmur; uma crista que corre para baixo na superfície posterior da diáfise do fêmur, desde o trocanter menor, na qual se insere o músculo pectíneo; continua superiormente com a linha intertrocantérica e, inferiormente, com o lábio medial da linha áspera. SIN linea pectinea femoris [TA].

pectineal l. of pubis, l. pectínea do púbis. SIN pecten pubis.

PICC l., l. PICC; acrônimo para *p*eripherally *i*nserted *c*entral *c*atheter; um cateter venoso central de demora, inserido por via periférica.

pleural l.'s, linhas pleurais; na radiografia de tórax, a imagem dos tecidos moles entre o pulmão aerado e os ossos do tórax. SIN Correra l., pleural stripe.

l.'s of pleural reflection, linhas de reflexão pleural; as linhas, geralmente projetadas na superfície da parede torácica, que indicam a alteração abrupta na direção da pleura parietal à medida que ela passa de uma parede da cavidade de pulmonar para outra. VER TAMBÉM vertebral l. of pleural reflection.

pleuroesophageal l., l. pleuroesofágica; em uma radiografia frontal do tórax, a imagem da interface entre o pulmão direito e o esôfago, o limite do recesso azigoesofágico.

Poirier l., l. de Poirier; uma l. que se estende desde o násio até o lambda.

popliteal l., l. do músculo sóleo. SIN soleal l.

postaxillary l., l. axilar posterior. SIN posterior axillary l.

posterior axillary l., l. axilar posterior; uma linha vertical que se estende inferiormente a partir da dobra axilar posterior. SIN linea axillaris posterior [TA], linea postaxillaris, postaxillary l.

posterior junction l., l. juncional posterior; a imagem radiográfica do septo mediastinal entre os lobos superiores atrás do esôfago, acima do arco aórtico.

posterior median l. [TA], l. mediana posterior; a linha da interseção do plano mesossagital com a superfície posterior do corpo. SIN linea mediana posterior [TA].

Poupart l., l. de Poupart; uma l. vertical que passa através do centro do ligamento inguinal de cada lado; separa o hipocôndrio, a região lombar e a região ilíaca das regiões epigástrica, umbilical e hipogástrica, respectivamente.

preaxillary l., l. axilar anterior. SIN anterior axillary l.

Reid base l., l. básica de Reid; uma l. traçada a partir da margem inferior da órbita até o ponto auricular (centro do orifício do meato acústico externo) e que se estende para trás até o centro do osso occipital. Usada como o plano zero na tomografia computadorizada.

retentive fulcrum l., (1) uma l. imaginária que une os pontos de retenção dos ramos das braçadeiras na manutenção de dentes adjacentes às bases da dentadura em contato com a mucosa; (2) uma linha imaginária que une os pontos de retenção das braçadeiras, ao redor da qual a dentadura tende a rodar quando sujeita a forças como a tração por alimentos grudentos.

l.'s of Retzius, linhas de Retzius. SIN calcification l.'s of Retzius.

Richter-Monro l., l. de Richter-Monro. SIN Monro-Richter l.

Roser-Nélaton l., l. de Roser-Nélaton. SIN Nélaton l.

rough l., l. áspera. SIN *linea* aspera.

sagittal l., l. sagital; qualquer l. imaginária paralela à linha média, indicando (ocorrendo dentro) de um plano sagital (sagittal *plane*).

Salter incremental l.'s, linhas de aumento de Salter; as linhas transversas por vezes observadas na dentina, devido calcificação imprópria.

S-BP l., l. S-BP; uma l. que conecta a sela com o ponto de Bolton; indica a porção posterior da base do crânio em cefalometria.

scapular l. [TA], l. escapular; uma linha vertical que passa através do ângulo inferior da escápula. SIN linea scapularis [TA].

Schreger l.'s, linhas de Schreger. SIN Hunter-Schreger *bands*, em *band.*

semicircular l., l. arqueada da bainha do músculo reto do abdome. SIN arcuate l. of rectus sheath.

semicircular l. of Douglas, l. semicircular de Douglas; uma l. em formato de crescente que define a extremidade da bainha fascial posterior do músculo reto do abdome.

semilunar l., l. semilunar. SIN *linea* semilunaris.

septal l.'s, linhas septais; imagens radiográficas de septos interlobulares espessados, mais freqüentemente ao longo da borda lateral do pulmão, estendendo-se até a pleura; linhas A e B de Kerley; geralmente causadas por edema septal e fibrose, e também por carcinomatose.

Sergent white l., l. branca de Sergent. SIN white l. (2).

Shenton l., l. de Shenton; uma l. curva formada pelo ápice do forame obturado e lado interno do colo do fêmur, observada em uma radiografia frontal ântero-posterior de uma articulação do quadril normal; está deformada nas lesões da articulação, como luxação ou fratura.

S-N l., linha S-N; uma l. conectando um ponto (S) que representa o centro da sela turca com a junção frontonasal (N); indica a porção anterior da base do crânio em cefalometria.

soleal l. [TA], l. do músculo sóleo; uma crista que se estende obliquamente para baixo e medialmente, através da parte posterior da tíbia, a partir da faceta articular fibular; dá origem ao músculo sóleo. SIN linea musculi solei [TA], l. for soleus muscle, linea poplitea, popliteal l.

l. for soleus muscle, l. do músculo sóleo. SIN soleal l.

Spigelius l., l. de Spigelius. SIN *linea* semilunaris.

spiral l., l. intertrocantérica. SIN intertrochanteric l.

stabilizing fulcrum l., l. estabilizadora do fulcro; uma l. imaginária que une os restos oclusivos, ao redor da qual a dentadura tende a rodar sob a força mastigatória.

sternal l. [TA], l. esternal; uma linha vertical que corresponde à margem lateral do esterno. SIN linea sternalis [TA].

sternal l. of pleural reflection, l. esternal de reflexão pleural; a projeção superficial da l. aguda ao longo da qual a parte costal da pleura parietal se torna contínua com a parte mediastinal anteriormente; as linhas esternais direita e esquerda de reflexão pleural são paralelas ao plano mediano, posteriores ao esterno, ao nível das cartilagens costais 2–4; ao nível da cartilagem costal 4, a l. esquerda vira-se lateralmente para ficar em paralelo com a margem esquerda do esterno, criando uma "incisura" mais rasa que a incisura cardíaca do pulmão esquerdo e uma área onde o saco pericárdico faz contato com a parede torácica anterior, sem o saco pleural interveniente — significativo para a pericardiocentese.

Stocker l., l. de Stocker; uma l. fina de pigmento no epitélio da córnea próximo à cabeça de um pterígio.

subcostal l., l. subcostal; uma l. transversa que transecciona a borda mais inferior do gradil torácico, indicando o plano subcostal. VER TAMBÉM subcostal *plane*. SIN linea subcostalis.

superior nuchal l. [TA], l. nucal superior; a crista que se estende lateralmente, desde a protuberância occipital externa para o ângulo lateral do osso occipital; fornece inserção para os músculos trapézio, esternocleidomastóideo e esplênio da cabeça. SIN linea nuchae superior [TA].

superior temporal l. of parietal bone [TA], l. temporal superior do osso parietal; a mais superior das duas linhas curvas no osso parietal; a fáscia temporal insere-se nela. SIN linea temporalis superior ossis parietalis [TA], temporal ridge.

supracrestal l., plano supracristal; uma l. transversa que transecciona o ponto mais elevado de ambas as cristas ilíacas, indicando o plano supracristal (supracristal *plane*). VER TAMBÉM supracristal *plane*. SIN linea supracristalis.

survey l., l. guia do grampo; (1) uma linha feita sobre um dente de apoio de um molde dentário por meio de um vigilante dentário, indicando a altura do contorno do dente de acordo com uma via de inserção específica; (2) uma l. que serve como guia na localização adequada de várias partes de um conjunto de grampos para uma dentadura parcial removível. SIN clasp guideline, Cummer guideline.

Sidney l., l. de Sidney. SIN Sidney *crease.*

sylvian l., l. de Sylvius; a l. do ramo posterior do sulco lateral (fissura de Sylvius) do córtex cerebral.

temporal l., l. temporal. VER inferior temporal l. of parietal bone, superior temporal l. of parietal bone.

temporal l. of frontal bone [TA], l. temporal da face externa do osso frontal; a continuação anterior da linha temporal inferior do osso temporal sobre a face lateral da superfície externa do osso frontal, demarcando a superfície temporal do osso. SIN linea temporalis ossis frontalis [TA].

tender l.'s, linhas sensíveis. SIN Head l.'s.

tension l.'s [TA], linhas de tensão, linhas de clivagem; as linhas que podem ser extrapoladas através da união das aberturas lineares feitas quando um pino redondo é introduzido na pele de um cadáver, resultantes do eixo principal de orientação das fibras do tecido conjuntivo subcutâneo (colágenas) da derme; a direção dessas linhas varia de acordo com a região da superfície do corpo. SIN lineae distractionis [TA], cleavage l.'s, Langer l.'s.

terminal l., l. terminal da pelve. SIN *linea* terminalis of pelvis.

Topinard l., l. de Topinard; uma l. que corre entre a glabela e o ponto mentual.

tram l.'s, trilhos de bonde; as imagens das paredes brônquicas em uma radiografia simples de tórax. Quando observadas distalmente, são indicativas de bronquiectasia ou bronquite crônica; usualmente espessadas; inglês coloquial. SIN radiographic parallel line shadow.

trapezoid l. [TA], l. trapezóide; a área na superfície inferior da clavícula, próximo à sua extremidade lateral, na qual se insere o ligamento trapezóide. SIN linea trapezoidea [TA], trapezoid ridge.

Ullmann l., l. de Ullmann; a l. de deslocamento na espondilolistese.

vertebral l. of pleural reflection, l. vertebral de reflexão pleural; a aproximação da reflexão mais gradual da parte costal da pleura parietal sobre o mediastino posteriormente.

Vesling l., l. de Vesling. SIN *raphe* of scrotum.

vibrating l., l. de vibração; a l. imaginária que cruza a parte posterior do palato, marcando a divisão entre os tecidos móveis e imóveis.

l. of vision, l. de visão. SIN visual *axis.*

Wegner l., l. de Wegner; uma l. estreita, esbranquiçada e discretamente curva, que representa uma área de calcificação preliminar na junção da epífise e diáfise de um osso longo, relacionada com a epifisite sifilítica.

white l., l. branca; (1) linha alba. SIN *linea* alba; (2) uma faixa pálida que aparece 30 a 60 segundos após passar a unha de um dedo da mão na pele e que dura vários minutos; considerado um sinal de tensão arterial diminuída. SIN Sergent white l.

white l. of anal canal, l. branca do canal anal; uma zona rosa-azulada, estreita e ondulada na mucosa do canal anal abaixo da l. pectinada no nível do intervalo entre a parte subcutânea do esfíncter externo e a borda inferior do esfíncter interno, considerada palpável. SIN Hilton white l.

white l. of Toldt, l. branca de Toldt; **(1)** a reflexão lateral da pleura parietal posterior do abdome sobre o mesentério dos colos ascendente e descendente. **(2)** a junção do peritônio parietal com a fáscia de Denonvilliers.

Z l., linha Z; uma estriação cruzada que divide em duas a faixa I de miofibrilas do músculo estriado e que serve como ponto de ancoragem dos filamentos de actina nas duas extremidades do sarcômero. SIN intermediate disk, Z band, Z disk.

l.'s of Zahn, linhas de Zahn; as marcas semelhantes a costelas observadas a olho nu na superfície dos trombos antes da morte; consistem em uma estrutura ramificada de plaquetas e fibrina que separa as células do sangue coagulado. SIN striae of Zahn.

Zöllner l.'s, linhas de Zöllner; figuras idealizadas para mostrar a possibilidade de ilusões ópticas; uma figura comum consiste em duas linhas paralelas que são ligadas por inúmeras linhas curtas obliquamente dispostas; as linhas paralelas parecem, então, convergir ou divergir.

LINEA

lin·ea, gen. e pl. **lin·e·ae** (lin'ē-ā, -ē-ē)[TA]. Linha. SIN line. [L.]

l. al'ba [TA], uma faixa fibrosa que corre verticalmente por toda a extensão da linha média da parede abdominal anterior, recebendo as inserções dos músculos transverso e oblíquo do abdome. SIN Hunter line, white line (1).

l. anorectalis [TA], l. anocutânea. SIN anocutaneous *line*.

l. arcua'ta [TA], l. arqueada. SIN arcuate *line*.

l. arcua'ta os'sis il'ii [TA], linha arqueada do ílio. SIN arcuate *line* of ilium.

l. arcua'ta vagi'nae mus'culi rec'ti abdom'inis [TA], l. arqueada da bainha do músculo reto do abdome. SIN arcuate *line* of rectus sheath. VER TAMBÉM rectus *sheath*, posterior *layer* of rectus sheath.

l. as'pera [TA], l. áspera; uma crista áspera, com dois lábios pronunciados, que corre pela superfície posterior da diáfise do fêmur; o lábio lateral da linha áspera é uma continuação da tuberosidade glútea, o lábio medial da linha intertrocantérica; essa crista permite a inserção dos músculos vasto medial, adutor longo, adutor magno, adutor curto, a porção curta do bíceps e vasto lateral, bem como para o septo intermuscular da coxa. SIN rough line.

lin'eae atroph'icae, estrias atróficas. SIN *striae* cutis distensae, em *stria*.

l. axilla'ris ante'rior [TA], l. axilar anterior. SIN anterior axillary *line*.

l. axilla'ris me'dia [TA], l. axilar média. SIN midaxillary *line*.

l. axilla'ris poste'rior [TA], l. axilar posterior. SIN posterior axillary *line*.

l. cor'neae seni'lis, arco senil. SIN *arcus* senilis.

lineae distractionis [TA], linhas de tensão. SIN tension *lines*, em *line*.

l. epiphysia'lis [TA], l. epifisial. SIN epiphysial *line*.

l. glu'tea ante'rior, l. glútea anterior. VER gluteal *lines*, em *line*.

lineae glu'teae [TA], linhas glúteas. SIN gluteal *lines*, em *line*.

l. glutea inferior, l. glútea inferior. VER gluteal *lines*, em *line*.

l. glutea posterior, l. glútea posterior. VER gluteal *lines*, em *line*.

l. intercondyla'ris fem'oris [TA], l. intercondilar do fêmur. SIN intercondylar *line* of femur.

l. interme'dia cris'tae ili'acae [TA], l. intermédia da crista ilíaca. SIN intermediate *zone* of iliac crest.

l. interspina'lis, l. interespinal. SIN interspinal *line*. VER TAMBÉM interspinous *plane*.

l. intertrochanter'ica [TA], l. intertrocantérica. SIN intertrochanteric *line*.

l. intertubercula'ris, l. intertubercular. SIN intertubercular *line*. VER TAMBÉM intertubercular *plane*.

l. mammilla'ris [TA], l. mamilar. SIN mammilary *line*.

l. media'na ante'rior [TA], l. mediana anterior. SIN anterior median *line*.

l. media'na poste'rior [TA], l. mediana posterior. SIN posterior median *line*.

l. medio-axilla'ris, l. axilar média. SIN midaxillary *line*.

l. medioclavicula'ris [TA], l. medioclavicular. SIN midclavicular *line*.

l. mus'culi sol'ei [TA], l. do músculo sóleo. SIN soleal *line*.

l. mylohyoi'dea [TA], l. milo-hióidea. SIN mylohyoid *line*.

l. ni'gra, l. negra; a l. alba na gestação que se torna pigmentada. SIN black line.

l. nu'chae infe'rior [TA], l. nucal inferior. SIN inferior nuchal *line*.

l. nu'chae media'na, crista occipital externa. SIN external occipital *crest*.

l. nu'chae supe'rior [TA], l. nucal superior. SIN superior nuchal *line*.

l. nu'chae supre'ma [TA], l. nucal suprema. SIN highest nuchal *line*.

l. obli'qua [TA], l. oblíqua. SIN oblique *line*.

l. obliqua cartilag'inis thyroi'deae [TA], l. oblíqua da cartilagem tireóidea. SIN oblique *line* of thyroid cartilage.

l. obliqua mandib'ulae [TA], l. oblíqua da mandíbula. SIN oblique *line* of mandible.

l. parasterna'lis [TA], l. paraesternal. SIN parasternal *line*.

l. paravertebra'lis [TA], l. paravertebral. SIN paravertebral *line*.

l. pectinata canalis analis [TA], l. pectinada. SIN pectinate *line*.

l. pecti'nea femoris [TA], l. pectínea do fêmur. SIN pectineal *line* of femur.

l. poplit'ea, l. do músculo sóleo. SIN soleal *line*.

l. postaxilla'ris, l. axilar posterior. SIN posterior axillary *line*.

l. preaxilla'ris, l. axilar anterior. SIN anterior axillary *line*.

l. scapula'ris [TA], l. escapular. SIN scapular *line*.

l. semicircula'ris, l. arqueada da bainha do músculo reto do abdome. SIN arcuate *line* of rectus sheath.

l. semiluna'ris [TA], l. semilunar; o sulco discreto na parede abdominal externa paralelo à borda lateral da bainha do reto. SIN semilunar line, Spigellius line.

l. spira'lis, l. intertrocantérica. SIN intertrochanteric *line*.

l. splen'dens, l. de Haller; uma faixa espessada da pia-máter ao longo da linha média da superfície anterior da medula espinal. SIN Haller line.

l. sterna'lis [TA], l. esternal. SIN sternal *line*.

l. subcosta'lis, l. subcostal. SIN subcostal *line*. VER TAMBÉM subcostal *plane*.

l. supracrista'lis, plano supracristal. SIN supracrestal *line*. VER TAMBÉM supracrestal *plane*.

l. tempora'lis infe'rior ossis parietalis [TA], l. temporal inferior do osso parietal. SIN inferior temporal *line* of parietal bone.

l. temporalis ossis frontalis [TA], l. temporal do osso frontal. SIN temporal *line* of frontal bone.

l. tempora'lis supe'rior ossis parietalis [TA], l. temporal superior do osso parietal. SIN superior temporal *line* of parietal bone.

l. termina'lis of pelvis [TA], l. terminal da pelve; uma crista oblíqua na superfície interna do ílio e que continua sobre o púbis, que forma o limite inferior da fossa ilíaca; separa a pelve verdadeira da falsa. SIN l. terminalis pelvis [TA], iliopectineal line, terminal line.

l. terminalis pelvis [TA], l. terminal da pelve. SIN l. terminalis of pelvis.

lineae transver'sae ossis sacri [TA], linhas transversais do sacro. SIN transverse *ridges* of sacrum, em *ridge*.

l. trapezoi'dea [TA], l. trapezóide. SIN trapezoid *line*.

lin·e·age (lĭn'aj, lin'ē-āj). Linhagem; o descendente de uma fonte ou progenitor comum. [Fr. ant. *ligne*, linha de descendência]

lin·e·ar (lin'ē-ăr). Linear; pertinente a ou que se assemelha a uma linha.

linearity (lin-ē-ar'ĭ-tē). Linearidade; uma relação entre duas quantidades na qual uma alteração em uma provoca uma alteração diretamente proporcional na outra. [L. *linearis*, linear, de *linea*, linha]

line·breed·ing. Cruzamento linear; a prática do cruzamento sucessivo de indivíduos intimamente relacionados com o objetivo de concentrar características genéticas desejáveis ou cientificamente interessantes de algum indivíduo ou grupo.

li·ner (lī'ner). Revestimento; uma camada de material de proteção.

asbestos l., r. de asbesto; uma camada de asbesto usada para revestir um anel de molde dentário, de modo que, durante o aquecimento e a expansão do revestimento, a compressão do revestimento livrará o revestimento da contenção do anel.

cavity l., r. de cavidade. SIN varnish (dental).

LINES Abreviatura para long interspersed *elements* (elementos interespaçados), em *element*.

Lineweaver, Hans, físico-químico norte-americano, *1907. VER L.-Burk *equation, plot*.

Ling, Per Henrik, sanitarista sueco, 1776–1839. VER L. *method*.

Lin·gel·sheim·ia (lin'jels-hīi'mē-ā). SIN *Acinetobacter*. [W. von *Lingelsheim*]

L. anitra'ta, SIN *Acinetobacter calcoaceticus*.

lin·gua, gen. e pl. **lin·guae** (ling'gwă, ling'gwē). Língua, língula. **1.** SIN tongue (1). **2.** SIN tongue (2). [L. língua]

l. cerebel'li, língula do cerebelo. SIN *lingula* of cerebellum.

l. fissura'ta, l. fissurada. SIN fissured *tongue*.

l. frena'ta, uma língua com um freio muito curto, constituindo a língua presa.

l. geograph'ica, l. geográfica. SIN geographic tongue.

l. ni'gra, l. negra. SIN black *tongue*.

l. plica'ta, l. sulcada. SIN fissured *tongue*.

lin·gual (ling'gwăl). Lingual. **1.** Relativo à língua ou a qualquer parte semelhante à língua. SIN glossal. **2.** Próximo a ou no sentido da língua.

Lin·guat·u·la (ling-gwat'ū-lă). Um gênero de artrópodos hematófagos endoparasitários (família Linguatulidae, classe Pentastomida), comumente conhecido como vermes da língua; outrora considerados ácaros (Acarina) degenerados, mas, atualmente, em geral considerados uma categoria inicial distinta, porém pequena, de artrópodes (Arthropoda). Os vermes adultos são encontrados nos pulmões ou vias aéreas de vários hospedeiros (p.ex., répteis, pássaros, carnívoros); vermes jovens são encontrados em uma grande variedade de hospedeiros, incluindo os seres humanos, mas principalmente em animais de caça. [L. *linguatu*, linguado, + *-ula*, sufixo diminutivo]

L. rhina'ria, SIN *L. serrata*.

L. serra'ta, uma espécie mais comum na Europa, mas também encontrada nos Estados Unidos, América do Sul e, provavelmente, em outros locais; o adulto é um verme esbranquiçado, liso, achatado, anelado, equipado com ganchos através dos quais ele se prende à mucosa nasal de cães e outros canídeos; as larvas desenvolvem-se no fígado e nos linfonodos de roedores, suínos, gado e, por vezes, em seres humanos e outros primatas. SIN *L. rhinaria*.

lin·guat·u·li·a·sis (ling - gwat - ū - lī′ă - sis). Linguatulíase; infecção por *Linguatula*. VER TAMBÉM halzoun.

Lin·gua·tu·li·dae (ling - gwat′ū - li - dē). Uma das famílias de Pentastomida de interesse médico, sendo a outra a Porocephalidae. As l. possuem corpos achatados; os adultos habitam as cavidades nasais de vários carnívoros, como o cão e o gato, e as formas larvais são encontradas em tecidos de roedores, herbívoros e outros animais; as larvas e os adultos foram reportados a partir dos seres humanos.

lin·gui·form (ling′gwi - fōrm). Lingüiforme; em formato de língua.

lin·gu·la, pl. **lin·gu·lae** (ling′gū - lă, - lē) [TA]. Língula. **1.** Um termo aplicado a vários processos em forma de língua. **2.** Quando não qualificado, a l. do cerebelo. [L. dim. de *lingua*, língua]

  l. cerebel′li [TA], l. do cerebelo. SIN l. of cerebellum.
  l. of cerebellum [TA], l. do cerebelo; uma seqüência de folhas cerebelares achatadas em forma de língua, formando o extremo anterior (ou superior) do verme do cerebelo, estendendo-se para diante, na superfície do véu medular superior, entre os dois pedúnculos cerebelares superiores emergentes. SIN l. cerebelli [TA], alae lingulae cerebelli, lingua cerebelli, tongue of cerebellum.
  l. of left lung [TA], l. do pulmão esquerdo; uma projeção inferomedial, a partir da face anterior do lobo superior do pulmão esquerdo, que limita inferiormente a incisura cardíaca. SIN l. pulmonis sinistri [TA].
  l. of mandible [TA], l. da mandíbula; uma língua afilada de osso que se sobrepõe ao forame da mandíbula, proporcionando inserção ao ligamento esfenomandibular. SIN l. mandibulae [TA], mandibular tongue, Spix spine.
  l. mandib'ulae [TA], l. da mandíbula. SIN l. of mandible.
  l. pulmo'nis sinis'tri [TA], l. pulmonar esquerda. SIN l. of left lung.
  sphenoidal l. [TA], l. esfenoidal; um processo delgado que se projeta posteriormente entre o corpo e a asa maior do osso esfenóide, dos dois lados, formando a margem lateral do sulco carotídeo. No crânio seco, projeta-se para dentro do forame lacerado. SIN l. sphenoidalis [TA].
  l. sphenoida'lis [TA], l. esfenoidal. SIN sphenoidal l.

lin·gu·lar (ling′gū - lăr). Lingular; pertinente a qualquer língula.

lin·gu·lec·to·my (ling′gū - lek′tō - mē). Lingulectomia; excisão da porção lingular do lobo superior esquerdo do pulmão.

△ **linguo-.** Forma combinante relativa à língua. [L. *lingua*]

lin·guo·cli·na·tion (ling′gwō - kli - nā′shŭn). Linguoclinação; inclinação axial de um dente quando a coroa está mais inclinada em direção à língua que o normal.

lin·guo·clu·sion (ling - gwō - kloo′zhŭn). Linguoclusão; deslocamento de um dente em direção ao interior do arco dentário ou no sentido da língua. VER TAMBÉM lingual *occlusion* (2). SIN lingual occlusion (1).

lin·guo·dis·tal (ling - gwō - dis′tăl). Linguodistal; relativo à parte lingual e distal do dente, p.ex., a cúspide l. VER TAMBÉM distolingual.

lin·guo·gin·gi·val (ling - gwō - jin′ji - văl). Linguogengival. **1.** Relativo ao terço gengival da superfície lingual de um dente. **2.** Relativo ao ângulo ou ponto de junção da borda lingual e à linha gengival na superfície mesial ou distal de um dente incisivo.

lin·guo·oc·clu·sal (ling′gwō - ŏ - kloo′săl). Linguoclusal; relativo à linha de junção das superfícies lingual e oclusal de um dente.

lin·guo·pap·il·li·tis (ling′gwō - pap′i - lī′tis). Linguopapilite; pequenas úlceras dolorosas que afetam as papilas nas margens linguais.

lin·guo·plate (ling′gwō - plāt). Placa lingual; um conector principal de uma dentadura parcial formada como uma barra lingual estendida para cobrir os cíngulos dos dentes anteriores inferiores. SIN lingual plate.

lin·guo·ver·sion (ling′gwō - ver - zhŭn). Linguoversão; a posição errônea de um dente lingual em relação à posição normal.

lin·i·ment (lin′i - ment). Linimento; uma preparação líquida para aplicação externa ou nas gengivas; os linimentos podem ser dispersões límpidas, suspensões ou emulsões, sendo freqüentemente aplicados por atrito na pele usados como contra-irritante, rubefaciente, anódino ou agentes de limpeza. [L., de *lino*, esfregar]

li·nin (lī′nin). Linina. **1.** Um glicosídeo amargo obtido a partir do *Linum catharticum* (família Linaceae). **2.** Uma proteína da semente do linho. **3.** Termo obsoleto para a substância filiforme, não-corável do núcleo da célula, na qual se acreditava que estivessem suspensos os grânulos de cromatina. [L. *linum*, de G. *linon*, linho]

lin·ing (līn′ing). Revestimento; uma cobertura aplicada às paredes pulposas de uma preparação dentária restauradora para proteger a polpa da irritação térmica ou química; usualmente um veículo que contém um verniz, resina e/ou hidróxido de cálcio.

li·ni·tis (li - nī′tis, lī - nī′tis). Linite; a inflamação do tecido celular, especificamente do tecido perivascular do estômago. [G. *linon*, linho, tecido de linho, + *-itis*, inflamação]

  l. plas'tica, l. plástica; originalmente considerada uma condição inflamatória, mas atualmente reconhecida como decorrente do carcinoma cirroso infiltrante que provoca espessamento extenso da parede do estômago; freqüentemente denominado estômago em odre.

link. Ligação; uma conexão.
  tip l.'s, ligações de extremidade; as conexões entre os estereocílios das células ciliadas auditivas e vestibulares.

link·age (lingk′ij). Ligação. **1.** Uma ligação covalente química. **2.** A relação entre *loci* sintênicos próximos o suficiente para que os respectivos alelos não sejam herdados de maneira independente pela prole; uma característica dos *loci*, não dos genes.
  genetic l., l. genética. VER linkage (2).
  medical record l., ligação entre registros médicos; a reunião de histórias clínicas individuais de muitos anos ou de toda a vida a partir de dados vitais e clínicos de múltiplas fontes.
  record l., l. de registro; um método de agrupamento das informações contidas em dois ou mais grupos de registros clínicos ou de um grupo de registros médicos e registros vitais, como certidões de nascimento ou atestados de óbito, e um procedimento para garantir que os registros de cada pessoa são compilados apenas uma vez; facilitado por um sistema de numeração único, como o número de Hogben ou o código soundex, para identificar com precisão as pessoas.
  sex l., l. sexual; a herança de um traço ou de um cromossoma sexual ou genossoma. Um homem recebe todos os seus genes ligados ao sexo de sua mãe e os transmite para todas as suas filhas, mas não para seus filhos; um caráter recessivo ligado ao sexo é muito mais provável de ser expresso no homem. VER TAMBÉM sex *chromosomes*, em *chromosome*.

linked. Ligado; diz-se de dois *loci* genéticos que exibem ligação genética.

link·er. Ligador; um fragmento do DNA sintético contendo um local de restrição que pode ser utilizado para unir os genes.

link·er scan·ning. Rastreamento de ligador; um tipo de mutagênese por deleção no qual a distância e/ou a estrutura de leitura entre regiões potencialmente importantes são mantidas pela substituição por um oligonucleotídeo sintético de seqüência conhecida.

Linné, Carl von, botânico e médico sueco, 1707–1778. VER linnaean *system* of nomenclature.

Li·nog·na·thus (li - nog′nă - thŭs). Um gênero de piolhos sugadores (ordem Anoplura, família Linognathidae) que inclui a espécie *L. africanus*, o piolho azul africano de carneiros e cabras; *L. ovillus*, o piolho do corpo do carneiro; *L. pedalis*, o piolho do pé do carneiro; *L. setosus*, o piolho sugador do cão e de outros canídeos; *L. stenopsis*, o piolho sugador de cabras; e *L. vituli*, o piolho sugador de "nariz comprido", o piolho do boi ou o piolho azul do gado. [G. *linon*, linho, fio, + *gnathos*, mandíbula]

li·no·le·ate (li - nō′lē - āt). Linoleato; sal do ácido linoleico.

lin·o·le·ic ac·id (lin - ō - lē′ik). Ácido linoleico; ácido 9,12-octadecadienóico; um ácido graxo duplamente insaturado, que ocorre amplamente nos glicerídeos vegetais, sendo essencial à nutrição em mamíferos. SIN linolic acid. [L. *linum*, linho, + *oleum*, óleo]

lin·o·len·ic ac·id (lin - ō - len′ik). Ácido linolênico; ácido 9,12,15-octadecatrienóico (também referido como α-1); um ácido graxo insaturado que é essencial à nutrição de mamíferos. O ácido γ-linolênico é o ácido 6,9, 12-octadecatrienóico.

linolic acid. Ácido linólico. SIN linoleic acid.

lin·seed (lin′sēd). Semente de linho; a semente madura dessecada do *Linum usitatissimum* (família Linaceae), linho, cuja fibra é usada na fabricação do linho; uma infusão era usada como demulcente nas afecções catarrais dos tratos respiratório e urogenital, e as sementes são empregadas na preparação de cataplasmas. SIN flaxseed. [G. *linon*, linho]
  l. oil, óleo de linho; um óleo graxo expresso das sementes maduras do *Linum usitatissimum*; usado na preparação do linimento. SIN flaxseed oil.

lint. Fibras de algodão; um material macio e absorvente raramente utilizado em compressas cirúrgicas, usualmente na forma de um material espesso, trançado frouxamente (folha ou tecido). [l. ant. *lin*, linho]

△ **lio-.** VER leio-.

LIP Acrônimo de lymphocytic interstitial pneumonia (pneumonia intersticial linfocítica) ou lymphoid interstitial pneumonia (pneumonia intersticial linfóide). VER lymphocytic interstitial *pneumonia*.

lip [TA]. Lábio. **1.** Uma das duas dobras musculares com uma membrana externa apresentando uma camada superficial epitelial escamosa estratificada que limita a boca anteriormente. **2.** Qualquer estrutura semelhante a um lábio que limita uma cavidade ou sulco. VER TAMBÉM labium, labrum. SIN labium (1) [TA]. [A. S. *lippa*]
  acetabular l., l. acetabular. SIN acetabular *labrum*.
  anterior l. of external os of uterus [TA], lábio anterior do óstio externo do útero; a porção da parte vaginal do colo uterino que limita o óstio anteriormente, localizada entre o óstio e o fórnice vaginal anterior. É um pouco mais curto que o lábio posterior. SIN labium anterius ostii uteri [TA], anterior l. of uterine os.

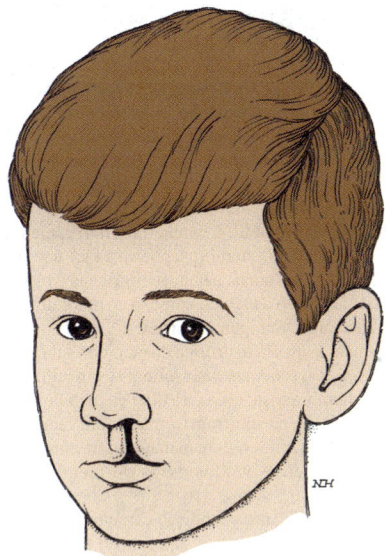

lábio leporino (fenda labial)

anterior l. of uterine os, l. anterior do óstio uterino. SIN anterior l. of external os of uterus.
articular l., l. articular. SIN labrum (3).
cleft l., l. fendido, fenda labial; uma anormalidade facial congênita do l. (usualmente do l. superior) que resulta da ausência de união das proeminências nasais medial e lateral com o processo maxilar; associado com freqüência, mas não necessariamente, ao alvéolo fendido e à fenda palatina. Em muitas famílias e em várias formas [MIM*119300, *119500, *119530, *119540 e 119550] parece ser uma herança autossômica dominante e, igualmente, para a herança ligada ao X [MIM*303400]. Mas, da mesma forma que com as supostas formas autossômicas recessivas, a genética é, em geral, mais confusa e pode representar um aspecto variável de uma síndrome. SIN harelip.
double l., l. duplo; excesso congênito ou adquirido de tecido na mucosa da face interna do l.; pode ser uma manifestação da síndrome de Ascher.
external l. of iliac crest, l. externo da crista ilíaca. SIN outer l. of iliac crest.
glenoidal l., l. glenóide. SIN glenoid labrum of scapula.
Hapsburg l., l. de Hapsburg. VER Hapsburg *jaw*.
inner l. of iliac crest [TA], l. interno da crista ilíaca; a margem interna áspera da crista que fornece a inserção para as partes dos músculos transverso do abdome, quadrado lombar e eretor da coluna. SIN labium internum cristae iliacae [TA], internal l. of iliac crest.
internal l. of iliac crest, l. interno da crista ilíaca. SIN inner l. of iliac crest.
large pudendal l., lábio maior do pudendo. SIN *labium* majus.
lateral l. of linea aspera [TA], l. lateral da linha áspera; a margem lateral da linha áspera do fêmur que fornece inserção para o septo intermuscular lateral e porção curta dos músculos bíceps femoral. SIN labium laterale lineae asperae [TA].
lower l. [TA], l. inferior; a dobra muscular que limita a abertura da boca inferiormente. SIN labium inferius oris [TA].
medial l. of linea aspera [TA], l. medial da linha áspera; a margem medial da linha áspera do fêmur que fornece inserção para parte do músculo vasto medial. SIN labium mediale lineae asperae [TA].
l.'s of mouth [TA], lábios da boca; as dobras carnosas com a pele, externamente, e a mucosa oral, internamente, que circundam a fissura oval e formam as paredes anteriores do vestíbulo oral; tendo envolto o orbicular da boca e vários músculos dilatadores, os lábios constituem o esfíncter craniano do trato alimentar. SIN labia oris [TA].
outer l. of iliac crest [TA], l. externo de crista ilíaca; a margem externa áspera da crista que fornece inserção para os músculos oblíquo externo e grande dorsal, acima, e para a fáscia lata e músculo tensor da fáscia lata, abaixo. SIN labium externum cristae iliacae [TA], external l. of iliac crest.
posterior l. of external os of uterus [TA], l. posterior do orifício externo do útero; a porção do colo uterino que se liga ao óstio, posteriormente. É discretamente mais longo que o lábio anterior, intervindo entre o canal cervical e o fórnice posterior da vagina. SIN labium posterius ostii uteri [TA].
rhombic l., l. rômbico; a placa alar espessada do rombencéfalo embrionário.
small pudendal l., lábio menor do pudendo. SIN *labium* minus.
tympanic l. of limbus of spiral lamina, l. do limbo timpânico do limbo espiral. SIN tympanic l. of spiral limbus.
tympanic l. of spiral limbus [TA], l. do limbo timpânico do limbo espiral [TA]; a extensão perióstea inferior longa do limbo da lâmina espiral óssea que repousa sobre a lâmina basal do órgão espiral (de Corti). SIN labium limbi tympanicum limbi spiralis ossei [TA], labium limbi tympanicum laminae spiralis ossei, tympanic labium of limbus of spiral lamina, tympanic l. of limbus of spiral lamina.
upper l. [TA], l. superior; a prega muscular que forma a borda superior da boca. SIN labium superius oris [TA].
vestibular l. of limbus of spiral lamina, l. do limbo vestibular do limbo espiral. SIN vestibular l. of spiral limbus.
vestibular l. of spiral limbus [TA], l. do limbo vestibular do limbo espiral; a extensão perióstea superior curta do limbo da lâmina espiral óssea que fornece a inserção central para a membrana tectória. SIN labium limbi vestibulare limbi spiralis ossei [TA], labium limbi vestibulare laminae spiralis ossei, lamina dentata, vestibular labium of limbus of spiral lamina, vestibular l. of limbus of spiral lamina.

lip-. Ver lipo-.
li·pan·cre·a·tin (li-pan′krē-ă-tin, krē′ă-tin). Lipancreatina. SIN pancrelipase.
lip·a·ro·cele (lip′ă-rō-sēl). Liparocele; uma hérnia omental. [G. *liparos*, gorduroso, + *kēlē*, tumor, hérnia]
li·pase (lip′ās). Lipase. **1.** Em geral, qualquer enzima lipolítica ou clivadora de lipídios; uma carboxilesterase; p.ex., triacilglicerol lipase, fosfolipase A$_2$, lipoproteína lipase. **2.** SIN *triacylglycerol* lipase.
lip·ec·to·my (lip-ek′tō-mē). Lipectomia; remoção cirúrgica de tecido adiposo, como nos casos de adiposidade. [lipo- + G. *ektomē*, excisão]
lip·e·de·ma (lip′e-dē′mă). Lipedema; inchação crônica, usualmente dos membros inferiores, particularmente nas mulheres de meia-idade, causada pela distribuição ampla e uniforme de líquido e gordura subcutânea. [lipo- + G. *oidēma*, inchação]
li·pe·mia (lip-ē′mē-ă). Lipemia; concentração anormalmente alta de lipídios no sangue circulante. SIN hyperlipidemia, hyperlipoidemia, lipidemia, lipoidemia. [lipid + G. *haima*, sangue]
alimentary l., l. alimentar; l. relativamente transitória que ocorre após a ingestão de alimentos com grande conteúdo de gorduras. SIN postprandial l.
diabetic l., l. diabética; o desenvolvimento do plasma lactescente após a ingestão de lipídios; uma rara manifestação do diabetes melito descontrolado causada pelo metabolismo defeituoso dos lipídios da dieta e abolida pela administração de insulina.
postprandial l., l. pós-prandial. SIN alimentary l.
l. retina'lis, l. retiniana; um aspecto cremoso dos vasos sanguíneos retinianos, que ocorre quando os lipídios do sangue excedem a 5%.
li·pe·mic (li-pē′mik). Lipêmico; relativo à lipemia.
lip·id (lip′id). Lipídio; "lipossolúvel", um termo operacional que descreve uma característica de solubilidade, não uma substância química, ou seja, indica as substâncias extraídas de células animais ou vegetais por solventes apolares; fazendo parte da coleção heterogênea dos materiais assim passíveis de extração, incluem-se os ácidos graxos, glicerídeos e éteres de gliceril, fosfolipídios, esfingolipídios, álcoois e ceras de cadeias longas, terpenos, esteróides e vitaminas "lipossolúveis", como A, D e E. [G. *lipos*, gordura]
l. A, l. A; o componente glicolipídio do lipopolissacarídeo responsável pela sua atividade endotóxica.
anisotropic l., l. anisotrópico; um l. na forma de gotículas duplamente refratárias.
anular l., l. anular; a camada de l. ligada a e/ou que circunda uma proteína integrante da membrana.
brain l., l. cerebral; a cefalina impura que possui ação hemostática acentuada, quando aplicada localmente.
compound l.'s, lipídios compostos; o l. que pode ser hidrolisado sob condições alcalinas para produzir constituintes menores.
isotropic l., l. isotrópico; um l. que ocorre na forma de gotículas com refração única.
simple l.'s, lipídios simples. SIN homolipids.
lip·i·de·mia (lip′i-dē′mē-ă). Lipidemia. SIN lipemia.
lip·i·do·ly·tic (lip′ī-dō-lit′ik). Lipidolítico; que provoca a ruptura do lipídio. [lipid + G. *lysis*, ruptura]
lip·i·do·sis, pl. **lip·i·do·ses** (lip-i-dō′sis, -sēz). Lipidose; anormalidade hereditária do metabolismo lipídico que resulta em deposição lipídica anormal; a classificação é tipicamente baseada na deficiência da enzima responsável e no tipo de lipídio envolvido. Essa atividade enzimática ocorre nos lisossomas, e os produtos anormais aparecem como doenças de armazenamento anormal. As esfingolipidoses constituem a maior porção de lipidoses reconhecidas, incluindo o metabolismo anormal de gangliosídeos, ceramidas e cerebrosídeos. [lipid + G. *-ōsis,* condição]
ceramide lactoside l., l. lactosídica ceramídica; um distúrbio herdado associado a um acúmulo de ceramida lactosídeo devido a uma deficiência de ceramida lactosidase; resulta em lesão cerebral progressiva com dilatação hepática e esplênica.

cerebral l., l. cerebral. SIN cerebral *sphingolipidosis.*
cerebroside l., l. cerebrosídica. SIN Gaucher *disease.*
ganglioside l., l. gangliosídica. SIN *gangliosidosis.*
glycolipid l., l. glicolipídica. SIN Fabry *disease.*
sphingomyelin l., l. esfingomielínica. SIN Niemann-Pick *disease.*
sulfatide l., l. sulfatídica. SIN metachromatic *leukodystrophy.*

Lipmann, Fritz A., bioquímico alemão radicado nos Estados Unidos e laureado com o Prêmio Nobel, 1899–1986. VER Warburg-L.-Dickens-Horecker *shunt.*

lipo-, lip-. Formas combinantes que se relacionam a gorduras ou lipídios. [G. *lipos*, gordura]

lip·o·am·ide (lip-ō-am′īd, -am′id). Lipoamida. VER lipoic acid.

lip·o·am·ide de·hy·dro·gen·ase. Lipoamida desidrogenase. SIN dihydrolipoamide dehydrogenase.

lip·o·am·ide di·sul·fide. Dissulfeto de lipoamida; o ácido lipóico oxidado em combinação amida com um grupamento ε-amino de um resíduo L-lisil da ácido pirúvico desidrogenase.

lip·o·am·ide re·duc·tase (NADH). Lipoamida redutase. SIN dihydrolipoamide dehydrogenase.

lip·o·ar·thri·tis (lip′ō-ar-thrī′tis). Lipoartrite; a inflamação dos tecidos adiposos periarticulares do joelho. [lipo- + arthritis]

lip·o·ate (lip′ō-āt). Lipoato; um sal ou éster do ácido lipóico.

lip·o·ate ace·tyl·trans·fer·ase. Lipoato-aceltransferase. SIN dihydrolipoamide *S-*acetyltransferase.

lip·o·a·tro·phia (lip-ō-a-trō′fē-ă). Lipoatrofia. SIN lipoatrophy.
    l. annula′ris, l. anular; uma rara afecção de etiologia desconhecida, caracterizada por panatrofia localizada, uma área deprimida que envolve o braço, com esclerose e atrofia do tecido adiposo.
    l. circumscrip′ta, l. circunscrita; atrofia adiposa localizada.

lip·o·at·ro·phy (lip-ō-at′rō-fē). Lipoatrofia; a perda do tecido subcutâneo, podendo ser total, congênita e associada a hepatomegalia, crescimento ósseo excessivo e diabetes insulino-resistente. SIN Lawrence-Seip syndrome, lipoatrophia, lipoatrophic diabetes. [G. *lipos*, gordura, + *a-*, priv. + *trophē*, nutrição]
    insulin l., l. insulínica. SIN insulin *lypodystrophy.*
    partial l., l. parcial. SIN progressive *lipodistrophy.*

lip·o·blast (lip′ō-blast). Lipoblasto; uma célula adiposa (adipócito) embrionária. [lipo- + G. *blastos*, germe]

lip·o·blas·to·ma (lip′ō-blas-tō′mă). Lipoblastoma; um tumor subcutâneo benigno composto de células adiposas embrionárias, separadas em lóbulos distintos, que geralmente ocorre em lactentes.

lip·o·blas·to·ma·to·sis (lip′ō-blas-tō-mă-tō′sis). Lipoblastomatose; uma forma difusa de lipoblastoma com infiltração local, mas que não gera metástases.

lip·o·car·di·ac (lip′ō-kar′dē-ak). Lipocardíaco. **1.** Relativo à esteatose cardíaca. **2.** Indica uma pessoa que sofre de degeneração gordurosa do coração. [lipo- + G. *kardia*, coração]

lip·o·cat·a·bol·ic (lip′ō-kat-ă-bol′ik). Lipocatabólico; relativo à clivagem (catabolismo) da gordura.

lip·o·cer·a·tous (lip-ō-ser′ă-tŭs). Liposeratoso. SIN adipoceratous.

lip·o·cere (lip′ō-sēr). Lipocera. SIN adipocere. [lipo- + L. *cera*, cera]

lip·o·chon·dria (lip′ō-kon′drē-ă). Lipocôndrias; vacúolos de armazenamento temporário de lipídios encontrados no aparelho de Golgi. VER TAMBÉM phytosterolemia. [lipo- + mitochondria]

lip·o·chon·dro·dys·tro·phy (lip′ō-kon-drō-dis′trō-fē). Lipocondrodistrofia. SIN Hurler *syndrome.*

lip·o·chrome (lip′ō-krōm). Lipocromo. **1.** Um lipídio pigmentado, p.ex., luteína, caroteno. SIN chromolipid. **2.** Um termo por vezes utilizado para designar os pigmentos de desgaste, p.ex., lipofucsina, hemofucsina, ceróide. Mais precisamente, os lipocromos são pigmentos amarelados que parecem idênticos ao caroteno e à xantofila, sendo freqüentemente encontrados no soro, na pele, no córtex da supra-renal, no corpo lúteo e nas placas ateroscleróticas, bem como no fígado, baço e tecido adiposo; os lipocromos não se coram com os corantes comuns para o tecido adiposo. **3.** O pigmento produzido por determinadas bactérias. [lipo- + G. *chroma*, cor]

li·poc·la·sis (li-pok′lă-sis). Lipoclase. SIN *lipolysis.* [lipo- + G. *klasis*, uma ruptura]

lip·o·clas·tic (lip-ō-klas′tik). Lipoclástico; SIN *lipolytic.*

lip·o·crit (lip′ō-krit). Lipócrito; um aparelho e procedimento para separar e analisar volumetricamente a concentração de lipídio no sangue ou em outro líquido corporal. [lipo- + G. *krino*, separar]

lip·o·cyte (lip′ō-sīt). Lipócito. SIN fat-storing *cell.* [lipo- + G. *kytos*, célula]

lip·o·der·moid (lip-ō-der′moyd). Lipodermóide; tumor adiposo benigno, congênito e amarelo-esbranquiçado, subconjuntival. [lipo- + dermoid]

lip·o·di·er·e·sis (lip′ō-dī-er′ē-sis). Lipodiérese, lipólise. SIN *lipolysis.* [lipo- + G. *diairesis*, divisão]

lip·o·dys·tro·phia (lip′ō-dis-trō′fē-ă). Lipodistrofia. SIN *lipodystrophy.*
    l. progressi′va supe′rior, l. progressiva superior. SIN progressive *lipodystrophy.*

lip·o·dys·tro·phy (lip-ō-dis′trō-fē). Lipodistrofia; metabolismo defeituoso da gordura. SIN lipodystrophia. [lipo- + G. *dys-*, ruim, difícil, + *trophē*, nutrição]
    congenital total l. [MIM*269700], l. congênita total; caracterizada por ausência quase total de tecido adiposo subcutâneo, crescimento e desenvolvimento esquelético acelerados durante os primeiros 3 a 4 anos de vida, hipertrofia muscular, cardiomegalia, hepatoesplenomegalia, acantose nigricans, hipertricose, dilatação renal, hipertrigliceridemia e hipermetabolismo; herança autossômica recessiva. SIN Berardinelli syndrome, Seip syndrome.
    familial partial l. [MIM*151660], l. parcial familial; caracterizada por lipoatrofia simétrica do tronco e dos membros, porém a face é poupada; com a face totalmente arredondada, xantomas, acantose nigricans e hiperglicemia insulino-resistente; existe acúmulo de tecido adiposo ao redor do pescoço, ombros e genitália. SIN Kobberling-Dunnigan syndrome.
    insulin l., l. insulínica; a atrofia distrófica dos tecidos subcutâneos no diabético no local das injeções freqüentes de insulina. SIN insulin lipoatrophy.
    membranous l., l. membranosa; uma rara doença metabólica em que as células adiposas da medula óssea são transformadas em membranas convolutas espessas, coráveis por PAS, que englobam material fracamente osmofílico; leva à reabsorção cística progressiva dos ossos do membro e demência com leucodistrofia sudanofílica.
    progressive l., l. progressiva; uma condição caracterizada por perda completa de tecido adiposo subcutâneo da parte superior do tronco, braços, pescoço e face, por vezes com aumento de gordura nos tecidos em torno e abaixo da pelve. SIN Barraquer disease, lipodystrophia progressiva superior, partial lipoatrophy, Simons disease.

lip·o·e·de·ma (lip′ō-e-dē′mă). Lipoedema; edema do tecido adiposo subcutâneo, provocando inchações dolorosas, principalmente das pernas nas mulheres. SIN cellulite (2).

lip·o·fec·tin (līp′o-fek′tin). Lipofectina; uma mistura predominantemente de fosfolipídios utilizada para auxiliar na transferência de DNA para dentro das células.

lip·o·fec·tion (līp′o-fek′shŭn). Lipofecção; o processo de injetar um DNA contido em ou associado a lipídios dentro das células eucarióticas. [lipo- + trans*fection*]

li·pof·er·ous (lip-of′er-ŭs). Lipófero; que transporta lipídios. [lipo- + L. *fero*, transportar]

lip·o·fi·bro·ma (lip′ō-fī-brō′mă). Lipofibroma; uma neoplasia benigna do tecido conjuntivo fibroso, com numerosas células adiposas.

lip·o·fus·cin (lip-ō-fūs′in). Lipofuscina; grânulos de pigmento acastanhado que representam os resíduos da digestão lipossomial contendo lipídios e considerados um dos pigmentos senescentes ou de "desgaste"; encontrados no fígado, rim, músculo cardíaco, supra-renal e células ganglionares.

lip·o·fus·ci·no·sis (lip′ō-fŭs-i-nō′sis). Lipofuscinose; o armazenamento anormal de qualquer um dos componentes de um grupo de pigmentos adiposos.
    ceroid l., l. ceróide. SIN Batten *disease.*
    neuronal ceroid l., l. ceróide neuronal; um grupo de doenças caracterizadas por acúmulo de pigmentos anormais no tecido (previamente classificadas como esfingolipidoses cerebrais). Os principais subtipos compreendem a forma juvenil crônica (doença de Batten), sintomas comportamentais e visuais lentamente progressivos, herança autossômica recessiva; forma infantil tardia aguda (doença de Bielschowsky); herança autossômica recessiva; forma adulta crônica (doença de Kufs), herança variável; forma infantil aguda (doença de Santavuori-Haltia), deterioração, — tanto mental como motora — fulminante, freqüentemente associada a convulsões mioclônicas. As formas mais brandas também foram descritas.

lip·o·gen·e·sis (lip-ō-jen′ē-sis). Lipogênese; a produção de gordura, por degeneração gordurosa ou por infiltração gordurosa; termo também aplicado à deposição normal de gordura ou à conversão de carboidrato ou proteína em lipídios. SIN adipogenesis. [lipo- + G. *genesis*, produção]

lip·o·gen·ic (lip-ō-jen′ik). Lipogênico; relativo à lipogênese. SIN adipogenic, adipogenous, lipogenous.

li·pog·e·nous (li-poj′ē-nŭs). Lipogênico. SIN lipogenic.

lip·o·gran·u·lo·ma (lip′ō-gran-ū-lō′mă). Lipogranuloma; um nódulo ou foco de inflamação granulomatosa (usualmente do tipo corpo estranho) em associação com material lipídico depositado nos tecidos, p.ex., após a injeção de determinados óleos. VER TAMBÉM paraffinoma. SIN eleoma, oil tumor, oleogranuloma, oleoma.

lip·o·gran·u·lo·ma·to·sis (lip′ō-gran′ū-lō-mă-tō′sis). Lipogranulomatose. **1.** Presença de lipogranulomas. **2.** Reação inflamatória local à necrose do tecido adiposo.
    disseminated l., l. disseminada; uma forma de mucolipidose que se desenvolve logo depois do nascimento, por causa da deficiência de ceramidase; caracterizada por articulações edemaciadas, nódulos subcutâneos, linfadenopatia e acúmulo nos lisossomas das células afetadas do lipídio PAS-positivo, consistindo em ceramida. SIN Farber disease, Farber syndrome.

lip·o·he·mia (lip-ō-hē′mē-ă). Lipoemia; termo obsoleto para lipemia.

li·po·ic ac·id (li-pō′ik). Ácido lipóico; funciona como a amida (lipoamida) na forma dissulfeto (–S–S–) na transferência do "aldeído ativo" (acetil), o fragmento de dois carbonos que resulta da descarboxilação do piruvato do pirofosfato de α-hidroxietiltiamina em acetil-CoA, ele mesmo sendo reduzido à forma ditiol (isto é, ácido diidrolipóico) no processo; presente em leveduras e extratos hepáticos, pode ser útil no tratamento da intoxicação por cogumelos. O ácido lipóico também é um componente essencial de outros complexos de desidrogenases de α-cetoácidos. SIN acetate replacement factor, ocoprotogen, protogen, protogen A, pyruvate oxidation factor, thioctic acid.

lip·oid (lip'oyd). Lipóide. **1.** Que se assemelha ao lipídio. **2.** Termo original para lipídio. SIN adipoid. [lipo- + G. *eidos*, aparência]

lip·oi·de·mia (lip-oy-dē'mē-ă). Lipoidemia, lipemia. SIN lipemia.

lip·oi·do·sis (lip-oy-do'sis). Lipoidose; a presença de lipóides anisotrópicos nas células.

 cerebroside l. (ser-ē'bro-sīd), l. cerebrosídeo; um grupo de doenças de armazenamento lisossômico caracterizadas por acúmulo de lipídios nas células do tecido afetado e comumente acompanhado por um distúrbio manifesto do desenvolvimento do sistema nervoso central; p.ex., doença de Gaucher (Gaucher *disease*) e doença de Krabbe (Krabbe *disease*).

 l. cor´neae, l. da córnea. SIN *arcus* senilis.

 l. cu´tis et muco´sae, l. mucocutânea. SIN lipoid *proteinosis*.

 galactosylceramide l., l. galactosilceramídica. SIN globoid cell *leukodystrophy*.

lip·o·in·jec·tion (lip-ō-in-jek'shun). Lipoinjeção; o aumento do tecido por células adiposas depois da atrofia, como na paralisia ou fibrose das cordas vocais.

lip·o·lip·oi·do·sis (lip'ō-lip-oy-dō'sis). Lipolipoidose; infiltração gordurosa, existindo gorduras neutras e lipóides anisotrópicos nas células. VER TAMBÉM liposis (2).

li·pol·y·sis (li-pol'i-sis). Lipólise; a clivagem (hidrólise) ou decomposição química da gordura. SIN lipoclasis, lipodieresis. [lipo- + G. *lysis*, dissolução]

lip·o·lyt·ic (lip-ō-lit'ik). Lipolítico; relativo a ou que causa lipólise. SIN lipoclastic.

li·po·ma (li-pō'mă). Lipoma; uma neoplasia benigna do tecido adiposo, composta de células adiposas maduras. SIN adipose tumor. [lipo- + G. *-oma*, tumor]

 l. annula´re col´li, l. anular do pescoço; um lipoma de crescimento envolvente (ou lipomas coalescentes) no pescoço, resultando em um aumento semelhante a um colarinho. VER TAMBÉM Madelung *neck*.

 l. arbores´cens, l. arborescente; um l. de formato irregular que envolve a membrana sinovial de uma articulação, resultando em pregas hiperplásicas semelhantes a dedos das mãos ou árvores nas vilosidades.

 atypical l., l. atípico; o l. que ocorre principalmente em homens idosos, na parte posterior do pescoço, ombros e costas, de natureza benigna, mas microscopicamente atípico, contendo células gigantes com múltiplos núcleos se superpondo, formando um círculo. SIN pleomorphic l.

 l. capsula´re, l. capsular; uma massa bem circunscrita que resulta de tecido adiposo muito aumentado adjacente à mama.

 l. caverno´sum, l. cavernoso. SIN angiolipoma.

 l. fibro´sum, l. fibroso. SIN fibrolipoma.

 l. myxomatodes, l. mixomatoso. SIN myxolipoma.

 l. ossif´icans, l. ossificante; um l. em que a metaplasia ocorre e se formam pequenos focos de osso.

 l. petri´ficans, l. petrificante; uma l. em que a degeneração e a necrose resultam em calcificação distrófica considerável.

 pleomorphic l., l. pleomórfica. SIN atypical l.

 spindle cell l., l. de células fusiformes; uma forma benigna de l., microscopicamente distinta, na qual o tecido adiposo está infiltrado por fibroblastos e colágeno; usualmente encontrado no ombro ou pescoço de homens idosos.

 telangiectasic l., l. telangiectásico. SIN angiolipoma.

li·po·ma·toid (li-pō'mă-toyd). Lipomatóide; que se assemelha a um lipoma, diz-se, com freqüência, dos acúmulos de tecido adiposo que não são considerados neoplásicos.

lip·o·ma·to·sis (lip'ō-mă-tō'sis). Lipomatose. SIN adiposis.

 encephalocraniocutaneous l., l. encefalocraniocutânea; uma rara síndrome de múltiplos fibrolipomas ou angiofibromas da face, couro cabeludo e pescoço presentes ao nascimento, por vezes com lipomas intracranianos sintomáticos.

 mediastinal l., l. mediastinal; o tecido adiposo mediastinal aumentado provocado pela ingestão de esteróides.

 multiple symmetric l., l. simétrica múltipla; acúmulo e aumento progressivo de coleções de tecido adiposo no tecido subcutâneo da cabeça, pescoço, parte superior do tronco e porções superiores dos membros superiores; observada principalmente nos homens adultos; sua etiologia é desconhecida. SIN Launnois-Bensaude syndrome, Madelung disease, symmetric adenolipomatosis.

 l. neurot´ica, l. neurótica. SIN *adiposis* dolorosa.

li·po·ma·tous (li-pō'mă-tus). Lipomatoso; pertinente a ou que manifesta os aspectos do lipoma, ou caracterizado pela presença de um lipoma (ou lipomas).

lip·o·me·nin·go·cele (lip'ō-mē-ning'gō-sēl). Lipomeningocele; um lipoma intra-espinal na cauda eqüina associado a espinha bífida. [lipo- + G. *mēninx*, membrana, + *kēlē*, tumor]

lip·o·mu·co·pol·y·sac·cha·ri·do·sis (lip'ō-mū'ko-pol-ē-sak'ă-ri-dō'sis). Lipomucopolissacaridose. SIN *mucolipidosis* I.

lip·o·nu·cle·o·pro·teins (lip'ō-noo'klē-ō-prō'tēnz). Liponucleoproteínas; associações ou complexos que contêm lipídios, ácidos nucleicos e proteínas.

Lip·o·nys·sus (lip-ō-nis'ŭs). Nome original para *Ornithonyssus*. [lipo- + G. *nysso*, espetar]

lip·o·pe·nia (lip-ō-pē'nē-ă). Lipopenia; quantidade anormalmente pequena, ou deficiência, de lipídios no corpo. [lipo- + G. *penia*, pobreza]

lip·o·pe·nic (lip-ō-pē'nik). Lipopênico. **1.** Relativo a ou caracterizado por lipopenia. **2.** Um agente ou medicamento que reduz a concentração dos lipídios no sangue.

lip·o·pep·tid, lip·o·pep·tide (lip-ō-pep'tid, lip-ō-pep'tīd). Lipopeptídeo; um composto ou complexo de lipídio e aminoácidos.

lip·o·phage (lip'ō-fāj). Lipófago; uma célula que fagocita gordura. [G. *lipos*, gordura, + *phago*, comer]

lip·o·phag·ic (lip-ō-fā'jik). Lipofágico; relativo à lipofagia.

lip·oph·a·gy (lip-of'ă-jē). Lipofagia; fagocitose de gordura por um lipófago. [lipo- + G. *phago*, comer]

lip·o·phan·er·o·sis (lip'ō-fan-er-ō'sis). Lipofanerose; uma alteração em determinadas células pela qual a gordura previamente invisível torna-se demonstrável como pequenas gotículas sudanofílicas. VER fatty *degeneration*. [lipo- + G. *phaneros*, visível, + *-osis*, condição]

lip·o·phil (lip'ō-fil). Lipófilo; uma substância com propriedades lipofílicas (hidrofóbicas). [lipo- + G. *philos*, gostar de]

lip·o·phil·ic (lip-ō-fil'ik). Lipofílico; capaz de dissolver, de ser dissolvido em ou de absorver lipídios.

lip·o·phos·pho·di·es·ter·ase I (lip'ō-fos'-fō-dī-es'ter-ās). Lipofosfodiesterase I. SIN *phospholipase* C.

lip·o·phos·pho·di·es·ter·ase II. Lipofosfodiesterase II. SIN *phospholipase* D.

lip·o·pol·y·sac·cha·ride (LPS) (lip'ō-pol'ē-sak'ă-rīd). Lipopolissacarídeo. **1.** Um composto ou complexo de lipídios e carboidratos. **2.** O l. (endotoxina) liberado pelas paredes celulares de microrganismos Gram-negativos que produz o choque séptico.

lip·o·pro·tein (lip-ō-prō'tēn, lī-pō-). Lipoproteína; qualquer complexo ou composto que contenha lipídios e proteína. As lipoproteínas são importantes constituintes das membranas biológicas e da mielina. A conjugação com a proteína facilita o transporte de lipídios, os quais são hidrofóbicos, no meio aquoso do plasma. As lipoproteínas plasmáticas podem ser separadas por ultracentrifugação, eletroforese ou imunoeletroforese; elas migram, na eletroforese, com as α- e β-globulinas, mas, em geral, são classificadas de acordo com suas densidades (constantes de flotação). As principais classes por densidade são os quilomícrons, que transportam o colesterol e os triglicerídeos da dieta do intestino até o fígado e outros tecidos; lipoproteínas de densidade muito baixa (VLDL), que transportam os triglicerídeos desde o intestino e fígado até o músculo e tecido adiposo; as lipoproteínas de baixa densidade (LDL), que transportam o colesterol para tecidos diferentes do fígado; e as lipoproteínas de alta densidade (HDL), que transportam o colesterol até o fígado para a excreção na bile. As propriedades dessas e de outras lipoproteínas plasmáticas são mostradas no quadro a seguir. A porção proteica de uma lipoproteína é chamada de apolipoproteína (ou apoproteína). Além de tornar solúveis os lipídios, algumas apolipoproteínas realizam funções bioquímicas, como a ativação de enzimas. As apolipoproteínas das lipoproteínas plasmáticas são sintetizadas pelo fígado e pelas células da mucosa intestinal e seu peso molecular varia de 7.000 a 500.000. A proteína constitui mais de 50% de algumas HDL, mas apenas 1% dos quilomícrons. À medida que aumenta a proporção de lipídio em uma lipoproteína, sua densidade aumenta. Uma partícula de lipoproteína plasmática é tipicamente esférica, com um cerne hidrofóbico de triacilglicerol, ésteres colesteril e resíduos de aminoácidos apolares circundados por estruturas de proteínas hidrofílicas e fosfolipídios.

 As concentrações de determinadas lipoproteínas séricas têm uma correlação importante com o risco de aterosclerose. Níveis de HDL-colesterol < 35 mg/dL (0,90 mmol/L), de LDL-colesterol > 160 mg/dL (4,15 mmol/L) e de triglicerídeos em jejum > 250 mg/dL são, sem exceção, fatores de risco independentes para a doença da artéria coronária. Embora os fatores nutricionais sejam importantes em algumas pessoas, os níveis basais de lipoproteínas, colesterol e triglicerídeos dependem principalmente da hereditariedade. Já foram identificados vários fenótipos de hiperlipoproteinemia associados ao risco de doença cardiovascular prematura e morte. VER hyperlipoproteinemia. O controle clínico de pacientes com a doença da artéria coronária (infarto do miocárdio, angina de peito, revascularização miocárdica ou angioplastia coronária) e outros distúrbios ateroscleróticos (doença arterial periférica, aneurisma de aorta abdominal, doença da artéria carótida) inclui a detecção e a correção da hipercolesterolemia e hiperlipoproteinemia. A redução do LDL-colesterol diminui o risco de doença da artéria coronária; além de conter a progressão da aterosclerose, pode até mesmo reduzir o tamanho de lesões ateroscleróticas estabelecidas. Dentre as pessoas com LDL-colesterol elevado, 75% conseguem atingir níveis normais com dieta, redução de peso e exercício; o restante precisa de tratamento medicamentoso. Os outros fatores, além da hiperlipoproteinemias familiais, que podem elevar o LDL-colesterol são diabetes melito, hipotireoidismo, síndrome nefrótica, doença hepática obstrutiva e medicamentos (progestogênios, esteróides anabólicos, corticosteróides, diuréticos tiazídicos). Os lipídios saturados da dieta aumentam o LDL-colesterol mais que qualquer outro componente dietético, não se excetuando o próprio colesterol.

l. (a), lipoproteína (a); uma l. que consiste em uma partícula de LDL à qual uma grande glicoproteína, apolipoproteina (a), está ligada de forma covalente. A elevação de sua concentração no soro foi identificada como um fator de risco para a doença da artéria coronária.

A elevação da lipoproteína (a) plasmática acima de 30 mg/dL é um forte fator de risco independente para a doença da artéria coronária e, possivelmente, para o acidente vascular cerebral. Um aspecto singular da lipoproteína (a) é a semelhança estrutural de sua porção não-lipídica, apolipoproteína (a), com o plasminogênio. Essa semelhança permite que ela se ligue ao endotélio e às proteínas das membranas celulares. Ela inibe a fibrinólise por competir com os locais de ligação do plasminogênio, favorecendo também a deposição de lipídios e estimulando a proliferação das células musculares lisas. A niacina e o estrogênio diminuem a Lp(a), mas os inibidores da HMG-CoA redutase, fibratos e seqüestradores de ácidos biliares não o fazem.

α_1**-l.,** lipoproteína α_1; uma fração de lipoproteína de peso molecular relativamente baixo, alta densidade, rica em fosfolipídios e encontrada na fração α_1-globulina do plasma humano.
β_1**-l.,** lipoproteína β_1; uma fração de lipoproteína com peso molecular relativamente alto, baixa densidade, rica em colesterol e encontrada na fração β-globulina do plasma humano.
intermediate density l. (IDL), l. de densidade intermediária; classe de lipoproteínas formada na degradação das lipoproteínas de densidade muito baixa; cerca da metade é rapidamente depurada do plasma para dentro do fígado, através da endocitose mediada por receptor; a outra metade é degradada em lipoproteínas de baixa densidade.
l. Lp(a), Lp (a) I; uma l. composta de uma partícula de LDL combinada com uma proteína adicional, proteína específica da Lp(a); os níveis elevados foram identificados como um fator de risco para a doença da artéria coronária; as elevações podem ser tratadas com niacina.
malondialdehyde-modified low-density l., l. de baixa densidade modificada por malondialdeído; molécula de IDL com resíduo(s) lisina substituído(s) por aldeído na porção apoproteína, resultante de reação oxidativa que acompanha a síntese de prostaglandinas e a agregação plaquetária.
l.-X, l. X; uma lipoproteína de baixa densidade anormal encontrada nos pacientes com icterícia obstrutiva.
lip·o·pro·tein li·pase. Lipoproteína lipase; uma enzima que hidrolisa um ácido graxo a partir de um triglicerídeo; sua atividade é estimulada pela heparina e inativada pela heparinase. É ativada pela apolipoproteína C-II; a deficiência de lipoproteína lipase está associada à hiperlipoproteinemia familial do tipo I. VER TAMBÉM familial lipoprotein lipase *inhibitor*, clearing *factors*, em *factor*. SIN diacylglycerol lipase, diglyceride lipase.

lip·o·sar·co·ma (lip′ō-sar-kō′mă). Lipossarcoma; uma neoplasia maligna de adultos que ocorre especialmente nos tecidos retroperitoneais e na coxa, em geral profundamente nos planos intermusculares ou periarticulares; histologicamente, o l. é um grande tumor que pode ser composto de células adiposas bem diferenciadas ou desdiferenciadas, sejam células mixóides, arredondadas ou pleiomórficas; usualmente em associação a uma rica rede de capilares; as recorrências são comuns, e o l. desdiferenciado gera metástases para os pulmões ou para as superfícies serosas. [lipo- + *sarx*, carne, + *-oma*, tumor]
li·po·sis (li-pō′sis). Lipose. **1.** SIN adiposis. **2.** Infiltração gordurosa, com lipídios neutros sendo encontrados nas células. VER TAMBÉM lipolipoidosis. [lipo- + G. *-osis*, corpo]
li·pos·i·tol (lip-os′i-tol). Lipositol. SIN inositol.
lip·o·sol·u·ble (lip-ō-sol′ū-bl). Lipossolúvel; solúvel em lipídios.
lip·o·some (lip′ō-sōm). Lipossoma. **1.** Uma partícula esférica da substância lipídica suspensa em um meio aquoso dentro de um tecido. **2.** Qualquer vesícula artificial pequena, aparentemente esférica, que consiste em uma dupla camada lipídica envolvendo parte do meio suspensor. [lipo- + G. *sōma*, corpo]
lip·o·suc·tion (lip′ō-sŭk-shun). Lipossucção, lipoaspiração; método de remoção de lipídios subcutâneos indesejados usando drenos de aspiração inseridos por via subcutânea.
 tumescent l., l. tumescente; realizada após a infusão subcutânea de solução de lidocaína e uso de microcânulas.
 wet-technique l., l. por técnica úmida; a l. realizada depois da infusão subcutânea de solução de epinefrina diluída.
lip·o·suc·tion·ing (lip′ō-sŭk′shŭn-ing). Lipoescultura; remoção de gordura por pressão elevada com vácuo; usada na modelagem do corpo.
lip·o·thi·am·ide py·ro·phos·phate (lip-ō-thī′am-īd). Pirofosfato de lipotiamida; nome outrora dado às coenzimas do complexo multienzimático que catalisa a formação da acetil-CoA a partir do piruvato e que envolve a lipoamida e pirofosfato de tiamina, na suposição de que eles eram um composto único. VER lipoic acid.
lip·o·tro·phic (lip-ō-trof′ik). Lipotrófico; relativo à lipotrofia.
li·pot·ro·phy (li-pot′rō-fē). Lipotrofia; aumento da gordura no corpo. [lipo- + G. *trophē*, nutrição]
lip·o·tro·pic (lip-ō-trop′ik). Lipotrópico. **1.** Pertinente às substâncias que impedem ou corrigem os depósitos excessivos de gorduras no fígado, como acontece na deficiência de colina. **2.** Relativo à lipotropia.
lip·o·tro·pin (li-pō-trō′pin). Lipotropina; hormônio hipofisário que mobiliza a gordura do tecido adiposo. A β-l. é um peptídeo de cadeia única com 91 resíduos aminoacil que contêm as seqüências de endorfinas, metencefalina e β-melanotropina; a γ-l. é mais curta e sua seqüência é idêntica à dos 58 resíduos N-terminais da β-lipoproteína; ambas contêm seqüências comuns ao ACTH e β-melanotropina. SIN lipid-mobilizing hormone, lipotropic hormone, lipotropic pituitary hormone.
li·pot·ro·py (li-pot′rō-pē). Lipotropia. **1.** Afinidade dos corantes básicos pelo tecido adiposo. **2.** Prevenção do acúmulo de gordura no fígado. **3.** Afinidade das substâncias apolares entre si. [lipo- + G. *tropē*, virada]
lip·o·vac·cine (lip′ō-vak-sēn). Lipovacina; uma vacina suspensa em óleo vegetal como solvente. VER adjuvant *vaccine*.
lip·o·vi·tel·lin (lip′ō-vi-tel′in). Lipovitelina. SIN vitellin.
li·pox·e·nous (li-pok′se-nŭs). Lipoxênico; pertinente à lipoxenia.

lipoproteínas plasmáticas						
classe	densidade (g/ml)	diâmetro (nm)	apolipoproteínas	proteína (%)	triglicerídeos (%)	colesterol (livre e esterificado) (%)
quilomícrons	<0,95	90–1.000	A-1, A-2, B-48, C-2, C-3, E	1–2	88	4
lipoproteínas de muito baixa densidade (VLDL)	0,95–1,006	30–90	B-100, C-1, C-2, C-3, E	7–10	56	23
lipoproteínas de densidade intermediária (IDL)	1,006–1,019	25–30	B-100	11	43	29
lipoproteínas de baixa densidade (LDL)	1,019–1,063	20–25	B-100	21	58	13
lipoproteínas de alta densidade (HDL)						
HDL$_2$	1,063–1,125	10–20	A-1, A-2, A-4, C-1, C-2, C-3, D	33	41	16
HDL$_3$	1,125–1,210	7,5–10		57	35	13

li·pox·e·ny (li - pok′sĕ - nē, lī-). Lipoxenia; deserção do hospedeiro por um parasita quando o desenvolvimento do último está completo. [G. *leipō*, deixar, + *xenos*, hospedeiro]

li·pox·i·dase (li - poks′i - dās). Lipoxidase. SIN lipoxygenase.

li·pox·y·ge·nase (li - pok′sē - jĕ - nās). Lipoxigenase; uma classe de enzimas que catalisa a oxidação de ácidos graxos insaturados com O_2 para fornecer hidroperóxidos dos ácidos graxos; a 5-lipoxigenase catalisa a primeira etapa na biossíntese de leucotrieno, atuando sobre o araquidonato. SIN carotene oxidase, lipoxidase.

lip·o·yl (lip′ō - il). Lipoil; o radical acil do ácido lipóico.

lip·o·yl de·hy·dro·gen·ase. Lipoil desidrogenase. SIN dihydrolipoamide dehydrogenase.

lip·ping (lip′ing). Labiação; a formação de uma estrutura semelhante ao lábio, como na extremidade articular de um osso na osteoartrite.

lip·pi·tude, lip·pi·tu·do (lip′i - tood, lip - i - too′dō). Borramento visual. SIN blear *eye*. [L., de *lippus*, vista turva]

Lipschütz, Benjamin, médico austríaco, 1878–1931. VER L. *cell*.

li·pu·ria (li - poo′rē - ă). Lipúria; presença de lipídios na urina. SIN adiposuria. [lipo- + G. *ouron*, urina]

li·pur·ic (li - poo′rik). Lipúrico; pertinente à lipúria.

liq·ue·fa·cient (lik′we - fā′shent). Liquefaciente. 1. Que torna líquido; que faz com que um sólido se torne líquido. 2. Que indica um solvente que provoca a resolução de um tumor sólido por liquefazer seu conteúdo. [L. *liquefacio*, pres. p. *-faciens*, tornar líquido, de *liqueo*, ser líquido]

liq·ue·fac·tion (lik - wĕ - fak′shŭn). Liquefação; o ato de tornar líquido; mudar da forma sólida para a líquida. [ver liquefacient]

liq·ue·fac·tive (lik - wĕ - fak′tiv). Liquefactivo; relativo à liquefação.

li·queur (li - ker′). Licor; um cordial, bebida revigorante; um destilado que contém açúcar e aromatizante. [Fr.]

liq·uid (l) (lik′wid). Líquido. 1. Uma substância inelástica, como a água, que não é sólida nem gasosa, e na qual as moléculas estão relativamente livres para se moverem entre si, embora ainda sejam restringidas pelas forças intermoleculares. 2. Que flui como a água. [L. *liquidus*]

Cotunnius l., l. de Cotunnius. SIN perilymph.

li·quor, gen. **li·quor·is,** pl. **li·quo·res** (lik′er, - wōr - is, - wō′rēs) [TA]. Líquido. 1. Qualquer líquido ou fluido. 2. Um termo utilizado para determinados líquidos corporais. 3. Um termo farmacopeico para qualquer solução aquosa (não uma decocção ou infusão) de uma substância não-volátil e para as soluções aquosas de gases. VER TAMBÉM solution. [L.]

l. am′nii, l. amniótico. SIN amnionic *fluid*.

l. cerebrospina′lis [TA], l. cefalorraquidiano. SIN cerebrospinal *fluid*.

l. cotun′nii, l. de Cotunnius. SIN perilymph.

l. enter′icus, l. entérico; secreções intestinais.

l. follic′uli, l. folicular; o líquido no antro do folículo ovariano.

malt l., licor de malte; uma bebida obtida do malte, como a cerveja ou *ale*.

Morgagni l., l. de Morgagni; um líquido encontrado após a morte entre o epitélio e as fibras da lente, resultando da liquefação de um material semilíquido existente durante a vida. SIN Morgagni humor.

mother l., l.-mãe; a solução saturada que permanece depois de uma cristalização ou precipitação.

Scarpa l., l. de Scarpa. SIN endolymph.

spirituous l., bebida alcoólica forte obtida por destilação, como o uísque.

vinous l., l. vinho. SIN wine (1).

li·quo·rice (lik′ŏ - ris). Alcaçuz. SIN glycyrrhiza.

li·quor·rhea (lik - ŏ - rē′a). Liquorréia; o fluxo de líquido. [L. *liquor*, líquido, + G. *rhoia*, fluxo]

Lisch, Karl, oftalmologista austríaco, *1907. VER L. *nodule*.

Lisfranc (de St. Martin), Jacques, cirurgião francês, 1790–1847. VER L. *amputation, joints,* em *joint, ligaments,* em *ligament, operation;* scalene *tubercle* of L.

lis·in·o·pril (līs - in′ō - pril). Lisinopril; um inibidor da enzima conversora de angiotensina usado no tratamento da hipertensão.

Lison, Lucien, cientista belga, *1907. VER L.-Dunn *stain*.

lisp·ing. Ceceio, sigmatismo; a pronúncia errônea das letras sibilantes *s* e *z*. SIN parasigmatism, sigmatism.

lis·sa·mine rho·da·mine B 200 (lis′să - mēn rō′dă - mēn). Lissamina rodamina B 200. SIN sulforhodamine B.

Lissauer, Heinrich, neurologista alemão, 1861–1891. VER L. *bundle, column, fasciculus, tract,* marginal *zone; column* of Spitzka-L.

lis·sen·ce·pha·lia (lis′en - sĕ - fā′lē - ă). Lissencefalia. SIN agyria. [G. *lissos*, liso, + *enkephalos*, cérebro]

lis·sen·ce·phal·ic (lis′en - sĕ - fal′ik). Lissencefálico; pertinente a ou caracterizado por lissencefalia.

lis·sen·ceph·a·ly (lis - en - sef′ă - lē). Lissencefalia. SIN agyria. [G. *lissos*, liso, + *enkephalos*, cérebro]

lis·sive (lis′iv). Que possui a propriedade de aliviar o espasmo muscular sem causar flacidez. [G. *lissos*, liso]

lis·so·sphinc·ter (lis′ō - sfingk′ter). Um esfíncter da musculatura lisa. SIN smooth muscular sphincter. [G. *lissos*, liso, + *sphincter*]

lis·so·trich·ic, lis·sot·ri·chous (lis - ō - trik′ik, - trik′ŭs). Lissótrico, liótrico; que possui pêlos retos. [G. *lissos*, liso, + *thrix (trich-)*, pêlo]

Lister, Joseph (Lord Lister), cirurgião inglês, 1827–1912. VER Listerella; Listeria; listerism; L. *dressing, method, tubercle*.

Lis·ter·el·la (lis′ter - el′ă). Em bacteriologia, um nome genérico rejeitado e, por vezes, citado como sinônimo de *Listeria*. A espécie típica é *L. hepatolytica*. [Joseph *Lister*]

Lis·te·ria (lis - tēr - ē - ă). Gênero de bactérias variando de aeróbicas a microaerofílicas, móveis e peritríquias, contendo pequenos bastonetes Grampositivos cocóides; esses microrganismos tendem a produzir cadeias de 3–5 células e, no estado rugoso, formas alongadas e filamentosas. As células com 18–24 horas de idade podem mostrar uma disposição em paliçada com algumas formas em V ou Y; as bactérias produzem ácido, mas nenhum gás, a partir da glicose e são encontradas nas fezes de seres humanos e de outros animais, na vegetação e na forragem, sendo parasitas em animais poiquilotérmicos e de sangue quente, inclusive seres humanos. A espécie típica é *L. monocytogenes*. [Joseph *Lister*]

L. denitri′ficans, uma espécie bacteriana reclassificada como *Jonesia denitrificans*.

L. gra′yi, uma espécie bacteriana encontrada nas fezes de chinchilas.

L. monocytog′enes, uma espécie bacteriana que provoca meningite, encefalite, septicemia, endocardite, aborto, abscessos e lesões purulentas locais; com freqüência, é fatal; é encontrada em furões sadios, insetos e fezes de chinchilas, ruminantes e seres humanos, bem como no esgoto, vegetação em decomposição, solo e fertilizantes. Por vezes envolvida em infecções em hospedeiros imunocomprometidos. Um agente causal de infecções perinatais, sepse neonatal e septicemia. Também ligada recentemente a doenças transmitidas por alimentos, principalmente associadas a carnes e laticínios.

lis·te·ri·o·sis (lis - tēr′ē - ō′sis). Listeriose; uma doença esporádica de animais e seres humanos, principalmente aqueles que estão imunocomprometidos ou gestantes, provocada pela bactéria *Listeria monocytogenes*. A infecção em carneiros e no gado bovino freqüentemente envolve o sistema nervoso central, causando vários sinais neurológicos; em animais monogástricos e aves domésticas, as principais manifestações são a septicemia e a necrose do fígado. Meningite, bacteriemia e doença metastática focal estão associadas a listeriose. SIN listeria meningitis. [do organismo *Listeria*]

lis·ter·ism (lis′ter - izm). Listerismo. SIN Lister *method*.

Listing, Johann B., fisiologista alemão, 1808–1882. VER L. reduced *eye, law*.

Liston, Robert, cirurgião inglês, 1794–1847. VER L. *knives,* em *knife, shears*.

li·sur·ide (lī′soor - īd). Lisurida; um derivado solúvel do esporão de centeio com efeitos endócrinos similares aos da bromocriptina; um inibidor da serotonina.

li·ter (L, l) (lē′ter). Litro; uma medida de capacidade de 1.000 centímetros cúbicos ou 1 decímetro cúbico; equivalente a 1,056688 quarto (medida de líquido norte-americana). [Fr., do G. *litra*, uma libra]

literature. Literatura.

gray l., relatos que contêm dados, p.ex., sobre saúde e doença em uma população, que não são publicados ou que possuem distribuição limitada. Os exemplos incluem os relatos de serviços de saúde municipais e teses de mestrado e doutourado existentes em bibliotecas de universidades.

△ **lith-.** VER litho-.

lith·a·gogue (lith′ă - gog). Litagogo; que causa o deslocamento ou a expulsão de cálculos, principalmente os cálculos urinários. [litho- + G. *agōgos*, empurrão]

lith·arge (lith′arj). Litargírio, monóxido de chumbo. SIN lead monoxide. [litho- + G. *argyros*, prata]

li·thec·to·my (li - thek′tō - mē). Litectomia, litotomia. SIN lithotomy. [litho- + G. *ektomē*, excisão]

li·thi·a·sis (li - thī′ă - sis). Litíase; formação de cálculos de qualquer tipo, especialmente de cálculos biliares ou urinários. [litho- + G. *-iasis*, condição]

l. conjunti′vae, l. conjuntival; nódulos endurecidos causados por deposição de material calcário nas áreas de degeneração celular nas glândulas de Henle.

2,8-dihydroxyadenine l., l. de 2,8-diidroxiadenina; formação de cálculos de 2,8-diidroxiadenina decorrente de deficiência ou atividade reduzida da adenina fosforribosiltransferase.

pancreatic l., l. pancreática; a formação de cálculos no pâncreas, usualmente associada a inflamação crônica e obstrução dos ductos pancreáticos.

lith·ic ac·id (lith′ik). Ácido lítico, ácido úrico. SIN uric acid.

lith·i·um (Li) (lith′ē - ŭm). Lítio; um elemento do grupo dos metais alcalinos, número atômico 3, peso atômico 6.941. Muitos de seus sais possuem aplicações clínicas. [L. mod. do G. *lithos*, uma pedra]

l. bromide, brometo de lítio; LiBr; um pó esbranquiçado deliqüescente, usado como sedativo e hipnótico.

l. carbonate, carbonato de lítio; agente anti-reumático e antilítico, também empregado no tratamento e na profilaxia das fases depressiva, hipomaníaca e maníaca dos distúrbios afetivos bipolares.

l. citrate, citrato de lítio; diurético e anti-reumático, também utilizado no tratamento das psicoses maníacas.

effervescent l. citrate, citrato de l. efervescente; uma preparação que contém citrato de lítio, bicarbonato de sódio, ácido tartárico e ácido cítrico; uso idêntico ao do citrato de potássio ou de sódio.

l. tungstate, tungstato de lítio; usado em microscopia eletrônica como um corante negativo.

litho-, lith-. Formas combinantes relacionadas a uma pedra, cálculo ou calcificação. [G. *lithos*]

Lith·o·bi·us (li-thō′bē-ŭs). Um gênero de centípedes caracterizado por 15 pares de pernas. As espécies comuns nos Estados Unidos incluem *L. multidentatus* e *L. fortificatus*. [litho- + G. *bios*, vida]

lith·o·cho·lic ac·id (lith-ō-kō′lik). Ácido litocólico; um dos ácidos isolados na bile humana, bem como a partir da bile de vacas, coelhos, carneiros e cabras.

lith·o·clast (lith′ō-klast). Litoclasto. SIN lithotrite. [litho- + G. *klastos*, quebrado]

lith·o·gen·e·sis, li·thog·e·ny (lith-ō-jen′ē-sis, lith-oj′ē-nē). Litogênese; litogenia; formação de cálculos. [litho- + G. *genesis*, produção]

lith·o·gen·ic (lith-ō-jen′ik). Litogênico; que promove a formação de cálculos.

lith·og·e·nous (lith-oj′ē-nŭs). Litogênico; que forma cálculo.

lith·oid (lith′oyd). Litóide; que se assemelha a um cálculo ou pedra. [litho- + G. *eidos*, semelhança]

lith·o·kel·y·pho·pe·di·on, lith·o·kel·y·pho·pe·di·um (lith-ō-kel′ē-fō-pē′dē-on, -ŭm). Litocelifopédio; um litopédio em que as partes fetais em contato com as membranas circunvizinhas, bem como estas, estão calcificadas. [litho- + G. *kelyphos*, concha, + *paidion*, criança]

lith·o·kel·y·phos (lith-ō-kel′ē-fos). Litocélifo; um tipo de litopédio em que apenas as membranas fetais sofrem calcificação. [litho- + G. *kelyphos*, concha]

lith·o·labe (lith′ō-lāb). Litolábio; instrumento obsoleto para fixar um cálculo biliar durante sua remoção. [litho- + G. *lambanō, labein*, agarrar]

li·thol·a·paxy (li-thol′ă-pak-sē). Litolapaxia; a técnica de esmagar um cálculo na vesícula e remover os fragmentos através de um cateter. [litho- + G. *lapaxis*, esvaziamento]

li·thol·y·sis (li-thol′i-sis). Litólise; a dissolução de cálculos urinários. [litho- + G. *lysis*, dissolução]

lith·o·lyte (lith′ō-līt). Litólito; um instrumento para injetar os solventes de cálculos.

lith·o·lyt·ic (li-thō-lit′ik). Litolítico. **1.** Que tende a dissolver os cálculos. **2.** Um agente que possui essas propriedades. [litho- + G. *lysis*, dissolução]

lith·o·myl (lith′ō-mil). Litômilo; um instrumento para pulverizar um cálculo na bexiga. [litho- + G. *mylē*, moinho]

lith·o·ne·phri·tis (lith′ō-ne-frī′tis). Litonefrite; a nefrite intersticial associada à formação de cálculo.

lith·o·pe·di·on, lith·o·pe·di·um (lith-ō-pē′dē-on, -ŭm). Litopédio; um feto retido, geralmente extra-uterino, que se tornou calcificado. [litho- + G. *paidion*, criança pequena]

lith·o·tome (lith′ō-tōm). Litótomo; um bisturi empregado na litotomia.

li·thot·o·mist (li-thot′ō-mist). Litotomista; uma pessoa habilitada na litotomia.

li·thot·o·my (li-thot′ō-mē). Litotomia; cirurgia de corte para remoção de um cálculo, em especial de um cálculo vesical. SIN lithectomy. [litho- + G. *tomē*, incisão]

high l., l. alta. SIN suprapubic l.

lateral l., l. lateral; l. em que o períneo é incisado em um lado da linha mediana.

marian l., l. mediana. SIN median l. [L. *mas* (*mar-*), masculino]

median l., l. mediana; a l. em que a incisão perineal é feita na rafe mediana. SIN marian l.

perineal l., l. perineal; a l. em que a bexiga é abordada por uma incisão no períneo.

prerectal l., l. pré-retal; a l. por uma incisão na linha média do períneo, anterior ao ânus.

suprapubic l., l. suprapúbica; a l. em que a bexiga é penetrada por uma incisão imediatamente acima da sínfise pubiana. SIN high l.

vaginal l., l. vaginal; a l. em que a bexiga ou o ureter é penetrado através de uma incisão na vagina.

vesical l., l. vesical. SIN cystolithotomy.

lith·o·tre·sis (lith-ō-trē′sis). Litotrese; a perfuração de orifícios em um cálculo para facilitar seu esmagamento. [litho- + G. *trēsis*, uma perfuração]

lith·o·trip·sy (lith′ō-trip-sē). Litotripsia; o esmagamento de um cálculo na pelve renal, ureter ou bexiga através de força mecânica ou da energia sonora focalizada. SIN lithotrity. [litho- + G. *tripsis*, um atrito]

electrohydraulic shock wave l. (ESWL), l. por onda de choque eletro-hidráulica; a destruição de cálculos (trato urinário ou em outro local) através de fragmentação usando ondas de choque de transdutores ultra-sônicos enviadas por via transcutânea.

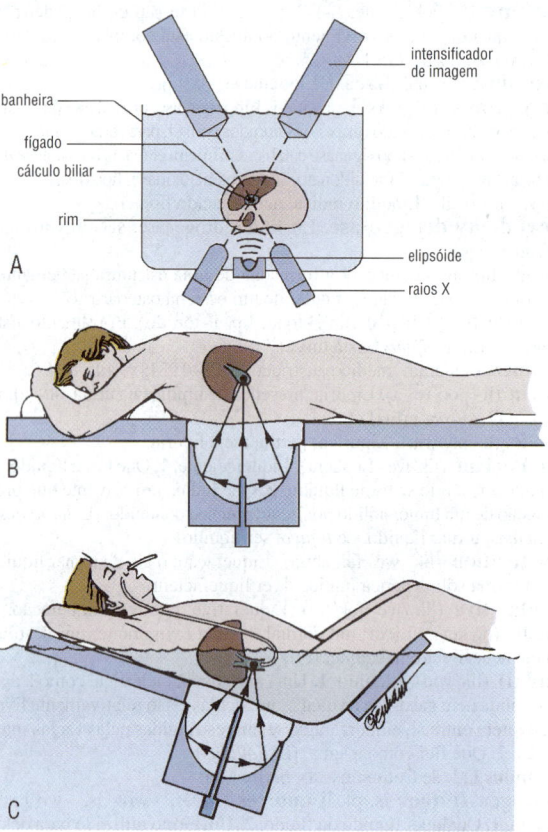

litotripsia por onda de choque extracorpórea: (A) o cálculo da vesícula biliar é localizado por método de imagem; as ondas de choque são produzidas no refletor elipsóide e transmitidas através da água até o cálculo; (B) o posicionamento do paciente para o tratamento dos cálculos localizados na vesícula biliar; a bolsa cheia de líquido é colocada em um recesso na mesa e transmite a onda de choque do gerador para a pele do paciente; (C) o posicionamento do paciente para o tratamento dos cálculos localizados no ducto biliar comum; o paciente é parcialmente submerso em uma banheira com água; o tubo nasobiliar é usado para introduzir contraste para permitir a visualização e a localização do cálculo e para descomprimir a árvore biliar

extracorporeal shock wave l. (ESWL) (lith′ō-trip′sē), l. por onda de choque extracorpórea; fragmentação de cálculos renais ou ureterais através da energia sonora focalizada.

shock wave l., l. por onda de choque; um método para fragmentar cálculos.

ultrasonic l., l. ultra-sônica; a destruição dos cálculos por ondas sonoras de alta freqüência.

lith·o·trip·tic (lith-ō-trip′tik). Litotríptico. **1.** Relativo à litotripsia. **2.** Um agente que empreende a dissolução de um cálculo.

lith·o·trip·tor (lith-ō-trip′tōr). Litotriptor; um aparelho utilizado para esmagar ou fragmentar um cálculo na litotripsia.

lith·o·trip·tos·co·py (lith′ō-trip-tos′kō-pē). Litotriptoscopia; esmagamento de um cálculo na bexiga sob visualização direta com um litotriptoscópio. [litho- + G. *tribō*, atritar, esmagar, + *skopeō*, visualizar]

lith·o·trite (lith′ō-trīt). Litótrito; um instrumento mecânico empregado para esmagar um cálculo urinário na litotripsia. SIN lithoclast. [litho- + L. *tero*, pp. *tritus*, atritar]

li·thot·ri·ty (li-thot′ri-tē). Litotripsia; SIN lithotripsy.

lith·o·troph (lith′ō-trof). Litótrofo; um organismo cujas necessidades de carbono são satisfeitas pelo dióxido de carbono. Cf. chemoautotroph.

lith·u·re·sis (lith′ū-rē′sis). Liturese; a eliminação de cálculos na urina. [litho- + G. *ourēsis*, micção]

li·thu·ri·a (li-thoo′rē-ă). Litúria; excreção de ácido úrico ou de uratos em grande quantidade na urina. [lithic (acid) + G. *ouron*, urina]

lit·mus (lit′mŭs) [C.I. antiga 1242]. Litmo; uma substância que colore azul obtida da *Roccella tinctoria* e outras espécies de liquens, cujo componente principal é a azolitmina; usado como indicador (avermelhado por ácidos e novamente corado em azul por bases). [uma corruptela de *lacmus*, do Hol. *lakmoes*]

lit·ter (lit′er). **1.** Padiola; uma padiola ou leito para mover a pessoa enferma ou lesionada. **2.** Ninhada; um grupo de animais dos mesmos genitores, nascidos ao mesmo tempo. SIN brood (1). [Fr. *litière*; de *lit*, leito]

Little, James, cirurgião norte-americano, 1836–1885. VER L. *area*.

Little, William J., cirurgião inglês, 1810–1894. VER L. *disease*.

Littré, Alexis, anatomista francês, 1658–1726. VER L. *glands*, em *gland, hernia.*
Litzmann, Karl K.T., ginecologista alemão, 1815–1890. VER L. *obliquity.*
live·birth, live birth (līv′berth). Nascido vivo; uma criança com sinais de vida depois do nascimento. VER TAMBÉM liveborn *infant.*
li·ve·do (li - vē′dō). Livedo; coloração azulada da pele, em placas limitadas ou generalizada. [L. *lividez,* de *liveo,* ficar preto ou azul]
  postmortem l., l. pós-morte, livores; coloração purpúrea das partes do corpo mais baixas, exceto nas áreas de pressão por contato, que aparece trinta minutos a duas horas depois da morte, em consequência do movimento gravitacional do sangue dentro dos vasos. SIN postmortem hypostasis, postmortem lividity, postmortem suggillation.
  l. reticula′ris, l. reticular; coloração cutânea purpúrea persistente, em padrão reticular, causada pela dilatação de capilares e vênulas decorrente da estase ou de alterações nos vasos sanguíneos subjacentes, incluindo hialinização; raramente aparece como um defeito do desenvolvimento. SIN dermatopathia pigmentosa reticularis.
  l. reticula′ris idiopath′ica, l. reticular idiopático; uma forma extensa e permanente de l. reticular; em raros casos associado à doença arterial central.
  l. reticula′ris symptomat′ica, l. reticular sintomático; coloração ou mosqueamento da pele com alguma causa demonstrável, como aquele observado no eritema *ab igne* e em determinadas tuberculides. VER TAMBÉM *cutis* marmorata.
  l. telangiectat′ica, l. telangiectásico; mosqueamento permanente da pele decorrente de uma anomalia, provavelmente congênita, dos capilares cutâneos; uma forma de l. reticular.
liv·e·doid (liv′ē - doyd). Livedóide; pertinente ou que se assemelha ao livedo.
liv·er (liv′er) [TA]. Fígado; a maior glândula do corpo, localiza-se sob o diafragma no hipocôndrio direito e na parte superior da região epigástrica; tem formato irregular e pesa de 1 a 2 kg ou cerca de 1/40 do peso corporal. Como glândula exócrina, secreta bile; a princípio, recebe a maior parte dos nutrientes absorvidos através da veia porta; ele detoxifica e também é muito importante nos metabolismos lipídico, proteico e de carboidratos e armazena glicogênio. SIN hepar [TA]. [A.S. *lifer*]
  cardiac l., cirrose cardíaca. SIN cardiac cirrhosis.
  desiccated l., f. dessecado; um pó seco e desengordurado, preparado a partir de fígados de mamíferos, empregado como alimento humano; contém riboflavina, ácido nicotínico e colina; usado no tratamento de anemias macrocíticas e como suplemento nutricional.
  fatty l., esteatose hepática; coloração amarelada do f. decorrente da degeneração gordurosa das células parenquimatosas do f. SIN hepatic steatosis.
  hobnail l., f. tacheado; na cirrose de Laënnec, a contração do tecido cicatricial e a regeneração celular hepática, provocando um aspecto nodular na superfície do fígado.
  lardaceous l., f. lardáceo. SIN waxy l.
  left l. [TA], f. esquerdo; a porção do fígado que recebe o sangue dos ramos esquerdos da artéria hepática e da veia porta, e a partir da qual a bile é drenada pelo canal hepático esquerdo; o plano da veia hepática média (demarcado externamente na superfície visceral, pelas fossas para a vesícula biliar e veia cava inferior e, na superfície diafragmática, por uma linha extrapolada a partir da vesícula biliar para a veia cava inferior terminal) separa o fígado esquerdo do direito. SIN pars hepatis sinistra [TA], left part of liver*.
  nutmeg l., f. em noz-moscada; a congestão passiva crônica do f., que gera acentuação do padrão lobar com zonas centrais avermelhadas e zonas periportais amareladas ou bronzeadas.
  pigmented l., f. pigmentado; f. que contém pigmento, como o que acontece na síndrome de Dubin-Johnson (Dubin-Johnson *syndrome*), hemocromatose, malária de longa duração.
  polycystic l., f. policístico; dilatação cística gradual dos ductos biliares intralobulares (complexos de Meyenburg) que não involuem no desenvolvimento embriológico do f.; freqüentemente associado a rins policísticos congênitos bilaterais e, ocasionalmente, ao envolvimento cístico do pâncreas, pulmões e outros órgãos. SIN polycystic liver disease.
  posterior l., f. posterior;* termo oficial alternativo para posterior hepatic *segment* I.
  right l. [TA], f. direito; a porção do f. que recebe sangue dos ramos direitos da artéria hepática e da veia porta, e a partir da qual a bile é drenada pelo ducto hepático direito; o plano da veia hepática média (demarcado externamente, na superfície visceral, pelas fossas para a vesícula biliar e para a veia cava inferior e, na superfície diafragmática, por uma linha traçada desde a vesícula biliar até a veia cava inferior terminal) separa o fígado direito do esquerdo. SIN pars hepatis dextra [TA], right part of liver*.
  wandering l., f. migratório. SIN hepatoptosis.
  waxy l., f. céreo; degeneração amilóide do f. SIN lardaceous l.
liv·e·tin (liv′ē - tin). Livetina; qualquer uma das três principais proteínas hidrossolúveis na gema do ovo: α-**livetina**, albumina sérica; β-**livetina**, α-glicoproteína; γ-**livetina**, γ-globulina sérica.
liv·id. Lívido; que possui uma coloração azul-escura ou acinzentada ou plúmbea, como na coloração de uma contusão, congestão ou cianose. [L. *lividus,* ser preto e azul]

li·vid·i·ty (li - vid′i - tē). Lividez; estar lívido.
  postmortem l., l. pós-morte, l. cadavérica. SIN postmortem *livedo.*
li·vor (lī′vor). Livor, lividez cadavérica; a descoloração lívida da pele nas partes de um cadáver. [L. uma mancha negra e azul]
lix·iv·i·um (lik - siv′ē - ŭm). Lixívia. SIN lye. [L. neutro de *lixivius,* transformado em lixívia]
LLAT Abreviatura de *lysolecithin*-lecithin acyltransferase (aciltransferase de lisolecitina-lecitina).
LLETZ. Abreviatura de large loop excision of transformation zone of the cervix of the uterus (excisão com alça grande de zona de transformação do colo do útero).
LLL Abreviatura de left lower lobe (of lung) (lobo inferior esquerdo [do pulmão]).
Lloyd, John Uri, farmacêutico norte-americano, 1849–1936. Destacou-se pelo trabalho de pesquisa na química e fotoquímica de vegetais, conforme aplicados a medicamentos, alcalóides e glicosídeos.
Lloyd re·a·gent. Reagente de Lloyd. Ver em reagent.
LLQ Abreviatura para left lower quadrant (of abdomen) (quadrante inferior esquerdo [do abdome]).
LM Abreviatura de licenciado em Obstetrícia.
lm Abreviatura para lumen (2).
LMA Abreviatura para left mentoanterior position (posição mentoanterior esquerda).
LMP 1. Abreviatura para left mentoposterior position (posição mentoposterior esquerda); last menstrual period (data da última menstruação); latent membrane *protein* (proteína de membrana latente); low molecular weight *proteins* (proteínas de baixo peso molecular), em *protein*. **2.** Produto genético do vírus Epstein-Barr (latent membrane protein).
LMT Abreviatura de left mentotransverse position (posição mentoanterior esquerda).
L-α-nar·co·tine. L-α-narcotina. SIN noscapine.
LNPF Abreviatura de lymph node permeability *factor* (fator de permeabilidade ganglionar).
Lo, L₀. VER Lo *dose*.
LOA Abreviatura de left occipitoanterior position (posição occipitoanterior esquerda).
load (lōd). **1.** Sobrecarga; desvio do conteúdo corporal normal, como de água, sal ou calor; as cargas positivas são quantidades superiores ao normal; as cargas negativas são quantidades em déficit. **2.** Carga; a quantidade de uma entidade mensurável transportada por um objeto ou organismo. [I.m. *lode,* do A.S. lād.]
  electronic pacemaker l., c. do marca-passo eletrônico; a impedância para o débito, sendo a c. padronizada a resistência de 500 ohms ± 1%.
  genetic l., c. genética; o agregado de genes mais ou menos perigosos que são transportados, em sua maior parte ocultos, no genoma e que podem ser transmitidos aos descendentes e provocar morbidade e doença; na dinâmica genética clássica, a c. genética pode ser vista como os débitos genéticos não descarregados que resultam de mutações prévias; acredita-se que cada um desses débitos exija um número médio de equivalentes letais dependentes apenas do padrão de herança, independentemente de quão brando ou grave possa ser o fenótipo.

  viral l., c. viral; o nível plasmático do RNA viral, conforme determinado por várias técnicas que incluem o ensaio de ampliação do alvo por reação da cadeia da polimerase com transcriptase reversa e tecnologia de DNA ramificado com amplificação de sinal. Como os níveis de detecção variam de acordo com o método, os resultados do exame por métodos diferentes não são comparáveis.

  > A determinação seriada da carga de HIV tornou-se um procedimento padronizado na monitoração da evolução da AIDS/SIDA. Reportado como o número de cópias de RNA viral por ml de plasma, a avaliação da carga viral proporciona importantes informações sobre o número de células linfóides ativamente infectadas pelo HIV. Esse procedimento laboratorial superou a contagem de CD4 como um indicador do prognóstico de pessoas infectadas pelo HIV, na determinação de quando iniciar a terapia anti-retroviral e na mensuração da resposta à terapia. Como a contagem de CD4 é considerada superior na determinação do nível de comprometimento imunológico e do risco de infecção oportunista, os dois exames são atualmente utilizados. A terapia anti-retroviral é iniciada quando a concentração plasmática de RNA do HIV excede 5.000 cópias/ml. Quando, em conseqüência do tratamento, o número de cópias de RNA viral cai abaixo do nível que pode ser detectado pelos métodos padronizados, considera-se a replicação do HIV como tendo sido suprimida. Entretanto, em nenhum caso a AIDS/SIDA foi curada ou a proliferação viral permaneceu interrompida após a cessação da terapia anti-retroviral.

load·ing (lōd′ing). Sobrecarga; administração de uma substância com a finalidade de testar a função metabólica.

carbohydrate l., s. de carboidratos; um procedimento, popular entre os corredores de longa distância e outros atletas, de "preencher" os músculos com uma grande reserva de glicogênio antes de um evento atlético; com freqüência, o atleta consome muito pouco carboidrato durante três dias, seguido por uma dieta rica em carboidratos durante os três últimos dias antes do evento.

salt l., s. de sais; a administração de 2 g de cloreto de sódio (com uma dieta regular), 3 vezes ao dia durante 4 dias; um teste diagnóstico no aldosteronismo primário, no qual a sobrecarga de sal produz um padrão hormonal e eletrolítico plasmático típico.

soda l., um procedimento adotado por inúmeros atletas que ingerem bicarbonato de sódio em uma tentativa de tamponar a produção de prótons durante o exercício.

Loa loa (lō'ă lō'ă). O verme ocular africano, uma espécie da família Onchocercidae (superfamília Filarioidea) que é própria da região oeste da África Equatorial, especialmente na região do rio Congo, sendo o agente etiológico da loíase. Os vermes adultos são brancos ou branco-acinzentados, cilindróides e filiformes, com os machos tendo em média 25–35 por 0,3–0,4 mm (com uma cauda curva), e as fêmeas, 50–60 por 0,4–0,6 mm; as microfilárias são embainhadas, com os núcleos estendendo-se até a extremidade da cauda. O ciclo de vida é algo similar ao das espécies de *Wuchereria*; os seres humanos são o único hospedeiro definitivo conhecido, e os parasitas são transmitidos por moscas *Chrysops* (família Tabanidae); as larvas infectantes precisam de 3 anos ou mais para amadurecer nos seres humanos, e as formas adultas podem persistir em um hospedeiro humano por até 17 anos. VER TAMBÉM loiasis.

lo·bar (lō'bar). Lobar; relativo a qualquer lobo.
l. nephronia, (1) uma massa renal focal relacionada à infecção aguda. **(2)** nefrite bacteriana focal aguda. **(3)** fleimão renal (não um abscesso; sem pus livre).

lo·bate (lō'bāt). Lobado. **1.** Dividido em lobos. **2.** Em formato de lobo; indicando uma colônia bacteriana com uma margem profundamente ondulada. SIN lobose, lobous.

lobe (lōb) [TA]. Lobo. **1.** Uma das subdivisões de um órgão ou de outra região, limitada por fissuras, sulcos, septos de tecido conjuntivo ou outras demarcações estruturais. **2.** Uma parte em projeção arredondada, como o l. da orelha. VER TAMBÉM lobule. **3.** Uma das divisões maiores da coroa de um dente, formada a partir de um ponto distinto de calcificação. SIN lobus [TA]. [G. *lobos*, lobo]

anterior l. of hypophysis, adeno-hipófise; * termo oficial alternativo para adenohypophysis.
az'ygos l. of right lung, l. ázigos do pulmão direito; um pequeno l. acessório formado acima do hilo do pulmão direito; separado do restante do l. superior por um sulco profundo que aloja a veia ázigos. SIN lobus azygos pulmonis dextri.
caudate l., l. caudado; * termo oficial alternativo para posterior hepatic *segment* I.
cerebral l.'s, lobos do cérebro. SIN *lobi* cerebri, em *lobus*.
cuneiform l., lóbulo biventre. SIN biventer *lobule*.
ear l., l. da orelha. SIN *lobule* of auricle.
falciform l., l. giro do cíngulo. SIN cingulate *gyrus*.
flocculonodular l. [TA], lóbulo flocculonodular; a pequena subdivisão posterior e inferior do córtex cerebelar que limita a linha de inserção do teto coróide da fossa rombóide, consistindo nos flóculos esquerdo e direito, juntamente com o nódulo isolado (o mais posterior da folha que compõe o verme do cerebelo). Suas principais conexões aferentes originam-se dos núcleos vestibulares e diretamente do nervo vestibular; projetam-se principalmente para os núcleos vestibulares, de maneira direta e por meio do núcleo fastigial. SIN lobus flocculonodularis [TA].
frontal l. [TA], l. frontal. SIN frontal l. of cerebrum.
frontal l. of cerebrum [TA], l. frontal do cérebro; a porção de cada hemisfério cerebral anterior ao sulco central. SIN frontal l. [TA], lobus frontalis [TA].
glandular l. of hypophysis, adeno-hipófise; SIN adenohypophysis.
Home l., l. de Home; o l. médio aumentado da glândula prostática.
inferior l. of (left/right) lung, l. inferior do pulmão (esquerdo/direito); localiza-se abaixo e atrás da fissura oblíqua e contém cinco segmentos broncopulmonares: superior (S VI), basal medial (S VII), basal anterior (S VIII), basal lateral (S IX) e basal posterior (S X). SIN lobus inferior pulmonis dextri et sinistri [TA], lower l. of lung*.
insular l., l. insular; * termo oficial alternativo para *lobus* insula.
kidney l.'s [TA], lobos renais; uma das subdivisões do rim, consistindo em uma pirâmide renal e no tecido cortical associado a ela. SIN lobus renalis [TA], renal l.
left l. [TA], lobo esquerdo; a subdivisão esquerda de várias glândulas, p.ex., próstata, tireóide, timo. SIN lobus sinister [TA].
left l. of liver [TA], l. hepático esquerdo; é separado do lobo direito muito maior, anterior e superior aos ligamentos falciforme e coronário, e dos lobos quadrado e caudado pela fissura do ligamento redondo e pela fissura do ligamento venoso. Os lobos do fígado não são unidades funcionais, sendo definidos por estruturas externas; a distribuição da veia porta, da artéria hepática e dos ductos biliares não corresponde às divisões lobares macroscópicas do fígado. SIN lobus hepatis sinister [TA], divisio lateralis sinistra*, lateral division of left liver*.

limbic l. [TA], l. límbico; conforme originalmente definido por P. Broca: o anel quase fechado de estruturas cerebrais que circundam o hilo, ou margem, do hemisfério cerebral nos mamíferos; é composto do giro fornicado (giro do cíngulo, giro fasciolar, giro para-hipocampal e tonsila) e do hipocampo. VER limbic *system*. SIN lobus limbicus [TA].
lingual l., l. cíngulo dos dentes. SIN *cingulum* of tooth.
lower l. of lung, l. inferior do pulmão; * termo oficial alternativo para inferior l. of (left/right) lung.
l.'s of mammary gland [TA], lobos da glândula mamária; as 15 a 20 porções separadas da glândula mamária que se irradiam da área central, profundamente ao mamilo, semelhantes a aros de roda, e que constituem o corpo da glândula mamária; cada um é drenado por um único ducto lactífero. SIN lobi glandulae mammariae [TA].
middle l. of prostate [TA], l. médio da próstata; a porção da próstata que se situa entre a uretra e os ductos ejaculatórios; indistinto, a menos que esteja hipertrofiado. SIN lobus medius prostatae [TA], Morgagni caruncle.
middle l. of right lung [TA], l médio do pulmão direito; localiza-se anteriormente, entre as fissuras horizontal e oblíqua, e inclui os segmentos broncopulmonares lateral (S IV) e medial (S V). SIN lobus medius pulmonis dextri [TA].
nervous l., neuro-hipófise. SIN neurohypophysis.
neural l. of hypophysis, neuro-hipófise; a parte bulbosa da neuro-hipófise ligada ao hipotálamo pelo infundíbulo. É composto de pituícitos, vasos sangüíneos e terminações das fibras nervosas a partir dos núcleos supra-óptico e paraventricular.
occipital l. [TA], l. occipital. SIN occipital l. of cerebrum.
occipital l. of cerebrum [TA], l. occipital do cérebro; a parte posterior com formato algo semelhante a uma pirâmide, em cada hemisfério cerebral, sem nenhuma marca nítida na superfície na convexidade lateral do hemisfério com os lobos parietal e temporal, mas nitidamente marcada a partir do lobo parietal pelo sulco parieto-occipital na superfície medial. SIN lobus occipitalis [TA], occipital l. [TA].
parietal l. [TA], l. parietal. SIN parietal l. of cerebrum.
parietal l. of cerebrum [TA], l. parietal do cérebro; a porção média de cada hemisfério cerebral, separada do lobo frontal pelo sulco central, do lobo temporal pelo sulco lateral em frente e por uma linha imaginária projetada posteriormente, e do lobo occipital apenas parcialmente pelo sulco parieto-occipital em sua face medial. SIN lobus parietalis [TA], parietal l. [TA].
placental l.'s, lobos placentários; os cotilédones da placenta humana, visualizados na superfície materna como elevações ou lobos com formatos irregulares.
polyalveolar l., l. polialveolar; um tipo de anomalia congênita no qual um aumento de várias vezes no número total de alvéolos leva a enfisema lobar congênito.
posterior l. of hypophysis, neuro-hipófise. SIN neurohypophysis.
l . of prostate [TA], l. da próstata; um dos lobos laterais (direito ou esquerdo) ou o lobo médio ou istmo da próstata; no adulto, os lobos são mal definidos. SIN lobus prostatae [TA].
pyramidal l. of thyroid gland [TA], l. piramidal da glândula tireóide; um lobo estreito e inconstante da glândula tireóide que se origina da borda superior do istmo e se estende para cima, por vezes até o osso hióide; marca o ponto de continuidade com o ducto tireoglosso. SIN lobus pyramidalis glandulae thyroideae [TA], Lallouette pyramid, Morgagni appendix, pyramid of thyroid.
quadrate l., (1) lobo quadrado do fígado; lobo na superfície interna do fígado localizado entre a fossa para a vesícula biliar e a fissura para o ligamento redondo; **(2)** lóbulo quadrangular. SIN quadrangular *lobule*; **(3)** pré-cúneo. SIN precuneus.
renal l., lobos renais. SIN kidney l.'s.
Riedel l., l. de Riedel um prolongamento ocasional, semelhante a uma língua, que se estende para baixo a partir do l. hepático direito, lateral à vesícula biliar; um prolongamento similar pode, embora raramente, originar-se do lobo esquerdo. SIN lobus appendicularis, lobus linguiformis.
right l. [TA], l. direito; a subdivisão direita de várias glândulas, p.ex., próstata, tireóide, timo. SIN lobus dexter [TA].
right l. of liver [TA], l. hepático direito do fígado; o maior lobo do fígado, separado do lobo esquerdo, anterior e superiormente, pelos ligamentos falciforme e coronário, e dos lobos quadrado e caudado pelo sulco para a veia cava e pela fossa para a vesícula biliar. SIN lobus hepatis dexter [TA].
Spigelius l., l. de Spigelius. SIN posterior hepatis *segment* I.
superior l. of (right/left) lung, l. superior do pulmão (direito/esquerdo); o lobo do pulmão direito que se localiza acima das fissuras oblíqua e horizontal, incluindo os segmentos broncopulmonares apical (S I), posterior (S II) e anterior (S III); no pulmão esquerdo, o lobo situa-se acima da fissura oblíqua e contém os segmentos apicoposterior (S I + II), anterior (S III), lingular superior (S IV) e lingular inferior (S V). SIN lobus superior pulmonis (dextri et sinistri) [TA], upper l. of lung*.
supplemental l., l. suplementar; em anatomia dentária, um l. extra; aquele que não está incluído na formação típica de um dente.
temporal l. [TA], l. temporal; um l. longo, a mais inferior das principais subdivisões do manto cortical, formando os dois terços posteriores da superfície

ventral do hemisfério cerebral, separada dos lobos frontal e parietal, acima, pelo sulco lateral, arbitrariamente delineado por um plano imaginário desde o l. occipital, com o qual é contínuo posteriormente. O l. temporal apresenta uma composição heterogênea; além de um grande componente neocortical que consiste nos giros superior, médio e inferior e nos giros occipitotemporais lateral e medial, ele inclui o giro para-hipocampal, em sua maior parte justacortical, com seu gancho paleocortical (olfativo) e, abaixo deste, a tonsila. SIN lobus temporalis [TA], temporal cortex.

l.'s of thyroid gland [TA], lobos da glândula tireóide; as duas principais divisões da glândula que se situam nos lados direito e esquerdo da traquéia, conectadas pelo istmo. Um lobo piramidal menor está freqüentemente presente como uma extensão para cima, a partir do istmo. SIN lobi glandulae thyroideae [TA].

upper l. of lung, l. superior do pulmão; * termo oficial alternativo para superior l. of (right/left) lung.

lo·bec·to·my (lō-bek'tō-mē). Lobectomia; a excisão de um lobo de qualquer órgão ou glândula. [G. *lobos*, lobo, + *ektomē*, excisão]

lo·be·lia (lō-bē'lē-ă). Lobélia. **1.** As folhas e extremidades secas da *Lobelia inflata* (família Lobeliaceae); contém vários alcalóides: lobelina, lobelamina, lobelanidina, lobelanina, norlobelanina, norlobelanidina e isolobelanina. O extrato líquido e a tintura têm sido utilizados como expectorante na asma e bronquite crônica. **2.** Um de uma classe de alcalóides isolados da l. (1). **3.** Qualquer vegetal do gênero *Lobelia*. SIN asthma-weed (1), wild tobacco.

lo·be·li·ne, lo·be·lin (lō'bĕ-lēn, lob'ĕ-lēn, -lin). Lobelina; uma piperidilacetofenona; um alcalóide da lobélia com as mesmas ações que a nicotina, porém menos potente.

l. sulfate, sulfato de l.; uma forma de l. que ocorre em massas amareladas friáveis, solúvel em água; usado na coqueluche e na asma; há muito sugerido como um redutor do fumo.

lo·bi (lō'bī). Lobos; plural de lobus. [L.]

lo·bi·tis (lō-bī'tis). Lobite; inflamação de um lobo.

Lobo, Jorge, médico brasileiro, 1900–1979. VER L. *disease*.

Lo·boa lo·boi (lō'bō'ă lō-bō'ē). Uma espécie de fungo que provoca a lobomicose. O microrganismo não se desenvolveu em cultura.

lo·bo·my·co·sis (lō-bō-mī-kō'sis). Lobomicose; micose crônica localizada da pele, reportada na América do Sul, que resulta em nódulos granulomatosos ou quelóides, os quais contêm células em brotamento, com paredes espessas, com aproximadamente 9 μm de diâmetro, ou seja, a forma tecidual da *Loboa loboi*, o fungo etiológico, que não foi cultivado. Também ocorre em golfinhos. SIN Lobo disease.

lo·bo·po·di·um, pl. **lo·bo·po·dia** (lō'bō-pō'dē-ŭm, -dē-ă). Lobopódio; um pseudópode loboso e espesso. [G. *lobos*, lobo, + *pous*, pé]

lo·bose, lo·bous (lō'bōs, lō'bŭs). Lobado; SIN lobate.

lo·bot·o·my (lō-bot'ō-mē). Lobotomia. **1.** A incisão dentro de um lobo. **2.** A divisão de um ou mais tratos nervosos em um lobo do cérebro. [G. *lobos*, lobo, + *tomē*, um corte]

prefrontal l., l. pré-frontal; a divisão de um ou mais tratos nervosos na área pré-frontal do cérebro para o tratamento cirúrgico da dor e distúrbio emocional. SIN prefrontal leukotomy.

transorbital l., l. transorbital; l. por uma abordagem através do teto da órbita, atrás do seio frontal. SIN transorbital leukotomy.

Lobry de Bruyn, Cornelius A., químico holandês, 1857–1904. VER L. de B.-van Ekenstein *transformation*.

Lobstein, Johann F. D., patologista alemão, 1777–1840. VER L. *ganglion*.

lob·u·lar (lob'ū-lăr). Lobular; relativo a um lóbulo.

lob·u·late, lob·u·lat·ed (lob'ū-lāt, -ed). Lobulado; dividido em lóbulos.

lob·ule (lob'ūl) [TA]. Lóbulo; um pequeno lobo ou subdivisão de um lobo. SIN lobulus [TA].

ala central l. [TA], asa do l. central. SIN wing of central lobule. SIN pars inferior alae lobuli centralis [TA], pars superior ali lobuli centralis [TA].

ansiform l., l. semilunar; compreende a parte maior do hemisfério do cerebelo; suas superfícies superior e inferior são separadas pela fissura horizontal em partes maiores conhecidas como lóbulo semiluar superior e lóbulo semilunar inferior.

anterior lunate l., l. semilunar superior. SIN superior semilunar l.

l. of auricle [TA], l. da orelha; a parte mais inferior da orelha; consiste em tecido adiposo e fibroso, não reforçado pela cartilagem da orelha; é freqüentemente utilizado como um local para se obter uma pequena amostra de sangue, usando-se uma lanceta. SIN lobulus auriculae [TA], ear lobe.

biventer l. [TA], l. biventre; um l. na superfície inferior de cada hemisfério cerebelar, dividido por um sulco curvo em uma porção lateral e uma medial; corresponde à pirâmide do verme. SIN lobulus biventer [TA], biventral l., cuneiform lobe, lobulus biventralis, lobulus cuneiformis.

biventral l., l. biventre; SIN biventer l.

central l. [TA], l. central do cerebelo. SIN central l. of cerebellum.

central l. of cerebellum, l. central do cerebelo; uma divisão do verme superior do cerebelo entre a língula e o cúlmen, consistindo nos lóbulos II e III. SIN central l. [TA], lobulus centralis corporis cerebelli [TA].

conical l.'s of epididymis, lóbulos do epidídimo; * termo oficial alternativo para l.'s of epididymis.

cortical l.'s of kidney, lóbulos corticais do rim; uma das subdivisões do rim, consistindo em um raio medular e aquela porção da parte contornada (corpúsculos renais e túbulos contornados) associada a seu ducto coletor. SIN lobulus corticalis renalis, renal cortical l., renculus (1), reniculus (1), renunculus (1).

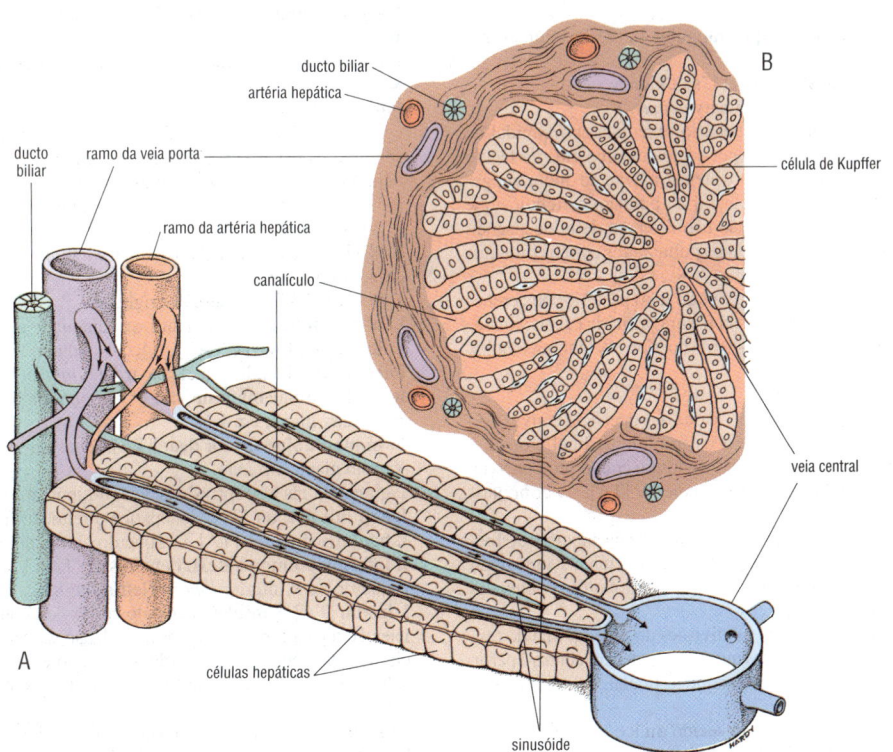

lóbulo hepático e sinusóides: (A) diagrama esquemático do corte do lóbulo hepático, (B) corte transversal de um lóbulo hepático

crescentic l.'s of the cerebellum, lóbulos semilunares do cerebelo; termo arcaico para *lobulus* semilunaris inferior e *lobulus* semilunaris superior.

l.'s of epididymis [TA], lóbulos do epidídimo; a porção espiralada dos canalículos eferentes que constituem a cabeça do epidídimo; estes formam o canal do epidídimo. SIN lobuli epididymidis [TA], coni epididymidis*, conical l.'s of epidimis*, coni vasculosi, Haller cones, vascular cones.

gracile l. [TA], l. paramediano; a porção anterior do lóbulo póstero-inferior do cerebelo, sendo sua parte posterior o l. semilunar inferior; os dois são contínuos com o tubérculo do verme. SIN lobulus paramedianus [TA], lobulus gracilis*, paramedian l.*, slender l.

hepatic l., lóbulos hepáticos. SIN l.'s of liver.

inferior parietal l. [TA], l. parietal inferior; a parte da superfície superior do hemisfério cerebelar que se situa atrás da fissura horizontal. SIN lobulus parietalis inferior [TA], inferior parietal gyrus.

inferior semilunar l. [TA], l. semilunar inferior; a parte da superfície superior do hemisfério cerebelar que se situa por trás da fissura horizontal. SIN lobulus semilunaris inferior [TA], crus II, posterior lunate l.

l.'s of liver [TA], lóbulos hepático; a unidade histológica poligonal conceitual do fígado, consistindo em massas de células hepáticas dispostas em torno de uma veia central, um ramo terminal de uma das veias hepáticas; na periferia estão localizados os ramos pré-terminal e terminal da veia porta, artéria hepática e canal biliar; os lóbulos hepáticos são unidades anatômicas no fígado suíno ou patologicamente nos seres humanos, quando existem septos fibrosos. SIN lobulus hepatis [TA], hepatic l.

l.'s of mammary gland [TA], lóbulos da glândula mamária; as subdivisões dos lobos da glândula mamária. SIN lobuli glandulae mammariae [TA].

paracentral l. [TA], l. paracentral; uma divisão da face medial do córtex cerebral, que se situa acima do sulco do cíngulo, sendo limitada pelo sulco paracentral, anteriormente, e pela parte marginal do sulco do cíngulo, posteriormente; esse l. é formado pelo giro paracentral anterior e pelo giro paracentral posterior. SIN lobulus paracentralis [TA].

paramedian l., l. paramediano; * termo oficial alternativo para gracile l.

portal l. of liver, l. porta do fígado; uma unidade conceitual do fígado, enfatizando sua função exócrina na secreção da bile, que compreende uma área de corte transversal com formato aproximadamente triangular, com um canal porta em seu centro e três ou mais veias hepáticas centrais em sua periferia.

posterior lunate l., l. semilunar posterior. SIN inferior semilunar l.

primary pulmonary l., ácino pulmonar. SIN pulmonary *acinus*.

quadrangular l., l. quadrangular; a porção principal da parte superior de cada hemisfério do cerebelo, correspondendo, na terminologia atual, ao lóbulo quadrangular anterior; as porções do hemisfério do cúlmen (lóbulos IV e V) do verme consistem em uma parte anterior (lóbulo HIV) e uma parte posterior (lóbulo HV); localizado entre as fissuras pré-culminal e primária. SIN lobulus quadrangularis, lobulus quadratus (1), lobus quadratus, quadrate lobe (2), quadrate l. (1).

quadrate l., (1) l. quadrangular. SIN quadrangular l.; (2) Pré-cúneo. SIN precuneus.

renal cortical l., l. cortical renal. SIN cortical l.'s of kidney.

respiratory l., ácino respiratório. SIN pulmonary *acinus*.

secondary pulmonary l., l. pulmonar secundário; uma massa piramidal de tecido pulmonar cujos lados são limitados por septos incompletos de tecido conjuntivo interlobular e cujas bases, que possuem 1 a 2 cm de diâmetro, geralmente estão voltadas para a superfície pleural do pulmão; os lóbulos que ocupam uma posição mais central no pulmão não são bem definidos, sendo considerados como consistindo em cinco ácinos pulmonares com os bronquíolos terminais proximais.

simple l. [TA], l. simples; a menor parte anterior do lobo posterior do cerebelo, separada rostralmente do lobo anterior pela fissura primária e, caudalmente, do grande lóbulo semilunar pela fissura póstero-superior. SIN lobulus simplex [TA].

slender l., l. paramediano. SIN gracile l.

superior parietal l. [TA], l. parietal superior; a área da superfície convexa do lobo parietal do cérebro que se situa entre a fissura longitudinal e o sulco interparietal caudalmente ao giro pós-central; é contínuo com o pré-cúneo na face medial do hemisfério. SIN lobulus parietalis superior [TA], superior parietal gyrus.

superior semilunar l. [TA], l. semilunar superior; a parte da superfície superior do hemisfério cerebelar que se situa entre as fissuras horizontal e lunográcil e que une as folhas e as partes do tubérculo do verme. SIN lobulus semilunaris superior [TA], anterior lunate l., crus I.

l.'s of testis [TA], lóbulos do testículo; as subdivisões do parênquima do testículo formadas por delicados septos fibrosos que se dirigem para dentro a partir da túnica albugínea, convergindo para o mediastino testicular. SIN lobuli testis [TA].

l.'s of thymus [TA], lóbulos do timo; áreas de tecido tímico, com 0,5 a 2 mm de diâmetro, com um córtex e medula. SIN lobuli thymi [TA].

l.'s of thyroid gland [TA], lóbulos da glândula tireóide; as subdivisões do lobo da glândula tireóide, consistindo em grupos irregulares, separados de maneira incompleta, de folículos tireóideos (em número de 20 a 40), agrupados por tecido conjuntivo delicado. SIN lobuli glandulae thyroideae [TA].

lob·u·let, lob·u·lette (lob′u-let′). Um lóbulo muito pequeno ou uma das menores subdivisões de um lóbulo.

lob·u·lus, gen. e pl. **lob·u·li** (lob′u-lus, u-li) [TA]. Lóbulo. SIN lobule. [L. Mod. dim. de *lobus*, lobo]

l. auric′ulae [TA], l. da orelha. SIN lobule of auricle.

l. biven′ter [TA], l. biventre. SIN biventer *lobule*.

l. biventra′lis, l. biventre. SIN biventer *lobule*.

l. centra′lis corporis cerebel′li [TA], l. central do cerebelo. SIN central *lobule* of cerebellum.

l. cli′vi, declive. SIN declive.

l. cortica′lis rena′lis, l. cortical renal. SIN cortical *lobules* of kidney, em *lobule*.

l. cul′minis, cúlmen. SIN culmen.

l. cune′iform′is, l. biventre. SIN biventer *lobule*.

lob′uli epididym′idis [TA], lóbulos do epidídimo. SIN lobules of epididymis, em *lobule*.

l. fo′lii, folha de verme; a parte do verme superior do cerebelo que se situa imediatamente atrás da fissura póstero-superior e caudal ao declive.

l. fusifor′mis, giro occipitotemporal lateral. SIN fusiform *gyrus*.

lob′uli glan′dulae mamma′riae [TA], lóbulos da glândula mamária. SIN lobules of mammary gland, em *lobule*.

lob′uli glan′dulae thyroi′deae [TA], lóbulos da glândula tireóide. SIN lobules of thyroid gland, em *lobule*.

l. grac′ilis, l. paramediano *termo oficial alternativo para gracile *lobule*.

l. hep′atis [TA], l. hepático. SIN lobules of liver, em *lobule*.

l. paracentra′lis [TA], l. paracentral. SIN paracentral *lobule*.

l. paramedianus [TA], l. paramediano. SIN gracile *lobule*.

l. parieta′lis infe′rior [TA], l. parietal inferior. SIN inferior parietal *lobule*.

l. parieta′lis supe′rior [TA], l. parietal superior. SIN superior parietal *lobule*.

l. quadrangula′ris, l. quadrangular. SIN quadrangular *lobule*.

l. quadra′tus, (1) lóbulo quadrangular. SIN quadrangular *lobule*. (2) Pré-cúneo. SIN precuneus.

l. semiluna′ris infe′rior [TA], l. semilunar inferior. SIN inferior semilunar *lobule*.

l. semiluna′ris supe′rior [TA], l. semilunar superior. SIN superior semilunar *lobule*.

l. sim′plex [TA], l. simples. SIN simple *lobule*.

lob′uli tes′tis [TA], lóbulos do testículo. SIN lobules of testis, em *lobule*.

lobuli thy′mi [TA], lóbulos do timo. SIN lobules of thymus, em *lobule*.

lo·bus, gen. e pl. **lo·bi** (lo′bus, lo′bi) [TA]. Lobo, lobos. SIN lobe. [L. ant. do G. *lobos*]

l. ante′rior hypophys′eos [TA], adeno-hipófise. SIN adenohypophysis.

l. appendicula′ris, l. de Riedel. SIN Riedel *lobe*.

l. azygos pulmonis dextri, l. ázigos do pulmão direito. SIN azygos *lobe* of right lung.

l. cauda′tus, l. caudado; *termo oficial alternativo para posterior hepatic *segment* l.

lobi cer′ebri [TA], lobos do cérebro; as principais divisões do hemisfério cerebral; incluem os lobos frontal, parietal, temporal e occipital, nomeados segundo os ossos suprajacentes do crânio, e o lobo límbico. A ínsula também pode ser considerada como um lobo (lobo insular [TA]) porque é separada dos opérculos frontal, parietal e temporal pelo sulco circular da ínsula [TA]. SIN cerebral lobes.

l. cli′vi, termo obsoleto para cúlmen e lóbulos semilunares do cerebelo, considerados como um lobo.

l. dex′ter [TA], l. direito. SIN right *lobe*.

l. falcifor′mis, giro do cíngulo. SIN cingulate *gyrus*.

l. flocculonodularis [TA], l. flóculo-nodular. SIN flocculonodular *lobe*.

l. fronta′lis [TA], l. frontal. SIN frontal *lobe* of cerebrum.

lo′bi glan′dulae mamma′riae [TA], lobos da glândula mamária. SIN lobes of mammary gland, em *lobe*.

lo′bi glan′dulae thyroi′deae [TA], lobos da glândula tireóide. SIN lobes of thyroid gland, em *lobe*.

l. glandula′ris hypophys′eos, adeno-hipófise. SIN adenohypophysis.

l. hep′atis dex′ter [TA], l. hepático direito. SIN right *lobe* of liver.

l. hep′atis sinis′ter [TA], l. esquerdo do fígado. SIN left *lobe* of liver.

l. inferior pulmonis dextri et sinistri [TA], l. inferior do pulmão (direito e esquerdo). SIN inferior *lobe* of (left/right) lung.

l. insula [TA], l. insular; a área do córtex cerebral localizada interna ao sulco lateral e separada dos opérculos frontal, parietal e temporal adjacentes pelo sulco circular da ínsula; composto do giro longo e dos giros curtos separados pelo sulco central da ínsula. VER TAMBÉM insula. SIN insular lobe*, l. insularis*, insular part, pars insularis.

l. insularis, l. insular; *termo oficial alternativo para l. insula.

l. limbicus [TA], l. límbico. SIN limbic *lobe*.

l. linguifor′mis, l. de Riedel. SIN Riedel *lobe*.

l. me′dius pro′statae [TA], l. médio da próstata. SIN middle *lobe* of prostate.

l. me'dius pulmo'nis dex'tri [TA], l. médio do pulmão direito. SIN middle *lobe* of right lung.
l. nervo'sus [TA], neuro-hipófise. SIN neurohypophysis.
l. occipita'lis [TA], l. occipital. SIN occipital *lobe* of cerebrum.
l. parieta'lis [TA], l. parietal. SIN parietal *lobe* of cerebrum.
l. poste'rior hypophys'eos, neuro-hipófise; *termo oficial alternativo para neurohypophysis. VER TAMBÉM pituitary *gland.*
l. pro'statae [TA], l. da próstata. SIN *lobe* of prostate.
l. pyramida'lis glan'dulae thyroi'deae [TA], l. piramidal da glândula tireóide. SIN pyramidal *lobe* of thyroid gland.
l. quadra'tus, l. lóbulo quadrangular. SIN quadrangular *lobule*.
l. rena'lis [TA], l. renal. SIN kidney *lobes*, em *lobe*.
l. sinis'ter [TA], l. esquerdo. SIN left *lobe*.
l. supe'rior pulmo'nis (dextri et sinistri) [TA], lobo superior do pulmão (direito e esquerdo). SIN superior *lobe* of (right/left) lung.
l. tempora'lis [TA], l. temporal. SIN temporal *lobe*.
LOCA Abreviatura de low osmolar contrast *agent* (contraste hipoosmolar).
lo·cal (lō′kăl). Local; que possui referência ou confinado a uma parte limitada; não generalizado ou sistêmico. [L. *localis,* de *locus,* lugar]
lo·cal·i·za·tion (lō′kăl-i-zā′shŭn). Localização. **1.** A limitação a uma área definida. **2.** A referência de uma sensação a seu ponto de origem. **3.** A determinação da localização de um processo mórbido.
auditory l., l. auditiva; na psicologia sensorial, a nomeação ou o ato de apontar para as direções de onde emanam os sons.
cerebral l., l. cerebral; **(1)** o mapeamento do córtex cerebral em áreas e a correlação das várias áreas com a função cerebral; **(2)** a determinação do local de uma lesão cerebral com base nos sinais e sintomas manifestados pelo paciente ou pelo neuroimageamento.
germinal l. l. germinativa. SIN fate *map*.
radiotherapy l., l. radioterápica; o planejamento do tamanho e alinhamento dos feixes de radiação para englobar a neoplasia a ser tratada.
spatial l., l. espacial; a referência de uma sensação visual para uma localidade definida no espaço.
stereotaxic l., l. estereotáxica; a l. dos núcleos intracerebrais por coordenadas com a referência dos marcos anatômicos no cérebro.
lo·cal·ized (lō′kăl-īzd). Localizado; restrito ou limitado a uma parte definida.
lo·cant (lō′kănt). Um número ou letra que antecede um nome substituinte no nome de uma substância química complexa, especificando a posição (localização) do substituinte na molécula original; p.ex., 5 em 5-metiluridina, *S* em *S*-adenosilmetionina.
lo·ca·tor (lō′kā-ter, tōr). Localizador; um instrumento ou aparelho para encontrar a posição de um objeto estranho no tecido.
lo·chia (lō′kē-ă). Lóquios; eliminação de muco, sangue e restos de tecidos através da vagina, após o parto. [G. neut. pl. de *lochios,* relativo ao parto, de *lochos,* parto]

lóquios

nome (coloração)	composição	períodos (varia para os indivíduos)
lóquios rubros (vermelha)	principalmente sanguíneo, resíduos teciduais, decíduas (ocasionalmente vérnix caseoso, lanugem, mecônio)	1.º–3.º dias (primeira semana)
lóquios foscos (acastanhada)	hemólise crescente, menos sangue; secreção serosa (linfa, leucócitos)	3.º–7.º dias (segunda semana)
lóquios serosos	leucócitos, células deciduais, muco cervical	7.º–14.º dias
lóquios amarelos (amarelada)	principalmente leucócitos, bactérias, restos celulares (a chamada endometrite fisiológica)	2.º–3.ª semanas
lóquios brancos (acinzentada)	declínio do fluxo semanal; epitelialização endometrial; secreção mucosa clara das glândulas uterinas	3.ª (4.ª) semana

l. al'ba, l. brancos; a última secreção que não está mais tinta de sangue.
l. ru'bra, l. rubros; a secreção inicial tinta de sangue.
l. sanguinolen'ta, l. sanguinolentos; a secreção vaginal espessa, vermelho-escura, observada alguns dias depois do parto.
l. sero'sa, l. serosos; os lóquios aquosos e pouco espessos.
lo·chi·al (lō′kē-ăl). Loquial; relativo aos lóquios.
lo·chi·o·me·tra (lō-kē-ō-mē′tră). Loquiometro; distensão do útero pelos lóquios retidos. [G. *mētra,* útero]
lo·chi·or·rha·gia (lō-kē-ō-rā′jē-ă). Loquiorragia. SIN lochiorrhea. [lochia + G. *rhēgnymi,* expulsar]
lo·chi·or·rhea (lō-kē-ō-rē′ă). Loquirréia; fluxo profuso de lóquios. SIN lochiorrhagia. [lochia + G. *rhoia,* um fluxo]
lo·ci (lō′sī). Locos; plural de *locus*.
lock (lok). Trava, fecho; um dispositivo para prender ou fechar.
English l., t. inglesa; a articulação das lâminas do fórceps obstétrico que consiste em um encaixe na haste na junção com o cabo em um encaixe similar na outra haste; usado no fórceps de Simpson.
sliding l., t. deslizante; uma fenda em uma haste do fórceps obstétrico (como no fórceps de Kjelland) permitindo que as hastes se movimentem para frente e para trás de forma independente.
Locke, Frank S., fisiologista britânico, 1871–1949. VER Cabot-L. *murmur*; L. *solutions,* em *solution*; L.-Ringer *solution*.
lock·jaw (lok′jaw). Trismo. SIN trismus.
Lockwood, Charles B., anatomista e cirurgião inglês, 1858–1914. VER L. *ligament*.
LOCM Abreviatura de low osmolar contrast *medium* (contraste hipoosmolar).
lo·co·mo·tive (lō-kō-mō′tiv). Locomotivo, locomotor. SIN locomotor.
lo·co·mo·tor (lō-kō-mō′ter). Locomotor; relativo à locomoção ou movimento de um local para outro. SIN locomotive, locomotory. [L. *locus,* place, + L. *moveo,* pp. *motus,* mover]
lo·co·mo·to·ri·al (lō-kō-mō-tō′rē-ăl). Locomotor; relativo ao aparelho locomotor.
lo·co·mo·to·ri·um (lō′kō-mō-tō′rē-ŭm). Locomotor; o aparelho locomotor do corpo. [L. *locus,* lugar + *motorius,* que movimenta]
lo·co·mo·to·ry (lō-kō-mō′tō-rē). Locomotor. SIN locomotor.
loc·u·lar (lok′ū-lăr). Locular; relativo a um lóculo.
loc·u·late (lok′ū-lāt). Loculado; que contém inúmeros lóculos.
loc·u·la·tion (lok-ū-lā′shŭn). Loculação. **1.** Uma região loculada em um órgão ou tecido, ou uma estrutura loculada formada entre as superfícies dos órgãos, mucosas ou serosas, e assim por diante. **2.** O processo que resulta na formação de um lóculo ou lóculos.
loc·u·lus, pl. **loc·u·li** (lok′ū-lŭs, -lī). Lóculo; uma pequena cavidade ou compartimento. [L. dim. de *locus,* lugar]
lo·cum ten·ant (lō′kum ten′ent). Uma substituição temporária de um médico por outro. SIN locum tenens. [anglicização parcial de *locum tenens*]
lo·cum ten·ens (lō′kum ten′ens). Substituto. SIN locum tenant. [L. aquele que ocupa uma posição]
lo·cus, pl. **lo·ci** (lō′kŭs, lō′sī). **1.** Um lugar; geralmente, um local específico. **2.** *Locus;* a posição que um gene ocupa em um cromossoma. **3.** A posição de um ponto, conforme definido pelas coordenadas em um gráfico. [L.]
l. caeru'leus [TA], *locus ceruleus;* uma depressão rasa, de coloração azulada no cérebro fresco, que se situa lateralmente na porção mais rostral da fossa rombóide, adjacente ao aqueduto do mesencéfalo; situa-se próximo à parede lateral do quarto ventrículo e consiste em aproximadamente 20.000 corpos neuronais pigmentados por melanina, cujos axônios contendo norepinefrina possuem uma distribuição notadamente ampla no cerebelo, bem como no hipotálamo e no córtex cerebral. SIN l. cinereus, l. ferrugineus, substantia ferruginea.
l. cine'reus, *locus ceruleus*. SIN l. caeruleus.
cis-**acting l.,** local de ação *cis*; uma seção do DNA que afeta a atividade das seqüências de DNA na mesma molécula de DNA.
complex l., *locus* complexo; um grupo de *loci* genéticos intimamente relacionados com uma função comum, como no *locus* do complexo de histocompatibilidade principal (MHC).
l. of control, local de controle; uma construção teórica destinada a avaliar o controle percebido de uma pessoa sobre seu próprio comportamento; classificado como *interno,* quando a pessoa se sente no controle dos eventos, e *externo* quando percebe que outros exercem esse controle.
l. ferrugin'eus, *locus ceruleus*. SIN l. caeruleus.
genetic l., *locus* genético; o grupo de partes homólogas de um par de cromossomas que pode ser ocupado por genes alélicos. Dessa maneira, o *locus* compreende um par de localizações (exceto no cromossoma X no sexo masculino). O conceito de um *locus* é algo idealizado, não levando em consideração os acidentes que podem ocorrer na meiose, como a duplicação dos locos, em conseqüência do cruzamento desigual, translocações, inversões, etc.
marker l., *locus* marcador; um l. em um cromossoma ou em um filamento de DNA que pode ser identificado (p.ex., um fragmento de restrição do comprimento do polimorfismo) e pode servir na análise de ligação e no isolamento de um gene da doença. VER TAMBÉM linkage *marker*.
l. ni'ger, substância negra. SIN *substantia* nigra.
l. perfora'tus anti'cus, substância perfurada anterior. SIN anterior perforated *substance*.

l. perfora'tus posti'cus, substância perfurada posterior. SIN posterior perforated substance.

sex-linked l., *locus* ligado ao sexo; qualquer l. que, nos cariótipos normais, é transportado em um heterossoma; aplicado em geral, mas de forma incorreta, a um *locus* ligado ao X.

X-linked l., *locus* ligado ao X; qualquer *locus* que, nos cariótipos normais, é transportado no cromossoma X.

Y-linked l., *locus* ligado ao Y; qualquer *locus* (haplóide) que, nos cariótipos normais, é transportado no cromossoma Y. O conteúdo conhecido é, até agora, pequeno.

lod score (lod skōr). Um número usado em estudos de ligação genética; o logaritmo (decádico) das chances a favor da ligação genética. [logarithm + *od*ds]

Loeb, Leo, patologista norte-americano, 1869–1959. VER L. *deciduoma*.

Loeffler, Friedrich A. J., bacteriologista e cirurgião alemão, 1852–1915. VER L. *bacillus*, blood culture *medium*, *stain*, caustic *stain*, *methylene blue*; Klebs-L *bacillus*; Loeffler *syndrome* I; Loeffler *syndrome* II.

Loevit, Moritz, patologista austríaco, 1851–1918. VER L. *cell*.

Loewenthal, Wilhelm, médico alemão, 1850–1894. VER L. *bundle*, *reaction*, *tract*.

lo·fen·ta·nil (lō-fen'tă-nil). Lofentanil; um poderoso narcótico e analgésico de ação prolongada quimicamente relacionado ao fentanil.

Löffler, Wilhelm, médico suíço, 1887–1972. VER L. *disease, endocarditis*, parietal fibroplastic *endocarditis*, *syndrome*.

♻ **log-.** VER logo-.

Logan, William H.G., cirurgião plástico norte-americano, do início do século XX. VER L. *bow*.

log·a·rithm (lŏg'ar-ridhm). Logaritmo; se um número, *x*, é expresso como uma potência de outro número, *y*, ou seja, se $x = y^n$, então se diz que n é o logaritmo de *x* para a base *y*. Os logaritmos comuns são de base 10; os logaritmos naturais ou de Napier são de base e, uma constante matemática. [G. *logos*, palavra, proporção, + *arithmos*, número]

log·e·tro·nog·ra·phy (log-ē-tron-og'ră-fē). Logetronografia; um método de impressão fotográfica em que os detalhes finos são enfatizados pela estimulação eletrônica de seus contrastes; originalmente utilizado para reproduzir as imagens radiográficas.

♻ **-logia.** Forma combinante que significa estudo. **1.** O estudo do tema contido no corpo da palavra, ou um tratado sobre o mesmo; o equivalente em inglês é -logy, ou com uma vogal de ligação, -ology. [G. *logos*, discurso, tratado]. **2.** Que colhe ou apanha. [G. *legō,* coletar]

lo·git (lŏg'it). O logaritmo da relação das freqüências de dois resultados de diferentes categorias ou mutuamente exclusivas, como saudável e doente.

♻ **logo-, log-.** Formas combinantes relativas à fala, palavras. [G. *logos*, palavra, discurso]

log·o·pe·dia (log-ō-pē'dē-ă). Logopedia. SIN logopedics.

log·o·pe·dics (log'ō-pē'diks). Logopedia; um ramo da ciência relacionado com a fisiologia e patologia dos órgãos da fala e com a correção dos defeitos da fala. SIN logopedia. [logo- G. *pais (paid-)*, criança]

log·or·rhea (log-ō-rē'ă). Logorréia; termo raramente utilizado para a loquacidade anormal ou patológica. [logo- + G. *rhoia*, um fluxo]

log·o·spasm (log'ō-spazm). Logoespasmo. **1.** Tartamudez. SIN stuttering. **2.** SIN explosive speech. [logo- + G. *spasmos*, spasm]

log·o·ther·a·py (log'ō-thār'ă-pē). Logoterapia; uma forma de psicoterapia que coloca ênfase especial na vida espiritual do paciente e sobre o médico como o "ministério médico". [logo- + G. *therapeia*, cura]

♻ **-logy.** VER -logia. [G. *logos*, tratado, discurso]

Lohlein-Baehr le·sion. Lesão de Lohlein-Baehr. Ver em lesion.

lo·i·a·sis (lō-ī'ă-sis). Loíase; doença crônica causada pelo nematódeo filarial *Loa loa*, com sintomas e sinais que ocorrem primeiramente em torno de 3 a 4 anos após a picada de uma mosca tabanídea infectada. Quando as larvas infectantes amadurecem, os vermes adultos seguem de forma irregular pelo tecido conjuntivo do corpo (com velocidade que chega a 1 cm/minuto), tornando-se, com freqüência, visíveis sob a pele e as mucosas; p.ex., nas costas, couro cabeludo, tórax, superfície interna do lábio e, especialmente, na conjuntiva. Os vermes provocam hiperemia e exsudação de líquido, freqüentemente uma resposta do hospedeiro aos produtos do verme, uma inchação fugaz ou do tipo Calabar que não provoca lesão grave e diminui à medida que o parasita se movimenta; o paciente fica importunado pelos movimentos "serpenteantes" nos tecidos e prurido intenso, bem como dor ocasional, especialmente quando a inchação está na região dos tendões e articulações. Muitos pacientes apresentam eosinofilia de 10 a 30 ou 40% no sangue circulante. SIN Calabar swelling, fugitive swelling.

loin (loyn). Flanco; a parte do lado e nas costas entre as costelas e a pelve. SIN lumbus. [Fr. *longe*; E. *lumbus*]

Lok, VER Luer-Lok *syringe*.

lo·li·ism (lō'li-izm). Lolismo; a intoxicação pelas sementes de uma gramínea, *Lolium temulentum* (na forma de farinha transformada em pão), caracterizada por tonteira, tremor, visão esverdeada, pupilas dilatadas, prostração e, por vezes, vômitos. [L. *lolium*, joio, ervilhaca]

Lombard, Etienne, médico francês, 1868–1920. VER L. voice-reflex *test*.

lo·mus·tine (lō-mŭs'tēn). Lomustina; um agente antineoplásico. SIN CCNU.

Long, John H., médico norte-americano, 1856–1927. VER L. *coefficient, formula*.

long-chain ac·yl-CoA de·hy·dro·gen·ase. Acil-CoA desidrogenase de cadeia longa. VER *acyl-CoA* dehydrogenase (NADPH).

long-chain fat·ty ac·id-CoA li·gase. Ligase do ácido graxo de cadeia longa – CoA; tiocinase do ácido graxo (cadeia longa), uma ligase que forma acil-CoA, AMP e pirofosfato a partir de ácidos graxos de cadeia longa, ATP e coenzima A. SIN acyl-activating enzyme (1), dodecanoyl-CoA synthetase.

lon·gev·i·ty (lon-jev'i-tē). Longevidade; duração de uma determinada vida além do normal para a espécie. VER TAMBÉM lifespan. SIN macrobiosis.

lon·gi·tu·di·nal (lon'ji-too'di-năl) [TA]. Longitudinal. **1.** Que se faz ao longo do comprimento; na direção do eixo longitudinal do corpo ou de qualquer uma de suas partes. SIN longitudinalis [TA]. **2.** Estudado durante um período de tempo, diacrônico; contraste com o transversal ou sincrônico, que fornece resultados equivalentes apenas sob determinadas condições estritas de estabilidade e equilíbrio. A atenção estrita a essas condições é da máxima importância no estudo da sobrevida, quer na demografia, quer na economia celular (como o padrão de sobrevida dos eritrócitos e plaquetas). [L. *longitudo*, comprimento]

lon·gi·tu·di·na·lis (lon'ji-too'di-nā'lis) [TA]. Longitudinal. SIN longitudinal (1).

lon·gi·type (lon'ji-tīp). Longitipo. SIN ectomorph.

Longmire, William P., Jr., cirurgião norte-americano, 1913–1977. VER L. *operation*.

Looney, Joseph M., bioquímico norte-americano, *1896. VER Folin-Looney *test*.

loop (loop). Alça. **1.** Uma curva aguda ou volta completa em um vaso, cordão ou outro corpo cilíndrico, que forma um anel oval ou circular. VER TAMBÉM ansa. **2.** Um fio (comumente de platina ou nicromo) fixado em um cabo em uma extremidade e curvado em um círculo na outra, esterilizado na chama e usado para transferir microrganismos. [I. m. *loupe*]

Biebl l., a. de Biebl; uma a. contínua do intestino delgado exteriorizada através da parede abdominal até uma localização subcutânea, para a observação da motilidade.

bulboventricular l., a. bulboventricular; a porção do tubo cardíaco embrionário no somito inicial que evolui para o ventrículo e bulbo cardíaco. SIN ventricular l.

capillary l., a. capilar; pequeno vaso sanguíneo nas papilas dérmicas.

cervical l., a. cervical. SIN *ansa* cervicalis.

cruciform l.'s, alças cruciformes; uma estrutura secundária de DNA formada pela ligação de hidrogênio de regiões autocomplementares.

D l., a. D; uma estrutura na replicação do DNA circular. SIN displacement l.

displacement l., a. de deslocamento. SIN D l.

gamma l., a. gama; o arco reflexo que consiste em pequenas células do corno anterior e neuroma, projetando suas pequenas fibras para o feixe intrafusal, produzindo sua contração; esta inicia os impulsos aferentes que atravessam a raiz posterior até as células do corno anterior, induzindo um reflexo de estiramento. SIN gamma motor neurons, gamma motor system, Granit l.

Gerdy interatrial l., a. interatrial de Gerdy; um fascículo muscular, no septo interatrial do coração, que passa para trás a partir do sulco atrioventricular.

Granit l., a. de Granit. SIN gamma l.

hairpin l.'s, a. em grampo de cabelo; DNA e RNA unifilamentares podem dobrar-se para trás, sobre si mesmos, sob as condições adequadas que formam alças de dupla hélice irregulares.

Henle l., a. de Henle. SIN nephronic l.

l. of hypoglossal nerve, a. cervical. SIN *ansa* cervicalis.

Hyrtl l., a. de Hyrtl; uma a. comunicante entre os nervos hipoglossos direito e esquerdo, situando-se entre os músculos gênio-hióideo e genioglosso ou na substância do gênio-hióideo; é encontrada em aproximadamente 1 de cada 10 pessoas. SIN Hyrtl anastomosis.

lenticular l., a. lenticular; as fibras pálidas eferentes que se curvam ao redor da borda medial da cápsula interna. SIN ansa lenticularis [TA], lenticular ansa.

memory l., a. de memória; um dispositivo eletrônico para lembrar os dados que foram armazenados e/ou demonstrados no osciloscópio em um momento anterior; usada para rever os eventos elétricos imediatamente anteriores a um distúrbio específico.

Meyer-Archambault l., a. de Meyer-Archambault; as fibras de radiação visual que formam uma alça ao redor da ponta do corno temporal.

nephronic l., a. nefrônica; a parte em forma de U do néfron que vai dos túbulos contornados proximais até os distais, consistindo nos ramos descendente e ascendente, localizados na medula renal e no raio medular. SIN Henle ansa, Henle l.

peduncular l., a. peduncular. SIN *ansa* peduncularis.

l.'s of spinal nerves, alças dos nervos espinais; as alças dos nervos espinais, fazendo a conexão dos ramos primários ventrais dos nervos espinais. SIN ansae nervorum spinalium.

subclavian l., a. subclávia. SIN *ansa* subclavia.

vector l., a. vetora; uma curva lisa ou irregular, usualmente elíptica, que representa a direção média e a magnitude da ação do coração, de um momento para outro, durante todo o ciclo cardíaco. VER TAMBÉM vector (2), vectorcardiogram.
ventricular l., a. ventricular. SIN bulboventricular l.
Vieussens l., a. de Vieussens. SIN *ansa subclavia.*

loos·en·ing of as·so·ci·a·tion. Afrouxamento de associação; uma manifestação de um grave distúrbio do raciocínio caracterizado pela falta de uma conexão evidente entre um pensamento ou frase e a seguinte, ou com a resposta a uma questão.

Looser, Emil, médico suíço, 1877–1936. VER L. *zones,* em *zone.*

LOP Abreviatura de left occipitoposterior position (posição occipitoposterior esquerda).

lop-ear (lop′ēr). Orelha pendente; anormalidade congênita da orelha externa, com o desenvolvimento deficiente da hélice e da antélice. SIN bat ear.

lo·per·am·ide hy·dro·chlo·ride (lō′per′ā - mīd). Cloridrato de loperamida; agente antiperistáltico prescrito para diarréia.

loph·o·dont (lof′ō - dont). Lofodonte; que possui as coroas dos dentes molares formadas nas cristas transversais ou longitudinais, em contraste com o bunodonte. [G. *lophos,* crista, + *odous,* dente]

Lo·phoph·o·ra wil·liam·sii (lō - fof′ō - rā wil – yăm′sē - ī). A origem botânica do peiote (mescal); contém uma dúzia de alcalóides, dos quais a mescalina é o mais importante; outros são pelotina, anhalomina, anhalonidina, anhalamina, anhalinina, anhalidina e lofoforina.

lo·phot·ri·chate (lō - fot′ri - kāt). Lofotríquio. SIN lophotrichous.

lo·phot·ri·chous (lō - fot′ri - kŭs). Lofotríquio; que se refere a uma célula bacteriana com dois ou mais flagelos em um ou ambos os pólos. SIN lophotrichate. [G. *lophos,* crista, + *thrix,* pelo]

lo·pre·mone (lō′pre - mōn). Lopremona; nome original para a protirelina.

Lorain, Paul, médico francês, 1827–1875. VER L. *disease;* L. -Lévi *dwarfism, infantilism, syndrome.*

lor·a·ze·pam (lō - rā′ze - pam). Lorazepam; ansiolítico do grupo benzodiazepínico.

lor·cai·nide (lor - kā - nīd). Lorcainida; agente antiarrítmico usado no tratamento das arritmias ventriculares; muito semelhante a um depressor cardíaco (antiarrítmico).

lor·do·sco·li·o·sis (lōr′dō - skō - lē - ō′sis). Lordoescoliose; curvatura para trás e lateral combinada da coluna vertebral. [G. *lordos,* curvado para trás, + *skoliōsis,* tortuosidade, de *skolios,* curvado, dobrado]

lor·do·sis (lōr - dō′sis) [TA]. Lordose; uma curvatura anteriormente convexa da coluna vertebral; as lordoses centrais das regiões cervical e lombar são curvaturas secundárias da coluna vertebral, adquirida no período pós-natal. SIN hollow back, saddle back. [G. *lordōsis,* uma curvatura para trás]
cervical l. [TA], l. cervical; a curvatura anteriormente convexa normal do segmento cervical da coluna vertebral; a lordose cervical é uma curvatura secundária da coluna vertebral, adquirida no período pós-natal, à medida que a criança levanta a cabeça. SIN l. cervicis [TA], l. colli*.
l. cervicis [TA], l. cervical. SIN cervical l.
l. colli [TA], l. cervical; *termo oficial alternativo para cervical l.
l. lumbalis [TA], l. lombar. SIN lumbar l.
lumbar l. [TA], l. lombar; a curvatura anteriormente convexa, normal, do segmento lombar da coluna vertebral; a l. lombar é uma curvatura secundária da coluna vertebral, adquirida no período pós-natal quando a postura ereta é adotada ao aprender a andar. SIN l. lumbalis [TA], lumbar flexure.

lor·dot·ic (lōr - dot′ik). Lordótico; pertinente a ou caracterizado por lordose.

Lorenz, Adolf, cirurgião austríaco, 1854–1946. VER L. *sign.*

Loschmidt, Joseph (Johann), químico e físico checo, 1821–1895. VER L. *number.*

LOT Abreviatura de left occipitotransverse position (posição occipitotransversa esquerda).

lo·tion (lō′shŭn). Loção; uma classe de preparações farmacêuticas que são suspensões líquidas ou dispersões para aplicação externa; algumas consistem em sólidos insolúveis, finamente pulverizados, mantidos em suspensão mais ou menos permanente por agentes de suspensão e/ou agentes tensoativos; os outros são emulsões de óleo em água estabilizadas por agentes tensoativos. [L. *lotio,* uma lavagem, de *lavo,* lavar]

Louis, Pierre C. A., médico francês, 1787–1872. VER L. *angle, law.*

Louis-Bar, Denise, médica francesa da metade do século XX. VER Louis-Bar *syndrome.*

loupe (loop). Lupa; uma lente de aumento. [Fr.]
binocular l., lupa binocular; um dispositivo de ampliação, preso a óculos ou a um suporte de crânio, usado como um auxílio visual quando realiza operações em pequenas estruturas.

louse, pl. **lice** (lows, līs). Piolho; nome comum para insetos ectoparasitários membros das ordens Anoplura (piolhos sugadores) e Mallophaga (piolhos picadores). Espécies importantes são *Felicola subrostrata* (piolho do gato), *Goniocotes gallinae* (p. de galináceos), *Goniodes dissimilis* (p. castanho da galinha), *Haemodipsus ventricosus* (p. do coelho), *Lipeurus caponis* (p. da asa),

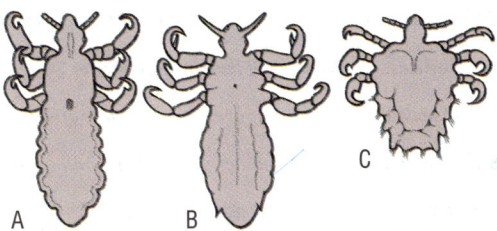

piolhos comuns dos seres humanos: (A) piolho da cabeça (*Pediculus humanus capitis*), (B) piolho do corpo (*Pediculus humanus humanus*), (C) piolho pubiano (*Pthirus pubis*)

Menacanthus stramineus (p. do corpo da galinha), *Pthirus pubis* (p. pubiano ou chato) e *Polyplax serratus* (p. do camundongo). [A.S. *lūs*]
biting l. chewing l., feather l., piolhos picadores; ectoparasitas (ordem Mallophaga) encontrados principalmente nos pássaros, nos quais se alimentam de penas, pêlos, resíduos epidérmicos e (menos amiúde) de sangue; possuem mandíbulas fortemente cornificadas, semelhantes a tenazes, e uma cabeça larga característica; muitas espécies são hospedeiro-específicas.
sea l., as larvas muito pequenas da água-viva *Linuche unguiculata.*
sucking l., p. sugador; os ectoparasitas hematófagos dos mamíferos (ordem Anoplura), caracterizados por uma cabeça estreita com presas perfurantes e sugadoras que se localizam em um saco preso na cabeça.

lousy (low′- sē). Pediculoso. SIN pediculous.

lo·va·stat·in (lō - vă - stat′in). Lovastatina; agente redutor do colesterol, isolado de uma cepa de *Aspergillus terreus,* que reduz tanto o colesterol sérico normal como o elevado. SIN mevinolin.

Lovén, Otto C., médico sueco, 1835–1904. VER L. *reflex.*

Lovibond, J.L., dermatologista inglês do século XX. VER Lovibond *angle,* Lovibond profile *sign.*

Lowe, Charles U., pediatra norte-americano, *1921. VER L. *syndrome;* L.-Terrey-MacLachlan *syndrome.*

Löwenberg, Benjamin B., laringologista francês, 1836–1905. VER L. *canal, forceps, scala.*

lower. Inferior. SIN inferior.

Lower, Richard, anatomista e fisiologista inglês. 1631–1691. VER L.'s *ring, tubercle.*

Lown, Bernard, cardiologista norte-americano, *1921. VER L.-Ganong-Levine *syndrome.*

Lowry, Oliver H., bioquímico norte-americano, *1910. VER L. -Folin *assay;* Lowry protein *assay.*

Lowry, R. Brian, geneticista clínico irlandês radicado no Canadá no século XX. VER Coffin-L. *syndrome.*

Lowsley, Oswald S., urologista norte-americano, 1884–1955. VER L. *tractor.*

lox·a·pine (lok′să - pēn). Loxapina; 2-cloro-11-(4-metil-1-piperazinil)-dibenz[*b,f*] [1,4]-oxazepina; agente neuroléptico antipsicótico usado como os sais succinato e cloridrato.

Lox·os·ce·les (lok - sos′ē - lēz). Um gênero de aranhas venenosas, as aranhas-marrons, caracterizadas por um padrão na forma de violino no cefalotórax e encontradas principalmente na América do Sul. Infligem uma lesão dérmica extremamente ulcerativa, disseminante, no local da picada (loxocelismo). As espécies importantes incluem *L. laeta,* a aranha-marrom reclusa chilena; *L. reclusus,* a aranha-marrom reclusa da América do Norte; e *L. rufipes,* a aranha-marrom do Peru. [G. *loxos,* oblíquo, + *skelos,* perna]

lox·os·ce·lism (lok - sos′ē - lizm). Loxocelismo; doença clínica produzida pela aranha-marrom reclusa, *Loxosceles reclusus,* da América do Norte; caracterizada por ulceração gangrenosa no local da picada, náuseas, indisposição, febre, hemólise e trombocitopenia.

Lox·o·tre·ma ova·tum (lok - sō - trē′mă ō - vā′tŭm). Nome original de *Metagonimus yokogawai.* [G. *loxos,* oblíquo, + *trēma,* um orifício; L. *ovatus,* em formato de ovo]

loz·enge (loz′enj). Pastilha, trocisco. SIN troche. [Fr. *losange,* de *lozangé,* rombico]

LPH Abreviatura de lipotropic *hormone* (hormônio lipotrópico).

L.P.N. Abreviatura de licensed practical *nurse.*

LPO Abreviatura de left posterior oblique (oblíqua posterior esquerda), uma incidência radiográfica.

LPS Abreviatura de lipopolysaccharide (lipopolissacarídeo).

Lr Símbolo de lawrencium (laurêncio).

Lr, Lr VER Lr *dose.*

L.R.C.P. Abreviatura de *Licentiate of the Royal College of Physicians* (of England).

L.R.C.P.(E) Abreviatura de *Licentiate of the Royal College of Physicians* (Edinburgh).

L.R.C.P.(I) Abreviatura de *Licentiate of the Royal College of Physicians* (Ireland).

L.R.C.S. Abreviatura de *Licentiate of the Royal College of Surgeons* (of England).

L.R.C.S.(E) Abreviatura de *Licentiate of the Royal College of Surgeons* (Edinburgh).

L.R.C.S.(I) Abreviatura de *Licentiate of the Royal College of Surgeons* (Ireland).

LRF Abreviatura de luteinizing hormone-releasing *factor*.

L.R.F.P.S. Abreviatura de *Licentiate of the Royal Faculty of Physicians and Surgeons*, uma instituição escocesa.

LRH Abreviatura de luteinizing hormone-releasing *hormone* (hormônio liberador do hormônio luteinizante).

LSA Abreviatura de left sacroanterior position (posição sacroanterior esquerda).

LSD Abreviatura de *lisergic acid* diethylamide (dietilamida do ácido lisérgico).

LSF Abreviatura de line spread *function* (função de ampliação de linha).

LSIL Abreviatura de low-grade squamous intraepithelial *lesion* (lesão intraepitelial escamosa de baixo grau).

LSP Abreviatura de left sacroposterior position (posição sacroposterior esquerda).

LST Abreviatura de left sacrotransverse position (posição sacrotransversa esquerda).

LT Abreviatura de leukotrienes (leucotrienos), usualmente seguido por outra letra com um algarismo subscrito; p.ex., LTA_4, LTC_4.

LTM Abreviatura de long-term *memory* (memória de longa data).

LTP Abreviatura de laser *trabeculoplasty* (trabeculoplastia a laser).

LTR Abreviatura de long terminal repeat *sequence* (seqüência repetida terminal longa), em *sequence*.

Lu Símbolo de lutetium (lutécio).

Lubarsch, Otto, patologista alemão, 1860–1933. VER L. *crystals*, em *crystal*.

Luc, Henri, laringologista francês, 1855–1925. VER L. *operation;* Caldwell-L. *operation*; Ogston-L. *operation*.

lu·can·thone hy·dro·chlo·ride (loo′kan′ - thōn). Cloridrato de lucantona; usado no tratamento da esquistossomose urinária (*Schistosoma haematobium*) e esquistossomose intestinal (*S. mansoni*).

Lucas, Richard C., anatomista e cirurgião inglês, 1846–1915. VER L. *groove*.

lu·cen·so·my·cin (loo - sen - sō - mī′sin). Lucensomicina; um antibiótico isolado de culturas de *Streptomyces lucensis*; um agente antifúngico. SIN lucimycin.

lu·cent (loo′sent). Claro, transparente. [L. *luceo*, brilhar]

lu·cid (loo′sid). Lúcido; brilhante; claro, não-obscurecido ou confuso, como em um momento l. ou uma expressão l. [L. *lucidus*, claro]

lu·cid·i·fi·ca·tion (loo - sid′i - fi - kā′shŭn). Clarificação, purificação. SIN clarification. [L. *lucidus*, claro, + *facio*, tornar]

lu·cid·i·ty (loo - sid′i - tē). Lucidez; a qualidade ou estado de ser lúcido.

lu·cif·er·as·es (loo - sif′er - ās - ēz). Luciferases; enzimas presentes em determinados organismos luminosos que desencadeiam a oxidação de luciferinas; a energia produzida no processo é liberada como bioluminescência; essas enzimas podem ser usadas para detectar concentrações muito reduzidas de metabólitos.

lu·cif·er·ins (loo - sif′er - inz). Luciferinas; substâncias químicas presentes em determinados organismos luminosos que, ao sofrerem a ação das luciferases, produzem bioluminescência. [L. *lux*, luz, + *fero*, transportar]

lu·cif·u·gal (loo - sif′ū - gǎl). Lucífugo; que evita a luz. [L. *lux*, luz, + *fugio*, fugir de]

Lu·cil·ia (loo - sil′ē - ă). Gênero de moscas-varejeiras (família Calliphoridae) cujas larvas alimentam-se de carniça ou excrementos; ocasionalmente infestam feridas (miíase).

L. cae′sar, uma espécie cujas larvas originalmente eram usadas no tratamento de feridas sépticas. VER TAMBÉM *Phormia regina*.

L. illus′tris, uma mosca-varejeira azul-esverdeada metálica amplamente distribuída na América do Norte; os ovos são depositados principalmente em carcaças de animais.

L. serica′ta, SIN Phaenicia sericata.

lu·ci·my·cin (loo - si - mī′sin). Lucimicina. SIN lucensomycin.

Lucio, R., médico mexicano, 1819–1866. VER L. *leprosy;* Lucio leprosy *phenomenon*.

lu·cip·e·tal (loo - sip′i - tǎl). Lucípeto; que procura a luz. [L. *lux*, luz, + *peto*, procurar]

Lucké, Balduin, patologista norte-americano, 1889–1954. VER L. *virus*.

Lücke, George H., cirurgião alemão, 1829–1894. VER L. *test*.

lüc·ken·schä·del (luk - en - shā′dl). Craniolacunia com meningocele ou encefalocele. [Ger. *Lücke*, intervalo + *Schädel*, crânio]

Ludwig, Daniel, anatomista alemão, 1625–1680. VER L. *angle*.

Ludwig, Karl F. W., anatomista e fisiologista alemão, 1816–1895. VER depressor *nerve* of L.; L. *ganglion, labyrinth, nerve, stromuhr*.

Ludwig, Kurt, anatomista alemão, *1922. VER Klinger-L. acid-thionin *stain* for sex chromatin.

Ludwig, Wilhelm Friedrich von, cirurgião alemão, 1790–1865. VER L. *angina*.

Luebering, J. VER Rapoport-Luebering *shunt*.

Luer, fabricante alemão de instrumentos, †1883. VER L. *syringe;* L.-Lok *syringe*.

lu·es (loo′ēz). Lues; uma praga ou peste; especificamente, sífilis. [L. pestilência]

l. vene′rea, l. venérea, sífilis. SIN syphilis.

lu·et·ic (loo - et′ik). Luético, sifilítico. SIN syphilitic.

Luft, John H., histologista norte-amerciano, *1927. VER L. potassium permanganate *fixative*.

Luft, Rolf, endocrinologista sueco, *1914. VER L. *disease*.

Lugol, Jean G. A., médico francês, 1786–1851. Ver Lugol iodine *solution*.

Lukes, L. J., patologista norte-americano do século XX, VER L.-Collins *classification*.

Lukes-Collins clas·si·fi·ca·tion. Classificação de Lukes-Collins. Ver em classification.

LUL Abreviatura de left upper lobe (of lung) (lobo superior esquerdo do pulmão).

lu·lib·er·in (loo - lib′er - in). Luliberina; um hormônio decapeptídeo originário do hipotálamo que estimula a adeno-hipófise a liberar o hormônio folículo-estimulante e o hormônio luteinizante; hormônio liberador de gonadotropina. SIN luteinizing hormone-releasing hormone. [*luteinizing hormone* + L. *libero*, liberar, + -in]

lum·ba·go (lŭm - bā′gō). Lumbago, lombalgia; dor nas regiões média e inferior das costas; um termo descritivo que não especifica a causa. [L. de *lumbus*, flanco]

ischemic l., l. isquêmico; uma forma isquêmica de dor nas costas caracterizada por cãibra dolorosa dos músculos na região lombar incitada pelo esforço de caminhar ou ficar em pé e prontamente aliviada pelo repouso.

lum·bar (lŭm′bar). Lombar; relativo aos flancos, ou à parte das costas e lados entre as costelas e a pelve. [L. *lumbus*, um flanco]

lum·bar·i·za·tion (lŭm′bar - i - zā′shŭn). Lombarização; uma anomalia congênita da junção lombossacra caracterizada pelo desenvolvimento da primeira vértebra sacral como uma vértebra lombar, resultando em seis vértebras lombares em lugar de cinco.

lum·bi (lŭm - bī). Lombos; Plural de lumbus. [L.]

lum·bo·ab·dom·i·nal (lŭm′bō - ab - dom′i - nǎl). Lomboabdominal; relativo aos lados e à parte frontal do abdome.

lum·bo·cos·tal (lŭm′bō - kos′tǎl). Lombocostal. 1. Relativo à região lombar e ao hipocôndrio. 2. Relativo às vértebras lombares e costelas; indicando um ligamento que une a primeira vértebra lombar com o colo da décima segunda costela. [L. *lumbus*, flanco, + *costa*, costela]

lum·bo·il·i·ac (lŭm - bō - il′ē - ak). Lomboilíaco. SIN lumboinguinal.

lum·bo·in·gui·nal (lŭm′bō - ing′gwi - nǎl). Lomboinguinal; relativo às regiões lombar e inguinal. SIN lumboiliac. [L. *lumbus*, flanco, + *inguen* (*inguin-*), virilha]

lum·bo·ova·ri·an (lŭm - bō - ō - vā′rē - an). Lombovariano; relativo ao ovário e às regiões lombares.

lum·bo·sa·cral (lŭm - bō - sā′krǎl). Lombossacro; relativo às vértebras lombares e ao sacro. SIN sacrolumbar.

lum·bri·cal (lŭm′bri - kǎl). Lombrical, lumbrical, lombricóide. SIN lumbricoid (1). [L. *lumbricus*, minhoca]

lum·bri·ca·lis. Lombrical. VER lumbricals (lumbrical *muscles*) of hand, em *muscle*, lumbricals (lumbrical *muscles*) of foot, em *muscle*.

lum·bri·ci·dal (lŭm - bri - sī′dǎl). Lombricida; destrutivo para os vermes lombricóides (intestinais).

lum·bri·cide (lŭm′bri - sīd). Lombricida; um agente que mata os vermes lombricóides (intestinais). [L. *lumbricus*, verme, + *caedo*, matar]

lum·bri·coid (lŭm′bri - koyd). Lombricóide. 1. Denota uma lombriga ou assemelha-se a esta, especialmente *Ascaris lumbricoides*. SIN lumbrical, lumbricus (1). VER TAMBÉM scolecoid (2), vermiform. 2. Nome comum obsoleto para *Ascaris lumbricoides*. [L. *lumbricus*, minhoca, + G. *eidos*, semelhança]

lum·bri·co·sis (lŭm′bri - kō′sis). Lombricose; a infecção por nematódeos intestinais.

lum·bri·cus (lŭm′bri - kŭs). 1. Lombricóide. SIN lumbricoid (1). 2. Lombriga; termo obsoleto para *Ascaris lumbricoides*. [L. minhoca]

lum·bus, gen. e pl. **lum·bi** (lŭm′bŭs, - bī). Lombo, a região lombar. SIN loin. [L.]

lu·men, pl. **lu·mi·na, lu·mens** (loo′men, - min - ă, - menz). 1. Luz, lúmen, cavidade de uma estrutura tubular, como uma artéria ou o intestino. 2 **(lm)**. Lúmen; a unidade de fluxo luminoso; o fluxo luminoso emitido em um ângulo sólido de 1 esteradiano por uma fonte pontual uniforme de luz que possui uma intensidade luminosa de 1 candela. 3. O volume contido pelas membranas de uma mitocôndria ou do retículo endoplasmático. 4. O cerne de um cateter ou agulha oca. [L. luz, janela]

false l., luz falsa; em um aneurisma dissecante, o canal anormal dentro da parede da artéria envolvida.

residual l., fenda residual. SIN residual *cleft*.

true l., luz verdadeira; em um aneurisma dissecante, o canal que representa a real artéria revestida pela camada íntima.

lu·mi·chrome (loo′mi-krōm). Lumícromo; 7,8-dimetilaloxazina; um fotoderivativo amarelo da riboflavina, portando um grupamento metila em vez de ribitil; produzido pela irradiação ultravioleta da riboflavina em solução alcalina.

lu·mi·fla·vin (loo′mi-flā-vin). Lumiflavina, 7,8,10-trimetilisoaloxazina; um fotoderivado da riboflavina, apresentando um grupamento metila em vez de ribitil; produzido por irradiação ultravioleta da riboflavina em solução alcalina.

lu·mi·na (loo′mi-nă). Luzes, lumens; plural de lumen. [L.]

lu·mi·nal (loo′mi-năl) [TA]. Luminal; relativo à luz de um vaso sanguíneo ou outra estrutura tubular. SIN luminalis [TA].

luminalis [TA]. Luminal. SIN luminal.

lu·mi·nance (loo′mi-năns). Luminância, brilhância; o brilho de um objeto, expresso como o fluxo luminoso por unidade de ângulo por unidade da área projetada, medida em lamberts ou em candelas por metro quadrado. [L. *lumino*, iluminar, de *lumen*, luz]

lu·mi·nes·cence (loo-mi-nes′ens). Luminescência; a emissão de luz de um corpo em consequência de uma reação química. VER bioluminescence. [L. *lumen*, luz]

lu·mi·nif·er·ous (loo-mi-nif′er-ŭs). Luminífero; que produz ou conduz a luz. [L. *lumen*, luz, + *fero*, carregar]

lu·mi·no·phore (loo′mi-nō-fōr). Luminóforo; um átomo ou agrupamento atômico em um composto orgânico que aumenta sua capacidade de emitir a luz. [L. *lumen*, luz, + G. *phoros*, condutor]

lu·mi·nous (loo′mi-nŭs). Luminoso; que emite luz, com ou sem calor associado. [L. *lumen*, luz]

lu·mi·rho·dop·sin (loo′mi-rō-dop′sin). Lumirodopsina; um intermediário entre a rodopsina e *all-trans*-retinal mais opsina durante o clareamento da rodopsina pela luz; formada a partir da batorodopsina e convertido em metarodopsina I com uma meia-vida de cerca de 20 µs. [L. *lumen*, luz, + G. *rhodon*, rosa, + *opsis*, visão]

lum·is·ter·ol (loom-ē-ster′ol). Lumisterol. **1.** Um subproduto na biossíntese do ergocalciferol. **2.** Um derivado fosforilado da ribulose que é um intermediário no *shunt* da pentose monofosfato.

lump·ec·to·my (lŭm-pek′tō-mē). Nodulectomia; a remoção de uma lesão benigna ou maligna a partir da mama com preservação da anatomia essencial da mama; tilectomia que envolve o tecido mamário. [lump + G. *ektomē*, excisão]

Luna, Lee G., tecnólogo médico norte-americano do século XX. VER L.-Ishak *stain*.

lu·na·cy (loo′nă-sē). Loucura. **1.** Um termo obsoleto para uma forma de insanidade caracterizada por alternância de períodos lúcidos e insanos, tida como influenciada pelas fases da lua. **2.** Qualquer forma de insanidade. **3.** Insanidade conforme definido variadamente por lei. [L. *luna*, lua]

lu·nar (loo′ner). **1.** Lunar; relativo à lua ou a um mês. **2.** Que se assemelha à lua em formato, especialmente uma meia-luz. SIN lunate (1) [TA], semilunar. VER TAMBÉM crescentic. **3.** Relativo à prata (a lua foi o símbolo da prata na alquimia). [L. *luna*, lua]

lunar caustic. Nitrato de prata. SIN toughened *silver* nitrate.

lu·na·re (loo-nā′re). Semilunar (osso). SIN lunate (*bone*).

lu·nate (loo′nāt) [TA]. Semilunar. **1.** SIN lunar (2). **2.** Relativo ao osso semilunar.

lu·na·tic (loo′nă-tik). Lunático; termo obsoleto para uma pessoa com transtornos mentais. [ver lunacy]

lu·na·to·ma·la·cia (loo-nā′tō-mă-lā′shē-ă). Lunatomalacia. SIN Kienböck *disease*.

lung (lŭng) [TA]. Pulmão; uma de um par de vísceras que ocupam as cavidades pulmonares do tórax, os órgãos da respiração em que ocorre a aeração do sangue. Em seres humanos, o p. direito é um pouco maior que o esquerdo e é dividido em três lobos (um superior, um médio e um inferior ou basal), enquanto o esquerdo possui apenas dois lobos (um superior e um inferior). Cada l. exibe forma irregularmente cônica, que apresenta uma extremidade superior cega (o ápice), uma base côncava seguindo a curvatura do diafragma, uma superfície externa convexa (superfície costal), uma superfície medial ou interna geralmente côncava (superfície mediastinal), uma borda anterior fina e aguda, e uma borda posterior arredondada. SIN pulmo [TA]. [A.S. *lungen*]

air-conditioner l., p. de ar condicionado; alveolite alérgica extrínseca causada por ar contaminado por actinomicetos termofílicos e outros microrganismos.

bird-breeder's l., bird-fancier's l., p. dos criadores de aves; alveolite alérgica extrínseca causada por inalação de emanações particuladas de aves; por vezes especificado segundo a espécie da ave, p.ex., p. do criador de pombos, p. de criadores de periquitos. SIN bird-breeder's disease.

black l., p. preto; uma forma de pneumoconiose, comum em mineiros de carvão, caracterizada por depósitos de partículas de carbono no pulmão. SIN miner's l. (2).

brown l., p. marrom; doença obstrutiva das vias aéreas com asma produzida por exposição à poeira do algodão, linho ou cânhamo. VER TAMBÉM byssinosis.

butterfly l., p. em borboleta; marcas hemorrágicas que aparecem no p. de um animal após a inoculação com *Leptospira interrogans* (*L. icterohaemorrhagiae*).

cardiac l., p. cardíaco; distúrbio na anatomia e fisiologia pulmonares secundário a doença valvular do coração ou a outros distúrbios da circulação inerentes a doença cardíaca.

cheese worker's l., p. do queijeiro; alveolite alérgica extrínseca causada por inalação dos esporos de *Penicillium casei* e queijos mofados.

collier l., p. do carvoeiro. SIN anthracosis.

cystic l., p. cístico. SIN honeycomb l.

endstage l., p. em estágio terminal; fibrose intersticial difusa grave e faveolamento.

farmer's l., p. de fazendeiro; pneumonite por hipersensibilidade caracterizada por febre e dispnéia, causada por inalação de poeira orgânica oriunda do feno mofado contendo esporos de actinomicetos termofílicos, como *Micromonospora vulgaris*, *M. faeni* e *Thermopolyspora polyspora*, que se desenvolvem nas temperaturas elevadas de silos e celeiros de feno; a exposição repetida pode resultar em sensibilização alveolar e, por fim, doença pulmonar granulomatosa com incapacidade grave. SIN thresher's l.

fibroid l., p. fibróide; pneumonia intersticial crônica em um pulmão.

honeycomb l., p. cístico, p. faveolado; o aspecto radiológico e macroscópico dos pulmões que resultam de fibrose intersticial e dilatação cística dos bronquíolos e dos alvéolos distais; de etiologia desconhecida ou uma seqüela de qualquer uma dentre diversas doenças, inclusive granuloma eosinofílico, sarcoidose e qualquer doença pulmonar intersticial. SIN cystic l.

hyperlucent l., p. hipertransparente; o achado radiográfico de que um pulmão ou parte dele é menos denso que o normal, como a partir de retenção de ar por um corpo estranho brônquico, enfisema assimétrico ou fluxo sanguíneo decrescente. VER unilateral hyperlucent l.

iron l., p. de ferro. SIN Drinker *respirator*.

malt-worker's l., p. do cervejeiro; alveolite alérgica extrínseca provocada pela inalação de esporos do *Aspergillus clavatus* e *A. fumigatus* a partir da cevada contaminada durante a fabricação da cerveja.

mason's l., p. do pedreiro; silicose que ocorre em pedreiros.

miner's l., p. do mineiro; **(1)** antracose. SIN anthracosis; **(2)** Pulmão preto. SIN black l.

mushroom-worker's l., p. dos trabalhadores com cogumelos; alveolite alérgica extrínseca causada pela inalação dos esporos do fungo *Thermopolyspora polyspora* ou *Micromonospora vulgaris* a partir de cogumelos contaminados sob cultivo.

postperfusion l., p. pós-perfusão; uma condição em que função pulmonar anormal se desenvolve em pacientes que sofreram cirurgia cardíaca envolvendo circulação extracorpórea; atualmente rara, graças aos avanços da técnica e do equipamento de perfusão.

pump l., p. de choque. SIN shock l.

quiet l., o colapso de um p. durante cirurgias torácicas, induzido para facilitar o procedimento cirúrgico através da ausência de movimento pulmonar.

shock l., p. de choque; no choque, o desenvolvimento de edema, perfusão comprometida e redução do espaço alveolar, como acontece no colapso alveolar. SIN pump l., wet l. (1), white l.

silo-filler's l., p. do trabalhador em silos; edema pulmonar (pulmonary *edema*), usualmente retardado em 1 a 4 horas, que acontece em um indivíduo exposto à silagem, provavelmente causado por dióxido de nitrogênio; pode progredir para bronquiolite obliterante.

thresher's l., p. do debulhador. SIN farmer's l.

unilateral hyperlucent l., p. hipertransparente unilateral; bronquiolite obliterante crônica predominando em um lado. VER unilateral lobar *emphysema*. VER TAMBÉM Swyer-James *syndrome* (2).

uremic l., p. urêmico; edema peri-hilar do pulmão associado a insuficiência renal e hipertensão; as partes periféricas do p. permanecem limpas. SIN uremic pneumonia (1), uremic pneumonitis.

vanishing l., p. evanescente. VER vanishing lung *syndrome*.

welder's l., p. do soldador; forma relativamente benigna de pneumoconiose, associada à soldagem, resultante do depósito de finas partículas metálicas no p.

wet l., white l., p. encharcado; p. branco; **(1)** pulmão de choque. SIN shock l; **(2)** síndrome de angústia respiratória do adulto (SARA). SIN adult respiratory distress *syndrome*.

lung·worms (lŭng′wermz). Vermes pulmonares; nematódeos que habitam as vias aéreas de animais, principalmente na família Metastrongylidae (ou Protostrongylidae). VER *Aelurostrongylus, Crenosoma vulpis, Metastrongylus, Muellerius capillaris*.

lu·nu·la, pl. **lu·nu·lae** (loo′noo-lă, -lē) [TA]. Lúnula. **1** [NA]. A área arqueada pálida na porção proximal da placa ungueal. **2.** Uma pequena estrutura semilunar. [L. dim. de *luna*, lua]

azure l. of nails, l. azul das unhas; a coloração azulada das lúnulas de todas as unhas, que não esmaece, na degeneração hepatolenticular.

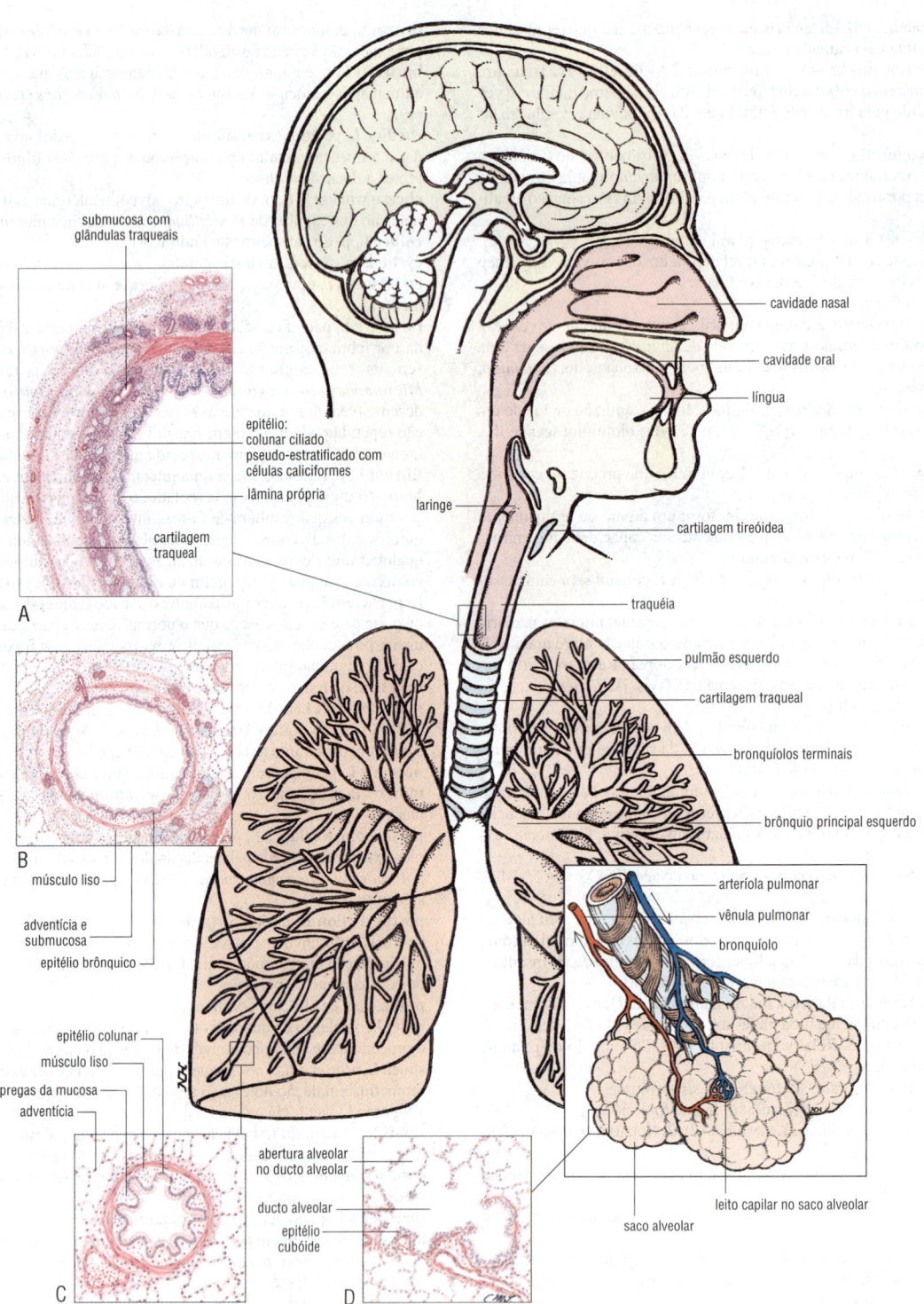

pulmões e anatomia respiratória: (A) traquéia (corte transversal, panorâmica); (B) brônquio intrapulmonar; (C) bronquíolo terminal; (D) bronquíolo respiratório com alvéolos

l. of semilunar cusps of aortic/pulmonary valves, l. das válvulas semilunares das valvas aórtica/pulmonar; a borda livre de uma válvula das valvas semilunares em cada lado dos nódulos das válvulas semilunares. SIN l. of semilunar valve, lunulae valvularum semilunarium valvae aortae/trunci pulmonalis.
l. of semilunar valve, l. das válvulas semilunares. SIN l. of semilunar cusps of aortic/pulmonary valves.
l. unguis, l. das unhas. SIN *lunule* of nail.
lunulae valvularum semilunarium valvae aortae/trunci pulmonalis, l. das válvulas semilunares das valvas aórtica/pulmonar. SIN l. of semilunar cusps of aortic/pulmonary valves.
lunule. Lúnula. **1** [TA]. Lúnula da unha. SIN l. of nail. **2.** Uma pequena estrutura semilunar.

l. of nail, l. da unha; a área arqueada pálida na porção proximal da placa ungueal. SIN arcus unguium, half-moon, lunula unguis, lunule (1), selene unguium.
lu·pin·i·dine (loo - pin′i - dēn). Lupinidina. SIN sparteine.
lu·pi·no·sis (loo - pi - nō′sis). Lupinose. SIN lathyrism. [L. *lupinus,* lupino, de *lupus,* lobo]
lu·poid (loo′poyd). Lupóide; que se assemelha ao lúpus. [L. *lupus* + G. *eidos,* semelhança]
lu·pu·lin (loo′poo - lin). Lupulina; um material granular, amarelado e viscoso, consistindo em pêlos glandulares multicelulares (tricomas) inteiros, oriundo do fruto e brácteas do lupo, *Humulus lupulus*; os óleos essenciais e resinas desses pêlos glandulares são responsáveis pelo característico paladar amargo

da cerveja ou de medicamentos feitos com o lupo; tem sido utilizado como um antiespasmódico e sedativo. SIN humulin.

lu·pus (loo′pŭs). Lúpus; um termo originalmente usado para descrever a erosão (como se fosse corroída) da pele, atualmente empregado com os termos modificadores que designam as várias doenças arroladas adiante. [L. lobo]

chilblain l., (1) SIN chilblain l. erythematosus; **(2)** lúpus pérnio que é uma manifestação da sarcoidose.

chilblain l. erythematosus, as lesões cutâneas observadas em pacientes com l. eritematoso, que se assemelham às pequenas áreas nodulares endurecidas de uma lesão por frio chamada geladura. SIN chilblain l. (1).

chronic discoid l. erythemato´sus, l. eritematoso discóide crônico. SIN discoid l. erythematosus.

cutaneous l. erythematosus, l. eritematoso cutâneo; **(1)** doença cutânea observada em pacientes com a forma discóide do l. eritematoso; **(2)** um termo para várias lesões cutâneas observadas no l. eritematoso sistêmico.

discoid l. erythemato'sus, l. eritematoso discóide; uma forma de l. eritematoso na qual existem lesões cutâneas; estas comumente aparecem na face e são placas atróficas com eritema, hiperceratose, rolhas foliculares e telangiectasia; em alguns casos, pode desenvolver-se o l. eritematoso sistêmico. SIN chronic discoid l. erythematosus.

disseminated l. erythemato'sus, l. eritematoso disseminado. SIN systemic l. erythematosus.

drug-induced l., l. fármaco-induzido; a síndrome do l. eritematoso sistêmico produzida pela exposição a medicamentos, especialmente procainamida ou hidralazina e caracterizada por anticorpos anti-histona. Mais benigna que a doença usual, com menor envolvimento renal. A síndrome desaparece após a interrupção do medicamento agressor. SIN hydralazine syndrome.

l. erythemato'sus (LE, L.E.), l. eritematoso; uma doença que pode ser crônica (caracterizada apenas por lesões cutâneas), subaguda (caracterizada por lesões cutâneas não-cicatrizantes superficiais recorrentes que são mais disseminadas e apresentam aspectos mais agudos tanto clínicos como histológicos, que os notados na fase discóide crônica), ou sistêmica ou disseminada (na qual há anticorpos antinucleares e, quase sempre, envolvimento de estruturas vitais). VER TAMBÉM discoid l. erythematosus, systemic l. erythematosus.

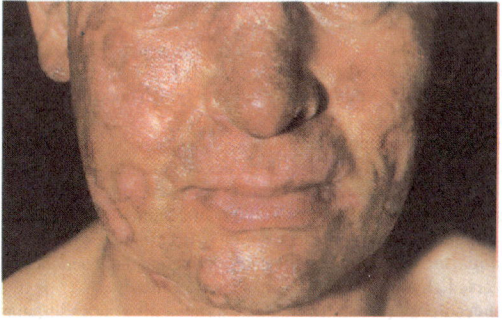

lúpus eritematoso

l. erythematosus, neonatal, l. eritematoso neonatal; o l. eritematoso presente ao nascimento como conseqüência de anticorpos transmitidos por via transplacentária de uma mãe com l. eritematoso sistêmico; caracterizado por lesões cutâneas e hematopoéticas transitórias e por anormalidades cardíacas permanentes.

l. erythemato'sus profun'dus, l. eritematoso profundo; paniculite subcutânea com acentuada infiltração linfocitária de lóbulos adiposos, originando nódulos elásticos, firmes e profundos, que, por vezes, tornam-se ulcerados, comumente na face; pode ocorrer no l. eritematoso sistêmico e localizado. SIN l. profundus.

l. livedo, l. lívido; lesões cianóticas persistentes nos membros, associadas a manifestações cutâneas da doença de Raynaud.

l. milia'ris dissemina'tus facie'i, l. miliar disseminado da face; erupção papular semelhante ao milho miúdo da face associada a infiltração perifolicular tuberculóide (no exame histopatológico), mas provavelmente relacionada a rosácea em vez de infecção tuberculosa.

neonatal l., l. neonatal; l. eritematoso que ocorre nos recém-nascidos de mulheres que tiveram lúpus durante a gravidez; os anticorpos anti-SSA geralmente devem ser pesquisados; cerca de 50% apresentam anticorpos antinucleares. São notadas várias lesões cutâneas, as quais podem resolver ou deixar cicatriz; a síndrome geralmente desaparece; no entanto, as manifestações cardíacas podem ser fatais. Algumas crianças desenvolvem lúpus sistêmico em uma fase mais tardia na vida.

l. per'nio, l. pérnio; a lesão cutânea granulomatosa, purpúrea, endurecida e crônica da sarcoidose, que se assemelha clinicamente à geladura, envolvendo orelhas, bochechas, nariz, lábios e fronte; geralmente associado a sarcoidose intratorácica.

l. profundus (pro-fŭn′dŭs), l. profundo. SIN l. erythematosus profundus. [L. profundo]

l. serpigino'sus, l. serpiginoso; lesão tuberculosa cutânea que se dissemina para a periferia, curando no centro, com formação de cicatriz.

systemic l. erythemato'sus (SLE), l. eritematoso sistêmico; doença inflamatória do tecido conjuntivo com aspectos variáveis, incluindo, com freqüência, febre, fraqueza muscular e fatigabilidade, dores articulares ou artrite, que se assemelha à artrite reumatóide; lesões eritematosas cutâneas difusas na face, pescoço ou membros superiores, com degeneração por liquefação da camada basal e atrofia epidérmica, linfadenopatia, pleurisia ou pericardite, lesões glomerulares, anemia, hiperglobulinemia e um teste positivo de células LE, com anticorpos séricos contra a proteína nuclear e, por vezes, para o DNA de filamento duplo e outras substâncias. SIN disseminated l. erythematosus.

l. vulga'ris, l. vulgar; tuberculose cutânea com as características lesões nodulares na face, em particular em torno do nariz e das orelhas.

LUQ Abreviatura de left upper quadrant (of abdomen) (quadrante superior esquerdo [do abdome]).

lu·ra (loo′ra). Lura; o término contraído do infundíbulo do cérebro. [L. o gargalo de uma garrafa]

lu·ral (loo′ral). Lural; pertinente à lura.

Luschka, Hubert, anatomista alemão, 1820–1875. VER L. *bursa, cartilage, ducts,* em *duct, gland,* cystic *glands,* em *gland, joints,* em *joint, ligaments,* em *ligament, sinus, tonsil; foramen* of L.

Luse, Sarah A., médica norte-americana, 1918–1970. VER L. *bodies,* em *body.*

lus·i·tropic (loos-e-tro′pik). Lusitrópico; relativo à lusitropia.

lus·it·ropy (loos-it′tro-pe). Lusitropia; as funções de relaxamento do músculo e compartimentos cardíacos.

lute (loot). Vedar ou reforçar com cera ou cimento. [L. *lutum,* lodo]

lu·te·al (loo′te-al). Lúteo; relativo ao corpo lúteo; células lúteas, hormônio luteinizante, etc. SIN luteus. [L. *luteus,* açafrão-amarelo]

lu·te·ci·um (loo-te′se-ŭm). Lutécio. SIN lutetium.

lu·te·in (loo′te-in). Luteína. **1.** O pigmento amarelo no corpo lúteo, na gema de ovos, ou qualquer lipocromo. **2.** SIN xanthophyll. **3.** O corpo lúteo de suíno, ressecado e pulverizado, originalmente utilizado como fonte de progesterona. [L. *luteus,* açafrão-amarelo]

lu·te·in·i·za·tion (loo′te-in-i-za′shŭn). Luteinização; a transformação do folículo ovariano maduro e sua teca interna em um corpo lúteo após a ovulação; a formação do tecido lúteo, que se mostra amarelo em algumas espécies.

lu·te·i·nize (loo′te-i-niz). Luteinizar; formar o tecido lúteo.

lu·te·i·no·ma (loo′te-i-no′ma). Luteinoma. SIN luteoma.

Lutembacher, René, cardiologista francês, 1887–1916. VER L. *syndrome.*

lu·te·o·gen·ic (loo′te-o-jen′ik). Luteogênico; luteinizante; que induz a produção ou o crescimento do corpo lúteo.

lu·te·o·hor·mone (loo′te-o-hor′mon). Hormônio luteínico, progesterona. SIN progesterone.

lu·te·ol, lu·te·ole (loo′te-ol, -ol). Luteol. SIN xanthophyll.

lu·te·o·lin (loo-te-o′lin). Luteolina; a aglicona da galuteolina e cinarosídeo. SIN cyanidenon.

lu·te·ol·y·sin (loo-te-ol′i-sin). Luteolisina; qualquer agente, natural ou composto, que destrói a função do corpo lúteo. [L. *luteus,* açafrão-amarelo + G. *lysis,* dissolução]

lu·te·ol·y·sis (loo-te-ol′i-sis). Luteólise; a degeneração ou destruição do tecido luteinizado do ovário.

lu·te·o·lyt·ic (loo-te-o-lit′ik). Luteolítico; que promove ou é característico da luteólise.

lu·te·o·ma (loo-te-o′ma). Luteoma; um tumor ovariano, originário das células granulosas ou da teca luteínica, que produz os efeitos da progesterona sobre a mucosa uterina. SIN luteinoma.

pregnancy l., l. da gravidez; um tumor de células luteínicas benigno do ovário.

lu·te·o·tro·pic, lu·te·o·tro·phic (loo′te-o-trop′ik, -trof′ik). Luteotrópico, luteotrófico; que possui ação estimulante sobre o desenvolvimento e função do corpo lúteo.

lu·te·ti·um (Lu) (loo-te′she-ŭm). Lutécio; um elemento de terras raras; número atômico 71, peso atômico 174,967. SIN lutecium. [L. *Lutetia,* Paris]

lu·te·us (loo-te′ŭs). Lúteo. SIN luteal. [L.]

Lu·ther·an Blood Group, Lu Blood Group. Grupo sanguíneo Lutheran. Ver Apêndice de Grupos Sanguíneos.

lu·tro·pin (loo′tro-pin). Lutropina; um dos dois hormônios glicoproteicos que estimulam o amadurecimento final dos folículos e a secreção de progesterona por eles, suas rupturas para a liberação do óvulo e a conversão do folículo rompido no corpo lúteo. SIN interstitial cell-stimulating hormone, luteinizing hormone, luteinizing principle.

lu·tu·trin (loo′too-trin). Lututrina; fração hidrossolúvel semelhante à proteína, extraída do corpo lúteo dos ovários da porca, que se assemelha à relaxina; provoca o relaxamento uterino e é usada na dismenorréia.

Lutz, Alfredo, médico brasileiro, 1855–1940. VER L.-Splendore-Almeida *disease*.

Lutz·o·my·ia (loot - zō - mī′ã). Um gênero de mosquitos-palha do Novo Mundo ou maruins hematófagos (família Psychodidae) que servem como vetores de leishmaniose e da febre de Oroyo; outrora associado ao gênero de mosquitos-palha do Velho Mundo *Phlebotomus*.
   L. flaviscutella′ta, uma espécie de mosquito-palha que é um vetor da *Leishmania mexicana*, o agente da úlcera do chiclero. SIN *Phlebotomus flaviscutellatus*.
   L. interme′dius, uma de um grupo de espécies de mosquitos-palha que são vetores da *Leishmania braziliensis*, o agente da espúndia.
   L. longipal′pis, SIN *Phlebotomus longipalpis*.
   L. peruen′sis, uma espécie de mosquito-palha que é um vetor da *Leishmania peruviana*, o agente da uta.

lux (lx) (lùks). Lux; uma unidade de luz ou iluminação; a recepção de um fluxo luminoso de 1 lúmen por metro quadrado de superfície. SIN candlemeter, meter-candle. [L. luz]

lux·a·tio (lŭk - sā′shē - ō). Luxação. VER luxation. [L. *luxo*, pp. *-atus*, deslocar]
   l. erec′ta, l. ereta; a luxação subglenóide da cabeça do úmero na qual o braço é elevado e abduzido e não pode ser abaixado.
   l. perinea′lis, l. perineal; uma condição em que a cabeça do fêmur é deslocada para o períneo.

lux·a·tion (lŭk - sā′shŭn). Luxação. **1.** SIN dislocation. **2.** Em odontologia, a luxação ou deslocamento do côndilo na fossa temporomandibular ou de um dente do alvéolo. [L. *luxatio*]
   Malgaigne l., l. de Malgaigne. SIN nursemaid's *elbow*.

Lux·ol fast blue. Azul resistente ao luxol; nome para um grupo de corantes intimamente relacionados da ftalocianina cúprica empregados para tingir (com PAS, PTAH, hematoxilina, nitrato de prata, etc.) a mielina nas fibras nervosas.

lux·us (lŭks′ŭs). Luxo; excesso de qualquer tipo. [L. extravagância, luxúria]

Luys, Jules Bernard, médico francês, 1828–1897. VER L. *body;* centre médian de L.; *corpus* luysi; *nucleus* of L.

LVET Abreviatura de left ventricular ejection *time* (tempo de ejeção do ventrículo esquerdo).

L.V.N. Abreviatura para licensed vocational *nurse*.

Lw Símbolo antigo do lawrencium (laurêncio).

lx Abreviatura de lux (luz).

ly·ase (lī′ās). Liase; nome de classe para as enzimas que removem grupamentos de forma não-hidrolítica (EC classe 4); prefixos como "hidro-" e "amonia-" são empregados para indicar o tipo de reação. Os nomes comuns para as liases incluem sintases, descarboxilases, aldolases, desidratases. Cf. synthase, synthetase.

ly·can·thro·py (lī - kan′thrō - pē). Licantropia; a ilusão mórbida de que alguém é um lobo, possivelmente um atavismo mental da superstição do lobisomem. [G. *lykos*, lobo, + *anthrōpos*, homem]

ly·coc·to·nine (lī - kok′tō - nēn). Licoctonina; um alcalóide, $C_{25}H_{41}NO_7$, obtido do *Aconitum lycoctonum*, uma espécie extremamente venenosa de acônito; também ocorre em outras espécies de *Aconitum* e *Delphinium*.

ly·co·pene (lī′kō - pēn). Licopeno; Ψ,Ψ-caroteno; o característico pigmento vermelho do tomate que pode ser considerado, quimicamente, como a substância original, da qual derivam todos os pigmentos carotenóides naturais; um hidrocarboneto insaturado constituído de oito unidades isopreno, duas das quais hidrogenadas, com 11 ligações duplas conjugadas.

ly·co·pe·ne·mia (lī′kō - pē - nē′mē - ã). Licopenemia; condição em que existe uma alta concentração de licopeno no sangue, produzindo pigmentação cutânea amarelada semelhante ao carotenóide; encontrada em pessoas que consomem quantidades excessivas de tomates ou suco de tomate, ou frutas e bagas contendo licopeno. [lycopene + G. *haima*, sangue]

Ly·co·per·don (līkō - per′don). Um gênero de fungos (família Lycoperdaceae), do qual algumas espécies têm sido utilizadas de modo medicinal, p.ex., na medicina popular, por inalação nasal para tratar a epistaxe. Os esporos do *L. bovista* (*L. gemmatum, L. caelatum*) e do *L. pyriforme* raramente podem produzir licoperdonose. SIN puffball. [G. *lykos*, lobo, + *perdomai*, romper]

ly·co·per·do·no·sis (lī′kō - per - don - ō′sis). Licoperdonose; pneumonite persistente após a inalação de esporos dos fungos *Lycoperdon pyriforme* e *L. bovista*.

ly·coph·o·ra (lī′kof′ō - rã). Licófora; a larva de 10 ganchos das solitárias primitivas da subclasse Cestodaria.

ly·co·po·di·um (lī - kō - pō′dē - ŭm). Licopódio; os esporos do *Lycopodium clavatum* (família Lycopodiaceae) e de outras espécies de *L*.; pó amarelado, insípido e inodoro, foi usado como um pó secante e em farmácia para evitar a aglutinação de comprimidos em um recipiente. SIN club moss, vegetable sulfur. [G. *lykos*, lobo, + *pous*, pé]

lye (lī). Lixívia; o líquido obtido pela lixiviação das cinzas da madeira. VER *potassium* hydroxide, *sodium* hydroxide. SIN lixivium. [A.S. *leáh*]

Lyell, Aian. VER L. *disease, syndrome*.

Lym·naea (lim - nē′ã). Um gênero de lesmas, cujas espécies são hospedeiros invertebrados para o verme do fígado do carneiro, *Fasciola hepatica* e outros trematódeos. [G. *limnē*, pântano]

lymph (limf) [TA]. Linfa; um líquido discretamente opalescente, claro, transparente, por vezes discretamente amarelado, que é coletado dos tecidos por todo o corpo, flui nos vasos linfáticos (através dos linfonodos) e, por fim, é acrescentado à circulação venosa. A l. consiste em uma porção líquida clara, com um número variável de leucócitos (principalmente linfócitos) e alguns eritrócitos. SIN lympha [TA]. [L. *lympha*, água límpida da fonte]
   aplastic l., l. aplásica; a l. que contém um número relativamente grande de leucócitos, mas uma quantidade relativamente pequena de fibrinogênio; essa l. não forma um bom coágulo e manifesta apenas uma discreta tendência para se tornar organizada. SIN corpuscular l.
   blood l., l. sanguínea; a l. exsudada dos vasos sanguíneos e não derivada do líquido nos espaços teciduais.
   corpuscular l., l. corpuscular. SIN aplastic l.
   croupous l., l. cruposa; uma forma de l. inflamatória com um conteúdo relativamente grande de fibrinogênio; em consequência da fibrina que é formada em camadas relativamente densa, é provável que uma pseudomembrana seja produzida.
   dental l., líquido dentinário. SIN dentinal *fluid*.
   euplastic l., l. euplásica; a l. que contém relativamente poucos leucócitos, mas uma concentração comparativamente alta de fibrinogênio; essa l. coagula muito bem e tende a se tornar organizada com o tecido fibroso.
   fibrinous l., l. fibrinosa; l. euplásica ou cruposa.
   inflammatory l., l. inflamatória; líquido levemente amarelado, usualmente coagulável (ou seja, l. euplásica) que se acumula na superfície de uma lesão cutânea ou de membrana agudamente inflamada.
   intercellular l., l. intercelular; o líquido nos espaços potenciais entre as células nos diversos órgãos e tecidos.
   intravascular l., l. intravascular; a l. nos vasos linfáticos, em contraste com a l. intercelular e a l. que foi exsudada dos vasos.
   plastic l., l. plástica; a l. inflamatória que tende a se tornar organizada.
   tissue l., l. tecidual; a l. verdadeira, ou seja, a l. derivada principalmente do líquido nos espaços teciduais (em contraste com a l. sanguínea).
   vaccine l., vaccinia l., l. vacínica; aquela coletada das vesículas da infecção da vacínia e usada para a imunização ativa contra a varíola.

lymph-. VER lympho-.

lym·pha (lim′fa) [TA]. Linfa. SIN lymph. [L.]

lym·pha·den (limf′a - den). Linfonodo. SIN lymph node. [lymph- + G. *adēn*, glândula]

lymphaden-. VER lymphadeno-.

lym·phad·e·nec·to·my (lim - fad - ē - nek′tō - mē). Linfadenectomia; excisão de linfonodos. [lymphadeno- + G. *ektomē*, excisão]

lym·phad·e·ni·tis (lim - fad′e - nī′tis). Linfadenite; inflamação de um linfonodo ou linfonodos. [lymphadeno- + G. *-itis*, inflamação]
   dermatopathic l., l. dermatopática. SIN dermatopathic *lymphadenopathy*.
   mesenteric l., l. mesentérica. SIN mesenteric *adenitis*.
   paratuberculous l., l. paratuberculosa; termo antigo para a inflamação crônica dos linfonodos, não especificamente tuberculosa (ou seja, os bacilos da tuberculose não são demonstráveis), mas estão associados a inflamação tuberculosa comprovada em outra parte ou órgão do corpo.
   regional l., l. regional; inflamação de um grupo de linfonodos que recebe a drenagem de um local de infecção.
   regional granulomatous l., l. granulomatosa regional. SIN catscratch *disease*.
   tuberculosis l., l. tuberculosa. SIN tuberculous l.
   tuberculous l., l. tuberculosa; l. que resulta da infecção por *Mycobacterium tuberculosis*; tuberculose ganglionar. SIN tuberculosis l.

lymphadeno-, lymphaden-. Linfadeno-; linfaden-; formas combinantes que significam os linfonodos. [L. *lympha*, água de fonte, + G. *adēn*, glândula]

lym·phad·e·nog·ra·phy (lim - fad′e - nog′ra - fē). Linfadenografia; visualização radiográfica dos linfonodos depois da injeção de um contraste; linfografia. [lymphadeno- + G. *graphō*, escrever]

lym·phad·e·noid (lim - fad′ē - noyd). Linfadenóide; relativo ou que se assemelha a ou derivado de um linfonodo. [lymphadeno- + G. *eidos*, semelhança]

lym·phad·e·no·ma (lim - fad′ē - nō′mã). Linfadenoma; termo obsoleto para: **1.** Um linfonodo aumentado. **2.** Doença de Hodgkin. SIN Hodgkin *disease*. [lymphadeno- + G. *-ōma*, tumor]

lym·phad·e·nop·a·thy (lim - fad - ē - nop′a - thē). Linfadenopatia; qualquer processo patológico que afeta um linfonodo ou linfonodos. [lymphadeno- + G. *pathos*, sofrimento]
   angioimmunoblastic l. with dysproteinemia (AILD), l. angioimunoblástica com disproteinemia; distúrbio linfoproliferativo caracterizado por l. generalizada, hepatoesplenomegalia, febre, sudorese, perda de peso, lesões cutâneas e prurido com hipergamaglobulinemia; ocorre principalmente em idosos, frequentemente levando à morte. Demonstrou-se a proliferação de células B e a deficiência de células T. SIN immunoblastic l.

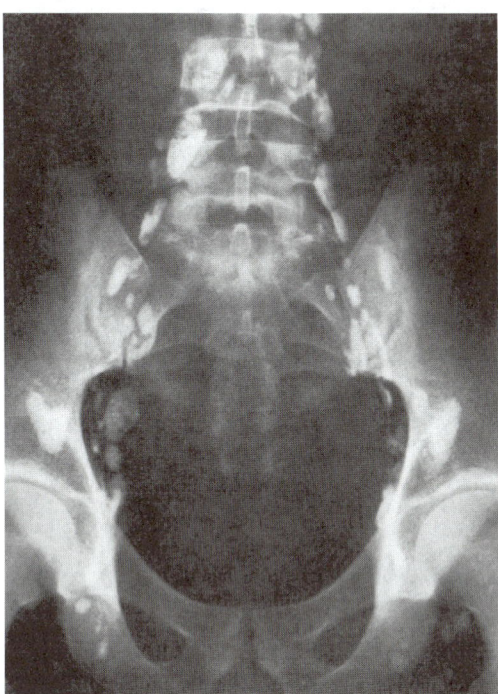

linfadenografia: fase de armazenamento

bulky l., l. volumosa. SIN bulky *disease.*

dermatopathic l., l. dermatopática; aumento dos linfonodos, com proliferação de células reticulares interdigitantes que se coram palidamente e macrófagos contendo lipídios e melanina; secundária a várias formas de dermatite. SIN dermatopathic lymphadenitis.

immunoblastic l., l. imunoblástica. SIN angioimmunoblastic l. with dysproteinemia.

persistent generalized l., l. generalizada persistente; síndrome caracterizada por hiperplasia reativa dos linfonodos (com duração mínima de um mês e em dois locais diferentes do corpo, não incluindo a área inguinal) em pacientes infectados pelo vírus da imunodeficiência humana. As lesões dos linfonodos progridem desde a hiperplasia reativa benigna, atravessando um estágio de hiperplasia folicular mista, até a involução folicular com depleção linfocítica. Muitas envolvem para um linfoma maligno não-Hodgkin.

lym·phad·e·no·sis (lim - fad´e - nō´sis). Linfadenose; o processo proliferativo subjacente básico que resulta em aumento dos linfonodos, como na leucemia linfocítica e em determinadas inflamações. [lymphadeno- + G. *-osis,* condição]

benign l., mononucleose infecciosa. SIN infectious *mononucleosis.*

lym·phad·e·no·va·rix (lim - fad´e - nō - vā´riks). Linfadenovariz; deformidade varicosa de um linfonodo associada à linfangiectasia. [lymphadeno- + L. *varix*]

lym·pha·gogue (limf´ă - gog). Linfagogo; um agente que aumenta a formação e o fluxo da linfa. [lymph + G. *agōgos,* que impele]

lym·phan·ge·i·tis (lim - fan´jē - ī´tis). Linfangeíte, linfangite. SIN lymphangitis.

lymphangi-. VER lymphangio-.

lym·phan·gi·al (lim - fan´jē - ăl). Linfangial; relativo a um vaso linfático.

lym·phan·gi·ec·ta·sis, lym·phan·gi·ec·ta·sia (lim - fan´jē - ek´tā - sis, - ek - tā´zē - a). Linfangiectasia; a dilatação dos vasos linfáticos, o processo básico que pode resultar na formação de um linfangioma. SIN lymphectasia, telangiectasia lymphatica. [lymphangio- + G. *ektasis,* um estiramento]

cavernous l., l. cavernosa. SIN lymphangioma cavernosum.
cystic l., l. cística. SIN lymphangioma cysticum.
intestinal l. [MIM*152800], l. intestinal; l. familial com perda intestinal de linfa, causando linfocitopenia e hipogamaglobulinemia.
simple l., l. simples. SIN lymphangioma simplex.

lym·phan·gi·ec·tat·ic (lim - fan´jē - ek - tat´ik). Linfangiectásico; relativo a, ou caracterizado por, linfangiectasia.

lym·phan·gi·ec·to·my (lim - fan´jē - ek´tō - mē). Linfangiectomia; a excisão de um canal linfático. [lymphangio- + G. *ektomē,* excisão]

lym·phan·gi·i·tis (lim - fan´jē - ī´tis). Linfangite. SIN lymphangitis.

lymphangio-, lymphangi-. Linfangio-, linfangi-; formas combinantes que indicam os vasos linfáticos. [L. *lympha,* água da fonte, + G. *angeion,* vaso]

lym·phan·gi·o·en·do·the·li·o·ma (lim - fan´jē - ō - en´dō - thē - lē - ō´mă). Linfangioendotelioma; termo antigo para a malformação linfático-venosa combinada. [lymphangio- + endothelium + -*oma,* tumor]

lym·phan·gi·og·ra·phy (lim - fan´jē - og´ră - fē). Linfangiografia; a demonstração radiográfica dos vasos linfáticos e linfonodos após a injeção de um contraste; linfografia. [lymphangio- + G. *graphō,* escrever]

lymphangioleiomyomatosis. Linfangioliomiomatose; distúrbio raro, de etiologia desconhecida, observado em mulheres em idade fértil e nos pacientes de ambos os sexos com esclerose tuberosa. As complicações pulmonares são decorrentes da proliferação hamartomatosa das células musculares lisas, preferencialmente ao longo das estruturas broncovasculares, resultando em obliteração das vias aéreas e desenvolvimento consecutivo de cistos nos pulmões. Geralmente progressivo, levando à morte por insuficiência respiratória. O tratamento por transplante pulmonar foi bem-sucedido. SIN lymphangiomyomatosis.

lym·phan·gi·ol·o·gy (lim - fan - jē - ol´ō - jē). Linfangiologia; o ramo da ciência médica relacionado com os vasos linfáticos. SIN lymphology. [lymphangio- + G. *logos,* estudo]

lym·phan·gi·o·ma (lim - fan´jē - ō´mă). Linfangioma; termo antigo para uma massa de vasos linfáticos anômalos ou canais que variam em tamanho, estão usualmente muito dilatados e são revestidos por células endoteliais normais; o tecido linfóide geralmente é encontrado nas porções periféricas das lesões, as quais estão presentes ao nascimento ou logo depois, e que, provavelmente, representam o desenvolvimento errôneo dos vasos linfáticos (em vez de neoplasias verdadeiras); ocorrem com maior freqüência no pescoço e na axila, mas também podem desenvolver-se no braço, mesentério, retroperitônio e em outros locais. [lymphangio- + G. *-oma,* tumor]

l. caverno´sum, l. cavernoso; uma condição de dilatação conspícua dos vasos linfáticos em uma região bastante circunscrita, geralmente com a formação de cavidades ou "lagos" cheios de linfa. SIN cavernous lymphangiectasis.
l. circumscrip´tum, l. circumscrito; lesão nevóide congênita que consiste em um grupo circunscrito de vesículas linfáticas tensas.
l. cys´ticum, l. cístico; condição caracterizada por um grupo muito bem circunscrito de vários ou inúmeros vasos dilatados, semelhantes a cistos, ou espaços revestidos por endotélio e cheios de linfa. SIN cystic lymphangiectasis.
l. sim´plex, l. simples; região circunscrita ou foco de vários ou inúmeros vasos linfáticos que estão moderadamente dilatados. SIN simple lymphangiectasis.
l. tubero´sum mul´tiplex, l. tuberoso múltiplo; lesão cutânea caracterizada por múltiplos nódulos cistiformes, discretamente avermelhados (localizados principalmente no tronco), resultantes de espaços e vasos linfáticos muito grandes e de grupos de células endoteliais proliferantes; a lesão apresenta alguma semelhança macroscópica com o espiradenoma, exceto pela localização característica.
l. xanthelasmoid´eum, l. xantelasmóide; l. capilar com degeneração colóide dos tecidos elásticos da pele, caracterizada por placas amarelo-acastanhadas ou cinza-acastanhadas que podem estar apenas discretamente acima da superfície cutânea.

lym·phan·gi·o·ma·tous (lim - fan´jē - ō´mă - tŭs). Linfangiomatoso; pertinente a, caracterizado por ou contendo o linfangioma.

lymph·an·gi·o·my·o·ma·to·sis (lim - fan´gē - ō - mī´ō - ma - tō´sis). Linfangiomiomatose. SIN lymphangioleiomyomatosis. [lymphangio- + myoma + -*osis,* condição]

lym·phan·gi·on (lim - fan´jē - on). Linfângio; um vaso linfático. VER lymph *vessels,* em *vessel.* [L. *lympha,* linfa, + G. *angeion,* vaso]

lym·phan·gi·o·phle·bi·tis (lim - fan´jē - ō - fle - bī´tis). Linfangioflebite; inflamação dos vasos linfáticos e veias.

lym·phan·gi·o·plas·ty (lim - fan´jē - ō - plas - tē). Linfangioplastia; alteração cirúrgica dos vasos linfáticos. [lymphangio- + G. *plastos,* formado]

lym·phan·gi·o·sar·co·ma (lim - fan´jē - ō - sar - kō´mă). Linfangiossarcoma; neoplasia maligna derivada do tecido vascular, ou seja, um angiossarcoma no qual as células neoplásicas se originam das células endoteliais dos vasos linfáticos, desenvolvendo-se usualmente no braço, vários anos depois da mastectomia radical.

lym·phan·gi·ot·o·my (lim - fan´jē - ot´ō - mē). Linfangiotomia; incisão dos vasos linfáticos. [lymphangio- + G. *tomē,* incisão]

lym·phan·gi·tis (lim - fan - jī´tis). Linfangite; inflamação dos vasos linfáticos. SIN lymphangeitis, lymphangiitis. [lymphangio- + G. *-itis,* inflamação]
l. carcinomato´sa, l. carcinomatosa: permeação linfática extensa por células tumorais, com fibrose circundante, produzindo cordões visíveis ou palpáveis, principalmente na pleura ou pele suprajacente a um carcinoma.

lym·pha·phe·re·sis (lim´fă - fe - rē´sis). Linfaférese. SIN lymphocytapheresis.

lym·phat·ic (lim - fat´ik). Linfático. **1.** Pertinente à linfa. **2.** Um canal vascular que transporta linfa. **3.** Por vezes utilizado para referir-se a uma característica preguiçosa ou fleumática. SIN vas lymphaticum. [L. *lymphaticus,* exaltado; L. mod. uso, de ou para linfa]

afferent l., l. aferente; um vaso l. que penetra ou conduz a linfa até um linfonodo. SIN afferent vessel (3), vas lymphaticum afferens.

efferent l., l. eferente. SIN vas efferens (1).

lym·phat·i·cos·to·my (lim-fat-i-kos′tō-mē). Linfaticostomia; que faz uma abertura em um canal linfático. [lymphatic + G. *stoma*, boca]
lymph·at·ics (lim-fat′iks). Linfáticos. SIN lymph *vessels*, em *vessel*.
lym·pha·ti·tis (lim-fă-tī′tis). Linfatite; termo obsoleto para inflamação dos vasos linfáticos ou linfonodos. [lymphatic + G. *-itis*, inflamação]
lym·pha·tol·o·gy (lim-fă-tol′ō-jē). Linfatologia; o estudo do sistema linfático. [lymphatic + G. *logos*, estudo]
lym·pha·tol·y·sis (lim′fă-tol′i-sis). Linfatólise; termo obsoleto para destruição dos vasos linfáticos e/ou do tecido linfóide. [lymphatic + G. *lysis*, destruição]
lym·pha·to·lyt·ic (lim′fă-tō-lit′ik). Linfatolítico; pertinente a ou caracterizado por linfatólise.
lym·phec·ta·sia (lim-fek-tā′zē-ă). Linfectasia. SIN lymphangiectasis. [lymph + G. *ektasis*, um estiramento]
lymph·e·de·ma (limf′e-dē′mă). Linfedema; inchação (especialmente nos tecidos subcutâneos) em consequência de obstrução dos vasos linfáticos ou linfonodos e do acúmulo de grandes quantidades de linfa na região afetada. VER TAMBÉM elephantiasis. [lymph + G. *oidēma*, uma inchação]
  congenital l., l. congênito. VER hereditary l.
  hereditary l., l. hereditário; edema depressível permanente, geralmente confinado às pernas; dois tipos, congênito (doença de Milroy [MIM*153100], causado por mutação no gene 4 da tirosina cinase semelhante ao FMS (FLT4) em 5q, ou com início em torno da puberdade (doença de Meige [MIM*153200]); herança autossômica dominante.
  l. prae′cox, l. precoce, l. primário. SIN primary l.
  primary l., l. primário; uma forma de l. observada principalmente em mulheres jovens e meninas, caracterizada por inchação difusa dos membros inferiores. SIN l. praecox.
lym·phe·mia (lim-fē′mē-ă). Linfemia; a presença de um número incomumente grande de linfócitos e/ou de seus precursores no sangue circulante. [lymph(ocyte) + G. *haima*, sangue]
lim·phi·za·tion (lim-fi-zā′shŭn). Linfização; a formação de linfa.

LYMPH NODE

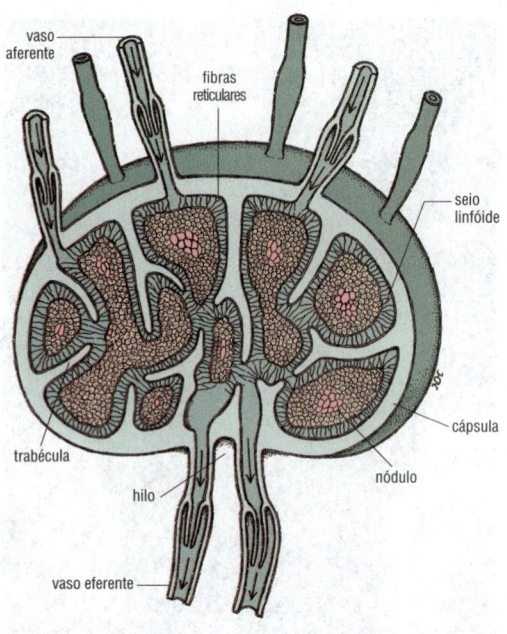

linfonodo

lymph node [TA]. Linfonodo; um dos numerosos corpúsculos arredondados, ovais ou em formato de ervilha localizados ao longo do trajeto dos vasos linfáticos, variando muito em tamanho (1–25 mm de diâmetro) e, em geral, apresentando uma área deprimida, o hilo, em um lado através do qual os vasos sanguíneos penetram e os vasos linfáticos eferentes saem. A estrutura consiste em uma cápsula fibrosa e trabéculas internas que sustentam o tecido linfóide e os seios linfáticos; o tecido linfóide é disposto em nódulos no córtex e cordões na medula de um linfonodo, com os vasos aferentes penetrando em muitos pontos da periferia. SIN nodus lymphoideus [TA], lymphonodus*, nodus lymphaticus*, lymph gland, lymphaden, lymphoglandula.
  abdominal l. n.'s [TA], linfonodos abdominais; os linfonodos parietais e viscerais do abdome, coletivamente. SIN nodi lymphoidei abdominis [TA].
  l. n.'s of abdominal organs, linfonodos dos órgãos abdominais. SIN visceral l. n.´s of abdomen.
  accessory l. n.'s '[TA], linfonodos acessórios; os linfonodos do grupamento cervical profundo lateral que estão localizados ao longo do nervo acessório; seus vasos eferentes passam para os linfonodos supraclaviculares. SIN nodi lymphoidei accessorii [TA], accessory nerve l. n.'s, companion l. n.'s of accessory nerve, nodi lymphatici comitantes nervi accessorii.
  accessory nerve l. n.'s, linfonodos do nervo acessório. SIN accessory l. n.´s.
  anorectal l. n.'s, linfonodos pararretais. SIN pararectal l. n.'s.
  anterior axillary l. n.'s, linfonodos axilares anteriores; *termo oficial alternativo para pectoral axillary l. n.'s.
  l. n. of anterior border of omental foramen [TA], l. do forame omental; um dos linfonodos hepáticos localizados adjacentes ao forame omental. SIN nodus lymphoideus foraminalis [TA], foraminal l. n., foraminal node.
  anterior cervical l. n.'s [TA], linfonodos cervicais anteriores; o grupo de linfonodos localizado na região anterior do pescoço, dividido nos grupos superficial e profundo. SIN nodi lymphoidei cervicales anteriores [TA].
  anterior deep cervical l. n.'s, linfonodos profundos cervicais anteriores. SIN deep anterior cervical l. n.'s.
  anterior jugular l. n.'s, linfonodos superficiais cervicais anteriores. SIN anterior superficial cervical l. n.'s.
  anterior mediastinal l. n.'s, linfonodos braquiocefálicos. SIN brachiocephalic l. n.
  anterior superficial cervical l. n.'s [TA], linfonodos superficiais cervicais anteriores; os linfonodos no tecido subcutâneo da região anterior do pescoço. SIN nodi lumphoidei cervicales anteriores superficiales [TA], anterior jugular l. n.'s, nodi lymphoidei jugulares anteriores.
  anterior tibial l. n. [TA], l. tibial anterior; um pequeno l. inconstante adiante da membrana interóssea, ao longo da parte superior dos vasos tibiais anteriores. SIN nodus tibialis anterior [TA], anterior tibial node.
  apical axillary l. n.'s [TA], linfonodos axilares apicais; o grupamento de linfonodos localizados no ápice da fossa axilar que recebem a drenagem linfática de outros grupos de linfonodos axilares e, em seguida, drenam, por sua vez, para o tronco linfático subclávio. SIN nodi lymphoidei axillares apicales [TA].
  appendicular l. n.'s [TA], linfonodos apendiculares; linfonodos viscerais ao longo dos vasos apendiculares no mesoapêndice; recebem os vasos aferentes do apêndice vermiforme e enviam vasos eferentes para os linfonodos ileocólicos. SIN nodi lymphoidei appendiculares [TA].
  l. n. of arch of azygos vein [TA], um l. visceral do grupo braquiocefálico direito adjacente ao arco da veia ázigo. SIN nodus lymphoideus arcus venae azygos [TA], l. n. of azygos arch, nodus lymphoideus arcus venae azygos.
  l. n.'s around cardia of stomach [TA], anel linfático do cárdia; um grupo de linfonodos ao redor do cárdia do estômago. SIN anulus lymphaticus cardiae [TA], cardiac lymphatic ring, lymphatic ring of cardiac part of stomach.
  axillary l. n.'s [TA], linfonodos axilares; numerosos linfonodos, ao redor das veias axilares, que recebem a drenagem linfática do membro superior, da região escapular e da região peitoral (incluindo a glândula mamária); drenam para o tronco subclávio. SIN nodi lymphoidei axillares [TA], axillary glands.
  l. n. of azygos arch, l. do arco da veia ázigo. SIN l. n. of arch of azygos vein.
  bifurcation l. n.'s, linfonodos traqueobronquiais inferiores. SIN inferior tracheobronchial l. n.'s.
  brachial l. n.'s, linfonodos axilares umerais, linfonodos axilares. SIN humeral axillary l. n.'s.
  brachiocephalic l. n., l. braquiocefálico; localizados no mediastino superior em relação aos grandes vasos, esses linfonodos recebem linfa do timo, pericárdio e lado direito do coração; seus vasos eferentes unem-se aos dos linfonodos traqueais para formar os troncos broncomediastinais. SIN nodi lymphoidei brachiocephalici [TA], anterior mediastinal l. n.'s, nodi lymphoidei mediastinales anteriores.
  bronchopulmonary l. n.'s [TA], linfonodos broncopulmonares; os linfonodos no hilo do pulmão que recebem linfa dos linfonodos intrapulmonares e drenam para os linfonodos traqueobronquiais. SIN nodi lymphoidei bronchopulmonales [TA], hilar l. n.'s.
  buccal l. n., l. bucinatório; um linfonodo da cadeia de linfonodos faciais localizados superficialmente ao músculo bucinador. SIN nodus lymphoideus buccinatorius [TA], buccinator node, buccal node, nodus buccinatorius.
  carinal l. n.'s, linfonodos traqueobronquiais inferiores. SIN inferior tracheobronchial l. n.'s.
  celiac l. n.'s [TA], linfonodos celíacos; linfonodos viscerais localizados ao longo do tronco celíaco que drenam a linfa oriunda do estômago, duodeno, pâncreas, baço e trato biliar e drenam para a cisterna do quilo, através dos troncos linfáticos intestinais direito e esquerdo. SIN nodi lymphoidei coeliaci [TA].
  central axillary l. n.'s [TA], linfonodos axilares centrais; linfonodos localizados ao redor da porção média da veia axilar; recebem os vasos aferentes dos grupos umerais (lateral), peitoral (anterior) e subescapular (posterior) de lin-

fonodos axilares e enviam vasos eferentes para o grupamento apical dos linfonodos axilares. SIN nodi lymphoidei axillares centrales [TA].
central mesenteric l. n.'s, linfonodos mesentéricos superiores centrais. SIN central superior mesenteric l. n.'s. VER TAMBÉM mesenteric l. n.'s.
central superior mesenteric l. n.'s [TA], linfonodos mesentéricos superiores centrais; os linfonodos mesentéricos localizados ao longo dos ramos intestinais (jejunal e ileal) da artéria mesentérica superior. SIN nodi lymphoidei superiores centrales [TA], central mesenteric l. n.'s, middle group of mesenteric l. n.'s.
colic l. n.'s, linfonodos cólicos. SIN nodi lymphatici colici. VER left colic l. n.'s, middle colic l. n.'s, right colic l. n.'s.
common iliac l. n.'s [TA], linfonodos ilíacos comuns; linfonodos parietais associados à veia ilíaca comum; são subdivididos em cinco grupos: linfonodos ilíacos comuns intermédios, entre a artéria e veia ilíacas comuns; linfonodos ilíacos comuns laterais, lateralmente à veia; linfonodos ilíacos comuns mediais, medialmente à veia; linfonodos ilíacos comuns do promontório, no promontório sacral; e linfonodos ilíacos comuns subaórticos, na bifurcação da aorta; todos eles recebem os vasos aferentes dos linfonodos ilíacos externos e internos e enviam vasos eferentes para os linfonodos lombares. SIN nodi lymphoidei iliaci communes [TA].
companion l. n.'s of accessory nerve, linfonodos acessórios. SIN accessory l. n.'s.
cubital l. n.'s [TA], linfonodos cubitais; dois grupos de linfonodos, superficial e profundo, que se situam ao longo da veia basílica acima do epicôndilo medial; recebem aferentes do lado ulnar do antebraço e mão, e enviam eferentes para os linfonodos braquiais. SIN nodi lymphoidei cubitales [TA], l. n.'s of elbow.
cystic l. n. [TA], l. cístico; um l. visceral no colo da vesícula biliar que drena a linfa para os linfonodos hepáticos. SIN nodus lymphoideus cysticus [TA], cystic node.
deep anterior cervical l. n.'s [TA], linfonodos cervicais anteriores profundos; os linfonodos próximos à laringe, traquéia e glândula tireóide. SIN anterior deep cervical l. n.'s, nodi lymphoidei cervicales anteriores profundi.
deep inguinal l. n.'s [TA], linfonodos inguinais profundos; vários linfonodos pequenos e inconstantes (proximais, intermédios e distais), profundos em relação à fáscia lata e mediais à veia femoral; recebem linfa das estruturas profundas do membro inferior, da glande do pênis e dos linfonodos inguinais superficiais; os eferentes dirigem-se para os linfonodos ilíacos externos. SIN nodi lymphoidei inguinales profundi.
deep lateral cervical l. n.'s [TA], linfonodos cervicais laterais profundos; os linfonodos localizados no triângulo posterior do pescoço profundamente à camada de revestimento da fáscia cervical; drenam para o tronco jugular no lado direito ou esquerdo; o grupamento é subdividido em quatro cadeias menores: linfonodos cervicais profundos superiores, linfonodos cervicais profundos inferiores, linfonodos acessórios e linfonodos supraclaviculares. SIN nodi lymphoidei cervicales laterales profundi [TA].
deep parotid l. n.'s [TA], linfonodos parotídeos profundos; o grupo de linfonodos associados à glândula parótida, que se situam profundamente à fáscia massetérica da parótida. SIN nodi lymphoidei parotidei profundi [TA].
l. n.'s of elbow, linfonodos cubitais. SIN cubital l. n.'s.
external iliac l. n.'s [TA], linfonodos ilíacos externos; linfonodos parietais associados à veia ilíaca externa; são subdivididos em três grupos: linfonodos ilíacos externos intermédios, entre a veia e a artéria ilíaca externa; linfonodos ilíacos externos laterais; e linfonodos ilíacos externos mediais, mediais à veia; todos recebem vasos aferentes dos linfonodos inguinais, da parede abdominal inferior e das vísceras pélvicas, enviando vasos eferentes para os linfonodos ilíacos comuns. SIN nodi lymphoidei iliaci externi [TA].
facial l. n.'s [TA], linfonodos da face; uma cadeia de linfonodos situados ao longo da veia facial que recebem os vasos aferentes das pálpebras, nariz, bochecha, lábio e gengivas, e enviam vasos eferentes para os linfonodos submandibulares. SIN nodi lymphoidei faciales [TA].
fibular l. n., l. fibular; um pequeno l. inconstante ao longo do trajeto da veia fibular (venae comitantes). SIN nodus lymphoideus fibularis [TA], fibular node, peroneal l. n.
foraminal l. n., l. do forame omental. SIN l. n. of anterior border of omental foramen.
gastroduodenal l. n.'s, linfonodos pilóricos. SIN pyloric l. n.'s.
gluteal l. n.'s [TA], linfonodos glúteos; linfonodos parietais dos linfonodos ilíacos internos; são subdivididos em dois grupos: linfonodos glúteos inferiores, localizados ao longo da veia glútea inferior; e linfonodos glúteos superiores, localizados ao longo da veia glútea superior. SIN nodi lymphoidei gluteales [TA].
l. n.'s of head and neck [TA], linfonodos da cabeça e do pescoço; linfonodos localizados na cabeça e no pescoço, que drenam essas regiões e, por fim, desembocam nos troncos linfáticos jugulares. SIN nodi lymphoidei capitis et colli [TA].
hepatic l. n.'s [TA], linfonodos hepáticos; linfonodos viscerais localizados ao longo da artéria hepática até a porta do fígado; drenam fígado, vesícula biliar, estômago, duodeno e pâncreas, enviando eferentes para os linfonodos celíacos. SIN nodi lymphoidei hepatici [TA].
hilar l. n.'s, linfonodos broncopulmonares; SIN bronchopulmonary l. n.'s.
humeral axillary l. n.'s [TA], linfonodos axilares umerais; os linfonodos ao longo da veia braquial, enviando vasos eferentes para os linfonodos axilares centrais. SIN nodi lymphoidei axillares humerales [TA], lateral axillary l. n.'s*, nodi lymphoidei axillares laterales*, brachial l. n.'s, nodi lymphoidei brachiales.
ileocolic l. n.'s [TA], linfonodos ileocólicos; linfonodos viscerais, localizados ao longo da artéria ileocólica, que drenam a linfa do colo ascendente até os linfonodos mesentéricos superiores. SIN nodi lymphoidei ileocolici [TA].
inferior epigastric l. n.'s [TA], linfonodos epigástricos inferiores; três ou quatro linfonodos parietais dispostos ao longo dos vasos epigástricos inferiores; recebem aferentes da parede abdominal inferior e desembocam nos linfonodos ilíacos externos. SIN nodi lymphoidei epigastrici inferiores [TA].
inferior mesenteric l. n.'s [TA], linfonodos mesentéricos inferiores; linfonodos viscerais localizados ao longo da artéria mesentérica inferior e seus ramos que drenam a parte superior do reto, colo sigmóide e colo descendente. SIN nodi lymphoidei mesenterici inferiores [TA].
inferior phrenic l. n.'s [TA], linfonodos frênicos inferiores; pequenos linfonodos associados aos vasos frênicos inferiores. SIN nodi lymphoidei phrenici inferiores [TA].
inferior tracheobronchial l. n.'s [TA], linfonodos traqueobronquiais inferiores; vários linfonodos grandes, inferiores à bifurcação traqueal; recebem aferentes dos linfonodos broncopulmonares e do coração, e enviam eferentes para os linfonodos traqueobronquiais superiores e paratraqueais. SIN bifurcation l. n.'s, carinal l. n.'s, nodi lymphoidei tracheobronchiales inferiores.
infraauricular deep parotid l. n.'s [TA], linfonodos parotídeos profundos infra-auriculares; pequenos linfonodos localizados profundamente à fáscia parotídea e abaixo da orelha. SIN infra-auricular subfascial parotid l. n.'s, nodi lymphoidei parotidei profundi infra-auriculares.
infraauricular subfascial parotid l. n.'s, linfonodos parotídeos profundos infra-auriculares. SIN infraauricular deep parotid l. n.'s.
intercostal l. n.'s [TA], linfonodos intercostais; um ou dois pequenos linfonodos localizados posteriormente em cada espaço intercostal; recebem linfa da pleura parietal, espaço intercostal e parede posterior do corpo; os linfonodos nos espaços superiores desembocam no ducto torácico, enquanto os linfonodos nos espaços inferiores formam um tronco intercostal descendente, que se abre para a cisterna do quilo. SIN nodi lymphoidei intercostales [TA].
interiliac l. n.'s [TA], linfonodos interilíacos; vários linfonodos localizados entre as artérias ilíacas externa e interna e a artéria obturadora; esses linfonodos são considerados por alguns como sendo parte dos linfonodos ilíacos externos. SIN nodi lymphoidei interiliaci [TA].
intermediate lacunar l. n. [TA], linfonodo lacunar intermédio; um linfonodo inconstante dos linfonodos ilíacos externos que, freqüentemente, ocorre entre a artéria e a veia ilíacas externas no espaço vascular do compartimento subinguinal. SIN nodus lymphoideus lacunaris intermedius [TA], intermediate lacunar node.
intermediate lumbar l. n.'s [TA], linfonodos lombares intermédios; a cadeia de linfonodos localizada entre a aorta e a veia cava inferior. SIN nodi lymphoidei lumbales intermedii [TA], lumbar l. n.'s.
internal iliac l. n.'s [TA], linfonodos ilíacos internos; os linfonodos ao longo da artéria ilíaca interna e seus ramos; recebem linfa das vísceras pélvicas, da região glútea e das partes profundas do períneo, e enviam vasos eferentes para os linfonodos ilíacos comuns. SIN nodi lymphoidei iliaci interni [TA].
interpectoral l. n.'s [TA], linfonodos interpeitorais; pequenos linfonodos localizados entre os músculos peitorais maior e menor; recebem linfa dos músculos e da glândula mamária, enviando-se para o plexo linfático axilar. SIN nodi lymphoidei interpectorales [TA].
intraglandular deep parotid l. n.'s [TA], linfonodos parotídeos profundos intraglandulares; pequenos linfonodos do grupo parotídeo profundo que se situam dentro da glândula parótida. SIN nodi lymphoidei parotidei intraglandulares [TA], intraglandular parotid l. n.'s.
intraglandular parotid l. n.'s [TA], linfonodos parotídeos profundos intraglandulares. SIN intraglandular deep parotid l. n.'s.
intrapulmonary l. n.'s [TA], linfonodos intrapulmonares; pequenos linfonodos que ocorrem ao longo dos brônquios dentro do parênquima do pulmão; recebem a drenagem de áreas localizadas do pulmão e enviam eferentes para os linfonodos broncopulmonares. SIN nodi lymphoidei intrapulmonales [TA], nodi lymphoidei pulmonales, pulmonary l. n.'s.
jugulodigastric l. n. [TA], linfonodo jugulodigástrico; um linfonodo proeminente no grupamento cervical lateral que se situa abaixo do músculo digástrico e anterior à veia jugular interna; recebe a drenagem linfática da faringe, tonsila palatina e língua. SIN nodus lymphoideus jugulodigastricus [TA], jugulodigastric node, subdigastric node.
juguloomohyoid l. n. [TA], l. jugulo-omo-hióideo; um l. do grupo cervical profundo lateral que se situa acima do tendão intermédio do músculo omo-hióideo e anterior à veia jugular interna; recebe a drenagem linfática dos linfonodos submentuais, submandibulares e cervicais anteriores profundos; seus

vasos eferentes dirigem-se para outros linfonodos cervicais laterais profundos. SIN nodus lymphoideus juguloomohyoideus [TA], juguloomohyoid node.

juxtaesophageal l. n.'s [TA], linfonodos justaglomerulares; vários linfonodos localizados ao longo de ambos os lados do esôfago; recebem linfa do esôfago e dos pulmões. SIN nodi lymphoidei juxtaesophageales [TA], nodi lymphoidei juxtaesophageales pulmonales.

juxta-intestinal mesenteric l. n.'s [TA], linfonodos mesentéricos superiores justa-intestinais; os linfonodos mesentéricos localizados nas proximidades imediatas do jejuno ou íleo. SIN nodi lymphoidei juxtaintestinales [TA].

lateral axillary l. n.'s, linfonodos axilares umerais; *termo oficial alternativo para humeral axillary l. n.'s.

lateral jugular l. n.'s, linfonodos cervicais profundos laterais; linfonodos profundos dos linfonodos cervicais laterais que se situam lateralmente à veia jugular interna; em geral, desembocam no tronco jugular. SIN nodi lymphoidei jugulares laterales.

lateral lacunar l. n., [TA], l. lacunar lateral; um l. do grupo ilíaco externo localizado lateralmente à artéria ilíaca externa no espaço vascular do compartimento sublingual. SIN nodus lymphoideus lacunaris lateralis [TA], lateral lacunar node.

lateral pericardial l. n.'s [TA], linfonodos pericárdicos laterais; pequenos linfonodos, localizados ao longo dos vasos pericardicofrênicos, que drenam o pericárdio. SIN nodi lymphoidei pericardiales laterales [TA].

left coli l. n.'s [TA], linfonodos cólicos esquerdos; pequenos linfonodos, ao longo da artéria cólica esquerda e seus ramos, que drenam a flexura esquerda e a parte superior do colo descendente; os vasos eferentes passam para os linfonodos mesentéricos inferiores. SIN nodi lymphoidei colici sinistri [TA].

left gastric l. n.'s [TA], linfonodos gástricos esquerdos; linfonodos localizados ao longo da artéria gástrica esquerda e seus ramos; são divididos nos grupamentos paracardíaco, superior e inferior. SIN nodi lymphoidei gastrici sinistri [TA], superior gastric l. n.'s.

left gastroepiploic l. n.'s, linfonodos gastromentais esquerdos. SIN left gastroomental l. n.'s.

left gastroomental l. n.'s [TA], linfonodos gastroomentais esquerdos; linfonodos localizados no omento maior, ao longo da artéria gastroepiplóica esquerda, que drenam parte da curvatura maior do estômago e do omento maior. SIN nodi lymphoidei gastroomentales sinistri [TA], left gastroepiploic l. n.'s.

left lumbar l. n.'s [TA], linfonodos lombares esquerdos; a cadeia de linfonodos associada à aorta no abdome; é dividida em três grupos: linfonodos aórticos laterais, à esquerda da aorta; linfonodos pré-aórticos, à frente da aorta; e linfonodos retroaórticos, por trás da aorta. SIN nodi lymphoidei lumbales sinistri [TA], lumbar l. n.'s.

l. n. of ligamentum arteriosum [TA], linfonodo do ligamento arterial; um l. inconstante do grupo mediastinal anterior adjacente ao ligamento arterial. SIN nodus lymphoideus ligamenti arteriosi [TA], node of ligamentum arteriosum.

lingual l. n.'s [TA], linfonodos linguais; um l., ao longo da veia lingual, que recebe a drenagem da língua (excetuando-se a ponta); drena para os linfonodos submandibulares. SIN nodi lymphoidei linguales [TA].

l. n.'s of lower limb [TA], linfonodos do membro inferior; os linfonodos localizados nos membros inferiores e que os drenam como um grupo; incluem os linfonodos inguinais, poplíteos, tibiais e fibulares. SIN nodi lymphoidei membri inferioris [TA].

lumbar l. n.'s, linfonodos lombares. SIN right lumbar l. n.'s, intermediate lumbar l. n.'s, left lumbar l. n.'s.

malar l. n. [TA], linfonodo zigomático; um dos linfonodos da face próximo ao músculo zigomático menor. SIN nodus lymphoideus malaris [TA], malar node.

mandibular l. n. [TA], l. mandibular; um dos linfonodos da face localizados pela artéria facial próximo ao ponto em que ela cruza a mandíbula. SIN nodus lymphoideus mandibularis [TA], mandibular nodes.

mastoid l. n.'s [TA], linfonodos mastóideos; dois ou três linfonodos na região do processo mastóide; recebem os vasos linfáticos aferentes do couro cabeludo e da orelha e enviam vasos eferentes para os linfonodos cervicais profundos superiores. SIN nodi lymphoidei mastoidei [TA], retroauricular l. n.'s.

medial lacunar l. n. [TA], l. lacunar medial; um l. do grupo ilíaco externo localizado medialmente à veia ilíaca externa no espaço vascular do compartimento sublingual. SIN nodus lymphoideus lacunaris medialis [TA], medial lacunar node.

mesenteric l. n.'s [TA], linfonodos mesentéricos; linfonodos localizados no mesentério; são de três classes: linfonodos ileocólicos, linfonodos mesentéricos justaintestinais e grupo superior central dos linfonodos mesentéricos. SIN nodi lymphoidei mesenterici [TA].

mesocolic l. n.'s [TA], linfonodos mesocólicos; linfonodos localizados no mesocolo; são de duas classes: linfonodos paracólicos, localizados nas proximidades imediatas ao colo; e linfonodos cólicos, situados ao longo das artérias que suprem o colo. SIN nodi lymphoidei mesocolici [TA], nodi lymphoidei paracolici.

middle colic l. n.'s [TA], linfonodos cólicos médios; linfonodos ao longo da artéria cólica média e seus ramos que drenam a flexura cólica direita e a maior parte do colo transverso. SIN nodi lymphoidei colici medii [TA].

middle group of mesenteric l. n.'s, linfonodos mesentéricos superiores centrais. SIN central superior mesenteric l. n.'s.

middle rectal l. n., l. retal médio; um l., ao longo da artéria retal média, que recebe aferentes dos linfonodos pararretais e envia eferentes para os linfonodos ilíacos internos. SIN middle rectal node, nodus lymphoideus rectalis medius.

nasolabial l. n. [TA], l. nasolabial; um dos linfonodos faciais localizados próximo à junção das artérias facial e labial superior. SIN nodus lymphoideus nasolabialis [TA], nasolabial node.

obturator l. n.'s [TA], linfonodos obturatórios; os linfonodos do grupo ilíaco interno localizados ao longo da artéria obturatória. SIN nodi lymphoidei obturatorii [TA].

occipital l. n.'s [TA], linfonodos occipitais; um ou dois pequenos linfonodos ao longo dos vasos occipitais, próximo ao músculo trapézio, que recebem aferentes da parte posterior do couro cabeludo e drenam para os linfonodos cervicais laterais profundos superiores; são os linfonodos mais posteriores do anel linfático pericervical da cabeça e pescoço, os quais recebem a drenagem da cabeça. SIN nodi lymphoidei occipitales [TA].

pancreatic l. n.'s [TA], linfonodos pancreáticos; linfonodos que drenam o corpo e a cauda do pâncreas; são subdivididos em dois grupos: linfonodos pancreáticos inferiores [TA] (nodi lymphoidei pancreatici inferiores [TA]), localizados ao longo da artéria pancreática inferior; e linfonodos pancreáticos superiores (nodi lymphoidei pancreatici superiores [TA]), localizados ao longo da artéria esplênica próximo à origem de seus ramos pancreáticos. SIN nodi lymphoidei pancreatici [TA].

pancreaticoduodenal l. n.'s [TA], linfonodos pancreaticoduodenais; linfonodos ao longo das artérias pancreaticoduodenais superior e inferior. SIN nodi lymphoidei pancreaticoduodenales [TA].

pancreaticosplenic l. n.'s [TA], linfonodos pancreaticosplênicos; linfonodos da cauda do pâncreas e do baço, recebendo aferentes dos dois órgãos além da curvatura maior do estômago; drenam para os linfonodos celíacos. SIN nodi lymphoidei pancreaticosplenales [TA], nodi lymphoidei pancreaticolienales.

parammary l. n.'s [TA], linfonodos paramamários; vários linfonodos na face lateral da glândula mamária que recebem aferentes da glândula mamária e enviam eferentes para o grupo peitoral axilar de linfonodos. Os linfonodos paramamários são comumente considerados parte dos linfonodos axilares peitorais. SIN nodi lymphoidei paramammarii [TA].

pararectal l. n.'s [TA], linfonodos pararretais; linfonodos localizados dos dois lados do reto; enviam eferentes para os linfonodos retais médios e superiores. SIN nodi lymphoidei pararectales [TA], anorectal l. n.'s, nodi lymphoidei anorectales.

parasternal l. n.'s [TA], linfonodos paraesternais; inúmeros linfonodos pequenos que se situam ao longo do trajeto dos vasos torácicos internal; a linfa entra nesses linfonodos proveniente dos espaços intercostais anteriores, pericárdio, diafragma, fígado e porção medial da glândula mamária; os vasos eferentes ascendem para se unirem ao tronco broncomediastinal do mesmo lado. SIN nodi lymphoidei parasternales [TA].

paratracheal l. n.'s [TA], linfonodos paratraqueais; linfonodos ao longo dos lados da traquéia no pescoço e no mediastino posterior; recebem a drenagem dos linfonodos traqueobronquiais superiores (e inferiores), traquéia e esôfago; drenam para o(s) tronco(s) linfático(s) broncomediastinal(is) e ducto torácico. SIN nodi lymphoidei paratracheales [TA], tracheal l. n.'s.

parauterine l. n.'s [TA], linfonodos parauterinos; linfonodos dos dois os lados do útero que drenam a linfa para os linfonodos ilíacos internos e linfonodos lombares, através de vasos linfáticos que seguem as artérias ováricas. SIN nodi lymphoidei parauterini [TA].

paravaginal l. n.'s [TA], linfonodos paravaginais; os linfonodos associados à vagina; drenam para os linfonodos ilíacos internos. SIN nodi lymphoidei paravaginales [TA].

paravesical l. n.'s, linfonodos paravesicais; os linfonodos localizados ao redor da bexiga urinária e, no homem, da próstata; existem três grupos: linfonodos pré-vesicais, à frente da bexiga; linfonodos vesicais laterais, nos lados direito e esquerdo; linfonodos retrovesicais, atrás da bexiga.

parietal l. n.'s [TA], linfonodos parietais; os linfonodos que drenam as paredes do abdome ou da pelve (em oposição aos linfonodos viscerais que drenam as vísceras abdominopélvicas). SIN nodi lymphoidei parietales [TA], parietal nodes.

pectoral axillary l. n.'s [TA], linfonodos axilares peitorais; os linfonodos localizados ao longo da veia torácica lateral; recebem a drenagem da região peitoral, inclusive a maior parte da drenagem da mama. SIN nodi lymphoidei axillares pectorales [TA], anterior axillary l. n.'s*, nodi lymphoidei axillares anteriores.

pelvic l. n.'s [TA], linfonodos da pelve; os linfonodos parietais e viscerais da pelve, coletivamente. SIN nodi lymphoidei pelvis [TA].

peroneal l. n., l. fibular. SIN fibular l. n.

popliteal l. n.'s [TA], linfonodos poplíteos; dois grupos de linfonodos localizados na fossa poplítea: os linfonodos poplíteos superficiais, localizados ao redor da terminação da veia safena menor, que drena a pele da parte posterior da perna e o lado lateral do pé; e os linfonodos poplíteos profundos, localizados ao redor dos vasos poplíteos, que drenam o grupo superficial, as estruturas profundas da perna e a articulação do joelho. SIN nodi lymphoidei popliteales [TA].

posterior axillary l. n.'s, linfonodos axilares posteriores; *termo oficial alternativo para subscapular axillary l. n.'s.

posterior mediastinal l. n.'s, linfonodos pré-vertebrais. SIN prevertebral l. n.'s.

posterior tibial l. n. [TA], l. tibial posterior; um pequeno l. inconstante localizado ao longo do trajeto da artéria tibial posterior. SIN nodus lymphoideus tibialis posterior [TA], posterior tibial node.

preauricular deep parotid l. n.'s [TA], linfonodos parotídeos profundos pré-auriculares; pequenos linfonodos localizados profundamente à fáscia parotídea e à frente da orelha. SIN nodi lymphoidei parotidei profundi preauriculares [TA].

prececal l. n.'s [TA], linfonodos pré-cecais; linfonodos localizados à frente do ceco que drenam a linfa para os linfonodos ileocólicos. SIN nodi lymphoidei precaecales [TA].

prelaryngeal l. n.'s [TA], linfonodos pré-laríngeos; linfonodos do grupo cervical anterior profundo que se situam à frente da laringe; drenam para os linfonodos cervicais laterais profundos. SIN nodi lymphoidei prelaryngeales [TA].

prepericardial l. n.'s [TA], linfonodos pré-pericárdicos; vários linfonodos pequenos localizados entre o pericárdio e o esterno, no mediastino anterior. SIN nodi lymphoidei prepericardiaci [TA].

pretracheal l. n.'s [TA], linfonodos pré-traqueais; linfonodos do grupo cervical anterior profundo que se situam à frente da traquéia; drenam para o grupo cervical lateral profundo ou para os linfonodos paraesternais. SIN nodi lymphoidei pretracheales [TA].

prevertebral l. n.'s [TA], linfonodos pré-vertebrais; os linfonodos localizados ao longo da aorta torácica; recebem os vasos do esôfago, diafragma, fígado e pericárdio, enviando eferentes para o ducto torácico e tronco linfático broncomediastinal. SIN nodi lymphoidei prevertebrales*, nodi lymphoidei mediastinales posteriores, posterior mediastinal l. n.'s.

proximal deep inguinal l. n. [TA], l. inguinal profundo proximal; um dos linfonodos inguinais profundos localizados no canal femoral ou adjacente a ele; por vezes confundido com uma hérnia femoral, quando aumentado. SIN nodus lymphoideus proximalis profundus [TA], node of Cloquet, Rosenmüller gland, Rosenmüller node.

pulmonary l. n.'s, linfonodos intrapulmonares. SIN intrapulmonary l. n.'s.

pyloric l. n.'s [TA], linfonodos pilóricos; grupo de linfonodos que circundam o piloro, drenando a linfa para os linfonodos gastroomentais direitos ou gástricos direitos; dividem-se em três grupos menores: linfonodos suprapilóricos, superiores ao piloro; linfonodos subpilóricos, abaixo do piloro; e linfonodos retropilóricos, posteriores ao piloro. SIN gastroduodenal l. n.'s, nodi lymphoidei pylorici.

retroauricular l. n.'s, linfonodos mastóideos. SIN mastoid l. n.'s.

retrocecal l. n.'s [TA], linfonodos retrocecais; linfonodos localizados atrás do ceco que drenam a linfa para os linfonodos ileocólicos. SIN nodi lymphoidei retrocecales [TA].

retropharyngeal l. n.'s [TA], linfonodos retrofaríngeos; os três grupos de linfonodos, um mediano e dois laterais, localizados entre a faringe e a camada pré-vertebral da fáscia cervical; recebem linfa da nasofaringe, tuba auditiva e articulações atlanto-occipital e atlanto-axial. SIN nodi lymphoidei retropharyngeales [TA].

retropyloric l. n.'s [TA], linfonodos retropilóricos; um grupo de linfonodos localizados atrás do piloro. SIN nodi lymphoidei retropylorici [TA], retropyloric nodes.

right colic l. n.'s [TA], linfonodos cólicos direitos; linfonodos localizados ao longo da artéria cólica direita que drenam a parte superior do colo ascendente. SIN nodi lymphoidei colici dextri [TA].

right gastric l. n.'s [TA], linfonodos gástricos direitos; pequenos linfonodos, ao longo do trajeto da artéria gástrica direita, que drenam parte da curvatura menor do estômago. SIN nodi lymphoidei gastrici dextri [TA].

right gastroepiploic l. n.'s, linfonodos gastroomentais direitos. SIN right gastroomental l. n.'s.

right gastromental l. n.'s [TA], linfonodos gastroomentais direitos; os linfonodos localizados ao longo da artéria gastroepiplóica direita que drenam parte da curvatura maior do estômago e do omento maior. SIN nodi lymphoidei gastroomentales dextri [TA], right gastroepiploic l. n.'s.

right lumbar l. n.'s [TA], linfonodos lombares direitos; a cadeia de linfonodos associada à veia cava inferior; dividem-se em três grupos: linfonodos cavais laterais, à direita da veia cava inferior; linfonodos pré-cavais, anterior à veia cava inferior; linfonodos retrocavais, posteriores à veia cava inferior. SIN nodi lymphoidei lumbales dextri [TA], lumbar l. n.'s.

sacral l. n.'s [TA], linfonodos sacrais; linfonodos na concavidade do sacro que drenam o reto e a parede pélvica posterior. SIN nodi lymphoidei sacrales [TA].

sentinel l. n., linfonodo sentinela; o primeiro linfonodo a receber a drenagem linfática de um tumor maligno; o linfonodo sentinela é identificado como o primeiro usando um radionuclídeo ou corante injetado no tumor; cada vez mais usado em cirurgias para melanoma e câncer de mama; quando o linfonodo sentinela está sem metástases, os linfonodos mais distais também estão. VER TAMBÉM signal l. n. SIN sentinel node.

sigmoid l. n.'s [TA], linfonodos sigmóideos; linfonodos do grupo mesentérico inferior, localizados ao longo das artérias sigmóides. SIN nodi lymphoidei sigmoidei [TA].

signal l. n., linfonodo sinalizador; um l. supraclavicular de consistência firme, especialmente no lado esquerdo, suficientemente aumentado, que é palpável a partir da superfície cutânea; esse l. é assim chamado porque seria a primeira evidência presuntiva reconhecida de uma neoplasia maligna em uma das vísceras. Um l. sinalizador que, sabidamente, contém uma metástase de uma neoplasia maligna é, por vezes, designado por um antigo epônimo, gânglio de Troisier (Troisier *ganglion*). VER TAMBÉM sentinel l. n. SIN jugular gland, Virchow node.

splenic l. n.'s [TA], linfonodos esplênicos; linfonodos próximos ao hilo do baço; recebem aferentes do baço e estômago, e enviam eferentes para os linfonodos pancreáticos pós-esplênicos e celíacos. SIN nodi lymphoidei splenici [TA], nodi lymphoidei lienales*.

subaortic l. n.'s [TA], linfonodos subaórticos; linfonodos do grupo ilíaco comum localizados na bifurcação da aorta. SIN nodi lymphoidei subaortici [TA].

submandibular l. n.'s [TA], linfonodos submandibulares; quatro ou cinco linfonodos que mantêm uma relação com a mandíbula e com a glândula submandibular; recebem vasos da face abaixo dos olhos e da língua e drenam para os linfonodos cervicais profundos superiores, principalmente o linfonodo jugulodigástrico; esses linfonodos fazem parte do anel linfático, pericervical, que, a princípio, recebe a drenagem da cabeça. SIN nodi lymphoidei submandibulares [TA].

submental l. n.'s [TA], linfonodos submentuais; pequenos linfonodos que se localizam superficialmente ao músculo milo-hióideo; recebem aferentes do lábio inferior, do queixo e da ponta da língua, e enviam eferentes para os linfonodos cervicais laterais profundos; esses linfonodos fazem parte do anel linfático pericervical, que, a princípio, recebe a drenagem da cabeça. SIN nodi lymphoidei submentales [TA].

subpyloric l. n.'s [TA], linfonodos subpilóricos; um grupo de linfonodos pilóricos localizados abaixo do piloro. SIN nodi lymphoidei subpylorici [TA], subpyloric node.

subscapular axillary l. n.'s [TA], linfonodos axilares subescapulares; os linfonodos da região axilar localizados ao longo da veia subescapular, e suas tributárias; recebem vasos aferentes da superfície dorsal do tórax e da região escapular e enviam vasos eferentes para o grupo central dos linfonodos. SIN nodi lymphoidei axillares subscapulares [TA], nodi lymphoidei axillares posteriores*, posterior axillary l. n.'s*.

superficial inguinal l. n.'s [TA], linfonodos inguinais superficiais; um grupo de 12 a 20 linfonodos que se situam no tecido subcutâneo abaixo do ligamento inguinal e ao longo da parte terminal da veia safena magna; drenam a pele e o tecido subcutâneo da parede abdominal inferior, do períneo, das nádegas, da genitália externa e do membro inferior; são subdivididos em três grupos: grupo inferior (vertical) dos linfonodos inguinais superficiais, localizados inferiormente à abertura da safena, recebendo a drenagem do membro inferior; linfonodos inguinais superficiais súpero-laterais (horizontal lateral) localizados lateralmente à abertura da safena, recebendo a drenagem da parte lateral da nádega e da parede abdominal anterior inferior; e os linfonodos inguinais superficiais súpero-mediais (horizontais mediais), localizados medialmente à abertura da safena, recebendo a drenagem do períneo e da genitália externa. SIN nodi lymphoidei inguinales superficiales [TA].

superficial lateral cervical l. n.'s [TA], linfonodos cervicais laterais superficiais; cerca de 1 a 4 linfonodos que se situam ao longo da veia jugular externa; drenam a pele e as estruturas superficiais sobre a região do músculo esternocleidomastóideo e enviam vasos eferentes para os linfonodos cervicais laterais profundos. SIN nodi lymphoidei cervicales laterales superficiales [TA].

superficial parotid l. n.'s, linfonodos parotídeos superficiais; vários pequenos linfonodos localizados no tecido subcutâneo na região parotídea. SIN nodi lymphoidei parotidei superficiales. [TA].

superior gastric l. n.'s, linfonodos gástricos esquerdos; SIN left gastric l. n.'s.

superior mesenteric l. n.'s [TA], linfonodos mesentéricos superiores; os numerosos linfonodos localizados no mesentério ao longo da artéria mesentérica superior; recebem linfa dos linfonodos mesentéricos centrais e drenam para o tronco linfático pulmonar. SIN nodi lymphoidei mesenterici superiores [TA], nodi lymphoidei centrales.

superior phrenic l. n.'s [TA], linfonodos frênicos superiores; três grupos de pequenos linfonodos, anterior, médio e posterior, na superfície superior do diafragma; recebem aferentes do fígado, diafragma e espaços intercostais, e enviam eferentes para os linfonodos paraesternais e pré-vertebrais. SIN nodi lymphoidei phrenici superiores [TA].

superior rectal l. n.'s [TA], linfonodos retais superiores; linfonodos do grupo mesentérico inferior, localizados ao longo da artéria retal superior. SIN nodi lymphoidei rectales superiores [TA].

superior tracheobronchial l. n.'s [TA], linfonodos traqueobronquiais superiores; vários linfonodos grandes do mediastino posterior localizados superiormente aos brônquios em suas uniões com a traquéia; recebem linfa dos linfonodos traqueobronquiais inferiores e dos linfonodos broncopulmonares; dre-

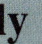

nam para os linfonodos paratraqueais. SIN nodi lymphoidei tracheobronchiales superiores [TA].

supraclavicular l. n.'s [TA], linfonodos supraclaviculares; a parte dos linfonodos cervicais laterais profundos inferiores localizada entre a porção carnosa inferior do músculo omo-hióideo e a clavícula; os vasos aferentes originam-se das regiões adjacentes, inclusive do mediastino; os vasos eferentes terminam no tronco subclávio. SIN nodi lymphoidei supraclaviculares [TA].

suprapyloric l. n. [TA], l. suprapilórico; um l. localizado acima do piloro. SIN nodus lymphoideus suprapyloricus [TA], suprapyloric node.

thoracic l. n.'s [TA], linfonodos do tórax; os linfonodos parietais e viscerais do tórax, coletivamente. SIN nodi lymphoidei thoracis [TA].

thyroid l. n.'s [TA], linfonodos tireóideos; linfonodos do grupo cervical anterior profundo localizados ao redor da glândula tireóide; drenam para o grupo cervical lateral profundo. SIN nodi lymphoidei thyroidei [TA].

tracheal l. n.'s, linfonodos paratraqueais. V. paratracheal l. n.

l. n.'s of upper limb [TA], linfonodos do membro superior; linfonodos localizados no membro superior e que o drenam, sendo, por fim, drenados pelo tronco linfático subclávio; incluídos estão os linfonodos axilares, interpeitorais, deltopeitorais braquiais e cubitais. SIN nodi lymphoidei membri superioris [TA].

visceral l. n.'s [TA], linfonodos viscerais; os linfonodos que drenam as vísceras do abdome ou da pelve em oposição aos linfonodos parietais, que drenam as paredes corporais. SIN nodi lymphoidei viscerales [TA], visceral nodes.

visceral l. n.'s of abdomen [TA], linfonodos viscerais do abdome; os numerosos linfonodos que recebem linfa dos órgãos abdominais associados aos ramos viscerais da aorta. SIN nodi lymphoidei abdominis viscerales [TA], l. n.'s of abdominal organs.

♻ **lympho-, lymph-.** Linfa. [L. *lympha*, água da fonte]

lym·pho·blast (lim'fō-blast). Linfoblasto; uma célula imatura (jovem) que amadurece em um linfócito e é caracterizada por citoplasma mais abundante que o de um linfócito, com um núcleo em que a cromatina é mais delgada que a de um linfócito (porém, mais rude que um mieloblasto) e um ou dois nucléolos algo proeminentes. SIN lymphocytoblast. [lympho- + G. *blastos*, germe]

lym·pho·blas·tic (lim-fō-blas'tik). Linfoblástico; pertinente à produção de linfócitos.

lym·pho·blas·to·ma (lim-fō-blas-tō'mă). Linfoblastoma. SIN lymphoblastic *lymphoma*. [lymphoblast + G. *-oma*, tumor]

giant follicular l., l. folicular gigante. SIN nodular *lymphoma*.

lym·pho·blas·to·sis (lim'fō-blas-tō'sis). Linfoblastose; a presença de linfoblastos no sangue periférico; por vezes usado como sinônimo de leucemia linfocítica aguda. [lymphoblast + G. *-osis*, condição]

lym·pho·cele (lim'fō-sēl). Linfocele; uma massa cística que contém linfa, usualmente oriunda de canais linfáticos enfermos ou lesionados. SIN lymphocyst. [lympho- + G. *kēlē*, tumor]

lym·pho·cer·as·tism (lim-fō-ser'as-tizm). Linfocerastismo; termo obsoleto para o processo de formação de células na série linfocítica. [lympho- + G. *kerastos*, misto, entremeado]

lym·pho·ci·ne·sis, lym·pho·ci·ne·sia (lim'fō-si-nē'sis, nē-zē-ă). Linfocinesia. SIN limphokinesis.

lym·pho·cyst (lim'fō-sist). Linfocisto, linfocele. SIN lymphocele. [lympho- + G. *kystis*, bexiga]

lym·pho·cy·ta·phe·re·sis (lim'fō-sīt-āf-ĕ-rē'sis). Linfocitoférese; separação e remoção dos linfócitos do sangue coletado, com o restante do sangue retransfundido para o doador. SIN lymphapheresis. [lymphocyte + G. *aphairesis*, uma retirada]

ℹ **lym·pho·cyte** (lim'fō-sīt). Linfócito; um leucócito formado no tecido linfático por todo o corpo (p.ex., linfonodos, baço, timo, tonsilas, placas de Peyer e, por vezes, na medula óssea) e que, nos adultos normais, constituem aproximadamente 22 a 28% do número total de leucócitos no sangue circulante. Os linfócitos geralmente são pequenos (7 a 8 μm), porém formas maiores são freqüentes (10-20 μm); com o método de Wright (ou um similar), o núcleo se cora intensamente (azul-purpúrico), sendo composto de densos agregados de cromatina envoltos por uma membrana nuclear bem definida; o núcleo é usualmente arredondado, porém pode ser discretamente indentado, e excêntrico em uma quantidade relativamente pequena de citoplasma azul-claro, o qual, em geral, não contém grânulos; principalmente nas formas maiores, o citoplasma pode ser muito abundante e inclui vários grânulos delicados e brilhantes, vermelho-violeta; em contraste com os grânulos da série mielóide de células, os grânulos nos linfócitos não fornecem uma reação de oxidase ou peroxidase positiva. Os linfócitos são divididos em 2 grupos principais, denominados células T e B, com base em suas moléculas de superfície, bem como em sua função. As células *natural killer* (destruidoras naturais), que são grandes linfócitos granulares, representam um pequeno percentual da população de linfócitos. SIN lymph cell, lympholeukocyte. [lympho- + G. *kytos*, célula]

B. l., l. B; um l. imunologicamente importante que não é timo-dependente, tem vida curta e assemelha-se ao l. bursa-derivado dos pássaros pelo fato de ser responsável pela produção de imunoglobulinas, ou seja, é o precursor dos plasmócitos e expressa imunoglobulinas em sua superfície, mas não as libera. Não desempenha uma função direta na imunidade celular. VER TAMBÉM T l. SIN B cell (2.)

pre-B l., l. pré-B; uma célula do tipo linfóide B inicial que é reconhecida por imunofluorescência como uma célula de medula óssea μ-positiva e negativa para a cadeia L.

Rieder l., l. de Rieder; uma forma anormal de l. que possui um núcleo muito indentado (ou lobulado) e discretamente torcido; essas células são usualmente observadas em determinados exemplares da leucemia linfocítica crônica.

T l., l. T; um l. timócito-derivado com importância imunológica que possui vida longa (meses a anos), sendo responsável pela imunidade celular. Os linfócitos T formam rosetas com eritrócitos de carneiro e, na presença de agentes transformadores (mitógenos), diferenciam-se e dividem-se. Essas células possuem marcadores de superfície CD3 característicos e podem ser subdivididas em subgrupos de acordo com a função, p. ex., auxiliares, citotóxicas, etc. VER TAMBÉM B. l. SIN T cell.

transformed l., l. transformado. VER lymphocyte *transformation.*

tumor-infiltrating l.'s (TIL, TILS) (lim'fō-sītz), linfócitos infiltrantes tumorais; linfócitos coletados de um tumor e expostos a IL-2 *in vitro* para expandir a população. Quando essas células são injetadas de volta no hospedeiro que alberga o tumor, matam especificamente o tumor do qual elas se originaram.

lym·pho·cy·the·mia (lim'fō-sī-thē'mē-ă). Linfocitemia, linfocitose. SIN lymphocytosis.

lym·pho·cyt·ic (lim-fō-sit'ik). Linfocítico; pertinente a, ou caracterizado por, linfócitos.

lym·pho·cy·to·blast (lim-fō-sī'tō-blast). Linfocitoblasto, linfoblasto. SIN lymphoblast. [lymphocyte + G. *blastos*, germe]

lym·pho·cy·to·ma (lim'fō-sī-tō'mă). Linfocitoma; um nódulo ou massa circunscrita de linfócitos maduros que se assemelha superficialmente a uma neoplasia. [lymphocyte + G. *-oma*, tumor]

	linfócitos	
	linfócitos T	**linfócitos B**
local de formação	medula (a partir das células primordiais indiferenciadas)	
regulando órgão ou local de diferenciação	timo	tecido linfóide do intestino (placa de Peyer); em pássaros, bursa de Fabricius
função	imunidade celular	imunidade humoral
formas de função celular	células T de memória, *killer*, auxiliadoras, supressoras	células B de memória, produtoras de anticorpos (plasmócitos)
interações	ver "imunidade" (e diagrama relacionado)	
características de superfície da membrana celular	estruturas de superfície, diferenciado por anticorpos monoclonais (ver "marcador")	
	receptor (antígeno) de célula T receptor para eritrócito de carneiro; o mostrado por teste de roseta	receptor para o fator C3 do complemento receptor de eritrócito de camundongo
estimulantes da transformação (blastogênese, mitose)	antígenos (p.ex., transplante ou tecido, antígeno bacteriano), mitógenos (p.ex., fito-hemaglutinina [PHA], concavalina A [con A])	antígenos (indireta), interleucina II, antígeno da erva-dos-cancros (PWM)
produtos solúveis dos linfócitos ativados	linfocinas	imunoglobulinas (anticorpos)
defeitos	ver "imunodeficiência"	
proliferação maligna	ver "linfoma" (diagrama), leucemia linfática	

benign l. cutis, l. cutâneo benigno; um nódulo cutâneo vermelho-claro a violáceo que, freqüentemente, afeta a cabeça, sendo causado por densa infiltração da derme por linfócitos e histiócitos, formando, com freqüência, folículos linfóides, separados da epiderme por uma estreita camada não-infiltrativa. SIN cutaneous pseudolymphoma, Spiegler-Fendt sarcoid.

lym·pho·cy·to·pe·nia (lim'fō-si-tō-pē'nē-ā). Linfocitopenia, linfopenia. SIN lymphopenia.

lym·pho·cy·to·poi·e·sis (lim'fō-sī-tō-poy-ē'sis). Linfocitopoese; a formação dos linfócitos. [lymphocyte + G. *poiēsis*, uma produção]

lym·pho·cy·to·sis (lim'fō-sī-tō'sis). Linfocitose; uma forma de leucocitose real ou relativa em que existe um aumento do número de linfócitos. SIN lymphocythemia, lymphocytic leukocytosis.

lym·pho·der·ma (lim'fō-der'mă). Linfoderma; uma condição que resulta de qualquer doença dos vasos linfáticos cutâneos. [lympho- + G. *derma*, pele]

lym·pho·duct (lim'fō-dŭkt). Linfoducto; um vaso linfático. VER lymph vessels, em *vessel*. [lympho- + L. *ductus*, um conduto]

lym·pho·gen·e·sis (lim-fō-gen'e-sis). Linfogênese; produção de linfa. [lympho- + G. *genesis*, produção]

lym·pho·gen·ic (lim-fō-jen'ik). Linfogênico. SIN lymphogenous (1).

lym·phog·e·nous (lim-foj'e-nŭs). Linfógeno. **1.** Que se origina da linfa ou do sistema linfático. SIN lymphogenic. **2.** Que produz linfa.

lym·pho·glan·du·la (lim-fō-glan'doo-lā). Linfonodo. SIN lymph node.

lym·pho·gran·u·lo·ma (lim'fō-gran-ū-lō'mă). Linfogranuloma; termo antigo e inespecífico usado com referência a algumas doenças basicamente diferentes, nas quais os processos patológicos resultam em granulomas ou lesões semelhantes a granulomas, em especial em vários grupos de linfonodos (que, em seguida, se tornam conspicuamente aumentados).
 l. benig'num, l. benigno; termo antigo para sarcoidose.
 l. inguina'le, linfogranuloma venéreo. SIN venereal l.
 l. malig'num, l. maligno; termo antigo para doença de Hodgkin.
 Schaumann l., l. de Schaumann; epônimo antigo para sarcoidose.
 venereal l., l. vene'reum, l. venéreo; uma infecção venérea usualmente causada por *Chlamydia trachomatis* e caracterizada por uma úlcera genital transitória e adenopatia inguinal no homem; na mulher, os linfonodos perirretais são envolvidos, sendo a estenose retal uma ocorrência comum. SIN Favre-Durand-Nicholas disease, l. inguinale, Nicolas-Favre disease, tropical bubo.

lym·pho·gran·u·lo·ma·to·sis (lim-fō-gran'ū-lō-ma-tō'sis). Linfogranulomatose; qualquer condição caracterizada por linfogranulomas múltiplos e amplamente distribuídos.

lym·phog·ra·phy (lim-fog'ră-fē). Linfografia; a visualização dos linfáticos (linfangiografia) e linfonodos (linfadenografia) por radiografia após a injeção intralinfática de um contraste, usualmente um óleo iodado. [lympho- + *graphō*, escrever]

lym·pho·his·ti·o·cy·to·sis (lim'fō-his'tē-ō-sī-tō'sis). Linfo-histiocitose; proliferação ou infiltração dos linfócitos e histiócitos.
 familial erythrophagocytic l. (FEL), l. eritrofagocítica familial, l. hemofagocítica familial. SIN familial hemophagocytic l.
 familial hemophagocytic l. (FMLH), l. hemofagocítica familial; uma doença extremamente rara, usualmente fatal, da infância, caracterizada por infiltração multiorgânica por macrófagos e linfócitos ativados. Com freqüência, a doença é familial e parece ser herdada como um traço autossômico recessivo. SIN familial erythrophagocytic l.

lym·phoid (lim'foyd). Linfóide; que se assemelha à linfa ou ao tecido linfático, ou que é pertinente ao sistema linfático. [lympho- + G. *eidos*, aparência]

lym·phoi·dec·to·my (lim-foy-dek'tō-mē). Linfoidectomia; a excisão do tecido linfóide. [lymphoid + G. *ektomē*, excisão]

lym·phoi·do·cyte (lim-foy'dō-sīt). Linfoidócito; uma célula mesenquimal primitiva considerada capaz de diferenciar-se em todos os tipos de células linfóides, incluindo linfócitos, células de revestimento e células reticulares dos linfonodos.

lym·pho·kine (lim'fō-kīne). Linfocinas; peptídeos semelhantes a hormônios, liberados por linfócitos ativados, que mediam a resposta imune; uma citocina obtida dos linfócitos. [*lympho*cyte + G. *kineō*, por em movimento]

lym·pho·ki·ne·sis (lim'fō-ki-nē'sis). Linfocinese. **1.** Circulação da linfa nos vasos linfáticos e através dos linfonodos. **2.** O movimento da endolinfa nos canais semicirculares da orelha interna. SIN lymphocinesis, lymphocinesia. [lympho- + G. *kinēsis*, movimento]

lym·pho·leu·ko·cyte (lim'fō-loo'kō-sīt). Linfoleucócito, linfócito. SIN lymphocyte.

lym·phol·o·gy (lim-fol'o-jē). Linfologia, linfangiologia. SIN lymphangiology. [lympho- + G. *logos*, estudo]

lym·pho·ma (lim-fō'mă). Linfoma; qualquer neoplasia de tecido linfóide; no uso geral, l. maligno, sinônimo de l. maligno. [lympho- + G. *-oma*, tumor]
 adult T-cell l. (ATL), l. de célula T adulta; uma doença aguda ou subaguda associada a um vírus de célula T humana, com linfadenopatia, hepatoesplenomegalia, lesões cutâneas, envolvimento sanguíneo periférico e hipercalcemia. SIN adult T-cell leukemia.
 anaplastic large cell l., l. de células anaplásicas grandes; uma forma de linfoma caracterizada por anaplasia das células, crescimento sinusoidal e imunorreatividade com CD30 (Ki-1 ou Ber-H2). SIN Ki-1 + l.
 benign l. of the rectum, l. benigno do reto; termo obsoleto para um pólipo retal composto de tecido linfóide com formação de folículos, cobertos por mucosa.
 Burkitt l., l. de Burkitt; uma forma de l. maligno descrita em crianças africanas, envolvendo freqüentemente a mandíbula e os linfonodos abdominais. A distribuição geográfica do l. de Burkitt sugere que ele é encontrado nas áreas com malária endêmica. É basicamente uma neoplasia das células B e acredita-se que seja causado pelo vírus Epstein-Barr, um membro da família Herpesviridae, que pode ser isolado das células tumorais em cultura, ocorrências ocasionais de l. com aspectos similares foram descritos nos Estados Unidos.
 chronic lymphocytic l., l. linfocítica crônica; um tipo de l. não-Hodgkin de baixo grau caracterizado por linfocitose, linfadenopatia e, nos estágios terminais, hepatoesplenomegalia; pode evoluir para a leucemia linfocítica crônica em alguns anos.
 diffuse small cleaved cell l., l. difuso de células clivadas pequenas; l. linfocítico difuso e mal diferenciado; l. de células centrais foliculares que não tem um padrão folicular; a malignidade é de grau intermediário.
 extranodal marginal zone l., l. de zona marginal extraganglionar. SIN MALToma.
 follicular l., l. folicular. SIN nodular l.
 follicular predominantly large cell l., l. de células foliculares predominantemente grandes; um l. de células B de malignidade intermediária.
 follicular predominantly small cleaved cell l., l. folicular de células clivadas predominantemente pequenas. SIN poorly differentiated lymphocytic l.
 histiocytic l., l. histiocítico; um tumor maligno do tecido reticular composto principalmente por histiócitos neoplásicos. VER TAMBÉM large cell l.
 Hodgkin l., l. de Hodgkin. SIN Hodgkin *disease*.
 immunoblastic l., l. imunoblástico; proliferação monomórfica de imunoblastos que envolve os linfonodos; pode desenvolver-se em alguns pacientes com linfadenopatia angio-imunoblástica.
 Ki-1 + l., Ki-1 +, l. de células anaplásicas grandes. SIN anaplastic large cell l.
 large cell l., l. de células grandes; l. composto de grandes células mononucleares do tipo indeterminado. Recentemente, constatou-se que muitos linfomas originalmente classificados como histiocíticos consistem em grandes histiócitos.
 Lennert l., l. de Lennert; l. maligno com uma alta proporção de células epitelióides difusamente espalhadas, envolvimento tonsilar e evolução imprevisível.
 lymphoblastic l., l. linfoblástica; l. difuso em crianças, com distribuição supradiafragmática e linfócitos T que apresentam núcleos convolutos; muitos pacientes desenvolvem leucemia linfoblástica aguda. SIN lymphoblastoma.
 malignant l., l. maligno; termo geral para neoplasias habitualmente malignas dos tecidos linfóides e reticuloendoteliais, que se apresentam como tumores sólidos aparentemente circunscritos, compostos de células que parecem primitivas ou se assemelham a linfócitos, plasmócitos ou histiócitos. Os linfomas aparecem mais amiúde nos linfonodos, no baço ou em outros locais normais de células linforreticulares; quando disseminados, os linfomas, em especial do tipo linfocítico, podem invadir o sangue periférico e manifestar-se como leucemia. Os linfomas são classificados pelo tipo celular, graus de diferenciação e pelo padrão nodular ou difuso; a doença de Hodgkin e o l. de Burkitt são formas especiais.
 mantle cell l., l. de células de revestimento; uma neoplasia de células B clínica e biologicamente distinta com uma anormalidade genética adquirida recorrente, a translocação t(11;14), e um aspecto histológico heterogêneo, que pode levar à confusão com distúrbios reativos ou outros distúrbios linfoproliferativos neoplásicos.
 marginal zone l., l. de zona marginal; um grupo heterogêneo de neoplasias que se originam de zonas ricas em células B nos linfonodos, no baço ou no tecido linfóide extraganglionar. Os tumores que se originam do tecido linfóide associado à mucosa (MALT) são denominados de MALTomas e ocorrem mais comumente no estômago, nos intestinos, nas glândulas salivares e nos pulmões.
 Mediterranean l., l. do Mediterrâneo. SIN immunoproliferative small intestinal *disease*.
 nodular l., l. nodular; l. maligno que se origina de células B foliculares linfóides, podendo ser pequenos ou grandes, crescendo em um padrão nodular. SIN follicular l., giant follicular lymphoblastoma.
 nodular histiocytic l., l. histiocítico nodular. SIN poorly differentiated lymphocytic l.
 non-Hodgkin l. (NHL), l. não-Hodgkin; um linfoma diferente da doença de Hodgkin, classificado por Rappaport em um padrão tumoral nodular ou difuso e pelo tipo celular; uma formulação internacional ou funcional separa esses linfomas em malignidade de grau baixo, intermediário ou alto e nos subtipos citológicos que refletem a origem na célula do centro folicular ou outra origem.

categoria WF*	freqüência (%)†	classificação REAL‡	
		neoplasias de célula B	neoplasias de célula T
comparação da formulação funcional (WF) e da classificação Revised European-American Lymphoma (REAL)			
A. linfocítico pequeno compatível com LLC plasmacitóide	4	LLC de células B/LLP/LPL zona marginal/MALT células de revestimento linfoplasmacitóide	LLC de células T/LPL LLG
B. células foliculares clivadas, predominantemente pequenas	26	centro folicular, folicular, grau I zona de revestimento zona marginal	
C. células foliculares grandes e pequenas clivadas mistas	9	centro folicular, folicular, grau II zona marginal/MALT	
D. folicular, células grandes	4	centro folicular, folicular, grau III	
E. difuso, células pequenas clivadas	8	células de revestimento centro folicular, pequenas células difusas zona marginal/MALT	LLC de célula T/LPL LLG célula T periférica, inespecífico L/LTA angioimunoblástica angiocêntrica
F. difuso, células pequenas e grandes mistas	7	linfoma de grandes células B (rico em células T) centro folicular, pequenas células difusas linfoplasmocitóide zona marginal/MALT células de revestimento	célula T periféricas, inespecífico L/LTA angioimunoblástica angiocêntrica
G. difuso, células grandes	22	linfoma de células B grandes difusas	célula T periférica, inespecífico L/LTA angioimunoblástica angiocêntrica
H. imunoblástica de grandes células	9	linfoma de células B grandes difusas	célula T periférica, inespecífico L/LTA angioimunoblástica angiocêntrica células grandes anaplásicas
I. linfoblástica	5	linfoblástica B precursora	linfoblástica T precursora
J. pequena célula não-clivada Burkitt não-Burkitt	6	Burkitt célula B de alto grau, semelhante ao linfoma de Burkitt	célula T periférica, inespecífico

*categorias A–C = baixo grau (sobrevida de 5–10 ou mais anos sem tratamento); D–G = grau intermediário (sobrevida de 2–5 anos sem tratamento); H–J = alto grau (sobrevida de 0,5–2 anos sem tratamento); categorias D–H também são chamadas de linfomas agressivos

†L/LTA, leucemia/linfoma de células T adultas; LLC, leucemia linfocítica crônica; LLG, leucemia de linfócitos granulares grandes; MALT, tecido linfóide associado à mucosa; LPL, leucemia pró-linfocítica; LLP, leucemia linfocítica pequena

‡linfoma

peripheral T-cell l., unspecified, l. de célula T periférica, inespecífico; um grupo heterogêneo de neoplasias de célula T que expressam marcadores de células T típicos como CD2, CD3, CD5 e os receptores α/β ou γ/δ da célula T.
poorly differentiated lymphocytic l., l. linfocítico mal diferenciado; um l. de células B com envolvimento nodular ou difuso da medula óssea ou dos linfonodos por células linfóides. SIN follicular predominantly small cleaved cell l., nodular histiocytic l.
small lymphocytic l., l. linfocítico pequeno. SIN well-differentiated lymphocytic l.
T-cell–rich, B-cell l., l. de células B, rico em células T; um l. de células B em que mais de 90% das células provêm da célula T, mascarando as grandes células que formam o componente de células B neoplásicas. VER TAMBÉM adult T-cell l.
well-differentiated lymphocytic l., l. linfocítico bem diferenciado; essencialmente a mesma doença que a leucemia linfocítica crônica, mas o número de linfócitos não está aumentado no sangue periférico; os linfonodos estão aumentados e outros tecidos linfóides ou a medula óssea estão infiltrados por pequenos linfócitos. SIN small lymphocytic l.
lym·pho·ma·toid (lim-fō′mă-toyd). Linfomatóide; que se assemelha a um linfoma.
lym·pho·ma·to·sis (lim′fō-mă-to′sis). Linfomatose; qualquer condição caracterizada por locais múltiplos e amplamente distribuídos de envolvimento por linfoma.
lym·pho·ma·tous (lim-fō′mă-tŭs). Linfomatoso; pertinente a, ou caracterizado por, linfoma.
lym·pho·no·dus. Linfonodo; *termo oficial alternativo para lymph node.
lym·pho·path·ia (lim-fō-path′ē-ă). Linfopatia. SIN lymphopathy.
lym·phop·a·thy (lim-fop′ă-thē). Linfopatia; qualquer doença dos vasos linfáticos ou linfonodos. SIN lymphopathia. [lympho- + G. *pathos*, sofrimento]
lym·pho·pe·nia (lim-fō-pē′nē-ă). Linfopenia; redução, relativa ou absoluta, do número de linfócitos no sangue circulante. SIN lymphocytic leukopenia, lymphocytopenia. [lympho- + G. *penia*, pobreza]
lym·pho·plas·ma·phe·re·sis (lim′fō-plaz′mă-fĕ-rē′sis). Linfoplasmaférese; separação e remoção dos linfócitos e plasma do sangue coletado, com o restante do sangue sendo retransfundido para o doador. [lymphocyte + plasma + G. *aphairesis*, uma retirada]
lym·pho·poi·e·sis (lim-fō-poy-ē′sis). Linfopoese; a formação de tecido linfático. [lympho- + G. *poiēsis*, uma produção]
lym·pho·poi·et·ic (lim-fō-poy-et′ik). Linfopoético; pertinente a, ou caracterizado por, linfopoese.
lym·pho·re·tic·u·lo·sis (lim′fō-rĕ-tik-ū-lō′sis). Linforreticulose; proliferação de células reticuloendoteliais (macrófagos) dos linfonodos.
 benign inoculation l., doença da arranhadura do gato. SIN catscratch *disease*.
lym·phor·rha·gia (lim-fō-rā′jē-ă). Linforragia. SIN lymphorrhea. [lympho- + G. *rhēgnymi*, impelir]

lym·phor·rhea (lim-fō-rē´ă). Linforréia; extravasamento de linfa para a superfície da pele a partir de vasos linfáticos rotos, lacerados ou seccionados. SIN lymphorrhagia. [lympho- + G. *rhoia*, um fluxo]

lym·phor·rhoid (lim´fo-royd). Linforróide; dilatação de um canal linfático, assemelhando-se a uma hemorróida. [lymph + -rrhoid, que tende a extravasar, em analogia com *hemorrhoid*]

lym·pho·scin·tig·ra·phy (lim´fo-sin-tig´ră-fē). Linfocintigrafia; a obtenção de imagens de vasos linfáticos ou linfonodos após a injeção intralinfática ou subcutânea de um radionuclídeo.

lym·pho·sis (lim-fō´sis). Linfose; termo obsoleto para lymphocytic *leukemia* (leucemia linfocítica).

lym·phos·ta·sis (lim-fos´tă-sis). Linfoestase; obstrução do fluxo normal de linfa. [lympho- + G. *stasis*, uma parada]

lym·pho·tax·is (lim-fō-tak´sis). Linfotaxia; o ato de exercer um efeito que atrai ou repele linfócitos. [lympho- + G. *taxis*, distribuição ordenada]

lym·pho·tox·ic·i·ty (lim´fo-tok-sis´i-tē). Linfotoxicidade; efeitos tóxicos exercidos contra linfócitos.

lym·pho·tox·in (lim´fo-tok-sin). Linfotoxina; linfocina oriunda dos linfócitos T que lisa ou compromete muitos tipos celulares.

lym·phot·ro·phy (lim-fot´rō-fē). Linfotrofia; a nutrição dos tecidos pela linfa nas regiões desprovidas de vasos sanguíneos. [lympho- + G. *trophē*, nutrição]

lym·phu·ria (lim-foo´rē-ă). Linfúria; eliminação de linfa na urina. [lympho- + G. *ouron*, urina]

Lynch, Henry T., oncologista norte-americano do século XX. VER L. *syndrome*.

lyn·es·tre·nol (lin-es´tren-ol). Linestrenol; agente progestacional, associado ao mestranol como contraceptivo oral. SIN ethinylestrenol.

lyo-. Forma combinante relativa a dissolução. VER TAMBÉM lyso-. [G. *lyō*, amolecer, dissolver]

ly·o·en·zyme (lī-ō-en´zim). Lioenzima. **1.** Qualquer enzima existente na célula na forma solúvel. **2.** Uma enzima solúvel.

ly·ol·y·sis (lī-ol´i-sis). Liólise; termo raramente empregado para solvólise.

Lyon, B. B. Vincent, médico norte-americano, 1880–1953. VER Meltzer-L. *test*.

Lyon, Mary F., citogeneticista inglesa, *1925. VER L. *hypothesis*; lyonization.

ly·on·i·za·tion (lī´on-i-zā´shŭn). Lionização; o fenômeno normal por meio do qual, onde quer que existam dois ou mais grupos haplóides de genes ligados ao X em cada célula, todos, excetuando-se um dos genes, são aparentemente inativados ao acaso e não exibem expressão fenotípica. A l. é comum, porém não é invariável, para todos os *loci*. Sua atuação ao acaso explica a expressividade dos traços ligados ao X mais variável nas mulheres que nos homens. A l. ocorre nos homens com o cariótipo Klinefelter (XXY). VER TAMBÉM gene dosage *compensation*. SIN Lyon hypothesis, X-inactivation. [M. *Lyon*]

ly·o·phil, ly·o·phile (lī´ō-fil, -fīl). Liófilo; uma substância que é liofílica.

ly·o·phil·ic (lī-ō-fil´ik). Liofílico. **1.** Em química odontológica, indica uma fase dispersa que possui uma afinidade pronunciada pelo meio de dispersão; quando a fase dispersa é l., o colóide é usualmente reversível. **2.** Indica uma preferência para o solvente. SIN lyotropic. [lyo- + G. *phileō*, amar]

ly·oph·i·li·za·tion (lī-of´i-li-zā´shŭn). Liofilização. **1.** O processo de isolamento de uma substância sólida de uma solução por meio de congelamento da solução e evaporação do gelo sob vácuo. **2.** O processo de conferir propriedades liofílicas a uma substância. SIN freeze-drying.

ly·o·phobe (lī´ō-fōb). Liófobo; uma substância que é liófoba.

ly·o·pho·bic (lī-ō-fo´bik). Liofóbico. **1.** Em química coloidal, indica uma fase dispersa que possui apenas afinidade discreta pelo meio de dispersão; quando a fase dispersa é l., o colóide geralmente é irreversível. **2.** Indica falta de preferência ou rejeição do solvente. [lyo- + G. *phobos*, medo]

ly·o·sorp·tion (lī-ō-sōrp´shŭn). Liosorção; a adsorção de um líquido a uma superfície sólida.

ly·o·tro·pic (lī-ō-trop´ik). Liotrópico, liofílico. SIN lyophilic. [lyo- + G. *tropē*, uma virada]

ly·pres·sin (lī´pres-in). Lipressina; a vasopressina que contém lisina na posição 8; um hormônio antidiurético e vasopressor. SIN 8-lysine vasopressin.

ly·ra (lī´ră). Lira; uma estrutura em formato de lira. [L. e G. lira]

l. davidis, lyre of David, lira de Davi; termo obsoleto para *commissura* fornicis.

l. uteri´na, l. pregas palmadas do canal do colo do útero. SIN palmate *folds* of cervical canal, em *fold*.

Lys Símbolo de lysine (lisina) ou lysyl (lisil).

lys-. VER lyso-.

ly·sate (lī´sāt). Lisado; material produzido pelo processo destrutivo da lise.

lyse (līz). Lisar, fragmentar, desintegrar, efetuar a lise. SIN lyze.

ly·se·mia (lī-sē´mē-ă). Lisemia; a desintegração ou dissolução dos eritócitos e a ocorrência de hemoglobina no plasma circulante e na urina. [lyso- + G. *haima*, sangue]

ly·serg·am·ide (lī-serj´ă-mīd). Lisergamida. SIN *lysergic acid* amide.

ly·ser·gic ac·id (lī-ser´jik). Ácido lisérgico; o D-isômero é o produto de clivagem da hidrólise alcalina dos alcalóides do esporão de centeio; ocorre como cristais brilhosos, discretamente hidrossolúveis; psicotomimético.

l. a. amide, amida do ácido lisérgico; lisergamida; agente presente na *Rivea corymbosa* e *Ipomoea tricolor*; possui menor potência alucinógena que a dietilamida do ácido lisérgico. SIN ergine, lysergamide.

l. a. diethylamide (LSD), dietilamida do ácido lisérgico (LSD); no nível periférico, um antagonista da serotonina; cerca de 1 a 2 μg por kg induzem estados alucinatórios de natureza visual em vez de auditiva; seu uso pode precipitar psicoses; foi ocasionalmente empregado no tratamento do alcoolismo crônico e de distúrbios psicóticos. SIN lysergide.

l. a. monoethylamide, monoetilamida do ácido lisérgico; um agente psicotomimético presente na *Rivea corymbosa* e *Ipomoea tricolor*; possui menor potência alucinatória que a dietilamida do ácido lisérgico.

ly·ser·gide (lī-ser´jid). Lisergida. SIN *lysergic acid* diethylamide.

ly·ser·gol (lī-sŭr´jol). Lisergol; um alcalóide semi-sintético do esporão de centeio.

ly·sin (lī´sin). Lisina. **1.** Um anticorpo fixador de complemento específico que atua de forma destrutiva sobre células e tecidos; os vários tipos são designados de acordo com a forma de antígeno que estimula a produção da l., p.ex., hemolisina, bacteriolisina. **2.** Qualquer substância que provoque lise.

ly·sine (K, Lys) (lī´sēn). Lisina; ácido 2,6-diamino-hexanóico; L-isômero é um α-aminoácido essencial na nutrição dos mamíferos, sendo encontrado em muitas proteínas; diferenciado por um grupamento ε-amino.

l. decarboxylase, lisina descarboxilase; uma enzima que catalisa a descarboxilação da L-l., com a produção de cadaverina e CO_2.

ly·si·ne·mia (lī-si-nē´mē-ă). Lisinemia. VER hyperlysinemia.

8-ly·sine va·so·pres·sin. 8-lisina vasopressina. SIN lypressin.

ly·sin·i·um (lī-in´ē-um). Lisínio; a forma de cátion da lisina, quer lisínio (+1) ou lisínio (+2).

ly·sin·o·gen (lī-sin´ō-jen). Lisinogênio; antígeno que estimula a formação de uma lisina específica.

ly·si·no·gen·ic (lī´si-nō-jen´ik). Lisinogênico; que possui a propriedade de um lisinogênio.

ly·sin·u·ria (lī-si-noo´rē-ă). Lisinúria; a presença de lisina na urina.

ly·sis (lī´sis). Lise. **1.** A destruição de eritrócitos, bactérias e outras estruturas por uma lisina específica, usualmente referida de acordo com a estrutura destruída (p.ex., hemólise, bacteriólise, nefrólise); pode ser causada por uma toxina direta ou por um mecanismo imune, como o anticorpo que reage com um antígeno na superfície de uma célula-alvo, usualmente por ligação e ativação de uma série de proteínas no sangue com atividade enzimática (sistema complemento). **2.** A diminuição gradual dos sintomas de uma doença aguda, uma forma de processo de recuperação, diferenciado da crise. [G. dissolução ou amolecimento]

bystander l., a l. das células adjacentes, mediada por complemento, nas proximidades de um local de ativação do complemento.

lyso-, lys-. Liso-, lis-; formas combinantes relativas a lise, destruição. VER TAMBÉM lyo-. [G. *lysis*, um amolecimento]

ly·so·ceph·a·lin (lī-sō-sef´ă-lin). Lisocefalina; um ácido lisofosfatídico esterificado com serina ou etanolamina, ou seja, uma lisofosfatidilserina ou lisoetanolamina; análoga à lisolecitina.

ly·so·gen (lī´sō-jen). Lisógeno. **1.** Aquele que é capaz de induzir a lise. **2.** Uma bactéria no estado de lisogenia. **3.** Qualquer antígeno que estimule a produção de lisina. [lysin + G. -gen, produtor]

ly·so·gen·e·sis (lī-sō-jen´ē-sis). Lisogênese; a produção de lisinas.

ly·so·gen·ic (lī-sō-jen´ik). Lisogênico. **1.** Que causa ou possui o poder de provocar lise, como a ação de determinados anticorpos e substâncias químicas. **2.** Pertinente às bactérias no estado de lisogenia.

ly·so·ge·nic·i·ty (lī´sō-jē-nis´i-tē). Lisogenicidade; a propriedade de ser lisogênico.

ly·so·ge·ni·za·tion (lī´sō-jē-ni-zā´shŭn, lī-soj´ē-ni-zā´shŭn). Lisogenização; o processo pelo qual uma bactéria se torna lisogênica.

ly·sog·e·ny (lī-soj´ē-nē). Lisogenia; o fenômeno pelo qual uma bactéria é infectada por um bacteriófago temperado, cujo DNA está integrado no genoma bacteriano e replica-se juntamente com o DNA bacteriano, mas que permanece latente ou não é expresso; a deflagração do ciclo lítico pode ocorrer de forma espontânea ou através de determinados agentes, resultando na produção do bacteriófago e na lise da célula bacteriana.

ly·so·ki·nase (lī-sō-kī´nās). Lisocinase, lisoquinase; termo para os agentes ativadores (p.ex., estreptocinase, uroquinase, estafilocinase) que produzem plasmina por ação indireta ou em múltiplos estágios sobre o plasminogênio.

ly·so·lec·i·thin (lī-sō-les´i-thin). Lisolecitina; uma lisofosfatidilcolina capaz de lisar eritrócitos.

l.-lecithin acyltransferase (LLAT), l.-lecitina aciltransferase; uma enzima que catalisa a reação reversível da l. e outro fosfolipídio (p.ex., fosfatidiletanolamina) para formar lecitina e lisofosfatidiletanolamina; uma importante na reconstrução da lecitina.

ly·so·lec·i·thin·ase (lī-sō-les´i-thin-ās). Lisolecitinase. SIN lysophospholipase.

ly·so·phos·pha·tid·ic ac·id (lī´-sō-fos´fă-tid´ik). Ácido lisofosfatídico; um ácido fosfatídico em que apenas um dos dois grupamentos hidroxila do

glicerofosfato está esterificado; mais amiúde, quando o carbono 1 do glicerol está esterificado (p.ex., 1-acilglicerol-3-fosfato).
l. a. acyltransferase, 1-acylglycerol-3-phosphate acyltransferase, aciltransferase do ácido lisofosfatídico, 1-acilglicerol-3-fosfato aciltransferase.

ly·so·phos·pha·ti·dyl·cho·line (lī′sō - fos′fă - tī′dil - kō′lēn). Lisofosfatidilcolina; uma fosfatidilcolina em que um ácido graxo foi removido da posição C2 do grupamento glicerol.

ly·so·phos·pha·ti·dyl·ser·ine (lī′sō - fos′fă - tī′dil - ser′ēn). Lisofosfatidilserina; a fosfatidilserina da qual um resíduo ácido graxo foi removido da porção glicerol, tipicamente no carbono 2. Cf. lysophosphatidic acid.

ly·so·phos·pho·li·pase (lī′sō - fos′fō - lip′ās). Lisofosfolipase; uma hidrolase que remove o único grupamento acil de uma lisolecitina, produzindo glicerofosfocolina e o ânion de ácido graxo livre. SIN lecithinase B, lysolecithinase, phospholipase B (1).

ly·so·some (lī′sō - sōm). Lisossoma; uma vesícula citoplasmática ligada à membrana, medindo 5–8 nm (l. primário) e que contém uma ampla variedade de enzimas de hidrólise de glicoproteína ativas em um pH ácido; serve para digerir o material exógeno, como bactérias, bem como as organelas esgotadas das células. [lyso- + G. *soma*, corpo]
definitive l.'s, lisossomas secundários. SIN secondary l.'s.
primary l.'s, lisossomas primários; lisossomas produzidos no aparelho de Golgi, onde as enzimas hidrolíticas são incorporadas; fundem-se com os fagossomas ou pinossomas para se transformarem em lisossomas secundários.
secondary l.'s, lisossomas secundários; lisossomas em que ocorre a lise devido à atividade das enzimas hidrolíticas; acredita-se que acabam se transformando, em corpúsculos residuais. SIN definitive l.'s, digestive vacuole.

ly·so·staph·in (lī - sō - staf′in). Lisoestafina; uma enzima do tipo peptidase produzida por determinadas cepas de estafilococos com atividade antiestafilocócica.

ly·so·type (lī′so - typ). Lisótipo; um tipo de uma espécie bacteriana determinado por sua reação a fagos específicos. [lyso + type]

ly·so·zyme (lī′sō - zīm). Lisozima; uma enzima que hidrolisa as ligações 1,4-β entre o ácido *N*-acetilmurâmico e a *N*-acetil-D-glicosamina, sendo, dessa maneira, destrutiva para as paredes celulares de determinadas bactérias; presente na lágrima e em alguns outros líquidos corporais, na clara do ovo e em alguns tecidos vegetais; usada na prevenção de cáries e no tratamento de leites artificiais para lactentes. SIN mucopeptide glycohydrolase, muramidase.

Lys·sa·vi·rus (lis′ă - vī - rŭs). Um gênero de vírus (família Rhabdoviridae) que inclui o grupo do vírus da raiva.
Australian bat L., L. do morcego australiano; uma espécie que provocou uma doença fatal, semelhante à raiva, em uma mulher na Austrália.
European bat L., L. do morcego europeu; duas espécies (1 e 2) que causam doenças semelhantes à raiva em seres humanos na Europa; transmitidos pela mordida de morcegos insetívoros.

ly·syl (K) (lī′sil). Lisil; o radical univalente da lisina.
l. hydroxylase, l. hidroxilase; uma enzima que atua sobre resíduos lisil específicos em determinadas proteínas (p.ex., colágenos) com α-cetoglutarato e O_2 para produzir resíduos δ-hidroxilisil, succinato e CO_2; há deficiência dessa enzima, que necessita de Fe^{2+} e ascorbato, na síndrome de Ehlers-Danlos do tipo VI. SIN l. 2-oxoglutarate dioxygenase.
l. oxidase, l. oxidase; uma enzima, exigindo Cu^{2+} e O_2, que oxida determinados resíduos lisil no colágeno em resíduos alisil e resíduos hidroxilisil em resíduos hidroxialisil; essa é uma etapa necessária para a ligação cruzada (através de condensações de aldol e rearranjos de Amadori) dos filamentos de colágeno; uma atividade menor dessa enzima está associada à síndrome do corno occipital.
l. 2-oxoglutarate dioxygenase, l. 2-oxoglutarato dioxigenase. SIN l. hydroxylase.

ly·syl-brad·y·ki·nin (lī′sil - brad - ē - kī′nin). Lisil-bradicinina. SIN kallidin.

Lyth·o·glyph·op·sis (lith - ō - glif - op′ - sis). Um gênero de lesmas operculadas anfíbias, de água doce, da família Hydrobiidae (subfamília Hydrobiinae; subclasse Prosobranchiata). No delta do rio Mekong, *Lythoglyphopsis aperta* serve como hospedeiro intermediário do trematódeo sanguíneo, *Schistosoma mekongi*.

lyt·ic (lit′ik). Lítico; pertinente à lise; usado coloquialmente como uma abreviatura para osteolítico.

lyx·i·tol (lik′si - tol). Lixitol; um pentitol (lixose reduzida) que ocorre na lixoflavina.

lyx·o·fla·vin (lik - sō - flā′vin). Lixoflavina; um composto similar à riboflavina, à exceção de que D-lixitol está presente em lugar do grupamento D-ribitol; existente em pequena quantidade no músculo cardíaco.

lyx·ose (lik′sōs). Lixose; uma aldopentose; a D-l. é epimérica com a D-arabinose e D-xilose; a L-l. é epimérica com a D-ribose.

lyx·u·lose (liks′ū - lōs). Lixulose; um 2-cetoderivado da lixose.

lyze (līz). Lisar. SIN lyse.

M

μ **1.** A 12.ª letra do alfabeto grego, mu. **2.** Símbolo de micro- (2); micron (mícron); viscosidade dinâmica (dynamic *viscosity*); momento de dipolo magnético ou elétrico de uma molécula; potencial químico (chemical *potential*); designa a posição de um substituinte localizado no 12.º átomo da carboxila ou de outro grupamento funcional.

μ_N Símbolo de nuclear *magneton* (magnéton nuclear).
μ_B **1.** Símbolo de Bohr *magneton* (magnéton de Bohr).
μμ micromicro-; micromícron.
μμg Símbolo de micromicrogram (micromicrograma).
μ Símbolo de microhm (microhm).
μC Símbolo de microcoulomb (microcoulomb).
μCi Símbolo de microcurie (microcurie).
μg Símbolo de microgram (micrograma).
μl, μL Símbolo de microliter (microlitro).
μm Símbolo de micrometer (micrômetro).
μmol Símbolo de micromole (micromol).
μmol/L Símbolo de micromolar (micromolar).
μV Símbolo de microvolt (microvolt).

M 1. Símbolo de mega- (2); morgan; molaridade (mols por litro, também escrito *M* ou M); miopia ou míope; metionina; ribonucleosídeo 6-mercaptopurina em um ácido nucleico; L. *misce*, mistura; metal. **2.** Símbolo de um fator sanguíneo. VER entradas no grupo sanguíneo MNS, Apêndice de Grupos Sanguíneos.

M. Abreviatura de L. *misce*, mistura.
M Símbolo de molarity (molaridade).
M_r Símbolo de molecular weight *ratio* (relação de peso molecular) ou relative molecular *mass* (massa molecular relativa).
m Símbolo de meter (metro); mili-; minim (mínimo, medida de capacidade); mass (massa); momento de dipolo magnético; molality (molalidade).
mμ Símbolo de millimicron (milimícron).
M Símbolo de mols por litro (também escrito M ou *M*).
m- Abreviatura de *meta-* (2).
MA Abreviatura de mental *age* (idade mental); mentoanterior *position* (posição mento-anterior).
ma, mA Abreviatura de milliampere (miliampère).
MAA Abreviatura de macroaggregated *albumin* (albumina macroagregada).
MAB Abreviatura de monoclonal *antibody* (anticorpo monoclonal).
MAC 1. Abreviatura de minimal anesthetic *concentration* (concentração anestésica mínima); minimal alveolar *concentration* (concentração alveolar mínima); membrane attack *complex* (complexo de ataque de membrana). **2.** Abreviatura de *Mycobacterium avium complex* (complexo do *Mycobacterium avium*). VER *Mycobacterium avium-intracellulare complex.*
Mac-. Quanto aos nomes próprios iniciados dessa forma, ver também Mc-.
Ma·ca·ca (mă-kah′kă). Grande gênero de macacos do Velho Mundo (família Cercopithecidae) que inclui o macaco comum e o macaco rhesus, e os macacos de Gibraltar e do norte da África. *M. mulatta*, o macaco rhesus, é usado como animal de pesquisa. [Pg. *macaco*, macaco]
ma·caque (mă-kahk′). Macaco. VER *Macaca*. [Fr.]
MacConkey, Alfred T., bacteriologista inglês, 1861–1931. VER MacConkey *agar.*
Mace, MACE Acrônimo de *m*etilclorofórmio 2-clor*ace*tofenona (o gás lacrimejante clássico) em um leve dispersante de petróleo e um propelente pressurizado.
mac·er·ate (mas′er-āt). Macerar; amolecer por meio de infusão ou embebição. [ver maceration]
mac·er·a·tion (mas-er-ā′shŭn). Maceração. **1.** Amolecimento pela ação de um líquido. **2.** Amolecimento dos tecidos após morte por autólise não-putrefativa (estéril); observado principalmente no natimorto, com descolamento da epiderme. [L. *macero*, pp. *-atus*, amolecer por embebição]
Macewen, Sir William, cirurgião escocês, 1848–1924. VER M. *sign, symptom, triangle.*
Mach, Ernst, cientista austríaco, 1838–1916. VER M. *band, number.*
ma·chine (mă-shēn′). Máquina; qualquer aparelho ou dispositivo mecânico. [L. *machina*, aparelho]
  anesthesia m., equipamento anestésico; equipamento usado para anestesia inalatória, incluindo fluxômetros, vaporizadores e fontes de gases comprimidos, mas que não inclui o circuito anestésico nem mecanismos para eliminação de dióxido de carbono.
  heart-lung m., máquina coração-pulmão artificial; aparelho que incorpora uma bomba sanguínea (coração artificial) e um oxigenador de sangue (pulmão artificial) para estabelecer circulação e oxigenação extracorpóreas do sangue durante uma cirurgia cardíaca.
  panoramic rotating m., m. de rotação panorâmica; um aparelho de raios X que usa um movimento alternado do tubo e filme extra-oral para obter uma radiografia de todos os dentes e das estruturas adjacentes. VER TAMBÉM tomography.

Mackay, Ralph Stuart, físico norte-americano, *1924. VER M.-Marg *tonometer.*
Mackenrodt, Alwin K., ginecologista alemão, 1859–1925. VER M. *ligament.*
Mackenzie, Sir James, médico escocês que trabalhava em Londres, 1853–1925. VER M. *polygraph.*
Mackenzie, Richard J., cirurgião escocês, 1821–1854. VER M. *amputation.*
MacLachlan, Elsie A., pesquisadora do século XX. VER Lowe-Terrey-MacL. *syndrome.*
Macleod, Roderick, médico escocês, 1795–1852. VER M. *rheumatism.*
Macleod, William Mathieson, médico inglês, 1911–1977. VER M. *syndrome;* Swyer-James-MacLeod *syndrome.*
ma·clur·in (mă-kloor′in) [C.I. 75240]. Maclurina; corante natural associado à morina e derivado da tatajuba; usado no tingimento de tecidos com vários mordentes metálicos. Torna-se verde-escuro com a adição de cloreto férrico.
MacNeal, Ward J., bacteriologista norte-americano, 1881–1946. VER M. tetrachrome blood *stain;* Novy and M. blood *agar.*
△ **macr-.** VER macro-.
Mac·ra·can·tho·rhyn·chus (mak′ră-kan-thō-ring′kŭs). Gênero de vermes gigantes com cabeça espiculada (classe Acanthocephala). [macro- + G. *akantha*, espinho, + *rhynchos*, focinho]
  M. hirudina′ceus, o verme gigante de cabeça espiculada do porco, aproximadamente do mesmo tamanho do nematódeo gigante (*Ascaris*); habita o tubo intestinal, onde surgem nódulos no local de penetração da probóscide espinhosa de cada verme; foi descrito ocasionalmente no homem; a transmissão se dá por ingestão de insetos infectados, freqüentemente besouros do estrume ou baratas que se alimentaram nas fezes de porcos infectados, contendo ovos viáveis, e desenvolveram o estágio de cistacanto infeccioso para o hospedeiro vertebrado, incluindo os seres humanos.
mac·ren·ceph·a·ly, mac·ren·ce·pha·lia (mak′ren-sef′ă-lē, -sē-fā-lē-ă). Macroencefalia; hipertrofia do encéfalo; a condição de possuir um encéfalo grande. [macro- + G. *enkephalos*, encéfalo]
△ **macro-, macr-.** Macro-, macr-; grande, longo. VER TAMBÉM mega-, megalo-. [G. *makros*]
mac·ro·ad·e·no·ma (mak′rō-ad-ĕ-nō′mă). Macroadenoma; um adenoma hipofisário com diâmetro > 10 mm.
mac·ro·am·y·lase (mak-rō-am′i-lās). Macroamilase; termo descritivo aplicado a uma forma de amilase sérica na qual a enzima está presente como um complexo unido a uma globulina; o peso molecular da enzima sozinha é de 50.000, enquanto o peso do complexo provavelmente é maior que 160.000; assim, a excreção renal do complexo não é considerável.
mac·ro·am·y·la·se·mia (mak′rō-am′i-lā-sē′mē-ă). Macroamilasemia; uma forma de hiperamilasemia, na qual uma parte da amilase sérica está na forma de macroamilase. [macroamylase + G. *haima*, sangue]
mac·ro·bac·te·ri·um (mak′rō-bak-tēr′ē-ŭm). Macrobactéria. SIN megabacterium.
mac·ro·bi·o·sis (mak′rō-bi-ō′sis). Macrobiose. SIN longevity. [macro- + G. *bios*, vida]
mac·ro·bi·ote (mak-rō-bī′ot). Macróbio; organismo que tem vida longa. [macro- + G. *bios*, vida]
mac·ro·bi·ot·ic (mak′rō-bī-ot′ik). Macrobiótico. **1.** De vida longa. **2.** Que tende a prolongar a vida.
mac·ro·bi·ot·ics (mak′rō-bī-ot′iks). Macrobiótica; o estudo do prolongamento da vida.
mac·ro·blast (mak′rō-blast). Macroblasto; um grande eritroblasto. [macro- + G. *blastos*, germe]
mac·ro·ble·pha·ron (mak′rō-blef′ar-on). Macroblefaria; pálpebra anormalmente grande. [macro- + G. *blepharon*, pálpebra]
mac·ro·bra·chia (mak-rō-brā′kē-ă). Macrobraquia; condição na qual os braços são anormalmente grossos ou longos. [macro- + G. *brachiōn*, braço]

△ Formas Combinantes
🅘 Indica que o termo é ilustrado, ver Índice de Ilustrações
SIN Sinônimo
Cf. Comparar, confrontar
[NA] *Nomina Anatomica*
[TA] *Terminologia Anatomica*

☆ Termo oficial alternativo para a *Terminologia Anatomica*

[MIM] Mendelian Inheritance in Man

I.C. Índice de Corantes

Termo de Alta Importância

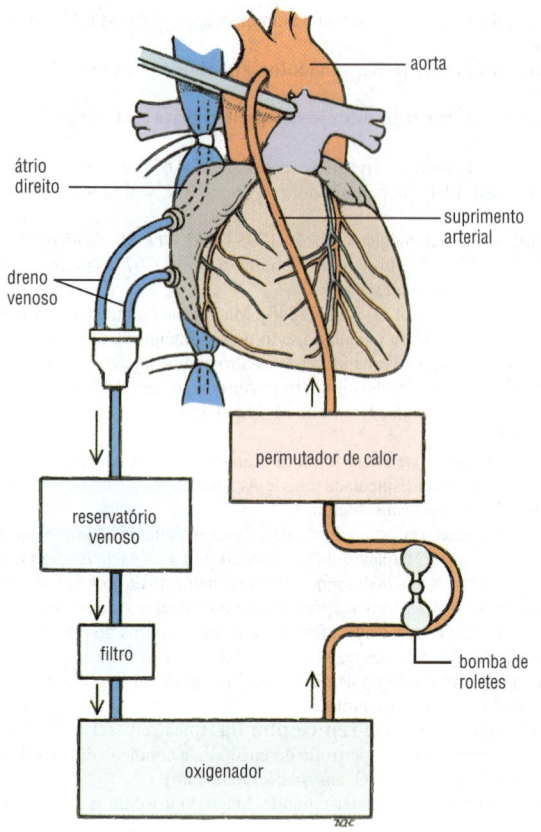

máquina coração–pulmão artificial

mac·ro·car·dia (mak-rō-kar'dē-ă). Macrocardia. SIN cardiomegaly.
mac·ro·ce·phal·ic, mac·ro·ceph·a·lous (mak'rō-se-fal'ik, -sef'ă-lŭs). Macrocefálico, macrocéfalo. SIN megacephalic. [macro- + G. kephalē, cabeça]
mac·ro·ceph·a·ly, mac·ro·ce·pha·lia (mak-rō-sef'ă-lē, -sē-fā'lē-ă). Macrocefalia. SIN megacephaly. [macro- + G. kephalē, cabeça]
mac·ro·chei·lia, mac·ro·chi·lia (mak-rō-kī'lē-ă). Macroquilia. 1. Aumento anormal dos lábios. SIN macrolabia. 2. Linfangioma cavernoso do lábio, uma condição de edema labial permanente, causada por grande distensão dos espaços linfáticos. [macro- + G. cheilos, lábio]
mac·ro·chei·ria, mac·ro·chi·ria (mak-rō-kī'rē-ă). Macroquiria; condição caracterizada por mãos anormalmente grandes. SIN cheiromegaly, chiromegaly, megalocheiria, megalochiria. [macro- + G. cheir, mão]
mac·ro·chem·is·try (mak-rō-kem'is-trē). Macroquímica; o uso de procedimentos químicos, cujas reações (mudança de cor, efervescência etc.) são visíveis a olho nu. Cf. microchemistry.
mac·ro·chy·lo·mi·cron (mak'rō-kī-lō-mī'kron). Macroquilomícron; quilomícron extraordinariamente grande.
mac·ro·cne·mia (mak-rō-nē'mē-ă). Macrocnemia; condição caracterizada por aumento das pernas abaixo do joelho. [macro- + G. knēmē, perna]
mac·ro·coc·cus (mak'rō-kok'ŭs). Macrococo. SIN megacoccus.
mac·ro·co·lon (mak-rō-kō'lon). Macrocólon; cólon sigmóide de comprimento incomum; uma variedade de megacólon.
mac·ro·co·nid·i·um, pl. **mac·ro·co·nid·ia** (mak'rō-kō-nid'ē-ŭm, -ă). Macroconídio. 1. Conídio, ou exosporo, grande. 2. Em fungos, o maior de dois tipos de conídios de tamanhos bem diferentes em uma única espécie, com paredes espessas ou finas e constituído por 2 a 10 células; característico da maioria dos dermatófitos e de alguns outros gêneros, como, p. ex., Histoplasma, Fusarium. [macro- + L. mod. dim. do G. konis, poeira]
mac·ro·cor·nea (mak-rō-kōr'nē-ă). Macrocórnea; córnea anormalmente grande.
mac·ro·cra·ni·um (mak-rō-krā'nē-ŭm). Macrocrânio; crânio aumentado, principalmente os ossos que contêm o encéfalo, como observado na hidrocefalia; a face parece relativamente pequena em comparação.
mac·ro·cry·o·glob·u·lin (mak-rō-krī-ō-glob'ū-lin). Macrocrioglobulina; macroglobulina que possui propriedades de uma crioglobulina.
mac·ro·cry·o·glob·u·li·ne·mia (mak-rō-krī-ō-glob'ū-lin-ē'mē-ă). Macrocrioglobulinemia; a presença de macroglobulinas precipitadas pelo frio no sangue periférico; essas macrocrioglobulinas freqüentemente são denominadas crioemaglutininas.
mac·ro·cyst (mak'rō-sist). Macrocisto; cisto de proporções macroscópicas.
mac·ro·cyte (mak'rō-sīt). Macrócito; eritrócito grande, como aquele observado na anemia perniciosa. SIN macroerythrocyte. [macro- + G. kytos, uma cavidade (célula)]
mac·ro·cy·the·mia (mak'rō-sī-thē'mē-ă). Macrocitemia; a ocorrência de um número extraordinariamente grande de macrócitos no sangue circulante. SIN macrocytosis, megalocythemia, megalocytosis. [macrocyte + G. haima, sangue]
  hyperchromatic m., m. hipercromática; termo inexato freqüentemente usado para designar macrócitos que contêm uma quantidade extraordinariamente grande de hemoglobina, mas são normocrômicos; embora a massa total de hemoglobina seja maior que o normal (devido às grandes células), a percentagem de hemoglobina nas células não é maior que o normal.
mac·ro·cy·to·sis (mak'rō-sī-tō'sis). Macrocitose. SIN macrocythemia. [macrocyte + G. -osis, condição]
mac·ro·dac·tyl·ia, mac·ro·dac·tyl·ism, mac·ro·dac·ty·ly (mak-rō-dak-til'ē-ă, -dak'til-izm, dak'ti-lē). Macrodactilia. SIN megadactyly.
mac·ro·dont (mak'rō-dont). Macrodonte. 1. Dente de proporções anormalmente grandes e, em geral, distorcidas; a condição pode ser localizada ou generalizada. 2. Designa um crânio com um índice dental acima de 44. SIN megadont, megalodont. [macro- + G. odous (odont-), dente]
mac·ro·don·tia, mac·ro·don·tism (mak-rō-don'shē-ă, -don'tizm). Macrodontia; o estado caracterizado por dentes anormalmente grandes. SIN megadontism, megalodontia.
mac·ro·dys·tro·phia li·po·ma·to·sa (mak'rō-dis-trō'fē-ă lip-ō-mă-tō'să). Macrodistrofia lipomatosa; doença não-familiar rara, caracterizada pelo aumento dos dedos das mãos por lipomas, com artropatia degenerativa dolorosa das articulações metacarpofalângicas e interfalângicas.
mac·ro·ele·ments (mak'rō-el'ē-ments). Macroelementos; nutrientes inorgânicos necessários em quantidades diárias relativamente altas (isto é, mais de 100 mg por dia), como p. ex., cálcio, fósforo, sódio, etc. SIN macrominerals.
mac·ro·en·ceph·a·lon (mak'rō-en-sef'ă-lon). Macroencéfalo. SIN megaloencephalon. [macro- + G. enkephalos, encéfalo]
mac·ro·e·ryth·ro·blast (mak'rō-ē-rith'rō-blast). Macroeritroblasto; um grande eritroblasto. SIN macronormochromoblast.
mac·ro·e·ryth·ro·cyte (mak'rō-ē-rith'rō-sīt). Macroeritrócito. SIN macrocyte.
mac·ro·es·the·sia (mak'rō-es-thē'zē-ă). Macroestesia; sensação subjetiva de que todos os objetos são maiores do que o são na verdade.
mac·ro·ga·mete (mak-rō-gam'ēt). Macrogameta; o elemento feminino na anisogamia; é a maior das duas células sexuais, com mais material de reserva e, geralmente, imóvel. SIN megagamete. [macro- + G. gametē, esposa]
mac·ro·ga·me·to·cyte (mak'rō-gă-mē'tō-sīt). Macrogametócito; o gametócito feminino ou célula-mãe, que dá origem ao macrogameta ou gameta feminino nos fungos ou protozoários que sofrem anisogamia. SIN macrogamont.
mac·ro·gam·ont (mak-rō-gam'ont). Macrogamonte. SIN macrogametocyte.
ma·crog·a·my (mă-krog'ă-mē). Macrogamia; conjugação de duas células adultas ou gametas. [macro- + G. gamos, casamento]
mac·ro·gas·tria (mak-rō-gas'trē-ă). Macrogastria. SIN megalogastria.
mac·ro·gen·i·to·so·mia (mak'rō-jen'i-tō-sō'mē-ă). Macrogenitossomia; desenvolvimento excessivo do corpo e dos órgãos genitais. [macro- + L. genitalis, genital, + G. sōma, corpo]
  m. prae'cox, m. precoce; distúrbio no qual a maturação gonádica (puberdade) e o estirão de crescimento do adolescente em relação à altura corporal ocorrem na primeira década de vida; freqüentemente associada a um tumor pineal ou a lesões em áreas hipotalâmicas que, sabidamente, regulam a secreção de gonadotrofina. SIN Pellizzi syndrome.
  m. prae'cox su'prarena'lis, m. precoce supra-renal; crescimento somático precoce e maturação isossexual de características sexuais secundárias, resultantes de um tumor do córtex supra-renal.
ma·crog·lia (ma-krog'lē-ă). Macróglia. SIN astrocyte. [macro- + G. glia, cola]
mac·ro·glob·u·lin·e·mia (mak'rō-glob'ū-li-nē'mē-ă). Macroglobulinemia; a presença de níveis aumentados de macroglobulinas no sangue circulante.
  Waldenström m., m. de Waldenström; macroglobulinemia que ocorre em pessoas idosas, caracterizada por proliferação de células semelhantes a linfócitos ou plasmócitos na medula óssea, anemia, aumento da velocidade de hemossedimentação e hiperglobulinemia com um pico estreito de γ-globulina ou $β_2$-globulina em cerca de 19 unidades S. Amiúde observa-se aumento do baço, fígado ou linfonodos, e, freqüentemente, há púrpura ou sangramento de mucosas. SIN hyperglobulinemic purpura, Waldenström purpura, Waldenström syndrome.

mac·ro·glob·u·lins (mak-rō-glob'ū-lins). Macroglobulinas; globulinas plasmáticas de peso molecular extraordinariamente grande, p. ex., até 1.000.000; a α_2-macroglobulina inibe a trombina e outras proteases.

mac·ro·glos·sia (mak-rō-glos'ē-ă). Macroglossia; aumento da língua, seja congênito ou secundário a uma neoplasia ou a um hamartoma vascular. SIN megaloglossia. [macro- + G. *glossa*, língua]

mac·ro·gna·thia (mak-rō-nā'thē-ă). Macrognatia, macrognatismo; aumento ou alongamento da mandíbula. SIN megagnathia. [macro- + G. *gnathos*, mandíbula]

ma·crog·ra·phy (mă-krog'ră-fē). Macrografia; termo raramente usado para designar a escrita com letras muito grandes. SIN megalographia. [macro- + G. *grapho*, escrever]

mac·ro·gy·ria (mak-rō-jī'rē-ă). Macrogiria. SIN pachygyria. [macro- + G. *gyros*, círculo (giro)]

mac·ro·la·bia (mak'rō-lā'bē-ă). Macroquilia. SIN macrocheilia (1). [macro- + L. *labium*, lábio]

mac·ro·leu·ko·blast (mak-rō-loo'kō-blast). Macroleucoblasto; leucoblasto notavelmente grande.

mac·ro·lide (mak'rō-līd). Macrolídeo; uma lactona natural, cujo anel é grande, geralmente com 14–20 átomos; vários antibióticos, incluindo a eritromicina, são macrolídeos. Eles inibem a biossíntese de proteínas.

mac·ro·lides (mak'rō-līdz). Macrolídeos; classe de antibióticos descobertos em estreptomicetos, caracterizada por moléculas compostas de lactonas de anel grande; p. ex., eritromicina, que inibem a biossíntese de proteínas.

mac·ro·mas·tia, mac·ro·ma·zia (mak-rō-mas'tē-a, -mā'zē-ă). Macromastia; mamas anormalmente grandes. VER TAMBÉM hypermastia (2). [macro- + G. *mastos*, mama]

mac·ro·mel·a·no·some (mak-rō-mel'ă-nō-sōm). Macromelanossoma. SIN giant melanosome.

mac·ro·me·lia (mak-rō-mē'lē-ă). Macromelia; tamanho anormal de um ou mais membros. SIN megalomelia. [macro- + G. *melos*, membro]

mac·ro·mere. Macrômero; blastômero grande, como nos anfíbios. [macro- + G. *meros*, parte]

mac·ro·mer·o·zo·ite (mak'rō-mer-ō-zō'īt). Macromerozoíta; um merozoíta grande. SIN megamerozoite. [macro- + G. *meros*, parte, + *zoon*, animal]

mac·ro·min·er·als (mak-rō-min-er-alz). Macrominerais. SIN macroelements.

mac·ro·mol·e·cule (mak-rō-mol'ē-kūl). Macromolécula; molécula de tamanho coloidal; p. ex., proteínas, ácidos polinucleicos, polissacarídeos.

mac·ro·mon·o·cyte (mak-rō-mon'ō-sīt). Macromonócito; monócito extraordinariamente grande.

mac·ro·my·e·lo·blast (mak-rō-mī'ē-lō-blast). Macromieloblasto; mieloblasto excepcionalmente grande.

mac·ro·nor·mo·blast (mak-rō-nōr'mō-blast). Macronormoblasto. **1.** Um normoblasto grande. **2.** Uma hemácia grande, incompletamente hemoglobinífera, nucleada, com um núcleo em forma de "roda de carroça".

mac·ro·nor·mo·chro·mo·blast (mak'rō-nōr-mō-krō'mō-blast). Macronormocromoblasto. SIN macroerythroblast.

mac·ro·nu·cle·us (mak-rō-noo'klē-ŭs). Macronúcleo. **1.** Núcleo que ocupa uma parte relativamente grande da célula, ou o núcleo maior quando uma célula possui dois ou mais núcleos. SIN meganucleus. **2.** O maior dos dois núcleos em ciliados, controlando as funções metabólicas vegetativas, e não a reprodução. SIN somatic nucleus, trophic nucleus, trophonucleus. VER TAMBÉM micronucleus (2).

mac·ro·nu·tri·ents (mak-rō-noo'trē-ents). Macronutrientes; nutrientes necessários em maior quantidade; p. ex., carboidratos, proteína, gorduras.

mac·ro·nych·ia (mak-rō-nik'ē-ă). Macroniquia; unhas excepcionalmente grandes nas mãos ou nos pés. [macro- + G. *onyx*, unha]

mac·ro·or·chid·ism (mak-rō-ōr'ki-dizm). Macroorquidismo; que possui testículos excepcionalmente grandes; observado em homens com a síndrome do X frágil. [macro- + G. *orchis (orchid-)*, testículo]

mac·ro·par·a·site (mak-rō-par'ă-sīt). Macroparasita; parasita, como um piolho ou um verme intestinal, visível a olho nu.

mac·ro·pa·thol·o·gy (mak'rō-pa-thol'ō-jē). Macropatologia; a fase da patologia que diz respeito às alterações anatômicas macroscópicas na doença.

mac·ro·pe·nis (mak-rō-pē'nis). Macropênis; pênis excepcionalmente grande. SIN macrophallus.

mac·ro·phage (mak'rō-faj). Macrófago; qualquer célula mononuclear, ativamente fagocitária, que se origina de células-tronco (células primordiais) monocíticas na medula óssea; essas células encontram-se amplamente distribuídas no corpo e variam em morfologia e motilidade, embora a maioria consista em células grandes, de longa vida, com um núcleo quase redondo, que possuem abundantes vacúolos endocíticos, lisossomas e fagolisossomas. A atividade fagocitária é tipicamente mediada por fatores de reconhecimento séricos, incluindo algumas imunoglobulinas e componentes do sistema complemento, mas também pode ser inespecífica para alguns materiais inertes e bactérias, como no caso dos macrófagos alveolares; os macrófagos também estão envolvidos na produção de anticorpos e em respostas imunes celulares, participam da apresentação de antígenos aos linfócitos e secretam várias moléculas imunorreguladoras. SIN macrophagocyte, rhagiocrine cell. [macro- + G. *phago*, comer]

activated m., m. ativado; macrófago maduro, em um estado metabólico ativo, citotóxico para células tumorais/alvo, geralmente após exposição a determinadas citocinas. SIN armed m.

alveolar m., m. alveolar; macrófago vigorosamente fagocitário na superfície epitelial dos alvéolos pulmonares, onde ingere partículas inaladas. SIN coniophage, dust cell.

armed m., m. ativado. SIN activated m.

fixed m., m. fixo; macrófago relativamente imóvel encontrado no tecido conjuntivo, linfonodos, baço e medula óssea. SIN resting wandering cell.

free m., m. livre; macrófago ativamente móvel, encontrado tipicamente em locais de inflamação.

Hansemann m., m. de Hansemann; termo obsoleto para designar grandes histiócitos com abundante citoplasma, que pode conter corpúsculos de Michaelis-Gutmann e um ou vários núcleos; descrito em lesões de malacoplaquia.

inflammatory m., m. inflamatório; macrófago encontrado em locais de inflamação.

tangible body m., macrófago que se especializa na fagocitose de células linfóides.

mac·ro·phag·o·cyte (mak-rō-fag'ō-sīt). Macrofagócito. SIN macrophage.

mac·ro·phal·lus (mak-rō-fal'lŭs). Macropênis. SIN macropenis. [macro- + G. *phallos*, pênis]

mac·roph·thal·mia (mak-rof-thal'mē-ă). Macroftalmia. SIN megalophthalmos. [macro- + G. *ophthalmos*, olho]

mac·ro·po·dia (mak-rō-pō'dē-ă). Macropodia; pés anormalmente grandes. SIN megalopodia, pes gigas. [macro- + G. *pous*, pé]

mac·ro·pol·y·cyte (mak-rō-pol'ē-sīt). Macropolícito; leucócito polimorfonuclear neutrofílico, excepcionalmente grande, que contém um núcleo multissegmentado (p. ex., 8, 10 ou mais lobos); o arranjo da cromatina é menos compacto que no neutrófilo normal, e os grânulos citoplasmáticos tendem a ser maiores e mais acidófilos. Essas alterações freqüentemente precedem alterações significativas nas hemácias, p. ex., como na anemia perniciosa e algumas outras formas de anemia. [macro- + G. *polys*, muitos, + *kytos*, célula]

mac·ro·pro·my·e·lo·cyte (mak'rō-prō-mī'ē-lō-sīt). Macropromielócito; um promielócito excepcionalmente grande.

mac·ro·pro·so·pia (mak'rō-prō-sō'pē-ă). Macroprosopia; condição na qual a face é grande demais em proporção ao tamanho da abóbada craniana. SIN megaprosopia. [macro- + G. *prosopon*, face]

mac·ro·pro·so·pous (mak-rō-prō'sō-pŭs, -prō-sō'pŭs). Macroprosópico; relativo a ou que exibe macroprosopia. SIN megaprosopous.

ma·crop·sia (mă-krop'sē-ă). Macropsia; percepção de objetos como sendo maiores do que realmente são. [macro- + G. *opsis*, visão]

mac·ro·rhin·ia (mak-rō-rin'ē-ă). Macrorrinia; tamanho excessivo do nariz, seja congênito ou patológico. [macro- + G. *rhis (rhin-)*, nariz]

mac·ro·sce·lia (mak-rō-sē'lē-ă). Macroscelia; aumento anormal do comprimento ou da espessura das pernas. [macro- + G. *skelos*, perna]

mac·ro·scop·ic (mak-rō-skop'ik). Macroscópico. **1.** De tamanho visível a olho nu ou sem o uso de um microscópio. **2.** Relativo à macroscopia.

ma·cros·co·py (mă-kros'kō-pē). Macroscopia; exame de objetos a olho nu. [macro- + G. *skopeo*, ver]

mac·ro·sig·moid (mak-rō-sig'moyd). Macrossigmóide; aumento ou dilatação do cólon sigmóide. SIN megasigmoid.

ma·cro·sis (mă-krō'sis). Macrose; aumento do comprimento ou volume. [G.]

mac·ros·mat·ic (mak'roz-mat'ik). Macrosmático; designa um sentido do olfato anormalmente aguçado. [macro- + G. *osme*, olfato]

mac·ro·so·mia (mak-rō-sō'mē-ă). Macrossomia; tamanho excepcionalmente grande do corpo. SIN megasomia. [macro- + G. *soma*, corpo]

mac·ro·splanch·nic (mak-rō-splangk'nik). Macroesplâncnico. SIN megalosplanchnic.

mac·ro·spore (mak'rō-spōr). Macrosporo; o maior de dois tipos de esporos de certos protozoários ou fungos. SIN megalospore, megaspore. [macro- + G. *sporos*, semente]

mac·ro·ster·e·og·no·sis (mak'rō-ster-ē-og-nō'sis). Macrostereognosia; erro de percepção no qual os objetos parecem maiores do que são. [macro- + G. *stereos*, sólido, + *gnosis*, reconhecimento]

mac·ro·sto·mia (mak-rō-stō'mē-ă). Macrostomia; tamanho anormalmente grande da boca, resultante de ausência de fusão entre os processos maxilar e mandibular na face do embrião. [macro- + G. *stoma*, boca]

mac·ro·tia (mak-rō'shē-ă). Macrotia; aumento congênito excessivo da orelha. [macro- + G. *ous*, orelha]

mac·ro·tome (mak'rō-tōm). Macrótomo; instrumento para fazer cortes anatômicos macroscópicos. [macro- + G. *tome*, que corta]

mac·u·la, pl. **mac·u·lae** (mak'ū-lă, -ū-lē). Mácula. **1** [TA]. Uma área plana circunscrita, com até 1,0 cm de diâmetro, de cor perceptivelmente diferente do tecido adjacente. **2.** Um ponto ou mancha pequena e descorada na pele,

macula   936   **maggot**

sem relevo nem depressão. VER TAMBÉM spot. **3.** Os receptores sensoriais neuroepiteliais do utrículo e sáculo do labirinto vestibular coletivamente. SIN maculae utriculosaccularis [TA]. VER TAMBÉM *neuroepithelium* of macula. SIN macule, spot (1). [L. uma mancha]
    mac'ulae acus'ticae, máculas acústicas. VER m. of saccule, m. of utricle.
    m. adher'ens, m. aderente; desmossoma. SIN desmosome.
    m. al'bida, pl. **mac'ulae al'bidae,** mácula álbida; placas ou manchas brancas ou branco-acinzentadas, arredondadas ou irregulares, ligeiramente opacas, observadas algumas vezes no epicárdio, após a morte, principalmente em pessoas de meia-idade ou idosas; resultam de espessamento fibroso e, algumas vezes, da hialinização do epicárdio; também pode haver lesões semelhantes na camada visceral do peritônio. SIN m. lactea, m. tendinea, tache blanche, tache laiteuse (2), tendinous spot, white spot.
    m. atroph'ica, m. atrófica; uma mancha branca brilhante, atrófica, na pele.
    m. ceru'lea, m. cerúlea; mancha azulada na pele causada pelas picadas de pulgas ou piolhos, principalmente na pediculose pubiana. SIN blue spot (1).
    m. commu'nicans, junção comunicante. SIN gap *junction*.
    m. commu'nis, m. comum; a área espessa na parede medial da vesícula auditiva que, posteriormente, se subdivide para formar as máculas do sáculo e utrículo, bem como as cristas das ampolas dos ductos semicirculares.
    m. cor'neae, m. córnea; uma opacidade moderadamente densa da córnea. SIN corneal spot.
    m. cribro'sa, pl. **mac'ulae cribro'sae** [TA], m. crivosa; uma das três áreas na parede do vestíbulo do labirinto, caracterizadas por numerosos forames que dão passagem a filamentos nervosos que suprem partes do labirinto membranáceo; **m. cribrosa inferior** [TA], m. crivosa inferior; localizada na ampola óssea posterior para passagem das fibras do nervo ampular posterior; **m. cribrosa media** [TA], c. crivosa média; área próxima da base da cóclea através da qual passam as fibras nervosas saculares; **m. cribrosa superior** [TA], m. crivosa superior; área perfurada acima do recesso elíptico para a passagem das fibras do nervo utriculoampular; quarta m. crivosa, nome aplicado algumas vezes à abertura para o nervo coclear.
    m. cribrosa quarta, quarta m. crivosa; nome aplicado algumas vezes à abertura para o nervo coclear.
    m. den'sa, m. densa; grupo de células aglomeradas, densamente coradas no epitélio tubular distal de um néfron, diretamente apostas às células justaglomerulares; podem funcionar como quimiorreceptores ou como barorreceptores enviando informações para as células justaglomerulares.
    false m., m. falsa; ponto de fixação fora da fóvea.
    m. fla'va, m. amarela; mancha amarelada na extremidade anterior da rima da glote, onde as duas pregas vocais se unem.
    m. gonorrho'ica, m. gonorreica; uma mancha de cor vermelha mais brilhante que a membrana adjacente, no orifício congestionado do ducto da glândula de Bartholin, algumas vezes observada na gonorréia.
    honeycomb m., m. alveolar; edema da região macular da retina.
    m. lac'tea, m. láctea. SIN m. albida.
    m. lu'tea [TA], m. lútea. SIN m. of retina.
    m. pellu'cida, m. pelúcida. SIN follicular *stigma*.
    m. of retina [TA], m. lútea; uma área oval da retina sensorial, de 3 a 5 mm, temporal ao disco óptico, que corresponde ao pólo posterior do olho; em seu centro está a fóvea central, que contém apenas os cones da retina. SIN m. lutea [TA], area centralis, m. retinae, macular area, punctum luteum, Soemmerring spot, yellow spot.
    m. ret'inae, m. lútea. SIN m. of retina.
    m. of saccule [TA], m. do sáculo; o receptor sensorial neuroepitelial oval na parede anterior do sáculo; as células ciliadas do neuroepitélio sustentam a membrana dos estatocônios e possuem arborizações terminais das fibras do nervo vestibular ao redor de seus corpos. SIN m. sacculi [TA], saccular spot.
    m. sac'culi [TA], m. do sáculo. SIN m. of saccule.
    m. tendin'ea, m. tendínea. SIN m. albida.
    m. of utricle [TA], m. do utrículo; o receptor sensorial neuroepitelial na parede ínfero-lateral do utrículo; as células pilosas do neuroepitélio sustentam a membrana dos estatocônios e possuem arborizações terminais das fibras do nervo vestibular ao redor de seus corpos; sensível à aceleração linear no eixo longitudinal do corpo e às influências da gravidade. SIN m. utriculi [TA], utricular spot.
    m. utric'uli [TA], m. do utrículo. SIN m. of utricle.
    maculae utriculosaccularis [TA], mácula. SIN macula (3).
mac·u·lar, mac·u·late (mak'ū-lăr, -lāt). Macular. **1.** Relativo a, ou caracterizado por, máculas. **2.** Designa a parte central da retina, principalmente a mácula da retina.
mac·ule (mak'ūl). Mácula; mancha. SIN macula. [L. *macula*, mácula]
    ash-leaf m., mancha em folha de freixo; mácula hipocrômica, freqüentemente com o formato de uma folha de freixo, que é encontrada por ocasião do nascimento em muitos pacientes com esclerose tuberosa.

mac·u·lo·ce·re·bral (mak'ū-lō-ser'e-brăl). Maculocerebral; relativo à mácula lútea e ao encéfalo; designa um tipo de doença nervosa caracterizada por lesões degenerativas na retina e no encéfalo.

mac·u·lo·er·y·the·ma·tous (mak'ū-lō-er-i-the'mă-tŭs). Maculoeritematosa; designa lesões eritematosas e maculares, que cobrem grandes áreas.
mac·u·lo·pap·ule (mak'ū-lō-pap'ūl). Maculopápula; lesão com uma base plana circundando uma pápula no centro.
mac·u·lop·a·thy (mak-ū-lop'ă-thē). Maculopatia; qualquer condição patológica da mácula lútea. SIN macular retinopathy.
    bull's-eye m., m. em olho de boi; condição ocular na qual o edema ou a degeneração da retina sensorial no pólo posterior do olho causa áreas claras e escuras alternadas, como em um alvo; observada em condições tóxicas, inflamatórias e hereditárias.
    cystoid m., m. cistóide; degeneração cística da retina central que pode ocorrer, após extração de catarata, na degeneração macular senil e em outras anormalidades da retina.
    familial pseudoinflammatory m., m. pseudo-inflamatória familiar; degeneração macular familiar semelhante a alterações inflamatórias.
    nicotinic acid m., m. por ácido nicotínico; maculopatia observada em pessoas que tomam 3.000 mg ou mais de ácido nicotínico diariamente; a visão normal retorna após a interrupção do uso do medicamento.
    solar m., m. solar; lesão da fóvea central da retina e da coróide adjacente devida à ação térmica dos raios infravermelhos, causada pela contemplação demorada do sol ou de um eclipse solar sem proteção ocular suficiente. VER TAMBÉM photoretinopathy. SIN eclipse blindness, solar blindness.
mad. Louco; termo pejorativo, não-médico para: **1.** Enfurecido, raivoso. **2.** Mentalmente doente; insano. [A.S. *gemād*]
mad·a·ro·sis (mad-ă-rō'sis). Madarose. **1.** SIN milphosis. **2.** SIN *alopecia adnata*. [G. queda dos cílios, de *madaō*, cair (de cabelos)]
mad·der (mad'ĕr). Garança; ruiva. **1.** A raiz seca e pulverizada da *Rubia tinctorum* (família Rubiaceae); contém vários glicosídeos que, após a fermentação, fornecem os corantes vermelhos, alizarina e purpurina. Quando a garança (ou alizarina) é usada como alimento de animais jovens, o cálcio no sal ósseo recém-depositado, hidroxiapatita, é corado de vermelho. **2.** Qualquer corante obtido de vegetais da família da garança (Rubiaceae). SIN turkey red. [A.S. *maedere*]
Maddox, Ernest E., oftalmologista inglês, 1860–1933. VER M. *rod*.
Madelung, Otto W., cirurgião alemão, 1846–1926. VER M. *deformity, disease, neck*.
Madlener, Max, cirurgião alemão, 1868–1951. VER M. *operation*.
mad·ness (mad'nes). Loucura; o estado de estar louco.
Madsen, Thorvald J.M., 1870–1957. VER Arrhenius-M. *theory*.
Mad·u·rel·la (mad'ū-rel'ă). Gênero de fungos que inclui várias espécies, como *M. grisea* e *M. mycetomi*, causadoras de micetoma. [*Madura*, Índia]
ma·du·ro·my·co·sis (mad'ū-rō-mī-kō'sis). Maduromicose. SIN mycetoma. [*Madura*, Índia, + mycosis]
MAF Abreviatura de macrophage-activating *factor* (fator ativador de macrófagos, FAM).
ma·fe·nide (mā'fe-nīd). Mafenida; agente antibacteriano tópico ativo contra patógenos anaeróbicos. O acetato de mafenida é o sal preferido para pomadas; o cloridrato de mafenida é o sal preferido para solução. SIN 4-homosulfanilamide.
Maffucci, Angelo, médico e anátomo-patologista italiano, 1847–1903. VER M. *syndrome*.
mag·al·drate (mag'al-drāt). Magaldrato; uma combinação química de hidróxido de alumínio e hidróxido de magnésio usada como antiácido.
Magendie, François, fisiologista francês, 1783–1855. VER *foramen* of M.; Bell-M. *law*; M. *law, spaces*, em *space*; M.-Hertwig *sign, syndrome*.
ma·gen·stras·se (mag'en-stras'e). Canal gástrico. SIN gastric *canal*. [Al. *Magen*, estômago, + *Strasse*, rua]
mag·got (mag'ot). Larva; uma larva de mosca ou de outro inseto.
    cheese m., larva do queijo. SIN *Philopia casei*.

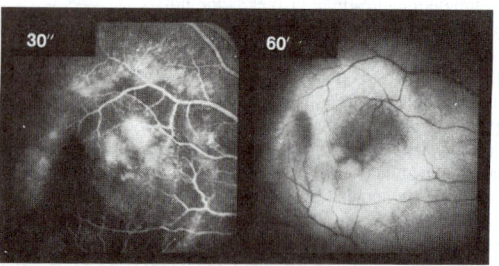

maculopatia em olho de boi: angiografia com fluoresceína mostrando degeneração macular do olho direito

surgical m., larva cirúrgica; larva de gastrófilo esterilizada usada em um tratamento obsoleto de desbridamento de feridas e remoção de tecidos necróticos.

Magill, Sir Ivan Whiteside, anestesiologista inglês, 1888–1975. VER M. *forceps*.

mag·is·tral (maj′is-trăl). Magistral; designa uma preparação aviada de acordo com a prescrição de um médico, ao contrário da oficinal (oriunda do estoque de um farmacêutico). [L. *magister*, mestre]

mag·ma (mag′mă). Magma. **1.** Uma massa de consistência mole que resta após a extração dos princípios ativos. **2.** Uma pomada ou pasta espessa. [G. massa pastosa ou pomada, de *massō*, amassar]

   m. reticula′re, m. reticular; filamentos acelulares delicados observados entre o saco vitelino e a parede externa do blastocisto, que é o saco coriônico incipiente.

Magnan, Valentin J.J., psiquiatra em Paris, 1835–1916. VER M. trombone *movement, sign*.

mag·ne·sia (mag-nē′zhŭh). Magnésia. SIN *magnesium oxide*. [ver magnesium]

   calcined m., m. calcinada. SIN *magnesium oxide*.

   m. magma, magma de magnésia. SIN *milk of magnesia*.

mag·ne·si·um (Mg) (mag-nē′zē-ŭm). Magnésio; elemento alcalino terroso, número atômico 12, peso atômico 24,3050, que oxida em magnésia; um bioelemento; muitos sais têm aplicações clínicas. [L. mod. do G. *Magnēsia*, uma região da Tessália]

   m. aluminum silicate, silicato de magnésio de alumínio; um antiácido. SIN aluminum magnesium silicate.

   m. bacteriopheophytinate, bacteriofeofitinato de magnésio. VER bacteriochrolophyll.

   m. benzoate, benzoato de magnésio; tem sido usado na gota e na artrite reumatóide.

   m. carbonate, carbonato de magnésio; usado na acidez gástrica e intestinal, e como laxante.

   m. chloride, cloreto de magnésio; foi usado como laxante.

   m. citrate, citrato de magnésio; laxante; geralmente administrado como uma bebida flavorizada efervescente.

   effervescent m. citrate, citrato de magnésio efervescente; carbonato de magnésio, ácido cítrico, bicarbonato de sódio e açúcar, umedecidos com álcool, peneirados e secos até formarem um pó granular grosso; usado como laxante.

   effervescent m. sulfate, sulfato de magnésio efervescente; sal de Epsom efervescente; sulfato de magnésio, bicarbonato de sódio, ácido tartárico e ácido cítrico, umedecidos, peneirados e secos até formarem um pó granular grosso; um purgante.

   m. hydroxide, hidróxido de magnésio; antiácido e laxante.

   m. lactate, lactato de magnésio; laxante.

   m. oxide, óxido de magnésio; usado como antiácido e laxante. SIN calcined magnesia, magnesia.

   m. peroxide, peróxido de magnésio; decompõe-se na água em peróxido de hidrogênio; usado como ingrediente em dentifrícios e no polvilho anti-séptico.

   m. phytinates, fitinatos de magnésio; clorofilas *a* e *b*. VER entradas em chlorophyll.

   m. salicylate, salicilato de magnésio; um derivado do salicilato sem sódio com propriedades antiinflamatórias, analgésicas e antipiréticas; usado para alívio da dor leve a moderada.

   m. stearate, estearato de magnésio; composto de magnésio com proporções variáveis de ácidos esteárico e palmítico; usado no preparo de comprimidos, como lubrificante e como ingrediente em alguns talcos para bebês.

   m. sulfate, sulfato de magnésio; sal de Epsom; ingrediente ativo da maioria das águas laxativas naturais; usado como catártico de ação imediata em alguns envenenamentos, no tratamento do aumento da pressão intracraniana e do edema, como anticonvulsivante na eclâmpsia (quando administrado por via intravenosa) e como antiinflamatório (quando aplicado localmente). SIN Epsom salts.

   tribasic m. phosphate, fosfato de magnésio tribásico; fosfato de magnésio terciário, é usado como antiácido, mas não produz alcalinização sistêmica; 1 g tem potencial neutralizante equivalente a cerca de 0,46 g de bicarbonato de sódio.

   m. trisilicate, trissilicato de magnésio; composto de óxido de magnésio e dióxido de silício com proporções variáveis de água; encontrado na natureza como sepiolita (magnesita), pararrepiolita e repiolita; um antiácido gástrico.

mag·net. Magneto; ímã. **1.** Um corpo que tem a propriedade de atrair partículas de ferro, cobalto, níquel ou qualquer de várias ligas metálicas e que, quando livremente suspenso, tende a assumir uma direção definida entre os pólos magnéticos da terra (polaridade magnética). **2.** Um pedaço de ferro ou aço, em forma de barra ou ferradura, que se tornou magnético por contato com outro magneto ou, como no caso de um eletromagneto, por passagem de corrente elétrica por um núcleo metálico (ferro). **3.** Um eletromagneto construído em configuração cilíndrica para acomodar um paciente em seu centro, para obtenção de imagens por ressonância magnética. [G. *magnēs*]

   superconducting m., m. supercondutor; magneto cujas bobinas são resfriadas, geralmente com hélio líquido, até uma temperatura na qual o metal se torne supercondutor, removendo efetivamente toda resistência elétrica.

mag·net·ic. Magnético. **1.** Relativo a, ou característico de, um magneto. **2.** Que possui magnetismo.

mag·ne·tism (mag′nĕ-tizm). Magnetismo; a propriedade de atração ou repulsão mútua observada nos magnetos.

   animal m., m. animal; uma força psíquica semelhante à propriedade de atração ou repulsão mútua presente em magnetos metálicos, e antes considerada o principal agente na hipnose, sendo assim denominada magnetismo animal. VER hypnosis, mesmerism.

mag·ne·to·car·di·og·ra·phy (mag′nĕ-tō-kar-dē-og′ră-fē). Magnetocardiografia; medida do campo magnético do coração, que é produzido pelas mesmas correntes iônicas que geram o eletrocardiograma, e exibindo ondas P, QRS, T e U características.

mag·ne·to·en·ceph·a·lo·gram (MEG) (mag-nē′tō-en-sef′ă-lō-gram). Magnetoencefalograma; um registro de tempo de Gauss do campo magnético do encéfalo.

mag·ne·to·en·ceph·a·log·ra·phy (mag-nē′tō-en-sef-ă-log′ră-fē). Magnetoencefalografia; o processo de registro do campo magnético do encéfalo.

mag·ne·tom·e·ter (mag-nĕ-tom′ĕ-ter). Magnetômetro; instrumento para detectar e medir o campo magnético.

mag·ne·ton (mag′nĕ-ton). Magnéton; unidade de medida do momento magnético de uma partícula (p. ex., átomo ou partícula subatômica).

   Bohr m. (μ_B), m. de Bohr; uma constante na equação relativa à diferença nas energias entre alinhamentos de rotações paralelas e antiparalelas de elétrons em um campo magnético; o momento magnético final de um elétron ímpar; usado em espectrometria de ressonância da rotação de elétrons para detecção e estimativa de radicais livres; a menor unidade de momento magnético (aproximadamente $9,274 \times 10^{-24}$ J T^{-1}). SIN electron m.

   electron m., m. de elétron. SIN Bohr m.

   nuclear m. (μ_N), m. nuclear; uma constante na equação relativa à diferença de energia entre alinhamentos de rotações paralelas e antiparalelas de núcleos atômicos em um campo magnético; usado em espectrometria de ressonância magnética nuclear; $5,05 \times 10^{-27}$ J T^{-1}.

mag·ne·to·ther·a·py (mag-nē′tō-thār′ă-pē). Magnetoterapia; tratamento experimental de doenças por aplicação de magnetos ou de campos magnéticos induzidos.

mag·ni·fi·ca·tion (mag′ni-fi-kā′shŭn). Ampliação. **1.** O aumento aparente no tamanho de um objeto visto ao microscópio; quando observado, esse aumento do tamanho é expresso por um número precedido por X, indicando o número de vezes de aumento do diâmetro. **2.** A amplitude aumentada de um traçado, como de uma contração muscular, causada pelo uso de uma alavanca com um braço de registro longo, isto é, um braço no qual o fulcro está mais próximo do músculo que da ponta registradora. [L. *magnifico*, pp. *-atus*, ampliar]

mag·ni·tude (mag′ni-tood). Magnitude; tamanho ou extensão.

   average pulse m., m. média do pulso; a amplitude média do pulso durante toda a sua duração; idêntica à amplitude máxima para uma onda quadrada ou pulso sem inclinação.

   peak m., m. máxima; a maior amplitude.

mag·no·cel·lu·lar (mag′nō-sel′ū-lar). Magnocelular; composto de células de grande tamanho. [L. *magnus*, grande, + cellular]

mag·num (mag′nŭm). Capitato, maior osso do carpo. SIN capitate (1). [L. *magnus*, grande]

Magnus, Rudolph, fisiologista alemão, 1873–1927. VER M. *sign*.

mag·nus (mag′nŭs). Magno; grande; designa uma estrutura de tamanho grande. [L.]

Mahaim, Ivan, cardiologista do século XX, 1897–1965. VER M. *fibers*, em *fiber*.

Ma-huang (mah-hwahng). Nome dado à *Ephedra equisetina*. [Chinês]

MAI Abreviatura de *Mycobacterium avium-intracellulare*. VER TAMBÉM *Mycobacterium avium-intracellulare complex*.

maidenhair tree. SIN *Ginkgo biloba*.

maid·en·head (mā′den-hed). Virgindade; termo obsoleto para designar o hímen intacto de uma virgem.

mai·dism (mā′dizm). Pelagra. SIN pellagra. [*Zea mays*, milho]

Maier, Rudolf, médico alemão, 1824–1888. VER M. *sinus*.

maim (mām). Mutilar; incapacitar ou inutilizar por meio de uma lesão.

main (man). Mão. SIN hand. [Fr.]

   m. succulente, mão suculenta. SIN *Marinesco succulent hand*.

main·frame (mān′frām). Servidor; grande computador digital, como o usado em um hospital para gerenciamento das informações. Cf. mini.

main·stream·ing (mān′strēm-ing). Integração; proporcionar o ambiente menos restritivo (quanto aos aspectos social, físico e educacional) para indivíduos cronicamente incapacitados, mediante sua introdução no ambiente natural, e não segregando-os em grupos homogêneos que vivem em ambientes protegidos sob supervisão constante.

main·tain·er (mān-tā′ner). Mantenedor; dispositivo utilizado para manter ou segurar os dentes em determinada posição.
  space m., m. de espaço; aparelho ortodôntico usado para evitar a perda de espaço ou o desvio de dentes após extração ou perda prematura de dentes. SIN space retainer.

main·te·nance (mān′ten-ans). Manutenção. **1.** Esquema terapêutico que visa preservar um benefício. Cf. compliance (2), adherence (2). **2.** O período durante o qual o paciente mantém práticas saudáveis sem supervisão, incorporando-as a um estilo de vida geral. Cf. compliance. [l.m., do Fr. ant., do L. mediev. *manuteneo*, segurar na mão]

maise oil (māz). Óleo de milho. SIN corn oil.

Maissiat, Jacques H., anatomista francês, 1805–1878. VER M. *band*.

Majocchi, Domenico, dermatologista italiano, 1849–1929. VER M. *granulomas*, em *granuloma*.

ma·jor (mā′jŏr). Maior; principal; importante; a maior de duas estruturas semelhantes. [L. comparativo de *magnus*, grande]

Makeham, William Matthew, atuário inglês,† 1892. VER M. *hypothesis*.

mal (mahl). Mal; uma doença ou distúrbio. [Fr. do L. *malum*, mal]
  m. de la rosa, m. rosso, pelagra. SIN pellagra.
  m. del pinto, pinta. SIN pinta.
  m. de Meleda, m. de Meleda; ceratodermia simétrica endêmica dos membros, observada na ilha de Meleda, na costa da Dalmácia, na Europa Oriental.
  m. de mer, enjôo marítimo. SIN seasickness.
  grand m. (grahn), grande mal. SIN generalized tonic-clonic *seizure*.
  m. morado (mal mō-rā′do), mal morado; coloração violácea da pele observada em crises agudas de oncodermatite causada por *Onchocerca volvulus* na América Central. [Esp. *mal*, doença, + *morado*, púrpura]
  petit m. (pĕ-tē′). Pequeno mal. VER petit mal *seizure*. [Fr. pequeno]

♻ **mal-.** Doente, mal; oposto de eu-. Cf. dys-, caco-. [L. *malus*, mau]

ma·la (mā′lă). Malar; maçã do rosto. **1.** Bochecha. SIN cheek. **2.** Osso zigomático. SIN zygomatic *bone*. [L. osso da bochecha]

ℹ **mal·ab·sorp·tion** (mal-ab-sōrp′shŭn). Má absorção, malabsorção; imperfeição, inadequação ou outro tipo de perturbação da absorção gastrointestinal.
  congenital selective glucose and galactose m., má absorção congênita seletiva de glicose e galactose; distúrbio hereditário no qual há acúmulo de D-glicose e D-galactose na luz intestinal, produzindo um efeito osmótico; leva à plenitude abdominal, dor abdominal e diarréia.
  enterocyte cobalamin m., má absorção de cobalamina pelos enterócitos; distúrbio hereditário de comprometimento do transporte transintestinal de cobalamina; os sintomas são semelhantes aos da deficiência de vitamina B_{12}.
  fructose m., má absorção de frutose; erro congênito do metabolismo no qual a D-frutose oral é absorvida incompletamente; resulta em sintomas abdominais e diarréia.
  hereditary folate m., má absorção hereditária de folato; distúrbio hereditário no qual o transporte de folatos no intestino e no plexo coróide está deficiente e resulta em anemia megaloblástica e anormalidades neurológicas.

Malacarne, Michele V.G., cirurgião italiano, 1744–1816. VER M. *pyramid, space*.

mal·a·chite green (mal′ă-kīt) [C.I. 42000]. Verde de malaquita; corante que foi usado como anti-séptico em feridas, como tratamento de infecções cutâneas micóticas, e na coloração biológica de tecidos e bactérias. [G. *malachē*, malva]

ma·la·cia (mă-lā′shē-ă). Malacia; amolecimento ou perda de consistência e contiguidade em qualquer órgão ou tecido. Também usado como forma combinante na posição de sufixo. SIN mollities (2). SIN malacosis. [G. *malakia*, amolecimento]

ma·la·cic (mă-lā′sik). Malácico. SIN malacotic.

♻ **malaco-.** Malaco-; mole, amolecimento. [G. *malakos*, mole; *malakia*, amolecimento]

mal·a·co·pla·kia, mal·a·ko·pla·kia (mal′ă-kō-plā′kē-ă, mal′ă-kō-plā′kē-a). Malacoplaquia; malacoplacia; lesão rara na mucosa da bexiga e de outros órgãos, mais freqüente em mulheres, caracterizada por numerosas placas e nódulos mosqueados, amarelos e cinza, de consistência mole, que consistem em numerosos macrófagos e calcosferitas (corpúsculos de Michaelis-Guttmann) que podem se formar ao redor de bactérias intracelulares, geralmente *Escherichia coli*. [malaco- + G. *plax*, lâmina, placa]

mal·a·co·sis (mal-ă-kō′sis). Malacose. SIN malacia.

mal·a·cot·ic (mal′ă-kot′ik). Malacótico; relativo a, ou caracterizado por, malacia. SIN malacic.

ma·lac·tic (mă-lak′tik). Maláctico; malático. SIN emollient. [G. *malaktikos*, amolecimento]

ma·la·die (mal′ă-dē′). Doença; enfermidade; mal-estar. SIN malady. [Fr.]
  m. de Roger, doença de Roger. SIN Roger *disease*. [Fr.]
  m. des jambes (mal′ă-dē′ dĕ zhamb′), doença das pernas; doença maldefinida observada em plantadores de arroz na Louisiana.

mal·ad·just·ment (mal-ad-jŭst′ment). Desajustamento; inadaptação; nas profissões relacionadas à saúde mental, uma incapacidade de enfrentar os problemas e desafios da vida diária. [mal- + *adjust*, do Fr. ant. *adjuster*, do L. ant. *adjuxto*, aproximar de, + -ment]
  social m., d. social; desajustamento sem transtorno psiquiátrico evidente, como aquele ocasionado por uma incapacidade de enfrentar situações sociais.

mal·a·dy (mal′ă-dē). Doença, enfermidade. SIN maladie. [Fr. *maladie*, enfermidade]

ma·lag·ma (mă-lag′mă). Malagma; cataplasma ou emoliente. [G. cataplasma]

mal·aise (mă-lāz′). Mal-estar; indisposição; sensação de desconforto ou embaraço generalizado, uma sensação de "indisposição", freqüentemente a primeira indicação de uma infecção ou outra doença. [Fr. desconforto]

mal·a·lign·ment (mal-ă-līn′ment). Desalinhamento; deslocamento de um dente ou dentes de uma posição normal no arco dental.

ma·lar (mā′lăr). Malar; relativo ao osso malar, à bochecha ou aos ossos da bochecha.

---

má digestão ou má absorção

Estágio Intraluminal

defeito no estágio secretor (pancreático)
  ausência de tripsina, lipase ou colipase (hereditária)
  fibrose cística*
  pancreatectomia
  pancreatite crônica
  carcinoma do pâncreas*
  defeito da estimulação devido a doença intestinal ou cirurgia gástrica
  obstrução do ducto pancreático
  síndrome de Zollinger-Ellison
  desnutrição

defeito no estágio biliar
  doença do parênquima hepático*
  obstrução biliar*
  doença do íleo terminal*
  ressecção do íleo terminal*
  administração de colestiramina
  ação bacteriana em virtude de estase ou supercrescimento bacteriano

Estágio do Intestino Delgado

defeito no estágio de superfície
  deficiência de enterocinase (hereditária)
  deficiências de dissacaridase (hereditária e adquirida)

defeito no estágio celular e de oferta
  defeitos do transporte de aminoácidos
  má absorção primária de vitamina B_{12}
  ressecção maciça
  enterite por radiação
  isquemia intestinal
  espru celíaco
  espru tropical*
  colite ulcerativa
  enterite regional
  doença de Whipple
  linfoma intestinal primário
  hipogamaglobulinemia
  alergia alimentar
  amiloidose
  parasitoses

Defeitos em Múltiplos Estágios

  pós-gastrectomia
  diabetes melito
  endocrinopatias
  doença do colágeno
  administração de neomicina

*doenças mais comuns

MALARIA

ma·lar·ia (mă-lār′ē-ă). Malária; doença causada pela presença do esporozoário *Plasmodium* nas hemácias humanas ou de outro vertebrado, geralmente transmitida para seres humanos pela picada de um mosquito fêmea infectado do gênero *Anopheles*, que anteriormente sugou o sangue de uma pessoa com malária. A infecção humana começa com o ciclo exoeritrocitário nas células do parênquima hepático, seguido por uma série de ciclos esquizogênicos eritrocitários repetidos a intervalos regulares; a produção de gametócitos em outras hemácias fornece os futuros gametas para a infecção de outro mosquito; caracterizada por fortes calafrios episódicos e febre alta, prostração, ocasionalmente morte fetal. VER tropical *diseases*, em *disease*. VER TAMBÉM *Plasmodium*. VER jungle fever, marsh fever, paludal fever. [It. *malo* (fem. *mala*), mau, + *aria*, ar, referente à antiga teoria da origem miasmática da doença]

acute m., m. aguda; forma de m. que pode ser intermitente ou remitente, consistindo em calafrio acompanhado e seguido por febre com seus sintomas gerais associados e terminando em um estágio de sudorese; os acessos, causados por liberação de merozoítas de células infectadas, tipicamente recorrem a cada 48 horas na malária terçã (vivax ou ovale), a cada 72 horas na malária quartã (malariae) e a intervalos indefinidos, mas freqüentes, geralmente cerca de 48 horas, na malária terçã maligna (falcíparo); em muitos casos, porém, a periodicidade não está bem estabelecida.

airport m., m. inadvertidamente importada por transporte de um mosquito anofelino infectado em um avião.

algid m., m. álgida; forma de m. falcípara que envolve principalmente o intestino e outras vísceras abdominais; a m. álgida gástrica é caracterizada por vômito persistente; a m. álgida disentérica é caracterizada por fezes diarreicas com sangue, nas quais é encontrado um número muito grande de hemácias infectadas.

autochthonous m., m. autóctone; doença adquirida através de transmissão por mosquito em uma área onde a malária ocorre regularmente.

benign tertian m., m. terçã benigna. SIN vivax m.

bilious remittent m., m. remitente biliosa; forma de m. falcípara caracterizada por vômito bilioso, diarréia biliosa, etc.

cerebral m., m. cerebral; forma de m. falcípara caracterizada por envolvimento cerebral, com extrema hipertermia e cefaléia, e uma taxa de fatalidade de aproximadamente 50%.

chronic m., m. crônica; m. que se desenvolve após crises repetidas freqüentes de uma das formas agudas, geralmente m. falcípara; é caracterizada por anemia intensa, esplenomegalia, emagrecimento, depressão mental, palidez, edema dos tornozelos, digestão difícil e fraqueza muscular. SIN limnemia, malarial cachexia.

m. comato·sa, m. comatosa; m. falcípara complicada por coma.

double tertian m., m. terçã dupla. VER quotidian m.

dysenteric algid m., m. álgida disentérica. VER algid m.

falciparum m., m. falcípara; m. causada por *Plasmodium falciparum* e caracterizada por acessos maláricos graves, que, tipicamente, ocorrem a cada 48 horas, com manifestações cerebrais, renais ou gastrointestinais agudas em casos graves, sendo causados principalmente pelo grande número de hemácias afetadas e pela tendência das hemácias infectadas de se tornarem viscosas e aglomeradas, bloqueando assim os capilares. VER TAMBÉM malarial *knobs*, em *knob*. SIN aestivoautumnal fever, falciparum fever, malignant tertian fever, malignant tertian m., pernicious m.

gastric algid m., m. álgida gástrica. VER algid m.

induced m., m. induzida; m. adquirida por meios artificiais, p. ex., transfusão sanguínea, uso compartilhado de seringas ou malarioterapia.

intermittent m., m. intermitente; febre malárica, geralmente do tipo terçã ou quartã, na qual há apirexia completa, com ausência dos outros sintomas, nos intervalos entre os acessos.

malariae m., m. por *Plasmodium malariae*; febre malárica com acessos que, tipicamente, recidivam a cada 72 horas ou a cada quatro dias, considerando-se o dia do acesso como o primeiro; devido à esquizogonia e liberação de merozoítas das células infectadas, com invasão de novos eritrócitos por *Plasmodium malariae*. SIN quartan fever, quartan m.

malignant tertian m., m. terçã maligna. SIN falciparum m.

monkey m., m. do macaco. SIN simian m.

nonan m., m. nonã; febre malárica com acessos que ocorrem a cada nove dias, isto é, a cada oito dias após o acesso prévio, sendo o dia de cada acesso incluído no cálculo.

ovale m., ovale tertian m., m. ovale, m. terçã ovale; malária causada por *Plasmodium ovale*.

pernicious m., m. perniciosa. SIN falciparum m.

quartan m., m. quartã. SIN malariae m.

quotidian m., m. cotidiana; m. na qual os acessos ocorrem diariamente; geralmente uma m. terçã dupla, na qual há uma infecção por dois grupos distintos de parasitas *Plasmodium vivax* que formam esporos alternadamente a cada 48 horas, mas também pode ser uma infecção pela forma perniciosa do parasita da malária, *P. falciparum*, combinado ao *P. vivax*, ou infecção por duas gerações distintas de *P. falciparum*, que amadurecem em dias diferentes; também pode desenvolver-se a partir da infecção por *P. knowlesi*. SIN quotidian fever.

relapsing m., m. recorrente; renovação da atividade clínica algum tempo após o ataque primário.

remittent m., m. remitente; febre malárica, geralmente do grave tipo falcíparo, na qual a temperatura cai, mas não chega a atingir o nível normal, durante o intervalo entre dois fortes acessos.

simian m., m. dos símios; infecção de macacos e símios por plasmódios, como a malária humana, transmitida principalmente por mosquitos anofelinos; é causada por várias espécies de *Plasmodium*, sendo o Sudeste Asiático e a África os aparentes centros de evolução; entre os 20 plasmódios descritos em primatas não-humanos, alguns se assemelham, induzindo uma infecção malárica semelhante à causada pelas quatro espécies de *Plasmodium* que acometem o homem, das quais os agentes da m. humana parecem ser derivados. SIN monkey m.

tertian m., m. terçã. SIN vivax m.

therapeutic m., m. terapêutica; malária induzida intencionalmente, outrora empregada contra a neurossífilis e algumas outras doenças paralíticas. SIN malariotherapy.

vivax m., m. vivax; febre malárica com acessos que, tipicamente, recorrem a cada 48 horas ou em dias alternados (a cada três dias, considerando-se como primeiro dia o do acesso); a febre é induzida por liberação de merozoítas e sua invasão de novas hemácias. SIN benign tertian fever, benign tertian m., tertian fever, tertian m., vivax fever.

ma·lar·i·al (mă-lār′ē-ăl). Malárico; relativo a, ou afetado por, malária.

ma·lar·i·ol·o·gy (mă-lār-ē-ol′ō-jē). Malariologia; estudo da malária em todos os aspectos, com referência particular à sua epidemiologia e controle.

ma·lar·i·o·ther·a·py (ma-lar-ē-ō-ther′a-pē). Malarioterapia. SIN therapeutic *malaria*.

ma·lar·i·ous (mă-lār′ē-ŭs). Malarioso; relativo a, ou caracterizado pela, prevalência de malária.

Malassez, Louis C., fisiologista francês, 1842–1910. VER *Malassezia*; M. epithelial *rests*, em *rest*.

Ma·las·sez·ia (mal-ă-sā′zē-ă). Gênero de fungos (família Cryptococcaceae) de baixa patogenicidade que não tem a capacidade de sintetizar ácidos graxos de cadeias média e longa, e requer um suprimento exógeno desses lipídios para seu crescimento, como se pode encontrar na pele. [L.C. *Malassez*]

M. fur·fur, espécie de fungo que pertence à flora cutânea normal, mas que pode causar tinha versicolor, foliculite ou fungemia em pacientes que recebem lipídios intravenosos. SIN *Pityrosporum orbiculare, Pityrosporum ovale*.

M. ova·lis, espécie de levedura encontrada nas escamas epidérmicas superficiais e nos folículos pilosos na pele oleosa, de patogenicidade limítrofe; pode causar dermatite seborreica associada à imunodeficiência.

M. pachydermatis, fungo ocasionalmente isolado de lesões cutâneas de seres humanos e animais; uma causa rara de fungemia em pacientes que recebem lipídios intravenosos.

mal·as·sim·i·la·tion (mal′ă-sim-i-lā′shŭn). Má assimilação; termo raramente usado para designar a assimilação incompleta ou imperfeita; má absorção.

ma·late (mal′āt). Malato; sal ou éster do ácido málico.

m. dehydrogenase, m. desidrogenase; enzima que catalisa, através do NAD^+ ou do $NADP^+$, a desidrogenação do malato em oxaloacetato, ou sua descarboxilação em piruvato e CO_2. São conhecidas pelo menos seis malato desidrogenases, diferenciadas por seus produtos, uso de NAD^+ ou $NADP^+$, e especificidade do substrato (uma atua sobre o D-malato; as outras atuam sobre o L-malato); uma é uma enzima do ciclo do ácido tricarboxílico. SIN malic acid dehydrogenase, malic dehydrogenase, malic enzyme, pyruvic-malic carboxylase.

m. synthase, m. sintase; enzima que catalisa a condensação reversível da acetil-CoA com glioxilato e água para formar L-malato e coenzima A; uma enzima no ciclo do glioxilato. SIN glyoxylate transacetylase, malate-condensing enzyme.

mal·a·thi·on (mal-ă-thī′on, mă-lā′thi-on). Malation; malatião; composto organofosforado usado como inseticida e ectoparasiticida veterinário; considerado menos tóxico que o paration.

mal·ax·a·tion (mal′ak-sā′shŭn). Malaxação. **1.** Formação de ingredientes em uma massa para comprimidos e emplastros. **2.** Um processo de fazer massagem. [L. *malaxo*, pp. *-atus*, amolecer]

mal·di·ges·tion (mal-dī-jes′chŭn). Má digestão; digestão imperfeita.

Mal·do·na·do-San Jo·se stain. Corante de Maldonado-São José. VER em *stain*.

male (māl). Macho. **1.** Em zoologia, designa o sexo ao qual pertencem aqueles que produzem espermatozóides; um indivíduo desse sexo. **2.** SIN masculine. [L. *masculus*, de *mas*, macho]
  genetic human m., m. genético humano; **(1)** um indivíduo cujo cariótipo contém um cromossoma Y; **(2)** um indivíduo cujos núcleos celulares não contêm os corpúsculos de cromatina sexual de Barr, que estão normalmente presentes nas fêmeas. Os pacientes com desenvolvimento sexual ambíguo e aqueles com síndrome de Turner são classificados como machos genéticos ou fêmeas genéticas de acordo com a ausência ou presença de corpúsculos de Barr, embora seu complemento cromossômico sexual possa sugerir outra coisa.
  XX m., m. XX; um fenótipo masculino evidente na presença de um cariótipo 46,XX; provavelmente, as partes vitais do cromossoma Y estão localizadas em outro lugar no genoma em virtude de translocação, ao menos em algumas dessas pessoas.
  XXY m., m. XXY. VER Klinefelter *syndrome*.
  XYY m., m. XYY. VER XYY *syndrome*.
Malecot, Achille-Etienne, cirurgião francês, *1852. VER M. *catheter*.
ma·le·ic ac·id (mā - lē'ik). Ácido maleico; ácido butenodióico; o isômero *cis* do ácido fumárico; usado no preparo de sais maleato de anti-histamínicos e substâncias semelhantes. SIN toxilic acid.
mal·e·mis·sion (mal - ē - mish'ŭn). Má emissão; incapacidade de ejetar sêmen do pênis durante o orgasmo. [mal- + L. *e-mitto*, pp. *missus*, emitir]
mal·e·rup·tion (mal - ē - rŭp'shŭn). Má erupção; erupção imperfeita dos dentes.
ma·ley·lac·e·to·ac·e·tate (mal'a - il - as'e - tō - as'ē - tāt). Maleilacetoacetato; intermediário no catabolismo da L-fenilalanina e L-tirosina; acumula-se em determinados distúrbios hereditários do metabolismo da tirosina.
  m. cis, trans-isomerase, m. *cis, trans*-isomerase; enzima que catalisa a conversão reversível de maleilacetoacetato em 4-fumarilacetoacetato; enzima que participa do catabolismo da L-tirosina; a deficiência dessa enzima está associada com tirosinemia tipo IB.
mal·for·ma·tion (mal - fōr - mā'shŭn). Má-formação; malformação; ausência de desenvolvimento apropriado ou normal; mais especificamente, um defeito estrutural primário que resulta de um erro localizado da morfogênese; p. ex., fenda labial. Cf. deformation.
  Arnold-Chiari m., m. de Arnold-Chiari; má-formação das estruturas da fossa posterior associada à tração caudal e ao deslocamento do rombencéfalo, causada por aprisionamento da medula espinal; pode ou não ser acompanhada por espina bífida e anomalias associadas como meningomielocele; essa má-formação geralmente tem herança multifatorial; há evidências muito fracas de herança autossômica recessiva [MIM*207950]. SIN Arnold-Chiari deformity, Arnold-Chiari syndrome, cerebellomedullary malformation syndrome.
  cystic adenomatoid m., m. adenomatóide cística; anormalidade congênita rara do broto pulmonar, que resulta em natimorto, doença respiratória progressiva aguda de recém-nascidos, ou pneumonias infantis prolongadas; essa má-formação combina aspectos de um hamartoma, crescimento displásico e crescimento tumoral. Já foram descritos três tipos, com base principalmente nos diâmetros do cisto: Tipo I: até 10 cm; Tipo II: menos de 1,2 cm; Tipo III: menos de 0,5 cm.
  mermaid m., m. da sereia; sirenomelia. SIN sirenomelia.
  Michel m., m. de Michel; hipoplasia da pirâmide petrosa e aplasia da orelha interna.
  venous m., m. venosa. SIN venous *angioma*.
mal·func·tion (mal - fŭnk'shŭn). Disfunção; função desordenada, inadequada ou anormal.
Malgaigne, Joseph F., cirurgião francês, 1806–1865. VER M. *amputation, fossa, hernia, luxation, triangle*.
Malherbe, Albert, 1845–1915. VER M. calcifying *epithelioma*.
mal·ic ac·id (mal'ik, mā'lik). Ácido málico; ácido hidroxissuccínico; um ácido encontrado em maçãs e em várias outras frutas ácidas; intermediário no ciclo do ácido tricarboxílico, no ciclo do glioxilato e em um sistema transportador bidirecional. SIN monohydroxysuccinic acid.
mal·ic ac·id de·hy·dro·gen·ase. Ácido málico desidrogenase. SIN malate dehydrogenase.
mal·ic de·hy·dro·gen·ase. Desidrogenase málica. SIN malate dehydrogenase.
ma·lig·nan·cy (ma - lig'nan - sē). Malignidade; a propriedade ou condição de ser maligno.
ma·lig·nant (mă - lig'nănt). Maligno. **1.** Resistente ao tratamento; que ocorre na forma grave e, freqüentemente, fatal; que tende a se agravar e cuja evolução é para pior. **2.** Em referência a uma neoplasia, que tem a propriedade de crescimento localmente invasivo e destrutivo e metástase. [L. *maligno*, p. pres. *-ans (ant-)*, realizar algo maliciosamente]
ma·lin·ger (mă - ling'ger). Simular; exercer a simulação.
ma·lin·ger·er (mă - ling'ger - er). Simulador; alguém que simula.
ma·lin·ger·ing (mă - ling'ger - ing). Simulação; fingimento de doença ou incapacidade para faltar ao trabalho, provocar simpatia ou obter recompensa. [Fr. *malingre*, inferior, fracamente]

mal·in·ter·dig·i·ta·tion (mal'in - ter - dij'i - tā'shŭn). Má interdigitação; interdigitação defeituosa das cúspides dentárias.
Mall, Franklin Paine, anatomista e embriologista norte-americano, 1862–1917. VER M. *formula, ridges,* em *ridge;* periportal *space* of M.
mal·le·a·ble (mal'ē - ă - bl). Maleável; capaz de ser moldado por batidas ou compressão; propriedade de alguns metais, como o ouro e a prata. [L. *malleus,* martelo]
mal·le·brin (mal'e - brin). Malebrina. SIN aluminum chlorate nonahydrate.
mal·le·o·in·cu·dal (mal'ē - ō - ing'koo - dăl). Maleoincudal; relativo ao martelo e à bigorna no tímpano.
mal·le·o·lar (mă - lē'ō - lăr). Maleolar; relativo a um ou a ambos os maléolos.
mal·le·o·lus, pl. **mal·le·o·li** (ma - lē'ō - lŭs, - lī) [TA]. Maléolo; proeminência óssea arredondada, como aquelas de cada lado da articulação do tornozelo. [L. dim. de *malleus,* martelo]
  external m., m. externo, m. lateral. SIN lateral m.
  inner m., m. interno, m. medial. SIN medial m.
  internal m., m. interno, m. medial. SIN medial m.
  lateral m. [TA], m. lateral; o processo na face lateral da extremidade inferior da fíbula, formando a projeção da parte lateral do tornozelo; o maléolo lateral estende-se mais inferiormente que o maléolo medial. SIN m. lateralis [TA], external m., extramalleolus, outer m.
  m. latera'lis [TA], m. lateral. SIN lateral m.
  medial m. [TA], m. medial; o processo na face medial da extremidade inferior da tíbia, formando a projeção da face medial do tornozelo; o maléolo medial situa-se superior ao nível do maléolo lateral. SIN m. medialis [TA], inner m., internal m.
  m. media'lis [TA], m. medial. SIN medial m.
  outer m., m. externo. SIN lateral m.
mal·le·ot·o·my (mal'ē - ot'ō - mē). Maleotomia; divisão do martelo. [malleus + G. *tomē,* incisão]
mal·le·us, gen. e pl. **mal·lei** (mal'ē - ŭs, mal'ē - ī) [TA]. Martelo; o maior dos três ossículos da audição, semelhante a uma clava, e não a um martelo; considera-se que possui uma cabeça, abaixo da qual está o colo, e deste diverge o cabo ou manúbrio, bem como o delgado processo anterior; da base do manúbrio origina-se o curto processo lateral. O manúbrio e o processo lateral estão firmemente fixados à membrana timpânica, e a cabeça articula-se com uma superfície em forma de sela no corpo da bigorna. SIN hammer. [L. martelo]
Mal·loph·a·ga (mă - lof'ă - gă). Ordem de piolhos picadores que causam irritação por se alimentarem nos pêlos, penas e pele, e de sangue e exsudatos quando presentes; a maioria das espécies é encontrada em aves, mas algumas são encontradas em animais domésticos comuns. Os gêneros *Menacanthus* e *Menopon* (família Menoponidae) atacam as aves domésticas, bem como *Columbicola, Chelopistes, Lipeurus* e outros gêneros da família Philopteridae, enquanto os gêneros *Bovicola, Felicola* e *Trichodectes* (família Trichodectidae) infestam mamíferos domésticos. [G. *mallos,* lã, + *phagein,* comer]
Mallory, Frank B., patologista norte-americano, 1862–1941. VER M. *bodies,* em *body;* picro-M. trichrome *stain*. VER entradas em stain.
Mallory, G. Kenneth, patologista norte-americano, *1926. VER M.-Weiss *lesion, syndrome, tear*.
mal·nu·tri·tion (mal - noo - trish'ŭn). Desnutrição; nutrição inadequada resultante de má absorção, dieta insatisfatória ou da ingestão excessiva.
  malignant m., d. maligna. SIN kwashiorkor.
  protein m., d. proteica; subnutrição resultante da ingestão inadequada de proteínas; as manifestações características incluem edema nutricional (nutritional *edema*), kwashiorkor.
mal·oc·clu·sion (mal - ō - kloo'zhŭn). Má oclusão. **1.** Qualquer desvio de um contato fisiologicamente aceitável de dentições opostas. **2.** Qualquer desvio de uma oclusão normal.
mal·on·ate (măl'on - āt). Malonato; o sal ou éster do ácido malônico.
mal·on·ate sem·i·al·de·hyde. Malonato semi-aldeído; o produto transaminado da β-alanina; elevado na hiper-β-alaninemia.
Maloney bou·gies. Velas de Maloney. VER em bougie.
ma·lo·nic ac·id (mă - lō'nik, - lon'ik). Ácido malônico; ácido dicarboxílico importante no metabolismo intermediário; um inibidor da succinato desidrogenase. SIN propanedioic acid.
mal·o·nyl (mal'ō - nil). Malonil; a porção divalente derivada do ácido malônico.
  m. transacylase, m. transacilase. SIN ACP-malonyltransferase.
mal·o·nyl-CoA. Malonil-CoA; o produto de condensação do ácido malônico e da coenzima A, um intermediário na biossíntese dos ácidos graxos. SIN malonylcoenzyme A.
mal·o·nyl·co·en·zyme A (mal'ō - nil - kō - en'zīm). Malonilcoenzima A. SIN malonyl-CoA.
mal·o·nyl·u·rea (mal'ō - nil - ū - rē'ă). Maloniluréia. SIN barbituric acid.
Malpighi, Marcello, anatomista, histologista e embriologista italiano, 1628–1694. VER malpighian *bodies,* em *body;* malpighian *capsule;* malpighian *cell;* malpighian *corpuscles,* em *corpuscle;* malpighian *glands,* em *gland;* malpighian

glomerulus; malpighian *layer;* malpighian *nodules,* em *nodule;* malpighian *pyramid;* malpighian *rete;* malpighian *stigmas,* em *stigma;* malpighian *stratum;* malpighian *tubules,* em *tubule;* malpighian *tuft;* malpighian *vesicles,* em *vesicle.*

mal·pi·ghi·an (mahl - pig′ē - an). De Malpighi; descrito por, ou atribuído a, Marcello Malpighi.

mal·po·si·tion (mal - pō - zish′ŭn). Posição anormal; posição anômala; distopia. SIN dystopia.

mal·prac·tice (mal - prak′tis). Tratamento errado de um paciente por imperícia, imprudência, negligência ou intenção criminal.

mal·pre·sen·ta·tion (mal′prē - sen - tā′shŭn). Apresentação anômala; apresentação anormal do feto; apresentação de qualquer outra parte, afora o occipúcio.

mal·ro·ta·tion (mal - rō - tā′shŭn). Má rotação; rotação anômala; falha, durante o desenvolvimento embrionário, da rotação normal completa ou parcial de um órgão ou sistema, como o tubo digestivo ou o rim.

MALT Abreviatura de mucosa-associated lymphoid *tissue* (tecido linfóide associado a mucosa).

malt (mawlt). Malte; a semente da cevada ou de outro cereal, artificialmente germinada e seca, que contém dextrina, maltose, pequenas quantidades de glicose e enzimas amilolíticas. Usado na forma de extrato como um agente digestivo e flavorizante. [A.S. *mealt*]

malt·ase (mawl - tās). Maltase. VER α-D-glicosidase.
  acid m., m. ácida. SIN exo-1,4-α-D-glucosidase.

mal·to·bi·ose (mawl - tō - bī′ōs). Maltobiose. SIN maltose.

MALToma. MALToma; linfoma de células B do tecido linfóide associado à mucosa. SIN extranodal marginal zone lymphoma.

mal·tose (mawl′ - tōs). Maltose; dissacarídeo formado na hidrólise do amido e que consiste em dois resíduos D-glicose mantidos juntos por uma ligação 1,4-α-glicosídeo. SIN malt sugar, maltobiose.

mal·to·tet·rose (mawl - tō - tet′rōs). Maltotetrose; sacarídeo composto por quatro unidades D-glicose na ligação α-1,4.

ma·lum (mā′lŭm). Mal; uma doença. [L. um mal]
  m. artic'ulorum seni'lis, mal senil das articulações; artrite no idoso.
  m. per'forans pe'dis, m. perfurante plantar; úlcera perfurante do pé que ocorre em algumas neuropatias.
  m. vene'reum, sífilis. SIN syphilis.

mal·un·ion (mal - ūn′yŭn). Consolidação viciosa; união das extremidades de um osso fraturado em posição defeituosa, resultando em deformidade ou curvatura do membro; freqüentemente usado como sinônimo de consolidação defeituosa. SIN vicious union.

ma·man·pi·an (mä - mon - pē - on′). Termo usado antigamente para boubamãe (mother *yaw*). [Fr. *maman,* mãe, + *pian,* bouba]

mam·e·lon (mam′e - lon). Mamelão; uma das proeminências arredondadas, em número de três, na borda de corte de um dente incisivo quando irrompe da gengiva. [Fr. mamilo]

mam·e·lon·at·ed (mam′e - lon - āt - ed). Mamelonado; que possui elevações arredondadas, mamiliformes; noduladas. [Fr. *mamelon,* mamilo]

mam·e·lo·na·tion (mam′e - lō - nā′shŭn). Mamelonação; a formação de projeções arredondadas ou nódulos em estruturas ósseas e outras.

⚠ **mamil-, mamilli-.** Os mamilos. VER TAMBÉM mammil-. Cf. thelo-. [L. *mamilla,* mamilo]

mam·ma, gen. e pl. **mam·mae** (mam′ă, mam′ē) [TA]. Mama. SIN breast. VER TAMBÉM mammary *gland.* [L.]
  m. accesso'ria [TA], m. acessória. SIN accessory *breast.*
  m. errat'ica, m. errática; uma mama supranumerária em localização aberrante, isto é, em alguma outra parte fora da linha láctea.
  m. masculi'na [TA], m. masculina. SIN male *breast.*
  supernumerary m., m. supranumerária. SIN accessory *breast.*
  m. viri'lis, m. masculina. SIN male *breast.*

mam·mal (mam′ăl). Mamífero; animal da classe Mammalia.

mam·mal·gia (mă - mal′jē - ă). Mamalgia. SIN mastodynia. [L. *mamma,* mama, + G. *algos,* dor]

Mam·ma·lia (mă - mā′lē - ă). A classe mais elevada de organismos vivos; inclui todos os animais vertebrados (monotremados, marsupiais e placentários) que amamentam seus filhotes, possuem pêlos e (exceto os monotremados que põem ovos) dão à luz filhos vivos, em vez de ovos. [L. *mamma,* mama]

mam·ma·plas·ty (mam′ă - plas - tē). Mamoplastia; cirurgia plástica da mama para modificar seu formato, tamanho ou posição, ou todos esses elementos. SIN mammoplasty, mastoplasty. [L. *mamma,* mama, + G. *plastos,* formado]
  augmentation m., m. de aumento; cirurgia plástica para aumentar a mama, freqüentemente por inserção de um implante.
  reconstructive m., m. reconstrutora; confecção de uma mama simulada por cirurgia plástica, para substituir uma mama que foi retirada.
  reduction m., m. redutora; cirurgia plástica da mama para reduzir seu tamanho e (freqüentemente) melhorar seu formato e posição.

mam·ma·ry (mam′ă - rē). Mamário; relativo às mamas.

mam·mec·to·my (ma - mek′tō - mē). Mamectomia. SIN mastectomy. [L. *mamma,* mama, + *ektomē,* excisão]

mam·mi·form (mam′i - form). Mamiforme; que se assemelha a uma mama; em formato de mama. SIN mammose (1). [L. *mama,* mama, + *forma,* forma]

⚠ **mammil-, mammilli-.** Mamil-, mamili-; os mamilos. VER TAMBÉM mamil-. Cf. thelo-. [L. *mammilla (mamilla),* mamilo]

mam·mil·la, pl. **mam·mil·lae** (mă - mil′ă, mă - mil′ē). **1.** Pequena elevação arredondada semelhante à mama feminina. **2.** Mamilo. SIN nipple. [L. mamilo]

mam·mil·la·plas·ty (ma - mil′ă - plas - tē). Mamiloplastia; cirurgia plástica do mamilo e da aréola. [L. *mammilla,* mamilo, + G. *plastos,* formado]

mam·mil·la·re (mam - i - lā′rē) [TA]. Mamilar. SIN mammillary. [L.]

mam·mil·lar·ia. VER mammillary *body.*

mam·mil·lary (mam′i - lār - ē) [TA]. Mamilar; relativo ou com o formato semelhante ao de um mamilo. SIN mammillare [TA].

mam·mil·late (mam′i - lāt). Mamilado; repleto de projeções semelhantes a mamilos.

mam·mi·la·tion (mam - i - lā′shŭn). Mamiloso. **1.** Projeção semelhante a um mamilo. **2.** A condição de possuir mamilo.

mam·mil·li·form (mă - mil′i - form). Mamiliforme; em forma de mamilo. [L. *mamilla,* mamilo, + *forma,* forma]

mam·mil·li·tis (mam - i - lī′tis). Mamilite; inflamação do mamilo. [L. *mamilla,* mamilo, + G. *-itis,* inflamação]

⚠ **mammo-.** Mamo-; as mamas. Cf. masto-. [L. *mamma,* mama]

ℹ **mam·mo·gram** (mam′ō - gram). Mamograma; o registro produzido por mamografia.

ℹ **mam·mog·ra·phy** (ma - mog′ră - fē). Mamografia; exame radiológico da mama feminina com equipamento e técnicas designados para rastreamento de câncer. [mammo- + G. *graphō,* escrever]

A mamografia consegue detectar carcinoma da mama algumas vezes até 2 anos antes de se tornar palpável e, em muitos casos, antes de haver metástase para linfonodos. Os achados mamográficos que constituem forte sugestão de carcinoma são microcalcificações e densidades mal definidas no tecido mamário. Entretanto, esses achados são inespecíficos e a probabilidade cumulativa de uma mulher ter uma mamografia falso-positiva durante 10 anos de exames anuais aproxima-se dos 50%. A cintimamografia após injeção intravenosa de sestamibi-Tc99m pode ser usada para acompanhamento de uma mamografia questionável. A tomografia por emissão de pósitrons (PET) mostrou-se promissora na discriminação entre massas benignas e malignas da mama, bem como na detecção de metástases para linfonodos axilares em pacientes com câncer de mama recém-diagnosticado e de metástases a distância em pacientes com carcinoma da mama avançado ou recorrente. Devido ao alto custo desse procedimento, seu uso atualmente é limitado a pacientes de alto risco e com mamas densas. A importância da mamografia na detecção precoce do câncer de mama foi bem estabelecida em mulheres de risco médio, entre 50 e 69 anos. Nesse grupo, a mamografia anual reduz em 30-40% a taxa de mortalidade por câncer de mama. A análise de muitos estudos clínicos revelou que a mamografia pode não salvar vidas de mulheres com menos de 50 anos (apenas 17% de todos os cânceres de mama ocorrem em mulheres com menos de 40 anos). A maior densidade do tecido mamário em mulheres jovens limita a capacidade da radiografia de identificar tumores em mulheres de 40 a 50 anos, situação em que é preferível usar a ultra-sonografia para avaliação de lesões mamárias palpáveis. A pesquisa sugeriu que, em uma pequena fração de mulheres, a exposição à radiação durante a mamografia pode, na verdade, deflagrar um câncer de mama. A *American Cancer Society,* o *National Cancer Institute* e o *American College of Radiology* recomendam uma mamografia aos 40 anos para ser tomada como referência e mamografias anuais após os 50 anos. No caso de mulheres sob risco especial em virtude de história familiar, deve-se começar a realizar mamografia aos 25 anos de idade. Como cerca de 10% dos cânceres de mama que podem ser percebidos ao exame não são detectados pela mamografia, também é recomendado o exame anual das mamas por um médico. A vigilância pela *Food and Drug Administration* mostrou um aumento da sensibilidade das mamografias nos últimos 5 anos, devido principalmente a aperfeiçoamentos nos sistemas de écran e filme. Uma técnica de exame digital aprovada em 1998 aumenta ainda mais a detecção de microcalcificações e massas espiculadas à mamografia. Entretanto, a mamografia ainda é um procedimento de rastreamento, e o diagnóstico de lesões mamárias depende do exame físico e dos achados à biopsia. Uma lei federal exige que todas as instituições nos Estados Unidos que realizam mamografia entreguem a cada paciente um laudo dos resultados em linguagem simples e clara no prazo de 30 dias após o exame, além de um laudo detalhado para o médico solicitante. VER TAMBÉM carcinoma of the breast.

Mam·mo·mon·o·ga·mus (mam′ō - mon - og′ă - mus). Gênero de trematódeo singamídeo (família Syngamidae) encontrado no sistema respiratório de ruminantes e ocasionalmente descrito em seres humanos; os vermes geralmente se juntam em uma formação em Y.

M. laryngeus, nematódeo encontrado nas vias respiratórias superiores de alguns mamíferos; já foram descritos aproximadamente 100 casos humanos, a maioria nas ilhas do Caribe; o verme é vermelho ou castanho-avermelhado; ao copularem, o macho e a fêmea assumem a forma de um Y; o ciclo vital não é conhecido.

mam·mo·plas·ty (mam′o - plas - tē). Mamoplastia. SIN mammaplasty. [mammo- + G. *plastos,* formado]

mam·mose (mam′mōs). Mamose. **1.** SIN mammiform. **2.** Que possui grandes mamas.

mam·mo·so·ma·to·troph (mam′o - sō - mat′o - trof). Mamossomatotrofo; uma célula da adeno-hipófise que produz prolactina e somatotropina.

mam·mot·o·my (ma - mot′o - mē). Mamotomia. SIN mastotomy. [mammo- + G. *tomē,* incisão]

mam·mo·troph (mam′o - trof). Mamotrofo; uma célula acidófila da adeno-hipófise que produz prolactina. SIN prolactin cell.

mam·mo·tro·pic, mam·mo·tro·phic (mam - ō - trop′ik, - trof′ik). Mamotrópico, mamotrófico; que possui um efeito estimulante sobre o desenvolvimento, crescimento ou função das glândulas mamárias. [mammo- + G. *tropos,* uma volta]

mam·mo·tro·pin, mam·mo·tro·phin (mam - ō - trō′pin, - trō′fin). Mamotropina, mamotrofina; termo obsoleto para prolactina.

Man Símbolo de mannose and mannosyl (manose e manosil).

management. Administração; gerenciamento; gestão.

case m., gerenciamento de casos; processo no qual são identificadas pessoas seguradas com necessidades de saúde específicas, e é formulado e implementado um plano de tratamento eficiente para produzir os resultados mais custo-efetivos.

component m., gerenciamento de componentes; a abordagem de contenção de custos em saúde que envolve a tentativa de controle de componentes individuais como custos de medicamentos, hospitalização ou testes laboratoriais. VER TAMBÉM managed *care.*

man·chette (man - shet′). Punho, bainha; arranjo cônico de microtúbulos que reveste o núcleo de uma espermátide; acredita-se que participe na moldagem do núcleo durante a espermatogênese. [Fr. punho, dim. de *manche,* manga, do L. *manicae;* de *manus,* mão]

man·del·ate (man′de - lāt). Mandelato; um sal ou éster do ácido mandélico.

man·del·ic ac·id (man - del′ik). Ácido mandélico; agente antibacteriano urinário (bactericida e bacteriostático). SIN hydroxytoluic acid, phenylglycolic acid. [Al. *Mandel,* amêndoa]

Mandelin re·a·gent. Reagente de Mandelin. VER em reagent.

man·de·lyt·ro·pine (man - de - lit′rō - pēn). Mandelitropina. SIN homatropine.

man·di·ble (man′di - bl) [TA]. Mandíbula; osso em formato de U (em vista superior), que forma o maxilar inferior, articulando-se por suas extremidades voltadas para cima com o osso temporal de cada lado. SIN mandibula [TA], jaw bone, lower jaw, mandibulum, submaxilla.

man·dib·u·la, pl. **man·dib·u·lae** (man - dib′u - lă, - lē) [TA]. Mandíbula. SIN mandible. [L. mandíbula, de *mando,* pp. *mansus,* mastigar]

man·dib·u·lar (man - dib′u - lăr). Mandibular; relativo à mandíbula. SIN inframaxillary, submaxillary (1).

man·dib·u·lec·to·my (man - dib - ū - lek′to - mē). Mandibulectomia; ressecção da mandíbula. [mandibula + G. *ektomē,* excisão]

man·dib·u·lo·fa·cial (man - dib′u - lō - fā′shăl). Mandibulofacial; relativo à mandíbula e à face.

man·dib·u·lo·oc·u·lo·fa·cial (man - dib′u - lō - ok′u - lō - fā′shăl). Mandibulo-oculofacial; relativo à mandíbula e à face.

man·dib·u·lo·pha·ryn·ge·al (man - dib′u - lō - fa - rin′jē - ăl). Mandibulofaríngeo; relativo à mandíbula e à faringe; designa a região entre a faringe e o ramo da mandíbula, na qual são encontrados a artéria carótida interna, a veia jugular interna e os nervos vago, glossofaríngeo, acessório e hipoglosso.

mand·ib·u·lum (man - dib′u - lŭm). Mandíbula. SIN mandible.

man·drag·o·ra (man - drag′o - ră). Mandrágora; a mandrágora européia, *Mandragora officinalis,* ou *Atropa mandragora* (família Solanaceae), a mandrágora da Bíblia; suas propriedades são semelhantes às do estramônio, hiosciamo e da beladona. [G. *mandragoras*]

man·drake (man′drāk). Mandrágora. **1.** VER mandragora. **2.** VER podophyllum. [pelo L., do G. *mandragoras*]

wild m., m. selvagem. SIN podophyllum *resin.*

man·drel, man·dril. Mandril. **1.** A haste ou eixo ao qual um instrumento é fixado, e por meio do qual é rodado. **2.** SIN mandrin. **3.** Em odontologia, um instrumento manual para segurar um disco, pedra ou taça, usado para moldar, polir ou fazer acabamento. [G. *mandra,* estável; um estábulo; o leito em que se coloca a pedra de um anel]

man·drill. Mandril; nome comum de uma espécie de macaco do gênero *Cynocephalus,* com cauda curta e cabeça semelhante à de um cão.

man·drin. Mandril; fio rígido ou estilete introduzido na luz de um cateter flexível para dar formato e firmeza na passagem através de uma estrutura tubular oca. SIN mandrel (2), mandril. [Fr. *mandrin,* mandril]

ma·neu·ver (mă - noo′ver). Manobra; movimento ou procedimento planejado. [Fr. *manoeuvre,* do L. *manu operari,* trabalhar com as mãos]

Adson m., m. de Adson. SIN Adson *test.*

Barlow m., m. de Barlow; pesquisa de instabilidade do quadril, havendo luxação quando é realizada flexão, adução e aplicada força posterior. SIN Barlow test.

Bill m., m. de Bill; rotação da cabeça fetal com um fórceps na região média da pelve antes da extração da cabeça.

Bracht m., m. de Bracht; desprendimento de um feto em posição pélvica por extensão das pernas e tronco do feto sobre a sínfise púbica e o abdome da mãe; a cabeça fetal se desprende espontaneamente enquanto as pernas e o tronco são levantados acima da pelve materna, e enquanto o corpo do lactente é estendido pelo operador.

Buzzard m., m. de Buzzard; teste do reflexo patelar com o paciente sentado fazendo firme pressão sobre o assoalho com os dedos dos pés.

Credé m.'s, manobras de Credé. SIN Credé *methods,* em *method.*

Dix-Hallpike m., m. de Dix-Hallpike; teste para produzir vertigem paroxística e nistagmo, no qual o paciente em posição sentada é colocado em decúbito dorsal com a cabeça pendente sobre a mesa de exame e virado para a direita ou esquerda; ocorrem vertigem e nistagmo quando a cabeça é rodada em direção ao ouvido afetado.

Ejrup m., m. de Ejrup; demonstração de circulação colateral por redução da proeminência da atividade das artérias maiores e reduzido volume de pulso após atividade muscular.

Hampton m., m. de Hampton; rolar um paciente em decúbito dorsal para o lado direito e, depois, para o lado esquerdo a fim de obter uma radiografia contrastada com ar do antro e duodeno, cheios de contraste na fluoroscopia gastrointestinal.

Heimlich m., m. de Heimlich; ação designada para expelir um bolo de alimento obstrutor da garganta colocando-se um punho sobre o abdome entre o umbigo e a margem costal, segurando o punho por detrás, com a outra mão, e empurrando-o para dentro e para cima de forma a forçar a subida do diafragma, levando o ar da traquéia para cima e deslocando a obstrução.

Hillis-Müller m., m. de Hillis-Müller; compressão manual do fundo uterino a termo enquanto um dedo na vagina determina a insinuação da cabeça na pelve.

Hueter m., m. de Hueter; compressão da língua do paciente para baixo e para diante com o dedo indicador esquerdo ao se introduzir uma sonda gástrica.

Jendrassik m., m. de Jendrassik; método para realçar o reflexo patelar; o indivíduo junta as mãos com os dedos entrelaçados e fletidos e puxa, tentando separá-las, com toda a força.

LeCompte m., m. de LeCompte; reparo de dupla via de saída do ventrículo direito com estenose pulmonar e outras anormalidades da junção ventrículo-arterial e comunicação interventricular, na qual o VE (ventrículo esquerdo) está ligado à aorta e o VD (ventrículo direito) à artéria pulmonar, utilizando uma técnica que não requer um conduto extracardíaco. SIN LeCompte operation.

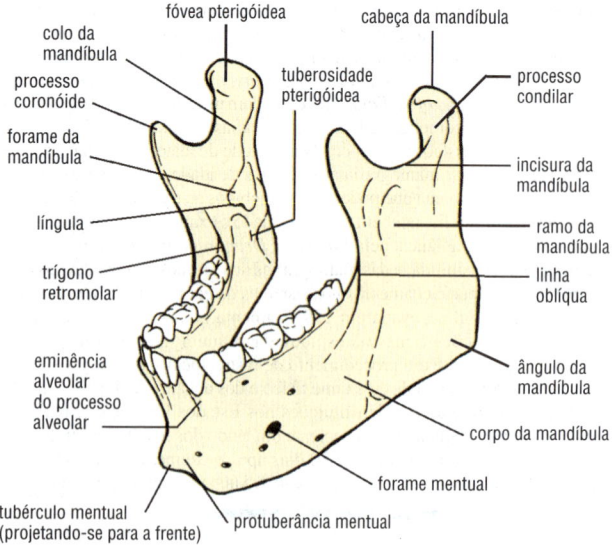

mandíbula: vista frontal esquerda

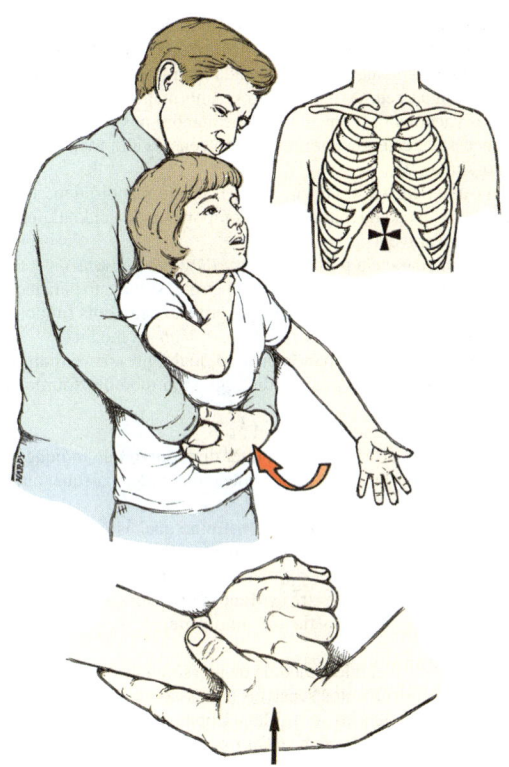

manobra de Heimlich

Leopold m.'s, manobras de Leopold; quatro manobras empregadas para determinar a posição fetal: 1) determinação do que se encontra no fundo; 2) avaliação do dorso e dos membros fetais; 3) palpação da parte de apresentação acima da sínfise; 4) determinação da direção e do grau de flexão da cabeça.
load-and-shift m., m. de pressão e deslocamento; teste para determinar a instabilidade do ombro, no qual a cabeça do úmero é empurrada contra a glenóide e deslocada para frente e para trás.
Mauriceau m., m. de Mauriceau; método de parto pélvico assistido no qual o corpo do lactente é montado sobre o antebraço direito, e o dedo médio da mão direita é colocado na boca do feto para manter a flexão enquanto se faz tração sobre os ombros com a outra mão. SIN Mauriceau-Levret m.
Mauriceau-Levret m., m. de Mauriceau-Levret. SIN Mauriceau m.
McDonald m., m. de McDonald; medida do útero da borda superior da sínfise até uma linha tangencial ao fundo sobre o abdome com uma fita para determinar a altura do útero; cada centímetro corresponde aproximadamente à idade gestacional em semanas entre 20 e 34 semanas de gestação.
McRoberts m., m. de McRoberts; manobra para reduzir uma distocia do ombro fetal por flexão dos quadris maternos.
Müller m., m. de Müller; após expiração forçada, é feita uma tentativa de inspiração com a boca e o nariz fechados ou com a glote fechada, pela qual a pressão negativa no tórax e nos pulmões se torna muito menor que a atmosférica; o inverso da manobra de Valsalva.
Ortolani m., m. de Ortolani; manobra para redução de luxação do quadril, utilizando flexão e abdução da coxa com movimento para a frente da cabeça do fêmur; a redução é acompanhada por reposicionamento palpável da cabeça do fêmur no acetábulo. SIN Ortolani test.
Phalen m., m. de Phalen; manobra pela qual o punho é mantido em flexão volar; a ocorrência de parestesia na distribuição do nervo mediano em 60 segundos pode indicar síndrome do túnel do carpo.
Pinard m., m. de Pinard; no tratamento de uma apresentação pélvica evidente, comprime-se o espaço poplíteo com o dedo indicador, enquanto os outros três dedos fletem a perna, fazendo-a deslizar ao longo da outra coxa, com o pé da perna fletida sendo trazido para baixo e para fora.
Ritgen m., m. de Ritgen; desprendimento da cabeça de uma criança por pressão sobre o períneo, enquanto se controla a velocidade do desprendimento por pressão com a outra mão sobre a cabeça.
Scanzoni m., m. de Scanzoni; rotação e tração com fórceps em um trajeto espiral, com reaplicação do fórceps para desprendimento.
Sellick m., m. de Sellick; pressão aplicada à cartilagem cricóide, para evitar regurgitação durante intubação traqueal no paciente anestesiado.
Valsalva m., m. de Valsalva; qualquer esforço ("tensão") expiratório contra vias aéreas fechadas, seja no nariz, na boca ou na glote, o inverso da manobra de Müller; como a pressão intratorácica impede o retorno venoso para o átrio direito, essa manobra é usada para estudar os efeitos cardiovasculares do aumento da pressão venosa periférica e da diminuição do enchimento cardíaco e do débito cardíaco, bem como as respostas pós-esforço.
Wigand m., m. de Wigand; um parto pélvico assistido com pressão acima da sínfise, enquanto o feto está montado sobre o outro braço do operador.
Zavanelli m., m. de Zavanelli. SIN cephalic *replacement.*
man·ga·nese (Mn) (mang′gă-nēz). Manganês; elemento metálico semelhante e freqüentemente associado, particularmente em minérios, ao ferro; número atômico 25, peso atômico 54,94; os sais de manganês às vezes são utilizados na medicina. SIN manganum. [L. mod. *manganesium, manganum,* forma alterada de *magnesium*]
man·gan·ic (mang-gan′ik). Mangânico; designa o cátion trivalente do manganês, Mn^{3+}.
man·ga·nous (mang′gă-nŭs). Manganoso; designa o cátion divalente do manganês, Mn^{2+}.
man·ga·num (man′gă-nŭm). Manganês. SIN manganese. [L.]
mange (mānj). Sarna; gafeira; doença cutânea de animais domésticos e selvagens causada por qualquer um dos vários gêneros de ácaros que escavam a pele; em seres humanos, as infestações por ácaros geralmente são denominadas escabiose. [Fr. *manger,* comer]
demodectic m., sarna demodécica; infestação dos folículos pilosos e das glândulas sebáceas por ácaros do gênero *Demodex;* eles são observados em seres humanos e em vários animais domesticados; embora sejam assintomáticos na maioria das espécies, esses ácaros podem causar dermatite grave e extensa ("sarna vermelha") em cães. VER *Demodex.*
sarcoptic m., s. sarcóptica; doença cutânea de animais causada por ácaros do gênero *Sarcoptes,* incluindo *Sarcoptes scabiei.*
Manhold, John H., dentista norte-americano, *1919. VER Volpe-M. *Index.*
ma·nia (mā′nē-ă). Mania; distúrbio emocional caracterizado por euforia ou irritabilidade, aumento da atividade psicomotora, fala rápida, mudança rápida de idéias (vôo de idéias), diminuição da necessidade de sono, falta de atenção, grandiosidade e comprometimento da capacidade de julgamento; em geral ocorre no transtorno bipolar. VER manic-depressive, manic *excitement.* [G. mania]
acute m., m. aguda. SIN manic *excitement.*
-mania. -mania; amor anormal por, ou tendência mórbida para algum objeto, lugar ou ação específica. [G. mania]
ma·ni·ac (mā′nē-ak). Maníaco. 1. Termo obsoleto para uma pessoa mentalmente doente ou perturbada. 2. Aquele que sofre de mania.
ma·ni·a·cal (mă-nī′ă-kăl). Maníaco; relativo a, ou caracterizado por mania. VER amok. SIN manic.
man·ic (man′ik, mā′nik). Maníaco. SIN maniacal.
man·ic-de·pres·sive. Maníaco-depressivo. 1. Relativo a uma psicose maníaco-depressiva (transtorno bipolar, bipolar *disorder*). 2. Aquele que sofre desse distúrbio.
manicky (man′i-kē). Maníaco; comportamento característico da fase maníaca do transtorno bipolar.
man·i·fes·ta·tion (man′i-fes-tā′shŭn). Manifestação; a exibição ou revelação de sinais ou sintomas característicos de uma doença. [L. *manifestus,* pego no ato]

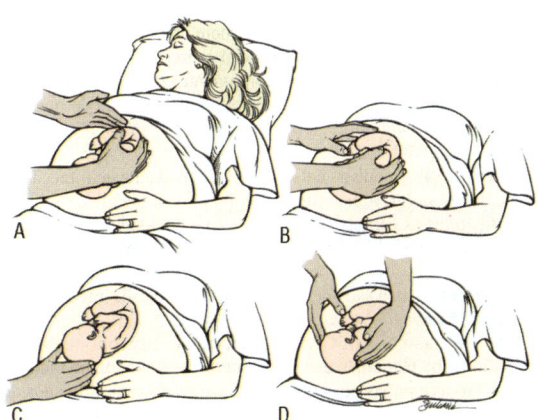

manobras de Leopold: (A) primeira manobra: palpar a superfície superior do fundo uterino; (B) segunda manobra: palpar as laterais do útero para determinar qual a direção do dorso fetal; (C) terceira manobra: palpar para descobrir o que está na abertura superior da pelve; (D) quarta manobra: supondo-se que o feto esteja em apresentação cefálica, deve-se determinar, então, a posição fetal (grau de flexão)

behavioral m., m. comportamental; m. caracterizada por defeitos na estrutura da personalidade e, conseqüentemente, do comportamento, com ansiedade mínima e com leve ou nenhum sentimento de angústia, indicativo de um transtorno psiquiátrico; ocasionalmente, a encefalite ou traumatismo craniano causarão o quadro clínico que é apropriadamente diagnosticado como distúrbio encefálico crônico com manifestações comportamentais.

neurotic m., m. neurótica; m. caracterizada por defesas como conversão, dissociação, deslocamento, formação de fobias ou pensamentos e atitudes repetitivos utilizados para lidar com a ansiedade; em contraste com as manifestações psicóticas, não há distorção grosseira nem falsificação da realidade e, geralmente, não se observa desintegração evidente da personalidade.

psychophysiologic m., m. psicofisiológica; m. caracterizada pela expressão visceral de afeto, sendo os sintomas um estado crônico e exagerado da expressão fisiológica da emoção com o sentimento reprimido; essas m. comumente são características de distúrbios psicossomáticos.

psychotic m., m. psicótica; m. caracterizada por pensamentos, sentimentos e comportamento que evidenciam um grau variável de desintegração da personalidade e distorção ou falsificação da realidade em várias esferas; as pessoas com essa manifestação não conseguem manter relacionamentos efetivos com outras pessoas ou com seu trabalho.

man·i·kin (man'i - kin). Manequim; um modelo do corpo humano ou de qualquer de suas partes, particularmente um que possua partes removíveis. VER TAMBÉM phantom (2). [dim. de *man*]

man·i·pha·lanx (man'i - fā'langks). Manifalange; uma falange da mão; um segmento ósseo de um dedo da mão; distinta da pedifalange. [L. *manus*, mão, + *phalanx*]

Mann, Frank C., cirurgião norte-americano, 1887–1962. VER M.-Bollman *fistula*; M.-Williamson *operation, ulcer.*

man·na (man'ă). Maná; exsudação sacarina da *Fraxinus ornus*, freixo florescente, uma árvore da costa do Mediterrâneo, usada como laxante, principalmente para crianças. É encontrada na forma de **m. cannellata,** m. em flocos; **m. in lacrimis,** m. em lágrimas ou pequenos flocos; e **m. communis** ou **m. in sortis,** m. natural. [L., do G. *manna*, do Heb. *mān*]

man·nans (man'anz). Mananas; manosanas. **1.** Polissacarídeos da manose, encontrados em vários legumes e na jarina. **2.** Polissacarídeos nos quais a manose é o monossacarídeo presente em maior proporção. SIN mannosans.

man·ner·ism (man'er - izm). Maneirismo; modo característico peculiar ou incomum de movimento, ação ou fala.

man·nite (man'īt). Manita, manitol. SIN mannitol.

man·ni·tol (man'i - tol). Manitol; o álcool hexáidrico, comum em plantas, obtido por redução da frutose; usado em provas de função renal para medir a filtração glomerular, bem como por via intravenosa como diurético osmótico. SIN manna sugar, mannite.

m. hexanitrate, hexanitrato de manitol; substância explosiva formada pela nitração do manitol; quando diluído com carboidratos (uma parte de hexanitrato de manitol para nove ou mais partes de carboidratos) não é explosivo, sendo usado como vasodilatador e agente hipotensor; sua ação é mais lenta que a da nitroglicerina; atua através da formação de óxido nítrico. SIN nitromannitol.

Mannkopf, Emil W., médico alemão, 1836–1918. VER M. *sign.*

Mann meth·yl blue-e·o·sin stain. Corante azul de metileno-eosina de Mann. VER em stain.

man·no·hep·tu·lose (man - ō - hep'too - lōs). Manoeptulose. VER D-*manno*-heptulose.

man·no·mus·tine (man - ō - mŭs'tēn). Manomustina; dicloridrato de 1,6-bis(2-cloroetilamino)-1,6-didesoxi-D-manitol; um agente antineoplásico.

man·no·pro·teins (man'ō - prō - tēnz). Manoproteínas; componentes da parede celular de leveduras que são proteínas com grandes números de grupos manose fixados; muito antigênicas.

man·no·sa·mine (man - ō - să - mēn). Manosamina; 2-amino-2-desoximanose; o D-isômero é um constituinte dos ácidos neuramínicos, bem como dos mucolipídios e das mucoproteínas.

man·no·sans (man'ō - sanz). Manosanas. SIN mannans.

man·nose (Man) (man'ōs). Manose; uma aldoexose obtida de várias fontes vegetais (isto é, das mananas); um epímero da glicose.

man·nose-1-phos·phate gua·nyl·yl·trans·fer·ase (GDP). Manose-1-fosfato guanililtransferase; uma transferase que catalisa a reação do GTP e da manose 1-fosfato para produzir GDP manose e pirofosfato. SIN GDPmannose phosphorylase.

man·nose·phos·phate isom·er·ase. Manosefosfato isomerase; enzima que catalisa a conversão reversível de D-manose 6-fosfato em D-frutose 6-fosfato; etapa fundamental na síntese de derivados da manose, bem como na entrada de manose nas vias centrais do metabolismo dos carboidratos.

man·no·si·dases (man - ō'si - dā'ses). Manosidases; grupo de enzimas que catalisam a hidrólise de resíduos D-manose não-redutores terminais de manosídeos (particularmente nas glicoproteínas e glicolipídios); as α-manosidases atuam sobre os α-D-manosídeos, enquanto as β-manosidases atuam sobre os β-D-manosídeos; uma deficiência de α-manosidase está associada à manosidose.

man·no·side (man'ō - sīd). Manosídeo; um glicosídeo da manose.

man·no·si·do·sis (man'ō - si - dō'sis) [MIM*248500]. Manosidose; deficiência congênita de α-manosidase; associada a características faciais grosseiras, aumento da língua, retardo mental, cifose, anormalidades ósseas radiográficas e linfócitos vacuolados, com acúmulo de manose nos tecidos; herança autossômica recessiva, causada por mutação no gene da alfa-manosidase (MANB) no cromossoma 19p.

man·nu·ron·ic ac·id (man - ū - ron'ik). Ácido manurônico; ácido urônico derivado da oxidação da manose; um componente do ácido algínico.

man-of-war. Caravela.

Portuguese m., caravela portuguesa. SIN *Physalia physalis.*

ma·nom·e·ter (mă - nom'e - ter). Manômetro; instrumento para indicar a pressão de qualquer fluido ou a diferença de pressão entre dois fluidos, sejam gases ou líquidos. [G. *manos*, fino, escasso, + *metron*, medida]

aneroid m., m. aneróide; manômetro no qual a pressão é indicada por um ponteiro que gira movido por um diafragma ou tubo de Bourdon exposto à pressão. SIN dial m.

dial m., m. de mostrador. SIN aneroid m.

differential m., m. diferencial; qualquer dispositivo que indique a diferença na pressão entre dois líquidos, independentemente de quaisquer alterações nas suas pressões absolutas.

mercurial m., m. de mercúrio; manômetro no qual as pressões variáveis são mostradas por diferenças de elevação em uma coluna de mercúrio.

man·o·met·ric (man - ō - met'rik). Manométrico; relativo a um manômetro.

ma·nom·e·try (mă - nom'e - trē). Manometria; medida da pressão de gases ou de líquidos por meio de um manômetro. SIN manoscopy. [ver manometer]

esophageal m., m. esofágica; medida de pressões intra-esofágicas, em um ou mais locais, por instrumentos sensíveis à pressão intraluminal.

ma·nos·co·py (mă - nos'kō - pē). Manoscopia. SIN manometry.

mam. pr. Abreviatura do L. *mane primo*, de manhã cedo, a primeira coisa pela manhã.

Manson, Sir Patrick, autoridade inglesa em medicina tropical, 1844-1922. VER *Mansonella; Mansonia;* M. *disease, schistosomiasis; Schistosoma mansoni; schistosomiasis* mansoni; M. *eye worm.*

Man·son·el·la (man - sō - nel'ă). Gênero de filárias, amplamente distribuídas na África tropical e na América do Sul, que infectam a cavidade peritoneal, as superfícies serosas ou a pele de seres humanos e de outros primatas com microfilárias sem bainha. Os importantes parasitas humanos *M. perstans* e *M. streptocerca* eram outrora classificados nos gêneros *Dipetalonema, Acanthocheilonema* e *Tetrapetalonema.*

M. demarqua'yi, SIN *M. ozzardi.*

M. ozzar'di, parasita filarióideo encontrado em Yucatan, Panamá, Colômbia, norte da Argentina, Guiana, Guiana Francesa e nas ilhas de São Vicente e Dominica, causando mansoneíase; as microfilárias não possuem bainha, e não há núcleos na cauda pontuda; o ciclo vital é semelhante ao da *Wuchereria bancrofti;* os seres humanos são o único hospedeiro definitivo conhecido, e os hospedeiros intermediários são mosquitos-pólvora, *Culicoides furens* e, possivelmente, *C. paraensis.* SIN *M. demarquayi, M. tucumana.*

M. per'stans, a "filária persistente," espécie extremamente prevalente na África tropical e no norte da América do Sul, onde infecta a cavidade peritoneal e outras cavidades corporais dos seres humanos, mas não é patogênica ou é pouco patogênica; são observadas microfilárias subperiódicas características no sangue periférico. Na África é transmitida pela picada dos mosquitos-pólvora *Culicoides austeni* e *C. grahami.*

M. streptocer'ca, espécie filarióide do homem que produz microfilárias sem bainha não-periódicas, encontradas no sangue circulante; pode causar um distúrbio liquenóide ou edema cutâneo; comumente encontrada no cório da pele de habitantes da África ocidental e transmitida pela picada do mosquito-pólvora, *Culicoides grahami.*

M. tucuma'na, SIN *M. ozzardi.*

man·so·nel·li·a·sis (man'sō - nel - ī'ă - sis). Mansoneliase; infecção por uma espécie de *Mansonella,* transmitida ao homem pela picada de mosquitos do gênero *Culicoides;* os vermes adultos vivem nas cavidades serosas, principalmente na cavidade peritoneal, no tecido adiposo mesentérico e perivisceral, e na pele.

man·son·el·lo·sis (man - sō - nel'lō - sis). Mansonelose; infecção pelo parasita filarióide *Mansonella ozzardi.*

Man·so·ni·a (man - sō'nē - ă). Gênero de mosquitos marrons ou pretos, de tamanho médio (tribo Culicini), que freqüentemente possuem abdome e pernas listrados; as larvas e pupas possuem tubos respiratórios modificados que lhes permitem perfurar plantas aquáticas para obter ar. Os mosquitos *M.* são encontrados em todo o mundo e, em áreas tropicais, são importantes vetores da *Brugia malayi;* em algumas áreas, também transmitem a *Wuchereria bancrofti.* [P. *Manson*]

Man·so·noi·des (man - sō - noy'dēz). Subgênero de *Mansonia.*

Mantel, Nathan, bioestatístico norte-americano, *1927. VER Mantel-Haenszel *test.*

man·tle (man′tl). Manto. **1.** Uma camada de revestimento. **2.** SIN cerebral *cortex.*
  brain m., córtex cerebral. SIN cerebral *cortex.*
  myoepicardial m., m. mioepicárdico; a parede dorsal do pericárdio primitivo que, no somito do embrião inicial, torna-se tanto o epicárdio quanto o miocárdio.
Mantoux, Charles, médico francês, 1877–1947. VER M. *pit, test.*
man·u·al Eng·lish. Inglês gestual; forma de comunicação em inglês com uma pessoa portadora de acentuada deficiência auditiva, por uma combinação de sinais, alfabeto manual e gestos.
ma·nu·bri·um, pl. **ma·nu·bria** (mă-noo′brē-ŭm, -ă) [TA]. Manúbrio; a porção do esterno ou do martelo que representa o cabo de uma espada ou martelo. [L. cabo]
  m. mal'lei, cabo do martelo. SIN m. of malleus.
  m. of malleus, cabo do martelo; a porção que se estende do colo do martelo para baixo, para dentro e para trás; está incrustada, em todo o seu comprimento, na membrana timpânica. SIN m. mallei.
  m. ster'ni [TA], manúbrio do esterno. SIN m. of sternum.
  m. of sternum [TA], manúbrio do esterno; o segmento superior do esterno, um osso plano, aproximadamente triangular, ocasionalmente fundido com o corpo do esterno, formando com ele um pequeno ângulo, o ângulo do esterno. SIN m. sterni [TA], episternum, presternum.
man·u·dy·na·mom·e·ter (man′ū-dī-nă-mom′ē-ter). Manodinamômetro; em odontologia, um dispositivo para medir a força exercida pelo impulso de um instrumento. [L. *manus,* mão, + G. *dynamis,* força, + *metron,* medida]
ma·nus, gen. e pl. **ma·nus** (mā′nŭs) [TA]. Mão. SIN hand. [L.]
MAO Abreviatura de monoamine oxidase (monoamina oxidase).
MAOI Abreviatura de monoamine oxidase *inhibitor* (inibidor da monoamina oxidase).
map. Mapa; representação de uma região ou estrutura; p. ex., de um trecho de DNA.
  choroplethic m., mapa coroplético; método de mapeamento para exibir informações quantitativas como taxas de mortalidade em jurisdições definidas (estados, condados, etc.) por códigos de cores ou sombreado. [G. *choros,* distrito, + *plethos,* multidão, + -ic]
  chromosome m., m. cromossômico; representação sistemática, semi-abstrata da posição física de *loci* em um cariótipo. Cf. genetic map.
  conformational m., m. de conformação; gráfico de Ramachandran. SIN Ramachandran *plot.*
  contig m., m. de contig; mapa físico de um cromossoma ou trecho de DNA construído a partir de blocos de clones superpostos (contigs).
  cytogenetic m., m. citogenético; mapa no qual é mostrado o padrão de ligação clássico de um cromossoma.
  fate m., m. do destino; determinação em embriões muito jovens da origem celular de órgãos ou estruturas específicas. SIN germinal localization.
  genetic m., m. genético; representação abstrata do conjunto ordenado de *loci* genéticos em que o intervalo entre as entradas possui sinais algébricos e magnitude proporcional ao número esperado de entrecruzamentos cromossômicos entre eles, e as distâncias são algebricamente aditivas; p. ex., em um mapa a distância combinada entre o *locus* A e o *locus* C é a soma algébrica das duas distâncias entre os *loci* A e B, e B e C.
  isodemographic m., m. isodemográfico; método diagramático de exibir países ou jurisdições administrativas de um país em mapas bidimensionais, sendo cada área diretamente proporcional à densidade populacional do país ou da jurisdição. [iso- + G. *dēmos,* povo, + *graphō,* escrever, + -ic]
  linkage m., m. de ligação; uma representação matemática abstrata de *loci* genéticos que conserva a ordem dos *loci* posicionados de tal forma que as distâncias são algebricamente aditivas; convencionalmente, um mapa é representado em escala de forma que as distâncias entre *loci* se tornem menores, a razão entre a distância no mapa e o valor da fração de recombinação se aproxima de 1 e *loci* de grupos distintos independentes estão muito distantes.
  physical m., m. físico; mapa de um trecho de DNA com marcos ordenados a uma distância conhecida entre si; o mapa físico final seria a seqüência básica de todo o cromossoma.
  restriction m., m. de restrição; a ordem de sítios de restrição ao longo de um cromossoma ou plasmídeo.
  sequence-tagged site (STS) m., m. de segmento marcado por sua seqüência; um mapa que representa a ordem e o intervalo de sítios com seqüências marcadas em um segmento de DNA.
  spot m., planta de situação; mapa que mostra a localização geográfica de pessoas com uma característica específica, p. ex., casos de uma doença infecciosa.
map dis·tance. Distância no mapa; o grau de separação de dois *loci* em um mapa de ligação, medido em morgans ou centimorgans.
map·pine (map′ēn). Mapina. SIN bufotenine.
map·ping (map′ing). Mapeamento; o processo de identificação da posição relativa de sítios ou elementos.

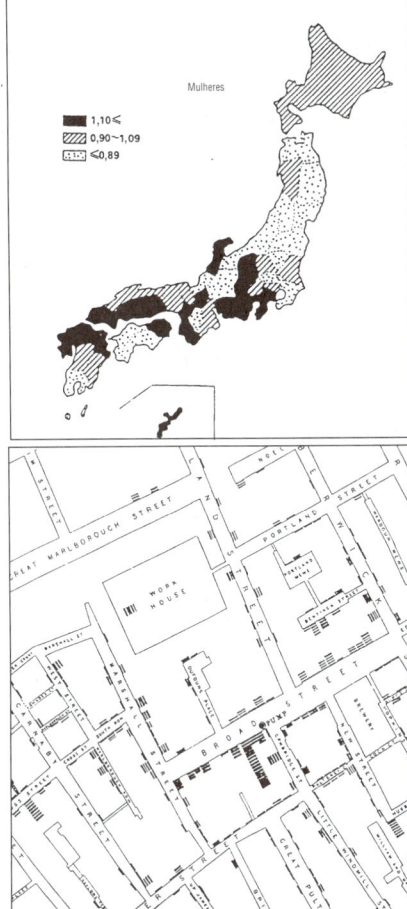

mapa coroplético e planta de situação: o mapa coroplético (superior) mostra diferenças regionais da incidência de fratura do quadril no Japão; planta de situação (inferior), parte do mapa do Soho, Londres, feito por John Snow, mostrando a distribuição dos casos de cólera em residências próximas da bomba da Broad Street em 1849

  cardiac m., m. cardíaco; um método pelo qual os potenciais cardíacos locais são representados espacialmente de forma integrada, em função do tempo (mapa isocrômico) ou do potencial (mapa isopotencial).
  chromosome m., m. cromossômico; o processo de determinar a posição de *loci* em cromossomas específicos e construir um diagrama de cada cromossoma mostrando as posições relativas de *loci*; as técnicas incluem estudos familiares com análise de ligação, hibridização de células somáticas e mapeamento da deleção cromossômica.
  gene m., m. genético. VER genetic *map.*
  S1 nuclease m., m. da nuclease S1; método para localizar a extremidade 5′ de um transcrito em uma mistura de RNA.
map·ping func·tion. Função de mapeamento; em análise de ligação, uma fórmula que converte a fração de recombinação (que está na escala de probabilidade) em distância do mapa (em morgans).
ma·pro·ti·line (ma-prō′ti-lēn). Maprotilina; antidepressivo tricíclico usado no tratamento de várias doenças depressivas e para alívio da ansiedade associada à depressão.
MAPs Abreviatura de microtubule-associated *proteins* (proteínas associadas a microtúbulos), em *protein.*
Marañón, Gregorio, endocrinologista espanhol, 1887–1960. VER M. *sign;* syndrome.
ma·ran·tic (mă-ran′tik). Marântico. SIN marasmic. [G. *marantikos,* debilitante]
ma·ras·mic (mă-raz′mik). Marásmico; relativo a, ou que sofre de, marasmo. SIN marantic.
ma·ras·moid (mă-raz′moyd). Marasmóide; semelhante ao marasmo. [G. *marasmos,* definhamento, + *eidos,* semelhança]
ma·ras·mus (mă-raz′mŭs). Marasmo; caquexia, principalmente em crianças pequenas, basicamente devida à deficiência alimentar prolongada de proteínas e calorias. SIN marantic atrophy, Parrot disease (2), pedatrophia, pedatrophy. [G. *marasmos,* definhamento]

nutritional m., m. nutricional; fraqueza e definhamento extremos, secundários à desnutrição.

marc (mark). Bagaço; o resíduo que permanece após percolação de uma droga. [Fr. de *marcher*, pisar]

Marcacci, Arturo, fisiologista italiano, 1854–1915. VER M. *muscle*.

Marchand, Felix J., patologista alemão, 1846–1928. VER M. *adrenals*, em *adrenal, rest*, wandering *cell*.

Marchant, Gérard T.J., cirurgião francês, 1850–1903. VER M. *zone*.

Marchesani, Oswald, 1900–1952. VER Weill-M. *syndrome*.

Marchetti, Andrew A., ginecologista e obstetra norte-americano, 1901–1970. VER Marshall-M. *test*; Marshall-M.-Krantz *operation*.

Marchi, Vittorio, médico italiano, 1851–1908. VER M. *fixative, reaction, stain, tract*.

Marchiafava, Ettore, patologista italiano, 1847–1935. VER M.-Bignami *disease*; M.-Micheli *anemia, syndrome*.

mar·cid (mar′sid). Emagrecedor; consuntivo. [L. *marcidus*; de *marceo*, murchar]

Marcille, Maurice, 1871–1941. VER M. *triangle*.

mar·cor (mar′kōr). Termo obsoleto para marasmo. [L. de *marceo*, murchar]

Marcus Gunn, Robert. VER Gunn.

Marek, Josef, veterinário e patologista húngaro, 1868–1952. VER M. disease *virus*.

marenostrin. Marenostrina, pirina. SIN pyrin.

Marey, Étienne Jules, fisiologista francês, 1830–1904. VER M. *law*.

Marfan, Antoine Bernard-Jean, pediatra francês, 1858–1942. VER M. *disease, law, syndrome*.

mar·fan·oid (mar′fan-oyd). Marfanóide; termo usado para designar aqueles cujo fenótipo guarda uma semelhança superficial com o fenótipo da síndrome de Marfan.

Marg, Elwin, físico norte-americano, *1918. VER Mackay-M. *tonometer*.

Mar·ga·ro·pus (mar-gar′ō-pŭs). Gênero de carrapatos ixodídeos muito semelhantes ao *Boophilus*, mas que não possuem festões nem ornamentos; são caracterizados por pernas posteriores muito aumentadas e por uma placa mediana longa. [G. *margaros*, ostra de pérolas, + *pous*, pé]

M. winthe′mi, o carrapato do cavalo, de inverno, sul-americano, de hospedeiro único; algumas vezes, também ataca bois e carneiros.

mar·gin (mar′jin) [TA]. Margem, limbo, limite ou borda, como de uma superfície ou estrutura. VER TAMBÉM border, edge. SIN margo [TA]. [L. *margo*, borda, margem]

acetabular m. [TA], limbo do acetábulo; a borda de osso ao redor do acetábulo à qual está fixado o lábio do acetábulo. SIN limbus acetabuli [TA], m. of acetabulum [TA], margo acetabularis*.

m. of acetabulum [TA], limbo do acetábulo. SIN acetabular m.

anterior m., m. anterior. SIN anterior *border*.

anterior palpebral m. [TA], limbo anterior da pálpebra; a borda anterior da margem livre de cada pálpebra, ao longo da qual estão presos os cílios. SIN limbus anterior palpebrae [TA], anterior border of eyelids.

articular m., lábio glenoidal da escápula. SIN glenoid *labrum* of scapula.

cavity m., m. cavitária; a periferia de um enchimento, a linha de junção entre uma restauração e a superfície externa de um dente.

cervical m., m. cervical; **(1)** SIN gingival m.; **(2)** fim de uma restauração na área gengival.

cervical m. of tooth, m. cervical do dente, colo do dente. SIN neck of tooth.

ciliary m. of iris [TA], m. ciliar da íris; a borda periférica da íris fixada ao corpo ciliar. SIN margo ciliaris iridis [TA], ciliary border of iris.

corneal m., limbo da córnea. SIN corneal *limbus*.

costal m. [TA], arco costal; aquela parte da abertura inferior do tórax formada pelas cartilagens articuladas da sétima a décima (falsa) costelas. SIN arcus costalis [TA], costal arch*, arcus costarum.

m.'s of eyelids, limbos das pálpebras. SIN palpebral m.'s.

falciform m. of saphenous opening [TA], m. falciforme do hiato safeno; a margem livre, acentuadamente curva, do hiato safeno na fáscia lata; medialmente, termina em um corno superior e um inferior. SIN margo falciformis hiatus sapheni [TA], margo arcuatus hiatus sapheni*.

fibular m. of foot, m. fibular do pé. SIN lateral *border* of foot.

m. of fossa ovalis, m. da fossa oval. SIN *limbus* fossae ovalis.

free m., m. livre. SIN free *border*.

free m. of eyelids, m. livre das pálpebras; a borda inferior não-fixada da pálpebra superior e a borda superior da pálpebra inferior, onde a superfície anterior (cutânea) da pálpebra encontra a superfície posterior (conjuntival) da pálpebra. As margens livres das pálpebras limitam a rima das pálpebras, e cada margem livre tem um limbo anterior e um posterior. VER TAMBÉM palpebral m.'s.

frontal m., m. frontal. SIN frontal *border*.

frontal m. of sphenoid [TA], m. frontal do esfenóide; a margem da asa maior do osso esfenóide, que se articula com o osso frontal. SIN margo frontalis ossis sphenoidalis [TA], frontal border of sphenoid bone.

gingival m., m. gengival; **(1)** a porção mais coronal da gengiva que circunda o dente; **(2)** a borda da gengiva livre. SIN cervical m. (1), gingival crest.

incisal m. [TA], m. incisal; a parte de um dente anterior mais distante do ápice da raiz. SIN margo incisalis [TA], cutting edge (2), incisal edge, incisal surface, shearing edge.

inferior m., m. inferior. SIN inferior *border*.

inferolateral m., m. ínfero-lateral. SIN inferolateral m. of cerebral hemisphere.

inferolateral m. of cerebral hemisphere [TA], m. ínfero-lateral do hemisfério cerebral; a margem irregular, descontínua do hemisfério cerebral na junção das superfícies inferior e súpero-lateral. SIN margo inferolateralis [TA], inferolateral m., margo inferior cerebri.

inferomedial m. of cerebral hemisphere [TA], m. ínfero-medial do hemisfério cerebral; a borda irregular do hemisfério cerebral na junção das superfícies inferior e medial. SIN margo inferomedialis hemispherii cerebri [TA], margo medialis cerebri.

infraorbital m., m. infra-orbital; a metade inferior da margem orbital, ou a margem inferior da órbita, formada pelo maxilar, medialmente, e pelo osso zigomático lateralmente. VER orbital m. SIN margo infraorbitalis.

interosseous m., m. interóssea. SIN interosseous *border*.

lacrimal m. of maxilla [TA], m. lacrimal da maxila; a margem da superfície nasal da maxila, que se articula com o osso lacrimal. SIN margo lacrimalis maxillae [TA], lacrimal border of maxilla.

lambdoid m. of occipital bone, m. lambdóidea do occipital. SIN lambdoid *border* of occipital bone.

lateral m., m. lateral. SIN lateral *border*.

mastoid m. of occipital bone, m. mastóidea do occipital. SIN mastoid *border* of occipital bone.

medial m., m. medial. SIN medial *border*.

mesovarian m. of ovary, m. mesovárica do ovário. SIN mesovarian *border* of ovary.

nasal m. of frontal bone [TA], m. nasal do osso frontal; a borda do osso frontal que se articula com os ossos nasais. SIN margo nasalis ossis frontalis [TA], nasal border of frontal bone.

occipital m., m. occipital. SIN occipital *border*.

occipital m. of temporal bone [TA], m. occipital do osso temporal; a parte do osso temporal que se articula com a escama occipital. SIN margo occipitalis ossis temporalis [TA], occipital border of temporal bone.

m. of orbit, m. orbital. SIN orbital m.

orbital m. [TA], m. orbital; a borda mais aguda da abertura orbital, que é a borda periférica da base da órbita piramidal. A metade superior da margem orbital é a margem supra-orbital; a metade inferior é a margem infra-orbital. Os ossos frontal, maxilar e zigomático contribuem para a margem orbital, que geralmente é forte para proteger o conteúdo da órbita. Os locais fracos, de possível fratura, da margem coincidem com as suturas entre os ossos participantes. SIN margo orbitalis [TA], m. of orbit, orbital rim.

orbital m. of eyelids, m. orbital das pálpebras; as bordas fixadas externas ou periféricas das pálpebras superior e inferior; a "raiz" das pálpebras, ao longo da qual a m. orbital das pálpebras está fixada à margem orbital.

palpebral m.'s [TA], limbos da pálpebra; as bordas anterior e posterior da margem livre das pálpebras superior e inferior. VER TAMBÉM anterior palpebral m., posterior palpebral m. SIN limbi palpebrales [TA], margo palpebrae [TA], borders of eyelids, m.'s of eyelids.

parietal m., m. parietal. SIN parietal *border*.

parietal m. of frontal bone [TA], m. parietal do osso frontal; a margem do osso frontal que se articula com o osso parietal. SIN margo parietalis ossis frontalis [TA], parietal border of frontal bone.

parietal m. of greater wing of sphenoid [TA], m. parietal da asa maior do esfenóide; a margem da asa maior do esfenóide que se articula com o osso parietal. SIN margo parietalis alaris majoris ossis sphenoidalis [TA], margo parietalis ossis sphenoidalis, parietal border of sphenoid bone.

posterior palpebral m. [TA], limbo posterior da pálpebra; a borda posterior da margem livre de cada pálpebra, que também é a borda da conjuntiva. SIN posterior border of eyelids.

psoas m., m. do psoas; nas radiografias de abdome, o aparecimento da faixa de gordura que define a margem lateral do músculo psoas; mostra um retroperitônio normal quando visível.

pupillary m. of iris [TA], m. pupilar da íris; a borda interna da íris que forma a margem da pupila. SIN margo pupillaris iridis [TA], pupillary border of iris.

right m. of heart, m. direita do coração. SIN right *border* of heart.

m. of safety, m. de segurança; a faixa entre a dose terapêutica mínima e a dose tóxica mínima de uma droga.

sphenoidal m. of temporal bone [TA], m. esfenoidal do osso temporal; a porção da borda da parte escamosa do osso temporal que se articula com a asa maior do esfenóide. SIN margo sphenoidalis ossis temporalis [TA], sphenoidal border of temporal bone.

squamosal m., m. escamosa. SIN squamosal border.

squamosal m. of greater wing of sphenoid [TA], m. escamosa da asa maior do esfenóide; a margem da asa maior do osso esfenóide que se articula com a parte escamosa do osso temporal. SIN margo squamous alaris majoris ossis sphenoidalis [TA], margo squamosus ossis sphenoidalis, squamous border of sphenoid bone.

squamous m., m. escamosa. SIN squamosal border.
superior m. of cerebral hemisphere [TA], m. superior do hemisfério cerebral; a margem curva do hemisfério cerebral na junção das superfícies súperolateral e medial. SIN margo superior hemispherii cerebri [TA], margo superomedialis, superomedial m.
superomedial m., m. superior do hemisfério cerebral. SIN superior m. of cerebral hemisphere.
supraorbital m. [TA], m. supra-orbital; a metade superior da borda orbital, que constitui a borda superior curva da abertura da órbita, formada pelo osso frontal. VER orbital m. SIN margo supraorbitalis [TA], supraorbital arch, supraorbital ridge.
m. of tongue [TA], m. da língua; a borda lateral que separa o dorso da superfície inferior da língua de cada lado, com as duas bordas se encontrando anteriormente no ápice. SIN margo linguae [TA].
ulnar m. of forearm, m. ulnar da região antebraquial. SIN ulnar border of forearm.
zygomatic m. of greater wing of sphenoid bone, m. zigomática da asa maior do esfenóide; a borda da asa maior do esfenóide que se articula com o osso zigomático. SIN margo zygomaticus alaris majoris ossis sphenoidalis [TA], margo zygomaticus alae majoris, zygomatic border of greater wing of sphenoid bone.

mar·gi·nal (mar′ji-năl). Marginal; relativo a uma margem.
Mar·gi·nal Line Cal·cu·lus In·dex (MLC). Índice de Cálculo da Linha Marginal; índice que classifica os cálculos (tártaro) supragengivais encontrados em áreas cervicais paralelas à gengiva marginal.
mar·gin·a·tion (mar′ji-nā′shŭn). Marginação; fenômeno que ocorre durante as fases relativamente iniciais da inflamação; em conseqüência da dilatação de capilares e lentificação da corrente sanguínea, os leucócitos tendem a ocupar a periferia da luz transversal e aderir às células endoteliais que revestem os vasos.
m. of placenta, m. da placenta. VER placenta marginata.
mar·gi·nes (mar′ji-nēz). Margens; plural de margo. [L.]
mar·go, gen. **mar·gi·nis,** pl. **mar·gi·nes** (mar′gō, mar′ji-nis, -nēz) [TA]. Margem. SIN margin, border. [L.]
m. acetabularis, limbo do acetábulo; *termo oficial alternativo para acetabular margin.
m. anterior [TA], m. anterior. SIN anterior border.
m. anterior corporis pancreatis [TA], m. anterior do corpo do pâncreas. SIN anterior border of body of pancreas.
m. anterior fibulae [TA], m. anterior da fíbula. SIN anterior border of fibula.
m. anterior pancreatis, m. anterior do corpo do pâncreas. SIN anterior border of body of pancreas.
m. anterior pulmonis [TA], m. anterior do pulmão. SIN anterior border of lung.
m. anterior radii [TA], m. anterior do rádio. SIN anterior border of radius.
m. anterior testis [TA], m. anterior do testículo. SIN anterior border of testis.
m. anterior tibiae [TA], m. anterior da tíbia. SIN anterior border of tibia.
m. anterior ulnae [TA], m. anterior da ulna. SIN anterior border of ulna.
m. arcuatus hiatus sapheni, m. falciforme do hiato safeno; *termo oficial alternativo para falciform margin of saphenous opening.
m. cilia′ris i′ridis [TA], m. ciliar da íris. SIN ciliary margin of iris.
m. dex′ter cor′dis [TA], margem direita do coração. SIN right border of heart.
m. falcifor′mis hiatus sapheni [TA], m. falciforme do hiato safeno. SIN falciform margin of saphenous opening.
m. fibula′ris pedis, m. fibular do pé; *termo oficial alternativo para lateral border of foot.
m. frontalis [TA], m. frontal. SIN frontal border.
m. frontalis ossis parietalis [TA], m. frontal do parietal. SIN frontal border of parietal bone.
m. frontalis ossis sphenoidalis [TA], m. frontal do esfenóide. SIN frontal margin of sphenoid.
m. incisa′lis [TA], m. incisal. SIN incisal margin.
m. inferior [TA], m. inferior. SIN inferior border.
m. inferior cer′ebri, m. ínfero-lateral do hemisfério cerebral. SIN inferolateral margin of cerebral hemisphere.
m. inferior corporis pancreatis [TA], m. inferior do corpo do pâncreas. SIN inferior border of body of pancreas.
m. inferior corporis splenis, m. inferior do baço. SIN inferior border of body of spleen.
m. inferior hep′atis [TA], m. inferior do fígado. SIN inferior border of liver.
m. inferior pancrea′tis, m. inferior do corpo do pâncreas. SIN inferior border of body of pancreas.
m. inferior pulmo′nis [TA], m. inferior do pulmão. SIN inferior border of lung.
m. inferior splenis [TA], m. inferior do baço. SIN inferior border of spleen.
m. inferolatera′lis [TA], m. ínfero-lateral do hemisfério cerebral. SIN inferolateral margin of cerebral hemisphere.
m. inferomedia′lis hemispherii cerebri [TA], m. ínfero-medial do hemisfério cerebral. SIN inferomedial margin of cerebral hemisphere.
m. infraorbita′lis, m. infra-orbital. SIN infraorbital margin.
m. interosseus [TA], m. interóssea. SIN interosseous border.
m. interos′seus fib′ulae [TA], m. interóssea da fíbula. SIN interosseous border of fibula.
m. interos′seus ra′dii [TA], m. interóssea do rádio. SIN interosseous border of radius.
m. interos′seus tib′iae [TA], m. interóssea da tíbia. SIN interosseous border of tibia.
m. interos′seus ul′nae [TA], m. interóssea da ulna. SIN interosseous border of ulna.
m. lacrima′lis maxillae [TA], m. lacrimal da maxila. SIN lacrimal margin of maxilla.
m. lambdoideus ossis occipitalis [TA], m. lambdóidea do occipital. SIN lambdoid border of occipital bone.
m. lambdoid′eus squa′mae occipita′lis, m. lambdóidea da escama occipital. SIN lambdoid border of occipital bone.
m. lateralis [TA], m. lateral. SIN lateral border.
m. latera′lis antebra′chii, m. radial do antebraço; *termo oficial alternativo para radial border of forearm.
m. latera′lis humer′i [TA], m. lateral do úmero. SIN lateral border of humerus.
m. latera′lis pe′dis [TA], m. lateral do pé. SIN lateral border of foot.
m. latera′lis re′nis [TA], m. lateral do rim. SIN lateral border of kidney.
m. latera′lis scap′ulae [TA], m. lateral da escápula. SIN lateral border of scapula.
m. latera′lis un′guis [TA], m. lateral da unha. SIN lateral border of nail.
m. liber [TA], m. livre. SIN free border.
m. li′ber ova′rii [TA], m. livre do ovário. SIN free border of ovary.
m. li′ber un′guis [TA], m. livre da unha. SIN free border of nail.
m. lin′guae [TA], m. da língua. SIN margin of tongue.
m. mastoideus ossis occipitalis [TA], m. mastóidea do occipital. SIN mastoid border of occipital bone.
m. mastoi′deus squa′mae occipita′lis, m. mastóidea da escama occipital. SIN mastoid border of occipital bone.
m. medialis [TA], m. medial. SIN medial border.
m. media′lis antebra′chii, m. medial do antebraço; *termo oficial alternativo para ulnar border of forearm.
m. media′lis cer′ebri, m. ínfero-medial do hemisfério cerebral. SIN inferomedial margin of cerebral hemisphere.
m. media′lis glan′dulae suprarena′lis [TA], m. medial da glândula suprarenal. SIN medial border of suprarenal gland.
m. media′lis humer′i [TA], m. medial do úmero. SIN medial border of humerus.
m. media′lis pe′dis [TA], m. medial do pé. SIN medial border of foot.
m. media′lis re′nis [TA], m. medial do rim. SIN medial border of kidney.
m. media′lis scap′ulae [TA], m. medial da escápula. SIN medial border of scapula.
m. media′lis tib′iae [TA], m. medial da tíbia. SIN medial border of tibia.
m. mesova′ricus ovarii, m. mesovárica do ovário. SIN mesovarian border of ovary.
m. nasa′lis os′sis fronta′lis [TA], m. nasal do osso frontal. SIN nasal margin of frontal bone.
m. occipita′lis [TA], m. occipital. SIN occipital border.
m. occipita′lis os′sis parieta′lis [TA], m. occipital do parietal. SIN occipital border of parietal bone.
m. occipita′lis os′sis tempora′lis [TA], m. occipital do temporal. SIN occipital margin of temporal bone.
m. occul′tus un′guis [TA], m. oculta da unha. SIN hidden border of nail.
m. orbitalis [TA], m. orbital. SIN orbital margin.
m. pal′pebrae [TA], limbos das pálpebras. SIN palpebral margins, em margin.
m. parieta′lis [TA], m. parietal. SIN parietal border.
m. parietalis alaris majoris ossis sphenoidalis [TA], m. parietal da asa maior do esfenóide. SIN parietal margin of greater wing of sphenoid.
m. parieta′lis os′sis fronta′lis [TA], m. parietal do frontal. SIN parietal margin of frontal bone.
m. parietá′lis os′sis sphenoida′lis. m. parietal do esfenóide. SIN parietal margin of greater wing of sphenoid.
m. parieta′lis os′sis tempora′lis, m. parietal do temporal. SIN parietal border of squamous part of temporal bone.
m. parietalis partis squamosae ossis temporalis [TA], m. parietal da parte escamosa do temporal. SIN parietal border of squamous part of temporal bone.
m. poste′rior fib′ulae [TA], m. posterior da fíbula. SIN posterior border of fibula.
m. poste′rior par′tis petro′sae os′sis tempora′lis [TA], m. posterior da parte petrosa do temporal. SIN parietal border of petrous part of temporal bone.
m. poste′rior ra′dii [TA], m. posterior do rádio. SIN posterior border of radius.
m. poste′rior tes′tis [TA], m. posterior do testículo. SIN posterior border of testis.
m. poste′rior ul′nae [TA], m. posterior da ulna. SIN posterior border of ulna.
m. pupilla′ris ir′idis [TA], m. pupilar da íris. SIN pupillary margin of iris.

margo

m. radia'lis antebra'chii [TA], m. radial do antebraço. SIN radial border of forearm.
m. sagitta'lis os'sis parieta'lis [TA], m. sagital do parietal. SIN sagittal border of parietal bone.
m. sphenoida'lis os'sis tempora'lis [TA], m. esfenoidal do temporal. SIN sphenoidal margin of temporal bone.
m. squamo'sus [TA], m. escamosa. SIN squamosal border.
m. squamosus alaris majoris ossis sphenoidalis [TA], m. escamosa da asa maior do esfenóide. SIN squamosal margin of greater wing of sphenoid.
m. squamo'sus os'sis parieta'lis [TA], m. escamosa do parietal. SIN squamosal border of parietal bone.
m. squamo'sus os'sis sphenoida'lis, m. escamosa do esfenóide. SIN squamosal margin of greater wing of sphenoid.
m. superior corporis pancreatis [TA], m. superior do corpo do pâncreas. SIN superior border of body of pancreas.
m. supe'rior glan'dulae suprarena'lis [TA], m. superior da glândula suprarenal. SIN superior border of suprarenal gland.
m. supe'rior hemispherii cer'ebri [TA], m. superior do hemisfério cerebral. SIN superior margin of cerebral hemisphere.
m. supe'rior pancrea'tis, m. superior do corpo do pâncreas. SIN superior border of body of pancreas.
m. superior par'tis petro'sae os'sis tempora'lis [TA], m. superior da parte petrosa do temporal. SIN superior border of petrous part of temporal bone.
m. supe'rior scap'ulae [TA], m. superior da escápula. SIN superior border of scapula.
m. supe'rior splenis [TA], m. superior do baço. SIN superior border of spleen.
m. superomedia'lis, m. superior do hemisfério cerebral. SIN superior margin of cerebral hemisphere.
m. supraorbita'lis [TA], m. supra-orbital. SIN supraorbital margin.
m. tibia'lis pe'dis, m. tibial do pé; *termo oficial alternativo para medial border of foot.
m. ulna'ris antebra'chii [TA], m. ulnar do antebraço. SIN ulnar border of forearm.
m. u'teri [TA], m. do útero. SIN border of uterus.
m. zygomat'icus a'lae majo'ris, m. zigomática da asa maior do esfenóide. SIN zygomatic margin of greater wing of sphenoid bone.
m. zygomaticus alaris majoris ossis sphenoidalis [TA], m. zigomática da asa maior do esfenóide. SIN zygomatic margin of greater wing of sphenoid bone.

Marie, Pierre, neurologista francês, 1853–1940. VER M. *ataxia*; Charcot-M.-Tooth *disease*; Bamberger-M. *disease, syndrome*; M.-Strümpell *disease*; Strümpell-M. *disease*; Brissaud-M. *syndrome*; Foix-Cavany-Marie *syndrome*.

mar·i·hua·na (mar-i-wah'na). Maconha; nome popular das folhas florescentes secas de *Cannabis sativa*, que são fumadas como cigarros, conhecidos nos Estados Unidos como "joints" ou "reefers". Nos Estados Unidos, a maconha inclui qualquer parte ou qualquer extrato da planta feminina. Grafias alternativas são mariguana, marijuana. VER TAMBÉM cannabis. [do Esp. *Maria-Juana*, Maria-Joana]

Marinesco, Georges, neurologista romeno, 1863–1938. VER M. succulent *hand*; M.-Garland *syndrome;* Marinesco-Sjögren *syndrome*.

mar·i·no·bu·fo·tox·in (mar'i-no-boo'fo-toks-in). Marinobufotoxina; veneno produzido pela parótida do *Bufo marinus* (família Bufonidae), um grande sapo nativo das Américas Central e do Sul; utilizado em países tropicais para controle de insetos.

Marion, Georges, urologista francês, 1869–1932. VER M. *disease*.
Mariotte, Edmé, físico francês, 1620–1684. VER M. *bottle, experiment, law,* blind *spot*.

mar·i·po·sia (mar-i-po'ze-a). Mariposia; talassoposia; termo raramente usado para designar o consumo anormal de água do mar em virtude de fatores psicogênicos. SIN thalassoposia. [L. *mare*, o mar, + G. *posis*, bebida]

Marjolin, Jean N., médico francês, 1780–1850. VER M. *ulcer*.

mar·jo·ram (mar'jo-ram). Manjerona; manjerona doce, manjerona da folha ou manjerona do jardim, cujas folhas, com e sem uma pequena porção dos topos florescentes de *Majorana hortensis* (*Origanum majorana*) (família Labiatae), são utilizadas como tempero e na medicina como estimulante, antifisético e emenagogo.

mark. Marca; qualquer mancha, linha ou outra figura na superfície cutânea ou cutaneomucosa, visível através da diferença de cor, elevação ou outra peculiaridade. [A.S. *mearc*]
alignment m., m. de alinhamento; marcas feitas em traçados enquanto o cimógrafo ou outro aparelho de registro está em repouso a fim de indicar as relações de tempo entre dois traçados inscritos um acima do outro, p. ex., pulsos jugular e radial.
stretch m.'s, SIN *striae cutis distensae*, em *stria*.

mark·er. Marcador. 1. Dispositivo usado para fazer uma marca ou indicar medida. 2. Uma característica ou fator pelo qual uma célula ou molécula pode ser reconhecida ou identificada. 3. Um *locus* que contém dois ou mais alelos que, sendo inofensivos, são comuns e, portanto, produzem altas freqüências de heterozigotos que facilitam a análise de ligação (linkage *analysis*).
allotypic m., m. alotípico. SIN allotype.
cell m., m. celular; característica de identificação de uma célula; p. ex., formação de rosetas com eritrócitos de carneiro como marcador de linfócitos T, ou a presença de imunoglobulina de superfície como m. de linfócitos B.
cell surface m., m. da superfície celular; proteína superficial, glicoproteína ou grupo de proteínas que distinguem uma célula ou um subgrupo de células de outro subgrupo definido de células.
genetic m., m. genético. SIN genetic *determinant*.
linkage m., m. de ligação; *locus* no qual há uma grande probabilidade de heterozigotos (estado indispensável para a análise de ligação), mas que talvez não tenha interesse clínico. VER TAMBÉM marker *locus*.
oncofetal m., m. oncofetal; m. tumoral produzido por tecido tumoral e por tecido fetal do mesmo tipo do tumor, mas não pelo tecido adulto normal que dá origem ao tumor.
polymorphic genetic m., m. genético polimórfico; característica hereditária que ocorre em determinada população como dois ou mais traços.
time m., m. de tempo; instrumento que marca o tempo, geralmente em segundos ou frações de segundos, em um registro por cimógrafo em experiências fisiológicas.
tumor m., m. tumoral; substância, liberada na circulação por tecido tumoral, cuja detecção no soro indica a existência de tumor.

Markov, Andrei, matemático russo, 1865–1922. VER Markov *process*.
Marme re·a·gent. Reagente de Marme. VER em reagent.
mar·mo·rat·ed (mar'mo-ra-ted). Marmoreado; mármoreo; designa uma condição na qual a aparência da pele é estriada como mármore. VER TAMBÉM *cutis* marmorata. [L. *marmoratus*, mármoreo]
mar·mot (mar'mot). Marmota; roedor hibernante que pode servir como hospedeiro reservatório do bacilo da peste na América do Norte. [Fr. *marmotte*]
Maroteaux, Pierre, geneticista médico francês, *1926. VER M.-Lamy *syndrome*.
Marquis re·a·gent. Reagente de Marquis. VER em reagent.
mar·row (mar'o) [TA]. Medula óssea. 1. Tecido conjuntivo hematopoético extremamente celular, que ocupa as cavidades medulares e as epífises esponjosas dos ossos; torna-se predominantemente adiposa com a idade, sobretudo nos ossos longos dos membros. 2. Qualquer material mole gelatinoso ou gorduroso semelhante à medula óssea. VER TAMBÉM medulla. [A.S. *mearh*]
bone m. [TA], m. óssea; o tecido mole, pulposo, que preenche as cavidades medulares dos ossos, que possui um estroma de fibras reticulares e células; sua consistência difere com a idade e localização. VER TAMBÉM gelatinous bone m., red bone m., yellow bone m. SIN medulla ossium [TA].
gelatinous bone m. [TA], m. óssea gelatinosa; m. óssea degenerada dos ossos do crânio na velhice.
red bone m. [TA], m. óssea vermelha; m. óssea cujo estroma contém basicamente eritrócitos, leucócitos e megacariócitos em fases de desenvolvimento; é encontrada em todo o esqueleto durante a vida fetal e ao nascimento. Após o quinto ano de vida, é gradualmente substituída, nos ossos longos, por medula óssea amarela. SIN medulla ossium rubra [TA].
spinal m., m. espinal. SIN spinal *cord*.
yellow bone m. [TA], m. óssea amarela; m. óssea na qual o estroma da rede reticular é basicamente preenchido por gordura; substitui a m. óssea vermelha nos ossos longos após o quinto ano de vida. SIN medulla ossium flava [TA].

Marshall, Don, oftalmologista norte-americano, *1905. VER M. *syndrome*.

| marcadores tumorais usados em diagnósticos primários ||
tipo de tumor	marcador
carcinoma testicular, coriocarcinoma	subunidade β da gonadotrofina coriônica humana (β-HCG) e α-1-fetoproteína (AFP)
mieloma múltiplo	imunoglobulinas, proteína de Bence Jones
neuroblastoma, feocromocitoma	catecolaminas, ácido vanililmandélico, metanefrinas
carcinóide, carcinoma primário dos hepatócitos	ácido 5-hidroxindoleacético α-1-fetoproteína
carcinoma medular da tireóide	calcitonina
linfoma maligno, leucemia	antígenos de superfície

Marshall, Eli K., farmacologista norte-americano, 1889–1966. VER M. *method*.
Marshall, John, anatomista inglês, 1818–1891. VER M. vestigial *fold*, oblique *vein*.
Marshall, Victor F., urologista norte-americano, *1913. VER M. *test*; M.-Marchetti *test*; M.-Marchetti-Krantz *operation*.
Mar·shal·la·gia mar·shalli (mar-sha-lā´jē-ă mar-shal´ī). Um dos vermes gástricos médios da família dos nematódeos Trichostrongylidae, encontrados no abomaso de ovinos, caprinos, camelos e de vários ruminantes selvagens.
marsh·mal·low root (marsh´mal-ō). Raiz de altéia; raiz de malvavisco. SIN althea.
mar·su·pi·al (mar-soo´pē-ăl). Marsupial. **1.** Membro da ordem Marsupalia, que inclui mamíferos como os cangurus, vombates, nesóquias e gambás, cujas fêmeas possuem uma bolsa abdominal para transportar os filhotes. **2.** De ou relativo a marsupiais. [L. *marsupium*, bolsa]
mar·su·pi·al·i·za·tion (mar-soo´pē-ăl-i-zā´shŭn). Marsupialização; exteriorização de um cisto ou outra cavidade fechada por ressecção da parede anterior e sutura das bordas seccionadas da parede remanescente às bordas cutâneas adjacentes, criando assim uma bolsa. [L. *marsupium*, bolsa]
mar·su·pi·um (mar-soo´pē-ŭm). Marsúpio; bolsa marsupial. **1.** SIN scrotum. **2.** Uma bolsa ou saco; p. ex., em marsupiais. [L. bolsa]
Martegiani, J., anatomista italiano do século XIX. VER M. *area, funnel*.
Martin, August E., ginecologista alemão, 1847–1933. VER M. *tube*; M.-Gruber *anastomosis*.
Martin, Henry A., cirurgião norte-americano, 1824–1884. VER M. *bandage, disease*.
Martin, J.E. VER Thayer-M. *medium*.
Martinotti, Giovanni, médico italiano, 1857–1928. VER M. *cell*.
mar·ti·us yel·low (marsh´ē-ŭs) [C.I. 10315]. Amarelo de Martius; corante ácido utilizado como corante plasmático em histologia vegetal e animal, e como filtro de luz para fotomicrografia. [Karl A. *Martius*, químico alemão, *1920]
Martorell, Fernando Otzet, cardiologista espanhol, 1906–1984. VER M. *syndrome*.
Mar·y·land co·ma scale. Escala de coma de Maryland. VER coma *scale*.
mas·cha·le (mas´kăl-ē). Axila. SIN axilla. [G.]
mas·chal·y·per·i·dro·sis (mas´kăl-i-per-i-drō´sis). Mascaliperidrose; sudorese excessiva nas axilas. [G. *maschalē,* axila, + *hyper,* hiper, + *hidrōs,* suor]
mas·cu·line (mas´kū-lin). Masculino; relativo ao sexo masculino, ou marcado pelas características desse sexo. SIN male (2), masculinus. [L. *masculus,* masculino, de *mas,* masculino]
mas·cu·line pro·test. Protesto masculino; termo de Adler para descrever o deslocamento de indivíduos de papéis passivos para ativos em um desejo de fugir do papel feminino.
mas·cu·lin·i·ty (mas-kū-lin´i-tē). Masculinidade; as qualidades e características de um macho.
mas·cu·lin·i·za·tion (mas´kū-lin-i-zā´shŭn). Masculinização; a condição caracterizada pelo surgimento de características masculinas, como pêlos faciais, seja fisiologicamente, como parte do amadurecimento masculino, ou patologicamente por indivíduos de qualquer sexo. [L. *masculus,* masculino]
mas·cu·li·nize (mas´kū-li-nīz). Masculinizar; conferir as qualidades ou características peculiares do macho.
mas·cu·li·nus (mas-kū-lī´nŭs). Masculino. SIN masculine, masculine. [L.]
Masini, Giulio, médico italiano, 1874–1937.
mask (mask). Máscara. **1.** Qualquer um dentre vários estados patológicos que produzem alteração ou mudança de coloração da pele da face. **2.** A aparência inexpressiva observada em algumas doenças; p. ex., fácies de Parkinson. **3.** Um curativo facial. **4.** Proteção destinada a cobrir a boca e o nariz para manter condições anti-sépticas. **5.** Dispositivo destinado a cobrir a boca e o nariz para administração de anestésicos inalatórios, oxigênio ou outros gases.
 ecchymotic m., m. equimótica; coloração pardacenta da cabeça e do pescoço que ocorre quando o tronco foi submetido a compressão súbita e extrema, como na asfixia traumática.
 Hutchinson m., m. de Hutchinson; a sensação experimentada na neurossífilis tabética, como se a face estivesse coberta por uma máscara ou por teias.
 laryngeal m., m. laríngea; cânula orofaríngea tubular com uma margem insuflável na extremidade distal que, quando inflada, cria uma vedação hermética imediatamente acima da laringe.
 nonrebreathing m., m. unidirecional; máscara que possui uma válvula de inalação e uma válvula de exalação, de forma que todo o gás expirado vai para a atmosfera externa, e o gás inalado vem apenas de um reservatório conectado à máscara.
 tropical m., m. tropical. SIN chloasma bronzinum.
masked (maskt). Mascarado; oculto; escondido.
mask·ing. Mascaramento. **1.** O uso de ruído de qualquer tipo para interferir com a audibilidade de outro som. Em qualquer intensidade, tons graves têm um maior efeito de mascaramento que os agudos. **2.** Em audiologia, o uso de um ruído aplicado a uma orelha enquanto se testa a audição da outra. **3.** O ocultamento de ritmos menores no registro de ondas cerebrais por ondas maiores e mais lentas cuja forma eles distorcem. **4.** Em odontologia, revestimento opaco usado para camuflar as partes metálicas de uma prótese. **5.** Em radiografia, a superposição de uma imagem positiva alterada sobre o negativo original para produzir uma cópia mais nítida fotograficamente. VER subtraction.
 unsharp m., m. indefinido; em radiografia, superposição de um negativo borrado de uma radiografia para ocultar grandes diferenças de densidade, deixando mais visíveis os detalhes finos.
Maslow, Abraham H., psicólogo norte-americano, 1908–1970. VER M. *hierarchy*.
mas·och·ism (mas´ō-kizm, maz´ō-). Masoquismo. **1.** Algolagnia passiva; forma de perversão, freqüentemente de natureza sexual, na qual uma pessoa tem prazer em ser vítima de abuso, humilhação ou maus-tratos. Cf. sadism. **2.** Orientação geral na vida de que o sofrimento pessoal alivia a culpa e conduz a uma recompensa. [Leopold von Sacher-*Masoch*, novelista austríaco, 1836–1895]
mas·och·ist (mas´ō-kist). Masoquista; a parte passiva na prática do masoquismo.
Mason, Edward E., cirurgião norte-americano, *1920.
MASS Acrônimo para *m*itral valve prolapse, *a*ortic anomalies, *s*keletal changes, and *s*kin changes (prolapso da valva mitral, anomalias aórticas, alterações ósseas e cutâneas). VER MASS *syndrome*.
mass (m). Massa. **1.** Tumoração ou agregação de material aderente. SIN massa [TA]. **2.** Em farmácia, preparação sólida macia contendo um agente medicinal ativo, com tal consistência que pode ser dividida em pequenas porções e transformada em comprimidos. **3.** Uma das sete quantidades fundamentais no sistema SI; sua unidade é o quilograma, definido como a massa do protótipo internacional do quilograma, que é feita de platina-irídio e encontra-se no *International Bureau of Weights and Measures*. **4.** A quantidade de matéria em um corpo ou substância. [L. *massa,* massa de bolo]
 apperceptive m., m. aperceptível; a base de conhecimento já existente em uma área semelhante ou relacionada, com a qual o novo material de percepção é articulado.
 filar m., m. filamentosa. SIN reticular *substance* (1).
 injection m., m. de injeção; soluções ou suspensões coloridas injetadas no sistema vascular para tornar os vasos e suas paredes proeminentes; útil em preparações macroscópicas e em estudo sob pequeno aumento após clareamento; a maioria dos fluidos contém gelatina morna, e os materiais corantes são o carmim, o azul de Berlim ou o carbono.

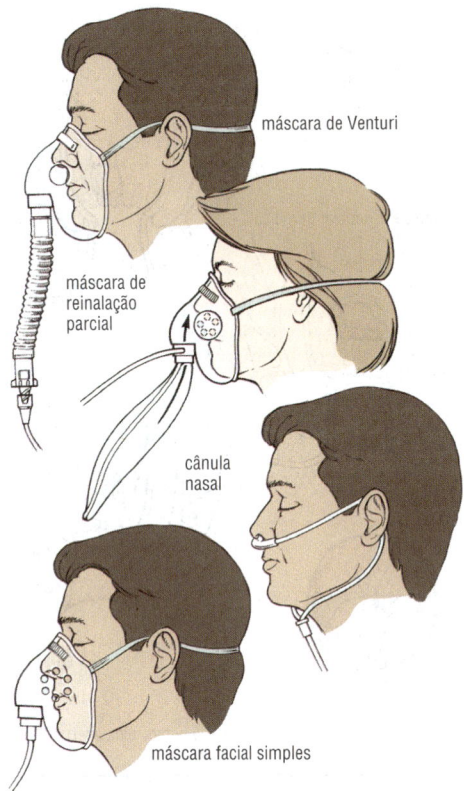

máscaras de oxigênio

massa (m). 950 **mastectomy**

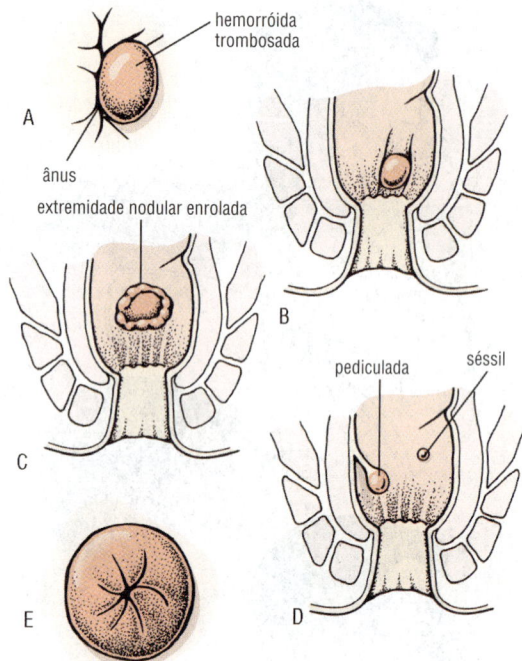

massas anais e retais: (A) hemorróida externa, (B) hemorróida interna, (C) tumor retal, (D) pólipos retais, (E) prolapso retal

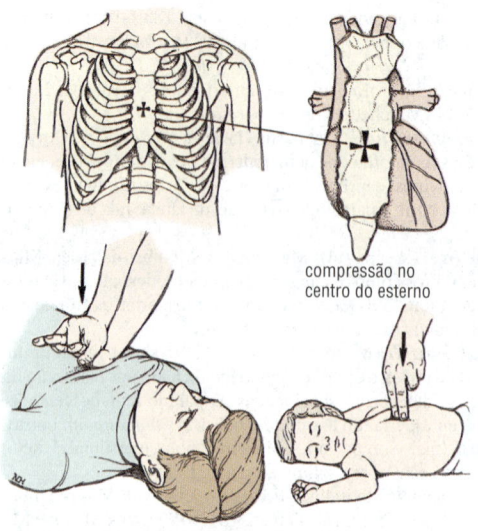

massagem torácica fechada

inner cell m., m. celular interna; as células no pólo embrionário do blastocisto relacionadas à formação do corpo do embrião em si. SIN embryoblast.
intermediate m., m. intermediária. SIN interthalamic adhesion.
lateral m. of atlas [TA], m. lateral do atlas; a parte lateral espessa, de sustentação de peso, situada de cada lado do atlas e que se articula, acima, com o côndilo occipital e, abaixo, com o áxis. SIN massa lateralis atlantis [TA].
lateral m. of ethmoid bone, m. lateral do etmóide. SIN ethmoidal labyrinth.
molar m., m. molar. VER molecular weight.
molecular m., m. molecular. SIN molecular weight.
pilular m., m. pilular; mistura de droga(s), excipientes, diluentes e ligantes com um volume adequado de líquido para formar uma massa plástica que pode ser enrolada em um longo cilindro e cortada no número apropriado de unidades para que sejam feitos comprimidos. SIN pill mass.
relative molecular m. (M_r), m. molecular relativa. SIN molecular weight.
sclerotic cemental m., m. cemento-esclerótica; displasia óssea florida; lesões fibro-ósseas benignas da mandíbula de etiologia desconhecida, encontradas predominantemente em mulheres negras de meia-idade, que se apresentam como massas radiopacas indolores grandes, que geralmente envolvem diversos quadrantes da mandíbula. SIN florid osseous dysplasia, cemental dysplasia.
tubular excretory m., m. excretora tubular; a massa de túbulos excretores funcionantes do rim, determinada a partir da excreção de substâncias mensuráveis processadas no rim basicamente por secreção tubular.
mas·sa, gen. e pl. **mas·sae** (mas'să, mas'sē) [TA]. Massa. SIN mass (1). [L.]
  m. interme'dia, aderência intertalâmica; *termo oficial alternativo para interthalamic adhesion.
  m. latera'lis atlan'tis [TA], m. lateral do atlas. SIN lateral mass of atlas.
mas·sage (mă-sahzh'). Massagem; método de manipulação do corpo ou de parte dele por meio de fricções, compressões, amassaduras, golpes leves, etc. SIN tripsis (2). [Fr. do G. massō, amassar]
  cardiac m., m. cardíaca. SIN heart m.
  closed chest m., m. cardíaca fechada; compressão rítmica do coração entre o esterno e a coluna vertebral por depressão da parte inferior do esterno com a parte inferior das mãos, com o paciente em decúbito dorsal. SIN external cardiac m.
  external cardiac m., m. cardíaca externa. SIN closed chest m.
  gingival m., m. gengival; estimulação mecânica da gengiva por fricção ou pressão.
  heart m., m. cardíaca; massagem rítmica do coração, seja com o tórax aberto ou através da parede torácica, para reiniciar a circulação ausente durante ressuscitação cardíaca. SIN cardiac m.
  open chest m., m. torácica aberta; compressão manual rítmica dos ventrículos cardíacos com a mão dentro da cavidade torácica.
  prostatic m., m. prostática; **(1)** expressão manual das secreções prostáticas por técnica digital retal; **(2)** o esvaziamento dos ácinos e ductos prostáticos por repetidas manobras de compressão descendentes, para tratamento de vários distúrbios congestivos e inflamatórios da próstata.
  vibratory m., m. vibratória; aplicação de golpes leves e muito rápidos à superfície por meio de um instrumento, geralmente com extremidade elástica. SIN seismotherapy, sismotherapy, vibrotherapeutics.
Masselon, Julián, médico francês, 1844–1917. VER M. spectacles.
mas·se·ter. Masseter. VER masseter (muscle).
mas·seur (mă-ser'). **1.** Massagista; homem que faz massagem. **2.** Massageador; instrumento usado na massagem mecânica. [Fr. ver massage]
mas·seuse (mă-sooz'). Massagista; mulher que faz massagem.
mas·si·cot (mas'i-kot). Monóxido de chumbo. SIN lead monoxide.
Masson, Pierre, patologista canadense, 1880–1959. VER M.-Fontana ammoniac silver stain. VER entradas em stain.
mas·so·ther·a·py (mas-ō-thār'ă-pē). Massoterapia; o uso terapêutico de massagem. [G. massō, amassar, + therapeia, tratamento]
MAST Abreviatura para military antishock trousers (vestes antichoque).
mast-. VER masto-.
mast·ad·e·ni·tis (mast'ad-ĕ-nī'tis). Mastadenite, mastite. SIN mastitis. [masto- + G. adēn, glândula, + -itis, inflamação]
mast·ad·e·no·ma (mast'ad-ĕ-nō'mă). Mastadenoma; um adenoma da mama. [masto- + G. adēn, glândula, + -ōma, tumor]
Mast·ad·e·no·vi·rus (mast-ad'e-nō-vī'rŭs). Gênero da família Adenoviridae, incluindo adenovírus que infectam mamíferos, com mais de 40 tipos antigênicos (espécies) infecciosos para os seres humanos. Causam infecções respiratórias em crianças, doença respiratória aguda epidêmica em recrutas, conjuntivite folicular aguda em adultos, ceratoconjuntivite epidêmica e gastroenterite; muitas infecções não são aparentes. [G. mastos, mama, daí mamífero, + adenovirus]
mas·tal·gia (mas-tal'jē-ă). Mastalgia. SIN mastodynia. [masto- + G. algos, dor]
mas·tat·ro·phy, mas·ta·tro·phia (mas-tat'rō-fē, mast-ă-trō'fē-ă). Mastatrofia; atrofia ou definhamento das mamas. [masto- + atrophy]
mas·tauxe (mas-tawk'sē). Mastauxe; hipertrofia da mama. [masto- + G. auxē, aumento]
mas·tec·to·my (mas-tek'tō-mē). Mastectomia; excisão da mama. SIN mammectomy. [masto- + G. ektomē, excisão]
  extended radical m., m. radical estendida; excisão de toda a mama, incluindo o mamilo, a aréola e a pele sobrejacente, bem como os músculos peitorais e os tecidos com linfáticos da axila e da parede torácica e a cadeia mamária interna de linfonodos.
  modified radical m., m. radical modificada; excisão de toda a mama, incluindo o mamilo, a aréola e a pele sobrejacente, bem como o tecido com linfáticos na axila, com preservação dos músculos peitorais.
  radical m., m. radical; excisão de toda a mama, incluindo o mamilo, a aréola e a pele sobrejacente, bem como dos músculos peitorais, do tecido com lin-

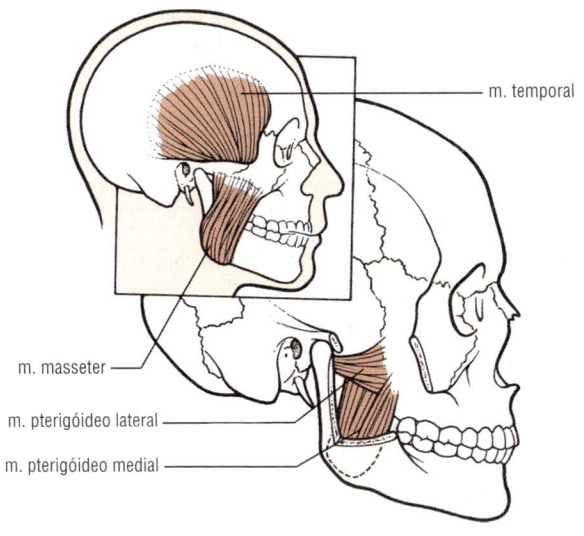

músculos da mastigação

fáticos na axila e de vários outros tecidos adjacentes. SIN Halsted operation (2).
simple m., m. simples; excisão da mama, incluindo o mamilo, a aréola e parte da pele sobrejacente. SIN total m.
subcutaneous m., m. subcutânea; excisão dos tecidos mamários, com preservação da pele, do mamilo e da aréola; geralmente é seguida por implantação de uma prótese.
total m., m. total. SIN simple m.

Master, Arthur M., médico norte-americano, 1895–1973. VER M. *test,* two-step exercise *test*.

Masters, William H., ginecologista norte-americano, *1915. VER Allen-M. *syndrome*.

mas·tic (mas′tik). Mástique; almécega; exsudato resinoso da *Pistacia lentiscus* (família Anacardiaceae), pequena árvore do litoral mediterrâneo; usada em goma de mascar, como revestimento entérico e como material de obturação temporária em odontologia. SIN mastich, mastiche. [G. *mastichē,* a resina da aroeira-da-praia]

mas·ti·cate (mas′ti-kāt). Mastigar; realizar mastigação.

mas·ti·ca·tion (mas-ti-kā′shŭn). Mastigação; o processo de mastigar o alimento, preparando-o para a deglutição e digestão; o ato de triturar ou fragmentar com os dentes. [L. *mastico,* pp. *-atus,* mastigar]

mas·ti·ca·to·ry (mas′ti-kā-tō-rē). Mastigatório; relativo à mastigação.

mas·tich, mas·ti·che (mas′tik, mas′ti-kē). Mástique. SIN mastic.

Mas·ti·goph·o·ra (mas′ti-gof′o-ră). Os flagelados, um subfilo do Protozoa que possui um ou mais flagelos para locomoção, um único núcleo vesicular e divisão binária simétrica; a reprodução sexuada é desconhecida em muitos grupos (p. ex., *Volvox, Trypanosoma, Euglena*). Possui duas classes: Phytomastigophorea (a que pertence a *Euglena*), que contém clorofila e, portanto, é fotossintética e holofítica (embora isso tenha sido secundariamente perdido em alguns grupos), e Zoomastigophorea (incluindo *Trypanosoma* e *Leishmania*), que não possui cromatóforos e é heterotrófico. [G. *mastix* (*mastig-*), flagelo, + *phoros,* portador]

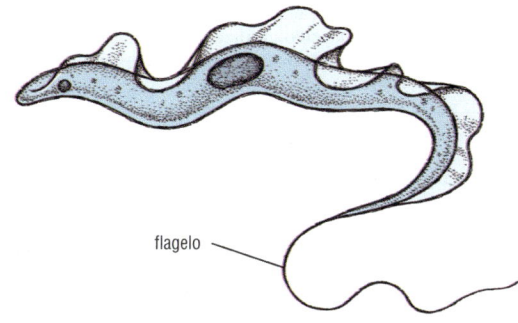

Mastigophora com flagelo

mas·ti·gote (mas′ti-gōt). Mastigota; um flagelado individual. [G. *mastix,* flagelo]

mas·ti·tis (mas-tī′tis). Mastite; inflamação da mama. SIN mastadenitis. [masto- + G. *–itis,* inflamação]
chronic cystic m., m. cística crônica; termo antigo que corresponde à doença fibrocística da mama (fibrocystic *condition* of the breast).
gargantuan m., m. gigantesca; termo obsoleto para inflamação crônica da mama com grande aumento da glândula.
glandular m., m. glandular. SIN parenchymatous m.
granulomatous m., m. granulomatosa; inflamação granulomatosa rara do tecido mamário lobular, com células gigantes multinucleadas; a sarcoidose é incluída pela presença freqüente de neutrófilos e ausência de envolvimento de outros tecidos.
interstitial m., m. intersticial; inflamação do tecido conjuntivo da glândula mamária.
lactational m., m. da lactação, m. puerperal. SIN puerperal m.
m. neonator'um, m. neonatal; mastite no tecido mamário secretor do recém-nascido, geralmente estafilocócica.
parenchymatous m., m. parenquimatosa; inflamação do tecido secretor da mama. SIN glandular m.
plasma cell m., m. de plasmócitos; doença das mamas caracterizada por massas endurecidas tumorais, contendo numerosos plasmócitos, geralmente resultante de ectasia dos ductos mamários; embora clinicamente seja semelhante à doença maligna (aderência à pele e aumento dos linfonodos axilares), não é neoplásica.
puerperal m., m. puerperal; mastite, geralmente supurativa, que ocorre na última parte do puerpério. SIN lactational m.
retromammary m., m. retromamária. SIN submammary m.
stagnation m., m. de estagnação; distensão dolorosa da mama, que ocorre durante os últimos dias da gravidez e nos primeiros dias da lactação.
submammary m., m. submamária; inflamação dos tecidos situados profundamente na glândula mamária. SIN retromammary m.
suppurative m., m. supurativa; inflamação da mama devida à infecção por bactérias piogênicas.

masto-, mast-. Masto-, mast-; a mama; o processo mastóide. Cf. mammo-, mazo-. [G. *mastos*]

mas·toc·cip·i·tal (mast′ok-sip′-i-tāl). Mastoccipital. SIN masto-occipital.
mas·to·cyte (mas′tō-sīt). Mastócito. SIN mast cell.
mas·to·cy·to·gen·e·sis (mas′tō-sī′tō-jen′e-sis). Mastocitogênese; formação e desenvolvimento de mastócitos. [mastocyte + G. *genesis,* produção]
mas·to·cy·to·ma (mas′tō-sī-tō′mă). Mastocitoma; acúmulo muito bem circunscrito ou foco nodular de mastócitos; macroscopicamente semelhante a uma neoplasia. [mastocyte + G. *-oma,* tumor]
mas·to·cy·to·sis (mas′tō-sī-tō′sis). Mastocitose; proliferação anormal de mastócitos em vários tecidos; pode ser sistêmica, envolvendo vários órgãos, ou cutânea (urticária pigmentosa). [mastocyte + G. *–osis,* condição]
diffuse m., m. difusa; infiltração de muitos órgãos ou sistemas por mastócitos com diversas manifestações clínicas, que podem incluir febre, emagrecimento, rubor, broncospasmo, rinorréia, palpitações, dispnéia, diarréia, hemorragia gastrointestinal e hipotensão. SIN systemic m.
diffuse cutaneous m., m. cutânea difusa; processo benigno que consiste em infiltrados cutâneos focais compostos de mastócitos; as lesões são planas ou ligeiramente elevadas, formam pápulas e são pruriginosas quando tocadas; pode haver lesões ósseas.
systemic m., m. sistêmica. SIN diffuse m.

mas·to·dyn·i·a (mas-tō-din′ē-ă). Mastodinia; dor na mama. VER TAMBÉM mammary *neuralgia*. SIN mammalgia, mastalgia. [masto- + G. *odynē,* dor]

mas·toid (mas′toyd). Mastóide. **1.** Semelhante a uma mama; que tem a forma de mama. **2.** Mastóideo; relativo ao processo mastóideo, antro mastóideo, células mastóideas, etc. SIN mastoidal. [masto- + G. *eidos,* semelhante]

mas·toi·dal (mas-toy′dăl). Mastóideo. SIN mastoid (2).

mas·toi·da·le (mas-toy-dā′lē). Mastóide; o ponto mais baixo no contorno do processo mastóide.

mas·toid·ec·to·my (mas′toy-dek′tō-mē). Mastoidectomia; um grupo de operações, no processo mastóide do osso temporal e na orelha média, para drenar, expor ou remover uma lesão infecciosa, inflamatória ou neoplásica. [mastóide (processo) + G. *ektomē,* excisão]
complete m., m. completa; cirurgia para extrair o sistema de células aéreas do processo mastóide do osso temporal para drenagem da supuração na mastoidite aguda. SIN simple m.
modified radical m., m. radical modificada; cirurgia para tratamento de colesteatoma situado lateral ao remanescente da membrana timpânica e dos ossículos da orelha média; envolve extração das células aéreas remanescentes do processo mastóide e retirada das paredes posterior e superior do canal auditivo externo para abrir o mastóide e o recesso epitimpânico da orelha média para o exterior e preservar a audição.
radical m., m. radical; cirurgia para o tratamento do colesteatoma extenso; envolve a extração das células aéreas mastóideas e a remoção das paredes

posterior e superior do canal auditivo externo e dos remanescentes da membrana timpânica e dos ossículos da orelha média, para exteriorizar a cavidade mastóidea e a orelha média através do canal auditivo externo. SIN tympanomastoidectomy.
  simple m., m. simples. SIN complete m.
mas·toid·i·tis (mas-toy-dī′tis). Mastoidite; inflamação de qualquer parte do processo mastóide. SIN mastoid empyema.
  sclerosing m., m. esclerosante; mastoidite crônica na qual as trabéculas se encontram muito espessas, tendendo a obliterar as células.
mas·ton·cus (mas-tong′kŭs). Mastoncose; tumor ou edema das mamas. [masto- + G. *onkos*, massa]
mas·to·oc·cip·i·tal (mas′tō-ok-sip′i-tăl). Masto-occipital; relativo à porção mastóidea do osso temporal e ao osso parietal, designando a sutura que os une.
mas·to·pa·ri·e·tal (mas′tō-pa-rī′e-tăl). Mastoparietal; relativo à porção mastóidea do osso temporal e ao osso parietal, designando a sutura que os une.
mas·top·a·thy (mas-top′a-thē). Mastopatia; qualquer doença das mamas. [masto- + G. *pathos*, que sofre]
mas·to·pexy (mas′tō-pek-sē). Mastopexia; cirurgia plástica para elevar uma mama ptótica para a posição normal, freqüentemente com alguma melhora do formato. [masto- + G. *pēxis*, fixação]
mas·to·pla·sia (mas-tō-plā′zē-ă). Mastoplasia; aumento da mama. [masto- + G. *plasis*, moldagem]
mas·to·plas·ty (mas′tō-plas-tē). Mastoplastia. SIN mammaplasty. [masto- + G. *plastos*, formado]
mas·top·to·sis (mas-top-tō′sis). Mastoptose; ptose ou queda da mama. [masto- + G. *ptōsis*, queda]
mas·tor·rha·gia (mas-tō-rā′jē-ă). Mastorragia; hemorragia da mama. [masto- + G. *rhēgnymi*, romper]
mas·to·squa·mous (mas′tō-skwā′mŭs). Mastoescamoso; relativo ao processo mastóide e às partes escamosas do osso temporal.
mas·to·syr·inx (mas′tō-sir′ingks). Mastossiringe; uma fístula da glândula mamária. [masto- + G. *syrinx*, tubo]
mas·tot·o·my (mas-tot′ō-mē). Mastotomia; incisão da mama. SIN mammotomy. [masto- + G. *tomē*, incisão]
mas·tur·bate (mas′ter-bāt). Masturbar; praticar masturbação. [L. *masturbari*, pp. *masturbatus*]
mas·tur·ba·tion (mas′ter-bā′shung). Masturbação; auto-estimulação da genitália para obter prazer erótico, freqüentemente resultando em orgasmo.
MAT Abreviatura de multifocal atrial *tachycardia* (taquicardia atrial multifocal).
Matas, Rudolph, cirurgião norte-americano, 1860–1957.
match·ing. Emparelhamento; o processo de tornar um grupo de estudo e um grupo de comparação em um estudo epidemiológico comparáveis em relação a fatores estranhos ou que geram confusão, como idade, sexo e peso.
  impedance m., casamento de impedância; a força aplicada através do favorecimento mecânico dos ossículos da audição e da razão entre a área da membrana timpânica e da janela oval, para superar a impedância acústica entre o ar ambiente e o fluido na orelha interna.
maté (mah-tā′). Erva-mate; mate; as folhas secas do *Ilex paraguayensis* e outras espécies de *Ilex* (família Aquifoliaceae), arbustos que crescem no Paraguai e no Brasil e que contêm cafeína e tanino; usada em países da América do Sul como bebida e por suas propriedades medicinais, como diurético e diaforético, e para o alívio de cefaléia. SIN Paraguay tea. [Esp. *maté*, um recipiente no qual as folhas são preparadas]
mat·er (mā′ter). Máter; os revestimentos "protetores" do sistema nervoso central. VER *arachnoid* mater, dura mater, pia mater. [L. mãe]
  arachnoidea mater cranialis [TA], aracnóide-máter, parte encefálica. SIN cranial *arachnoid* mater.
  arachnoidea mater encephali, aracnóide-máter, parte encefálica; *termo oficial alternativo para cranial *arachnoid* mater.
  cranial pia mater [TA], pia-máter, parte encefálica; a pia-máter encontrada especificamente ao redor do encéfalo; contígua com a aracnóide-máter através das trabéculas aracnóideas. VER TAMBÉM pia mater. SIN pia mater encephali*.
  pia mater encephali, pia-máter, parte encefálica; *termo oficial alternativo para cranial pia mater.
  pia mater spinalis [TA], pia-máter, parte espinal. SIN spinal pia mater; VER TAMBÉM pia mater.
  spinal arachnoid mater [TA], aracnóide-máter, parte espinal. VER spinal *arachnoid* mater; VER TAMBÉM *arachnoid* mater.
  spinal pia mater [TA], pia-máter, parte espinal; a pia-máter encontrada especificamente em torno da medula espinal; inclui especializações como os ligamentos denticulados. VER TAMBÉM pia mater. SIN pia mater spinalis [TA].
ma·te·ria (mă-tē′rē-ă). Matéria ou substância. [L. substância]
  m. al′ba, matéria alba; placa bacteriana; acúmulo ou agregação de microrganismos, células epiteliais descamadas, células do sangue e restos de alimentos frouxamente aderidos a superfícies de placas, dentes, gengiva ou aparelhos dentários. [L. matéria branca]

  m. med′ica, matéria médica; (**1**) ramo da ciência médica que trata da origem e do preparo de medicamentos, suas doses e sua forma de administração; (**2**) qualquer agente usado terapeuticamente. VER TAMBÉM pharmacognosy, pharmacology. [L. matéria médica]
ma·te·ri·al (mă-tēr′ē-ăl). Material; substância da qual algo é feito ou composto; o elemento constituinte de uma substância. [L. *materialis*, de *materia*, substância]
  base m., m. de base; qualquer substância com a qual pode ser feita a base de uma dentadura, como goma-laca, resina acrílica, ebonite, poliestireno, metal, etc.
  by-product m., subproduto nuclear; material radioativo produzido por fissão nuclear ou por irradiação de nêutrons em um reator nuclear ou dispositivo semelhante.
  certified reference m. (CRM), m. de referência certificado; material de referência documentado ou descoberto por um certificado ou publicação de uma fonte confiável e que declara os valores das propriedades envolvidas.
  contrast m., m. de contraste. SIN contrast *medium*.
  cross-reacting m. (CRM), m. de reação cruzada; substância suficientemente diferente de uma substância de referência (R) para ter uma função perceptivelmente diferente de R, mas semelhante o suficiente para reagir com anticorpos anti-R.
  dental m., m. dental; qualquer material usado em odontologia.
  genetic m., m. genético; o portador das informações hereditárias; em organismos superiores é o DNA duplo.
  impression m., m. de impressão; qualquer substância ou combinação de substâncias usada para fazer uma reprodução negativa ou impressão.
  plastic restoration m., m. de restauração plástica; em odontologia, qualquer material que possa ser moldado diretamente na cavidade do dente, tal como amálgama, cimento ou resina.
  restorative dental m.'s, materiais dentários de restauração; materiais usados para substituir tecidos orais em odontologia; p. ex., amálgama, ligas de ouro, cimentos, porcelana, plástico e materiais para dentadura.
ma·te·ri·es mor·bi (mă-tē′rē-ēz mōr′bī). A substância que age como causa imediata de uma doença. [L. a matéria da doença]
ma·ter·nal (mă-ter′năl). Materno; relativo a ou derivado da mãe. [L. *maternus*, de *mater*, mãe]
ma·ter·ni·ty (mă-ter′ni-tē). Maternidade. [ver maternal]
mat·ing (māt′ing). Acasalamento; a união de macho e fêmea para reprodução.
  assortative m., a. concordante; seleção de um parceiro com preferência por (ou aversão a) um genótipo específico, isto é, acasalamento não-aleatório. SIN nonrandom m.
  cross m., cruzamento. VER cross.
  nonrandom m., a. não-aleatório. SIN assortative m.
  random m., a. aleatório; prática de acasalamento na qual todos os óvulos têm oportunidades iguais de serem fertilizados por qualquer espermatozóide; assim, a chance de um genótipo em um determinado *locus* de se combinar a outro genótipo nesse *locus* é aleatória. SIN panmixis.
mat·rass (mat′răs). Matraz; vaso de vidro com colo longo usado para aquecer substâncias secas em manipulações químicas. [Fr. *matras*]
mat·ri·cal (mat′ri-kăl). Matricial; relativo a qualquer matriz. SIN matricial.
mat·ri·ca·ria (mat-ri-kā′rē-ă). Camomila; matricária; camomila comum; camomila da Alemanha; as flores da *Matricaria chamomilla* (família Compositae); usada internamente como tônico e, externamente, como contra-irritante. VER TAMBÉM chamomile. [L. *matrix*, útero]
ma·tri·ces (mā′tri-sēz, mat′rī-sēz). Matrizes, plural de matrix. [L.]
ma·tri·cial (mă-trish′ăl). Matricial. SIN matrical.
mat·ri·cide (mat′ri-sīd). **1.** Matricídio; assassinato da própria mãe. Cf. patricide. **2.** Matricida; aquele que comete tal ato. [L. *mater*, mãe, + *caedo*, matar]
mat·ri·lin·e·al (mat-ri-lin′ē-ăl). Matrilinear; indica a ascendência através da linha materna. [L. *mater*, mãe, + *linea*, linha]
ma·trix, pl. **ma·tri·ces** (mā′triks, mat′riks; mā′tri-sēz, mat′ri-sēz). Matriz. **1** [NA]. Matriz; a porção formadora de um dente ou de uma unha. **2.** substância intercelular de um tecido. **3.** Uma substância adjacente na qual há alguma coisa contida ou incrustada, p. ex., o tecido adiposo no qual há vasos sanguíneos ou linfonodos; proporciona uma matriz para essas estruturas incrustadas. **4.** Molde no qual algo é vertido para modelagem ou forjado; contramolde; instrumento de formato especial, material plástico ou tira metálica usada para reter e modelar o material usado na obturação de uma cavidade dentária. **5.** Conjunto retangular de números ou quantidades simbólicas que simplificam a execução de operações lineares de complexidade tediosa, p. ex., o método ITO; a teoria da matriz é amplamente usada para a resolução de equações simultâneas e em genética da população. [L. útero; animal de procriação do sexo feminino]
  amalgam m., m. de amálgama; dispositivo usado durante a colocação da massa de amálgama em uma preparação de cavidade composta, daí facilitando a condensação e o contorno apropriados por proporcionar uma parede limitante.

bone m., m. óssea; a substância intercelular de tecido ósseo que consiste em fibras de colágeno, substância fundamental e sais ósseos inorgânicos.

cartilage m., m. de cartilagem; a substância intercelular de cartilagem que consiste em fibras e substância fundamental.

cell m., m. celular. SIN cytoplasmic m.

cytoplasmic m., m. citoplasmática; substância citoplasmática fluida que preenche os interstícios do citoesqueleto. SIN cell m., cytomatrix.

external m., m. externa; a substância que ocupa o espaço entre as membranas interna e externa de qualquer organela (p. ex., mitocôndria) com uma membrana dupla.

identity m., m. de identidade; matriz quadrada na qual as quantidades na diagonal do ângulo superior esquerdo ao ângulo inferior direito são iguais a 1 e todas as outras variáveis são iguais a 0.

mitochondrial m., m. mitocondrial. SIN m. mitochondrialis.

m. mitochondria'lis, m. mitocondrial; a substância que ocupa o espaço limitado pela membrana interna de uma mitocôndria; contém enzimas, filamentos de DNA, ribossomas, grânulos e inclusões de cristais de proteínas, glicogênio e lipídios. SIN mitochondrial m.

nail m. [TA], m. da unha; a área da derme na qual está apoiada a unha; é extremamente sensível e apresenta muitas cristas longitudinais em sua superfície. Segundo alguns anatomistas, a matriz da unha é apenas a parte na qual a raiz da unha se apóia. SIN m. unguis [TA], keratogenous membrane, nail bed, onychostroma.

nuclear m., m. nuclear; a rede de fibras proteicas situada em torno e dentro do núcleo.

square m., m. quadrada; matriz na qual os números de linhas e colunas são iguais.

territorial m., m. territorial. SIN cartilage capsule.

m. un'guis [TA], m. da unha. SIN nail m.

mat·ter. Matéria; substância. SIN substance. VER TAMBÉM substance. [L. *materies*, substância]

gray m. [TA], substância cinzenta; as regiões do encéfalo e da medula espinal formadas basicamente pelos corpos celulares e dendritos das células nervosas, em vez de axônios mielinizados. SIN gray substance [TA], substantia grisea [TA], substantia cinerea.

pontine gray m., núcleos da ponte. SIN pontine *nuclei*, em *nucleus*.

white m. [TA], substância branca; as regiões do encéfalo e da medula espinal formadas, em grande parte ou totalmente, de fibras nervosas e que contêm poucos (ou nenhum) corpos celulares neuronais ou dendritos. SIN alba, substantia alba, white substance.

mat·u·rate (mat'u-rāt). Amadurecer; supurar. [L. *maturo*, pp. *-atus*, tornar maduro, de *maturus*, maduro]

mat·u·ra·tion (mat-u-rā'shŭn). Maturação; amadurecimento. **1.** Conquista de desenvolvimento ou crescimento completo. **2.** Alterações do desenvolvimento que levam à maturidade. **3.** Processamento de uma macromolécula, p. ex., modificação pós-transcricional de RNA ou modificação pós-tradução de proteínas. **4.** O processo geral que leva à incorporação de um genoma viral a um capsídeo e ao desenvolvimento de um virion completo. [L. *maturatio*, amadurecimento, de *maturus*, maduro]

ma·ture (mă-choor', -toor). **1.** Maduro; totalmente desenvolvido. **2.** Amadurecer; tornar-se totalmente desenvolvido. [L. *maturus*, maduro]

ma·tu·ri·ty (mă-choor'i-tē). Maturidade; estado de desenvolvimento completo ou crescimento concluído.

Mauchart (Mauchard), Burkhard D., anatomista alemão, 1696–1751. VER M. *ligaments,* em *ligament.*

Maurer, Georg, médico alemão em Sumatra, *1909. VER M. *clefts,* em *cleft, dots,* em *dot.*

Mauriac, Pierre, médico francês, *1882. VER M. *syndrome.*

Mauriceau, François, obstetra francês, 1637–1709. VER M. *maneuver;* M.-Levret *maneuver.*

Mauthner, Ludwig, oftalmologista austríaco, 1840–1894. VER M. *sheath.*

max·il·la, gen. e pl. **max·il·lae** (mak-sil'ă, mak-sil'ē) [TA]. Maxila; osso pneumatizado de forma irregular, que sustenta os dentes superiores e toma parte na formação da órbita, do palato duro e da cavidade nasal e contém o seio maxilar. SIN upper jaw bone, upper jaw. [L. maxilar]

max·il·lary (mak'si-lār-ē). Maxilar; relativo à maxila.

max·il·lec·to·my (mak-sil-ek'tō-mē). Maxilectomia; ressecção da maxila. [maxilla + G. *ektomē*, excisão]

max·il·li·tis (mak'si-lī'tis). Maxilite; inflamação da maxila.

max·il·lo·den·tal (mak-sil'ō-den'tăl). Maxilodental; relativo à maxila e a seus dentes associados.

max·il·lo·fa·cial (mak-sil'ō-fā'shăl). Maxilofacial; relativo à maxila e mandíbula e à face, particularmente em referência à cirurgia especializada dessa região.

max·il·lo·ju·gal (mak-sil'ō-joo'găl). Maxilojugal; relativo à maxila e ao osso zigomático.

max·il·lo·man·dib·u·lar (mak-sil'ō-man-dib'u-lăr). Maxilomandibular; relativo à maxila e à mandíbula.

max·il·lo·pal·a·tine (mak-sil'ō-pal'ă-tīn). Maxilopalatino; relativo à maxila e ao palatino.

max·il·lot·o·my (mak-si-lot'ō-mē). Maxilotomia; secção cirúrgica da maxila para permitir movimento de parte do maxilar ou de todo ele até a posição desejada. [maxilla + G. *tomē,* incisão]

max·il·lo·tur·bi·nal (mak-sil'lō-ter'bi-năl). Maxiloturbinal; relativo à concha nasal inferior.

Maximow, Alexander A., médico russo nos Estados Unidos, 1874–1928. VER M. *stain* for bone marrow.

max·i·mum (mak'si-mŭm). Máximo; a maior quantidade, valor ou grau alcançado ou alcançável. [L. neuter of *maximus,* máximo]

glucose transport m., transporte máximo de glicose; a taxa máxima de reabsorção de glicose do filtrado glomerular; é de aproximadamente 320 mg/min em seres humanos.

transport m. (Tm), transporte máximo; a taxa máxima de secreção ou reabsorção de uma substância pelos túbulos renais. SIN tubular m.

tubular m. (Tm), tubular máximo. SIN transport m.

May, Richard, médico alemão. VER M.-Hegglin *anomaly.*

May ap·ple. Podofilo. SIN podophyllum.

Mayer, Karl, neurologista austríaco, 1862–1932. VER M. *reflex.*

Mayer, Karl, W., ginecologista alemão, 1795–1868. VER M. *pessary;* M.-Rokitansky-Küster-Hauser *syndrome.*

Mayer, Paul, histologista alemão, 1848–1923. VER M. hemalum *stain,* mucicarmine *stain,* muchematein *stain.*

May-Grünwald stain. Corante de May-Grünwald. VER em stain.

may·id·ism (mā'id-izm). Pelagra. SIN pellagra. [*Zea mays,* milho]

Mayo, Charles H., cirurgião norte-americano, 1865–1939. VER M. *bunionectomy.*

Mayo, William J. cirurgião norte-americano, 1861–1939. VER M. *operation, vein.*

Mayo-Robson, Sir Arthur W., cirurgião inglês, 1853–1933. VER Mayo-Robson *point;* Mayo-Robson *position.*

Mayou, Marmaduke Stephen, oftalmologista inglês, 1876–1934. VER Batten-M. *disease.*

ma·za·mor·ra (maz-ă-mōr'ă). Mazamorra; nome dado em Porto Rico a uma dermatite causada por penetração cutânea de larvas de anciloóstomo.

maze (māz). Labirinto; freqüentemente usado para estudar funções superiores do sistema nervoso em ratos. [I. m. *masen,* confundir]

ma·zin·dol (mā'zin-dol). Mazindol; anorexiante isoindol distinto por não possuir a cadeia fenetilamina comum às aminas simpaticomiméticas.

♻ **mazo-.** A mama. VER TAMBÉM masto-. [G. *mazos*]

Mazzoni, Vittorio, médico italiano, 1880–1940. VER M. *corpuscle;* Golgi-M. *corpuscle.*

Mazzotti, Luigi, médico mexicano especializado em medicina tropical em meados do século XX. VER Mazzotti *reaction,* Mazzotti *test.*

Mb, MbCO, MbO$_2$ Mioglobina e suas combinações com CO e O$_2$ (oximioglobina), respectivamente.

MBC Abreviatura de maximum breathing *capacity* (capacidade respiratória máxima).

M.C. Abreviatura de *Magister Chirurgiae,* Mestre em Cirurgia; Medical Corps.

mc Abreviatura antiga de millicurie (milicurie).

MCAD Abreviatura de medium-chain acyl-CoA dehydrogenase (desidrogenase da acil-CoA de cadeia média).

McArdle, Brian, neurologista inglês do século XX. VER McA. *disease;* McA.-Schimid-Pearson *disease;* McA. *syndrome.*

McBurney, Charles, cirurgião norte-americano, 1845–1913. VER McB. *incision, point, sign.*

McCall, M.L., ginecologista norte-americano do século XX. VER M. culdoplasty *procedure.*

McCarthy, Daniel J., neurologista norte-americano, 1874–1958. VER McC. *reflexes,* em *reflex.*

McClintock, Barbara, 1902–1992, ganhadora do Prêmio Nobel em 1993 pelo seu trabalho na genética do milho.

McCrea, Lowrain E., urologista norte-americano, *1896. VER McC. *sound.*

McCune, Donovan James, pediatra norte-americano, 1902–1976. VER M.-Albright *syndrome.*

McDonald, Ellice, ginecologista norte-americano, 1876–1955. VER McD. *maneuver.*

McGoon, Dwight C., cirurgião norte-americano, *1925. VER McG. *technique.*

MCH Abreviatura de mean corpuscular *hemoglobin* (hemoglobina corpuscular média).

M.Ch. Abreviatura de *Magister Chirurgiae,* Mestre em Cirurgia.

MCHC Abreviatura de mean corpuscular hemoglobin *concentration* (concentração de hemoglobina corpuscular média).

mCi Abreviatura de millicurie (milicurie).

McKee, George Kenneth, cirurgião ortopédico inglês, *1930. VER McK. *line.*

McKusick, Victor Almon, médico norte-americano, *1921. VER McKusick metaphyseal *dysplasia.*

McLean, Malcolm, obstetra norte-americano, 1848–1924. VER Tucker-McL. *forceps.*

MCMI Abreviatura de Millon clinical multiaxial *inventory* (inventário multiaxial clínico de Millon).

McMurray, Thomas P., cirurgião inglês, 1887–1949. VER McM. *test.*

m-cone. Cone m; cone sensível ao comprimento de onda médio (cone verde).

MCP-1. Abreviatura de monocyte chemoattractant *protein*-1 (proteína 1 quimioatrativa de monócitos).

McPhail, M.K., fisiologista canadense, *1907. VER McP. *test.*

MCR Abreviatura de steroid metabolic clearance *rate* (taxa de depuração metabólica de esteróides).

McReynolds, John O., oftalmologista norte-americano, 1865–1942.

M-CSF Abreviatura de macrophage colony-stimulating *factor* (fator estimulante de colônias de macrófagos).

MCV Abreviatura de mean corpuscular *volume* (volume corpuscular médio).

McVay, Chester B., cirurgião norte-americano, *1911. VER McV. *operation.*

MD Abreviatura de methyldichloroarsine (metildicloroarsina).

M.D. Abreviatura de *Medicinae Doctor,* Doutor em Medicina.

Md Símbolo de mendelevium (mendelévio).

MDF Abreviatura de myocardial depressant *factor* (fator depressor do miocárdio).

m. dict. Abreviatura de [L.] *more dicto,* conforme orientado.

MDMA Um derivado da fenetilamina, de ação central, relacionado à anfetamina e metanfetamina, com propriedades alucinógenas e de excitação do sistema nervoso central. SIN 3,4-methylenedioxymethamphetamine.

MDNCF Abreviatura de monocyte-derived neutrophil chemotactic *factor* (fator quimiotático de neutrófilos derivado de monócito).

M'Dowel, Benjamin G., anatomista irlandês, 1829–1885. VER *frenulum* of M.

M.D.S. Abreviatura de Master of Dental Surgery, Mestre em Cirurgia Dentária.

Me Símbolo de methyl (metila).

Meadows, William Robert, cardiologista norte-americano, *1919. VER M. *syndrome.*

meal (mēl). **1.** Refeição; o alimento consumido a intervalos regulares ou em um horário específico. **2.** Farinha de um cereal.
  Boyden m., consiste em três ou quatro gemas de ovo, batidas com leite e temperadas com açúcar, vinho do porto, etc.; usada para testar o tempo de evacuação da vesícula biliar; dois terços a três quartos do conteúdo serão normalmente evacuados em 40 minutos.
  Lundh m., refeição de leite desnatado em pó misturado com óleo de milho e dextrose, usada para avaliar a função pancreática.
  test m., r. de teste; **(1)** chá com torrada ou chá com biscoitos tipo *cracker,* ou mingau ou outro alimento brando, administrada para estimular a secreção gástrica antes da coleta do conteúdo gástrico para análise; **(2)** administração de alimento contendo uma substância considerada responsável pelos sintomas, como em uma reação alérgica.

mean (mēn). Média; uma medida estatística da tendência central ou distribuição de um conjunto de valores, geralmente compreendida como a média aritmética, exceto se houver especificação em contrário. [I.m., *mene,* do Fr. ant., do L. *medianus,* no meio]
  arithmetic m., m. aritmética; a média calculada somando-se um conjunto de valores, e depois, dividindo-se a soma pelo número de valores.
  geometric m., m. geométrica; a média calculada como o antilogaritmo da média aritmética dos logaritmos dos valores individuais; também pode ser calculada como a enésima raiz do produto de *n* valores.
  harmonic m., m. harmônica; a média calculada dividindo-se o número de valores cuja média será calculada pela soma de suas recíprocas.
  regression of the m., regressão da média; se, para uma população simétrica com uma moda única, uma medida, selecionada devido ao seu extremo, é repetida, em geral a segunda leitura será mais próxima da média que a primeira.
  standard error of the m. (SEM), erro padrão da média; índice estatístico da probabilidade de que a média de determinada amostra seja representativa da média populacional na qual a amostra foi colhida.

mea·sle (mē´zl). **1.** A larva (*Cysticercus cellulosae*) da *Taenia solium,* a tênia do porco; *C. cellulosae* é um termo menos usado para designar cisticercos de *T. solium.* **2.** A larva (*Cysticercus bovis*) de *Taenia saginata,* a tênia bovina; o termo *C. bovis* é usado com menor freqüência para designar cisticercos de *T. bovis.*

mea·sles (mē´zlz). **1.** Sarampo; doença exantematosa aguda, causada pelo vírus do sarampo (gênero Morbilivirus), um membro da família Paramyxoviridae, e caracterizada por febre e outros distúrbios constitucionais, inflamação catarral das mucosas respiratórias e erupção maculopapular generalizada e de cor vermelho-escura; a erupção surge cedo na mucosa bucal sob a forma de manchas de Koplik, uma manifestação utilizada no diagnóstico precoce; o período de incubação médio é de 10–12 dias. A recuperação geralmente é rápida, mas complicações respiratórias e otite média causada por infecções bacterianas secundárias são comuns. Raramente há encefalite. Mais tarde pode haver pan-encefalite esclerosante subaguda associada à infecção crônica. SIN morbilli. **2.** Doença de suínos causada pela presença de *Cysticercus cellulosae,* a tênia ou larva da *Taenia solium,* a tênia do porco. **3.** Uma doença de bovinos causada pela presença de *Cysticercus bovis,* a tênia ou larva da *Taenia saginata,* a tênia da carne de boi que infesta o homem. [D. *maselen*]
  atypical m., s. atípico; manifestação clínica incomum, algumas vezes grave, da infecção natural pelo vírus do sarampo em pessoas com diminuição da imunidade produzida pela vacina, particularmente naquelas pessoas que receberam vacina inativada por formaldeído; uma reação alérgica acelerada, aparentemente resultante de uma resposta anamnéstica dos anticorpos, caracterizada por febre alta, ausência de manchas de Koplik, redução do período prodrômico, exantema atípico e pneumonia.
  black m., (1) Sarampo hemorrágico. SIN hemorrhagic m.; **(2)** Febre maculosa das Montanhas Rochosas. SIN Rocky Mountain spotted *fever.*
  German m., rubéola. SIN rubella.
  hemorrhagic m., s. hemorrágico; forma grave na qual a erupção tem cor escura devida ao extravasamento de sangue para as áreas da pele afetadas. SIN black m. (1).
  three-day m., rubéola. SIN rubella.
  tropical m., s. tropical; doença de caráter incerto, um pouco semelhante à rubéola, observada no sul da China.

mea·sly (mēz´lē). Relativo à carne de porco ou de boi infectada pelos cisticercos de *Taenia solium* ou *Taenia saginata,* respectivamente.

mea·sure (mezh´er). **1.** Medir; determinar a magnitude ou quantidade de uma substância mediante sua comparação com algum padrão aceito ou por cálculo. **2.** Medida; magnitude específica de uma quantidade física. **3.** Instrumento graduado usado para medir um objeto ou substância. [Fr. ant. *mesure,* do L. *mensura,* de *metior,* medir]
  Geneva lens m., dispositivo para medir os raios da curvatura de uma lente de óculos. SIN lens clock. [*Geneva,* Suíça]

mea·sure·ment (mezh´ur-ment). Medida; determinação de uma dimensão ou quantidade.
  end-point m., m. final; medida analítica no fim de uma reação química, em oposição à medida feita durante a reação.
  kinetic m., m. cinética; monitorização contínua ou freqüente das leituras durante uma reação química para determinar sua velocidade.
  nasion-pogonion m., m. násio-pogônio. SIN facial *plane.*

mea·sures of cen·tral ten·den·cy. Medidas de tendência central; termo geral para designar várias características da distribuição de um conjunto de medidas ou valores em torno de um valor ou valores no meio do grupo ou próximos do meio; as principais medidas de tendência central são média, mediana e moda.

me·a·tal (mē-ā´tal). Meatal; relativo a um meato.

meato-. Meato. [L. *meatus,* passagem]

me·a·tom·e·ter (mē-ă-tom´ē-ter). Meatômetro; instrumento para medir o tamanho de um meato, principalmente do meato uretral. [meato- + G. *metron,* medida]

me·a·to·plas·ty (mē´ă-tō-plas-tē). Meatoplastia; aumento ou outra reconfiguração cirúrgica de um meato ou canal, p. ex., o meato acústico externo ou o óstio da uretra.

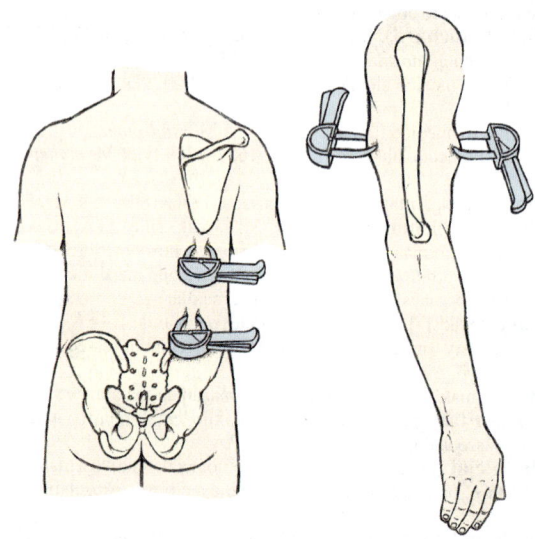

medida da prega cutânea: o uso de compasso em locais padrões permite uma estimativa acurada da gordura subcutânea

me·a·tor·rha·phy (mē-ă-tōr'ă-fē). Meatorrafia; fechamento por sutura da ferida feita por meatomia. [meato- + G. *rhaphē*, sutura]

me·at·o·scope (mē-ăt'ō-skōp). Meatoscópio; forma de espéculo para examinar um meato, principalmente o meato da uretra. [meato- + G. *skopeō*, ver]

me·a·tos·co·py (mē-ă-tos'kō-pē). Meatoscopia; inspeção, em geral com instrumentos, de qualquer meato, principalmente do meato uretral. [meato- + G. *skopeō*, ver]

me·at·o·tome (mē-at'ō-tōm). Meatótomo; bisturi com borda cortante curta para uso em meatotomia.

me·a·tot·o·my (mē-ă-tot'ō-mē). Meatotomia; incisão feita para aumentar um meato, p. ex., da uretra ou ureter. [meato- + G. *tomē*, incisão]

me·a·tus, pl. **me·a·tus** (mē-ā'tŭs) [TA]. Meato; passagem ou canal, em especial a abertura externa de um canal. SIN external opening. [L. um caminho, uma passagem, de *meo*, pp. *meatus*, ir, passar]
  acoustic m., m. acústico externo. SIN external acoustic m.
  m. acus'ticus exter'nus [TA], m. acústico externo. SIN external acoustic m.
  m. acus'ticus inter'nus [TA], m. acústico interno. SIN internal acoustic m.
  external acoustic m. [TA], m. acústico externo; a passagem que segue para dentro, atravessando a parte timpânica do osso temporal, da orelha até a membrana timpânica; consiste em uma parte óssea (interna) e uma parte fibrocartilaginosa (externa), o meato acústico externo cartilagíneo. SIN m. acusticus externus [TA], acoustic m., antrum auris, auditory canal, ear canal, external auditory m.
  external auditory m., m. acústico externo. SIN external acoustic m.
  external urinary m., óstio externo da uretra; *termo oficial alternativo para external urethral orifice.
  fish-mouth m., m. em boca de peixe; eritema e edema do óstio da uretra (meato urinário) na gonorréia.
  internal acoustic m. [TA], m. acústico interno; canal que começa na abertura do meato acústico interno na fossa posterior do crânio, seguindo lateralmente através da parte petrosa do osso temporal, terminando no fundo, onde uma fina lâmina de osso o separa do vestíbulo; dá passagem aos nervos facial e vestibulococlear juntamente com a artéria e as veias do labirinto. SIN m. acusticus internus [TA], internal auditory m.
  internal auditory m., m. acústico interno. SIN internal acoustic m.
  nasal m. [TA], m. nasal; qualquer das quatro passagens na cavidade nasal formadas pela projeção das conchas: meato nasal inferior [TA] (meatus nasi inferior [TA]), situado abaixo da concha nasal inferior; meato nasal médio [TA] (meatus nasi medius [TA]), situado entre as conchas média e inferior; meato nasal superior [TA] (meatus nasi superior [TA]), situado entre as conchas superior e média; meato nasal comum [TA] (meatus nasi communis [TA]), que é a parte da cavidade nasal entre as conchas e o septo nasal. SIN m. nasi [TA].
  m. na'si [TA], m. nasal. SIN nasal m.
  nasopharyngeal m. [TA], m. nasofaríngeo; a parte posterior da cavidade nasal, desde os limites posteriores das conchas até os cóanos. SIN m. nasopharyngeus [TA], nasopharyngeal passage.
  m. nasopharyn'geus [TA], m. nasofaríngeo. SIN nasopharyngeal m.
  ureteral m., óstio do ureter. SIN ureteric orifice.
  m. urina'rius, m. urinário. SIN external urethral orifice.

me·ban·a·zine (mē-ban'ă-zēn). Mebanazina; antidepressivo com efeito inibitório sobre a monoamina oxidase.

me·ben·da·zole (mē-ben'dă-zōl). Mebendazol; agente nematicida de amplo espectro, efetivo contra nematódeos intestinais, como os oxiúros, ancilóstomos duodenais, *Trichuris* e *Ascaris*.

me·bev·er·ine hy·dro·chlo·ride (mē-bev'er-ēn). Cloridrato de mebeverina; antiespasmódico intestinal.

me·bro·phen·hy·dra·mine (mē-brō-fen-hī'dră-mēn). Mebrofenidramina; anti-histamínico H_1.

me·but·a·mate (mē-bū'tă-māt). Mebutamato; quimicamente, difere discretamente do meprobamato e possui propriedades depressoras do SNC semelhantes.

mec·a·myl·a·mine hy·dro·chlo·ride (mek'ă-mil'ă-mēn). Cloridrato de mecamilamina; uma amina secundária que bloqueia a transmissão de impulsos em gânglios autônomos (semelhante, porém mais efetivo que o hexametônio); usado no tratamento da hipertensão grave.

me·chan·i·cal (mē-kan'i-kăl). Mecânico. **1.** Realizado por meio de algum aparelho, não manualmente. **2.** Que explica fenômenos em termos de mecânica. **3.** Automático. [G. *mechanikos*, relativo a uma máquina, de *mēchanē*, aparelho, máquina]

me·chan·i·co·re·cep·tor (mē-kan'i-kō-rē-sep'ter, tōr). Mecanorreceptor. SIN mechanoreceptor.

me·chan·ics (mē-kan'iks). Mecânica; a ciência da ação de forças na promoção de movimento ou equilíbrio. [ver mechanical]
  body m., m. do corpo; o estudo da ação dos músculos na produção de movimento ou postura corporal.

mech·a·nism (mek'ă-nizm). Mecanismo. **1.** Um arranjo ou agrupamento das partes de qualquer coisa com uma ação definida. **2.** O meio pelo qual é obtido um efeito. **3.** A cadeia de eventos em determinado processo. **4.** A descrição detalhada de uma via de reação. [G. *mēchanē*, aparelho]
  association m., m. de associação; o mecanismo cerebral pelo qual a memória de sensações passadas pode ser comparada ou associada às presentes.
  countercurrent m., m. de contracorrente; sistema na medula renal que facilita a concentração da urina à medida que esta atravessa os túbulos renais. VER countercurrent exchanger, countercurrent multiplier.
  defense m., m. de defesa; **(1)** meio psicológico de enfrentar um conflito ou ansiedade, p. ex., conversão, negação, dissociação, racionalização, repressão, sublimação; **(2)** a estrutura psíquica subjacente a uma estratégia de enfrentamento; **(3)** mecanismo imunológico *versus* mecanismo de defesa inespecífico.
  double displacement m., m. de deslocamento duplo. SIN ping-pong m.
  Douglas m., m. de Douglas; mecanismo de evolução espontânea em situação transversa; flexão lateral extrema da coluna vertebral com saída da face lateral antes das nádegas.
  Duncan m., m. de Duncan; saída da placenta do útero com a face áspera em primeiro lugar.
  gating m., m. de comporta; m. de portal; **(1)** ocorrência do período refratário máximo entre células de condução cardíacas aproximadamente 2 mm proximais às fibras de Purkinje terminais no músculo ventricular, além das quais o período refratário é reduzido através de uma seqüência de células de Purkinje, células de transição e células musculares; o mecanismo de sincronização pode ser uma causa de aberração ventricular, taquicardia bidirecional e extra-sístoles ocultas; **(2)** mecanismo pelo qual impulsos dolorosos podem ter bloqueada sua entrada na medula espinal. Cf. gate-controle *theory*.
  immunologic m., m. imunológico; os grupos de células (principalmente linfócitos e células do sistema reticuloendotelial) que funcionam no estabelecimento de imunidade adquirida ativa (sensibilidade induzida, alergia).
  ordered m., m. ordenado; esquema de ligação de substrato e liberação de produto para enzimas que atuam sobre múltiplos substratos; para uma enzima com dois substratos e dois produtos com um mecanismo ordenado, um substrato específico deve primeiro se ligar à enzima, seguido pelo outro substrato; há então uma reação química, e os produtos são formados e liberados da enzima em uma ordem distinta. Existem esquemas mais complexos para enzimas que possuem mais de dois substratos. Algumas das desidrogenases possuem esse mecanismo. SIN ordered.
  ordered on-random off m., m. ordenado ativado-aleatório desativado; esquema para ligação de substrato e liberação de produto para enzimas com múltiplos substratos; para uma enzima com dois substratos e dois produtos com esse mecanismo, os reagentes devem se ligar à enzima em uma ordem distinta; entretanto, quando os produtos estão formados, podem se dissociar da enzima em qualquer ordem. Foi sugerido que a piruvatocinase tem esse mecanismo. O mecanismo aleatório ativado-ordenado desativado é simplesmente o inverso desse mecanismo.
  ping-pong m., m. de pingue-pongue; reação especial com múltiplos substratos na qual, para um sistema com dois substratos e dois produtos (ou seja, bi-bi), uma enzima reage com um substrato para formar um produto e uma enzima modificada, e esta última então reage com um segundo substrato para formar um segundo produto, final, havendo recuperação da enzima original. Um exemplo desse mecanismo é encontrado nas aminotransferases. Existem mecanismos de pingue-pongue mais complexos para enzimas que possuem mais de dois substratos. SIN double displacement m.
  pressorreceptive m., m. pressurreceptor; o sistema pressurreceptor, principalmente dos seios carotídeos e do arco aórtico.
  proprioceptive m., m. proprioceptivo; o mecanismo do sentido de posição e movimento pelo qual os movimentos musculares podem ser ajustados, com manutenção de alto grau de acurácia e equilíbrio.
  random m., m. aleatório; esquema para ligação de substrato e liberação de produto por uma enzima com múltiplos substratos; para uma enzima com dois substratos e dois produtos com esse mecanismo, qualquer um dos substratos pode se ligar primeiro e, após a reação, qualquer um dos produtos pode ser o primeiro a se dissociar da enzima. A hexocinase encefálica tem um mecanismo aleatório. Existem mecanismos aleatórios mais complexos para enzimas que possuem mais de dois substratos.
  re-entrant m., m. reentrante; a provável base da maioria das arritmias, exigindo pelo menos três critérios no coração: 1. um circuito em alça, 2. bloqueio unidirecional e 3. lentificação da condução. Os impulsos entram no circuito em alça e dividem-se em ambas as direções (bloqueados apenas em uma direção), transpõem o circuito em alça até à área de bloqueio, onde a condução mais lenta permitiu que o impulso chegasse num momento em que o tecido proximal ao bloqueio unidirecional já havia se recuperado e permitirá sua passagem na direção oposta.
  Schultze m., m. de Schultze; expulsão da placenta com a superfície fetal primeiro.

mech·a·no·car·di·og·ra·phy (mek'ă-nō-kar-dē-og'ră-fē). Mecanocardiografia; uso de traçados gráficos que refletem os efeitos mecânicos do batimento cardíaco, como o traçado do pulso carotídeo ou do apicecardiograma; a fonocardiografia geralmente também é considerada uma forma de mecanocardiografia.

mech·a·no·cyte (mek'ă-nō-sīt). Mecanócito; cultura tecidual *in vitro* de fibroblastos.

mech·a·no·pho·bia (mek'ă-nō-fō'bē-ă). Mecanofobia; medo mórbido de máquinas. [G. *mēchanē*, máquina, + *phobos*, medo]

mech·a·no·re·cep·tor (mek'ă-nō-rē-sep'tŏr). Mecanorreceptor; receptor que responde à pressão ou distorção mecânica; p. ex., receptores nos seios carotídeos, receptores táteis na pele. SIN mechanicoreceptor.

mech·a·no·re·flex (mek'ă-nō-rē'fleks). Mecanorreflexo; reflexo deflagrado por estimulação de um mecanorreceptor.

mech·a·no·ther·a·py (mek'ă-nō-thar'ă-pē). Mecanoterapia; tratamento de doença por meio de aparelho ou dispositivos mecânicos de qualquer tipo. [G. *mēchanē*, máquina, + *therapeia*, tratamento]

mèche (māsh). Mecha; tira de gaze ou outro material usado como sonda ou dreno. [Fr. mecha]

mech·lor·eth·a·mine hy·dro·chlo·ride (mek'lōr-eth'ă-mēn). Cloridrato de mecloretamina; é citotóxico para todas as células, mas com uma afinidade especial pela medula óssea, tecidos linfáticos e células rapidamente proliferativas de algumas neoplasias. Usado para o tratamento paliativo da doença de Hodgkin, linfossarcoma e algumas leucemias crônicas. SIN mustine hydrochloride.

me·cism (mē'sizm). Mecismo; alongamento anormal do corpo ou de uma ou mais de suas partes. [G. *mēkos*, comprimento, *-ismos*, condição]

Me·cis·to·cir·rus (mē-sis-tō-sir'ŭs). Gênero monotípico de nematódeos tricostrongilídeos (subfamília Mecistocirrinae), com uma única espécie, *M. digitatus*; não se distingue macroscopicamente do *Haemonchus contortus* e tem quase o mesmo efeito sobre o hospedeiro. O *M*. é encontrado principalmente na Ásia em bovinos, ovinos, búfalos, bisões, no estômago de porcos e, ocasionalmente, em seres humanos. [G. *mēkistos*, muito longo, + L. *cirrus*, espiral, o órgão masculino protruso de um nematóideo]

Meckel, Johann F., o jovem, anatomista comparativo e embriologista alemão, 1781–1833. VER M. *scan, syndrome, cartilage, diverticulum, plane;* M.-Gruber *syndrome.*

Meckel, Johann F., o velho, anatomista e obstetra alemão, 1714–1774. VER M. *band, cavity, ganglion, ligament, space.*

Mecke re·a·gent. Reagente de Mecke. VER em reagent.

me·clas·tine (mē-klas'tēn). Meclastina. SIN clemastine.

mec·li·zine hy·dro·chlo·ride (mek'li-zēn). Cloridrato de meclizina; anti-histamínico H₁ útil na prevenção e no alívio da cinetose e dos sintomas causados por distúrbios vestibulares. SIN meclozine hydrochloride.

mec·lo·fen·a·mate so·di·um (mek-lō-fen'ă-māt). Meclofenamato sódico; agente antiinflamatório não-esteróide com atividades analgésicas e antipiréticas.

mec·lo·fen·a·mic ac·id (mē-klō-fen-am'ik). Ácido meclofenâmico; AINE usada no tratamento de distúrbios inflamatórios e dismenorréia; também antipirético.

mec·lo·fen·ox·ate (mek'lō-fen-ok'sāt). Meclofenoxato; analéptico.

mec·lo·zine hy·dro·chlo·ride (mek'lō-zēn). Cloridrato de meclozina. SIN meclizine hydrochloride.

me·com·e·ter (mē-kom'ĕ-ter). Mecômetro; instrumento, semelhante a um compasso de calibre com uma escala, para medida de recém-nascidos. [G. *mēkos*, comprimento, + *metron*, medida]

mec·o·nate (mek'ō-nāt). Meconato; um sal ou éster do ácido mecônico. [G. *mēkōn*, papoula]

me·con·ic ac·id (me-kon'ik). Ácido mecônico; obtido do ópio; forma sais solúveis (meconatos) com muitos dos alcalóides do ópio.

mec·o·nin (mek'ō-nin). Meconina; $C_{10}H_{10}O_4$; a lactona do ácido mecônico, encontrada também na *Hydrastis canadensis*; um hipnótico. SIN opianyl.

me·co·ni·or·rhea (mē-kō'nē-ō-rē'ă). Meconiorréia; eliminação, pelo recém-nascido, de uma quantidade anormalmente grande de mecônio. [meconium + G. *rhoia*, fluxo]

me·co·ni·um (mē-kō'nē-ŭm). Mecônio. **1.** A primeira descarga intestinal do recém-nascido, de cor verde e consistindo em células epiteliais, muco e bile. **2.** SIN opium. [L., do G. *mēkonion*, dim. de *mēkon*, papoula]

me·daz·e·pam hy·dro·chlo·ride (mē-daz'ĕ-pam). Cloridrato de medazepam; agente ansiolítico.

med·fal·an (med'fal-an). Medfalam. SIN medphalan.

me·dia (mē'dē-ă). **1.** Média. SIN tunica media. **2.** Meios; plural de medium. [L. fem. de *medius*, meio]

me·di·ad (mē'dē-ad). Medial; em direção à linha média.

me·di·al (mē'dē-ăl) [TA]. Medial; relativo ao meio ou centro; mais próximo do plano mediano ou mediossagital. SIN medialis [TA]. [L. *medialis*, meio]

me·di·a·lec·i·thal (mē-dē-ă-les'i-thăl). Mediolécito; designa um ovo com quantidade moderada de vitelo, como em anfíbios. [L. *medialis*, medial, + G. *lekithos*, vitelo de ovo]

me·di·a·lis (mē-dē-ā'lis). [TA]. Medial. SIN medial. [L.]

med·i·al·i·za·tion (mēd-ē-al-ī-zā'shun). Medialização; operação para mover uma parte em direção à linha média, como a cartilagem aritenóide ou a prega vocal na paralisia das pregas vocais.

me·di·an (mē'dē-an). Mediano. **1.** Central; médio; situado na linha média. SIN medianus. **2.** O valor médio em um grupo de medidas; como a média, uma medida da tendência central. [L. *medianus*, médio]

me·di·a·nus (mē-dē-ā'nŭs). Mediano. SIN median (1). [L.]

me·di·as·ti·nal (mē'dē-as-tī'năl). Mediastinal; relativo ao mediastino.

me·di·as·ti·ni·tis (mē'dē-as-ti-nī'tis). Mediastinite; inflamação do tecido celular do mediastino.

fibrosing m., m. fibrosante. SIN mediastinal *fibrosis.*
fibrous m., m. fibrosa; fibrose das estruturas mediastinais de origem desconhecida ou devida à infecção.
idiopathic fibrous m., m. fibrosa idiopática. SIN mediastinal *fibrosis.*

me·di·as·ti·nog·ra·phy (mē'dē-as-ti-nog'ră-fē). Mediastinografia; radiografia do mediastino. [mediastinum + G. *graphō*, escrever]

gaseous m., m. gasosa; radiografia do mediastino após injeção de ar (pneumomediastino artificial), um procedimento obsoleto.

me·di·as·tin·o·per·i·car·di·tis (mē'dē-as'tin-ō-per'i-kar-dī'tis). Mediastinopericardite; inflamação do pericárdio e do tecido celular mediastínico adjacente.

me·di·as·tin·o·scope (mē-dē-as'tin'-ō-skōp). Mediastinoscópio; endoscópio para inspeção do mediastino através de uma incisão supra-esternal.

me·di·as·ti·nos·co·py (mē'dē-as-ti-nos'kŏ-pē). Mediastinoscopia; exame endoscópico do mediastino através de uma incisão supra-esternal, geralmente para biopsia de linfonodos paratraqueais. [mediastinum + G. *skopeō*, ver]

anterior m., m. anterior; modificação do procedimento de Chamberlain (Chamberlain *procedure*) na qual é usado um mediastinoscópio para exploração das regiões do mediastino anterior e subaórtica.
extended m., m. estendida; mediastinoscopia cervical na qual, além da exploração pré-traqueal e paratraqueal padrão, o mediastinoscópio é introduzido anteriormente à artéria inominada e ao arco aórtico para permitir acesso aos linfonodos subaórticos (janela aortopulmonar) e mediastínicos anteriores; uma alternativa ao procedimento de Chamberlain (Chamberlain *procedure*).

me·di·as·ti·not·o·my (mē'dē-as-ti-not'ō-mē). Mediastinotomia; incisão do mediastino. [mediastinum + G. *tomē*, incisão]

anterior m., m. anterior. SIN Chamberlain *procedure.*

me·di·as·ti·num (mē'dē-as-tī'nŭm). Mediastino. **1.** Um septo entre duas partes de um órgão ou cavidade. **2.** [TA]. A divisão mediana da cavidade torácica, coberta pela parte mediastinal da pleura parietal e contém todas as vísceras e estruturas torácicas, exceto os pulmões. É dividida arbitrariamente em duas partes principais: o mediastino superior [TA] (mediastinum superius [TA]), situado diretamente superior a um plano horizontal que cruza o ângulo esternal e aproximadamente o disco intervertebral T4–5, e o mediastino inferior [TA] (mediastinum inferius [TA]) inferior a esse plano; este último, por sua vez, é subdividido em 3 partes: o mediastino médio [TA] (mediastinum medium [TA]), adjacente ao saco pericárdico que contém o coração; um mediastino anterior [TA] quase virtual (mediastinum anterius [TA]), situado na frente; e um mediastino posterior [TA] (mediastinum posterius [TA]), atrás, contendo o esôfago, a aorta descendente e o ducto torácico. SIN interpleural space, interpulmonary septum, mediastinal space, septum mediastinale. [L. mod. um septo médio, do L. mediev. *mediastinus*, medial, do L. *mediastinus*, servo inferior, de *medius*, meio]

anterior m. [TA], m. anterior; o espaço estreito, quase virtual, entre o pericárdio, posteriormente, e o esterno, anteriormente, que contém o timo ou seus remanescentes, alguns linfonodos e vasos e ramos da artéria torácica interna. SIN m. anterius [TA].
m. ante'rius [TA], m. anterior. SIN anterior m.
inferior m. [TA], m. inferior; a região abaixo de um plano horizontal que cruza aproximadamente o disco intervertebral T4–5, posteriormente, e o ângulo esternal, anteriormente, demarcando o limite inferior do mediastino superior. É subdividido em três regiões: média, anterior e posterior. SIN m. inferius [TA].
m. infe'rius [TA], m. inferior. SIN inferior m.
m. me'dium [TA], m. médio. SIN middle m.
middle m. [TA], m. médio; a grande porção central do mediastino inferior, que inclui o pericárdio e o coração por ele contidos, bem como os nervos frênicos e os vasos cardiofrênicos. SIN m. medium [TA].
posterior m. [TA], m. posterior; situado entre o pericárdio, anteriormente, e a coluna vertebral, posteriormente, e abaixo do plano que cruza o ângulo esternal e o disco intervertebral T4–5. Contém a aorta descendente, o ducto torácico, esôfago, as veias ázigos e os nervos vagos. SIN m. posterius [TA], postmediastinum.
m. poste'rius [TA], m. posterior. SIN posterior m.
superior m. [TA], m. superior; parte do mediastino situada acima do plano horizontal que cruza o ângulo esternal e aproximadamente o disco intervertebral T4–5 (isto é, acima do pericárdio); contém o arco da aorta e os vasos que dele se originam, as veias braquiocefálicas e a porção superior da veia cava superior, a traquéia, o esôfago, o ducto torácico, o timo e os nervos frênico, vago, cardíaco e laríngeo recorrente esquerdo. SIN m. superius [TA].
m. supe'rius [TA], m. superior. SIN superior m.

m. tes'tis [TA], m. do testículo. SIN m. of testis.

m. of testis [TA], m. do testículo; massa de tecido fibroso contínua com a túnica albugínea, que se projeta de sua borda posterior para o testículo; os séptulos do testículo irradiam-se como continuações circundando os lóbulos do testículo. SIN m. testis [TA], corpus highmori, corpus higmorianum, Highmore body, septum of testis.

me·di·ate. 1 (mē'dē-it). Intermediário; situado entre. **2** (mē'dē-āt). Mediar; realizar algo por meio de uma substância intermediária, como na fagocitose mediada por complemento. [L. *mediatus*, de *medio*, pp. *-atus*, dividir ao meio]

me·di·a·tion (mē-dē-ā'shŭn). Mediação; a ação de uma substância intermediária (mediador).

me·di·a·tor (mē'dē-ā-ter, -tōr). Mediador; substância ou coisa intermediária.

pharmacologic m.'s of anaphylaxis, mediadores farmacológicos da anafilaxia; substâncias liberadas de mastócitos (e outras células) pela reação de antígeno e anticorpo homocitotrópico específico em suas superfícies; incluem a histamina, a substância de reação lenta da anafilaxia (SRS-A), bradicinina e (em algumas espécies de animais) serotonina.

med·i·ca·ble (med'i-kă-bl). Medicável; tratável, com esperança de cura.

med·i·cal (med'i-kăl). **1.** Médico; relativo à medicina ou à prática da medicina. SIN medicinal (2). **2.** Medicinal. SIN medicinal (1). [L. *medicalis*, de *medicus*, médico]

med·i·cal corps. Corpo médico; a subdivisão de uma organização militar, como o Exército norte-americano, dedicada ao tratamento médico das tropas.

med·i·cal tran·scrip·tion·ist. Transcricionista médico; indivíduo que realiza a transcrição de relatórios ditados pelo médico acerca do tratamento de um paciente, que passam a fazer parte do prontuário médico permanente do paciente; um transcricionista médico registrado (TMR) atendeu às exigências de certificação da *American Association for Medical Transcription* (*Associação Americana de Transcrição Médica*).

me·dic·a·ment (me-dik'ă-ment, med'i-kă-ment). Medicamento; um remédio, uma aplicação medicinal. [L. *medicamentum*, medicamento]

med·i·ca·men·to·sus (med'i-kă-men-tō'sŭs). Medicamentoso; relativo a um medicamento; designa uma erupção cutânea causada por um medicamento. [L.]

med·i·cate (med'i-kāt). Medicar. **1.** Tratar doença mediante administração de medicamentos. **2.** Impregnar com uma substância medicinal. [L. *medico*, pp. *-atus*, cicatrizar]

med·i·cat·ed (med'i-kāt-ed). Medicado; impregnado com substância medicinal.

med·i·ca·tion (med-i-kā'shŭn). Medicação. **1.** O ato de medicar. **2.** Uma substância medicinal ou medicamento.

ionic m., m. iônica. SIN iontophoresis.

maintenance medication, m. de manutenção; medicação usada para estabilizar uma doença ou os sintomas de uma doença.

preanesthetic m., m. pré-anestésica; medicamentos administrados antes de um anestésico para reduzir a ansiedade e obter indução, manutenção e saída mais suaves da anestesia.

sublingual m., m. sublingual; forma de apresentação de um medicamento para ser usada sob a língua; o medicamento (p. ex., nitroglicerina) é absorvido pelos tecidos da mucosa e não passa pelo trato gastrointestinal, onde pode ser parcial ou totalmente degradado.

med·i·ca·tor (med'i-kā-ter, -tōr). **1.** Medicador; instrumento usado para fazer aplicações terapêuticas em partes mais profundas do corpo. **2.** Aquele que administra medicamentos para o alívio da doença; algumas vezes, o termo é usado com a intenção de menosprezar aquele que prescreve medicamentos em excesso para pequenos males.

me·dic·e·phal·ic (mē'dē-se-fal'ik). Medicefálico; cefálico mediano; designa o vaso comunicante entre as veias intermédia e cefálica do antebraço.

me·dic·i·nal (mē-dis'i-năl). Medicinal. **1.** Relativo a medicamento que tem propriedades curativas. SIN medical (2). **2.** SIN medical (1).

me·dic·i·nal scar·let red. Vermelho-escarlate medicinal. SIN scarlet red.

med·i·cine (med'i-sin). **1.** Medicamento; um remédio. **2.** Medicina; a arte de prevenir ou curar doenças; a ciência que estuda a doença em todas as suas relações. **3.** O estudo e o tratamento das doenças gerais ou daquelas que afetam as partes internas do corpo, principalmente aquelas que, geralmente, não necessitam de intervenção cirúrgica. [L. *medicina*, de *medicus*, médico (ver medicus)]

adolescent m., medicina do adolescente; o ramo da medicina relacionado ao tratamento dos jovens na faixa dos 13 aos 21 anos. SIN hebiatrics.

aerospace m., medicina aeroespacial; ramo da medicina que combina as áreas de interesse da medicina de aviação e da medicina espacial.

alternative m., medicina alternativa; termo que se refere a um grupo heterogêneo de filosofias e práticas de higiene, diagnóstico e terapêutica, cujas bases teóricas e técnicas divergem daquelas da medicina científica moderna. Algumas diferem da medicina tradicional apenas pela preferência por métodos higiênicos e terapêuticos naturais em lugar da farmacoterapia e da cirurgia; alguns desses métodos são sobrenaturais, mágicos ou religiosos, com raízes em sistemas filosóficos ou religiosos antigos ou modernos; alguns são baseados em conhecimentos crédulos, falsos ou inconsistentes de anatomia, fisiologia, psicologia, patologia e farmacologia; e alguns são esquemas fraudulentos destinados a explorar pacientes inocentes e aqueles cujas supostas necessidades médicas não foram atendidas pela medicina científica. As práticas de medicina alternativa foram trazidas para algumas partes dos Estados Unidos por populações migrantes, particularmente asiáticos e hispânicos. Muitos ramos da medicina alternativa têm em comum uma visão holística da saúde humana, enfatizando a integração de corpo, mente e espírito. Nenhum deles conseguiu ser aceito como parte da medicina prevalente porque não possuem base científica plausível nem evidências de eficácia. SIN complementary m., holistic m. (2).

Os norte-americanos têm um maior número de consultas anuais com profissionais de medicina alternativa (MA) que com médicos de atendimento primário, e o custo total da MA, nos EUA, ultrapassa 21 bilhões de dólares por ano. Três quintos dos adultos entrevistados tinham procurado a MA no ano anterior, mas apenas 5% confiam exclusivamente nela. A MA é atraente sobretudo para pessoas de maior escolaridade, que acreditam fortemente no papel da mente na saúde e na doença, e para aquelas com interesse em formas esotéricas de espiritualidade e psicologia de crescimento espiritual. Os usuários da MA tendem a estar em piores condições gerais de saúde que os outros e a possuir algumas doenças crônicas (incluindo ansiedade, depressão, cefaléia e dor nas costas), mas a insatisfação com a medicina convencional parece ser menos importante na sua escolha que uma preferência por um sistema de saúde compatível com suas crenças e valores pessoais. Os profissionais de algumas formas de MA são publicamente hostis à medicina tradicional e costumam contestar a competência e a integridade dos profissionais de saúde legítimos. Por outro lado, alguns médicos utilizam métodos alternativos, como acupuntura e hipnose, sobretudo aqueles que adotam uma visão holística da prática médica. Alguns planos de seguro cobrem determinadas terapias alternativas, como acupuntura, *biofeedback* e massoterapia. Embora o uso da MA possa beneficiar algumas pessoas por fornecer esperança e o apoio emocional necessário, exercer efeitos placebo ou aliviar sintomas através de mecanismos ainda não-compreendidos, ela impede que muitas pessoas tenham um diagnóstico e um tratamento apropriados. Além disso, as terapias alternativas podem interagir adversamente com muitas formas ortodoxas de tratamento, e algumas são inerentemente perigosas para a saúde. Em 1992, o Congresso norte-americano criou o *Office of Alternative Medicine* (OAM) (*Departamento de Medicina Alternativa*) dentro da Diretoria do *National Institutes of Health* (*Instituto Nacional de Saúde*) para facilitar a completa avaliação científica das terapias alternativas, estabelecer um local para a troca de informações e para apoiar treinamento de pesquisa em tópicos relacionados à MA que não costumam ser incluídos no currículo de treinamento dos profissionais de saúde correntes. Em 1998, o OAM foi renomeado como *National Center for Complementary and Alternative Medicine* (NCCAM) (*Centro Nacional de Medicina Complementar e Alternativa*), sendo destinado a ele um orçamento anual de 50 milhões de dólares. As filosofias ou métodos de diagnóstico ou tratamento alternativo populares nos Estados Unidos incluem acupressão, acupuntura, aromaterapia, *biofeedback*, quelação, quiropraxia, Ciência Cristã, fitoterapia, homeopatia, hidroterapia, hipnoterapia, iridologia, macrobiótica, massoterapia, meditação, tratamento megavitamínico, moxibustão, naturopatia, osteopatia, técnicas de relaxamento, Rolfing (integração estrutural), shiatsu, tai chi e yoga.

aviation m., medicina da aviação; o estudo e prática da medicina aplicado a problemas fisiológicos peculiares da aviação. SIN aeromedicine.

behavioral m., medicina comportamental; campo interdisciplinar relacionado com o desenvolvimento e com a integração do conhecimento e das técnicas da ciência comportamental e biomédica relevantes para a saúde e para a doença, e com sua aplicação e prevenção, diagnóstico, tratamento e reabilitação.

clinical m., medicina clínica; o estudo e a prática da medicina em relação ao tratamento dos pacientes; a arte da medicina, distinta da ciência laboratorial.

community m., medicina comunitária; o estudo da saúde e da doença em uma comunidade definida; a prática da medicina nessa situação.

comparative m., medicina comparativa; campo de estudo que se concentra nas semelhanças e diferenças entre medicina veterinária e medicina humana.

complementary m., medicina complementar. SIN alternative m.

defensive m., medicina defensiva; medidas diagnósticas ou terapêuticas realizadas basicamente como proteção contra possível ação judicial subseqüente por imperícia.

desmoteric m., medicina desmotérica; ramo da medicina que lida com problemas de saúde que ocorrem em prisioneiros. [G. *desmōtērion*, prisão, de *deo*, ligar, + *-ic*]

electrodiagnostic m., medicina eletrodiagnóstica; a área específica da prática médica na qual médicos especialmente treinados usam informações da história clínica e do exame físico, juntamente com o método científico de registro e análise de potenciais elétricos biológicos, para diagnosticar e tratar distúrbios neuromusculares.

evidence-based m., medicina baseada em evidências (MBE); o processo de aplicar informações relevantes obtidas na literatura médica revista por colegas para tratar um problema clínico específico; a aplicação de regras simples da ciência e do bom senso para determinar a validade das informações e a aplicação dessas informações ao problema clínico. VER TAMBÉM Cochrane *collaboration,* clinical practice *guidelines,* em *guideline.*

experimental m., medicina experimental; a investigação científica de problemas clínicos por experiência com animais ou por pesquisa clínica.

family m., medicina de família; a especialidade clínica relacionada ao atendimento contínuo e abrangente de todas as faixas etárias, desde o primeiro contato com o paciente até a assistência terminal, com ênfase especial no atendimento à família como uma unidade.

folk m., medicina popular; tratamento de doenças fora da medicina organizada por meio de remédios e medidas simples com base na experiência e no conhecimento transmitido de uma geração para outra.

forensic m., medicina forense; m. legal; (1) a relação e aplicação de fatos médicos a questões legais; (2) a lei em suas aplicações na prática da medicina. SIN legal m., medical jurisprudence.

geriatric m., medicina geriátrica; especialidade da medicina relacionada com doenças e problemas de saúde das pessoas idosas, geralmente aquelas com mais de 65 anos de idade. Considerada uma subespecialidade da medicina interna.

holistic m., medicina holística; (1) abordagem assistencial que enfatiza o estudo de todos os aspectos de saúde de uma pessoa, principalmente o fato de que ela deve ser considerada como uma unidade, incluindo influências psicológicas, sociais e econômicas sobre a saúde. (2) SIN alternative m.

hyperbaric m., medicina hiperbárica; o uso medicinal da pressão barométrica elevada, geralmente em câmaras especialmente construídas, para aumentar o conteúdo de oxigênio do sangue e dos tecidos.

internal m. (IM), medicina interna; o ramo da medicina relacionado com doenças não-cirúrgicas em adultos, mas que não inclui doenças limitadas à pele ou ao sistema nervoso.

legal m., medicina legal. SIN forensic m.

maternal-fetal m., medicina materno-fetal; subespecialidade da obstetrícia/ginecologia dedicada ao estudo das complicações obstétricas, clínicas e cirúrgicas da gravidez. SIN fetology.

military m., medicina militar; a prática da medicina aplicada às circunstâncias especiais associadas à vida militar.

neonatal m., medicina neonatal. SIN neonatology.

nuclear m., medicina nuclear; a disciplina clínica relacionada com os usos diagnósticos e terapêuticos dos radionuclídeos, incluindo fontes de radiação fechadas.

osteopathic m., medicina osteopática. SIN osteopathy (2).

patent m., medicamento registrado; medicamento, em geral originalmente patenteado, anunciado para o público.

perinatal m., medicina perinatal. SIN perinatology.

physical m., medicina física; fisiatria; o estudo e o tratamento de doenças, principalmente por meios mecânicos ou outros meios físicos. SIN physiatry.

podiatric m., medicina podiátrica. SIN podiatry.

preventive m., medicina preventiva; o ramo da ciência médica relacionado com a prevenção de doenças e promoção da saúde física e mental, através do estudo da etiologia e epidemiologia dos processos patológicos.

proprietary m., medicamento patenteado; medicamento cuja fórmula e modo de fabricação são propriedades do fabricante.

psychosomatic m., medicina psicossomática; o estudo e o tratamento de doenças, distúrbios ou estados anormais nos quais se acredita que processos psicológicos que resultam em reações fisiológicas tenham papel proeminente.

quack m., medicamento de curandeiro; composto falsamente anunciado como curativo de determinada doença ou doenças. Cf. nostrum.

social m., medicina social; campo especializado do conhecimento médico que se concentra no impacto social, cultural e econômico de fenômenos médicos.

socialized m., medicina socializada; a organização e o controle da prática médica por um órgão do governo, sendo os profissionais empregados pela organização, da qual recebem uma remuneração padronizada por seus serviços, e para a qual a população geralmente contribui na forma de tributação, e não de honorário por serviço.

space m., medicina espacial; o campo da medicina relacionado com doenças fisiológicas ou distúrbios resultantes das condições peculiares das viagens espaciais.

sports m., medicina desportiva; campo da medicina que usa uma abordagem holística, ampla e multidisciplinar para o tratamento das pessoas que realizam atividades desportivas ou de lazer.

tropical m., medicina tropical; o ramo da medicina relacionado com doenças, principalmente de origem parasitária, em áreas de clima tropical.

veterinary m., medicina veterinária; o campo relacionado com as doenças e com a saúde de todas as espécies de animais além do ser humano.

medico-. Medico-; médico. Cf. iatro-. [L. *medicus,* médico]

med·i·co·bi·o·log·ic, med·i·co·bi·o·log·i·cal (med'i-kō-bī-ō-loj'ik, -loj'i-kăl). Médico-biológico; relativo aos aspectos biológicos da medicina.

med·i·co·chi·rur·gi·cal (med'i-kō-kī-rŭr'ji-kăl). Clínico-cirúrgico; relativo à medicina interna e à cirurgia, ou aos clínicos e cirurgiões. [medico- + G. *cheirourgia,* cirurgia]

med·i·co·le·gal (med'i-kō-lē'găl). Médico-legal; relativo à medicina e à lei. VER TAMBÉM forensic *medicine.* [medico- + L. *legalis,* legal]

med·i·co·me·chan·i·cal (med'i-kō-mē-kan'i-kăl). Médico-mecânico; relativo a medidas medicinais e mecânicas em terapêutica.

med·i·co·phys·i·cal (med'i-kō-fiz'i-kăl). Médico-físico; relativo à doença e à condição do corpo em geral; p. ex., um exame médico-físico, no qual uma pessoa é examinada a fim de determinar a presença ou ausência de doença, e também observar a condição física geral.

med·i·co·psy·chol·o·gy (med'i-kō-sī-kol'ō-jē). Psicologia médica; psicologia em sua relação com a medicina. VER medical *psychology,* health *psychology.*

medio-, medi-. Medio-, medi-; meio, médio. [L. *medius*]

me·di·o·car·pal (mē'dē-ō-kar'păl). Mediocarpal; mesocarpal. SIN midcarpal.

me·di·oc·cip·i·tal (mē'dē-ok-sip'i-tăl). Médio-occipital. SIN midoccipital.

me·di·o·dens (mē'dē-ō-dens). Mediodente; dente supranumerário localizado entre os dois incisivos centrais maxilares. [medio- + L. *dens,* dente]

me·di·o·dor·sal (mē'dē-ō-dōr'săl). Mediodorsal; relativo aos planos mediano e dorsal.

me·di·o·lat·er·al (mē'dē-ō-lat'er-ăl). Mediolateral; relativo ao plano mediano e a um lado.

me·di·o·ne·cro·sis (mē'dē-ō-ne-krō'sis). Medionecrose; necrose da túnica média.
  m. of the aorta, necrose cística da média. SIN cystic medial *necrosis.*
  m. aor'tae idiopath'ica cys'tica, m. idiopática cística da aorta. SIN cystic medial *necrosis.*

me·di·o·tar·sal (mē'dē-ō-tar'săl). Mediotarsal; mesotarsal. SIN midtarsal.

me·di·o·tru·sion (mē'dē-ō-troo'zhŭn). Mediotrusão; impulso do côndilo mandibular em direção à linha média durante o movimento da mandíbula. [medio- + L. *trudo,* pp. *trusus,* empurrar]

me·di·o·type (mē'dē-ō-tīp). Mesomórfico. SIN mesomorph.

me·di·sect (mē'di-sekt). Cortar ao meio; realizar incisão na linha média. [L. *medius,* médio, + *seco,* pp. *sectus,* cortar]

me·di·um, pl. **me·dia** (mē'dē-ŭm, -ă). Meio. 1. Um meio; aquele através do qual é realizada uma ação. 2. Substância através da qual são transmitidos impulsos ou impressões. 3. Meio de cultura. SIN culture m. 4. O líquido que contém uma substância em solução ou suspensão. 5. Qualquer uma das substâncias em que é realizada uma separação cromatográfica ou eletroforética. [L. neutro de *medius,* médio]

Acanthamoeba **m.,** m. para *Acanthamoeba;* placas de ágar não-nutritivas com uma cobertura de *E. coli* usadas para detectar a presença de *Acanthamoeba* ou *Naegleria* em amostras de tecido ou de solo.

Balamuth aqueous egg yolk infusion m., m. de infusão de gema de ovo aquosa de Balamuth; meio usado para detectar amebas intestinais, basicamente *Entamoeba histolytica.*

Boeck and Drbohlav Locke-egg-serum m., m. de soro e ovo de Boeck e Drbohlav Locke; meio de cultura contendo ovos inteiros, soro humano e pó de arroz, usado para detectar amebas intestinais, basicamente *Entamoeba histolytica.*

clearing m., m. de clarificação; meio usado em histologia para fazer amostras translúcidas ou transparentes.

complete m., m. completo; meio de cultura *in vitro* que contém os nutrientes suplementares, bem como os nutrientes básicos, para satisfazer as necessidades de crescimento exigentes ou mutantes.

contrast m., m. de contraste; qualquer substância administrada internamente que possui uma opacidade diferente dos tecidos moles à radiografia ou tomografia computadorizada; inclui bário, usado para opacificar partes do trato gastrointestinal; compostos iodados hidrossolúveis, usados para opacificar vasos sanguíneos ou o trato genitourinário; pode referir-se ao ar presente naturalmente ou introduzido no corpo; também, substâncias paramagnéticas usadas em ressonância magnética. SIN contrast agent, contrast material.

culture m., m. de cultura; substância, sólida ou líquida, usada para o cultivo, isolamento, identificação ou armazenamento de microrganismos. SIN growth m., medium (3), nutrient m.

Czapek-Dox m., m. de Czapek-Dox. SIN Czapek solution *agar.*

Diamond TYM m., m. de Diamond TYM; meio de tripticase, extrato de levedura, maltose e soro usado para detectar *Trichomonas vaginalis.*

dispersion m., m. de dispersão. SIN external *phase.*

Dorset culture egg m., m. de cultura com ovo de Dorset; meio para cultivar *Mycobacterium tuberculosis*; consiste nas claras e gemas de quatro ovos frescos e uma solução de cloreto de sódio.
Eagle basal m., m. basal de Eagle; uma solução de vários sais contendo 13 aminoácidos naturais, várias vitaminas, dois antibióticos e vermelho fenol; usado como meio de cultura tecidual.
Eagle minimum essential m. (MEM), m. essencial mínimo de Eagle; meio de cultura tecidual semelhante ao meio basal de Eagle, mas com diferentes quantidades e algumas exclusões (p. ex., antibióticos e vermelho fenol).
Endo m., m. de Endo. SIN Endo *agar.*
external m., fase externa. SIN external *phase.*
growth m., m. de cultura. SIN culture m.
high osmolar contrast m. (HOCM), contraste de alta osmolaridade. SIN high osmolar contrast *agent.*
Lash casein hydrolysate-serum m., m. com hidrolisado de caseína-soro de Lash; usado para detectar *Trichomonas vaginalis.*
Loeffler blood culture m., m. para hemocultura de Loeffler; meio de cultura que consiste em soro sanguíneo bovino, soro sanguíneo ovino e caldo de carne contendo peptona, glicose e cloreto de sódio; usado para isolamento de *Corynebacterium diphtheriae.*
Lowenstein-Jensen m., m. de Lowenstein-Jensen. SIN Lowenstein-Jensen culture m.
Lowenstein-Jensen culture m., m. de cultura de Lowenstein-Jensen; meio de isolamento de micobactérias primárias, composto de ovos inteiros frescos, sais definidos, glicerol, fécula de batata e verde malaquita (como agente inibidor). SIN Lowenstein-Jensen m.
low osmolar contrast m. (LOCM), contraste de baixa osmolaridade. SIN low osmolar contrast *agent.*
McCarey-Kaufmann media, meio de McCarey-Kaufmann; solução de cultura usada para armazenamento de olhos enucleados para transplante de córnea (corneal *transplantation*).
motility test m., m. para prova de motilidade; meio de cultura com uma concentração de ágar que produz uma consistência menos sólida que a habitual e permite que microrganismos móveis cresçam distantes da linha de inoculação; usado para diferenciar espécies de bactérias.
mounting m., m. de montagem; substância, geralmente resinosa, usada para montar uma lamínula sobre suspensões histológicas.
Mueller-Hinton m., m. de Mueller-Hinton; meio com base de ágar composto de infusão bovina, casaminoácidos e amido; o meio recomendado para antibiogramas para bactérias aeróbicas e anaeróbicas facultativas mais comuns.
NNN m., m. NNN; ágar inclinado com sangue de coelho desfibrinado superposto usado para detectar *Leishmania* ou *Trypanosoma cruzi.*
nutrient m., m. nutriente. SIN culture m.
passive m., m. passivo; meio que não produz alteração nas amostras nele colocadas.
selective m., m. seletivo; meio de cultura contendo ingredientes que inibem o crescimento de contaminantes ou outros microrganismos além dos desejados.
separating m., m. de separação; (1) qualquer revestimento que sirva para impedir a aderência de uma superfície a outra; (2) em odontologia, material geralmente aplicado a um molde para facilitar separação da base da dentadura de resina após a cura; um revestimento sobre impressões para facilitar a remoção do molde.
Simmons citrate m., m. de citrato de Simmons; meio diagnóstico usado na diferenciação de espécies de Enterobacteriaceae, baseado em sua capacidade de utilizar o citrato de sódio como única fonte de carbono.
support m., m. de suporte; o material no qual ocorre separação, como na separação de componentes na eletroforese.
Thayer-Martin m., m. de Thayer-Martin. SIN Thayer-Martin *agar.*
transport m., m. de transporte; meio para transporte de amostras clínicas para exame em laboratório.
TY1-S-33 m., m. TY1-S-33; meio de biosato, peptona, dextrose, vitaminas e soro bovino usado para detectar *Entamoeba histolytica.*
TYSGM-9 m, m. TYSGM-9; meio de mucina gástrica, caldo nutritivo, soro bovino e amido de arroz usado para detectar *Entamoeba histolytica.*
me·di·um-chain ac·yl-CoA de·hy·dro·gen·ase (MCAD). Desidrogenase da acil-CoA de cadeia média. VER *acyl-CoA* dehydrogenase (NADPH).
me·di·us (mē'dē-ŭs). Médio. VER middle. [L.]
MEDLARS Abreviatura de *Medical Literature Analysis and Retrieval System*, um sistema de indexação por computador da *U.S. National Library of Medicine.*
MEDLINE. [MEDLARS-on-line]. Contato telefônico e pela internet, utilizando um computador, com a MEDLARS para consulta rápida de bibliografia médica.
med·pha·lan (med'fă-lan). Medfalan; agente antineoplásico. SIN medfalan.
med·ro·ges·tone (med-rō-jes'tōn). Medrogestona; uma progestina oral.
me·drox·y·pro·ges·ter·one ac·e·tate (med-rok'sē-prō-jes'ter-ōn). Acetato de medroxiprogesterona; agente progestacional ativo por via oral e parenteral, mais potente que a progesterona; usado no controle do sangramento uterino e, associado ao etinil estradiol, como contraceptivo oral.

med·ryl·a·mine (med-ril'ă-mēn). Medrilamina; anti-histamínico H₁.
med·ry·sone (med'ri-sōn). Medrisona; glicocorticóide usado topicamente como antiinflamatório, geralmente no olho.
me·dul·la, pl. **me·dul·lae** (me-dool'ă, me-dool'ē) [TA]. Medula; qualquer estrutura de consistência mole, semelhante à medula óssea, especialmente no centro de uma parte. VER TAMBÉM m. oblongata. SIN substantia medullaris (1). [L. medula óssea, de *medius*, meio]
    m. of adrenal gland, m. da glândula supra-renal; *termo oficial alternativo para m. of suprarenal gland.
    m. glan'dulae suprarena'lis [TA], m. da glândula supra-renal. SIN m. of suprarenal gland.
    m. of hair shaft, m. da haste do cabelo; o eixo central de alguns pêlos, que contém uma coluna de grandes células vacuoladas e queratinizadas; a porção medular é circundada pelo córtex.
    m. of kidney, m. renal. SIN renal m.
    m. of lymph node [TA], m. do linfonodo; a porção central de um linfonodo que consiste em massas de linfócitos, plasmócitos e macrófagos semelhantes a cordões, em um estroma de fibras reticulares separado por seios linfáticos; atinge a superfície do linfonodo no hilo. SIN m. nodi lymphoidei [TA].
    m. no'di lymphoidei [TA], m. do linfonodo. SIN m. of lymph node.
    m. oblonga'ta [TA], m. oblonga; bulbo; mielencéfalo; a subdivisão mais caudal do tronco encefálico, imediatamente contínua com a medula espinal, que se estende da borda inferior da decussação da pirâmide até a ponte; sua superfície ventral se assemelha à da medula espinal, exceto pela proeminência bilateral da oliva inferior; a superfície dorsal de sua metade superior forma parte do assoalho do quarto ventrículo. Os núcleos motores da medula oblonga incluem o núcleo do nervo hipoglosso, o núcleo motor dorsal, o núcleo salivatório inferior e o núcleo ambíguo; os núcleos sensoriais incluem os núcleos da coluna posterior (grácil e cuneiforme), os núcleos cocleares e vestibulares, as partes média e caudal do núcleo espinal do nervo trigêmeo e o núcleo do trato solitário. VER TAMBÉM medulla. SIN myelencephalon [TA], oblongata.
    m. os'sium [TA], m. óssea. SIN bone *marrow.*
    m. os'sium fla'va [TA], m. óssea amarela. SIN yellow bone *marrow.*
    m. os'sium ru'bra [TA], m. óssea vermelha. SIN red bone *marrow.*
    renal m., [TA], m. renal; a porção mais interna e escura do parênquima renal; consiste nas pirâmides renais. SIN m. renalis [TA], m. of kidney.
    m. rena'lis [TA], m. renal. SIN renal m.
    m. spina'lis [TA], m. espinal. SIN spinal *cord.*
    suprarenal m., m. da glândula supra-renal. SIN m. of suprarenal gland.
    m. of suprarenal gland [TA], m. da glândula supra-renal; é composta principalmente de cordões anastomosantes de células no cerne da glândula; as células exibem uma reação cromafin por causa da epinefrina e da norepinefrina existentes em seus grânulos. SIN m. glandulae suprarenalis [TA], m. of adrenal gland*, suprarenal m.
me·dul·lar (med-ool'ăr). Medular. SIN medullary.
med·ul·lary (med'ul-er-ē, med'oo-lăr-ē). Medular; relativo à medula ou medula óssea. SIN medullar.
med·ul·lat·ed (med'ŭ-lā-ted, med'oo-). 1. Medulado; que tem uma medula ou substância medular. 2. Mielinizado. SIN myelinated.
med·ul·la·tion (med'ŭ-lā'shŭn, med'oo-). 1. Medulação; a aquisição, ou o ato de formação de medula óssea ou de outro tipo. 2. Mielinização. SIN myelination.
med·ul·lec·to·my (med-oo-lek'tō-mē, med-ŭ-). Medulectomia; excisão de qualquer substância medular. [medulla + G. *ektomē*, excisão]
med·ul·li·za·tion (med'ŭ-li-zā'shŭn, med'ŭ-). Medulização; aumento dos espaços medulares no tratamento de vários distúrbios ósseos.
medullo-. Medulo-; medula. Cf. myel-. [L. *medulla*]
me·dul·lo·ar·thri·tis (med-ŭ-lō-ar-thrī'tis). Meduloartrite; inflamação da extremidade articular esponjosa de um osso longo.
me·dul·lo·blas·to·ma (med'ŭ-lō-blas-tō'mă). Meduloblastoma; tumor que consiste em células neoplásicas semelhantes às células indiferenciadas do tubo medular primitivo; os meduloblastomas geralmente estão localizados no verme do cerebelo e podem implantar-se de forma distinta ou coalescente nas superfícies do cerebelo, tronco encefálico e medula espinal; representam aproximadamente 3% das neoplasias intracranianas e são mais freqüentes em crianças; as células neoplásicas são células redondas ou ovóides, com núcleos hipercromáticos e citoplasma relativamente escasso, dispostas compactamente e em grupos pequenos e mal definidos, ou, algumas vezes, em um padrão de pseudo-roseta (roseta de Homer-Wright). Um tipo de tumor primitivo do neuroectoderma.
    desmoplastic m., m. desmoplásico; subtipo de meduloblastoma com padrão bifásico de folhas compactas de células indiferenciadas, alternadas com ilhotas de células menos coesas; geralmente ocorre no adolescente e no adulto jovem, e tem melhor prognóstico que o meduloblastoma habitual.
    melanotic m., m. melanótico; variante rara de meduloblastoma na qual há células pigmentadas com melanina.
me·dul·lo·cell (med'ŭ-lō-sel, med'oo-). Mielócito. SIN myelocyte (2).

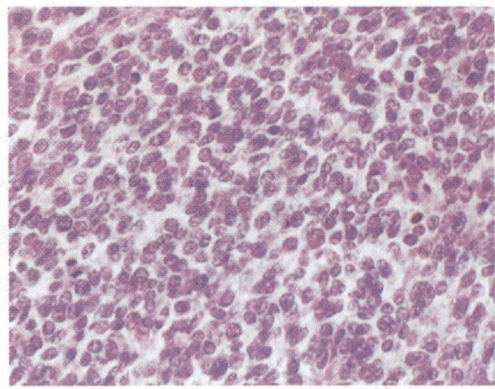
meduloblastoma: observe a proliferação difusa das células indiferenciadas

me·dul·lo·ep·i·the·li·o·ma (me′dŭ-lo-ep′ĭ-thē-lē-ō′mă). Meduloepitelioma; neoplasia intracraniana rara, primitiva, de crescimento rápido, que parece ter origem nas células do canal medular embrionário e, portanto, é incluída com os ependimoblastomas por alguns neuropatologistas; também foram descritas células ganglionares e maturação de astrócitos. Os tumores que ocorrem no corpo ciliar são denominados meduloepiteliomas embrionários. [medullo- + epithelium + -oma, tumor]
  adult m., m. do adulto. SIN malignant ciliary *epithelioma*.
  embryonal m., m. embrionário; tumor epiteliomatoso da camada não-pigmentada do epitélio ciliar. SIN embryonal tumor of ciliary body.

me·dul·lo·my·o·blas·to·ma (med′ŭ-lo-mī′o-blas-tō′mă). Medulomioblastoma; variante histológica rara de meduloblastoma, com células musculares lisas e estriadas dispersas incorporadas à neoplasia.

Meeh, K., fisiologista alemão do século XIX. VER M. *formula*; M.-Dubois *formula*.

Mees, R.A., médico holandês do século XX. VER M. *lines*, em *line, stripes*, em *stripe*.

Meesman, A., oftalmologista alemão, 1888–1969. VER M. *dystrophy*.

mef·e·nam·ic ac·id (me-fĕ-nam′ik). Ácido mefenâmico; analgésico semelhante ao ácido acetilsalicílico, com propriedades antiinflamatórias.

me·fen·o·rex hy·dro·chlo·ride (me-fen′ō-reks). Cloridrato de mefenorex; medicamento simpaticomimético com atividade anorética.

me·fex·a·mide (mĕ-fekʹa-mīd). Mefexamida; um antidepressivo.

mef·lo·quine (mef′lō-kwin). Mefloquina; antimalárico semelhante à quinina e à cloroquina.

MEG Abreviatura de magnetoencephalogram (magnetoencefalograma).

mega-. Mega-. **1.** Forma combinante que significa grande; oposto de micro-. VER TAMBÉM macro-, megalo-. **2 (M).** Prefixo usado no SI e no sistema métrico para designar múltiplos de um milhão (10⁶). [G. *megas*, grande]

meg·a·bac·te·ri·um (meg′a-bak-tēr′ē-ŭm). Megabactéria; uma bactéria de tamanho incomumente grande. SIN macrobacterium.

meg·a·ca·ly·co·sis (meg′a-kal-ĭ-kō′sis). Megacalicose. **1.** Aumento congênito, não-obstrutivo, dos cálices renais. **2.** Número excessivamente grande de cálices. [mega- + G. *kalyx*, cálice de uma flor, + -*osis*, condição]

meg·a·car·di·a (meg-ă-kar′dē-ă). Megacardia; cardiomegalia. SIN cardiomegaly.

meg·a·car·y·o·blast (meg-ă-karʹē-ō-blast). Megacarioblasto. SIN megakaryoblast.

meg·a·car·y·o·cyte (meg-ă-karʹē-ō-sīt). Megacariócito. SIN megakaryocyte.

meg·a·ce·pha·lia (meg-ă-se-faʹlē-ă). Megacefalia; megalocefalia. SIN megacephaly.

meg·a·ce·phal·ic (megʹă-se-falʹik). Megacefálico; megalocefálico; relativo à, ou caracterizado por, megalocefalia. SIN macrocephalic, macrocephalous, megacephalous.

meg·a·ceph·a·lous (meg-ă-sefʹa-lŭs). Megacéfalo; megalocéfalo. SIN megacephalic.

meg·a·ceph·a·ly (meg-ă-sefʹa-lē). Megacefalia; megalocefalia; condição, congênita ou adquirida, na qual a cabeça é anormalmente grande; termo geralmente aplicado a um crânio de adulto com capacidade maior que 1.450 ml. SIN leontiasis ossea, macrocephaly, macrocephalia, megacephalia, megalocephaly, megalocephalia, Virchow disease. [mega- + G. *kephalē*, cabeça]

meg·a·cins (megʹa-sinz). Megacinas; proteínas antibacterianas produzidas por cepas de *Bacillus megaterium*.

meg·a·coc·cus, pl. **meg·a·coc·ci** (megʹă-kokʹŭs, -kokʹsī). Megacoco; coco de tamanho incomumente grande. SIN macrococcus.

meg·a·co·lon (megʹă-kō′lon). Megacolo; condição de extrema dilatação do colo. SIN giant colon.
  acquired m., m. adquirido; megacolo que ocorre com base em uma doença adquirida; ocorre na doença intestinal inflamatória (m. tóxico) e na doença de Chagas (Chagas *disease*) (tripanossomíase sul-americana) (South American *trypanosomiasis*).
  congenital m., m. congen′itum, m. congênito; dilatação e hipertrofia congênitas do colo devidas à ausência (aganglionose) ou grande redução (hipoganglionose) do número de células ganglionares do plexo mioentérico do reto e de uma extensão variável, porém contínua, do intestino acima do reto; também observada em cães. SIN Hirschsprung disease.
  idiopathic m., m. idiopático; megacolo adquirido observado em crianças e adultos, sem obstrução distal ou ausência de células ganglionares; o músculo do colo dilatado é fino.
  toxic m., m. tóxico; dilatação não-obstrutiva aguda do colo, observada na colite ulcerativa fulminante e na doença de Crohn.

meg·a·cy·cle (megʹă-sī-kl). Megaciclo; um milhão de ciclos por segundo.

meg·a·cys·tis (megʹă-sis-tis). Megacisto; megabexiga; bexiga patologicamente grande em crianças. SIN megalocystis. [mega- + *kystis*, bexiga]

meg·a·dac·ty·ly, meg·a·dac·tyl·ia, meg·a·dac·tyl·ism (meg-ă-dakʹti-lē, -dak-tilʹē-ă, -dakʹtil-izm). Megalodactilia; condição caracterizada por aumento de um ou mais dedos (das mãos ou dos pés). SIN dactylomegaly, macrodactylia, macrodactylism, macrodactyly, megalodactylia, megalodactylism, megalodactyly. [mega- + G. *daktylos*, dedo]

meg·a·dol·i·cho·co·lon (megʹă-dolʹi-kō-kō′lon). Megadolicocolo; comprimento e dilatação excessivos do cólon. [mega- + G. *dolichos*, longo, + *kōlon*, colo]

meg·a·dont (megʹă-dont). Megalodonte. SIN macrodont. [mega- + G. *odous* (*odont*-), dente]

meg·a·don·tism (meg-ă-donʹtizm). Megalodontismo. SIN macrodontia.

meg·a·dyne (megʹă-dīn). Megadina; um milhão de dinas.

meg·a·e·soph·a·gus (megʹă-ē-sofʹa-gŭs, megʹă-e-sofʹ). Megaesôfago; grande aumento da parte inferior do esôfago, observado em pacientes com acalásia e doença de Chagas.

meg·a·ga·mete (meg-ă-gamʹēt). Megagameta. SIN macrogamete.

meg·a·gna·thia (meg-ă-nāʹthē-ă). Megalognatia; macrognatia. SIN macrognathia.

meg·a·hertz (MHz) (megʹă-hertz). Megahertz; um milhão de hertz.

meg·a·kar·y·o·blast (meg-ă-karʹē-ō-blast). Megacarioblasto; o precursor de um megacariócito. SIN megacaryoblast.

meg·a·kar·y·o·cyte (meg-ă-karʹē-ō-sīt). Megacariócito; uma célula grande (com até 100 μm de diâmetro), com um núcleo poliplóide, geralmente multilobulado; os megacariócitos estão normalmente presentes na medula óssea, não no sangue circulante, e dão origem às plaquetas sanguíneas. SIN megacaryocyte, megalokaryocyte, thromboblast. [mega- + G. *karyon*, noz (núcleo), + *kytos*, vaso oco (célula)]

megal-. VER megalo-.

meg·a·lec·i·thal (meg-ă-les-i-thăl). Megalécito; designa um ovo rico em vitelo, como nos peixes ósseos, répteis e aves. [mega- + G. *lekithos*, vitelo]

meg·al·gia (meg-alʹjē-ă). Megalgia; dor muito forte. [mega- + G. *algos*, dor]

megalo-, megal-. Megalo-, megal-; grande; oposto de micro-. VER TAMBÉM macro-, megа-. [G. *megas* (*megal*-)]

meg·a·lo·blast (megʹă-lō-blast). Megaloblasto; tipo de célula embrionária, grande, nucleada, que é um precursor de eritrócitos em um processo eritropoético anormal observado na anemia perniciosa; os quatro estágios de desenvolvimento de um megaloblasto são os seguintes: 1) pró-megaloblasto, 2) megaloblasto basófilo, 3) megaloblasto policromático, 4) megaloblasto ortocromático. VER TAMBÉM erythroblast. [megalo- + G. *blastos*, + germe, broto]

meg·a·lo·car·di·a (megʹă-lō-karʹdē-ă). Megalocardia. SIN cardiomegaly. [megalo- + G. *kardia*, coração]

meg·a·lo·ceph·a·ly, meg·a·lo·ce·pha·lia (megʹă-lō-sefʹă-lē, -sĕ-faʹlē-ă). Megalocefalia. SIN megacephaly.

meg·a·lo·chei·ria, meg·a·lo·chi·ria (megʹă-lō-kīʹrē-ă). Megaloquiria. SIN macrocheiria. [megalo- + G. *cheir*, mão]

meg·a·lo·cor·nea (megʹă-lō-korʹnē-ă). Megalocórnea. SIN keratoglobus.

meg·a·lo·cys·tis (megʹă-lō-sisʹtis). Megabexiga. SIN megacystis. [megalo- + G. *kystis*, bexiga]

meg·a·lo·cyte (megʹă-lō-sīt). Megalócito; uma hemácia grande (10–20 μm), não-nucleada. [megalo- + G. *kytos*, célula]

meg·a·lo·cy·the·mi·a (megʹă-lō-sī-thēʹmē-ă). Megalocitemia. SIN macrocythemia.

meg·a·lo·cy·to·sis (megʹă-lō-sī-tōʹsis). Megalocitose. SIN macrocythemia.

meg·a·lo·dac·tyl·ia, meg·a·lo·dac·tyl·ism, meg·a·lo·dac·ty·ly (megʹă-lō-dak-tilʹē-ă, dakʹtil-izm, -dakʹti-lē). Megalodactilia. SIN megadactyly.

meg·a·lo·dont (megʹă-lō-dont). Megalodonte. SIN macrodont.

meg·a·lo·don·tia (megʹă-lō-donʹshē-ă). Megalodontia. SIN macrodontia.

meg·a·lo·en·ce·phal·ic (meg′ă-lō-en′sĕ-fal′ik). Megaloencefálico; designa um encéfalo anormalmente grande.

meg·a·lo·en·ceph·a·lon (meg′ă-lō-en-sef′ă-lon). Megaloencéfalo; um encéfalo anormalmente grande. [megalo- + G. *enkephalos*, encéfalo]

meg·a·lo·en·ceph·a·ly (meg′ă-lō-en-sef′ă-lē). Megaloencefalia; tamanho anormalmente grande do encéfalo. [megalo- + G. *enkephalon*, encéfalo]

meg·a·lo·en·ter·on (meg′ă-lō-en′ter-on). Enteromegalia; tamanho anormalmente grande do intestino. SIN enteromegaly, enteromegalia. [megalo- + G. *enteron*, intestino]

meg·a·lo·gas·tria (meg′ă-lō-gas′trē-ă). Megalogastria; tamanho anormalmente grande do estômago. SIN macrogastria. [megalo- + G. *gaster*, estômago]

meg·a·lo·glos·sia (meg′ă-lō-glos′sē-ă). Megaloglossia. SIN macroglossia. [megalo- + G. *glōssa*, língua]

meg·a·lo·graph·ia (meg′ă-lō-graf′ē-ă). Megalografia. SIN macrography.

meg·a·lo·kar·y·o·cyte (meg′ă-lō-kar′ē-ō-sīt). Megalocariócito. SIN megakaryocyte.

meg·a·lo·ma·nia (meg′ă-lō-mā′nē-ă). Megalomania. **1.** Tipo de delírio no qual o indivíduo se considera grandioso. Ele acredita ser Cristo, Deus, Napoleão, etc., ou todos e tudo, incluindo um advogado, médico, clérigo, mercador, príncipe, melhor atleta em todas as divisões do esporte, etc. **2.** Superavaliação verbalizada mórbida de si próprio ou de algum aspecto próprio. [megalo- + G. *mania*, mania]

meg·a·lo·ma·ni·ac (meg′ă-lō-mā′nē-ak). Megalomaníaco; uma pessoa que exibe megalomania.

meg·a·lo·me·lia (meg′ă-lō-mē′lē-ă). Megalomelia. SIN macromelia.

meg·a·loph·thal·mos (meg′ă-lof-thal′mŭs). Megaloftalmo; bulbo do olho grande, congênito. SIN macrophthalmia, megophthalmus. [megalo- + G. *ophthalmos*, olho]

anterior m., m. anterior. SIN keratoglobus.

meg·a·lo·po·dia (meg′ă-lō-pō′dē-ă). Megalopodia. SIN macropodia. [megalo- + G. *pous*, pé]

meg·a·lo·splanch·nic (meg′ă-lō-splangk′nik). Megaloesplâncnico; que possui vísceras anormalmente grandes. SIN macrosplanchnic. [megalo- + G. *splanchnon*, víscera]

meg·a·lo·sple·nia (meg′ă-lō-splē′nē-ă). Esplenomegalia. SIN splenomegaly.

meg·a·lo·spore (meg′ă-lō-spōr). Megalosporo. SIN macrospore.

meg·a·lo·syn·dac·ty·ly, meg·a·lo·syn·dac·tyl·ia (meg′ă-lō-sin-dak′ti-lē, -dak-til′ē-ă). Megalossindactilia; condição de dedos das mãos ou artelhos unidos por membrana ou fundidos. [megalo- + G. *syn*, juntos, + *daktylos*, dedo]

meg·a·lo·u·re·ter (meg′ă-lō-ū-rē′ter). Megaloureter. SIN ureterectasia. SIN megaureter.

meg·a·lo·u·re·thra (meg′ă-lō-ū-rē′thră). Megalouretra; dilatação congênita da uretra.

-megaly. -megalia; grande. [G. *megas* (*megal-*)]

meg·a·mer·o·zo·ite (meg′ă-mer-ō-zō′īt). Megamerozoíta. SIN macromerozoite.

meg·a·nu·cle·us (meg-ă-noo′klē-ŭs). Meganúcleo. SIN macronucleus (1).

megapoietin (meg′ă-poy′ē-tin). Megapoetina, trombopoetina. SIN thrombopoietin. [mega- + G. *poiētēs*, produtor, + -in]

meg·a·pro·so·pia (meg′ă-prō-sō′pē-ă). Megaprosopia. SIN macroprosopia. [mega- + G. *prosōpon*, face]

meg·a·pros·o·pous (meg-ă-pros′ō-pŭs). Megaprosópico. SIN macroprosopous.

meg·a·rec·tum (meg-ă-rek′tŭm). Megarreto; dilatação extrema do reto.

meg·a·seme (meg′ă-sēm). Megassemo; designa uma abertura orbital com um índice superior a 89. [mega- + G. *sēma*, sinal]

meg·a·sig·moid (meg-ă-sig′moyd). Megassigmóide. SIN macrosigmoid.

meg·a·so·mia (meg-ă-sō′mē-ă). Megassomia. SIN macrosomia.

meg·a·spore (meg′ă-spōr). Megaesporo. SIN macrospore.

meg·a·throm·bo·cyte (meg-ă-throm′bō-sīt). Megatrombócito; uma grande plaqueta sanguínea, principalmente uma plaqueta jovem, recentemente liberada da medula óssea. [mega- + G. *thrombos*, coágulo, + *kytos*, célula]

meg·a·u·re·ter (meg′ă-ū-rē′ter). Megaureter. SIN megaloureter.

primary m., m. primário; dilatação ureteral independente; pode ser não-obstrutiva ou estar relacionada à obstrução ureteral distal congênita.

secondary m., m. secundário; hidroureter secundário ao refluxo vesicoureteral ou à obstrução distal.

meg·a·volt (meg′ă-vōlt). Megavolt; um milhão de volts.

meg·a·volt·age (meg′ă-vol′tij). Megavoltagem; em radioterapia, um termo para designar voltagem acima de um milhão de volts.

me·ges·trol ac·e·tate (me-jes′trol). Acetato de megestrol; uma progestina sintética com efeitos progestacionais semelhantes aos da progesterona; seus empregos atuais incluem o tratamento paliativo no câncer de mama e a estimulação do apetite na neoplasia maligna avançada.

meg·lit·in·ides (meg-lit′in-īdz). Meglitinidas; classe de fármacos hipoglicemiantes orais, que atuam fechando os canais de potássio ATP-dependentes nas células beta pancreáticas, assim causando abertura dos canais de cálcio e subseqüente liberação de insulina.

meg·lu·mine (meg′loo-mēn). Meglumina; contração de *N*-metilglucamina, aprovada pela USAN.

m. acetrizoate, acetrizoato de m.; meio de contraste radiológico. VER acetrizoate sodium.

m. diatrizoate, diatrizoato de m.; composto de iodo orgânico hidrossolúvel, usado antigamente na urografia excretora, na visualização do sistema cardiovascular com contraste, e por via oral para opacificação do trato gastrointestinal. SIN methylglucamine diatrizoate.

m. iothalamate, iotalamato de m.; sal *N*-metilglucamina de ácido iotalâmico (solução a 60%); um contraste radiopaco diagnóstico para uso intravascular em angiografia e urografia.

meg·ohm (meg′ōm). Megohm; um milhão de ohms.

meg·oph·thal·mus (meg-of-thal′mŭs). Megoftalmo. SIN megalophthalmos.

meg·ox·y·cyte (meg-oks′ē-sīt). Megoxicito. SIN megoxyphil.

meg·ox·y·phil, meg·ox·y·phile (meg-oks′ē-fil, -fīl). Megoxicito; leucócito eosinofílico que contém grânulos grosseiros. SIN megoxycyte. [mega- + G. *oxys*, ácido, + *phileō*, gostar]

me·grim (mē′grim). Termo obsoleto para enxaqueca (migraine).

Meibom (Meibomius), Hendrik (Heinrich), anatomista alemão, 1638–1700. VER meibomian cyst, meibomian *glands*, em *gland*, meibomian *sty*.

mei·bo·mi·an (mī-bō′mē-an). Meibomiano; atribuído a, ou descrito por, Meibom.

mei·bo·mi·tis, mei·bo·mi·a·ni·tis (mī′bō-mī′tis, mī-bō′mē-ă-nī′tis). Meibomite, meibomianite; inflamação das glândulas de Meibomio (glândulas tarsais).

Meier, Georg, sorologista alemão, *1875. VER Porges-M. *test*.

Meige, Henri, médico francês, 1866–1940. VER M. *disease*.

Meigs, Joe V., ginecologista norte-americano, 1892–1963. VER M. *syndrome*.

Meinicke, Ernst, médico alemão, 1878–1945. VER M. *test*.

meio-. Quanto às palavras que começam assim e não são encontradas aqui, ver mio-.

mei·o·sis (mī-ō′sis). Meiose; um processo especial de divisão celular que compreende duas divisões nucleares em rápida sucessão, que produz quatro gametócitos, cada um contendo metade do número de cromossomas encontrados nas células somáticas. SIN meiotic division. [G. *meiōsis*, redução]

mei·ot·ic (mī-ot′ik). Meiótico; relativo à meiose.

Meissel. VER Wachstein-Meissel *stain* for calcium-magnesium-ATPase.

Meissner, Georg, histologista alemão, 1829–1905. VER M. *corpuscle, plexus*.

mel. **1.** Mel. SIN honey. **2.** Mel; unidade de altura ou intensidade do som; uma intensidade de 1.000 mels resulta de um tom simples na freqüência de 1.000 Hz a 40 dB acima do limiar normal de audibilidade.

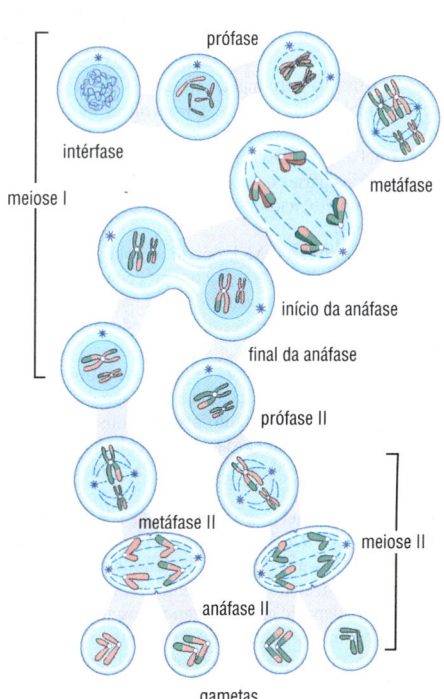

meiose celular

mel-, melo-. Mel-, melo-. **1.** Membro. [G. *melos*] **2.** Uma bochecha. [G. *mēlon*]. **3.** Mel, açúcar. VER TAMBÉM meli-. [L. *mel, mellis*, G. *meli, melitos*]. **4.** Carneiro. [G. *mēlon*]

me·lag·ra (mē - lag'ră). Melagra; dores reumáticas ou miálgicas nos braços ou pernas. [G. *melos*, membro, + *agra*, convulsão]

me·lal·gia (mē - lal'jē - ă). Melalgia; dor em um membro; especificamente, dor em queimação nos pés que ascende na perna, chegando até mesmo à coxa. [G. *melos*, um membro, + *algos*, dor]

mel·a·mine form·al·de·hyde (mel'ă - mēn). Formaldeído de melamina. SIN melamine resin.

melan-, melano-. Melan-, melano-; preto, coloração extremamente escura. [G. *melas*]

mel·an·cho·lia (mel - an - kō'lē - ă). Melancolia. **1.** Forma grave de depressão caracterizada por anedonia, insônia, alterações psicomotoras e culpa. **2.** Um sintoma que ocorre em outros distúrbios, caracterizado por depressão espiritual e por um processo de raciocínio lento e doloroso. [melan- + G. *cholē*, bile. VER humoral *doctrine*]

hypochondriacal m., m. hipocondríaca; melancolia com muitas queixas físicas associadas, freqüentemente com pouca base nos fatos.

involutional m., m. involutiva; distúrbio depressivo da meia-idade, comumente associado ao climatério.

mel·an·chol·ic (mel - an - kol'ik). Melancólico. **1.** Relativo a, ou característico de, melancolia. **2.** Antigamente designava um temperamento caracterizado por irritabilidade e uma perspectiva pessimista. **3.** Pessoa que exibe melancolia.

mel·an·choly (mel'an - kol - ē). Melancolia. SIN melancholia.

mel·a·ne·mia (mel - ă - nē'mē - ă). Melanemia; a presença de grânulos castanho-escuros, quase pretos ou pretos, de pigmento insolúvel (melanina) no sangue circulante. [melan- + G. *haima*, sangue]

mel·a·nif·er·ous (mel - ă - nif'er - ŭs). Melanífero; que contém melanina ou outro pigmento preto. [melan- (melanina) + L. *ferro*, conduzir]

mel·a·nin (mel'ă - nin). Melanina; qualquer um dos polímeros castanho-escuros ou pretos de indol-5,6-quinona e/ou ácido 5,6-diidroxiindol 2-carboxílico normalmente presentes na pele, pêlos, camada pigmentada da retina e, inconstantemente, na medula e na zona reticular da glândula supra-renal. A melanina pode ser formada *in vitro* ou biologicamente por oxidação da L-tirosina ou do L-triptofano, sendo o mecanismo habitual a oxidação enzimática da L-tirosina em 3,4-diidroxi-L-fenilalanina (dopa) e dopaquinona pela monofenol monooxigenase, e a oxidação adicional (provavelmente espontânea) desse intermediário em melanina. Cf. eumelanin, pheomelanin. SIN melanotic pigment. [G. *melas* (*melan-*), preto]

artificial m., factitious m., m. artificial; m. factícia. SIN melanoid.

mel·a·nism (mel'ă - nizm). Melanismo; pigmentação por melanina difusa, incomumente acentuada, dos pêlos e da pele (geralmente não afetando a íris). VER TAMBÉM melanosis.

Melano-. Melano. VER melan-.

mel·a·no·ac·an·tho·ma (mel'ă - nō - ak - an - thō'mă). Melanoacantoma; ceratose seborreica, com pigmentação por melanina, associada à proliferação de melanócitos intra-epidérmicos. [melano- + G. *akantha*, espinho, + sufixo *-ōma*, tumor]

mel·a·no·am·e·lo·blas·to·ma (mel'ă - nō - am'ē - lō - blas - tō'mă). Melanoameloblastoma. SIN melanotic neuroectodermal *tumor* of infancy. [melano- + ameloblastoma]

mel·a·no·blast (mel'ă - nō - blast). Melanoblasto; célula derivada da crista neural; migra para várias partes do corpo no início da vida embrionária, e depois se torna um melanócito maduro capaz de produzir melanina. [melano- + G. *blastos*, germe, broto]

mel·a·no·cyte (mel'ă - nō - sīt). Melanócito; célula produtora de pigmento localizada na camada basal da epiderme, com processos ramificados, por meio dos quais os melanossomas são transferidos para as células epidérmicas, resultando em pigmentação da epiderme. SIN melanodendrocyte, pigment cell of skin. [melano- + G. *kytos*, célula]

mel·a·no·cy·to·ma (mel'ă - nō - sī - tō'mă). Melanocitoma. **1.** Tumor pigmentado do estroma uveal. **2.** Melanoma do disco óptico, geralmente benigno, que aparece em indivíduos muito pigmentados como um pequeno tumor intensamente pigmentado na borda do disco, algumas vezes estendendo-se até a retina e coróide; a neoplasia maligna é rara. [megalo- + cyto- + G. *-ōma*, tumor]

mel·a·no·den·dro·cyte (mel'ă - nō - den'drō - sīt). Melanodendrócito. SIN melanocyte. [melano- + G. *dendron*, árvore, + *kytos*, uma cavidade (célula)]

mel·a·no·der·ma (mel'ă - nō - der'mă). Melanodermia. **1.** Escurecimento anormal da pele por deposição de melanina em excesso. **2.** Hiperpigmentação da pele por melanina ou deposição de substâncias escuras como a prata, o ferro e os derivados de fármacos. [melano- + G. *derma*, pele]

m. cachectico'rum, m. dos caquéticos; ocorre em algumas doenças crônicas, como malária e tuberculose.

parasitic m., m. parasitária; escoriações e melanodermia causadas por coçadura das picadas do piolho do corpo, *Pediculus corporis*. SIN vagabond's disease, vagrant's disease.

racial m., m. racial; a pele normalmente escura de membros de algumas raças não-brancas.

senile m., m. senil; pigmentação cutânea que ocorre nos idosos. SIN melasma universale.

mel·a·no·der·ma·ti·tis (mel'ă - nō - der - mă - tī'tis). Melanodermatite; depósito excessivo de melanina na área de dermatite.

me·la·no·gen (mē - lan'ō - jen, mel'ă - nō - jen). Melanogênio; substância incolor que pode ser convertida em melanina; p. ex., alguns pacientes com metástases disseminadas de melanoma excretam melanogênio em sua urina, e a melanina é formada quando a urina é exposta ao ar (isto é, oxidada) por algumas horas. [melanin + G. *-gen*, que produz]

mel·a·no·ge·ne·mia (mel'ă - nō - je - nē'mē - ă). Melanogenemia; a presença de precursores da melanina no sangue; pode ocorrer no melanoma maligno com metástase. [melanogen + G. *haima*, sangue]

mel·a·no·gen·e·sis (mel'ă - nō - jen'ē - sis). Melanogênese; formação de melanina. [melanin + G. *genesis*, produção]

mel·a·no·glos·sia (mel'ă - nō - glos'ē - ă). Melanoglossia. SIN black *tongue*. [melano- + G. *glōssa*, língua]

mel·a·noid (mel'ă - noyd). Melanóide; pigmento escuro, semelhante à melanina, formado a partir de glucosaminas na quitina. SIN artificial melanin, factitious melanin.

mel·a·no·ker·a·to·sis (mel'ă - nō - ker - ă - tō'sis). Melanoceratose; migração de melanoblastos conjuntivais para a córnea. [melano- + kerato- + G. *-osis*, condição]

mel·a·no·leu·ko·der·ma (mel'ă - nō - loo - kō - der'mă). Melanoleucodermia; pele marmórea ou marmorizada. [melano- + G. *leukos*, branco, + *derma*, pele]

m. col'li, m. do colo. SIN syphilitic leukoderma.

mel·an·o·lib·er·in (mel'ă - nō - lib'er - in). Melanoliberina; hexapeptídeo semelhante à ocitocina; estimula a liberação de melanotropina. SIN melanotropin-releasing factor, melanotropin-releasing hormone. [melanotropin + L. *libero*, libertar, + -in]

mel·a·no·ma (mel'ă - nō'mă). Melanoma; neoplasia maligna derivada de células capazes de produzir melanina, originada principalmente na pele de qualquer parte do corpo, ou no olho, e, raramente, nas mucosas da genitália, do ânus, da cavidade oral ou de outros locais; ocorre principalmente em adultos e pode originar-se *de novo* ou de um nevo pigmentado ou de um lentigo maligno. Nas fases iniciais, a forma cutânea é caracterizada por proliferação de células na junção dérmico-epidérmica, que logo invadem os tecidos adjacentes. As células variam em número e na pigmentação do citoplasma; os núcleos são relativamente grandes e freqüentemente têm formato bizarro, com nucléolos acidófilos proeminentes; e as figuras de mitose tendem a ser numerosas. O prognóstico está relacionado à profundidade da invasão cutânea. Os melanomas freqüentemente dão amplas metástases; linfonodos regionais, pele, fígado, pulmões e encéfalo tendem a ser envolvidos. A exposição intermitente e intensa ao sol, principalmente de crianças de pele clara, aumenta o risco de melanoma mais tarde. SIN malignant m. [melano- + G. *-ōma*, tumor]

acral lentiginous m., m. lentiginoso das extremidades; forma de lentigo maligno que ocorre nas regiões plantares e palmares e áreas subungueais.

amelanotic m., m. amelanótico; melanoma anaplásico, que consiste em células derivadas dos melanócitos, mas que não produzem melanina.

benign juvenile m., m. juvenil benigno. SIN Spitz *nevus*.

Cloudman m., m. de Cloudman; melanoma transplantável que surgiu espontaneamente em um camundongo da cepa DBA, e que cresce e metastatiza em camundongos de cepas relacionadas.

desmoplastic malignant m. (dez - mō - plas - mik), m. maligno desmoplásico; melanoma com acentuada fibrose adjacente aos melanócitos fusiformes atípicos na derme, que tende a apresentar ampla invasão ao redor de pequenos nervos.

Harding-Passey m., m. de Harding-Passey; tumor formador de melanina que surgiu espontaneamente em um camundongo não-endogâmico, e que é transplantável para camundongos de muitas cepas; mas, comumente, não se metastatiza.

malignant m., m. maligno. SIN melanoma.

malignant lentigo m., m. lentiginoso maligno; melanoma originado (em casos incomuns) de um lentigo maligno.

malignant m. in situ, m. maligno *in situ*; melanoma limitado à epiderme e composto de ninhos de melanócitos atípicos e células isoladas dispersas que se estendem até a parte superior da epiderme; a excisão local é curativa, embora a lesão, se não for tratada, possa logo invadir a derme. O lentigo maligno pode ser considerado um tipo lentamente progressivo de melanoma maligno *in situ*.

minimal deviation m., m. de desvio mínimo; melanoma maligno que exibe menor atipia citológica que o habitual nas células do melanoma, que, todavia, demonstram invasão expansiva assimétrica da derme ou metástase.

nodular m., m. nodular; melanoma cutâneo primário que se apresenta como nódulos de crescimento rápido, esferóides, lisos ou ulcerados, nos quais as células tumorais invadem microscopicamente a derme sob todas as margens epidérmicas laterais de envolvimento.

subungual m., m. subungueal; melanoma que começa na pele na borda da unha ou sob a mesma, geralmente do tipo lentiginoso das extremidades (q.v.).

superficial spreading m., m. disseminado superficial; melanoma cutâneo primário caracterizado por crescimento intra-epidérmico que se estende lateralmente além do local de invasão dérmica.

mel·a·no·ma·to·sis (mel′ă - nō - mă - tō′sis). Melanomatose; condição caracterizada por inúmeras lesões disseminadas de melanoma. [melanoma + G. *-osis*, condição]

mel·a·no·nych·i·a (mel′ă - nō - nik′ē - ă). Melanoníquia; pigmentação preta das unhas. [melano- + G. *onyx* (*onych-*), unha]

mel·a·nop·a·thy (mel′ă - nop′ă - thē). Melanopatia; qualquer doença caracterizada por pigmentação anormal da pele. [melano- + G. *pathos*, que sofre]

mel·a·no·phage (mel′ă - nō - fāj, mē - lan′ō - fāj). Melanófago; histiócito que fagocitou melanina. [melano- + G. *phagein*, comer]

mel·a·no·phore (mel′ă - nō - fōr, mē - lan′ō - fōr). Melanóforo; célula dérmica com pigmento, que não secreta seus grânulos de pigmento, mas participa das rápidas alterações da cor por agregação e dispersão intracelular dos melanossomas; é bem desenvolvida nos peixes, anfíbios e répteis, mas ausente em seres humanos. [melano- + G. *phoros*, que possui]

mel·a·no·pla·kia (mel′ă - nō - plā′kē - ă). Melanoplaquia; a ocorrência de placas pigmentadas na língua e na mucosa oral. [melano- + G. *plax*, lâmina, placa]

mel·a·no·pro·tein (mel′ă - nō - prō′tēn). Melanoproteína; um complexo proteico que contém melanina.

mel·a·nor·rha·gia (mel′ă - nō - rā′jē - ă). Melanorragia. SIN melena. [melano- + G. *rhēgnymi*, explodir]

mel·a·nor·rhea (mel′ă - nō - rē′ă). Melanorréia. SIN melena. [melano- + G. *rhoia*, fluxo]

mel·a·no·sis (mel - ă - nō′sis). Melanose; pigmentação castanho-escura ou castanho-preta anormal de vários tecidos ou órgãos, em virtude de melanina ou, em algumas situações, de outras substâncias semelhantes à melanina em vários graus; p. ex., a melanose cutânea pode ocorrer no melanoma metastático disseminado, na queimadura solar, durante a gravidez e em virtude de infecções crônicas. [melano- + G. *-osis*, condição]

m. co'li, m. do colo; melanose da mucosa do intestino grosso devido ao acúmulo de pigmento de composição incerta nos macrófagos na lâmina própria.

neurocutaneous m., m. neurocutânea; nevos pigmentados gigantes cutâneos associados à melanose das leptomeninges; melanomas malignos podem surgir na pele ou nas meninges.

oculodermal m., m. oculodérmica; pigmentação da esclera e da pele ao redor dos olhos, geralmente unilateral; observada principalmente em mulheres de ascendência asiática. SIN Ota nevus.

pustular m., m. pustular; exantema pustular, benigno, transitório, de etiologia desconhecida, observado em recém-nascidos; deixa uma base hiperpigmentada quando a pústula resolve.

Riehl m., m. de Riehl; condição pigmentar castanha das partes expostas da pele do pescoço e da face, com melanina em macrófagos dérmicos, considerada resultante de fotodermatite por materiais, tais como cosméticos ou óleos encontrados em várias ocupações.

mel·a·no·some (mel′ă - nō - sōm). Melanossoma; o grânulo de pigmentos, geralmente oval (0,2 por 0,6 μm), produzido por melanócitos. SIN eumelanosome. [melano- + G. *sōma*, corpo]

giant m., m. gigante; grande melanossoma esférico (1 a 6 μ de diâmetro) formado no citoplasma de melanócitos nas manchas café-com-leite e em outros distúrbios melanocíticos. SIN macromelanosome.

mel·an·o·sta·tin. Melanostatina; inibe a síntese e a liberação de melanotropina; neuropeptídeo Y. SIN melanotropin release-inhibiting hormone. [melanotropin + G. *states*, estacionário, + -in]

mel·a·not·ic (mel′ă - not′ik). Melanótico. **1.** Relativo à presença, normal ou patológica, de melanina. **2.** Relativo a, ou caracterizado por, melanose.

mel·a·no·ton·in (mel′ă - nō - tō - nin). Melanotonina. VER melatonin.

mel·a·not·ri·chous (mel - ă - not′ri - kŭs). Melanotríquio; que possui pêlos negros. [melano- + G. *thrix* (*trich-*), pêlo]

mel·a·no·troph (mel′ă - nō - trōf). Melanotrofo; uma célula do lobo intermediário da hipófise que produz melanotropina. [melano- + G. *trophē*, nutrição]

mel·a·no·tro·phin (mel′ă - nō - trō′fin). Melanotropina. SIN melanotropin. [melano- + G. *trophē*, nutrição, + -in]

mel·a·no·tro·pin (mel′ă - nō - trō′pin). Melanotropina; hormônio polipeptídico secretado pelo lobo intermediário da hipófise em seres humanos (na neuro-hipófise em algumas outras espécies), que causa dispersão de melanina pelos melanóforos, resultando em escurecimento da pele, provavelmente por promoção da síntese de melanina; esse efeito é facilmente demonstrado em alguns vertebrados inferiores, tais como as rãs e os peixes; a α-melanotropina é um peptídeo *N*-acetilado com 13 aminoácidos; a β-melanotropina tem 22 aminoácidos. SIN intermedin, melanocyte-stimulating hormone, melanophore-expanding principle, melanotrophin.

mel·a·nu·ria (mel - ă - noo′rē - ă). Melanúria; a excreção de urina escura, resultante da presença de melanina ou outros pigmentos, ou da ação do fenol, creosoto, resorcina e outros derivados do alcatrão. [melano- + G. *ouron*, urina]

mel·a·nu·ric (mel - ă - noo′rik). Melanúrico; relativo a, ou caracterizado por, melanúria.

mel·ar·so·prol (me - lar′sō - prol). Melarsoprol; usado no tratamento dos estágios meningoencefalíticos da tripanossomíase; pode produzir uma encefalopatia reativa fatal.

MELAS Acrônimo para *m*iopatia mitocondrial, *e*ncefalopatia, acidose *l*áctica (*l*actic *a*cidosis) e acidente vascular cerebral (*s*troke); um distúrbio hereditário da cadeia respiratória, seja uma deficiência do NADH:ubiquinona oxidorredutase (complexo I da cadeia) ou da citocromo *c* oxidase.

MELAS Acrônimo para miopatia *m*itocondrial, *e*ncefalopatia, acidose *l*áctica (*l*actic *a*cidosis) e episódios semelhantes a acidentes vasculares cerebrais (*s*trokelike episodes). Um dos distúrbios mitocondriais, essa condição geralmente é hereditária, com uma mutação no genoma mitocondrial no *locus* 3243.

me·las·ma (mĕ - laz′mă). Melasma; pigmentação segmentar da pele exposta ao sol, mais comum na gravidez. VER TAMBÉM chloasma. [G. uma cor preta, uma mancha preta]

m. gravida'rum, m. da gravidez; cloasma que ocorre na gravidez.

m. universa'le, m. universal. SIN senile *melanoderma.*

mel·a·ton·in (mel - ă - tōn′in). Melatonina; *N*-acetil-5-metoxitriptamina; substância formada pela glândula pineal dos mamíferos, que parece deprimir a função gonadal em mamíferos e causa contração dos melanóforos dos anfíbios; um precursor é a serotonina; a melatonina é rapidamente metabolizada e captada por todos os tecidos; está envolvida nos ritmos circadianos. [melanophore + G. *tonos*, contração, + -in]

A secreção de melatonina está ligada aos ciclos sono-vigília e claro-escuro. Foi demonstrado que a percepção ocular de que a luz ambiente está diminuindo deflagra, através de vias neurais que envolvem o hipotálamo, um aumento da secreção de melatonina pela glândula pineal. Os níveis séricos aumentam 10 vezes antes do sono e atingem seu máximo por volta da meia-noite. A secreção em 24 horas é maior no inverno que no verão. A diminuição da secreção de melatonina com a idade foi culpada pela tendência à insônia nos idosos. Como a melatonina atua como antioxidante na neutralização dos radicais livres, foi promovida como forma de retardar o envelhecimento e evitar câncer, cardiopatia e demência de Alzheimer. Também foi proposta como antidepressivo porque a serotonina (5-hidroxitriptamina), cujo metabolismo está perturbado na depressão clínica, é um precursor químico da melatonina. Não existem estudos em grande escala, adequadamente controlados, da eficácia, segurança e dosagem ideal da melatonina. Há evidências experimentais de que a administração prolongada pode reajustar o marcapasso circadiano. Relatos de casos sugerem que cursos mais breves podem acelerar a recuperação do *jet lag* e facilitar a adaptação a turnos de trabalho noturno. Em um estudo controlado de 15 médicos emergencistas, a melatonina não melhorou o sono quando eles retomaram o padrão de sono normal após plantões noturnos. O efeito soporífero direto da melatonina varia muito de uma pessoa para outra. Estudos limitados sugerem que a melatonina pode aumentar a duração do sono noturno repousante nos idosos. Altas doses de melatonina resultam em elevação prolongada do nível sérico de melatonina e em aumento da produção de prolactina pela hipófise. Ao contrário da maioria dos hormônios, a melatonina é rapidamente absorvida pelo trato digestivo, e é um componente de alguns alimentos. Assim, as formulações terapêuticas não estão sujeitas às regulamentações federais dos medicamentos ou a padrões de pureza. O teste de preparações de melatonina encontradas à venda indicou variação na potência e a presença de contaminantes possivelmente prejudiciais.

Melchior, J.C., médico dinamarquês. VER Dyggve-Melchior-Clausen *syndrome.*

me·le·na (me - lē′nă). Melena; eliminação de fezes escuras, semelhantes a alcatrão, devido à presença de sangue alterado pelos sucos intestinais. Cf. hematochezia. SIN melanorrhagia, melanorrhea. [G. *melaina*, fem. de *melas*, preto]

m. neonato'rum, m. neonatal; melena do recém-nascido; melena que ocorre em lactentes pequenos.

m. spu'ria, m. espúria; eliminação fecal de sangue que foi ingerido, principalmente aquele ingerido ao mamar em um mamilo fissurado.

m. ve'ra, m. verdadeira; distinta da melena espúria.

mel·e·nem·e·sis (mel - ĕ - nem′ĕ - sis). Melenêmese; vômito de material escuro ou enegrecido. VER TAMBÉM black *vomit.* [G. *melas*, preto, + *emesis*, vômito]

Meleney, Frank L., cirurgião norte-americano, 1889–1963. VER M. *gangrene, ulcer.*

mel·en·ges·trol ac·e·tate (mel-en-jes'trōl). Acetato de melengestrol; um agente progestacional.

mel·e·tin (mel'ē-tin). Meletina. SIN quercetin.

♻ **meli-.** Meli-; mel, açúcar. VER TAMBÉM mel- (3). [G. *meli*]

mel·i·bi·ase (mel-i-bī'ās). Melibiase. SIN α-D-galactosidase.

mel·i·bi·ose (mel-i-bī'ōs). Melibiose; dissacarídeo formado pela hidrólise da rafinose pela β-frutofuranosidase; também presente em sucos vegetais.

mel·i·ce·ra, mel·i·ce·ris (mel-i-sē'rā, mel-i-sē'ris). Melicéris; um higroma ou outro tipo de cisto que contém um material semilíquido, viscoso, relativamente espesso. [G. *meli- kēris*, um tumor, de *melikēron*, favo de mel, de *meli*, mel, + *kēros*, cera]

mel·i·oi·do·sis (mel'ē-oy-dō'sis). Melioidose; doença infecciosa de roedores na Índia e no sudeste asiático, causada por *Pseudomonas pseudomallei* e transmissível para seres humanos. A lesão característica é um pequeno nódulo caseoso, geralmente encontrado em todo o corpo, que se rompe em um abscesso; os sinais e sintomas variam de acordo com os tratos ou órgãos envolvidos. SIN pseudoglanders, Whitmore disease. [G. *mēlis*, perturbação, + *eidos*, semelhança, + *osis*, condição]

me·lis·sa (me-lis'ā). Melissa; erva cidreira verdadeira; as folhas da *Melissa officinalis* (família Labiatae), uma planta do sul da Europa; um diaforético. SIN sweet balm. [G. abelha]

me·lis·sic ac·id (me-lis'ik). Ácido melíssico; ácido graxo saturado de cadeia longa encontrado em ceras. [G. *melissa*, abelha + *-ic*]

me·lis·so·pho·bia (mē-lis'ō-fō'bē-ā). Melissofobia. SIN apiphobia. [G. *melissa*, abelha, + *phobos*, medo]

me·li·tis (mē-lī'tis). Melite; inflamação da bochecha. [G. *mēlon*, bochecha, + *-itis*, inflamação]

mel·i·tose (mel'i-tōs). Melitose. SIN raffinose.

mel·i·tra·cen hy·dro·chlo·ride (mel-i-trā'sen). Cloridrato de melitraceno; antidepressivo.

mel·i·tri·ose (mel-i-trī'ōs). Melitriose. SIN raffinose.

mel·it·tin (mel'i-tin). Melitina; o principal componente do veneno de abelha; a melitina é uma amida peptídica que contém 26 aminoácidos e é uma hemolisina. [G. *melitta*, abelha, + *-in*]

Melkersson, Ernst G., médico sueco, 1898–1932. VER M.-Rosenthal *syndrome*.

mel·li·tum, gen. **mel·li·ti,** pl. **mel·li·ta** (me-lī'tŭm,-tī, tā). Melito; preparado farmacêutico que usa mel como excipiente. [L. neutro de *mellitus*, melado]

Melnick, John C., radiologista norte-americano, *1928. VER Melnick-Needles *osteodysplasty*; M.-Needles *syndrome*.

♻ **melo-.** Melo-. VER melo-.

mel·o·did·y·mus (mel'ō-did'ī-mus). Melodídimo; feto com um membro supranumerário. [melo- + G. *didymos*, gêmeo]

mel·o·ma·nia (mel-ō-mā'nē-ā). Melomania; uma fascinação anormal pela música, ou devoção a ela. [L. *melos*, música + *mania*, mania]

mel·o·me·lia (mel-ō-mē'lē-ā). Melomelia; malformação na qual o feto tem um ou mais membros rudimentares além dos membros normais. Cf. micromelia. [G. *melos*, membro]

mel·o·plas·ty (mel'ō-plas-tē). Meloplastia; termo antigo para cirurgia plástica da bochecha; também usado para "*facelift*". [melo- + G. *plastos*, formado]

mel·o·rhe·os·to·sis (mel'ō-rē-os-tō'sis). Melorreostose; reostose limitada aos ossos longos. [G. *melos*, membro, + *rheos*, corrente, + *osteon*, osso, + *-ōsis*]

me·los·chi·sis (me-los'ki-sis). Melosquise; fenda congênita na face. [G. *mēlon*, bochecha, + *schisis*, uma clivagem]

me·lo·tia (me-lō'shē-ā). Melotia; deslocamento congênito da orelha para a bochecha. [G. *mēlon*, bochecha, + *ous*, orelha]

mel·pha·lan (mel'fā-lan). Melfalan; L-fenilalanina mostarda; L-sarcolisina; L-3-[*p*-[*bis*(2-cloroetil)amino]fenil]alanina; um derivado fenilalanina da mostarda nitrogenada; um agente antineoplásico alquilante.

melt. Desnaturar; usado para descrever a ação da RNA polimerase no desacoplamento dos pares de bases de DNA.

Meltzer, Samuel J., fisiologista norte-americano, 1851–1920. VER M. *law*; M.-Lyon *test*.

MEM Abreviatura de Eagle minimum essential *medium* (meio essencial mínimo de Eagle).

mem·ber. Membro. SIN limb (1). [L. *membrum*]
   inferior m. [TA], m. inferior. SIN lower *limb*.
   superior m. [TA], m. superior. SIN upper *limb*.
   virile m., termo obsoleto para pênis.

mem·bra (mem'brā). Membros; plural de membrum. [L.]

MEMBRANA

---

mem·bra·na, gen. e pl. **mem·bra·nae** (mem-brā'nă, -brā'nē) [TA]. Membrana. SIN membrane (1). [L.]

m. abdom'inis, peritônio. SIN peritoneum.
m. adamanti'na, m. adamantina. SIN enamel *cuticle*.
m. adventi'tia, m. adventícia; (1) SIN adventitia; (2) SIN *decidua* capsularis.
m. atlan'to-occipita'lis ante'rior [TA], m. atlantoccipital anterior. SIN anterior atlanto-occipital *membrane*.
m. atlan'to-occipita'lis poste'rior [TA], m. atlantoccipital posterior. SIN posterior atlanto-occipital *membrane*.
m. basa'lis duc'tus semicircula'ris, lâmina basilar do ducto semicircular. SIN basal *membrane* of semicircular duct.
m. basila'ris, lâmina basilar do ducto coclear. SIN basal *lamina* of cochlear duct.
m. capsula'ris, m. capsular; a rede vascular hialóide ao redor do pólo posterior ou da lente no embrião.
m. capsulopupilla'ris, m. capsulopupilar; a porção lateral da túnica vascular da lente do olho no embrião.
m. carno'sa, m. superficial do escroto. SIN dartos *fascia*.
m. cer'ebri, m. cerebral; qualquer uma das meninges cerebrais.
m. choriocapilla'ris, lâmina capilar da corióide. SIN capillary *lamina* of choroid.
m. cor'dis, pericárdio. SIN pericardium.
m. cricothyroi'dea, m. cricotireóidea. SIN cricothyroid *membrane*.
m. decid'ua, m. decídua. SIN deciduous *membrane*.
m. e'boris, m. ebúrnea; a m. de revestimento da cavidade pulpar de um dente que consiste na camada odontoblástica. SIN ivory *membrane*.
m. fibroelas'tica laryn'gis [TA], m. fibroelástica da laringe. SIN fibroelastic *membrane* of larynx.
m. fibro'sa capsulae articularis [TA], camada fibrosa da cápsula articular. SIN fibrous *layer* of joint capsule.
m. flac'cida, parte flácida da m. timpânica. SIN flaccid *part* of tympanic *membrane*.
m. fus'ca, lâmina supracorióide da esclera. SIN suprachoroid *lamina* of sclera.
m. germinati'va, m. germinativa. SIN blastoderm.
m. granulo'sa, m. granulosa. SIN *stratum* granulosum folliculi ovarici vesiculosi.
m. hyaloi'dea, lâmina limitante posterior da córnea. SIN posterior limiting *lamina* of cornea.
m. hyothyroi'dea, m. tíreo-hióidea. SIN thyrohyoid *membrane*.
membran'ae intercosta'les [TA], membranas intercostais. SIN intercostal *membranes*, em *membrane*.
m. intercosta'lis exter'na [TA], m. intercostal externa. SIN external intercostal *membrane*.
m. intercosta'lis inter'na [TA], m. intercostal interna. SIN internal intercostal *membrane*.
m. interos'sea antebra'chii [TA], m. interóssea do antebraço. SIN interosseous *membrane* of forearm.
m. interos'sea cru'ris [TA], m. interóssea da perna. SIN interosseous *membrane* of leg.
m. lim'itans, m. limitante; (1) SIN limiting *membrane* of retina; (2) membrana limitante que separa o parênquima neural da pia-máter e dos vasos sanguíneos.
m. lim'itans gli'ae, m. limitante da glia. SIN glial limiting *membrane*.
m. muco'sa, mucosa. SIN mucosa.
m. nic'titans, prega semilunar da conjuntiva. SIN *plica* semilunaris of conjunctiva (2).
m. obturato'ria [TA], m. obturadora. SIN obturator *membrane*.
m. perine'i [TA], m. do períneo. SIN perineal *membrane*.
m. pituito'sa, m. do nariz. SIN *mucosa* of nose.
m. preformati'va, m. pré-formadora; a m. espessa formada por fusão de fibras de Korff e da m. basal dos ameloblastos em um dente em desenvolvimento.
m. pro'pria duc'tus semicircula'ris, m. própria do ducto semicircular. SIN proper *membrane* of semicircular duct.
m. propria of semicircular duct, m. própria do ducto semicircular. SIN proper *membrane* of semicircular duct.
m. pupilla'ris, m. pupilar. SIN pupillary *membrane*.
m. quadrangula'ris [TA], m. quadrangular. SIN quadrangular *membrane*.
m. reticula'ris organi spiralis [TA], m. reticular do órgão espiral. SIN reticular *membrane* of spiral organ.
m. sero'sa, m. serosa; (1) SIN serosa, chorion; (2) SIN serosa (2).
m. seroti'na, m. serotina; sinônimo obsoleto de *decidua* basalis.
m. spira'lis, superfície timpânica do ducto coclear; *termo oficial alternativo para tympanic *surface* of cochlear duct.
m. stape'dis [TA], m. estapedial. SIN stapedial *membrane*.
m. statoconio'rum [TA], m. dos estatocônios. SIN otolithic *membrane*.
m. ster'ni [TA], m. do esterno. SIN sternal *membrane*.
m. stria'ta, zona estriada. SIN *zona* striata.
m. succin'gens, m. pleural. SIN pleura. [L. *succingere*, circundar]
m. suprapleura'lis [TA], m. suprapleural. SIN suprapleural *membrane*.
m. synovia'lis [TA], m. sinovial. SIN synovial *membrane*.

m. tecto'ria (articulationis atlantoaxialis medianae) [TA], m. tectória (articulações atlantoaxiais medianas). SIN tectorial membrane (of median atlantoaxial joint).
m. tecto'ria duc'tus cochlea'ris [TA], m. tectória do ducto coclear. SIN tectorial membrane of cochlear duct.
m. ten'sa, m. tensa. SIN tense part of the tympanic membrane.
m. thyrohyoi'dea [TA], m. tíreo-hióidea. SIN thyrohyoid membrane.
m. tym'pani [TA], m. timpânica. SIN tympanic membrane.
m. tym'pani secunda'ria [TA], m. timpânica secundária. SIN secondary tympanic membrane.
m. versic'olor, tapete. SIN tapetum (2).
m. vestibula'ris ductus cochlearis, superfície vestibular do ducto coclear; *termo oficial alternativo para vestibular surface of cochlear duct.
m. vi'brans, parte tensa da membrana timpânica. SIN tense part of the tympanic membrane.
m. vitelli'na, m. vitelina; **(1)** a membrana que envolve o vitelo; especificamente, a membrana celular espessa de ovos com grande vitelo. SIN ovular membrane, vitelline membrane. **(2)** Termo usado algumas vezes para designar a zona pelúcida de um óvulo de mamífero. SIN yolk membrane.
m. vit'rea, m. vítrea. SIN posterior limiting lamina of cornea.

mem·bra·na·ceous (mem - brā - nā'shŭs). Membranáceo. SIN membranous.
mem·bra·nate (mem'brā - nāt). Membranoso; da natureza de uma membrana.

MEMBRANE

mem·brane (mem'brān). **1.** Membrana; uma fina lâmina ou camada de tecido elástico que serve como revestimento ou envoltório de uma parte, como o revestimento de uma cavidade, como uma divisão ou um septo, ou unindo duas estruturas. SIN membrana [TA]. **2.** Biomembrana. SIN biomembrane. [L. *membrana*, uma pele ou membrana que cobre partes do corpo, de *membrum*, um membro]
adamantine m., m. adamantina. SIN enamel cuticle.
allantoid m., m. alantóide. SIN allantois.
alveolocapillary m., m. alveolocapilar; a barreira à difusão pulmonar.
alveolodental m., m. alveolodentária. SIN periodontium.
anal m., m. anal; a porção dorsal da membrana cloacal embrionária após sua divisão pelo septo urorretal.
anterior atlanto-occipital m. [TA], m. atlantoccipital anterior; a camada fibrosa que se estende do arco anterior do atlas até a margem anterior do forame magno do osso occipital. SIN membrana atlanto-occipitalis anterior [TA].
arachnoid m., m. aracnóide, aracnóide-máter. SIN arachnoid mater.
atlanto-occipital m., m. atlantoccipital. VER anterior atlanto-occipital m., posterior atlanto-occipital m.
Barkan m., m. de Barkan; um revestimento tecidual teórico que cobre a rede trabecular (trabecular *meshwork*); acredita-se que obstrua a saída de humor aquoso (aqueous *humor* outflow) e seja responsável pelo glaucoma congênito.
basal m. of semicircular duct, lâmina basilar do ducto semicircular; a membrana basilar subjacente ao epitélio do ducto semicircular. SIN basal lamina of semicircular duct, membrana basalis ductus semicircularis.
basement m., m. basal; uma camada extracelular amorfa intimamente aplicada à superfície basal do epitélio e que também reveste as células musculares, adipócitos e células de Schwann; considerada um filtro seletivo e possui funções estruturais e morfogênicas. É composta de três camadas sucessivas (lâmina lúcida, lâmina densa e lâmina fibrorreticular), uma matriz de colágeno (cujo tipo IV é exclusivo dessa membrana) e várias glicoproteínas. SIN basement lamina, basilemma.
basilar m. of cochlear duct, m. basilar do ducto coclear. SIN basal lamina of cochlear duct.
Bichat m., m. de Bichat; a membrana elástica interna das artérias.
Bogros serous m., m. serosa de Bogros; uma membrana do espaço episcleral (de Tenon).
Bowman m., m. de Bowman, camada limitante anterior da córnea. SIN anterior limiting layer of cornea.
Bruch m., m. de Bruch. SIN lamina basalis choroideae.
Brunn m., m. de Brunn; o epitélio da região olfatória do nariz.
bucconasal m., m. buconasal; lâmina epitelial fina, transitória, que separa a cavidade nasal primitiva do estomódio no embrião humano de 7 semanas. SIN oronasal m.
buccopharyngeal m., m. bucofaríngea; uma membrana bilaminar (ectoderma e endoderma) derivada da placa pré-cordal; após o desenvolvimento da prega da cabeça embrionária, situa-se no limite caudal do estomódio. SIN oral m., oropharyngeal m.

cell m., m. celular; o limite protoplásmico de todas as células que controla a permeabilidade e pode ter outras funções através de especializações da superfície; p. ex., absorção por transporte iônico ativo pela formação de vesículas pinocitóticas; reconhecimento de antígenos mediado por receptor etc.; sua ultraestrutura é trilaminar e consiste na lâmina externa elétron-densa e na lâmina interna com uma lâmina intermediária elétron-transparente. SIN cytolemma, cytomembrane, plasma m., plasmalemma, plasmolemma, Wachendorf m. (2).
chorioallantoic m., m. corioalantóide; membrana extra-embrionária formada por fusão do córion com a alantóide.
choroid m. [TA], tela corióidea. SIN tela choroidea.
cloacal m., m. cloacal; uma membrana transitória, na área caudal do embrião, que separa o proctódio da cloaca; é dividida em membranas anal e genitourinária, que se rompem durante a 8.ª à 9.ª semana do desenvolvimento embrionário para estabelecer a abertura externa para os tratos alimentar e genitourinário.
closing m.'s, membranas de fechamento; folhetos finos, compostos de ectoderma externamente e endoderma internamente, que separam as bolsas faríngeas das fendas branquiais sobrejacentes no embrião inicial. SIN pharyngeal m.'s.
Corti m., m. de Corti. SIN tectorial m. of cochlear duct.
cricothyroid m., m. cricotireóidea; uma das membranas bilaterais que se estendem entre o arco da cartilagem cricóide e a borda inferior da lâmina tireóide de cada lado da linha média, ocupada pelo ligamento cricotireóide mediano, mais espesso. VER TAMBÉM *conus* elasticus, median cricothyroid ligament. SIN membrana cricothyroidea.
cricotracheal m., ligamento cricotraqueal. SIN cricotracheal ligament.
cricovocal m., cone elástico; *termo oficial alternativo para *conus* elasticus.
croupous m., m. falsa, pseudomembrana. SIN false m.
deciduous m., m. decídua; a mucosa do útero grávido que já sofreu certas alterações, sob a influência do ciclo ovulatório, para se preparar para a implantação e nutrição do ovo; assim denominada porque a membrana é eliminada após o trabalho de parto. SIN caduca, decidua, Hunter m., membrana decidua.
Descemet m., m. de Descemet. SIN posterior limiting lamina of cornea.
diphtheritic m., m. diftérica; a membrana falsa que se forma sobre as mucosas na difteria.
double m., m. dupla; duas camadas de biomembrana, com um espaço intermembrana que circunda determinadas organelas (p. ex., mitocôndrias) ou estruturas.
drum m., m. timpânica. SIN tympanic m.
Duddell m., m. de Duddell. SIN posterior limiting lamina of cornea.
dysmenorrheal m., m. dismenorreica; membrana semelhante à decídua, eliminada em casos de dismenorréia membranosa.
egg m., m. do ovo; o invólucro que reveste o ovo; uma **primary egg m.** (m. primária do ovo) é produzida pelo citoplasma ovariano (p. ex., uma membrana vitelina); uma **secondary egg m.** (m. secundária do ovo) é o produto do folículo ovariano (p. ex., a zona pelúcida); uma **tertiary egg m.** (m. terciária do ovo) é secretada pelo revestimento do oviduto (p. ex., uma casca).
elastic m., m. elástica; membrana formada de tecido conjuntivo elástico, presente na forma de lâminas fenestradas no revestimento das artérias e em outros locais.
embryonic m., m. embrionária, m. fetal. SIN fetal m.
enamel m., m. de esmalte; a camada interna do órgão do esmalte formada pelas células de esmalte.
epipapillary m., m. epipapilar; **(1)** membrana congênita que cobre o disco óptico; **(2)** os remanescentes gliais da papila de Bergmeister (Bergmeister *papilla*).
epiretinal m., m. epirretiniana; membrana, geralmente adquirida, que cobre uma parte da retina e é composta de tecido fibroso da metaplasia das células epiteliais do pigmento retiniano ou da glia.
exocelomic m., m. exocelômica; uma camada de células separada da superfície interna do citotrofoblasto blastocítico e do envoltório do saco vitelino primário durante a segunda semana de vida embrionária. SIN Heuser m.
external intercostal m. [TA], m. intercostal externa; a membrana que substituiu o músculo intercostal externo anteriormente, entre as cartilagens costais. SIN membrana intercostalis externa [TA].
extraembryonic m., m. extra-embrionária, m. fetal. SIN fetal m.
false m., m. falsa, pseudomembrana; exsudato fibrinoso, firme, espesso ou tecido necrosado na superfície de uma mucosa ou da pele, como o observado na difteria. SIN croupous m., pseudomembrane.
fenestrated m., m. fenestrada; membrana elástica, como nas lâminas elásticas das artérias.
fertilization m., m. de fecundação; membrana viscosa que se forma na superfície interna da membrana vitelina do citoplasma do óvulo após a penetração do espermatozóide, impedindo a entrada de outros espermatozóides.
fetal m., m. fetal; estrutura ou tecido que se desenvolve a partir do ovo fecundado, mas não faz parte do embrião propriamente dito. SIN embryonic m., extraembryonic m.
fibroelastic m. of larynx [TA], m. fibroelástica da laringe; uma camada de fibras fibrosas e elásticas que toma o lugar da submucosa na laringe. É divi-

dida em duas partes pelo ventrículo da laringe: a membrana quadrangular, superiormente, e o cone elástico, inferiormente. SIN membrana fibroelastica laryngis [TA].
fibrous m. of joint capsule, camada fibrosa da cápsula articular; *termo oficial alternativo para fibrous layer of joint capsule.
Fielding m., m. de Fielding, tapete. SIN tapetum (2).
flaccid m., parte flácida da m. timpânica. SIN flaccid part of tympanic membrane.
germ m., germinal m., m. germinativa. SIN blastoderm.
glassy m., (1) a m. basal presente entre o estrato granuloso e a teca interna de um folículo ovariano vesicular; torna-se muito proeminente em grandes folículos atrésicos; **(2)** a membrana basal e o tecido conjuntivo associado do folículo piloso. SIN hyaline m. (2).
glial limiting m., m. limitante da glia; uma m. elástica, densa, que forma a verdadeira cápsula do encéfalo e da medula espinal, composta dos processos de astrócitos (células da macróglia) e totalmente coberta pela pia-máter, que adere firmemente a ela; as duas m. são coletivamente denominadas m. pio-glial. SIN membrana limitans gliae.
Henle m., m. de Henle, lâmina basilar da corióide. SIN lamina basalis choroideae.
Henle fenestrated elastic m., lâminas elásticas fenestradas de Henle. SIN elastic laminae of arteries, em lamina.
Heuser m., m. de Heuser. SIN exocelomic m.
Hunter m., m. de Hunter. SIN deciduous m.
Huxley m., camada de Huxley. SIN Huxley layer.
hyaline m., m. hialina; **(1)** a m. basal clara e fina situada sob determinados epitélios; **(2)** SIN glassy m. (2).
hyaloid m., lâmina limitante posterior da córnea. SIN posterior limiting lamina of cornea.
hyoglossal m., m. hioglossa; alargamento posterior do septo da língua que une a raiz da língua ao osso hióide; as fibras inferiores do músculo genioglosso inserem-se nele e, dessa forma, ao corpo ântero-superior do osso hióide próximo à linha média.
inner m., m. interna; a menor das duas membranas de uma membrana dupla.
intercostal m.'s [TA], membranas intercostais; a porção membranosa das camadas musculares intercostais entre as costelas. SIN membranae intercostales [TA], intercostal ligaments, ligamenta intercostalia.
internal intercostal m. [TA], m. intercostal interna; a membrana que substitui o músculo intercostal interno posteriormente, medial aos ângulos das costelas. SIN membrana intercostalis interna [TA].
interosseous m. of forearm [TA], m. interóssea do antebraço; a membrana densa que une as margens interósseas do rádio e da ulna, formando a sindesmose radioulnar, e com esses ossos separando os compartimentos flexor e extensor do antebraço. SIN membrana interossea antebrachii [TA].
interosseous m. of leg [TA], m. interóssea da perna; a camada fibrosa densa que une as margens interósseas da tíbia e da fíbula, formando a porção superior da sindesmose tibiofibular e, com os ossos e septos intermusculares, criando os compartimentos anterior e posterior da perna. SIN membrana interossea cruris [TA], ligamentum tibiofibulare medium.
ivory m., m. ebúrnea. SIN membrana eboris.
Jackson m., m. de Jackson; uma membrana vascular fina ou aderência semelhante a um véu, cobrindo a superfície anterior do colo ascendente desde o ceco até a flexura direita; pode causar obstrução por torção do intestino. SIN Jackson veil.
keratogenous m., matriz ungueal. SIN nail matrix.
limiting m. of retina, m. limitante da retina; uma das duas camadas da retina:
internal limiting m. (m. limitante interna), formada pelas extremidades internas expandidas das fibras de Müller; **outer limiting m.** (m. limitante externa), que não é uma membrana, mas uma fileira de complexos juncionais. SIN membrana limitans (1).
medullary m., endósteo. SIN endosteum.
mitochondrial m., m. mitocondrial; a biomembrana dupla que circunda a mitocôndria.
mucous m.'s, mucosas; *termo oficial alternativo para mucosa.
mucous m. of bronchus, mucosa do brônquio; *termo oficial alternativo para mucosa of bronchi.
mucous m. of ductus deferens, mucosa do ducto deferente; *termo oficial alternativo para mucosa of ductus deferens.
mucous m. of esophagus, mucosa do esôfago; *termo oficial alternativo para mucosa of esophagus.
mucous m. of female urethra, mucosa da uretra feminina; *termo oficial alternativo para mucosa of female urethra.
mucous m. of gallbladder, mucosa da vesícula biliar; *termo oficial alternativo para mucosa of gallbladder.
mucous m. of large intestine, mucosa do intestino grosso; *termo oficial alternativo para mucosa of large intestine.
mucous m. of larynx, mucosa da laringe; *termo oficial alternativo para mucosa of larynx.
mucous m. of male urethra, mucosa da uretra masculina. SIN mucosa of male urethra.
mucous m. of nose, mucosa do nariz; *termo oficial alternativo para mucosa of nose.
mucous m. of pharyngotympanic auditory tube, mucosa da tuba auditiva faringotimpânica; *termo oficial alternativo para mucosa of pharyngotympanic (auditory) tube.
mucous m. of pharynx, mucosa da faringe. SIN mucosa of pharynx.
mucous m. of small intestine, mucosa do intestino delgado; *termo oficial alternativo para mucosa of small intestine.
mucous m. of stomach, mucosa do estômago; *termo oficial alternativo para mucosa of stomach.
mucous m. of tongue, mucosa da língua; *termo oficial alternativo para mucosa of tongue.
mucous m. of trachea, mucosa da traquéia; *termo oficial alternativo para mucosa of trachea.
mucous m. of tympanic cavity, mucosa da cavidade timpânica; *termo oficial alternativo para mucosa of tympanic cavity.
mucous m. of ureter, mucosa do ureter; *termo oficial alternativo para mucosa of ureter.
mucous m. of urinary bladder, mucosa da bexiga; *termo oficial alternativo para mucosa of (urinary) bladder.
mucous m. of uterine tube, mucosa da tuba uterina; *termo oficial alternativo para mucosa of uterine tube.
mucous m. of vagina, mucosa da vagina; *termo oficial alternativo para mucosa of vagina.
Nasmyth m., m. de Nasmyth. SIN enamel cuticle.
nictitating m., prega semilunar da conjuntiva. SIN plica semilunaris of conjunctiva (2).
Nitabuch m., m. de Nitabuch; uma camada de fibrina entre a zona limite de endométrio compacto e o revestimento citotrofoblástico na placenta. SIN Nitabuch layer, Nitabuch stria.
nuclear m., envoltório nuclear. SIN nuclear envelope.
obturator m. [TA], m. obturadora; a membrana fina de fibras entrelaçadas fortes que preenchem o forame obturado e com o osso circundante, dando origem aos músculos obturadores externo e interno. SIN membrana obturatoria [TA].
olfactory m., região olfatória do nariz. SIN olfactory region of nose.
oral m., m. oral. SIN buccopharyngeal m.
oronasal m., m. oronasal. SIN bucconasal m.
oropharyngeal m., m. orofaríngea. SIN buccopharyngeal m.
otolithic m., m. dos estatocônios; membrana gelatinosa sustentada por pêlos das células ciliadas das máculas do sáculo e utrículo do ouvido interno; aderidas à superfície, há muitas partículas cristalinas denominadas otólitos (estatocônios). SIN membrana statoconiorum [TA], statoconial m.
outer m., m. externa; a maior das duas membranas de uma membrana dupla.
ovular m., m. vitelina. SIN membrana vitellina (1).
Payr m., m. de Payr; uma prega de peritônio que cruza sobre a flexura esquerda do colo.
pericardiopleural m., prega pericardiopleural. SIN pleuropericardial fold.
peridental m., periodôntio. SIN periodontium.
perineal m. [TA], m. do períneo; a camada de fáscia que se estende entre os ramos isquiopúbicos inferiores ao esfíncter uretral e os músculos transversos profundos do períneo. SIN membrana perinei [TA], Camper ligament, ligamentum triangulare, triangular ligament.
periodontal m., periodôntio; *termo oficial alternativo para periodontium.
periorbital m., m. periorbital. SIN periorbita.
pharyngeal m.'s, membranas faríngeas. SIN closing m.'s.
pial-glial m., m. pio-glial; o revestimento externo duplo do encéfalo e da medula espinal, composto da membrana limitante glial e da pia-máter.
pituitary m., m. do nariz. SIN mucosa of nose.
placental m., m. placentária; a camada semipermeável de tecido fetal que separa o sangue materno do sangue fetal na placenta; composta de: 1) endotélio dos vasos fetais nas vilosidades coriônicas, 2) estroma das vilosidades, 3) citotrofoblasto (negligenciável após o quinto mês de gestação) e 4) trofoblasto sincicial cobrindo as vilosidades; a membrana placentária atua como uma membrana seletiva que regula a passagem de substâncias do sangue materno para o sangue fetal. SIN placental barrier.
plasma m., m. plasmática. SIN cell m.
pleuropericardial m., prega pleuropericárdica. SIN pleuropericardial fold.
pleuroperitoneal m., prega pleuroperitoneal. SIN pleuroperitoneal fold.
posterior atlanto-occipital m. [TA], m. atlantoccipital posterior; a membrana fibrosa que se fixa entre o arco posterior do atlas e a margem posterior do forame magno. SIN membrana atlanto-occipitalis posterior [TA].
postsynaptic m., m. pós-sináptica; a parte da membrana plasmática de um neurônio ou fibra muscular com a qual uma terminação axônica forma uma junção sináptica; em muitos casos, ao menos parte dessa pequena placa da membrana pós-sináptica exibe modificações morfológicas características como

maior espessura e maior elétron-densidade, que parece corresponder ao sítio receptor sensível ao transmissor dessas sinapses.

presynaptic m., m. pré-sináptica; a parte da membrana plasmática de uma terminação axônica voltada para a membrana plasmática do neurônio ou fibra muscular com a qual a terminação axônica estabelece uma junção sináptica; muitas junções sinápticas exibem características pré-sinápticas estruturais, como protrusões internas cônicas, elétron-densas, que as distinguem do restante do plasma do axônio. VER TAMBÉM synapse.

primary egg m., m. primária do ovo. VER egg m.

proligerous m., m. prolígera. SIN cumulus oöphorus.

proper m. of semicircular duct [TA], m. própria do ducto semicircular; a rede de fibras de tecido conjuntivo entre o ducto semicircular e o canal semicircular ósseo; forma uma delicada rede no espaço perilinfático comumente cheio de perilinfa. SIN membrana propria ductus semicircularis, membrana propria of semicircular duct.

prophylactic m., m. profilática. SIN pyogenic m.

pupillary m., m. pupilar; remanescentes da porção central da camada anterior do estroma da íris (a lâmina iridopupilar), que oclui a pupila na vida fetal e, normalmente, sofre atrofia por volta do sétimo mês de gestação. Os filamentos persistentes geralmente se distendem através da pupila de uma colarete da íris até a outra, sem tocar a margem pupilar. A incapacidade de regredir é uma causa rara de cegueira congênita. SIN membrana pupillaris, Wachendorf m. (1).

pyogenic m., m. piogênica; uma camada de piócitos que reveste a cavidade de um abscesso que ainda não foi autolisada. SIN prophylactic m.

quadrangular m. [TA], m. quadrangular; parte da membrana fibroelástica da laringe, situada acima do ventrículo laríngeo; sua borda inferior ligeiramente espessada, o ligamento vestibular, está situada sob a prega vestibular da laringe; fixa-se, anteriormente, à epiglote e, posteriormente, à margem lateral das cartilagens aritenóidea e corniculada; sua porção superior situa-se sob a mucosa da prega ariepiglótica, que separa o vestíbulo laríngeo da fossa piriforme da laringofaringe. SIN membrana quadrangularis [TA], Tourtual m.

Reissner m., m. de Reissner. SIN vestibular surface of cochlear duct.

reticular m. of spiral organ, m. reticular do órgão espiral; a membrana formada por lâminas cuticulares das células do órgão espiral de Corti; assemelha-se a uma rede quando vista de cima. SIN membrana reticularis organi spiralis [TA].

Rivinus m., m. de Rivinus. SIN flaccid part of tympanic membrane.

round window m., m. timpânica secundária. SIN secondary tympanic m.

Ruysch m., m. de Ruysch. SIN capillary lamina of choroid.

Scarpa m., m. de Scarpa. SIN secondary tympanic m.

schneiderian m., m. de Schneider. SIN mucosa of nose.

Schultze m., m. de Schultze. SIN olfactory region of nasal mucosa.

secondary egg m., m. secundária do ovo. VER egg m.

secondary tympanic m. [TA], m. timpânica secundária; a membrana que fecha a janela redonda (janela da cóclea). SIN membrana tympani secundaria [TA], round window m., Scarpa m.

semipermeable m., m. semipermeável; membrana relativamente permeável ao solvente, mas relativamente impermeável a todos os solutos, ou pelo menos a alguns, em uma ou em ambas as soluções separadas pela membrana.

serous m., m. serosa. SIN serosa.

Shrapnell m., m. de Shrapnell. SIN flaccid part of tympanic membrane.

spiral m., superfície timpânica do ducto coclear; *termo oficial alternativo para tympanic surface of cochlear duct.

stapedial m. [TA], m. estapedial; a delicada camada de mucosa que une o espaço entre os ramos e a base do estribo. SIN membrana stapedis [TA].

statoconial m., m. dos estatocônios. SIN otolithic m.

sternal m. [TA], m. do esterno; fibras entrelaçadas dos ligamentos costoesternais anteriores, cobrindo a superfície anterior do esterno. SIN membrana sterni [TA].

striated m., zona estriada. SIN zona striata.

suprapleural m., m. suprapleural; a porção espessada da fáscia endotorácica que se estende sobre a cúpula da pleura e a reforça; fixa-se à borda interna da primeira costela e ao processo transverso da sétima vértebra cervical. SIN membrana suprapleuralis [TA], Sibson aponeurosis, Sibson fascia.

synovial m. [TA], m. sinovial; o tecido conjuntivo que reveste a cavidade de uma articulação sinovial e produz o líquido sinovial; reveste todas as superfícies internas da cavidade, exceto a cartilagem articular dos ossos. SIN membrana synovialis [TA], stratum synoviale, synovium.

tectorial m. of cochlear duct [TA], m. tectória do ducto coclear; uma membrana gelatinosa sobrejacente ao órgão espiral (de Corti) no ouvido interno. SIN membrana tectoria ductus cochlearis [TA], Corti m., tectorium (2).

tectorial m. (of median atlantoaxial joint) [TA], m. tectória (da articulação atlantoaxial mediana); a continuação superior da parte anterior do ligamento longitudinal posterior fixada (atravessada entre) à superfície superior da porção basilar do osso occipital e aos corpos da segunda e terceira vértebras cervicais; forma um "teto" sobre a articulação atlantoaxial mediana. SIN membrana tectoria (articulationis atlantoaxialis medianae) [TA], apparatus ligamentosus weitbrechti, posterior occipitoaxial ligament.

tertiary egg m., m. terciária do ovo. VER egg m.

thyrohyoid m. [TA], m. tíreo-hióidea; uma lâmina membranosa, fibrosa e fina que preenche o espaço entre o osso hióide e a cartilagem tireóidea. SIN membrana thyrohyoidea [TA], membrana hyothyroidea.

Toldt m., m. de Toldt; a camada anterior da fáscia renal.

Tourtual m., m. de Tourtual. SIN quadrangular m.

tympanic m. [TA], m. timpânica; uma membrana fina e tensa que forma a maior parte da parede lateral da cavidade timpânica e a separa do meato acústico externo; constitui o limite entre a orelha externa e a orelha média; é uma membrana trilaminar coberta por pele em sua superfície externa, mucosa em sua superfície interna, sendo recoberta, em ambas as superfícies, por epitélio e, na parte tensa, apresenta uma camada intermediária de fibras colágenas radiais externas e circulares internas. SIN membrana tympani [TA], drum m., drum, drumhead, m. of tympanum, myringa, myrinx.

m. of tympanum, m. timpânica. SIN tympanic m.

undulating m., undulatory m., m. ondulante, m. ondulatória; uma organela locomotora de alguns parasitas flagelados (tripanossomas e tricomonas), que consiste em uma extensão da membrana limitante com a bainha do flagelo, em forma de barbatana; o encrespamento em forma de onda da membrana ondulante produz um movimento característico.

unit m., m. unitária; a estrutura trilaminar do plasmalema e de outras membranas intercelulares, quando observada em corte transversal ao microscópio eletrônico, composta de duas lâminas elétron-densas com aproximadamente 20 Å de espessura separadas por uma lâmina menos densa, com espessura de 35 Å.

urogenital m., m. urogenital; a porção ventral da membrana cloacal embrionária após sua divisão pelo septo urorretal.

urorectal m., m. urorretal; no embrião, o septo urorretal que separa a cloaca em seio urogenital e reto. SIN urorectal fold.

uteroepichorial m., m. uteroepicorial; termo raramente usado para *decidua parietalis*.

vaginal synovial m., bainha do tendão sinovial. SIN synovial tendon sheath.

vestibular m., superfície vestibular do ducto coclear; *termo oficial alternativo para vestibular surface of cochlear duct.

virginal m., m. virginal; termo obsoleto para hímen.

vitelline m., m. vitelina. SIN membrana vitellina (1).

vitreous m., (1) lâmina limitante posterior da córnea. SIN posterior limiting lamina of cornea; (2) uma condensação de fibras colágenas finas em locais no córtex do corpo vítreo; anteriormente se acreditava que formasse uma membrana ou cápsula em sua periferia; (3) lâmina basilar da corióide. SIN lamina basalis choroideae.

Wachendorf m., m. de Wachendorf; (1) SIN pupillary m.; 2) SIN cell m.

yolk m., m. vitelina. SIN membrana vitellina.

Zinn m., m. de Zinn; a camada anterior da íris.

mem·bra·nec·to·my (mem - bră - nek′tō - mē). Membranectomia; remoção das membranas de um hematoma subdural. [membrane + G. *ektomē*, excisão]

mem·bra·nelle (mem - bră - nel′). Membranela; uma pequena membrana formada por cílios fundidos, encontrada em determinados protozoários ciliados.

mem·bra·ni·form (mem - brā′ni - fōrm). Membraniforme; que possui a aparência ou característica de uma membrana. SIN membranoid.

mem·bra·no·car·ti·lag·i·nous (mem′brā - nō - kar - ti - laj′i - nŭs). Membranocartilaginoso. 1. Parcialmente membranoso e parcialmente cartilaginoso. 2. Derivado tanto de uma membrana mesenquimal quanto de cartilagem; designando certos ossos.

mem·bra·noid (mem′brā - noyd). Membranóide. SIN membraniform.

mem·bra·nous (mem′brā - nŭs). Membranoso; relativo a, ou que possui a forma de, uma membrana. SIN hymenoid (1), membranaceous.

mem·brum, pl. **mem·bra** (mem′brŭm, mem′brā). Membro. [L. membro]
 m. infe′rius [TA], m. inferior. SIN lower limb.
 m. mulieb′re, termo obsoleto para clitóris.
 m. supe′rius [TA], m. superior. SIN upper limb.
 m. vir′ile, pênis. SIN penis.

mem·o·ry (mem′o - rē). Memória. 1. Termo genérico para designar a recordação daquilo que já foi experimentado ou aprendido. 2. O sistema de processamento de informações mentais que recebe (registra), modifica, armazena e recupera os estímulos informativos; composto de três estágios: codificação, armazenamento e recuperação. [L. *memoria*]

affect m., m. afetiva; o elemento emocional que recorre sempre que é lembrada uma experiência importante.

anterograde m., m. anterógrada; m. para o que ocorreu após um evento como uma lesão do encéfalo.

long-term m. (LTM), m. a longo prazo; a fase do processo mnemônico considerada como o depósito permanente de informações registradas, codificadas, passadas para a memória a curto prazo, codificadas, enumeradas e, finalmente, transferidas e armazenadas para futura recuperação; o material e a informação retidos na LTM fundamentam as habilidades cognitivas.

remote m., m. remota; memória para eventos antigos, em oposição aos recentes.

memory   968   **meningitis**

retrograde m., m. retrógrada; memória para aquilo que ocorreu antes de um evento como uma lesão do encéfalo.
screen m., m. falsa; em psicanálise, uma m. conscientemente tolerável que serve inconscientemente como disfarce para outra memória associada que seria emocionalmente dolorosa se lembrada.
selective m., m. seletiva; recepção ou recuperação de apenas alguns dos eventos de uma experiência.
senile m., m. senil; memória boa para acontecimentos antigos, freqüentemente em contraste com os eventos atuais; observada caracteristicamente em pessoas idosas ou dementes.
short-term m. (STM), m. a curto prazo; aquela fase do processo de memória na qual estímulos que foram reconhecidos e registrados são armazenados por breve período; há rápida perda, algumas vezes em segundos, mas pode ser armazenada indefinidamente pelo uso da enumeração como processo de conservação para reciclar o material repetidas vezes na memória a curto prazo. SIN temporary m.
subconscious m., m. subconsciente; informação não disponível imediatamente para lembrança.
temporary m., m. temporária. SIN short-term m.
MEN Abreviatura de multiple endocrine *neoplasia* (neoplasia endócrina múltipla).
MEN1 Abreviatura de multiple endocrine *neoplasia*, type 1 (neoplasia endócrina múltipla, tipo 1).
MEN2A Abreviatura de multiple endocrine *neoplasia*, type 2A (neoplasia endócrina múltipla, tipo 2A).
men·ac·me (me-nak′me). Menacma; o período de atividade menstrual na vida de uma mulher. [G. *mēn*, mês, + *akmē*, auge]
men·a·di·ol di·ac·e·tate (men-ā-dī′ol). Acetato de menadiol; menadiol acetilado em ambos os grupamentos hidroxila; uma vitamina pró-trombogênica. SIN acetomenaphthone, vitamin K₄.
men·a·di·ol so·di·um di·phos·phate. Difosfato sódico de menadiol; um derivado diidro da menadiona, com atividade semelhante à da vitamina K.
men·a·di·one (men-ā-dī′on). Menadiona; a raiz de substâncias que são derivadas 3-multiprenil da menadiona, e conhecidas como menaquinonas ou vitaminas K₂. SIN menaphthone, vitamin K₃.
  m. reductase, m. redutase. SIN NADPH dehydrogenase (quinone).
  m. sodium bisulfite, bissulfito sódico de menadiona; possui a mesma ação e é usada para os mesmos fins que a menadiona ou vitamina K; entretanto, difere da menadiona por ser hidrossolúvel.
men·aph·thone (men-ā-naf′thōn). Menaftona. SIN menadione.
men·a·quin·one (MK, MQ) (men′ā-kwin′ōn, -kwī′nōn). Menaquina; o nome da classe de uma série de 2-metil-3-*all-trans*-poliprenil)-1,4-naftoquinonas (vitaminas K₂).
men·a·quin·one-6 (MK-6). Menaquinona-6; hexaprenilmenaquinona; prenilmenaquinona-6; isolada da carne de peixe pútrida; a potência corresponde a aproximadamente 60% da potência da filoquinona (vitamina K₁). SIN farnoquinone, vitamin K₂, vitamin K₂ (30).
men·a·quin·one-7 (MK-7). Menaquinona-7; menaquinona-6 com uma cadeia lateral 3-heptaprenil. SIN vitamin K₂(35).
men·ar·che (me-nar′kē). Menarca; estabelecimento da função menstrual; o momento do primeiro período menstrual. [G. *mēn*, mês, + *archē*, início]
men·ar·che·al, men·ar·chi·al (me-nar′kē-ăl). Menárquico; relativo à menarca.
Mendel, Gregor J., geneticista austríaco, 1822–1884. VER mendelian *character*; mendelian *inheritance*; mendelian *ratio*; M. first *law*, second *law*.
Mendel, Kurt, neurologista alemão, 1874–1946. VER M. instep *reflex*; Bechterew-M. *reflex*.
Mendeléeff (Mendeleev), Dimitri (Dmitri) I., químico russo, 1834–1907. VER mendelevium; M. *law*.
men·de·le·vi·um (Md) (men-dĕ-lē′vē-ŭm). Mendelévio; um elemento, número atômico 101, peso atômico 258,1, preparado em 1955 por bombardeio do einstênio com partículas alfa. [D. Mendeléeff]
men·de·li·an (men-dē′lē-ăn). Mendeliano; atribuído a, ou descrito por, Gregor Mendel; geralmente refere-se ao comportamento e ao mecanismo da transmissão genética de traços de *locus* único.
***Men·de·li·an In·her·i·tance in Man* (MIM).** Fonte de referência padronizada, abrangente, atualizada regularmente, para traços humanos comprovadamente mendelianos ou que se supõe serem mendelianos com fundamentação razoável. Cada entrada tem um número de seis dígitos catalogado. Aqueles estabelecidos com certeza (por biologia molecular ou por estudos clínicos extensos) são marcados com um asterisco.
men·del·ism (men′del-izm). Mendelismo; os princípios hereditários de traços genéticos isolados derivados das leis de Mendel.
men·del·iz·ing (men′del-īz-ing). Mendelização; designa um padrão de herança de um traço que corresponde fenotipicamente à segregação de genes conhecidos ou supostos em um *locus* genético.
Mendelson, Curtis L., médico norte-americano, *1913.
Ménétrier, Pierre E., médico francês, 1859–1935. VER M. *disease, syndrome*.

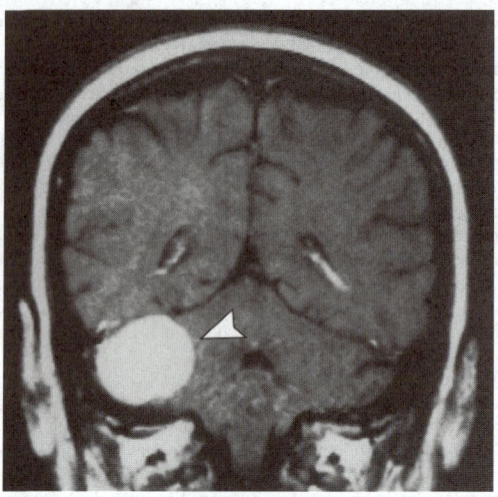

meningioma: meningioma no ângulo cerebelopontino direito (RM, após injeção de contraste)

Menge, Karl, ginecologista alemão, 1864–1945. VER M. *pessary*.
Ménière, Prosper, médico francês, 1799–1862. VER M. *disease, syndrome*.
mening-. VER meningo-.
me·nin·ge·al (mĕ-nin′jē-ăl, men′in-jē′ăl). Meníngeo; relativo às meninges.
me·nin·ge·o·cor·ti·cal (mĕ-nin′jē-ō-kōr′ti-kăl). Meningeocortical. SIN meningocortical.
me·nin·ge·or·rha·phy (mĕ-nin′jē-ōr′ă-fē). Meningeorrafia; sutura das meninges cranianas ou espinais ou de qualquer membrana. [G. *mēninx (mēning-)*, membrana, + *rhaphē*, sutura]
me·nin·ges (mĕ-nin′jēz) [TA]. Meninges; plural de meninx.
me·nin·gi·o·an·gi·o·ma·to·sis (mĕ-nin′jē-ō-an′jē-ō-mă-tō-sis). Meningioangiomatose; proliferação de vasos e células meningoteliais, associada à epilepsia e neurofibromatose.
me·nin·gi·o·ma (mĕ-nin′jē-ō′mă). Meningioma; neoplasia encapsulada benigna de origem aracnóide, mais freqüente em adultos; a forma mais freqüente consiste em células alongadas, fusiformes em espirais e pseudolóbulos com corpos psamomatosos freqüentes; os meningiomas tendem a ocorrer ao longo do seio sagital superior, ao longo da crista esfenóide ou na vizinhança do quiasma óptico; além do meningotelial, são conhecidas as formas fibrosa, de transição, metaplásica, psamomatosa, secretora, de células claras, papilar, cordóide e linfoplasmocítica. [mening- + G. *-oma*, tumor]
  cutaneous m., m. cutâneo; uma lesão na pele e no tecido subcutâneo, composta de células meníngeas; ocorre como uma lesão congênita em crianças ou como extensão de um meningioma intracraniano em adultos.
  malignant m., m. maligno; meningioma que invade o parênquima encefálico ou metastatiza.
  psammomatous m., m. psamomatoso; uma neoplasia celular firme, derivada do tecido fibroso das meninges, plexo coróide e algumas outras estruturas associadas ao encéfalo, caracterizada pela formação de múltiplos corpos calcários, concentricamente laminados, distintos (corpos psamomatosos); a maioria dessas neoplasias é histologicamente benigna, mas podem levar a sintomas graves em virtude da compressão do encéfalo. SIN sand tumor, Virchow psamoma.
me·nin·gi·o·ma·to·sis (mĕ-nin′jē-ō-mă-tō′sis). Meningiomatose; a presença de múltiplos meningiomas, algumas vezes observada na doença de von Recklinghausen.
me·nin·gism (men′in-jizm, mĕ-nin′jizm). Meningismo; uma condição na qual os sinais e sintomas simulam uma meningite, mas em que não há inflamação real dessas membranas. SIN pseudomeningitis.
men·in·git·ic (men′in-jit′ik). Meningítico; relativo a, ou caracterizado por, meningite.
men·in·gi·tis, pl. **men·in·git·i·des** (men-in-jī′tis, -jit′i-dēz). Meningite; inflamação das membranas do encéfalo ou da medula espinal. VER TAMBÉM arachnoiditis, leptomeningitis. SIN cerebrospinal m. [mening- + G. *itis*, inflamação]
  basilar m., m. basilar; meningite na base do encéfalo, geralmente devida a tuberculose, sífilis ou qualquer processo granulomatoso crônico de baixo grau; pode resultar em hidrocefalia interna.
  cerebrospinal m., m. cerebroespinal. SIN meningitis.
  eosinophilic m., m. eosinofílica. SIN angiostrongylosis.
  epidemic cerebrospinal m., m. cerebroespinal epidêmica. SIN meningococcal m.
  epidural m., m. epidural. SIN pachymeningitis externa.

external m., m. externa. SIN *pachymeningitis* externa.
internal m., m. interna. SIN *pachymeningitis* interna.
listeria m., m. por *Listeria*. SIN listeriosis.

meningococcal m., m. meningocócica; doença infecciosa aguda de crianças e adultos jovens, causada por *Neisseria meningitidis*, caracterizada por febre, cefaléia, fotofobia, vômitos, rigidez de nuca, convulsões, coma e erupção cutânea purpúrica; mesmo na ausência de meningite, a meningococcemia pode induzir fenômenos tóxicos como vasculite, coagulação intravascular disseminada, choque e síndrome de Waterhouse-Friderichsen devida à hemorragia supra-renal; as complicações tardias incluem paralisia, retardo mental e gangrena dos membros. SIN cerebrospinal fever, epidemic cerebrospinal m.

Aproximadamente 2.500 casos de doença meningocócica invasiva ocorrem anualmente nos Estados Unidos, com uma taxa de mortalidade de 10-15%. A incidência de doença meningocócica endêmica é máxima entre o final do inverno e o início da primavera. As taxas de acometimento e as taxas de mortalidade são maiores em crianças de 6–12 meses. A exposição domiciliar à fumaça do tabaco é um fator de risco para doença meningocócica em crianças. Os microrganismos são transmitidos de uma pessoa para outra por contato direto e pela saliva e secreções respiratórias. A epidemiologia da doença meningocócica é mal compreendida. A taxa de portadores nasofaríngeos na população geral é de 5–10%. Esse estado de portador assintomático pode persistir por meses ou anos e pode conferir proteção contra doença invasiva. Durante epidemias de meningite meningocócica, a taxa de portadores pode aproximar-se de 95%, porém menos de 1% pode desenvolver a doença. O diagnóstico é estabelecido pela constatação de meningococos no líquido cerebroespinal ou no sangue. Como a meningococcemia pode evoluir de forma fulminante para um estágio irreversível, é instituído o uso de penicilina G intravenosa, ampicilina ou cloranfenicol logo que se suspeita do diagnóstico, geralmente antes da confirmação laboratorial. O suporte intensivo das funções vitais é fundamental durante a fase aguda. Contactantes íntimos de casos conhecidos são tratados profilaticamente com rifampina ou ciprofloxacina; a profilaxia em massa pode ser apropriada em um surto institucional confirmado. Uma vacina quadrivalente tem sido efetiva na prevenção da doença meningocócica causada pelos sorogrupos A, C, W-135 e Y. As desvantagens da vacina são que não protege contra o sorogrupo B, que causa 30–40% das doenças meningocócicas nos Estados Unidos; não interrompe o estado de portador; não induz imunidade com velocidade suficiente para proteger uma pessoa já infectada; e protege apenas durante 4–5 anos. A imunização rotineira só é recomendada para recrutas militares, pessoas que viajam para áreas endêmicas e outras que estão sob alto risco por longo período. Uma importante objeção à vacinação do lactente foi a indução insatisfatória de imunidade nessa faixa etária contra o sorotipo C, que causa 45% dos casos de meningite nos Estados Unidos. O uso de uma vacina meningocócica C conjugada à proteína produziu altos títulos iniciais de anticorpos anticapsulares e bactericidas em lactentes e crianças pequenas, bem como proteção mais longa e melhor resposta às doses de reforço.

Mollaret m., m. de Mollaret; meningite asséptica recorrente; doença febril acompanhada por cefaléia, mal-estar, sinais de irritação meníngea e monócitos no líquido cerebroespinal.
neoplastic m., m. neoplásica; infiltração do espaço subaracnóide por células neoplásicas, tipicamente meduloblastoma ou carcinoma metastático. SIN neoplastic arachnoiditis.
occlusive m., m. oclusiva; leptomeningite que causa oclusão das vias de líquido espinal.
otitic m., m. otítica; infecção das meninges secundária à otite média ou mastoidite.
serous m., m. serosa; meningite aguda com hidrocefalia externa secundária.
tuberculous m., m. tuberculosa; inflamação das leptomeninges cerebrais caracterizada por inflamação granulomatosa; geralmente é limitada à base do encéfalo (m. basilar, hidrocefalia interna) e é acompanhada em crianças por um acúmulo de liquor nos ventrículos (hidrocefalia aguda). SIN cerebral tuberculosis (1).
meningo-, mening-. Meningo-, mening-; as meninges. [G. *mēninx*, membrana]
me·nin·go·cele (mē - ning'gō - sēl). Meningocele; protrusão das membranas do medula espinal através de um defeito no crânio ou na coluna vertebral. [meningo- + G. *kēlē*, tumor]
spurious m., m. espúria; acúmulo extracraniano ou extravertebral de líquido cerebroespinal, devido à ruptura da meninge. SIN traumatic m.
traumatic m., m. traumática. SIN spurious m.
me·nin·go·coc·ce·mia (mē - ning'gō - kok - sē'mē - ă). Meningococcemia; presença de meningococos (*N. meningitidis*) no sangue circulante.
acute fulminating m., m. fulminante aguda; infecção sistêmica rápida por *Neisseria meningitidis*, geralmente sem meningite, caracterizada por erupção cutânea, geralmente petequial ou purpúrica, febre alta e hipotensão. Pode causar morte em horas.

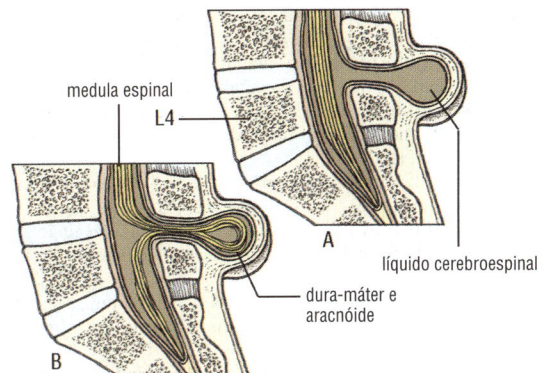

meningocele (A) e **meningomielocele:** entre as vértebras L4 e L5

me·nin·go·coc·cus, pl. **me·nin·go·coc·ci** (mē - ning'gō - kok'ŭs, - kok'sī). Meningococo. SIN *Neisseria meningitidis*. [meningo- + G. *kokkos*, baga]
me·nin·go·cor·ti·cal (mē - ning'gō - kōr'ti - kăl). Meningocortical; relativo às meninges e ao córtex do encéfalo. SIN meningeocortical.
me·nin·go·cyte (mē - ning'gō - sīt). Meningócito; uma célula epitelial mesenquimal do espaço subaracnóide; pode tornar-se um macrófago. [meningo- + G. *kytos*, célula]
me·nin·go·en·ceph·a·li·tis (mē - ning'gō - en - sef'ăl - ī'tis). Meningoencefalite; inflamação do encéfalo e de suas membranas. SIN cerebromeningitis, encephalomeningitis. [meningo- + G. *enkephalos*, encéfalo, + -itis, inflamação]
acute primary hemorrhagic m., m. hemorrágica primária aguda. SIN acute epidemic *leukoencephalitis*.
biundulant m., m. biondulante. SIN tick-borne *encephalitis* (Central European subtype).
chronic progressive syphilitic m., m. sifilítica progressiva crônica. SIN paretic *neurosyphilis*.
eosinophilic m., m. eosinofílica; doença causada por infecção pelo nematódeo pulmonar do rato, *Angiostrongylus cantonensis*, cujas larvas, ingeridas com lesmas ou caracóis terrestres (ou algum hospedeiro transportador não identificado), migram do intestino para as meninges do encéfalo, onde a doença é produzida; geralmente é leve, de curta duração e caracterizada por febre, eosinofilia e leucócitos (raramente larvas de nematódeos) no líquido espinal.
herpetic m., m. herpética; forma grave de meningococcemia causada pelo herpesvírus tipo 1 e associada a uma alta taxa de mortalidade.
mumps m., m. da caxumba; infecção do sistema nervoso, geralmente benigna, que surge durante a fase ativa da caxumba clínica (parotidite).
primary amebic m., m. amebiana primária; infecção cerebral invasiva, rapidamente fatal, por amebas do solo, principalmente *Naegleria fowleri,* encontrada em seres humanos e outros primatas e, experimentalmente, em roedores; a doença é caracterizada por febre alta, rigidez de nuca e sintomas associados à infecção respiratória alta, como tosse e náuseas; embora tenham sido cultivados organismos provenientes de vários órgãos, o encéfalo é o foco primário, principalmente os lobos olfatórios e o córtex cerebral, que primeiro são atacados pelas amebas que entram na mucosa nasal através da lâmina cribriforme; geralmente o paciente morre dois a três dias após o início dos sintomas.
syphilitic m., m. sifilítica; uma manifestação do estágio secundário ou terciário da sífilis; raramente fatal.
me·nin·go·en·ceph·a·lo·cele (mē - ning'ō - en - sef'ă - lō - sēl). Meningoencefalocele; protrusão das meninges e do encéfalo através de um defeito congênito no crânio, geralmente na região frontal ou occipital. SIN encephalomeningocele. [meningo- + G. *enkephalos*, encéfalo, + *kēlē*, hérnia]
me·nin·go·en·ceph·a·lo·my·e·li·tis (mē - ning'gō - en - sef'ă - lō - mī - ĕ - lī'tis). Meningoencefalomielite; inflamação do encéfalo e da medula espinal juntamente com suas membranas. [meningo- + G. *enkephalos*, encéfalo, + *myelos*, medula óssea, + -itis, inflamação]
me·nin·go·en·ceph·a·lop·a·thy (mē - ning'gō - en - sef - ă - lop'ă - thē). Meningoencefalopatia; distúrbio que afeta as meninges e o encéfalo. SIN encephalomeningopathy. [meningo- + G. *enkephalos*, encéfalo, + *pathos*, que sofre]
me·nin·go·my·e·li·tis (mē - ning'gō - mī'ĕ - lī'tis). Meningomielite; inflamação da medula espinal e da aracnóide e pia-máter que a revestem, e, menos comumente, também da dura-máter. [meningo- + G. *myelos*, medula óssea, + -itis, inflamação]
me·nin·go·my·e·lo·cele (mē - ning - gō - mī'ĕ - lō - sēl). Meningomielocele; protrusão da medula espinal e de suas membranas através de um defeito na

coluna vertebral. SIN myelocystomeningocele, myelomeningocele. [meningo- + G. *myelos*, medula óssea, + *kēlē*, tumor]

me·nin·go-os·te·o·phle·bi·tis (mē-ning′gō′os-tē-ō-flē-bī′tis). Meningoosteoflebite; inflamação das veias do periósteo.

me·nin·go·ra·dic·u·lar (mē-ning′gō-ra-dik′ū-lar). Meningorradicular; relativo às meninges que cobrem as raízes dos nervos cranianos ou espinais. [meningo- + L. *radix*, raiz]

me·nin·go·ra·dic·u·li·tis (mē-ning′gō-ra-dik-ū-lī′tis). Meningorradiculite; inflamação das meninges e das raízes dos nervos.

me·nin·gor·rha·chid·i·an (mē-ning′gō-ra-kid′ē-an). Meningorraquidiano; relativo à medula espinal e suas membranas. [meningo- + G. *rhachis*, coluna vertebral]

me·nin·gor·rha·gia (mē-ning′gō-rā′jē-ā). Meningorragia; hemorragia para as meninges cerebrais ou espinais, ou sob estas. [meningo- + G. *rhēgnymi*, romper]

men·in·go·sis (men′ing-gō′sis). Meningose; união membranosa dos ossos, como no crânio do recém-nascido. [meningo- + G. *-ōsis*, condição]

me·nin·go·vas·cu·lar (mē-ning′gō-vas′kū-lar). Meningovascular; relativo aos vasos sanguíneos nas meninges; ou às meninges e aos vasos sanguíneos.

men·in·gu·ria (men-ing-goo′rē-ā). Meningúria; a eliminação de fragmentos membraniformes na urina. [meningo- + G. *ouron*, urina]

me·ninx, gen. **me·nin·gis,** pl. **me·nin·ges** (mē′ninks, -jēz; men′ingks; mē-nin′jes) [TA]. Meninge; qualquer membrana; especificamente, um dos revestimentos membranosos do encéfalo e da medula espinal. VER TAMBÉM *arachnoid* mater, dura mater, pia mater, leptomeninx. [L. mod. do G. *mēninx*, membrana]
   m. fibro'sa, termo raramente usado para designar a dura-máter.
   m. primiti'va, m. primitiva. SIN primitive m.
   primitive m., m. primitiva; o tecido mesenquimatoso frouxo embrionário que circunda o encéfalo e a medula espinal; dela são derivadas as três meninges definidas (aracnóide-máter, dura-máter e pia-máter). SIN m. primitiva.
   m. ten'uis, leptomeninge. SIN leptomeninx.
   vascular m., termo raramente usado para pia-máter. SIN m. vasculosa.
   m. vasculo'sa, pia-máter. SIN vascular m.

men·is·cec·to·my (men′i-sek′tō-mē). Meniscectomia; excisão de um menisco, geralmente da articulação do joelho. [G. *mēniskos*, crescente (menisco) + *ektomē*, excisão]

me·nis·ci (mē-nis′sī). Meniscos; plural de meniscus.

men·is·ci·tis (men′i-sī′tis). Meniscite; inflamação de um menisco fibrocartilaginoso. [G. *mēniskos*, crescente (menisco), + *-itis*, inflamação]

me·nis·co·cyte (mē-nis′kō-sīt). Célula falciforme. SIN sickle *cell*. [G. *mēniskos*, um crescente, + *kytos*, uma cavidade (célula)]

me·nis·co·pexy (mē-nis′kō-pek-sē). Meniscopexia; procedimento cirúrgico que ancora o menisco medial em sua antiga fixação. SIN meniscorrhaphy. [menisco- + G. *pēxis*, fixação]

men·is·cor·rha·phy (men-is-kōr′ā-fē). Meniscorrafia. SIN meniscopexy. [menisco- + G. *rhaphē*, sutura]

me·nis·co·tome (mē-nis′kō-tōm). Meniscótomo; instrumento usado na remoção de um menisco. [G. *mēniskos*, crescente (menisco) + *tomē*, incisão]

me·nis·cus, pl. **me·nis·ci** (mē-nis′kus, mē-nis′sī). Menisco. **1.** m. articular. SIN meniscus *lens*. **2** [TA]. Uma fibrocartilagem intra-articular em forma de crescente em algumas articulações. **3.** Uma estrutura fibrocartilaginosa em forma de crescente no joelho, as articulações acromioclavicular, esternoclavicular e temporomandibular. [G. *mēniskos*, crescente]
   articular m., m. articular. SIN meniscus *lens*.
   m. articula'ris, m. articular. SIN meniscus *lens*.
   converging m., m. convergente; uma lente convexo-côncava na qual o grau da convexidade é maior que o da concavidade. SIN positive m.
   diverging m., m. divergente; uma lente convexo-côncava na qual o grau da concavidade é maior que o da convexidade. SIN negative m.
   lateral m. [TA], m. lateral; cartilagem intra-articular em forma de crescente na articulação do joelho, fixada à borda lateral da superfície articular superior da tíbia, ocupando o espaço que circunda as superfícies de contato do fêmur e da tíbia. SIN m. lateralis [TA], external semilunar fibrocartilage.
   m. latera'lis [TA], m. lateral. SIN lateral m.
   medial m. [TA], m. medial; cartilagem intra-articular em forma de crescente na articulação do joelho, fixada à borda medial da superfície articular superior da tíbia, que ocupa o espaço que circunda as superfícies de contato do fêmur e da tíbia. SIN m. medialis [TA], falciform cartilage, internal semilunar fibrocartilage of knee joint.
   m. media'lis [TA], m. medial. SIN medial m.
   negative m., m. negativo. SIN diverging m.
   periscopic m., m. periscópico. SIN aplanatic *lens*.
   positive m., m. positivo. SIN converging m.
   tactile m., m. tátil; uma terminação nervosa sensorial tátil especializada na epiderme, caracterizada por expansão caliciforme terminal de um axônio intra-epidérmico em contato com a base de um único ceratinócito modificado. SIN m. tactus, Merkel corpuscle, Merkel tactile cell, Merkel tactile disk, tactile disk.
   m. tac'tus, m. tátil. SIN tactile m.

Menkes, John H., neurologista norte-americano, *1928. VER M. *syndrome*.

meno-. Meno-; a menstruação. [G. *mēn*, mês]

men·o·ce·lis (men-ō-sē′lis). Menocelidose; uma erupção macular escura ou petequial que ocorre algumas vezes em casos de amenorréia. [meno- + G. *kēlis*, mancha]

men·o·me·tror·rha·gia (men′ō-mē-trō-rā′jē-ā). Menometrorragia; hemorragia irregular ou excessiva durante a menstruação e entre os períodos menstruais. [meno- + G. *mētra*, útero, + *rhēgnymi*, romper]

men·o·pau·sal (men′ō-paw-zāl). Menopáusico; associado à, ou causado pela, menopausa.

men·o·pause (men′ō-pawz). Menopausa; interrupção permanente da menstruação; interrupção da vida menstrual. [meno- + G. *pausis*, cessação]
   premature m., m. prematura; falha da função ovariana cíclica antes de 40 anos de idade. SIN premature ovarian failure.

men·o·pha·nia (men-ō-fā′nē-ā). Menofania; primeiro sinal da menstruação na puberdade. [meno- + G. *phainō*, mostrar]

Men·o·pon (men′ō-pon). Gênero de piolhos hematófagos (família Menoponidae, ordem Mallophaga) encontrados em aves; inclui pestes importantes que infectam aves domésticas, como *M. gallinae* (*M. pallidum*), o piolho das aves domésticas, um piolho amarelo-claro, que mede cerca de 1,7 a 2,0 mm de comprimento, encontrado em aves de quintal, patos e pombos.

men·or·rha·gia (men-ō-ral′jē-ā). Menorragia. SIN hypermenorrhea. [meno- + G. *rhēgnymi*, romper]

men·or·rhal·gia (men-ō-rajē-ā). Menorralgia. SIN dysmenorrhea. [meno- + G. *algos*, dor]

men·o·tro·pins (men-ō-trō′pinz). Menotropinas; extrato de urina pós-menopausa contendo basicamente o hormônio folículo-estimulante. VER TAMBÉM human menopausal *gonadotropin*, urofollitropin.

men·o·u·ria (men-ō-ū′rē-ā). Menoúria; menstruação que ocorre através da bexiga em virtude de fístula vesicouterina. [meno- + G. *ouron*, urina , + *-ia*, condição]

men·o·xe·nia (men-ō-zē′nē-ā, men′ok-sē′nē-ā). Menoxenia; qualquer anormalidade da menstruação. [meno- + G. *xenos*, estranho]

men·ses (men′sēz). Menstruação; hemorragia fisiológica periódica, que ocorre aproximadamente a intervalos de 4 semanas, com origem na mucosa uterina; geralmente a hemorragia é precedida por ovulação e alterações pré-deciduais no endométrio. VER TAMBÉM menstrual *cycle*. SIN menstrual period. [L. pl. de *mensis*, mês]

men·stru·al (men′stroo-āl). Menstrual; relativo à menstruação. [L. *menstrualis*]

men·stru·ant (men′stroo-ant). Menstruante; que menstrua.

men·stru·ate (men′stroo-āt). Menstruar; apresentar menstruação. [L. *menstruo*, pp. *-atus*, menstruar]

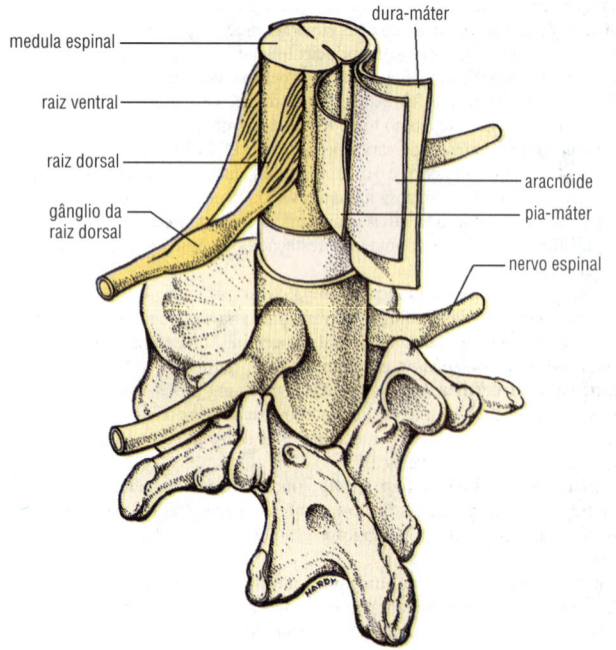

medula espinal e meninges

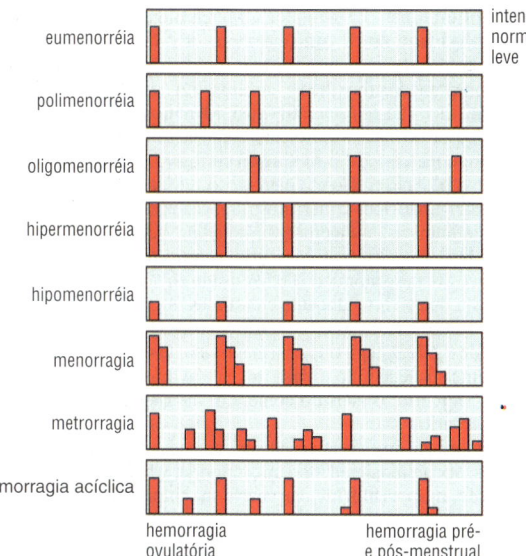

menstruação: anormalidades mostradas no gráfico de Kaltenbach

---

men·stru·a·tion (men-stroo-a′shŭn). Menstruação; descamação cíclica do endométrio e eliminação de líquido sanguinolento do útero durante o ciclo menstrual. [VER menstruate]
 anovular m., m. anovular; sangramento menstrual sem ovulação recente; também ocorre em primatas subumanos. SIN anovulational m., nonovulational m.
 anovulational m., m. anovulatória. SIN anovular m.
 nonovulational m., m. anovulatória. SIN anovular m.
 retained m., m. retida. SIN hematocolpos.
 retrograde m., m. retrógrada; refluxo de sangue menstrual através das tubas de Falópio; algumas vezes leva consigo células endometriais.
 supplementary m., m. suplementar; sangramento do umbigo ou vias urinárias devido à endometriose que ocorre no momento da menstruação.
 supressed m., m. suprimida; não-aparecimento do sangramento menstrual por qualquer causa.
 vicarious m., m. vicariante; hemorragia de qualquer superfície além da mucosa da cavidade uterina, que ocorre periodicamente no momento em que deve ocorrer a menstruação normal.
men·stru·um, pl. **men·strua** (men′stroo-ŭm, -stroo-ă). Mênstruo; termo antigo para designar solvente. [L. mediev. líquido menstrual, que se acreditava que possuísse algumas propriedades solventes, neutro do L. *menstruus*, mensalmente]
men·su·al (men′soo-ăl, -shoo-ăl). Mensal. [L. *mensis*, mês]
men·su·ra·tion (men-soo-ra′shŭn). Mensuração; o ato ou processo de medir. [L. *mensuratio*, de *mensuro*, medir]
men·tal. Mental. 1. Relativo à mente. [L. *mens* (*ment*-), mente] 2. Mentual; mentoniano; relativo ao queixo. SIN genial, genian. [L. *mentum*, queixo]
men·ta·lis (men-ta′lis). Músculo mental. VER mentalis (*muscle*). [L.]
men·tal·i·ty (men-tal′i-te). Mentalidade; as características funcionais da mente; atividade mental.
men·ta·tion (men-ta′shŭn). Atividade mental; o processo de raciocínio e pensamento.
Menten, Maud L., patologista canadense radicado nos Estados Unidos, 1879–1960. VER Michaelis-M. *constant, hypothesis*.
Men·tha (men′thă). Gênero de plantas da família Labiatae. *M. piperita* é a hortelã-pimenta; *M. pulegium*, poejo-das-hortas; *M. viridis*, hortelã verde. SIN mint. [L.]
men·thane (men′thān). Mentano; o terpeno monocíclico, origem de álcoois como o mentol e a terpina.
men·thol. Mentol; um álcool obtido do óleo de hortelã-pimenta ou outros óleos de menta, ou preparado sinteticamente; usado como antipruriginoso e anestésico tópico, em *sprays* nasais, remédio para tosse e inalações nasais, e como agente flavorizante. SIN peppermint camphor.
 camphorated m., m. canforado; líquido obtido pela titulação de partes iguais de cânfora e mentol; foi aplicado localmente como contra-irritante e (diluído) na forma de *spray* na rinite e faringite.
men·thyl sa·lic·y·late. Salicilato de mentila; usado como protetor solar para filtrar a luz ultravioleta em preparados para proteger a pele de queimaduras solares.
men·to·la·bi·a·lis (men′to-lā-bē-ā′lis). Mentolabial; os músculos mentual e abaixador do lábio inferior considerados como um músculo. [L.]

men·ton. Mento; em cefalometria, a parte mais inferior na imagem da sínfise, observada em uma incidência lateral da mandíbula. [L. *mentum*, queixo]
men·to·plas·ty (men′to-plas-te). Mentoplastia; cirurgia plástica do queixo, na qual é alterado seu formato ou tamanho. [L. *mentum*, queixo, + G. *plastos*, formado]
men·tum, gen. **men·ti** (men′tŭm, -tī) [TA]. Mento, queixo. SIN chin. [L.]
men·yan·thes (men-yan′thez). Trevo d'água. SIN buckbean.
mep·a·crine hy·dro·chlo·ride (mep′ă-krēn). Cloridrato de mepacrina. SIN quinacrine hydrochloride.
mep·a·zine ac·e·tate (mep′ă-zēne). Acetato de mepazina; um derivado fenotiazínico com ações e empregos semelhantes aos da clorpromazina. Também encontrado na forma de cloridrato de acetato de mepazina.
me·pen·zo·late bro·mide (me-pen′zō-lāt). Brometo de mepenzolato; um anticolinérgico.
me·per·i·dine hy·dro·chlo·ride (me-per′i-dēn). Cloridrato de meperidina; analgésico narcótico amplamente usado. SIN pethidine.
me·phen·e·sin (me-fen′ē-sin). Mefenesina; um relaxante do músculo esquelético de ação central; também disponível como carbamato de mefenesina.
me·phen·ter·mine (me-fen′ter-mēn). Mefentermina; uma amina simpaticomimética.
 m. sulfate, sulfato de mefentermina; usado topicamente como descongestionante nasal e sistemicamente por seus efeitos pressores em estados hipotensivos agudos.
me·phen·y·to·in (me-fen′i-tō-in). Mefenitoína; anticonvulsivante usado quando agentes mais seguros são inadequados; usado em estudos do metabolismo de drogas.
me·phit·ic (me-fit′ik). Mefítico; fétido, tóxico ou nocivo. [L. *mephitis*, uma exalação nociva]
meph·o·bar·bi·tal (mef-ō-bar′bi-tawl). Mefobarbital; usado como sedativo e hipnótico de ação prolongada, e como anticonvulsivante no tratamento da epilepsia; convertido em fenobarbital no corpo.
me·piv·a·caine hy·dro·chlo·ride (me-piv′ă-kān). Cloridrato de mepivacaína; um anestésico local.
me·pro·ba·mate (me-prō′bă-māt). Meprobamato; um relaxante do músculo esquelético com ação semelhante à produzida pela mefenesina, mas de maior duração; usado no tratamento de alguns distúrbios associados à atividade motora anormal, como um hipnótico leve, e como ansiolítico.
mep·ta·zi·nol (mep-taz′i-nol). Meptazinol; analgésico narcótico agonista/antagonista misto (como a pentazocina) cuja potência corresponde a aproximadamente um décimo da potência da morfina na produção de analgesia. Embora seu potencial de abuso seja menor que o de agonistas puros, a droga pode precipitar uma síndrome de abstinência em pessoas dependentes de opióides.
me·pyr·a·mine ma·le·ate (me-pir′ă-mēn). Maleato de mepiramina. SIN pyrilamine maleate.
me·pyr·a·pone (me-pir′ă-pōn). Mepirapona. SIN metyrapone.
mEq, meq Abreviatura de milliequivalent (miliequivalente).
-mer. 1. Sufixo químico ligado a um prefixo como mono-, di-, poli-, tri-, etc., para indicar a menor unidade de uma estrutura repetitiva; p. ex., um polímero. 2. Sufixo que designa um membro de um grupo específico; p. ex., isômero, enantiômero.
me·ral·gia (me-ral′jē-ă). Meralgia; dor na coxa; especificamente, meralgia parestésica. [G. *meros*, coxa, + *algos*, dor]
 m. paresthet′ica, m. parestésica; dor em queimação, sensação de picadas, prurido ou formigamento na face lateral da coxa, na distribuição do nervo cutâneo femoral lateral devido ao aprisionamento deste; freqüentemente há hiperestesia da área cutânea afetada. SIN Bernhardt disease, Bernhardt-Roth syndrome.
mer·al·lu·ride (mer-al′ū-rīd). Meralurida; um diurético mercurial.
mer·bro·min (mer-brō′min). Merbromina; o sal dissódico da 2,7-dibromo-4-hidroximercurifluoresceína; um anti-séptico mercurial orgânico que também possui propriedades de coloração semelhantes às da eosina e floxina, com grande afinidade por estruturas citoplasmáticas; também usada histoquimicamente para corar grupamentos sulfidril e dissulfeto ligados à proteína para microscopia de campo claro e de fluorescência. SIN mercurochrome.
mer·cap·tal (mer-kap′tal). Mercaptal; substância derivada de um aldeído pela substituição do oxigênio bivalente por dois grupamentos tioalquil (—SR).
mer·cap·tan (mer-kap′tan). Mercaptana. 1. Uma classe de substâncias nas quais o oxigênio de um álcool foi substituído por enxofre (p. ex., cisteína). SIN thioalcohol. VER thiol. 2. Em odontologia, uma classe de compostos de impressão elástica, algumas vezes denominados materiais de base de borracha.
 methyl m., mercaptano de metil; formado no intestino pela ação bacteriana sobre proteínas que contêm enxofre, e aparece na urina após a ingestão de aspargos (contribuindo para o odor característico); também na fabricação de vários fungicidas e pesticidas orgânicos que contêm enxofre.
mercapto-. Mercapto-; prefixo que indica a presença de um grupamento tiol, —SH.
mer·cap·to·a·ce·tic ac·id (mer-kap′to-ā-sē′tik). Ácido mercaptoacético. SIN thioglycolic acid.

mer·cap·to·eth·a·nol (mer - kap′tō - eth′ā - nol). Mercaptoetanol; agente redutor comumente usado.

β-mercaptoethanol. β-mercaptoetanol. SIN 2-mercaptoethanol.

2-mer·cap·to·eth·a·nol (mer - kap′tō - eth - an - ol). 2-mercaptoetanol; reagente usado para reduzir ligações dissulfeto, particularmente em proteínas, e para evitar sua formação. SIN β-mercaptoethanol.

mer·cap·tol (mer - kap′tol). Mercaptol; substância derivada de uma cetona pela substituição do oxigênio bivalente por dois grupamentos tioalquil (—SR).

3-mer·cap·to·lac·tate (mer - kap′tō - lak - tāt). 3-Mercaptolactato; um produto do catabolismo da cisteína; formado pela ação da lactato desidrogenase sobre o 3-mercaptopiruvato que, por sua vez, foi formado por transaminação da cisteína; presente na urina humana normal como um dissulfeto misto com a cisteína; elevado na urina em indivíduos com mercaptolacto-cisteína dissulfidúria.

mer·cap·to·lac·tate-cys·te·ine di·sul·fid·u·ria. Mercaptolactato-cisteína dissulfidúria; níveis elevados do dissulfeto misto de 3-mercaptolactato e cisteína na urina.

mer·cap·tom·er·in so·di·um (mer - kap - tom′e - rin, mer - kap - tō - mer′in). Mercaptomerina sódica; um diurético mercurial.

6-mer·cap·to·pu·rine (Shy) (mer - kap - tō - poor′ēn). 6-Mercaptopurina; um análogo da hipoxantina e da adenina; um agente antineoplásico.

3-mer·cap·to·py·ru·vate ((mer - kap′tō - pī - roo - vāt). 3-Mercaptopiruvato; o produto transaminado da cisteína; formado no catabolismo da cisteína; elevado em indivíduos com deficiência de 3-mercaptopiruvato sulfurtransferase.

3-m. sulfurtransferase, 3-m. sulfurtransferase; uma enzima que faz parte da via catabólica da cisteína; catalisa a conversão do 3-mercaptopiruvato em piruvato e H_2S; a deficiência dessa enzima resultará em concentração urinária elevada de 3-mercaptopiruvato bem como de 3-mercaptolactato, ambos na forma de dissulfetos com cisteína.

mer·cap·tu·ric ac·id (mer - kap - tūr′ik). Ácido mercaptúrico; um produto da condensação da L-cisteína com compostos aromáticos, como bromobenzeno, e geralmente acetilado; formado biologicamente através da glutationa no fígado e excretado na urina; uma L-cisteína N-acetilada com substituição do S. Cf. mercapturic acid *pathway.*

Mercier, Louis A., urologista francês, 1811–1882. VER M. *bar, sound, valve;* median *bar* of M.

mer·co·cre·sols (mer - kō - krē′solz). Mercocresóis; mistura que consiste em partes iguais por peso de *sec*-amiltricresol e cloreto de *o*-hidroxi-fenilmercúrico; possui ações fungicida, germicida e bacteriostática.

mer·cu·ma·til·in (mer′kū - mă - til′in, - mat′i - lin). Mercumatilina; um diurético mercurial; também encontrado na forma mercumatilina sódica.

mer·cu·ra·mide (mer - koo′ra - mīd). Mercuramida. SIN mersalyl.

mer·cu·ri·al (mer - kū′rē - ăl). Mercurial. **1.** Relativo ao mercúrio. **2.** Qualquer sal de mercúrio usado medicinalmente. **3.** Que possui a característica de rápida mudança do humor.

mer·cu·ri·a·len·tis (mer - kū′rē - ă - len′tis). Mercurialente; coloração castanha da cápsula anterior da lente, causada por mercúrio; sinal precoce de intoxicação por mercúrio.

mer·cu·ri·a·lism (mer - kū′rē - ă - lizm). Mercurialismo. SIN mercury poisoning.

***p*-mer·cur·i·ben·zo·ate** (mer - kūr - i - ben′zō - āt). *p*-Mercuribenzoato; um inibidor enzimático comumente usado devido à sua reação com grupamentos sulfidrila; geralmente é usado *p*-cloromercuribenzoato ou *p*-hidroximercuribenzoato.

mer·cu·ric (mer - kū′rik). Mercúrico; designa um sal de mercúrio no qual o íon do metal é bivalente, como no sublimado corrosivo, cloreto mercúrico, $HgCl_2$; o cloreto mercuroso é o calomelano, HgCl.

mer·cu·ric chlo·ride. Cloreto mercúrico; anti-séptico tópico e desinfetante para objetos inanimados. SIN corrosive sublimate, mercury bichloride, mercury perchloride, corrosive mercury chloride.

ammoniated m. c., cloreto de mercúrio amoniacal. SIN ammoniated *mercury.*

mer·cu·ric io·dide, red. Iodeto vermelho de mercúrio; foi usado como anti-séptico e como desinfetante para objetos inanimados. SIN mercury biniodide, mercury deutoiodide.

mer·cu·ric ole·ate. Oleato de mercúrio; preparado semelhante a uma pomada, usado em parasitoses cutâneas.

mer·cu·ric ox·ide, red. Óxido vermelho de mercúrio; o precipitado vermelho do HgO; foi usado externamente como anti-séptico em doenças cutâneas crônicas e infecções fúngicas. SIN red precipitate.

mer·cu·ric ox·ide, yel·low. Óxido amarelo de mercúrio; o precipitado amarelo do HgO; usado externamente como anti-séptico no tratamento de afecções inflamatórias das pálpebras e conjuntivas. SIN yellow precipitate.

mer·cu·ric sa·lic·y·late. Salicilato de mercúrio; pó aplicado externamente no tratamento de doenças parasitárias e fúngicas da pele. SIN mercury subsalicylate.

mer·cu·ro·chrome (mer - kur′ō - krōm). Mercurocromo. SIN merbromin.

mer·cu·ro·phen (mer - kū′ - rō - fen). Mercurofeno; anti-séptico local.

mer·cu·ro·phyl·line so·di·um (mer - kūr - of′i - lēn). Mercurofilina sódica; o sal sódico da β-metoxi-γ-hidroximercuripropilamida do ácido trimetilciclopentanodicarboxílico e teofilina; um diurético mercurial.

mer·cu·rous (mer - kū′rŭs, mer′kū - rŭs). Mercuroso; designa um sal de mercúrio no qual o íon do metal é univalente, como no calomelo, cloreto mercuroso, HgCl; o cloreto mercúrico é o sublimado corrosivo, $HgCl_2$.

mer·cu·rous chlo·ride. Cloreto mercuroso. SIN calomel.

mer·cu·rous io·dide. Iodeto mercuroso; aplicado externamente como pomada em doenças oftálmicas. SIN mercury protoiodide, yellow mercury iodide.

mer·cu·ry (Hg) (mer′kū - rē). Mercúrio; elemento metálico líquido, denso, de n.° atômico 80, peso atômico 200,59; usado em termômetros, barômetros, manômetros e outros instrumentos científicos; alguns sais e mercuriais orgânicos são usados na medicina; deve-se ter cuidado no seu manuseio: o Hg^{197} (meia-vida de 2,672 dias) e o Hg^{203} (meia-vida de 46,61 dias) têm sido usados em exames do encéfalo e dos rins. SIN hydrargyrum, quicksilver. [L. *Mercurius,* Mercúrio, o deus do comércio, mensageiro dos deuses; em L. Mediev., mercúrio]

ammoniated m., m. amoniacal; usado em pomadas para tratamento de doenças cutâneas. SIN ammoniated mercuric chloride, white mercuric precipitate.

m. bichloride, m. perchloride, corrosive m. chloride, bicloreto de mercúrio. SIN mercuric chloride.

m. biniodide, biodeto de mercúrio. SIN mercuric iodide, red.

m. deutoiodide, deutoiodeto de mercúrio. SIN mercuric iodide, red.

m. protoiodide, protoiodeto de mercúrio. SIN mercurous iodide.

m. subsalicylate, subsalicilato de mercúrio. SIN mercuric salicylate.

yellow m. iodide, iodeto amarelo de mercúrio. SIN mercurous iodide.

⌂ **mere-, mero-.** Parte; também indicam uma série de partes semelhantes. VER TAMBÉM -mer. [G. *mēros,* parte]

Merendino, K. Alvin, cirurgião norte-americano, 1914–1985. VER M. *technique.*

mer·e·prine (mer′ē - prēn). Mereprina. SIN doxylamine succinate.

Meretoja, J., médico finlandês. VER Meretoja *syndrome.*

me·rid·i·an (mē - rid′ - ē - an). Meridiano. **1** [TA]. Uma linha que circunda um corpo globular em ângulos retos com seu equador e que toca ambos os pólos, ou a metade desse círculo que se estende de um pólo ao outro. SIN meridianus [TA]. **2.** Em acupuntura, as linhas que ligam diferentes pontos anatômicos. [L. *meridianus,* pertinente ao meio-dia, no lado sul, meridional]

m. of cornea, m. da córnea; qualquer linha que divida a córnea em duas partes, atravessando seu ápice.

m.'s of eyeball [TA], meridianos do bulbo do olho; linhas que circundam a superfície do bulbo do olho, atravessando os pólos anterior e posterior. SIN meridiani bulbi oculi [TA].

me·rid·i·a·ni (mē - rid - ē - ā′nī). Meridianos; plural de meridianus.

me·rid·i·a·nus, pl. **me·rid·i·a·ni** (mē - rid′ē - ā′nŭs, -nī) [TA]. Meridiano. SIN meridian (1). [L.]

meridiani bul′bi oc′uli [TA], meridianos do bulbo do olho. SIN *meridians* of *eyeball,* em *meridian.*

me·rid·i·o·nal (mē - rid′ē - ō - năl). Meridional; relativo a um meridiano.

mer·i·spore (mer′i - spōr). Merisporo; um esporo secundário, resultante da segmentação de outro esporo (composto ou septado). [G. *meros,* uma parte, + *sporos,* semente]

mer·i·ste·mat·ic (mer′is - tĕ - mat′ik). Meristemático; relativo (em fungos) a uma área (meristema) das hifas ou de outras estruturas especializadas a partir das quais ocorre novo crescimento. [G. *merizein,* dividir]

me·ris·tic (mē - ris′tik). Merístico; simétrico; que pode ser dividido igualmente; designa simetria bilateral ou longitudinal no arranjo de partes em um organismo. [G. *meristikos,* adequado para divisão]

Merkel, Friedrich S., anatomista e fisiologista alemão, 1845–1919. VER M. *cell tumor, corpuscle,* tactile *cell,* tactile *disk.*

Merkel, Karl L., anatomista e laringologista alemão, 1812–1876. VER M. *filtrum ventriculi, fossa, muscle.*

Mer·mis (mer′mis). Gênero de nematódeos opacos, longos; os estágios larvares são eliminados na cavidade hemocílica de insetos, particularmente gafanhotos, enquanto os adultos têm vida livre no solo. A ingestão acidental por seres humanos causa infecção.

M. nigrescens, espécie de nematódeo encontrada no solo que deposita ovos em plantas acima do solo; os hospedeiros normais são os gafanhotos; foi isolado nos tratos alimentar e urogenital dos seres humanos, mas as infecções são raras.

⌂ **mero-.** VER mere-.

mer·o·a·cra·nia (mer′ō - ă - krā′nē - ă). Meroacrania; ausência congênita de uma parte do crânio, afora o osso occipital. [mero- + G. *a-* priv. + *kranion,* crânio]

mer·o·an·en·ceph·a·ly (mer′ō - an - en - sef′ă - lē). Meroanencefalia; tipo de anencefalia em que o encéfalo e o crânio estão presentes na forma rudimentar. [mero- + G. *an-* priv. + *enkephalos,* encéfalo]

mer·o·crine (mer′ō - krin, - krīn, - krēn). Merócrino. VER merocrine *gland.* [mero- + G. *krino,* separar]

mer·o·di·a·stol·ic (mer′ō-dī-ă-stol′ik). Merodiastólico; parcialmente diastólico; relativo a uma parte da diástole do coração. [mero- + diastole]

mer·o·gas·tru·la (mer′ō-gas′troo-lă). Merogástrula; a gástrula de um ovo meroblástico.

mer·o·gen·e·sis (mer-ō-jen′ĕ-sis). Merogênese. 1. Reprodução por segmentação. 2. Clivagem de um ovo. [mero- + G. *genesis*, origem]

mer·o·ge·net·ic, mer·o·gen·ic (mer-ō-jĕ-net′ik, -ō-jen′ik). Merogenético, merogênico; relativo à merogênese.

me·rog·o·ny (mĕ-rog′o-nē). Merogonia. 1. O desenvolvimento incompleto de um óvulo que foi desorganizado. 2. Uma forma de esquizogonia assexuada, típica de protozoários esporozoários, na qual o núcleo divide-se várias vezes antes de o citoplasma se dividir; o esquizonte divide-se para formar merozoítas nessa fase assexuada do ciclo vital. [mero- + G. *gonē*, geração]

mer·o·me·lia (mer-ō-mē′lē-ă). Meromelia; ausência parcial de um membro livre (exclusivo do cíngulo); p. ex., hemimelia, focomelia. [mero- + G. *melos*, membro]

mer·o·mi·cro·so·mia (mer′ō-mī′krō-sō′mē-ă). Meromicrossomia; pequenez anormal de alguma parte do corpo; local dwarfism. [mero- + G. *mikros*, pequeno, + *sōma*, corpo]

mer·o·my·o·sin (mer-ō-mī′ō-sin). Meromiosina; uma subunidade da digestão tríptica da miosina; são produzidos dois tipos: H-m e L-m.
  H-m, heavy-m., m. pesada; um dos produtos relativamente pesados (peso molecular de aproximadamente 350.000) da ação da tripsina sobre a miosina; possui a atividade ATPase da miosina.
  L-m, light-m., m. leve; o produto, de peso molecular relativamente baixo (peso molecular de aproximadamente 120.000), da digestão tríptica da miosina.

mer·ont (mer′ont). Meronte; um estágio no ciclo vital de esporozoários em que ocorrem múltiplas divisões assexuadas (esquizogonia), resultando na produção de merozoítas. VER TAMBÉM schizont.

mer·o·ra·chis·chi·sis, mer·or·rha·chis·chi·sis (mer′ō-ră-kis′ki-sis). Merorraquisquise; fissura de uma parte da medula espinal. SIN rachischisis partialis. [mero- + G. *rhachis*, coluna vertebral, + *schisis*, fissura]

me·ros·mia (me-roz′mē-ă). Merosmia; condição na qual a percepção de alguns odores é deficiente; análoga à cegueira para cores. [mero- + G. *osmē*, olfato]

mer·o·spor·an·gi·um (mer′ō-spōr-ran′-jē-ŭm). Merosporângio; um pequeno esporângio cilíndrico contendo poucos esporos e encontrado em alguns zigomicetos. [G. *meros*, parte, + sporangium]

mer·o·sys·tol·ic (mer′ō-sis-tol′ik). Merossistólico; parcialmente sistólico; relativo a uma parte da sístole cardíaca. [mero- + systole]

me·rot·o·my (me-rot′ō-mē). Merotomia; o procedimento de cortar em partes, como o corte de uma célula em partes distintas para estudar sua capacidade de sobrevida e desenvolvimento. [mero- + G. *tomē*, incisão]

mer·o·zo·ite (mer-ō-zō′īt). Merozoíta; o estágio infeccioso móvel de protozoários esporozoários que resulta de esquizogonia ou de um tipo semelhante de reprodução assexuada; p. ex., endodiogenia ou endopoligenia. Os merozoítas formam-se na superfície de esquizontes, blastóforos ou em invaginações nos esquizontes, e são responsáveis pelas grandes forças reprodutivas dos parasitas esporozoários; isso é observado na malária humana, na qual a produção cíclica de merozoítas causa a síndrome típica de febre e calafrios. SIN endodyocyte (2). [mero- + G. *zōon*, animal]

me·ro·zy·gote (mĕ-rō-zī′gōt). Merozigoto; em genética microbiana, um organismo que, além de seu próprio genoma original (endogenoto), contém um fragmento (exogenoto) de um genoma de outro organismo; o tamanho relativamente pequeno do exogenoto permite uma condição diplóide apenas para uma região limitada do endogenoto. [mero- + *zygōtos*, que tem vitelo]

mer·pha·lan (mer′fă-lan). Merfalan; a mistura racêmica de melfalan e medfalan; um agente antineoplásico. SIN sarcolysine.

MERRF Acrônimo para *myoclonic epilepsy* with *ragged red fiber myopathy* (epilepsia mioclônica com miopatia com fibras vermelhas anfractuosas). Distúrbio mitocondrial causado por uma mutação pontual do *locus* 8344 do genoma da mitocôndria, onde é codificado o RNA de transferência.

Merrifield, R. Bruce, bioquímico e Prêmio Nobel norte-americano, *1921. VER M. synthesis.

Merrifield knife. Bisturi de Merrifield. VER em knife.

Merritt, Katharine K., pediatra norte-americana, *1886. VER Kasabach-M. syndrome.

mer·sa·lyl (mer′să-lil). Mersalil; sal sódico do ácido (3-hidroximercúrico-2-metoxipropil)salicilamida-*O*-acético; um diurético mercurial. SIN mercuramide.
  m. acid, ácido mersálico; mistura de *o*-carboximetilsalicil-(3-hidroximercúrico-2-metoxipropil)amida e seus anidridos; mesmo uso do mersalil.
  m. theophylline, teofilina mersalil; mersalil mais teofilina adicionada para inibir a decomposição do mersalil.

Méry, Jean, anatomista francês, 1645–1722. VER M. *gland*.

Merzbacher, Ludwig, médico alemão na Argentina, 1875-1942. VER M.-Pelizaeus *disease*; Pelizaeus-M. *disease*.

⚠ **mes-.** VER meso-.

me·sad (mē′zad, mē′sad). Mesial; que passa pelo, ou que se estende em direção ao plano mediano do corpo ou de uma parte. SIN mesiad. [G. *mesos*, meio, + L. *ad*, para]

me·sal (mē′zal, -mē′sal). Termo raramente usado para designar o plano mediano do corpo ou de uma parte. [G. *mesos*, meio]

mes·a·me·boid (mez-ă-mē′boyd). Mesamebóide; termo de Minot para uma célula primitiva, "migratória", derivada do mesoderma, provavelmente um hemocitoblasto. [mes- + G. *amoibē*, modificação (ameba), + *eidos*, semelhança]

mes·an·gi·al (mes-an′jē-ăl). Mesangial; referente ao mesângio.

mes·an·gi·um (mes-an′jē-ŭm). Mesângio; uma parte central do glomérulo renal entre capilares; as células mesangiais são fagocíticas e estão, na maior parte, separadas da luz capilar por células endoteliais. [mes- + G. *angeion*, vaso]
  extraglomerular m., m. extraglomerular; células mesangiais que ocupam o espaço triangular entre a mácula densa e as arteríolas aferentes e eferentes do aparelho justaglomerular. SIN polkissen of Zimmermann.

mes·a·or·ti·tis (mes-ā-ōr-tī′tis). Mesaortite; inflamação da túnica média ou muscular da aorta. [mes- + aortitis]

mes·a·re·ic, mes·a·ra·ic (mes-ă-rā′ik). Mesaraico. SIN mesenteric. [G. *mesaraion*, mesentério, de *mesos*, médio, + *araia*, flanco, ventre]

mes·ar·ter·i·tis (mes-ar-ter-ī′tis). Mesarterite; inflamação da túnica média (muscular) de uma artéria. [mes- + arteritis]

me·sat·i·ce·phal·ic (mĕ-sat′i-se-fal′ik). Mesaticefálico. SIN mesocephalic. [G. *mesatos*, o mais central, + *kephalē*, cabeça]

me·sat·i·pel·lic, me·sat·i·pel·vic (mĕ-sat′i-pel′ik, -pel′vik). Mesatipélico, mesatipélvico; designa um indivíduo com um índice pélvico entre 90 e 95; o estreito superior tem um aspecto arredondado, com o diâmetro transverso maior que o ântero-posterior em 1 cm ou menos. [G. *mesatos*, o mais central, + *pellis*, pelve]

mes·ax·on (mez-ak′son, mes-). Mesaxônio; a membrana plasmática do neurolema preguada para circundar o axônio de um nervo. Em microfotografias eletrônicas, essa camada dupla tem aparência semelhante à de um mesentério.

mes·cal but·tons (mes′kal). Botões de mescal; as folhas secas do cactus *Lophophora williamsii* contendo mescalina e alcalóides relacionados.

mes·ca·line (mes′kă-lēn). Mescalina; o alcalóide mais ativo presente nos botões do cactus mescal, *Lophophora williamsii*. O mescal produz efeitos psicotomiméticos semelhantes aos produzidos pelo LSD: alteração do humor, alterações da percepção, devaneios, alucinações, visões, delírios, despersonalização, midríase, atetose pupilar e aumento da temperatura corporal e do peso ao nascimento; há desenvolvimento de dependência psíquica, tolerância e tolerância cruzada ao LSD e à psilocibina; o principal componente do peiote.

mes·ec·to·derm (mez-ek′tō-derm). Mesectoderma. 1. Células na área ao redor do lábio dorsal do blastoporo onde o mesoderma e o ectoderma sofrem um processo de separação. 2. A parte do mesênquima derivada do ectoderma, principalmente da crista neural na região cefálica em embriões muito jovens. SIN ectomesenchyme. [mes- + ectoderm]

mes·en·ce·phal·ic (mez-en-se-fal′ik). Mesencefálico; relativo ao mesencéfalo.

mes·en·ceph·a·li·tis (mez′en-sef′ă-lī′tis). Mesencefalite; inflamação do mesencéfalo.

mes·en·ceph·a·lon (mez-en-sef′ă-lon) [TA]. Mesencéfalo; a parte do tronco encefálico que se desenvolve a partir do meio das três vesículas cerebrais primárias do embrião (sendo a caudal o rombencéfalo ou metencéfalo, e a rostral, o prosencéfalo ou encéfalo anterior). No adulto, o mesencéfalo é caracterizado pela conformação única de sua lâmina do teto [TA], composta pelo par de colículos superiores e inferiores bilaterais e pelo grande par de proeminências dos pilares do cérebro em sua superfície ventral. Ao corte transversal, seu canal central pérvio, o aqueduto do mesencéfalo, é circundado por um anel proeminente de substância cinzenta pobre em fibras mielinizadas; a substância cinza periaquedutal é unida ventral e lateralmente pelo tegmento mesencefálico rico em mielina, e coberta dorsalmente pela lâmina do teto do mesencéfalo. Grupos celulares proeminentes do mesencéfalo incluem os núcleos motores dos nervos troclear e oculomotor, o núcleo vermelho e a substância negra. SIN midbrain vesicle,* midbrain*. [mes- + G. *enkephalos*, encéfalo]

mes·en·ceph·a·lot·o·my (mez′en-sef′ă-lot′ō-mē). Mesencefalotomia. 1. A secção de qualquer estrutura no mesencéfalo, principalmente dos tratos espinotalâmicos para alívio de dor intratável, ou do pedúnculo cerebral para tratamento das discinesias. 2. Uma tractotomia espinotalâmica mesencefálica. [mesencephalon + G. *tomē*, incisão]

me·sen·chy·ma (mĕ-seng′ki-mă, mĕ-zeng′). Mesênquima. SIN mesenchyme.

me·sen·chy·mal (mē-seng′ki-măl, mez-eng-kī′măl). Mesenquimatoso, mesenquimal; relativo ao mesênquima.

mes·en·chy·me (mez′en-kim). Mesênquima. 1. Uma agregação de células mesenquimais ou fibroblásticas. 2. Tecido conjuntivo embrionário primordial que consiste em células mesenquimais, geralmente de forma estrelada, sustentadas na geléia interlaminar. SIN mesenchyma. [mes- + G. *enkyma*, infusão]

interzonal m., m. interzonal; uma área de m. avascular entre elementos ósseos adjacentes no embrião; designa a região de articulações futuras.

synovial m., m. sinovial; m. vascular circundando o m. interzonal; transforma-se na membrana sinovial de uma articulação.

mes·en·chy·mo·ma (mez′en-kī-mō′ma). Mesenquimoma; termo raramente usado para uma neoplasia na qual há uma mistura de derivados mesenquimais, além do tecido fibroso. Um **m. benigno** pode conter focos de tecido vascular, muscular, adiposo, osteóide, ósseo e cartilaginoso; essas neoplasias algumas vezes são classificadas sob um nome composto, p. ex., angioleiomiolipoma e semelhantes, mas pode ser preferido o termo mais amplo. Um **m. maligno** também pode ocorrer como uma mistura semelhante de dois tipos ou mais de células mesenquimais malignas (além das células de tecido fibroso).

mes·en·ter·ic (mez-en-ter′ik). Mesentérico; relativo ao mesentério. SIN mesareic, mesaraic.

mes·en·ter·i·o·lum (mez-en-ter-ē′ō-lum). Mesenteríolo; um pequeno mesentério, como o de um divertículo intestinal. SIN mesoenteriolum. [L. mod. dim. de *mesenterium*, mesentério]

m. proces′sus vermifor′mis, mesoapêndice. SIN mesoappendix.

mes·en·ter·i·o·pexy (mes′en-ter-ē-ō-pek′sē). Mesenteriopexia; fixação de um mesentério roto ou incisado. SIN mesopexy. [mesentery + G. *pēxis*, fixação]

mes·en·ter·i·or·rha·phy (mez′en-ter-ē-ōr′a-fē). Mesenteriorrafia; sutura do mesentério. SIN mesorrhaphy. [mesentery + G. *rhaphē*, sutura]

mes·en·ter·i·pli·ca·tion (mez′en-ter-i-pli-kā′shun). Mesenteriplicatura; redução da redundância de um mesentério fazendo nele uma ou mais pregas. [mesentery + L. *plico*, pp. *-atus*, preguear]

mes·en·ter·i·tis (mez′en-ter-ī′tis). Mesenterite; inflamação do mesentério.

mes·en·te·ri·um (mez′en-ter′ē-um). [TA]. Mesentério. SIN mesentery, mesentery. [L. mod.]

m. dorsa′le commu′ne, m. dorsal comum. SIN mesentery (2).

mes·en·ter·on (mez-en′ter-on). Mesêntero; a porção média do canal alimentar dos insetos e local de digestão; o mesêntero pode possuir projeções digitiformes anteriores, os cecos gástricos, e um intestino médio anterior tubular, seguido posteriormente pelo ventrículo sacular ou estômago. [mes- + G. *enteron*, intestino]

mes·en·tery (mes′en-ter-ē). [TA]. Mesentério. **1.** Uma camada dupla de peritônio fixada à parede abdominal e encerrando em sua prega uma parte das vísceras abdominais, ou todas elas, conduzindo seus vasos e nervos. **2.** A prega de peritônio, em forma de leque, que suspende a maior parte do intestino delgado (jejuno e íleo) e fixa-o à parede abdominal anterior na raiz do mesentério. SIN mesenterium dorsale commune, mesostenium. SIN mesenterium [TA]. [L. mod. *mesenterium*, do G. *mesenterion*, do G. *mesos*, meio, + *enteron*, intestino]

m. of appendix, mesoapêndice. SIN mesoappendix.

m. of cecum, m. do ceco. SIN mesocecum.

m. of lung, m. pulmonar. SIN mesopneumonium.

m. of sigmoid colon, mesocolo sigmóide. VER mesocolon.

m. of transverse colon. mesocolo transverso. VER mesocolon.

urogenital m., m. urogenital. SIN diaphragmatic ligament of the mesonephros.

mesh·work. Rede. VER network.

trabecular m., tecido trabecular da esclera. SIN trabecular tissue of sclera.

me·si·ad (mē′zē-ad, mes′ē-ad). Mesial. SIN mesad.

me·si·al (mē′zē-al, mes′ē-al). [TA]. Proximal. SIN proximal. [G. *mesos*, meio]

△ **mesio-.** Mesial (particularmente em odontologia). [G. *mesos*, meio]

me·si·o·buc·cal (mē′zē-ō-buk′al). Mesiobucal; relativo às superfícies mesial e bucal de um dente; designando principalmente o ângulo formado pela junção dessas duas superfícies.

me·si·o·buc·co·oc·clu·sal (mē′zē-ō-buk′ō-ō-kloo′sal). Mesiobucoclusal; relativo ao ângulo formado pela junção das superfícies mesial, bucal e oclusal de um dente bicúspide ou molar.

me·si·o·buc·co·pul·pal (mē′zē-ō-buk′ō-pul′pal). Mesiobucopulpar; relativo ao ângulo que designa a junção das superfícies mesial, bucal e pulpar em uma preparação da cavidade do dente.

me·si·o·cer·vi·cal (mē′zē-ō-ser′vi-kal). Mesiocervical. **1.** Relativo ao ângulo de uma preparação cavitária na junção das paredes mesial e cervical. **2.** Relativo à área de um dente na junção da superfície mesial e da região cervical.

me·si·o·clu·sion (mē′zē-ō-kloo′zhun). Mesioclusão; uma má oclusão na qual o arco mandibular articula-se com o arco maxilar em uma posição mesial à normal; na classificação de Angle, uma má oclusão classe III. SIN mesial occlusion (2).

me·si·o·dens (mē′zē-ō-denz). Mesiodente; um dente supranumerário localizado na linha média das maxilas anteriores, entre os dentes incisivos centrais maxilares. [mesio- + L. *dens*, dente]

me·si·o·dis·tal (mē′zē-ō-dis′tal). Mesiodistal; designa o plano ou diâmetro de um dente, cortando suas superfícies mesial e distal.

me·si·o·dis·toc·clu·sal (MOD) (mē′zē-ō-dist′ō-kloo′sal,-zal). Mesiodistoclusal; designa cavidade, ou preparação cavitária ou restauração, de três superfícies (classe 2, classificação de Black) nos pré-molares (bicúspides) e molares.

me·si·o·gin·gi·val (mē′zē-ō-jin′ji-val). Mesiogengival; relativo ao ângulo formado pela junção da superfície mesial com a linha gengival de um dente.

me·si·o·gnath·ic (mē′zē-ō-nath′ik). Mesiognático; designa a má posição de uma ou de ambas as mandíbulas à frente de sua posição normal.

me·si·o·in·ci·sal (mē′zē-ō-in-sī′sal,-zal). Mesioincisal; relativo às superfícies mesial e incisal de um dente; designa o ângulo formado por sua junção.

me·si·o·la·bi·al (mē′zē-ō-lā′bē-al). Mesiolabial; relativo às superfícies mesial e labial de um dente; designa principalmente o ângulo formado por sua junção.

me·si·o·lin·gual (mē′zē-ō-ling′gwal). Mesiolingual; relativo às superfícies mesial e lingual de um dente; designa principalmente o ângulo formado por sua junção.

me·si·o·lin·guo·oc·clu·sal (mē′zē-ō-ling′gwō-ō-kloo′sal,-zal). Mesiolinguoclusal; designa o ângulo formado pela junção das superfícies mesial, lingual e oclusal de um dente bicúspide ou molar.

me·si·o·lin·guo·pul·pal (mē′zē-ō-ling′gwō-pul′pal). Mesiolinguopulpar; relativo ao ângulo que designa a junção das superfícies mesial, lingual e pulpar na preparação da cavidade em um dente.

me·sio-oc·clu·sal (mē′zē-ō-ō-kloo′sal,-zal). Mesioclusal; designa o ângulo formado pela junção das superfícies mesial e oclusal de um dente bicúspide ou molar.

me·sio-oc·clu·sion (mē′zē-ō-ō-kloo′zhun). Mesioclusão. SIN mesial occlusion (1).

me·si·o·place·ment (mē′zē-ō-plās′ment). Mesiodeslocamento. SIN mesioversion.

me·si·o·pul·pal (mē′zē-ō-pul′pal). Mesiopulpar; relativo à parede interna ou assoalho da preparação da cavidade na face mesial de um dente.

me·si·o·ver·sion (mē′zē-ō-ver-zhun). Mesioversão; má posição de um dente mesial à normal, em uma direção anterior seguindo a curvatura do arco dentário. SIN mesial displacement, mesioplacement.

Mesmer, F.A., médico austríaco, 1733–1815. VER mesmerism.

mes·mer·ism (mes′mer-izm). Mesmerismo; um sistema terapêutico a partir do qual se desenvolveram o hipnotismo e a sugestão terapêutica. [F.A. *Mesmer*, médico austríaco, 1733–1815]

mes·mer·ize (mes′mer-īz). Mesmerizar; termo obsoleto para hipnotizar. [ver mesmerism]

△ **meso-, mes-. 1.** Meio, médio, intermediário. **2.** Um mesentério, uma estrutura semelhante ao mesentério. **3.** Prefixo que designa uma substância, contendo mais de um centro quiral, que possui um plano interno de simetria; essas substâncias não exibem atividade óptica (p. ex., *meso*-cistina). [G. *mesos*]

mes·o·ap·pen·dix (mez′ō-a-pen′diks). [TA]. Mesoapêndice; o mesentério curto do apêndice situado através do íleo terminal, no qual segue a artéria apendicular. SIN mesenteriolum processus vermiformis, mesentery of appendix.

mes·o·ar·i·um (mez-ō-ar′ē-um). Mesovário. SIN mesovarium.

mes·o·bi·lane (mez-ō-bī′lān). Mesobilano; uma mesobilirrubina reduzida sem ligações duplas entre os anéis pirróis e, conseqüentemente, incolor. VER TAMBÉM bilirubinoids. SIN mesobilirubinogen, urobilinogen IXα.

mes·o·bi·lene, mesobilene- (mez-ō-bī′lēn). Mesobileno; um bilirrubinóide. VER bilirubin. SIN urobilin IXα.

mes·o·bil·i·ru·bin (mez′ō-bil-i-roo′bin). Mesobilirrubina; uma substância diferente da bilirrubina apenas porque os grupamentos vinila da bilirrubina são reduzidos a grupamentos etila. VER TAMBÉM bilirubinoids.

mes·o·bil·i·ru·bin·o·gen (mez′ō-bil-i-roo-bin′ō-jen). Mesobilirrubinogênio. SIN mesobilane.

mes·o·bil·i·vi·o·lin (mez′ō-bil-i-vī-ō′lin). Mesobiliviolina; um bilirrubinóide.

mes·o·blast (mez′ō-blast). Mesoblasto. SIN mesoderm. [meso- + G. *blastos*, germe]

mes·o·blas·te·ma (mez′ō-blas-tē′ma). Mesoblastema; todas as células que, coletivamente, constituem o mesoderma indiferenciado inicial. [meso- + G. *blastēma*, broto]

mes·o·blas·tem·ic (mez′ō-blas-tē′mik). Mesoblastêmico; relativo a ou derivado do mesoblastema.

mes·o·blas·tic (mez′ō-blas′tik). Mesoblástico; relativo a ou derivado do mesoderma.

mes·o·car·dia (mez′ō-kar′dē-a). Mesocardia. **1.** Posição atípica do coração em uma posição central no tórax, como no início da vida embrionária. **2.** Mesocárdios; plural de mesocardium. [meso- + G. *kardia*, coração]

mes·o·car·di·um, pl. **mes·o·car·dia** (mez-ō-kar′dē-um). Mesocárdio; a dupla camada de mesoderma esplâncnico que sustenta o coração embrionário na cavidade pericárdica. Desaparece antes do nascimento. [meso- + G. *kardia*, coração]

dorsal m., m. dorsal; a parte do mesocárdio dorsal ao coração embrionário; divide-se para formar o seio transverso do pericárdio.

ventral m., m. ventral; a parte do mesocárdio ventral ao tubo cardíaco embrionário; transitório em todos os vertebrados; nos mamíferos superiores, surge assim que suas camadas constituintes do epicárdio entram em contato entre si.

mes·o·car·pal (mez′ō - kar′pal). Mesocarpal. SIN midcarpal.

mes·o·ce·cal (mez′ō - sē′kal). Mesocecal; relativo ao mesoceco.

mes·o·ce·cum (mez′ō - sē′kum). Mesoceco; parte do mesocolo que sustenta o ceco e, ocasionalmente, persiste quando o colo ascendente torna-se retroperitoneal durante a vida fetal. SIN mesentery of cecum. [meso- + cecum]

mes·o·ce·phal·ic (mez′ō - se - fal′ik). Mesocefálico; que possui uma cabeça de comprimento médio; designa um crânio com um índice cefálico entre 75 e 80 e com uma capacidade de 1.350 a 1.450 ml, ou um indivíduo com esse crânio. SIN mesaticephalic, mesocephalous, normocephalic. [meso- + G. kephalē, cabeça]

mes·o·ceph·a·lous (mez′ō - sef′a - lŭs). Mesocéfalo. SIN mesocephalic.

Mes·o·ces·toi·des (mez - ō - ses - toy′dēz). Gênero de tênia encontrado em mamíferos carnívoros, como raposas; os ácaros provavelmente são hospedeiros intermediários; alguns casos humanos foram identificados no Japão, nos Estados Unidos e na China.

mes·o·col·ic (mez′ō - kol′ik). Mesocólico; relativo ao mesocolo.

mes·o·co·lon (mez′ō - kō′lon). [TA]. Mesocolo; a prega de peritônio que fixa o colo à parede abdominal posterior; o m. ascendente [TA], m. transverso [TA], m. descendente [TA] e m. sigmóide [TA] correspondem às respectivas divisões do colo; as porções ascendente e descendente geralmente são fundidas ao peritônio da parede abdominal posterior, mas podem ser mobilizadas. [meso- + kolon, colo]

mes·o·co·lo·pexy (mez′ō - kō′lō - pek - sē). Mesocolopexia; uma operação para encurtar o mesocolo, para corrigir mobilidade indevida e ptose. SIN mesocoloplication. [meso- + G. kolon, colo, + pēxis, fixação]

mes·o·co·lo·pli·ca·tion (mes′ō - kō′lō - pli - kā′shŭn). Mesocoloplicatura. SIN mesocolopexy. [meso- + G. kolon, colo, + L. plico, pp. -atus, dobrar]

mes·o·cord (mez′ō - kōrd). Mesocórdio; uma prega de âmnio que algumas vezes une um segmento do cordão umbilical à placenta.

mes·o·cu·ne·i·form (mez′ō - koo′nē - i - fōrm). Mesocuneiforme. SIN intermediate cuneiform (bone).

mes·o·derm (mez′ō - derm). Mesoderma; a camada intermediária das três camadas germinativas primárias do embrião (sendo as outras o ectoderma e o endoderma); o m. é a origem dos tecidos conjuntivos, mioblastos, sangue, sistemas cardiovascular e linfático, a maior parte do sistema urogenital e o revestimento das cavidades pericárdica, pleural e peritoneal. SIN mesoblast. [meso- + G. derma, pele]

branchial m., m. branquial; m. que circunda o estomódio primitivo e a faringe; contribui para a formação dos arcos faríngeos.

extraembryonic m., m. extra-embrionário; células extra-embrionárias que, embora sejam derivadas do zigoto, não são parte do embrião propriamente dito e contribuem para a formação das membranas fetais (p. ex., âmnio). SIN primary m.

gastral m., m. gástrico; m. nos vertebrados inferiores formado por constrição do teto do arquêntero ou do saco vitelino.

intermediate m., m. intermediário; uma faixa contínua de m. entre o m. paraxial segmentado medialmente e o m. da lâmina lateral lateralmente; a partir dele se desenvolve o cordão nefrogênico.

intraembryonic m., m. intra-embrionário; m. derivado da estria primitiva e situado entre o ectoderma e o endoderma. SIN secondary m.

lateral m., m. lateral. SIN lateral plate m.

lateral plate m., m. da lâmina lateral; a porção periférica do m. intra-embrionário, contínua com o m. extra-embrionário além das margens do disco embrionário; forma os m. somático e esplâncnico entre os quais se desenvolve o celoma intra-embrionário. SIN lateral m.

paraxial m., m. paraxial; o m. situado de cada lado da notocorda embrionária mediana; após segmentação, forma o par de somitos.

primary m., m. primário. SIN extraembryonic m.

prostomial m., m. prostômico; m. que surge em vertebrados inferiores por proliferação contínua nos lábios laterais do blastoporo.

secondary m., m. secundário. SIN intraembryonic m.

somatic m., m. somático; m. adjacente ao ectoderma no embrião inicial, após formação do celoma intra-embrionário; os membros e a parede do corpo são parcialmente derivados dele.

somitic m., m. somítico; m. derivado de células situadas nos somitos ou derivadas deles.

splanchnic m., m. esplâncnico; a camada de m. da lâmina lateral adjacente ao endoderma.

visceral m., m. visceral; o m. esplâncnico ou branquial.

mes·o·der·mal (mez - ō - der′mal). Mesodérmico; relativo ao mesoderma.

mes·o·der·mic (mez - ō - der′mik). Mesodérmico; relativo ao mesoderma.

mes·o·di·a·stol·ic (mez - ō - dī - ā - stol′ik). Mesodiastólico.

mes·o·dont (mez′ō - dont). Mesodonte; que possui dentes de tamanho médio; designa um crânio com um índice dentário entre 42 e 43,9. [meso- + G. odous, dente]

mes·o·du·o·de·nal (mez′ō - doo - ō - dē′nal). Mesoduodenal; relativo ao mesoduodeno.

mes·o·du·o·de·num (mez′ō - doo′ō - dē′nŭm, - doo - od′ē - nŭm). Mesoduodeno; o mesentério do duodeno.

mes·o·en·te·ri·o·lum (mes′ō - en - ter - ē′ō - lŭm). Mesoenteríolo. SIN mesenteriolum.

mes·o·ep·i·did·y·mis (mez - ō - ep - i - did′i - mis). Mesoepidídimo; uma prega ocasional da túnica vaginal unindo o epidídimo ao testículo. [meso- + epididymis]

mes·o·gas·ter (mez - ō - gas′ter). Mesogástrio. SIN mesogastrium.

mes·o·gas·tric (mez - ō - gas′trik). Mesogástrico; relativo ao mesogástrio.

mes·o·gas·tri·um (mez - ō - gas′trē - ŭm). Mesogástrio; no embrião, o mesentério da porção dilatada do canal entérico que é o futuro estômago; dá origem ao omento maior e, conseqüentemente, está envolvido na formação da bolsa omental. O baço e o corpo do pâncreas se desenvolvem em seu interior, e, assim, os ligamentos esplenorrenal e gastroesplênico são derivados do mesogástrio (dorsal). SIN dorsal m., mesogaster. [meso- + G. gastēr, estômago]

dorsal m., m. dorsal. SIN mesogastrium.

ventral m., m. ventral; o mesentério primitivo da linha média que se estende entre o futuro estômago e porção proximal do duodeno e a parede abdominal anterior, superior ao umbigo (veia umbilical). O fígado desenvolve-se em seu interior, e, consequentemente, o omento menor, os ligamentos coronário e falciforme são derivados dele. A veia umbilical segue em sua borda livre caudal, tornando-se o ligamento redondo do fígado após o nascimento.

mes·o·gen·ic (mez - ō - jen′ik). Mesogênico; designa a virulência de um vírus capaz de induzir infecção letal em embriões hospedeiros, após um breve período de incubação, e uma infecção inaparente em hospedeiros imaturos e adultos; usado na caracterização do vírus da doença de Newcastle, particularmente cepas usadas na vacinação parenteral de galinhas. [meso- + G. –gen, que produz]

me·sog·li·a (me - sog′lē - ă). Mesóglia; células neurogliais de origem mesodérmica. VER TAMBÉM microglia. SIN mesoglial cells. [meso- + G. glia, cola]

mes·o·glu·te·al (mez′ō - gloo′tē - ăl). Mesoglúteo; relativo ao músculo glúteo médio.

mes·o·glu·te·us (mez′ō - gloo - tē′ŭs). Glúteo médio. SIN gluteus medius (muscle).

mes·o·gnath·ic (mez - ō - nath′ik, - og - nath′ik). Mesognático. **1.** Relativo ao mesognátio. **2.** SIN mesognathous.

mes·o·gna·thi·on (mez′ō - nā′thē - on, -og - nā′thē - on, nath′ē - on). Mesognátio; o segmento lateral do osso pré-maxilar ou incisivo externo ao endognátio. [meso- + G. gnathos, mandíbula]

me·sog·na·thous (me - zog′nă - thŭs). Mesognático; que possui uma face com a mandíbula discretamente projetada, com um índice gnático de 98 a 103. SIN mesognathic (2).

mes·o·il·e·um (mez - ō - il′ē - ŭm). Mesoíleo; o mesentério do íleo.

mes·o·je·ju·num (mez′ō - je - joo′nŭm). Mesojejuno; o mesentério do jejuno.

me·sol·o·bus (me - sol′ō - bŭs). Mesolobo; termo obsoleto para corpo caloso (corpus callosum). [meso- + L. lobus, lobo]

mes·o·lym·pho·cyte (mez - ō - lim′fō - sit). Mesolinfócito; um leucócito mononuclear de tamanho médio, provavelmente um linfócito, com um núcleo grande de coloração intensa, mas relativamente menor que na maioria dos linfócitos. [meso- + lymphocyte]

mes·o·me·li·a (mez - ō - mē′lē - ă). Mesomelia; a condição de apresentar encurtamento anormal dos antebraços e da parte inferior das pernas. [meso- + G. melos, membro]

mes·o·mel·ic (mez - ō - me′lik). Mesomélico; relativo ao segmento médio de um membro.

mes·o·mere (mez′ō - mēr). Mesômero. **1.** Blastômero de tamanho intermediário entre um macrômero e um micrômero. **2.** A zona entre um epímero e um hipômero. [meso- + G. meros, parte]

mes·o·mer·ic (mez - ō - mēr′ik). Mesomérico; relativo a mesomerismo.

me·som·er·ism (mē - som′er - izm). Mesomerismo; deslocamento de elétrons em uma molécula, de forma a criar cargas elétricas fracionárias em diferentes partes da molécula; ressonância.

mes·o·me·tri·um (mez′ō - mē′trē - ŭm). Mesométrio; o ligamento largo do útero, abaixo da mesossalpinge. [meso- + G. mētra, útero]

mes·o·morph (mez′ō - morf). Mesomorfo; tipo ou construção constitucional do corpo (biotipo ou somatotipo) em que prevalecem os tecidos originados do mesoderma; do ponto de vista morfológico, há um equilíbrio entre troncos e membros. VER TAMBÉM hypermorph, hypomorph, ectomorph, endomorph. SIN mediotype. [meso- + G. morphē, forma]

mes·o·mor·phic (mez - ō - morf′ik). Mesomórfico; relativo ao mesomorfismo.

me·son (mez′on, mē′zon, mes′on). Meson; uma partícula elementar que possui uma massa em repouso de valor intermediário entre a massa de um elétron e a massa de um próton. [G. neutro de mesos, médio]

mes·o·neph·ric (mez-ō-nef′rik). Mesonéfrico; relativo ao mesonefro.

mes·o·neph·roi (mez-ō-nef′roy). Mesonefros; plural de mesonephros.

mes·o·ne·phro·ma (mez′ō-ne-frō′mă). Mesonefroma; termo obsoleto para uma neoplasia maligna relativamente rara do ovário e do corpo do útero, sendo considerada originada em estruturas mesonéfricas deslocadas do tecido ovariano durante o desenvolvimento embrionário; caracterizado por um padrão tubular, com proliferação focal de células epiteliais com citoplasma claro ou em forma de cravo; são descritas estruturas glomerulóides, isto é, pequenas convoluções ou tufos de pequenas formações tubulares com capilares estendendo-se até o interior dos espaços. SIN clear cell carcinoma, mesonephric adenocarcinoma, mesonephroid tumor, wolffian duct carcinoma. [mesonephros + -oma, tumor]

mes·o·neph·ros, pl. **mes·o·neph·roi** (mez′ō-nef′ros, -roy). Mesonefro; um dos três órgãos excretores que aparecem na evolução de vertebrados; nas formas de vida com um metanefro, o mesonefro está localizado entre o pronefro em regressão e o metanefro, cefálico em relação a este último. Em embriões jovens de mamíferos, o mesonefro é bem desenvolvido e funciona brevemente até o estabelecimento do metanefro, o rim definitivo; em embriões mais velhos, o mesonefro sofre regressão como órgão excretor, mas seu sistema ductal é mantido no homem como epidídimo e ducto deferente. SIN middle kidney, wolffian body. [meso- + G. *nephros,* rim]

mes·o·neu·ri·tis (mez′ō-noo-rī′tis). Mesoneurite; inflamação de um nervo ou de seu tecido conjuntivo sem envolvimento de sua bainha.

   nodular m., m. nodular; inflamação do tecido conjuntivo sob a bainha nervosa, com a formação de espessamentos fibrosos circunscritos.

meso-on·to·morph (mez-ō-on′tō-mōrf). Mesontomorfo; um indivíduo largo e atarracado. [meso- + G. *on,* sendo, + *morphē,* forma]

mes·o·pexy (mez′ō-pek-sē). Mesopexia. SIN mesenteriopexy.

mes·o·phil, mes·o·phile (mez′ō-fil, -fīl). Mesófilo; um microrganismo com uma temperatura ideal entre 25°C e 40°C, mas que cresce dentro dos limites de 10°C e 45°C. [meso- + G. *philos,* amigo]

mes·o·phil·ic (mez′ō-fil′ik). Mesofílico; relativo a um mesófilo.

mes·o·phle·bi·tis (mez′ō-fle-bī′tis). Mesoflebite; inflamação da túnica média de uma veia. [meso- + phlebitis]

mes·o·phrag·ma (mez-ō-frag′mă). Mesofragma. SIN M *line.* [meso- + G. *phragma,* cerca]

me·soph·ry·on (mez-of′ri-on). Mesófrio. SIN glabella (2). [meso- + Gr. *ophrys,* supercílio]

me·sop·ic (me-zō′pik). Mesópico; relativo à iluminação entre as faixas fotópica e escotópica. [meso- + G. *opsis,* visão]

mes·o·pneu·mo·ni·um (mez′ō-noo-mō′nē-um). Mesopneumônio; a reflexão da pleura que circunda a raiz do pulmão (incluindo o ligamento pulmonar inferiormente), enquanto a pleura parietal torna-se contínua com a pleura visceral do pulmão. SIN mesentery of lung, pleural isthmus.

mes·o·por·phy·rins (mez-ō-pōr′fi-rinz). Mesoporfirinas; compostos porfirínicos semelhantes às protoporfirinas, exceto pelo fato de as cadeias laterais vinila desta última serem reduzidas a cadeias laterais etila; p. ex., mesobilano.

mes·o·proc·ton. Fáscia retossacral. SIN rectosacral *fascia.*

mes·o·pro·sop·ic (mez′ō-prō-sop′ik). Mesoprosópico; que possui a face de largura moderada, isto é, com um índice facial de aproximadamente 90. [meso- + G. *prosōpon,* face]

mes·o·pul·mon·um (mez-ō-pŭl′mon-ŭm). Mesopulmão; o mesentério do pulmão embrionário. [meso- + L. *pulmo,* pulmão]

me·sor·chi·al (mez-ōr′kē-ăl). Mesórquico; relativo ao mesórquio.

me·sor·chi·um (mez-ōr′kē-ŭm). Mesórquio. **1.** No feto, uma prega de túnica vaginal do testículo que sustenta o mesonefro e o testículo em desenvolvimento. **2.** No adulto, uma prega de túnica vaginal testicular entre o testículo e o epidídimo. [meso- + G. *orchis,* testículo]

mes·o·rec·tum (mez-ō-rek′tŭm). Mesorreto; o revestimento peritoneal do reto, cobrindo apenas a parte superior.

mes·o·rid·a·zine be·syl·ate (mez-ō-rid′ă-zēn). Besilato de mesoridazina; um produto da biotransformação da tioridazina; um antipsicótico.

mes·or·rha·phy (mez-ōr′ă-fē). Mesorrafia. SIN mesenteriorrhaphy.

mes·or·rhine (mez′ō-rīn). Mesorríneo; que possui um nariz de largura moderada. Designa um crânio com um índice nasal de 47 a 51 (acordo de Frankfort) ou de 48 a 53 (Broca). [meso- + G. *rhis* (rhin-), nariz]

mes·o·sal·pinx (mez′ō-sal′pinks). [TA]. Mesossalpinge; a parte do ligamento largo que reveste a tuba uterina (de Falópio). [meso- + G. *salpinx,* trompa]

mes·o·scope (mez′ō-skōp). Mesoscópio; instrumento para observação de objetos maiores que os microscópicos, mas que não podem ser observados distintamente a olho nu. [meso- + G. *skopeō,* ver]

mes·o·seme (mez′ō-sēm). Mesossema; designa uma abertura orbitária com um índice entre 84 e 89; característico da raça branca. [meso- + G. *sēma,* sinal]

mes·o·sig·moid (mez′ō-sig′moyd). Mesossigmóide; mesocolo sigmóide. VER mesocolon.

mes·o·sig·moid·i·tis (mes′ō-sig-moy-dī′tis). Mesossigmoidite; inflamação do mesossigmóide.

mes·o·sig·moid·o·pexy (mez-ō-sig-moy′dō-pek-sē). Mesossigmoidopexia; fixação cirúrgica do mesossigmóide.

mes·o·so·ma·tous (mez′ō-sō′mă-tŭs). Mesossomático; designa uma pessoa de altura média.

mes·o·some (mez′ōsom). Mesossomo; um corpo membranoso convoluto formado por involução das membranas plasmáticas de determinadas bactérias; atua na respiração celular e na formação do septo. [meso- + G. *soma,* corpo]

mes·o·so·mia (mez′ō-sō′mē-ă). Mesossomia; altura média. [meso- + G. *sōma,* corpo]

mes·o·ste·ni·um (mez′ō-stē′nē-ŭm). Mesostênio. SIN mesentery (2).

mes·o·ster·num (mez′ō-ster′nŭm). Mesosterno. SIN body of sternum. [meso- + G. *sternon,* tórax]

mes·o·sys·tol·ic (mez′ō-sis-tol′ik). Mesossistólico.

mes·o·tar·sal (mez′ō-tar′săl). Mesotársico. SIN midtarsal.

mes·o·ten·di·ne·um (mez′ō-ten-din′ē-ŭm) [TA]. Mesotendíneo. SIN mesotendon.

mes·o·ten·don (mez′ō-ten′don) [TA]. Mesotendão; as camadas sinoviais que seguem de um tendão até a parede de uma bainha tendínea em determinados lugares onde os tendões se situam no interior de canais osteofibrosos. Na maioria dos casos, o mesotendão degenera-se, deixando apenas os vínculos. SIN mesotendineum [TA].

mes·o·the·lia (mez-ō-thē′lē-ă). Mesotélios; plural de mesothelium.

mes·o·the·li·al (mez-ō-thē′lē-ăl). Mesotelial; relativo ao mesotélio.

mes·o·the·li·o·ma (mez′ō-thē-lē-ō′mă). Mesotelioma; uma neoplasia rara das células de revestimento da pleura e periósteo, crescendo como um folheto espesso que cobre as vísceras; é composto de células fusiformes ou tecido fibroso que pode encerrar espaços glandulares revestidos por células cúbicas. [mesothelium + G. *-oma,* tumor]

   benign m., m. benigno. SIN solitary fibrous *tumor.*

   benign m. of genital tract, m. benigno do sistema genital. SIN adenomatoid *tumor.*

mes·o·the·li·um, pl. **mes·o·the·lia** (mez-ō-thē′lē-ŭm, -lē-ă). Mesotélio; uma camada única de células achatadas formando um epitélio que reveste cavidades serosas; p. ex., peritônio, pleura, pericárdio. [meso- + epithelium]

mes·o·tho·ri·um (mez′ō-thōr′ē-ŭm). Mesotório; os primeiros dois produtos da desintegração do tório; o mesotório 1 é Ra^{228}, um emissor beta com meia-vida de 6,7 anos, que se decompõe em mesotório 2, que é Ac^{228}, um emissor beta com uma meia-vida de 6,13 h, que se desintegra em radiotório (Th^{228}).

mes·o·tro·pic (mez′ō-trop′ik). Mesotrópico; voltado para o plano mediano. [meso- + G. *tropē,* uma volta]

mes·o·tym·pan·um (mez-ō-tim′pan-ŭm). Mesotímpano; a parte da orelha média medial à membrana timpânica.

mes·o·u·ran·ic (mes′ō-ū-ran′ik). Mesourânico; que possui um índice palatino entre 110 e 115. SIN measuranic. [meso- + G. *ouranos,* palato]

mes·o·va·ri·um, pl. **mes·o·va·ria** (mez′ō-vā′rē-ŭm, -ă) [TA]. Mesovário; parte do ligamento largo do útero que se reflete sobre o ovário e o suspende. SIN mesoarium. [meso- + L. *ovarium,* ovário]

Mes·o·zoa (mez-ō-zō′ă). Pequeno filo com aproximadamente 50 espécies de parasitas de invertebrados marinhos, com ciclos vitais complexos. Os Mesozoa são classificados com os Metazoa, mas alguns observadores os consideram intermediários entre animais unicelulares e multicelulares; outros os consideram um grupo degenerado de platelmintos. Os Mesozoa são divididos em duas ordens muito distintas: a Orthonectida e a Dicyemida; estes últimos são parasitas nefrídios de lulas, polvos e moluscos. [meso- + G. *zōon,* animal]

mes·sen·ger (mes′en-jer). Mensageiro. **1.** Aquele que conduz uma mensagem. **2.** Que possui propriedades de condução de mensagem.

   first m., primeiro m.; hormônio que se liga a um receptor na superfície da célula e, ao fazê-lo, comunica-se com processos metabólicos intracelulares.

   second m., segundo m.; uma molécula intermediária gerada em conseqüência de interação hormônio-receptor; p. ex., ver adenosine 3′,5′-cyclic monophosphate (3′5′-monofosfato cíclico de adenosina), guanosine 3′,5′-cyclic monophosphate (3′5′-monofosfato cíclico de guanosina), calcium (cálcio), inositide (inositida).

mes·sen·ger RNA (mRNA). RNA mensageiro. VER em ribonucleic acid.

mes·tan·o·lone (mes-tan′ō-lōn). Mestanolona; esteróide androgênico com propriedades anabólicas.

mes·tene·di·ol (mes-tēn′dī-ol). Mestenediol. SIN methandriol.

mes·tra·nol (mes′tră-nōl). Mestranol; o éter 3-metil do etinil estradiol; um estrogênio usado em muitos contraceptivos orais.

me·sul·phen (mē-sŭl′fen). Messulfeno; escabicida tópico com propriedades antipruriginosas.

me·su·ran·ic (mez′ū-ran′ik). Mesurânico. SIN mesouranic.

MET Abreviatura de metabolic *equivalent* (equivalente metabólico).

Met Símbolo de methionine (metionina) ou methionyl (metionil).

meta-. Meta-; em medicina e biologia, um prefixo que designa o conceito de após, subseqüente a, atrás ou posterior. Cf. post-. [G. após, entre, sobre]

meta-. *Meta-.* **1.** Em química, um prefixo em itálico que designa junta, compartilhamento de ação. **2** (*m-*). Em química, um prefixo em itálico que designa uma substância formada por duas substituições no anel benzeno separadas por um átomo de carbono, isto é, ligado ao primeiro e terceiro, segundo e quarto, etc., átomos de carbono do anel. Quanto aos termos que começam com *meta-* ou *m-*, ver o nome específico. [G. após, entre, sobre]

met·a·nal·y·sis (met′ă - năl′ĭ - sĭs). Metaanálise; o processo de usar métodos estatísticos para combinar os resultados de diferentes estudos; avaliação sistemática, organizada e estruturada de um problema utilizando informações, comumente na forma de quadros estatísticos, de vários estudos diferentes de um problema.

me·tab·a·sis (mĕ - tăb′ă - sĭs). Metabase; termo raramente usado para uma modificação de qualquer tipo nos sintomas ou na evolução de uma doença. [G. passagem sobre, mudança, de *metabaino*, passar sobre]

met·a·bi·o·sis (met′ă - bī - ō′sĭs). Metabiose; dependência de um organismo de outro para sua existência. VER TAMBÉM commensalism, mutualism, parasitism. [meta- + G. *biosis*, forma de vida]

met·a·bol·ic (met - ă - bŏl′ĭk). Metabólico; relativo ao metabolismo.

met·a·bo·lim·e·ter (met′ă - bō - lĭm′ĕ - ter). Metabolímetro; calorímetro modificado para medir a taxa de metabolismo basal.

me·tab·o·lin (mĕ - tăb′ō - lĭn). Metabolina. SIN metabolite.

me·tab·o·lism (mĕ - tăb′ō - lĭzm). Metabolismo. **1.** A soma das alterações químicas e físicas que ocorrem no tecido, e consistem em anabolismo, reações que convertem pequenas moléculas em grandes moléculas, e catabolismo, reações que convertem grandes moléculas em pequenas, incluindo tanto grandes moléculas endógenas quanto a biodegradação de xenobióticos. **2.** Freqüentemente é usado incorretamente como sinônimo de anabolismo ou catabolismo. [G. *metabole*, alteração]

basal m., m. basal; utilização de oxigênio de um indivíduo durante atividade fisiológica mínima em vigília; um teste obsoleto determinado por medida do consumo de oxigênio de um indivíduo em jejum, em completo repouso corporal e mental, e a uma temperatura ambiente de 20°C. SIN basal metabolic rate.

carbohydrate m., m. dos carboidratos; oxidação, degradação e síntese de carboidratos nos tecidos.

electrolyte m., m. eletrolítico; as alterações químicas que vários minerais essenciais (p. ex., sódio, potássio, cálcio, magnésio) sofrem nos tecidos.

energy m., m. energético; reações metabólicas cujo papel é liberar ou fornecer energia.

fat m., m. de lipídios; oxidação, decomposição e síntese de gorduras nos tecidos.

first-pass m., m. na primeira passagem; a degradação ou alteração intestinal e hepática de uma droga ou substância ingerida, após absorção, removendo parte da substância ativa do sangue antes de entrar na circulação geral. SIN first-pass effect.

inborn error of m., erro congênito do metabolismo; distúrbio bioquímico genético de uma enzima específica que forma um bloqueio metabólico, p. ex., fenilcetonúria.

intermediary m., m. intermediário; a soma de todas as reações metabólicas entre absorção de alimentos e formação de produtos excretores.

oxidative m., m. oxidativo. SIN ventilation (2).

primary m., m. primário; processos metabólicos fundamentais para a maioria das células; p. ex., biossíntese de macromoléculas, produção de energia, renovação, etc.

protein m., m. das proteínas; decomposição e síntese de proteínas nos tecidos. SIN proteometabolism.

respiratory m., m. respiratório; a troca de gases respiratórios nos pulmões, oxidação de alimentos nos tecidos e produção de dióxido de carbono e água.

secondary m., m. secundário; processos metabólicos nos quais substâncias (como pigmentos, alcalóides, terpenos, etc.) só são sintetizadas em determinados tipos de tecidos ou células ou só são sintetizadas em determinadas condições.

me·tab·o·lite (mĕ - tăb′ō - līt). Metabólito; qualquer produto ou substrato (alimentar, intermediário, residual) do metabolismo, principalmente do catabolismo. SIN metabolin.

primary m., m. primário; metabólito sintetizado em uma etapa no metabolismo primário.

secondary m., m. secundário; metabólito sintetizado em uma etapa no metabolismo secundário.

me·tab·o·lize (mĕ - tăb′ō - līz). Metabolizar; sofrer as alterações químicas do metabolismo.

met·a·car·pal (met′ă - kăr′păl). Metacarpal. **1.** Relativo ao metacarpo. **2.** Qualquer um dos ossos do metacarpo. VER metacarpal (*bones*) [I–V], em *bone*.

met·a·car·pec·to·my (met′ă - kăr - pĕk′tō - mē). Metacarpectomia; excisão de um ou de todos os metacarpais. [metacarpus + G. *ektome*, excisão]

met·a·car·po·pha·lan·ge·al (met′ă - kăr′pō - fă - lăn′jē - ăl). Metacarpofalângico; relativo ao metacarpo e às falanges; designa as articulações entre eles.

met·a·car·pus, pl. **met·a·car·pi** (met′ă - kăr′pŭs, - kăr′pī). Metacarpo; os cinco ossos da mão entre o carpo e as falanges. [meta- + G. *karpos*, punho]

met·a·cen·tric (met - ă - sen′trĭk). Metacêntrico; que possui o centrômero aproximadamente eqüidistante das extremidades, refere-se a um cromossomo. [meta- + G. *kentron*, círculo]

met·a·cer·ca·ria, pl. **met·a·cer·ca·ri·ae** (met′ă - ser - kar′ē - ă, - ē). Metacercária; a fase encistada pós-cercariana no ciclo biológico de um trematódeo, antes da transferência para o hospedeiro definitivo. Algumas cercárias fixam-se à grama ou a outra vegetação, formam metacercárias e, depois, são ingeridas por herbívoros, como a *Fasciola* e formas semelhantes; outras encistam-se nos músculos de peixes, como o *Clonorchis*, ou no camarão de água doce, como o *Paragonimus*. [meta- + G. *kerkos*, cauda]

met·a·ces·tode (met - ă - sĕs′tōd). Metacestódeo; as fases larvares de uma tênia, incluindo a metamorfose da oncosfera como primeiro sinal de sexualidade no verme adulto, diferenciação do escólex e início da formação de proglotes; inclui as fases pró-cercóide e plerocercóide de cestódeos pseudofilídeos e as fases de cisticerco, cisticercóide, ceuro e hidátide de cestódeos ciclofilídeos.

met·a·chlo·ral (met - ă - klō′răl). Metacloral. SIN m-cloral.

met·a·chro·ma·sia (met′ă - krō - mā′zē - ă). Metacromasia. **1.** A condição na qual uma célula ou um componente tecidual adquire uma cor diferente do corante com que é corado. SIN metachromatism (2). **2.** Uma alteração na cor característica de determinados corantes tiazina básicos, como azul de toluidina, quando as moléculas de corante são unidas em sucessão imediata aos polímeros polianiônicos teciduais, como as glicosaminoglicanas. [meta- + G. *chroma*, cor]

met·a·chro·mat·ic (met′ă - krō - mat′ĭk). Metacromático; designa células ou corantes que exibem metacromasia. SIN metachromophil, metachromophile.

met·a·chro·ma·tism (met - ă - krō′mă - tĭzm). Metacromatismo. **1.** Qualquer mudança de cor, seja natural ou produzida por corantes anilina básicos. **2.** SIN metachromasia (1). [meta- + G. *chroma*, cor]

met·a·chrom·ing (met′ă - krō′mĭng). Metacromagem; o processo de misturar um mordente metálico com um corante antes de aplicá-lo em um tecido.

met·a·chro·mo·phil, met·a·chro·mo·phile (met - ă - krō′mō - fĭl, - fīl). Metacromófilo. SIN metachromatic. [meta- + G. *chroma*, cor, + *philos*, amigo]

me·tach·ro·nous (mĕ - tăk′rō - nŭs). Metacrônico; não-sincrônico; múltiplas ocorrências separadas, como múltiplos cânceres primários que se desenvolvem de tempo em tempo. [meta- + G. *chronos*, tempo]

met·a·chro·sis (met - ă - krō′sĭs). Metacrose; uma mudança de cor, como a que ocorre em determinados animais, p. ex., o camaleão, por expansão e contração dos cromatóforos. [meta- + G. *chrosis*, coloração]

met·a·cone (met′ă - kōn). Metacone; a cúspide distobucal de um dente molar superior. [meta- + G. *konos*, cone]

met·a·co·nid (met - ă - kon′ĭd, - kō′nĭd). Metaconídio; a cúspide mesolingual de um dente molar inferior.

met·a·con·trast (met - ă - kon′trast). Metacontraste; inibição do brilho de iluminação quando um campo visual adjacente é iluminado.

met·a·con·ule (met - ă - kon′ŭl). Metacônulo; a cúspide intermediária distal de um dente molar superior. [meta- + G. *konos*, cone]

met·a·cre·sol (met - ă - krē′sol). Metacresol. SIN m-cresol.

met·a·cryp·to·zo·ite (met′ă - krĭp - tō - zō′ĭt). Metacriptozoíta; o estágio exoeritrocítico que se desenvolve a partir de merozoítas formados pela primeira geração, ou criptozoíta; as gerações criptozoíta e metacriptozoíta compreendem os estágios exoeritrocíticos primários de desenvolvimento da malária (período pré-patente) antes da infecção das hemácias. [meta- + G. *kryptos*, oculto, + *zoon*, animal]

met·a·dys·en·tery (met - ă - dĭs′en - tăr - ē). Metadisenteria; termo antigo para bacillary *dysentery* (disenteria bacilar).

Met·a·gon·i·mus (met - ă - gon′ĭ - mŭs). Gênero de trematódeos (superfamília Heterophyundea) que se encistam no peixe e infectam vários animais que comem peixe, incluindo seres humanos. *M. yokogawai*, um trematódeo intestinal amplamente distribuído no Extremo Oriente e nos Bálcãs e um dos menores trematódeos (1–2,5 mm) que infectam o homem, passa dos caramujos *Semisulcospira* para os peixes ciprinóides e, depois, para os seres humanos e outros mamíferos e aves que comem peixe. [meta- + G. *gonimos*, produtivo]

met·a·ic·ter·ic (met - ă - ĭk′tĕr - ĭk). Metaictérico; que ocorre como uma seqüela de icterícia. [meta- + G. *ikterikos*, ictérico]

met·a·in·fec·tive (met′ă - ĭn - fek′tĭv). Metainfeccioso; que ocorre após uma infecção; designa especificamente uma condição febril observada algumas vezes durante a convalescença de uma doença infecciosa.

met·a·ki·ne·sis, met·a·ki·ne·sia (met′ă - ki - nē′sĭs, - ki - nē′sē - ă). Metacinesia; movimento de afastamento; a separação das duas cromátides de cada cromossoma e seu movimento para pólos opostos na anáfase da mitose. [meta- + G. *kinesis*, movimento]

met·al (M) (met′ăl). Metal; um dos elementos eletropositivos, anfotérico ou básico, geralmente caracterizado por propriedades como brilho, maleabilidade, ductilidade, capacidade de conduzir eletricidade e tendência a perder, ao invés de ganhar, elétrons em reações químicas. [L. *metallum*, mina, mineral, do G. *metallon*, mina, poço de mina]

metal (M)   978   **metaplasia**

alkali m., m. alcalino; um álcali da família Li, Na, K, Rb, Cs e Fr, todos os quais possuem hidróxidos muito ionizados. SIN alkali (3).
alkali earth m., m. alcalino-terroso. VER alkaline earth *elements*, em *element*.
Babbitt m., m. de Babbitt; uma liga de antimônio, cobre e estanho; usada ocasionalmente em odontologia.
base m., basic m., m. de base, m. básico; metal facilmente oxidado; p. ex., ferro, cobre.
colloidal m., m. coloidal; solução coloidal de um metal obtida pela passagem de centelhas elétricas entre terminais do metal em água destilada. SIN electrosol.
d'Arcet m., m. d'Arcet; liga de chumbo, bismuto e estanho; usada em odontologia.
fusible m., m. fusível; metal com baixo ponto de fusão.
heavy m., m. pesado; metal com alta densidade específica, tipicamente maior que 5; p. ex., Fe, Co, Cu, Mn, Mo, Zn, V.
light m., m. leve; metal com densidade específica menor que 4.
noble m., m. nobre; metal que não pode ser oxidado apenas pelo calor, nem é facilmente dissolvido por ácido; p. ex., ouro, platina. SIN noble element.
rare earth m., m. terras-raras. VER lanthanides.
respiratory m., m. respiratório; metal presente em certos pigmentos respiratórios; p. ex., ferro, manganês, cobre, vanádio.
met·al·de·hyde (met - al′dĕ - hīd). Metaldeído; polímero do acetaldeído. [meta- + aldehyde]
me·tal·lic (mĕ - tal′ik). Metálico; relativo a, composto de ou semelhante a metal.
♻ **metallo-.** Metalo-; metal, metálico. [ver metal]
me·tal·lo·cy·a·nide (mĕ - tal - ō - sī′ă - nīd). Metalocianeto; composto de cianogênio com um metal, formando um radical iônico que se combina a um elemento básico para formar um sal; p. ex., ferricianeto de potássio, $K_3Fe(CN)_6$.
me·tal·lo·en·zyme (mĕ - tal - ō - en′zīm). Metaloenzima; uma enzima que contém um metal (íon) como parte integrante de sua estrutura ativa; p. ex., citocromos (Fe, Cu), aldeído oxidase (Mo), catecol oxidase (Cu), anidrase carbônica (Zn).
me·tal·lo·fla·vo·de·hy·dro·ge·nase (mĕ - tal′ō - flā′vō - dē - hī′drō - jen - ās). Metaloflavodesidrogenase; um tipo de enzima oxidante que contém os nucleotídeos flavina como coenzima mais um íon metálico, também necessário para a ação; o metal pode ser Fe (como na succinato desidrogenase), Cu (como na urato oxidase) ou Mo (como na xantina oxidase).
me·tal·lo·fla·vo·en·zyme (mĕ - tal′ō - flā - vō - en′zīm). Metaloflavoenzima; enzima que contém um dos nucleotídeos flavina e, pelo menos, um íon metálico como uma parte necessária de sua estrutura ativa.
me·tal·lo·fla·vo·pro·tein (mĕ - tal′ō - flā′vō - prō - tēn). Metaloflavoproteína; uma proteína que contém um elemento flavina e, pelo menos, um íon metálico.
met·al·loid (met′ă - loyd). Metalóide; semelhante a um metal em, pelo menos, uma forma anfotérica; p. ex., o silício e o germânio como semicondutores. [metal- + G. *eidos*, semelhança]
me·tal·lo·phil·ia (mĕ - tal′ō - fil′ē - ă). Metalofilia; afinidade por sais metálicos; p. ex., a afinidade do citoplasma de células do sistema reticuloendotelial pela coloração com carbonato de prata e sais de ouro e ferro. [metallo- + G. *philos*, amigo]
me·tal·lo·pho·bia (mĕ - tal′ō - fō′bē - ă). Metalofobia; medo mórbido de objetos metálicos. [G. *metallon*, metal, + *phobos*, medo]
me·tal·lo·por·phy·rin (mĕ - tal - ō - pōr′fi - rin). Metaloporfirina; combinação de uma porfirina com um metal, p. ex., Fe (heme), Mg (como na clorofila), Cu (na hemocianina), Zn.
me·tal·lo·pro·tein (mĕ - tal - ō - prō′tēn). Metaloproteína; uma proteína com um íon ou íons metálicos firmemente ligados; p. ex., hemoglobina.
metalloproteinase (met′a - lō - prō′tēn - āz). Metaloproteinase; família de endopeptidases que hidrolisam proteínas e contêm íons zinco como parte da estrutura ativa.
matrix m., m. matriz; subfamília de endopeptidases que hidrolisam proteínas extracelulares, principalmente colágenos e elastina. Regulando a integridade e a composição da matriz extracelular, essas enzimas desempenham um papel fundamental no controle de sinais emitidos por moléculas da matriz que regulam a proliferação, a diferenciação e a morte celular.
me·tal·lo·thi·o·nein (mĕ - tal - ō - thī′ō - nēn). Metalotioneína; qualquer elemento de um grupo de proteínas pequenas, ricas em resíduos cisteinil, sintetizadas no fígado e no rim em resposta à presença de íons divalentes (zinco, mercúrio, cádmio, cobre, etc.), que se liga firmemente a esses íons; importante no transporte iônico e na detoxificação; a apoproteína é a tioneína.
met·a·lu·et·ic (met′ă - loo - et′ik). Metaluético. **1.** SIN metasyphilitic (1). **2.** SIN metasyphilitic (2). **3.** SIN parasyphilitic. [meta- + L. *lues*, pestilência]
met·a·mer (met′ă - mer). Metamérico. **1.** Elemento semelhante a, mas finalmente diferenciável de, outro elemento. **2.** Isômero estrutural. [meta- + -mer]
met·a·mere (met′ă - mēr). Metâmero; elemento de uma série de segmentos homólogos no corpo. VER TAMBÉM somite. [meta- + G. *meros*, parte]
met·a·mer·ic (met - ă - mer′ik). Metamérico. **1.** Relativo a, ou que exibe metamerismo, ou que ocorre em um metâmero. **2.** Referente a um metâmero.

me·tam·er·ism (me-tam′er-izm). Metamerismo. **1.** Tipo de estrutura anatômica que exibe metâmeros seriadamente homólogos; em formas primitivas, como os anelídeos, os metâmeros possuem estrutura quase semelhante; em vertebrados, a especialização na região cefálica mascara o metamerismo subjacente, que ainda é claramente evidente nas vértebras seriadamente repetidas, costelas, músculos intercostais e nervos espinais, e em embriões vertebrados jovens. **2.** Em química, sinônimo raramente usado de isomerismo estrutural.
met·a·mor·phop·sia (met′ă - mōr - fop′sē - ă). Metamorfopsia; distorção de imagens visuais. [meta- + G. *morphē*, formato, + *opsis*, visão]
met·a·mor·pho·sis (met - ă - mōr′fō - sis, - mōr - fō′sis). Metamorfose. **1.** Modificação na forma, estrutura ou função. **2.** Transição de um estágio do desenvolvimento para outro. SIN allaxis, transformation (1). [G. *metamorphosos*, transformação de *meta*, além, sobre, + *morphē*, forma]
complete m., m. completa; desenvolvimento do inseto a partir do ovo, através de sucessivos instares larvares, pupa e adulto; este último é diferente das duas primeiras formas do inseto, permitindo especialização das funções de alimentação (larvar) e de reprodução-vôo (adulto); característica das ordens superiores de insetos, como Coleoptera (besouros), Hymenoptera (abelhas, vespas, formigas), Diptera (moscas de duas asas) e Siphonaptera (pulgas). SIN holometabolous m.
fatty m., m. gordurosa; o aparecimento de gotículas de gordura visíveis microscopicamente no citoplasma das células. VER TAMBÉM *degeneration*. SIN fatty change.
heterometabolous m., m. heterometabólica. SIN incomplete m.
holometabolous m., m. holometabólica. SIN complete m.
incomplete m., m. incompleta; o desenvolvimento de uma ninfa em imago, que, em muitos aspectos, assemelha-se à primeira; característico de ordens de insetos mais primitivas, como Heteroptera (percevejos verdadeiros), Orthoptera (gafanhotos) e Blatteria (baratas). SIN heterometabolous m.
retrograde m., m. retrógrada. SIN degeneration (3); **(1)** SIN cataplasia.
met·a·mor·phot·ic (met′ă - mōr - fot′ik). Metamorfótico; relativo a, ou caracterizado por, metamorfose.
met·a·my·e·lo·cyte (met - ă - mī′el - ō - sīt). Metamielócito; forma de transição de mielócito com construção nuclear intermediária entre o mielócito maduro (mielócito C de Sabin) e o leucócito granular bilobulado. SIN juvenile cell. [meta- + G. *myelos*, medula óssea, + *kytos*, célula]
met·a·neph·ric (met - ă - nef′rik). Metanéfrico; de ou relativo ao metanefro.
met·a·neph·rine (met - ă - nef′rin). Metanefrina; um catabólito da epinefrina encontrado, juntamente com a normetanefrina, na urina e em alguns tecidos, resultante da ação da catecol-*O*-metiltransferase sobre a epinefrina; não tem ações simpaticomiméticas.
met·a·neph·ro·gen·ic, met·a·ne·phrog·e·nous (met′ă - nef - rō - jen′ik, - nĕ - froj′ĕ - nŭs). Metanefrogênico; aplicado à parte mais caudal do mesoderma intermediário que, sob a ação indutiva do divertículo metanéfrico, tem a capacidade de formar túbulos metanéfricos. [meta- + G. *nephros*, rim, + -gen, que produz]
met·a·neph·ros, pl. **met·a·neph·roi** (met - ă - nef′ros, - roy). Metanefro; o mais caudalmente localizado dos três órgãos excretores que aparecem na evolução dos vertebrados (sendo os outros o pronefro e o mesonefro); em embriões de mamíferos, o metanefro desenvolve-se caudal ao mesonefro durante sua regressão, tornando-se o rim permanente. SIN hind kidney. [meta- + G. *nephros*, rim]
met·a·neu·tro·phil, met·a·neu·tro·phile (met - ă - noo′trō - fil, - fīl). Metaneutrófilo; que não se cora normalmente com corantes neutros. [meta- + L. *neuter*, nenhum, G. *philos*, amigo]
met·a·nil yel·low (met′ă - nil) [C.I. 13065]. Amarelo de metanila; um corante ácido monoazo, $C_{18}H_{14}N_3O_3SNa$, usado como corante citoplasmático e do tecido conjuntivo.
metaperiodic acid. Ácido metaperiódico. SIN periodic acid (1).
met·a·phase (met′ă - fās). Metáfase; o estágio de mitose ou meiose no qual os cromossomas são alinhados na placa equatorial da célula, separando os centrômeros. Na mitose e na segunda divisão meiótica, os centrômeros de cada cromossoma dividem-se, e os dois centrômeros-filhos estão voltados para pólos opostos da célula; na primeira divisão da meiose, os centrômeros não se dividem, mas os centrômeros de cada par de cromossomas homólogos estão direcionados para pólos opostos. [meta- + G. *phasis*, aspecto]
met·a·phos·phor·ic ac·id (met′ă - fos - fōr′ik). Ácido metafosfórico. SIN glacial phosphoric acid.
met·a·phy·si·al, met·a·phy·se·al (met - ă - fiz′ē - ăl). Metafisário; relativo a uma metáfise.
me·taph·y·sis, pl. **me·taph·y·ses** (mĕ - taf′i - sis, - sēz) [TA]. Metáfise; uma secção cônica de osso entre a epífise e a diáfise dos ossos longos. [meta- + G. *physis*, crescimento]
me·taph·y·si·tis (mĕ - taf′i - sī′tis). Metafisite; inflamação da metáfise.
met·a·pla·sia (met - ă - plā′zē - ă). Metaplasia; transformação anormal de um tecido adulto, totalmente diferenciado de um tipo em um tecido diferenciado de outro tipo; uma condição adquirida, ao contrário da heteroplasia. SIN metaplasis (2). [G. *metaplasis*, transformação]

agnogenic myeloid m., m. mielóide agnogênica. SIN primary myeloid m.
apocrine m., m. apócrina; alteração do epitélio acinar do tecido mamário para assemelhar-se às glândulas sudoríparas apócrinas; comumente observada na doença fibrocística das mamas.
autoparenchymatous m., m. autoparenquimatosa; metaplasia que ocorre nas células parenquimatosas próprias do tecido.
Barrett m., m. de Barrett. SIN Barrett *syndrome.*
coelomic m., m. celômica; potencial do epitélio celômico de se diferenciar em vários diferentes tipos celulares histológicos.
intestinal m., m. intestinal; a transformação da mucosa, particularmente do estômago, em mucosa glandular semelhante à do intestino, embora geralmente sem vilosidades.
myeloid m., m. mielóide; síndrome caracterizada por anemia, esplenomegalia, hemácias nucleadas e granulócitos imaturos no sangue circulante, e focos visíveis de hematopoese extramedular no baço e no fígado; pode desenvolver-se no curso da policitemia rubra vera; há uma alta incidência de desenvolvimento de leucemia mielóide.
primary myeloid m., m. mielóide primária; metaplasia mielóide que ocorre como condição primária, freqüentemente associada à mielofibrose. SIN agnogenic myeloid m.
secondary myeloid m., m. mielóide secundária; metaplasia mielóide que ocorre em pessoas com outra doença. SIN symptomatic myeloid m.
squamous m., m. escamosa; a transformação de epitélio glandular ou mucoso em epitélio escamoso estratificado. SIN epidermalization.
squamous m. of amnion, m. escamosa do âmnio. SIN *amnion* nodosum.
symptomatic myeloid m., m. mielóide sintomática. SIN secondary myeloid m.
me·ta·pla·sis (mĕ - tap′lă - sis). Metaplasia. **1.** O estágio de completo crescimento ou desenvolvimento do indivíduo. **2.** SIN metaplasia. [G. uma transformação]
met·a·plas·tic (met - ă - plas′tik). Metaplásico; relativo à metaplasia.
met·a·plex·us (met′ă - plek′sŭs). Metaplexo; o plexo coróide no quarto ventrículo do encéfalo. [meta- + L. *plexus,* entrelaçamento]
met·a·poph·y·sis (met′ă - pof′i - sis). Metapófise. SIN mammillary *process of lumbar vertebra.* [meta- + G. *apophysis,* processo]
met·a·pore (met′ă - pōr). Metaporo; termo raramente usado para *apertura mediana ventriculi quarti* (abertura mediana do quarto ventrículo). [meta- + G. *poros,* poro]
met·a·pro·tein (met - ă - prō′tēn). Metaproteína; termo não-descritivo para uma proteína derivada obtida pela ação de ácidos ou álcalis, solúveis em ácidos ou álcalis fracos, mas insolúveis em soluções neutras; p. ex., albuminato.
met·a·pro·ter·e·nol sul·fate (met′ă - prō - ter′ē - nol). Sulfato de metaproterenol; broncodilatador simpaticomimético usado no tratamento do broncospasmo na asma e na doença pulmonar obstrutiva crônica. Tem efeito relativamente maior sobre os receptores β$_2$-adrenérgicos que B$_1$, conferindo alguma seletividade no relaxamento da musculatura lisa bronquiolar em comparação com a estimulação cardíaca. SIN orciprenaline sulfate.
met·a·psy·chol·o·gy (met′ă - sī - kol′ō - jē). Metapsicologia. **1.** Tentativa sistemática de discernir e descrever o que se encontra além dos fatos empíricos e leis da psicologia, como as relações entre corpo e mente, ou relacionado ao lugar da mente no universo. **2.** Em psicanálise, ou metapsicologia psicanalítica, a psicologia relacionada às suposições fundamentais da teoria freudiana da mente, que impõem cinco pontos de vista: 1) dinâmico, relacionado com as forças psicológicas; 2) econômico, relacionado com a energia psicológica; 3) estrutural, relacionado com as configurações psicológicas; 4) genético, relacionado com as origens psicológicas; 5) adaptativo, referentes às relações psicológicas com o ambiente. [G. *meta,* além, transcendendo, + psychology]
met·a·py·ret·ic (met′ă - pī - ret′ik). Metapirético. SIN postfebrile. [meta- + G. *pyretos,* febre]
met·a·py·ro·cat·e·chase (met′ă - pī - rō - kat′ē - kās). Metapirocatecase. SIN catechol 2,3-dioxygenase.
met·a·ram·i·nol bi·tar·trate (met - ă - ram′i - nol). Bitartarato de metaraminol; uma potente amina simpaticomimética usada para a elevação e manutenção da pressão arterial em estados de hipotensão aguda e, topicamente, como descongestionante nasal.
met·a·rho·dop·sin (met - ă - rō - dop′sin). Metarrodopsina; forma de rodopsina ativada pela luz; a metarrodopsina I é formada a partir da lumirrodopsina e convertida em metarrodopsina II; a metarrodopsina II é a forma de rodopsina que libera retinal todo-*trans.*
met·ar·te·ri·ole (met′ar - tēr′ē - ōl). Metarteríola; um dos pequenos vasos sangüíneos periféricos entre as arteríolas e os capilares verdadeiros, contendo grupos dispersos de fibras musculares lisas em suas paredes. [meta- + arteriole]
met·a·ru·bri·cyte (met - ă - roo′bri - sīt). Metarrubricito; normoblasto ortocromático. VER normoblast.
pernicious anemia type m., m. típico da anemia perniciosa; megaloblasto ortocromático. VER megaloblast.
met·a·sta·ble (met′ă - stā - bl). Metaestável. **1.** Que possui estabilidade incerta; em condição de passar para outra fase quando levemente perturbado; p. ex., a água, quando resfriada abaixo do ponto de congelamento, pode permanecer líquida, mas congelará imediatamente se lhe for acrescentado um pedaço de gelo. **2.** Designa a condição excitada do núcleo de um radionuclídeo isômero que atinge um estado de menor energia pelo processo de decaimento transicional isomérico sem alteração do seu número ou peso atômico; p. ex., $^{99m}_{43}Tc \rightarrow {^{99}_{43}Tc} + \gamma$. [meta- + L. *stabilis,* estável]

ℹ me·tas·ta·sis, pl. **me·tas·ta·ses** (mĕ - tas′tă - sis, - sēz). Metástase. **1.** O deslocamento de uma doença ou de suas manifestações locais, de uma parte do corpo para outra, como na caxumba quando os sintomas referentes à glândula parótida cessam e o testículo é acometido. **2.** A disseminação de um processo patológico de uma parte do corpo para outra, como no surgimento de neoplasias em partes do corpo distantes do local do tumor primário; resulta da disseminação de células tumorais pelos linfáticos ou vasos sangüíneos, ou por extensão direta através das cavidades serosas ou subaracnóide ou outros espaços. **3.** O transporte de bactérias de uma parte do corpo para outra, através da corrente sanguínea (metástase hematogênica) ou através da rede linfática (metástase linfogênica). SIN secondaries (1). [G. uma remoção, de *meta,* no meio de, + *stasis,* colocação]
biochemical m., m. bioquímica; o transporte e a indução de especificidades imunoquímicas anormais em órgãos aparentemente normais.
calcareous m., m. calcária; depósito de material calcário em tecidos distantes no caso de extensa reabsorção de tecido ósseo em cáries, neoplasias malignas, e assim por diante.
hematogenous m., m. hematogênica. VER metastasis.
in-transit m., m. em trânsito; no melanoma, depósito metastático que ocorre na via linfática entre o tumor primário e seus linfonodos de drenagem.
lymphogenous m., m. linfogênica. VER metastasis.
pulsating metastases, metástases pulsáteis; metástases para o osso, geralmente de hipernefromas, mas ocasionalmente de tumores da tireóide; a vascularização considerável pode apresentar pulsação expansiva e um sopro contínuo.
satellite m., m. satélite; metástase na vizinhança imediata de uma neoplasia maligna primária; p. ex., pele adjacente a um melanoma.
me·tas·ta·size (mĕ - tas′tă - sīz). Metastatizar; entrar ou invadir por metástase.
met·a·stat·ic (met - ă - stat′ik). Metastático; relativo à metástase.
met·a·ster·num (met′ă - ster′nŭm). Processo xifóide. SIN xiphoid *process.*
met·a·stron·gyle (met - ă - stron′jīl). Metaestrôngilo; nome comum de membros do gênero *Metastrongylus* ou da família Metastrongylidae.
Met·a·stron·gy·lus (met - ă - stron′ji - lŭs). Gênero de nematódeos pulmonares (família Metastrongylidae), o único gênero em sua subfamília (Metastrongylinae). As quatro espécies conhecidas são encontradas apenas em porcos; a transmissão é feita por hospedeiros intermediários, como a minhoca. [meta- + G. *strongylos,* redondo]
met·a·syph·i·lis (met - ă - sif′i - lis). Metassífilis. **1.** O estado constitucional devido à sífilis congênita sem lesões locais. **2.** SIN parasyphilis.
met·a·syph·i·lit·ic (met′ă - sif - i - lit′ik). Metassifilítico. **1.** Relativo à metassífilis. SIN metaluetic (1). **2.** Subseqüente ou que ocorre como seqüela da sífilis. SIN metaluetic (2). **3.** SIN parasyphilitic.
met·a·tar·sal (met′ă - tar′săl). Metatarsal. **1.** Relativo ao metatarso ou a um dos ossos metatarsais. VER metatarsal (*bones*) [I–V], em *bone.* **2.** Qualquer um dos ossos metatarsais.
met·a·tar·sal·gia (met′ă - tar - sal′jē - ă). Metatarsalgia; dor na parte anterior do pé na região das cabeças dos metatarsais. [meta- + G. *algos,* dor]
Morton m., m. de Morton. SIN Morton *neuralgia.*
met·a·tar·sec·to·my (met′ă - tar - sek′tō - mē). Metatarsectomia; excisão do metatarso. [metatarsus + G. *ektomē,* excisão]
met·a·tar·so·pha·lan·ge·al (met′ă - tar′sō - fă - lan′jē - ăl). Metatarsofalângico; relativo aos ossos metatarsais e às falanges; designa as articulações entre eles.
met·a·tar·sus, pl. **me·ta·tar·si** (met′ă - tar′sŭs, - sī). Metatarso; a porção distal do pé entre o dorso do pé e os dedos, tendo como seu esqueleto os cinco ossos longos (ossos metatarsais) que se articulam, proximalmente, com os ossos cubóide e cuneiforme, distalmente, com as falanges. [meta- + G. *tarsos,* tarso]
m. adductova′rus, m. adutovaro; deformidade fixa do pé na qual os vétores adutor e varo contribuem para a postura resultante do pé.
m. adduc′tus, m. aduto; deformidade fixa do pé na qual o antepé forma um ângulo com o eixo longitudinal principal do pé em direção à linha média; geralmente é congênito. SIN intoe.
m. atav′icus, m. atávico; encurtamento anormal do primeiro osso metatarsal em comparação com o segundo.
m. la′tus, pé transversoplano; deformidade causada pelo afundamento do arco transverso do pé. SIN talipes transversoplanus.
m. va′rus, m. varo; deformidade fixa do pé na qual o antepé é rodado sobre o eixo longitudinal do pé, ficando a superfície plantar voltada para a linha média do corpo.
met·a·thal·a·mus (met′ă - thal′ă - mŭs) [TA]. Metatálamo; a parte caudoventral do tálamo, que consiste nos corpos geniculados medial e lateral. [meta- + G. *thalamos,* tálamo]
me·tath·e·sis (mĕ - tath′ē - sis). Metátese. **1.** Transferência de um produto patológico (p. ex., um cálculo) de um lugar para outro, onde cause menor inconveniência ou lesão, quando não é possível ou viável removê-lo do corpo. **2.**

Em química, uma decomposição dupla, na qual uma substância, A-B, reage com outra substância, C-D, para produzir A-C + B-D, ou A-D + B-C. [meta- + G. *thesis*, colocação]

met·a·troph (met'ă-trof). Metatrofo; organismo que precisa de fontes orgânicas complexas de carbono e nitrogênio para seu crescimento.

met·a·tro·phic (met-ă-trof'ik). Metatrófico; designa a capacidade de realizar anabolismo ou obter nutrição de várias fontes, isto é, tanto de matéria orgânica nitrogenada quanto carbonácea. [meta- + G. *trophē*, nutrição]

met·a·tro·pic (met-ă-trop'ik). Metatrópico; designa uma reversão para um estado anterior. [meta- + G. *tropē*, volta]

met·a·typ·i·cal (met-ă-tip'i-kăl). Metatípico; relativo ao tecido que é formado por elementos idênticos aos encontrados num local em condições normais, mas os vários elementos não estão dispostos no padrão normal habitual.

me·tax·a·lone (mē-tak'să-lōn). Metaxalona; relaxante muscular esquelético.

Met·a·zoa (met-ă-zō'ă). Sub-reino do reino Animalia, incluindo todos os animais multicelulares, nos quais as células são diferenciadas e formam tecidos; distinta do sub-reino Protozoa, ou animais unicelulares. [meta- + G. *zōon*, animal]

met·a·zo·o·no·sis (met'ă-zō-ō-nō'sis). Metazoonose; zoonose que requer um hospedeiro vertebrado e um invertebrado para concluir seu ciclo biológico; p. ex., as infecções de seres humanos e de outros vertebrados por arbovírus. [meta- + G. *zōon*, animal, + *nosos*, doença]

Metchnikoff, Elie, biólogo russo em Paris e prêmio Nobel, 1845–1916. VER M. *theory*.

met·en·ce·phal·ic (met'en-se-fal'ik). Metencefálico; relativo ao metencéfalo.

met·en·ceph·a·lon (met'en-sef'ă-lon)[TA]. Metencéfalo; a anterior das duas subdivisões principais do rombencéfalo (sendo a posterior o mielencéfalo ou bulbo), constituído pela ponte e pelo cerebelo. [meta- + G. *enkephalos*, encéfalo]

Metenier sign. Sinal de Metenier. VER em sign.

met·en·keph·a·lin (met-en-kef'ă-lin). Metencefalina. VER enkephalins.

me·te·or·ism (mē'tē-ō-rizm). Meteorismo. SIN tympanites. [G. *meteōrismos*, elevação]

me·te·or·op·a·thy (mē'tē-ōr-op'ă-thē). Meteoropatia; termo raramente usado para doenças decorrentes das condições climáticas. [G. *meteōra*, coisas elevadas, no firmamento, + *pathos*, sofrimento]

me·te·or·o·tro·pic (mē'tē-ōr-ō-trop'ik). Meteorotrópico; denota doenças cuja incidência é afetada pelo clima. [G. *meteōra*, coisas elevadas, no firmamento + G. *tropos*, uma volta]

me·ter (m) (mē'ter). **1.** Metro; a unidade fundamental de comprimento nos sistemas SI e métrico, equivalente a 39,37007874 polegadas. Definido como a distância percorrida pela luz no vácuo em 1/299792458 s. **2.** Medidor; aparelho usado para medir a quantidade daquilo que o atravessa. [Fr. *metre*; G. *metron*, medida]

potential acuity m. (PAM), medidor da acuidade potencial; instrumento usado para projetar uma imagem como os optótipos de Snellen (Snellen *test types*) na retina, através de uma lente com catarata, a fim de prever a função visual provável se fosse removida a catarata.

rate m., medidor de razão; aparelho que exibe continuamente a magnitude de eventos cuja média é calculada durante intervalos de tempo variáveis.

ventilation m., medidor de ventilação; medidor usado para determinar os volumes ventilatórios corrente e minuto.

Venturi m., medidor de Venturi; aparelho para medir o fluxo de um líquido em termos da queda de pressão quando o líquido flui para a constrição de um tubo de Venturi.

me·ter-can·dle (mē'ter-kan'dl). Lux. SIN lux.

met·er·ga·sia (met-er-gā'zē-ă). Mudança de função. [G. *meta*, designa mudança, + *ergasia*, trabalho]

me·ter·go·line (mē'ter-gō-lēn). Metergolina; um derivado do esporão do centeio com perfil farmacológico semelhante à metissergida; bloqueador não-seletivo dos receptores da serotonina. Usada como analgésico na enxaqueca. SIN methergoline.

met·es·trus, met·es·trum (met-es'trŭs, -trŭm). Metaestro; o período entre o estro e o diestro no ciclo estral. [meta- + estrus]

met·for·min (met-fōr'min). Metformina; agente hipoglicemiante oral.

♻ **meth-, metho-.** Met-, meto-; prefixos químicos que geralmente designam um grupo metila, metoxi.

meth·a·cho·line chlo·ride (meth'ă-kō-lēn). Cloreto de metacolina; derivado da acetilcolina; agente parassimpaticomimético usado como broncoconstritor no teste de hiper-reatividade brônquica.

meth·a·cryl·ic ac·id (meth'ă-kril'ik). Ácido metacrílico; encontrado no óleo de camomila romana; usado na fabricação de resinas e plásticos de metacrilato. SIN methylacrylic acid.

meth·a·cy·cline hy·dro·chlo·ride (meth-ă-sī'klēn). Cloridrato de metaciclina; agente antimicrobiano.

meth·a·done hy·dro·chlo·ride (meth'ă-dōn). Cloridrato de metadona; narcótico sintético; analgésico efetivo por via oral, com ação semelhante à da morfina, mas com potência um pouco maior e duração mais prolongada. Causa dependência física e psíquica como a morfina, mas os sintomas de abstinência são um pouco mais leves; usado como substituto (via oral) da morfina e da heroína; também é usado durante o tratamento da abstinência no vício em morfina e heroína.

meth·al·len·es·tril (meth'ă-len-es'tril). Metalenestril; composto estrogênico não-esteróide, efetivo por via oral.

meth·am·phet·a·mine hy·dro·chlo·ride (meth-am-fet'ă-mēn). Cloridrato de metanfetamina; agente simpaticomimético que exerce maiores efeitos estimulantes sobre o sistema nervoso central que a anfetamina (daí o nome popular: "speed" (velocidade)); amplamente usado por via oral e intravenosa; pode causar forte dependência psíquica. Quando convertido em base livre (metanfetamina), pode ser fumado como o "crack", sendo denominado "ICE". SIN methylamphetamine hydrochloride.

meth·am·py·rone (meth-am-pī'rōn). Metampirona. SIN dipyrone.

meth·an·di·e·none (meth-an-dī'ĕ-nōn). Metandienona. SIN methandrostenolone.

meth·an·dri·ol (meth-an'drē-ol). Metandriol; o derivado metila do androstenediol, com ações e empregos semelhantes. SIN mestenediol.

meth·an·dro·sten·o·lone (meth-an-drō-sten'ō-lōn). Metandrostenolona; esteróide anabólico efetivo por via oral, que pode promover retenção de nitrogênio quando associado a uma dieta adequada; além disso, pode exercer tipicamente efeitos androgênicos. SIN methandienone.

meth·ane (meth'ān). Metano; CH_4; gás inodoro produzido pela decomposição de matéria orgânica; explosivo quando misturado a 7 ou 8 volumes de ar, constituindo então o gás inflamável nas minas de carvão. SIN marsh gas.

Meth·a·no·bac·te·ri·a·ce·ae (meth'ă-nō-bak-tēr-ē-ā'sē-ē). Bactérias Archaea contendo bastonetes e cocos Gram-negativos e Gram-positivos, móveis ou imóveis, estritamente anaeróbicos, que obtêm energia pela redução do dióxido de carbono para formar metano ou pela fermentação de substâncias como acetato e metanol, com a produção de metano e dióxido de carbono; são encontrados em hábitats anaeróbicos como sedimentos de águas naturais, solo, digestores anaeróbicos de esgoto e o trato gastrointestinal de animais.

meth·a·no·gen (meth-an'ō-jen). Metanógeno; qualquer bactéria produtora de metano da família Methanobacteriaceae.

meth·a·nol (meth'ă-nol). Metanol. SIN methyl alcohol.

meth·an·the·line bro·mide (meth-an'thē-lēn). Brometo de metantelina; anticolinérgico.

meth·a·pyr·i·lene (meth-ă-pir'i-lēn). Metapirileno; anti-histamínico H_1. O fumarato de metapirileno é administrado topicamente sobre a pele; o cloridrato de metapirileno é o sal preferido para uso oral ou parenteral.

meth·a·qua·lone (meth-ă-kwā'lōn). Metaqualona; sedativo e hipnótico, também é uma droga ilícita; disponível na forma de cloridrato.

meth·ar·bi·tal (meth-ar'bi-tahl). Metarbital; derivado *N*-metilado do barbital, com propriedades anticonvulsivantes semelhantes às do fenobarbital; convertido em barbital no corpo.

meth·ar·gen (meth'ar-jen). Metargeno; anti-séptico tópico.

meth·a·zo·la·mide (meth-ă-zol'ă-mīd). Metazolamida; inibidor da anidrase carbônica com empregos semelhantes aos da acetazolamida.

metHb Abreviatura de methemoglobin (metemoglobina).

meth·dil·a·zine hy·dro·chlo·ride (meth-dil'ă-zēn). Cloridrato de metidilazina; composto fenotiazina com atividade anti-histamínica; usado no tratamento de várias dermatoses para aliviar o prurido.

met·hem·al·bu·min (met'hĕm-al-boo'min, -hem-al'boo-min). Metemalbumina; composto anormal formado no sangue por combinação do heme com a albumina plasmática.

met·hem·al·bu·mi·ne·mia (met'hĕm-al-boo-min-ē'mē-ă). Metemalbuminemia; a presença de metemalbumina no sangue circulante, indicativa de hemólise intravascular com rápida decomposição da hemoglobina; encontrada em alguns pacientes com febre hemoglobinúrica ou hemoglobinúria paroxística noturna; descrita como uma forma de diferenciar a pancreatite grave (hemorrágica) da leve (edematosa), e também foi descrita em outros distúrbios agudos, tais como obstrução por estrangulamento do intestino e oclusão da artéria mesentérica.

met·he·mo·glo·bin (metHb) (met-hē-mō-glō'bin). Metemoglobina; produto da transformação da oxi-hemoglobina devido à oxidação do Fe^{2+} normal em Fe^{3+}, assim convertendo a ferroprotoporfirina em ferriprotoporfirina; contém água em união firme com o ferro férrico, assim sendo quimicamente diferente da oxi-hemoglobina e inútil para a respiração; encontrada em derrames sanguíneos e no sangue circulante após intoxicação por acetanilida, clorato de potássio e outras substâncias. SIN ferrihemoglobin.

m. reductase, m. redutase; uma flavoenzima que catalisa a redução de metemoglobina em hemoglobina na hemácia.

met·he·mo·glo·bi·ne·mia (met-hē'mō-glō-bi-nē'mē-ă, meth'ē-mō-). Metemoglobinemia; a presença de metemoglobina no sangue circulante; quando acentuada, há oxigenação inadequada dos tecidos. A metemoglobina faz com que o sangue adquira uma coloração acastanhada, que pode ser confundida com cianose. [methemoglobin + G. *haima*, sangue]

acquired m., m. adquirida; metemoglobinemia causada por vários agentes químicos, como os nitritos ou os anestésicos tópicos. SIN enterogenous m., secondary m.
congenital m., m. congênita; (1) metemoglobinemia devida à formação de qualquer um de um grupo de hemoglobinas anormais de cadeia α [MIM*141800] ou cadeia β [MIM*141900], coletivamente conhecidas como hemoglobina M. Há cianose acinzentada nos primeiros meses de vida, sem doença pulmonar ou cardíaca, que é resistente ao tratamento com ácido ascórbico ou azul de metileno; herança autossômica dominante; (2) metemoglobinemia devida à deficiência da citocromo b_5 redutase [MIM*250790] ou de metemoglobina redutase [MIM*250700], a enzima responsável pela redução da metemoglobina intra-eritrocitária; a cianose melhora com a administração de ácido ascórbico ou azul de metileno; herança autossômica recessiva. SIN hereditary m., hereditary methemoglobinemic cyanosis, primary m.
enterogenous m., m. enterógena. SIN acquired m.
hereditary m., m. hereditária. SIN congenital m.
primary m., m. primária. SIN congenital m.
secondary m., m. secundária. SIN acquired m.

met·he·mo·glo·bi·nu·ria (met-hē′mō-glō-bi-noo′rē-ă, meth′ē-mō-). Metemoglobinúria; a presença de metemoglobina na urina. [methemoglobin + G. *ouron*, urina]

meth·en·a·mine (me-then′a-mēn). Metenamina; produto de condensação obtido pela ação da amônia sobre o formaldeído; em uma urina ácida, decompõe-se para produzir formaldeído, um anti-séptico urinário. SIN hexamine.
m. hippurate, hipurato de m.; anti-séptico urinário.
m. mandelate, mandelato de m.; anti-séptico urinário.
m. salicylate, salicilato de m.; solvente do ácido úrico e anti-séptico urinário.

meth·en·a·mine-sil·ver. Metenamina de prata; metenamina argêntica; complexo de hexametilenotetramina-prata preparado pela adição de nitrato de prata à metenamina; surge um precipitado branco na solução, que se dissolve com a agitação e é estável sob refrigeração; usado em vários métodos de coloração histológica e histoquímica. VER TAMBÉM Gomori methenamine-silver *stain*, em stain.

meth·ene (meth′ēn). Meteno; a porção =CH–.

N⁵,N¹⁰-meth·e·nyl·tet·ra·hy·dro·fol·ic ac·id. Ácido N^5,N^{10}-metiltetraidrofólico. SIN anhydroleucovorin.

N⁵,N¹⁰-meth·e·nyl·tet·ra·hy·dro·fo·la·te. N^5,N^{10}-metiltetraidrofolato; um derivado do tetraidrofolato que contém um carbono; usado na biossíntese de purinas.

meth·er·go·line. Metergolina. SIN metergoline.

meth·i·cil·lin so·di·um (meth-i-sil′in). Meticilina sódica; sal semi-sintético da penicilina para administração parenteral; é recomendada a restrição de seu uso a infecções causadas por estafilococos resistentes à penicilina G; é menos eficaz que a penicilina G em infecções causadas por estreptococos hemolíticos, pneumococos, gonococos e estafilococos sensíveis à penicilina G. SIN sodium methicilin.

meth·im·a·zole (me-thim′ă-zōl). Metimazol; medicamento anti-tireóideo com ação semelhante à do propiltiouracil.

me·thi·o·dal so·di·um (meth-ī′ō-dăl). Metiodal sódico; contraste radiopaco contendo iodo, CH_2ISO_3Na ou metanessulfonato de sódio, usado outrora para exame das vias urinárias.

me·thi·o·nine (Met, M) (me-thī′ō-nēn). Metionina; ácido 2-amino-4-(metiltio)butírico; o isômero L é um aminoácido essencial e a fonte natural mais importante de grupos "metil ativos" no corpo, por isso geralmente envolvidos em metilações *in vivo*; a forma DL é usada como auxiliar no tratamento de hepatopatias.
active m., m. ativa. SIN S-adenosyl-L-methionine.
m. adenosyltransferase, m. adenosiltransferase; enzima que catalisa a condensação de L-metionina e ATP, formando S-adenosil-L-metionina, ortofosfato e pirofosfato; a deficiência da enzima hepática resultará em hipermetionemia. SIN methionine-activating enzyme.
m. sulfoxime, sulfoxima de m.; derivado tóxico da metionina formado quando proteínas que a contêm são tratadas com cloreto de nitrogênio para produzir $-SO(NH)-CH_3$ no lugar de $-SCH_3$.
m. synthase, m. sintase; tetraidropteroilglutamato metiltransferase; metionina-homocisteína metiltransferase; enzima que catalisa a reação de N^5-metiltetraidrofolato com L-homocisteína para formar tetraidrofolato e L-metionina; uma enzima que precisa de cobalamina; a deficiência dessa enzima resulta em acúmulo de L-homocisteína e anormalidades neurológicas. SIN tetrahydrofolate methyltransferase.

me·this·a·zone (mē-this′ă-zōn). Metisazona; um agente antiviral.

meth·i·tu·ral (me-thit′t-oo-ral). Metitural; tiobarbiturato intravenoso semelhante ao tiopental e usado para indução de anestesia; exerce um breve efeito devido à rápida redistribuição no corpo após uma única injeção.

me·thix·ene hy·dro·chlo·ride (me-thik′sēn). Cloridrato de metixeno; agente anticolinérgico.

metho-. VER meth-.

meth·o·car·ba·mol (meth-ō-kar′bă-mol). Metocarbamol; relaxante muscular esquelético de ação central, quimicamente relacionado ao carbamato de mefenesina; tem início de ação mais lento, porém maior duração, e pode ser administrado por via intravenosa, intramuscular ou oral.

METHOD

meth·od (meth′ŏd). Método; modo, maneira ou seqüência ordenada de eventos de um processo ou procedimento. VER TAMBÉM fixative, operation, procedure, stain, technique. [G. *methodos*; de *meta*, após, + *hodos*, forma]

Abell-Kendall m., m. de Abell-Kendall; m. de referência padrão para estimativa do colesterol sérico total, envolvendo saponificação do éster de colesterol por hidróxido, extração com éter de petróleo e desenvolvimento de cor com anidrido acético-ácido sulfúrico; o método evita interferência por bilirrubina, proteína e hemoglobina.

activated sludge m., m. da lama ativada; m. de descarte do esgoto no qual este é tratado com lama líquida, com atividade bacteriana de 15%, produzida por aeração vigorosa repetida de esgoto fresco para formar flóculos ou sedimento; quando esse processo de floculação está completo, a lama ativada resultante contém numerosas bactérias, juntamente com leveduras, mofos e protozoários, que realizam ativamente a oxidação de substâncias orgânicas; essa mistura é canalizada até um tanque de sedimentação, cujo efluente é o esgoto completamente tratado.

Altmann-Gersh m., m. de Altmann-Gersh; o m. de congelar rapidamente um tecido e desidratá-lo em um vácuo.

Anel m., m. de Anel; ligadura de uma artéria imediatamente acima (no lado proximal) de um aneurisma.

Antyllus m., m. de Antyllus; ligadura da artéria acima e abaixo de um aneurisma, seguida por incisão e esvaziamento do saco.

aristotelian m., m. aristotélico; m. de estudo que enfatiza a relação entre uma categoria geral e um objeto em particular.

Ashby m., m. de Ashby; m. de aglutinação diferencial para estimar o tempo de vida do eritrócito; o sangue compatível possuindo um fator de grupo que falta ao receptor é transferido para o receptor; após a transfusão, soros com potentes aglutininas para as hemácias do receptor são adicionados às amostras de sangue do receptor, e as hemácias não-aglutinadas são contadas; utilizando essa técnica, o tempo de vida das hemácias em pessoas normais é de 110 a 120 dias.

auxanographic m., m. auxanográfico; método para estudo de enzimas bacterianas no qual o ágar é misturado com o material (p. ex., amido ou leite) que servirá como indicador da ação enzimática e é inoculado e colocado em placas; se as bactérias produzem enzimas que digerem o material misturado, haverá uma zona de clareamento no meio de cultura em torno de cada colônia. SIN diffusion m.

Barraquer m., m. de Barraquer. SIN zonulolysis.

Beck m., m. de Beck; abertura permanente para o estômago feita em sua curvatura maior.

Bier m., m. de Bier; (1) SIN intravenous regional *anesthesia*; (2) tratamento de vários distúrbios cirúrgicos por hiperemia reativa.

Billings m., m. de Billings; m. contraceptivo que envolve períodos de abstinência determinados por alterações no muco cervical.

Born m. of wax plate reconstruction, m. de Born de reconstrução com placa de cera; confecção de modelos tridimensionais de estruturas a partir de cortes seriados; depende da construção de uma série de placas de cera, moldadas em aumentos em escala dos cortes individuais componentes da região a ser reconstruída.

Brasdor m., m. de Brasdor; tratamento de aneurisma por ligadura da artéria imediatamente abaixo (no lado distal) do tumor.

Callahan m., m. de Callahan. SIN chloropercha m.

capture-recapture m., m. de captura-recaptura; originalmente, uma técnica desenvolvida por biólogos para rastrear populações de animais selvagens; agora adaptada para estudos epidemiológicos de populações humanas esquivas (p. ex., prostitutas, adolescentes fugitivos, usuários de drogas IV).

Charters m., m. de Charters; m. para escovar os dentes utilizando um movimento circular restrito com as cerdas inclinadas coronalmente em um ângulo de 45°.

Chayes m., m. de Chayes; m. para substituição de dentes perdidos utilizando um aparelho mecânico para a fixação e estabilização de próteses dentárias que permite "movimento coerente" com os dentes vizinhos.

chloropercha m., m. de cloropercha; m. de obturação dos canais radiculares dos dentes por dissolução de cones de guta-percha em um meio de resina de clorofórmio dentro do canal radicular. SIN Callahan m., Johnson m.

closed circuit m., m. de circuito fechado; m. para medir o consumo de oxigênio no qual o indivíduo reinala uma quantidade inicial de oxigênio através de um absorvedor de dióxido de carbono, observando-se a diminuição do volume de oxigênio reinalado.

Cobb m., m. de Cobb; técnica usada na escoliose para determinar o grau de curvatura da coluna vertebral; a medida é feita traçando-se uma linha perpendicular à linha que passa pela borda superior da vértebra final superior (mais inclinada) e outra linha perpendicular à linha que passa pela borda inferior da vértebra final inferior; o ângulo formado pela intersecção das duas linhas perpendiculares é o ângulo de Cobb, que mede a magnitude da curva.
combined m.'s, métodos combinados; combinações variadas do m. auditivo oral e do m. visual manual de educação de crianças surdas. VER TAMBÉM oral auditory m., manual visual m., total *communication.*
confrontation m., m. de confrontação; m. de perimetria; o examinador compara os campos visuais do paciente com o próprio campo visual do examinador ficando de frente para o paciente, que tem um olho coberto e o outro fixado no olho correspondente (confrontante) do examinador. O examinador então coloca um dedo a meio caminho entre eles e move-o lentamente, em diferentes direções, até que o paciente não o veja mais. Em cada caso, o dedo é movido novamente em direção à posição original até o exato momento em que o paciente possa vê-lo.
cooled-knife m., m. do bisturi congelado; a realização de cortes por congelamento com um bisturi resfriado até alguns graus abaixo do ponto de congelamento.
copper sulfate m., m. do sulfato de cobre; m. para determinação da densidade específica do sangue ou plasma, no qual o sangue ou plasma é administrado por gotas em soluções de sulfato de cobre graduadas em densidade por aumentos de 0,004, estando cada um dos frascos de solução dentro da faixa esperada da amostra de sangue ou plasma; a densidade da solução de sulfato de cobre na qual a gota de sangue ou plasma permanece suspensa indefinidamente indica a densidade da amostra.
correlational m., m. correlacional; m. estatístico, usado mais freqüentemente na clínica e em outras áreas aplicadas da psicologia, para estudar a relação existente entre uma característica e outra em um indivíduo.
Credé m.'s, métodos de Credé; **(1)** instilação de uma gota de uma solução a 2% de nitrato de prata em cada olho do recém-nascido, para evitar oftalmia neonatal; **(2)** apoio da mão sobre o fundo do útero a partir do momento da expulsão do feto, e realização de massagem delicada no caso de hemorragia ou ausência de contração; então, quando as secundinas estiverem soltas, são expelidas por compressão firme ou espremendo-se o fundo com a mão; **(3)** uso de pressão manual sobre a bexiga, particularmente uma bexiga paralisada, para expelir a urina. SIN Credé maneuvers.
cross-sectional m., m. de corte transversal; em psicologia do desenvolvimento, o estudo do tempo de vida que envolve a comparação de grupos de indivíduos em diferentes faixas etárias. Cf. longitudinal m.
Deaver m., m. de Deaver; método de reeducação motora.
definitive m., m. definitivo; procedimento analítico para medida de um analisado específico em um material específico que, sabidamente, fornece o verdadeiro valor para a concentração do analisado.
Dick m., m. de Dick. SIN Dick *test.*
diffusion m., m. de difusão. SIN auxanographic m.
direct m. for making inlays, m. direto para fazer incrustações; em odontologia, uma técnica de incrustação pela qual o molde de cera é feito diretamente na cavidade preparada no dente. SIN direct technique.
disk sensitivity m., m. de sensibilidade do disco; procedimento para testar a efetividade relativa de vários antibióticos; pequenos discos de papel (ou de outro material adequado) são impregnados com quantidades conhecidas e apropriadas de antibiótico e, depois, colocados na superfície de meio semi-sólido previamente inoculado com o organismo testado; após períodos de incubação adequados a 37°C, a ausência de crescimento em zonas ao redor dos vários discos indica a efetividade relativa do antibiótico.
double antibody m., m. do anticorpo duplo. SIN double antibody *precipitation.*
Edman m., m. de Edman. VER phenilisothiocyanate.
Eggleston m., m. de Eggleston; termo obsoleto para digitalização rápida por meio de grandes doses de folha ou tintura de digital repetidas com freqüência.
Eicken m., m. de Eicken; facilitação de hipofaringoscopia por meio de tração anterior da cartilagem cricóidea por uma sonda laríngea.
encu m., m. encu; forma de simplificar o cálculo do risco em aconselhamento genético para traços autossômicos dominantes por conversão de todas as evidências pertinentes em unidades encu (*encu*).
ensu m., m. ensu; forma de simplificar o cálculo do risco em aconselhamento genético para traços ligados ao X por conversão de todas as evidências pertinentes em unidades ensu (*ensu*).
experimental m., m. experimental; em psicologia experimental, controle de fatores ambientais, fisiológicos ou de atitude para observar alterações dependentes nos aspectos de experiência e comportamento.
Fick m., m. de Fick; em 1870, A. Fick propôs que o débito cardíaco pode ser calculado como o quociente do consumo total de oxigênio pelo corpo dividido pela diferença no conteúdo de oxigênio do sangue arterial e do sangue venoso misto. No método de Fick direto são medidas todas as variáveis. O método de Fick indireto emprega vários meios para evitar medir o conteúdo de oxigênio no sangue venoso misto. Por extensão, o método de Fick pode ser usado para medir o débito cardíaco ou o fluxo sanguíneo em um órgão com qualquer substância indicadora cuja taxa de captação ou consumo e as concentrações arteriais e venosas mistas podem ser medidas, desde que o indicador não entre no sistema nem o deixe por qualquer via medida. SIN Fick principle.
flash m., m. rápido de pasteurização; esterilização do leite por elevação rápida de sua temperatura até 81°C, mantendo-a por um curto período e reduzindo-a rapidamente para 4°C.
flotation m., m. de flutuação; qualquer dos vários procedimentos de concentração de ovos de helmintos para obter resultados mais fidedignos quando é difícil encontrar ovos ao exame direto; os métodos de flutuação dependem da flutuação de ovos de helminto na superfície de um líquido com densidade suficientemente alta, aproximadamente 1:180; 1 parte de fezes misturada a aproximadamente 10 partes de solução salina saturada exibirá flutuação da maioria dos cistos de protozoários e de ovos de helminto não-operculados. VER TAMBÉM zinc sulfate flotation centrifugation.
Gärtner m., m. de Gärtner; m. de medida da pressão venosa, baseado no fenômeno venoso de Gärtner; com o paciente sentado ereto, é selecionada uma veia no dorso da mão, com esta mantida um pouco abaixo do nível do átrio direito, sendo então elevada lentamente; quando se observa colapso da veia, a distância entre seu nível e o do átrio é medida com uma régua milimétrica; essa distância fornece a pressão venosa em mililitros de sangue; assim, a própria veia é usada como manômetro comunicando-se com o átrio direito; muito impreciso, principalmente em idosos.
Gerota m., m. de Gerota; injeção nos linfáticos de um corante solúvel em clorofórmio ou éter, mas não em água; a alcanina, o sulfeto vermelho de mercúrio e o azul da Prússia são adequados para esse objetivo.
glucose oxidase m., m. da glicose oxidase; método muito específico para medida da glicose no soro ou no plasma por reação com a glicose oxidase, na qual são formados o ácido glucônico e o peróxido de hidrogênio.
Gruber m., m. de Gruber; modificação do método de Politzer no qual o paciente não engole, mas diz "hoc" no momento da compressão da bolsa colocada na cavidade nasal.
Hamilton-Stewart m., m. de Hamilton-Stewart; fórmula para calcular o débito cardíaco após a injeção intravenosa do indicador; o fluxo sanguíneo em litros por minuto é obtido dividindo-se a dose de material injetado em miligramas pelo produto da concentração média de corante na curva inicial da concentração de corante obtida em determinado ponto na circulação e multiplicado pela dose de corante (em miligramas) para escrever a curva do surgimento ao desaparecimento (na ausência de qualquer recirculação). SIN Hamilton-Stewart formula, indicator dilution m., Stewart-Hamilton m.
Hammerschlag m., m. de Hammerschlag; m. hidrométrico para determinação da densidade específica do sangue, deixando-se cair uma gota de sangue em cada um de uma série de tubos contendo misturas de clorofórmio e benzeno com densidades específicas graduadas conhecidas; a densidade específica da mistura na qual a gota permanece exatamente suspensa, não aumentando nem caindo, corresponde à densidade específica da amostra de sangue.
hexokinase m., m. de hexokinase; o método mais específico para medida da glicose no soro ou no plasma, no qual a hexokinase mais o ATP transforma glicose em glicose-6-fosfato mais ADP; a glicose-6-fosfato reage então com NADP e glicose-6-fosfato desidrogenase para formar NADP, que é medido espectrofotometricamente.
Hilton m., m. de Hilton; divisão dos nervos que suprem uma parte, para alívio da dor nas úlceras.
Hirschsberg m., m. de Hirschsberg; método de medida do desvio de um olho estrábico, observando-se o reflexo de uma luz fixada pelo olho sem desvio na córnea do olho que apresenta desvio.
Hung method, método de Hung. SIN Wilson m.
immunofluorescence m., m. de imunofluorescência; qualquer método no qual se usa um anticorpo com marcação fluorescente para detectar a presença ou determinar a localização do antígeno correspondente.
impedance m., m. da impedância; método para localização de estruturas encefálicas medindo-se a impedância da corrente elétrica.
indicator dilution m., m. de diluição do indicador. SIN Hamilton-Stewart m.
indirect m. for making inlays, m. indireto para fazer incrustações; método pelo qual a incrustação é construída inteiramente sobre um modelo feito a partir de uma impressão do dente ou dentes preparados na boca. SIN indirect technique.
indophenol m., m. do indofenol; m. para determinar a quantidade de vitamina C em tecidos vegetais e animais com base na rápida redução de uma solução de indofenol padronizada em um composto incolor pela vitamina C em solução ácida.
introspective m., m. introspectivo; no funcionalismo, o estudo sistemático de fenômenos mentais pela contemplação dos processos em suas próprias experiências conscientes.
ITO m., m. ITO; m. de matriz conciso para calcular a distribuição dos genótipos de parentes que, em um *locus*, podem não ter genes em comum, um ou ambos.
Johnson m., m. de Johnson. SIN chloropercha m.

Keating-Hart m., m. de Keating-Hart; fulguração no tratamento do câncer externo ou do campo de operação após a retirada de um tumor maligno.

Kety-Schmidt m., m. de Kety-Schmidt; m. para medida do fluxo sanguíneo para um órgão, aplicado pela primeira vez ao encéfalo em 1944 por C.F. Schmidt e S.S. Kety. Um gás indicador quimicamente inerte é equilibrado com o tecido do órgão de interesse, sendo medida a taxa de desaparecimento do órgão. O fluxo sanguíneo é calculado com base na suposição de que as concentrações do gás indicador no tecido e no sangue venoso estão em equilíbrio de difusão em todas as velocidades de fluxo sanguíneo, e de que a velocidade de desaparecimento do indicador do tecido é uma função da quantidade existente no tecido naquele momento, isto é, supõe-se que seja um desaparecimento exponencial.

Kjeldahl m., m. de Kjeldahl. VER macro-Kjeldahl m., micro-Kjeldahl m.

Lamaze m., m. de Lamaze; técnica de preparo psicoprofilático para o parto, com o objetivo de minimizar a dor do trabalho de parto.

Langendorff m., m. de Langendorff; perfusão do coração de mamífero isolado pelo transporte de líquido sob pressão para o interior da aorta seccionada e, depois, para o sistema coronário.

Lee-White m., m. de Lee-White; m. para determinar o tempo de coagulação do sangue venoso em tubos de calibre padronizado à temperatura corporal.

Liborius m., m. de Liborius; m. para cultura de bactérias anaeróbicas; é feita uma cultura por agulha em ágar apropriado, depois liquefaz-se um pouco mais do mesmo meio e despeja-se no tubo de ensaio, sobre a cultura por agulha, vedando-a hermeticamente.

Ling m., m. de Ling; exercícios físicos (como nos movimentos suecos) sem uso de aparelhos.

Lister m., m. de Lister; cirurgia anti-séptica, defendida pela primeira vez por Lister em 1867; suas operações eram realizadas sob uma névoa de aerossol de ácido carbólico diluído, os instrumentos eram imersos em uma solução carbólica antes do uso, e a ferida era coberta por uma camada espessa de gaze carbolisada; a partir daí foi desenvolvida a prática atual de cirurgia asséptica. SIN listerism.

lod m., m. de lod; método de análise de ligação que utiliza um exame do logaritmo comum da razão de probabilidade para determinado valor da fração de recombinação e a probabilidade se a fração de recombinação fosse igual a 0,5 (isto é, não houver ligação); assim, um escore lod de 3 com uma fração de recombinação de 0,2 significa que os dados são 1.000 vezes mais facilmente explicados supondo-se uma fração de recombinação 0,2 do que supondo-se que os *loci* não estejam ligados e que a fração de recombinação seja 0,5. [logaritmo dos produtos cruzados]

longitudinal m., m. longitudinal; em psicologia do desenvolvimento, o estudo do tempo de vida de um indivíduo envolvendo comparações de diferentes faixas etárias. Cf. cross-sectional m.

macro-Kjeldahl m., m. de macro-Kjeldahl; procedimento para analisar o conteúdo dos compostos nitrogenados na urina, soro ou outras amostras, geralmente para determinar quantidades relativamente grandes de nitrogênio (p. ex., 20-100 mg); a amostra é tratada com uma mistura de digestão (sulfato de cobre e ácido sulfúrico), completamente aquecida e alcalinizada com uma solução de hidróxido de sódio; a seguir, a amônia é destilada da mistura, retida em uma solução indicadora de ácido bórico e titulada com ácido clorídrico ou sulfúrico padrão.

manual visual m., m. visual-manual; uma abordagem para a educação de crianças surdas que enfatiza o papel da visão na comunicação e o uso precoce e consistente da linguagem americana de sinais (ASL) ou de outras linguagens nacionais de sinais. VER TAMBÉM oral auditory m. combined m.'s, total *communication*.

Marshall m., m. de Marshall; procedimento quantitativo para estimar a sulfanilamida livre e conjugada nos líquidos corporais.

micro-Astrup m., m. micro-Astrup; técnica de interpolação para medida ácido-básica, baseada no pH e no uso do nomograma de Siggaard-Andersen para determinar o déficit de bases como uma expressão da acidose metabólica e a P_{CO_2} arterial como uma expressão da acidose ou alcalose respiratória.

micro-Kjeldahl m., m. micro-Kjeldahl; uma modificação do método macro-Kjeldahl designada para análise de compostos nitrogenados em quantidades relativamente pequenas, p. ex., amostras nas quais o conteúdo total de nitrogênio está na faixa de 1 a alguns miligramas.

microsphere m., m. das microsferas; método para medida do fluxo sanguíneo para um órgão por diluição do indicador, porém, mais importante, um método para medir a distribuição do débito cardíaco ou a distribuição do fluxo sanguíneo no órgão. Para medir a distribuição do fluxo, microsferas quimicamente inertes, flutuantes neutras que possuem uma propriedade indicadora (p. ex., radioatividade) são injetadas em uma câmara cardíaca ou no sangue arterial. Presume-se que sejam distribuídas proporcionalmente à distribuição do fluxo sanguíneo arterial. O tamanho da esfera injetada é selecionado de forma a ser grande o suficiente para fornecer amostras estatisticamente significativas e pequeno o suficiente para não alterar o fluxo sanguíneo para o órgão que está sendo investigado. São colhidas amostras do órgão para quantificar a distribuição das microsferas e, portanto, o fluxo. VER Fick m., Stewart-Hamilton m.

Moore m., m. de Moore; tratamento de aneurisma por introdução de um fio de prata ou zinco no saco para induzir a deposição de fibrina.

Needles split cast m., m. de divisão do molde de Needles. SIN split cast m.

Nikiforoff m., m. de Nikiforoff; a fixação de esfregaços sanguíneos por imersão por 5 a 15 minutos em álcool absoluto, uma mistura de partes iguais de álcool e éter, ou éter puro.

Ochsner m., m. de Ochsner; tratamento obsoleto para apendicite (por repouso peristáltico), quando não é aconselhável realizar cirurgia.

open circuit m., m. do circuito aberto; método para medir o consumo de oxigênio e a produção de dióxido de carbono colhendo-se o gás expirado durante um período conhecido e medindo-se seu volume e composição.

oral auditory m., m. auditivo-oral; conduta para a educação de crianças surdas que enfatiza o treinamento auditivo precoce, a fala e a leitura labial, e o uso precoce e consistente de amplificação de alta qualidade para utilizar a audição residual. VER TAMBÉM manual visual m., combined m.'s, total *communication*.

Orsi-Grocco m., m. de Orsi-Grocco; percussão palpatória do coração.

Ouchterlony method, método de Ouchterlony. SIN Ouchterlony *test.*

Pachon m., m. de Pachon; cardiografia realizada com o paciente em decúbito lateral esquerdo.

paracelsian m., m. de Paracelso; tratamento de doença utilizando apenas agentes químicos.

parallax m., m. da paralaxe; localização de um corpo estranho, por observação da direção de seu movimento em uma tela fluoroscópica, enquanto se movimenta o tubo de raios X ou a tela.

Pavlov m., m. de Pavlov; o método para estudo da atividade reflexa condicionada pela observação de um indicador motor, como a resposta salivar ou eletroencefalográfica.

Politzer m., m. de Politzer; insuflação da tuba auditiva (de Eustáquio) e da membrana timpânica forçando a entrada de ar na cavidade nasal no momento em que o paciente engole.

Porges m., m. de Porges; método de destruição das cápsulas bacterianas por aquecimento com ácido clorídrico N/4 e neutralização com NaOH.

Purmann m., m. de Purmann; tratamento de aneurisma por extirpação do saco.

Quick m., m. de Quick. SIN prothrombin *test.*

reference m., m. de referência; procedimento analítico suficientemente livre de erro aleatório ou sistemático, útil para validar novos procedimentos analíticos propostos para o mesmo analisado.

Rehfuss m., m. de Rehfuss; método de medida fracional da atividade gástrica; um tubo fino com ponta de metal fenestrada é introduzido no estômago após uma refeição de teste, e pequenos volumes (6 ou 8 ml) do conteúdo gástrico são removidos a intervalos de 15 minutos e examinados.

rhythm m., m. de ritmo; método contraceptivo natural que programa as relações sexuais humanas para evitar o período fértil do ciclo menstrual. SIN rhythm (2).

Rideal-Walker m., m. de Rideal-Walker. VER Rideal-Walker *coefficient*.

Roux m., m. de Roux; divisão da mandíbula na linha média, para facilitar a operação de ablação da língua.

Sanger m., m. de Sanger; o método para seqüenciamento de DNA empregando uma enzima que consegue polimerizar o DNA e os nucleotídeos marcados.

Scarpa m., m. de Scarpa; cura de aneurisma por ligadura da artéria a alguma distância acima do saco.

Schäfer m., m. de Schäfer; método obsoleto de ressuscitação em casos de afogamento ou asfixia; o paciente é colocado com a face voltada para baixo e a respiração natural é imitada por compressão suave intermitente da parte inferior do tórax na freqüência de, aproximadamente, 15 vezes por minuto.

Schede m., m. de Schede; enchimento do defeito no osso, após remoção de um seqüestro ou raspagem de material cariado, permitindo que a cavidade se encha de sangue, que pode tornar-se organizado (coágulo de Schede).

Schick m., m. de Schick. SIN Schick *test.*

Schmidt-Thannhauser m., m. de Schmidt-Thannhauser; método para fracionamento de ácidos nucleicos baseado no fato de que o RNA, mas não o DNA, é hidrolisado em nucleotídeos por álcalis; o RNA pode ser hidrolisado em cerca de 2 h em NaOH 0,75 N, mas geralmente são usadas 18 h e NaOH 0,3 N.

Schweninger m., m. de Schweninger; método sugerido para reduzir a obesidade por restrição da ingestão de líquido.

Shaffer-Hartmann m., m. de Shaffer-Hartmann; método obsoleto para determinação quantitativa de glicose nos líquidos biológicos, baseado na redução do cobre pelo grupo redutor do açúcar.

Somogyi m., m. de Somogyi. VER Somogyi *unit*.

split cast m., m. de divisão do molde; (1) um procedimento para colocação de moldes indexados em um articulador para facilitar sua remoção e substituição no instrumento; (2) o procedimento de verificar a capacidade de um articulador de receber ou estar ajustado para registro de uma relação maxilomandibular. SIN Needles split cast m.

Stas-Otto m., m. de Stas-Otto; método de extração de alcalóides de vegetais e corpos de animais: a substância é digerida em álcool e ácido tartárico; os materiais gordurosos e resinosos são precipitados com água, o líquido é tornado alcalino e os alcalóides são extraídos com éter ou clorofórmio.

Stewart-Hamilton m., m. de Stewart-Hamilton. SIN Hamilton-Stewart m.

method 984 **methyl bromide.**

Thane m., m. de Thane; método para indicar a posição do sulco central (fissura de Rolando) do encéfalo; a extremidade superior do sulco corresponde ao ponto médio de uma linha desenhada da glabela até o ínio.

Theden m., m. de Theden; tratamento de aneurismas ou de grandes derrames sanguíneos por compressão de todo o membro com uma atadura cilíndrica.

Thezac-Porsmeur m., m. de Thezac-Porsmeur; tratamento térmico de feridas infectadas por concentração de raios solares em área supurativa por meio de uma lente montada em um cilindro de lona.

thiochrome m., m. do tiocromo; método para determinação da tiamina baseado na produção de tiocromo quando a vitamina é oxidada por ferricianeto alcalino para produzir o composto fluorescente tiocromo.

twin m., m. gemelar; forma geral de análise genética que se beneficia do fato de que, embora os gêmeos tenham a mesma idade e estejam no mesmo ambiente intra-uterino, os gêmeos idênticos (monozigóticos) possuem o mesmo genótipo, mas os gêmeos dizigóticos não são mais semelhantes do que irmãos e podem ter sexos diferentes.

ultropaque m., m. ultra-opaco; método rápido para exame de cortes espessos (1–3 mm) de tecido fresco com o ultramicroscópio, que utiliza um objeto construído em um iluminador de forma que a luz seja refletida sobre o tecido.

u-score m., m. u-score; um método mais antigo, mais simples, porém um pouco menos eficiente de análise de ligação que por estimativa da probabilidade máxima.

Wardrop m., m. de Wardrop; tratamento de aneurisma por ligadura da artéria a alguma distância além do saco, deixando um ou mais ramos da artéria entre o saco e a ligadura.

Westergren m., m. de Westergren; procedimento para estimar a velocidade de hemossedimentação (VHS) misturando-se o sangue venoso com uma solução aquosa de citrato de sódio, e permitindo que repouse em uma pipeta padrão vertical (200 mm de comprimento) cheia até a marca zero; observa-se, então, a queda das hemácias, em milímetros, em 1 hora; a VHS normal para homens é de 0–15 mm (média, 4 mm) e, para mulheres, 0–20 mm (média, 5 mm).

Wheeler m., m. de Wheeler; procedimento cirúrgico para correção de ectrópio cicatricial.

Wilson m., m. de Wilson; método de flutuação simples em solução salina para concentração de ovos de helmintos nas fezes. VER flotation m. SIN Hung method.

zinc sulfate flotation centrifugation m., m. de centrifugação com flutuação em sulfato de zinco; m. de flutuação no qual a amostra de fezes é suspensa em água de torneira, coada através de uma gaze úmida, centrifugada, ressuspensa em água de torneira, lavada e recentrifugada várias vezes e, depois, suspensa em solução de sulfato de zinco a 33% e centrifugada em velocidade máxima por 45–60 segundos; pode-se usar uma alça bacteriológica para apanhar a camada superficial, que contém cistos de protozoários e ovos de helmintos.

---

meth·od·ism (meth′od - izm). Metodismo. SIN solidism.
meth·o·dol·o·gy (meth′u - dol - ō - jē). Metodologia; o estudo científico ou a análise lógica de métodos.
meth·o·hex·i·tal so·di·um (meth - ō - heks′i - tawl). Metoexital sódico; um barbitúrico de ação ultracurta, usado por via intravenosa para indução e para anestesia geral de curta duração.
meth·o·phen·a·zine (me - thō - fen′a - zēn). Metofenazina; antipsicótico.
meth·o·pho·line (me - thō - fō′lēn). Metofolina; analgésico.
meth·op·ter·in (meth - op′ter - in). Metopterina; antagonista do ácido fólico.
meth·or·phi·nan (meth - ōr′fi - nan). Metorfinano. VER dextromethorphan hydrobromide, levorphanol tartrate.
meth·o·ser·pi·dine (meth - ō - ser′pi - dēn). Metosserpidina; anti-hipertensivo com ações semelhantes às da reserpina.
meth·o·trex·ate (meth - ō - trek′sāt). Metotrexato; antagonista do ácido fólico usado como antineoplásico; usado no tratamento da psoríase e da artrite reumatóide. SIN amethopterin.
meth·o·tri·mep·ra·zine (meth′ō - trī - mep′ra - zēn). Metotrimeprazina; um analgésico fenotiazínico.
me·thox·a·mine hy·dro·chlo·ride (me - thok′sa - mēn). Cloridrato de metoxamina; uma amina simpaticomimética.
me·thox·sa·len (me - thok′sa - len). Metoxissaleno; derivado do metoxipsoraleno que aumenta a produção de melanina na pele quando exposta à luz ultravioleta; usado por via oral e tópica no tratamento do vitiligo idiopático, e também como acelerador do bronzeamento e protetor solar.
⚠ **methoxy-.** Prefixo químico que designa substituição de um grupo metoxila.
4-me·thox·y·ben·zo·ic ac·id (meth - ok′sē - ben - zō′ik). Ácido 4-metoxibenzóico. SIN anistic acid.
me·thox·y·chlor (me - thok′sē - klōr). Metoxicloro; inseticida semelhante ao DDT; ectoparasiticida.
me·thox·y·flu·rane (me - thok - sē - floor′an). Metoxiflurano; potente anestésico inalatório não mais usado devido à insuficiência renal de alto débito causada por aumento das concentrações plasmáticas de fluoreto inorgânico, um produto da decomposição metabólica do metoxiflurano.

3-me·thox·y-4-hy·drox·y·man·del·ic ac·id. Ácido 3-metoxi-4-hidroximandélico. VER vanillylmandelic acid.
5-me·thox·y·in·dole-3-ac·e·tate (meth - oks′ē - in - dōl). 5-Metoxindol-3-acetato; intermediário da degradação do triptofano e da serotonina; excretado como conjugados.
me·thox·yl (me-thok′sil). Metoxil; o grupamento –OCH$_3$.
me·thox·y·phen·a·mine hy·dro·chlo·ride (me - thok - sē - fen′a - mēn). Cloridrato de metoxifenamina; uma amina simpaticomimética.
5-me·thox·y·trypt·a·mine (meth - oks′ē - trip - ta - mēn). 5-Metoxitriptamina; um intermediário na degradação do L-triptofano e da serotonina.
meth·sco·pol·a·mine bro·mide (meth - skō - pol′a - mēn). Brometo de metescopolamina; agente parassimpaticolítico semelhante à atropina; o nitrato de metila tem a mesma ação e empregos.
meth·sux·i·mide (meth - sŭk′si - mīd). Metossuximida; antiepiléptico efetivo contra o pequeno mal e a epilepsia psicomotora; semelhante à etossuximida.
meth·y·clo·thi·a·zide (meth′i - klō - thī′a - zīd). Meticlotiazida; diurético e anti-hipertensivo do grupo tiazida, eficaz por via oral.
meth·yl (Me) (meth′il). Metila; o radical –CH$_3$. [G. *methy*, vinho, + *hylē*, madeira]
  active m., m. ativa; grupamento metila fixado a um íon amônio quaternário ou a um íon sulfônio terciário que pode tomar parte nas reações de transmetilação; p. ex., grupamentos metila na colina e na *S*-adenosil-L-metionina, que, assim, são doadores de metila.
  m. aldehyde, aldeído metílico. SIN formaldehyde.
  angular m., m. angular; grupamento metila fixado ao carbono 10 (entre os anéis A e B) ou ao carbono 13 (entre os anéis C e D) do núcleo esteróide.
  m. chloride, cloreto de metila. SIN chloromethane.
  m. cysteine hydrochloride, cloridrato de m. cisteína; o éster metil do cloridrato de cisteína; um agente mucolítico.
  m. hydroxybenzoate, hidroxibenzoato de metila. SIN methylparaben.
  m. isobutyl ketone, cetona metil isobutílica; em altas concentrações, possui ação narcótica, em concentrações relativamente baixas, pode causar irritação dos olhos e mucosas.
  m. methacrylate, metacrilato de metila; material termoplástico usado para bases de dentaduras e como material de incrustação para microscopia eletrônica.
  m. nicotinate, nicotinato de metila; éster metílico do ácido nicotínico, usado como rubefaciente.
2-meth·yl·a·ce·to·a·ce·tyl-CoA thi·o·lase. 2-Metilacetoacetil-CoA tiolase; enzima que faz parte da via de degradação da L-isoleucina; catalisa a conversão da 2-metilacetoacetil-CoA em acetil-CoA e propionil-CoA. A deficiência dessa enzima leva ao acúmulo de 2-metilacetoacetil-CoA, causando episódios de acidose metabólica grave e cetose.
meth·yl·a·cryl·ic ac·id (meth′il - ă - kril′ik). Ácido metilacrílico. SIN methacrylic acid.
meth·yl·am·phet·a·mine hy·dro·chlo·ride (meth′il - am - fet′a - mēn). Cloridrato de metilanfetamina. SIN methamphetamine hydrochloride.
N-methyl D-aspartic acid. Ácido *N*-metil D-aspártico. SIN NMDA.
meth·yl·ate (meth′i - lāt). **1.** Metilar; misturar com metanol. **2.** Introduzir um grupo metil. **3.** Metilato; composto em que um íon metálico metil substitui o hidrogênio alcoólico do álcool.
meth·yl·a·tion (meth - i - lā′shŭn). Metilação; adição de grupos metila; em histoquímica, usado para esterificar grupamentos carboxila e remover grupos sulfato por tratamento de cortes de tecido com metanol quente na presença de ácido clorídrico; o efeito final é a redução da basofilia tecidual e a extinção da metacromasia.
  restriction m., m. de restrição; a adição enzimática de grupamentos metila a resíduos adenina e citosina selecionados para proteger da hidrólise por algumas enzimas de restrição.
meth·yl·at·ro·pine bro·mide (meth - il - at′rō - pēn, - pin). Brometo de metilatropina; derivado quaternário da atropina menos lipossolúvel e que, portanto, produz menos ações no sistema nervoso central; um ciclopégico. SIN atropine methylbromide.
meth·yl·ben·zene (meth - il - ben′zēn). Metilbenzeno. SIN toluene.
meth·yl·ben·ze·tho·ni·um chlo·ride (meth′il - ben - zē - thō′nē - ŭm). Cloreto de metilbenzetônio; composto de amônio quaternário que possui uma ação superficial semelhante à de outros detergentes catiônicos; geralmente germicida e bacteriostático; usado na limpeza de fraldas de crianças e lençóis na prevenção da dermatite amoniacal.
meth·yl blue [C.I. 42780]. Azul de metila; corante trifenilrosanilina sulfatado usado como corante do citoplasma, colágeno e corpúsculos de Negri, e como anti-séptico.
meth·yl bro·mide. Brometo de metila; usado nas câmaras de ionização; para retirar a gordura da lã; extrair óleos de nozes, sementes, flores; usado como fumigante de insetos em moinhos, armazéns, cofres, navios, vagões de carga; também é usado como fumigante do solo.

N-meth·yl·car·no·sine (meth - il - kar′nō - sēn). N-metilcarnosina. SIN anserine (2).

meth·yl-CCNU. Metil-CCNU; agente antineoplásico nitrosuréia semelhante à carmustina (BCNU) e à lomustina (CCNU). SIN semustine.

meth·yl·cel·lu·lose (meth - il - sel′ū - lōs). Metilcelulose; éster metílico da celulose que forma um líquido viscoso incolor quando dissolvido em água, álcool ou éter; usado para aumentar o volume do conteúdo intestinal para aliviar a constipação, ou do conteúdo gástrico para reduzir o apetite na obesidade; também é usada dissolvida em água na forma de *spray* para cobrir áreas queimadas e como agente suspensor em medicamentos e alimentos.

meth·yl·chlo·ro·form (meth - il - chlōr′ō - form). Metilclorofórmio. SIN trichloroethane.

3-meth·yl·chol·an·threne, 20-meth·yl·chol·an·threne (meth′il - kōl - an′thrēn). 3-Metilcolantreno, 20-metilcolantreno; hidrocarboneto muito carcinógeno que pode ser formado quimicamente a partir dos ácidos desoxicólico ou cólico, ou do colesterol; induz a síntese de RNAm do citocromo P-450; a escolha entre 3- ou 20- para o grupamento metila depende da escolha de numeração do hidrocarboneto (interno) ou do esteróide (externo); no último caso, a relação formal entre os ácidos cólicos e o colesterol é clara.

meth·yl·cit·rate (meth - il - sit′trāt). Metilcitrato; metabólito menor que se acumula em indivíduos com acidemia propiônica.

meth·yl·co·bal·a·min (meth - il - kō - bal′a - mēn). Metilcobalamina. SIN vitamin B$_{12}$.

3-meth·yl·cro·ton·yl-CoA (meth - il - krō′ton - il). 3-Metilcrotonil-CoA; um intermediário na degradação da L-leucina; acumula-se na deficiência de 3-metilcrotonil-CoA carboxilase.

3-methylcrotonyl-CoA carboxylase, 3-metilcrotonil-CoA carboxilase; enzima dependente de biotina na via da degradação da L-leucina que catalisa a reação da 3-metilcrotonil-CoA com CO_2, ATP e água para formar ADP, ortofosfato e 3-metilcrotonil-CoA; uma deficiência dessa enzima causa episódios de acidose metabólica grave.

5-meth·yl·cy·to·sine (meth′il - sī′tō - sēn). 5-Metilcitosina; base menor que está presente no DNA bacteriano e humano.

meth·yl·di·chlo·ro·ar·sine (MD) (meth′il - dī - klōr - ō - ar′sēn). Metildicloroarsina; vesicante; causa irritação das vias respiratórias e produz lesão pulmonar e lesão oftálmica; foi usado em algumas operações militares.

meth·yl·do·pa (meth - il - dō′pä). Metildopa; agente anti-hipertensivo, também usado como cloridrato de éster etílico, com a mesma ação e empregos. SIN alpha methyl dopa.

meth·yl·ene (meth′i - lēn). Metileno; o radical –CH_2–.

meth·yl·ene az·ure. Azur de metileno. SIN azure I.

meth·yl·ene blue [C.I. 52015]. Azul de metileno; corante básico facilmente oxidado em azur, com misturas de corantes; usado em histologia e microbiologia para corar protozoários intestinais em preparações a fresco, rastrear RNA e RNase na eletroforese, e como antídoto para metemoglobinemia; suas propriedades indicadoras redox são úteis na bacteriologia do leite.

Kühne m. b., azul de metileno de Kühne; azul de metileno em solução de álcool absoluto e fenol.

Loeffler m. b., azul de metileno de Loeffler; corante para organismos da difteria que contêm azul de metileno em etanol diluído mais uma pequena quantidade de hidróxido de potássio; a solução do corante oferece melhores resultados quando envelhecida até um estado policromo.

new m. b. [C.I. 52030], azul de metileno novo; corante tiazínico básico usado para coloração supravital de reticulócitos em esfregaços sanguíneos.

polychrome m. b., azul de metileno policromo; solução alcalina de azul de metileno que sofre desmetilação oxidativa progressiva com o envelhecimento (amadurecimento) para produzir uma mistura de azul de metileno, azures e violeta de metileno; a fervura com bicarbonato de sódio ou outros agentes oxidantes leva rapidamente a esse resultado, embora isso não seja muito levado em consideração.

meth·yl·ene chlo·ride. Cloreto de metileno; líquido volátil com odor acre; vapor nocivo. Solvente orgânico usado no plástico de acetato de celulose; em líquidos desengordurantes e de limpeza; e no processamento de alimentos. Auxiliar farmacêutico (solvente).

3,4-meth·yl·ene·di·oxy·meth·am·phet·a·mine. 3,4-Metilenodioximetanfetamina. SIN MDMA.

meth·yl·ene·suc·cin·ic ac·id (meth′il - ēn - sŭk′sin - ik). Ácido metilenossuccínico. SIN itaconic acid.

N^5,N^{10}-meth·yl·ene·tet·ra·hy·dro·fo·late re·duc·tase. N^5,N^{10}-metilenotetraidrofolato redutase; enzima que converte N^5,N^{10}-metilenotetraidrofolato em N^5,N^{10}-metiniltetraidrofolato utilizando $NADP^+$; a deficiência dessa enzima resulta em acúmulo de L-homocisteína e em distúrbios neurológicos graves.

meth·yl·ene white. Branco de metileno. SIN leucomethylene blue.

meth·yl·en·o·phil, meth·yl·en·o·phile (meth - i - lēn′ō - fil, - fīl). Metilenófilo; que se cora facilmente com azul de metileno; designa determinadas células e estruturas histológicas. SIN methylenophilic, methylenophilous. [methylene + G. *philos*, amigo]

meth·yl·en·o·phil·ic, meth·yl·e·noph·i·lous (meth′i - lē - nō - fil′ik, meth′ - il - ē - nof′i - lŭs). Metilenofílico. SIN methylenophil.

meth·yl·er·go·met·rine ma·le·ate (meth′il - er - gō - met′rēn). Maleato de metilergometrina. SIN methylergonovine maleate.

meth·yl·er·go·no·vine ma·le·ate (meth′il - er - gō - nō′vēn). Maleato de metilergonovina; derivado do ácido lisérgico, parcialmente sintetizado, com ação ocitócica, usado para prevenir ou tratar atonia e hemorragia uterina pósparto. SIN methylergometrine maleate.

meth·yl·glu·ca·mine (meth - il - gloo′kă - mēn). Metilglucamina; cátion comumente usado em contrastes radiológicos iodados hidrossolúveis. SIN N-methylglucamine.

m. diatrizoate, diatrizoato de metilglucamina. SIN meglumine diatrizoate.

N-meth·yl·glu·ca·mine. N-metilglucamina. SIN metylglucamine.

3-meth·yl·glu·ta·con·ic ac·i·du·ria (meth - il - gloo - ta - kon′ik). 3-Metilglutacônico acidúria; níveis elevados de ácido 3-metilglutacônico na urina. Distúrbio hereditário cuja forma leve é resultado da deficiência de 3-metilglutaconil-CoA hidratase, levando ao atraso no desenvolvimento da fala.

3-meth·yl·glu·ta·con·yl-CoA hy·dra·tase. 3-Metilglutaconil-CoA hidratase; enzima que catalisa a reação de *trans*-3-metilglutaconil-CoA e água para formar 3-hidroxi-3-metilglutaconil-CoA; essa enzima participa da via para degradação da L-leucina; uma deficiência dessa enzima resultará em 3-metilglutacônico acidúria.

meth·yl·gly·ox·al (meth′il - glī - ok′sal). Metilglioxal; piruvaldeído; o aldeído do ácido pirúvico; intermediário do metabolismo dos carboidratos em alguns organismos. SIN pyruvic aldehyde.

m. bis(guanylhydrazone), m. bis(guanil-hidrazona); agente antineoplásico.

meth·yl·gly·ox·a·lase (meth′il - glī - oks′ă - lās). Metilglioxalase. SIN lactoylglutathione lyase.

meth·yl green [C.I. 42585]. Verde de metila; corante trifenilmetano básico usado como corante da cromatina e, combinado à pironina, para coloração diferencial de RNA (vermelho) e DNA (verde); também usado como corante de rastreamento do DNA na eletroforese.

meth·yl·hex·ane·a·mine (meth′il - hek - sān′ă - mēn, - min). Metilexanoamina; base amina simpática volátil, usada como descongestionante nasal por via inalatória.

N-meth·yl·his·tid·ine (meth′il - his′ti - dēn). N-metilistidina; derivado metilado da histidina encontrado na actina; na degradação da actina e miosina, a N-metilistidina é liberada na urina; o débito urinário da N-metilistidina é um índice fidedigno da taxa de degradação das proteínas miofibrilares na musculatura.

meth·yl·ki·nase (meth′il - kī′nās). Metilcinase. SIN methyltransferase.

meth·yl·mal·o·nate sem·i·al·de·hyde (meth′il - mă - lon - āt). Semi-aldeído de metilmalonato; intermediário no catabolismo da L-valina; elevado em alguns distúrbios congênitos.

meth·yl·ma·lon·ic ac·id (meth′il - mă - lon′ik). Ácido metilmalônico; ácido 2-metil-propanedióico, importante intermediário no metabolismo dos ácidos graxos; observado em níveis elevados em casos de deficiência de vitamina B$_{12}$. Observe que o metilmalonato não é o mesmo que malonato de metila, que é o éster dimetílico do malonato. SIN isosuccinic acid.

meth·yl·ma·lon·ic ac·i·de·mia. Acidemia metilmalônica. SIN ketotic hyperglycinemia.

meth·yl·ma·lon·ic ac·i·du·ria. Acidúria metilmalônica; excreção de quantidades excessivas de ácido metilmalônico na urina devido à atividade deficiente de metilmalonil-CoA mutase ou deficiência de cobalamina redutase. Existem dois tipos: 1) um erro congênito do metabolismo que resulta em cetoacidose grave logo após o nascimento, com cetonas urinárias de cadeia longa; herança autossômica recessiva, causada por mutações no gene da metilmalonil-CoA mutase (MCM) no cromossoma 6p [MIM*251000]; 2) adquirido, um tipo de deficiência de vitamina B$_{12}$ [MIM*251110] devido à deficiência da síntese de adenosilcobalamina.

meth·yl·mal·o·nyl-CoA. Metilmalonil-CoA; intermediário na degradação de vários metabólitos (p. ex., valina, metionina, ácidos graxos de ímpar, treonina); está elevada em casos de anemia perniciosa.

m.-CoA epimerase, m.-CoA epimerase; enzima que catalisa a interconversão de D-metilmalonil-CoA e L-metilmalonil-CoA.

m.-CoA mutase, m.-CoA mutase; enzima que catalisa uma interconversão reversível de L-metilmalonil-CoA e succinil-CoA; uma enzima cobalamina-dependente; a deficiência dessa enzima resultará em acidemia metilmalônica.

meth·yl·mer·cu·ry. Metilmercúrio. SIN dimethylmercury.

meth·yl·mor·phine (meth - il - mōr′fēn). Metilmorfina. SIN codeine.

meth·yl·ol (meth′i-lol). Metilol; hidroximetil; o radical –CH_2OH.

meth·yl or·ange. Laranja de metila; corante fracamente ácido usado como indicador do pH (vermelho a 3,2; amarelo a 4,4). SIN helianthine.

meth·y·lose (meth′i - lōs). Metilose; açúcar no qual o átomo de carbono mais distante do grupamento carbonila é uma metila (CH_3).

meth·yl·par·a·ben (meth - il - par′ă - ben). Metilparabeno; um preservativo antifúngico. SIN methyl hydroxybenzoate.

meth·yl·pen·tose (meth - il - pen′tōs). Metilpentose; uma hexose (6-desoxiexose) na qual o carbono 6 é parte de um grupo metila; p. ex., ramnose, fucose.

meth·yl·phen·i·date hy·dro·chlo·ride (meth - il - fen′i - dāt). Cloridrato de metilfenidato; estimulante do sistema nervoso central usado para produzir estimulação cortical leve em vários tipos de depressões; comumente usado no tratamento de crianças hipercinéticas ou hiperativas (distúrbio do déficit de atenção).

meth·yl·pred·nis·o·lone (meth′il - pred - nis′ō - lōn). Metilprednisolona; glicocorticóide antiinflamatório.
   m. acetate, acetato de m.; possui as mesmas ações e empregos da metilprednisolona; as suspensões aquosas são adequadas para injeção intra-sinovial e nos tecidos moles.
   sodium m. succinate, succinato sódico de m.; possui as mesmas ações metabólicas e antiinflamatórias que a substância original, metilprednisolona; devido à sua solubilidade, pode ser administrado em pequenos volumes.

meth·yl red. Vermelho de metila; corante fracamente ácido usado como indicador do pH (vermelho a 4,8; amarelo a 6,0); facilmente reduzido com a perda de cor, e as leituras de pH devem ser feitas rapidamente.

5-meth·yl·res·or·cin·ol (meth′il - rē - sōr′sin - ol). 5-Metilresorcinol. SIN orcinol.

meth·yl·ros·an·i·line chlo·ride (meth′il - rō - zan′i - lēn, - lin). Cloreto de metilrosanilina. SIN crystal violet.

meth·yl sa·lic·y·late. Salicilato de metila; o éster metílico do ácido salicílico, produzido sinteticamente ou destilado da *Gaultheria procumbens* (família Ericaceae) ou da *Betula lenta* (família Betulaceae); usado externa e internamente para tratamento de várias formas de reumatismo. SIN checkerberry oil, gaultheria oil, sweet birch oil, wintergreen oil.

methyl-*tert*-butyl ether (MTBE). Éter de metil-*tert*-butil; usado para dissolver cálculos biliares.

meth·yl·tes·tos·ter·one (meth′il - tes - tos′ter - ōn). Metiltestosterona; derivado metil da testosterona, com as mesmas ações e empregos, exceto por ser ativo quando administrado por via oral ou sublingual. Usado no tratamento do hipogenitalismo. SIN 17α-methyltestosterone.

17α-meth·yl·tes·tos·ter·one. 17α-Metiltestosterona. SIN methyltestosterone.

N⁵-meth·yl·tet·ra·hy·dro·fo·late (meth - il - tet′ra - hī - drō - fōl - āt). N⁵-metiltetraidrofolato; derivado ativo do tetraidrofolato, contendo um carbono, e que participa da S-metilação da L-homocisteína.
   N⁵-m.:homocysteine methyltransferase, N⁵-m.:homocisteína metiltransferase. VER methionine synthase.

meth·yl·thi·o·a·den·o·sine (meth′il - thī′ō - a - den′ō - sēn). Metiltioadenosina; adenosina que possui um grupamento –SCH₃ no lugar do OH na posição 5′; o grupamento –SCH₃ é transferido para o ácido α-aminobutírico para formar L-metionina em algumas bactérias. A metiltioadenosina é formada a partir da S-adenosil-L-metionina no curso da síntese da espermidina por perda do grupamento alanina. SIN thiomethyladenosine.

meth·yl·thi·o·u·ra·cil (meth′il - thī - ō - ū′ra - sil). Metiltiouracil; composto antitireóideo com a mesma ação do propiltiouracil, mas que exige dose menor.

meth·yl·to·col (meth - il - tō′kol). Metiltocol; tocol metilado; p. ex., tocotrienol, os tocoferóis.

meth·yl·trans·fer·ase (meth - il - trans′fer - ās). Metiltransferase; qualquer enzima que transfira grupamentos metila de uma substância para outra. SIN demethylase, methylkinase, transmethylase.

meth·yl vi·o·let [C.I. 42535]. Violeta de metila; misturas de tetra-, penta- ou pararrosanilina que variam em tons de violeta, dependendo do grau de metilação (designada R para tons avermelhados e B para tons azulados); o composto hexametil é conhecido como violeta cristal, o composto pentametil como violeta de metila 6B. Como corante, o violeta de metila tem muitas aplicações bacteriológicas, histológicas e citológicas.

meth·yl·xan·thines (meth′il-zan′thinz). Metilxantinas; grupo químico de substâncias derivadas da xantina (derivado da purina); os membros do grupo incluem teofilina, cafeína e teobromina.

meth·yl yel·low. Amarelo de metila. SIN butter yellow.

meth·y·pry·lon, meth·y·pry·lone (meth - i - prī′lon, - lōn). Metiprilona; sedativo e hipnótico.

meth·y·ser·gide ma·le·ate (meth - i - ser′jīd). Maleato de metisergida; antagonista da serotonina, fracamente adrenolítico, quimicamente relacionado com a metilergonovina; usado no tratamento profilático da cefaléia vascular (enxaqueca); é comum haver efeitos indesejados.

me·thys·ti·cum (mē - this′ti - kŭm). Kawa kawa; a raiz da *Piper methysticum* (família Piperaceae), uma planta das ilhas do Pacífico, usada pelos nativos como inebriante. Foi usada na diarréia e na afecção inflamatória do sistema urogenital. SIN kava (1).

metMb Abreviatura de metmyoglobin (metemioglobina).

met·my·o·glo·bin (metMb) (met′mī - ō - glō′bin). Metemioglobina; mioglobina na qual o íon ferroso do grupo prostético heme é oxidado em íon férrico; ferrimyoglobin.

met·o·clo·pra·mide hy·dro·chlo·ride (met′ō - klō - pram′īd). Cloridrato de metoclopramida; agente antiemético.

met·o·cur·ine io·dide (met - ō - kūr′ēn). Iodeto de metocurina; bloqueador neuromuscular não-despolarizante, usado para produzir relaxamento durante cirurgias. SIN dimethyl *d*-tubocurarine, dimethyl tubocurarine iodide.

me·tol·a·zone (me - tol′a - zōn). Metolazona; diurético com atividade anti-hipertensiva.

me·top·a·gus (mē - top′a - gŭs). Metópago; metopópago; gêmeos conjugados unidos pela fronte. VER conjoined *twins*, em *twin*. [G. *metōpon*, fronte, + *pagos*, algo fixo]

me·top·ic (me - tō′pik, me - top′ik). Metópico; relativo à fronte ou à porção anterior do crânio. [G. *metōpon*, fronte]

me·to·pi·on (mē - tō′pē - on). Um ponto craniométrico a meio caminho entre as eminências frontais. SIN ponto metópico. [G. *metōpon*, fronte]

met·o·pism (met′ō - pizm). Metopismo; persistência da sutura frontal no adulto. [G. *metōpon*, fronte]

met·o·po·plas·ty (met′ō - pō - plas - tē, me - top′ō - plas - tē). Metopoplastia; cirurgia plástica da pele ou osso da fronte. [G. *metōpon*, fronte, + *plastos*, formado]

met·o·pos·co·py (met′ō - pos′kō - pē). Metoposcopia; o estudo da fisiognomia. [G. *metōpon*, fronte, + *skopeō*, ver]

me·to·pro·lol tar·trate (me - tō′prō - lol). Tartarato de metoprolol; bloqueador β-adrenérgico usado no tratamento da hipertensão; exibe alguma cardiosseletividade.

Met·or·chis (met - ōr′kis). Gênero de trematódeos de peixes opistorquídeos parasitas da vesícula biliar de mamíferos e aves que se alimentam de peixe, comum nas regiões temperadas do norte. *M. conjunctus* é uma espécie encontrada em cães e gatos e, algumas vezes, em seres humanos na América do Norte. [G. *meta*, atrás, + *orchis*, testículo]

me·tox·e·nous (me - tok′sē - nŭs). Metóxeno. SIN heterecious. [G. *meta*, além, + *xenos*, hospedeiro]

me·tox·e·ny (me - tok′sē - nē). Metoxenia. **1.** SIN heterecism. **2.** Alteração do hospedeiro por um parasita. [G. *meta*, além, + *xenos*, hospedeiro]

⚠ **metr-, metra-, metro-.** O útero. VER TAMBÉM hystero- (1), utero. [G. *mētra*]

me·tra (mē′tra). Útero. SIN uterus. [G. uterus]

me·tra·to·nia (mē - tra - tō′nē - ă). Metratonia, atonia pós-parto. SIN postpartum *atony*. [metra- + G. *a-* priv. + *tonos*, tensão]

me·tria (mē′trē - ă). Celulite pélvica ou outra afecção inflamatória no período puerperal. [G. *mētra*, útero]

met·ric (met′rik). Métrico; quantitativo; relativo a medida. VER metric *system*. [G. *metrikos*, de *metron*, medida]

me·tri·fo·nate (me - tri′fō - nāt). Metrifonato. SIN trichlorfon.

met·ri·o·ce·phal·ic (met′rē - ō - se - fal′ik). Metriocefálico; que possui uma cabeça proporcional à altura; designa um crânio com índice entre 72 e 77. VER TAMBÉM orthocephalic. [G. *metrios*, moderado, de *metron*, medida, + *kephalē*, cabeça]

me·tri·tis (mē - trī′tis). Metrite; inflamação do útero. [G. *mētra*, útero, + *-itis*, inflamação]

me·triz·a·mide (me - triz′a - mīd). Metrizamida. SIN metrizoate sodium.

met·ri·zo·ate so·di·um (met - ri - zō′āt). Metrizoato sódico; meio radiopaco para diagnóstico. SIN metrizamide.

⚠ **metro-.** VER metr-. [G. *mētra*, útero]

me·tro·cyte (mē′trō - sīt). Metrócito, célula-mãe. SIN mother *cell*. [G. *mētēr*, mãe, + *kytos*, uma cavidade (célula)]

me·tro·dy·na·mom·e·ter (mē - trō - dī′na - mom′e - ter). Metrodinamômetro; instrumento para medir a força das contrações uterinas. [metro- + G. *dynamis*, força, + *metron*, medida]

me·tro·dyn·ia (mē - trō - dī′nē - ă). Metrodinia. SIN hysteralgia. [metro- + G. *odynē*, dor]

me·tro·lym·phan·gi·tis (mē′trō - lim - fan - jī′tis). Metrolinfangite; inflamação dos linfáticos uterinos. [metro- + lymphangitis]

met·ro·ni·da·zole (met - rō - ni′da - zōl). Metronidazol; tricomonicida efetivo por via oral, usado no tratamento de infecções causadas por *Trichomonas vaginalis* e *Entamoeba histolytica* e bactérias anaeróbicas Gram-negativas. Pode causar uma reação do tipo dissulfiram quando combinado ao álcool.

me·tron·o·scope (me′tron′ō - skōp). Metronoscópio; aparelho taquistoscópico que expõe, durante intervalos determinados, curtas seleções de material impresso para leitura; usado no teste e no desenvolvimento da velocidade de leitura. [G. *metron*, medida, + *skopeō*, ver]

me·tro·path·ia (mē - trō - path′ē - ă). Metropatia. SIN metropathy. [L.]
   m. hemorrhag′ica, m. hemorrágica; hemorragia uterina anormal, excessiva, freqüentemente contínua, devida à persistência e exagero da fase folicular do ciclo menstrual; o endométrio é a sede de hiperplasia glandular com formação de cisto. VER Swiss cheese *endometrium*.

me·tro·path·ic (mē - trō - path′ik). Metropático; relativo a, ou causado por, doença uterina.

me·trop·a·thy (mē - trop′ă - thē). Metropatia; qualquer doença uterina, principalmente do miométrio. SIN metropathia. [metro- + G. *pathos*, que sofre]

me·tro·per·i·to·ni·tis (mē′trō - per - i - tō - nī′tis). Metroperitonite. SIN perimetritis. [metro- + peritonitis]

me·tro·phle·bi·tis (mē′trō - fle - bī′tis). Metroflebite; inflamação das veias uterinas, geralmente após o parto. [metro- + G. *phleps*, veia, + *-itis*, inflamação]

met·ro·plas·ty (met′trō - plas - tē, mē′trō-). Metroplastia. SIN uteroplasty.
me·tror·rha·gia (mē - trō - rā′jē - ă). Metrorragia; qualquer hemorragia irregular, acíclica do útero entre os períodos menstruais. [metro- + G. *rhē̄gnymi*, romper]
me·tror·rhea (mē′trō - rē′ă). Metrorréia; secreção ou eliminação de muco ou pus do útero. [metro- + G. *rhoia*, fluxo]
me·tro·sal·pin·gi·tis (mē′trō - sal - pin - jī′tis). Metrossalpingite; inflamação do útero e de uma ou ambas as tubas uterinas (de Falópio). [metro- + G. *salpinx*, tuba (oviduto), + *-itis*, inflamação]
me·tro·stax·is (mē - trō - stak′sis). Metrostaxe; hemorragia pequena, mas contínua, da mucosa uterina. [metro- + G. *staxis*, gotejamento]
me·tro·ste·no·sis (mē′trō - stē - nō′sis). Metroestenose; estreitamento da cavidade uterina. [metro- + G. *stenō̄sis*, estreitamento]
me·trot·o·my (mē - trot′ō - mē). Metrotomia. SIN hysterotomy. [metro- + G. *tomē̄*, incisão]
me·tyr·a·pone (mē - tir′ă - pōn). Metirapona; inibidor da β-hidroxilação do esteróide adrenocortical C-11, administrado por via oral ou intravenosa para determinar a capacidade da hipófise de aumentar sua secreção de corticotropina; como os 11-desoxicorticosteróides, em virtude da administração de metirapona, causam apenas fraca inibição da secreção hipofisária de corticotropina, a hipófise normal aumentará consideravelmente a liberação desse hormônio. SIN mepyrapone.
me·ty·ro·sine (mē - tī′rō - sin, - sēn). Metirosina; inibidor da tirosina hidroxilase e, portanto, um potente inibidor da síntese de catecolaminas; usado para controle das manifestações de feocromocitoma, no preparo pré-operatório, ou em casos em que a ressecção cirúrgica é contra-indicada ou incompleta.
Mev Símbolo de 1 milhão de elétron-volts.
mev·a·lo·nate (mev - ă - lon′at). Mevalonato; o sal ou éster do ácido mevalônico.
  m. kinase, mevalonatocinase; enzima que catalisa a reação do mevalonato e ATP para formar ADP e 5-fosfato de mevalonato; essa enzima participa da via para síntese de esteróides; a deficiência dessa enzima levará à acidúria mevalônica e à ausência de desenvolvimento.
mev·a·lon·ic ac·id (mev - ă - lon′ik). Ácido mevalônico; precursor do esqualeno, esteróides, terpenos e dolicol.
mev·a·lon·ic ac·i·du·ria. Mevalônico acidúria; níveis elevados de ácido mevalônico na urina; associada a deficiência de mevalonatocinase.
mev·a·sta·tin (mev′ă - stat - in). Mevastatina; metabólito fúngico que é um potente inibidor da HMG-CoA redutase, a enzima controladora da velocidade na biossíntese do colesterol. A m., assim como a lovastatina, pravastatina e sinvastatina, é usada no tratamento da hiperlipidemia.
me·vin·o·lin (me - vin′ - ō - lin). Mevinolina. SIN lovastatin.
mex·e·none (mek′se - nōn). Mexenona; agente protetor solar.
mex·il·e·tine (meks - il′ē - tēn). Mexiletina; antiarrítmico cardíaco usado no tratamento de arritmias ventriculares; possui ações semelhantes à da lidocaína, mas é efetiva por via oral.
mex·il·e·tine hy·dro·chlo·ride (meks - il′ē - tēn). Cloridrato de mexiletina; antiarrítmico ativo por via oral para suprimir arritmias ventriculares sintomáticas; possui ações semelhantes às da lidocaína, mas é efetivo por via oral.
Meyenburg, H. von, patologista suíço, *1877. VER M. *complex, disease*; M.-Altherr-Uehlinger *syndrome*.
Meyer, Adolf, psiquiatra norte-americano, 1866–1950. VER M.-Archambault *loop*.
Meyer, Edmund V., laringologista alemão, 1864–1931. VER M. *cartilages*, em *cartilage*.
Meyer, Georg H., anatomista suíço, 1815–1892. VER M. *line, sinus*.
Meyer, Hans H., farmacologista alemão, 1853–1939. VER M.-Overton *rule, theory* of narcosis.
Meyer, Willy, cirurgião norte-americano, 1858–1932. VER M. *reagent*.
Meyer-Betz, Friedrich, médico alemão do século XX. VER Meyer-Betz *disease*; Meyer-Betz *syndrome*.
Meyerhof, Otto F., bioquímico e Prêmio Nobel alemão-norte-americano, 1884–1951. VER Embden-M. *pathway*; Embden-M.-Parnas *pathway*; M. oxidation *quotient*.
Meyer-Schwickerath, Gerhard Rudolph Edmund, oftalmologista alemão, *1920.
Meynert, Theodor H., neurologista de Viena, 1833–1892. VER retroflex *bundle* of Meynert; M. *cells*, em *cell, commissure, decussation; fasciculus* of Meynert; M. *layer*.
mez·lo·cil·lin so·di·um (mez - lō - sil′in). Mezlocilina sódica; $C_{21}H_{24}NaN_5O_8S_2$; uma penicilina de amplo espectro usada por via intravenosa e intramuscular.
Mg Símbolo de magnesium (magnésio).
mg Símbolo de milligram (miligrama).
MGP Abreviatura de matrix Gla *protein* (proteína Gla da matriz).
MGUS Abreviatura de monoclonal *gammopathy* of unknown significance (gamopatia monoclonal de importância desconhecida).

MHC Abreviatura de major histocompatibility *complex* (complexo de histocompatibilidade principal), minor histocompatibility *complex* (complexo de histocompatibilidade menor).
mho (mō). Siemens. SIN siemens. [*ohm* invertido]
MHz Símbolo de megahertz.
MI Abreviatura de myocardial *infarction* (infarto do miocárdio).
mi·an·ser·in hy·dro·chlo·ride (mē - an′ser - in). Cloridrato de mianserina; anti-histamínico H₁ com atividade anti-serotonina.
mibefradil (mib - ef′ra - dil). Mibefradil; derivado do tetralol em uma nova classe de antagonistas do cálcio que bloqueiam os canais tipo T; usado no tratamento da hipertensão leve a moderada e da angina de peito.
Mibelli, Vittorio, dermatologista italiano, 1860–1910. VER M. *angiokeratomas*, em *angiokeratoma, disease*.
MIC Abreviatura de minimal inhibitory *concentration* (concentração inibitória mínima).
mi·ca·to·sis (mī′kă - tō - sis). Micatose; pneumoconiose causada pela inalação de partículas de mica.
mi·cel·lar (mī - sel′er, mi-). Micelar; que possui as propriedades de um conjunto de micelas, isto é, de um gel.
mi·celle (mi - sel′, mī - sel′). Micela. **1.** Termo de Nägeli para partículas submicroscópicas (ópticas), alongadas, detectadas em hidrogéis, de caráter supramolecular e estrutura cristalina; agora definidas como uma dentre duas classes de partícula coloidal; aquelas que consistem em muitas moléculas, sendo a outra classe constituída de macromoléculas isoladas observadas à microscopica óptica ou submicroscópicas. Assim, uma micela é uma unidade estrutural da fase dispersa em um gel, uma unidade cuja repetição em três dimensões constitui a estrutura micelar do gel; não designa as partículas individuais em suspensão livre ou solução, nem a estrutura unitária de um cristal. **2.** Qualquer agregado hidrossolúvel, formado de forma espontânea e reversível a partir de moléculas anfifílicas. **3.** Uma região ordenada hipotética em uma fibra natural como a celulose. [L. *micella*, pequeno pedaço, dim. de *mica*, pedaço, grão]
Michaelis, Leonor, químico alemão radicado nos EUA, 1875–1949. VER M.-Guttmann *body*; M. *constant*; M.-Menten *constant, equation, hypothesis*.
Michel, Gaston, cirurgião francês, 1874–1937. VER Michel *spur*.
Michel, M., médico francês do século XIX. VER M. *malformation*.
Micheli, Ferdinando, médico italiano, 1872–1936. VER Marchiafava-M. *anemia, syndrome*.
mi·con·a·zole ni·trate (mī - kon′ă - zōl). Nitrato de miconazol; agente antifúngico.
♻ **micr-.** VER micro-.
mi·cren·ce·pha·lia (mī′kren - se - fā′lē - ă). Microencefalia. SIN micrencephaly.
mi·cren·ceph·a·lous (mī - kren - sef′ă - lŭs). Microencéfalo; que possui um encéfalo pequeno.
mi·cren·ceph·a·ly (mī - kren - sef′ă - lē). Microencefalia; tamanho pequeno anormal do encéfalo. SIN micrencephalia, microencephaly. [micro- + G. *enkephalos*, encéfalo]
♻ **micro-, micr-.** Micro-, micr-. **1.** Prefixo que designa tamanho pequeno. **2.** (μ) Prefixo usado no sistema SI e métrico para indicar submúltiplos de um milionésimo (10^{-6}) dessa unidade. **3.** Em química, prefixo de termos que designam exame químico, métodos, etc., que utilizam quantidades mínimas da substância a ser examinada; p. ex., uma gota ou duas no lugar de 1 ml ou mais. **4.** Formas combinantes que significam microscópico; oposto de macro-, megalo-. [G. *mikros*, pequeno]
mi·cro·ab·scess (mī′krō - ab′ses). Microabscesso; coleção muito pequena e circunscrita de leucócitos em tecidos sólidos.
  Munro m., m. de Munro; coleção microscópica de leucócitos polimorfonucleares encontrada no estrato córneo na psoríase. SIN Munro abscess.
  Pautrier m., m. de Pautrier; lesão microscópica na epiderme, observada na micose fungóide; é composta do mesmo tipo de células mononucleares atípicas como as que formam o infiltrado no cório. SIN Pautrier abscess.
mi·cro·ad·e·no·ma (mī′krō - ad - ĕ - nō′mă). Microadenoma; adenoma hipofisário com menos de 10 mm de diâmetro.
mi·cro·ae·ro·bi·on (mī′krō - ā - rō′bī - on). Microaeróbio; microrganismo microaerófilo.
mi·cro·aer·o·phil, mi·cro·aer·o·phile (mī - krō - ār′ō - fil, - fīl). Microaerófilo. **1.** Bactéria aeróbica que precisa de oxigênio, porém em menor quantidade do que a presente no ar, e cresce melhor em condições atmosféricas modificadas. **2.** Relativo a esse microrganismo. SIN microaerophilic, microaerophilous. [micro- + G. *aēr*, ar, + *philos*, amigo]
mi·cro·aer·o·phil·ic (mī′krō - ār - ō - fil′ik). Microaerófilo. SIN microaerophil (2).
mi·cro·aer·oph·i·lous (mī′krō - ār - of′i - lŭs). Microaerófilo. SIN microaerophil (2).
mi·cro·aer·o·sol (mī - krō - ār′ō - sol). Microaerossol; suspensão no ar de partículas submicrônicas ou, na maioria das vezes, com 1–10 μm de diâmetro.
microalbuminuria (mī′krō - al - boo - min - ū′rē - ă). Microalbuminúria; pequeno aumento da excreção urinária de albumina que pode ser detectada utilizan-

do-se imunoensaios, mas não utilizando medidas convencionais das proteínas na urina; um marcador precoce de doença renal em pacientes com diabetes. [micro- + albuminuria]

mi·cro·a·nal·y·sis (mī'krō - ā - nal'i - sis). Microanálise; técnicas analíticas que envolvem amostras incomumente pequenas.

mi·cro·a·nas·to·mo·sis (mī'krō - a - nas - tō - mō'sis). Microanastomose; anastomose de pequenas estruturas realizadas sob microscopia.

mi·cro·a·nat·o·mist (mī'krō - ā - nat'ō - mist). Microanatomista, histologista. SIN histologist.

mi·cro·a·nat·o·my (mī'krō - ā - nat'ō - mē). Microanatomia. SIN histology.

mi·cro·an·eu·rysm (mī'krō - an'ū - rizm). Microaneurisma; dilatação focal de capilares retinianos que ocorre no diabetes melito, na obstrução da veia retiniana e no glaucoma absoluto, ou das junções arteriolocapilares em muitos órgãos na púrpura trombocitopênica trombótica.

mi·cro·an·gi·og·ra·phy (mī'krō - an - jē - og'ra - fē). Microangiografia; radiografia dos vasos mais finos de um órgão após a injeção de um contraste e aumento da radiografia resultante. SIN microarteriography. [micro- + angiography]

mi·cro·an·gi·op·a·thy (mī'krō - an - jē - op'a - thē). Microangiopatia. SIN capillaropathy.

 thrombotic m., m. trombótica; trombose nos pequenos vasos sanguíneos, como na púrpura trombocitopênica trombótica.

mi·cro·an·gi·os·co·py (mī'krō - an - jē - os'kō - pē). Microangioscopia. SIN capillarioscopy.

mi·cro·ar·te·ri·og·ra·phy (mī'krō - ar - tēr - ē - og'ra - fē). Microarteriografia. SIN microangiography.

microatelectasis. Microatelectasia. SIN adhesive *atelectasis*.

mi·cro·bal·ance (mī'krō - bal - ans). Microbalança; balança destinada ao uso na pesagem de amostras muito pequenas de material.

mi·crobe (mī'krōb). Micróbio; qualquer organismo muito pequeno. Originalmente, a palavra deveria ser usada como um termo coletivo para a grande variedade de microrganismos conhecidos no século XIX; o uso moderno preservou o significado coletivo original, mas ampliou-o para incluir organismos microscópicos e ultramicroscópicos (espiroquetas, bactérias, riquétsias e vírus). Esses organismos são considerados formadores de um grupo biologicamente distinto, porque o material genético não é circundado por uma membrana nuclear, e não há mitose durante a replicação. [Fr., do G. *mikros*, pequeno, + *bios*, vida]

mi·cro·bi·al (mī - krō'bē - al). Microbiano; relativo a um micróbio ou micróbios. SIN microbic, microbiotic (2).

mi·cro·bi·al as·so·ci·ates (mī - krō'bē - al ā - sō'shē - āts). SIN flora (2).

mi·cro·bic (mī - krō'bik). Microbiano. SIN microbial.

mi·cro·bi·ci·dal (mī - krō'bi - sī'dal). Microbicida; destrutivo para os micróbios. SIN microbicide (1).

mi·cro·bi·cide (mī - krō'bi - sīd). Microbicida. 1. SIN microbicidal. 2. Agente destrutivo para micróbios; germicida; anti-séptico. [microbe + L. *caedo*, matar]

mi·cro·bi·o·log·ic (mī'krō - bī - ō - loj'ik). Microbiológico; relativo à microbiologia.

mi·cro·bi·ol·o·gist (mī'krō - bī - ol'ō - jist). Microbiologista; aquele que se especializa na ciência da microbiologia.

mi·cro·bi·ol·o·gy (mī'krō - bī - ol'ō - jē). Microbiologia; a ciência que estuda os microrganismos, incluindo fungos, protozoários, bactérias e vírus. [Fr. *microbiologie*]

mi·cro·bi·ot·ic (mī'krō - bī - ot'ik). Microbiótico. 1. De vida curta. 2. SIN microbial.

mi·cro·bism (mī'krō - bizm). Microbismo; infecção por micróbios.

 latent m., m. latente; a presença de microrganismos patogênicos no corpo que não produzem sintomas; a condição de portador de patógenos.

mi·cro·blast (mī'krō - blast). Microblasto; hemácia pequena, nucleada. [micro- + G. *blastos*, broto, germe]

mi·cro·ble·pha·ria (mī'krō - ble - far'ē - ā). Micrbléfaro. SIN microblepharon.

mi·cro·bleph·a·rism (-blef'ar - izm). Microbléfaro. SIN microblepharon.

mi·cro·bleph·a·ron (-blef'a - ron). Microbléfaro; pálpebras com dimensões verticais anormalmente curtas. SIN microblepharia, microblepharism. [micro- + G. *blepharon*, pálpebra + *-ia*, condição]

mi·cro·body (mī'krō - bod - ē). Microcorpo; organela citoplasmática, limitada por uma única membrana e contendo enzimas oxidativas. Os microcorpos incluem os peroxissomas e os glioxissomas.

mi·cro·bra·chia (mī - krō - bra'kē - ā). Microbraquia; tamanho anormalmente pequeno dos braços. [micro- + G. *brachion*, braço]

mi·cro·bren·ner (mī - krō - bren'er). Cautério elétrico com ponta em forma de agulha. [micro- + Al. *Brenner*, queimador]

mi·cro·cal·ci·fi·ca·tions (mī'krō - kal - si - fi - kā'shuns). Microcalcificações; calcificações com menos de 1 mm de diâmetro observadas à mamografia; freqüentemente associadas a lesões malignas. [micro- + calcification]

mi·cro·car·dia (mī - krō - kar'dē - ā). Microcardia; tamanho anormalmente pequeno do coração. [micro- + G. *kardia*, coração]

mi·cro·cen·trum (mī - krō - sen'trum). Microcentro. SIN cytocentrum. [micro- + G. *kentron*, centro]

mi·cro·ce·pha·lia (mī - krō - se - fā'lē - ā). Microcefalia. SIN microcephaly.

mi·cro·ce·phal·ic (mī'krō - sē - fal'ik). Microcefálico; nanocefálico; que tem cabeça pequena. SIN microcephalous, nanocephalous, nanocephalic.

mi·cro·ceph·a·lism (mī - krō - sef'a - lizm). Microcefalismo. SIN microcephaly.

mi·cro·ceph·a·lous (mī - krō - sef'a - lŭs). Microcéfalo. SIN microcephalic.

mi·cro·ceph·a·ly (mī - krō - sef'a - lē). Microcefalia. Tamanho anormalmente pequeno da cabeça; aplicado a um crânio com capacidade inferior a 1.350 ml. Geralmente associada a retardo mental. SIN microcephalia, microcephalism, nanocephalia, nanocephaly. [micro- + G. *kephale*, cabeça]

 encephaloclastic m., m. encefaloclástica; distúrbios do crescimento complexos no encéfalo em virtude de alterações regressivas na vida fetal.

 schizencephalic m., m. esquizencefálica; processo disgênico que resulta em defeitos cerebrais focais.

mi·cro·chei·lia, mi·cro·chi·lia (mī - krō - kī'lē - ā). Microquilia; tamanho pequeno dos lábios. [micro- + G. *cheilos*, lábio]

mi·cro·chei·ria, mi·cro·chi·ria (mī - krō - kī'rē - ā). Microquiria; tamanho pequeno das mãos. [micro- + G. *cheir*, mão]

mi·cro·chem·is·try (mī - krō - kem'is - trē). Microquímica; o uso de procedimentos químicos envolvendo pequenas quantidades ou reações não-visíveis a olho nu. Cf. macrochemistry.

micro·chim·er·ism (mī - krō - kim'er - izm). Microquimerismo; a presença de células doadoras em um receptor de enxerto, ou de células fetais remanescentes na circulação materna, que podem ser detectadas por métodos moleculares, mas não por citometria de fluxo.

mi·cro·cide (mī'krō - sīd). Microcida. SIN *glucose* oxidase.

mi·cro·cin·e·ma·tog·ra·phy (mī'kro - sin - ē - ma - tog'ra - fē). Microcinematografia; a aplicação de imagens em movimento feitas através de lentes de aumento para o estudo de um órgão ou sistema em movimento; p. ex., a circulação em embriões vivos. [micro- + G. *kinema*, movimento, + *grapho*, escrever]

mi·cro·cir·cu·la·tion (mī'krō - sir - kū - lā'shŭn). Microcirculação; passagem de sangue nos menores vasos, a saber: arteríolas, capilares e vênulas.

Mi·cro·coc·ca·ce·ae (mī'krō - kok - ā'sē - ē). Família de bactérias (ordem Eubacteriales) contendo células esféricas Gram-positivas, que ocorrem isoladamente ou em pares, tétrades, aglomerados, massas irregulares ou até mesmo cadeias. Raramente esses organismos são móveis. Ocorrem espécies de vida livre, saprofíticas, parasitárias e patogênicas. O gênero típico é o *Micrococcus*.

mi·cro·coc·ci (mī'krō - kok'sī). Micrococos; plural de micrococcus.

Mi·cro·coc·cus (mī'krō - kok - ŭs). Gênero de bactérias (família Micrococcaceae) que contém células esféricas, Gram-positivas observadas em massas irregulares. Algumas espécies são móveis ou produzem mutantes móveis. Esses microrganismos são saprofíticos, parasitas facultativos ou parasitas, mas não são realmente patogênicos. A espécie típica é *M. luteus*. É o gênero típico da família Micrococcaceae. [micro- + G. *kokkos*, baga]

 M. conglomera'tus, espécie de bactéria encontrada em infecções, leite, laticínios, utensílios da indústria de laticínios e água.

 M. lu'teus, espécie saprofítica encontrada no leite e laticínios ou em partículas de poeira; causou meningite em seres humanos; é a espécie típica do gênero *Micrococcus*.

 M. var'ians, nome antigo da *Kocuria varians*.

mi·cro·coc·cus, pl. **mi·cro·coc·ci** (mī'krō - kok'ŭs, - kok'sī). Micrococo; termo usado para se referir a qualquer membro do gênero *Micrococcus*.

mi·cro·co·li·tis (mī'krō - ko - lī'tis). Microcolite; colite não observada por endoscopia, mas na qual o exame microscópico das biopsias mostra inflamação inespecífica da mucosa.

mi·cro·co·lon (mī'krō - kō - lon). Microcolo; colo não-usado, de pequeno calibre, observado no recém-nascido ao enema contrastado; geralmente uma conseqüência da atresia intestinal ou do íleo meconial.

mi·cro·col·o·ny (mī'krō - kol - ō - nē). Microcolônia; colônia de bactérias visível apenas ao microscópio em pequeno aumento.

mi·cro·co·nid·i·um, pl. **mi·cro·co·nid·ia** (mī'krō - kō - nid'ē - ŭm, - ā). Microconídio; em fungos, o menor de dois tipos de conídios de tamanhos muito diferentes em uma única espécie, geralmente de células isoladas e esféricos, ovóides, piriformes ou claviformes.

mi·cro·co·ria (mī - krō - kō'rē - ā). Microcoria; pupila pequena congênita com incapacidade de dilatar. [micro- + G. *kore*, pupila]

mi·cro·cor·nea (mī - krō - kōr'nē - a). Microcórnea; córnea anormalmente pequena.

mi·cro·cou·lomb (µC) (mī - krō - koo'lom). Microcoulomb; a milionésima parte de um coulomb.

mi·cro·crys·tal·line (mī - krō - krys'tā - lin). Microcristalino; que ocorre em pequenos cristais.

mi·cro·cu·rie (µCi) (mī'krō - kū'rē). Microcurie; a milionésima parte de um curie; quantidade de qualquer radionuclídeo com $3,7 \times 10^4$ desintegrações por segundo.

mi·cro·cyst (mī′krō-sist). Microcisto; cisto pequeno, freqüentemente de dimensões tais que é necessária uma lente de aumento ou microscópio para sua observação.

mi·cro·cyte (mī′krō-sīt). Micrócito; hemácia anucleada pequena (5 μm ou menos). SIN microerythrocyte. [micro- + G. *kytos*, célula]

mi·cro·cy·the·mia (mī′krō-sī-thē′mē-ă). Microcitemia; a presença de muitos micrócitos no sangue circulante. SIN microcytosis. [microcyte + G. *haima*, sangue]

mi·cro·cy·to·sis (mī′krō-sī-tō′sis). Microcitose. SIN microcythemia. [microcyte + G. *-osis*, condição]

mi·cro·dac·tyl·ia (mī′krō-dak-til′ē-ă). Microdactilia. SIN microdactyly.

mi·cro·dac·ty·lous (mī-krō-dak′ti-lŭs). Microdáctilo; relativo à, ou caracterizado por, microdactilia.

mi·cro·dac·ty·ly (mī-krō-dak′ti-lē). Microdactilia; pequenez ou encurtamento dos dedos das mãos ou dos pés. SIN microdactylia. [micro- + G. *dactylos*, dedo]

microdialysis. Microdiálise; método de estudo da composição do líquido extracelular e da resposta a agentes exógenos, utilizando uma diminuta sonda tubular, com uma membrana de diálise e velocidade do fluxo de líquido de 1–3 μl/min, introduzido nos tecidos.

mi·cro·dis·sec·tion (mī′krō-dī-sek′shŭn). Microdissecção; dissecção de tecidos com microscópio ou lente de aumento, geralmente realizado afastando os tecidos com agulhas.

mi·cro·dont (mī′krō-dont). Microdonte; que possui dentes pequenos; designa um crânio com índice dentário abaixo de 41,9. [micro- + G. *odous* (*odonto-*), dente]

mi·cro·don·tia, mi·cro·don·tism (mī-krō-don′shē-ă, -don′tizm). Microdontia; condição na qual um único dente, ou pares de dentes ou toda a dentição, pode apresentar tamanho desproporcionalmente pequeno. [micro- + G. *odous*, dente]

mi·cro·dose (mī′krō-dōs). Microdose; uma dose muito pequena.

mi·cro·drep·a·no·cy·to·sis (mī′krō-drep′ă-nō-sī-tō′sis). Microdrepanocitose; anemia hemolítica crônica resultante da interação dos genes para anemia falciforme e talassemia. [microcytosis + drepanocytosis]

mi·cro·dys·ge·ne·sia (mī′krō-dis-ge-nē′sē-ă). Microdisgenesia; aumento de neurônios parcialmente distópicos no estrato zonal, substância branca, hipocampo e córtex cerebelar, produzindo uma borda indistinta entre o córtex e a substância branca subcortical e um arranjo colunar de neurônios corticais; observada em pacientes com epilepsia generalizada primária. [micro- + dys- + G. *genesis*, produção]

mi·cro·e·lec·trode (mī′krō-ē-lek′trōd). Microeletrodo; eletrodo muito fino, geralmente consistindo em um fio fino ou tubo de vidro de diâmetro capilar (10 μm a 1 mm) esticado até formar uma ponta fina e cheio com solução salina ou com um metal como gálio ou índio (enquanto fundido); usado em experiências fisiológicas para estimular ou registrar correntes de ação de origem extracelular ou intracelular.

microelements (mī′krō-el′ē-ments). Microelementos. SIN trace elements, em element.

mi·cro·en·ceph·a·ly (mī′krō-en-sef′ă-lē). Microencefalia. SIN micrencephaly.

mi·cro·e·ryth·ro·cyte (mī′krō-ē-rith′rō-sīt). Microeritrócito. SIN microcyte.

mi·cro·ev·o·lu·tion (mī′krō-ev-ō-loo′shŭn). Microevolução; a evolução de bactérias e outros microrganismos através de mutações.

mi·cro·fi·bril (mī-kro-fī′bril). Microfibrila; fibrila muito pequena que possui um diâmetro médio de 13 nm; pode ser um feixe de elementos ainda menores: os microfilamentos.

mi·cro·fil·a·ment (mī-krō-fil′ă-ment). Microfilamento; o elemento filamentoso mais fino do citoesqueleto, que possui um diâmetro de aproximadamente 5 nm e consiste basicamente em actina. VER TAMBÉM actin *filament*.

mi·cro·fil·a·re·mia (mī′krō-fil-ă-rē′mē-ă). Microfilaremia; infecção do sangue por microfilárias. A microfilaremia causada por *Wuchereria brancofti* é caracterizada por periodicidade noturna bem definida, aparentemente associada aos hábitos noturnos dos mosquitos vetores; em áreas geográficas onde os vetores não são estritamente picadores noturnos (como em partes da Polinésia), a periodicidade das microfilárias é modificada ou ausente. VER TAMBÉM periodic *filariasis*.

mi·cro·fi·lar·ia, pl. **mi·cro·fi·lar·i·ae** (mī′krō-fi-lar′ē-ă, -ē). Microfilária; termo para embriões de nematódeos filarianos da família Onchocercidae. No passado, esse termo foi usado como uma designação genérica (p. ex., *Microfilaria bancrofti, M. malaya*). VER *Filaria*.

mi·cro·film (mī′krō-film). **1.** Microfilme; filme fotográfico com imagens muito reduzidas de registros impressos. **2.** Microfilmar; registrar em microfilme.

mi·cro·flo·ra (mī′krō-flō-ră). Microflora; as bactérias e fungos que habitam uma área.

mi·cro·ga·mete (mī-krō-gam′ēt). Microgameta; o elemento masculino na anisogamia, ou conjugação de células de tamanhos diferentes; é a menor das duas células e apresenta mobilidade ativa. [micro- + G. *gametēs*, marido]

mi·cro·ga·me·to·cyte (mī-krō-gam′ē-tō-sīt). Microgametócito; a célula-mãe que produz os microgametas, ou elementos masculinos de reprodução sexuada em protozoários de esporozoários e fungos. SIN microgamont.

mi·cro·gam·ont (mī-krō-gam′ont). Microgamonte. SIN microgametocyte.

mi·crog·a·my (mī-krog′ă-mē). Microgamia; conjugação entre duas células jovens, o produto recente da esporulação ou de alguma outra forma de reprodução. [micro- + G. *gamos*, casamento]

mi·cro·gas·tria (mī-krō-gas′trē-ă). Microgastria; tamanho pequeno do estômago. [micro- + G. *gaster*, estômago]

mi·cro·gen·ia (mī-krō-jēn′ē-ă). Microgenia; tamanho pequeno anormal do queixo resultante do subdesenvolvimento da sínfise mental. [micro- + G. *geneion*, queixo]

mi·cro·gen·i·tal·ism (mī-krō-jen′i-tal-izm). Microgenitalismo; tamanho pequeno anormal dos órgãos genitais externos.

mi·crog·lia (mī-krog′lē-ă). Micróglia; pequenas células da neuróglia, possivelmente de origem mesodérmica, que podem tornar-se fagocíticas, em áreas de lesão ou inflamação neural. SIN Hortega cells, microglia cells, microglial cells. [micro- + G. *glia*, cola]

mi·crog·li·a·cyte (mī-krog′lē-ă-sīt). Microgliácito; uma célula, particularmente uma célula embrionária, da micróglia. [micro- + G. *glia*, cola, + *kytos*, célula]

mi·crog·li·o·ma (mī-krog′lē-ō′mă). Microglioma; termo obsoleto para uma neoplasia intracraniana com origem nas células da micróglia, estruturalmente semelhante ao linfoma. [microglia + G. *-oma*, tumor]

mi·crog·li·o·ma·to·sis (mī-krog′lē-ō-mă-tō′sis). Microgliomatose; termo obsoleto para designar uma condição caracterizada pela presença de microgliomas múltiplos.

mi·crog·li·o·sis (mī-krog′lē-ō′sis). Microgliose; presença de micróglia no tecido nervoso secundária à lesão. [microglia + G. *-osis*, condição]

mi·cro·glob·u·lin (mī′krō-glob′oo-lin). Microglobulina. **1.** Qualquer globulina sérica ou urinária de massa molecular abaixo de 40 kd, incluindo proteínas de Bence Jones (Bence Jones *proteins*, em *protein*). **2.** Algumas vezes, um termo usado para se referir às imunoglobulinas 7S (p. ex., IgG).

β-m., β-m.; polipeptídeo de 11.600 Da que forma a cadeia leve dos antígenos de histocompatibilidade maiores classe 1 e, portanto, pode ser detectado em todas as células que possuem esses antígenos. É encontrada β-microglobulina livre no sangue e na urina de pacientes com determinadas doenças, incluindo doença de Wilson (Wilson *disease*), intoxicação por cádmio e acidose tubular renal (renal tubular *acidosis*).

β$_2$-m., β$_2$-m.; a cadeia leve da molécula de histocompatibilidade classe I. Essa cadeia é invariável em determinada espécie; é encontrada em níveis elevados em indivíduos com doença de Wilson e na cirrose hepática induzida por álcool.

mi·cro·glos·sia (mī-krō-glos′ē-ă). Microglossia; tamanho pequeno da língua. [micro- + G. *glossa*, língua]

mi·cro·gna·thia (mī-krō-nā′thē-ă, mī-krog-nath′ē-ă). Micrognatia; tamanho anormalmente pequeno da maxila e, principalmente, da mandíbula. [micro- + G. *gnathos*, mandíbula]

m. with peromelia, m. com peromelia; hipoplasia da mandíbula com dentes malformados e ausentes, face de pássaro e deformidades graves das mãos e antebraços, algumas vezes também dos pés e das pernas. SIN Hanhart syndrome.

mi·cro·gram (μg, γ). (mī′krō-gram). Micrograma; a milionésima parte de um grama.

mi·cro·graph (mī′krō-graf). Micrógrafo. **1.** Instrumento que amplia os movimentos microscópicos de um diafragma por meio de interferência na luz e os registra em um filme fotográfico em movimento; pode ser usado para registrar várias curvas de pulso, ondas sonoras e quaisquer formas de movimento que possam ser comunicadas através do ar para um diafragma. **2.** Microfotografia. SIN photomicrograph. [micro- + G. *graphō*, escrever]

electron m., m. eletrônica; a imagem produzida pelo feixe de elétrons de um microscópio eletrônico, registrado em uma placa ou filme elétron-sensível.

light m., m. óptica; fotografia produzida por meio de um microscópio óptico.

mi·crog·ra·phy (mī-krog′ră-fē). Micrografia. **1.** Escrita com letras muito pequenas, algumas vezes observada em psicoses e na paralisia agitante. **2.** Uma descrição de objetos observados com um microscópio. **3.** SIN photomicrography. [micro- + G. *graphō*, escrever]

mi·cro·gy·ria (mī-krō-jī′rē-ă). Microgiria; estreitamento anormal dos giros do cérebro. [micro- + G. *gyros*, giro]

mi·cro·he·pat·ia (mī-krō-he-pat′ē-ă). Microepatia; tamanho anormalmente pequeno do fígado. [micro- + G. *hepar* (*hepat-*), fígado]

mi·cro·het·er·o·ge·ni·ty (mī′krō-het′er-ō-jē-nē′i-tē; nē′i-tē). Microeterogeneidade; pequenas diferenças na estrutura entre moléculas essencialmente idênticas; p. ex., na porção sacarídeo de uma glicoproteína.

mi·crohm (μΩ) (mī′krōm). Microhm; a milionésima parte de um ohm. SIN micro-ohm.

mi·cro·in·cin·er·a·tion (mī′krō-in-sin′ē-rā′shŭn). Microincineração; combustão, em um forno, de constituintes orgânicos em um corte de tecido de forma que as cinzas minerais restantes possam ser examinadas microscopicamente. SIN spodography.

mi·cro·in·cis·ion (mī - krō - in - sizh'ŭn). Microincisão; incisão feita com a ajuda de um microscópio.

mi·cro·in·jec·tor (mī'krō - in - jek - tor). Microinjetor; instrumento para infusão de quantidades muito pequenas de líquidos ou drogas em animais ou seres humanos.

mi·cro·in·va·sion (mī'krō - in - vā'zhŭn). Microinvasão; invasão de tecido imediatamente adjacente a um carcinoma *in situ*, o primeiro estágio de invasão neoplásica maligna.

mi·cro·kat·al (mī'krō - kat'al). Microkatal; a milionésima parte de um katal.

mi·cro·ky·mat·o·ther·a·py (mī'krō - kī - mat'ō - thār'a - pē). Microquimatoterapia; tratamento com radiações de alta freqüência de 3.000.000.000 Hz (3.000 MHz), em um comprimento de onda de 10 cm. SIN microwave therapy. [micro- + G. *kyma*, onda, + *therapeia*, tratamento]

mi·cro·leu·ko·blast (mī - krō - loo'kō - blast). Microleucoblasto. SIN micromyeloblast.

mi·cro·li·ter (μl, μL) (mī'krō - lē - ter). Microlitro; a milionésima parte de um litro.

mi·cro·lith (mī'krō - lith). Micrólito; um pequeno cálculo, geralmente múltiplo, algumas vezes constituindo uma areia grossa. [micro- + G. *lithos*, cálculo]

mi·cro·li·thi·a·sis (mī - krō - li - thī'a - sis). Microlitíase; a formação, presença ou eliminação de pequenas concreções ou areia, p. ex., microlitíase testicular.

pulmonary alveolar m., m. alveolar pulmonar; grânulos microscópicos de cálcio ou osso disseminados pelos pulmões.

mi·crol·o·gy (mī - krol'ō - jē). Micrologia; a ciência que estuda objetos microscópicos, dos quais a histologia é um ramo. [micro- + G. *logos*, estudo]

mi·cro·ma·nip·u·la·tion (mī'krō - ma - nip'ū - lā'shŭn). Micromanipulação; dissecção, afastamento, estimulação etc., sob microscopia, de pequenas estruturas; p. ex., células teciduais ou organismos unicelulares.

mi·cro·ma·nip·u·la·tor (mī'krō - ma - nip'ū - lā'ter, - tor). Micromanipulador; instrumento usado em micromanipulação, pelo qual são realizadas microdissecção, microinjeção e outras manobras, geralmente com a ajuda de um microscópio.

mi·cro·ma·zia (mī - krō - mā'zē - a). Micromazia; condição na qual as mamas são rudimentares e não-funcionantes. [micro- + G. *mazos*, mama]

mi·cro·me·lia (mī - krō - mē'lē - a). Micromelia; presença de membros desproporcionalmente curtos ou pequenos. VER TAMBÉM achondroplasia. SIN nanomelia. [micro- + G. *melos*, membro]

mi·cro·mere (mī'krō – mer). Micrômero; blastômero de tamanho pequeno; p. ex., um dos blastômeros no pólo animal de um ovo de anfíbio. [micro- + G. *meros*, parte]

mi·cro·mer·o·zo·ite (mī'krō - mer - ō - zō'īt). Micromerozoíta; um merozoíta pequeno.

mi·cro·me·tas·ta·sis (mī'krō - mē - tas'tā - sis). Micrometástase; estágio de metástase em que os tumores secundários são pequenos demais para serem clinicamente detectados, como na doença micrometastática.

mi·cro·met·a·stat·ic (mī'krō - met - a - stat'ik). Micrometastático; que designa ou é caracterizado por micrometástase, como na doença micrometastática.

mi·crom·e·ter (μm) (mī - ktom'e - ter). Micrômetro. **1.** A milionésima parte de um metro; antes denominado mícron. **2.** Dispositivo para medir diversos tipos de objetos de forma exata e precisa; em medicina e biologia, o termo geralmente é usado em referência a uma lâmina de vidro ou lente, que é marcada exatamente para medir formas microscópicas. [micro- + G. *metron*, medida]

caliper m., m. de calibre; escala com um parafuso micrométrico calibrado para medida de objetos finos, como lâminas e lamínulas microscópicas.

filar m., m. filar; micrômetro ocular com uma linha movida por uma membrana graduada, de tal forma que possa ser feito um movimento da linha de 5 μm ou menos em relação a linhas paralelas fixas.

ocular m., m. ocular; disco de vidro que se encaixa na ocular de um microscópio e que possui uma escala marcada; quando calibrado com um micrômetro de lâmina, podem-se fazer medidas diretas de um objeto microscópico.

slide m., m. de lâmina; escala feita em uma lâmina microscópica com linhas marcadas em divisões, geralmente de 0,01 mm; tipicamente usado para calibrar um micrômetro ocular.

mi·crom·e·try (mī - krom'e - trē). Micrometria; medida de objetos com algum tipo de micrômetro e um microscópio.

♻ **micromicro-** (μμ). Prefixo usado antigamente para designar um trilionésimo (10^{-12}); atualmente usa-se pico-.

mi·cro·mi·cro·gram (μμg) (mī'krō - mī'krō - gram). Micromicrograma; termo antigo para picograma.

mi·cro·mi·cron (μμ) (mī – krō – mī'kron). Designação antiga de picômetro.

mi·cro·min·er·als (mī - krō - min'er - ālz). Microminerais. SIN trace elements, em element.

mi·cro·mo·lar (μmol/L) (mī - krō - mō'lar). Micromolar; designa uma concentração de 10^{-6} mol/L.

mi·cro·mole (μmol) (mī'krō - mōl). Micromol; a milionésima parte de um mol.

mi·cro·mo·to·scope (mī'krō - mō'tō - skōp). Micromotoscópio; cinematoscópio para representar os movimentos de amebas e outros objetos microscópicos móveis. [micro- + L. *motus*, movimento, + G. *skopeō*, ver]

mi·cro·my·e·lia (mī - krō - mī - ē'lē - a). Micromielia; pequenez ou encurtamento anormal da medula espinal. [micro- + G. *myelos*, medula óssea]

mi·cro·my·el·o·blast (mī - krō - mī'el - ō - blast). Micromieloblasto; um mieloblasto pequeno, freqüentemente a célula predominante na leucemia mieloblástica. SIN microleukoblast.

mi·cron (μ) (mī'kron). Mícron; termo antigo para micrômetro.

mi·cro·nee·dle (mī'krō – nē'dl). Microagulha; uma pequena agulha de vidro usada em manipulação cirúrgica.

mi·cro·neme (mī'krō – nēm). Micronema, pequena organela torcida como uma corda, osmiófila, encontrada na região anterior de muitos esporozoários; uma das características que ajuda a definir o subfilo Apicomplexa. SIN sarconeme. [micro- + G. *nēma*, fio]

mi·cron·ic (mī - kron'ik). Micrônico; do tamanho de 1 mícron (micrômetro).

mi·cro·nod·u·lar (mī'krō - nod'ū - lār). Micronodular; caracterizado pela presença de pequenos nódulos; designa um aspecto um pouco mais grosseiro que o de um tecido ou substância granular. [G. *mikros*, pequeno]

mi·cro·nu·cle·us (mī – krō – noo'klē – ŭs). Micronúcleo. **1.** Um núcleo pequeno em uma célula grande, ou os núcleos menores em células que possuem duas ou mais dessas estruturas. **2.** O menor dos dois núcleos em ciliados que se dividem por mitose e possuem material hereditário específico. SIN gametic nucleus, germ nucleus, gonad nucleus, karyogonad, reproductive nucleus. VER TAMBÉM macronucleus (2).

mi·cro·nu·tri·ents (mī - krō - noo'trē - ents). Micronutrientes; fatores alimentares essenciais necessários apenas em pequenas quantidades pelo organismo; p. ex., vitaminas, oligoelementos. SIN trace nutrient.

mi·cro·nych·ia (mī - krō - nik'ē - a). Microníquia; pequenez anormal das unhas. [micro- + G. *onyx*, unha]

mi·cro·nys·tag·mus (mī'krō - nis - tag'mŭs). Micronistagmo; nistagmo de amplitude tão pequena que não é detectado pelos testes clínicos habituais. SIN minimal amplitude nystagmus. [micro- + G. *nystagmos*, oscilação]

mi·cro-ohm (mī'krō - ōm). Micro-ohm. SIN microhm.

mi·cro·or·gan·ism (mī - krō - ōr'gan - izm). Microrganismo; um organismo microscópico (vegetal ou animal).

mi·cro·par·a·site (mī - krō – par'a – sīt). Microparasita; um microrganismo parasita.

mi·cro·pa·thol·o·gy (mī'krō - pa - thol'ō - jē). Micropatologia; termo obsoleto para estudo microscópico de alterações patológicas. [micro- + G. *pathos*, que sofre, + *logos*, estudo]

mi·cro·pe·nis (mī – krō – pē'nis). Micropênis; pênis anormalmente pequeno. SIN microphallus.

mi·cro·phage (mī'krō - fāj). Micrófago; leucócito polimorfonuclear que é fagocítico. VER TAMBÉM phagocyte. SIN microphagocyte. [micro- + phag(ocyte)]

mi·cro·phag·o·cyte (mī – krō – fāj'ō – sīt). Microfagócito. SIN microphage.

mi·cro·phal·lus (mī - krō - fal'ŭs). Microfalo. SIN micropenis.

mi·cro·pho·bia (mī - krō - fō'bē - a). Microfobia; medo de objetos pequenos, microrganismos, germes etc. [micro- + G. *phobos*, medo]

mi·cro·phone (mī'krō - fōn). Microfone; instrumento para converter sons em impulsos elétricos. [micro- + G. *phōnē*, som]

mi·cro·pho·nia, mi·croph·o·ny (mī - krō - fō'nē - a, mī - krof'ō - nē). Microfonia. SIN hypophonia. [micro- + G. *phōnē*, voz]

mi·cro·pho·no·scope (mī - krō - fō'nō - skōp). Microfonoscópio; um estetoscópio com fixação de um diafragma para amplificar o som.

mi·cro·pho·to·graph (mī – krō - fō'tō - graf). Microfotografia; fotografia pequena de qualquer objeto, distinta de uma fotomicrografia.

mi·croph·thal·mia (mī'krof - thal'mē - a). Microftalmia. SIN microphthalmos.

colobomatous m., m. colobomatosa; defeito congênito que ocorre ao longo de uma fissura embrionária em um olho pequeno, algumas vezes associado a cistos.

mi·croph·thal·mos (-thal'mos). Microftalmia; tamanho anormalmente pequeno do olho. SIN microphthalmia, nanophthalmia, nanophthalmos. [micro- + G. *ophthalmos*, olho]

mi·cro·pi·pette, mi·cro·pi·pet (mī'krō - pi - pet', - pī - pet'). Micropipeta; pipeta designada para a medida de volumes muito pequenos.

mi·cro·pla·nia (mī – krō – plā'nē – a). Microplania; diminuição do diâmetro horizontal das hemácias. [micro- + L. *planus*, plano]

mi·cro·pla·sia (mī - krō - plā'zē - a). Microplasia; interrupção do crescimento, como no nanismo. [micro- + G. *plasis*, moldagem, formação]

mi·cro·pleth·ys·mog·ra·phy (mī - krō - pleth - iz - mog'ra - fē). Micropletismografia; a técnica de medir pequenas alterações no volume de uma parte em virtude do fluxo sanguíneo que entra e sai.

mi·cro·po·dia (mī - krō - pō'dē - a). Micropodia; pequenez anormal dos pés. [micro- + G. *pous*, pé]

mi·cro·pore (mī'krō-pōr). Microporo; organela formada pela película de todos os estágios dos protozoários esporozoários do subfilo Apicomplexa, também encontrada em estágios do desenvolvimento que podem não possuir a película interna; é composto de dois anéis concêntricos (em corte transversal), com o anel interno correspondendo a uma invaginação da película externa. Os microporos observados até agora parecem servir como organelas de alimentação; seu papel nas formas evolutivas não-alimentares é desconhecido. [micro- + G. *poros*, poro]

mi·cro·pro·my·el·o·cyte (mī'krō-prō-mī'el-ō-sīt). Micropromielócito; uma célula derivada de um pró-mielócito.

mi·cro·pro·so·pia (mī'krō-prō-sō'pē-ă). Microprosopia; condição caracterizada por uma face anormalmente pequena ou imperfeitamente desenvolvida. [micro- + G. *prosōpon*, face]

mi·crop·sia (mī-krop'sē-ă). Micropsia; percepção dos objetos como menores do que são. [micro- + G. *opsis*, visão].

mi·cro·punc·ture (mī'krō-pŭnk-choor). Micropunção; pequena punção feita com a ajuda de um microscópio.

mi·cro·pyle (mī'krō-pīl). Micrópila. **1.** Pequena abertura que se supõe existir na membrana de revestimento de certos ovos como ponto de entrada para o espermatozóide. [micro- + G. *pylē*, portão]. **2.** Nome antigo de microporo.

mi·cro·ra·di·og·ra·phy (mī'krō-rā-dē-og'ră-fē). Microrradiografia; realização de radiografias de cortes histológicos de tecido para aumento. **ver também** historadiography.

mi·cro·re·frac·tom·e·ter (mī'krō-rē-frak-tom'ĕ-ter). Microrrefratômetro; refratômetro usado no estudo das células do sangue.

mi·cro·res·pi·rom·e·ter (mī'krō-res-pi-rom'ĕ-ter). Microrrespirômetro; aparelho para medir a utilização de oxigênio por pequenas partículas de tecidos isolados ou células ou partículas de células.

mi·cro·sac·cades (mī'krō-să-kădz'). Microssacadas; pequenos movimentos de vaivém dos olhos. [micro- + Fr. *saccade*, súbito refreamento (de um cavalo)]

mi·cro·scin·tig·ra·phy (mī'krō-sin-tig'ră-fē). Microcintigrafia; estudo por imagem de pequenas estruturas anatômicas por uso de um radionuclídeo em conjunto com um colimador especial que "amplia" a imagem; p. ex., o uso de tecnécio-99m em conjunto com um colimador puntiforme para mostrar a drenagem lacrimal. [micro- + scintigraphy]

mi·cro·scope (mī'krō-skōp). Microscópio; instrumento que produz uma imagem aumentada de um objeto ou substância pequena ou invisível a olho nu; geralmente, o termo designa um microscópio composto; para os pequenos aumentos, são usados os termos microscópio simples ou lente de aumento. [micro- + G. *shopeō*, ver]

binocular m., m. binocular; microscópio que tem duas oculares; pode ser um microscópio composto ou um microscópio estereoscópico.

color-contrast m., m. de contraste de cores; tipo de microscópio no qual o obturador do condensador é de uma cor e o anel é um complemento dele, de forma que objetos não-corados são observados em uma cor sobre um campo de outra.

comparator m., m. de comparação; dispositivo construído com um ou mais microscópios que possuem oculares micrométricas usadas para medir alterações dimensionais durante alterações de ambiente ou de temperatura.

compound m., m. composto; microscópio que possui duas ou mais lentes de aumento.

confocal m., m. confocal; microscópio que permite ao observador visualizar objetos em um único plano de foco, assim produzindo uma imagem mais nítida (geralmente, os objetos são moléculas fluorescentes); um aperfeiçoamento dessa microscopia usa o seccionamento óptico e um computador para registrar cortes seriados. Isso permite reconstrução tridimensional.

dark-field m., m. de campo escuro; microscopia que tem um condensador especial e objetiva com um diafragma ou obturador que dispersa a luz do objeto observado, resultando em uma imagem de um objeto brilhante sobre fundo escuro.

electron m., m. eletrônico; microscopia visual e fotográfica na qual feixes de elétrons com comprimentos de onda milhares de vezes mais curtos que a luz visível são utilizados no lugar da luz, assim permitindo resolução e ampliação muito maiores; por essa técnica, os elétrons são transmitidos através de um corte muito fino de uma amostra incrustada e desidratada mantida em um vácuo.

fluorescence m., m. de fluorescência. VER fluorescence *microscopy*.

flying spot m., m. de ponto móvel; microscópio no qual um ponto de luz móvel é focalizado no plano do objeto, a energia transmitida pela amostra sendo detectada com uma célula fotoelétrica; a fonte luminosa pode ser um tubo de raios catódicos, um disco ou cilindro de cintilação, ou um espelho oscilante.

infrared m., m. infravermelho; microscópio equipado com óptica de transmissão de raios infravermelhos e que mede a absorção de infravermelho por pequenas amostras com a ajuda de células fotoelétricas; as imagens podem ser observadas com conversores de imagem ou televisão.

interference m., m. de interferência; microscópio especialmente construído no qual a luz que entra é dividida em dois feixes que atravessam a amostra e se reúnem no plano de imagem, onde os efeitos de interferência tornam os detalhes do objeto refrátil transparente (invisível) visíveis como diferenças de intensidade; permite medidas do retardo da luz, do índice de refração e da espessura e massa da amostra; é útil no exame de células vivas ou não-coradas.

laser m., m. de laser; microscópio no qual um feixe de laser é focalizado sobre um campo microscópico, causando sua vaporização; a radiação emitida é analisada por meio de um microespectrofotômetro; em baixa intensidade, o laser é empregado como a fonte luminosa em um microscópio de interferência.

light m., m. óptico; uma classe de microscópio que forma uma imagem ampliada utilizando luz visível.

opaque m., epimicroscópio. SIN epimicroscope.

operating m., m. cirúrgico. SIN surgical m.

phase m., phase-contrast m., m. de fase, m. de contraste de fase; microscópio especialmente construído que possui um condensador especial e objetiva contendo um anel de desvio de fase, em que pequenas diferenças no índice de refração tornam-se visíveis como diferenças de intensidade ou de contraste na imagem, particularmente útil para examinar detalhes estruturais em amostras transparentes, como células e tecidos vivos ou não-corados.

polarizing m., m. de polarização; microscópio equipado com um filtro polarizante abaixo e acima da amostra, que forma uma imagem pela influência de birrefringência da amostra à luz polarizada; tipicamente, a direção de polarização dos dois filtros é ajustável, o que, juntamente com uma platina giratória graduada, permite medida do valor angular de diferentes índices de refração em amostras biológicas ou químicas.

Rheinberg m., m. de Rheinberg; forma modificada de microscopia de campo escuro na qual o obturador opaco central no condensador é substituído por um filtro colorido, produzindo um fundo de cor contrastante contra o qual a amostra é iluminada.

scanning electron m., m. eletrônico de varredura; microscópio no qual o objeto no vácuo é examinado em um amplo padrão por um feixe de elétrons fino, gerando elétrons refletidos e secundários da superfície da amostra, que são usados para modular a imagem em um tubo de raios catódicos examinado sincronicamente; com esse método é obtida uma imagem tridimensional, com alta resolução e grande profundidade de foco.

simple m., single m., m. simples; microscópio que possui uma única lente de aumento.

stereoscopic m., m. estereoscópico; microscópio que possui oculares e objetivas duplas e, assim, trajetos luminosos independentes, produzindo uma imagem tridimensional.

stroboscopic m., m. estroboscópico; microscópio que tem uma fonte de luz que pisca em uma freqüência constante, de forma que se possa analisar a motilidade de um objeto; pode ser usado para cinefotomicrografia de alta velocidade ou de baixa velocidade (lapso de tempo).

surgical m., m. cirúrgico; microscópio binocular usado para obter boa visualização de estruturas finas no campo cirúrgico; no tipo padrão de microscópio, um sistema de lentes com "zoom" motorizado operado por controles manuais ou por pedais permite ajustar a distância de trabalho; nos modelos de cabeça, oculares intercambiáveis produzem o aumento necessário. SIN operating m.

television m., m. de televisão; microscópio em que a imagem é observada por uma câmera de televisão que produz uma imagem; é usado para estudos quantitativos, exibição para uma grande audiência ou exames em regiões ultravioleta e infravermelha do espectro.

ultra-m., ultramicroscópio. VER ultramicroscope.

ultrasonic m., m. ultra-sônico; microscópio que possui lentes destinadas a usar energia acústica, de forma que possam ser utilizados os comprimentos de onda ultra-sônicos; por meio de transdutores, a informação é traduzida em uma forma que possa ser visualizada ou registrada.

ultraviolet m., m. de ultravioleta; microscópio com a parte óptica de quartzo e fluoreto que permite a transmissão de ondas luminosas mais curtas que aquelas do espectro visível, isto é, abaixo de 400 nm; a imagem é tornada visível por fotografia, fluorescência de lentes especiais, ou televisão; em um instrumento de varredura, o receptor é um fototubo multiplicador.

x-ray m., m. de raios X; microscópio no qual as imagens são obtidas utilizando-se raios X como fonte de energia, sendo registradas em um filme finamente granulado, ou a imagem é ampliada por projeção; se for usado filme, ele pode ser examinado com o microscópio óptico em ampliações muito grandes.

mi·cro·scop·ic, mi·cro·scop·i·cal (mī-krō-skop'ik, -i-kăl). Microscópico. **1.** De tamanho diminuto; visível apenas com o auxílio do microscópio. **2.** Relativo a um microscópio.

mi·cros·co·py (mī-kros'kŏ-pē). Microscopia; investigação de objetos diminutos por meio de um microscópio. VER TAMBÉM microscope.

electron m., m. eletrônica; exame de pequenos objetos por uso de um microscópio eletrônico.

epiluminescence m., m. de epiluminescência; dermatoscopia; microscopia de pequeno aumento (×50–×100), comumente um microscópio de televisão (television *microscope*), aplicada a uma lâmina de vidro sobre óleo mineral na superfície de uma lesão cutânea, p. ex., para determinar malignidade em lesões pigmentadas. SIN surface m.

fluorescence m., m. de fluorescência; procedimento baseado no fato de que os materiais fluorescentes emitem luz visível quando são irradiados com raios ultravioleta ou raios azul-violeta visíveis; alguns materiais apresentam essa propriedade naturalmente, enquanto outros podem ser tratados com soluções fluorescentes (de modo um pouco semelhante à coloração); quando a absorção da amostra está na faixa relativamente longa do ultravioleta, é usado um filtro que deixa passar essas radiações, e um filtro amarelo é colocado sobre a ocular ou no seu interior; o campo de fundo então é escuro, e qualquer fluorescência amarela ou vermelha torna-se visível.

immersion m., m. de imersão. VER immersion.

immune electron m., m. imunoeletrônica; microscopia eletrônica de amostras biológicas às quais foi ligado anticorpo específico.

immunofluorescence m., m. de imunofluorescência. VER immunofluorescence.

Nomarski interference m., m. de interferência de Nomarski. VER Nomarski optics.

surface m., m. de superfície. SIN epiluminescence m.

time-lapse m., m. em lapso de tempo; microscopia na qual o mesmo objeto (p. ex., uma célula) é fotografado a intervalos regulares durantes várias horas.

mi·cro·seme (mī′krō-sēm). Microssema; designa um crânio com índice orbitário abaixo de 84. [micro- + G. *sēma*, sinal]

mi·cro·sides (mī′krō-sīdz). Microsídeos; ésteres de ácidos graxos da trealose e manose isolados de bacilos da difteria.

mi·cros·mat·ic (mī′kroz-mat′ik). Microsmático; que possui um sentido do olfato pouco desenvolvido. [micro- + G. *osmē*, sentido do olfato]

mi·cro·some (mī′krō-sōm). Microssoma; uma das pequenas vesículas esféricas derivadas do retículo endoplasmático após ruptura das células e ultracentrifugação. [micro- + G. *sōma*, corpo]

mi·cro·so·mia (mī-krō-sō′mē-ă). Microssomia; tamanho anormalmente pequeno do corpo, tal como no nanismo ou em um feto. SIN nanocormia. [micro- + G. *sōma*, corpo]

mi·cro·spec·tro·pho·tom·e·try (mī′krō-spek-trō-fō-tom′ĕ-trē). Microespectrofotometria; técnica para caracterizar e quantificar nucleoproteínas em células isoladas ou organelas celulares por seus espectros naturais de absorção (ultravioleta) ou após ligação estoiquiométrica em reações de coloração citoquímica seletiva, como na coloração de Feulgen para DNA. VER TAMBÉM cytophotometry.

mi·cro·spec·tro·scope (mī-krō-spek′trō-skōp). Microespectroscópio; instrumento para observar o espectro óptico de objetos microscópicos.

micro·sphere (mī′krō-sfēr). Microsfera; diminutos glóbulos de material radiomarcado, como albumina macroagregada, medindo cerca de 15 mícrons.

mi·cro·sphe·ro·cy·to·sis (mī′krō-sfēr′ō-sī-tō′sis). Microesferocitose. SIN spherocytosis.

mi·cro·sphyg·my (mī′krō-sfig′mē). Microsfigmia; tamanho pequeno do pulso. SIN microsphyxia. [micro- + G. *sphygmos*, pulso]

mi·cro·sphyx·ia (mī-krō-sfik′sē-ă). Microsfigmia. SIN microsphygmy. [micro- + G. *sphyxis*, pulso]

mi·cro·splanch·nic (mī-krō-splangk′nik). Microesplâncnico; referente ao tamanho pequeno das vísceras abdominais. [micro- + G. *splanchna*, víscera]

mi·cro·sple·nia (mī-krō-splē′nē-ă). Microsplenia; tamanho anormalmente pequeno do baço.

Mi·cro·spo·ra (mī-krō-spōr′ă). Filo de protozoários que inclui o gênero *Nosema* e *Encephalitozoon*, e é caracterizado pela presença de esporos unicelulares com uma parede imperfurada e um aparelho de extrusão que possui um tubo polar e um capuz polar; não há mitocôndrias. São parasitas intracelulares de invertebrados e vertebrados inferiores, com raros exemplos nos vertebrados superiores. SIN Cnidospora. [micro- + G. *sporos*, semente]

Mi·cro·spo·ra·si·da (mī′krō-spōr-as′ī-dă). SIN Microsporida.

Mi·cro·spo·ri·da (mī-krō-spō′rī-dă). Ordem da classe de protozoários Microsporea e filo Microspora, caracterizada por pequenos esporos com um único filamento tubular, espiralado, longo, que encerra a célula infecciosa ou esporoplasma. São tipicamente parasitas de invertebrados e vertebrados inferiores, embora tenham sido infectados peixes e vertebrados superiores (incluindo o homem). A ordem inclui gêneros como *Encephalitozoon* e *Nosema*. SIN Cnidosporidia, Microsporasida.

mi·cro·spor·id·ia (mī′krō-spōr-id′ē-ă). Microsporídios; nome comum dado aos membros do filo de protozoários Microspora. Inclui cerca de 80 gêneros que parasitam todas as classes de vertebrados e muitos invertebrados, principalmente os insetos. Vários gêneros, como *Encephalitozoon, Enterocytozoon, Nosema, Vittaforma, Pleistophora* e *Trachipleistophora*, foram implicados na infecção de seres humanos imunodeprimidos.

mi·cro·spor·id·i·a·sis (mī′krō-spō-ri-dī′a-sis). Microsporidiose. VER microsporidiosis.

mi·cro·spo·rid·i·o·sis, mi·cro·spo·rid·i·a·sis (mī-krō-spō-rid-ē-ō′sis, mī′krō-spō-ri-dī′a-sis). Microsporidiose; infecção por um membro do filo Microspora, os microsporídios.

Mi·cros·po·rum (mī-kros′pō-rŭm, mī-krō-spō′rŭm). Gênero de fungos patogênicos causadores de dermatofitose. Em meio de cultura apropriado, são observados macroconídios característicos; os microconídios são raros na maioria das espécies. [micro- + G. *sporos*, semente]

M. audoui'nii, espécie de fungo antrofílica que costuma causar dermatofitose da cabeça epidêmica em crianças.

M. ca'nis, a principal causa de dermatofitose em cães e gatos e uma espécie fúngica zoofílica que causa dermatofitose esporádica em seres humanos, principalmente dermatofitose da cabeça em crianças que convivem com gatos e cães.

M. canis, var. distor'tum, espécie fúngica zoofílica que causa dermatofitose em seres humanos e animais; observada em pessoas que lidam com animais de laboratório.

M. ferrugin'eum, espécie fúngica antropofílica que causa dermatofitose, basicamente no Japão e no Extremo Oriente.

M. ful'vum, espécie fúngica geofílica que causa dermatofitose em seres humanos e é um membro do complexo *M. gypseum*, cujo estado ascomiceto a eleva à posição de espécie-específica.

M. galli'nae, espécie fúngica que causa dermatofitose em aves domésticas e, algumas vezes, em seres humanos; devido aos seus macroconídios claviformes, foi erroneamente classificada como uma espécie de *Trichophyton*.

M. gyp'seum, causa de dermatofitose em cães e cavalos, e algumas vezes em outras espécies de animais; um complexo geofílico de espécies fúngicas que causam dermatofitose esporádica em seres humanos.

M. na'num, espécie fúngica geofílica que é a principal causa de dermatofitose em porcos; raramente causa dermatofitose em seres humanos.

M. persic'olor, espécie fúngica geofílica que causa dermatofitose em ratazanas, ratos do campo e, ocasionalmente, em seres humanos; seu estado ascomiceto é a *Nannizzia persicolor*.

M. vanbreusegh'emi, espécie fúngica zoofílica que causa dermatofitose em cães e esquilos e, algumas vezes, em seres humanos.

mi·cro·steth·o·phone (mī-krō-steth′ō-fōn). Microstetofone. SIN microstethoscope. [micro- + G. *stethos*, tórax, + *phōnē*, som]

mi·cro·steth·o·scope (mī-krō-steth′ō-skōp). Microstetoscópio; estetoscópio muito pequeno que amplifica os sons ouvidos. SIN microstethophone.

mi·cro·sto·mia (mī-krō-stō′mē-ă). Microstomia; tamanho pequeno da abertura oral. [micro- + G. *stoma*, boca]

mi·cro·sur·gery (mī-krō-ser′jer-ē). Microcirurgia; procedimentos cirúrgicos realizados sob a ampliação de um microscópio cirúrgico.

mi·cro·su·ture (mī-krō-soo′choor). Fio para microssutura; material de sutura de pequeno calibre, freqüentemente 9–0 ou 10–0, com uma agulha de tamanho correspondente fixada, para uso em microcirurgia.

mi·cro·sy·ringe (mī′krō-si-rinj′). Microsseringa; seringa hipodérmica que tem um parafuso micrométrico acoplado ao êmbolo, por meio do qual podem ser injetadas quantidades pequenas precisas de líquido.

mi·cro·the·lia (mī-krō-thē′lē-ă). Microtelia; pequenez dos mamilos. [micro- + G. *thēlē*, mamilo]

mi·cro·tia (mī-krō′shē-ă). Microtia; pequenez da orelha, com um meato auditivo externo cego ou ausente. [micro- + G. *ous*, orelha]

Mi·cro·ti·nae (mī-krot′in-ē). A subfamília de roedores que compreende ratazanas ou lemingues.

mi·cro·tine (mī′krō-tēn). Relativo às ratazanas ou lemingues.

mi·cro·tome (mī′krō-tōm). Micrótomo; instrumento para fazer cortes de tecido biológico para exame microscópico. VER TAMBÉM ultramicrotome. SIN histotome.

mi·crot·o·my (mī-krot′ō-mē). Microtomia; a realização de cortes finos de tecidos para exame microscópico. SIN histotomy. [micro- + G. *tomē*, incisão]

mi·cro·to·nom·e·ter (mī′krō-tō-nom′ĕ-ter). Microtonômetro; pequeno tonômetro inventado por Krogh, originalmente destinado a animais, mas depois adaptado para seres humanos, para determinar as tensões de oxigênio e dióxido de carbono no sangue arterial; proporciona a forma de colocar uma pequena bolha de ar em equilíbrio gasoso com uma amostra de sangue obtida por punção arterial. [micro- + G. *tonos*, tônus, + *metron*, medida]

Mi·cro·trom·bid·i·um (mī′krō-trom-bid′ē-ŭm). Gênero de micuins ou ácaros que causam forte prurido devido à presença do estágio larvar (micuim) na pele. [micro- + L. mod. *trombidium*, tímido]

mi·cro·tro·pia (mī-krō-trō′pē-ă). Microtropia; estrabismo menor que quatro graus, associado a ambliopia, fixação excêntrica ou correspondência retiniana anômala. [micro- + G. *tropē*, volta]

mi·cro·tu·bule (mī-krō-too′bŭl). Microtúbulo; elemento citoplasmático cilíndrico, oco, com 20–27 nm de diâmetro e de comprimento variável, amplamente encontrado no citoesqueleto, cílios e flagelos das células; os microtúbulos participam na manutenção do formato da célula e aumentam em número durante a mitose e a meiose, onde estão relacionados ao movimento dos cromossomas pelo fuso nuclear.

subpellicular m., m. subpelicular; microtúbulo situado sob a unidade de membrana (película) de muitos protozoários, freqüentemente como uma paliçada de fibrilas dispostas longitudinalmente e unidas por finas pontes laterais que sustentam a forma celular externa; em determinados estágios de esporozoários, é encontrado um número fixo de microtúbulos, estendendo-se longitudinalmente do anel polar. SIN subpellicular fibril.

mi·cro·ves·i·cle (mī - krō - ves′i - kl). Microvesícula; espaço cheio de líquido formado na epiderme, pequeno demais para ser reconhecido como uma vesícula.

mi·cro·vil·lus, pl. **mi·cro·vil·li** (mī - krō - vil′ŭs, - vil′ī). Microvilosidade; uma das pequenas projeções das membranas celulares que aumentam muito a área da superfície; as microvilosidades formam as bordas estriadas ou em escova de algumas células.

Mi·cro·vir·i·dae (mī - krō - vir′i - dē). Família de vírus bacterianos esféricos, pequenos, com um genoma de DNA monofilamentar (PM $1,7 \times 10^6$).

mi·cro·volt (μv) (mī′krō - vōlt). Microvolt; a milionésima parte de um volt.

mi·cro·waves (mī - krō - wāvz). Microondas; a parte do espectro de ondas de rádio que possui o menor comprimento de onda, incluindo a região com comprimentos de onda de 1 mm a 30 cm (1.000–300.000 megaciclos por segundo). SIN microelectric waves.

mi·cro·weld·ing (mī - krō - weld′ing). Microssolda; método de fixação ou união de fios de sutura de aço inoxidável ou desses fios a agulhas.

mi·crox·y·phil (mī - krok′si - fil). Microxífilo; leucócito oxífilo multinuclear. [micro- + G. *oxys*, ácido, + *philos*, amigo]

mi·cro·zo·on (mī - krō - zō′on). Microzoário; forma microscópica do reino animal; um protozoário. [micro- + G. *zōon*, animal]

mi·crur·gi·cal (mī - krer′ji - kăl). Microcirúrgico; relativo a procedimentos microscópicos realizados em pequenas estruturas. [micro- + G. *ergon*, trabalho]

mic·tion (mik′shŭn). Micção. SIN urination.

mic·tu·rate (mik′choo - rāt). Urinar. SIN urinate. [ver micturition]

mic·tu·ri·tion (mik - choo - rish′ŭn). Micção. **1.** SIN urination. **2.** O desejo de urinar. **3.** Freqüência de micção. [L. *micturo*, desejar produzir água]

MID Abreviatura de minimal infecting *dose* (dose infectante mínima).

♲ **mid-.** Meio. [A.S. *mid, midd*]

mi·daz·o·lam hy·dro·chlo·ride. Cloridrato de midazolam; benzodiazepínico injetável, de ação curta, depressor do sistema nervoso central, usado para sedação pré-operatória.

mid·body (mid′bod′ē). Corpo médio; pedículo denso de fibras fusiformes interzonais residuais (microtúbulos) e filamentos contendo actina, formado durante a anáfase da mitose e que une células-filhas durante a telófase; corpos médios são freqüentemente observados entre espermátides. SIN intermediate body of Flemming.

mid·brain (mid′brān). Mesencéfalo; *termo oficial alternativo para mesencephalon.

mid·car·pal (mid′kar′ - păl). Mesocarpal. **1.** Relativo à parte central do carpo. **2.** Designa a articulação entre as duas fileiras de ossos do carpo. SIN carpocarpal. SIN mediocarpal, mesocarpal.

mid·dle (mid′el). Médio; designa uma estrutura anatômica situada entre duas outras estruturas semelhantes ou que está a meio caminho. SIN medius.

midge (midj). Mosquito-pólvora; o menor dos mosquitos que picam, do gênero *Culicoides*; enxames podem atacar os seres humanos e outros animais; vetores de infecções por filárias. [I. ant. *mycg*]

mid·grac·ile (mid-gras′il). Mesográcil; designa uma fissura ocasional que divide o lobo grácil do cerebelo em duas partes.

mid·gut (mid′gŭt). Intestino médio. **1.** A porção central do tubo digestivo; a porção distal do duodeno, intestino delgado e porção proximal do cólon. **2.** A porção do tubo intestinal embrionário situada entre o intestino anterior e o intestino posterior que, originalmente, se abre para o saco vitelino.

mid·men·stru·al (mid′men′stroo - ăl). Mesomenstrual; designa os vários dias entre dois períodos menstruais.

mid·oc·cip·i·tal (mid′ok - sip′i - tăl). Mesoccipital; relativo à porção central do occipúcio. SIN medioccipital.

mid·pain (mid′pān). Dor intermenstrual. SIN intermenstrual *pain* (1).

mid·plane (mid′plān). Plano médio. SIN pelvic *plane* of least dimensions.

mid·riff (mid′rif). Diafragma. SIN diaphragm (1). [A.S. *mid*, meio, + *hrif*, ventre]

mid·sec·tion (mid′sek - shŭn). Secção média; corte ou secção através do meio de um órgão.

mid·ster·num (mid′ster′nŭm). Mesoesterno. SIN body of sternum.

mid·tar·sal (mid′tar′săl). Mesotarsal; relativo ao meio do tarso. SIN mediotarsal, mesotarsal.

mid·wife (mid′wīf). Parteira; pessoa qualificada para realizar partos, que possui treinamento especializado em obstetrícia e cuidados com crianças. [A.S. *mid*, com, + *wif*, esposa]

mid·wife·ry (mid′wīf′rē, mid - wif′ē - rē). Trabalho de parteira; obstetrícia; tratamento independente de mulheres e lactentes saudáveis, essencialmente normais, por uma parteira no período pré-parto, durante e após o parto, e/ou obstetricamente em um hospital, centro obstétrico ou em casa, e incluindo o parto normal do lactente, com consulta ao médico, conduta colaborativa e encaminhamento dos casos em que surgem anormalidades; é dada grande ênfase ao preparo educacional dos pais com respeito ao parto e à criação dos filhos, com orientação voltada para o parto como um processo fisiológico normal que exige intervenção mínima.

Miescher, Johann F., patologista suíço, 1811–1887. VER M. *elastoma, granuloma, tubes,* em *tube.*

MIF Abreviatura de migration-inhibitory *factor* (fator inibidor da migração).

mife·pris·tone (mif′pris - tōn). Mifepristona; composto químico sintético com propriedades antiprogesterona usado na interrupção precoce da gravidez; a substância liga-se a receptores glicocorticóides, resultando em aumento da secreção pela supra-renal. SIN RU-486.

mi·graine (mī′grăn, mi - grăn′). Enxaqueca; complexo de sintomas que ocorre periodicamente e é caracterizado por dor na cabeça (geralmente unilateral), vertigem, náuseas e vômitos, fotofobia e escotomas cintilantes. Classificada como enxaqueca clássica, enxaqueca comum, cefaléia histamínica, enxaqueca hemiplégica, enxaqueca oftalmoplégica e enxaqueca oftálmica. SIN bilious headache, blind headache, hemicrania (1), sick headache, vascular headache. [através do Fr. ant., do G. *hēmi-krania,* dor de um lado da cabeça, de *hēmi-*, metade, + *kranion*, crânio]

abdominal m., e. abdominal; **(1)** enxaqueca em crianças acompanhada por dor abdominal paroxística. Esta deve ser distinguida de sintomas semelhantes que exigem cuidados cirúrgicos. **(2)** Um distúrbio que causa dor abdominal intermitente e se supõe estar relacionado à enxaqueca; a enxaqueca abdominal possui algumas das características de enxaqueca, p. ex., pode haver uma forte história familiar de enxaqueca, e a condição pode ser aliviada pelo sono; entretanto, pode não haver cefaléia. O diagnóstico depende da exclusão de outras causas de dor abdominal.

acephalgic m., e. acefálgica; episódio de enxaqueca clássica no qual a teicopsia não é seguida por cefaléia. SIN m. without headache.

basilar m., e. basilar; enxaqueca acompanhada por sinais transitórios referentes ao tronco encefálico (vertigem, zumbido, parestesia perioral, diplopia, etc.) considerados causados pelo estreitamento vasoespástico da artéria basilar.

classic m., e. clássica; forma de hemicrania precedida por escotomas cintilantes (teicopsia).

common m., e. comum; forma de enxaqueca sem o pródromo visual, que não é limitada a um lado da cabeça, mas que, todavia, é reconhecida como enxaqueca devido à evolução estereotipada; há tendência a náuseas, fotofobia e fonofobia; e o alívio é produzido pelo sono.

complicated m., e. complicada; crise de enxaqueca durante a qual ocorre um infarto tecidual.

fulgurating m., e. fulgurante; enxaqueca caracterizada por seu início abrupto e pela gravidade do episódio.

Harris m., e. de Harris. SIN periodic migrainous *neuralgia.*

hemiplegic m., e. hemiplégica; forma associada à hemiplegia transitória.

ocular m., e. ocular; forma de enxaqueca com amaurose monocular transitória, tipicamente em adultos jovens, que pode ou não estar associada a cefaléia ao nervo dos olhos.

ophthalmoplegic m., e. oftalmoplégica; forma de enxaqueca associada a paralisia dos músculos extra-oculares.

retinal m., e. retiniana. SIN ocular m.

m. without headache, e. sem cefaléia. SIN acephalgic m.

mi·gra·tion (mī - grā′shŭn). Migração. **1.** Que passa de uma parte para outra, diz-se de determinados processos mórbidos ou sintomas. **2.** SIN diapedesis. **3.** Movimento de um dente ou dentes para fora da posição normal. **4.** Movimento de moléculas durante eletroforese, centrifugação ou difusão. [L. *migro,* pp. *-atus,* mover-se de um local para outro]

branch m., processo no qual a conexão cruzada, em torno da posição onde duas hélices de DNA se unem, move-se ao longo dos filamentos.

epithelial m., m. epitelial; desvio apical da fixação epitelial, expondo mais a coroa do dente.

m. of ovum, m. do óvulo; a passagem transperitoneal de um óvulo do folículo ovariano para a tuba uterina.

MIH Abreviatura de melanotropin release-inhibiting *hormone* (hormônio inibidor da liberação de melanotropina).

Mikity, Victor G., radiologista norte-americano, *1919. VER Wilson-M. *syndrome.*

Mikulicz, Johannes von-Radecki, cirurgião polonês radicado na Alemanha, 1850–1905. VER M. *aphthae,* em *aphtha, cells,* em *cell, clamp disease, drain, operation, syndrome;* M.-Vladimiroff *amputation;* Vladimiroff-M. *amputation;* Heineke-Mikulicz *pyloroplasty.*

Miles, William E., cirurgião inglês, 1869–1947. VER M. *operation.*

mil·ia (mil′ē - ă). Plural de milium.

mil·i·a·ria (mil - ē - ā′rē - ă). Miliária; erupção de pequenas vesículas e pápulas devidas à retenção de líquido nos orifícios das glândulas sudoríparas. SIN miliary fever (2). [L. *miliarius,* relativo ao milho miúdo, de *milium,* milho miúdo, painço]

m. al'ba, m. alba; miliária com vesículas contendo um líquido leitoso.

apocrine m., m. apócrina. SIN Fox-Fordyce *disease.*

m. crystalli'na, m. cristalina; forma não-inflamatória de miliária na qual as vesículas subcórneas frágeis, com cerca de 100 mm de diâmetro, estão cheias de líquido claro. SIN crystal rash, sudamina (2).

m. profun'da, m. profunda; pápulas firmes, pálidas, mais comumente no tronco; a miliária profunda é assintomática e resulta de lesão grave dos ductos sudoríparos após episódios repetidos de miliária rubra. O estresse do calor pode causar colapso devido à alta proporção de glândulas sudoríparas não-funcionais.

m. ru'bra, m. rubra; erupção de máculas pruriginosas com pequenas vesículas centrais nos orifícios das glândulas sudoríparas, acompanhada por eritema e reação inflamatória da pele. SIN heat rash, prickly heat, summer rash, wildfire rash.

mil·i·a·ry (mil'ē-ā-rē, mil'yă-rē). Miliar. **1.** Semelhante, em tamanho, à semente do painço (cerca de 2 mm). **2.** Caracterizado pela presença de nódulos do tamanho da semente de painço sobre qualquer superfície. [ver miliaria]

mil·ieu (mēl'ū'). Meio. **1.** Vizinhança; ambiente. **2.** Em psiquiatria, ambiente social do paciente mental, p. ex., a unidade familiar ou uma unidade hospitalar. [Fr. *mi*, do L. *medius*, meio, + *lieu*, do L. *locus*, local]

m. intérieur, m. inter'ne, m. interno; o ambiente interno; os líquidos que banham as células teciduais de animais multicelulares.

mil·i·tar·y an·ti·shock trou·sers (MAST). Calça militar antichoque. SIN pneumatic antishock garment.

mil·i·um, pl. **mil·ia** (mil'ē-ŭm, -ē-ă). Pequeno cisto queratinoso subepidérmico, geralmente múltiplo e, portanto, comumente referido no plural. Pode ser primário (congênito), ocorrendo predominantemente na face em lactentes e adultos, ou podem ser cistos de retenção secundários a causas de fibrose ou vesículas subepidérmicas envolvendo o epitélio dos anexos. SIN whitehead (1). [L. milho miúdo]

milk. Leite. **1.** Líquido branco, contendo proteínas, açúcar e lipídios, secretado pelas glândulas mamárias e destinado à nutrição dos bebês. SIN lac (1). **2.** Qualquer líquido leitoso esbranquiçado, p. ex., o leite do coco ou uma suspensão de vários óxidos metálicos. **3.** Preparação da farmacopéia que é uma suspensão de fármacos insolúveis em um meio aquoso; diferente dos géis, principalmente porque as partículas suspensas do leite são maiores. **4.** SIN strip (1). [A.S. *meolc*]

acidophilus m., l. acidófilo; leite inoculado com uma cultura de *Bacillus acidophilus*.

m. of bismuth, l. de bismuto; suspensão de hidróxido de bismuto e subcarbonato de bismuto em água; usado em distúrbios gastrointestinais como agente protetor.

buddeized m., VER Budde *process*.

certified m., l. certificado; leite de vaca que não possui mais que o limite máximo permissível de 10.000 bactérias/mL em qualquer momento antes da venda ao consumidor, e que tem de ser resfriado a 10°C ou menos e mantido a essa temperatura até a venda.

certified pasteurized m., l. pasteurizado certificado; leite de vaca no qual o limite permissível máximo de bactérias não deve ser maior que 10.000 bactérias/mL antes da pasteurização e não mais de 500 bactérias/mL após a pasteurização; tem de ser resfriado a 7,2°C ou menos e mantido a essa temperatura até a venda.

condensed m., l. condensado; líquido espesso preparado pela evaporação parcial do leite de vaca, com ou sem a adição de açúcar.

fortified m., l. enriquecido; leite ao qual foi adicionado algum nutriente essencial, geralmente vitamina D.

fortified vitamin D m., l. enriquecido com vitamina D; leite produzido com adição direta de vitamina D; padronizado em 400 unidades USP por 0,95 L.

irradiated vitamin D m., leite de vaca exposto em fina película de luz ultravioleta e padronizado em 400 unidades USP de vitamina D por 0,95 L.

lactobacillary m., l. com lactobacilos; leite inoculado com uma cultura de *Bacillus acidophilus, B. bulgaricus* ou outro microrganismo formador de ácido láctico.

m. of magnesia, l. de magnésia; mistura de hidróxido de magnésia; solução aquosa de hidróxido de magnésio, usado como antiácido e laxante. SIN magnesia magma.

metabolized vitamin D m., l. metabolizado com vitamina D; leite produzido por alimentação de vacas com levedo irradiado; padronizado para conter não menos que 400 unidades USP por 0,95 L.

modified m., l. modificado; leite de vaca alterado pelo acréscimo de gordura e redução da quantidade de proteínas, para sua composição tornar-se semelhante à do leite humano.

perhydrase m., l. peridrase; leite tratado pela adição de peróxido de hidrogênio. VER Budde *process*.

skim m., skimmed m., l. desnatado; a parte aquosa (não-cremosa) do leite, da qual é isolada a caseína.

m. of sulfur, leite de enxofre. SIN precipitated *sulfur*.

vitamin D m., l. com vitamina D; leite de vaca ao qual foi adiciona vitamina D para conter 400 unidades USP de vitamina D por 0,95 L.

witch's m., l. de bruxa; secreção de leite semelhante ao colostro que, algumas vezes, ocorre nas glândulas de recém-nascidos de ambos os sexos 3 a 4 dias após o nascimento, durando uma ou duas semanas; devido à estimulação endócrina da mãe antes do nascimento.

Milkman, Louis A., radiologista norte-americano, 1895–1951. VER M. *syndrome*.

milk·pox (milk'poks). Alastrim. SIN alastrim.

Millard, Auguste L.J., médico francês, 1830–1915. VER M.-Gubler *syndrome*.

Miller, Thomas Grier, médico norte-americano, *1886. VER M.-Abbott *tube*.

Miller, Willoughby D., dentista norte-americano, 1853–1907. VER M. chemicoparasitic *theory*.

mil·let seed (mil'et). Semente de painço; a semente de uma gramínea, usada antigamente como designação de tamanho aproximado de 2 mm.

milli- (m). Mili-; prefixo usado nos sistemas SI e métrico para indicar submúltiplos de um milésimo (10^{-3}). [L. *mille*, um milésimo]

mil·li·am·pere (ma, mA) (mil'ē-am'pēr). Miliampère; a milésima parte de um ampère.

mil·li·bar (mil'i-bar). Milibar; a milésima parte de um bar; 100 newtons/m^2; 0,75006 mm Hg; a pressão atmosférica padrão é de 1.013 milibars.

mil·li·cu·rie (mc, mCi) (mil'i-kū'rē). Milicurie; unidade de radioatividade equivalente a $3,7 \times 10^7$ desintegrações por segundo.

mil·li·e·quiv·a·lent (mEq, meq) (mil'i-ē-kwiv'ă-lent). Miliequivalente; equivalente a um milésimo; 10^{-3} mol dividido pela valência.

mil·li·gram (mg) (mil'i-gram). Miligrama; a milésima parte de um grama.

mil·li·lam·bert (mil-i-lam'bert). Mililambert; a milésima parte de um lambert; unidade de brilho igual a 0,929 lumens por pé quadrado (aproximadamente 1 equivalente de pé-vela).

mil·li·li·ter (mil'i-lē-ter). Mililitro; a milésima parte de um litro.

mil·li·me·ter (mm) (mil'i-mē-ter). Milímetro; a milésima parte de um metro.

millimicro-. Milimicro-; prefixo usado antigamente para indicar submúltiplos de um bilionésimo (10^{-9}); agora se usa nano-.

mil·li·mi·cron (mμ) (mil'i-mī-kron). Milimícron; termo antigo para nanômetro.

mil·li·mole (mmol) (mil'i-mōl). Milimol; a centésima parte de uma molécula-grama.

mil·ling-in (mil'ing-in). Polimento; aprimoramento da oclusão dos dentes pelo uso de abrasivos entre suas superfícies oclusais, enquanto as dentaduras são friccionadas uma contra a outra na boca ou no articulador.

mil·li·os·mole (mil'i-oz-mōl). Miliosmol; a milésima parte de um osmol.

mil·li·pede (mil'i-pēd). Milípede; artrópode não-predador, venenoso, da ordem Diplopoda, caracterizado por dois pares de pernas por segmento portador de pernas. O veneno é puramente defensivo, escorrendo ou esguichando de poros ao longo do corpo, causando irritação da pele ou inflamação intensa se atingir os olhos. [milli- + L. *pes, pedis*, pé]

	densidade específica	proteína %	gordura %	carboidratos (lactose) %	cinzas %	joule/ 100 ml	conteúdo mineral, mg%						ácido cítrico
							Na	K	Ca	Mg	Fe	Cl	P	
leite humano	1,030	1,1-1,5	2,5-4,8	6-7,1	0,20	293	14	53	30	4	0,15	30	15	120
leite de vaca	1,031	3,1-4,0	3,5-4,8	4-4,8	0,75	285	45	160	126	12	0,18	126	98	250
leite de cabra	1,031	3,7-4,0	4,0-4,8	4-4,8	0,80	293	79	145	128	12	0,21	128	100	150

mil·li·sec·ond (ms, msec) (mil′i-sek′ŏnd). Milissegundo (ms); a milésima parte de um segundo.

mil·li·volt (mV) (mil′i-vōlt). Milivolt; a milésima parte de um volt.

Millon, Auguste N.E., químico francês, 1812–1867. VER M. *reaction, reagent*; M.-Nasse *test*.

mil·pho·sis (mil-fō′sis). Milfose; perda dos cílios. SIN madarosis (1). [G. *milphōsis*]

mil·ri·none (mil′rĭ-nōn). Milrinona; inibidor da xantina oxidase que aumenta a força de contração do coração; usado na insuficiência cardíaca congestiva; assemelha-se à anrinona; cardiotônico.

Milroy, William F., médico norte-americano, 1855–1942. VER M. *disease*.

MIM Abreviatura de *Mendelian Inheritance in Man* (Herança Mendeliana no Homem).

mi·me·sis (mi-mē′sis, mī-). Mimese. **1.** Simulação histérica de doença orgânica. **2.** A imitação sintomática de uma doença orgânica por outra. [G. *mimēsis*, imitação, de *mimeomai*, imitar]

mi·met·ic (mi-met′ik, mī-). Mimético; relativo à mimese. [G. *mimētikos*, imitativo]

mim·ic (mim′ik). Imitar ou simular. [G. *mimikos*, imitativo, de *mimos*, mímica]

mim·ma·tion (mi-mā′shŭn). Mimação; forma de gagueira em que o som m é atribuído a várias letras. [Ar. *mim*, a letra m]

min. Abreviatura de minute (minuto).

mind. Mente. **1.** O órgão ou sede da consciência e das funções superiores do encéfalo humano, como a cognição, o raciocínio, o desejo e a emoção. **2.** A totalidade organizada de todos os processos mentais e atividades físicas, com ênfase na relação dos fenômenos. [A.S. *gemynd*]
   prelogical m., pensamento pré-lógico. SIN prelogical *thinking*.
   subconscious m., m. subconsciente. SIN subliminal *self*.

mind-read·ing. Leitura da mente, telepatia. SIN telepathy.

min·er·al (min′er-ăl). Mineral; qualquer material inorgânico homogêneo geralmente encontrado na crosta terrestre. [L. *mineralis*, pertinente a minas, de *mino*, escavar]

min·er·al·i·za·tion (min′er-al-i-zā′shŭn). Mineralização; a introdução de minerais em uma estrutura, como na mineralização normal dos ossos e dentes ou a mineralização patológica dos tecidos, isto é, calcificação distrófica ou metastática.

min·er·al·o·coid (min-er-al′ō-koyd). Mineralocorticóide. SIN mineralocorticoid.

min·er·al·o·cor·ti·coid (min′er-al-ō-kōr′ti-koyd). Mineralocorticóide; um dos esteróides do córtex supra-renal que influenciam o metabolismo e o equilíbrio hidroeletrolítico (particularmente de íons sódio e potássio). SIN mineralocoid.

min·er·al oil. Óleo mineral; mistura de hidrocarbonetos líquidos obtidos do petróleo, usados como veículo em preparações farmacêuticas; algumas vezes é usado como lubrificante intestinal; pode interferir com a absorção de vitaminas lipossolúveis. SIN heavy liquid petrolatum, liquid paraffin, liquid petroleum.

min·er·al·o·tro·pic (min-er-al′ō-trō′pik). Mineralotrópico; relativo aos mineralocorticóides ou à ação destes.

mini (mi′nē). Computador de tamanho médio que pode servir a muitos usuários em um departamento, ou que é dedicado a uma função computacional completa, como tomografia computadorizada ou ressonância magnética; menores e mais lentos que um servidor, mais complexos e potentes que um computador pessoal. [It. *miniatura*, decoração de manuscritos, do L. *minium*, chumbo vermelho]

min·i·lap·a·rot·o·my (min′ē-lap-ă-rot′ō-mē). Minilaparotomia; técnica para esterilização por ligadura cirúrgica das tubas de Falópio, realizada através de uma pequena incisão suprapúbica ou infra-umbilical.

min·im (m). Mínimo. **1.** Medida de líquido, 1/60 de uma dracma líquida; no caso da água, cerca de uma gota. **2.** Que é o menor; a menor de várias estruturas semelhantes. [L. *minimus*, mínimo]

min·i·mum (min-i-mum). Mínimo; a menor quantidade ou o limite mais baixo. [L. o menor]

min·i·my·o·sin (min-ē-mī′ō-sin). Minimiosina; proteína semelhante à miosina por possuir um domínio globular de ligação à actina e uma cauda curta que pode ligar-se a membranas, mas que não possui uma longa cauda α-helicoidal; acredita-se que tenha um papel na extensão do filopódio no cone de crescimento de neurônios.

minithoracotomy. Minitoracotomia; ver em thoracotomy.

min·o·cy·cline (min-ō-sī′klēn). Minociclina; substituto da naftacenocarboxamida; antibacteriano relacionado à tetraciclina.

mi·nor (mī′ner). Menor; designa a menor de duas estruturas semelhantes. [L.]

mi·nox·i·dil (mi-nok′si-dil). Minoxidil; anti-hipertensivo usado no tratamento da calvície prematura; algumas vezes é usado topicamente no couro cabeludo para aumentar o crescimento do cabelo.

mint. Menta. SIN Mentha. [G. *mintha*]

△ **mio-.** Mio-; menos. [G. *meiōn*]

mi·o·did·y·mus, mi·od·y·mus (mī-ō-did′i-mŭs, mī-od′i-mŭs). Miodídimo; gêmeos conjugados desiguais, com a cabeça do gêmeo menor unida à região occipital da cabeça do gêmeo maior. VER conjoined *twins*, em *twin*. [mio- + G. *didymos*, gêmeo]

mi·o·lec·i·thal (mī-ō-les′i-thal). Miolécito; designa um ovo com pouco vitelo, uniformemente disperso em todo o ovo. [mio- + G. *lekithos*, vitelo]

mi·o·pra·gia (mī-ō-prā′jē-ă). Miopragia; diminuição da atividade funcional de uma parte. [mio- + G. *prassō*, fazer]

mi·o·pus (mī-ō′pŭs). Miopo; gêmeos conjugados desiguais com cabeças unidas de tal forma que uma face é rudimentar. VER conjoined *twins*, em *twin*. [mio- + *ōps*, olho]

mi·o·sis (mī-ō′sis). **1.** Miose; contração da pupila. **2.** Ortografia alternativa errada de meiose. [G. *meiōsis*, diminuição]
   paralytic m., m. paralítica; miose devida à paralisia do músculo dilatador da pupila.
   spastic m., m. espástica; miose devida à contração espasmódica do esfíncter da pupila.

mi·ot·ic (mī-ot′ik). Miótico. **1.** Relativo a, ou caracterizado por, constrição da pupila. **2.** Agente que causa contração da pupila de forma que esta fique pequena.

MIP Abreviatura de maximum intensity *projection* (projeção de intensidade máxima).

MIP Abreviatura de macrophage inflammatory *protein* (proteína inflamatória de macrófagos).

mi·ra·cid·i·um, pl. **mi·ra·cid·ia** (mī-ră-sid′ē-ŭm, -ă). Miracídio; a larva ciliada em primeiro estágio de um trematódeo que emerge do ovo e deve penetrar nos tecidos de um caramujo hospedeiro intermediário adequado para continuar seu ciclo biológico; seguido pelo desenvolvimento em um esporocisto-mãe e pela produção de vários produtos de sucessivas gerações de larvas. VER TAMBÉM sporocyst (1). [G. *meirakidion*, menino]

Mirchamp sign. Sinal de Mirchamp. VER em sign.

mire (mēr). Mira; um dos objetos de teste no oftalmômetro; sua imagem (também denominada mira), espelhada na superfície da córnea, é medida para determinar os raios de curvatura da córnea. [L. *mirror*, pp. *-atus*, admirar]

mi·rex (mī′reks). Mirex; derivado do benzeno usado como inseticida e para retardar o fogo em plásticos, borracha, tinta, papel, material elétrico; provavelmente é carcinógeno.

Mirizzi, P.L., médico argentino do século XX. VER M. *syndrome*.

mir·ror (mir′or). Espelho; superfície polida que reflete os raios luminosos refletidos de objetos à sua frente. [Fr. *miroir*, do L. *miror*, admirar]
   concave m., e. côncavo; superfície refletora esférica que constitui um segmento do interior de uma esfera.
   convex m., e. convexo; superfície refletora esférica que constitui um segmento do exterior de uma esfera.
   head m., e. de cabeça; espelho côncavo circular, fixado a uma faixa na cabeça, usado para projetar um feixe luminoso em uma cavidade, como o nariz ou laringe, para fins de exame e para permitir visão binocular.
   mouth m., e. de boca; pequeno espelho em um cabo usado para facilitar a visualização no exame dos dentes.
   van Helmont m., e. de van-Helmont; termo obsoleto para designar o tendão central do diafragma (central *tendom* of diaphragm).

mir·ror-writ·ing (mir′or-rit′ing). Escrita em espelho; escrita para trás, da direita para a esquerda, com as letras assemelhando-se a uma escrita comum vista em um espelho. SIN retrography.

mir·yach·it (mir-yach′it). Afecção nervosa observada na Sibéria. VER jumping *disease*.

MIS Abreviatura de müllerian inhibiting *substance* (substância inibidora mülleriana).

mis·an·dry (mis′an-drē). Misandria; aversão ou ódio aos homens. [G. *miseō*, odiar, + *anēr, andros*, homem]

mis·an·thro·py (mis-an′thrō-pē). Misantropia; aversão e ódio aos seres humanos. [G. *miseō*, odiar, + *anthrōpos*, homem]

mis·car·riage (mis-kar′ij). Abortamento; expulsão espontânea dos produtos da gravidez antes do meio do segundo trimestre. SIN spontaneous abortion.

mis·car·ry (mis-kar′ē). Abortar; sofrer um aborto.

mis·ce·ge·na·tion (mis′e-jē-nā′shŭn). Miscigenação; casamento ou cruzamento de indivíduos de diferentes raças. [L. *misceo*, misturar, + *genus*, descendência, raça]

mis·ci·ble (mis′i-bl). Miscível; capaz de ser misturado e assim permanecer após cessar o processo de mistura. [L. *misceo*, misturar]

mis·di·ag·no·sis (mis′dī-ag-nō′sis). Diagnóstico errado; um diagnóstico errado ou equivocado.

mi·sog·a·my (mi-sog′ă-mē). Misogamia; aversão ao casamento. [G. *miseō*, odiar, + *gamos*, casamento]

mi·sog·y·ny (mi-soj′i-nē). Misoginia; aversão ou ódio às mulheres. [G. *miseō*, odiar, + *gynē*, mulher]

mis·o·pe·dia, mis·op·e·dy (mis-ō-pē′dē-ă, -op′e-dē). Misopedia; aversão ou ódio às crianças. [G. *miseō*, odiar, + *pais* (*paid*-), criança]

mi·so·pros·tol (mī - sō - prost′ol). Misoprostol; análogo da prostaglandina usado no tratamento da úlcera; particularmente útil em pessoas que usam antiinflamatórios não-esteróides; antiulcerativo.

mis·sense (mis′ens). Sentido incorreto; como usado em genética, uma mutação que causa uma seqüência de forma que há uma substituição de um resíduo aminoácido por outro.

  m. supression, supressão de sentido incorreto; mutação no RNAt que permite a incorporação de um resíduo aminoácido que possibilita a função completa do produto genético.

mis·tle·toe (mis′l - tō). Visco; visgo. SIN viscum (1).

MIT Abreviatura de monoiodotyrosine (monoiodotirosina).

Mitchell. VER Weir Mitchell.

mite (mīt). Ácaro; artrópode diminuto da ordem Acarina, amplo conjunto de organismos parasitários e (basicamente) de vida livre. A maioria ainda não foi descrita, e apenas um número relativamente pequeno tem importância médica ou veterinária como vetores ou hospedeiros intermediários de agentes patogênicos, causando diretamente dermatite ou lesão tecidual, ou causando perda de sangue ou de líquido tecidual. As larvas de seis pernas dos a. trombiculídeos, os ácaros terrestres (*Trombicula*), são parasitas de seres humanos e de muitos mamíferos e aves, e são importantes vetores do tifo rural (doença de tsutsugamushi) e outras riquétsias. Alguns outros a. importantes são *Acarus hordei* (a. da cevada), *Demodex folliculorum* (a. folicular ou a. da sarna), *Dermanyssus gallinae* (a. das galinhas), *Ornithonyssus bacoti* (a. do rato tropical), *m. sylviarum* (a. das aves domésticas do norte), *Pyemotes tritici* (a. da palha ou de cereais) e *Sarcoptes scabiei* (a. da sarna). [A.S.]

mith·ra·my·cin (mith - rā - mī′sin). Mitramicina; antibiótico produzido por *Streptomyces argillaceus* e *S. tanashiensis*; possui atividade antineoplásica. SIN aureolic acid, mitramycin.

mith·ri·da·tism (mith′ri - dā′tizm, mith - rid′ă - tizm). Mitridatismo; imunidade contra a ação de um veneno adquirida pela administração de doses pequenas e crescentes dele. [*Mithridates*, Rei do Ponto (132–63 a.C.), supostamente um suicida malsucedido (por veneno) devido às pequenas doses repetidas tomadas para se tornar invulnerável ao assassinato por veneno]

mi·ti·ci·dal (mī - ti - sī′dăl). Acaricida; destrutivo para ácaros.

mi·ti·cide (mī′ti - sīd). Acaricida; agente destrutivo para ácaros. [mite + L. *caedo*, matar]

mit·i·gate (mit′i - gāt). Mitigar; aliviar. SIN palliate. [L. *mitigo*, pp. *-atus*, tornar leve ou suave, de *mitis*, leve, + *ago*, fazer]

mi·tis (mī′tis). Leve. [L.]

mi·to·chon·dria (-ă). Mitocôndrias; plural de mitochondrion.

mi·to·chon·dri·al (mī - tō - kon′drē - ăl). Mitocondrial; relativo às mitocôndrias.

mi·to·chon·dri·on, pl. **mi·to·chon·dria** (mī - tō - kon′drē - on, - ă). Mitocôndria; organela do citoplasma celular que consiste em dois grupos de membranas, uma camada externa lisa e uma membrana interna disposta em túbulos ou, na maioria das vezes, em pregas que formam membranas duplas semelhantes a lâminas denominadas cristas; as mitocôndrias são a principal fonte de energia da célula e contêm as enzimas do citocromo do transporte de elétron terminal e as enzimas do ciclo do ácido cítrico, oxidação dos ácidos graxos e fosforilação oxidativa. SIN Altmann granule (2). [G. *mitos*, fio, + *chondros*, grânulo, areia]

  m. of hemoflagellates, m. dos hemoflagelados; a "mitocôndria-mãe", da qual parecem originar-se mitocôndrias menores.

mi·to·gen (mī′tō - jen). Mitógeno; substância freqüentemente derivada de vegetais que estimula a mitose e a transformação de linfócitos; inclui não apenas lectinas, como as fitoemaglutininas e a concanavalina A, mas também substâncias derivadas de estreptococos (associadas à estreptolisina S) e de cepas de estafilococos produtores de α-toxina. SIN transforming agent (1). [mitosis + G. *-gen*, que produz]

  pokeweed m. (PWM), m. do caruru-de-cacho, erva-do-canadá; um mitógeno (lectina) da *Phytolacca americana* (caruru-de-cacho), que estimula principalmente os linfócitos B.

mi·to·gen·e·sis (mī - tō - jen′ē - sis). Mitogênese; o processo de indução de mitose ou transformação de uma célula. [mitosis + G. *genesis*, origem]

mi·to·ge·net·ic (mī′tō - jĕ - net′ik). Mitogenético; relativo ao fator ou fatores que promovem mitose celular.

mi·to·gen·ic (mī - tō - jen′ik). Mitogênico; que causa mitose ou transformação.

mi·to·my·cin (mī - tō - mī′sin). Mitomicina; antibiótico produzido por *Streptomyces caespitosus*, cujas variantes são designadas m. A, m. B, etc.; a m. C é um agente antineoplásico e bactericida; inibe a síntese de DNA.

mi·to·plast (mī′tō - plast). Mitoplasto; mitocôndria sem sua membrana externa.

mi·to·sis, pl. **mi·to·ses** (mī - tō′sis, - sēz). Mitose; o processo habitual de reprodução somática de células que consistem em uma seqüência de modificações do núcleo (prófase, prometáfase, metáfase, anáfase, telófase) que resultam na formação de duas células-filhas exatamente com o mesmo conteúdo de DNA cromossomial e nuclear que o da célula original. VER TAMBÉM cell *cycle*. SIN indirect nuclear division, mitotic division. [G. *mitos*, fio]

  heterotype m., m. heterotípica; várias mitoses nas quais as metades cromossômicas são unidas em suas extremidades, formando figuras anulares. Ocorre na primeira divisão da meiose.

  multipolar m., m. multipolar; forma patológica na qual o fuso tem três ou mais pólos, resultando na formação de um número correspondente de núcleos.

  somatic m., m. somática; o processo comum de mitose, como ocorre nas células somáticas ou do corpo, caracterizado pela formação do número definido de cromossomas apropriado para a espécie (no homem, o número é 46).

mi·to·tane (mī′tō - tān). Mitotano; agente antineoplásico.

mi·tot·ic (mī - tot′ik). Mitótico; relativo a, ou caracterizado por, mitose.

mi·to·xan·trone hy·dro·chlo·ride (mī - tō - zan′trōn). Cloridrato de mitoxantrona; antineoplásico sintético usado por via intravenosa no tratamento inicial da leucemia não-linfocítica aguda em adultos.

mi·tral (mī′trăl). Mitral. **1.** Relativo à valva mitral ou bicúspide. **2.** Com a forma de mitra de bispo; designando uma estrutura com formato semelhante ao de uma faixa de cabeça ou turbante. [L. *mitra*, coifa ou turbante]

mi·tral·i·za·tion (mī′tră - li - zā′shŭn). Mitralização; retificação da borda esquerda do coração em uma radiografia do tórax devido à proeminência do apêndice atrial esquerdo ou do trato de saída pulmonar; uma indicação não-confiável de doença da valva mitral.

mit·ra·my·cin (mit - ră - mī′sin). Mitramicina. SIN mithramycin.

Mitrofanoff, Paul, cirurgião pediátrico francês, *1934. VER Mitrofanoff *principle*.

Mitsuda, Kensuke, médico japonês, 1876–1964. VER M. *antigen, reaction*.

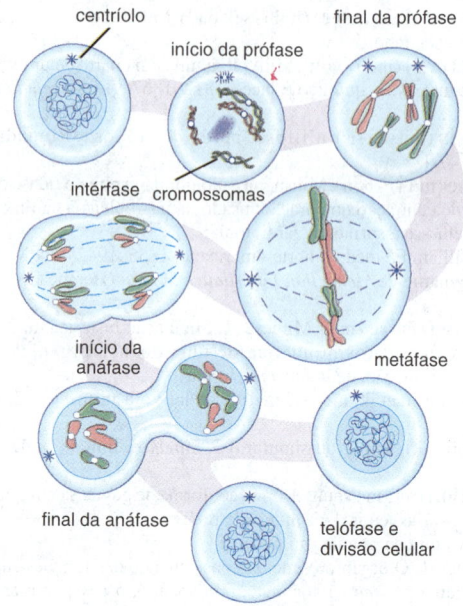

mitose celular

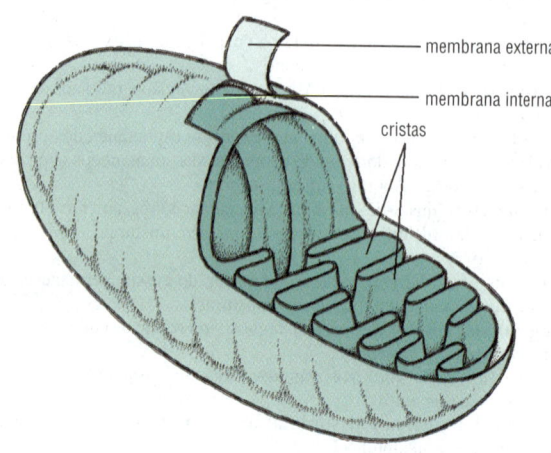

mitocôndria

Mitsuo, Gentaro, oftalmologista japonês, 1876–1913. VER M. *phenomenon*.

mit·tel·schmerz (mit′el‑schmārts). Dor intermenstrual; dor abdominal que ocorre no momento da ovulação, resultante da irritação do peritônio por hemorragia no local da ovulação. SIN intermenstrual pain (2), middle pain. [Al. Mittelschmerz, meio + pain]

mi·vac·ur·i·um (mī′vă‑kūr′ē‑ŭm). Mivacúrio; bloqueador neuromuscular semelhante à *d*-tubocurarina, mas que possui menor duração de ação.

mix·ing (mik′sing). Mistura; a mistura ou reunião de partículas ou componentes, principalmente de diferentes tipos.
  phenotypic m., m. fenotípica; interação não-genética na qual partículas virais liberadas de uma célula infectada por dois vírus diferentes possuem componentes de ambos os agentes infecciosos, mas com um genoma de um deles.

mix·o·tro·phy (miks‑o′trō‑fē). Mixotrofia; a propriedade de alguns microrganismos que podem assimilar compostos orgânicos como fontes de carbono, mas não como fontes de energia. [G. *mixis*, mistura, de *mignumi*, misturar, + *trophē*, nutrição]

mix·ture (miks′chŭr). Mistura. **1.** Incorporação mútua de duas ou mais substâncias, sem união química, sendo preservadas as características físicas de cada um dos componentes. Uma **mistura mecânica** (mechanical m.) é uma mistura de partículas ou massas distinguíveis ao exame microscópico ou de outras formas; uma **mistura física** (physical mixture) é uma mistura mais "íntima" de moléculas, como no caso dos gases e de muitas soluções. **2.** Em química, uma mistura de duas ou mais substâncias sem a ocorrência de uma reação pela qual elas perderiam suas propriedades individuais, isto é, sem ganho ou perda permanente de elétrons. **3.** Em farmácia, uma preparação consistindo em um líquido que mantém uma substância medicinal insolúvel em suspensão por meio de acácia, açúcar ou algum outro material viscoso. [L. *mixtura* ou *mistura*]
  Bordeaux m., m. de Bordeaux; mistura fungicida vegetal que consiste em sulfato de cobre (5 partes) e óxido de cálcio (5 partes) em água (400 partes) recém-misturada; o CaO é adicionado à solução de $CuSO_4$.
  extemporaneous m., m. extemporânea; mistura preparada no momento determinado, de acordo com as orientações de uma prescrição, distinta de um preparado estocado.
  Seidlitz m., m. de Seidlitz; uma mistura de 3 partes de sal Rochelle e 1 parte de bicarbonato de sódio. Dez gramas da mistura são empregados com 2,17 g de ácido tartárico para uma de pó de Seidlitz. O pó, que efervesce quando colocado em água, foi amplamente usado como catártico.

Miyagawa, Yoneji, bacteriologista japonês, 1885–1959. VER *Miyagawanella*; M. *bodies*, em *body*.

Mi·ya·ga·wa·nel·la (mē′yă‑gah′wă‑nel′ă). Anteriormente considerado um gênero de Chlamydiaceae, mas agora sinônimo de *Chlamydia*. [Y. *Miyagawa*]

MK Abreviatura de menaquinone (menaquinona).

MK-6 Abreviatura de menaquinone-6 (menaquinona-6).

MK-7 Abreviatura de menaquinone-7 (menaquinona-7).

MLC Abreviatura de Marginal Line Calculus Index (Índice de Cálculo da Linha Marginal).

MLD, mld Abreviatura de minimal lethal *dose* (dose letal mínima).

mlRNA Abreviatura de messengerlike RNA (RNA semelhante ao RNA mensageiro).

mM, mM Abreviatura de millimolar (milimolar).

mm Abreviatura de millimeter (milímetro).

MMMT Abreviatura de malignant mixed müllerian *tumor* (tumor mülleriano misto maligno) ou malignant mixed mesodermal tumor (tumor mesodérmico misto maligno).

M-mode. Modo M; apresentação ultra-sonográfica diagnóstica das alterações temporais em ecos nos quais a profundidade de interfaces produtoras de eco é exibida ao longo de um eixo com o tempo (T) ao longo do segundo eixo; é exibido o movimento (M) nas interfaces aproximando-se e afastando-se do transdutor. SIN TM-mode.

mmol Abreviatura de millimole (milimol).

MMPI Abreviatura de Minnesota Multiphasic Personality Inventory *test*.

MMR Abreviatura de measles, mumps and rubella *vaccine* (vacina para sarampo, caxumba e rubéola).

Mn Símbolo do manganese (manganês).

M'Naghten, Daniel, criminoso inglês, julgado em março de 1843. VER M. *rule*.

MND Abreviatura de motor neuron *disease* (doença do neurônio motor).

mne·me (nē′mē). Memória; a qualidade duradoura na mente responsável pelos fatos da memória; o engrama de uma experiência específica. [G. *mnēmē*, memória]

mne·men·ic, mne·mic (nē‑men′ik, nē′mik). Mnemônico; relativo à memória.

mne·mism (nē′mizm). Mnemismo. SIN mnemic *hypothesis*. [G. *mnēmē*, memória]

mne·mon·ic (nē‑mon′ik). Mnemônico. SIN anamnestic (1).

mne·mon·ics (nē‑mon′iks). Mnemônica; a arte de melhorar a memória; sistema para ajudar a memória. [G. *mnēmonikos*, mnemônico, relativo à memória]

MNSs blood group. Grupo sanguíneo MNS. VER Apêndice de Grupos Sanguíneos.

M.O. Abreviatura de Medical Officer.

Mo Símbolo do molybdenium (molibdênio).

⁹⁹Mo. Abreviatura de molybdenium-99 (molibdênio-99).

MoAb Abreviatura de monoclonal *antibody* (anticorpo monoclonal).

mo·bi·li·za·tion (mō′bi‑li‑zā′shŭn). Mobilização. **1.** Tornar móvel; restaurar a capacidade de movimento em uma articulação. **2.** O ato ou resultado do ato de mobilização; excitar um processo até então quiescente em atividade fisiológica. VER TAMBÉM mobilize. **3.** O processo pelo qual um plastídeo conjugador efetua a transferência de DNA de uma célula para outra.
  stapes m., m. do estribo; operação para remobilizar a plataforma do estribo a fim de aliviar os distúrbios de condução da audição causados por sua imobilização devida a otosclerose ou a outra doença do ouvido médio.

mo·bi·lize (mō′bi‑līz). Mobilizar. **1.** Liberar material armazenado no corpo; mais especificamente, deslocar uma substância dos depósitos teciduais para a corrente sanguínea. **2.** Excitar material quiescente para atividade fisiológica. [Fr. *mobiliser*, liberar, deixar pronto, do L. *mobilis*, móvel]

Mobitz, Woldemar, cardiologista alemão, *1889. VER M. types of atrioventricular *block*.

Möbius, Paul J. médico alemão, 1853–1907. VER M. *sign, syndrome;* Leyden-M. muscular *dystrophy*.

MOD Abreviatura de mesiodistocclusal (mesiodistobucal).

mo·dal·i·ty (mō‑dal′i‑tē). Modalidade. **1.** Forma de aplicação ou emprego de um agente ou regime terapêutico. **2.** Várias formas de sensibilidade, p. ex., tato, visão, etc. [L. Mediev. *modalitas*, do L. *modus*, modo]

mode (mōd). Moda; em um conjunto de medidas, o valor que aparece com maior freqüência. [L. *modus*, medida, quantidade]

mod·el (mod′el). Modelo. **1.** Representação de alguma coisa, freqüentemente idealizada ou modificada para torná-la conceitualmente mais fácil de compreender. **2.** Algo a ser imitado. **3.** Em odontologia, um modelo. **4.** Representação matemática de determinado fenômeno. **5.** Animal usado para imitar uma condição patológica. [It. *midello*, do L. *modus*, medida, padrão]
  Adair-Koshland-Némethy-Filmer m. (AKNF), m. de Adair-Koshland-Némethy-Filmer. SIN Koshland-Némethy-Filmer m.
  additive m., m. aditivo; m. no qual o efeito combinado de vários fatores é a soma dos efeitos que seriam produzidos por cada um dos fatores na ausência dos outros.
  animal m., m. animal; estudo em uma população de animais de laboratório que usa condições de animais análogas às condições de seres humanos para simular processos comparáveis àqueles que ocorrem em populações humanas.
  Armitage-Doll m., m. de Armitage-Doll; m. de carcinogênese com a premissa de que a principal variável que determina modificação do risco não é a idade, mas o tempo.
  Bingham m., m. de Bingham; m. que representa o comportamento do fluxo de um plástico de Bingham; no caso idealizado.
  biomedical m., m. biomédico; m. conceitual de doença que exclui fatores psicológicos e sociais, e inclui apenas fatores biológicos em uma tentativa de compreender a doença ou distúrbio de uma pessoa.
  biopsychosocial m., m. biopsicossocial; m. conceitual que supõe que fatores psicológicos e sociais também devem ser incluídos, juntamente com os biológicos, na compreensão da doença ou distúrbio de uma pessoa.
  cloverleaf m., m. em trevo; modelo para a estrutura de RNAt; assim denominado porque a estrutura lembra um pouco um trevo.
  computer m., m. computadorizado; representação matemática do funcionamento de um sistema, apresentada na forma de um programa de computador. SIN computer simulation.
  concerted m., m. combinado. SIN Monod-Wyman-Changeux m.
  cooperativity m., m. de cooperatividade; m. usado para explicar a propriedade de cooperatividade observada em algumas enzimas; p. ex., alosterismo ou histerese.
  fluid mosaic m., m. do mosaico fluido; m. para a estrutura de uma biomembrana com capacidade de difusão lateral dos constituintes e pouco, ou nenhum, movimento de oscilação.
  genetic m., m. genético; hipótese formalizada sobre o comportamento de uma estrutura hereditária na qual os termos componentes devem ter interpretação literal como estruturas padronizadas de genética empírica.
  induced fit m., m. do ajuste induzido; **(1)** um modelo que sugere um modo de ação das enzimas no qual o substrato liga-se ao sítio ativo da proteína, causando uma alteração da conformação da proteína; **(2)** SIN Koshland-Némethy-Filmer m.
  Koshland-Némethy-Filmer m. (KNF model), m. de Koshland-Némethy-Filmer; um modelo para explicar a forma alostérica de cooperatividade; nesse modelo, na ausência de ligantes, a proteína existe em apenas uma conformação; quando ocorre a ligação, o ligante induz uma alteração na configuração que pode ser transmitida para outras subunidades. SIN Adair-Koshland-Némethy-Filmer m., induced fit m. (2).
  lock-and-key m., m. chave-e-fechadura; m. usado para sugerir o modo de operação de uma enzima no qual o substrato se liga ao sítio ativo da proteína, como uma chave em uma fechadura.

logistic m., m. logístico; um m. estatístico; em epidemiologia, um m. de risco como uma função da exposição a um fator de risco.
mathematical m., m. matemático; representação de um sistema, processo ou relação na forma matemática, utilizando equações para simular o comportamento do sistema ou processo em estudo.
medical m., m. médico; conjunto de suposições que vê anormalidades do comportamento na mesma estrutura que doença ou anormalidades físicas.
Monod-Wyman-Changeux m. (MWCm.), m. de Monod-Wyman-Changeux; m. usado para explicar a forma alostérica de cooperatividade; nesse modelo, pode haver uma proteína oligomérica em dois estados de configuração na ausência do ligante; esses estados estão em equilíbrio, e o predominante tem uma menor afinidade pelo ligante (que se liga à proteína em uma forma de equilíbrio rápido). SIN concerted m.
multiplicative m., m. multiplicativo; m. no qual o efeito conjunto de duas ou mais causas é o produto de seus efeitos se estivessem agindo isoladamente.
multistage m., m. em estágios múltiplos; m. matemático, principalmente para carcinogênese, baseado na teoria de que um carcinógeno específico pode afetar um dentre vários estágios no desenvolvimento do câncer.
MWC m., m. MWC, abreviatura de Monod-Wyman-Changeux m.
pathologic m., m. patológico; um animal, ou grupo de animais, que, por herança ou manipulação artificial, desenvolve um distúrbio semelhante a alguma doença de interesse e, portanto, fornece, diretamente, ou por analogia, evidências de sua patogenia, podendo ser usado como m. para estudo de medidas preventivas ou terapêuticas.
Reed-Frost m., m. de Reed-Frost; m. matemático de transmissão de doenças infecciosas e imunidade de grupo. O m. fornece o número de novos casos de uma infecção que podem ser esperados em determinado período em uma população fechada, de cruzamento livre de indivíduos imunes e suscetíveis, com várias suposições sobre freqüência de contato.
Sartwell incubation m., m. de incubação de Sartwell; m. matemático, baseado em observações empíricas, mostrando que os períodos de incubação de doenças transmissíveis têm uma distribuição log-normal; o modelo é válido para determinados tipos de cânceres com causas externas bem definidas.
statistical m., m. estatístico; representação formal de uma classe de processos que permite uma forma de analisar resultados a partir de estudos experimentais, como o m. de Poisson ou o m. linear geral; não precisa propor um processo literalmente interpretável no contexto do caso individual.
mod·el·ing (mod′ĕl-ing). Modelagem. **1.** Na teoria da aprendizagem, a aquisição e o aprendizado de uma nova habilidade através da observação e imitação do comportamento de outro indivíduo. **2.** Em modificação do comportamento, um procedimento de tratamento pelo qual o terapeuta ou outra pessoa importante apresenta (modela) o comportamento alvo que o aprendiz deve imitar e que deve fazer parte do repertório. **3.** Processo contínuo pelo qual um osso tem seu tamanho e formato alterados durante o crescimento, mediante reabsorção e formação de osso em diferentes locais e taxas. **4.** Processo pelo qual é formada a representação de uma entidade.
mod·i·fi·ca·tion (mod′i-fi-kā′shŭn). Modificação. **1.** Alteração não-hereditária de um organismo; p. ex., a adquirida em decorrência de sua própria atividade ou ambiente. **2.** Alteração química ou estrutural de uma molécula.
behavior m., m. do comportamento; o uso sistemático de princípios de condicionamento e aprendizado, em particular o condicionamento operante e instrumental, para ensinar determinadas habilidades ou extinguir comportamentos, atitudes ou fobias indesejáveis.
chemical m., m. química; alteração na estrutura de uma molécula, tipicamente uma macromolécula, como uma proteína, por meios químicos; freqüentemente, a adição covalente por algum reagente.
covalent m., m. covalente; alteração na estrutura de uma macromolécula por meios enzimáticos, resultando em modificação das propriedades dessa macromolécula; amiúde, esse tipo de modificação é fisiologicamente relevante.
mod·i·fi·er (mod′ĭ-fī-er). Modificador; aquilo que altera ou limita.
biologic response modifier, m. da resposta biológica; agente que modifica as respostas do hospedeiro a neoplasias mediante o fortalecimento do sistema imune ou a reconstituição de mecanismos imunes comprometidos.
mo·di·o·lus, pl. **mo·di·o·li** (mō-dī′ō-lŭs, -ō-lī). **1.** [TA] Modíolo; o centro cônico do osso esponjoso em torno do qual gira o canal espiral do modíolo. **2.** SIN m. of angle of mouth. [L. o cubo de uma roda].
m. of angle of mouth [TA], modíolo do ângulo da boca; um ponto próximo do ângulo da boca para o qual convergem vários músculos da expressão facial. SIN m. anguli oris [TA], columella cochleae, m. labii, modiolus (2).
m. anguli oris [TA], modíolo do ângulo da boca. SIN m. of angle of mouth.
m. la'bii, modíolo do ângulo da boca. SIN m. of angle of mouth.
mod·u·la·tion (mod-ū-lā′shŭn). Modulação. **1.** A flutuação funcional e morfológica de células em resposta a mudanças das condições ambientais. **2.** Variação sistemática de uma característica (p. ex., freqüência, amplitude) de uma oscilação mantida para codificar outras informações. **3.** Uma modificação na cinética de uma enzima ou via metabólica. **4.** A regulação da taxa de tradução do RNAm por um códon modulador. [L. *modulor*, medir adequadamente]

biochemical m., m. bioquímica; termo que descreve a modulação (seja estimulação da atividade ou redução da toxicidade) de um agente quimioterápico por outro agente, que pode ou não possuir atividade antineoplásica própria.
mod·u·la·tor. Modulador; aquilo que regula ou ajusta.
selective estrogen receptor modulator (SERM), modulador do receptor estrogênico seletivo; agente farmacêutico com afinidade seletiva pelo receptor estrogênico; as preparações atuais possuem um efeito primário sobre os tecidos ósseo e cardiovascular e menor efeito sobre os tecidos endometriais, genitais e mamários.
mo·du·lus (moj′ū-lŭs, mod′ū-). Módulo; coeficiente que expressa a magnitude de uma propriedade física por um valor numérico. [L. dim. de *modus*, medida, quantidade]
bulk m., m. de compressibilidade, m. hidrostático. SIN m. of volume elasticity.
m. of elasticity, m. de elasticidade; coeficiente que expressa a razão entre a tensão por área unitária que age deformando um corpo e o grau de deformação resultante.
m. of volume elasticity, m. de elasticidade do volume; coeficiente que expressa a razão entre a pressão que age modificando o volume de uma substância e o grau de alteração resultante. SIN bulk m.
Young m., m. de Young; tipo de m. de elasticidade que especifica a força aplicada a um corpo em uma direção, por unidade de área transversal do corpo perpendicular a essa direção, dividida pela alteração fracional no comprimento do corpo nessa direção.
Moeller, Alfred, bacteriologista alemão, *1868. VER M. grass *bacillus*.
Moeller, Julius O.L., cirurgião alemão, 1819–1887. VER M. *glossitis*.
mo·fe·bu·ta·zone (mof-e-bū′tă-zōn). Mofebutazona; antiinflamatório usado no tratamento da artrite.
mog·i·ar·thria (moj-i-ar′thrē-ă). Mogiartria; disartria causada por deficiência da coordenação muscular. [G. *mogis*, com dificuldade, + *arthroō*, articular]
mog·i·la·lia (moj-i-lā′lē-ă). Mogilalia; gagueira, tartamudez ou qualquer distúrbio da fala. SIN molilalia. [G. *mogis*, com dificuldade, + *lalia*, fala]
mog·i·pho·nia (moj-i-fō′nē-ă). Mogifonia; espasmo laríngeo que ocorre nos oradores em virtude do uso excessivo da voz. [G. *mogis*, com dificuldade, + *phōnē*, voz]
Mohrenheim, Joseph J. Freiherr von, cirurgião austríaco-russo, 1755–1799. VER M. *fossa, space*.
Mohs, Frederic E., cirurgião norte-americano, *1910, que, quando estudante de medicina, projetou um sistema de remoção de tumores cutâneos controlado por microscopia. VER M. fresh tissue chemosurgery *technique, chemosurgery*.
Mohs, Friedrich, mineralogista alemão, 1773–1839. VER M. *scale*.
moi·e·ty (moy′i-tē). Metade; porção. **1.** Originalmente, metade; agora, livremente, uma porção de algo. **2.** Grupamento funcional. [I.m. *moite*, metade]
mol Abreviatura de mole (4) (mol).
mo·lal (mō′lăl). Molal; designa 1 mol de soluto dissolvido em 1.000 g de solvente; essas soluções possuem uma razão definida entre moléculas de soluto e solvente. Cf. molar (4).
mo·lal·i·ty (m) (mō-lăl′i-tē). Molalidade; moles de soluto por quilograma de solvente; a molaridade é igual a mρ/(1 + mM), na qual m é a molalidade, ρ é a densidade da solução e M é a massa molar do soluto. Cf. molarity.
mo·lar (mō′lăr). Molar. **1.** Designa um triturador, abrasivo ou desgastante. [L. *molaris*, relativo a um moinho, pedra de moinho]. **2.** Dente molar. SIN molar *tooth*. **3.** Maciço; relativo a uma massa; não molecular. [L. *moles*, massa]. **4.** Designa uma concentração de peso molecular de 1 grama (1 mol) de soluto por litro de solução, a unidade comum de concentração em química. Cf. molal. **5.** Designa quantidade específica, p. ex., volume molar (volume de 1 mol).

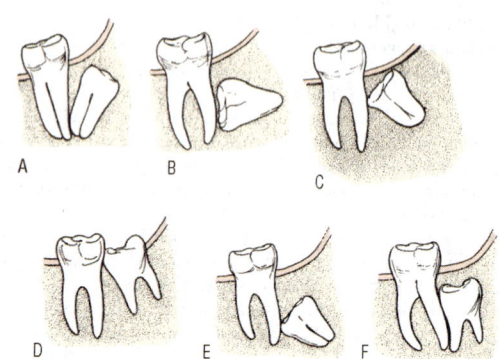

impactação do terceiro molar mandibular: (A) distoangular; (B) horizontal; (C) mesioangular; (D) nível alto; (E) nível baixo; (F) vertical

first m., first permanent m., primeiro molar, primeiro molar permanente; sexto dente permanente ou quarto dente decíduo na maxila e na mandíbula de cada lado do plano mediano sagital da cabeça acompanhando a forma do arco.
Moon m.'s, molares de Moon; primeiros molares pequenos, em forma de abóbada, observados na sífilis congênita.
mulberry m., m. em amora; dente molar com depressões não-anatômicas e nódulos de esmalte arredondados alternados na superfície de sua coroa, geralmente associado à sífilis congênita.
second m., segundo molar; sétimo dente permanente ou quinto dente decíduo na maxila e na mandíbula de cada lado do plano mediano sagital da cabeça, seguindo a forma do arco.
sixth-year m., m. dos seis anos; o primeiro dente molar permanente.
third m., terceiro molar. SIN third-year molar *tooth.*
twelfth-year m., m. dos 12 anos; o segundo dente molar permanente.

mo·lar·i·form (mō-lar′i-fōrm). Molariforme; que possui a forma de um dente molar. [molar (dente) + L. *forma,* forma]

mo·lar·i·ty (M, m) (mō-lar′i-tē). Molaridade; moles por litro de solução (mol/L). Cf. molality.

mold (mōld). **1.** Mofo; bolor; fungo filamentar, geralmente uma colônia circular que pode ser algodonosa, lanuginosa, etc., ou glabra, mas com filamentos não-organizados em grandes espóforos, como cogumelos. **2.** Forma; matriz; molde; receptáculo moldado no qual é pressionada a cera ou derramado o gesso líquido para se fazer um modelo. **3.** Moldar; modelar uma massa de material plástico de acordo com um padrão definido. **4.** Modificar o formato; designa principalmente a adaptação da cabeça do feto ao canal pélvico. **5.** Termo usado para especificar o formato de um dente (ou dentes) artificial. SIN mould.
pink bread m., bolor vermelho do pão. SIN *Neurospora.*

mold·ing (mōld′ing). Modelagem; moldagem; forma obtida por meio de um molde.
border m., moldagem periférica; a moldagem de um material de impressão pela manipulação dos tecidos adjacentes às bordas de uma impressão. SIN muscle-trimming, tissue m., tissue-trimming.
compression m., m. por compressão; **(1)** o ato de comprimir ou espremer para dar forma a um molde; **(2)** a adaptação de um material plástico à forma negativa de um molde dividido por compressão. VER TAMBÉM injection m.
injection m., m. por injeção; a adaptação de um material plástico à forma negativa de um molde fechado, forçando-se a entrada do material no molde através de aberturas apropriadas. VER TAMBÉM compression m. (2).
tissue m., m. tecidual. SIN border m.

mole (mōl). **1.** Nevo. SIN nevus (2). **2.** Nevo pigmentoso. SIN *nevus* pigmentosus. [A.S. *māel* (L. *macula*), uma mancha]. **3.** Mola; massa intra-uterina formada pela degeneração dos produtos da concepção parcialmente desenvolvidos. [L. *moles,* massa] **4 (mol).** Mol; no sistema SI, a unidade de quantidade de substância, definida como a quantidade de uma substância que contém tantas "entidades elementares" quantos são os átomos em 0,0120 kg de carbono-12; "entidades elementares" podem ser átomos, moléculas, íons ou qualquer entidade discernível ou mistura definida de entidades, e devem ser especificadas quando for usado esse termo; na prática, o mol corresponde a $6,0221367 \times 10^{23}$ "entidades elementares". VER TAMBÉM Avogadro *number.*
carneous m., mola carnosa. SIN *fleshy m.*
cystic m., mola cística. SIN *hydatidiform m.*
fleshy m., mola carnosa; massa uterina encontrada após a morte fetal e que consiste em coágulos sanguíneos, membranas fetais e placenta. SIN carneous m.
hairy m., nevo piloso. SIN *nevus* pilosus.
hydatidiform m., hydatid m. [MIM*231090], mola hidatiforme; massa vesicular ou policística, resultante da proliferação do trofoblasto, com degeneração hidrópica e avascularidade das vilosidades coriônicas; o tecido anormal tipicamente resulta da expressão de cromossomas paternos e da perda dos cromossomas maternos. SIN cystic m., gestational trophoblastic disease.
invasive m., m. invasiva. SIN *chorioadenoma* destruens.

mo·lec·u·lar (mō-lek′ū-lär). Molecular; relativo a moléculas.

mo·lec·u·lar·i·ty (mō-lek′ū-lär′i-tē). Molecularidade; número de reagentes em uma reação elementar. Por exemplo, uma reação que envolve um reagente é unimolecular; reações que envolvem duas substâncias são bimoleculares. Molecularidade e ordem não são sinônimos. Cf. order (2).

mol·e·cule (mol′ē-kūl). Molécula; a menor quantidade possível de uma substância di-, tri- ou poliatômica que preserva as propriedades químicas da substância. [L. Mod. *molecula,* dim. de L. *moles,* massa]
accessory m.'s, moléculas acessórias; moléculas de adesão à superfície celular nas células T, envolvidas na ligação da ativação de uma célula para outra célula e na transdução de sinais, p. ex., CD4.
adhesion m.'s, moléculas de adesão; moléculas envolvidas nas interações entre células T auxiliares — células acessórias, células T auxiliares — células B e células T citotóxicas — células-alvo; proteínas da matriz extracelular que atraem leucócitos da circulação.
cell adhesion m. (CAM), m. de adesão celular; proteínas que mantêm as células unidas, p. ex., uvomorulina, e as prendem aos seus substratos, p. ex., laminina.
chimeric m., m. quimérica; molécula (geralmente um biopolímero) que contém seqüências derivadas de dois genes diferentes; especificamente, de duas espécies diferentes. Cf. chimera.
classe I m., m. classe I; um antígeno do complexo principal de histocompatibilidade (MHC) constituído de duas cadeias polipeptídicas com ligação não-covalente, uma glicosilada, pesada e com especificidade antigênica variável; a outra cadeia é a β_2-microglobulina.
classe II m., m. classe II; um antígeno do complexo principal de histocompatibilidade (MHC) que perfura a membrana, constituído de duas cadeias polipeptídicas com ligação não-covalente, designadas α e β.
costimulatory m., m. co-estimulatória; produto ligado à membrana ou secretado de células acessórias, que é necessário para a transdução de sinais.
endothelial-leukocyte adhesion m. (E-LAM), m. de adesão de leucócitos ao endotélio; glicoproteína na superfície de células endoteliais envolvida na adesão dos leucócitos do sangue às paredes dos vasos, bem como na emigração dos vasos para os tecidos.
gram-molecule, molécula-grama; a quantidade de uma substância com uma massa em gramas igual a seu peso molecular; p. ex., uma molécula de hidrogênio pesa 2,016 g, e uma molécula de água, 18,015 g.
intercellular adhesion m.-1 (ICAM-1), m. de adesão intercelular-1; glicoproteína expressa em várias células. É o ligante para o LFA-1 bem como o receptor dos rinovírus.
lectin pathway m., m. da via da lectina; a ligação de proteína de ligação à manose a carboidratos bacterianos, resultando na ativação da via do complemento.

mol·i·la·lia (mol′i-lā′lē-ä). Molilalia, SIN mogilalia. [G. *molis*, com dificuldade (uma forma posterior de *mogis*), + *lalia,* falar]

mo·li·men (mo-li′men). Molímen; o conjunto de fenômenos interiores que têm lugar antes da manifestação de qualquer função orgânica normal.

mo·lim·i·na (-lim′i-nä). Plural de molimen.
menstrual m., molímen hemorrágico. SIN premenstrual *syndrome.*

mo·lin·done hy·dro·chlo·ride (mō-lin′dōn). Cloridrato de molindona; um antipsicótico.

Molisch, Hans, químico austríaco, 1856–1937. VER M. *test.*

Moll, Jacob A., oculista holandês, 1832–1914. VER M. *glands,* em gland.

mol·li·ti·es (mo-lish′i-ēz). Amolecimento. **1.** Caracterizado por uma consistência mole. **2.** SIN malacia. [L. *mollis,* mole]

mol·lusc (mol′ŭsk). Molusco. SIN mollusk.

Mol·lus·ca (mo-lŭs′kä). Filo do sub-reino Metazoa, com corpos moles, não segmentados, que consistem em uma cabeça anterior, uma massa visceral dorsal e um pé ventral. A maioria das formas está encerrada em uma concha calcária protetora. O filo Mollusca inclui as classes Gastropoda (caracóis, búzios, lesmas), Pelecypoda (ostras, mariscos, mexilhões), Cephalopoda (lulas, polvos), Amphineura (quítons), Scaphopoda (conchas dentadas) e a classe de moluscos metaméricos primitivos, Monoplacophora. [L. *mollusca,* uma noz com uma casca fina, de *mollis,* mole]

Mol·lus·ci·pox·vi·rus (mol′lusk-′e-poks-vī-rus). Gênero da família Poxviridae; causa lesões cutâneas verrucosas localizadas. SIN molluscum contagiosum.

mol·lus·cum (mo-lŭs′kŭm). Molusco; doença caracterizada pela ocorrência de tumores arredondados moles da pele. [L. *molluscus,* mole]
m. contagio'sum, m. contagioso. SIN *Molluscipoxvirus.*

mol·lusk (mol′ŭsk). Molusco; nome comum dado aos membros do filo Mollusca, embora geralmente seja restrito aos gastrópodes e bivalves. SIN mollusc.

Moloney, John B., oncologista norte-americano do século XX. VER M. *virus.*
Moloney, Paul J., médico canadense, 1870–1939. VER M. *test.*
Moloy, Howard C., obstetra norte-americano, 1903–1953. VER Caldwell-M. *classification.*

molt (mōlt). Muda; deixar cair as penas, pêlos ou a epiderme; sofrer ecdise. VER TAMBÉM desquamate. SIN moult. [L. *muto,* mudar]

mol wt Abreviatura de molecular *weight* (peso molecular).

mo·lyb·date (mō-lib′dāt). Molibdato; sal do ácido molíbdico.

mo·lyb·den·ic, mo·lyb·de·nous (mō-lib′den-ik, -den-ŭs). Molibdênico; relativo ao molibdênio.

mo·lyb·de·num (Mo) (mō-lib′dē-nŭm). Molibdênio; elemento metálico branco prateado, n.º atômico 42, peso atômico 95,94; bioelemento encontrado em várias proteínas (p. ex., xantina oxidase). VER molybdenum target *tube.* [G. *molybdaina,* pedaço de chumbo; um metal, provavelmente a galena, de *molybdos,* chumbo]

mo·lyb·de·num-99 (^{99}Mo). Molibdênio-99; radioisótopo do molibdênio produzido em reator, com meia-vida de 2,7476 dias, usado em geradores de radionuclídeos para a produção de tecnécio-99m.

mo·lyb·dic (mō-lib′dik). Molíbdico; designa o molibdênio no estado 6+, como no MoO_3.

moléculas de adesão envolvidas na migração dos leucócitos

molécula	estrutura	localização	ligante(s)	função
P-selectina	selectina	endotélio neutrófilos plaquetas	sLeX = sialil Lewis X (carboidrato)	inflamação aguda adesão de neutrófilos hemostasia
E-selectina	selectina	endotélio	sialil Lewis X (p. ex., CD15)	lentificação dos leucócitos
L-selectina	selectina	linfócitos neutrófilos	sialil Lewis X	lentificação da ligação às HEV (vênulas do endotélio)
ICAM-1	família Ig	endotélio (indutível)	LFA-1 CR3, CR4	adesão e migração
ICAM-2	família Ig	endotélio	LFA-1	adesão e migração
VCAM-1	família Ig	endotélio (indutível)	VLA-4 LPAM	adesão
MAdCAM-1	família Ig sialilada	endotélio linfóide	LPAM L-selectina	linfócito residente
PECAM	família Ig	endotélio linfócitos	PECAM ?	ativação da adesão orientação da migração
LFA-1	$\alpha_L\beta_2$ integrina	leucócitos	ICAM-1, ICAM-2 CR3	migração
CR3	$\alpha_M\beta_2$ integrina	fagócitos	ICAM-1, ICAM-2 C3bi fibronectina	migração captação de imunocomplexo
CR4	$\alpha_X\beta_2$ integrina	fagócitos	ICAM-1 ICAM-2 C3bi	adesão captação de imunocomplexo
VLA-4	$\alpha_4\beta_1$ integrina	linfócitos	VCAM-1 LPAM fibronectina	adesão em sítios inflamatórios e nas HEVs (vênulas do endotélio)
LPAM	$\alpha_4\beta_7$ integrina	linfócitos	MAdCAM-1	migração para o tecido linfóide
GlyCAM-1	sialoglicoproteína (solúvel)	vênulas endoteliais altas	L-selectina	controle da adesão
PSGL-1	sialoglicoproteína	neutrófilos	P-selectina	lentificação na inflamação aguda
CLA	glicoproteína	linfócitos	E-selectina	migração dos linfócitos para a pele

mo·lyb·dic ac·id. Ácido molíbdico; $MoO_3 \cdot H_2O$; ácido cristalino amarelado, que forma molibdatos; usado na determinação do fósforo ou fosfato.

mo·lyb·do·en·zymes (mō - lib'dō - en'zīmz). Molibdoenzimas; enzimas que necessitam de um íon molibdênio como componente (p. ex., xantina oxidase).

mo·lyb·do·fla·vo·pro·teins (mō - lib'dō - flā'vō - prō'tēnz). Molibdoflavoproteínas; proteínas que necessitam de um íon molibdênio e de um nucleotídeo flavina como parte de sua estrutura natural (p. ex., aldeído desidrogenase).

mo·lyb·dop·ter·in (mō - lib - op'ter - in). Molibdopterina; derivado pterina que se associa ao molibdênio para formar o co-fator molibdênio exigido por várias enzimas.

mo·lyb·dous (mō - lib'dŭs). Molibdoso; designa o molibdênio no estado 4+, como no MoO_2.

mo·lys·mo·pho·bia (mō - liz - mō - fō'bē - ă). Molismofobia; temor mórbido de infecção. [G. *molysma*, sujeira, infecção, + *phobos*, medo]

mo·ment (mō'ment). Momento; o produto de uma quantidade por uma distância. [L. *momentum* (para *movimentum*), movimento, momento, de *moveo*, mover]

dipole m., momento dipolo; o produto de uma das duas cargas de um dipolo pela distância que as separa; medida importante do grau de polaridade de muitas biomoléculas.

mom·ism (mom'izm). Momismo; termo relativo aos cuidados maternos excessivos ou dominadores, principalmente quando atribuídos aos estereótipos culturais norte-americanos.

△ **mon-**. VER mono-.

mo·nad (mō'nad, mon'ad). Mônada. **1.** Elemento ou radical univalente. **2.** Organismo unicelular. **3.** Em meiose, o único cromossoma derivado de uma tétrade após a primeira e a segunda divisões de maturação. [G. *monas*, o número um, unidade]

Monakow, Constantin von, histologista suíço, 1853–1930. VER M. *bundle, nucleus, syndrome, tract.*

mon·am·ide (mon-am'id). Monamida. SIN monoamide.

mon·am·ine (mon-am'in). Monamina. SIN monoamine.

mon·am·i·nu·ria (mon'am - i - noo'rē - ă). Monaminúria. SIN monoaminuria.

mon·an·gle (mon'ang-gl). Que possui apenas um ângulo, designa um instrumento dental que tem apenas um ângulo entre o cabo ou haste e a porção funcionante (lâmina ou ponta).

mon·ar·da (mon - ar'dă). Monarda; as folhas da *Monarda punctata* (família Labiatae), hortelã americana, uma planta labiada dos EUA ao leste do Mississippi; a principal fonte comercial de timol natural; usado como carminativo na cólica.

mon·ar·thric (mon - ar'thrik). Monártrico. SIN monarticular.

mon·ar·thri·tis (mon - ar - thrī'tis). Monartrite; artrite de uma única articulação.

mon·ar·tic·u·lar (mon - ar - tik'ū - lăr). Monarticular; relativo a uma única articulação. SIN monarthric, uniarticular.

mon·as·ter (mon-as'ter). Monáster; a figura de estrela única no fim da prófase, na mitose. SIN mother star. [mono- + G. *astēr*, estrela]

mon·a·tom·ic (mon - ă - tom'ik). Monoatômico. **1.** Relativo a, ou que contém apenas, um átomo. **2.** SIN monovalent (1).

mon·au·ral (mon-aw′răl). Monaural; relativo a uma orelha. [mono- + L. *auris*, orelha]

mon·ax·on·ic (mon-aks-on′ik). Monoaxônico. **1.** Que possui apenas um eixo, sendo, assim, alongado e fino. **2.** Que possui um axônio. [mono- + G. *axōn*, eixo]

Mönckeberg, Johann G., patologista alemão, 1877–1925. VER M. *arteriosclerosis, calcification, degeneration, sclerosis.*

Mondini, C., médico italiano, 1729–1803. VER Mondini *hearing impairment,* Mondini *dysplasia.*

Mondonesi, Filippo, médico italiano. VER M. *reflex.*

Mondor, Henri, cirurgião francês, 1885–1962. VER M. *disease.*

-mone. Sufixo que designa um hormônio ou uma substância semelhante a um hormônio. [Fr. hormônio]

Mo·ne·ra (mō-nē′ră). Os procariotos, um reino de organismos microbianos primitivos caracterizados por ausência de núcleo ou cromossomas definidos; DNA não-ligado à membrana; e ausência de centríolos, fuso mitótico, microtúbulos e mitocôndrias; a divisão da zona nuclear mal definida (nucleóide) é feita por separação de duas massas fixadas a partes da membrana celular, que, depois, crescem separadas (uma forma de mitose). O reino Monera inclui as algas verde-azuladas e as bactérias; os vírus, que não possuem uma célula verdadeira, podem ter se originado como "ácidos nucleicos fugitivos" ou "genes selvagens" a partir de células eucarióticas e não estão incluídos. [pl. do L. Mod. *moneron*, do G. *monērēs*, solitário]

mo·ne·ran (mō-nē′ran). Membro do reino procarioto Monera.

mon·es·trous (mon-es′trŭs). Monestro; que tem apenas um ciclo estral em uma estação de acasalamento.

Monge Medrano, Carlos, professor de medicina peruano e especialista em grandes altitudes, 1884–1970. VER Monge *disease.*

mon·go·li·an (mon-gō′lē-ăn). Mongólico. **1.** Relativo a um membro da raça mongólica. **2.** *Obsoleto.* Relativo à síndrome de Down (devido à fácies de aspecto asiático).

mo·nil·e·thrix (mō-nil′ē-thriks). Moniletrix; tricodistrofia autossômica dominante na qual pêlos frágeis exibem uma série de constrições, geralmente sem uma medula. SIN beaded hair, moniliform hair. [L. *monile*, colar, + G. *thrix*, pêlo]

Mo·nil·i·a (mo-nil′ē-ă). Termo genérico para designar um grupo de fungos comumente conhecidos como mofo das frutas; o estado sexual é *Neurospora.* Alguns organismos patogênicos intimamente relacionados, antes classificados nesse gênero, agora são apropriadamente denominados *Candida.* [L. *monile*, colar]

Mo·nil·i·a·ce·ae (mō-nil-ē-ā′sē-ē). Família de fungos imperfeitos (ordem Moniliales) que inclui *Sporothrix schenckii,* o agente causador da esporotricose.

mo·nil·i·al (mō-nil′ē-ăl). Monilial; a rigor, refere-se à *Monilia,* mas, em medicina, amiúde é usado erradamente em relação ao gênero *Candida.*

mon·i·li·a·sis (mō-ni-lī′ă-sis). Moníliase. SIN candidiasis.

mo·nil·i·form (mō-nil′i-fōrm). Moniliforme; que possui o formato de um cordão de contas ou colar de rosário. [L. *monile,* colar, + *forma,* aparência]

Mo·nil·i·for·mis (mō-nil-i-fōr′mis). Gênero da classe (ou filo) Acanthocephala, os vermes com cabeça espinhosa. *M. dubius,* o verme de cabeça espinhosa comum de ratos domésticos, é transmitido por baratas, *Periplaneta americana,* infectadas; foram descritas algumas infecções em seres humanos. *M. moniliformis* é uma espécie normalmente encontrada em roedores, sendo um raro parasita de seres humanos. [L. *monile,* colar, + *forma,* aparência]

mon·ism (mō′nizm). Monismo; sistema metafísico no qual toda a realidade é concebida como um todo unificado. [G. *monos,* único]

mo·nis·tic (mo-nis′tik). Monístico; relativo ao monismo.

mon·i·tor (mon′i-ter, -tōr). Monitor; dispositivo que exibe e/ou registra dados especificados para uma determinada série de eventos, operações ou circunstâncias. [L., aquele que adverte, de *moneo,* pp. *monitum,* advertir]

cardiac m., m. cardíaco; monitor eletrônico que, quando conectado ao paciente, assinala cada batimento cardíaco com um piscar de luz, uma curva eletrocardiográfica, um sinal audível ou de todas essas três maneiras.

electronic fetal m., m. fetal eletrônico; instrumento para monitorização contínua do coração fetal antes ou no decorrer do trabalho de parto.

Holter m., m. Holter; técnica para registro prolongado, contínuo, geralmente ambulatorial, de sinais eletrocardiográficos em fita magnética para exame e seleção de alterações significativas, mas transitórias, que poderiam não ser notadas de outra forma.

home m., m. domiciliar; monitor para freqüência cardíaca e respiratória, geralmente usado em lactentes considerados em risco de síndrome de morte súbita do lactente ou apnéia.

mon·i·tor·ing. Monitorização. **1.** Realização e análise de medidas de rotina com o objetivo de detectar uma mudança no ambiente ou na condição de saúde de uma população. **2.** Medida contínua da prestação de um serviço de saúde. **3.** Supervisão contínua da implementação de uma atividade.

mon·key-paw (mong′kē-paw). Garra de macaco. SIN ape *hand.*

mon·key·pox (mŏng′kē-poks). Varíola do macaco; doença de macacos e, raramente, de seres humanos, causada pelo vírus da varíola do macaco, um membro da família Poxviridae; a doença humana é grave e assemelha-se clinicamente à varíola.

monks·hood (monks′hud). Acônito. VER aconite.

mono-, mon-. Mono, mon-; a participação ou envolvimento de um único elemento ou de uma única parte. Cf. uni-. [G. *monos,* único]

mon·o·ac·yl·glyc·er·ol (mon-ō-ăs-il-gli′ser-ol). Monoacilglicerol; glicerol com uma porção acil esterificada na posição 1 (isto é, 1-monoacilglicerol) ou na posição 2 (isto é, 2-monoacilglicerol); um intermediário na degradação e síntese de lipídios; os 2-monoacilgliceróis são um importante produto final da degradação do triacilglicerol. SIN monoglyceride.

m. acyltransferase, m. aciltransferase; enzima intestinal que catalisa a reação da 2-monoacilglicerol e acil-CoA para formar coenzima A e 1,2-diacilglicerol.

m. lipase, m. lipase; enzima que catalisa a hidrólise do monoacilglicerol para produzir um ânion do ácido graxo e glicerol; uma parte da degradação lipídica.

mon·o·a·me·li·a (mon-ō-ă-mē′lē-ă). Monoamelia; ausência de um membro.

mon·o·am·ide (mon-ō-am′īd, -id). Monoamida; molécula que contém um grupo amida. SIN monamide.

mon·o·am·ine (mon-ō-am′īn, -in). Monoamina; molécula que contém um grupo amina. SIN monamine.

mon·o·am·ine ox·i·dase (MAO). Monoamina oxidase. SIN *amine* oxidase (flavin-containing).

mon·o·am·i·ner·gic (mon′ō-am-i-ner′jik). Monoaminérgico; refere-se às células ou fibras nervosas que transmitem impulsos nervosos por meio de uma catecolamina ou indolamina. [monoamine + G. *ergon,* trabalho]

mon·o·am·i·nu·ri·a (mon′ō-am-i-noo′rē-ă). Monoaminúria; a excreção de qualquer monoamina na urina. SIN monaminuria.

mon·o·am·ni·ot·ic (mon′ō-am-nē-ot′ik). Monoamniótico; designa dois ou mais produtos de uma gravidez múltipla que compartilhavam um saco amniótico comum.

mon·o·as·so·ci·at·ed (mon′ō-ă-sō′shē-ā-tĕd). Monoassociado; designa um organismo livre de germes colonizado por uma única espécie microbiana.

mon·o·aux·o·troph (mon-ō-auks′ō-troph). Monoauxotrofo; microrganismo mutante que requer um nutriente específico, não requerido pelo organismo do tipo selvagem. Cf. auxotroph, polyauxotroph.

mon·o·bac·tam (mon-ō-bak′tam). Monobactâmico; classe de antibiótico que possui um núcleo β-lactâmico monocíclico, estruturalmente diferente dos outros β-lactâmicos; p. ex., aztreonam.

mon·o·ba·sic (mon-ō-bā′sik). Monobásico; designa um ácido com apenas um átomo de hidrogênio substituível, ou apenas um átomo de hidrogênio substituído.

mon·o·ben·zone (mon-ō-ben′zōn). Monobenzona; agente inibidor do pigmento melanina; usada topicamente no tratamento da hiperpigmentação causada pela formação de melanina.

mon·o·blast (mon′ō-blast). Monoblasto; uma célula imatura que se transforma em um monócito. [mono- + G. *blastos,* germe]

mon·o·bra·chi·us (mon-ō-brā′kē-ŭs). Monobráquio; a condição de ter apenas um braço. [mono- + G. *brachiōn,* braço]

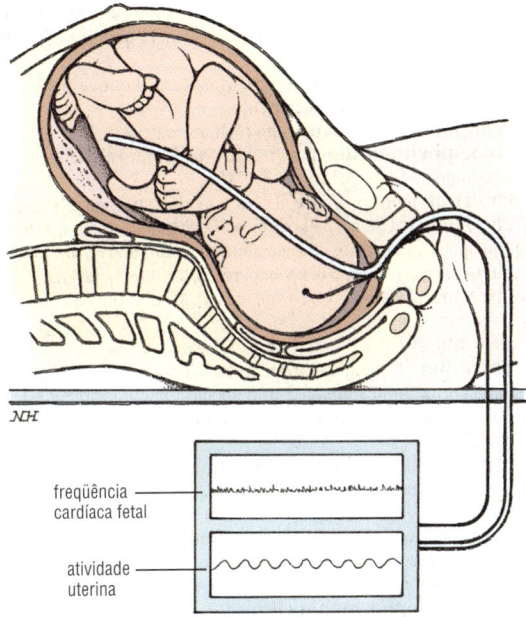

freqüência cardíaca fetal

atividade uterina

monitorização fetal eletrônica

mon·o·bro·mat·ed, mon·o·bro·mi·nat·ed (mon-ō-brō'māt-ed, -brō'-min-āt-ed). Monobromato; designa uma substância química com um átomo de bromo por molécula.

mon·o·car·di·an (mon-ō-kar'dē-an). Monocardíaco; que possui um coração com apenas um átrio e um ventrículo.

mon·o·ceph·a·lus (mon-ō-sef'a-lŭs). Monocéfalo. SIN syncephalus.

mon·o·chlor·phen·am·ide (mon'ō-klōr-fen'a-mīd). Monoclorfenamida. SIN clofenamide.

mon·o·cho·ri·al (mon-ō-kō-rē'al). Monocorial. SIN monochorionic.

mon·o·cho·ri·on·ic (mon'-ō-kōr-ē-on'ik). Monocoriônico; relativo a, ou que possui apenas, um córion; designa gêmeos monovulares. SIN monochorial.

mon·o·chro·ic (mon-ō-krō'ik). Monocróico. SIN monochromatic.

mon·o·chro·ma·sia (mon'ō-krō-mā'zē-a). Monocromasia. SIN achromatopsia.

mon·o·chro·ma·sy (mon-ō-krō'ma-sē). Monocromasia. SIN achromatopsia.

mon·o·chro·mat·ic (mon'ō-krō-mat'ik). Monocromático. 1. Que possui apenas uma cor. 2. Indica uma luz com apenas um comprimento de onda. 3. Relativo a, ou caracterizado por, monocromatismo. SIN monochroic, monochromic.

mon·o·chro·ma·tism (mon-ō-krō'ma-tizm). Monocromatismo. 1. O estado de possuir ou exibir apenas uma cor. 2. SIN achromatopsia. [mono- + G. *chrōma*, cor]

blue cone m., m. de cone azul. VER incomplete *achromatopsia*.
pi cone m., VER incomplete *achromatopsia*.
rod m., m. de bastonetes. SIN complete achromatopsia.

mon·o·chro·mat·o·phil, mon·o·chro·mat·o·phile (mon'-ō-krō-mat'ō-fil, -fīl). Monocromatófilo. 1. Que absorve apenas um corante. 2. Uma célula, ou qualquer elemento histológico, apenas com um tipo de corante. SIN monochromophil, monochromophile. [mono- + G. *chrōma*, cor, + *philos*, amigo]

mon·o·chro·ma·tor (mon-ō-krō'mā-ter, -tōr). Monocromador; um prisma ou gradil de difração usado em espectrofotometria para isolar uma faixa espectral estreita.

mon·o·chro·mic (mon-ō-krō'mik). Monocrômico. SIN monochromatic.

mon·o·chro·mo·phil, mon·o·chro·mo·phile (mon-ō-krō'mō-fil, -fīl). Monocromófilo. SIN monochromatophil.

mon·o·cis·tron·ic (mon-ō-sis-tron'ik). Monocistrônico; que se refere ao RNAm totalmente processado que codifica uma única proteína.

mon·o·cle (mon'ō-kl). Monóculo; lente usada em um olho, geralmente na correção da presbiopia.

mon·o·clin·ic (mon-ō-klin'ik). Monoclínico; relativo a cristais com uma única inclinação oblíqua. [mono- + G. *klinō*, inclinar]

mon·o·clo·nal (mon-ō-klō'nal). Monoclonal; em imunoquímica, relativo a uma proteína de um único clone de células, das quais todas as moléculas são iguais; p. ex., no caso da proteína de Bence Jones, as cadeias são todas κ ou λ.

mon·o·cra·ni·us (mon-ō-krā'nē-ŭs). Monocrânio. SIN syncephalus. [mono- + G. *kranion*, crânio]

mon·o·crot·ic (mon'ō-krot'ik). Monocrótico; designa um pulso cuja curva não exibe entalhes ou onda subsidiária em sua linha descendente. [mono- + G. *krotos*, batimento]

mon·oc·ro·tism (mon-ok'rō-tizm). Monocrotismo; o estado no qual o pulso é monocrótico. [mono- + G. *krotos*, batimento]

mo·noc·u·lar (mon-ok'ū-lar). Monocular; relativo a, que afeta ou é visível apenas por um olho. [mono- + L. *oculus*, olho]

mo·no·cu·lus (mon-ok'ū-lŭs). Monóculo. 1. Ciclope. SIN cyclops. 2. Bandagem aplicada apenas a um olho. [L. homem de um olho, uma palavra híbrida do G. *monos*, único, + L. *oculus*, olho]

mon·o·cyte (mon'ō-sīt). Monócito; leucócito mononuclear relativamente grande (16–22 μm de diâmetro) que, normalmente, constitui 3–7% dos leucócitos do sangue circulante, sendo normalmente encontrado em linfonodos, no baço, na medula óssea e no tecido conjuntivo frouxo. Quando tratado com os corantes habituais, os monócitos exibem um citoplasma abundante, azul-pálido ou cinza-azulado, que contém numerosos grânulos finos, vermelho-azulados, semelhantes a poeira; freqüentemente há vacúolos; o núcleo geralmente é entalhado, ou discretamente preguneado, e tem uma estrutura de cromatina filamentar que parece mais condensada no local onde os filamentos delicados estão em contato. VER TAMBÉM monocytoid *cell*, endothelial *leukocyte*. [mono- + G. *kytos*, célula]

mon·o·cy·to·pe·nia (mon'ō-sī-tō-pē'nē-a). Monocitopenia; diminuição do número de monócitos no sangue circulante. SIN monocytic leukopenia, monopenia. [mono- + G. *kytos*, célula, + *penia*, pobreza]

mon·o·cy·to·sis (mon-ō-sī-tō'sis). Monocitose; aumento anormal do número de monócitos no sangue circulante. SIN monocytic leukocytosis.

Monod, Jacques L., bioquímico francês e ganhador do Prêmio Nobel, 1910–1976. VER Monod-Wyman-Changeux *model*.

mon·o·dac·ty·ly, mon·o·dac·tyl·ism (mon-ō-dak'ti-lē, -dak'-ti-lizm). Monodactilia; a presença de apenas um dedo na mão ou no pé. [mono- + G. *daktylos*, dedo]

mon·o·dis·perse (mon'ō-dis-pers). Monodisperso; de tamanho relativamente uniforme; diz-se de suspensões de aerossóis com variação do tamanho menor que ± 20%.

mon·o·eth·a·nol·a·mine (mon'ō-eth-a-nol'a-mēn). Monoetanolamina; um surfactante; o oleato é usado como agente esclerosante no tratamento de veias varicosas.

mon·o·ga·met·ic (mon'ō-ga-met'ik). Monogamético. SIN homogametic.

mo·nog·a·my (mon-og'a-mē). Monogamia; o sistema de casamento ou acasalamento no qual cada parceiro tem apenas um parceiro. [mono- + G. *gamos*, casamento]

mon·o·gen·e·sis (mon-ō-jen'ē-sis). Monogênese. 1. A produção de organismos semelhantes em cada geração. 2. A produção de filhotes por apenas um genitor, como na geração assexuada ou partenogênese. 3. O processo de parasitar apenas um hospedeiro, no qual ocorre o ciclo biológico do parasita; p. ex., *Boophilus annulatus*, o carrapato que tem o gado bovino como único hospedeiro, ou alguns trematódeos da ordem Monogenea. [mono- + G. *genesis*, origem, produção]

mon·o·ge·net·ic (mon'ō-je-net'ik). Monogenético; relativo à monogênese. SIN monoxenous.

mon·o·gen·ic (mon-ō-jen'ik). Monogênico; relativo a uma doença ou síndrome hereditária, ou a uma característica hereditária, controlada por alelos em um único *locus* genético.

mo·nog·e·nous (mō-noj'ē-nŭs). Monogenético; produzido de forma assexuada, como por fissão, gemação ou esporulação.

mon·o·ger·mi·nal (mon-ō-jer'mi-nal). Monogerminal. SIN unigerminal.

mon·o·glyc·er·ide (mon-ō-gli'ser-īd). Monoglicerídeo. SIN monoacylglycerol.

mon·o·graph (mon'ō-graf). Monografia; tratado sobre determinado assunto ou sobre aspecto específico de um assunto. [mono- + G. *graphē*, escrita]

mon·o·hy·drat·ed (mon-ō-hī'drā-ted). Monoidratado; que contém ou é unido a uma única molécula de água por molécula de substância.

mon·o·hy·dric (mon-ō-hī'drik). Monoídrico; que possui apenas um átomo de hidrogênio na molécula.

mon·o·hy·drox·y·succinic ac·id (mon-ō-hī-droks'ē-suk-sin'ik). Ácido monoidroxissuccínico. SIN malic acid.

mon·o·i·de·ism (mon'ō-ī-dē'izm). Monoideísmo; preocupação acentuada com uma idéia ou assunto; pequeno grau de monomania. [mono- + G. *idea*, forma, idéia]

mon·o·in·fec·tion (mon'ō-in-fek'shoon). Monoinfecção; infecção simples por um único tipo de microrganismo.

mon·o·i·o·do·ty·ro·sine (MIT) (mon'ō-ī-ō'dō-tī-rō-sēn). Monoiodotirosina (MIT); intermediário na síntese do hormônio tireóideo.

mon·o·i·so·ni·tro·so·ac·e·tone (mon-ō-ī'sō-nī-trō'sō-as'ē-tōn). Monoisonitrosoacetona. SIN isonitrosoacetone.

mon·o·kine (mon'ō-kin). Monocina; citocinas secretadas por monócitos e macrófagos. Essas substâncias influenciam a atividade de outras células. VER cytokine. [monocyte + G. *kineō*, colocar em movimento]

mon·o·lay·ers (mon-ō-lā'erz). Monocamadas. 1. Películas, com espessura de uma molécula, formadas sobre a água por determinadas substâncias, como proteínas e ácidos graxos, caracterizadas por moléculas que contêm alguns grupamentos atômicos hidrossolúveis e outros grupos atômicos insolúveis em água. 2. Uma lâmina confluente de células, com profundidade de uma célula, que cresce sobre uma superfície em uma cultura celular.

mon·o·loc·u·lar (mon-ō-lok'ū-lar). Monolocular; que possui uma cavidade ou câmara. SIN unicameral, unicamerate. [mono- + L. *loculus*, um local pequeno]

mon·o·ma·nia (mon-ō-mā'nē-a). Monomania; obsessão ou entusiasmo anormalmente extremo por uma única idéia ou assunto; uma psicose caracterizada pela limitação dos sintomas rigorosamente a um grupo, como o delírio na paranóia. [mono- + G. *mania*, mania]

mon·o·ma·ni·ac (mon-ō-mā'nē-ak). Monomaníaco. 1. Aquele que exibe monomania. 2. Caracterizado por, ou relativo à, monomania.

mon·o·mas·ti·gote (mon-ō-mas'ti-gōt). Monomastigota; mastigota que possui apenas um flagelo. [mono- + Romano *mastix*, flagelo]

mon·o·mel·ic (mon-ō-mel'ik). Monomélico; relativo a um membro. [mono- + G. *melos*, membro]

mon·o·mer (mon'ō-mer). Monômero. 1. A unidade molecular que, por repetição, constitui uma grande estrutura ou polímero; p. ex., etileno, $H_2C=CH_2$, é o monômero do polietileno, $H(CH_2)_nH$. VER TAMBÉM subunit (1). 2. A unidade estrutural proteica de um capsídeo de víron. VER virion. 3. A subunidade proteica de uma proteína composta de várias dessas unidades livremente associadas, geralmente ligadas de forma não-covalente. [mono- + -mer]

mon·o·mer·ic (mon-ō-mer'ik). Monomérico. 1. Aquilo que consiste em um único componente. 2. Em genética, relativo a uma doença hereditária ou característica controlada por genes em um único *locus*. 3. Que consiste em monômeros. [mono- + G. *meros*, parte]

mon·o·me·tal·lic (mon'ō-mē-tal'ik). Monometálico; que contém um átomo de um metal por molécula.

mon·o·mi·cro·bic (mon′o-mī-krō′bik). Monomicrobiano; designa uma monoinfecção.

mon·o·mo·lec·u·lar (mon′o-mō-lek′u-lăr). Monomolecular. **1.** SIN unimolecular. **2.** Relativo a uma única molécula.

mon·o·mor·phic (mon-ō-mōr′fik). Monomorfo; que tem uma única forma; de formato inalterável. [mono- + G. *morphē*, formato]

mon·om·pha·lus (mon-om′fă-lŭs). Monônfalo. SIN omphalopagus. [mono- + G. *omphalos*, umbigo]

mon·o·my·o·ple·gia (mon′o-mī′o-plē′jē-ă). Monomioplegia; paralisia limitada a um músculo. [mono- + G. *mys*, músculo, + *plēgē*, golpe]

mon·o·my·o·si·tis (mon′o-mī-o-sī′tis). Monomiosite; inflamação de um único músculo.

mon·o·neme (mon′o-nēm). Mononema; uma hélice ímpar de ácido nucleico, como se observa em uma cromátide.

mon·o·neu·ral, mon·o·neu·ric (mon′o-noo′răl, -noo′rik). Mononeural. **1.** Que possui apenas um neurônio. **2.** Suprido por apenas um nervo.

mononeuritis multiplex. Mononeurite múltipla. SIN mononeuropathy multiplex.

mon·o·neu·rop·a·thy (mon′o-noo-rop′ă-thē). Mononeuropatia; distúrbio que envolve apenas um nervo.

 m. mul′tiplex, m. múltipla; envolvimento atraumático de duas ou mais partes do sistema nervoso periférico (p. ex., raízes, elementos do plexo, troncos nervosos), geralmente de forma seqüencial e em diferentes áreas do corpo; na maioria das vezes, a conseqüência de vasculites. SIN mononeuritis multiplex.

mon·o·nu·cle·ar (mon-ō-noo′klē-ăr). Mononuclear; que possui apenas um núcleo; usado principalmente em referência às células do sangue.

mon·o·nu·cle·o·sis (mon′o-noo-klē-ō′sis). Mononucleose; número anormalmente grande de leucócitos mononucleares no sangue circulante, principalmente em relação às formas que não são normais.

 infectious m., m. infecciosa; doença febril aguda de adultos jovens, causada pelo vírus Epstein-Barr, um membro da família Herpesviridae; freqüentemente transmitida por transferência de saliva; caracterizada por febre, dor de garganta, aumento dos linfonodos e do baço e por leucopenia, que se modifica para uma linfocitose durante a segunda semana; o sangue circulante geralmente contém linfócitos T grandes, anormais, que se assemelham a monócitos, embora as células B sejam infectadas, e há anticorpo heterófilo que pode ser completamente adsorvido em eritrócitos bovinos, mas não no antígeno renal de cobaia. Pode haver coleções dos linfócitos anormais característicos não apenas nos linfonodos e no braço, mas em vários outros locais, como as meninges, o encéfalo e o miocárdio. SIN benign lymphadenosis, glandular fever.

mon·o·nu·cle·o·tide (mon-ō-noo′klē-ō-tīd). Mononucleotídeo. SIN nucleotide.

mon·o·oc·tan·o·in (mon′o-ok′-ta′nō′in). Monoctanoína; glicerol esterificado semi-sintético usado como agente solubilizante para cálculos biliares radiotransparentes retidos nas vias biliares após colecistectomia.

mon·o·ox·y·gen·a·ses (mon-ō-ok′si-jĕ-nā-sez). Monoxigenases; oxidorredutases que induzem a incorporação de um átomo de oxigênio do O_2 à substância oxidada.

mon·o·pa·re·sis (mon′o-pa-rē′sis, -par′ĕ-sis). Monoparesia; paresia que afeta um único membro ou parte de um membro.

mon·o·par·es·the·sia (mon′o-par-es-thē′zē-ă). Monoparestesia; parestesia que afeta apenas uma região.

mon·o·path·ic (mon-ō-path′ik). Monopático; relativo à monopatia.

mo·nop·a·thy (mon-op′ă-thē). Monopatia. **1.** Doença isolada, sem complicações. **2.** Uma doença local que afeta apenas um órgão ou uma parte. [mono- + G. *pathos*, que sofre]

mon·o·pe·nia (mon-ō-pē′nē-ă). Monopenia. SIN monocytopenia.

mo·noph·a·gism (mō-nof′ă-jizm). Monofagismo; ingestão habitual apenas de um tipo de alimento ou apenas de uma refeição por dia quando esta última é claramente uma aberração. [mono- + G. *phagō*, comer]

mon·o·pha·sia (mon-ō-fā′zē-ă). Monofasia; incapacidade de falar outra coisa além de uma única palavra ou frase. [mono- + G. *phasis*, fala]

mon·o·pha·sic (mon-ō-fā′zik). Monofásico. **1.** Caracterizado por monofasia. **2.** Que ocorre apenas em, ou é caracterizado apenas por, uma fase ou estágio. **3.** Que flutua apenas em uma direção a partir da linha de base.

mon·o·phe·nol mon·o·ox·y·gen·ase (mon-ō-fē′nol). Monofenol monoxigenase. **1.** Uma oxidorredutase que contém cobre e catalisa a oxidação de *o*-difenóis em *o*-quinonas pelo O_2, com a incorporação de um dos dois átomos de oxigênio no produto; também catalisa a oxidação de monofenóis, como L-tirosina, em diidroxi-L-fenilalanina (dopa), um precursor da melanina e da adrenalina (catecolaminas), e pode atuar como uma catecol oxidase; uma deficiência dessa enzima é observada em várias formas de albinismo. SIN cresolase, monophenol oxidase, tyrosinase. **2.** SIN laccase.

mon·o·phe·nol ox·i·dase. Monofenol oxidase. SIN monophenol monooxygenase (1).

mon·o·pho·bia (mon-ō-fō′bē-ă). Monofobia; medo mórbido da solidão ou de ser deixado sozinho. [mono- + G. *phobos*, medo]

mon·oph·thal·mos (mon-of-thal′mos). Monoftalmia; falha de crescimento de uma vesícula óptica primária, com ausência dos tecidos oculares; o olho remanescente freqüentemente é mal desenvolvido. [mono- + G. *ophthalmos*, olho]

mon·oph·thal·mus (mon′of-thal′mŭs). Monoftalmo. SIN cyclops. [mono- + G. *ophthalmos*, olho]

mon·o·phy·let·ic (mon-ō-fī-let′ik). Monofilético. **1.** Que se origina de um único tipo celular; derivado de uma linha de descendência, ao contrário do polifilético. **2.** Em hematologia, relativo a monofiletismo. [mono- + G. *phylē*, tribo]

mon·o·phy·le·tism (mon-ō-fī′lĕ-tizm). Monofiletismo; em hematologia, a teoria de que todas as células do sangue derivam de uma célula-tronco comum ou histioblasto. SIN monophyletic theory. [mono- + G. *phylē*, tribo]

mon·o·phy·o·dont (mon-ō-fī′o-dont). Monofiodonte; que possui apenas um conjunto de dentes; sem dentição decídua. [mono- + G. *phyō*, crescer, + *odous* (*odont*-), dente]

mon·o·plas·mat·ic (mon-ō-plas-mat′ik). Monoplasmático; formado apenas por um tecido. [mono- + G. *plasma*, algo formado]

mon·o·plast (mon′ō-plast). Monoplasto; organismo unicelular que preserva a mesma estrutura ou formato durante toda a sua existência. [mono- + G. *plastos*, formado]

mon·o·plas·tic (mon-ō-plas′tik). Monoplástico; que não sofre alteração na estrutura; relativo a um monoplasto.

mon·o·ple·gia (mon-ō-plē′jē-ă). Monoplegia; paralisia de um membro. [mono- + G. *plēgē*, golpe]

 m. masticato′ria, m. mastigatória; paralisia unilateral dos músculos da mastigação (masseter, temporal, pterigóide).

mon·o·ploid (mon′o-ployd). Monoplóide. SIN haploid. [mono- + G. *ploides*, na forma]

mon·o·po·dia (mon-ō-pō′dē-ă). Monopodia; malformação na qual apenas um pé é externamente reconhecível. [mono- + G. *pous*, pé]

mon·ops (mon′ops). Monope. SIN cyclops. [mono- + G. *ops*, olho]

mon·o·pty·chi·al (mon-ō-tī′kē-al). Monoptíquico; disposto em uma camada única, mas preguada, como as células no epitélio da vesícula biliar ou de determinadas glândulas. [mono- + G. *ptychē*, prega]

mon·or·chia (mon-ōr′kē-ă). Monorquia. SIN monorchism.

mon·or·chid·ic, mon·or·chid (mon-ōr-kid′ik, mon-ōr′kid). Monorquídico. **1.** Que possui apenas um testículo. **2.** Que, aparentemente, possui apenas um testículo, com o outro não-descido.

mon·or·chid·ism (mon-ōr′ki-dizm). Monorquidismo. SIN monorchism.

mon·or·chism (mon′ōr-kizm). Monorquismo; condição na qual apenas um testículo é aparente, estando o outro ausente ou não-descido. SIN monorchia, monorchidism. [mono- + G. *orchis*, testículo]

mon·o·rec·i·dive (mon-o-res′i-dēv). Monorrecidiva; designa uma manifestação tardia ou terciária de sífilis, que assume a forma de uma pápula ulcerada, no local do cancro original. [mono- + L. *recidivus*, recidivante]

mon·o·rhin·ic (mon-ō-rin′ik). Monorrínico; que tem apenas um nariz; usado para caracterizar gêmeos conjugados nos quais há apenas uma cavidade nasal evidente. [mono- + G. *rhis* (*rhin*-), nariz]

mon·o·sac·cha·ride (mon-ō-sak′ă-rīd). Monossacarídeo; carboidrato que não pode formar qualquer açúcar mais simples apenas por hidrólise; p. ex., pentoses, hexoses. SIN monose.

mon·o·scel·ous (mon-ō-sel′ŭs, -skel′ŭs). Monóscelo; que tem apenas uma perna. [mono- + G. *skelos*, perna]

mon·o·sce·nism (mon-ō-sē′nizm). Monoscenismo; concentração mórbida em alguma experiência passada. [mono- + G. *skēnē*, tenda (queda de estrado)]

mon·ose (mon′ōs). Monose. SIN monosaccharide.

mon·o·so·di·um glu·ta·mate (MSG) (mon-ō-sō′dē-ŭm gloo′tă-māt). Glutamato monossódico; o sal monossódico da forma L natural do ácido glutâmico; usado como flavorizante, que causa ou contribui para a síndrome do "restaurante chinês"; também usado por via intravenosa como auxiliar no tratamento de encefalopatias associadas à doença hepática.

mon·o·some (mon′ō-sōm). **1.** Cromossoma acessório. SIN accessory chromosome. **2.** Termo obsoleto para ribossoma. **3.** Monossoma; estrutura que consiste em um ribossoma único ligado a uma molécula de RNAm. [mono- + chromosome]

mon·o·so·mia (mon-ō-sō′mē-ă). Monossomia; em gêmeos conjugados, condição na qual há duas cabeças e um único tronco. VER conjoined *twins*, em *twin*. [mono- + G. *sōma*, corpo]

mon·o·so·mic (mon-ō-sō′mik). Monossômico; relativo à monossomia.

mon·o·so·mous (mon-ō-sō′mŭs). Monossômico; caracterizado por ou relativo à monossomia.

mon·o·so·my (mon′ō-sō-mē). Monossomia; ausência de um cromossoma de um par de cromossomas homólogos. VER TAMBÉM chromosomal *deletion*. [ver monosome]

mon·o·sper·my (mon′o-sper-mē). Monospermia; fertilização pela entrada apenas de um espermatozóide no óvulo. [mono- + G. *sperma*, semente]

Mon·o·spo·ri·um ap·i·o·sper·mum (mon-ō-spō'rē-ŭm ap'ē-ō-sper'-mŭm). Nome antigo do *Scedosporium apiospermum*. Telemorph é *Pseudallescheria boydii*.

Mo·nos·to·ma (mō-nos'tō-mă, mon-ō-stō'mă). Nome arcaico de um gênero de trematódeos, baseado na presença de uma única ventosa. [mono- + G. *stoma*, boca]

mon·o·stome (mon'ō-stōm). Monostoma; nome comum dado a trematódeos digenéticos que possuem apenas uma ventosa, oral ou ventral, em vez de ambas. VER TAMBÉM *Monostoma*. [mono- + G. *stoma*, boca]

mon·o·stot·ic (mon-os-tot'ik). Monostótico; que envolve apenas um osso. [mono- + G. *osteon*, osso]

mon·o·stra·tal (mon-ō-strā'tăl). Monoestrático; composto apenas de uma camada. [mono- + L. *stratum*, camada]

mon·o·sub·sti·tut·ed (mon-ō-sŭb'sti-too-tĕd). Monossubstituído; em química, designa um elemento ou radical do qual só se encontra um átomo ou unidade em cada molécula de um composto de substituição.

mon·o·symp·to·mat·ic (mon'ō-simp-tō-mat'ik). Monossintomático; designa uma doença ou condição mórbida que se manifesta apenas por um sintoma acentuado.

mon·o·sy·nap·tic (mon'ō-si-nap'tik). Monossináptico; refere-se a conexões neurais diretas (aquelas que não envolvem um neurônio internuncial); p. ex., a conexão direta entre células nervosas sensoriais primárias e neurônios motores que caracterizam o arco reflexo monossináptico.

mon·o·syph·i·lide (mon-o-sif'i-lid). Monossifílide; caracterizado pela ocorrência de uma única lesão sifilítica.

mon·o·ter·penes (mon-ō-ter'pĕnz). Monoterpenos; hidrocarbonetos ou seus derivados formados pela condensação de duas unidades isopreno e, portanto, contendo 10 átomos de carbono; p. ex., cânfora; freqüentemente contendo uma estrutura cíclica.

mon·o·ther·mia (mon-ō-ther'mē-ă). Monotermia; uniformidade da temperatura corporal; ausência de uma elevação noturna da temperatura corporal. [mono- + G. *thermē*, calor]

mon·o·thi·o·glyc·er·ol (mon'ō-thī-ō-glis'er-ol). Monotioglicerol; usado para promover a cicatrização de feridas. SIN thioglycerol.

mo·not·o·cous (mŏ-not'ō-kŭs). Monótoco; que produz apenas um descendente em cada parto. [mono- + G. *tokos*, parto]

Mon·o·tre·ma·ta (mon-ō-trē'mă-tă). Ordem de mamíferos que depositam ovos e que possuem uma cloaca ou uma câmara comum para receber produtos digestivos, urinários e reprodutivos; apenas a Austrália possui estas formas: o ornitorrinco, com bico-de-pato (*Ornithorhynchus*), e a eqüidna (*Tachyglossus*). [mono- + G. *trēma*, um orifício]

mon·o·treme (mon'ō-trēm). Monotremo; um membro da ordem Monotremata.

mo·not·ri·chate (mŏ-not'ri-kāt). Monotríquio. SIN monotrichous.

mo·not·ri·chous (mŏ-not'ri-kŭs). Monotríquio; designa um microrganismo que possui um único flagelo ou cílio. SIN monotrichate, uniflagellate.

mon·o·va·lence, mon·o·va·len·cy (mon-ō-vā'lens, -vā'len-sē). Monovalência; capacidade de combinação (valência) igual à do átomo de hidrogênio. SIN univalence, univalency.

mon·o·va·lent (mon-ō-vā'lent). Monovalente. **1.** Que possui a capacidade de combinação (valência) de um átomo de hidrogênio. SIN monatomic (2), univalent. **2.** Relativo a um anti-soro monovalente (específico) contra um único antígeno ou organismo.

mon·ox·e·nous (mon-oks'ē-nŭs). Monoxeno. SIN monogenetic. [mono- + G. *xenos*, estrangeiro]

mon·ox·ide (mon-ok'sīd). Monóxido; qualquer óxido que possui apenas um átomo de oxigênio; p. ex., CO.

mon·o·zo·ic (mon-ō-zō'ik). Monozóico; unissegmentado, como nas tênias cestódeas. VER polyzoic.

mon·o·zy·got·ic, mon·o·zy·gous (mon-ō-zī-got'ik, -zī'gŭs). Monozigótico. SIN uniserminal. VER monozygotic *twins*, em *twin*. [mono- + G. *zygōtos*, que tem vitelo]

Monro, Alexander, Jr., anatomista escocês, 1733–1817. VER M. *doctrine, foramen, line, sulcus;* M.-Kellie *doctrine;* M.-Richter *line;* Richter-M. *line.*

Monro, Alexander Sr., anatomista e cirurgião escocês, 1697–1767. VER *bursa* of M.

mons, gen. **mon·tis,** pl. **mon·tes** (monz, mon'tis, mon'tēz) [TA]. Monte; proeminência anatômica ou pequena elevação acima do nível geral da superfície. [L. montanha]

m. pu'bis [TA], monte do púbis; a proeminência causada por um coxim de tecido adiposo sobre a sínfise púbica na mulher. SIN pubes (2) [TA], m. veneris, pubic bone.

m. ure'teris, m. do ureter; proeminência rosa na parede da bexiga, marcando cada óstio do ureter.

m. ven'eris, m. de Vênus. SIN m. pubis. [L. *Venus*]

Monson, George S., dentista norte-americano, 1869–1933. VER M. *curve;* anti-M. *curve.*

mon·ster. Monstro; termo obsoleto para designar um embrião, feto ou indivíduo malformado. VER entradas que começam com terato-. VER teras. [L. *monstrum*, um mau presságio, uma monstruosidade, um assombro]

mon·tan·ic ac·id (mon-tan'ik). Ácido montânico. SIN octacosanoic acid. [(cera) montanha]

Monteggia, Giovanni B., cirurgião italiano, 1762–1815. VER M. *fracture.*

montelukast sodium (mon-te-loo'kast). Montelucaste sódico (MSD); antagonista competitivo e seletivo do receptor Cys-LT$_1$, que atua como bloqueador dos leucotrienos, potentes broncoconstritores endógenos. Profilático; inútil no tratamento de um ataque de asma em curso.

Montgomery, William F., obstetra irlandês, 1797–1859. VER M. *follicles,* em *follicle, glands,* em *gland, tubercles,* em *tubercle.*

mon·tic·u·lus, pl. **mon·tic·u·li** (mon-tik'ū-lŭs, -lī). Montículo. **1.** Qualquer pequena projeção arredondada acima de uma superfície. **2.** A porção central do verme superior que forma uma projeção sobre a superfície do cerebelo; sua porção anterior e mais proeminente é denominada cúlmen, sua porção oblíqua posterior, o declive. [L. dim. de *mons*, montinha]

palmar monticuli, montículo palmar; três pequenas elevações na parte distal da palma da mão, correspondentes a deficiências semelhantes a janelas na aponeurose palmar distal entre os quatro feixes longitudinais e proximal ao ligamento metacarpiano transverso superficial.

mood (mood). Humor; o sentimento difuso, o espírito e o estado emocional interno de um indivíduo que, quando comprometido, pode influenciar, de forma significativa, praticamente todos os aspectos do comportamento de uma pessoa ou sua percepção de eventos externos.

mood swing. Variação de humor; oscilação do tom de sentimento emocional de uma pessoa entre períodos de euforia e depressão.

Moon, Henry, cirurgião inglês, 1845–1892. VER M. *molars,* em *molar.*

Moon, Robert C., oftalmologista norte-americano, 1844–1914. VER Laurence-M. *syndrome.*

Moore, Charles H., cirurgião inglês, 1821–1870. VER M. *method.*

Moore, Robert Foster, oftalmologista inglês, 1878–1963. VER M. lightning *streaks,* em *streak.*

Mooren, Albert, oftalmologista alemão, 1828–1899. VER M. *ulcer.*

Mooser, Hermann, patologista suíço no México, 1891–1971. VER M. *bodies,* em *body.*

MOPP Acrônimo para *m*ecloretamina, *o*ncovina (vincristina), *p*rocarbazina e *p*rednisona, esquema quimioterápico usado no tratamento da doença de Hodgkin.

Morand, Sauveur F., cirurgião francês, 1697–1773. VER M. *foot, spur.*

Morax, Victor, oftalmologista francês, 1866–1935. VER *Moraxella.*

Mor·ax·el·la (mōr'ak-sel'ă). Gênero de bactérias imóveis, obrigatoriamente aeróbicas (família Neisseriaceae), contendo cocóides ou bastonetes curtos Gram-negativos, que geralmente ocorrem em pares. Não produzem ácido a partir de carboidratos, são oxidase-positivos e suscetíveis à penicilina, e infectam as mucosas dos seres humanos e de outros mamíferos. A espécie típica é a *M. lacunata*. [V. *Morax*]

M. anatipes'tifer, espécie de bactéria que causa doença respiratória em filhotes de patos.

M. catarrha'lis, espécie de bactéria que causa infecções respiratórias altas, particularmente em hospedeiros imunodeprimidos; a espécie típica do gênero *M.* SIN *Branhamella catarrhalis.*

M. kingae, SIN *Kingella kingae.*

M. lacuna'ta, espécie de bactéria que causa conjuntivite em seres humanos; é a espécie típica do gênero *M.*

M. nonliquefa'ciens, espécie de bactéria encontrada no sistema respiratório de seres humanos, principalmente no nariz; geralmente não é patogênica, mas algumas vezes causa sinusite.

M. osloen'sis, espécie de bactéria encontrada no sistema genitourinário, no sangue, nos líquidos espinais e torácicos e no nariz; raramente encontrada nas vias respiratórias; geralmente não é patogênica, embora tenham sido isoladas algumas cepas de patologias graves em seres humanos.

M. phenylpyru'vica, espécie de bactéria de patogenicidade desconhecida encontrada no sistema genitourinário, sangue, líquido cerebroespinal e no pus de várias lesões.

mor·bid (mōr'bid). Mórbido. **1.** Doente ou patológico. **2.** Em psicologia, anormal ou divergente. [L. *morbidus*, doente, de *morbus*, doença]

mor·bid·i·ty (mōr-bid'i-tē). Morbidade. **1.** Um estado patológico. **2.** A razão entre doença e bem-estar em uma comunidade. SIN morbility. VER TAMBÉM morbidity *rate.* **3.** A freqüência do surgimento de complicações após um procedimento cirúrgico ou outro tratamento.

maternal m., m. materna; complicações médicas em uma mulher causadas por gravidez, trabalho de parto ou parto.

puerperal m., m. puerperal; doença que surge durante os primeiros 10 dias do período pós-parto, isto é, uma temperatura de 38°C ou mais em quaisquer dois dias dos 10 primeiros, excluindo as primeiras 24 horas.

mor·bif·ic (mōr-bif'ik). Morbífico. SIN pathogenic. [L. *morbus*, doença, + *facio*, fazer]

mor·big·e·nous (mor - bij'ē - nŭs). Morbígeno. SIN pathogenic. [L. *morbus,* doença, + G. *-gen,* que produz]
mor·bil·i·ty (mor - bil'i - tē). Morbilidade. SIN morbidity (2).
mor·bil·li (mor - bil'ī). Sarampo. SIN measles (1). [L. Mediev. *morbillus,* dim. do L. *morbus,* doença]
mor·bil·li·form (mor - bil'i - form). Morbiliforme; semelhante ao sarampo (1). [ver morbilli]
Mor·bil·li·vi·rus (mor - bil'i - vī'rŭs). Gênero da família Paramyxoviridae, incluindo os vírus do sarampo, da raiva canina e da peste bovina.
  equine M., M. eqüino; uma espécie que causa uma doença respiratória fatal em cavalos e seres humanos na Austrália, também sendo observada encefalite em alguns casos humanos. SIN Hendra virus.
mor·bi·lous (mor - bil'ŭs). Relativo ao sarampo (1). [ver morbilli]
mor·bus (mor'bŭs). Morbo. SIN disease (1). [L. doença]
mor·bus Ad·di·so·nii (mor'bŭs ad'ĭ - son - ē). SIN chronic adrenocortical insufficiency.
mor·cel (mor - sel'). Remover aos pedaços. [Fr. *morceler,* subdividir]
mor·cel·la·tion (mor - se - lā'shŭn). Divisão em pedaços pequenos e remoção destes, como de um tumor. SIN morcellement. [Fr. *morceler,* subdividir]
mor·celle·ment (mor - sel - maw'). SIN morcellation. [Fr.]
mor·dant (mor'dant). Mordente. **1.** Substância capaz de se combinar com um corante e com o material a ser corado, assim aumentando a afinidade ou ligação do corante; p. ex., um mordente comumente usado para promover coloração com hematoxilina é o alúmen. **2.** Tratar com um mordente. [L. *mordeo,* morder]
mor.dict. Abreviatura do L. *more dicto,* conforme orientado.
Morel, Benedict A., psiquiatra francês, 1809–1873. VER M. *ear;* Stewart-M. *syndrome.*
Mo·re·ra·stron·gy·lus cos·tar·i·cen·sis (mor'er - ă - stron'ji - lŭs kos'tar - i - sen'sis). SIN *Angiostrongylus costaricensis.*
mo·res (mo'rāz). Costumes; conceito usado nas ciências do comportamento e sociais para se referir a culturas populares importantes e aceitas, e a padrões culturais que incorporam as opiniões morais fundamentais de um grupo. [L. pl. de *mos,* costume]
Morgagni, Giovanni B., anatomista e patologista italiano, 1682–1771. VER morgagnian *cyst;* M. *appendix, cartilage, caruncle, cataract, columns,* em *column, concha, crypts,* em *crypt, disease, foramen;* Morgagni foramen *hernia;* M. *fossa, fovea, frenum, globules,* em *globule, humor, hydatid, lacuna, liquor, nodule, prolapse, retinaculum, sinus, spheres,* em *sphere, syndrome, tubercle, valves,* em *valve, ventricle;* M.-Adams-Stokes *syndrome; frenulum* of M.
Morgan, Harry de R., médico inglês, 1863–1931. VER M. *bacillus.*
mor·gan (M) (mor'găn). Morgan; a unidade padrão de distância genética no mapa genético: a distância entre dois *loci,* de forma que ocorrerá, em média, um cruzamento por meiose; para fins de trabalho, é usado o centimorgan (0,01 M). [T.H. *Morgan,* geneticista norte-americano, 1866–1945]
Mor·gan·el·la (mor'gan - el' - ah). Gênero (família Enterobacteriaceae) de bastonetes Gram-negativos, anaeróbicos facultativos, quimioorganotróficos, retos, que se movem por meio de flagelos peritríquios; encontrado nas fezes de seres humanos, de outros animais e répteis; pode causar infecções oportunistas do sangue, vias respiratórias, feridas e vias urinárias.
  M. morganii, espécie típica do gênero *M.* SIN Morgan bacillus.
morgue (morg). Morgue; necrotério. **1.** Uma construção ou uma sala em um hospital ou outra unidade onde os mortos são mantidos enquanto aguardam necrópsia, sepultamento ou cremação. **2.** Uma construção onde mortos não identificados são mantidos enquanto aguardam a identificação antes do sepultamento. SIN mortuary (2). [Fr.]
Mori, O., patologista japonês do século XX. VER Harada-M. filter paper strip *culture.*
mo·ria (mor'ē - ă). Moria. **1.** Termo raramente usado que significa loucura ou diminuição da compreensão. SIN hebetude. **2.** Termo raramente usado para designar um estado mental caracterizado por frivolidade, jovialidade, tendência patológica a gracejar e incapacidade de levar qualquer coisa a sério. [G. *moria,* loucura, de *moros,* estúpido, tolo]
mor·i·bund (mor'i - bŭnd). Moribundo; agonizante; às portas da morte. [L. *moribundus,* agonizante, de *morior,* morrer]
mo·rin (mor'in). [C.I. 75660]. Morina; corante amarelo natural obtido da tatajuba e de outros membros da família da amora e freqüentemente associado ao corante maclurina; usado como fluorocromo para detecção de metais, particularmente alumínio. Também são formados morinatos fluorescentes com berílio, gálio, índio, escândio, tório, titânio e zircônio.
Morison, James R., cirurgião inglês, 1853–1939. VER M. *pouch.*
Mörner, Karl A.H. químico sueco, 1855–1917. VER M. *test.*
morn·ing glo·ry (mor'ning glo'rē). Ipoméia; glória da manhã; boa-noite. **1.** SIN *Ipomoea rubrocoerulea* var. *praecox.* **2.** SIN *Rivea corymbosa.*
morn·ing glo·ry seeds. Sementes de ipoméia; as sementes da *Rivea corymbosa,* que foram usados para alteração da mente; alucinógeno; intoxicante.
Moro, Ernst, médico alemão, 1874–1951. VER M. *reflex.*

mo·ron (mor'on). Idiota; débil mental; termo obsoleto para designar uma subclasse de retardo mental ou o indivíduo nela classificado. [G. *moros,* estúpido]
mo·rox·y·dine (mo - rok'si - dēn). Moroxidina; agente antiviral.
△ **morph-.** VER morpho-.
mor·phea (mor - fē'a). Morféia; lesão ou lesões cutâneas caracterizadas por placas endurecidas, discretamente deprimidas, de tecido fibroso dérmico espessado, de cor esbranquiçada ou branco-amarelada circundadas por um halo róseo ou púrpura. As lesões ocorrem em qualquer idade, sem envolvimento sistêmico, e geralmente resolvem após alguns anos. SIN localized scleroderma. [G. *morphē,* forma, figura]
  m. gut·ta'ta, m. em gota; forma de morféia com lesões endurecidas, céreas, brancas, distintas e pequenas. SIN white spot disease.
  m. line·a'ris, m. linear. SIN linear *scleroderma.*
mor·pheme (mor'fēm). Morfema; a menor unidade lingüística provida de significado. [G. *morphē,* forma, + *-eme,* de *phoneme,* G. *phēmē,* expressão vocal]
mor·phine (mor'fēn, mor - fēn'). Morfina; o principal alcalóide fenantreno do ópio, que contém 9–14% de morfina anidra. Produz uma combinação de depressão e excitação no sistema nervoso central e em alguns tecidos periféricos; o predomínio da estimulação ou depressão central depende da espécie e da dose; a administração repetida leva ao desenvolvimento de tolerância, dependência física e (se houver abuso) dependência psíquica. Usada como analgésico, sedativo e ansiolítico. [L. *Morpheus,* deus dos sonhos ou do sono]
  m. hydrochloride, cloridrato de m.; cristais brancos aculeiformes ou cúbicos, de sabor amargo, solúveis em aproximadamente 25 partes de água.
  m. sulfate (MS), sulfato de m.; morfina usada para formulação de comprimidos e, também, de soluções para injeção parenteral, peridural ou intratecal para alívio da dor.
△ **morpho-, morph-.** Morfo-, morf-; forma, formato, estrutura. [G. *morphē*]
mor·pho·gen·e·sis (mor - fō - jen'ē - sis). Morfogênese. **1.** Diferenciação de células e tecidos no embrião inicial que estabelece a forma e a estrutura dos vários órgãos e partes do corpo. **2.** A capacidade de uma molécula ou de um grupo de moléculas (particularmente macromoléculas) de assumir determinado formato. [morpho- + G. *genesis,* produção]
mor·pho·ge·net·ic (mor'fō - jē - net'ik). Morfogenético; relativo à morfogênese.
mor·pho·log·ic (mor - fō - loj'ik). Morfológico; relativo à morfologia.
mor·phol·o·gy (mor - fol'ō - jē). Morfologia; a ciência que estuda a configuração ou a estrutura de animais e vegetais. [morpho- + G. *logos,* estudo]
mor·pho·met·ric (mor'fō - met'rik). Morfométrico; relativo à morfometria.
mor·phom·e·try (mor - fom'ē - trē). Morfometria; a medida do formato de organismos ou de suas partes. [morpho- + G. *metron,* medida]
mor·phon (mor'fon). Morfon; qualquer uma das estruturas individuais que entram na formação de um organismo; um elemento morfológico, como uma célula. [G. *morphē,* forma]
mor·pho·phys·i·ol·o·gy (mor - fō - fiz - ē - ol'ō - jē). Morfofisiologia. SIN functional *anatomy.*
mor·pho·sis (mor - fō'sis). Morfose; modalidade de desenvolvimento de uma parte. [G. formação, ato de formar]
mor·pho·syn·the·sis (mor - fō - sin'thē - sis). Morfossíntese; consciência do espaço e do esquema corporal representado nos lobos parietais do córtex cerebral. [morpho- + synthesis]
mor·pho·type (mor'fō - tīp). Morfotipo; um grupo infra-subespecífico de cepas bacterianas, distinguível de outras cepas da mesma espécie com base nas características morfológicas que podem ou não estar associadas a uma alteração do estado sorológico. [morpho- + G. *typos,* modelo]
Morquio, Louis, médico uruguaio, 1867–1935. VER M. *disease, syndrome;* M.-Ullrich *disease;* Brailsford-Morquio *disease.*
mor·rhu·ate so·di·um (mor'roo - āt). Morruato de sódio; os sais sódicos dos ácidos graxos do óleo de fígado de bacalhau; agente esclerosante usado no tratamento das veias varicosas, misturado com um anestésico local. [de *Gadus morrhua,* bacalhau]
Morrison, Ashton B., patologista irlandês radicado nos EUA, *1922. VER Verner-M. *syndrome.*
mors, gen. **mor·tis** (morz, mor'tis). Morte. SIN death. [L.]
  m. thy'mica, m. tímica; termo obsoleto para designar morte súbita em crianças pequenas, geralmente resultante de infecção; antes era erroneamente atribuída ao aumento do timo. VER TAMBÉM sudden infant death *syndrome.*
mor·si·ca·tio (mor - sik'ă - tē - ō). Mordiscar habitual dos lábios (labiorum), língua (linguae) ou mucosa bucal (buccarum); freqüentemente produz uma lesão branca irregular. [L. que morde, de *mordeo,* morder]
  morsicatio buccarum, elevações brancas da mucosa bucal causadas pela pressão dos dentes molares. [L. mastigação das bochechas]
mor. sol. Abreviatura do L. *more solito,* como habitual, como de costume.
mor·su·lus (mor'soo - lŭs). Morsolo; trocisco. SIN troche. [L. Mod. dim. do L. *morsus,* mordida]
mor·tal (mor'tăl). Mortal. **1.** Relativo a, ou que causa, morte. **2.** Destinado a morrer. [L. *mortalis,* de *mors,* morte]

mor·tal·i·ty (mōr-tal'i-tē). Mortalidade. **1.** A condição de ser mortal. **2.** SIN death rate. **3.** Evolução fatal. [L. *mortalitas*, de *mors* (*mort-*), morte]
   perinatal m. (per'ē-nā-tal). Mortalidade perinatal; mortalidade próxima ao nascimento, convencionalmente limitada ao período que vai da 28.ª semana de gestação até 1 semana após o nascimento.

mor·tar (mōr'tar). Almofariz; gral; recipiente com interior arredondado no qual drogas brutas e outras substâncias são trituradas ou amassadas por meio de um pilão. [L. *mortarium*]

Mor·ti·er·el·la (mōr'tē-ē-rel'ā). Gênero de fungos saprófitas (classe Zygomycetes, família Mucoraceae) comumente encontrados na natureza; a patogenicidade é questionável.

mor·ti·fi·ca·tion (mōr'ti-fi-kā'shŭn). Mortificação. SIN gangrene (1). [L. *mors*, (*mort-*), morte, + *facio*, fazer]

mor·tise (mōr'tēs). Encaixe; o encaixe para o tálus formado pela união da parte distal da fíbula e da tíbia na articulação do tornozelo. [I.m., do Fr. ant. do Ar. *murtazz*, ajustado]

Morton, Dudley J., ortopedista norte-americano, 1884–1960. VER M. *syndrome*.

Morton, Samuel G., médico norte-americano, 1799–1851. VER M. *plane*.

Morton, Thomas G., médico norte-americano, 1835–1903. VER M. *neuralgia*; Morton *metatarsalgia*.

mor·tu·ary (mōr'tū-ār-ē). Mortuário. **1.** Relativo à morte ou ao funeral. **2.** SIN morgue. [L. *mortuus*, morte, part. adj. de *morior*, pp. *mortuus*, morrer]

mor·u·la (mōr'oo-lā, mōr'ū-). Mórula; a massa sólida de blastômeros resultante das primeiras divisões de clivagem do zigoto. Em ovos com pouco vitelo, a mórula é uma massa esferóide de células; nas formas com vitelo considerável, a configuração do estágio de mórula é muito modificada. [L. mod. dim do L. *morus*, amora]

mor·u·la·tion (mōr-oo-lā'shŭn, mōr-ū-). Morulação; formação da mórula.

mor·u·loid (mōr'oo-loyd, mōr'ū-). Morulóide. **1.** Semelhante a uma mórula. **2.** Que tem o formato de uma amora.

Morvan, Augustin, médico francês, 1819–1897. VER M. *chorea, disease*.

mo·sa·ic (mō-zā'ik). Mosaico. **1.** Marchetado; incrustado; semelhante ao trabalho marcheteado. **2.** A justaposição, em um organismo, de tecidos geneticamente diferentes; pode ocorrer normalmente (como na lionização, *q.v.*), ou patologicamente, como um fenômeno ocasional. A partir da mutação somática (mosaicismo genético), uma anomalia da divisão cromossomial resultando em dois ou mais tipos de células contendo diferentes números de cromossomas (mosaicismo cromossomial), ou quimerismo (mosaicismo celular). [L. mod. *mosaicus, musaicus*, relativo às Musas, artístico]

mo·sa·i·cism (mō-zā'i-sizm). Mosaicismo; condição de ser mosaico (2).
   cellular m., m. celular; quimerismo no qual um tecido contém células de diferentes zigotos, p. ex., em seres humanos, envolvendo eritrócitos.
   chromosome m., m. cromossomial. VER mosaic (2).
   gene m., m. genético. VER mosaic (2).
   germinal m., gonadal m., m. germinativo, m. gonadal; estado no qual algumas das células germinativas da gônada são de uma forma não-presente em qualquer genitor, devido à mutação em um progenitor intermediário dessas células.

Moschcowitz, Eli, médico norte-americano, 1879–1964. VER Moschcowitz *test*.

mos·chus (mos'kŭs). Almíscar. [G. *moschos*, almíscar]

Mosenthal, Herman Otto, médico americano, 1878–1954. VER Mosenthal *test*.

Mosler, Karl F., médico alemão, 1831–1911. VER M. *diabetes, sign*.

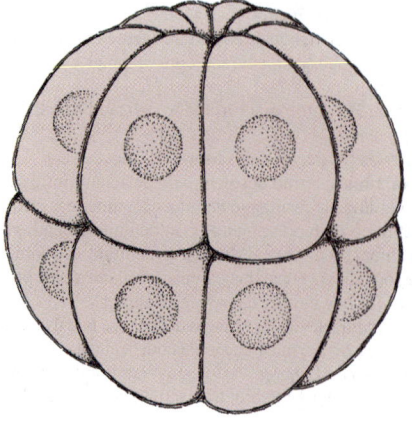

mórula

mos·qui·to, pl. **mos·qui·toes** (mŭs-kē'tō, -tōs). Mosquito; inseto díptero hematófago da família Culicidae. *Aedes, Anopheles, Culex, Mansonia* e *Stegomyia* são os gêneros que contêm a maioria das espécies envolvidas na transmissão de protozoários e de outros parasitas causadores de doença. [Esp. dim. de *mosca*, mosca, do L. *musca*, mosca]

Moss, Gerald, médico norte-americano, 1931–1973. VER M. *tube*.

Moss, Melvin L., patologista oral norte-americano, *1923. VER Gorlin-Chaudhry-M. *syndrome*.

moss. Musgo. **1.** Qualquer vegetal criptógamo, delicado, baixo, da classe Musci. **2.** Popularmente, qualquer um dentre vários liquens e algas marinhas. [A.S. *meōs*]
   Ceylon m., m. do Ceilão; alga marinha vermelha; fonte de ágar.
   club m., licopódio. SIN lycopodium.
   Iceland m., líquen-da-islândia; cetrária. SIN cetraria.
   Irish m., SIN chondrus (2).
   muskeag m., m. almiscarado. SIN sphagnum m.
   pearl m., SIN chondrus (2).
   peat m., m. da turfa. SIN sphagnum m.
   sphagnum m., esfagno; musgo bastante absorvente, usado como substituto de algodão ou gaze absorvente em curativos cirúrgicos e em absorventes íntimos. SIN muskeag m., peat m.

Mosso, Angelo, fisiologista italiano, 1846–1910. VER M. *ergograph, sphygmomanometer*.

Motais, Ernst, oftalmologista francês, 1845–1913. VER M. *operation*.

mote (mōt). Argueiro; cisco; uma pequena partícula; um grânulo. [A.S. *mot*]
   blood m.'s, hemocônia. SIN hemoconia.

moth·er (mŭth'er). Mãe. **1.** O genitor do sexo feminino. **2.** Qualquer célula ou outra estrutura a partir da qual são formados outros corpos semelhantes. [A.S. *mōdor*]
   surrogate m., m. de aluguel; mulher contratada para engravidar para uma outra mulher ou um casal.

mo·tile (mō'til). Móvel. **1.** Que é capaz de movimentar-se espontaneamente. **2.** Indica o tipo de fantasia mental em que a pessoa aprende e recorda-se mais facilmente daquilo que sentiu, isto é, que possui um sistema de representação cinestésico. Cf. audile. **3.** Uma pessoa que tem essa fantasia mental. [ver motion]

mo·til·in (mō-til'in). Motilina; polipeptídeo com 22 aminoácidos encontrado na mucosa duodenal como controlador da atividade motora gastrointestinal normal; em pequenas doses (ng) induz grandes aumentos da atividade motora na área glandular do fundo e nas bolsas do antro do estômago, com um aumento da secreção de pepsina pela primeira. [motility + -in]

mo·til·i·ty (mō-til'i-tē). Motilidade; a capacidade de realizar movimento espontâneo.

mo·tion (mō'shŭn). **1.** Movimento; mudança de lugar ou posição. Cf. movement (1). **2.** Defecação. SIN defecation. **3.** Fezes. SIN stool. [L. *motio*, movimento, de *moveo*, pp. *motus*, mover]
   brownian m., m. browniano. SIN brownian movement. [R. Brown, botânico inglês, 1773–1858]
   continuous passive m. (CPM), m. passivo contínuo; técnica pela qual uma articulação, geralmente o joelho, é movimentada constantemente em amplitude de movimento variável para evitar rigidez e aumentar a amplitude de movimento; na maioria das vezes é realizado utilizando-se um aparelho motorizado específico para esse fim.

mo·ti·va·tion (mō-ti-vā'shŭn). Motivação; em psicologia, a reunião de todos os motivos, necessidades e impulsos individuais que atuam em um indivíduo em qualquer momento, influenciando a vontade e determinando a conduta. [LM. *motivus*, propulsor]
   extrinsic m., m. extrínseca; a busca de satisfação, ou a fuga da insatisfação, através de aspectos não-trabalhosos do ambiente, como buscar conforto, segurança e proteção de outros ou através dos esforços de outros.
   intrinsic m., m. intrínseca; obtenção de satisfação pessoal através de realização e comportamento auto-iniciado.
   personal m., m. pessoal; predisposições e expectativas individuais que dão significado e direção à personalidade.

mo·tive (mō'tiv). Motivo. **1.** Predisposição adquirida, necessidade ou estado específico de tensão em um indivíduo que desperta, mantém e orienta o comportamento para um objetivo. SIN learned drive. **2.** A razão atribuída a um indivíduo, ou por ele fornecida, para um comportamento. Cf. instinct. [L. *moveo*, mover, colocar em movimento]
   achievement m., m. de realização; uma necessidade adquirida, crônica, de obter sucesso na presença de obstáculos reconhecíveis; sua intensidade geralmente é diagnosticada a partir de assuntos recorrentes em histórias contadas pelo indivíduo ao realizar um teste de apercepção temática ou por outros instrumentos de avaliação usados por psicólogos clínicos.
   mastery m., m. de superioridade; necessidade adquirida de ser positivo, de destacar-se na multidão, de dominar.

mo·to·fa·cient (mō-tō-fā'shent). Que causa movimento; designa a segunda fase da atividade muscular na qual é produzido movimento real. [L. *motus*, movimento, + *facio*, fazer]

mo·to·neu·ron (mō′tō - noo′ron). Motoneurônio. SIN motor neuron.
mo·tor (mō′ter). Motor. **1.** Em anatomia e fisiologia, designa aquelas estruturas neurais que, pelos impulsos gerados e transmitidos por elas, causam contração das fibras musculares ou das células de pigmento, ou secreção glandular. VER TAMBÉM motor *cortex*, motor *endplate*, motor *neuron*. **2.** Em psicologia, designa a reação evidente do organismo a um estímulo (resposta motora). [L. que move, de *movere*, mover]
   m. oc'uli, nervo oculomotor [3.º par craniano]. SIN oculomotor nerve [CN III].
   plastic m., m. plástico; um ponto artificial de fixação em um coto de amputação ao qual se prende o fio ou extensor pelo qual o movimento é transmitido para um membro artificial; usado em cinematização.
mo·tor·i·al (mō - tōr′ē - ăl). Motor; relativo ao movimento, a um nervo motor ou ao núcleo motor.
mo·tor·me·ter (mō′ter - mē′ter). Motômetro; aparelho para determinar a quantidade, a força e a velocidade do movimento.
MOTT Termo usado para descrever outras micobactérias além do *Mycobacterium tuberculosis*, *M. bovis* e *M. africanum* (complexo *M. tuberculosis*).
mot·tle (mot′tl). Mancha; fina heterogeneidade de uma área de opacidade geralmente uniforme em uma fotografia ou radiografia; ruído. [de *motley*, do I.m. *mot*, grânulo]
   quantum m., ruído quântico; manchas causadas pela flutuação estatística do número de fótons absorvidos pelos écrans intensificadores para formar a imagem clara no filme; écrans mais rápidos produzem maior ruído quântico.
mot·tling (mot′ling). Mosqueamento; área de pele composta de lesões maculares de vários tons ou cores. [I. *motley*, de cor variada]
Motulsky dye re·duc·tion test. Teste de redução do corante de Motulsky. VER test.
mou·lage (moo-lazh′). Moldagem; reprodução em cera de uma lesão cutânea, tumor ou outro estado patológico da pele. [F. moldagem]
mould (mōld). Molde. SIN mold.
moult (mōlt). Muda. SIN molt.
mound·ing (mownd′ing). Mioedema. SIN myoedema.
Mounier-Kuhn, Pierre, médico francês, *1901. VER Mounier-Kuhn *syndrome*.
mount (mownt). Montar. **1.** Preparar para exame microscópico. **2.** Subir com o objetivo de copular. **3.** Organizar e apresentar, como uma febre, uma resposta imunológica, etc.
mount·ing (mownt′ing). Montagem; em odontologia, o procedimento laboratorial de fixar um modelo da maxila e/ou mandíbula a um articulador.
   split cast m., m. de modelo dividido; **(1)** um modelo com sulcos-chave em sua base, montado sobre um articulador para fácil remoção e substituição precisa; podem ser usadas placas metálicas de remontagem divididas, em vez de sulcos nos modelos; **(2)** forma de testar a precisão do ajuste do articulador.
mourn (mōrn). Prantear; lamentar; expressar pesar ou sofrimento por uma perda. Em psicanálise, o luto é o processo, freqüentemente não expresso, de responder à perda de um objeto querido que, ao contrário da melancolia, geralmente não envolve perda da auto-estima. [I. ant. *murnan*]
mouse (mows). Camundongo; pequeno roedor pertencente ao gênero *Mus*.
   joint m.'s, artrófitos; corpos móveis articulares; pequenos corpos livres fibrosos, cartilaginosos ou ósseos na cavidade sinovial de uma articulação.
   knockout m., camundongo nocaute; camundongo de cujo genoma foi deletado artificialmente um único gene.

> Os animais experimentais que não possuem genes específicos tornaram-se instrumentos de pesquisa úteis em muitos ramos da medicina, incluindo genética, fisiologia, farmacologia, imunologia, biologia celular e oncologia. Um animal transgênico é aquele em cujo genoma foi deliberadamente introduzido um gene estranho, construído por tecnologia de DNA recombinante. O posicionamento do gene inserido em um *locus* específico no genoma é possibilitado pela sua incorporação em um vetor no qual é flanqueado por seqüências de DNA específicas do local alvo. O material genético artificial é introduzido em um embrião, que então se transforma em uma quimera cujos tecidos contêm células normais e células contendo o transgene. Acasalamentos entre esses animais produzem alguns descendentes homozigotos para o transgene. Se o gene introduzido for um alelo não-funcional (nulo), remove ou "nocauteia" o alelo selvagem, normal. Não apenas o gene deletado não é expresso, como também os descendentes de acasalamentos entre homozigotos constituem uma raça pura, na qual o gene está ausente em todos os membros. Embora, teoricamente, qualquer animal possa ser submetido à técnica de nocaute, foram usados quase exclusivamente camundongos. Estes são pequenos e facilmente mantidos, reproduzem-se rapidamente e possuem um período de vida curto. Além disso, há uma semelhança surpreendente entre os genomas do camundongo e os do ser humano, com aproximadamente 75% de correspondência dos genes. O fato de camundongos nocaute que não possuem vários genes serem fenotipicamente normais indica que o genoma do camundongo, como o dos seres humanos, freqüentemente possui redundância suficiente para compensar a ausência de um único par de alelos. Camundongos nocaute que não possuem o gene supressor tumoral p53 são usados em estudos de carcinogênese, enquanto aqueles que não possuem o gene para o receptor LDL constituem um modelo animal de hipercolesterolemia familiar humana. Os camundongos nocaute mostraram-se úteis na revelação das funções de genes para os quais ainda não existiam raças mutantes.

   multimammate m., roedor africano, *Praomys natalensis*, amplamente usado na pesquisa do câncer.
   New Zealand mice, camundongos da Nova Zelândia; cepas endogâmicas de camundongos, pretos (NZB) ou brancos (NZW), únicas entre as cepas usadas em imunologia experimental devido à sua tendência a anormalidades imunológicas espontâneas e distúrbios, incluindo o lúpus eritematoso sistêmico, semelhantes aos encontrados nos seres humanos.
   nude m., c. atímico; camundongo mutante sem pêlos, com hipoplasia tímica, que não possui células T.
   transgenic m.'s (tranz′jen-ik), camundongos transgênicos; camundongos que possuem um pedaço de DNA estranho integrado ao seu genoma.
mouth (mowth). Boca. **1.** SIN oral cavity. **2.** A abertura, geralmente externa, de uma cavidade ou canal. VER os (2), ostium, orifice, stoma (2). [A.S. *mūth*]
   carp m., boca de carpa; boca semelhante à de uma carpa, com ângulos descendentes; observada na síndrome de Cornelia de Lange e no nanismo de Silver-Russell.
   denture sore m., eritema da mucosa subjacente à base de uma dentadura, geralmente representando inflamação causada por dentaduras mal ajustadas, má higiene oral ou *Candida albicans*.
   scabby m., SIN orf.
   sore m., VER soremouth.
   tapir m., boca de tapir; protrusão labial devida à fraqueza dos músculos orbiculares da boca; observada em algumas distrofias. SIN bouche de tapir.
   trench m., gengivite ulcerativa necrotizante. SIN necrotizing ulcerative gingivitis.
   m. of the womb, orifício externo do útero. SIN external *os* of uterus.
mouth guard. Protetor de boca; aparelho de plástico flexível, adaptado para cobrir os dentes maxilares, usado para reduzir possível lesão das estruturas orais durante a participação em esportes de contato.
mouth stick. Prótese segura pelos dentes e utilizada por pessoas deficientes para realizar atos como datilografar, pintar e levantar pequenos objetos.
mouth·wash. Colutório; medicamento líquido usado para limpeza da boca e tratamento de estados patológicos de suas mucosas. SIN collutorium, collutory.
move·ment (moov′ment). Movimento. **1.** O ato de movimentar; diz-se de todo o corpo ou de um ou mais de seus membros ou partes. **2.** Fezes. SIN stool. **3.** Defecação. SIN defecation. [L. *moveo*, pp. *motus*, mover]

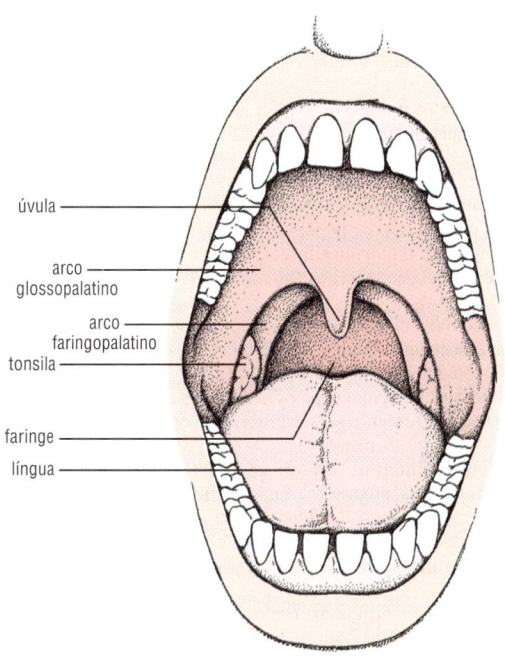

boca

active m., m. ativo; (1) movimento realizado pelo próprio organismo, sem auxílio de influências externas; (2) em fisioterapia, movimento realizado totalmente pelos músculos do paciente, amiúde com a orientação do terapeuta.

adversive m., m. adverso; rotação dos olhos, cabeça ou tronco em torno do eixo longitudinal do corpo.

after-m., pós-movimento. VER aftermovement.

ameboid m., m. amebóide; a forma de movimento característica do protoplasma de leucócitos, amebas e outros organismos unicelulares; envolve a aglomeração do protoplasma em um ponto onde a pressão superficial é menor e sua extrusão na forma de um pseudópode; o protoplasma pode retornar ao corpo da célula, resultando na retração do pseudópode, ou toda a massa pode fluir para este último e, assim, resultar em locomoção da célula. SIN streaming m.

assistive m., m. de assistência; em fisioterapia, movimento realizado com a ajuda graduada do terapeuta.

associated m.'s, movimentos associados; movimentos involuntários normais do membro que acompanham o movimento voluntário, p. ex., oscilação do braço ao caminhar.

Bennett m., m. de Bennett; o movimento lateral do corpo ou o desvio lateral da mandíbula durante um movimento laterotrusivo.

border m.'s, movimentos marginais; qualquer extensão extrema do movimento mandibular limitada por osso, ligamentos ou tecidos moles; geralmente é aplicado aos movimentos horizontais da mandíbula.

border tissue m.'s, movimentos dos tecidos periféricos; a ação dos músculos e de outros tecidos adjacentes às bordas de uma dentadura.

bowel m., m. intestinal; defecação.

brownian m., m. browniano; movimento errático, não-direcionado, em ziguezague, observado ao ultramicroscópio em algumas soluções colóides e ao microscópio em suspensões de partículas leves, resultante de impulsos ou colisões das partículas maiores pelas moléculas no meio de suspensão consideradas em movimento contínuo. SIN brownian motion, brownian-Zsigmondy m., molecular m., pedesis.

brownian-Zsigmondy m., m. browniano de Zsigmondy. SIN brownian m.

cardinal ocular m.'s, movimentos oculares cardinais; rotações oculares para a direita e esquerda, ascendentes para a direita e esquerda e descendentes para a direita e esquerda, para diagnosticar posições do olhar.

choreic m., m. coreico; contração espasmódica ou espasmo involuntário em grupos de músculos não-associados na produção de movimentos intencionais definidos.

ciliary m., m. ciliar; movimento de varredura, rítmico, dos cílios das células epiteliais, de protozoários ciliados ou o movimento oscilante de flagelos, realizado possivelmente pela contração e relaxamento alternados de filamentos contráteis (mióides) de um lado do cílio ou flagelo.

circus m., m. circular; onda de contração ou excitação que segue continuamente em formato circular em torno de um anel de músculo ou através da parede do coração. SIN circus rhythm.

cogwheel ocular m.'s, movimentos oculares em roda dentada; rotações oculares espasmódicas, frouxas, que substituem as rotações de acompanhamento suaves.

conjugate m. of eyes, m. conjugado dos olhos; rotação dos dois olhos em direções opostas, como na convergência ou divergência. VER TAMBÉM version (4).

decomposition of m., decomposição do m., uma manifestação da doença cerebelar na qual um movimento muscular não é realizado como um todo, mas em uma série de componentes.

disconjugate m. of eyes, m. desconjugado dos olhos, rotação dos dois olhos em direções opostas, como na convergência ou divergência.

drift m.'s, movimentos de impulso. SIN drifts.

fetal m., m. fetal; o movimento característico do feto no útero; geralmente começa entre a décima sexta e a décima oitava semanas de gravidez. VER TAMBÉM quickening.

fixational ocular m., m. ocular de fixação; rotação dos olhos durante a fixação voluntária em um objeto; ocorrem tremores, estalidos e impulsos.

flick m.'s, movimentos rápidos. SIN flicks.

free mandibular m.'s, movimentos livres da mandíbula; (1) quaisquer movimentos mandibulares feitos sem interferência dos dentes; (2) quaisquer movimentos não-inibidos da mandíbula.

functional mandibular m.'s, movimentos funcionais da mandíbula; todos os movimentos naturais, próprios ou característicos da mandíbula feitos durante a fala, mastigação, bocejo, deglutição e outros movimentos associados.

fusional m., m. de fusão; movimento reflexo que tende a deslocar os eixos visuais para o objeto de fixação, de forma que seja possível a visão estereoscópica.

hinge m., m. de dobradiça; movimento de abertura ou fechamento da mandíbula no eixo de dobradiça.

intermediary m.'s, movimentos intermediários; em odontologia, todos os movimentos entre os extremos das excursões mandibulares.

lateral m., m. lateral; em odontologia, movimento da mandíbula para o lado.

Magnan trombone m., m. do trombone de Magnan; movimento involuntário da língua para frente e para trás quando é trazida para fora da boca; pode ser observada em vários distúrbios dos gânglios da base.

mandibular m., m. mandibular; (1) movimentos da mandíbula; (2) todas as alterações na posição de que a mandíbula é capaz.

mass m., m. de massa. SIN mass peristalsis.

molecular m., m. molecular. SIN brownian m.

morphogenetic m., m. morfogenético; o fluxo de células no embrião inicial para formar tecidos ou órgãos.

muscular m., m. muscular; movimento causado pela contração das miofibrilas das células musculares.

neurobiotactic m., m. neurobiotático; o fluxo de células nervosas em direção à área da qual elas recebem a maioria dos estímulos.

non-rapid eye m. (NREM), m. não-rápido dos olhos; lenta oscilação dos olhos durante o sono.

opening m., m. de abertura; em odontologia, o movimento da mandíbula executado durante a separação da maxila e da mandíbula.

paradoxical m. of eyelids, m. paradoxal das pálpebras, elevação ou abaixamento involuntário e espontâneo das pálpebras, associado ao movimento dos músculos extra-oculares ou dos músculos da mastigação (pterigóides externos). VER jaw winking.

paradoxical vocal cord m., m. paradoxal das pregas vocais; adução das cordas vocais à inspiração, resultando em estridor e obstrução das vias aéreas.

passive m., m. passivo; (1) movimento conferido a um organismo ou a qualquer de suas partes por agentes externos; (2) em fisioterapia, movimento totalmente realizado pelo terapeuta sem a ajuda dos músculos do paciente.

pendular m., m. pendular; movimento de vaivém do intestino, sem qualquer ação propulsora ou peristáltica, pelo qual o conteúdo é agitado e totalmente misturado aos fermentos intestinais.

protoplasmic m., m. protoplásmico; movimento produzido pela capacidade inerente de contração e relaxamento do protoplasma; esses movimentos são de três tipos: muscular, em defluxo e ciliar.

rapid eye m.'s (REM), movimentos rápidos dos olhos; movimentos de varredura rápidos e simétricos dos olhos que ocorrem muitas vezes durante o sono em períodos de 5 a 60 minutos; associados aos sonhos.

reflex m., m. reflexo; movimento involuntário resultante de um estímulo sensorial.

resistive m., m. de resistência; em fisioterapia, movimento feito pelo paciente contra os esforços do terapeuta, ou movimento forçado pelo operador contra a resistência do paciente.

saccadic m., m. sacádico; (1) rotação rápida dos olhos de um ponto de fixação para outro, como na leitura; (2) o rápido movimento de correção de um nistagmo espasmódico, como no nistagmo labiríntico e optocinético.

streaming m., m. de corrente. SIN ameboid m.

Swedish m.'s, movimentos suecos; forma de cinesiterapia na qual alguns movimentos sistemáticos do corpo e dos membros são regulados por resistência feita por um auxiliar.

translatory m., m. de translação; o movimento do corpo em qualquer momento, quando todos os pontos no corpo estão se movendo na mesma velocidade e na mesma direção.

vermicular m., m. vermicular. SIN peristalsis.

moxa (mok'sa). Moxa; cone ou cilindro de algodão ou outro material combustível, colocado sobre a pele e queimado a fim de produzir contra-irritação. VER TAMBÉM moxibustion. [Jap. *moe kusa*, erva que queima]

mox·a·lac·tam (moks-a-lak'tam). Moxalactam; cefalosporina de terceira geração com ação antibacteriana de amplo espectro; causa distúrbios hemorrágicos, que limitam seu uso.

mox·i·bus·tion (mok-sī-bŭs'chŭn). Moxabustão; combustão de ervas, como moxa, sobre a pele como contra-irritante no tratamento da doença; um componente da tradicional medicina chinesa e japonesa.

mox·i·sy·lyte (mok-sī'si-līt). Moxisilita; usado como bloqueador α-adrenérgico para tratamento de doença vascular periférica. SIN thymoxamine.

MP Abreviatura de mentoposterior *position* (posição mentoposterior).

m.p. 1. Abreviatura de melting *point* (ponto de derretimento). **2.** Abreviatura do [L.] *modo praescripto*, da forma prescrita.

MPD Abreviatura de maximum permissible *dose* (máxima dose permissível).

MPR Abreviatura de mannose-6-phosphate *receptors* (receptores de manose-6-fosfato) em *receptor*.

MPS Abreviatura de mononuclear phagocyte *system* (sistema fagocitário mononuclear).

MPTP Derivado da piperidina que causa sintomas irreversíveis de parkinsonismo em seres humanos e macacos. Um produto intermediário da meperidina, fabricada ilegalmente, que causou numerosos casos de parkinsonismo. Usado como instrumento experimental na pesquisa do parkinsonismo.

MQ Abreviatura antiga de menaquinone (menaquinona); agora MK.

MRA Abreviatura de MR *angiography* (angiorressonância nuclear).

M.R.C.P. Abreviatura de *Member of the Royal College of Physicians* (da Inglaterra).

M.R.C.P.(E) Abreviatura de *Member of the Royal College of Physicians* (Edimburgo).

M.R.C.P.(I) Abreviatura de *Member of the Royal College of Physicians* (Irlanda).

M.R.C.S. Abreviatura de *Member of the Royal College of Surgeons* (Inglaterra).

M.R.C.S.(E) Abreviatura de *Member of the Royal College of Surgeons* (Edimburgo).

M.R.C.S.(I) Abreviatura de *Member of the Royal College of Surgeons* (Irlanda).

MRD, mrd Abreviatura de minimal reacting *dose* (dose reativa mínima).

MRF Abreviatura de melanotropin-releasing *factor* (fator liberador de melanotropina).

MRH Abreviatura de melanotropin-releasing *hormone* (hormônio liberador de melanotropina).

MRI Abreviatura de magnetic resonance *imaging* (imagem por ressonância magnética).

mRNA Abreviatura de messenger RNA (RNA mensageiro). ver entradas em ribonucleic acid.

MS Abreviatura de multiple *sclerosis* (esclerose múltipla); *morphine* sulfate (sulfato de morfina); mitral *stenosis* (estenose mitral); e myasthenic *syndrome* (Lambert-Eaton syndrome; síndrome miastênica ou de Lambert-Eaton).

ms Abreviatura de millisecond (milissegundo).

M.S.D. Abreviatura de Master of Science in Dentistry.

msec Abreviatura de millisecond (milissegundo).

MSG Abreviatura de monosodium glutamate (glutamato monossódico).

MSH Abreviatura de melanocyte-stimulating *hormone* (hormônio estimulante de melanócitos).

MTBE Abreviatura de methyl-*tert*-butyl ether (metil-*tert*-butil éter).

MTF Abreviatura de modulation transfer *function* (função de transferência de modulação).

m.u. Abreviatura de mouse *unit* (unidade de camundongo).

mu (mū). Décima segunda letra do alfabeto grego, μ.

mu·case (mū′kās). Mucase. SIN mucinase.

Much, Hans C.R., médico alemão, 1880–1932. VER M. *bacillus*.

Mucha, Victor, dermatologista austríaco, 1877–1919. VER M.-Habermann *disease*.

muci-. Mucoso, mucina. VER TAMBÉM muco-, myxo-. [L. *mucus*]

mu·ci·car·mine (mū - si - kar′mĭn). Mucicarmina; corante vermelho que contém cloreto de alumínio e carmim; usado para detectar mucinas epiteliais e adenocarcinomas secretores de mucina; também é usado para demonstrar a cápsula de *Cryptococcus neoformans* e outros fungos.

mu·cid (mū′sĭd). Múcide. SIN muciparous.

mu·cif·er·ous (mū - sĭf′er - ŭs). Mucífero. SIN muciparous.

mu·ci·fi·ca·tion (mū′si - fi - kā′shŭn). Mucificação; alteração produzida na mucosa vaginal de animais experimentais castrados, após estimulação com estrogênio; caracterizada pela formação de células colunares altas secretoras de muco. [L. *mucus* + *facio*, fazer]

mu·ci·form (mū′si - form). Muciforme; semelhante a muco. SIN blennoid, mucoid (2).

mu·cig·e·nous (mū - sĭj′ē - nŭs). SIN muciparous.

mu·ci·he·ma·te·in (mū - si - hē′mă - tē - in). Muciematína; líquido corante azul-violeta que contém cloreto de alumínio e hemateína; usado para detectar mucinas no tecido conjuntivo.

mu·ci·lage (mū′si - lij). Mucilagem; preparação da farmacopéia que consiste em uma solução aquosa dos princípios mucilaginosos de substâncias vegetais; usada como aplicação calmante das mucosas e no preparo de misturas oficiais e extemporâneas. [L. *mucilago*]

mu·ci·lag·i·nous (mū - si - lăj′i - nŭs). Mucilaginoso. **1.** Semelhante à mucilagem; isto é, adesivo, viscoso. **2.** SIN muciparous.

mu·cin (mū′sin). Mucina; secreção que contém glicoproteínas ricas em carboidratos, como aquela das células caliciformes do intestino, as glândulas submaxilares e outras células glandulares mucosas; também é encontrada na substância fundamental de tecido conjuntivo, principalmente do tecido conjuntivo mucoso, é solúvel em água alcalina e precipitada pelo ácido acético; as mucinas atuam como lubrificantes e protetores dos revestimentos das cavidades corporais.

   gastric m., m. gástrica; pó branco ou amarelado que forma um líquido opalescente viscoso com água, preparado a partir da mucosa do estômago de porco pela digestão com pepsina-ácido clorídrico e precipitação do líquido sobrenadante com álcool a 60%; usado na úlcera péptica por sua ação protetora e lubrificante.

mu·cin·ase (mū′si - nās). Mucinase; termo aplicado especificamente à hialuronato liase, hialuronoglucosaminidase e hialuronoglucuronidase (hialuronidases), porém é aplicado mais livremente a qualquer enzima que hidrolise substâncias mucopolissacarídicas (mucinas). SIN mucase, mucopolysaccharidase.

mu·ci·ne·mia (mū - si - nē′mē - ă). Mucinemia; a presença de mucina no sangue circulante. SIN myxemia. [mucin- + G. *haima*, sangue]

mu·cin·o·gen (mū′sin - ō - jen). Mucinogênio; glicoproteína que forma mucina através de embebição em água. [mucin + G. *-gen*, que produz]

mu·ci·noid (mū′si - noyd). Mucinóide. **1.** SIN mucoid (1). **2.** Semelhante à mucina.

mu·ci·no·lyt·ic (mū′si - nō - lĭt′ĭk). Mucinolítico; capaz de produzir hidrólise de mucina, como por uma mucinase.

mu·ci·no·sis (mū - si - nō′sis). Mucinose; condição na qual a mucina está presente na pele em quantidades excessivas, ou em distribuição anormal; classificada como: **metabolic m.,** m. metabólica; mixedema difuso ou pré-tibial, líquen mixedematoso, gargoilismo; **secondary m.,** m. secundária; degeneração em tumores; **localized m.,** m. localizada; cisto folicular, papular, em placa, focal e mixóide ou sinovial. [mucin + G. *-osis*, condição]

   cutaneous focal m., m. focal cutânea; pápulas cutâneas cor de carne, compostas de material mucinoso homogêneo com fibroblastos dispersos.

   follicular m., m. folicular; erupção benigna, relativamente incomum, de lesões eritematosas distintas que progridem para alopecia na face ou no couro cabeludo, geralmente em pessoas jovens, na qual há alterações mucinosas císticas no epitélio dos folículos pilosos da área envolvida; também podem desenvolver-se na micose fungóide.

   oral focal m., m. focal oral; área de tecido conjuntivo mixomatoso; o equivalente mucoso da mucinose focal cutânea.

   papular m., m. papular. SIN lichen myxedematosus.

   reticular erythematous m. (REM), m. eritematosa reticular. SIN REM *syndrome*.

mu·ci·nous (mū′si - nŭs). Mucinoso; relativo a, ou que contém, mucina. SIN mucoid (3).

mu·ci·nu·ria (mū - si - nū′rē - ă). Mucinúria; a presença de mucina na urina. [mucin + G. *ouron*, urina]

mu·cip·a·rous (mū - sĭp′ă - rŭs). Mucíparo; que produz ou secreta muco. SIN blennogenic, blennogenous, mucid, muciferous, mucigenous, mucilaginous (2). [mucin + L. *pario*, produzir, levar]

mu·ci·tis (mū - sī′tis). Mucite; inflamação de uma mucosa.

Muckle, T.J., pediatra canadense do século XX. VER M.-Wells *syndrome*.

muco-. Muco, mucoso (mucosa). VER TAMBÉM muci-, myxo-. [L. *mucus*]

mu·co·cele (mū′kō - sēl). Mucocele. **1.** SIN mucous *cyst*. **2.** Cisto de retenção da glândula salivar, saco lacrimal, seios paranasais, apêndice, vesícula biliar ou outro local. [muco- + G. *kēlē*, tumor, hérnia]

mu·co·cil·i·ary (mū′kō - sĭl′ē - ă - rē). Mucociliar; relativo à interação entre o muco e o epitélio ciliado.

mu·coc·la·sis (mū - kok′lă - sis). Mucoclase; termo obsoleto para designar a desnudação de qualquer superfície mucosa. [muco- + G. *klasis*, separação]

mu·co·co·li·tis (mū′kō - kō - lī′tis). Mucocolite. SIN mucous *colitis*.

mu·co·col·pos (mū - kō - kol′pos). Mucocolpo; presença de muco na vagina. [muco- + G. *kolpos*, vagina]

mu·co·cu·ta·ne·ous (mū′kō - kū - tā′nē - ŭs). Mucocutâneo; cutâneo-mucoso; relativo à mucosa e pele; designa a linha de junção das duas nos orifícios nasal, oral, vaginal e anal. SIN cutaneomucosal.

mu·co·en·ter·i·tis (mū′kō - en - ter - ī′tis). Mucoenterite. **1.** Inflamação da mucosa intestinal. **2.** SIN mucomembranous *enteritis*.

mu·co·ep·i·der·moid (mū′kō - ep - i - der′moyd). Mucoepidermóide; designa uma mistura de células secretoras de muco e epiteliais, como no carcinoma mucoepidermóide.

mu·co·glob·u·lin (mū - kō - glob′ū - lin). Mucoglobulina; glicoproteína ou mucoproteína na qual o componente proteico é uma globulina.

mu·coid (mū′koyd). Mucóide. **1.** Termo geral para mucina, mucoproteína ou glicoproteína. SIN mucinoid (1). **2.** SIN muciform. **3.** SIN mucinous. [mucus + G. *eidos*, aspecto]

mu·co·lip·i·do·sis, pl. **mu·co·lip·i·do·ses** (mū′kō - lip - i - dō′sis, - sēz). Mucolipidose; qualquer uma de um grupo de doenças de depósito lisossômico nas quais há sinais e sintomas de armazenamento visceral e mesenquimal de mucopolissacarídeos, glicoproteínas, oligossacarídeos ou glicolipídios; clinicamente, possuem uma semelhança superficial com as mucopolissacaridoses; herança autossômica recessiva. [muco- + lipid + *-osis*, condição]

   m. I [MIM*256550], m. I; mucolipidose um pouco semelhante a uma forma leve de síndrome de Hurler (Hurler *syndrome*) com características faciais grosseiras, máculas vermelho-cereja, epilepsia mioclônica, disostose leve múltipla e retardo mental moderado devido à deficiência de neuraminidase; herança autossômica recessiva causada por mutação no gene da neuraminidase (NEU) em 6p. SIN lipomucopolysaccharidosis.

   m. II [MIM*252500], m. II; distúrbio metabólico que se instala nos primeiros anos de vida, caracterizado por achados clínicos e radiológicos semelhantes aos observados na síndrome de Hurler (Hurler *syndrome*), incluindo hipertrofia gengival, displasia torácica, luxação congênita do quadril e retardo mental; são encontrados linfócitos vacuolados e corpúsculos de inclusão incomuns em fibroblastos cultivados (células I); as enzimas lisossômicas estão aumentadas no soro, no líquido espinal e na urina; os mucopolissacarídeos urinários são normais; associada a deficiência de *N*-acetilglucosaminil-1-fosfotransferase; herança autossômica recessiva. SIN I-cell disease, inclusion cell disease.

m. III [MIM*252600], m. III; mucolipidose com sintomas leves semelhantes aos da síndrome de Hurler, restrição da mobilidade articular, baixa estatura, retardo mental leve e alterações ósseas displásicas, principalmente do quadril; freqüentemente há doença das valvas aórtica e mitral; associada a deficiência de N-acetil-α-glucosaminidase ou outras deficiências enzimáticas, de forma que a enzima lisossômica N-acetilglucosaminil-1-fosfotransferase em fibroblastos mutantes não consegue reconhecer enzimas lisossômicas e substratos específicos para fosforilação; herança autossômica recessiva. SIN pseudo-Hurler polydystrophy, pseudopolydystrophy.

m. IV [MIM*252650], m. IV; retardo psicomotor com córneas turvas e degeneração da retina com células de inclusão em fibroblastos cultivados; a patogenia é incerta; herança autossômica recessiva.

mu·col·y·sis (mū - kol′i - sis). Mucólise; a solução, digestão ou liquefação de muco. [muco- + G. *lysis*, dissolução]

mu·co·lyt·ic (mū - kō - lit′ik). Mucolítico; capaz de dissolver, digerir ou liquefazer o muco.

mu·co·mem·bra·nous (mū′kō - mem′bră - nŭs). Mucomembranoso; relativo a uma mucosa.

mu·co·pep·tide (mū - kō - pep′tīd). Mucopeptídeo. **1.** Peptídeo encontrado em combinação com polissacarídeos que contêm ácidos murâmico ou siálico. **2.** SIN peptidoglycan.

m. glycohydrolase, m. glicoidrolase. SIN lysozyme.

mu·co·per·i·os·te·al (mū′kō - per - ē - os′tē - al). Mucoperiosteal; relativo ao mucoperiósteo.

mu·co·per·i·os·te·um (mū′kō - per - ē - os′tē - ŭm). Mucoperiósteo; mucosa e periósteo unidos tão intimamente a ponto de formarem praticamente uma membrana única, como a que cobre o palato duro.

mu·co·pol·y·sac·cha·ri·dase (mū′kō - pol - ē - sak′ă - ri - dās). Mucopolissacaridase. SIN mucinase, β-*d*-glucuronidase deficiency.

mu·co·pol·y·sac·cha·ride (mū′kō - pol - ē - sak′ă - rīd). Mucopolissacarídeo; termo geral para um complexo de proteínas e polissacarídeos obtido a partir de proteoglicanas e contendo até 95% de polissacarídeos; os mucopolissacarídeos incluem as substâncias dos grupos sanguíneos. Um termo mais moderno é glicosaminoglicana, pois todas as seis classes conhecidas contêm grandes quantidades de D-glucosamina e D-galactosamina.

mu·co·pol·y·sac·cha·ri·do·sis, pl. **mu·co·pol·y·sac·cha·ri·do·ses** (mū′kō - pol - ē - sak′ă - ri - dō′sis, - sēz). Mucopolissacaridose; qualquer uma doença de um grupo de doenças de depósito lisossômico que têm em comum um distúrbio do metabolismo dos mucopolissacarídeos, conforme evidenciado pela excreção de vários mucopolissacarídeos na urina e infiltração dessas substâncias no tecido conjuntivo, resultando em vários defeitos nos ossos, cartilagem, tecido conjuntivo e outros órgãos.

type IH m., m. tipo I-H. SIN Hurler syndrome.
type I H/S m., m. tipo I H/S. SIN Hurler-Scheie syndrome.
type II m., m. tipo II. SIN Hunter syndrome.
type III m., m. tipo III. SIN Sanfilippo syndrome.
type IS m., m. tipo IS. SIN Scheie syndrome.
type IVA, B m., m. tipo IVA, B. SIN Morquio syndrome.
type V m., m. tipo V; designação anterior de Scheie syndrome.
type VI m., m. tipo IV. SIN Maroteaux-Lamy syndrome.
type VII m., m. tipo VII; **(1)** SIN Sly syndrome; **(2)** SIN Di Ferrante syndrome.

mu·co·pol·y·sac·cha·ri·du·ria (mū′kō - pol - ē - sak′ă - ri - doo′rē - ă). Mucopolissacaridúria; a excreção de mucopolissacarídeos na urina.

mu·co·pro·tein (mū - kō - prō′tēn). Mucoproteína; termo geral para um complexo proteína-polissacarídeo, geralmente indicando que o componente proteína é a principal parte do complexo, ao contrário do mucopolissacarídeo; as mucoproteínas incluem as $α_1$- e $α_2$-globulinas do soro (e outras). Algumas vezes denominadas glicoproteínas, embora este termo geralmente se refira àquelas mucoproteínas que contêm menos de 4% de carboidratos.

Tamm-Horsfall m., m. de Tamm-Horsfall; a matriz de cilindros urinários derivada da secreção das células tubulares renais.

mu·co·pu·ru·lent (mū - kō - poo′roo - lent). Mucopurulento; relativo a um exsudato que é principalmente purulento (pus), mas que contém proporções relativamente visíveis de material mucoso. SIN puromucous.

mu·co·pus (mū′kō - pŭs). Mucopus; secreção mucopurulenta; mistura de material mucoso e pus. SIN mycopus.

Mu·cor (mū′kor). Gênero de fungos (classe Zygomycetes, família Mucoraceae), a maioria de suas espécies é sapróbia; algumas espécies são patogênicas e causam zigomicose em seres humanos.

Mu·co·ra·ce·ae (mū′kor - a′sē - ē). Uma família de fungos (classe Zygomycetes) que compreende organismos terrestres, aquáticos e, algumas vezes, parasitas; inclui os gêneros *Mucor, Absidia, Rhizopus, Rhizomucor, Apophysomyces* e *Mortierella.* Embora as várias espécies dos gêneros sejam comumente formas sapróbias, de vida livre, algumas delas causam mucormicose em seres humanos. [L. *mucor*, mofo]

Mucorales (moo-kor-al′ez). Ordem da classe de fungos Zygomycetes que contém todas as espécies causadoras da mucormicose em seres humanos. Os gêneros incluem *Cunninghamella, Rhizopus, Absidia, Rhlizomucor, Mucor,*

Apophysomyces, Saksenaea, Syncepthalastrum e *Cokeromyces.* As espécies de *Mortierella* são incluídas, mas sua patogenicidade para seres humanos é questionável.

mu·cor·my·co·sis (mū′kor - mī - kō′sis). Mucormicose; infecção por fungos da ordem Mucorales; para ser distinguida da zigomicose, termo mais amplo que inclui infecções causadas por fungos da ordem Entomophthorales.

mu·co·sa (mū - kō′să) [TA]. Mucosa; tecido mucoso que reveste várias estruturas tubulares, consistindo em epitélio, lâmina própria e, no sistema digestivo, em uma camada de músculo liso (muscular da mucosa). SIN tunica mucosa [TA], mucous membranes*, membrana mucosa, mucosal tunics, mucous tunics. [L. fem. de *mucosus*, mucoso]

alveolar m., m. alveolar; a mucosa apical à gengiva fixada.
m. of bronchi [TA], túnica mucosa dos brônquios; o revestimento interno de um brônquio. SIN tunica mucosa bronchi [TA], mucous membrane of bronchus*, bronchial m.
bronchial m., m. brônquica. SIN m. of bronchi.
m. of colon, m. do colo; o revestimento do colo. SIN tunica mucosa coli.
m. of ductus deferens [TA], túnica mucosa do ducto deferente; a camada interna do ducto deferente. SIN tunica mucosa ductus deferentis [TA], mucous membrane of ductus deferens*.
esophageal m., m. do esôfago. SIN m. of esophagus.
m. of esophagus [TA], túnica mucosa do esôfago; a camada interna do esôfago. SIN tunica mucosa esophagi [TA], mucous membrane of esophagus*, esophageal m.
m. of female urethra [TA], túnica mucosa da uretra feminina; a camada mucosa interna da uretra feminina. SIN tunica mucosa urethrae femininae [TA], mucous membrane of female urethra*.
m. of gallbladder [TA], túnica mucosa da vesícula biliar; a camada interna da vesícula biliar. SIN tunica mucosa vesicae biliaris [TA], mucous membrane of gallbladder*, tunica mucosa vesicae felleae*.
gastric m., m. gástrica. SIN m. of stomach.
gingival m., m. gengival; a parte da mucosa oral que cobre os colos dos dentes e está fixada a eles e ao processo alveolar da mandíbula e maxila; é demarcada da mucosa de revestimento, no lado facial, por uma linha bem definida que marca a junção mucogengival, e, ao contrário da mucosa de revestimento, é queratinizada e tem cor mais clara; na superfície palatina, a gengiva funde-se imperceptivelmente à mucosa palatina.
m. of large intestine [TA], túnica mucosa do intestino grosso; o revestimento mucoso (epitélio, lâmina própria e muscular da mucosa) da parede de todas as partes do intestino grosso (ceco, colo, reto e canal anal) coletivamente. SIN tunica mucosa intestini crassi [TA], mucous membrane of large intestine*.
laryngeal m., m. da laringe. SIN m. of larynx.
m. of larynx [TA], túnica mucosa da laringe; o revestimento mucoso da laringe. SIN tunica mucosa laryngis [TA], mucous membrane of larynx*, laryngeal m.
lingual m., m. da língua. SIN m. of tongue.
m. of male urethra [TA], túnica mucosa da uretra masculina; camada mais interna da uretra, incluindo um epitélio típico das vias urinárias (um epitélio de transição ou urotélio) proximal às aberturas dos ductos ejaculatórios e típico do sistema genital (epitélio colunar estratificado) distalmente, que continua através da uretra intermediária e da maior parte da uretra esponjosa, mudando novamente para um epitélio escamoso estratificado na região da fossa navicular; há muitos recessos na mucosa da porção esponjosa que continuam nas glândulas mucosas ramificadas tubulares. SIN tunica urethrae masculinae [TA], mucous membrane of male urethra.
m. of mouth [TA], túnica mucosa da boca; a mucosa da cavidade oral, incluindo a gengiva. SIN oral m. [TA], tunica mucosa oris [TA].
nasal m., m. nasal. SIN m. of nose.
m. of nose [TA], túnica mucosa do nariz; o revestimento da cavidade nasal, contínuo com a pele no vestíbulo do nariz e com a mucosa da nasofaringe, seios paranasais e ducto nasolacrimal e contém células caliciformes; é subdividida na região olfatória e região respiratória. SIN tunica mucosa nasi [TA], mucous membrane of nose*, membrana pituitosa, nasal m., pituitary membrane, schneiderian membrane.
olfactory m. m. olfatória. SIN olfactory region of mucosa of nose.
oral m. [TA], túnica mucosa da boca. SIN m. of mouth.
pharyngeal m., túnica mucosa da faringe. SIN m. of pharynx.
m. of pharyngotympanic (auditory) tube [TA], túnica mucosa da tuba auditiva (faringotimpânica); o revestimento da tuba auditiva. SIN tunica mucosa tubae auditivae [TA], mucous membrane of pharyngotympanic auditory tube*, tunica mucosa tubae auditoriae.
m. of pharynx [TA], túnica mucosa da faringe; o revestimento mucoso da faringe. SIN tunica mucosa pharyngis [TA], mucous membrane of pharynx*, pharyngeal m.
m. of renal pelvis [TA], túnica mucosa da pelve renal; a mais interna das três camadas da parede da pelve renal, com estrutura idêntica à do ureter, isto é, consistindo em um epitélio de transição (urotélio) e uma lâmina própria subjacente. SIN tunica mucosa pelvis renalis [TA].

respiratory m., m. respiratória; epitélio colunar ciliado pseudo-estratificado com células caliciformes e uma lâmina própria contendo, além do tecido conjuntivo, numerosas glândulas soromucosas e, em algumas regiões, muitas veias de paredes finas que revestem as vias aéreas; inclui a parte respiratória da túnica mucosa do nariz [TA] (pars respiratoria tunicae mucosa nasi [TA]), túnica mucosa da traquéia [TA] (tunica mucosa tracheae [TA]) e túnica mucosa dos brônquios [TA] (tunica mucosa bronchi [TA]). VER respiratory *region* of mucosa of nasal cavity.

m. of seminal gland [TA], túnica mucosa da glândula seminal; a mucosa que reveste a glândula (vesícula) seminal. SIN tunica mucosa vesiculae seminalis*, m. of seminal vesicle.

m. of seminal vesicle, túnica mucosa da glândula seminal. SIN m. of seminal gland.

m. of small intestine [TA], túnica mucosa do intestino delgado; a mucosa que reveste o intestino delgado. SIN tunica mucosa intestini tenuis [TA], mucous membrane of small intestine*.

m. of stomach [TA], túnica mucosa do estômago; a camada mucosa do estômago. SIN tunica mucosa gastrica [TA], mucous membrane of stomach*, gastric m.

m. of tongue [TA], túnica mucosa da língua; a mucosa que forma a superfície da língua; a mucosa do dorso da língua parece aveludada devido à presença de numerosas papilas; a mucosa da superfície inferior é lisa e mais fina. SIN tunica mucosa linguae [TA], mucous membrane of tongue*, lingual m.

m. of trachea [TA], túnica mucosa da traquéia; a camada mucosa interna da traquéia. SIN tunica mucosa tracheae [TA], mucous membrane of trachea*, tracheal m.

tracheal m., túnica mucosa da traquéia. SIN m. of trachea.

m. of tympanic cavity [TA], túnica mucosa da cavidade timpânica; a mucosa que reveste a cavidade timpânica e as estruturas nela contidas. SIN tunica mucosa cavitatis tympani [TA], mucous membrane of tympanic cavity*.

m. of ureter [TA], túnica mucosa do ureter; a camada mucosa interna do ureter. SIN tunica mucosa ureteris [TA], mucous membrane of ureter*.

m. of urethra [TA], túnica mucosa da uretra. VER m. of female urethra, m. of male urethra.

m. of (urinary) bladder [TA], túnica mucosa da bexiga; a camada interna da bexiga. SIN tunica mucosa vesicae urinariae [TA], mucous membrane of urinary bladder*.

m. of uterine tube [TA], túnica mucosa da tuba uterina; a camada mucosa interna da tuba uterina. SIN tunica mucosa tubae uterinae [TA], mucous membrane of uterine tube*.

m. of vagina [TA], túnica mucosa da vagina; a camada mucosa da vagina. SIN tunica mucosa vaginae [TA], mucous membrane of vagina*, vaginal m.

vaginal m., mucosa da vagina. SIN m. of vagina.

mu·co·sal (mū-kō′sǎl). Mucoso; relativo à mucosa ou membrana mucosa.

mu·co·san·guin·e·ous, mu·co·san·guin·o·lent. (mū′-kō-săng-gwin′e-ŭs, -ō-lent). Mucossanguíneo, mucossanguinolento; relativo a um exsudato ou a outro material líquido que possui um conteúdo relativamente alto de sangue e muco. [muco- + L. *sanguis,* sangue]

mu·co·sec·to·my (mū-kō-sek′to-me). Mucossectomia; excisão da mucosa, geralmente do reto, antes de anastomose ileoanal. [mucosa- + G. *ektome,* excisão]

mu·co·se·rous (mū-kō-sē′rŭs). Mucosseroso; relativo a um exsudato ou secreção que consiste em muco e soro ou em um componente aquoso.

mu·co·stat·ic (mū-kō-stat′ik). Mucostático. **1.** Designa a condição relaxada normal dos tecidos mucosos que revestem a mandíbula e a maxila. **2.** Que interrompe a secreção de muco. [muco- + G. *stasis,* imobilidade]

mu·cous (mū′kŭs). Mucoso; relativo ao muco ou a uma mucosa. [L. *mucosus,* mucoso, de *mucus*]

mu·co·vis·ci·do·sis (mū′kō-vis-i-dō′sis). Mucoviscidose. SIN cystic fibrosis. [mycro- + G. *toxikon,* veneno, + -osis, condição]

mu·cro, pl. **mu·cron·es** (mū′krō-, mū-krō′nēz). Mucro; termo aplicado à extremidade pontiaguda de uma estrutura. [L. ponta, espada]

m. cor′dis, m. do coração; termo obsoleto para *apex* of heart.

m. ster′ni, processo xifóide. SIN xiphoid *process.*

mu·cron (mū′kron). Mucron; organela de fixação de gregarinas asseptadas, semelhante a um epimerito; este último é separado do resto do corpo da gregarina por um septo.

mu·cro·nate (mū′krō-nāt). Mucronado, xifóide. SIN xiphoid. [L. *mucronatus,* pontiagudo]

mu·cus (mū′kŭs). Muco; a secreção viscosa clara das mucosas, que consiste em mucina, células epiteliais, leucócitos e vários sais inorgânicos dissolvidos em água. [L.]

glairy m., m. viscoso. SIN pituita.

Muehrcke, Robert C., nefrologista norte-americano do século XX. VER Muehrcke *bands,* em *band;* M. *lines,* em *line;* Muehrcke *sign.*

Mueller. Fabricante norte-americano de instrumentos cirúrgicos. VER Mueller electronic *tonometer.*

Muel·le·ri·us cap·il·la·ris (mū-ler′ē-ŭs kap-i-lā′ris). Uma das espécies mais comuns de vermes pulmonares capilares (subfamília Protostrongylinae) de ovinos, caprinos e cervídeos. É menor que o *Dictyocaulus,* habita os brônquios menores e o parênquima pulmonar, e é relativamente não-patogênico para seu hospedeiro.

MUGA Acrônimo para multiple-gated acquisition *scan.*

Muir, Edward G., cirurgião britânico, 1906–1973. VER M.-Torre *syndrome.*

Mules, Philip H., oftalmologista inglês, 1843–1905. VER M. *operation.*

mu·li·e·bria (moo′le-ē′brē-ă). Os órgãos genitais femininos. [L. neutro pl. de *muliebris,* relativo a *mulier,* uma mulher]

Müller, Friedrich von, médico alemão, 1858–1941. VER M. *sign.*

Müller, Heinrich, anatomista alemão, 1820–1864. VER M. radial *cells,* em *cell, fibers,* em *fiber, muscle, trigone.*

Müller, Hermann F., histologista alemão, 1866–1898. VER formol-M. *fixative;* M. *fixative.*

Müller, Johannes P., anatomista, fisiologista e patologista alemão, 1801–1858. VER M. *capsule, duct, law, maneuver, tubercle;* müllerian *agenesis.*

Müller, Leopold, oftalmologista tchecoslovaco, 1862–1936.

Müller, Peter, obstetra alemão, 1836–1922. VER Hillis-M. *maneuver.*

Müller, Walther, físico alemão do século XX. VER Geiger-M. *counter, tube.*

mül·le·ri·an (mū-ler′ē-an). Mülleriano; atribuído a, ou descrito por, Johannes Müller.

mul·ling (mŭl′ing). Em odontologia, a etapa final de mistura do amálgama dentário, quando a massa triturada é amassada para completar a amalgamação.

mult·ang·u·lar (mŭl-tang′gū-lăr). Multiangular; que possui muitos ângulos.

△ **multi-.** Multi-; muitos. VER TAMBÉM pluri-. Cf. poly-. [L. *multus,* muito]

mul·ti·ar·tic·u·lar (mŭl′tē-ar-tik′ū-lăr). Multiarticular; relativo a, ou envolve, muitas articulações. SIN polyarthric, polyarticular. [multi- + L. *articulus,* articulação]

mul·ti·bac·il·lary (mŭl-tē-bas′i-lār-ē). Multibacilar; constituído de, ou que indica existir, muitos bacilos.

mul·ti·cap·su·lar (mŭl-tē-kap′soo-lăr). Multicapsular; que possui numerosas cápsulas.

mul·ti·cel·lu·lar (mŭl-tē-sel′ū-lăr). Multicelular; composto de muitas células.

Mul·ti·ceps (mŭl′ti-seps). Gênero de vermes teníedeos no qual as formas larvares em herbívoros ocorrem na forma de cenuro (múltiplos escólices invaginados em um único cisto). [multi- + L. *caput,* cabeça]

M. mul′ticeps, espécie cuja forma madura é encontrada no intestino de cães; o cenuro desenvolve-se nos encéfalos de animais herbívoros, principalmente ovinos; o cisto freqüentemente é denominado *Coenurus cerebralis.*

M. seria′lis, espécie cuja forma madura é encontrada no intestino de cães; o cenuro é encontrado nos tecidos subcutâneos de coelhos.

mul·ti·col·lin·e·ar·i·ty (mŭl′tē-kol′in-ē-ar′i-tē). Multicolinearidade; em análise de regressão múltipla, situação na qual pelo menos algumas variáveis independentes em um conjunto estão altamente correlacionadas entre si. [multi- + L. *col·lineo,* alinhar]

mul·ti-CSF Abreviatura de multicolony-stimulating *factor* (fator estimulante de múltiplas colônias).

mul·ti·cus·pid (mŭl-tē-kŭs′pid). Multicúspide. SIN multicuspidate (2).

mul·ti·cus·pi·date (mŭl-tē-kŭs′pi-dāt). Multicuspidado. **1.** Que possui mais de duas cúspides. **2.** Dente molar com três ou mais cúspides ou projeções na coroa. SIN multicuspid.

mul·ti·en·zyme (mŭl′tī-en′zīm, mŭl′tē-). Multienzimático; referente a várias enzimas; p. ex., complexo multienzimático.

mul·ti·fe·ta·tion (mŭl-tē-fe-tā′shŭn). Multifetação. SIN superfetation.

mul·ti·fid (mŭl′tē-fid). Multifido; dividido em muitas fendas ou segmentos. SIN multifidus (1). [L. *multifidus,* de *multus,* muito, + *findo,* clivar]

mul·tif·i·dus (mŭl-tif′i-dŭs). Multífido. **1.** SIN multifid. **2.** VER multifidus (*muscle*). [L.]

mul·ti·fo·cal (mŭl-tē-fō′kăl). Multifocal; relativo a, ou que se origina de, muitos focos.

mul·ti·form (mŭl′ti-fōrm). Multiforme. SIN polymorphic.

mul·ti·glan·du·lar (mŭl-tē-glan′dū-lăr). Multiglandular. SIN pluriglandular.

mul·ti·grav·i·da (mŭl-tē-grav′i-dă). Multigrávida; mulher grávida que já esteve grávida uma ou mais vezes antes. [multi- + L. *gravida,* grávida]

mul·ti·in·fec·tion (mŭl′tē-in-fek′shŭn). Multiinfecção; infecção mista por duas ou mais formas de microrganismos que se desenvolvem simultaneamente.

mul·ti·lo·bar, mul·ti·lo·bate, mul·ti·lobed (mŭl-tē-lō′bar, -lō′bāt, -lōbd′). Multilobar; que possui vários lobos.

mul·ti·lob·u·lar (mŭl-tē-lob′ū-lăr). Multilobular; que possui muitos lóbulos.

mul·ti·lo·cal (mŭl-tē-lō′kăl). Multilocal; designa traços com uma etiologia que compreende os efeitos de múltiplos *loci* genéticos que operam juntos e simultaneamente. Cf. galtonian.

mul·ti·loc·u·lar (mŭl-tē-lok′ū-lăr). Multilocular; que tem muitas células; que possui muitos compartimentos ou lóculos. SIN plurilocular.

mul·ti·mam·mae (mŭl-tē-mam′ē). Polimastia. SIN polymastia. [multi- + L. *mamma,* mama]

multinodal   1012   **murmur**

mul·ti·no·dal (mŭl - tē - nō′dăl). Multinodal; que possui muitos nodos.
mul·ti·nod·u·lar, mul·ti·nod·u·late (mŭl - tē - nŏd′u - lăr, - ū - lāt). Multinodular; que possui muitos nódulos.
mul·ti·nu·cle·ar, mul·ti·nu·cle·ate (mŭl - tē - noo′klē - ăr, - āt). Multinuclear; multinucleado; que possui dois ou mais núcleos. SIN plurinuclear, polynuclear, polynucleate.
mul·ti·nu·cle·o·sis (mool′tē - nook - lē - ō′sis). Multinucleose. SIN polynucleosis.
mul·tip·a·ra (mŭl - tip′a - ra). Multípara; mulher que deu à luz, pelo menos duas vezes, um lactente, vivo ou não, pesando 500 g ou mais, ou com uma duração estimada da gestação de, pelo menos, 20 semanas. [multi- + L. *pario*, produzir, trazer]
    grand m., grande m.; multípara que deu à luz cinco vezes ou mais.
mul·ti·par·i·ty (mŭl - tē - par′i - tē). Multiparidade; condição de ser uma multípara.
mul·tip·a·rous (mŭl - tip′a - rŭs). Multíparo; relativo a uma multípara.
mul·ti·par·tial (mŭl′tē - par′shal). Polivalente, em relação a um anti-soro.
mul·ti·ple (mŭl′ti - pl). Múltiplo; repetido várias vezes; que ocorre em várias partes ao mesmo tempo, como a artrite múltipla, neurite múltipla. [L. *multiplex*, de *multus*, muitos, + *plico*, pp. -*atus*, dobrar]
mul·ti·po·lar (mŭl - tē - pō′lar). Multipolar; que possui mais de dois pólos; designa uma célula nervosa na qual os ramos se projetam de vários pontos.
mul·ti·root·ed (mŭl - tē - root′ed). Multirradicular; que tem mais de duas raízes.
mul·ti·ro·ta·tion (mŭl - tē - rō - tā′shŭn). Multirrotação. SIN mutarotation.
mul·ti·sub·strate (mŭl - ti - sub′stăt, mŭl - tē′-). Multissubstrato; que se refere a uma enzima, receptor ou proteína aceptora que precisa de dois ou mais substratos.
mul·ti·syn·ap·tic (mŭl′tē - si - nap′tik). Multissináptico. SIN polysynaptic.
mul·ti·va·lence, mul·ti·va·len·cy (mŭl - tē - vā′lens, - vā′len - sē). Multivalência, polivalência; o estado de ser multivalente (polivalente).
mul·ti·va·lent (mŭl - tē - vā′lent). Multivalente. **1.** Em química, que possui um poder combinatório (valência) de mais de um átomo de hidrogênio. **2.** Eficaz em mais de uma direção. **3.** Anti-soro específico para mais de um antígeno ou organismo. **4.** Antígeno ou anticorpo com um poder combinatório maior que dois. SIN polyvalent (1).
mum·mi·fi·ca·tion (mŭm′i - fi - kā′shŭn). Mumificação. **1.** Gangrena seca. SIN dry gangrene. **2.** Enrugamento de um feto morto retido. **3.** Em odontologia, tratamento da polpa dentária inflamada com substâncias fixadoras (geralmente derivados do formaldeído) a fim de reter os dentes assim tratados por períodos relativamente curtos; geralmente aceitável apenas para dentes primários (decíduos). [mummy- + L. *facio*, fazer]
mumps (mŭmps). Caxumba; doença infecciosa aguda e contagiosa causada por um vírus do gênero Rubulavirus e caracterizada por febre, inflamação e edema da glândula parótida, algumas vezes de outras glândulas salivares, e, ocasionalmente, por inflamação do testículo, ovário, pâncreas ou meninges. SIN epidemic parotiditis. [Inglês dialético, *mump*, inchação ou ressalto]
    metastatic m., caxumba metastática; caxumba complicada por envolvimento de outros órgãos além das glândulas parótidas, como o testículo, a mama ou o pâncreas.
mumpvirus. SIN Rubulavirus.
Münchhausen, Barão Karl F.H. von, nobre, soldado e contador de histórias alemão, 1720–1797. VER Munchausen *syndrome*; Munchausen *syndrome* by proxy.
Munro, John C., cirurgião norte-americano, 1858–1910. VER M. *point*.
Munro, William J., dermatologista australiano, 1863–1908. VER M. *abscess, microabscess*.
Munsell, Albert H., artista norte-americano, 1858–1918. VER Farnsworth-M. color *test*.
Munsell, Hazel E., químico norte-americano, *1891. VER Sherman-M. *unit*.
Munson, Edward Sterling, oftalmologista norte-americano, *1933. VER Munson *sign*.
Münzer, Egmont, médico austríaco, 1865–1924. VER *tract* of M. and Wiener.
Mur Abreviatura de muramic acid (ácido murâmico).
mu·ral (mū′răl). Mural; relativo à parede de qualquer cavidade. [L. *muralis;* de *murus*, parede]
mu·ram·ic ac·id (Mur) (mū - ram′ik). Ácido murâmico; 2-amino-3-*O*-(1-carboxietil)-2-desoxi-D-glicose; D-glucosamina e lactato em ligação éter entre as posições 3 e 2, respectivamente; um constituinte das mureínas nas paredes celulares bacterianas.
mu·ram·i·dase (mū - ram′i - dās). Muramidase. SIN lysozyme.
mu·reins (mūr′enz). Mureínas; peptidoglicanos que compõem o sáculo ou célula que cobre as bactérias e que consistem em polissacarídeos lineares de unidades alternadas de *N*-acetil-D-glucosamina e ácido *N*-acetilmurâmico, a cujas cadeias laterais lactato estão ligados oligopeptídeos; as cadeias independentes estão ligadas de forma cruzada em três dimensões através dos peptídeos ou dos grupos 6-OH (estes últimos podem estar ligados, via fosfato, a um ácido teicóico). [L. *murus*, parede]
Muret, Paul-Louis, médico francês, *1878. VER Quénu-M. *sign*.

mu·rex·ide (mū - rek′sīd, - sid). Murexida; o sal amoniacal do ácido purpúrico, antigamente usado como corante, mas substituído pelos corantes anilina.
mu·ri·ate (mū′rē - āt). Muriato; termo antigo para cloreto. [L. *muria*, salmoura]
mu·ri·at·ic (mū - rē - at′ik). Muriático; relacionado a salmoura. [L. *muriaticus*, conservado em salmoura, de *muria*, salmoura]
mu·ri·at·ic ac·id. Muriático, ácido clorídrico. SIN hydrochloric acid.
Mu·ri·dae (mū′ri - dē). A maior família de Rodentia e de mamíferos, compreendendo os camundongos e ratos do Velho Mundo. [L. *mus* (*mur*-), camundongo]
mu·ri·form (mūr′i - fōrm). Muriforme; multicelular com septos transversais e longitudinais; designa um agregado de células que se encaixam como pedras em uma parede de pedra. [L. *murus*, parede, + -form]
mu·rine (mū′rīn, - rin, - rēn). Murino; relativo a animais da família Muridae. [L. *murinus*, relativo a camundongos, de *mus* (*mur*-), camundongo]
mur·mur (mer′mer). Sopro. **1.** Ruído suave, como aquele produzido pela expiração algo forçada com a boca aberta, ouvido à ausculta do coração, pulmões ou vasos sanguíneos. SIN susurrus. **2.** Outro som além do sopro, que pode ser alto, áspero, friccional, etc.; p. ex., sopros cardíacos orgânicos podem ser suaves ou fortes e ásperos; os sopros pericárdicos geralmente são de atrito e mais apropriadamente descritos como "atritos" que como sopros. [L.]
    accidental m., s. acidental; sopro cardíaco evanescente não causado por lesão valvar.
    anemic m., s. anêmico; sopro não-valvar ouvido à ausculta do coração e dos grandes vasos sanguíneos em casos de anemia profunda, associado principalmente ao fluxo sanguíneo turbulento devido à diminuição da viscosidade sanguínea.
    aneurysmal m., s. aneurismático; sopro sistólico ou diastólico ouvido sobre alguns aneurismas cardíacos.
    aortic m., s. aórtico; sopro produzido no orifício aórtico, seja obstrutivo ou regurgitante.
    arterial m., s. arterial; sopro ouvido ao auscultar uma artéria.
    atriosystolic m., s. pré-sistólico. SIN presystolic m.
    Austin Flint m., s. de Austin Flint. SIN Austin Flint *phenomenon*, Flint m.
    bellows m., s. de fole; ruído soprado.
    brain m., s. encefálico; sons produzidos por aneurismas intracranianos ou aneurismas arteriovenosos na angiomatose displásica congênita.
    Cabot-Locke m., s. de Cabot-Locke; um sopro protodiastólico, como o da insuficiência aórtica, mais bem auscultado na borda esternal inferior esquerda na anemia grave.

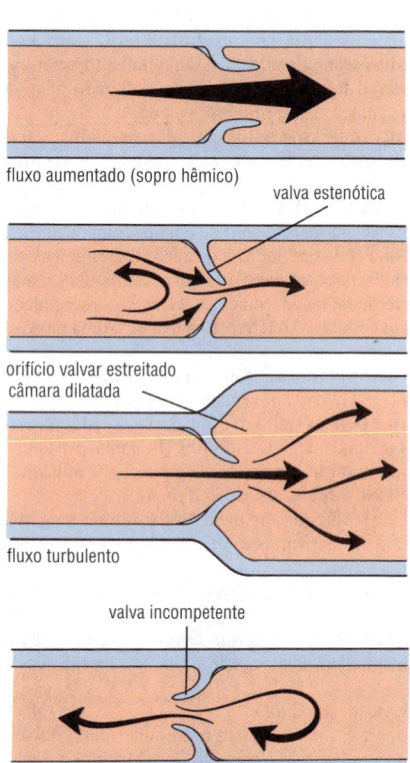

origem dos sopros cardíacos

cardiac m., s. cardíaco; sopro produzido no coração, em um de seus orifícios valvares ou através de comunicações interventriculares.

cardiopulmonary m., s. cardiopulmonar; sopro extracardíaco inocente, sincrônico com o batimento cardíaco, mas que desaparece quando a respiração é interrompida, considerado devido ao movimento de ar em um segmento pulmonar comprimido pela contração cardíaca.

cardiorespiratory m., s. cardiorrespiratório. SIN cardiopulmonary m.

Carey Coombs m., s. de Carey Coombs; sopro mesodiastólico apical bolhoso, que ocorre no estágio agudo da valvulite mitral reumática e desaparece quando cessa a valvulite. SIN Coombs m.

Cole-Cecil m., s. de Cole-Cecil; o sopro diastólico da insuficiência aórtica quando ouvido bem ou predominantemente na axila esquerda.

continuous m., s. contínuo; sopro ouvido sem interrupção durante toda a sístole e a diástole.

cooing m., s. em arrulho; sopro, geralmente de regurgitação mitral, de intensidade muito alta, semelhante ao arrulho de um pombo ou de uma pomba.

Coombs m., s. de Coombs. SIN Carey Coombs m.

crescendo m., s. em crescendo; sopro que aumenta em intensidade e cessa subitamente; o sopro pré-sistólico da estenose mitral é um exemplo comum.

Cruveilhier-Baumgarten m., s. de Cruveilhier-Baumgarten; sopro venoso ouvido sobre veias colaterais que unem os sistemas venosos porta e cava, na parede abdominal. VER TAMBÉM Cruveilhier-Baumgarten *sign.*

diamond-shaped m., s. em diamante; sopro em crescendo-decrescendo, recebe esse nome devido ao formato da curva de intensidade de freqüência do fonocardiograma, freqüentemente audível dessa forma.

diastolic m. (DM), s. diastólico; sopro ouvido durante a diástole.

Duroziez m., s. de Duroziez; sopro bifásico sobre artérias periféricas, principalmente a artéria femoral, devido ao fluxo e refluxo de sangue durante insuficiência aórtica. SIN Duroziez sign.

dynamic m., s. dinâmico; sopro cardíaco devido à anemia ou a qualquer outra causa além de uma lesão valvar.

early diastolic m., s. protodiastólico; sopro que começa com a segunda bulha, como o sopro da insuficiência aórtica.

ejection m., s. de ejeção; sopro sistólico, em forma de diamante, produzido pela ejeção de sangue para a aorta ou artéria pulmonar e terminando no momento do componente da segunda bulha, produzido, respectivamente, pelo fechamento da valva aórtica ou pulmonar.

endocardial m., s. endocárdico; sopro, de qualquer causa, originado no coração.

extracardiac m., s. extracardíaco; sopro audível sobre o precórdio, ou próximo dele, originado de outras estruturas além do coração; o termo inclui atritos pericárdicos e sopros cardiopulmonares.

Flint m., s. de Flint; sopro diastólico, semelhante ao da estenose mitral, mais bem auscultado no ápice cardíaco em alguns casos de insuficiência aórtica livre; possivelmente causado pelo fluxo regurgitante turbulento da aorta misturando-se ao fluxo proveniente do átrio esquerdo, que entra simultaneamente através da valva mitral, causando movimento posterior da válvula anterior da valva mitral com aceleração transitória do fluxo sanguíneo através dela. SIN Austin Flint m.

Fräntzel m., s. de Fräntzel; sopro de estenose mitral quando mais alto em seu início e fim que em sua porção média.

friction m., atrito. SIN friction *sound.*

functional m., s. funcional; sopro cardíaco não associado a uma lesão cardíaca significativa. SIN innocent m., inorganic m.

Gibson m., s. de Gibson; o sopro "em maquinaria" contínuo, típico da persistência do canal arterial.

Graham Steell m., s. de Graham Steell; sopro protodiastólico de insuficiência pulmonar secundária à hipertensão pulmonar, como na estenose mitral e em vários defeitos congênitos associados à hipertensão pulmonar. SIN Steell m.

Hamman m., s. de Hamman; crepitação precordial, sincrônica com o batimento cardíaco; ouvida no enfisema pulmonar; também conhecida como crepitação de Hamman.

hemic m., s. hêmico; sopro cardíaco ou vascular auscultado em pessoas anêmicas sem lesão valvular, provavelmente devido ao aumento da velocidade do sangue e à turbulência que caracterizam a anemia.

Hodgkin-Key m., s. de Hodgkin-Key; sopro diastólico musical associado à retroversão de uma cúspide aórtica; ouvido e muito alto.

holosystolic m., s. holossistólico. SIN pansystolic m.

hourglass m., s. em ampulheta; sopro no qual há duas áreas de intensidade máxima, diminuindo até um ponto médio entre as duas.

innocent m., s. inocente. SIN functional m.

inorganic m., s. inorgânico. SIN functional m.

late apical systolic m., s. telessistólico apical; sopro previamente considerado benigno, ou mesmo extracardíaco, com uma possível relação com doença pericárdica; freqüentemente representa insuficiência mitral, muitas vezes localizada e de intensidade moderada, mas com propensão a desenvolver endocardite bacteriana, e amiúde está associado a estalido sistólico e prolapso mitral (síndrome de Barlow; abaulamento ou ondulação da cúspide da valva mitral), muitas vezes produzindo um estalido e/ou sopro, como quando prolapsa para o átrio esquerdo durante a sístole.

late diastolic m., s. telediastólico, s. pré-sistólico. SIN presystolic m.

machinery m., s. "em maquinaria"; o sopro retumbante "contínuo" longo da persistência do canal arterial.

middiastolic m., s. mesodiastólico; sopro que começa após a abertura das valvas A-V na diástole, isto é, um período considerável após a segunda bulha, como o sopro da estenose mitral.

mill wheel m., s. em roda de moinho; sopro cardíaco semelhante produzido por embolia gasosa cardíaca; também é ouvido no pneumoidropericárdio. SIN water wheel m.

mitral m., s. mitral; sopro produzido na valva mitral, seja obstrutivo ou regurgitante.

musical m., s. musical; sopro cardíaco ou vascular que possui um tom musical agudo.

nun's m., zumbido venoso. SIN venous *hum.*

obstructive m., s. obstrutivo; sopro causado por estreitamento de um dos orifícios valvares.

organic m., s. orgânico; sopro causado por uma lesão orgânica.

pansystolic m., s. pansistólico; sopro que ocupa todo o intervalo sistólico, da primeira até a segunda bulha. SIN holosystolic m.

pericardial m., s. pericárdico; som de atrito, sincrônico com os movimentos cardíacos, ouvido em alguns casos de pericardite.

pleuropericardial m., s. pleuropericárdico; som de atrito pleural sobre a região pericárdica, sincrônico com a atividade cardíaca e simulando um sopro pericárdico (atrito).

presystolic m., s. pré-sistólico; sopro auscultado no final da diástole ventricular (durante a sístole atrial se estiver em ritmo sinusal), geralmente devido à obstrução em um dos orifícios atrioventriculares. SIN atriosystolic m., late diastolic m.

pulmonary m., pulmonic m., s. pulmonar; sopro produzido no orifício pulmonar do coração, seja obstrutivo ou regurgitante.

regurgitant m., s. regurgitante; sopro devido ao extravasamento ou fluxo retrógrado em um dos orifícios valvulares do coração.

respiratory m., s. respiratório. SIN vesicular *respiration.*

Roger m., s. de Roger; sopro pansistólico alto, máximo na borda esternal esquerda, causado por uma pequena comunicação interventricular. SIN bruit de Roger, Roger bruit.

sea gull m., pio de gaivota; sopro que imita o pio de uma gaivota, quase sempre devido à estenose aórtica ou regurgitação mitral.

seesaw m., s. de vaivém. SIN to-and-fro m.

Steell m., s. de Steell. SIN Graham-Steell m.

stenosal m., s. estenótico; sopro arterial devido ao estreitamento do vaso por pressão ou alteração orgânica.

Still m., s. de Still; sopro musical inocente, semelhante ao ruído produzido por uma corda tensa; ouvido quase exclusivamente em crianças pequenas, de origem incerta e acaba por desaparecer.

systolic m., s. sistólico; sopro ouvido durante a sístole ventricular.

to-and-fro m., s. de vaivém; sopro auscultado na sístole e na diástole cardíacas, como na estenose e na insuficiência aórticas. SIN seesaw m.

tricuspid m., s. tricúspide; sopro produzido no orifício tricúspide, seja obstrutivo ou regurgitante.

vascular m., s. vascular; sopro originado em um vaso sanguíneo.

venous m., s. venoso; sopro auscultado sobre uma veia.

vesicular m., s. vesicular. SIN vesicular *respiration.*

water wheel m., s. em moinho de água. SIN mill wheel m.

mu·ro·mo·nab-CD3 (mū - rō - mō'nab). Muromonab-CD3; anticorpo monoclonal murino contra o antígeno T3 (CD3) de linfócitos T humanos, usado como imunossupressor no tratamento da rejeição aguda de aloenxerto após transplante renal.

Murphy, John B., cirurgião norte-americano, 1857–1916. VER M. *drip, button, percussion.*

Mus (mŭs). Gênero da família Muridae que inclui cerca de 16 espécies de camundongos; as raças domesticadas são numerosas e geneticamente bem definidas, sendo as mais populares as raças albina e malhada. [L. *mus* (mur-), camundongo]

Mus·ca (mŭs'kă). Gênero de moscas (família Muscidae, ordem Diptera) que inclui a mosca doméstica comum, *M. domestica*, espécie universalmente associada aos seres humanos, particularmente em condições precárias de higiene; reproduz-se na sujeira e no lixo orgânico, e está envolvida na transferência mecânica de numerosos patógenos. [L. mosca]

mus·cae vol·i·tan·tes (mŭs'sē, mŭs'kē vol - i - tan'tēs). Moscas volantes; surgimento de pontos móveis diante dos olhos, originados de remanescentes do sistema vascular hialóide embriológico no humor vítreo. [L. pl. de *musca,* mosca; pres. ppl. de *volito,* voar de um lado para outro]

mus·ca·rine (mŭs'kă - rēn, - rin). Muscarina; toxina com efeitos neurológicos, isolada pela primeira vez da *Amanita muscaria* (agárico das moscas) e também presente em algumas espécies de *Hebeloma* e *Inocybe*. O sal trimetilamônio quaternário do 2-metil-3-hidroxi-5-(aminometil)-tetraidrofurano é uma substância colinérgica cujos efeitos farmacológicos assemelham-se aos da acetilcolina e da estimulação parassimpática pós-ganglionar (inibição cardíaca, vasodilatação, salivação, lacrimejamento, broncoconstrição, estimulação gastrointestinal).

mus·ca·rin·ic (mŭs-kă-rin′ik). Muscarínico. **1.** Que possui uma ação semelhante à da muscarina, isto é, que produz efeitos semelhantes à estimulação parassimpática pós-ganglionar. **2.** Um agente que estimula o receptor parassimpático pós-ganglionar. VER TAMBÉM muscarine, nicotinic.

mus·ca·rin·ism (mŭs′kă-rin-izm). Muscarinismo. SIN mycetism.

Mus·ci (mŭs′sī). A classe de plantas que inclui os musgos. [L. pl. de *muscus*, musgo]

mus·ci·cide (mŭs′ĭ-sīd). Muscicida; agente destrutivo para moscas. [L. *musca*, mosca, + *caedo*, matar]

Mus·ci·dae (mŭs′ĭ-dē). A família de moscas (ordem Diptera) que inclui as moscas domésticas (*Musca*) e as moscas do estábulo (*Stomoxys*). [L. *musca*, mosca]

mus·ci·mol (mus′ĭ-mol). Muscimol; alcalóide extraído do cogumelo venenoso *Amanita muscaria*; estimula seletivamente receptores do ácido γ-aminobutírico (GABA) e é usado como sonda molecular para estudo dos receptores GABA; potente depressor do SNC, o muscimol inibe a função motora e pode levar à psicose.

MUSCLE

ℹ️ **mus·cle** (mŭs′el)[TA]. Músculo; tecido primário que consiste predominantemente em células contráteis bastante especializadas, que podem ser classificadas como m. esquelético, m. cardíaco ou m. liso; microscopicamente, este último não possui as estriações transversais características dos outros dois tipos; um dos órgãos contráteis do corpo pelo qual são realizados os movimentos dos vários órgãos e partes; o músculo típico é uma massa de fibras musculares (ventre), inserida em cada extremidade, por meio de um tendão, a um osso ou outra estrutura; a inserção mais proximal ou mais fixa é denominada origem (*origin*); a inserção mais distal ou mais móvel é a inserção (*insertion*); a parte mais estreita do ventre fixada ao tendão de origem é denominada cabeça. Ver a descrição anatômica macroscópica em musculus. SIN musculus [TA]. [L. *musculus*]

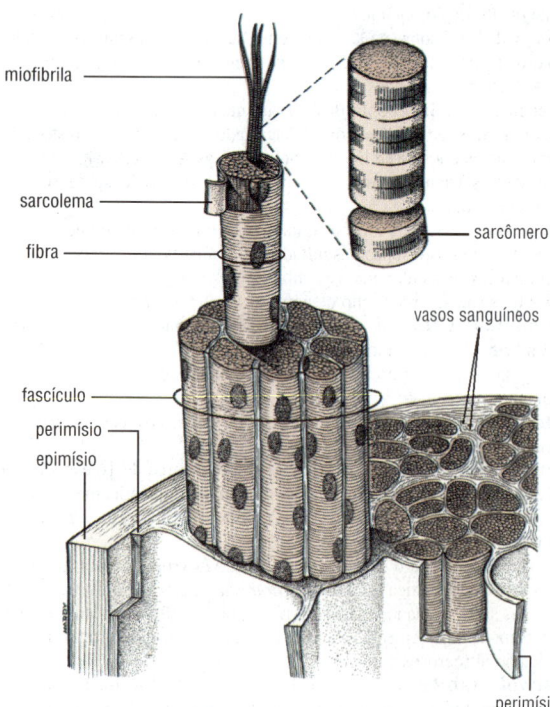

músculo esquelético: diagrama dos componentes do tecido conjuntivo; também são indicadas as relações entre um feixe muscular (fascículo), uma única célula muscular (fibra) e uma miofibrila

m.'s of abdomen [TA], músculos do abdome; músculos que formam a parede do abdome, incluindo os músculos reto, oblíquos externo e interno e transverso do abdome e quadrado do lombo. SIN musculi abdominis.

abdominal external oblique (m.), m. oblíquo externo do abdome. SIN external oblique (m.).

abdominal internal oblique m., m. oblíquo interno do abdome. SIN internal oblique (m.).

abductor (m.) [TA], m. abdutor; m. que causa movimento de afastamento do plano mediano do corpo, eixo do dedo médio da mão ou eixo do segundo dedo do pé, ou, no caso do polegar, anterior ao plano da palma da mão. SIN musculus abductor [TA], abductor.

abductor digiti minimi (m.) of foot [TA], m. abdutor do dedo mínimo do pé; m. da primeira camada de músculos plantares; *origem*, processos lateral e medial da tuberosidade do calcâneo; *inserção*, face lateral da falange proximal do quinto dedo do pé; *ação*, abduz e flete o dedo mínimo do pé; *inervação*, nervo plantar lateral. SIN musculus abductor digiti minimi pedis [TA], abductor m. of little toe, musculus abductor digiti quinti (2).

abductor digiti minimi (m.) of hand [TA], m. abdutor do dedo mínimo da mão; m. hipotenar superficial da palma da mão; *origem*, osso pisiforme e ligamento piso-hamato; *inserção*, face medial da base da falange proximal do dedo mínimo; *ação*, abduz e flete o dedo mínimo; *inervação*, ramo profundo do nervo ulnar. SIN musculus abductor digiti minimi manus [TA], abductor m. of little finger, musculus abductor digiti quinti (1).

abductor m. of great toe, m. abdutor do hálux. SIN abductor hallucis (m.).

abductor hallucis (m.) [TA], m. abdutor do hálux; m. da terceira camada dos músculos plantares; *origem*, processo medial da tuberosidade do calcâneo, retináculo dos músculos flexores e aponeurose plantar; *ação*, abduz o hálux; *inervação*, nervo plantar medial. SIN musculus abductor hallucis [TA], abductor m. of great toe.

abductor m. of little finger, m. abdutor do dedo mínimo da mão. SIN abductor digiti minimi (m.) of hand.

abductor m. of little toe, m. abdutor do dedo mínimo do pé. SIN abductor digiti minimi (m.) of foot.

abductor pollicis brevis (m.) [TA], m. abdutor curto do polegar; m. tenar superficial; *origem*, tubérculo do trapézio e retináculo dos músculos flexores; *inserção*, face lateral da falange proximal do polegar; *ação*, abduz o polegar; *inervação*, nervo mediano. SIN musculus abductor pollicis brevis [TA], short abductor m. of thumb.

abductor pollicis longus (m.) [TA], m. abdutor longo do polegar; m. que aflora do compartimento posterior do antebraço; *origem*, membrana interóssea e superfícies posteriores do rádio e ulna; *inserção*, face lateral da base do primeiro osso metacarpal; *ação*, abduz e ajuda na extensão do polegar; *inervação*, nervo radial. SIN musculus abductor pollicis longus [TA], long abductor m. of thumb, musculus extensor ossis metacarpi pollicis.

accessory flexor m. of foot, m. quadrado plantar. SIN quadratus plantae (m.).

adductor m. [TA], m. adutor; m. que causa movimento em direção ao plano mediano do corpo, ao eixo do terceiro dedo da mão ou segundo dedo do pé, ou, no caso do polegar, ao plano da palma da mão. SIN musculus adductor [TA], adductor.

adductor brevis (m.) [TA], m. adutor curto; m. do compartimento medial (adutor) da coxa; *origem*, ramo superior do púbis; *inserção*, terço superior do lábio medial da linha áspera; *ação*, aduz a coxa; *inervação*, nervo obturatório. SIN musculus adductor brevis [TA], short adductor m.

adductor m. of great toe, m. adutor do hálux. SIN adductor hallucis (m.).

adductor hallucis (m.) [TA], m. adutor do hálux; m. da terceira camada de músculos plantares; *origem*, por duas cabeças: a cabeça transversa, das cápsulas das quatro articulações metatarsofalângicas laterais, e a cabeça oblíqua, do cuneiforme lateral e das bases do terceiro e quarto ossos metatarsais; *inserção*, face lateral da base da falange proximal do hálux; *ação*, aduz o hálux; *inervação*, nervo plantar lateral. SIN musculus adductor hallucis [TA], adductor m. of great toe.

adductor longus (m.) [TA], m. adutor longo; m. do compartimento medial (adutor) da coxa; *origem*, sínfise e crista do púbis; *inserção*, terço médio do lábio medial da linha áspera; *ação*, aduz a coxa; *inervação*, nervo obturatório. SIN musculus adductor longus [TA], long adductor m.

adductor magnus (m.) [TA], m. adutor magno; m. do compartimento medial (adutor) da coxa; *origem*, tuberosidade isquiática e ramo isquiopúbico; *inserção*, linha áspera e tubérculo adutor do fêmur; *ação*, aduz e estende a coxa; *inervação*, nervos obturatório e ciático. SIN musculus adductor magnus [TA], great adductor m.

adductor minimus (m.) [TA], m. adutor mínimo; pequeno m. plano do compartimento medial (adutor) da coxa que consiste na porção superior do adutor magno; *inserção*, o espaço acima da linha áspera. SIN musculus adductor minimis [TA].

adductor pollicis (m.) [TA], m. adutor do polegar; m. intrínseco da palma; *origem*, por duas cabeças: a cabeça transversa origina-se da diáfise do terceiro metacarpal, e a cabeça oblíqua da frente da base do segundo metacarpal, dos ossos trapezóide e capitato; *inserção*, face medial da base da falange proximal

muscle

do polegar; *ação*, aduz o polegar; *inervação*, nervo ulnar. SIN musculus adductor pollicis [TA], adductor m. of thumb.
adductor m. of thumb, m. adutor do polegar. SIN adductor pollicis (m.).
Albinus m., m. de Albinus; **(1)** SIN risorius (m.); **(2)** scalenus minimus (m.).
m.'s of anal triangle [TA], músculos do trígono anal; músculos voluntários da região posterior ao corpo do períneo e músculos transversos do períneo e anteriores às margens inferiores dos músculos glúteos máximos; inclui o músculo levantador do ânus (incluindo o puborretal) e todas as partes do esfíncter externo do ânus. SIN musculi regionis analis [TA].
anconeus m. [TA], m. ancôneo; *origem*, dorso do côndilo lateral do úmero; *inserção*, olécrano e superfície posterior da ulna; *ação*, estende o antebraço e abduz a ulna (em pronação) do punho; *inervação*, nervo radial. SIN musculus anconeus [TA], anconeus.
anorectoperineal m.'s [TA], músculos anorretoperineais; fibras musculares lisas que seguem da camada muscular longitudinal do reto para a frente, até a parte membranácea da uretra no homem. SIN musculi anorectoperineales [TA], musculi rectourethrales*, rectourethral m.'s*.
antagonistic m.'s, músculos antagonistas; dois ou mais músculos que produzem movimentos (funções) opostos, e, teoricamente, a contração de um pode "neutralizar" a do outro; entretanto, ao fazê-lo, eles frequentemente estão agindo de forma sinérgica na fixação da parte em movimento.
anterior auricular m., m. auricular anterior. SIN auricularis anterior (m.).
anterior cervical intertransversarii (m.'s) [TA], músculos intertransversários anteriores do pescoço; m. profundo do dorso; *origem*, tubérculos anteriores dos processos transversos cervicais; *inserção*, tubérculo anterior do próximo processo transverso superior; *ação*, abduz as vértebras cervicais; *inervação*, ramo ventral dos nervos cervicais. SIN musculi intertransversarii anteriores cervicis [TA], anterior cervical intertransverse m.'s.
anterior cervical intertransverse m.'s, músculos intertransversários anteriores do pescoço. SIN anterior cervical intertransversarii (m.'s).
anterior rectus m. of head, m. reto anterior da cabeça. SIN rectus capitis anterior (m.).
anterior scalene m., m. escaleno anterior; *termo oficial alternativo para scalenus anterior (m.).
anterior serratus m., m. serrátil anterior. SIN serratus anterior (m.).
anterior tibial m., m. tibial anterior. SIN tibialis anterior (m.).
antigravity m.'s, músculos antigravitacionais; os músculos que mantêm a postura característica de determinada espécie de animal. Na maioria dos mamíferos são os músculos extensores.
antitragicus (m.) [TA], m. antitrágico; faixa de fibras musculares transversas na superfície externa do antitrago, originada da borda da incisura antitrágica e inserida na antélice e na cauda da hélice. SIN musculus antitragicus [TA], m. of antitragus.
m. of antitragus, m. antitrágico. SIN antitragicus (m.).
appendicular m., m. dos membros; um dos músculos esqueléticos dos membros.
arrector m. of hair [TA], m. eretor do pêlo; feixes de fibras musculares lisas, fixados à parte mais profunda dos folículos passivos, seguindo para fora ao longo das glândulas sebáceas até a camada papilar da derme; causam ereção dos pêlos, produzindo aspecto de "pele de galinha" (cútis anserina) nos seres humanos, mas aumentam a profundidade (eficiência) da pele/pêlo da maioria dos animais. SIN musculus arrector pili [TA], arrector pili m.'s, erector m. of hair.
arrector pili m.'s, músculos eretores dos pêlos. SIN arrector m. of hair.
articular m., m. articular; m. que se insere diretamente na cápsula de uma articulação, retraindo a cápsula em determinados movimentos. SIN musculus articularis.
articular m. of elbow, m. articular do cotovelo. SIN articularis cubiti (m.).
articularis cubiti (m.) [TA], m. articular do cotovelo; nome dado a uma pequena faixa da cabeça medial do tríceps que se insere na cápsula da articulação do cotovelo. SIN musculus articularis cubiti [TA], articular m. of elbow, subanconeus m.
articularis genus (m.) [TA], m. articular do joelho; porção profunda, distal do m. vasto intermédio; *origem*, quarto inferior da superfície anterior da diáfise do fêmur; *inserção*, bolsa suprapatelar da articulação do joelho; *ação*, retrai a bolsa suprapatelar durante a extensão do joelho; *inervação*, nervo femoral. SIN musculus articularis genus [TA], articular m. of knee, Dupré m., subcrural m., subcruralis, subcrureus, subquadricipital m.
articular m. of knee, m. articular do joelho. SIN articularis genus (m.).
aryepiglottic m., m. ariepiglótico; parte ariepiglótica do m. aritenóideo oblíquo. SIN aryepiglottic *part* of oblique arytenoid muscle.
m.'s of auditory ossicles [TA], músculos dos ossículos da audição; o músculo estapédio e o músculo tensor do tímpano. SIN musculi ossiculorum auditus [TA], musculi ossiculorum auditoriorum*.
auricular m.'s [TA], músculos auriculares; pequenos músculos associados à orelha que têm pouca função nos seres humanos. SIN musculi auriculares [TA].
auricularis anterior (m.) [TA], m. auricular anterior; *origem*, aponeurose epicrânica; *inserção*, cartilagem da orelha; *ação*, puxa a orelha para cima e para frente; *inervação*, nervo facial. Alguns o consideram a parte anterior do m. temporoparietal. SIN anterior auricular m., musculus attrahens aurem, musculus attrahens auriculam, musculus auricularis anterior, zygomaticoauricularis.
auricularis posterior (m.) [TA], m. auricular posterior; m. facial da orelha externa; *origem*, processo mastóide; *inserção*, porção posterior da raiz da orelha; *ação*, puxa a orelha para trás; *inervação*, nervo facial. SIN musculus auricularis posterior [TA], musculus retrahens aurem, musculus retrahens auriculam, posterior auricular (m.).
auricularis superior (m.) [TA], m. auricular superior; m. facial associado à orelha externa; *origem*, gálea aponeurótica; *inserção*, cartilagem da orelha; *ação*, leva a orelha para cima e para trás; *inervação*, nervo facial. Alguns o consideram a parte posterior do músculo temporoparietal. SIN musculus auricularis superior [TA], attollens aurem, attollens auriculam, musculus attollens aurem, musculus attollens auriculam, superior auricular m.
axial m., m. axial; um dos músculos esqueléticos do tronco ou da cabeça.
axillary arch m., m. do arco axilar. SIN pectorodorsalis m.
m.'s of back [TA], músculos do dorso; os músculos do dorso em geral, incluindo os músculos toracoapendiculares que fixam o cíngulo do membro superior ao tronco posteriormente, os músculos serráteis posteriores e os músculos eretor da espinha e espinotransversais. SIN musculi dorsi [TA], dorsal m.'s.
m.'s of back proper [TA], músculos próprios do dorso; músculos do dorso inervados pelos ramos primários dorsais dos nervos espinais; incluem os músculos eretor da espinha, espinotransversais, interespinais e intertransversários anteriores e laterais; excluem os músculos superficiais do dorso, que são apendiculares e inervados por ramos ventrais, e o trapézio, inervado pelo nervo acessório espinal. SIN musculi dorsi proprii [TA], deep m.'s of back, true m.'s of back.
Bell m., m. de Bell; faixa de fibras musculares que forma uma pequena prega na parede da bexiga, seguindo da úvula até a abertura do ureter de cada lado, limitando o trígono.
biceps m. of arm, m. bíceps braquial. SIN biceps brachii (m.).
biceps brachii (m.) [TA], m. bíceps braquial; m. superficial do compartimento anterior (flexor) do braço; *origem*, a cabeça longa origina-se do tubérculo supraglenoidal da escápula, e a cabeça curta origina-se do processo coracóide; *inserção*, tuberosidade do rádio; *ação*, flexão do cotovelo e supinação do antebraço (é o supinador primário do antebraço); *inervação*, nervo musculocutâneo. SIN musculus biceps brachii [TA], biceps m. of arm.
biceps femoris (m.) [TA], m. bíceps femoral; m. do jarrete do compartimento posterior da coxa; *origem*, a cabeça longa (caput longum) origina-se do túber isquiático, e a cabeça curta (caput breve) origina-se da metade inferior do lábio lateral da linha áspera; *inserção*, cabeça da fíbula; *ação*, flete o joelho e roda a perna fletida lateralmente; *inervação*, cabeça longa, nervo tibial; cabeça curta, nervo fibular. SIN musculus biceps femoris [TA], biceps m. of thigh, musculus biceps flexor cruris.
biceps m. of thigh, m. bíceps femoral. SIN biceps femoris (m.).
bipennate m., m. peniforme. SIN pennate m.
Bochdalek m., m. de Bochdalek. SIN *musculus* triticeoglossus.
Bowman m., m. de Bowman. SIN ciliary m.
brachial m., m. braquial. SIN brachialis (m.).
brachialis (m.) [TA], m. braquial; m. profundo do compartimento anterior (flexor) do braço; *origem*, dois terços inferiores da superfície anterior do úmero; *inserção*, processo coronóide da ulna; *ação*, flete o cotovelo; *inervação*, nervo musculocutâneo, geralmente com uma pequena contribuição do nervo radial. SIN musculus brachialis [TA], brachial m.
brachioradial m., m. braquiorradial. SIN brachioradialis (m.).
brachioradialis (m.) [TA], m. braquiorradial; m. do compartimento posterior (extensor) do antebraço; *origem*, crista supra-epicondilar lateral do úmero; *inserção*, face anterior da base do processo estilóide do rádio; *ação*, flete o cotovelo e ajuda no retorno do membro em pronação ou supinação à posição neutra; *inervação*, nervo radial (comum). SIN musculus brachioradialis [TA], brachioradial m.
branchiomeric m.'s, músculos branquioméricos; os músculos associados aos arcos branquiais; fornecem uma grande parte da musculatura para a face e pescoço; os mioblastos para esses músculos originam-se do mesoderma paroxial, enquanto a crista neural fornece seu tecido conjuntivo.
Braune m., m. de Braune. SIN puborectalis (m.).
broadest m. of back, m. latíssimo do dorso. SIN latissimus dorsi (m.).
bronchoesophageal m., m. broncoesofágico. SIN bronchoesophageus (m.).
bronchoesophageus (m.). [TA], m. broncoesofágico; fascículos musculares, originados da parede do brônquio esquerdo, que reforçam a musculatura do esôfago. SIN musculus bronchoesophageus [TA], bronchoesophageal m.
Brücke m., m. de Brücke; a parte do m. ciliar formada pelas fibras meridionais. SIN Crampton m.
buccinator (m.) [TA], m. bucinador; m. facial da bochecha; *origem*, porção posterior da parte alveolar da maxila e mandíbula e rafe pterigomandibular; *inserção*, ângulo da boca; também é interposto com partes mais horizontais do músculo orbicular da boca; *ação*, achata a bochecha, retrai o ângulo da boca; é importante na mastigação, trabalhando com a língua e com o m. orbicular da

boca para manter o alimento entre os dentes; quando está paralisado, como na paralisia de Bell, o alimento acumula-se no vestíbulo da boca; *inervação*, nervo facial. SIN musculus buccinator [TA], cheek m.

bulbocavernosus m., m. bulboesponjoso. SIN bulbospongiosus (m.).

bulbospongiosus (m.) [TA], m. bulboesponjoso; m. perineal; no homem: *origem*, a fáscia da membrana do períneo no dorso do bulbo do pênis; *inserção*, tendão central do períneo e rafe mediana na superfície livre do bulbo; *ação*, contração voluntária da uretra bulbar ao se tentar expelir as últimas gotas após a micção, ou espasmodicamente, durante e após a ejaculação, para expelir o sêmen. Na mulher: *origem*, o dorso do clitóris, o corpo cavernoso e a membrana perineal; *inserção*, tendão central do períneo; *ação*, atua como um fraco esfíncter da vagina; quando desenvolvido, é uma parte da "musculatura do membro cruzado" do assoalho pélvico que resiste ao prolapso das vísceras pélvicas; circunda e comprime a glândula vestibular maior, principalmente durante a ereção do bulbo do vestíbulo, emitindo a secreção. *Inervação*, nervo pudendo (ramo perineal profundo). SIN musculus bulbospongiosus [TA], bulbocavernosus m., musculus bulbocavernosus, musculus ejaculator seminis, musculus sphincter vaginae, sphincter vaginae.

cardiac m., m. cardíaco; o m. involuntário, compreendendo o miocárdio e as paredes das veias pulmonares e da veia cava superior, que consiste em fibras de músculos estriados que se anastomosam transversalmente, formados de células unidas a discos intercalados; os núcleos (um ou dois) de cada célula estão localizados centralmente, e as miofibrilas, dispostas em sentido longitudinal, apresentam considerável sarcoplasma ao seu redor; o tecido conjuntivo é limitado às fibras reticulares e colágenas finas; a contração é rítmica e intrinsecamente estimulada. SIN m. of heart.

Casser perforated m., m. perfurado de Casser; m. coracobraquial. SIN coracobrachialis m.

ceratocricoid (m.) [TA], m. ceratocricóideo; fascículo inconstante do m. cricoaritenóideo posterior, inserido no corno inferior da cartilagem tireóidea. SIN musculus ceratocricoideus [TA], Merkel m.

ceratoglossus (m.) [TA], m. ceratoglosso; parte posterior, principal, do m. hioglosso (*vs.* condroglosso), originada no corno maior do osso hióide. SIN musculus ceratoglossus [TA].

cervical iliocostal m., m. iliocostal do pescoço. SIN iliocostalis cervicis (m.).

cervical interspinal m., m. interespinal do pescoço. SIN interspinales cervicis (m.'s).

cervical interspinales m.'s, músculos interespinais do pescoço. SIN interspinales cervicis (m.'s).

cervical longissimus m., m. longuíssimo do pescoço. SIN longissimus cervicis (m.).

cervical rotator m.'s, músculos rotadores do pescoço. SIN rotatores cervicis (m.'s).

cheek m., m. bucinador. SIN buccinator (m.).

chin m., m. mentual. SIN mentalis (m.).

chondroglossus m. [TA], m. condroglosso; parte menor do m. hioglosso, originada como fibras do corno menor do osso hióide, que são separadas da parte principal do m. hioglosso (o ceratoglosso) por faixas de m. genioglosso. SIN musculus chondroglossus.

ciliary m., [TA], m. ciliar; o m. liso intrínseco do corpo ciliar do bulbo do olho; consiste em fibras circulares [TA] (fibrae circulares [TA]), fibras radiais [TA] (fibrae radialis [TA]), fibras meridionais [TA] (fibrae meridoneales [TA]) e fibras longitudinais [TA] (fibrae longitudinales [TA]); *ação*, na contração, seu diâmetro é reduzido (como o de um esfíncter), reduzindo as forças tênseis (de estiramento) sobre a lente, permitindo que esta se torne mais espessa para visão de perto (acomodação). SIN musculus ciliaris [TA], Bowman m., ciliary ligament.

coccygeal m., m. isquiococcígeo. SIN coccygeus m.

coccygeus m. [TA], m. isquiococcígeo; m. pélvico estriado associado à face profunda (pélvica) do ligamento sacroespinal, formando parte do diafragma pélvico; *origem*, espinha isquiática e ligamento sacroespinal; *inserção*, laterais da parte inferior do sacro e parte superior do cóccix; *ação*, com o ligamento sacroespinal ajuda a sustentar o assoalho pélvico, teoricamente de forma progressiva quando as pressões intra-abdominais aumentam; *inervação*, terceiro e quarto nervos sacrais. SIN musculus coccygeus [TA], coccygeal m., ischiococcygeus, musculus ischiococcygeus.

m.'s of coccyx, músculos do cóccix; os músculos do cóccix considerados como um grupo, incluindo o músculo isquiococcígeo e os músculos sacrococcígeos ventral e dorsal inconstantes. SIN musculi coccygei.

Coiter m., m. de Coiter. SIN corrugator supercilii (m.).

compressor urethra (m.) [TA], m. compressor da uretra; parte do complexo muscular do esfíncter externo da uretra; consiste em uma faixa muscular fina, que se estende entre as faces mais posteriores dos ramos isquiopúbicos, mas forma uma faixa anterior à uretra de forma que sua contração puxa a uretra para trás, comprimindo sua parede anterior contra a parede posterior, fechando a uretra como uma pequena dobra em uma mangueira; a *Terminologia Anatomica* apresenta esse m. apenas na mulher, mas já foi descrita uma estrutura semelhante no homem. SIN musculus compressor urethrae [TA].

coracobrachial m., m. coracobraquial. SIN coracobrachialis m.

coracobrachialis m. [TA], m. coracobraquial; m. do compartimento anterior (flexor) do braço; *origem*, processo coracóide da escápula; *inserção*, meio da borda medial do úmero; *ação*, aduz e flete o braço; atua como um m. de afastamento para resistir ao deslocamento para baixo da articulação do ombro; *inervação*, nervo musculocutâneo. SIN musculus coracobrachialis [TA], Casser perforated m., coracobrachial m.

corrugator m., m. corrugador do supercílio. SIN corrugator supercilii (m.).

corrugator cutis m. of anus, m. corrugador da pele do ânus; m. do trígono anal com fibras musculares que se irradiam da porção superficial do esfíncter externo até a face profunda da pele perianal, diz-se que causa pregueamento dessa pele, que contribui para a "vedação" ao ar/água do canal anal. SIN musculus corrugator cutis ani.

corrugator supercilii (m.) [TA], m. corrugador do supercílio; m. facial da fronte; *origem*, da parte orbital do músculo orbicular do olho e da proeminência do nariz; *inserção*, pele do supercílio; *ação*, leva a extremidade medial do supercílio para baixo e enruga a fronte verticalmente, produzindo a expressão de pensamento profundo, preocupação ou interesse; *inervação*, nervo facial. SIN musculus corrugator supercilii [TA], Coiter m., corrugator m., wrinkler m. of eyebrow.

cowl m., m. trapézio. SIN trapezius (m.).

Crampton m., m. de Crampton. SIN Brücke m.

cremaster m. [TA], m. cremaster; *origem*, continuação de fibras do músculo oblíquo interno mais inferior e tiras originadas do ligamento inguinal; *inserção*, torna-se interposto na fáscia cremastérica do cordão espermático e revestimento intermediário do testículo; na mulher, o ligamento redondo do útero; *ação*, eleva o testículo; *inervação*, ramo genital do nervo genitofemoral. SIN musculus cremaster [TA], Riolan m. (2).

cricopharyngeus m., m. cricofaríngeo; *termo alternativo oficial para cricopharyngeal part of inferior constrictor (muscle) of pharynx.

cricothyroid m. [TA], m. cricotireóideo; m. intrínseco da laringe; *origem*, superfície anterior do arco da cartilagem cricóidea; *inserção*, a parte anterior ou reta ascende até a asa da tireóide; a parte posterior ou oblíqua segue mais para fora até o corno inferior da tireóide; *ação*, age na articulação cricotireóidea, unindo as faces anteriores das cartilagens tireóidea e cricóidea, rodando a porção superior da lâmina da cartilagem cricóidea e a cartilagem aritenóidea posteriormente, causando tensão das pregas vocais, aumentando a altura do tom da voz; o antagonista desse movimento é o m. tireoaritenóideo; *inervação*, ramo laríngeo externo do nervo laríngeo superior (do vago). SIN musculus cricothyroideus [TA].

cruciate m., m. cruzado; tipo geral de m. no qual os músculos ou feixes de fibras musculares se cruzam formando um X; p. ex., os músculos aritenóideos oblíquos. SIN musculus cruciatus.

cutaneous m. [TA], m. cutâneo; m. situado no tecido subcutâneo e que se fixa à pele; pode ou não possuir uma fixação óssea. Os músculos da expressão são os principais exemplos de músculos cutâneos no ser humano. SIN musculus cutaneus [TA].

dartos m., m. dartos; fibras musculares lisas interpostas na fáscia do dartos (fáscia superficial do escroto), causando contração do escroto, como durante a exposição a uma baixa temperatura ambiental. VER TAMBÉM dartos *fascia*.

deep m.'s of back, músculos profundos do dorso. SIN m.'s of back proper.

deep flexor (m.) of fingers, m. flexor profundo dos dedos da mão. SIN flexor digitorum profundus (m.).

deep transverse perineal m. [TA], m. transverso profundo do períneo; *origem*, ramo do ísquio; *inserção*, com seu companheiro no corpo do períneo; *ação*, com o m. transverso superficial do períneo na formação do elemento transverso do membro cruzado (sendo o elemento sagital formado pelos músculos bulboesponjoso e esfíncter externo do ânus), que proporciona sustentação do períneo e do diafragma pélvico acima durante aumento da pressão abdominopélvica; em homens, aumenta a sustentação do bulbo do pênis; *inervação*, nervo pudendo (nervo dorsal do pênis/clitóris). SIN musculus transversus perinei profundus [TA], deep transverse m. of perineum.

deep transverse m. of perineum, m. transverso profundo do períneo. SIN deep transverse perineal m.

deltoid (m.) [TA], m. deltóide; m. intrínseco (escapuloumeral) da articulação do ombro; *origem*, terço lateral da borda anterior da clavícula, borda lateral e posterior do acrômio, borda inferior da espinha da escápula; *inserção*, face lateral da diáfise do úmero (tuberosidade deltóide), um pouco acima de seu meio; *ação*, suas porções anterior, média e posterior atuam independentemente para realizar abdução, flexão, extensão e rotação do úmero na articulação do ombro; *inervação*, axilar (quinto e sexto segmentos da medula espinal cervical através do plexo braquial). SIN musculus deltoideus [TA].

depressor anguli oris (m.) [TA], m. abaixador do ângulo da boca; m. facial da boca; *origem*, base ântero-lateral da mandíbula anteriormente; *inserção*, funde-se a outros músculos no lábio inferior próximo ao ângulo da boca; *ação*, abaixa os ângulos da boca; *inervação*, nervo facial. SIN musculus depressor anguli oris [TA], musculus triangularis (2) [TA], triangular m. (2) [TA], musculus triangularis labii inferioris.

depressor m. of epiglottis, m. abaixador da epiglote; parte tireoepiglótica do m. tireoaritenóideo. SIN thyroepiglottic *part* of thyroarytenoid (muscle).

depressor m. of eyebrow, m. abaixador do supercílio. SIN depressor supercilii (m.).

depressor labii inferioris (m.) [TA], m. abaixador do lábio inferior; m. facial da boca; *origem,* porção anterior da base da mandíbula; *inserção,* interdigita-se com fibras do m. orbicular da boca para alcançar a pele do lábio inferior; *ação,* abaixa o lábio inferior; *inervação,* nervo facial. SIN musculus depressor labii inferioris [TA], depressor m. of lower lip, musculus quadratus labii inferioris, musculus quadratus menti.

depressor m. of lower lip, m. abaixador do lábio inferior. SIN depressor labii inferioris (m.).

depressor septi nasi (m.) [TA], m. abaixador do septo nasal; m. facial do nariz; fascículo vertical da maxila superior ao incisivo central, seguindo para cima ao longo da linha média do lábio superior, para se inserir na parte móvel do septo nasal; *ação,* atua com a parte alar (dilatadora) do m. nasal para alargar as narinas durante a inspiração profunda; abaixa o septo; *inervação,* ramo bucal do nervo facial. SIN musculus depressor septi nasi [TA], depressor (m.) of septum.

depressor (m.) of septum, m. abaixador do septo. SIN depressor septi nasi (m.).

depressor supercilii (m.) [TA], m. abaixador do supercílio; m. facial originado na parte nasal do osso frontal, medial ao m. corrugador do supercílio, e inserindo-se na pele subjacente ao meio do supercílio; *ação,* abaixa o supercílio; *inervação,* nervo facial. SIN musculus depressor supercilii [TA], depressor m. of eyebrow.

detrusor (m.) [TA], m. detrusor da bexiga; a túnica muscular da bexiga, que, juntamente com a gravidade e o aumento da pressão intra-abdominal, facilita o esvaziamento da bexiga durante a micção por sua contração. SIN musculus detrusor urinae [TA].

digastric (m.) [TA], m. digástrico; (1) um m. do grupo de músculos supra-hióideos que consiste em dois ventres unidos por um tendão central que atravessa uma alça de fáscia unida ao corpo do osso hióide; *origem,* pelo ventre posterior, do sulco digástrico medial ao processo mastóide; *inserção,* pelo ventre anterior, na borda inferior da mandíbula, próximo da linha média; *ação,* eleva o osso hióide quando a mandíbula está fixa; abaixa a mandíbula quando o hióide está fixo; *inervação,* ventre posterior pelo nervo facial e ventre anterior pelo nervo milo-hióideo da divisão mandibular do trigêmeo. SIN musculus biventer [TA], musculus digastricus [TA], two-bellied m. [TA], biventer mandibulae, musculus biventer mandibulae. (2) m. com dois ventres carnosos separados por uma inserção fibrosa.

dilator m. [TA], m. dilatador; m. que abre um orifício ou dilata a luz de um órgão; é o componente de dilatação ou abertura de um piloro (o outro componente é o músculo esfíncter). SIN musculus dilatator [TA], musculus dilator.

dilator (m.) of ileocecal sphincter, m. dilatador do esfíncter ileocecal; as fibras musculares longitudinais que abrem o orifício ileal ao nível da junção cecocólica. SIN musculus dilator pylori ilealis.

dilator pupillae (m.) [TA], m. dilatador da pupila; "músculo" intrínseco do bulbo do olho; camada radialmente disposta de processos musculares das células mioepiteliais que formam o epitélio da superfície posterior da íris, que se estende da margem pupilar até a margem ciliar; a estimulação simpática causa contração, que dilata lentamente a pupila para permitir que mais luz atinja a retina. SIN musculus dilator pupillae [TA], dilator iridis, dilator of pupil, musculus dilator iridis.

dilator (m.) of pylorus, m. dilatador do piloro; as fibras musculares longitudinais que abrem a junção gastroduodenal. SIN musculus dilator pylori gastroduodenalis.

dorsal m.'s, músculos dorsais. SIN m's of back.

dorsal interossei (interosseous m.'s) of foot [TA], músculos interósseos dorsais plantares; quatro músculos intrínsecos da quarta camada de músculos plantares; *origem,* das laterais dos ossos metatarsais adjacentes; *inserção,* o primeiro insere-se na face medial, o segundo na face lateral da falange proximal do segundo dedo, o terceiro e o quarto inserem-se na face lateral da falange proximal do terceiro e quarto dedos; *ação,* abduz o 2.º, 3.º e 4.º dedos a partir de um eixo através do segundo dedo; *inervação,* nervo plantar lateral. SIN musculi interossei dorsalis pedis [TA].

dorsal interossei (interosseous m.'s) of hand [TA], músculos interósseos dorsais palmares; quatro músculos intrínsecos da mão; *origem,* laterais dos ossos metacarpais adjacentes; *inserção,* falanges proximais e expansão extensora, o primeiro na face radial do indicador, o segundo na face radial do dedo médio, o terceiro na face ulnar do dedo médio, o quarto na face ulnar do dedo anular; *ação,* abduz o 2.º, 3.º e 4.º dedos da mão a partir do eixo do dedo médio; *inervação,* nervo ulnar. SIN musculi interossei dorsalis manus [TA].

dorsal sacrococcygeal m., m. sacrococcígeo dorsal. SIN dorsal sacrococcygeus m.

dorsal sacrococcygeus m., m. sacrococcígeo dorsal; m. inconstante e pouco desenvolvido nas superfícies dorsais do sacro e cóccix, o remanescente de uma parte da musculatura da cauda de animais inferiores. SIN dorsal sacrococcygeal m., musculus extensor coccygis, musculus sacrococcygeus dorsalis, musculus sacrococcygeus posterior.

Dupré m., m. de Dupré. SIN articularis genus (m.).

Duverney m., m. de Duverney. SIN lacrimal *part* of orbicularis oculi muscle. VER orbicularis oculi (m.).

elevator m. of anus, m. levantador do ânus. SIN levator ani (m.).

elevator (m.) of prostate, m. levantador da próstata; m. puboprostático. SIN puboprostaticus (m.).

elevator m. of rib, m. levantador da costela. SIN levatores costarum (m.'s).

elevator (m.) of scapula, m. levantador da escápula. SIN levator scapulae (m.).

(elevator) m. of soft palate, m. levantador do véu palatino. SIN levator veli palatini (m.).

elevator (m.) of thyroid gland, m. levantador da glândula tireóide. SIN levator (m.) of thyroid gland.

elevator (m.) of upper eyelid, m. levantador da pálpebra superior. SIN levator palpebrae superioris (m.).

elevator m. of upper lip, m. levantador do lábio superior. SIN levator labii superioris (m.).

elevator m. of upper lip and wing of nose, m. levantador do lábio superior e da asa do nariz. SIN levator labii superioris alaeque nasi (m.).

epicranial m., m. epicrânico. SIN epicranius (m.).

epicranius (m.) [TA], m. epicrânico; músculo facial (couro cabeludo) composto formado pela aponeurose epicrânica e pelos músculos que nela se inserem, isto é, o m. occipitofrontal e o m. temporoparietal. SIN musculus epicranius [TA], epicranial m., scalp m.

erector m. of hair, m. eretor do pêlo. SIN arrector m. of hair.

erector m. spinae (m.'s) [TA], músculos eretores da espinha; músculos próprios do dorso; *origem,* no sacro, ílio e espinhas das vértebras lombares; divide-se em três colunas: m. iliocostal, m. longuíssimo e m. espinal, que se inserem nas costelas e vértebras com faixas de músculo adicionais que se unem às colunas em níveis sucessivamente mais altos; *ação,* estende e flete lateralmente a coluna vertebral; *inervação,* ramos primários dorsais dos nervos espinais. SIN musculus erector spinae [TA], erector m. of spine, musculus sacrospinalis.

erector m. of spine, m. eretor da espinha. SIN erector spinae (m.'s).

extensor m. [TA], m. extensor; m. que realiza extensão, isto é, um movimento que produz retificação, ou um aumento do ângulo de uma articulação. SIN musculus extensor [TA].

extensor carpi radialis brevis (m.) [TA], m. extensor radial curto do carpo; m. do compartimento posterior do antebraço; *origem,* epicôndilo lateral do úmero; *inserção,* base do terceiro osso metacarpal; *ação,* estende e abduz a mão na articulação do punho; *inervação,* nervo radial profundo. SIN musculus extensor carpi radialis brevis [TA], short radial extensor m. of wrist.

extensor carpi radialis longus (m.) [TA], m. extensor radial longo do carpo; m. do compartimento posterior (extensor) do antebraço; *origem,* crista supracondilar lateral do úmero; *inserção,* face posterior da base do segundo osso metacarpal; *ação,* estende e abduz a mão na articulação do punho; *inervação,* nervo radial. SIN musculus extensor carpi radialis longus [TA], long radial extensor m. of wrist.

extensor carpi ulnaris (m.) [TA], m. extensor ulnar do carpo; m. do compartimento posterior (extensor) do antebraço; *origem,* epicôndilo lateral do úmero (cabeça umeral) e linha oblíqua e borda posterior da ulna (cabeça ulnar); *inserção,* base do quinto metacarpal; *ação,* estende e aduz a mão na articulação do punho; *inervação,* nervo radial (interósseo posterior). SIN musculus extensor carpi ulnaris [TA], ulnar extensor (m.) of wrist.

extensor digiti minimi (m.) [TA], m. extensor do dedo mínimo; m. do compartimento posterior (extensor) do antebraço; *origem,* epicôndilo lateral do úmero; *inserção,* dorso das falanges proximal, média e distal do dedo mínimo; *ação,* estende o dedo mínimo; *inervação,* nervo radial (interósseo posterior). SIN musculus extensor digiti minimi [TA], extensor (m.) of little finger, musculus extensor digiti quinti proprius, musculus extensor minimi digiti.

extensor digitorum m. [TA], m. extensor dos dedos; m. do compartimento posterior (extensor) do antebraço; *origem,* epicôndilo lateral do úmero; *inserção,* por quatro tendões na base das falanges proximal e média e na base da falange distal; *ação,* estende os dedos da mão, principalmente na articulação metacarpofalângica; *inervação,* nervo radial (interósseo posterior). SIN musculus extensor digitorum [TA], extensor (m.) of fingers, musculus extensor digitorum communis.

extensor digitorum brevis (m.) [TA], m. extensor curto dos artelhos; m. intrínseco do dorso do pé; *origem,* superfície dorsal do calcâneo; *inserção,* por quatro tendões que se fundem com os do músculo extensor longo dos artelhos e por uma faixa fixada de forma independente à base da falange proximal do hálux; *ação,* estende os quatro artelhos laterais (II–V); *inervação,* nervo fibular profundo. SIN musculus extensor digitorum brevis [TA], musculus extensor brevis digitorum, short extensor (m.) of toes.

extensor digitorum brevis (m.) of hand, m. extensor curto dos dedos da mão; m. extensor curto dos dedos da mão raro e comparável ao extensor curto dos artelhos. SIN musculus extensor digitorum brevis manus, Pozzi m.

extensor digitorum longus (m.) [TA], m. extensor longo dos artelhos; m. do compartimento anterior (extensor/dorsiflexor) da perna; *origem,* côndilo lateral da tíbia, dois terços superiores da margem anterior da fíbula; *inserção,* por quatro tendões, nas superfícies dorsais das bases das falanges proximal, média e distal do segundo ao quinto dedos; *ação*, estende os quatro dedos laterais; *inervação*, nervo fibular profundo. SIN musculus extensor digitorum longus [TA], long extensor (m.) of toes, musculus extensor longus digitorum.

extensor (m.) of fingers, m. extensor dos dedos da mão. SIN extensor digitorum m.

extensor hallucis brevis (m.) [TA], m. extensor curto do hálux; m. intrínseco do dorso do pé, considerado por alguns anatomistas como o ventre medial do músculo extensor curto dos artelhos, cujo tendão está inserido na base da falange proximal do hálux; *origem*, face dorsal do calcâneo; *inserção*, através de uma face firme da base da falange proximal do hálux; *ação*, estende o hálux; *inervação*, nervo fibular profundo. Seu tendão está inserido na base da falange proximal do hálux. SIN musculus extensor hallucis brevis [TA], short extensor (m.) of great toe.

extensor hallucis longus (m.) [TA], m. extensor longo do hálux; m. do compartimento anterior (extensor/dorsiflexor) da perna; *origem*, superfície anterior da fíbula e membrana interóssea; *inserção*, face dorsal da base da falange distal do hálux; *ação*, estende o hálux; *inervação*, nervo fibular profundo. SIN musculus extensor hallucis longus [TA], long extensor (m.) of great toe.

extensor indicis (m.) [TA], m. extensor do indicador; m. do compartimento posterior (extensor) do antebraço; *origem*, superfície dorsal da parte distal da ulna e membrana interóssea adjacente; *inserção*, expansão extensora do dedo indicador; *ação*, estende independentemente o dedo indicador e ajuda a estender a mão na articulação do punho; *inervação*, nervo radial (interósseo posterior). SIN musculus extensor indicis [TA], index extensor (m.), musculus extensor indicis proprius.

extensor (m.) of little finger, m. extensor do dedo mínimo. SIN extensor digiti minimi (m.).

extensor pollicis brevis (m.) [TA], m. extensor curto do polegar; m. do compartimento posterior (extensor) do antebraço; *origem*, superfície dorsal da parte distal do rádio e membrana interóssea adjacente; *inserção*, face posterior da base da falange proximal do polegar; *ação*, estende e abduz o polegar na articulação metacarpofalângica; *inervação*, nervo radial (interósseo posterior). SIN musculus extensor pollicis brevis [TA], musculus extensor brevis pollicis, short extensor (m.) of thumb.

extensor pollicis longus (m.) [TA], m. extensor longo do polegar; m. do compartimento posterior (extensor) do antebraço; *origem*, superfície posterior da parte média da diáfise da ulna; *inserção*, face dorsal da base da falange distal do polegar; *ação*, estende a falange distal do polegar; *inervação*, nervo radial (interósseo posterior). SIN musculus extensor pollicis longus [TA], long extensor (m.) of thumb, musculus extensor longus pollicis.

external intercostal (m.) [TA], m. intercostal externo; m. plano do tórax originado da borda inferior de uma costela, e que segue obliquamente para baixo e para frente a fim de se inserir na borda superior da costela, abaixo; *ação*, contrai durante a inspiração para levantar as costelas; também para manter a tensão nos espaços intercostais, resistindo assim ao movimento para dentro durante a inspiração; *inervação*, nervo intercostal. SIN musculus intercostales externi [TA].

external oblique (m.) [TA], m. oblíquo externo; m. plano do abdome; *origem*, superfícies externas da quinta a décima segunda costelas; *inserção*, metade anterior do lábio lateral da crista ilíaca e ligamento inguinal, inferiormente, e continua medialmente como parte da camada anterior da bainha do m. reto; *ação*, sustenta e comprime as vísceras abdominais; flete e roda o tronco; *inervação*, nervos toracoabdominais. SIN musculus obliquus externus abdominis [TA], abdominal external oblique (m.).

external obturator m., m. obturador externo. SIN obturator externus (m.).

external pterygoid m., m. pterigóideo lateral. SIN lateral pterygoid (m.).

external m. of anus, m. esfíncter externo do ânus. SIN external anal *sphincter*.

extraocular m.'s [TA], músculos extrínsecos do bulbo do olho; os músculos situados dentro da órbita, mas fora do bulbo do olho, incluindo os quatro músculos retos (superior, inferior, medial e lateral); dois músculos oblíquos (superior e inferior) e o levantador da pálpebra superior (levator palpebrae superioris). SIN musculi externi bulbi oculi [TA], extrinsic m.'s of eyeball*, m.'s of eyeball, musculi bulbi, ocular m.'s.

extrinsic m.'s, músculos extrínsecos; músculos originados fora da estrutura em consideração, mas que agem sobre ela. Por exemplo, os músculos que operam a mão, mas apresentando ventres carnosos localizados no antebraço.

extrinsic m.'s of eyeball, músculos extrínsecos do bulbo do olho; *termo oficial alternativo para extraocular m.'s.

🛈 **m.'s of eyeball,** músculos do bulbo do olho. SIN extraocular m.'s.

facial m.'s [TA], músculos faciais; os inúmeros músculos supridos pelo nervo facial que estão fixados à pele da face e a movimentam. A *Terminologia Anatomica* inclui o m. bucinador nesse grupo devido à sua inervação e origem embrionária, embora ele atue basicamente na mastigação. SIN mimetic m.'s, m.'s of facial expression, musculi faciei.

m.'s of facial expression, músculos da expressão facial. SIN facial m.'s.

femoral m., m. femoral. SIN vastus intermedius (m.).

fibularis brevis (m.) [TA], m. fibular curto; *origem*, dois terços inferiores da superfície lateral da fíbula; *inserção*, base do quinto osso metatarsal; *ação*, everte o pé; *inervação*, nervo fibular superficial. SIN musculus fibularis brevis [TA], musculus peroneus brevis*, peroneus brevis (m.)*, short fibular m., short peroneal m.

fibularis longus (m.) [TA], m. fibular longo; *origem*, dois terços superiores da superfície externa da fíbula e côndilo lateral da tíbia; *inserção*, por tendão que passa atrás do maléolo lateral e através da planta do pé até o cuneiforme medial e base do primeiro metatarsal; *ação*, flexão plantar e eversão do pé; *inervação*, nervo fibular superficial. SIN musculus fibularis longus [TA], musculus peroneus longus*, peroneus longus (m.)*, long fibular m., long peroneal m.

fibularis tertius (m.) [TA], m. fibular terceiro; *origem*, em comum com o m. extensor longo dos dedos; *inserção*, dorso da base do quinto osso metatarsal; *inervação*, ramo profundo do nervo fibular; *ação*, ajuda na dorsiflexão e eversão do pé. SIN musculus fibularis tertius [TA], musculus peroneus tertius*, peroneus tertius (m.)*, third peroneal m.

fixator m., m. fixador; m. que atua como estabilizador de uma parte do corpo durante o movimento de outra parte.

flat m. [TA], m. plano; m. largo, relativamente fino, semelhante a uma folha, p. ex., músculos da parede abdominal ântero-lateral (oblíquos externo e interno, transverso do abdome). SIN musculus plana [TA].

flexor m. [TA], m. flexor; m. que produz flexão, isto é, um movimento que curva ou diminui o ângulo das articulações. SIN musculus flexor [TA].

flexor accessorius (m.), m. flexor acessório; m. quadrado plantar; *termo oficial alternativo para quadratus plantae (m.).

flexor carpi radialis (m.) [TA], m. flexor radial do carpo; m. do compartimento anterior (flexor) do antebraço; *origem*, origem flexora comum do côndilo medial do úmero; *inserção*, superfície anterior da base do segundo osso metacarpal, na maioria das vezes enviando uma faixa até a base do terceiro metacarpal; *ação*, flete e abduz o punho; *inervação*, nervo mediano; seu tendão segue em seu próprio canal coberto por uma camada do ligamento transverso do carpo. SIN musculus flexor carpi radialis [TA], radial flexor (m.) of wrist.

flexor carpi ulnaris (m.) [TA], m. flexor ulnar do carpo; m. do compartimento anterior (flexor) do antebraço; *origem*, através de uma cabeça umeral do

movimentos dos olhos e músculos empregados				
movimento lateral (abdução e adução)	**movimento vertical**	**movimento oblíquo**		**movimento de rolagem**
dextroversão	elevação	dextroelevação	levoelevação	torção para fora (rolagem externa)
olho direito: reto lateral	reto superior	olho direito: reto superior	olho esquerdo: reto superior	reto inferior
olho esquerdo: reto medial	oblíquo inferior	olho esquerdo: oblíquo inferior	olho direito: oblíquo inferior	oblíquo inferior
levoversão	depressão	dextrodepressão	levodepressão	torção para dentro (rolagem interna)
olho direito: reto medial	reto inferior	olho direito: reto inferior	olho esquerdo: reto inferior	reto superior
olho esquerdo: reto lateral	oblíquo inferior	olho esquerdo: oblíquo superior	olho direito: oblíquo superior	oblíquo superior

côndilo medial do úmero e uma cabeça ulnar do olécrano e três quintos superiores da borda posterior da ulna; *inserção*, osso pisiforme, mas é contínuo até o quinto metacarpal através do ligamento pisometacarpal; *ação*, flete e aduz a mão na articulação do punho em direção ulnar; *inervação*, nervo ulnar. SIN musculus flexor carpi ulnaris [TA], ulnar flexor (m.) of wrist.

flexor digiti minimi brevis (m.) of foot [TA], m. flexor curto do dedo mínimo do pé; m. da terceira camada de músculos plantares; *origem*, base do osso metatarsal do dedo mínimo e bainha do m. fibular longo; *inserção*, superfície lateral da base da falange proximal do dedo mínimo; *ação*, flete o dedo mínimo na articulação metacarpofalângica; *inervação*, nervo plantar lateral. SIN musculus flexor digiti minimi brevis pedis [TA], short flexor (m.) of little toe.

flexor digiti minimi brevis (m.) of hand [TA], m. flexor curto do dedo mínimo da mão; m. hipotenar palmar; *origem*, gancho do osso hamato; *inserção*, face medial da falange proximal do dedo mínimo; *ação*, flete o dedo mínimo na articulação metacarpofalângica; *inervação*, ramo profundo do nervo ulnar. SIN musculus flexor digiti minimi brevis manus [TA], short flexor (m.) of little finger.

flexor digitorum brevis (m.) [TA], m. flexor curto dos dedos; m. da primeira camada de músculos plantares; *origem*, tubérculo medial do calcâneo e aponeurose plantar; *inserção*, falanges médias dos quatro artelhos laterais por tendões perfurados por aqueles do flexor longo dos artelhos; *ação*, flete os quatro artelhos laterais; *inervação*, nervo plantar medial. SIN musculus flexor digitorum brevis [TA], musculus flexor brevis digitorum, short flexor (m.) of toes.

flexor digitorum longus (m.) [TA], m. flexor longo dos artelhos; m. do compartimento posterior profundo ou flexor (flexor plantar) da perna; *origem*, terço médio da superfície posterior da tíbia; *inserção*, por quatro tendões, perfurando aqueles do flexor curto, nas bases das falanges distais de quatro dedos laterais; *ação*, flete do segundo ao quinto dedos; *inervação*, nervo tibial. SIN musculus flexor digitorum longus [TA], long flexor (m.) of toes, musculus flexor longus digitorum.

flexor digitorum profundus (m.) [TA], m. flexor profundo dos dedos; m. da camada profunda do compartimento anterior (flexor) do antebraço; *origem*, superfície anterior do terço proximal da ulna; *inserção*, por quatro tendões, perfurando aqueles do flexor superficial dos dedos até a face anterior da base da falange distal de cada dedo; *ação*, flete a articulação interfalângica distal dos dedos; *inervação*, nervos ulnar e mediano (músculo interósseo anterior). SIN musculus flexor digitorum profundus [TA], deep flexor (m.) of fingers, musculus flexor profundus.

flexor digitorum superficialis (m.) [TA], m. flexor superficial dos dedos; m. intermediário do compartimento anterior (flexor) do antebraço; *origem*, via cabeça umeroulnar do epicôndilo medial do úmero, a borda medial do processo coronóide e um arco tendíneo entre esses pontos, e cabeça radial da linha oblíqua e terço médio da borda lateral do rádio; *inserção*, por quatro tendões divididos, que passam de cada lado dos tendões do flexor profundo dos dedos da mão até as laterais da falange média de cada dedo da mão; *ação*, flete a articulação interfalângica proximal de cada dedo da mão; *inervação*, nervo mediano. SIN musculus flexor digitorum superficialis [TA], musculus flexor digitorum sublimis, musculus flexor sublimis, superficial flexor (m.) of fingers.

flexor hallucis brevis (m.) [TA], m. flexor curto do hálux; m. tenar plantar; *origem*, superfície medial dos ossos cubóide e cuneiformes medial e lateral; *inserção*, por dois tendões, circundando o tendão do flexor longo do hálux, nas laterais da base da falange proximal do hálux; *ação*, flete o hálux; *inervação*, nervos plantares medial e lateral. SIN musculus flexor hallucis brevis [TA], musculus flexor brevis hallucis, short flexor (m.) of great toe.

flexor hallucis longus (m.) [TA], m. flexor longo do hálux; m. do compartimento posterior profundo (flexor plantar) da perna; *origem*, dois terços inferiores da superfície posterior da fíbula; *inserção*, base da falange distal do hálux; *ação*, flete o hálux; *inervação*, nervo plantar medial. SIN musculus flexor hallucis longus [TA], long flexor (m.) of great toe, musculus flexor longus hallucis.

flexor pollicis brevis (m.) [TA], m. flexor curto do polegar; m. tenar da palma; *origem*, a cabeça superficial origina-se do retináculo dos músculos flexores do punho, e a cabeça profunda origina-se da face ulnar do primeiro osso metacarpal; *inserção*, face palmar da base da falange proximal do polegar; *ação*, flete a falange proximal do polegar; *inervação*, nervo mediano (cabeça superficial) e ramo profundo do nervo ulnar (cabeça profunda). Alguns autores consideram que a cabeça profunda é a primeira em uma série de quatro músculos interósseos palmares da mão. SIN musculus flexor pollicis brevis [TA], short flexor (m.) of thumb.

flexor pollicis longus (m.) [TA], m. flexor longo do polegar; m. da camada profunda do compartimento anterior (flexor) do antebraço; *origem*, superfície anterior do terço médio do rádio; *inserção*, face palmar da falange distal do polegar; *ação*, flete o polegar na articulação interfalângica; *inervação*, nervo mediano (interósseo anterior). SIN musculus flexor pollicis longus [TA], long flexor m. of thumb, musculus flexor longus pollicis.

four-headed m. [TA], m. quadríceps; que tem quatro cabeças; designa um m. da coxa, m. femoral, e — raramente — um da panturrilha, o m. sural, ou os músculos gastrocnêmio (com duas cabeças), sóleo e plantar, mais comumente denominado m. tríceps sural, sendo o m. plantar considerado um músculo separado. SIN quadríceps.

frontalis m., m. frontal. SIN frontal *belly* of occipitofrontalis muscle.

fusiform m. [TA], m. fusiforme; aquele que possui um ventre carnoso, afilando em uma das extremidades. SIN musculus fusiformis [TA], spindle-shaped m.

Gantzer m., m. de Gantzer; um m. acessório que se estende do flexor superficial dos dedos até o flexor profundo dos dedos.

gastrocnemius (m.) [TA], m. gastrocnêmio; m. superficial do compartimento posterior (flexor plantar) da perna; *origem*, por duas cabeças (lateral e medial) dos côndilos lateral e medial do fêmur; *inserção*, com o m. sóleo, através do tendão do calcâneo, na metade inferior da superfície posterior do calcâneo; *ação*, flexão plantar do pé; *inervação*, nervo tibial. SIN musculus gastrocnemius [TA], gastrocnemius.

Gavard m., m. de Gavard; fibras oblíquas na túnica muscular do estômago.

genioglossal m., m. genioglosso. SIN genioglossus (m.).

genioglossus (m.) [TA], m. genioglosso; um músculo do par de músculos linguais; *origem*, espinha geniana da mandíbula; *inserção*, fáscia lingual sob a mucosa e epiglote; *ação*, abaixa e protrai a língua; *inervação*, nervo hipoglosso. SIN musculus genioglossus [TA], genioglossal m., genioglossus, musculus geniohyoglossus.

geniohyoid (m.) [TA], m. genio-hióideo; um dos músculos supra-hióideos do pescoço; *origem*, espinha geniana da mandíbula; *inserção*, corpo do osso hióide; *ação*, leva o hióide para frente, ou abaixa a mandíbula quando o hióide está fixo; *inervação*, fibras dos ramos primários ventrais do primeiro e segundo nervos espinais cervicais conduzidas pelo nervo hipoglosso. SIN musculus geniohyoideus [TA], geniohyoid, geniohyoideus.

gluteus maximus (m.) [TA], m. glúteo máximo; m. superficial da região glútea; *origem*, ílio atrás da linha glútea posterior, superfície posterior do sacro e cóccix, e ligamento sacrotuberal; *inserção*, trato iliotibial da fáscia lata (três quartos superficiais) e tuberosidade glútea (quarto inferior profundo) do fêmur; *ação*, estende a coxa, principalmente a partir da posição fletida, como ao subir escadas ou ao se levantar estando em posição sentada; *inervação*, nervo glúteo inferior. SIN musculus gluteus maximus [TA].

gluteus medius (m.) [TA], m. glúteo médio; m. intermediário da região glútea; *origem*, ílio entre as linhas glúteas anterior e posterior; *inserção*, superfície lateral do trocânter maior; *ação*, abduz e roda medialmente a coxa; *inervação*, nervo glúteo superior. SIN musculus gluteus medius [TA], mesogluteus.

gluteus minimus (m.) [TA], m. glúteo mínimo; m. profundo da região glútea; *origem*, ílio entre as linhas glúteas anterior e inferior; *inserção*, trocânter maior do fêmur; *ação*, abduz e roda medialmente a coxa; *inervação*, nervo glúteo superior. SIN musculus gluteus minimus [TA].

gracilis (m.) [TA], m. grácil; m. do compartimento medial da coxa; *origem*, ramo do púbis próximo da sínfise; *inserção*, diáfise da tíbia abaixo da tuberosidade medial (ver *pes* anserinus); *ação*, aduz a coxa, flete o joelho, roda a perna medialmente; *inervação*, nervo obturatório. SIN musculus gracilis [TA], gracilis (2).

great adductor m., m. adutor magno. SIN adductor manus (m.).

great pectoral m., m. peitoral maior. SIN pectoralis major (m.).

greater posterior rectus m. of head, m. reto posterior maior da cabeça. SIN rectus capitis posterior major (m.).

greater psoas m., m. psoas maior. SIN psoas major (m.).

greater rhomboid m., m. rombóide maior. SIN rhomboid major (m.).

greater zygomatic m., m. zigomático maior. SIN zygomaticus major (m.).

Guthrie m., m. de Guthrie. SIN external urethral *sphincter*.

hamstring m.'s, músculos do jarrete; os músculos situados no dorso da coxa, compreendendo a cabeça longa do bíceps, o semitendíneo e o semimembranáceo; os músculos do jarrete originam-se no túber isquiático, agem através das articulações do quadril e do joelho, sendo inervados pelo nervo tibial.

m.'s of head [TA], músculos da cabeça; os músculos da expressão, da mastigação e os músculos suboccipitais em geral. SIN musculi capitis [TA].

m. of heart, m. cardíaco. SIN cardiac m.

helicis major (m.) [TA], m. maior da hélice; m. da orelha que se apresenta como uma faixa estreita de fibras musculares na borda anterior da hélice da orelha, originado na espinha e inserido no ponto onde a hélice torna-se transversa. SIN musculus helicis major [TA], large m. of helix.

helicis minor (m.) [TA], m. menor da hélice; m. da orelha que se apresenta como uma faixa de fibras oblíquas cobrindo o ramo da hélice da orelha. SIN musculus helicis minor [TA], smaller m. of helix.

Horner m., m. de Horner. SIN lacrimal *part* of orbicularis oculi muscle. VER orbicularis oculi (m.).

Houston m., m. de Houston. SIN compressor venae dorsalis penis.

hyoglossal m., m. hioglosso. SIN hyoglossus (m.).

hyoglossus (m.) [TA], m. hioglosso; músculo da língua; *origem*, corpo e corno maior do osso hióide; *inserção*, lateral da língua; *ação*, retrai e puxa para baixo o lado da língua; *inervação*, motora pelo nervo hioglosso e sensitiva pelo nervo lingual. SIN musculus hyoglossus [TA], hyoglossal m., hyoglossus.

iliac m., m. ilíaco. SIN iliacus (m.).
iliacus (m.). [TA], m. ilíaco; *origem*, fossa ilíaca; *inserção*, através de um tendão comum com o psoas maior na superfície anterior do trocânter menor do fêmur e cápsula da articulação do quadril; *ação*, flete a coxa e roda-a medialmente; *inervação*, plexo lombar. SIN musculus iliacus [TA], iliac m.
iliacus minor (m.), m. ilíaco menor; as fibras do m. ilíaco originadas da espinha ilíaca ântero-inferior e inseridas no ligamento iliofemoral, algumas vezes está bem separado do restante do músculo. SIN musculus iliacus minor, musculus iliocapsularis.
iliococcygeal m., m. iliococcígeo. SIN iliococcygeus (m.).
iliococcygeus (m.) [TA], m. iliococcígeo; a parte posterior do levantador do ânus; *origem*, arco tendíneo do m. levantador do ânus (fáscia obturatória); *inserção*, ligamento anococcígeo e cóccix; *ação*, resistência ao aumento da pressão intrapélvica e elevação do canal anal após a defecação. SIN musculus iliococcygeus [TA], iliococcygeal m.
iliocostal m., m. iliocostal. SIN iliocostalis (m.).
iliocostalis (m.) [TA], m. iliocostal; a divisão lateral do m. eretor da espinha, que possui três subdivisões: m. iliocostal do lombo, m. iliocostal do tórax e m. iliocostal do pescoço. SIN musculus iliocostalis [TA], iliocostal m.
iliocostalis cervicis (m.) [TA], m. iliocostal do pescoço; m. profundo do dorso (eretor da espinha); *origem*, ângulos das seis costelas superiores; *inserção*, processos transversos das vértebras cervicais médias; *ação*, estende, abduz e roda as vértebras cervicais; *inervação*, ramos dorsais dos nervos torácicos superiores. SIN musculus iliocostalis cervicis [TA], cervical iliocostal m., cervicalis ascendens (1), musculus cervicalis ascendens.
iliocostalis lumborum (m.) [TA], m. iliocostal do lombo; m. profundo do dorso (eretor da espinha); *origem*, face posterior do sacro e fáscia toracolombar; *inserção*, os ângulos das seis costelas inferiores; *ação*, estende, abduz e roda as vértebras lombares; *inervação*, ramos dorsais dos nervos torácicos e lombares. SIN musculus iliocostalis lumborum [TA], lumbar iliocostal m., musculus sacrolumbalis.
iliocostalis thoracis (m.) [TA], m. iliocostal do tórax; m. profundo do dorso (eretor da espinha); *origem*, face medial dos ângulos das seis costelas inferiores; *inserção*, ângulos das seis costelas superiores; *ação*, estende, abduz e roda as vértebras torácicas; *inervação*, ramos dorsais dos nervos torácicos. SIN musculus iliocostalis thoracis [TA], musculus iliocostalis dorsi.
iliopsoas (m.) [TA], m. iliopsoas; m. composto que consiste nos músculos ilíaco e psoas maior, inserindo-se através de um tendão comum na superfície anterior do trocânter menor do fêmur. SIN musculus iliopsoas [TA].
index extensor (m.), m. extensor do indicador. SIN extensor indicis (m.).
inferior constrictor (m.) of pharynx [TA], m. constritor inferior da faringe; parte inferior da camada muscular "circular" externa da faringe; *origem*, superfícies externas das cartilagens tireóidea (parte tireofaríngea [TA]) e cricóidea (parte cricofaríngea [TA], músculo cricofaríngeo [TA]); m. esfíncter esofágico superior ou inferior); *inserção*, rafe da faringe na porção posterior da parede da faringe; *ação*, estreita a parte inferior da faringe na deglutição, e a parte cricofaríngea possui uma função de esfíncter para o esôfago, permitindo algum controle voluntário da eructação e do refluxo; *inervação*, plexo faríngeo (raiz craniana do nervo acessório via vago) e ramos dos nervos laríngeos externo e recorrente. SIN musculus constrictor pharyngis inferior [TA], laryngopharyngeus, musculus laryngopharyngeus, superior esophageal sphincter.
inferior gemellus (m.) [TA], m. gêmeo inferior; m. profundo da região glútea; *origem*, túber isquiático; *inserção*, tendão do m. obturador interno; *ação*, roda a coxa lateralmente; *inervação*, plexo sacral. SIN musculus gemellus inferior [TA], gemellus.
inferior lingual m., m. inferior da língua; m. longitudinal inferior da língua. SIN inferior longitudinal m. of tongue.
inferior longitudinal m. of tongue [TA], m. longitudinal inferior da língua; um m. intrínseco da língua, de formato cilíndrico, que ocupa a parte inferior de cada lado; *ação*, encurta a parte inferior da língua; *inervação*, motora pelo nervo hipoglosso e sensitiva pelo nervo lingual. SIN musculus longitudinalis inferior linguae [TA], inferior lingual m.
inferior oblique (m.) [TA], m. oblíquo inferior; m. extra-ocular na órbita; *origem*, lâmina orbital da maxila lateral ao sulco lacrimal; *inserção*, esclera entre os músculos retos superior e lateral; *ação*, primária, torção para fora; secundária, elevação e abdução; *inervação*, nervo oculomotor (ramo inferior). SIN musculus obliquus inferior [TA].
inferior oblique m. of head, m. oblíquo inferior da cabeça. SIN obliquus capitis inferior (m.).
inferior posterior serratus m., m. serrátil posterior inferior. SIN serratus posterior inferior (m.).
inferior rectus (m.) [TA], m. reto inferior; m. extra-ocular na órbita; *origem*, parte inferior do anel tendíneo comum; *inserção*, parte inferior da esclera do olho; *ação*, primária, depressão; secundária, adução e extorsão; *inervação*, nervo oculomotor (ramo inferior). SIN musculus rectus inferior [TA].
inferior tarsal m. [TA], m. tarsal inferior; m. liso, pouco desenvolvido na pálpebra inferior, que atua alargando a fissura palpebral. SIN musculus tarsalis inferior [TA].

infrahyoid m.'s [TA], músculos infra-hióideos; os pequenos músculos planos inferiores ao osso hióide, incluindo os músculos esterno-hióideo, omo-hióideo, esternotireóideo, tireo-hióideo e levantador da glândula tireóide. SIN musculi infrahyoidei [TA], strap m.'s;
infraspinatus (m.) [TA], m. infra-espinal; m. intrínseco (escapouloumeral) da articulação do ombro, cujo tendão contribui para a formação do manguito rotador; *origem*, fossa infra-espinal da escápula; *inserção*, face média do tubérculo maior do úmero; *ação*, estende o braço e roda-o lateralmente; sua contração tônica ajuda a manter a cabeça do úmero na fossa glenóide rasa; *inervação*, nervo supra-escapular (do quinto a sexto nervos espinais cervicais). SIN musculus infraspinatus [TA].
innermost intercostal (m.) [TA], m. intercostal íntimo; m. plano do tórax observado como uma camada paralela ao músculo intercostal interno, sendo inerentemente parte deste, mas separado pelos vasos e nervos intercostais. Ver também entradas em internal intercostal muscle para fixação, ação e inervação. SIN musculus intercostalis intimus [TA].
intermediate great m., m. vasto intermédio. SIN vastus intermedius (m.).
intermediate vastus (m.), m. vasto intermédio. SIN vastus intermedius (m.).
internal intercostal (m.) [TA], m. intercostal interno; m. plano do tórax originado na borda inferior da costela, seguindo obliquamente para baixo e para trás, para se inserir na borda superior da costela inferior; *ação*, contrai durante a expiração, também mantém a tensão nos espaços intercostais para resistir ao movimento mediolateral; *inervação*, nervo intercostal. SIN musculus intercostalis internus [TA].
internal oblique (m.) [TA], m. oblíquo interno do abdome; m. plano da parede ântero-lateral do abdome; *origem*, fáscia ilíaca profunda à parte lateral do ligamento inguinal, metade anterior da crista ilíaca e fáscia lombar; *inserção*, décima à décima segunda costelas, com a aponeurose contribuindo para a bainha do reto; algumas das fibras do ligamento inguinal terminam no tendão conjunto; *ação*, diminui a capacidade do abdome e flete a coluna vertebral lombar (curva o tórax para frente); *inervação*, nervo torácico inferior. SIN musculus obliquus internus abdominalis [TA], abdominal internal oblique m.
internal obturator m., m. obturador interno. SIN obturator internus (m.).
internal pterygoid m., m. pterigóideo interno; m. pterigóideo medial. SIN medial pterygoid (m.).
internal m. of anus, esfíncter interno do ânus. SIN internal anal sphincter.
interosseous m.'s [TA], músculos interósseos; músculos que se originam dos ossos longos da mão e do pé (metacarpais e metatarsais) e correm entre eles, estendendo-se até os dedos e movimentando-os. VER TAMBÉM dorsal interossei (interosseous m.'s) of foot, dorsal interossei (interosseous m.'s) of hand, palmar interossei (interosseous m.'s), plantar interossei (interosseous m.'s). SIN musculi interossei [TA].
interspinal m.'s, músculos interespinais. SIN interspinales (m.'s).
interspinales (m.'s) [TA], m. interespinais; o par de músculos entre os processos espinhosos de vértebras adjacentes; subdivididos em músculos cervicais, torácicos e lombares. SIN musculi interspinales [TA], interspinal m.'s.
interspinales cervicis (m.'s) [TA], músculos interespinais do pescoço; continuação do m. profundo do dorso até o pescoço; *origem*, tubérculo do processo espinhoso da vértebra cervical; *inserção*, tubérculo do processo espinhoso da próxima vértebra superior; *ação*, estende o pescoço; *inervação*, ramos dorsais dos nervos cervicais. SIN cervical interspinal m., cervical interspinales m.'s, musculus interspinalis cervicis.
interspinales lumborum (m.'s) [TA], músculos interespinais do lombo; m. profundo da região lombar; *origem*, margem superior do processo espinhoso lombar; *inserção*, margem inferior do próximo processo espinhoso superior; *ação*, estende as vértebras lombares; *inervação*, ramos primários dorsais dos nervos espinais lombares. SIN musculus interspinalis lumborum [TA], lumbar interspinal m.
interspinales thoracis (m.'s) [TA], músculos interespinais do tórax; músculos profundos do dorso, freqüentemente pouco desenvolvidos ou ausentes entre os processos espinhosos das vértebras torácicas; *ação*, estende as vértebras torácicas; *inervação*, ramos primários dorsais dos nervos torácicos. SIN musculus interspinalis thoracis [TA], thoracic interspinal m., thoracic interspinales m.'s.
intertransversarii (m.'s) [TA], músculos intertransversários; o par de músculos entre os processos transversos de vértebras adjacentes; há músculos anteriores e posteriores na região cervical; músculos laterais e mediais na região lombar; e músculos únicos na região torácica. SIN musculi intertransversarii [TA], intertransverse m.'s.
intertransverse m.'s, músculos intertransversários. SIN intertransversarii (m.'s).
intrinsic m.'s, músculos intrínsecos; músculos totalmente contidos (origem, ventre e inserção) na estrutura em consideração. Por exemplo, os músculos interósseos e lumbricais são músculos intrínsecos da mão.
intrinsic m.'s of foot, músculos intrínsecos do pé; músculos totalmente contidos (origem, ventre, inserção) no pé e nos artelhos. Esses músculos estão dispostos em quatro camadas, sendo todos inervados pelos ramos plantares do nervo tibial. Embora possam ser capazes de produzir as ações descritas em suas

descrições individuais, como um grupo a função primária dos músculos intrínsecos do pé é proporcionar sustentação dinâmica do arco longitudinal do pé, resistindo às forças que atuam momentaneamente para expandir o arco ao caminhar e correr.

involuntary m.'s, músculos involuntários; músculos que, normalmente, não estão sob controle voluntário; exceto no caso do coração, são compostos de fibras musculares lisas (não-estriadas) e inervados pelo sistema nervoso autônomo.

ischiocavernous (m.) [TA], m. isquiocavernoso; m. do trígono urogenital; *origem*, ramo do ísquio; *inserção*, corpo cavernoso do pênis (ou clitóris); *ação*, comprime o ramo do pênis (ou clitóris), forçando a passagem do sangue em seus seios para a parte distal do corpo cavernoso e diminuindo a saída de sangue venoso; *inervação*, nervo pudendo (perineal). SIN musculus ischiocavernosus [TA], musculus erector clitoridis, musculus erector penis.

Jung m., m. de Jung. SIN pyramidal m. of auricle.

Kohlrausch m., m. de Kohlrausch; os músculos longitudinais da parede retal.

Landström m., m. de Landström; fibras musculares microscópicas na fáscia atrás e ao redor do bulbo do olho, fixadas anteriormente às pálpebras e fáscia anterior da órbita; sua ação é levar o bulbo do olho para frente e as pálpebras para trás, resistindo à tração dos quatro músculos da órbita.

Langer m., m. de Langer. SIN pectorodorsalis m.

large m. of helix, m. maior da hélice. SIN helicis major (m.).

m.'s of larynx [TA], músculos da laringe; músculos intrínsecos que regulam o comprimento, a posição e a tensão das pregas vocais, e servem como esfíncteres e dilatadores das vias aéreas, ajustando o tamanho das aberturas entre as pregas ariepiglóticas, ventriculares e vocais. SIN musculi laryngis [TA].

lateral cricoarytenoid (m.) [TA], m. cricoaritenóideo lateral; m. intrínseco da laringe; *origem*, margem superior do arco da cartilagem cricóidea; *inserção*, processo muscular da cartilagem aritenóidea; *ação*, aduz as pregas vocais (estreita a rima da glote); *inervação*, nervo laríngeo recorrente. SIN musculus cricoarytenoideus lateralis [TA].

lateral great m., m. vasto lateral. SIN vastus lateralis (m.).

lateral lumbar intertransversarii (m.'s) [TA], músculos intertransversários laterais do lombo; m. profundo da parte inferior do dorso; *origem*, processos transversos das vértebras lombares; *inserção*, processo transverso superior subseqüente; *ação*, abduz as vértebras lombares; *inervação*, ramos ventrais dos nervos lombares. SIN musculi interstransversarii laterales lumborum [TA], lateral lumbar intertransverse m.'s.

lateral lumbar intertransverse m.'s, músculos intertransversários laterais do lombo. SIN lateral lumbar intertransversarii (m.'s).

lateral posterior cervical intertransversarii m.'s [TA], músculos intertransversários posteriores laterais do pescoço. VER posterior cervical intertransversarii (m.'s).

lateral pterygoid (m.) [TA], m. pterigóideo lateral; m. da mastigação da fossa infratemporal; *origem*, a cabeça inferior origina-se da lâmina lateral do processo pterigóide; a cabeça superior origina-se da crista infratemporal e da asa maior do esfenóide adjacente; *inserção*, na fóvea pterigóidea da mandíbula e no disco articular e cápsula da articulação temporomandibular; *ação*, protrai a mandíbula para permitir abertura da boca; a contração unilateral desvia o queixo lateralmente, permitindo movimento de trituração para a mastigação; *inervação*, nervo pterigóideo lateral da divisão mandibular do nervo trigêmeo. SIN musculus pterygoideus lateralis [TA], external pterygoid m., musculus pterygoideus externus.

lateral rectus (m.) [TA], m. reto lateral; m. extra-ocular na órbita; *origem*, parte lateral do anel tendíneo comum que une a fissura orbital superior; *inserção*, parte lateral da esclera do olho; *ação*, abdução; *inervação*, nervo abducente. SIN musculus rectus lateralis [TA], abducens oculi, musculus rectus externus.

lateral rectus m. of the head, m. reto lateral da cabeça. SIN rectus capitis lateralis (m.).

lateral vastus (m.), m. vasto lateral. SIN vastus lateralis (m.).

latissimus dorsi (m.) [TA], m. latíssimo do dorso; m. toracoapendicular (m. superficial do dorso); *origem*, processos espinhosos das cinco ou seis vértebras torácicas inferiores e vértebras lombares; *inserção*, com o m. redondo maior no lábio posterior do sulco bicipital do úmero; *ação*, aduz o braço, roda-o medialmente e estende-o; *inervação*, nervo toracodorsal. SIN musculus latissimus dorsi [TA], broadest m. of back.

lesser rhomboid m., m. rombóide menor. SIN rhomboid minor (m.).

lesser zygomatic m., m. zigomático menor. SIN zygomaticus minor (m.).

levator anguli oris (m.) [TA], m. levantador do ângulo da boca; m. facial do lábio superior; *origem*, fossa canina da maxila; *inserção*, músculo orbicular da boca e pele no ângulo da boca; *ação*, levanta o ângulo da boca; *inervação*, nervo facial. SIN musculus levator anguli oris [TA], musculus caninus, musculus triangularis labii superioris.

levator ani (m.) [TA], m. levantador do ânus; m. composto da pelve; formado pelos músculos pubococcígeo e iliococcígeo; *origem*, corpo posterior do púbis, arco tendíneo do levantador do ânus (fáscia obturatória) e espinha isquiática; *inserção*, ligamento anococcígeo, laterais da parte inferior do sacro e do cóccix; *ação*, resiste às forças de prolapso e leva o ânus para cima após a defecação; sustenta as vísceras pélvicas; *inervação*, nervo para o levantador do ânus (quarto nervo espinal sacral). SIN musculus levator anis [TA], elevator m. of anus.

levatores costarum longi (m.'s) [TA], músculos levantadores longos das costelas; músculos vertebrotorácicos (costovertebrais); *inserção*, a segunda costela abaixo de sua origem; *ação*, levantam as costelas; *inervação*, nervo intercostal. SIN musculi levatores costarum longi [TA], long levatores costarum (m.'s).

levatores costarum (m.'s) [TA], músculos levantadores das costelas; m. do tórax; *origem*, extremidades dos processos transversos às vértebras C7 e T1-T11; *inserção*, costelas, entre o tubérculo e o ângulo; *ação*, elevam as costelas na inspiração profunda; *nervo*, ramos dorsais dos nervos espinais C8-T11. VER levatores costarum longi (m.'s), levatores costarum breves (m.'s). SIN musculi levatores costarum [TA], elevator m. of rib, musculus levator costae.

levatores costarum breves (m.'s) [TA], músculos levantadores curtos das costelas; *origem*, os processos transversos da última vértebra cervical e de onze vértebras torácicas; *inserção*, costelas imediatamente abaixo, entre o ângulo e o tubérculo. SIN musculi levatores costarum breves [TA], short levatores costarum (m.'s).

levatores labii superioris (m.) [TA], m. levantador do lábio superior; m. facial do lábio superior; *origem*, maxila abaixo do forame infra-orbital; *inserção*, interposta com o m. orbicular da boca para alcançar a pele do lábio superior; *ação*, eleva o lábio superior; *inervação*, nervo facial. SIN musculus levator labii superioris [TA], caput infraorbitale quadrati labii superioris, elevator m. of upper lip.

levator labii superioris alaeque nasi (m.) [TA], m. levantador do lábio superior e da asa do nariz; m. facial do lábio superior e do nariz; *origem*, raiz do processo nasal da maxila; *inserção*, asa do nariz e músculo orbicular da boca do lábio superior; *ação*, eleva o lábio superior e a asa do nariz; *inervação*, nervo facial. SIN musculus levator labii superioris alaeque nasi [TA], caput angulare quadrati labii superioris, elevator m. of upper lip and wing of nose.

levator palati (m.), m. levantador do véu palatino. SIN levator veli palatini (m.).

levator palpebrae superioris (m.) [TA], m. levantador da pálpebra superior; m. extra-ocular na órbita; *origem*, superfície orbital da asa menor do esfenóide, acima e anterior ao canal óptico; *inserção*, pele da pálpebra, tarso e paredes da órbita, por expansões mediais e laterais da aponeurose de inserção; *ação*, levanta a pálpebra superior; *inervação*, nervo oculomotor. SIN musculus levator palpebrae superioris [TA], elevator (m.) of upper eyelid, musculus orbitopalpebralis, palpebralis.

levator prostatae (m.), m. levantador da próstata; m. puboprostático; *termo oficial alternativo para puboprostaticus (m.).

levator scapulae (m.) [TA], m. levantador da escápula; m. extrínseco do ombro; *origem*, dos tubérculos posteriores dos processos transversos de quatro vértebras cervicais superiores; *inserção*, no ângulo superior da escápula; *ação*, levanta a escápula; *inervação*, nervo escapular dorsal. SIN musculus levator scapulae [TA], elevator (m.) of scapula, musculus levator anguli scapulae.

levator (m.) of thyroid gland [TA], m. levantador da glândula tireóide; fascículo que, ocasionalmente, passa do m. tireo-hióideo até o istmo da glândula tireóide. SIN musculus levator glandulae thyroideae [TA], elevator (m.) of thyroid gland, Soemmerring m.

levator veli palatini (m.) [TA], m. levantador do véu palatino; m. do palato mole; *origem*, ápice da porção petrosa do osso temporal e parte inferior da tuba auditiva (faringotimpânica) cartilaginosa; *inserção*, aponeurose do palato mole; *ação*, levanta o palato mole; através da expansão de seu ventre carnoso durante a contração, ajuda a "abrir" a tuba auditiva para equilíbrio da pressão; *inervação*, plexo faríngeo (raiz craniana do nervo acessório). SIN musculus levator veli palatini [TA], (elevator) m. of soft palate, levator palati (m.), musculus levator palati, musculus petrostaphylinus.

lingual m.'s, músculos da língua. SIN m.'s of tongue.

long abductor m. of thumb, m. abdutor longo do polegar. SIN abductor pollicis longus (m.).

long adductor m., m. adutor longo. SIN adductor longus (m.).

long extensor (m.) of great toe, m. extensor longo do hálux. SIN extensor hallucis longus (m.).

long extensor (m.) of thumb, m. extensor longo do polegar. SIN extensor pollicis longus (m.).

long extensor (m.) of toes, m. extensor longo dos dedos do pé. SIN extensor digitorum longus (m.).

long fibular m., m. fibular longo. SIN fibularis longus (m.).

long flexor (m.) of great toe, m. flexor longo do hálux. SIN flexor hallucis longus (m.).

long flexor m. of thumb, m. flexor longo do polegar. SIN flexor pollicis longus (m.).

long flexor (m.) of toes, m. flexor longo dos dedos do pé. SIN flexor digitorum longus (m.).

long m. of head, m. longo da cabeça. SIN longus capitis (m.).

longissimus (m.) [TA], m. longuíssimo; a divisão intermediária do m. eretor da espinha que possui três subdivisões: m. longuíssimo da cabeça, m. longuíssimo do pescoço e m. longuíssimo do tórax. SIN musculus longissimus [TA].

longissimus capitis (m.) [TA], m. longuíssimo da cabeça; m. eretor da espinha intermediário no pescoço; *origem*, dos processos transversos das vértebras torácicas superiores e dos processos transversos e articulares das vértebras cervicais inferiores e médias; *inserção*, no processo mastóide; *ação*, mantém a cabeça ereta, leva-a para trás ou para um lado; *inervação*, ramos primários dorsais dos nervos espinais cervicais. SIN musculus longissimus capitis [TA], musculus complexus minor, musculus trachelomastoideus, musculus transversalis capitis.

longissimus cervicis (m.) [TA], m. longuíssimo do pescoço; m. eretor da espinha intermediário no pescoço; *origem*, processos transversos das vértebras torácicas superiores; *inserção*, processos transversos das vértebras cervicais médias e superiores; *ação*, estende as vértebras cervicais; *inervação*, ramos primários dorsais dos nervos espinais cervicais inferiores e torácicos superiores. SIN musculus longissimus cervicis [TA], cervical longissimus m., musculus transversalis cervicis, musculus transversalis colli.

longissimus thoracis (m.) [TA], m. longuíssimo do tórax; m. eretor da espinha intermediário do dorso; *origem*, com o m. iliocostal e dos processos transversos das vértebras torácicas inferiores; *inserção*, por tiras laterais, na maioria das costelas ou em todas elas, entre os ângulos e tubérculos e nas extremidades dos processos transversos das vértebras lombares superiores, e por tiras mediais nos processos acessórios das vértebras lombares superiores e nos processos transversos das vértebras torácicas; *ação*, estende a coluna vertebral; *inervação*, ramos primários dorsais dos nervos espinais torácicos e lombares. SIN musculus longissimus thoracis [TA], musculus longissimus dorsi, thoracic longissimus m.

long levatores costarum (m.'s), músculos levantadores longos das costelas. SIN levatores costarum longi (m.'s).

long m. of neck, m. longo do pescoço. SIN longus colli (m.).

long palmar m., m. palmar longo. SIN palmaris longus (m.).

long peroneal m., m. fibular longo. SIN fibularis longus (m.).

long radial extensor m. of wrist, m. extensor radial longo do carpo. SIN extensor carpi radialis longus (m.).

longus capitis (m.) [TA], m. longo da cabeça; m. pré-vertebral do pescoço; *origem*, tubérculos anteriores dos processos transversos da terceira à sexta vértebras cervicais; *inserção*, processo basilar do osso occipital; *ação*, gira ou flete o pescoço anteriormente; *inervação*, plexo cervical. SIN musculus longus capitis [TA], long m. of head, musculus rectus capitis anticus major.

longus colli (m.) [TA], m. longo do pescoço; m. pré-vertebral do pescoço; parte medial: *origem*, corpos da terceira vértebra torácica até a quinta vértebra cervical; *inserção*, corpos da segunda à quarta vértebras cervicais; parte súperolateral: *origem*, tubérculos anteriores dos processos transversos da terceira à quinta vértebras cervicais; *inserção*, tubérculo anterior do atlas; parte ínferolateral: *origem*, corpos da primeira à terceira vértebras torácicas; *inserção*, tubérculos anteriores dos processos transversos da quinta e sexta vértebras cervicais; *ação*, de todas as três partes, gira o pescoço e flete o pescoço anteriormente; *inervação*, de todas as três partes, ramos primários ventrais dos nervos espinais cervicais (plexo cervical). SIN musculus longus colli [TA], long m. of neck.

lumbar iliocostal m., m. iliocostal do lombo. SIN iliocostalis lumborum (m.).

lumbar interspinal m., m. interespinal do lombo. SIN interspinales lumborum (m.'s).

lumbar quadrate m., m. quadrado do lombo. SIN quadratus lumborum (m.).

lumbar rotator m.'s, músculos rotadores do lombo. SIN rotatores lumborum (m.'s).

lumbricals (lumbrical m.'s) of foot [TA], músculos lumbricais do pé; quatro músculos intrínsecos da segunda camada e músculos plantares; *origem*, primeiro: da face tibial do tendão para o segundo dedo do flexor longo dos dedos; segundo, terceiro e quarto: das faces adjacentes de todos os quatro tendões desse músculo; *inserção*, face tibial do tendão extensor no dorso de cada um dos quatro dedos laterais; *inervação*, nervo plantar lateral (segundo ao quarto lumbricais) e medial (primeiro lumbrical). SIN musculus lumbricalis pedis [TA].

lumbricals (lumbrical m.'s) of hand [TA], músculos lumbricais da mão; quatro músculos intrínsecos da palma; *origem*, os dois laterais: da face radial dos tendões do flexor profundo dos dedos que vai para os dedos indicador e médio; os dois mediais: das faces adjacentes do segundo e terceiro, e terceiro e quarto tendões; *inserção*, face radial do tendão extensor no dorso de cada um dos quatro dedos; *ação*, flete a articulação metacarpofalângica e estende a articulação interfalângica proximal e distal; *inervação*, os dois músculos radiais pelo nervo mediano, os dois músculos ulnares pelo nervo ulnar. SIN musculus lumbricalis manus [TA].

Marcacci m., m. de Marcacci; uma lâmina de fibras de m. liso situada sob a aréola e mamilo da glândula mamária.

masseter (m.) [TA], m. masseter; m. da mastigação da porção posterior da bochecha; *origem*, parte superficial: borda inferior dos dois terços anteriores do arco zigomático; parte profunda, borda inferior e superfície medial do arco zigomático; *inserção*, superfície lateral do ramo e processo coronóide da mandíbula; *ação*, eleva a mandíbula (fecha a mandíbula); *inervação*, ramo massetérico da divisão mandibular do nervo trigêmeo. SIN musculus masseter [TA].

m.'s of mastication, músculos da mastigação. SIN masticatory m.'s.

masticatory m.'s [TA], músculos da mastigação; músculos derivados do primeiro arco (mandibular) usados na mastigação; todos são inervados pela raiz motora do nervo trigêmeo através de sua divisão mandibular; inclui m. masseter, m. temporal, m. pterigóideo lateral e m. pterigóideo medial. SIN m.'s of mastication.

medial great m., m. vasto medial. SIN vastus medialis (m.).

medial lumbar intertransversarii (m.'s) [TA], músculos intertransversários mediais do lombo; parte dos músculos profundos do dorso; *origem*, processos acessórios e mamilares das vértebras lombares; *inserção*, processos correspondentes da vértebra superior seguinte; *ação*, abduz as vértebras lombares; *inervação*, ramos primários dorsais dos nervos espinais lombares. SIN musculi intertransversarii mediales lumborum [TA], medial lumbar intertransverse m.'s.

medial lumbar intertransverse m.'s, músculos intertransversários mediais do lombo. SIN medial lumbar intertransversarii (m.'s).

medial posterior cervical intertransversarii (m.'s), músculos intertransversários posteriores mediais do pescoço. VER posterior cervical intertransversarii (m.'s).

medial pterygoid (m.) [TA], m. pterigóideo medial; m. da mastigação da fossa infratemporal; *origem*, fossa pterigóidea do esfenóide e tuberosidade da maxila; *inserção*, superfície medial da mandíbula entre o ângulo e o sulco milohióideo; *ação*, eleva a mandíbula, fechando a boca; *inervação*, nervo para o m. pterigóideo medial da divisão mandibular do nervo trigêmeo. SIN musculus pterygoideus medialis [TA], internal pterygoid m., musculus pterygoideus internus.

medial rectus (m.) [TA], m. reto medial; m. extra-ocular na órbita; *origem*, parte medial do anel tendíneo comum; *inserção*, parte medial da esclera do olho; *ação*, adução; *inervação*, nervo oculomotor. SIN musculus rectus medialis [TA], musculus rectus internus.

medial vastus (m.), m. vasto medial. SIN vastus medialis (m.).

mentalis (m.) [TA], m. mentual; m. facial do queixo; *origem*, fossa incisiva da mandíbula; *inserção*, pele do queixo; *ação*, eleva e enruga a pele do queixo, assim elevando o lábio inferior; *inervação*, nervo facial. SIN musculus mentalis [TA], chin m., musculus levator labii inferioris.

Merkel m., m. de Merkel. SIN ceratocricoid (m.).

middle constrictor (m.) of pharynx [TA], m. constritor médio da faringe; parte intermediária da túnica muscular "circular" externa da faringe; *origem*, ligamento estilo-hióideo, corno menor do osso hióide (parte condrofaríngea [TA]) e corno maior do osso hióide (parte ceratofaríngea [TA]); *inserção*, rafe faríngea na parede posterior da faringe; *ação*, estreita a faringe no ato da deglutição; *inervação*, plexo faríngeo. SIN musculus constrictor pharyngis medius [TA].

middle scalene m., m. escaleno médio; *termo oficial alternativo para scalenus medius (m.).

mimetic m.'s, músculos faciais. SIN facial m.'s.

Müller m., m. de Müller; **(1)** SIN orbitalis (m.); **(2)** SIN circular *fibers*, em *fiber*; **(3)** SIN superior tarsal m.

multifidus (m.) [TA], m. multífido; camada intermediária de músculos mais profundos (transverso-espinais) do dorso; *origem*, do sacro, ligamento sacroilíaco, processos mamilares das vértebras lombares, processos transversos das vértebras torácicas e processos articulares das quatro últimas vértebras cervicais; *inserção*, nos processos espinhosos de todas as vértebras até o áxis, inclusive; *ação*, gira a coluna vertebral; *inervação*, ramos primários dorsais dos nervos espinais. SIN musculus multifidus [TA], musculus multifidus spinae.

multipennate m. [TA], m. multipeniforme; m. com vários tendões centrais em cuja direção as fibras musculares convergem como filamentos de penas. SIN musculus multipennatus [TA].

mylohyoid (m.) [TA], m. milo-hióideo; m. do assoalho da boca; *origem*, linha milo-hióidea da mandíbula; *inserção*, borda superior do osso hióide e rafe que separa o músculo de seu companheiro; *ação*, eleva o assoalho da boca e a língua, deprime a mandíbula quando o osso hióide está fixo; *inervação*, nervo para o milo-hióideo da divisão mandibular do trigêmeo. SIN musculus mylohyoideus [TA], diaphragm of mouth, diaphragma oris, mylohyoideus.

nasal m., m. nasal. SIN nasalis (m.).

nasalis (m.) [TA], m. nasal; m. facial do nariz; m. composto que consiste em: uma parte transversa [TA] (pars transversa [TA], musculus compressor naris), que se origina da maxila acima da raiz do dente canino de cada lado, formando uma aponeurose através da ponte do nariz; e uma parte alar [TA] (pars alaris [TA], musculus dilator naris), que se origina da maxila acima do incisivo lateral e se fixa à asa do nariz; a parte alar dilata a narina; *inervação*, facial. SIN musculus nasalis [TA], nasal m.

m.'s of neck [TA], músculos do pescoço; os músculos ântero-laterais do pescoço, incluindo platisma, esternocleidomastóideo, supra-hióideo, infra-hióideo, longo do pescoço e escaleno. SIN musculi colli [TA], musculi cervicis*.

m. of notch of helix, m. da incisura terminal. SIN m. of terminal notch.

oblique arytenoid m. [TA], m. aritenóideo oblíquo; m. intrínseco da laringe; *origem*, processo muscular da cartilagem aritenóide; *inserção*, cume da cartilagem aritenóide do lado oposto e continua como o músculo ariepiglótico na prega ariepiglótica até a epiglote; *ação*, estreita ou fecha a porção interaritenóidea da rima da glote; *inervação*, nervo laríngeo recorrente. SIN musculus arytenoideus obliquus [TA], arytenoideus.

oblique m. of auricle [TA], m. oblíquo da orelha; uma faixa fina de fibras musculares oblíquas que se estendem da parte superior da eminência da concha até a convexidade da hélice, atravessando o sulco que corresponde ao ramo inferior da antélice. SIN musculus obliquus auriculae [TA], oblique auricular m., Tod m.

oblique auricular m., m. oblíquo da orelha. SIN oblique m. of auricle.

obliquus capitis inferior (m.) [TA], m. oblíquo inferior da cabeça; m. suboccipital que, apesar do seu nome, não se fixa ao crânio; *origem*, processo espinhoso do áxis; *inserção*, processo transverso do atlas; *ação*, roda a cabeça; *origem*, processo espinhoso do áxis; *inserção*, processo transverso do atlas; *inervação*, nervo suboccipital. VER TAMBÉM suboccipital m.'s. SIN musculus obliquus capitis inferior [TA], inferior oblique m. of head.

obliquus capitis superior (m.) [TA], m. oblíquo superior da cabeça; m. suboccipital; *origem*, processo transverso do atlas; *inserção*, terço lateral da linha nucal inferior; *ação*, roda a cabeça; *inervação*, nervo suboccipital VER TAMBÉM suboccipital m.'s. SIN musculus obliquus capitis superior [TA], superior oblique m. of head.

obturator externus (m.) [TA], m. obturador externo; m. do compartimento medial (adutor) da coxa; *origem*, metade inferior do forame obturado e parte adjacente da superfície externa da membrana obturadora; *inserção*, fossa trocantérica do trocânter maior; *ação*, roda a coxa lateralmente; *inervação*, nervo obturatório. SIN musculus obturator externus [TA], external obturator m.

obturator internus (m.) [TA], m. obturador interno; m. intrapélvico que se estende até a região glútea; *origem*, superfície pélvica da membrana obturadora e margem do forame obturado; *inserção*, sai da pelve através do forame ciático menor e, ao fazê-lo, descreve uma curva de 90° para se inserir na superfície medial do trocânter maior; *ação*, roda a coxa lateralmente; *inervação*, nervo para o obturador interno (sacral plexus). SIN musculus obturator internus [TA], internal obturator m.

occipitalis m., m. occipital. SIN occipital *belly* of occipitofrontalis muscle.

occipitofrontal m., m. occipitofrontal. SIN occipitofrontalis (m.).

occipitofrontalis (m.) [TA], m. occipitofrontal; m. facial composto do músculo epicrânico; o ventre occipital (m. occipital) origina-se do osso occipital e insere-se na gálea aponeurótica; o ventre frontal (m. frontal) origina-se da gálea e insere-se na pele do supercílio e do nariz; *ação*, mover o couro cabeludo; *inervação*, nervo facial. SIN musculus occipitofrontalis [TA], occipitofrontal m.

ocular m.'s, músculos oculares. SIN extraocular m.'s.

Oehl m.'s, músculos de Oehl; filamentos de fibras musculares nas cordas tendíneas da valva atrioventricular esquerda.

omohyoid (m.) [TA], m. omo-hióideo; m. infra-hióideo; formado por dois ventres fixados ao tendão intermediário; *origem*, pelo ventre inferior, da borda superior da escápula, entre o ângulo superior e a incisura; *inserção*, pelo ventre superior, no osso hióide; *ação*, abaixa o osso hióide; *inervação*, nervos espinais cervicais superiores através da alça cervical. SIN musculus omohyoideus [TA], omohyoid.

opponens m., m. oponente; m. que facilita a oposição da polpa da falange distal do polegar às polpas dos outros dedos, principalmente do dedo mínimo. SIN musculus opponens [TA].

opponens digiti minimi (m.) [TA], m. oponente do dedo mínimo; m. hipotenar da palma; *origem*, hâmulo do osso hamato e ligamento transverso do carpo; *inserção*, diáfise do quinto metacarpal; *ação*, põe a mão em concha, levando a face ulnar da mão em direção ao centro da palma; *inervação*, nervo ulnar. SIN musculus opponens digiti minimi [TA], musculus opponens digiti quinti, musculus opponens digiti, opposer (m.) of little finger.

opponens pollicis (m.) [TA], m. oponente do polegar; m. tenar da palma; *origem*, crista do trapézio e ligamento transverso do carpo (retináculo dos músculos flexores); *inserção*, superfície anterior de toda a extensão da diáfise do primeiro osso metacarpal; *ação*, atua na articulação carpometacarpal para colocar a mão em concha, permitindo que se oponha o polegar a outros dedos; *inervação*, nervo mediano. SIN musculus opponens pollicis [TA], opposer (m.) of thumb.

opposer (m.) of little finger, m. oponente do dedo mínimo da mão. SIN opponens digiti minimi (m.).

opposer (m.) of thumb, m. oponente do polegar. SIN opponens pollicis (m.).

orbicular m. [TA], m. orbicular; lâmina de m. semelhante a um esfíncter, que circunda um orifício como a boca ou as fissuras palpebrais. SIN musculus orbicularis [TA], orbicularis m., orbicularis (2).

orbicular m. of eye, m. orbicular do olho. SIN orbicularis oculi (m.).

orbicularis m., m. orbicular. SIN orbicular m.

orbicularis oculi (m.) [TA], m. orbicular do olho; m. facial das pálpebras; consiste em três partes: parte orbital, ou porção externa, que se origina do processo frontal da maxila e do processo nasal do osso frontal, circunda a abertura da órbita e está inserido próximo da origem; parte palpebral, ou porção interna, que se origina do ligamento palpebral medial, atravessa cada pálpebra e insere-se na rafe palpebral lateral; a parte lacrimal (músculo tensor do tarso, ou músculo de Duverney ou Horner) origina-se da crista lacrimal posterior e atravessa o saco lacrimal para se unir à parte palpebral; *ação*, fecha o olho, enruga a fronte verticalmente; *inervação*, ramos zigomático e temporal do nervo facial. SIN musculus orbicularis oculi [TA], musculus orbicularis palpebrarum, orbicular m. of eye, sphincter oculi.

orbicularis oris (m.) [TA], m. orbicular da boca; m. facial da boca; *origem*, por faixa nasolabial do septo do nariz, por feixe incisivo superior da fossa incisiva da maxila, por feixe incisivo inferior da mandíbula de cada lado da sínfise; *inserção*, fibras circundam a boca entre a pele e a mucosa dos lábios e das bochechas, e estão fundidas com outros músculos; *ação*, fecha os lábios; *inervação*, nervo facial. SIN musculus orbicularis oris [TA], musculus sphincter oris, orbicular m. of mouth, sphincter oris.

orbicular m. of mouth, m. orbicular da boca. SIN orbicularis oris (m.).

orbital m., m. orbital. SIN orbitalis (m.).

orbitalis (m.) [TA], m. orbital; m. não-estriado rudimentar que cruza o sulco infra-orbital e a fissura esfenomaxilar, intimamente unido ao periósteo da órbita. SIN musculus orbitalis [TA], Müller m. (1), orbital m.

palatoglossus (m.) [TA], m. palatoglosso; m. palatino que forma o pilar anterior da fossa tonsilar; *origem*, superfície oral do palato mole; *inserção*, lateral da língua; *ação*, eleva o dorso da língua e estreita as fauces; *inervação*, plexo faríngeo (raiz craniana do nervo acessório). SIN musculus palatoglossus [TA], glossopalatinus, musculus glossopalatinus, palatoglossus.

palatopharyngeal (m.), m. palatofaríngeo. SIN palatopharyngeus (m.).

palatopharyngeus (m.) [TA], m. palatofaríngeo; *origem*, palato mole; forma o pilar posterior das fauces ou fossa tonsilar; *inserção*, borda posterior da cartilagem tireóidea e aponeurose da faringe quando se torna parte da camada muscular longitudinal interna da faringe; *ação*, estreita as fauces, abaixa o palato mole, eleva a faringe e a laringe; *inervação*, plexo faríngeo (raiz craniana do nervo acessório). SIN musculus palatopharyngeus [TA], musculus pharyngopalatinus, palatopharyngeal (m.), palatopharyngeus, pharyngopalatinus, pharyngostaphylinus.

palatouvularis m., m. da úvula. SIN m. of uvula.

palmar interossei (interosseous m.'s) [TA], músculos interósseos palmares; três músculos intrínsecos na mão; *origem*, primeiro: face ulnar do segundo metacarpal; segundo e terceiro: faces radiais do quarto e quinto metacarpais; *inserção*, primeiro: na face ulnar do indicador; segundo e terceiro: nas faces radiais do quarto e quinto dedos; *ação*, aduz os dedos em direção ao eixo do terceiro dedo; *inervação*, nervo ulnar. VER TAMBÉM flexor pollicis brevis (m.) SIN musculus interosseus palmaris [TA], musculus interosseus volaris.

palmaris brevis (m.) [TA], m. palmar curto; m. cutâneo da mão; *origem*, face ulnar da porção central da aponeurose palmar; *inserção*, pele da face ulnar da mão; *ação*, enruga a pele na face medial da palma; *inervação*, nervo ulnar. SIN musculus palmaris brevis [TA], short palmar m.

palmaris longus (m.) [TA], m. palmar longo; m. da camada superficial do compartimento anterior (flexor) do antebraço; *origem*, epicôndilo medial do úmero; *inserção*, retináculo dos músculos flexores do punho e fáscia palmar; *ação*, tensiona a fáscia palmar e flete a mão e o antebraço; está ausente em cerca de 20% dos casos; quando tensionado, seu tendão sobressai nitidamente no punho e fica sobre o nervo mediano; *inervação*, nervo mediano. SIN musculus palmaris longus [TA], long palmar m.

panniculus carnosus m., panículo carnoso; (1) camada de m., situada sob a pele, através da qual pode-se fazer a pele arrepiar; é particularmente bem desenvolvida em cavalos; (2) em seres humanos, platisma.

papillary m. [TA], m. papilar; m. do grupo de feixes miocárdicos que terminam na corda tendínea, fixando-se às cúspides das valvas atrioventriculares; cada ventrículo tem um m. papilar anterior e um posterior; o ventrículo direito algumas vezes apresenta um m. papilar septal. SIN musculus papillaris [TA].

pectinate m.'s [TA], músculos pectíneos; cristas proeminentes de miocárdio atrial localizadas na superfície interna de grande parte do átrio direito e de ambas as aurículas. SIN musculi pectinati [TA], pectinate fibers.

pectineal m., m. pectíneo. SIN pectineus (m.).

pectineus (m.) [TA], m. pectíneo; *origem*, crista do púbis; *inserção*, linha pectínea do fêmur; *ação*, aduz a coxa e ajuda na flexão; *inervação*, nervo obturatório e femoral. SIN musculus pectineus [TA], pectineal m.

pectoralis major m. [TA], m. peitoral maior; m. toracoapendicular superficial do tórax; *origem*, parte clavicular [TA] (pars clavicularis [TA]), metade medial da clavícula; parte esternocostal [TA] (pars sternocostalis [TA]), superfície anterior do manúbrio e corpo do esterno e cartilagens da primeira a sexta costelas; parte abdominal [TA] (pars abdominalis [TA]), aponeurose do oblíquo externo; *inserção*, crista do tubérculo maior do úmero; *ação*, aduz e roda medialmente o braço; *inervação*, nervo torácico anterior. SIN musculus pectoralis major [TA], greater pectoral m.

pectoralis minor (m.) [TA], m. peitoral menor; m. toracoapendicular profundo do tórax; *origem*, terceira à quinta costelas nas articulações costocondrais;

inserção, extremidade do processo coracóide da escápula; *ação*, abaixa a escápula ou eleva as costelas; *inervação*, nervo peitoral medial. SIN musculus pectoralis minor [TA], smaller pectoral m.

pectorodorsal m., m. pectorodorsal. SIN pectorodorsalis m.

pectorodorsalis m., m. pectorodorsal; m. anômalo ou tira tendínea que atravessa a axila a partir do m. peitoral maior para se inserir com o m. latíssimo do dorso no úmero. Considerado um vestígio do panículo carnoso de animais inferiores. SIN axillary arch m., axillary arch, Langer arch, Langer m., pectorodorsal m.

pennate m. [TA], m. peniforme; m. com um tendão central em direção ao qual as fibras convergem de cada lado, como os filamentos de uma pena. SIN musculus pennatus [TA], bipennate m., musculus bipennatus. VER semipennate m.

perineal m.'s [TA], músculos perineais; os músculos situados na região perineal; estes são o esfíncter externo do ânus, o m. transverso superficial do períneo, m. isquiocavernoso, m. bulboesponjoso, m. transverso profundo do períneo e esfíncter da uretra. SIN musculi perinei [TA].

peroneus brevis (m.), m. fibular curto; *termo oficial alternativo para fibularis brevis (m.).

peroneus longus (m.), m. fibular longo; *termo oficial alternativo para fibularis longus (m.).

peroneus tertius (m.), m. fibular terceiro; *termo oficial alternativo para fibularis tertius (m.).

piriform m., m. piriforme. SIN piriformis (m.).

piriformis (m.) [TA], m. piriforme; m. que se estende da pelve até a região glútea; *origem*, margens dos forames sacrais pélvicos e incisura isquiática maior do ílio; *inserção*, borda superior do trocânter maior; *ação*, roda a coxa lateralmente; *inervação*, nervo para o músculo piriforme (plexo ciático). SIN musculus piriformis [TA], musculus pyriformis, piriform m.

plantar m., m. plantar. SIN plantaris (m.).

plantar interossei (interosseous m.'s), músculos interósseos plantares; três músculos intrínsecos do pé; *origem*, a face medial do terceiro, quarto e quinto ossos metatarsais; *inserção*, face correspondente da falange proximal dos mesmos dedos; *ação*, aduz três dedos laterais; *inervação*, nervo plantar lateral. SIN musculi interosseus plantaris [TA].

plantaris (m.) [TA], m. plantar; pequeno m. do compartimento superficial posterior (flexor plantar) da perna; *origem*, crista supracondilar lateral; *inserção*, margem medial do tendão de Aquiles e fáscia profunda do tornozelo; *ação*, tradicionalmente descrita como flexão plantar do pé; muitos pesquisadores agora acreditam que o m. plantar é basicamente um órgão proprioceptivo; *inervação*, nervo tibial. SIN musculus plantaris [TA], musculus tibialis gracilis, plantar m.

plantar quadrate m., m. quadrado plantar. SIN quadratus plantae (m.).

platysma (m.) [TA], platisma; m. facial na região do pescoço; *origem*, camada subcutânea e fáscia que cobre os músculos peitoral maior e deltóide ao nível da primeira ou segunda costela; *inserção*, borda inferior da mandíbula, risório e platisma do lado oposto; *ação*, abaixa o lábio inferior, forma estrias na pele do pescoço e da parte superior do tórax quando a mandíbula é cerrada, indicando estresse, raiva; *inervação*, ramo cervical do nervo facial. SIN platysma [TA], musculus platysma myoides, musculus platysma, musculus subcutaneus colli, musculus tetragonus.

pleuroesophageal (m.), m. pleuroesofágico. SIN pleuroesophageus (m.).

pleuroesophageus (m.) [TA], m. pleuroesofágico; fascículos musculares, originados da pleura mediastinal, que reforçam a musculatura do esôfago. SIN musculus pleuroesophageus [TA], pleuroesophageal (m.).

popliteal m., m. poplíteo. SIN popliteus (m.).

popliteus (m.) [TA], m. poplíteo; m. que forma o assoalho da fossa poplítea; *origem*, côndilo lateral do fêmur; *inserção*, superfície posterior da tíbia acima da linha oblíqua; *ação*, a partir da posição de extensão completa e "travada", roda o fêmur medialmente, sobre o platô tibial fixo cerca de 5°, com o "destravamento" do joelho permitindo a flexão; *inervação*, nervo tibial. SIN musculus popliteus [TA], popliteal m., popliteus (3).

posterior auricular (m.), m. auricular posterior. SIN auricularis posterior (m.).

posterior cervical intertransversarii (m.'s) [TA], músculos intertransversários posteriores do pescoço; *origem*, músculos laterais: tubérculo posterior do processo transverso cervical; músculos mediais: processo transverso; *inserção*, partes correspondentes do próximo processo transverso superior; *ação*, abduz as vértebras cervicais; *inervação*, parte lateral: ramos primários ventrais dos nervos espinais cervicais; parte medial: ramos primários dorsais dos nervos espinais cervicais. SIN musculi intertransversarii posteriores cervicis [TA], posterior cervical intertransverse m.'s.

posterior cervical intertransverse m.'s, músculos intertransversários posteriores do pescoço. SIN posterior cervical intertransversarii (m.'s).

posterior cricoarytenoid (m.) [TA], m. cricoaritenóideo posterior; m. intrínseco da laringe; *origem*, depressão na superfície posterior da lâmina da cricóide; *inserção*, processo muscular da aritenóide; *ação*, abduz as pregas vocais, alargando a rima da glote como para realizar uma inspiração profunda; *inervação*, nervo laríngeo recorrente. SIN musculus cricoarytenoideus posterior [TA].

posterior scalene m., m. escaleno posterior; *termo oficial alternativo para scalenus posterior (m.).

posterior tibial m., m. tibial posterior. SIN tibialis posterior (m.).

Pozzi m., m. de Pozzi. SIN estensor digitorum brevis (m.) of hand.

procerus (m.) [TA], m. prócero; m. facial da parte central da fronte; *inserção*, no frontal; *ação*, ajuda o frontal; *origem*, da membrana que cobre a ponte do nariz; *inervação*, ramo do nervo facial. SIN musculus procerus [TA], musculus pyramidalis nasi, procerus.

pronator (m.) [TA], m. pronador; m. que gira o antebraço em torno de um eixo longitudinal, da posição de supinação ou neutra em direção a uma posição na qual o dorso da mão está voltado anteriormente em relação à posição anatômica. SIN musculus pronator (m.).

pronator quadratus (m.) [TA], m. pronador quadrado; m. da camada profunda do compartimento anterior (flexor) do antebraço; *origem*, quarto distal da superfície anterior da ulna; *inserção*, quarto distal da superfície anterior do rádio; *ação*, realiza a pronação do antebraço; *inervação*, nervo interósseo anterior. SIN musculus pronator quadratus [TA], quadrate pronator m.

pronator teres (m.) [TA], m. pronador redondo; m. da camada superficial do compartimento anterior do antebraço; *origem*, a cabeça superficial (umeral), da origem do flexor comum no epicôndilo medial do úmero; a cabeça profunda (ulnar), da face medial do processo coronóide da ulna; *inserção*, meio da superfície lateral do rádio; *ação*, realiza a pronação do antebraço; *inervação*, nervo mediano. SIN musculus pronator teres [TA], musculus pronator radii teres, round pronator m.

psoas major (m.) [TA], m. psoas maior; m. inguinal; *origem*, corpos das vértebras e discos intervertebrais da décima segunda vértebra torácica até a quinta vértebra lombar, e processos transversos das vértebras lombares; *inserção*, forma uma inserção comum com os músculos ilíacos no trocânter menor do fêmur; *ação*, flexão primária da articulação do quadril; *inervação*, plexo lombar (ramos ventrais do primeiro, segundo e, geralmente, terceiro nervos espinais lombares). SIN musculus psoas major [TA], greater psoas m.

psoas minor (m.) [TA], m. psoas menor; m. inconstante, ausente em cerca de 40% das pessoas; *origem*, corpos da décima segunda vértebra torácica e primeira vértebra lombar e disco entre elas; *inserção*, eminência iliopúbica através do arco iliopectíneo (fáscia ilíaca); *ação*, ajuda na flexão da coluna lombar; *inervação*, plexo lombar. SIN musculus psoas minor [TA], smaller psoas (m.).

puboanalis (m.) [TA], m. puboanal; parte do m. pubococcígeo cujas fibras se inserem na superfície externa do canal anal. SIN musculus puboanalis [TA].

pubococcygeal m., m. pubococcígeo. SIN pubococcygeus (m.).

pubococcygeus (m.) [TA], m. pubococcígeo; parte anterior do m. levantador do ânus, originada na superfície pélvica do corpo do púbis e arco tendíneo adjacente da fáscia obturatória, fixando-se ao cóccix. SIN musculus pubococcygeus [TA], pubococcygeal m.

puboperinealis (m.) [TA], m. puboperineal; parte do m. pubococcígeo cujas fibras se inserem no corpo perineal. SIN musculus puboperinealis [TA].

puboprostatic (m.), m. puboprostático. SIN puboprostaticus (m.).

puboprostaticus (m.) [TA], m. puboprostático; fibras musculares lisas no ligamento puboprostático. SIN musculus puboprostaticus [TA], levator prostatae (m.)*, musculus levator prostatae*, elevator (m.) of prostate, puboprostatic (m.).

puborectal m., m. puborretal. SIN puborectalis (m.).

puborectalis (m.) [TA], m. puborretal; a parte medial do m. pubococcígeo (levantador do ânus) que passa do corpo do púbis ao redor da face posterior do ânus, para formar uma tira muscular ao nível da junção anorretal; contrai para aumentar a flexura anorretal (perineal) durante uma peristalse, a fim de manter a continência fecal, e relaxa para permitir a defecação. SIN musculus puborectalis [TA], Braune m., puborectal m.

pubovaginal m., m. pubovaginal. SIN pubovaginalis (m.).

pubovaginalis (m.) [TA], m. pubovaginal; na mulher, as fibras mais mediais do m. pubococcígeo (levantador do ânus), que se estendem do púbis até as paredes laterais da vagina. SIN musculus pubovaginalis [TA], pubovaginal m.

pubovesical m., m. pubovesical. SIN pubovesicalis (m.).

pubovesicalis (m.) [TA], m. pubovesical; fibras musculares lisas no ligamento pubovesical na mulher. SIN musculus pubovesicalis [TA], pubovesical m.

pyramidal m., m. piramidal. SIN pyramidalis (m.).

pyramidal m. of auricle [TA], m. piramidal da orelha; um prolongamento ocasional das fibras do m. trágico até a espinha da hélice. SIN musculus pyramidalis auriculae [TA], Jung m., pyramidal auricular m.

pyramidal auricular m., m. piramidal da orelha. SIN pyramidal m. of auricle.

pyramidalis (m.) [TA], m. piramidal; m. da parte inferior do abdome; *origem*, crista do púbis; *inserção*, parte inferior da linha alba; *ação*, tensiona a linha alba; *inervação*, nervo subcostal. SIN musculus pyramidalis [TA], pyramidal m.

quadrate m. [TA], m. quadrado; m. aproximadamente quadrado ou com quatro lados. SIN musculus quadratus [TA], quadratus m.

quadrate m. of loins, m. quadrado do lombo. SIN quadratus lumborum (m.).

quadrate pronator m., m. pronador quadrado. SIN pronator quadratus (m.).

quadrate m. of sole, m. quadrado plantar. SIN quadratus plantae (m.).

quadrate m. of thigh, m. quadrado femoral. SIN quadratus femoris (m.).
quadrate m. of upper lip, m. quadrado do lábio superior. SIN *musculus quadratus labii superioris.*
quadratus m., m. quadrado. SIN quadrate m.
quadratus fem'oris (m.) [TA], m. quadrado femoral; m. profundo da região glútea inferior (nádega); *inserção,* crista intertrocantérica; *origem,* borda lateral do túber isquiático; *ação,* roda a coxa lateralmente; *inervação,* nervo para o m. quadrado femoral (plexo sacral). SIN musculus quadratus femoris [TA], quadrate m. of thigh.
quadratus lumborum (m.) [TA], m. quadrado do lombo; m. plano da parede abdominal posterior; *origem,* crista ilíaca, ligamento iliolombar e processos transversos das vértebras lombares inferiores; *inserção,* décima segunda costela e processos transversos das vértebras lombares superiores; *ação,* abduz o tronco; *inervação,* ramos primários ventrais dos nervos espinais lombares superiores. SIN musculus quadratus lumborum [TA], lumbar quadrate m., quadrate m. of loins.
quadratus plantae (m.) [TA], m. quadrado plantar; m. da segunda camada de músculos plantares; *origem,* por duas cabeças, das bordas lateral e medial da superfície inferior do calcâneo; *inserção,* tendões do músculo flexor longo dos dedos; *ação,* ajuda o flexor longo; *inervação,* nervo plantar lateral. SIN musculus quadratus plantae [TA], flexor accessorius (m.)*, musculus flexor accessorius*, accessory flexor m. of foot, caro quadrata sylvii, musculus pronator pedis, plantar quadrate m., quadrate m. of sole.
quadriceps fem'oris (m.) [TA], m. quadríceps femoral; músculos anteriores da coxa; *origem,* por quatro cabeças: reto femoral, vasto lateral, vasto intermédio e vasto medial; *inserção,* patela e, portanto, pelo ligamento patelar à tuberosidade tibial; *ação,* estende a perna; flete a coxa por ação do reto femoral; *inervação,* nervo femoral. SIN musculus quadriceps femoris [TA], musculus quadriceps [TA], musculus quadriceps extensor femoris, quadriceps m. of thigh.
quadriceps m. of thigh, m. quadríceps femoral. SIN quadriceps femoris (m.).
radial flexor (m.) of wrist, m. flexor radial do carpo. SIN flexor carpi radialis (m.).
rectococcygeal m., m. retococcígeo. SIN rectococcygeus (m.).
rectococcygeus (m.) [TA], m. retococcígeo; faixa de fibras musculares lisas que segue da superfície posterior do reto até a superfície anterior do segundo ou terceiro segmento coccígeo. SIN musculus rectococcygeus [TA], rectococcygeal m.
rectourethral m.'s, músculos retouretrais; *termo oficial alternativo para anorectoperineal m.'s.
rectouterine m., m. retouterino. SIN rectouterinus (m.).
rectouterinus (m.) [TA], m. retouterino; faixa de tecido fibroso e fibras musculares lisas que passam entre o colo do útero e o reto na prega retouterina, de cada lado. SIN musculus rectouterinus [TA], rectouterine m.
rectovesical m., m. retovesical. SIN rectovesicalis (m.).
rectovesicalis (m.) [TA], m. retovesical; fibras musculares lisas na prega sacrogenital no homem; elas correspondem ao m. retouterino da mulher. SIN musculus rectovesicalis [TA], rectovesical m.
rectus m. of abdomen, m. reto do abdome. SIN rectus abdominis (m.).
rectus abdominis (m.) [TA], m. reto do abdome; m. da parede abdominal ventral, ao lado da linha alba, e caracterizado por intersecções tendíneas que separam seu comprimento em múltiplos ventres; *origem,* crista e sínfise púbicas; *inserção,* processo xifóide e quinta à sétima cartilagens costais; *ação,* flete a coluna vertebral lombar, puxa o tórax para baixo em direção ao púbis; *inervação,* nervos toracoabdominais. SIN musculus rectus abdominis [TA], rectus m. of abdomen.
rectus capitis anterior (m.) [TA], m. reto anterior da cabeça; m. suboccipital (pré-vertebral); *origem,* processo transverso e massa lateral do atlas; *inserção,* processo basilar do osso occipital; *ação,* roda e inclina a cabeça para a frente; *inervação,* ramo primário ventral do primeiro e segundo nervos espinais cervicais. SIN musculus rectus capitis anterior [TA], anterior rectus m. of head, musculus rectus capitis anticus minor.
rectus capitis lateralis (m.) [TA], m. reto lateral da cabeça; m. suboccipital (pré-vertebral) da parte superior do pescoço; *origem,* processo transverso do atlas; *inserção,* processo jugular do osso occipital; *ação,* inclina a cabeça para um lado; *inervação,* ramo primário ventral do primeiro nervo espinal cervical. SIN musculus rectus capitis lateralis [TA], lateral rectus m. of the head.
rectus capitis posterior major (m.) [TA], m. reto posterior maior da cabeça; m. do triângulo suboccipital; *origem,* processo espinhoso do áxis; *inserção,* meio da linha nucal inferior do osso occipital; *ação,* roda e leva a cabeça para trás; *inervação,* ramo dorsal do primeiro nervo cervical (suboccipital). VER TAMBÉM suboccipital m.'s. SIN musculus rectus capitis posterior major [TA], greater posterior rectus m. of head, musculus rectus capitis posticus major.
rectus capitis posterior minor (m.) [TA], m. reto posterior menor da cabeça; m. do triângulo suboccipital; *origem,* do tubérculo posterior do atlas; *inserção,* terço medial da linha nucal inferior do osso occipital; *ação,* roda e leva a cabeça para trás; *inervação,* ramo dorsal do primeiro nervo cervical (suboccipital). VER TAMBÉM suboccipital m.'s. SIN musculus rectus capitis posterior minor [TA], musculus rectus capitis posticus minor, smaller posterior rectus m. of head.
rectus femoris (m.) [TA], m. reto femoral; cabeça anterior (superficial) média do m. quadríceps femoral; *origem,* espinha ântero-inferior do ílio e margem superior do acetábulo; *inserção,* através do tendão comum do quadríceps femoral, na patela, e através do ligamento patelar à tuberosidade tibial. SIN musculus rectus femoris [TA], rectus m. of thigh.
rectus m. of thigh, m. reto femoral. SIN rectus femoris (m.).
red m., m. vermelho; m. de contração lenta, no qual predominam pequenas fibras musculares "vermelhas" de tom escuro; a mioglobina é abundante e há numerosas mitocôndrias, caracterizado por contração lenta e mantida (tônica). Contrasta com o m. branco.
Reisseisen m.'s, músculos de Reisseisen; fibras musculares lisas microscópicas nos menores tubos brônquicos.
rhomboid major (m.) [TA], m. rombóide maior; m. toracoapendicular; *origem,* processos espinhosos e ligamentos supra-espinais correspondentes das quatro primeiras vértebras torácicas; *inserção,* borda medial da escápula abaixo da espinha; *ação,* move a escápula em direção à coluna vertebral; *inervação,* nervo dorsal da escápula. SIN musculus rhomboideus major [TA], greater rhomboid m.
rhomboid minor (m.) [TA], m. rombóide menor; m. toracoapendicular; *origem,* processos espinhosos da sexta e sétima vértebras cervicais; *inserção,* margem medial da escápula sobre a espinha; *ação,* movimenta a escápula em direção à coluna vertebral e ligeiramente para cima; *inervação,* nervo dorsal da escápula. SIN musculus rhomboideus minor [TA], lesser rhomboid m.
rider's m.'s, músculos de montaria; os músculos adutores da coxa, que entram em ação especialmente ao se montar a cavalo.
Riolan m., m. de Riolan; **(1)** fibras marginais da parte palpebral do m. orbicular do olho; **(2)** SIN cremaster m.
risorius (m.) [TA], m. risório; m. facial da boca; *origem,* do platisma e da fáscia do masseter; *inserção,* orbicular da boca e pele no ângulo da boca; *ação,* movimenta o ângulo da boca lateralmente, alongando a rima da boca; *inervação,* nervo facial. SIN musculus risorius [TA], Albinus m. (1), Santorini m.
rotator m., m. rotador; **(1)** um dos músculos rotadores; **(2)** m. que produz uma rotação, isoladamente ou em conjunto com outros rotadores, em torno de um eixo, p. ex., músculos rotadores da coluna vertebral. SIN musculus rotator [TA], rotator.
rotatores (m.'s) [TA], músculos rotadores; a mais profunda das três camadas de músculos transverso-espinais, desenvolvida sobretudo na região torácica; originam-se do processo transverso de uma vértebra e estão inseridos na raiz do processo espinhoso de duas ou três vértebras subseqüentes acima; *ação,* tradicionalmente descrito como uma coluna, é mais provável que esses músculos, que possuem uma densidade muito alta de fusos musculares, sejam órgãos de propriocepção; *inervação,* ramos primários dorsais dos nervos espinais. SIN musculi rotatores [TA].
rotatores cervicis (m.'s) [TA], músculos rotadores do pescoço; os músculos rotadores fixados às vértebras cervicais. SIN musculi rotatores cervicis [TA], cervical rotator m.'s.
rotatores lumborum (m.'s) [TA], músculos rotadores do lombo; os músculos rotadores das vértebras lombares. SIN musculi rotatores lumborum [TA], lumbar rotator m.'s.
rotatores thoracis (m.'s) [TA], músculos rotadores do tórax; os rotadores das vértebras torácicas. SIN musculi rotatores thoracis [TA], thoracic rotator m.'s.
Rouget m., m. de Rouget. SIN circular *fibers,* em *fiber.*
round pronator m., m. pronador redondo. SIN pronator teres (m.).
Ruysch m., m. de Ruysch; o tecido muscular do fundo do útero.
salpingopharyngeal m., m. salpingofaríngeo. SIN salpingopharyngeus (m.).
salpingopharyngeus (m.) [TA], m. salpingofaríngeo; *origem,* lâmina medial da parte cartilaginosa da tuba auditiva; *inserção,* camada muscular longitudinal da faringe associada ao m. palatofaríngeo; *ação,* ajuda na elevação da faringe e, de acordo com alguns, ajuda na abertura da tuba auditiva durante a deglutição; *inervação,* plexo faríngeo. SIN musculus salpingopharyngeus [TA], salpingopharyngeal m.
Santorini m., m. de Santorini. SIN risorius (m.).
sartorius (m.) [TA], m. sartório; m. anterior superficial da coxa; *origem,* espinha ântero-superior do ílio; *inserção,* borda medial da tuberosidade da tíbia; *ação,* flete a coxa e a perna, roda a perna medialmente e a coxa lateralmente; *inervação,* nervo femoral. SIN musculus sartorius [TA], tailor's m.
scalenus anterior (m.) [TA], m. escaleno anterior; m. lateral da metade inferior do pescoço; *origem,* tubérculos anteriores dos processos transversos da terceira à sexta vértebras cervicais; *inserção,* tubérculo escaleno da primeira costela; *ação,* eleva a primeira costela; *inervação,* plexo cervical. SIN musculus scalenus anterior [TA], anterior scalene m.*, musculus scalenus anticus.
scalenus medius (m.) [TA], m. escaleno médio; m. lateral da metade inferior do pescoço; *origem,* lamelas costotransversas dos processos transversos da segunda à sexta vértebras cervicais; *inserção,* primeira costela posterior à artéria subclávia; *ação,* eleva a primeira costela; *inervação,* plexo cervical. SIN musculus scalenus medius [TA], middle scalene m.*

scalenus minimus (m.) [TA], m. escaleno mínimo; fascículo muscular independente ocasional entre os músculos escaleno anterior e médio, tendo a mesma ação e inervação. SIN musculus scalenus minimus [TA], Albinus m. (2), Sibson m., smallest scalene m.

scalenus posterior (m.) [TA], m. escaleno posterior; m. lateral da metade inferior do pescoço; *origem*, tubérculos posteriores de processos transversos da quarta à sexta vértebras cervicais; *inserção*, superfície lateral da segunda costela; *ação*, eleva a segunda costela; *inervação*, plexos cervical e braquial. SIN musculus scalenus posterior [TA], posterior scalene m.*, musculus scalenus posticus.

scalp m., m. epicrânico. SIN epicranius (m.).

scapulohumeral m.'s [TA], músculos escapuloumerais; músculos intrínsecos da articulação do ombro originados na escápula, que se inserem no úmero e atuam sobre ele, produzindo movimento da articulação glenoumeral; incluem os músculos supra-espinal, infra-espinal, redondos menor e maior e subescapular. SIN musculi scapulohumerales [TA].

Sebileau m., m. de Sebileau; fibras profundas da túnica dartos que entram no septo escrotal.

second tibial m., m. tibial segundo. SIN musculus tibialis secundus.

semimembranosus (m.) [TA], m. semimembranóseo; m. profundo do jarrete do compartimento posterior (flexor) da coxa; *origem*, túber isquiático; *inserção*, côndilo medial da tíbia e pela membrana ao ligamento colateral tibial da articulação do joelho, fáscia poplítea e, através de seu tendão refletido de inserção (ligamento poplíteo oblíquo), ao côndilo lateral do fêmur; *ação*, flete o joelho e roda a perna medialmente quando o joelho está fletido; e contribui para a estabilidade do joelho estendido tensionando a cápsula articular do joelho; *inervação*, nervo tibial. SIN musculus semimembranosus [TA].

semipennate m. [TA], m. semipeniforme; m. com um tendão lateral ao qual as fibras estão fixadas obliquamente, como a metade de uma pena. SIN musculus semipennatus [TA], musculus unipennatus*, unipennate m.*.

semispinal m., m. semi-espinal. SIN semispinalis m.

semispinal m. of head, m. semi-espinal da cabeça. SIN semispinalis capitis (m.).

semispinalis m. [TA], m. semi-espinal; a camada mais superficial das três camadas do m. transverso-espinal; formado pelos músculos semi-espinal da cabeça, semi-espinal do pescoço e semi-espinal do tórax. SIN musculus semispinalis [TA], semispinal m.

semispinalis capitis (m.) [TA], m. semi-espinal da cabeça; *origem*, processos das cinco ou seis vértebras torácicas superiores e processos articulares das quatro vértebras cervicais inferiores; *inserção*, osso occipital entre as linhas nucal superior e inferior; *ação*, roda a cabeça e movimenta-a para trás; *inervação*, ramos primários dorsais dos nervos espinais cervicais. SIN musculus semispinalis capitis [TA], musculus complexus, semispinal m. of head.

semispinalis cervicis (m.) [TA], m. semi-espinal do pescoço; contínuo com o m. semi-espinal do tórax; *origem*, processos transversos da segunda à quinta vértebras torácicas; *inserção*, processos espinhosos do áxis e da terceira à quinta vértebras cervicais; *ação*, estende a coluna cervical; *inervação*, ramos primários dorsais dos nervos espinais cervicais e torácicos. SIN musculus semispinalis cervicis [TA], musculus semispinalis colli*, semispinal m. of neck.

semispinalis thoracis (m.) [TA], m. semi-espinal do tórax; *origem*, processos transversos da quinta à décima primeira vértebras torácicas; *inserção*, processos espinhosos das quatro primeiras vértebras torácicas e da quinta e sétima vértebras cervicais; *ação*, estende a coluna vertebral; *inervação*, ramos primários dorsais dos nervos espinais cervicais e torácicos. SIN musculus semispinalis thoracis [TA], musculus semispinalis dorsi, semispinal m. of thorax.

semispinal m. of neck, m. semi-espinal do pescoço. SIN semispinalis cervicis (m.).

semispinal m. of thorax, m. semi-espinal do tórax. SIN semispinalis thoracis (m.).

semitendinosus (m.) [TA], m. semitendíneo; m. do jarrete medial superficial do compartimento posterior (flexor) da coxa; *origem*, túber isquiático; *inserção*, superfície medial do quarto superior da diáfise da tíbia; *ação*, estende a coxa, flete a perna e roda-a medialmente; *inervação*, nervo tibial. SIN musculus semitendinosus [TA].

serratus anterior (m.) [TA], m. serrátil anterior; m. toracoapendicular (escapulotorácico); *origem*, do centro da face lateral das oito ou nove primeiras costelas; *inserção*, ângulos superior e inferior e a margem medial interveniente da escápula; *ação*, roda e empurra a escápula para frente, eleva as costelas; *inervação*, nervo torácico longo do plexo braquial. SIN musculus serratus anterior [TA], anterior serratus m., costoscapularis, musculus serratus magnus.

serratus posterior inferior (m.) [TA], m. serrátil posterior inferior; m. intermediário inferior do dorso; *origem*, com o latíssimo do dorso, dos processos espinhosos das duas vértebras torácicas inferiores e das duas vértebras lombares superiores; *inserção*, nas bordas inferiores das quatro últimas costelas; *ação*, leva as costelas inferiores para trás e para baixo; *inervação*, nono ao décimo segundo nervos intercostais. SIN musculus serratus posterior inferior [TA], inferior posterior serratus m.

serratus posterior superior (m.) [TA], m. serrátil posterior superior; m. intermediário superior do dorso; *origem*, dos processos espinhosos das duas vértebras cervicais inferiores e duas vértebras torácicas superiores; *inserção*, na face lateral dos ângulos da segunda à quinta costelas; *inervação*, primeiro ao quarto nervos intercostais. SIN musculus serratus posterior superior [TA], superior posterior serratus m.

shawl m., m. do xale; designação obsoleta do m. trapézio (trapezius (m.)).

short abductor m. of thumb, m. abdutor curto do polegar. SIN abductor pollicis brevis (m.).

short adductor m., m. adutor curto. SIN adductor brevis (m.).

short extensor (m.) of great toe, m. extensor curto do hálux. SIN extensor hallucis brevis (m.).

short extensor (m.) of thumb, m. extensor curto do polegar. SIN extensor pollicis brevis (m.).

short extensor (m.) of toes, m. extensor curto dos dedos do pé. SIN extensor digitorum brevis (m.).

short fibular m., m. fibular curto. SIN fibularis brevis (m.).

short flexor (m.) of great toe, m. flexor curto do hálux. SIN flexor hallucis brevis (m.).

short flexor (m.) of little finger, m. flexor curto do dedo mínimo da mão. SIN flexor digiti minimi brevis (m.) of hand.

short flexor (m.) of little toe, m. flexor curto do dedo mínimo do pé. SIN flexor digiti minimi brevis (m.) of foot.

short flexor (m.) of thumb, m. flexor curto do polegar. SIN flexor pollicis brevis (m.).

short flexor (m.) of toes, m. flexor curto dos dedos do pé. SIN flexor digitorum brevis (m.).

short levatores costarum (m.'s), músculos levantadores curtos das costelas. SIN levatores costarum breves (m.'s).

short palmar m., m. palmar curto. SIN palmaris brevis (m.).

short peroneal m., m. fibular curto. SIN fibularis brevis (m.).

short radial extensor m. of wrist, m. extensor radial curto do carpo. SIN extensor carpi radialis brevis (m.).

shunt m. [TA], m. que, em vez de produzir movimento observável, contrai para resistir às forças de deslocamento que ocorrem nas articulações, p. ex., o músculo coracobraquial, a cabeça curta do bíceps e a cabeça longa do tríceps contraem-se para resistir às forças de deslocamento para baixo na articulação do ombro, como ao carregar bagagem.

Sibson m., m. de Sibson. SIN scalenus minimus (m.).

skeletal m., m. esquelético; macroscopicamente, um conjunto de fibras musculares estriadas unidas em uma ou ambas as extremidades com o arcabouço ósseo do corpo; pode ser um músculo apendicular ou axial; histologicamente, um m. que consiste em fibras musculares esqueléticas alongadas, multinucleadas, com estriações transversais, juntamente com tecido conjuntivo, vasos sanguíneos e nervos; fibras musculares individuais são circundadas por finas fibras reticulares e colágenas (endomísio); feixes (fascículos) de fibras musculares são circundados por tecido conjuntivo irregular (perimísio); todo o m. é circundado, exceto na junção do tendão muscular, por um tecido conjuntivo denso (epimísio). SIN musculus skeleti.

smaller m. of helix, m. menor da hélice. SIN helicis minor (m.).

smaller pectoral m., m. peitoral menor. SIN pectoralis minor (m.).

smaller posterior rectus m. of head, m. reto posterior menor da cabeça. SIN rectus capitis posterior minor (m.).

smaller psoas (m.), m. psoas menor. SIN psoas minor (m.).

smallest scalene m., m. escaleno mínimo. SIN scalenus minimus (m.).

smooth m., m. liso; uma das fibras musculares dos órgãos internos, vasos sanguíneos, folículos pilosos, etc.; os elementos contráteis são células alongadas, geralmente fusiformes, com núcleos centrais e um comprimento de 20 a 200 μm, ou ainda maiores no útero grávido; embora não haja estriações transversais, há miofibrilas espessas e finas; as fibras musculares lisas estão unidas em folhetos ou feixes por fibras reticulares, e, freqüentemente, também há redes de fibras elásticas abundantes. VER TAMBÉM involuntary m.'s. SIN unstriated m., unstriped m., visceral m.

Soemmerring m., m. de Soemmerring. SIN levator (m.) of thyroid gland.

soleus (m.) [TA], m. sóleo; m. do compartimento posterior superficial (flexor plantar) da perna; *origem*, superfície posterior da cabeça e terço superior da diáfise da fíbula, linha oblíqua e terço médio da margem medial da tíbia, e um arco tendíneo que passa entre a tíbia e a fíbula sobre os vasos poplíteos; *inserção*, com o gastrocnêmio, pelo tendão do calcâneo (de Aquiles), na tuberosidade do calcâneo; *ação*, flexão plantar do pé; *inervação*, nervo tibial. SIN musculus soleus [TA].

sphincter m. [TA], esfíncter. SIN sphincter.

m. m. of commom bile duct, m. esfíncter do ducto colédoco. SIN sphincter of (common) bile duct.

sphincter m. of pancreatic duct, esfíncter do ducto pancreático. SIN sphincter of pancreatic duct.

sphincter m. of pupil, esfíncter da pupila. SIN sphincter pupillae.

sphincter m. of pylorus, esfíncter do piloro. SIN pyloric sphincter.

sphincter m. of urethra, esfíncter da uretra. SIN external urethral sphincter.

sphincter m. of urinary bladder, esfíncter vesical; esfíncter interno da uretra. SIN internal urethral sphincter.

spinal m., m. espinal. SIN spinalis (m.).
spinal m. of head, m. espinal da cabeça. SIN spinalis capitis (m.).
spinalis (m.) [TA], m. espinal; o componente medial do m. eretor da espinha; é formado pelos músculos espinal da cabeça, espinal do pescoço e espinal do tórax. SIN musculus spinalis [TA], spinal m.
spinalis capitis (m.) [TA], m. espinal da cabeça; extensão inconstante do m. espinal do pescoço até o osso occipital, algumas vezes fundindo-se com o m. semi-espinal da cabeça. SIN musculus spinalis capitis [TA], biventer cervicis, spinal m. of head.
spinalis cervicis (m.) [TA], m. espinal do pescoço; m. inconstante ou rudimentar; *origem*, processos espinhosos da sexta e sétima vértebras cervicais; *inserção*, processos espinhosos do áxis e da terceira vértebra cervical; *ação*, estende a coluna cervical; *inervação*, ramos primários dorsais do nervo cervical. SIN musculus spinalis cervicis [TA], musculus spinalis colli, spinal m. of neck.
spinalis thoracis (m.) [TA], m. espinal do tórax; *origem*, processos espinhosos das vértebras lombares superiores e duas vértebras torácicas inferiores; *inserção*, processos espinhosos das vértebras torácicas médias e superiores; *ação*, sustenta e estende a coluna vertebral; *inervação*, ramos primários dorsais do nervo torácico e lombar superior. SIN musculus spinalis thoracis [TA], musculus spinalis dorsi, spinal m. of thorax.
spinal m. of neck, m. espinal do pescoço. SIN spinalis cervicis (m.).
spinal m. of thorax, m. espinal do tórax. SIN spinalis thoracis (m.).
spindle-shaped m., m. fusiforme. SIN fusiform m.
splenius (m.'s) [TA], músculos esplênios. SIN musculi splenii [TA].
splenius capitis (m.) [TA], m. esplênio da cabeça; m. superficial plano da parte posterior do pescoço, distinto do m. esplênio do pescoço basicamente por sua inserção no crânio; *origem*, do ligamento nucal das quatro últimas vértebras cervicais e do ligamento supra-espinal da primeira e segunda vértebras torácicas; *inserção*, metade lateral da linha nucal superior e processo mastóide; *ação*, roda a cabeça e estende o pescoço; *inervação*, ramos primários dorsais do segundo ao sexto nervos espinais cervicais. SIN musculus splenius capitis [TA], splenius m. of head.
splenius cervicis (m.) [TA], m. esplênio do pescoço; m. superficial plano da parte posterior do pescoço, distinto do m. esplênio da cabeça basicamente por sua inserção nas vértebras cervicais; *origem*, do ligamento supra-espinal e dos processos espinhosos da terceira à quinta vértebras torácicas; *inserção*, tubérculos posteriores dos processos transversos da primeira e segunda (algumas vezes da terceira) vértebras cervicais; *ação*, roda e estende o pescoço; *inervação*, ramos primários dorsais do quarto ao oitavo nervos espinais cervicais. SIN musculus splenius cervicis [TA], musculus splenius colli, splenius m. of neck.
splenius m. of head, m. esplênio da cabeça. SIN splenius capitis (m.).
splenius m. of neck, m. esplênio do pescoço. SIN splenius cervicis (m.).
stapedius (m.) [TA], m. estapédio; um dos músculos dos ossículos da audição; *origem*, paredes internas da eminência piramidal na cavidade timpânica; *inserção*, colo do estribo; *ação*, amortece a vibração do estribo, levando a sua cabeça para trás, em virtude de um reflexo protetor estimulado pelo ruído alto; *inervação*, nervo facial. SIN musculus stapedius [TA], stapedius.
sternal m., m. esternal. SIN sternalis (m.).
sternalis (m.) [TA], m. esternal; m. inconstante, que segue paralelo ao esterno, através da origem costoesternal do músculo peitoral maior, e geralmente ligado aos músculos esternocleidomastóideo e reto do abdome devido à sua origem comum. SIN musculus sternalis [TA], musculus rectus thoracis, sternal m.
sternochondroscapular m., m. esternocondroescapular; m. ocasional que se origina no manúbrio do esterno e na primeira cartilagem costal, seguindo lateralmente e para trás para se inserir na borda superior da escápula. SIN musculus sternochondroscapularis.
sternoclavicular m., m. esternoclavicular; m. ocasional que é uma porção do músculo subclávio, seguindo da parte superior do esterno até a clavícula sob o músculo peitoral maior. SIN musculus sternoclavicularis.
sternocleidomastoid (m.) (SCM) [TA], m. esternocleidomastóideo; m. superficial da face ântero-lateral do pescoço; *origem*, por duas cabeças, da superfície anterior do manúbrio do esterno e extremidade esternal da clavícula; *inserção*, processo mastóide e metade lateral da linha nucal superior; *ação*, roda a cabeça obliquamente para o lado oposto; quando age em conjunto, flete o pescoço e estende a cabeça; *inervação*, motora pelo nervo acessório, sensitiva pelo plexo cervical. SIN musculus sternocleidomastoideus [TA], sternomastoid m.
sternocostalis m., m. esternocostal. SIN transversus thoracis (m.).
sternohyoid m. [TA], m. esterno-hióideo; m. infra-hióideo da parte anterior do pescoço; *origem*, superfície posterior do manúbrio do esterno e primeira cartilagem costal; *inserção*, corpo do osso hióide; *ação*, abaixa o osso hióide; *inervação*, nervo cervical superior através dos nervos espinais (alça cervical). SIN musculus sternohyoideus [TA].
sternomastoid m., m. esternocleidomastóideo. SIN sternocleidomastoid (m.).
sternothyroid (m.) [TA], m. esternotireóideo; m. infra-hióideo da parte anterior do pescoço; *origem*, superfície posterior do manúbrio do esterno e primeira ou segunda cartilagem costal; *inserção*, linha oblíqua da cartilagem tireóidea; *ação*, abaixa a laringe; *inervação*, nervo cervical superior através dos nervos espinais (alça cervical). SIN musculus sternothyroideus [TA].
straight m. [TA], m. reto; membro(s) de um grupo de músculos que seguem mais diretamente ou em uma direção mais próxima do eixo vertical ou horizontal que outros músculos do grupo, p. ex., músculos retos dos músculos extra-oculares ou suboccipitais. SIN musculus rectus [TA].
strap m.'s, músculos infra-hióideos. SIN infrahyoid m.'s.
striated m., m. estriado; m. esquelético ou voluntário no qual há estriações cruzadas nas fibras em virtude de superposição regular de miofilamentos grossos e finos; contrasta com o músculo liso. Embora o m. cardíaco (que não é um músculo voluntário) também tenha aspecto estriado, o termo "músculo estriado" é comumente usado como sinônimo de m. esquelético, voluntário.
styloauricular (m.), m. estiloauricular; pequeno m. ocasional que se estende da raiz do processo estilóide até a cartilagem do meato acústico. SIN musculus styloauricularis.
styloglossus (m.) [TA], m. estiloglosso; m. extrínseco da língua; *ação*, retrai a língua; *origem*, extremidade inferior do processo estilóide; *inserção*, face lateral e inferior da língua; *inervação*, nervo hipoglosso. SIN musculus styloglossus [TA].
stylohyoid (m.) [TA], m. estilo-hióideo; *origem*, processo estilóide do osso temporal; *inserção*, osso hióide por duas porções de cada lado do tendão intermediário do digástrico; *ação*, eleva o osso hióide; *inervação*, nervo facial. SIN musculus stylohyoideus [TA].
stylopharyngeal m., m. estilofaríngeo. SIN stylopharyngeus (m.).
stylopharyngeus (m.) [TA], m. estilofaríngeo; *origem*, raiz do processo estilóide; *inserção*, cartilagem tireóidea e parede da faringe (torna-se parte da túnica longitudinal); *ação*, eleva a faringe e a laringe; *inervação*, nervo glossofaríngeo. SIN musculus stylopharyngeus [TA], stylopharyngeal m.
subanconeus m., m. articular do cotovelo. SIN articularis cubiti (m.).
subclavian m., m. subclávio. SIN subclavius (m.).
subclavius (m.) [TA], m. subclávio; m. toracoapendicular; *origem*, primeira cartilagem costal; *inserção*, superfície inferior da extremidade acromial da clavícula; *ação*, fixa a clavícula ou eleva a primeira costela; *inervação*, nervo subclávio do plexo braquial. SIN musculus subclavius [TA], subclavian m.
subcostal m. [TA], m. subcostal; um dentre vários músculos inconstantes da parede torácica póstero-lateral, que segue a mesma direção que os músculos intercostais internos, mas estende-se através de (profundamente a) uma ou mais costelas. SIN musculus subcostalis [TA], musculus infracostalis.
subcrural m., m. articular do joelho. SIN articularis genus (m.).
suboccipital m.'s [TA], músculos suboccipitais; grupo de músculos localizados imediatamente abaixo do osso occipital; são eles: m. reto anterior da cabeça, músculos retos posteriores maior e menor da cabeça, m. reto lateral da cabeça; músculos oblíquos superior e inferior da cabeça; inervados pelo nervo suboccipital; embora as ações sejam descritas, muitos especialistas afirmam que esses músculos atuam basicamente como órgãos da propriocepção. SIN musculi suboccipitales [TA].
subquadricipital m., m. articular do joelho. SIN articularis genus (m.).
subscapular m., m. subescapular. SIN subscapularis (m.).
subscapularis (m.) [TA], m. subescapular; m. intrínseco (escapuloumeral) da articulação do ombro, cujo tendão contribui para a formação do manguito rotador; *origem*, fossa subescapular; *inserção*, tuberosidade menor do úmero; *ação*, roda o braço medialmente; sua contração tônica ajuda a manter a cabeça do úmero na fossa glenóide rasa; *inervação*, nervos subescapulares superior e inferior da divisão posterior do plexo braquial (quinto e sexto nervos espinais cervicais). SIN musculus subscapularis [TA], subscapular m.
superficial back m.'s, músculos superficiais do dorso; músculos originados na coluna vertebral e que possuem seus ventres carnosos localizados no dorso, mas inserindo-se no esqueleto apendicular do membro superior ou nas costelas. Eles não são inervados por ramos primários dorsais dos nervos espinais, como os músculos profundos ou verdadeiros do dorso; incluem o m. trapézio (inervado pelo nervo acessório espinal) e os músculos latíssimo do dorso, rombóides, levantador da escápula e torácicos (inervados por ramos primários ventrais dos nervos espinais, ou derivados deles).
superficial flexor (m.) of fingers, m. flexor superficial dos dedos da mão. SIN flexor digitorum superficialis (m.).
superficial lingual m., m. superficial da língua. SIN superior longitudinal m. of tongue.
superficial transverse perineal m. [TA], m. transverso superficial do períneo; m. inconstante do trígono urogenital; *origem*, ramo do ísquio; *inserção*, tendão central do períneo que atua com outros músculos perineais para resistir ao aumento da pressão intrapélvica; *ação*, leva para trás e fixa o tendão central do períneo; *inervação*, nervo pudendo (perineal). SIN musculus transversus perinei superficialis [TA], superficial transverse m. of perineum, Theile m.
superficial transverse m. of perineum, m. transverso superficial do períneo. SIN superficial transverse perineal m.
superior auricular m., m. auricular superior. SIN auricularis superior (m.).

superior gemellus (m.) [TA], m. gêmeo superior; m. profundo da região glútea; *origem*, espinha isquiática e margem da incisura isquiática menor; *inserção*, tendão do músculo obturador interno; *ação*, roda a coxa lateralmente; *inervação*, plexo sacral. SIN musculus gemellus superior [TA], gemellus.

superior longitudinal m. of tongue [TA], m. longitudinal superior da língua; músculo intrínseco da língua, que vai da base até a extremidade no dorso, logo abaixo da mucosa; *ação*, encurta a parte superior da língua; *inervação*, motora pelo nervo hipoglosso, sensorial pelo nervo lingual. SIN musculus longitudinalis superior linguae [TA], superficial lingual m.

superior oblique (m.) [TA], m. oblíquo superior; m. extra-ocular na órbita; *origem*, acima da margem medial do canal óptico; *inserção*, por um tendão que atravessa a tróclea, sendo depois refletido para trás, para baixo e lateralmente até a esclera entre os músculos retos superior e lateral; *ação*, primária, torção interna; secundária, depressão e abdução; *inervação*, nervo troclear. SIN musculus obliquus superior [TA].

superior oblique m. of head, m. oblíquo superior da cabeça. SIN obliquus capitis superior (m.).

superior pharyngeal constrictor (m.) [TA], m. constritor superior da faringe; componente mais superior da camada muscular "circular" externa da faringe; *origem*, lâmina pterigóidea medial (parte pterigofaríngea [TA]), rafe pterigomandibular (parte bucofaríngea [TA]), linha milo-hióidea da mandíbula (parte milofaríngea [TA]) e a mucosa do assoalho da boca e a lateral da língua (parte glossofaríngea [TA]); *inserção*, rafe faríngea na parede posterior da faringe; *ação*, estreita a faringe; ajuda a fechar a nasofaringe da orofaringe e contrai de forma peristáltica durante a deglutição; *inervação*, plexo faríngeo. SIN musculus constrictor pharyngis superior [TA], musculus cephalopharyngeus.

superior posterior serratus m., m. serrátil posterior superior. SIN serratus posterior superior (m.).

superior rectus (m.) [TA], m. reto superior; m. extra-ocular na órbita; *origem*, parte superior do anel tendíneo; *inserção*, parte superior da esclera do olho; *ação*, primária, elevação; secundária, adução e torção interna; *inervação*, nervo oculomotor. SIN musculus rectus superior [TA], attollens oculi.

superior tarsal m. [TA], m. tarsal superior; camada bem definida de m. liso que se estende da aponeurose do músculo levantador da pálpebra superior até o tarso superior; é inervado por nervos simpáticos e atua mantendo a pálpebra superior em uma posição elevada; sua paralisia na síndrome de Horner resulta em ptose. SIN musculus tarsalis superior [TA], Müller m. (3).

supinator (m.) [TA], m. supinador; **(1)** m. da camada profunda da parte proximal do compartimento posterior do antebraço; *origem*, epicôndilo lateral do úmero, ligamentos colateral radial e anular do rádio, e crista do músculo supinador da ulna; *inserção*, superfície anterior e lateral do rádio; *ação*, supina o antebraço; *inervação*, nervo radial (interósseo posterior); **(2)** m. que realiza supinação, isto é, gira o antebraço em torno de um eixo longitudinal, da posição de pronação ou neutra em direção àquela na qual as palmas ficam voltadas anteriormente (na posição anatômica). SIN musculus supinator [TA], supinator [TA], musculus supinator radii brevis.

supraclavicular m., m. supraclavicular; faixa muscular anômala que segue lateralmente a partir da borda superior do manúbrio do esterno até, aproximadamente, o meio da superfície superior da clavícula. SIN musculus supraclavicularis.

suprahyoid m.'s [TA], músculos supra-hióideos; o grupo de músculos fixados à parte superior do osso hióide, incluindo os músculos digástrico, estilo-hióideo, milo-hióideo e gênio-hióideo. SIN musculi suprahyoidei [TA].

supraspinalis (m.), m. supra-espinhoso; uma dentre várias faixas musculares que passam entre as extremidades dos processos espinhosos das vértebras cervicais. SIN musculus supraspinalis.

supraspinatus (m.) [TA], m. supra-espinal; m. intrínseco (escapouloumeral) da articulação do ombro cujo tendão contribui para o manguito rotador; *origem*, fossa supra-espinal da escápula; *inserção*, tuberosidade maior do úmero; *ação*, inicia a abdução do braço; sua contração tônica ajuda a manter a cabeça do úmero na fossa glenóide superficial; *inervação*, nervo supra-escapular do quinto e sexto nervos cervicais. SIN musculus supraspinatus [TA], supraspinous m.

supraspinous m., m. supra-espinal. SIN supraspinatus (m.).

suspensory m. of duodenum [TA], m. suspensor do duodeno; faixa plana e larga de m. liso e tecido fibroso, fixada ao pilar direito do diafragma e ao duodeno em sua junção com o jejuno. SIN musculus suspensorius duodeni [TA], ligamentum suspensorium duodeni*, suspensory ligament of duodenum*, Treitz ligament, Treitz m.

synergistic m.'s, músculos sinérgicos; músculos que têm função ou ação semelhante e mutuamente útil.

tailor's m., m. sartório. SIN sartorius (m.).

temporal m., m. temporal. SIN temporalis (m.).

temporalis (m.) [TA], m. temporal; m. da mastigação mais superior; *origem*, fossa temporal; *inserção*, processo coronóide da mandíbula e borda anterior do ramo; *ação*, eleva a mandíbula (fecha a boca); suas fibras posteriores, orientadas quase horizontalmente, são os afastadores primários da mandíbula protrusa; *inervação*, ramos temporais profundos da divisão mandibular do nervo trigêmeo. SIN musculus temporalis [TA], temporal m., temporalis.

temporoparietal m., m. temporoparietal. SIN temporoparietalis (m.).

temporoparietalis (m.) [TA], m. temporoparietal; a parte do m. epicrânico que se origina da parte lateral da aponeurose epicrânica e insere-se na cartilagem da orelha. SIN musculus temporoparietalis [TA], temporoparietal m.

tensor fasciae latae (m.) [TA], m. tensor da fáscia lata; m. anterior da região glútea (compartimento abdutor da coxa); *origem*, espinha ântero-superior e superfície lateral adjacente do ílio; *inserção*, faixa iliotibial da fáscia lata; *ação*, tensiona a fáscia lata; flete, abduz e roda medialmente a coxa; *inervação*, nervo glúteo superior. SIN musculus tensor fasciae latae [TA], tensor (m.) of fascia lata*, musculus tensor fasciae femoris.

tensor (m.) of fascia lata, m. tensor da fáscia lata; *termo oficial alternativo para tensor fasciae latae (m.).

tensor (m.) of soft palate, m. tensor do véu palatino. SIN tensor veli palati (m.).

tensor tarsi m., m. tensor do tarso; parte lacrimal do m. orbicular do olho. VER orbicularis oculi (m.).

tensor tympani (m.) [TA], m. tensor do tímpano; m. dos ossículos da audição; *origem*, a parte cartilaginosa da tuba faringotimpânica (auditiva) e as paredes de seu hemicanal logo acima da porção óssea da tuba faringotimpânica; *inserção*, cabo do martelo; *ação*, movimenta o cabo do martelo medialmente, tensionando o tímpano para protegê-lo da vibração excessiva produzida por sons altos; *inervação*, ramos do nervo trigêmeo através do gânglio ótico. SIN musculus tensor tympani [TA], tensor (m.) of tympanic membrane, Toynbee m.

tensor (m.) of tympanic membrane, m. tensor do tímpano. SIN tensor tympani (m.).

tensor veli palati (m.) [TA], m. tensor do véu palatino; m. que tensiona o palato mole de forma a permitir que a língua comprima o bolo alimentar contra ele durante a deglutição, forçando a entrada da massa na orofaringe; *origem*, fossa escafóide do esfenóide, parte cartilagínea e membranácea da tuba auditiva (faringotimpânica) e espinha do esfenóide; *inserção*, borda posterior do palato duro e aponeurose do palato mole; *ação*, tensiona o palato mole para deglutição; contribui para a abertura da tuba auditiva para permitir equilíbrio da pressão; *inervação*, ramos do nervo trigêmeo através do gânglio ótico. SIN musculus tensor veli palatini [TA], musculus palatosalpingeus, tensor (m.) of soft palate.

teres major (m.) [TA], m. redondo maior; m. intrínseco (escapouloumeral) da articulação do ombro; *origem*, ângulo inferior e terço inferior da borda da escápula; *inserção*, borda medial do sulco intertubercular do úmero; *ação*, aduz e estende o braço e roda-o medialmente; *inervação*, nervo subescapular inferior da divisão posterior do plexo braquial (quinto e sexto nervos espinais cervicais). SIN musculus teres major [TA].

teres minor (m.) [TA], m. redondo menor; m. intrínseco (escapouloumeral) da articulação do ombro, cujo tendão contribui para a formação do manguito rotador; *origem*, dois terços superiores da borda lateral da escápula; *inserção*, faceta inferior da tuberosidade maior do úmero; *ação*, aduz e roda o braço lateralmente; sua contração tônica ajuda a manter a cabeça do úmero na fossa glenóide superficial; *inervação*, nervo axilar (quinto e sexto nervos espinais cervicais). SIN musculus teres minor [TA].

m. of terminal notch [TA], m. da incisura terminal; um m. ocasional na superfície craniana da orelha que cobre a fissura antitrago-helicina. SIN musculus incisurae helicis [TA], m. of notch of helix, musculus intertragicus.

Theile m., m. de Theile. SIN superficial transverse perineal m.

third peroneal m., m. fibular terceiro. SIN fibular tertius (m.).

thoracic interspinal m., m. interespinal do tórax. SIN interspinales thoracis (m.'s).

thoracic interspinales m.'s, músculos interespinais do tórax. SIN interspinales thoracis (m.'s).

thoracic intertransversarii (m.'s) [TA], músculos intertransversários do tórax; músculos profundos da parte superior do dorso; *origem*, processos transversos das vértebras torácicas; *inserção*, processo transverso superior subseqüente; *ação*, abduz vértebras torácicas; *inervação*, ramos primários dorsais dos nervos torácicos. SIN musculi intertransversarii thoracis [TA], thoracic intertransverse m.'s.

thoracic intertransverse m.'s, músculos intertransversários do tórax. SIN thoracic intertransversarii (m.'s).

thoracic longissimus m., m. longuíssimo do tórax. SIN longissimus thoracis (m.).

thoracic rotator m.'s, músculos rotadores do tórax. SIN rotatores thoracis (m.'s).

thoracoappendicular m.'s [TA], músculos toracoapendiculares; músculos extrínsecos do membro superior que se originam no esqueleto axial do tronco (costelas e processos espinhosos das vértebras cervicotorácicas) e inserem-se no esqueleto apendicular do membro superior. SIN musculi thoracoappendiculares [TA].

m.'s of thorax [TA], músculos do tórax; os músculos fixados à caixa torácica, incluindo os músculos peitorais, serrátil anterior, subclávio, músculos levantadores, músculos intercostais, músculo transverso do tórax, músculos subcostais e diafragma. SIN musculi thoracis [TA].

three-headed m. [TA], m. tríceps; m. complexo no qual três cabeças distintas de origem convergem para se inserirem através de um tendão comum, p. ex., tríceps braquial, tríceps da coxa ou tríceps sural. SIN musculus triceps [TA], triceps (m.) [TA]. [L. de *tri-*, três, + *caput*, cabeça]

thyroarytenoid (m.) [TA], m. tireoaritenóideo; m. intrínseco da laringe; *origem*, superfície interna da cartilagem tireóidea; *inserção*, processo muscular e superfície externa da aritenóide; *ação*, diminui a tensão sobre (relaxa) as pregas vocais, reduzindo a intensidade do tom de voz; é antagonista do m. cricotireóideo nessa ação; *inervação*, nervo laríngeo recorrente. SIN musculus thyroarytenoideus [TA], musculus thyroarytenoideus externus.

thyroepiglottic m., thyroepiglottidean m., m. tireoepiglótico; parte tireoepiglótica do m. tireoaritenóideo. SIN thyroepiglottic part of thyroarytenoid (muscle).

thyrohyoid (m.) [TA], m. tíreo-hióideo; m. infra-hióideo da parte anterior do pescoço, que parece ser uma continuação do esternotireóideo; *origem*, linha oblíqua da cartilagem tireóidea; *inserção*, corpo do osso hióide; *ação*, aproxima o osso hióide da laringe; *inervação*, nervos espinais cervicais superiores conduzidos pelo nervo hipoglosso. SIN musculus thyrohyoideus [TA].

tibialis anterior (m.) [TA], m. tibial anterior; m. medial do compartimento anterior (dorsiflexor) da perna; *origem*, dois terços superiores da superfície lateral da tíbia, membrana interóssea e fáscia crural sobrejacente; *inserção*, cuneiforme medial e base do primeiro metatarsal; *ação*, dorsiflexão e inversão do pé; proporciona sustentação dinâmica dos arcos longitudinal e transverso do pé; *inervação*, nervo fibular profundo. SIN musculus tibialis anterior [TA], anterior tibial m., musculus tibialis anticus.

tibialis posterior (m.) [TA], m. tibial posterior; m. mais anterior (profundo) do compartimento posterior profundo (flexor plantar) da perna; *origem*, linha do m. sóleo e superfície posterior da tíbia, a cabeça e diáfise da fíbula entre a crista medial e a borda interóssea, e a superfície posterior da membrana interóssea; *inserção*, navicular, três cuneiformes, cubóide e segundo, terceiro e quarto ossos do metatarso; *ação*, flexão plantar e inversão do pé; *inervação*, nervo tibial. SIN musculus tibialis posterior [TA], musculus tibialis posticus, posterior tibial m.

Tod m., m. de Tod. SIN oblique m. of auricle.

m.'s of tongue [TA], músculos da língua; os músculos extrínsecos incluem os músculos genioglosso, hioglosso, condroglosso e estiloglosso; os músculos intrínsecos são o vertical, transverso e o longitudinal superior e inferior; todos são inervados pelo nervo hipoglosso. SIN musculi linguae [TA], lingual m.'s.

Toynbee m., m. de Toynbee. SIN tensor tympani (m.).

trachealis (m.) [TA], m. traqueal; a faixa de fibras musculares lisas, dispostas mais transversalmente na membrana fibrosa, que une, na parte posterior, as extremidades dos anéis traqueais; *ação*, reduz o calibre da traquéia. SIN musculus trachealis [TA].

tracheloclavicular m., m. traqueloclavicular; m. anômalo que, ocasionalmente, se origina das vértebras cervicais e está inserido na extremidade lateral da clavícula. SIN musculus tracheloclavicularis.

tragicus (m.) [TA], m. trágico; um dos músculos da orelha que ocorrem como uma faixa de fibras musculares verticais na superfície externa do trago da orelha. SIN musculus tragicus [TA], m. of tragus, Valsalva m.

m. of tragus, m. trágico. SIN tragicus (m.).

transverse m. of abdomen, m. transverso do abdome. SIN transversus abdominis (m.).

transverse arytenoid (m.) [TA], m. aritenóideo transverso; m. intrínseco da laringe; uma faixa de fibras musculares que passa entre as duas cartilagens aritenóideas posteriormente; *ação*, estreita a parte intercartilagínea da rima da glote; *inervação*, nervo laríngeo recorrente. SIN musculus arytenoideus transversus [TA], arytenoideus.

transverse m. of auricle [TA], m. transverso da orelha; faixa de fibras musculares esparsas, na superfície craniana da orelha, que se estende da eminência da concha até a eminência da escafa. SIN musculus transversus auriculae [TA], transverse auricular m*.

transverse auricular m., m. transverso da orelha; *termo oficial alternativo para transverse m. of auricle.

transverse m. of chin, m. transverso do mento. SIN transversus menti (m.).

transverse m. of nape, m. transverso da nuca. SIN transversus nuchae (m.).

transverse m. of thorax, m. transverso do tórax. SIN transversus thoracis (m.).

transverse m. of tongue [TA], m. transverso da língua; m. intrínseco da língua, cujas fibras se originam do septo e irradiam-se para o dorso e para as laterais; *ação*, diminui a dimensão lateral da língua; *inervação*, motora pelo nervo hipoglosso, sensitiva pelo nervo lingual. SIN musculus transversus linguae [TA].

transversospinal m., m. transverso-espinal. SIN transversospinales (m.'s).

transversospinales (m.'s) [TA], músculos transverso-espinais; o grupo de músculos profundos do dorso que se originam dos processos transversos das vértebras e seguem até os processos espinhosos das vértebras mais altas; atuam como rotadores e incluem os músculos semi-espinal (da cabeça, do pescoço, do tórax), multífido e rotadores (do pescoço, do tórax, do lombo). Todos são inervados pelos ramos primários dorsais dos nervos espinais. SIN musculi transversospinales [TA], transversospinal m., transversospinales.

transversus abdominis (m.) [TA], m. transverso do abdome; camada mais profunda de músculos planos da parede ântero-lateral do abdome; *origem*, sétima à décima segunda cartilagens costais, fáscia lombar, crista ilíaca e ligamento inguinal; *inserção*, cartilagem xifóide e linha alba e, através do tendão conjunto, tubérculo púbico e pécten; *ação*, comprime o conteúdo abdominal; roda e flete o tronco; *inervação*, nervo torácico inferior. SIN musculus transversus abdominis [TA], musculus transversalis abdominis, transverse m. of abdomen.

transversus menti (m.) [TA], m. transverso do mento; m. do queixo formado quando fibras inconstantes do músculo depressor do ângulo da boca continuam até o pescoço e cruzam para o lado oposto abaixo do queixo. SIN musculus transversus menti [TA], transverse m. of chin.

transversus nuchae (m.) [TA], m. transverso da nuca; m. ocasional que passa entre os tendões do trapézio e esternocleidomastóideo, possivelmente um fascículo do músculo auricular posterior. SIN musculus transversus nuchae [TA], transverse m. of nape.

transversus thoracis (m.) [TA], m. transverso do tórax; m. interno do tórax; *origem*, superfície dorsal do processo xifóide e porção inferior da superfície dorsal do corpo do esterno; *inserção*, segunda à sexta cartilagens costais; *ação*, contribui para a depressão das costelas, estreitando o tórax; *inervação*, nervo intercostal. SIN musculus transversus thoracis [TA], musculus triangularis sterni, sternocostalis m., transverse m. of thorax.

trapezius (m.) [TA], m. trapézio; m. extrínseco (toracoapendicular) do ombro; *origem*, terço medial da linha nucal superior, protuberância occipital externa, ligamento nucal, processos espinhosos da sétima vértebra cervical e das vértebras torácicas e ligamentos supra-espinais correspondentes; *inserção*, terço lateral da superfície posterior da clavícula, face anterior do acrômio e borda superior e medial da espinha da escápula; *ação*, quando as escápulas estão fixas, partes do músculo podem agir independentemente: a parte cervical eleva a escápula, a parte torácica contribui para a depressão da escápula; as partes superior e inferior atuam simultaneamente para rodar a fossa glenóide superiormente; quando todo o músculo, especialmente a parte média, se contrai, as escápulas se retraem; movimenta a cabeça para um lado ou para trás; *inervação*, motora pelo nervo acessório, sensitiva pelo plexo cervical. SIN musculus trapezius [TA], cowl m., trapezius.

Treitz m., m. de Treitz. SIN suspensory m. of duodenum.

triangular m. [TA], m. triangular; **(1)** m. de três lados. SIN musculus triangularis (1) [TA]. **(2)** SIN depressor anguli oris (m.).

triceps (m.) [TA], m. tríceps. SIN three-headed m.

triceps m. of arm, m. tríceps braquial. SIN triceps brachii (m.).

triceps brachii (m.) [TA], m. tríceps braquial; m. de três cabeças do compartimento posterior (extensor) do braço; *origem*, cabeça longa ou escapular: borda lateral da escápula abaixo da fossa glenóide, cabeça lateral: superfície lateral e posterior do úmero abaixo do tubérculo maior, cabeça medial: superfície posterior do úmero abaixo do sulco radial; *inserção*, olécrano da ulna; *ação*, estende o cotovelo; *inervação*, nervo radial. SIN musculus triceps brachii [TA], triceps m. of arm.

triceps (m.) of calf, m. tríceps sural. SIN triceps surae (m.).

triceps coxae (m.), m. tríceps da coxa; o m. obturador interno e os músculos gêmeos superior e inferior, considerados como um músculo, inserindo-se através de um tendão comum único no trocânter maior do fêmur. SIN musculus triceps coxae, triceps m. of hip.

triceps (m.) of hip, m. tríceps da coxa. SIN triceps coxae (m.).

triceps surae (m.) [TA], m. tríceps sural; os dois ventres dos músculos gastrocnêmio e sóleo, considerados como um músculo inserindo-se, através do tendão calcâneo, na tuberosidade do calcâneo. SIN musculus triceps surae [TA], triceps (m.) of calf.

true m.'s of back, músculos próprios do dorso. SIN m.'s of back proper

two-bellied m. [TA], m. digástrico. SIN digastric (m.) (1).

two-headed m. [TA], m. bíceps; m. com duas origens ou cabeças. Comumente usado para se referir ao músculo bíceps braquial.

ulnar extensor (m.) of wrist, m. extensor ulnar do carpo. SIN extensor carpi ulnaris (m.).

ulnar flexor (m.) of wrist, m. flexor ulnar do carpo. SIN flexor carpi ulnaris (m.).

unipennate m., m. semipeniforme; *termo oficial alternativo para semipennate m.

unstriated m., unstriped m., m. liso. SIN smooth m.

m.'s of urogenital triangle [TA], músculos do trígono urogenital; músculos localizados entre os ramos isquiopúbicos e anteriores a uma linha que une os túberes isquiáticos; incluem os músculos bulboesponjoso, isquicavernoso e transverso do períneo e o esfíncter externo da uretra. SIN musculi regionis urogenitalis [TA].

m. of uvula [TA], m. da úvula; m. intrínseco do palato mole; *origem*, espinha nasal posterior; *inserção*, forma o principal volume da úvula; *ação*, eleva a úvula; *inervação*, plexo faríngeo. SIN musculus uvulae [TA], musculus azygos uvulae, palatouvularis m., uvular m., uvularis.

muscle   1030   **musculus**

uvular m., m. da úvula. SIN m. of uvula.
Valsalva m., m. de Valsalva, m. da úvula. SIN tragicus (m.).
vastus intermedius (m.) [TA], m. vasto intermédio; cabeça profunda central do m. quadríceps do compartimento anterior (extensor) da coxa; *origem*, três quartos superiores da superfície anterior da diáfise do fêmur; *inserção*, tuberosidade tibial através do tendão comum do quadríceps femoral e ligamento patelar; *ação*, estende a perna; *inervação*, nervo femoral. SIN musculus vastus intermedius [TA], crureus, femoral m., intermediate great m., intermediate vastus (m.).
vastus lateralis (m.) [TA], m. vasto lateral; cabeça lateral do m. quadríceps do compartimento anterior (extensor) da coxa; *origem*, lábio lateral da linha áspera até o trocânter maior; *inserção*, tuberosidade tibial através do tendão comum do músculo quadríceps femoral e ligamento patelar; *ação*, estende a perna; *inervação*, nervo femoral. SIN musculus vastus lateralis [TA], lateral great m., lateral vastus (m.), musculus vastus externus.
vastus medialis (m.) [TA], m. vasto medial; cabeça medial do m. quadríceps do compartimento anterior (extensor) da coxa; *origem*, lábio medial da linha áspera; *inserção*, tuberosidade tibial através do tendão comum do quadríceps femoral e ligamento patelar; *ação*, estende a perna; *inervação*, nervo femoral. SIN musculus vastus medialis [TA], medial great m., medial vastus (m.), musculus vastus internus.
ventral sacrococcygeal m., m. sacrococcígeo ventral. SIN ventral sacrococcygeus (m.).
ventral sacrococcygeus (m.), m. sacrococcígeo ventral; m. inconstante nas superfícies pélvicas do sacro e cóccix, os remanescentes de uma parte da musculatura da cauda de animais inferiores. SIN musculus sacrococcygeus anterior, musculus sacrococcygeus ventralis, ventral sacrococcygeal m.
vertical m. of tongue [TA], m. vertical da língua; m. intrínseco da língua, consistindo em fibras que passam da aponeurose do dorso até a aponeurose da superfície inferior; *ação*, diminui a dimensão súpero-inferior da língua (achatando-a); *inervação*, motora pelo nervo hipoglosso, sensorial pelo nervo lingual. SIN musculus verticalis linguae [TA].
vestigial m., m. vestigial; estrutura imperfeita em seres humanos que corresponde a um músculo funcionante nos animais inferiores.
visceral m., m. visceral; m. liso. SIN smooth m.
vocal m., m. vocal. SIN vocalis (m.).
vocalis (m.) [TA], m. vocal; m. intrínseco da laringe formado por várias fibras mais mediais e mais finas do músculo tireoaritenóideo, fixadas diretamente à face externa do ligamento vocal; *origem*, depressão entre as duas lâminas da cartilagem tireóidea; *inserção*, partes do ligamento vocal e processo vocal da aritenóide; *ação*, encurta e relaxa partes das pregas vocais; *inervação*, nervo laríngeo recorrente. SIN musculus vocalis [TA], musculus thyroarytenoideus internus, vocal m.
voluntary m., m. voluntário; m. cuja ação está sob controle voluntário; todos os músculos estriados, exceto o coração, são músculos voluntários.
white m., m. branco; m. de contração rápida no qual há predomínio de fibras "brancas" grandes e pálidas; as mitocôndrias e a mioglobulina são relativamente escassas em comparação com o músculo vermelho; envolvido na contração fásica.
Wilson m., m. de Wilson; **(1)** esfíncter uretral externo. SIN external urethral sphincter; **(2)** algumas fibras do músculo levantador do ânus.
wrinkler m. of eyebrow, m. corrugador do supercílio. SIN corrugator supercilii (m.).
zygomaticus major (m.) [TA], m. zigomático maior; m. facial da porção anterior da bochecha que se estende até o lábio superior; *origem*, osso zigomático anterior à sutura temporozigomática; *inserção*, músculos no ângulo da boca; *ação*, movimenta o lábio superior para cima e lateralmente; *inervação*, nervo facial. SIN musculus zygomaticus major [TA], greater zygomatic m., musculus zygomaticus.
zygomaticus minor (m.) [TA], m. zigomático menor; m. facial da parte anterior da bochecha, que se estende até o lábio superior; *origem*, osso zigomático posterior à sutura zigomaticomaxilar; *inserção*, orbicular da boca do lábio superior; *ação*, movimenta o lábio superior para cima e para fora; *inervação*, nervo facial. SIN musculus zygomaticus minor [TA], caput zygomaticum quadrati labii superioris, lesser zygomatic m.

---

mus·cle-bound (mŭs'el-bownd). Designa uma condição na qual os músculos individuais são superdesenvolvidos, porém dissinérgicos na ação conjunta.
mus·cle·trim·ming. Moldagem periférica; impressão periférica. SIN border molding.
mus·cone (mŭs'kōn). Muscona.
mus·cu·la·mine (mŭs'kūl-ă-mēn). Musculamina. SIN spermine.
mus·cu·lar (mŭs'kū-lăr). **1.** Muscular; relativo a um músculo ou músculos. **2.** Musculoso; que possui musculatura bem desenvolvida.
mus·cu·la·ris (mŭs-kū-lā'ris). Muscular; a túnica muscular de um órgão oco ou de uma estrutura tubular. [L. mod. muscular]

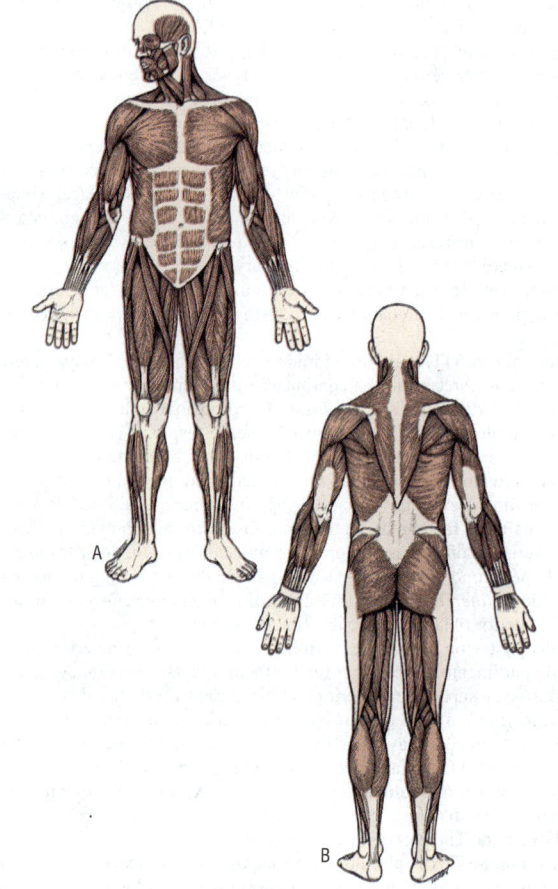

musculatura: (A) vista anterior, (B) vista posterior

m. muco'sae, m. da mucosa; a fina camada de músculo liso encontrada na maior parte do tubo digestivo, localizada fora da muscular própria da mucosa e adjacente à tela submucosa. SIN lamina muscularis mucosae, muscular layer of mucosa.
mus·cu·lar·i·ty (mŭs'kū-lar'i-tē). Muscularidade; o estado ou condição de possuir músculos bem desenvolvidos.
mus·cu·la·ture (mŭs'kū-lă-choor). Musculatura; o arranjo dos músculos em uma parte do corpo ou no corpo como um todo.
mus·cu·lo·ap·o·neu·rot·ic (mŭs'kū-lō-ap'ō-noo-rot'ik). Musculoaponeurótico; relativo ao tecido muscular e a uma aponeurose de origem ou inserção.
mus·cu·lo·cu·ta·ne·ous (mŭs'kū-lō-kū-tā'nē-ŭs). Musculocutâneo; relativo ao músculo e à pele. SIN myocutaneous, myodermal.
mus·cu·lo·mem·bra·nous (mŭs'kū-lō-mem'brā-nŭs). Musculomembranáceo; relativo ao tecido muscular e à membrana; designa determinados músculos, como o occipitofrontal, que são extremamente membranáceos.
mus·cu·lo·phren·ic (mŭs'kū-lō-fren'ik). Músculofrênico; relativo à porção muscular do diafragma; designando uma artéria que supre essa parte.
mus·cu·lo·skel·e·tal (mŭs'kū-lō-skel'ĕ-tăl). Músculo-esquelético; relativo aos músculos e ao esqueleto, como, por exemplo, o sistema muscular.
mus·cu·lo·spi·ral (mŭs'kū-lō-spī'ral). Musculoespiral; designa o nervo musculoespiral. VER radial *nerve*.
mus·cu·lo·ten·di·nous (mŭs'kū-lō-ten'di-nŭs). Musculotendíneo; relativo aos tecidos muscular e tendíneo.
mus·cu·lo·tro·pic (mŭs'kū-lō-trop'ik). Musculotrópico; que afeta, age sobre ou é atraído pelo tecido muscular.

MUSCULUS

mus·cu·lus, gen. e pl. **mus·cu·li** (mŭs'kū-lŭs, -kū-li) [TA]. Músculo. SIN muscle. Ver a descrição histológica em muscle. [L. um camundongo pequeno, um músculo, de *mus* (*mur-*), camundongo]

mus'culi abdom'inis, músculos abdominais. SIN *muscles* of abdomen, em *muscle*.
m. abductor [TA], m. abdutor. SIN *abductor* (*muscle*).
m. abduc'tor dig'iti min'imi ma'nus [TA], m. abdutor do dedo mínimo da mão. SIN *abductor digiti minimi* (*muscle*) of hand.
m. abduc'tor dig'iti min'imi pe'dis [TA], m. abdutor do dedo mínimo do pé. SIN *abductor digiti minimi* (*muscle*) of foot.
m. abduc'tor dig'iti quin'ti, m. abdutor do quinto dedo; (**1**) SIN *abductor digiti minimi* (*muscle*) of hand; (**2**) SIN *abductor digiti minimi* (*muscle*) of foot.
m. abduc'tor hal'lucis [TA], m. abdutor do hálux. SIN *abductor hallucis* (*muscle*).
m. abduc'tor pol'licis bre'vis [TA], m. abdutor curto do polegar. SIN *abductor pollicis brevis* (*muscle*).
m. abduc'tor pol'licis lon'gus [TA], m. abdutor longo do polegar. SIN *abductor pollicis longus* (*muscle*).
m. adductor [TA], m. adutor. SIN *adductor muscle*.
m. adduc'tor bre'vis [TA], m. adutor curto. SIN *adductor brevis* (*muscle*).
m. adduc'tor hal'lucis [TA], m. adutor do hálux. SIN *adductor hallucis* (*muscle*).
m. adduc'tor lon'gus [TA], m. adutor longo. SIN *adductor longus* (*muscle*).
m. adduc'tor mag'nus [TA], m. adutor magno. SIN *adductor magnus* (*muscle*).
m. adduc'tor min'imus [TA], m. adutor mínimo. SIN *adductor minimus* (*muscle*).
m. adduc'tor pol'licis [TA], m. adutor do polegar. SIN *adductor pollicis* (*muscle*).
m. anco'neus [TA], m. ancôneo. SIN *anconeus muscle*.
musculi anorectoperineales [TA], músculos anorretoperineais. SIN *anorectoperineal muscles*, em *muscle*.
m. antitrag'icus [TA], m. antitrágico. SIN *antitragicus* (*muscle*).
m. arrector pili [TA], m. eretor do pêlo. SIN *arrector muscle* of hair.
m. articula'ris, m. articular. SIN *articular muscle*.
m. articula'ris cu'biti [TA], m. articular do cotovelo. SIN *articularis cubiti* (*muscle*).
m. articula'ris ge'nus [TA], m. articular do joelho. SIN *articularis genus* (*muscle*).
m. aryepiglot'ticus, m. ariepiglótico. SIN *aryepiglottic part* of oblique arytenoid muscle.
m. arytenoi'deus obli'quus [TA], m. aritenóideo oblíquo. SIN *oblique arytenoid muscle*.
m. arytenoi'deus transver'sus [TA], m. aritenóideo transverso. SIN *transverse arytenoid* (*muscle*).
m. aryvoca'lis, m. arivocal; várias fibras mais profundas do músculo vocal fixadas diretamente à face externa da prega vocal.
m. attol'lens au'rem, m. attol'lens auric'ulam, m. auricular superior. SIN *auricularis superior* (*muscle*).
m. a'ttrahens au'rem, m. a'ttrahens auric'ulam, m. auricular anterior. SIN *auricularis anterior* (*muscle*).
musculi auriculares [TA], músculos auriculares. SIN *auricular muscles*, em *muscle*.
m. auricula'ris ante'rior, m. auricular anterior. SIN *auricularis anterior* (*muscle*).
m. auricula'ris poste'rior [TA], m. auricular posterior. SIN *auricularis posterior* (*muscle*).
m. auricula'ris supe'rior [TA], m. auricular superior. SIN *auricularis superior* (*muscle*).
m. az'ygos u'vulae, m. da úvula. SIN *muscle* of uvula.
m. bi'ceps bra'chii [TA], m. bíceps braquial. SIN *biceps brachii* (*muscle*).
m. bi'ceps fem'oris [TA], m. bíceps femoral. SIN *biceps femoris* (*muscle*).
m. bi'ceps flex'or cru'ris, m. bíceps femoral. SIN *biceps femoris* (*muscle*).
m. bipenna'tus, m. peniforme. SIN *pennate muscle*.
m. biventer [TA], m. digástrico. SIN *digastric* (*muscle*) (1).
m. biven'ter mandib'ulae, m. digástrico. SIN *digastric* (*muscle*) (1).
m. brachia'lis [TA], m. braquial. SIN *brachialis* (*muscle*).
m. brachioradia'lis [TA], m. braquiorradial. SIN *brachioradialis* (*muscle*).
m. bronchoesopha'geus [TA], m. broncoesofágico. SIN *bronchoesophageus* (*muscle*).
m. buccina'tor [TA], m. bucinador. SIN *buccinator* (*muscle*).
m. buccopharyn'geus, m. bucofaríngeo. VER *superior pharyngeal constrictor* (*muscle*).
mus'culi bul'bi, músculos extra-oculares. SIN *extraocular muscles*, em *muscle*.
m. bulbocaverno'sus, m. bulbocavernoso. SIN *bulbospongiosus* (*muscle*).
m. bulbospongio'sus [TA], m. bulboesponjoso. SIN *bulbospongiosus* (*muscle*).
m. cani'nus, m. levantador do ângulo da boca. SIN *levator anguli oris* (*muscle*).
mus'culi cap'itis [TA], músculos da cabeça. SIN *muscles* of head, em *muscle*.
m. cephalopharyn'geus, m. cefalofaríngeo. SIN *superior pharyngeal constrictor* (*muscle*).
m. ceratocricoi'deus [TA], m. ceratocricóideo. SIN *ceratocricoid* (*muscle*).
m. ceratoglossus [TA], m. ceratoglosso. SIN *ceratoglossus* (*muscle*).

m. ceratopharyn'geus, m. ceratofaríngeo. VER *middle constrictor* (*muscle*) of pharynx.
m. cervica'lis ascen'dens, m. cervical ascendente; m. iliocostal do pescoço. SIN *iliocostalis cervicis* (*muscle*).
musculi cervicis, músculos do pescoço; *termo oficial alternativo para *muscles* of neck, em *muscle*.
m. chondroglos'sus, m. condroglosso. SIN *chondroglossus muscle*.
m. chondropharyn'geus, m. condrofaríngeo. VER *middle constrictor* (*muscle*) of pharynx.
m. cilia'ris [TA], m. ciliar. SIN *ciliary muscle*.
m. cleidoepitrochlea'ris, m. cleidoepitroclear; a porção anterior do deltóide que se origina da clavícula.
m. cleidomastoi'deus, m. cleidomastóideo; a parte do músculo esternocleidomastóideo que passa entre a clavícula e o processo mastóide.
m. cleido-occipita'lis, m. cleido-occipital; a porção do músculo esternocleidomastóideo entre a clavícula e a linha nucal superior.
mus'culi coccyg'ei, músculos coccígeos. SIN *muscles* of coccyx, em *muscle*.
m. coccyg'eus [TA], m. coccígeo; m. isquiococcígeo. SIN *coccygeus muscle*.
mus'culi col'li [TA], músculos do pescoço. SIN *muscles* of neck, em *muscle*.
m. complex'us, m. complexo; m. semi-espinal da cabeça. SIN *semispinalis capitis* (*muscle*).
m. complex'us mi'nor, m. complexo menor; m. longuíssimo da cabeça. SIN *longissimus capitis* (*muscle*).
m. compres'sor na'ris, m. nasal. VER *nasalis* (*muscle*).
m. compressor urethrae [TA], m. compressor da uretra. SIN *compressor urethra* (*muscle*).
m. constric'tor pharyn'gis infe'rior [TA], m. constritor inferior da faringe. SIN *inferior constrictor* (*muscle*) of pharynx.
m. constric'tor pharyn'gis me'dius [TA], m. constritor médio da faringe. SIN *middle constrictor* (*muscle*) of pharynx.
m. constric'tor pharyn'gis supe'rior [TA], m. constritor superior da faringe. SIN *superior pharyngeal constrictor* (*muscle*).
m. constric'tor ure'thrae, m. constritor da uretra; esfíncter externo da uretra. SIN *external urethral sphincter*.
m. coracobrachia'lis [TA], m. coracobraquial. SIN *coracobrachialis muscle*.
m. corruga'tor cu'tis a'ni, m. corrugador do ânus. SIN *corrugator cutis muscle* of anus.
m. corruga'tor supercil'ii [TA], m. corrugador do supercílio. SIN *corrugator supercilii* (*muscle*).
m. cremas'ter [TA], m. cremaster. SIN *cremaster muscle*.
m. cricoarytenoi'deus latera'lis [TA], m. cricoaritenóideo lateral. SIN *lateral cricoarytenoid* (*muscle*).
m. cricoarytenoi'deus poste'rior [TA], m. cricoaritenóideo posterior. SIN *posterior cricoarytenoid* (*muscle*).
m. cricopharyn'geus, m. cricofaríngeo; parte cricofaríngea do m. constritor inferior da faringe. VER *inferior constrictor* (*muscle*) of pharynx.
m. cricothyroi'deus [TA], m. cricotireóideo. SIN *cricothyroid muscle*.
m. crucia'tus, m. cruzado. SIN *cruciate muscle*.
m. cuta'neus [TA], m. cutâneo. SIN *cutaneous muscle*.
m. deltoi'deus [TA], m. deltóide. SIN *deltoid* (*muscle*).
m. depres'sor an'guli o'ris [TA], m. abaixador do ângulo da boca. SIN *depressor anguli oris* (*muscle*).
m. depres'sor la'bii inferio'ris [TA], m. abaixador do lábio inferior. SIN *depressor labii inferioris* (*muscle*).
m. depres'sor sep'ti [TA], m. abaixador do septo nasal. SIN *depressor septi nasi* (*muscle*).
m. depres'sor supercil'ii [TA], m. abaixador do supercílio. SIN *depressor supercilii* (*muscle*).
m. detru'sor uri'nae [TA], m. detrusor da bexiga. SIN *detrusor* (*muscle*).
m. diaphrag'ma, diafragma. VER *diaphragm*.
m. digas'tricus [TA], m. digástrico. SIN *digastric* (*muscle*) (1).
m. dilata'tor [TA], m. dilatador. SIN *dilator muscle*.
m. dila'tor, m. dilatador. SIN *dilator muscle*.
m. dila'tor i'ridis, m. dilatador da pupila. SIN *dilatador pupillae muscle*.
m. dila'tor na'ris, m. dilatador de nariz. VER *nasalis* (*muscle*).
m. dila'tor pupil'lae [TA], m. dilatador da pupila. SIN *dilator pupillae muscle*.
m. dila'tor pylo'ri gastroduodena'lis, m. dilatador do piloro. SIN *dilator* (*muscle*) of pylorus.
m. dila'tor pylo'ri ilea'lis, m. dilatador do esfíncter ileocecal. SIN *dilator* (*muscle*) of ileocecal sphincter.
m. dila'tor tu'bae, m. dilatador da tuba; parte do músculo tensor do véu palatino que se fixa à mucosa da tuba auditiva; antigamente descrito como um músculo distinto.
mus'culi dor'si [TA], músculos do dorso. SIN *muscles* of back, em *muscle*.
musculi dorsi proprii [TA], músculos próprios do dorso. SIN *muscles* of back proper, em *muscle*.
m. ejacula'tor sem'inis, m. ejaculador do sêmen; m. bulboesponjoso. SIN *bulbospongiosus* (*muscle*).

m. epicra'nius [TA], m. epicrânico. SIN epicranius (*muscle*).
m. epitrochleoanco'neus, m. epitrocleoancôneo; um músculo ocasional; *origem,* do dorso do côndilo medial do úmero; *inserção,* na face medial do olécrano.
m. erec'tor clitor'idis, m. eretor do clitóris; m. isquiocavernoso. SIN ischiocavernous (*muscle*).
m. erec'tor pe'nis, m. eretor do pênis; m. isquiocavernoso. SIN ischiocavernous (*muscle*).
m. erec'tor spi'nae [TA], m. eretor da espinha. SIN erector spinae (*muscles*), em *muscle*.
m. extensor [TA], m. extensor. SIN extensor *muscle*.
m. exten'sor bre'vis digito'rum, m. extensor curto dos dedos. SIN extensor digitorum brevis (*muscle*).
m. exten'sor bre'vis pol'licis, m. extensor curto do polegar. SIN extensor pollicis brevis (*muscle*).
m. exten'sor car'pi radia'lis bre'vis [TA], m. extensor radial curto do carpo. SIN extensor carpi radialis brevis (*muscle*).
m. exten'sor car'pi radia'lis lon'gus [TA], m. extensor radial longo do carpo. SIN extensor carpi radialis longus (*muscle*).
m. exten'sor car'pi ulna'ris [TA], m. extensor ulnar do carpo. SIN extensor carpi ulnaris (*muscle*).
m. exten'sor coccyg'is, m. extensor do cóccix. SIN dorsal sacrococcygeus *muscle*.
m. exten'sor dig'iti min'imi [TA], m. extensor do dedo mínimo. SIN extensor digiti minimi (*muscle*).
m. exten'sor dig'iti quin'ti pro'prius, m. extensor do dedo mínimo. SIN extensor digiti minimi (*muscle*).
m. exten'sor digito'rum [TA], m. extensor dos dedos. SIN extensor digitorum *muscle*.
m. exten'sor digito'rum bre'vis [TA], m. extensor curto dos dedos. SIN extensor digitorum brevis (*muscle*).
m. exten'sor digito'rum bre'vis ma'nus, m. extensor curto dos dedos da mão. SIN extensor digitorum brevis (*muscle*) of hand.
m. exten'sor digito'rum commu'nis, m. extensor dos dedos. SIN extensor digitorum *muscle*.
m. exten'sor digito'rum lon'gus [TA], m. extensor longo dos dedos. SIN extensor digitorum longus (*muscle*).
m. exten'sor hal'lucis bre'vis [TA], m. extensor curto do hálux. SIN extensor hallucis brevis (*muscle*).
m. exten'sor hal'lucis lon'gus [TA], m. extensor longo do hálux. SIN extensor hallucis longus (*muscle*).
m. exten'sor in'dicis [TA], m. extensor do indicador. SIN extensor indicis (*muscle*).
m. exten'sor in'dicis pro'prius, m. extensor do indicador. SIN extensor indicis (*muscle*).
m. exten'sor lon'gus digito'rum, m. extensor longo dos dedos. SIN extensor digitorum longus (*muscle*).
m. exten'sor lon'gus pol'licis, m. extensor longo do polegar. SIN extensor pollicis longus (*muscle*).
m. exten'sor min'imi dig'iti, m. extensor do dedo mínimo. SIN extensor digiti minimi (*muscle*).
m. exten'sor os'sis metacar'pi pol'licis, m. abdutor longo do polegar. SIN abductor pollicis longus (*muscle*).
m. exten'sor pol'licis bre'vis [TA], m. extensor curto do polegar. SIN extensor pollicis brevis (*muscle*).
m. exten'sor pol'licis lon'gus [TA], m. extensor longo do polegar. SIN extensor pollicis longus (*muscle*).
musculi externi bulbi oculi [TA], músculos extrínsecos do bulbo do olho. SIN extraocular *muscles,* em *muscle*.
mus'culi faciei, músculos da face. SIN facial *muscles,* em *muscle*.
m. fibula'ris brev'is [TA], m. fibular curto. SIN fibularis brevis (*muscle*).
m. fibula'ris long'us [TA], m. fibular longo. SIN fibularis longus (*muscle*).
m. fibula'ris ter'tius [TA], m. fibular terceiro. SIN fibularis tertius (*muscle*).
m. flexor [TA], m. flexor. SIN flexor *muscle*.
m. flex'or accesso'rius, m. flexor acessório; m. quadrado plantar; *termo oficial alternativo para quadratus plantae (*muscle*).
m. flex'or bre'vis digito'rum, m. flexor curto dos dedos. SIN flexor digitorum brevis (*muscle*).
m. flex'or bre'vis hal'lucis, m. flexor curto do hálux. SIN flexor hallucis brevis (*muscle*).
m. flex'or car'pi radia'lis [TA], m. flexor radial do carpo. SIN flexor carpi radialis (*muscle*).
m. flex'or car'pi ulna'ris [TA], m. flexor ulnar do carpo. SIN flexor carpi ulnaris (*muscle*).
m. flex'or dig'iti min'imi brev'is ma'nus [TA], m. flexor curto do dedo mínimo da mão. SIN flexor digiti minimi brevis (*muscle*) of hand.
m. flex'or dig'iti min'imi brev'is pe'dis [TA], m. flexor curto do dedo mínimo do pé. SIN flexor digiti minimi brevis (*muscle*) of foot.

m. flex'or digito'rum bre'vis [TA], m. flexor curto dos dedos. SIN flexor digitorum brevis (*muscle*).
m. flex'or digito'rum lon'gus [TA], m. flexor longo dos dedos. SIN flexor digitorum longus (*muscle*).
m. flex'or digito'rum profun'dus [TA], m. flexor profundo dos dedos. SIN flexor digitorum profundus (*muscle*).
m. flex'or digito'rum subli'mis, m. flexor superficial dos dedos. SIN flexor digitorum superficialis (*muscle*).
m. flex'or digito'rum superficia'lis [TA], m. flexor superficial dos dedos. SIN flexor digitorum superficialis (*muscle*).
m. flex'or hal'lucis bre'vis [TA], m. flexor curto do hálux. SIN flexor hallucis brevis (*muscle*).
m. flex'or hal'lucis lon'gus [TA], m. flexor longo do hálux. SIN flexor hallucis longus (*muscle*).
m. flex'or lon'gus digito'rum, m. flexor longo dos dedos. SIN flexor digitorum longus (*muscle*).
m. flex'or lon'gus hal'lucis, m. flexor longo do hálux. SIN flexor hallucis longus (*muscle*).
m. flex'or lon'gus pol'licis, m. flexor longo do polegar. SIN flexor pollicis longus (*muscle*).
m. flex'or pol'licis bre'vis [TA], m. flexor curto do polegar. SIN flexor pollicis brevis (*muscle*).
m. flex'or pol'licis lon'gus [TA], m. flexor longo do polegar. SIN flexor pollicis longus (*muscle*).
m. flex'or profun'dus, m. flexor profundo dos dedos. SIN flexor digitorum profundus (*muscle*).
m. flex'or subli'mis, m. flexor superficial dos dedos. SIN flexor digitorum superficialis (*muscle*).
m. fronta'lis, m. frontal. VER occipitofrontalis (*muscle*).
m. fusifor'mis [TA], m. fusiforme. SIN fusiform *muscle*.
m. gastrocne'mius [TA], m. gastrocnêmio. SIN gastrocnemius (*muscle*).
m. gemel'lus infe'rior [TA], m. gêmeo inferior. SIN inferior gemellus (*muscle*).
m. gemel'lus supe'rior [TA], m. gêmeo superior. SIN superior gemellus (*muscle*).
m. genioglos'sus [TA], m. genioglosso. SIN geniogiossus (*muscle*).
m. geniohyoglos'sus, m. genioglosso. SIN genioglossus (*muscle*).
m. geniohyoi'deus [TA], m. genio-hióideo. SIN geniohyoid (*muscle*).
m. glossopalati'nus, m. palatoglosso. SIN palatoglossus (*muscle*).
m. glossopharyn'geus, m. glossofaríngeo; parte glossofaríngea do m. constritor superior da faringe. VER superior pharyngeal constrictor (*muscle*).
m. glu'teus max'imus [TA], m. glúteo máximo. SIN gluteus maximus (*muscle*).
m. glu'teus me'dius [TA], m. glúteo médio. SIN gluteus medius (*muscle*)
m. glu'teus min'imus [TA], m. glúteo mínimo. SIN gluteus minimus (*muscle*).
m. grac'ilis [TA], m. grácil. SIN gracilis (*muscle*).
m. hel'icis ma'jor [TA], m. maior da hélice. SIN helicis major (*muscle*).
m. hel'icis mi'nor [TA], m. menor da hélice. SIN helicis minor (*muscle*).
m. hyoglos'sus [TA], m. hioglosso. SIN hyoglossus (*muscle*)
m. hypopharyn'geus, m. hipofaríngeo. VER middle constrictor (*muscle*) of pharynx.
m. ili'acus [TA], m. ilíaco. SIN iliacus (*muscle*).
m. ili'acus mi'nor, m. ilíaco menor. SIN iliacus minor (*muscle*).
m. iliocapsula'ris, m. iliocapsular. SIN iliacus minor (*muscle*).
m. il'iococcyg'eus [TA], m. iliococcígeo. SIN iliococcygeus (*muscle*).
m. iliocosta'lis [TA], m. iliocostal. SIN iliocostalis (*muscle*).
m. iliocosta'lis cer'vicis [TA], m. iliocostal do pescoço. SIN iliocostalis cervicis (*muscle*).
m. iliocosta'lis dor'si, m. iliocostal do tórax. SIN iliocostalis thoracis (*muscle*).
m. iliocosta'lis lumbo'rum [TA], m. iliocostal do lombo. SIN iliocostalis lumborum (*muscle*).
m. iliocosta'lis thora'cis [TA], m. iliocostal do tórax. SIN iliocostalis thoracis (*muscle*).
m. iliopso'as [TA], m. iliopsoas. SIN iliopsoas (*muscle*).
m. incisi'vus la'bii inferio'ris, m. incisivo do lábio inferior; feixe incisivo inferior da origem do músculo orbicular da boca.
m. incisi'vus la'bii superio'ris, m. incisivo do lábio superior; feixe incisivo superior da origem do músculo orbicular da boca.
m. incisu'rae hel'icis [TA], m. da incisura terminal. SIN *muscle* of terminal notch.
m. infracosta'lis, pl. **musculi infracosta'les,** m. subcostal. SIN subcostal *muscle*.
mus'culi infrahyoi'dei [TA], músculos infra-hióideos. SIN infrahyoid *muscles,* em *muscle*.
m. infraspina'tus [TA], m. infra-espinal. SIN infraspinatus (*muscle*).
m. intercosta'les exter'ni, pl. **mus'culi intercosta'les exter'ni** [TA], m. intercostal externo. SIN external intercostal (*muscle*).
m. intercosta'lis inter'nus, pl. **mus'culi intercosta'les inter'ni** [TA], m. intercostal interno. SIN internal intercostal (*muscle*).
m. intercosta'lis in'timus, pl. **mus'culi intercosta'les in'timi** [TA], m. intercostal íntimo. SIN innermost intercostal (*muscle*).

musculi interos'sei [TA], músculos interósseos. SIN interosseous *muscles*, em *muscle*.
musculi interos'sei dorsa'lis ma'nus, pl. **mus'culi interos'sei dorsa'les ma'nus** [TA], m. interósseo dorsal da mão. SIN dorsal interossei (interosseous *muscles*) of hand, em *muscle*.
musculi interos'sei dorsa'lis pe'dis, pl. **mus'culi interos'sei dorsa'les pe'dis** [TA], m. interósseo dorsal do pé. SIN dorsal interossei (interosseous *muscles*) of foot, em *muscle*.
musculi interos'seus planta'ris [TA], músculos interósseos plantares. SIN plantar interossei (interosseous *muscles*), em *muscle*.
m. interos'seus palma'ris, pl. **mus'culi interos'sei palma'res** [TA], músculos interósseos palmares. SIN palmar interossei (interosseous *muscles*), em *muscle*.
m. interos'seus vola'ris, músculos interósseos palmares. SIN palmar interossei (interosseous *muscles*), em *muscle*.
mus'culi interspina'les [TA], músculos interespinais. SIN interspinales (*muscles*), em *muscle*.
m. interspina'lis cer'vicis, m. interespinal do pescoço. SIN interspinales cervicis (*muscles*), em *muscle*.
m. interspina'lis lumbo'rum [TA], m. interespinal do lombo. SIN interspinales lumborum (*muscles*), em *muscle*.
m. interspina'lis thora'cis [TA], m. interespinal do tórax. SIN interspinales thoracis (*muscles*), em *muscle*.
m. intertra'gicus, m. intertrágico; m. da incisura terminal. SIN *muscle* of terminal notch.
mus'culi intertransversa'rii [TA], músculos intertransversários. SIN intertransversarii (*muscles*), em *muscle*.
mus'culi intertransversa'rii anterio'res cer'vicis [TA], músculos intertransversários anteriores do pescoço. SIN anterior cervical intertransversarii (*muscles*), em *muscle*.
mus'culi intertransversa'rii latera'les lumbo'rum [TA], músculos intertransversários laterais do lombo. SIN lateral lumbar intertransversarii (*muscles*), em *muscle*.
mus'culi intertransversa'rii media'les lumbo'rum [TA], músculos intertransversários mediais do lombo. SIN medial lumbar intertransversarii (*muscles*), em *muscle*.
mus'culi intertransversa'rii posterio'res cer'vicis [TA], músculos intertransversários posteriores do pescoço. SIN posterior cervical intertransversarii (*muscles*), em *muscle*.
mus'culi intertransversa'rii thora'cis [TA], músculos intertransversários do tórax. SIN thoracic intertransversarii (*muscles*), em *muscle*.
m. ischiocaverno'sus [TA], m. isquicavernoso. SIN ischiocavernous (*muscle*).
m. ischiococcyg'eus, m. isquicoccígeo. SIN coccygeus *muscle*.
m. keratopharyn'geus, m. ceratofaríngeo; parte ceratofaríngea do músculo constritor médio da faringe. VER middle constrictor (*muscle*) of pharynx.
mus'culi laryn'gis [TA], músculos da laringe. SIN *muscles* of larynx, em *muscle*.
m. laryngopharyn'geus, m. laringofaríngeo. SIN inferior constrictor (*muscle*) of pharynx.
m. latis'simus dor'si [TA], m. latíssimo do dorso. SIN latissimus dorsi (*muscle*).
m. leva'tor a'lae na'si, m. levantador da asa do nariz; parte do m. levantador do lábio superior e da asa do nariz que se insere na asa do nariz.
m. leva'tor an'guli o'ris [TA], m. levantador do ângulo da boca. SIN levator anguli oris (*muscle*).
m. leva'tor an'guli scap'ulae, m. levantador da escápula. SIN levator scapulae (*muscle*).
m. leva'tor a'ni [TA], m. levantador do ânus. SIN levator ani (*muscle*).
m. leva'tor cos'tae, pl. **mus'culi levato'res costa'rum,** m. levantador das costelas. SIN levatores costarum (*muscles*), em *muscle*.
mus'culi levato'res costa'rum [TA], músculos levantadores das costelas. SIN levatores costarum (*muscles*), em *muscle*.
musculi levatores costa'rum breves [TA], músculos levantadores curtos das costelas. SIN levatores costarum breves (*muscles*), em *muscle*.
musculi levatores costa'rum longi [TA], músculos levantadores longos das costelas. SIN levatores costarum longi (*muscles*), em *muscle*.
m. leva'tor glan'dulae thyroi'deae [TA], m. levantador da glândula tireóide. SIN levator (*muscle*) of thyroid gland.
m. leva'tor la'bii inferio'ris, m. levantador do lábio inferior; m. mentual. SIN mentalis (*muscle*).
m. leva'tor la'bii superio'ris [TA], m. levantador do lábio superior. SIN levator labii superioris (*muscle*).
m. leva'tor la'bii superio'ris alae'que na'si [TA], m. levantador do lábio superior e da asa do nariz. SIN levator labii superioris alaeque nasi (*muscle*).
m. leva'tor pala'ti, m. levantador do véu palatino. SIN levator veli palatini (*muscle*).
m. leva'tor pal'pebrae superio'ris [TA], m. levantador da pálpebra superior. SIN levator palpebrae superioris (*muscle*).
m. leva'tor pro'statae, m. levantador da próstata; m. puboprostático; *termo oficial alternativo para puboprostaticus (*muscle*).

m. leva'tor scap'ulae [TA], m. levantador da escápula. SIN levator scapulae (*muscle*).
m. leva'tor ve'li palati'ni [TA], m. levantador do véu palatino. SIN levator veli palatini (*muscle*).
mus'culi lin'guae [TA], músculos da língua. SIN *muscles* of tongue, em *muscle*.
m. longis'simus [TA], m. longuíssimo. SIN longissimus (*muscle*).
m. longis'simus cap'itis [TA], m. longuíssimo da cabeça. SIN longissimus capitis (*muscle*).
m. longis'simus cer'vicis [TA], m. longuíssimo do pescoço. SIN longissimus cervicis (*muscle*).
m. longis'simus dor'si, m. longuíssimo do tórax. SIN longissimus thoracis (*muscle*).
m. longis'simus thora'cis [TA], m. longuíssimo do tórax. SIN longissimus thoracis (*muscle*).
m. longitudina'lis infe'rior linguae [TA], m. longitudinal inferior da língua. SIN inferior longitudinal *muscle* of tongue.
m. longitudina'lis supe'rior linguae [TA], m. longitudinal superior da língua. SIN superior longitudinal *muscle* of tongue.
m. lon'gus cap'itis [TA], m. longo da cabeça. SIN longus capitis (*muscle*).
m. lon'gus col'li [TA], m. longo do pescoço. SIN longus colli (*muscle*).
m. lumbrica'lis ma'nus, pl. **mus'culi lumbrica'les ma'nus** [TA], m. lumbrical da mão. SIN lumbricals (lumbrical *muscles*) of hand, em *muscle*.
m. lumbrica'lis pe'dis, pl. **mus'culi lumbrica'les pe'dis** [TA], m. lumbrical do pé. SIN lumbricals (lumbrical *muscles*) of foot, em *muscle*.
m. masse'ter [TA], m. masseter. SIN masseter (*muscle*).
m. menta'lis [TA], m. mentual. SIN mentalis (*muscle*).
m. multif'idus [TA], m. multífido. SIN multifidus (*muscle*).
m. multif'idus spi'nae, m. multífido. SIN multifidus (*muscle*).
m. multipenna'tus [TA], m. multipeniforme. SIN multipennate *muscle*.
m. mylohyoi'deus [TA], m. milo-hióideo. SIN mylohyoid (*muscle*).
m. mylopharyn'geus, m. milofaríngeo; parte milofaríngea do músculo constritor superior da faringe. VER superior pharyngeal constrictor (*muscle*).
m. nasa'lis [TA], m. nasal. SIN nasalis (*muscle*).
m. obli'quus auric'ulae [TA], m. oblíquo da orelha. SIN oblique *muscle* of auricle.
m. obli'quus cap'itis infe'rior [TA], m. oblíquo inferior da cabeça. SIN obliquus capitis inferior (*muscle*).
m. obli'quus capi'tis supe'rior [TA], m. oblíquo superior da cabeça. SIN obliquus capitis superior (*muscle*).
m. obli'quus exter'nus abdom'inis [TA], m. oblíquo externo do abdome. SIN external oblique (*muscle*).
m. obli'quus infe'rior [TA], m. oblíquo inferior. SIN inferior oblique (*muscle*).
m. obli'quus inter'nus abdom'inis [TA], m. oblíquo interno do abdome. SIN internal oblique (*muscle*).
m. obli'quus supe'rior [TA], m. oblíquo superior. SIN superior oblique (*muscle*).
m. obtura'tor exter'nus [TA], m. obturador externo. SIN obturator externus (*muscle*).
m. obtura'tor inter'nus [TA], m. obturador interno. SIN obturator internus (*muscle*).
m. occipita'lis, m. occipital; m. occipitofrontal. VER occipitofrontalis (*muscle*).
m. occipitofronta'lis, m. occipitofrontal. SIN occipitofrontalis (*muscle*).
m. omohyoi'deus [TA], m. omo-hióideo. SIN omohyoid (*muscle*).
m. oppo'nens [TA], m. oponente. SIN opponens *muscle*.
m. oppo'nens dig'iti min'imi [TA], m. oponente do dedo mínimo. SIN opponens digiti minimi (*muscle*).
m. oppo'nens dig'iti quin'ti, m. oponente do dedo mínimo. SIN opponens digiti minimi (*muscle*).
m. oppo'nens min'imi dig'iti, m. oponente do dedo mínimo. SIN opponens digiti minimi (*muscle*).
m. oppo'nens pol'licis [TA], m. oponente do polegar. SIN opponens pollicis (*muscle*).
m. orbicula'ris [TA], m. orbicular. SIN orbicular *muscle*.
m. orbicula'ris oc'uli [TA], m. orbicular do olho. SIN orbicularis oculi (*muscle*).
m. orbicula'ris o'ris [TA], m. orbicular da boca. SIN orbicularis oris (*muscle*).
m. orbicula'ris palpebra'rum, m. orbicular do olho. SIN orbicularis oculi (*muscle*).
m. orbita'lis [TA], m. orbital. SIN orbitalis (*muscle*).
m. orbitopalpebra'lis, m. orbitopalpebral. SIN levator palpebrae superioris (*muscle*).
musculi ossiculorum auditoriorum, músculos dos ossículos da audição. *termo oficial alternativo para *muscles* of auditory ossicles, em *muscle*.
mus'culi ossiculo'rum audi'tus [TA], músculos dos ossículos da audição. SIN *muscles* of auditory ossicles, em *muscle*.
m. palatoglos'sus [TA], m. palatoglosso. SIN palatoglossus (*muscle*).
m. palatopharyn'geus [TA], m. palatofaríngeo. SIN palatopharyngeus (*muscle*).
m. palatosalpin'geus, m. tensor do véu palatino. SIN tensor veli palati (*muscle*).

m. palatostaphyli'nus, m. palatoestafilino; feixe de fibras musculares do tensor do véu palatino que se unem ao m. da úvula.
m. palma'ris bre'vis [TA], m. palmar curto. SIN palmaris brevis (*muscle*).
m. palma'ris lon'gus [TA], m. palmar longo. SIN palmaris longus (*muscle*).
m. papilla'ris [TA], m. papilar. SIN papillary *muscle*.
mus'culi pectina'ti [TA], músculos pectíneos. SIN pectinate *muscles*, em *muscle*.
m. pectin'eus [TA], m. pectíneo. SIN pectineus (*muscle*).
m. pectora'lis ma'jor [TA], m. peitoral maior. SIN pectoralis major (*muscle*).
m. pectora'lis mi'nor [TA], m. peitoral menor. SIN pectoralis minor (*muscle*).
m. pennatus [TA], m. peniforme. SIN pennate *muscle*.
mus'culi perine'i [TA], músculos do períneo. SIN perineal *muscles*, em *muscle*.
m. peroneocalca'neus, m. fibulocalcâneo; músculo ocasional que se origina da diáfise da fíbula e se insere no calcâneo.
m. perone'us bre'vis, m. fibular curto; *termo oficial alternativo para fibularis brevis (*muscle*).
m. perone'us lon'gus, m. fibular longo; *termo oficial alternativo para fibularis longus (*muscle*).
m. perone'us ter'tius, m. fibular terceiro; *termo oficial alternativo para fibularis tertius (*muscle*).
m. petropharyn'geus, m. petrofaríngeo; músculo levantador acessório ocasional da faringe, que se origina da superfície inferior da porção petrosa do osso temporal e se insere na faringe.
m. petrostaphyli'nus, m. levantador do véu palatino. SIN levator veli (*muscle*).
m. pharyngopalati'nus, m. faringopalatino. SIN palatopharyngeus (*muscle*).
m. pirifor'mis [TA], m. piriforme. SIN piriformis (*muscle*).
m. plana [TA], m. plano. SIN flat *muscle*.
m. planta'ris [TA], m. plantar. SIN plantaris (*muscle*).
m. platys'ma, platisma. SIN platysma (*muscle*).
m. platys'ma myoi'des, platisma. SIN platysma (*muscle*).
m. pleuroesopha'geus [TA], m. pleuroesofágico. SIN pleuroesophageus (*muscle*).
m. poplit'eus [TA], m. poplíteo. SIN popliteus (*muscle*).
m. proce'rus [TA], m. prócero. SIN procerus (*muscle*).
m. prona'tor [TA], m. pronador. SIN pronator (*muscle*).
m. prona'tor pe'dis, m. pronador do pé. SIN quadratus plantae (*muscle*).
m. prona'tor quadra'tus [TA], m. pronador quadrado. SIN pronator quadratus (*muscle*).
m. prona'tor ra'dii te'res, m. pronador redondo. SIN pronator teres (*muscle*).
m. prona'tor te'res [TA], m. pronador redondo. SIN pronator teres (*muscle*).
m. prostat'icus, m. prostático. SIN muscular *substance* of prostate.
m. pso'as ma'jor [TA], m. psoas maior. SIN psoas major (*muscle*).
m. pso'as mi'nor [TA], m. psoas menor. SIN psoas minor (*muscle*).
m. pterygoi'deus exter'nus, m. pterigóideo lateral. SIN lateral pterygoid (*muscle*).
m. pterygoi'deus inter'nus, m. pterigóideo medial. SIN medial pterygoid (*muscle*).
m. pterygoi'deus latera'lis [TA], m. pterigóideo lateral. SIN lateral pterygoid (*muscle*).
m. pterygoi'deus media'lis [TA], m. pterigóideo medial. SIN medial pterygoid (*muscle*).
m. pterygopharyn'geus, m. pterigofaríngeo; parte pterigofaríngea do músculo constritor superior da faringe. VER superior pharyngeal constrictor (*muscle*).
m. pterygospino'sus, m. pterigoespinhoso; uma porção de músculo, ocasionalmente presente, que passa entre a espinha do osso esfenóide e a margem posterior da lâmina pterigóidea lateral.
m. puboanalis [TA], m. puboanal. SIN puboanalis (*muscle*).
m. pubococcyg'eus [TA], m. pubococcígeo. SIN pubococcygeus (*muscle*).
m. puboperinealis [TA], m. puboperineal. SIN puboperinealis (*muscle*).
m. puboprostat'icus [TA], m. puboprostático. SIN puboprostaticus (*muscle*).
m. puborecta'lis [TA], m. puborretal. SIN puborectalis (*muscle*).
m. pubovagina'lis [TA], m. pubovaginal. SIN pubovaginalis (*muscle*).
m. pubovesica'lis [TA], m. pubovesical. SIN pubovesicalis (*muscle*).
m. pyramida'lis [TA], m. piramidal. SIN pyramidalis (*muscle*).
m. pyramida'lis auric'ulae [TA], m. piramidal da orelha. SIN pyramidal *muscle* of auricle.
m. pyramida'lis na'si, m. prócero. SIN procerus (*muscle*).
m. pyrifor'mis, m. piriforme. SIN piriformis (*muscle*).
m. quadra'tus [TA], m. quadrado. SIN quadrate *muscle*.
m. quadra'tus fem'oris [TA], m. quadrado femoral. SIN quadratus femoris (*muscle*).
m. quadra'tus la'bii inferio'ris, m. quadrado do lábio inferior. SIN depressor labii inferioris (*muscle*).
m. quadra'tus la'bii superio'ris, m. quadrado do lábio superior; composto de três cabeças, geralmente descritas como três músculos distintos; são elas a cabeça angular ou músculo levantador do lábio superior e da asa do nariz; cabeça infra-orbital ou músculo levantador do lábio superior; cabeça zigomática ou músculo zigomático menor. SIN quadrate muscle of upper lip.

m. quadra'tus lumbo'rum [TA], m. quadrado do lombo. SIN quadratus lumborum (*muscle*).
m. quadra'tus men'ti, m. quadrado do mento; m. abaixador do lábio inferior. SIN depressor labii inferioris (*muscle*).
m. quadra'tus plan'tae [TA], m. quadrado plantar. SIN quadratus plantae (*muscle*).
m. quadriceps [TA], m. quadríceps. SIN quadriceps femoris (*muscle*).
m. quad'riceps exten'sor fem'oris, m. quadríceps femoral. SIN quadriceps femoris (*muscle*).
m. quad'riceps fem'oris [TA], m. quadríceps femoral. SIN quadriceps femoris (*muscle*).
m. rectococcyg'eus [TA], m. retococcígeo. SIN rectococcygeus (*muscle*).
musculi rectourethra'les, músculos retouretrais; *termo oficial alternativo para anorectoperineal *muscles*, em *muscle*.
m. rectouteri'nus [TA], m. retouterino. SIN rectouterinus (*muscle*).
m. rectovesica'lis [TA], m. retovesical. SIN rectovesicalis (*muscle*).
m. rectus [TA], m. reto. SIN straight *muscle*.
m. rec'tus abdom'inis [TA], m. reto do abdome. SIN rectus abdominis (*muscle*).
m. rec'tus cap'itis ante'rior [TA], m. reto anterior da cabeça. SIN rectus capitis anterior (*muscle*).
m. rec'tus cap'itis anti'cus ma'jor, m. longo da cabeça. SIN longus capitis (*muscle*).
m. rec'tus cap'itis anti'cus mi'nor, m. reto anterior da cabeça. SIN rectus capitis anterior (*muscle*).
m. rec'tus cap'itis latera'lis [TA], m. reto lateral da cabeça. SIN rectus capitis lateralis (*muscle*).
m. rec'tus cap'itis poste'rior ma'jor [TA], m. reto posterior maior da cabeça. SIN rectus capitis posterior major (*muscle*).
m. rec'tus cap'itis poste'rior mi'nor [TA], m. reto posterior menor da cabeça. SIN rectus capitis posterior minor (*muscle*).
m. rec'tus cap'itis posti'cus ma'jor, m. reto posterior maior da cabeça. SIN rectus capitis posterior major (*muscle*).
m. rec'tus cap'itis posti'cus mi'nor, m. reto posterior menor da cabeça. SIN rectus capitis posterior minor (*muscle*).
m. rec'tus exter'nus, m. reto lateral. SIN lateral rectus (*muscle*).
m. rec'tus fem'oris [TA], m. reto femoral. SIN rectus femoris (*muscle*).
m. rec'tus infe'rior [TA], m. reto inferior. SIN inferior rectus (*muscle*).
m. rec'tus inter'nus, m. reto medial. SIN medial rectus (*muscle*).
m. rec'tus latera'lis [TA], m. reto lateral. SIN lateral rectus (*muscle*).
m. rec'tus media'lis [TA], m. reto medial. SIN medial rectus (*muscle*).
m. rec'tus supe'rior [TA], m. reto superior. SIN superior rectus (*muscle*).
m. rec'tus thora'cis, m. reto do tórax; m. esternal. SIN sternalis (*muscle*).
musculi regionis analis [TA], músculos do trígono anal. SIN *muscles* of anal triangle, em *muscle*.
musculi regionis urogenitalis [TA], músculos do trígono urogenital. SIN *muscles* of urogenital triangle, em *muscle*.
m. ret'rahens au'rem, m. ret'rahens auric'ulam, m. auricular posterior. SIN auricularis posterior (*muscle*).
m. rhomboatloi'deus, m. romboatlóideo; musculo ocasional que se origina das vértebras cervicais e torácicas com os músculos rombóides e se insere no atlas.
m. rhomboi'deus ma'jor [TA], m. rombóide maior. SIN rhomboid major (*muscle*).
m. rhomboi'deus mi'nor [TA], m. rombóide menor. SIN rhomboid minor (*muscle*).
m. riso'rius [TA], m. risório. SIN risorius (*muscle*).
m. rotator [TA], m. rotador. SIN rotator (*muscle*).
mus'culi rotato'res [TA], músculos rotadores. SIN rotatores (*muscles*), em *muscle*.
mus'culi rotato'res cer'vicis [TA], músculos rotadores do pescoço. SIN rotatores cervicis (*muscles*), em *muscle*.
mus'culi rotato'res lumbo'rum [TA], músculos rotadores do lombo. SIN rotatores lumborum (*muscles*), em *muscle*.
mus'culi rotato'res thora'cis [TA], músculos rotadores do tórax. SIN rotatores thoracis (*muscles*), em *muscle*.
m. sacrococcyg'eus ante'rior, m. sacrococcígeo anterior. SIN ventral sacrococcygeus (*muscle*).
m. sacrococcyg'eus dorsa'lis, m. sacrococcígeo dorsal. SIN dorsal sacrococcygeus *muscle*.
m. sacrococcyg'eus poste'rior, m. sacrococcígeo posterior. SIN dorsal sacrococcygeus *muscle*.
m. sacrococcyg'eus ventra'lis, m. sacrococcígeo ventral. SIN ventral sacrococcygeus (*muscle*).
m. sacrolumba'lis, m. sacrolombar; m. iliocostal do lombo. SIN iliocostalis lumborum (*muscle*).
m. sacrospina'lis, m. sacroespinal; m. eretor da espinha. SIN erector spinae (*muscles*), em *muscle*.
m. salpingopharyn'geus [TA], m. salpingofaríngeo. SIN salpingopharyngeus (*muscle*).

m. sarto'rius [TA], m. sartório. SIN sartorius (muscle).
m. scale'nus ante'rior [TA], m. escaleno anterior. SIN scalenus anterior (muscle).
m. scale'nus anti'cus, m. escaleno anterior. SIN scalenus anterior (muscle).
m. scale'nus me'dius [TA], m. escaleno médio. SIN scalenus medius (muscle).
m. scale'nus min'imus [TA], m. escaleno mínimo. SIN scalenus minimus (muscle).
m. scale'nus poste'rior [TA], m. escaleno posterior. SIN scalenus posterior (muscle).
m. scale'nus posti'cus, m. escaleno posterior. SIN scalenus posterior (muscle).
musculi scapulohumerales [TA], músculos escapuloumerais. SIN scapulohumeral muscles, em muscle.
m. semimembrano'sus [TA], m. semimembranáceo. SIN semimembranosus (muscle).
m. semipennatus [TA], m. semipeniforme. SIN semipennate muscle.
m. semispina'lis [TA], m. semi-espinal. SIN semispinalis muscle.
m. semispina'lis cap'itis [TA], m. semi-espinal da cabeça. SIN semispinalis capitis (muscle).
m. semispina'lis cer'vicis [TA], m. semi-espinal do pescoço. SIN semispinalis cervicis (muscle).
m. semispina'lis col'li, m. semi-espinal do pescoço; *termo oficial alternativo para semispinalis cervicis (muscle).
m. semispina'lis dor'si, m. semi-espinal do tórax. SIN semispinalis thoracis (muscle).
m. semispina'lis thora'cis [TA], m. semi-espinal do tórax. SIN semispinalis thoracis (muscle).
m. semitendino'sus [TA], m. semitendíneo. SIN semitendinosus (muscle).
m. serra'tus ante'rior [TA], m. serrátil anterior. SIN serratus anterior (muscle).
m. serra'tus mag'nus, m. serrátil anterior. SIN serratus anterior (muscle).
m. serra'tus poste'rior infe'rior [TA], m. serrátil posterior inferior. SIN serratus posterior inferior (muscle).
m. serra'tus poste'rior supe'rior [TA], m. serrátil posterior superior. SIN serratus posterior superior (muscle).
m. skel'eti, m. esquelético. SIN skeletal muscle.
m. sol'eus, m. sóleo. SIN soleus (muscle).
m. sphinc'ter, esfíncter. SIN sphincter.
m. sphinc'ter ampullae biliaropancrea'ticae, m. esfíncter da ampola hepatopancreática; *termo oficial alternativo para sphincter of hepatopancreatic ampulla.
m. sphinc'ter ampullae, m. esfíncter da ampola; *termo oficial alternativo para sphincter of hepatopancreatic ampulla.
m. sphinc'ter ampullae hepatopancrea'ticae [TA], m. esfíncter da ampola hepatopancreática. SIN sphincter of hepatopancreatic ampulla.
m. sphinc'ter a'ni exter'nus [TA], m. esfíncter externo do ânus. SIN external anal sphincter.
m. sphinc'ter a'ni inter'nus [TA], m. esfíncter interno do ânus. SIN internal anal sphincter.
m. sphinc'ter ductus biliaris, m. esfíncter do ducto colédoco; *termo oficial alternativo para sphincter of (common) bile duct.
m. sphinc'ter duc'tus chole'dochi [TA], m. esfíncter do ducto colédoco. SIN sphincter of (common) bile duct.
m. sphinc'ter duc'tus pancrea'tici [TA], m. esfíncter do ducto pancreático. SIN sphincter of pancreatic duct.
m. sphinc'ter o'ris, m. orbicular da boca. SIN orbicularis oris (muscle).
m. sphinc'ter palatopharyn'geus, m. esfíncter palatofaríngeo; *termo oficial alternativo para posterior fascicle of palatopharyngeus muscle.
m. sphinc'ter pupil'lae [TA], m. esfíncter da pupila. SIN sphincter pupillae.
m. sphinc'ter pylo'ri [TA], m. esfíncter do piloro. SIN pyloric sphincter.
m. sphinc'ter ure'thrae externus, m. esfíncter externo da uretra. SIN external urethral sphincter.
m. sphinc'ter ure'thrae externus femininae [TA], m. esfíncter externo da uretra feminina. SIN external urethral sphincter of female.
m. sphinc'ter urethrae externus masculinae [TA], m. esfíncter externo da uretra masculina. SIN external urethral sphincter of male.
m. sphinc'ter urethrae internus, m. esfíncter interno da uretra; *termo oficial alternativo para internal urethral sphincter.
m. sphinc'ter urethrovaginalis [TA], m. esfíncter uretrovaginal. SIN urethrovaginal sphincter.
m. sphinc'ter vagi'nae, m. esfíncter da vagina; m. bulboesponjoso. SIN bulbospongiosus (muscle).
m. sphinc'ter vesi'cae, m. esfíncter da bexiga; m. esfíncter interno da uretra. SIN internal urethral sphincter.
m. spina'lis [TA], m. espinal. SIN spinalis (muscle).
m. spina'lis cap'itis [TA], m. espinal da cabeça. SIN spinalis capitis (muscle).
m. spina'lis cer'vicis [TA], m. espinal do pescoço. SIN spinalis cervicis (muscle).
m. spina'lis col'li, m. espinal do pescoço. SIN spinalis cervicis (muscle).
m. spina'lis dor'si, m. espinal do tórax. SIN spinalis thoracis (muscle).

m. spina'lis thora'cis [TA], m. espinal do tórax. SIN spinalis thoracis (muscle).
musculi splenii [TA], músculos esplênios. SIN splenius (muscles), em muscle.
m. sple'nius cap'itis [TA], m. esplênio da cabeça. SIN splenius capitis (muscle).
m. sple'nius cer'vicis [TA], m. esplênio do pescoço. SIN splenius cervicis (muscle).
m. sple'nius col'li, m. esplênio do pescoço. SIN splenius cervicis (muscle).
m. stape'dius [TA], m. estapédio. SIN stapedius (muscle).
m. sterna'lis [TA], m. esternal. SIN sternalis (muscle).
m. sternochondroscapula'ris, m. esternocondroescapular. SIN sternochondroscapular muscle.
m. sternoclavicula'ris, m. esternoclavicular. SIN sternoclavicular muscle.
m. sternocleidomastoi'deus [TA], m. esternocleidomastóideo. SIN sternocleidomastoid (muscle).
m. sternofascia'lis, m. esternofascial; uma porção ocasional de músculo que se origina do manúbrio do esterno e insere-se na fáscia do pescoço.
m. sternohyoi'deus [TA], m. esterno-hióideo. SIN sternohyoid (muscle).
m. sternothyroi'deus [TA], m. esternotireóideo. SIN sternothyroid (muscle).
m. styloauricula'ris, m. estiloauricular. SIN styloauricular (muscle).
m. styloglos'sus [TA], m. estiloglosso. SIN styloglossus (muscle).
m. stylohyoi'deus [TA], m. estilo-hióideo. SIN stylohyoid (muscle).
m. stylolaryn'geus, m. estilolaríngeo; a parte do músculo estilofaríngeo que está inserida na cartilagem tireóidea.
m. stylopharyn'geus [TA], m. estilofaríngeo. SIN stylopharyngeus (muscle).
m. subcla'vius [TA], m. subclávio. SIN subclavius (muscle).
m. subcosta'lis, pl. **mus'culi subcosta'les** [TA], músculos subcostais. SIN subcostal muscle.
m. subcuta'neus col'li, m. subcutâneo do pescoço; platisma. SIN platysma (muscle).
mus'culi suboccipita'les [TA], músculos suboccipitais. SIN suboccipital muscles, em muscle.
m. subscapula'ris [TA], m. subescapular. SIN subscapularis (muscle).
m. supina'tor [TA], m. supinador. SIN supinator (muscle).
m. supina'tor lon'gus, m. supinador longo; designação obsoleta e não-acurada para o músculo braquiorradial (brachioradialis muscle).
m. supina'tor ra'dii brev'is, m. supinador curto do rádio. SIN supinator (muscle).
m. supraclavicula'ris, m. supraclavicular. SIN supraclavicular muscle.
mus'culi suprahyoi'dei [TA], músculos supra-hióideos. SIN suprahyoid muscles, em muscle.
m. supraspina'lis, m. supra-espinhoso. SIN supraspinalis (muscle).
m. supraspina'tus [TA], m. supra-espinal. SIN supraspinatus (muscle).
m. suspenso'rius duode'ni [TA], m. suspensor do duodeno. SIN suspensory muscle of duodenum.
m. tarsa'lis infe'rior [TA], m. tarsal inferior. SIN inferior tarsal muscle.
m. tarsa'lis supe'rior [TA], m. tarsal superior. SIN superior tarsal muscle.
m. tempora'lis [TA], m. temporal. SIN temporalis (muscle).
m. temporoparieta'lis [TA], m. temporoparietal. SIN temporoparietalis (muscle). VER TAMBÉM auricularis anterior (muscle), auricularis superior (muscle).
m. ten'sor fas'ciae fem'oris, m. tensor da fáscia lata. SIN tensor fasciae latae (muscle).
m. ten'sor fas'ciae la'tae [TA], m. tensor da fáscia lata. SIN tensor fasciae latae (muscle).
m. ten'sor tar'si, m. tensor do tarso. SIN lacrimal part of orbicularis oculi muscle. VER orbicularis oculi (muscle).
m. ten'sor tym'pani [TA], m. tensor do tímpano. SIN tensor tympani (muscle).
m. ten'sor ve'li palati'ni [TA], m. tensor do véu palatino. SIN tensor veli palati (muscle).
m. te'res ma'jor [TA], m. redondo maior. SIN teres major (muscle).
m. te'res mi'nor [TA], m. redondo menor. SIN teres minor (muscle).
m. tetrago'nus, platisma. SIN platysma (muscle).
mus'culi thora'cis [TA], músculos do tórax. SIN muscles of thorax, em muscle.
musculi thoracoappendiculares [TA], músculos toracoapendiculares. SIN thoracoappendicular muscles, em muscle.
m. thyroarytenoi'deus [TA], m. tireoaritenóideo. SIN thyroarytenoid (muscle).
m. thyroarytenoi'deus exter'nus, m. tireoaritenóideo externo. SIN thyroarytenoid (muscle).
m. thyroarytenoi'deus inter'nus, m. tireoaritenóideo interno. SIN vocalis (muscle).
m. thyroepiglot'ticus, m. tireoepiglótico. SIN thyroepiglottic part of thyroarytenoid (muscle).
m. thyrohyoi'deus [TA], m. tireo-hióideo. SIN thyrohyoid (muscle).
m. thyropharyn'geus, m. tireofaríngeo. VER inferior constrictor (muscle) of pharynx.
m. tibia'lis ante'rior [TA], m. tibial anterior. SIN tibialis anterior (muscle).
m. tibia'lis anti'cus, m. tibial anterior. SIN tibialis anterior (muscle).
m. tibia'lis gra'cilis, m. plantar. SIN plantaris (muscle).
m. tibia'lis poste'rior [TA], m. tibial posterior. SIN tibialis posterior (muscle).

m. tibia'lis posti'cus, m. tibial posterior. SIN tibialis posterior (*muscle*).
m. tibia'lis secun'dus, m. tibial segundo; músculo inconstante, de tamanho pequeno, que se origina na face posterior da tíbia e se insere na cápsula articular do tornozelo. SIN second tibial muscle.
m. tibiofascia'lis ante'rior, m. tibiofascia'lis anti'cus, m. tibiofascial anterior; fibras distintas do músculo tibial anterior, inseridas na fáscia do dorso do pé.
m. trachea'lis [TA], m. traqueal. SIN trachealis (*muscle*).
m. tracheloclavicula'ris, m. traqueoclavicular. SIN tracheloclavicular *muscle*.
m. trachelomastoi'deus, m. traqueomastóideo; m. longuíssimo da cabeça. SIN longissimus capitis (*muscle*).
m. tra'gicus [TA], m. trágico. SIN tragicus (*muscle*).
m. transversa'lis abdom'inis, m. transverso do abdome. SIN transversus abdominis (*muscle*).
m. transversa'lis cap'itis, m. transverso da cabeça; m. longuíssimo da cabeça. SIN longissimus capitis (*muscle*).
m. transversa'lis cer'vicis, m. transversa'lis col'li, m. longuíssimo do pescoço. SIN longissimus cervicis (*muscle*).
m. transversa'lis na'si, m. transverso do nariz. VER nasalis (*muscle*).
musculi transversospina'les [TA], músculos transverso-espinais. SIN transversospinales (*muscles*), em *muscle*.
m. transver'sus abdom'inis [TA], m. transverso do abdome. SIN transversus abdominis (*muscle*).
m. transver'sus auric'ulae [TA], m. transverso da orelha. SIN transverse *muscle* of auricle.
m. transver'sus lin'guae [TA], m. transverso da língua. SIN transverse *muscle* of tongue.
m. transver'sus men'ti [TA], m. transverso do mento. SIN transversus menti (*muscle*).
m. transver'sus nu'chae [TA], m. transverso da nuca. SIN transversus nuchae (*muscle*).
m. transver'sus perine'i profun'dus [TA], m. transverso profundo do períneo. SIN deep transverse perineal *muscle*.
m. transver'sus perine'i superficia'lis [TA], m. transverso superficial do períneo. SIN superficial transverse perineal *muscle*.
m. transver'sus thora'cis [TA], m. transverso do tórax. SIN transversus thoracis (*muscle*).
m. trape'zius [TA], m. trapézio. SIN trapezius (*muscle*).
m. triangula'ris [TA], m. triangular; **(1)** [NA], SIN triangular *muscle* (1); **(2)** SIN depressor anguli oris (*muscle*).
m. triangula'ris la'bii inferior'is, m. triangular do lábio inferior; m. abaixador do ângulo da boca. SIN depressor anguli oris (*muscle*).
m. triangula'ris la'bii superior'is, m. triangular do lábio superior; m. levantador do ângulo da boca. SIN levator anguli oris (*muscle*).
m. triangula'ris ster'ni, m. triangular do esterno; m. transverso do tórax. SIN transversus thoracis (*muscle*).
m. tri'ceps [TA], m. tríceps. SIN three-headed *muscle*.
m. tri'ceps bra'chii [TA], m. tríceps braquial. SIN triceps brachii (*muscle*).
m. tri'ceps cox'ae, m. tríceps da coxa. SIN triceps coxae (*muscle*).
m. tri'ceps su'rae [TA], m. tríceps sural. SIN triceps surae (*muscle*).
m. triticeoglos'sus, m. triticeoglosso; uma porção fina ocasional de fibras musculares que passam entre a raiz da língua e a cartilagem tritícea. SIN Bochdalek muscle.
m. unipenna'tus, m. semipeniforme; *termo oficial alternativo para semipennate *muscle*.
m. u'vulae [TA], m. da úvula. SIN *muscle* of uvula.
m. vas'tus exter'nus, m. vasto lateral. SIN vastus lateralis (*muscle*).
m. vas'tus interme'dius [TA], m. vasto intermédio. SIN vastus intermedius (*muscle*).
m. vas'tus inter'nus, m. vasto medial. SIN vastus medialis (*muscle*).
m. vas'tus latera'lis [TA], m. vasto lateral. SIN vastus lateralis (*muscle*).
m. vas'tus media'lis [TA], m. vasto medial. SIN vastus medialis (*muscle*).
m. ventricula'ris, m. ventricular; fibras do músculo tireoaritenóideo que entram na prega vestibular (falsa corda vocal).
m. vertica'lis lin'guae [TA], m. vertical da língua. SIN vertical *muscle* of tongue.
m. voca'lis [TA], m. vocal. SIN vocalis (*muscle*).
m. zygomat'icus, m. zigomático. SIN zygomaticus major (*muscle*).
m. zygomat'icus ma'jor [TA], m. zigomático maior. SIN zygomaticus major (*muscle*).
m. zygomat'icus mi'nor [TA], m. zigomático menor. SIN zygomaticus minor (*muscle*).

mush·bite (mŭsh′bīt). Registro maxilomandibular feito introduzindo-se uma massa de cera mole na boca do paciente e instruindo-o a mordê-la até o grau desejado; não é um procedimento aceito por todos.

mu·si·co·ther·a·py (mū′sik-ō-thār′a-pē). Musicoterapia; tratamento auxiliar de transtornos mentais por meio da música.

Musset, L.C., Alfred de, poeta francês, 1810–1857; pessoa na qual foi estudado o sinal de Musset. VER M. *sign*.

mus·si·ta·tion (mŭs-i-tā′shŭn). Mussitação; movimentos dos lábios como se estivesse falando, mas sem emitir som; observado no delírio, no semicoma e na doença de Parkinson grave. [L. *mussito*, murmurar constantemente, de *musso*, pp. -*atus*, sussurrar]

Mussy. VER Guéneau de Mussy.

must (mŭst). Mosto; suco não-fermentado de uva ou de outras frutas. [L. *mustum*, vinho novo, neutro de *mustus*, fresco]

Mustard, William T., cirurgião torácico canadense, 1914–1987. VER M. *operation, procedure*.

mus·tard (mŭs′tard). Mostarda. **1.** As sementes maduras secas da *Brassica alba* (mostarda branca) e *B. nigra* (mostarda negra) (família Cruciferae). **2.** SIN mustard gas. [Fr. ant. *moustarde*, do L. *mustum*, mosto]
black m., m. negra; a semente madura e seca da *Brassica nigra* ou da *B. juncea*; é a fonte de alil isotiocianato; contém sinigrina (mironato de potássio); mirosina; sulfocianato de sinapina; ácidos erúcico, beênico e sinapólico; e óleo fixo; um emético imediato, rubefaciente e condimento.
m. chlorohydrin, m. cloridrina. SIN hemisulfur m.
hemisulfur m., m. hemi-sulfúrica; agente antineoplásico. SIN m. chlorohydrin, semisulfur m.
nitrogen m.'s (HN2), mostardas nitrogenadas; compostos que possuem a fórmula geral R—N(CH$_2$CH$_2$Cl), o protótipo é a m. nitrogenada HN-2, mecloretamina, na qual o R é CH$_3$. Algumas foram usadas terapeuticamente por sua ação destrutiva sobre o tecido linfóide no linfossarcoma, leucemia, doença de Hodgkin e em alguns outros cânceres; a maioria é agente vesicante. VER TAMBÉM mechlorethamine hydrochloride.
semisulfur m., m. semi-sulfúrica. SIN hemisulfur m.
sulfur m., m. de enxofre; gás de mostarda. SIN mustard gas.
uracil m., m. de uracil. VER *uracil* mustard.
white m., m. branca; as sementes maduras da *Brassica* (*Sinapis*) *alba*; menos picante que a m. negra, mas com os mesmos constituintes e empregos.

mus·tard oil. Óleo de mostarda; termo aplicado a qualquer um dos isotiocianatos orgânicos em geral, porém mais especificamente ao alil isotiocianato; esses óleos podem ser convertidos metabolicamente em tiocianatos e, assim, causar bócio.
expressed m. o., o. de mostarda espremido; o óleo fixo espremido das sementes de *Brassica alba* e *B. nigra*; contém os glicerídeos dos ácidos oleico, araquídico e outros ácidos graxos; usado como óleo de salada e na fabricação de oleomargarina.
volatile m. o., o. de mostarda volátil. SIN allyl isothiocyanate.

mus·tine hy·dro·chlo·ride (mŭs′tēn). Cloridrato de mustina. SIN mechlorethamine hydrochloride.

mu·ta·cism (mū′ta-sizm). Mutacismo. SIN mytacism.

mu·ta·gen (mū′ta-jen). Mutagênico; qualquer agente que promove uma mutação ou causa um aumento da freqüência de eventos mutacionais, p. ex., substâncias radioativas, raios X ou algumas substâncias químicas. [L. *muto*, modificar, + G. -*gen*, que produz]
frame-shift m., m. da fase de leitura; mutagênico, como um derivado da acridina, que causa uma mutação por deslocamento da estrutura de leitura; os códons (trincas de bases) são lidos fora de fase e são utilizados diferentes aminoácidos.

mu·ta·gen·e·sis (mū-tă-jen′ĕ-sis). Mutagênese. **1.** Produção de uma mutação. **2.** Produção de alteração genética através do uso de substâncias químicas ou radiação.
cassette m., m. de cassete; a produção de mutantes em uma região (freqüentemente limitada por locais de restrição únicos) pelo uso de oligonucleotídeos sintéticos que preenchem a abertura com mutantes designados no material genético sintético.
insertional m., m. insercional; mutação causada por inserção de novo material genético em um gene normal, particularmente de retrovírus no DNA cromossomial.
site-directed m., m. sítio-dirigida; as alterações controladas de regiões selecionadas de uma molécula de DNA.

mu·ta·gen·ic (mū-tă-jen′ik). Mutagênico; que promove mutação.

mu·tant (myū′tant). Mutante. **1.** Fenótipo no qual se manifesta uma mutação. **2.** Um gene que é raro e geralmente prejudicial, em contraste com um gene do tipo selvagem, não necessariamente gerado recentemente.
active m., m. ativo; mutante com expressão fenotípica evidente.
amber m., m. âmbar; mutante com uma mutação que resulta em um códon UAG.
auxotrophic m., m. auxotrófico; mutante com uma exigência nutricional que não existe no organismo do tipo selvagem. SIN defective organism, deficiency m.
cold-sensitive m., m. sensível ao frio; mutante que é defeituoso em baixa temperatura, mas funcional em temperatura normal. Cf. temperature-sensitive m.
conditional-lethal m., m. letal condicional. SIN conditionally lethal m.
conditionally lethal m., m. letal condicional; mutante viral que consegue se replicar em algumas condições permissivas, mas não em outras condições (res-

tritivas ou não-permissivas), sendo a cepa original (selvagem) capaz de se replicar em ambas as condições. VER suppressor-sensitive m., temperature-sensitive m. SIN conditional-lethal m.

deficiency m., m. auxotrófico. SIN auxotrophic m.
inactive m., m. inativo; mutante que não se manifesta fenotipicamente. SIN silent m.
petite m., m. pequeno; mutante com uma mutação que fez com que o microrganismo crescesse muito lentamente ou formasse colônias pequenas. [Fr. pequeno]
quick-stop m., mutante bacteriano que interrompe sua replicação imediatamente quando a temperatura atinge determinado nível. Cf. temperature-sensitive m.
silent m., m. silencioso. SIN inactive m.
suppressor-sensitive m., m. sensível ao supressor; mutante bacteriófago, com um espectro de hospedeiros, letal condicional, que produz códons sem sentido e só consegue se replicar em uma bactéria hospedeira capaz de traduzir o códon sem sentido; os efeitos da mutação são letais (isto é, impedem a replicação do vírus) em uma bactéria sem esse mecanismo supressor.
temperature-sensitive m., m. termossensível; mutante viral capaz de se replicar em uma parte de uma faixa de temperatura, mas não em outra; a cepa original (selvagem) é capaz de se replicar em toda a faixa de temperatura; geralmente não se obtém um produto em temperatura elevada. Cf. cold-sensitive m., quick-stop m.
uninducible m., m. não-indutível; mutante que não pode ser induzido.
virulent phage m., m. de fago virulento; mutante de um fago incapaz de estabelecer lisogenia.

mu·ta·ro·tase (mū′tă-rō-tās). Mutarrotase. SIN aldose 1-epimerase.
mu·ta·ro·ta·tion (mū′tă-rō-tā′shŭn). Mutarrotação; o processo de modificar a rotação específica em determinado comprimento de onda; p. ex., uma solução de α-D-glicose recristalizada a partir de sua solução em ácido acético e recém-dissolvida em água produz uma rotação de $[\alpha]_D^{20} = +112,2°$, mas, quando recristalizada a partir de uma solução aquosa fervente (como a forma β), exibe uma rotação inicial de $[\alpha]_D^{20} = +18,7°$; ambas as soluções em repouso têm sua rotação específica lentamente modificada para um valor de $[\alpha]_D^{20} = +52,7°$, indicando uma mistura das duas formas de D-glicose. SIN birotation, multirotation.
mu·tase (mū′tās). Mutase; qualquer enzima que catalisa a aparente migração de grupamentos dentro de uma molécula, p. ex., fosfoglicerato fosfomutase; algumas vezes, a transferência se dá de uma molécula para outra, p. ex., fosfoglucomutase, fosfogliceromutase (ambas fosfotransferases).
mu·ta·tion (mū-tā′shŭn). Mutação. **1.** Alteração na química de um gene, perpetuada nas divisões subseqüentes da célula em que ocorre; uma alteração na seqüência de pares de bases na molécula cromossomial. **2.** Termo cunhado por De Vries para a súbita produção de uma espécie, distinta da variação. [L. *muto*, pp. *-atus*, modificar]
addition m., m. por adição. SIN reading-frame-shift m.
addition-deletion m., m. por adição-deleção. SIN reading-frame-shift m.
amber m., m. âmbar; mutação que resulta na formação do códon UAG, que resulta na interrupção prematura de uma cadeia polipeptídica. Cf. supressor m.
back m., m. retrógrada; reversão de um gene a uma forma ancestral devido à mutação adicional para o códon original ou a uma codificação para o mesmo aminoácido. SIN reverse m.
deletion m., m. por deleção. SIN reading-frame-shift m.
frame-shift m., m. da fase de leitura. SIN reading-frame-shift m.
induced m., m. induzida; mutação causada por exposição a um mutágeno.
lethal m., m. letal; traço mutante que leva a um fenótipo incompatível com a reprodução efetiva.
missense m., m. de sentido incorreto; mutação na qual a alteração ou substituição de uma base resulta em um códon que causa inserção de um aminoácido diferente na cadeia polipeptídica em crescimento, dando origem a uma proteína alterada. [missense por analogia com non-sense]
natural m., m. natural. SIN spontaneous m.
neutral m., m. neutra; mutação com impacto negligenciável sobre a aptidão genética.
new m., m. nova; termo redundante para um traço hereditário encontrado na prole, mas que não existe em nenhum dos pais, isto é, não é uma forma mutante preexistente hereditária.
nonsense m., m. sem sentido. SIN supressor m.
ochre m., m. ocre; mutação que produz o códon de terminação UAA, resultando em terminação prematura de uma cadeia polipeptídica. Cf. suppressor m.
opal m., m. opala. SIN umber m.
point m., m. pontual; mutação que envolve apenas um nucleotídeo; pode consistir na perda de um nucleotídeo, substituição de um nucleotídeo por outro, ou inserção de um nucleotídeo adicional.
reading-frame-shift m., m. da fase de leitura; mutação resultante da inserção ou da deleção de um único nucleotídeo na seqüência de DNA normal; como o código genético é lido com três nucleotídeos de uma vez, todos os trinucleotídeos distais à mutação estarão fora de fase e serão lidos incorretamente e, portanto, traduzidos em diferentes aminoácidos. SIN addition m., addition-deletion m., deletion m., frame-shift m.
reverse m., m. reversa. SIN back m.
silent m., m. silenciosa; a forma de um traço genético distinguível ao nível do genótipo, mas não ao nível do fenótipo arbitrário (p. ex., clínico, imunológico ou eletroforético).
site specific m., m. sítio-específica; alteração da estrutura de um gene em uma seqüência específica, geralmente referindo-se às alterações produzidas experimentalmente na seqüência genética.
somatic m., m. somática; mutação que ocorre nas células do corpo em geral (em oposição às células germinativas) e, portanto, não são transmitidas à prole.
spontaneous m., m. espontânea; mutação que ocorre naturalmente, e não em virtude da exposição a mutágenos. SIN natural m.
suppressor m., m. supressora; **(1)** mutação secundária que altera o anticódon em um RNAt, de forma que ele possa reconhecer um códon sem sentido, assim suprimindo a terminação da cadeia de aminoácidos. SIN amber m., ochre m., umber m; **(2)** alterações genéticas tais que o efeito de uma mutação em um local pode ser mascarado por uma segunda mutação em outro local. Há dois tipos: supressão intergênica (que ocorre em um gene diferente) e supressão intragênica (que ocorre no mesmo gene, mas em um local diferente). SIN nonsense m.
transition m., m. de transição; mutação pontual que envolve a substituição de um par de base por outro, isto é, a substituição de uma purina por outra e de uma pirimidina por outra pirimidina, sem alteração na orientação purina-pirimidina.
transversion m., m. por transversão; mutação pontual que envolve substituição de base, na qual a orientação da purina e da pirimidina está invertida, ao contrário da mutação de transição.
umber m., m. umbra; mutação que produz o códon de terminação UGA, resultando em terminação prematura de uma cadeia polipeptídica. Cf. supressor m. SIN opal m.
up promoter m., mutação que aumenta a freqüência de início da transcrição.

mute (mūt). Mudo. **1.** Incapaz ou sem vontade de falar. **2.** Pessoa que não é capaz de falar. [L. *mutus*]
mu·tein (mū′tēn). Muteína; termo usado para designar uma proteína que se origina em virtude de uma mutação. [*mut*ation + prot*ein*]
mu·ti·la·tion (mū-ti-lā′shŭn). Mutilação; desfiguramento ou lesão por remoção ou destruição de qualquer parte visível ou essencial do corpo. [L. *mutilatio*, de *mutilo*, pp. *-atus*, mutilar]
mut·ism (mū′tizm). Mutismo. **1.** O estado de ser silencioso. **2.** Ausência orgânica ou funcional da capacidade de falar. [L. *mutus*, mudo]
akinetic m., m. acinético; estado subagudo ou crônico de alteração da consciência no qual o paciente parece estar alerta intermitentemente, mas não reage aos estímulos, embora suas vias motoras descendentes pareçam intactas; devido a lesões de várias estruturas cerebrais. SIN coma vigil.
elective m., m. eletivo; mutismo devido a causas psicogênicas. SIN voluntary m.
voluntary m., m. voluntário. SIN elective m.
mu·ton (mū′ton). Muton; em genética, a menor unidade de um cromossoma na qual a alteração pode ser efetiva na produção de uma mutação (alteração de um único nucleotídeo). [*mut*ation + *-on*]
mu·tu·al·ism (mū′tū-ăl-izm). Mutualismo; relação simbiótica na qual ambas as espécies se beneficiam. Cf. commensalism, metabiosis, parasitism.
mu·tu·al·ist (mū′tū-ăl-ist). Mutualista. SIN symbion. [L. *mutuus*, em retorno, mútuo]
Mv Abreviatura obsoleta de mendelevium (mendelévio).
mV Abreviatura de millivolt (milivolt).
MVV Abreviatura de maximum voluntary *ventilation* (ventilação voluntária máxima).
MW Abreviatura de molecular *weight* (peso molecular, PM).
my·al·gia (mī-al′jē-ă). Mialgia; dor muscular. SIN myodynia. [G. *mys*, músculo, + *algos*, dor]
epidemic m., m. epidêmica. SIN epidemic *pleurodynia*.
m. ther'mica, m. térmica. SIN heat *cramps*, em *cramp*.
my·as·the·nia (mī-as-thē′nē-ă). Miastenia; fraqueza muscular. [G. *mys*, músculo, + *astheneia*, fraqueza]
m. angiosclerot'ica, m. angiosclerótica. SIN intermittent *claudication*.
m. gravis, m. grave; distúrbio da transmissão neuromuscular caracterizado por fraqueza e fadiga variáveis de alguns músculos voluntários, incluindo aqueles inervados por núcleos motores do tronco encefálico; causado por uma redução acentuada do número de receptores da acetilcolina na membrana pós-sináptica da junção neuromuscular, resultante de um mecanismo auto-imune. SIN Goldflam disease.
my·as·then·ic (mī′as-then′ik). Miastênico; relativo à miastenia.
my·a·to·nia, my·at·o·ny (mī-ă-tō′nē-ă, mī-at′ō-nē). Miatonia; extensibilidade anormal de um músculo. [G. *mys*, músculo, + *a* priv. + *tonos*, tônus]

m. congen'ita, m. congênita. SIN *amyotonia* congenita.
my·at·ro·phy (mī-atʹrō-fē). Miatrofia. SIN muscular *atrophy.*
my·ce·lia (mī-sēʹlē-ă). Micélios; plural de mycelium (micélio).
my·ce·li·an (mī-sēʹlē-an). Miceliano; relativo a um micélio.
my·ce·li·oid (mī-sēʹlē-oyd). Micelióide; semelhante a um micélio. [mycelium + G. *eidos,* semelhança]
my·ce·li·um, pl. **my·ce·lia** (mī-sēʹlē-ŭm, -ă). Micélio; a massa de hifas que constituem uma colônia de fungos. [G. *mykēs,* fungo, + *hēlos,* unha, verruga, excrescência em animal ou vegetal]
  aerial m., m. aéreo; a parte do micélio que cresce da superfície do substrato para cima ou para fora, e da qual se desenvolvem esporos propagadores em estruturas características, ou sobre elas, que são distintos para vários grupos genéricos.
  nonseptate m., m. não-septado; micélio sem septos, ou "paredes cruzadas", nas hifas; como estas últimas não estão divididas em numerosas células individuais, o protoplasma multinucleado pode fluir através de estruturas tubulares.
  septate m., m. septado; aquele no qual septos, ou "paredes cruzadas", dividem as hifas em numerosas células uninucleadas ou multinucleadas.
mycet-, myceto-. Micet-, miceto-; fungo. VER TAMBÉM myco-. [G. *mykēs,* fungo]
my·cete (mīʹsēt). Miceto; um fungo. [G. *mykēs,* fungo]
my·ce·tism, my·ce·tis·ʹmus (mīʹsē-tizm, -tizʹmŭs). Micetismo; envenenamento por algumas espécies de cogumelos. SIN muscarinism. [G. *mykēs,* fungo]
  m. cerebraʹlis, m. cerebral; condição caracterizada por sintomas alucinógenos transitórios após a ingestão de cogumelos como *Psilocybe* e *Panaeolus.*
  m. choliforʹmis, m. coliforme; doença grave, algumas vezes fatal, causada pelo consumo de *Amanita phalloides* e outras espécies de cogumelos venenosos.
  m. gastrointestinaʹlis, m. gastrointestinal; tipo relativamente leve de intoxicação por cogumelo, caracterizado por náuseas, vômitos e diarréia, e causado pela ingestão de algumas espécies de *Boletus, Lactarius, Entoloma* e *Lepiota.*
  m. nervoʹsa, m. nervoso; envenenamento por cogumelos que envolve o sistema nervoso e causa desconforto gastrointestinal, após consumo de espécies como *Amanita, Inocybe* e *Clitocybe.*
  m. sanguinaʹreus, m. sanguinário; hemoglobinúria transitória e icterícia causadas pela ingestão do cogumelo *Helvella esculenta,* cru ou cozido.
my·ce·to·ge·net·ic, my·ce·to·gen·ic (mī-sēʹtō-je-netʹik, mīʹsē-tō-;-jenʹik).Micetogenético, micetogênico; causado por fungos. SIN mycetogenous. [G. *mykēs,* fungo, + *gennētos,* gerado]
my·ce·tog·e·nous (mī-sē-tojʹe-nŭs). Micetógeno. SIN mycetogenetic.
my·ce·to·ma (mī-sē-tōʹmă). Micetoma; infecção crônica que envolve o tecido subcutâneo, a pele e o osso contíguo; caracterizado pela formação de lesões localizadas, com tumefações e múltiplos seios de drenagem. O exsudato contém grânulos que podem ser amarelos, brancos, vermelhos, castanhos ou pretos, dependendo do agente causador. O micetoma é causado por dois grupos principais de microrganismos: 1) o actinomicetoma é causado por actinomicetos, incluindo espécies de *Streptomyces, Actinomadurae* e *Nocardia,* 2) o eumicetoma é causado por fungos verdadeiros, incluindo espécies de *Madurella, Exophiala, Pseudallescheria, Curvularia, Neotestudina, Pyrenochaeta, Aspergillus, Leptosphaeria, Plemodomus, Polycytella, Fusarium, Phialophora, Corynespora, Cylindrocarpon, Pseudochaetosphaeronema, Bipolaris* e *Acremonium.* SIN Madura boil, Madura foot, maduromycosis.
myco-. Mico-; fungo. VER TAMBÉM mycet-. [G. *mykēs,* fungo]
my·co·bac·te·ria (mīʹkō-bak-tērʹē-ă). Micobactérias; microrganismos que pertencem ao gênero *Mycobacterium.*
  atypical m., m. atípicas; outras espécies de micobactérias além do *M. tuberculosis* ou *M. bovis,* que podem causar doença em seres humanos imunodeprimidos; esse termo está sendo substituído pela designação MOTT [Mycobacteria Other Than Tuberculosis (Outras Micobactérias Além da *M. tuberculosis*)].
  Runyon group I m., m. do grupo I de Runyon; micobactérias que produzem uma cor amarelo brilhante quando cultivadas na presença de luz. Os microrganismos pertencentes a esse grupo incluem *Mycobacterium kansasii.* SIN photochromogens.
  Runyon group II m., m. do grupo II de Runyon; micobactérias que produzem um pigmento amarelo mesmo quando cultivadas no escuro; quando cultivadas na presença de luz, o pigmento é laranja. Esses microrganismos comportam-se como saprófitas em seres humanos e, geralmente, não são patogênicos para animais de laboratório. SIN scotochromogens.
  Runyon group III m., m. do grupo III de Runyon; micobactérias incolores ou que produzem lentamente um pigmento amarelo claro quando cultivadas na presença de luz. Os microrganismos que pertencem a esse grupo incluem *Mycobacterium avium* e *M. intracellulare.* SIN nonchromogens.
  Runyon group IV m., m. do grupo IV de Runyon; micobactérias que crescem rapidamente e que não produzem pigmento. Os microrganismos desse grupo pertencem a espécies como *Mycobacterium ulcerans* e *M. marinum.*
My·co·bac·te·ri·a·ce·ae (mīʹkō-bak-tēr-e-āʹsē-ē). Família de bactérias aeróbicas (ordem Actinomycetales) contendo células esféricas a bacilares, Gram-positivas. Não há ramificação em condições comuns de cultura. Geralmente são álcool-ácido-resistentes. São encontradas no solo e em laticínios, e como parasitas em seres humanos e outros animais. O gênero típico é o *Mycobacterium.*
my·co·bac·te·ri·o·sis (mīʹkō-bak-tērʹē-ōʹsis). Micobacteriose; infecção por micobactérias.
My·co·bac·te·ri·um (mīʹkō-bak-tērʹē-ŭm). Gênero de bactérias aeróbicas, imóveis (família Mycobacteriaceae) contendo bastonetes retos ou levemente curvos, delgados, álcool-ácido-resistentes, Gram-positivos; algumas vezes, há filamentos delgados, mas raramente são produzidas formas ramificadas. Existem espécies parasitárias e saprófitas. Várias espécies estão associadas a infecções em pessoas imunodeprimidas, principalmente aquelas com AIDS/SIDA. A espécie típica é *M. tuberculosis.* É o gênero típico da família Mycobacteriaceae. [myco- + bacterium]
  M. **abscesʹsus,** SIN *M. chelonae* subsp. *abscessus.*
  M. **aʹvium,** espécie bacteriana causadora de tuberculose em aves domésticas e outras aves. Causa infecções oportunistas em seres humanos.
  M. avium-intracellulare **complex,** complexo *M. avium-intracellulare;* agente oportunista de infecção, sobretudo em pessoas com AIDS/SIDA. O tratamento é difícil porque *M. avium-intracellulare* é resistente a muitos antibióticos. O microrganismo também pode causar infecções respiratórias inferiores crônicas em pacientes sem comprometimento grave, principalmente aqueles com anormalidade subjacente do parênquima pulmonar.
  M. **boʹvis,** espécie bacteriana que é a causa primária de tuberculose no gado bovino; transmissível para seres humanos e outros animais, causando tuberculose. SIN tubercle bacillus (2).
  M. **cheloʹnae,** microrganismo de crescimento rápido (grupo IV de Runyon) que provoca infecção esporádica em qualquer tecido ou sistema de órgãos em seres humanos após cirurgia cardiotorácica, hemodiálise ou diálise peritoneal, mamoplastia ampliadora, artroplastia e imunocomprometimento.
  M. **cheloʹnae** subsp. **abscesʹsus,** espécie bacteriana originalmente encontrada em uma infecção traumática do joelho. SIN *M. abscessus.*
  M. **fortuiʹtum,** espécie bacteriana saprofítica encontrada no solo e em infecções de seres humanos, bois e animais de sangue frio. Causa abscessos cutâneos.
  M. **intracellulaʹre,** espécie bacteriana encontrada em lesões pulmonares e no escarro de seres humanos; pode causar lesões ósseas e da bainha tendínea em coelhos; algumas cepas são patogênicas para camundongos. Recentemente relacionada a infecções oportunistas em seres humanos. SIN Battey bacillus.
  M. **kansasʹii,** espécie bacteriana causadora de doença pulmonar semelhante à tuberculose; foi constatado que causa infecções raras (e geralmente lesões) no líquido espinal, baço, fígado, pâncreas, testículos, articulação do quadril, articulação do joelho, dedo da mão, punho e linfonodos.
  M. **lepʹrae,** espécie bacteriana que causa hanseníase; uma micobactéria intracelular obrigatória que ainda não foi propagada em laboratório, mas que sobreviverá no tatu-galinha (*Dasypus novemcinctus*). SIN Hansen bacillus, leprosy bacillus.
  M. **mariaʹnum,** denominação antiga do *M. scrofulaceum.*
  M. **mariʹnum,** espécie bacteriana que causa tuberculose espontânea em peixes de águas salgadas; também ocorre em outros animais de sangue frio, em alguns aquários e piscinas, nos quais pode causar infecção cutânea humana (ver swimming pool *granuloma*), valas e canais de irrigação e praias oceânicas.
  M. **microʹti,** espécie bacteriana que causa tuberculose generalizada em ratazanas; transmissível para cobaias, coelhos e bezerros, causando infecções localizadas.
  M. **paratuberculoʹsis,** espécie bacteriana que causa a doença de Johne, uma enterite crônica em bois.
  M. **phleʹi,** espécie bacteriana encontrada no solo e na poeira e em vegetais. SIN Moeller grass bacillus.
  M. **scrofulaʹceum,** espécie bacteriana freqüentemente associada a adenite cervical em crianças.
  M. **smegʹmatis,** espécie bacteriana saprofítica encontrada no esmegma da genitália de seres humanos e de muitos animais inferiores; também é encontrada no solo, na poeira e na água.
  M. **tuberculoʹsis,** espécie bacteriana que causa tuberculose em seres humanos; é a espécie típica do gênero *M.* SIN Koch bacillus, tubercle bacillus (1).
  M. **ulʹcerans,** espécie bacteriana que causa úlceras de Buruli em seres humanos; transmissível a partir do solo, geralmente após uma lesão e, possivelmente, por um inseto vetor.
  M. **vaccae,** espécie escotocromogênica, não-patogênica, de crescimento rápido, amplamente distribuída na natureza.
  M. **xenʹopi,** espécie bacteriana encontrada em uma lesão cutânea de um animal de sangue frio, *Xenopus laevis;* causa rara de tuberculose pulmonar humana hospitalar.
my·co·bac·tin (mīʹkō-bakʹtin). Micobactina; fator lipídico complexo descrito como necessário para o crescimento de *Mycobacterium tuberculosis* no plasma humano; parece ser idêntico ao fator lipídico extraído do *M. phlei* e essencial para o crescimento do *M. johnei.*

my·co·cide (mī′kō-sīd). Fungicida. SIN fungicide. [myco- + L. *caedo*, matar]

my·co·der·ma·ti·tis (mī′kō-der-mă-tī-tis). Micodermatite; termo obsoleto para designar uma erupção cutânea de origem micótica (fungo, levedura, bolor).

my·co·gas·tri·tis (mī′kō-gas-trī′tis). Micogastrite; inflamação do estômago decorrente da presença de um fungo. [myco- + G. *gastēr*, estômago, + *-itis*, inflamação]

my·col·ic ac·ids (mī-kol′ik). Ácidos micólicos; ácidos ciclopropanocarboxílicos de cadeia longa (C_{19}–C_{21}), substituídos posteriormente por alcanos de cadeia longa (C_{24}–C_{30}), contendo grupamentos hidroxila livres, encontrados em determinadas bactérias; essas substâncias céreas parecem ser responsáveis pela álcool-ácido-resistência das bactérias que as contêm. SIN mykol.

my·col·o·gist (mī-kol′ō-jist). Micologista; pessoa especializada em micologia.

my·col·o·gy (mī-kol′ō-jē). Micologia; o estudo dos fungos: sua classificação, comestibilidade, cultivo e biologia. [myco- + G. *logos*, estudo]
  medical m., m. médica; o estudo de fungos que produzem doença em seres humanos e outros animais, e das doenças que eles produzem, sua ecologia e sua epidemiologia.

my·co·phage (mī′kō-fāj). Micófago; vírus cujo hospedeiro é um fungo, ao contrário de um bacteriófago, cujo hospedeiro é uma bactéria. VER TAMBÉM mycovirus. [myco- + G. *phagō*, comer]

My·co·plas·ma (mī′kō-plaz′mă). Gênero de bactérias aeróbicas ou anaeróbicas facultativas (família Mycoplasmataceae), que contêm células Gram-negativas sem uma parede celular verdadeira, mas limitadas por uma membrana de três camadas; não revertem a bactérias contendo paredes celulares ou fragmentos de paredes celulares. As unidades reprodutivas mínimas desses microrganismos têm 0,2–0,3 μm de diâmetro. As células são pleomórficas e, em meio líquido, apresentam-se como corpos cocóides, anéis ou filamentos. As colônias da maioria das espécies consistem em um núcleo central, que penetra no meio de cultura, circundado por crescimento periférico superficial; necessitam de esterol para crescer, assim como enriquecimento com soro ou líquido ascítico. Esses microrganismos são encontrados em seres humanos e em outros animais e podem ser patogênicos. A espécie típica é *M. mycoides*. SIN Asterococcus. [myco- + G. *plasma*, algo formado (plasma)]
  M. bucca′le, espécie que é um parasita pouco freqüente, habitante da orofaringe humana; é o micoplasma predominante na orofaringe de primatas não-humanos.
  M. fau′cium, espécie bacteriana que é um membro raro da flora normal da orofaringe humana; é encontrada ocasionalmente na orofaringe de primatas não-humanos.
  M. fermen′tans, espécie bacteriana encontrada em lesões genitais ulcerativas associadas a bactérias fusiformes e espirilos, sendo também encontrada na mucosa genital aparentemente normal de seres humanos.
  M. genita′lium, espécie bacteriana que pode causar uretrite; exibe reação cruzada imunológica com *M. pneumoniae*; pode causar infecções graves envolvendo as vias respiratórias, o coração, a corrente sanguínea, o sistema nervoso central e próteses valvares e articulares.
  M. hom′inis, espécie bacteriana que é o agente causal da doença inflamatória pélvica e de outras infecções genitourinárias; também pode causar corioamnionite e febre pós-parto; pode ser um comensal orofaríngeo e já causou infecções de feridas hospitalares.
  M. laidla′wii, SIN Acholeplasma laidlawii.
  M. ora′le, espécie bacteriana de *M.* associada às cavidades bucal e faríngea de seres humanos e animais.
  M. pharyn′gis, espécie bacteriana encontrada como comensal na orofaringe humana.
  M. pneumo′niae, espécie bacteriana causadora de otite e de doença das vias respiratórias superiores e inferiores, incluindo pneumonia atípica primária em seres humanos. SIN Eaton agent.
  M. saliva′rium, espécie bacteriana encontrada na faringe humana.

my·co·plas·ma, pl. **my·co·plas·ma·ta** (mī′kō-plaz′mă, -plaz′mah-tă). Micoplasma; termo usado apenas para se referir a qualquer membro do gênero *Mycoplasma*.

My·co·plas·ma·ta·les (mī′kō-plaz′mă-tā′lēz). Ordem de bactérias Gram-negativas contendo células limitadas por uma membrana de três camadas, mas que não possuem uma parede celular verdadeira. As unidades reprodutivas mínimas apresentam 0,2 a 0,3 μm de diâmetro. Existem espécies patogênicas e saprofíticas. Esses microrganismos reproduzem-se através da quebra de filamentos ramificados em cocóides, corpúsculos elementares filtráveis. A ordem inclui os denominados microrganismos semelhantes aos da pleuropneumonia (pleuropneumonia-like *organisms*, em *organism*) (PPLO).

my·co·pus (mī′kō-pūs). Mucopus. SIN mucopus.

my·cose (mī′kōs). Trealose. SIN trehalose.

my·co·sis, pl. **my·co·ses** (mī-kō′sis, -sēz). Micose; qualquer doença causada por um fungo (filamentoso ou leveduriforme). [myco- + G. *-osis*, condição]
  m. framboesioi′des, framboesia tropical; bouba. SIN yaws.

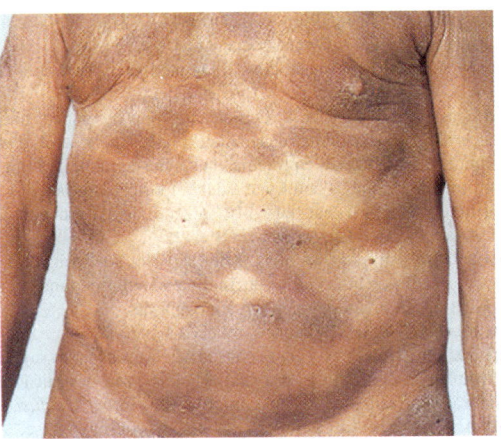

micose fungóide

  m. fungoi′des, m. fungóide; linfoma progressivo crônico, originado na pele, que, inicialmente, simula o eczema ou outras dermatoses inflamatórias; o aspecto das placas está associado a acantose e infiltração em faixa da derme superior por um infiltrado pleomórfico, incluindo linfócitos T auxiliares com grandes núcleos convolutos que também se acumulam em espaços claros na epiderme inferior (microabscessos de Pautrier); em casos avançados, pode haver tumores ulcerados e infiltração dos linfonodos.
  m. intestina′lis, m. intestinal; forma gastrointestinal de antraz, cujos sinais e sintomas são aqueles de gastroenterite seguidos por toxemia e depressão geral.

my·co·stat·ic (mī-kō-stat′ik). Micostático. SIN fungistatic.

my·cos·ter·ols (mī-kos′ter-olz). Micosteróis; esteróides obtidos de fungos.

my·cot·ic (mī-kot′ik). Micótico; relativo a, ou causado por, fungos.

my·co·tox·i·co·sis (mī′kō-tok-si-kō′sis). Micotoxicose; intoxicação causada pela ingestão de substâncias pré-formadas produzidas pela ação de alguns fungos sobre determinados alimentos ou ingestão dos próprios fungos; p. ex., ergotismo. [myco- + G. *toxikon*, veneno, + *-osis*, condição]

my·co·tox·in (mī′kō-tok-sinz). Micotoxina; toxina produzida por alguns fungos; algumas são usadas para fins medicinais; p. ex., muscarina, psilocibina.

my·co·vi·rus (mī′kō-vī-rŭs). Micovírus; vírus que infecta fungos.

my·da·le·ine (mī-dā′lē-ēn). Midaleína; ptomaína venenosa formada no fígado e em outras vísceras em putrefação; atua especificamente sobre o coração, causando parada de sua atividade em diástole. [G. *mydaleos*, mofado, de *mydos*, umidade]

my·da·tox·in (mī-dă-tok′sin). Midatoxina; ptomaína de vísceras e carne em putrefação. [G. *mydos*, umidade, decaimento, + *toxikon*, veneno]

my·dri·a·sis (mi-drī′ă-sis). Midríase; dilatação da pupila. [G.]
  alternating m., m. alternante; midríase que afeta alternadamente cada olho.
  amaurotic m., m. amaurótica; alargamento moderado de ambas as pupilas resultante do comprometimento da entrada visual em um ou em ambos os olhos.
  paralytic m., m. paralítica; dilatação pupilar causada por paralisia do músculo esfíncter da pupila induzida por agentes anticolinérgicos administrados topica ou sistemicamente, ou resultante de lesões do núcleo ou nervo oculomotor, contusão do bulbo do olho ou glaucoma.
  spastic m., m. espástica; dilatação pupilar devida à contração do músculo dilatador da pupila induzida por agentes adrenérgicos ou por estimulação da via simpática.

myd·ri·at·ic (mi-drē-at′ik). Midriático. **1.** Que causa midríase ou dilatação da pupila. **2.** Um agente que dilata a pupila.

my·ec·to·my (mī-ek′tō-mē). Miectomia; excisão de parte de um músculo. [G. *mys*, músculo, + *ektomē*, excisão]

my·ec·to·py, my·ec·to·pia (mī-ek′tō-pē, mī-ek-tō′pē-ă). Miectopia; termo raramente usado para designar o deslocamento de um músculo. [G. *mys*, músculo, + *ektopos*, fora de lugar]

myel-, myelo-. Miel-, mielo-. **1.** A medula óssea. **2.** A medula espinal e o bulbo. Cf. medullo-. **3.** A bainha de mielina das fibras nervosas. [G. *myelos*, medula, medula óssea]

my·el·ap·o·plexy (mī′el-ap′ō-plek′sē). Mielapoplexia. SIN hematomyelia. [myel- + G. *apoplexia*, apoplexia]

my·el·a·te·lia (mī′el-ă-tē′lē-ă). Mielatelia; defeito do desenvolvimento da medula espinal. [myel- + G. *ateleia*, incompleto]

my·el·auxe (mī-el-awk′sē). Mielauxe; hipertrofia da medula espinal. [myel- + G. *auxē*, aumento]

my·e·le·mia (mī-ĕ-lē′mē-ă). Mielemia; termo raramente usado para mielocitose. [myel- + G. *haima*, sangue]

myelencephalon (mī′el-en-sef′ă-lon) [TA]. Mielencéfalo. SIN *medulla oblongata*. [myel- + G. *enkephalos*, encéfalo]

myelic (mī-el′ik). Miélico; relativo à (1) medula espinal ou à (2) medula óssea.

myelin (mī′ĕ-lin). Mielina. **1.** O material lipoproteináceo, composto de membranas alternadas regulares de lamelas lipídicas (colesterol, fosfolipídios, esfingolipídios, fosfatidatos) e proteína, da bainha de mielina. **2.** Gotículas de lipídios formadas durante a autólise e a decomposição *postmortem*.

myelinated (mī′ĕ-li-nāt-ed). Mielinizado; que possui uma bainha de mielina. SIN medullated (2).

myelination (mī′ĕ-li-nā′shŭn). Mielinização; a aquisição, desenvolvimento ou formação de uma bainha de mielina ao redor de uma fibra nervosa. SIN medullation (2), myelinization, myelinogenesis.

myelinic (mī′ĕ-lin′ik). Mielínico; relativo à mielina.

myelinization (mī′ĕ-li-nī-zā′shŭn). Mielinização. SIN *myelination*.

myelinoclasis (mī′ĕ-li-nok′lă-sis). Mielinoclasia; destruição da mielina. VER TAMBÉM demyelination, dysmyelination. [myelin- + G. *klasis*, quebra]

myelinogenesis (mī′ĕ-lin-ō-jen′ĕ-sis). Mielinogênese. SIN *myelination*. [myelin- + G. *genesis*, produção]

myelinolysis (mī′ĕ-li-nol′i-sis). Mielinólise; dissolução das bainhas de mielina das fibras nervosas. [myelin- + G. *lysis*, dissolução]

    central pontine m., m. pontina central; perda localizada de mielina na metade da base da ponte; relacionada à desnutrição e, freqüentemente, ao alcoolismo.

myelinopathy (mī′ĕ-lin-op′ă-thē). Mielinopatia; distúrbio que afeta a mielina das fibras nervosas periféricas, ao contrário daquele que afeta axônios (axonopatia).

myelitic (mī-ĕ-lit′ik). Mielítico; relativo a, ou afetado por, mielite.

myelitis (mī-ĕ-lī′tis). Mielite. **1.** Inflamação da medula espinal. **2.** Inflamação da medula óssea. [myel- + G. *-itis*, inflamação]

    acute necrotizing m., m. necrotizante aguda; distúrbio da medula espinal, provavelmente uma doença desmielinizante, que afeta pessoas de todas as idades e de ambos os sexos. Apresenta início abrupto ou mais gradual, com anormalidades sensoriais e fraqueza referente ao neurônio motor superior; logo sobrevém uma paralisia motora flácida reflexa e paralisia do esfíncter, que é permanente. Em alguns, mas não em todos os casos, há neurite óptica bilateral ou unilateral associada. No líquido cerebroespinal, há aumento do nível de proteínas, e são encontradas células mononucleares. À necropsia, a lesão foi identificada como sendo uma leucomielite hemorrágica necrotizante.

    acute transverse m., m. transversa aguda; inflamação aguda e amolecimento da medula espinal; envolve toda a espessura da medula espinal, mas sua extensão longitudinal é limitada; múltiplas etiologias.

    ascending m., m. ascendente; inflamação progressiva envolvendo áreas sucessivamente mais altas da medula espinal.

    bulbar m., m. bulbar; inflamação do bulbo.

    concussion m., m. por concussão; mielopatia traumática.

    demyelinated m., m. desmielinizada; esclerose múltipla aguda que se apresenta como mielite.

    Foix-Alajouanine m., m. de Foix-Alajouanine. SIN subacute necrotizing m.

    funicular m., m. funicular; **(1)** inflamação que envolve qualquer uma das colunas da medula espinal; **(2)** SIN subacute combined *degeneration* of the spinal cord.

    postinfectious m., m. pós-infecciosa; inflamação da medula espinal que sucede de uma infecção viral, geralmente exantemática.

    postvaccinal m., m. pós-vacinação; inflamação da medula espinal que sucede a vacinação.

    radiation m., m. por radiação. SIN radiation *myelopathy*.

    subacute necrotizing m., m. necrotizante aguda; distúrbio da parte inferior da medula espinal, em homens adultos, que resulta em paraplegia progressiva. SIN angiodysgenetic myelomalacia, Foix-Alajouanine m.

    systemic m., m. sistêmica; inflamação limitada a tratos especiais da medula espinal.

    transverse m., m. transversa; processo inflamatório que envolve as substâncias cinzenta e branca da medula espinal.

△ **myelo-.** VER myel-.

myeloarchitectonics (mī′ĕ-lō-ar′ki-tek-ton′iks). Mieloarquitetônico; o padrão de fibras nervosas mielinizadas no encéfalo, diferente do citoarquitetônico.

myeloblast (mī′ĕ-lō-blast). Mieloblasto; uma célula imatura (10 a 18 μm de diâmetro) da série granulocítica, que ocorre normalmente na medula óssea, mas não no sangue circulante (exceto em algumas doenças). Quando corado pelos métodos habituais, o citoplasma é azul claro, não-granular, e sua quantidade é variável, algumas vezes sendo apenas uma fina orla ao redor do núcleo; este último é azul-púrpura escuro, com cromatina filiforme, pontilhada, finamente dividida, um pouco condensada na periferia. Alguns nucléolos azul-claros geralmente estão presentes no núcleo, e costumam desaparecer à medida que o m. amadurece e transforma-se em pró-mielócito e, depois, em mielócito. Comumente, os m. produzem uma reação negativa com a peroxidase. [myelo- + G. *blastos*, germe]

myeloblastemia (mī′ĕ-lō-blas-tē′mē-ă). Mieloblastemia; a presença de mieloblastos no sangue circulante. [myeloblast + G. *haima*, sangue]

myeloblastoma (mī′ĕ-lō-blas-tō′mă). Mieloblastoma; foco nodular ou acúmulo razoavelmente bem circunscrito de mieloblastos, como se observa algumas vezes na leucemia mieloblástica aguda e na clorose. [myeloblast + G. *-oma*, tumor]

myeloblastosis (mī′ĕ-lō-blas-tō′sis). Mieloblastose; a presença de um número incomumente grande de mieloblastos no sangue circulante e/ou tecidos (como na leucemia aguda).

myelocele (mī′ĕ-lō-sēl). Mielocele. **1.** Protrusão da medula espinal na espinha bífida. [myelo- + G. *kēlē*, hérnia] **2.** O canal central da medula espinal. [G. *myelos*, medula óssea, + *koilia*, cavidade]

myelocyst (mī′ĕ-lō-sist). Mielocisto; qualquer cisto (geralmente revestido por células colunares ou cúbicas) que se desenvolve a partir de um canal central rudimentar no sistema nervoso central. [myelo- + G. *kystis*, bexiga]

myelocystic (mī′ĕ-lō-sist′ik). Mielocístico; relativo a, ou caracterizado pela presença de, um mielocisto.

myelocystocele (mī′ĕ-lō-sis′tō-sēl). Mielocistocele; espinha bífida contendo substância da medula espinal. [myelo- + G. *kystis*, bexiga, + *kēlē*, tumor]

myelocystomeningocele (mī′ĕ-lō-sis′tō-mĕ-ning′gō-sēl). Mielocistomeningocele. SIN *meningomyelocele*. [myelo- + G. *kystis*, bexiga, + *mēninx* (*mēning-*), membrana, + *kēlē*, hérnia]

ℹ **myelocyte** (mī′ĕ-lō-sīt). Mielócito. **1.** Célula jovem da série granulocítica que ocorre normalmente na medula óssea, mas não no sangue circulante (exceto em algumas doenças). Quando corado com os corantes habituais, o citoplasma é distintamente basófilo e relativamente mais abundante que em mieloblastos ou pró-mielócitos, embora os mielócitos sejam células menores; há numerosos grânulos citoplasmáticos (isto é, neutrofílicos, eosinofílicos ou basofílicos) nas formas mais maduras de mielócitos, e os dois primeiros tipos são peroxidase-positivos. A cromatina nuclear é mais grosseira que a observada em mieloblastos, mas é relativamente pouco corada e não possui uma membrana bem definida; o núcleo tem contorno razoavelmente regular (isto é, não entalhado) e parece estar "sepultado" sob os numerosos grânulos citoplasmáticos. **2.** Uma célula nervosa da substância cinzenta do encéfalo ou da medula espinal. SIN medullocell. [myelo- + G. *kytos*, célula]

    m. A, m. A; a forma mais jovem de mielócito, caracterizada por apenas alguns (não mais de 10) grânulos citoplasmáticos, demonstrados de forma mais fidedigna por meio de coloração com vermelho neutro; as mitocôndrias são numerosas e assemelham-se às do mieloblasto.

    m. B, m. B; a forma intermediária de mielócito, caracterizada por aproximadamente 30–100 (ou mais) grânulos citoplasmáticos dispersos entre as mitocôndrias; as mitocôndrias são menos numerosas que nos mielócitos do estágio A e, freqüentemente, são deslocadas em direção à periferia da célula.

    m. C, m. C; o mais maduro dos mielócitos, caracterizado por numerosos grânulos citoplasmáticos, reconhecíveis como neutrofílicos, eosinofílicos e basofílicos; com vermelho neutro, coram-se, respectivamente, de vermelho, amarelo brilhante e marrom forte; os mielócitos C freqüentemente são maiores que as formas anteriores; se o núcleo estiver entalhado, o mielócito está amadurecendo para metamielócito.

myelocythemia (mī′ĕ-lō-sī-thē′mē-ă). Mielocitemia; a presença de mielócitos no sangue circulante, principalmente em número persistentemente alto (como na leucemia mielocítica). [myelocyte + G. *haima*, sangue]

myelocytic (mī′ĕ-lō-sit′ik). Mielocítico; relativo a, ou caracterizado por, mielócitos.

myelocytoma (mī′ĕ-lō-sī-tō′mă). Mielocitoma; foco nodular ou acúmulo relativamente denso de mielócitos, razoavelmente bem circunscrito, como em determinados tecidos de pessoas com leucemia mielocítica. [myelocyte + G. *-oma*, tumor]

myelocytomatosis (mī′ĕ-lō-sī′tō-mă-tō′sis). Mielocitomatose; forma de tumor que envolve principalmente os mielócitos.

myelocytosis (mī′ĕ-lō-sī-tō′sis). Mielocitose; a ocorrência de um número anormalmente grande de mielócitos no sangue circulante e/ou nos tecidos. [myelocyte + G. *-osis*, condição]

myelodiastasis (mī′ĕ-lō-dī-as′tă-sis). Mielodiástase; amolecimento e destruição da medula espinal. [myelo + G. *diastasis*, separação]

myelodysplasia (mī′ĕ-lō-dis-plā′zē-ă). Mielodisplasia. **1.** Anormalidade do desenvolvimento da medula espinal, principalmente a parte inferior da medula. **2.** Termo impreciso para espinha bífida oculta. [myelo- + G. *dys-*, difícil, + *plasis*, moldagem]

myelofibrosis (mī′ĕ-lō-fi-brō′sis). Mielofibrose; fibrose da medula óssea, particularmente generalizada, associada a metaplasia mielóide do baço e de outros órgãos, anemia leucoeritroblástica e trombocitopenia, embora a medula óssea freqüentemente contenha muitos megacariócitos. SIN myelosclerosis, osteomyelofibrotic syndrome.

myelogenesis (mī′ĕ-lō-jen′ĕ-sis). Mielogênese. **1.** Desenvolvimento de medula óssea. **2.** Desenvolvimento do sistema nervoso central. **3.** Formação de mielina ao redor de um axônio.

my·e·lo·ge·net·ic, my·e·lo·gen·ic (mī'ĕ-lō-jĕ-net'ik, -jen'ik). Mielogênico. **1.** Relativo à mielogênese. **2.** Produzido pela, ou que se origina na, medula óssea. SIN myelogenous.

my·e·log·e·nous (mī-ĕ-loj'ĕ-nŭs). Mielógeno. SIN myelogenetic (2).

my·e·lo·gone, my·e·lo·go·ni·um (mī'ĕ-lō-gōn, mī'ĕ-lo-gō'nē-ŭm). Mielogônio; leucócito imaturo da série mielóide, caracterizado por um núcleo relativamente grande, corado de forma razoavelmente intensa, finamente reticulado, que contém nucléolos pálidos e uma pequena quantidade de citoplasma não-granular, moderadamente basófilo, semelhante a uma orla. É difícil distinguir os mielogônios dos linfoblastos e monoblastos, exceto se forem avaliados em relação às formas mais maduras geralmente associadas às células mais jovens. [myelo- + G. *gonē*, semente]

my·e·lo·gram (mī'ĕ-lō-gram). Mielograma; radiografia contrastada do espaço subaracnóide espinal e seu conteúdo.

   cervical m., m. cervical; contraste introduzido diretamente no espaço subaracnóide cervical, ou deslocado da região lombar com a ajuda da gravidade, para delinear a medula cervical e as raízes dos nervos.

   lumbar m., m. lombar; estudo mais comum na hérnia do núcleo pulposo ou na protrusão do disco intervertebral.

my·e·log·ra·phy (mī'ĕ-log'ră-fē). Mielografia; radiografia da medula espinal e das raízes nervosas após a injeção de um contraste no espaço subaracnóide espinal. [myelo- + G. *graphē*, desenho]

my·e·lo·ic (mī-ĕ-lō'ik). Mielóico; relativo ao tecido e às células precursoras das quais são derivados os neutrófilos, eosinófilos e basófilos.

my·e·loid (mī'ĕ-loyd). Mielóide. **1.** Relativo a, derivado de, ou que apresenta algumas características da medula óssea. **2.** Algumas vezes usado em relação à medula espinal. **3.** Relativo a algumas características de formas mielocíticas, mas que não indicam necessariamente a origem na medula óssea. [myel- + oid]

my·e·loi·do·sis (mī'ĕ-loy-dō'sis). Mieloidose; hiperplasia geral do tecido mielóide.

myelokathexis. Mielocatexia. SIN kathexis.

my·e·lo·leu·ke·mia (mī'ĕ-lō-loo-kē'mē-ă). Mieloleucemia; forma de leucemia na qual as células anormais são derivadas do tecido mielopoético.

my·e·lo·li·po·ma (mī'ĕ-lō-li-pō'mă). Mielolipoma; acúmulos nodulares de células derivadas da proliferação localizada de tecido reticuloendotelial nos seios sanguíneos das glândulas supra-renais; macroscopicamente, os nódulos podem parecer tecido adiposo, mas, na verdade, são focos de medula óssea contendo células eritropoéticas ou mielóides.

my·e·lo·lym·pho·cyte (mī'ĕ-lō-lim'fō-sīt). Mielolinfócito; designação obsoleta de uma forma anormal da série linfocítica na medula óssea, presumidamente formada nesse tecido.

my·e·lol·y·sis (mī-ĕ-lol'i-sis). Mielólise; decomposição da mielina.

my·e·lo·ma (mī-ĕ-lō'mă). Mieloma. **1.** Tumor composto de células derivadas dos tecidos hemopoéticos da medula óssea. **2.** Tumor de plasmócitos. [myelo- + G. *-oma*, tumor]

   Bence Jones m., m. de Bence Jones; um tipo de m. múltiplo no qual os plasmócitos malignos excretam apenas cadeias leves de um tipo (κ ou λ); ocorrem lesões ósseas líticas em cerca de 60% dos casos, e são encontradas cadeias leves (proteína de Bence-Jones) na urina; a amiloidose e a insuficiência renal grave são mais comuns que no m. múltiplo. SIN L-chain disease, L-chain m.

   endothelial m., m. endotelial. SIN Ewing *tumor.*

   giant cell m., m. de células gigantes. SIN giant cell *tumor* of bone.

   L-chain m., m. da cadeia L. SIN Bence Jones m.

   multiple m., m. mul'tiplex, m. múltiplo; doença incomum, ocorrendo mais amiúde em homens que em mulheres; associada a anemia, hemorragia, infecções recorrentes e fraqueza. Comumente, é considerada uma neoplasia maligna que se origina na medula óssea e envolve principalmente o esqueleto, com características clínicas atribuíveis aos locais de envolvimento e às anormalidades na formação da proteína plasmática; caracterizado por muitos focos difusos ou acúmulos nodulares de plasmócitos anormais ou malignos na medula óssea de vários ossos (principalmente o crânio), causando tumefações palpáveis dos ossos e, ocasionalmente, em locais extra-ósseos; radiologicamente, as lesões ósseas apresentam aspecto em saca-bocado característico. As células do mieloma produzem proteínas anormais no soro e na urina; aquelas formadas em qualquer exemplo de mieloma múltiplo são diferentes das outras proteínas do mieloma, bem como das proteínas séricas normais, sendo as anormalidades mais freqüentes no metabolismo das proteínas: 1) a ocorrência de proteinúria de Bence Jones, 2) um grande aumento da γ-globulina monoclonal no plasma, 3) a formação ocasional de crioglobulina e 4) uma forma de amiloidose primária. A proteína de Bence Jones não é um derivado da proteína sérica anormal, mas parece ser formada *de novo* a partir dos aminoácidos precursores. VER TAMBÉM plasma cell m. SIN multiple myelomatosis, myelomatosis multiplex, plasma cell m. (1).

   nonsecretory m., m. não-secretor; um tipo de m. múltiplo em que não há paraproteinemia ou paraproteinúria detectável.

   plasma cell m., m. de plasmócitos; **(1)** SIN multiple m.; **(2)** plasmacitoma do osso, que geralmente é uma lesão solitária e não associada à ocorrência de proteína de Bence Jones ou outros distúrbios no metabolismo da proteína (observado no mieloma múltiplo). Alguns observadores enfatizam que a lesão solitária provavelmente representa uma fase inicial do m. múltiplo clássico, ou um exemplo deste último no qual é reconhecido apenas um foco.

my·e·lo·ma·la·cia (mī'ĕ-lō-ma-lā'shē-ă). Mielomalacia; amolecimento da medula espinal. [myelo- + G. *malakia*, amolecimento]

   angiodysgenetic m., m. angiodisgenética. SIN subacute necrotizing *myelitis.*

my·e·lo·ma·to·sis (mī'ĕ-lō-ma-tō'sis). Mielomatose; doença caracterizada pela ocorrência de mieloma em vários locais.

   multiple m., m. mul'tiplex, m. múltipla. SIN multiple *myeloma.*

my·e·lo·me·ning·o·cele (mī'ĕ-lō-mĕ-ning'gō-sēl). Mielomeningocele. SIN meningomyelocele. [myelo- + G. *mēninx*, membrana, + *kēlē*, hérnia]

my·e·lo·mere (mī'ĕ-lō-mēr). Mielômero; neurômero do encéfalo ou da medula espinal. [myelo- + G. *meros*, parte]

my·e·lo·mono·cyte (mī'ĕ-lō-mon'ō-sīt). Mielomonócito; leucócito que parece assemelhar-se aos mielócitos e monócitos porque a cromatina nuclear é menos condensada que no mielócito e o citoplasma tem poucos grânulos neutrofílicos; essas células representam maturação aberrante, como ocorre na leucemia mielomonocítica.

my·e·lo·neu·ri·tis (mī'ĕ-lō-noo-rī'tis). Mieloneurite. SIN neuromyelitis.

my·e·lon·ic (mī-ĕ-lon'ik). Mielônico; relativo à medula espinal. [G. *myelon*, de *myelos*, medula óssea]

my·e·lo·pa·ral·y·sis (mī'ĕ-lō-pă-ral'i-sis). Mieloparalisia. SIN spinal *paralysis.*

my·e·lo·path·ic (mī'ĕ-lō-path'ik). Mielopático; relativo à mielopatia.

my·e·lop·a·thy (mī-ĕ-lop'ă-thē). Mielopatia. **1.** Distúrbio da medula espinal. **2.** Uma doença dos tecidos mielopoéticos. [myelo- + G. *pathos*, que sofre]

   carcinomatous m., m. carcinomatosa; degeneração ou necrose da medula espinal associada a um carcinoma. SIN paracarcinomatous m.

   compressive m., m. compressiva; destruição do tecido da medula espinal causada por pressão de neoplasias, hematomas ou outras massas.

   diabetic m., m. diabética; alterações degenerativas do tecido da medula espinal que ocorrem como uma complicação do diabetes melito.

   paracarcinomatous m., m. paracarcinomatosa. SIN carcinomatous m.

   radiation m., m. por radiação; lesão da medula espinal por exposição a raios X ou a outro tipo de radiação de alta energia; geralmente mielite por radiação. SIN radiation myelitis.

my·e·lo·per·ox·i·dase (mī'el-ō-per-oks'i-dās). Mieloperoxidase; uma peroxidase de ocorrência em células fagocíticas que conseguem oxidar íons halogênio (p. ex., I⁻) em halogênio livre; a deficiência autossômica recessiva de mieloperoxidase leva a comprometimento da destruição bacteriana.

my·e·lop·e·tal (mī-ĕ-lop'ĕ-tăl). Mielópeto; que prossegue em direção à medula espinal; diz-se de diferentes impulsos nervosos. [myelo- + L. *peto*, buscar]

my·e·lo·phthis·ic (mī'ĕ-lō-tiz'ik, -thiz'ik). Mielotísico; relativo a, ou que sofre de, mielotísica.

my·e·loph·thi·sis (mī'ĕ-lof'thi-sis, mī'ĕ-lō-tī'sis, -tē'sis). Mielotísica. **1.** Definhamento ou atrofia da medula espinal como no tabes dorsal. **2.** Substituição de tecido hemopoético na medula óssea por tecido anormal, geralmente tecido fibroso ou tumores malignos que são, na maioria das vezes, carcinomas metastáticos. SIN panmyelophthisis. [myelo- + G. *phthisis*, desgaste]

my·e·lo·plast (mī'ĕ-lō-plast). Mieloplasto; qualquer uma das séries leucocitárias na medula óssea, principalmente formas jovens. [myelo- + G. *plastos*, formado]

my·e·lo·ple·gia (mī'ĕ-lō-plē'jē-ă). Mieloplegia. SIN spinal *paralysis.* [myelo- + G. *plēgē*, ataque]

my·e·lo·poi·e·sis (mī'ĕ-lō-poy-ē'sis). Mielopoese; formação dos elementos teciduais da medula óssea, ou qualquer um dos tipos de células sanguíneas derivados da medula óssea; ou ambos os processos. [myelo- + G. *poiēsis*, formado]

my·e·lo·poi·et·ic (mī'ĕ-lō-poy-et'ik). Mielopoético; relativo à mielopoese.

my·e·lo·pro·lif·er·a·tive (mī'ĕ-lō-prō-lif'er-ă-tiv). Mieloproliferativo; relativo a, ou caracterizado por, proliferação incomum de tecido mielopoético.

my·e·lo·ra·dic·u·li·tis (mī'ĕ-lō-ra-dik-ū-lī'tis). Mielorradiculite; inflamação da medula espinal e das raízes nervosas. [myelo- + L. *radicula*, raiz, + G. *-itis*, inflamação]

my·e·lo·ra·dic·u·lo·dys·pla·sia (mī'ĕ-lō-ra-dik'ū-lō-dis-plā-zē-ă). Mielorradiculodisplasia; deficiência congênita do desenvolvimento da medula espinal e das raízes dos nervos espinais. [myelo- + L. *radicula*, raiz, + dysplasia]

my·e·lo·ra·dic·u·lop·a·thy (mī'ĕ-lō-ră-dik'ū-lop'ă-thē). Mielorradiculopatia; doença que envolve a medula espinal e as raízes nervosas. SIN radiculomyelopathy. [myelo- + L. *radicula*, raiz, + G. *pathos*, doença]

my·e·lo·ra·dic·u·lo·pol·y·neu·ron·i·tis (mī'ĕ-lō-ra-dik'ū-lō-pol'ē-noo-ron-ī'tis). Mielorradiculopolineurite. SIN Guillain-Barré *syndrome.*

my·e·lor·rha·gia (mī'ĕ-lō-rā'jē-ă). Mielorragia. SIN hematomyelia. [myelo- + G. *rhēgnymi*, eclodir]

myelorrhaphy (mī-ē-lōr′a-fē). Mielorrafia; sutura de uma ferida da medula espinal. [myelo- + G. *rhaphē*, sutura]

myeloschisis (mī-ē-los′ki-sis). Mielosquise; fenda na medula espinal resultante da falha do fechamento normal das pregas neurais na formação do tubo neural; inevitavelmente a espinha bífida é uma seqüela. [myelo- + G. *schisis*, clivagem]

myelosclerosis (mī′ē-lō-skle-rō′sis). Mielosclerose. SIN myelofibrosis. [myelo- + G. *sklērōsis*, endurecimento]

myelosis (mī-ē-lō′sis). Mielose. **1.** Condição caracterizada por proliferação anormal de tecido ou de elementos celulares da medula óssea, p. ex., mieloma múltiplo, leucemia mielocítica, mielofibrose. **2.** Uma condição em que há proliferação anormal do tecido medular na medula espinal, como em um glioma.
 aleukemic m., m. aleucêmica; m. sem elementos celulares anormais no sangue periférico.
 chronic nonleukemic m., m. não-leucêmica crônica; condição na qual há proliferação anormal de tecido leucopoético que resulta em leucócitos imaturos no sangue circulante, mas a contagem total está dentro da faixa normal.
 erythremic m., m. eritrêmica; processo neoplásico que envolve o tecido eritropoético, caracterizado por anemia, febre irregular, esplenomegalia, hepatomegalia, distúrbios hemorrágicos e numerosos eritroblastos em todos os estágios de maturação (com um número desproporcionalmente grande de formas menos maduras) no sangue circulante; estudos *postmortem* revelam eritroblastos primitivos e células reticuloendoteliais, não apenas em órgãos hemopoéticos, mas também nos rins, glândulas supra-renais e outros locais. São reconhecidas formas agudas e crônicas, mas, nestas últimas, há menor proeminência das células imaturas; a primeira também é denominada doença de Di Guglielmo e eritremia aguda.
 funicular m., m. funicular; degeneração da substância branca da medula espinal.
 leukemic m., m. leucêmica; (**1**) SIN granulocytic *leukemia*; (**2**) SIN myeloblastic *leukemia*.
 leukopenic m., **subleukemic m.**, m. leucopênica, m. subleucêmica. SIN subleukemic *leukemia*.

myelospongium (mī′ē-lō-spŭn′jē-ŭm). Mielospôngio; a rede fibrocelular na medula espinal do embrião, a partir da qual se desenvolve a neuróglia. [myelo- + G. *spongos*, esponja]

myelosyphilis (mī′e-lō-sif′i-lis). Mielossífilis. SIN tabetic *neurosyphilis*.

myelotome (mī′e-lō-tōm). Mielótomo; instrumento usado para fazer cortes seriados da medula espinal ou para realizar a incisão da medula espinal. [myelo- + G. *tomos*, que corta]

myelotomography (mī′e-lō-tō-mog′ra-fē). Mielotomografia; tomografia do espaço subaracnóide espinal opacificado com contrastes; um procedimento obsoleto.

myelotomy (mī-e-lot′o-mē). Mielotomia; incisão da medula espinal. [myelo- + G. *tomē*, incisão]
 Bischof m., m. de Bischof; incisão longitudinal da medula espinal através da coluna lateral para tratamento da espasticidade dos membros inferiores.
 commissural m., m. comissural. SIN midline m.
 midline m., m. na linha média; secção das fibras transversais medianas da medula espinal para alívio de dor intratável. SIN commissural m., commissurotomy (2).
 T m., m. em T; mielotomia mediana com cortes laterais nos cornos anteriores.

myelotoxic (mī′e-lō-tok′sik). Mielotóxico. **1.** Inibidor, depressor ou destrutivo para um ou mais componentes da medula óssea. **2.** Relativo a, derivado de, ou que manifesta as características da medula óssea acometida.

myenteric (mī-en-ter′ik). Mientérico; relativo ao mienteron.

myenteron (mī-en′ter-on). Mienteron; a túnica muscular do intestino. [G. *mys*, músculo, + *enteron*, intestino]

myesthesia (mī-es-thē′zē-a). Miestesia. SIN kinesthetic *sense*. [G. *mys*, músculo, + *aisthēsis*, sensação]

myiasis (mī-ī′a-sis). Miíase; qualquer infecção causada por invasão dos tecidos ou cavidades do corpo por larvas de insetos dípteros. [G. *myia*, mosca]
 accidental m., m. acidental; m. gastrointestinal por ingestão de alimento contaminado.
 African furuncular m., m. furuncular africana. SIN cordylobiasis.
 aural m., m. da orelha; invasão da orelha externa, média ou interna por larvas de insetos dípteros.
 human botfly m., dermatobíase. SIN dermatobiasis.
 intestinal m., m. intestinal; presença de larvas de determinados insetos dípteros no trato gastrointestinal, como de *Musca domestica* (mosca doméstica), o ácaro do queijo e *Fannia canicularis* (mosca doméstica menor).
 nasal m., m. nasal; invasão das vias nasais por larvas de moscas, causadas mais comumente, nos Estados Unidos, por larvas primárias de *Cochliomyia hominivorax*, que se desenvolvem na cavidade nasal ou da orelha.
 ocular m., m. ocular; invasão do saco conjuntival ou do bulbo do olho por larvas de moscas, p. ex., *Hypoderma bovis*, *H. lineata*, *Sarcophaga* ou *Gasterophilus intestinalis*. SIN ophthalmomyiasis.
 tumbu dermal m., cordilobíase. SIN cordylobiasis.
 wound m., m. de ferida; a infestação de uma ferida superficial ou outra lesão aberta por larvas de moscas.

mykol (mī′kol). Micol. SIN mycolic acids.

mylabris (mil′a-bris). Milabris; o besouro *Mylabris phalerata* seco; um vesicante semelhante à cantárida. [G. uma barata encontrada em moinhos e padarias, de *mylē*, moinho]

mylohyoid (mī′lō-hī′oyd). Milo-hióideo; relativo aos dentes molares, ou à porção posterior da mandíbula e ao osso hióide; designa várias estruturas. VER *nerve* to mylohyoid, muscle, region, sulcus. [G. *mylē*, um moinho, no pl. *mylai*, dentes molares]

mylohyoideus (mī-lō-hī-oy′dē-ŭs). Milo-hióideo. SIN mylohyoid (*muscle*).

△ **myo-**. Mio-; músculo. [G. *mys*, músculo]

myoadenylate deaminase (mī′o-a-den-il-āt). Mioadenilato desaminase; AMP desaminase muscular. VER AMP deaminase.

myoalbumin (mī′o-al-bū′min). Mioalbumina; albumina no tecido muscular, possivelmente igual à albumina sérica.

myoarchitectonic (mī′o-ar′ki-tek-ton′ik). Mioarquitetônico; relativo ao arranjo estrutural do músculo ou das fibras em geral. [myo- + G. *architektonikos*, relativo à construção]

myoatrophy (mī-o-at′rō-fē). Mioatrofia. SIN muscular *atrophy*.

myoblast (mī′o-blast). Mioblasto; uma célula muscular primitiva com a potencialidade de se transformar em uma fibra muscular. SIN sarcoblast, sarcogenic cell. [myo- + G. *blastos*, germe]

myoblastic (mī-o-blas′tik). Mioblástico; relativo a um mioblasto ou ao modo de formação das células musculares.

myoblastoma (mī′o-blas-tō′ma). Mioblastoma; tumor de células musculares imaturas. [myo- + G. *blastos*, germe, + *-oma*, tumor]
 granular cell m., m. de células granulares; designação obsoleta de tumor de células granulares (granular cell *tumor*).

myobradia (mī-o-brā′dē-a). Miobradia; reação lenta do músculo após estímulo. [myo- + G. *bradys*, lento]

myocardia (mī-o-kar′dē-a). Miocárdios; plural de myocardium.

myocardial (mī-o-kar′dē-al). Miocárdico; relativo ao miocárdio.

myocardiograph (mī′o-kar′dē-ō-graf). Miocardiógrafo; instrumento composto de um tambor com fixação a uma alavanca de registro, por meio da qual é feito um traçado dos movimentos do músculo cardíaco. [myo- + G. *kardia*, coração, + *graphō*, registrar]

myocardiopathy (mī′o-kar-dē-op′a-thē). Miocardiopatia. SIN cardiomyopathy. [myocardium + G. *pathos*, que sofre]
 alcoholic m., m. alcoólica. SIN alcoholic *cardiomyopathy*.
 chagasic m. (cha′ga-sik); m. chagásica; doença do músculo cardíaco devida à doença de Chagas (causada por *Trypanosoma cruzi*), na qual é comum haver bloqueio do ramo direito.

myocardiorrhaphy (mī′o-kar-dē-ōr′a-fē). Miocardiorrafia; sutura do miocárdio. [myocardium + G. *rhaphē*, sutura]

myocarditic (mī′o-kar-dī′ik). Miocardítico; relacionado à miocardite (adjetivo).

myocarditis (mī′o-kar-dī′tis). Miocardite; inflamação das paredes musculares do coração.
 acute isolated m., m. isolada aguda; m. intersticial aguda de causa desconhecida, sem acometimento do endocárdio e do pericárdio. SIN Fiedler m.
 Fiedler m., m. de Fiedler. SIN acute isolated m.
 giant cell m., m. de células gigantes; m. isolada aguda caracterizada por infiltração por granulomas contendo células gigantes.
 idiopathic m., m. idiopática; inflamação do músculo cardíaco de origem desconhecida.
 indurative m., m. indurativa; m. crônica que causa enrijecimento da parede muscular do coração.
 toxic m., m. tóxica; inflamação do músculo cardíaco causada por qualquer substância química nociva, p. ex., álcool, metais pesados.

myocardium, pl. **myocardia** (mī-o-kar′dē-ŭm, -kar′dē-a) [TA]. Miocárdio; a túnica média do coração, que consiste no músculo cardíaco. [myo- + G. *kardia*, coração]
 hibernating m., m. hibernante; disfunção ventricular após meses ou anos de isquemia reversível quando o fluxo sanguíneo é restabelecido. É preciso distingui-lo cuidadosamente da disfunção causada por necrose ou fibrose do miocárdio.
 stunned m., m. atordoado; comprometimento do desempenho contrátil miocárdico após um período de isquemia e, finalmente, reversível.

myocele (mī′o-sēl). Miocele. **1.** Protrusão da substância muscular através de uma abertura em sua bainha. [myo- + G. *kēlē*, hérnia] **2.** A pequena cavidade que aparece em alguns somitos. SIN somite cavity. [myo- + G. *koilia*, cavidade]

myocelialgia (mī′o-sē-lē-al′jē-a). Miocelialgia; designação obsoleta de celiomialgia. [myo- + G. *koilia*, o ventre, + *algos*, dor]

myocelitis (mī′o-sē-lī′tis). Miocelite; inflamação dos músculos abdominais. [myo- + G. *koilia*, ventre, + *-itis*, inflamação]

my·o·cel·lu·li·tis (mī′ō-sel-ū-lī′tis). Miocelulite; inflamação do músculo e do tecido celular. [myo- + L. Mod. *cellularis*, celular (tecido), + G. *-itis*, inflamação]

my·o·ce·ro·sis (mī′ō-sē-rō′sis). Miocerose; degeneração cérea dos músculos. SIN myokerosis. [myo- + G. *kēros*, cera]

my·o·chrome (mī′ō-krōm). Miocromo; termo raramente usado para o citocromo encontrado no tecido muscular.

my·o·chron·o·scope (mī-ō-kron′ō-skōp). Miocronoscópio; instrumento para determinar o momento de um impulso muscular, isto é, o intervalo entre a aplicação do estímulo e o movimento muscular em resposta. [myo- + G. *chronos*, tempo, + *skopeō*, examinar]

my·o·ci·ne·sim·e·ter (mī′ō-sin-ē-sim′ē-ter). Miocinesímetro. SIN myokinesimeter.

my·o·clo·nia (mī′ō-klō′nē-ă). Mioclonia; qualquer distúrbio caracterizado por mioclônus. [myo- + G. *klonos*, tumulto]

  fibrillary m., m. fibrilar; a contração de uma parte ou grupo limitado de fibras de um músculo.

my·o·clon·ic (mī-ō-klon′ik). Mioclônico; que exibe mioclônus.

my·oc·lo·nus (mī-ok′lō-nŭs, mī-ō-klō′nŭs). Mioclônus; uma contração ou uma série de contrações de um grupo de músculos, semelhantes a choques, de regularidade, sincronismo e simetria variáveis, geralmente causadas por lesão do sistema nervoso central. [myo- + G. *klonos*, tumulto]

  benign m. of infancy, m. benigno do lactente. SIN benign infantile m.

  benign infantile m., m. benigno do lactente; distúrbio convulsivo do lactente no qual ocorrem movimentos mioclônicos no pescoço, no tronco e nos membros; o EEG é normal, e as convulsões não persistem após os 2 anos de idade. SIN benign m. of infancy.

  m. mul′tiplex, m. múltiplo; distúrbio mal definido, caracterizado por contrações musculares rápidas e difusas. SIN paramyoclonus multiplex, polyclonia, polymyoclonus.

  nocturnal m., m. noturno; contrações musculares repetidas freqüentemente, que ocorrem no momento em que se adormece.

  palatal m., m. palatino; contrações rítmicas do palato mole, dos músculos da face e do diafragma, relacionadas a lesões das vias olivocerebelares. VER TAMBÉM palatal *nystagmus*.

  stimulus sensitive m., m. sensível a estímulos; mioclônus induzido por vários estímulos, p. ex., fala, cálculo, ruídos altos, pancadinhas, etc.

my·o·col·pi·tis (mī-ō-kol-pī′tis). Miocolpite; inflamação do tecido muscular da vagina. [myo- + G. *kolpos*, vagina, + *-itis*, inflamação]

my·o·com·ma, pl. **my·o·com·ma·ta** (mī-ō-kom′ă, -kom′ă-tă). Miosepto; o septo de tecido conjuntivo que separa miótomos adjacentes. SIN myoseptum. [myo- + G. *komma*, uma moeda ou a estampa de uma moeda]

my·o·cris·mus (mī-ō-kris′mŭs). Miocrismo; um som de rangido algumas vezes ouvido à ausculta de um músculo em contração. [myo- + G. *krizō*, ranger]

my·o·cu·ta·ne·ous (mī-ō-kū-tā′nē-ŭs). Miocutâneo. SIN musculocutaneous. [myo- + L. *cutis*, pele]

my·o·cyte (mī′ō-sīt). Miócito; uma célula muscular. [myo- + G. *kytos*, célula]

  Anitschkow m., m. de Anitschkow. SIN cardiac histiocyte.

my·o·cy·tol·y·sis (mī-ō-sī-tol′i-sis). Miocitólise; dissolução da fibra muscular. [myo- + G. *kytos*, célula, + *lysis*, afrouxamento]

  m. of heart, m. do coração; perda focal de sincício miocárdico em virtude de um desequilíbrio metabólico, insuficiente em intensidade ou duração (ou ambos) para causar lesão do estroma ou para produzir qualquer exsudação reativa.

  m. cor′dis, m. do coração; m. das paredes cardíacas.

my·o·cy·to·ma (mī′ō-sī-tō′mă). Miocitoma; neoplasia benigna derivada do músculo.

my·o·de·gen·er·a·tion (mī′ō-dē-jen-ē-rā′shŭn). Miodegeneração; degeneração muscular.

my·o·de·mia (mī-ō-dē′mē-ă). Miodemia; degeneração gordurosa do músculo. [myo- + G. *dēmos*, sebo]

my·o·der·mal (mī-ō-der′mal). Miodérmico. SIN musculocutaneous. [myo- + G. *derma*, pele]

my·o·di·as·ta·sis (mī′ō-dī-as′tă-sis). Miodiástase; separação do músculo. [myo- + G. *diastasis*, separação]

my·o·dy·na·mia (mī′ō-dī-nā′mē-ă). Miodinamia; força muscular. [myo- + G. *dynamis*, força]

my·o·dy·nam·ics (mī′ō-dī′nam′iks). Miodinâmica; a dinâmica da ação muscular.

my·o·dy·na·mom·e·ter (mī′ō-dī-nă-mom′ē-ter). Miodinamômetro; instrumento para determinar a força muscular. [myo- + G. *dynamis*, força, + *metron*, medida]

my·o·dyn·ia (mī′ō-din′ē-ă). Miodinia. SIN myalgia. [myo- + G. *odynē*, dor]

my·o·dys·to·ny (mī-ō-dis′tō-nē). Miodistonia; condição de relaxamento lento, interrompido por uma sucessão de pequenas contrações, após estimulação elétrica de um músculo. [myo- + G. *dys-*, difícil, + *tonos*, tônus, tensão]

my·o·dys·tro·phy, my·o·dys·tro·phia (mī-ō-dis′trō-fē, mī′-ō-dis-trō′fē-ă). Miodistrofia. SIN muscular dystrophy. [myo- + G. *dys-*, difícil, deficiente, + *trophē*, nutrição]

my·o·e·de·ma (mī-ō-e-dē′mă). Mioedema; constrição localizada de um músculo em degeneração, que ocorre no ponto de um golpe agudo, independentemente da inervação. SIN idiomuscular contraction, mounding, myoidema. [myo- + G. *oidēma*, tumefação]

my·o·e·las·tic (mī′ō-ē-las′tik). Mioelástico; relativo a fibras musculares lisas intimamente associadas e ao tecido conjuntivo elástico.

my·o·e·lec·tric (mī′ō-ē-lek′trik). Mioelétrico; relativo às propriedades elétricas do músculo.

my·o·en·do·car·di·tis (mī′ō-en′dō-kar-dī′tis). Mioendocardite; inflamação da parede muscular e da membrana de revestimento do coração. [myo- + G. *endon*, dentro, + *kardia*, coração, + *-itis*, inflamação]

my·o·ep·i·the·li·al (mī′ō-ep-i-thē′lē-al). Mioepitelial; relativo ao miopitélio.

my·o·ep·i·the·li·o·ma (mī′ō-ep-i-thē-lē-ō′mă). Mioepitelioma; um tumor benigno das células mioepiteliais. [myo- + epithelium, + G. *-ōma*, tumor]

my·o·ep·i·the·li·um (mī′ō-ep-i-thē′lē-ŭm). Mioepitélio; células fusiformes, contráteis, semelhantes às células musculares lisas, de origem epitelial, dispostas longitudinal ou obliquamente ao redor das glândulas sudoríparas e dos alvéolos secretores da glândula mamária; há células mioepiteliais ao redor das unidades secretoras das glândulas lacrimais e de algumas glândulas salivares. SIN muscle epithelium. [myo- + epithelium]

my·o·es·the·sis, my·o·es·the·sia (mī′ō-es-thē′sis, -thē′zē-ă). Miestesia. SIN kinethetic sense.

my·o·fas·ci·al (mī-ō-fash′ē-al). Miofascial; de ou relativo à fáscia que circunda e separa o tecido muscular.

my·o·fas·ci·tis (mī′ō-fă-sī′tis). Miofascite. SIN myositis fibrosa.

my·o·fi·bril (mī-ō-fī′bril). Miofibrila; uma das finas fibrilas longitudinais encontradas em uma fibra muscular esquelética ou cardíaca que constitui muitos miofilamentos espessos e finos ultramicroscópicos regularmente superpostos. SIN muscular fibril, myofibrilla. [myo- + L. *fibrilla*, fibrila]

my·o·fi·bril·la, pl. **my·o·fi·bril·lae** (mī-ō-fī-bril′ă, -bril′ē). Miofibrila. SIN myofibril.

my·o·fib·ril·lar (mī-ō-fī-bril-ar). Miofibrilar; pertinente ou relativo a miofibrila.

my·o·fi·bro·blast (mī-ō-fī′brō-blast). Miofibroblasto; uma célula considerada responsável pela contratura de feridas; essas células possuem algumas características de músculo liso, como propriedades contráteis e fibrilas, e também parecem produzir, temporariamente, colágeno tipo III.

my·o·fi·bro·ma (mī′ō-fī-brō′mă). Miofibroma; neoplasia benigna que consiste, principalmente, em tecido conjuntivo fibroso, com um número variável de células musculares formando partes da neoplasia.

my·o·fi·bro·ma·to·sis (mī-′yō-fī-brō-ma-tō′sis). Miofibromatose; tumores solitários ou múltiplos de tecido muscular e fibroso, ou tumores compostos por miofibroblastos. [myo- + L. *fibra*, fibra, + G. sufixo, *-ōma*, tumor, + sufixo *-osis*, condição]

  infantile myofibromatosis, miofibromatose do lactente; m. observada ao nascimento ou em lactentes, com múltiplas lesões ósseas líticas e envolvendo os tecidos moles ou com envolvimento visceral.

my·o·fi·bro·sis (mī′ō-fī-brō′sis). Miofibrose; miosite crônica com hiperplasia difusa do tecido conjuntivo intersticial pressionando e causando atrofia do tecido muscular.

my·o·fi·bro·si·tis (mī′ō-fī-brō-sī′tis). Miofibrosite; inflamação do perimísio.

my·o·fil·a·ments (mī-ō-fil′ă-ments). Miofilamentos; os filamentos ultramicroscópicos das proteínas filamentares que formam miofibrilas no músculo estriado. Os m. espessos contêm miosina e os finos actina; m. grossos e finos também são encontrados nas fibras musculares lisas, mas não são dispostos regularmente em miofibrilas distintas e, assim, não conferem um aspecto estriado a essas células.

my·o·func·tion·al (mī′ō-fŭnk′shŭn-al). Miofuncional. **1.** Relativo à função dos músculos. **2.** Em odontologia, relativo ao papel da função muscular na etiologia ou correção de problemas ortodônticos.

my·o·gen (mī′ō-jen). Miógeno; proteínas extraídas do músculo esquelético com água fria, principalmente as enzimas que promovem glicólise; do resíduo, o KCl alcalino 0,6 mol L^{-1} extrai actina e miosina como actomiosina, sendo a miosina ainda separável em duas meromiosinas por tratamento com proteinase. SIN myosinogen. [myo- + G. *-gen*, que produz]

my·o·gen·e·sis (mī-ō-jen′ē-sis). Miogênese; formação embrionária de células ou fibras musculares. [myo- + G. *genesis*, origem]

my·o·ge·net·ic, my·o·gen·ic (mī-ō-jē-net′ik, -jen′ik). Miogênico. **1.** Que se origina ou começa no músculo. **2.** Relativo à origem das células ou fibras musculares. SIN myogenous.

my·og·e·nous (mī-oj′ē-nŭs). Miogênico. SIN myogenetic.

my·o·glo·bin (Mb, MbCO, MbO$_2$) (mī-ō-glō′bin). Mioglobina; a proteína de transporte de oxigênio e armazenamento do músculo, com função semelhante à da hemoglobina sanguínea, mas que contém apenas uma subunidade e um heme como parte da molécula (em vez dos quatro da hemoglobina) e com um peso molecular que corresponde a, aproximadamente, um quarto do peso molecular da hemoglobina. SIN muscle hemoglobin, myohemoglobin. [myo- + hemoglobin]
  carbonmonoxy m., carboxiemoglobina. SIN carboxyhemoglobin.
my·o·glo·bi·nu·ria (mī′ō-glō-bi-noo′rē-ă). Mioglobinúria; excreção de mioglobina na urina; resulta da degeneração muscular, que libera mioglobina no sangue; ocorre em determinados tipos de trauma (síndrome de esmagamento), isquemia avançada ou prolongada do músculo, ou como um processo paroxístico de etiologia desconhecida. SIN idiopathic paroxysmal rhabdomyolysis, Meyer-Betz disease, Meyer-Betz syndrome.
my·o·glob·u·lin (mī-ō-glob′ū-lin). Mioglobulina; globulina presente no tecido muscular.
my·o·glob·u·li·nu·ria (mī′ō-glob′ū-li-noo′rē-ă). Mioglobulinúria; a excreção de mioglobulina na urina.
my·og·na·thus (mī-og′nă-thŭs, mī-ō-năth′ŭs). Miognato; gêmeo conjugado desigual em que a cabeça rudimentar do parasita está fixada à mandíbula do autósito apenas por músculo e pele. VER conjoined *twins*, em *twin*. [myo- + G. *gnathos*, mandíbula]
my·o·gram (mī′ō-gram). Miograma; o traçado feito por um miógrafo. SIN muscle curve. [myo- + G. *gramma*, desenho]
my·o·graph (mī′ō-graf). Miógrafo; instrumento de registro pelo qual são feitos traçados das contrações musculares. [myo- + G. *graphō*, escrever]
  palate m., m. palatino. SIN palatograph.
my·o·graph·ic (mī-ō-graf′ik). Miográfico; relativo a um miograma, ou ao registro de um miógrafo.
my·og·ra·phy (mī-og′ră-fē). Miografia. **1.** O registro de movimentos musculares pelo miógrafo. **2.** Uma descrição ou tratado sobre os músculos. SIN descriptive myology.
my·o·he·mo·glo·bin (mī′ō-hēm-ō-glō′bin). Mioglobina. SIN myoglobin.
my·oid (mī′oyd). Mióide. **1.** Semelhante a músculo. **2.** Um dos elementos protoplasmáticos filiformes, contráteis, finos, encontrados em algumas células epiteliais em animais inferiores. **3.** Uma parte contrátil dos cones retinianos em alguns peixes e anfíbios. Em mamíferos, o mióide é a parte interna do segmento interno dos bastonetes e cones; contém microtúbulos, o aparelho de Golgi, retículo endoplasmático e ribossomas, mas não há miofibrilas. [myo- + G. *eidos*, aspecto]
my·oi·de·ma (mī-oy-dē′mă). Mioedema. SIN myoedema. [myo- + G. *oidēma*, edema]
my·o·in·o·si·tol (mī-ō-in-o′-si-tōl). Mioinositol. VER *myo*-inositol.
my·o·is·che·mia (mī′ō-is-kē′mē-ă). Mioisquemia; condição de deficiência ou ausência localizada de suprimento sanguíneo no tecido muscular.
my·o·ke·ro·sis (mī′ō-kē-rō′sis). Miocerose. SIN myocerosis.
my·o·ki·nase (mī-ō-kī′nās). Miocinase. SIN adenylate kinase.
my·o·kin·e·sim·e·ter (mī-ō-kin-ĕ-sim′ĕ-ter). Miocinesímetro; dispositivo para registro do momento exato e da extensão da contração dos maiores músculos do membro inferior em resposta à estimulação elétrica. SIN myocinesimeter. [myo- + G. *kinesis*, movimento, + *metron*, medida]
my·o·ky·mia (mī-ō-kī′mē-ă). Mioquimia; agitação ou tremor involuntário contínuo de músculos em repouso, causado por deflagração espontânea, repetitiva de potenciais da unidade motora. SIN fibrillary chorea, Morvan chorea. [myo- + G. *kyma*, onda]
  facial m., m. facial; m. que aparece nos músculos da face, causando estreitamento da fissura palpebral e ondulação contínua da superfície da pele facial; esta última é denominada aspecto de "saco de vermes", sendo mais bem observada com luz refletida; causada por lesão intrínseca do tronco cerebral, como glioma pontino ou esclerose múltipla.
  generalized m., m. generalizada; m. disseminada, presente em múltiplos membros e freqüentemente na face; tem várias causas, incluindo síndrome de Isaac, uremia, tireotoxicose e intoxicação por ouro (síndrome do ouro-mioquimia).
  hereditary m. [MIM*160100], m. hereditária; síndrome que consiste em contrações musculares e cãibras noturnas; herança autossômica dominante.
  limb m., m. do membro; m. presente em um ou mais membros; várias causas, uma das mais comuns sendo irradiação prévia de plexo.
my·o·lem·ma (mī-ō-lem′ă). Miolema. SIN sarcolemma.
my·o·li·po·ma (mī′ō-li-pō′mă). Miolipoma; neoplasia benigna que consiste, principalmente, em células de gordura (tecido adiposo), com números variáveis de células musculares formando partes da neoplasia.
my·o·lo·gia (mī-ō-lō′jē-ă). Miologia. SIN myology.
my·ol·o·gist (mī-ol′ō-jist). Miologista; indivíduo versado no conhecimento dos músculos.
my·ol·o·gy (mī-ol′ō-jē). Miologia; o ramo da ciência que estuda os músculos e suas partes acessórias, tendões, aponeuroses, bursas e fáscias. SIN myologia, sarcology (1). [myo- + G. *logos*, estudo]
  descriptive m., m. descritiva. SIN myography (2).

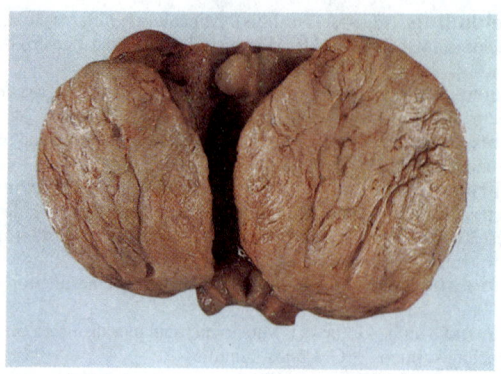

mioma uterino: corte transversal mostrando estreitamento da cavidade uterina

my·ol·y·sis (mī-ol′i-sis). Miólise; dissolução ou liquefação do tecido muscular, freqüentemente precedida por alterações degenerativas, como infiltração de gordura, atrofia e degeneração gordurosa. [myo- + G. *lysis*, dissolução]
  cardiotoxic m., m. cardiotóxica; cardiomalacia que ocorre na febre e em várias infecções sistêmicas.
my·o·ma (mī-ō′mă). Mioma; neoplasia benigna do tecido muscular. VER TAMBÉM leiomyoma, rhabdomyoma. [myo- + G. -*oma*, tumor]
my·o·ma·la·cia (mī′ō-mă-lā′shē-ă). Miomalacia; amolecimento patológico do tecido muscular. [myo- + G. *malakia*, amolecimento]
my·o·ma·tous (mī-ō′mă-tŭs). Miomatoso; relativo aos, ou caracterizado pelos, aspectos de um mioma.
my·o·mec·to·my (mī-ō-mek′tō-mē). Miomectomia; remoção cirúrgica de um mioma, especificamente de um mioma uterino. SIN fibroidectomy, fibromectomy, hysteromyomectomy. [myoma + G. *ektomē*, excisão]
  abdominal m., m. abdominal; remoção de um mioma uterino através de uma incisão abdominal.
  left ventricular m., m. ventricular esquerda; ressecção do tecido miocárdico usada em casos de estenose subaórtica hipertrófica idiopática.
  vaginal m., m. vaginal; remoção de um mioma uterino através da vagina. SIN colpomyomectomy.
my·o·mel·a·no·sis (mī′ō-melă-nō′sis). Miomelanose; pigmentação escura anormal do tecido muscular. VER TAMBÉM melanosis. [myo- + G. *melanōsis*, que se torna preto]
my·o·mere (mī′ō-mēr). Miômero. SIN myotome (4). [myo- + G. *meros*, uma parte]
my·om·e·ter (mī-om′ĕ-ter). Miômetro; instrumento para medir a extensão de uma contração muscular. [myo- + G. *metron*, medida]
my·o·me·tri·al (mī-ō-mē′trē-ăl). Miometrial; relativo ao miométrio.
my·o·me·tri·tis (mī-ō-mē-trī′tis). Miometrite; inflamação da parede muscular do útero. [myo- + G. *mētra*, útero, + -*itis*, inflamação]
my·o·me·tri·um (mī′ō-mē′trē-ŭm) [TA]. Miométrio; a parede muscular do útero. SIN tunica muscularis uteri [TA], muscular coat of uterus. [myo- + G. *mētra*, útero]
my·o·mi·to·chon·dri·on, pl. **my·o·mi·to·chon·dria** (mī′ō-mī′tō-kon′drē-on, -drē-ă). Miomitocôndria; uma mitocôndria de uma fibra muscular.
my·o·mot·o·my (mī-ō-mot′ō-mē). Miomotomia; incisão de um mioma. [myoma + G. *tomē*, incisão]
my·on (mī′on). Mion; uma unidade muscular individual. [G. *mys*, músculo]
my·o·ne·cro·sis (mī′ō-nĕ-krō′sis). Mionecrose; necrose do músculo.
  clostridial m., m. por clostrídios. SIN gas gangrene.
my·o·neme (mī′ō-nēm). Mionema. **1.** Uma fibrila muscular. **2.** Uma das fibrilas contráteis de alguns protozoários; acredita-se que funcione de forma análoga às fibras musculares dos metazoários. [myo- + G. *nēma*, filamento]
my·o·neu·ral (mī-ō-noo′răl). Mioneural; relativo ao músculo e ao nervo; designa, especificamente, a sinapse do neurônio motor com as fibras musculares estriadas: junção mioneural ou placa terminal motora. VER TAMBÉM neuromuscular. [myo- + G. *neuron*, nervo]
my·o·neu·ro·ma (mī′ō-noo-rō′mă). Mioneuroma; uma tumefação que consiste, principalmente, em células de Schwann de proliferação anormal, com um número variável de células musculares formando partes da massa; os músculos provavelmente são malformações, em vez de neoplasias verdadeiras. [myo- + G. *neuron*, nervo, + -*oma*, tumor]
my·on·y·my (mī-on′i-mē). Mionimia; nomenclatura dos músculos. [myo- + G. *onyma* ou *onoma*, nome]
my·o·pa·chyn·sis (mī′ō-pă-kin′sis). Hipertrofia muscular. [myo- + G. *pachynsis*, espessamento]

my·o·pal·mus (mī-ō-palʹmŭs). Espasmo muscular. [myo- + G. *palmos*, estremecimento]

my·o·path·ic (mī-ō-pathʹik). Miopático; designa um distúrbio que envolve o tecido muscular.

my·op·a·thy (mī-opʹa-thē). Miopatia; qualquer condição anormal ou doença dos tecidos musculares; comumente designa um distúrbio que envolve o músculo esquelético. [myo- + G. *pathos*, que sofre]

carcinomatous m., m. carcinomatosa. SIN Lambert-Eaton *syndrome.*

centronuclear m., m. centronuclear; fraqueza e atrofia muscular generalizadas, lentamente progressivas, que começam na infância; à biopsia do músculo esquelético, os núcleos da maioria das fibras musculares são observados próximos ao centro de uma fibra pequena (a posição normal em um embrião de 10 semanas), e não na periferia da fibra; incidência familiar. Existem formas autossômica dominante [MIM*160150], recessiva [MIM*255200] e ligada ao X [310400]. A forma ligada ao X é causada por mutação no gene da miopatia miotubular (MTM1) em Xq28. SIN myotubular m.

distal m., m. distal; miopatia que afeta predominantemente as porções distais dos membros; o início geralmente se dá após os 40 anos de idade, com fraqueza e definhamento dos pequenos músculos das mãos; a forma do lactente [MIM*160300] e a forma sueca de início tardio [MIM*160500] são autossômicas dominantes. Há um tipo japonês de início tardio [MIM*254130] que é recessivo e causado por mutação no gene que codifica a disferilina em 2p13.

dysthyroid m., m. tireotóxica. SIN thyrotoxic m.

minicore-multicore m., miopatia não-progressiva incomum, com início precoce, fraqueza proximal e hipotonia. As fibras musculares exibem defeitos focais de enzimas oxidativas e adenosina trifosfatase miofibrilar, com desorganização da ultra-estrutura da miofibrila.

mitochondrial m., m. mitocondrial; fraqueza e hipotonia dos músculos, basicamente do pescoço, cínglos do membro superior e do membro inferior, com início nos primeiros anos da vida; à biopsia, são observadas mitocôndrias gigantes, bizarras, situadas entre fibrilas musculares logo abaixo do sarcolema. Há formas autossômica dominante [MIM*251900] e recessiva devidas a deleções ou duplicações do DNA mitocondrial, com uma forma recessiva [MIM*252010] associada a uma deficiência de complexo 1 da cadeia respiratória mitocondrial.

myotubular m., m. miotubular. SIN centronuclear m.

nemaline m., m. da nemalina; fraqueza muscular congênita, não-progressiva, mais evidente nos músculos proximais; assim denominada devido aos bastonetes de nemalina (filiformes) característicos observados nas células musculares compostas de material da banda Z. Há duas formas: dominante [MIM*161800], causada por mutação no gene da tropomiosina-3 (TPM3) em 1q22-q23, e recessiva [MIM*256030], que são clinicamente indistinguíveis. SIN rod m.

ocular m., m. ocular. SIN chronic progressive external *ophthalmoplegia.*

proximal myotonic m. (PROMM), m. miotônica proximal; distúrbio multissistêmico, autossômico dominante, com início na vida adulta jovem, caracterizado por miotonia e fraqueza proximal, dor muscular, calvície, catarata, distúrbios da condução cardíaca e atrofia testicular. Ao contrário da distrofia miotônica, as características desse distúrbio não incluem fraqueza facial e ptose, fraqueza e definhamento dos membros distais, e expansão da repetição do trinucleotídeo nos *loci* genéticos para distrofia miotônica.

rod m., m. de bastonete. SIN nemaline m.

thyrotoxic m., m. tireotóxica; fraqueza muscular extrema, na tireotoxicose grave, que afeta músculos dos membros e do tronco, bem como aqueles usados na fala e na deglutição. SIN dysthyroid m.

my·o·per·i·car·di·tis (mīʹō-per-i-kar-dīʹtis). Miopericardite; inflamação da parede muscular do coração e do pericárdio que o reveste; também, perimiocardite — a escolha do termo é determinada de acordo com o envolvimento principal, se pericárdico ou miocárdico. [myo- + pericarditis]

my·o·per·i·to·ni·tis (mīʹō-per-i-tō-nīʹtis). Mioperitonite; inflamação do peritônio parietal com miosite da parede abdominal.

my·o·phone (mīʹō-fōn). Miofone; instrumento que permite ouvir o som das contrações musculares. [myo- + G. *phōnē*, som]

my·o·phos·phor·y·lase (mī-ō-fus-fōrʹi-lās). Miofosforilase; fosforilase muscular.

my·o·pia (M) (mī-ōʹpē-ă). Miopia; a condição óptica na qual apenas raios a uma distância finita do olho são focalizados na retina. SIN near sight, nearsightedness, short sight, shortsightedness. [G. de *myo*, fechar, + *ōps*, olho]

axial m., m. axial; m. devida a alongamento do bulbo do olho.

curvature m., m. por curvatura; m. devida a erros de refração resultante de curvatura excessiva da córnea.

degenerative m., m. degenerativa. SIN pathologic m.

index m., m. decorrente do aumento da refratividade da lente, como na esclerose nuclear.

malignant m., m. maligna. SIN pathologic m.

night m., m. noturna; na adaptação ao escuro, o olho torna-se mais sensível a menores comprimentos de onda (desvio de Purkinje), e a acuidade visual depende dos cones azuis parafoveais. Menores comprimentos de onda entram em foco na frente da retina, e essa aberração cromática é responsável por parte da m. relativa que um olho normal apresenta à noite; a maioria do restante é decorrente de aumento do tom acomodativo no escuro.

pathologic m., m. patológica; m. progressiva caracterizada por alterações do fundo, estafiloma posterior e acuidade corrigida subnormal. SIN degenerative m., malignant m.

prematurity m., m. da prematuridade; m. observada em bebês com baixo peso ao nascimento ou associada à fibroplasia retrolenticular.

senile lenticular m., m. lenticular senil. SIN second *sight.*

simple m., m. simples; m. originada da ausência de correlação entre a capacidade refrativa do segmento anterior e o comprimento do bulbo do olho.

space m., m. espacial; tipo de m. que se origina quando não se forma qualquer contorno de imagem na retina.

transient m., m. transitória; m. observada no espasmo acomodativo secundário à iridociclite ou contusão ocular.

my·o·pic (M) (mī-opʹik, -ōʹpik). Miópico; relativo a, ou que sofre de, miopia.

my·o·plasm (mīʹō-plazm). Mioplasma; a porção contrátil da célula muscular, distinta do sarcoplasma. [myo- + G. *plasma*, algo formado]

my·o·plas·tic (mī-ō-plasʹtik). Mioplástico; relativo à cirurgia plástica dos músculos, ou ao uso de tecido muscular para corrigir um defeito.

my·o·plas·ty (mīʹō-plas-tē). Mioplastia; cirurgia plástica do tecido muscular. [myo- + G. *plastos*, formado]

my·o·po·lar (mī-ō-pōʹlăr). Miopolar; relativo à polaridade muscular, ou à parte de músculo entre dois eletrodos.

my·o·pro·tein (mī-ō-prōʹtēn). Mioproteína; proteína que ocorre no músculo.

my·or·rha·phy (mī-ōrʹa-fē). Miorrafia; sutura de um músculo. [myo- + G. *rhaphē*, sutura]

my·or·rhex·is (mī-ō-rekʹsis). Miorrexe; laceração de um músculo. [myo- + G. *rhēxis*, ruptura]

my·o·sal·pin·gi·tis (mīʹō-sal-pin-jīʹtis). Miossalpingite; inflamação do tecido muscular da tuba uterina. [myosalpinx + G. *-itis*, inflamação]

my·o·sal·pinx (mīʹō-salʹpingks). Miossalpinge; a túnica muscular da tuba uterina. [myo- + salpinx]

my·o·sar·co·ma (mīʹō-sar-kōʹmă). Miossarcoma; termo genérico que designa uma neoplasia maligna derivada do tecido muscular. VER TAMBÉM leiomyosarcoma, rhabdomyosarcoma.

my·o·scle·ro·sis (mīʹō-skle-rōʹsis). Miosclerose; miosite crônica com hiperplasia do tecido conjuntivo intersticial.

my·o·sep·tum (mī-ō-sepʹtŭm). Miossepto. SIN myocomma. [myo- + L. *saeptum*, uma barreira]

my·o·sin (mīʹō-sin). Miosina; uma globulina presente no músculo e que possui atividade ATPase; em combinação com a actina, forma actomiosina; a m. forma os filamentos espessos no músculo.

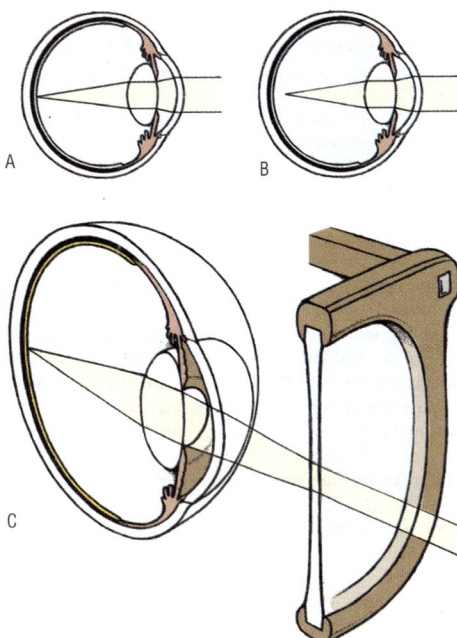

miopia: (A) visão normal (20/20), raio de luz focalizando com precisão na retina; (B) miopia, raio de luz de um ponto distante focaliza em frente à retina; (C) miopia corrigida com lentes côncavas

m. light chain kinase, cinase da cadeia leve de miosina; uma enzima dependente de cálcio/calmodulina, que fosforila as cadeias leves de miosina do músculo liso e inicia a contração. No músculo esquelético, a fosforilação modula a tensão durante a contração.

my·o·sin·o·gen (mī-ō-sin′ō-jen). Miosinogênio. SIN myogen.

my·o·si·nose (mī′ō-si-nōs). Miosinose; proteose formada pela hidrólise parcial da miosina.

my·o·sit·ic (mī-ō-sit′ik). Miosítico; relativo à miosite.

my·o·si·tis (mī-ō-sī′tis). Miosite; inflamação de um músculo. SIN initis (2). [myo- + G. -itis, inflamação]

  cervical m., m. cervical. VER posttraumatic neck *syndrome*.

  epidemic m., m. epidem'ica acu'ta, m. epidêmica, m. epidêmica aguda. SIN epidemic *pleurodynia*.

  m. fibro'sa, m. fibrosa; endurecimento de um músculo decorrente do crescimento intersticial de tecido fibroso. SIN interstitial m., myofascitis.

  infectious m., m. infecciosa; inflamação dos músculos voluntários, caracterizada por edema e dor, que geralmente afeta os ombros e os braços, embora quase todo o corpo possa ser envolvido.

  interstitial m., m. intersticial. SIN m. fibrosa.

  m. ossif'icans, m. ossificante; ossificação ou depósito de osso no músculo com fibrose, causando dor e edema nos músculos.

  m. ossif'icans circumscrip'ta, m. ossificante circunscrita; depósito local de osso em um músculo, geralmente após trauma prolongado; p. ex., osso dos cavaleiros.

  m. ossif'icans progressi'va, m. ossificante progressiva; uma mutação rara e freqüentemente fatal, que começa no início da vida, caracterizada por ossificação progressiva dos músculos; não é rigorosamente uma miosite, mas uma ossificação não-inflamatória.

  proliferative m., m. proliferativa; nódulo fibroso infiltrante benigno, de crescimento rápido no músculo esquelético, contendo células gigantes características semelhantes a células ganglionares.

  m. purulen'ta trop'ica, m. purulenta tropical. SIN tropical *pyomyositis*.

  tropical m., m. tropical. SIN tropical *pyomyositis*.

my·o·spasm, my·o·spas·mus (mī′ō-spazm, mī-ō-spaz′mŭs). Mioespasmo; contração muscular espasmódica.

  cervical m., m. cervical. VER posttraumatic neck *syndrome*.

my·o·spher·u·lo·sis (mī-ō-sfēr-oo-lō′sis). Mioesferulose; reação granulomatosa crônica a estruturas esféricas indeterminadas, freqüentemente contidas em um cisto microscópico; descrita pela primeira vez em lesões císticas no músculo esquelético na África oriental e, subseqüentemente, em infecções nasais nos Estados Unidos. [myo- + L. *sphaerula*, esfera pequena, + G. -osis, condição]

my·o·sthe·nom·e·ter (mī′ō-sthē-nom′ē-ter). Mioestenômetro; instrumento para medir a força dos grupos musculares. [myo- + G. *sthenos*, força, + *metron*, medida]

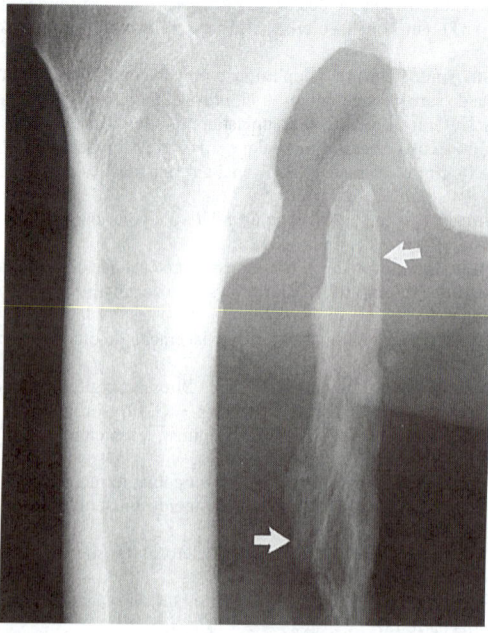

miosite ossificante: hematoma ossificante bem organizado no músculo adutor maior (setas)

my·o·stro·ma (mī-ō-strō′mă). Mioestroma; o tecido conjuntivo ou estrutura de sustentação do tecido muscular. [myo- + G. *stroma*, colchão]

my·o·stro·min (mī-ō-strō′min). Miostromina; proteína encontrada no estroma muscular.

my·o·tac·tic (mī-ō-tak′tik). Miotático; relativo à sensibilidade muscular. [myo- + L. *tactus*, tato]

my·ot·a·sis (mī-ot′ă-sis). Miotasia; estiramento de um músculo. [myo + G. *tasis*, estiramento]

my·o·tat·ic (mī-ō-tat′ik). Miotático; relativo à miotase.

my·o·ten·o·si·tis (mī′ō-te-nō-sī′tis). Miotenosite; inflamação de um músculo com seu tendão. [myo- + G. *tenōn*, tendão, + -itis, inflamação]

my·o·te·not·o·my (mī′ō-te-not′ō-mē). Miotenotomia; secção através do tendão principal de um músculo, com divisão do próprio músculo no todo ou em parte. SIN tenomyotomy, tenontomyotomy. [myo- + G. *tenōn*, tendão, + *tomē*, incisão]

my·o·ther·mic (mī-ō-ther′mik). Miotérmico; relativo à temperatura aumentada no tecido muscular resultante de sua contração. [myo- + G. *thermē*, calor]

my·o·tome (mī′ō-tōm). Miótomo. **1.** Um bisturi para dividir o músculo. **2.** Em embriões, aquela parte do somito que se transforma no músculo esquelético. SIN muscle plate. **3.** Todos os músculos derivados de um somito e inervados por um nervo espinal segmentar. **4.** Em vertebrados primitivos, a parte muscular de um metâmero. SIN myomere. [myo- + G. *tomos*, um corte]

my·ot·o·my (mī-ot′ō-mē). Miotomia. **1.** Anatomia ou dissecção dos músculos. **2.** Divisão cirúrgica de um músculo. [myo- + G. *tomē*, excisão]

  cricopharyngeal m., m. cricofaríngeo; divisão da porção cefálica do músculo cricofaríngeo, geralmente para tratamento do divertículo esofágico de Zenker.

  Heller m., m. de Heller; esofagomiotomia distal, geralmente para o tratamento de acalasia.

my·o·tone (mī′ō-tōn). Miotônus. SIN myotony.

my·o·to·nia (mī-ō-tō′nē-ă). Miotonia; relaxamento tardio de um músculo após uma contração forte, que contração prolongada após estimulação mecânica (como por percussão) ou breve estimulação elétrica; devida a anormalidade da membrana muscular, especificamente dos canais iônicos. [myo- + G. *tonos*, tensão, estiramento]

  m. acquisi'ta, m. adquirida; m. adquirida após exposição a algumas toxinas.

  m. atroph'ica, m. atrófica. SIN myotonic *dystrophy*.

  m. congen'ita [MIM*160800], m. congênita; distúrbio muscular incomum, com início nos primeiros anos de vida, caracterizado por hipertrofia muscular, miotonia e evolução não-progressiva; herança autossômica dominante; causada por mutações no gene do canal de cloreto do músculo esquelético (CLCN1) no cromossoma 7q. SIN Thomsen disease.

  m. dystroph'ica, m. distrófica. SIN myotonic *dystrophy*.

  m. neonato'rum, m. neonatal. SIN neonatal *tetany*.

my·o·ton·ic (mī-ō-ton′ik). Miotônico; relativo a ou que exibe miotonia.

my·ot·o·noid (mī-ot′ō-noyd). Miotonóide; designa uma reação muscular, excitada de forma natural ou elétrica, caracterizada por contração lenta e, principalmente, relaxamento lento. [myo- + G. *tonos*, tônus, tensão, + *eidos*, semelhança]

my·ot·o·nus (mī-ot′ō-nŭs). Miotônus; espasmo tônico ou rigidez temporária de um músculo ou grupo de músculos. [myo- + G. *tonos*, tensão, estiramento]

my·ot·o·ny (mī-ot′ō-nē). Miotônus; tônus ou tensão muscular. SIN myotone. [myo- + G. *tonos*, tensão]

my·ot·ro·phy (mī-ot′rō-fē). Miotrofia; nutrição do tecido muscular. [myo- + G. *trophē*, nutrição]

my·o·tube (mī-ō-toob). Miotubo; fibra muscular esquelética formada pela fusão de mioblastos durante um estágio do desenvolvimento; algumas miofibrilas ocorrem na periferia, e o centro é ocupado por núcleos e sarcoplasma, de forma que a fibra possui um aspecto tubular.

my·o·tu·bule (mī-ō-too′bool). Miotúbulo; designação antiga de miotubo.

My·o·vir·i·dae (mī-ō-vir′i-dē). Família de vírus bacterianos relativamente grandes com caudas contráteis complexas, cabeças geralmente alongadas, mas isométricas em algumas espécies, e um genoma de DNA de duplo filamento (PM 21–190 × 10^6). Inclui o grupo fago T-uniforme e, provavelmente, outros gêneros.

myr·i·ca (mir′i-kă). Mirica; a casca da *Myrica cerifera* (família Myricaceae); usada na diarréia e na icterícia e, externamente, na dor de garganta. SIN bayberry bark.

myr·i·cin (mir′i-sin). Miricina; palmitato de miricil, uma substância sólida, branca, quase inodora, que é o principal constituinte da cera de abelha.

♻ **myring-.** VER myringo-.

my·rin·ga (mi-ring′gă). Miringe. SIN tympanic *membrane*. [L. mod. membrana timpânica]

myr·ing·gec·to·my (mir-in-jek′tō-mē). Miringectomia; excisão da membrana timpânica. [myring- + G. *ektomē*, excisão]

myr·in·gi·tis (mir-in-jī′tis). Miringite; inflamação da membrana timpânica. SIN tympanitis. [myring- + G. -itis, inflamação]

m. bulbo'sa, m. bulbosa. SIN myringodermatitis.
bullous m., m. bolhosa; inflamação dolorosa da membrana timpânica acompanhada por bolhas.

myringo-, myring-. Miringo-, miring-; a membrana timpânica. [L. mod. *myringa*]

my·rin·go·der·ma·ti·tis (mi-ring'gō-der-mă-tī'tis). Miringodermatite; inflamação da superfície meatal ou externa da membrana timpânica e da pele adjacente do canal auditivo externo. SIN myringitis bulbosa.

my·rin·go·plas·ty (mi-ring'gō-plas'tē). Miringoplastia; reparo cirúrgico de uma membrana timpânica lesada. [myringo- + G. *plassō*, formar]

my·rin·go·scler·o·sis (mi-ring'gō-skler-ō'sis). Miringosclerose; formação de tecido conjuntivo denso na membrana timpânica, geralmente não associada à perda auditiva. [myringo- + sclerosis]

my·rin·go·sta·pe·di·o·pexy (mi-ring'gō-stā-pē'dē-ō-pek'sē). Miringoestapediopexia; técnica de timpanoplastia na qual a membrana timpânica ou um enxerto de membrana timpânica é colocado em conexão funcional com o estribo. [*myringo-* + L. *stapes*, estribo, + G. *pēxis*, fixação]

my·rin·go·tome (mi-ring'gō-tōm). Miringótomo; bisturi usado para paracentese da membrana timpânica. [myringo +G. *tomē*, excisão]

myr·in·got·o·my (mir-ing-got'ō-mē). Miringotomia; incisão da membrana timpânica. SIN tympanotomy. [myringo- + G. *tomē*, excisão]

my·rinx (mī'ringks, mir'ringks). Miringe, membrana timpânica. SIN tympanic *membrane*. [L. mod. *myringa*, membrana timpânica]

my·ris·ti·ca (mi-ris'ti-kă). Noz-moscada. SIN nutmeg. [G. *myrizō*, untar, de *myron*, ungüento]
m. oil, óleo de noz-moscada. SIN nutmeg oil.

my·ris·tic ac·id (mi-ris'tik). Ácido mirístico; ácido graxo saturado presente na forma de um acilglicerol no leite, em gorduras vegetais, no óleo de fígado de bacalhau e em ceras. SIN tetradecanoic acid.

my·ris·ti·cin (mī-ris'ti-sin). Miristicina; um constituinte da noz-moscada considerado responsável, ao menos em parte, pelos sintomas bizarros do sistema nervoso central produzidos pela ingestão de grandes quantidades de noz-moscada.

my·ris·to·le·ic ac·id (mi-ris-tō-lē'ik). Ácido miristoleico; um ácido graxo insaturado de 14 carbonos, com uma ligação dupla entre os carbonos 9 e 10; o análogo de 14 carbonos do ácido oleico.

myr·me·cia (mir-mē'shē-ă). Mirmécia; forma de verruga viral na qual a lesão tem uma superfície abobadada (isto é, uma configuração de formigueiro) e está associada à coloração pálida intranuclear e a corpúsculos de inclusão intracitoplasmáticos anfofílicos nas células epidérmicas. [G. *murmex*, formiga]

my·ro·si·nase (mī-rō'si-nās). Mirosinase. SIN thioglucosidase.

myrrh (mer). Mirra; resina gomosa da *Commiphora molmol* e *C. abyssinica* (família Burseraceae) e outras espécies de *C.*, um arbusto da Arábia e do Leste da África; usada como adstringente, tônico e estimulante e, localmente, nas doenças da cavidade oral e em colutórios; acredita-se que tenha sido usada no Antigo Egito na medicina e na embalsamação. [G. *myrrha*]

my·so·phil·ia (mī-sō-fil'ē-ă). Misofilia. SIN coprophilia (2). [G. *mysos*, sujeira, + *philos*, amigo]

my·so·pho·bia (mī-sō-fō'bē-ă). Misofobia; medo mórbido de sujeira ou imundície decorrente do contato com objetos familiares. SIN rhyophobia. [G. *mysos*, sujeira, + *phobos*, medo]

my·ta·cism (mī'tă-sizm). Mitacismo; uma forma de gagueira na qual a letra *m* é freqüentemente substituída por outras consoantes. SIN mutacism. [G. *my*, a letra μ]

my·ur·ous (mī-ū'rŭs). Que diminui gradualmente em espessura, como a cauda de um camundongo; termo raramente usado que designa alguns sintomas no processo de cessação, ou o batimento cardíaco em alguns casos nos quais ele se torna cada vez mais fraco por um período e, depois, se fortalece. [G. *mys*, camundongo, + *ouros*, cauda]

myx·ad·e·ni·tis la·bi·a·lis. Mixadenite labial. SIN cheilitis glandularis.

myx·as·the·nia (mik-sas-thē'nē-ă). Mixastenia; secreção deficiente de muco. [myx- + G. *astheneia*, fraqueza]

myx·e·de·ma (mik-se-dē'mă). Mixedema; hipotireoidismo caracterizado por edema relativamente duro do tecido subcutâneo, com aumento do conteúdo de mucinas (proteoglicanas) no líquido; caracterizado por sonolência, raciocínio lento, ressecamento e perda de cabelo, aumento de líquido em cavidades como o saco pericárdico, temperatura subnormal, rouquidão, fraqueza muscular e lento retorno de um músculo à posição neutra após a estimulação de um reflexo tendinoso; geralmente é causado por remoção ou perda do tecido tireóideo funcionante. [myx- + G. *oidēma*, edema]
congenital m., m. congênito. SIN infantile *hypothyroidism.*
infantile m., m. do lactente. SIN infantile *hypothyroidism.*
operative m., m. cirúrgico; mixedema que se desenvolve após tireoidectomia.
pituitary m., m. hipofisário; mixedema resultante da secreção inadequada do hormônio tireotrópico; comumente ocorre associado à secreção inadequada de outros hormônios da hipófise anterior.

myx·e·de·ma·toid (mik-se-dem'ă-toyd). Mixedematóide; semelhante ao mixedema.

myx·e·dem·a·tous (mik-se-dem'ă-tŭs). Mixedematoso; relativo a mixedema.

myx·e·mia (mik-sē'mē-ă). Mixemia. SIN mucinemia. [myx- + G. *haima*, sangue]

myxo-, myx-. Mixo-, mix-; muco. VER TAMBÉM muci-, muco-. [G. *myxa*, muco]

myx·o·chon·dro·fi·bro·sar·co·ma (mik'sō-kon'drō-fī'brō-sar-kō'mă). Mixocondrofibrossarcoma; neoplasia maligna derivada do tecido conjuntivo fibroso, isto é, um fibrossarcoma no qual há focos intimamente associados de tecido cartilaginoso e mixomatoso. [myxo- + G. *chondros*, cartilagem, + L. *fibra*, fibra, + G. *sarx*, carne, + *-ōma*, tumor]

myx·o·chon·dro·ma (mik'sō-kon-drō'mă). Mixocondroma; neoplasia benigna do tecido cartilaginoso, isto é, um condroma no qual o estroma assemelha-se ao tecido mesenquimal relativamente primitivo. SIN myxoma enchondromatosum. [myxo- + G. *chondros*, cartilagem, + *-ōma*, tumor]

Myx·o·coc·cid·i·um steg·o·my·i·ae (mik'sō-kok-sid'ē-ŭm steg-ō-mī'ē-ē). Protozoário que foi encontrado há algum tempo no corpo de um mosquito, *Stegomyia calopus*, que se alimentou do sangue de um paciente com febre amarela; foi então postulado, erradamente, como o agente causador da febre amarela.

myx·o·cyte (mik'sō-sīt). Mixócito; uma das células estreladas ou poliédricas presentes no tecido mucoso. [myxo- + G. *kytos*, célula]

myx·o·fi·bro·ma (mik'sō-fī-brō'mă). Mixofibroma; neoplasia benigna do tecido conjuntivo fibroso semelhante ao tecido mesenquimal primitivo. SIN fibroma myxomatodes, myxoma fibrosum. [myxo- + L. *fibra*, fibra, + G. *-ōma*, tumor]

myx·o·fi·bro·sar·co·ma (mik'sō-fī'brō-sar-kō'mă). Mixofibrossarcoma; histiocitoma fibroso maligno com predomínio de áreas mixóides que se assemelham ao tecido mesenquimal primitivo. [myxo- + L. *fibra*, fibra, + G. *sarx*, carne, + *-ōma*, tumor]

myx·oid (mik'soyd). Mixóide; semelhante a muco. [myxo- + G. *eidos*, semelhança]

myx·o·li·po·ma (mik'sō-li-pō'mă). Mixolipoma; neoplasia benigna de tecido adiposo na qual partes do tumor assemelham-se ao tecido mesenquimal mucóide. SIN lipoma myxomatodes, myxoma lipomatosum. [myxo- + G. *lipos*, gordura, + *-ōma*, tumor]

myx·o·ma (mik-sō'mă). Mixoma; neoplasia benigna, derivada do tecido conjuntivo, que consiste, principalmente, em células poliédricas e estreladas, frouxamente incrustadas em uma matriz mucóide mole, assemelhando-se assim ao tecido mesenquimal primitivo; freqüentemente é intramuscular (onde pode ser confundida com um sarcoma), mas também ocorre nos ossos da mandíbula e encistada na pele (mucinose focal e cisto dorsal do punho). [myxo- + G. *-ōma*, tumor]
atrial m., m. atrial; neoplasia cardíaca primária que se origina, na maioria das vezes, no átrio esquerdo como uma massa polipóide mole fixada por um pedículo ao septo interatrial; pode assemelhar-se a um trombo mural organizado, e os sinais e sintomas podem incluir sopros cardíacos, que se modificam com a mudança de posição do corpo e sinais de estenose ou insuficiência mitral, com risco contínuo de embolia por fragmentos do tumor ou de toda a sua massa.
m. enchondromato'sum, m. encondromatoso. SIN myxochondroma.
m. fibro'sum, m. fibroso. SIN myxofibroma.
m. lipomato'sum, m. lipomatoso. SIN myxolipoma.
odontogenic m., m. odontogênico; neoplasia radiotransparente multilocular, expansiva, benigna, das mandíbulas, que consiste em tecido conjuntivo fibroso mixomatoso; provavelmente é derivado dos componentes mesenquimais do aparelho odontogênico.
m. sarcomato'sum, m. sarcomatoso. SIN myxosarcoma.

myx·o·ma·to·sis (mik'sō-mă-tō'sis). Mixomatose. **1.** SIN mucoid *degeneration*. **2.** Mixomas múltiplos.

my·xo·ma·tous (mik-sō'mă-tŭs). Mixomatoso. **1.** Relativo a ou com características de um mixoma. **2.** Diz-se do tecido que se assemelha ao tecido mesenquimal primitivo.

myx·o·my·cete (mik'sō-mī-sēt). Mixomiceto; um membro da classe Myxomycetes.

Myx·o·my·ce·tes (mik'sō-mī-sē'tēz). Classe de fungos na qual se incluem os mofos do lodo, que ocorrem em vegetação putrefeita, mas não são patogênicos para seres humanos. [myxo- + G. *mykēs*, fungo]

myx·o·neu·ro·ma (mik'sō-noo-rō'mă). Mixoneuroma. **1.** Termo obsoleto para uma tumefação resultante da proliferação anormal de células de Schwann, na qual alterações degenerativas focais ou difusas resultam em partes semelhantes ao tecido mesenquimal primitivo. **2.** Termo obsoleto para um neurilemoma, meningioma ou glioma no qual o estroma é de natureza mixomatosa. [myxo- + G. *neuron*, nervo, + *-ōma*, tumor]

myx·o·pap·il·lo·ma (mik'sō-pap-i-lō'mă). Mixopapiloma; neoplasia benigna do tecido epitelial na qual o estroma assemelha-se ao tecido mesenquimal primitivo. [myxo- + L. *papilla*, mamilo, + G. *-ōma*, tumor]

myx·o·poi·e·sis (mik'sō-poy-ē'sis). Mixopoese; produção de muco. [myxo- + G. *poiēsis*, produção]

myxorrhea gas·'tri·ca. Gastromixorréia. SIN gastromyxorrhea.

myx·o·sar·co·ma (mik'sō-sar-kō'ma). Mixossarcoma; sarcoma, geralmente um lipossarcoma ou histiocitoma fibroso maligno, com um componente abundante de tecido mixóide semelhante ao mesênquima primitivo, que contém mucina do tecido conjuntivo. SIN myxoma sarcomatosum. [myxo- + G. *sarx*, carne, + *-ōma*, tumor]

Myx·o·spo·ra (mik-sō-spō'ra). Subfilo do filo Protozoa, caracterizado por esporos de origem multicelular, geralmente com duas ou três válvulas, dois ou mais filamentos polares e um esporoplasma amebóide; parasita em vertebrados inferiores, particularmente comum em peixes. Gêneros importantes incluem *Ceratomyxa*, *Hanneguya*, *Leptotheca*, *Myxidium* e *Myxobolus*. [myxo- + G. *sporos*, semente]

Myx·o·spo·rea (mik'sō-spō-rē'a). Classe de Myxozoa com esporos contendo uma a seis cápsulas polares (geralmente duas), cada uma contendo um filamento polar espiralado; parasita no celoma ou nos tecidos de vertebrados de sangue frio, principalmente peixes. Os gêneros importantes incluem *Ceratomyxa*, *Hanneguya*, *Leptotheca*, *Myxidium* e *Myxobolus*.

myx·o·vi·rus (mik'sō-vī'rus). Mixovírus; termo usado antigamente para vírus com uma afinidade por mucinas, agora incluídos nas famílias Orthomyxoviridae e Paramyxoviridae. Os mixovírus incluíram vírus influenza, vírus parainfluenza, vírus sincicial respiratório, vírus do sarampo e vírus da caxumba.

Myx·o·zoa (mik-sō-zō'a). Filo do sub-reino Protozoa, caracterizado por esporos de origem multicelular (geralmente com duas ou três válvulas), uma a seis cápsulas polares ou nematocistos (cada um com um filamento oco espiralado), e um esporoplasma amebóide com um ou muitos núcleos; parasita em anelídeos e outros invertebrados (classe Actinosporea; subclasse Actinomyxa) e em vertebrados inferiores (classe Myxosporea). [myxo- + G. *zōon*, animal]

N

v 1. Décima terceira letra do alfabeto grego, nu. **2.** Símbolo de kinematic *viscosity* (*viscosidade* cinemática); freqüência; stoichiometric *number* (número estequiométrico). **3.** Em química, indica a posição de um substituto localizado no décimo terceiro átomo a partir do grupamento carboxilase ou outro grupamento funcional.

N 1. Símbolo de newton; nitrogênio; asparagina; nucleosídeo; solução normal; número cromossômico haplóide. **2.** Designação de um fator sanguíneo herdado. Ver grupo sanguíneo MNS no apêndice de Grupos Sanguíneos.

N/2 Símbolo de seminormal.

^{15}N Símbolo do nitrogênio-15 (N^{15}).

^{13}N Símbolo do nitrogênio-13 (N^{13}).

^{14}N Símbolo do nitrogênio-14 (N^{14}).

N_A Símbolo de Avogadro *number* (número de avogadro).

n Símbolo de nano- (2); ordem da reação.

N Símbolo de normal *concentration* (concentração normal). VER normal (3).

n 1. Número em um estudo científico. Tamanho da amostra. **2.** Símbolo de refractive *index* (índice de refração).

n_0 Abreviatura de Loschmidt *number* (número de Loschmidt).

NA Abreviatura de *Nomina Anatomica*.

N.A. Abreviatura de numerical *aperture* (abertura numérica).

Na Símbolo do sódio (natrium).

^{24}Na. Símbolo do sódio-24 (Na^{24}).

nab·i·lone (nab′i - lōn). Nabilona. Canabinóide sintético utilizado no tratamento das náuseas e dos vômitos associados à quimioterapia do câncer.

Naboth, Martin, anatomista e médico alemão, 1675–1721. VER nabothian *cyst; follicle*.

na·cre·ous (nā′krē - ŭs). Nacarado. Lustroso, semelhante a madrepérola, termo descritivo utilizado para colônias bacterianas. [Fr. *nacre*, madrepérola]

NAD NAD. Abreviatura de nicotinamide adenine dinucleotide (nicotinamida adenina dinucleotídeo).

N.A.D. Abreviatura de no appreciable disease (sem doença digna de nota); nothing abnormal detected (nada de anormal detectado). Usada na Grã-Bretanha.

NAD$^+$ Abreviatura de nicotinamide adenine dinucleotide (nicotinamida adenina dinucleotídeo) (forma oxidada).

NAD$^+$ nucleosidase, NAD$^+$ nucleosidase; enzima que hidroliza o NAD$^+$ a nicotinamida e adenosina difosforribose. SIN NADase.

NAD$^+$ pyrophosphorylase, NAD$^+$ pirofosforilase; enzima que participa na síntese de NAD$^+$; catalisa a reação do nicotinamida mononucleotídeo com ATP, produzindo NAD$^+$ e pirofosfato; atua também sobre o nicotinato mononucleotídeo.

NAD$^+$ synthetase, NAD$^+$ sintetase; enzima que catalisa a reação do ATP, da L-glutamina e do nicotinato adenina dinucleotídeo para formar NAD$^+$, ADP e L-glutamato.

NADase. NADase. SIN *NAD$^+$ nucleosidase.*

NADH NADH. Abreviatura de nicotinamide adenine dinucleotide (nicotinamida adenina dinucleotídeo) (forma reduzida).

NADH dehydrogenase, NADH desidrogenase; uma flavoproteína contendo ferro-enxofre que oxida reversivelmente NADH a NAD$^+$; a deficiência hereditária desse complexo resulta em acidose avassaladora. SIN cytochrome *c* reductase (citocromo c redutase).

NADH dehydrogenase (quinone), NADH desidrogenase (quinona); enzima que oxida o NADH com quinonas (p. ex., menaquinona) como aceptores.

NADH-hydroxylamine reductase, NADH-hidroxilamina-redutase; enzima que catalisa a reação da hidroxilamina e do NADH para formar amônia, NAD$^+$ e água; utilizada em diversos ensaios clínicos.

na·dide (nā′dĭd). Nadida. Composto de nicotinamida adenina dinucleotídeo utilizado como antagonista do álcool e de narcóticos.

nadir (nā′dēr). Nadir. O valor mais baixo das contagens hematológicas após quimioterapia. [I.M., L. Med., ponto mais baixo, do árabe *nazīr*, oposto (ao zênite)]

Nadi re·ac·tion. Reação de Nadi. Ver em reaction.

na·do·lol (nā′dō - lol). Nadolol. Agente bloqueador β-adrenérgico com ações semelhantes às do propranolol.

NADP NADP. Abreviatura de nicotinamide adenine dinucleotide phosphate (fosfato de nicotinamida adenina dinucleotídeo).

NADP$^+$ Abreviatura de nicotinamide adenine dinucleotide phosphate (fosfato de nicotinamida adenina dinucleotídeo) (forma oxidada).

NAD(P)$^+$ nu·cle·o·si·dase. NAD(P)$^+$ nucleosidase. Enzima que hidrolisa o NAD(P)$^+$, liberando nicotinamida livre e adenosina difosforribose (fosfato).

NADPH Abreviatura de nicotinamide adenine dinucleotide phosphate (fosfato de nicotinamida adenina dinucleotídeo) (forma reduzida).

NADPH-cytochrome c_2 reductase, NADPH-citocromo c_2 redutase; enzima que catalisa a reação de 2ferricitocromo c_2 a 2ferrocitocromo c_2 à custa de NADPH. SIN cytochrome c_2 reductase.

NADPH dehydrogenase, NADPH desidrogenase; flavoproteína que oxida o NADPH a NADP$^+$. SIN NADPH diaphorase, old yellow enzyme, Warburg old yellow enzyme.

NADPH dehydrogenase (quinone), NADPH desidrogenase (quinona); flavoproteína que oxida o NADH ou NADPH a NAD$^+$ ou NADP$^+$ com quinonas (p. ex., menadiona) como aceptores de hidrogênio. SIN DT-diaphorase, menadione reductase, phylloquinone reductase, quinone reductase.

NADPH diaphorase, NADPH diafarose. SIN NADPH dehydrogenase.

NADPH-ferrihemoprotein reductase (fer′ī - hē - mō - prō′tēn, fer′ē-). NADPH-ferriemoproteína redutase; enzima que catalisa a redução de 2ferricitocromo pelo NADPH a 2ferrocitocromo; o aceptor fisiológico é provavelmente o citocromo P-450; por conseguinte, participa nas hidroxilações dos esteróides. SIN cytochrome reductase.

Naegeli, Otto, médico suíço, 1871–1938. VER N. type of monocytic *leukemia*.

Naegeli, Oskar, médico suíço, 1885–1959. VER N. *syndrome*.

Nae·gle·ria (nā - glē′rē - ā). *Naegleria*. Gênero de ameba de vida livre encontrada no solo, na água e em esgotos (ordem Schizopyrenida, família Vahlkampfiidae), cuja espécie *N. fowleri*, foi implicada como agente etiológico da meningoencefalite amebiana rapidamente fatal. A infecção foi atribuída a piscinas (incluindo piscinas internas cloradas); a entrada ocorre pela mucosa nasal, a partir da qual as amebas alcançam as meninges e o cérebro através da placa cribriforme e dos nervos olfatórios. Outras amebas do solo que foram implicadas, embora de muito menor importância epidemiológica, incluem os gêneros *Acanthamoeba* e *Hartmanella*, sendo esta última um agente causal suspeito, mas não comprovado.

naf·cil·lin (naf′sil′in). Nafcilina. Penicilina semi-sintética derivada do ácido 6-aminopenicilânico; resistente à penicilinase e efetiva contra *Staphylococcus aureus*.

n. sodium, n. sódica; penicilina resistente à penicilinase.

Naffziger, Howard C., cirurgião norte-americano, 1884–1961. VER N. *operation, syndrome*.

naf·ti·fine hy·dro·chlo·ride (naf′ti - fēn). Cloridrato de naftifina. Agente antifúngico de amplo espectro utilizado no tratamento tópico da tinha.

NAG Abreviatura de *N*-acetylglutamate (*N*-acetilglutamato).

na·ga·na (nah-gah′nah). Nagana. Doença aguda ou crônica de bovinos, cães, suínos, cavalos, ovinos e caprinos na África sub-Saariana; caracteriza-se por febre, anemia e caquexia, variando a sua gravidade de acordo com o parasita e o hospedeiro. Termo coletivo para referir-se a doenças causadas pelos protozoários parasitas *Trypanosoma brucei brucei*, *T. congolense* e *T. vivax*.

Nagel, Willibald A., oftalmologista e fisiologista alemão, 1870–1911. VER N. *test*.

Nägele, Franz K., obstetra alemão, 1777–1851. VER N. *obliquity, pelvis, rule*.

Nägeli, Karl W. von, botânico suíço, 1817–1891. VER micelle.

Nageotte, Jean, histologista francês, 1866–1948. VER N. *cells*, em *cell*.

nail (nāl). Unha. **1.** Placa fina, córnea e semitransparente que recobre a superfície dorsal da extremidade distal de cada falange terminal dos dedos das mãos e dos pés. A unha consiste em um corpo, a parte visível, e em uma raiz na extremidade proximal, oculta sob uma dobra de pele. A parte inferior da unha é formada pelo estrato germinativo da epiderme, superfície livre do estrato lúcido, sendo o estrato córneo representado pela delgada prega cuticular superposta à lúnula. SIN unguis [TA], nail plate, onyx. **2.** Pino. Bastonete fino de metal, osso ou outra substância sólida, utilizado em operações para fixar firmemente os fragmentos de um osso fraturado. [A.S. *naegel*]

egg shell n., u. em casca de ovo. SIN hapalonychia.

half and half n., u. meio a meio; divisão da unha por uma linha transversal em uma parte proximal branca e uma parte distal rosada ou castanha; observada na uremia.

Hippocratic n.'s, unhas hipocráticas; unhas rugosas e que se curvam, cobrindo dedos em baqueta de tambor.

ingrown n., u. encravada; unha de dedo do pé, cuja borda prolifera pela prega ungueal, produzindo granuloma piogênico; decorrente do corte incorreto das unhas ou de compressão por um calçado apertado. SIN ingrowing toenail, onychocryptosis, unguis aduncus, unguis incarnatus.

Küntscher n., pino de Küntscher; pino intramedular utilizado para fixação interna de uma fratura.

parrot-beak n., u. em bico de papagaio; unha acentuadamente encurvada dos dedos das mãos.

△ Formas Combinantes	☆ Termo oficial alternativo para a *Terminologia Anatomica*
🛈 Indica que o termo é ilustrado, ver Índice de Ilustrações	[MIM] Mendelian Inheritance in Man
SIN Sinônimo	I.C. Índice de Corantes
Cf. Comparar, confrontar	
[NA] *Nomina Anatomica*	Termo de Alta Importância
[TA] *Terminologia Anatomica*	

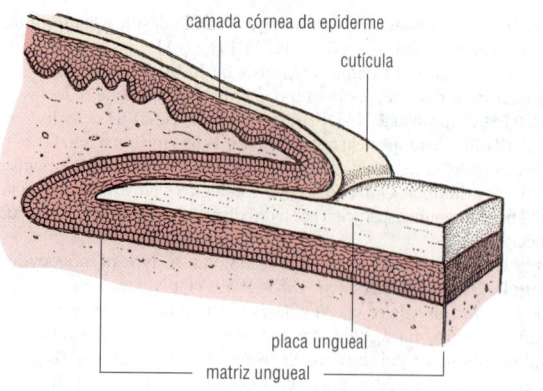
estrutura da unha (ungueal)

pincer n., u. em pinça; encurvamento transversal exagerado da unha que aumenta distalmente, fazendo com que suas bordas laterais pincem o tecido mole, com conseqüente hipersensibilidade; pode resultar de uma anomalia de desenvolvimento ou de exostose subungueal.
racket n., u. em raquete; unha do polegar larga e achatada, resultante de uma falange distal do polegar congenitamente mais curta e mais larga.
reedy n., u. juncosa; unha caracterizada por cristas e depressões longitudinais.
shell n., u. em concha; distrofia ungueal que acompanha o baqueteamento dos dedos na bronquiectasia, com excessiva curvatura longitudinal da placa ungueal e atrofia do leito ungueal e do osso subjacente.
Smith-Petersen n., pino de Smith-Petersen; um pino de três flanges para fixação interna de uma fratura do colo do fêmur.
spoon n., u. em colher. SIN koilonychia.
yellow n., u. amarela; interrupção completa ou quase completa de todo crescimento ungueal, com espessamento das unhas, aumento da convexidade, perda da cutícula e amarelamento; a onicólise resultante pode acarretar a perda de algumas unhas; com freqüência, a condição está associada a doença pulmonar, porém difere do baqueteamento, visto que não ocorre hipertrofia dos tecidos moles. A drenagem linfática pode estar reduzida, mesmo na ausência de linfedema. SIN yellow nail syndrome.
nail·ing (nāl'ing). Encravamento. Ato de inserir ou orientar um pino nas extremidades de um osso fraturado.
Najjar, Victor A., médico e bioquímico norte-americano, *1914. VER Crigler-N. *syndrome.*
Nakanishi, Kazuhiro, médico japonês, *1945. VER N. *stain.*
nal·bu·phine hy·dro·chlo·ride (nal - bū'fēn). Cloridrato de nalbufina. Analgésico opióide sintético, quimicamente relacionado à oximorfina, um narcótico, e à naloxona, um antagonista narcótico, com propriedades narcóticas tanto agonistas quanto antagonistas.
na·li·dix·ic ac·id (nal - i - dik'sik). Ácido nalidíxico. Agente antibacteriano efetivo por via oral, utilizado no tratamento de infecções do trato genitourinário.
nal·or·phine (nal - ōr'fēn). Nalorfina. Um dos primeiros antagonistas da maioria dos efeitos depressores e estimulantes da morfina e analgésicos narcóticos relacionados; precipita graves sintomas de abstinência em dependentes de morfina; é utilizada no diagnóstico de suspeita de dependência de morfina e neutraliza a depressão respiratória produzida pela morfina e compostos correlatos; quando administrada na ausência de narcóticos, a nalorfina exerce efeitos analgésicos e depressores respiratórios leves em não-dependentes; suplantada pela naloxona. SIN *N*-allyl-normorphine.
nal·ox·one hy·dro·chlo·ride (nal - ok'sōn). Cloridrato de naloxona. Poderoso antagonista de endorfinas e narcóticos, incluindo a pentazocina; desprovido de ação farmacológica quando administrado sem narcóticos.
nal·trex·one (nal - treks'ōn). Naltrexona. Antagonista narcótico ativo por via oral; desprovida de ação farmacológica quando administrada na ausência de narcóticos.
NAME Acrônimo de *nevi, atrial myxoma, myxoid neurofibromas, e ephilides (nevos, mixoma atrial, neurofibromas mixóides e efélides).* SIN NAME *syndrome.*
NANDA Acrônimo de *North American Nursing Diagnosis Association (Associação Norte-Americana de Diagnóstico de Enfermagem).*
nan·dro·lone (nan'drō - lōn). Nandrolona. Esteróide androgênico anabólico semi-sintético, administrado por via parenteral.
 n. decanoate, decanoato de n.; androgênio anabólico.
 n. phenpropionate, fenpropionato de n.; androgênio anabólico sintético de ação moderadamente prolongada. SIN n. phenylpropionate.
 n. phenylpropionate, fenilpropionato de n. SIN n. phenpropionate.

nan·ism (nan'izm). Nanismo. Termo obsoleto para dwarfism. [G. *nanos*; L. *nanus,* anão]
 mulibrey n. (mū'li - brā), n. "mulibrey"; distúrbio autossômico recessivo com defeitos no fígado, cérebro, músculo e olhos. [de *mu*scle, *li*ver, *br*ain e *ey*es]
 renal n., n. renal; osteodistrofia renal infantil.
 symptomatic n., n. sintomático; nanismo com defeitos no desenvolvimento do osso e da dentição e desenvolvimento sexual.
Nan·niz·zia (nā - niz'ē - ā). *Nannizzia.* Gênero de fungos ascomicetos, que compreende espécies de *Microsporum* em seu estado perfeito.
△ **nano-.** Nano-. **1.** Forma combinante relativa a nanismo. **2. (n).** Prefixo utilizado nos sistemas SI e métrico para indicar submúltiplos da ordem de um bilionésimo (10^{-9}). [G. *nanos,* anão]
nan·o·ce·pha·lia (nan'ō - se - fā'lē - ā). Nanocefalia. SIN microcephaly.
nan·o·ceph·a·lous, nan·o·ce·phal·ic (nan - ō - sef'ā - lŭs, - se - fal'ik). Nanocéfalo, nanocefálico. SIN microcephalic.
nan·o·ceph·a·ly (nan - ō - sef'ā - lē). Nanocefalia. SIN microcephaly. [nano- +G. *kephalē,* cabeça]
nan·o·cor·mia (nan - ō - kōr'mē - ā). Nanocormia. SIN microsomia. [nano- G. *kormos,* tronco]
nan·o·gram (ng) (nan'ō - gram). Nanograma. Um bilionésimo de grama (10^{-9} g).
nan·o·ka·tal (nkat) (nan - ō - ka - tāl'). Nanokatal. Um bilionésimo de um katal (10^{-9} kat).
nan·o·me·lia (nan - ō - mē'lē - ā). Nanomelia. SIN micromelia. [nano- +G. *melos,* membro]
nan·o·me·ter (nm) (nan - om'ē - ter). Nanômetro. Um bilionésimo de um metro (10^{-9} m).
nan·oph·thal·mia, nan·oph·thal·mos (nan - of - thal'mē - ā, - mos). Nanoftalmia. SIN microphthalmos. [nano- +G. *ophthalmos,* olho]
Na·no·phy·e·tus sal·min·co·la (na - nō'fī - e - tŭs sal - min'kō - lā). *Nanophyetus salmincola.* Trematódeo transmitido por peixe, digenético (família Nanophyetidae) de cães e outros mamíferos que se alimentam de peixe; vetor de *Neorickettsia helmintheca,* o agente da intoxicação por salmão. SIN *Troglotrema salmincola.*
Nanta. Nanta. VER Gandy-Nanta *disease.*
na·nu·ka·ya·mi (nā - noo - kā - yah'mē). Nanukayami. SIN nanukayami *fever.*
nape (nāp). Nuca. SIN nucha.
na·pex (nā'peks). Napex. A região do couro cabeludo imediatamente abaixo da protuberância occipital.
naph·az·o·line hy·dro·chlo·ride (nā - faz'ō - lēn, naf - az'-). Cloridrato de nafazolina. Amina simpaticomimética, utilizada como vasoconstritor tópico; disponível na forma de nitrato de cloridrato de nafazolina, com as mesmas aplicações. SIN naphthazoline hydrochloride.
naph·tha (naf'thā). Nafta. SIN *petroleum* benzin. [G.]
 coal tar n., n. de alcatrão. SIN benzene.
 •**wood n.,** n. de madeira. SIN methyl *alcohol.*
naph·tha·lene (naf'thā - lēn). Naftaleno. Hidrocarboneto carcinogênico e tóxico obtido do alcatrão; utilizado para muitas sínteses na indústria e em alguns repelentes contra traças; o naftaleno pode causar um episódio de anemia hemolítica em indivíduos com deficiência de glicose-6-fosfato desidrogenase. SIN naphthalin, tar camphor.
naph·thal·e·nol (naf - thal'ē - nol). Naftalenol. SIN naphthol.
naph·tha·lin (naf'thā - lin). Naftalina. SIN naphthalene.
naph·thaz·o·line hy·dro·chlo·ride (naf - thaz'ō - lēn). Cloridrato de naftazolina. SIN naphazoline hydrochloride.
naph·thol (naf'thol). Naftol. Fenol do naftaleno, que ocorre em duas formas: o α-naftol, um corante intermediário utilizado em citoquímica para a localização da L-arginina; e o β-naftol, também conhecido como isonaftol, utilizado como anti-helmíntico e anti-séptico. As duas formas são também utilizadas na fabricação de corantes, substâncias químicas orgânicas e produtos da borracha. SIN naphthalenol.
naph·tho·late (naf'thō - lāt). Naftolato. Composto de naftol em que o hidrogênio no radical hidroxila é substituído por uma base.
naph·thol yel·low S [C.I. 10316]. Naftol amarelo S. Corante ácido empregado como corante para proteínas básicas na microspectrofotometria.
naph·tho·qui·none (naf - thō - kwin'ōn). Naftoquinona. **1.** Derivado quinônico do naftaleno, passível de redução a naftoidroquinona; os derivados 1,4-naftoquinona possuem atividade de vitamina K (p. ex., menaquinona). **2.** Classe de compostos contendo a estrutura n. (1).
naph·thyl (naf'thil). Naftil, naftila. Radical do naftaleno, $C_{10}H_7$-.
α-naph·thyl·thi·o·u·rea (ANTU) (naf'thil - thī'ō - ū - rē'ā). α-naftiltiouréia. Derivado da tiouréia; agente antitireóideo extremamente tóxico, particularmente para pequenos mamíferos, que provoca edema pulmonar, degeneração gordurosa do fígado e baixa temperatura corporal; utilizado como raticida.
na·pi·er (nā'pē - er). Napier. SIN neper. [John *Napier,* matemático escocês, 1550–1617]
na·prox·en (nā - prok'sēn). Naproxeno. Analgésico antiinflamatório não-esteróide, utilizado no tratamento de condições reumáticas.

nap·syl·ate (nap′si - lāt). Napsilato. Contração aprovada pelos USAN para 2-naftalenossulfonato.

nar·ce·ine (nar′sē - ēn). Narceína. Alcalóide do ópio; $C_{23}H_{27}NO_8$. A etilnarceína é um narcótico, analgésico e antitussígeno.

nar·cis·sism (nar - sis′izm, nar′si - sizm). Narcisismo. **1.** Estado em que o indivíduo interpreta e encara todas as coisas em relação a si próprio, e não em relação a outras pessoas ou coisas. **2.** Auto-estima, que pode incluir atração sexual por si próprio. VER TAMBÉM autoeroticism. SIN self-love. [Narkissos, G. personagem da mitologia grega]
 primary n., n. primário; em psicanálise, a energia psíquica original incorporada ou investida no ego.
 secondary n., n. secundário; em psicanálise, a energia psíquica uma vez ligada a objetos externos, porém removida desses objetos e reinvestida no ego.

narco-. Narco-. Torpor, narcose. [G. narkoō, entorpecer, amortecer]

nar·co·a·nal·y·sis (nar′kō - ā - nal′i - sis). Narcoanálise. Tratamento psicoterápico sob anestesia leve, originalmente utilizado em casos agudos de combate durante a II Guerra Mundial; também utilizada no tratamento de traumatismo da infância. VER TAMBÉM narcotherapy. SIN narcosynthesis.

nar·co·hyp·nia (nar - kō - hip′nē - ā). Narco-hipnia. Dormência geral algumas vezes experimentada no momento de acordar. [narco- + G. hypnos, sono]

nar·co·hyp·no·sis (nar′kō - hip - nō′sis). Narco-hipnose. Torpor ou sono profundo induzido por hipnose. [narco- + G. hypnos, sono]

nar·co·lep·sy (nar′kō - lep - sē). Narcolepsia. Transtorno do sono que habitualmente aparece em adultos jovens; consiste em episódios recorrentes de sono durante o dia e em sono noturno freqüentemente interrompido; muitas vezes acompanhada de cataplexia, paralisia do sono e alucinações hipnagógicas; doença geneticamente determinada. SIN Gélineau syndrome, paroxysmal sleep. [narco- + G. lēpsis, convulsão]

nar·co·lep·tic (nar′kō - lep′ - tik). Narcoléptico. **1.** Substância que induz sono. **2.** Indivíduo com narcolepsia.

nar·co·sis (nar - kō′sis). Narcose. Depressão reversível, geral e inespecífica da excitabilidade neuronal, produzida por diversos agentes físicos e químicos, resultando habitualmente mais em torpor do que em anestesia (da qual a narcose já foi sinônimo). [G. entorpecimento]
 CO_2 n., n. por CO_2. SIN hypoventilation coma.
 intravenous n., n. intravenosa; administração de medicação opiácea por via intravenosa.
 nitrogen n., n. por nitrogênio; **(1)** narcose produzida por materiais nitrogenados, como ocorre em certas formas de uremia e coma hepático; **(2)** condição torporosa, caracterizada por desorientação e perda do discernimento e habilidade, atribuída a um aumento da pressão parcial de nitrogênio do ar inspirado em mergulhadores de profundidade durante operações submarinas. Comumente conhecida como "êxtase das profundezas". SIN rapture of the deep.

nar·co·syn·the·sis (nar - kō - sin′thē - sis). Narcossíntese. SIN narcoanalysis.

nar·co·ther·a·py (nar - kō - thār′a - pē). Narcoterapia. Psicoterapia conduzida com o paciente sob a influência de um sedativo ou narcótico.

nar·cot·ic (nar - kot′ik). Narcótico. **1.** Originalmente, qualquer substância derivada do ópio ou de compostos semelhantes ao ópio com potentes efeitos analgésicos associados a uma alteração significativa do humor e do comportamento, com potencial de dependência e tolerância. **2.** Mais recentemente, qualquer substância, sintética ou de ocorrência natural, com efeitos semelhantes aos do ópio e derivados, incluindo meperidina e fentanil e seus derivados. **3.** Capaz de induzir um estado de analgesia torporosa. [G. narkōtikos, entorpecimento]

nar·co·tism (nar′kō - tizm). Narcotismo. **1.** Analgesia torporosa induzida por um narcótico. **2.** Dependência de narcótico.

na·ris, pl. **na·res** (nā′ris, - res). [TA]. Narina. Abertura anterior da cavidade nasal. SIN anterior n., external n., nostril, prenaris. [L.]
 anterior n., n. anterior. SIN naris.
 external n., n. externa. SIN naris.
 internal n., n. interna; termo obsoleto para referir-se às coanas (choanae).
 posterior nares, narinas posteriores. SIN choanae.

NARP Acrônimo de neuropathy, ataxia, retinitis pigmentosa syndrome (síndrome de neuropatia, ataxia, retinite pigmentar), um dos distúrbios hereditários das mitocôndrias, causado por mutação puntiforme, resultando na substituição de um único aminoácido na posição 8993 do DNA mitocondrial. Uma expressão mais grave da mesma mutação puntiforme manifesta-se clinicamente como doença de Leigh (q.v.).

nar·row·band. Banda estreita. Banda limitada de freqüências sonoras, em oposição à banda larga de freqüências, também conhecida como ruído branco; utilizada para mascarar a audição no ouvido não submetido a teste na medição da audição.

na·sal (nā′zal). Nasal. Relativo ao nariz. SIN rhinal. [L. nasus, nariz]

nas·cent (nas′ent, nā′sent). Nascente. **1.** Principiante; que está nascendo ou sendo produzido. **2.** Indica o estado de um elemento químico no momento em que é liberado de um de seus compostos. [L. nascor, pres. p. nascens, nascer]

na·si·o·in·i·ac (nā′zē - ō - in′ē - ak). Nasioiníaco. Relativo ao násio e ínio; indica a distância, em linha reta, entre a sutura frontonasal e a protuberância occipital externa.

na·si·on (nā′zē - on) [TA]. Násio. Ponto no crânio que corresponde ao meio da sutura nasofrontal. SIN nasal point. [L. nasus, nariz]

Nasmyth, Alexander, dentista londrino, 1789–1849. VER N. cuticle, membrane.

naso-. Naso-. Forma combinante que significa nariz. [L. nasus]

na·so·an·tral (nā′zō - an′tral). Nasoantral. Relativo ao nariz e ao seio maxilar.

na·so·cil·i·ary. Nasociliar. Relativo ao nariz e às pálpebras. VER nasociliary nerve.

na·so·fron·tal (nā - zō - frŭn′tal). Nasofrontal. Relativo ao nariz e à fronte ou à cavidade nasal e seios frontais.

na·so·gas·tric (nā - zō - gas′trik). Nasogástrico. Relativo a ou que envolve as vias nasais e o estômago, como na intubação nasogástrica.

na·so·la·bi·al (nā - zō - lā′bē - al). Nasolabial. Relativo ao nariz e ao lábio superior. [naso- + L. labium, lábio]

na·so·lac·ri·mal (nā - zō - lak′ri - mal). Nasolacrimal. Relativo aos ossos nasal e lacrimal ou à cavidade nasal e ductos lacrimais.

na·so·oral (nā - zō - ō′ral). Naso-oral. Relativo ao nariz e à boca.

na·so·pal·a·tine (nā′zō - pal′a - tēn, - tin). Nasopalatino. Relativo ao nariz e ao palato.

na·so·pha·ryn·ge·al (nā′zō - fa - rin′jē - al). Nasofaríngeo. Relativo ao nariz ou à cavidade nasal e à faringe. SIN rhinopharyngeal (1).

na·so·pha·ryn·go·la·ryn·go·scope (nā′zō - fa - ring′gō - lā - ring′gō - skōp). Nasofaringolaringoscópio. Instrumento, freqüentemente do tipo de fibra óptica, utilizado para visualizar as vias aéreas superiores e a faringe.

na·so·pha·ryn·go·scope (nā′zō - fa - ring′gō - skōp). Nasofaringoscópio. Instrumento telescópico, iluminado eletricamente, para o exame das vias nasais e da nasofaringe.

na·so·pha·ryn·gos·co·py (nā′zō - fa - ring - gos′kō - pē). Nasofaringoscopia. Exame da nasofaringe por instrumentos ópticos rígidos ou flexíveis ou com espelho. [nasofaringe + G. skopeō, ver, examinar]

na·so·pha·rynx (nā′zō - far′ingks) [TA]. Nasofaringe. A parte da faringe localizada acima do palato mole; anteriormente, abre-se na cavidade nasal através das coanas; inferiormente, comunica-se com a orofaringe através do istmo faríngeo; lateralmente, comunica-se com a cavidade timpânica através da tuba faringotimpânica (auditiva). SIN pars nasalis pharyngis [TA], epipharynx, nasal parte of pharynx, nasal pharynx, pharyngonasal cavity, rhinopharynx.

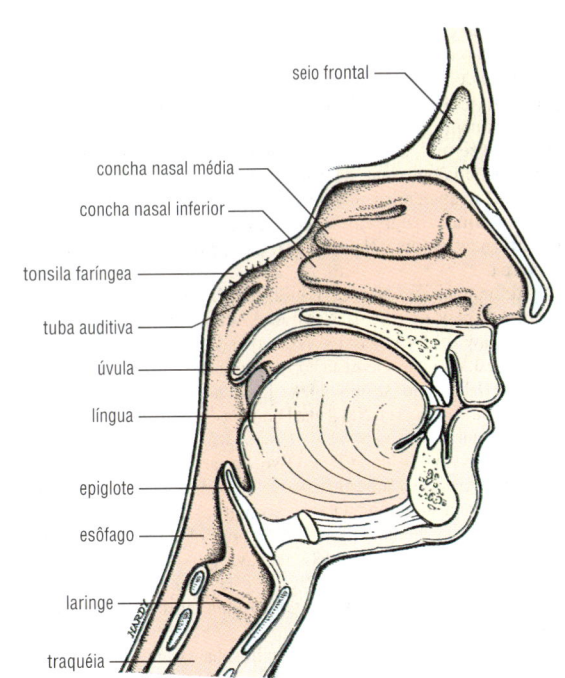

nasofaringe e estruturas circundantes

na·so·ros·tral (nā′zō - ros′tral). Nasorrostral. Relativo à cavidade nasal e ao rostro do osso esfenóide.

na·so·si·nu·si·tis (nā′zō - sī - nū - sī′tis). Nasossinusite. Inflamação das cavidades nasais e dos seios acessórios.

Nasse, Christian Friedrich, médico alemão, 1788–1851.

Nasse law. Lei de Nasse. Ver em law.

na·sus (na'sŭs). **1.** Porção externa do nariz. SIN external *nose*. **2.** Nariz. SIN nose. [L.]

n. exter'nus, porção externa do nariz. SIN external *nose*.

na·tal (na'tăl). Natal. **1.** Relativo ao nascimento. (L. *natalis,* de *nascor,* pp. *natus,* nascer]. **2.** Relativo às nádegas. [L. *nates,* nádegas]

na·tal·i·ty (na - tal'ĭ - tē). Natalidade. O índice (a taxa) de nascimento; o número de nascimentos em relação à população geral. [ver natal (1)]

na·ta·my·cin (na - tă - mī'sin). Natamicina. SIN pimaricin.

na·tes (na'tēz)[TA]. Nádegas. SIN buttocks. [L.pl. de *natis*]

Na·tion·al For·mu·lary (NF). Compêndio oficial antigamente publicado pela *American Pharmaceutical Association,* porém atualmente publicado pela *United States Pharmacopeial Convention* com o objetivo de fornecer padrões e especificações que possam ser utilizados para avaliar a qualidade dos produtos farmacêuticos e agentes terapêuticos.

na·tre·mia, na·tri·e·mia (na - trē'mē - ă, na'trē - ē'mē - ă). Natremia, natriemia. Presença de sódio no sangue. [natrium, sódio + G. *haima,* sangue]

na·trex·one hy·dro·chlo·ride (na - treks'on).Cloridrato de natrexona. Antagonista narcótico ativo por via oral, utilizado na terapia de manutenção de pacientes desintoxicados, anteriormente dependentes de opióides.

na·trif·er·ic (na - trif'er - ik). Natriférico. Que tende a aumentar o transporte de sódio. [natrium + L. *fero,* transportar]

na·tri·um (Na) (na'trē - ŭm). Sódio. SIN sodium. [Ar. *natrŭn,* do G. *nitron,* do carbonato de sódio]

na·tri·u·re·sis (na'trē - ū - rē'sis). Natriurese. Excreção urinária de sódio; designa comumente a excreção aumentada de sódio, que pode ocorrer em certas doenças ou em consequência da administração de agentes diuréticos. [natrium + G. *ouron,* urina]

na·tri·u·ret·ic (na'trē - ū - ret'ik). Natriurético. **1.** Relativo a ou caracterizado por natriurese. **2.** Substância que aumenta a excreção urinária de sódio, geralmente em consequência da reabsorção tubular diminuída de íons sódio do filtrado glomerular.

Nattrassia mangiferae. *Nattrassia mangiferae.* Fungo dematiáceo, anteriormente conhecido como *Hendersonula toruloidea,* que causa onicomicose e feoipomicose. *Scytalidium dimidiatum* é um fungo sinanamorfo. SIN *Hendersonula toruloidea.*

na·tur·o·path (na'choor - ō - path). Naturopata. Aquele que pratica a naturopatia.

na·tur·o·path·ic (na'choor - ō - path'ik). Naturopático. Relativo à, ou por meio da, naturopatia.

na·tur·op·a·thy (na - choor - op'ă - thē). Naturopatia. Sistema de terapêutica em que não são utilizados agentes medicinais ou cirúrgicos, que depende exclusivamente de forças da natureza (não-medicinais).

nau·path·ia (naw - path'ē - ă). Naupatia. SIN seasickness. [G. *naus,* navio + *pathos,* sofrimento]

nau·sea (naw'zē - ă, - zhă). Náusea. Inclinação a vomitar. SIN sicchasia (1). [L. do G. *nausia,* enjôo do mar, de *naus,* navio]

epidemic n., n. epidêmica. SIN epidemic *vomiting.*

n. gravida'rum, n. da gravidez. SIN morning *sickness.*

nau·se·ant (naw'zē - ănt). Nauseante. **1.** Que causa náusea. **2.** Agente que provoca náusea.

nau·se·ate (naw'zē - āt). Náusea. Causar tendência a vômitos.

nau·se·at·ed (naw'zē - ā - ted). Nauseado. Acometido de náusea. SIN sick (2).

nau·seous (naw'zē - ŭs, naw'shŭs). Nauseoso. **1.** Enjoado. **2.** Que causa náusea.

Nauta, Walle J.H., neurocientista norte-americano, *1916. VER N. stain.

na·vel (na'vel). Umbigo. SIN umbilicus. [A.S. *nafela*]

na·vic·u·la (na - vik'ū - lă). Navícula. Pequena estrutura em forma de barco. [L. dim de *navis,* navio]

na·vic·u·lar (na - vik'ū - lăr)[TA]. Osso do tarso achatado, de localização medial, côncavo em sua superfície posterior, para acomodar a cabeça do tálus, e convexo em sua superfície anterior, para articular-se com os três ossos cuneiformes. SIN os naviculare [TA], central bone of ankle, navicular (bone), os centrale tarsi. [L. *navicularis,* relativo a navio]

Nb Símbolo do nióbio.

NBT NBT. Abreviatura de nitroblue *tetrazolium* (nitro azul de tetrazólio).

Nd Símbolo de neodímio.

NDP NDP. Abreviatura de *nucleoside* diphosphate (nucleosídeo difosfato).

Ne Símbolo de neônio.

near·sight·ed·ness (nēr'sĭt - ed - nes). Miopia. SIN myopia.

ne·ar·thro·sis (nē - ar - thrō'sis). Neartrose. Nova articulação; p. ex., pseudoartrose que surge numa fratura não-consolidada, ou articulação artificial resultante de substituição cirúrgica total de uma articulação. SIN neoarthrosis. [G. *neos,* novo + *arthrōsis,* articulação]

neb·ra·my·cin (neb - ră - mī'sin).Nebramicina. Complexo de substâncias produzidas por *Streptomyces tenebrarius;* agente antibacteriano.

nebul. Abreviatura de nebula (nébula).

neb·u·la (nebul.), pl. **neb'u·lae** (neb'ū - lă, - lē).Nébula. **1.** Opacidade translúcida semelhante à névoa da córnea. **2.** Classe de preparações oleosas para aplicação por meio de atomização. VER spray. **3.** Spray. [L. nevoeiro, nuvem, neblina]

neb·u·la·rine (neb - ū - lăr'in). Nebularina. Nucleosídeo tóxico isolado do cogumelo *Agaricus nebularis* e de *Streptomyces* sp. SIN 9-β-ribofuranosylpurine, purine ribonucleoside, ribosylpurine.

neb·u·lin (neb'ū - lin). Nebulina. Proteína muito grande, representando cerca de 3% da proteína do músculo esquelético; ajuda na organização dos filamentos de actina, bem como na sua polimerização. [L. *nebula,* nevoeiro, neblina, do G. *nephelē* + -in]

neb·u·li·za·tion (neb'ū - li - za'shŭn). Nebulização. Pulverização ou vaporização. [L. *nebula,* névoa]

neb·u·lize (neb'ū - līz). Nebulizar. Pulverizar um líquido em finos borrifos ou vapor; vaporizar. [L. *nebula,* névoa]

neb·u·liz·er (neb'ū - līz - er). Nebulizador. Dispositivo utilizado para reduzir uma medicação líquida a partículas nebulosas extremamente finas; útil para levar uma medicação às partes mais profundas do trato respiratório. VER TAMBÉM atomizer, vaporizer.

jet n., n. a jato; atomizador que utiliza uma corrente de ar ou de gás para transformar um líquido em pequenas partículas.

spinning disk n., n. de disco giratório; nebulizador em que a água é transformada em pequenas partículas à medida que é atirada de um disco giratório por força centrífuga.

ultrasonic n., n. ultra-sônico; umidificador que utiliza eletricidade de alta freqüência para energizar um transdutor que vibra 1.350.000 vezes por segundo e transforma a água em partículas de 0,5–3 μm de tamanho em sua câmara nebulizadora; utilizado para inaloterapia.

Ne·ca·tor (nē - kā'tŏr). *Necator.* Gênero de ancilóstomos nematódeos (família Ancylostomatidae, subfamília Necatorinae) caracterizado por duas placas cortantes quitinosas na cavidade bucal e por espículas copulatórias fundidas no macho. As espécies incluem *N. americanus,* o denominado ancilóstomo do Novo Mundo (embora também seja prevalente nos trópicos da África, sul da Ásia e Polinésia); os adultos dessa espécie fixam-se às vilosidades do intestino delgado e sugam sangue, causando desconforto abdominal, diarréia (geralmente com melena) e cólicas, anorexia, perda de peso e anemia microcítica hipocrômica, que pode ocorrer num estágio avançado da doença. VER TAMBÉM *Ancylostoma.* [L. assassino]

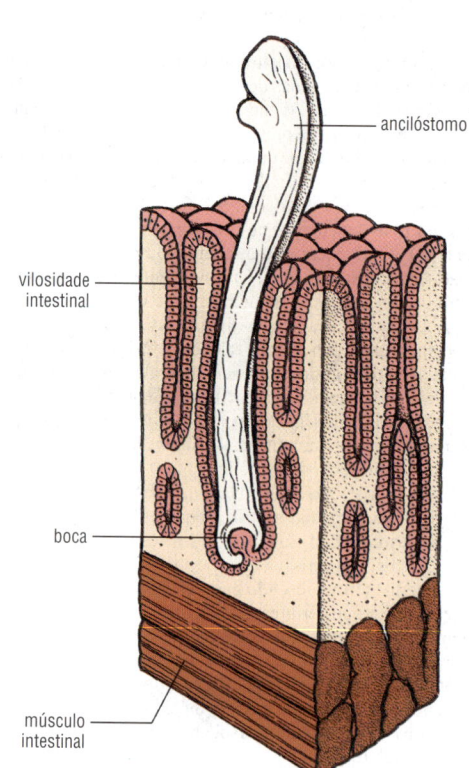

nematódeo: ancilóstomo do Novo Mundo (*Necator americanus*)

ne·ca·to·ri·a·sis (nē - kă - tō - rī'ă - sis). Necatoríase. Doença causada por *Necator,* em que a anemia resultante é, em geral, menos grave do que a observada na ancilostomíase.

neck (nek) [TA]. Pescoço, colo. **1.** Parte do corpo que une a cabeça ao tronco: estende-se da base do crânio até a parte superior dos ombros. **2.** Em anatomia, qualquer porção estreitada tendo semelhança com o pescoço de um animal. **3.**

A porção germinativa de uma tênia adulta, a partir da qual se desenvolvem os segmentos ou proglotes; a região de segmentação dos seis cestóides atrás do escólex. SIN cervix (1) [TA], collum*. [A.S. *hnecca*]

anatomical n. of humerus [TA], colo anatômico do úmero; sulco que separa a cabeça do úmero das tuberosidades, proporcionando uma inserção para cápsula articular. SIN collum anatomicum humeri [TA].

buffalo n., corcova de búfalo, giba de búfalo; combinação de cifose moderada com coxim gorduroso espesso no pescoço, observada principalmente em indivíduos com doença ou síndrome de Cushing.

bull n., p. bovino; pescoço espesso e maciço causado por hipertrofia muscular ou aumento dos linfonodos cervicais.

dental n., colo dentário. SIN n. of tooth.

n. of femur [TA], colo do fêmur; barra curta, estreita e forte que se projeta em ângulo obtuso (cerca de 125°) a partir da extremidade superior da diáfise do fêmur e que sustenta a sua cabeça. SIN collum femoris [TA], collum ossis femoris, n. of thigh bone.

n. of fibula [TA], colo da fíbula; região discretamente estreitada entre a cabeça e o corpo da fíbula. SIN collum fibulae [TA].

n. of gallbladder [TA], colo da vesícula biliar; porção estreita situada entre o corpo da vesícula biliar e o começo do ducto cístico. SIN collum vesicae biliaris [TA], collum vesicae felleae*.

n. of glans [TA], colo da glande do pênis; constrição atrás da coroa da glande peniana. SIN collum glandis [TA].

n. of hair follicle, colo do folículo piloso; parte estreitada do folículo piloso, entre o bulbo e a superfície da pele. SIN collum folliculi pili.

n. of humerus, c. do úmero. VER anatomical n. of humerus, surgical n. of humerus.

Madelung n., pescoço de Madelung; lipomatose múltipla simétrica (doença de Madelung), limitada ao pescoço.

n. of malleus [TA], colo do martelo; porção estreitada do martelo, entre a cabeça e o manúbrio. SIN collum mallei [TA].

n. of mandible [TA], colo da mandíbula; parte estreitada do processo condilar, abaixo da cabeça da mandíbula. SIN collum mandibulae [TA].

n. of pancreas [TA], colo do pâncreas; segmento do pâncreas, de aproximadamente 2 cm de comprimento, que une a cabeça ao corpo do pâncreas; interposta entre o duodeno, anteriormente, e a junção das veias esplênica e mesentérica superior, formando o início da veia porta, posteriormente. SIN collum pancreaticus [TA].

n. of radius [TA], colo do rádio; porção estreita da diáfise, imediatamente abaixo da cabeça. SIN collum radii [TA].

n. of rib [TA], c. da costela; porção achatada de uma costela entre a cabeça e a tuberosidade. SIN collum costae [TA].

n. of scapula [TA], colo da escápula; discreta constrição que marca a separação da parte que contém a cavidade glenóide e o processo coracóide do restante da escápula. SIN collum scapulae [TA].

stiff n., pescoço rígido; termo inespecífico para referir-se à mobilidade limitada do pescoço, freqüentemente causada por cãibras musculares e acompanhada de dor.

surgical n. of humerus [TA], colo cirúrgico do úmero; parte estreita situada abaixo da cabeça e das tuberosidades. SIN collum chirurgicum humeri [TA].

n. of talus [TA], colo do tálus; constrição que separa a cabeça ou porção anterior do corpo do tálus. SIN collum tali [TA].

n. of thigh bone, colo do fêmur. SIN n. of femur.

n. of tooth [TA], colo dentário; parte discretamente estreitada de um dente, entre a coroa e a raiz. SIN cervix dentis [TA], cervix of tooth*, cervical margin of tooth, cervical zone of tooth, collum dentis, dental n.

turkey gobbler n., pescoço de peru; grandes dobras de pele que pendem sob o queixo.

n. of (urinary) bladder [TA], colo da bexiga urinária; a parte mais baixa da bexiga, formada pela junção do fundo e das superfícies ínfero-laterais. SIN cervix vesicae urinariae [TA], collum vesicae*.

n. of uterus, colo uterino. SIN cervix of uterus.

webbed n., pescoço alado; o pescoço largo devido a pregas laterais de pele que se estendem da clavícula até a cabeça, mas que não contém músculos, ossos ou outras estruturas; ocorre na síndrome de Turner e na síndrome de Noonan.

n. of womb, colo do útero. SIN cervix of uterus.

wry n., torcicolo. SIN torticollis.

neck·lace (nek′lās). Colar. Termo utilizado para descrever uma erupção cutânea que circunda o pescoço.

Casal n., c. de Casal; dermatite que circunda parcial ou completamente a parte inferior do pescoço na pelagra.

necr-. Necr-. VER necro-.

nec·rec·to·my (ne - krek′tō - mē). Necrectomia. Remoção cirúrgica de qualquer tecido necrosado. [necr- + G. *ektomē*, excisão]

necro-, necr-, Necro-, necr-. Morte, necrose [G. *nekros*, cadáver, defunto]

nec·ro·ba·cil·lo·sis (nek′rō - bas - il - ō′sis). Necrobacilose. Qualquer doença em que está associada a bactéria *Fusobacterium necrophorum*.

nec·ro·bi·o·sis (nek′rō - bī - ō′sis). Necrobiose. **1.** Morte fisiológica ou normal de células ou tecidos, em conseqüência de alterações associadas ao desenvolvimento, envelhecimento ou uso. **2.** Necrose de uma pequena área de tecido. [necro- + G. *bios*, vida]

n. lipoid′ica, n. lipoid′ica diabetico′rum, n. lipóide, n. lipóide diabética; condição, associada em muitos casos ao diabetes melito, em que se verifica o desenvolvimento de uma ou mais lesões amarelas, atróficas e brilhantes nas pernas (tipicamente pré-tibiais); caracteriza-se, histologicamente, por áreas indistintas de necrose na pele.

nec·ro·bi·ot·ic (nek′rō - bī - ot′ik). Necrobiótico. Relativo a ou caracterizado por necrobiose.

nec·ro·cy·to·sis (nek′rō - sī - tō′sis). Necrocitose. Processo que resulta em, ou condição caracterizada por, morte anormal ou patológica de células. [necro- + G. *kytos*, célula + *-osis*, condição]

nec·ro·gen·ic (nek - rō - jen′ik). Necrogênico. Relativo a, que vive na ou que se origina de matéria morta. SIN necrogenous. [necro- + G. *genesis*, origem]

ne·crog·e·nous (nē - kroj′e - nŭs). Necrógeno. SIN necrogenic.

nec·ro·gran·u·lo·ma·tous (nek′rō - gran - ū - lō′mă - tŭs). Necrogranulomatoso. Termo obsoleto para referir-se às características de um granuloma com necrose central.

ne·crol·o·gist (nē - krol′ō - jist). Necrologista. Estudante ou especialista em necrologia.

ne·crol·o·gy (nē - krol′ō - jē). Necrologia. A ciência da colheita, classificação e interpretação da estatística da mortalidade. [necro- + G. *logos*, estudo]

ne·crol·y·sis (nē - krol′i - sis). Necrólise. Necrose e dissolução de tecido. [necro- + G. *lysis*, dissolução]

toxic epidermal n. (TEN), n. epidérmica tóxica (NET); síndrome em que grande parte da pele torna-se intensamente eritematosa com necrose epidérmica e desprende-se à semelhança de uma queimadura de segundo grau, freqüentemente de modo simultâneo com a formação de bolhas flácidas, em decorrência de sensibilidade a drogas ou de causa desconhecida; o nível de separação é subepidérmico, em contraste com a síndrome da pele escaldada estafilocócica, em que ocorre alteração subcórnea. SIN Lyell syndrome.

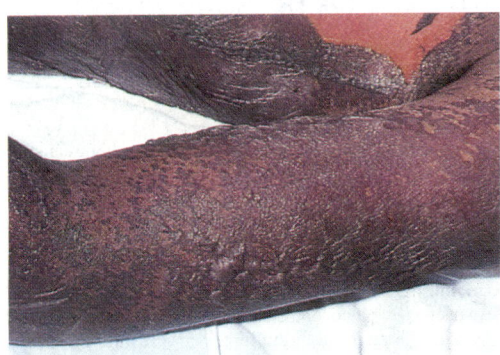

necrólise epidérmica tóxica

nec·ro·ma·nia (nek - rō - mā′nē - ă). Necromania. **1.** Tendência mórbida a viver desejando a morte. **2.** Atração mórbida por cadáveres. [necro- + G. *mania*, mania]

ne·crom·e·ter (nē - krom′e - ter). Necrômetro. Instrumento para medir um cadáver ou qualquer uma de suas partes ou órgãos. [necro- + G. *metron*, medida]

nec·ro·par·a·site (nek - rō - par′ă - sīt). Necroparasita, saprófita. SIN saprophyte.

ne·crop·a·thy (nē - krop′ă - thē). Necropatia. Tendência à morte tecidual ou gangrena. [necro- + G. *pathos*, doença]

ne·croph·a·gous (nē - krof′ă - gŭs). Necrófago. **1.** Que se alimenta de carne putrefata. **2.** SIN necrophilous. [necro- + G. *phago*, comer]

nec·ro·phil·ia, nec·roph·i·lism (nek - rō - fil′ē - ă, ne - krof′i - lizm). Necrofilia. **1.** Tendência mórbida a estar na presença de cadáveres. **2.** Impulso de ter contato sexual ou o contato com um cadáver, habitualmente de homens com cadáveres de mulheres. [necro- + G. *phileō*, amar]

ne·croph·i·lous (nē - krof′i - lŭs). Necrófilo. Que tem preferência por tecido morto; refere-se a certas bactérias. SIN necrophagous (2). [necro- + G. *philos*, amigo]

nec·ro·pho·bia (nek - rō - fō′bē - ă). Necrofobia. Medo mórbido de cadáveres. [necro- + G. *phobos*, medo]

ne·crop·sy (nek′rop - sē). Necropsia. SIN autopsy (1). [necro- + G. *opsis*, visão]

nec·ro·sa·dism (nek - rō - sād′izm). Necrossadismo. Gratificação sexual obtida com a mutilação de cadáveres. [necro- + sadismo]

ne·cros·co·py (nē - kros′kō - pē). Necroscopia. Termo raramente utilizado para necropsia. [necro- + G. *skopeō*, examinar]

ne·crose (nē - krōz′). Necrosar. **1.** Produzir necrose. **2.** Tornar-se o local de necrose.

nec·ro·sec·to·my (nē - krō′sek - tō - mē). Necrossectomia. Ressecção de tecido necrótico.

ne·cro·sis (ne - krō′sis). Necrose. Morte patológica de uma ou mais células ou de parte de tecido ou órgão, em conseqüência de lesão irreversível; as primeiras alterações irreversíveis são mitocondriais e consistem em aumento de volume e depósitos granulares de cálcio observados à microscopia eletrônica; as alterações visíveis mais freqüentes são nucleares: picnose, contração e coloração basofílica anormalmente escura; cariólise, aumento de volume de coloração basofílica anormalmente pálida; ou cariorrexe, ruptura e fragmentação do núcleo. Depois dessas alterações, os contornos de cada célula tornam-se indistintos, e as células afetadas podem fundir-se, formando algumas vezes um foco de material grosseiramente granular, amorfo ou hialino. [G. *nekrōsis*, morte, de *nekroō*, matar]

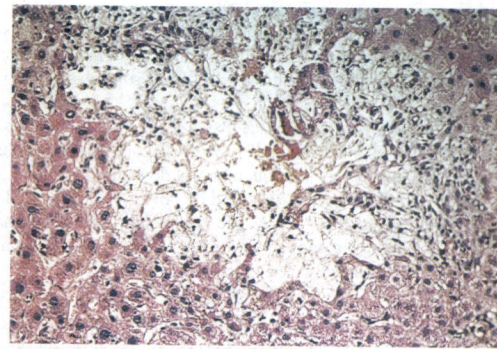

necrose hepática (centrilobular): corte microscópico mostrando a transformação reticular do citoplasma, com degeneração e fragmentação celulares

acute massive liver n., necrose hepática maciça aguda; lesão caracterizada por morte rápida e substancial de células parenquimatosas do fígado, algumas vezes com degeneração gordurosa de todo o órgão; a necrose pode resultar de infecção viral fulminante ou de intoxicação química; associada a icterícia. SIN acute parenchymatous hepatitis, acute yellow atrophy of the liver, Rokitansky disease (1).

acute retinal n. (ARN), necrose retiniana aguda (NRA); síndrome viral observada em pacientes imunocompetentes, caracterizada por destruição retiniana periférica, que se torna circunferencial e resulta em descolamento (*detachment*) da retina.

aseptic n., n. asséptica; necrose que ocorre na ausência de infecção.

avascular n., n. avascular; necrose devido à deficiência de suprimento sangüíneo.

bridging hepatic n., n. hepática coalescente; área de necrose hepática que forma uma ponte entre áreas porta adjacentes e veias centrais; é provável que o colapso e a fibrose pós-necróticos subseqüentes resultem em cirrose.

caseous n., caseation n., n. caseosa, n. de caseação; necrose característica de certas inflamações (p. ex., tuberculose, histoplasmose), que representa a necrose com perda de estruturas independentes dos vários elementos celulares e histológicos; o tecido afetado exibe a consistência friável e fragmentável e a qualidade opaca e fosca observadas no queijo. SIN caseous degeneration.

central n., n. central; necrose que acomete as porções mais profundas ou internas de um tecido, órgão ou suas unidades.

coagulation n., n. de coagulação; tipo de necrose em que as células ou os tecidos afetados são convertidos numa massa eosinofílica seca, fosca e bastante homogênea sem coloração nuclear, em conseqüência da coagulação da proteína, como ocorre num infarto; microscopicamente, o processo necrótico envolve principalmente as células, e podem ser identificados remanescentes de elementos histológicos (p. ex., elastina, colágeno, fibras musculares), bem como "fantasmas" de células e fragmentos de membranas celulares; pode ser causada por calor, isquemia e outros agentes que destroem o tecido, incluindo enzimas que continuariam a alterar a substância celular desvitalizada.

colliquative n., n. coliquativa; termo obsoleto para referir-se à necrose liquefativa.

contraction band n., n. de faixas de contração. SIN contraction *band.*

cystic medial n., n. cística da média; perda de fibras elásticas e musculares na camada média da aorta, com acúmulo de mucopolissacarídeos, algumas vezes em espaços cistiformes entre as fibras; doença de causa desconhecida, que pode ser hereditária e que predispõe a aneurismas dissecantes. SIN Erdheim disease, medionecrosis aortae idiopathica cystica, medionecrosis of the aorta, mucoid medial degeneration.

epiphysial aseptic n., n. asséptica epifisária; necrose asséptica de epífises ósseas em crianças ou adultos, provavelmente devido a isquemia; pode afetar a extremidade superior do fêmur (doença de Legg-Calvé-Perthes), o tubérculo tibial (doença de Osgood-Schlatter), o osso navicular do tarso ou a patela (doença de Köhler), a cabeça do segundo metatarso (doença de Freiberg), corpos vertebrais (doença de Scheuermann) ou o capítulo do úmero (doença de Panner).

fat n., n. gordurosa; morte do tecido adiposo, caracterizada pela formação de pequenos focos (1–4 mm) brancos ou cinzentos, foscos e da consistência do giz, que representam pequenas quantidades de sabões de cálcio formados no tecido afetado, quando a gordura é hidrolisada a glicerol e ácidos graxos. SIN steatonecrosis.

fibrinoid n., n. fibrinóide; necrose em que o tecido necrótico exibe algumas reações de coloração que se assemelham à fibrina e tornam-se profundamente eosinofílicas, homogêneas e refráteis.

focal n., n. focal; ocorrência de numerosas porções de tecido habitualmente esferóides, relativamente pequenas ou diminutas e razoavelmente bem circunscritas, que manifestam necrose coagulativa, caseosa ou gomatosa, tipicamente associadas a agentes de disseminação hematogênica; com freqüência, é observada apenas em cortes histológicos, porém os focos podem ser grandes (até 1–3 mm) e macroscopicamente visíveis; arbitrariamente, os focos maiores que esses não costumam ser denominados necrose focal.

ischemic n., n. isquêmica; necrose causada por hipoxia em decorrência da privação local de suprimento sangüíneo, como ocorre no infarto.

laminar cortical n., n. cortical laminar; degeneração de uma camada celular definida no córtex cerebral, observada tipicamente após parada cardíaca temporária ou hipoxia perinatal.

liquefactive n., n. liquefativa; tipo de necrose caracterizada por lesão bem circunscrita, microscópica ou macroscopicamente visível, que consiste em remanescentes foscos, opacos ou turvos, branco-acinzentados ou amarelo-acinzentados, moles ou parcial ou totalmente líquidos de tecido que se tornou necrótico e foi digerido por enzimas, especialmente enzimas proteolíticas liberadas de leucócitos em desintegração; classicamente observada nos abscessos e, com freqüência, em infartos do cérebro.

progressive emphysematous n., n. enfisematosa progressiva. SIN gas *gangrene.*

progressive outer retinal n. (PORN), n. retiniana externa progressiva (NERP); síndrome viral que ocorre em pacientes com AIDS/SIDA, causada por herpesvírus e caracterizada pela destruição da retina periférica.

renal papillary n., n. papilar renal; necrose das papilas renais, que ocorre na pielonefrite aguda, especialmente em diabéticos ou na nefropatia por analgésicos; pode acarretar insuficiência renal. SIN necrotizing papillitis.

simple n., n. simples; estágio da necrose de coagulação; ocorrência de alteração grosseiramente granular ou hialina no citoplasma e ausência de núcleo reconhecível, com uma configuração geral relativamente inalterada das células mortas.

subcutaneous fat n. of newborn, n. gordurosa subcutânea do recém-nascido; placas e nódulos endurecidos que aparecem habitualmente alguns dias ou algumas semanas após o nascimento e que costumam regredir em alguns meses; caracterizada, microscopicamente, por cristais birrefringentes em forma de agulha no interior das células adiposas necróticas; a condição permanece localizada, ao contrário do esclerema do recém-nascido, embora possa haver desenvolvimento de hipercalcemia.

suppurative n., n. supurativa; necrose liquefativa com formação de pus.

total n., n. total; **(1)** necrose completa dos elementos citológicos e histológicos numa porção de tecido, como na necrose caseosa; **(2)** morte completa ou parcial de um órgão.

zonal n., n. zonal; necrose que afeta predominantemente, ou que se limita a, uma zona anatômica, especialmente partes dos lóbulos hepáticos definidos de acordo com a proximidade aos tratos porta ou veias centrais (hepáticas).

nec·ro·sper·mia (nek - rō - sper′mē - a). Necrospermia. Condição em que existem espermatozóides mortos ou imóveis no sêmen. [necro- + G. *sperma*, semente]

ne·cros·te·on, ne·cros·te·o·sis (nē - kros′tē - on, nē - kros - tē - ō′sis). Necrosteose. Gangrena do osso. [necro- + G. *osteon*, osso]

ne·crot·ic (nē - krot′ik). Necrótico. Relativo a ou acometido por necrose.

ne·crot·o·my (ne - krot′ō - mē). Necrotomia. **1.** SIN dissection. **2.** Operação para a remoção de uma porção necrosada de osso (seqüestro). [necro- + G. *tomē*, corte]

osteoplastic n., n. osteoplástica; remoção de um seqüestro ósseo através de uma janela articulada de osso, que é posteriormente recolocada.

nee·dle (nē′dl). Agulha. **1.** Instrumento fino, sólido e habitualmente pontiagudo utilizado para a perfuração de tecidos, suturas ou realização de ligadura em redor ou através de um vaso. **2.** Agulha oca utilizada para injeção, aspiração, biópsia ou para orientar a introdução de um cateter num vaso ou outro espaço. **3.** Separar os tecidos por meio de uma ou duas agulhas na dissecção de pequenas partes. **4.** Efetuar a discissão de uma catarata através de bisturi com ponta em agulha. [I.M. *nedle*, de A.S. *nǣdl*]

aneurysm n., artery n., a. de aneurisma, a. arterial; agulha de ponta romba, curva, colocada num cabo, com o olho na ponta, utilizada para efetuar uma ligadura em torno de uma artéria.

aspirating n., a. de aspiração; agulha oca utilizada para retirar líquido de uma cavidade, quando associada a um tubo aspirador fixado em uma extremidade.

atraumatic n., a. atraumática; agulha cirúrgica sem olho com o fio de sutura permanentemente fixado numa extremidade oca.

biopsy n., a. de biópsia; agulha oca utilizada para obter um fragmento de tecido para estudo histológico.

cataract n., a. de catarata. SIN knife n.

cutting n., a. cortante; agulha cirúrgica com superfície angulada para a punção de tecido.

Deschamps n., a. de Deschamps; agulha longa para sutura em tecidos profundos.

Emmet n., a. de Emmet; agulha forte com olho na ponta, tendo uma ampla curva e fixada a um cabo; utilizada para efetuar uma ligadura em torno de uma estrutura não-dissecada.

exploring n., a. exploradora; agulha forte com sulco longitudinal, que é colocada num tumor ou cavidade para determinar se existe líquido, que escapa ao longo do sulco.

Francke n., a. de Francke; pequena agulha em forma de lanceta, ativada por mola, utilizada para a evacuação de pequeno derrame de sangue.

Frazier n., a. de Frazier; agulha para drenagem dos ventrículos laterais do cérebro.

Gillmore n., a. de Gillmore; dispositivo para obter o tempo de colocação de cimento dentário.

Hagedorn n., a. de Hagedorn; agulha cirúrgica curva, achatada nos lados.

hypodermic n., a. hipodérmica; agulha oca, semelhante a uma agulha de aspiração, porém menor, fixada a uma seringa; utilizada primariamente para injeção.

knife n., a. de bisturi; bisturi muito estreito com ponta em agulha, utilizado na discissão de uma catarata. SIN cataract n.

lumbar puncture n., a. de punção lombar; agulha provida de estilete para penetrar no canal raquiano ou na cisterna magna, com um orifício de pelo menos 1 mm e comprimento de 40 mm ou mais.

Millner n., a. de Millner; agulha fina não-cortante com olho para a passagem de fio, freqüentemente utilizada para sutura da pele.

Salah sternal puncture n., a. de Salah para punção esternal; agulha de grande calibre para obtenção de amostras de medula vermelha do esterno.

spatula n., a. da espátula; agulha muito pequena com superfície côncava achatada (não-cortante), utilizada em cirurgia ocular.

stop-n., a. de interrupção; agulha cirúrgica com olho na extremidade, cuja haste possui uma saliência que se projeta para deter a agulha quando atingiu a distância desejada através dos tecidos.

Tuohy n., a. de Tuohy; agulha com abertura lateral na extremidade distal, destinada à passagem de um cateter através da luz da agulha para sair lateralmente, num ângulo de 45°; utilizada para a colocação de cateteres no espaço subaracnóide ou epidural.

Veress n., a. de Veress; agulha equipada com obturador com mola, utilizada para insuflação do abdome em cirurgia laparoscópica.

nee·dle-hold·er, nee·dle-car·ri·er, nee·dle-driv·er. Porta-agulha. Instrumento para segurar uma agulha durante a sutura. SIN needle forceps.

Needles, Carl F., pediatra norte-americano. *1935. VER Melnick-Needles *osteodystoplasty;* Melnick-N. *syndrome.*

Needles, J.W., dentista norte-americano. VER N split cast *method.*

nee·dling (nēd′ling). Discissão de uma catarata mole ou secundária.

Neelsen, Friedrich K.A., patologista alemão, 1854–1894. VER Ziehl-N. *stain.*

ne·en·ceph·a·lon (nē-en-sef′ă-lon). Neoencéfalo. Termo de Edinger para os níveis superiores do sistema nervoso central, superposto ao sistema metamérico ou proprioespinhal (paloencéfalo). SIN neoencephalon. [G. *neos,* novo + *enkephalos,* cérebro]

NEEP Abreviatura de negative end-expiratory *pressure* (pressão expiratória final negativa).

nef·o·pam hy·dro·chlo·ride (nef′ō-pam). Cloridrato de nefopam. Agente analgésico.

Neftel, William B., neurologista norte-americano, 1830–1906.

ne·ga·tion (nē-gā′shŭn). Negação. SIN denial.

neg·a·tive (neg′ă-tiv). Negativo, negativo. **1.** Não-afirmativo; refutativo; não-positivo; não-anormal. **2.** Indica ausência de resposta, ausência de reação ou ausência de entidade ou condição em questão. [L. *negativus,* de *nego,* negar]

neg·a·tive G. G. negativa. Gravidade na direção cefálica durante o vôo ou ao ficar de cabeça para o chão; oposto da G. positiva.

neg·a·tive S. Constante de flutuação. SIN flotation *constant.*

neg·a·tiv·ism (neg′ă-tiv-izm). Negativismo. Tendência a fazer o oposto daquilo solicitado ou resistência teimosa sem razão aparente; observado em estados catatônicos, bem como em crianças com 1 a 3 anos de idade.

neg·a·tron (neg′ă-tron). Negatron. Termo utilizado para um elétron, a fim de salientar a sua carga elétrica negativa em oposição à carga elétrica positiva apresentada pelo positron semelhante nos demais aspectos.

Negri, Adelchi, médico italiano, 1876–1912. VER N. *bodies,* em *body, corpuscles,* em *corpuscle.*

Negro, Camillo, neurologista italiano, 1861–1927. VER N. *phenomenon.*

Neisser, Albert L.S., médico alemão, 1855–1916. VER *Neisseria;* N. *coccus, syringe.*

Neisser, Max, bacteriologista alemão, 1869–1938. VER N. *stain.*

Neis·se·ria (nī-sē′rē-ă). *Neisseria.* Gênero de bactérias aeróbicas (família Neisseriaceae) contendo cocos Gram-negativos, que ocorrem em pares, com os lados adjacentes achatados. Esses microrganismos são parasitas de animais. A espécie típica é *N. gonorrhoeae.* [A. *Neisser*]

N. catarrhalis, termo antigo para *Moraxella catarrhalis.*

N. ca'viae, espécie encontrada na região faríngea de cobaias; pode ocorrer também em outros animais.

N. fla'va, espécie bacteriana encontrada nas mucosas das vias respiratórias humanas; facilmente confundida com *N. meningitidis.* SIN *N. subflava.*

N. flaves'cens, espécie encontrada no líquido cefalorraquidiano em casos de meningite; ocorre provavelmente nas mucosas das vias respiratórias humanas.

N. gonorrhoe'ae, espécie que causa gonorréia e outras infecções em seres humanos; a espécie típica do gênero *N.* SIN gonococcus, Neisser coccus.

N. haemol'ysans, nome antigo para *Gemella haemolysans.* VER *Gemella.*

N. meningi'tidis, espécie encontrada na nasofaringe de seres humanos, mas não em outros animais; agente etiológico da meningite meningocócica e da meningococcemia; os microrganismos purulentos são fortemente Gram-negativos e ocorrem isoladamente ou aos pares; no último caso, os cocos são alongados e dispostos com os eixos longitudinais paralelos e lados em forma de rim; os grupos caracterizados por polissacarídeos capsulares sorologicamente específicos são designados por letras maiúsculas (sendo os principais sorogrupos A, B, C e D). SIN meningococcus, Weichselbaum coccus.

N. sic'ca, espécie encontrada nas mucosas das vias respiratórias humanas.

N. subfla'va, SIN *N. flava.*

neis·se·ria, pl. **neis·se·ri·ae** (nī-sē′rē-ă, nī-sē′rē-ē). *Neisseria.* Termo vernacular utilizado para referir-se a qualquer membro do gênero *Neisseria.*

Nélaton, Auguste, cirurgião francês, 1807–1873. VER N. *catheter, fibers,* em *fiber, line, sphincter;* Roser-N. *line.*

Nelson, Don H., internista norte-americano, *1925. VER N. *syndrome, tumor.*

nem. Unidade nutricional definida como 1 grama de leite materno de componentes nutricionais específicos, com valor calórico equivalente a 2/3 de calorias. [Ger. *Nahrungseinheit Milch,* unidade de nutrição láctea]

△ **nema-, nemat-, nemato-.** Nema-, nemat-, nemato-. Fio, filiforme. [G. *nēma*]

nem·a·thel·minth (nem-ă-thel′minth). Nematelminto. Membro do antigo filo Nemathelminthes.

Nem·a·thel·min·thes (nem′-ă-thel-min′thēz). Nemathelminthes. Antigamente considerado um filo para incorporar os organismos pseudocelomados, que atualmente são divididos nos filos distintos Acanthocephala, Entoprocta, Rotifera, Gastrotricha, Kinorhyncha, Nematoda e Nematomorpha. [nemat- + G. *helmins, helminthos,* verme]

nem·a·ti·ci·dal, nem·a·to·ci·dal (nem′ă-ti-sī′dăl, -tō-sī′dăl). Nematocida. Destrutivo para vermes nematódeos.

nem·a·ti·cide, nem·a·to·cide (nē-mat′i-sīd, -ō-sīd). Nematocida. Agente que mata nematódeos. [nematode + L. *caedo,* matar]

nem·a·ti·za·tion (nem′ă-ti-zā′shŭn). Nematização. Infestação por nematódeos.

nem·a·to·blast (nem′ah-to-blast). Nematoblasto. SIN spermatid. [G. *nēma,* fio + *blastos,* germe]

nem·a·to·cyst (nem′ă-tō-sist). Nematocisto. Célula de celenterados provida de ferrão, que consiste num saco de veneno e num ferrão espiralado capaz de ser ejetado e de penetrar na pele de um animal quando este entra em contato; de considerável conseqüência nas grandes medusas e na caravela, em que o grande número dessas células providas de ferrão podem causar dor intensa e até mesmo morte. SIN cnida, cnidocyst. [nemato- + G. *kystis,* bexiga]

Nem·a·to·da (nem-ă-tō′dă). Nematoda. Vermes cilíndricos; grande filo que inclui muitos dos helmintos parasitas de seres humanos e um número ainda maior de parasitas vegetais e espécies não-parasitárias de vida livre no solo e na água. Para fins práticos, os nematódeos parasitas podem ser classificados em dois grupos, com base no *habitat* do verme adulto no corpo humano: 1) nematódeos intestinais (p. ex., os gêneros *Ascaris, Trichuris, Ancylostoma, Necator, Strongyloides, Enterobius* e *Trichinella*) e 2) nematódeos filariais do sangue, tecidos linfáticos e vísceras (p. ex., os gêneros *Wuchereria, Mansonella, Loa, Onchocerca* e *Dracunculus*). [nemat- + G. *eidos,* forma]

nem·a·tode (nem′ă-tōd). Nematódeo. Termo comum para referir-se a qualquer verme cilíndrico do filo Nematoda.

nem·a·to·di·a·sis (nem′ă-tō-dī′ă-sis). Nematodíase. Infestação por parasitas nematódeos.

cerebrospinal n., n. cefalorraquidiana; invasão do sistema nervoso central por larvas migratórias de nematódeos; p. ex., *Angiostrongylus cantonensis,* em ratos e seres humanos.

Nem·a·to·di·rel·la lon·gi·spi·cu·la·ta (nē′mă-tō-di-rel′ă lon′gi-spik-ū-lā′ta). Um dos nematódeos tricostrôngilos de pescoço filiforme, encontrado no intestino delgado de carneiros, cabras, renas, alce americano, boi almiscarado e antilocabra.

nem·a·toid (nem'ā - toyd). Nematóide. Relativo a nematódeos.

nem·a·tol·o·gist (nem - ă - tol'ō - jist). Nematologista. Especialista em nematologia.

nem·a·tol·o·gy (nem - ă - tol'ō - jē). Nematologia. Ciência relacionada com todos os aspectos dos nematódeos, sua biologia e sua importância para o homem. [nematode + G. *logos*, estudo]

nem·a·to·sper·mia (nem'a - tō - sper'mē - ă). Nematospermia. Espermatozóides com cauda alongada, como nos seres humanos, em contraste com a esferospermia. [nemat- G. *sperma*, semente]

Némethy, George, bioquímico húngaro-norte-americano, *1934. VER Adair-Koshland-Némethy-Filmer *model;* Koshland-N.-Filmer *model.*

neo-. Neo-. Novo, recente. [G. *neos*]

neoadjuvant (nē - ō - ad'joo - vant). Neo-adjuvante. Quimioterapia ou radioterapia administrada antes de cirurgia para câncer. [neo- + adjuvant]

ne·o·an·ti·gens (nē - ō - an'ti - jenz). Neo-antígenos. SIN tumor antigens, em antigen.

ne·o·ars·phen·a·mine (nē'ō - ar - sfen'a - mēn). Neo-arsfenamina. Antigamente utilizada como agente anti-sifilítico.

ne·o·ar·thro·sis (nē - ō - ar - thrō'sis). Neo-artrose. SIN nearthrosis.

Ne·o·as·ca·ris vi·tu·lo·rum (nē - ō - as'kă - ris vit - ū - lō'rŭm). O grande verme cilíndrico que ocorre no intestino delgado de bovinos, búfalo aquático e (raramente) ovinos; embora seja incomum nos Estados Unidos, trata-se de um grave parasita do gado bovino em muitas outras áreas. Já foi produzida uma infestação experimental em roedores e seres humanos.

ne·o·bi·o·gen·e·sis (nē'ō - bī - ō - jen'ē - sis). Neobiogênese. Teoria segundo a qual a vida pode originar-se de matéria não-viva. [neo- + G. *bios*, vida + *genesis*, origem]

neo·bladder (nē'ō - blad'er). Neobexiga. Reposição cirurgicamente constrita (utilizando habitualmente o estômago do intestino) da bexiga urinária.

ne·o·blas·tic (nē - ō - blas'tik). Neoblástico. Que se desenvolve em novo tecido ou que tem a característica de tecido novo. [neo- + G. *blastos*, germe, descendente]

ne·o·cer·e·bel·lum (nē'ō - ser - ē - bel'ŭm) [TA]. Neocerebelo. Termo filogenético para referir-se à porção lateral maior do hemisfério cerebelar, recebendo seu impulso dominante dos núcleos pontinos que, por sua vez, são dominados por nervos aferentes que se originam de todas as partes do córtex cerebral; do ponto de vista filogenético, tem origem mais recente do que o arquicerebelo e o paleocerebelo, q.v., o neocerebelo atinge o seu maior desenvolvimento no homem e em outros primatas. SIN corticocerebellum.

ne·o·chy·mo·tryp·sin·o·gen (nē - ō - kī'mō - trip - sin'ō - jen). Neoquimiotripsinogênio. Intermediário na conversão da quimiotripsina em α-quimiotripsina por clivagem da quimiotripsina.

ne·o·cin·cho·phen (nē - ō - sin'kō - fen). Neocincofeno. Éster etílico do ácido 6-metil-2-fenilquinolina-4-carboxílico; sua ação e usos são semelhantes aos do cincofeno.

ne·o·cor·tex (nē - ō - kōr'teks) [TA]. Neocórtex. SIN isocortex.

ne·o·cys·tos·to·my (nē'ō - sis - tos'tō - mē). Neocistostomia. SIN ureteroneocystostomy. [neo- + G. *kystis*, bexiga + *stoma*, boca]

ne·o·dym·i·um (Nd) (nē - ō - dim'ē - ŭm). Neodímio. Um dos raros elementos terrosos; número atômico 60, peso atômico 144,24. [*neo-*, novo, + G. *didymos*, gêmeo (de lantano)]

ne·o·en·ceph·a·lon (nē - ō - en - sef'ă - lon). Neo-encéfalo. SIN neencephalon.

ne·o·fe·tal (nē - ō - fē'tal). Neofetal. Relativo ao neofeto ou à transição entre os períodos embrionário e fetal de desenvolvimento.

ne·o·fe·tus (nē - ō - fē'tŭs). Neofeto. Organismo intra-uterino de cerca de 8 semanas de desenvolvimento.

ne·o·for·ma·tion (nē'ō - fōr - mā'shŭn). Neoformação. **1.** Formação de neoplasia ou neoplasma. **2.** Termo algumas vezes utilizado para indicar o processo de regeneração ou de tecido ou parte regenerada.

ne·o·gen·e·sis (nē - ō - jen'ē - sis). Neogênese. SIN regeneration (1). [neo- + G. *genesis*, origem]

ne·o·ge·net·ic (nē'ō - je - net'ik). Neogenético. Relativo a, ou caracterizado por, neogênese.

ne·o·ki·net·ic (nē'ō - ki - net'ik). Neocinético. Indica uma das divisões do sistema motor, cuja função consiste na transmissão de movimentos sinérgicos isolados de origem voluntária; representa uma forma mais especializada de movimento do que a função paleocinética. [neo- + G. *kinētikos*, relativo a movimento]

ne·o·lal·ism (nē - ō - lal'izm). Neolalismo. Uso anormal de neologismos na fala. [neo- + G. *laleō*, tagarelar]

ne·ol·o·gism (nē - ol'ō - jizm). Neologismo. Palavra ou frase nova elaborada pelo próprio paciente, que ocorre freqüentemente na esquizofrenia (p. ex., "sapato da cabeça" para referir-se a um chapéu) ou palavra já existente utilizada com novo sentido; em psiquiatria, esses usos podem ter significado apenas para o paciente ou indicar a sua condição. [neo- + G. *logos*, palavra]

ne·o·morph, ne·o·mor·phism (nē'ō - morf, nē'ō - mōr'fizm). Neomorfo, neomorfismo. Formação nova; estrutura encontrada em organismos superiores, ausente ou presente apenas em traços leves em ordens inferiores. [neo- + G. *morphē*, forma]

ne·o·my·cin sul·fate (nē - ō - mī'sin). Sulfato de neomicina. Sulfato de uma substância antibiótica antibacteriana produzida pelo crescimento de *Streptomyces fradiae,* ativa contra várias bactérias Gram-positivas e Gram-negativas.

ne·on (Ne) (nē'on). Néon, neônio. Gás inerte na atmosfera, separado do argônio por W. Ramsay e M. Travers em 1898; número atômico 10, peso atômico 20,1797. [G. *neos,* novo]

ne·o·na·tal (nē - ō - nā'tal). Neonatal. Relativo ao período que sucede imediatamente ao nascimento, que se estende durante os primeiros 28 dias de vida extra-uterina. SIN newborn. [neo- + L. *natalis*, relativo ao nascimento]

ne·o·nate (nē'ō - nāt). Neonato, recém-nascido. Lactente de 1 mês ou menos. SIN newborn. [neo- + L. *natus*, nascido, de *nascor*, nascer]

ne·o·na·tol·o·gist (nē'ō - nā - tol'ō - jist). Neonatologista. Especialista em neonatologia.

ne·o·na·tol·o·gy (nē'ō - nā - tol'ō - jē). Neonatologia. Subespecialidade pediátrica relacionada com os distúrbios do neonato. SIN neonatal medicine. [neo- + L. *natus,* pp. nascido + G. *logos,* teoria]

ne·o·neu·rot·i·za·tion (nē - ō - noo - rot'ī - zā'shun). Neoneurotização. Fenômeno raramente observado de retorno da função motora facial após transecção deliberada do nervo facial; acredita-se que representa a reinervação trigêmea dos músculos faciais.

ne·o·pal·li·um (nē - ō - pal'ē - ŭm). Neopálio. SIN isocortex.

ne·o·pho·bia (nē - ō - fō'bē - ă). Neofobia. Aversão mórbida a ou medo de novidades ou do desconhecido. [neo- + G. *phobos,* medo]

ne·o·pla·sia (nē - ō - plā'zē - ă). Neoplasia. Processo patológico que leva à formação e ao crescimento de neoplasia. [neo- + G. *plasis,* moldagem]

cervical intraepithelial n., n. intra-epitelial cervical; alterações displásicas que começam na junção escamocolunar do colo uterino, podendo constituir precursores do carcinoma de células escamosas: grau 1, displasia leve afetando o terço inferior ou menos da espessura epitelial; grau 2, displasia moderada com um a dois terços de comprometimento; grau 3, displasia grave ou carcinoma *in situ*, com comprometimento de dois terços a toda a espessura.

lobular n., n. lobular. SIN noninfiltrating lobular carcinoma.

multiple endocrine n. (MEN), n. endócrina múltipla (NEM); grupo de distúrbios caracterizados por tumores funcionais em mais de uma glândula endócrina. SIN familial multiple endocrine adenomatosis, multiple endocrine adenomatosis.

multiple endocrine n. 1 [MIM*131100], n. endócrina múltipla 1; síndrome caracterizada por tumores da hipófise, de células das ilhotas pancreáticas e das glândulas paratireóides, podendo estar associada à síndrome de Zollinger-Ellison; herança autossômica dominante, causada pela mutação do gene NEM1 no cromossomo 11q.

multiple endocrine n. 2 [MIM*171400], n. endócrina múltipla 2; síndrome associada a feocromocitoma, adenoma das paratireóides e carcinoma medular da tireóide; herança autossômica dominante, causada por mutação no oncogene RET, no cromossoma 10q.

multiple endocrine n. 3 [MIM*162300], n. endócrina múltipla 3; síndrome caracterizada por tumores encontrados na NEM2, constituição alta e magra, lábios proeminentes e neuromas na língua e nas pálpebras; herança autossômica dominante, causada por mutação no oncogene RET, no cromossoma 10q. SIN multiple endocrine n. 2B.

multiple endocrine n. 2B, n. endócrina múltipla 2B. SIN multiple endocrine n. 3.

multiple endocrine n., type 1, n. endócrina múltipla, tipo 1. SIN multiple endocrine neoplasia *syndrome, type 1.*

multiple endocrine n., type 2A (MEN2A), n. end na múltipla tipo 2A (NEM2A). SIN multiple endocrine neoplasia *syndrome, type 2A.*

prostatic intraepithelial n. (PIN), n. intra-epitelial prostática (NIP); alterações displásicas das glândulas e ductos da próstata, que podem constituir um precursor do adenocarcinoma; grau baixo (NIP 1), displasia leve com aglomeração celular, variação no tamanho e na forma do núcleo e espaçamento celular irregular; grau alto (NIP 2 e 3); displasia moderada a grave com aglomeração celular, nucleomegalia e nucleolomegalia e espaçamento celular irregular.

vaginal intraepithelial n., n. intra-epitelial vaginal; carcinoma de células escamosas pré-invasivo (carcinoma *in situ*), limitado ao epitélio vaginal; a exemplo da neoplasia intra-epitelial vulvar ou cervical, graduação histológica numa escala de 1 a 3 ou subdivisão em neoplasia maligna intra-epitelial de baixo grau e alto grau; em geral, relacionada à infecção por papilomavírus humano (HPV); pode evoluir para o carcinoma invasivo.

vulvar intraepithelial n., n. intra-epitelial vulvar; carcinoma de células escamosas pré-invasivo (carcinoma *in situ*), limitado ao epitélio vulvar; a exemplo da neoplasia intra-epitelial vaginal ou cervical, graduação histológica numa escala de 1 a 3 ou subdivisão em neoplasia maligna intra-epitelial de baixo grau e alto grau; em geral, relacionada à infecção por papilomavírus humano (HPV); pode evoluir para o carcinoma invasivo.

TERMOS DE RELAÇÃO

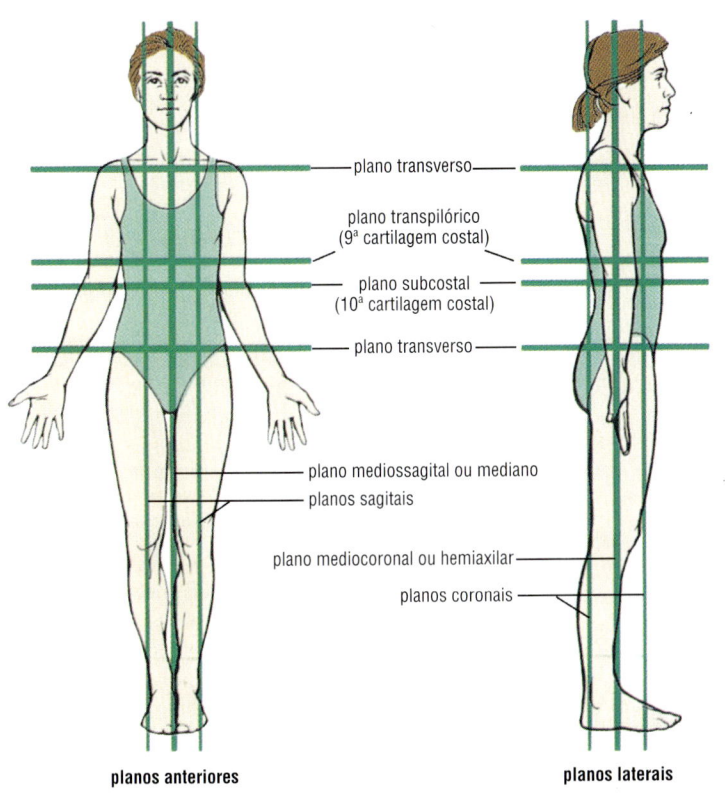

planos anteriores

planos laterais

Planos Anatômicos

Plano longitudinal:	obtido por corte ao longo do eixo longitudinal do corpo ou de uma parte do corpo; em posição ortostática, esse plano é denominado *vertical* e é perpendicular ao horizontal
Plano transverso:	obtido por corte através do corpo ou parte do corpo (em ângulo reto com o eixo longitudinal); se o paciente estiver de pé, esse plano é denominado *horizontal* (paralelo ao horizonte)
Plano mediossagital ou mediano:	plano longitudinal obtido por corte da frente (anterior) para trás (posterior) ao longo da linha mediana do corpo e ao longo da sutura sagital do crânio
Plano sagital:	plano longitudinal obtido por corte da frente (anterior) para trás (posterior) de cada lado da sutura sagital e paralelo ao plano mediossagital ou mediano
Plano coronal:	plano longitudinal obtido por corte longitudinal de um lado ao outro através da cabeça e do corpo (ou parte do corpo) ao longo da sutura coronal do crânio ou paralelo a ela
Plano transpilórico:	plano transverso obtido por corte através de um lado ao outro ao nível das 9as cartilagens costais; o nome desse plano reflete o fato de que deve atravessar o piloro do estômago
Plano mediocoronal (axilar médio):	plano longitudinal obtido por corte através da cabeça e do corpo ao longo da sutura coronal da cabeça e extensão descendente do corte pelo corpo

Terminologia das Partes do Corpo

Anterior:	na frente de (em direção à frente do corpo ou de uma estrutura dentro dele); algumas vezes é denominado *ventral*
Posterior:	na parte de trás de (em direção à parte de trás do corpo ou de uma estrutura dentro dele); algumas vezes é denominado *dorsal*
Proximal:	mais próximo do ponto de fixação ou origem; nas extremidades, mais próximo do tronco
Distal:	mais distante do ponto de fixação ou origem; nas extremidades, mais distante do tronco
Cefálico, superior:	em direção à cabeça ou parte superior de uma estrutura
Caudal, inferior:	em direção oposta à cabeça ou parte superior de uma estrutura (literalmente significa "em direção à cauda")

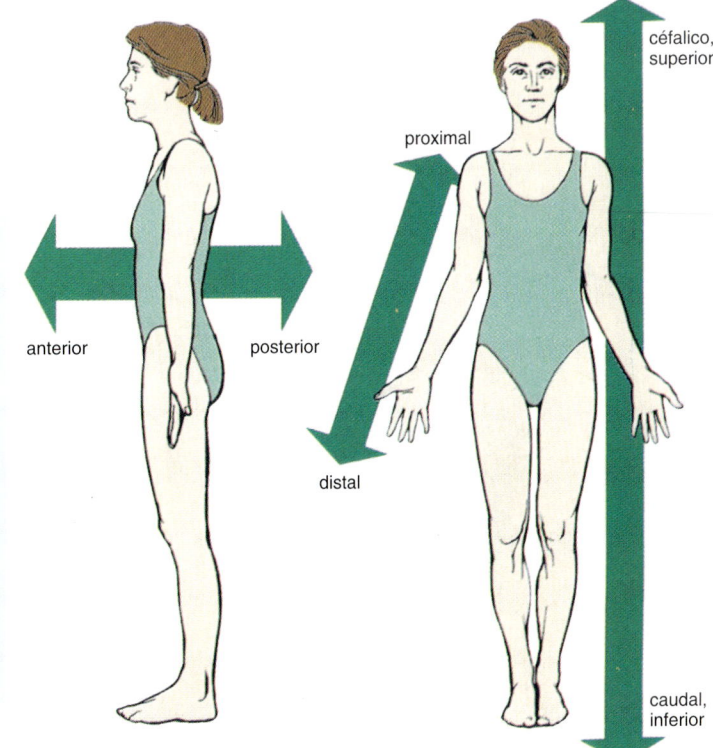

Diagnóstico por Imagens

TERMOS DE MOVIMENTO

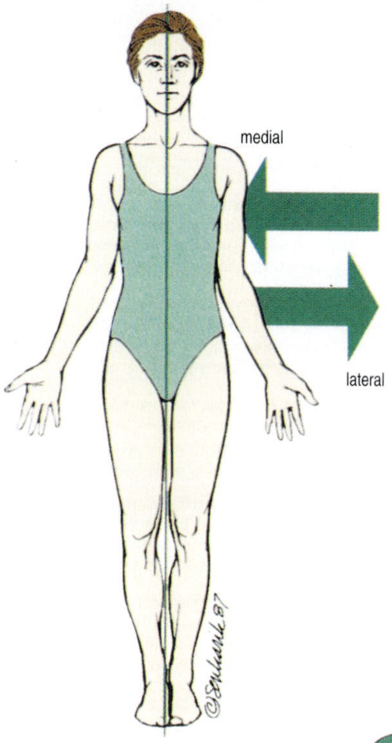

Terminologia das Partes do Corpo (*continuação*)

Medial: em direção à linha média do corpo

Lateral: que se afasta da linha média do corpo (para o lado)

Movimento do Corpo

Abdução: movimento de afastamento de um membro ou parte do corpo em relação à linha média do corpo

Adução: movimento de aproximação de um membro ou parte do corpo em direção à linha média do corpo

Extensão: retificação de uma articulação ou extremidade de forma que o ângulo entre ossos contíguos (adjacentes) esteja aumentado

Flexão: curvatura de uma articulação ou extremidade de forma que o ângulo entre ossos contíguos (adjacentes) esteja diminuído

Eversão: movimento de rotação de uma parte do corpo para fora (afastando-se da linha média)

Inversão: movimento de rotação de uma parte do corpo para dentro (em direção à linha média)

Pronação: movimento de rotação de uma parte do corpo para ficar voltada para baixo, ou rotação da mão de forma que a palma fique voltada para baixo

Supinação: movimento de rotação de uma parte do corpo para ficar voltada para cima, ou de rotação da mão de forma que a palma fique voltada para cima

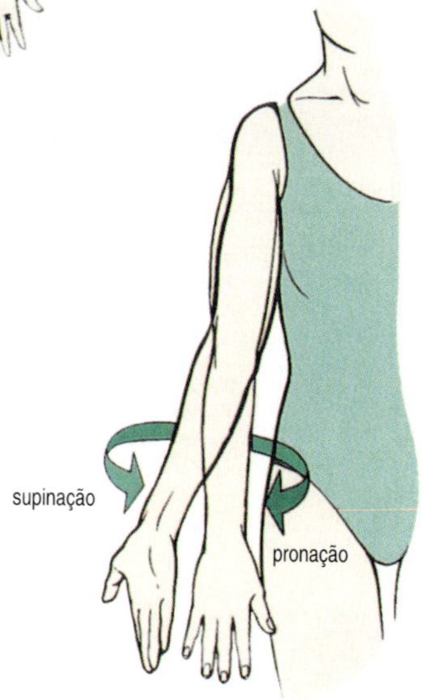

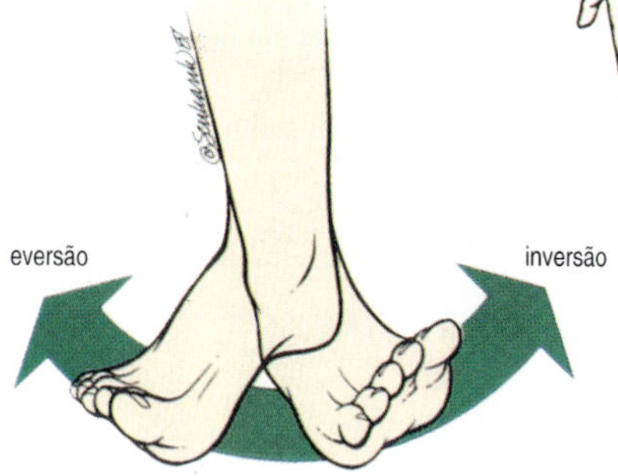

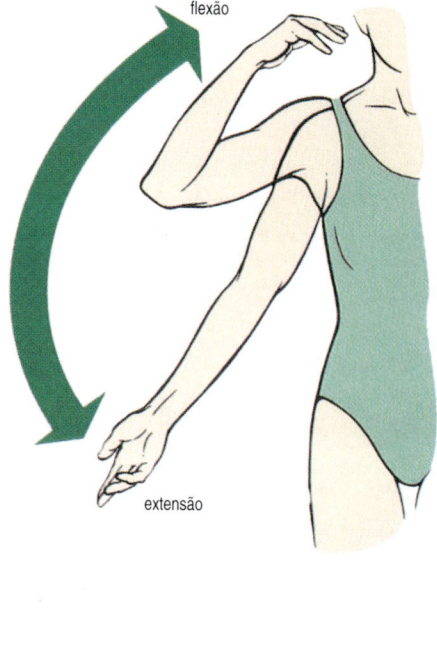

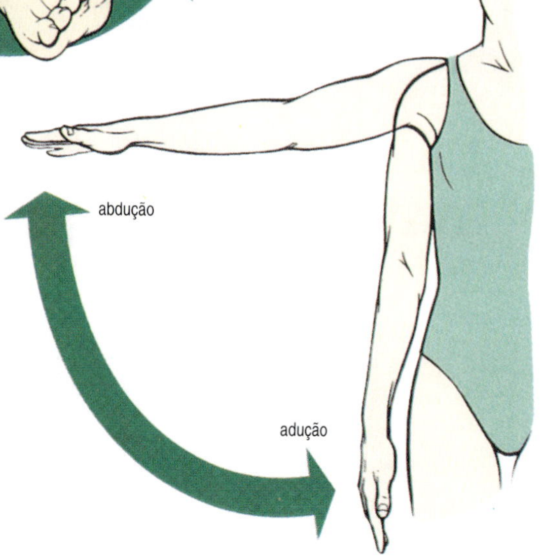

POSICIONAMENTO

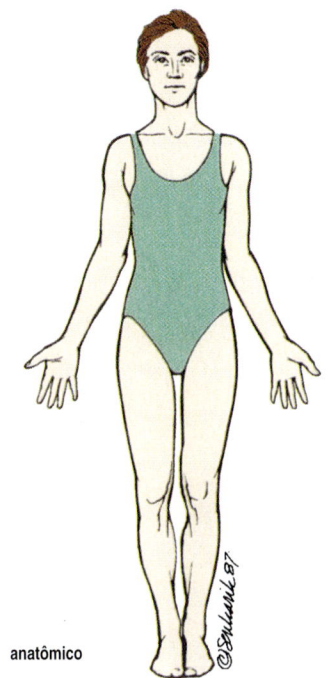

anatômico

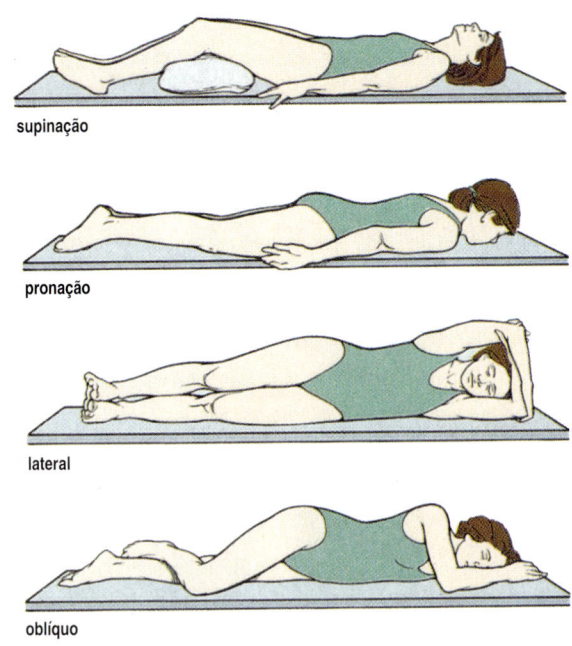

supinação

pronação

lateral

oblíquo

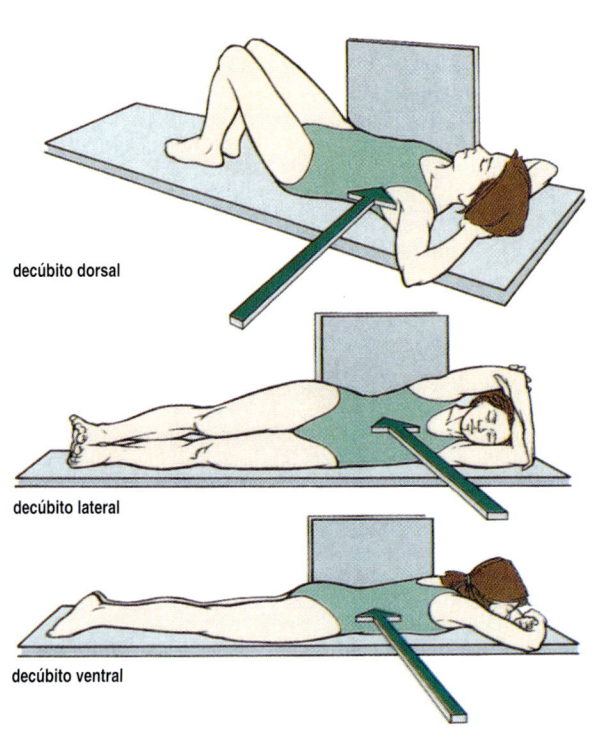

decúbito dorsal

decúbito lateral

decúbito ventral

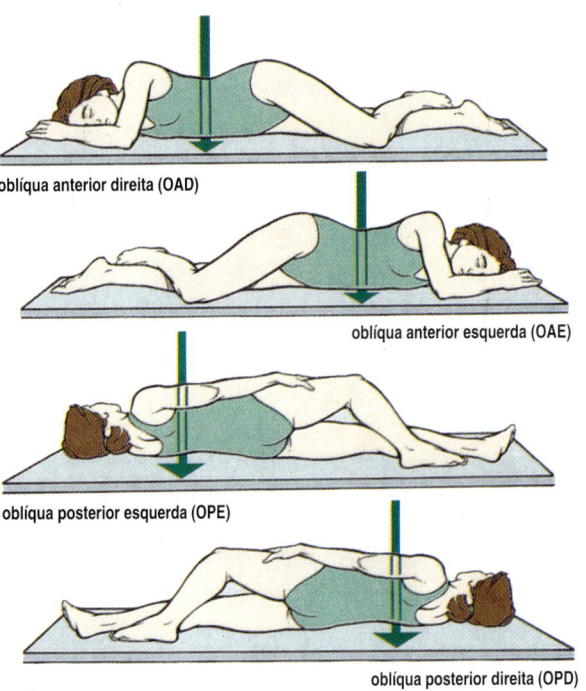

oblíqua anterior direita (OAD)

oblíqua anterior esquerda (OAE)

oblíqua posterior esquerda (OPE)

oblíqua posterior direita (OPD)

Diagnóstico por Imagens

OFTALMOSCOPIA

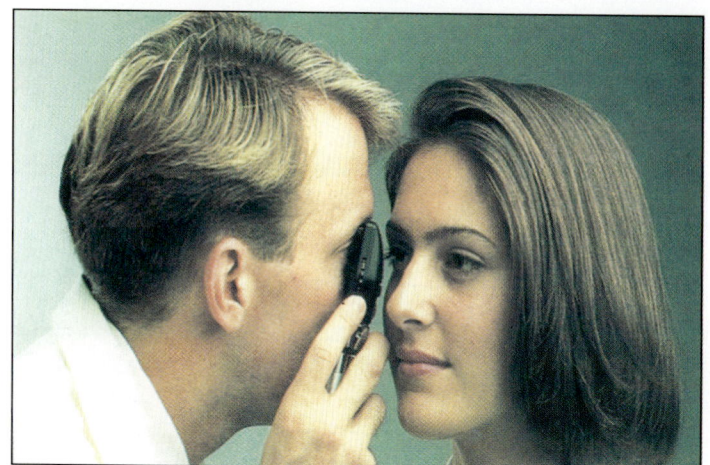
médico examinando paciente usando oftalmoscópio

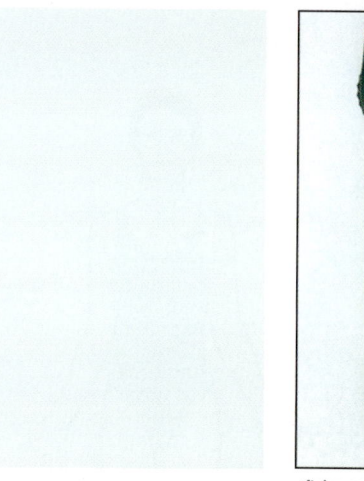
oftalmoscópio

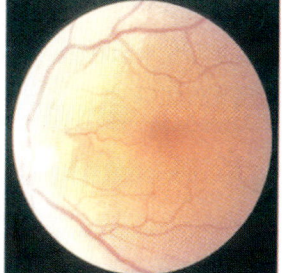
fundo normal

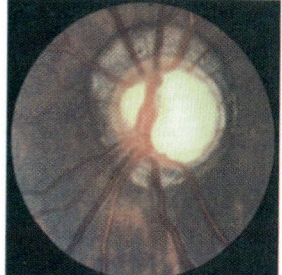
cálice glaucomatoso do disco

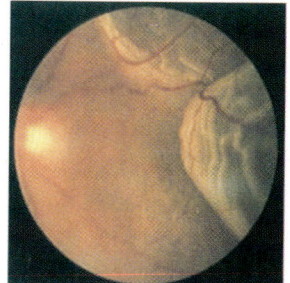
descolamento da retina

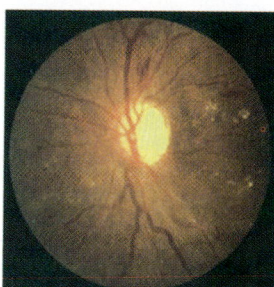
retinopatia diabética não-proliferativa

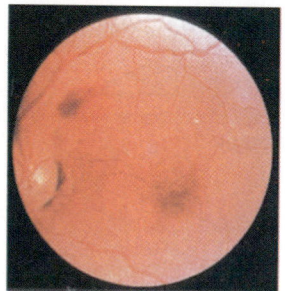
retinopatia hipertensiva

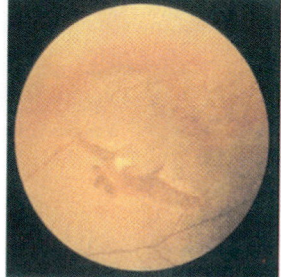
ruptura da retina

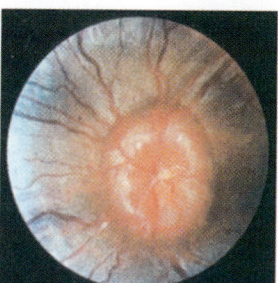
papiledema

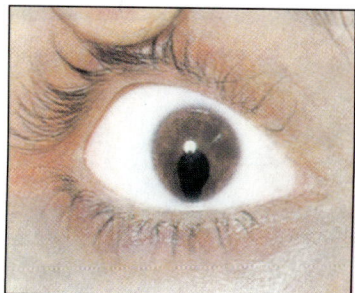
coloboma

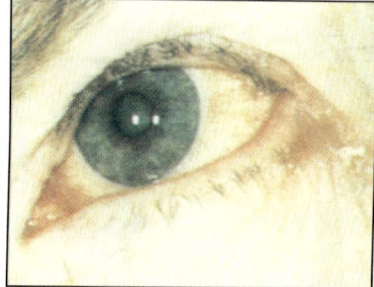
blefarite angular (*Staphylococcus aureus*)

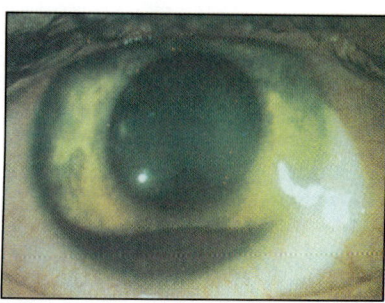
hifema

OTOSCOPIA

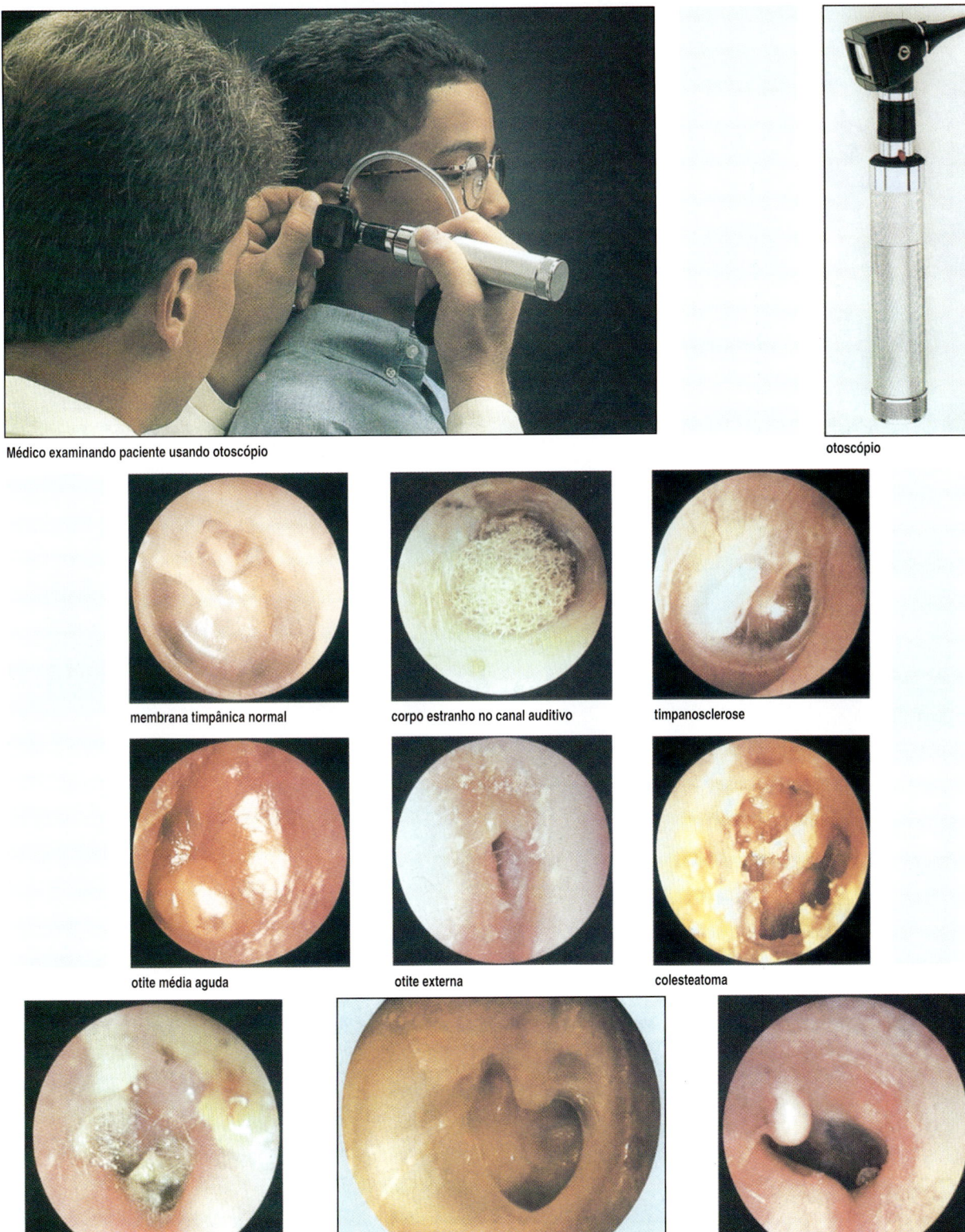

ESTUDO DOS DENTES POR IMAGENS

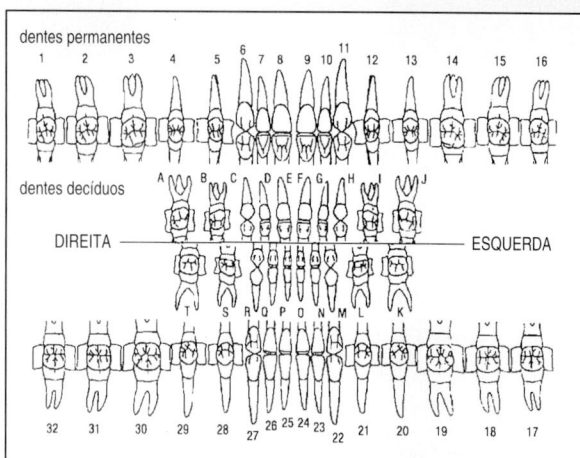

ficha odontológica: mostrando todas as superfícies dos dentes permanentes e decíduos; os dentes numerados de 1–16 são dentes permanentes maxilares, de 17–32 são dentes permanentes mandibulares; os dentes designados A–J e K–T são, respectivamente, dentes decíduos maxilares e mandibulares

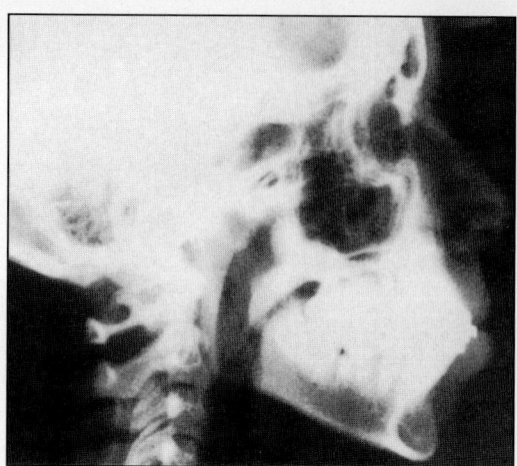

radiografia cefalométrica: mostrando estruturas ósseas e tecidos moles sobrejacentes

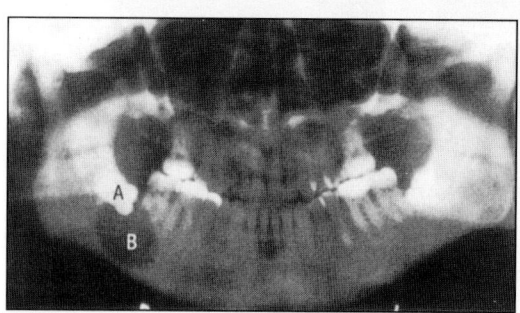

radiografia panorâmica: dentição de adulto, terceiro molar mandibular incluso (A) e grande cisto no osso mandibular ao redor da coroa do molar (B)

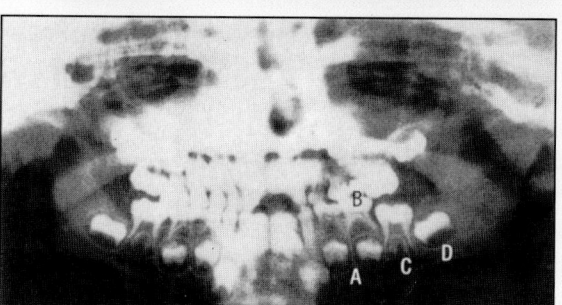

radiografia panorâmica: dentição mista; molares mandibulares permanentes parcialmente formados (A) irrompendo abaixo dos molares decíduos (B); primeiro molar permanente irrompido com raízes incompletamente formadas (C); coroa do segundo molar permanente, incluso, incompletamente formado (D)

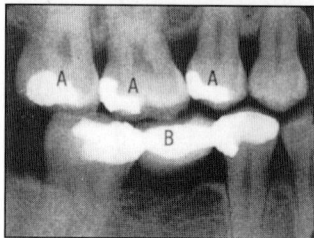

restaurações de amálgama (A) e ponte fixa (B); radiografia interproximal (*bitewing*)

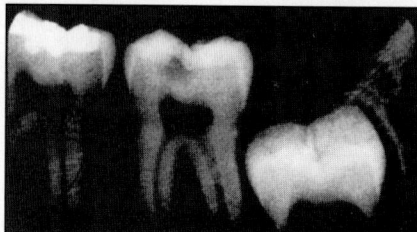

3º molar não-irrompido: a coroa está formada, mas as raízes estão incompletas

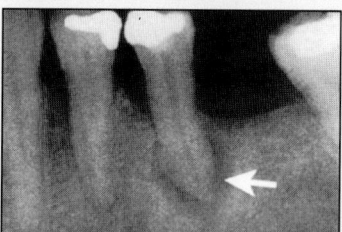

área radiotransparente (seta) ao redor da raiz do pré-molar mandibular indicando processo patológico

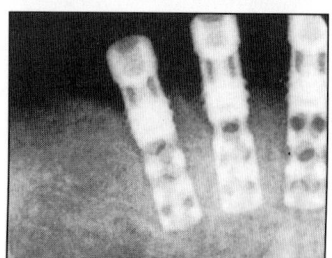

implantes endosteais: no osso alveolar; as coroas ainda não estão no lugar

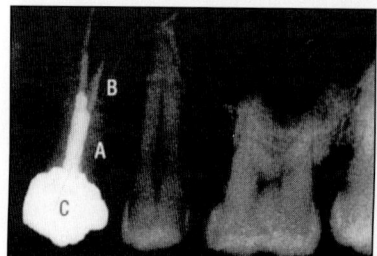

obturação do canal da raiz (A); pinos para retenção (B) para coroa protética revestida de metal (C)

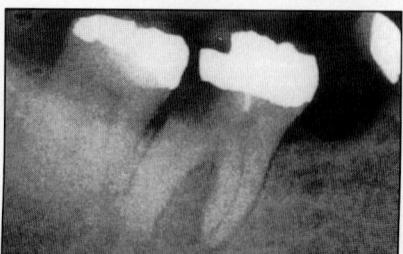

cárie recorrente após uma restauração metálica em um molar

ODONTOLOGIA ESTÉTICA

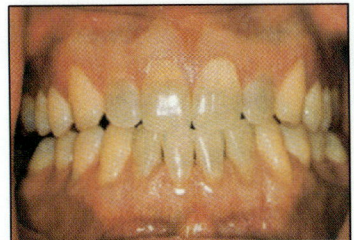
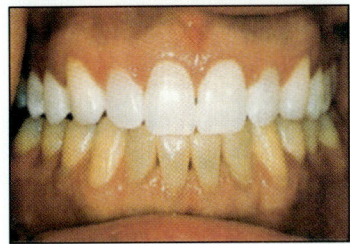

clareamento vital dos dentes para remover manchas causadas por tetraciclina; (em cima) antes, (embaixo) depois

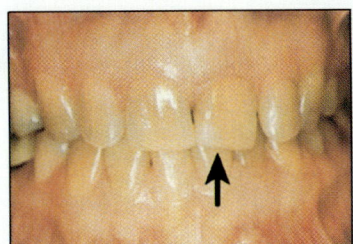
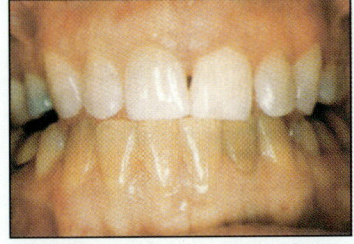

restauração imperfeita (seta em cima): os dentes maxilares foram clareados (embaixo) para remover manchas causadas por tetraciclina e a restauração foi substituída

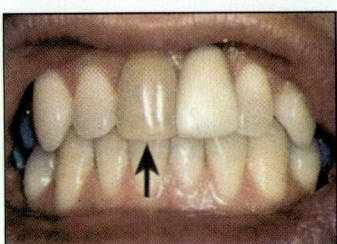
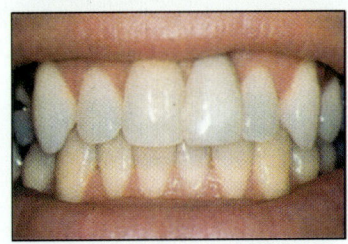

incisivo central submetido a coloração não-vital (seta em cima): clareado para fins estéticos (embaixo)

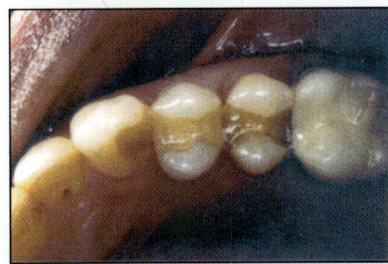
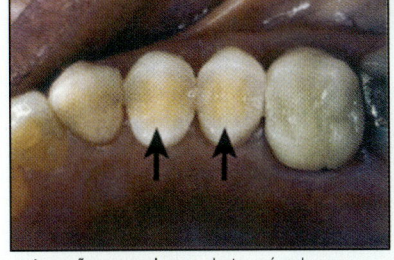

restaurações por resina: em dentes pré-molares e cúspides (em cima); restaurações de aspecto desagradável substituídas por restaurações de resina estéticas (setas na imagem inferior)

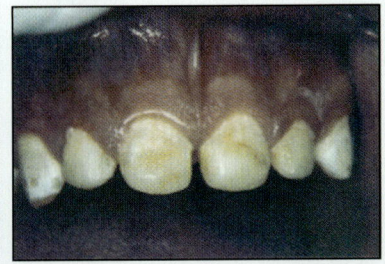
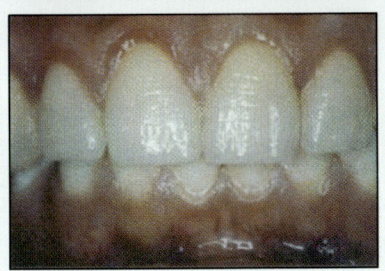
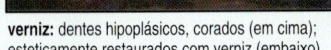

verniz: dentes hipoplásicos, corados (em cima); esteticamente restaurados com verniz (embaixo)

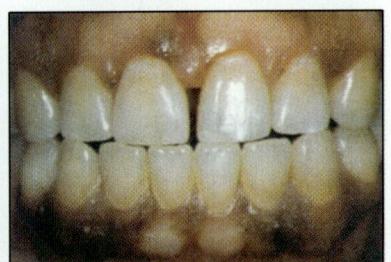
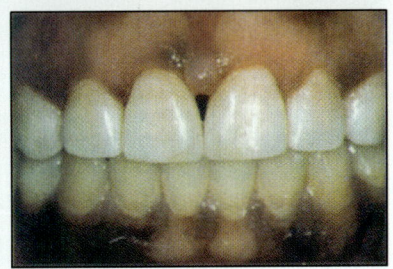

diastema (em cima): entre dentes fechados por verniz composto de resina (embaixo)

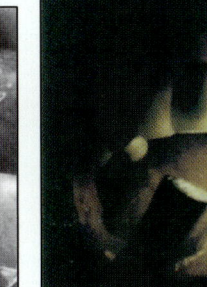

ponte estética unida por resina: (à extrema esquerda) a estrutura metálica está ligada a dentes naturais, sem coroa, de apoio e segura à prótese dental (seta)

coroas de porcelana: (esquerda) transiluminadas, mostrando como as coroas podem ser feitas para preservar a transparência natural

Diagnóstico por Imagens

ENDOSCOPIA

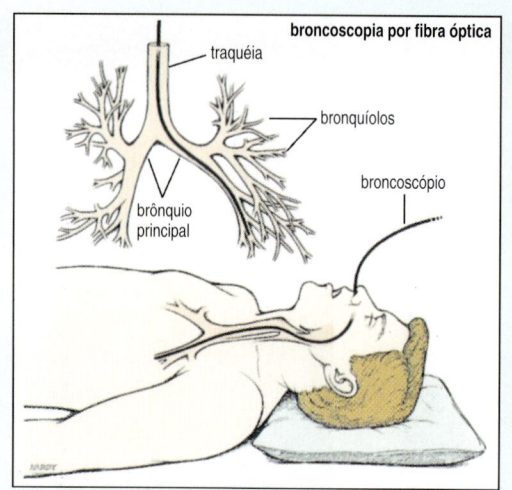

broncoscopia por fibra óptica
- traquéia
- bronquíolos
- brônquio principal
- broncoscópio

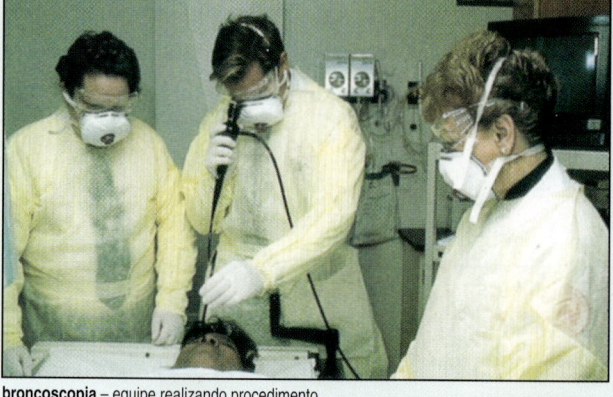

broncoscopia – equipe realizando procedimento

broncoscopia é o exame do aparelho respiratório com um broncoscópio flexível para fins de diagnóstico ou tratamento; o broncoscópio é introduzido por via nasal e lentamente levado para a traquéia até se chegar ao nível desejado; as fotografias nesta página foram feitas com uma câmera acoplada à extremidade do instrumento que fica com o examinador

carcinoma laríngeo
- prega vocal
- carcinoma

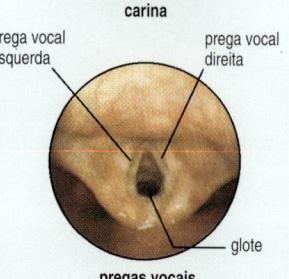

- toda a traquéia e a carina — carina
- carina — brônquio principal esquerdo, carina, brônquio principal direito
- brônquio lobar superior direito — B¹, B², B³
- pregas vocais — prega vocal esquerda, prega vocal direita, glote

esofagogastroduodenoscopia é o exame do esôfago, estômago e parte superior do intestino delgado utilizando um esofagogastroduodenoscópio flexível; as fibras ópticas no instrumento permitem a passagem de luz fria, brilhante por um trajeto curvo, permitindo a iluminação dos tecidos e estruturas dentro do corpo; o escópio freqüentemente contém pequenos instrumentos como alças para biopsia

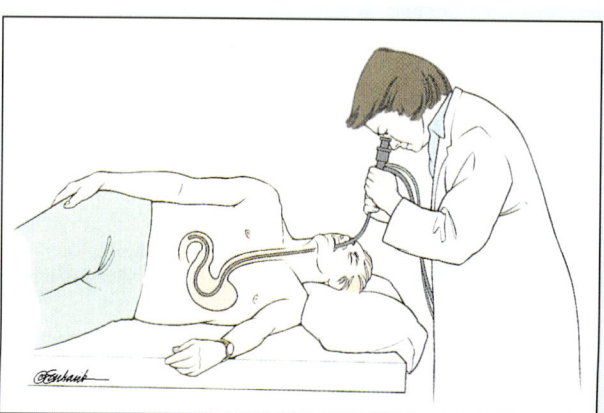

esofagoduodenoscópio é introduzido por via nasal ou oral e levado lentamente pelo esôfago e trato gastrointestinal até que se chegue ao nível desejado

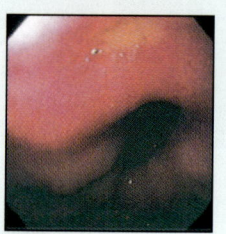

gastrite

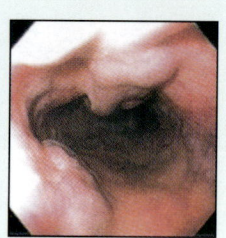

varizes esofágicas

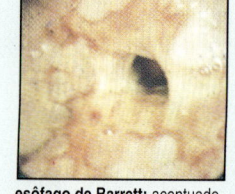

esôfago de Barrett: acentuado estreitamento esofágico

pólipo gástrico hiperplásico pediculado

ENDOSCOPIA

cistoscopia é a inspeção do interior da bexiga utilizando um cistoscópio, um tubo flexível que contém fibra óptica e pequenos instrumentos; o cistoscópio é introduzido através da uretra e lentamente avançado até chegar à bexiga; a cistoscopia pode ser usada em procedimentos de diagnóstico e em pequenos procedimentos cirúrgicos, conforme se observa nas duas imagens cistoscópicas abaixo

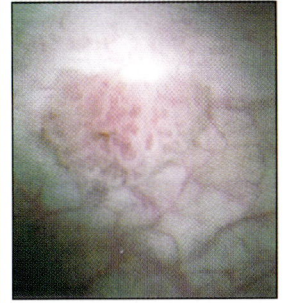

tumor vesical: na superfície interna da bexiga

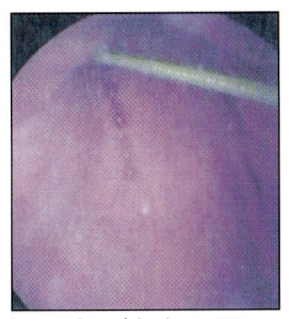

imagem cistoscópica de um cateter sendo introduzido em um ureter

colangiografia intra-operatória: está sendo feito um corte limpo na parede lateral do ducto cístico de forma que possa ser introduzido um cateter

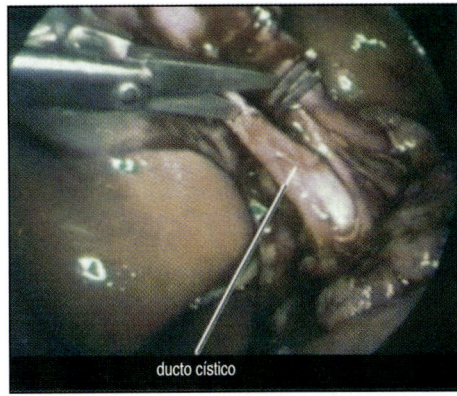

ducto cístico

laparoscopia envolve a introdução de um laparoscópio na cavidade peritoneal através de uma incisão de 2 cm abaixo do umbigo para permitir visualização das estruturas pélvicas (abaixo, à esquerda); as indicações de laparoscopia são diagnósticas; a laparoscopia também pode facilitar pequenos procedimentos cirúrgicos, como a ligadura tubária, a biopsia ovariana e a lise de aderências; nesse caso, uma pinça é introduzida através do escópio para segurar a tuba uterina; a insuflação de gás cria uma bolsa de ar (pneumoperitônio), e a pelve é elevada, o que força a elevação dos intestinos no abdome

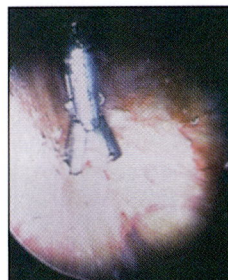

biopsia laparoscópica

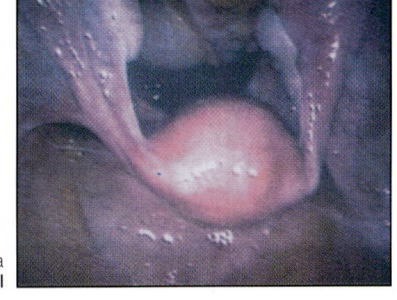

imagem laparoscópica da **pelve normal**

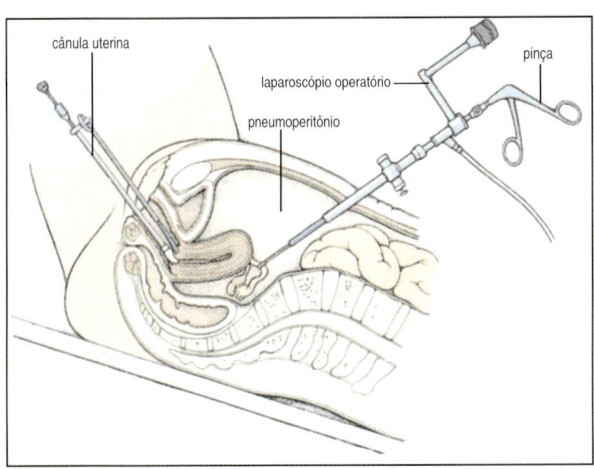

cânula uterina — laparoscópio operatório — pinça — pneumoperitônio

toracoscopia é um procedimento diagnóstico no qual a cavidade pleural é examinada com um endoscópio (direita); são feitas pequenas incisões na cavidade pleural em um espaço intercostal; o uso de instrumentos de fibra óptica e de equipamento de vídeo miniaturizado permite a visualização das estruturas torácicas; o tecido pode ser excisado para biopsia, e pode ser realizado tratamento de alguns distúrbios torácicos

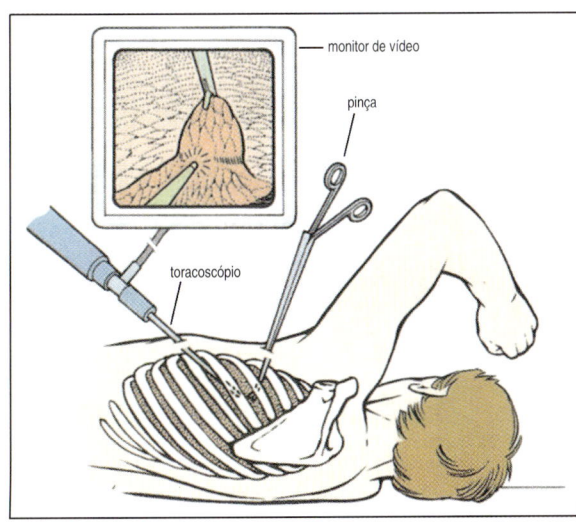

monitor de vídeo — pinça — toracoscópio

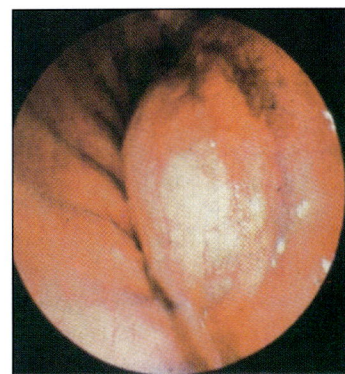

cavidade pleural: imagem toracoscópica; os vasos intercostais podem ser observados à esquerda e a pleura retraída medialmente à direita

Diagnóstico por Imagens

ENDOSCOPIA

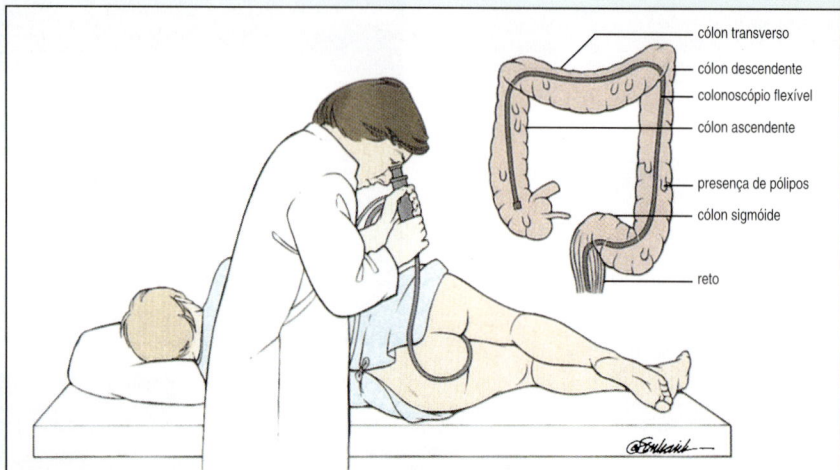

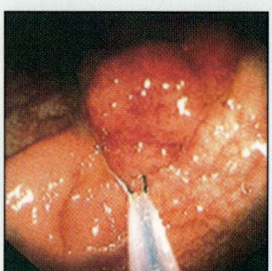
polipectomia do cólon

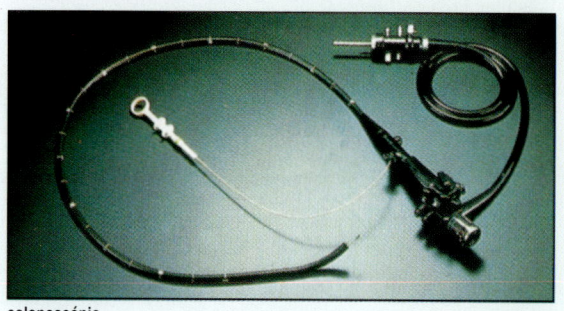
colonoscópio

colonoscopia é o exame e diagnóstico de afecções do cólon; o colonoscópio flexível atravessa o reto e o cólon sigmóide até o cólon descendente, transverso e ascendente (acima); pequenos instrumentos podem ser introduzidos pelo colonoscópio e usados para facilitar pequenos procedimentos cirúrgicos; as imagens à direita foram feitas por uma câmera acoplada ao colonoscópio

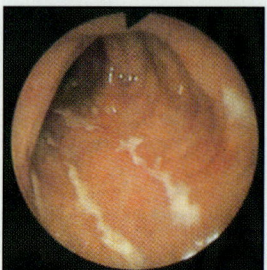
colite ulcerativa

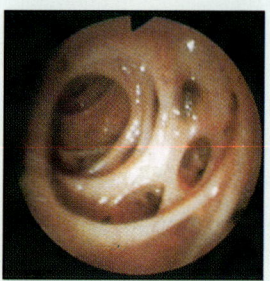
diverticulose

artroscopia é o exame endoscópico do interior de uma articulação; são feitas pequenas incisões, conhecidas como portais, para a introdução do artroscópio e de outros instrumentos; o artroscópio contém fibras ópticas e uma minicâmera de vídeo que projeta a anatomia e o procedimento em um monitor de vídeo (direita); uma segunda cânula contém instrumentos e equipamento motorizado usados para reparar estruturas e remover o tecido lesado; freqüentemente é introduzida solução salina através de uma terceira cânula para expandir a articulação e remover qualquer sangue ou fragmento; as imagens abaixo foram capturadas utilizando-se uma câmera artroscópica

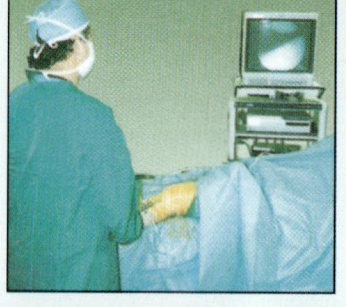
artroscopia do joelho: o cirurgião usa o monitor de vídeo para observar o progresso

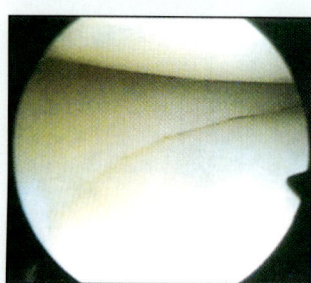
menisco lateral normal do joelho

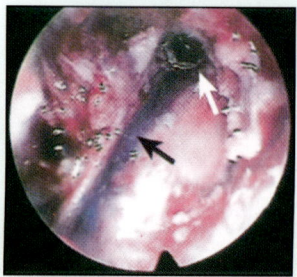
enxerto do LCA (seta preta) com parafuso de interferência femoral visível (seta branca)

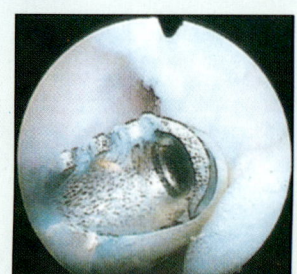
desbastamento de um menisco lateral roto

ULTRA-SONOGRAFIA

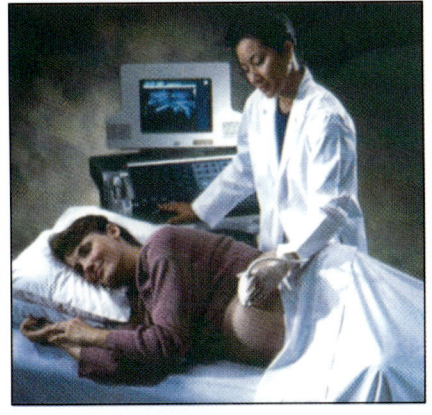

durante a **ultra-sonografia** (direita), a energia na forma de ondas sonoras é refletida pelos órgãos internos ou, durante a gravidez, pelo feto, sendo transformada em imagem em um monitor tipo TV; no caso de ultra-sonografia obstétrica (esquerda), é feita uma imagem ultra-sonográfica do útero grávido para determinar o desenvolvimento fetal

ultra-sonografia obstétrica realizada em uma gestante

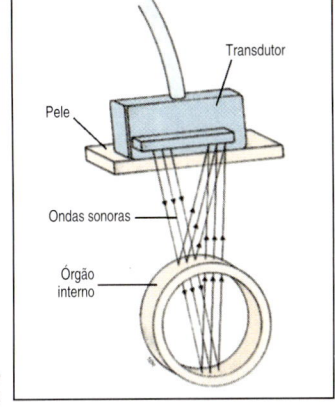

princípio de ultra-sonografia

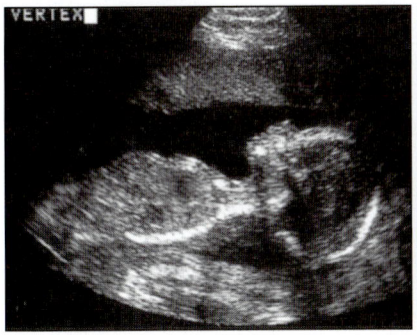

feto em posição pélvica: imagem sagital

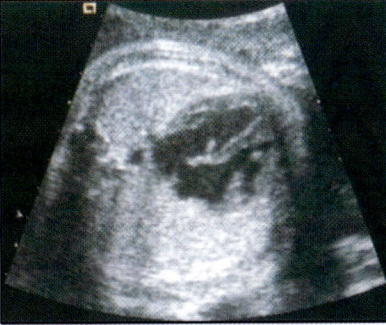

coração fetal: imagem transversa, as câmaras são áreas escuras circundadas pelos pulmões

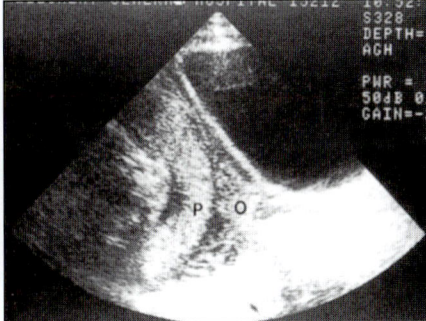

placenta prévia: imagem longitudinal mostra a placenta (P) situada logo acima do óstio cervical (O)

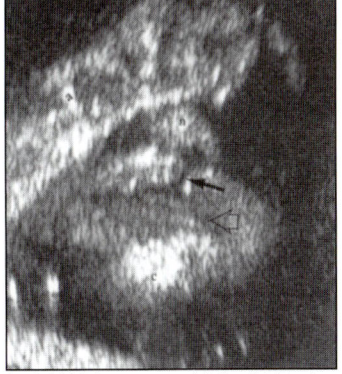

fenda labial: imagem coronal da face fetal mostra uma fenda (seta), no lábio esquerdo, que se estende até a narina esquerda; boca (seta aberta), nariz (n), queixo (c)

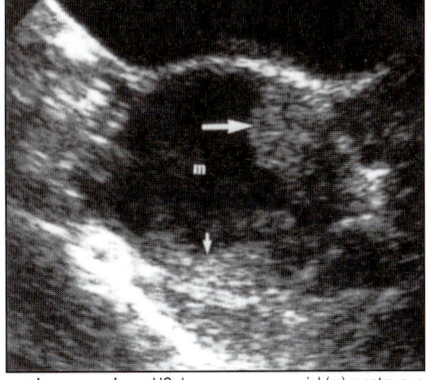

carcinoma ovariano: US de uma massa anexial (m) mostra que esta é predominantemente cística, mas possui uma parede espessa (seta pequena) e um nódulo sólido proeminente (seta grande)

durante **ultra-sonografia Doppler,** um instrumento emite um feixe de ultra-som para o interior do corpo; o ultra-som refletido pelas estruturas em movimento modifica sua freqüência (efeito Doppler); a ultra-sonografia Doppler freqüentemente é usada no diagnóstico de doença vascular periférica e cardíaca

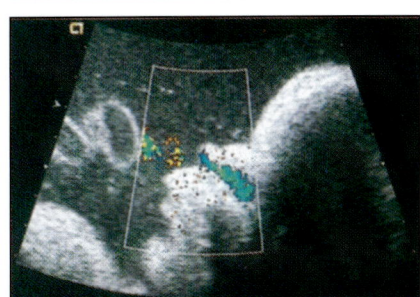

ultra-sonografia Doppler de fluxo mostrando o fluxo de líquido amniótico para a cavidade nasal do feto

ecocardiografia é o uso de ultra-som na investigação do coração e dos grandes vasos e no diagnóstico de lesões vasculares (esquerda e extrema esquerda)

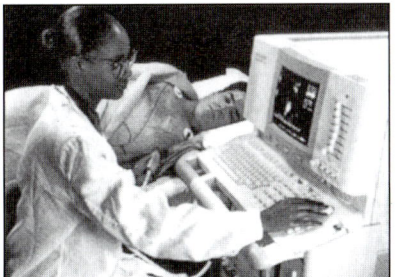

técnica de ecocardiografia

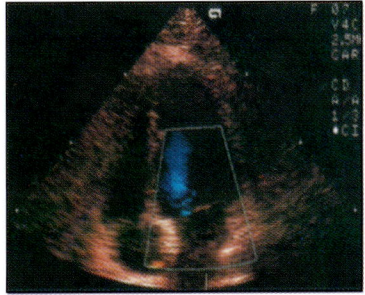

ecocardiograma: normal, imagem bidimensional, apical das quatro câmaras

Diagnóstico por Imagens

RADIOGRAFIA

radiografia é o exame de qualquer parte do corpo para fins diagnósticos por meio de raios X com o registro dos achados geralmente impresso em um filme fotográfico

como mostrado no gráfico adiante, a absorção diferencial de raios X depende da composição de vários tecidos, o tecido mais denso (como o osso) absorve mais raios X, o tecido menos denso (como a gordura subcutânea) transmite mais raios X; a maior absorção produz menor escurecimento no filme, enquanto a menor absorção produz maior escurecimento; a imagem radiográfica resultante é essencialmente um "exame de imagens"

as imagens da **radiografia de tórax simples** nestas duas páginas mostram várias condições patológicas do tórax e do sistema respiratório

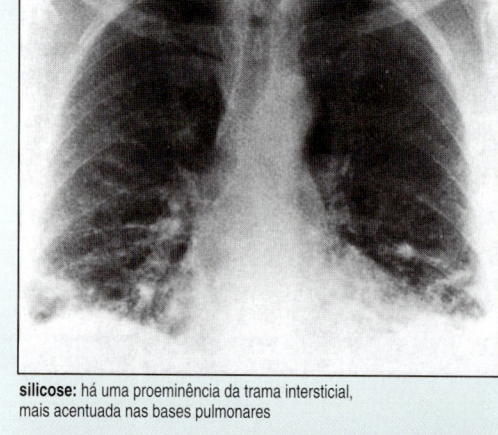

silicose: há uma proeminência da trama intersticial, mais acentuada nas bases pulmonares

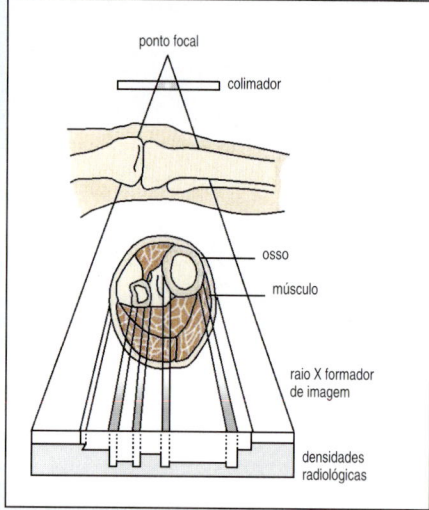

raios X atravessam a parte do corpo, com as estruturas mais densas absorvendo mais raios X, resultando nas áreas mais claras na radiografia

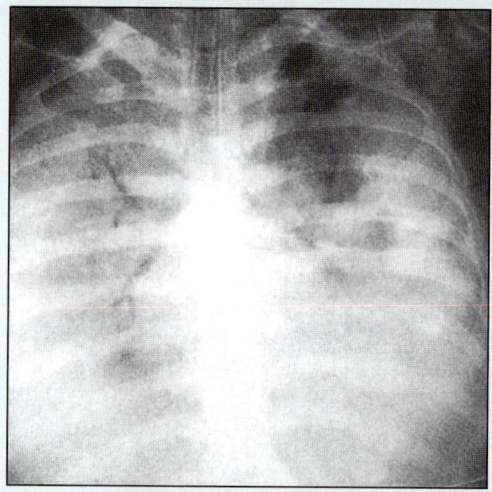

síndrome de angústia respiratória do adulto (SARA)

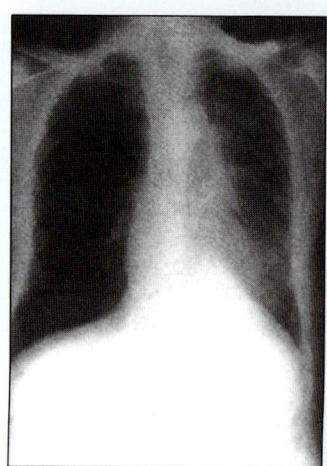 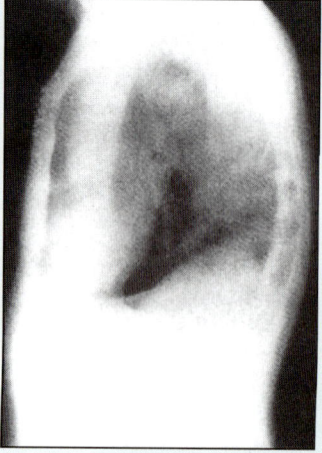

colapso do lobo superior esquerdo: incidência póstero-anterior (esquerda) e lateral (direita)

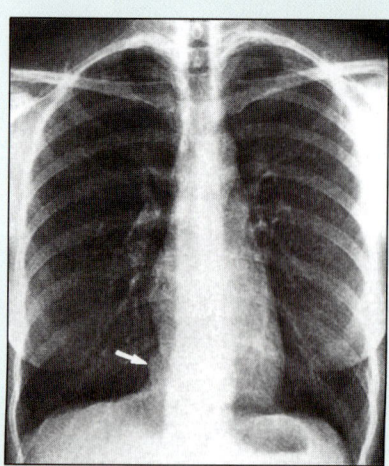

cisto pericárdico: (seta)

RADIOGRAFIA

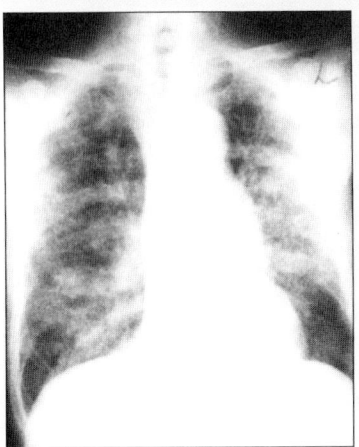
doença pulmonar intersticial

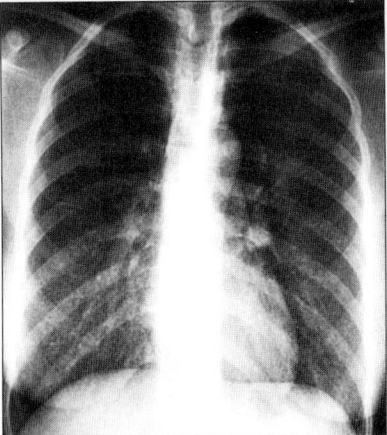
tuberculose miliar: em pacientes com AIDS/SIDA mostrando padrão nodular difuso fino em ambos os lobos inferiores

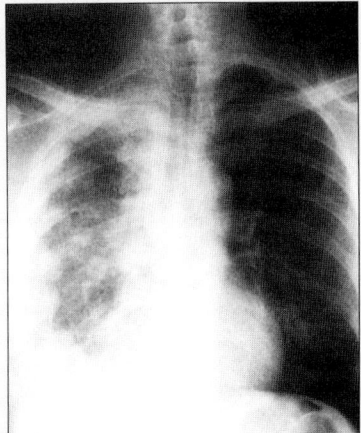
mesotelioma maligno: observe o espessamento pleural direito lobulado, compreendendo o pulmão direito

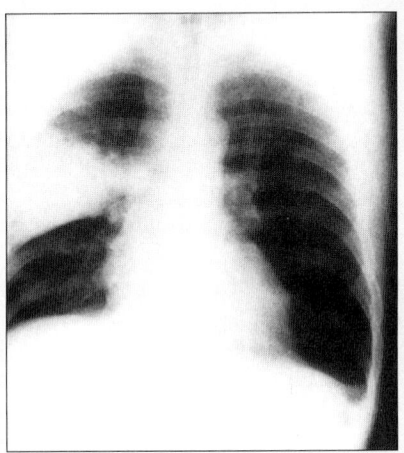
pneumonia bacteriana: no lobo superior direito

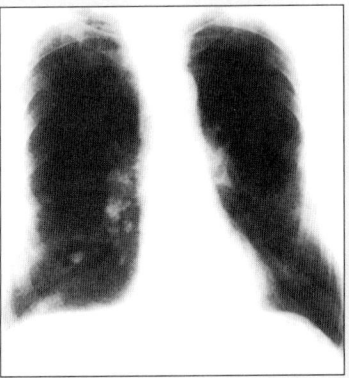
complexo de Ranke: com foco de Ghon no lado direito secundário à tuberculose cicatrizada

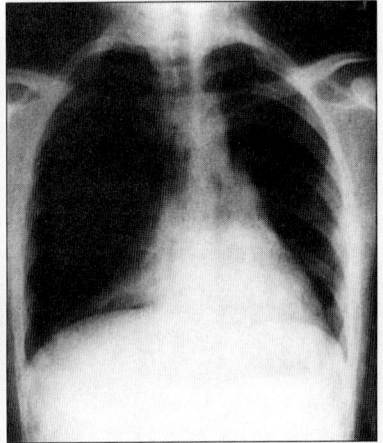
pneumotórax do lado direito: com evidência de desvio do mediastino (tensão)

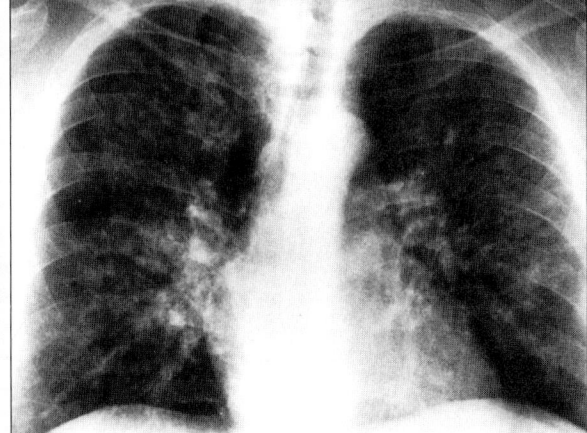
pneumonia por *Pneumocystis carinii* (PPC): em paciente aidético mostrando densidades pneumônicas bilaterais

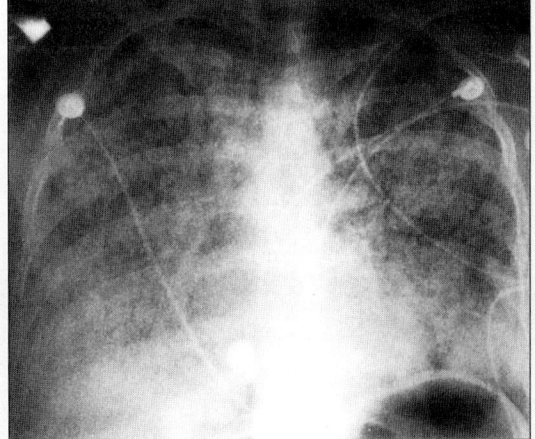
edema pulmonar: há densidades alveolares algodonosas difusas nos dois pulmões

Diagnóstico por Imagens

TOMOGRAFIA COMPUTADORIZADA E MAMOGRAFIA

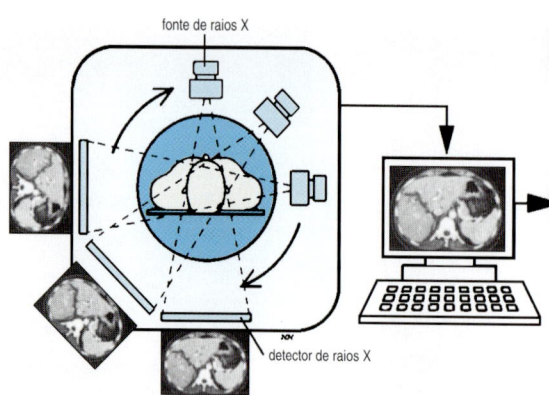

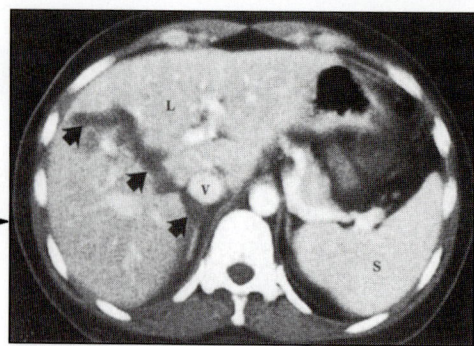

imagem de TC de um paciente que sofreu um acidente automobilístico mostra uma laceração irregular (setas) que se estende desde a porção posterior até a veia cava inferior (V), atravessando o lobo direito do fígado (L); (S) baço

tomografia computadorizada (TC) é um procedimento radiológico que utiliza um aparelho denominado *scanner* para examinar um local do corpo pela realização de uma série de imagens transversais, uma fatia (corte) de cada vez em uma rotação circular completa; um computador então calcula e converte as taxas de absorção e densidade dos raios X em uma imagem em uma tela

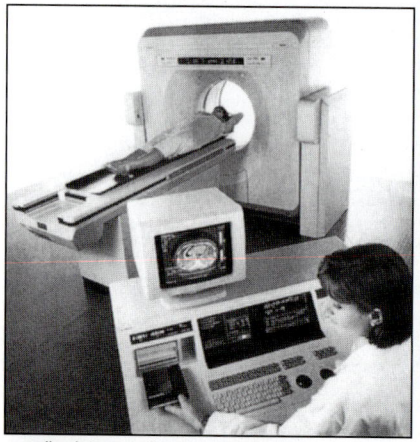

aparelho de tomografia computadorizada

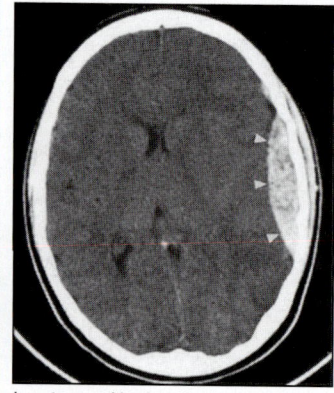

hematoma peridural agudo: observe o formato lentiforme do hematoma (setas)

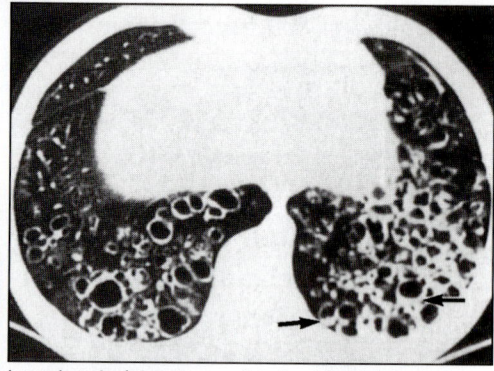

bronquiectasia cística: observe a dilatação crônica dos brônquios e bronquíolos (setas)

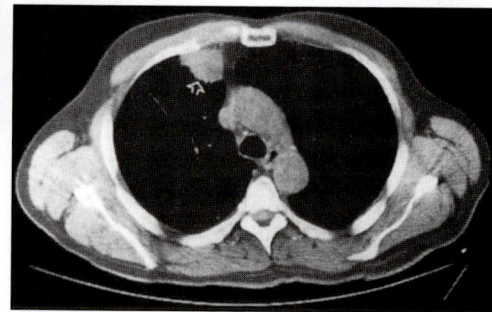

carcinoma pulmonar: corte de TC mostra massa localizada no segmento anterior do lobo superior direito (seta) adjacente à pleura

mamografia é o exame por imagens da mama por meio de raios X, ultra-som e ressonância magnética nuclear, usada para rastreamento e diagnóstico de doença da mama; a mamografia por raios X mostrou ser a mais eficaz na detecção de câncer de mama oculto

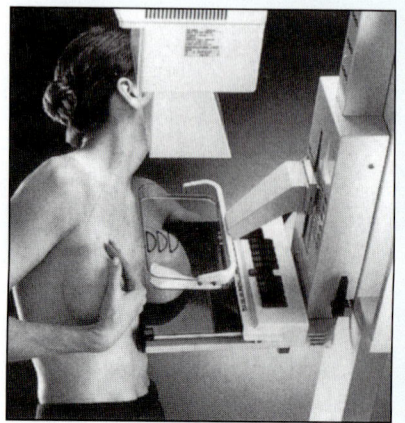

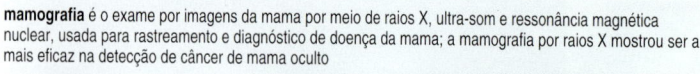

posicionamento da paciente para uma incidência MLO (extrema esquerda)

mamografia: incidência CC da mama esquerda; o mamilo está em perfil e o músculo peitoral (setas) é observado posteriormente (esquerda)

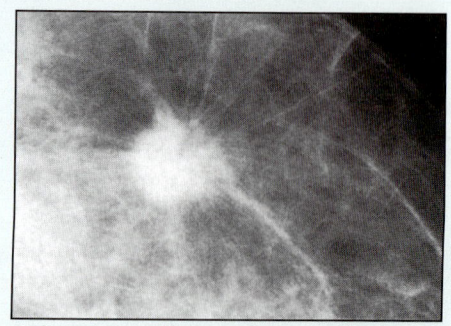

carcinoma de mama clássico: essa massa mamária espiculada é um carcinoma ductal infiltrativo

RESSONÂNCIA MAGNÉTICA

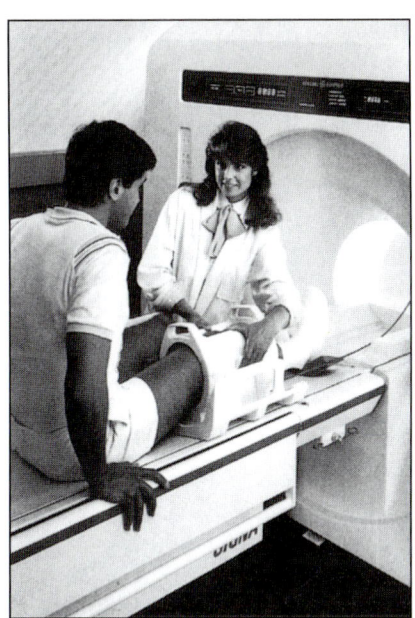

unidade de RM

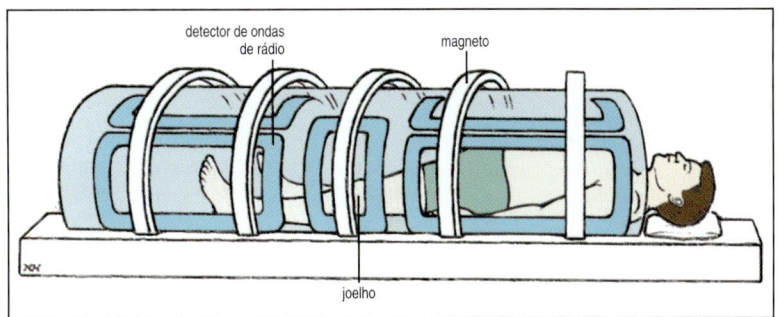

ressonância magnética (RM) é uma técnica não-ionizante (não utiliza raios X) que emprega campos magnéticos e ondas de radiofreqüência para visualizar estruturas anatômicas – útil na detecção de distúrbios das articulações, tendões e vértebras; o paciente é posicionado dentro do campo magnético (acima) à medida que sinais de onda de rádio são conduzidos através da parte do corpo selecionada; a energia é absorvida pelos tecidos e depois liberada

computador processa a energia liberada e forma a imagem

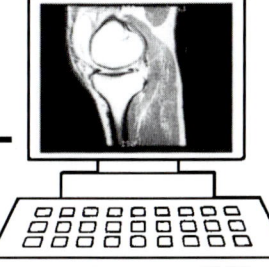

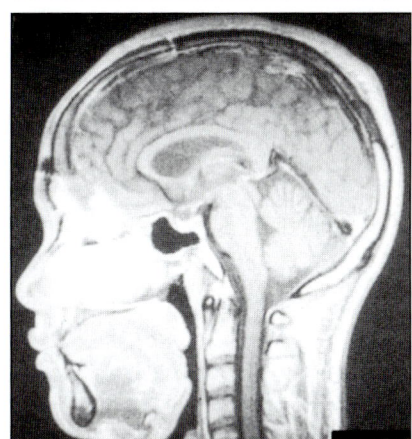

imagem de RM do cérebro normal: corte sagital

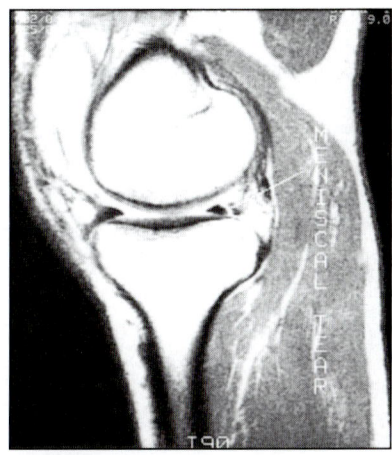

ressonância magnética do joelho (incidência lateral) identificando um menisco roto

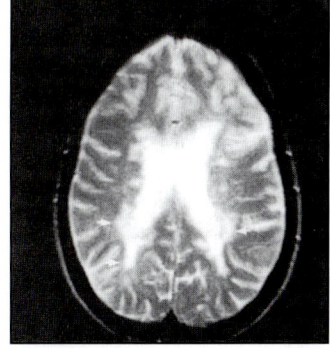

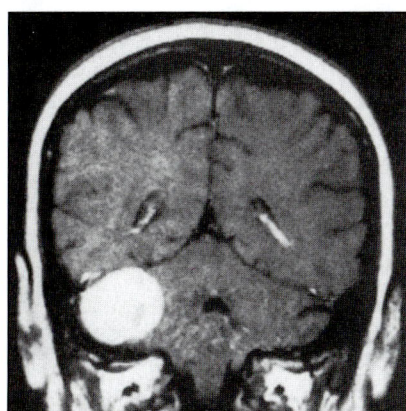

meningioma no cerebelo

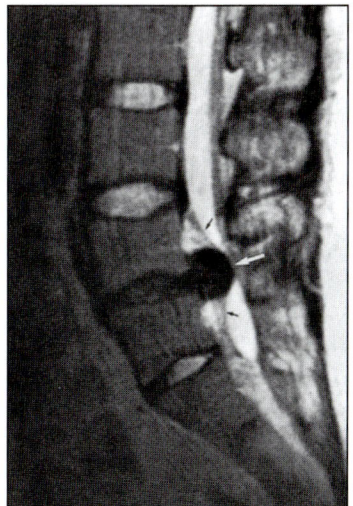

herniação do núcleo pulposo: RM sagital mostra uma grande herniação posterior (setas) no espaço do disco L4; observe o deslocamento posterior do saco tecal (setas pequenas)

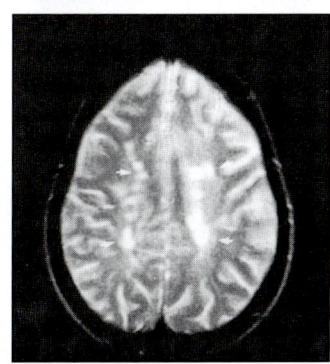

esclerose múltipla: imagens de RM ponderadas em T2, contíguas, mostram áreas de placas ventriculares de sinal elevado (setas)

Diagnóstico por Imagens

MEDICINA NUCLEAR

a formação de imagens por **medicina nuclear** é uma técnica diagnóstica que utiliza isótopos radioativos injetados ou ingeridos e uma câmera gama para determinar o tamanho, o formato, a localização e a função de várias partes do corpo

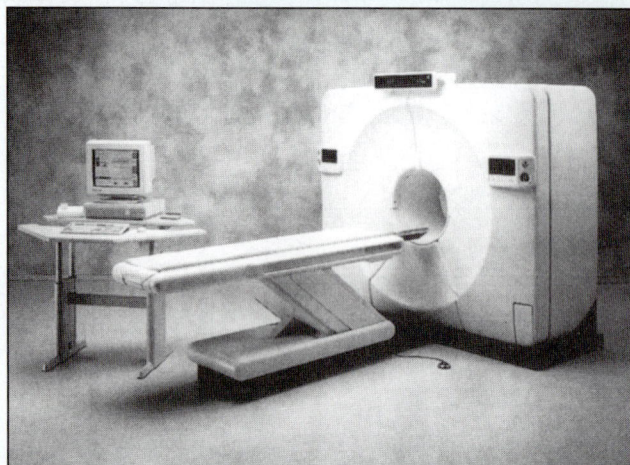

a **tomografia por emissão de pósitrons** (TEP) combina a medicina nuclear e a tomografia computadorizada para produzir imagens da anatomia encefálica e da fisiologia correspondente – é usada para estudar condições como acidente vascular cerebral, doença de Alzheimer (direita), epilepsia, distúrbios encefálicos metabólicos e bioquímica da função neural

as cores quentes (vermelho e amarelo) indicam uma maior taxa de metabolismo e de atividade encefálica no encéfalo normal (A) quando comparadas ao encéfalo de um paciente com doença de Alzheimer (B)

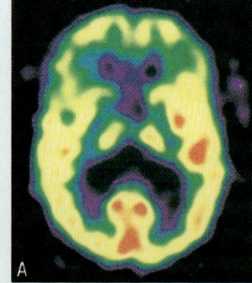
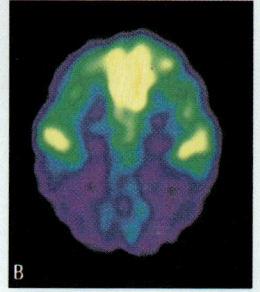

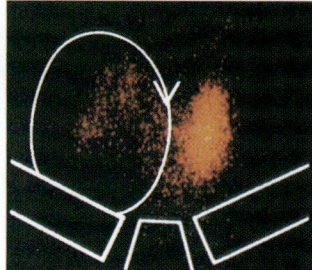

a **captação e a imagem da tireóide** são um estudo nuclear que envolve o escaneamento da glândula tireóide para visualizar acúmulo radioativo de isótopos previamente injetados para detectar nódulos ou tumores na tireóide

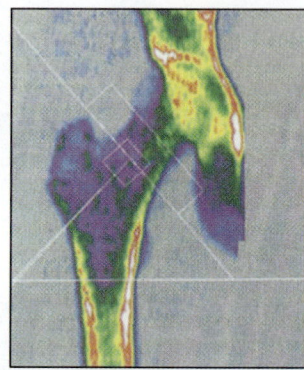

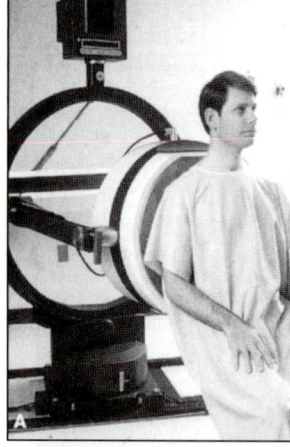
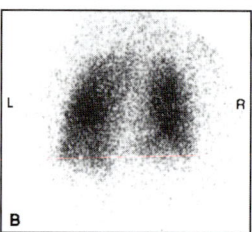
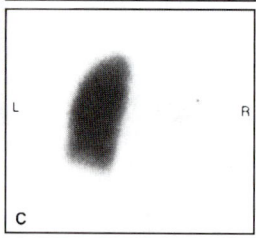

a **cintigrafia pulmonar nuclear** é usada para detectar anormalidades de perfusão (fluxo sanguíneo) ou ventilação (respiração); comumente denominada cintigrafia V/Q (ventilação/perfusão); (A) câmera gama usada para produzir cintigrafia pulmonar; neste paciente uma cintigrafia pulmonar posterior mostra um êmbolo no pulmão direito; a cintigrafia de ventilação (B) mostra um padrão normal; a ausência de fluxo sanguíneo para o pulmão direito é aparente à cintigrafia de perfusão (C)

Exame pelo **método DEXA** (em cima, à direita) de um fêmur para verificar a densidade óssea; as cores mais quentes (amarelo, vermelho) indicam áreas de baixa densidade

cintigrafia hepática: (direita) mostrando resultados normais

cintigrafia óssea: cintigrafia nuclear de tecido ósseo para detectar anormalidades como tumores malignos; abaixo é mostrado um exemplo de uma cintigrafia óssea de todo o corpo

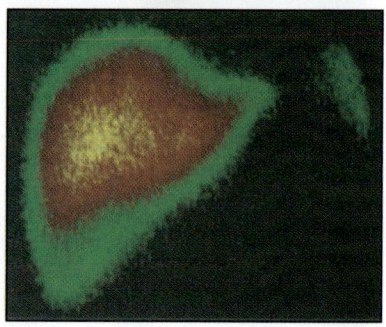

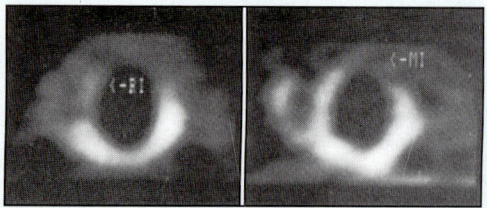

a **cintigrafia de perfusão miocárdica com estresse** é uma cintigrafia nuclear do coração feita antes e depois de exercício físico controlado (esteira ou bicicleta) ou da administração de um fármaco que produz os efeitos de estresse do exercício em pacientes incapazes de caminhar

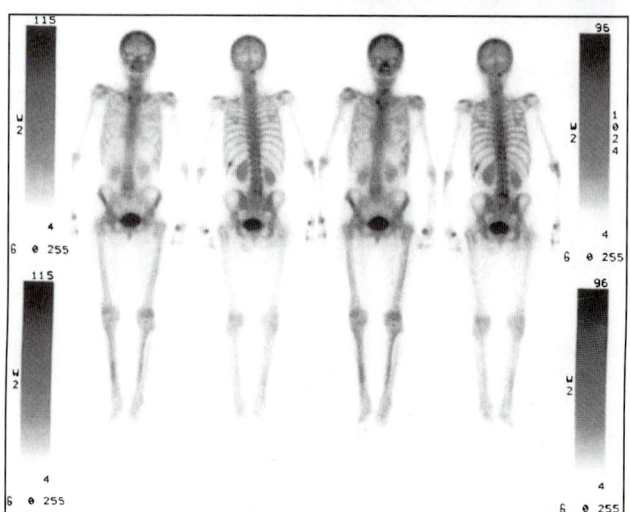

International Lymphoma Study Group
(Grupo de Estudo Internacional do Linfoma)

neoplasias de células B

I.	neoplasia de células precursoras B; linfoma/leucemia linfoblástica de células precursoras B
II.	neoplasias de células periféricas
	1. leucemia linfocítica crônica de células B/leucemia pró-linfocítica/linfoma linfocítico pequeno
	2. linfoma linfoplasmocitóide/imunocitoma
	3. linfoma de células do manto
	4. linfoma de centro folicular, folicular graus citológicos provisórios: I (pequenas células), II (pequenas e grandes células mistas), III (grandes células) subtipo provisório: difuso, predominantemente de pequenas células
	5. linfoma de células B da zona marginal extranodal (tipo MALT +/− células B monocitóides) subtipo provisório: ganglionar (+/− células B monocitóides)
	6. entidade provisória: linfoma de zona marginal esplênico (+/− linfócitos de vilosidades)
	7. leucemia de células pilosas
	8. plasmocitoma/mieloma de plasmócitos
	9. linfoma difuso de grandes células B* subtipo: linfoma mediastinal (tímico) primário de células B
	10. linfoma de Burkitt
	11. entidade provisória: linfoma de células B de alto grau Burkitt-símile*

neoplasias de células T e supostas células *natural killer* (NK)

I.	neoplasia de células precursoras T: leucemia/linfoma linfoblástico de células precursoras T
II.	neoplasias de células T e células NK periféricas
	1. leucemia linfocítica crônica de células T/leucemia prolinfocítica
	2. leucemia linfocítica granular (LLG) grande tipo celular T tipo celular NK
	3. micose fungóide/síndrome de Sézary
	4. linfomas de células T periféricas, não-especificados* categorias citológicas provisórias: células de tamanho médio, células mistas de tamanhos médio e grande, grandes células, células linfoepitelióides subtipo provisório: linfoma de células T hepatoesplênico subtipo provisório: linfoma de células T da paniculite subcutânea
	5. linfoma de células T angioimunoblástico (LTAI)
	6. linfoma angiocêntrico
	7. linfoma de células T intestinal (+/− associado a enteropatia)
	8. linfoma/leucemia de células T do adulto (L/LTA)
	9. linfoma anaplásico de grandes células (LAGC), tipos celulares CD30*, T e nulo
	10. entidade provisória: linfoma anaplásico de grandes células Hodgkin-símile

doença de Hodgkin (DH)

I.	predomínio linfocítico
II.	esclerose nodular
III.	celularidade mista
IV.	depleção de linfócitos
V.	entidade provisória: DH clássica rica em linfócitos

*acredita-se que essas categorias provavelmente incluem mais de uma entidade mórbida

ne·o·plasm (nē′ō - plazm). Neoplasma. Tecido anormal que cresce por proliferação celular mais rapidamente do que o normal e continua crescendo após a interrupção dos estímulos que iniciaram o neocrescimento. Os neoplasmas caracterizam-se por falta parcial ou completa de organização estrutural e coordenação funcional com o tecido normal e, em geral, formam uma massa distinta de tecido, que pode ser benigna (*tumor* benigno [benign *tumor*]) ou maligna (câncer). SIN new growth, tumor (2). [neo- + G. *plasma,* coisa formada]

histoid n., n. históide; termo antigo para um neoplasma caracterizado por padrão cisto-histológico que se assemelha estreitamente ao tecido do qual derivam as células neoplásicas.

ne·o·plas·tic (nē - ō - plas′tik). Neoplásico. Relativo a, ou caracterizado por, neoplasia ou que contém uma neoplasia.

ne·op·ter·in (nē - op′trin). Neopterina. Pteridina presente nos líquidos corporais; os níveis elevados resultam de ativação do sistema imune, doença maligna, rejeição de aloenxerto e infecções virais (especialmente como ocorre na AIDS/SIDA). [neo- + G. *pteron,* asa + -in]

ne·o·pyr·i·thi·a·min (nē′ō - pir - i - thī′a - min). Neopiritiamina. SIN pyrithiamin.

ne·o·ret·i·nal b (nē - ō - ret′in - al). Neorretinal b. SIN 11-*cis*-retinal.

ne·o·ret·i·nene B (nē - ō - ret′i - nēn). Neorretineno B. SIN 11-*cis*-retinol.

Ne·o·spo·ra ca·ni·um (nē - ō - spōr - ā kān′ - ē - um). Protozoário parasita de cães do filo Apicomplexa, um patógeno intracelular formador de cistos no tecido neural e outros tecidos. Sua epidemiologia e seu ciclo de vida não são conhecidos.

ne·o·stig·mine (nē - ō - stig′min). Neostigmina. Composto sintético, com ação semelhante à fisostigmina (eserina); inibidor reversível da colinesterase, utilizado na forma de sais brometo ou metilssulfato no tratamento da miastenia grave, distensão pós-operatória, retenção urinária e antagonista de drogas bloqueadoras neuromusculares estabilizantes.

ne·os·to·my (nē - os′tō - mē). Neostomia. Construção cirúrgica de uma abertura nova ou artificial. [neo- + G. *stoma,* boca]

ne·o·stri·a·tum (nē - ō - strī - ā′tūm). Neostriado. *Termo oficial alternativo para striatum.

ne·ot·e·ny (nē - ot′e - nē). Neotenia. Prolongamento do estado larvário, como ocorre na salamandra mexicana ou axolotl ou em certas castas de cupins mantidas no estágio larvário para futuras substituições da rainha. Cf. pedogenesis. [neo- + G. *teinō,* estirar]

Ne·o·tes·tu·di·na ro·sa·ti (nē′o - tes - too - dī′nā rō - sā′tī). Espécie de fungo que provoca o micetoma do cereal branco na Somália e em outras regiões da África.

ne·o·thal·a·mus (nē - ō - thal′ā - mŭs). Neotálamo. Porção do tálamo que se projeta para o neocórtex.

ne·o·ty·ro·sine (nē - ō - tī′rō - sēn). Neotirosina. Dimetiltirosina; um antimetabólito da tirosina.

ne·o·vas·cu·lar·i·za·tion (nē′ō - vas′kū - lar - i - zā′shŭn). Neovascularização. Proliferação de vasos sanguíneos no tecido que normalmente não os contém, ou proliferação de vasos sanguíneos de um tipo diferente do habitualmente observado no tecido.

choroidal n., n. coróide; crescimento de novos vasos da lâmina coriocapilar no epitélio pigmentar sub-retiniano e retina; espaço associado a lesão da retina externa.

classic choroidal n., n. coróide clássica; áreas bem demarcadas de hiperfluorescência observadas nas fases iniciais da angiografia retiniana.

occult choroidal n., n. coróide oculta; área de extravasamento de origem indeterminada, observada nas fases tardias da angiografia retiniana.

Type 1 choroidal n., n. coróide tipo 1; crescimento de novos vasos da lâmina coriocapilar no espaço epitelial pigmentar sub-retiniano; associado a lesão da retina externa.

Type 2 choroidal n., n. coróide tipo 2; crescimento de novos vasos a partir da lâmina coriocapilar para o espaço sub-retiniano; associado a lesão da retina externa.

ne·per (Np). Neper. Unidade para comparar a magnitude de duas forças, geralmente em eletricidade ou acústica; corresponde à metade do logaritmo natural da relação entre as duas forças. SIN napier. [de *neperus,* forma latinizada de (John) *Napier*]

neph·e·lom·e·ter (nef - ē - lom′e - ter). Nefelômetro. Instrumento utilizado em nefelometria. [G. *nephelē,* nuvem + *metron,* medida]

neph·e·lom·e·try (nef - ē - lom′e - trē). Nefelometria. Técnica para estimar o número e o tamanho de partículas numa suspensão ao medir a luz dispersa de uma fonte luminosa passando através da solução.

△ **nephr-.** Nepr-. VER nephro-.

ne·phral·gia (ne - fral′jē - ā). Nefralgia. Termo raramente utilizado para referir-se à ocorrência de dor no rim. [nephr- + G. *algos,* dor]

ne·phral·gic (ne - fral′jik). Nefrálgico. Relativo à nefralgia.

ne·phrec·to·my (ne - frek′tō - mē). Nefrectomia. Remoção de um rim. [nephr- + G. *ektomē,* excisão]

abdominal n., n. abdominal; remoção transperitoneal do rim por uma incisão feita através da parede abdominal anterior.

laparoscopic n., n. laparoscópica; remoção de um rim por técnica endoscópica percutânea.

lumbar n., n. lombar; nefrectomia extraperitoneal através do flanco ou incisão lombar posterior.

morcellated n., n. por fragmentação; remoção de um rim em fragmento.

posterior n., n. posterior; remoção retroperitoneal de um rim através de uma incisão feita nos músculos lombares posteriores, em geral com o paciente em decúbito ventral. SIN lumbotomy incision.

neph·re·de·ma (nef-re-dē'mă). Nefredema. Edema causado por doença renal; raramente, edema do rim. [nephr- + G. *oidēma*, intumescimento]

neph·rel·co·sis (nef-rel-kō'sis). Nefrelcose. Ulceração da mucosa da pelve ou dos cálices renais. [nephr- + G. *helkōsis*, ulceração]

neph·ric (nef'rik). Néfrico. Relativo ao rim. SIN renal.

ne·phrid·i·um, pl. **ne·phrid·ia** (ne-frid'ē-ŭm, -ă). Nefrídio. Um dos túbulos excretores de distribuição segmentar, pares, encontrados em invertebrados, como os anelídeos. [G. *nephros*, rim + L. Mod. *idium*, dim. sufixo, de G. *-idion*]

ne·phrit·ic (ne-frit'ik). Nefrítico. Relativo a, ou que sofre de, nefrite.

ne·phri·tis, pl. **ne·phrit·i·des** (ne-frī'tis, -frit'i-dēz). Nefrite. Inflamação dos rins. [nephr- + G. *-itis*, inflamação]
  acute n., n. aguda. SIN acute glomerulonephritis.
  acute intersticial n., n. interticial aguda; nefrite interticial com lesão tubular variável e infiltração por numerosos neutrófilos, devido a infecção bacteriana, obstrução das vias urinárias ou outras causas (incluindo medicamentos/drogas), que podem representar reações de hipersensibilidade; acompanhada de insuficiência renal, febre, eosinofilia sanguínea ou tecidual e erupção cutânea.
  analgesic n., n. por analgésicos; nefrite intersticial crônica com necrose papilar renal, que ocorre em pacientes com história de consumo excessivo e prolongado de analgésicos, particularmente os que contêm fenacetina. SIN analgesic nephropathy.
  anti-basement membrane n., n. antimembrana basal; glomerulonefrite produzida por anticorpos autólogos ou heterólogos dirigidos contra as membranas basais dos capilares glomerulares, sendo esta última conhecida como nefrite por anti-soro renal.
  anti-kidney serum n., n. por anti-soro renal; glomerulonefrite experimental produzida pela injeção de anti-soro no rim.
  chronic n., n. crônica. SIN chronic *glomerulonephritis*.
  focal n., n. focal. SIN focal *glomerulonephritis*.
  glomerular n., n. glomerular. SIN *glomerulonephritis*.
  n. gravida'rum, n. da gravidez; nefrite que se desenvolve durante a gravidez.
  hemorrhagic n., n. hemorrágica; glomerulonefrite aguda acompanhada de hematúria.
  hereditary n. [MIM*161900], n. hereditária; doença renal familiar que ocorre na vida adulta, caracterizada por proteinúria, hematúria e hipertensão, evoluindo para a insuficiência renal crônica. Não há defeito ocular nem surdez; herança autossômica dominante. VER TAMBÉM Alport *syndrome*.
  immune complex n., n. por imunocomplexos; doença por imunocomplexos resultantes de depósitos glomerulares, conforme observado no lúpus eritematoso sistêmico.
  interstitial n., n. intersticial; forma de nefrite em que o tecido conjuntivo intersticial é principalmente afetado.
  lupus n., n. do lúpus; glomerulonefrite que ocorre em alguns pacientes com lúpus eritematoso sistêmico, caracterizada por hematúria e evolução progressiva, culminando em insuficiência renal, freqüentemente na ausência de hipertensão; algumas vezes, o termo refere-se também à síndrome nefrótica observada em pacientes com lúpus sistêmico. As biópsias renais em pacientes com evolução progressiva revelam glomerulonefrite proliferativa difusa; nos casos mais leves, ocorrem lesões glomerulares proliferativas focais ou nefrite mesangial.
  mesangial n., n. mesangial; glomerulonefrite com aumento das células mesangiais glomerulares ou da matriz ou depósitos mesangiais.
  salt-losing n., n. perdedora de sal; distúrbio raro, resultante de lesão tubular renal de várias etiologias; simula a insuficiência supra-renal, devido à perda renal anormal de cloreto de sódio, acompanhada de hiponatremia, azotemia, acidose, desidratação e colapso vascular. SIN salt-losing syndrome, Thorn syndrome.
  scarlatinal n., n. por escarlatina; glomerulonefrite aguda que ocorre como complicação da escarlatina.
  serum n., n. sérica; glomerulonefrite que ocorre na doença do soro ou em animais aos quais são injetadas proteínas séricas estranhas.
  subacute n., n. subaguda. SIN subacute *glomerulonephritis*.
  suppurative n., n. supurativa; glomerulonefrite focal com formação de abscesso no rim.
  syphilitic n., n. sifilítica; complicação rara da sífilis congênita e secundária, com síndrome nefrótica, em decorrência de depósitos glomerulares de imunocomplexos.
  transfusion n., n. de transfusão; insuficiência renal e lesão tubular em conseqüência de transfusão de sangue incompatível; a hemoglobina dos eritrócitos hemolisados deposita-se sob a forma de cilindros nos túbulos renais.
  tuberculous n., n. tuberculosa; nefrite, principalmente intersticial, devida ao bacilo da tuberculose.
  tubulointerstitial n., n. tubulointersticial; nefrite que afeta os túbulos renais e o tecido intersticial, com infiltração por plasmócitos e células mononucleares; observada na nefrite lúpica, rejeição de aloenxerto e sensibilização à meticilina.
  uranium n., n. por urânio; nefrite experimental produzida pela administração de nitrato de urânio.

ne·phrit·o·gen·ic (nef'ri-tō-jen'ik). Nefritogênico. Que causa nefrite; refere-se a condições ou agentes. [nefrite + G. *genesis*, produção]

nephro-, nephr-. Nefro-, nefr-. Rim. VER TAMBÉM reno-. [G. *nephros*, rim]

neph·ro·blas·te·ma (nef'rō-blas-tē'mă). Nefroblastema. SIN nephric *blastema*. [nephro- + G. *blastēma*, broto]

neph·ro·blas·to·ma (nef'rō-blas-tō'mă). Nefroblastoma. SIN Wilms *tumor*.

neph·ro·cal·ci·no·sis (nef'rō-kal-si-nō'sis). Nefrocalcinose. Forma de litíase renal, caracterizada por focos difusamente dispersos de calcificação no parênquima renal; em geral, presença de depósitos radiologicamente demonstráveis de fosfato de cálcio, oxalato de cálcio monoidratado e compostos semelhantes. [nephro- + calcinose]

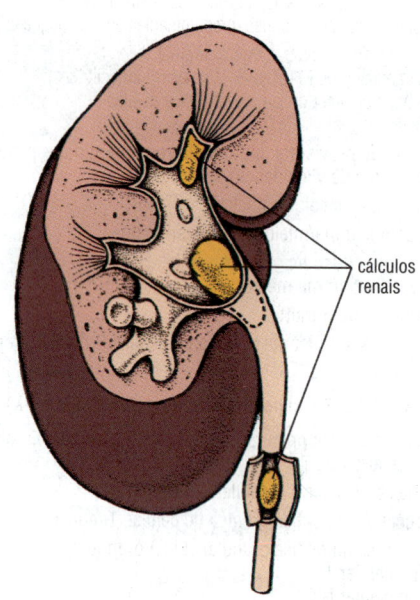

nefrolitíase

neph·ro·cap·sec·to·my (nef'rō-kap-sek'tō-mē). Nefrocapsectomia. Operação obsoleta para descorticação ou descapsulação do rim. [nephro- + L. *capsula*, pequena caixa + G. *ektomē*, excisão]

neph·ro·car·di·ac (nef'rō-kar'dē-ak). Nefrocardíaco. SIN cardiorenal. [nephro- + G. *kardia*, coração]

neph·ro·cele (nef'rō-sēl). Nefrocele. **1.** Deslocamento herniário de um rim. [nephro- + G. *kēlē*, hérnia]. **2.** Cavidade do nefrótomo. SIN nephrotomic *cavity*. [nephro- + G. *koilōma*, cavidade (celoma)]

neph·ro·cys·to·sis (nef'rō-sis-tō'sis). Nefrocistose. Formação de cistos renais. [nephro- + G. *kystis*, cisto + *-osis*, condição]

neph·ro·ge·net·ic, neph·ro·gen·ic (nef'rō-jĕ-net'ik, -jen'ik). Nefrogenético, nefrogênico. Que se desenvolve em tecido renal. [nephro- + G. *genesis*, origem]

ne·phrog·e·nous (ne-froj'ĕ-nŭs). Nefrógeno. Que se desenvolve a partir do tecido renal.

neph·ro·gram (nef'rō-gram). Nefrograma. **1.** Exame radiográfico do rim após a injeção intravenosa de contraste iodado hidrossolúvel. **2.** Opacificação difusa do parênquima renal após essa injeção, fornecendo uma indicação do fluxo sanguíneo renal e da filtração glomerular. Um nefrograma persistente indica obstrução da drenagem renal.

ne·phrog·ra·phy (ne-frog'ră-fē). Nefrografia. Radiografia do rim. [nephro- + G. *graphō*, escrever]

neph·roid (nef'royd). Nefróide. Em forma de rim; semelhante a um rim. SIN reniform. [nephro- + G. *eidos*, semelhança]

neph·ro·lith (nef'rō-lith). Nefrólito. SIN renal *calculus*. [nephro- + G. *lithos*, pedra]

neph·ro·li·thi·a·sis (nef'rō-li-thī'ă-sis). Nefrolitíase. Presença de cálculos renais.

neph·ro·li·thot·o·my (nef'rō-li-thot'ō-mē). Nefrolitotomia. Incisão efetuada no rim para remoção de cálculo renal. [nephro- + G. *lithos*, pedra + *tomē*, incisão]

ne·phrol·o·gy (ne-frol'ō-jē). Nefrologia. Ramo da ciência médica relacionado com as doenças dos rins. [nephro- + G. *logos*, estudo]

ne·phrol·y·sin (ne - frol′i - sin). Nefrolisina. Anticorpo que causa destruição das células renais, produzido em resposta à injeção de uma emulsão do parênquima renal; específico para a espécie a partir da qual foi preparado o antígeno.

ne·phrol·y·sis (ne - frol′i - sis). Nefrólise. **1.** Liberação do rim de aderências inflamatórias, com preservação da cápsula. **2.** Destruição de células renais. [nephro- + G. *lysis*, dissolução]

neph·ro·lyt·ic (nef - rō - lit′ik). Nefrolítico. Relativo a, caracterizado por ou que causa nefrólise. SIN nephrotoxic (2).

ne·phro·ma (ne - frō′mă). Nefroma. Tumor que se origina do tecido renal. [nephro- + G. *-oma*, tumor]

   mesoblastic n., n. mesobástico. Neoplasia de células fusiformes do rim de lactente e, raramente, do adulto com túbulos renais aprisionados.

neph·ro·ma·la·cia (nef′rō - ma - lā′shē - ă). Nefromalacia. Amolecimento dos rins. [nephro- + G. *malakia*, amolecimento]

neph·ro·meg·a·ly (nef - rō - meg′ă - lē). Nefromegalia. Hipertrofia extrema de um ou de ambos os rins. [nephro- + G. *megas*, grande]

neph·ro·mere (nef′rō - mēr). Nefrômero. Porção do mesoderma intermediário a partir do qual se desenvolvem os túbulos renais segmentados. VER nephrotome. [nephro- + G. *meros*, parte]

neph·ron (nef′ron). Néfron. Longa estrutura tubular contornada do rim, consistindo no corpúsculo renal, túbulo contornado proximal, alça nefrônica e túbulo contornado distal. VER TAMBÉM uriniferous *tubule*. [G. *nephros*, rim]

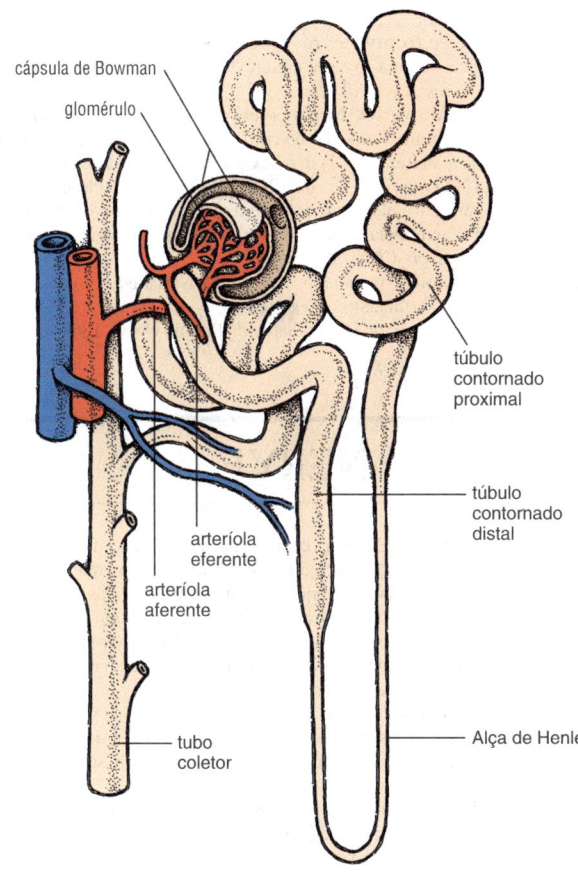

néfron

neph·ro·path·ia (nef′rō - path′e - ă). Nefropatia. SIN nephropathy.

   n. epidemica, n. epidêmica; forma geralmente benigna de febre hemorrágica epidêmica relatada na Escandinávia.

neph·ro·path·ic (nef′rō - path′ik). Nefropático. Que causa doença renal orgânica ou comprometimento da função renal.

ne·phrop·a·thy (ne - frop′ă - thē). Nefropatia. Qualquer doença do rim. SIN nephropathia, nephrosis (1). [nephro- + G. *pathos*, sofrimento]

   analgesic n., n. por analgésicos. SIN analgesic *nephritis*.

   Balkan n., n. dos Balcãs; nefrite crônica intersticial de etiologia desconhecida, originalmente descrita como doença endêmica nos Balcãs, caracterizada por início insidioso, achados urinários escassos, anemia e acidose. SIN Danubian endemic familial n.

   Danubian endemic familial n., n. familiar endêmica do Danúbio. SIN Balkan n.

   diabetic n., n. diabética; síndrome que ocorre em indivíduos com diabetes melito, caracterizada por albuminúria, hipertensão e insuficiência renal progressiva.

A nefropatia diabética constitui uma importante causa de morbidade e mortalidade em indivíduos com diabetes melito (DM). Os pacientes com diabetes constituem a maior parcela (> 25%) de pacientes que iniciam a diálise renal anualmente nos Estados Unidos para doença renal terminal (DRT). A incidência de DRT aproxima-se de 40% em indivíduos que tiveram DM tipo 1 durante 20 anos. O risco de nefropatia diabética é maior em homens, negros, hispânicos e americanos nativos. Nos 3 anos seguintes ao diagnóstico de DM, os estudos histológicos revelam espessamento da membrana basal glomerular e expansão mesangial, alterações características da glomerulosclerose diabética (doença de Kimmelstiel-Wilson). Os rins aumentam de tamanho e de peso devido à hipertrofia e hiperplasia das células parenquimatosas, e verifica-se um aumento no fluxo sangüíneo renal e na taxa de filtração glomerular (TFG); em conseqüência, os níveis séricos de creatinina e de uréia estão um pouco reduzidos. Depois de 10-15 anos, podem surgir os primeiros sinais de lesão renal na forma de microalbuminúria, excreção persistente de albumina em concentrações que não são detectadas por testes habituais de proteína urinária. Uma taxa de excreção de albumina de 20–200 μg/min (30–300 mg/dia) é um prenúncio de nefropatia diabética e indica fortemente o posterior desenvolvimento de DRT. A progressão contínua da lesão renal resulta em albuminúria franca e declínio da taxa de filtração glomerular e da depuração de nitrogênio. A prevalência da hipertensão é bem maior em indivíduos com microalbuminúria, e a hipertensão acelera a progressão da doença renal. A nefropatia diabética pode resultar em hiperpotassemia, acidose metabólica, síndrome nefrótica, necrose papilar e maior suscetibilidade à insuficiência renal aguda após exposição a contrastes radiográficos. As diretrizes atuais para tratamento do DM exigem avaliação anual da excreção de albumina de 24 horas, tratamento imediato das infecções das vias urinárias e contra-indicação de agentes nefrotóxicos e contrastes radiográficos. Nenhuma intervenção reverte comprovadamente a nefropatia diabética clínica. Entretanto, estudos randomizados prospectivos estabeleceram que a melhora do controle metabólico, mantendo-se sempre o nível plasmático de glicose o mais próximo possível do normal, pode reduzir sobremaneira o desenvolvimento e a progressão da nefropatia diabética, bem como outras complicações microvasculares em longo prazo do diabetes (retinopatia e neuropatia). Além disso, foi constatado que o controle agressivo da hipertensão com inibidores da ECA ou bloqueadores dos receptores de angiotensina II retarda a progressão da nefropatia por mecanismos que não dependem do controle da pressão arterial, e verificou-se que a limitação da ingestão diária de proteína para 0,8 g/kg de peso corporal (não apropriada durante a gravidez) retarda a progressão da doença renal tanto diabética quanto não-diabética. A DRT é tratada com transplante renal, hemodiálise ou diálise peritoneal. Como a retinopatia e a neuropatia diabéticas evoluem mais rapidamente com o início da insuficiência renal, a diálise costuma ser instituída precocemente (quando o nível sérico de creatinina atinge cerca de 6 mg/dl) na nefropatia diabética.

   hypokalemic n., n. hipopotassêmica; vacuolização do citoplasma epitelial dos túbulos contornados renais em pacientes com grave depleção de potássio; os vacúolos não contêm gordura nem glicogênio, a capacidade de concentração está afetada, é comum a ocorrência de poliúria e polidipsia e pode haver desenvolvimento de pielonefrite. SIN vacuolar nephrosis.

   IgA n., n. por IgA. SIN focal *glomerulonephritis*.

   IgM n., n. por IgM. SIN mesangial proliferative *glomerulonephritis*.

   reflux n., n. por refluxo; lesão do parênquima renal secundária ao refluxo vesicoureteral de urina infectada.

neph·ro·pexy (nef′rō - pek - sē). Nefropexia. Fixação cirúrgica de um rim flutuante ou móvel. VER TAMBÉM nephrorrhaphy. [nephro- + G. *pēxis*, fixação]

neph·roph·thi·sis (nef - rof′thi - sis, - tī - sis). Nefrotísica. **1.** Nefrite supurativa com perda da substância do órgão. **2.** Tuberculose renal. [nephro- + G. *phthisis*, consunção]

   familial juvenile n., n. juvenil familiar; doença cística da medula renal, caracterizada por poliúria, polidipsia, anemia e insuficiência renal. Existem duas formas: uma forma hereditária autossômica recessiva [MIM*256100], causada por uma mutação no gene NPHP1, no cromossoma 2q13; a segunda é uma forma autossômica dominante [MIM*174000].

neph·rop·to·sis, neph·rop·to·sia (nef - rop - tō′sis, - tō′sē - ă). Nefroptose. Prolapso do rim. [nephro- + G. *ptōsis*, queda]

neph·ro·py·o·sis (nef′rō - pī - ō′sis). Nefropiose. SIN pyonephrosis. [nephro- + G. *pyōsis*, supuração]

neph·ror·rha·phy (nef - ror′ă - fē). Nefrorrafia. Nefropexia através de sutura do rim. [nephro- + G. *rhaphē*, sutura]

neph·ros (nef′ros). Rim. SIN kidney.

neph·ro·scle·ro·sis (nef′rō - skle - rō′sis). Nefrosclerose. Fibrose do rim em conseqüência de crescimento excessivo e contração do tecido conjuntivo intersticial. [nephro- + G. *sklērōsis*, endurecimento]

  arterial n., n. arterial; fibrose atrófica irregular do rim devido ao estreitamento arteriosclerótico da luz dos grandes ramos da artéria renal, que ocorre em indivíduos idosos ou hipertensos e que, em certas ocasiões, provoca hipertensão. SIN arterionephrosclerosis, senile n.

  arteriolar n., n. arteriolar; fibrose renal devido à esclerose arteriolar decorrente de hipertensão prolongada; os rins apresentam-se finamente granulares e exibem contração leve a moderada, com espessamento hialino das paredes das arteríolas glomerulares aferentes e fibrose hialina de glomérulos disseminados; raramente ocorre desenvolvimento de insuficiência renal crônica. SIN arteriolonephrosclerosis, benign n.

  benign n., n. benigna. SIN arteriolar n.

  malignant n., n. maligna; alterações renais na hipertensão maligna; evolução terminal comum consiste em petéquias subcapsulares, necrose nas paredes das arteríolas glomerulares aferentes disseminadas e presença de eritrócitos e cilindros na urina, com uremia.

  senile n., n. senil. SIN arterial n.

neph·ro·scle·rot·ic (nef′rō - skle - rot′ik). Nefrosclerótico. Relativo a ou que causa nefrosclerose.

neph·ro·scope (ne - frō′skŏp). Nefroscópio. Endoscópio introduzido na pelve renal para sua visualização. A via de acesso pode ser percutânea, através de rim cirurgicamente exposto, ou retrógrada, através do ureter.

ne·phro·sis (ne - frō′sis). Nefrose. 1. SIN nephropathy. 2. Degeneração do epitélio tubular renal. 3. SIN nephrotic *syndrome*. [nephro- + G. *-osis*, condição]

  acute n., n. aguda; insuficiência renal oligúrica aguda, especialmente aquela causada por certos venenos.

  acute lobar n., n. lobar aguda; infecção bacteriana grave, porém localizada, do parênquima renal, que pode produzir um efeito expansivo (simulando um abscesso renal).

  amyloid n., n. amilóide; **(1)** SIN renal *amyloidosis;* **(2)** síndrome nefrótica devido à deposição de amilóide no rim.

  familial n. [MIM*256300], n. familiar; síndrome nefrótica que aparece em irmãos no primeiro ano de vida, sem surdez nervosa; herdada como caráter autossômico recessivo, em que o tipo finlandês é devido a uma mutação no gene da nefrina no cromossoma 19q.

  hemoglobinuric n., n. hemoglobinúrica; insuficiência renal oligúrica aguda associada a hemoglobinúria, devido a hemólise intravascular maciça, como, p. ex., após transfusão de sangue incompatível; os rins exibem as alterações morfológicas da nefrose hipóxica.

  hypoxic n., n. hipóxica; insuficiência renal oligúrica aguda que ocorre após hemorragia, queimaduras, choque ou outras causas de hipovolemia e redução do fluxo sanguíneo renal; freqüentemente associada a necrose tubular irregular, tubulorrexe e cilindros tubulares distais de hemoglobina.

  lipoid n., n. lipóide; síndrome nefrótica idiopática que ocorre mais comumente em crianças, nas quais os glomérulos exibem alterações mínimas, sem espessamento das membranas basais, vacúolos de gordura no epitélio tubular e fusão dos podócitos glomerulares. SIN minimal-change disease, nil disease.

  osmotic n., n. osmótica; edema do epitélio tubular renal associado a filtração glomerular de açúcares e dextrose; o edema é devido à formação de vesículas citoplasmáticas por pinocitose e é reversível, provavelmente sem disfunção, quando produzido por glicose ou manitol.

  toxic n., n. tóxica; insuficiência renal oligúrica aguda, devido a venenos químicos, septicemia ou toxemia bacteriana; freqüentemente associada a necrose extensa dos túbulos contornados proximais.

  vacuolar n., n. vacuolar. SIN hypokalemic *nephropathy.*

ne·phros·to·gram (ne - fros′tō - gram). Nefrostograma. Radiografia do rim após opacificação da pelve renal mediante injeção de um contraste através de um tubo de nefrostomia. [nefrostomia + G. *gramma*, escrita]

neph·ros·to·ma, neph·ro·stome (ne - fros′tō - mă, nef′rō - stōm). Nefróstoma. Uma das aberturas ciliadas em forma de funil, através das quais os túbulos pronéfricos e alguns túbulos mesonéfricos primitivos se comunicam com o celoma. [nephro- + G. *stoma*, boca]

ne·phros·to·my (ne - fros′tō - mē). Nefrostomia. Estabelecimento de uma abertura entre o sistema coletor do rim, através de seu parênquima, e o exterior do corpo; pode ser efetuada por incisão cirúrgica ou por via percutânea. [nephro- + G. *stoma*, boca]

  percutaneous n., n. percutânea; drenagem do sistema coletor através de um cateter inserido na pele do flanco, sob controle fluoroscópico, utilizando habitualmente a técnica de Seldinger.

neph·rot·ic (nef - rot′ik). Nefrótico. Relativo a, causado por ou semelhante a nefrose.

neph·ro·tome (nef′rō - tōm). Nefrótomo. O mesoderma intermediário segmentado que se desenvolve em primórdios néfricos. [nephro- + G. *tomē*, corte]

neph·ro·tom·ic (nef - rō - tom′ik). Nefrotômico. Relativo ao nefrótomo.

neph·ro·to·mo·gram (nef - rō - tō′mō - gram). Nefrotomograma. Exame tomográfico dos rins após a administração intravenosa de contraste com o objetivo de melhorar a visualização de anormalidades do parênquima renal. [nephro- + G. *tomos*, corte + *gramma*, escrita]

neph·ro·to·mog·ra·phy (nef′rō - tō - mog′ră - fē). Nefrotomografia. Exame tomográfico do rim.

ne·phrot·o·my (ne - frot′ō - mē). Nefrotomia. Incisão no rim. [nephro- + G. *tomē*, incisão]

  anatrophic n., n. anatrófica; incisão no parênquima renal póstero-lateral, dando acesso ao sistema calicial através de um plano avascular, entre os ramos anterior e posterior da artéria renal; utilizada para a remoção de cálculos caliciais e renais ramificados, com exposição máxima, porém com sangramento ou lesão parenquimatosa mínima. SIN Smith-Boyce operation.

neph·ro·tox·ic (nef - rō - tok′sik). Nefrotóxico. **1.** Relativo à nefrotoxina; tóxico para as células renais. **2.** SIN nephrolytic.

neph·ro·tox·ic·i·ty (nef′rō - tok - sis′i - tē). Nefrotoxicidade. Qualidade ou estado de ser tóxico para as células renais.

neph·ro·tox·in (nef - rō - tok′sin). Nefrotoxina. Citotoxina específica para as células do rim.

neph·ro·troph·ic (nef - rō - trof′ik). Nefrotrófico. SIN renotrophic.

neph·ro·tro·pic (nef - rō - trop′ik). Nefrotrópico. SIN renotrophic.

neph·ro·tu·ber·cu·lo·sis (nef′rō - too - ber - kū - lō′sis). Nefrotuberculose. Tuberculose do rim.

neph·ro·u·re·ter·ec·ta·sis (nef′rō - ū - rē′ter - dk - ta′sis). Nefroureterectasia. SIN ureterohydronephrosis.

neph·ro·u·re·ter·ec·to·my (nef′rō - ū - rē′ter - ek′tō - mē). Nefroureterectomia. Remoção cirúrgica de um rim e seu ureter. SIN ureteronephrectomy. [nephro- + ureter + G. *ektomē*, excisão]

neph·ro·u·re·ter·o·cys·tec·to·my (nef′rō - ū - rē′ter - ō - sis - tek′tō - mē). Nefroureterocistectomia. Remoção do rim, do ureter e de parte ou de toda a bexiga. [nephro- + ureter + G. *kystis*, bexiga + *ektomē*, excisão]

nep·tu·ni·um (Np) (nep - too′nē - ŭm). Netúnio. Elemento radioativo; número atômico 93; primeiro elemento da série transuraniana (não encontrado na natureza). O Np^{237} tem meia-vida de $2{,}14 \times 10^6$ anos. [do planeta Netuno]

ne·ral (nē′ral). Neral. *cis*-Citral. VER citral.

Néri, Vincenzo, neurologista italiano, *1882. VER Néri *sign*.

ne·ri·ne (nē′ri - ēn). Neriína. SIN conessine.

Nernst, Walther, médico alemão e ganhador do Prêmio Nobel, 1864–1941. VER N. *equation*.

NERVE

nerve (nerv) [TA]. Nervo. Estrutura esbranquiçada em forma de cordão, composta de um ou mais feixes (fascículos) de fibras nervosas mielinizadas ou não-mielinizadas ou, com mais freqüência, misturas de ambas, que se estendem fora do sistema nervoso central, juntamente com tecido conjuntivo no interior dos fascículos e ao redor do neurolema de fibras nervosas individuais (endoneuro), ao redor de cada fascículo (perineuro) e ao redor de todo o nervo e seus vasos sanguíneos nutridores (epineuro), através da qual os estímulos são transmitidos do sistema nervoso central para uma parte do corpo, ou inversamente. Os ramos nervosos aparecem na definição do nervo principal; muitos estão também relacionados e definidos em branch. SIN nervus [TA]. [L. *nervus*].

  abdominopelvic splanchnic n.'s, nervos esplâncnicos abdominopélvicos; ramos viscerais dos troncos simpáticos que contêm fibras simpáticas pré-sinápticas para os gânglios pré-vertebrais e plexos paraórticos/hipogástricos e fibras aferentes viscerais para inervação das vísceras localizadas abaixo do diafragma. Pertencem a esse grupo os nervos esplâncnicos maior, menor, mínimo, lombares e sacros.

  abducens n., n. abducente; *termo oficial alternativo para abducent n. [CN VI].

  abducent n. [CN VI] [TA], n. abducente [NC VI]; pequeno nervo motor que supre o músculo reto lateral do olho; origina-se na parte dorsal do tegmento da ponte, imediatamente abaixo da superfície da fossa rombóide, e emerge do cérebro na fissura entre o bulbo e a borda posterior da fonte (sulco medulopontino); penetra na dura do clivo e passa através do seio cavernoso, penetrando na órbita através da fissura orbitária superior. SIN nervus abducens [CN VI] [TA], abducens n.*, abducent (2), sixth cranial n. [CN VI].

  accelerator n.'s, nervos aceleradores; alguns dos nervos esplâncnicos cardiopulmonares que estabelecem a inervação simpática do coração; as fibras eferentes não-mielinizadas dos nervos aceleradores estimulam um aumento da freqüência cardíaca e originam-se de células ganglionares do gânglio cervical superior, médio e inferior do tronco simpático.

accessory n. [CN XI] [TA], n. acessório [NC XI]; origina-se de dois conjuntos de raízes: a presumida raiz craniana, que surge do lado da medula oblonga, e a raiz espinal, que emerge da parte ventrolateral dos primeiros cinco segmentos cervicais da medula espinal; essas raízes unem-se para formar o tronco do nervo acessório, que se divide em dois ramos: interno e externo; o ramo interno, que transporta fibras da raiz craniana, une-se com o vago no forame jugular e supre os músculos da faringe, laringe e palato mole; o ramo externo continua independente através do forame jugular para suprir os músculos esternocleidomastóideo e trapézio. Embora, a princípio, se acreditasse que o nervo acessório tivesse raízes craniana e espinal, a noção geral atualmente é que a denominada raiz craniana constitui, na verdade, uma porção do nervo vago. SIN nervus accessorius [CN XI] [TA], accessorius willisii, eleventh cranial n. [CN XI], spinal accessory n.

accessory phrenic n.'s [TA], nervos frênicos acessórios; faixas nervosas acessórias que se originam do quinto nervo cervical, freqüentemente como ramos do nervo para o subclávio, descendo para unir-se ao nervo frênico. SIN nervi phrenici accessorii [TA].

acoustic n., n. acústico; termo arcaico algumas vezes utilizado para referir-se ao n. vestibulococlear [NC VIII].

afferent n., n. aferente; nervo que envia impulsos da periferia para o sistema nervoso central. SIN centripetal n., esodic n.

Andersch n., n. de Andersch. SIN tympanic n.

anococcygeal n., n. anococcígeo; pequeno nervo que se origina do plexo coccígeo e supre a pele sobre o cóccix. SIN nervus anococcygeus.

anterior ampullary n. [TA], n. ampular anterior; ramo do nervo utriculoampular que supre a crista ampular do ducto semicircular anterior. SIN nervus ampullaris anterior [TA].

anterior antebrachial n., n. antebraquial anterior. SIN anterior interosseous n.

anterior auricular n.'s [TA], nervos auriculares anteriores; ramos do nervo auriculotemporal que supre o trago e a parte superior da aurícula. SIN nervi auriculares anteriores [TA].

anterior crural n., n. crural anterior. SIN femoral n.

anterior cutaneous n.'s of abdomen, nervos cutâneos anteriores do abdome. SIN thoracoabdominal n.'s.

anterior ethmoidal n. [TA], n. etmoidal anterior; ramo do nervo nasociliar; passa através do forame etmoidal anterior sobre a parede superomedial da aorta na cavidade craniana, dando origem aos nervos meníngeos anteriores; em seguida, passa através das placas cribriformes na cavidade nasal, suprindo a mucosa nasal ântero-superior. SIN nervus ethmoidalis anterior [TA].

anterior femoral cutaneous n.'s, nervos cutâneos femorais anteriores. SIN anterior cutaneous branches of femoral nerve, em branch.

anterior interosseous n. [TA], n. interósseo anterior; ramo do nervo mediano que se origina na região do cotovelo, percorre a membrana interóssea e supre os músculos flexor longo do polegar, parte do flexor profundo dos dedos e pronador quadrado, bem como as articulações radiocarpais e intercarpais. SIN nervus interosseus antebrachii anterior [TA], anterior antebrachial n., nervus antebrachii anterior, volar interosseous n.

anterior labial n.'s [TA], nervos labiais anteriores; ramos do nervo ilioinguinal que se distribuem para os grandes lábios, monte pubiano e parte adjacente da coxa. SIN nervi labiales anteriores [TA].

anterior scrotal n.'s [TA], nervos escrotais anteriores; ramos do nervo ilioinguinal que se distribuem para a pele da raiz do púbis, monte pubiano, parte adjacente da coxa e superfície anterior do escroto. SIN nervi scrotales anteriores [TA].

anterior superior alveolar n.'s [TA], nervos alveolares superiores anteriores; ramos do nervo alveolar superior que suprem os incisivos, os caninos, os pré-molares e o primeiro molar em virtude de sua contribuição para o plexo dental superior. SIN anterior superior alveolar branches of infraorbital nerve, rami alveolares superiores anteriores nervi infraorbitalis.

anterior supraclavicular n., n. supraclavicular anterior. SIN medial supraclavicular n.

anterior tibial n., n. tibial anterior. SIN deep fibular n.

aortic n., n. aórtico; ramo do vago que termina no arco aórtico e na base do coração; constituído inteiramente de fibras aferentes; sua estimulação desencadeia um reflexo do tronco cerebral que causa redução da freqüência cardíaca, dilatação dos vasos periféricos e queda da pressão arterial. SIN Cyon n., depressor n. of Ludwig, Ludwig n.

Arnold n., n. de Arnold. SIN auricular branch of vagus nerve.

articular n., n. articular; ramo de um nervo que supre uma articulação. SIN nervus articularis.

auditory n., n. auditivo. SIN cochlear n.

augmentor n.'s, nervos ampliadores. SIN cervical splanchnic n.'s.

auriculotemporal n. [TA], n. auriculotemporal; ramo do mandibular que surge, habitualmente, através de duas raízes envolvendo a artéria meníngea média; passa através da glândula parótida, transportando fibras parassimpáticas pós-sinápticas secretomotoras do gânglio ótico; termina na pele da têmpora e do couro cabeludo; envia também ramos para o meato acústico externo, membrana timpânica e aurícula, bem como um ramo comunicante para o nervo facial. SIN nervus auriculotemporalis [TA].

autonomic n., n. autônomo; feixe de fibras nervosas autônomas, fora do sistema nervoso central, que pertencem ou que estão relacionadas ao sistema nervoso autônomo (motor visceral). SIN nervus autonomicus [TA].

axillary n. [TA], n. axilar; origina-se do cordão posterior do plexo braquial na axila, segue lateral e posteriormente através do espaço quadrangular com a artéria umeral circunflexa posterior, curva-se ao redor do colo cirúrgico do úmero para suprir os músculos deltóide e redondo menor, terminando como nervo cutâneo braquial lateral superior. SIN nervus axillaris [TA], circumflex n.

baroreceptor n., n. barorreceptor. SIN pressoreceptor n.

Bell respiratory n., n. respiratório de Bell. SIN long thoracic n.

Bock n., n. de Bock. SIN pharyngeal n.

buccal n. [TA], n. bucal; ramo sensitivo da divisão mandibular do nervo trigêmeo; segue para baixo, emergindo da parte inferior do ramo da mandíbula e seguindo para diante, sobre o músculo bucinador, atravessando-o (sem inervá-lo) para suprir a mucosa bucal e pele da bochecha, próximo ao ângulo da boca. SIN nervus buccalis [TA], buccinator n., long buccal n.

buccinator n., n. bucinador. SIN buccal n.

cardiopulmonary splanchnic n.'s, nervos esplâncnicos cardiopulmonares; ramos viscerais dos troncos simpáticos que contêm fibras simpáticas pós-sinápticas e fibras aferentes viscerais das vísceras localizadas acima do diafragma, principalmente através dos plexos cardíaco, pulmonar e esofágico. Pertencem a esse grupo os nervos esplâncnicos cervical e torácico superior.

caroticotympanic n., n. caroticotimpânicos; dois ramos simpáticos do plexo carótido interno para o plexo timpânico. SIN nervi caroticotympanicus, small deep petrosal n.

carotid sinus n., n. do seio carotídeo. SIN carotid branch of glossopharyngeal nerve (CN IX).

n. to carotid sinus, n. do seio carotídeo. SIN carotid branch of glossopharyngeal nerve (CN IX).

cavernous n.'s of clitoris [TA], nervos cavernosos do clitóris; nervos que correspondem aos nervos cavernosos do pênis no sexo masculino; originam-se da porção vesicular do plexo pélvico. SIN nervi cavernosi clitoridis [TA], cavernous plexus of clitoris.

cavernous n.'s of penis [TA], nervos cavernosos do pênis; dois nervos, maior e menor, derivados da porção prostática do plexo pélvico que supre as fibras simpáticas e parassimpáticas para as artérias helicinas e anastomoses arteriovenosas do corpo cavernoso, estimulando a ereção. SIN nervi cavernosi penis [TA], cavernous plexus of penis.

centrifugal n., n. centrífugo. SIN efferent n.

centripetal n., n. centrípeto. SIN afferent n.

cervical n.'s [C1–C8], nervos cervicais; nervos espinais que surgem dos segmentos cervicais da medula espinal. SIN nervi cervicales [C1–C8].

cervical splanchnic n.'s, nervos esplâncnicos cervicais; ramos viscerais que surgem dos gânglios cervicais superior, médio e inferior (estrelado); incluem os nervos cardíacos cervicais superior, médio e inferior e fazem parte dos nervos esplâncnicos cardiopulmonares. SIN augmentor n.'s.

circumflex n., n. circumflexo. SIN axillary n.

coccygeal n. [Co] [TA], n. coccígeo; pequeno nervo, o mais baixo dos nervos espinais, que entra na formação do plexo coccígeo. SIN nervus coccygeus [Co] [TA].

cochlear n. [TA], n. coclear; parte do nervo vestibulococlear [NC VIII] perifericamente à raiz coclear; composto dos processos nervosos centrais dos neurônios bipolares do gânglio espiral, que possuem seus processos periféricos em quatro séries de células neuroepiteliais (células pilosas) do órgão espiral. VER TAMBÉM cochlear root of VIII nerve. SIN nervus cochlearis [TA], auditory n., cochlear part of vestibulocochlear nerve, inferior part of vestibulocochlear nerve, pars cochlearis nervi vestibulocochlearis.

common fibular n. [TA], n. fibular comum; uma das divisões terminais do nervo ciático, que se afasta do nervo tibial na extremidade superior da fossa poplítea; a seguir, segue seu trajeto com o tendão do bíceps ao longo da porção lateral do espaço poplíteo para curvar-se ao redor do colo da fíbula, onde se divide em nervos peroneais superficial e profundo. O nervo fibular comum ou seu ramo profundo constitui o nervo mais comumente lesado, estando localizado numa posição subcutânea lateral no colo da fíbula; a ocorrência de lesão provoca perda da capacidade de dorsiflexão do pé ("pé caído"). SIN nervus fibularis communis, common peroneal n.*, nervus peroneus communis*.

common palmar digital n.'s [TA], nervos digitais palmares comuns; quatro nervos na região palmar que enviam ramos (nervos digitais palmares próprios) para os lados adjacentes de dois dedos; três consistem em ramos do nervo mediano, um do nervo ulnar. SIN nervi digitales palmares communes [TA].

common peroneal n., n. fibular comum; *termo oficial alternativo para common fibular n.

common plantar digital n.'s [TA], nervos digitais plantares comuns; três nervos derivados do nervo plantar medial e um do nervo plantar lateral, que suprem a pele sobre os metatarsos, terminando como nervos digitais plantares próprios para o lado de cada dedo do pé. SIN nervi digitales plantares communes [TA].

cranial n.'s [TA], n. cranianos; nervos que emergem do, ou penetram no, crânio, em contraste com os nervos espinais, que emergem da coluna vertebral. Os doze pares de nervos cranianos são os nervos olfatório [NC I], óptico [NC II], oculomotor [NC III], troclear [NC IV], trigêmeo [NC V], abducente [NC VI], facial [NC VII], vestibulococlear [NC VIII], glossafaríngeo [NC IX], vago [NC X], acessório [NC XI] e hipoglosso [NC XII]. SIN nervi craniales [TA].

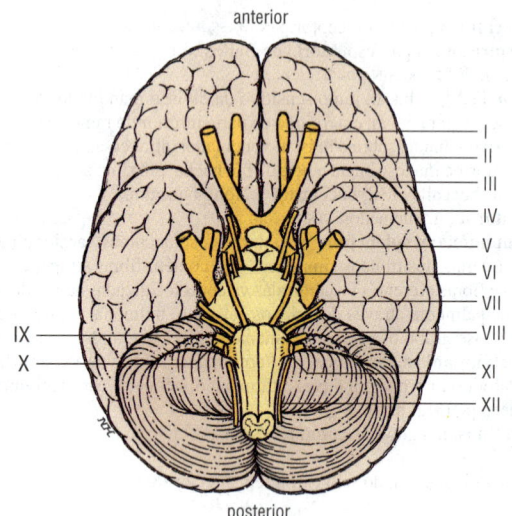

nervos cranianos: (vista inferior): (I) olfatório, (II) óptico, (III) oculomotor, (IV) troclear, (V) trigêmeo, (VI) abducente, (VII) facial, (VIII) vestibulococlear, (IX) glossofaríngeo, (X) vago, (XI) acessório, (XII) hipoglosso

crural interosseous n. [TA], n. interósseo da perna; nervo que se origina de um dos ramos musculares do nervo tibial que desce sobre a superfície posterior da membrana interóssea, inervando-a e inervando os dois ossos da perna. SIN nervus interosseus cruris [TA], interosseous n. of leg.
cubital n., n. cubital. SIN ulnar n.
cutaneous n. [TA], n. cutâneo; nervo misto que supre uma região da pele, incluindo suas terminações sensoriais, vasos sanguíneos, músculos lisos e glândulas. SIN nervus cutaneus [TA].
cutaneous cervical n., n. cervical cutâneo. SIN transverse cervical n.
Cyon n., n. de Cyon. SIN aortic n.
dead n., n. morto; termo incorreto para referir-se à polpa morta de um dente.
deep fibular n. [TA], n. fibular profundo; um dos ramos terminais do nervo fibular comum, que surge no colo fibular e passa no compartimento anterior da perna; inerva os músculos tibial anterior, extensor longo do hálux, extensor longo dos dedos e fibular terceiro na perna; a seguir, cruza a articulação do tornozelo para suprir os músculos no dorso do pé (extensores do hálux e extensor curto dos dedos), passando a ser cutâneo para inervar os lados adjacentes do hálux e do segundo artelho. SIN nervus fibularis profundi [TA], deep peroneal n.*, nervus peroneus profundus*, anterior tibial n.
deep peroneal n., n. peroneal profundo; *termo oficial alternativo para deep fibular n.
deep petrosal n. [TA], n. petroso profundo; ramo petroso profundo do plexo carotídeo interno, que se une ao nervo petroso maior na entrada do canal pterigóide, formando o nervo do canal pterigóide e, assim, fornecendo fibras póssinápticas para o gânglio pterigopalatino. SIN nervus petrosus profundus [TA], radix sympathica ganglii pterygopalatini*, sympathetic root of pterygopalatine ganglion*.
deep temporal n.'s [TA], nervos temporais profundos; dois ramos, anterior e posterior, provenientes do nervo mandibular, que suprem o músculo temporal e o periósteo da fossa temporal. SIN nervi temporales profundi [TA].
dental n., n. dentário; (**1**) termo leigo para referir-se à polpa dentária; (**2**) ramos dos nervos alveolares inferior e superior dos dentes. VER inferior alveolar n., superior alveolar n.'s.
depressor n. of Ludwig, n. depressor de Ludwig. SIN aortic n.
dorsal n. of clitoris [TA], n. dorsal do clitóris; ramo terminal profundo do pudendo, que inerva especialmente a glande do clitóris após passar pela musculatura perínea profunda, seguindo seu trajeto ao longo do dorso do corpo do clitóris. SIN nervus dorsalis clitoridis [TA].
dorsal digital n.'s, nervos digitais dorsais. SIN dorsal digital n.'s of hand.

dorsal digital n.'s of deep fibular nerve [TA], nervos digitais dorsais do nervo fibular profundo; porção sensorial terminal do nervo fibular profundo no dorso do pé, que permanece após terem sido supridos os ramos motores dos músculos extensor curto dos dedos do pé e extensor curto do hálux; fornece a inervação cutânea para uma pequena área em forma de cunha que inclui os lados adjacentes do hálux e segundo dedo do pé. SIN nervi digitales dorsales nervi fibularis profundi [TA].
dorsal digital n.'s of foot [TA], nervos digitais dorsais do pé; nervos que suprem a pele da face dorsal das falanges proximal e média dos dedos dos pés. VER dorsal digital n.'s of superficial fibular nerve, dorsal digital n.'s of deep fibular nerve. SIN nervi digitales dorsales pedis [TA], dorsal n.'s of toes.
dorsal digital n.'s of hand [TA], nervos digitais dorsais da mão; ramos terminais dos nervos radial e ulnar da mão que suprem a pele da face dorsal das falanges proximal e média dos dedos. VER dorsal digital n.'s of ulnar nerve. SIN dorsal digital n.'s, nervi digitales dorsales.
dorsal digital n.'s of superficial fibular nerve [TA], nervos digitais dorsais do nervo fibular superficial; nervos que surgem no compartimento fibular lateral da perna e que passam para o dorso do pé, suprindo a pele da maior parte do dorso do pé e face dorsal dos dedos, à exceção de uma pequena área em forma de cunha, incluindo os lados adjacentes do hálux e segundo dedo do pé. SIN nervi digitales dorsales nervi fibularis superficialis [TA].
dorsal digital n.'s of ulnar nerve [TA], nervos digitais dorsais do nervo ulnar; nervos que surgem do ramo dorsal do nervo ulnar, suprindo a pele da face dorsal do quinto dedo e metade ulnar do dedo anular e área adjacente do dorso da mão. SIN nervi digitales dorsales nervi ulnaris [TA].
dorsal interosseous n., n. interósseo dorsal. SIN posterior interosseous n.
dorsal lateral cutaneous n., n. cutâneo dorsal lateral. SIN lateral dorsal cutaneous n.
dorsal medial cutaneous n., n. cutâneo dorsal medial. SIN medial dorsal cutaneous n.
dorsal n. of penis [TA], n. dorsal do pênis; ramo terminal profundo dos nervos pudendos, que corre através dos músculos períneos profundos, emitindo ramos e seguindo ao longo do dorso do pênis, para inervar a pele do pênis, o prepúcio, os corpos cavernosos e a glande. SIN nervus dorsalis penis [TA].
dorsal n. of scapula, n. dorsal da escápula. SIN dorsal scapular n.
dorsal scapular n. [TA], n. dorsal da escápula; origina-se dos ramos primários ventrais do quinto ao sétimo nervo cervical e passa para baixo, inervando o elevador da escápula e os músculos rombóides maior e menor. SIN nervus dorsalis scapulae [TA], dorsal n. of scapula n. to rhomboid, posterior scapular n.
dorsal n.'s of toes, n. nervos dorsais dos artelhos. SIN dorsal digital n.'s of foot.
efferent n., n. eferente; nervo que envia impulsos do sistema nervoso central para a periferia. SIN centrifugal n., exodic n.
eighth n., oitavo nervo craniano. SIN vestibulocochlear n. [CN VIII].
eighth cranial n. [CN VIII], oitavo nervo craniano [NC VIII]. SIN vestibulocochlear n. [CN VIII].
eleventh cranial n. [CN XI], décimo primeiro nervo craniano [NC XI]. SIN accessory n. [CN XI].
esodic n., n. exódico. SIN afferent n.
excitor n., n. excitador; nervo condutor de impulsos que estimulam o aumento de uma função.
excitoreflex n., n. excitor reflexo; nervo visceral cuja função especial é provocar uma ação reflexa.
exodic n., n. exódico. SIN efferent n.
n. to external acoustic meatus [TA], n. do meato acústico externo; ramo do nervo auriculotemporal que supre o revestimento do meato acústico externo. SIN nervus meatus acustici externi [TA].
external carotid n.'s [TA], nervos carótidos externos; ramo arterial cefálico do tronco simpático que emite diversas fibras nervosas simpáticas desde o gânglio cervical superior até a artéria carótida externa, formando o plexo carótido externo. SIN nervi carotici externi [TA].
external respiratory n. of Bell, n. respiratório externo de Bell. SIN long thoracic n.
external saphenous n., n. safeno externo. SIN sural n.
external spermatic n., n. espermático externo. SIN genital branch of genitofemoral nerve.
facial n. [CN VII] [TA], n. facial [NC VII]; nervo que tem a sua origem no tegmento da porção inferior da ponte; emerge do cérebro na borda posterior da ponte; deixa a cavidade craniana através do meato acústico interno, onde se une ao nervo intermediário, atravessa o canal facial na porção petrosa do osso temporal e sai através do forame estilomastóide; após suprir os músculos estapédio, occipital, auricular, estiloióideo e o ventre posterior dos músculos digástricos, seu tronco principal ramifica-se no interior da glândula parótida, formando o plexo intraparótido, cujos vários ramos se estendem até os músculos da expressão facial. SIN nervus facialis [CN VII] [TA], motor n. of face, seventh cranial n. [CN VII].

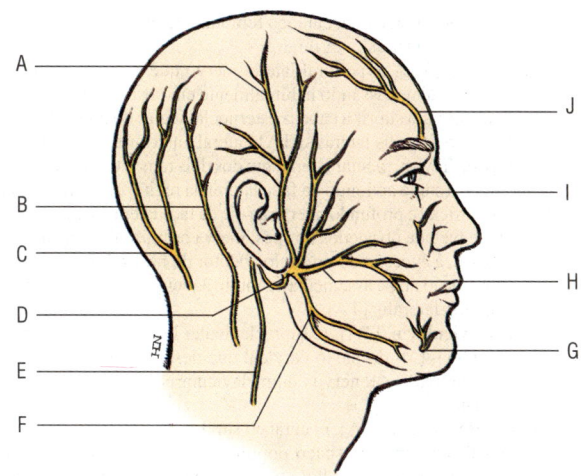

nervo facial e outros nervos que suprem a cabeça e o pescoço: (A) ramo auriculotemporal do nervo facial; (B) nervo occipital menor; (C) nervo occipital maior; (D) nervo facial; (E) grande nervo auricular; (F) ramo mandibular do nervo facial; (G) nervo mentual; (H) ramo bucal do nervo facial; (I) ramo temporal do nervo facial; (J) nervo supra-orbital

femoral n. [TA], n. femoral; origina-se como ramo do plexo lombar, transportando fibras do segundo, terceiro e quarto nervos lombares através da substância do músculo psoas, e penetra na coxa através do espaço do músculo retroinguinal, posteriormente ao ligamento inguinal, lateralmente aos vasos femorais; no interior do triângulo femoral, ramifica-se em ramos musculares para os músculos sartório, pectíneo e quadríceps, em ramos cutâneos femorais anteriores para a pele e região anterior e medial da coxa; seu ramo terminal é o nervo safeno, através do qual supre a pele da face medial da perna e do pé. SIN nervus femoralis [TA], anterior crural n.

fifth cranial n. [CN V], quinto nervo craniano [NC V]. SIN trigeminal n. [CN V].

first cranial n. [CN I], primeiro nervo craniano [NC I]. SIN olfactory n.'s [CN I].

fourth cranial n. [CN IV], quarto nervo craniano [NC IV]. SIN trochlear n. [CN IV].

fourth lumbar n. [L4] [TA], quarto nervo lombar [L4]; o ramo ventral do nervo bifurca-se para penetrar na formação dos plexos lombar e sacro. SIN furcal n., nervus furcalis.

frontal n. [TA], n. frontal; ramo do nervo oftálmico que se divide no interior da órbita nos nervos supratroclear e supra-orbital. SIN nervus frontalis [TA].

furcal n., n. furcal. SIN fourth lumbar n. [L4].

Galen n., n. de Galeno. SIN communicating branch of internal laryngeal nerve with recurrent laryngeal nerve.

gangliated n., n. ganglionar; um nervo simpático.

genitocrural n., n. genitocrural. SIN genitofemoral n.

genitofemoral n. [TA], n. genitofemoral; origina-se do primeiro e do segundo nervos lombares, passa distalmente ao longo da superfície anterior do músculo psoas maior e divide-se nos ramos genital e femoral. SIN nervus genitofemoralis [TA], genitocrural n.

glossopharyngeal n. [CN IX] [TA], n. glossofaríngeo [NC IX]; nono nervo craniano que emerge da extremidade rostral do bulbo e passa através do forame jugular para suprir a sensação, incluindo paladar na faringe e terço posterior da língua; transporta também fibras motoras somáticas para o músculo estilofaríngeo e fibras parassimpáticas pré-sinápticas secretomotoras para o gânglio ótico para inervação da glândula parótida. SIN nervus glossopharyngeus [CN IX] [TA], ninth cranial n. [CN IX].

great auricular n. [TA], n. auricular grande; origina-se como ramo do plexo cervical, transportando fibras dos ramos primários ventrais do segundo e terceiro nervos espinais cervicais; supre a pele de parte da orelha, porção adjacente do couro cabeludo e ângulo da mandíbula; inerva também a bainha da parótida, transportando as fibras para dor estimuladas pelo estiramento da bainha na parotidite (caxumba). SIN nervus auricularis magnus [TA].

greater occipital n. [TA], n. occipital maior; ramo medial do ramo primário dorsal do segundo nervo cervical; envia ramos para os músculos semi-espinhal da cabeça e multífido cervical, porém é principalmente sensitivo, inervando a parte posterior do couro cabeludo, ramos meníngeos para a fossa craniana posterior e ramos para dor e proprioceptivos para o primeiro nervo cervical para os músculos suboccipitais. SIN nervus occipitalis major [TA].

greater palatine n. [TA], n. palatino maior; ramo do gânglio pterigopalatino que segue inferiormente através do canal palatino maior para suprir a mucosa e as glândulas do palato duro e a parte anterior do palato mole. SIN nervus palatinus major [TA].

greater petrosal n. [TA], n. petroso maior; ramo do joelho do nervo facial que sai através do hiato do canal facial e segue seu trajeto num sulco da superfície anterior da parte petrosa do osso temporal, ao lado do forame lácero, para unir-se ao nervo petroso profundo, formando assim o nervo do canal pterigóide, que passa através do canal pterigóide para alcançar o gânglio pterigopalatino. SIN nervus petrosus major [TA], parasympathetic root of pterygopalatine ganglion*, greater superficial petrosal n.

greater splanchnic n. [TA], n. esplâncnico maior; o mais alto dos nervos esplâncnicos abdominopélvicos que se origina do quinto ou sexto ao nono ou décimo gânglio simpático torácico, no tórax, e segue seu trajeto inferiormente ao longo dos corpos das vértebras torácicas, penetrando no diafragma para unir-se ao plexo celíaco; transporta fibras simpáticas pré-sinápticas para os gânglios celíacos e fibras aferentes viscerais a partir do plexo celíaco. SIN nervus splanchnicus major [TA].

greater superficial petrosal n., n. petroso superficial maior. SIN greater petrosal n.

great sciatic n., grande n. isquiático. SIN sciatic n.

hemorrhoidal n.'s, nervos hemorroidários. VER superior rectal (nervous) *plexus,* middle rectal (nervous) *plexus,* inferior anal n.'s.

Hering sinus n., n. sinusal de Hering. SIN carotid *branch* of glossopharyngeal nerve (CN IX).

hypogastric n. [TA], n. hipogástrico; um dos dois troncos nervosos (direito e esquerdo) que se dirigem do plexo hipogástrico superior (nervo pré-sacro) para a pelve, unindo-se aos plexos hipogástricos inferiores. SIN nervus hypogastricus [TA].

hypoglossal n. [CN XII] [TA], n. hipoglosso [NC XII]; origina-se de um núcleo oblongo no bulbo e emerge por diversos filamentos radiculares entre a pirâmide e a oliva, através do sulco pré-olivar; passa através do canal hipoglosso, segue seu trajeto para baixo e para diante, suprindo os músculos intrínsecos e quatro dos cinco músculos extrínsecos da língua. SIN nervus hypoglossus [CN XII] [TA], twelfth cranial n. [CN XII].

iliohypogastric n. [TA], n. ilioipogástrico; ramo terminal, com o nervo ilioinguinal, do primeiro nervo lombar; supre os músculos abdominais e a pele da parte inferior da parede abdominal anterior. SIN nervus iliohypogastricus [TA].

ilioinguinal n. [TA], n. ilioinguinal; ramo terminal, com o nervo ilioipogástrico, do primeiro nervo lombar; passa através do canal inguinal e anel inguinal superficial para inervar a pele da parte medial superior da coxa, monte pubiano e escroto ou grandes lábios. SIN nervus ilioinguinalis [TA].

inferior alveolar n. [TA], n. alveolar inferior; um dos ramos terminais do mandibular, penetra no canal mandibular e distribui-se para os dentes inferiores, periósteo e gengiva da mandíbula; um ramo, o nervo mentual, passa através do forame mentual para suprir a pele e a mucosa do lábio inferior e do queixo. SIN nervus alveolaris inferior [TA], inferior dental n.

inferior anal n.'s [TA], n. anais inferiores; diversos ramos do nervo pudendo que passam para o esfíncter anal externo e pele da região anal. SIN nervi anales inferiores [TA], inferior rectal n.'s*, nervi rectales inferiores*, inferior hemorrhoidal n.'s.

inferior cervical cardiac n. [TA], n. cardíaco cervical inferior; nervo que passa do gânglio estrelado para o plexo cardíaco. SIN nervus cardiacus cervicalis inferior [TA].

inferior clunial n.'s [TA], nervos clúnios inferiores; ramos do nervo cutâneo femoral posterior que emergem por debaixo da borda inferior do músculo glúteo máximo para suprir a pele da metade inferior da região glútea. SIN nervi clunium inferiores [TA].

inferior dental n., n. dental inferior. SIN inferior alveolar n.

inferior gluteal n. [TA], n. glúteo inferior; origina-se como ramo do plexo sacro, transportando fibras do quinto nervo lombar e do primeiro e segundo nervos sacros, suprindo o músculo glúteo máximo. É propenso a sofrer lesão por compressão e isquemia nos indivíduos sedentários, resultando em dificuldade em levantar de uma posição sentada e de subir escadas. SIN nervus gluteus inferior [TA].

inferior hemorrhoidal n.'s, nervos hemorroidários inferiores. SIN inferior anal n.'s.

inferior laryngeal n. [TA], n. laríngeo inferior; ramo terminal do nervo laríngeo recorrente quando este último passa profundamente no constritor faríngeo inferior; inerva a mucosa laríngea inferiormente às pregas vocais e todos os músculos laríngeos, à exceção do cricotireóideo. SIN nervus laryngeus inferior [TA].

inferior lateral brachial cutaneous n., n. cutâneo lateral inferior do braço; *termo oficial alternativo para inferior lateral cutaneous n. of arm.

inferior lateral cutaneous n. of arm [TA], n. cutâneo lateral inferior do braço; ramo cutâneo do nervo radial que supre a pele da face lateral inferior do braço; com freqüência, surge como ramo do nervo antebraquial posterior. SIN nervus cutaneus brachii lateralis inferior [TA], inferior lateral brachial cutaneous n.*

inferior maxillary n., n. maxilar inferior. SIN mandibular n. [CN V3].

inferior rectal n.'s, nervos retais inferiores; *termo oficial alternativo para inferior anal n.'s.

infraorbital n. [TA], n. infra-orbital; continuação do nervo maxilar [NC V2] após atravessar a fossa pterigopalatina e penetrar na órbita, através da fissura infra-orbital; a seguir, passa pelo canal infra-orbital para alcançar a face; supre a mucosa do seio maxilar, os incisivos, os caninos e os pré-molares superiores, a gengiva superior, a pálpebra inferior e a conjuntiva, parte do nariz e o lábio superior. SIN nervus infraorbitalis [TA].

infratrochlear n. [TA], n. infratroclear; ramo terminal do nervo nasociliar que segue seu trajeto abaixo da polia do músculo oblíquo superior para frente da órbita, inervando a pele das pálpebras e raiz do nariz. SIN nervus infratrochlearis [TA].

inhibitory n., n. inibitório; nervo que envia impulsos que diminuem a atividade funcional em determinada parte.

intercarotid n., n. intercarotídeo. SIN carotid branch of glossopharyngeal nerve (CN IX).

intercostal n.'s [TA], nervos intercostais; ramos primários ventrais dos nervos torácicos [T1–T11]. SIN nervi intercostales.

intercostobrachial n.'s [TA], nervos intercostobraquiais; ramos cutâneos laterais do segundo e terceiro nervos intercostais que passam para a pele do lado medial do braço. SIN nervi intercostobrachiales [TA], intercostohumeral n.'s.

intercostohumeral n.'s, nervos intercostoumerais. SIN intercostobrachial n.'s.

intermediary n., n. intermediário. SIN intermediate n.

intermediate n. [TA], n. intermediário; uma raiz do nervo facial que contém fibras sensitivas para o paladar nos 2/3 anteriores da língua, cujos corpos celulares estão localizados no gânglio geniculado, e fibras autônomas parassimpáticas pré-sinápticas, cujos corpos celulares localizam-se no núcleo salivatório superior, isto é, as fibras acabam sendo transportadas através da corda do tímpano do nervo facial para o nervo lingual. SIN nervus intermedius [TA], intermediary n., portio intermedia, Wrisberg n. (2).

intermediate dorsal cutaneous n. [TA], n. cutâneo dorsal intermédio; ramo terminal lateral do nervo fibular superficial, que supre o dorso do pé e nervos dorsais para os dedos do pé (exceto para partes adjacentes do hálux e segundo artelho). SIN nervus cutaneus dorsalis intermedius [TA].

intermediate supraclavicular n. [TA], n. supraclavicular intermédio; um dos vários nervos que se originam da parte C-3—C-4 do plexo cervical, que seguem seu trajeto através da parte superior do ombro e descem através da clavícula para suprir a pele da parte superior do ombro e na região infraclavicular. SIN nervus supraclavicularis intermedius [TA], middle supraclavicular n.

internal carotid n. [TA], n. carótido interno; ramo arterial cefálico que transporta fibras simpáticas pós-sinápticas do gânglio cervical superior para a artéria carótida interna, formando o plexo carotídeo interno. SIN nervus caroticus internus [TA].

internal saphenous n., n. safeno interno. SIN saphenous n.

interosseous n. of leg, n. interósseo da perna. SIN crural interosseous n.

Jacobson n., n. de Jacobson. SIN tympanic n.

jugular n. [TA], n. jugular; ramo comunicante entre o gânglio cervical superior do nervo simpático, o gânglio superior do nervo vago e o gânglio inferior do nervo glossofaríngeo. SIN nervus jugularis [TA].

lacrimal n. [TA], n. lacrimal; ramo do nervo oftálmico [NC V1] que supre fibras sensitivas para a parte lateral da pálpebra superior, conjuntiva e glândula lacrimal. As fibras secretomotoras desta última são transportadas para o nervo lacrimal pelo ramo comunicante do nervo zigomático (um ramo do nervo maxilar [NC V2]). SIN nervus lacrimalis [TA].

Latarget n., n. de Latarget; **(1)** SIN superior hypogastric (nervous) *plexus;* **(2)** ramo terminal do tronco vagal anterior que segue seu percurso ao longo da pequena curvatura do estômago para alguns centímetros da junção gastroduodenal, mas que, aparentemente, nunca atinge o esfíncter pilórico.

lateral ampullar n. [TA], n. ampular lateral; ramo do nervo utriculoampular que inerva a crista ampular do ducto semicircular lateral. SIN nervus ampullaris lateralis [TA].

lateral antebrachial cutaneous n., n. cutâneo lateral do antebraço; *termo oficial alternativo para lateral cutaneous n. of forearm.

lateral anterior thoracic n., n. torácico anterior lateral. SIN lateral pectoral n.

lateral cutaneous n. of calf, n. cutâneo lateral da panturrilha. SIN lateral sural cutaneous n.

lateral cutaneous n. of forearm [TA], n. cutâneo lateral do antebraço; ramo cutâneo terminal do nervo musculocutâneo que emerge entre os músculos bíceps do braço e braquial para suprir a pele do lado radial do antebraço. SIN nervus cutaneus antebrachii lateralis [TA], lateral antebrachial cutaneous n.*.

lateral cutaneous n. of thigh [TA], n. cutâneo lateral da coxa; origina-se do plexo lombar, transmitindo fibras do segundo e terceiro nervos lombares; supre a pele das superfícies ântero-lateral e lateral da coxa. SIN nervus cutaneus femoris lateralis [TA], lateral femoral cutaneous n.*.

lateral dorsal cutaneous n. [TA], n. cutâneo dorsal lateral; continuação do nervo sural do pé, que supre a margem lateral e o dorso. SIN nervus cutaneus dorsalis lateralis [TA], dorsal lateral cutaneous n.

lateral femoral cutaneous n., n. cutâneo femoral lateral; *termo oficial alternativo para lateral cutaneous n. of thigh.

lateral pectoral n. [TA], n. peitoral lateral; nervo que se origina do cordão lateral do plexo braquial, passando habitualmente em posição medial ao músculo peitoral menor para suprir a cabeça esternoclavicular do músculo peitoral maior. SIN nervus pectoralis lateralis [TA], lateral anterior thoracic n.

lateral plantar n. [TA], n. plantar lateral; um dos dois ramos terminais do nervo tibial; segue seu percurso ao longo da face lateral da região plantar, dividindo-se em ramos superficial e profundo; inerva a pele da face lateral da região plantar e a parte lateral e metade dos dedos dos pés; inerva os músculos intrínsecos da parte plantar do pé, à exceção do músculo abdutor do hálux e flexor curto dos dedos; sua distribuição no pé assemelha-se muito àquela do nervo ulnar na mão. SIN nervus plantaris lateralis [TA].

lateral supraclavicular n. [TA], n. supraclavicular lateral; um dos vários ramos da porção C-3—C-4 do plexo cervical que descem para a pele sobre o acrômio e região deltóide. SIN nervus supraclavicularis lateralis [TA], posterior supraclavicular n.

lateral sural cutaneous n. [TA], n. cutâneo sural lateral; origina-se do nervo fibular (peroneal) comum no espaço poplíteo e distribui-se para a pele da superfície ínfero-lateral da panturrilha. SIN nervus cutaneus surae lateralis [TA], lateral cutaneous n. of calf.

least splanchnic n. [TA], n. esplâncnico mínimo; um dos nervos esplâncnicos abdominopélvicos que surgem no tórax e penetram no diafragma para suprir fibras simpáticas pré-sinápticas ao plexo renal; freqüentemente combinado com o nervo esplâncnico menor; todavia, em certas ocasiões, ocorre como nervo independente. SIN nervus splanchnicus imus [TA], lowest splanchnic n.*, smallest splanchnic n.

lesser internal cutaneous n., n. cutâneo interno menor. SIN medial cutaneous n. of arm.

lesser occipital n. [TA], n. occipital menor; origina-se do plexo cervical, transportando fibras dos ramos primários ventrais do segundo e terceiro nervos cervicais; supre a pele da superfície posterior da aurícula e porção adjacente do couro cabeludo até a aurícula. SIN nervus occipitalis minor [TA].

lesser palatine n.'s [TA], nervos palatinos menores; geralmente em número de dois; esses nervos emergem através dos forames palatinos menores e suprem a mucosa e as glândulas do palato mole e úvula; são ramos do gânglio pterigopalatino e contêm fibras sensoriais e parassimpáticas pós-sinápticas do nervo maxilar. SIN nervi palatini minores [TA].

lesser petrosal n. [TA], n. petroso menor; a raiz parassimpática do gânglio ótico, derivada do plexo timpânico; deixa a cavidade timpânica através do canal para o nervo petroso menor e passa dentro do crânio para a fissura esfenopetrosa ou para o forame oval ou para o forame petroso, através do qual desce para alcançar o gânglio ótico; transporta fibras parassimpáticas pré-sinápticas do nervo glossofaríngeo relacionado com a inervação secretomotora da glândula parótida. SIN nervus petrosus minor [TA], parasympathetic root of otic ganglion*, radix parasympathica ganglii otici*, lesser superficial petrosal n.

lesser splanchnic n. [TA], n. esplâncnico menor; um dos nervos esplâncnicos abdominopélvicos que surgem no tórax a partir dos dois últimos gânglios simpáticos torácicos, passando através do diafragma para o gânglio aórtico renal; transporta fibras simpáticas pré-sinápticas e fibras aferentes viscerais. SIN nervus splanchnicus minor [TA].

lesser superficial petrosal n., n. petroso superficial menor. SIN lesser petrosal n.

lingual n. [TA], n. lingual; um dos ramos do nervo mandibular [NC V3], que passa medialmente ao músculo pterigóide lateral, entre o pterigóide medial e a mandíbula, e por debaixo da mucosa do assoalho da boca para o lado da língua, onde se distribui em seus dois terços anteriores; supre também a mucosa do assoalho da boca. Passa próximo ao lado lingual das raízes do segundo e terceiro molares inferiores e corre risco de comprometimento durante extrações dentárias. SIN nervus lingualis [TA].

long buccal n., n. bucal longo. SIN buccal n.

long ciliary n. [TA], n. ciliar longo; um de dois ou três ramos do nervo nasociliar que contornam o gânglio ciliar, suprindo fibras simpáticas pós-sinápticas para o músculo dilatador da pupila e fibras sensoriais para os músculos ciliares, íris e córnea. SIN nervus ciliaris longus [TA].

long saphenous n., n. safeno longo. SIN saphenous n.

long subscapular n., n. subescapular longo. SIN thoracodorsal n.

long thoracic n. [TA], n. torácico longo; origina-se do quinto, sexto e sétimo nervos cervicais (raízes do plexo braquial), desce pelo pescoço atrás do plexo braquial e distribui-se para o músculo serrátil anterior; é um pouco singular por seguir seu trajeto sobre a face superficial do músculo por ele inervado; sua paralisia resulta em "escápula alada". SIN nervus thoracicus longus [TA], Bell respiratory n., external respiratory n. of Bell, posterior thoracic n.

lowest splanchnic n., n. esplâncnico mínimo; *termo oficial alternativo para least splanchnic n.

Ludwig n., n. de Ludwig. SIN aortic n.

lumbar n.'s [L1-L5], nervos lombares [L1-L5]; cinco nervos espinais bilaterais que emergem da porção lombar da medula espinal; os primeiros quatro nervos entram na formação do plexo lombar, o quarto e o quinto entram na formação do plexo sacro. SIN nervi lumbales.

lumbar splanchnic n.'s [TA], nervos esplâncnicos lombares; ramos que se originam da face medial dos troncos simpáticos lombares que passam anterior e medialmente para transportar fibras simpáticas pré-sinápticas para os plexos celíaco, intermesentérico, aórtico e hipogástrico superior e fibras aferentes viscerais a partir desses plexos. SIN nervi splanchnici lumbales [TA].

lumboinguinal n., n. lomboinguinal; ramo femoral do nervo genitofemoral. VER genitofemoral n.

mandibular n. [CN V3] [TA], n. mandibular [NC V3]; a terceira divisão do nervo trigêmeo, pela união de fibras sensitivas provenientes do gânglio trigêmeo e raiz motora do nervo trigêmeo no forame oval, através do qual surge o nervo; seus ramos são o meníngeo, massetérico, temporal profundo, pterigóide lateral e medial, bucal, aurículo temporal, lingual e alveolar inferior; suas fibras sensitivas distribuem-se para a aurícula, meato acústico externo, membrana timpânica, região temporal, bochecha, pele sobre a mandíbula (exceto o seu ângulo), 2/3 anteriores da língua, assoalho da boca, dentes inferiores e gengiva; suas fibras motoras inervam todos os músculos da mastigação mais o músculo milo-hióide, o ventre anterior do digástrico e os tensores do palato mole e da membrana timpânica. SIN nervus mandibularis [CN V3 [TA], inferior maxillary n.

masseteric n. [TA], n. massetérico; ramo muscular do nervo mandibular [NC V3], que passa através da incisura mandibular para a superfície medial do músculo masseter que ele inerva e articulação temporomandibular. SIN nervus massetericus [TA].

masticator n., n. mastigador. SIN motor root of trigeminal nerve.

maxillary n. [CN V2], n. maxilar [NC V2]; a segunda divisão do nervo trigêmeo, que passa do gânglio trigêmeo na fossa craniana média, através do forame redondo, para dentro da fossa pterigopalatina, onde emite ramos ganglionares para o gânglio pterigopalatino e prossegue para diante, emitindo o nervo zigomático e penetrando na órbita, onde continua como nervo infra-orbitário. Suas fibras sensoriais distribuem-se para a pele e conjuntiva da pálpebra inferior, pele e mucosa do lábio superior e bochecha, palato, dentes e gengiva superiores, seio maxilar, asas do nariz e cavidade nasal posterior/interior. SIN nervus maxillaris [CN V2] [TA], superior maxillary n.

medial antebrachial cutaneous n., n. cutâneo medial do antebraço; *termo oficial alternativo para medial cutaneous n. of forearm.

medial anterior thoracic n., n. torácico anterior medial. SIN medial pectoral n.

medial brachial cutaneous n., n. cutâneo medial do braço; *termo oficial alternativo para medial cutaneous n. of arm.

medial clunial n.'s [TA], n. clúnios médios; ramos terminais dos ramos dorsais primários dos nervos sacros, que suprem a pele da região glútea média. SIN nervi clunium medii [TA], middle cluneal n.'s.

medial crural cutaneous n., n. cutâneo medial da perna; *termo oficial alternativo para medial cutaneous n. of leg.

medial cutaneous n. of arm [TA], n. cutâneo medial do braço; origina-se do cordão medial do plexo braquial, une-se na axila com o ramo cutâneo lateral do segundo nervo intercostal e supre a pele do lado medial do braço. SIN nervus cutaneus brachii medialis [TA], medial brachial cutaneous n.*, lesser internal cutaneous n., Wrisberg n. (1).

medial cutaneous n. of forearm [TA], n. cutâneo medial do antebraço; origina-se do cordão medial do plexo braquial, passa para baixo junto com a artéria braquial e, em seguida, com a veia basílica, inervando a pele das superfícies anterior e ulnar do antebraço. SIN nervus cutaneus antebrachii medialis [TA], medial antebrachial cutaneous n.*.

medial cutaneous n. of leg [TA], n. cutâneo medial da perna; ramos do nervo safeno que se distribuem para a pele do lado medial da perna. SIN rami cutanei cruris mediales nervi sapheni [TA], medial crural cutaneous n.*, medial crural cutaneous branches of saphenous nerve.

medial dorsal cutaneous n. [TA], n. cutâneo dorsal medial; ramo terminal medial do nervo fibular superficial que inerva o dorso do pé e nervos dorsais para os artelhos (exceto os lados adjacentes do hálux e segundo dedo do pé). SIN nervus cutaneus dorsalis medialis [TA], dorsal medial cutaneous n.

medial pectoral n. [TA], n. peitoral medial; nervo que se origina do cordão medial do plexo braquial para inervar os músculos peitorais; em geral, perfura o músculo peitoral menor e, a seguir, prossegue para inervar principalmente a porção esternocostal do músculo peitoral maior. SIN nervus pectoralis medialis [TA], medial anterior thoracic n.

medial plantar n. [TA], n. plantar medial; um dos dois ramos terminais do nervo tibial; segue um percurso ao longo da face medial da região plantar para inervar os músculos abdutor do hálux e flexor curto dos dedos e, por meio dos ramos digitais comum e próprio, a pele da parte medial do pé e dos três e meio artelhos mediais. SIN nervus plantaris medialis [TA].

medial popliteal n., n. n. poplíteo medial. SIN tibial n.

medial supraclavicular n. [TA], n. supraclavicular medial; um dos vários nervos que se originam da alça C3–C4 do plexo cervical, que inervam a pele sobre a extremidade medial da clavícula e parte medial superior do tórax. SIN nervus supraclavicularis medialis [TA], anterior supraclavicular n.

medial sural cutaneous n. [TA], n. cutâneo medial da perna; origina-se do nervo tibial no espaço poplíteo, passa por baixo da panturrilha entre as duas cabeças do músculo gastrocnêmio e une-se, no meio da perna, com o ramo comunicante do peroneiro comum para formar o nervo sural, que se distribui para a pele das superfícies distal e lateral da perna e do tornozelo. SIN nervus cutaneus surae medialis [TA], popliteal communicating n., tibial communicating n.

median n. [TA], n. mediano; formado pela união das raízes medial e lateral dos cordões medial e lateral do plexo braquial, respectivamente; proporciona a inervação de todos os músculos no compartimento anterior do antebraço, à exceção do flexor ulnar do punho e metade ulnar do flexor profundo dos dedos; passa através do túnel do carpo para suprir os músculos tenares (à exceção do adutor do polegar e cabeça profunda do flexor curto do polegar) através de seu ramo tenar recorrente; suas fibras sensoriais distribuem-se para a pele da face palmar e face dorsal distal dos três dedos e meio radiais e região palmar adjacente. O nervo mediano é mais comumente lesado por compressão na síndrome do túnel do carpo, resultando em perda da capacidade de oposição do polegar ("mão de macaco") e perda da sensação na porção radial da mão. SIN nervus medianus [TA].

mental n. [TA], n. mentoniano; ramo do nervo alveolar inferior, que se origina no canal mandibular e passa através do forame mentoniano para o queixo e lábio inferior. SIN nervus mentalis [TA].

middle cervical cardiac n. [TA], n. cardíaco cervical médio; um dos nervos esplâncnicos cardiopulmonares que transportam fibras simpáticas pós-sinápticas que correm para baixo do gânglio cervical médio, ao longo da artéria subclávia (à esquerda) ou braquiocefálica (do lado direito), para unir-se ao plexo cardíaco. SIN nervus cardiacus cervicalis medius [TA].

middle cluneal n.'s, n. clúnios médios. SIN medial clunial n.'s.

middle meningeal n., n. meníngeo médio. SIN meningeal branch of maxillary nerve.

middle supraclavicular n., n. supraclavicular médio. SIN intermediate supraclavicular n.

mixed n. [TA], n. misto; nervo que contém fibras tanto aferentes quanto eferentes. SIN nervus mixtus [TA].

motor n. [TA], n. motor; nervo composto, em grande parte ou totalmente, de fibras nervosas eferentes (motoras) que transportam impulsos, excitando a contração muscular; os nervos motores no sistema nervoso autônomo também estimulam a secreção dos epitélios glandulares.

motor n. of face, n. motor da face. SIN facial n. [CN VII].

musculocutaneous n. [TA], n. musculocutâneo; origina-se a partir do cordão lateral do plexo braquial, passa através do músculo coracobraquial e, a seguir, desce entre os músculos braquial e bíceps, inervando esses músculos e prosseguindo distalmente como nervo cutâneo lateral do antebraço. SIN nervus musculocutaneus [TA].

musculocutaneous n. of leg, n. musculocutâneo da perna. SIN superficial fibular n.

musculospiral n., n. musculoespiral. SIN radial n.

myelinated n., n. mielinizado; nervo periférico cujos axônios são circundados por bainhas de membranas de células de Schwann que formam a bainha de mielina; também denominado nervo medulado.

mylohyoid n., n. miloióideo. SIN n. to mylohyoid.

n. to mylohyoid [TA], n. para o miloióideo; pequeno ramo do nervo alveolar inferior que se origina posteriormente, antes de o nervo penetrar no forame mandibular, distribuindo-se para o ventre anterior do músculo digástrico e para o músculo miloióideo. SIN nervus mylohyoideus [TA], mylohyoid n.

nasal n., n. nasal. SIN nasociliary n.

nasociliary n. [TA], n. nasociliar; ramo do nervo oftálmico [NC V1] na fissura orbitária superior, que passa através da órbita, dando origem ao ramo comunicante do gânglio ciliar, aos nervos ciliares longos, nervos etmoidal anterior e etmoidal posterior e terminando como ramos infratroclear e nasal, que inervam a mucosa do nariz, a pele da extremidade nasal e a conjuntiva. SIN nervus nasociliaris [TA], nasal n.

nasopalatine n. [TA], n. nasopalatino; ramo do gânglio pterigopalatino que passa através do forame esfenopalatino, cruzando e, a seguir, descendo pelo septo nasal e através do forame incisivo para inervar a mucosa do palato duro. SIN nervus nasopalatinus [TA].

ninth cranial n. [CN IX], nono n. craniano [NC IX]. SIN glossopharyngeal n. [CN IX].

obturator n. [TA], n. obturador; origina-se do plexo lombar, transportando fibras do segundo, do terceiro e do quarto nervos lombares no músculo psoas; cruza a borda da pelve e penetra na coxa através do canal obturador; inerva os músculos do compartimento medial da coxa (adutores da coxa na articulação do quadril) e termina como ramo cutâneo do nervo obturador, suprindo uma pequena área da face medial da coxa, acima do joelho. SIN nervus obturatorius [TA].

oculomotor n. [CN III] [TA], n. oculomotor [NC III]; terceiro nervo craniano; supre todos os músculos extrínsecos do olho, exceto o reto lateral e o oblíquo superior; inerva também o elevador da pálpebra superior e transporta fibras parassimpáticas pré-sinápticas para o gânglio ciliar, para inervação do músculo ciliar e esfíncter da pupila; sua origem é no mesencéfalo, abaixo do aqueduto cerebral; emerge do cérebro na fossa interpeduncular, perfura a dura-máter para o lado do processo clinóide posterior, passa na parede lateral do seio cavernoso e penetra na órbita através da fissura orbitária superior. SIN nervus oculomotorius [CN III] [TA], motor oculi, oculomotorius, third cranial n. [CN III].

olfactory n.'s [CN I] [TA], nervos olfatórios [NC I]; termo coletivo para referir-se aos numerosos filamentos olfatórios: fascículos delgados compostos, cada um, de finos axônios amielínicos de 8 a 12 das células receptoras olfatórias bipolares na porção olfatória da mucosa nasal; os filamentos olfatórios passam através da placa cribriforme do osso etmóide e penetram no bulbo olfatório, onde terminam em contato sináptico com células mitrais, células em tufos e células granulares. VER TAMBÉM olfactory tract. SIN fila olfactoria [TA], nervus olfactorii [CN I] [TA], first cranial n. [CN I], n. of smell, olfactory fila.

ophthalmic n. [CN V1] [TA], n. oftálmico [NC V1]; ramo do nervo trigêmeo que passa para diante do gânglio trigêmeo da parede lateral do seio cavernoso, penetrando na órbita através da fissura orbitária superior; através de seus ramos frontal, lacrimal e nasociliar, fornece a sensibilidade para a órbita e seu conteúdo, a parte anterior da cavidade nasal e a pele do nariz e da testa. SIN nervus ophthalmicus [CN V1] [TA].

optic n. [CN II] [TA], n. óptico; embora seja classificado como nervo craniano, trata-se, na verdade, de uma extensão do prosencéfalo; transporta fibras aferentes das células ganglionares da retina, sai da órbita através do canal óptico para o quiasma, onde parte das fibras cruza para o lado oposto e passa através do trato óptico para os corpos geniculados, colículo superior e pré-teto. SIN nervus opticus [CN II] [TA], second cranial n. [CN II].

orbital n., n. orbitário. SIN zygomatic n.

parasympathetic n., n. parassimpático; um dos nervos do sistema nervoso parassimpático.

pathetic n., n. patético. SIN trochlear n. [CN IV].

pelvic splanchnic n.'s [TA], nervos esplâncnicos pélvicos; ramos viscerais dos ramos primários ventrais do segundo, terceiro e quarto nervos sacros que se unem ao plexo hipogástrico inferior para formar os plexos pélvicos, a partir dos quais e para os quais transportam fibras parassimpáticas pré-sinápticas e sensoriais, respectivamente. SIN nervi pelvici splanchnici [TA], parasympathetic root of pelvic ganglia*, radices parasympathicae gangliorum pelvicorum*, nervi erigentes.

perineal n.'s [TA], nervos perineais; ramos terminais superficiais do nervo pudendo que inervam a maioria dos músculos do períneo (ramo profundo), bem como a pele dessa região (ramo superficial). SIN nervi perineales [TA].

peroneal communicating n., n. comunicante do peroneal. SIN sural communicating branch of common fibular nerve.

pharyngeal n. [TA], n. faríngeo; ramo do gânglio pterigopalatino que passa posteriormente, através do canal faríngeo, para suprir fibras parassimpáticas pós-sinápticas das glândulas mucosas da nasofaringe. SIN nervus pharyngeus [TA], Bock n., pharyngeal branch of pterygopalatine ganglion, ramus pharyngeus ganglii pterygopalatini.

phrenic n. [TA], n. frênico; origina-se do plexo cervical, transportando principalmente fibras do quarto nervo cervical; passa por debaixo, na frente do músculo escaleno anterior, e penetra no tórax, entre a artéria e a veia subclávias, atrás da articulação esternoclavicular; a seguir, passa em frente da raiz do pulmão para o diafragma; é principalmente o nervo motor do diafragma, porém envia fibras sensoriais para a pleura parietal mediastínica, pericárdio, pleura diafragmática e peritônio, e ramos (ramos frenicoabdominais) que se comunicam com ramos do plexo celíaco. SIN nervus phrenicus [TA].

pneumogastric n., n. pneumogástrico. SIN vagus n. [CN X].

popliteal communicating n., n. comunicante poplíteo. SIN medial sural cutaneous n.

posterior ampullar n. [TA], n. ampular posterior; ramo da parte vestibular o oitavo nervo que supre a crista ampular do ducto semicircular posterior. SIN nervus ampullaris posterior [TA].

posterior antebrachial n., n. antebraquial posterior. SIN posterior interosseous n.

posterior antebrachial cutaneous n., n. cutâneo posterior do antebraço; *termo oficial alternativo para posterior cutaneous n. of forearm.

posterior auricular n. [TA], n. auricular posterior; o primeiro ramo extracraniano do nervo facial; passa por detrás da orelha, inervando os músculos auricular posterior e intrínseco da aurícula e, através de seu ramo occipital, o ventre occipital do músculo occipitofrontal. SIN nervus auricularis posterior [TA].

posterior brachial cutaneous n., n. cutâneo posterior do braço; *termo oficial alternativo para posterior cutaneous n. of arm.

posterior cutaneous n. of arm [TA], n. cutâneo posterior do braço; ramo do nervo radial que supre a pele da superfície posterior do braço. SIN nervus cutaneus brachii posterior [TA], posterior brachial cutaneous n.*

posterior cutaneous n. of forearm [TA], n. cutâneo posterior do antebraço; ramo do nervo radial que supre a pele da superfície dorsal do antebraço. SIN nervus cutaneus antebrachii posterior [TA], posterior antebrachial cutaneous n.*

posterior cutaneous n. of thigh [TA], n. cutâneo posterior da coxa; origina-se como ramo do plexo sacro, transportando fibras dos ramos ventrais dos três primeiros nervos sacros; inerva a pele da superfície posterior da coxa e da região poplítea (componentes S1 e S2); dá origem a um ramo perineal (componente S3) que passa para a face lateral do escroto ou do lábio maior do pudendo. SIN nervus cutaneus femoris posterior [TA], posterior femoral cutaneous n.*, small sciatic n.

posterior ethmoidal n. [TA], n. etmoidal posterior; ramo do nervo nasociliar que fornece inervação sensorial para o seio esfenoidal e células etmoidais posteriores. SIN nervus ethmoidalis posterior [TA].

posterior femoral cutaneous n., n. cutâneo posterior femoral da coxa; *termo oficial alternativo para posterior cutaneous n. of thigh.

posterior inferior nasal n.'s [TA], nervos nasais posteriores inferiores; ramos do nervo palatino maior para a parede lateral posterior e inferior da cavidade nasal, incluindo a face posterior da mucosa sobre a porção posterior da concha e meato nasal inferior; podem surgir independentemente do gânglio pterigopalatino. SIN rami nasales posteriores inferiores nervi palatini majoris [TA], posterior inferior nasal branches of greater palatine nerve.

posterior interosseous n. [TA], n. interósseo posterior; porção terminal do ramo profundo do nervo radial; surge na região cubital, penetrando e suprindo o músculo supinador e continuando seu trajeto com a artéria interóssea posterior para inervar todos os músculos extensores do antebraço. SIN nervus interosseus antebrachii posterior [TA], dorsal interosseous n., nervus antebrachii posterior, nervus interosseous dorsalis, nervus interosseous posterior, posterior antebrachial n.

posterior labial n.'s [TA], nervos labiais posteriores; ramos terminais do nervo perineal superior que inervam a pele da porção posterior dos lábios e o vestíbulo da vagina, correspondendo aos nervos escrotais posteriores no sexo masculino. SIN nervi labiales posteriores [TA].

posterior scapular n., n. escapular posterior. SIN dorsal scapular n.

posterior scrotal n.'s [TA], nervos escrotais posteriores; diversos ramos terminais do nervo perineal superficial que inervam a pele da porção posterior do escroto, correspondendo aos nervos labiais posteriores no sexo feminino. SIN nervi scrotales posteriores [TA].

posterior supraclavicular n., n. supraclavicular posterior. SIN lateral supraclavicular n.

posterior thoracic n., n. torácico posterior. SIN long thoracic n.

presacral n., n. pré-sacro; *termo oficial alternativo para superior hypogastric (nervous) plexus.

pressor n., n. pressor; nervo aferente cujo estímulo excita uma vasoconstrição reflexa, elevando, conseqüentemente, a pressão arterial.

pressoreceptor n., n. pressorreceptor; nervo composto de fibras aferentes cujas terminações são sensíveis a aumentos da pressão mecânica; o termo refere-se, especificamente, a nervos sensoriais que inervam as paredes de órgãos ocos. SIN baroreceptor n.

proper palmar digital n.'s [TA], nervos digitais palmares próprios; os nervos palmares dos dedos da mão derivados dos nervos digitais palmares comuns; cada nervo supre um quadrante palmar de um dedo e uma parte da superfície dorsal da falange distal. SIN nervi digitales palmares proprii [TA].

proper plantar digital n.'s [TA], nervos digitais plantares próprios; os dez nervos derivados dos nervos digitais plantares comuns; cada nervo supre um quadrante plantar de um artelho e parte da superfície dorsal da falange distal. SIN nervi digitales plantares proprii [TA].

pterygoid n. [TA], n. pterigóideo; um de dois ramos motores, os nervos para os músculos pterigóideos lateral e medial, do nervo mandibular, inervando os músculos com fibras da raiz motora do nervo trigêmeo. SIN nervus pterygoideus [TA].

n. of pterygoid canal [TA], n. do canal pterigóideo; o nervo que constitui as raízes parassimpática e simpática do gânglio pterigopalatino; formado na região do forame lácero pela união dos nervos petroso maior e petroso profundo, seguindo seu percurso através do canal pterigóideo para a fossa pterigopalatina. SIN nervus canalis pterygoidei [TA], facial root, radix facialis, vidian n.

pterygopalatine n.'s, nervos pterigopalatinos. SIN sensory root of pterygopalatine ganglion.

pudendal n. [TA], n. pudendo; ramos do plexo sacro formado por fibras dos ramos primários ventrais do segundo, terceiro e quarto nervos sacros; deixa a pelve através do forame isquiático maior, passa posteriormente ao ligamento sacro espinoso e acompanha a artéria pudenda interna, penetrando no períneo através do forame isquiático menor; dá origem aos nervos retais inferiores; a seguir, segue através do canal pudendo na parede lateral da fossa isquiorretal, terminando no nervo dorsal do pênis ou do clitóris. SIN nervus pudendus [TA], plexus pudendus nervosus, pudic n.

pudic n., n. pudendo. SIN pudendal n.

radial n. [TA], n. radial; origina-se do cordão posterior do plexo braquial, transportando fibras de todas as raízes do plexo; curva-se ao redor da superfície posterior do úmero e desce para a fossa cubital, onde se divide em seus dois ramos terminais, o ramo cutâneo superficial e o ramo motor profundo; inerva os músculos dos compartimentos posteriores do braço e do antebraço e a pele sobrejacente. O nervo radial é mais comumente lesado por fraturas do terço médio do úmero, resultando em perda da extensão do punho ("punho caído"). SIN nervus radialis [TA], musculospiral n.

recurrent n., n. recorrente. SIN recurrent laryngeal n.

recurrent laryngeal n. [TA], n. laríngeo recorrente; ramo do nervo vago que se curva para cima, no lado direito ao redor da raiz da artéria subclávia, no lado esquerdo ao redor do arco da aorta, passando, a seguir, para cima, posteriormente à artéria carótida comum, entre a traquéia e o esôfago, para a laringe; supre os ramos cardíaco, traqueal e esofágico e termina como nervo laríngeo inferior. SIN nervus laryngeus recurrens [TA], recurrent n.

recurrent meningeal n., n. meníngeo recorrente; ramos meníngeos dos nervos 1) mandibular, 2) maxilar, 3) oftálmico e 4) espinal.

n. to rhomboid, n. para o rombóide. SIN dorsal scapular n.

saccular n., [TA], n. sacular; ramo da parte inferior do nervo vestibular que se dirige para a mácula do sáculo. SIN nervus saccularis [TA].

sacral splanchnic n.'s [TA], n. nervos esplâncnicos sacros; ramos do tronco simpático do sacro que passam para o plexo hipogástrico inferior; parte dos nervos esplâncnicos abdominopélvicos (simpáticos), embora sua função específica não esteja bem definida. Tendem a ser confundidos com os nervos esplâncnicos pélvicos, que são estruturas muito mais importantes. SIN nervi splanchnici sacrales [TA].

sacral n.'s [S1–S5], nervos sacros [S1–S5]; cinco nervos que saem do forame sacro de cada lado; os ramos ventrais dos três primeiros entram na formação do plexo sacro, e os dois últimos, na formação do plexo coccígeo. SIN nervi sacrales [S1–S5].

saphenous n. [TA], n. safeno; ramo do nervo femoral; estende-se do triângulo femoral para o pé, tornando-se subcutâneo no lado medial do joelho; supre ramos cutâneos para a pele da perna e do pé, através dos ramos infrapatelar e crural medial. SIN nervus saphenus [TA], internal saphenous n., long saphenous n.

sciatic n. [TA], n. isquiático; origina-se como principal produto do plexo sacro, sai da pelve através do forame isquiático maior e desce no compartimento posterior da coxa, profundamente à cabeça longa do músculo bíceps da coxa; no ápice da fossa poplítea, divide-se nos nervos fibular comum e tibial, embora os dois possam se separar em níveis mais altos. SIN nervus ischiadicus [TA], great sciatic n., nervus sciaticus.

second cranial n. [CN II], segundo n. craniano [NC II]. SIN optic n. [CN II].

secretomotor n., n. secretomotor. SIN secretory n.

secretory n., n. secretor; nervo que envia impulsos que excitam a atividade funcional numa glândula. SIN secretomotor n.

sensory n., n. sensitivo; nervo aferente que envia impulsos processados pelo sistema nervoso central, de modo que se tornam parte da percepção do organismo de si próprio e de seu ambiente.

seventh cranial n. [CN VII], sétimo n. craniano [NC VII]. SIN facial n. [CN VII].

short ciliary n. [TA], n. ciliar curto; um de diversos ramos que passam do gânglio ciliar para o globo ocular, inervando os músculos ciliares, a íris e as túnicas do globo ocular. SIN nervus ciliaris brevis [TA].

short saphenous n., n. safeno curto. SIN sural n.

sinus n. of Hering, n. sinusal de Hering. SIN carotid branch of glossopharyngeal nerve [CN IX].

sinuvertebral n.'s, nervos sinovertebrais. SIN meningeal branch of spinal nerves.

sixth cranial n. [CN VI], sexto n. craniano [NC VI]. SIN abducent n. [CN VI].

small deep petrosal n., pequeno n. petroso profundo. SIN caroticotympanic n.'s.

smallest splanchnic n., n. esplâncnico mínimo. SIN least splanchnic n.

small sciatic n., pequeno n. isquiático. SIN posterior cutaneous n. of thigh.

n. of smell, n. do olfato. SIN olfactory n.'s [CN I].

somatic n., n. somático; um dos nervos da sensação parietal ou movimento voluntário, distinto dos nervos sensoriais viscerais, motores involuntários e secretores.

spinal n.'s [TA], nervos espinais; os nervos que saem da medula espinal; existem 31 pares, originando-se, cada um deles, do cordão por radículas que convergem para formar duas raízes, a anterior (ventral ou motora) e a posterior (dorsal ou sensorial); esta última apresenta um aumento de volume circunscrito, o gânglio espinal (raiz dorsal); as duas raízes unem-se no forame intervertebral, e o nervo espinal misto quase imediatamente divide-se de novo em ramos anterior e posterior (primário), inervando o primeiro a parte ântero-lateral do tronco e os membros, e o segundo, os músculos e a pele sobrejacente do dorso. SIN nervi spinales [TA].

spinal accessory n., n. espinal acessório. SIN accessory n. [CN XI].

splanchnic n., n. esplâncnico; um dos nervos que suprem as vísceras. Existem três grupos de nervos esplâncnicos: os nervos esplâncnicos cardiopulmonares, que enviam fibras simpáticas pós-sinápticas para as vísceras torácicas; os nervos abdominopélvicos, que enviam fibras simpáticas pré-sinápticas para os gânglios simpáticos da cavidade abdominopélvica; e os nervos esplâncnicos pélvicos, que enviam fibras parassimpáticas pré-sinápticas para os gângli-

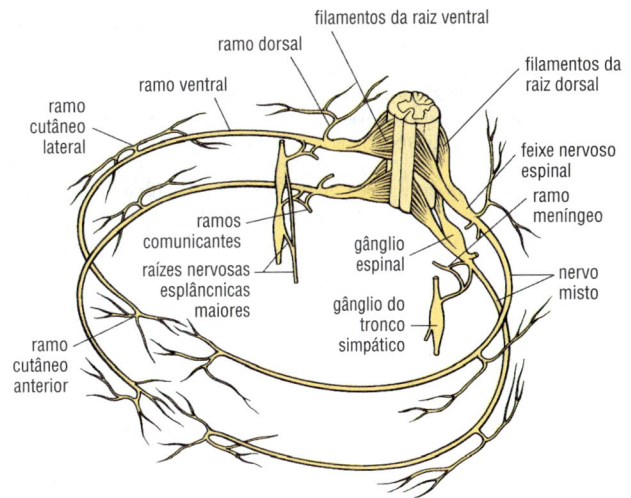

nervos espinais com suas raízes e ramos

os pélvicos. Ver também as entradas nos nomes individuais dos nervos esplâncnicos mencionados.

n. to stapedius muscle [TA], n. para o músculo estapédio; ramo do nervo facial que se origina no canal facial e inerva o músculo estapédio. SIN nervus stapedius [TA].

statoacoustic n., n. estatoacústico. SIN vestibulocochlear n. [CN VIII].

subclavian n. [TA], n. subclávio; ramo do tronco superior do plexo braquial que inerva o músculo subclávio. SIN nervus subclavius [TA].

subcostal n. [TA], n. subcostal; ramo ventral do décimo nervo torácico; segue um percurso abaixo da última costela, paralelamente aos nervos intercostais superiores a ele; inerva partes dos músculos abdominais e dá origem a ramos cutâneos para a pele da parede abdominal ventrolateral inferior e região glútea súpero-lateral. SIN nervus subcostalis [TA].

sublingual n. [TA], n. sublingual; ramo do nervo lingual para a glândula sublingual e mucosa do assoalho da boca. SIN nervus sublingualis [TA].

suboccipital n. [TA], n. suboccipital; ramo dorsal do primeiro nervo cervical, que passa através do triângulo suboccipital e envia ramos para os músculos reto posterior maior da cabeça e reto posterior menor da cabeça, oblíquo superior da cabeça e oblíquo inferior da cabeça, reto lateral da cabeça e semi-espinal da cabeça; o primeiro nervo espinal cervical é geralmente considerado como tendo apenas fibras motoras, porém o nervo suboccipital recebe fibras sensitivas para a propriocepção através de um ramo comunicante do segundo nervo cervical. SIN nervus suboccipitalis [TA].

subscapular n.'s [TA], nervos subescapulares; dois ramos do cordão posterior do plexo braquial, um superior e outro inferior, que inervam o músculo subescapular; o nervo subescapular inferior inerva também o músculo redondo maior. SIN nervi subscapulares [TA].

sudomotor n.'s, nervos sudomotores; nervos que contêm fibras autônomas (eferentes viscerais gerais–pós-ganglionares) que inervam as glândulas sudoríparas.

superficial cervical n., n. cervical superficial. SIN transverse cervical n.

superficial fibular n. [TA], n. fibular superficial; ramo do nervo fibular (peroneal) comum que desce no compartimento lateral da perna para inervar os músculos fibular longo e fibular curto, terminando como nervos cutâneos dorsal intermédio e dorsal medial que inervam a pele do dorso do pé e artelhos (exceto os lados adjacentes do hálux e segundo artelho). SIN nervus fibularis superficialis [TA], nervus peroneus superficialis*, superficial peroneal n.*, musculocutaneous n. of leg.

superficial peroneal n., n. peroneal superficial; *termo oficial alternativo para superficial fibular n.

superior alveolar n.'s [TA], nervos alveolares superiores; três ramos (posterior, médio e anterior) do nervo maxilar (ou de sua continuação como nervo infra-orbitário) que penetram na maxila para inervar a mucosa do seio maxilar, dentes superiores e gengiva. SIN nervi alveolares superiores [TA], superior dental n.'s.

superior cervical cardiac n. [TA], n. cardíaco cervical superior; o mais alto dos nervos esplâncnicos cardiopulmonares, originando-se da parte inferior do gânglio cervical superior e descendo para formar, com ramos do vago, o plexo cardíaco. SIN nervus cardiacus cervicalis superior [TA].

superior clunial n.'s [TA], nervos clúneos superiores; ramos terminais dos ramos primários dorsais dos nervos lombares, que inervam a pele da metade superior da região glútea. SIN nervi clunium superiores [TA].

superior dental n.'s, nervos dentais superiores. SIN superior alveolar n.'s.

superior gluteal n. [TA], n. glúteo superior; origina-se do plexo sacro, enviando fibras do quarto e do quinto nervos lombares e do primeiro nervo sacro; inerva os músculos glúteo médio e glúteo mínimo e o tensor da fáscia lata (abdutores e rotadores mediais da articulação do quadril). A lesão desse nervo provoca queda da pelve do lado não-sustentado quando o pé é elevado do solo (sinal de Trendelenburg). SIN nervus gluteus superior [TA].

superior laryngeal n. [TA], n. laríngeo superior; ramo do nervo vago no gânglio inferior; na cartilagem tireóide, divide-se em dois ramos: o nervo laríngeo interno, um ramo sensorial que inerva a mucosa da laringe acima das pregas vocais, e o nervo laríngeo externo, um ramo motor que inerva o músculo constritor inferior da faringe e o músculo cricotireóide. SIN nervus laryngeus superior [TA].

superior lateral brachial cutaneous n., n. cutâneo lateral superior do braço; *termo oficial alternativo para upper lateral cutaneous n. of arm.

superior maxillary n., n. maxilar superior. SIN maxillary n. [CN V2].

supraorbital n. [TA], n. supra-orbitário; ramo do nervo frontal que deixa a órbita através do forame ou incisura supra-orbitária e divide-se em ramos que se distribuem para a testa e couro cabeludo, pálpebra superior e seio frontal. SIN nervus supraorbitalis [TA].

suprascapular n. [TA], n. supra-escapular; origina-se do tronco superior do plexo braquial (quinto e sexto nervos cervicais), desce paralelamente aos cordões do plexo braquial, em seguida através da incisura escapular, inervando os músculos supra-espinal e infra-espinal, enviando também ramos para a articulação do ombro. É sujeito a lesão nas fraturas do terço médio da clavícula; a lesão do nervo supra-escapular resulta em perda da rotação lateral do ombro, de modo que, quando relaxado, o membro faz rotação medial (posição inclinada do garçom); a capacidade de iniciar a abdução também está afetada. SIN nervus suprascapularis [TA].

supratrochlear n. [TA], n. supratroclear; ramo do nervo frontal que inerva a parte medial da pálpebra superior, a parte central da pele da testa e a raiz do nariz. SIN nervus supratrochlearis [TA].

sural n. [TA], n. sural; formado pela união do nervo cutâneo sural medial a partir do tibial e do ramo comunicante fibular do nervo fibular comum, geralmente na porção média da panturrilha, embora isso seja muito variável; a partir daí, acompanha a pequena veia safena ao redor do maléolo lateral para o dorso do pé como nervo cutâneo dorsal lateral. SIN nervus suralis [TA], external saphenous n., short saphenous n.

sympathetic n., n. simpático; um dos nervos do sistema nervoso simpático.

temporomandibular n., n. temporomandibular. SIN zygomatic n.

n. to tensor tympani (muscle) [TA], n. para o tensor do tímpano; ramo do nervo mandibular que envia fibras da raiz motora do nervo trigêmeo que passam através do gânglio ótico, sem fazer sinapse para inervar o músculo tensor do tímpano. SIN nervus musculi tensoris tympani [TA].

n. to tensor veli palatini (muscle) [TA], n. para o tensor do véu palatino; ramo do nervo mandibular que envia fibras da raiz motora do nervo trigêmeo, que passam através do gânglio ótico sem fazer sinapse para inervar o músculo tensor do véu palatino. SIN nervus musculi tensoris veli palatini [TA].

tenth cranial n. [CN X], décimo n. craniano [NC X]. SIN vagus n. [CN X].

tentorial n. [TA], n. tentorial; ramo meníngeo originado de modo recorrente da porção intracraniana do nervo oftálmico que inerva o tentório e a foice do cérebro supratentorial. SIN ramus meningeus recurrens nervi ophthalmici [TA], ramus tentorii*, nervus tentorii.

terminal n. [TA], n. terminal; delicada faixa nervosa plexiforme que passa paralela e medialmente aos tratos olfatórios, distribuindo-se perifericamente com os nervos olfatórios e passando centralmente na substância perfurada anterior; acredita-se que tenham uma função autônoma, porém a natureza exata dessa função não é conhecida. SIN nervus terminalis [TA].

third cranial n. [CN III], terceiro n. craniano [NC III]. SIN oculomotor n. [CN III].

third occipital n. [TA], n. terceiro occipital; ramo medial do ramo primário dorsal do terceiro nervo cervical; em geral, une-se com o nervo occipital maior, mas pode existir como nervo independente, suprindo ramos cutâneos para o couro cabeludo e nuca. SIN nervus occipitalis tertius [TA].

thoracic cardiac n.'s, nervos cardíacos torácicos. SIN thoracic cardiac branches of thoracic ganglia, em branch.

thoracic splanchnic n.'s, nervos esplâncnicos torácicos; nervos esplâncnicos que se originam da porção torácica dos troncos simpáticos; os nervos esplâncnicos torácicos superiores (de T1 a T4 ou 5) passam para as vísceras acima do diafragma (principalmente coração, pulmões e esôfago) e, portanto, são nervos esplâncnicos cardiopulmonares; os nervos esplâncnicos torácicos inferiores formam os nervos esplâncnicos maior, menor e inferior e inervam as vísceras abaixo do diafragma, de modo que são nervos esplâncnicos abdominopélvicos.

thoracic n.'s [T1–T12] [TA], nervos torácicos [T1–T12]; doze nervos de cada lado, motores e sensoriais mistos, que suprem os músculos e a pele das paredes torácica e abdominal. SIN nervi thoracici [T1–T12].

thoracoabdominal n.'s, nervos toracoabdominais; ramos primários ventrais dos nervos espinais T7–T11 (do sétimo ao décimo primeiro nervo intercostal), que suprem a parede abdominal, bem como a parede torácica; inervam os músculos intercostal, subcostal, serrátil ínfero-posterior, abdominal transverso, oblíquo externo e oblíquo interno e reto do abdome, e fornecem ramos sensitivos para a periferia do diafragma e pleura parietal e peritônio. SIN anterior cutaneous n.'s of abdomen, pectoral and abdominal anterior cutaneous branch of intercostal nerves, rami cutanei anteriores pectoralis et abdominalis nervorum intercostalium, ramus cutaneus anterior (pectoralis et abdominalis) nervorum thoracicorum.

thoracodorsal n. [TA], n. toracodorsal; origina-se do cordão posterior do plexo braquial; contém fibras do sexto, sétimo e oitavo nervos cervicais e inerva o músculo grande dorsal. SIN nervus thoracodorsalis [TA], long subscapular n.

n. to thyrohyoid muscle, n. para o músculo tireoióideo. SIN thyrohyoid branch of ansa cervicalis.

tibial n. [TA], n. tibial; uma das duas principais divisões do nervo isquiático; desce pela parte posterior da perna, terminando como nervos plantares medial e lateral do pé; inerva os músculos posteriores da coxa, os músculos da parte posterior da perna (os dorsiflexores e inversores do pé) e a face plantar do pé, bem como a pele na parte posterior da perna e região plantar do pé. SIN nervus tibialis [TA], medial popliteal n.

tibial communicating n., n. comunicante tibial. SIN medial sural cutaneous n.

Tiedemann n., n. de Tiedemann; nervo simpático que acompanha a artéria central da retina no nervo óptico.

transverse cervical n. [TA], n. transverso do pescoço; ramo do plexo cervical que inerva a pele sobre o triângulo anterior do pescoço. SIN nervus transversus colli [TA], nervus transversus cervicalis*, cutaneous cervical n., nervus cervicalis superficialis, superficial cervical n., transverse n. of neck.

transverse n. of neck, n. transverso do pescoço. SIN transverse cervical n.

trifacial n., n. trifacial. SIN trigeminal n. [CN V].

trigeminal n. [CN V] [TA], n. trigêmeo [NC V]; o principal nervo sensitivo da face e o nervo motor dos músculos da mastigação; seus núcleos encontram-se no mesencéfalo e na ponte e bulbo, estendendo-se para a porção cervical da medula espinal; emerge por duas raízes, sensorial e motora, a partir da porção lateral da superfície da ponte, e penetra numa cavidade da dura-máter, a cavidade do trigêmeo, no ápice da porção petrosa do osso temporal, onde a raiz sensorial se expande para formar o gânglio trigêmeo; a partir daí, originam-se três divisões (oftálmica [NC V1], maxilar [NC V2] e mandibular [NC V3]). SIN nervus trigeminus [CN V] [TA], fifth cranial n. [CN V], trifacial n.

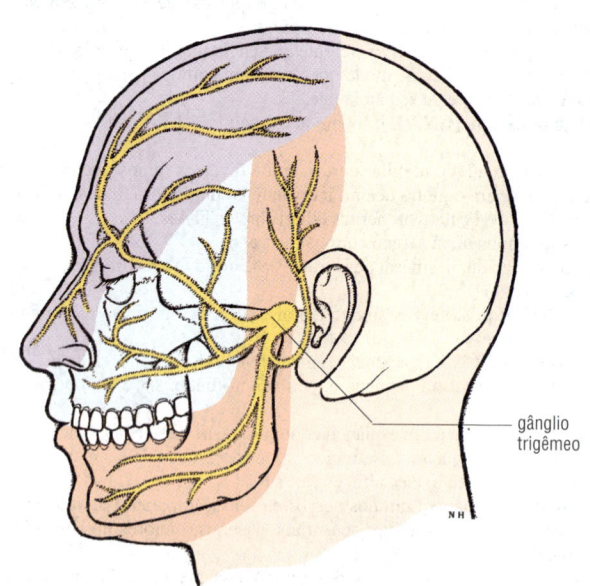

nervo trigêmeo: os três ramos sensoriais originam-se do gânglio trigêmeo e inervam as áreas mostradas em cores; (violeta) nervo oftálmico NC V¹; (azul) nervo maxilar, NC V²; (vermelho) nervo mandibular, NC V³

trochlear n. [CN IV] [TA], n. troclear [NC IV]; inerva o músculo oblíquo superior do olho; sua origem é no mesencéfalo, abaixo do aqueduto cerebral, e suas fibras decussam no véu medular superior e emergem do cérebro ao lado do frênulo; trata-se do único nervo craniano que se origina da face dorsal do tronco cerebral; por conseguinte, tem o maior percurso intracraniano, penetrando na dura na borda livre do tentório, próximo ao processo clinóide posterior, passando na parede lateral do seio cavernoso para penetrar na órbita através da fissura orbitária superior. SIN nervus trochlearis [CN IV] [TA], fourth cranial n. [CN IV], pathetic n.

twelfth cranial n. [CN XII], décimo segundo n. craniano [NC XII]. SIN hypoglossal n. [CN XII].
tympanic n. [TA], n. timpânico; um nervo do gânglio inferior do nervo glossofaríngeo, que passa através do canalículo timpânico para a cavidade timpânica, onde forma o plexo timpânico que supre a mucosa da cavidade timpânica, as células mastóide e a tuba auditiva; as fibras parassimpáticas pré-sinápticas também passam através do nervo timpânico pelo nervo petroso superficial menor até o gânglio ótico, onde fazem sinapse com fibras pós-sinápticas que prosseguem para inervar a glândula parótida. SIN nervus tympanicus [TA], Andersch n., Jacobson n.
n. of tympanic membrane, n. da membrana timpânica. SIN branches of auriculotemporal nerve to tympanic membrane, em branch.
ulnar n. [TA], n. ulnar; origina-se do cordão medial do plexo braquial que envia fibras principalmente dos nervos C8 e T1; desce pelo braço, atrás do epicôndilo medial do úmero e pelo lado ulnar do compartimento anterior do antebraço para a mão; dá origem a ramos musculares no antebraço para o músculo flexor ulnar do punho e porção ulnar do músculo flexor profundo dos dedo e inerva a eminência hipotenar, os músculos interósseos, lumbrical medial, adutor do polegar e cabeça profunda do plexo curto do hálux e músculos intrínsecos da mão, pele do quinto dedo e lado medial do quarto dedo, além de porções adjacentes da palma da mão. O nervo ulnar é mais vulnerável a lesões no local onde passa subcutaneamente por trás do epicôndilo medial do úmero. Nesse local, a ocorrência de lesão leve produz a sensação de "osso louco". A lesão do nervo ulnar nessa região resulta em perda da flexão das articulações metacarpofalangianas e da extensão nas articulações interfalangianas ("mão em garra"). SIN nervus ulnaris [TA], cubital n.
unmyelinated n., n. não-mielinizado; nervo constituído, em grande parte ou exclusivamente, de fibras não-mielinizadas; nervo composto de axônios e que não tem bainha de mielina, ficando em depressões nas células de Schwann; nervo condutor lento.
upper lateral cutaneous n. of arm [TA], n. cutâneo lateral superior do braço; ramo terminal do nervo axilar que inerva a pele sobre a porção inferior do músculo deltóide e por uma distância abaixo de sua inserção. SIN nervus cutaneus brachii lateralis superior [TA], superior lateral brachial cutaneous n.*.
upper subscapular n., n. subescapular superior. VER subscapular n.'s.
upper thoracic splanchnic n.'s, nervos esplâncnicos torácicos superiores. SIN thoracic cardiac branches of thoracic ganglia, em branch.
utricular n. [TA], n. utricular; ramo do nervo utriculoampular, que inerva a mácula do utrículo. SIN nervus utricularis [TA].
utriculoampullar n. [TA], n. utriculoampular; divisão da parte vestibular do oitavo nervo craniano; dá origem a ramos para a mácula do utrículo (nervo utricular) e para as cristas das ampolas dos ductos semicirculares anterior e lateral (nervos ampulares anterior e lateral). SIN nervus utriculoampullaris [TA].
vaginal n.'s [TA], nervos vaginais; diversos nervos que passam do plexo uterovaginal para a vagina. SIN nervi vaginales [TA].
vagus n. [CN X] [TA], n. vago [NC X]; nervo misto que se origina como numerosas raízes pequenas do lado do bulbo, entre o nervo glossofaríngeo, acima, e o nervo acessório, abaixo; deixa a cavidade craniana pelo forame jugular e desce para inervar a faringe, a laringe, a traquéia, os pulmões, o coração e o trato gastrintestinal até a flexura cólica (esplênica) esquerda; trata-se do único nervo craniano que não se origina do cérebro, porém é classificado como tal por sair do crânio. SIN nervus vagus [CN X] [TA], pneumogastric n., tenth cranial n. [CN X], vagus.
Valentin n., n. de Valentin; nervo que une o gânglio pterigopalatino com o nervo abducente.
vascular n.'s [TA], nervos vasculares; pequeno filamento nervoso que supre a parede de um vaso sanguíneo. SIN nervi vascularorum [TA].
vasomotor n., n. vasomotor; nervo motor que efetua ou inibe a contração dos vasos sanguíneos.
vertebral n., n. vertebral; ramo do gânglio estrelado que sobe ao longo da artéria vertebral até o nível do áxis ou do atlas, dando origem a ramos para os nervos cervicais e meninges. SIN nervus vertebralis.
vestibular n. [TA], n. vestibular; parte do nervo vestibulococlear [NC VIII] periférica à raiz vestibular; é composto dos processos nervosos centrais de neurônios bipolares que têm suas terminações dos processos periféricos sobre as células pilosas das ampolas dos ductos semicirculares e das máculas do sáculo e utrículo, e corpos celulares do gânglio vestibular. VER TAMBÉM vestibular *root*. SIN nervus vestibularis [TA], pars vestibularis nervi vestibulocochlearis, superior part of vestibulocochlear nerve, vestibular part of vestibulocochlear nerve.
vestibulocochlear n. [CN VIII] [TA], n. vestibulococlear [NC VIII]; nervo sensitivo composto que inerva as células receptoras do labirinto membranoso; consiste em dois componentes principais, distintos do ponto de vista anatômico e funcional, tendo cada um deles diferentes conexões centrais: o nervo vestibular e o nervo coclear. SIN nervus vestibulocochlearis [CN VIII] [TA], eighth cranial n. [CN VIII], eighth n., nervus acusticus, nervus octavus, nervus statoacusticus, octavus, statoacoustic n.
vidian n., n. vidiano. SIN n. of pterygoid canal.

visceral n., n. visceral; termo que descreve nervos que enviam fibras autônomas (eferentes viscerais gerais).
volar interosseous n., n. interósseo volar. SIN anterior interosseous n.
Wrisberg n., n. de Wrisberg; **(1)** SIN medial cutaneous n. of arm; **(2)** SIN intermediate n.
zygomatic n. [TA], n. zigomático; ramo do nervo maxilar [NC V2] na fissura orbitária inferior através da qual passa; divide-se em dois ramos sensitivos, o zigomático temporal e o zigomático facial, que inervam a pele das regiões temporal e zigomática, continuando-se como ramo comunicante do nervo lacrimal com o nervo zigomático. SIN nervus zygomaticus [TA], orbital n., temporodibular n.

nerve root sleeve. Bainha da raiz nervosa. Em mielografia, extensão afunilada do espaço subaracnóide opacificado que circunda cada raiz nervosa quando entra no forame neural.
ner·vi (ner'vī). Nervos. Plural de nervus. [L.]
ner·vi·mo·til·i·ty (ner - vi - mō - til'i - tē). Nervomotilidade. Capacidade de movimento em resposta a um estímulo nervoso. SIN neurimotility.
ner·vi·mo·tion (ner - vi - mō'shŭn). Nervimovimento. Movimento em resposta a um estímulo nervoso.
ner·vi·mo·tor (ner - vi - mō'ter). Neuromotor. Relativo a um nervo motor. SIN neurimotor.
ner·vine (ner'vīn). Nervino, neural. Que atua terapeuticamente, em particular como sedativo, sobre o sistema nervoso.
ner·vone (ner'vōn). Nervona. Cerebrosídeo contendo um radical nervonil.
ner·von·ic ac·id (ner - von'- ik). Ácido nervônico. Ácido graxo de cadeia retilínea de 24 carbonos, insaturado entre C-15 e C-16; ocorre em cerebrosídeos como a nervona.
ner·vous (ner'vŭs). Nervoso. **1.** Relativo a um nervo ou nervos. **2.** Facilmente excitado ou agitado, que sofre de instabilidade mental ou emocional; tenso ou ansioso. **3.** Antigamente, termo utilizado para referir-se a um temperamento caracterizado por excessiva atividade mental e física, pulso rápido, excitabilidade, freqüente volubilidade, mas nem sempre persistência nos propósitos. [L. *nervosus*]
ner·vous break·down. Esgotamento nervoso; termo não-médico para referir-se a uma doença emocional ou mental; com freqüência, eufemismo para um distúrbio psiquiátrico.
ner·vous·ness (ner'vŭs - nes). Nervosismo; condição de estar nervoso (2).

NERVUS

ner·vus, gen. e pl. **ner·vi** (ner'vŭs, - vī). [TA]. Nervo. SIN nerve. [L.]
n. abdu'cens [CN VI] [TA], n. abducente [NC VI]. SIN abducent *nerve* [CN VI].
n. accesso'rius [CN XI] [TA], n. acessório [NC XI]. SIN accessory *nerve* [CN XI].
n. acu'sticus, n. acústico. SIN vestibulocochlear *nerve* [CN VIII].
ner'vi alveola'res superio'res [TA], nervos alveolares superiores. SIN superior alveolar *nerves*, em *nerve*.
nervi alveolares superiores anteriores [TA], ramos alveolares superiores anteriores. SIN anterior superior alveolar branches, em branch.
n. alveola'ris infe'rior [TA], n. alveolar inferior. SIN inferior alveolar *nerve*.
n. ampulla'ris ante'rior [TA], n. ampular anterior. SIN anterior ampullary *nerve*.
n. ampulla'ris latera'lis [TA], n. ampular lateral. SIN lateral ampullar *nerve*.
n. ampulla'ris poste'rior [TA], n. ampular posterior. SIN posterior ampullar *nerve*.
nervi anales inferiores [TA], nervos anais inferiores. SIN inferior anal *nerves*, em *nerve*.
n. anococcyg'eus, n. anococcígeo. SIN anococcygeal *nerve*.
n. antebra'chii ante'rior, n. antebraquial anterior. SIN anterior interosseous *nerve*.
n. antebra'chii poste'rior, n. antebraquial posterior. SIN posterior interosseous *nerve*.
n. articula'ris, n. articular. SIN articular *nerve*.
ner'vi auricula'res anterio'res [TA], nervos auriculares anteriores. SIN anterior auricular *nerves*, em *nerve*.
n. auricula'ris mag'nus [TA], n. auricular magno. SIN great auricular *nerve*.
n. auricula'ris poste'rior [TA], n. auricular posterior. SIN posterior auricular *nerve*.
n. auriculotempora'lis [TA], n. auriculotemporal. SIN auriculotemporal *nerve*.
n. autonomicus [TA], n. autônomo. SIN autonomic *nerve*.
n. axilla'ris [TA], n. axilar. SIN axillary *nerve*.

n. bucca'lis [TA], n. bucal. SIN buccal nerve.
n. cana'lis pterygoi'dei [TA], n. do canal pterigóideo. SIN nerve of pterygoid canal.
ner'vi cardi'aci thora'cici, nervos cardíacos torácicos. SIN thoracic cardiac branches of thoracic ganglia, em branch.
n. cardi'acus cervica'lis infe'rior [TA], n. cardíaco cervical inferior. SIN inferior cervical cardiac nerve.
n. cardi'acus cervica'lis me'dius [TA], n. cardíaco cervical médio. SIN middle cervical cardiac nerve.
n. cardi'acus cervica'lis supe'rior [TA], n. cardíaco cervical superior. SIN superior cervical cardiac nerve.
ner'vi carot'ici exter'ni [TA], nervos caróticos externos. SIN external carotid nerves, em nerve.
nervi caroticotympan'icus, nervos caroticotimpânicos. SIN caroticotympanic nerves, em nerve.
n. carot'icus inter'nus [TA], n. carótico interno. SIN internal carotid nerve.
ner'vi caverno'si clitor'idis [TA], nervos cavernosos do clitóris. SIN cavernous nerves of clitoris, em nerve.
ner'vi caverno'si pe'nis [TA], nervos cavernosos do pênis. SIN cavernous nerves of penis, em nerve.
ner'vi cervica'les [C1–C8], nervos cervicais [C1-C8]. SIN cervical nerves [C1–C8], em nerve.
n. cervica'lis superficia'lis, n. cervical superficial. SIN transverse cervical nerve.
n. cilia'ris bre'vis, pl. **ner'vi cilia'res bre'ves** [TA], n. ciliar curto. SIN short ciliary nerve.
n. cilia'ris lon'gus, pl. **ner'vi cilia'res lon'gi** [TA], n. ciliar longo. SIN long ciliary nerve.
ner'vi clu'nium inferio'res [TA], nervos clúnios inferiores. SIN inferior clunial nerves, em nerve.
ner'vi clu'nium me'dii [TA], nervos clúnios médios. SIN medial clunial nerves, em nerve.
ner'vi clu'nium superio'res [TA], nervos clúnios superiores. SIN superior clunial nerves, em nerve.
n. coccyg'eus [Co] [TA], n. coccígeo. SIN coccygeal nerve [Co].
n. cochlea'ris [TA], n. coclear. SIN cochlear nerve. VER TAMBÉM cochlear root of VIII nerve.
n. commu'nicans fibula'ris, ramo comunicante do n. fibular. SIN sural communicating branch of common fibular nerve.
n. commu'nicans perone'us, ramo comunicante do n. fibular. SIN sural communicating branch of common fibular nerve.
ner'vi crania'les [TA], nervos cranianos. SIN cranial nerves, em nerve.
n. cuta'neus [TA], n. cutâneo. SIN cutaneous nerve.
n. cuta'neus antebra'chii latera'lis [TA], n. cutâneo lateral do antebraço. SIN lateral cutaneous nerve of forearm.
n. cuta'neus antebra'chii media'lis [TA], n. cutâneo medial do antebraço. SIN medial cutaneous nerve of forearm.
n. cuta'neus antebra'chii poste'rior [TA], n. cutâneo posterior do antebraço. SIN posterior cutaneous nerve of forearm.
n. cuta'neus bra'chii latera'lis infe'rior [TA], n. cutâneo lateral inferior do braço. SIN inferior lateral cutaneous nerve of arm.
n. cuta'neus bra'chii latera'lis supe'rior [TA], n. cutâneo lateral superior do braço. SIN upper lateral cutaneous nerve of arm.
n. cuta'neus bra'chii media'lis [TA], n. cutâneo medial do braço. SIN medial cutaneous nerve of arm.
n. cuta'neus bra'chii poste'rior [TA], n. cutâneo posterior do braço. SIN posterior cutaneous nerve of arm.
n. cuta'neus dorsa'lis interme'dius [TA], n. cutâneo dorsal intermédio. SIN intermediate dorsal cutaneous nerve.
n. cuta'neus dorsa'lis latera'lis [TA], n. cutâneo lateral dorsal. SIN lateral dorsal cutaneous nerve.
n. cuta'neus dorsa'lis media'lis [TA], n. cutâneo dorsomedial. SIN medial dorsal cutaneous nerve.
n. cuta'neus fem'oris latera'lis [TA], n. cutâneo lateral da coxa. SIN lateral cutaneous nerve of thigh.
n. cuta'neus fem'oris poste'rior [TA], n. cutâneo posterior da coxa. SIN posterior cutaneous nerve of thigh.
n. cuta'neus su'rae latera'lis [TA], n. cutâneo lateral da perna. SIN lateral sural cutaneous nerve.
n. cuta'neus su'rae media'lis [TA], n. cutâneo medial da perna. SIN medial sural cutaneous nerve.
ner'vi digita'les dorsa'les, nervos digitais dorsais. SIN dorsal digital nerves of hand, em nerve.
nervi digitales dorsales nervi fibularis profundi [TA], nervos digitais dorsais do nervo fibular profundo. SIN dorsal digital nerves of deep fibular nerve, em nerve.
nervi digitales dorsales nervi fibularis superficialis [TA], nervos digitais dorsais do nervo fibular superficial. SIN dorsal digital nerves of superficial fibular nerve, em nerve.
nervi digitales dorsales nervi ulnaris [TA], nervos digitais dorsais do nervo ulnar. SIN dorsal digital nerves of ulnar nerve, em nerve.
ner'vi digita'les dorsa'les pe'dis [TA], nervos digitais dorsais do pé. SIN dorsal digital nerves of foot, em nerve.
ner'vi digita'les palma'res commu'nes [TA], nervos digitais palmares comuns. SIN common palmar digital nerves, em nerve.
ner'vi digita'les palma'res pro'prii [TA], nervos digitais palmares próprios. SIN proper palmar digital nerves, em nerve.
ner'vi digita'les planta'res commu'nes [TA], nervos digitais plantares comuns. SIN common plantar digital nerves, em nerve.
ner'vi digita'les planta'res pro'prii [TA], nervos digitais plantares próprios. SIN proper plantar digital nerves, em nerve.
n. dorsa'lis clitor'idis, n. dorsal do clitóris. SIN dorsal nerve of clitoris.
n. dorsa'lis pe'nis [TA], n. dorsal do pênis. SIN dorsal nerve of penis.
n. dorsa'lis scap'ulae [TA], n. dorsal da escápula. SIN dorsal scapular nerve.
ner'vi erigen'tes, nervos eretores. SIN pelvic splanchnic nerves, em nerve.
n. ethmoida'lis ante'rior [TA], n. etmoidal anterior. SIN anterior ethmoidal nerve.
n. ethmoida'lis poste'rior [TA], n. etmoidal posterior. SIN posterior ethmoidal nerve.
n. facia'lis [CN VII] [TA], n. facial [NC VII]. SIN facial nerve [CN VII].
n. femora'lis [TA], n. femoral. SIN femoral nerve.
n. fibula'ris commu'nis [TA], n. fibular comum. SIN common fibular nerve.
n. fibula'ris profun'dus [TA], n. fibular profundo. SIN deep fibular nerve.
n. fibula'ris superficia'lis [TA], n. fibular superficial. SIN superficial fibular nerve.
n. fronta'lis [TA], n. frontal. SIN frontal nerve.
n. furca'lis, quarto n. lombar. SIN fourth lumbar nerve [L4].
n. genitofemora'lis [TA], n. genitofemoral. SIN genitofemoral nerve.
n. glossopharyn'geus [CN IX] [TA], n. glossofaríngeo [NC IX]. SIN glossopharyngeal nerve [CN IX].
n. glu'teus infe'rior [TA], n. glúteo inferior. SIN inferior gluteal nerve.
n. glu'teus supe'rior [TA], n. glúteo superior. SIN superior gluteal nerve.
n. hemorrhoida'lis, n. hemorroidário. VER superior rectal (nervous) plexus, inferior anal nerves, em nerve.
n. hypogas'tricus [TA], n. hipogástrico. SIN hypogastric nerve.
n. hypoglos'sus [CN XII] [TA], n. hipoglosso [NC XII]. SIN hypoglossal nerve [CN XII].
n. iliohypogas'tricus [TA], n. ilioipogástrico. SIN iliohypogastric nerve.
n. ilioinguina'lis [TA], n. ilioinguinal. SIN ilioinguinal nerve.
n. im'par. SIN terminal filum.
n. infraorbita'lis [TA], n. infra-orbitário. SIN infraorbital nerve.
n. infratrochlea'ris [TA], n. infratroclear. SIN infratrochlear nerve.
ner'vi intercosta'les [TA], nervos intercostais. SIN intercostal nerves, em nerve.
ner'vi intercostobrachia'les [TA], nervos intercostobraquiais. SIN intercostobrachial nerves, em nerve.
n. interme'dius [TA], n. intermédio. SIN intermediate nerve.
n. interos'seus antebrachii ante'rior [TA], n. interósseo anterior do antebraço. SIN anterior interosseous nerve.
n. interosseous antebrachii posterior [TA], n. interósseo posterior do antebraço. SIN posterior interosseous nerve.
n. interos'seus cru'ris [TA], n. interósseo da perna. SIN crural interosseous nerve.
n. interos'seus dorsa'lis, n. interósseo dorsal. SIN posterior interosseous nerve.
n. interos'seus poste'rior, n. interósseo posterior. SIN posterior interosseous nerve.
n. ischia'dicus [TA], n. isquiático. SIN sciatic nerve.
n. jugula'ris [TA], n. jugular. SIN jugular nerve.
ner'vi labia'les anterio'res [TA], nervos labiais anteriores. SIN anterior labial nerves, em nerve.
ner'vi labia'les posterio'res [TA], nervos labiais posteriores. SIN posterior labial nerves, em nerve.
n. lacrima'lis [TA], n. lacrimal. SIN lacrimal nerve.
n. laryn'geus infe'rior [TA], n. laríngeo inferior. SIN inferior laryngeal nerve.
n. laryn'geus recur'rens [TA], n. laríngeo recorrente. SIN recurrent laryngeal nerve.
n. laryn'geus supe'rior [TA], n. laríngeo superior. SIN superior laryngeal nerve.
n. lingua'lis [TA], n. lingual. SIN lingual nerve.
ner'vi lumba'les, nervos lombares. SIN lumbar nerves [L1–L5], em nerve.
n. mandibula'ris [CN V3] [TA], n. mandibular [NC V3]. SIN mandibular nerve [CN V3].
n. masseter'icus [TA], n. massetérico. SIN masseteric nerve.
n. maxilla'ris [CN V2] [TA], n. maxilar [NC V2]. SIN maxillary nerve [CN V2].
n. mea'tus acus'tici exter'ni [TA], n. para o meato acústico externo. SIN nerve to external acoustic meatus.

n. media'nus [TA], n. mediano. SIN median nerve.
n. menta'lis [TA], n. mentual. SIN mental nerve.
n. mixtus [TA], n. misto. SIN mixed nerve.
n. musculi tenso'ris tym'pani [TA], n. para o músculo tensor do tímpano. SIN nerve to tensor tympani (muscle).
n. musculi tenso'ris ve'li palati'ni [TA], n. para o músculo tensor do véu palatino. SIN nerve to tensor veli palatini (muscle).
n. musculocuta'neus [TA], n. musculocutâneo. SIN musculocutaneous nerve.
n. mylohyoi'deus [TA], n. milo-hióideo. SIN nerve to mylohyoid.
n. nasocilia'ris [TA], n. nasociliar. SIN nasociliary nerve.
n. nasopalati'nus [TA], n. nasopalatino. SIN nasopalatine nerve.
ner'vi nervo'rum, nervos do nervo; nervos distribuídos para as bainhas de troncos nervosos.
n. obturato'rius [TA], n. obturatório. SIN obturator nerve.
n. occipita'lis ma'jor [TA], n. occipital maior. SIN greater occipital nerve.
n. occipita'lis mi'nor [TA], n. occipital menor. SIN lesser occipital nerve.
n. occipita'lis ter'tius [TA], nervo occipital terceiro. SIN third occipital nerve.
n. octa'vus, nervo vestibulococlear. SIN vestibulocochlear nerve [CN VIII].
n. oculomoto'rius [CN III] [TA], n. oculomotor [NC III]. SIN oculomotor nerve [CN III].
n. olfacto'rii [CN I] [TA], n. olfatório [NC I]. SIN olfactory nerves [CN I], em nerve; VER TAMBÉM olfactory tract.
n. ophthal'micus [CN V1] [TA], n. oftálmico [NC V1]. SIN ophthalmic nerve [CN V1].
n. op'ticus [CN II] [TA], n. óptico [NC II]. SIN optic nerve [CN II].
ner'vi palati'ni mino'res [TA], nervos palatinos menores. SIN lesser palatine nerves, em nerve.
n. palati'nus ma'jor [TA], n. palatino maior. SIN greater palatine nerve.
n. pectora'lis lateral'is [TA], n. peitoral lateral. SIN lateral pectoral nerve.
n. pectoral'is medial'is [TA], n. peitoral medial. SIN medial pectoral nerve.
ner'vi pel'vici splanch'nici [TA], nervos esplâncnicos pélvicos. SIN pelvic splanchnic nerves, em nerve.
ner'vi perinea'les [TA], nervos perineais. SIN perineal nerves, em nerve.
n. perone'us commu'nis, n. fibular comum; *termo oficial alternativo para common fibular nerve.
n. perone'us profun'dus, n. fibular profundo; *termo oficial alternativo para deep fibular nerve.
n. perone'us superficia'lis, n. fibular superficial; *termo oficial alternativo para superficial fibular nerve.
n. petro'sus ma'jor [TA], n. petroso maior. SIN greater petrosal nerve.
n. petro'sus mi'nor [TA], n. petroso menor. SIN lesser petrosal nerve.
n. petro'sus profun'dus [TA], n. petroso profundo. SIN deep petrosal nerve.
n. pharyngeus [TA], n. faríngeo. SIN pharyngeal nerve.
ner'vi phren'ici accesso'rii [TA], nervos frênicos acessórios. SIN accessory phrenic nerves, em nerve.
n. phren'icus [TA], n. frênico. SIN phrenic nerve.
n. planta'ris latera'lis [TA], n. plantar lateral. SIN lateral plantar nerve.
n. planta'ris media'lis [TA], n. plantar medial. SIN medial plantar nerve.
n. presacra'lis, plexo hipogástrico superior; *termo oficial alternativo para superior hypogastric (nervous) plexus.
n. pterygoi'deus [TA], n. pterigóideo. SIN pterygoid nerve.
ner'vi pterygopalati'ni, nervos pterigopalatinos. SIN sensory root of pterygopalatine ganglion.
n. puden'dus [TA], n. pudendo. SIN pudendal nerve.
n. radia'lis [TA], n. radial. SIN radial nerve.
ner'vi recta'les inferio'res, nervos retais inferiores; *termo oficial alternativo para inferior anal nerves, em nerve.
n. saccula'ris [TA], n. sacular. SIN saccular nerve.
ner'vi sacra'les [S1–S5], nervos sacrais [S1–S5]. SIN sacral nerves [S1–S5], em nerve.
n. saphe'nus [TA], n. safeno. SIN saphenous nerve.
n. sciaticus, n. isquiático. SIN sciatic nerve.
ner'vi scrota'les anterio'res [TA], nervos escrotais anteriores. SIN anterior scrotal nerves, em nerve.
ner'vi scrota'les posterio'res [TA], nervos escrotais posteriores. SIN posterior scrotal nerves, em nerve.
n. spermat'icus exter'nus, n. espermático externo. SIN genital branch of genitofemoral nerve.
ner'vi sphenopalati'ni, nervos esfenopalatinos. SIN sensory root of pterygopalatine ganglion.
ner'vi spina'les [TA], nervos espinais. SIN spinal nerve, em nerve.
n. spinosus, n. espinhoso; *termo oficial alternativo para meningeal branch of mandibular nerve.
ner'vi splanch'nici lumba'les [TA], nervos esplâncnicos lombares. SIN lumbar splanchnic nerves, em nerve.
ner'vi splanch'nici sacra'les [TA], nervos esplâncnicos sacrais. SIN sacral splanchnic nerves, em nerve.
n. splanch'nicus i'mus [TA], n. esplâncnico mínimo. SIN least splanchnic nerve.
n. splanch'nicus ma'jor [TA], n. esplâncnico maior. SIN greater splanchnic nerve.
n. splanch'nicus mi'nor [TA], n. esplâncnico menor. SIN lesser splanchnic nerve.
n. stape'dius [TA], n. para o músculo do estapédio. SIN nerve to stapedius muscle.
n. statoacus'ticus, n. vestibulococlear. SIN vestibulocochlear nerve [CN VIII].
n. subcla'vius [TA], n. subclávio. SIN subclavian nerve.
n. subcosta'lis [TA], n. subcostal. SIN subcostal nerve.
n. sublingua'lis [TA], n. sublingual. SIN sublingual nerve.
n. suboccipita'lis [TA], n. suboccipital. SIN suboccipital nerve.
nervi subscapula'res [TA], nervos subescapulares. SIN subscapular nerves, em nerve.
n. supraclavicula'ris interme'dius [TA], n. supraclavicular intermédio. SIN intermediate supraclavicular nerve.
n. supraclavicula'ris latera'lis [TA], n. supraclavicular lateral. SIN lateral supraclavicular nerve.
n. supraclavicula'ris media'lis [TA], n. supraclavicular medial. SIN medial supraclavicular nerve.
n. supraorbita'lis [TA], n. supra-orbital. SIN supraorbital nerve.
n. suprascapula'ris [TA], n. supra-escapular. SIN suprascapular nerve.
n. supratrochlea'ris [TA], n. supratroclear. SIN supratrochlear nerve.
n. sura'lis [TA], n. sural. SIN sural nerve.
ner'vi tempora'les profun'di [TA], nervos temporais profundos. SIN deep temporal nerves, em nerve.
n. tento'rii, n. do tentório. SIN tentorial nerve.
n. termina'lis [TA], n. terminal. SIN terminal nerve.
ner'vi thora'cici [T1-12], nervos torácicos [T1–12]. SIN thoracic nerves [T1–T12], em nerve.
n. thora'cicus lon'gus [TA], n. torácico longo. SIN long thoracic nerve.
n. thoracodorsa'lis [TA], n. toracodorsal. SIN thoracodorsal nerve.
n. tibia'lis [TA], n. tibial. SIN tibial nerve.
n. transversus cervicalis, n. cervical transverso; *termo oficial alternativo para transverse cervical nerve.
n. transver'sus col'li [TA], n. cervical transverso. SIN transverse cervical nerve.
n. trigem'inus [CN V] [TA], n. trigêmeo [NC V]. SIN trigeminal nerve [CN V].
n. trochlea'ris [CN IV] [TA], n. troclear [NC IV]. SIN trochlear nerve [CN IV].
n. tympan'icus [TA], n. timpânico. SIN tympanic nerve.
n. ulna'ris [TA], n. ulnar. SIN ulnar nerve.
n. utricula'ris [TA], n. utricular. SIN utricular nerve.
n. utriculoampulla'ris [TA], n. utriculoampular. SIN utriculoampullar nerve.
ner'vi vagina'les [TA], nervos vaginais. SIN vaginal nerves, em nerve.
n. va'gus [CN X] [TA], n. vago [NC X]. SIN vagus nerve [CN X].
nervi vascula'rorum [TA], nervos vasculares. SIN vascular nerves, em nerve.
n. vertebra'lis, n. vertebral. SIN vertebral nerve.
n. vestibula'ris [TA], n. vestibular. SIN vestibular nerve; VER TAMBÉM vestibular root of vestibulocochlear nerve.
n. vestibulocochlea'ris [CN VIII] [TA], n. vestibulococlear [NC VIII]. SIN vestibulocochlear nerve [CN VIII]. Ver entradas em radix.
n. zygomat'icus [TA], n. zigomático. SIN zygomatic nerve.

ne·sid·i·ec·to·my (nē-sid′ē-ek′tō-mē), Nesidiectomia. Excisão do tecido das ilhotas do pâncreas. [G. nēsidion, ilhota, dim. de nēsos, ilha + ektomē, excisão]

ne·sid·i·o·blast (nē-sid′ē-ō-blast). Nesidioblasto. Célula formadora das ilhotas pancreáticas. [G. nēsidion, dim. de nēsos, ilha + blastos, germe]

ne·sid·i·o·blas·to·sis (ne-sid′ē-ō-blas-tō′sis). Nesidioblastose. Hiperplasia das células das ilhotas de Langerhans. [nesidioblasto + G. -osis, tumor]

Nessler, A. químico alemão, 1827–1905. VER N. reagent.

ness·ler·ize (nes′ler-īz). Nesselerizar. Tratar com reagente de Nessler; utilizado na determinação da uréia no sangue e na urina.

nest. Ninho, coleção, nicho. Grupo ou coleção de objetos semelhantes. VER TAMBÉM nidus. [A.S.]

Brunn n., n. de Brunn; invaginação semelhante a uma glândula do epitélio de transição superficial no epitélio das vias urinárias inferiores.

cell n., n. celular; pequeno foco ou acúmulo de um tipo de células diferentes das outras células no tecido.

epithelial n., n. epitelial. SIN keratin pearl.

isogenous n., n. isogênico; clone de células cartilaginosas todas provenientes de uma célula progenitora, ocorrendo em agregado.

net. Rede, sistema reticulado. SIN network (1).

Chiari n., r. de Chiari; faixas fibrosas anormais no átrio direito, que se estendem das margens das válvulas coronárias ou cavas e que se fixam na parede atrial, ao longo da linha da crista terminal; surgem quando a reabsorção do septo espúrio é bem menor do que o normal.

chromidial n., r. cromidial; retículo de material basófilo no citoplasma de certas células.

Netherton, Earl W., dermatologista norte-americano do século XX. VER N. *syndrome.*

net·il·mi·cin sul·fate (net - il - mī′sin). Sulfato de netilmicina. Antibiótico aminoglicosídico parenteral utilizado no tratamento em curto prazo de infecções bacterianas graves ou potencialmente fatais.

net·tle (net′l). Urtiga. SIN urtica. [A.S. *netele*]

net·work (net′werk). Rede, sistema reticulado, entrelaçamento **1.** Estrutura que se assemelha a um tecido. Rede de fibras nervosas ou pequenos vasos. SIN net, rete (1). VER TAMBÉM reticulum. **2.** As pessoas presentes no ambiente de um paciente, especialmente quando são importantes para a evolução da doença.
  acromial arterial n., r. arterial acromial. SIN acromial *anastomosis* of the thoracoacromial artery.
  arteriolar n., r. arteriolar. SIN arterial *plexus*.
  articular n., r. articular. SIN articular vascular *plexus*. VER plane *joint*.
  articular vascular n., n. vascular articular. SIN articular vascular *plexus*.
  articular vascular n. of elbow, r. vascular articular do cotovelo. SIN cubital *anastomosis*.
  articular vascular n. of knee, r. vascular articular do joelho. SIN genicular *anastomosis*.
  calcaneal arterial n., r. arterial do calcanhar. SIN calcaneal *anastomosis*.
  chromatin n., r. de cromatina; o aparecimento de material basofílico nos núcleos de muitas células após fixação. VER TAMBÉM chromatin.
  dorsal carpal n., r. carpal dorsal. SIN dorsal carpal arterial *arch*.
  dorsal venous n. of foot [TA], r. venosa dorsal do pé; rede superficial de finas veias no dorso do pé. SIN rete venosum dorsale pedis [TA].
  dorsal venous n. of hand [TA], r. venosa dorsal da mão; rede superficial de veias no dorso da mão que deságuam nas veias cefálica e basílica. SIN rete venosum dorsale manus [TA].
  lateral malleolar n. [TA], r. maleolar lateral; rede sobre o maléolo lateral, formada por ramos das artérias maleolar lateral posterior, maleolar lateral anterior, fibular e tarsal lateral. SIN rete malleolare laterale [TA].
  linin n., r. de linina; VER linin (3).
  medial malleolar n. [TA], r. maleolar medial; rede sobre o maléolo medial, formada por ramos das artérias maleolar medial anterior e posterior e társica medial. SIN rete malleolare mediale [TA].
  neurofibrillar n., n. neurofibrilar; padrões entrelaçados formados por neurofibrilas no neurônio.
  patellar n., r. patelar. SIN patellar *anastomosis*.
  peritarsal n., r. peritarsal; vasos linfáticos ao longo da margem palpebral.
  plantar venous n. [TA], r. venosa plantar; delicada rede venosa superficial na planta do pé. SIN rete venosum plantare [TA].
  Purkinje n., r. de Purkinje; rede formada pelas fibras de Purkinje por baixo do endocárdio.
  subpapillary n., r. subpapilar; vasos sanguíneos capilares nas camadas mais profundas da pele.
  trabecular n., r. trabecular. SIN trabecular *tissue* of sclera.

NeuAc NeuAc. Abreviatura de *N*-acetylneuraminic acid (ácido *N*-acetilneuramínico).

Neubauer, Johann E., anatomista alemão, 1742–1777. VER N. *artery*.

Neufeld, Fred, bacteriologista alemão, 1869–1945. VER N. *reaction,* capsular *swelling.*

Neumann, Ernst F.C., histologista, anatomista e patologista alemão, 1834–1918. VER N. *sheath*; Rouget-N. *sheath*.

Neumann, Franz E., físico alemão, 1798–1895. VER N. *law*.

Neumann, Isidor Edler von Heilwart, dermatologista austríaco, 1832–1906. VER N. *disease.*

♺ **neur-, neuri-, neuro-.** Neur-, neuri-, neuro-. Nervo, tecido nervoso, sistema nervoso. [G. *neuron*]

neu·ral (noor′ăl). Neural. **1.** Relativo a qualquer estrutura composta de células nervosas ou seus prolongamentos, ou que, durante o seu desenvolvimento, evolui, transformando-se em células nervosas. **2.** Refere-se ao lado dorsal dos corpos vertebrais ou seus precursores, onde se localiza a medula espinhal, em oposição ao hemal (2). [G. *neuron*, nervo]

neu·ral·gia (noo - ral′jē - ă). Neuralgia. Dor intensa, de caráter pulsátil ou em punhalada no trajeto ou na distribuição de um nervo. SIN neurodynia (neurodinia). [neur- + G. *algos*, dor]
  atypical facial n., n. facial atípica. SIN atypical trigeminal n.
  atypical trigeminal n., n. do trigêmeo atípica; dor periódica em qualquer região da face, nos dentes, na língua e, em certas ocasiões, na área occipital ou do ombro, de vários minutos a vários dias de duração, mas que não tem nenhum ponto de deflagração e carece da natureza paroxística do tique doloroso. SIN atypical facial n.
  epileptiform n., n. epileptiforme. SIN trigeminal n.
  facial n., n. facial. SIN trigeminal n.
  n. facia′lis ve′ra, n. facial verdadeira. SIN geniculate n.
  Fothergill n., n. de Fothergill. SIN trigeminal n.
  geniculate n., n. geniculada; dor lancinante paroxística intensa profundamente no ouvido, na parede anterior do meato externo e na pequena área imediatamente em frente ao pavilhão da orelha. SIN geniculate otalgia, Hunt n., n. facialis vera.
  glossopharyngeal n., n. glossofaríngea; dor lancinante paroxística na garganta ou no palato. SIN glossopharyngeal tic.
  hallucinatory n., n. alucinatória; impressão de dor local que persiste após ter cessado uma crise de neuralgia.
  Hunt n., n. de Hunt. SIN geniculate n.
  idiopathic n., n. idiopática; dor nervosa que não é devida a qualquer causa aparente.
  intercostal n., n. intercostal; dor na parede torácica devido à neuralgia de um ou mais nervos intercostais.
  mammary n., n. mamária; neuralgia do nervo ou nervos intercostais que inervam a mama.
  Morton n., n. de Morton; neuralgia de um nervo interdigital, habitualmente o ramo anastomótico entre os nervos plantares medial e lateral, em decorrência da compressão do nervo pela articulação metatarsofalângica. SIN Morton metatarsalgia, Morton neuroma.
  occipital n., n. occipital; VER posttraumatic neck *syndrome*.
  periodic migrainous n., n. enxaquecosa periódica; dor facial recorrente e cefaléia, mais comum nos homens do que nas mulheres. SIN Harris migraine.
  sciatic n., n. isquiática. SIN sciatica.
  Sluder n., n. de Sluder. SIN sphenopalatine n.
  sphenopalatine n., n. esfenopalatina; neuralgia na metade inferior da face, com dor referida para a raiz do nariz, dentes superiores, olhos, orelhas, mastóide e occipício, associada a congestão nasal e rinorréia que ocorrem na infecção dos seios nasais; produzida por lesões do gânglio esfenopalatino; podem ocorrer hiperemia ocular e lacrimejamento excessivo. SIN Sluder n.
  stump n., n. do coto; dor percebida como proveniente de uma parte ausente, causada pela irritação de neuromas no tecido cicatricial de um coto de amputação.
  suboccipital n., n. suboccipital. VER posttraumatic neck *syndrome*.
  supraorbital n., n. supra-orbital; neuralgia do nervo supra-orbital.
  symptomatic n., n. sintomática; neuralgia que ocorre como sintoma de alguma doença local ou sistêmica, que não afeta primariamente estruturas nervosas.
  trifacial n., n. trifacial. SIN trigeminal n.
  trigeminal n., n. do trigêmeo; surtos paroxísticos intensos de dor em um ou mais ramos do nervo trigêmeo; freqüentemente induzida pelo toque de pontos-gatilho na boca ou ao seu redor. SIN epileptiform n., facial n., Fothergill *disease* (1), Fothergill n., tic douloureux, trifacial n.

neu·ral·gic (noo-ral′jik). Neurálgico. Relativo a, que se assemelha à ou da natureza da neuralgia.

neu·ral·gi·form (noo - ral′ji - fōrm). Neuralgiforme. Que se assemelha à ou que tem o caráter da neuralgia.

neur·am·e·bim·e·ter (noor′am - ē - bim′ē - ter). Neuramebímetro. Instrumento para medir a velocidade de resposta de um nervo a qualquer estímulo. [neur- + G. *amoibē*, troca, retorno, resposta + *metron*, medida]

neur·a·min·ic ac·id (noor′ā - min′ik). Ácido neuramínico. Produto aldólico da D-manosamina e do ácido pirúvico, ligando o C-1 da primeira ao C-3 do último. Os derivados *N*- e *O*-acila do ácido neuramínico são conhecidos como ácidos siálicos e são componentes de gangliosídeos e dos componentes polissacarídicos de mucoproteínas e glicoproteínas de numerosos tecidos, secreções e espécies. SIN prehemataminic acid.

neur·a·min·i·dase (noor - ă - min′i - dās). Neuraminidase. SIN sialidase.

α₂-neur·a·mi·no·gly·co·pro·tein (noor - ā - min′ō - glī - kō - prō′tēn). α₂-neuraminoglicoproteína. Glicoproteína que contém ácido neuramínico e que, durante a eletroforese, migra para a porção α₂ das proteínas séricas. VER TAMBÉM C1 esterase *inhibitor.*

neur·an·a·gen·e·sis (noor′an - ă - jen′ē - sis). Neuranagênese. Regeneração de um nervo. [neur- + G. *ana*, para cima, de novo + *genesis*, origem]

neu·ra·poph·y·sis (noor - ă - pof′i - sis), Neurapófise. SIN lamina of vertebral arch. [neur- + G. *apophysis*, ramo]

neu·ra·prax·ia (noor - ă - prak′sē - ă). Neurapraxia. O tipo mais leve de lesão nervosa focal que provoca déficits clínicos; perda localizada da condução ao longo de um nervo sem degeneração axonal; causada por uma lesão focal, habitualmente desmielinizante e seguida de recuperação completa. O termo é freqüentemente pronunciado de forma errada (neuropraxia) e utilizado incorretamente como sinônimo de lesão nervosa. VER TAMBÉM axonotmesis. [neur- + G. *a-* priv. + *praxis*, ação]

neur·ar·chy (noor′ar - kē). Neurarquia. A ação dominante do sistema nervoso sobre os processos físicos do organismo. [neur- + G. *archē*, domínio]

neur·as·the·nia (noor - as - thē′nē - ă). Neurastenia. Condição mal definida, que acompanha ou ocorre comumente após a depressão, caracterizada por fadiga vaga possivelmente produzida por fatores psicológicos. [neur- + G. *astheneia*, fraqueza]

neurasthenia

angiopathic n., angioparalytic n., n. angiopática, n. angioparalítica; termo obsoleto para referir-se a uma forma de neurastenia leve em que a queixa principal consiste em pulsação universal ou sensação de pulsação por todo o corpo.
gastric n., n. gástrica; condição caracterizada por atonia epigástrica vaga e distensão e por sintomas neurastênicos discretos.
n. gra'vis, n. grave; termo obsoleto para referir-se a uma condição de neurastenia extrema e duradoura.
n. prae'cox, n. precoce; termo obsoleto para referir-se a uma forma de exaustão nervosa que aparece no período da adolescência.
primary n., n. primária; termo obsoleto para referir-se à neurastenia precoce.
pulsating n., n. pulsátil; termo obsoleto para referir-se à neurastenia angiopática.
sexual n., n. sexual; termo obsoleto para referir-se a uma forma em que o eretismo, a fraqueza ou a perversão sexual constituem um sintoma dominante.
traumatic n., n. traumática; termo obsoleto para referir-se à síndrome pós-traumática.
neur·as·then·ic (noor-as-then'ik). Neurastênico. Relativo a, ou que sofre de, neurastenia.
neur·ax·is (noo-rak'sis). Neuroeixo. Porção axial e não-pareada do sistema nervoso central: medula espinal, rombencéfalo, mesencéfalo e diencéfalo, em contraste com o hemisfério cerebral pareado ou o telencéfalo.
neur·ax·on, neur·ax·one (noo-rak'son, -sōn). Neuraxônio, neuroaxônio. Termo obsoleto para referir-se ao axônio. [neur- + G. *axōn*, eixo]
neur·ec·ta·sis, neur·ec·ta·sia, neur·ec·ta·sy (noo-rek'tă-sis, noor-ek-tā'zē-ă, -ek'tă-sē). Neurectasia. Cirurgia para estiramento de um nervo ou tronco nervoso. SIN neurotension. [neur- + G. *ektasis*, extensão]
neu·rec·to·my (noo-rek'tō-mē). Neurectomia. Excisão de um segmento de um nervo. SIN neuroectomy. [neur- + G. *ektomē*, excisão]
occipital n., n. occipital; excisão do nervo occipital maior para tratamento da neuralgia occipital.
presacral n., n. pré-sacra; secção do plexo hipogástrico superior para aliviar a dismenorréia intensa. SIN Cotte operation, presacral sympathectomy.
retrogasserian n., n. retrogasseriana. SIN trigeminal *rhizotomy*.
vestibular n., n. vestibular; transecção da divisão vestibular do oitavo nervo craniano.
neur·ec·to·pia, neur·ec·to·py (noor-ek-tō'pē-ă, -ek'tō-pē). Neurectopia. Condição em que um nervo segue um trajeto anormal. [neur- + G. *ektopos*, de *ek*, fora de + *topos*, lugar]
neur·ep·i·the·li·um (noor'ep-i-thē'lē-ŭm). Neurepitélio. SIN neuroepithelium.
neuri-. Neuri-. VER neur-.
neu·ri·dine (noor'i-dēn). Neuridina. SIN spermine.
neu·ri·lem·ma (noor-i-lem'ă). Neurilema. Célula que envolve um ou mais axônios do sistema nervoso periférico; nas fibras mielinizadas, sua membrana plasmática forma as lamelas de mielina. SIN neurolemma, sheath of Schwann. [neuri + G. *lemma*, palha de milho]
neu·ri·le·mo·ma (noor'i-lē-mō'mă). Neurilemoma. SIN schwannoma. [neurilemma + G. -*oma*, tumor]
acoustic n., n. acústico; schwanoma que se origina do nervo craniano VIII.
Antoni type A n., n. de Antoni tipo A; tecido neoplásico de organização relativamente sólida ou compacta, que consiste em células de Schwann dispostas em feixes espiralados e associadas a fibras de reticulina delicadas; os núcleos das células de Schwann estão freqüentemente agrupados em fileiras paralelas (as denominadas paliçadas), e os núcleos e as fibras formam, algumas vezes, corpúsculos táteis exagerados, denominados corpúsculos de Verocay.
Antoni type B n., n. de Antoni tipo B; tecido neoplásico de organização relativamente mole ou frouxa, que consiste em células de Schwann dispostas de modo aleatório entre fibras de reticulina em minúsculos focos semelhantes a cistos; macrófagos repletos de gordura podem ser observados em algumas das neoplasias maiores.
neu·ril·i·ty (noo-ril'i-tē). Neurilidade. Propriedade, inerente aos nervos, de conduzir estímulos.
neu·ri·mo·til·i·ty (noor'i-mō-til'i-tē). Neurimotilidade. SIN nervimotility.
neu·ri·mo·tor (noor-i-mō'ter). Neuromotor. SIN nervimotor.
neu·rine (noor'ēn). Neurina. Amina tóxica, produto de decomposição de matéria animal (desidratação da colina) e constituinte venenoso de cogumelos.
neu·ri·no·ma (noor-i-nō'mă). Neurinoma. Termo obsoleto para referir-se ao schwanoma.
acoustic n., n. do acústico. SIN vestibular *schwannoma*.
neu·rit·ic (noo-rit'ik). Neurítico. Relativo a neurite.
neu·ri·tis, pl. **neu·ri·ti·des** (noo-rī'tis, noo-rit'i-dēz). Neurite. **1.** Inflamação de um nervo. **2.** SIN neuropathy. [neuri- + G. -*itis*, inflamação]
adventitial n., n. adventícia; inflamação da bainha de um nervo. VER TAMBÉM perineuritis.
ascending n., n. ascendente; inflamação que progride para cima, ao longo de um tronco nervoso, afastando-se da periferia.

neuroblastoma

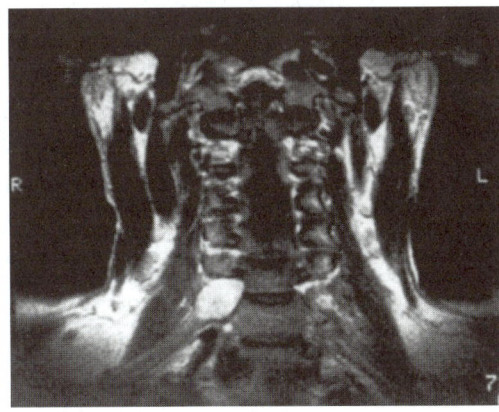

neurinoma da raiz nervosa de C$_7$: RMN, após injeção de contraste

axial n., n. axial. SIN parenchymatous n.
brachial n., n. braquial. SIN neuralgic *amyotrophy*.
central n., n. central. SIN parenchymatous n.
descending n., n. descendente; inflamação que progride ao longo de um tronco nervoso em direção à periferia.
Eichhorst n., n. de Eichhorst. SIN interstitial n.
endemic n., n. endêmica. SIN beriberi.
fallopian n., n. de Falópio. SIN facial *paralysis*.
interstitial n., n. intersticial; inflamação do arcabouço de tecido conjuntivo de um nervo. SIN Eichhorst n.
intraocular n., n. intra-ocular; inflamação da porção retiniana do nervo óptico.
Leyden n., n. de Leyden; degeneração gordurosa das fibras do nervo afetado.
multiple n., n. múltipla. SIN polyneuropathy.
occipital n., n. occipital. VER posttraumatic neck *syndrome*.
optic n., n. óptica; inflamação do nervo óptico. VER TAMBÉM *neuromyelitis optica*, retrobulbar n., papillitis.
parenchymatous n., n. parenquimatosa; inflamação da substância nervosa propriamente dita, dos axônios e da mielina. SIN axial n., central n.
retrobulbar n., n. retrobulbar; neurite óptica sem edema do disco óptico.
sciatic n., n. isquiática. SIN sciatica.
segmental n., n. segmentar; **(1)** inflamação que ocorre em diversos pontos ao longo do trajeto de um nervo; **(2)** neuropatia desmielinizante segmentar.
suboccipital n., n. suboccipital. VER posttraumatic neck *syndrome*.
toxic n., n. tóxica; neurite causada por uma toxina endógena ou exógena.
traumatic n., n. traumática; inflamação de nervo após lesão.
neuro-. Neuro-. VER neur-.
neu·ro·al·ler·gy (noor-ō-al'er-jē). Neuroalergia. Reação alérgica no tecido nervoso.
neu·ro·an·as·to·mo·sis (noor'ō-an-as-tō-mō'sis). Neuroanastomose. Formação cirúrgica de uma junção entre nervos.
neu·ro·a·nat·o·my (noor'ō-ă-nat'ō-mē). Neuroanatomia. A anatomia do sistema nervoso, geralmente específica do sistema nervoso central.
neu·ro·ar·throp·a·thy (noor'ō-ar-throp'ă-thē) Neuroartropatia. Distúrbio articular causado pela perda da sensação articular. VER Charcot *joint*. [neuro- + G. *arthron*, articulação + *pathos*, sofrimento, doença]
neu·ro·aug·men·ta·tion (noor'ō-awg-men-tā'shoon). Neuroaumento. Uso de estimulação elétrica para suplementar a atividade do sistema nervoso.
neu·ro·aug·men·tive (noor'ō-awq-men'tiv). Neuroaumentativo. Relativo a neuroaumento.
neur·o·bi·ol·o·gy. Neurobiologia. Biologia do sistema nervoso.
neu·ro·bi·o·tax·is. Neurobiotaxia. A teoria segundo a qual os corpos das células nervosas podem migrar para a — ou seus axônios podem crescer em direção à — área a partir da qual recebem a maioria dos estímulos. [G. *neuron*, nervo + *bios*, vida + *taxis*, distribuição]
neu·ro·blast (noor'ō-blast). Neuroblasto. Célula nervosa embrionária. [neuro- + G. *blastos*, germe]
neu·ro·blas·to·ma (noor'ō-blas-tō'mă). Neuroblastoma. Neoplasia maligna caracterizada por células nervosas imaturas e apenas um pouco diferenciadas, do tipo embrionário, isto é, neuroblastos; as células típicas são relativamente pequenas (10–15 μm de diâmetro) com núcleos vesiculares desproporcionalmente grandes e intensamente corados e citoplasma escasso e palidamente acidófilo; podem distribuir-se em lâminas, agregados irregulares ou grupos semelhantes a cordões; também podem ocorrer individualmente e em pseudo-rosetas (com os núcleos de distribuição periférica ao redor de processos cito-

plasmáticos centralmente dirigidos); em geral, o estroma é disperso, e não é raro observar focos de necrose e hemorragia. Os neuroblastomas ocorrem freqüentemente em lactentes e crianças nas regiões mediastinal e retroperitoneal (cerca de 30% estão associados às glândulas supra-renais); é muito comum a ocorrência de metástases disseminadas para o fígado, pulmões, linfonodos, cavidade craniana e esqueleto.
  olfactory n., n. olfatório; tumor maligno raro e, com freqüência, de crescimento lento de células nervosas primitivas, que habitualmente se origina na área olfatória da cavidade nasal. SIN olfactory esthesioneuroblastoma.
neu·ro·bor·re·li·o·sis (noor-ō-bōr-rel′ē-ō′sis). Neuroborreliose. Inflamação ou doença causada pela infecção do sistema nervoso central por um membro do gênero *Borrelia*. Com freqüência, constitui um estágio tardio do processo mórbido, sobretudo em indivíduos imunossuprimidos, como pacientes com AIDS/SIDA.
neu·ro·car·di·ac (noor-ō-kar′dē-ak). Neurocardíaco. **1.** Relativo à inervação do coração. **2.** Relativo à neurose cardíaca. [neuro- + G. *kardia*, coração]
neu·ro·cele (noor′ō-sēl). Neurocele. Termo coletivo raramente utilizado para referir-se à cavidade central do eixo cerebroespinal; os ventrículos combinados do cérebro e o canal central da medula espinal. [neuro- + G. *koilos*, cavidade]
neu·ro·chem·is·try (noor-ō-kem′is-trē). Neuroquímica. A ciência relacionada aos aspectos químicos da estrutura e da função do sistema nervoso.
neu·ro·chi·tin (noor-ō-kī′tin). Neuroquitina. SIN neurokeratin. [neuro- + G. *chitōn*, túnica]
neu·ro·cho·ri·o·ret·i·ni·tis (noor-ō-kōr′ē-ō-ret-in-ī′tis). Neurocoriorretinite. Inflamação da coróide, da retina e do nervo óptico.
neu·ro·cho·roi·di·tis (noor′ō-kō-roy-dī′tis). Neurocoroidite. Inflamação da coróide e do nervo óptico.
neu·roc·la·dism (noo-rok′lā-dizm). Neurocladismo. Proliferação de axônios a partir do coto central para preencher a lacuna num nervo seccionado. SIN odogenesis. [neuro- + G. *klados*, ramo jovem]
neu·ro·cra·ni·um (noor-ō-krā′nē-ŭm) [TA]. Neurocrânio. Os ossos do crânio que encerram o cérebro, em oposição aos ossos da face. SIN brain box*, braincase, cranial vault, cranium cerebrale, cerebral cranium. [neuro- + G. *kranion*, crânio]
  cartilaginous n., n. cartilaginoso; no embrião, a parte da base do crânio "moldada" primeiro em cartilagem e, a seguir, ossificada.
  membranous n., n. membranoso; a abóbada do crânio embrionário que está ossificada em membrana.
neu·ro·cris·top·a·thy (noor′ō-kris-top′ă-thē). Neurocristopatia. Anomalia de desenvolvimento que decorre do desenvolvimento incorreto das células da crista neural. [neuro- + L. *crista*, crista + G. *pathos*, sofrimento]
neu·ro·cyte (noor′ō-sīt) Neurócito. SIN neuron. [neuro- + G. *kytos*, célula]
neu·ro·cy·tol·y·sis (noor′ō-sī-tol′i-sis). Neurocitólise. Destruição de neurônios. [neuro- + G. *kytos*, célula + *lysis*, dissolução]
neu·ro·cy·to·ma (noor′ō-sī-tō′mă). Neurocitoma. Tumor de diferenciação neuronal, habitualmente de localização intraventricular, que consiste em lâminas de células com núcleos uniformes e formação ocasional de pseudo-rosetas perivasculares. [neuro- + G. *kytos*, célula + *-oma*, tumor]
neu·ro·den·drite (noor-ō-den′drīt). Neurodendrito. SIN dendrite (1).
neu·ro·den·dron (noor-ō-den′dron). Neurodendro. SIN dendrite (1).
neu·ro·der·ma·ti·tis (noor′ō-der-mă-tī′tis). Neurodermatite. Lesão cutânea liquenificada crônica, localizada ou disseminada. [neuro- + G. *derma*, pele + *-itis*, inflamação]
neu·ro·dy·nam·ic (noor′ō-dī-nam′ik). Neurodinâmico. Relativo à energia nervosa. [neuro- + G. *dynamis*, força]
neu·ro·dyn·ia (noor-ō-din′ē-ă). Neurodinia. SIN neuralgia. [neuro- + G. *odynē*, dor]
neu·ro·ec·to·derm (noor-ō-ek′tō-derm). Neuroectoderma. A região central do ectoderma embrionário inicial que, durante o desenvolvimento posterior, forma o cérebro e a medula espinal, bem como as células da crista neural que se transformam nas células nervosas e neurilema ou células de Schwann do sistema nervoso periférico.
neu·ro·ec·to·der·mal (noor′ō-ek-tō-der′măl). Neuroectodérmico. Relativo ao neuroectoderma.
neu·ro·ec·to·my (noor-ō-ek′tō-mē). Neuroectomia. SIN neurectomy.
neu·ro·en·ceph·a·lo·my·e·lop·a·thy (noor′ō-en-sef′ă-lō-mī-ĕ-lop′ă-thē). Neuroencefalomielopatia. Doença do cérebro, da medula espinal e dos nervos.
neu·ro·en·do·crine (noor-ō-en′dō-krin). Neuroendócrino. **1.** Referente às relações anatômicas e funcionais entre o sistema nervoso e o sistema endócrino. **2.** Descreve as células que liberam um hormônio no sangue circulante em resposta a um estímulo neural. Essas células podem formar uma glândula endócrina periférica (p. ex., as células beta secretoras de insulina das ilhotas de Langerhans no pâncreas e as células cromafins secretoras de adrenalina da medula supra-renal); outras consistem em neurônios no cérebro (p. ex., os neurônios do núcleo supra-óptico que liberam o hormônio antidiurético de suas terminações axonais no lobo posterior da hipófise).

neu·ro·en·do·crin·ol·o·gy (noor-ō-en′dō-krin-ol′ō-jē). Neuroendocrinologia. A especialidade envolvida com as relações anatômicas e funcionais entre o sistema nervoso e o sistema endócrino.
neu·ro·ep·i·the·li·al (noor′ō-ep-i-thē′lē-ăl). Neuroepitelial. Relativo ao neuroepitélio.
ℹ **neu·ro·ep·i·the·li·um** (noor′ō-ep-i-thē′lē-oom). Neuroepitélio. Células epiteliais especializadas na recepção de estímulos externos. A maioria das células neuroepiteliais, notavelmente as células ciliadas do ouvido interno e as células receptoras das papilas gustativas, não são neurônios verdadeiros, mas células transdutoras que estão em contato sináptico com as terminações periféricas de células ganglionares sensitivas. Por outro lado, as células receptoras neuroepiteliais do epitélio olfatório são verdadeiros neurônios periféricos, cujos axônios não-mielinizados e extremamente delgados formam os filamentos olfatórios que penetram no bulbo olfatório do hemisfério cerebral. A NA aplica também o termo aos bastonetes e cones da retina. SIN neurepithelium, neuroepithelial cells.

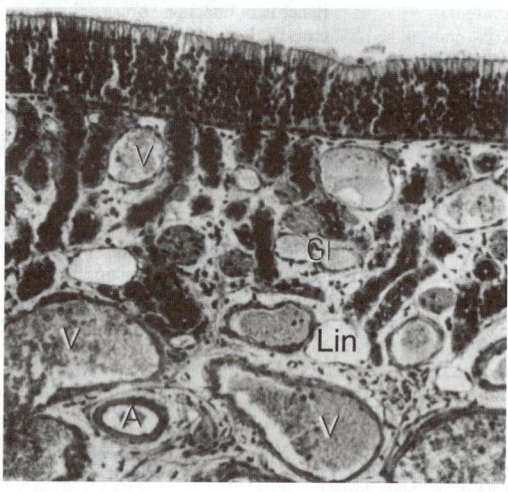

neuroepitélio: fotomicrografia da mucosa olfatória incluindo o epitélio olfatório e o tecido conjuntivo subjacente que se estende até o osso (não mostrado); A, artéria; V, veias; Lin, vasos linfáticos; N, nervos; Gl, glândulas de Bowman; 160x

  n. of ampullary crest, n. da crista ampular; as células ciliadas sensoriais especializadas na crista ampular da ampola de cada ducto semicircular.
  n. of macula, n. da mácula; as células ciliadas sensoriais especializadas do epitélio da mácula do sáculo e da mácula do utrículo. VER TAMBÉM macula.
neu·ro·fi·bra. Neurofibra. Fibra nervosa: um prolongamento delicado de um neurônio; o termo é freqüentemente usado como sinônimo de axônio.
  neurofibrae autonomicae [TA], neurofibras autônomas. SIN autonomic nerve *fibers*, em *fiber*.
  neurofibrae postganglionicae, neurofibras pós-ganglionares. SIN postganglionic.
  neurofibrae preganglionicae, neurofibras pré-ganglionares. SIN preganglionic nerve *fibers*, em *fiber*.
  neurofibrae somaticae [TA], neurofibras somáticas. SIN somatic nerve *fibers*, em *fiber*.
neu·ro·fi·bril (noor-ō-fī′bril). Neurofibrila. Estrutura filamentosa observada ao microscópio óptico no corpo das células nervosas, nos dendritos, axônios e, algumas vezes, nas terminações sinápticas, como agregados de elementos ultramicroscópicos muito mais finos, os neurofilamentos e os microtúbulos; sua importância funcional ainda não foi estabelecida.
neu·ro·fi·bril·lar (noor-ō-fī′bri-lĕr). Neurofibrilar. Relativo a neurofibrilas.
neu·ro·fi·bro·ma (noor′ō-fi-brō′mă). Neurofibroma. Tumor encapsulado benigno, de consistência moderadamente firme, resultante da proliferação de células de Schwann num padrão desordenado, incluindo porções de fibras nervosas; na neurofibromatose, os neurofibromas são múltiplos. SIN fibroneuroma.
  plexiform n., n. plexiforme; tipo de neurofibroma que representa mais uma anomalia do que uma verdadeira neoplasia, em que a proliferação de células de Schwann ocorre a partir da face interna da bainha nervosa, produzindo, assim, uma estrutura sinuosa, deformada e irregularmente espessada; em alguns casos, o processo estende-se ao longo do trajeto do nervo e pode acabar envolvendo as raízes espinais e a medula espinal; observado mais freqüentemente na neurofibromatose. SIN fibrillary neuroma, plexiform neuroma.

storiform n., dermatofibrossarcoma protuberante pigmentado. SIN pigmented *dermatofibrosarcoma protuberans.*

neu·ro·fi·bro·ma·to·sis (noor´o-fi-bro-mă-to´sis). Neurofibromatose. Esse termo abrange dois distúrbios hereditários distintos, antigamente denominados neurofibromatose (NF) periférica e neurofibromatose central, que, hoje em dia, receberam a designação de neurofibromatose tipo 1 e tipo 2. A neurofibromatose tipo 1 (periférica) [MIM*162200], que constitui, sem dúvida alguma, a mais comum dos dois tipos, caracteriza-se clinicamente pela combinação de placas de hiperpigmentação e tumores cutâneos e subcutâneos. As áreas cutâneas hiperpigmentadas, presentes desde o nascimento e encontradas em qualquer parte da superfície corporal, podem variar acentuadamente quanto a seu tamanho e cor — as que têm coloração castanho-escura são denominadas manchas café-com-leite (*café-au-lait*). Os tumores cutâneos e subcutâneos múltiplos, que consistem em neoplasias das bainhas nervosas, denominadas neurofibromas, podem surgir em qualquer parte ao longo das fibras dos nervos periféricos, desde as raízes distalmente. Os neurofibromas podem tornar-se muito grandes, causando desfiguração significativa, erosão dos ossos e compressão de várias estruturas nervosas periféricas; um pequeno hamartoma (nódulo de Lisch) pode ser encontrado na íris de quase todos os pacientes. A NF tipo 1, também denominada doença de van Recklinghausen, é de herança autossômica dominante, estando o *locus* gênico situado no cromossoma 17q11; é causada pela mutação do gene NF1 que codifica a neurofibromina. A neurofibromatose tipo 2 (central) [MIM*101000] apresenta poucas manifestações cutâneas e caracteriza-se, primariamente, por neuromas do acústico bilaterais (e, com menor freqüência, unilaterais) que causam surdez, freqüentemente acompanhados de outras neoplasias intracranianas e paraespinais, como meningiomas e gliomas. A NF tipo 2 também é um distúrbio de herança autossômica dominante, com *locus* gênico situado no cromossoma 22q11, causada pela mutação do gene NF2 que codifica o produto merlina. SIN elephant man's disease (2).

abortive n., n. abortiva. SIN incomplete n.
central type n., n. de tipo central; neurofibromatose tipo 2. VER neurofibromatosis.
incomplete n., n. incompleta; neurofibromas múltiplos com manifestações mínimas, talvez limitadas a manchas café-com-leite; os indivíduos com lesões mínimas podem ter descendentes com comprometimento grave. SIN abortive n.
neu·ro·fil·a·ment (noor-o-fil´ă-ment). Neurofilamento. Classe de filamentos intermediários encontrados em neurônios.
neu·ro·gang·li·on (noor-o-gang´le-on). Neurogânglio. SIN ganglion (1).
neu·ro·gas·tric (noor-o-gas´trik). Neurogástrico. Relativo à inervação do estômago.
neu·ro·gen·e·sis (noor-o-jen´e-sis). Neurogênese. Formação do sistema nervoso. [neuro- + G. *genesis*, produção]
neu·ro·gen·ic, neu·ro·ge·net·ic (noor-o-jen´ik, -je-net´ik). Neurogênico, neurogenético. 1. Que se origina, começa no ou é causado pelo sistema nervoso ou impulsos nervosos. SIN neurogenous. 2. Relativo à neurogênese.
neu·rog·e·nous (noo-roj´e-nŭs). Neurogênico. SIN neurogenic (1).
neu·rog·li·a (noo-rog´le-ă). Neuróglia. Elementos celulares não-neuronais dos sistemas nervosos central e periférico; antigamente, acreditava-se que fossem apenas células do sustentação, mas, hoje em dia, acredita-se que desempenhem funções metabólicas importantes, visto que estão invariavelmente interpostas entre os neurônios e os vasos sanguíneos que suprem o sistema nervoso. No tecido nervoso central, incluem as células da oligodendróglia, os astrócitos, as células ependimárias e as células da micróglia. As células-satélites dos gânglios e neurolema ou as células de Schwann ao redor das fibras nervosas periféricas podem ser interpretadas como células da oligodendróglia do sistema nervoso periférico. SIN reticulum (2) [TA], glia, Kölliker reticulum. [neuro- + G. *glia*, cola]
neu·rog·li·a·cyte (noo-rog´le-ă-sīt). Neurogliócito. Célula da neuróglia. VER neuroglia. [neuro- + G. *glia*, cola + *kytos*, célula]
neu·rog·li·al, neu·rog·li·ar (noo-rog´le-ăl, -le-ăr). Neuroglial. Relativo à neuróglia.
neu·rog·li·o·ma·to·sis (noo-rog´le-o-mă-to´sis). Neurogliomatose. SIN gliomatosis.
neu·ro·gram (noor´o-gram). Neurograma. A impressão (*imprint*) na substância cerebral que, teoricamente, persiste após cada experiência mental, isto é, o engrama ou registro físico da experiência mental, cujo estímulo leva à recuperação e reprodução da experiência original, produzindo, assim, o processo da memória. [neuro- + G. *gramma*, algo escrito]
neu·rog·ra·phy (noo-rog´ră-fe). Neurografia. Método para descrever o estado de um nervo periférico, como um registro elétrico ou a visualização radiográfica por contraste. [neuro- + G. *graphō*, escrever]
neu·ro·he·mal (noor-o-he´măl). Neuro-hemal. Relativo a estruturas contendo neurônios neurossecretores, cujos axônios não formam sinapses com outros neurônios e cujas terminações axonais são modificadas para permitir o armazenamento e a liberação, na circulação, de material neurossecretor. [neuro- + G. *haima*, sangue + sufixo -in, material]

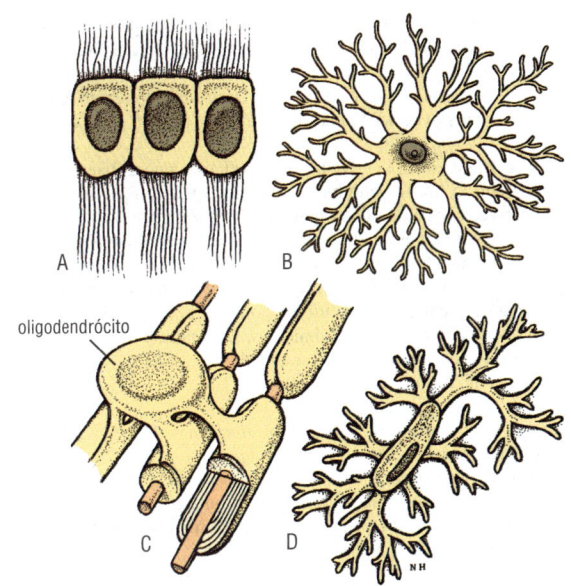

neuróglia: (A) células ependimárias, (B) astrócito, (C) oligodendrócito, (D) micróglia

neu·ro·his·tol·o·gy (noor-o-his-tol´o-je). Neuro-histologia. A anatomia microscópica do sistema nervoso. SIN histoneurology.
neu·ro·hor·mone (noor-o-hor´mōn). Neuro-hormônio. Hormônio formado por células neurossecretoras e liberado por impulsos nervosos (p. ex., norepinefrina).
neu·ro·hy·po·phys·i·al (noor-o-hī-po-fiz´e-ăl). Neuro-hipofisário. Relativo à neuro-hipófise.
neu·ro·hy·poph·y·sis (noor-o-hī-pof´i-sis) [TA]. Neuro-hipófise. Formada pelo infundíbulo e lobo nervoso da hipófise. VER TAMBÉM pituitary *gland.* SIN lobus nervosus [TA], lobus posterior hypophyseos*, pars nervosa hypophyseos*, nervous lobe, neural part of hypophysis, posterior lobe of hypophysis. [neuro- + hypophysis]
neu·roid (noor´oyd). Neuróide. Semelhante a um nervo. [neuro- + G. *eidos*, semelhança]
neu·ro·ker·a·tin (noor-o-kăr´ă-tin). Neuroceratina. 1. Rede proteinácea que permanece da bainha de mielina dos axônios após fixação e remoção do material lipídico; o aspecto reticular representa, provavelmente, um artefato de fixação. 2. A matéria proteica insolúvel do cérebro que permanece após extração com solventes e digestão proteolítica; não tem nenhuma relação com as ceratinas. SIN neurochitin. [neuro- + G. *keras*, corno]
neu·ro·lem·ma (noor-o-lem´ă). Neurolema. SIN neurilemma. [neuro- + G. *lemma*, invólucro]
neu·ro·lept·an·al·ge·sia (noor-o-lept-an-ăl-je´ze-ă). Neuroleptanalgesia. Intenso estado analgésico e amnésico produzido pela administração de analgésicos narcóticos e agentes neurolépticos; pode ocorrer ou não inconsciência, e pode haver alteração da função cardiorrespiratória.
neu·ro·lept·an·es·the·sia (noor-o-lept-an-es-the´ze-ah). Neuroleptanestesia. Técnica de anestesia geral, baseada na administração intravenosa de agentes neurolépticos, juntamente com inalação de um anestésico fraco com ou sem relaxantes musculares.
neu·ro·lep·tic (noor-o-lep´tik). Neuroléptico. Qualquer membro de uma classe de agentes psicotrópicos utilizados no tratamento da psicose, sobretudo a esquizofrenia; inclui os derivados de fenotiazina, tioxanteno e butirofenona, bem como as diidroindolonas. SIN neuroleptic agent. VER TAMBÉM antipsychotic *agent.* [neuro- + G. *lēpsis*, crise]
neu·ro·lin·guis·tics (nur´o-ling-gwis´tiks). Neurolingüística. Ramo da ciência médica relacionado com a base neuroanatômica da fala e seus distúrbios.
neu·rol·o·gist (noo-rol´o-jist). Neurologista. Especialista no diagnóstico e no tratamento de doenças do sistema neuromuscular: os sistemas nervosos central, periférico e autônomo, a junção neuromuscular e os músculos.
neu·rol·o·gy (noo-rol´o-je). Neurologia. Ramo da ciência médica relacionado com os vários sistemas nervosos (central, periférico e autônomo), juntamente com a junção neuromuscular e os músculos e seus distúrbios. [neuro- + G. *logos*, estudo]
neu·ro·lymph (noor´o-limf). Neurolinfa. Termo obsoleto para referir-se ao *líquido* cefalorraquidiano. [neuro- + L. *lympha*, água clara]
neu·ro·lym·pho·ma·to·sis (noor´o-lim-fo-mă-to´sis). Neurolinfomatose. Invasão linfoblástica de um nervo.

neu·rol·y·sin (nū-rol'i-sin). Neurolisina. Anticorpo que provoca destruição de células ganglionares e corticais, obtido pela injeção de substância cerebral. SIN neurotoxin (1).

neu·rol·y·sis (noo-rol'i-sis). Neurólise. **1.** Destruição do tecido nervoso. **2.** Liberação de um nervo de aderências inflamatórias. [neuro- + G. *lysis*, dissolução]

neu·ro·lyt·ic (noor-ō-lit'ik). Neurolítico. Relativo à neurólise.

neu·ro·ma (noo-rō'mă). Neuroma. Termo geral para referir-se a qualquer neoplasia derivada de células do sistema nervoso; com base nos conhecimentos mais recentes relativos às características citológicas e histológicas, várias neoplasias, antigamente incluídas na categoria geral de neuroma, podem ser atualmente classificadas em categorias mais específicas, como, p. ex., ganglioneuroma, neurilemoma, pseudoneuroma e outros. [neuro- + G. *-oma*, tumor]
   acoustic n., n. do acústico. SIN vestibular *schwannoma*.
   amputation n., n. de amputação. SIN traumatic n.
   n. cu'tis, n. cutâneo; neurofibroma da pele.
   false n., n. falso. SIN traumatic n.
   fibrillary n., n. fibrilar. SIN plexiform *neurofibroma*.
   Morton n., n. de Morton. SIN Morton *neuralgia*.
   plexiform n., n. plexiforme. SIN plexiform *neurofibroma*.
   n. telangiecto'des, n. telangiectóide; neurofibroma com número notável de vasos sanguíneos, alguns dos quais apresentam luz inusitadamente grande (em proporção à espessura das paredes).
   traumatic n., n. traumático; massa proliferativa não-neoplásica de células de Schwann e neurite que pode ocorrer na extremidade proximal de um nervo lesado ou seccionado. SIN amputation n., false n., pseudoneuroma.

neu·ro·ma·la·cia (noor'ō-mă-lā'shē-ă). Neuromalacia. Amolecimento patológico do tecido nervoso. [neuro- + G. *malakia*, amolecimento]

neu·ro·ma·to·sis (noor'ō-mă-tō'sis). Neuromatose. Presença de múltiplos neuromas, como na neurofibromatose.

neu·ro·mel·a·nin (noor-ō-mel'ă-nin). Neuromelanina. Forma modificada do pigmento melanina normalmente encontrado em certos neurônios do sistema nervoso, especialmente na substância negra e no *locus ceruleus*.

neu·ro·men·in·ge·al (noor-ō-mĕ-nin'jē-al). Neuromeníngeo. Relativo ao comprometimento do tecido nervoso e das meninges.

neu·ro·mere (noor'ō-mēr). Neurômero. Elevações na parede do tubo neural em desenvolvimento que dividem a medula espinal em formação (neurômero) em porções às quais se fixam as raízes dorsal e ventral ou que dividem o rombencéfalo em desenvolvimento em porções associadas primariamente a porções motoras dos nervos cranianos do bulbo e da ponte. SIN encephalomere, neural segment, neurotome (2). [neuro- + G. *meros*, parte]

neu·ro·mi·met·ic (noor'ō-mi-met'ik). Neuromimético. Relativo à ação de uma substância que imita a resposta de um órgão efetor a impulsos nervosos.

neu·ro·mus·cu·lar (noor-ō-mŭs'kū-lăr). Neuromuscular. Refere-se à relação entre nervo e músculo, em particular à inervação motora dos músculos esqueléticos e sua patologia (p. ex., distúrbios neuromusculares). VER TAMBÉM myoneural.

neu·ro·my·as·the·nia (noor'ō-mī-as-thē'nē-ă). Neuromiastenia. Termo obsoleto para referir-se à fraqueza muscular, habitualmente de origem emocional. [neuro- + G. *mys*, músculo + *a-* priv. + *sthenos*, força]
   epidemic n., n. epidêmica; doença epidêmica, caracterizada por rigidez da nuca e das costas, cefaléia, diarréia, febre e fraqueza muscular localizada; restrita quase exclusivamente a adultos, afetando mais as mulheres do que os homens; provavelmente de origem viral. SIN benign myalgic encephalomyelitis, epidemic myalgic encephlomyelitis, Iceland disease.

neu·ro·my·e·li·tis (noor'ō-mī-el-ī'tis). Neuromielite. Neurite associada a inflamação da medula espinal. SIN myeloneuritis. [neuro- + G. *myelos*, medula + *-itis*, inflamação]
   n. op'tica, n. óptica; distúrbio desmielinizante, consistindo em mielopatia transversa e neurite óptica. SIN Devic disease.

neu·ro·my·op·a·thy (noor'ō-mī-op'ă-thē). Neuromiopatia. **1.** Distúrbio do músculo devido ao comprometimento de sua inervação. **2.** Distúrbio simultâneo do nervo e do músculo. [neuro- + G. *mys*, músculo + *pathos*, doença]
   carcinomatous n., n. carcinomatosa; neuromiopatia associada a carcinoma, especialmente do pulmão.

neu·ro·my·o·si·tis (noor'ō-mī-ō-sī'tis). Neuromiosite. Termo obsoleto para referir-se à polimiosite. [neuro- + G. *mys*, músculo + *-itis*, inflamação]

ℹ **neu·ron** (noor'on). Neurônio. A unidade morfológica e funcional do sistema nervoso, consistindo no corpo das células nervosas, nos dendritos e no axônio. SIN nerve cell, neurocyte, neurone. [G. *neuron*, nervo]
   autonomic motor n., n. motor autônomo. VER motor n.
   bipolar n., n. bipolar; neurônio que possui dois processos que se originam dos polos opostos do corpo celular.
   gamma motor n.'s, neurônios motores gama. SIN gamma *loop*.
   ganglionic motor n., n. motor ganglionar. VER motor n.
   Golgi type I n., n. de Golgi tipo I; células nervosas cujos axônios longos deixam a substância cinzenta da qual fazem parte.

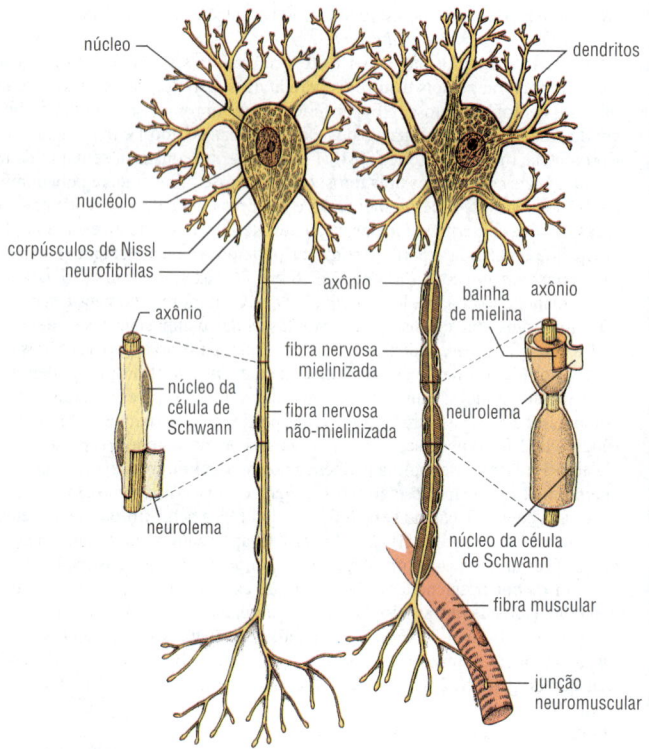

neurônios eferentes típicos: (à esquerda) fibra não-mielinizada, (à direita) fibra mielinizada

Golgi type II n., n. de Golgi tipo II; células nervosas com axônios curtos que se ramificam na substância cinzenta.
intercalary n., n. intercalar. SIN internuncial n.
internuncial n., n. internuncial; neurônio interposto entre dois outros neurônios, estabelecendo a sua conexão. SIN intercalary n.
lower motor n., n. motor inferior; termo clínico utilizado para indicar os neurônios motores finais que inervam os músculos esqueléticos; distingue-se do neurônio motor superior do córtex motor que contribui para o trato corticospinal. VER TAMBÉM motor n.
motor n., n. motor; célula nervosa na medula espinal, no rombencéfalo ou no mesencéfalo, caracterizada por um axônio que deixa o sistema nervoso central para estabelecer uma conexão funcional com um tecido efetor (músculo ou glândula); os **neurônios motores somáticos** fazem sinapse diretamente com fibras musculares estriadas através de placas terminais motoras; por outro lado, os **neurônios motores viscerais** ou **neurônios motores autônomos** (neurônios motores pré-ganglionares) inervam as fibras musculares lisas ou glândulas apenas por intermédio de um segundo neurônio periférico (neurônio motor pós-ganglionar) localizado num gânglio motor visceral ou autônomo. VER TAMBÉM motor *endplate*, autonomic *division* of nervous system. SIN anterior horn cell, motoneuron.
multipolar n., n. multipolar; neurônio com diversos processos, geralmente um axônio e três ou mais dendritos.
NANC n., n. NANC; abreviatura de neurônio não-adrenérgico, não-colinérgico.
nonadrenergic, noncholinergic n. (NANC n.), n. não-adrenérgico, não-colinérgico (n. NANC); neurônio eferente autônomo cuja transmissão não é bloqueada pelo bloqueio da transmissão adrenérgica e colinérgica. O óxido nítrico seria o transmissor em alguns casos.
polymorphic n., n. polimórfico; neurônio que apresenta muitas formas. VER TAMBÉM multipolar *cell*.
postganglionic motor n., n. motor pós-ganglionar. VER motor n.
preganglionic motor n., n. motor pré-ganglionar. VER motor n.
pseudounipolar n., n. pseudo-unipolar. SIN unipolar n.
sensory n., n. sensorial; neurônio que envia a informação proveniente de receptores sensoriais ou terminações nervosas; neurônio aferente, pode ser sensorial geral ou especial.
somatic motor n., n. motor somático. VER motor n.
ℹ **unipolar n.,** n. unipolar; neurônio cujo corpo celular emite um único prolongamento axonal resultante da fusão de dois processos polares durante o desenvolvimento; a uma distância variável do corpo celular, esse prolongamento divide-se num ramo axonal periférico, que se estende para fora como fibra

neuron | neuropathy

nervosa aferente (sensorial) periférica, e num ramo axonal central, que entra em contato sináptico com neurônios na medula espinal ou no tronco cerebral. Com a única exceção conhecida dos neurônios que compõem o núcleo mesencefálico do trigêmeo, os neurônios unipolares constituem os elementos neurais exclusivos dos gânglios sensoriais. A ausência de processos dendríticos desses neurônios sensitivos primários é apenas aparente: o pólo dendrítico do neurônio unipolar é representado pelas ramificações terminais não-mielinizadas do ramo axonal periférico. SIN pseudounipolar cell, pseudounipolar n., unipolar cell.

upper motor n., n. motor superior; termo clínico indicando os neurônios do córtex motor que contribuem para a formação dos tratos corticospinal e corticonuclear (corticobulbar), em contraste com os neurônios motores inferiores, que inervam os musculos esqueléticos. Embora não sejam neurônios motores no sentido estrito, esses neurônios corticais passaram a ser classificados coloquialmente como neurônios motores, visto que a sua estimulação produz movimento e a sua destruição causa distúrbios moderados a graves do movimento. VER TAMBÉM n., motor *cortex*.

visceral motor n., n. motor visceral. VER motor n.

neu·ro·nal (noor′ō-năl, noo-rō′năl). Neuronal. Relativo a um neurônio.

neu·rone (noor′ōn). Neurônio. SIN neuron.

neu·ro·neph·ric (noor-ō-nef′rik). Neuronéfrico. Relativo à inervação do rim. [neuro- + G. *nephros*, rim]

neu·ro·ne·vus (noor-ō-nē′vŭs). Neuronevo. Variedade de nevo intradérmico, em adultos, em que os ninhos de células do nevo atróficas na derme inferior estão hialinizados e assemelham-se a feixes nervosos.

neu·ron·i·tis (noor-ō-nī′tis). Neuronite. Distúrbio inflamatório do neurônio.

vestibular n., n. vestibular; ataque paroxístico de vertigem intensa, não acompanhada de surdez ou tinido, que afeta adultos jovens a indivíduos de meia-idade, ocorrendo freqüentemente após infecção respiratória superior inespecífica; devido à disfunção vestibular unilateral. SIN endemic paralytic vertigo, epidemic vertigo, Gerlier disease, kubisagari, kubisagaru, paralyzing vertigo.

neu·ro·nop·a·thy (noor-ō-nop′ă-thē). Neuronopatia. Distúrbio, freqüentemente tóxico, do neurônio (1).

sensory n., n. sensorial; neuronopatia limitada aos gânglios da raiz dorsal e de Gasser.

X-linked recessive bulbospinal n., n. bulboespinal recessiva ligada ao X. SIN Kennedy *disease*.

neu·ron·o·phage (noo-ron′ō-fāj). Neuronófago. Fagócito que ingere elementos neuronais. VER microglia. [neuron + G. *phagō*, comer]

neu·ron·o·pha·gia, neu·ro·noph·a·gy (noor′on′ō-fā′jē-ă, noor-ō-nof′ă-jē). Neuronofagia. Fagocitose de células nervosas. [neuron + G. *phagō*, comer]

neu·ro·nyx·is (noor-ō-nik′sis). Neuronixe. Acupuntura de um nervo. [neuro- + G. *nyxis*, punção]

neu·ro·on·col·o·gy (noor′ō-on-kol′ō-jē). Neuroncologia. Ramo da medicina relacionado com os efeitos diretos e indiretos de neoplasias sobre o sistema nervoso, junção neuromuscular e músculo. [neuro- + G. onco- + G. *logos*, estudo]

neu·ro-oph·thal·mol·o·gy (noor′ō-of-thal-mol′ō-jē). Neuroftalmologia. Ramo da medicina relacionado com os aspectos neurológicos do aparelho visual.

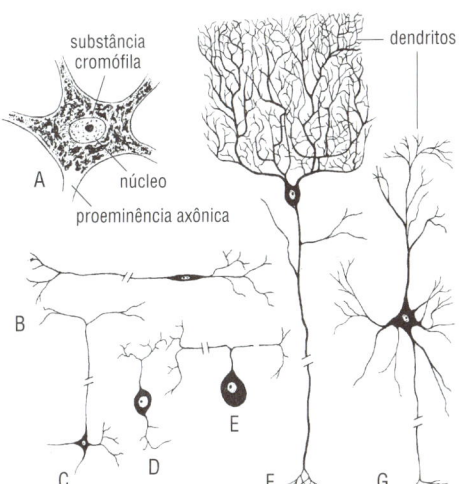

neurônios típicos: (A) corpo celular nervoso típico mostrando a estrutura interna; (B) célula horizontal (de Cajal) do córtex cerebral; (C) célula de Martinotti, (D) célula bipolar, (E) célula unipolar (gânglio da raiz posterior), (F) célula de Purkinje, (G) célula piramidal da área motora do córtex cerebral. As bainhas não são mostradas

neu·ro·otol·o·gy (noor′ō-ō-tol′ō-jē). Neurotologia. Ramo da medicina interessado no sistema nervoso relacionado com os sistemas auditivo e vestibular.

neu·ro·pa·ral·y·sis (noor′ō-pă-ral′i-sis). Neuroparalisia. Paralisia resultante de doença da inervação da parte afetada.

neu·ro·par·a·lyt·ic (noor′ō-pă-ră-lit′ik). Neuroparalítico. Relativo a, ou caracterizado por, neuroparalisia.

neu·ro·path (noor′ō-path). Neuropata. Que sofre de, ou tem predisposição a, alguma doença do sistema nervoso.

neuropathia (noo-rō-path′ē-ă). Neuropatia. SIN neuropathy.

n. epidemica, n. epidêmica; febre hemorrágica com complicações renais, causada pelo vírus Puumala.

neu·ro·path·ic (noor-ō-path′ik). Neuropático. Relativo à neuropatia.

neu·ro·path·o·gen·e·sis (noor′ō-path-ō-jen′ĕ-sis). Neuropatogenia. A origem ou causa de uma doença do sistema nervoso. [neuro- + G. *pathos*, sofrimento + *genesis*, origem]

neu·ro·pa·thol·o·gy (noor′ō-pa-thol′ō-jē). Neuropatologia. **1.** Patologia do sistema nervoso. **2.** Ramo da patologia relacionado com o sistema nervoso.

neu·rop·a·thy (noo-rop′ă-thē). Neuropatia. **1.** Termo clássico que designa qualquer distúrbio afetando qualquer segmento do sistema nervoso. **2.** No uso contemporâneo, refere-se a uma doença que acomete os nervos cranianos ou o sistema nervoso periférico ou autônomo. SIN neuritis (2), neuropathia. [neuro- + G. *pathos*, sofrimento]

acute motor axonal n., n. axonal motora aguda; tipo de polirradiculoneuropatia aguda motora pura, de degeneração dos axônios, variante da síndrome de Guillain-Barré; segue principalmente um padrão sazonal (primavera ou verão) em crianças na China rural após epidemia de diarréia causada por *Campylobacter jejuni*.

acute sensory motor axonal n., n. axonal motora sensorial aguda; polirradiculoneuropatia aguda de degeneração axonal, que afeta fibras tanto motoras quanto sensoriais; variante da síndrome de Guillain-Barré.

asymmetric motor n., n. motora assimétrica; **(1)** neuropatia em que a perda da função é mais acentuada nos membros de um lado do corpo; **(2)** manifestação da amiotrofia diabética (*amyotrophy*).

auditory n., n. auditiva; distúrbio da audição em crianças, caracterizado por perda da audição sensorioneural para tons puros, redução da discriminação das palavras desproporcional à perda dos tons puros, função normal das células ciliadas externas, determinada por medida de emissões otoacústicas e ausência ou anormalidade da resposta auditiva do tronco cerebral.

brachial plexus n., n. do plexo braquial. SIN neuralgic *amyotrophy*.

compression n., n. por compressão; lesão nervosa focal produzida por aplicação persistente de pressão a uma porção localizada do nervo, de fonte externa ou interna; a principal fonte de lesão consiste no diferencial de pressão existente entre uma porção do nervo e outra.

dapsone n., n. por dapsona; polineuropatia que se desenvolve em pacientes que fazem uso de dapsona (4,4-diaminodifenilsulfona); as manifestações incomuns consistem em neuropatia motora pura que começa nas mãos, algumas vezes de modo assimétrico. SIN motor dapsone n.

diabetic n., n. diabética; termo genérico para referir-se a qualquer distúrbio do sistema nervoso periférico, do sistema nervoso autônomo e de alguns nervos cranianos associado ao diabetes melito.

A neuropatia diabética, que é a mais comum das complicações crônicas do diabetes, pode acometer o sistema nervoso periférico e/ou o sistema nervoso autônomo. As neuropatias periféricas podem causar hipestesia, hiperestesia, parestesia, perda da sensação da temperatura e da percepção vibratória ou causalgia bilateralmente simétricas. O comprometimento do sistema nervoso autônomo pode manifestar-se como hipotensão postural, gastroparesia, diarréia alternando com constipação e impotência. A patogenia da neuropatia diabética crônica não está bem esclarecida. Os sintomas tendem a progredir, e a resposta ao tratamento é imprevisível. Em contrapartida, a paralisia de nervos cranianos devido à microangiopatia no diabetes melito freqüentemente sofre resolução espontânea.

diphtheritic n., n. diftérica; polineuropatia de desenvolvimento rápido, causada por uma toxina elaborada por *Corynebacterium diphtheriae*.

entrapment n., n. por encarceramento, n. compressiva; lesão nervosa focal produzida por constrição ou deformação mecânica do nervo, no interior de um túnel fibroso ou fibro-ósseo, ou por uma faixa fibrosa; nessas lesões, o estiramento e a angulação do nervo podem ser tão importantes quanto a compressão como causa de lesão; a neuropatia por encarceramento tende a ocorrer em determinados locais do corpo.

familial amyloid n. [MIM*105120, vários tipos], n. amilóide familiar; distúrbio em que vários nervos periféricos estão infiltrados por amilóide e têm as suas funções comprometidas; ocorre também formação de uma pré-albumina anormal, que é encontrada no sangue; tipicamente, surge durante a meia-ida-

de, sendo encontrada, na maioria dos casos, em indivíduos de origem portuguesa; herança autossômica dominante. Ocorrem outros tipos clínicos raros. SIN familial amyloidosis, hereditary amyloidosis.
giant axonal n., n. axonal gigante; distúrbio raro que começa no terceiro ano de vida ou depois; clinicamente, manifesta-se por cabelos crespos, incapacitação indolor progressiva, fraqueza e atrofia muscular, perda sensorial e arreflexia. Do ponto de vista patológico, as fibras nervosas tanto mielinizadas quanto não-mielinizadas contêm esferóides axonais aglomerados com neurofilamentos; de natureza esporádica.
Graves optic n., n. óptica de Graves; disfunção visual em decorrência da compressão do nervo óptico na orbitopatia de Graves.
heavy metal n., n. por metais pesados; distúrbios do sistema nervoso periférico atribuídos à intoxicação por um dos metais pesados: arsênico, ouro, chumbo, mercúrio, platina e tálio.
hereditary hypertrophic n. [MIM*145900], n. hipertrófica hereditária. SIN Dejerine-Sottas disease.
hereditary sensory radicular n. [MIM*162400], n. radicular sensorial hereditária; polineuropatia caracterizada pela ocorrência de graves ulcerações recidivantes do pé de origem neuropática, destruição das porções terminais dos dedos dos pés e das mãos e perda da sensação; a herança autossômica dominante está associada ao início da doença na segunda década de vida ou posteriormente.
hypertrophic interstitial n., n. intersticial hipertrófica; polineuropatia sensoriomotora, caracterizada histopatologicamente por coleções de processos de células de Schwann de distribuição concêntrica ao redor de uma ou mais fibras nervosas. Não foi identificado nenhum fator genético na sua etiologia. Para os tipos hereditários, ver hereditary hypertrophic neuropathy.
ischemic n., n. isquêmica; neuropatia decorrente de isquemia aguda ou crônica dos nervos acometidos.
ischemic optic n., n. óptica isquêmica; neuropatia do nervo óptico secundária à hipoperfusão das artérias ciliares posteriores de baixa pressão que suprem a cabeça do nervo óptico (não-arterítica) ou à arterite temporal (arterítica).
isoniazid n., n. por isoniazida; perda dos axônios; tipo de polineuropatia observado em alguns pacientes tratados com isoniazida.
lead n., n. por chumbo; polineuropatia observada na intoxicação crônica por chumbo; supostamente caracterizada por punho caído, porém sem nenhum relato moderno convincente dessa ocorrência.
leprous n., n. leprosa; neuropatia granulomatosa de desenvolvimento lento, comumente observada na lepra, causada por *Mycobacterium leprae*.
motor dapsone n., n. motora por dapsona. SIN dapsone n.
onion bulb n., n. em bulbo de cebola; designação de qualquer uma de várias polineuropatias desmielinizantes, em que os nervos estão aumentados devido à formação de bulbos de cebola — espirais de processos de células de Schwann superpostos circundando axônios insuficientemente medulados; p. ex., polineuropatia hipertrófica progressiva. VER hypertrophic interstitial n.
symmetric distal n., n. distal simétrica. SIN polyneuropathy.
vitamin B₁₂ n., n. por vitamina B₁₂. SIN subacute combined degeneration of the spinal cord.
neu·ro·pep·tide (noor - ō - pep′tĭd). Neuropeptídeo. Qualquer um de inúmeros peptídeos encontrados no tecido neural; p. ex., endorfinas, encefalinas.
n. Y, n. Y; neurotransmissor peptídico de 36 aminoácidos, encontrado no cérebro e no sistema nervoso autônomo. Aumenta os efeitos vasoconstritores de neurônios noradrenérgicos.
neu·ro·phar·ma·col·o·gy (noor′ō - far′mă - kol′ō - jē). Neurofarmacologia. O estudo das substâncias que afetam o tecido neuronal.
neu·ro·phil·ic (noor - ō - fil′ik). Neurófilo. SIN neurotropic. [neuro- + G. *philos*, amigo]
neu·ro·pho·nia (noor - ō - fō′nē - ă). Neurofonia. Espasmo ou tique dos músculos da fonação, causando sons ou gritos involuntários. [neuro- + G. *phonē*, voz]
neu·ro·phy·sins (noor - ō - fiz′inz). Neurofisinas. Família de proteínas sintetizadas no hipotálamo como parte da grande proteína precursora que inclui a vasopressina e a oxitocina nos grânulos neurossecretores; as neurofisinas atuam como carreadoras no transporte e no armazenamento dos hormônios neuro-hipofisários.
neu·ro·phys·i·ol·o·gy (noor′ō - fiz - ē - ol′ō - jē). Neurofisiologia. Fisiologia do sistema nervoso.
neu·ro·pil, neu·ro·pile (noor′ō - pil, - pīl). Neurópilo. Rede complexa e semelhante a feltro de arborizações axonais, dendríticas e gliais que forma a massa da substância cinzenta do sistema nervoso central e na qual estão mergulhados os corpos das células nervosas. [neuro- + G. *pilos*, feltro]
neu·ro·plasm (noor′ō - plazm). Neuroplasma. O protoplasma de uma célula nervosa.
neu·ro·plas·ty (noor′ō - plas - tē). Neuroplastia. Cirurgia dos nervos. [neuro- + G. *plastos*, formado]
neu·ro·ple·gic (noor - ō - plē′jik). Neuroplégico. Que se refere à paralisia decorrente de doença do sistema nervoso. [neuro- + G. *plēgē*, golpe]
neu·ro·plex·us (noo′rō - plek′sus). Neuroplexo. Plexo ou rede de células ou fibras nervosas.

neu·ro·po·dia (noor - ō - pō′dē - ă). Neurópodos. SIN axon terminals, em terminal. [pl. de *neuropodium* ou *neuropodion*, de neuro- + G. *podion*, pé pequeno]
neu·ro·pore (noor′ō - pōr). Neuroporo. Abertura no embrião que leva do canal central do tubo neural para o exterior do tubo. [neuro- + G. *poros*, poro]
anterior n., n. anterior. SIN rostral n.
caudal n., n. caudal; abertura temporária na extremidade caudal do tubo neural em embriões em fase inicial de desenvolvimento; ocorre fechamento aproximadamente no estágio do 25.º somito nos seres humanos. SIN posterior n.
cranial n., n. cranial. SIN rostral n.
posterior n., n. posterior. SIN caudal n.
rostral n., n. rostral; abertura temporária na extremidade rostral (cefálica) do prosencéfalo no embrião em fase de desenvolvimento inicial; ocorre fechamento aproximadamente no estágio do 20.º somito nos seres humanos. SIN anterior n., cranial n.
neu·ro·prax·ia. Neuropraxia. Erro de ortografia comumente cometido para neurapraxia.
neu·ro·psy·chi·a·try (noor′ō - sī - kī′ă - trē). Neuropsiquiatria. A especialidade que trata de distúrbios do sistema nervoso tanto orgânicos quanto psíquicos; termo mais antigo para a psiquiatria.
neu·ro·psy·cho·log·ic, neu·ro·psy·cho·log·i·cal (noor′ō - sī - kō - loj′ik, - loj′i - kal). Neuropsicológico. Relativo à neuropsicologia.
neu·ro·psy·chol·o·gy (noor′ō - sī - kol′ō - jē). Neuropsicologia. Especialidade da psicologia que trata do estudo das relações entre o cérebro e o comportamento, incluindo o uso de testes psicológicos e técnicas de avaliação para diagnosticar déficits cognitivos e comportamentais específicos e prescrever estratégias de reabilitação para a sua correção.
neu·ro·psy·cho·path·ic (noor′ō - sī - kō - path′ik). Neuropsicopático. Relativo à neuropsicopatia.
neu·ro·psy·chop·a·thy (noor′ō - sī - kop′ă - thē). Neuropsicopatia. Doença emocional de origem neurológica.
neu·ro·psy·cho·phar·ma·col·o·gy (noor′ō - sī′kō - far - mă - kol′ō - jē). Neuropsicofarmacologia. SIN psychopharmacology.
neu·ro·ra·di·ol·o·gy (noor′rō - rā - dē - ol′ō - jē). Neurorradiologia. A subespecialidade clínica relacionada com a radiologia diagnóstica de doenças do sistema nervoso central, da cabeça e pescoço.
neu·ro·reg·u·la·tor (noor′ō - reg′u - lā - tor). Neurorregulador. Fator químico que estende um efeito modulador sobre um neurônio.
neu·ro·re·lapse (noor′ō - rē - laps′). Neurorrecidiva. Termo obsoleto para referir-se à recorrência de sintomas neurológicos após o início do tratamento, especialmente com fármacos anti-sifilíticos.
neu·ro·ret·i·ni·tis (noor′ō - ret - i - nī′tis). Neurorretinite. Inflamação que afeta a cabeça do nervo óptico e o pólo posterior da retina, com células no vítreo adjacente, produzindo geralmente uma estrela macular. SIN papilloretinitis.
diffuse unilateral subacute n. (DUSN), n. subaguda unilateral difusa (NSUD); inflamação da retina neurossensorial causada por infiltração de nematódeo, como espécies de *Baylisascaris* ou *Ancylostoma*.
Leber idiopathic stellate n., n. estrelada idiopática de Leber. SIN stellate n.
stellate n., n. estrelada; neurorretinite unilateral com exsudatos perifoveais na camada de fibras do nervo de Henle, produzindo uma estrela macular, com regressão espontânea em alguns meses. SIN Leber idiopathic stellate n.
neu·ror·rha·phy (noor - ōr′ă - fē). Neurorrafia. União, geralmente através de sutura, das duas partes de um nervo seccionado. SIN nerve suture, neurosuture. [neuro- + G. *rhaphē*, sutura]
neu·ro·sar·co·clei·sis (noor′ō - sar - kō - klī′sis). Neurossarcocleise. Operação para alívio da neuralgia, consistindo na ressecção de uma das paredes de um canal ósseo atravessado pelo nervo e transposição do nervo para os tecidos moles. [neuro- + G. *sarx*, carne + *kleisis*, fechamento]
neu·ro·sar·coid·o·sis (noor′ō - sar - koy - dō′sis). Neurossarcoidose. Doença granulomatosa de etiologia desconhecida, que afeta o sistema nervoso central, geralmente com comprometimento sistêmico concomitante.
neu·ro·sar·co·ma (noo′rō - sar - kō′mă). Neurossarcoma. Sarcoma com elementos neuromatosos; inclui o neurofibrossarcoma, o sarcoma neurogênico e o schwanoma maligno.
neu·ro·schwan·no·ma (noor′ō - shwah - nō′mă). Neuroschwanoma. SIN schwanoma.
neu·ro·sci·enc·es (noor - ō - sī′en - sez). Neurociência. Disciplina científica que trata do desenvolvimento, da estrutura, da função, da química, da farmacologia, da avaliação clínica e da patologia do sistema nervoso.
neu·ro·se·cre·tion (noor′ō - sē - krē′shun). Neurossecreção. A liberação de uma substância secretora das terminações axônicas de certas células nervosas no cérebro para o sangue circulante. O produto secretor pode ser um hormônio verdadeiro, como, p. ex., o hormônio antidiurético liberado pelas terminações axônicas dos neurônios que compõem o núcleo supra-óptico do hipotálamo; no caso do denominado fator de liberação dos neurônios do hipotálamo, o produto celular não é um hormônio sistêmico propriamente dito, mas desencadeia a liberação de hormônios tróficos pelo lobo anterior da hipófise, os quais, por sua vez, estimulam as glândulas endócrinas periféricas a liberar seus hormônios sistemicamente ativos.

neu·ro·se·cre·to·ry (noor′ō-sē′krē-tōr-ē, -sē-krē′tōr-ē). Neurossecretor. Relativo à neurossecreção.

neu·ro·sis, pl. **neu·ro·ses** (noo-rō′sis, -sēz). Neurose. **1.** Distúrbio psicológico ou comportamental cuja característica primária consiste em ansiedade; os mecanismos de defesa ou qualquer uma das fobias constituem as técnicas de ajustamento que o indivíduo aprende com a finalidade de conviver com essa ansiedade subjacente. Ao contrário das psicoses, os indivíduos com neurose não apresentam deformação visível da realidade nem desorganização de sua personalidade. **2.** Doença nervosa funcional ou doença em que não há lesão evidente. **3.** Estado peculiar de tensão ou irritabilidade do sistema nervoso; qualquer forma de nervosismo. SIN neurotic disorder. [neuro- + G. *-osis*, condição]
  accident n., n. de acidente. SIN traumatic n.
  anxiety n., n. de ansiedade; angústia e preocupação anormais e crônicas a ponto de ficar em estado de pânico, seguidas de tendência a evitar a situação temida ou fugir dela, associadas a hiperatividade do sistema nervoso simpático.
  cardiac n., n. cardíaca. Ansiedade relacionada ao estado do coração, em conseqüência de palpitações, dor torácica ou outros sintomas que não são devidos a cardiopatia; forma de hipocondríase. SIN cardioneurosis.
  character n., n. de caráter; subclasse de distúrbios da personalidade.
  combat n., n. de combate. VER battle *fatigue*, posttraumatic stress *disorder*.
  compensation n., n. de compensação; desenvolvimento de sintomas de neurose que se acredita sejam motivados pelo desejo e esperança de ganho monetário ou interpessoal.
  compulsive n., n. compulsiva. SIN obsessive-compulsive n.
  conversion n., n. de conversão. SIN conversion *hysteria*.
  conversion hysteria n., n. da histeria de conversão. SIN conversion *hysteria*.
  depressive n., n. depressiva. VER depression, dysthymia.
  experimental n., n. experimental; distúrbio de comportamento produzido experimentalmente, como, p. ex., quando um organismo é obrigado a fazer uma discriminação extremamente difícil e "sofre colapso" no processo.
  hypochondriacal n., n. hipocondríaca. SIN hypochondriasis.
  hysterical n., n. histérica; distúrbio genuíno caracterizado por alteração ou perda de funcionamento físico, como borramento visual, dormência ou paralisia dos membros, dificuldades de coordenação, etc., sugerindo um distúrbio físico, mas que constitui, aparentemente, a expressão de um conflito ou necessidade psicológica. Também denominada distúrbio de conversão. VER TAMBÉM hysteria.
  noogenic n., n. noogênica; em psiquiatria existencial, sintomatologia neurótica resultante de frustração existencial.
  obsessional n., n. obsessiva. SIN obsessive-compulsive n.
  obsessive-compulsive n., n. obsessivo-compulsiva; distúrbio caracterizado pela intrusão persistente e repetida de pensamentos, impulsos ou atos que o indivíduo é incapaz de evitar; os pensamentos compulsivos podem consistir em palavras isoladas, idéias ou ruminações freqüentemente percebidas pela pessoa afetada como desprovidas de sentido; os impulsos ou atos repetitivos variam desde movimento simples a rituais complexos; a ansiedade ou a angústia constitui a expressão subjacente ou o estado de impulso, e o comportamento ritualista é um método aprendido para reduzir a ansiedade. VER TAMBÉM obsessive-compulsive *disorder*. SIN compulsive n., obsessional n.
  oedipal n., n. edipiana; continuação do complexo de Édipo na idade adulta.
  pension n., n. de pensão; tipo de neurose de compensação motivada pelo desejo de aposentadoria prematura.
  posttraumatic n., n. pós-traumática. SIN traumatic n.
  torsion n., n. de torção. SIN *dysbasia* lordotica progressiva.
  transference n., n. de transferência; em psicanálise, o fenômeno de desenvolvimento de um forte relacionamento emocional do paciente com o analista, simbolizando um relacionamento emocional com um membro da família; a análise dessa neurose constitui uma importante parte do tratamento psicanalítico.
  traumatic n., n. traumática; qualquer distúrbio nervoso funcional após um acidente ou lesão. VER posttraumatic stress *disorder*. SIN accident n., posttraumatic n.

neu·ro·splanch·nic (noor-ō-splangk′nik). Neuroesplâncnico. SIN neurovisceral. [neuro- + G. *splanchnon*, víscera]

neu·ro·spon·gi·um (noor-ō-spon′jē-ŭm, noor-ō-spŭn′jē-ŭm). Neuroespôngio. **1.** Termo obsoleto para referir-se ao plexo de neurofibrilas no interior das células nervosas. **2.** Designação obsoleta para camada reticular da retina. [neuro- + G. *spongium*, pequena esponja]

Neu·ros·po·ra (noo-ros′pōr-ă). *Neurospora*. Gênero de fungos (classe Ascomycetes) que cresce em culturas, utilizado em pesquisa em bioquímica genética e celular. SIN pink bread mold. [neuro- + G. *spora*, semente]

neurosteroid (nūr-ō-stēr′oyd). Neuroesteróide. Esteróide produzido no cérebro.

neu·ro·stim·u·la·tor (noor-ō-stim′ū-lā-ter). Neuroestimulador. Dispositivo para excitação elétrica do sistema nervoso central ou periférico.

neu·ro·sur·geon (noor-ō-ser′jŭn). Neurocirurgião. Cirurgião especializado em operações do cérebro, da medula espinal, da coluna vertebral e dos nervos periféricos.

neu·ro·sur·gery (noor-ō-ser′jer-ē). Neurocirurgia. Cirurgia do sistema nervoso.
  functional n., n. funcional; destruição ou excitação crônica de uma parte do cérebro para tratar distúrbios comportamentais ou funcionais.

neu·ro·su·ture (noor-ō-soo′choor). Neurossutura. SIN neurorrhaphy.

neu·ro·syph·i·lis (noor-ō-sif′i-lis). Neurossífilis. Infecção do sistema nervoso central por *Treponema pallidum*, ou sífilis; existem várias subdivisões, incluindo neurossífilis assintomática, neurossífilis meníngea, neurossífilis meningovascular, neurossífilis parética e neurossífilis tabética.
  asymptomatic n., n. assintomática; infecção sifilítica das meninges clinicamente inaparente (à exceção de possível anormalidade das pupilas), diagnosticada com base no exame do líquido cefalorraquidiano; quando não tratada, evolui freqüentemente para alguma forma de neurossífilis sintomática.
  meningeal n., n. meníngea; infecção sifilítica das meninges, produzindo meningite clínica afebril com cefaléia, rigidez da nuca, obtusão, etc., além de achados anormais do LCR. Com mais freqüência, desenvolve-se nos 2 anos seguintes à infecção inicial.
  meningovascular n., n. meningovascular; infecção sifilítica das meninges acompanhada de alterações (inflamação, espessamento fibroso) nas paredes das artérias subaracnóides, manifestada na forma de acidente vascular cerebral, com aparecimento súbito de sintomas, incluindo hemiplegia, afasia, distúrbios visuais, etc., e achados anormais do LCR.
  paretic n., n. parética; infecção sifilítica manifestada na forma de demência (freqüentemente com características de delírio), disartria, convulsões, contrações mioclônicas, tremor de intenção, comprometimento da marcha e permanência em pé, anormalidades pupilares e achados anormais do LCR. SIN chronic progressive syphilitic meningoencephalitis, general paresis.
  tabetic n., n. tabética; tipo de neurossífilis em que as raízes posteriores da medula espinal, especialmente na área lombossacra, constituem os principais locais de infecção, resultando em ataxia, hipotonia, impotência, constipação, bexiga hipotônica, arreflexia e sinal de Romberg; outros achados incluem dor lancinante (mais freqüentemente nas pernas), crises viscerais, pupilas de Argyll Robertson, atrofia óptica e articulações de Charcot; na maioria dos pacientes, o LCR está anormal. SIN myelosyphilis, posterior sclerosis, posterior spinal sclerosis.

neu·ro·tax·is (noor′ō-tak′sis). Neurotaxia. Alongamento neuronal em direção a um alvo. [neuro- + *taxis*, arranjo]

neu·ro·ten·di·nous (noor-ō-ten′di-nŭs). Neurotendinoso. Relativo tanto a nervos quanto a tendões.

neu·ro·ten·sin (noo-rō-ten′sin). Neurotensina. Neurotransmissor peptídico de 13 aminoácidos encontrado nos sinapsomas do hipotálamo, amígdala, gânglios da base e substância cinzenta dorsal da medula espinal; desempenha um papel na percepção da dor, porém seus efeitos analgésicos não são bloqueados por antagonistas de opióides; afeta também a liberação de hormônios hipofisários e a função gastrintestinal.

neu·ro·ten·sion (noor-ō-ten′shŭn). Neurotensão. SIN neurectasis.

neu·ro·the·ke·o·ma (noor-ō-thē-kē-ō′mă). Neurotecoma. Mixoma benigno que se origina na bainha de nervo cutâneo. [neuro- + G. *thēkē*, caixa, bainha + *-oma*, tumor]

neu·ro·the·le (noor′ō-thēl). Neurotélio. SIN nerve papilla. [neuro- + G. *thēlē*, mamilo]

neu·ro·ther·a·peu·tics, neu·ro·ther·a·py (noor′ō-thār′ă-pū′tiks, -thār′ă-pē). Neuroterapêutica, neuroterapia. Termo mais antigo para referir-se ao tratamento de transtornos psicológicos, psiquiátricos e nervosos.

neu·ro·tic (noo-rot′ik). Neurótico. Relativo a, ou que sofre de, neurose. VER neurosis.

neu·rot·i·cism (noo-rot′i-sizm). Neuroticismo. Condição ou traço psicológico de ser neurótico.

neu·rot·i·za·tion (noor′ō-ti-zā′shŭn). Neurotização. Aquisição de substância nervosa; regeneração de um nervo.

neu·ro·tize (noor′ō-tīz). Neurotizar. Fornecer substância nervosa.

neu·rot·me·sis. Neurotmese. Tipo de perda axônica decorrente de lesão focal de nervos periféricos em que, no local da lesão, o estroma nervoso é lesado em graus variáveis, bem como o axônio e a mielina, que degeneram distalmente; nas lesões mais graves, ocorre ruptura da continuidade do nervo. VER axonotmesis, neurapraxia.

neu·ro·tome (noor′ō-tōm). Neurótomo. **1.** Bisturi muito fino ou agulha utilizados para separar fibras nervosas na microdissecção. **2.** SIN neuromere. [neuro- + G. *tomē*, um corte]

neu·rot·o·my (noo-rot′o-mē). Neurotomia. Secção cirúrgica de nervo. [neuro- + G. *tomē*, um curto]
  retrogasserian n., n. retrogasseriana. SIN trigeminal *rhizotomy*.

neu·ro·ton·ic (noor-ō-ton′ik). Neurotônico. **1.** Relativo à neurotonia. **2.** Que fortalece ou estimula a ação nervosa comprometida. **3.** Agente que melhora o tônus ou a força do sistema nervoso.

neu·ro·tox·ic (noor-ō-tok′sik). Neurotóxico. Tóxico para a substância nervosa.

neu·ro·tox·in (noor-ō-tok′sin). Neurotoxina. **1.** SIN neurolysin. **2.** Qualquer toxina capaz de atuar especificamente sobre o tecido nervoso.

neu·ro·trans·mis·sion (noor′o-trans-mish′ŭn). Neurotransmissão. SIN neurohumoral transmission.

neu·ro·trans·mit·ter (noor′ō-trans-mit′er). Neurotransmissor. Qualquer agente químico específico (incluindo acetilcolina, cinco aminas, quatro aminoácidos, duas purinas e mais de 28 peptídeos) liberado por uma célula pré-sináptica, em consequência de excitação, que atravessa a sinapse para estimular ou inibir a célula pós-sináptica. Pode ocorrer liberação de mais de um neurotransmissor em qualquer sinapse. O neurotransmissor liberado por células pré-sinápticas pode modular a liberação de transmissores de células pré-sinápticas. O óxido nítrico (NO) pode ser um neurotransmissor retrógrado, liberado por células pós-sinápticas, atuando sobre células pré-sinápticas. [neuro- + L. *transmitto*, transmitir]

  adrenergic n., n. adrenérgico; neurotransmissor formado em sinapses pós-ganglionares simpáticas (p. ex., norepinefrina).

  cholinergic n., n. colinérgico; neurotransmissor formado em sinapses pré e pós-ganglionares do sistema nervoso parassimpático (p. ex., acetilcolina).

neu·ro·trau·ma (noor-o-traw′mă). Neurotrauma. 1. Traumatismo do sistema nervoso. 2. Traumatismo ou ferimento de um nervo. SIN neurotrosis. [neuro- + G. *trauma*, lesão]

neu·ro·trip·sy (noor-o-trip′sē). Neurotripsia. Esmagamento cirúrgico de um nervo. [neuro- + G. *tripsis*, atrito]

neu·ro·tro·phic (noor-ō-trof′ik). Neurotrófico. Relativo à neurotrofia.

neu·rot·ro·phy (noo-rot′rō-fē). Neurotrofia. Nutrição e metabolismo dos tecidos sob a influência nervosa. [neuro- + G. *trophe*, nutrição]

neu·ro·tro·pic (noor-o-trop′ik). Neurotrópico. Que tem afinidade pelo sistema nervoso. SIN neurophilic.

neu·rot·ro·py, neu·rot·ro·pism (noo-rot′rō-pē, -pizm). Neurotropia, neurotropismo. 1. Afinidade de corantes básicos para o tecido nervoso. 2. Atração de certos microrganismos patogênicos, venenos e substâncias nutritivas para os centros nervosos. [neuro- + G. *trope*, uma volta]

neu·ro·tro·sis (noor-ō-trō′sis). Neurotrose. SIN neurotrauma (2). [neuro- + G. *trosis*, ferimento]

neu·ro·tu·bule (noor′o-too-būl). Neurotúbulo. Um dos microtúbulos com cerca de 24 nm de diâmetro que ocorrem no corpo celular, nos dendritos, no axônio e em algumas terminações sinápticas de neurônios.

neu·ro·vac·cine (noor-ō-vak′sēn). Neurovacina. Vírus vacínico fixo ou padronizado de concentração definida, obtido por passagem contínua através do cérebro de coelhos; antigo método de preparação da vacina anti-rábica.

neu·ro·var·i·co·sis, neu·ro·var·i·cos·i·ty (noor′ō-var-i-kō′sis, -var-i-kos′i-tē). Neurovaricose, neurovaricosidade. Condição caracterizada por múltiplas tumefações ao longo do trajeto de um nervo. [neuro- + L. *varix*, varicose]

neu·ro·vas·cu·lar (noor-ō-vas′kū-lăr). Neurovascular. Relativo tanto ao sistema nervoso quanto ao sistema vascular; relativo aos nervos que suprem as paredes dos vasos sanguíneos, os nervos vasomotores.

neu·ro·veg·e·ta·tive (noor-ō-vej′e-tā-tiv). Neurovegetativo. SIN neurovisceral.

neu·ro·vi·rus (noor-ō-vī′rŭs). Neurovírus. Vírus vacínico modificado por meio de passagem e crescimento no tecido nervoso.

neu·ro·vis·cer·al (noor-ō-vis′er-ăl). Neurovisceral. Refere-se à inervação dos órgãos internos pelo sistema nervoso autônomo (motor visceral). SIN neurosplanchnic, neurovegetative. [neuro- + L. *viscera*, órgãos internos]

neu·ru·la, pl. **neu·ru·lae** (noor′oo-lă, -lē). Nêurula. Estágio no desenvolvimento embrionário em que os processos proeminentes consistem na formação da placa neural e fechamento da placa para formar o tubo neural. [neur- + L. *-ulus*, pequeno]

neu·ru·la·tion (noor-oo-lā′shŭn). Neurulação. Formação da placa neural e seu fechamento para formar o tubo neural. [ver neurula]

Neusser, Edmund von, médico austríaco, 1852–1912. VER N. *granules*, em *granule*.

neu·tral (noo′trăl). Neutro. 1. Que não apresenta propriedades positivas; indiferente. 2. Em química, nem ácido nem alcalino, isto é, [OH$^-$] = [H$^+$]. 3. Que tem o mesmo número de cargas elétricas positivas e negativas. [L. *neutralis*, de *neuter*, nenhum]

neu·tral·i·za·tion (noo′trăl-i-zā′shŭn). Neutralização. 1. Mudança na reação de uma solução de ácido ou alcalino para neutro através da adição de uma quantidade suficiente de uma substância alcalina ou ácida, respectivamente. 2. O ato de tornar inefetiva qualquer ação, processo ou potencial.

  viral n., n. viral; eliminação da infectividade viral, como no caso de anticorpos específicos.

neu·tra·lize (noo′tră-līz). Neutralizar. Efetuar a neutralização.

neu·tral red [C.I. 50040]. Vermelho neutro. Usado como indicador (vermelho em pH de 6,8, amarelo em 8,0), como corante vital para corar grânulos e vacúolos em células vivas, no exame da secreção de ácido pelo estômago (administrado com uma refeição de prova) e na coloração histológica em geral. SIN toluylene red.

neutro-, neutr-. Neutro-, neutr-. Neutro. [L. *neutralis*, de *neuter*, nenhum]

neu·tro·clu·sion (noo-trō-kloo′zhŭn). Neutroclusão. Má oclusão em que existe uma relação ântero-posterior normal entre o maxilar e a mandíbula; na classificação de Angle, má oclusão da Classe I. SIN neutral occlusion (2). [neuro- + occlusion]

neu·tron (noo′tron). Nêutron. Partícula eletricamente neutra nos núcleos de todos os átomos (exceto o hidrogênio-1) com massa um pouco maior que a de um próton; isoladamente, possui meia-vida de cerca de 10,3 minutos. [L. *neuter*, nenhum]

  epithermal n., n. epitérmico; nêutron que possui uma energia na faixa térmica, isto é, que tem uma energia entre alguns centésimos e cerca de 100 ev.

neu·tro·pe·nia (noo-trō-pē′nē-ă). Neutropenia. Presença de um número anormalmente pequeno de neutrófilos no sangue circulante. SIN neutrophilic leukopenia, neutrophilopenia. [neutrophil + G. *penia*, pobreza]

  cyclic n., n. cíclica. SIN periodic n.

  periodic n., n. periódica; neutropenia que sofre recidiva a intervalos regulares (14–45 dias), associada a vários tipos de doenças infecciosas, como, p. ex., estomatite, úlceras cutâneas, furúnculos, artrite e outras. SIN cyclic n.

neu·tro·phil, neu·tro·phile (noo′trō-fil, -fīl). Neutrófilo. 1. Leucócito maduro da série granulocítica, formado pelo tecido mielopoético da medula óssea (algumas vezes também em locais extramedulares) e liberado no sangue circulante, onde normalmente representa 54–65% do número total de leucócitos. Quando corados com os tipos habituais de corantes de Romanovsky, os neutrófilos caracterizam-se por 1) um núcleo azul-púrpura escuro, lobulado (três a cinco lobos distintos, unidos por filamentos delgados de cromatina), com uma rede bastante grosseira de cromatina densa; e 2) um citoplasma fracamente róseo (em nítido contraste com o núcleo) que contém numerosos grânulos róseos ou róseo-violeta finos, isto é, nem acidófilos nem basófilos (como nos eosinófilos ou basófilos). Os precursores dos neutrófilos, por ordem de maturidade crescente, são os seguintes: mieloblastos, promielócitos, mielócitos, metamielócitos e formas em bastão. Embora os termos leucócitos neutrófilos e granulócitos neutrófilos incluam células mais jovens nas quais são identificados grânulos neutrófilos, as duas expressões são frequentemente utilizadas como sinônimos de neutrófilos, que constituem formas maduras, a não ser que indicado diferentemente por um termo específico, como neutrófilo imaturo. VER TAMBÉM leukocyte, leukocytosis. 2. Qualquer célula ou tecido que não manifesta afinidade especial para corantes ácidos ou básicos, isto é, o citoplasma cora-se aproximadamente igual com ambos os tipos de corantes. [neutro- + G. *philos*, amigo]

  band n., n. em bastão. SIN band cell.

  hypersegmented n., n. hipersegmentado; neutrófilo senescente e degenerado, no qual pode haver 6 a 10 lobos no núcleo.

  immature n., n. imaturo; neutrófilo jovem; o termo é habitualmente empregado para referir-se a neutrófilos em bastão (ou a outros neutrófilos "juvenis"), granulócitos neutrófilos em que o núcleo está indentado, mas não nitidamente segmentado.

  juvenile n., n. juvenil; qualquer célula da série granulocítica, em que os grânulos neutrófilos são identificáveis e o núcleo é indentado (primeira fase da segmentação).

  mature n., n. maduro. SIN segmented n.

  segmented n., n. segmentado; neutrófilo totalmente maduro que tem pelo menos 2 (e até 5) lobos distintos no núcleo e exibe movimento amebóide ativo. SIN mature n.

  stab n., n. em bastão. SIN band *cell*.

neu·tro·phil·ia (noo-trō-fil′ē-ă). Neutrofilia. Aumento dos leucócitos neutrófilos no sangue ou nos tecidos; o termo também é utilizado frequentemente como sinônimo de leucocitose, visto que esta última decorre geralmente de um aumento do número de granulócitos neutrófilos no sangue circulante (ou nos tecidos ou em ambos). A neutrofilia costuma ser absoluta, isto é, ocorre aumento no número total de leucócitos, bem como na percentagem de neutrófilos; em alguns casos, a neutrofilia pode ser relativa (isto é, ocorre aumento na percentagem de neutrófilos), porém o número total de todos os tipos de leucócitos pode estar situado dentro da faixa normal. SIN neutrophilic leukocytosis.

neu·tro·phil·ic (noo-trō-fil′ik). Neutrofílico. 1. Relativo a ou caracterizado por neutrófilos, como, p. ex., um exsudato em que as células predominantes consistem em granulócitos neutrófilos. 2. Caracterizado por uma falta de afinidade para corantes ácidos ou básicos, isto é, cora-se aproximadamente igual com ambos os tipos. SIN neutrophilous.

neu·tro·phil·o·pe·nia (noo-trō-fil-ō-pē′nē-ă). Neutrofilopenia. SIN neutropenia. [neutrophil + G. *penia*, pobreza]

neu·troph·i·lous (noo-trof′i-lŭs). Neutrófilo. SIN neutrophilic (2).

neu·tro·tax·is (noo-trō-tak′sis). Neutrotaxia. Fenômeno em que os leucócitos neutrófilos são estimulados por uma substância, de tal modo que são atraídos e movem-se em direção a ela (**neutrotaxia positiva**) ou são repelidos, afastando-se da substância (**neutrotaxia negativa**); em alguns casos, não há nenhum efeito (algumas vezes denominado **neutrotaxia indiferente**). [neutrophil + G. *taxis*, arranjo, distribuição]

ne·vi (nē′vī). Nevos. Plural de nevus. [L.]

ne·vo·cyte (nē′vō-sīt). Nevócito. SIN nevus *cell*.

ne·void (nē′voyd). Nevóide. Que se assemelha a um nevo. [L. *naevus*, mola (nevo), + G. *eidos*, semelhança]

ne·vo·xan·tho·en·do·the·li·o·ma (nē′vō - zan′thō - en′dō - thē - lē - ō′mä). Nevoxantoendotelioma. SIN juvenile *xanthogranuloma*. [nevus + G. *xanthos*, amarelo + endothelioma]

ne·vus, pl. **ne·vi** (nē′vŭs, -vī). Nevo. **1.** Malformação circunscrita da pele, especialmente quando colorida por hiperpigmentação ou por vascularidade aumentada; o nevo pode ser predominantemente epidérmico, anexial, melanocítico, vascular ou mesodérmico ou pode consistir numa proliferação mista desses tecidos. **2.** Proliferação localizada benigna de células formadoras de melanina da pele, presente por ocasião do nascimento ou que aparece no início da vida. SIN mole (1). [L. *naevus*, mola, marca de nascimento]

acquired n., n. adquirido; nevo melanocítico que não é visível ao nascimento, mas que aparece na infância ou na vida adulta.

n. ane'micus, n. anêmico; defeito de desenvolvimento funcional no enchimento vascular, caracterizado por lesões pálidas, arredondadas ou ovais, achatadas, indistinguíveis da pele normal circundante na diascopia.

n. ara'neus, n. arâneo. SIN spider *angioma*.

balloon cell n., n. de células em balão; nevo em que muitas das células são grandes, com citoplasma claro.

basal cell n. [MIM*109400], n. de células basais, n. basocelular; doença hereditária observada na lactância ou adolescência, caracterizada por lesões das pálpebras, nariz, bochechas, pescoço e axilas, que aparecem como pápulas de cor da carne não-erosadas, algumas das quais se tornam pedunculadas e histologicamente indistinguíveis do epitelioma de células basais; são também observadas lesões ceratóticas puntiformes nas regiões palmares e plantares; em geral, as lesões permanecem benignas; todavia, em alguns casos, ocorrem ulceração e invasão, constituindo uma evidência de alteração maligna; herança autossômica dominante; causada por mutação do PTCH humano, o homólogo do "gene patched" de *Drosophila*. O PTCH encontra-se no cromossoma 9q22.

bathing trunk n., n. em calção de banho; grande nevo pigmentado congênito piloso, com predileção por toda a parte inferior do tronco; pode ocorrer desenvolvimento de melanoma maligno na infância. SIN giant pigmented n.

Becker n., n. de Becker; nevo observado pela primeira vez como pigmentação irregular dos ombros, parte superior do tórax ou área escapular, aumentando gradualmente e de forma irregular e tornando-se espessado e piloso. SIN pigmented hair epidermal n.

blue n., n. azul; nevo azul-escuro ou preto-azulado coberto por pele lisa e formado por melanócitos fusiformes ou dendríticos intensamente pigmentados na derme reticular.

blue rubber-bleb nevi, nevos azuis; síndrome caracterizada por nódulos hemangiomatosos eréteis, facilmente compressíveis e de paredes finas, presentes ao nascimento e que se distribuem amplamente na pele e no canal alimentar e, algumas vezes, em outros tecidos; as lesões no intestino podem perfurar ou causar hemorragia, e o paciente pode tornar-se anêmico em decorrência de sangramento contínuo.

capillary n., n. capilar; hemangioma capilar da pele.

n. caverno'sus, n. cavernoso. SIN cavernous *angioma*.

cellular blue n., n. celular azul; grande nevo azul adquirido, em que os melanócitos são freqüentemente claros e grandes, alternando com células fusiformes pigmentadas, podendo estender-se profundamente na subcutis; é muito raro haver alteração maligna.

n. comedon'icus, n. comedônico; invaginações císticas ceratinosas lineares congênitas ou da infância na epiderme, sem desenvolvimento de folículos pilossebáceos normais.

compound n., n. composto; nevo caracterizado por ninhos de melanócitos na junção dermoepidérmica e na derme.

congenital n., n. congênito; nevo melanocítico, visível por ocasião do nascimento, em geral maior do que um nevo adquirido e que costuma envolver estruturas mais profundas. Os nevos congênitos com mais de 20,0 cm de diâmetro, denominados nevos congênitos gigantes, apresentam um risco de 6–12% de desenvolvimento de melanoma durante a vida do indivíduo. VER TAMBÉM bathing trunk n.

dysplastic n., n. displásico; nevo com diâmetro de mais de 5 mm e bordas irregulares, indistintas ou chanfradas, de cor preto-acastanhada e róseo-avermelhada mista. Ao microscópio, trata-se de melanócitos intra-epidérmicos de localização basal e dispersos, com núcleos hipercromáticos maiores do que os núcleos dos ceratinócitos basais. Quando múltiplos e associados a uma história familiar de melanoma, esses nevos implicam alto risco de transformação maligna; entretanto, os nevos displásicos isolados na ausência de história familiar de melanoma são menos freqüentemente pré-malignos. VER TAMBÉM malignant mole *syndrome*. VER dysplastic nevus *syndrome*.

epithelioid cell n., n. de células epitelióides. SIN Spitz n.

faun tail n., n. em cauda de fauno; proliferação circunscrita de pêlos na área lombossacra associada a diastematomielia.

n. flam'meus, flame n., n. flâmeo; grande nevo vascular congênito de cor violácea; em geral, ocorre na cabeça e no pescoço e persiste durante toda a vida. VER TAMBÉM Sturge-Weber *syndrome*. SIN port-wine stain.

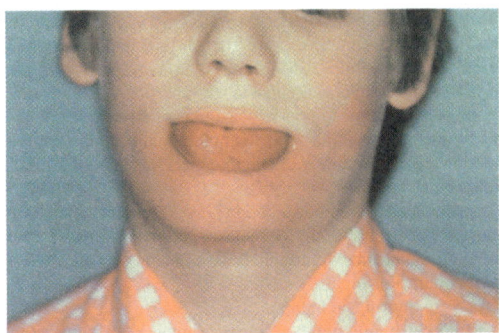

nevo flâmeo

giant pigmented n., n. pigmentado gigante. SIN bathing trunk n.

halo n., n. com halo; nevo melanocítico benigno, algumas vezes múltiplo, em que ocorre involução, com mola castanha central circundada por uma zona ou halo de despigmentação uniforme. SIN leukoderma acquisitum centrifugum, Sutton n.

inflammatory linear verrucous epidermal n., n. epidérmico verrucoso linear inflamatório; pápulas eritematosas escamosas e confluentes, pruriginosas, de distribuição linear, que habitualmente aparecem em um dos membros no início da infância, regredindo antes da vida adulta.

intradermal n., n. intradérmico; nevos em que são encontrados ninhos de melanócitos na derme, mas não na junção dermoepidérmica; nos adultos, os nevos pigmentados benignos são mais comumente intradérmicos.

Ito n., n. de Ito; pigmentação da pele inervada pelos ramos laterais do nervo supraclavicular e nervo cutâneo lateral do braço, devido a melanócitos dendríticos intensamente pigmentados espalhados na derme.

Jadassohn n., n. de Jadassohn. SIN n. sebaceus.

junction n., n. juncional; nevo que consiste em aglomerados de melanócitos na zona de células basais, na junção da epiderme com a derme, aparecendo como pequeno tumor pigmentado não-piloso achatado e discretamente elevado (castanho ou preto).

linear epidermal n., n. epidérmico linear. SIN n. unius lateris.

n. lymphat'icus, n. linfático; linfangioma cutâneo.

nape n., n. da nuca; marca de nascimento vascular pálida encontrada na nuca de 25–50% dos indivíduos normais.

oral epithelial n., n. epitelial oral. SIN white sponge n.

Ota n., n. de Ota. SIN oculodermal *melanosis.*

n. papillomato'sus, n. papilomatoso; mola verrucosa proeminente.

pigmented hair epidermal n., n. epidérmico piloso pigmentado. SIN Becker n.

n. pigmento'sus, n. pigmentado; proliferação melanocítica pigmentada benigna; elevado ou ao nível da pele, presente por ocasião do nascimento ou que surge no início da vida. SIN mole (2).

n. pilo'sus, n. piloso; mola coberta por proliferação abundante de pêlos. SIN hairy mole.

n. seba'ceus, n. sebáceo; acantose papilar congênita da epiderme, com hiperplasia das glândulas sebáceas, que se desenvolve na puberdade, e presença de glândulas apócrinas em áreas não-apócrinas da pele (comumente o couro cabeludo). Vários tumores epiteliais podem desenvolver-se a partir do nevo sebáceo na vida adulta, mais comumente o carcinoma basocelular. SIN Jadassohn n.

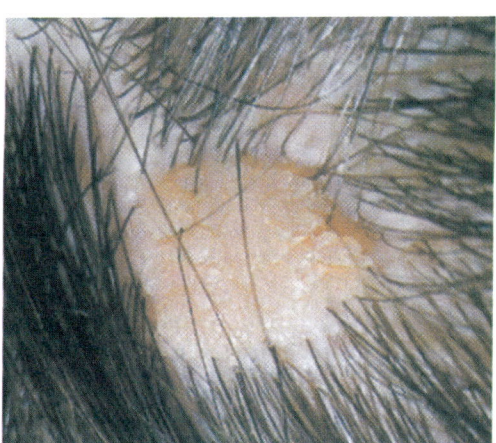

nevo sebáceo

spider n., angioma aracneiforme. SIN spider angioma.
n. spi'lus, n. *spilus;* forma de nevo pigmentar (achatado). SIN spilus.
spindle cell n., n. de células fusiformes. SIN Spitz n.
Spitz n., n. de Spitz; pequeno tumor cutâneo superficial benigno, discretamente pigmentado ou vermelho, composto de células fusiformes, epitelióides e multinucleadas, que podem exibir aspecto atípico; mais comum em crianças, embora também ocorra em adultos. SIN benign juvenile melanoma, epithelioid cell n., spindle cell n.
strawberry n., n. em morango; pequeno nevo vascular (hemangioma capilar) que se assemelha a um morango quanto ao tamanho, forma e cor; em geral, desaparece espontaneamente no início da infância. VER capillary *hemangioma.* SIN strawberry birthmark.
Sutton n., n. de Sutton. SIN halo n.
n. u'nius lat'eris, n. unilateral; n. linear sistematizado congênito, limitado a um lado do corpo ou a porções dos membros em um lado; as lesões são freqüentemente extensas, formando faixas semelhantes a ondas no tronco e listas espiraladas nos membros. SIN linear epidermal n.
Unna, n. de Unna; mancha capilar na nuca; forma persistente do nevo flâmeo da nuca. SIN erythema nuchae.
n. vascula'ris, n. vasculo'sus, n. vascular. SIN capillary *hemangioma.*
n. veno'sus, n. venoso; nevo formado por uma placa de vênulas dilatadas.
verrucous n., n. verrucoso; lesão verrucosa, freqüentemente linear, da cor da pele ou mais escura, que aparece por ocasião do nascimento ou na infância e que ocorre em tamanhos e locais variáveis, isolada ou múltipla.
white sponge n. [MIM*193900], n. esponjoso branco; condição autossômica dominante da cavidade oral, caracterizada por pregas macias, brancas ou opalescentes, espessadas ou enrugadas da mucosa; em certas ocasiões, ocorre comprometimento simultâneo de outros locais mucosos; distúrbio causado pela mutação do gene da ceratina mucosa K4 no cromossoma 12 ou do gene da ceratina-13 no cromossoma 17. SIN familial white folded dysplasia, oral epithelial n.
woolly hair n. [MIM*194300], n. lanoso; placa circunscrita de cabelos crespos e finos no couro cabeludo, normal sob os demais aspectos, que aparece na infância e aumenta durante um período de 2–3 anos; herança autossômica dominante. Existe outra forma principalmente esporádica, que pode ser autossômica recessiva [MIM*278150].
new·bery·ite (noo'ber-e-īt). New berita. O triidrato de fosfato de hidrogênio e magnésio; encontrado em alguns cálculos renais. Cf. bobierrite, struvite. [J. Cosmo *Newberry,* mineralogista australiano + -ite]
new·born (noo'bōrn). Recém-nascido. SIN neonatal, neonate.
Newcomer fix·a·tive. Fixador de Newcomer. ver em fixative.
Newton, Sir Isaac, físico inglês, 1642–1727. VER newton; newtonian *aberration;* Newtonian *constant* of gravitation; newtonian *flow;* newtonian *viscosity;* N. *disk, law.*
new·ton (N) (noo'tŏn). Newton. Unidade derivada de força no sistema SI, expressa em metros-quilogramas por segundo quadrado. (mg·kg s^{-2}); equivalente a 10^5 dinas no sistema CGS. [I. *Newton*]
new·ton·me·ter. Newton-metro; unidade do sistema MKS, expressa como força despendida ou trabalho realizado por uma força de 1 N atuando por uma distância de 1 m; igual a 1 J = 10^7 ergs.
nex·ins (neks'inz). Nexinas. Proteínas que unem pares de microtúbulos adjacentes do axonema dos cílios e flagelos. [L. *nexus,* ligação, de *necto,* ligar + -in]
nex·us, pl. **nex·us** (nek'sŭs). Nexo. SIN gap junction. [L. interconexão]
Nezelof, C., patologista francês, *1922. VER N. *syndrome,* type of thymic *alymphoplasia.*
NF NF. Abreviatura de National Formulary.
ng ng. Abreviatura de nanograma.
NGF FCN. Abreviatura de nerve growth *factor* (fator de crescimento do nervo).
NHL LNH. Abreviatura de non-Hodgkin *lymphoma* (linfoma não-Hodgkin).
N.H.S. NHS. Abreviatura de National Health Service (Inglaterra).
NH$_2$-ter·mi·nal. NH$_2$-terminal. SIN amino-terminal.
Ni Ni. Símbolo do níquel.
ni·a·cin (nī'a-sin). Niacina. SIN nicotinic acid.
ni·a·cin·a·mide (nī'ă-sin-am'īd). Niacinamida. SIN nicotinamide.
ni·al·a·mide (nī-al'ă-mīd). Nialamida. Inibidor da monoamina oxidase utilizado no tratamento de distúrbios depressivos.
nib. Bico. Em odontologia, a porção de um instrumento de condensação que entra em contato com o material restaurador a ser condensado; sua extremidade, a face, é lisa e serrilhada.
ni·car·di·pine (nī-kar'dē-pēn). Nicardipina. Bloqueador dos canais de cálcio da série diidropiridina; utilizada como agente anti-hipertensivo e antianginoso.
niche (nitch, nēsh). Nicho. **1.** Em radiografia contrastada, uma área erosada ou ulcerada, particularmente gastrointestinal ou vascular, que pode ser detectada quando preenchida por contraste. **2.** Termo ecológico para referir-se à posição ocupada por uma espécie numa comunidade biótica, particularmente suas relações com várias outras espécies competitivas, predadoras, de rapina e parasitas. [Fr.]
enamel n., n. de esmalte. SIN enamel *crypt.*
Haudek n., n. de Haudek; termo arcaico para designar o aspecto radiográfico de contraste preenchendo uma úlcera gástrica na parede do estômago.
nick (nik). Chanfradura, entalhe. Em biologia molecular, clivagem hidrolítica de uma ligação fosfodiester num filamento de ácido polinucleico de filamento duplo. Cf. cut.
nick·el (Ni) (nik'l). Níquel. Bioelemento metálico, de número atômico 28, peso atômico 58,6934, que se assemelha bastante ao cobalto e freqüentemente associado a ele. Protege a estrutura dos ribossomas contra desnaturação pelo calor. A deficiência de níquel provoca alterações na ultra-estrutura do fígado. Trata-se de um co-fator de diversas enzimas (p. ex., urease). [abreviatura do al. *kupfernickel,* nome do minério de cobre a partir do qual o níquel foi obtido pela primeira vez; *nickel,* palavra alemã que significa duende, diabrete]
Raney n., n. de Raney. SIN Raney Nickel.
nick·el·o·plas·min (nik'l-ō-plas-mēn). Niqueloplasmina. Proteína contendo níquel encontrada no soro humano.
Nickerson-Kveim test. Teste de Nickerson-Kveim. Ver em test.
nick·ing (nik'ing). Chanfradura, entalhe. Constrições localizadas nos vasos sanguíneos da retina.
arteriovenous n., e. arteriovenoso; constrição de uma veia da retina em um cruzamento arteriovenoso.
ni·clo·sa·mide (ni-klō'să-mīd). Niclosamida. Tenicida efetivo contra cestóides intestinais.
ni·co·fu·ra·nose (ni-kō-fū'ră-nōs). Nicofuranose. Vasodilatador periférico.
Nicol, William, físico escocês, 1768–1851. VER N. *prism.*
Nicolas, Joseph, médico francês, *1878. VER N.-Favre *disease.*
Nicolle, Charles J.H., microbiologista francês e ganhador do Prêmio Nobel, 1866–1936. VER N. *stain* for capsules.
nic·o·tin·a·mide (nik-ō-tin'ă-mīd). Nicotinamida. A amida biologicamente ativa do ácido nicotínico, utilizada na profilaxia e no tratamento da pelagra. SIN niacinamide, nicotinic acid amide.
nic·o·tin·a·mide ad·e·nine di·nu·cle·o·tide (NAD, NAD$^+$, NADH). Nicotinamida adenina dinucleotídeo (NAD, NAD$^+$, NADH). Ribosilnicotinamida 5'-fosfato (NMN) e adenosina 5'-fosfato (AMP) ligadas por uma ligação fosfoanidrido entre os dois grupamentos fosfóricos; liga-se como coenzima a proteínas, atuando no metabolismo respiratório (aceptor e doador de hidrogênio) através de oxidação e redução alternada (NAD$^+$ $\rightleftharpoons$ NADH). Ver também entradas em NAD$^+$ e NADP$^+$.
nic·o·tin·a·mide ad·e·nine di·nu·cle·o·tide phos·phate (NADP, NADP$^+$, NADPH). Fosfato de nicotinamida adenina dinucleotídeo (NADP, NADP$^+$, NADPH). Coenzima de muitas oxidases (desidrogenases), em que ocorre a reação NADP$^+$ + 2H $\rightleftharpoons$ NADPH + H$^+$; o terceiro grupamento fosfórico esterifica a 2'-hidroxila da adenosina do NAD$^+$.
nic·o·tin·a·mide mon·o·nu·cle·o·tide (NMN). Mononucleotídeo de nicotinamida (NMN). Produto de condensação da nicotinamida e ribose 5-fosfato, ligando o N da nicotinamida ao (β) C-1 da ribose; no NAD$^+$, o anel está ligado pelo resíduo 5'-fosforil da ribose ao resíduo 5'-fosforil do AMP; precursor na síntese de NAD$^+$.
nic·o·tin·ate (nik'ō-ti-nāt). Nicotinato. Sal ou éster do ácido nicotínico; alguns nicotinatos são utilizados em pomadas como rubefacientes.

nic·o·tine (nik'ō-tēn). Nicotina. 1-Metil-2-(3-piridil)pirrolidina; alcalóide volátil tóxico derivado do tabaco (*Nicotiana* spp.) e responsável por muitos dos efeitos deste; a princípio, estimula (em pequenas doses) e, a seguir, deprime (em grandes doses) ao nível dos gânglios autônomos e junções mioneurais; seu principal metabólito urinário é a cotinina. A nicotina constitui uma importante ferramenta na investigação fisiológica e farmacológica, é utilizada como inseticida e fumegante e forma sais com a maioria dos ácidos. VER TAMBÉM tobacco. [*Nicotiana,* nome de gênero de origem botânica + -ine]

> A nicotina na fumaça de tabaco inalada ou no tabaco sem fumaça, aplicada à mucosa bucal ou nasal, penetra na circulação em alguns segundos, causando aumento da freqüência cardíaca, do volume sistólico ventricular e consumo de oxigênio do miocárdio, bem como euforia, maior prontidão e sensação de relaxamento. O uso da nicotina provoca forte dependência, resultando rapidamente em habituação, tolerância e dependência. A abstinência da nicotina provoca inquietação, irritabilidade, ansiedade, dificuldade de concentração e intenso desejo de nicotina. A dependência da nicotina é a razão do uso de tabaco, sendo, portanto, diretamente responsável pela conseqüente morbidade e mortalidade.

nic·o·tine·hy·drox·am·ic ac·id me·thi·o·dide (nik'ō-tēn-hī'drok-sam'ik as'id-mē-thī'ō-dīd). Metiodida do ácido nicotino-hidroxâmico. Reativador efetivo da colinesterase, com ações mais pronunciadas na junção neuromuscular esquelética; os efeitos antídotos são menos notáveis nos locais efetores autônomos, sendo insignificantes no sistema nervoso central.

nic·o·tin·ic (nik-ō-tin′ik). Nicotínico. Relativo à ação estimulante da acetilcolina e de outros agentes semelhantes à nicotina sobre os gânglios autônomos, medula supra-renal e placa terminal motora do músculo estriado.

nic·o·tin·ic ac·id. Ácido nicotínico. Ácido piridino-3-carboxílico; parte do complexo da vitamina B; utilizado na profilaxia e no tratamento da pelagra, como vasodilatador, e na hiperlipidemia, onde reduz os níveis de colesterol e atua como agente que aumenta os níveis de HDL. SIN anti-black-tongue factor, antipellagra factor, niacin, pellagra-preventing factor, vitamin PP.

nic·o·tin·ic ac·id am·ide. Amida do ácido nicotínico. SIN nicotinamide.

nic·o·tin·ic al·co·hol. Álcool nicotínico. SIN nicotinyl alcohol.

nic·o·tin·o·mi·met·ic (nik-ō-tin′ō-mi-met′ik). Nicotinomimético. Que imita a ação da nicotina.

nic·o·ti·nyl al·co·hol (nik-ō-tin′il). Álcool nicotinílico. Tem a mesma ação e o mesmo uso que o tartarato de nicotinil. SIN nicotinic alcohol.

nic·o·ti·nyl tar·trate. Tartarato de nicotinil. Vasodilatador periférico relativamente fraco relacionado ao ácido nicotínico; utilizado em distúrbios vasculares periféricos, como doença de Raynaud, acrocianose e eritema pérnio.

ni·cou·ma·lone (ni-koo′ma-lōn). Nicumalona. SIN acenocoumarol.

nic·ta·tion (nik-tā′shŭn). Nictação. SIN nictitation.

nic·ti·tate ((nik′ti-tāt). Piscar. [ver nictitation]

nic·ti·ta·tion (nik-ti-tā′shŭn). Nictitação. Que pestaneja. SIN nictation. [L. *nicto*, pp, *-atus*, piscar, de *nico*, fazer sinal, acenar]

ni·dal (nī′dăl). Nidal. Relativo a um ninho.

ni·da·tion (nī-dā′shŭn). Nidação. Implantação do embrião em fase inicial de desenvolvimento no endométrio uterino. [L. *nidus*, ninho]

NIDDM DMNID. Abreviatura de non-insulin-dependent *diabetes* mellitus (diabetes melito não-insulino-dependente).

ni·do·gen (nī′dō-jen). Nidogene. SIN entactin. [L. *nidus*, ninho + -gen 1.]

ni·dus, pl. **ni·di** (nī′dŭs, nī′dī). Ninho, nicho. **1.** Ninho. **2.** Núcleo ou ponto central de origem de um nervo. **3.** Foco de infecção. **4.** O núcleo de um cristal; a coalescência de moléculas ou pequenas partículas que constituem o início de um cristal ou depósito sólido semelhante. **5.** O foco de densidade reduzida no centro de um osteoma osteóide em radiografias de osso. [L. nest]

 n. a′vis, n. de ave; depressão profunda em cada lado da superfície inferior do cerebelo, entre a úvula e o lobo biventral, onde repousa a amígdala. SIN n. hirundinis. [L. ninho de ave]

 n. hirun′dinis, n. de andorinha. SIN n. avis. [L. ninho de andorinha]

Niemann, Albert, médico alemão, 1880–1921. VER N.-Pick *cell, disease;* N. *disease, splenomegaly.*

Niewenglowski, Gaston H., cientista francês do século XIX. VER N. *rays,* em *ray.*

ni·fed·i·pine (ni-fed′i-pēn). Nifedipina. Agente bloqueador dos canais de cálcio do tipo diidropiridina; dilatador coronário.

ni·fen·a·zone (ni-fen-ā-zōn). Nifenazona. Analgésico e antipirético.

ni·fur·al·de·zone (nī-fŭr-al′dē-zōn). Nifuraldezona. Agente antibacteriano.

ni·fu·ra·tel (nī-fū′ra-tel). Nifuratel. Tricomonicida.

ni·fu·rox·ime (nī-fū-rok′sēm, -sim). Nifuroxima. Derivado do furano, efetivo principalmente contra *Candida albicans*.

ni·ge·rose (nī′je-rōs). Nigerose. Dissacarídeo obtido pela hidrólise de amilopectinas, que consistem em dois resíduos de D-glicose unidos por uma ligação α1–3. [de *nigeran*, polissacarídeo sintetizado pelo *Aspergillus niger*]

night guard (nīt′gard). Aparelho utilizado para estabilizar os dentes e reduzir os efeitos traumáticos do bruxismo.

Nightingale, Florence, 1820–1910. Enfermeira inglesa; fundadora da moderna enfermagem.

night·mare (nīt′mār). Sonho aterrorizante, em que o indivíduo é incapaz de pedir socorro ou de escapar de uma calamidade aparentemente iminente. VER TAMBÉM incubus, succubus. [A.S. *nyht*, noite + *mara*, demônio]

night·shade (nīt′shād). Meimendro. Qualquer uma de numerosas plantas do gênero *Solanum* (família Solanaceae) e de alguns outros gêneros da família Solanaceae.

 deadly n., beladona. SIN belladonna.

night ter·rors (nīt′tăr-erz). Terrores noturnos. Distúrbio que ocorre em crianças, em que a criança acorda gritando com pavor, persistindo o distúrbio por algum tempo durante um estado de semiconsciência. SIN pavor nocturnus, sleep terror.

nig·ra (nī′gră). Negra. Em neuroanatomia, a substância negra. [L. de *niger*, negro]

ni·gri·ti·es (nī-grish′i-ēz). Nigricante. Pigmentação preta. [L. escuridão, de *niger*, preto]

 n. lin′guae, língua negra. SIN black *tongue.*

ni·gro·sin, ni·gro·sine (nī′grō-sin, -sēn). [C.I. 50420]. Nigrosina. Mistura variável de corantes de anilina azul-pretos; utilizada como corante histológico para o tecido nervoso e como corante negativo para o estudo de bactérias e espiroquetas; também utilizada para discriminar entre células vivas e mortas na coloração por exclusão de corante.

Ni·gros·po·ra (nī-gros′pōr-ă). *Nigrospora.* Gênero de fungos de crescimento rápido, que produz conídios negros e brilhantes em culturas; trata-se de um contaminante comum em culturas de laboratórios, não sendo patogênico para os seres humanos.

ni·gro·stri·a·tal (nī′grō-strī-ā′tăl). Nigroestriatal. Que se refere à conexão eferente da substância negra com o estriado. VER *substantia nigra.*

NIH NIH. Abreviatura de *National Institutes of Health* (Serviço de Saúde Pública dos Estados Unidos)

ni·hil·ism (nī′i-lizm, nī′hi-lizm) Niilismo. **1.** Em psiquiatria, a ilusão da inexistência de tudo, especialmente do *self* ou de parte dele. **2.** Empenho em atos que são totalmente destrutivos para os próprios objetivos e para aqueles de um grupo. [L. *nihil*, nada]

 therapeutic n., n. terapêutico; descrença na eficácia ou no valor da terapia, como farmacoterapia, psicoterapia, etc.

ni·keth·a·mide (nī-keth′ă-mīd). Niquetamida. Substância que atua principalmente sobre o sistema nervoso central, como estimulante respiratório e cardiovascular.

Nikiforoff, Mikhail, dermatologista russo, 1858–1915. VER N. *method.*

Nikolsky, Pyotr V., dermatologista russo, 1858–1940. VER N. *sign.*

Nile blue A [C.I. 51180]. Nilo azul A. Corante oxazínico básico, utilizado como corante de gordura e corante vital, bem como na coloração de Kittrich; como indicador, passa do azul para o vermelho violáceo em pH de 10–11.

ni·mo·di·pine (nī-mō′di-pēn). Nimodipina. Bloqueador dos canais de cálcio da série diidropiridina, utilizado como vasodilatador.

ni·mus·tine (nī′mŭs-tīn). Nimustina. Nitrosouréia antineoplásica semelhante à carmustina (BCNU).

nin·hy·drin (nin-hī′drin). Ninidrina. Reage com aminoácidos livres, produzindo CO_2, NH_3 e um aldeído; o NH_3 produzido fornece um produto colorido (dicetoidrindilideno-dicetoidranamina, um derivado bi-indanediona). VER TAMBÉM ninhydrin *reaction.*

ni·o·bi·um (Nb) (nī-ō′bē-ŭm). Nióbio. Elemento metálico raro, de número atômico 41, peso atômico 92,90638, geralmente encontrado com o tântalo. [*Niobe*, filha de tântalo]

nip·ple (nip′l) [TA]. Mamilo. Projeção verruciforme no ápice da mama, em cuja superfície se abrem os ductos lactíferos; é circundada por uma área pigmentar circular, a aréola. SIN papilla mammae [TA], mammilla (2), papilla of breast, teat (1), thele, thelium (3). [dim. de A.S. *neb*, bico, nariz (?)]

 accessory n., m. acessório; mamilo supranumerário que ocorre na linha mamária.

 aortic n., m. aórtico; termo coloquial para o aspecto radiográfico da veia intercostal superior esquerda ou da veia hemiázigo acessória como proeminência no bulbo aórtico.

ni·ri·da·zole (nī-rid′ă-zōl). Niridazol. Agente utilizado no tratamento da esquistossomose, amebíase e dracontíase.

nisin (nī′sin). Nisina. Antibiótico polipeptídico produzido por *Streptococcus lactis;* ativa contra certos estreptococos, *Mycobacterium tuberculosis*, *Clostridium difficile* e outras bactérias.

nisol·di·pine (nī-sol′dī-pēn). Nisoldipina. Bloqueador dos canais de cálcio da série diidropiridina; utilizada como agente anti-hipertensivo e antianginoso.

Nissen, Rudolf, cirurgião suíço, 1896–1981. VER Collis-Nissen *fundoplication;* Nissen *fundoplication;* N. *operation.*

Nissl, Franz, neurologista alemão, 1860–1919. VER N. *bodies*, em *body, degeneration, granules* em *granule, substance, stain.*

nit (nit). **1.** Lêndea; o ovo ou ovo eclodido de um piolho do corpo, da cabeça ou do púbis; o ovo fixa-se aos cabelos e pêlos humanos ou as roupas por uma camada de quitina. **2.** Nit, nepit; uma unidade de luminância; uma intensidade luminosa de uma candela por metro quadrado de superfície projetada ortogonalmente. [A. S. *knitu*]

Nitabuch, Raissa, médico alemão do século XIX. VER N. *layer membrane, stria.*

ni·ter (nī′ter). Nitro, salitre, nitrato de potássio. SIN *potassium* nitrate. [G. *nitron*, soda, antigamente não diferenciada da potassa]

 cubic n., nitrato de sódio. SIN *sodium* nitrate.

ni·ton (nī′ton). Niton. Termo arcaico para radon.

ni·trate (nī′trāt). Nitrato. Sal do ácido nítrico.

ni·tra·ze·pam (nī-tră′zĕ-pam). Nitrazepam. Hipnótico e sedativo da classe dos benzodiazepínicos.

ni·tren·di·pine (nī-tren′-di-pēn). Nitrendipina. Bloqueador dos canais de cálcio da série diidropiridina; utilizada como agente anti-hipertensivo.

ni·tric ac·id (nī′trik). Ácido nítrico. Ácido oxidante e corrosivo forte.

 fuming n. a., a. nítrico fumegante; contém cerca de 91% de ácido nítrico; utilizado como cáustico.

ni·tric ox·ide (NO·). Óxido nítrico (NO·). Gás sem radicais, incolor, que reage rapidamente com O_2 para formar outros óxidos de nitrogênio (p. ex., NO_2, N_2O_3 e N_2O_4), sendo finalmente convertido em nitrito (NO_2^-) e nitrato (NO_3^-). Mediador gasoso da comunicação intercelular e potente vasodilatador, formado a partir da L-arginina no osso, cérebro, endotélio, granulócitos, células beta do pâncreas e nervos periféricos por uma óxido nítrico sintase constitutiva, bem como nos hepatócitos, células de Kupffer, macrófagos e músculo liso por uma óxido nítrico sintase induzível (p. ex., induzida por endotoxina). O NO· ativa a guanilato ciclase solúvel, medeia a ereção do pênis e seria o primeiro neurotransmissor retrógrado conhecido.

A molécula de NO· de vida curta é um produto de vários tecidos, que desempenha um papel em diversos processos. O NO· elaborado pelo endotélio, que é idêntico ao fator de relaxamento derivado do endotélio, dilata os vasos ao relaxar o músculo liso vascular; os nitritos utilizados na coronariopatia e doença vascular periférica induzem ou imitam essa ação. O Prêmio Nobel de Medicina ou Fisiologia de 1998 foi concedido a três farmacologistas norte-americanos, Robert F. Furchgott, Ferid Murad e Louis J. Ignarro, pelas suas descobertas independentes do papel desempenhado pelo óxido nítrico na fisiologia cardiovascular. No sistema imune, os macrófagos utilizam o NO· como agente citotóxico. A deficiência ou inativação do NO· contribuiria para a patogenia da hipertensão e da aterosclerose. O NO· em excesso, que é um radical livre, é tóxico para as células cerebrais, e o NO· também é responsável pela queda precipitada e freqüentemente fatal da pressão arterial que acompanha o choque séptico. O NO· livre na corrente sanguínea é rapidamente reduzido pelo ferro da hemoglobina.

nitric oxide reductase, óxido nítrico redutase; enzima que oxida o N_2 com algum aceptor para 2NO·, a primeira etapa na fixação do nitrogênio atmosférico por bactérias.
nitric oxide synthase (NO synthase), óxido nítrico sintase (NO sintetase); enzima que cataliza a reação da L-arginina com $2O_2$ e 1,5NADPH para formar NO, L-citrulina, $1,5NADP^+$ e $2H_2O$; existem uma forma induzível e duas formas constitutivas dessa enzima: as formas constitutivas têm papéis significativos na regulação do tônus vascular, fluxo sanguíneo tecidual, função renal, etc.; no osso, no cérebro, no endotélio, nos granulócitos, nas células Z do pâncreas e nos nervos periféricos, as formas constitutivas são dependentes de cálcio-calmodulina; no cérebro, a enzima é citosólica; no endotélio, está ligada à membrana; a forma induzível da enzima (p. ex., por endotoxina) nos hepatócitos, nas células de Kupffer, nos macrófagos e no músculo liso não depende de calmodulina.
ni·trid·a·tion (nī-tri-dā′shŭn). Nitridação. Formação de nitritos; formação de compostos nitrogenados através da ação da amônia (análogo à oxidação).
ni·tride (nī′trīd). Nitreto. Composto de nitrogênio e outro elemento, como, p. ex., nitreto de magnésio, Mg_3N_2.
ni·tri·fi·ca·tion (nī′tri-fi-kā′shŭn). Nitrificação, salitrização. **1.** Conversão bacteriana de matéria nitrogenada em nitratos. **2.** Tratamento de um material com ácido nítrico.
ni·trile (nī′tril). Nitrila. Cianeto alquílico. As nitrilas individuais são denominadas de acordo com o ácido formado na hidrólise; p. ex., a CH_3CN é mais uma acetonitrila do que cianeto de metila.
nitrilo-. Nitrilo-. Prefixo indicando um átomo de nitrogênio tervalente (trivalente) fixado a três grupamentos idênticos; p. ex., ácido nitrilotriacético, $N(CH_2COOH)_3$.
ni·tri·mu·ri·at·ic ac·id (nī′tri-mū-rē-at′ik). Ácido nitrimuriático. SIN nitrohydrochloric acid.
ni·trite (nī′trīt). Nitrito. Sal do ácido nitroso.
ni·tri·tu·ria (nī-tri-too′rē-ă). Nitritúria. Presença de nitritos na urina, em conseqüência da ação de *Escherichia coli*, *Proteus vulgaris* e outros microrganismos capazes de reduzir os nitratos.
nitro-. Nitro-. Prefixo que indica o grupamento $-NO_2$. [G. *nitron*, carbonato de sódio]
ni·tro·cel·lu·lose (nī-trō-sel′ū-lōs). Nitrocelulose. SIN pyroxylin.
ni·tro·chlo·ro·form (nī-trō-klōr′ō-form). Nitroclorofórmio. SIN chloropicrin.
ni·tro·fu·rans (nī-trō-fū′ranz). Nitrofuranos. Agentes antimicrobianos (p. ex., nitrofurasona) efetivos contra microrganismos Gram-positivos e Gram-negativos.
ni·tro·fu·ran·to·in (nī′trō-fū-ran′tō-in). Nitrofurantoína. Agente antibacteriano urinário com ampla faixa de atividade contra microrganismos Gram-positivos e Gram-negativos; também disponível na forma de nitrofurantoína sódica para injeção.
ni·tro·fu·ra·zone (nī-trō-fū′ră-zōn). Nitrofurazona. Agente bacteriostático e bactericida tópico freqüentemente utilizado em queimaduras.
ni·tro·gen (N). 1. Nitrogênio. Elemento gasoso de número atômico 7, peso atômico 14,00674; o N_2 forma cerca de 78,084% por volume da atmosfera seca. **2.** Forma molecular do nitrogênio, N_2. **3.** Grau farmacêutico N_2 contendo não menos que 99,0% por volume de N_2; utilizado como diluente de gases medicinais, bem como para substituição do ar em preparações farmacêuticas. [L. *nitrum*, nitro + *-gen*, produzir]

principais componentes do nitrogênio não-proteico
(valores normais expressos em mEq/100 mL)

	sangue total	plasma/soro
nitrogênio não-proteico total	20–40	18–29 (40)
nitrogênio não-proteico, não-uréia	16–26	6–18
compostos nitrogenados não-identificados	5–18	—
aminoácidos livres (aminoácidos não-proteicos)	4,6–6,8	3,4–5,9
Amônia	0,07–0,1	0,1–0,2
Creatina	1,0–1,6	—
Creatinina	—	0,5–1,3
Ergotioneína	0,03	—
Glutationa	4,6	—
ácido úrico	0,3–1,3	0,7–1,3
uréia (nitrogênio sanguíneo)	8,5–15	9,6–17,6
nucleotídeos	4,4–7,4	—

blood urea n. (BUN), uréia sanguínea; nitrogênio na forma de uréia no sangue; o mais prevalente dos compostos nitrogenados não-proteicos no sangue; normalmente, o sangue contém 10-15 mg de uréia/100 mL. É comum efetuar determinações no laboratório como medida da função renal. VER TAMBÉM urea n.
filtrate n., n. filtrado; nitrogênio não-proteico em vários compostos que, normalmente, passam através da filtração glomerular ou através de um filtro no laboratório (após precipitação das proteínas).
heavy n., n. pesado. SIN nitrogen-15.
n. monoxide, monóxido de n. SIN nitrous oxide.
nonprotein n. (NPN), n. não-proteico (NNP); conteúdo de nitrogênio de outros compostos diferentes das proteínas; p. ex., cerca da metade do nitrogênio não-proteico no sangue está contida na uréia. SIN rest n.
rest n., n. residual. SIN nonprotein n.
undetermined n., n. indeterminado; nitrogênio do sangue, da urina, etc., que pode ser estimado diretamente, diferente daquele contido na uréia, no ácido úrico, nos aminoácidos, etc.; no sangue, corresponde a cerca de 25 mg/100 mL.
urea n., n. ureico; a porção de nitrogênio numa amostra biológica, como o sangue ou urina, que provém de seu teor de uréia. VER TAMBÉM blood urea n.
urinary n., n. urinário; nitrogênio excretado como uréia, aminoácidos, ácido úrico, etc., na urina; 1 g de nitrogênio urinário indica a degradação de 6,25 g de proteína no organismo. VER TAMBÉM nitrogen *equivalent*.
ni·tro·gen-13 (^{13}N). Nitrogênio-13 (N^{13}). Radioisótopo do nitrogênio produzido no ciclotron, emissor de positrons, com meia-vida de 9,97 minutos; utilizado em estudos do metabolismo proteico e na tomografia com emissão de positrons.
ni·tro·gen-14 (^{14}N). Nitrogênio-14 (N^{14}). O isótopo comum do nitrogênio, que constitui 99,63% do nitrogênio natural.
ni·tro·gen-15 (^{15}N). Nitrogênio-15 (N^{15}). O isótopo estável menos comum do nitrogênio, que representa 0,37% do nitrogênio natural. SIN heavy nitrogen.
ni·tro·ge·nase (nī′trō-jĕ-nās). Nitrogenase. Antigamente, termo genérico utilizado para descrever sistemas enzimáticos que catalisam a redução do nitrogênio molecular à amônia nas bactérias fixadoras de nitrogênio; hoje em dia, aplica-se especificamente a enzimas que efetuam esta reação com ferredoxina reduzida e ATP; tipicamente, a nitrogenase consiste em dois componentes: o primeiro reduz o N_2, enquanto o segundo transfere elétrons.
ni·tro·gen dis·tri·bu·tion. Distribuição do nitrogênio. SIN nitrogen partition.
ni·tro·gen group. Grupo de nitrogênio. Cinco elementos trivalentes ou pentavalentes cujos compostos hidrogenados são básicos e cujos oxiácidos variam de monobásicos a tetrabásicos: nitrogênio, fósforo, arsênico, antimônio e bismuto.
ni·tro·gen lag. Latência do nitrogênio. Período de tempo após a ingestão de determinada proteína, antes que tenha sido excretada na urina a quantidade de nitrogênio igual àquela contida na proteína.
ni·trog·e·nous (nī-troj′ĕ-nŭs). Nitrogenoso. Relativo ao, ou que contém, nitrogênio.
ni·tro·gen par·ti·tion. Distribuição do nitrogênio. Determinação da distribuição do nitrogênio na urina entre os vários constituintes. SIN nitrogen distribution.
ni·tro·glyc·er·in (nī-trō-glis′er-in). Nitroglicerina. Líquido oleoso amarelado explosivo, formado pela ação dos ácidos sulfúrico e nítrico sobre a glice-

rina; utilizado como vasodilatador, especialmente na angina de peito; produz óxido nítrico. SIN glyceryl trinitrate, trinitroglycerin.

ni·tro·hy·dro·chlo·ric ac·id (nī'trō - hī - drō - klōr'ik). Ácido nitroclorídrico, água-régia, ácido nitromuriático; mistura extremamente cáustica que contém 18 partes de ácido nítrico e 82 partes de ácido clorídrico. SIN aqua regia, aqua regalis, nitrimuriatic acid.

ni·tro·man·ni·tol (nī - trō - man'i - tol). Nitromanitol. SIN *mannitol* hexanitrate.

ni·tro·mer·sol (nī - trō - mer'sol). Nitromersol. O anidro do 4-nitro-3-hidroximercuriortocresol; composto mercurial orgânico sintético utilizado como anti-séptico para a pele e mucosas.

ni·trom·e·ter (nī - trom'e - ter). Nitrômetro. Aparelho para colher e medir o nitrogênio liberado numa reação química. [nitrogen + G. *metron*, medida]

ni·tron (nī'tron). Nítron. Reagente para determinação do ácido nítrico, perclorato e rênio, por ser uma das poucas substâncias a formar um nitrato insolúvel.

ni·tro·phen·yl·sul·fen·yl (Nps) (nī'trō - fen'il - sul - fen'il). Nitrofenilsulfenil. $O_2N-C_6H_4-S-$; nitrofeniltio; radical facilmente fixado a grupamentos amino; utilizado na síntese de peptídeos e na química das proteínas.

ni·tro·prus·side (nī - trō - prus'īd). Nitroprussiato. O ânion $[Fe(CN)_5NO]^=$; como no nitroprussiato de sódio; utilizado como vasodilatador por via intravenosa.

ni·tros·a·mines (nī - trōs'am - ēnz). Nitrosaminas. Aminas substituídas por um grupamento nitroso (NO), geralmente num átomo de nitrogênio, produzindo *N*-nitrosaminas (R–NH–NO ou R_2N–NO); podem ser formadas pela combinação direta de uma amina e ácido nitroso (podem ser formadas a partir de nitritos no suco gástrico ácido); algumas delas são mutagênicas e/ou carcinogênicas.

△ **nitroso-.** Nitroso-. Prefixo que indica um composto contendo nitrosil. [L. *nitrosus*]

S-nitrosohemoglobin (nī - trō'sō - hē'mōglō'bin). *S*-nitroso hemoglobina. Composto formado pela ligação do óxido nítrico com a hemoglobina; a liberação e a captação do óxido nítrico produzem alterações na resistência vascular e no fluxo sanguíneo, que ajudam na homeostasia do oxigênio.

ni·tro·sou·rea (nī - trō'sō - oor'ē - ā). Nitrosouréia. Agente alquilante utilizado no tratamento de numerosas neoplasias; um exemplo é a BCNU [*N,N*'-bis(2-cloroetil)-*N*-nitrosouréia; carmustina]

ni·tro·syl (nī'trō - sil). Nitrosil. Radical ou grupamento atômico univalente, –N=O, formando os compostos nitrosos.

ni·trous (nī'trŭs). Nitroso. Refere-se a um composto nitrogenado contendo menos um átomo de oxigênio do que os compostos nítricos; composto em que o nitrogênio está presente em seu estado trivalente.

ni·trous ac·id. Ácido nitroso. HNO_2; reagente laboratorial biológico e clínico padrão.

ni·trous ox·ide. Óxido nitroso. N_2O; gás não-inflamável, não-explosivo que sustenta a combustão (comburente); amplamente utilizado como analgésico inalatório de ação rápida, rapidamente reversível, não-depressivo e atóxico para suplementar outros anestésicos e analgésicos; seu potencial anestésico isolado não é adequado para produzir anestesia cirúrgica. SIN dinitrogen monoxide, nitrogen monoxide.

ni·tro·xan·thic ac·id (nī - trō - zan'thik). Ácido nitroxântico. SIN picric acid.

ni·trox·o·line (nī - trok'sō - lēn). Nitroxolina. Agente antibacteriano.

ni·troxy (nī - trok'sē). Nitroxi. Radical –O–NO_2. [contração de nitriloxi]

ni·trox·yl (nī - trok'sil). Nitroxila. Hidreto de nitrosila, HNO.

ni·tryl (nī'tril). Nitrila. O radical –NO_2 dos compostos nitro.

ni·zat·i·dine (ni - zat'i - den). Nizatidina. Antagonista histamínico H_2 utilizado no tratamento de úlceras duodenais ativas.

njo·ve·ra (nyō - ver'ā). Niovera. Doença não-venérea de crianças em Zimbabwe, indistinguível da sífilis, causada por um microrganismo aparentemente idêntico ao *Treponema pallidum*; provavelmente idêntica ao bejel. [termo do Zimbabwe]

N.K. N.K. Abreviatura de Nomenklatur Kommission (Comissão de Nomenclatura).

nkat Nkat. Abreviatura de nanokatal.

Nle Nle. Abreviatura de norleucine (norleucina).

NLN. NLN. Abreviatura de National League for Nursing (Liga Nacional de Enfermagem).

nM nM. Abreviatura de nanomolar.

nm nm. Abreviatura de nanômetro.

NMDA NMDA. Abreviatura de *N*-methyl D-aspartate (*N*-metil D-aspartato). Aminoácido excitotóxico utilizado para identificar um subgrupo específico de receptores de glutamato (um aminoácido excitatório). SIN *N*-methyl D-aspartic acid.

NMN NMN. Abreviatura de nicotinamide mononucleotide (mononucleotídeo de nicotinamida).

NMP NMP. Abreviatura de nucleoside 5'-monophosphate (nucleosídeo 5'-monofosfato).

NMR RMN. Abreviatura de nuclear magnetic *resonance* (ressonância magnética nuclear).

NO· NO·. Símbolo do óxido nítrico.
No No. Símbolo de nobélio.
Noack, M., médico alemão do século XX. VER N. *syndrome*.
no·bel·i·um (No) (nō - bel'ē - ŭm). Nobélio (No). Elemento transurânico instável, de número atômico 102, preparado pelo bombardeio do cúrio com núcleos de carbono 12 e íons pesados semelhantes sobre outros elementos da série transurânica. [Instituto *Nobel* de Física e A.B. Nobel, inventor sueco, 1833–1896]
Noble, Robert L., fisiologista canadense, *1910. VER N.-Collip *procedure*.
Noble, Charles P., ginecologista norte-americano, 1863–1935. VER N. *position*.
Noble stain. Corante de Noble. ver em stain.
Nocard, Edmund I.E., veterinário francês, 1850–1903. VER *Nocardia*; *Nocardiaceae*.
No·car·dia (nō - kar'dē - ā). *Nocardia*. Gênero de actinomicetos aeróbicos (família Nocardiaceae, ordem Actinomycetales), bactérias superiores, contendo filamentos ou bastonetes delgados fracamente álcool-ácido-resistentes, muitas vezes dilatados e, em certas ocasiões, ramificados, formando um micélio. As formas de cocos ou bacilares são produzidas por esses microrganismos, que são principalmente saprófitas, mas que podem constituir uma causa de micetoma ou nocardiose. [E. *Nocard*]
N. asteroi'des, espécie de microrganismos aeróbicos, Gram-positivos, parcialmente álcool-ácido-resistentes e ramificados, que causam nocardiose e, possivelmente, micetoma nos seres humanos.
N. brasilien'sis, espécie de bactéria que se assemelha bastante à *N. asteroides*, constituindo uma causa de micetoma e nocardiose nos seres humanos.
N. ca'viae, nome antigo de *N. otitidiscaviarum*.
N. fasci'nica, espécie que causa farcinose bovina; trata-se da espécie típica do gênero *Nocardia*.
N. gibso'nii, SIN *Streptomyces gibsonii*.
N. lu'rida, nome antigo de *Amycolatopsis orientalis* subespécie *lurida*.
N. ma'durae, nome antigo de *Actinomadura madurae*.
N. mediterra'nei, espécie de bactéria que produz a rifamicina.
N. nova, espécie de bactéria comumente isolada de infecções humanas.
N. orienta'lis, espécie de bactéria que produz a vancomicina.
N. otitidiscaviarum, bactéria superior (antes denominada *Nocardia cavae*) que vive no solo e constitui uma das causas de nocardiose e actinomicetoma.
N. transvalensis, actinomiceto aeróbico; uma das causas de nocardiose.
no·car·dia, pl. **no·car·di·ae** (nō - kar'dē - ā, nō - kar'dē - ē). Nocardia. Termo vernacular utilizado para referir-se a qualquer membro do gênero *Nocardia*.
No·car·di·a·ce·ae (nō - kar - dē - ā'sē - ē). Família de bactérias aeróbicas Gram-positivas álcool-ácido-resistentes (ordem Actinomycetales) que inclui o gênero *Nocardia*. [E. *Nocard*]
no·car·di·a·sis (nō - kar - dī'a - sis). Nocardíase. SIN nocardiosis.
no·car·di·o·form (nō - kar'dē - ō - fōrm). Nocardioforme. Refere-se a um microrganismo que se assemelha, morfologicamente e quanto à sua cultura, a membros do gênero *Nocardia*.
Nocardiopsis (nō - kar - dē - op'sis). *Nocardiopsis*. Gênero de bactéria superior que vive no solo e causa pneumonia subaguda ou crônica, infecção subcutânea ou doença disseminada, geralmente em pacientes imunossuprimidos.
N. dassonvillei, actinomiceto aeróbico, antigamente conhecido como *Nocardia dassonvillei*; uma das causas de actinomicetoma.
no·car·di·o·sis (nō - kar - dē - ō'sis). Nocardiose. Doença generalizada nos seres humanos e em outros animais, causada por *Nocardia asteroides*, *N. otitidiscaviarum, N. transvalensis* e *N. brasiliensis*, e caracterizada por lesões pulmonares primárias que podem ser subclínicas ou crônicas, com disseminação hematogênica para vísceras profundas, incluindo o sistema nervoso central; ocorre mais comumente em pacientes imunossuprimidos. SIN nocardiasis.
granulomatous n., n. granulomatosa; forma de nocardiose caracterizada por emagrecimento, distensão abdominal e substituição do tecido linfóide nos linfonodos e no baço por tecido granulomatoso.
nocebo (nō - sē'bō). Nocebo. Efeito desagradável atribuível à administração de placebo; jargão. [L. prejudico, de *noceo*, prejudicar, por analogia a *placebo*, placebo, agrado]
△ **noci-.** Noci-. Ferimento, dor, lesão. [L. *noceo*]
no·ci·cep·tive (nō - si - sep'tiv). Nociceptivo. Capaz de avaliar ou transmitir dor. [ver nociceptor]
no·ci·cep·tor (nō - si - sep'ter, - tōr). Nociceptor. Mecanismo ou órgão nervoso periférico para a recepção e transmissão de estímulos dolorosos ou lesivos. [noci- + L. *capio*, tomar]
no·ci·fen·sor (nō - si - fen'ser). Nocifensor. Indica processos ou mecanismos que atuam para proteger o corpo de lesões; especificamente, um sistema de nervos na pele e nas mucosas que reage a uma lesão adjacente, causando vasodilatação. [noci- + L. *fendo* (apenas em compostos), combater, evitar]
△ **noct-.** Noct-. Noturno. VER TAMBÉM nycto-. [L. *nox*, noite]
noc·tal·bu·min·ur·ia (nok'tal - boo'mi - nū'rē - ā). Noctalbuminúria. Aumento patológico da albumina na urina excretada à noite, um evento raramente observado. [L. *nox*, noite + albuminúria]

noc·ti·pho·bia (nok′tē-fō′bē-ă). Noctifobia. Medo mórbido da noite, do escuro e do silêncio. [noct- + phobia]

noct. maneq. Abreviatura do L. *nocte maneque*, à noite e pela manhã.

noc·to·graph (nok′tō-graf). Noctógrafo. SIN scotograph. [noct- + G. *graphō*, escrever]

noc·tu·ria (nok-too′rē-ă). Noctúria, nictúria. Micção voluntária à noite, após acordar do sono; tipicamente causada por secreção noturna aumentada de urina resultante da incapacidade de supressão da produção de urina em decúbito ou de esvaziamento incompleto da bexiga devido a lesões obstrutivas nas vias urinárias inferiores ou instabilidade do músculo detrusor. SIN nycturia. [noct- + G. *ouron*, urina]

noc·tur·nal (nok-ter′nal). Noturno. Relativo às horas de escuridão; oposto a diurnal (1) (diurno). [L. *nocturnus*, da noite]

no·dal (nō′dăl). Nodal. Relativo a qualquer nodo.

NODE

node (nōd) [TA]. Nodo, linfonodo. **1.** Nódulo ou nodosidade; aumento de volume circunscrito; em anatomia, massa circunscrita de tecido. **2.** Massa circunscrita de tecido diferenciado. **3.** Nódulo ou articulação do dedo. SIN nodus [TA]. [L. *nodus*, um nó]

anterior tibial n., linfonodo tibial anterior. SIN anterior tibial lymph node.

n. of Aschoff and Tawara, nodo de Aschoff e Tawara. SIN atrioventricular n.

atrioventricular n. (AV n.) [TA], n. atrioventricular; **(1)** pequeno nodo de fibras musculares cardíacas modificadas, localizado próximo ao óstio do seio coronário; dá origem ao feixe atrioventricular do sistema de condução cardíaca; **(2)** tecido de condução frouxamente circunscrito, com células esparsas semelhantes a marcapasso (P) na junção atrioventricular. SIN nodus atrioventricularis [TA], n. of Aschoff and Tawara, Tawara n.

Babès n.'s, nodos de Babès; coleção de linfócitos no sistema nervoso central encontrada na raiva.

buccinator n., buccal n., n. linfonodo bucinador, linfonodo bucal. SIN buccal lymph node.

n. of Cloquet, n. de Cloquet. SIN proximal deep inguinal lymph node.

coronary n., n. coronário; a parte mais elevada do nodo atrioventricular.

cystic n., n. cístico. SIN cystic lymph node.

delphian n., n. linfonodo de Delfos; linfonodo pré-laríngeo na linha mediana, adjacente à glândula tireóide, cujo aumento indica a existência de doença da tireóide ou metástase precoce da laringe subglótica.

Dürck n.'s, nodos de Dürck; infiltrados inflamatórios crônicos perivasculares no cérebro, que ocorrem na tripanossomíase humana.

fibular n., linfonodo fibular. SIN fibular lymph node.

Flack n., n. de Flack. SIN sinuatrial n.

foraminal n., linfonodo foraminal. SIN lymph node of anterior border of omental foramen.

Haygarth n.'s, nodos de Haygarth; exostoses das margens das superfícies articulares e do periósteo e osso na vizinhança das articulações dos dedos das mãos, resultando em anciloses e associadas a deflexão cubital dos dedos das mãos para o lado ulnar, ocorrendo na artrite reumatóide.

Heberden n.'s, nodos de Heberden; exostoses aproximadamente do tamanho de uma ervilha ou menores, encontradas nas falanges terminais dos dedos das mãos na osteoartrite, que consistem em aumentos dos tubérculos nas extremidades articulares das falanges distais. SIN tuberculum arthriticum (1).

hemal n., n. hêmico; estrutura linfóide em que os seios sanguíneos estão presentes no local de seios linfáticos; os nodos hêmicos ocorrem em ruminantes e em alguns outros mamíferos, porém a sua presença nos seres humanos é duvidosa. SIN hemal gland, hemolymph gland, hemolymph n., vascular gland.

hemolymph n., n. hemolinfático. SIN hemal n.

Hensen n., n. de Hensen. SIN primitive n.

intermediate lacunar n., n. lacunar intermediário. SIN intermediate lacunar lymph node.

jugulodigastric n., n. jugulodigástrico. SIN jugulodigastric lymph node.

juguloomohyoid n., n. jugulomoióideo. SIN juguloomohyoid lymph node.

Keith n., n. de Keith. SIN sinuatrial n.

Keith and Flack n., n. de Keith e Flack. SIN sinuatrial n.

Koch n., n. de Koch. SIN sinuatrial n.

lateral lacunar n., n. lacunar lateral. SIN lateral lacunar lymph node.

n. of ligamentum arteriosum, n. do ligamento arterioso. SIN lymph node of ligamentum arteriosum.

lymph n., linfonodo. VER lymph node.

malar n., linfonodo malar. SIN malar lymph node.

mandibular n.'s, linfonodos mandibulares. SIN mandibular lymph node.

medial lacunar n., linfonodo lacunar medial. SIN medial lacunar lymph node.

middle rectal n., linfonodo retal médio. SIN middle rectal lymph node.

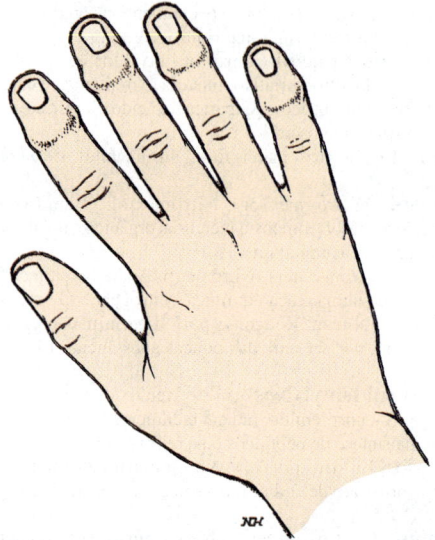

nodos de Heberden

milkers' n.'s, nodos dos leiteiros. SIN milkers' nodules, em nodule.

nasolabial n., linfonodo nasolabial. SIN nasolabial lymph node.

Osler n., n. de Osler; na endocardite bacteriana subaguda, aumentos de volume eritematosos circunscritos e indolores, cujo tamanho varia desde a cabeça de um alfinete até uma ervilha, observados na pele e tecidos subcutâneos das mãos e dos pés. SIN Osler sign.

parietal n.'s, linfonodos parietais. SIN parietal lymph nodes, em lymph node.

posterior tibial n., linfonodo tibial posterior. SIN posterior tibial lymph node.

primitive n., n. primitivo; espessamento local do blastoderma na extremidade cefálica da linha primitiva do embrião. SIN Hensen knot, Hensen n., Hubrecht protochordal knot, primitive knot, protochordal knot.

promontorial common iliac n.'s [TA], linfonodos ilíacos comuns do promontório; linfonodos do grupo ilíaco comum localizados no promontório do sacro. SIN nodi lymphoidei iliaci communes promontorii [TA], nodi lymphoidei promontorii.

n. of Ranvier, n. de Ranvier; curto intervalo na bainha de mielina de uma fibra nervosa, que ocorre entre dois segmentos sucessivos da bainha de mielina; no nodo, o axônio é apenas revestido por curtos processos citoplasmáticos digitiformes das duas células de Schwann vizinhas, ou, no sistema nervoso central, por células da oligodendróglia. VER TAMBÉM myelin *sheath*.

retropyloric n.'s, linfonodos retropilóricos. SIN retropyloric lymph nodes, em lymph node.

Rosenmüller n., n. linfonodo de Rosenmüller. SIN proximal deep inguinal lymph node.

n. of Rouviere, n. de Rouviere; um do grupo lateral de linfonodos retrofaríngeos. VER retropharyngeal lymph nodes, em lymph node.

S-A n., n. S-A. Abreviatura de sinoatrial n.

sentinel n., linfonodo sentinela. SIN sentinel lymph node.

signal n., linfonodo sentinela. VER signal lymph node.

singer's n.'s, nódulos do cantor. SIN vocal cord nodules, em nodule.

sinoatrial n. (S-A n.), n. sinoatrial (n. S-A). SIN sinuatrial n.

sinuatrial n. [TA], n. sinoatrial; a massa de fibras musculares cardíacas especializadas que, normalmente, atua como "marcapasso" do sistema de condução cardíaca; localiza-se sob o epicárdio, na extremidade superior do sulco terminal. SIN nodus sinuatrialis [TA], atrionector, Flack n., Keith and Flack n., Keith n., Koch n., sinoatrial n., sinus n.

sinus n., n. sinusal. SIN sinuatrial n.

subdigastric n., linfonodo subdigástrico. SIN jugulodigastric lymph node.

subpyloric n., linfonodo subpilórico. SIN subpyloric lymph nodes, em lymph node.

suprapyloric n., linfonodo suprapilórico. SIN suprapyloric lymph node.

Tawara n., n. Tawara. SIN atrioventricular n.

teacher's n.'s, nódulos do professor. SIN vocal cord nodules, em nodule.

Troisier n., n. de Troisier. SIN Troisier ganglion.

Virchow n., n. de Virchow. SIN signal lymph node.

visceral n.'s, linfonodos viscerais. SIN visceral lymph nodes, em lymph node.

vital n., n. vital. SIN noeud vital.

no·di (nō′dī). Nodos. Plural de nodus. [L.]

no·dose (nō′dōs). Nodoso. Que apresenta nodos ou aumentos de volume nodular. [L. *nodosus*]

nod·u·la·tion (nod-ū-lā′shŭn). Nodulação. Formação ou presença de nódulos.

nod·ule (nod′ūl) [TA]. Nódulo. Pequeno nó; na pele, nodo de até 1,0 cm de diâmetro, sólido, de profundidade palpável. SIN nodulus (1) [TA]. [L. *nodulus*, dim. de *nodus*, nó]

aggregated lymphatic n.'s, linfonodos agregados. SIN aggregated lymphoid n.'s of small intestine.

aggregated lymphoid n.'s [TA], nódulos linfóides agregados; massas de tecido linfóide no revestimento submucoso do apêndice vermiforme. SIN noduli lymphoidei aggregati appendicis vermiformis [TA], aggregated lymphatic follicles of vermiform appendix, folliculi lymphatici aggregati appendicis vermiformis.

aggregated lymphoid n.'s of small intestine [TA], nódulos linfóides agregados do intestino delgado; coleções de muitos folículos linfóides densamente agrupados, formando elevações oblongas sobre a mucosa do íleo oposta à fixação do mesentério. SIN aggregate glands, aggregated lymphatic follicles of small intestine, aggregated lymphatic n.'s, agmen peyerianum, agminate glands, agminated glands, folliculi lymphatici aggregati, Peyer glands, Peyer patches.

Albini n.'s, nódulos de Albini; diminutos nódulos fibrosos nas margens das valvas mitral e tricúspide do coração, algumas vezes presentes no recém-nascido, que representam remanescentes teciduais fetais; descritos previamente por Cruveilhier. Cf. n.'s of semilunar cusps.

apple jelly n.'s, nódulos em geléia de maçã; termo descritivo para as células papulares do lúpus vulgar, como aparecem na diascopia.

Arantius n., n. de Arantius. SIN n.'s of semilunar cusps.

Aschoff n.'s, nódulos de Aschoff. SIN Aschoff *bodies,* em *body*.

benign rheumatoid n.'s, nódulos reumatóides benignos. SIN pseudorheumatoid n.'s.

Bianchi n., n. de Bianchi. SIN n.'s of semilunar cusps.

Bohn n.'s, nódulos de Bohn; cistos minúsculos e múltiplos em recém-nascidos. São encontrados na junção do palato duro e palato mole, bem como ao longo das partes bucal e lingual das cristas dentais; derivam de remanescentes epiteliais de tecido glandular mucoso.

Busacca n.'s, nódulos de Busacca; nódulos granulomatosos inflamatórios localizados longe da margem pupilar da íris.

Caplan n.'s, nódulos de Caplan. SIN Caplan *syndrome*.

cold n., n. frio; nódulo tireóideo com captação muito menor de iodo radioativo do que o parênquima circundante; cerca de um em quatro mostra-se maligno.

Dalen-Fuchs n.'s, nódulos de Dalen-Fuchs; coleções de células epiteliais localizadas entre a membrana de Bruch e o epitélio pigmentar retiniano na exoftalmia simpática e, raramente, em outras inflamações intra-oculares granulomatosas.

enamel n., n. de esmalte. SIN enameloma.

Gamna-Gandy n.'s, nódulos de Gamna-Gandy. SIN Gamna-Gandy *bodies,* em *body*.

gastric lymphoid n.'s, nódulos linfóides gástricos; tecido linfóide no interior da lâmina própria que, especialmente no início da vida, agrupa-se em pequenas massas semelhantes a folículos linfáticos solitários intestinais. SIN folliculi lymphatici gastrici.

Hoboken n.'s, nódulos de Hoboken; dilatações macroscópicas na superfície externa das artérias umbilicais. VER TAMBÉM Hoboken *valves,* em *valve*. SIN Hoboken gemmules.

hot n., n. quente; nódulo tireóideo com captação muito maior de iodo radioativo do que o parênquima circundante; habitualmente benigno, porém causa algumas vezes hipertireoidismo.

Jeanselme n.'s, nódulos de Jeanselme; forma de bouba terciária, caracterizada pela ocorrência de nódulos nos braços e nas pernas, situados habitualmente próximos às articulações. SIN juxta-articular n.'s.

juxta-articular n.'s, nódulos justa-articulares. SIN Jeanselme n.'s.

laryngeal lymphoid n.'s, nódulos linfóides laríngeos; pequenos folículos localizados na face posterior da epiglote e no ventrículo da laringe. SIN folliculi lymphatici laryngei, laryngeal tonsils, lymphatic follicles of larynx.

Lisch n., n. de Lisch; hamartomas da íris tipicamente observados na neurofibromatose tipo 1. SIN Sakurai-Lisch n.

lymph n., linfonodo. SIN lymphoid n.

lymphatic n., n. linfático. SIN lymphoid n.

lymphoid n., linfonodo; uma das massas esféricas de células linfóides que, freqüentemente, exibem um centro com coloração mais clara. VER solitary lymphatic n.'s, aggregated lymphoid n.'s of small intestine. SIN folliculus lymphaticus, lymph n., lymphatic n., nodulus lymphaticus.

malpighian n.'s, nódulos de Malpighi. SIN splenic lymph *follicles,* em *follicle*.

milkers' n.'s, nódulos dos leiteiros; infecção dos úberes da vaca pelo vírus da vacínia, um membro dos Poxviridae, que é transmitido aos dedos e mãos dos leiteiros, produzindo nódulos e linfangite e, em certas ocasiões, erupções papulares ou papulovesiculares disseminadas; a infecção humana é transferível por vacas não-infectadas. SIN milkers' nodes, paravaccinia, pseudocowpox.

Morgagni n., n. de Morgagni. SIN n.'s of semilunar cusps.

picker's n.'s, nódulos do colhedor; nódulos cutâneos liquenificados observados no prurido nodular.

primary n., n. primário; linfonodo que apresenta pequenos linfócitos e carece de centro germinativo.

pseudorheumatoid n.'s, nódulos pseudo-reumatóides; nódulos subcutâneos benignos, de etiologia desconhecida, que se assemelham aos nódulos reumatóides, mas que não estão associados a doença reumática; podem ocorrer em múltiplos locais, como dorso dos pés ou das mãos, cotovelos, couro cabeludo e área pré-tibial. Os testes sorológicos para doença vascular do colágeno são negativos. SIN benign rheumatoid n.'s.

pulp n., n. da polpa. SIN endolith.

rheumatoid n.'s, nódulos reumatóides; nódulos subcutâneos que ocorrem mais comumente sobre proeminências ósseas em alguns pacientes com artrite reumatóide; ao exame microscópico, os nódulos consistem em focos de necrose fibrinóide, circundados por uma paliçada de fibroblastos.

Sakurai-Lisch n., n. de Sakurai-Lisch. SIN Lisch n.

Schmorl n., n. de Schmorl; prolapso do núcleo pulposo através da placa terminal do corpo vertebral para a camada esponjosa de uma vértebra adjacente.

secondary n., n. secundário; linfonodo com centro germinativo.

n.'s of semilunar cusps [TA], n. da valva semilunar; nódulo no centro da borda livre de cada valva semilunar no início da artéria pulmonar e aorta. SIN noduli valvularum semilunarium [TA], Arantius n., Bianchi n., corpus arantii, Morgagni n., n. of semilunar valve.

n. of semilunar valve, n. da válvula semilunar. SIN n.'s of semilunar cusps.

siderotic n., nódulos sideróticos. SIN Gamna-Gandy *bodies,* em *body*.

singer's n.'s, nódulos do cantor. SIN vocal cord n.'s.

solitary n.'s of intestine, nódulos solitários do intestino. SIN solitary lymphatic n.'s.

solitary lymphatic n.'s [TA], nódulos linfáticos solitários; coleções minúsculas de tecido linfóide na mucosa dos intestinos delgado e grosso, especialmente numerosas no ceco e no apêndice. SIN noduli lymphoidei solitarii [TA], folliculi lymphatici solitarii, solitary follicles, solitary glands, solitary lymphatic follicles, solitary n.'s of intestine.

splenic lymph n.'s, linfonodos esplênicos. SIN splenic lymph *follicles,* em *follicle*.

vocal cord n.'s, nódulos das cordas vocais; pequenas proliferações circunscritas, bilaterais e em forma de rosário na borda livre das cordas vocais, na junção do terço anterior e dos dois terços posteriores, causadas pelo uso exagerado ou abuso da voz; freqüentemente reversíveis com terapia da voz. SIN singer's nodes, singer's n.'s, teacher's nodes.

no·du·lus, pl. **no·du·li** (nod′ū-lŭs, nod′ū-lī) [TA]. Nódulo. **1.** SIN nodule. **2.** A extremidade posterior do verme inferior do cerebelo, formando com o véu medular posterior a porção central do lobo floculonodular. [L. dim. de *nodus*]

n. carot′icus, n. carótico. SIN carotid *body*.

n. lymphat′icus, n. linfático. SIN lymphoid *nodule*.

noduli lymphoidei aggregati appendicis vermiformis [TA], nódulos linfóides agregados do apêndice vermiforme. SIN aggregated lymphoid *nodules,* em *nodule*.

noduli lymphoidei solitarii [TA], nódulos linfóides solitários. SIN solitary lymphatic *nodules,* em *nodule*.

noduli val′vularum semiluna′rium [TA], nódulos da válvula semilunar. SIN *nodules* of semilunar cusps, em *nodule*.

no·dus, pl. **no·di** (nō′dŭs, -dī) [TA]. Nó. SIN node. [L. um nó]

n. atrioventricula′ris [TA], n. atrioventricular. SIN atrioventricular *node*.

n. buccinato′rius, n. bucinador. SIN buccal *lymph node*.

n. sinuatria′lis [TA], n. sinuatrial. SIN sinuatrial *node*.

n. tibia′lis ante′rior [TA], n. tibial anterior. SIN anterior tibial *lymph node*.

NODUS LYMPHATICUS

no·dus lym·pha·ti·cus, pl. **no·di lym·pha·ti·ci** (nō′dŭs lim′fat′ĕ-kus, -nō′dī). Linfonodo. *Termo oficial alternativo para lymph node. [lympho- + L. *nodus*, nodo]

nodi lymphatici col′ici, linfonodos cólicos. SIN colic *lymph nodes,* em *lymph node*.

nodi lymphatici comitan′tes ner′vi accesso′rii, linfonodos satélites do nervo acessório. SIN accessory *lymph nodes,* em *lymph node*.

nodi lymphatici iliaci communes media′les, linfonodos ilíacos comuns mediais. VER common iliac *lymph nodes,* em *lymph node*.

nodi lymphatici iliaci externi latera′les, linfonodos ilíacos externos laterais. VER external iliac *lymph nodes,* em *lymph node*.

nodi lymphatici iliaci externi media′les, linfonodos ilíacos externos mediais. VER external iliac *lymph nodes,* em *lymph node*.

nodi lymphatici prancrea′tici superio′res, linfonodos pancreáticos superiores. VER pancreatic *lymph nodes,* em *lymph node*.

nodi lymphatici paravesiculares, linfonodos paravesicais. VER paravesical *lymph nodes,* em *lymph node*.

nodi lymphatici postcavales, linfonodos lombares direitos inferiores. VER right lumbar *lymph nodes,* em *lymph node.*
nodi lymphatici postvesiculares, linfonodos paravesicais. VER paravesical *lymph nodes,* em *lymph node.*
nodi lymphatici prevesiculares, linfonodos pré-vesicais. VER paravesical *lymph nodes,* em *lymph node.*
nodi lymphatici vesicales laterales, linfonodos vesicais laterais. VER paravesical *lymph nodes,* em *lymph node.*

---

nodus lymphoideus, pl. **nodi lymphoidei** [TA], linfonodo. SIN *lymph node.*
nodi lymphoidei abdominis [TA], linfonodos abdominais. SIN abdominal *lymph nodes,* em *lymph node.*
nodi lymphoidei accessorii [TA], linfonodos acessórios. SIN accessory *lymph nodes,* em *lymph node.*
nodi lymphoidei anorecta'les, linfonodos anorretais. SIN pararectal *lymph nodes,* em *lymph node.*
nodi lymphoidei appendicula'res [TA], linfonodos apendiculares. SIN appendicular *lymph nodes,* em *lymph node.*
n. l. ar'cus ve'nae az'ygos, linfonodo do arco da veia ázigo. SIN *lymph node* of arch of azygos vein.
nodi lymphoidei axilla'res [TA], linfonodos axilares. SIN axillary *lymph nodes,* em *lymph node.*
nodi lymphoidei axillares anteriores, linfonodos axilares anteriores. SIN pectoral axillary *lymph nodes,* em *lymph node.*
nodi lymphoidei axillares apicales [TA], linfonodos axilares apicais. SIN apical axillary *lymph nodes,* em *lymph node.*
nodi lymphoidei axillares centrales [TA], linfonodos axilares centrais. SIN central axillary *lymph nodes,* em *lymph node.*
nodi lymphoidei axillares humerales [TA], linfonodos axilares umerais. SIN humeral axillary *lymph nodes,* em *lymph node.*
nodi lymphoidei axillares laterales, linfonodos axilares laterais; *termo oficial alternativo para humeral axillary *lymph nodes,* em *lymph node.*
nodi lymphoidei axillares posteriores, linfonodos axilares posteriores; *termo oficial alternativo para subscapular axillary *lymph nodes,* em *lymph node.*
nodi lymphoidei axillares subscapulares [TA], linfonodos axilares subescapulares. SIN subscapular axillary *lymph nodes,* em *lymph node.*
nodi lymphoidei axillares pectorales [TA], linfonodos axilares peitorais. SIN pectoral axillary *lymph nodes,* em *lymph node.*
nodi lymphoidei brachia'les, linfonodos braquiais. SIN humeral axillary *lymph nodes,* em *lymph node.*
nodi lymphoidei brachiocephalici [TA], linfonodos braquiocefálicos. SIN brachiocephalic *lymph nodes.*
nodi lymphoidei bronchopulmona'les [TA], linfonodos broncopulmonares. SIN bronchopulmonary *lymph nodes,* em *lymph node.*
n. l. buccinatorius [TA], linfonodo bucinatório. SIN buccal *lymph node.*
nodi lymphoidei capitis et colli [TA], linfonodos da cabeça e pescoço. SIN *lymph nodes* of head and neck, em *lymph node.*
nodi lymphoidei centra'les, linfonodos centrais. SIN superior mesenteric *lymph nodes,* em *lymph node.*
nodi lymphoidei cervicales anterio'res [TA], linfonodos cervicais anteriores. SIN anterior cervical *lymph nodes,* em *lymph node.*
nodi lymphoidei cervicales anterio'res profun'di, linfonodos cervicais anteriores profundos. SIN deep anterior cervical *lymph nodes,* em *lymph node.*
nodi lymphoidei cervicales anterio'res superficia'les [TA], linfonodos cervicais laterais superficiais. SIN anterior superficial cervical *lymph nodes,* em *lymph node.*
nodi lymphoidei cervicales laterales profundi [TA], linfonodos cervicais laterais profundos. SIN deep lateral cervical *lymph nodes,* em *lymph node.*
nodi lymphoidei cervicales laterales superficiales [TA], linfonodos cervicais laterais superficiais. SIN superficial lateral cervical *lymph nodes,* em *lymph node.*
nodi lymphoidei coeliaci [TA], linfonodos celíacos. SIN celiac *lymph nodes,* em *lymph node.*
nodi lymphoidei col'ici dex'tri [TA], linfonodos cólicos direitos. SIN right colic *lymph nodes,* em *lymph node.*
nodi lymphoidei col'ici me'dii [TA], linfonodos cólicos médios. SIN middle colic *lymph nodes,* em *lymph node.*
nodi lymphoidei col'ici sinis'tri [TA], linfonodos cólicos esquerdos. SIN left colic *lymph nodes,* em *lymph node.*
nodi lymphoidei cubitales [TA], linfonodos cubitais. SIN cubital *lymph nodes,* em *lymph node.*
n. l. cys'ticus [TA], linfonodo cístico. SIN cystic *lymph node.*
nodi lymphoidei epigastrici inferiores [TA], linfonodos epigástricos inferiores. SIN inferior epigastric *lymph nodes,* em *lymph node.*
nodi lymphoidei faciales [TA], linfonodos faciais. SIN facial *lymph nodes,* em *lymph node.*
n. l. fibula'ris [TA], linfonodo fibular. SIN fibular *lymph node.*
n. l. foraminalis [TA], linfonodo do forame. SIN *lymph node* of anterior border of omental foramen.
nodi lymphoidei gastrici dextri [TA], linfonodos gástricos direitos. SIN right gastric *lymph nodes,* em *lymph node.*
nodi lymphoidei gastrici sinistri [TA], linfonodos gástricos esquerdos. SIN left gastric *lymph nodes,* em *lymph node.*
nodi lymphoidei gastroomentales dextri [TA], linfonodos gastroomentais direitos. SIN right gastroomental *lymph nodes,* em *lymph node.*
nodi lymphoidei gastroomentales sinistri [TA], linfonodos gastroomentais esquerdos. SIN left gastroomental *lymph nodes,* em *lymph node.*
nodi lymphoidei gluteales [TA], linfonodos glúteos. SIN gluteal *lymph nodes,* em *lymph node.*
nodi lymphoidei hepatici [TA], linfonodos hepáticos. SIN hepatic *lymph nodes,* em *lymph node.*
nodi lymphoidei ileocolici [TA], linfonodos ileocólicos. SIN ileocolic *lymph nodes,* em *lymph node.*
nodi lymphoidei iliaci communes [TA], linfonodos ilíacos comuns. SIN common iliac *lymph nodes,* em *lymph node.*
nodi lymphoidei iliaci communes promonto'rii [TA], linfonodos ilíacos comuns do promontório. SIN promontorial common iliac *nodes,* em *node.*
nodi lymphoidei iliaci externi [TA], linfonodos ilíacos externos. SIN external iliac *lymph nodes,* em *lymph node.*
nodi lymphoidei iliaci interni [TA], linfonodos ilíacos internos. SIN internal iliac *lymph nodes,* em *lymph node.*
nodi lymphoidei inguinales profundi, linfonodos inguinais profundos. SIN deep inguinal *lymph nodes,* em *lymph node.*
nodi lymphoidei inguinales superficiales [TA], linfonodos inguinais superficiais. SIN superficial inguinal *lymph nodes,* em *lymph node.*
nodi lymphoidei intercostales [TA], linfonodos intercostais. SIN intercostal *lymph nodes,* em *lymph node.*
nodi lymphoidei interiliaci [TA], linfonodos interilíacos. SIN interiliac *lymph nodes,* em *lymph node.*
nodi lymphoidei interpectorales [TA], linfonodos interpeitorais. SIN interpectoral *lymph nodes,* em *lymph node.*
nodi lymphoidei intrapulmonales [TA], linfonodos intrapulmonares. SIN intrapulmonary *lymph nodes,* em *lymph node.*
nodi lymphoidei jugulares anteriores, linfonodos cervicais anteriores. SIN anterior superficial cervical *lymph nodes,* em *lymph node.*
nodi lymphoidei jugulares laterales, linfonodos cervicais laterais. SIN lateral jugular *lymph nodes,* em *lymph node.*
n. l. jugulodigas'tricus [TA], linfonodo jugulodigástrico. SIN jugulodigastric *lymph node.*
n. l. juguloomohyoi'deus [TA], linfonodo jugulomo-hióideo. SIN juguloomohyoide *lymph node.*
nodi lymphoidei juxtaesophageales [TA], linfonodos justaesofágicos. SIN juxtaesophageal *lymph nodes,* em *lymph node.*
nodi lymphoidei juxtaesophageales pulmonales, linfonodos pulmonares justaesofágicos. SIN juxtaesophageal *lymph nodes,* em *lymph node.*
nodi lymphoidei juxtaintestinales [TA], linfonodos justaintestinais. SIN juxtaintestinal mesenteric *lymph nodes,* em *lymph node.*
n. l. lacuna'ris interme'dius [TA], linfonodo lacunar intermédio. SIN intermediate lacunar *lymph node.*
n. l. lacuna'ris latera'lis [TA], linfonodo lacunar lateral. SIN lateral lacunar *lymph node.*
n. l. lacuna'ris media'lis [TA], linfonodo lacunar medial. SIN medial lacunar *lymph node.*
nodi lymphoidei lienales, linfonodos esplênicos; *termo oficial alternativo para splenic *lymph nodes,* em *lymph node.*
n. l. ligamen'ti arterio'si [TA], linfonodo do ligamento arterioso. SIN *lymph node* of ligamentum arteriosum.
nodi lymphoidei linguales [TA], linfonodos linguais. SIN lingual *lymph nodes,* em *lymph node.*
nodi lymphoidei lumbales dextri [TA], linfonodos lombares direitos. SIN right lumbar *lymph nodes,* em *lymph node.*
nodi lymphoidei lumbales intermedii [TA], linfonodos lombares intermédios. SIN intermediate lumbar *lymph nodes,* em *lymph node.*
nodi lymphoidei lumbales sinistri [TA], linfonodos lombares esquerdos. SIN left lumbar *lymph nodes,* em *lymph node.*
nodi lymphoidei abdom'inis viscera'les [TA], linfonodos viscerais abdominais. SIN visceral *lymph nodes* of abdomen, em *lymph node.*
n. l. mala'ris [TA], linfonodo malar. SIN malar *lymph node.*
n. l. mandibula'ris [TA], linfonodo mandibular. SIN mandibular *lymph node.*
nodi lymphoidei mastoidei [TA], linfonodos mastóideos. SIN mastoid *lymph node.*
nodi lymphoidei mediastinales anteriores, linfonodos braquiocefálicos. SIN brachiocephalic *lymph nodes.*
nodi lymphoidei mediastinales posteriores, linfonodos pré-vertebrais. SIN prevertebral *lymph nodes,* em *lymph node.*

nodi lymphoidei membri inferioris [TA], linfonodos dos membros inferiores. SIN *lymph nodes of lower limb*, em *lymph node*.
nodi lymphoidei membri superioris [TA], linfonodos dos membros superiores. SIN *lymph nodes of upper limb*, em *limph node*.
nodi lymphoidei mesenterici [TA], linfonodos mesentéricos. SIN *mesenteric lymph nodes*, em *lymph node*.
no'di lymphoidei mesenter'ici inferio'res [TA], linfonodos mesentéricos inferiores. SIN *inferior mesenteric lymph nodes*, em *lymph node*.
no'di lymphoidei mesenter'ici superio'res [TA], linfonodos mesentéricos superiores. SIN *superior mesenteric lymph nodes*, em *lymph node*.
nodi lymphoidei mesocolici [TA], linfonodos mesocólicos. SIN *mesocolic lymph nodes*, em *lymph node*.
n. l. nasolabia'lis [TA], linfonodo nasolabial. SIN *nasolabial lymph node*.
nodi lymphoidei obturatorii [TA], linfonodos obturadores. SIN *obturator lymph nodes*, em *lymph node*.
nodi lymphoidei occipitales [TA], linfonodos occipitais. SIN *occipital lymph nodes*, em *lymph node*.
nodi lymphoidei pancrea'tici [TA], linfonodos pancreáticos. SIN *pancreatic lymph nodes*, em *lymph node*.
nodi lymphoidei pancreaticoduodenales [TA], linfonodos pancreaticoduodenais. SIN *pancreaticoduodenal lymph nodes*, em *lymph node*.
nodi lymphoidei pancreaticolienales, linfonodos pancreaticoesplênicos. SIN *pancreaticosplenic lymph nodes*, em *lymph node*.
nodi lymphoidei pancreaticosplenales [TA], linfonodos pancreaticoesplênicos. SIN *pancreaticosplenic lymph nodes*, em *lymph node*.
nodi lymphoidei paracolici, linfonodos paracólicos. SIN *mesocolic lymph nodes*, em *lymph node*.
nodi lymphoidei paramammarii [TA], linfonodos paramamários. SIN *paramammary lymph nodes*, em *lymph node*.
nodi lymphoidei pararectales [TA], linfonodos pararretais. SIN *pararectal lymph nodes*, em *lymph node*.
nodi lymphoidei parasternales [TA], linfonodos paraesternais. SIN *parasternal lymph nodes*, em *lymph node*.
nodi lymphoidei paratracheales [TA], linfonodos paratraqueais. SIN *paratracheal lymph nodes*, em *lymph node*.
nodi lymphoidei parauterini [TA], linfonodos parauterinos. SIN *parauterine lymph nodes*, em *lymph node*.
nodi lymphoidei paravaginales [TA], linfonodos paravaginais. SIN *paravaginal lymph nodes*, em *lymph node*.
no'di lymphoidei parieta'les [TA], linfonodos parietais. SIN *parietal lymph nodes*, em *lymph node*.
nodi lymphoidei parotid'ei intraglandulares [TA], linfonodos parotídeos intraglandulares. SIN *intraglandular deep parotid lymph nodes*, em *lymph node*.
nodi lymphoidei parotid'ei profundi [TA], linfonodos parotídeos profundos. SIN *deep parotid lymph nodes*, em *lymph node*.
nodi lymphoidei parotid'ei profundi infra-auricula'res, linfonodos parotídeos profundos infra-auriculares. SIN *infraauricular deep parotid lymph nodes*, em *lymph node*.
nodi lymphoidei parotidei profundi preauriculares [TA], linfonodos parotídeos profundos pré-auriculares. SIN *preauricular deep parotid lymph nodes*, em *lymph node*.
nodi lymphoidei parotid'ei superficiales [TA], linfonodos parotídeos superficiais. SIN *superficial parotid lymph nodes*, em *lymph node*.
nodi lymphoidei pelvis [TA], linfonodos pélvicos. SIN *pelvic lymph nodes*, em *lymph node*.
nodi lymphoidei pericardiales laterales [TA], linfonodos pericárdicos laterais. SIN *lateral pericardial lymph nodes*, em *lymph node*.
nodi lymphoidei phrenici inferiores [TA], linfonodos frênicos inferiores. SIN *inferior phrenic lymph nodes*, em *lymph node*.
nodi lymphoidei phrenici superiores [TA], linfonodos frênicos superiores. SIN *superior phrenic lymph nodes*, em *lymph node*.
nodi lymphoidei popliteales [TA], linfonodos poplíteos. SIN *popliteal lymph nodes*, em *lymph node*.
nodi lymphoidei precaecales [TA], linfonodos pré-cecais. SIN *prececal lymph nodes*, em *lymph node*.
nodi lymphoidei prelaryngeales [TA], linfonodos pré-laríngeos. SIN *prelaryngeal lymph nodes*, em *lymph node*.
nodi lymphoidei prepericardiaci [TA], linfonodos pré-pericárdicos. SIN *prepericardial lymph nodes*, em *lymph node*.
nodi lymphoidei pretracheales [TA], linfonodos pré-traqueais. SIN *pretracheal lymph nodes*, em *lymph node*.
nodi lymphoidei prevertebrales, linfonodos pré-vertebrais; *termo oficial alternativo para *prevertebral lymph nodes*, em *lymph node*.
nodi lymphoidei promontorii, linfonodos do promontório. SIN *promontorial common iliac nodes*, em *lymph node*.
n. l. proximalis profundus [TA], linfonodo proximal profundo. SIN *proximal deep inguinal lymph node*.
nodi lymphoidei pulmonales, linfonodos pulmonares. SIN *intrapulmonary lymph nodes*, em *lymph node*.
nodi lymphoidei pylorici, linfonodos pilóricos. SIN *pyloric lymph nodes*, em *lymph node*.
nodi lymphoidei rectales superiores [TA], linfonodos retais superiores. SIN *superior rectal lymph nodes*, em *lymph node*.
n. l. recta'lis me'dius, linfonodo retal médio. SIN *middle rectal lymph node*.
nodi lymphoidei retrocecales [TA], linfonodos retrocecais. SIN *retrocecal lymph nodes*, em *lymph node*.
nodi lymphoidei retropharyngeales [TA], linfonodos retrofaríngeos. SIN *retropharyngeal lymph nodes*, em *lymph node*.
no'di lymphoidei retropylo'rici [TA], linfonodos retropilóricos. SIN *retropyloric lymph nodes*, em *lymph node*.
nodi lymphoidei sacrales [TA], linfonodos sacros. SIN *sacral lymph nodes*, em *lymph node*.
nodi lymphoidei sigmoidei [TA], linfonodos sigmóideos. SIN *sigmoid lymph nodes*, em *lymph node*.
nodi lymphoidei splenici [TA], linfonodos esplênicos. SIN *splenic lymph nodes*, em *lymph node*.
nodi lymphoidei subaortici [TA], linfonodos subaórticos. SIN *subaortic lymph nodes*, em *lymph node*.
nodi lymphoidei submandibulares [TA], linfonodos submandibulares. SIN *submandibular lymph nodes*, em *lymph node*.
nodi lymphoidei submentales [TA], linfonodos submentuais. SIN *submental lymph nodes*, em *lymph node*.
no'di lymphoidei subpylo'rici [TA], linfonodos subpilóricos. SIN *subpyloric lymph nodes*, em *lymph node*.
nodi lymphoidei superiores centrales [TA], linfonodos centrais superiores. SIN *central superior mesenteric lymph nodes*, em *lymph node*.
nodi lymphoidei supraclaviculares [TA], linfonodos supraclaviculares. SIN *supraclavicular lymph nodes*, em *lymph node*.
n. l. suprapylo'ricus [TA], linfonodo suprapilórico. SIN *suprapyloric lymph node*.
nodi lymphoidei thoracis [TA], linfonodos torácicos. SIN *thoracic lymph nodes*, em *lymph node*.
nodi lymphoidei thyroidei [TA], linfonodos tireóideos. SIN *thyroid lymph nodes*, em *lymph node*.
n. l. tibia'lis poste'rior [TA], linfonodo tibial posterior. SIN *posterior tibial lymph node*.
nodi lymphoidei tracheobronchiales inferiores, linfonodos traqueobronquiais inferiores. SIN *inferior tracheobronchial lymph nodes*, em *lymph node*.
nodi lymphoidei tracheobronchiales superiores [TA], linfonodos traqueobronquiais superiores. SIN *superior tracheobronchial lymph nodes*, em *lymph node*.
nodi lymphoidei viscerales [TA], linfonodos viscerais. SIN *visceral lymph nodes*, em *lymph node*.

NOE NOE. Abreviatura de nuclear Overhauser *effect* (efeito nuclear de Overhauser).

no·e·mat·ic (nō-ē-mat′ik). Noemático. Termo raramente utilizado para referir-se aos processos mentais. [G. *noēma*, percepção, pensamento]

no·e·sis (nō-ē′sis). Noese. Cognição, especialmente através do conhecimento direto e auto-evidente. [G. *noēsis*, pensamento, inteligência]

no·et·ic (nō-et′ik). Noético. Relativo à noese.

no·eud vi·tal (noo vē-tal′). Nó vital. Região circunscrita na parte inferior da medula oblonga, próxima ao ápice do *calamus scriptorius* (ventrículo de Arantius); interpretado por M. Flourens (1858) como um centro nervoso que controla a respiração. SIN vital knot, vital node. [Fr.]

No·gu·chia (nō-goo′chē-ā). *Noguchia*. Gênero de bactérias peritríquias (família Brucellaceae) aeróbicas a facultativamente anaeróbicas e móveis, contendo pequenos bastonetes Gram-negativos, encapsulados e delgados. Esses microrganismos estão presentes na conjuntiva dos seres humanos e de outros animais acometidos por um tipo folicular de doença. A espécie típica é *N. granulosis*. [Hideyo *Noguchi*, bacteriologista japonês, 1876–1928]

N. granulo'sis, espécie considerada por alguns como causa de tracoma nos seres humanos; provoca conjuntivite granular em macacos e monos; trata-se da espécie típica do gênero *N.*

noise (noyz). Ruído. **1.** Som indesejável, particularmente um som complexo que carece de qualidade musical, visto que as várias freqüências das quais é composto não constituem múltiplos inteiros ou parciais (harmônicos) entre si. **2.** Acréscimos indesejáveis a um sinal que não provém de sua fonte; p. ex., a onda de freqüência de 60 ciclos num eletrocardiograma; em grande parte eliminado das modernas máquinas (após 1980) (inclui ruído visual em estudos de imageamento). VER *signal-to-noise ratio*. **3.** Variáveis externas não-controladas que influenciam a distribuição de medidas num conjunto de dados. [I.E., de O.Fr., de L.L. *nausea*, enjôo]

structured n., r. estruturado; em radiologia, os sinais de estruturas anatômicas que interferem na detecção de patologia significativa.

white n., r. branco; som complexo que consiste em muitas freqüências numa ampla faixa de freqüências; freqüentemente utilizado para impedir a audição no ouvido não-testado na audiometria.

no·ma (nō′mă). Noma. Estomatite gangrenosa que, habitualmente, surge na mucosa do canto da boca ou bochecha e, a seguir, progride com bastante rapidez, acometendo toda a espessura dos lábios e/ou das bochechas, com necrose evidente e descamação completa do tecido. Em geral, observada em crianças desnutridas e em adultos debilitados, especialmente nos grupos socioeconômicos inferiores; com freqüência, precedido de outra doença, como, p. ex., calazar, disenteria ou escarlatina. Um processo semelhante (noma pudendo, noma vulvar) também pode acometer os lábios maiores do pudendo. Em geral, são encontrados diversos microrganismos no material necrótico, porém os mais freqüentemente observados incluem bacilos fusiformes, *Borrelia*, estafilococos e estreptococos anaeróbicos. SIN cancrum oris, stomatonecrosis, water canker. [G. *nomē*, disseminação (úlcera)]

Nomarski, Georges, inventor óptico francês do século XX. VER N. *optics*.

no·men·cla·ture (nō′men-klă-choor, nō-men′klă-choor). Nomenclatura. Sistema de nomes, como os de estruturas anatômicas, organismos, etc., utilizado em qualquer ciência. [L. *nomenclatura*, lista de nomes, de *nomen*, nome + *calo*, proclamar]

  binary n., binomial n., n. binária, n. binominal. SIN linnaean system of nomenclature.

  Cleland n., n. de Cleland; nomenclatura para referir-se aos mecanismos de ligação de reações catalisadas por enzimas; nessa nomenclatura, os substratos são representados pelas letras A, B, C, etc., enquanto os produtos representados por P, Q, R, etc., a enzima por E, e as formas modificadas da enzima por F, G; além disso, o número de substratos ou produtos é representado por uni, bi, ter (tri), etc.; assim, uma reação de aminotransferase (p. ex., alanina transaminase) possui um mecanismo bi bi em pingue-pongue, enquanto a glutamina sintetase tem um mecanismo ter ter randômico. Ver também as subentradas em mechanism.

No·men·kla·tur Kom·mis·sion (N. K.). Comitê sobre Nomenclatura da Sociedade Anatômica Alemã, indicado para rever ou suplementar a BNA (1895).

no·mi·fen·sine ma·le·ate (nō-mi-fen′sēn). Maleato de nomifensina. Antidepressivo.

Nom·i·na An·a·tom·i·ca (NA) (nom′i-nă an-ă-tom′i-kă, nō′mi-nă an′ă-tō′mi-kă). Nomenclatura Anatômica. A modificação da *Basle Nomina Anatomica* ou sistema BNA de terminologia anatômica adotada em 1955 pelo Congresso Internacional de Anatomistas em Paris, França. O Comitê Internacional de Nomenclatura Anatômica foi responsável por revisões contínuas da NA, que são revistas e adotadas pelo Congresso Internacional de Anatomistas que se reúne a intervalos de cinco anos, desde 1955 a 1985. A NA foi substituída pela *Terminologia Anatomica* [TA] em 1998, fundada pelo Comitê Federativo de Terminologia Anatômica.

🛈 **nom·o·gram** (nōm′ō-gram). Nomograma. Forma de gráfico linear mostrando escalas para as variáveis envolvidas em determinada fórmula, de modo que os valores correspondentes para cada variável situam-se numa reta fazendo intersecção em todas as escalas. SIN nomograph (2). [G. *nomos*, lei + *gramma*, algo escrito]

  blood volume n, n. do volume sanguíneo; nomograma utilizado para medir o volume sanguíneo com base no peso e na altura do indivíduo.

  cartesian n., n. cartesiano; nomograma baseado em coordenadas retangulares, representando duas variáveis, em que uma família de isopletas é superposta para cada uma das variáveis adicionais envolvidas. [de R. Descartes, filósofo e matemático francês, 1596–1650]

  d'Ocagne n., n. d'Ocagne; gráfico de alinhamento que consiste na distribuição de três ou mais linhas graduadas (retas ou curvas), constituindo, cada uma delas, uma escala de valores de determinada variável, construída de tal modo que qualquer reta cruzando essas escalas liga os valores simultaneamente compatíveis; a partir dos valores de quaisquer duas variáveis, podem-se determinar os valores de todas as outras variáveis.

  Radford n., n. de Radford; nomograma utilizado para prever o volume corrente necessário para respiração artificial, baseando-se na freqüência respiratória, no peso corporal e no sexo; são fornecidos fatores de correção relativos à atividade, presença de febre, altitude, acidose metabólica e alterações do espaço morto.

  Siggaard-Andersen n., n. de Siggaard-Andersen; nomograma utilizado para prever a composição ácido-básica do sangue pela inclinação e posição de uma linha tampão construída quando a P_{CO_2} numa escala logarítmica é representada graficamente contra o pH.

nom·o·graph (nom′ō-graf). Nomografia. **1.** Gráfico que consiste em três curvas coplanares, habitualmente paralelas, cada uma graduada para uma variável diferente, de modo que uma linha reta cortando todas essas curvas cruza os valores relacionados de cada variável. **2.** SIN nomogram. [G. *nomos*, lei + *graphō*, escrever]

nom·o·thet·ic (nom-ō-thet′ik). Nomotético. Refere-se a generalizações relativas ao comportamento de grupos de indivíduos como grupos, em oposição a idiográfico. [G. *nomos*, lei + *thesis*, colocação]

no·mo·top·ic (nō-mō-top′ik). Nomotópico. Relativo ao, ou que ocorre no, local usual ou normal. [G. *nomos*, lei, costume + *topos*, local]

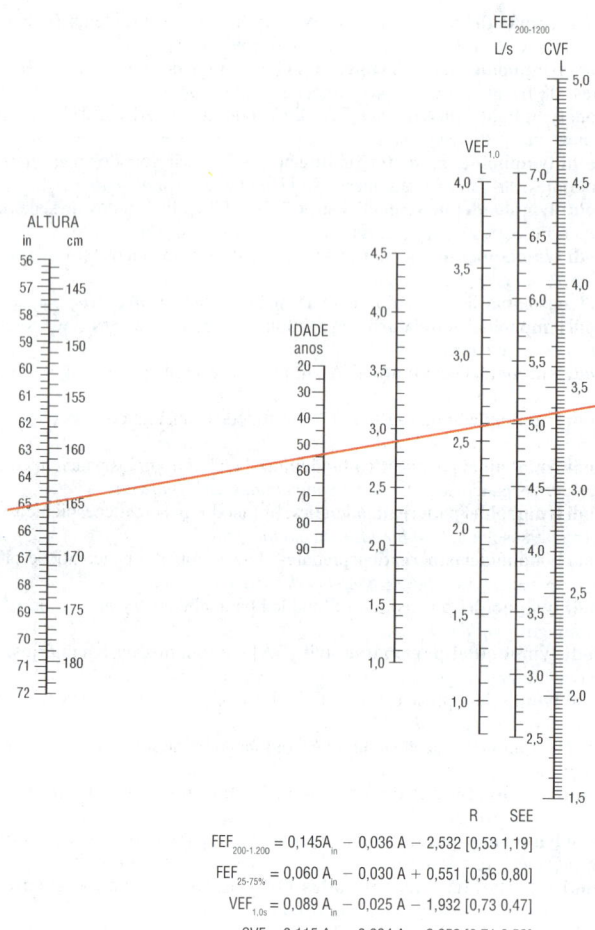

nomograma: prevendo o fluxo expiratório (mulheres)

non·al·lele (non′ă-lēl′). Não-alelo. Refere-se a genes que não competem no mesmo *locus*; o grau com que irão comportar-se independentemente irá depender de seus *loci* estarem ou não ligados. Pelo menos quando inicialmente formados (p. ex., em conseqüência de *crossing-over* desigual), os dois não-alelos podem ser idênticos.

no·nan (nō′nan). Que ocorre no nono dia. [L. *nonus*, nono]

***n*-non·a·no·ic ac·id** (non-ă-nō′ik). Ácido *n*-nonanóico. SIN pelargonic acid.

non·a·pep·tide (non-a-pep′tĭd). Nonapeptídeo. Oligopeptídeo contendo nove resíduos de aminoácidos (p. ex., oxitocina).

non·bur·sate (non-ber′sāt). Refere-se a uma divisão não-taxonômica dos Nematoda, incluindo as espécies em que a bolsa copuladora do macho consiste apenas numa dobra da pele sem nenhuma costela carnosa, conforme observado nos ancilóstomos e outros nematódeos com bolsa. [L. *non*, não + L. Mediev. *bursa*, bolsa]

non·car·i·o·gen·ic (nor-kā′rē-ō-jen′ik). Não-cariogênico, que não produz cárie.

non·cel·lu·lar (non-sel′ū-lăr). Não-celular. **1.** Que carece de organização celular, como os vírus, que só podem replicar-se no interior de uma célula, seja ela procariótica ou eucariótica. SIN subcellular. **2.** SIN acellular (1).

non·chro·mo·gens (non-krō′mō-jenz). Não-cromógenos. SIN Runyon group III mycobacteria.

non·com·e·do·gen·ic (non-kom′e-dō-jen′ik). Não-comedogênico. Que não tende a promover a formação de comedones.

non com·pos men·tis (non kom′pos men′tis). Que não tem uma mente sadia; mentalmente incapaz de administrar seus próprios negócios. [L. *non*, não + *compos*, participante, competente, + *mens*, gen. *mentis*, mente]

non·dis·ease (non′dis-ēz). Sem doença. Ausência de doença quando se suspeita de uma doença específica, mas esta não é encontrada.

non·dis·junc·tion (non-dis-jŭnk′shŭn). Não-disjunção; incapacidade de separação de um ou mais pares de cromossomas na fase meiótica da cariocinese, de modo que ambos os cromossomas são transportados para uma célula-filha e nenhum para a outra.

  primary n., não-disjunção primária; não-disjunção que ocorre numa célula previamente normal.

secondary n., não-disjunção secundária; não-disjunção que ocorre numa célula aneuplóide, resultado de uma não-disjunção primária.

non·e·lec·tro·lyte (non - ē - lek′trō - līt). Não-eletrólito. Substância cujas moléculas, em solução, não se dissociam em íons e, portanto, não conduzem uma corrente elétrica.

non·es·tro·gen·ic (non - es - trō - jen′ik). Não-estrogênico. **1.** Que não causa estro em animais. **2.** Que não possui ação semelhante à de um estrogênio. Cf. nonuterotropic. SIN nonoestrogenic.

non·im·mune (non - i - mūn′). Não-imune. Relativo a um indivíduo que não está imunizado ou ao soro desse indivíduo.

non·im·mun·i·ty (non - i - mūn′i - tē). Não-imunidade. SIN aphylaxis.

non·in·fec·tious (non′in - fek′shŭs). Não-infeccioso. Que não é infeccioso; incapaz de transmitir doença.

non·in·va·sive (non - in - vā′siv). Não-invasivo. Indica um procedimento que não exige a introdução de um instrumento ou dispositivo através da pele ou de um orifício corporal para diagnóstico ou tratamento.

non·ion·ic (non - ī - on′ik). Não-iônico. Classe de contrastes radiográficos que não sofrem ionização e solução, diminuindo, assim, a osmolalidade efetiva e a toxicidade. VER TAMBÉM low osmolar contrast *agent*.

non·ma·lef·i·cence (non - mal′ef - ī - sens). Não-maleficência. Princípio ético de não prejudicar, baseado no aforismo de Hipócrates, *primum non nocere*, em primeiro lugar, não prejudicar. [non- + L. *maleficencia*, malefício, de *male*, ruim, erradamente + *facio*, fazer, atuar]

non·med·ul·lat·ed (non - med′ū - lāt - ed). Não-medulado. SIN unmyelinated.

non·my·e·li·nat·ed (non - mī′e - li - nāt′ed). Não-mielinizado. SIN unmyelinated.

non·ne·o·plas·tic (non′nē - ō - plas′tik). Não-neoplásico. Que não apresenta neoplasia.

non·nu·cle·at·ed (non - noo′klē - ā - ted). Não-nucleado. Que não possui núcleo.

non·oc·clu·sion (non - ō - kloo′shŭn). Não-oclusão. Incapacidade de um dente de entrar em contato com o dente oposto.

non·oes·tro·gen·ic. Não-estrogênico. SIN nonestrogenic.

non·ose (non′ōs). Nonose. Açúcar com nove átomos de carbono. [L. *nonus*, nono]

non·ox·y·nol 9 (non′noks - ī - nol). Nonoxinol 9. Grupo de compostos tensoativos, utilizados em preparações espermicidas, como espuma contraceptiva e geléia para diafragma.

nonparametric (non - par′ā - met′rik). Não-paramétrico. Grupo de manobras estatísticas que podem ser efetivamente aplicadas a dados não-normais ou de distribuição outra que não a de Gauss.

non·par·ous (non - par′ŭs). Nulípara. SIN nulliparous.

non·pen·e·trance (non - pen′ĕ - trans). Não-penetrância. O estado no qual um traço genético, apesar de estar presente no genótipo apropriado (isto é, homozigoto, hemizigoto ou heterozigoto, de acordo com o estado de dominância e modo de herança), é incapaz de manifestar-se no fenótipo, devido a fatores modificadores. Cf. hypostasis.

non·pro·pri·e·tar·y name (non - prō - prī′e - tār - ē). Não-comercial. Nome curto (freqüentemente conhecido como nome genérico) de uma substância química, medicamento ou outra substância que não está sujeita aos direitos de marca registrada, mas que é, ao contrário do nome trivial, reconhecida ou recomendada por departamentos governamentais (p. ex., a *Federal Food and Drug Administration*) e por organizações quase oficiais (p. ex., *U.S. Adopted Names Council*) para uso público geral. À semelhança do nome comercial, trata-se quase sempre de uma designação derivada sem se basear em critérios estabelecidos. Cf. trivial name, proprietary name, semisystematic name, systematic name.

non·pro·te·o·gen·ic (non - prō′tē - ō - jen′ik). Não-proteogênico. Que não leva à produção de proteínas.

non·re·set no·dus si·nu·a·tri·a·lis (non - rē′set nō′dŭs sī′noo - ā - trē - ā′lis). Não-reajuste do nodo sinoatrial. Condição produzida por uma despolarização atrial prematura quando a soma da duração do ciclo prematuro e do ciclo de retorno é totalmente compensatória, isto é, duas vezes a duração do comprimento do ciclo espontâneo. Cf. reset nodus sinuatrialis.

non·ro·ta·tion (non - rō - tā′shŭn). Não-rotação. Ausência de rotação normal.
n. of intestine, não-rotação do intestino; anomalia de desenvolvimento que faz com que o intestino delgado fique localizado no lado direito do abdome e o cólon, no lado esquerdo.
n. of kidney, não-rotação do rim; anomalia em desenvolvimento em que o hilo do rim mantém a sua posição original, com a pelve renal voltada ventralmente.

non·sa·pon·i·fi·a·ble (non - sā - pon - i - fī′a - bl). Não-saponificável. Não-sujeito a saponificação; p. ex., os triacilgliceróis são saponificáveis, enquanto o colesterol é não-saponificável.

non·se·cre·tor (non - sē - krē′tor, - tor). Não-secretor. Indivíduo cuja saliva não contém antígenos do grupo sanguíneo ABO. VER TAMBÉM secretor.

non·sense. Sem sentido. Termo utilizado em genética para referir-se a uma mutação que causa uma seqüência tal que ocorre terminação da cadeia peptídica em crescimento, freqüentemente após a incorporação de resíduos aminoácido incorretos.

nonsense suppression, supressão sem sentido; tRNA mutante que faz a leitura de um códon de terminação de cadeia como sinal para a incorporação de um resíduo aminoácido específico.

non·un·ion (non′ŭn - yŭn). Não-união. Incapacidade de consolidação normal de um osso fraturado.

non·uter·o·tro·pic (non - ū - ter - ō - trō′pik). Não-uterotrópico. Que não produz efeito sobre o útero. Cf. nonestrogenic.

non·va·lent (non - vā′lent). Não-valente. Que não possui valência. Incapaz de entrar numa composição química.

non·vas·cu·lar (non - vas′kū - lăr). Não-vascular. SIN avascular.

non·ver·bal (non - ver′bl). Não-verbal. Denota a comunicação sem palavras, como, p. ex., através de sinais, símbolos, expressões faciais, gestos, postura.

non·vi·a·ble (non - vī′ă - bl). Não-viável. **1.** Incapaz de existência independente; com freqüência, indica um feto nascido prematuramente. **2.** Refere-se a um microrganismo ou parasita incapaz de ter atividade metabólica ou reprodutiva.

Noonan, Jacqueline A., cardiologista pediatra norte-americana. *1921. VER N. *syndrome*.

nor-. Nor-. **1.** Prefixo químico que indica: 1) eliminação de um grupamento metileno de uma cadeia, sendo utilizado o locante mais alto permissível; 2) contração de um anel (esteróide por uma unidade CH_2, sendo o locante a letra maiúscula que identifica o anel. A eliminação de dois grupos metileno é indicada pelo prefixo dinor-; de três grupos, por trinor-, etc. **2.** Prefixo químico que indica "normal", isto é, cadeia não-ramificada de átomos de carbono em compostos alifáticos, em oposição à cadeia ramificada com o mesmo número de átomos de carbono; p. ex., norleucina *vs.* leucina.

nor·a·dren·a·line (nor - ă - dren′ă - lin). Norepinefrina. SIN norepinephrine.
n. acid tartrate, tartarato ácido de n. SIN norepinephrine bitartrate.
n. bitartrate, bitartarato de n. SIN norepinephrine bitartrate.

nor·da·ze·pam (nor′daz - pam). Nordazepam. Sedativo-hipnótico ativo da classe dos benzodiazepínicos; metabólito ativo do diazepam, do clorazepato e de vários outros benzodiazepínicos; possui meia-vida biológica prolongada (40–80 horas).

nor·def·rin hy·dro·chlo·ride (nōr - def′rin). Cloridrato de nordefrina. Simpaticomimético e vasoconstritor.

nor·ep·i·neph·rine (nōr′ep - i - nef′rin). Norepinefrina. Álcool L-(−)-α-(aminometil)-3,4-diidroxibenzílico; hormônio catecolamínico cuja forma natural é D, apesar de a forma L exibir alguma atividade; a base é considerada o mediador adrenérgico pós-ganglionar, atuando sobre os receptores α e β; é armazenada em grânulos cromafins na medula supra-renal, em quantidades muito menores do que a epinefrina, e secretada em resposta à hipotensão e ao estresse físico; em contraste com a epinefrina, exerce pouco efeito sobre o músculo liso brônquico, processos metabólitos e débito cardíaco, porém possui efeitos vasoconstritores pronunciados e é utilizada farmacologicamente como vasopressor, primariamente na forma do sal bitartarato. SIN levarterenol, noradrenaline.
n. bitartrate, n. bitartarato de n.; tartarato do álcool (-)-α-(aminometil)-3,4-diidroxibenzílico. Para suas ações e usos, ver n. SIN levarterenol bitartrate, noradrenaline acid tartrate, noradrenaline bitartrate.

nor·eth·an·dro·lone (nōr - eth - an′drō - lōn). Noretandrolona. Esteróide androgênico química e farmacologicamente semelhante à testosterona.

nor·eth·in·drone (nōr - eth′in - drōn). Noretindrona. Poderoso agente progestacional efetivo por via oral, com alguma atividade estrogênica e androgênica; utilizada como substituto da progesterona e, em combinação com um estrogênio, como anticoncepcional oral. SIN norethisterone.
n. acetate, acetato de n.; progestina ativa por via oral, com alguma atividade estrogênica e androgênica, utilizada no tratamento da endometriose e, com um estrogênio, como anticoncepcional oral.

nor·eth·is·ter·one (nōr - eth - is′ter - ōn). Noretisterona. SIN norethindrone.

nor·e·thyn·o·drel (nōr - ē - thī′nō - drel). Noretinodrel. Progestina ativa por via oral, com alguma atividade estrogênica; utilizado como agente progestacional e, em combinação com mestranol, como anticoncepcional oral.

nor·flox·a·cin (nōr - floks′ă - sin). Norfloxacina. Agente antibacteriano quinolínico oral de amplo espectro, utilizado no tratamento de infecções das vias urinárias.

nor·ges·trel (nōr - jes′trel). Norgestrel. Progestina utilizada em produtos anticoncepcionais orais.

nor·leu·cine (Nle) (nōr - loo′sin). Norleucina. Ácido α-amino-*n*-capróico; ácido 2-amino-hexanóico; α-aminoácido, isômero da leucina e da isoleucina, mas não encontrado em proteínas, produto de desaminação da L-lisina, a qual está ligado nos colágenos. SIN glycoleucine.

norm. Norma. **1.** O valor usual. **2.** O valor ou comportamento desejável.

nor·ma, pl. **nor·mae** (nōr′mă, nōr′mē). **1.** Face, expressão. SIN aspect. **2.** Perfil. SIN profile (1). **3.** Projeção. SIN projection. [L. esquadro de carpinteiro]
n. ante′rior, n. anterior. SIN facial *aspect*.
n. basilaris, n. basilar. SIN external *surface* of cranial base.

n. facia′lis [TA], n. facial. SIN facial *aspect*.
n. fronta′lis, n. frontal; *termo oficial alternativo para facial *aspect*.
n. infe′rior, n. inferior. SIN external *surface* of cranial base.
n. latera′lis [TA], n. lateral. SIN lateral *aspect*.
n. occipita′lis [TA], n. occipital. SIN occipital *aspect*.
n. poste′rior, n. posterior. SIN occipital *aspect*.
n. sagitta′lis, n. sagital; o contorno de um corte sagital através do crânio.
n. supe′rior [TA], n. superior. SIN superior *aspect*.
n. tempora′lis, n. temporal. SIN lateral *aspect*.
n. ventra′lis, n. ventral. SIN external *surface* of cranial base.
n. vertica′lis, n. vertical; *termo oficial alternativo para superior *aspect*.
nor·mal (N) (nōr′măl). Normal. **1.** Típico; usual; de acordo com a regra ou o padrão. **2.** Em bacteriologia, não-imune; não-tratado; refere-se a um animal ou ao soro ou substância nele contida, que não foi experimental ou naturalmente imunizado contra qualquer microrganismo ou seus produtos. **3.** Refere-se a uma solução contendo 1 eq de hidrogênio (ou hidroxila substituível) por litro; p. ex., 1 mol/L de HCl é 1N, porém 1 mol/L de H_2SO_4 é 2 N. **4.** Em psiquiatria e psicologia, indica um nível de funcionamento efetivo que é satisfatório tanto para o indivíduo quanto para seu meio social. **5.** Refere-se a uma linha reta (ou plano) em ângulo reto com outra linha (ou plano). **6.** Sem doença ou que não foi submetido a procedimento experimental. [L. *normalis*, de acordo com o padrão]
nor·mal·i·za·tion (nōr′mal - i - zā′shŭn). Normalização. **1.** Que está se tornando normal ou de acordo com o padrão. **2.** Redução ou concentração de uma solução para torná-la normal. **3.** Ajuste de uma curva para outra através da multiplicação dos pontos de uma por algum fator arbitrário.
nor·mal·ize (nōr′măl - īz). Normalizar. Efetuar a normalização.
nor·ma·tive. Normativo. Relativo ao normal ou usual.
nor·me·per·i·dine (nōr - mep′er - ĭ - dīn). Normeperidina. Metabólito da meperidina em que foi removido o grupamento *N*-metil. O composto possui propriedades convulsivantes.
nor·met·a·neph·rine (nōr - met′ă - nef′rin). Normetanefrina. Catabólito da norepinefrina encontrado, juntamente com a metanefrina, na urina e em alguns tecidos, resultante da ação da catecol-*O*-metiltransferase sobre a norepinefrina; não possui ações simpaticomiméticas.
nor·meth·a·done (nōr - meth′ă - dōn). Normetadona. Antitussígeno com propriedades narcóticas.
♻ **normo-.** Normo-. Normal, usual. [L. *normalis*, de acordo com o padrão]
nor·mo·bar·ic (nōr - mō - bar′ik). Normobárico. Refere-se a uma pressão barométrica equivalente à pressão ao nível do mar. [normo- + G. *baros*, peso]
nor·mo·blast (nōr′mō - blast). Normoblasto. Eritrócito nucleado, precursor imediato do eritrócito normal nos seres humanos. Seus quatro estágios de desenvolvimento são: 1) pronormoblasto, 2) normoblasto basófilo, 3) normoblasto policromático e 4) normoblasto ortocromático. VER erythroblast. [normo- + G. *blastos*, broto, germe]
nor·mo·blas·to·sis. Normoblastose. Produção excessiva de normoblastos pela medula óssea.
nor·mo·cap·nia (nōr - mō - kap′nē - ă). Normocapnia. Estado em que a pressão arterial de dióxido de carbono é normal, de cerca de 40 mm Hg. VER TAMBÉM eucapnia. [normo- + G. *kapnos*, vapor]
nor·mo·ce·phal·ic (nōr′mō - se - fal′ik). Normocefálico. SIN mesocephalic. [normo- + G. *kephalē*, cabeça]
nor·mo·chro·mia (nōr - mō - krō′mē - ă). Normocromia. Cor normal; refere-se ao sangue em que a quantidade de hemoglobina nos eritrócitos é normal. [normo- + G. *chrōma*, cor]
nor·mo·chro·mic (nōr - mō - krō′mik). Normocrômico. Normal quanto à cor; refere-se especialmente a eritrócitos que possuem uma quantidade normal de hemoglobina.
nor·mo·cyte (nōr′mō - sīt). Normócito. Eritrócito não-nucleado de tamanho normal (em média 7,5 μm); eritrócito sadio normal. SIN normoerythrocyte. [normo- + G. *kytos*, célula]
nor·mor·cy·to·sis (nōr′mō - sī - tō′sis). Normocitose. Estado normal do sangue em relação a seus elementos figurados.
nor·mo·e·ryth·ro·cyte (nōr′mō - ĕ - rith′rō - sīt). Normoeritrócito. SIN normocyte.
nor·mo·gly·ce·mia (nōr′mō - glī - sē′mē - ă). Normoglicemia. SIN euglycemia.
nor·mo·gly·ce·mic (nōr′mō - glī - sē′mik). Normoglicêmico. SIN euglycemic.
nor·mo·ka·le·mia, nor·mo·ka·li·e·mia (nōr′mō - kā - lē′mē - ă, - ka - lē - ē′mē - ă). Normocaliemia, normopotassemia. Nível normal de potássio no sangue.
nor·mo·sthe·nu·ria (nōr′mō - sthĕ - noo′rē - ă). Normostenúria. Condição em que a densidade da urina é normal. [normo- + G. *sthenos*, força + *ouron*, urina]
nor·mo·ten·sive (nōr - mō - ten′siv). Normotenso. Refere-se a uma pressão arterial normal. SIN normotonic (2).
nor·mo·ther·mia (nōr - mō - ther′mē - ă). Normotermia. Temperatura ambiental que não produz aumento nem redução da atividade das células corporais. [normo- + G. *thermē*, calor]

nor·mo·ton·ic (nōr - mō - ton′ik). **1.** Normotônico; relativo a, ou caracterizado por, tônus muscular normal. SIN eutonic. **2.** Normotenso. SIN normotensive.
nor·mo·to·pia (nōr - mō - tō′pē - ă). Normotopia. O estado de estar no lugar normal; utilizado para referir-se à posição normal de um órgão. [normo- + G. *topos*, lugar]
nor·mo·top·ic (nōr - mō - top′ik). Normotópico. Relativo à normotopia; no lugar certo.
nor·mo·vol·e·mia (nōr′mō - vol - ē′mē - ă). Normovolemia. Volume sanguíneo normal. [normo- + volume, + G. *haima*, sangue]
nor·mox·ia (nōr - mok′sē - ă). Normoxia. Estado em que a pressão parcial de oxigênio no gás inspirado é igual à do ar ao nível do mar, de cerca de 150 mm Hg. [normo- + oxigênio]
nor·oph·thal·mic ac·id (nōr′of - thal - mik). Ácido noroftálmico. Análogo tripeptídico da glutationa (L-cisteína substituída por L-alanina), encontrado na lente do olho.
nor·pi·pa·none (nōr - pip′ă - nōn). Norpipanona. Agente analgésico.
Norrie, Gordon, oftalmologista holandês, 1855–1941. VER N. *disease*.
Norris, Richard, fisiologista inglês, 1830–1916. VER N. *corpuscles*, em *corpuscle*.
nor·ster·oids (nōr - stēr′oydz). Noresteróides. Esteróides em que falta um grupamento metila angular; mais comumente, o grupamento entre os anéis A e B (C-19).
nor·sym·pa·tol (nōr - sim′pă - tōl). Norsimpatol. SIN octopamine.
nor·sy·neph·rine (nōr - si - nef′rin). Norsinefrina. SIN octopamine.
Norton, Larry, oncologista norte-americano do século XX. VER N.-Smon *hypothesis*.
Norton, U.F., obstetra norte-americano. VER N. *operation*.
nor·trip·ty·line hy·dro·chlo·ride (nōr - trip′ti - lēn). Cloridrato de nortriptilina. Antidepressivo.
nor·val·ine (Nva) (nōr - val′ēn, - vā′lēn). Ácido α-aminovalérico; análogo de cadeia retilínea da valina; não encontrado em proteínas.
nos·ca·pine (nos′ka - pēn). Noscapina. Alcalóide isoquinolínico, que ocorre no ópio, com ação semelhante à da papaverina sobre o músculo liso; suprime o reflexo da tosse e é utilizado como antitussígeno; parece não apresentar risco de dependência. SIN L-α-narcotine, opianine.
nose (nōz). Nariz. A porção das vias respiratórias acima do palato duro; inclui tanto o nariz externo quanto a cavidade nasal. SIN nasus (2). [A.S. *nosu*]
brandy n., rinofima. SIN rhinophyma.
cleft n., fenda nasal; nariz com fenda causada pela falta de convergência completa dos primórdios embrionários.
copper n., rinofima. SIN rhinophyma.
dog n., goundou. SIN goundou.
external n., n. externo; a porção visível do nariz que forma um aspecto proeminente da face; consiste numa raiz, no dorso e no ápice de cima para baixo, sendo perfurado inferiormente por duas narinas separadas por um septo. SIN nasus externus, nasus (1).
hammer n., rinofima. SIN rhinophyma.
potato n., rinofima. VER rhinophyma.
rum n., rinofima. SIN rhinophyma.
saddle n., n. em sela; nariz com acentuada depressão da ponte, observado na sífilis congênita, após lesão por traumatismo, cirurgia ou infecção do septo nasal.
toper's n., rinofima. SIN rhinophyma.
nose·bleed (nōz′blēd). Sangramento nasal, epistaxe. SIN epistaxis.
No·se·ma (nō - sē′mă). Nosema. Gênero de protozoários (família Nosematidae, ordem Microsporida, filo Microspora) com espécies (*N. apis*, *N. bombycis* e outras) patogênicas para invertebrados de importância econômica (abelhas, bicho-da-seda); outras estão sendo estudadas como possíveis agentes de controle biológico de pragas ou outros invertebrados. *N. connori* infecta o tecido adiposo, o diafragma, o miocárdio, o fígado e outros tecidos de indivíduos imunossuprimidos. [G. *nosēma*, peste, de *noseō*, estar doente, de *nosos*, doença]
N. corneum, *N. corneum*; causa de ceratoconjuntivite e de ceratopatia puntiforme difusa em pacientes com AIDS/SIDA.
No·se·mat·i·dae (nō - sē - mat′i - dē). Nosematidae. Família da classe Microsporida que inclui os gêneros *Encephalitozoon* e *Nosema*, contendo diversas espécies patogênicas e economicamente importantes.
no·sem·a·to·sis (nō - sē′ma - tō′sis). Nosematose. Infecção de coelhos pelo protozoário parasita *Encephalitozoon cuniculi*, que pode causar nefrite intersticial focal; foi relatado caso de nosematose em seres humanos.
nose·piece (nōz′pēs). Porta-objetiva. Acessório de microscópio que consiste em diversas objetivas em torno de um pivô central.
nos·e·ti·ol·o·gy (nōs′ē - tē - ol′ō - jē). Nosetiologia. Termo raramente utilizado para referir-se ao estudo das causas da doença. [G. *nosos*, doença + *aitia*, causa + *logòs*, estudo]
♻ **noso-.** Noso-. Doença. VER TAMBÉM path-. [G. *nosos*]
no·so·ac·u·sis (nō - sō - ak - ū′sis). Nosoacusia. Perda da audição devido a doença, em oposição ao envelhecimento. [nosso- + G. *akousis*, audição]

nos·och·tho·nog·ra·phy (nos'ok-thō-nog'ră-fē). Nosoctonografia. SIN geomedicine. [noso- + G. *chthōn*, a terra + *graphē*, descrição]

nos·o·co·mi·al (nos-ō-kō'mē-ăl). Nosocomial, hospitalar. **1.** Relativo a um hospital. **2.** Refere-se a um novo distúrbio (mas não à condição original do paciente) associado ao tratamento hospitalar, como uma infecção adquirida em hospital. [G. *nosokomeion*, hospital, de *nosos*, doença + *komeō*, cuidar]

nos·o·gen·e·sis, no·sog·e·ny (nos-ō-jen'e-sis, no-soj'e-nē). Nosogênese, nosogenia. Termos raramente utilizados para patogenis. [noso- + G. *genesis*, produção]

nos·o·gen·ic (nos-ō-jen'ik). Nosogênico. SIN pathogenic.

nos·o·ge·og·ra·phy (nos'ō-jē-og'rā-fē). Nosogeografia. SIN geomedicine.

nos·o·graph·ic (nos-ō-graf'ik). Nosográfico. Relativo à nosografia ou descrição de doenças.

no·sog·ra·phy (nō-sog'rā-fē). Nosografia. **1.** Nomes dados a cada entidade mórbida num grupo que foi classificado de acordo com uma nosologia sistemática. **2.** Tratado de patologia ou prática de medicina. [noso- + G. *graphē*, descrição]

nos·o·log·ic (nos-ō-loj'ik). Nosológico. Relativo à nosologia.

no·sol·o·gy (nō-sol'ō-jē). Nosologia. A ciência da classificação das doenças. SIN nosonomy, nosotaxy. [noso- + G. *logos*, estudo]

psychiatric n., n. psiquiátrica. SIN psychonosology.

nos·o·ma·ni·a (nos-ō-mā'nē-ă). Nosomania. Termo raramente utilizado para referir-se a uma crença mórbida, infundada, de que se está sofrendo de alguma doença especial. [noso- + G. *mania*, mania]

nos·om·e·try (nō-som'e-trē). Nosometria. Medida da morbidade ou da taxa de doença em condições profissionais e sociais. [noso- + G. *metron*, medida]

nos·o·my·co·sis (nos'ō-mī-kō'sis). Nosomicose. Qualquer doença causada por fungo. [noso- + G. *mykēs*, fungo]

no·son·o·my (nō-son'ō-mē). Nosonomia. SIN nosology. [noso- + G. *nomos*, lei]

nos·o·phil·i·a (nos-ō-fil'ē-ă). Nosofilia. Desejo mórbido de estar doente. [noso- + G. *phileō*, gostar]

nos·o·pho·bi·a (nos-ō-fō'bē-ă). Nosofobia. Medo e pavor incomum de doença. SIN pathophobia. [noso- + G. *phobos*, medo]

nos·o·phyte (nos'ō-fīt). Nosófito. Microrganismo patogênico do reino vegetal. [noso- + G. *phyton*, planta]

nos·o·poi·et·ic (nos'ō-poy-et'ik). Nosopoético. SIN pathogenic. [noso- + G. *poiēsis*, produção]

Nos·o·psyl·lus (nos-ō-sil'ŭs). *Nosopsyllus.* Gênero de pulga comumente encontrado em roedores. *N. fasciatus*, a pulga do rato do norte, é uma espécie que raramente transmite o bacilo da peste a seres humanos. [noso- + G. *psylla*, pulga]

nos·o·tax·y (nos'ō-tak-sē). Nosotaxia. SIN nosology. [noso- + G. *taxis*, distribuição]

nos·o·tox·ic (nos-ō-tok'sik). Nosotóxico. Relativo a uma nosotoxina ou à nosotoxicose.

nos·o·tox·i·co·sis (nos'ō-tok-si-kō'sis). Nosotoxicose. Estado mórbido causado por uma toxina. VER TAMBÉM toxicosis. [noso- + G. *toxikon*, veneno]

nos·o·tox·in (nos-ō-tok'sin). Nosotoxina. Termo raramente empregado para referir-se a qualquer toxina associada a uma doença.

no·sot·ro·phy (nō-ot'rō-fē). Nosotropia. Termo raramente utilizado para designar o cuidado com o paciente. [noso- + G. *trophē*, nutrição]

nos·o·tro·pic (nos-ō-trop'ik). Nosotrópico. Dirigido contra alterações patológicas ou sintomas de uma doença. [noso- + G. *tropē*, uma volta]

nos·tal·gia (nos-tal'jē-ă). Nostalgia. Ânsia para regressar ao lar, para retornar a um período anterior da vida ou para pessoas e ambiente familiares. [G. *nostos*, regresso (ao lar) + *algos*, dor]

nos·to·ma·ni·a (nos-tō-ma'nē-ă). Nostomania. Termo raramente utilizado para referir-se ao interesse obsessivo ou anormal em nostalgia, especialmente como manifestação extrema de saudades. [G. *nostos*, regresso, volta ao lar + *mania*, mania]

nos·to·pho·bi·a (nos-tō-fō'bē-ă). Nostofobia. Medo mórbido de regressar ao lar. [G. *nostos*, regresso, retorno ao lar + *phobos*, medo]

nos·tril. Narina. SIN naris.

internal n., n. interna. SIN secondary choana.

nos·trum (nos'trŭm). Nostro. Termo genérico para referir-se a um agente terapêutico, algumas vezes registrado, mas habitualmente de composição secreta, oferecido ao público como remédio específico para qualquer doença ou classe de doenças. O termo tem atualmente uma conotação pejorativa. [L. neutro de *noster*, nosso, "nosso próprio remédio"]

NO syn·thase NO sintase. Abreviatura de *nitric oxide* synthase (óxido nítrico sintase).

no·tal (nō'tăl). Notal. Relativo às costas. [G. *nōtos*, costas]

no·tan·ce·pha·li·a (nō'tan-se-fā'lē-ă). Notancefalia. Malformação fetal caracterizada pela ausência do osso occipital do crânio. [G. *nōtos*, costas + *an-* priv. + *kephalē*, cabeça]

no·tan·en·ce·pha·li·a (nō'tan-en-se-fā'lē-ă). Notanencefalia. Ausência do cérebro. [G. *nōtos*, costas + *an-* priv. + *enkephalos*, cérebro]

no·ta·tin (nō-tā'tin). Notatina. Proteína (glicose oxidase) que foi especificamente isolada de *Penicillium notatum*. [de *Penicillium notatum*]

NOTCH

notch [TA]. Incisura, chanfradura. **1.** Indentação na borda de qualquer estrutura. **2.** Qualquer desvio curto, estreito, em forma de V, seja positivo ou negativo, num traçado linear. SIN incisura [TA], emargination, incisure.

acetabular n. [TA], i. acetabular; hiato na parte inferior da margem do acetábulo. SIN incisura acetabuli [TA], cotyloid n.

angular n., i. angular. SIN angular *incisure*.

antegonial n., i. antegonial; o ponto mais elevado da incisura ou concavidade da borda inferior do ramo, onde se une ao corpo da mandíbula.

anterior n. of auricle [TA], i. anterior da orelha; chanfradura entre o tubérculo supratragal e a cruz da hélice. SIN anterior auricular groove, anterior n. of ear, auricular n. (1), incisura anterior auris, sulcus auriculae anterior.

anterior cerebellar n., i. anterior do cerebelo; chanfradura superficial e larga na superfície anterior do cerebelo, ocupada lateralmente pelos pedúnculos cerebelares superiores e, medialmente, pelos corpos quadrigêmeos inferiores. SIN anterior n. of cerebellum, incisura cerebelli anterior, semilunar n. (1).

anterior n. of cerebellum, i. anterior do cerebelo. SIN anterior cerebellar n.

anterior n. of ear, i. anterior da orelha. SIN anterior n. of auricle.

aortic n., i. aórtica; a chanfradura no traçado esfingmográfico causada por rebote após fechamento das válvulas aórticas.

n. of apex of heart, i. do ápice cardíaco. SIN n. of cardiac apex.

auricular n., i. auricular; **(1)** SIN anterior n. of auricle; **(2)** SIN terminal n. of auricle.

cardiac n., i. da cárdia. SIN cardial n.

n. of cardiac apex [TA], i. do ápice cardíaco; discreta chanfradura próxima ao ápice do coração, onde o sulco interventricular anterior alcança a superfície diafragmática do coração. SIN incisura apicis cordis [TA], n. of apex of heart.

cardiac n. of left lung [TA], i. cardíaca do pulmão esquerda; a chanfradura na borda anterior do lobo superior do pulmão esquerdo, que acomoda o pericárdio. SIN incisura cardiaca pulmonis sinistri [TA].

cardial n. [TA], i. da cárdia; chanfradura profunda entre o esôfago e o fundo do estômago. SIN cardiac n., incisura cardiaca.

n. in cartilage of acoustic meatus [TA], i. na cartilagem do meato acústico; (em geral) duas fissuras verticais na porção anterior da cartilagem do meato auditivo externo, preenchidas por tecido fibroso. SIN incisura cartilaginis meatus acustici [TA], Duverney fissures, incisura santorini, Santorini fissures, Santorini incisures.

clavicular n. of sternum [TA], i. clavicular do esterno; depressão em cada lado da superfície superior do manúbrio do esterno, que se articula com a clavícula. SIN incisura clavicularis [TA], clavicular facet.

costal n.'s [TA], i. costal; chanfraduras ou facetas na borda lateral do esterno para articulação com uma cartilagem costal. SIN incisurae costales [TA].

cotyloid n., i. cotilóide. SIN acetabular n.

dicrotic n. (dī-krot-ik), i. dicrótica; a queda aguda seguida de elevação nas curvas de pulso da pressão arterial após o pico sistólico, correspondendo à incisura do deslocamento da curva de pulso.

digastric n., i. digástrica. SIN mastoid n.

ethmoidal n. [TA], i. etmoidal; hiato oblongo entre as partes orbitárias do osso frontal onde se aloja o osso etmóide. SIN incisura ethmoidalis [TA].

fibular n. [TA], i. fibular; depressão na superfície lateral da extremidade inferior da tíbia, onde se aloja a fíbula. SIN incisura fibularis [TA].

frontal n. [TA], i. frontal; pequena chanfradura, algumas vezes um forame, na margem orbitária do osso frontal, medialmente à chanfradura supra-orbitária. SIN incisura frontalis [TA].

greater sciatic n. [TA], i. isquiática maior; a indentação profunda na borda posterior do ilíaco, no ponto de união do íleo com o ísquio. SIN incisura ischiadica major [TA], ilioscatic n., sacrosciatic n.

hamular n., i. hamular. SIN *groove* of pterygoid hamulus.

Hutchinson crescentic n., i. em crescente de Hutchinson; a chanfradura semilunar na borda incisiva dos dentes de Hutchinson, observada na sífilis congênita.

iliosciatic n., i. ilioisquiática. SIN greater sciatic n.

inferior thyroid n. [TA], i. tireóidea inferior; chanfradura superficial no meio da borda inferior da cartilagem tireóidea. SIN incisura thyroidea inferior [TA].

interarytenoid n. [TA], i. interaritenóidea; indentação da abertura superior da laringe entre as duas cartilagens aritenóideas. SIN incisura interarytenoidea [TA].

interclavicular n., i. interclavicular. SIN jugular n. of sternum.

intercondyloid n., n. intercondilóide. SIN intercondylar *fossa*.

intertragic n. [TA], i. intertrágica; chanfradura profunda na parte inferior da aurícula, entre o trago e antitrago. SIN incisura intertragica [TA], incisura tragica.

intervertebral n., i. intervertebral. SIN vertebral n.
ischiatic n., i. isquiática. VER greater sciatic n., lesser sciatic n.
jugular n. of occipital bone [TA], i. jugular do osso occipital; a chanfradura no osso occipital que forma um limite do forame jugular. SIN incisura jugularis ossis occipitalis [TA].
jugular n. of petrous part of temporal bone [TA], i. jugular da parte petrosa do osso temporal; a chanfradura na parte petrosa do osso temporal que forma um limite do forame jugular. SIN incisura jugulares ossis temporalis [TA].
jugular n. of sternum [TA], i. jugular do esterno; a grande chanfradura na margem superior do esterno. SIN incisura jugularis sternalis [TA], suprasternal n.*, interclavicular n., presternal n., sternal n.
Kernohan n., i. de Kernohan; uma incisura no pedúnculo cerebral causada pelo deslocamento do tronco cerebral contra a incisura do tentório por uma herniação transtentorial.
lacrimal n. [TA], i. lacrimal; a chanfradura no processo frontal do maxilar dentro da qual se encaixa o osso lacrimal. SIN incisura lacrimalis [TA].
lesser sciatic n. [TA], i. isquiática menor; chanfradura na borda posterior do ísquio, abaixo da espinha isquiática. SIN incisura ischiadica minor [TA].
n. for ligamentum teres [TA], i. para o ligamento redondo; a chanfradura na borda inferior do fígado, que acomoda o ligamento redondo. SIN incisura ligamenti teretis hepatis [TA], incisura umbilicalis, n. for round ligament of liver, umbilical n.
mandibular n. [TA], i. da mandíbula; chanfradura profunda nos processos condilar e coronóide da mandíbula. SIN incisura mandibulae [TA], sigmoid n.
marsupial n., i. marsupial. SIN posterior cerebellar n.
mastoid n. [TA], i. do mastóide; sulco medial ao processo mastóide do osso temporal, do qual se origina o músculo digástrico. SIN incisura mastoidea [TA], digastric groove, digastric n., mastoid groove.
nasal n. [TA], i. nasal; a chanfradura na borda medial do maxilar, anteriormente, que, com sua companheira, forma a maior parte da abertura piriforme da cavidade nasal. SIN incisura nasalis [TA].
pancreatic n. [TA], i. pancreática; chanfradura que separa o processo uncinado da cabeça do pâncreas do colo. SIN incisura pancreatis [TA].
parietal n. [TA], i. parietal; ângulo posterior entre as partes escamosa e petrosa do osso temporal. SIN incisura parietalis [TA].
parotid n., i. parótida; o espaço entre o ramo da mandíbula e o processo mastóide do osso temporal.
popliteal n., i. poplítea. SIN intercondylar fossa.
posterior cerebellar n., i. posterior do cerebelo; chanfradura estreita entre os hemisférios cerebelares posteriormente, ocupada pela foice do cerebelo. SIN incisura cerebelli posterior, marsupial n., posterior n. of cerebellum.
posterior n. of cerebellum, i. posterior do cerebelo. SIN posterior cerebellar n.
preoccipital n. [TA], i. pré-occipital; indentação na borda ventrolateral do lobo temporal do hemisfério cerebral. SIN incisura preoccipitalis [TA].
presternal n., i. pré-esternal. SIN jugular n. of sternum.
pterygoid n. [TA], i. pterigóide; a fenda entre as placas medial e lateral do processo pterigóide do osso esfenóide, onde se aloja o processo piramidal do osso palatino. SIN fissura pterygoidea, incisura pterygoidea, pterygoid fissure.
pterygomaxillary n., i. pterigomaxilar. SIN groove of pterygoid hamulus.
radial n. [TA], i. radial; a concavidade na face lateral do processo coronóide da ulna, que se articula com a cabeça do rádio. SIN incisura radialis [TA].
Rivinus n., i. de Rivinus. SIN tympanic n.
n. for round ligament of liver, i. para o ligamento redondo do fígado. SIN n. for ligamentum teres.
sacrosciatic n., i. sacroisquiática. SIN greater sciatic n.
scapular n., i. escapular. SIN suprascapular n.
semilunar n., i. semilunar; **(1)** SIN anterior cerebellar n; **(2)** SIN trochlear n.
sigmoid n., i. sigmóide. SIN mandibular n.
sphenopalatine n. [TA], i. esfenopalatina; chanfradura profunda entre os processos orbitário e esfenóide do osso palatino, que é convertida no forame do mesmo nome pela superfície inferior do osso esfenóide. SIN incisura sphenopalatina [TA].
sternal n., i. esternal. SIN jugular n. of sternum.
superior thyroid n. [TA], i. tireóidea superior; chanfradura profunda no meio da borda superior da cartilagem tireóidea. SIN incisura thyroidea superior [TA].
supraorbital n. [TA], i. supra-orbitária; sulco na margem orbitária do osso frontal, próximo à junção dos terços medial e intermédio, através do qual passam o nervo e a artéria supra-orbitária. VER TAMBÉM supraorbital foramen. SIN incisura supraorbitalis [TA].
suprascapular n., i. supra-escapular; chanfradura na borda superior da escápula, através da qual passa o nervo supra-escapular. SIN incisura scapulae [TA], scapular n.
suprasternal n., i. supra-esternal; *termo oficial alternativo para jugular n. of sternum.
tentorial n. [TA], i. tentorial; a abertura triangular no tentório do cerebelo através da qual o tronco cerebral se estende da fossa craniana posterior a fossa média. SIN incisura tentorii [TA], incisura of tentorium*, n. of tentorium.
n. of tentorium, i. do tentório. SIN tentorial n.
terminal n. of auricle [TA], i. terminal da aurícula; chanfradura profunda que separa a lâmina do trago e a cartilagem do meato auditivo externo da cartilagem auricular principal, estando os dois ligados abaixo pelo istmo. SIN incisura terminalis auricularis [TA], auricular n. (2), incisura terminalis auris.
trochlear n. [TA], i. da tróclea; grande chanfradura semicircular na extremidade proximal da ulna, entre o olecrânio e os processos coronóides, que se articula com a tróclea do úmero. SIN incisura trochlearis [TA], incisura semilunaris ulnae, semilunar n. (2).
tympanic n. [TA], i. timpânica; chanfradura na parte superior do anel timpânico transposta pela parte flácida da membrana do tímpano. SIN incisura tympanica [TA], incisura rivini, Rivinus incisure, Rivinus n., tympanic incisure.
ulnar n. [TA], i. da ulna; superfície côncava no lado medial da extremidade distal do rádio, que se articula com a cabeça da ulna. SIN incisura ulnaris [TA].
umbilical n., i. umbilical. SIN n. for ligamentum teres.
vertebral n. [TA], i. vertebral; uma das duas concavidades acima (superior) e abaixo (inferior) do pedículo de uma vértebra; as chanfraduras de duas vértebras adjacentes (mais o disco intervertebral) formam um forame intervertebral. SIN incisura vertebralis [TA], intervertebral n.

notched. Chanfrado. SIN emarginate.
no·ten·ceph·a·lo·cele (nō-ten-sef′a-lō-sēl). Notencefalocele. Malformação na porção occipital do crânio, com protrusão da substância cerebral. [G. nōtos, dorso, costas + enkephalos, cérebro + kēlē, hérnia]
Nothnagel, C.W. Hermann, médico austríaco, 1841–1905. VER N. syndrome.
no·to·chord (nō′tō-kōrd). Notocorda. **1.** Nos vertebrados primitivos, refere-se à estrutura de suporte axial primário do corpo, derivada do processo notocordal ou da cabeça do embrião em fase inicial de desenvolvimento; trata-se de um importante organizador na determinação da forma final do sistema nervoso e estruturas correlatas. **2.** Nos embriões, refere-se à corda fibrocelular axial ao redor da qual se desenvolvem os primórdios vertebrais; persistem vestígios no adulto na forma dos núcleos pulposos dos discos intervertebrais. SIN chorda dorsalis. [G. nōtos, dorso, costas + chordē, corda, cordão]
no·to·chor·dal (nō-tō-kōr′dal). Notocordal. Relativo à notocorda.
No·to·ed·res cati (nō-tō-ed′rēz kā′tī). *Notoedres cati.* Ácaro da sarna sarcóptica de gatos.
nou·men·al (noo′men-al). Numênico. Intelectualmente, e não por meio dos sentidos, da emoção ou da intuição; refere-se ao objeto de pensamento puro, divorciado de todos os conceitos de tempo ou espaço. [G. nooumenos, percebido, de noeō, perceber, pensar]
nour·ish·ment (ner′ish-ment). Alimento. Substância utilizada para alimentar ou sustentar a vida e o crescimento de um organismo. SIN aliment (1).
nous (noos, nows). Nous. Palavra originalmente utilizada por Anaxágoras para referir-se a um espírito ou a uma força que tudo sabe e penetra; na filosofia grega posterior, passou a designar apenas a mente, a razão ou o intelecto. [G. mente, razão]
no·vo·bi·o·cin (nō-vō-bī′ō-sin). Novobiocina. Substância antibacteriana que atua como antibiótico, produzido por fermentação de culturas de *Streptomyces niveus* ou *S. spheroides,* efetiva contra *Staphylococcus* e *Proteus* resistentes à penicilina; também disponível na forma de novobiocina cálcica e novobiocina sódica. SIN streptonivicin.
Novy, Frederick George, bacteriologista norte-americano, 1864–1957. VER N. e MacNeal blood *agar.*
noxa (nok′sä). Noxa. Tudo que exerce uma influência prejudicial, como traumatismo, veneno, etc. [L. lesão, de *noceo,* lesar]
nox·ious (nok′shŭs). Nocivo. Lesivo; prejudicial. [L. *noxius,* lesivo, de *noceo,* lesar]
nox·y·thi·o·lin (nok-sē-thī′ō-lin). Noxitiolina. Agente antibacteriano e antifúngico.
Np 1. Np. Símbolo do netúnio. **2.** Abreviatura de neper.
NPC NPC. Abreviatura de Niemann-Pick C1 *disease* (doença de Niemann-Pick C1).
NPN NNP. Abreviatura de nonprotein *nitrogen* (nitrogênio não-proteico).
NPO, n.p.o.. Dieta zero. Abreviatura do L. *non per os* ou *nil per os,* nada pela boca.
Nps Nps. Abreviatura de nitrophenylsulfenyl (nitrofenilsulfenil).
NREM Abreviatura de nonrapid eye movement (movimento ocular não-rápido).
nRNA nRNA. Abreviatura de nuclear RNA (RNA nuclear).
NSAID AINE. Abreviatura de nonsteroidal anti-inflammatory *drugs* (antiinflamatórios não-esteróides), em *drug;* p. ex., ácido acetilsalicílico, ibuprofeno.
NSF Abreviatura de National Science Foundation.
NSILA Abreviatura de nonsuppressible insulinlike *activity* (atividade insulinosímile não-supressível).
NTMI Abreviatura de nontransmural myocardial *infarction* (infarto do miocárdio não-transmural).
NTNG Abreviatura de nontoxic nodular goiter (bócio nodular atóxico).
NTP NTP. Abreviatura de nucleoside 5′-triphosphate (nucleosídeo 5′-trifosfato).

nu (noo). Nu. Décima terceira letra do alfabeto grego, ν (q.v.).

nu·bec·u·la (noo-bek'ŭ-lă). Nubécula. Pequena mancha ou turvação. [L. dim. de *nubes*, nuvem]

Nuc Abreviatura de nucleoside (nucleosídeo).

nu·cha (noo'kă). Nuca. Parte posterior do pescoço. SIN nape (nuca). [Fr. *nuque*]

nu·chal (noo'kăl). Nucal. Relativo à nuca.

Nuck, Anton, anatomista holandês, 1650–1692. VER N. *diverticulum, hydrocele; canal* of N.

nucl-. Nucl-. VER nucleo-.

nu·cle·ar (noo'klē-er). Nuclear. Relativo a um núcleo, seja ele celular ou atômico; neste último sentido, o termo refere-se habitualmente à irradiação que emana dos núcleos atômicos (α, β e γ) ou à fissão atômica.

Nuclear Regulatory Commission. Comissão Federal dos Estados Unidos que supervisiona o uso de material radioativo para fins comerciais e médicos; sucessora da Atomic Energy Commission, juntamente com o U.S. Department of Energy.

nu·cle·ase (noo'klē-ās). Nuclease. Termo genérico para designar enzimas que catalisam a hidrólise do ácido nucleico em nucleotídeos ou oligonucleotídeos pela clivagem das ligações fosfodiéster. Para as nucleases não relacionadas a seguir, ver o termo específico. Cf. exonuclease, endonuclease.

azotobacter n., azotobacter n.; endonuclease (*Serratia marcescens*).

micrococcal n., n. micrócica. SIN micrococcal *endonuclease.*

mung bean n., endonuclease S$_1$ (*Aspergillus*).

nu·cle·ate (noo'klē-āt). Nucleato. Sal de um ácido nucleico.

nu·cle·at·ed (noo'klē-ā-ted). Nucleado. Que possui um núcleo, uma característica de todas as células verdadeiras.

nu·cle·a·tion (noo-klē-ā'shŭn). Nucleação. Processo de formação de um ninho [nidus (4)].

heterogeneous n., n. heterogênea; nucleação ao redor de um ninho composto de material diferente do material precipitante.

homogeneous n., n. homogênea; nucleação ao redor de um ninho composto de material idêntico ao material precipitante.

nu·clei (noo'klē-ī). Núcleos. Plural de nucleus.

nu·cle·ic ac·id (noo-klē'ik, -klā'ik). Ácido nucleico. Família de macromoléculas de massas moleculares a partir de 25.000, encontradas nos cromossomas, nucléolos, mitocôndrias e citoplasma de todas as células, bem como nos vírus; quando formam complexos com proteínas, são denominadas nucleoproteínas. Na hidrólise, produzem purinas, pirimidinas, ácido fosfórico e uma pentose, que pode ser D-ribose ou D-desoxirribose; com base nestas últimas, os ácidos nucleicos recebem designações mais específicas: ácido ribonucleico e ácido desoxirribonucleico. Os ácidos nucleicos são cadeias lineares (isto é, não-ramificadas) de nucleotídeos, em que o grupamento 5′-fosfórico de cada um é esterificado com a 3′-hidroxila do nucleotídeo adjacente.

infectious n. a., ácido nucleico infeccioso; ácido nucleico viral capaz de infectar células e permitir a produção de vírus.

nu·cle·i·form (noo'klē-i-form). Nucleiforme. Que tem a forma semelhante a, ou o aspecto de, um núcleo. SIN nucleoid (1).

nucleo-, nucl-. Nucleo-, nucl-. Núcleo, nuclear. VER TAMBÉM karyo-, caryo-. [L. *nucleus*]

nu·cle·o·cap·sid (noo'klē-ō-kap'sid). Nucleocapsídeo. VER virion.

nu·cle·o·chy·le·ma (noo-klē-ō-kī-lē'mă). Nucleoquilema. SIN karyolymph. [nucleo- + G. *chylos*, suco]

nu·cle·o·chyme (noo'klē-ō-kīm). Nucleoquimo. SIN karyolymph.

nu·cle·o·fil·a·ments (noo'klē-ō-fil'-a-ments). Nucleofilamentos. Forma filamentar de cromossoma formada em soluções de força iônica baixa; as fibras têm cerca de 100 Å de largura e possuem um aspecto em cordão de pérolas.

nu·cle·o·his·tone (noo'klē-ō-his'tōn). Núcleo-histona. Complexo de histona e ácido desoxirribonucleico, a forma na qual este último é habitualmente encontrado nos núcleos das células; a núcleo-histona pode ser considerada como um sal entre a proteína básica e o ácido nucleico ácido.

nu·cle·oid (noo'klē-oyd). Nucleóide. **1.** SIN nucleiform. **2.** Corpúsculo de inclusão nuclear. **3.** SIN nucleus (2). [nucleo- + G. *eidos*, semelhança]

Lavdovsky n., n. de Lavdovsky. SIN astrosphere.

nu·cle·o·lar (noo-klē'ō-lăr). Nucleolar. Relativo a um nucléolo.

nu·cle·o·li (noo-klē'ō-lī). Nucléolos. Plural de nucleolus.

nu·cle·o·li·form (noo-klē'ō-lē-form). Nucleoliforme. Semelhante a um nucléolo. SIN nucleoloid.

nu·cle·o·loid (noo-klē'ō-loyd). Nucleolóide. SIN nucleoliform. [nucleolus + G. *eidos*, semelhança]

nu·cle·o·lo·ne·ma (noo-klē'ō-lō-nē'mă). Nucleolonema. Rede irregular ou fileiras de finos grânulos ribonucleoproteicos ou microfilamentos que formam a maior parte do nucléolo. [nucleolus + G. *nēma*, fio]

nu·cle·o·lus, pl. **nu·cle·o·li** (noo-klē'ō-lŭs, -lī). Nucléolo. **1.** Pequena massa arredondada no interior do núcleo da célula, onde é produzida a ribonucleoproteína; em geral, é único, mas podem ser observados diversos nucléolos acessórios além do principal. O nucléolo é composto de uma rede (nucleolonema) de microfilamentos e grânulos e da parte amorfa, atualmente considerada como possuindo também microfilamentos. **2.** Corpúsculo mais ou menos central existente no núcleo vesicular de certos protozoários nos quais falta um endossoma, porém com presença de um ou mais nucléolos Feulgen-positivos (DNA+); característica de certos esporozoários, flagelados, opaliníeos, dinoflagelados e radiolários entre os Protozoários. A cromatina distribui-se por todo o núcleo, mais do que perifericamente, como no tipo de endossoma do núcleo de *Entamoeba*. [L. dim de *nucleus,* núcleo, semente]

chromatin n., n. de cromatina. SIN karyosome.

false n., n. falso. SIN karyosome.

nu·cle·o·mi·cro·some (noo'klē-ō-mī'krō-sōm). Nucleomicrossoma. SIN karyomicrosome.

nu·cle·on (noo'klē-on). Nucleon. **1.** Uma das partículas subatômicas do núcleo atômico, isto é, um próton ou um nêutron. **2.** Termo jargão para referir-se ao especialista em medicina nuclear. [nucleus + -on]

Nu·cle·oph·a·ga (noo-klē-of'a-gă). *Nucleophaga.* Parasita do filo microspora de amebas, que destrói o núcleo de seu hospedeiro. [nucleo- + G. *phagō,* fago]

nu·cle·o·phil, nu·cle·o·phile (noo'klē-ō-fil, -fīl). Nucleófilo. **1.** O átomo doador de um par de elétrons numa reação química, em que o par de elétrons é capturado por um eletrófilo; qualquer reagente ou substância atraída para uma região de baixa densidade eletrônica. **2.** Relativo a um nucleófilo. SIN nucleophilic (1). [nucleo- + G. *philos*, amigo]

nu·cle·o·phil·ic (noo'klē-ō-fil'ik). Nucleofílico. **1.** SIN nucleophil (2). **2.** Reação que envolve um nucleófilo.

nu·cle·o·phos·pha·tas·es (noo'klē-ō-fos'fă-tās-ez). Nucleofosfatases. SIN nucleotidases.

nu·cle·o·plasm (noo'klē-ō-plazm). Nucleoplasma. O protoplasma do núcleo de uma célula.

nu·cle·o·plas·min (noo'klē-ō-plas'min). Nucleoplasmina. Conteúdo do núcleo em repouso (interfase). [nucleo- + plasma + -in]

nu·cle·o·pro·tein (noo'klē-ō-prō'tēn) Nucleoproteína. Complexo de proteína e ácido nucleico, a forma na qual praticamente todos os ácidos nucleicos existem na natureza; os cromossomas e os vírus são, em grande parte, nucleoproteínas.

nu·cle·o·re·tic·u·lum (noo'klē-ō-re-tik'ŭ-lŭm). Nucleorretículo. A rede intranuclear de cromatina ou linina. [nucleo- + L. *reticulum,* dim. de *rete*, rede]

nu·cle·or·rhex·is (noo'klē-ō-rek'sis). Nucleorrexe. Fragmentação de um núcleo celular. [nucleo- + G. *rhēxis*, ruptura]

nu·cle·o·si·das·es (noo'klē-ō-sī'dās-ez). Nucleosidases. Enzimas (particularmente do subgrupo EC 3.2.2) que catalisam a hidrólise ou fosforólise de nucleosídeos, liberando a base purina ou pirimidina.

nu·cle·o·side (Nuc, N) (noo'klē-ō-sīd). Nucleosídeo. Composto de um açúcar (habitualmente ribose ou desoxirribose) com uma base de purina ou pirimidina através de uma ligação *N*-glicosil.

n. bisphosphate, n. bisfosfato; nucleosídeo que transporta dois resíduos fosfóricos independentes (isto é, não ligados entre si). Cf. n. diphosphate.

n. diphosphate (NDP), n. difosfato; o éster pirofosfórico de um nucleosídeo, isto é, um nucleosídeo em que o H de uma das hidroxilas da ribose (geralmente a 5′) é substituído por um radical pirofosfórico (difosfórico); p. ex., adenosina 5′-difosfato. Cf. n. bisphosphate.

n. monophosphate, n. monofosfato; nucleosídeo que contém apenas um grupo fosforil, como, p. ex., AMP.

n. triphosphate, n. trifosfato; nucleosídeo em que o H de uma das hidroxilas da ribose (geralmente a 5′) é substituído por um grupamento trifosfórico, –PO–(OH)–O–PO(OH)–O–PO(OH)$_2$ ou pela base conjugada correspondente; p. ex., trifosfato de adenosina.

nu·cle·o·side di·phos·phate ki·nase. Nucleosídeo difosfato cinase. Fosfotransferase que catalisa reversivelmente a transferência de um grupamento fosforil do ATP para um nucleosídeo difosfato, produzindo um nucleosídeo trifosfato e ADP.

nu·cle·o·side di·phos·phate sug·ars. Açúcares de nucleosídeo difosfato. Nucleosídeos difosfatos ligados através do grupamento 5′-difosfórico com carboidratos simples ou complexos; p. ex., GDP-manose, UDP-glicose (UDPG), dTDP-glicosamina.

nu·cle·o·skel·e·ton (noo'klē-ō-skel'ē-ton). Nucleoesqueleto. Proteínas que formam uma subestrutura fibrilar da matriz nuclear à qual está ligado o DNA.

nu·cle·o·some (noo'klē-ō-sōm). Nucleossoma. Agregação localizada de histona e DNA, que se torna evidente quando a cromatina está no estágio não-condensado. [nucleo- + G. *sōma*, corpo]

nu·cleo·spin·dle (noo'klē-ō-spin'dl). Fusonuclear. O corpo fusiforme na mitose.

nu·cle·o·ti·das·es (noo'klē-ō-tī-dās-ez). Nucleotidases. Enzimas (EC 3.1.3.x) que catalisam a hidrólise de nucleotídeos em ácido fosfórico e nucleosídeos; as especificidades estão indicadas pelos prefixos 3′- e 5′-. SIN nucleophosphatases.

nu·cle·o·tide (noo'klē-ō-tīd). Nucleotídeo. Originalmente, uma combinação de (ácido nucleico) purina ou pirimidina, um açúcar (em geral, ribose ou desoxirribose) e um grupo fosfórico, por extensão, qualquer composto contendo

um composto heterocíclico ligado a um açúcar fosforilado por uma ligação N-glicosil (p. ex., adenosina monofosfato, NAD$^+$). Para os nucleotídeos individuais, ver os nomes específicos. SIN mononucleotide.
cyclic n., n. cíclico; nucleosídeo monofosfato em que o grupo fosforil está ligado duas vezes ao açúcar; p. ex., adenosina 3′,5′-monofosfato cíclico (AMPc).
flavin n., n. de flavina. VER flavin.
nu·cle·o·tid·yl·trans·fer·as·es (noo′klē-ō-ti′dil-trans′fer-ās-ez). Nucleotidiltransferases. Enzimas (EC 2.7.7.x) que transferem resíduos de nucleotídeos (nucleotidilas) de nucleosídeo di ou trifosfatos em formas diméricas ou poliméricas. Algumas dessas enzimas possuem nomes específicos (p. ex., adenililtransferases), nomes triviais que indicam a ligação hidrolisada na síntese (pirofosforilases, fosforilases) ou nomes do material sintetizado (RNA ou DNA polimerase).
nu·cle·o·tox·in (noo′klē-ō-tok′sin). Nucleotoxina. Toxina que atua sobre os núcleos das células.

NUCLEUS

nu·cle·us, pl. **nu·clei** (noo′klē-ŭs, noo′klē-ī). Núcleo. **1.** Em citologia, refere-se tipicamente a uma massa arredondada ou oval de protoplasma no interior do citoplasma de uma célula vegetal ou animal; é circundado por um envoltório nuclear, que encerra eucromatina, heterocromatina e um ou mais nucléolos; sofre mitose durante a divisão celular. SIN karyon. **2.** Por extensão, em virtude de sua função semelhante, refere-se ao genoma de microrganismos (micróbios), que é relativamente simples na sua estrutura, carece de membrana nuclear e não sofre mitose durante a replicação. SIN. nucleoid (3). VER TAMBÉM virion. **3.** [TA]. Em neuroanatomia, grupo de corpos de células nervosas no cérebro ou na medula espinal que pode ser demarcado de grupos vizinhos baseando-se em diferenças no tipo celular ou na presença de uma zona circundante de fibras nervosas ou neurópilo pobre em células. **4.** Qualquer substância (p. ex., corpo estranho, muco, cristal) ao redor da qual se forma um cálculo urinário ou outro cálculo. **5.** Porção central de um átomo (composto de prótons e nêutrons) onde estão concentradas a maior parte da massa e toda a carga elétrica positiva. **6.** Partícula sobre a qual ocorre formação de cristal, gotícula ou bolha. **7.** Disposição característica de átomos numa série de moléculas; p. ex., o núcleo benzeno é uma série de compostos aromáticos. [L. pequena noz, semente, caroço de frutas, o interior de uma coisa, dim. de *nux*, noz]
abducens n., n. abducen'tis, n. of abducens nerve, n. abducente, n. do nervo abducente; grupo de neurônios motores, na parte inferior da ponte, que inerva o músculo reto lateral ipsolateral do olho; singular entre os núcleos dos nervos cranianos motores pelo fato de consistir em duas populações distintas de neurônios: os neurônios que dão origem a fibras formadoras da raiz nervosa abducente e os neurônios internucleares cujos processos cruzam a linha média, ascendem ao fascículo longitudinal medial oposto e terminam em neurônios oculomotores específicos; considerado um centro primário para mecanismos que controlam o olhar horizontal conjugado. SIN nervi abducentis [TA].
nuclei accessorii tractus optici [TA], núcleos acessórios do trato óptico. SIN accessory nuclei of optic tract.
accessory cuneate n. [TA], n. cuneiforme acessório; grupo de células lateralmente ao n. cuneiforme, que recebe fibras radiculares posteriores correspondentes à inervação proprioceptiva do braço e da mão; projeta-se para o cerebelo através do trato cuneiforme-cerebelar e pode ser considerado o equivalente do n. torácico no membro superior. SIN n. cuneatus accessorius [TA], external cuneate n., lateral cuneate n., Monakow n.
n. of accessory nerve, n. do nervo acessório; delgada coluna de neurônios motores que se estende longitudinalmente através das partes central e lateral do corno ventral dos seis segmentos superiores da medula espinal, dando origem ao nervo acessório. SIN n. nervi accessorii [TA].
accessory olivary nuclei, núcleos olivares acessórios. VER dorsal accessory olivary n., medial accessory olivary n.
accessory nuclei of optic tract [TA], núcleos acessórios do trato óptico; pequenos grupos de corpos celulares de neurônios localizados ao longo do trajeto das fibras ópticas no mesencéfalo. Consistem no núcleo posterior [TA] (nucleus posterior [TA]), no núcleo medial [TA] (nucleus medialis [TA]) e no núcleo lateral [TA] (nucleus lateralis [TA]), que também são denominados núcleos terminais posterior, medial e lateral. As conexões desses núcleos, juntamente com o núcleo do trato óptico, formam o sistema óptico acessório, que parece estar relacionado com o deslizamento da retina em direções específicas. SIN nuclei accessorii tractus optici [TA].
n. accum'bens [TA], *nucleus accumbens*; a região de fusão entre a cabeça do núcleo caudado e o putame, recoberto o lado ventral pelo tubérculo olfatório. O nome antigo nucleus accumbens septi ("um núcleo inclinado contra o septo") refere-se a uma expansão medial em forma de gancho dessa região ântero-ventral do estriado, que se curva sob o assoalho do corno ventral do ventrículo

lateral e ascende, por alguma distância, à metade ventral da região septal. Composto de uma pars lateralis [TA] (parte lateral [TA] ou região central [TAalt]) e de uma pars medialis [TA] (parte medial [TA] ou região da concha [TAalt]).
n. acu'sticus, n. acústico; termo obsoleto para os núcleos vestibular e coclear combinados.
n. a'lae cine'reae, n. posterior do nervo vago. SIN posterior n. of vagus nerve.
ambiguus n., n. ambíguo. SIN n. ambiguus.
n. ambig'uus [TA], n. ambíguo; coluna longitudinal e muito delgada de neurônios motores na porção ventrolateral do bulbo; suas fibras eferentes saem com o vago e nervo glossofaríngeo e inervam as fibras musculares estriadas da faringe (incluindo o músculo levantador do véu palatino) e os músculos das cordas vocais da laringe. SIN ambiguus n.
n. amyg'dalae, corpo amigdalóide. SIN amygdaloid *body*.
n. amygdalae basalis lateralis [TA], corpo amigdalóide basolateral. SIN basolateral amygdaloid n.
n. amygdalae basalis medialis [TA], corpo amigdalóide basomedial. SIN basomedial amygdaloid n.
n. amygdalae centralis [TA], corpo amigdalóide central. SIN central amygdaloid n.
n. amygdalae corticalis [TA], corpo amigdalóide cortical. SIN cortical amygdaloid n.
n. amygdalae interstitialis [TA], corpo amigdalóide intersticial. SIN interstitial amygdaloid n.
n. amygdalae lateralis [TA], corpo amigdalóide lateral. SIN lateral amygdaloid n.
n. amygdalae medialis [TA], corpo, amigdalóide medial. SIN medial amygdaloid n.
amygdaloid n., corpo amigdalóide. SIN amygdaloid *body*.
n. ansae lenticularis [TA], n. das alças lenticulares. SIN n. of the ansa lenticularis; VER dorsal hypothalamic *area*.
n. of the ansa lenticularis [TA], n. da alça lenticular; VER dorsal hypothalamic *area*. SIN n. ansae lenticularis [TA].
n. anterior [TA], n. anterior. VER anterior *horn*.
anterior n. [TA], n. anterior. VER anterior *horn*.
n. anterior corporis trapezoidei [TA], n. anterior do corpo trapezóide. SIN anterior n. of trapezoid body; VER nuclei of trapezoid body.
nu'clei anterio'res thal'ami [TA], núcleos anteriores do tálamo. SIN anterior nuclei of thalamus.
n. anterior hypothalami [TA], n. hipotalâmico anterior. SIN anterior hypothalamic n; VER anterior hypothalamic *area*.
anterior hypothalamic n. [TA], n. hipotalâmico anterior. VER anterior hypothalamic *area*. SIN n. anterior hypothalami [TA].
anterior interpositus n. [TA], n. interposto anterior; um de dois núcleos cerebelares interposto entre os núcleos dentado e fastigial. SIN n. interpositus anterior [TA].
anterior olfactory n. [TA], n. olfatório anterior; núcleo localizado no trato olfatório e proeminente em animais microsmáticos; recebe impulsos do bulbo olfatório e projeta-se para o bulbo, para outros alvos de fibras olfatórias e para sua parte contralateral. SIN n. olfactorius anterior [TA].
anterior periventricular n. [TA], n. periventricular anterior. VER anterior hypothalamic *area*. SIN n. periventricularis ventralis [TA].
anterior nuclei of thalamus [TA], núcleos anteriores do tálamo; termo coletivo para três grupos de células nervosas que, em seu conjunto, formam o tubérculo anterior do tálamo: o n. ântero-ventral [TA], um núcleo relativamente grande; o n. ântero-medial [TA]; e o n. ântero-dorsal [TA], um núcleo pequeno (mas com células grandes). Esses núcleos recebem o trato mamilotalâmico do corpo mamilar e aferentes adicionais através do fórnice; projetam-se coletivamente para o córtex dos giros singulado e para-hipocampal. SIN nuclei anteriores thalami [TA].
anterior n. of trapezoid body [TA], n. anterior do corpo trapezóide. VER nuclei of trapezoid body. SIN n. anterior corporis trapezoidei [TA].
n. anterodorsa'lis [TA], n. ântero-dorsal. SIN anterodorsal n. of thalamus; VER anterior nuclei of thalamus.
anterodorsal n. of thalamus, n. ântero-dorsal do tálamo. SIN n. anterodorsalis [TA]. VER anterior nuclei of thalamus.
n. anterolatera'lis [TA], n. ântero-lateral. VER anterior *horn*.
anteromedial n. [TA], n. ântero-medial. VER anterior *horn*.
n. anteromedia'lis [TA], n. ântero-medial. SIN anteromedial n. of thalamus; VER anterior nuclei of thalamus.
anteromedial n. of thalamus, n. ântero-medial do tálamo. SIN n. anteromedialis [TA]. VER anterior nuclei of thalamus.
n. anteroventra'lis [TA], n. ântero-ventral. SIN anteroventral n. of thalamus; VER anterior nuclei of thalamus.
anteroventral n. of thalamus, n. ântero-ventral do tálamo. SIN n. anteroventralis [TA]. VER anterior nuclei of thalamus.
arcuate n. [TA], n. arqueado; (**1**) SIN n. arcuatus of intermediate hypothalamic area [TA], posterior periventricular n. [TA] SIN arcuate n. of thalamus; (**2**) grupo de células no hipotálamo, localizado na parte mais inferior do infundíbulo,

adjacente à eminência mediana. SIN. n. arcuatus of medulla oblongata [TA]. **(3)** conjunto variável de pequenos grupos de células, provavelmente componentes dos núcleos da ponte, nas faces ventral e medial da pirâmide na medula oblonga (bulbo). SIN n. arcuatus [TA].

arcuate n. of thalamus, n. arqueado do tálamo; a pequena região ventral do núcleo ventral póstero-medial do tálamo, em que as fibras dos tratos do lemnisco gustatório e trigeminal secundário terminam; projeta-se para a parte inferior do giro pós-central do córtex cerebral. SIN arcuate n. (1) [TA], n. arcuatus thalami, semilunar n. of Flechsig, thalamic gustatory n.

n. arcuatus [TA], n. arqueado. SIN arcuate n; VER intermediate hypothalamic area.

n. arcua'tus of intermediate hypothalamic area [TA], n. arqueado da área hipotalâmica intermediária. SIN arcuate n. (1).

n. arcuatus of medulla oblongata [TA], n. arqueado da medula oblonga (bulbo). SIN arcuate n. (2).

n. arcua'tus thal'ami, n. arqueado do tálamo. SIN arcuate n. of thalamus.

auditory n., n. auditivo. VER nuclei nervi vestibulocochlearis.

autonomic (visceral motor) nuclei, núcleos autônomos (motores viscerais); núcleos localizados na medula espinal (T1–L2, S2–S4) e no tronco cerebral (n. de Edinger-Westphal, núcleos salivares superior e inferior, núcleo dorsal do vago e partes do núcleo ambíguo) a partir dos quais surgem fibras pré-ganglionares eferentes viscerais gerais; podem ser simpáticos (T1–L2) ou parassimpáticos (craniossacrais); as áreas/núcleos hipotalâmicos funcionam em conjunto com os núcleos autônomos.

basal nuclei [TA], núcleos basais; núcleos do hemisfério cerebral que originalmente incluíam os núcleos caudado e lenticular, o claustro e o corpo (complexo) amigdalóide; funcionalmente, o termo núcleos basais específica, hoje em dia, os núcleos caudado e lenticular e grupos celulares adjacentes que possuem importantes conexões (núcleo subtalâmico; substância negra e partes compacta e reticulada); hoje em dia, sabe-se que o complexo amigdalóide faz parte do sistema límbico; VER TAMBÉM basal *ganglia,* em ganglion. SIN nuclei basales [TA].

nuclei basales [TA], núcleos basais. SIN basal nuclei.

basal n. of Ganser, n. basal de Ganser; grande grupo de grandes células na substância inominada, ventralmente ao núcleo lentiforme. SIN n. basalis of Ganser.

n. basa'lis of Ganser, n. basal de Ganser. SIN basal n. of Ganser.

basket n., n. em cesto; estrutura nuclear que pode ser observada em cistos de *Iodamoeba bütschlii* e, em certas ocasiões, em trofozoítas; em preparações coradas, podem-se observar fibrilas que se estendem entre o cariossoma e os grânulos de cromatina.

basolateral amygdaloid n. [TA], corpo amigdalóide basolateral. VER amygdaloid *body*. SIN n. amygdalae basalis lateralis [TA].

basomedial amygdaloid n. [TA], corpo amigdalóide basomedial. VER amygdaloid *body*. SIN n. amygdalae basalis medialis [TA].

Bechterew n., n. de Bechterew; **(1)** VER vestibular nuclei; **(2)** SIN n. centralis tegmenti superior.

benzene n., n. do benzeno; os seis átomos de carbono conjugados do anel benzeno.

Blumenau n., n. de Blumenau; o núcleo cuneiforme acessório [TA] da medula oblonga.

branchiomotor nuclei, núcleos branquiomotores; termo coletivo para designar os núcleos motoneuronais do tronco cerebral (n. ambíguo, n. motor facial, n. motor do trigêmeo) que se desenvolvem a partir da coluna branquiomotora do embrião e inervam as fibras dos músculos estriados (músculos da mastigação, musculatura facial, músculos da faringe e das cordas vocais) associadas aos arcos branquiais. SIN special visceral efferent nuclei, special visceral motor nuclei.

Burdach n., n. de Burdach. SIN cuneate n.

caeruleun n. [TA], n. cerúleo; termo amplamente utilizado para designar o *locus ceruleus*. VER *locus* caeruleus.

n. caeruleus [TA], n. cerúleo; depressão superficial, de cor azul no cérebro fresco, situada lateralmente na porção mais rostral da fossa rombóide, próximo ao aqueduto cerebral; localiza-se próximo à parede lateral do quarto ventrículo e consiste em cerca de 20.000 corpos celulares neuronais pigmentados de melanina, cujos axônios contendo norepinefrina apresentam uma distribuição notavelmente ampla no córtex cerebral, tálamo dorsal, complexo amigdalóide e hipocampo, tegmento mesencefálico, núcleos cerebelares e córtex, vários núcleos na fonte e no bulbo e substância cinzenta da medula espinal.

n. campi dorsalis [TA], núcleos dos campos dorsais. SIN n. of dorsal field; VER nuclei of perizonal fields.

n. campi medialis [TA], n. do campo medial. SIN n. of medial field; VER nuclei of perizonal fields.

nuclei camporum perizonalium [TA], núcleos do campo perizonal. SIN nuclei of perizonal fields.

n. campi ventralis [TA], n. do campo ventral. SIN. n. of ventral field; VER nuclei of perizonal fields.

caudal pontine reticular n. [TA], núcleos reticulares caudais da ponte. VER reticular nuclei of pons. SIN n. reticularis pontis caudalis [TA].

caudate n. [TA], n. caudado; massa curva alongada de substância cinzenta, consistindo numa porção anterior espessa, o caput [TA] ou cabeça [TA], que faz protrusão no interior do corno anterior do ventrículo lateral, uma porção que se estende ao longo do assoalho do corpo do ventrículo lateral, conhecido como corpus [TA] ou corpo [TA], e uma porção curva fina e alongada, a cauda [TA], que se curva para baixo, para trás e para diante no lobo temporal na parede dorsolateral do ventrículo lateral. SIN n. caudatus [TA], caudate (2), caudatum.

n. cauda'tus [TA], n. caudado. SIN caudate n.

central n. [TA], n. central. VER anterior horn.

central amygdaloid n. [TA], corpo amigdalóide central. VER amygdaloid *body*. SIN n. amygdalae centralis [TA].

n. centralis [TA], n. central. VER anterior horn.

n. centra'lis latera'lis [TA], n. central lateral. SIN central lateral n. of thalamus.

n. centra'lis tegmen'ti supe'rior, n. central do tegmento superior; um dos núcleos da rafe. SIN Bechterew n. (2).

central lateral n. of thalamus [TA], n. central lateral do tálamo; o mais lateral dos núcleos intralaminares do tálamo. SIN n. centralis lateralis [TA].

centromedian n. [TA], n. centromediano; um grande grupo de células em forma de lentilha, o maior e mais caudal dos núcleos intralaminares, localizado dentro da lâmina medular interna do tálamo, entre o núcleo médio-dorsal e o núcleo ventrobasal, assim denominado por Luys em virtude de sua aparência proeminente em cortes frontais, a meio caminho entre o pólo anterior e o pólo posterior do tálamo humano. O núcleo recebe numerosas fibras provenientes do segmento interno do globo pálido através do fascículo talâmico, da alça lenticular e do fascículo lenticular, bem como projeções da área 4 do córtex motor; sua principal conexão eferente ocorre com o putame, embora as colaterais alcancem áreas largas do córtex cerebral. SIN n. centromedianus [TA], centre médian de Luys, centrum medianum.

n. centromedia'nus [TA], n. centromediano. SIN centromedian n.

cerebellar nuclei [TA], núcleos cerebelares; termo coletivo que abrange os núcleos dentado, globoso e emboliforme, bem como os núcleos do teto e do fastígio do cerebelo. SIN nuclei cerebelli [TA].

nuclei cerebelli [TA], núcleos do cerebelo. SIN cerebellar nuclei.

Clarke n., n. de Clarke. SIN posterior thoracic n.

cochlear nuclei [TA], núcleos cocleares. SIN nuclei cochleares.

nu'clei cochlea'res [TA], núcleos cocleares, o nucleus cochlearis posterior [TA] (núcleo coclear posterior [TA] ou núcleo coclear dorsal [TAalt]) e o nucleus cochlearis anterior [TA] (núcleo coclear anterior [TA] ou núcleo coclear ventral [TAalt]) estão localizados nas superfícies dorsal e lateral do pedúnculo cerebelar inferior, no assoalho do recesso lateral da fossa rombóide. Os núcleos cocleares anteriores podem ser divididos numa parte anterior [TA] (pars anterior [TA]) e numa parte posterior [TA] (pars posterior [TA]); recebem as fibras da parte coclear do nervo vestibulococlear e constituem a principal fonte de origem do lemnisco ventral ou via auditiva central. SIN cochlear nuclei [TA], nuclei nervi cochlearis.

n. cochlearis anterior [TA], n. coclear anterior. VER nuclei cochleares.

n. cochlearis posterior [TA], n. coclear posterior. VER nuclei cochleares.

nuclei collic'uli inferio'ris [TA], núcleos do colículo inferior. SIN nuclei of inferior colliculus.

n. commissurae posterioris [TA], n. da comissura posterior. SIN n. of posterior commissure.

convergence n. of Perlia, n. de convergência de Perlia. SIN Perlia n.

nuclei cor'poris genicula'ti media'lis [TA], núcleos do corpo geniculado medial. SIN medial geniculate nuclei.

nu'clei cor'poris mamilla'ris, núcleos do corpo mamilar. SIN nuclei of mammillary body.

n. corporis mammillaris lateralis [TA], n. lateral do corpo mamilar. SIN nuclei of mammillary body.

n. corporis mammillaris medialis [TA], n. medial do corpo mamilar. SIN nuclei of mammillary body.

nuclei corporis trapezoidei [TA], núcleos do corpo trapezóide. SIN nuclei of trapezoid body.

cortical amygdaloid n. [TA], corpo amigdalóide cortical. VER amygdaloid *body*. SIN n. amygdalae corticalis [TA].

nuclei of cranial nerves, núcleos dos nervos cranianos; grupos de células nervosas associados aos nervos cranianos na forma de núcleos motores (núcleos de origem) ou núcleos sensoriais (núcleos terminais). SIN n. nervi cranialis [TA].

cuneate n. [TA], n. cuneiforme; o maior núcleo de Burdach; um dos três núcleos da coluna posterior da medula espinal; localizado próximo à superfície dorsal da medula oblonga ao nível do óbex (e abaixo dele), o núcleo recebe fibras radiculares posteriores que correspondem à inervação sensorial do braço e da mão do mesmo lado; consiste numa pars centralis [TA] (parte central [TA]), região de ninho celular [TAalt] e numa pars rostralis [TA] (parte rostral [TA]), região da concha [TAalt]; juntamente com seu "companheiro" me-

dial, o núcleo grácil, constitui a principal fonte de origem do lemnisco medial. SIN n. cuneatus pars rostralis [TA], n. cuneatus, pars centralis [TA], n. cuneatus [TA], Burdach n., n. funiculi cuneati, n. of cuneate fasciculus.
n. of cuneate fasciculus, n. do fascículo cuneiforme. SIN cuneate n.
n. cunea'tus [TA], n. cuneiforme. SIN cuneate n.
n. cunea'tus accesso'rius [TA], n. cuneiforme acessório. SIN accessory cuneate n.
n. cuneatus, pars centralis [TA], n. cuneiforme, parte central. SIN cuneate n.
n. cuneatus, pars rostralis [TA], n. cuneiforme, parte rostral. SIN cuneate n.
cuneiform n. [TA], n. cuneiforme. VER reticular nuclei of mesencephalon. SIN n. cuneiformis [TA].
n. cuneiformis [TA], n. cuneiforme. SIN cuneiform n; VER reticular nuclei of mesencephalon.
n. of Darkschewitsch, n. de Darkschewitsch; grupo de células ovóides na substância cinzenta central ventral, rostralmente ao núcleo oculomotor, que recebe fibras provenientes dos núcleos vestibulares através do fascículo longitudinal medial; as projeções não são conhecidas, embora algumas cruzem na comissura posterior.
Deiters n., n. de Deiters. VER vestibular nuclei.
dentate n. of cerebellum, n. denteado do cerebelo; o mais lateral e maior dos núcleos cerebelares; recebe os axônios das células de Purkinje da área lateral do córtex cerebelar (o denominado neocerebelo) e vias colaterais de fibras aferentes cerebelares em direção ao córtex cerebelar sobrejacente; juntamente com os núcleos globoso e emboliforme de localização mais medial, constitui a principal fonte de fibras que compõem o pedúnculo cerebelar superior maciço ou braquio conjuntivo. SIN n. dentatus [TA], n. lateralis cerebelli*, corpus dentatum, dentatum.
n. denta'tus [TA], n. denteado. SIN dentate n. of cerebellum.
descending n. of the trigeminus, n. descendente do trigêmeo. SIN spinal n. of trigeminal nerve.
diploid n., n. diplóide; núcleo que contém o número diplóide ou complemento duplo normal de cromossomas para uma célula somática.
dorsal n. [TA], n. dorsal. VER medial geniculate nuclei. SIN n. dorsalis hypothalami [TA], n. dorsalis [TA].
dorsal accessory olivary n., n. olivar dorsal acessório; parte destacada do núcleo olivar dorsalmente ao corpo principal deste último. SIN n. olivaris accessorius posterior [TA], posterior accessory olivary n. [TA].
n. dorsales thalami [TA], n. dorsal do tálamo. SIN dorsal n. of thalamus.
n. of dorsal field [TA], n. do campo dorsal. VER nuclei of perizonal fields. SIN n. campi dorsalis [TA].
n. dorsalis [TA], n. dorsal. SIN dorsal n; VER medial geniculate nuclei.
n. dorsalis corporis geniculati lateralis [TA], n. dorsal do corpo geniculado lateral. SIN dorsal lateral geniculate n.
n. dorsa'lis cor'poris trapezoi'dei, n. dorsal do corpo trapezóide. SIN dorsal n. of trapezoid body.
n. dorsalis hypothalami [TA], n. dorsal do hipotálamo. SIN dorsal n; VER intermediate hypothalamic *area.*
n. dorsalis lateralis [TA], n. dorsal lateral. SIN lateral dorsal n. VER dorsal n. of thalamus.
n. dorsa'lis ner'vi va'gi, n. dorsal dos nervos vagos; *termo oficial alternativo para posterior n. of vagus nerve.
dorsal lateral geniculate n. [TA], n. dorsal do corpo geniculado lateral; principal divisão do *corpo* geniculado lateral; consiste em duas camadas magnocelulares [TA] (strata magnocellularia [TA]) e quatro camadas parvocelulares [TA] (strata parvocellularia [TA]), que atuam como estação de processamento da principal via que se estende da retina até o córtex cerebral, recebendo fibras do trato óptico e dando origem à irradiação geniculocalcarina para o córtex visual do lobo occipital. SIN n. dorsalis corporis geniculati lateralis [TA].
dorsal motor n. of vagus, n. motor dorsal do vago. SIN posterior n. of vagus nerve.
dorsal premammillary n. [TA], n. pré-mamilar dorsal. VER posterior hypothalamic *area.* SIN n. premammillaris dorsalis [TA].
dorsal septal n. [TA], n. septal dorsal. VER septal *area.*
dorsal n. of thalamus, n. dorsal do tálamo; uma das principais subdivisões do tálamo; o núcleo dorsal composto inclui o núcleo lateral anterior ou dorsal, o núcleo lateral intermédio, o núcleo lateral posterior e o pulvinar; em conjunto, esses grupos celulares formam a maior parte da superfície dorsal livre da metade posterior do tálamo e projetam-se para uma região muito grande do córtex parietal, occipitoparietal e temporal; suas conexões aferentes são, em grande parte, obscuras, porém o núcleo lateral posterior e o pulvinar recebem uma projeção do colículo superior. SIN n. dorsales thalami [TA].
dorsal thoracic n., n. torácico dorsal; *termo oficial alternativo para posterior thoracic n.
dorsal n. of trapezoid body, n. dorsal do corpo trapezóide; termo algumas vezes utilizado para designar o núcleo olivar superior localizado ventrolateralmente no tegmento pontino inferior, imediatamente dorsal ao corpo trapezóide; o núcleo recebe fibras dos núcleos cocleares ipsilateral e contralateral e contribui com fibras para o lemnisco lateral (auditivo) de ambos os lados.

Acredita-se que esteja proeminentemente envolvido na função de localização espacial do som. SIN n. dorsalis corporis trapezoidei, oliva superior, superior olive.
dorsal vagal n., n. dorsal do vago. SIN posterior n. of vagus nerve.
dorsal n. of vagus, n. dorsal do vago. SIN posterior n. of vagus nerve.
dorsolateral n., n. dorsolateral. VER anterior *horn.*
dorsomedial n. [TA], n. dorsomedial. VER dorsal hypothalamic *area.* SIN n. dorsomedialis [TA].
dorsomedial hypothalamic n., n. hipotalâmico dorsomedial. SIN dorsomedial n. of hypothalamus.
dorsomedial n. of hypothalamus [TA], n. dorsomedial do hipotálamo; aglomerado oval de células localizadas dorsalmente ao núcleo hipotalâmico ventromedial. SIN n. dorsomedialis hypothalami [TA], dorsomedial hypothalamic n.
n. dorsomedialis [TA], n. dorsomedial. SIN dorsomedial n; VER intermediate hypothalamic *area.*
n. dorsomedia'lis hypothal'ami [TA], n. dorsomedial do hipotálamo. SIN dorsomedial n. of hypothalamus.
droplet nuclei, núcleos de gotículas; partículas de 1–10 µm de diâmetro, implicadas na disseminação das infecções transmitidas pelo ar; resíduo seco formado pela evaporação de gotículas expelidas com a tosse ou espirro na atmosfera ou por aerossolização de material infectante.
Edinger-Westphal n., n. de Edinger-Westphal; pequeno grupo de neurônios motores parassimpáticos pré-ganglionares na linha mediana, próximo ao pólo rostral do núcleo oculomotor do mesencéfalo; os axônios desses neurônios motores deixam o cérebro com o nervo oculomotor e fazem sinapse nas células do gânglio ciliar que, por sua vez, inervam o esfíncter da pupila e o músculo ciliar. A destruição desse núcleo ou de suas fibras eferentes provoca dilatação paralítica máxima da pupila; já se constatou também que o núcleo projeta fibras para níveis inferiores do tronco cerebral e para todos os níveis espinais. SIN visceral nuclei of oculomotor nerve [TA].
emboliform n., n. emboliforme; um de dois núcleos cerebelares interpostos entre os núcleos denteado e do fastígio; pequeno núcleo em forma de cunha na substância branca central do cerebelo, imediatamente interno ao hilo do núcleo denteado; recebe axônios das células de Purkinje da área intermediária do córtex cerebral; os axônios dessas células deixam o cerebelo através do pedúnculo cerebelar superior. SIN n. emboliformis*, embolus (2).
n. embolifor'mis, n. emboliforme; *termo oficial alternativo para emboliform n.
endolemniscal n. [TA], n. endolemniscal; pequenos aglomerados de corpos celulares neuronais localizados na face lateral do lemnisco medial na medula oblonga ou insinuados no interior dos fascículos desse feixe de fibras. SIN n. endolemniscalis [TA].
n. endolemniscalis [TA], n. endolemniscal. SIN endolemniscal n.
endopeduncular n. [TA], n. endopeduncular. VER dorsal hypothalamic *area.* SIN n. endopeduncularis [TA].
n. endopeduncularis [TA], n. endopeduncular. SIN endopeduncular n; VER dorsal hypothalamic *area.*
external cuneate n., n. cuneiforme acessório. SIN accessory cuneate n.
facial n., n. facial; grupo de neurônios motores localizados na região ventrolateral do tegmento pontino inferior, que inervam os músculos faciais, o músculo estapédio do ouvido médio, o ramo posterior do músculo digástrico e o músculo estiloióideo. SIN motor n. of facial nerve [TA], n. nervi facialis [TA], facial motor n., n. facialis.
n. facia'lis, n. facial. SIN facial n.
facial motor n., n. motor facial. SIN facial n.
n. fascic'uli gra'cilis, n. do fascículo grácil. SIN gracile n.
fastigial n. [TA], n. do fastígio; o mais medial dos núcleos cerebelares, localizado medialmente ao núcleo interposto, próximo à linha média, na substância branca abaixo do verme do córtex cerebelar. Recebe os axônios das células de Purkinje de todas as partes do verme do cerebelo. Sua principal projeção é para os núcleos vestibulares e formação reticular bulbar. SIN n. fastigii [TA], n. medialis cerebelli*, fastigatum n. tecti, roof n., tectal nucleus.
n. fasti'gii [TA], n. do fastígio. SIN fastigial n.
filiform n., n. filiforme. SIN paraventricular n. [TA] of hypothalamus.
n. filifor'mis, n. filiforme. SIN paraventricular n. [TA] of hypothalamus.
n. funic'uli cunea'ti, n. do funículo cuneado. SIN cuneate n.
n. funic'uli gra'cilis, n. do funículo grácil. SIN gracile n.
gametic n., n. gamético. SIN micronucleus (2).
n. gelatino'sus, n. pulposo. SIN n. pulposus.
gelatinous n., n. pulposo. SIN n. pulposus.
geniculatus lateralis n., n. do geniculado lateral. VER lateral geniculate *body.*
germ n., n. germinativo. SIN micronucleus (2).
n. gigantocellula'ris medul'lae oblonga'tae [TA], n. gigantocelular da medula oblonga. SIN gigantocellular n. of medulla oblongata.
gigantocellular n. of medulla oblongata [TA], n. gigantocelular da medula oblonga; um dos três principais núcleos da formação reticular do tronco cerebral; sua pequena porção ventromedial é denominada pars alpha [TA]. SIN n. gigantocellularis medullae oblongatae [TA].

n. globo'sus, n. globoso; *termo oficial alternativo para globosus n.
globosus n., n. globoso; um de dois núcleos cerebelares interposto entre os núcleos do fastígio e denteado; um grupo de duas ou três pequenas massas de substância cinzenta no núcleo central branco do cerebelo, medialmente ao núcleo emboliforme; recebe axônios das células de Purkinje da área intermediária do córtex cerebelar; os axônios dessas células deixam o cerebelo através do pedúnculo cerebelar superior. SIN n. globosus*, spherical n.
n. of Goll, n. de Goll. SIN gracile n.
gonad n., n. gonádico. SIN micronucleus (2).
gracile n. [TA], n. grácil; o núcleo medial dos três núcleos da coluna dorsal, sendo os dois outros o núcleo cuneiforme e o núcleo cuneiforme acessório, que corresponde ao tubérculo grácil; pode ser dividido numa pars centralis [TA] (parte central [TA]), região de ninho de células [TAalt]) numa pars rostralis [TA] (parte rostral [TA], região da concha [TAalt]) e num subnucleus rostrodorsalis [TA] (subnúcleo rostrodorsal [TA], grupo de células z [TAalt]); recebe fibras radiculares dorsais que enviam a inervação sensorial da perna e parte inferior do tronco e projeta-se, por meio de lemnisco medial, para o núcleo póstero-lateral ventral do tálamo. SIN n. gracilis [TA], n. fasciculi gracilis, n. funiculi gracilis, n. of Goll.
n. gra'cilis [TA], n. grácil. SIN gracile n.
Gudden tegmental nuclei, núcleos tegmentares de Gudden. SIN tegmental nuclei.
gustatory n., n. gustatório. VER rhombencephalic gustatory n., thalamic gustatory n.
habenular nuclei, núcleos habenulares; a substância cinzenta da habênula, composta de um núcleo habenular medial de células pequenas [TA] (nucleus habenularis medialis [TA]) e de um núcleo habenular lateral de grandes células [TA] (nucleus habenularis lateralis [TA]); ambos os núcleos recebem fibras das regiões basais do prosencéfalo (septo, núcleo basal, núcleo pré-óptico lateral); o núcleo habenular lateral recebe uma projeção adicional do segmento medial do globo pálido. Ambos os núcleos projetam-se através do fascículo retroflexo para o núcleo interpeduncular e uma zona medial do tegmento mesencefálico. SIN ganglion habenulae.
n. habenularis lateralis [TA], n. habenular lateral. SIN lateral habenular n; VER habenular nuclei.
n. habenularis medialis [TA], n. habenular medial. SIN medial habenular n; VER habenular nuclei.
hypoglossal n., n. hipoglosso; o núcleo motor que inerva o músculo intrínseco e quatro dos cinco músculos extrínsecos da língua; localiza-se na medula oblonga, próximo à linha mediana, imediatamente abaixo do assoalho do recesso inferior da fossa rombóide. SIN n. nervi hypoglossi [TA], n. of hypoglossal nerve [TA].
n. of hypoglossal nerve [TA], n. do nervo hipoglosso. SIN hypoglossal n.
nuclei of inferior colliculus [TA], núcleos do colículo inferior; os grupos de células nervosas que compõem o colículo inferior, consistindo num núcleo central [TA] (nucleus centralis [TA]), núcleo externo [TA] (nucleus externus [TA] ou nucleus lateralis [TAalt]) e núcleo pericentral [TA] (nucleus pericentralis [TA]). SIN nuclei colliculi inferioris [TA].
inferior olivary n., n. olivar inferior; grande agregado de pequenas células nervosas densamente agrupadas, que consiste em núcleos olivares acessórios medial e dorsal e num núcleo olivar principal, disposto em lâminas pregueadas que se assemelham a uma bolsa com a abertura (hilo) voltada medialmente. Corresponde, em posição, à oliva, projeta-se para todas as partes da metade contralateral do córtex cerebelar através do trato olivocerebelar e constitui a única fonte de fibras ascendentes cerebelares. Suas conexões aferentes incluem fibras da medula espinal, do núcleo denteado e do córtex motor, porém seu principal impulso parece ser o trato tegmentar central, que se origina de múltiplos núcleos em níveis mesencefálicos. SIN n. olivaris inferior.
inferior salivary n., n. salivar inferior. SIN inferior salivatory n.
inferior salivatory n. [TA], n. salivar inferior; grupo de neurônios motores parassimpáticos pré-ganglionares, localizados na formação reticular da medula oblonga, dorsalmente ao núcleo ambíguo; seus axônios deixam o cérebro com o nervo glossofaríngeo e controlam a secreção da glândula parótida por intermédio do gânglio ótico; as células do núcleo inferior e núcleo superior estão espalhadas e superpostas nas regiões laterais da formação reticular. SIN n. salivatorius inferior [TA], inferior salivary n.
inferior vestibular n. [TA], n. vestibular inferior. VER TAMBÉM vestibular nuclei. SIN n. vestibularis inferior [TA].
intercalated n. [TA], n. intercalado; pequena coleção de células nervosas na medula oblonga, situada lateralmente ao núcleo hipoglosso. SIN n. intercalatus [TA], Staderini n.
n. intercala'tus [TA], n. intercalado. SIN intercalated n.
intermediolateral n. [TA], n. intermédio lateral; coluna de células que forma o corno lateral da substância cinzenta da medula espinal. Estendendo-se do primeiro segmento torácico até o segundo lombar, a coluna contém os neurônios motores autônomos que dão origem às fibras pré-ganglionares do sistema simpático. SIN n. intermediolateralis [TA], intermediolateral cell column of spinal cord.
n. intermediolatera'lis [TA], n. intermédio lateral. SIN intermediolateral n.
intermediomedial n. [TA], n. intermédio medial; pequeno grupo de neurônios motores viscerais espalhados, imediatamente ventrais ao núcleo torácico nos segmentos torácico e dois lombares superiores da medula espinal; acredita-se que recebe fibras aferentes viscerais em todos os níveis espinais. SIN n. intermediomedialis [TA].
n. intermediomedia'lis [TA], n. intermédio medial. SIN intermediomedial n.
interpeduncular n. [TA], n. interpeduncular; grupo de células ovóides, mediano, não-pareado, na base do tegmento mesencefálico, entre os pedúnculos cerebrais; recebe o fascículo retroflexo da habênula e projeta-se para a região da rafe (núcleos da rafe) e substância cinzenta periaqueductal do mesencéfalo. SIN n. interpeduncularis [TA], ganglion isthmi, Gudden ganglion, intercrural ganglion, interpeduncular ganglion.
n. interpeduncula'ris [TA], n. interpeduncular. SIN interpeduncular n.
n. interpos'itus, n. interposto. SIN interpositus n.
interpositus n., n. interposto; termo coletivo que indica o núcleo globoso e o núcleo emboliforme do cerebelo. SIN n. interpositus.
n. interpositus anterior [TA], n. interposto anterior. SIN anterior interpositus n.
n. interpositus posterior [TA], n. interposto posterior. SIN posterior interpositus n.
interstitial n. [TA], n. intersticial; grupo de neurônios de tamanho médio, bem espaçados, na região dorsomedial do tegmento mesencefálico superior, imediatamente lateral ao núcleo de Darkschewitsch; juntamente com este último, o núcleo intersticial está intimamente associado ao fascículo longitudinal medial, através do qual recebe fibras dos núcleos vestibulares e projeta fibras cruzadas através da comissura posterior para o núcleo oculomotor; projeta também fibras para todos os níveis espinais. Acredita-se que esteja envolvido na integração dos movimentos da cabeça e dos olhos, sobretudo os movimentos oculares de natureza vertical ou oblíqua. SIN n. interstitialis [TA], interstitial n. of Cajal.
interstitial amygdaloid n. [TA], n. amigdalóide intersticial. VER amygdaloid *body*. SIN n. amygdalae interstitialis [TA].
interstitial nuclei of anterior hypothalamus [TA], núcleos intersticiais do hipotálamo anterior. VER anterior hypothalamic *area*. SIN nuclei interstitiales hypothalami anterioris [TA].
interstitial n. of Cajal, n. intersticial de Cajal. SIN interstitial n.
n. interstitiales fasciculi longitudinalis medialis [TA], núcleos intersticiais do fascículo longitudinal medial. SIN interstitial n. of medial longitudinal fasciculus.
nuclei interstitiales hypothalami anterioris [TA], núcleos intersticiais do hipotálamo anterior. SIN interstitial nuclei of anterior hypothalamus; VER anterior hypothalamic *area*.
n. interstitia'lis [TA], n. intersticial. SIN interstitial n.
interstitial n. of medial longitudinal fasciculus [TA], n. intersticial do fascículo longitudinal medial; pequenos grupos de células localizados lateralmente, adjacentes ao fascículo longitudinal medial na área do núcleo oculomotor; envolvidos no movimento ocular através de conexões com os núcleos oculomotor e troclear. Essas conexões são primariamente ipsilaterais, porém têm um componente bilateral. SIN n. interstitiales fasciculi longitudinalis medialis [TA].
nu'clei intralamina'res thal'ami [TA], núcleos intralaminares do tálamo. SIN intralaminar nuclei of thalamus.
intralaminar nuclei of thalamus [TA], núcleos intralaminares do tálamo; termo coletivo para referir-se a diversos grupos de células mergulhados na lâmina medular interna do tálamo: o núcleo central lateral [TA], o núcleo paracentral [TA] (nucleus paracentralis [TA]), o núcleo central medial [TA] (nucleus centralis medialis [TA]), o núcleo centromediano e o núcleo parafascicular [TA] (nucleus parafascicularis [TA]). O central lateral e o paracentral recebem aferentes do córtex cerebral, do tronco cerebral, da formação reticular, do cerebelo e da medula espinal e projetam-se, de forma mais ou menos difusa, para grandes regiões do córtex frontal e parietal. O núcleo centromediano recebe impulsos do segmento interno do globo pálido e córtex motor e projeta-se para o estriado e córtex motor. VER TAMBÉM centromedian n. SIN nuclei intralaminares thalami [TA].
Klein-Gumprecht shadow nuclei, núcleos fantasmas de Klein-Gumprecht; núcleos fantasmas em linfócitos e macrolinfócitos em processo de degeneração na leucemia.
lateral n. [TA], n. lateral. VER accessory nuclei of optic tract. SIN n. lateralis [TA].
lateral amygdaloid n. [TA], corpo amigdalóide lateral. VER amygdaloid *body*. SIN n. amygdalae lateralis [TA].
lateral cervical n. [TA], n. cervical lateral; núcleo difusamente disposto, localizado nas porções dorsais do funículo lateral aproximadamente dos níveis cervicais C1–C3; estação sináptica para o trato espinocervicotalâmico.
lateral cuneate n., n. cuneiforme lateral. SIN accessory cuneate n.
lateral dorsal n. [TA], n. dorsal lateral. VER dorsal n. of thalamus. SIN n. dorsalis lateralis [TA].
lateral geniculate n., n. geniculado lateral. VER dorsal lateral geniculate n.

n. of lateral geniculate body, n. do corpo geniculado lateral. VER dorsal lateral geniculate n.
lateral habenular n. [TA], n. habenular lateral. VER habenular nuclei. SIN n. habenularis lateralis [TA].
n. lateralis [TA], n. lateral. SIN lateral n; VER accessory nuclei of optic tract.
n. lateralis cerebelli, n. lateral do cerebelo; *termo oficial alternativo para dentate n. of cerebellum.
n. lateralis corporis trapezoidei [TA], n. lateral do corpo trapezóide. SIN lateral n. trapezoid body; VER nuclei of trapezoid body.
n. latera'lis medu'lae oblonga'tae, n. lateral da medula oblonga. SIN lateral n. of medulla oblongata.
n. lateralis posterior [TA], n. lateral posterior. SIN lateral posterior n; VER dorsal n. of thalamus.
nuclei of lateral lemniscus [TA], núcleos do lemnisco lateral; massa significativa de células mergulhada no lemnisco lateral, imediatamente abaixo da entrada deste no colículo inferior; pode ser dividido em núcleo posterior do lemnisco lateral [TA] (núcleo dorsal do lemnisco lateral [TAalt], nucleus posterior lemnisci lateralis [TA]), num núcleo intermédio do lemnisco lateral [TA] (nucleus intermedius lemnisci lateralis [TA]) e num núcleo anterior do lemnisco lateral [TA] (nucleus anterior lemnisci lateralis [TA], núcleo ventral do lemnisco lateral [TAalt]; o núcleo representa uma estação sináptica para parte das fibras do lemnisco lateral. SIN nuclei lemnisci lateralis [TA].
lateral n. of mammillary body [TA], n. lateral do corpo mamilar; VER posterior hypothalamic *area.*
lateral n. of medulla oblongata, n. lateral da medula oblonga. SIN lateral reticular n. SIN lateralis medullae oblongate.
n. of the lateral olfactory tract [TA], n. do trato olfatório lateral. VER amygdaloid *body.* SIN n. tractus olfactorii lateralis [TA].
lateral parabrachial n., n. parabraquial lateral; grupo de células localizado lateralmente ao pedúnculo cerebelar superior em regiões rostrais da ponte; pode ser dividido em pars lateralis [TA] (parte lateral [TA]), pars medialis [TA] (parte medial [TA]), pars posterior [TA] (parte posterior [TA]) e pars anterior [TA] (parte anterior [TA]). VER TAMBÉM parabrachial nuclei. SIN n. parabrachialis lateralis [TA].
lateral pericuneate n. [TA], n. pericuneiforme lateral; pequeno grupo achatado de corpos celulares neuronais de localização ventrolateral ao núcleo cuneiforme e insinuado entre o fascículo cuneiforme e o núcleo cuneiforme acessório e trato espinal do nervo trigêmeo. SIN n. pericuneatus lateralis [TA].
lateral posterior n. [TA], n. lateral posterior. VER dorsal n. of thalamus. SIN n. lateralis posterior [TA].
lateral preoptic n. [TA], n. pré-óptico lateral; grupo vagamente definido de células nervosas na zona lateral da região pré-óptica. VER TAMBÉM anterior hypothalamic *area.* SIN n. preopticus lateralis [TA].
lateral reticular n., n. reticular lateral; grupo de células na medula oblonga, localizado entre a oliva inferior e o núcleo trigêmeo descendente e trato; composto de uma parte magnocelular [TA] (pars magnocellularis [TA]), uma parte parvocelular [TA] (pars parvocellularis [TA]) e uma parte subtrigêmea [TA] (pars subtrigeminalis [TA]); recebe fibras da medula espinal e do córtex motor e projeta-se para o cerebelo. SIN lateral n. of medulla oblongata.
lateral septal n. [TA], n. septal lateral. VER septal *area.*
lateral superior olivary n. [TA], n. olivar superior lateral. VER superior olivary n. SIN n. olivaris superior lateralis [TA].
lateral n. of thalamus, n. lateral do tálamo. VER dorsal n. of thalamus.
lateral n. of trapezoid body [TA], n. lateral do corpo trapezóide. VER nuclei of trapezoid body. SIN n. lateralis corporis trapezoidei [TA].
lateral tuberal nuclei [TA], núcleos tuberais laterais. VER intermediate hypothalamic *area.*
lateral vestibular n. [TA], n. vestibular lateral. VER vestibular nuclei. SIN n. vestibularis lateralis [TA].
nuclei lemnis'ci latera'lis [TA], núcleos do lemnisco lateral. SIN nuclei of lateral lemniscus.
n. of lens [TA], n. da lente. SIN n. lentis.
lenticular n., n. da lente. SIN n. lentis.
n. lentifor'mis [TA], n. da lente. SIN lentiform *nucleus.*
n. len'tis [TA], n. da lente; porção densa central ou interna da lente. SIN n. of lens [TA].
n. of Luys, n. de Luys. SIN subthalamic n.
nuclei of mammillary body, núcleos do corpo mamilar; esse grupo de núcleos, localizado na área hipotalâmica posterior, consiste num núcleo lateral de grandes células do corpo mamilar e em núcleos mediais maiores do corpo mamilar, núcleos pré-mamilares dorsal e ventral e núcleo supramamilar; os dois primeiros formam a elevação observada na face ventral do diencéfalo, o corpo mamilar. SIN n. corporis mammillaris lateralis [TA], n. corporis mammillaris medialis [TA], nuclei corporis mamillaris.
n. masticato'rius, n. mastigatório. SIN motor n. of trigeminal nerve.
masticatory n., n. mastigatório. SIN motor n. of trigeminal nerve.
medial n. [TA], n. medial. VER accessory nuclei of optic tract. SIN n. medialis [TA].

medial accessory olivary n. [TA], n. olivar acessório medial; parte destacada do núcleo olivar medial ao corpo principal deste último, contra a face lateral do lemnisco medial e trato piramidal. SIN n. olivaris accessorius medialis [TA].
medial amygdaloid n. [TA], corpo amigdalóide medial. VER amygdaloid *body.* SIN n. amygdalae medialis [TA].
medial central n. of thalamus, n. central medial do tálamo; pequeno grupo de células na adesão intertalâmica do tálamo, ocupando a região da linha média da lâmina medular interna, entre os núcleos paracentrais esquerdo e direito. SIN n. medialis centralis thalami.
medial dorsal n. [TA] **of thalamus,** n. dorsomedial do tálamo; grande grupo de células compostas na região dorsomedial do tálamo, apresentando conexões recíprocas com toda a extensão do córtex frontal anteriormente ao córtex motor (área 4) e ao córtex pré-motor (área 6). As conexões aferentes do núcleo dorsomedial também incluem projeções do córtex olfatório e da amígdala. Composto de uma pars parvocellularis lateralis [TA] (núcleo lateral [TA] ou núcleo parvocelular [TAalt], pars magnocellularis medialis [TA] (núcleo medial [TA] ou núcleo magnocelular [TAalt] e pars paralaminaris [TA] (parte paralaminar [TA] ou pars laminaris [TAalt]. SIN mediodorsal n., n. medialis thalami, n. mediodorsalis.
nuclei mediales thalami [TA], núcleos mediais do tálamo. SIN medial nuclei of thalamus.
n. of medial field [TA], n. do campo medial. VER nuclei of perizonal fields. SIN n. campi medialis [TA].
medial geniculate nuclei, núcleos do corpo geniculado medial; grupos de corpos celulares que funcionam como a última de uma série de estações de processamento ao longo da via de condução auditiva para o córtex cerebral, recebendo o braço do colículo inferior e dando origem à irradiação auditiva para o córtex auditivo no giro temporal superior. SIN nuclei corporis geniculati medialis, n. of medial geniculate body.
medial geniculate nuclei [TA], núcleos do corpo geniculado medial; células nervosas que, em seu conjunto, formam uma elevação superficial, o corpo geniculado medial; compreendem um núcleo principal ventral [TA], um núcleo dorsal [TA] e um pequeno núcleo magnocelular medial; transmissão do impulso auditivo para o córtex auditivo.
n. of medial geniculate body, n. do corpo geniculado medial. SIN medial geniculate nuclei.
medial habenular n. [TA], n. habenular medial. VER habenular nuclei. SIN n. habenularis medialis [TA]
n. medialis [TA], n. medial. SIN medial n; VER accessory nuclei of optic tract.
n. media'lis centra'lis thal'ami, n. medial central do tálamo. SIN medial central n. of thalamus.
n. medialis cerebelli, n. medial do cerebelo; *termo oficial alternativo para fastigial n.
n. medialis corporis trapezoidei [TA], n. medial do corpo trapezóide. SIN medial n. of trapezoid body; VER nuclei of trapezoid body.
n. medialis magnocellularis, n. magnocelular medial. SIN medial magnocellular n; VER medial geniculate nuclei.
n. media'lis thal'ami, n. medial do tálamo. SIN medial dorsal n. [TA] of thalamus.
medial magnocellular n., n. magnocelular medial. VER medial geniculate nuclei. SIN n. medialis magnocellularis.
medial parabrachial n. [TA], n. parabraquiais mediais; grupo de células localizado medialmente ao braço conjuntivo em áreas rostrais da ponte; pode ser dividido em pars medialis [TA] (parte medial [TA]) e pars lateralis [TA] (parte lateral [TA]). VER TAMBÉM parabrachial nuclei. SIN n. parabrachialis medialis [TA].
medial pericuneate n. [TA], n. pericuneiforme medial; pequeno grupo de corpos celulares neuronais de localização imediatamente ventromedial ao núcleo cuneado, insinuado numa camada difusa de células, a matriz pericuneada. SIN n. pericuneatus medialis [TA].
medial preoptic n. [TA], n. pré-óptico medial; grupo de células nervosas que formam a zona medial da região pré-óptica. SIN n. preopticus medialis [TA].
medial septal n. [TA], n. septal medial. VER septal *area.*
medial superior olivary n. [TA], n. olivar superior medial. VER superior olivary n. SIN n. olivaris superior medialis [TA].
medial nuclei of thalamus [TA], núcleos mediais do tálamo; grupo coletivo de células que formam o grande núcleo dorsal medial (ou núcleo dorsomedial) e suas subdivisões (núcleo lateral ou núcleo parvocelular, núcleo medial ou núcleo magnocelular, parte paralaminar ou *pars paralaminaris*) e o núcleo ventral medial [TA] (núcleo medioventral [TA]). SIN nuclei mediales thalami [TA].
medial n. of trapezoid body [TA], n. medial do corpo trapezóide. VER nuclei of trapezoid body. SIN n. medialis corporis trapezoidei [TA].
medial ventral n. [TA], n. ventral medial. VER medial nuclei of thalamus. SIN n. medioventralis [TA].
medial vestibular n. [TA], n. vestibular medial. VER vestibular nuclei. SIN n. vestibularis medialis [TA].
median preoptic n. [TA], n. pré-óptico mediano. VER anterior hypothalamic *area.* SIN n. preopticus medianus [TA].
mediodorsal n., n. médio dorsal. SIN medial dorsal n. [TA] of thalamus.

n. mediodorsalis, n. médio dorsal. SIN medial dorsal n. [TA] of thalamus.
n. medioventralis [TA], n. medioventral. SIN medial ventral n; VER medial nuclei of thalamus.
mesencephalic n. of trigeminal nerve [TA], n. mesencefálico do nervo trigêmeo; longa placa estreita de neurônios unipolares que se estende através do comprimento do mesencéfalo, dentro e ao longo do ângulo lateral da substância cinzenta central. O núcleo é o único caso conhecido de neurônios sensoriais primários incluídos no sistema nervoso central, em vez de estarem num gânglio sensorial periférico. Seus processos axonais periféricos passam com o nervo trigêmeo, emitem colaterais para o núcleo motor trigêmeo e terminam nos músculos da mastigação. SIN n. mesencephalicus nervi trigemini [TA].
n. mesenceph'alicus ner'vi trigem'ini [TA], n. mesencefálico do nervo trigêmeo. SIN mesencephalic n. of trigeminal nerve.
Monakow n., n. de Monakow. SIN accessory cuneate n.
motor nuclei, núcleos motores. SIN nuclei of origin.
motor n. of facial nerve [TA], n. motor do nervo facial. SIN facial n.
n. moto'rius ner'vi trigem'ini [TA], n. motor do nervo trigêmeo. SIN motor n. of trigeminal nerve.
motor n. of trigeminal nerve [TA], n. motor do nervo trigêmeo; grupo de neurônios motores que inervam os músculos da mastigação (músculos massé-ter, temporal e pterigóides interno e externo) e os músculos tensor do tímpano e tensor do véu palatino. O núcleo localiza-se no tegmento pontino superior, medialmente ao núcleo sensorial principal do nervo trigêmeo. SIN n. motorius nervi trigemini [TA], masticatory n., motor n. of trigeminus, n. masticatorius.
motor n. of trigeminus, n. motor do trigêmeo. SIN motor n. of trigeminal nerve.
n. ner'vi abducen'tis [TA], n. dos nervos abducentes. SIN abducens n.
n. ner'vi accesso'rii [TA], n. dos nervos acessórios. SIN n. of accessory nerve.
nu'clei ner'vi cochlea'ris, núcleos do nervo nuclear. SIN nuclei cochleares.
n. nervi crania'lis [TA], n. dos nervos cranianos. SIN nuclei of cranial nerves.
n. ner'vi facia'lis [TA], n. do nervo facial. SIN facial n.
n. ner'vi hypoglos'si [TA], n. do nervo hipoglosso. SIN hypoglossal n.
n. ner'vi oculomoto'rii [TA], n. do nervo oculomotor. SIN oculomotor n.
n. nervi phrenici [TA], n. do nervo frênico. SIN n. of phrenic nerve.
n. ner'vi trochlea'ris [TA], n. do nervo troclear. SIN n. of trochlear nerve.
nu'clei ner'vi vestibulocochlea'ris, núcleos do nervo vestibulococlear. SIN vestibulocochlear nuclei.
n. ni'ger, n. negro. SIN substantia nigra.
oculomotor n., n. oculomotor; o grupo composto de neurônios motores que inervam todos os músculos externos dos olhos, exceto o músculo reto lateral e o músculo oblíquo superior, incluindo o músculo levantador da pálpebra superior; o componente mais rostral do núcleo é o núcleo de Edinger-Westphal, que inerva os músculos esfincteriano da pupila e ciliar através do gânglio ciliar. O núcleo oculomotor localiza-se na metade rostral do mesencéfalo, próximo à linha medial na parte mais ventral da substância cinzenta central; as fibras do fascículo longitudinal medial formam suas bordas laterais. SIN n. nervi oculomotorii [TA], n. of oculomotor nerve [TA].
n. of oculomotor nerve [TA], n. do nervo oculomotor. SIN oculomotor n.
n. olfactorius anterior [TA], n. olfatório anterior. SIN anterior olfactory n.
n. oliva'ris accesso'rius media'lis [TA], n. olivar acessório medial. SIN medial accessory olivary n.
n. oliva'ris accesso'rius posterior [TA], n. olivar acessório posterior. SIN dorsal accessory olivary n.
n. oliva'ris inferior, n. olivar inferior. SIN inferior olivary n.
n. olivaris principalis [TA], n. olivar principal. SIN principal olivary n.
n. olivaris superior [TA], n. olivar superior. SIN superior olivary n.
n. olivaris superior lateralis [TA], n. olivar superior lateral. SIN lateral superior olivary n.
n. olivaris superior medialis [TA], n. olivar superior medial. SIN medial superior olivary n; VER superior olivary n.
Onuf n., n. de Onuf; grupo de pequenos neurônios motores somáticos no corno ventral da medula espinal, ao nível sacral 2, que inervam os esfíncteres vesicorretais, isto é, o esfíncter anal externo e o uretral; o núcleo de Onuf foi identificado no gato, no cão e nos seres humanos. SIN n. of pudendal nerve [TA]. [Onufrowicz, Wladislaus, anatomista suíço.]
oral pontine reticular n. [TA], n. reticular pontino oral. VER reticular nuclei of pons. SIN n. reticularis pontis oralis [TA].
nuclei of origin, núcleos de origem; coleções de neurônios motores (formando uma coluna contínua na medula espinal, descontínua no bulbo e na ponte), dando origem aos nervos motores espinais e cranianos. SIN n. originis [TA], motor nuclei.
n. ori'ginis [TA], núcleos de origem. SIN nuclei of origin.
parabigeminal n. [TA], n. parabigeminal; grupo de corpos celulares neuronais localizado na posição lateral do mesencéfalo, na área das fibras espinotalâmicas; adjacente, ventrolateralmente, ao colículo inferior, com o qual estabelece interconexões. SIN n. parabigeminalis [TA].
n. parabigeminalis [TA], n. parabigeminal. SIN parabigeminal n.
parabrachial nuclei [TA], núcleos parabraquiais; os grupos celulares que flanqueiam o pedúnculo cerebelar superior em níveis imediatamente caudais ao colículo inferior; atuam como estações intermediárias nas vias ascendentes do núcleo do trato solitário para o tálamo e hipotálamo e recebem fibras aferentes do hipotálamo e do corpo amigdalóide. SIN nuclei parabrachiales [TA].
nuclei parabrachia'les [TA], núcleos parabraquiais. SIN parabrachial nuclei.
n. parabrachialis lateralis [TA], n. parabraquial lateral. SIN lateral parabrachial n.
n. parabrachialis medialis [TA], n. parabraquial medial. SIN medial parabrachial n.
n. paracentra'lis thal'ami [TA], n. paracentral do tálamo. SIN paracentral n. of thalamus.
paracentral n. of thalamus [TA], n. paracentral do tálamo; um dos núcleos intralaminares do tálamo, medial ao núcleo central lateral. SIN n. paracentralis thalami [TA].
paralemniscal n. [TA], n. paralemniscal. VER reticular nuclei of pons. SIN n. paralemniscalis [TA].
n. paralemniscalis [TA], n. paralemniscal. SIN paralemniscal n; VER reticular nuclei of pons.
paramedial reticular n. [TA], n. reticular paramedial. VER reticular nuclei of pons.
paranigral n. [TA], n. paranigral; pequeno agregado de células localizado nas regiões ventromediais do mesencéfalo e insinuado entre a face medial da substância negra e o núcleo interpeduncular. SIN n. paranigralis [TA].
n. paranigralis [TA], n. paranigral. SIN paranigral n.
parapeduncular n. [TA], n. parapeduncular. VER reticular nuclei of mesencephalon. SIN n. parapeduncularis [TA].
n. parapeduncularis [TA], n. parapeduncular. SIN parapeduncular n; VER reticular nuclei of mesencephalon.
paraventricular n. [TA], n. paraventricular. VER anterior hypothalamic *area*.
n. paraventricula'ris hypothalami, n. paraventricular do hipotálamo. SIN paraventricular n. [TA] of hypothalamus.
paraventricular n. [TA] of hypothalamus, n. paraventricular do hipotálamo; grupo triangular de grandes neurônios magnocelulares na zona periventricular da metade anterior do hipotálamo. As células do núcleo assemelham-se às do núcleo supra-óptico; os axônios de cerca de 20% dessas células unem-se na formação do trato supra-óptico-hipofisário e estão funcionalmente associados ao lobo posterior da hipófise; projetam fibras para os núcleos do tronco cerebral (núcleo motor dorsal e núcleo solitário) e para a coluna de células intermédias laterais da medula espinal nos níveis torácico, lombar e espinal; fibras autônomas descendentes semelhantes originam-se dos núcleos hipotalâmicos lateral e posterior. SIN filiform n., n. filiformis, n. paraventricularis hypothalami.
pedunculopontine tegmental n. [TA], n. pedunculopontino do tegmento. VER reticular nuclei of mesencephalon. SIN n. tegmentalis pedunculopontinus [TA].
n. pericuneatus lateralis [TA], n. pericuneiforme lateral. SIN lateral pericuneate n.
n. pericuneatus medialis [TA], n. pericuneiforme medial. SIN medial pericuneate n.
perifornical n. [TA], n. perifornicial. VER lateral hypothalamic *area*. SIN n. perifornicalis [TA].
n. perifornicalis [TA], n. perifornicial. SIN perifornical n.
perihypoglossal nuclei [TA], núcleos peri-hipoglossais; núcleos encontrados no assoalho do quarto ventrículo em relação ao núcleo hipoglosso; o termo inclui os núcleos prepósito e intercalado e o núcleo de Roller.
nuclei perioliva'res [TA], núcleos perioliva res. SIN periolivary nuclei; VER superior olivary n.
periolivary nuclei [TA], núcleos periolivares; VER superior olivary n. SIN nuclei periolivares [TA].
peripeduncular n. [TA], n. peripeduncular; grupo de corpos celulares neuronais que formam uma fina configuração semelhante a uma coifa sobre a face dorsolateral do pedúnculo cerebral; muitas de suas células são acetilcolinesterase-positivas. SIN n. peripeduncularis [TA].
n. peripeduncularis [TA], n. peripeduncular. SIN peripeduncular n.
peritrigeminal n. [TA], n. peritrigeminal; pequenos agrupamentos difusos de células localizados principalmente na face lateral do trato espinal do nervo trigêmeo ou insinuados no interior desse feixe de fibras ao nível do óbex e caudalmente a ele. SIN n. peritrigeminalis [TA].
n. peritrigeminalis [TA], n. peritrigeminal. SIN peritrigeminal n.
n. periventricularis posterior [TA], n. periventricular posterior. SIN posterior periventricular n; VER intermediate hypothalamic *area*.
n. periventricularis ventralis [TA], n. periventricular lateral. SIN anterior periventricular n; VER anterior hypothalamic *area*.
periventricular preoptic n. [TA], n. pré-óptico periventricular; VER anterior hypothalamic *area*. SIN n. preopticus periventricularis [TA].
nuclei of perizonal fields [TA], núcleos dos campos perizonais; pequenos grupos de células distribuídos ao longo do trajeto das fibras palidofugais e insinuados dentro delas, que formam o fascículo lenticular (núcleo do campo ventral [TA], nucleus campi ventralis [TA], núcleo do campo H2), que se arqueiam através do campo pré-rubro (núcleo do campo medial [TA], nucleus

campi medialis [TA], núcleo do campo H) e o fascículo talâmico (núcleo do campo dorsal [TA], nucleus campi dorsalis [TA], núcleo do campo H1). VER TAMBÉM *fields* of Forel, em *field*. SIN. nuclei camporum perizonalium [TA].

Perlia n., n. de Perlia; pequeno grupo celular localizado entre as colunas de células somáticas dos núcleos oculomotores. Devido à sua localização entre os grupos de neurônios motores, inervando, respectivamente, os músculos retos mediais esquerdo e direito, o núcleo é considerado como representando, possivelmente, um mecanismo de integração para convergência ocular. SIN convergence n. of Perlia, Spitzka n.

phenanthrene n., n. fenantrênico; termo incorreto para referir-se ao núcleo esteróide tetracíclico.

phrenic n., n. frênico; *termo oficial alternativo para n. of phrenic nerve.

n. of phrenic nerve [TA], n. do nervo frênico; corpos celulares neuronais, localizados nas porções mais mediais do corno anterior nos níveis cervicais C3 a C7, que inervam o diafragma através do nervo frênico. VER TAMBÉM phrenic n. SIN n. nervi phrenici [TA], phrenic n.*.

pontine nuclei [TA], núcleos pontinos; a substância cinzenta maciça, composta de núcleos individuais, que preenche a ponte basilar. Esses núcleos apresentam uma arquitetura razoavelmente homogênea e projetam-se primariamente para o lado contralateral do cerebelo, através do pedúnculo cerebelar médio; existe uma projeção pontocerebelar ipsilateral modesta. Seus aferentes principais provêm de toda a extensão do neocórtex cerebral através das fibras corticopontinas (feixes pontinos longitudinais); assim, os núcleos pontinos formam uma importante estação intermediária na condução de impulsos do córtex cerebral de um hemisfério para o lobo posterior do cerebelo oposto. Os núcleos pontinos incluem os seguintes: nucleus anterior [TA] (núcleo anterior [TA]), núcleo ventral [TAalt]), nucleus lateralis [TA] (núcleo lateral [TA]), nucleus medianus [TA] (núcleo mediano [TA]), nucleus paramedianus [TA] (núcleo paramediano [TA]), nucleus peduncularis [TA] (núcleo peduncular [TA], núcleo peripeduncular [TAalt]), nucleus posterior lateralis [TA] (núcleo póstero-lateral [TA], núcleo dorsolateral [TAalt]) e nucleus posterior medialis [TA] (núcleo póstero-medial [TA], núcleo dorsomedal [TAalt]). O nucleus reticularis tegmenti pontis [TA] (núcleo reticulotegmentar [TA]) localiza-se na interface das porções tegmentar e basilar da ponte, sendo algumas vezes reunido com os núcleos pontinos. SIN nuclei pontis [TA], pontine gray matter.

nu'clei pon'tis [TA], núcleos pontinos. SIN pontine nuclei.

pontobulbar n. [TA], n. pontobulbar; camada de células de forma irregular, localizada dorsal e lateralmente ao corpo restiforme, a meio caminho dos níveis rostrais da medula oblonga; torna-se maior imediatamente ventrolateral ao corpo restiforme na junção bulbopontina; essas células assemelham-se àquelas dos núcleos pontinos basilares. SIN n. pontobulbaris [TA].

n. pontobulbaris [TA], n. pontobulbar. SIN pontobulbar n.

n. posterior [TA], n. posterior. SIN posterior n; VER accessory nuclei of optic tract.

posterior n. [TA], n. posterior. VER accessory nuclei of optic tract. SIN n. posterior [TA].

posterior accessory olivary n. [TA], n. olivar posterior acessório. SIN dorsal accessory olivary n.

n. of posterior commissure [TA], n. da comissura posterior; grupo de células localizado imediatamente adjacente à comissura posterior na junção mesencéfalo-diencéfalo; pode ser dividido em parte ventral [TA] (subdivisão ventral [TA]), parte dorsal [TA] (subdivisão dorsal [TA]) e parte intersticial [TA] (subdivisão intersticial [TA]). SIN n. commissurae posterioris [TA].

n. poste'rior hypothal'mi [TA], n. posterior do hipotálamo. SIN posterior hypothalamic n.

posterior hypothalamic n. [TA], n. posterior do hipotálamo; grande núcleo hipotalâmico periventricular localizado dorsalmente ao corpo mamilar, contínuo com a substância cinzenta central do mesencéfalo. SIN n. posterior hypothalami [TA].

n. posterior hypothalamic [TA], n. posterior do hipotálamo. SIN posterior n. of hypothalamus.

posterior n. of hypothalamus [TA], n. posterior do tálamo; VER posterior hypothalamic *area*. SIN n. posterior hypothalamic [TA].

posterior interpositus n. [TA], n. interposto posterior; um de dois núcleos cerebelares interposto entre os núcleos fastigial e denteado. VER TAMBÉM globosus n. SIN n. interpositus posterior [TA].

n. posterior nervi vagi [TA], n. posterior do nervo vago. SIN posterior n. of vagus nerve.

posterior periventricular n. [TA], n. periventricular posterior. SIN arcuate n. (1). SIN n. periventricularis posterior [TA].

posterior thoracic n. [TA], n. torácico posterior; coluna de grandes neurônios localizada na base da coluna cinzenta posterior da medula espinal, estendendo-se do primeiro segmento torácico até o segundo lombar; dá origem ao trato espinocerebelar do mesmo lado. SIN n. thoracicus posterior [TA], dorsal thoracic n.*, Clarke column, Clarke n., Stilling column, Stilling n.

posterior n. of vagus nerve, n. posterior do nervo vago; o núcleo motor visceral localizado no trígono vagal (asa cinérea) do assoalho do quarto ventrículo. Dá origem às fibras parassimpáticas do nervo vago que inervam o músculo cardíaco e a musculatura lisa e glândulas dos tratos respiratório e intestinal. SIN n. posterior nervi vagi [TA], n. dorsalis nervi vagi*, dorsal motor n. of vagus, dorsal n. of vagus, dorsal vagal n., n. alae cinereae.

posterolateral n. [TA], n. póstero-lateral; VER anterior horn.

n. posterolateralis [TA], n. póstero-lateral; VER anterior horn.

posteromedial n. [TA], n. póstero-medial; VER anterior horn.

n. posteromedialis [TA], n. póstero-medial; VER anterior horn.

precommissural septal n. [TA], n. septal pré-comissural; camada verticalmente orientada de corpos celulares neuronais de localização rostral à comissura anterior na base do septo pelúcido. SIN n. septalis precommissuralis [TA].

pregeniculate n., n. pré-geniculado; *termo oficial alternativo para ventral lateral geniculate n.

n. premammillaris dorsalis [TA], n. pré-mamilar dorsal. SIN dorsal premammillary n.

n. premammillaris ventralis [TA], n. pré-mamilar ventral. SIN ventral premammillary n.

n. preop'ticus latera'lis [TA], n. pré-óptico lateral. SIN lateral preoptic n.

n. preop'ticus media'lis [TA], n. pré-óptico medial. SIN medial preoptic n.

n. preopticus medianus [TA], n. pré-óptico mediano. SIN median preoptic n; VER anterior hypothalamic *area*.

n. preopticus periventricularis [TA], n. pré-óptico periventricular. SIN periventricular preoptic n.; VER anterior hypothalamic *area*.

prerubral n., n. pré-rubro; a matéria cinzenta do campo H$_2$; VER *fields* of Forel, em *field*.

pretectal nuclei [TA], núcleos pré-tetais; grupos de células que formam diversos subnúcleos, localizados rostralmente ao colículo superior na área "pré-tetal"; recebem impulsos de células do gânglio retiniano (através do trato óptico) e projetam-se bilateralmente para o núcleo de Edinger-Westphal; centro de retransmissão para a via de reflexo de luz pupilar; consistem no nucleus pretectalis anterior [TA] (núcleo pré-tetal anterior [TA]), nucleus pretectalis olivaris [TA] (núcleo pré-tetal olivar [TA]) e nucleus pretectalis posterior [TA] (núcleo pré-tetal posterior [TA]). O nucleus tractus optici [TA] (núcleo do trato óptico) também costuma ser agrupado como um dos núcleos da área prétetal. SIN nuclei pretectales [TA].

nuclei pretectales, núcleos pré-tetais. SIN pretectal nuclei.

n. principa'lis ner'vi trigem'ini [TA], n. principal do nervo trigêmeo. SIN principal sensory n. of trigeminal nerve.

principal olivary n. [TA], n. olivar principal; a maior parte do complexo olivar inferior, consistindo numa camada ondulante de células formada por uma lâmina dorsal [TA] (lamella posterior [TA]) e lâmina ventral [TA] (lamella anterior [TA]), conectadas entre si lateralmente por uma lâmina lateral [TA] (lamella lateralis [TA]). A abertura medialmente dirigida dessa camada celular contínua é o hilo. SIN n. olivaris principalis [TA].

principal sensory n. of trigeminal nerve [TA], n. sensorial principal do nervo trigêmeo; termo comumente utilizado para designar o núcleo pontino do nervo trigêmeo; localizado na ponte, lateralmente ao n. trigêmeo motor; recebe impulsos sensoriais primários (toque e pressão) através do nervo trigêmeo e projeta-se para o núcleo ventral póstero-medial do tálamo. SIN n. principalis nervi trigemini [TA], n. sensorius superior nervi trigemini, principal sensory n. of the trigeminus.

principal sensory n. of the trigeminus, n. sensorial principal do trigêmeo. SIN principal sensory n. of trigeminal nerve.

n. of pudendal nerve [TA], n. do nervo pudendo. SIN Onuf n.

n. pulpo'sus [TA], n. pulposo; porção central de fibrocartilagem macia do disco intervertebral; considerado como derivado da notocorda. SIN gelatinous n., n. gelatinosus, vertebral pulp.

pulvinar nuclei [TA], núcleos pulvinares; a grande porção caudal do grupo de núcleos laterais do tálamo; podem ser divididos em quatro núcleos com base na citoarquitetura e conexões: o nucleus pulvinaris anterior [TA] (núcleo pulvinar anterior [TA]), o nucleus pulvinaris inferior [TA] (núcleo pulvinar inferior [TA]), o nucleus pulvinaris lateralis [TA] (núcleo pulvinar lateral [TA]) e o nucleus pulvinaris medialis [TA] (núcleo pulvinar medial [TA]); funcionalmente relacionados ao sistema visual. SIN nuclei pulvinaris [TA].

nuclei pulvinares [TA], núcleos pulvinares. SIN pulvinar nuclei.

n. pyramida'lis, n. piramidal; termo obsoleto para o núcleo olivar acessório medial.

pyrrole n., n. pirrólico; núcleo de porfirinas, um tetrapirrol cíclico; quatro grupamentos de pirrol unem-se numa estrutura em anel através de pontes –CH= (metilidina) entre a posição α (2) de um pirrol e a posição α' (5) de outro pirrol, sendo o quarto pirrol unido ao primeiro. VER TAMBÉM porphin, porphyrin.

raphe nuclei [TA], núcleos da rafe; termo coletivo para referir-se a vários grupos de células nervosas no plano mediano da medula oblonga e ao longo dele [n. raphes obscurus [TA] (núcleo da rafe obscuro [TA]), n. raphes pallidus [TA] (núcleo da rafe pálida [TA]) e porções caudais do n. raphes magnus [TA] (núcleo da rafe magna [TA]); da ponte [porções rostrais do n. raphes magnus [TA] (núcleo da rafe magna [TA]), n. raphes pontis [TA] (núcleo da rafe pontina [TA]), n. raphes medianus [TA] (núcleo da rafe mediana [TA] ou núcleo superior central [TAalt]) e porções caudais do n. raphes posterior [TA] (nú-

cleo da rafe posterior [TA]) ou núcleo da rafe dorsal [TAalt]; e do mesencéfalo [porções rostrais do n. raphe posterior [TA] (núcleo da rafe posterior [TA]), n. linearis inferioris [TA] (núcleo linear inferior [TA]), n. linearis intermedius [TA] (núcleo linear intermédio [TA]) e n. linearis superior [TA] (núcleo linear superior [TA]). Esses núcleos incluem neurônios caracterizados pelo seu conteúdo do agente transmissor indolamínico, a serotonina; seus axônios, que transportam a serotonina, estendem-se rostralmente até o hipotálamo, septo, hipocampo e giro do cíngulo, incluindo projeções para o tronco cerebral, cerebelo e medula espinal. SIN nuclei raphes [TA].
nu'clei raph'es [TA], núcleos da rafe. SIN raphe nuclei.
red n., n. rubro; grande massa celular bem definida e um tanto alongada, de tonalidade cinza-avermelhado no cérebro fresco, localizada no tegmento mesencefálico rostral. Esse núcleo é composto de uma pars magnocellularis [TA] caudal (parte magnocelular [TA]), de uma pars parvocellularis [TA] rostral (parte parvocelular [TA]) e de uma pequena pars posteromedialis [TA] (parte póstero-medial [TA], parte dorsomedial [TAalt]). O núcleo recebe uma projeção maciça da metade contralateral do cerebelo através do pedúnculo cerebelar superior e uma projeção adicional do córtex motor ipsilateral. As projeções do núcleo interposto anterior e do córtex motor para o núcleo vermelho são organizadas somatotopicamente. Suas conexões eferentes são feitas com a formação reticular rombencefálica contralateral e com a medula espinal através dos tratos rubrobulbar e rubroespinal. As fibras rubroespinais têm origem somatotópica. SIN n. ruber [TA].
reduction n., n. de redução; um núcleo que degenera na célula durante as alterações associadas à fertilização.
reproductive n., n. reprodutor. SIN micronucleus (2).
reticular nuclei of the brainstem, núcleos reticulares do tronco cerebral; grupos celulares vagamente delineados que compõem a substância cinzenta da formação reticular da medula oblonga, ponte e mesencéfalo. Em geral, os territórios de células grandes ocupam os dois terços mediais da formação reticular; alguns exemplos incluem o núcleo gigantocelular da medula oblonga, os núcleos do tegmento da ponte caudal e oral. São encontrados grupos menores de núcleos reticulares lateralmente e em localizações paramedianas; os núcleos laterais recebem colaterais sensoriais e projetam-se medialmente; os núcleos reticulares paramedianos projetam-se, em grande parte, para o cerebelo. VER TAMBÉM reticular *formation*.
n. reticulares medullae oblongatae [TA], núcleos reticulares da medula oblonga. SIN reticular nuclei of medulla oblongata.
nuclei reticulares mesencephali [TA], núcleos reticulares do mesencéfalo. SIN reticular nuclei of mesencephalon.
nuclei reticulares pontis [TA], núcleos reticulares da ponte. SIN reticular nuclei of pons.
n. reticularis pontis caudalis [TA], n. reticular da porção caudal da ponte. SIN caudal pontine reticular n; VER reticular nuclei of pons.
n. reticularis pontis oralis [TA], n. reticular da ponte oral. SIN oral pontine reticular n; VER reticular nuclei of pons.
n. reticularis tegmenti pontis [TA], n. reticular do tegmento da ponte; VER reticular nuclei of pons.
n. reticula'ris thal'ami [TA], n. reticular do tálamo. SIN reticular n. of thalamus.
reticular nuclei of medulla oblongata [TA], núcleos reticulares da medula oblonga; grupos de corpos celulares neuronais localizados geralmente nas porções mais centrais de cada metade da medula oblonga; nem todos estão bem separados uns dos outros, embora tenham conexões específicas. Esses núcleos são: o núcleo reticular gigantocelular [TA] e sua pars alpha [TA] (n. gigantocellularis [TA]) de localização ventromedial (n. gigantocelular [TA]), o núcleo reticular gigantocelular anterior [TA] ou núcleo reticular gigantocelular ventral [TAalt] (n. gigantocellularis anterior [TA]), o núcleo reticular paragigantocelular lateral [TA] (n. paragigantocellularis lateralis [TA]), o núcleo interfascicular do nervo hipoglosso [TA] (n. interfasciccullaris nervi hypoglossi [TA]), o núcleo reticular intermédio [TA] (n. reticularis intermedius [TA]), o núcleo reticular parvocelular [TA] (n. reticularis parvocellularis [TA]), o núcleo reticular paragigantocelular posterior [TA] ou núcleo reticular paragigantocelular dorsal [TAalt] (n. paragigantocellularis posterior [TA]) e o núcleo reticular medial [TA] (n. reticularis medialis [TA]). O núcleo reticular central [TA] (n. reticulairs centralis [TA]) pode ser dividido em uma parte dorsal [TA] e outra ventral [TA] (pars dorsalis [TA], pars ventralis [TA]). O núcleo reticular lateral [TA] localiza-se na área ventrolateral da medula oblonga e pode ser dividido nas partes magnocelular [TA] (pars magnocellularis [TA]), parvocelular [TA] (pars parvocellularis [TA] e subtrigêmea [TA] (pars subtrigeminalis [TA]). VER TAMBÉM reticular nuclei of the brainstem. SIN n. reticulares medullae oblongatae [TA].
reticular nuclei of mesencephalon [TA], núcleos reticulares do mesencéfalo; grupos celulares de distribuição difusa localizados na área dorsal e mais medial do tegmento do mesencéfalo. Esses núcleos são: o núcleo cuneiforme [TA] (n. cuneiformis [TA]), o núcleo subcuneiforme [TA] (n. subcuneiformis [TA]), o núcleo parapeduncular [TA] (n. parapeduncularis [TA]) e o núcleo tegmentar pedunculopontino [TA] (n. tegmentalis pedunculopontinus [TA]). Este último núcleo pode ser dividido numa parte compacta [TA] ou subnúcleo compacto [TAalt] (pars compacta [TA]) e numa parte dispersa [TA] ou subnúcleo disperso [TAalt] (pars dissipata [TA]). SIN nuclei reticulares mesencephali [TA].
reticular nuclei of pons [TA], núcleos reticulares da ponte; grupos de células localizados no tegmento da ponte, que não estão claramente separados uns dos outros, mas que apresentam, em alguns casos, conexões distintas. Esses núcleos são: o núcleo reticular da ponte caudal [TA] (n. reticularis pontis caudalis [TA]), o núcleo reticular da ponte oral [TA] (n. reticularis pontis oralis [TA]), o núcleo paralemniscal [TA] (n. paralemniscalis [TA]) e o núcleo reticular paramediano [TA] (n. reticularis paramedianus [TA]). O núcleo reticulotegmentar [TA] (n. reticularis tegmenti pontis [TA]) localiza-se na porção ventromedial do tegmento da ponte e é corretamente parte do complexo reticular da ponte; algumas vezes, está também associado à extensão dorsal dos núcleos da ponte basilar. SIN nuclei reticulares pontis [TA].
reticular n. of thalamus [TA], n. reticular do tálamo; lâmina de neurônios bastante grandes que recobre as superfícies lateral, ventral e rostral do tálamo; seu aspecto reticular é produzido pelos numerosos fascículos dos pedúnculos talâmicos que atravessam o núcleo. O núcleo recebe numerosas fibras do córtex cerebral, mas não possui nenhuma projeção cortical. SIN n. reticularis thalami [TA].
retroposterior lateral n., n. lateral retroposterior; VER anterior *horn*.
n. reuniens [TA], n. de reunião; pequeno grupo celular pertencente ao grupo de núcleos talâmicos da linha mediana, que se estende para a aderência intertalâmica (massa intermédia) quando esta última está presente.
rhombencephalic gustatory n., n. gustatório rombencefálico; o terço rostral do núcleo do trato solitário, que recebe aferentes dos nervos facial, glossofaríngeo e vago, transmitindo impulsos que se originam das células receptoras dos botões gustativos.
Roller n., n. de Roller; (1) núcleo lateral do nervo acessório; (2) pequeno núcleo bulbar de localização imediatamente anterior ao núcleo hipoglosso, considerado um dos núcleos peri-hipoglossais. VER subhypoglossal nucleus.
roof n., n. do fastígio. SIN fastigial n.
n. ru'ber [TA], n. rubro. SIN red n.
n. saguli [TA], n. ságulo. SIN sagulum n.
sagulum n. [TA], n. ságulo; grupo de corpos celulares neuronais localizado entre o lemnisco lateral e a superfície lateral do tronco cerebral, imediatamente caudal ao colículo inferior; associado funcionalmente ao sistema auditivo. SIN n. saguli [TA].
n. salivato'rius infe'rior [TA], n. salivatório inferior. SIN inferior salivatory n.
n. salivato'rius supe'rior [TA], n. salivatório superior. SIN superior salivatory n.
Schwalbe n., n. de Schwalbe; VER vestibular nuclei.
secondary sensory nuclei, núcleos sensoriais secundários. SIN terminal n.
segmentation n., n. de segmentação; (1) o núcleo composto no ovo fecundado, formado pela conjugação dos núcleos do óvulo e do espermatozóide (pronúcleos feminino e masculino); (2) o núcleo do zigoto após iniciar a primeira divisão de clivagem.
semilunar n. of Flechsig, n. semilunar de Flechsig, n. arqueado. SIN arcuate n. of thalamus.
n. senso'rius supe'rior ner'vi trigem'ini, n. sensorial superior do nervo trigêmeo. SIN principal sensory n. of trigeminal nerve.
sensory nuclei, núcleos sensoriais; grupo de corpos celulares que recebem impulsos aferentes (sensoriais) da periferia.
n. septalis precommissuralis [TA], n. septal pré-comissural. SIN precommissural septal n.
septofimbrial n. [TA], n. septofimbrial; VER septal *area*.
shadow n., n. fantasma; núcleo que perdeu seu pigmento e suas propriedades tintoriais.
sole nuclei, núcleos solitários; acúmulo de núcleos de fibras musculares esqueléticas na junção mioneural.
nuclei of solitary tract, núcleos do trato solitário; delgada coluna celular que se estende sagitalmente através da parte dorsal da medula oblonga, por baixo do assoalho da fossa rombóide, imediatamente lateral ao sulco limitante. Essa coluna de células é composta de núcleos individuais menores, que coletivamente constituem os núcleos sensoriais viscerais (aferentes viscerais) do tronco cerebral, recebendo as fibras aferentes dos nervos vago, glossofaríngeo e facial através do trato solitário. Os dois terços caudais do núcleo solitário processam impulsos provenientes da faringe, laringe, trato intestinal, trato respiratório e coração e grandes vasos sanguíneos; seu terço rostral recebe impulsos das papilas gustativas e é conhecido como núcleo gustatório rombencefálico. Os núcleos individuais que, coletivamente, formam o núcleo comumente denominado solitário são: o núcleo parassolitário [TA] (nucleus parasolitarius [TA]), o núcleo solitário comissural [TA] (nucleus commissuralis [TA]), o núcleo solitário gelatinoso [TA] (nucleus gelatinosus solitarius [TA]), o núcleo solitário intermediário [TA] (nucleus intermedius solitarius [TA]), o núcleo solitário intersticial [TA] (nucleus interstitialis solitarius [TA]), núcleo solitário medial [TA] (nucleus medialis solitarius [TA]), o núcleo solitário paracomissural [TA]

nucleus

(nucleus paracommissuralis solitarius [TA]), o núcleo solitário posterior [TA] ou núcleo solitário dorsal [TAalt] (nucleus solitarius posterior [TA]), o núcleo solitário póstero-lateral [TA] ou núcleo solitário dorsolateral [TAalt] (nucleus solitarius posterolateralis [TA]), o núcleo solitário anterior [TA] ou núcleo solitário ventral [TAalt] (nucleus solitarius anterior [TA]) e o núcleo solitário ântero-lateral [TA] ou núcleo solitário ventrolateral [TA] (nucleus solitarius anterolateralis [TA]). SIN nuclei tractus solitarii [TA].

somatic n., n. somático. SIN macronucleus (2).

somatic motor nuclei, núcleos motores somáticos; termo coletivo indicando os núcleos motores que inervam a musculatura da língua (n. hipoglosso) e os músculos extra-oculares do olho (n. abducente, n. troclear e n. oculomotor), os músculos esternocleidomastóide e trapézio (nervo acessório) e os músculos esqueléticos do corpo (raízes ventrais dos nervos espinais).

special visceral efferent nuclei, núcleos eferentes viscerais especiais. SIN branchiomotor nuclei.

special visceral motor nuclei, núcleos motores viscerais especiais. SIN branchiomotor nuclei.

sperm n., n. do espermatozóide; o núcleo na cabeça do espermatozóide, que se transforma no pró-núcleo masculino após penetrar no óvulo. VER TAMBÉM pronucleus.

spherical n., n. globoso. SIN globosus n.

n. spina'lis ner'vi trigem'ini [TA], n. espinal do nervo trigêmeo. SIN spinal n. of trigeminal nerve.

spinal trigeminal n., n. espinal do trigêmeo; VER spinal n. of trigeminal nerve.

spinal n. of trigeminal nerve [TA], n. espinal do nervo trigêmeo; o longo núcleo sensorial que se estende da borda caudal do núcleo sensorial pontino do trigêmeo, através da região lateral do rombencéfalo, para os três segmentos superiores do corno dorsal da medula espinal; recebe as fibras da raiz sensorial do nervo trigêmeo que descem ao longo de sua borda lateral na forma do trato espinal do nervo trigêmeo [TA]. Esse núcleo é dividido em pars caudalis [TA] (parte caudal [TA]), pars interpolaris [TA] (parte interpolar [TA]) e subnucleus oralis [TA] (subnúcleo oral [TA]). A pars caudalis é ainda organizada em subnucleus zonalis [TA] (subnúcleo zonal [TA]), subnucleus gelatinosus [TA] (subnúcleo gelatinoso [TA]) e subnucleus magnocellularis [TA] (subnúcleo magnocelular [TA]). SIN n. spinalis nervi trigemini [TA], descending n. of the trigeminus, spinal n. of the trigeminus.

spinal n. of the trigeminus, n. espinal do trigêmeo. SIN spinal n. of trigeminal nerve.

Spitzka n., n. Spitzka. SIN Perlia n.

Staderini n., n. de Staderini, n. intercalado. SIN intercalated n.

steroid n., n. de esteróides. SIN tetracyclic steroid n.

Stilling n., n. de Stilling. SIN posterior thoracic n.

subcaeruleus n., n. subcerúleo; núcleo difusamente organizado de células noradrenérgicas localizado ventralmente ao núcleo cerúleo.

subcuneiform n. [TA], n. subcuneiforme; VER reticular nuclei of mesencephalon. SIN n. subcuneiformis [TA].

n. subcuneiformis [TA], n. subcuneiforme. SIN subcuneiform n; VER reticular nuclei of mesencephalon.

subhypoglossal n. [TA], n. sub-hipoglossal; pequeno núcleo bulbar de localização imediatamente ventral (anterior) ao núcleo do nervo hipoglosso; considerado um dos núcleos peri-hipoglossais. SIN n. subhypoglossalis [Ta].

n. subhypoglossalis [TA], n. sub-hipoglossal. SIN subhypoglossal n.

n. subparabrachialis [TA], n. subparabraquial. SIN subparabrachial n.

subparabrachial n. [TA], n. subparabraquial. SIN grupo de células localizado ventralmente ao pendúnculo cerebelar superior, na área geral onde os núcleos parabraquiais medial e lateral entram em contato, deslocando-se para a posição um pouco mais lateral em direção rostral. VER TAMBÉM parabrachial nuclei. SIN n. subparabrachialis [TA].

subthalamic n. [TA], n. subtalâmico; núcleo circunscrito, de forma semelhante a uma lente biconvexa, localizado na parte ventral do subtálamo, na superfície dorsal da parte peduncular da cápsula interna, imediatamente rostral à substância negra. O núcleo recebe uma projeção topográfica maciça do segmento lateral do globo pálido e uma projeção organizada somatotopicamente do córtex motor ipsolateral; um feixe menor de aferentes do núcleo centromediano do tálamo termina na parte rostral do núcleo. O núcleo subtalâmico projeta-se para ambos os segmentos pálidos, para a parte reticulada da substância negra e, num pequeno trajeto, para o núcleo pedunculopontino ipsolateral. SIN n. subthalamicus [TA], corpus luysi, Luys body, n. of Luys.

n. subthalam'icus [TA], n. subtalâmico. SIN subthalamic n.

superior central tegmental n., n. da rafe. SIN median raphe nucleus; VER raphe nuclei.

superior olivary n. [TA], n. olivar superior; grupo de células circunscritas localizado ventrolateralmente no tegmento pontino inferior, imediatamente dorsal ao corpo trapezóide; o núcleo recebe fibras dos núcleos cocleares ipsolateral e contralateral e contribui com fibras para o lemnisco lateral de ambos os lados. Está proeminentemente envolvido na função da localização espacial do som. O núcleo (também denominado complexo olivar superior) consiste num núcleo olivar superior lateral [TA] (n. olivaris superior lateralis [TA]), num núcleo olivar superior medial [TA] (n. olivaris superior medialis [TA]) e nos núcleos periolivares [TA] (nuclei periolivares [TA]), que são habitualmente divididos em núcleos mediais [TA] e núcleos laterais [TA] (nuclei mediales [TA] e nuclei laterales [TA]). SIN n. olivaris superior [TA], superior olivary complex*.

superior salivary n., n. salivatório superior. SIN superior salivatory n.

superior salivatory n. [TA], n. salivatório superior; grupo de neurônios motores parassimpáticos pré-ganglionares situado rostral e lateralmente ao núcleo salivar inferior; governa a secreção das glândulas lacrimal, sublingual e submaxilar através do nervo facial e dos gânglios esfenopalatino e submandibular. SIN n. salivatorius superior [TA], superior salivary n.

superior vestibular n. [TA], n. vestibular superior; VER vestibular nuclei. SIN n. vestibularis superior [TA].

suprachiasmatic n. [TA], n. supraquiasmático; VER anterior hypothalamic area.

n. suprachiasmaticus [TA], n. supraquiasmático; pequeno núcleo localizado dorsalmente ao quiasma óptico; recebe impulsos da retina e influencia a função neuroendócrina do hipotálamo; estreitamente associado à regulação da ritmicidade circadiana. VER TAMBÉM anterior hypothalamic area.

supralemniscal n. [TA], n. supralemniscal; pequeno grupo de neurônios localizado dorsalmente ao lemnisco medial, insinuando-se entre as fibras do trato trigeminotalâmico ventral entre os níveis rostrais da ponte. SIN n. supralemniscalis [TA].

n. supralemniscalis [TA], n. supralemniscal. SIN supralemniscal n.

n. supramammillaris [TA], n. supramamilar. SIN supramammillary n.

supramammillary n. [TA], n. supramamilar. VER posterior hypothalamic area. SIN n. supramammillaris [TA].

supraoptic n. [TA], n. supra-óptico. SIN supraoptic n. [TA] of hypothalamus.

supraoptic n. [TA] of hypothalamus, n. supra-óptico do hipotálamo; núcleo neurossecretor de células grandes no hipotálamo, localizado sobre a borda lateral do trato óptico, a partir do qual se origina o trato supra-óptico-hipofisário; seus neurônios produzem e transportam a vasopressina liberada na circulação geral a partir das terminações axonais no trato supra-óptico hipofisário. Esse núcleo pode ser dividido em parte dorsolateral [TA], parte dorsomedial [TA] e parte ventromedial [TA]. SIN n. supraopticus [TA], supraoptic n. [TA].

n. supraop'ticus [TA], n. supra-óptico. SIN supraoptic n. [TA] of hypothalamus.

n. tec'ti, n. do fastígio. SIN fastigial n.

tegmental nuclei, núcleos tegmentais; termo coletivo para referir-se aos grupos celulares na porção caudal do mesencéfalo e na porção média e rostral da ponte, com um deles (núcleo do tegmento ventral) associado aos núcleos mamilares através do pedúnculo mamilar e trato mamilotegmentar. Os neurônios nesses núcleos são ricos em acetilcolinesterase. O núcleo tegmental anterior [TA], também denominado núcleo do tegmento ventral [TAalt] (n. tegmentalis anterior [TA]), localiza-se no tegmento da ponte, adjacente ao fascículo longitudinal medial ao nível do núcleo motor trigêmeo. O núcleo do tegmento posterior [TA], também denominado núcleo do tegmento dorsal [TAalt], localiza-se na ponte rostral, na área da substância cinzenta central. O núcleo tegmental póstero-lateral [TA], também conhecido como núcleo tegmental dorsolateral [TAalt] (n. tegmentalis posterolateralis [TA]), é um grupo celular maior, localizado parcialmente na substância cinzenta central e parcialmente ventrolateral a esta última, ao nível da ponte rostral. O núcleo do tegmento pedunculopontino [TA] (nucleus tegmentalis pedunculopontinus [TA]) localiza-se na ponte rostral e mesencéfalo caudal e consiste numa parte compacta [TA] (pars compacta [TA] ou subnúcleo compacto [TAalt]) e numa parte dispersa [TA] (pars dissipata [TA] ou subnúcleo disperso [TAalt]). SIN Gudden tegmental nuclei, nuclei tegmenti.

n. tegmentalis pedunculopontinus [TA], n. tegmental pedunculopontino [TA]. SIN pedunculopontine tegmental n; VER reticular nuclei of mesencephalon.

nu'clei tegmen'ti, núcleos tegmentais. SIN tegmental nuclei.

terminal n., n. termina'lis, n. terminal; termo coletivo que indica os grupos de células nervosas no rombencéfalo e na medula espinal, onde terminam as fibras aferentes dos nervos espinais e cranianos. SIN n. terminationis [TA], secondary sensory nuclei.

n. terminatio'nis [TA], n. terminal. SIN terminal n.

tetracyclic steroid n., n. de esteróides tetracíclicos; o grupo de quatro anéis fundidos que formam o arcabouço ou a substância original dos esteróides. SIN perhydrocyclopenta[a]phenanthrene, steroid n.

thalamic gustatory n., n. arqueado do tálamo. SIN arcuate n. of thalamus.

n. thorac'icus posterior [TA], n. torácico posterior. SIN posterior thoracic n.

n. tractus olfactorii lateralis [TA], n. do trato olfatório lateral. SIN n. of the lateral olfactory tract.

nuclei trac'tus solita'rii [TA], núcleos do trato solitário. SIN nuclei of solitary tract.

nuclei of trapezoid body [TA], núcleos do corpo trapezóide; pequenos grupos de neurônios associados ao corpo trapezóide, formando o núcleo lateral do corpo trapezóide [TA] (n. lateralis corporis trapezoidei [TA]), o núcleo medial do corpo trapezóide [TA] (n. medialis corporis trapezoidei [TA]) e o

núcleo anterior do corpo trapezóide [TA] ou núcleo ventral do corpo trapezóide [TA] (n. anterior corporis trapezoidei [TA]). Esses grupos celulares indistintos estão envolvidos na retransmissão do aporte auditivo. SIN nuclei corporis trapezoidei [TA].
triangular n., n. triangular; termo alternativo para medial vestibular nucleus (núcleo vestibular medial).
triangular n. of septum [TA], n. triangular do septo. VER septal *area*.
trochlear n., n. troclear. SIN n. of trochlear nerve.
n. of trochlear nerve, n. do nervo troclear; grupo de neurônios motores que inervam o músculo oblíquo superior do olho contralateral. O núcleo localiza-se na metade caudal do mesencéfalo, atrás do núcleo oculomotor, na parte mais ventral da substância cinzenta central, próximo à linha média. SIN n. nervi trochlearis [TA], trochlear n.
trophic n., n. trófico. SIN macronucleus (2).
tuberal nuclei, núcleos tuberais laterais; dois ou três pequenos agrupamentos redondos ou ovóides e encapsulados de células na área hipotalâmica lateral, ao longo da superfície da tuberosidade cinérea; suas conexões e importância funcional não são conhecidas. SIN nuclei tuberales laterales [TA].
nu′clei tubera′les laterales [TA], núcleos tuberais laterais. SIN tuberal nuclei.
n. tuberomammillaris [TA], n. túbero-mamilar. SIN tuberomammillary n.
tuberomammillary n. [TA], n. túbero-mamilar; VER lateral hypothalamic *area*. SIN n. tuberomammillaris [TA].
ventral anterior n. [TA] of thalamus, n. ventral anterior do tálamo; a mais rostral das subdivisões do núcleo ventral, que recebe projeções do globo pálido e projeta-se para o córtex pré-motor e frontal. Esse núcleo pode ser dividido numa porção magnocelular (pars magnocellularis [TA]) e numa divisão principal [TA] (pars principalis [TA]). SIN n. ventralis anterior [TA].
nuclei ventra′les thal′ami [TA], núcleos ventrais do tálamo. SIN ventral nuclei of thalamus.
n. of ventral field [TA], n. do campo ventral; VER nuclei of perizonal fields. SIN n. campi ventralis [TA].
ventral intermediate n. [TA] of thalamus, n. ventral intermédio do tálamo; o terço médio composto do núcleo ventral, que recebe em suas várias partes projeções distintas da metade contralateral do cerebelo (por meio do pedúnculo cerebelar superior) e globo pálido ipsolateral; quase todas as partes do núcleo projetam-se para o córtex motor. SIN n. ventralis intermedius [TA], n. ventralis lateralis, ventral lateral n. of thalamus.
n. ventralis [TA], n. ventral. SIN ventral principal n; VER medial geniculate nuclei.
n. ventra′lis ante′rior [TA], n. ventral anterior. SIN ventral anterior n. [TA] of thalamus.
n. ventralis corporis geniculi lateralis [TA], n. ventral do corpo geniculado lateral. SIN ventral lateral geniculate n.
n. ventra′lis interme′dius [TA], n. ventral intermédio. SIN ventral intermediate n. [TA] of thalamus.
n. ventra′lis latera′lis, n. ventral lateral. SIN ventral intermediate n. [TA] of thalamus.
n. ventra′lis poste′rior interme′dius thal′ami, n. ventral posterior intermédio do tálamo; parte intermediária do complexo nuclear ventrobasilar. VER ventral posterior n. of thalamus. SIN ventral posterior intermediate n. of thalamus.
n. ventra′lis poste′rior thal′ami, n. ventral posterior do tálamo. SIN ventrobasal *complex*.
n. ventra′lis posterolatera′lis [TA], n. ventral póstero-lateral. SIN ventral posterolateral n. [TA] of thalamus.
n. ventra′lis posteromedia′lis [TA], n. ventral póstero-medial. SIN ventral posteromedial n. [TA] of thalamus.
ventral lateral geniculate n. [TA], n. ventral do corpo geniculado lateral; pequeno grupo de células localizado rostralmente ao núcleo dorsal do corpo geniculado lateral. SIN n. ventralis corporis geniculi lateralis [TA], pregeniculate n.*.
ventral lateral n. of thalamus [TA], n. ventral lateral do tálamo. SIN ventral intermediate n. [TA] of thalamus.
ventral posterior intermediate n. of thalamus, n. ventral posterior intermédio do tálamo. SIN n. ventralis posterior intermedius thalami; VER ventral posterior n. of thalamus.
ventral posterior n. of thalamus [TA], n. ventral posterior do tálamo; VER ventrobasal *complex*.
ventral posterolateral n. [TA] of thalamus, ventral posterior lateral n. of thalamus, n. ventral póstero-lateral do tálamo; parte lateral do complexo nuclear ventrobasal. VER ventrobasal *complex*. SIN n. ventralis posterolateralis [TA].
ventral posteromedial n. [TA] of thalamus, posterior medial n. of thalamus, n. ventral póstero-medial do tálamo, n. póstero-medial do tálamo; parte medial do complexo nuclear ventrobasal. VER ventrobasal *complex*. SIN n. ventralis posteromedialis [TA].
ventral premammillary n. [TA], n. pré-mamilar ventral; VER posterior hypothalamic *area*. SIN n. premammillaris ventralis [TA].

ventral principal n. [TA], n. principal ventral; SIN medial geniculate nuclei. SIN n. ventralis.
ventral nuclei of thalamus [TA], núcleos ventrais do tálamo; grande massa celular complexa, cuja borda externa forma o limite ventral e grande parte do limite lateral, bem como a borda rostral do tálamo; os núcleos que compõem essa grande área do diencéfalo são o núcleo ventral anterior [TA] (nucleus ventralis anterior [TA]) o complexo ventral lateral [TA] (nuclei ventrales laterales [TA]), o complexo ventral medial [TA] (nuclei ventrales medialis [TA]), o núcleo ventral intermediário [TA] (nucleus ventralis intermedius [TA]), o complexo ventrobasilar [TA] (nuclei ventrobasales [TA]), o ventroposterior inferior [TA] (nucleus ventroposterior internus [TA]) e o núcleo ventroposterior parvocelular [TA] (nucleus ventroposterior parvocellularis [TA]). Em geral, essa área pode ser subdividida em partes anterior, intermediária e posterior. SIN nuclei ventrales thalami [TA].
ventral tier thalamic nuclei, núcleos talâmicos ventrais; termo coletivo para referir-se aos núcleos na parte ventral do grupo nuclear lateral, p. ex., os núcleos ventral anterior, lateral, póstero-lateral e póstero-medial e os núcleos do corpo geniculado medial e núcleo dorsal do corpo geniculado lateral. O complexo nuclear basoventral constitui a parte caudal dos núcleos talâmicos ventrais.
ventral n. of trapezoid body, n. ventral do corpo trapezóide; grupo de células mergulhado entre as fibras do corpo trapezóide, a principal decussação da via auditiva central, na porção inferior da ponte. O núcleo recebe fibras dos núcleos cocleares contralaterais e contribui com fibras para o sistema auditivo ascendente ou lemnisco lateral.
ventrobasal nuclei (complex) [TA], núcleos (complexo) ventrobasais. SIN ventrobasal *complex*.
nuclei ventrobasales [TA], núcleos ventrobasilares. SIN ventrobasal *complex*.
ventrolateral n. [TA], n. ventral lateral; VER anterior *horn*.
ventromedial n. [TA], n. ventral medial; VER intermediate hypothalamic *area*.
ventromedial n. of hypothalamus [TA], n. ventral medial do hipotálamo; grupo ovóide circunscrito de pequenos neurônios na zona medial da região tuberal do hipotálamo. A destruição bilateral desse núcleo no rato resulta em grave obesidade. O núcleo recebe numerosas fibras da amígdala através da estria terminal; suas conexões eferentes são obscuras. SIN n. ventromedialis hypothalami [TA].
n. ventromedia′lis hypothal′ami [TA], n. ventral medial do hipotálamo. SIN ventromedial n. of hypothalamus; VER intermediate hypothalamic *area*.
vestibular nuclei [TA], núcleos vestibulares; grupo de quatro núcleos principais localizados na região lateral do rombencéfalo, abaixo do assoalho da fossa rombóide. Esses núcleos incluem: o núcleo vestibular inferior, o núcleo vestibular medial (núcleo de Schwalbe), o núcleo vestibular lateral (núcleo de Deiter) e o núcleo vestibular superior (núcleo de Bechterew). O núcleo inferior contém um grupo de grandes células, a parte magnocelular do núcleo vestibular inferior [TA] ou grupo celular F [TAalt] (pars magnocellularis nuclei vestibularis inferioris [TA]), de localização caudal no núcleo. Um grupo de neurônios de tamanho médio localiza-se nas porções laterais do núcleo lateral, a parte parvocelular [TA] ou grupo celular I [TAalt] (pars parvocellularis [TA]). Esses núcleos recebem fibras primárias do nervo vestibular, estão reciprocamente ligadas com o lobo floconodular do cerebelo e projetam-se através do fascículo longitudinal medial para os núcleos abducente, troclear e oculomotor e para o corno ventral da medula espinal. O núcleo vestibular lateral projeta-se para o corno ventral ipsolateral da medula espinal pelo trato vestibuloespinal. SIN. nuclei vestibulares [TA].
nu′clei vestibula′res [TA], núcleos vestibulares. SIN vestibular nuclei.
n. vestibularis inferior [TA], n. vestibular inferior. SIN inferior vestibular n; VER vestibular nuclei.
n. vestibularis lateralis [TA], n. vestibular lateral. SIN lateral vestibular n; VER vestibular nuclei.
n. vestibularis medialis [TA], n. vestibular medial. SIN medial vestibular n; VER vestibular nuclei.
n. vestibularis superior [TA], n. vestibular superior. SIN superior vestibular n; VER vestibular nuclei.
vestibulocochlear nuclei, núcleos vestibulococleares; os núcleos cocleares e vestibulares combinados, no tronco cerebral, que recebem as fibras do oitavo nervo craniano. VER vestibular nuclei. SIN nuclei nervi vestibulocochlearis.
nuclei viscerales nervi oculomotorii, núcleos viscerais do nervo oculomotor; o núcleo motor visceral do nervo oculomotor, também denominado núcleo de Edinger-Westphal, que pode ser dividido em núcleo anterior medial [TA] (n. anteromedialis [TA]) e núcleo posterior [TA] (n. dorsalis [TA]). VER TAMBÉM Edinger-Westphal n.
visceral nuclei of oculomotor nerve [TA], núcleos viscerais do nervo oculomotor. SIN Edinger-Westphal n.

nu·clide (noo′klīd). Nuclídeo. Espécie nuclear particular (atômica), com massa atômica e número atômico definidos. VER TAMBÉM isotope.
Nuel, Jean Pierre, oftalmologista e otologista belga, 1847–1920. VER N. *space*.
NUG GUN. Abreviatura de necrotizing ulcerative *gingivitis* (gengivite ulcerativa necrosante).

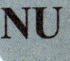

Nuhn, Anton, anatomista alemão, 1814–1889. VER N. *gland.*

nul·li·grav·i·da (nŭl-i-grav′i-dă). Nuligrávida. Mulher que nunca concebeu um filho. [L. *nullus,* nenhum + *gravida,* grávida].

nul·lip·a·ra (nŭ-lip′a-ră). Nulípara. Mulher que nunca deu à luz. [L. *nullus,* nenhum + *pario,* parir]

nul·li·par·i·ty (nŭl-i-par′i-tē). Nuliparidade. Condição da mulher que nunca deu à luz.

nul·lip·a·rous (nŭl-ip′a-rŭs). Nulípara. Que nunca deu à luz. SIN nonparous.

num·ber (nŭm′ber). Número. **1.** Símbolo que expressa um certo valor ou uma quantidade específica determinada por cálculo. **2.** Lugar de qualquer unidade numa série.

atomic n. (Z), n. atômico; o número de prótons no núcleo de um átomo; indica a posição do elemento no sistema periódico.

Avogadro n. (Λ, N_A), n. de Avogadro; o número de moléculas em uma molécula-grama de peso (1 mol) de qualquer composto; definido como o número de átomos em 0,0120 kg de carbono-12 puro; equivalente a $6,0221367 \times 10^{23}$. SIN Avogadro constant.

Brinell hardness n. (BHN), n. de dureza de Brinell; número relacionado ao tamanho da impressão permanente produzida por um indentador esférico de dimensão especificada (em geral, 10 mm de diâmetro) comprimido sobre a superfície do material, exercendo uma carga específica:

$$BHN = \frac{P}{\frac{\pi D}{2}(D - \sqrt{D^2 - d^2})}$$

onde P = a carga aplicada em kg; D = diâmetro da bola em mm, e d = diâmetro da impressão em mm.

CT n., n. TC; valor normalizado do coeficiente calculado de absorção de raios X de um pixel (elemento do quadro) numa tomografia computadorizada, expresso em unidades Hounsfield, onde o n. TC do ar é de −1.000 e o da água é 0. SIN Hounsfield n..

electronic n., n. eletrônico; o número de elétrons na órbita mais externa (camada de valência) de um elemento.

gold n., n. de ouro. SIN gold *equivalent.*

Hehner n., n. de Hehner; o peso ou percentagem dos ácidos graxos não-voláteis produzidos por 5 g de um óleo ou gordura saponificada. SIN Hehner value.

Hogben n., n. de Hogben; número exclusivo de identificação pessoal obtido para utilizar uma seqüência de dígitos referentes à data do nascimento, sexo, local de nascimento e outros identificadores; inventado por Lancelot Hogben, matemático inglês; o número de Hogben constitui a base para os números de identificação em muitos estabelecimentos de assistência primária e são utilizados em muitos sistemas de ligação de registros.

Hounsfield n., n. de Hounsfield. SIN CT n.

hydrogen n., n. de hidrogênio; quantidade de hidrogênio absorvida por 1 g de gordura; trata-se de uma medida da quantidade de ácidos graxos insaturados na gordura. VER TAMBÉM iodine n.

iodine n., n. de iodo; indicação da quantidade de ácidos graxos insaturados presente na gordura; representa o número de gramas de iodo absorvido por cada 100 g de gordura. VER TAMBÉM hydrogen n. SIN iodine value.

Kestenbaum n., n. de Kestenbaum; a diferença entre os diâmetros das duas pupilas quando cada olho é medido à luz brilhante estando o outro olho totalmente coberto; indicador do defeito pupilar aferente relativo em pacientes com duas íris de inervação normal.

Knoop hardness n. (KHN), n. de dureza de Knoop; número obtido ao dividir a carga em kg aplicada a um diamante em forma de pirâmide de dimensão específica pela área projetada da impressão: KHN = *L/A,* onde A = a área projetada da impressão em mm^2 e L = a carga em kg; utilizado para medidas de dureza de qualquer material, especialmente substâncias muito duras e quebradiças, como a dentina e o esmalte do dente.

Koettstorfer n., n. de Koettstorfer. SIN saponification n.

linking n. (L), n. de ligação; propriedade de um biopolímero longo (como DNA de filamento duplo) igual ao número de voltas (relacionado à freqüência de voltas em torno do eixo central da hélice) mais o número de torção.

Loschmidt n. (n_0), n. de Loschmidt; número de moléculas em 1 cm^3 de gás ideal a 0°C e 1 atm de pressão; o número de Avogadro dividido por 22.414 (isto é, $2,6868 \times 10^{19}$ cm^{-3}).

Mach n., n. de Mach; número que representa a relação entre a velocidade de um objeto que se move através de um meio fluido, como o ar, e a velocidade do som no mesmo meio.

mass n., n. de massa; a massa do átomo de um isótopo particular em relação ao hidrogênio-1 (ou a 1/12 da massa do carbono-12), geralmente muito próximo ao número total representado pela soma dos prótons e dos nêutrons no núcleo atômico do isótopo (indicado no número ou símbolo do isótopo; p. ex., oxigênio-16, O^{16}); não deve ser confundido com o peso atômico de um elemento, que pode incluir um número de isótopos em proporção natural.

MIM n., n. MIM; classificação de 1-mendeliano no sistema MIM. Se o número inicial for 1, o traço é considerado autossômico dominante; se for 2, autossômico recessivo; e 3, ligado ao cromossoma X. Sempre que um traço definido nesse dicionário tiver um número MIM, o número da décima segunda edição do MIM é fornecido entre colchetes, com ou sem asterisco (o asterisco indica que o modo de herança é conhecido; o símbolo # antes de um número significa que o fenótipo pode ser causado por mutação em quaisquer 2 ou mais genes), quando apropriado; p. ex., a doença de Pelizaeus-Merzbacher [MIM*169500] é um distúrbio mendeliano autossômico dominante bem estabelecido.

Polenské n., n. de Polenské; número de mililitros de KOH 0,1 N necessários para neutralizar os ácidos graxos não-voláteis obtidos de 5 g de gordura ou óleo saponificado.

Reichert-Meissl n., n. de Reichert-Meissl; índice do conteúdo de ácidos voláteis de uma gordura; o número de mililitros de KOH 0,1 N necessários para neutralizar os ácidos graxos voláteis solúveis existentes em 5 g de gordura que foi saponificada, acidificada para liberar os ácidos graxos e, a seguir, destilada na forma de vapor. SIN volatile fatty acid n.

Reynolds n., n. de Reynolds; número sem dimensão que descreve a tendência de um líquido que flui, como o sangue, a passar do fluxo laminar para o fluxo turbulento, ou vice-versa.

saponification n., n. de saponificação; o número de miligramas de KOH necessários para saponificar 1 g de gordura; medida aproximada do peso molecular médio de uma gordura, com o qual varia inversamente. SIN Koettstorfer n.

stoichiometric n. (V), n. estequiométrico; o número associado a um reagente ou produto que participa numa reação química definida; em geral, número inteiro.

thiocyanogen n., n. de tiocianogênio; número de gramas de tiocianogênio captados por 100 g de gordura; análogo ao número de iodo, exceto que o tiocianógeno não irá adicionar-se a todas as ligações duplas nos ácidos graxos poliinsaturados, como o iodo. SIN thiocyanogen value.

transport n., n. de transporte; fração da corrente total transportada através de uma solução por um tipo particular de íon presente na solução.

turnover n. (k_{cat}), n. de renovação; o número de moléculas de substrato convertidas em produto numa reação catalisada por enzima em condições de saturação por unidade de tempo por unidade de quantidade de enzima; p. ex., $k_{cat} = V_{máx}/[E_{total}]$.

volatile fatty acid n., n. de ácidos graxos voláteis. SIN Reichert-Meissl n.

wave n., n. de ondas; o número de ondas (ou de qualquer forma de ondas, como a luz ou o som) por unidade de comprimento.

writhing n., n. de torção; número de vezes que o eixo de DNA de filamento duplo cruza a si próprio no espaço.

numb·ness (nŭm′nes). Entorpecimento. Termo indefinido para referir-se a uma sensação anormal, incluindo ausência ou redução de percepção de estímulos, bem como parestesias.

num·mi·form (nŭm′i-form). Numiforme. SIN nummular.

num·mu·lar (nŭm′ū-ler). Numular, numismal. **1.** Discóide ou em forma de moeda; refere-se ao escarro mucopurulento ou mucoso espesso em certas doenças respiratórias, assim denominado em virtude da forma discóide adotada quando achatado no fundo de uma escarradeira contendo água ou desinfetante transparente. **2.** Disposição em pilhas de moedas, indicando a associação dos eritrócitos na formação de *rouleaux.* SIN nummiform. [L. *nummulus,* pequena moeda, dim. de *nummus,* moeda]

num·mu·la·tion (nŭm-ū-lā′shŭn). Numulação. Formação de massas numulares.

nun·na·tion (nŭ-nā′shŭn). Distúrbio da fala em que o som *n* é dado a outras consoantes. [Ar. *nūn,* a letra n.]

nurse (ners). **1.** Amamentar. **2.** Prestar assistência aos enfermos. **3.** Enfermeira(o); pessoa treinada na base científica da enfermagem sob padrões definidos de formação e envolvida no diagnóstico e tratamento das respostas humanas a problemas reais ou potenciais de saúde. [Fr. antigo *nourice,* do L. *nutrix,* ama-de-leite, de *nutrio,* amamentar, cuidar de]

certified registered n. anesthetist (C.R.N.A.), enfermeira com formação em anestesiologia; enfermeira com treinamento adicional na administração de anestésicos. O certificado é obtido através de um programa de estudo reconhecido pela *American Association of Nurse Anesthetists.*

charge n., enfermeira encarregada; enfermeira responsável, do ponto de vista administrativo, por uma enfermaria de hospital, habitualmente com 8 horas de trabalho. SIN head n. (2).

clinical n. specialist, enfermeira com formação em clínica; enfermeira com pelo menos um grau de mestre, que recebeu treinamento avançado numa determinada área de prática clínica, como oncologia ou psiquiatria. Geralmente empregada num estabelecimento clínico, como hospital.

community n., enfermeira de comunidade, enfermeira de saúde pública. SIN public health n.

community health n., enfermeira sanitária da comunidade. SIN public health n.

dry n., ama-seca; mulher encarregada de cuidar de recém-nascidos sem amamentá-los, em oposição a ama-de-leite.

n. epidemiologist, enfermeira com formação em epidemiologia; enfermeira registrada com treinamento adicional na monitorização e prevenção de infec-

ções hospitalares na população de clientes num estabelecimento. SIN infection control n.
flight n., enfermeira de aviação; enfermeira que atende os clientes durante o seu transporte em qualquer tipo de aeronave.
general duty n., enfermeira geral; enfermeira que aceita a sua colocação em qualquer unidade de um hospital, à exceção da unidade de tratamento intensivo.
graduate n., enfermeira formada; enfermeira que recebeu um grau, mais freqüentemente de bacharelado, de uma escola ou de enfermagem.
head n., enfermeira-chefe; (1) enfermeira responsável, do ponto de vista administrativo, por uma unidade particular do hospital, turno de 24 horas; (2) SIN charge n.
home health n., n. domiciliar; enfermeira responsável por um grupo de clientes no ambiente domiciliar. Visita os clientes de forma regular, atendendo aos clientes e às suas famílias, conforme a necessidade e treinando a família nos cuidados necessários, de modo que o cliente possa permanecer em casa. SIN visiting n.
hospital n., enfermeira hospitalar; enfermeira que trabalha em hospital.
infection control n., enfermeira com formação em epidemiologia. SIN n. epidemiologist.
licensed practical n. (L.P.N.), técnico de enfermagem; graduando de uma escola reconhecida de enfermagem (vocacional) que se submeteu ao exame para licenciatura e que recebeu licença para praticar por uma autoridade estadual. O programa é, em geral, de 1 ano de duração. SIN licensed vocational n.
licensed vocational n. (L.V.N.), técnico de enfermagem. SIN licensed practical n.
practical n., auxiliar de enfermagem; graduando num programa de treinamento específico que prepara a pessoa para a carreira de enfermagem com menos responsabilidade do que uma enfermeira.
private n., enfermeira particular. SIN private duty n.
private duty n., enfermeira particular; (1) enfermeira que não é membro de uma equipe hospitalar, mas contratada, sem vínculo empregatício, pelo cliente ou família para cuidar do cliente; (2) enfermeira que se especializa nos cuidados de pacientes com doenças de determinado tipo, como, p. ex., casos cirúrgicos, tuberculose, doenças infantis. SIN private n.
public health n., enfermeira de saúde pública; enfermeira que presta assistência a indivíduos ou grupos numa comunidade fora de instituições. Em geral, trabalha sob os auspícios de um departamento sanitário do estado ou da cidade. SIN community health n., community n.
registered n. (R.N.), enfermeira graduada em uma faculdade reconhecida que prestou exame estadual para obter a licenciatura; registrada e licenciada para a prática por uma autoridade estadual.
school n., enfermeira de escola; geralmente uma enfermeira que trabalha numa escola ou instituição semelhante.
scrub n., enfermeira instrumentadora; enfermeira que escova as mãos e os braços, coloca luvas esterilizadas e, em geral, avental esterilizado e auxilia o cirurgião no centro cirúrgico, principalmente passando-lhe os instrumentos.
special n., enfermeira particular; enfermeira que pode ser uma enfermeira ou auxiliar de enfermagem, com funções limitadas e especializadas; em geral, sinônimo de enfermeira particular.
student n., estudante de enfermagem; estudante num programa que leva a um certificado numa forma de enfermagem; refere-se habitualmente a estudantes num programa para enfermeira ou auxiliar de enfermagem.
visiting n., enfermeira visitadora. SIN home health n.
wet n., ama-de-leite; mulher que amamenta uma criança que não é sua.

nurse prac·ti·tion·er (ners prak-tish'ū-ner). Enfermeira com pelo menos um grau de mestre em enfermagem e treinamento avançado no atendimento primário de determinados grupos de clientes; capaz de exercer uma prática independente em vários tipos de ambientes.

Os enfermeiros passaram a ser reconhecidos nos Estados Unidos a partir de 1955. As leis estaduais regulam o âmbito de sua ação e grau de autonomia. Ao assumir a responsabilidade pelo atendimento preventivo, educação sanitária, vigilância rotineira e manejo de doenças crônicas, os enfermeiros permitem aos médicos fornecer serviços diagnósticos e terapêuticos mais sofisticados ou elaborados. Em áreas de baixa densidade populacional, tornam possível o tratamento para a maioria dos problemas clínicos sem a necessidade de os pacientes percorrerem longas distâncias. Alguns observadores assinalaram que a busca dos enfermeiros por aumento de sua autonomia e sua popularidade com as organizações de atendimento gerenciado (*managed care*) ameaça diminuir a qualidade do atendimento médico primário.

nurs·ing (ner'sing). **1.** Amamentar uma criança. Zelar e cuidar de uma criança. **2.** A aplicação científica dos princípios de assistência relacionada à prevenção da doença e cuidados durante a doença.

n. assignment, incumbência de enfermagem; método ou métodos pelos quais o ônus do atendimento é distribuído entre a equipe de enfermagem disponível para fornecer os cuidados.
n. audit, auditoria de enfermagem; procedimento definido utilizado para avaliar a qualidade do cuidado de enfermagem oferecido por um estabelecimento a seus clientes.
n. model, modelo de enfermagem; conjunto de declarações teóricas e gerais sobre os conceitos que servem para proporcionar um arcabouço na organização de idéias sobre clientes, seu ambiente, sua saúde e enfermagem.
n. plan of care, plano de cuidado de enfermagem; a estrutura redigida que fornece orientação para os cuidados de enfermagem.
n. process, processo de enfermagem; método sistemático de tomada de decisões em cinco partes, enfocando a identificação e as respostas terapêuticas dos indivíduos ou grupos de indivíduos a alterações verdadeiras ou potenciais de sua saúde. Inclui a avaliação de enfermagem, o diagnóstico de enfermagem, o planejamento, a implementação e evolução. A primeira fase do processo de enfermagem é a avaliação inicial de enfermagem, que consiste na coleta de dados por diversos meios, como entrevista, exame físico e observação. Exige a coleta de dados tanto objetivos quanto subjetivos. A segunda fase é o diagnóstico de enfermagem, um julgamento clínico sobre as respostas da pessoa, da família ou da comunidade aos problemas de saúde/processos da vida reais ou potenciais. Fornece a base para a seleção da intervenção de enfermagem para obter resultados pelos quais a enfermeira é responsável (NANDA, 1990). A terceira fase é o planejamento, que exige o estabelecimento de critérios de metas para o atendimento ao cliente. A quarta fase é a implementação (intervenção). Essa fase envolve a demonstração das atividades que serão executadas (nos pacientes e com os clientes) para permitir a concretização dos resultados esperados do atendimento. A avaliação da evolução é a quinta fase e a etapa final do processo de enfermagem. Exige a comparação do estado atual do cliente com os resultados esperados e fixados, redundando na revisão do plano de atendimento para acelerar o progresso em direção aos resultados fixados.
nurs·ing home. Clínica de repouso. Clínica ou estabelecimento particular de convalescença para o cuidado de indivíduos que não necessitam de hospitalização, mas que não podem receber cuidados em casa.
Nussbaum, Johann H.R. von, cirurgião alemão, 1829–1890.
nu·ta·tion (noo-tā'shŭn). Nutação. O ato de menear a cabeça, especialmente de modo involuntário. [L. *annuo*, cabecear]
nut·gall (nŭt'gahl). Noz-de-galha, bugalho. Excrescência no carvalho, *Quercus infectoria* (família Fagaceae) e de outras espécies de *Quercus*, causada pela deposição dos ovos de uma mosca *Cynips gallae tinctorae*; adstringente e estíptico, em virtude do tanino que contém. SIN gall (3), galla, oak apple.
nut·meg (nŭt'meg). Noz-moscada. Semente madura e seca de *Myristica fragrans* (família Myristicaceae), desprovida da casca e arilódio; estimulante aromático, carminativo, condimento e fonte de óleos voláteis e espremidos de noz-moscada; é consumida pelos seus efeitos bizarros sobre o sistema nervoso central. VER TAMBÉM myristicin. SIN myristica.
nut·meg oil. Óleo de noz-moscada. Óleo volátil destilado das sementes (grãos) secas e maduras de *Myristica fragrans*; usado como aromatizante carminativo; em grandes quantidades, pode produzir narcose e delírio; o óleo fixo extraído de *M. fragrans* é utilizado como rubefaciente. SIN myristica oil.
nu·tri·ent (noo'trē-ent). Nutriente. Constituinte do alimento necessário para a função fisiológica normal. [L. *nutriens*, de *nutrio*, nutrir]

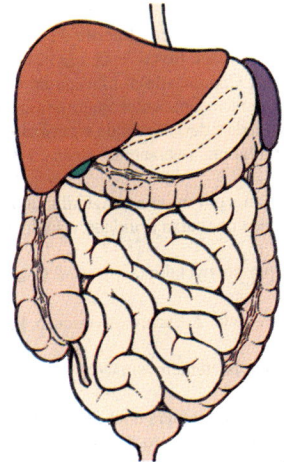

duodeno e jejuno
água
ácidos graxos livres
aminoácidos
monossacarídeos
minerais, incluindo ferro
vitaminas, exceto a vitamina B_{12}

íleo
água
principais substratos remanescentes
minerais
ácidos biliares
vitamina B_{12}

cólon
água
eletrólitos
ácidos graxos de cadeia curta
vitamina K

absorção de nutrientes: locais no trato gastrointestinal

essential n., nutrientes essenciais; substâncias nutricionais necessárias para a saúde ótima. Esses elementos têm de ser obtidos na dieta, já que não são formados metabolicamente no organismo.
trace n., micronutrientes. SIN micronutrients.

nu·tri·lites (noo′tri-līts). Nutrílitos. Fatores nutricionais essenciais. [L. *nutrio*, amamentar, nutrir]

nu·tri·tion (noo-trish′ŭn). Nutrição. **1.** Função dos vegetais e animais vivos, consistindo na captação e metabolismo de material alimentar através do qual o tecido é formado e a energia liberada. SIN trophism (2). **2.** O estudo das necessidades de alimentos e líquidos dos seres humanos ou animais para o desempenho da função fisiológica normal, incluindo as necessidades de energia, manutenção, crescimento, atividade, reprodução e lactação. [L. *nutritio*, de *nutrio*, nutrir]

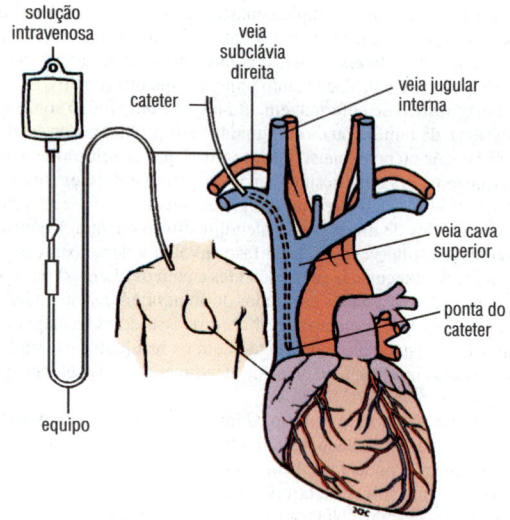

nutrição parenteral total: o cateter é introduzido na circulação através da veia subclávia direita

total parenteral n. (TPN), n. parenteral total (NPT); nutrição mantida totalmente por injeção intravenosa ou outra via não-gastrintestinal.

nu·tri·tive (noo′tri-tiv). Nutritivo. **1.** Relativo à nutrição. **2.** Capaz de nutrir. SIN alible.

nu·tri·ture (noo′tri-choor). Estado ou condição da nutrição do corpo; estado do corpo em relação à nutrição. [L. *nutritura*, enfermeira, de *nutrio*, nutrir]

Nuttall, G.H.F., biólogo norte-americano, 1862–1937. VER *Nuttallia*.

Nut·tal·lia (nŭ-tal′ē-ă). Nome antigo de *Babesia*.

nux vom·i·ca (nŭks vom′i-kă). Noz-vômica. A semente de *Strychnos nux-vomica* (família Logeniaceae), uma árvore da Ásia tropical; contém dois alcalóides, estricnina e a brucina; tem sido utilizada como tônico amargo e estimulante do sistema nervoso central. [L. Mod. noz emética, do L. *nux*, noz + *vomo*, vomitar]

Nva. Nva. Abreviatura de norvaline (norvalina).

nyct-. Nict-. VER nycto-.

nyc·tal·gia (nik-tal′jē-ă). Nictalgia. Refere-se especialmente às dores osteocópicas da sífilis durante a noite. SIN night pain. [nyct- + G. *algos*, dor]

nyc·ta·lo·pia (nik-tă-lō′pē-ă). Nictalopia. Capacidade diminuída de ver com iluminação reduzida. Observada em pacientes com comprometimento da função dos bastonetes; freqüentemente associada a deficiência de vitamina A. SIN day sight, night blindness, nocturnal amblyopia, nyctanopia. [nyct- + G. *alaos*, obscuro + *ōps*, olho]

n. with congenital myopia [MIM*310500], n. com miopia congênita; anormalidade de herança ligada ao X, caracterizada por baixa acuidade visual, estrabismo ou nistagmo.

nyc·ta·no·pia (nik-tă-nō′pē-ă). Nictanopia. SIN nyctalopia. [nyct- + G. *an-* priv. + *opsis*, visão]

nyc·ter·ine (nik′ter-in, -in). Nicterino. **1.** À noite. **2.** Escuro ou obscuro. [G. *nykterinos*]

nyc·ter·o·hem·er·al (nik′ter-ō-hĕ′mer-ăl). Nictêmero. SIN nyctohemeral. [G. *nykteros*, à noite, noturno + *hēmera*, dia]

nycto-, nyct-. Nicto-, nict-. À noite, noturno. VER TAMBÉM noct-. [G. *nyx*]

nyc·to·hem·e·ral (nik-tō-hē′mer-ăl). Nictêmero. Tanto de dia quanto de noite. SIN nycterohemeral. [nycto- + G. *hēmera*, dia]

nyc·to·phil·ia (nik-tō-fil′ē-ă). Nictofilia. Preferência pela noite ou escuridão. SIN scotophilia. [nycto- + G. *philos*, amigo]

nyc·to·pho·bia (nik-tō-fō′bē-ă). Nictofobia. Medo mórbido da noite ou da escuridão. SIN scotophobia. [nycto- + G. *phobos*, medo]

Nyc·to·the·rus (nik-tō-thē′rus). *Nyctotherus*. Gênero de Ciliophora, cuja espécie *N. faba*, tem sido encontrada, ainda que raramente, no intestino humano; em geral, ocorre em anfíbios. [G. *nyktothēras*, que caça à noite, de *thēraō*, caçar, de *thēr*, animal selvagem]

nyc·tu·ria (nik-too′rē-ă). Nictúria. SIN nocturia.

Nyhan, William L., pediatra norte-americano, *1926. VER Lesch-N. *syndrome*.

ny·li·drin hy·dro·chlo·ride (nī′li-drin, nil′). Cloridrato de nilidrina. Agente simpaticomimético, semelhante ao isoproterenol, que produz dilatação das arteríolas dos músculos esqueléticos e aumenta o fluxo sanguíneo muscular; utilizado no tratamento de doenças vasculares periféricas.

nymph (nimf). Ninfa. **1.** Série mais precoce de estágios na metamorfose após a eclosão no desenvolvimento dos insetos hemimetabólicos (p. ex., gafanhoto); a ninfa assemelha-se ao adulto em muitos aspectos, porém faltam-lhe asas completas ou desenvolvimento dos órgãos genitais; cresce através de transformações sucessivas sem qualquer estágio intermediário ou culpa na forma de imago ou adulta. VER TAMBÉM incomplete *metamorphosis*, complete *metamorphosis*. **2.** O terceiro estágio no ciclo de vida de um carrapato, entre a larva e o adulto. [G. *nymphē*, donzela]

nym·pha, pl. **nym·phae** (nim′fă, nim′fē). Ninfa. Um dos lábios pequenos do pudendo. [L. Mod. do G. *nymphē*, noiva]

nym·phal (nim′făl). Ninfal. **1.** Relativo ou pertinente a ninfa. **2.** Relativo aos pequenos lábios do pudendo (ninfas).

nym·phec·to·my (nim-fek′tō-mē). Ninfectomia. Remoção cirúrgica dos pequenos lábios do pudendo hipertrofiados. [nympha + G. *ektomē*, excisão]

nym·phi·tis (nim-fī′tis). Ninfite. Inflamação dos pequenos lábios do pudendo. [nympha + G. *-itis*, inflamação]

nympho-, nymph-. Ninfo-, ninf-. Ninfas (pequenos lábios do pudendo). [L. *nympha*]

nym·pho·la·bi·al (nim′fō-lā′bē-ăl). Ninfolabial. Relativo aos pequenos (ninfas) e grandes lábios do pudendo; indica um sulco entre os dois lábios do pudendo de cada lado.

nym·pho·lep·sy (nim-fō-lep′sē). Ninfolepsia. Frenesi demoníaco, especialmente de natureza erótica. [nympho- + G. *lēpsis*, convulsão]

nym·pho·ma·nia (nim-fō-mā′nē-ă). Ninfomania. Impulso insaciável ao comportamento sexual numa mulher; o correspondente da satiríase no homem. [nympho- + G. *mania*, frênesi, loucura]

nym·pho·ma·ni·ac (nim-fō-mā′nē-ak). Ninfomaníaca. Mulher que exibe ninfomania.

nym·pho·ma·ni·a·cal (nim′fō-mă-nī′ă-kăl). Ninfomaníaca. Relativo à, ou que exibe, ninfomania.

nym·phon·cus (nim-fong′kŭs). Ninfoncose. Edema ou hipertrofia de um ou de ambos os pequenos lábios. [nympho- + G. *onkos*, tumor]

nym·phot·o·my (nim-fot′ō-mē). Ninfotomia. Incisão nos pequenos lábios ou no clitóris. [nympho- + G. *tomē*, incisão]

nys·tag·mic (nis-tag′mik). Nistagmo. Relativo ao, ou que sofre de, nistagmo.

nys·tag·mi·form (nis-tag′mi-fōrm). Nistagmiforme. SIN nystagmoid.

nys·tag·mo·gram (nis-tag′mō-gram). Nistagmograma. Traçado produzido por um nistagmógrafo.

nys·tag·mo·graph (nis-tag′mō-graf). Nistagmógrafo. Aparelho para medir a amplitude, a periodicidade e a velocidade dos movimentos oculares no nistagmo, medindo-se a alteração no potencial de repouso do olho durante o movimento ocular. [nystagmus + G. *graphō*, escrever]

nys·tag·mog·ra·phy (nis-tag-mog′ră-fē). Nistagmografia. Técnica de registro do nistagmo.

nys·tag·moid (nis-tag′moyd). Nistagmóide. Que se assemelha ao nistagmo. SIN nystagmiform. [nystagmus + G. *eidos*, semelhança]

nys·tag·mus (nis-tag′mŭs). Nistagmo. Oscilação rítmica involuntária dos globos oculares, seja pendular ou com componente lento ou rápido. [G. *nystagmos*, oscilação, de *nystazō*, estar sonolento, cabecear]

after-n, n. tardio; nistagmo que ocorre após cessação súbita de rotação na direção oposta do nistagmo rotatório.

amaurotic n., n. amaurótico. SIN ocular n.

Bruns n., n. de Bruns; nistagmo rítmico fino (vestibular) no olhar horizontal em uma direção, juntamente com nistagmo mais lento, de maior amplitude (olhar fixo, parético) ao olhar na direção oposta; devido à compressão lateral do tronco cerebral, geralmente por uma massa no ângulo cerebelo-pontino, como neuroma do acústico.

caloric n., n. calórico; nistagmo com componentes lento e rápido induzido por estimulação do labirinto com água quente ou fria no ouvido. VER TAMBÉM Bárány *sign*.

cervical n., n. cervical; nistagmo que se origina de uma lesão do mecanismo proprioceptivo do pescoço.

compressive n., n. compressivo; nistagmo rítmico resultante de alterações unilaterais da pressão nos canais semicirculares.

congenital n., n. congênito; **(1)** nistagmo presente por ocasião do nascimento ou causado por lesões que ocorrem *in utero* ou no momento do nascimento;

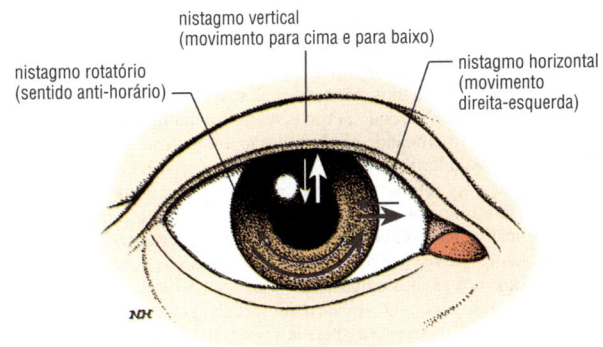

nistagmo: as setas mais espessas indicam a primeira fase (mais lenta)

(2) nistagmo hereditário, habitualmente ligado ao X, sem lesões neurológicas associadas e não-progressivo; podem ocorrer todos os três padrões de herança mendeliana: autossômico dominante [MIM*164100, *164150], autossômico recessivo [MIM*257400] ou recessivo ligado ao X [MIM*310800, *310700]; (3) nistagmo associado a albinismo, acromatopsia e hipoplasia da mácula.
conjugate n., n. conjugado; nistagmo em que os dois olhos movem-se simultaneamente na mesma direção.
convergence-retraction n., nistagmo de convergência–retração; nistagmo rítmico irregular combinando convergência e retração do olho na órbita, especialmente no olhar para cima. SIN Koerber-Salus-Elschnig syndrome.
deviational n., n. de desvio. SIN end-point n.
dissociated n., n. dissociado; nistagmo em que os movimentos dos dois olhos têm direção, amplitude e periodicidade diferentes. SIN dysjunctive n., incongruent n., irregular n.
downbeat n., n. de batimento descendente; nistagmo vertical com componente rápido para baixo, observado em lesões da parte inferior do tronco cerebral ou do cerebelo.
dysjunctive n., n. disjuntivo, n. dissociado. SIN dissociated n.
end-point n., n. de posição terminal; n. rítmico fisiológico que ocorre no indivíduo normal ao tentar fixar um ponto no limite do campo de fixação. SIN deviational n.
fast component of n., componente rápido do nistagmo; movimento compensatório dos olhos no reflexo vestibuloocular.
fixation n., n. de fixação; nistagmo agravado ou induzido por fixação ocular; que se origina como nistagmo optocinético, ou resultante de lesões do mesencéfalo.
galvanic n., n. galvânico; nistagmo que envolve a estimulação galvânica do labirinto.
gaze paretic n., n. do olhar parético; nistagmo que ocorre na paralisia parcial do olhar, quando se tenta olhar na direção da paresia.
incongruent n., n. incongruente, n. dissociado. SIN dissociated n.
irregular n., n. irregular. SIN dissociated n.
jerky n., n. rítmico; nistagmo em que existe um deslocamento lento dos olhos em uma direção, seguido de rápido movimento de recuperação, sempre descrito na direção do movimento de recuperação; em geral, origina-se de lesões ou estímulos labirínticos ou neurológicos.
labyrinthine n., n. labiríntico, n. vestibular. SIN vestibular n.
latent n., n. latente; nistagmo rítmico que é produzido ao se cobrir um dos olhos. A fase rápida é sempre afastando-se do olho coberto.
miner's n., n. dos mineiros; nistagmo que ocorria em mineiros de carvão no século XIX e considerado, naquela época, relacionado à falta de iluminação, bem como a outros fatores. SIN miner's disease (1).
minimal amplitude n., n. de amplitude mínima. SIN micronystagmus.
ocular n., n. ocular; nistagmo pendular ou raramente rítmico, observado na visão gravemente reduzida. SIN amaurotic n.
opticokinetic n., n. opticocinético, n. optocinético. SIN optokinetic n.
optokinetic n., n. optocinético; nistagmo induzido ao olhar para estímulos visuais móveis. SIN opticokinetic n., railroad n.
palatal n., n. palatal; espasmo clônico do músculo levantador do palato, causando um clique audível. VER TAMBÉM palatal *myoclonus*.
pendular n., n. pendular; nistagmo que, na maioria das posições do olhar, exibe oscilações de velocidade e amplitude iguais, originando-se em geral de um distúrbio visual.
positional n., n. de posição; nistagmo que só ocorre quando a cabeça está numa posição particular.
railroad n., n. optocinético. SIN optokinetic n.
rotational n., n. rotacional; nistagmo rítmico que se origina da estimulação do labirinto pela rotação da cabeça ao redor de qualquer eixo e induzido por uma mudança do movimento.
rotatory n., n. rotatório; movimento dos olhos ao redor do eixo visual.
seesaw n., n. em gangorra; nistagmo em que um dos olhos se move para cima à medida que o outro se move para baixo, freqüentemente combinado com uma rotação de torção (para baixo e para fora, para cima e para dentro — como numa gangorra).
slow component of n., componente lento do nistagmo; o movimento fundamental dos olhos no reflexo vestibuloocular.
upbeat n., n. espasmódico; nistagmo vertical espasmódico, com componente rápido para cima, que ocorre em lesões do tronco cerebral.
vertical n., n. vertical; oscilação para cima e para baixo dos olhos.
vestibular n., n. vestibular; nistagmo resultante de estímulos fisiológicos do labirinto. Esses estímulos podem ser rotatórios, lineares, calóricos, compressivos ou galvânicos, ou devido a lesões do labirinto. VER TAMBÉM Bárány *sign*. SIN labyrinthine n.
voluntary n., n. voluntário; nistagmo pendular em que o indivíduo produz uma oscilação horizontal extremamente fina e rápida dos olhos. O nistagmo consiste em movimentos sacádicos e raramente é mantido por mais de alguns segundos de cada vez.
nys·tat·in (nī-stat′in, nis′tă-tin). Nistatina. Substância antibiótica isolada de culturas de *Streptomyces noursei*, efetiva no tratamento de todas as formas de candidíase, particularmente nas infecções do intestino, da pele e das mucosas por *Candida*. SIN fungicidin. [*New York State* + *-in*]
Nysten, Pierre H., médico francês, 1771–1818. VER N. *law*.
nyx·is (nik′sis). Punção, paracentese. [G.]

O

Ω 1. A 24.ª e última letra do alfabeto grego, ômega. **2.** Símbolo de ohm.
O 1. Símbolo de oxygen (oxigênio); orotidine (orotidina). **2.** Abreviatura de *opening* (abertura, nas fórmulas para reações elétricas). **3.** Símbolo de um grupo sanguíneo no sistema ABO. Ver grupo sanguíneo ABO, Apêndice de Grupos Sanguíneos. **4.** Uma abreviatura derivada de *ohne Hauch* (sem fôlego), usada para designar: 1) antígenos que acontecem na célula bacteriana, em contraste com aqueles nos flagelos; 2) anticorpos específicos para esses antígenos somáticos; 3) a reação de aglutinação entre um antígeno somático e seu anticorpo.
^{15}**O** Símbolo de oxygen-15 (oxigênio-15).
^{16}**O** Símbolo de oxygen-16 (oxigênio-16).
^{17}**O** Símbolo de oxygen-17 (oxigênio-17).
^{18}**O** Símbolo de oxygen-18 (oxigênio-18).
o- Em química, a abreviatura de *ortho-* (orto-) (2).
OA Abreviatura para occipitoanterior *position* (posição occipitoanterior).
oak ap·ple. Bugalho, noz-de-galha. SIN nutgall.
oari-, oario-. Formas combinantes obsoletas para indicar um ovário. VER oo,- oophor-, ovario-. [G. ōarion, um pequeno ovo, dim. de ōon, ovo]
oath (ōth). Juramento; uma afirmação ou declaração solene.
OB Abreviatura de obstetrics (obstetrícia).
O'Beirne, James, cirurgião irlandês, 1786–1862. VER O'B. *sphincter*.
obe·li·ac (ō - bē′lē - ak). Obeliáco; relativo ao obélio.
obe·li·ad (ō - bē′lē - ad). Em direção ao obélio.
obe·li·on (ō - bē′lē - on). Obélio, obélion; um ponto craniométrico na sutura sagital entre os forames parietais, próximo à sutura lambdóidea. [G. *obelos*, uma lança]
Obermayer, Friedrich, médico austríaco, 1861–1925. VER O. *test*.
Obermeier, Otto H.F., médico alemão, 1843–1873. VER O. *spirillum*.
Obersteiner, Heinrich, neurologista austríaco, 1847–1922. VER O.-Redlich *line, zone*.
obese (ō - bēs′). Obeso; excessivamente gordo. SIN corpulent. [L. *obesus*, gordo, adj. partic. de *ob-edo*, pp. *-esus*, comer demais, devorar]

obe·si·ty (ō - bē′si - tē). Obesidade; excesso de tecido adiposo subcutâneo em relação à massa corporal magra. O acúmulo excessivo de tecido adiposo está associado a aumento tanto no tamanho (hipertrofia) como no número (hiperplasia) das células do tecido adiposo. A o. é definida em termos de peso absoluto, proporção peso-altura, distribuição de tecido adiposo subcutâneo e normas sociais e estéticas. As medidas de peso em relação à altura incluem o peso relativo (PR, peso do corpo dividido pelo peso mediano desejável para uma pessoa com a mesma altura e estrutura mediana de acordo com as tabelas atuariais), índice de massa corporal (IMC, kg/m^2) e índice ponderal (kg/m^3). Essas medidas não diferenciam a adiposidade excessiva da massa corporal magra aumentada. Por outro lado, as medidas das pregas cutâneas subescapular e do tríceps e a determinação da relação cintura–quadril ajudam a definir a deposição regional de gordura e diferenciam a o. central, com maior importância clínica, da o. periférica nos adultos. Nenhuma causa isolada consegue explicar todos os casos de o. Em última instância, resulta do desequilíbrio entre o aporte energético e o gasto de energia. Embora hábitos alimentares errados relacionados com a falência dos mecanismos normais de retroalimentação da saciedade possam ser responsáveis por alguns casos, muitas pessoas obesas não consomem mais calorias, nem ingerem proporções diferentes de alimentos que as pessoas não-obesas. Contrário à crença popular, a o. não é causada por distúrbios do metabolismo da hipófise, da tireóide ou das glândulas suprarenais. Entretanto, com freqüência, está associada a hiperinsulinismo e à resistência relativa à insulina. Estudos com gêmeos obesos sugerem fortemente a existência de influências genéticas sobre a taxa metabólica em repouso, comportamento alimentar, alterações no dispêndio energético em resposta à alimentação excessiva, atividade da lipase da lipoproteína e taxa basal de lipólise. Os fatores ambientais associados à o. incluem nível socioeconômico, raça, local de residência, estação do ano, vida urbana e fazer parte de uma família menor. A prevalência da o. é maior quando o peso é determinado durante o inverno que no verão. A o. é muito mais comum no Nordeste e Meio-Oeste dos Estados Unidos que no Sul e no Oeste, um fenômeno independente de raça, densidade populacional e estação do ano. SIN adiposity (1), corpulence, corpulency. [L. *obesus*, pp. de *obedo*, comer demais, + *-ity*]

> A obesidade constitui um importante problema de saúde pública e consiste no principal distúrbio nutricional nos Estados Unidos. Uma definição amplamente aceita de obesidade é o peso corporal que está 20% ou mais acima do peso ideal para a altura, de acordo com as tabelas atuariais. Por essa definição, 34% dos adultos nos Estados Unidos são obesos, e há evidências de que a prevalência da obesidade está aumentando tanto em crianças como em adultos. O *National Institutes of Health* definiu a obesidade como um IMC de 30 kg/m^2 ou mais, e excesso de peso (sobrepeso) como um IMC entre 25 e 30 kg/m^2. Por esses critérios, aproximadamente 55% dos adultos estão com excesso de peso ou obesos. A obesidade é um fator de risco independente para hipertensão, hipercolesterolemia, diabetes melito do tipo 2, infarto do miocárdio, determinados processos malignos (câncer de cólon, reto e próstata nos homens; da mama, colo uterino, endométrio e ovário em mulheres), apnéia obstrutiva do sono, síndrome de hipoventilação, osteoartrite e outros distúrbios ortopédicos, infertilidade, doença por estase venosa em membro inferior, doença por refluxo gastroesofágico e incontinência urinária por esforço. Graus menores de obesidade podem constituir um risco de saúde significativo na vigência do diabetes melito, hipertensão, cardiopatia ou seus fatores de risco associados. A distribuição da gordura corporal em depósitos nos tecidos adiposos centrais (padrão abdominal ou masculino, com relação cintura–quadril aumentada) *versus* periféricos (padrão glúteo ou feminino) está associada a riscos mais elevados de muitos desses distúrbios. As pessoas obesas estão mais sujeitas a lesão, são mais difíceis de examinar por palpação e técnicas de imagens, além de ser mais provável a ocorrência de fracasso e complicações de intervenções cirúrgicas. Com a mesma importância, dentre os efeitos adversos da obesidade estão a estigmatização social, a auto-imagem deteriorada e o estresse psicológico. A redução do peso está associada à melhora da maioria dos riscos de saúde gerados pela obesidade. Todos os tratamentos para a obesidade (exceto os procedimentos cirúrgicos cosméticos nos quais a gordura subcutânea é mecanicamente removida) exigem a criação de um déficit de energia, seja pela diminuição da ingestão calórica e/ou aumento do exercício físico. Os programas básicos de redução de peso envolvem o consumo de uma dieta hipolipídica e hipocalórica e a realização de pelo menos 30 minutos de atividade física do tipo resistência com intensidade pelo menos moderada quase todos os dias e, de preferência, todos os dias da semana. A terapia de modificação comportamental, a hipnose, os medicamentos anorexígenos e os procedimentos cirúrgicos para reduzir a capacidade gástrica ou a absorção intestinal de nutrientes são úteis em alguns casos, mas a ênfase deve ser dada às modificações permanentes no estilo de vida. Não se recomenda a diminuição do peso durante a gestação ou quando os pacientes têm osteoporose, colelitíase, doença mental grave englobando a anorexia nervosa, ou doença terminal.

android o., o. andróide; o. central (formato de maçã) com excesso de gordura principalmente na parede abdominal e mesentério visceral; associada à intolerância à glicose, diabetes, diminuição da globulina de ligação de hormônios sexuais, níveis aumentados de testosterona livre e risco cardiovascular aumentado.
gynecoid o., o. ginecóide; o. com excesso de gordura principalmente na região femoro-glútea (formato de pêra).
hypothalamic o., o. hipotalâmica; o. causada por doença do hipotálamo.
hypothalamic o. with hypogonadism, o. hipotalâmica com hipogonadismo. SIN adiposogenital *dystrophy*.
morbid o., o. mórbida; o. suficiente para impedir atividades ou funções fisiológicas normais, ou para causar o estabelecimento de uma condição patológica.
simple o., o. simples; o. quando a ingestão calórica excede o dispêndio energético.
obex (ō′beks) [TA]. Óbex; o ponto na linha média da superfície dorsal do bulbo que marca o ângulo caudal da fossa rombóide ou quarto ventrículo. Corresponde a uma pequena prega bulbar transversa que pende sobre a porção inferior da fossa rombóide (*calamus scriptorius*). [L. barreira]
ob·fus·ca·tion (ob - fus - kā′shŭn). Ofuscação. **1.** Que torna escuro ou obscurece. **2.** Uma tentativa deliberada para confundir ou evitar a compreensão. [L. *ob-fusco*, pp. *-atus*, escurecer, de *fuscus*, escuro, fulvo]
OB/GYN Abreviatura de obstetrics and gynecology (obstetrícia e ginecologia).
ob·i·dox·ime chlo·ride (ob′ē - dok - sēm). Cloreto de obidoxima; um reativador da colinesterase muito similar ao 2-PAM (2-pralidoxima).
ob·ject (ob′jekt). Objeto. **1.** Qualquer coisa para a qual o pensamento ou ação é direcionado. **2.** Em psicanálise, aquilo através do qual um instinto pode al-

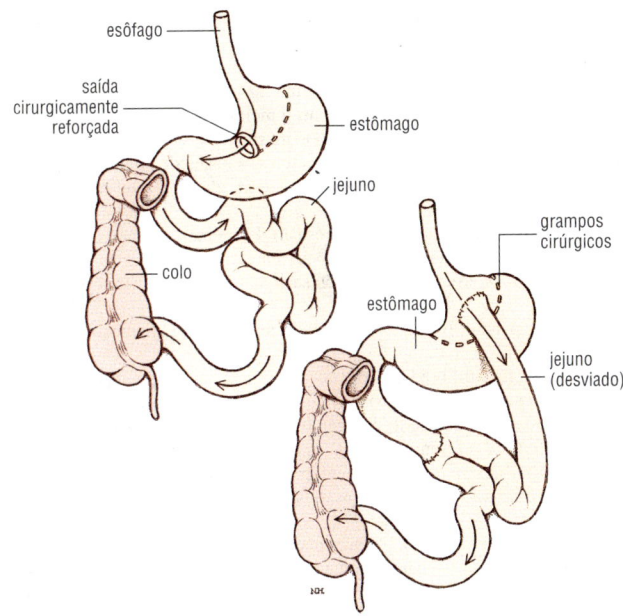

procedimentos cirúrgicos para controlar a obesidade: (A) gastroplastia com ligadura vertical, (B) derivação (*bypass*) gástrica (gastrojejunostomia)

cançar seu objetivo. **3.** Em psicanálise, freqüentemente utilizado como sinônimo para pessoa.
  good o., o. bom; em psicanálise, os aspectos bons ou de sustentação de uma pessoa importante na vida do paciente, em especial de um pai ou alguém que o substitui.
  sex o., o. sexual; uma pessoa pela qual outra sente atração sexual; um termo mais empregado por uma mulher para indicar que um homem a vê estritamente como um veículo para o sexo, enquanto desconsidera por completo o restante de sua pessoa.
  test o., o. de teste; **(1)** um o. que possui marcas superficiais muito delicadas, montadas sobre uma lâmina, usado para determinar o poder de definição da objetiva de um microscópio; **(2)** o alvo na mensuração do campo visual.
  transitional o., o. de transição; um o. utilizado por muitas crianças como um substituto para um genitor que está ausente (em geral, temporariamente), de modo a ajudá-las a lidar com a separação; tipicamente, um cobertor ou brinquedo de pelúcia.
ob·ject choice. Escolha do objeto; em psicanálise, o objeto (geralmente uma pessoa) sobre o qual é centrada a energia psíquica.
ob·jec·tive (ob-jek'tiv). Objetivo, objetiva. **1.** A lente ou lentes na extremidade inferior do tubo de um microscópio, por meio das quais os raios oriundos do objeto examinado são trazidos até um foco. SIN object glass. **2.** Visualizar eventos ou fenômenos como existem no mundo exterior, de maneira impessoal ou de forma não-preconceituosa, aberto para a observação pela própria pessoa e por outras. Cf. subjective. [L. *ob-jicio*, pp. *-jectus*, arremessar para frente]
  achromatic o., o. acromática; uma o. que é corrigida cromaticamente para duas cores e esfericamente para uma cor.
  apochromatic o., o. apocromática; uma o. em que a aberração cromática é corrigida para três cores e a aberração esférica é corrigida para duas.
  immersion o., o. de imersão; uma o. de alta potência usada com uma gota de óleo entre a lente e a amostra na lâmina, permitindo uma maior abertura numérica; lentes similares estão disponíveis para o uso com água como o líquido de imersão.
ob·jec·tive as·sess·ment da·ta. Dados de avaliação objetiva; aqueles fatos que são passíveis de observação e mensuração pela enfermagem.
ob·li·gate (ob'li-gāt). Obrigatório; sem um sistema ou via alternativa. [L. *obligo*, pp. *-atus*, ligar a]
ob·lique (ob-lēk'). Oblíquo; inclinado; que se desvia do plano perpendicular, horizontal, sagital ou coronal do corpo. Na radiografia, uma incidência que não é frontal nem lateral. [L. *obliquus*]
ob·liq·ui·ty (ob-lik'wi-tē). Obliquidade, assinclitismo. SIN asynclitism.
  Litzmann o., o. de Litzmann; a inclinação da cabeça fetal de modo que o diâmetro biparietal fique oblíquo em relação ao plano da borda pélvica, com a porção posterior do osso parietal apresentando-se ao canal de parto. SIN posterior asynclitism.
  Nägele o., o. de Nägele; a inclinação da cabeça fetal nos casos de pelve plana, de modo que o diâmetro biparietal fique oblíquo em relação ao plano da borda pélvica, com a porção anterior do osso parietal apresentando-se ao canal de parto. SIN anterior asynclitism.
ob·li·qu·us (ob-lī'kwūs). Oblíquo; indica uma estrutura que possui uma direção ou trajeto oblíquo; um nome conferido, com qualificação adicional, a diversos músculos. VER muscle. [L. inclinado, oblíquo]
ob·lit·er·a·tion (ob-lit-er-ā'shūn). Obliteração; obscurecimento, em especial por preenchimento de um espaço natural ou luz por fibrose ou inflamação. Em radiologia, o desaparecimento do contorno de um órgão quando o tecido adjacente possui a mesma absorção dos raios X. VER silhouette *sign* of Felson. [L. *oblittero*, obscurecer]
  osteoplastic o. of frontal sinus, o. osteoplástica do seio frontal; operação para remover o conteúdo enfermo, inclusive a mucosa, do seio frontal e para obliterar esse seio com um enxerto de gordura livre sem alterar o contorno externo do mesmo.
ob·lon·ga·ta (ob-long-gah'tā). Medula oblonga; bulbo. SIN medulla oblongata. [L. fem. de *oblongatus*, de *oblongus*, muito longo]
ob·nu·bi·la·tion (ab-noo'bil-ā'shun). Obnubilação; estado mental obscurecido. [L. *ob-nubilo*, turvar, obscurecer, de *nubes*, turvo]
OBS Abreviatura de organic brain *syndrome* (síndrome cerebral orgânica).
ob·serv·er (ob-zer'ver). Observador; aquele que percebe, nota ou observa; na pesquisa comportamental com seres humanos, o pesquisador ou seu substituto. [L. *observo*, observar]
  nonparticipant o., o. não-participante; um pesquisador que estuda um grupo de pessoas engajadas em determinadas atividades, mas que não participa diretamente nessas atividades, sendo presumivelmente capaz de estudá-las de maneira mais objetiva.
  participant o., o. participante; um investigador que, enquanto estuda as atividades de um grupo de indivíduos, também participa em suas atividades, sendo presumivelmente capaz de obter informações mais detalhadas e relevantes, porém com menor objetividade.
ob·ses·sion (ob-sesh'ūn). Obsessão; uma idéia, pensamento ou impulso recorrente e persistente para realizar um ato que é egodistônico, que é experimentado como sem sentido ou repugnante, e que o indivíduo não consegue suprimir voluntariamente. [L. *obsideo*, pp. *-sessus*, cercar, de *sedeo*, sentar]
  impulsive o., o. impulsiva; o. acompanhada por ação e que, por vezes, se transforma em uma mania.
  inhibitory o., o. inibitória; o. que envolve um impedimento à ação, representando, em geral, uma fobia.
ob·ses·sive-com·pul·sive. Obsessivo-compulsivo; que tende a realizar determinados atos repetitivos ou comportamento ritualista para aliviar a ansiedade, como na neurose obsessivo-compulsiva (p.ex., uma necessidade compulsiva ritualista para lavar as mãos muitas dúzias de vezes por dia).
ob·so·les·cence (ob-sō-les'ens). Obsolescência; cair em desuso; indica a abolição de uma função. [L. *obsolesco*, sair de uso]
ob·stet·ric, ob·stet·ri·cal (ob-stet'rik, -ri-kāl). Obstétrico; relativo à obstetrícia.
ob·ste·tri·cian (ob-stē-tri-sh'ūn). Obstetra; médico que se especializa no cuidado médico de mulheres durante a gestação e o parto. [ver obstetrics]
ob·stet·rics (OB) (ob-stet'riks). Obstetrícia; a especialidade da medicina relacionada com a assistência à mulher durante a gestação, o parto e o puerpério. SIN tocology. [L. *obstetrix*, uma parteira, de *ob-sto*, ficar em pé diante de, indicando a posição originalmente tomada pela parteira]
ob·sti·nate (ob'sti-nāt). Obstinado. **1.** Que adere firmemente aos próprios objetivos ou opiniões, mesmo quando errado; que não cede a argumentação, persuasão ou solicitação. SIN intractable (2), refractory (2). **2.** Resistente, refratário. SIN refractory (1). [L. *obstinatus*, determinado]
ob·sti·pa·tion (ob-sti-pā'shūn). Obstipação; obstrução intestinal; constipação grave. [L. *ob*, contra, + *stipo*, pp. *-atus*, aglomerar]
ob·struc·tion (ob-strŭk'shŭn). Obstrução; bloqueio, tamponamento ou comprometimento de fluxo, p.ex., por oclusão ou estenose. [L. *obstructio*]
  closed loop o., o. de alça fechada; o. de um segmento do intestino por rotação sobre um ponto fixo (volvo) ou por herniação através de uma abertura fibrosa (como sob uma aderência ou dentro de uma hérnia); freqüentemente associada a comprometimento da perfusão, resultando, por fim, em gangrena.
  ureteropelvic junction o., o. da junção ureteropélvica; um impedimento da drenagem da urina a partir do rim, geralmente provocada pelo bloqueio parcial ou intermitente do sistema coletor renal na junção da pelve renal com o ureter.
  ureterovesical o., o. ureterovesical; a o. da parte inferior do ureter em sua entrada na bexiga.
ob·stru·ent (ob'stroo-ent). Obstrutivo. **1.** Termo raramente utilizado para aquilo que obstrui ou oclui. **2.** Termo raramente empregado para um agente que obstrui ou evita secreção normal, especialmente quando proveniente do intestino. [L. *obstruo*, construir contra, obstruir]
ob·tund (ob-tŭnd'). Obtundir; embotar ou abrandar, especialmente sensações ou dor. [L. *ob-tundo*, pp. *-tusus*, bater contra, embotar]
ob·tu·ra·tion (ob-too-rā'shūn). Obturação; obstrução ou oclusão. [ver obturator]

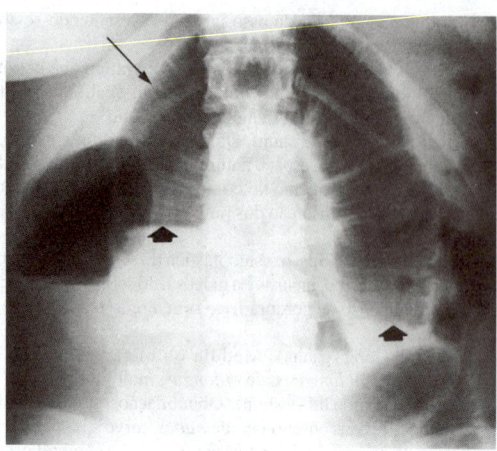

obstrução do intestino delgado: radiografia simples do abdome, em posição ortostática, revela alças do intestino delgado dilatadas e cheias de ar (setas); a obstrução é decorrente de aderências

intermittent self-o., auto-o. intermitente; introdução de um objeto rombudo em um lúmen ou meato para ocluí-lo ou dilatá-lo.

ob·tu·ra·tor (ob'too-rā-tor). Obturador. **1.** Qualquer estrutura que oclua uma abertura. **2.** Indica o forame obturado, a membrana obturadora ou qualquer uma das diversas partes em relação a esse forame. **3.** Prótese empregada para fechar uma abertura do palato duro, usualmente uma fenda palatina. **4.** Estilo (buril) ou tampão removível usado durante a inserção de muitos instrumentos tubulares. [L. *obturo*, pp. *-atus*, ocluir ou tampar]

ob·tuse (ob-toos'). Obtuso. **1.** Embotado no intelecto; de compreensão lenta. **2.** Rombudo; não-agudo. [ver obtund.]

ob·tu·sion (ob-too'zhŭn). Obtusão. **1.** Lentidão de sensibilidade. **2.** Turvação ou embotamento da sensibilidade.

Occam's ra·zor. O princípio da parcimônia científica. William de Occam (filósofo do século XIV) afirmou isto: "As suposições introduzidas para explicar uma coisa não devem ser multiplicadas além do necessário."

oc·cip·i·tal (ok-sip'i-tăl). Occipital; relativo ao occipital; que se refere ao osso occipital ou à parte posterior da cabeça. SIN occipitalis.

oc·ci·pi·ta·lis (ok'sip-i-tā'lis). Occipital. SIN occipital. [L.]

oc·cip·i·tal·i·za·tion (ok'sip'i-tăl-i-zā'shŭn). Occipitalização; anquilose óssea entre o atlas e o osso occipital.

occipito-. Formas combinantes relativas ao occipício e às estruturas occipitais. [L. *occiput*]

oc·cip·i·to·at·loid (ok-sip'i-tō-at'loyd). Occipitoatlóide; relativo ao osso occipital e ao atlas; indica a articulação entre os dois ossos.

oc·cip·i·to·ax·i·al, oc·cip·i·to·ax·oid (ok-sip'i-tō-ak'sē-ăl, -ak'soyd). Occipitoaxial, occipitoaxóide; relativo ao osso occipital e ao áxis.

oc·cip·i·to·breg·mat·ic (ok-sip'i-tō-breg-mat'ik). Occipitobregmático; relativo ao occipício e bregma; indica uma medida em craniometria.

oc·cip·i·to·fa·cial (ok-sip'i-tō-fā'shăl). Occipitofacial; relativo ao occipício e à face.

oc·cip·i·to·fron·tal (ok-sip'i-tō-frŭn-tăl). Occipitofrontal. **1.** Relativo ao occipício e à fronte. **2.** Relativo aos lobos occipital e frontal do córtex cerebral e às vias de associação que interligam essas regiões.

oc·cip·i·to·fron·ta·lis (ok-sip'i-tō-frŭn-tā'lis). Occipitofrontal. VER occipitofrontalis (*muscle*). [L.]

oc·cip·i·to·mas·toid (ok-sip'i-tō-mas'toyd). Occipitomastóide; relativo ao osso occipital e ao processo mastóide.

oc·cip·i·to·men·tal (ok-sip'i-tō-men'tăl). Occipitomentual; relativo ao occipício e ao queixo.

oc·cip·i·to·pa·ri·e·tal (ok-sip'i-tō-pă-rī'ĕ-tăl). Occipitoparietal; relativo ao occipício e aos ossos parietais.

oc·cip·i·to·tem·po·ral (ok-sip'i-tō-tem'pŏ-răl). Occipitotemporal; relativo ao occipício e à têmpora, ou aos ossos occipital e temporal.

oc·cip·i·to·tha·lam·ic (ok-sip'i-tō-tha-lam'ik). Occipitotalâmico; relativo às fibras nervosas que vão do lobo occipital do córtex cerebral até o tálamo.

oc·ci·put, gen. **oc·cip·i·tis** (ok'si-put, ok-sip'i-tis) [TA]. Occipício; o dorso da cabeça. [L.]

oc·clude (ŏ-klood). Ocluir. **1.** Fechar ou unir. **2.** Envolver, como em um vírus ocluído (occluded *virus*). [ver occlusion]

oc·clud·er (ŏ-klood'er). Oclusor; em odontologia, um nome dado a alguns articuladores.

oc·clu·sal (ŏ-kloo'zăl). Oclusal. **1.** Pertinente à oclusão ou fechamento. **2.** Em odontologia, pertinente às superfícies de contato de unidades oclusais opostas (bordas dentárias ou de oclusão) ou às superfícies de mastigação dos dentes posteriores.

oc·clu·sion (ŏ-kloo'zhŭn). Oclusão. **1.** O ato de fechar ou o estado de ser fechado. **2.** Em química, a absorção de um gás por um metal ou a inclusão de uma substância em outra (como em um precipitado gelatinoso). **3.** Qualquer contato entre as superfícies incisivas ou mastigatórias dos dentes superiores e inferiores. **4.** A relação entre as superfícies oclusais dos dentes maxilares e mandibulares quando estão em contato. [L. *oc-cludo*, pp. *-clusus*, fechar, de *ob-*, contra, + *claudo*, fechar]

abnormal o., o. anormal; uma disposição dos dentes que não é considerada como dentro dos limites normais de variação.

afunctional o., o. afuncional; maloclusão que não permite a função normal da dentição.

anterior o., o. anterior; **(1)** a o. dos dentes anteriores; **(2)** o. mesial. SIN mesial o. (1).

balanced o., o. equilibrada; o contato simultâneo dos dentes superiores e inferiores à direita e à esquerda e nas áreas de oclusão anteriores e posteriores em posições cêntricas e excêntricas dentro dos limites funcionais; termo usado basicamente em referência à boca, mas também arranjado e observado em articuladores, desenvolvido para evitar a inclinação ou rotação das bases da dentadura em relação às estruturas de sustentação. SIN balanced articulation, balanced bite.

bimaxillary protrusive o., o. protrusiva bimaxilar; o. em que a maxila e a mandíbula projetam-se para a frente, fazendo com que os eixos longitudinais dos dentes maxilares anteriores fiquem em um ângulo extremamente agudo com os dentes mandibulares; pode ser secundária a uma deformidade esquelética e/ou dentária; observada comumente em negros.

buccal o., o. bucal; **(1)** posicionamento errado de um dente em relação à bochecha; **(2)** o. observada a partir do lado bucal dos dentes.

centric o., o. cêntrica; **(1)** a relação das superfícies de oclusão opostas que fornece o contato planejado máximo entre as cúspides de dentes opostos; **(2)** a o. dos dentes quando a mandíbula está em relação cêntrica com a maxila. SIN centric contact.

coronary o., o. coronária; o bloqueio de um vaso coronário, usualmente por trombose ou ateroma, levando, com freqüência, ao infarto do miocárdio.

distal o., o. distal; **(1)** um dente que oclui em uma posição distal à normal. SIN disto-occlusion, postnormal o., retrusive o. (2). **(2)** SIN distoclusion.

eccentric o., o. excêntrica; qualquer o. diferente da cêntrica.

edge-to-edge o., o. borda-a-borda; o. em que os dentes anteriores das mandíbulas se encontram ao longo de suas bordas de incisão quando os dentes estão em o. cêntrica. SIN edge-to-edge bite, end-to-end bite, end-to-end o.

end-to-end o., o. borda-a-borda; SIN edge-to-edge o.

functional o., o. funcional; **(1)** qualquer contato dentário feito dentro dos limites funcionais das superfícies dentárias opostas; **(2)** a o. que ocorre durante a função.

gliding o., o. deslizante. SIN dental *articulation*.

hyperfunctional o., o. hiperfuncional; estresse oclusal do dente ou dentes que excede as demandas fisiológicas normais.

labial o., o. labial; **(1)** posição errada de um dente em uma direção labial; **(2)** a o. quando observada a partir do lado labial dos arcos.

lateral o., o. lateral; o posicionamento errado de um dente ou de toda a arcada dentária em uma direção oposta à linha média.

lingual o., o. lingual; **(1)** SIN linguoclusion; **(2)** interdigitação dos dentes conforme observado a partir da face interna ou lingual.

mechanically balanced o., o. mecanicamente equilibrada; uma o. equilibrada sem referência às considerações fisiológicas, como em um articulador.

mesenteric artery o., o. da artéria mesentérica; obstrução do fluxo arterial na circulação mesentérica por um êmbolo ou trombo; geralmente se refere à o. da artéria mesentérica superior, embora o estreitamento aterosclerótico possa afetar todos os três ramos esplâncnicos principais (celíaco, mesentéricos superior e inferior).

mesial o., o. mesial; **(1)** o. em que os dentes mandibulares se articulam com os dentes maxilares em uma posição anterior à normal. SIN anterior o. (2), mesio-occlusion. **(2)** SIN mesioclusion.

neutral o., o. neutra; **(1)** disposição dos dentes de modo que os primeiros molares permanentes maxilares e mandibulares se encontram em uma relação ântero-posterior normal. SIN normal o. (2). **(2)** SIN neutroclusion.

normal o., o. normal; **(1)** o arranjo dos dentes e de suas estruturas de sustentação que, em geral, é encontrado na saúde e que se aproxima de uma disposição ideal ou padronizada. SIN normal bite. **(2)** SIN neutral o. (1).

pathogenic o., o. patogênica; uma relação oclusal capaz de produzir alterações patológicas nos tecidos de sustentação.

physiologic o., o. fisiológica; a o. em harmonia com as funções do sistema mastigatório.

physiologically balanced o., o. fisiologicamente equilibrada; uma o. equilibrada que está em harmonia com as articulações temporomandibulares e com o sistema neuromuscular.

posterior o., o. posterior; o contato mais efetivo dos dentes molares e bicúspi-

occlusion

des da maxila e da mandíbula que permite todos os movimentos naturais essenciais à mastigação e ao fechamento normais. SIN posteroclusion.

postnormal o., o. pós-normal. SIN distal o. (1).

protrusive o., o. protrusiva; a o. que resulta quando a mandíbula se projeta para diante a partir da posição cêntrica.

o. of pupil, o. da pupila; a presença de uma membrana opaca que fecha a área pupilar.

retrusive o., o. retrusiva; (1) relação de mordedura em que a mandíbula é colocada de maneira forçada ou habitual em uma posição mais distal que a o. cêntrica do paciente; (2) SIN distal o. (1)

spherical form of o., forma esférica de o.; um arranjo dos dentes que coloca suas superfícies de oclusão sobre a superfície de uma esfera imaginária (comumente de 20 cm de diâmetro) com seu centro acima do nível dos dentes. VER TAMBÉM Monson curve.

torsive o., o. por torção. SIN torsiversion.

traumatic o., o. traumática. SIN traumatogenic o.

traumatogenic o., o. traumatogênica; uma maloclusão capaz de produzir lesão para os dentes e/ou estruturas associadas. SIN traumatic o.

working o., o. funcional. SIN working contacts, em contact.

oc·clu·sive (ŏ-kloo′siv) Oclusivo; que serve para fechar; indica uma atadura ou curativo que fecha uma ferida e a separa do ar.

oc·clu·som·e·ter (ok-loo-som′ĕ-ter) Oclusômetro. SIN gnathodynamometer.

oc·cult (ō-kŭlt′, ok′ŭlt) Oculto. 1. Escondido; não manifesto; dissimulado. 2. Indica uma hemorragia oculta, estando o sangue inaparente ou localizado em um local onde não é visível. VER occult blood. 3. Em oncologia, um tumor primário clinicamente não-identificado com metástases reconhecidas. [L. *occulo,* pp. -*cultus,* cobrir, ocultar]

Oce·an·o·spi·ril·lum (ō′shen-ō-spī-ril′ŭm) Um gênero de bactérias aeróbicas, móveis e não-formadoras de esporos (família Spirillaceae) contendo células Gram-negativas, rígidas e helicoidais, que são de 0,3–1,2 μm de diâmetro. As células móveis contêm fascículos bipolares dos flagelos. Não há crescimento anaeróbico com nitrato. Esses microrganismos são quimiorganotróficos e possuem um metabolismo estritamente anaeróbico; não oxidam nem fermentam carboidratos; encontradas em ambientes marinhos. Existem, no momento, cinco espécies nesse gênero, das quais a espécie típica é O. linum. [L. *oceanus,* oceano, + *spirillum,* mola]

ocel·lus, pl. **ocel·li** (ō-sel′ŭs, -lī) Ocelo. 1. O olho simples encontrado em muitos invertebrados. SIN eyespot (2). 2. Faceta do olho composto de um inseto. [L. dim. de *oculus,* olho]

och·lo·pho·bia (ok-lō-fō′bē-ă) Oclofobia; temor mórbido de multidões. [G. *ochlos,* uma multidão, + *phobos,* medo]

Ochoa, Severo, bioquímico hispano-americano e laureado com o prêmio Nobel, 1905–1993. VER O. *law.*

ochra·tox·in (ō-kra-toks′ins) Ocratoxina; uma micotoxina produzida por *Aspergillus ochraceus* que cresce em grãos de cereais armazenados. Afeta aves e outros animais que se alimentam desses grãos.

ochratoxin A, ocratoxina A; a ocratoxina produzida por algumas espécies de *Aspergillus* e *Penicillium* que podem contaminar grãos de cereais e alimentos, principalmente após armazenamento impróprio; um potente carcinógeno em roedores.

Ochrobactrum (ō-krō-bak′trum) Um gênero de bactérias Gram-negativas semelhante às espécies de *Alcaligenes* e *Pseudomonas* em sua distribuição em fontes ambientais e de água e suas características de cultura. Já foram isoladas de inúmeras fontes clínicas e parecem ser uma causa de bacteriemia nosocomial.

ochro·der·mia (ō-krō-der′mē-ă) Ocrodermia; coloração amarelada da pele. [G. *ōchros,* amarelo-pálido, + *derma,* pele]

ochrom·e·ter (ō-krom′ĕ-ter) Ocrômetro; um instrumento para determinar a pressão arterial capilar; um de dois dedos adjacentes é comprimido por um balão de borracha até que ocorra o clareamento da pele, depois do que a força necessária para efetuar essa alteração da coloração é lida em milímetros de mercúrio. [G. *ōchros,* amarelo-pálido, + *metron,* medida]

ochro·no·sis (o-kron-ō′sis) Ocronose; uma rara doença autossômica recessiva caracterizada por alcaptonúria com pigmentação das cartilagens e, por vezes, de tecidos como músculo, células epiteliais e tecido conjuntivo denso; pode afetar também escleróticas, mucosa dos lábios e pele das orelhas, face e mãos, além de tornar a urina em repouso escura e com cilindros pigmentados; acredita-se que a pigmentação decorra do ácido homogentísico oxidado, e a degeneração da cartilagem resulta em osteoartrite, sobretudo da coluna vertebral. [G. *ōchros,* amarelo-pálido, + *nosos,* doença]

exogenous o., o. exógena; a pigmentação da pele da face e de outros pontos em decorrência da exposição tópica prolongada a cremes de alvejantes contendo hidroquinona.

ochro·not·ic (ō-kron-ot′ik) Ocronótico; relativo a, ou caracterizado por, ocronose.

Ochsner, Albert John, cirurgião norte-americano, 1858–1925. VER O. *clamp, method.*

oc·ry·late (ok′ri-lāt) Ocrilato; um adesivo tecidual para cirurgia.

oculo-.

△ **oct-, octi-, octo-, octa-.** Formas combinantes que significam oito. [G. *oktō,* L. *octo*]

OCTA (ok′ta) Uma seqüência de oito pares de bases no DNA que possui uma função regulamentadora; por exemplo, quando é artificialmente aposta a um gene, fará com que o gene seja expresso de maneira preferencial nas células da linhagem do linfócito B.

oc·tac·o·san·o·ic ac·id (ok-tă-kō′san-ō-ik) Ácido octacosanóico; um ácido graxo de cadeia longa; encontrado em ceras. SIN montanic acid.

oc·tad (ok′tad) 1. Octavalente. SIN octavalent. 2. Um elemento ou radical octavalente. [L. *octo,* oito]

octafluoropropane (ok′ta-flōr′ō-prō-pān) Octafluoropropano; substância utilizada para acentuar o contraste durante a ultra-sonografia.

oc·ta·meth·yl py·ro·phos·phor·a·mide (OMPA) (ok-tă-meth′il pī′rō-fos-fōr′ă-mid) Octametil pirofosforamida. SIN schradan.

oc·ta·myl·a·mine (ok-tă-mil′ă-mēn) Octamilamina; um agente anticolinérgico.

oc·tan (ok′tan) Octã; aplica-se à febre cujos paroxismos ocorrem a cada oito dias, sendo o dia do paroxismo contado como o primeiro dia. [L. *octo,* oito]

oc·tan·di·o·ic ac·id Ácido octanodióico. SIN suberic acid.

oc·ta·no·ate (ok′tă-nō′at) Octanoato. SIN caprylate.

oc·ta·no·ic ac·id (ok′tă-nō′ik) Ácido octanóico. SIN caprylic acid.

oc·ta·no·yl-CoA syn·the·tase (ok′tăn-ō-il sin′thē-tās) Octanoil-CoA sintetase. SIN butyrate-CoA ligase.

oc·ta·pep·tide (ok′tă-pep′tīd) Octapeptídeo; um peptídeo constituído de oito resíduos aminoácidos.

oc·ta·ploi·dy (ok′tă-ploy′dē) Octaploidia. VER polyploidy.

oc·ta·pres·sin (ok′tă-pres′in) Octapressina. SIN felypressin.

oc·ta·va·lent (ok′tă-vā′lent, ok-tav′ă-lent) Octavalente; indica um elemento químico ou radical com potência de combinação (valência) de oito. SIN octad (1).

oc·ta·vus (ok-tā′vŭs) Oitavo nervo craniano. SIN vestibulocochlear *nerve* [CN VIII]. [L.]

△ **octi-.** VER oct-.
△ **octo-.** VER oct-.

Oc·to·mit·i·dae (ok-tō-mit′i-dē) Uma família na classe de protozoários Zoomastigophorea; os flagelados com seis a oito flagelos dispostos aos pares e um corpo com simetria bilateral; inclui o parasita intestinal humano comum *G. lamblia.* [octo- + G. *mitos,* filamento]

Oc·tom·i·tus hom·i·nis (ok-tom′i-tŭs hom′i-nis) *Pentatrichomonas hominis.*

oc·to·pa·mine (ok-tō′pă-mēn) Octopamina; uma amina simpaticomimética; um falso neurotransmissor produzido por neurônios noradrenérgicos na presença de inibidores da monoamina oxidase. SIN norsympatol, norsynephrine.

oc·tose (ok′tōs) Octose; um açúcar que contém oito átomos de carbono.

oc·tox·y·nol (ok-tok′si-nol) Octoxinol; um surfactante.

oc·tu·lose (ok′too-lōs) Octulose; uma monocetose com oito carbonos.

oc·tu·lo·son·ic ac·id (ok′too-lō-son′ik) Ácido octulossônico; o ácido-ônico formalmente produzido pela oxidação do átomo de carbono 1 da octulose em um grupamento de ácido carboxílico; um produto de condensação da D-arabinose e fosfoenolpiruvato análogo ao ácido neuramínico. Forma parte da unidade de repetição dos polissacarídeos dos lipopolissacarídeos complexos das Enterobacteriaceae, constituindo os característicos antígenos octose somáticos.

oc·tyl gal·late (ok′til gal′āt) Octilgalato; um antioxidante.

oc·tyl·phe·noxy pol·y·eth·ox·y·eth·a·nol (ok′til-fe-nok′sē pol′ē-eth-ok′sē-eth′ă-nol) Octilfenoxi polietoxietanol; mono-*p*-isooctil feniléter do polietilenoglicol; um agente tensoativo (umidificante).

oc·u·lar (ok′ū-lăr) Ocular. 1. SIN ophthalmic. 2. A ocular de um microscópio, a lente ou lentes na extremidade do observador de um microscópio, por meio da qual a imagem focalizada pela objetiva é visualizada. [L. *oculus,* olho]

compensating o., o. compensadora; uma o. que compensa e corrige os efeitos da aberração cromática na objetiva.

Huygens o., o. de Huygens; a o. composta de um microscópio, formada de duas lentes planoconvexas dispostas de tal forma que o lado plano de cada uma fique direcionado para o observador.

o. motor, o. motora; relativo a ou que causa os movimentos do globo ocular.

Ramsden o., o. de Ramsden; uma ocular de um microscópio, consistindo em duas lentes planoconvexas com as convexidades voltadas uma para a outra.

wide field o., o. de campo amplo; uma o. que fornece um campo de visão maior que o usual e um foco alto.

oc·u·lar·ist (ok′ū-lăr-ist) Uma pessoa especializada no desenho, fabricação e ajuste de olhos artificiais e na elaboração de próteses associadas à aparência ou função dos olhos. [L. *oculus,* olho]

o·cu·len·tum, pl. **o·cu·len·ta** (ok-ū-len′tŭm, -tă) Pomada oftálmica. SIN ophthalmic *ointment.* [L. mod., de L. *oculus,* olho]

oc·u·li (ok′ū-lī) Óculos; plural de oculus. [L.]

oc·u·list (ok′ū-list) Oculista. SIN ophthalmologist. [L. *oculus,* olho]

△ **oculo-.** Forma combinante que indica olho, ocular. VER TAMBÉM ophthalmo-. [L. *oculus*]

oc·u·lo·au·ric·u·lo·ver·te·bral (okū-lō-aw-rikū-lō-ver'tĕ-brăl). Oculoauriculovertebral; relativo aos olhos, orelhas e vértebras.

oc·u·lo·car·di·ac (okū-lō-kar'dē-ak). Oculocardíaco; relativo aos olhos e ao coração.

oc·u·lo·cer·e·bro·re·nal (okū-lō-ser'ē-brō-rē'nal). Oculocerebrorrenal; relativo aos olhos, cérebro e rins.

oc·u·lo·cu·ta·ne·ous (okū-lō-kū-tā'nē-ŭs). Oculocutâneo; relativo aos olhos e à pele.

oc·u·lo·den·to·dig·i·tal (okū-lō-den'tō-dij'i-tăl). Oculodentodigital; relativo aos olhos, dentes e dedos.

oc·u·lo·der·mal (okū-lō-der'măl). Oculodérmico; relativo aos olhos e à pele.

oc·u·lo·dyn·ia. Oculodinia; dor no globo ocular. SIN ophthalmalgia. [ophthalmo- + G. *algos*, dor]

oc·u·lo·fa·cial (ok-ū-lō-fā'shăl). Oculofacial; relativo aos olhos e à face.

oc·u·log·ra·phy (ok-ū-log'ră-fē). Oculografia; um método para registrar a posição e os movimentos dos olhos. [oculo- + G. *graphē*, uma escrita]
   photosensor o., o. fotossensora; o. em que as fotocélulas são direcionadas para a superfície do olho, de modo a registrar as rotações.

oc·u·lo·gy·ria (okū-lō-jī'rē-ă). Oculogiria; os limites da rotação dos globos oculares. [oculo- + G. *gyros*, círculo]

oc·u·lo·gy·ric (okū-lō-jī'rik). Oculogírico; referente à rotação dos globos oculares; caracterizado por oculogiria.

oc·u·lo·man·dib·u·lo·dys·ceph·a·ly (okū-lō-man-dibū-lō-dis-sef'ă-lē). Oculomandibulodiscefalia. SIN dyscephalia mandibulo-oculofacialis.

oc·u·lo·mo·tor (okū-lō-mō'tŏr). Oculomotor; pertinente ao nervo craniano o. [L. *oculomotorius*, de oculo- + L. *motorius*, movimento]

o·cu·lo·mo·to·ri·us (okū-lō-mō-tō'rē-ŭs). Oculomotor. SIN oculomotor nerve [CN III]. [L.]

oc·u·lo·na·sal (okū-lō-nā'săl). Oculonasal; relativo aos olhos e ao nariz. [oculo- + L. *nasus*, nariz]

oc·u·lop·a·thy (ok-ū-lop'ă-thē). Oculopatia. SIN ophthalmopathy.

oc·u·lo·pleth·ys·mog·ra·phy (okū-lō-pleth-iz-mog'ră-fē). Oculopletismografia; a medição indireta da importância hemodinâmica da oclusão ou estenose da artéria carótida interna através da demonstração de retardo ipsolateral na chegada da pressão ocular transmitida a partir dos ramos da artéria oftálmica. [oculo- + G. *plēthymos*, aumento, + *graphein*, escrever]

oc·u·lo·pneu·mo·pleth·ys·mog·ra·phy (okū-lō-noo'mō-pleth-iz-mog'ră-fē). Oculopneumopletismografia; um método de medição bilateral da pressão da artéria oftálmica que reflete a pressão e o fluxo na artéria carótida interna. VER oculoplethysmography.

oc·u·lo·pu·pil·lary (okū-lō-poo'pi-lār-ē). Oculopupilar; pertinente à pupila do olho.

oc·u·lo·sym·pa·thet·ic (okoo-lō-sim-pa-the'tik). Oculossimpático; pertinente à via simpática para o olho, cujo comprometimento provoca a síndrome de Horner (Horner *syndrome*).

oc·u·lo·ver·te·bral (okū-lō-ver'tĕ-brăl). Oculovertebral; relativo aos olhos e vértebras.

oc·u·lo·zy·go·mat·ic (okū-lō-zī-gō-mat'ik). Oculozigomático; relativo à órbita ou sua margem e ao osso zigomático.

oc·u·lus, gen. e pl. **oc·u·li** (okū-lŭs, -lī) [TA]. Olho. SIN eye (1). [L.]

△ **ocy-.** VER oxy-.

ocy·toc·in (ō-si-tō'sin). Ocitocina; SIN oxytocin. [G. *okytokos*, parto rápido, delivramento imediato]

OD Abreviatura de overdose; optic *density* (densidade óptica, ver absorbance).

O.D. 1. Abreviatura de L. *oculus dexter*, olho direito. 2. Abreviatura de Doctor of Optometry (Doutor em Optometria). VER optometrist.

o.d. Abreviatura de L. *omni die*, diariamente.

odax·es·mus (ō'dak-sez'mŭs). Sensação de mordedura; uma forma de parestesia. [G. *odaxēsmos*, uma irritação, de *odax* (adv.), por mordedura]

odax·et·ic (ō'dak-set'ik). 1. Que causa formigamento ou prurido. 2. Uma substância ou agente que causa formigamento ou prurido. [G. *odaxēsmos*, irritação]

Oddi, Ruggero, médico italiano; 1864–1913. VER O. *sphincter*.

odds. Chance; a relação entre a probabilidade de ocorrência e a de não-ocorrência de um evento. [pl. de *odd*, de I.m. *odde*, de O. Norse *oddi*, número ímpar]

△ **-odes.** -óide; que tem a forma de, assemelha-se a. [G. *eidos*, forma, semelhança]

Odland body. Corpúsculo de Odland, queratinossoma. VER em body.

odo·gen·e·sis (ō-dō-jen'ē-sis). Odogênese. SIN neurocladism. [G. *hodos*, trajeto, + *genesis*, fonte]

△ **odont-, odonto-.** Formas combinantes relativas ao dente ou dentes. [G. *odous* (*odont-*)]

odon·tag·ra (ō-don-tag'ră). Termo obsoleto para a odontalgia que se acreditava ter origem gotosa. [odonto- + G. *agra*, convulsão]

odon·tal·gia (ō-don-tal'jē-ă). Odontalgia. SIN toothache. [odont- + G. *algos*, dor]

   o. denta'lis, dor reflexa no ouvido decorrente de doença dentária, usualmente propagada ao longo do nervo auriculotemporal.

odon·tal·gic (ō-don-tal'jik). Odontálgico; relativo a, ou caracterizado por, odontalgia.

odon·tec·to·my (ō-don-tek'tō-mē). Odontectomia; remoção dos dentes através da reflexão de um retalho mucoperiósteo e excisão do osso ao redor da raiz ou raízes antes da aplicação da força para efetuar a remoção do dente. [odont- + G. *ektomē*, excisão]

odon·ter·ism (ō-don'ter-izm). Odonterismo; ranger dos dentes. [odont- + G. *erismos*, discussão]

odon·ti·a·sis (ō-don-tī'ă-sis). Odontíase. SIN teething.

odon·ti·noid (ō-don'ti-noyd). Odontinóide. 1. Que se assemelha à dentina. 2. Uma pequena excrescência de um dente, mais comum na raiz ou no colo. 3. Semelhante ao dente.

odon·ti·tis (ō-don-tī'tis). Odontite. SIN pulpitis.

△ **odonto-.** Odonto-. VER odont-.

odon·to·am·e·lo·blas·to·ma (ō-don'tō-am'ē-lō-blas-tō'mă). Odontoameloblastoma. SIN ameloblastic *odontoma*.

odon·to·blast (ō-don'tō-blast). Odontoblasto; uma das células formadoras de dentina, derivadas do mesênquima originário da crista neural, que revestem a cavidade da polpa de um dente; os odontoblastos estão dispostos em uma camada periférica na polpa dentária, cada qual com um prolongamento odontoblástico que se estende através da espessura da dentina; em geral, as células são colunares na polpa coronal, mas são mais cubóides na área radicular e adjacente à dentina terciária. [odonto- + G. *blastos*, germe, broto]

odon·to·blas·to·ma (ō-don'tō-blas-tō'mă). Odontoblastoma. 1. Um tumor composto de células mesenquimatosas e epiteliais neoplásicas que podem diferenciar-se em células capazes de produzir substâncias dentárias calcificadas. 2. Um odontoma em seu estágio de formação inicial. [odontoblast + G. *-oma*, tumor]

odon·to·clast (ō-don'tō-klast). Odontoclasto; uma das células que se acredita promovam a reabsorção das raízes dos dentes decíduos. [odonto- + G. *klastos*, quebrado]

odon·to·dyn·ia (ō-don-tō-din'ē-ă). Odontodinia. SIN toothache. [odonto- + G. *odynē*, dor]

odon·to·dys·pla·sia (ō-don'tō-dis-plā'zē-ă). Odontodisplasia; um distúrbio do desenvolvimento de um ou vários dentes adjacentes, de etiologia desconhecida, caracterizado por formação deficiente do esmalte e dentina, o que resulta em uma câmara da polpa anormalmente grande e que confere uma imagem radiográfica semelhante a um fantasma ao dente; esses dentes exibem uma erupção tardia para a cavidade oral. SIN odontogenesis imperfecta, odontogenic dysplasia.

odon·to·gen·e·sis (ō-don-tō-jen'ē-sis). Odontogênese; o processo de desenvolvimento dos dentes. SIN odontogeny, odontosis. [odonto- + G. *genesis*, produção]

   o. imperfec'ta, o. imperfeita. SIN odontodysplasia.

odon·tog·e·ny (ō-don-toj'ē-nē). Odontogenia. SIN odontogenesis.

odon·toid (ō-don'toyd). Odontóide. 1. Com formato semelhante a um dente. SIN dentoid. 2. Relativo ao processo o., semelhante a um dente, da segunda vértebra cervical. [odonto- + G. *eidos*, semelhança]

odon·tol·o·gy (ō-don-tol'ō-jē). Odontologia. SIN dentistry. [odonto- + G. *logos*, estudo]

   forensic o., o. forense. SIN forensic *dentistry*.

odon·to·lox·ia, odon·to·loxy (ō-don-tō-lok'sē-ă, ō-don-tol'ok-sē). Odontoloxia. SIN odontoparallaxis. [odonto- + G. *loxos*, inclinação]

odon·tol·y·sis (ō-don-tol'i-sis). Odontólise. SIN erosion (3). [odonto- + G. *lysis*, destruição]

odon·to·ma (ō-don-tō'mă). Odontoma. 1. Um tumor de origem odontogênica. 2. Um tumor odontogênico hamartomatoso composto de esmalte, dentina, cimento e tecido da polpa, que pode estar organizado, ou não, na forma de um dente. [odonto- + G. *-oma*, tumor]

   ameloblastic o., o. ameloblástico; um tumor odontogênico misto benigno, composto de um componente indiferenciado histologicamente idêntico a um ameloblastoma e um componente bem-diferenciado idêntico a um odontoma; aparece como uma lesão radiotransparente-radiopaca mista e que se apresenta clinicamente como um ameloblastoma. SIN odontoameloblastoma.

   complex o., o. complexo; um o. em que os vários tecidos odontogênicos estão organizados de forma aleatória, sem nenhuma semelhança com os dentes.

   compound o., o. composto; um o. em que os tecidos odontogênicos estão organizados de forma semelhante a dentes anômalos.

odon·to·neu·ral·gia (ō-don'tō-noo-ral'jē-ă). Odontoneuralgia; neuralgia facial causada por um dente cariado.

odon·ton·o·my (ō-don-ton'ō-mē). Odontonomia; nomenclatura dentária. [odonto- + G. *onoma*, nome]

odon·to·no·sol·o·gy (ō-don-tō-nō-sol'ō-jē). Odontonosologia. SIN dentistry. [odonto- + G. *nosos*, doença, + *logos*, estudo]

odon·to·par·al·lax·is (ō-don'tō-par-ă-lak'sis). Odontoparalaxe; irregularidade dos dentes. SIN odontoloxia, odontoloxy. [odonto- + G. *parallax*, alternadamente]

odon·top·a·thy (ō-don-top′ă-thē). Odontopatia; qualquer doença dos dentes ou de seus alvéolos. [odonto- + G. *pathos*, sofrimento]

odon·to·pho·bia (ō-don-tō-fō′bē-ă). Odontofobia; temor mórbido de dentes. [odonto- + G. *phobos*, medo]

odon·to·plas·ty (ō-don′tō-plas-tē). Odontoplastia; contorno cirúrgico da superfície do dente para estimular o controle da placa e a morfologia gengival. [odonto- + G. *plassō*, modelar]

odon·top·ri·sis (ō-don-top′ri-sis). Odontoprise; ranger dos dentes. VER TAMBÉM bruxism. [odonto- + G. *prisis*, uma serra, um ranger]

odon·top·to·sis (ō-don-top-tō′sis, -tō-tō′sis). Odontoptose; movimento para baixo de um dente superior devido à perda de seu antagonista inferior. VER TAMBÉM supereruption. [odonto- + G. *ptōsis*, uma queda]

odon·tor·rha·gia (ō-don-tō-rā′jē-ă). Odontorragia; sangramento profuso, a partir do alvéolo, após a extração de um dente. [odonto- + G. *rhēgnymi*, eclodir]

odon·to·schism (ō-don′tō-skizm, -sizm). Odontosquismo; fissura de um dente. [odonto- + G. *schisma*, uma fenda]

odon·to·scope (ō-don′tō-skōp). Odontoscópio; um dispositivo óptico, similar a um sistema de circuito fechado de televisão, que projeta uma imagem da cavidade oral em uma tela para o exame múltiplo.

odon·tos·co·py (ō-don-tos′kō-pē). Odontoscopia. **1.** Exame da cavidade oral por meio do odontoscópio. **2.** Exame das marcas nas impressões das bordas cortantes dos dentes; usado, como impressões digitais, como um método de identificação pessoal. [odonto- + G. *skopeō*, visualizar]

odon·to·sis (ō-don-tō′sis). Odontose. SIN odontogenesis.

odon·to·ther·a·py (ō-don-tō-thar′ă-pē). Odontoterapia; tratamento das doenças dos dentes.

odon·tot·o·my (ō-don-tot′ō-mē). Odontotomia; o corte na coroa de um dente. [odonto- + G. *tomē*, incisão]

   prophylactic o., o. profilática; uma cirurgia preventiva em que sulcos de desenvolvimento, fóveas e fissuras formados de modo imperfeito são abertos por meio de uma broca e preenchidos para evitar futuras cáries.

odor (ō′dŏr). Odor; emanação de qualquer substância que estimula as células sensoriais olfatórias. SIN scent, smell (3). [L.]

odor·ant (ō′dŏr-ant). Odorante; uma substância com odor.

odor·a·tism (ō′dŏr′ă-tizm). Odoratismo. VER lathyrism. [de *Lathyrus odoratus*, ervilha-de-cheiro]

odor·if·er·ous (ō-dō-rif′er-ŭs). Odorífero; que possui aroma, perfume ou odor. SIN odorous. [odor + L. *fero*, possuir]

odor·im·e·ter (ō′dō-rim′e-ter). Odorímetro; instrumento para realizar a odorimetria.

odo·rim·e·try (ō′dō-rim′e-trē). Odorimetria; a determinação da potência comparativa de diferentes substâncias na estimulação de sensações olfatórias. [odor + G. *metron*, medida]

odor·i·vec·tion (ō′dŏr-i-vek′shŭn). Odorivecção; que transmite ou transporta um odor, como no ar. [odor + L. *vector*, um transportador]

odor·og·ra·phy (ō′dŏ-rog′ră-fē). Odorigrafia; descrição dos odores. [odor + G. *graphē*, uma descrição]

odor·ous (ō′dŏr-ŭs). Odorífero. SIN odoriferous.

O'Dwyer, Joseph P., médico norte-americano, 1841–1898. VER O′D. *tube*.

odyn-, odyno-. Odino-, odin-; formas combinantes que indicam dor. [G. *odynē*]

odyn·a·cu·sis (ō-din′ă-koo′sis). Odinacusia; hipersensibilidade do órgão da audição, de modo que os sons provocam dor real. [odyn- + G. *akouō*, ouvir]

odyn·o·pha·gia (ō-din-o-fā′jē-ă). Odinofagia; dor à deglutição. [odyno- + G. *phagō*, comer]

odyn·o·pho·nia (ō-din-ō-fō′nē-ă). Odinofonia; dor ao usar a voz. [odyno- + G. *phonē*, som, voz]

Oe Símbolo de oersted (unidade de intensidade magnética).

oe-. Para as palavras assim iniciadas e não encontradas aqui, ver e-.

oe·di·pism (ed′i-pizm). Edipismo. **1.** Manifestação do complexo de Édipo. **2.** Termo raramente utilizado para a auto-inflição de lesão nos olhos, geralmente em uma tentativa de tirá-los. [*Oedipus*, pers. mit. G.]

Oehl, Eusebio, anatomista italiano, 1827–1903. VER O. *muscles*, em *muscle*.

oe·nan·thal (ē-nan′thăl). Enantol. SIN heptanal.

oer·sted (**Oe**) (er′sted). Uma unidade de intensidade de campo magnético; a intensidade do campo magnético que exerce uma força de 1 dina sobre uma unidade de pólo magnético; igual a $(1.000/4\pi)$ A m^{-1}. [Hans-Christian *Oersted*, físico dinamarquês, 1777–1851]

oe·soph·a·go·sto·mi·a·sis (ē-sof′ă-gō-stō-mī′ă-sis). Esofagostomíase; infecção por parasitas nematódeos do gênero *Oesophagostomum*. SIN esophagostomiasis. [G. *oi-sophagos*, goela (esôfago), + *stoma*, boca, + *-iasis*, condição]

Oe·soph·a·gos·to·mum (ē-sof-ă-gos′tō-mŭm). Um gênero de nematódeos estrongilóides (subfamília Oesophagostominae) que encistam na parede intestinal de herbívoros e primatas, causando doença nodular. As larvas parecem estimular uma reação do hospedeiro na parede intestinal, formando nódulos nos quais os vermes completam seu desenvolvimento (a menos que o hospedeiro seja imune); eles deixam, então, o nódulo e alimentam-se como adultos na luz do intestino grosso. [G. *oisophagos*, goela (esôfago), + *stoma*, boca]

O. apios′tomum, uma espécie de nematódeo relatado no norte da Nigéria e na África Central que se encista sob a submucosa do intestino humano e, ocasionalmente, provoca disenteria; um parasita comum de macacos e símios em cativeiro e selvagens.

O. brevicau′dum, uma espécie de nematódeo que ocorre no ceco e no colo de porcos na América do Norte e Índia.

O. brump′ti, uma espécie de nematódeo descrita em macacos africanos e relatados ocasionalmente em seres humanos.

O. columbia′num, uma espécie de nematódeo que ocorre em carneiros, cabras e antílopes selvagens africanos; exceto quando presente em grande número, não parece afetar gravemente a saúde do hospedeiro.

O. denta′tum, uma espécie de nematódeo que afeta o colo de suínos; as lesões são similares às encontradas no carneiro.

O. georgia′num, uma espécie de nematódeo que ocorre no ceco e colo de porcos nos Estados Unidos.

O. quadrispinula′tum, uma espécie que ocorre no ceco e colo de porcos nas Américas, na Europa e no Sudeste Asiático.

O. radia′tum, uma espécie que ocorre por todo o mundo no gado bovino e búfalo; as lesões são semelhantes às encontradas nos carneiros.

O. stephanos′tomum, uma espécie de nematódeo que ocorre em chimpanzés, macacos e gorilas na África, mas também descrita em seres humanos e macacos no Brasil.

O. venulo′sum, uma espécie que ocorre por todo o mundo no ceco e colo do gado bovino, cabras, cervos e muitos outros ruminantes.

oes·tra·di·ol (es-tră-dī′ol). Estradiol. SIN estradiol.

oes·trids (est′ridz). Estrídeos; nome comum de moscas-varejeiras da família Oestridae, como *Oestrus*. [G. *oistros*, moscardo]

oes·tri·ol (es′trē-ol). Estriol. SIN estriol.

oes·tro·gen (es′trō-jen). Estrogênio. SIN estrogen.

oes·trone (es′trōn). Estrona. SIN estrone.

oes·tro·sis (es-trō′sis). Estrose; a infecção de pequenos ruminantes e, raramente, seres humanos por larvas da mosca *Oestrus ovis*.

Oes·trus (es′trŭs). Um gênero de moscas invasoras de tecidos que provocam miíase em carneiros; os gasterófilos da cabeça na família Oestridae. *O. ovis* (mosca-varejeira do nariz) é um gasterofílideo semelhante a uma abelha, peludo, robusto e castanho-acinzentado, importado da Europa e, atualmente, uma peste grave em regiões dos Estados Unidos; as larvas são depositadas pela mosca adulta nas narinas do carneiro, e larvas com 2,5 cm de comprimento desenvolvem-se nos seios paranasais, provocando considerável secreção mucosa e sofrimento em carneiros fracos ou idosos. [G. *oistros*, moscardo]

of·fi·cial (ō-fish′ăl). Oficial; indica um medicamento ou preparação química ou farmacêutica reconhecida como padronizada na farmacopéia. Cf. officinal. [L. *officialis*, de *officium*, um favor, serviço, de *opus*, trabalho, + *facio*, fazer]

of·fic·i·nal (ō-fis′i-năl). Oficinal; indica um medicamento ou preparação farmacêutica mantida em estoque em contraste com a magistral (aviada na hora segundo a prescrição de um médico); uma preparação o. é com freqüência, embora não necessariamente, oficial. [L. *officina*, loja]

Ogino, Kyusaka, médico japonês do século XX. VER O.-Knaus *rule*.

Ogston, Sir Alexander, cirurgião escocês, 1844–1929. VER O. *line;* O.-Luc *operation*.

Oguchi, Chita, oftalmologista japonês, 1875-1945. VER O. *disease*.

Ogura, Joseph H., otorrinolaringologista norte-americano, 1915–1983. VER O. *operation*.

O'Hara, Michael, Jr., cirurgião norte-americano, 1869–1926. VER O′H. *forceps*.

OHI Abreviatura de Oral Hygiene Index (Índice de Higiene Oral).

OHI-S Abreviatura de Simplified Oral Hygiene Index (Índice de Higiene Oral Simplificado).

Ohm, Georg S., físico alemão, 1787–1854. VER ohm; O. *law*.

ohm (Ω) (ōm). A unidade prática de resistência elétrica; a resistência de qualquer condutor que permite que 1 A de corrente passe sob a força eletromotiva de 1 V. [G.S. *Ohm*]

ohm·am·me·ter (ōm-am′e-ter). Ohmamperímetro; um ohmômetro e amperímetro combinados.

ohm·me·ter (ōm′e-ter). Ohmômetro; um instrumento para determinar a resistência elétrica, em ohms, de um condutor.

oh·ne Hauch (ō′nă howch). Termo empregado para indicar o crescimento não-disseminador de bactérias não-flageladas em meios com ágar; também aplicado à aglutinação somática. VER TAMBÉM O *antigen*. [Al. sem fôlego]

Ohngren line. Linha de Ohngren. Ver em line.

OI Abreviatura de *osteogenesis* imperfecta (osteogênese imperfeita).

oi-. Para as palavras assim começadas e não encontradas aqui, ver e-.

-oid. -óide; sufixo que designa semelhante a, equivalente em inglês a -form. [G. *eidos*, forma, semelhança]

oid·ia (ō-id′ēă). Oídios; plural de oidium.

oid·i·um, pl. **oid·ia** (ō-id′ē-ŭm, ō-id′ē-ă). Oídio; termo originalmente empregado para artroconídio. [L. mod. dim. de G. *ōon*, ovo]

oil (oyl). Óleo; um líquido inflamável, de consistência gordurosa e sensação untuosa, que é insolúvel em água, solúvel ou insolúvel em álcool e livremente solúvel em éter. Os óleos são classificados como animais, vegetais e minerais, de acordo com suas origens (os óleos minerais provavelmente têm origem animal e vegetal remota); em óleos gordurosos (fixos) e voláteis (essenciais); e em óleos secantes e não-secantes (gordurosos), tornando-se os primeiros mais espessos quando expostos ao ar e, finalmente, secando até um verniz, com os últimos não secando, mas tornando-se rançosos na exposição. Muitos dos óleos, fixos e voláteis, são utilizados em medicina. Para os óleos individuais, ver os nomes específicos. [L. *oleum*; G. *elaion*, originalmente óleo de oliva]

absolute o.'s, óleos absolutos; óleos essenciais que são obtidos pela remoção de compostos insolúveis de óleos concretos.

o. of American wormseed, o. da erva-de-santa-maria. SIN o. of chenopodium.

o. of anise, o. de anis; o. volátil derivado do fruto maduro e seco de *Pimpinella anisum* (família Umbelliferae) ou *Illicium verum* (família Magnoliaceae) (anis-estrela chinês); possui o característico aroma de anis, assemelhando-se à erva-doce. Usado na fabricação de licores e como flavorizante para doces, biscoitos, dentifrícios. Base farmacêutica (sabor). Carminativo.

o. of bay, o. de louro; o. volátil derivado da destilação a vapor das folhas secas da *Pimenta (Myrcia) acris* (família Myrtaceae); usado como aromático na fabricação de loção pós-barba e como base farmacêutica.

o. of bergamot, o. de bergamota; o. volátil derivado da destilação a vapor da casca do fruto fresco do *Citrus aurantium* ou *C. bergamia*; contém L-linalil acetato; L-linalol; D-limoneno, dipenteno, bergapteno; usado como desodorante em preparações que contêm ingredientes com odores fétidos e como aromático em perfumes, laquês e pomadas.

betula o., o. de bétula, o. de vidoeiro; o. de bétula-doce, um o. volátil obtido por destilação da casca da *Betula lenta* (bétula-doce); usado como agente flavorizante e como linimento contra-irritante. VER TAMBÉM methyl salicylate.

o. of bitter almond, o. de amêndoa amarga; o. volátil obtido da semente madura seca de amêndoas amargas ou de outras sementes que contêm amigdalina, como damasco, pêssegos, ameixas e cerejas; obtido por destilação a vapor subseqüente à maceração da semente com água. Originalmente utilizado como antipruriginoso; tóxico — libera ácido cianídrico (cianeto de hidrogênio). Apenas o óleo sem cianeto de hidrogênio pode ser utilizado como flavorizante de licores e alimentos.

o. of bitter orange, o. de laranja amarga; o. volátil obtido por destilação a vapor da casca fresca da *Citrus aurantium* (família Rutaceae). Material aromático empregado como agente flavorizante em produtos farmacêuticos, alimentos e licores; também utilizado em perfumes.

o. of cardamom, o. de cardamomo; o. volátil obtido por destilação a vapor de sementes de *Elettaria cardamomum* (família Zingiberacea). Agente flavorizante em produtos farmacêuticos (xaropes), licores, molhos, confeitos e alimentos assados; originalmente utilizado como carminativo.

o. of chenopodium, o. de quenopódio; o. volátil obtido das partes aéreas frescas da flor da erva de santa-maria, *Chenopodium ambrosioides*, ou *C. anthelminticum*. Usado como anti-helmíntico. SIN o. of American wormseed.

o. of cherry laurel, o. de loureiro-cereja; o. volátil obtido por destilação a vapor do *Prunus laurocerasus* (família Rosaceae); semelhante ao o. de amêndoa amarga; extremamente tóxico por causa do conteúdo de cianeto de hidrogênio.

o. of cinnamon, o. de canela; o. volátil obtido por destilação a vapor das folhas e galhos finos da *Cinnamomum cassia* (família Lauracea); flavorizante em alimentos e perfumes.

o. of citronella, o. de citronela; o. volátil obtido por destilação a vapor de folhas frescas do limão. Contém citranelol; usado como repelente de insetos, quer sobre a pele, quer na forma de incenso; também empregado como perfume.

o. of clove, o. de cravo-da-índia; o. volátil obtido por destilação a vapor de brotos de flores secos da *Eugenia caryophyllata* (família Myrtacea). Contém cerca de 85% de eugenol, juntamente com outros constituintes. Usado em odontologia como anestésico local e componente de obturações temporárias dos dentes. Também utilizado para temperar alimentos; odor forte e pungente. SIN clove oil.

concrete o.'s, óleos concretos; óleos essenciais obtidos por extração com solventes orgânicos; contêm ceras e parafinas.

o. of coriander, o. de coentro; o. volátil do fruto maduro seco do *Coriandrum sativum* (família Umbelliferae). Flavorizante em alimentos e bebidas alcoólicas.

oil of crispmint, o. de hortelã-verde; SIN o. of spearmint.

o. of cubeb, o. de cubeba; o. volátil do fruto não-maduro da *Piper cubeba* (família Piperaceae). Originalmente utilizado como um anti-séptico urinário.

oil of curled mint, o. de hortelã-verde. SIN o. of spearmint.

o. of dwarf pine needles, o. de folha de pinheiro anão; o. volátil das folhas frescas do *Pinus montana* (família Pinaceae). Odor de pinho agradável; usado como base farmacêutica (flavorizante e perfume). Foi utilizado como expectorante.

essential o.'s, óleos essenciais; produtos vegetais, geralmente algo voláteis, fornecendo odores e sabores característicos da planta em questão, possuindo, assim, a essência, p.ex., citral, pineno, cânfora, mentano, terpenos; em geral, os destilados a vapor de plantas ou óleos de plantas obtidos ao espremer as cascas de determinada planta. VER TAMBÉM volatile o.

ethereal o., o. etéreo. SIN volatile o.

o. of eucalyptus, o. de eucalipto; o. volátil obtido das folhas frescas de *Eucalyptus globulus* (família Myrtacea) e algumas outras espécies de *Eucalyptus*; oriundo da Austrália; o. pungente com sabor refrescante e picante. Tem sido empregado como um aromatizante em inalantes, como expectorante, anti-helmíntico e anti-séptico local.

fatty o., o. graxo; o. derivado de animais e vegetais; quimicamente, um glicerídeo de um ácido graxo que, por substituição da glicerina por uma base alcalina, é convertido em um sabão; um o. graxo, em contraste com um o. volátil, é permanente, deixando uma mancha em uma superfície absorvente e, portanto, não pode ser destilado; é obtido por expressão ou extração; a consistência varia com a temperatura, com alguns sendo líquidos (óleos próprios), outros semi-sólidos (gorduras) e outros sólidos (sebos) nas temperaturas comuns; tanto os óleos líquidos como os semi-sólidos são solidificados pelo frio e os sólidos são liquefeitos pelo calor. SIN fixed o.

o. of fennel, o. de funcho; o. volátil do fruto seco da *Foeniculum vulgare* (família Umbelliferae). Um o. aromático com o odor e o paladar da erva-doce, semelhante ao anis; usado como agente flavorizante em produtos farmacêuticos. Tem sido empregado como carminativo.

fixed o., o. fixo. SIN fatty o.

fusel o., o. de fúsel; uma mistura de produtos secundários da fermentação alcoólica; consiste principalmente em álcoois (p.ex., álcool de amila, propila, isoamila e isobutila).

joint o., líquido sinovial. SIN synovial *fluid*.

jojoba o., o. de jojoba; uma mistura de éster de cera líquida extraída de sementes moídas ou amassadas da *Simmondsia chinensis* e *S. californica* (família Buxaceae), arbustos desérticos nativos do Arizona, Califórnia e norte do México. Muito usado em cosméticos por suas supostas propriedades de lubrificação e hidratação da pele; também empregado como lubrificante, combustível, caldos de alimentos artificiais, substitutos para o óleo de baleia. SIN oil of jojoba.

oil of jojoba, óleo de jojoba. SIN jojoba o.

o. of juniper, o. de zimbro; o. volátil do fruto maduro seco (bagas) da *Juniperus communis* (família Cupressaceae). Originalmente utilizado como diurético. Usado em perfumaria. SIN juniper berry oil.

o. of lavender, o. de alfazema; o. volátil dos caules floridos frescos da *Lavandula officinalis* (família Labiatae). O. aromático usado em perfume e como agente flavorizante. Tem sido utilizado como carminativo.

o. of lemon, o. de limão; o. volátil espremido da casca fresca do *Citrus limonum* (família Rutaceae). O. aromático usado para dar sabor a produtos farmacêuticos, licores, massas, alimentos e bebidas, bem como em perfumes.

o. of lemon grass, o. de capim-limão; o. volátil de *Cymbopogon citratus* e *C. flexuosus* (família Gramineae). Usado em perfumaria e como fonte de citral para a síntese de vitamina A.

Lorenzo o., o. de Lorenzo; uma mistura de quatro partes de glicerílico trioleato e uma parte de glicerílico trierucato; usado no tratamento da adrenoleucodistrofia. [em homenagem a Lorenzo Odone, uma criança com adrenoleucodistrofia, cuja descoberta e suporte desse agente pela família foram dramatizados no filme norte-americano *Lorenzo's Oil* (1992)]

olive o., azeite; o óleo espremido do fruto da *Olea europaea*; usado como colagogo, laxativo e emoliente na preparação de linimentos e na preparação de alimentos.

palm o., o. de palma, azeite de dendê; o. obtido das sementes da *Elaeis guineensis* (família Palmae); usado na fabricação de sabão, linimentos e pomadas, bem como em alimentos.

o. of pennyroyal, o. de poejo; quer americano, quer europeu. O primeiro é um o. volátil derivado das copas floridas e folhas do poejo norte-americano (*Hedeoma pulegioides*, da família Labiatae). Contém pulegona e cetonas. O segundo é o o. de poejo-das-hortas ou poejo-europeu; um o. volátil obtido de *Mentha pulegium* (família Labiatae); contém cerca de 85% de pulegona. Tem sido utilizado como carminativo aromático, abortifaciente e repelente de insetos.

o. of peppermint, o. de hortelã-pimenta; o. volátil que contém mentol (não menos que 50% do total) obtido por destilação a vapor do vegetal florido fresco *Mentha piperita* (família Labiatae). Usado como auxiliar farmacológico (sabor) e na flavorização de licores; um carminativo.

red o. [C.I. 26125], o. vermelho; um corante diazo fracamente ácido e solúvel em óleo, empregado na demonstração histológica de gorduras neutras.

rock o. (rok oyl), petróleo. SIN petroleum.

o. of rose, o. de rosas; o. volátil obtido de flores frescas de *Rosa gallica* e *R. damascena*, bem como de outros membros da família Rosaceae. Usado em grande escala em perfumaria, pomadas e preparações de banheiro. SIN attar of rose, essence of rose, otto of rose.

o. of spearmint, o. de hortelã-verde; o. volátil obtido das copas floridas da *Mentha spicata* (família Labiatae), auxiliar farmacêutico (flavorizante) e carminativo. SIN oil of crispmint, oil of curled mint.

sweet birch o., o. de bétula-doce. SIN methyl salicylate.

o. of turpentine, o. de terebintina; o. volátil destilado da oleoresina e obtido da *Pinus palastrus* (família Pinaceae) e de outras espécies de *Pinus* que fornecem óleos de terpenos. Solvente para óleos, resinas e vernizes; também empregado como veículo, tíner e removedor de tintas à base de óleo; rubefaciente; tem sido utilizado como contra-irritante em linimentos.

volatile o., o. volátil; uma substância de consistência e sensação oleosa, derivada de um vegetal e contendo os princípios dos quais se originam o odor e o sabor do vegetal (o. essencial); em contraste com um o. graxo, um o. volátil evapora quando exposto ao ar e, dessa maneira, pode ser destilado; também pode ser obtido por expressão ou extração; muitos óleos voláteis, idênticos ou que se assemelham muito aos óleos naturais, podem ser sintetizados. Os óleos voláteis são empregados em medicina como estimulantes, estomáquicos, corretivos e carminativos, e para fins de flavorização (p.ex., óleo de hortelã). SIN ethereal o.

o. of wormwood, o. de absinto; o. volátil obtido das folhas e copas da *Artemisia absinthium* (família Compositae). Acetato e álcool de tujol; tujona (um poderoso convulsivante), felandreno, cadineno; também um o. azul. Usado na flavorização do vermute e, originalmente, no absinto.

oil of vit·ri·ol. ácido sulfúrico. SIN sulfuric acid.

oint·ment (oynt'ment). Bálsamo, ungüento, pomada; uma preparação semi-sólida que, geralmente, contém substâncias medicinais e destinada à aplicação externa. As bases dessa preparação, usadas como veículos, estão dispostas em quatro classes gerais: 1) As bases de hidrocarboneto (bases oleaginosas) mantêm os medicamentos em contato prolongado com a pele, atuando como curativos compressivos, e são utilizadas principalmente por seus efeitos emolientes. 2) As bases de absorção permitem a incorporação de soluções aquosas com a formação de uma emulsão de água-em-óleo, ou são emulsões de água-em-óleo que permitem a incorporação de quantidades adicionais de soluções aquosas; essas bases permitem a melhor absorção de alguns medicamentos e são úteis como emolientes. 3) As bases removíveis por água (cremes) são emulsões de óleo em água que contém vaselina, lanolina anidra ou ceras; podem ser retiradas da pele com água e, dessa forma, são mais aceitáveis por motivos cosméticos; elas favorecem a absorção de secreções serosas nas afecções dermatológicas. 4) As bases hidrossolúveis (bases de pomada sem gordura) contêm apenas substâncias hidrossolúveis. VER TAMBÉM cerate. SIN salve, uncture, unguent. [Fr. ant. *oignement*; L. *unguo*, pp. *unctus*, esfregar]

blue o., uma pomada de base oleosa que contém 20% de mercúrio metálico finamente dividido, outrora muito utilizada topicamente na pele para a destruição dos piolhos do corpo. O risco está associado à absorção transdérmica de mercúrio e a uma dermatite local. SIN mild mercurial ointment.

eye o., pomada oftálmica. SIN ophthalmic o.

hydrophilic o., pomada hidrofílica; uma base de pomada que contém 25% de vaselina e álcool esteárilico, 12% de propil glicol emulsificado em 37% de água por 1% de lauril sulfato; preservado com parabeno. Adequado para a incorporação de inúmeros medicamentos destinados a aplicação local; uma base de pomada lavável.

mild mercurial ointment, pomada mercurial branda. SIN blue o.

ophthalmic o., pomada oftálmica; uma pomada especial para a aplicação no olho que tem de estar isenta de partículas e não deve ser irritante para o olho. SIN eye o., oculentum.

Okazaki, Reiji (1930–1975) e Tuneko, biólogos moleculares japoneses do século XX. VER O. *fragment*.

-ol. -ol; sufixo que indica que uma substância é um álcool ou um fenol.

ol·a·mine (ōl'a-mēn). Olamina; contração de etanolamina aprovada pela USAN.

Oldfield, Michael C., médico inglês do século XX. VER O. *syndrome*.

o·le·ag·i·nous (ō-lē-aj'i-nŭs). Oleaginosa; oleosa ou gordurosa. [L. *oleagineus*, pertinente a *olea*, a oliveira]

ole·an·der (ō-lē-an'der). Oleandro; a casca e as folhas da *Nerium oleander* (família Apocynaceae), um arbusto do leste do Mediterrâneo; originalmente empregado como diurético e cardiotônico.

ole·an·do·my·cin phos·phate (ō-lē-an-dō-mī'sin). Fosfato de oleandomicina; uma substância antibiótica produzida por espécies de *Streptomyces antibioticus*; efetiva contra estafilococos, estreptococos, pneumococos e algumas bactérias Gram-negativas.

ole·ate (ō'lē-āt). Oleato. 1. Um sal do ácido oleico. 2. Uma preparação farmacológica que é uma combinação ou solução de um alcalóide ou base metálica em ácido oleico, usada como unção.

olec·ra·non (ō-lek'ră-non, ō'lē-kră'non) [TA]. Olécrano; a extremidade curva proximal proeminente da ulna; em suas superfícies superior e posterior está a inserção do tendão do músculo tríceps, com a superfície anterior entrando na formação da incisura troclear. SIN elbow bone, olecranon process, point of elbow, tip of elbow. [G. a cabeça ou ponta do cotovelo, de ōlenē, ulna, + kranion, crânio, cabeça]

ole·fin (ō'lē-fin). Olefina. SIN alkene.

ole·ic ac·id (ō-lē'ik). Ácido oleico; um ácido graxo insaturado que é o ácido graxo mais abundante e amplamente distribuído na natureza; usado comercialmente na preparação de oleatos e loções, e como solvente farmacêutico. Cf. elaidic acid. [L. *oleum*, óleo]

ole·in (ō'lē-in). Oleína; trioleoil glicerol; trioleato de glicerila; um triacilglicerol, contendo apenas moléculas de oleíla, encontrado em gorduras e óleos. SIN triolein.

oleo-. Forma combinante relativa a óleo. VER TAMBÉM eleo-. [L. *oleum*]

ole·o·gom·en·ol (ō'lē-ō-gō'men-ol). Oleogomenol. SIN gomenol.

ole·o·gran·u·lo·ma (ō'lē-ō-gran-ū-lō'mă). Oleogranuloma. SIN lipogranuloma.

ole·o·ma (ō-lē-ō'mă). Oleoma. SIN lipogranuloma.

ole·om·e·ter (ō-lē-om'e-ter). Oleômetro; um instrumento, similar a um hidrômetro, para determinar a densidade específica dos óleos. SIN eleometer. [oleo- + G. *metron*, medida]

ole·o·pal·mi·tate (ō'lē-ō-pal'mi-tāt). Oleopalmitato; um sal duplo dos ácidos oleico e palmítico.

ole·o·res·in (ō'lē-ō-rez'in). Oleorresina. 1. Um composto de um óleo essencial e resina, presente em determinados vegetais. 2. Uma preparação farmacêutica. VER aspidium, capsicum, ginger. 3. Bálsamo. SIN balsam.

ole·o·sac·cha·rum, pl. **ole·o·sac·cha·ra** (ō'lē-ō-sak'ă-rŭm). Açúcar de óleo; uma classe de preparações feitas pela trituração de um óleo volátil (como de anis, erva-doce ou limão) com açúcar; usado como diluente ou corretivo de medicamentos com sabor ruim ou intenso na forma de pó. SIN oil sugar. [oleo- + G. *saccharon*, açúcar]

ole·o·ste·a·rate (ō'lē-ō-stē'ă-rāt). Oleostearato; um sal duplo dos ácidos oleico e esteárico.

ole·o·sus (ō-lē-ō'sŭs). Oleoso; gorduroso; relativo à anormalidade do aparelho sebáceo. [L., de *oleum*, óleo]

ole·o·ther·a·py (ō'lē-ō-thar'ă-pē). Oleoterapia; tratamento da doença por um óleo administrado por via interna ou externa. SIN eleotherapy. [oleo- + G. *therapeia*, terapia]

ole·o·vi·ta·min (ō'lē-ō-vī'tă-min). Oleovitamina; solução de uma vitamina em um óleo comestível.

o. A and D, o. A e D; uma solução de vitaminas A e D em óleo de fígado de peixe ou em um óleo vegetal comestível.

ole·um ter·e·bin·thin·ae (ō'lē-ŭm ter-ē-ben'thin-ī). Óleo de terebintina. SIN turpentine oil.

ole·yl al·co·hol (ō-lē'il). Álcool oleílico; uma mistura de álcoois alifáticos que consiste principalmente em $CH_3(CH_2)_7CH=CH(CH_2)_7CH_2OH$; usado como emulsificante e na preparação de cremes de beleza; encontrado em óleos de peixe.

ole·yl-CoA (ō-lē'il). Oleil-CoA; um produto do sistema da enzima Δ^9-dessaturase na biossíntese de ácidos graxos monoinsaturados. SIN oleyl-coenzyme A.

ole·yl-co·en·zyme A. Oleil-coenzima A. SIN oleyl-CoA.

ol·fac·tie, ol·fac·ty (ol-fak'tē). Olfatia; a unidade do olfato; o limiar da estimulação olfatória, ou o ponto em que o olfato acabou de ser recebido no olfatômetro. [ver olfaction]

ol·fac·tion (ol-fak'shŭn). Olfação. 1. A sensação do olfato. SIN smell (2). 2. O ato de cheirar. SIN osmesis, osphresis. [L. *ol- facio*, pp. *-factus*, cheirar]

ol·fac·tol·o·gy (ol'fak-tol'ō-jē). Olfatologia; o estudo da sensação do olfato. [olfaction + G. *logos*, estudo]

ol·fac·tom·e·ter (ol'fak-tom'e-ter). Olfatômetro; um dispositivo para estimar a sensibilidade a odorantes. [L. *olfactus*, olfato, + G. *metron*, medida]

ol·fac·tom·e·try (ol'fak-tom'e-trē). Olfatometria; determinação do grau de sensibilidade a odorantes.

ol·fac·to·pho·bia (ol-fak-tō-fō'bē-ă). Olfatofobia; temor mórbido a odores. SIN osmophobia, osphresiophobia. [L. *olfactus*, olfato, + G. *phobos*, medo]

ol·fac·to·ry (ol-fak'tō-rē). Olfatório; relativo ao sentido do olfato. SIN osmatic, osphretic. [ver olfaction]

olib·a·num (ō-lib'ă-nŭm). Olíbano; uma goma resina de várias árvores do gênero *Boswellia* (família Burseraceae); tem sido empregado como expectorante estimulante na bronquite, para fumigações e como incenso. SIN frankincense, thus. [Ar. *al*, o, + *lubān*, incenso]

olig-. VER oligo-.

ol·i·gam·ni·os (ol-i-gam'nē-os). Oligâmnio. SIN oligohydramnios.

ol·i·ge·mia (ol-i-gē'mē-ă). Oligemia; volume de sangue diminuído no corpo ou em qualquer órgão ou tecido. [oligo- + G. *haima*, sangue]

ol·i·ge·mic (ol-i-gē'mik). Oligêmico; pertinente a, ou caracterizado por, oligemia.

ol·ig·hid·ria, ol·ig·id·ria (ol-ig-hid'rē-ă, -id'rē-ă). Oligidria; transpiração escassa. [oligo- + G. *hidrōs*, suor]

oligo (ol'i-gō). Oligo; em genética molecular, o oligonucleotídeo.

oligo-, olig-. 1. Formas combinantes que indicam algum, um pouco; alguns. 2. Em química, usado em contraste com "poli-" na descrição de polímeros, p.ex., oligossacarídeo. [G. *oligos*, pouco]

ol·i·go·am·ni·os (ol'i-gō-am'nē-os). Oligoâmnio. SIN oligohydramnios. [oligo- + amnion]

ol·i·go·cho·lia (ol'i-gō-kō'lē-ă). Oligocolia; secreção deficiente de bile. [oligo- + G. *cholē*, bile]

ol·i·go·chy·li·a (ol'i-gō-kī'lē-ă). Oligoquilia; deficiência de suco gástrico. [oligo- + G. *chylos*, suco]

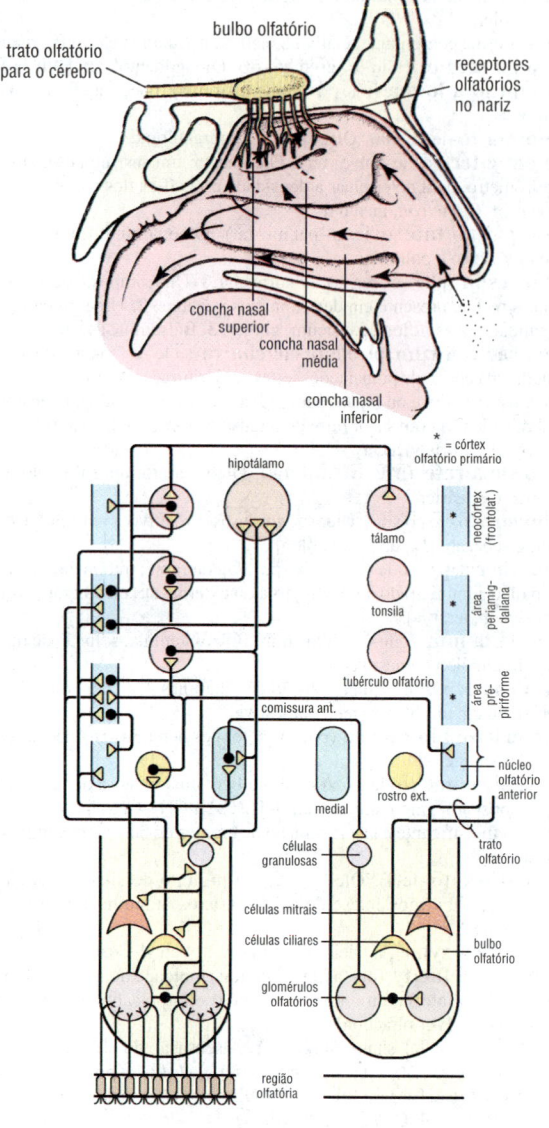

olfação

ol·i·go·chy·mia (ol′i‑gō‑kī′mē‑ă). Oligoquimia; deficiência de quimo. [oligo- + G. *chymos*, suco]

ol·i·go·cys·tic (ol′i‑gō‑sis′tik). Oligocístico; consiste apenas em alguns cistos, como ocasionalmente observado em determinados exemplos de mola hidatiforme e de outras lesões que comumente possuem inúmeros cistos. [oligo- + G. *kystis*, bexiga, cisto]

ol·i·go·dac·ty·ly, ol·i·go·dac·tyl·ia (ol′i‑gō‑dak′ti‑lē, ‑dak′til′ē‑ă). Oligodactilia; presença de menos de cinco dedos em um ou mais membros. [oligo- + G. *daktylos*, dedo ou artelho]

ol·i·go·den·dria (ol′i‑gō‑den′drē‑ă). Oligodendria, oligodendróglia. SIN oligodendroglia.

ol·i·go·den·dro·blast (ol′i‑gō‑den′drō‑blast). Oligodendroblasto; uma célula glial primitiva que é a célula precursora normal do oligodendrócito.

ol·i·go·den·dro·blas·to·ma (ol′i‑gō‑den′drō‑blas‑tō′mă). Oligodendroblastoma; termo obsoleto para o oligodendroglioma. [oligo- + G. *dendron*, árvore, + *blastos*, germe, + -oma]

ol·i·go·den·dro·cyte (ol′i‑gō‑den′drō‑sīt). Oligodendrócito; uma célula da oligodendróglia.

ol·i·go·den·drog·lia (ol′ī‑gō‑den‑drog′lē‑ă). Oligodendróglia; um dos três tipos de células gliais (as outras duas são a macróglia ou astrócitos e a micróglia), juntamente com as células nervosas, compõem o tecido do sistema nervoso central. As células da o. caracterizam-se por um número variável de prolongamentos semelhantes a véus ou lâminas que se enrolam ao redor de axônios individuais para formar a bainha de mielina das fibras nervosas no sistema nervoso central (comparados com as células de Schwann no sistema nervoso periférico); formam a mielina no sistema nervoso central; dessa maneira, são mais numerosas na substância branca que na substância cinzenta. SIN oligodendria. [oligo- + G. *dendron*, árvore, + *glia*, cola]

ol·i·go·den·dro·gli·o·ma (ol′i‑gō‑den′drō‑glī‑ō′mă). Oligodendroglioma; um glioma relativamente raro e com crescimento relativamente lento, derivado dos oligodendrócitos, que ocorre com maior freqüência no cérebro de pessoas adultas; a neoplasia é macroscopicamente homogênea, razoavelmente bem circunscrita, moderadamente firme e com uma consistência algo granulosa, com calcificação intersticial suficientemente densa, para ser detectada em radiográficas do crânio. À microscopia, um o. caracteriza-se por inúmeras células oligodendrogliais pequenas, redondas ou ovóides, com núcleos pequenos e intensamente corados (raramente observados em mitoses), e citoplasma indistinto e pouco corado; as células neoplásicas distribuem-se de maneira uniforme em um estroma fibrilar escasso, com corpúsculos calcificados disseminados e vascularização arqueada frequentemente saliente. [oligo- + G. *dendron*, árvore, + gli, + -oma]

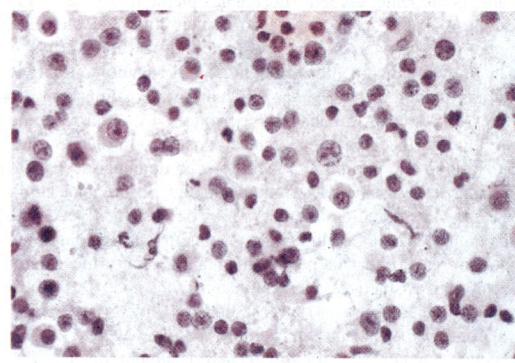

oligodendroglioma: corte mostrando células tumorais com núcleos arredondados uniformes, sem nenhum nucléolo nem prolongamentos celulares

anaplastic o., o. anaplásico; o. agressivo caracterizado por pleomorfismo nuclear evidente, mitoses e celularidade aumentada. SIN pleomorphic o.

pleomorphic o., o. pleomórfico. SIN anaplastic o.

ol·i·go·dip·sia (ol′i‑gō‑dip′sē‑ă). Oligodipsia; ausência anormal de sede. VER TAMBÉM hypodipsia. [oligo- + G. *dipsa*, sede]

ol·i·go·don·tia (ol′i‑gō‑don′shē‑ă). Oligodontia. SIN hypodontia. [oligo- + G. *odous*, dente]

ol·i·go·dy·nam·ic (ol′i‑gō‑dī‑nam′ik). Oligodinâmico; ativo em quantidade muito pequena; p.ex., o efeito germicida de uma solução excessivamente diluída (como 1 para 100 milhões) de cobre em água destilada. [oligo- + G. *dynamis*, potência]

ol·i·go·ga·lac·tia (ol′i‑gō‑gă‑lak′tē‑ă, ‑shē‑ă). Oligogalactia; secreção escassa ou discreta de leite. [oligo- + G. *gala*, leite]

ol·i·go·glu·can-branch·ing gly·co·syl·trans·fer·ase (ol′i‑gō‑gloo′kan). Oligoglicanorramificante glicosiltransferase. SIN 1,4-α-D-glucan 6-α-D-glucosyltransferase.

ol·i·go-α-1,6-glu·co·si·dase. Oligo-α-1,6-glicosidase; uma glicano-hidrolase que cliva as ligações α-1,6 na isomaltose e dextrinas produzidas a partir do amido e glicogênio por uma α-amilase; secretada no duodeno; a deficiência dessa enzima leva a defeitos na digestão intestinal de dextrinas terminais. VER TAMBÉM sucrose α-D-glucohydrolase. SIN isomaltase, limit dextrinase (2).

ol·i·go·hy·dram·ni·os (ol′i‑gō‑hī‑dram′nē‑os). Oligoidrâmnio; volume insuficiente de líquido amniótico (menos de 300 ml no termo). SIN hypamnion, hypamnios, oligamnios, oligoamnios. [oligo- + G. *hydor*, água, + amnion]

ol·i·go·hy·dru·ria (ol′i‑gō‑hī‑droo′rē‑ă). Oligoidrúria; termo obsoleto para a excreção de pequenos volumes de urina, como ocorre na desidratação. [oligo- + G. *hydor*, água, + *ouron*, urina]

ol·i·go·lec·i·thal (ol′i‑gō‑les′i‑thal). Oligolécito; que possui pouca gema; indica um ovo em que existe apenas um pequeno deutoplasma disperso. [oligo- + G. *lekithos*, gema]

ol·i·go·men·or·rhea (ol′i‑gō‑men‑ō‑rē′ă). Oligomenorréia; menstruação escassa. [oligo- + menorrhea]

ol·i·go·mer (ol′i‑gō‑mer). Oligômero; um polímero que contém apenas algumas unidades repetidas, sendo esse "algumas" geralmente considerado como menos de 20.

ol·i·go·mor·phic (ol′‑i‑gō‑mōr′fik). Oligomórfico; que apresenta poucas alterações da forma; não-polimórfico. [oligo- + G. *morphe*, forma]

ol·i·go·neph·ron·ic (ol′i‑gō‑nef‑ron′ik). Oligonefrônico; caracterizado por um número reduzido de néfrons.

ol·i·go·nu·cle·o·tide (ol′i-gō-noo′klē-ō-tīd). Oligonucleotídeo; um composto constituído da condensação de um número pequeno (tipicamente menos de 20) de nucleotídeos. Cf. polynucleotide.

ol·i·go·pep·sia (ol′i-gō-pep′sē-ā). Oligopepsia. SIN hypopepsia.

ol·i·go·pep·tide (ol′igō-pep-tīd). Um peptídeo cuja molécula contém até cerca de 20 resíduos aminoácidos.

ol·i·go·phre·nia (ol′i-go-frē′nē-ā). Oligofrenia. SIN mental retardation. **phenylpyruvate oligophrenia,** oligofrenia fenilpirúvica. SIN phenylketonuria.

ol·i·go·plas·tic (ol′i-gō-plas′tik). Oligoplásico; deficiente em termos de força de reparação. [oligo- + G. plasso, formar]

ol·i·gop·nea (ol′i-gop-nēā, -gop′nē-ā). Oligopnéia. SIN hypopnea. [oligo- + G. pnoē, respiração]

ol·i·go·pty·a·lism (ol′i-gō-tī′a-lizm, ol′i-gop-tī′). Oligoptialismo; secreção escassa de saliva. SIN oligosialia. [oligo- + G. ptyalon, saliva]

ol·i·gor·ia (ol-i-gōr′ē-ā). Oligoria; um termo raramente utilizado para indiferença anormal ou aversão a pessoas ou coisas. [G. oligōria, negligência, estima discreta, de oligos, pouco, + ōra, cuidados, consideração]

ol·i·go·sac·cha·ride (ol′i-gō-sak′ā-rīd). Oligossacarídeo; um composto constituído da condensação de um pequeno número de unidades monossacarídicas. Cf. polysaccharide.

ol·i·go·si·a·lia (ol′i-gō-sī-ā′lē-ā). Oligossialia. SIN oligoptyalism. [oligo- + G. sialon, saliva]

ol·i·go·sper·mia, ol·i·go·sper·ma·tism (ol-i-gō-sper′mē-ā, -mā-tizm). Oligospermia, oligozoospermia. SIN oligozoospermia. [oligo- + G. sperma, semente]

ol·i·go·symp·to·mat·ic (ol′i-gō-simp-tō-mat′ik). Oligossintomático; que possui poucos sintomas ou sintomas menores.

ol·i·go·sy·nap·tic (ol′i-gō-si-nap′tik). Oligossináptico; refere-se às vias de condução neural que são interrompidas apenas por algumas junções sinápticas, ou seja, constituída por uma seqüência de apenas algumas células nervosas, em contraste com as vias polissinápticas. SIN paucisynaptic.

ol·i·go·thy·mia (ol′i-gō-thī′mē-ā). Oligotimia; termo raramente utilizado para privação ou falta de afeto. [oligo- + -thymia]

ol·i·go·trich·ia (ol′i-gō-trik′ē-ā). Oligotriquia. SIN hypotrichosis.

ol·i·go·tri·cho·sis (ol′i-gō-tri-kō′sis). Oligotricose. SIN hypotrichosis.

ol·i·go·tro·phia, ol·i·got·ro·phy (ol′i-gō-trō′fē-ā, -got′rō-fē). Oligotrofia; nutrição deficiente. [oligo- + G. trophē, nutrição]

ol·i·go·zo·o·sper·ma·tism (ol′i-gō-zō′ō-sper′mā-tizm). Oligozoospermia. SIN oligozoospermia. [oligo- + G. zōon, animal, + sperma, semente]

ol·i·go·zo·o·sper·mia (ol′i-gō-zō′ō-sperm′ē-ā). Oligozoospermia; concentração subnormal de espermatozóides no sêmen ejaculado. SIN oligospermia, oligospermatism, oligozoospermatism. [oligo- + G. zōos, viver, + sperma, semente, sêmen, + -ia]

ol·i·gu·ria (ol-i-goo′rē-ā). Oligúria; produção diminuída de urina. [oligo- + G. ouron, urina]

oli·va, pl. **oli·′vae** (ō-lī′vā) [TA]. Oliva; uma proeminência oval e lisa da superfície ventrolateral do bulbo, lateral ao trato piramidal, correspondendo ao complexo olivar inferior. SIN corpus olivare, inferior olive, olivary body, olivary eminence, olive (1). [L.]
  o. infe′rior, o. inferior; a oliva.
  o. supe′rior, núcleo olivar superior. SIN dorsal nucleus of trapezoid body.

ol·i·vary (ol′i-vār-ē). Olivar. 1. Relativo à oliva. 2. Relativo a ou em formato de uma oliva.

ol·ive (ol′iv). 1. Oliva, núcleo olivar inferior. SIN oliva. 2. Oliva, azeitona; nome comum para uma árvore do gênero Olea (família Oleaceae) ou seu fruto. [L. oliva]
  inferior o. núcleo olivar inferior. SIN oliva.
  superior o., núcleo olivar superior. SIN dorsal nucleus of trapezoid body.

ol·ive oil. Azeite de oliva. Ver em oil.

ol·i·vif·u·gal (ol′i-vif′u-găl). Olivífugo; em sentido contrário ao da oliva. [oliva + L. fugio, fugir]

ol·i·vip·e·tal (ol′i-vip′ē-tăl). Olivípeto; em direção à da oliva. [oliva + L. peto, procurar]

ol·i·vo·co·chle·ar (ol′i-vō-kok′lē-ăr). Olivococlear. VER olivocochlear tract.

ol·i·vo·pon·to·cer·e·bel·lar (ol′i-vo-pon′tō-sār-ĕ-bel′ar). Olivopontocerebelar; relativo ao núcleo olivar, base da ponte e cerebelo.

Ollendorf, Helene, dermatologista alemã, fl. 1928. VER Buschke-O. syndrome.

Ollier, Louis X.E.L., cirurgião francês, 1830–1900. VER O. graft, disease, theory; O.-Thiersch graft.

Olmsted, H. C., pediatra norte-americano do século XX. VER O. syndrome.

△ **-ology.** VER -logia.

olo·liu·qui (ō-lō-lū′kē). Ololiúqui; alucinógeno usado em cerimônias pelos índios astecas no México; contém alcalóides do esporão de centeio e derivados do ácido lisérgico. VER TAMBÉM Rivea corymbosa, Ipomoea rubrocoerulea var. praecox.

olo·pho·nia (ol′ō-fō′nē-ā). Olofonia; fala comprometida causada por um defeito anatômico nos órgãos vocais. [G. oloos, destruído, perdido, + phōnē, voz]

Olszewski, Jerzy, neuropatologista polonês, naturalizado canadense, 1913–1964. VER Steele-Richardson-O. disease, syndrome.

△ **-oma.** Sufixo que indica um tumor ou neoplasia. [G. -ōma, sufixo que forma substantivos a partir de alguns troncos verbais]

△ **-omata.** Plural de -oma.

Ombrédanne, Louis, cirurgião francês, 1871–1956. VER O. operation.

om·bro·pho·bia (om-brō-fō′bē-ā). Ombrofobia; medo mórbido de chuva. [G. ombros, tempestade, + phobos, medo]

Omenn, Gilbert S., clínico norte-americano, *1941. VER O. syndrome.

omen·tal (ō-men′tăl). Omental; relativo ao omento. SIN epiploic.

omen·tec·to·my (ō-men-tek′tō-mē). Omentectomia; ressecção ou excisão do omento. SIN omentumectomy. [omentum + G. ektomē, excisão]

omen·ti·tis (ō-men-tī′tis). Omentite; peritonite envolvendo o omento. [L. omentum + G. -itis, inflamação]

△ **omento-, oment-.** Formas combinantes relativas ao omento. VER TAMBÉM epiplo-. [L. omentum]

omen·to·fix·a·tion (ō-men′tō-fik-sā′shŭn). Omentofixação, omentopexia. SIN omentopexy.

omen·to·pexy (ō-men′tō-pek-sē). Omentopexia. 1. Sutura do omento maior na parede abdominal para induzir a circulação porta colateral. 2. Sutura do omento a outro órgão para aumentar a circulação arterial. VER TAMBÉM omentoplasty. SIN omentofixation. [omento- + G. pēxis, fixação]

omen·to·plas·ty (ō-men′tō-plas-tē). Omentoplastia; uso do omento maior para cobrir ou preencher um defeito, aumentar a circulação arterial ou venosa porta, absorver derrames ou aumentar a drenagem linfática. VER TAMBÉM omentopexy. [omento- + G. plastos, formado]

omen·tor·rha·phy (ō-men-tōr′ă-fē). Omentorrafia; sutura de uma abertura no omento. [omento- + G. rhaphē, sutura]

omen·to·vol·vu·lus (ō-men-tō-vol′vū-lŭs). Omentovólvulo; torção do omento em torno de um pedículo.

omen·tu·lum (ō-men′tū-lŭm). Omento menor. SIN lesser omentum. [L. mod. dim. de omentum]

omen·tum, pl. **omen·ta** (ō-men′tŭm, -tăl) [TA]. Omento; uma dobra do peritônio que vai do estômago até outro órgão abdominal. [L. a membrana que reveste o intestino]
  gastrocolic o., o. maior. SIN greater o.
  gastrohepatic o., o. menor. SIN lesser o.
  gastrosplenic o., ligamento gastroesplênico. SIN gastrosplenic ligament.
  greater o. [TA], o. maior; uma dobra peritoneal areolar, com quatro camadas, formada pelo mesentério dorsal do estômago de dupla camada (mesogástrio dorsal) que desce desde a curvatura maior do estômago para dobrar sob si mesma e ascender até o colo transverso; as porções ascendente e descendente fundem-se, obliterando o recesso inferior da bolsa omental, resultando na estrutura de quatro camadas que, em geral, pende sobre a face anterior dos intestinos, como uma avental; os componentes incluem os seguintes ligamentos peritoneais: gastrofrênico, gastroesplênico, esplenorrenal e gastrocólico. SIN o. majus [TA], caul (2), cowl, epiploon, gastrocolic o., pileus, velum (3).
  lesser o. [TA], o. menor; uma dobra peritoneal fina de dupla camada formada pelo mesentério ventral do estômago (mesogástrio ventral) que vai da curvatura menor do estômago e da borda superior até a porção proximal do duodeno (2 cm distal ao piloro) e até o fígado (margens da porta do fígado e profundamente na fissura do canal venoso); os principais componentes incluem o ligamento hepatogástrico (porção principal semelhante a uma lâmina) e o ligamento hepatoduodenal (borda direita livre espessada, que engloba a artéria hepática, a veia porta e o ducto colédoco). SIN o. minus [TA], gastrohepatic o., omentulum.
  o. ma′jus [TA], o. maior. SIN greater o.
  o. mi′nus [TA], o. menor. SIN lesser o.

omen·tum·ec·to·my (ō-men-tū-mek′tō-mē). Omentectomia. SIN omentectomy.

ome·pra·zole (ō-me′pră-zol). Omeprazol; um medicamento que bloqueia o transporte de íons hidrogênio no estômago e é usado como antiulcerativo e no tratamento da síndrome de Zollinger-Ellison.

Ommaya, Ayub K., neurocirurgião norte-americano, *1930. VER O. reservoir.

omn. hor. Abreviatura para L. omni hora, a cada hora.

om·nip·o·tence of thought (om-nip′ō-tens). Onipotência do pensamento; um processo mental infantil ou mágico por meio do qual se acredita que a gratificação instantânea das fantasias e desejos seja iminente.

om·niv·o·rous (om-niv′ō-rŭs). Onívoro; viver de todos os tipos de alimento, animais e vegetais. [L. omnis, todo, + voro, comer]

△ **omo-.** Forma combinante que indica a relação com o ombro (por vezes incluindo o braço). [G. ōmos, ombro]

omo·cla·vic·u·lar (ō′mō-kla-vik′ū-lăr). Omoclavicular; relativo ao ombro e à clavícula; indica um músculo anômalo inserido no processo coracóide da escápula ou borda superior da escápula e na clavícula.

omo·hy·oid (ō-mō-hi′oyd). Omo-hióideo. SIN omohyoid (muscle).

omo·pha·gia (ō-mō-fa′jē-ā). Omofagia; que come alimentos crus, especialmente carne crua. [G. ōmos, cru, + phago, comer]

omo·thy·roid (ō-mō-thī′royd). Omotireóideo; indica uma faixa de fibras

omothyroid musculares que passa entre o corno superior da cartilagem tireóide e o músculo omo-hióideo.

OMP Abreviatura de oligo-*N*-methylmorpholinium propylene oxide (óxido de oligo-*N*-metilmorfolínio propileno); orotidylic acid (ácido orotidílico); orotidylate (orotidilato); *orotidine* 5′-monophosphate (5′-monofosfato de orotidina).

OMPA Abreviatura de octamethyl pyrophosphoramide (octametil pirofosforamida).

OMP de·car·box·yl·ase. OMP-descarboxilase. SIN orotidylic acid decarboxylase.

♻ **omphal-, omphalo-.** Formas combinantes que indicam o umbigo. [G. *omphalos*, umbigo]

om·pha·lec·to·my (om-fă-lek′tō-mē). Onfalectomia; excisão do umbigo ou de uma neoplasia ligada a ele. [omphal- + G. *ektomē*, excisão]

om·phal·el·co·sis (om′fal-el-kō′sis). Onfalelcose; ulceração no umbigo. [omphal- + G. *helkōsis*, ulceração]

om·phal·ic (om-fal′ik). Onfálico; que diz respeito ao umbigo. SIN umbilical. [G. *omphalos*, umbigo]

om·pha·li·tis (om-fă-lī′tis). Onfalite; inflamação do umbigo e partes circunvizinhas.

♻ **omphalo-.** VER omphal-.

om·pha·lo·an·gi·op·a·gus (om′fă-lō-an-jē-op′ă-gŭs). Onfaloangiópago; gêmeos conjuntos desiguais em que o parasita deriva seu aporte sanguíneo da placenta do autósito. VER conjoined *twins*, em *twin*. SIN allantoidoangiopagus. [omphalo- + G. *angeion*, vaso, + *pagos*, algo fixo]

om·phal·o·cele (om′fal-ō-sēl, om′fă-lō-). Onfalocele; herniação congênita das vísceras para dentro da base do cordão umbilical, com um saco membranoso de revestimento de peritônio–âmnio. O cordão umbilical está inserido no saco nesse caso, ao contrário de sua inserção na gastrosquise. VER TAMBÉM umbilical *hernia*. SIN amniocele, exomphalos (3), exumbilication (3). [omphalo- + G. *kēlē*, hérnia]

om·pha·lo·en·ter·ic (om′fă-lō-en-tār-ik). Onfaloentérico; relativo ao umbigo e ao intestino.

om·pha·lo·mes·en·ter·ic (om-fă-lō-mez-en-tār′ik). Onfalomesentérico. **1.** Termo que indica a relação do intestino com o saco vitelino. À medida que as pregas craniana e caudal do embrião continuam a se formar, essa relação diminui e é representada por um pedículo vitelino ou ducto vitelino estreito. **2.** Relativo ao ducto vitelino.

om·pha·lop·a·gus (om′fă-lop′ă-gŭs). Onfalópago; gêmeos conjuntos unidos em suas regiões umbilicais. VER conjoined *twins*, em *twin*. SIN monomphalus. [omphalo- + G. *pagos*, algo fixo]

om·pha·lo·phle·bi·tis (om′fă-lō-fle-bī′tis). Onfaloflebite; inflamação das veias umbilicais. [omphalo- + G. *phleps*, veia, + *-itis*, inflamação]

om·pha·lor·rha·gia (om′fă-lō-rā′jē-ă). Onfalorragia; sangramento a partir do umbigo. [omphalo- + G. *rhēgnymi*, eclodir]

om·pha·lor·rhea (om′fă-lō-rē′ă). Onfalorréia; secreção serosa a partir do umbigo. [omphalo- + G. *rhoia*, fluxo]

om·pha·lor·rhex·is (om′fă-lō-rek′sis). Onfalorrexe; ruptura do cordão umbilical durante o parto. [omphalo- + G. *rhēxis*, ruptura]

om·pha·los (om′fă-los). Termo raramente utilizado para umbigo. [G. umbigo]

om·pha·lo·site (om′fă-lō-sīt). Onfalosito; gêmeo subdesenvolvido de gêmeos alantóide-angiópagos; unidos por vasos umbilicais. SIN placental parasitic twin. [omphalo- + G. *sitos*, alimento]

om·pha·lo·spi·nous (om′fă-lō-spī′nŭs). Onfaloespinhoso; indica uma linha que liga o umbigo e a espinha ântero-superior do ílio, sobre a qual se situa o ponto de McBurney.

om·pha·lot·o·my (om-fă-lot′ō-mē). Onfalotomia; corte do cordão umbilical no nascimento. [omphalo- + G. *tomē*, incisão]

om·pha·lo·trip·sy (om′fă-lō-trip′sē). Onfalotripsia; esmagamento, em vez de corte, do cordão umbilical depois do parto. [omphalo- + G. *tripsis*, uma fricção]

om·pha·lo·ves·i·cal (om′fă-lō-ves′i-kăl). Onfalovesical. SIN vesicoumbilical.

om·pha·lus (om′fă-lŭs). Termo raramente utilizado para umbigo. [G. *omphalos*, umbigo]

OMP py·ro·phos·pho·ryl·ase. OMP pirofosforilase. SIN orotate phosphoribosyl-transferase.

♻ **oncho-.** VER onco-.

On·cho·cer·ca (ong-kō-ser′kă). Um gênero de nematódeos filariformes alongados (família Onchocercidae) que habita o tecido conjuntivo de seus hospedeiros, usualmente dentro de nódulos firmes em que esses parasitas estão espiralados e entrelaçados. SIN *Oncocerca*. [G. *onkos*, gancho, + *kerkos*, cauda] ***O. vol′vulus***, espécie que causa a oncocercíase.

on·cho·cer·ci·a·sis (ong′kō-ser-kī′ă-sis). Oncocercíase; infecção por *Onchocerca* (especialmente *O. volvulus*, um nematódeo filarial transmitido de uma pessoa para outra por moscas do gênero *Simulium*), caracterizada por tumorações nodulares que formam um cisto fibroso, envolvendo este os parasitas espiralados (oncocercoma); as microfilárias movimentam-se livremente para fora do nódulo e escapam para a linfa intercelular na derme. Com freqüência, desenvolvem-se alterações dermatológicas, em especial na África, resultando em prurido intenso, pele liquenóide ou descamativa, despigmentação e destruição das fibras elásticas. Mais importantes são as complicações oculares, que podem desenvolver-se após um curso longo e crônico, com a cegueira freqüentemente ocorrendo em casos avançados, provocada por microfilárias vivas ou mortas observadas por biomicroscopia com lâmpada de fenda. SIN blinding disease, onchocercosis, volvulosis.

ocular o., o. ocular; as complicações oculares, como ceratite, iridociclite ou neurite retrobulbar, causadas por microfilárias da *Onchocerca volvulus*. SIN river blindness.

on·cho·cer·cid (ong-kō-ser′kid). Oncocercídeo; nome comum para os membros da família Onchocercidae.

On·cho·cer·ci·dae (ong-kō-ser′ki-dē). Uma família de parasitas nematódeos (superfamília Filaroidea) caracterizada por produção de microfilárias; inclui os gêneros *Onchocerca*, *Wuchereria*, *Brugia*, *Loa* e *Mansonella*.

onchocercoma (on′kō-ser-kō′ma). Oncocercoma; nódulo contendo vermes adultos do *Onchocera volvulus*. [*Onchocerca*, termo taxonômico, + -oma]

on·cho·cer·co·sis (ong′kō-ser-kō′sis). Oncocercose. SIN onchocerciasis.

♻ **onco-, oncho-.** Formas combinantes relativas a um tumor. [G. *onkos*, volume, massa]

On·co·cer·ca (ong-kō-ser′kă). SIN *Onchocerca*.

on·co·cyte (ong′kō-sīt). Oncócito; uma célula tumoral grande, granular, acidófila, que contém numerosas mitocôndrias; uma célula oxifílica neoplásica. [onco- + G. *kytos*, célula]

on·co·cy·to·ma (ong′kō-sī-tō′mă). Oncocitoma; um tumor glandular composto de grandes células com citoplasma granular e eosinofílico devido à presença de mitocôndrias abundantes; ocorre raramente no rim, nas glândulas salivares e nas glândulas endócrinas. SIN oxyphil adenoma. [onco- + G. *kytos*, célula, + *-oma*, tumor]

on·co·fe·tal (ong-kō-fē′tăl). Oncofetal; relativo às substâncias associadas ao tumor presentes no tecido fetal, como os antígenos oncofetais.

🅘 **on·co·gene** (ong′kō-jēn). Oncogene. **1.** Qualquer um de uma família de genes que, normalmente, codificam as proteínas envolvidas na regulação ou crescimento da célula (p.ex., proteinoquinases, GTPases, proteínas nucleares, fatores de crescimento), mas que podem fomentar os processos malignos, quando mudados ou ativados pelo contato com retrovírus. Os oncogenes identificados incluem *ras*, originalmente percebido nos tumores de bexiga, e p53, uma versão que sofreu mutação de um gene no cromossomo 17 que já se constatou estar envolvido em mais da metade de todos os cânceres humanos. Os oncogenes podem trabalhar em conjunto para produzir o câncer, e sua ação pode ser exacerbada por retrovírus, genes saltadores ou mutações genéticas herdadas. VER TAMBÉM tumor suppressor *gene*. **2.** Um gene encontrado em determinados DNA vírus tumorais. É necessário para a replicação viral. SIN transforming gene. [onco- + gene]

> Os genes cujas mutações podem permitir ou induzir a proliferação celular descontrolada e a alteração maligna são de 2 tipos: proto-oncogenes e genes supressores tumorais (antioncogenes). Os proto-oncogenes codificam proteínas que estimulam a síntese de DNA e a divisão celular, incluindo os fatores de crescimento de peptídeos e seus receptores de membrana celular; proteínas da cascata de segundos mensageiros, que transmitem informações da membrana celular para o núcleo; e fatores de transcrição nuclear, que controlam a expressão do gene por meio de ligação ao DNA. A conversão de um proto-oncogene em um oncogene por amplificação, translocação ou mutação pontual pode levar à proliferação celular irrestrita e alteração maligna. Apenas 1 cópia (alelo) de um proto-oncogene precisa sofrer mutação para induzir a formação tumoral. Os proto-oncogenes não estão envolvidos nas síndromes de câncer hereditárias, com a exceção do proto-oncogene RET na neoplasia endócrina múltipla (NEM). Os genes supressores tumorais (antioncogenes), que codificam proteínas que normalmente refreiam a proliferação celular, podem ser inativados por mutação pontual, deleção ou perda de expressão. Uma mutação herdada em 1 cópia de um gene supressor tumoral é a base da maioria das predisposições familiais ao câncer. A proliferação celular maligna não ocorre até que a cópia funcional remanescente do gene seja inativada por mutação ou por deleção de parte do seu cromossoma ou de todo ele. Em uma pessoa nascida com 2 cópias normais de um gene supressor tumoral, ambas têm de ser inativadas por mutação antes que ocorra a formação do tumor. BRCA1 e BRCA2, que estão associados ao câncer de mama familial de início precoce e câncer de ovário, são genes supressores tumorais.

ras o., o. ras; mutações pontuais descritas pela primeira vez em células de sarcoma de rato que, comprovadamente, têm atividade transformadora em cultu-

oncogenes celulares representativos

classe geral	nome do oncogene	origem		produto proteico	
		retrovírus protótipo	espécie do hospedeiro[1]	propriedade	localização subcelular
não tem receptores tirosinoquinases	src	vírus do sarcoma Rous	galinha	tem receptores tirosinoquinases	membrana plasmática
	abl	vírus da leucemia murina Abelson	camundongo		membrana plasmática, citoplasma
	fes	vírus do sarcoma felino ST	gato		membrana plasmática, citoplasma
proteína receptora de tirosinoquinase	fms	vírus do sarcoma felino McDonough	gato	relacionado com o receptor do fator estimulador de colônia	membrana plasmática, retículo endoplasmático
	erb-B	vírus da eritroblastose das aves	galinha	receptor do fator de crescimento epidérmico (truncado)	membrana plasmática
	neu	nenhum	rato (neuroglioblastomas)	relacionado com o receptor do fator de crescimento epidérmico	membrana plasmática, retículo endoplasmático
serina/treonina proteinoquinase	mos	vírus do sarcoma murino Moloney	camundongo		citoplasma
fatores de crescimento	sis	vírus do sarcoma de símios	macacos	semelhante ao fator de crescimento derivado de plaquetas	citoplasma, secretado
	int-2	nenhum	camundongo	relacionado ao fator de crescimento de fibroblastos	
proteínas G associadas à membrana	Ha-ras	vírus do sarcoma murino Harvey	rato	ligação guanosina difosfato/trifosfato; guanosina trifosfatase	membrana plasmática
	Ki-ras	vírus do sarcoma murino Kirsten			
	N-ras	nenhum	seres humanos (neuroblastomas)		
fatores de transcrição nuclear	myb	vírus da mieloblastose das aves	galinha	ligação ao DNA	núcleo
	myc	vírus da mielocitomatose MC29			
	fos	vírus do osteossarcoma FBJ	camundongo	parte do fator de transição Ap-1	
	jun	vírus-17 do sarcoma de aves	galinha	ligação ao DNA; parte do fator de transcrição AP-1	
	erb-A	vírus da eritroblastose de aves	galinha	receptor do hormônio tireóideo mutante	citoplasma, núcleo

[1] As seqüências de proto-oncogenes são conservadas entre muitas espécies; a coluna indica o isolamento inicial do oncogene

ra, bem como em modelos de tumorigênese em camundongos; a família do gene ras é composta por três genes intimamente correlatos em três cromossomas diferentes; já foram identificadas anormalidades em vários tumores humanos.
on·co·gen·e·sis (ong-kō-jen′ē-sis). Oncogênese; origem e crescimento de uma neoplasia. [onco- + G. *genesis*, produção]

on·co·gen·ic (ong-kō-jen′ik). Oncogênico. SIN oncogenous.
on·cog·en·ous (ong-koj′ĕ-nŭs). Oncogênico; que causa, induz ou é adequado para a formação e o desenvolvimento de uma neoplasia. SIN oncogenic.
on·co·graph (ong′kō-graf). Oncógrafo; um oncômetro registrador, ou parte de registro de um oncômetro. [onco- + G. *graphē*, um registro]

on·cog·ra·phy (ong'kog'rǎ - fē). Oncografia; representação gráfica, por meio de um aparelho especial, do tamanho e configuração de um órgão.

on·coi·des (ong - koy'dēz). Intumescência ou turgescência. [onco- + G. *eidos*, semelhança]

on·col·o·gist (ong - kol'ō - jist). Oncologista; um especialista em oncologia.
radiation o., radioncologista. SIN radiotherapist.

on·col·o·gy (ong - kol'ō - jē). Oncologia; o estudo ou a ciência que lida com as propriedades físicas, químicas e biológicas e os aspectos de neoplasias, incluindo a causa, a patogenia e o tratamento. [onco- + G. *logos*, estudo]
radiation o., radioncologia; (1) a especialidade médica relacionada com o uso de radiação ionizante no tratamento da doença; (2) a especialidade médica da radioterapia (radiation *therapy*); (3) o uso da radiação no tratamento de neoplasias. SIN radiotherapy, therapeutic radiology.

on·col·y·sis (ong - kol'i - sis). Oncólise; destruição de uma neoplasia; por vezes utilizado com referência à redução de qualquer tumefação ou massa. [onco- + G. *lysis*, dissolução]

on·co·lyt·ic (ong - kō - lit'ik). Oncolítico; pertinente a, caracterizado por ou que causa oncólise.

On·co·me·la·nia (ong'kō - mē - lā'ni - ǎ). Um gênero de caramujos operculados anfíbios, de água-doce, com importância médica, da família Hydrobiidae (subfamília Hydrobiinae; subclasse Prosobranchiata). Na Ásia, várias subespécies de *O. hupensis* servem como hospedeiros intermediários do trematódeo sanguíneo oriental, *Schistosoma japonicum*. [onco- + G. *melas (melan-)*, negro]

on·com·e·ter (ong - kom'ě - ter). Oncômetro. 1. Um instrumento para medir o tamanho e a configuração dos rins e de outros órgãos. 2. O medidor, em contraste com a parte de registro do oncógrafo. [onco- + G. *metron*, medida]

on·com·et·ric (ong - kō - met'rik). Oncométrico; relativo à oncometria.

on·com·e·try (ong - kom'ě - trē). Oncometria; a medida do tamanho de um órgão.

on·co·sis (ong - kō'sis). Oncose; uma condição caracterizada pela formação de uma ou mais neoplasias ou tumores. [G. *onkōsis*, inchação, de *onkos*, massa, volume]

on·co·sphere (ong' - kō - sfēr). Oncosfera. SIN hexacanth. [onco- + G. *sphaira*, esfera]

oncostatin M (onk'ō - stat'in em). Oncostatina M; uma interleucina-6. [onco- + -stat + -in]

on·co·ther·a·py (ong - kō - thǎr'ǎ - pē). Oncoterapia; tratamento de tumores.

on·cot·ic (ong - kot'ik). Oncótico; relativo a, ou causado por, edema ou qualquer tumefação (oncose).

on·cot·o·my (ong - kot'ō - mē). Oncotomia; termo raramente utilizado para a incisão de um abscesso, cisto ou outro tumor. [onco- + G. *tomē*, incisão]

on·co·trop·ic (ong'kō - trop'ik). Oncotrópico; que manifesta uma afinidade especial por neoplasias ou células neoplásicas. [onco- + G. *tropē*, uma volta]

On·co·vir·i·nae (ong - kō - vir'i - nē). Termo originalmente utilizado para designar uma subfamília atualmente obsoleta de vírus (família Retroviridae), composta de RNA vírus tumorais que contêm duas moléculas de RNA idênticas com filamentos positivos. Os subgrupos baseiam-se em antigenicidade, gama de hospedeiros e tipo de malignidade induzida (complexo leucemia–sarcoma aviário, felino, de *hamsters* ou murino; vírus do tumor mamário murino; oncovírus de primatas). Semelhante a outros retrovírus, eles contêm DNA polimerases RNA-dependentes (transcriptases reversas). Um aspecto importante desses vírus parece ser o uso da transcriptase reversa viral para produzir DNA que pode ser integrado ao DNA da célula do hospedeiro e irá replicar-se junto com o DNA celular. VER TAMBÉM retrovírus.

on·co·vi·rus (ong'kō - vī'rǔs). Oncovírus; termo originalmente empregado para descrever qualquer vírus da subfamília Oncovirinae. VER TAMBÉM oncogenic *virus*.

on·dan·se·tron (on - dan'sě - tron). Ondansetron; antagonista do receptor 5-HT$_3$ de serotonina usado como antiemético, principalmente em pacientes submetidos a quimioterapia ou radioterapia para câncer.

Ondine, Ondina, personagem mitológico alemão. VER Ondine *curse*.

△ **-one**. -Ona; sufixo que indica um grupamento cetona (–CO–).

onei·ric (ō - nī'rik). Onírico. 1. Pertinente aos sonhos. 2. Pertinente ao estado clínico da onirofrenia. SIN oniric. [G. *oneiros*, sonho]

onei·rism (ō - nī'rizm). Onirismo; sensação de irrealidade, como em um sonho. [G. *oneiros*, sonho]

onei·ro·crit·i·cal (ō - nī - rō - krit'i - kǎl). Onirocrítico; termo raramente utilizado relativo à lógica dos sonhos. [G. *oneiros*, sonho, + *kritikos*, habilitado no julgamento]

onei·ro·dyn·ia (ō - nī - rō - din'ē - ǎ). Onirodinia; termo raramente utilizado para um sonho desagradável ou doloroso. [G. *oneiros*, sonho, + *odynē*, dor]
o. acti'va, o. ativa. SIN somnambulism (1).

onei·rol·o·gy (ō - nī - rol'ō - jē). Onirologia; o estudo de sonhos e seu conteúdo. [G. *oneiros*, sonho, + *logos*, estudo]

onei·ro·phre·nia (ō - nī - rō - frē'nē - ǎ). Onirofrenia; um termo raramente empregado para um estado em que ocorrem alucinações, causadas por certas condições como a privação prolongada do sono, isolamento sensorial e vários medicamentos. [G. *oneiros*, sonho, + *phrēn*, mente]

oni·o·ma·nia (ō'nē - ō - mā'nē - ǎ). Oniomania, oneomania; termo raramente utilizado para a urgência ou necessidade morbidamente exagerada de comprar além das necessidades realistas do indivíduo. [G. *ōnios*, para vender, + *mania*, insanidade]

oni·ric (ō - nī'rik). Onírico. SIN oneiric.

△ **-onium**. -ônio; sufixo que indica um radical positivamente carregado; p.ex., amônio, NH_4^+.

△ **onko-**. VER onco-.

on·lay (on'lā). 1. Uma restauração metálica (usualmente de ouro) da superfície oclusal de um dente posterior ou da superfície lingual de um dente anterior, cuja superfície inteira está na dentina, sem paredes laterais; a retenção no dente anterior se faz por pinos e, no posterior, por pinos e/ou compartimentos nos sulcos de retenção nas paredes bucal e lingual. 2. Um enxerto aplicado ao exterior de um osso. 3. Um enxerto aplicado na pele na uretra original na reparação de hipospadia ou de estenose.

Onodi, Adolf, laringologista húngaro, 1857–1920. VER Onodi *cell*.

on·o·mat·o·ma·nia (on'ō - mat - ō - mā'nē - ǎ). Onomatomania; obsessão caracterizada pela busca angustiante de uma palavra e seu suposto significado, ou por tentar freneticamente lembrar uma determinada palavra. [G. *onoma*, nome, + *mania*, frenesi]

on·o·mat·o·pho·bia (on'ō - mat - ō - fō'bē - ǎ). Onomatofobia; temor anormal de determinadas palavras ou nomes por causa de seu suposto significado. [G. *onoma*, nome, + *phobos*, medo]

on·o·mat·o·poi·e·sis (on'ō - mat'ō - poy - ē'sis). Onomatopoese; a criação de um nome ou palavra, especialmente para expressar ou imitar um som natural (p.ex., "siii", "crash", "bum"); em psiquiatria, diz-se que a tendência para criar novas palavras desse tipo caracteriza algumas pessoas com esquizofrenia. VER TAMBÉM neologism. [G. *onoma*, nome, + *poiēsis*, criação]

on·to·gen·e·sis (on - tō - jen'ě - sis). Ontogênese. SIN ontogeny.

on·to·ge·net·ic, on·to·gen·ic (on'tō - jě - net'ik, - jen'ik). Ontogenético, ontogênico; relativo à ontogenia.

on·tog·e·ny (on - toj'ě - nē). Ontogenia; o desenvolvimento do indivíduo, conforme diferenciado da filogenia, que é o desenvolvimento evolutivo da espécie. SIN ontogenesis. [G. *on*, ser, + *genesis*, origem]

on·tol·o·gy (on - tol'ō - jē). Ontologia; um ramo tradicional da metafísica que lida com os problemas do ser, da existência, da natureza interna, significado, etc. É fundamental para os problemas que envolvem a normalidade e a doença, individualidade, responsabilidade e a análise de valores. Nos últimos anos, vem assumindo aos poucos um lugar como um ramo da própria medicina.

Onufrowicz, Wladislaus, anatomista suíço, 1836–1900. VER Onuf *nucleus*.

on·y·al·ai (on - i - al'ǎ). Akembe; kafindo; doença aguda que aflige os nativos da África Central, caracterizada por vesículas sanguinolentas na boca e em outras superfícies mucosas, hematúria e melena; a nutrição deficiente pode ser a causa. SIN akembe, kafindo.

△ **onych-**. VER onycho-.

on·y·chal·gia (on - i - kal'jē - ǎ). Onicalgia; dor nas unhas. [onycho- + G. *algos*, dor]

on·y·cha·tro·phia, on·ych·at·ro·phy (on'i - kǎ - trō'fē - ǎ, on - ik - at'rō - fē). Onicatrofia; atrofia das unhas. [onycho- + G. *atrophia*, atrofia]

on·y·chaux·is (on - i - kawk'sis). Onicauxe; crescimento excessivo e acentuado das unhas dos dedos das mãos ou dos artelhos. [onycho- + G. *auxē*, aumento]

on·y·chec·to·my (on - i - kek'tō - mē). Oniquectomia; ablação de uma unha do artelho ou dedo da mão. [onycho- + G. *ektomē*, excisão]

onych·ia (ō - nik'ē - ǎ). Oníquia; inflamação da matriz da unha. [onycho- + G. *-ia*, condição]
o. malig'na, o. maligna; o. aguda que ocorre espontaneamente em pacientes debilitados ou em resposta a trauma leve.
o. sic'ca, o. seca; condição caracterizada por unhas quebradiças.

△ **onycho-, onych-**. Formas combinantes que indicam uma unha do dedo da mão ou artelho. [G. *onyx*, unha]

on·y·choc·la·sis (on - i - kok'lǎ - sis). Onicoclase; quebra das unhas. [onycho- + G. *klasis*, quebra]

on·y·cho·cryp·to·sis (on'i - kō - krip - tō'sis). Onicocriptose. SIN ingrown *nail*.

on·y·cho·dys·tro·phy (on'i - kō - dis'trō - fē). Onicodistrofia; alterações distróficas nas unhas que acontecem como um defeito congênito ou em decorrência de qualquer doença ou lesão que possa gerar uma unha malformada. [onycho- + G. *dys-*, ruim, + *trophē*, nutrição]

on·y·cho·graph (on'i - kō - graf). Onicógrafo; um instrumento para o registro da pressão arterial capilar, conforme demonstrado pela circulação sob a unha. [onycho- + G. *graphō*, escrever]

on·y·cho·gry·po·sis (on'i - kō - gri - pō'sis). Onicogripose; aumento das unhas dos dedos das mãos ou artelhos com espessamento e curvatura aumentados. [onycho- + G. *grypōsis*, uma curvatura]

on·y·cho·het·er·o·to·pia (on'i - kō - het - er - ō - tō'pē - ǎ). Onicoeteropia; posicionamento anormal das unhas.

on·y·choid (on'i - koyd). Onicóide; que se assemelha a uma unha do dedo da mão em estrutura ou forma. [onycho- + G. *eidos*, semelhança]

on·y·chol·o·gy (on-i-kol'ō-jē). Onicologia; estudo das unhas. [onycho- + G. *logos*, tratado]

on·y·chol·y·sis (on-i-kol'i-sis). Onicólise; afrouxamento das unhas, começando na borda livre e, em geral, incompleto. [onycho- + G. *lysis*, afrouxamento]

on·y·cho·ma·de·sis (on'i-kō-mă-dē'sis). Onicomadese; perda completa das unhas, usualmente associada a doença sistêmica. [onycho- + G. *madēsis*, calvície progressiva, de *madaō*, estar molhado, (do cabelo) queda]

on·y·cho·ma·la·cia (on'i-kō-mă-lā'shē-ă). Onicomalacia; amolecimento anormal das unhas. [onycho- + G. *malakia*, amolecimento]

on·y·cho·my·co·sis (on'i-kō-mī-kō'sis). Onicomicose; infecções fúngicas muito comuns das unhas, provocando espessamento, aspereza e rachaduras, freqüentemente causadas por *Trichophyton rubrum* ou *T. mentagrophytes*, *Candida* e, às vezes, mofos. SIN ringworm of nails. [onycho- + G. *mykēs*, fungo, + *-osis*, condição]

on·y·cho·pa·thol·o·gy (on'i-kō-pă-thol'ō-jē). Onicopatologia; estudo das doenças das unhas.

on·y·chop·a·thy (on-i-kop'ă-thē). Onicopatia; qualquer doença das unhas. SIN onychosis. [onycho- + G. *pathos*, sofrimento]

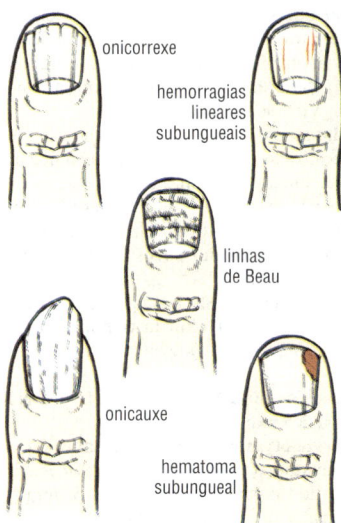

anormalidades nas unhas

on·y·choph·a·gy, on·y·cho·pha·gia (on-i-kof'ă-jē, on'i-kō-fā'jē-ă). Onicofagia; hábito de roer unhas. [onycho- + G. *phagō*, comer]

on·y·cho·pho·sis (on'i-kō-fō'sis). Onicofose; crescimento de epitélio córneo no leito ungueal. [onycho- + G. *phōs*, luz, + *-osis*, condição]

on·y·chop·to·sis (on'i-kop-tō'sis). Onicoptose; a queda das unhas. [onycho- + G. *ptōsis*, queda]

on·y·chor·rhex·is (on'i-kō-rek'sis). Onicorrexia; fragilidade anormal das unhas com rachadura da borda livre. [onycho- + G. *rhēxis*, uma quebra]

on·y·cho·schiz·ia (on'i-kō-skiz'ē-ă). Onicosquizia; rachadura das unhas em camadas. [onycho- + G. *schizo*, dividir, + *-ia*, condição]

on·y·cho·sis (on-i-kō'sis). Onicose, onicopatia. SIN onychopathy.

on·y·cho·stro·ma (on'i-kō-strō'mă). Matriz da unha. SIN nail *matrix*. [onycho- + G. *stroma*, fundamento]

on·y·chot·il·lo·ma·nia (on'i-kot'i-lō-mā'nē-ă). Onicotilomania; tendência a roer as unhas. [onycho- + G. *tillō*, arrancar, + *mania*, insanidade]

on·y·chot·o·my (on-i-kot'ō-mē). Onicotomia; incisão na unha do artelho ou dedo da mão. [onycho- + G. *tomē*, corte]

on·y·chot·ro·phy (on-i-kot'rō-fē). Onicotrofia; nutrição das unhas. [onycho- + G. *trophē*, nutrição]

on·yx (on'iks). Unha. SIN nail (1). [G. *unha*]

oo-. Forma combinante que indica ovo, ovário. VER TAMBÉM oophor-, ovario-, ovi-, ovo-. [G. *ōon*, ovo]

oo·cy·e·sis (ō-ō-sī-ē'sis). Gravidez ovariana. SIN ovarian *pregnancy*. [G. *ōon*, ovo, + *kyēsis*, gravidez]

oo·cyst (ō'ō-sist). Oocisto; a forma encistada do macrogameta fertilizado, ou zigoto, nos coccídeos Sporozoea em que ocorre a multiplicação esporogônica; resulta na formação de esporozoítos, os agentes infecciosos para o próximo estágio do ciclo de vida dos esporozoários. [G. *ōon*, ovo, + *kystis*, bexiga]

oo·cyte (ō'ō-sīt). Ovócito, oocito; o óvulo imaturo. SIN ovocyte. [G. *ōon*, ovo, + *kytos*, uma cavidade (célula)]

primary o., o. primário; um o. durante sua fase de crescimento e antes que complete a primeira divisão de maturação.

secondary o., o. secundário; um o. em que a primeira divisão meiótica é completada; a segunda divisão meiótica geralmente pára logo antes do término, a menos que ocorra fertilização.

oo·gen·e·sis (ō-ō-jen'ĕ-sis). Ovogênese; processo de formação e desenvolvimento do ovo. SIN ovigenesis, ovogenesis. [G. *ōon*, ovo, + *genesis*, origem]

oo·ge·net·ic (ō-ō-jĕ-net'ik). Ovogenético; que produz ovos. SIN oogenic, oogenous, ovigenetic, ovigenic, ovigenous.

oo·gen·ic, oog·e·nous (ō-ō-jen'ik, ō-oj'ĕ-nŭs). Ovogênico. SIN oogenetic.

oo·go·ni·um, pl. **oo·go·nia** (ō-ō-gō'nē-ŭm, -ă). **1.** Ovogônia; células germinativas primitivas; proliferam por divisão mitótica. Todas as ovogônias evoluem para ovócitos primários antes do nascimento; não há ovogônias depois do nascimento. **2.** Oogônio; em fungos, o gametângio feminino contendo um ou mais ovosporos. [G. *ōon*, ovo, + *gonē*, produção]

oo·ki·ne·sis, oo·ki·ne·sia (ō'ō-ki-nē'sis, -zē-ă). Ovocinese, ovocinesia; movimentos cromossomiais do ovo durante a maturação e fertilização. [G. *ōon*, ovo, + *kinēsis*, movimento]

oo·ki·nete (ō'ō-ki-nēt', -kī'nēt'). Oocineto; o zigoto móvel do plasmódio que penetra no estômago do mosquito para formar um oocisto sob o revestimento externo do interno; o conteúdo do oocisto divide-se, subseqüentemente, para produzir inúmeros esporozoítos. SIN vermicule (2). [G. *ōon*, ovo, + *kinētos*, móvel]

oo·lem·ma (ō-ō-lem'ă). Oolema; membrana plasmática do oócito. [G. *ōon*, ovo, + *lemma*, bainha]

oo·my·co·sis (ō'ō-mī-kō'sis). Oomicose; micose causada por fungos pertencentes à classe dos Oomycetes; p.ex., rinosporidiose.

oo·pha·gia, ooph·a·gy (ō-ō-fā'jē-ă, of'ă-jē). Oofagia; a ingestão habitual de ovos; que subsiste principalmente à base de ovos. [G. *ōon*, ovo, + *phagō*, comer]

oophor-, oophoro-. Oofor-, ooforo-; formas combinantes que designam o ovário. VER TAMBÉM oo-, ovario-. [L. mod. *oophoron*, ovário, de G. *ōophoros*, que possui ovos]

ooph·or·al·gia (ō-of-ōr-al'jē-ă). Ooforalgia. SIN ovarialgia. [oophor- + G. *algos*, dor]

ooph·o·rec·to·my (ō-of-ōr-ek'tō-mē). Ooforectomia. SIN ovariectomy. [G. *ōon*, ovo, + *phoros*, que transporta, + *ektomē*, excisão]

ooph·or·i·tis (ō-of-ōr-ī'tis). Ooforite; inflamação de um ovário. SIN ovaritis. [G. *ōon*, ovo, + *phoros*, um transporte, + *-itis*, inflamação]

oophoro-. VER oophor-.

ooph·or·o·cys·tec·to·my (ō-of'ōr-ō-sis-tek'tō-mē). Ooforocistectomia; excisão de um cisto ovariano.

ooph·or·o·cys·to·sis (ō-of'ōr-ō-sis-tō'sis). Ooforocistose; formação de cisto ovariano.

ooph·or·on (ō-of'ōr-on). Oóforo; termo raramente utilizado para ovário. [G. *ōon*, ovo, + *phoros*, que transporta]

ooph·or·op·a·thy (ō-of-ōr-op'ă-thē). Ooforopatia. SIN ovariopathy.

ooph·or·o·pexy (ō-of'ōr-ō-pek'sē). Ooforopexia; fixação cirúrgica ou suspensão de um ovário. [oophoro- + G. *pēxis*, fixação]

ooph·or·o·plas·ty (ō-of'ōr-ō-plas-tē). Ooforoplastia; cirurgia plástica em um ovário. [oophoro- + G. *plastos*, formado, moldado]

ooph·o·ror·rha·phy (ō-of-ō-rōr'ă-fē). Oofororrafia; suspensão do ovário por meio de inserção na parede pélvica. [oophoro- + G. *rhaphē*, sutura]

ooph·or·o·sal·pin·gec·to·my (ō-of'ōr-ō-sal-pin-jek'tō-mē). Ooforossalpingectomia. SIN ovariosalpingectomy.

ooph·or·o·sal·pin·gi·tis (ō-of'ōr-ō-sal-pin-jī'tis). Ooforossalpingite. SIN ovariosalpingitis. [oophoro- + salpingitis]

ooph·or·ot·o·my (ō-of-ōr-ot'ō-mē). Ooforotomia. SIN ovariotomy. [oophoro- + G. *tomē*, incisão]

ooph·or·rha·gia (ō-of-ōr-rā'jē-ă). Oofororragia; hemorragia ovariana. [oophoro- + G. *rhēgnymi*, eclodir]

oo·plasm (ō'ō-plazm). Ooplasma; porção protoplásmica do ovo. [G. *ōon*, ovo, + *plasma*, uma coisa formada]

oo·some (ō'ō-sōm). Oossoma; um corpúsculo citoplasmático no ovo que passa para a célula germinativa. [G. *ōon*, ovo, + *sōma*, corpo]

oo·spo·ran·gi·um (ō'ō-spō-ran'jē-ŭm). Oosporângio; termo obsoleto para oogonium (2). [oospore + G. *angeion*, vaso]

oo·spore (ō'ō-spōr). Oosporo; um esporo de fungo de parede espessa que se desenvolve a partir de um gameta feminino, quer através da fertilização, quer por partenogênese em um oogônio. [ver *Oospora*]

oo·the·ca (ō-oth-ē'kă). Ooteca. **1.** Uma cápsula do ovo encontrada em alguns animais inferiores. **2.** Termo raramente utilizado para ovário. [G. *ōon*, ovo, + *thēkē*, caixa, cápsula]

oo·tid (ō'ō-tid). Oótide; o ovo quase maduro após a primeira divisão meiótica ter sido completada e a segunda iniciada; na maioria dos animais superiores, a segunda divisão meiótica não é completada, a menos que ocorra a fertilização. [G. *ōotidion*, um ovo diminuto. Ver -id (2)]

oo·type (ō'ō-tīp). Oótipo; a porção central do complexo ovariano dos trematódeos e cestódeos em que a fertilização ocorre e os materiais vitelinos ou da casca do ovo cobrem o ovo; isso ocorre em uma seqüência rápida, depois da qual os ovos vão para o útero, para curtimento da casca, armazenamento e eliminação para o poro genital. [G. ōon, ovo, + typos, selo, impressão]

OP Abreviatura para occipitoposterior *position* (posição occipitoposterior).

opa·ci·fi·ca·tion (ō-pas′i-fi-kā′shun). Opacificação. **1.** O processo de tornar opaco. **2.** A formação de opacificações. [L. *opacus*, sombreado]

opa·ci·ty (ō-pas′i-tē). Opacidade. **1.** A falta de transparência; uma área opaca ou não-transparente. **2.** Em uma radiografia, uma área menos transparente (hipotransparência) é interpretada como uma o. **3.** Embotamento mental. [L. *opacitas*, opacidade]

   nodular o., o. nodular; uma imagem solitária, arredondada e circunscrita encontrada no pulmão na radiografia de tórax; as causas incluem granuloma, carcinoma primário ou metastático, tumor benigno, malformação vascular. SIN coin lesion of lungs.

   snowball o., o. em bola de neve; um corpo esférico, esbranquiçado, observado no humor vítreo na hialose asteróide.

opal·es·cent (ō-pā-les′ent). Opalescente; que se assemelha a uma opala na demonstração de várias cores; indica determinadas culturas bacterianas. [Fr. do L. *opalus*, opala]

Opalski, Adam, médico polonês, 1897–1963. VER O. *cell.*

opaque (ō-pāk′). Opaco; impermeável à luz; não-translúcido ou apenas um pouco translúcido. Cf. radiopaque. [Fr. do L. *opacus*, opaco]

open (ō′pen). **1.** Aberto; não fechado; exposto, diz-se de uma ferida. **2.** Abrir; penetrar ou expor, como uma ferida ou cavidade. [A. S.]

open·ing (ō′pen-ing) [TA]. Abertura; orifício; óstio; uma abertura ou entrada para um órgão, tubo ou cavidade. VER TAMBÉM aperture, fossa, ostium, orifice, pore.

   access o., a. de acesso. SIN access.
   aortic o., hiato aórtico. SIN aortic *hiatus*.
   o. of aqueduct of midbrain [TA], a. do aqueduto do mesencéfalo; entrada para o aqueduto cerebral; o ponto em que a parte caudal do terceiro ventrículo se continua com o aqueduto cerebral do mesencéfalo; localizado na linha média imediatamente ventral à comissura posterior. SIN apertura aqueductus mesencephali [TA], apertura aqueductus cerebri*, o. of cerebral aqueduct*, aditus ad aqueductum cerebri, Bartholin anus.
   cardiac o., óstio cárdico. SIN cardial *orifice*.
   o.'s of carotid canal [TA], aberturas do canal carótico; a abertura em cada extremidade do canal carotídeo na porção petrosa piramidal do osso temporal; a abertura externa do canal carotídeo localiza-se na superfície inferior da pirâmide; a abertura interna do canal localiza-se no ápice da porção petrosa. SIN carotid foramen.
   caval o. of diaphragm [TA], forame da veia cava; uma abertura no lobo direito do tendão central do diafragma que permite a passagem da veia cava inferior e dos ramos do nervo frênico direito. SIN foramen of vena cava, foramen quadratum, foramen venae cavae, vena caval foramen.
   o. of cerebral aqueduct, abertura do aqueduto do mesencéfalo;* termo oficial alternativo para o. of aqueduct of midbrain.
   o. of coronary sinus [TA], óstio do seio coronário; o orifício pelo qual o seio coronário entra e drena para o átrio direito do coração. SIN ostium sinus coronarii [TA].
   esophageal o., hiato esofágico. SIN esophageal *hiatus*.
   external o., meato. SIN meatus.
   o. of external acoustic meatus, poro acústico externo. SIN external acoustic *pore*.
   external o. of cochlear canaliculus [TA], abertura do canalículo da cóclea; a abertura externa do aqueduto da cóclea no osso temporal medial à fossa jugular. SIN apertura canaliculi cochleae, external aperture of cochlear canaliculus.
   external o. of urethra, óstio externo da uretra. SIN external urethral *orifice*.
   femoral o., hiato dos adutores. SIN adductor *hiatus*.
   o. of frontal sinus [TA], Abertura do seio frontal; cada uma das aberturas de um par localizado no assoalho dos seios frontais na porção nasal do osso frontal, através das quais os seios frontais se comunicam com o infundíbulo etmoidal por meio do ducto frontonasal. SIN apertura sinus frontalis [TA], frontal sinus aperture.
   ileocecal o., o. ileocecal. SIN ileal *orifice*.
   o. of inferior vena cava [TA], óstio da veia cava inferior; o orifício através do qual a veia cava inferior desemboca no átrio direito. SIN ostium venae cavae inferioris [TA], orifice of inferior vena cava.
   internal acoustic o. [TA], poro acústico interno. SIN internal acoustic *pore*.
   o. of internal acoustic meatus, poro acústico interno. SIN internal acoustic *pore*.
   internal urethral o., óstio interno da uretra;* termo oficial alternativo para internal urethral *orifice*.
   lacrimal o., ponto lacrimal. SIN lacrimal *punctum*.
   oral o., rima da boca;* termo oficial alternativo para oral *fissure*.
   orbital o. [TA], ádito orbital; a entrada anterior da órbita, algo quadrangular, que forma a base da cavidade orbital com formato de pirâmide. É limitada pelas bem definidas margens supra-orbital, infra-orbital e orbital lateral e uma margem medial menos evidente em cada lado da parte superior do nariz. SIN aditus orbitae [TA], aperture of orbit.
   o.'s of papillary ducts [TA], forames papilares; numerosas aberturas diminutas, as aberturas dos ductos papilares que convergem para o pólo apical de cada papila renal. SIN foramina papillaria renis [TA], papillary foramina of kidney.
   pharyngeal o. of eustachian tube, óstio faríngeo da tuba auditiva. SIN pharyngeal o. of pharyngotympanic (auditory) tube.
   pharyngeal o. of pharyngotympanic (auditory) tube [TA], óstio faríngeo da tuba auditiva; uma abertura na parte superior da nasofaringe cerca de 1,2 cm atrás da extremidade posterior da concha nasal inferior em cada lado. SIN ostium pharyngeum tubae auditivae [TA], ostium pharyngeum tubae auditoriae*, pharyngeal o. of eustachian tube.
   piriform o., abertura piriforme. SIN piriform *aperture*.
   o. of pulmonary trunk [TA], óstio do tronco pulmonar; o óstio do tronco pulmonar no ventrículo direito, protegido pela valva pulmonar. SIN ostium trunci pulmonalis [TA], pulmonary orifice.
   o.'s of pulmonary veins [TA], óstios das veias pulmonares; os orifícios das veias pulmonares, usualmente dois em cada lado, na parede do átrio esquerdo. SIN ostia venarum pulmonalium [TA]
   saphenous o. [TA], hiato safeno; a abertura na fáscia lata inferior à parte medial do ligamento inguinal através do qual a veia safena passa para entrar na veia femoral. SIN hiatus saphenus [TA], fossa ovalis (2), saphenous hiatus.
   o.'s of smallest cardiac veins [TA], forames das veias mínimas; inúmeras fossas na parede do átrio direito, contendo as aberturas de diminutas veias intramurais. SIN foramina of the smallest veins of heart, foramina of the venae minimae, foramina venarum minimarum cordis, Lannelongue foramina, thebesian foramina, Vieussens foramina.
   o. of the sphenoidal sinus [TA], abertura do seio esfenoidal; cada uma das aberturas do par localizado no corpo do osso esfenóide através das quais os seios esfenoidais se comunicam com o recesso esfenoetmoidal da cavidade nasal. SIN apertura sinus sphenoidalis [TA], sphenoidal sinus aperture.
   o. of superior vena cava [TA], óstio da veia cava superior; o ponto de entrada da veia cava superior no átrio direito. SIN ostium venae cavae superioris [TA], orifice of superior vena cava.
   tendinous o., hiato dos adutores. SIN adductor *hiatus*.
   tympanic o. of canaliculus for chorda tympani, abertura timpânica do canalículo da corda do tímpano. SIN tympanic *aperture* of canaliculus for chorda tympani.
   tympanic o. of eustachian tube, óstio timpânico da tuba auditiva. SIN tympanic o. of pharyngotympanic (auditory) tube.
   tympanic o. of pharyngotympanic (auditory) tube [TA], óstio timpânico da tuba auditiva; uma abertura na parte anterior da cavidade timpânica abaixo do canal para o tensor do tímpano (músculo). SIN ostium tympanicum tubae auditivae [TA], tympanic o. of eustachian tube.
   ureteral o., óstio do ureter. SIN ureteric *orifice*.
   urethral o.'s, óstios da uretra. VER external urethral *orifice*, internal urethral *orifice*.
   uterine o. of uterine tubes, óstio uterino da tuba uterina. SIN uterine *ostium* of uterine tubes.
   o. of uterus, óstio do útero. SIN external *os* of uterus.
   vaginal o., óstio da vagina. SIN vaginal *orifice*.
   vertical o., dimensão vertical. SIN vertical *dimension*.
   o. of vestibular canaliculus [TA], abertura do canalículo do vestíbulo; a abertura externa do aqueduto do vestíbulo na superfície posterior da porção petrosa do osso temporal próximo ao sulco para o seio sigmóideo. SIN apertura canaliculi vestibuli, external aperture of vestibular aqueduct.

op·er·a·ble (op′er-ā-bl). Operável; indica um paciente ou condição em que se pode realizar um procedimento cirúrgico com uma expectativa razoável de cura ou alívio.

op·er·ant (op′er-ănt). Resposta desejada, comportamento desejado; no condicionamento, qualquer comportamento ou resposta específica escolhida pelo experimentador; sua freqüência deve aumentar ou diminuir por meio de seu pareamento criterioso com um reforçador, quando ocorre. SIN target behavior (1), target response.

op·er·ate (op′er-āt). **1.** Operar; exercer uma ação no corpo por meio das mãos ou através de instrumentos de corte ou outros instrumentos. **2.** Operar; realizar um procedimento cirúrgico. **3.** Provocar a defecação; diz-se de um laxativo ou catártico. [L. *operor*, pp. *-atus*, trabalhar, de *opus*, trabalho]

OPERATION

---

op·er·a·tion (op-er-ā′shun). Operação. **1.** Qualquer procedimento cirúrgico. **2.** O ato, a maneira ou o processo de funcionamento. VER TAMBÉM method, procedure, technique.

   Altemeier o., o. de Altemeier; cirurgia para o prolapso retal que envolve uma ressecção em manga do reto e do cólon prolapsados, com uma anastomose primária realizada por via transanal.

Arlt o., o. de Arlt; transplante de cílios para trás da borda da pálpebra na triquíase.

arterial switch o., o. de troca arterial; o. para a transposição completa das grandes artérias; o meio mais comum de reparar esse defeito consiste na troca da aorta e das artérias pulmonares e no implante das artérias coronárias na nova aorta (a artéria pulmonar original).

Ball o., o. de Ball; divisão dos troncos nervosos sensoriais que suprem o ânus, para alívio do prurido anal.

Barkan o., o. de Barkan; goniotomia para o glaucoma congênito sob observação direta do ângulo da câmara anterior.

Bassini o., o. de Bassini. SIN Bassini *herniorrhaphy*.

Battista o., o. de Battista. SIN left ventricular volume reduction *surgery*.

Belsey Mark o., o. de Belsey Mark. SIN Belsey *fundoplication*.

Billroth o. I, o. de Billroth I; excisão do piloro e do antro e fechamento parcial da extremidade gástrica com anastomose término-terminal do estômago e duodeno.

Billroth o. II, o. de Billroth II; excisão do piloro e antro com fechamento das extremidades seccionadas do duodeno e estômago, seguida por gastrojejunostomia.

Blalock-Hanlon o., o. de Blalock-Hanlon; a criação de um grande defeito no septo interatrial como um procedimento paliativo para a transposição completa das grandes artérias.

Blalock-Taussig o., o. de Blalock-Taussig; o. para malformações congênitas do coração, na qual um volume anormalmente pequeno de sangue passa através do circuito pulmonar; o sangue da circulação sistêmica é dirigido para os pulmões por meio de anastomose da artéria subclávia direita ou esquerda com a artéria pulmonar direita ou esquerda.

bloodless o., o. sem sangue; uma cirurgia realizada com perda desprezível de sangue.

Bozeman o., o. de Bozeman; cirurgia para fístula uterovaginal, sendo o colo uterino preso à bexiga e abrindo-se em sua cavidade.

Bricker o., o. de Bricker; o. que utiliza um segmento isolado do íleo para coletar a urina proveniente dos ureteres e levando-a até a superfície cutânea.

Brock o., o. de Brock; valvotomia transventricular para alívio da estenose da valva pulmonar. Procedimento obsoleto.

Brunschwig o., o. de Brunschwig. SIN total pelvic *exenteration*.

Caldwell-Luc o., o. de Caldwell-Luc; um procedimento intra-oral para a abertura para o seio maxilar através da fossa canina acima dos dentes pré-molares maxilares. SIN intraoral antrostomy, Luc o.

Carmody-Batson o., o. de Carmody-Batson; redução de fraturas do zigoma e do arco zigomático através de uma incisão intra-oral acima dos dentes molares maxilares.

cesarean o., cesariana. VER cesarean *section*, cesarean *hysterectomy*.

commando o., o. de comando. SIN commando *procedure*.

concrete o.'s, operações concretas; na psicologia de Piaget, um estágio de desenvolvimento no pensamento, que ocorre aproximadamente entre 7 e 11 anos de idade, durante o qual uma criança se torna capaz de raciocinar a respeito de situações concretas.

Cotte o., o. de Cotte. SIN presacral *neurectomy*.

cricoid split o., o. de divisão da cricóide; cirurgia de reparo de estenose subglótica por meio de corte transversal das faces anterior e posterior do anel da cartilagem cricóide, com ou sem a inserção de enxertos para reconstruir a luz subglótica.

Dana o., o. de Dana. SIN posterior *rhizotomy*.

Dandy o., o. de Dandy. VER third *ventriculostomy*, trigeminal *rhizotomy*.

Daviel o., o. de Daviel; extração extracapsular de catarata.

debulking o., o. citorredutora; excisão de uma parte importante de um tumor maligno que não pode ser completamente removido.

decompression o., o. de descompressão. VER decompression.

Doyle o., o. de Doyle; desnervação uterina paracervical.

Elliot o., o. de Elliot; trepanação do globo ocular na margem corneoesclerótica para aliviar a tensão no glaucoma.

Emmet o., o. de Emmet. SIN trachelorrhaphy.

endolymphatic shunt o., o. de derivação endolinfática; cirurgia para estabelecer uma comunicação entre o saco endolinfático e o espaço do líquido cefalorraquidiano para o tratamento da doença de Ménière.

Estes o., o. de Estes; o. para a esterilidade em que uma porção de um ovário é implantada em um corno uterino.

fenestration o., o. de fenestração; um procedimento cirúrgico raramente utilizado que cria uma abertura do canal auditivo externo para o labirinto membranoso, visando melhorar a audição no comprometimento auditivo de condução decorrente de otoesclerose.

filtering o., o. de filtração; procedimento cirúrgico para a criação de uma fístula entre a câmara anterior do olho e o espaço subconjuntival no tratamento do glaucoma.

Finney o., o. de Finney; gastroduodenostomia que cria, através da técnica de fechamento, uma grande abertura para garantir o livre esvaziamento do estômago.

flap o., o. de retalho; (1) SIN flap *amputation*; (2) na cirurgia dentária, o. em que uma porção dos tecidos mucoperiósteos é cirurgicamente descolada do osso subjacente ou do dente impactado para melhor acesso e visibilidade na exploração da área coberta pelo tecido. VER TAMBÉM flap.

Fontan o., o. de Fontan. SIN Fontan *procedure*.

formal o.'s, operações formais; na psicologia de Piaget, um estágio de desenvolvimento no pensamento, ocorrendo aproximadamente entre 11 e 15 anos de idade, durante o qual uma criança se torna capaz de raciocinar a respeito de situações abstratas; o raciocínio nesse estágio é comparável ao de adultos normais, porém menos sofisticado.

Fothergill o., o. de Fothergill. SIN Manchester o.

Frazier-Spiller o., o. de Frazier-Spiller. VER trigeminal *rhizotomy*.

Fredet-Ramstedt o., o. de Fredet-Ramstedt. SIN pyloromyotomy.

Freund o., o. de Freund; (1) histerectomia abdominal total para o câncer de útero; (2) condrotomia para aliviar a anomalia de Freund.

Gilliam o., o. de Gilliam; cirurgia para a retroversão do útero por meio de sutura dos ligamentos redondos à fáscia da parede abdominal.

Gillies o., o. de Gillies; uma técnica para a redução de fraturas do zigoma e do arco zigomático através de uma incisão na região temporal acima da linha de implantação do cabelo.

Gil-Vernet o., o. de Gil-Vernet. SIN extended *pyelotomy*.

Glenn o., o. de Glenn; anastomose entre a veia cava superior e a artéria pulmonar direita para aumentar o fluxo sanguíneo pulmonar, como uma correção paliativa para a atresia tricúspide.

Graefe o., o. de Graefe; (1) remoção da catarata por uma incisão com capsulotomia e iridectomia. Ambas as cirurgias foram marcos no campo da cirurgia oftálmica; (2) iridectomia para o glaucoma.

Gritti o., o. de Gritti. SIN Gritti-Stokes *amputation*.

Halsted o., o. de Halsted; (1) cirurgia para a correção radical da hérnia inguinal; (2) mastectomia radical. SIN radical *mastectomy*.

Hartmann o., o. de Hartmann; ressecção do colo sigmóide que começa na reflexão peritoneal, ou logo acima dela, e se estende proximalmente, com fechamento do coto retal e colostomia terminal.

Heaney o., o. de Heaney; técnica de histerectomia vaginal.

Heller o., o. de Heller; esofagomiotomia logo acima da junção gastroesofágica.

Hill o., o. de Hill; reparo de hérnia de hiato; fixação da junção esofagogástrica no abdome ao prendê-lo ao ligamento arqueado medial.

Hoffa o., o. de Hoffa; na luxação congênita do quadril, uma cirurgia raramente utilizada que consiste na escavação do acetábulo e redução da cabeça do fêmur após seccionar os músculos inseridos na porção superior do osso.

Hofmeister o., o. de Hofmeister; gastrectomia parcial com o fechamento de uma porção da curvatura menor e anastomose retrocólica do restante do jejuno.

Hummelsheim o., o. de Hummelsheim; transplante de um músculo reto do bulbo do olho normal para substituir um músculo paralisado.

Hunter o., o. de Hunter; laqueadura de artéria proximal e distal a um aneurisma.

interval o., o. de intervalo; cirurgia realizada durante um período de quiescência na condição que necessita de cirurgia.

Jacobaeus o., o. de Jacobaeus; termo obsoleto para pleurólise.

Jansen o., o. de Jansen; uma cirurgia para a doença do seio frontal; a parede inferior e a porção inferior da parede anterior são removidas e a mucosa é curetada.

Kasai o., o. de Kasai. SIN portoenterostomy.

Kazanjian o., o. de Kazanjian; extensão cirúrgica do sulco vestibular das cristas edêntulas para aumentar sua altura e melhorar a retenção da dentadura. VER TAMBÉM ridge *extension*.

Keen o., o. de Keen; remoção de partes dos ramos posteriores dos nervos espinais para os músculos afetados, e da raiz espinal do nervo acessório, como uma cura para o torcicolo.

Keller-Madlener o., o. de Keller-Madlener; cirurgia para o tratamento da úlcera gástrica que envolve gastrectomia (75% do estômago) e gastrojejunostomia.

Kelly o., o. de Kelly; (1) correção da retroversão do útero por plicatura dos ligamentos uterossacrais; (2) correção da incontinência urinária por esforço através da colocação de suturas sob o colo da bexiga (por via vaginal).

Killian o., o. de Killian; cirurgia para doença do seio frontal em que toda a parede anterior é removida e a mucosa é curetada; as células etmoidais são removidas através de uma abertura no processo frontal do osso maxilar, sendo a porção superior da parede medial da órbita também removida.

Koerte-Ballance o., o. de Koerte-Ballance; anastomose cirúrgica dos nervos facial e hipoglosso para o tratamento da paralisia facial.

Kondoleon o., o. de Kondoleon; a excisão de faixas de tecido conjuntivo subcutâneo para o alívio da elefantíase.

Kraske o., o. de Kraske; remoção do cóccix e excisão da asa esquerda do sacro para possibilitar a abordagem para ressecção do reto por causa de câncer ou estenose.

Krönlein o., o. de Krönlein; descompressão orbital através da parede lateral anterior da órbita.

Ladd o., o. de Ladd; divisão da faixa de Ladd para aliviar a obstrução duodenal na má rotação do intestino.
Lambrinudi o., o. de Lambrinudi; uma forma de artrodese tríplice feita de forma a evitar o pé em gota, como acontece na poliomielite.
Laroyenne o., o. de Laroyenne; a punção do fundo-de-saco de Douglas (escavação retouterina) para evacuar o pus e assegurar a drenagem em casos de supuração pélvica.
Lash o., o. de Lash; remoção de uma cunha do óstio interno do útero com sutura do mesmo a uma estrutura de canal mais apertada.
LeCompte o., o. de LeCompte. SIN LeCompte *maneuver*.
Leriche o., o. de Leriche. SIN *periarterial sympathectomy*.
Lisfranc o., o. de Lisfranc. SIN Lisfranc *amputation*.
Longmire o., o. de Longmire; colangiojejunostomia intra-hepática com hepatectomia parcial para obstrução biliar.
Luc o., o. de Luc. SIN Caldwell-Luc o.
Madlener o., o. de Madlener; esterilização tubária por clampeamento e laqueadura.
major o., o. de grande porte; um procedimento cirúrgico relativamente difícil, que envolve órgãos vitais e/ou que em si é perigosa para a vida.
Manchester o., o. de Manchester; o. vaginal para o prolapso do útero, consistindo em amputação do colo do útero e fixação parametrial (ligamentos transversos do colo) anterior ao útero. SIN Fothergill o. [*Manchester*, Inglaterra]
Mann-Williamson o., o. de Mann-Williamson; o. realizada em animais de laboratório (cães) na pesquisa da úlcera péptica, sendo o duodeno, com suas secreções alcalinas, transplantado para o íleo e a extremidade seccionada do jejuno é anastomosada ao piloro; os animais desenvolvem úlceras no jejuno, o qual recebe diretamente o suco gástrico.
Marshall-Marchetti-Krantz o., o. de Marshall-Marchetti-Krantz; uma o. para a incontinência urinária de esforço, realizada por via retropúbica.
Mayo o., o. de Mayo; o. para a cura radical da hérnia umbilical; o colo do saco é exposto por duas incisões elípticas, o intestino é devolvido para dentro do abdome, o saco e o omento aderente são seccionados e retirados e as bordas fasciais da abertura são superpostas com suturas em colchoeiro.
McIndoe o., o. de McIndoe; o. para a criação de uma neovagina usando um enxerto cutâneo de espessura parcial sobre um molde vaginal.
McVay o., o. de McVay; reparo de hérnias inguinais e femorais através da sutura do músculo transverso do abdome e suas fáscias associadas (camada transversa) ao ligamento pectíneo.
mika o., o estabelecimento de uma fístula permanente na porção bulbosa da uretra para tornar o homem incapaz de procriar; diz-se que é uma prática entre determinados aborígenes australianos. [termo dos aborígenes australianos]
Mikulicz o., o. de Mikulicz; a excisão do intestino em dois estágios: 1) exteriorização da área enferma, sutura dos ramos aferente e eferente, em conjunto, e fechamento do abdome ao redor deles, depois do que a parte enferma é excisada; 2) mais tarde, o corte da porção que sobressai do abdome com um enterótomo e o fechamento do estoma extraperitonealmente.
Miles o., o. de Miles; ressecção abdominoperineal combinada para carcinoma do reto.
minor o., o. menor; um procedimento cirúrgico de porte relativamente pequeno e que não é prejudicial à vida por si só.
morcellation o., o. de fragmentação; histerectomia vaginal em que o útero é removido em múltiplos pedaços depois de ser dividido ou seccionado.
Motais o., o. de Motais; transplante do terço médio do tendão do músculo reto superior do bulbo do olho para a pálpebra superior, entre o tarso e a pele, visando suplementar a ação do músculo levantador da pálpebra superior na ptose.
Mules o., o. de Mules; evisceração do bulbo do olho seguida por inserção na esclera de uma prótese esférica para apoiar um olho artificial.
Mustard o., o. de Mustard; correção, no nível atrial, da anormalidade hemodinâmica causada pela transposição das grandes artérias por um anteparo intra-atrial para direcionar o sangue venoso pulmonar, através do orifício tricúspide, para o ventrículo direito e o sangue venoso sistêmico, através da válvula mitral, para o ventrículo esquerdo. SIN Mustand procedure.
Naffziger o., o. de Naffziger; descompressão orbital para a exoftalmia maligna grave por remoção das paredes orbitais lateral e superior.
Nissen o., o. de Nissen. SIN Nissen *fundoplication*.
Norton o., o. de Norton; cesariana extraperitoneal por via paravesical.
Norwood o., o. de Norwood; uma o. realizada em lactentes com estenose subaórtica e atresia tricúspide; a artéria pulmonar é dividida e as duas extremidades são fixadas à aorta, sendo a extremidade distal fixada por meio de uma prótese.
Ogston-Luc o., o. de Ogston-Luc; o. para a doença do seio frontal; uma incisão cutânea é feita desde o terço interno da borda da órbita até a raiz do nariz ou para fora; o periósteo é empurrado para cima e para fora, sendo o seio aberto no lado externo da linha mediana; em seguida, é feita uma ampla abertura por curetagem do ducto frontonasal, do seio frontal e das células etmoidais anteriores.
Ogura o., o. de Ogura; descompressão orbital através da retirada do assoalho da órbita por uma abertura feita na fossa canina.

Ombrédanne o., o. de Ombrédanne; uma técnica por meio da qual o testículo mobilizado é trazido para a bolsa escrotal e através do septo escrotal, para ser fixado aos tecidos na bolsa escrotal contralateral. SIN transseptal orchiopexy.
Payne o., o. de Payne; derivação (*bypass*) jejunoileal realizada para obesidade mórbida, utilizando a anastomose término-lateral da porção superior do jejuno ao íleo terminal, com o fechamento da extremidade proximal do intestino desviado.
Pólya o., o. de Pólya. SIN Pólya *gastrectomy*.
Pomeroy o., o. de Pomeroy; a excisão de uma porção ligada das tubas uterinas.
Potts o., o. de Potts; anastomose látero-lateral direta entre a aorta e a artéria pulmonar como um procedimento paliativo na malformação congênita do coração. SIN Potts anastomosis.
pubovaginal o., o. pubovaginal; procedimento cirúrgico para a incontinência urinária. Uma faixa de tecido, geralmente a fáscia do reto abdominal autólogo, é usada para suspender ou elevar o colo da bexiga e a porção posterior da uretra em direção à sínfise pubiana.
Putti-Platt o., o. de Putti-Platt; procedimento para a luxação anterior recorrente da articulação do ombro. SIN Putti-Platt procedure.
radical o. for hernia, o. radical para hérnia; o. pela qual a hérnia não é apenas reduzida, mas também é reparado o defeito herniário.
Ramstedt o., o. de Ramstedt. SIN pyloromyotomy.
Rastelli o., o. de Rastelli; para o reparo "anatômico" da transposição das grandes artérias (discordância ventriculoarterial) com defeito do septo interventricular e obstrução do trato de saída do ventrículo esquerdo; são usados condutos para criar continuidade entre o ventrículo esquerdo e a aorta e continuidade entre o ventrículo direito e a artéria pulmonar. Todos os defeitos septais são obliterados, bem como qualquer derivação (*shunt*) paliativa previamente construída.
Récamier o., o. de Récamier; curetagem do útero.
Ridell o., o. de Ridell; a remoção das paredes anterior e inferior (por inteiro) do seio frontal, por causa de inflamação crônica dessa cavidade.
Ripstein o., o. de Ripstein; o. para o prolapso retal que envolve uma abordagem transabdominal com dissecção ao redor do reto e colocação de uma tela de sustentação, de modo a impedir o prolapso do intestino através do ânus.
Roux-en-Y o., o. em Y de Roux; anastomose da extremidade distal do jejuno superior dividido ao estômago, esôfago, trato biliar ou outra estrutura e anastomose da extremidade proximal ao lado do jejuno em uma posição um pouco mais distal.
Saenger o., o. de Saenger; cesariana seguida por cuidadoso fechamento da ferida uterina por três fileiras de suturas.
Schauta vaginal o., o. vaginal de Schauta; extirpação extensa do útero e dos anexos, usando a abordagem vaginal facilitada pela o. de Schuchardt.
Schroeder o., o. de Schroeder; excisão da mucosa endocervical com alterações.
Schuchardt o., o. de Schuchardt; uma incisão de deslocamento retal paravaginal, a técnica cirúrgica de tornar acessível a parte superior da vagina para o fechamento da fístula ou cirurgia radical através da vagina.
scleral buckling o., o. de encurvamento da esclerótica; uma cirurgia realizada no descolamento da retina para fazer uma indentação na parede esclerocoroidal.
Scott o., o. de Scott; derivação (*bypass*) jejunoileal para a obesidade mórbida, utilizando a anastomose término-terminal do jejuno superior com o íleo terminal, com o intestino desviado fechado proximalmente e anastomosado distalmente ao cólon.
second-look o., o. de revisão; celiotomia exploradora um ano após a ressecção aparentemente curativa do câncer intra-abdominal, nos pacientes sem sinal ou sintoma de recidiva, para ressecar um tumor oculto, quando existente.
Senning o., o. de Senning; um desvio atrial para pacientes com transposição das grandes artérias que emprega um retalho septal em lugar da excisão do septo atrial como na o. de Mustard, minimizando, dessa maneira, o material estranho e possibilitando o crescimento.
seton o., cirurgia para o glaucoma avançado; a introdução de um tubo ou sedenho na câmara anterior para agir como um dreno.
Shirodkar o., o. de Shirodkar; procedimento de cerclagem feito por uma sutura em cordão de bolsa de um óstio cervical incompetente com fios de sutura não-absorventes.
Sistrunk o., o. de Sistrunk; excisão do cisto e ducto tireoglosso, incluindo a porção média do osso hióide através ou próximo do trajeto do ducto.
Smith o., o. de Smith. SIN Smith-Indian o.
Smith-Boyce o., o. de Smith-Boyce. SIN anatrophic *nephrotomy*.
Smith-Indian o., o. de Smith-Indian; técnica cirúrgica para a remoção da catarata dentro da cápsula. SIN Smith o.
Soave o., o. de Soave; tração endorretal para tratamento do megacólon congênito.
Spinelli o., o. de Spinelli; uma cirurgia de divisão da parede anterior do útero prolapsado e inversão do órgão antes da redução.
stapes mobilization o., o. de mobilização do estribo; cirurgia raramente usada em nossos dias, envolvendo a fratura do tecido otoesclerótico que imobiliza o estribo para restaurar a audição.

Stoffel o., o. de Stoffel; divisão de determinados nervos motores para o alívio da paralisia espástica.
Stookey-Scarff o., o. de Stookey-Scarff. VER third *ventriculostomy*.
Sturmdorf o., o. de Sturmdorf; remoção cônica do colo do útero.
subcutaneous o., o. subcutânea; uma cirurgia, como aquela para a divisão de um tendão, realizada com a incisão da pele restringindo-se a uma pequena abertura feita pela penetração do bisturi.
Syme o., o. de Syme. SIN Syme *amputation.*
talc o., uma cirurgia obsoleta na qual o silicato de magnésio em pó (talco) é aplicado ao epicárdio para criar uma pericardite granulomatosa estéril e, dessa maneira, promover anastomoses pericárdicas com a circulação coronariana. SIN poudrage (2).
TeLinde o., o. de TeLinde. SIN modified radical *hysterectomy.*
Torek o., o. de Torek; cirurgia em duas etapas para trazer para baixo um testículo não-descido.
Trendelenburg o., o. de Trendelenburg; embolectomia pulmonar.
Urban o., o. de Urban; mastectomia radical estendida, incluindo a ressecção em bloco dos linfonodos mamários internos, de parte do esterno e das cartilagens costais.
Waters o., o. de Waters; cesariana extraperitoneal com abordagem supravesical.
Waterston o., o. de Waterston; anastomose criada por meios cirúrgicos entre a artéria pulmonar e a aorta ascendente para aliviar a tetralogia de Fallot em adultos.
Wertheim o., o. de Wertheim; uma cirurgia radical para o carcinoma do útero em que a maior parte possível da vagina é excisada e há ampla excisão de linfonodos.
Whipple o., o. de Whipple. SIN pancreatoduodenectomy.
Whitehead o., o. de Whitehead; excisão de hemorróidas por meio de duas incisões circulares, acima e abaixo das veias envolvidas, permitindo que a mucosa normal seja puxada para baixo e suturada na pele anal.

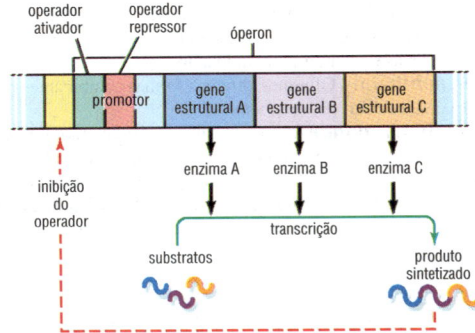

óperon: o produto sintetizado exerce retroalimentação negativa e inibe a função do óperon, controlando automaticamente, dessa maneira, a concentração do próprio produto

op·er·a·tive (op′er-ā-tiv). **1.** Operatório. relativo a, ou efetuado por meio de uma operação. **2.** Operante, operacional, ativo ou efetivo.
op·er·a·tor (op′er-ā-tor). Operador. **1.** Aquele que realiza uma operação ou opera equipamentos. **2.** Em genética, uma seqüência do DNA que interage com um repressor do óperon para controlar a expressão de genes estruturais adjacentes. VER operator *gene*. **3.** Um símbolo que representa uma operação matemática. [L. trabalhador, de *operor*, trabalhar]
oper·cu·lar (ō-per′kū-lar). Opercular; relativo a um opérculo.
oper·cu·lat·ed (ō-per′kū-lā-ted). Operculado; provido de opérculo; indica os moluscos membros da classe Gastropoda (os caramujos), subclasse Prosobranchiata (caramujos operculados), e os ovos de determinados vermes parasitas, como os trematódeos digenéticos (exceto os esquistossomas) e a grande tênia do peixe, *Diphyllobothrium latum*.
oper·cu·li·tis (ō-perk-ū-lī′tis). Operculite; que se origina sob um opérculo. [operculum + G. *-itis*, inflamação]
oper·cu·lum, gen. **oper·cu·li,** pl. **oper·cu·la** (ō-per′kū-lŭm, -lī, -lā). Opérculo. **1.** Qualquer coisa que se assemelha à pálpebra ou tampa. **2** [TA]. Em anatomia, as porções dos lobos frontais (operculum frontale [TA], frontal operculum [TA]), parietal (operculum parietale [TA], parietal operculum [TA]) e temporal (operculum temporale [TA], temporal operculum [TA]) que margeiam o sulco lateral e cobrem a ínsula. **3.** Em parasitologia, o opérculo ou cobertura semelhante a uma tampa da abertura da concha de caramujos operculados de água doce na subclasse Prosobranchiata e dos ovos de determinados parasitas trematódeos e cestódeos. **4.** O retalho preso na laceração do descolamento de retina. **5.** O retalho de mucosa que cobre, parcial ou completamente, um dente não-rompido. [L. cobertura ou pálpebra, de *operio*, pp. *opertus*, cobrir]
o. il′ei, óstio ileal. SIN ileal *sphincter.*
occipital o., o. occipital; uma porção do lobo occipital do cérebro demarcada pela fissura símia (*sulco* semilunar) quando presente em seres humanos.
trophoblastic o., o. trofoblástico; um tampão de fibrina em forma de cogumelo que preenche a abertura no endométrio feita pelo ovo em implantação.
op·er·on (op′er-on). Óperon; uma unidade funcional genética que controla a produção de um RNA mensageiro; consiste em um gene operador e dois ou mais genes estruturais localizados em seqüência na posição *cis* em um cromossoma. [L. *operor*, trabalhar, agir, + -on]
Lac o., o. Lac; uma coleção de genes bacterianos adjacentes responsável pela entrada e metabolismo da lactose; contém os genes que codificam três enzimas e é flanqueado por um repressor e uma região promotora para controlar expressão.
ophi·a·sis (ō-fī′ă-sis). Ofíase; uma forma de alopecia em áreas ou circunscrita em que a perda de cabelos acontece em faixas serpiginosas ao longo da margem do couro cabeludo, as quais circundam, de maneira parcial ou completa, a cabeça. [G., de *ophis*, cobra]
Ophid·ia (ō-fid′ē-ă). Ofídios; as cobras, uma subordem da classe Reptilia, incluindo as famílias Colubridae, Crotalidae, Elapidae, Hydrophyidae e Viperidae. [G. *ophidion*, dim. de *ophis*, uma serpente]

ophi·di·a·sis (ō′fi-dī′ă-sis). Ofidíase; envenenamento por uma cobra. SIN ophidism. [G. *ophidion*, dim. de *ophis*, uma serpente]
ophid·i·o·pho·bia (ō-fid′ē-ō-fō′bē-ă). Ofidiofobia; medo mórbido de cobras. [G. *ophidion*, uma pequena cobra, + *phobos*, medo]
ophid·ism (ō-fid-izm). Ofidismo. SIN ophidiasis.
oph·ri·tis (of-rī′tis). Ofrite; dermatite na região das sobrancelhas. SIN ophryitis. [G. *ophrys*, sobrancelha, + *-itis*, inflamação]
oph·ry·i·tis (of-rē-ī′tis). Ofrite. SIN ophritis.
oph·ry·og·e·nes (of′rē-yō-jen-′enz). Ofriogênese; relativo às sobrancelhas. [L. mod., de G. *ophrys*, sobrancelha, + sufixo *-genēs*, que se origina de]
oph·ry·on (of′rē-on). Ófrio; o ponto na linha média da fronte logo acima da glabela (1). SIN supranasal point, supraorbital point. [G. *ophrys*, sobrancelha]
Oph·ry·o·sco·lec·i·dae (of′rē-ō-skō-les′i-dē). Uma família de protozoários ciliados que ocorrem no rúmen e retículo de animais ruminantes, caracterizados por cílios dispostos em membranelas espiraladas ao redor da boca (adoral) e, em alguns gêneros, também em uma posição dorsal (metoral). Os gêneros mais importantes são *Entodinium, Diplodinium, Epidinium* e *Ophryoscolex*. Acredita-se que contribuem para a nutrição dos ruminantes ao converter a celulose existente nos vegetais ingeridos pelos ruminantes em proteína animal prontamente digerível por seus corpos. [G. *ophrys*, sobrancelha, + *skōlēx*, um verme]
oph·ry·o·sis (of-rē-ō′sis). Ofriose; a contratura espasmódica da parte palpebral do músculo orbicular do olho, provocando enrugamento da sobrancelha. [G. *ophrys*, sobrancelha, + *-osis*, condição]
ophthalm-. VER ophthalmo-.
ophthalmalgia (of′thal-mal′jē-ă). Oftalmalgia. SIN oculodynia. [ophthalmo- + G. *algos*, dor]
oph·thal·mia (of-thal′mē-ă). Oftalmia. **1.** Conjuntivite grave, freqüentemente purulenta. **2.** Inflamação das estruturas mais profundas do olho. [G.]
catarrhal o., o. catarral; uma forma branda de conjuntivite com secreção mucopurulenta.
caterpillar-hair o., o. nodosa. SIN o. nodosa.
Egyptian o., tracoma. SIN trachoma.
gonorrheal o., o. gonorreica; conjuntivite purulenta aguda provocada por *Neisseria gonorrhoeae*. SIN blennophthalmia (2), blennorrhea conjunctivalis, gonorrheal conjunctivitis.
granular o., tracoma. SIN trachoma.
metastatic o., o. metastática; **(1)** o. simpática; **(2)** coroidite na septicemia.
o. neonato′rum, o. neonatal; inflamação conjuntival que ocorre nos primeiros 10 dias de vida; as causas incluem *Neisseria gonorrhoeae, Staphylococcus, Streptococcus pneumoniae* e *Chlamydia trachomatis*. SIN blennorhea neonatorum, infantile purulent conjunctivitis, neonatal conjunctivitis.
o. niva′lis, ceratoconjuntivite por ultravioleta. SIN ultraviolet *keratoconjunctivitis.*
o. nodo′sa, o. nodosa; a presença de tumefações nodulares na conjuntiva, causadas pela penetração, nos tecidos oculares, de pêlos de lagarta. SIN caterpillar-hair o.
phlyctenular o., conjuntivite flictenular. SIN phlyctenular *conjunctivitis.*
purulent o., o. purulenta; conjuntivite purulenta, usualmente de origem gonorreica.
spring o., conjuntivite vernal. SIN vernal *conjunctivitis.*
sympathetic o., o. simpática; uveíte serosa ou plástica causada por uma ferida perfurante na úvea, seguida por uma reação grave similar no outro olho, podendo levar a cegueira bilateral. SIN transferred o.
transferred o., o. simpática. SIN sympathetic o.
oph·thal·mic (of-thal′mik). Oftálmico; relativo ao olho. SIN ocular (1). [G. *ophthalmikos*]
oph·thal·mic ac·id. Ácido oftálmico; um tripeptídeo que ocorre na lente do

olho, similar à glutationa, porém difere na substituição da cisteína pelo ácido α-amino-n-butírico (ou seja, na substituição do –SH por –CH$_3$); um potente inibidor de glioxalase. Cf. norophthalmic acid.

△ **ophthalmo-, ophthalm-.** Oftalmo-, oftalm-; formas combinantes relativas ao olho. VER TAMBÉM oculo-. [G. *ophthalmos*]

oph·thal·mo·dy·na·mom·e·ter (of - thal′mō - dī - nă - mom′e - ter). Oftalmodinamômetro; um instrumento para medir a pressão arterial nos vasos retinianos. [ophthalmo- + G. *dynamis*, força, + *metron*, medida]
   Bailliart o., o. de Bailliart; um instrumento utilizado para medir a pressão na artéria central da retina; valioso no diagnóstico da oclusão da artéria carótida proximal.
   suction o., o. de sucção; um o. com um disco de sucção que aumenta a pressão ocular durante a observação oftalmoscópica da artéria da retina.

oph·thal·mo·dy·na·mom·e·try (of - thal′mō - dī - nă - mom′e - trē). Oftalmodinamometria; a medição da pressão arterial nos vasos retinianos por meio de um oftalmodinamômetro. [ophthalmo- + G. *dynamis*, força, + *metron*, medida]

oph·thal·mo·lith (of - thal′mō - lith). Oftalmolito, dacriolito. SIN dacryolith. [ophthalmo- + G. *lithos*, pedra]

oph·thal·mol·o·gist (of - thal - mol′ō - jist). Oftalmologista; um especialista em oftalmologia. SIN oculist.

oph·thal·mol·o·gy (of - thal - mol′ō - jē). Oftalmologia; a especialidade médica relacionada com o olho, suas doenças e erros de refração. [ophthalmo- + G. *logos*, estudo]

oph·thal·mo·ma·la·cia (of - thal′mō - mă - lā′shē - ă). Oftalmomalacia; amolecimento anormal do bulbo do olho. [ophthalmo- + G. *malakia*, amolecimento]

oph·thal·mo·mel·a·no·sis (of - thal′mō - mel - ă - nō′sis). Oftalmomelanose; coloração melanótica da conjuntiva e dos tecidos adjacentes.

oph·thal·mom·e·ter (of - thal - mom′e - ter). Oftalmômetro, ceratômetro. SIN keratometer. [ophthalmo- + G. *metron*, medida]

oph·thal·mo·my·co·sis (of - thal′mō - mī - kō′sis). Oftalmomicose; qualquer doença do olho ou de seus apêndices causada por um fungo. [ophthalmo- + G. *mykēs*, fungo, + -*osis*, condição]

oph·thal·mo·my·i·a·sis (of - thal′mō - mī - ī′ă - sis). Oftalmomiíase. SIN ocular *myiasis.*

oph·thal·mop·a·thy (of - thal - mop′ă - thē). Oftalmopatia; qualquer doença dos olhos. SIN oculopathy. [ophthalmo- + G. *pathos*, sofrimento]
   endocrine o., o. endócrina. SIN Graves o.
   external o., o. externa; qualquer doença da conjuntiva, córnea ou anexos do olho.
   Graves o., o. de Graves; exoftalmia provocada pelo conteúdo hídrico aumentado dos tecidos orbitais retro-oculares; associada a doença tireóidea, usualmente ao hipertireoidismo. SIN endocrine o., Graves orbitopathy.
   internal o., o. interna; qualquer doença das estruturas internas do bulbo do olho.

oph·thal·mo·ple·gia (of - thal - mō - plē′jē - ă). Oftalmoplegia; paralisia de um ou mais dos músculos oculares. [ophthalmo- + G. *plēgē*, golpe]
   chronic progressive external o. (CPEO), o. externa progressiva crônica; um tipo específico de fraqueza dos músculos oculares que se agrava lentamente, associada em geral a retinopatia pigmentar. VER Kearns-Sayre *syndrome*, oculopharyngeal *dystrophy*. SIN ocular myopathy.
   exophthalmic o., o. exoftálmica; o. com protrusão do bulbo do olho devido ao conteúdo hídrico aumentado eventual dos tecidos orbitários nos distúrbios da tireóide, usualmente no hipertireoidismo.
   o. exter′na, o. externa; paralisia que afeta um ou mais músculos extrínsecos do olho. SIN external o.
   external o., o. externa. SIN o. externa.
   fascicular o., o. fascicular; o. decorrente de uma lesão no tronco cerebral.
   fibrotic o. [MIM*135700], o. fibrótica; o. que pode ser congênita em associação a blefaroptose; um distúrbio autossômico dominante.
   o. inter′na, o. interna; paralisia que afeta apenas o músculo esfíncter da pupila e o músculo ciliar. SIN internal o.
   internal o., o. interna. SIN o. interna.
   internuclear o. (INO), o. internuclear; o. nas lesões do fascículo longitudinal medial, com falha da adução na mirada horizontal, mas com conservação da convergência.
   nuclear o., o. nuclear; o. devido a uma lesão nos núcleos de origem dos nervos motores oculares.
   orbital o., o. orbital; o. decorrente de uma lesão na órbita.
   Parinaud o., o. de Parinaud. SIN Parinaud *syndrome*.
   o. partia′lis, o. parcial; o. incompleta que envolve apenas um ou dois dos músculos oculares extrínsecos ou intrínsecos.
   o. progressi′va, o. progressiva; paralisia bulbar superior progressiva, decorrente de degeneração dos núcleos dos nervos motores do olho.
   o. tota′lis, o. total; paralisia dos músculos oculares extrínsecos e intrínsecos.
   wall-eyed bilateral internuclear o. (WEBINO), o. internuclear bilateral exotrópica; uma forma de o. internuclear associada a exotropia.

oph·tha·mo·ple·gic (of - thal - mō - plē′jik). Oftalmoplégico; relativo a ou caracterizado por, oftalmoplegia.

ℹ **oph·thal·mo·scope** (of - thal′mō - skōp). Oftalmoscópio; um dispositivo para estudar o interior do bulbo do olho através da pupila. SIN fundoscope. [ophthalmo- + G. *skopeō*, examinar]
   binocular o., o. binocular; o. que fornece uma visão estereoscópica do fundo do olho.
   demonstration o., o. de demonstração; o. por meio do qual o fundo de olho pode ser observado simultaneamente por mais de uma pessoa.
   direct o., o. direto; um instrumento destinado a visualizar o interior do olho, sendo posicionado relativamente perto do olho da pessoa, com o observador visualizando uma imagem amplificada normal.
   indirect o., o. indireta; um instrumento destinado a visualizar o interior do olho, com o instrumento a uma distância equivalente ao comprimento do braço do olho da pessoa e o observador visualizando uma imagem invertida através de uma lente convexa localizada entre o instrumento e o olho da pessoa.

oph·thal·mo·scop·ic (of′thal - mō - skop′ik). Oftalmoscópico; relativo ao exame do interior do olho.

ℹ **oph·thal·mos·co·py** (of - thal - mos′kō - pē). Oftalmoscopia; exame do fundo de olho por meio do oftalmoscópio. SIN fundoscopy.

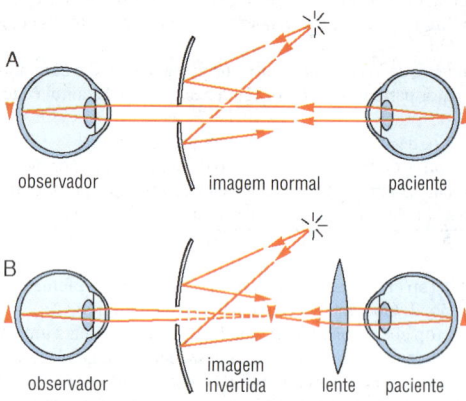

oftalmoscopia: a trajetória dos raios luminosos na oftalmoscopia (A) direta e (B) indireta, com imagem normal ou invertida, respectivamente

   direct o., o. direta; o. realizada com um oftalmoscópio direto.
   indirect o., o. indireta; o. realizada com um oftalmoscópio indireto.
   o. with reflected light, o. com luz refletida; exame da parte do fundo de olho adjacente a uma área iluminada por uma luz bem focalizada.

oph·thal·mo·trope (of - thal′mō - trōp). Oftalmótropo; um modelo dos dois olhos, com cada um deles estando preso a cordas que tracionam na direção dos seis músculos extrínsecos do olho; usado para mostrar a ação dos músculos oculares isoladamente ou em várias combinações. [ophthalmo- + G. *tropos*, uma virada]

oph·thal·mo·vas·cu·lar (of - thal′mō - vas′kū - lăr). Oftalmovascular; relativo aos vasos sanguíneos do olho.

△ **-opia.** Sufixo que significa visão. [G. *ōps*, olho]

opi·a·nine (ō - pī′ă - nēn). Opianina. SIN noscapine.

opi·a·nyl (ō - pī′ă - nil). Opianil. SIN meconin.

opi·ate (ō′pē - āt). Opiáceo; qualquer preparação ou derivado do ópio.

opine. (ō′pēn). Opina; um derivado de aminoácidos básicos, produzido por tumores da copa e galha em vegetais.

opi·o·cor·tin (ō′pē - ō - kōr′tin). Opiocortina. SIN opiomelanocortin.

opi·oid (ō′pē - oyd). Opióide; originalmente, um termo que indica narcóticos sintéticos semelhantes aos opiáceos, mas que é cada vez mais utilizado para se referir tanto aos opiáceos como aos narcóticos sintéticos.

opi·o·mel·a·no·cor·tin (ō′pē - ō - mel′ă - nō - kōr′tin). Opiomelanocortina; um polipeptídeo linear da hipófise que contém, em sua seqüência, as seqüências das endorfinas, MSH, ACTH e similares, que são decompostas enzimaticamente; a codificação da seqüência de nucleotídeo já foi determinada para várias espécies. SIN opiocortin.

opip·ra·mol hy·dro·chlo·ride (ō - pip′ră - mōl). Cloridrato de opipramol; dicloridrato de 4-[3-(5*H*-dibenz[*b.f*]azepin-5-il)propil]-1-piperazinetanol; um agente antidepressivo.

opis·the·nar (ō - pis′thē - nar). Opistenar; o dorso da mão. [G. as costas da mão, de *opisthen*, atrás, + *thenar*, palma da mão]

opis·thi·o·ba·si·al (ō - pis′thē - ō - bā′sē - ăl). Opistiobasial; relativo ao opístio e ao básio; indica uma linha que une os dois, ou a distância entre eles.

opis·thi·on (ō - pis′thē - on). Opístio; o ponto médio na margem posterior do forame magno, oposto ao básio. [G. *opisthios*, posterior]

opis·thi·o·na·si·al (ō-pis-thē-ō-nā′zē-āl). Opistionasal; relativo ao opístio e ao násio; indica a distância entre os dois pontos.

△ **opistho-**. Opisto-; forma combinante que indica para trás, por trás, dorsal. [G. *opisthen*, na retaguarda, por trás]

op·is·tho·chei·lia, op·is·tho·chi·lia (op′is-thō-kī′lē-ā). Opistoquilia; recessão dos lábios. [opistho- + G. *cheilos*, lábio]

opis·tho·mas·ti·gote (ō-pis-thō-mas′ti-gōt). Opistomastigota; termo atualmente utilizado, em lugar de herpetomônade, para o estágio de desenvolvimento de determinados flagelados que parasitam insetos e vegetais, de modo a evitar a confusão entre o estágio e o gênero *Herpetomonas*. Nesse estágio, o flagelo origina-se do cinetoplasto localizado atrás do núcleo e emerge da extremidade anterior do organismo; não há membrana ondulante. [opistho- + G. *mastix*, chicote]

op·is·thor·chi·a·sis (op′is-thōr-kī′a-sis). Opistorquíase; infecção pelo trematódeo hepático asiático, *Opisthorchis viverrini*, ou outros opistorquídeos.

op·is·thor·chid (op-is-thōr′kid). Opistorquídeo; nome comum para os membros da família Opisthorchiidae.

Opis·thor·chi·i·dae (op′is-thōr-kē′i-dē). Uma família de trematódeos que inclui os gêneros *Opisthorchis* e *Clonorchis*.

Opis·thor·chis (op-is-thōr′kis). Gênero de trematódeos digenéticos (família Opisthorchiidae) encontrado nos ductos biliares ou vesícula biliar de mamíferos que se alimentam de peixes, em pássaros e peixes. [opistho- + G. *orchis*, testículo]

 O. felin′eus, trematódeo do fígado do gato, uma espécie freqüentemente encontrada como parasita humano no leste europeu, Sibéria, Índia, Japão e Sudeste Asiático; os adultos exibem formato de lanceta, são finos, relativamente transparentes e hermafroditas, com os tamanhos variando de 7–12 por 2–3 mm; os ovos ingeridos eclodem em caramujos *Bithynia* e as cercárias encistam em várias espécies de peixes de água doce; os seres humanos adquirem a infecção ao ingerir peixe cru ou inadequadamente cozidos; os parasitas não causam, por vezes, nenhuma evidência de doença, mas podem ocorrer colangite, cirrose biliar e pancreatite crônica.

 O. sinen′sis, SIN *Clonorchis sinensis*.

 O. viverri′ni, uma espécie de trematódeo intimamente relacionada com *O. felineus*, muito comum em seres humanos na Tailândia; causa a opistorquíase.

op·is·thotic (op-is-thō′tik). Opistótico; por trás do ouvido. [opistho- + G. *ous*, (*ōt*-), ouvido]

op·is·thot·on·ic (op-is-thot′ō-nik, ō-pis′thō-ton′ik). Opistotônico; relativo a, ou caracterizado por, opistótono.

op·is·thot·o·noid (op-is-thot′ō-noyd). Opistotonóide; que se assemelha ao opistótono.

op·is·thot·o·nos, op·is·thot·o·nus (op-is-thot′ō-nŭs). Opistótono; espasmo tetânico em que a coluna vertebral e os membros apresentam convexidade para cima, com o corpo apoiando-se na cabeça e nos calcanhares. [opistho- + G. *tonos*, tensão, estiramento]

Opitz, John M., pediatra norte-americano, *1935. VER Smith-Lemli-O. *syndrome*; Opitz BBB *syndrome*; Opitz G *syndrome*.

opi·um (ō′pē-ŭm). Ópio; o exsudato leitoso seco ao ar livre obtido pela incisão de cápsulas verdes da *Papaver somniferum* (família Papaveraceae) ou de sua variedade, *P. album*. Contém cerca de 20 alcalóides, incluindo morfina, 9–14%; noscapina, 4–8%; codeína, 0,8–2,5%; papaverina, 0,5–2,5%, e tebaína, 0,5–2%. Usado como analgésico, hipnótico e diaforético, bem como na diarréia e nas condições espasmódicas. SIN gum opium, meconium (2). [L. de G. *opion*, suco de papoula]

 Boston o., o. de Boston; o. tão diluído após a importação, a ponto de mal satisfazer às exigências oficiais. SIN pudding o.

 deodorized o., denarcotized o., o. desodorizado, o. desnarcotizado; o. pulverizado tratado com benzina de petróleo purificada que remove determinados constituintes nauseantes e odorosos.

 granulated o., o. granulado; o. seco e reduzido a um pó grosseiro; contém 10 a 10,5% de morfina anidra.

 powdered o., o. pulverizado; o. seco e finamente pulverizado que contém 10% de morfina.

 pudding o., o. de Boston. SIN Boston o.

△ **opo-**. Opo-. 1. A face; um olho. VER TAMBÉM facio-. 2. Suco, bálsamo. [G. *ōps*]

op·o·bal·sa·mum (op-ō-bal′sa-mŭm). Opobálsamo. SIN *balm of Gilead*. [G. *opobalsamon*, o suco da árvore do bálsamo, de *opos*, suco, + *balsamon*]

op·o·did·y·mus (op-o-did′i-mŭs). Opodídimo; gêmeos unidos com um único corpo e duas cabeças fundidas nas costas com as regiões faciais parcialmente separadas. VER conjoined *twins*, em twin. [G. *ōps*, olho, face, + *didymos*, gêmeo]

Oppenheim, Hermann, neurologista de Berlim, 1858–1919. VER O. *disease, reflex, syndrome*; Ziehen-O. *disease*.

op·pi·la·tive (op-i-lā′tiv). Opilativo; que causa opilação (obstrução ou bloqueio) ou que tende a obstruir.

op·po·nens (ŏ′pō-nens). Oponente; um nome dado a diversos músculos dos dedos ou artelhos, cujas ações fazem com que esses dedos se oponham a outros. Os músculos oponentes das mãos atuam nas articulações carpometacarpais, fazendo com que a mão assuma um formato de concha; isso permite a flexão nas articulações metacarpofalângicas e a oposição do polegar com o dedo mínimo, ou vice-versa. Embora músculos comparáveis no pé sejam chamados de "oponentes", nenhuma oposição ocorre no pé. [L. *op-pono (obp-)*, part. pres. -*ens*, colocar contra, opor-se]

op·por·tun·is·tic (op′ōr-too-nis′tik). Oportunista. 1. Indica um organismo capaz de provocar doença apenas em um hospedeiro, cuja resistência está diminuída, p.ex., por outras doenças ou por medicamentos. 2. Indica uma doença causada por esse organismo.

op·po·sure (op′pō-shūr). Oposição; a junção dos tecidos durante a sutura.

op·sin. Opsina; a porção proteica da molécula da rodopsina; pelo menos três opsinas distintas estão localizadas nos cones.

op·sin·o·gen (op-sin′ō-jen). Opsinogênio; uma substância que estimula a formação de opsonina, como o antígeno contido em uma suspensão de bactérias usada para a imunização. SIN opsogen. [opsonin + -gen]

op·si·u·ria (op-sē-oo′rē-ā). Opsiúria; excreção mais rápida da urina durante o jejum que depois de uma refeição plena. [G. *opsi*, tardio, + *ouron*, urina]

op·so·clo·nus (op′sō-klō′nŭs). Opsoclono; movimentos do olho rápidos, irregulares e não-rítmicos nas direções horizontal e vertical. [G. *ōps, ōpos*, olho, + *klonos*, movimento confuso]

op·so·gen (op′sō-jen). Opsogênio. SIN opsinogen.

op·so·ma·nia (op′sō-mā′nē-ā). Opsomania; termo raramente utilizado para o desejo por determinado item da dieta ou para o alimento muito condimentado. [G. *opson*, condimento, + *mania*, loucura]

op·son·ic (op-son′ik). Opsônico; relativo às opsoninas ou à sua utilização.

op·so·nin (op′sō-nin). Opsonina; qualquer proteína sérica sanguínea que se liga a antígenos, estimulando a fagocitose (p.ex., C3b do sistema complemento, anticorpos específicos). [G. *opson*, carne fervida, provisões, de *hepsō*, ferver, + -*in*]

 common o., o. comum ou normal. SIN *normal o*.

 immune o., o. imune. SIN *specific o*.

 normal o., o. normal; o. normalmente existente no sangue, ou seja, sem estimulação por um antígeno específico conhecido, como determinados componentes do complemento; é relativamente termolábil e reage com vários organismos. SIN common o., thermolabile o.

 specific o., o. específica; anticorpos formados em resposta à estimulação por um antígeno específico, seja como resultado de um ataque de uma doença ou como conseqüência de injeções de uma suspensão adequadamente preparada do microrganismo específico. SIN immune o., thermostable o.

 thermolabile o., o. termolábil. SIN *normal o*.

 thermostable o., o. termoestável. SIN *specific o*.

op·son·i·za·tion (op′sō-nī-zā′shŭn). Opsonização; o processo pelo qual as bactérias e outras células são alteradas, de tal modo que sejam fagocitadas com maior rapidez e eficiência pelos fagócitos.

op·so·no·cy·to·pha·gic (op′sō-nō-sī′tō-fā′jik). Opsonocitofágico; pertinente à eficiência aumentada da atividade fagocítica dos leucócitos no sangue que contém opsonina específica. [opsonin + G. *kytos*, uma cavidade (célula), + *phagō*, comer]

op·so·nom·e·try (op-sō-nom′e-trē). Opsonometria; determinação do índice opsônico ou da atividade opsonocitofágica.

op·so·no·phil·ia (op-sō-nō-fil′ē-ā). Opsonofilia; a condição em que as bactérias se unem prontamente às opsoninas, sensibilizando-as para a fagocitose mais efetiva. [opsonin + G. *phileō*, amar]

op·so·no·phil·ic (op-sō-nō-fil′ik). Opsonofílico; pertinente a, caracterizado por ou que resulta em opsonofilia.

op·tic, op·ti·cal (op′tik, op′ti-kăl). Óptico; relativo ao olho, visão ou óptica. [G. *optikos*]

op·ti·cian (op-tish′an). Oculista; aquele que pratica a oculística.

op·ti·cian·ry (op-tish′an-rē). Oculística; a prática profissional de aviar prescrições de lentes oftálmicas, venda de óculos e fabricação e adaptação de lentes de contato.

△ **optico-**. VER opto-.

op·ti·co·cil·i·a·ry (op′ti-kō-sil′ē-ār-ē). Opticociliar; relativo aos nervos óptico e ciliar.

op·ti·co·pu·pil·lary (op′ti-kō-pū′pi-lār-ē). Opticopupilar; relativo ao nervo óptico e à pupila.

op·tics (op′tiks). Óptica; a ciência relacionada com as propriedades da luz, sua refração e absorção, e os meios de refração do olho nessa relação. [G. *optikos*, de *ōps*, olho]

 Nomarski o., o. de Nomarski; um sistema óptico para a microscopia de contraste de interferência diferencial.

 schlieren o., um sistema óptico, freqüentemente utilizado em estudos de difusão e centrifugação, que observa o gradiente do índice de refração nas soluções contendo macromoléculas.

op·ti·mism (op′ti-mizm). Otimismo; a tendência a ver o lado bom de todas as coisas, acreditar que existe algo bom em cada coisa. [L. *optimus*, melhor]

 therapeutic o., o. terapêutico; crença na eficácia dos medicamentos e outros agentes usados no tratamento das doenças.

op·ti·mum (op'ti-mŭm). Ótimo; o melhor ou o mais adequado; p.ex., indica a dose de um remédio que, provavelmente, proporciona o benefício máximo com efeitos colaterais mínimos, temperatura ou pH em que uma enzima apresenta a atividade máxima. [L. neut. sing. de *optimus*, melhor]

opto-, optico-. Formas combinantes que significam óptico, ocular. [G. *optikos*, óptico, de *ōps*, olho]

op·to·ki·net·ic (op'tō-ki-net'ik). Optocinético. VER optokinetic *nystagmus*. [opto- + G. *kinēsis*, movimento]

op·to·me·ninx (op'tō-mē'ninks). Retina. SIN retina. [opto- + G. *mēninx*, membrana]

op·tom·e·ter (op-tom'ĕ-ter). Optômetro; um instrumento para determinar a refração do olho. [opto- + G. *metron*, medida]
   objective o., refratômetro. SIN refractometer.

op·tom·e·trist (op-tom'ĕ-trist). Optometrista; aquele que pratica a optometria.

op·tom·e·try (op-tom'ĕ-trē). Optometria. **1.** A profissão relacionada com o exame dos olhos e estruturas correlatas para determinar se existem problemas de visão e distúrbios oculares e com a prescrição e ajuste das lentes e de outros auxílios ópticos ou uso de treinamento visual para a eficiência visual máxima. **2.** O uso de um optômetro.

op·to·my·om·e·ter (op'tō-mī-om'ĕ-ter). Optomiômetro; um instrumento para determinar a força relativa dos músculos extrínsecos do olho. [opto- + G. *mys*, músculo, + *metron*, medida]

op·to·types (op'tō-tīps). Optótipos; letras de teste. VER test types. [opto- + G. *typos*, tipo]

OPV Abreviatura para oral poliovirus *vaccine* (vacina oral para pólio). VER poliovirus *vaccines*, em *vaccine*.

ora, pl. **orae** (ō'ră, ō'rē). Uma orla ou uma margem. [L.]
   o. serra'ta retinae, ora serrata da retina; a extremidade serrilhada da parte óptica da retina, localizada um pouco atrás do corpo ciliar e marcando os limites da porção percipiente da membrana.

ora (ō'ră). Bocas; plural de L. *os*. [L.]

or·ad (ōr'ad). Adoral. **1.** Em direção à boca. **2.** Situado mais próximo à boca em relação a um ponto de referência específico; oposto a aboral. [L. *os* (*or*-), boca, + *ad*, para]

oral (ōr'ăl). Oral; relativo à boca. [L. *os* (*or*-), boca]

ora·le (ō-rā'lē). Ponto oral; ponto no lado lingual da terminação alveolar da sutura pré-maxilar. [L. mod. punctum *orale*, ponto oral, de L. *os* (*or*-), boca]

Oral Hy·giene In·dex (OHI). Índice de Higiene Oral; um índice utilizado em estudos epidemiológicos da doença dental para avaliar a placa dentária e o cálculo dental (tártaro) separadamente.

oral·i·ty (ōr-al'i-tē). Oralidade; na psicologia freudiana, um termo empregado para indicar a organização psíquica derivada, e característica, do período oral do desenvolvimento psicossexual.

Oram, Samuel, cardiologista inglês do século XX. VER Holt-O. *syndrome*.

or·ange (ōr'enj). Laranja. **1.** O fruto da laranjeira, *Citrus aurantium* (família Rutaceae). **2.** Uma cor entre o amarelo e o vermelho no espectro. Para corantes laranja individuais, ver o nome específico. [Fr. ant. *orenge*, do Ar. *nāranj*, com o *n* inicial sendo absorvido no artigo francês *une*]
   bitter o. peel, casca de l. amarga; a casca seca do fruto verde, porém plenamente desenvolvido; um agente flavorizante.
   bitter o. peel, dried, casca de l. amarga, seca; a parte externa seca do pericarpo do fruto maduro ou quase maduro; contém não menos que 2,5% de volume por peso do óleo volátil.
   bitter o. peel, fresh, casca de l. amarga, fresca; a parte externa do pericarpo do fruto maduro ou quase maduro; usada para preparar a tintura e o xarope.
   bitter o. peel oil, óleo de casca de l. amarga; óleo volátil obtido pela expressão da casca fresca da l. amarga.

or·ange G [C.I. 16230]. Laranja ou orange G; um azocorante, usado como corante citoplasmático em técnicas histológicas.

or·ange wood. Madeira da laranjeira; madeira macia utilizada em odontologia para a colocação de pontes, coroas, etc., através da pressão da mordedura, também empregada como um ponto de brilho no polimento de superfícies de raízes.

Orbeli, Leon A., fisiologista russo, 1882–1958. VER O. *effect*.

or·bic·u·lar (or-bik'ū-lăr). Orbicular; com formato semelhante a um olho; de forma circular. [L. *orbiculus*, um pequeno disco, dim. de *orbis*, círculo]

or·bic·u·la·re (ōr-bik-ū-lā'rē). Processo lenticular da bigorna. SIN lenticular *process* of incus. [L., de *orbiculus*, um pequeno disco]

or·bi·cu·la·ris (ōr-bik'ū-lā'ris). Orbicular. **1.** Circular; indicando uma estrutura circular ou em forma de disco. **2.** Músculo orbicular. SIN orbicular *muscle*. [L. de *orbiculus*, um pequeno disco]

or·bi·cu·lus cil·i·ar·is (ōr-bik'ū-lŭs sil-ē-ār'is) [TA]. Orbículo ciliar; a zona posterior intensamente pigmentada do corpo ciliar contínua com a retina na ora serrata. SIN ciliary disk, ciliary ring, pars plana. [L. mod.]

or·bit (ōr'bit) [TA]. Órbita; a cavidade óssea que contém o bulbo do olho e seus anexos; é formada de partes de sete ossos: os ossos frontal, maxilar, esfenóide, lacrimal, zigomático, etmóide e palatino. SIN orbita [TA], eye socket, orbital cavity.

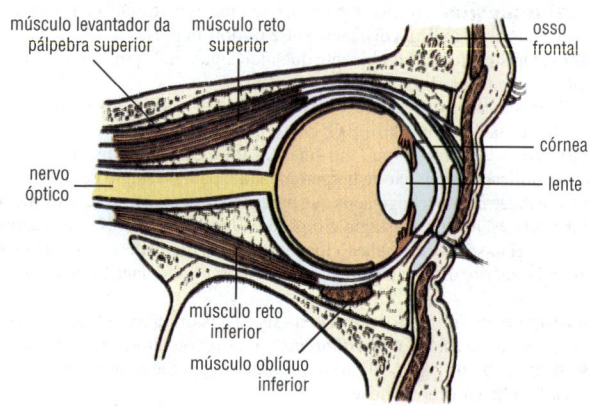

órbita: contendo o bulbo do olho e os músculos oculares

or·bi·ta, gen. **or·bi·tae** (ōr'bi-tă, -tē) [TA]. Órbita. SIN orbit. [L. um caminho circular, de *orbis*, círculo]

or·bi·tal (ōr'bi-tăl). Orbital; relativo à órbita.

or·bi·ta·le (ōr-bi-tā'lē). Em cefalometria, o ponto mais inferior na margem inferior da órbita óssea que pode ser palpado sob a pele. [L. de uma órbita]

or·bi·tog·ra·phy (ōr'bi-tog'ră-fē). Orbitografia; avaliação radiográfica da órbita. [L. *orbita*, órbita, + G. *graphō*, escrever]
   positive contrast o., o. de contraste positivo; a o. com injeção de um composto iodado hidrossolúvel no cone muscular ou ao longo do assoalho da órbita.

or·bi·to·na·sal (ōr'bi-tō-nā'săl). Orbitonasal; relativo à órbita e ao nariz ou cavidade nasal.

or·bi·to·nom·e·ter (ōr'bi-tō-nom'ĕ-ter). Orbitonômetro; um instrumento que mede a resistência oferecida à compressão do bulbo do olho para dentro de sua cavidade. [L. *orbita*, órbita, + G. *metron*, medida]

or·bi·to·nom·e·try (ōr'bi-tō-nom'ĕ-trē). Orbitonometria; a medição por meio do orbitonômetro.

or·bi·top·a·gus (ōr-bi-top'ă-gŭs). Orbitópago; gêmeos unidos desiguais nos quais o parasita, geralmente desenvolvido de maneira muito imperfeita, está ligado a uma órbita ao autósito. VER conjoined *twins*, em *twin*. SIN teratoma orbitae. [L. *órbita*, órbita, + G. *pagos*, algo fixo]

or·bi·top·a·thy. Orbitopatia; doença da órbita e de seu conteúdo.
   dysthyroid orbitopathy, orbitopatia tireoidiana; inflamação da órbita na doença de Graves.
   Graves orbitopathy, orbitopatia de Graves. SIN Graves *ophthalmopathy*.

or·bi·to·sphe·noid (ōr'bi-tō-sfē'noyd). Orbitoesfenóide; relativo à órbita e ao osso esfenóide.

or·bi·tot·o·my (ōr-bi-tot'ō-mē). Orbitotomia; incisão cirúrgica na órbita. [L. *orbita*, órbita, + *tomē*, uma incisão]

Or·bi·vi·rus (ōr'bi-vī-rŭs). Um gênero de vírus dos vertebrados (família Reoviridae) que se multiplica em artrópodes, incluindo determinados vírus originariamente incluídos com os arbovírus. Eles são antigenicamente distintos dos outros grupos de vírus e caracterizados por uma camada externa indistinta, porém algo grande, de capsômeros que fornecem a aparência de anéis (daí o nome). O gênero inclui, entre outros, o vírus da língua azul de carneiros e o vírus da doença eqüina africana. [L. *orbis*, anel, + virus]

or·ce·in (ōr'sē-in) [antigo C.I. 1242]. Orceína; corante natural derivado do orcinol por tratamento com ar e amônia, que, como um corante púrpura complexo, é empregado em vários métodos de coloração histológica.

orch·al·gia (ork-al'-jē-ă). Orquialgia. SIN orchialgia.

or·chec·to·my (ōr'kek'tō-mē). Orquiectomia. SIN orchiectomy.

or·chel·la (ōr-kel'ă). [antigo C.I. 1242] Rocelina. SIN archil.

orcheo-. VER orchio-.

orchi-, orchido-, orchio-. Orqui-, orquido-, orquio-; formas combinantes relativas aos testículos. [G. *orchis*, testículo]

or·chi·al·gia (ōr-kē-al'jē-ă). Orquialgia; dor no testículo. SIN orchalgia, orchiodynia, orchioneuralgia, testalgia. [orchi- + G. *algos*, dor]

or·chi·cho·rea (ōr'kē-kō-rē'ă). Orquicoréia; movimentos involuntários de subida e descida do testículo. [orchi- + G. *choreia*, uma dança]

or·chi·dec·to·my (ōr-ki-dek'tō-mē). Orquidectomia. SIN orchiectomy.

or·chid·ic (ōr-kid'ik). Orquídico; relativo ao testículo.

or·chi·di·tis (ōr-ki-dī'tis). Orquite. SIN orchitis.

orchido-. VER orchi-.

or·chi·dom·e·ter (ōr-ki-dom'ĕ-ter). Orquidômetro. **1.** Um dispositivo calibrador usado para medir o tamanho dos testículos. **2.** Um grupo de modelos de testículo de tamanho padronizado para comparação do desenvolvimento testicular. [orchido- + G. *metron*, medida]

or·chi·do·pexy (or-kid′o-peks-e). Orquidopexia. SIN orchiopexy.
or·chi·dop·to·sis (or′ki-dop-to′sis). Orquidoptose; ptose das gônadas masculinas. [orchido- + G. *ptōsis*, queda]
or·chi·dor·ra·phy (or-ki-dor′a-fe). Orquidorrafia. SIN orchiopexy.
or·chi·ec·to·my (or-ke-ek′to-me). Orquiectomia; remoção de um ou de ambos os testículos. SIN orchectomy, orchidectomy, testectomy. [orchi- + G. *ektomē*, excisão]
or·chi·ep·i·did·y·mi·tis (or′ke-ep′i-did′i-mi′tis). Orquiepididimite; inflamação dos testículos e epidídimo. [orchi- + epidídimo + G. *-itis*, inflamação]
or·chil (or′kil) [antigo C.I. 1242]. Rocelina. SIN archil.
orchio-. VER orchi-.
or·chi·o·cele (or′ke-o-sel). Orquiocele; um testículo retido no canal inguinal. [orchio- + G. *kēlē*, tumor]
or·chi·o·dyn·ia (or′ke-o-din′e-a). Orquiodinia. SIN orchialgia. [orchi- + G. *odynē*, dor]
or·chi·on·cus (or-ke-ong′kus). Orquioncose; uma neoplasia do testículo. [orchio- + G. *onkos*, volume, massa]
or·chi·o·neu·ral·gia (or′ke-o-noo-ral′je-a). Orquioneuralgia. SIN orchialgia. [orchio- + G. *neuron*, nervo, + *algos*, dor]
or·chi·op·a·thy (or′ke-op′a-the). Orquiopatia; doença de um testículo. [orchio- + G. *pathos*, sofrimento]
or·chi·o·pexy (or′ke-o-pek′se). Orquiopexia. **1.** Tratamento cirúrgico de um testículo não-descido com o propósito de liberá-lo e implantá-lo dentro da bolsa escrotal. **2.** Fixação de um testículo suscetível à torção na bolsa escrotal. SIN orchidopexy, orchidorraphy, orchiorrhaphy. [orchio- + G. *pēxis*, fixação]
transseptal o., o. transseptal. SIN Ombrédanne operation.
or·chi·o·plas·ty (or′ke-o-plas-te). Orquioplastia; reconstrução cirúrgica do testículo. [orchio- + G. *plastos*, formado]
or·chi·or·rha·phy (or-ke-or′a-fe). Orquiorrafia. SIN orchiopexy. [orchio- + G. *rhaphē*, uma sutura]
or·chi·o·ther·a·py (or′ke-o-thar′a-pe). Orquioterapia; tratamento com extratos testiculares.
or·chi·ot·o·my (or-ke-ot′o-me). Orquiotomia; incisão em um testículo. SIN orchotomy. [orchio- + G. *tomē*, incisão]
or·chis, pl. **or·chis·es** (or′kis, or′ki-sez). Testículo. SIN testis. [G. testículo, uma orquídea]
or·chit·ic (or-kit′ik). Orquítico; indica a orquite.
or·chi·tis (or-ki′tis). Orquite; inflamação do testículo. SIN orchiditis, testitis. [orchi- + G. *-itis*, inflamação]
o. parotid′ea, o. associada a caxumba.
traumatic o., o. traumática; inflamação simples do testículo causada por lesão mecânica.
o. vario′sa, o. variolosa; o. que é uma complicação da varíola.
or·chot·o·my (or-kot′o-me). Orquiotomia. SIN orchiotomy.
or·cin (or′sin). Orcinol. VER orcinol.
or·cin·ol (or′sin-ol). Orcinol; 3,5-diidroxitolueno; a substância-mãe do corante natural orceína, obtido de determinados líquens incolores (*Lecanora tinctoria, Rocella tinctoria*) através do tratamento com água fervente; usada como anti-séptico externo em inúmeras afecções cutâneas e em química como um reagente para pentoses. SIN 5-methylresorcinol, orcin.
or·ci·pren·a·line sul·fate (or-si-pren′a-len). Sulfato de orciprenalina. SIN metaproterenol sulfate.
ORD Abreviatura de optic rotatory *dispersion* (dispersão óptica rotatória).
Ord Símbolo para orotidina (orotidine).
or·deal bean (or′de-al). Fava de ordálio. SIN physostigma.
or·der (or′der). Ordem. **1.** Na classificação biológica, a divisão logo abaixo de classe (ou subclasse) e acima de família. **2.** Em uma reação, a o. é o somatório dos expoentes de todos os termos de concentração nessa expressão da velocidade da reação. Por exemplo, para a decomposição natural do pentóxido de nitrogênio, a expressão da velocidade é $v = -d[N_2O_5]/dt = k_1[N_2O_5]$. Portanto, essa é uma reação de primeira ordem. Uma reação que envolve dois compostos diferentes é, com freqüência, uma reação de segunda ordem (mas não necessariamente). As pseudo-reações de primeira ordem são reações de múltiplas ordens em que um dos reagentes existe em quantidades subestoquiométricas. Cf. molecularity. **3.** A seqüência de resíduos em um heteropolímero. [L. *ordo*, arranjo regular]
pecking o., o. de bicada; em algumas espécies de pássaros e primatas, o estabelecimento de uma dominância graduada entre os membros de um grupo através da agressão.
or·dered (ord′erd). Ordenado. SIN ordered mechanism.
or·der·ly (or′der-le). Um atendente em uma unidade hospitalar que auxilia no cuidado de pacientes.
or·di·nate (or′di-nat). Ordenada; em um sistema de coordenadas cartesiano, o eixo vertical (*y*). Cf. abscissa.
orec·tic (o-rek′tik). Oréctico; pertinente a, ou caracterizado por, orexia.
orex·ia (o-rek′se-a). Orexia. **1.** Os aspectos afetivo e instintivo de um ato, em contraste com o aspecto cognitivo. **2.** Apetite. SIN appetite. [G. *orexis*, apetite]
orex·i·gen·ic (o-rek-si-jen′ik). Orexígeno; que estimula o apetite.

orf. Orf; uma doença específica de carneiros e cabras, causada pelo vírus orf, família Poxviridae. Esse vírus é transmissível para os seres humanos e caracteriza-se por causar vesiculação e ulceração no local infectado. SIN contagious ecthyma, scabby mouth, soremouth. [I. ant. *orfcwealm*, gafeira, de *orf*, gado, + *cwealm*, destruição]
or·gan (or′gan) [TA]. Órgão; qualquer parte do corpo que exerce uma função específica, como da respiração, secreção ou digestão. SIN organum [TA], organon. [L. *organum*, do G. *organon*, um instrumento]
accessory o.'s, órgãos acessórios; **(1)** SIN accessory *structures*, em *structure*; **(2)** SIN supernumerary o.'s.
accessory o.'s of the eye, órgãos acessórios do olho. SIN accessory visual *structures*, em *structure*.
annulospiral o., o. anulospiral. SIN annulospiral *ending*.
auditory o., o. auditivo; termo arcaico para o o. de Corti.
Chievitz o., o. de Chievitz; uma estrutura epitelial normal, possivelmente um neurotransmissor, encontrada no ângulo da mandíbula com ramos do nervo bucal.
circumventricular o.'s, órgãos circumventriculares; quatro pequenas áreas na base do cérebro ou próximas a ela, que possuem capilares fenestrados e são externas à barreira hematoencefálica. Elas são a neuro-hipófise, área postrema [TA], órgão vascular da lâmina terminal [TA] e o órgão subfornicial [TA] (OSF). A neuro-hipófise é um órgão neuro-hemal. As outras três são quimiorreceptoras: a área postrema deflagra o vômito em resposta a alterações químicas no plasma, o órgão vascular da lâmina terminal percebe a osmolalidade e altera a secreção de vasopressina e o OSF inicia a ingestão de líquido em resposta à angiotensina II.
Corti o., o. de Corti. SIN spiral o.
critical o., o. crítico; o o. ou sistema fisiológico que, para uma determinada fonte de radiação, alcançaria em primeiro lugar sua exposição permissível máxima à radiação, legalmente definida, à medida que a dose de radiação é aumentada; p.ex., o rim é o órgão crítico, recebendo a radiação máxima, quando se administra o ácido dimetilsuccínico com Tc-99m.
enamel o., o. do esmalte; uma massa circunscrita de células ectodérmicas que brotam da lâmina dentária; assume um formato de taça, e, em sua face interna, surge a camada ameloblástica das células que produzem o revestimento do esmalte de um dente em desenvolvimento.
end o., o. terminal; a estrutura especial que contém a terminação de uma fibra nervosa em tecidos periféricos, como músculo, tecido, pele, mucosa ou glândulas. VER TAMBÉM ending.
external female genital o.'s, órgãos genitais femininos externos. SIN female external *genitalia*.
external male genital o.'s, órgãos genitais masculinos externos. SIN male external *genitalia*.
floating o., o. flutuante. SIN wandering o.
flower-spray o. of Ruffini, o. de Ruffini. SIN flower-spray *ending*.
genital o.'s, órgãos genitais. SIN genitalia.
Golgi tendon o., o. do tendão de Golgi; uma terminação nervosa sensorial proprioceptiva embebida entre as fibras de um tendão, freqüentemente próxima à junção musculotendinosa; é comprimido e ativado por qualquer aumento da tensão do tendão, provocada por contração ativa ou por estiramento passivo do músculo correspondente. SIN neurotendinous o., neurotendinous spindle.
gustatory o. [TA], o. gustatório; localizado nas papilas da mucosa da língua, principalmente nas papilas circunvaladas. SIN organum gustatorium [TA], organum gustus [TA], o. of taste.
o. of hearing, o. da audição. SIN cochlear *labyrinth*.
internal female genital o.'s, órgãos genitais femininos internos. SIN female internal *genitalia*.

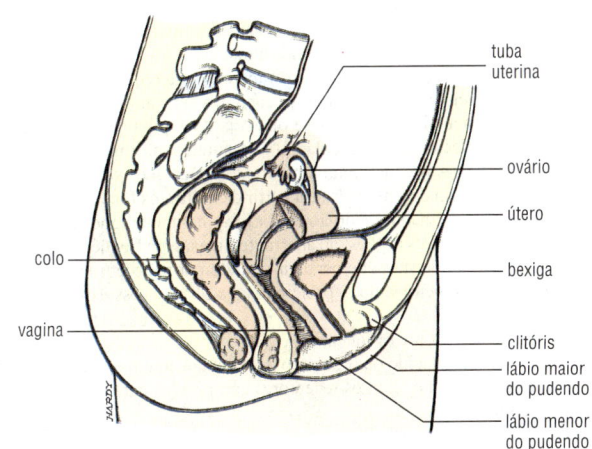

órgãos reprodutores femininos

internal male genital o.'s, órgãos genitais masculinos internos. SIN male internal *genitalia.*

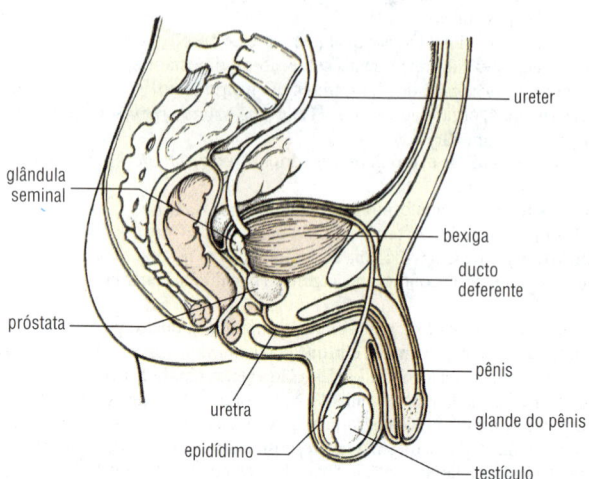

órgãos reprodutores masculinos

intromittent o., pênis. SIN penis.
Jacobson o., o. de Jacobson. SIN vomeronasal o.
neurohemal o.'s, órgãos neuro-hemais; áreas cerebrais a partir das quais as substâncias penetram no sangue, p.ex., a neuro-hipófise, a partir da qual a ocitocina e a vasopressina penetram no sangue.
neurotendinous o., o. neurotendinoso. SIN Golgi tendon o.
olfactory o. [TA], o. do olfato; a região olfatória na porção superior da cavidade nasal. SIN organum olfactus [TA], o. of smell.
otolithic o.'s, órgãos otolíticos; o utrículo e o sáculo da orelha interna que possuem otólitos e respondem à aceleração e desaceleração lineares, inclusive à gravidade.
ptotic o., o. migratório. SIN wandering o.
o. of Rosenmüller, o. de Rosenmüller. SIN epoophoron.
sense o.'s, órgãos dos sentidos; os órgãos de sentidos especiais, incluindo olho, ouvido, órgão do olfato, órgãos do paladar e as estruturas associadas a esses órgãos. SIN organa sensuum.
o. of smell, o. do olfato. SIN olfactory o.
spiral o. [TA], o. espiral; uma crista proeminente do epitélio extremamente especializado no assoalho do ducto coclear que se sobrepõe à membrana basilar da cóclea, contendo uma fileira interna e três fileiras externas de células ciliares ou células de Corti (as células receptoras auditivas inervadas pelo nervo coclear) sustentadas por várias células colunares; os pilares de Corti, células de Hensen e células de Claudius; o o. espiral fica parcialmente suspenso por uma projeção semelhante a um toldo, a membrana tectória, cuja zona marginal livre é coberta por uma substância gelatinosa na qual estão embebidos os estereocílios das células ciliares externas. SIN organum spirale [TA], acoustic papilla, Corti o.
subcommissural o. [TA], o. subcomissural; um órgão microscópico constituído de células ependimárias ciliadas colunares, localizado no aqueduto do mesencéfalo abaixo da comissura posterior; acredita-se que tenha uma função neurossecretora. SIN organum subcommissurale.
subfornical o. (SFO), o. subfornicial; o tubérculo intercolunar. Um dos órgãos circunventriculares. O SFO possui capilares fenestrados e é externo à barreira hematoencefálica. Acredita-se que seja uma zona quimiorreceptora envolvida na regulação cardiovascular. SIN organum subfornicale [TA].
supernumerary o.'s, órgãos supranumerários; órgãos que excedem o número normal, que podem desenvolver-se a partir de múltiplos focos de organização em um campo formador de órgão maior (originalmente) que aquele do o. principal definitivo; esses órgãos são aberrantes, mas, com freqüência, não são causa de doença; a doença pode persistir quando permanecem no corpo depois da remoção terapêutica do o. principal, p.ex., baço acessório. SIN accessory o.'s (2).
tactile o., o. do tato. SIN o. of touch.
target o., o.-alvo; um tecido ou o. sobre o qual um hormônio exerce sua ação; em geral, um tecido ou o. com os receptores apropriados para um hormônio. SIN target (3).
o. of taste, o. do paladar. SIN gustatory o.
o. of touch, o. do tato; qualquer um dos órgãos terminais sensoriais. SIN organum tactus, tactile o.

urinary o.'s, órgãos urinários; os órgãos envolvidos com a formação, armazenamento e excreção da urina. VER TAMBÉM urinary *system.* SIN organa urinária.
vascular o. of lamina terminalis [TA], o. vascular da lâmina terminal. VER circumventricular o.'s. SIN organum vasculosum laminae terminalis [TA].
vestibular o., o. vestibular. SIN vestibular *labyrinth.*
vestibulocochlear o. [TA], o. vestibulococlear; os ouvidos externo, médio e interno. SIN organum vestibulocochleare [TA].
vestigial o., o. vestigial; uma estrutura rudimentar, em seres humanos, que corresponde a uma estrutura funcional ou o. em animais inferiores.
o. of vision, o. da visão. SIN visual o.
visual o., o. visual; o olho e seus anexos. SIN o. of vision, organum visus.
vomeronasal o. [TA], o. vomeronasal; um fino canal horizontal vestigial, terminando em uma bolsa cega, na mucosa do septo nasal, começando exatamente atrás e acima do canal do incisivo; uma estrutura que geralmente regride depois do 6.º mês de gestação. Em muitos animais inferiores, funciona como um órgão olfatório acessório. SIN organum vomeronasale [TA], Jacobson o.
wandering o., o. migratório; um o. com inserções frouxas, permitindo seu deslocamento. SIN floating o., ptotic o.
Weber o., o. de Weber. SIN prostatic *utricle.*
o.'s of Zuckerkandl, órgãos de Zuckerkandl. SIN paraaortic *bodies*, em *body.*
or·ga·na (or'gă-nă). Órgãos; plural de organum.
or·gan·elle (or'gă-nel). Organela; uma das partes especializadas de um protozoário ou célula tecidual; essas unidades subcelulares incluem as mitocôndrias, o aparelho de Golgi, o núcleo e o centríolo, retículo endoplasmático granular e agranular, vacúolos, microssomas, lisossomas, membrana plasmática e determinadas fibrilas, bem como os plastídeos das células vegetais. SIN cell o., organoid (3). [G. *organon*, órgão, + Fr. *-elle*, dim. sufixo, do L. *-ella*]

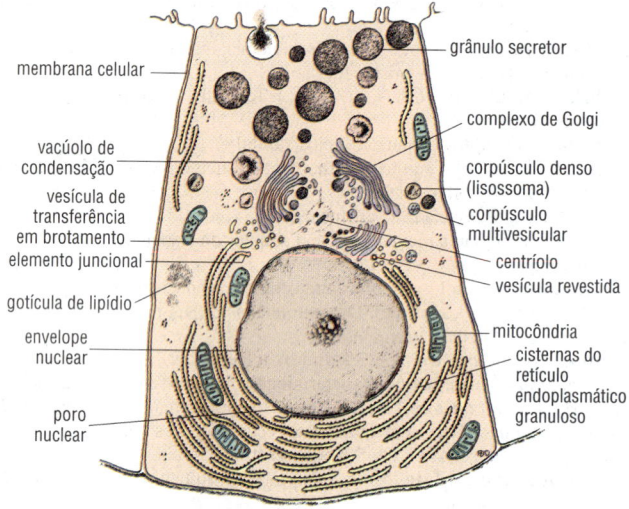

organelas: uma célula secretora como apareceria em um corte fino (microscopia eletrônica)

cell o., organela. SIN organelle.
paired o., o. pareada. SIN rhoptry.
or·gan·ic (or-gan'ik). Orgânico. **1.** Relativo a um órgão. **2.** Relativo a ou formado por um organismo. **3.** Organizado; estrutural. **4.** VER organic *compound.* [G. *organikos*]
or·gan·i·cism (or-gan'i-sizm). Organicismo; uma teoria que atribui a todas as doenças, em particular a todos os transtornos mentais, uma origem orgânica.
or·gan·i·cist (or-gan'i-sist). Organicista; aquele que acredita nos pontos de vista do organismo ou os subscreve.
or·gan·i·din. Nome comercial do glicerol iodado. SIN iodinated *glycerol.*
or·ga·nism (or'gă-nizm). Organismo; qualquer ser vivo, vegetal ou animal, considerado como um todo.
calculated mean o. (CMO), o. médio calculado; um o. hipotético cujas características são as médias das características positivas e negativas dos organismos que pertencem ao mesmo grupo taxonômico que o CMO, em oposição ao o. médio hipotético.
defective o., o. defeituoso. SIN auxotrophic *mutant.*
fastidious o., o. exigente; uma bactéria que possui requisitos nutricionais complexos.
hypothetical mean o. (HMO), o. médio hipotético; um o. hipotético cujas características são as médias das características positivas dos organismos que

pertencem ao mesmo grupo taxonômico que o HMO, em oposição ao o. médio calculado.

pleuropneumonia-like o.'s (PPLO), organismos semelhantes aos da pleuropneumonia; o nome original dado a um grupo de bactérias que não possuíam paredes celulares; esses organismos, isolados de seres humanos e outros animais, solo e esgoto, são atualmente classificados na ordem Mycoplasmatales.

or·ga·ni·za·tion (ōr'gan-i-zā'shŭn). Organização. **1.** Uma disposição de partes distintas, porém mutuamente dependentes. **2.** A conversão do sangue coagulado, exsudato ou tecido morto em tecido fibroso.

---

health maintenance o. (HMO), o. de manutenção da saúde; um sistema pré-pago e abrangente de assistência de saúde que enfatiza a prevenção e a detecção precoce da doença, bem como a continuidade dos cuidados; freqüentemente usado como sinônimo de "plano de atendimento gerenciado".

O termo HMO refere-se a um sistema de atendimento de saúde caracterizado pela multiplicidade de serviços (médicos de atendimento primário e especialistas, laboratório, radiologia, farmácia e hospitalização); pela restrição dos serviços aos conveniados e dos benefícios aos profissionais de saúde participantes, tipicamente confinados a determinada área geográfica; e por um sistema de contribuição baseado no pré-pagamento em lugar de honorários por serviços. Uma HMO pode ser uma instituição beneficente ou uma organização comercial. Durante os últimos 25 anos do século XX, as HMO surgiram como uma importante alternativa para os planos de saúde tradicionais, e os suplantaram. As HMO tiveram um profundo efeito sobre todos os aspectos da prática da medicina: profissional, científico, social, econômico e legal. Nos EUA, alguns estados, ao constatarem que as HMO controlavam quais serviços seriam apropriados para determinadas ciscunstâncias clínicas, promulgaram leis que tornaram a HMO passível de processo por mau exercício da medicina. VER TAMBÉM managed care.

---

preferred provider o. (PPO), o. com prestadores credenciados; um modelo de prestação de cuidados de saúde que utiliza um painel de médicos credenciados.
pregenital o., o. pré-genital; em psicanálise, a o. ou disposição da libido nos estágios anteriores ao da supremacia genital.
or·ga·nize (ōr'gan-īz). Organizar; prover com ou adquirir uma estrutura.
or·ga·niz·er (ōr'gan-ī-zer). Organizador. **1.** Originalmente aplicado a um grupo de células no lábio dorsal do blastóporo, que induzem a diferenciação das células no embrião e controlam o crescimento e desenvolvimento de partes adjacentes. **2.** Qualquer grupo de células que possui uma influência controladora desse tipo, sendo os efeitos produzidos através da ação de um evocador.
  nucleolar o., o. nucleolar; a região dos satélites nos cromossomas acrocêntricos que é ativa na formação do nucléolo. SIN nucleolar zone, nucleolus o.
  nucleolus o., o. do nucléolo. SIN nucleolar o.
  primary o., o. primário; o o. situado no lábio dorsal do blastóporo.
  procentriole o., deuterossoma. SIN deuterosome.
organo-. Forma combinante que designa órgão ou orgânico. [G. *organon*]
or·ga·no·ax·i·al (or-gā'nō-aks'ē-ăl). Organoaxial; rotação em torno do eixo longitudinal do órgão; um tipo de volvo gástrico.
or·gan·o·fer·ric (or-ga-nō-fār'ik). Organoférrico; relativo a um composto orgânico que contém ferro.
or·gan·o·gel (or-gan'ō-jel). Organogel; um hidrogel com um líquido orgânico em lugar da água como o meio de dispersão.
or·ga·no·gen·e·sis (ōr-gă-nō-jen'ĕ-sis). Organogênese; a formação de órgãos durante o desenvolvimento. SIN organogeny. [organo- + G. *genesis*, origem]
or·ga·no·ge·net·ic, or·ga·no·gen·ic (ōr'gă-nō-jĕ-net'ik, -jen'ik). Organogenético, organogênico; relativo à organogênese.
or·ga·nog·e·ny (ōr-gan-oj'ĕ-nē). Organogenia. SIN organogenesis.
or·ga·nog·ra·phy (ōr'gă-nog'ră-fē). Organografia; um tratado sobre os órgãos do corpo ou descrição desses órgãos. [organo- + G. *graphē*, uma escrita]
or·gan·oid (ōr'gă-noyd). Organóide. **1.** Que se assemelha superficialmente, em aspecto ou estrutura, a qualquer um dos órgãos ou glândulas do corpo. **2.** Composto de elementos glandulares ou orgânicos e não de um único tecido; pertinente a determinadas neoplasias (p.ex., um adenoma) que contêm elementos citológicos e histológicos dispostos em um padrão que se assemelha bastante ou é quase idêntico a um órgão normal. VER TAMBÉM histoid. **3.** SIN organelle. [organo- + G. *eidos*, semelhança]
or·ga·no·lep·tic (ōr'gă-nō-lep'tik). Organoléptico. **1.** Que estimula qualquer um dos órgãos da sensibilidade. **2.** Suscetível a um estímulo sensorial. [organo- + G. *lēptikos*, disposto a aceitar]
or·ga·nol·o·gy (ōr-gă-nol'ō-jē). Organologia; ramo da ciência relacionado com a anatomia, fisiologia, desenvolvimento e funções de vários órgãos. VER TAMBÉM splanchnology. [organo- + G. *logos*, estudo]
or·ga·no·meg·a·ly (ōr-gă-nō-meg'ă-lē). Organomegalia. SIN visceromegaly.
or·gan·o·mer·cu·ri·al (ōr-gan'ō-mer-kū'rē-ăl). Organomercurial; qualquer composto mercurial orgânico; p.ex., merbromina, timerosal.
or·ga·no·me·tal·lic (ōr'gă-nō-me-tal'ik). Organometálico; indica um composto orgânico que contém um ou mais átomos metálicos em sua estrutura.
or·ga·non, pl. **or·ga·na** (ōr-gă-non, ōr'gă-nă). Órgão, órgãos. SIN organ. [G. *órgão*]
or·ga·non·o·my (or-gă-non'ō-mē). Organonomia; o corpo de leis que regulam os processos de vida dos seres organizados. [organo- + G. *nomos*, lei]
or·ga·non·y·my (ōr'gă-non'i-mē). Organonimia; a nomenclatura dos órgãos do corpo, conforme diferenciado de toponimia. [organo- + G. *onyma*, nome]
or·ga·nop·a·thy (ōr-gă-nop'ă-thē). Organopatia; qualquer doença que afeta especialmente um dos órgãos do corpo. [organo- + G. *pathos*, sofrimento]
or·ga·no·pex·y, or·ga·no·pex·ia (ōr'gă-nō-pek-sē, -pek'sē-ă). Organopexia; fixação por sutura ou outro meio de um órgão flutuante ou migratório. [organo- + G. *pēxis*, fixação]
or·ga·no·phil·ic (ōr'gă-nō-fil'ik). Organofílico; pertinente à organofilia.
or·ga·no·phi·lic·i·ty (ōr'gă-nō-fi-lis'i-tē). Organofilia; atração das substâncias apolares (moléculas orgânicas) entre si.
or·ga·no·phos·phates (or-gă-nō-fos'fāts). Organofosforados; uma série de compostos orgânicos contendo fósforo que geralmente também contêm um íon halóide que reage com a colinesterase. Os organofosforados fosforilam a colinesterase e, dessa maneira, inibem-na de maneira irreversível. Usados como inseticidas; também já foram usados como gases de guerra.
or·gan·o·sol (or-gan'ō-sol). Organossol; um hidrossol com um líquido orgânico em lugar da água como o meio de dispersão.
or·ga·no·tax·is (ōr'gă-nō-tak'sis). Organotaxia; tendência a migrar seletivamente para determinado órgão. [organo- + G. *taxis*, disposição ordenada]
or·ga·no·ther·a·py (ōr'gă-nō-thăr'ă-pē). Organoterapia; tratamento da doença por preparações feitas a partir de órgãos de animais; agora freqüentemente são usadas preparações sintéticas em lugar de extratos de uma glândula.
or·ga·no·troph·ic (ōr'gă-nō-trof'ik). Organotrófico. **1.** Relativo à nutrição de um órgão. **2.** Pertinente a um microrganismo que utiliza os recursos orgânicos como uma força redutora. [organo- + G. *trophē*, nutrição]
or·ga·no·tro·pic (ōr'gă-nō-trop'ik). Organotrópico; pertinente a, ou caracterizado por, organotropismo.
or·ga·not·ro·pism (ōr'gă-not'rō-pizm). Organotropismo; a afinidade especial de determinados medicamentos, patógenos ou tumores metastáticos por determinados órgãos ou seus componentes. Cf. parasitotropism. SIN organotropy. [organo- + G. *tropē*, uma virada]
or·ga·not·ro·py (ōr-gă-not'rō-pē). Organotropia. SIN organotropism.
or·gan-spe·cif·ic. Órgão-específico. **1.** Indica, ou tem relação com, um soro produzido pela injeção das células de determinado órgão ou tecido que, quando injetado em outro animal, destrói as células do órgão correspondente. **2.** Indica um antígeno específico para determinado órgão.
or·ga·num, pl. **or·ga·na** (ōr'gă-num, ōr'gă-nă) [TA]. Órgão, órgãos. SIN organ, organ. [L. instrumento]
  o. audi'tus, o. da audição; termo arcaico para vestibulocochlear *organ* (órgão vestibulococlear).
  or'gana genita'lia [TA], órgãos genitais. SIN genitalia.
  organa genita'lia femini'na exter'na, órgãos genitais femininos externos. SIN female external *genitalia*.
  organa genita'lia femini'na inter'na, órgãos genitais femininos internos. SIN female internal *genitalia*.
  organa genita'lia masculi'na exter'na, órgãos genitais masculinos externos. SIN male external *genitalia*.
  organa genita'lia masculi'na inter'na, órgãos genitais masculinos internos. SIN male internal *genitalia*.
  o. gustatorium [TA], o. gustatório. SIN gustatory *organ*.
  o. gus'tus [TA], o. gustatório. SIN gustatory *organ*.
  or'gana oc'uli accesso'ria, órgãos acessórios do olho. SIN accessory visual *structures*, em *structure*.
  o. olfac'tus [TA], o. do olfato. SIN olfactory *organ*.
  or'gana sen'suum, órgãos dos sentidos. SIN sense *organs*, em *organ*.
  o. spira'le [TA], o. espiral. SIN spiral *organ*.
  o. subcommissurale, o. subcomissural. SIN subcommissural *organ*.
  o. subfornicale [TA], o. subfornicial. SIN subfornical *organ*. VER circumventricular *organs*, em *organ*.
  o. tac'tus, o. do tato. SIN *organ* of touch.
  or'gana urina'ria, órgãos urinários. SIN urinary *organs*, em *organ*.
  o. vasculosum laminae terminalis [TA], o. vascular da lâmina terminal. SIN vascular *organ* of lamina terminalis; VER circumventricular *organs*, em *organ*.
  o. vestibulocochlea're [TA], o. vestibulococlear. SIN vestibulocochlear *organ*.
  o. vi'sus, o. da visão. SIN visual *organ*.
  o. vomeronasa'le [TA], o. vomeronasal. SIN vomeronasal *organ*.
or·gasm (ōr-gazm). Orgasmo; o acme do ato sexual. SIN climax (2). [G. *orgaō*, dilatar-se, ficar excitado]

or·gas·mic, or·gas·tic (ōr-gaz′mik, -gas′tik). Orgástico; relativo a, característico do, ou que tende a produzir um orgasmo.

or·i·en·ta·tion (ōr-ē-en-tā′shŭn). Orientação. **1.** O reconhecimento das relações temporal, espacial e pessoal entre o indivíduo e o ambiente. **2.** A posição relativa de um átomo em relação a outro ao qual está ligado, ou seja, a direção da ligação que os une. [Fr. *orienter*, colocar em direção ao leste, portanto em uma posição definida]
  sexual o., o. sexual; o conceito que inclui as permutas entre a morfologia corporal, identidade sexual, função sexual e preferência sexual.

Orientia (ōr-ē-en′-ă). Um membro da família bacteriana Rickettsiae.
  O. tsutsugamushi, o único membro de seu gênero, essa espécie é o agente etiológico do tifo rural, transmitido por ácaros; originalmente chamada de *Rickettsia tsutsugamushi*.

or·i·en·to·my·cin (ōr′ē-en-tō-mī′sin). Nome comercial da ciclosserina. SIN cycloserine.

or·i·fice (or′i-fis) [TA]. Óstio, meato, poro; qualquer abertura ou hiato. VER TAMBÉM aperture, opening, os, ostium, meatus. SIN orificium [TA]. [L. *orificium*]
  anal o., ânus. SIN anus.
  aortic o. [TA], o. da aorta; a abertura a partir do ventrículo esquerdo para a aorta ascendente; é protegido pela valva aórtica. SIN ostium aortae [TA], aortic ostium.
  cardiac o., o. cárdico. SIN cardial o.
  cardial o. [TA], o. cárdico; a abertura do esôfago em formato de corneta para o estômago. SIN ostium cardiacum [TA], cardiac opening, cardiac o., esophagogastric o.
  esophagogastric o., o. cárdico. SIN cardial o.
  o. of external acoustic meatus, poro acústico externo. SIN external acoustic pore.
  external urethral o. [TA], o. externo da uretra; **(1)** a abertura da uretra semelhante a uma fenda na glande do pênis; **(2)** o orifício externo da uretra (na mulher) no vestíbulo, geralmente em uma pequena elevação, a papila uretral. SIN ostium urethrae externum [TA], external urinary meatus*, external opening of urethra, meatus urinarius, orificium urethrae externum.
  filling internal urethral o. [TA], o. interno da uretra no enchimento; o óstio interno da uretra quando a bexiga começa a ser distendida pela urina, estando os músculos do trígono contraídos e o músculo detrusor relaxado; durante esse estágio, o orifício localiza-se em um nível mais elevado e é limitado por uma porção da mucosa que não aquela durante a micção. VER TAMBÉM voiding internal urethral o. SIN ostium urethrae internum accipiens [TA].
  gastroduodenal o., o. pilórico. SIN pyloric o.
  golf-hole urethral o., o. uretral em buraco de golfe; um o. uretral circular e, com freqüência, muito lateral que pode estar associado a refluxo vesicoureteral, cirurgia vesical prévia ou tuberculose.
  ileal o. [TA], o. ileal; a abertura do íleo terminal para o intestino grosso na transição entre o ceco e o colo ascendente. SIN ostium ileale [TA], o. of ileal papilla*, ileocecal opening, ileocecal o., ostium ileocecale.
  o. of ileal papilla, o. ileal;* termo oficial alternativo para ileal o.
  ileocecal o., o. ileal. SIN ileal o.
  o. of inferior vena cava, o. da veia cava inferior. SIN opening of inferior vena cava.
  o. of internal acoustic meatus, poro acústico interno. SIN internal acoustic pore.
  internal urethral o. [TA], o. interno da uretra; a abertura ou orifício interno da uretra no ângulo anterior e inferior do trígono. SIN ostium urethrae internum [TA], internal urethral opening*.
  left atrioventricular o. [TA], o. atrioventricular esquerdo; uma abertura atrioventricular que leva do átrio esquerdo para o ventrículo esquerdo do coração. SIN ostium atrioventriculare sinistrum [TA], mitral o., ostium arteriosum.
  mitral o., o. atrioventricular esquerdo. SIN left atrioventricular o.
  pulmonary o., óstio do tronco pulmonar. SIN opening of pulmonary trunk.
  pyloric o. [TA], o. pilórico; a abertura entre o estômago e a parte superior do duodeno. SIN ostium pyloricum [TA], gastroduodenal o.
  right atrioventricular o. [TA], o. atrioventricular direito; uma abertura atrioventricular que leva do átrio direito para dentro do ventrículo direito do coração. SIN ostium atrioventriculare dextrum [TA], ostium venosum cordis, tricuspid o.
  root canal o., o. do canal radicular; uma abertura no compartimento pulpar que leva ao canal radicular.
  o. of superior vena cava, o. da veia cava superior. SIN opening of superior vena cava.
  tricuspid o., o. atrioventricular direito. SIN right atrioventricular o.
  ureteric o. [TA], o. do ureter; a abertura do ureter em cada ângulo lateral do trígono da bexiga; um o. muito dilatado geralmente indica o refluxo vesicoureteral. SIN ostium ureteris [TA], orificium ureteris, ureteral meatus, ureteral opening.
  o. of uterus, o. do útero. SIN external os of uterus.
  vaginal o. [TA], o. da vagina; a porção mais estreita do canal, no assoalho do vestíbulo posterior ao óstio da uretra. SIN ostium vaginae [TA], orificium vaginae, vaginal opening.
  o. of vermiform appendix [TA], o. do apêndice vermiforme; a abertura do apêndice vermiforme para a luz do ceco. SIN ostium appendicis vermiformis [TA], ostium of vermiform appendix.
  voiding internal urethral o. [TA], o. interno da uretra no esvaziamento; o óstio interno da uretra quando a bexiga está sendo esvaziada, os músculos do trígono estão relaxados e o músculo detrusor está contraindo; durante esse estágio, o óstio ocorre em um nível mais baixo, sendo limitado por uma porção da mucosa que não aquela durante o enchimento e o acúmulo de urina. VER TAMBÉM filling internal urethral o. SIN ostium urethrae internum evacuans [TA].

or·i·fi·cial (ōr-i-fish′ăl). Relativo a um orifício de qualquer tipo.

or·i·fi·ci·um, pl. **or·i·fi·cia** (ōr-i-fish′ē-ŭm, -ă) [TA]. Óstio. SIN orifice, orifice [L.].
  o. exter′num u′teri, o. externo do útero. SIN external os of uterus.
  o. inter′num u′teri, o. interno do útero. SIN isthmus of uterus.
  o. ure′teris, o. do ureter. SIN ureteric orifice.
  o. ure′thrae exter′num, o. externo da uretra. SIN external urethral orifice.
  o. vagi′nae, o. da vagina. SIN vaginal orifice.

orig·a·num oil (ō-rig′ă-nŭm). Óleo de manjerona; o óleo volátil (que contém carvacrol) obtido de diversas espécies de *Origanum* (família Labiatae); usado como rubefaciente, como um constituinte em linimentos veterinários e em técnicas microscópicas.

or·i·gin (ōr′i-jin). Origem. **1.** O menos móvel dos dois pontos de inserção de um músculo, aquele que está preso à parte mais fixa do esqueleto. **2.** O ponto inicial de um nervo craniano ou espinal. O primeiro apresenta duas origens: a **o. interna, o. profunda** ou **o. real**, o grupo celular no cérebro ou bulbo, de onde se originam as fibras do nervo, e a **o. externa, o. superficial** ou **o. aparente**, o ponto em que o nervo emerge do cérebro. [L. *origo*, fonte, início, de *orior*, levantar]
  o. of replication, o. da replicação; uma seqüência do genoma bacteriano necessária para o início da duplicação por meio da síntese do filamento condutor.

ori·za·ba jal·ap root (ō-riz′ă-bă ja′lap). Raiz seca de *Ipomoea orizabensis*. SIN ipomea.

Ormond, John K., urologista norte-americano, *1886. VER O. disease.

Orn Símbolo de ornithine (ornitina) ou seu radical.

or·nate (ōr′nāt). Adornado; um termo que se refere ao padrão do escudo (marcas cinza ou brancas em um fundo escuro) de carrapatos ixodídeos. [L. *ornatus*, decorado]

Ornish, Dean, médico norte-americano, *1953. VER O. reversal *diet*.

or·ni·thine (Orn) (ōr′ni-thēn, -thin). Ornitina; ácido 2,5-diaminovalérico; o L-isômero é o aminoácido formado quando a L-arginina é hidrolisada pela arginase; não é um constituinte de proteínas, mas é um importante intermediário no ciclo da uréia; níveis elevados são observados em determinados defeitos do ciclo da uréia.
  o. acetyltransferase, o. acetiltransferase. SIN glutamate acetyltransferase.
  o. δ-aminotransferase, o. δ-aminotransferase; enzima que catalisa de maneira reversível a reação do α-cetoglutarato e L-o. para formar L-glutamato e L-glutamato γ-semialdeído; a deficiência dessa enzima resultará em atrofia circinada da coróide e retina. SIN o. transaminase.
  o. carbamoyltransferase, o. carbamoiltransferase; enzima que catalisa a formação de L-citrulina e ortofosfato a partir de L-ornitina e carbamoil fosfato; uma parte do ciclo da uréia; a deficiência dessa enzima resultará em intoxicação por amônia e comprometimento da formação da uréia. SIN o. transcarbamoylase.
  o. decarboxylase, o. descarboxilase; enzima que catalisa a descarboxilação de L-o. em putrescina e CO_2; primeira etapa na biossíntese da poliamina.
  o. transaminase, o. transaminase. SIN o. δ-aminotransferase.
  o. transcarbamoylase, o. transcarbamoilase. SIN o. carbamoyltransferase.

or·ni·thi·ne·mia (ōr′ni-thi-nē′mē-ă). Ornitinemia; condição tóxica que, ocasionalmente, provoca edema cerebral localizado; causada por níveis anormais de ornitina no sangue. [ornithine + G. *haima*, sangue]

or·ni·thi·nu·ria (ōr′ni-thi-noo′rē-ă). Ornitinúria; excreção exagerada de ornitina pela urina.

Or·ni·thod·o·ros (ōr-ni-thod′ō-rŭs). Um gênero de carrapatos de casca mole (família Argasidae), da qual várias espécies são vetores de patógenos de diversas febres recidivantes. Caracterizam-se por um capítulo oculto sob o capuz e por discos e mamilas de tegumento que são contínuos desde a superfície dorsal até a ventral, em vários padrões. [G. *ornis* (*ornith-*), pássaro, + *doros*, uma bolsa de couro]
  O. coria′ceus, uma espécie de carrapato comum em áreas costeiras montanhosas da Califórnia; os adultos atacam facilmente o cervo, o gado bovino e os seres humanos; sua picada é irritante, dolorosa e, por vezes, tóxica. Transmite o aborto bovino epizoótico para o gado bovino. SIN pajaroello.
  O. errat′icus, uma espécie de carrapato da qual a variedade pequena é o vetor da *Borrelia crocidurae* na África, no Oriente Próximo e Ásia Central; a variedade grande é o vetor da *B. hispanica* na península hispânica e Norte da África.
  O. herm′si, uma espécie de carrapato que é um parasita de roedores e vetor dos espiroquetas da febre recidivante, como *Borrelia hermsii*, no Oeste dos Estados Unidos e Canadá.

O. lahoren'sis, uma espécie de carrapato que transmite a *Borrelia persica*, o agente da febre recidivante persa.

O. mouba'ta complex, um grupo de quatro espécies de carrapatos; a taxonomia e a ecologia desse complexo são muito importantes porque seus membros são vetores dos espiroquetas das febres recidivantes; os membros do complexo incluem *O. moubata* (vários hospedeiros), *O. compactus* (tartarugas), *O. apertus* (porco-espinho) e *O. porcinus* (javalis africanos); uma subespécie doméstica de *O. porcinus*, por sua vez, forma três cepas que se alimentam principalmente em seres humanos, aves e suínos.

O. pappil'ipes, o "percevejo persa", uma espécie de carrapato encontrada na Ásia Central e no Oriente Próximo que transmite *Borrelia persica*, o patógeno na febre recidivante persa no Irã.

O. par'keri, uma espécie de carrapato encontrado no oeste dos Estados Unidos e um vetor da *Borrelia parkeri*.

O. ru'dis, uma espécie de carrapato que é um vetor importante de espiroquetas da febre recidivante nas Américas Central e do Sul; possivelmente outro complexo similar ao complexo do *O. moubata*.

O. savi'gni, uma espécie de carrapato que transmite *Borrelia*, um agente da febre recidivante do leste da África, sul do Egito, Etiópia e sudoeste da Ásia.

O. talajé, uma espécie de carrapato encontrada no México e nas Américas Central e do Sul, onde se alimenta em roedores selvagens, animais domésticos e seres humanos; sua picada é dolorosa e irritante, sendo um vetor da *Borrelia mazzottii*, uma causa de febre recidivante.

O. tholoza'ni, uma espécie de carrapato que transmite a *Borrelia persica*, um agente da febre recidivante no Oriente Médio e Ásia Central.

O. turica'ta, uma espécie de carrapato que ataca prontamente os seres humanos e outros animais na porção sul dos Estados Unidos e México; é um vetor da *Borrelia turicatae*, um agente de febre recidivante; a picada é dolorosa e irritante.

O. venezuelen'sis, uma espécie de carrapato que é o vetor da *Borrelia venezuelensis*, o agente da febre recidivante na Colômbia, Venezuela e regiões montanhosas da América do Sul.

O. verruco'sus, uma espécie de carrapato, o vetor da *Borrelia caucasica*.

Or·ni·tho·nys·sus (ōr-ni-thon′i-sŭs). Um gênero de ácaros de pássaros e roedores; as espécies incluem *O. bacoti*, o ácaro do rato tropical, um possível vetor do tifo murino e uma causa de dermatite em seres humanos; *O. bursa*, o ácaro de aves tropicais; e o *O. sylviarum*, o ácaro das aves do norte. [G. *ornis* (*ornith-*), pássaro, + *nyssus*, bicar]

or·ni·tho·sis (ōr-ni-thō′sis). Ornitose; originalmente, uma doença em aves não-psitacídeas (galináceos domésticos, patos, pombos, perus e muitos pássaros selvagens) causada pela *Chlamydia psittaci*; agora, geralmente referido como a psitacose. [G. *ornis* (*ornith-*), pássaro, + *-osis*, condição]

Oro Símbolo de orotic acid (ácido orótico) ou orotate (orotato).

oro-. **1.** Forma combinante relativa a boca. [L. *os, oris*, boca] **2.** A ortografia alternativa obsoleta é orrho-. VER sero-. [G. *orrhos*, soro]

or·o·dig·i·to·fa·cial (ōr′o-dij′i-tō-fā′shăl). Orodigitofacial; relativo a boca, aos dedos da mão e à face.

or·o·fa·cial (ōr-ō-fā′shăl). Orofacial; relativo à boca e à face.

or·o·lin·gual (ōr-ō-ling′gwăl). Orolingual; relativo à boca e à língua.

or·o·na·sal (ōr-ō-nā′săl). Oronasal; relativo à boca e ao nariz.

or·o·pha·ryn·ge·al (ōr-ō-fă-rin′jē-ăl). Orofaríngeo; relativo à orofaringe.

or·o·phar·ynx (ōr′ō-far′ingks) [TA]. Orofaringe; a porção da faringe que se situa posterior à boca; é contínua, acima, com a nasofaringe através do istmo da faringe e, abaixo, com a laringofaringe. SIN pars oralis pharyngis [TA], oral part of pharynx, oral pharynx. [L. *os* (*or-*), boca]

or·o·so·mu·coid (ōr′ō-sō-mū′koyd). Orosomucóide; glicoproteína α₁-ácida; um subgrupo da fração α₁-globulina do sangue; níveis plasmáticos aumentados estão associados a inflamação. SIN α₁-acid glycoprotein, acid seromucoid.

or·o·tate (Oro) (ōr′ō-tāt). Orotato; um sal ou éster do ácido orótico.

o. phosphoribosyltransferase, o. fosforribosiltransferase; uma fosforribosiltransferase que sintetiza orotidilato e pirofosfato a partir de orotato e 5-fosfo-α-D-ribosil-1-pirofosfato; essa enzima é uma parte da biossíntese de pirimidina; a deficiência dessa enzima está associada a acidúria orótica do tipo I. Cf. *uridylic acid* synthase. SIN OMP pyrophosphorylase, orotidylic acid phosphorylase, orotidylic acid pyrophosphorylase.

orot·ic ac·id (Oro) (ōr-ot′ik) Ácido orótico; 6-carboxiuracil; ácido uracil-6-carboxílico; um importante intermediário na formação das pirimidinas nucleotídeos; elevado em determinados defeitos hereditários da biossíntese da pirimidina. SIN uracil-6-carboxylic acid.

orot·ic ac·i·du·ria [MIM*258900]. Acidúria orótica; um raro distúrbio do metabolismo da pirimidina caracterizado por anemia hipocrômica com alterações megaloblásticas na medula óssea, leucopenia, retardo do crescimento e excreção urinária de ácido orótico; herança autossômica recessiva, causada por mutação do gene da uridina monofosfatato sintase (MMPS) em 3q13. [orotic acid + G. *ouron*, urina]

orot·i·dine (O, Ord) (ō-rot′i-dēn) Orotidina; ácido-3-β-D-ribonucleosídeo; ácido uridina-6-carboxílico; elevada nos casos de orotidinúria. SIN 1-ribosylorotate.

o. 5′-monophosphate (OMP), 5′-monofosfato de o. SIN orotidylic acid.

orot·i·di·nu·ria (ō-rot′i-dĕn-ū′rē-ă). Orotidinúria; níveis urinários elevados de orotidina; foi observada nos defeitos da descarboxilase do ácido orotidílico e em sua inibição.

orot·i·dyl·ate (OMP) (ō-rot-i-dil′āt). Orotidilato; um sal ou éster do ácido orotidílico.

orot·i·dyl·ic ac·id (OMP) (ō-rot-i-dil′ik). Ácido orotidílico; 5′-monofosfato de orotidina; um intermediário na biossíntese dos nucleosídeos pirimidinas (citidina e uridina) que são encontrados em ácido nucleico. SIN orotidine 5′-monophosphate.

o. a. decarboxylase, descarboxilase do ácido orotidílico; uma enzima que catalisa a conversão do OMP em UMP e CO₂; um defeito ou inibição dessa enzima resultará em acidúria orótica e orotidinúria; essa enzima faz parte da biossíntese da pirimidina. Cf. *uridylic acid* synthase. SIN OMP decarboxylase.

o. a. phosphorylase, fosforilase do ácido orotidílico. SIN orotate phosphoribosyltransferase.

o. a. pyrophosphorylase, pirofosforilase do ácido orotidílico. SIN orotate phosphoribosyltransferase.

or·phan (ōr′făn). Órfão. VER orphan *products*, em *product*. [G. *orphanos*]

or·phen·a·drine cit·rate (ōr-fen′ă-drēn). Citrato de orfenadrina; um anti-histamínico que também possui a mesma ação e uso do cloridrato de orfenadrina.

or·phen·a·drine hy·dro·chlo·ride. Cloridrato de orfenadrina; reduz o espasmo de músculos voluntários, provavelmente por ação sobre as áreas motoras cerebrais; usado no tratamento sintomático da paralisia agitante e do parkinsonismo fármaco-induzido.

orrho-. Orro-; forma combinante que indica soro. VER sero-. [G. *orrhos, oros*, soro]

or·ris (ōr′is). Íris. SIN iris.

Orsi, Francesco, médico italiano, 1828–1890. VER O.-Grocco *method*.

Orth, Johannes J., patologista alemão, 1847–1923. VER O. *fixative, stain*.

orth-. VER ortho-.

or·the·sis (ōr-thē′sis). Órtese; termo raramente utilizado para um suporte, tala ou aparelho ortopédico. [ortho- + -esis, processo]

or·thet·ics (ōr-thet′iks). Ortóptica. SIN orthotics.

ortho-, orth-. Orto-, ort-. **1.** Prefixo que indica reto, normal, na ordem adequada. **2** (*o-*). Em química, prefixo em itálico que indica que um composto possui duas substituições nos átomos de carbono adjacentes em um anel benzênico. Para os termos que começam com *ortho*- ou *o-*, veja o nome específico. **3.** O mais hidratado de uma série de oxoácidos, p.ex., ácido ortofosfórico, H₃PO₄. [G. *orthos*, correto]

or·tho·ac·id (ōr′thō-as′id). Ortoácido; um ácido em que o número de grupamentos hidroxila iguala-se à valência do elemento formador do ácido; p.ex., C(OH)₄, ácido ortocarbônico. Quando não existe esse ácido, aquele que mais se aproxima dessa condição é por vezes chamado de o.; p.ex., OP(OH)₃, ácido ortofosfórico.

or·tho·caine (ōr′thō-kān). Ortocaína; o éster metílico do ácido 3-amino-4-hidroxibenzóico; agente anestésico de superfície geralmente utilizado na forma de pó.

or·tho·ce·phal·ic (ōr′thō-sĕ-fal′ik). Ortocefálico; que possui uma cabeça proporcional à altura; indica um crânio com um índice vertical entre 70 e 75. VER TAMBÉM metriocephalic. SIN orthocephalous. [ortho- + G. *kephalē*, cabeça]

or·tho·ceph·a·lous (ōr-thō-sef′ă-lŭs). Ortocéfalo. SIN orthocephalic.

or·tho·chro·mat·ic (ōr′thō-krō-mat′ik). Ortocromático; indica qualquer tecido ou célula que adquire a cor do corante empregado, ou seja, a mesma coloração da solução usada no processo. SIN euchromatic (1), orthochromophil, orthochromophile. [ortho- + G. *chrōma*, cor]

or·tho·chro·mo·phil, or·tho·chro·mo·phile (ōr-thō-krō′mō-fil, -fil). Ortocromófilo. SIN orthochromatic. [ortho- + G. *chrōma*, cor, + *philos*, ligação]

or·tho·cra·sia (ōr-thō-krā′sē-ă). Ortocrasia; termo obsoleto para a condição em que existe uma reação normal a drogas, componentes da dieta, etc. [ortho- + G. *krasis*, uma mistura, temperamento]

or·tho·cy·to·sis (ōr′thō-si-tō′sis). Ortocitose; uma condição em que todos os elementos celulares no sangue circulante são formas maduras, independentemente das proporções dos vários tipos e do número total. [ortho- G. *kytos*, célula, + -osis, condição]

or·tho·den·tin (ōr-thō-den′tin). Ortodentina; dentina tubular reta conforme se observa nos dentes de mamíferos.

or·tho·de·ox·ia. Ortodeoxia; queda no oxigênio arterial ao ficar de pé. Geralmente causada por derivação (*shunt*) vascular ou cardíaca da direita para a esquerda, com queda na pressão do lado esquerdo induzida pela postura, possibilitando um gradiente correspondente através da derivação.

or·tho·di·gi·ta (or-tho-dij′i-tah). Ortodigitismo; correção das malformações dos dedos das mãos ou artelhos. [ortho- + L. *digitus*, dedo ou artelho]

or·tho·don·tia (ōr-thō-don′shē-ă). Ortodontia. SIN orthodontics.

or·tho·don·tics (ōr-thō-don′tiks). Ortodontia; o ramo da odontologia relacionado com a correção e prevenção das irregularidades e má oclusão dos dentes. SIN dental orthopedics, orthodontia. [orhto- + G. *odous*, dente]

surgical o., o. cirúrgica; a correção das anormalidades de oclusão através do reposicionamento cirúrgico de segmentos da mandíbula ou maxila que contêm um ou mais dentes; ou o reposicionamento corporal de toda a mandíbula para melhorar a função e a estética. SIN orthognathic surgery.

or·tho·dont·ist. Ortodontista; um odontólogo que pratica a ortodontia.

or·tho·dro·mic (or - thō - drō'mik). Ortodrômico; indica a propagação de um impulso ao longo de um sistema de condução (p.ex., fibra nervosa) na direção em que ele viaja normalmente. Cf. antidromic. [ortho- + G. *dromos*, trajeto]

or·tho·gen·e·sis (or - thō - jen'e - sis). Ortogênese; a doutrina em que que a evolução é governada por fatores intrínsecos e ocorre em sentidos previsíveis. [ortho- + G. *genesis*, origem]

or·tho·gen·ic (or - thō - jen'ik). Ortogênico; relativo à ortogênese.

or·tho·gen·ics (or - thō - jen'iks). Ortogênica. SIN eugenics.

or·tho·gnath·ia (or - thō - nath'e - a, or - thog - nath'e - a). Ortognatismo; o estudo das causas e tratamento das condições relacionadas com a posição errônea dos ossos das mandíbulas. [ortho- + G. *gnathos*, mandíbula]

or·tho·gnath·ic, or·thog·na·thous (or - thō - nath'ik, or - thog'nathus). Ortognático. 1. Relativo ao ortognatismo. 2. Que possui uma face sem a mandíbula projetada; aquele com um índice gnático abaixo de 98. [ortho- + G. *ganthos*, mandíbula]

or·tho·grade (or'thō - grad). Ortógrado; caminhar ou ficar em pé ereto; indica a postura de seres humanos; oposto ao pronógrado. [ortho- + L. *gradior*, pp. *gressus*, caminhar]

or·tho·ker·a·tol·o·gy (or'thō - ker - a - tol'o - je). Ortoceratologia; um método de modelar a córnea com lentes de contato para melhorar a visão a olho nu. [ortho- + G. *keras*, corno (córnea), + *logos*, ciência]

or·tho·ker·a·to·sis (or - thō - ker - a - tō'sis). Ortoceratose; formação de uma camada de ceratina anuclear, como na epiderme normal. [ortho- + G. *keras*, corno, + *-osis*, condição]

or·tho·ki·net·ics (or - thō - ki - net'iks). Ortocinética; um método avançado para o tratamento da osteoartrite hipertrófica em que é feita uma tentativa para mudar a ação muscular de um grupo de músculos para outro grupo de músculos para proteger a articulação enferma. [ortho- + G. *kinētikos*, móvel, de *kineō*, mover]

or·tho·me·chan·i·cal (or - thō - me - kan'i - kal). Ortomecânico; pertinente aos suportes, próteses, dispositivos ortóticos e aparelhos. [ortho- + mechanical]

or·tho·me·chan·o·ther·a·py (or'thō - me - kan - o - thar'a - pē). Ortomecanoterapia; tratamento com suportes, próteses, órteses ou aparelhos. [ortho- + G. *mechanē*, máquina, + *therapeia*, tratamento médico]

or·tho·me·lic (or - thō - mē'lik). Ortomélico; malformações dos braços ou pernas. [ortho- + G. *melos*, membro]

or·thom·e·ter (or - thom'e - ter). Ortômetro. SIN exophthalmometer. [ortho- + G. *metron*, medida]

or·tho·mo·lec·u·lar (or'thō - mō - lek'u - lar). Ortomolecular; termo de L. C. Pauling que indica uma abordagem terapêutica destinada a fornecer um ambiente molecular ótimo para as funções corporais, com referência especial às concentrações ótimas das substâncias normalmente presentes no corpo humano, quer formadas no meio endógeno, quer ingeridas.

Or·tho·myx·o·vir·i·dae (or'thō - mik - sō - vir'i - dē). A família de vírus que contém os 3 gêneros de vírus influenza, os tipos A e B, C e "vírus Thogotosímiles". Os vírions são quase esféricos ou filamentares, tendo os primeiros (a forma mais comum) 80–120 mm de diâmetro e são éter-sensíveis; os envelopes são crivados de projeções de superfície; os nucleocapsídeos exibem simetria helicoidal, 6–9 nm de diâmetro e contêm RNA segmentado e com filamento único. O antígeno nucleoproteico de cada tipo de vírus é comum a todas as cepas do tipo, mas é distinto daqueles dos outros tipos; o mosaico dos antígenos de superfície varia de uma cepa para outra. Os nucleocapsídeos parecem ser formados nos núcleos das células infectadas, hemaglutinina e neuraminidase no citoplasma; a maturação viral acontece durante o brotamento da membrana celular. Os tipos A e B do vírus influenza estão sujeitos a mutação, resultando em epidemia. O vírus influenza C difere dos tipos A e B (p.ex., carece de neuraminidase) e pertence a um gênero separado. VER TAMBÉM Influenza virus.

or·tho·pae·dic, or·tho·pe·dic (or - thō - pē'dik). Ortopédico; relativo à ortopedia.

or·tho·pae·dics (or - thō - pē'diks). Ortopedia. SIN orthopedics. [ortho- + G. *pais (paid-)*, criança]

or·tho·pae·dist, or·tho·pe·dist (or - thō - pē'dist). Ortopedista; aquele que pratica a ortopedia.

or·tho·pe·dics. Ortopedia; a especialidade médica relacionada à preservação, restauração e desenvolvimento da forma e função do sistema musculoesquelético, membros, coluna vertebral e estruturas associadas através de métodos clínicos, cirúrgicos e físicos. SIN orthopaedics.

dental o., ortodontia. SIN orthodontics.

functional jaw o., o. mandibular funcional; a utilização das forças musculares para efetuar as alterações na posição da mandíbula e alinhamento dentário através de aparelhos removíveis. SIN functional orthodontic therapy.

or·tho·per·cus·sion (or'thō - per - kush'un). Ortopercussão; percussão muito leve do tórax feita em um sentido sagital (ou seja, no sentido ântero-posterior, e não no perpendicular, à parede do tórax); usado para determinar o tamanho do coração, com um som de percussão suave que desaparece quando o coração é alcançado, ainda que possa estar sobreposto por uma camada do pulmão.

or·tho·pho·ria (or - thō - fōr'ē - a). Ortoforia; ausência de heteroforia; a condição da fixação binocular em que as linhas da visão se encontram em um ponto distante ou próximo da referência na ausência de um estímulo de fusão. [ortho- + G. *phora*, movimento]

or·tho·pho·ric (or - thō - fōr'ik). Ortofórico; pertinente à ortoforia.

or·tho·phos·phate (or - thō - fos'fāt). Ortofosfato; um sal ou éster de ácido ortofosfórico.

inorganic o. (P_i), o. inorgânico; qualquer forma de íon ou sal de ácido fosfórico. SIN inorganic phosphate.

or·tho·phos·phor·ic ac·id (or'thō - fos - fōr'ik). Ácido ortofosfórico; ácido fosfórico, $O=P(OH)_3$, distinguido dos ácidos meta e pirofosfórico, $(HPO_3)_n$ e $OP(OH_2)OP(OH_2)O$, respectivamente, que são anidridos do H_3PO_4; o anidrido final é o pentóxido de fósforo, P_2O_5.

or·tho·phre·nia (or - thō - frē'nē - a). Ortofrenia. 1. Termo raramente utilizado para a integridade da mente. 2. Termo raramente empregado para relações interpessoais normais. [ortho- + G. *phrēn*, mente]

or·thop·nea (or - thop - nē - a, or - thop'nē - a). Ortopnéia; desconforto na respiração que é gerado ou agravado pelo decúbito. Cf. platypnea. [ortho- + G. *pnoē*, uma respiração]

or·thop·ne·ic (or'thop - nē'ik). Ortopneico; relativo a, ou caracterizado por, ortopnéia.

Or·tho·pox·vi·rus (or - thō - poks'vī - rus). O gênero da família Poxvoridae, que compreende os vírus do alastrim, da vacínia, varíola, varíola bovina, ectromelia, varíola do macaco e varíola do coelho.

or·tho·pros·the·sis (or'thō - pros - thē - sis, - pros - thē'sis). Ortoprótese; um aparelho empregado no controle de problemas protéticos relacionados com o alinhamento dos dentes.

or·tho·psy·chi·a·try (or'thō - sī - kī'a - trē). Ortopsiquiatria; uma ciência interdisciplinar que combina a psiquiatria infantil, psicologia do desenvolvimento, pediatria e cuidados familiares devotada à descoberta, prevenção e tratamento dos distúrbios mentais e psicológicos em crianças e adolescentes.

Or·thop·ter·a (or - thop - ter - a). Uma grande ordem de insetos hemimetabólicos que inclui gafanhotos, louva-a-deus, bicho-pau e formas correlatas. [ortho- + G. *pteron*, uma asa]

or·thop·tic (or - thop'tik). Relativo à ortóptica.

or·thop·tics (or - thop'tiks). Ortóptica; o estudo e tratamento da visão binocular defeituosa, de defeitos na ação dos músculos oculares, ou de hábitos visuais defeituosos. [*ortho-*, reto, + G. *optikos*, visão]

or·thop·tist (or - thop'tist). Técnico em ortóptica; aquele habilitado em ortóptica.

Or·tho·re·o·vi·rus (or - thō - rē'o - vī - rus). Um gênero na família Reoviridae, associado a várias doenças respiratórias e entéricas, porém sua relação causal não está comprovada.

or·tho·scope (or - thō - skōp). Ortoscópio. 1. Um instrumento por meio do qual se consegue desenhar os contornos de várias normas do crânio. [ortho- + G. *skopeō*, visualizar]

or·tho·sis, pl. or·tho·ses (or - thō - sis, - sēz). Órtese; um dispositivo ortopédico externo, como um suporte ou tala, que impede ou que assiste o movimento da coluna vertebral ou dos membros. [G. *orthōsis*, que faz reto]

ankle-foot o., o. de tornozelo-pé; uma o. que começa nos artelhos, cruzando o tornozelo e terminando na panturrilha.

cervical o., o. cervical; uma o. destinada a limitar a movimentação da coluna vertebral cervical em vários graus, p.ex., um colar cervical macio.

cervicothoracic o., o. cérvico-torácica; um dispositivo destinado a limitar a movimentação da coluna vertebral cervical que se estende e cobre mais a porção superior das costas que uma o. cervical padronizada.

knee-ankle-foot o., o. de joelho–tornozelo–pé; uma o. que se estende desde a porção superior da coxa, cruzando o joelho e o tornozelo, e que termina nos artelhos; destinada a controlar o movimento do joelho e tornozelo.

thoracolumbosacral o., o. toracolombossacral; um dispositivo externo aplicado ao tronco e que se estende desde a porção superior de coluna vertebral torácica até a pelve; destinada a imobilizar a coluna vertebral torácica.

wrist-hand o., o. de punho–mão; uma o. que começa nos dedos, cruza o punho e termina na porção distal do antebraço; usada para permitir a preensão e liberação, apesar de algum grau de paralisia da mão.

or·tho·stat·ic (or - thō - stat'ik). Ortostático; relativo a uma postura ou posição de pé.

or·tho·ster·e·o·scope (or'thō - ster'ē - ō - skōp). Ortoestereoscópio; um instrumento raramente utilizado para visualizar as radiografias estereoscópicas.

or·tho·tha·na·sia (or'thō - tha - nā'zē - a). Ortotanasia. 1. Uma maneira normal ou natural de morte e de morrer. 2. Por vezes usada para indicar a interrupção deliberada de meios artificiais ou heróicos para manter a vida. [ortho- + G. *thanatos*, morte]

or·thot·ics (ōr-thot′iks). A ciência preocupada com a manufatura e adaptação de aparelhos ortopédicos. SIN orthetics.
or·tho·tist (ōr′thō′tist). Um fabricante e adaptador de aparelhos ortopédicos.
or·tho·tol·i·dine (ōr-thō-tō′li-dēn). Ortotolidina; na presença de peroxidase, a o. (semelhante à benzidina) é oxidada em uma coloração azul; como a hemoglobina se comporta como uma peroxidase, a o. tem sido utilizada como um auxílio *in vitro* para a detecção de sangue oculto nas fezes.
or·thot·o·nos, or·thot·o·nus (ōr-thot′o-nos, -ō-nŭs). Ortótono; uma forma de espasmo tetânico em que o pescoço, os membros e o corpo são mantidos fixos em uma linha reta. [ortho- + G. *tonos*, tensão]
or·tho·top·ic (ōr-thō-top′ik). Ortotópico; na posição normal ou usual. [ortho- + G. *topos*, lugar]
or·tho·tro·pic (ōr-thō-trop′ik). Ortotrópico; que se estende ou cresce em uma direção reta, especialmente na vertical. [ortho- + G. *tropē*, uma volta]
or·tho·vol·tage (ōr-thō-vōl′tij). Ortovoltagem; na radioterapia, um termo para a voltagem entre 400 e 600 kV.
Ortolani, Marius, cirurgião ortopédico italiano do século XX. VER Ortolani *maneuver*, Ortolani *test*.
Orton, Samuel T., neurologista norte-americano, 1879–1975. VER Wolf-O. *bodies*, em *body*.
or·y·ce·nin (ōr-ē-sen′in). Oricenina; uma glutelina no arroz. [G. *oryza*, arroz, + -in]
O.S. Abreviatura de L. *oculus sinister*, olho esquerdo.
Os Símbolo de osmium (ósmio).

OS

os, gen. **os·sis,** pl. **os·sa** (os, os′is, os′ā) [TA]. Osso. SIN bone. Para a descrição histológica, ver bone. [L. osso]
 o. acromia′le, o. acromial; um acrômio que está unido à espinha escapular por união fibrosa em lugar de óssea.
 o. basila′re, o. basilar. SIN basilar *bone*.
 o. bre′ve [TA], o. curto. SIN short *bone*.
 o. cal′cis, calcâneo. SIN calcaneus (1).
 o. capita′tum [TA], o. capitato. SIN capitate (1).
 os′sa car′pi [TA], ossos carpais. SIN carpal *bones*, em *bone*.
 o. centra′le [TA], o. central; um pequeno osso ocasionalmente encontrado na face dorsal do punho entre o escafóide, capitato e trapezóide; desenvolve-se como uma cartilagem independente no início da vida fetal, mas geralmente se funde com o escafóide; ocorre normalmente na maioria dos macacos. SIN central bone.
 o. centra′le tar′si, o. navicular. SIN navicular.
 o. clitor′idis, o. do clitóris; um pequeno osso localizado no clitóris de muitos mamíferos carnívoros. É homólogo com o o. do pênis de muitos mamíferos machos.
 o. coc′cygis [TA], cóccix. SIN coccyx.
 o. costa′le, costela. SIN rib.
 o. cox′ae [TA], o. do quadril. SIN hip *bone*.
 ossa cra′nii [TA], ossos do crânio. SIN *bones of cranium*, em *bone*.
 o. cuboi′deum, o. cubóide. SIN cuboid (*bone*).
 o. cuneifor′me interme′dium, o. cuneiforme intermédio. SIN intermediate cuneiform (*bone*).
 o. cuneifor′me latera′le [TA], o. cuneiforme lateral. SIN lateral cuneiform (*bone*).
 o. cuneifor′me media′le [TA], o. cuneiforme medial. SIN medial cuneiform (*bone*).
 os′sa digito′rum, ossos dos dedos;* termo alternativo oficial para *bones of digits*, em *bone*. VER TAMBÉM phalanx (1).
 o. ethmoida′le [TA], o. etmóide. SIN ethmoid.
 os′sa facie′i, ossos da face. SIN facial *bones*, em *bone*.
 o. fem′oris, fêmur;* termo alternativo oficial para thigh.
 o. fronta′le [TA], o. frontal. SIN frontal *bone*.
 o. hama′tum, o. hamato. SIN hamate (*bone*).
 o. hyoi′deum, osso hióide. SIN hyoid *bone*. VER TAMBÉM hyoid *apparatus*.
 o. iliacum, ílio. SIN ilium.
 o. il′ium [TA], ílio. SIN ilium.
 o. in′cae, o. interparietal. SIN interparietal *bone*.
 o. incisi′vum, o. incisivo. SIN incisive *bone*.
 o. innomina′tum, o. do quadril. SIN hip *bone*.
 o. intermaxilla′re, o. incisivo. SIN incisive *bone*.
 o. interme′dium, o. semilunar. SIN lunate (*bone*).
 o. intermetatar′seum, o. intermetatarsal; um osso supranumerário na base do primeiro metatársico, ou entre o primeiro e segundo metatársicos, usualmente fundido com um ou outro ou com o osso cuneiforme medial. SIN intermetatarseum.
 o. interparieta′le [TA], o. interparietal. SIN interparietal *bone*.
 o. irregula′re [TA], o. irregular. SIN irregular *bone*.
 o. is′chii [TA], ísquio. SIN ischium.
 o. japoni′cum, um osso zigomático bipartido ou tripartido, encontrado com maior freqüência em japoneses que em outras raças.
 o. lacrima′le [TA], o. lacrimal. SIN lacrimal *bone*.
 o. lon′gum [TA], o. longo. SIN long *bone*.
 o. luna′tum [TA], o. semilunar. SIN lunate (*bone*).
 o. mag′num, capitato. SIN capitate (1).
 o. mala′re, o. zigomático. SIN zygomatic *bone*.
 os′sa mem′bri inferio′ris [TA], ossos do membro inferior. SIN *bones of lower limb*, em *bone*.
 os′sa mem′bri superio′ris [TA], ossos do membro superior. SIN *bones of upper limb*, em *bone*.
 ossa metacarpalia I-V, ossos metacarpais I-V. SIN metacarpal (*bones*) [I-V], em *bone*.
 ossa metacarpi, pl. **os′sa metacarpa′lia** [TA], ossos metacarpais. SIN metacarpal (*bones*) [I-V], em *bone*.
 ossa metatarsalia I-V, ossos metatarsais I-V. SIN metatarsal (*bones*) [I-V], em *bone*.
 ossa metatarsi, pl. **os′sa metatarsa′lia** [TA], ossos metatarsais. SIN metatarsal (*bones*) [I-V], em *bone*.
 o. multan′gulum ma′jus, o. trapézio. SIN trapezium *bone*.
 o. multan′gulum mi′nus, o. trapezóide. SIN trapezoid (*bone*).
 o. nasa′le [TA], o. nasal. SIN nasal *bone*.
 o. navicula′re [TA], o. navicular. SIN navicular.
 o. navicula′re ma′nus, o. escafóide. SIN scaphoid (*bone*).
 o. occipita′le [TA], o. occipital. SIN occipital *bone*.
 o. odontoi′deum, o dente do áxis quando, de forma anômala, não se funde com o corpo do eixo.
 o. orbicula′re, processo lenticular da bigorna. SIN lenticular *process* of incus.
 o. palati′num [TA], o. palatino. SIN palatine *bone*.
 o. parieta′le [TA], o. parietal. SIN parietal *bone*.
 ossa pedis [TA], ossos do pé. SIN *bones of foot*, em *bone*.
 o. pisifor′me [TA], o. pisiforme. SIN pisiform (*bone*).
 o. pla′num [TA], o. chato. SIN flat *bone*.
 o. pneumat′icum [TA], o. pneumático. SIN pneumatized *bone*.
 o. premaxilla′re, o. incisivo. SIN incisive *bone*.
 o. pterygoi′deum, processo pterigóideo do osso esfenóide. SIN pterygoid *process* of sphenoid bone.
 o. pu′bis, púbis. SIN pubis.
 o. pyramida′le, o. piramidal. SIN triquetrum.
 o. sa′crum [TA], o. sacro. SIN sacrum.
 o. scaphoi′deum [TA], o. escafóide. SIN scaphoid (*bone*).
 o. sesamoi′deum, pl. **os′sa sesamoi′dea** [TA], o. sesamóide. SIN sesamoid *bone*.
 o. sphenoida′le [TA], o. esfenóide. SIN sphenoid (*bone*).
 o. subtibia′le, o. subtibial; um osso inconstante encontrado muito raramente na extremidade articular distal da tíbia.
 ossa suprasterna′lia [TA], ossos supra-esternais. SIN suprasternal *bones*, em *bone*.
 o. sutura′rum [TA], suturas do crânio. SIN sutural *bones*, em *bone*.
 o. syl′vii, o. de Sylvius. SIN lenticular *process* of incus.
 ossa tarsalia, ossos tarsais;* termo oficial alternativo para tarsal *bones*, em *bone*.
 os′sa tar′si [TA], ossos tarsais. SIN tarsal *bones*, em *bone*.
 o. tempora′le [TA], o. temporal. SIN temporal *bone*.
 o. tibia′le poste′rius, o. tibia′le posti′cum, o. tibial posterior; um osso sesamóide no tendão do músculo tibial posterior, ocasionalmente fundido com a tuberosidade do navicular. SIN tibiale posticum.
 o. trape′zium, o. trapézio. SIN trapezium *bone*.
 o. trapezoi′deum, o. trapezóide. SIN trapezoid (*bone*).
 o. triangula′re, o. piramidal. SIN triquetrum.
 o. tribasila′re, o. tribasilar; o osso único que resulta da fusão, na infância, dos ossos occipital e temporal na base da cavidade craniana.
 o. trigo′num [TA], o. trígono; um ossículo independente por vezes presente no tarso; geralmente forma parte do talo, constituindo o tubérculo lateral do processo posterior. SIN triangular bone.
 o. trique′trum [TA], o. piramidal. SIN triquetrum.
 o. un′guis, o. lacrimal. SIN lacrimal *bone*.
 o. vesalia′num, o. de Vesalius; a tuberosidade do quinto osso metatarsal que, por vezes, existe como um osso separado. SIN vesalianum, Vesalius bone.
 o. zygomat′icum [TA], o. zigomático. SIN zygomatic *bone*.

os, gen. **o′ris,** pl. **ora. 1** [NA]. A boca. **2.** Termo por vezes aplicado a uma abertura para dentro de um órgão oco ou canal, principalmente com bordas espessas ou carnosas. VER TAMBÉM mouth (2), ostium, orifice, opening. [L. boca]
 anatomical internal o. of uterus [TA], óstio anatômico interno do útero; a

abertura no estreitamento da cavidade uterina demarcando e fornecendo comunicação entre a luz do corpo (cavidade uterina) e do colo (canal cervical) do útero. SIN ostium anatomicum [TA].
  external o. of uterus [TA], óstio externo do útero; a abertura vaginal do útero. SIN ostium uteri [TA], mouth of the womb, opening of uterus, orifice of uterus, orificium externum uteri, o. uteri externum, ostium uteri externum.
  histological internal o. of uterus [TA], óstio histológico interno do útero; local de transição da mucosa do útero (endométrio) para a do colo; pode ou não corresponder ao óstio anatômico interno. SIN ostium histologicum [TA].
  incompetent cervical o., óstio cervical incompetente; um defeito na força do o. interno que permite a dilatação prematura do colo.
  o. u'teri exter'num; óstio externo do útero. SIN external o. of uterus.
  o. u'teri inter'num, óstio interno do útero. SIN isthmus of uterus.
osa·zone (ō'sa - zōn). Osazona; o composto formado por determinados açúcares (p.ex., glicose, galactose, frutose) com excesso de hidrazinas, possuindo duas hidrazonas nos carbonos 1 e 2 em lugar de apenas uma em C-1, como na hidrazona comum, assim, RNH–N=CR'–CR''=N–NHR'''; osazonas formadas com fenilidrazina (fenilasazonas) são usadas para caracterizar e identificar determinados açúcares. SIN dihydrazone.
♺ **osche-, oscheo-.** Osque-, osqueo-; formas combinantes que significam escroto. [G. oschē]
os·che·al (os'kē - ăl). Escrotal. SIN scrotal.
os·che·o·plas·ty (os'kē - ō - plas - tē). Osqueoplastia. SIN scrotoplasty. [oscheo- + plastos, formado]
os·cil·la·tion (os - i - lā'shŭn). Oscilação. 1. Um movimento de um lado para outro. 2. Um estágio nas alterações vasculares na inflamação em que o acúmulo de leucócitos nos pequenos vasos paralisa a passagem do sangue e existe apenas um movimento de vaivém em cada contração cardíaca. [L. oscillatio, de oscillo, oscilar]
os·cil·la·tor (os'si - lā - ter). Oscilador. 1. Um aparelho semelhante a um vibrador, usado para dar uma forma de massagem mecânica. 2. Um circuito elétrico destinado a produzir corrente alternada em determinada freqüência. 3. Qualquer dispositivo que produza oscilação.
os·cil·lo·graph (ō - sil'ō - graf). Oscilógrafo; um instrumento que registra as oscilações, geralmente elétrico.
os·cil·log·ra·phy (os - i - log'rǎ - fē). Oscilografia; o estudo dos registros feitos por um oscilógrafo.
os·cil·lom·e·ter (os - i - lom'ĕ - ter). Oscilômetro; o aparelho para medir as oscilações de qualquer tipo, especialmente aquelas da corrente sanguínea na esfigmometria. VER TAMBÉM sphygmo-oscillometer. [L. oscillo, oscilar, + G. metron, medir]
os·cil·lo·met·ric (os'i - lō - met'rik). Oscilométrico; relativo ao oscilômetro ou aos registros feitos pelo mesmo.
os·cil·lom·e·try (os - i - lom'ĕ - trē). Oscilometria; a medida das oscilações de qualquer tipo com um oscilômetro.
os·cil·lop·sia (os - i - lop'sē - ă). Osciopsia; a sensação subjetiva de oscilação dos objetos visualizados. SIN oscillating vision. [L. oscillo, oscilar, + G. opsis, visão]
os·cil·lo·scope (ō - sil'ō - skōp). Osciloscópio; um oscilógrafo em que o registro das oscilações é continuamente visível.
  cathode ray o. (CRO), o. de raios catódicos; a forma comum de o., em que um sinal elétrico variado (y) deflete verticalmente um feixe de elétrons colidindo sobre uma tela fluorescente, enquanto alguma outra função (x ou tempo) deflete horizontalmente o feixe; o resultado é um gráfico visual de y plotado contra x ou tempo com distorção desprezível pela inércia.
  storage o., o. de armazenamento; um o. de raios catódicos em que o registro visual das oscilações persiste sobre a tela fluorescente até que seja apagado eletricamente.
os·ci·tate (os'i - tāt). Bocejar. [L. oscito, de os, boca, + cieo, colocar em movimento]
os·ci·ta·tion (os'i - tā'shŭn). Bocejo. SIN yawning. [L. oscitatio]
os·cu·lum, pl. **os·cu·la** (os'kū - lŭm, - lă). Ósculo; um poro ou abertura diminuta. [L. dim. de os, boca]
♺ **-ose. 1.** Em química, uma terminação que geralmente indica um carboidrato. **2.** Sufixo acrescentado a algumas raízes latinas que significa o mais comum -ous (2). [L. -osus, cheio de, abundante]
♺ **-oses.** Plural de -osis.
Osgood, Robert B., cirurgião ortopédico norte-americano, 1873–1956. VER O.-Schlatter disease.
OSHA Abreviatura de Occupational Safety and Health Administration (Administração de Segurança e Saúde Ocupacional) do Department of Labor dos EUA, responsável por estabelecer e cumprir os padrões de segurança e saúde no local de trabalho.
♺ **-osis,** pl. **-oses.** Sufixo que significa um processo, condição ou estado geralmente anormal ou enfermo; a produção ou aumento, fisiológico ou patológico; uma invasão ou infestação; no último sentido, é similar a e, com freqüência, usado como sinônimo do G. -iasis, conforme observado em triquinose, triquiníase. [G.]

Osler, Sir William, médico canadense nos Estados Unidos e Inglaterra, 1849–1919. VER O. disease, node, sign; Rendu-O.-Weber syndrome.
os·mate (os'māt). Osmato; um sal de ácido ósmico.
os·mat·ic (oz - ma - tik). Olfatório. SIN olfactory. [G. osmē, olfato]
OSMED condrodistrofia com surdez sensorioneural. SIN chondrodystrophy with sensorineural deafness.
os·me·sis (oz - mē'sis). Olfação. SIN olfaction. [G. osmēsis, olfação]
os·mic ac·id (oz'mik). Ácido ósmico; OsO$_4$; um agente cáustico volátil e oxidante forte; cristais incolores, pouco solúveis em água, mas solúveis em solventes orgânicos; a solução aquosa é um corante de gordura e mielina, além de ser um fixador geral para a microscopia eletrônica. SIN osmium tetroxide.
os·mi·cate (oz'mi - kāt). Corar ou fixar com ácido ósmico.
os·mi·ca·tion, os·mi·fi·ca·tion (os'mi - kā'shŭn, os'mi - fi - kā'shŭn). Osmicação; osmificação; a fixação do tecido com uma solução de ácido ósmico; também serve como corante para a microscopia óptica e eletrônica.
os·mics (oz'miks). Ósmica; a ciência da olfação. [G. osmē, olfato]
os·mi·o·phil·ic (oz'mi - ō - fil'ik). Osmiófilo; prontamente corado com ácido ósmico. [osmium + G. phileō, amar]
os·mi·o·pho·bic (oz'mi - ō - fō'bik). Osmiofóbico; não prontamente corado com ácido ósmico. [osmium + G. phobos, medo]
os·mi·um (Os) (oz'mē - ŭm). Ósmio; um elemento metálico do grupo da platina, número atômico 76, peso atômico 190,2. [G. osmē, olfato, por causa do forte odor do tetróxido]
  o. tetroxide, tetróxido de o. SIN osmic acid.
♺ **osmo-. 1.** Forma combinante que significa osmose. [G. ōsmos, impulsão] **2.** Olfato, odor. [G. osmē]
os·mo·cep·tor (os - mō - sep'ter, tōr). Osmoceptor. SIN osmoreceptor.
os·mo·dys·pho·ria (oz'mō - dis - fōr'ē - ă). Osmodisforia; ojeriza anormal a determinados odores. [G. osmē, olfato, + dys-, ruim, + phora, um transportador]
os·mo·gram (oz'mō - gram). Osmograma. SIN electroolfactogram. [G. osmē, olfato, + gramma, um desenho]
os·mo·lal·i·ty (os - mō - lal'i - tē). Osmolalidade; a concentração de uma solução expressa em osmoles de partículas do soluto por quilograma do solvente.
  calculated serum osmolality, osmolalidade sérica calculada; o cálculo da osmolalidade sérica a partir dos valores de sódio, glicose e uréia séricas através de diversas fórmulas, das quais a mais comum é: $1,86 \times$ [Na] (mmol/L) + glicose (mg/dL)/18 + uréia (mg/dL)/2,8.
os·mo·lar (os - mō - lar). Osmolar, osmótico. SIN osmotic.
os·mo·lar·i·ty (os - mō - lār'i - tē). Osmolaridade; a concentração osmótica de uma substância osmoticamente ativa na solução, expressa como osmoles das partículas do soluto por litro da solução.
os·mole (os'mōl). Osmol; o peso molecular de um soluto, em gramas, dividido pelo número de íons ou partículas em que ele se dissocia na solução.
os·mol·o·gy (os - mol'ō - jē). Osmologia. 1. O estudo dos odores, sua produção e seus efeitos. SIN osphresiology. 2. O estudo da osmose.
os·mom·e·ter (os - mom'ĕ - ter). Osmômetro. 1. Um instrumento para medir a osmolalidade por depressão do ponto de congelamento ou técnicas de elevação da pressão de vapor. 2. Um aparelho para medir a sensibilidade do olfato.
os·mom·e·try (os - mom'ĕ - trē). Osmometria; a medição da osmolalidade através do uso de um osmômetro.
os·mo·phil, os·mo·phil·ic (os'mō - fil, - fil'ik). Osmófilo, osmofílico; que se desenvolve em um meio com pressão osmótica alta. [osmo(sis) + G. phileō, amar]
os·mo·pho·bia (oz - mō - fō'bē - ă). Osmofobia. SIN olfactophobia. [G. osmē, olfato, + phobia]
os·mo·phore (oz'mō - fōr). Osmóforo; o grupo de átomos na molécula de um composto que é responsável pelo odor característico do composto. [G. osmē, olfato, + phonos, carregar]
os·mo·re·cep·tor (os'mō - rē - sep'ter, - tōr). Osmorreceptor. 1. Um receptor no sistema nervoso central (provavelmente o hipotálamo) que responde às alterações na pressão osmótica do sangue. [G. osmos, impulsão] 2. Um receptor que recebe os estímulos olfatórios. [G. osmē, olfato]. SIN osmoceptor.
os·mo·reg·u·la·to·ry (os - mō - reg'ū - lă - tōr - ē). Osmorregulador; que influencia o grau e a rapidez da osmose.
os·mose (os'mōs). Atravessar uma membrana por osmose.
os·mo·sis (os - mō'sis) Osmose; o processo pelo qual o solvente tende a atravessar uma membrana semipermeável a partir de uma solução de menor concentração osmolar dos solutos para uma de maior concentração dos solutos, aos quais a membrana é relativamente impermeável. [G. ōsmos, um empurrão, uma impulsão]
  reverse o., o. inversa; o movimento do solvente na direção oposta da osmose, isto é, filtração do solvente através de uma membrana semipermeável que reterá os solutos; comumente substituída por filtração ou ultrafiltração quando se fala de membranas capilares, como no glomérulo renal.
os·mos·i·ty (os - mos'i - tē). Osmosidade; uma medida indireta das características indiretas de uma solução, em relação a uma solução comparável de clo-

osmosity   1139   **osteitis**

reto de sódio, agora tornada obsoleta pelo termo definido com maior precisão: osmolalidade.

os·mo·ther·a·py (os′mō-thār′a-pē). Osmoterapia; desidratação por meio de injeções intravenosas de soluções hipertônicas de cloreto de sódio, glicose, uréia, manitol ou outras substâncias osmoticamente ativas, ou através da administração oral de glicerina, isosorbida, glicina etc.; usada no tratamento do edema cerebral e da pressão intracraniana aumentada. [osmosis + therapy]

os·mot·ic (os-mot′ik). Osmótico; relativo à osmose. SIN osmolar.

osphresio-. Osfresio-; forma combinante que significa odor ou o sentido do olfato. [G. *osphrēsis*, olfato]

os·phre·si·o·log·ic (os-frē-zē-ō-loj′ik). Osfresiológico; relativo à osfresiologia.

os·phre·si·ol·o·gy (os-frē′zē-ol′ō-jē). Osfresiologia. SIN osmology (1). [osphresio- + G. *logos*, estudo]

os·phre·si·o·phil·ia (os-frē′zē-ō-fil′ē-a). Osfresiofilia; um interesse incomum por odores. [osphresio- + G. *phileō*, amar]

os·phre·si·o·pho·bia (os-frē′zē-ō-fō′bē-a). Osfresiofobia. SIN olfactophobia. [osphresio- + G. *phobos*, medo]

os·phre·sis (os-frē′sis). Olfato. SIN olfaction. [G. *osphrēsis*, olfato]

os·phret·ic (os-fret′ik). Osfrético. SIN olfactory.

os·sa (os′a). Plural de L. *os*, osso. [L.]

os·se·in, os·se·ine (os′ē-in). Colágeno. SIN collagen. [L. *os*, osso]

osseo-. Forma combinante que significa ósseo. VER TAMBÉM ossi-, osteo-. [L. *osseus*]

os·se·o·car·ti·lag·i·nous (os′ē-ō-kar-ti-laj′i-nŭs). Osteocartilaginoso; relativo a, ou composto de, osso e cartilagem. SIN osteocartilaginous, osteochondrous.

os·se·o·mu·cin (os′ē-ō-mū′sin). Osseomucina; a substância fundamental do tecido ósseo.

os·se·o·mu·coid (os′ē-ō-mū′koyd). Osseomucóide; um mucóide derivado da osseína.

os·se·ous (os′ē-ŭs). Ósseo; com consistência ou estrutura semelhante ao osso. SIN osteal. [L. *osseus*]

ossi-. Forma combinante que significa osso. VER TAMBÉM osseo-, osteo-. [L. *os*]

os·si·cle (os′i-kl) [TA]. Ossículo; um pequeno osso; especificamente, um dos ossos da cavidade timpânica ou do ouvido médio. SIN ossiculum [TA], bonelet. [L. *ossiculum*, dim. de *os*, osso]

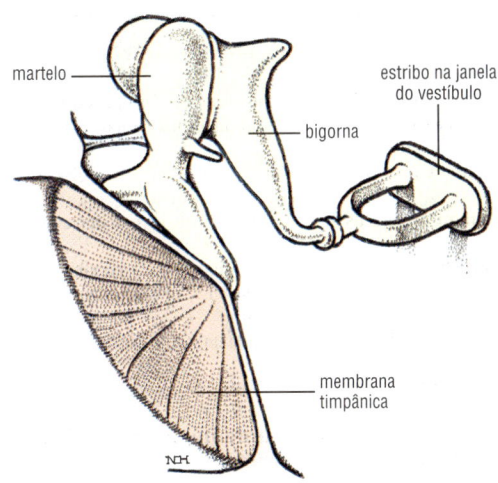

ossículos auditivos

    Andernach o.'s, ossículos de Andernach. SIN sutural *bones,* em *bone.*
    auditory o.'s [TA], ossículos da audição; os pequenos ossos da orelha média; são articulados para formar uma cadeia para a transmissão do som desde a membrana timpânica até a janela oval. SIN ossicula auditus [TA], ear bones, ossicular chain.
    Bertin o.'s, ossículos de Bertin. SIN sphenoidal *conchae,* em *concha.*
    epactal o.'s, suturas do crânio. SIN sutural *bones,* em *bone.*
    Kerckring o., o. de Kerckring. SIN Kerckring *center.*

os·sic·u·la (o-sik′ū-la). Ossículos; plural de ossiculum. [L.]

os·sic·u·lar (o-sik′ū-lar). Ossicular; pertinente a um ossículo.

os·sic·u·lec·to·my (os′i-kū-lek′tō-mē). Ossiculectomia; remoção de um ou mais ossículos da orelha média. [L. *ossiculum*, ossículo, + G. *ektomē*, excisão]

os·sic·u·lot·o·my (os′i-kū-lot′ō-mē). Ossiculotomia; divisão de um dos ossículos da orelha média. [L. *ossiculum*, ossículo, + G. *tomē*, incisão]

os·sic·u·lum, pl. **os·sic·u·la** (o-sik′ū-lŭm, -la) [TA]. Ossículo, ossículos. SIN ossicle. [L. dim. de *os*, osso]
    ossicula audi′tus [TA], ossículos da audição. SIN auditory *ossicles,* em *ossicle.*
    ossic′ula menta′lia, ossículos do mento; pequenos nódulos ósseos que aparecem na sínfise mental um pouco antes do nascimento e se fundem com a mandíbula depois do nascimento.

os·sif·er·ous (o-sif′er-ŭs). Ossífero; que contém ou produz osso. [ossi- + L. *fero*, trazer]

os·sif·ic (o-sif′ik). Relativo a uma alteração no osso ou na sua formação.

os·si·fi·ca·tion (os′i-fi-kā′shŭn). Ossificação. **1.** A formação do osso. **2.** Transformação em osso. [L. *ossificatio*, de *os*, osso, + *facio*, fazer]
    endochondral o., o. endocondral; a formação de tecido ósseo através da substituição da cartilagem endocondral; os ossos longos crescem em comprimento por o. endocondral na placa de cartilagem epifisária onde os osteoblastos formam trabéculas ósseas sobre um arcabouço de cartilagem calcificada.
    intramembranous o., o. intramembranosa. SIN membranous o.
    membranous o., o. membranosa; desenvolvimento do tecido ósseo no tecido mesenquimatoso sem formação prévia de cartilagem, como ocorre nos ossos frontal e parietal. SIN intramembranous o.
    metaplastic o., o. metaplásica; a formação de focos irregulares de osso (por vezes, inclusive a medula óssea) em várias estruturas macias, como músculos, pulmões, cérebro e outros locais onde o tecido ósseo é anormal.

os·si·form (os′i-fōrm). Ossiforme. SIN osteoid (1). [ossi- + L. *forma*, forma]

os·si·fy (os′i-fī). Ossificar; formar osso ou converter em osso. [ossi- + L. *facio*, fazer]

ost-. VER osteo-.

os·te·al (os′tē-al). Ósseo. SIN osseous. [G. *osteon*, osso]

os·te·al·gia (os-tē-al′jē-a). Ostealgia; dor em um osso. SIN osteodynia. [osteo- + G. *algos*, dor]

os·te·an·a·gen·e·sis (os′tē-an-a-jen′ē-sis). Osteanagênese. SIN osteoanagenesis.

os·te·a·naph·y·sis (os′tē-a-naf′i-sis). Osteanáfise. SIN osteoanagenesis. [osteo- + G. *anaphysis*, um novo crescimento]

os·tec·to·my (os-tek′tō-mē). Ostectomia. **1.** Remoção cirúrgica do osso. **2.** Em odontologia, a ressecção da estrutura óssea de sustentação para eliminar bolsas periodontais. SIN osteoectomy. [osteo- + G. *ektomē*, excisão]

os·te·in, os·te·ine (os′tē-in). Osteína. SIN collagen. [G. *osteon*, osso]

os·te·it·ic (os-tē-it′ik). Osteítico; relativo a, ou afetado por, osteíte. SIN ostitic.

os·te·i·tis (os-tē-ī′tis). Osteíte; inflamação do osso. SIN ostitis. [osteo- + G. *-itis*, inflamação]
    alveolar o., o. alveolar. SIN alveoalgia.
    caseous o., o. caseosa; cárie tuberculosa no osso.
    central o., o. central; **(1)** SIN osteomyelitis; **(2)** SIN endosteitis.
    o. condensans ilii (con-den′sanz il′ē-ī), o. condensante do ílio; osteoesclerose benigna simétrica da porção dos ossos ilíacos adjacentes às articulações sacroilíacas.
    condensing o., o. condensante. SIN sclerosing o.

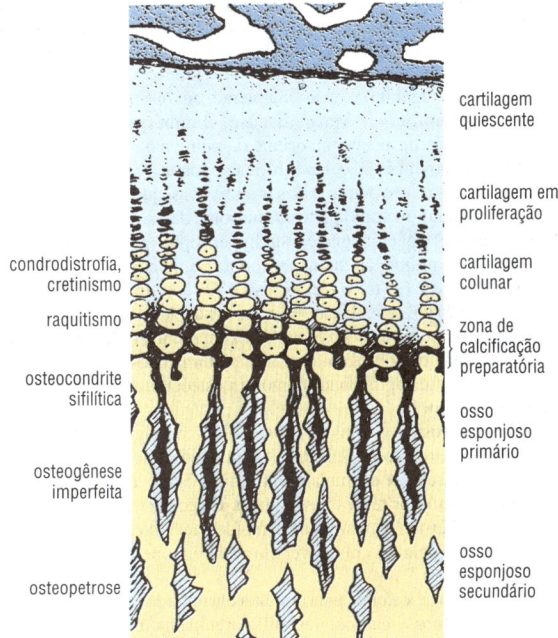

ossificação: ossificação endocondral e locais de anormalidades em diversos distúrbios

cortical o., o. cortical; periostite com envolvimento da camada superficial do osso.
o. defor'mans, o. deformante. SIN Paget disease (1).
o. fibro'sa cir'cumscrip'ta, o. fibrosa circunscrita. SIN monostotic fibrous dysplasia.
o. fibro'sa cys'tica, o. fibrosa cística; reabsorção osteoclástica aumentada do osso calcificado com substituição por tecido fibroso, causada por hiperparatireoidismo primário ou por outras causas de mobilização rápida de sais minerais. SIN parathyroid osteosis, Recklinghausen disease of bone.
o. fibro'sa disseminat'a, o. fibrosa disseminada. SIN polyostotic fibrous dysplasia.
focal condensing o., o. condensante focal. SIN chronic focal sclerosing osteomyelitis.
hematogenous o., o. hematogênica; qualquer o. causada por infecção realizada na corrente sanguínea.
localized o. fibro'sa, o. fibrosa localizada. SIN monostotic fibrous dysplasia.
multifocal o. fibro'sa, o. fibrosa multifocal. SIN polyostotic fibrous dysplasia.
o. pubis, o. pubiana; osteoesclerose do osso pubiano próximo à sínfise, causada por trauma nessa região, decorrente de gestação ou instrumentação.
renal o. fibro'sa, raquitismo renal. SIN renal rickets.
sclerosing o., o. esclerosante; espessamento fusiforme ou densidade aumentada dos ossos, de etiologia desconhecida; tem sido considerada uma forma de osteomielite crônica não-supurativa. SIN condensing o., Garré disease.
o. tuberculo'sa mul'tiplex cys'tica, o. tuberculosa múltipla cística; uma o. de origem tuberculosa, caracterizada por inúmeras pequenas cavidades na substância óssea. SIN Jüngling disease.

os·te·mia (os-tē'mē-ă). Ostemia; congestão ou hiperemia de um osso. [osteo- + G. *haima*, sangue]
os·tem·py·e·sis (os'tem-pī-ē'sis). Ostempiese; supuração no osso. [osteo- + G. *empyēsis*, supuração]
osteo-, ost-, oste-. Formas combinantes que significam osso. VER TAMBÉM osseo, ossi-. [G. *osteon*]
os·te·o·an·a·gen·e·sis (os'tē-ō-an-ă-jen'ē-sis). Osteoanagênese; regeneração do osso. SIN osteanagenesis, osteanaphysis. [osteo- + G. *ana*, novamente, + *genesis*, produção]
os·te·o·ar·thri·tis (os'tē-ō-ar-thrī'tis). Osteoartrite; artrite caracterizada por erosão da cartilagem articular, quer primária, quer secundária a traumatismo ou outras condições, a qual se torna amolecida, desgastada e adelgaçada, com eburnação do osso subcondral e crescimentos de osteófitos marginais; resultam dor e perda da função; afeta principalmente as articulações de sustentação de peso, sendo mais comum nas pessoas idosas. SIN arthrosis (2), degenerative arthritis, degenerative joint disease, osteoarthrosis.
hyperplastic o., o. hiperplásica. SIN hypertrophic pulmonary osteoarthropathy.
os·te·o·ar·throp·a·thy (os'tē-ō-ar-throp'ă-thē). Osteoartropatia; um distúrbio que afeta os ossos e articulações. [osteo- + G. *arthron*, articulação, + *pathos*, sofrimento].
hypertrophic pulmonary o., o. pulmonar hipertrófica; a expansão das extremidades distais, ou de toda a diáfise, dos ossos longos, por vezes com erosões das cartilagens articulares e espessamento e proliferação vilosa das membranas sinoviais, e, com freqüência, baqueteamento dos dedos das mãos; o distúrbio acontece em algumas doenças pulmonares crônicas, na cardiopatia (mais freqüentemente congênita) e, ocasionalmente, em outros distúrbios agudos e crônicos. SIN Bamberger-Marie disease, Bamberger-Marie syndrome, hyperplastic osteoarthritis, pneumogenic o., pulmonary o.
idiopathic hypertrophic o., o. hipertrófica idiopática; a o. que não é secundária a lesão pulmonar ou a outras lesões progressivas, que pode acontecer isoladamente (acropatia) ou uma parte da síndrome da paquidermoperiostose.
pneumogenic o., o. pneumogênica. SIN hypertrophic pulmonary o.
pulmonary o., o. pulmonar. SIN hypertrophic pulmonary o.
os·te·o·ar·thro·sis (os'tē-ō-ar-thrō'sis). Osteoartrose. SIN osteoarthritis. [osteo- + G. *arthron*, articulação, + *-osis*, condição]
os·te·o·blast (os'tē-ō-blast). Osteoblasto; uma célula formadora de osso que deriva das células osteoprogenitoras mesenquimatosas e forma uma matriz óssea em que ela fica aprisionada como um osteócito. SIN osteoplast. [osteo- + G. *blastos*, germe]
os·te·o·blas·tic (os'tē-ō-blas'tik). Osteoblástico; relativo aos osteoblastos; descreve qualquer região de densidade óssea radiográfica aumentada, em particular as metástases que estimulam a atividade osteoblástica.
os·te·o·blas·to·ma (os'tē-ō-blas-tō'mă). Osteoblastoma; um tumor benigno raro de osteoblastos com áreas de osteóide e tecido calcificado, ocorrendo com maior freqüência na coluna vertebral de uma pessoa jovem. SIN giant osteoid osteoma.
os·te·o·cal·cin. Osteocalcina; uma proteína encontrada em osteoblastos e dentina; contém resíduos γ-carboxiglutamil; participa na mineralização e homeostasia do íon cálcio. SIN bone Gla protein.
os·te·o·car·ti·lag·i·nous (os'te-ō-kar-ti-laj'i-nŭs). Osteocartilaginoso. SIN osseocartilaginous.

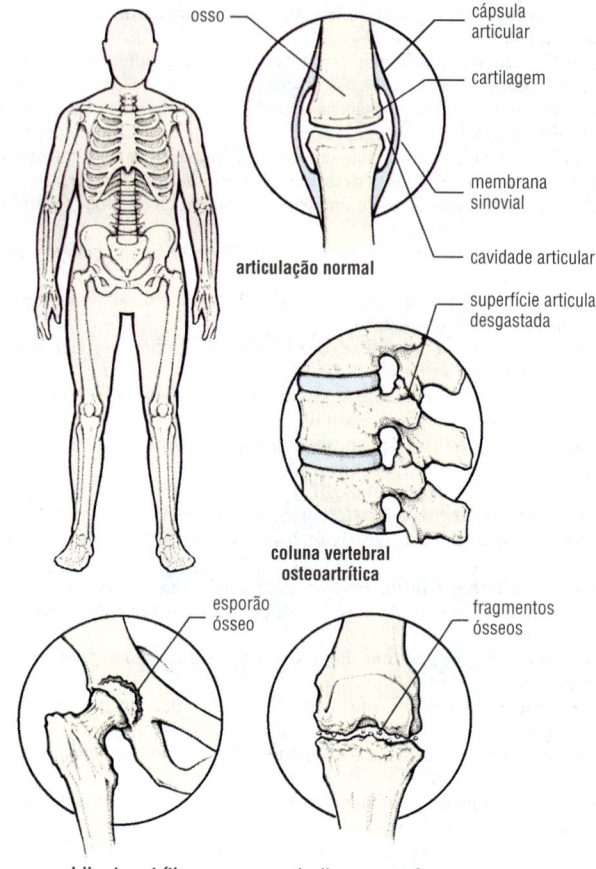

osteoartrite: problemas associados à osteoartrite e alguns locais onde geralmente ocorrem; uma articulação normal é mostrada no canto superior direito

os·te·o·chon·dri·tis (os'tē-ō-kon-drī'tis).. Osteocondrite; inflamação de um osso e sua cartilagem articular suprajacente. [osteo- + G. *chondros*, cartilagem, + *-itis*, inflamação]
o. defor'mans juveni'lis, o. deformante juvenil. SIN Legg-Calvé-Perthes disease.
o. defor'mans juveni'lis dor'si, o. deformante juvenil dorsal. SIN Scheurmann disease.
o. dis'secans, o. dissecante; separação completa ou incompleta de uma porção da cartilagem articular e do osso subjacente, envolvendo geralmente o joelho, associado a necrose asséptica epifisária.
syphilitic o., o. sifilítica; inflamação da linha epifisária associada à sífilis congênita. SIN Wegner disease.
os·te·o·chondro·dys·pla·sia. Osteocondrodisplasia. SIN camptomelic syndrome.
os·te·o·chon·dro·dys·tro·phia de·for·mans (os'tē-ō-kon'drō-dis-trō'fē-ă dē-for'manz). Osteocondrodistrofia deformante. SIN chondro-osteodystrophy.
os·te·o·chon·dro·dys·tro·phy (os'tē-ō-kon'drō-dis'trō-fē). Osteocondrodistrofia. SIN chondro-osteodystrophy.
os·te·o·chon·dro·ma (os'tē-ō-kon-drō'mă). Osteocondroma; uma neoplasia cartilaginosa benigna que consiste em um pedículo de osso normal (que se projeta do córtex) revestido por uma borda de células cartilaginosas proliferantes; pode originar-se em qualquer osso que é pré-formado em cartilagem, porém é mais freqüente próximo às extremidades dos ossos longos, usualmente nos pacientes com 10 a 25 anos de idade; a lesão não é freqüentemente percebida, a menos que sofra traumatismo ou seja grande; os osteocondromas múltiplos são herdados e referidos como exostoses múltiplas hereditárias. SIN solitary osteocartilaginous exostosis. [osteo- + G. *chondros*, cartilagem, + *-oma*, tumor]
os·te·o·chon·dro·ma·to·sis (os'tē-ō-kon-drō-mă-tō'sis). Osteocondromatose. SIN hereditary multiple exostoses, em exostosis.
synovial o., o. sinovial. SIN synovial chondromatosis.
os·te·o·chon·dro·sar·co·ma (os'tē-ō-kon'drō-sar-kō'-mă). Osteocondrossarcoma; o condrossarcoma que se origina no osso. Os sarcomas ósseos que contêm focos de cartilagem neoplásica, bem como osso, são classificados

como sarcomas osteogênicos. [osteo- + G. *chondros*, cartilagem, + *sarx*, carne, + *-oma*, tumor]

os·te·o·chon·dro·sis (os'tē-ō-kon-drō'sis). Osteocondrose; qualquer um de um grupo de distúrbios de um ou mais centros de ossificação em crianças, caracterizado por degeneração ou necrose asséptica seguida por reossificação; inclui as várias formas de necrose asséptica epifisária. [osteo- + G. *chondros*, cartilagem, + *-osis*, condição]

os·te·o·chon·drous (os'tē-ō-kon'drŭs). Osteocondroso. SIN osseocartilaginous. [osteo- + G. *chondros*, cartilagem]

os·te·oc·la·sis, os·te·o·cla·sia (os'tē-ok'lă-sis, os'tē-ō-klā'zē-ă). Osteoclasia; a fratura intencional em um osso para corrigir uma deformidade. SIN diaclasis, diaclasia. [osteo- + G. *klasis*, fratura]

os·te·o·clast (os'tē-ō-klast). Osteoclasto. **1.** Uma grande célula multinucleada, possivelmente da origem monocítica, com citoplasma acidófilo abundante, que atua na absorção e remoção do tecido ósseo. SIN osteophage. **2.** Um instrumento usado para fraturar um osso para corrigir uma deformidade. [osteo- + G. *klastos*, quebrado]

os·te·o·clas·tic (os'tē-ō-klas'tik). Osteoclástico; pertinente aos osteoclastos, especialmente com referência às suas atividades na absorção e remoção do tecido ósseo.

os·te·o·clas·to·ma (os'tē-ō-klas-tō'mă). Osteoclastoma. SIN giant cell *tumor* of bone.

os·te·o·cra·ni·um (os'tē-ō-krā'nē-ŭm). Osteocrânio; o crânio do feto após a ossificação do crânio membranoso que o torna rígido. [osteo- + G. *kranion*, crânio]

os·te·o·cys·to·ma (os'tē-ō-sis-tō'mă). Osteocistoma; SIN solitary bone *cyst*.

os·te·o·cyte (os'tē-ō-sīt). Osteócito; uma célula de tecido ósseo que ocupa uma lacuna e possui prolongamentos citoplasmáticos que se estendem para os canalículos e que fazem contato, por meio de junções comunicantes, com os prolongamentos de outros osteócitos. SIN bone cell, bone corpuscle, osseous cell. [osteo- + G. *kytos*, célula]

os·te·o·den·tin (os'tē-ō-den'tin). Osteodentina; dentina terciária rapidamente formada que contém odontoblastos aprisionados e poucos túbulos de dentina, assemelhando-se, assim, superficialmente ao osso. [osteo- + L. *dens*, dente]

os·te·o·der·ma·to·poi·ki·lo·sis (os'tē-ō-der'mă-tō-poy-ki-lō'sis). [MIM*166700]. Osteodermatopecilose; osteopecilose com lesões cutâneas, mais amiúde pequenos nódulos fibrosos elásticos sobre as faces posteriores das coxas e das nádegas; herança autossômica dominante irregular. SIN Buschke-Ollendorf syndrome. [osteo- + G. *derma*, pele, + *poikilos*, salpicado, + *-osis*, condição]

os·te·o·des·mo·sis (os'tē-ō-dez-mō'sis). Osteodesmose; transformação do tendão em tecido ósseo. [osteo- + G. *desmos*, uma faixa (tendão), + *-osis*, condição]

os·te·o·di·as·ta·sis (os'tē-ō-dī-as'tă-sis). Osteodiástase; separação de dois ossos adjacentes, como do crânio. [osteo- + G. *diastasis*, uma separação]

os·te·o·dyn·ia (os-tē-ō-din'ē-ă). Osteodinia. SIN ostealgia. [osteo- + G. *odynē*, dor]

os·te·o·dys·plas·ty (os'tē-ō-dis'plas-tē). Osteodisplasia. SIN Melnick-Needles *o*. [osteo- + G. *dys-*, ruim, + *plastos*, formado]

Melnick-Needles o., o. de Melnick-Needles; uma displasia esquelética generalizada com fronte proeminente e mandíbula pequena; nas radiografias, há constrições irregulares, semelhantes a laços de fita, das costelas e ossos tubulares; provavelmente ligada ao X [MIM*309350]. As heranças autossômicas dominante e recessiva [MIM*249420] também foram sugeridas. SIN osteodysplasty.

os·te·o·dys·tro·phia (os'tē-ō-dis-trō'fē-ă). Osteodistrofia. SIN osteodystrophy.

os·te·o·dys·tro·phy (os'tē-ō-dis'trō-fē). Osteodistrofia; formação defeituosa do osso. SIN osteodystrophia. [osteo- + G. *dys*, difícil, imperfeito, + *trophē*, nutrição]

Albright hereditary o., o. hereditária de Albright; uma forma hereditária de hiperparatireoidismo associada a calcificação e ossificação ectópicas e a defeitos esqueléticos, notadamente nos pequenos quartos metacarpos; a inteligência pode ser normal ou subnormal. A herança é heterogênea; a forma autossômica [MIM*103580] é causada por mutação no gene da proteína de fixação da guanina nucleotídeo (GNAS1) em 20q. Também existem as formas recessiva [MIM*203330] e ligada ao X [MIM*300800]. VER TAMBÉM pseudohypoparathyroidism. SIN Albright syndrome (2).

renal o., o. renal; alterações ósseas generalizadas que se assemelham à osteomalacia e ao raquitismo ou osteíte fibrosa, ocorrendo em crianças ou adultos com insuficiência renal crônica.

os·te·o·ec·to·my (os-tē-ō-ek'tō-mē). Ostectomia. SIN ostectomy.

os·te·o·e·piph·y·sis (os'tē-ō-e-pif'i-sis). Osteoepífise; a epífise de um osso.

os·te·o·fi·bro·ma (os'tē-ō-fi-brō'mă). Osteofibroma; uma lesão benigna do osso, não sendo provavelmente uma neoplasia verdadeira, que consiste principalmente em tecido conjuntivo fibroso, bastante denso, moderadamente celular, em que existem pequenos focos de osteogênese. Muitos exemplos dessa condição, principalmente na maxila e na mandíbula, provavelmente representam focos de displasia fibrosa; alguns exemplos de lesões fibrosas com focos de osteogênese, principalmente nos corpos vertebrais, podem ser neoplasias.

os·te·o·fi·bro·sis (os'tē-ō-fi-brō'sis). Osteofibrose; fibrose do osso, afetando principalmente a medula óssea vermelha.

periapical o., o. periapical. SIN periapical cemental *dysplasia.*

os·te·o·gen (os'tē-ō-jen). Osteógeno; uma camada ou tecido produtor de matriz óssea. [osteo- + G. *-gen*, que produz]

os·te·o·gen·e·sis (os'tē-ō-jen'ĕ-sis). Osteogênese; a formação do osso. SIN osteogeny, osteosis (2), ostosis(2). [osteo- + G. *genesis*, produção]

distraction o., o. por tração; uma técnica de induzir a formação de neo-osso através da divisão de um osso e aplicação de tração através de um dispositivo de fixação externa para aumentar o comprimento do osso.

o. imperfec'ta (OI), o. imperfeita; um grupo de distúrbios do tecido conjuntivo do colágeno do tipo I, caracterizados por fragilidade óssea, fraturas por traumatismos insignificantes, deformidade esquelética, escleróticas azuladas, frouxidão ligamentar e perda da audição. O sistema Sillence, que é uma classificação clínica, radiográfica e genética, mostra quatro tipos; herança autossômica dominante, causada por mutação no gene alfa 1 do colágeno do tipo I (COL1A1) no cromossoma 17q ou no gene alfa–2 (COL1A2) em 7q. SIN brittle bones.

o. imperfecta congenita, o. imperfeita congênita; uma forma grave [MIM 166230], com as fraturas ocorrendo antes do ou no nascimento.

o. imperfecta tarda, o. imperfeita tardia; uma forma menos grave, com as fraturas acontecendo em um período mais adiante na infância.

Type I o. imperfecta [MIM*166200], o. imperfeita do tipo I; uma forma branda caracterizada por escleróticas azuladas, perda da audição, equimoses fáceis, fragilidade óssea pré-púbere e baixa estatura.

Tipe II o. imperfecta [MIM*166210], o. imperfeita do tipo II; uma forma letal perinatal associada a natimortalidade ou tempo de sobrevida menor que 1 ano; tecido conjuntivo muito frágil, e achados radiográficos de fraturas *in utero*, crânio grande e mole, micromelia, ossos longos tubulares e costelas com nodosidades.

Type III o. imperfecta [MIM*259420], o. imperfeita do tipo III; uma forma deformante progressiva com fragilidade óssea grave, fraturas fáceis, fácies triangular com macrocefalia relativa, deformidades esqueléticas com escoliose, arqueamento dos membros, nanismo e achados radiográficos de alargamento metafisário dos ossos longos com formação de osso sutural. Muitos casos são distúrbios autossômicos recessivos, mas também já foi descrita herança autossômica recessiva.

Type IV o. imperfecta [MIM*166220], o. imperfeita do tipo IV; uma forma moderadamente grave, caracterizada por baixa estatura, fragilidade óssea, fraturas pré-deambulação e arqueamento dos ossos longos.

os·te·o·gen·ic, os·te·o·ge·net·ic (os'tē-ō-jen'ik, -jĕ-net'ik). Osteogênico, osteogenético; relativo à osteogênese. SIN osteogenous, osteoplastic (1).

os·te·og·e·nous (os-tē-oj'ĕ-nŭs). Osteogênico. SIN osteogenic.

os·te·og·e·ny (os-tē-oj'ĕ-nē). Osteogênese. SIN osteogenesis.

os·te·og·ra·phy (os'tē-og'ră-fē). Osteografia; um tratado sobre os ossos ou uma descrição dos ossos. [osteo- + G. *graphē*, uma escrita]

os·te·o·ha·lis·te·re·sis (os'tē-ō-hal'is-ter-ē'sis). Osteoalisterese; amolecimento dos ossos através da absorção ou aporte insuficiente da porção mineral. [osteo- + G. *hals*, salt, + *sterēsis*, privação]

os·te·o·hy·per·tro·phy (os'tē-ō-hī-per'trō-fē). Osteoipertrofia; condição caracterizada por crescimento excessivo dos ossos. [osteo- + G. *hyper*, excesso, + *trophē*, nutrição]

os·te·oid (os'tē-oyd). Osteóide. **1.** Relativo ou que se assemelha ao osso. SIN ossiform. **2.** Matriz óssea orgânica recentemente formada antes da calcificação. [osteo- + G. *eidos*, semelhança]

os·te·o·lip·o·chon·dro·ma (os'tē-ō-lip'ō-kon-drō'mă). Osteolipocondroma; uma neoplasia benigna do tecido cartilaginoso, na qual ocorre metaplasia e são formados focos de células adiposas e tecido ósseo. [osteo- + G. *lipos*, adiposo, + *chondros*, cartilagem, + *-oma*, tumor]

os·te·o·lo·gia (os-tē-ō-lō'jē-ă). Osteologia. SIN osteology, osteology. [L.]

os·te·ol·o·gist (os'tē-ol'ō-jist). Osteologista; um especialista em osteologia.

os·te·ol·o·gy (os'tē-ol'ō-jē). Osteologia; a anatomia dos ossos; a ciência relacionada com os ossos e suas estruturas. SIN osteologia. [osteo- + G. *logos*, estudo]

os·te·ol·y·sis (os-tē-ol'i-sis). Osteólise; amolecimento, absorção e destruição de tecido ósseo, decorrente da ação dos osteoclastos. [osteo- + G. *lysis*, dissolução]

os·te·o·lyt·ic (os-tē-ō-lit'ik). Osteolítico; pertinente a, caracterizado por ou que causa osteólise.

os·te·o·ma (os-tē-ō'mă). Osteoma; uma massa benigna e de crescimento lento de osso maduro, predominantemente lamelar, que geralmente se origina no crânio ou na mandíbula. [osteo- + G. *-oma*, tumor]

o. cu'tis, o. cutâneo; ossificação cutânea geralmente secundária à calcificação nos focos de degeneração nos tumores ou lesões inflamatórias ou, raramente, a formação primária de osso novo na pele normal, freqüentemente associada à osteodistrofia hereditária de Albright.

dental o., o. dentária; uma exostose que se origina da raiz de um dente.
giant osteoid o., o. osteóide gigante. SIN osteoblastoma.
o. medulla're, o. medular; um o. que contém espaços que são preenchidos (ou parcialmente preenchidos) por vários elementos da medula óssea.
osteoid o., o. osteóide; uma neoplasia benigna dolorosa que, em geral, se origina em um dos ossos dos membros inferiores, principalmente no fêmur ou na tíbia de adolescentes e adultos jovens; caracterizado por um nicho (geralmente não superior a 1 cm de diâmetro) que consiste em material osteóide, estroma osteogênico vascularizado e osso malformado; ao redor do nicho, existe uma zona relativamente grande de espessamento reativo do córtex.
o. spongio'sum, o. esponjoso; um o. que consiste principalmente em tecido ósseo esponjoso.

os·te·o·ma·la·cia (os'tē-ō-mā-lā'shē-ā). Osteomalacia; uma doença caracterizada por amolecimento e curvatura graduais dos ossos com intensidade variada da dor; o amolecimento acontece porque os ossos contêm tecido osteóide que não se calcifica por causa da carência de vitamina D ou disfunção tubular renal; mais comum em mulheres que nos homens, a o. freqüentemente começa durante a gestação. SIN adult rickets, late rickets, rachitis tarda. [osteo- + G. *malakia*, amolecimento]

etiologia da osteomalacia

deficiência de vitamina D

desnutrição (nos países em desenvolvimento, favelas, vegetarianos, idosos)

absorção reduzida devido à digestão comprometida (gastrectomia, secreção reduzida de bile, insuficiência pancreática, má absorção (espru, ressecções intestinais)

formação reduzida de vitamina D_3 devido à falta de luz UV (raquitismo em crianças)

metabolismo comprometido da vitamina D

defeitos hereditários no receptor para a 1,25(OH)$_2$D nos tecidos-alvo

comprometimento da formação de calcidiol no fígado (terapia antiepiléptica, cirrose hepática)

comprometimento da 1-hidroxilação nos rins (insuficiência renal, deficiência de pseudovitamina D, raquitismo)

metabolismo comprometido do fosfato

fosfatúria (diabetes com fosfato, congênita e adquirida)

cistinose (congênita e adquirida)

acidose tubular renal

formas induzidas por tumor (com tumores ósseos e tumores mesenquimatosos)

deficiência de fosfato

hipofosfatasia (congênita; autossômica recessiva)

infantile o., juvenile o., raquitismo. SIN rickets.
senile o., o. senil; a osteoporose no idoso.

os·te·o·ma·lac·ic (os'tē-ō-mā-lā'sik). Osteomalácico; relativo a ou que sofre de osteomalacia.

os·te·o·ma·toid (os-tē-ō'mă-toyd). Osteomatóide; um nódulo anormal ou pequena massa de crescimento exagerado do osso, que geralmente acontece de maneira bilateral e simétrica, nas regiões justaepifisárias, principalmente nos ossos longos dos membros inferiores; as lesões não são realmente em neoplasias, mas representam desenvolvimentos anômalos nos quais existem saliências no córtex (em contraste com um crescimento superposto ao córtex), e são mais adequadamente denominadas exostoses. [osteoma + G. *eidos*, aparência, forma]

os·te·o·mere (os'tē-ō-mēr). Osteômero; um de uma série de segmentos ósseos, como as vértebras. [osteo- + G. *meros*, uma parte]

os·te·om·e·try (os-tē-om'ĕ-trē). Osteometria; o ramo da antropometria relacionado com o tamanho relativo de diferentes partes do esqueleto. [osteo- + G. *metron*, medida]

os·te·o·my·e·li·tis (os'tē-ō-mī-ĕ-lī'tis). Osteomielite; inflamação da medula óssea e osso adjacente. SIN central osteitis (1). [osteo- + G. *myelos*, medula, + *-itis*, inflamação]
chronic diffuse sclerosing o., o. esclerosante difusa crônica; uma reação proliferativa do osso a uma infecção de baixa intensidade das mandíbulas; mais freqüentemente observada em mulheres negras idosas ou de meia-idade como extensas radiopacificações, freqüentemente bilaterais, da mandíbula e da maxila.
chronic focal sclerosing o., o. esclerosante focal crônica; uma reação do osso a uma infecção bacteriana discreta, com freqüência o resultado de um dente cariado, nas pessoas com um alto grau de resistência tecidual; resulta em uma radiopacificação localizada. SIN focal condensing osteitis.
Garré o., o. de Garré; o. crônica com periostite proliferativa. Um espessamento focal macroscópico do periósteo com formação óssea reativa periférica decorrente da infecção branda.
***Pseudomonas* o.**, o. por *Pseudomonas*. SIN malignant external otitis.

os·te·o·my·e·lo·dys·pla·sia (os'tē-ō-mī'ē-lō-dis-plā'-zē-ā). Osteomielodisplasia; uma doença caracterizada pela dilatação das cavidades medulares dos ossos, adelgaçamento do tecido ósseo, espaços vasculares grandes e com paredes finas, leucopenia e febre irregular. [osteo- + G. *myelos*, medula, + dysplasia]

os·te·on, os·te·one (os'tē-on, -ōn). Ósteon; um canal central que contém capilares sanguíneos e as lamelas ósseas concêntricas ao seu redor existentes no osso compacto. SIN haversian system. [G. *osteon*, osso]

os·te·on·cus (os-tē-ong'kŭs). Osteoncose; um osteoma, por vezes utilizado com referência a qualquer neoplasia de um osso. [osteo- + G. *onkos*, massa (inchação)]

os·te·o·ne·cro·sis (os'tē-ō-ne-krō'sis). Osteonecrose; a morte do osso em massa, conforme diferenciado da cárie ("morte molecular") ou focos relativamente pequenos de necrose no osso. [osteo- + G. *nekrōsis*, morte]

os·te·o·nec·tin. Osteonectina; uma proteína (PM 39.000-40.000) encontrada no osso e nos tecidos não-mineralizados e que se acredita ter uma participação na mineralização.

os·te·o·path (os'tē-ō-path). Médico osteopata. SIN osteopathic physician.
os·te·o·path·ia (os'tē-ō-path'ē-ā). Osteopatia. SIN osteopathy (1).
o. conden'sans, o. condensante. SIN osteopoikilosis.
o. hemorrha'gica infan'tum, escorbuto infantil. SIN infantile scurvy.
o. stria'ta, o. estriada; as estriações lineares observadas por meios radiográficos nas metáfises de ossos longos e, também, em ossos chatos; pode ser uma variante da osteopecilose. SIN Voorhoeve disease.

os·te·o·path·ic (os-tē-ō-path'ik). Osteopático; relativo à osteopatia.

os·te·o·pa·thol·o·gy (os'tē-ō-pa-thol'ō-jē). Osteopatologia; o estudo das doenças do osso.

os·te·op·a·thy (os-tē-op'ă-thē). Osteopatia. **1.** Qualquer doença do osso. SIN osteopathia. **2.** Uma escola de medicina baseada em um conceito do corpo normal como uma máquina vital capaz, quando no "ajuste correto", de produzir seus próprios remédios contra as infecções e contra outras condições tóxicas; os profissionais utilizam as medidas diagnósticas e terapêuticas da medicina convencional, além de medidas de manipulação. SIN osteopathic medicine. [osteo- + G. *pathos*, sofrimento]
alimentary o., o. alimentar; doença óssea decorrente da deficiência nutricional.

os·te·o·pe·di·on (os-tē-ō-pē'dē-on). Termo obsoleto para litopédio. [osteo- + G. *paidion*, dim. de *pais*, uma criança]

os·te·o·pe·nia (os'tē-ō-pē'nē-ā). Osteopenia. **1.** Calcificação ou densidade óssea diminuída; um termo descritivo aplicável a todos os sistemas esqueléticos em que tal condição é percebida; não comporta implicação sobre causalidade. **2.** Massa óssea reduzida devido à síntese inadequada de osteóide. [osteo- + G. *penia*, pobreza]

os·te·o·per·i·os·ti·tis (os'tē-ō-per'ē-os-tī'tis). Osteoperiostite; inflamação do periósteo e do osso subjacente.

os·te·o·pe·tro·sis (os'tē-ō-pe-trō'sis). [MIM*166600]. Osteopetrose; a formação excessiva de osso trabecular denso e cartilagem calcificada, em especial nos ossos longos, levando à obliteração de espaços medulares e a anemia com metaplasia mielóide e hepatoesplenomegalia, começando na fase de lactente, à fragilidade óssea e à surdez e cegueira progressivas; herança autossômica dominante. Também existem formas autossômicas recessivas, que podem ser branda [MIM*259710], grave [MIM*259700] ou letal [MIM*259720], e, por vezes, envolve um defeito tubular renal [MIM*259730]. Uma forma autossômica dominante mais branda apresenta início na infância e nenhuma seqüela neurológica. SIN Albers-Schönberg disease, marble bone disease, marble bones. [osteo- + G. *petra*, pedra, + *-osis*, condição]
o. ac'ro-osteoly'tica, o. acro-osteolítica. SIN piknodysostosis.
o. with renal tubular acidosis, o. com acidose tubular renal. SIN carbonic anhydrase II deficiency syndrome.

os·te·o·pe·trot·ic (os'tē-ō-pe-trot'ik). Osteopetrótico; relativo à osteopetrose.

os·te·o·phage (os'tē-ō-fāj). Osteoclasto. SIN osteoclast (1). [osteo- + G. *phagō*, comer]

os·te·o·phle·bi·tis (os′tē - ō - fle - bī′tis). Osteoflebite; inflamação das veias de um osso. [osteo- + G. *phleps*, veia, + *-itis*, inflamação]

os·te·oph·o·ny (os′tē - of′ō - nē). Condução óssea. SIN bone *conduction.*

os·te·o·phyte (os′tē - ō - fīt). Osteófito; crescimento ou protuberância óssea. [osteo- + G. *phyton*, vegetal]

os·te·o·plaque (os′tē - ō - plak). Osteoplaca; qualquer camada óssea. [osteo- + Fr. *plaque*, placa]

os·te·o·plast (os′tē - ō - plast). Osteoblasto. SIN osteoblast. [osteo- + G. *plastos*, formado]

os·te·o·plas·tic (os - tē - ō - plas′tik). Osteoplásico. **1.** SIN osteogenic. **2.** Relativo à osteoplastia.

os·te·o·plas·ty (os′tē - ō - plas - tē). Osteoplastia. **1.** Enxerto ósseo; cirurgia reparadora ou plástica dos ossos. **2.** Em odontologia, a ressecção da estrutura óssea para alcançar um contorno gengival aceitável. [osteo- + G. *plastos*, formado]

os·te·o·poi·ki·lo·sis (os′tē - ō - poy - ki - lō′sis). Osteopecilose; ossos mosqueados ou manchados causados por pequenos focos disseminados de osso compacto na substância esponjosa; herança autossômica dominante [MIM*166700]. VER TAMBÉM *osteopathia* striata, dermatofibrosis lenticularis disseminata. SIN osteopathia condensans. [osteo- + G. *poikilos*, mosqueado, + *-osis*, condição]

os·te·o·po·nin. Osteoponina; uma proteína produzida por osteoblastos de função desconhecida.

os·te·o·pon·tin. Osteopontina; uma fosfoproteína secretada, produzida por muitos tipos de células epiteliais, com substancial carga elétrica negativa e freqüentemente associada a processos de mineralização. É encontrada no plasma, na urina, no leite e na bile. As células transformadas expressam a o. em níveis elevados. SIN bone sialoprotein I.

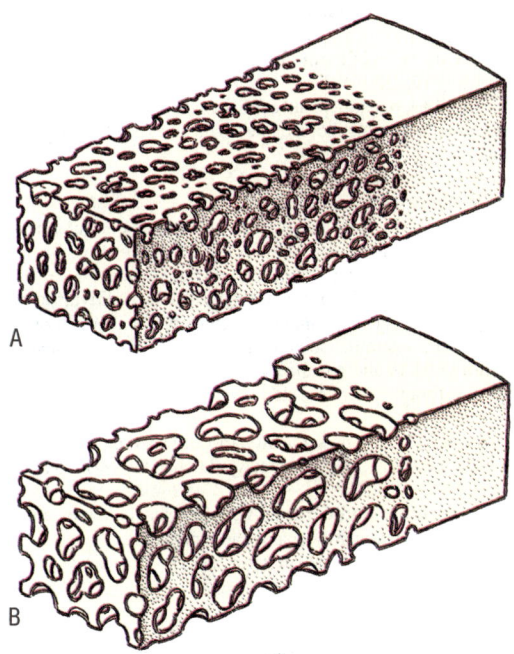

osteoporose: (A) osso normal; (B) osso osteoporótico

os·te·o·po·ro·sis (os′tē - ō - pō - rō′sis). Osteoporose; redução na quantidade de osso ou atrofia do tecido esquelético; um distúrbio relacionado com a idade caracterizado por massa óssea diminuída e suscetibilidade aumentada às fraturas. [osteo- + G. *poros*, poro, + *-osis*, condição]

> A osteoporose afeta 20 milhões de norte-americanos, dos quais 80% são mulheres, e custa até U$3,8 bilhões ao ano à sociedade norte-americana. Cerca de 1,3 milhão de fraturas atribuíveis à osteoporose ocorrem a cada ano em pessoas com 45 anos de idade ou mais, e essa condição é responsável por 50% das fraturas que ocorrem em mulheres com mais de 50 anos de idade. Embora todos os ossos sejam afetados, as fraturas vertebrais por compressão e as fraturas traumáticas do punho e do colo do fêmur são as mais comuns. A compressão vertebral assintomática gradual pode ser detectável apenas no exame radiográfico. A perda da altura corporal e o desenvolvimento de cifose podem ser os únicos sinais de colapso vertebral. Depois da fratura de quadril, a maioria dos pacientes idosos não recupera a atividade normal e a taxa de mortalidade em 1 ano se aproxima de 20%. As fraturas no idoso levam, com freqüência, à perda da mobilidade e da independência, à alienação social, ao medo de novas quedas e fraturas e à depressão. A osteoporose ocorre quando a reabsorção óssea supera a formação de osso. Os mecanismos subjacentes à osteoporose são complexos e provavelmente diversos. Os ossos passam constantemente por ciclos de reabsorção e formação (remodelação) para manter a concentração de cálcio e fosfato no líquido extracelular. Quando a concentração sérica de cálcio cai, aumenta a secreção de paratormônio (PTH), e esse hormônio estimula a reabsorção óssea por osteoclastos para restaurar os níveis séricos de cálcio à normalidade. A massa óssea diminui com a idade, sendo isso influenciado por sexo, raça, menopausa e pela relação entre peso e altura. A ingestão de cálcio e vitamina D nos alimentos, bem como as funções intestinal e renal, afeta a homeostasia de cálcio e fosfato. O risco de osteoporose é mais elevado nas mulheres após a menopausa. Parecem constituir fatores de risco independentes: raça asiática ou branca, baixo peso, ingestão insatisfatória de cálcio, sedentarismo, etilismo e tabagismo. O declínio do nível de vitamina D_3 com o envelhecimento resulta em má absorção de cálcio, que, por sua vez, estimula a reabsorção óssea. A deficiência de estrogênio exacerba esse problema por aumentar a sensibilidade do osso aos agentes de reabsorção. As mulheres amenorreicas em decorrência do exercício atlético rigoroso e restrição dietética ou de distúrbios alimentares correm risco de osteoporose. A formação e a reabsorção de osso também são influenciadas por fatores físicos externos, como o peso corporal e a prática de exercícios físicos. A imobilidade e o repouso prolongado no leito produzem perda óssea rápida, enquanto a prática de exercícios envolvendo levantamento de peso comprovadamente reduz a perda óssea e aumenta a massa óssea. A osteoporose é comum em adultos jovens com fibrose cística, principalmente aqueles que usam corticosteróides há muito tempo. O diagnóstico da osteoporose primária é confirmado pela documentação da redução da densidade óssea depois da exclusão das causas conhecidas de perda óssea excessiva. As radiografias são indicadores insensíveis da perda óssea, pois a densidade óssea precisa estar diminuída em, pelo menos, 20 a 30% antes que a redução possa ser apreciada. Os procedimentos diagnósticos padronizados são a determinação da densidade mineral óssea na porção ultradistal do rádio e na porção média da diáfise por meio da absorciometria fotônica única, e no quadril e na coluna lombar por absorciometria por raios X com energia dupla (DEXA). Um procedimento quantitativo com ultra-som recentemente aprovado pela FDA é comparável às mensurações da densidade óssea por DEXA na previsão de fraturas decorrentes da osteoporose. A terapia na osteoporose visa a prevenção de fraturas nos pacientes suscetíveis. A regulação temporal apropriada e o uso correto de agentes, como cálcio, vitamina D, estrogênio, bifosfonatos, calcitonina e raloxifeno, bem como a prática de exercícios físicos, geraram importantes esforços de pesquisa e considerável controvérsia. A ingestão de cotas adequadas de cálcio e vitamina D e a continuação de exercícios moderados de sustentação de peso constituem as medidas preventivas básicas para pessoas de todas as idades. A administração de estrogênio na menopausa, bem como depois dela, não somente interrompe a perda de osso, como, na verdade, aumenta a massa óssea. A reposição de estrogênio permanece como a prevenção e o tratamento mais efetivos para a osteoporose pós-menopausa. Acredita-se que seja mais apropriado iniciar o estrogênio ao sinal mais precoce da menopausa, pois a perda óssea provavelmente começa antes da cessação da menstruação. A terapia com estrogênio tem de ser mantida até a velhice, de modo a manter a densidade óssea ótima. Não há evidências convincentes de que o início da terapia com estrogênio em mulheres idosas evitará a osteoporose. Os benefícios da terapia com estrogênio têm de ser pesados contra o risco aumentado de hiperplasia endometrial e de carcinoma de endométrio (que pode ser contrabalançado pela administração concomitante de progestogênio) e, possivelmente, de carcinoma de mama. O modulador seletivo do receptor de estrogênio raloxifeno foi aprovado pela FDA para a prevenção da osteoporose. Ele não provoca hiperplasia endometrial, porém é menos efetivo que o estrogênio na conservação da massa óssea. O hormônio calcitonina, administrado por injeção ou *spray* nasal, inibe a reabsorção óssea e possui outros efeitos sobre o metabolismo mineral. Demonstrou-se que os bifosfonatos, como o alendronato e etidronato, que se ligam aos cristais ósseos, tornando-os mais resistentes à hidrólise enzimática e inibindo a ação dos osteoclastos, aumentam a densidade mineral óssea. As estratégias para evitar quedas são importantes nos pacientes idosos. VER TAMBÉM estrogen replacement therapy, raloxifene.

o. circumscrip′ta cra′nii, o. craniana circunscrita; a o. craniana localizada, freqüentemente observada na doença de Paget.

juvenile o., o. juvenil; o. idiopática com início antes da puberdade, levando a dor ou fraturas, com remissão espontânea em alguns anos.

posttraumatic o., o. pós-traumática. SIN Sudeck atrophy.
os·te·o·po·rot·ic (os'tē-ō-pō-rot'ik). Osteoporótico; pertinente a, caracterizado por o que causa uma condição porosa dos ossos.
osteoprotegerin (os'tē-ō-prō-teg'er-in). Osteoprotegerina; uma proteína secretada que inibe a diferenciação do osteoclasto.
os·te·o·ra·di·ol·o·gist (os'tē-ō-rā-dē-ol'ō-jist). Osteorradiologista; um médico que se especializa em radiologia dos ossos e articulações. [osteo- + radiologist]
os·te·o·ra·di·ol·o·gy. Osteorradiologia; a subespecialidade clínica da radiologia óssea diagnóstica.
os·te·o·ra·di·o·ne·cro·sis (os'tē-ō-rā'dē-ō-ne-krō'sis). Osteorradionecrose; a necrose do osso produzida por radiação ionizante; pode ser planejada ou não-planejada. [osteo- + radionecrosis]
os·te·or·rha·phy (os-tē-or'ă-fē). Osteorrafia; a união de fragmentos de um osso fraturado por meio de fios. [osteo- + G. *rhaphē*, sutura]
os·te·o·sar·co·ma (os'tē-ō-sar-kō'mă). Osteossarcoma. SIN osteogenic sarcoma.
  parosteal o., o. paraosteal; o o. de baixo grau que surge na superfície do osso sem envolvimento da medula subjacente, geralmente ocorrendo como uma massa maciçamente ossificada na porção distal do fêmur em mulheres na terceira e quarta décadas de vida.
  periosteal o., o. periosteal; o. condroblástico que ocorre na superfície dos ossos sem o envolvimento da medula; geralmente ocorre em adolescentes e adultos jovens como um defeito radiotransparente, com as espículas ósseas estendendo-se para os tecidos moles. Histologicamente, o tumor é de grau intermediário a alto, e a cartilagem se mostra lobulada.
os·te·o·scle·ro·sis (os'tē-ō-skle-rō'sis). Osteosclerose; endurecimento anormal ou eburnação do osso. [osteo- + G. *sklērōsis*, endurecimento]
os·te·o·scle·rot·ic (os'tē-ō-skle-rot'ik). Osteoesclerótico; relativo a, devido a ou caracterizado por endurecimento da substância óssea.
os·te·o·sis (os-tē-ō'sis). 1. Osteopatia; processo mórbido no osso. SIN ostosis (1). 2. Osteose. SIN osteogenesis. [osteo- + G. *osis*, condição]
  parathyroid o., osteíte fibrosa cística. SIN osteítis fibrosa cystica.
  renal fibrocystic o., raquitismo renal. SIN renal rickets.
os·te·o·spon·gi·o·ma (os'tē-ō-spon'jē-ō'mă). Osteoespongioma; termo inespecífico geral para uma neoplasia no osso que resulta em adelgaçamento e fragmentação (dessa maneira, em amolecimento) do córtex. [osteo- + G. *spongos*, esponja, + *-oma*, tumor]
os·te·o·ste·a·to·ma (os'tē-ō-stē'ă-tō'mă). Osteoesteatoma; uma massa benigna, geralmente um lipoma ou cisto sebáceo, no qual há pequenos focos de elementos ósseos. [osteo- + G. *stear*, sebo, gordura, + *-oma*, tumor]
os·te·o·su·ture (os-tē-ō-soo'choor). Osteorrafia. SIN osteorrhaphy.
os·te·o·syn·the·sis (os-tē-ō-sin'thē-sis). Osteossíntese; fixação interna de uma fratura por meio de um dispositivo mecânico, como um pino, parafuso ou placa.
os·te·o·throm·bo·sis (os'tē-ō-throm-bō'sis). Osteotrombose; trombose em uma ou mais veias de um osso.
os·te·o·tome (os'tē-ō-tōm). Osteótomo; um instrumento para uso no corte do osso. [osteo- + G. *tomē*, incisão]
os·te·ot·o·my (os-tē-ot'ō-mē). Osteotomia; corte de um osso, geralmente por meio de uma serra ou osteótomo. [osteo- + G. *tomē*, incisão]
  "C" sliding o., o. deslizante em forma de C; o. extra-oral na forma de um "C" realizada bilateralmente nos ramos mandibulares, visando a correção de retrognatismo e/ou apertognatia.
  Dwyer o., o. de Dwyer; um procedimento para o pé em gota.
  horizontal o., o. horizontal; o. realizada no nível intra-oral para genioplastia; a face inferior da porção anterior da mandíbula é avançada ou retraída por movimento do segmento livre.
  Le Fort o., o. de Le Fort; o. realizada ao longo das linhas clássicas de fratura, conforme descrito por Le Fort, a fim de corrigir uma deformidade esquelética maxilar; classificada como o. de Le Fort I, maxilar baixa; II, nasoorbitomaxilar piramidal; ou III, maxilar alta, dependendo da localização.
  sagittal split mandibular o., o. mandibular com divisão sagital; procedimento cirúrgico intra-oral para correção de retrognatismo, apertognatismo e prognatismo; os ramos mandibulares e a porção posterior da mandíbula são seccionados no plano sagital.
  segmental alveolar o., o. alveolar segmentar; procedimento cirúrgico intraoral em que os segmentos do osso alveolar que contêm os dentes são seccionados entre os dentes, bem como em um plano apical, para o reposicionamento dos alvéolos e dentes; pode ser maxilar ou mandibular, podendo ser combinada à ostectomia.
  sliding oblique o., o. por deslizamento oblíquo; um procedimento cirúrgico oral em que o ramo mandibular é cortado verticalmente desde a incisura da mandíbula até o ângulo para facilitar o reposicionamento posterior da mandíbula na correção da prognatia mandibular; pode ser realizada por via extra-oral ou intra-oral, sendo similar à o. vertical.
  vertical o., o. vertical; procedimento cirúrgico oral similar à o. por deslizamento oblíquo.

os·te·o·tribe (os'tē-ō-trīb). Osteótribo; um instrumento para a raspagem de pedaços de osso necrosado ou corroído. [osteo- + G. *tribō*, raspar, desgastar]
os·te·o·trite (os'tē-ō-trīt). Osteótrito; um instrumento com extremidade cônica ou olivar que possui uma superfície de corte, assemelhando-se a uma broca dentária, usado para a remoção do osso corroído. [osteo- + L. *tritus*, raspagem, desgaste]
os·te·ot·ro·phy (os-tē-ot'rō-fē). Osteotrofia; nutrição do tecido ósseo. [osteo- + G. *trophē*, nutrição]
os·te·o·tym·pan·ic (os'tē-ō-tim-pan'ik). Osteotimpânico. SIN otocranial. [osteo- + G. *tympanon*, tímpano]
os·tia (os'tē-ă). Óstios; plural de ostium. [L.]
os·ti·al (os'tē-ăl). Ostial; relativo a qualquer orifício ou óstio.
os·ti·tic (os-ti'tik). Osteítico. SIN osteitic.
os·ti·tis (os-ti'tis) Osteíte. SIN osteitis.
os·ti·um, pl. **os·tia** (os'tē-ŭm, -ă) [TA]. Óstio, óstios; uma pequena abertura, especialmente aquela da entrada para o interior de um órgão oco ou canal. VER TAMBÉM orifice, opening, os, mouth (2). [L. porta, entrada, boca]
  o. abdomina'le tu'bae uteri'nae [TA], o. abdominal da tuba uterina. SIN abdominal o. of uterine tube.
  abdominal o. of uterine tube [TA], o. abdominal da tuba uterina; uma extremidade fimbriada ou ovariana de um oviducto. SIN o. abdominale tubae uterinae [TA].
  o. anatomicum [TA], o. anatômico interno do útero. SIN anatomical internal *os* of uterus.
  o. aor'tae [TA], o. da aorta. SIN aortic *orifice*.
  aortic o., o. da aorta. SIN aortic *orifice*.
  o. appen'dicis vermifor'mis [TA], o. do apêndice vermiforme. SIN *orifice* of vermiform appendix.
  o. arterio'sum, o. atrioventricular esquerdo. SIN left atrioventricular *orifice*.
  o. atrioventricula're dex'trum [TA], o. atrioventricular direito. SIN right atrioventricular *orifice*.
  o. atrioventricula're sinis'trum [TA], o. atrioventricular esquerdo. SIN left atrioventricular *orifice*.
  o. cardi'acum [TA], o. cárdico. SIN cardiac *orifice*.
  o. histologicum [TA], o. histológico interno do útero. SIN histological internal *os* of uterus.
  o. ileale [TA], o. ileal. SIN ileal *orifice*.
  o. ileoceca'le, o. ileal. SIN ileal *orifice*.
  o. inter'num, o. uterino das tubas uterinas. SIN uterine o. of uterine tubes.
  o. pharyn'geum tu'bae auditi'vae [TA], o. faríngeo da tuba auditiva. SIN pharyngeal *opening* of pharyngotympanic (auditory) tube.
  o. pharyngeum tubae auditoriae, o. faríngeo da tuba auditiva;* termo oficial alternativo para pharyngeal *opening* of pharyngotympanic (auditory) tube.
  o. pri'mum. forame interatrial do tipo *primum*. SIN interatrial *foramen primum*.
  o. pylor'icum [TA], o. pilórico. SIN pyloric *orifice*.
  o. secun'dum, forame interatrial do tipo *secundum*. SIN interatrial *foramen* secundum.
  o. sinus coronarii [TA], o. do seio coronário. SIN *opening* of coronary sinus.
  o. trun'ci pulmona'lis [TA], o. do tronco pulmonar. SIN *opening* of pulmonary trunk.
  o. tympan'icum tu'bae auditi'vae [TA], o. timpânico da tuba auditiva. SIN tympanic *opening* of pharyngotympanic (auditory) tube.
  o. ure'teris [TA], o. do ureter. SIN ureteric *orifice*.

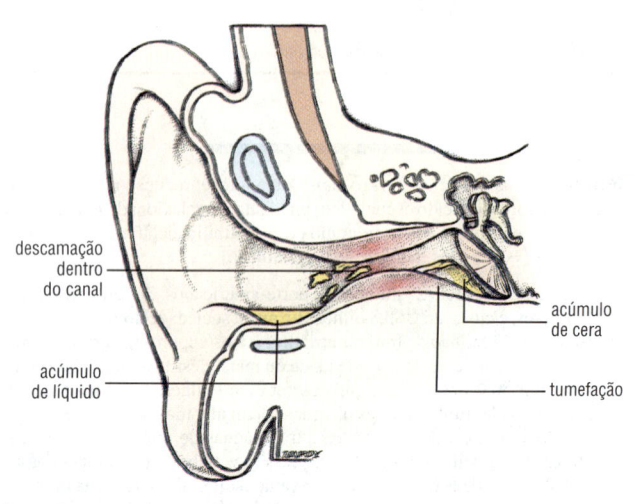

otite externa

o. ure'thrae exter'num [TA], o. externo da uretra. SIN external urethral *orifice*.
o. ure'thrae inter'num [TA], o. interno da uretra. SIN internal urethral *orifice*.
o. urethrae internum accipiens [TA], o. interno da uretra no enchimento. SIN filling internal urethral *orifice*.
o. urethrae internum evacuans [TA], o. interno da uretra no esvaziamento. SIN voiding internal urethral *orifice*.
o. u'teri [TA], o. do útero. SIN external *os* of uterus.
o. u'teri exter'num, o. externo do útero. SIN external *os* of uterus.
o. u'teri inter'num, o. interno do útero. SIN *isthmus* of uterus.
uterine o. of uterine tubes [TA], o. uterino das tubas uterinas; a abertura uterina do oviducto. SIN o. uterinum tubae uterinae [TA], o. internum, uterine opening of uterine tubes.
o. uteri'num tu'bae uterinae [TA], o. uterino das tubas uterinas. SIN uterine o. of uterine tubes.
o. vagi'nae [TA], o. da vagina. SIN vaginal *orifice*.
o. ve'nae ca'vae inferio'ris [TA], o. da veia cava inferior. SIN *opening* of inferior vena cava.
o. ve'nae ca'vae superio'ris [TA], o. da veia cava superior. SIN *opening* of superior vena cava.
os'tia vena'rum pulmona'lium [TA], óstios das veias pulmonares. SIN *openings* of pulmonary veins, em *opening*.
o. veno'sum cordis, o. atrioventricular direito. SIN right atrioventricular *orifice*.
o. of vermiform appendix, o. do apêndice vermiforme. SIN *orifice* of vermiform appendix.
os·to·mate (os'tō-māt). Ostomizado; termo para aquele que possui uma ostomia. [L. *ostium*, boca]
os·to·my (os'tō-mē) Ostomia. **1.** Um estoma ou abertura artificial para o canal urinário ou gastrointestinal, ou para a traquéia. **2.** Qualquer operação pela qual uma abertura permanente é criada entre dois órgãos ocos ou entre uma víscera oca e a pele, externamente, como na traqueostomia. [L. *ostium*, boca]
-ostomy. -ostomia. VER -stomy.
os·to·sis (os-tō'sis). **1.** Osteopatia SIN osteosis (1). **2.** Osteose. SIN osteogenesis.
os·tra·ceous (os-trā-shŭs). Ostráceo; indica o acúmulo de escamas observado na psoríase, que se assemelha à estratificação das conchas de ostra. [*Ostraeacea*, grupo que inclui as ostras]
os·tre·o·tox·ism (os-trē-ō-tok'sizm). Ostreotoxismo; intoxicação a partir da ingestão de ostras infectadas ou contaminadas. [G. *ostreon*, ostra, + *toxikon*, veneno]
Ostwald, Friedrich Wilhelm, físico-químico alemão e laureado com o prêmio Nobel, 1853–1932. VER O. solubility *coefficient*.
OT Abreviatura para *occupational therapist* ou *therapy* (terapeuta ou terapia ocupacional); Koch old *tuberculin* (tuberculina antiga de Koch).
ot-. Forma combinante que significa orelha. VER TAMBÉM auri-. [G. *ous*]
Ota, Masao T., dermatologista japonês, 1885–1945. VER Ota *nevus*.
otal·gia (ō-tal'jē-ă). Otalgia. SIN earache. [ot- + G. *algos*, dor]
geniculate o., neuralgia geniculada. SIN geniculate *neuralgia*.
reflex o., o. reflexa; dor referida à orelha decorrente de doença em outra região, mais amiúde dentes, seio maxilar, nasofaringe, tonsila, faringe ou laringe.
otal·gic (ō-tal'jik). **1.** Relativo à otalgia ou dor de ouvido. **2.** Um remédio para a otalgia.
OTC Abreviatura para *over the counter*, pertinente a uma droga vendida sem receita médica.
oth·er-di·rect·ed (odh'er-di-rek'ted). Dirigido por outro; pertinente a uma pessoa prontamente influenciada pela atitude de outras.
otic (ō'tik). Ótico; relativo à orelha. [G. *otikos*, de *ous*, ouvido]
Otis, Arthur Brooks, fisiologista respiratório norte-americano, *1913. VER Rahn-O. *sample*.
otit·ic (ō-tit'ik). Otítico; relativo à otite.
oti·tis (o-tī'tis), Otite; inflamação da orelha. [ot- + G. *-itis*, inflamação]
adhesive o., o. adesiva; a inflamação da orelha média causada pela disfunção prolongada da tuba auditiva, resultando em retração permanente da membrana timpânica e obliteração do espaço da orelha média.
o. desquamati'va, o. descamativa; o. externa com descamação copiosa.
o. exter'na, o. externa; inflamação do canal auditivo externo. SIN swimmer's ear.
o. inter'na, o. interna. SIN labyrinthitis.
malignant external o., o. externa maligna; osteomielite do osso temporal por *Pseudomonas* com risco de vida nos idosos diabéticos; começa com otalgia e inchação e secreção a partir do meato acústico externo. SIN *Pseudomonas* osteomyelitis.
o. me'dia, o. média; inflamação da orelha média ou da membrana timpânica.
reflux o. me'dia, o. média por refluxo; a o. média causada pela passagem de um líquido ingerido (usualmente leite) ou secreções nasofaríngeas através da tuba auditiva.
secretory o. media, o. média secretora. SIN middle-ear *effusion*.
serous o. media, o. média serosa. SIN middle-ear *effusion*.
oto-. Forma combinante que significa orelha. VER TAMBÉM auri-. [G. *ous*]
oto·acous·tic (ō'tō-a-koo-stik). Otoacústico; que se refere a sons muito suaves produzidos pela orelha; acredita-se que representem vibrações mecânicas na cóclea.

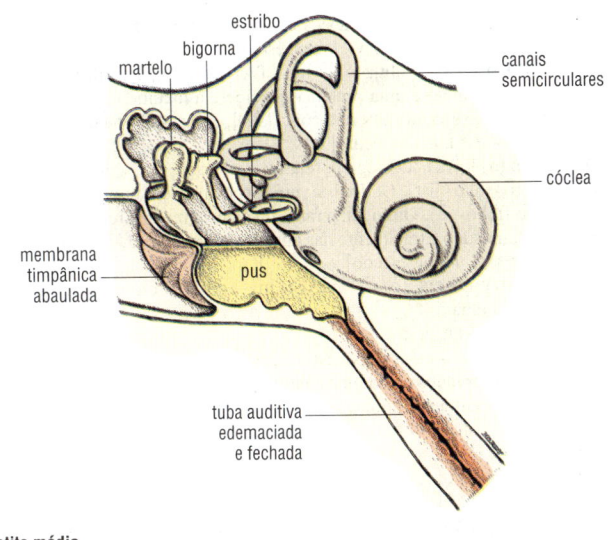

otite média

oto·bi·o·sis (ō'tō-bī-ō'sis). Otobiose; presença de larvas e as características ninfas espinhosas do carrapato *Otobius megnini* no canal auditivo externo do gado bovino, cavalos, gatos, cães, cervos, coiotes e outros animais domésticos e selvagens; podem permanecer na orelha durante vários meses antes de se transformarem em pupas e amadurecerem. São conhecidos vários registros de infestação em seres humanos.
Oto·bi·us (ō-tō'bē-ŭs). Um gênero de carrapatos argasídeos semelhantes ao *Ornithodoros*, mas caracterizados por um tegumento granulado, um hipostoma que é vestigial no adulto, mas bem desenvolvido nas ninfas espinhosas, e por ausência de olhos e capuz. Duas espécies são reconhecidas: *O. lagophilus* (o carrapato da face dos coelhos) e *O. megnini*, o carrapato espinhoso da orelha que provoca otobiose em cavalos, gado bovino, carneiro, cães e alguns animais selvagens; ocorrem nas regiões do sudoeste dos Estados Unidos, onde é uma peste importante, e também está distribuído mundialmente.
oto·ceph·a·ly (ō-tō-sef'ă-lē). Otocefalia; malformação caracterizada por desenvolvimento acentuadamente defeituoso da mandíbula (micrognatismo ou agnatismo) e a união ou grande aproximação das orelhas (sinotia) na frente do pescoço. [oto- + G. *kephalē*, cabeça]
oto·cer·e·bri·tis (ō-tō-ser-ē-brī'tis). Otocerebrite. SIN otoencephalitis.
oto·co·nia, sing. **oto·co·ni·um** (ō-to-kō'ne-ă, -ŭm). Otólitos; otólito. SIN otoliths.
oto·cra·ni·al (ō-tō-krā'nē-ăl). Otocraniano; relativo ao otocrânio. SIN osteotympanic.
oto·cra·ni·um (ō'tō-krā'nē-ŭm). Otocrânio; o arcabouço ósseo das orelhas interna e média, consistindo na porção petrosa do osso temporal. [oto- + G. *kranion*, crânio]
oto·cyst (ō'tō-sist). Otocisto. **1.** Vesícula auditiva embrionária. **2.** Um órgão do equilíbrio, análogo ao utrículo dos mamíferos, existente em determinados invertebrados e que contém grãos de material calcário ou de areia. [oto- + G. *kystis*, uma bexiga]
Oto·dec·tes (ō-tō-dek'tēz). Um gênero de ácaros da orelha (família Psoroptidae) que consiste em uma única espécie, *O. cynotis*, a causa da sarna octodética em cães, gatos e outros carnívoros; toda a vida desse ácaro se passa nas orelhas (raramente no corpo) do hospedeiro, onde ele se alimenta de resíduos epidérmicos; pode ser encontrado no material incrustado raspado de orelhas infectadas. [oto- + *dēktēs*, pedinte, receptor]
oto·dec·tic (ō-tō-dek'tik). Otodético; de, relativo a ou causado por ácaros do gênero *Otodectes*.
oto·dyn·ia (ō-tō-din'ē-ă). Otodinia. SIN earache. [oto- + G. *odynē*, dor]
oto·en·ceph·a·li·tis (ō-tō-en-sef-ă-lī'tis). Otoencefalite; inflamação do cérebro por extensão do processo a partir da orelha média e células da mastóide. SIN otocerebritis. [oto- + G. *enkephalos*, cérebro, + *-itis*, inflamação]
oto·gang·li·on (ō-tō-gang'glē-on). Gânglio ótico. SIN otic *ganglion*.
oto·gen·ic, otog·e·nous (ō'tō-jen'ik, ō-toj-ē-nŭs). Otogênico; de origem ótica; que se origina na orelha, em especial a partir de inflamação do ouvido. [oto- + G. *-gen*, que produz]
oto·lar·yn·gol·o·gist (ō-tō-lar-ing-gol'ō-jist). Otolaringologista; um médico que se especializa em otolaringologia.
oto·lar·yn·gol·o·gy (ō'tō-lar-ing-gol'ō-jē). Otolaringologia; as especialidades combinadas das doenças da orelha e laringe, incluindo o trato respira-

tório superior e as doenças da cabeça e pescoço, árvore traqueobrônquica e esôfago. [oto- + G. *larynx*, + G. *logos*, estudo]

oto·liths, oto·lites (ō′tō-lith, o′tō-līt) [TA]. Otólito; partículas cristalinas de carbonato de cálcio e uma proteína que adere à membrana gelatinosa da mácula do utrículo e sáculo. SIN statoconia [TA], ear crystals, otoconia, sagitta, statoliths. [oto- + G. *lithos*, pedra]

oto·log·ic (ō′tō-loj′ik). Otológico; relativo à otologia.

otol·o·gist (ō-tol′ō-jist). Otologista; um especialista em otologia.

otol·o·gy (ō-tol′ō-jē). Otologia; o ramo da ciência médica relacionado com o estudo, diagnóstico e tratamento das doenças da orelha e das estruturas correlatas. [oto- + G. *logos*, estudo]

oto·mu·cor·my·co·sis (ō-tō-mū′kŏr-mī-kō′sis). Otomucormicose; mucormicose da orelha.

-otomy. -Otomia. VER -tomy.

oto·my·co·sis (ō′tō-mī-kō′sis). Otomicose; infecção na qual os micélios fúngicos são observados no cerume e nas células descamadas no meato acústico externo, usualmente unilateral, com descamação, prurido e dor como manifestações básicas. O fungo não invade o tecido e tem pouca função na patogenicidade.

oto·neu·ral·gia (ō′tō-noo-ral′jē-ă). Otoneuralgia; otalgia de origem neurálgica, não provocada por inflamação. [oto- + G. *neuron*, nervo, + *algos*, dor]

oto·pal·a·to·dig·i·tal (ō′tō-pal′ă-tō-dij′i-tăl). Otopalatodigital; relativo às orelhas, ao palato e aos dedos das mãos.

otop·a·thy (ō-top′ă-thē). Otopatia; qualquer doença da orelha. [oto- + G. *pathos*, sofrimento]

oto·pha·ryn·ge·al (ō′tō-fă-rin′jē-ăl). Otofaríngeo; relativo à orelha média e à faringe.

oto·plas·ty (ō′tō-plas-tē). Otoplastia; cirurgia plástica construtiva ou reparadora da orelha. [oto- + G. *plastos*, formado]

oto·rhi·no·lar·yn·gol·o·gy (ō′tō-rī′nō-lar-ing-gol′ō-jē). Otorrinolaringologia; as especialidades combinadas das doenças da orelha, nariz, faringe e laringe; incluindo doenças da cabeça e do pescoço, árvore traqueobrônquica e esôfago. VER TAMBÉM otolaringology. [oto- + G. *rhis*, nariz, + *larynx*, laringe, + *logos*, estudo]

otor·rhea (ō-tō-rē′ă). Otorréia; secreção orinda da orelha. [oto- + G. *rhoia*, fluxo]

cerebrospinal fluid o., o. liquórica; eliminação de líquido cefalorraquidiano através do meato acústico externo ou através da tuba auditiva para a nasofaringe.

oto·sal·pinx (ō-tō-sal′pingks). Tuba auditiva. SIN pharyngotympanic (auditory) tube. [oto- + G. *salpinx*, trompa]

oto·scle·ro·sis (ō′tō-sklē-rō′sis). Otosclerose; uma doença da cápsula ótica (labirinto ósseo) caracterizada pela formação do osso vascular macio e que resulta na perda auditiva de condução progressiva, devido à fixação do estribo, e perda auditiva sensorial por causa do envolvimento do ducto coclear. [oto- + G. *sklērōsis*, endurecimento]

oto·scope (ō′tō-skōp). Otoscópio; um instrumento para examinar a membrana timpânica. [oto- + G. *skopeō*, visualizar]

Siegle o., o. de Siegle; um o. com uma inserção bulbosa através da qual pode ser variada a pressão do ar, conferindo, assim, movimento à membrana timpânica, quando intacta, durante a inspeção.

otos·co·py (ō-tos′kŏ-pē). Otoscopia; a inspeção da orelha, especialmente da membrana timpânica. [oto- + G. *skopeō*, visualizar]

pneumatic o., o. pneumática; inspeção da orelha com um dispositivo capaz de variar a pressão do ar exercida sobre a membrana timpânica. O movimento conferido à membrana timpânica sugere complacência normal da orelha média; a falta de movimento indica impedância aumentada (p. ex., presença de líquido na orelha média ou perfuração da membrana timpânica).

oto·spon·gi·o·sis (ot-ō-spun-jē′ō′sis). Otoespongiose; um termo que descreve com maior acurácia as alterações patológicas na otosclerose.

otos·te·al (ō-tos′tē-ăl). Otosteal; relativo aos ossículos da orelha. [oto- + G. *osteon*, osso]

oto·tox·ic (ō′tō-tok′sik). Ototóxico; relativo à ototoxicidade.

oto·tox·ic·i·ty (ō-tō-tok-sis′i-te). Ototoxicidade; a propriedade de ser lesivo para a orelha. [oto- + G. *toxikon*, veneno]

familial aminoglycoside o., o. familial por aminoglicosídeo; suscetibilidade hereditária à perda auditiva sensorial perante a administração de antibióticos aminoglicosídeos em decorrência de uma mutação no genoma mitocondrial.

Otto, Adolph W., cirurgião alemão, 1786–1845. VER O. *pelvis*, *disease*.

ot·to of rose. Óleo de rosa. SIN oil of rose.

Ottoson, David, fisiologista sueco, *1918. VER O. *potential*.

O. U. Abreviatura do latim *oculus uterque*, cada olho ou os dois olhos.

oua·ba·gen·in (wă′bă-jen-in). Ouabagenina; a aglicona obtida a partir da hidrólise do glicosídeo cardíaco ouabaína; exerce atividade cardiotônica.

oua·ba·in (wah′băn, wah′bah-in). Ouabaína; um glicosídeo e veneno africano para flechas obtido do ouabaio, da madeira da *Acocanthera ouabaio* ou das sementes da *Strophantus gratus*; sua ação é qualitativamente idêntica à do estrofanto e dos glicosídeos digitálicos; usada para digitalização rápida; freqüentemente empregada em estudos farmacológicos por causa de sua hidrossolubilidade.

Ouchterlony, Orjan, bacteriologista sueco, *1914. VER O. *method*, *technique*, *test*, *technique*.

oul-. Para as palavras assim iniciadas, ver ulo-.

ounce (oz.) (owns). Onça; um peso que contém 480 g ou 1/12 do peso da libra no sistema para metais preciosos e gemas e no sistema farmacêutico, ou 437,5 g, 1/16 do peso da libra *avoirdupois*. A onça farmacêutica (usada na USP) contém 8 dracmas e é equivalente a 31,10349 g; a libra *avoirdupois* equivale a 28,35 g. [L. *uncia*, a décima segunda parte (de uma libra ou pé), portanto, também polegada]

-ous. 1. Sufixo químico ligado ao nome de um elemento em uma de suas menores valências. Cf. -ic (1). **2.** Que possui muito de. [L. *-osus*, cheio de, abundante]

out·let (owt′let) [TA]. Abertura; entrada ou saída de uma passagem. VER TAMBÉM aperture.

pelvic o. [TA], abertura inferior da pelve; a abertura inferior da pelve verdadeira, limitada anteriormente pelo arco pubiano, lateralmente pelos ramos do ísquio e pelo ligamento sacrotuberal em ambos os lados, e, posteriormente, por esses ligamentos e pela extremidade do cóccix. SIN apertura pelvis inferior [TA], apertura pelvis minoris, fourth parallel pelvic plane, inferior pelvic aperture, pelvic plane of outlet, plane of outlet.

thoracic o., abertura torácica; **(1)** SIN inferior thoracic aperture; **(2)** SIN superior thoracic aperture.

out·li·er (owt′lē-er). Uma observação que difere bastante de todas as outras em um conjunto, como se fosse para justificar a conclusão de que ocorreu um erro grosseiro ou de que se origina de uma população diferente.

out·pa·tient (owt′pā′shent). Paciente externo; um paciente tratado em um ambulatório hospitalar ou clínica, em vez de em uma enfermaria ou quarto.

out of phase. Fora de fase; que se move em direções opostas ao mesmo tempo; 180° fora de fase; uma característica possível de duas oscilações simultâneas de freqüência semelhante.

out·put (owt′poot). Débito; a quantidade produzida, ejetada ou excretada de uma entidade específica em determinado período de tempo ou por unidade de tempo, p.ex., d. urinário de sódio; o oposto de ingestão ou aporte.

cardiac o., d. cardíaco; o volume de sangue ejetado pelo coração em uma unidade de tempo (ou seja, o volume por minuto), geralmente expressa em litros por minuto. SIN minute o.

maximum power o., d. de intensidade máxima; o maior som resultante da amplificação daquele que o instrumento consegue produzir; uma indicação do desempenho do aparelho auditivo.

minute o., d. cardíaco. SIN cardiac o.

pacemaker o., d. do marcapasso; a energia elétrica liberada em uma carga-padrão (resistência de 500 Ω).

stroke o., volume sistólico. SIN stroke volume.

ova (ō′vă). Ovos; plural de *ovum*. [L.]

oval (ō′văl). **1.** Relativo a um ovo. **2.** Oval; com formato de ovo, assemelhando-se no contorno ao corte longitudinal de um ovo.

ov·al·bu·min (ō-văl-bū′min). Ovalbumina; a principal proteína que ocorre na clara do ovo e que se assemelha à albumina sérica; também encontrada na forma fosforilada. SIN albumen, egg albumin.

oval·o·cy·to·sis (ō′vă-lō-sī-tō′sis). Ovalocitose. SIN elliptocytosis.

ovar·i·al·gia (ō-var′ē-ăl′jē-ă). Ovarialgia; dor em um ovário. SIN oophoralgia. [ovario- + G. *algos*, dor]

ovar·i·an (ō-var′ē-an). Ovariano; relativo ao ovário.

ovar·i·ec·to·my (ō-var-ē-ek′tō-mē). Ovariectomia; a excisão de um ou de ambos os ovários. SIN oophorectomy. [ovario- + G. *ektomē*, excisão]

ovario-, ovari. Formas combinantes que significam ovário. VER TAMBÉM oo-, oophor-. [L. *ovarium*]

ovar·i·o·cele (ō-var′ē-ō-sēl). Ovariocele; hérnia de um ovário. [ovario- + G. *kēlē*, hérnia]

ovar·i·o·cen·te·sis (ō-var′ē-ō-sen-tē′sis). Ovariocentese; punção de um ovário ou de um cisto ovariano. [ovario- + G. *kentēsis*, punção]

ovar·i·o·cy·e·sis (ō-var′ē-ō-sī-ē′sis). Gravidez ovariana. SIN ovarian pregnancy. [ovario- + G. *kyēsis*, gravidez]

ovar·i·o·dys·neu·ria (ō-var′ē-ō-dis-noo′rē-ă). Ovariodisneuria; dor ou neuralgia ovariana. [ovario- + G. *dys*, ruim, + *neuron*, nervo]

ovar·i·o·gen·ic (ō-var′ē-ō-jen′ik). Ovariogênico; que se origina no ovário. [ovario- + G. *-gen*, produção]

ovar·i·o·lyt·ic (ō-var′ē-ō-lit′ik). Ovariolítico; destrutivo para o ovário. [ovario- + G. *lysis*, dissolução]

ovar·i·op·a·thy (ō-var′ē-op′ă-thē). Ovariopatia; qualquer doença do ovário. SIN oophoropathy. [ovario- + G. *pathos*, sofrimento]

ovar·i·or·rhex·is (ō-var′ē-ō-rek′sis). Ovariorrexe; ruptura de um ovário. [ovario- + G. *rhēxis*, ruptura]

ovar·i·o·sal·pin·gec·to·my (ō-var′ē-ō-sal-pin′jek′tō-mē). Ovariossalpingectomia; remoção cirúrgica de um ovário e do oviducto correspondente. SIN oophorosalpingectomy. [ovario- + salpingectomy]

ovar·i·o·sal·pin·gi·tis (ō-var´ē-ō-sal-pin-jī´tis). Ovariossalpingite; inflamação do ovário e do oviducto. SIN oophorosalpingitis. [ovario- + salpingitis]

ovar·i·os·to·my (ō-var-ē-os´tŏ-mē). Ovariostomia; a criação de uma fístula temporária para a drenagem de um cisto do ovário. [ovario- + G. *stoma*, boca]

ovar·i·ot·o·my (ō-var-ē-ot´ŏ-mē). Ovariotomia; uma incisão em um ovário, p.ex., uma biópsia ou uma excisão em cunha. SIN oophorotomy. [ovário- + G. *tomē*, incisão]

ova·ri·tis (ō-vă-rī´tis) Ovarite, ooforite. SIN oophoritis.

ovar·i·um, pl. **ova·ria** (ō-var´ē-ŭm, -ă). [TA]. Ovário, ovários. SIN ovary. [L. mod. de *ovum*, ovo]

  o. biparti´tum, o. bipartido; um ovário separado em duas partes distintas.

  o. disjunc´tum, o. dividido; um ovário dividido, de maneira parcial ou completa, em duas partes.

  o. gyra´tum, o. circinado; um ovário que mostra sulcos ou estrias curvas ou irregulares.

  o. loba´tum, o. lobado; um ovário demarcado por estrias profundas em dois ou mais lobos.

  o. masculi´num, apêndice do testículo. SIN *appendix* of testis.

ova·ry (o´vă-rē) [TA]. Ovário; uma de um par de glândulas reprodutoras femininas que contêm os ovos ou células germinativas; o estroma do o. é um tecido conjuntivo vascular contendo inúmeros folículos ovarianos que encerram os ovos; ao redor desse estroma existe uma camada mais condensada de estroma, denominada túnica albugínea. SIN ovarium [TA], female gonad, genital gland (2). [L. mod. *ovarium*, de *ovum*, ovo]

  mulberry o., o. em amora; o tipo de o. produzido pela administração de extratos de hipófise anterior a ratos imaturos; esse o. contém um número muito maior de folículos que o normal, com os folículos apresentando-se em vários estágios de desenvolvimento e com o corpo lúteo proeminente em suas superfícies, daí a semelhança com uma amora.

  polycystic o., o. policístico; ovários císticos aumentados, com coloração branco-perolada, com a túnica albugínea espessada, característico da síndrome de Stein-Leventhal; as manifestações clínicas são menstruação anormal, obesidade e evidências de masculinização, como hirsutismo.

  third o., terceiro o.; um o. acessório.

over·bite (ō´ver-bīt). Sobremordida, superposição vertical. SIN vertical *overlap*.

over·clo·sure (ō´ver-klō-zher). Sobrefechamento; diminuição na dimensão oclusal vertical.

over·com·pen·sa·tion (ō´ver-kom-pen-sā´shŭn). Supercompensação. **1.** Um exagero da capacidade pessoal por meio do qual uma pessoa supera uma inferioridade real ou imaginária. **2.** O processo pelo qual uma deficiência psicológica inspira correção exagerada. VER compensation.

over·cor·rec·tion (ō´ver-kŏ-rek´shŭn). Hipercorreção; nos programas de tratamento de modificação do comportamento, principalmente aqueles que envolvem os indivíduos com retardo mental, o aprendizado excessivo do comportamento-alvo desejado além do critério estabelecido, de forma a garantir que o comportamento continuará a satisfazer o critério estabelecido quando ocorrerem as diminuições pós-aprendizado e o esquecimento.

over·den·ture (ō-ver-den´choor). Prótese dentária híbrida. SIN overlay *denture*.

over·de·ter·mi·na·tion (o´ver-dē-ter´min-ā´shŭn). Superdeterminação; em psicanálise, atribuir a causa de uma única reação emocional ou comportamental, sintoma mental ou sonho à operação de duas ou mais forças, ou seja, é superdeterminada (p.ex., atribuir a natureza de um surto emocional não somente ao fator precipitante imediato, mas também a um complexo de inferioridade persistente).

over·dom·i·nance (ō-ver-dom´i-nans). Superdominância; aquele estado em que o heterozigoto possui fenótipo de maior valor e, talvez, é mais adequado que o estado homozigoto para ambos os alelos que ele compreende. Cf. balanced *polymorphism*.

over·dom·i·nant (ō-ver-dom´i-nant). Superdominante; indica os estados heterozigóticos que exibem superdominância.

over·drive (ō-ver-drĭv). Superestímulo. **1.** Uma técnica de estimulação eletrofisiológica para superar a freqüência de um marcapasso anormal e, dessa maneira, capturar o território controlado por esse marcapasso (geralmente atrial). **2.** Um estado de RNA polimerase eucariótica em que há resistência aos sinais de pausa, parada ou término. VER TAMBÉM hesitant, antitermination.

over·e·rup·tion (ō´ver-ē-rŭp´shŭn). Supererupção; projeção oclusal de um dente além da linha de oclusão.

over·ex·ten·sion (ō-ver-eks-ten´shŭn). Hiperextensão. SIN hyperextension.

over·graft·ing (ō´ver-graft´ing). Sobreenxerto; colocar um segundo enxerto ou enxertos adicionais sobre um enxerto previamente curado, a partir do qual foi removido o epitélio, como por meio da dermabrasão, para fortalecer e espessar um enxerto de espessura dividida.

over·hang (ō´ver-hang). Ressalto; excesso de material de enchimento dentário além da margem da cavidade ou do contorno normal do dente.

over·head pro·jec·tor. Retroprojetor. SIN epidiascope.

over·hy·dra·tion (ō´ver-hī-drā´shŭn). Superidratação. SIN hyperhydration.

over·jet, over·jut (ō´ver-jet, o´ver-jŭt). Superposição horizontal. SIN horizontal *overlap*.

over·lap (ō´ver-lap). Superposição. **1.** Sutura de uma camada de tecido sobre ou sob outra para ganhar força. **2.** Uma extensão ou projeção de um tecido sobre outro.

  horizontal o., s. horizontal; a projeção dos dentes superiores anteriores e/ou posteriores além de seus antagonistas em uma direção horizontal. SIN overjet, overjut.

  vertical o., s. vertical; **(1)** a extensão dos dentes superiores sobre os dentes inferiores em uma direção vertical quando os dentes posteriores opostos estão em contato na oclusão cêntrica; **(2)** a distância segundo a qual os dentes se sobrepõem a seus antagonistas verticalmente, em especial a distância da qual as bordas dos incisivos superiores caem abaixo das bordas dos inferiores, mas também pode descrever as relações verticais de cúspides opostas; **(3)** sobremordida; a relação dos incisivos maxilares com os incisivos mandibulares quando as bordas dos incisivos passam uma pela outra na oclusão cêntrica. SIN overbite.

over·lay (ō´ver-lā). Fator agravante; um acréscimo a uma condição já existente.

  emotional o., fator agravante emocional; o ônus emocional ou psicológico que acompanha uma incapacidade orgânica.

over·learn·ing (ō´ver-lern´ing). Hiperaprendizado; na psicologia da memória, a continuação da prática além do ponto em que alguém é capaz de executar de acordo com o critério especificado; tipicamente, a retenção ocorre por mais tempo depois do hiperaprendizado em comparação com a retenção após prática apenas até o ponto de desempenho que satisfaz o critério especificado.

over·re·sponse (ō´ver-rē-spons´) Hiper-resposta; uma reação anormalmente forte a um estímulo.

over·rid·ing (ō´ver-rī´ding). Acavalgamento. **1.** Deslizamento do fragmento inferior de um osso longo fraturado para cima e ao longo da porção proximal. **2.** Termo obsoleto que indica que uma cabeça fetal é palpável acima da sínfise por causa da desproporção céfalo-pélvica. **3.** O deslizamento dos ossos fetais do crânio que ocorre depois de uma morte fetal *in utero*.

over·sens·ing (ō´ver-sen´sing). Hiperdetecção; a percepção dos sinais elétricos ou magnéticos, que normalmente não devem ser detectados por um marcapasso, mas que resultam na inibição inadequada do débito do marcapasso.

over·shoot (ō´ver-shoot). Ultrapassagem, sobreimpulso. **1.** Geralmente, qualquer alteração inicial, em resposta a uma súbita mudança de etapa em algum fator, que é maior que a resposta do estado de equilíbrio dinâmico ao novo nível desse fator; comum nos sistemas em que a inércia ou um retardo temporal na retroalimentação negativa supera qualquer amortecedor que possa estar presente. As alterações em uma direção negativa são por vezes distinguidas pelo termo *undershoot*, podendo as duas alternar-se de uma maneira oscilatória, como nas oscilações transitórias de um pêndulo quando liberado de um deslocamento inicial. **2.** A reversão momentânea do potencial de membrana de uma célula (com a face interna tornando-se positiva em vez de negativa em relação ao exterior) durante um potencial de ação; considerado uma forma de ultrapassagem (1) porque, antes da descoberta da ultrapassagem (2), acreditava-se que a excitação ocorria apenas para despolarizar a membrana até o potencial transmembrana zero.

Overton, Charles E., biólogo alemão na Suécia, 1865–1933. VER Meyer-O. *rule*, *theory* of narcosis.

over·tone (ō´ver-tōn). Sobretom, harmônico; qualquer um dos tons, que não o tom fundamental ou mais baixo, dos quais se compõe um som complexo.

  psychic o., s. psíquico; as associações mentais relacionadas com qualquer estímulo.

over·ven·ti·la·tion (ō´ver-ven-ti-lā´shŭn). Hiperventilação. SIN hyperventilation.

over·win·ter·ing (ō´ver-win´ter-ing). Persistência de um agente infeccioso em seu vetor por períodos demorados, como os meses mais frios do inverno, durante os quais o vetor não tem oportunidade de ser reinfectado ou de infectar outro hospedeiro.

ovi-. Forma combinante que significa ovo. VER TAMBÉM oo-, ovo-. [L. *ovum*]

ovi·ci·dal (ō´vi-sī-dăl). Ovicida; que causa a morte de um ovo. [ovi- + L. *caedo*, matar]

ovi·du·cal (ō-vi-doo´kăl). Oviductal. SIN oviductal.

ovi·duct (ō´vi-dŭkt). Tuba uterina, oviducto. SIN uterine *tube*. [ovi- + L. *ductus*, um conduto, de *duco*, pp. *ductus*, conduzir]

ovi·duc·tal (ō-vi-dŭk´tăl). Oviductal; relativo a uma tuba uterina. SIN oviducal.

ovif·er·ous (ō-vif´er-ŭs). Ovífero; que transporta, contém ou produz ovos. SIN ovigerous. [ovi- + L. *fero*, carregar]

ovi·form (ō´vi-fōrm). Oviforme. SIN ovoid (2).

ovi·gen·e·sis (ō-vi-jen´e-sis). Ovigênese. SIN oogenesis.

ovi·ge·net·ic, ovi·gen·ic (ō-vi-jĕ-net´ik, -jen´ik). Ovigenético, ovigênico. SIN oogenetic.

ovig·e·nous (ō-vij´ē-nŭs). Ovígeno. SIN oogenetic.

ovig·er·ous (ō-vij´er-ŭs). Ovígero. SIN oviferous.

ovi·ge·rus. Disco prolígero, membrana prolígera. SIN *cumulus oöphorus.*
ovine (ō'vin). Ovino; relativo a ovelhas, carneiros e cordeiro; com formato de carneiro. [L. *ovinus*, relativo a um carneiro]
ovi·par·i·ty (ō-vi-par'i-tē). Oviparidade; estado ou qualidade de ser ovíparo. [ovi- + L. *pario*, trazer]
ovip·a·rous (ō-vip'ā-rŭs). Ovíparo; que produz e põe ovos; indica aqueles pássaros, peixes, anfíbios, répteis, mamíferos monotremos e invertebrados cujos filhotes se desenvolvem em ovos fora do corpo materno. [L. *oviparus*, de *ovum*, ovo, + *pario*, trazer]
ovi·pos·it (ō'vi-poz'it). pôr ovos; aplicado especialmente aos insetos. [ovi- + L. *pono*, pp. *positus*, colocar]
ovi·po·si·tion (ō'vi-pō-zish'ŭn). Oviposição; o ato da deposição de ovos por fêmeas de insetos.
ovi·pos·i·tor (ō'vi-poz'i-tŏr, -tōr). Ovipositor, ovopositor; um órgão feminino especializado e especialmente bem desenvolvido nos insetos para ovipor ou depositar os ovos.
ovist (ō'vist). Um adepto da teoria da pré-formação segundo a qual a célula sexual feminina continha uma miniatura do corpo que crescia quando estimulada pelo sêmen. Cf. spermist.
ovo-. Forma combinante que significa ovo. VER TAMBÉM oo-, ovi-. [L. *ovum*]
ovo·cyte (ō'vō-sīt). Ovócito, oócito. SIN oocyte. [ovo- + G. *kytos*, um oco (célula)]
ovo·fla·vin (ō-vō-flā'vin). Ovoflavina; riboflavina encontrada nos ovos.
ovo·gen·e·sis (ō-vō-jen'ē-sis). Ovogênese, oogênese. SIN oogenesis.
ovo·glob·u·lin (ō-vō-glob'ū-kin). Ovoglobulina; globulina na clara do ovo.
ovoid (ō'voyd). Ovóide. **1.** Com a forma de um ovo ou oval. **2.** Que se assemelha a um ovo. SIN oviform. [ovo- + G. *eidos*, semelhança]
  fetal o., o. fetal; a forma do feto *in utero;* seu comprimento é cerca de metade do comprimento do feto esticado.
  Manchester o., o. de Manchester; aplicador de rádio ovóide para colocação nos fórnices vaginais laterais. [University of *Manchester*, England]
ovo·lar·vip·a·rous (ō'vō-lar-vip'ā-rŭs). Ovolarvíparo; indica determinados nematódeos e outros invertebrados nos quais os ovos se rompem dentro da fêmea e as larvas estão desenvolvidas ou protegidas dentro do útero até o momento correto de sua emergência. [ovo- + L. *larva*, uma máscara, + *pario*, trazer]
ovo·mu·cin (ō'vō-mū'sin). Ovomucina; uma glicoproteína na clara do ovo.
ovo·mu·coid (ō-vō-mū'koyd). Ovomucóide; uma mucoproteína obtida da clara de ovo.
ovo·plasm (ō'vō-plazm). Ovoplasma; protoplasma de um ovo não-fertilizado.
ovo·pro·to·gen (ō-vō-prō'tō-jen). Ácido lipóico. SIN lipoic acid.
ovo·sis·ton (ō-vō-sis'ton). Nome comercial de contraceptivo oral que consiste em uma associação de uma progestina e um estrogênio.
ovo·tes·tis (ō'vō-tes'tis). Ovotestículo; gônada em que existem os componentes testicular e ovariano; uma forma de hermafroditismo.
ovo·trans·fer·rin (ō'vō-trans-far'in). Ovotransferrina. SIN conalbumin.
ovo·vi·tel·lin (ō'vō-vi-tel'in). Vitelina. SIN vitellin. [ovo- + L. *vitellus*, gema]
ovo·vi·vip·ar·ous (ō'vō-vī-vip'ā-rŭs). Ovovivíparo; indica os peixes, anfíbios e répteis que produzem ovos que se rompem dentro do corpo do genitor. [ovo- + L. *viviparus*, que reproduz seres vivos, de *vivus*, vivo, + *pario*, parir]
o·vu·lar (ov'ū-lar, ō'vū-) Ovular; relativo a um óvulo.
o·vu·la·tion (ov'ū-lā'shun, ō'vū-) Ovulação; a liberação de um ovo a partir de um folículo ovariano.

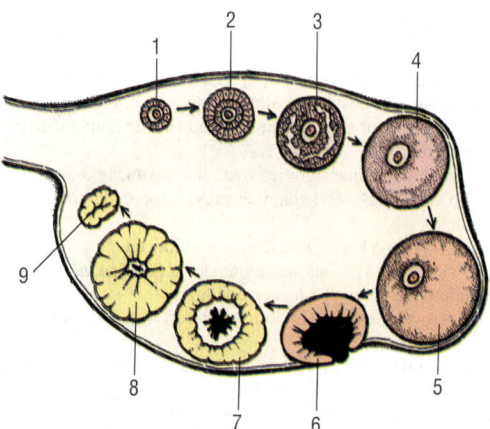

ovulação: (1) folículo primário; (2) folículo com dupla camada; (3) folículo no início da formação do antro; (4) folículo aproximando-se da maturidade; (5) folículo maduro; (6) corpo hemorrágico; (7) corpo lúteo jovem; (8) corpo lúteo; (9) corpo albicante

  anestrous o., o. anestra; a liberação de ovos que ocorre em animais sem estro.
  paracyclic o., o. paracíclica; termo obsoleto para a o. que acontece no ciclo menstrual em qualquer momento diferente daquele normalmente previsto.
o·vu·la·to·ry (ov'ū-lā-tō-rē, ō'vū-). Ovulatório; relativo à ovulação.
o·vule (ov'ūl, ō'vū-). Óvulo. **1.** O ovo de um mamífero, especialmente enquanto ainda no folículo ovariano. **2.** Uma pequena estrutura semelhante a uma conta que tem uma semelhança imaginária com um o. SIN ovulum. [L. mod. *ovulum*, dim. de L. *ovum*, ovo]
o·vu·lo·cy·clic (ov'ū-lō-sī'klik, ō'vū-). Ovulocíclico; indica qualquer fenômeno recorrente associado a e que ocorre em determinado momento no ciclo ovulatório, como, por exemplo, a porfíria ovulocíclica.
o·vu·lum, pl. **ovu·la** (ov'ū-lŭm, ō'vu-; -lă). Óvulo, óvulos. SIN ovule.
ovum, gen. **ovi,** pl. **ova** (ō'vŭm, -vī, -vă). Ovo; a célula sexual feminina. Quando fertilizado por um espermatozóide, um o. é capaz de se desenvolver em um novo indivíduo da mesma espécie; durante a maturação, o o., como o espermatozóide, sofre uma divisão pela metade de seu complemento cromossomial, de modo que, em sua união com o gameta masculino, o número de cromossomas da espécie (46 em seres humanos) se mantém; o vitelo contido nos ovos de diferentes espécies varia muito em quantidade e distribuição, o que influencia o padrão das divisões iniciais. [L. ovo]
  alecithal o., o. alécito; um o. em que o vitelo está quase ausente, consistindo apenas em algumas partículas.
  blighted o., o. anembrionado; um o. fertilizado cujo desenvolvimento cessou em um estágio inicial.
  centrolecithal o., o. centrolécito; o vitelo se localiza, em sua maior parte, próximo ao centro do ovo, como nos artrópodes.
  fertilized o., o. fertilizado; um o. fecundado por um espermatozóide.
  isolecithal o., o. isolécito; um o. em que o vitelo está uniformemente distribuído por todo o citoplasma.
  Peters o., o. de Peters; um o. com uma idade de fertilização presuntiva de cerca de 13 dias; durante muitos anos, um dos pouquíssimos embriões humanos jovens recuperados em boas condições, e seu estudo forneceu muitos fatos sobre as alterações embrionárias iniciais.
  telolecithal o., o. telolécito; um o. em que existe uma grande quantidade de vitelo concentrado no pólo vegetativo, como nos ovos de aves e répteis.
Owen, Sir Richard, anatomista inglês, 1804–1892. VER O. *lines,* em *line;* contour *lines* of O., em *line;* interglobular *space* of O.
Owren, Paul A., hematologista norueguês, *1905. VER O. *disease.*
oxa-. Forma combinante inserida em nomes de compostos orgânicos para significar a presença ou adição de átomo(s) de oxigênio a uma cadeia ou anel (como em éteres), não anexada a qualquer deles (como em cetonas e aldeídos). VER TAMBÉM hydroxy-, oxo-, oxy-. [Inglês. *oxygen*]
ox·a·cil·lin so·di·um (ok-să-sil'in). Oxacilina sódica; uma penicilina semi-sintética usada na terapia oral de infecções por estafilococos resistentes à penicilina.
ox·al·al·de·hyde (ok-să-lal'dĕ-hīd). Oxalaldeído. SIN glyoxal.
ox·a·late (ok'să-lāt). Oxalato; um sal de ácido oxálico.
ox·a·le·mia (ok-să-lē'mē-ă). Oxalemia; a presença de uma concentração anormalmente grande de oxalatos no sangue. [oxalate + G. *haima*, sangue]
ox·al·ic ac·id (ok'sal'ik). Ácido oxálico; um ácido, HOOC–COOH, encontrado em muitos vegetais e plantas, principalmente no trigo sarraceno (família Polygoniaceae) e *Oxalis* (família Oxalidaceae); usado como hemostático em medicina veterinária, mas tóxico em níveis elevados quando ingerido por seres humanos; também utilizado na remoção de nanquim e outros corantes, e como agente redutor geral; os sais de ácido oxálico são encontrados em cálculos renais; acumula-se nos casos de hiperoxalúria primária.
ox·a·lo (ok'să-lō). Oxalo-; o radical monoacil, HOOC–C(O)–.
ox·a·lo·ac·e·tate trans·ac·e·tase (ok'să-lō-as'ē-tāt trans-as'ē-tās) Oxaloacetato transacetase. SIN *citrate synthase.*
ox·a·lo·a·ce·tic ac·id (ok'să-lō-ā-sē'tik). Ácido oxaloacético; um ácido cetodicarboxílico e importante intermediário no ciclo do ácido tricarboxílico; o produto formado quando o ácido L-aspártico atua como doador de amina nas reações de transaminação. SIN ketosuccinic acid, oxosuccinic acid.
ox·a·lo·sis (ok-să-lō'sis). Oxalose; deposição disseminada de cristais de oxalato de cálcio nos rins, ossos, camada média das artérias e miocárdio, com excreção urinária aumentada de oxalato; pode ser um distúrbio adquirido, como na intoxicação por oxalato, ou representa um aspecto da hiperoxalúria primária e o. [oxalate + -osis, condição]
ox·a·lo·suc·cin·ic ac·id (ok'să-lō-sŭk-sin'ik). Ácido oxalossuccínico; o produto da desidrogenação do ácido isocítrico sob a influência catalítica da isocitrato desidrogenase; um intermediário ligado à enzima do ciclo do ácido tricarboxílico.
ox·a·lo·suc·cin·ic car·box·yl·ase. Oxalossuccínico carboxilase. SIN *isocitrate* dehydrogenase.
ox·a·lo·u·rea (ok'să-lō-ū-rē'ă). Oxalouréia. SIN oxalylurea.
ox·a·lu·ria (ok'să-loo'rē-ă). Oxalúria. SIN hyperoxaluria. [oxalate + G. *ouron*, urina]

ox·a·lur·ic ac·id (ok-să-loor′ik). Ácido oxalúrico; a ureída do ácido oxálico, derivada do ácido úrico ou da oxaliluréia.

ox·a·lyl (ok′să-lil). Oxalil; o radical diacil, –CO–CO–.

ox·a·lyl·u·rea (ok′să-lil-ū-rē′ă). Oxaliluréia; o anidrido da amida cíclica do ácido oxalúrico; um produto de oxidação do ácido úrico. SIN oxalourea, parabanic acid.

ox·am·ni·quine (oks-am′ni-quin). Oxamniquina; um derivado tetraidroquinolínico, semelhante à hicantona e lucantona, efetivo contra *Schistosoma mansoni*; atualmente superado pelo praziquantel, medicamento anti-helmíntico de amplo espectro.

ox·an·a·mide (ok-san′ă-mīd). Oxanamida; um sedativo.

ox·an·dro·lone (ok-san′drō-lōn). Oxandrolona; 17β-hidroxi-17α-metil-2-oxa-5α-androstan-3-ona (C-2 substituído por O no núcleo androstano); esteróide anabólico androgênico.

ox·a·phen·a·mide (ok-să-fen′ă-mīd). Oxafenamida; um colerético.

ox·a·ze·pam (ok-să′zē-pam). Oxazepam; uma benzodiazepina química e farmacologicamente relacionada ao clordiazepóxido e diazepam; agente ansiolítico.

ox·a·zin (ok′să-zin). Oxazina; substância-mãe de uma série de corantes biológicos, p.ex., galocianina, azul-cresil brilhante, acetato de violeta-cresil.

ox·a·zole (ok′să-zōl). Oxazol; o sistema anelar fundamental das piranoses.

ox·a·zo·li·dine·di·ones (ok-să-zō-lid′in-dē-onz). Oxazolidinedionas; uma classe química obsoleta de substâncias antiepilépticas úteis no tratamento das crises de ausência (pequeno mal); os exemplos incluem trimetadiona e parametadiona.

ox·a·zo·li·di·nones (oks′ă-zō-lid′i-nōnz). Oxazolidinonas; uma nova classe de antibióticos antibacterianos.

ox·el·a·din (ok-sel′ă-din). Oxeladina; agente antitussígeno.

ox·i·con·a·zole (ok′sē-kō′nă-zōl). Oxiconazol; agente antifúngico que se assemelha ao cetoconazol.

ox·i·dant (ok′si-dant). Oxidante; a substância que é reduzida e que, portanto, oxida o outro componente de uma reação de oxirredução.

ox·i·dase (ok′si-dās). Oxidase; classicamente, um de um grupo de enzimas, atualmente denominadas oxirredutases (EC classe 1), que desencadeiam oxidação pela adição de oxigênio a um metabólito ou pela remoção de hidrogênio ou de um ou mais elétrons. A o. é atualmente utilizada para aqueles casos em que o O_2 atua como um aceptor (de H ou de elétrons); aquelas que removem hidrogênio são atualmente denominadas desidrogenases. Para as oxidases individuais, veja os nomes específicos.

direct o., o. direta; originalmente, uma o. que catalisa a transferência de O_2 diretamente para outros corpos; atualmente denominada oxigenase.

indirect o., o. indireta; originalmente, uma o. que age através da redução de um peróxido; atualmente denominada peroxidase.

terminal o., o. terminal; a última proteína no transporte de elétrons, cadeia respiratória. Nos mamíferos, esta é a citocromo *c* oxidase.

ox·i·da·sis (ok-si-dā′sis). Oxidação por uma oxidase.

ox·i·da·tion (ok-si-dā′shun). Oxidação. **1.** Combinação com oxigênio. **2.** Aumento da valência de um átomo ou íon através da perda de hidrogênio ou de um ou mais elétrons, tornando-o mais eletropositivo, como quando o ferro é modificado do estado ferroso (2+) para o férrico (3+). **3.** Em bacteriologia, o catabolismo aeróbico dos substratos com produção de energia e água; em contraste com a fermentação, a transferência de elétrons no processo de o. é realizada através da cadeia respiratória, a qual utiliza o oxigênio como o aceptor final de elétrons.

alpha-o., α-**oxidation**, alfa-oxidação; α-oxidação; uma forma de o. de ácidos graxos em que os carbonos são removidos um de cada vez na forma de CO_2; o carbono α é primeiramente hidroxilado e, em seguida, convertido em carbonila; a deficiência dessa via está associada à doença de Refsum.

beta-o., β-**oxidation**, beta-oxidação, β-oxidação; **(1)** o. do carbono β (carbono 3) de um ácido graxo, formando o análogo β-ceto (β-oxo) ácido; importante no catabolismo dos ácidos graxos; **(2)** toda a via do catabolismo de ácidos graxos saturados que contêm um número par de átomos de carbono; a beta-o. (1) faz parte dessa via; a acetil-CoA é um importante produto dessa via.

end o., o. terminal; a última etapa da oxidação em uma via catabólica. SIN terminal o.

omega-o., ω-**oxidation**, oxidação ômega, ω-oxidação; a o. no átomo de carbono removido mais distante (carbono ω) de um grupamento carboxílico (carbono 1); dessa maneira, nessa via, é formado um ácido dicarboxílico; uma importante via na degradação de prostaglandinas.

terminal o., o. terminal. SIN end o.

ox·i·da·tion-re·duc·tion. Oxirredução, oxidorredução; qualquer reação química de oxidação ou redução, que precisa, *in toto*, abranger tanto a oxidação como redução; a base para a denominação de todas as enzimas oxidativas (originalmente oxidases) oxidorredutases. Freqüentemente encurtado para "redox".

ox·i·da·tive (ok-si-dā′tiv). Oxidative; que ou o oxida; indica um processo que envolve a oxidação.

ox·ide (ok′sīd). Óxido; um composto de oxigênio com outro elemento ou um radical; p.ex., o. de mercúrio; HgO.

acid o., o. ácido; um anidrido ácido; um o. de um elemento ou radical eletronegativo; pode combinar-se com a água para formar um ácido.

basic o., o. básico; um anidrido básico; um o. de um elemento ou radical eletropositivo; pode combinar-se com a água para formar uma base.

indifferent o., o. neutro. SIN neutral o.

neutral o., o. neutro; um o. que não é ácido nem básico; p.ex., água (óxido de hidrogênio, H_2O). SIN indifferent o.

ox·i·dize (ok′si-dīz). Oxidar; combinar-se com ou fazer com que um elemento ou radical se combine com oxigênio ou perca elétrons.

ox·i·do·re·duc·tase (ok′si-dō-rē-dŭk′tās). Oxirredutase; uma enzima (EC classe 1) que catalisa uma reação de oxirredução. Os nomes comuns para as oxirredutases incluem desidrogenase, redutase, oxidase (na qual O_2 é o aceptor de H), oxigenase (na qual O_2 é incorporado ao substrato), peroxidase (H_2O_2 é o aceptor; catalase é uma exceção) e hidroxilase (oxidação acoplada de dois doadores). VER TAMBÉM oxidase.

ox·ime (ok′sēm). Oxima; um composto que resulta da ação da hidroxilamina, NH_2OH, sobre uma cetona ou um aldeído para fornecer o grupamento =N–OH ligado ao átomo de carbono da carbonila original.

amide o.'s, amidoximas. SIN amidoximes.

ox·im·e·ter (ok-sim′e-ter). Oxímetro; um instrumento para determinar, por meios fotoelétricos, a saturação de oxigênio de uma amostra de sangue.

cuvette o., o. de cubeta; um o. que lê o percentual de saturação de oxigênio do sangue à medida que ele passa através de uma cubeta fora do corpo.

ox·im·e·try (oks-im-a-tree). Oximetria; o procedimento que emprega um dispositivo para medir a saturação de oxigênio através das flutuações da absorção da luz no tecido bem vascularizado durante a sístole e a diástole. O princípio fundamental é a lei de Beer, ou a relação entre a luz absorvida por um soluto em solução e a concentração do soluto desconhecida.

pulse o., o. de pulso; o. realizada de maneira não-invasiva, geralmente no dedo da mão ou lóbulo da orelha, na qual o pequeno aumento na absorção da luz durante o pulso sistólico é usado para calcular a saturação de oxigênio.

oxi·rane (oks′e-rān). óxido de etileno. SIN ethylene oxide.

oxo-. Prefixo que indica a adição de oxigênio; usado em lugar de ceto- na nomenclatura sistemática. VER TAMBÉM hydroxy-, oxa-, oxy-.

oxo·ace·tic ac·id (ok′sō-a-sē′tik). Ácido oxoacético. SIN glyoxylic acid.

oxo ac·id (ok′sō). cetoácido, oxoácido. SIN keto acid.

3-ox·o·ac·id-CoA trans·fer·ase. 3-oxoácido-CoA transferase; uma enzima que catalisa a conversão reversível de acetoacetil-CoA, e succinato em succinil-CoA e acetoacetato; a malonil-CoA pode substituir a succinil-CoA, e alguns outros 3-oxoácidos podem substituir o acetoacetato; uma importante etapa para que os corpos cetônicos sirvam como fonte de energia para os tecidos extra-hepáticos. SIN 3-ketoacid-CoA transferase, acetoacetyl-succinic thiophorase.

3-ox·o·ac·yl-ACP re·duc·tase (ok′sō-as′il). 3-oxoacil-ACP redutase; uma parte do complexo da sintase de ácidos graxos; uma enzima que faz 3-oxoacil-ACP (ACP = proteína transportadora de acil) reagir reversivelmente com NADPH para formar D-3-hidroxiacil-ACP e $NADP^+$. SIN β-ketoacyl-ACP reductase.

3-ox·o·ac·yl-ACP syn·thase. 3-oxoacil-ACP sintase; uma enzima que condensa o malonil-ACP (ACP = proteína transportadora de acil) e a acil-Cis-proteína em 3-oxoacil-ACP + Cis-proteína + CO_2 e reações similares, como etapas na síntese de ácidos graxos; Cis-proteína também é uma parte do complexo da sintase de ácidos graxos. SIN acyl-malonil-ACP synthase, β-ketoacyl-ACP synthase.

2-ox·o·glu·tar·ate de·hy·dro·gen·ase (ok′sō-gloo-tar′āt). 2-oxoglutarato desidrogenase. SIN α-*ketoglutarate* dehydrogenase.

2-ox·o·glu·tar·ic ac·id (oks′ō-gloo-tar-ik). Ácido 2-oxoglutárico. SIN α-ketoglutaramic acid.

2-oxo-5-guanidovaleric ac·id (gwan-ē′dō-va-ler′ik). Ácido 2-oxo-5-guanidovalérico; o derivado desaminado de arginina.

ox·ol·a·mine (ok-sol′ă-mēn). Oxolamina; usada para o tratamento de infecções broncopulmonares.

ox·o·lin·ic ac·id (ok′sō-lin′ik). Ácido oxolínico; um agente antibacteriano quinolona usado no tratamento de infecções do trato urinário.

ox·o·phen·ar·sine hy·dro·chlo·ride (ok′sō-fen-ar′sēn). Cloridrato de oxofenarsina; um agente anti-sifilítico e antitripanossoma.

5-ox·o·pro·lin·ase. 5-oxoprolinase; uma enzima que catalisa a hidrólise ATP-dependente da L-5-oxoprolina (ATP + L-5-oxoprolina → ADP + ortofosfato + L-glutamato); a deficiência dessa enzima resultará em 5-oxoprolinúria.

5-ox·o·pro·line (Glp) (oks′ō-prō′lēn). 5-oxoprolina; um cetoderivado da prolina que é formado de maneira não-enzimática a partir de glutamato, glutamina e peptídeos γ-glutamilados; também é produzido pela ação de γ-glutamilciclotransferase; os níveis elevados de 5-o. estão freqüentemente associados a problemas do metabolismo de glutamina ou glutationa. SIN 5-pyrrolidone-2-carboxylic acid, pyroglutamic acid, pyrrolidone-5-carcoxylate.

4-ox·o·pro·line re·duc·tase. 4-oxoprolina redutase. SIN 4-*hydroxyproline* oxidase.

5-ox·o·pro·lin·u·ria (oks′ō-prō′lēn-ūr-ē-ă). 5-oxoprolinúria; níveis elevados de 5-oxoprolina na urina.

17-ox·o·ste·roids (ok-sō-stēr′oydz). 17-oxoesteróides. SIN 17-ketosteroids.

ox·o·suc·cin·ic ac·id (ok′sō-sŭk-sin′ik). Ácido oxossuccínico. SIN oxaloacetic acid.

ox·o·tre·mo·rine (ok′sō-trem′er-ēn). Oxotremorina; um metabólito ativo da tremorina. Usada para provocar, farmacologicamente, tremor parkinsoniano.

ox·pren·o·lol hy·dro·chlo·ride (oks-pren′ō-lol). Cloridrato de oxiprenolol; um agente bloqueador do receptor β com atividade dilatadora coronariana.

OXT Abreviatura de oxytocin (ocitocina).

ox·tri·phyl·line (oks-trī′fi-lin, oks′trī-fil′in). Oxitrifilina; um sal verdadeiro da teofilina; possui ações diurética leve, vasodilatadora estimulante do miocárdio e broncodilatadora, com os mesmos usos que a teofilina; porém é mais bem absorvida e menos irritante. SIN choline theophyllinate.

⚠ **oxy-. 1.** Forma combinante que indica agudo, afilado, pontiagudo; rápido (incorretamente utilizado no lugar de ocy-, de G. ōkys, rápido). **2.** Em química, a forma combinante que indica a presença de oxigênio, quer acrescentado, quer substituído, em uma substância. VER TAMBÉM hydroxi-, oxa-, oxo-. [G. *oxys*, agudo]

ox·y·a·coia, ox·y·a·koia (ok′sē-ā-koy′ā). Oxiacóia; sensibilidade aumentada aos sons, ocorrendo na paralisia facial, em especial quando há paralisia do músculo estapédio. [G. *oxys*, agudo, + *akoē*, audição]

ox·y·a·phia (ok-sē-ā′fē-ā). Oxiafia. SIN hyperaphia. [G. *oxys*, agudo, + *haphē*, tato]

ox·y·bar·bi·tu·rates (ok′sē-bar-bit′ur-āts). Oxibarbitúricos; hipnóticos do grupo dos barbitúricos em que o átomo ligado na posição do carbono 2 é o oxigênio; quase todos os barbitúricos hipnóticos são oxibarbitúricos.

ox·y·ben·zone (ok-sē-ben′zōn). Oxibenzona; um filtro de luz ultravioleta para uso em pomadas e loções para pele.

ox·y·bi·o·tin (ok-sē-bī′ō-tin). Oxibiotina; análogo e antimetabólito da biotina, em que o átomo de enxofre é substituído por oxigênio.

ox·y·bu·ty·nin chlo·ride (ok-sē-bū′ti-nin). Cloreto de oxibutinina; antiespasmódico intestinal.

ox·y·cal·o·rim·e·ter (ok′sē-kal-ō-rim′e-ter). Oxicalorímetro; um calorímetro que mede o conteúdo energético das substâncias em relação ao oxigênio consumido.

ox·y·cel·lu·lose (ok′sē-sel′ū-lōs). Oxicelulose; a celulose que foi oxidada por NO_2 ou outros agentes oxidantes até o ponto em que todos os resíduos glicose, ou sua maioria, foram convertidos em resíduos ácido glicurônico; usado como absorvente em cromatografia ou outros processos de adsorção. VER TAMBÉM oxidized *cellulose*.

ox·y·ce·pha·lia (ok′sē-se-fā′lē-ā). Oxicefalia. SIN oxycephaly.

ox·y·ce·phal·ic, ox·y·ceph·a·lous (ok-sē-se-fal′ik, -sef′ā-lŭs). Oxicefálico; relativo a, ou caracterizado por, oxicefalia. SIN acrocephalic, acrocephalous.

ox·y·ceph·a·ly (ok-sē-sef′ā-lē). Oxicefalia; um tipo de craniossinostose em que existe fechamento prematuro das suturas lambdóidea e coronal, resultando em um crânio anormalmente alto, apiculado ou cônico. SIN acrocephalia, acrocephaly, hypsicephaly, hypsocephaly, oxycephalia, steeple skull, tower skull, turricephaly. [G. *oxys*, afilado, + *kephalē*, cabeça]

ox·y·chlo·ride (ok-sē-klōr′īd). Oxicloreto; um composto de oxigênio com um cloreto metálico; p.ex., um clorato ou perclorato.

ox·y·chro·mat·ic (ok′sē-krō-mat′ik). Oxicromático. SIN acidophilic. [G. *oxys*, azedo, ácido + *chrōma*, coloração]

ox·y·chro·ma·tin (ok-sē-krō′mā-tin). Oxicromatina; cromatina que se cora com corantes ácidos, como nos núcleos em interfase. SIN oxyphil chromatin.

ox·y·co·done (ok-sē-kō′dōn). Oxicodona; analgésico narcótico freqüentemente combinado ao ácido acetilsalicílico ou acetaminofeno.

11-ox·y·cor·ti·coids (ok-sē-kōr′ti-koydz). 11-oxicorticóides; corticosteróides que têm um grupamento álcool ou cetônico no carbono 11; p.ex., cortisona, cortisol.

ox·y·gen (O) (ok′sē-jen). Oxigênio. **1.** Um elemento gasoso, número atômico 8, peso atômico 15,9994 na base do C^{12} = 12,0000; um elemento químico abundante e amplamente distribuído, que se combina com a maioria dos outros elementos para formar óxidos e é essencial à vida de animais e vegetais. **2.** A forma molecular de o., O_2. **3.** Um gás medicinal que contém não menos que 99,0% por volume de O_2. [G. *oxys*, agudo, ácido e *genes*, formador]
heavy o., o. pesado. SIN oxygen-18.
hyperbaric o., high pressure o., o. hiperbárico, o. de alta pressão; o. em uma pressão superior a 1 atm. VER TAMBÉM hyperbaric *oxygenation*.
singlet o., o. singleto (O_2^1); uma forma excitada ou de alta energia de o. caracterizada pela rotação de um par de elétrons em direções opostas, enquanto a rotação do elétron é unidirecional no o. molecular normal. Por causa de sua grande reatividade, essa forma de o. é um provável intermediário na maioria das reações de foto-oxidação. Embora não exista por mais de 0,1 segundo, reage com poluentes atmosféricos para fomentar a formação de *smog* e tem efeitos biológicos prejudiciais.
triplet o., o. tripleto; o estado normal não-excitado do O_2 na atmosfera, em que o par de elétrons ímpar está tão deslocado que seus campos magnéticos estão orientados na mesma direção, resultando em paramagnetismo; cada uma das linhas pectrais geradas pelo calor dessa forma de o. pode ser dividida por um campo magnético em um tripleto. Cf. singlet o.

ox·y·gen-15 (^{15}O). Oxigênio-15; um radioisótopo do oxigênio, emissor de positrons e produzido por ciclotron, com uma meia-vida de 122,2 segundos; usado em estudos da função respiratória e na tomografia com emissão de positrons.

ox·y·gen-16 (^{16}O). Oxigênio-16; o isótopo comum do oxigênio, constituindo cerca de 99,76% do oxigênio natural.

ox·y·gen-17 (^{17}O). Oxigênio-17; o mais raro dos isótopos estáveis do oxigênio, constituindo 0,04% do oxigênio natural.

ox·y·gen-18 (^{18}O). Oxigênio-18; um isótopo estável do oxigênio compondo 0,20% do oxigênio natural; usado na espectrometria de massa e nos estudos dos tecidos com ressonância magnética nuclear (RMN). SIN heavy oxygen.

ox·y·gen·ase (ok-sē-jē-nās). Oxigenase; uma de um grupo de enzimas (EC subclasse 1,13) que catalisam a incorporação direta de O_2 em substratos; p.ex., triptofano 2,3-dioxigenase (triptofano pirrolase) que catalisa a reação entre O_2 e L-triptofano para formar *N*-L-formilquilurenina. Cf. dioxygenase, monooxygenases.
mixed function o., o. de função mista; qualquer monooxigenase que catalise $AH + O_2 + DH_2 \rightarrow AOH + H_2O + D$.

ox·y·gen·ate (ok′sē-jē-nāt). Oxigenar; realizar a oxigenação.

ox·y·gen·a·tion (ok′sē-jē-nā′shŭn). Oxigenação; a adição de oxigênio a qualquer sistema químico ou físico.
apneic o., respiração por difusão. SIN diffusion *respiration*.
hyperbaric o., o. hiperbárica; volume aumentado de oxigênio em órgãos e tecidos resultante da administração de oxigênio em uma câmara de compressão em uma pressão ambiental superior a 1 atm.

ox·y·gen·ic (ok-sē-jen′ik). Oxigênico; pertinente a ou que contém oxigênio.

ox·y·gen·ize (ok′sē-jen-īz). Oxigenar; oxidar com oxigênio.

ox·y·heme (ok′sē-hēm). Hematina. SIN hematin.

ox·y·he·mo·chro·mo·gen (ok-sē-hēm′ō-krō′mō-jen). Hematina. SIN hematin.

ox·y·he·mo·glo·bin (HbO₂) (ok′sē-hē-mō-glō′bin). Oxiemoglobina; hemoglobina em combinação com oxigênio, a forma de hemoglobina presente no sangue arterial, vermelho-escarlate ou vivo, quando dissolvido em água. SIN oxygenated hemoglobin.

ox·y·i·o·dide (ok-sē-ī′ō-dīd). Oxiiodeto; um composto de oxigênio com um iodeto metálico, p.ex., um iodato ou periodato.

ox·y·krin·in (ok-sē-krin′in). Secretina. SIN secretin.

ox·y·luc·i·fer·in (oks′ē-loo-si′fer-in). Oxiluciferina; o derivado ativado da luciferina formado na bioluminescência.

ox·y·mes·ter·one (ok-sē-mes′te-rōn). Oximesterona; esteróide anabólico.

ox·y·met·az·o·line hy·dro·chlo·ride (ok′sē-mē-taz′ō-lēn). Cloridrato de oximetazolina; vasoconstritor usado topicamente para reduzir a tumefação e a congestão da mucosa nasal.

ox·y·meth·o·lone (ok-sē-meth′ō-lōn). Oximetolona; esteróide anabólico androgênico.

ox·y·mor·phone hy·dro·chlo·ride (ok-sē-mōr′fōn). Cloridrato de oximorfona; analgésico narcótico semi-sintético com substancial correlação química com o cloridrato de hidromorfona; suas ações são similares às da morfina, porém mais potentes.

ox·y·my·o·glo·bin (MbO₂) (ok′sē-mī-ō-glō′bin). Oximioglobina; mioglobina em sua forma oxigenada, análoga em estrutura à oxiemoglobina.

ox·y·ner·vone (ok′sē-ner′vōn). Oxinervona. SIN hydroxynervone.

ox·yn·tic (ok-sin′tik). Oxíntico; que forma ácido, p.ex., as células parietais das glândulas gástricas. [G. *oxynō*, afiar, tornar azedo, ácido]

ox·y·per·tine (ok-sē-per′tēn). Oxipertina; um agente ansiolítico; também disponível como cloridrato.

ox·y·phen·bu·ta·zone (ok′sē-fen-boo′tā-zōn). Oxifembutazona; um agente antiinflamatório e analgésico efetivo por via oral, prescrito (geralmente em cursos curtos) para artrite reumatóide e gota.

ox·y·phen·cy·cli·mine hy·dro·chlo·ride (ok′sē-fen-sī′klī-mēn). Cloridrato de oxifenciclimina; o cloridrato de 1,4,5,6-tetraidro-1-metilpirimidina-2-ilmetil-α-cicloexil-α-hidroxi-L-fenilacetato; um agente anticolinérgico.

ox·y·phen·i·sa·tin ac·e·tate (ok′sē-fe-nī′sa-tin). Acetato de oxifenisatina; um catártico com propriedades farmacológicas que se assemelham às da fenolftaleína, mas não é absorvido pelo trato gastrointestinal.

ox·y·phe·no·ni·um bro·mide (ok′sē-fe-nō′nē-ŭm). Brometo de oxifenônio; um composto de amônio quaternário com ação anticolinérgica.

ox·y·phil, ox·y·phile (ok′sē-fil, -fīl). **1.** Célula oxifílica, célula oxífila. VER oxyphil *cell*. **2.** Leucócito eosinofílico. SIN eosinophilic *leukocyte*. **3.** Oxifílico, oxífilo. SIN oxyphilic. [G. *oxys*, azedo, ácido, + *philos*, ligação]

ox·y·phil·ic (ok-sē-fil′ik). Oxifílico; oxífilo; que possui afinidade por corantes ácidos; indica determinados elementos celulares ou teciduais. SIN oxyphil (3), oxyphile.

ox·y·pho·nia (ok-sē-fō′nē-ā). Oxifonia; voz estridente ou aguda e penetrante. [G. *oxys*, agudo, + *phōnē*, voz]

ox·y·pol·y·gel·a·tin (ok'sē-pol-ē-jel'ā-tin). Oxipoligelatina; uma gelatina modificada usada como expansor plasmático em transfusões.

ox·y·pu·rine (ok-sē-pūr'ēn). Oxipurina; uma purina que contém oxigênio; p.ex., hipoxantina, xantina, ácido úrico.

ox·y·pu·ri·nol (ok'sē-poor'ī-nol). Oxipurinol; aloxantina e inibidor da xantina oxidase; um metabólito ativo do alopurinol. Inibe a formação de ácido úrico e é prescrita para a gota.

ox·y·rhine (ok'sē-rīn). Oxirrino; que possui um nariz com a extremidade afilada. [G. *oxys*, agudo, + *rhis* (*rhin-*), nariz]

ox·y·ryg·mia (ok-sē-rig'mē-ā). Oxirregmia; termo obsoleto para a eructação de líquido ácido. [G. *oxys*, ácido, + *erygmos*, eructação]

Ox·y·spi·ru·ra man·so·ni (ok'-sē-spī-roo'rā man-sō'nī). Um parasita nematódeo espiruróide amplamente distribuído encontrado sob a membrana nictitante nos olhos de perus, galinhas, pavões, codornas e galos silvestres; as larvas desenvolvem-se até o estágio infeccioso em baratas. SIN Manson eye worm.

ox·y·ta·lan (ok-sit'ā-lan). Oxitalano; um tipo de fibra de tecido conjuntivo histoquimicamente distinto do colágeno ou das fibras elásticas descritas no ligamento periodontal e gengivas. [G. *oxys*, acid, + *talas*, sofrimento, que resiste; termo provavelmente cunhado com a intenção de significar "resistente à hidrólise ácida"]

ox·y·tet·ra·cy·cline (ok'sē-tet-rā-sī'klēn). Oxitetraciclina; um antibiótico produzido pelo actinomiceto, *Streptomyces rimosus*, presente no solo; suas ações e usos são similares aos da tetraciclina; disponível como diidrato, cloridrato e cálcica.

ox·y·thi·a·min (ok-sē-thī'ā-min). Oxitiamina; uma molécula similar à tiamina, mas com um grupamento hidroxila que substitui o grupamento amino no anel pirimidina; antagonista da tiamina capaz de induzir sintomas da deficiência de tiamina quando administrado; aumenta a excreção de tiamina.

ox·y·to·cia (ok-sē-tō'sē-ā). Oxitocia; parto rápido. [G. *okytokos*, parto rápido]

ox·y·to·cic (ok-sē-tō'sik). Oxitócico, ocitócico; **1.** Que acelera o parto. **2.** SIN parturifacient (2).

ox·y·to·cin (OXT) (ok-sē-tō'sin). Ocitocina, oxitocina; um hormônio nonapeptídico da neuro-hipófise que difere da vasopressina humana por possuir leucina na posição 8 e isoleucina na posição 3, que causa contrações miométricas ao termo e promove a liberação de leite durante a lactação; usado para a indução ou estimulação do trabalho de parto, no controle da hemorragia pós-parto e atonia, e para aliviar o ingurgitamento mamário doloroso. SIN ocytocin. [G. *okytokos*, parto rápido]

arginine o., arginina ocitocina; o. com arginina na posição 8 (idêntica à arginina vasotocina). VER TAMBÉM arginine *vasopressin*.

ox·y·u·ri·cide (ok'sē-ū'ri-sīd). Oxiuricida; um agente que destrói oxiúros. [oxyurid + L. *caedo*, matar]

ox·y·u·rid (ok-sē-ū'rid). Oxiurídeo; nome comum para os membros da família Oxyuridae. [ver *Oxyuris*]

Ox·y·u·ri·dae (ok-sē-ū'ri-dē). Uma família de nematódeos parasitas (superfamília Oxyuroidea) encontrada no intestino grosso ou ceco de vertebrados e no intestino de invertebrados, especialmente insetos e milípedes; inclui os gêneros *Aspiculurus, Enterobius, Oxyuris, Passalurus, Syphacia* e *Thelandros*.

Ox·y·u·ris (ok'sē-ū'ris). Um gênero de nematódeos comumente denominados de oxiúros (embora o oxiúro do homem seja a forma correlata, *Enterobius vermicularis*). *O. equi,* o oxiúro eqüino, é um parasita comum em cavalos em todas as regiões do mundo, habitando o intestino grosso. [G. *oxys*, agudo, + *oura*, cauda]

-oyl. -Oil; sufixo que indica um radical acil; -il substitui -ic em nomes de ácidos.

oz. Abreviatura para ounce (onça).

oze·na (ō-zē'nā). Ozena. SIN atrophic *rhinitis*. [G. *ozaina*, um pólipo fétido, de *ozō*, cheirar]

oze·nous (ō'zē-nŭs). Ozenoso; relativo à ozena.

ozo·ce·rite (ō-zō-sē'rīt). Ozocerita. SIN ozokerite.

ozo·ke·rite (ō-zō-kēr'īt). Ozocerita; espécie de resina, uma mistura de hidrocarbonetos parafínicos e cicloparafínicos que ocorre na natureza; possui um ponto de fusão mais elevado que a parafina sintética, sendo utilizado como substituto para a cera de abelha. SIN ozocerite.

purified o., o. purificado, ceresina, SIN ceresin.

ozon·a·tor (ō'zō-nā-ter, -tōr). Ozonador, ozonizador; um aparelho para produzir ozônio e difundi-lo na atmosfera de uma sala.

ozone (ō'zōn). Ozônio; O_3; um poderoso agente oxidante; o ar que contém um volume perceptível de O_3 formado por uma descarga elétrica ou pela lenta combustão do fósforo, e possui um odor sugestivo de Cl_2 ou SO_2; também formado pela ação da radiação UV solar sobre o O_2 atmosférico. [G. *ozō*, cheirar]

ozo·nide (ō-zō-nīd). Ozonide; o intermediário instável formado pela reação do ozônio com um composto orgânico insaturado, especialmente com ácidos graxos insaturados.

ozon·ol·y·sis (ō-zō-nol'ī-sis). Ozonólise; a divisão de uma dupla ligação em uma cadeia de hidrocarbonetos sob tratamento com ozônio, com a formação de dois aldeídos (uma ozonide é o intermediário instável); tem sido utilizado para determinar a estrutura de ácidos graxos insaturados. [ozone + G. *lysis*, dissolução]

ozon·om·e·ter (ō-zō-nom'e-ter). Ozonômetro; uma forma modificada do ozonoscópio, na qual pode ser estimada, através de uma série de papéis de teste, a quantidade de ozônio na atmosfera.

ozo·no·scope (ō-zō'nō-skōp). Ozonioscópio; papel de filtro saturado com amido e iodeto de potássio ou com tornassol e iodeto de potássio; fica azul na presença de ozônio.

ozo·sto·mia (ō-zō-stō'mē-ā). Ozostomia. SIN halitosis. [G. *ozō*, cheirar, + *stoma*, boca]

P

π. **1.** A 16.ª letra do alfabeto grego, pi. **2.** Símbolo da razão entre a circunferência de um círculo e seu diâmetro, aproximadamente 3,14159; símbolo da pressão osmótica [osmotic *pressure* (Π)]

Π. VER π.

Φ A 21.ª letra do alfabeto grego, fi. Símbolo de fenil (phenyl); símbolo de rendimento quântico [quantum *yield* (π)]

φ VER Φ.

Ψ, Ψ**rd. 1.** Psi maiúsculo, a 23.ª letra do alfabeto grego. **2.** Símbolo de pseudouridine (pseudouridina); psychology (psicologia).

P-170. SIN P-glycoprotein.

P 1. Símbolo de peta-; phosphorus (fósforo); proline (prolina); proline (produto); poise; power (força); freqüentemente com subscritos indicando a localização e/ou a espécie química. **2.** Seguido por um subscrito: 1) refere-se à concentração plasmática da substância indicada pelo subscrito; 2) constante de permeabilidade (permeability *constant*). **3.** Designação de um grupo sanguíneo. Ver grupo sanguíneo P, no Apêndice de Grupos Sanguíneos. **4.** Símbolo de probability (probabilidade); quando seguido pelo sinal "menor que" (<), indica que uma estatística, p. ex., um teste do qui quadrado, fornece um resultado que provavelmente não é ocasional.

P_{O_2}, pO_2 Símbolo da pressão (tensão) parcial de oxigênio. VER partial *pressure*.

P **1.** Em terminologia do ácido nucleico, símbolo do resíduo fosfórico. **2.** Símbolo de pressão; partial *pressure* (pressão parcial).

p 1. Abreviatura de pupil (pupila); optic *papilla* (disco óptico). **2.** No simbolismo dos polinucleotídeos, éster fosfórico ou fosfato. **3.** Símbolo de pico- (2); o logaritmo na base 10 negativo; próton; protein (proteína); *momentum* (em itálico). **4.** Em citogenética, símbolo do braço curto de um cromossoma. [do Fr. *petit*, pequeno]

P_{CO_2}, pCO_2 Símbolo da pressão (tensão) parcial de dióxido de carbono. VER partial *pressure*.

P_i Símbolo de inorganic *orthophosphate* (ortofosfato inorgânico; não deve ser usado quando ligado de forma covalente a outra porção).

P_1 Abreviatura de parental *generation* (geração parental).

^{32}P Símbolo de phosphorus-32 (fósforo-32).

^{33}P Símbolo de phosphorus-33 (fósforo-33).

P_{700} O pigmento nos cloroplastos descorado pela luz em comprimentos de onda de aproximadamente 700 nm.

P_B Símbolo de barometric *pressure* (pressão barométrica).

p53. Gene supressor tumoral, localizado no braço curto do cromossoma 17, que codifica uma nucleofosfoproteína, a qual se liga ao DNA e regula negativamente a divisão celular; freqüentemente é medido como um marcador de doenças malignas.

P_{870} O pigmento nos cromatóforos bacterianos descorados pela luz em comprimentos de onda de aproximadamente 870 nm.

△ *p-.* Abreviatura de *para-* (4).

P.A. Abreviatura de physician assistant (auxiliar de serviços médicos).

Pa Símbolo de pascal; protactinium (protactínio).

Paas, H.R., médico alemão, *1900. VER P. *disease*.

PABA Abreviatura de *p*-aminobenzoic acid (ácido *p*-aminobenzóico).

pab·lum (pab'lŭm). Cereais para bebês; alimento pré-cozido para lactentes, uma mistura de trigo, aveia e milho, germe de trigo, folhas de alfafa, lêvedo de cerveja, ferro e cloreto de sódio. [L. *pabulum*, nutrição, de *pasco*, nutrir]

pab·u·lar (pab'ū-lăr). Pabular; relativo ao pábulo ou da natureza deste.

pab·u·lum (pab'ū-lŭm). Pábulo; alimento ou nutriente. [L.]

Pacchioni, Antonio, anatomista italiano, 1665–1726. VER pacchionian *bodies*, em *body*, pacchionian *corpuscles*, em *corpuscle*, pacchionian *depressions*, em *depression*, pacchionian *glands*, em *gland*, pacchionian *granulations*, em *granulation*.

pac·chi·o·ni·an (pak-ē-ō'nē-an). Atribuído a, ou descrito por, Antonio Pacchioni (1665–1726).

pace-fol·low·er (pās'fawl-ō-er). Qualquer célula em tecido excitável que responde aos estímulos de um marcapasso.

pace-mak·er (pās'mā-ker). Marcapasso. **1.** Biologicamente, qualquer centro rítmico que estabeleça a velocidade da atividade. **2.** Um regulador artificial da velocidade de reação. **3.** Em química, a substância cuja velocidade de reação comanda a velocidade de uma série de reações em cadeia; a própria reação limitadora da velocidade; p. ex., em uma via metabólica, a enzima que catalisa a reação mais lenta ou limitadora de velocidade naquela via. [L. *passus*, passo, ritmo]

artificial p., m. artificial; qualquer dispositivo que substitua o m. normal e controle o ritmo do órgão; em especial, um m. cardíaco eletrônico, que pode ser implantado no tórax, com eletrodos fixados à superfície cardíaca externa, ou passados através da circulação venosa até o lado direito do coração (marcapasso pervenoso).

demand p., m. de demanda; uma forma de m. artificial que geralmente é implantado no tecido cardíaco porque os seus estímulos elétricos podem ser inibidos por atividade elétrica cardíaca endógena.

diaphragmatic p., m. diafragmático; dispositivo que estimula o diafragma, usado em pacientes com insuficiência ventilatória crônica resultante de tetraplegia ou de determinados tipos de disfunção do nervo frênico.

ectopic p., m. ectópico; qualquer m. que não o nó sinoatrial.

electric cardiac p., m. cardíaco elétrico; aparelho elétrico que consegue substituir o m. cardíaco normal, controlando o ritmo cardíaco por descargas elétricas artificiais. SIN electronic p.

electronic p., m. eletrônico. SIN electric cardiac p.

external p., m. externo, m. transtorácico; m. cardíaco artificial cujos eletrodos que levam os estímulos elétricos rítmicos para o coração são colocados sobre a parede torácica. SIN transthoracic p.

fixed-rate p., m. com freqüência fixa; m. artificial que emite estímulos elétricos a uma freqüência constante.

nuclear p., m. nuclear; unidade alimentada por energia nuclear, usada para gerar a corrente elétrica que estimula artificialmente o coração; substituída por unidades que usam bateria de níquel-cádmio de longa duração e outras fontes de energia.

pervenous p., m. pervenoso; m. artificial introduzido através da circulação venosa até o lado direito do coração.

runaway p., m. de fuga; freqüências cardíacas elevadas, acima de 140/min, causadas por instabilidade do circuito eletrônico em um gerador de pulsos implantado.

shifting p., m. migratório. SIN wandering p.

subsidiary atrial p., m. atrial acessório; fonte secundária para controle rítmico do coração, disponível para controle da atividade cardíaca se o m. sinoatrial falhar; geralmente localizado na crista terminal e na parede atrial livre próxima da veia cava inferior.

transthoracic m., m. transtorácico, m. externo. SIN external p.

wandering p., m. migratório; distúrbio do ritmo cardíaco normal no qual o local do m. controlador muda de um batimento para outro, geralmente entre os nós sinoatrial e AV, freqüentemente com alterações seqüenciais graduais na onda P entre positiva e negativa em determinada derivação ECG. SIN shifting p.

pa·chom·e·ter (pa-kom'e-ter). Paquímetro. SIN pachymeter.

Pachon, Michel V., fisiologista francês, 1867–1938. VER P. *method, test*.

△ **pachy-.** Paqui-; espesso. [G. *pachys*, espesso]

pach·y·bleph·a·ron (pak'ē-blef'ă-ron). Paquiblefarose; espessamento da margem tarsal da pálpebra. SIN tylosis ciliaris. [pachy- + G. *blepharon*, pálpebra]

pach·y·ce·pha·lia (pak'ē-se-fā'lē-ă). Paquicefalia. SIN pachycephaly.

pach·y·ce·phal·ic, pach·y·ceph·a·lous (pak'ē-se-fal'ik, -sef'ă-lŭs). Paquicefálico; relativo a, ou caracterizado por, paquicefalia.

pach·y·ceph·a·ly (pak-i-sef'ă-lē). Paquicefalia; espessamento anormal do crânio. SIN pachycephalia. [pachy- + G. *kephalē*, cabeça]

pach·y·chei·lia, pach·y·chi·lia (pak-i-kī'lē-ă). Paquiquilia; edema ou espessamento anormal dos lábios. [pachy- + G. *cheilos*, lábio]

pach·y·cho·lia (pak-i-kō'lē-ă). Paquicolia; espessamento da bile. [pachy- + G. *cholē*, bile]

pach·y·chro·mat·ic (pak'ē-krō-mat'ik). Paquicromático; que possui um retículo de cromatina grosseiro.

pach·y·chy·mia (pak-i-kī'mē-ă). Paquiquimia; espessamento do quimo. [pachy- + G. *chymos*, suco]

pach·y·dac·tyl·ia (pak'ē-dak-til'ē-ă). Paquidactilia. SIN pachydactyly.

pach·y·dac·ty·lous (pak-i-dak'ti-lŭs). Paquidáctilo; relativo a, ou caracterizado por, paquidactilia.

pach·y·dac·ty·ly (pak-i-dak'ti-lē). Paquidactilia. Espessamento dos dedos das mãos ou dos pés, sobretudo das pontas; comum na neurofibromatose. [pachy- + G. *daktylos*, dedo da mão ou do pé]

pach·y·der·ma (pak-i-der'mă). Paquidermia; espessamento anormal da pele. VER TAMBÉM elephantiasis. SIN pachydermatosis. [pachy- + G. *derma*, pele]

p. laryn'gis, p. da laringe; hiperplasia epitelial circunscrita na comissura posterior da laringe.

p. lymphangiectat'ica, p. linfangiectásica; elefantíase causada por estase linfática.

p. verruco'sa, p. verrucosa; elefantíase crônica semelhante a verrugas.

△ Formas Combinantes	☆ Termo oficial alternativo para a Terminologia Anatomica
🄸 Indica que o termo é ilustrado, ver Índice de Ilustrações	
SIN Sinônimo	[MIM] Mendelian Inheritance in Man
Cf. Comparar, confrontar	I.C. Índice de Corantes
[NA] Nomina Anatomica	Termo de Alta Importância
[TA] Terminologia Anatomica	

p. vesi'cae, p. vesiculosa; elefantíase com nódulos compostos de vesículas linfáticas na superfície cutânea.

pach·y·der·ma·to·sis (pak'i-der'mă-tō'sis). Paquidermia. SIN pachyderma.

pachydermodactyly. Paquidermodactilia; edema digital, devido a fibromatose difusa, que ocorre nas articulações interfalângicas proximais do segundo, terceiro e quarto dedos da mão (algumas vezes envolvendo o quinto dedo, raramente o polegar); existe uma forma familiar [MIM 600356].

pach·y·der·mo·per·i·os·to·sis (pak-i-der'mō-per'ē-os-tō'sis) [MIM*-167100]. Paquidermoperiostose; síndrome de baqueteamento digital, neosteogênese periosteal, principalmente nas extremidades distais dos ossos longos (osteoartropatia hipertrófica idiopática), e as feições tornam-se grosseiras, com espessamento, sulcos e oleosidade da pele da face e fronte (*cutis verticis gyrata*); há hiperplasia seborreica, com poros sebáceos abertos cheios de tampões de sebo; freqüentemente, de herança autossômica dominante, em geral mais grave em homens. SIN acropachyderma. [pachy- + G. *derma*, pele, + *periostosis*]

pach·y·glos·sia (pak-i-glos'ē-ă). Paquiglossia; língua espessa e aumentada de tamanho. [pachy- + G. *glōssa*, língua]

pa·chyg·na·thous (pă-kig'nath-ŭs). Paquignático; caracterizado por uma mandíbula grande ou espessa. [pachy- + G. *gnathos*, mandíbula]

pach·y·gy·ria (pak-i-jī'rē-ă). Paquigiria; condição na qual as convoluções do córtex cerebral são anormalmente grandes; há menos sulcos que o normal e, em alguns casos, a quantidade de substância encefálica está um pouco aumentada. SIN macrogyria. [pachy- + G. *gyros*, círculo]

pach·y·lep·to·men·in·gi·tis (pak'i-lep'tō-men-in-jī'tis). Paquileptomeningite; inflamação de todas as membranas do encéfalo ou da medula espinal. [G. *pachys*, espesso, + *leptos*, fino, + *mēninx* (*mēning-*), membrana, + -*itis*, inflamação]

pach·y·men·in·gi·tis (pak'i-men'in-jī'tis). Paquimeningite; inflamação da dura-máter. SIN perimeningitis. [pachy- + G. *mēninx*, membrana, + -*itis*, inflamação]

p. exter'na, p. externa; inflamação da superfície externa da dura-máter. SIN epidural meningitis, external meningitis.

hemorrhagic p., p. hemorrágica; hemorragia subdural (subdural *hemorrhage*) associada à paquimeningite. VER TAMBÉM subdural *hemorrhage*.

hypertrophic cervical p., p. cervical hipertrófica; espessamento fibrótico e inflamatório das paquimeninges espinais, sobretudo na região cervical, resultando em radiculopatia de nervos espinais; considerada de etiologia sifilítica.

p. inter'na, p. interna; inflamação da superfície interna da dura-máter. SIN internal meningitis.

pyogenic p., p. piogênica; inflamação supurativa da dura-máter, que freqüentemente se dissemina a partir de uma osteomielite adjacente.

pach·y·me·nin·gop·a·thy (pak'ē-mē-ning-gop'ă-thē). Paquimeningopatia; doença da dura-máter. [pachy- + G. *mēninx* (*mēning-*), membrana, + *pathos*, doença]

pach·y·me·ninx (pak'i-mē'ningks) [TA]. Paquimeninge. SIN dura mater. [pachy- + G. *mēninx*, membrana]

pa·chym·e·ter (pa-kim'e-ter). Paquímetro; instrumento para medir a espessura de qualquer objeto, principalmente de objetos finos como uma lâmina óssea ou uma membrana. SIN pachometer. [pachy- + G. *metron*, medida]

optical p., p. óptico; uma lente e/ou espelho usado para medir a espessura da córnea.

pach·y·ne·ma (pak-ē-nē'mă). Paquinema. SIN pachytene. [pachy- + G. *nēma*, filamento]

pa·chyn·sis (pă-kin'sis). Paquinse; termo obsoleto para designar qualquer espessamento patológico. [G. espessamento]

pa·chyn·tic (pa-kin'tic). Paquíntico; relativo à paquinse.

pach·y·o·nych·ia (pak'ē-ō-nik'ē-ă). Paquioníquia; espessamento anormal das unhas dos dedos das mãos ou dos pés. [pachy- + G. *onyx*, unha]

p. congen'ita [MIM*167200], p. congênita; síndrome de displasia ectodérmica de espessura anormal e elevação das lâminas ungueais com hiperceratose palmar e plantar; a língua é esbranquiçada e brilhante devido à atrofia papilar; herança autossômica dominante causada por mutação no gene 16 da queratina (KRT16) no cromossoma 17q ou no gene 6A da queratina (KRT6A) em 12q. SIN Jadassohn-Lewandowski syndrome.

pach·y·o·tia (pak-i-ō'shē-ă). Paquiotia; espessamento e embrutecimento da orelha externa. [pachy- + G. *ous*, orelha]

pach·y·per·i·os·ti·tis (pak'i-per'ē-ōs-tī'tis). Paquiperiostite; espessamento proliferativo do periósteo causado por inflamação. [pachy- + *periostitis*]

pach·y·per·i·to·ni·tis (pak'i-per'i-tō-nī'tis). Paquiperitonite; designação obsoleta da inflamação do peritônio com espessamento da membrana. SIN productive peritonitis. [pachy- + *peritonitis*]

pach·y·pleu·ri·tis (pak'ē-ploo-rī'tis). Paquipleurite; termo obsoleto para designar inflamação da pleura com espessamento da membrana. SIN productive pleurisy. [pachy- + *pleura* + G. -*itis*, inflamação]

pa·chyp·o·dous (pă-kip'ō-dŭs). Paquípode; que possui pés grandes e espessos. [pachy- + G. *pous*, pé]

pach·y·so·mia (pak-i-sō'mē-ă). Paquissomia; espessamento patológico das partes moles do corpo, notavelmente na acromegalia. [pachy- + G. *sōma*, corpo]

pach·y·tene (pak'i-tēn). Paquíteno; o estágio da prófase na meiose no qual o pareamento dos cromossomas homólogos é completo e os homólogos pareados podem entrelaçar-se enquanto continuam a encurtar; há clivagem longitudinal em cada cromossoma para formar duas cromátides-irmãs, de forma que cada par de cromossomas homólogos torna-se um conjunto de quatro cromátides entrelaçadas. SIN pachynema. [pachy- + G. *tainia*, faixa, fita]

pach·y·vag·i·nal·i·tis (pak'i-vaj'i-năl-ī'tis). Paquivaginalite; termo obsoleto para inflamação crônica com espessamento da túnica vaginal do testículo. [pachy- + L. mod. (tunica) *vaginalis*, + G. -*itis*, inflamação]

pach·y·vag·i·ni·tis (pak'i-vaj'i-nī'tis). Paquivaginite; designação obsoleta de vaginite crônica com espessamento e endurecimento das paredes vaginais. [pachy- + *vagina* + G. -*itis*, inflamação]

p. cys'tica, p. cística. SIN vaginitis emphysematosa.

Pacini, Filippo, anatomista italiano, 1812–1883. VER pacinian *corpuscles*, em *corpuscle*; Vater-P. *corpuscles*, em *corpuscle*.

pa·ci·ni·an (pa-sin'ē-an, pa-chin'). Paciniano; atribuído a, ou descrito por, Pacini.

pa·cin·i·tis (pa-sin-ī'tis, pa-chin-). Inflamação dos corpúsculos de Pacini.

pack (pak). 1. Encher, abarrotar ou tamponar. 2. Envolver ou revestir o corpo com um lençol, cobertor ou outro tipo de cobertura. 3. Aplicar um curativo ou uma compressa a um local cirúrgico. 4. Os artigos usados em curativos de feridas. [I.m. *pak*, do Alemão]

cold p., compressa fria; compressa de tecido ou outro material embebido em água fria ou servindo como envoltório para gelo.

dry p., compressa seca; envolvimento de uma pessoa com cobertores secos e aquecidos para induzir transpiração abundante.

hot p., compressa quente; compressa de tecido ou outro material embebido em água quente ou que produz calor úmido por outro meio.

wet p., compressa úmida; a forma habitual de compressa utilizando calor ou frio úmido.

pack·er (pak'er). 1. Instrumento para tamponamento. 2. Obturador. SIN plugger.

pack·ing (pak'ing). 1. Tamponamento; enchimento de uma cavidade natural, uma ferida ou um molde com algum material. 2. O material assim usado. 3. A aplicação de uma compressa.

denture p., enchimento e compressão do material da base de uma dentadura no molde em uma moldeira.

pac·li·tax·el (pac-lē-taks'el). Paclitaxel; agente antitumoral que promove reunião dos microtúbulos por impedir a despolimerização; atualmente é usado no tratamento de salvamento do carcinoma metastático do ovário.

PACS Acrônimo de *p*icture *a*rchive and *c*ommunication *s*ystem (sistema de arquivamento e transmissão de imagens), uma rede computadorizada para imagens e laudos radiológicos digitalizados.

pad. 1. Compressa; tampão; material de consistência mole, que forma um coxim, usado para aplicar ou aliviar a pressão em uma parte, ou no enchimento de uma depressão de forma que os curativos possam se encaixar bem. 2. Coxim; corpo mais ou menos encapsulado de gordura ou de algum outro tecido que serve para encher um espaço ou agir como um amortecedor no corpo. (isto é, o coxim do calcanhar).

abdominal p., compressa abdominal. SIN laparotomy p.

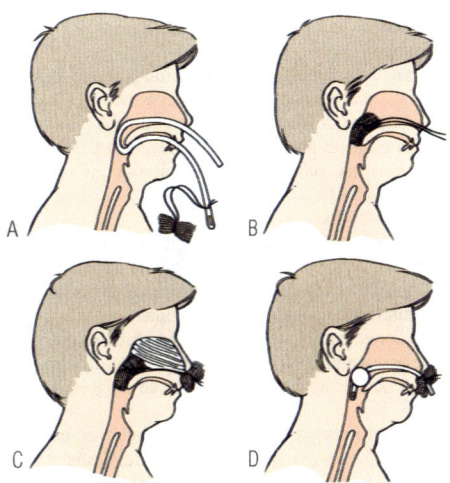

tamponamento nasal: tamponamento para controlar hemorragia da parte posterior do nariz, (A) o cateter é introduzido e a compressa fixada; (B) a compressa é posicionada enquanto o cateter é removido; (C) a fita é amarrada em um suporte para manter a compressa no lugar, com a compressa anterior instalada no formato sanfonado; (D) método alternativo, utilizando cateter com balão em vez de compressa com gaze

dinner p., almofada de espessura média, colocada sobre a região epigástrica antes da aplicação de um colete gessado; após o gesso secar, a almofada é retirada, deixando espaço para graus variáveis de distensão abdominal.
fat p., coxim gorduroso, corpo adiposo. VER fat-pad.
fat p. of ischioanal fossa, corpo adiposo da fossa isquioanal. SIN fat body of ischioanal fossa.
heel p., coxim do calcanhar; corpo adiposo encapsulado, sob a superfície plantar do calcâneo, que atua como amortecedor durante a sustentação de peso e a deambulação.
knuckle p.'s, (1) um traço autossômico dominante, no qual coxins espessos de pele surgem sobre as articulações interfalângicas proximais; ocasionalmente associado a leuconíquia e surdez ou contratura de Dupuytren; **(2)** uma reação de calo resultante de traumatismo ocupacional ou auto-infligido.
laparotomy p., compressa de laparotomia; compressa feita com várias camadas de gaze dobrada em formato retangular; usada como esponja, para proteger as vísceras em cirurgias abdominais, e de outras formas. SIN abdominal p.
Passavant p., crista de Passavant; crista palatofaríngea. SIN Passavant ridge.
periarterial p., corpúsculo justaglomerular. SIN juxtaglomerular body.
pharyngoesophageal p.'s, coxins faringoesofágicos. SIN pharyngoesophageal cushions, em cushion.
retromolar p., coxim retromolar; massa acolchoada de tecido, freqüentemente piriforme, localizada no processo alveolar da mandíbula atrás da área do último dente molar natural; é de particular interesse na adaptação de dentaduras. SIN pear-shaped area.
sucking p., suctorial p., corpo adiposo da bochecha. SIN buccal fat-pad.
threshold p.'s of anal canal, coxins anais. SIN anal cushions, em cushion.

Padykula-Herman stain for my·o·sin ATPase. Coloração de Padykula-Herman para miosina ATPase. Ver em stain.

Pae·ci·lo·my·ces (pē-sil-ō-mī′sēz). Gênero de fungos imperfeitos saprófitas, cujas hifas com conídios lembram superficialmente o penicilo do *Penicillium*; isolados como contaminantes, patógenos ocasionais.
P. lilacinus, um bolor; uma causa rara de paecilomicose; foi implicado em infecções oftálmicas humanas devidas a lentes intra-oculares implantadas contaminadas. SIN Penicillium lilacinum.

pae·ci·loy·co·sis (pē-sil′ō-ē-cō′sis). Peciloicose; micose sistêmica (principalmente pulmonar) dos seres humanos e de vários animais inferiores, causada por fungos do gênero *Paecilomyces*.

paed-. VER ped-.

PAF Abreviatura de platelet-activating *factor* (fator ativador de plaquetas).

PAGE Abreviatura de polyacrylamide gel *electrophoresis* (eletroforese em gel de poliacrilamida).

Pagenstecher, Alexander, oftalmologista alemão, 1828–1879. VER P. circle.

Paget, Sir James, cirurgião inglês, 1814–1899. VER P. cells, em *cell, disease*; extramammary P. *disease*; Paget-von Schrötter *syndrome*.

Paget-Eccleston stain. Coloração de Paget-Eccleston. Ver em stain.

pa·get·ic (pa-jet′ik). Pagético; relativo à doença de Paget ou que sofre dessa doença.

pag·et·oid (paj′ē-toyd). Pagetóide; semelhante à, ou característico da, doença de Paget.

pa·go·pha·gia (pā-gō-fā′jē-ă). Pagofagia; ingestão compulsiva e repetida de gelo; algumas vezes associada à anemia ferropriva. [G. *pagos*, gelo, + *phagō*, comer]

-pagus. -pago; gêmeos conjugados, o primeiro elemento da palavra designa as partes fundidas. VER TAMBÉM -didymus, -dymus. [G. *pagos*, algo fixo, de *pēgnymi*, unir]

PAH Abreviatura de *p*-aminohippuric acid (ácido *p*-amino-hipúrico).

pain (pān). Dor. **1.** Uma sensação desagradável associada a lesão tecidual real ou potencial e mediada por fibras nervosas específicas para o encéfalo, onde sua valorização consciente pode ser modificada por vários fatores. **2.** Termo usado para designar uma contração uterina dolorosa que ocorre no parto. [L. *poena*, multa, penalidade]
after-p.'s, dores pós-parto. VER afterpains.
bearing-down p., contração uterina acompanhada por esforço para defecar e tenesmo; geralmente ocorre no segundo estágio do trabalho de parto.
expulsive p.'s, dores do período expulsivo; dores efetivas do trabalho de parto associadas à contração da musculatura uterina.
false p.'s, falsas dores; contrações uterinas não-efetivas, que precedem e, algumas vezes, se assemelham ao trabalho de parto verdadeiro, mas distinguíveis dele pela ausência de apagamento e dilatação progressivos do colo uterino.
girdle p., dor em cinta; sensação dolorosa que circunda o corpo como uma cinta, ocorre no tabes dorsal ou em outra doença da medula espinal.
growing p.'s, dores do crescimento; dores, freqüentemente sentidas à noite, nos membros das crianças; a causa é obscura, mas o distúrbio é benigno.
hunger p., dor de fome; cólica epigástrica associada à fome.
intermenstrual p., dor intermenstrual; **(1)** desconforto pélvico que ocorre na época da ovulação, geralmente no meio do ciclo menstrual. SIN midpain. **(2)** SIN mittelschmerz.
intractable p., dor intratável; dor resistente ou refratária a analgésicos comuns.
labor p.'s, dores do parto; contrações uterinas rítmicas que, em condições normais, aumentam em intensidade, freqüência e duração, culminando em parto vaginal. SIN parodynia.
middle p., dor intermenstrual. SIN mittelschmerz.
night p., dor noturna. SIN nyctalgia.
organic p., dor orgânica; dor causada por uma lesão orgânica.
periodic bone p., artralgia periódica. SIN periodic arthralgia.
phantom limb p., d. do membro-fantasma; a sensação de que um membro amputado ainda está presente, freqüentemente associada a parestesia dolorosa. SIN phantom limb, pseudesthesia (3), pseudoesthesia (3), stump hallucination.
postprandial p., dor pós-prandial; d. que ocorre após a alimentação, típica de neoplasia maligna no esôfago ou estômago.
psychogenic p., d. psicogênica; d. somatiforme; d. associada ou relacionada a um estímulo psicológico, emocional ou comportamental. SIN psychalgia (2), somatoform p.
referred p., dor referida; dor de estruturas profundas, percebida como originando-se de uma área superficial distante de sua origem real; a área onde a dor é sentida é inervada pelo(s) mesmo(s) segmento(s) espinal(is) que a estrutura profunda. SIN telalgia.
respirophasic p., dor, amiúde erroneamente denominada pleurítica, que ocorre ou se agrava sincronicamente com o ciclo respiratório. [L. *respiro*, respirar, + G. *phasis*, aparecimento recorrente, como de uma estrela, de *phaino*, aparecer, + -ic]
rest p., dor em repouso; dor que geralmente ocorre nos membros, durante o repouso na posição sentada ou deitada.
somatoform p., dor psicogênica. SIN psychogenic p.

paint (pānt). Tintura; uma solução ou suspensão de um ou mais medicamentos, aplicada à pele com um pincel ou um aplicador grande; geralmente usada no tratamento de erupções disseminadas.
carbol-fuchsin p., t. de carbol-fucsina; tintura contendo ácido bórico, fenol, resorcinol, fucsina, acetona e álcool em água; usada no tratamento de infecções micóticas superficiais. SIN Castellani p.
Castellani p., t. de Castellani. SIN carbol-fuchsin p.

pair (pār). Par; dois objetos considerados juntos devido à semelhança, para um fim comum, ou devido a alguma força de atração entre eles.
base p. (b.p.), par de bases; o complexo de duas bases de ácido nucleico heterocíclicas, sendo uma pirimidina e a outra uma purina, mantido por pontes de hidrogênio entre a purina e a pirimidina; o pareamento das bases é o elemento essencial na estrutura do DNA proposta por J. Watson e F. Crick em 1953; geralmente a guanina forma par com a citosina (G-C), e a adenina com a timina (A-T) ou o uracil (A-U). SIN nucleoside p., nucleotide p.
buffer p., par tamponado; um ácido e sua base conjugada (ânion).
chromosome p., par de cromossomas; dois cromossomas do cariótipo diplóide completo, semelhantes em forma e função, mas que geralmente diferem em conteúdo, sendo um normalmente herdado de cada genitor e um transmitido a cada filho; no sexo heteromórfico (nos seres humanos, o homem), um par, os cromossomas sexuais, difere significativamente em aspecto, conteúdo e função.
conjugate acid-base p., par ácido-básico conjugado; em solventes prototônicos (p. ex., H_2O, NH_3, ácido acético), duas espécies moleculares diferindo apenas pela presença ou ausência de um íon hidrogênio (p. ex., ácido carbônico/íon bicarbonato ou íon amônio/amônia); a base da atividade tampão.
line p.'s, pares de linha; uma unidade de resolução de écrans e filmes radiográficos ou filmes fotográficos; o maior número de pares de linha por cm que pode ser definido.
nucleoside p., nucleotide p., par de nucleotídeos. SIN base p.
p. production, produção de pares; criação de um positron e elétron, cada um com massa 0,511 MeV, quando um fóton incidente de energia maior que 1,02 meV é absorvido pela matéria; ocorre na radioterapia de alta energia.

pa·ja·roe·llo (pah-har-wā′o). SIN *Ornithodoros coriaceus*. [Esp. am. *pajahuello*, do Esp. *paja*, palha, + *huello*, superfície inferior do casco]

Palade, George E., biólogo celular romeno-norte-americano e ganhador do Prêmio Nobel, *1912. VER P. *granule*; Weibel-P. *bodies*, em *body*.

pal·a·tal (pal′ă-tăl). Palatino; relativo ao palato ou ao osso do palato. SIN palatine.

pal·ate (pal′ăt) [TA]. Palato; a porção óssea e muscular entre as cavidades oral e nasal. SIN palatum [TA], root of mouth, uraniscus. [L. *palatum*, palato]
bony p. [TA], palato ósseo; lâmina óssea elíptica, côncava, que forma o teto da cavidade oral, formada pelo processo palatino da maxila e pela lâmina horizontal do osso palatino de cada lado. SIN palatum osseum [TA].
Byzantine arch p., p. em arco bizantino; fusão incompleta do processo palatino com a espinha nasal.
cleft p., fenda palatina; fissura congênita na linha média do palato, freqüentemente associada à fenda labial. Freqüentemente é uma manifestação de uma síndrome ou condição generalizada, p. ex., nanismo diastrófico ou displasia espondiloepifisária congênita; seu comportamento genético geral assemelha-se ao da fenda labial (cleft *lip*). SIN palatoschisis, palatum fissum.

avaliação da dor torácica

doença	caráter, localização e radiação	duração	condições precipitantes	medidas de alívio
angina de peito	dor subesternal ou retroesternal que se propaga através do tórax; pode irradiar-se para a face interna do braço, pescoço ou mandíbula	5–15 min	geralmente relacionada a esforços, emoção, alimentação, frio	repouso, nitroglicerina, oxigênio
infarto do miocárdio	dor subesternal ou precordial; pode disseminar-se por todo o tórax; pode haver incapacidade dolorosa dos ombros e das mãos	> 15 min	ocorre espontaneamente, mas pode ser seqüela de angina instável	sulfato de morfina, reperfusão bem-sucedida da artéria coronária obstruída
pericardite	dor subesternal aguda, forte ou dor à esquerda do esterno; pode ser sentida no epigástrio e referida para o pescoço, braços e dorso	intermitente	início súbito; a dor aumenta à inspiração, deglutição, tosse e rotação do tronco	o ato de sentar, analgesia, medicamentos antiinflamatórios
dor pulmonar	a dor se origina na parte inferior da pleura; pode ser referida para as margens costais ou parte superior do abdome; paciente pode ser capaz de localizar a dor	± 30 min	freqüentemente é espontânea; a dor ocorre ou aumenta à inspiração	repouso, tempo; tratamento da causa subjacente, broncodilatação
dor esofágica (hérnia de hiato, esofagite de refluxo ou espasmo)	dor subesternal; pode ser projetada em torno do tórax até os ombros	5–60 min	decúbito, líquidos frios, exercício; pode ocorrer espontaneamente	alimento, antiácido; a nitroglicerina alivia o espasmo
ansiedade	dor no hemitórax esquerdo; pode ser variável; não se irradia; paciente pode se queixar de dormência e formigamento nas mãos e na boca	2–3 min	estresse, taquipnéia emocional	retirada de estímulo, relaxamento

falling p., uvuloptose. SIN uvuloptosis.
Gothic p., p. gótico; palato anormalmente apiculado.
hard p. [TA], p. duro; (1) a parte anterior do palato, que consiste no palato ósseo coberto, acima, pela mucosa do assoalho da cavidade nasal e, abaixo, pelo mucoperiósteo do teto da boca, que contém os vasos, nervos e glândulas mucosas do palato. SIN palatum durum [TA]. (2) Em cefalometria, uma linha que une as espinhas nasais anterior e posterior, representando a posição do palato ósseo.
pendulous p., úvula palatina. SIN *uvula* of soft palate.
primary p., p. primário; no embrião inicial, a prateleira, formada pelos processos nasais mediais, que separa anteriormente a cavidade oral, abaixo, das cavidades nasais primitivas, acima. SIN primitive p.
primitive p., p. primitivo. SIN primary p.
secondary p., p. secundário; a porção do palato embrionário, posterior ao palato primário, que se forma a partir dos processos palatinos da maxila embrionária e se transforma nos palatos duro e mole.
soft p. [TA], p. mole; a porção muscular posterior do palato, que forma um septo incompleto entre a boca e a orofaringe, e entre a orofaringe e a nasofaringe. SIN palatum molle [TA], velum palatinum*, velum pendulum palati.

pa·lat·i·form (pă-lat′i-form). Palatiforme; em forma de palato; semelhante ao palato.
pa·lat·i·nase (pă-lat′i-nās). Palatinase; maltase na mucosa intestinal que hidrolisa palatinose; provavelmente oligo-1,6-glucosidase.
pal·a·tine (pal′ă-tīn). Palatino. SIN palatal.
pa·lat·i·nose (pă-lat′i-nōs). Palatinose; dissacarídeo que consiste em D-glicose e D-frutose na ligação α-1,6 (sacarose é α-1,2).
pal·a·ti·tis (pal-ă-tī′tis). Palatite; inflamação do palato. SIN uranisconitis.
palato-. Palato. [L. *palatum*, palato]
pal·a·to·glos·sal (pal′ă-tō-glos′ăl). Palatoglosso; relativo ao palato e à língua ou ao músculo palatoglosso.
pal·a·to·glos·sus (pal-ă-tō-glos′ŭs). Músculo palatoglosso. SIN palatoglossus (*muscle*).
pal·a·tog·na·thous (pal′ă-tog′nă-thŭs). Palatognato; que possui uma fenda palatina. [palato- + G. *gnathos*, mandíbula]
pal·a·to·gram (pal′ă-tō-gram). Palatograma; registro da atividade da língua contra o palato, feito pela colocação de cera mole ou de um pó sobre uma placa de base.

pal·a·to·graph (pal'ă-tō-graf). Palatógrafo; instrumento usado no registro dos movimentos do palato mole ao falar e durante a respiração. SIN palate myograph, palatomyograph. [palato- + G. *graphō*, registrar]

pal·a·to·max·il·lary (pal'ă-tō-mak'si-lār-ē). Palatomaxilar; relativo ao palato e à maxila.

pal·a·to·my·o·graph (pal'ă-tō-mī'ō-graf). Palatomiógrafo. SIN palatograph. [G. palato- + *mys*, músculo, + *graphō*, registrar]

pal·a·to·na·sal (pal-ă-tō-nā'sal). Palatonasal; relativo ao palato e à cavidade nasal.

pal·a·to·pha·ryn·ge·al (pal'ă-tō-fa-rin'jē-ăl). Palatofaríngeo; relativo ao palato e à faringe.

pal·a·to·pha·ryn·ge·us (pal'ă-tō-far-in-jē'ŭs). Músculo palatofaríngeo. SIN palatopharyngeus (*muscle*). [L.]

pal·a·to·pha·ryn·go·plas·ty (pal'ă-tō-fa-rin'gō-plas-tē). Palatofaringoplastia; ressecção cirúrgica de tecido palatino e orofaríngeo desnecessário em casos selecionados de ronco, com ou sem apnéia do sono. SIN uvulopalatopharyngoplasty. [palato- + pharynx, + *plastos*, formado]

pal·a·to·pha·ryn·gor·rha·phy (pal'ă-tō-far'in-gōr'ă-fē). Palatofaringorrafia. SIN staphylopharyngorrhaphy. [palato- + pharynx, + G. *rhaphē*, sutura]

pal·a·to·plas·ty (pal'ă-tō-plas-tē). Palatoplastia; cirurgia do palato para restaurar sua forma e função. SIN staphyloplasty, uraniscoplasty, uranoplasty, uvulopalatoplasty. [palato- + G. *plassō*, formar]

pal·a·to·ple·gia (pal'ă-tō-plē'jē-ă). Palatoplegia; paralisia dos músculos do palato mole. [palato- + G. *plēgē*, ataque]

pal·a·tor·rha·phy (pal-ă-tōr'ă-fē). Palatorrafia; sutura de uma fenda palatina. SIN staphylorrhaphy, uraniscorrhaphy, uranorrhaphy, velosynthesis. [palato- + G. *rhaphē*, sutura]

pal·a·tos·chi·sis (pal-ă-tos'ki-sis). Palatosquise. SIN cleft *palate*. [palato- + G. *schisis*, fissura]

pa·la·tum, pl. **pa·la·'ti** (pă-lā'tŭm). [TA]. Palato. SIN palate [L.]
  p. du'rum [TA], p. duro. SIN hard *palate* (1).
  p. fis'sum, fenda palatina. SIN cleft *palate*.
  p. mol'le [TA], p. mole. SIN soft *palate*.
  p. os'seum [TA], p. ósseo. SIN bony *palate*.

pa·le·en·ceph·a·lon (pā'lē-en-sef'ă-lon). Palencéfalo; termo cunhado por L. Edinger para designar o sistema nervoso metamérico (metameric nervous system). Exclui o córtex cerebral. [paleo- + G. *enkephalos*, encéfalo]

♻ **paleo-, pale-.** Paleo-, pale-; antigo, primitivo, primário, inicial. [G. *palaios*, antigo]

pa·le·o·cer·e·bel·lum (pā'lē-ō-ser'ē-bel'ŭm) [TA]. Paleocerebelo; termo filogenético referente à parte do cerebelo que inclui a maior parte do verme e as zonas adjacentes dos hemisférios cerebelares rostrais à fissura primária; o paleocerebelo equivale ao lobo anterior e corresponde à zona de distribuição dos tratos espinocerebelares, e algumas vezes é denominado espinocerebelo; no período filogenético, é considerado intermediário entre o arquicerebelo [TA] e o neocerebelo [TA]. SIN spinocerebellum [TA]. [paleo- + L. *cerebellum*]

pa·le·o·cor·tex (pā'lē-ō-kōr'teks) [TA]. Paleocórtex; a parte filogeneticamente mais antiga do manto cortical do hemisfério cerebral, representada pelo córtex olfatório.

pa·le·o·ki·net·ic (pā'lē-ō-ki-net'ik). Paleocinético; designa os mecanismos motores primitivos subjacentes aos reflexos musculares e aos movimentos automáticos, estereotipados. [paleo- + G. *kinētikos*, relativo ao movimento]

pa·le·o·pa·thol·o·gy (pā'lē-ō-pa-thol'ō-jē). Paleopatologia; a ciência da doença em tempos pré-históricos, revelada em ossos, múmias e artefatos arqueológicos. [paleo- + pathology]

pa·le·o·stri·a·tal (pā'lē-ō-strī-ā'tăl). Paleoestriado; relativo ao globo pálido (paleostriatum).

pa·le·o·stri·a·tum (pā'lē-ō-strī-ā'tŭm). Paleoestriado; termo que designa o globo pálido e expressa a hipótese de que, na evolução, esse componente do corpo estriado se desenvolveu antes do "neoestriado" ou estriado (núcleo caudado e putame) e que é um derivado diencefálico. VER TAMBÉM *globus* pallidus. [paleo- + L. *striatum*]

pa·le·o·thal·a·mus (pā'lē-ō-thal'ă-mŭs). Paleotálamo; os núcleos intralaminares, considerados os primeiros componentes do tálamo a se desenvolver; não possuem conexões recíprocas com o isocórtex.

Palfyn (Palfin), Jean, cirurgião e anatomista belga, 1650–1730. VER P. *sinus*.

pal·i·ki·ne·sia, pal·i·ci·ne·sia (pal-i-ki-nē'zē-ă, -si-nē'zē-ă). Palicinesia; repetição involuntária de movimentos. [G. *palin*, novamente, + *kinēsis*, movimento]

pal·i·nal (pal'i-năl). Movimento para trás. [G. *palin*, para trás]

pal·in·drome (pal'in-drōm). Palíndrome; em biologia molecular, uma seqüência de ácido nucleico autocomplementar; uma seqüência idêntica a seu filamento complementar, se ambos forem "lidos" na mesma direção 5′ para 3′, ou seqüências repetitivas invertidas em direções opostas (p. ex., 5′-AGT-TGA-3′) de cada lado de um eixo de simetria; os palíndromos ocorrem em locais de reações importantes (p. ex., locais de ligação, locais clivados por enzimas de restrição); existem palíndromos imperfeitos, como os palíndromos interrompidos que permitem a formação de alças. [G. *palindromos*, corrida para trás]

pal·in·dro·mia (pal-in-drō'mē-ă). Palindromia; recidiva ou recorrência de uma doença. [G. *palindromos*, corrida para trás, + *-ia*, condição]

pal·in·drom·ic (pal-in-drom'ik). Palindrômico; recorrente.

pal·i·sade (pal'i-sād). Paliçada; em patologia, uma fileira de núcleos alongados paralelos entre si. [Fr. *palissade*, do L. *palus*, estaca, paliçada]

pal·la·di·um (Pd) (pă-lā'dē-ŭm). Paládio; elemento metálico semelhante à platina, n.º atômico 46, peso atômico, 106,42. [do asteróide Pallas; G. *Pallas*, deusa da sabedoria]

pall·an·es·the·sia (pal'an-es-thē'zē-ă). Palanestesia; ausência de palestesia. SIN apallesthesia. [G. *pallō*, tremer, + *anaisthēsia*, insensibilidade]

pall·es·the·sia (pal'es-thē'zē-ă). Palestesia; a percepção da vibração, uma forma de sensibilidade à pressão; mais aguda quando se apóia um diapasão vibrando sobre uma proeminência óssea. SIN bone sensibility, pallesthetic sensibility, vibratory sensibility. [G. *pallō*, tremer, + *aisthēsis*, sensação]

pall·es·thet·ic (pal-es-thet'ik). Palestésico; relativo à palestesia.

pal·li·al (pal'ē-ăl). Relativo ao córtex cerebral (*pallium*).

pal·li·ate (pal'ē-āt). Paliar; reduzir a intensidade de; aliviar ligeiramente. SIN mitigate. [L. *palliatus* (adj.), vestido com um manto (*pallium*), escondido]

pal·li·a·tive (pal'ē-ă-tiv). Paliativo; que reduz a intensidade de; designa o alívio de sintomas sem curar a doença subjacente.

pal·li·dal (pal'i-dăl). Pálido; relativo ao globo pálido.

pal·li·dec·to·my (pal'i-dek'tō-mē). Palidectomia; excisão ou destruição do globo pálido, geralmente por estereotaxia; um prefixo pode indicar o método usado, p. ex., quimiopalidectomia (destruição por um agente químico), criopalidectomia (destruição pelo frio). [pallidum + G. *ektomē*, excisão]

pal·li·do·a·myg·da·lot·o·my (pal'i-dō-ă-mig'dă-lot'ō-mē). Palidoamigdalotomia; produção de lesões no globo pálido e nos núcleos amigdalóides. [pallidum + amygdala (1) + G. *tomē*, corte]

pal·li·do·an·sot·o·my (pal'i-dō-an-sot'ō-mē). Produção de lesões no globo pálido e na alça lenticular.

pal·li·dot·o·my (pal-i-dot'ō-mē). Palidotomia; operação destrutiva no globo pálido, realizada para aliviar movimentos involuntários ou rigidez muscular. [pallidum + G. *tomē*, incisão]

pal·li·dum (pal'i-dŭm) [TA]. Globo pálido. SIN *globus* pallidus. [L. *pallidus*, pálido]
  dorsal p. [TA], globo pálido dorsal; aquelas partes do globo pálido situadas geralmente dorsais ao plano da comissura anterior; juntamente com o estriado dorsal, participa de atividades motoras com origens cognitivas; também forma parte dos gânglios da base dorsais. SIN p. dorsale [TA].
  p. dorsale [TA], p. dorsal. SIN dorsal p.
  ventral p. [TA], p. ventral; aquelas partes do globo pálido localizadas ventrais à comissura anterior; inclui partes da substância inominada; acredita-se que funciona, juntamente com o estriado ventral, em atividades motoras com fortes constructos motivacionais ou emocionais. SIN p. ventrale [TA].
  p. ventrale [TA], p. ventral. SIN ventral p.

pal·li·um (pal'ē-ŭm) [TA]. Córtex cerebral. SIN cerebral *cortex*. [L. manto]

pal·lor (pal'ŏr). Palidez, como a palidez cutânea. [L.]
  cachectic p., p. caquética. SIN achromasia (1).

palm (pahm, pawlm) [TA]. Palma; palma da mão; a parte plana da mão; a superfície flexora ou anterior da mão, excluindo os dedos; o oposto do dorso da mão. SIN palma [TA]. [L. *palma*]
  liver p., p. hepática; eritema exagerado nas eminências tenar e hipotenar.

pal·ma, pl. **pal·mae** (pawl'mă, pawl'mē). [TA]. Palma. SIN palm, palm. [L.]
  p. ma'nus, p. da mão. VER palm.

pal·mar (pawl'măr). [TA]. Palmar; referente à palma da mão; volar. SIN palmaris [TA]. [L. *palmaris*, de *palma*]

pal·mar·is (pawl-mār'is) [TA]. Palmar. SIN palmar [L.]

pal·mel·lin (pal'mel-in). Palmelina; corante vermelho formado por uma alga, *Palmella cruenta*.

Palmer, Walter L., médico norte-americano, *1896. VER P. *acid test* for peptic ulcer.

palm·ic (pal'mik). Batimento; pulsátil; relativo à palpitação.

pal·mi·tal·de·hyde (pal-mi-tal'dē-hīd). Palmitaldeído; hexadecanal; o aldeído de 16 carbonos, análogo do ácido palmítico; constituinte dos plasmalogênios.

pal·mi·tate (pal'mi-tāt). Palmitato; um sal do ácido palmítico.

pal·mit·ic ac·id (pal-mit'ik). Ácido palmítico; ácido graxo saturado comum encontrado no azeite-de-dendê e no azeite de oliva, bem como em muitas outras gorduras e ceras; o produto final da ácido graxo sintetase dos mamíferos. SIN hexadecanoic acid.

pal·mi·tin (pal'mi-tin). Palmitina; o triglicerídeo do ácido palmítico que ocorre no azeite-de-dendê. SIN tripalmitin.

pal·mit·o·le·ic ac·id (pal'mi-tō-lē'ik). Ácido palmitoleico; ácido 9-hexadecanóico; um ácido monoinsaturado com 16 carbonos; um dos constituintes comuns dos triacilgliceróis do tecido adiposo humano. SIN zoomaric acid.

pal·mi·tyl al·co·hol (pal'mi-til). Álcool palmitílico. SIN cetyl *alcohol*.

pal·mod·ic (pal - mod′ik). Relativo ao tique facial palmus (1).
pal·mos·co·py (pal - mos′ko - pē). Palmoscopia; exame da pulsação cardíaca. [G. *palmos*, pulsação, + *skopeō*, examinar]
pal·mus, pl. **pal·mi** (pal′mŭs, - mī). **1.** Tique facial. SIN facial *tic.* **2.** Contrações fibrilares rítmicas em um músculo. VER TAMBÉM jumping *disease.* **3.** O batimento cardíaco. [G. *palmos*, pulsação, palpitação]
pal·pa·ble (pal′pă - bl). Palpável. **1.** Perceptível ao toque; capaz de ser palpado. **2.** Evidente; puro. [ver palpation]
pal·pate (pal′pāt). Palpar; examinar por meio do tato e da pressão com as palmas das mãos e os dedos.
pal·pa·tion (pal - pā′shŭn). Palpação. **1.** Exame com as mãos, palpação de órgãos, massas ou infiltração de uma parte do corpo, sentindo os batimentos cardíacos ou os pulsos, vibrações no tórax, etc. **2.** Toque, palpação ou percepção pelo sentido do tato. [L. *palpatio*, de *palpo*, pp. *-atus*, tocar, afagar]
  bimanual p., p. bimanual; uso de ambas as mãos para sentir órgãos ou massas, principalmente no abdome ou na pelve.
  light-touch p., p. delicada; método para determinar os contornos de órgãos ou massas por palpação delicada da superfície com a ponta de um dedo.

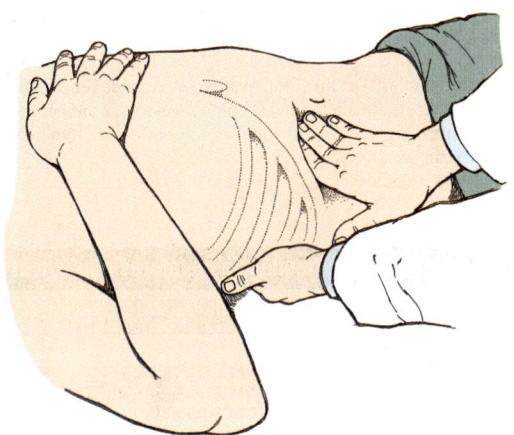

palpação do fígado

pal·pa·to·per·cus·sion (pal′pă - tō - per - kŭsh′ŭn). Exame por meio de palpação e percussão combinadas.
pal·pe·bra, pl. **pal·pe·brae** (pal - pē′bră, pē′brē) [TA]. Pálpebra. SIN eyelid. [L.]
  p. III, prega semilunar da túnica conjuntiva. SIN *plica* semilunaris of conjunctiva (2).
  p. infe′rior [TA], p. inferior. SIN inferior *eyelid.*
  p. supe′rior [TA], p. superior. SIN superior *eyelid.*
  p. ter′tia, prega semilunar da túnica conjuntiva. SIN *plica* semilunaris of conjunctiva (2).
pal·pe·bral (pal′pē - brăl). Palpebral; relativo a uma pálpebra ou às pálpebras.
pal·pe·bra·lis (pal′pē - brā′lis). Músculo levantador da pálpebra. SIN levator palpebrae superioris (*muscle*). [L.]
pal·pe·brate (pal′pē - brāt). **1.** Palpebrado; que tem pálpebras. **2.** Piscar. [L. *palpebra*, pálpebra]
pal·pe·bra·tion (pal - pē - brā′shŭn). Piscadela. [L. *palpebratio*]
pal·pi·ta·tio cor·dis (pal - pi - tā′shē - ō kōr′dis). Palpitação cardíaca.
pal·pi·ta·tion (pal - pi - tā′shŭn). Palpitação; pulsação vigorosa ou irregular do coração, percebida pelo paciente, geralmente com aumento da frequência ou força, com ou sem irregularidade do ritmo. SIN trepidatio cordis. [L. *palpito*, pulsar]
PALS Abreviatura de periarterial lymphatic *sheath* (bainha linfática periarterial).
pal·sy (pawl′zē). Paralisia ou paresia. [uma corrupção do Fr. ant. do L. e G. *paralysis*]
  Bell p., paresia ou paralisia de Bell, geralmente unilateral, dos músculos faciais, causada por disfunção do 7.º nervo craniano; provavelmente decorrente de infecção viral; geralmente do tipo desmielinizante. SIN peripheral facial paralysis.
  birth p., paresia ou paralisia por tocotraumatismo; déficits motores e sensitivos que resultam de lesão das fibras nervosas associada ao parto (tocotraumatismo); o plexo braquial é a região mais afetada. Os exemplos incluem paralisia ou paresia de Erb e paralisia ou paresia de Klumpke.
  brachial birth p., paresia ou paralisia por tocotraumatismo. SIN obstetric p.
  bulbar p., paralisia bulbar progressiva. SIN progressive bulbar *paralysis.*
  cerebral p., paralisia cerebral; termo genérico que designa vários tipos de disfunção motora não-progressiva, presentes ao nascimento ou no início da infância. As causas são hereditárias e adquiridas; dependendo da causa, é classificada como intra-uterina, natal e pós-natal inicial; os distúrbios motores incluem diplegia, hemiplegia, tetraplegia, coreoatetose e ataxia.
  crutch p., paralisia da muleta. SIN crutch *paralysis.*
  Dejerine-Klumpke p., paralisia de Dejerine-Klumpke. SIN Klumpke p.
  diver's p., doença descompressiva. SIN decompression *sickness.*
  double elevator p., paresia dupla do levantador; elevação limitada de um olho em abdução e adução, indicando paresia dos músculos reto superior e oblíquo inferior, embora muitos casos sejam decorrentes de restrição do músculo reto inferior.
  Erb p., paralisia de Erb; tipo de paralisia obstétrica na qual há paralisia dos músculos do braço e do cíngulo do membro superior (músculos deltóide, bíceps, braquial e braquiorradial) causada por lesão da parte superior do tronco do plexo braquial ou das raízes do quinto e sexto nervos cervicais. SIN Duchenne-Erb paralysis, Erb paralysis.
  extrapyramidal cerebral p., atetose. SIN athetosis.
  facial p., paralisia facial. SIN facial *paralysis.*
  Klumpke p., paralisia de Klumpke; tipo de paralisia obstétrica na qual há paralisia dos músculos da parte distal do antebraço e da mão (todos os músculos inervados pelo nervo ulnar, e também os músculos mais distais inervados pelos nervos radial e mediano), causada por uma lesão do tronco inferior do plexo braquial, ou das raízes cervicais de C8 e T1. SIN Dejerine-Klumpke p., Dejerine-Klumpke syndrome, Klumpke paralysis.
  lead p., paresia pelo chumbo; tipo peculiar de neuropatia supostamente tóxica, resultante da intoxicação pelo chumbo, consistindo em fraqueza bilateral dos músculos extensores do punho e dos dedos da mão, que, provavelmente, deve-se a neuropatias radiais bilaterais. Embora seja freqüentemente mencionada, aparentemente não foram descritos casos confirmados na literatura médica moderna. SIN lead paralysis.
  obstetric p., p. obstétrica; lesão do plexo braquial sofrida pelo feto durante o parto; são reconhecidos três tipos: 1) plexo superior, que afeta o ombro e a parte superior do braço (paralisia de Erb, q.v., sem dúvida a forma mais comum); 2) plexo total, envolvendo todo o braço; 3) plexo inferior, que envolve o antebraço e a mão (paralisia de Klumpke, q.v.). SIN brachial birth p., obstetric paralysis.
  posticus p., paralisia do músculo cricoaritenóideo posterior; fazendo com que a prega vocal seja mantida na linha média ou próxima desta.
  pressure p., paralisia por compressão. SIN pressure *paralysis.*
  progressive bulbar p., p. bulbar progressiva; um dos subgrupos da doença do neurônio motor; distúrbio degenerativo progressivo dos neurônios motores, basicamente do tronco encefálico, que se manifesta como fraqueza (e definhamento) dos vários músculos bulbares, resultando em disartria e disfagia — a regurgitação de líquido é uma manifestação proeminente e pode causar aspiração; geralmente a fraqueza e o definhamento da língua são evidentes, e freqüentemente há potenciais de fasciculação nos músculos da língua e da face. SIN glossopalatolabial paralysis, glossopharyngeolabial paralysis.
  progressive supranuclear p., paralisia supranuclear progressiva; distúrbio neurológico progressivo na sexta década de vida, caracterizado por paralisia supranuclear do olhar vertical, retração das pálpebras, exoforia sob oclusão, disartria e demência. SIN Steele-Richardson-Olszewski disease, Steele-Richardson-Olszewski syndrome.
  scrivener's p., cãibra do escrivão. SIN writer's *cramp.*
  shaking p., trembling p., p. agitante. SIN parkinsonism (1).
pal·u·dal (pal′oo - dăl). Palustre; sinônimo obsoleto de malárico. [L. *palus*, pântano]
PAM Acrônimo para potential acuity *meter* (medidor da acuidade potencial).
2-PAM Abreviatura de 2-pralidoxime (2-pralidoxima).
pam·a·quine (pam′ă - kwēn). Pamaquina; agente antimalárico, ativo contra a malária das aves e contra os gametócitos de todas as formas maláricas em seres humanos; é mais tóxica que a cloroquina ou primaquina e foi substituída pela primaquina.
pam·o·ate (pam′ō - āt). Pamoato; contração, aprovada pelo USAN, de 4,4′-metilenobis(3-hidroxi-2-naftoato).
pam·pin·i·form (pam - pin′i - fōrm). Pampiniforme; que possui o formato de uma gavinha; designa uma estrutura semelhante a uma videira. [L. *pampinus*, uma gavinha, + *forma*, forma]
pam·pin·o·cele (pam - pin′ō - sēl). Pampinocele. SIN varicocele. [L. *pampinus*, gavinha, + G. *kēlē*, tumor]
Pan. Gênero de macacos antropóides, incluindo o gorila e o chimpanzé. *P. panisus* e *P. troglodytes* são espécies de chimpanzé usadas em experiências biológicas. [deus da floresta na mitologia grega]
pan-. Pan-; todo, inteiro. VER TAMBÉM pant-. [G. *pas*, todo]
pan·a·cea (pan - ă - sē′ă). Panacéia; um cura-tudo; remédio que se diz ser capaz de curar todas as doenças. [G. *panakeia*, remédio universal, de Panacea, filha de Esculápio]
pan·ag·glu·ti·na·ble (pan - ă - gloo′ti - nă - bl). Pan-aglutinável; aglutinável com todos os tipos de soro humano; designa eritrócitos que possuem essa propriedade.

pan·ag·glu·ti·nins (pan-ă-gloo'ti-ninz). Pan-aglutininas; aglutininas que reagem com todos os eritrócitos humanos. [pan + L. *agglutino*, colar]

pan·an·gi·i·tis (pan'an-jē-ī'tis). Pan-angeíte; inflamação que envolve todas as túnicas de um vaso sanguíneo. [pan- + angiitis]

pan·ar·ter·i·tis (pan'ar-ter-ī'tis). Pan-arterite; distúrbio inflamatório das artérias, caracterizado por envolvimento de todas as camadas estruturais dos vasos. SIN endoperiarteritis. [pan- + L. *arteria*, artéria, + G. *-itis*, inflamação]

pan·ar·thri·tis (pan-ar-thrī'tis). Pan-artrite. **1.** Inflamação envolvendo todos os tecidos de uma articulação. **2.** Inflamação de todas as articulações do corpo.

pan·at·ro·phy (pan-at'rō-fē). Pan-atrofia. **1.** Atrofia de todas as partes de uma estrutura. **2.** Atrofia geral do corpo. SIN pantatrophia, pantatrophy.

pan·blas·tic (pan-blas'tik). Pan-blástico; relativo a todas as camadas germinativas primárias. [pan- + G. *blastos*, germe]

pan·bron·chi·ol·i·tis (pan'bron-kē-ō-lī'tis). Pan-bronquiolite; inflamação idiopática e obstrução dos bronquíolos, finalmente acompanhada por bronquiectasia; quase todos os casos descritos ocorreram no Japão. SIN diffuse panbronchiolitis.
diffuse panbronchiolitis, pan-bronquiolite difusa. SIN panbronchiolitis.

pan·car·di·tis (pan-kar-dī'tis). Pancardite. SIN endoperimyocarditis.

Pancoast, Henry K., radiologista norte-americano, 1875–1939. VER P. *syndrome, tumor.*

pan·co·lec·to·my (pan'kō-lek'tō-mē). Pancolectomia; extirpação de todo o colo.

pan·cre·as, pl. **pan·cre·a·ta** (pan'krē-as, pan-krē-ā'tă).[TA]. Pâncreas; glândula retroperitoneal lobulada e alongada, sem cápsula, que se estende da concavidade do duodeno até o baço; consiste em uma cabeça achatada na concavidade duodenal, um corpo alongado com três faces, que atravessa o abdome, e uma cauda em contato com o baço. A parte exócrina da glândula secreta suco pancreático, que é liberado para o intestino, e sua parte endócrina produz as secreções internas insulina e glucagon. [G. *pankreas*, moleja, de *pas* (*pan*), todos, + *kreas*, carne]

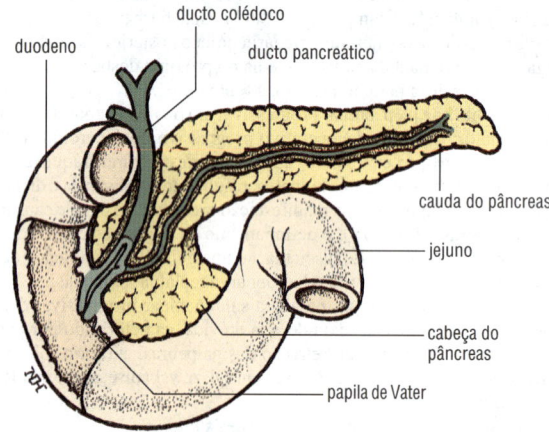

pâncreas (e parte do duodeno)

p. accesso'rium [TA], p. acessório. SIN accessory p.
accessory p. [TA], p. acessório; porção separada de tecido pancreático, geralmente o processo uncinado, e, portanto, na maioria das vezes, encontrada nas vizinhanças da cabeça do pâncreas, mas pode ocorrer na parede intestinal (estômago ou duodeno). SIN p. accessorium [TA].
anular p., p. anular; anel de p. circundando o duodeno, produzido pela ausência de migração do pâncreas ventral embriológico para a direita do duodeno.
Aselli p., p. de Aselli. SIN Aselli *gland*.
p. divi'sum, p. bífido; p. dividido, resultante de uma ausência congênita da fusão completa dos primórdios embrionários; cada uma das partes tem seu próprio ducto.
dorsal p., p. dorsal; aquela parte do primórdio pancreático do embrião originada como um broto dorsal do endoderma do intestino anterior acima do divertículo hepático.
lesser p., processo uncinado do pâncreas. SIN uncinate *process* of pancreas.
p. mi'nus, p. uncinado do pâncreas. SIN uncinate *process* of pancreas.
small p., p. uncinado do pâncreas. SIN uncinate *process* of pancreas.
uncinate p., unciform p., p. uncinado do pâncreas. SIN uncinate *process* of pancreas.
ventral p., p. ventral; aquela parte do primórdio do pâncreas que se desenvolve, juntamente com o divertículo hepático, como um broto ventral a partir do endoderma do intestino anterior.

Willis p., p. de Willis. SIN uncinate *process* of pancreas.
Winslow p., p. de Winslow. SIN uncinate *process* of pancreas.

pancreat-, pancreatico-, pancreato-, pancreo-. Pancreat-, pancreatico-, pancreato-, pancreo-; o pâncreas. [G. *pankreas*, pâncreas]

pan·cre·a·tal·gia (pan'krē-ă-tal'jē-ă). Pancreatalgia; termo raramente usado para designar a dor que se origina no pâncreas ou é sentida na região do pâncreas ou próxima dela. [pancreat- + G. *algos*, dor]

pan·cre·a·tec·to·my (pan'krē-ă-tek'tō-mē). Pancreatectomia; excisão do pâncreas. SIN pancreectomy. [pancreat- + G. *ektomē*, excisão]

pan·cre·at·em·phrax·is (pan'krē-at-em-frak'sis). Pancreatenfraxe; obstrução do ducto pancreático, que causa edema da glândula. [pancreat- + G. *emphraxis*, interrupção]

pan·cre·at·ic (pan-krē-at'ik). Pancreático; relativo ao pâncreas.

pancreatico-. VER pancreat-.

pan·cre·at·i·co·du·o·de·nal (pan-krē-at'i-kō-doo'ō-dē'năl, -doo-od'ē-năl). Pancreaticoduodenal; relativo ao pâncreas e ao duodeno.

pancreaticoduodenectomy (pan-krē-at'ĭ-kō-doo-od'en-ek'tō-mē). Pancreatoduodenectomia. SIN pancreatoduodenectomy.

pylorus-preserving p., p. com preservação do piloro; excisão de todo o pâncreas, ou de parte dele, e do duodeno, com preservação da parte distal do estômago e do piloro inervado; geralmente limitada à cabeça e ao colo do pâncreas, e na maioria das vezes, realizada para tratamento do carcinoma do pâncreas.

pan·cre·a·tin (pan'krē-ă-tin). Pancreatina; mistura das enzimas do pâncreas de boi ou porco, usada internamente como digestivo, e também como agente peptonizante no preparo de alimentos pré-digeridos; contém tripsina proteolítica, amilopsina amilolítica e esteapsina lipolítica.

pan·cre·a·ti·tis (pan'krē-ă-tī'tis). Pancreatite; inflamação do pâncreas.

pancreatite aguda: freqüência de fatores etiológicos	
I.	**principais causas**
1.	colecistolitíase, coledocolitíase
2.	alcoolismo
3.	cirurgia abdominal — pancreatite pós-operatória
4.	endoscopia dos ductos biliares e pancreáticos
5.	traumatismo abdominal não-penetrante
II.	**causas menos freqüentes**
1.	doenças endócrinas (poliadenomatose, hiperparatireoidismo, síndrome de Cushing)
2.	gravidez, hiperlipoproteinemia, pancreatite causada por ingestão de pílulas anticoncepcionais
3.	efeitos farmacológicos (corticosteróides, diuréticos)
4.	causas imunoalérgicas
5.	pancreatite neurogênica
6.	pancreatite hereditária
7.	pancreatite viral
8.	pancreatite parasitária
III.	**pancreatite causada por choque e acidose**

acute hemorrhagic p., p. hemorrágica aguda; inflamação aguda do pâncreas acompanhada pela formação de áreas necróticas e hemorragia na substância da glândula; clinicamente caracterizada por dor abdominal forte e súbita, náuseas, febre e leucocitose; existem áreas de necrose gordurosa na superfície do pâncreas e no omento devido à ação da enzima pancreática extravasada (tripsina e lipase).

calcareous p., p. calcárea; p. crônica com áreas de calcificação, observada por raios X. SIN calcific p.

calcific p. (kal'sif-ik), p. calcificada. SIN calcareous p.

chronic p., p. crônica; episódios recorrentes de doença inflamatória do pâncreas, caracterizada por fibrose e vários graus de perda irreversível da função exócrina e, por fim, da função endócrina.

chronic fibrosing p., p. fibrosante crônica; inflamação do pâncreas que consiste em fibrose, atrofia acinar e calcificação. Clinicamente, tem uma evolução prolongada, com recidivas e remissões, e geralmente deve-se ao abuso de álcool ou à desnutrição.

chronic relapsing p., p. recidivante crônica; exacerbações repetidas de p. em paciente com pancreatite crônica do pâncreas. As recidivas geralmente são causadas pela persistência do fator etiológico ou pela exposição repetida a ele, como ocorre na obstrução ductal parcial ou no alcoolismo crônico.

pancreato-. Pancreato-. VER pancreat-.

pan·cre·a·to·cho·le·cys·tos·to·my (pan-krē-at′ō-kō-lē-sis-tos′tō-mē, pan′krē-ă-tō-). Pancreatocolecistostomia; anastomose cirúrgica raramente realizada entre um cisto ou fístula pancreática e a vesícula biliar.

pan·cre·at·o·du·o·de·nec·to·my (pan-krē-at′ō-doo-ō-dē-nek′tō-mē, pan′krē-ă-tō-). Pancreatoduodenectomia; excisão de todo o pâncreas, ou de parte dele, juntamente com o duodeno e, geralmente, com a parte distal do estômago. SIN pancreaticoduodenectomy, Whipple operation.

pan·cre·at·o·du·o·de·nos·to·my (pan-krē-at′ō-doo-ō-dē-nos′tō-mē, pan′krē-ă-tō-). Pancreatoduodenostomia; anastomose cirúrgica de um ducto, cisto ou fístula pancreática com o duodeno.

pan·cre·at·o·gas·tros·to·my (pan-krē-at′ō-gas-tros′tō-mē, pan′krē-ă-tō-). Pancreatogastrostomia; anastomose cirúrgica entre um cisto ou fístula pancreática e o estômago.

pan·cre·a·to·gen·ic, pan·cre·a·tog·en·ous (pan′krē-ă-tō-jen′ik, -toj′ē-nŭs). Pancreatogênico; de origem pancreática; formado no pâncreas. [pancreato- + G. *genesis*, origem]

pan·cre·a·tog·ra·phy (pan′krē-ă-tog′ră-fē). Pancreatografia; demonstração radiográfica dos ductos pancreáticos, após injeção retrógrada de material radiopaco no ducto distal. [pancreato- + G. *graphō*, escrever]

pan·cre·a·to·je·ju·nos·to·my (pan-krē-at′ō-je-joo-nos′tō-mē, pan′krē-ă-tō-). Pancreatojejunostomia; anastomose cirúrgica de um ducto, cisto ou fístula pancreática ao jejuno.

pan·cre·at·o·lith (pan-krē-at′ō-lith). Pancreatólito. SIN pancreatic *calculus*. [pancreato- + G. *lithos*, cálculo]

pan·cre·at·o·li·thec·to·my (pan-krē-at′ō-li-thek′tō-mē, pan′krē-ă-tō-). Pancreatolitectomia. SIN pancreatolithotomy. [pancreato- + G. *lithos*, cálculo, + *ektomē*, excisão]

pan·cre·at·o·li·thi·a·sis (pan-krē-at′ō-li-thī′ă-sis, pan′krē-ă-tō-). Pancreatolitíase; cálculos no pâncreas, geralmente encontrados no sistema ductal pancreático.

pan·cre·at·o·li·thot·o·my (pan-krē-at′ō-li-thot′ō-mē, pan′krē-ă-tō-). Pancreatolitotomia; remoção de uma concreção pancreática. SIN pancreatolithectomy. [pancreato- + G. *lithos*, cálculo, + *tomē*, incisão]

pan·cre·a·tol·y·sis (pan′krē-ă-tol′i-sis). Pancreatólise; destruição do pâncreas. [pancreato- + G. *lysis*, dissolução]

pan·cre·a·to·lyt·ic (pan′krē-ă-tō-lit′ik). Pancreatolítico; designa a pancreatólise.

pan·cre·a·to·meg·a·ly (pan′krē-ă-tō-meg′ă-lē). Pancreatomegalia; aumento anormal do pâncreas. [pancreato- + G. *megas*, grande]

pan·cre·a·to·my (pan′krē-at′ō-mē). Pancreatomia. SIN pancreatotomy.

pan·cre·a·top·a·thy (pan′krē-ă-top′ă-thē). Pancreatopatia; qualquer doença do pâncreas. SIN pancreopathy. [pancreato- + G. *pathos*, que sofre]

pan·cre·a·to·pep·ti·dase E (pan′krē-ă-tō-pep′ti-dās). Pancreatopeptidase E. VER elastase.

pan·cre·a·tot·o·my (pan′krē-ă-tot′ō-mē). Pancreatotomia; incisão do pâncreas. SIN pancreatomy. [pancreato- + G. *tomē*, incisão]

pan·cre·a·tro·pic (pan′krē-ă-trop′ik). Pancreatrópico; que exerce uma ação sobre o pâncreas. [pancreat- + G. *tropikos*, relativo a um desvio]

pan·cre·ec·to·my (pan-krē-ek′tō-mē). Pancreatectomia. SIN pancreatectomy.

pan·cre·li·pase (pan-krē-lip′ās, -lī′pās). Pancrelipase; concentrado de enzimas pancreáticas padronizadas por seu teor de lipase; lipolítico usado em terapia de reposição. SIN lipancreatin.

pancreo-. VER pancreat-.

pan·cre·o·lith (pan′krē-ō-lith). Pancreólito. SIN pancreatic *calculus*. [pancreo- + G. *lithos*, cálculo]

pan·cre·op·a·thy (pan-krē-op′ă-thē). Pancreatopatia. SIN pancreatopathy.

pan·cre·o·zy·min (pan′krē-ō-zī′min). Pancreozimina. SIN cholecystokinin.

pan·cu·ro·ni·um bro·mide (pan-kūr-ō′nē-ŭm). Brometo de pancurônio; bloqueador neuromuscular esteróide não-despolarizante, semelhante ao curare, mas sem seu potencial de bloqueio ganglionar, liberação de histamina ou hipotensão.

pan·cy·to·pe·nia (pan′sī-tō-pē′nē-ă). Pancitopenia; redução acentuada do número de eritrócitos, de todos os tipos de leucócitos e das plaquetas no sangue circulante. [pan- + G. *kytos*, célula, + *penia*, escassez]

  congenital p., p. congênita. SIN Fanconi *anemia*.

  Fanconi p., p. de Fanconi. SIN Fanconi *anemia*.

pan·dem·ic (pan-dem′ik). Pandêmico; designa uma doença que afeta ou acomete a população de uma grande região, país, continente, global; extensamente epidêmica. [pan- + G. *dēmos*, o povo]

pan·de·mic·i·ty (pan-dē-mis′i-tē). Pandemicidade; o estado ou condição de ser pandêmico.

pan·dic·u·la·tion (pan-dik-ū-lā′shŭn). Pandiculação; o ato de espreguiçar-se, como ao acordar. [L. *pandiculor*, espreguiçar-se, de *pando*, espalhar-se]

Pandy, Kalman, neurologista húngaro, 1868–1945. VER P. *test, reaction*.

pan·en·ceph·a·li·tis (pan′en-sef-ă-lī′tis). Panencefalite; inflamação difusa do encéfalo.

  nodular p., p. nodular; provavelmente, uma forma de p. esclerosante subaguda. SIN Pette-Döring disease.

  subacute sclerosing p. (SSPE), p. esclerosante subaguda; encefalite progressiva, crônica, rara, que afeta basicamente crianças e adultos jovens, causada pelo vírus do sarampo. Caracterizada por uma história de infecção primária por sarampo antes dos 2 anos de idade, seguida por vários anos assintomáticos, e, depois, por deterioração psiconeurológica progressiva, gradual, que consiste em alteração da personalidade, convulsões, mioclônus, ataxia, fotossensibilidade, anormalidades oculares, espasticidade e coma. É observada atividade periódica característica ao EEG; histopatologicamente, a substância branca de ambos os hemisférios e a do tronco cerebral são afetadas, bem como o córtex cerebral, e há corpúsculos de inclusão eosinofílicos nos núcleos citoplasmáticos dos neurônios e das células gliais. A morte geralmente ocorre em 3 anos. SIN Bosin disease, Dawson encephalitis, inclusion body encephalitis, sclerosing leukoencephalitis, subacute inclusion body encephalitis, subacute sclerosing leukoencephalitis, van Bogaert encephalitis.

pan·en·do·scope (pan-en′dō-skōp). Pan-endoscópio; instrumento iluminado para inspeção do interior da uretra, bem como da bexiga, por meio de um sistema de lentes telescópico. [pan- + G. *endon*, dentro, + *skopeō*, ver]

pan·es·the·sia (pan-es-thē′zē-ă). Panestesia; o somatório de todas as sensações experimentadas por uma pessoa em um momento. VER TAMBÉM cenesthesia. [pan- + G. *aisthēsis*, sensação]

Paneth, Josef, médico austríaco, 1857–1890. VER P. granular *cells*, em *cell*.

pang (pang). Dor aguda, súbita e breve.

  breast p., angina de peito. SIN angina *pectoris*.

pan·hi·dro·sis (pan-hi-drō′sis). Panidrose. SIN panidrosis.

pan·hy·drom·e·ter (pan-hī-drom′ē-ter). Pan-hidrômetro; um hidrômetro para determinar a densidade específica de qualquer líquido. [pan- + G. *hydōr*, água, + *metron*, medida]

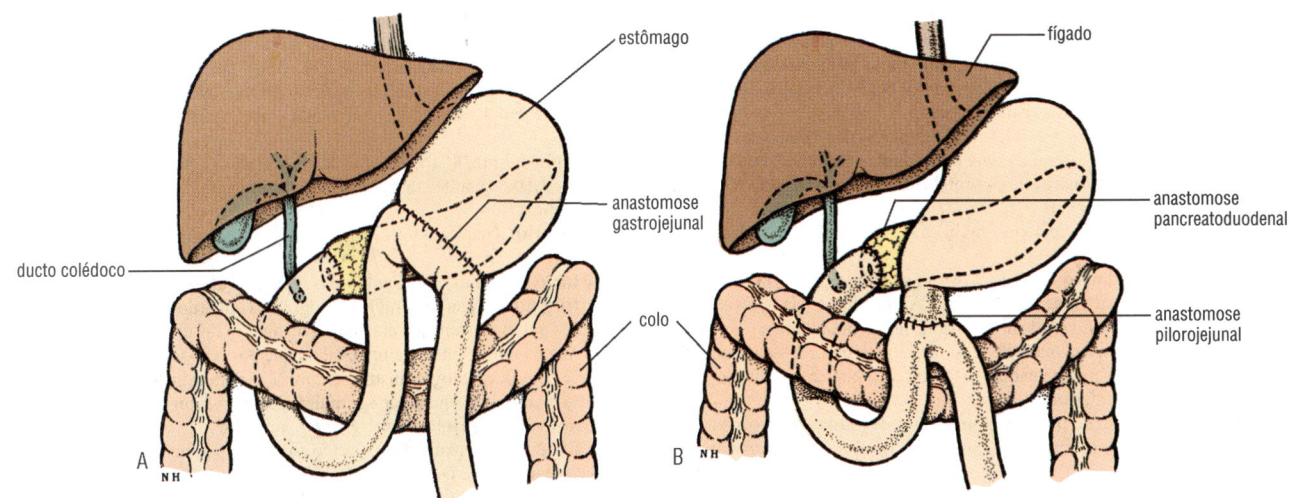

pancreatoduodenectomia: (A) operação de Whipple, (B) procedimento de Whipple com preservação do piloro

pan·hy·per·e·mia (pan′hī-per-ē′mē-ă). Pan-hiperemia; congestão ou hiperemia universal. [pan- + G. *hyper*, em excesso, + *haima*, sangue]

pan·hy·po·pi·tu·i·tar·ism (PHP) (pan-hī′pō-pi-tooʹi-tă-rizm). Pan-hipopituitarismo; estado no qual a secreção de todos os hormônios da adeno-hipófise é inadequada ou ausente; causado por vários distúrbios que resultam em destruição ou perda de função de toda a adeno-hipófise, ou de sua maior parte. Formas raras de PHP são herdadas de forma autossômica recessiva [MIM*262600] ou de forma recessiva ligada ao X [MIM*312000]. SIN ateliotic dwarfism, hypophyseal cachexia, hypophysial cachexia.

pan·ic (pan′ik). Pânico; ansiedade e medo extremos e ilógicos, freqüentemente acompanhados por distúrbio da respiração, aumento da atividade cardíaca, alterações vasomotoras, sudorese e sensação de pavor. VER anxiety. [personagem da mit. grega, *Pan*]

homosexual p., pânico homossexual; ataque agudo e intenso de ansiedade baseado em conflitos inconscientes acerca da homossexualidade.

pan·i·dro·sis (pan-i-drō′sis). Panidrose; sudorese de toda a superfície do corpo. SIN panhidrosis. [pan- + G. *hidros*, suor]

pan·im·mu·ni·ty (pan-i-mū′ni-tē). Pan-imunidade; imunidade geral contra muitas doenças infecciosas.

pan·mix·is (pan-mik′sis). Pan-mixia, acasalamento aleatório. SIN random mating. [pan- + G. *mixis*, relação sexual]

pan·my·e·loph·thi·sis (pan′mī-ĕ-lof′thi-sis). Pan-mieloftise. SIN myelophthisis (2).

pan·my·e·lo·sis (pan′mī-ĕ-lō′sis). Panmielose; metaplasia mielóide com células sangüíneas imaturas anormais no baço e no fígado, associada a mielofibrose. [pan- + G. *myelos*, medula óssea, + *-osis*, condição]

Panner, H.J., radiologista dinamarquês, 1871–1930. VER P. *disease*.

pan·ni (pan′ī). Panos; plural de pannus.

pan·nic·u·lec·to·my (pa-nik-ū-lek′tō-mē). Paniculectomia; excisão cirúrgica de panículo adiposo redundante, geralmente do abdome. [panniculus + G. *ektomē*, extirpação]

pan·nic·u·li·tis (pă-nik′ū-līʹtis). Paniculite; inflamação do tecido adiposo subcutâneo. [panniculus + G. *-itis*, inflamação]

α₁-**antitrypsin deficiency p.,** p. por deficiência de α₁-antitripsina; múltiplos nódulos subcutâneos dolorosos que ocorrem em pacientes com acentuada deficiência de antitripsina; as biopsias exibem paniculite lobular com neutrófilos e histiócitos espumosos. Alguns pacientes anteriormente diagnosticados com doença de Weber-Christian exibem essa deficiência.

cytophagic histiocytic p., p. histiocítica citofágica; termo obsoleto para designar a p. lobular crônica com infiltração por histiócitos que fagocitaram hemácias, leucócitos e plaquetas; pode haver diátese hemorrágica ou um linfoma de células T.

lupus erythematosus p., p. do lúpus eritematoso; p. caracterizada por nódulos eritematosos ou cor de carne, associada ao lúpus eritematoso, principalmente do tipo discóide, na face, nos membros superiores e no tronco, e com infiltração nodular por linfócitos e plasmócitos dos lóbulos de gordura.

poststeroid p., p. pós-esteróide; nódulos subcutâneos que se desenvolvem em crianças nos 30 dias após a suspensão dos corticosteróides administrados para tratar a síndrome nefrótica ou a febre reumática; microscopicamente idêntica à necrose de gordura subcutânea do recém-nascido, a condição resolve espontaneamente ou com readministração de esteróides.

relapsing febrile nodular nonsuppurative p., p. não-supurativa nodular febril recidivante; nódulos subcutâneos recorrentes acompanhados por febre e seguidos por depressão da pele à involução. Os nódulos exibem p. lobular neutrofílica com necrose, fagocitose de lipídios e fibrose subseqüente. A maioria dos casos pode ser classificada como artificial, ou secundária à deficiência de α₁-antitripsina, lúpus profundo, necrose adiposa pancreática (enzimática) ou p. histiocítica citofágica. Casos de causa indeterminada foram denominados doença ou síndrome de Weber-Christian (Weber-Christian *disease*). SIN Christian disease (2), Weber-Christian disease.

subacute migratory p., p. migratória subaguda; placas não-fibrosadas de configuração mutável na face lateral de uma ou de ambas as pernas, com muitos meses de duração. A biopsia revela p. septal com fibrose e células gigantes. SIN erythema nodosum migrans.

pan·nic·u·lus, pl. **pan·nic·u·li** (pă-nik′ū-lŭs, -lī). Panículo. SIN layer. [L. dim. de *pannus*, pano]

p. adiposus [TA], p. adiposo. SIN fatty layer of subcutaneous tissue.

p. adiposus telae subcutaneae abdominis [TA], p. adiposo da tela subcutânea do abdome. SIN fatty layer of subcutaneous tissue of abdomen.

p. carno′sus, p. carnoso; a camada de músculo esquelético, na fáscia superficial, representada, nos seres humanos, pelo músculo platisma; é muito mais extensa em mamíferos inferiores.

pan·ning (pan′ing). Uso de placas ou superfícies de plástico revestidas com antígeno ou anticorpo para separar ou concentrar células específicas com receptores apropriados.

pan·nus, pl. **pan·ni** (pan′ŭs, pan′ī). *Pannus*, pano; membrana de tecido de granulação que cobre uma superfície normal. **1.** O tecido sinovial inflamatório, encontrado em articulações reumatóides, que cobre as cartilagens articulares e destrói progressivamente as cartilagens articulares subjacentes; também encontrado em outra doença granulomatosa crônica, incluindo tuberculose. **2.** A córnea no tracoma. VER TAMBÉM corneal p. [L. cloth]

corneal p., p. corneano; tecido conjuntivo fibrovascular que prolifera nas camadas anteriores da córnea periférica na doença inflamatória da córnea, sobretudo no tracoma, no qual o *pannus* envolve a córnea superior. Existem três formas: **p. crassus** (espesso), no qual há muitos vasos sanguíneos e a opacidade é muito densa; **p. siccus** (seco), panículo com superfície seca, brilhante; e **p. tenuis** (fino), no qual há poucos vasos sanguíneos e a opacidade é leve.

phlyctenular p., p. flictenular; p. que ocorre na conjuntivite flictenular.

trachomatous p., p. tracomatoso; p. da córnea superior associado ao tracoma.

pan·oph·thal·mi·tis (pan′of-thal-mī′tis). Pan-oftalmite; inflamação purulenta de todas as camadas do olho. [pan- + G. *ophthalmos*, olho]

pan·op·tic (pan-op′tik). Pan-óptico; que tudo revela; designa o efeito da coloração múltipla ou diferencial. [pan- + G. *optikos*, relativo à visão]

pan·o·ste·i·tis. Pan-osteíte; inflamação de um osso inteiro.

pan·o·ti·tis (pan′ō-tī′tis). Pan-otite; inflamação geral de todas as partes da orelha; especificamente, uma doença que começa como uma otite interna, com a inflamação subseqüentemente estendendo-se até a orelha média e estruturas adjacentes. [pan- + G. *ous*, orelha, + *-itis*, inflamação]

pan·pho·bia (pan-fō′bē-ă). Panfobia; medo de tudo. [pan- + G. *phobos*, medo]

Pansch, Adolf, anatomista alemão, 1841–1887. VER P. *fissure*.

pan·scle·ro·sis (pan-skle-rō′sis). Pan-esclerose; esclerose universal de um órgão ou de uma parte.

pan·sin·u·i·tis (pan-sin-ū-ī′tis). Pansinusite. SIN pansinusitis.

pan·si·nu·si·tis (pan-sī-nū-sī′tis). Pansinusite; inflamação de todos os seios acessórios do nariz de um ou de ambos os lados. SIN pansinuitis.

pan·sper·mia, pan·sper·ma·tism (pan-sper′mē-ă, -sper′mă-tizm). Pan-espermia; a doutrina hipotética da onipresença de diminutas formas e esporos de vida animal e vegetal, assim contribuindo para a aparente geração espontânea. [pan- + G. *sperma*, semente]

pan·spor·o·blast (pan-spō′rō-blast). Pan-esporoblasto; o esporoblasto reprodutivo que dá origem a mais de um esporo na ordem Myxosporida (classe Myxosporea, filo Myxozoa). [pan- + G. *sporos*, semente, + *blastos*, germe]

pan·spo·ro·blas·tic (pan′spō-rō-blas′tik). Pan-esporoblástico; referente a um pan-esporoblasto.

pan·sys·tol·ic (pan′sis-tol′ik). Pansistólico; que dura toda a sístole, estendendo-se da primeira até a segunda bulha. SIN holosystolic.

pant. Ofegar; respirar de forma rápida e superficial. [Fr. *panteler*, arfar]

△ **pant-, panto-.** Pant-, panto-; todo. VER TAMBÉM pan-. [G. *pas*, todo]

pan·tal·gia (pan-tal′jē-ă). Pantalgia; dor que envolve todo o corpo. [pant- + G. *algos*, dor]

pan·ta·mor·phia (pan-tă-mōr′fē-ă). Pantamorfismo; sem forma; malformação generalizada. [pant- + G. *a-* priv. + *morphē*, formato]

pan·ta·mor·phic (pan-tă-mōr′fik). Pantamórfico; relacionado com, ou caracterizado por, pantamorfia.

pan·tan·en·ceph·a·ly, pan·tan·en·ce·pha·lia (pan′tan-en-sef′ă-lē, -se-fā′lē-ă). Pantanencefalia; ausência congênita do encéfalo. [pant- + G. *an-* priv. + *enkephalos*, encéfalo]

pan·ta·pho·bia (pan-tă-fō′bē-ă). Pantafobia; destemor absoluto. [pant- + G. *a-* priv. + *phobos*, medo]

pan·ta·tro·phia, pan·tat·ro·phy (pan-tă-trō′fē-ă, pan-tat′rō-fē). Pan-atrofia. SIN panatrophy. [pant- + atrophy]

pan·te·the·ine (pan-te-thē′in). Panteteína; o produto da condensação do ácido pantotênico e aminoetanetiol; N-pantotenil-2-aminoetanetiol; um intermediário na biossíntese da coenzima A através da 4′-fosfopanteteína (fosforil no grupamento –CH₂O terminal) e ATP. SIN *Lactobacillus bulgaricus* factor.

p. kinase, p. cinase, p. quinase; enzima que catalisa a fosforilação da panteteína pelo ATP em 4′-fosfato de panteteína; uma etapa na biossíntese da coenzima A.

p. 4′-phosphate, 4′-fosfato de panteteína. SIN 4′-phosphopantetheine.

pan·te·thine (pan′tē-thin). Pantetina; o dissulfeto formado a partir de duas panteteínas.

pan·the·nol (pan′thĕ-nol). Pantenol. SIN dexpanthenol.

△ **panto-.** VER pant-.

pan·to·ate (pan′tō-āt). Pantoato; sal ou éster do ácido pantóico.

pan·to·graph (pan′tō-graf). Pantógrafo. **1.** Instrumento para reproduzir desenhos por um sistema de alavancas, no qual se faz com que um lápis de registro siga os movimentos de um estilete que passa ao longo das linhas do original. **2.** Em odontologia, instrumento usado para registrar os movimentos da borda mandibular, que pode ser transferido para fazer ajustes equivalentes em um articulador. [panto- + G. *graphō*, registrar]

pan·to·ic ac·id (pan-tō′ik). Ácido pantóico; precursor da coenzima A, cuja β-alanina amida é o ácido pantotênico.

pan·to·mo·gram (pan′tō-mō-gram). Pantomograma; registro radiográfico panorâmico dos arcos dentais maxilar e mandibular e de suas estruturas associadas, obtido por um pantomógrafo. [pan- + tomogram]

pan·to·mo·graph (pan′tō-mō-graf). Pantomógrafo; instrumento radiográfico panorâmico que permite visualizar toda a dentição, o osso alveolar e estruturas contíguas em uma única radiografia extra-oral.

pan·to·mog·ra·phy (pan-tō-mog′rǎ-fē). Pantomografia; método de radiografia pelo qual se pode obter uma radiografia (pantomograma) dos arcos dentais maxilar e mandibular e de suas estruturas contíguas em um único filme.

pan·to·mor·phia (pan-to-mōr′fē-ǎ). Pantomorfismo. **1.** A condição de um organismo, como uma ameba, capaz de assumir todos os formatos. **2.** Simetria perfeita. [panto- + G. *morphē*, forma]

pan·to·mor·phic (pan-tō-mōr′fik). Pantomórfico; capaz de assumir todas as formas.

pan·to·nine (pan′tō-nēn). Pantonina; um aminoácido identificado na *Escherichia coli* que seria um intermediário na biossíntese do ácido pantotênico por esse microrganismo, contendo NH_2 no lugar do grupamento α-OH do ácido pantotênico.

pan·to·scop·ic (pan-tō-skop′ik). Pantoscópico; projetado para observar objetos a qualquer distância; designa lentes bifocais. [panto- + G. *skopeō*, ver]

pan·to·the·nate (pan-tō-then′āt). Pantotenato; um sal ou éster do ácido pantotênico.
  p. synthetase, p. sintetase; enzima que converte pantoato e β-alanina em pantotenato com clivagem do ATP em AMP e pirofosfato; uma etapa fundamental na biossíntese da coenzima A. SIN pantoate-activating enzyme.

pan·to·then·ic ac·id (pan-tō-then′ik). Ácido pantotênico; a β-alanina amida do ácido pantóico. Uma substância incentivadora do crescimento, amplamente encontrada em tecidos vegetais e animais, e essencial para o crescimento de vários organismos; sua deficiência na dieta causa dermatite em pintos e ratos e acromotríquia em ratos; um precursor da coenzima A. SIN antidermatitis factor.

pan·to·then·yl (pan-tō-then′il). Pantotenil; o radical acil do ácido pantotênico.
  p. alcohol, álcool pantotenílico. SIN dexpanthenol.

pan·to·yl (pan′tō-il). Pantoil; o radical acil do ácido pantóico.

pan·to·yl·tau·rine (pan′tō-il-taw′rin, -rēn). Pantoiltaurina; ácido pantotênico no qual o grupamento carboxila é substituído por um grupamento ácido sulfônico; possui estrutura análoga à do ácido pantotênico, exceto pelo fato de a taurina substituir a β-alanina na molécula. SIN thiopanic acid.

Panum, Peter L., fisiologista dinamarquês, 1820–1885. VER P. *area*.

pan·zer·herz (pahn′zer-hārtz). Coração blindado. SIN armored heart. [Al. *Panzerherz*]

PAP Acrônimo para *p*eroxidase *a*ntiperoxidase com*p*lex (complexo peroxidase antiperoxidase). Abreviatura de 3′-*p*hosphoadenosine 5′-*p*hosphate (3′-fosfoadenosina 5′-fosfato). VER PAP *technique*.

pap. Papa; alimento de consistência mole, como migalhas de pão embebidas em leite ou água.

pa·pa·in, pa·pa·in·ase (pa-pā′in, -ās). Papaína, papainase; uma cisteína endopeptidase, ou um extrato bruto contendo a mesma, obtido do látex do mamão. Possui atividades esterase, tiolase, transamidase e transesterase, e é usada como digestor de proteínas, amaciante para carnes e para evitar aderências. Tem sido usada para liquefazer o conteúdo dos discos intervertebrais herniados, de forma que esse conteúdo possa ser removido por aspiração. SIN papayotin.

Papanicolaou, George N., médico, anatomista e citologista grego radicado nos Estados Unidos, 1883–1962. VER Pap *smear;* Pap *test;* P. *examination, smear, smear test, stain.*

Pa·pav·er (pǎ-pā′ver, pǎ-pav′er). Gênero de plantas; uma espécie, *P. somniferum* (família Papaveraceae), fornece o ópio. SIN poppy. [L. *papoula*]

pa·pav·er·e·tum (pǎ-pav-er-ē′tum). Preparação de alcalóides do ópio hidrossolúveis, incluindo morfina anidra a 50%. [L. *papaver*, papoula]

pa·pav·er·ine (pa-pav′er-ēn). Papaverina; alcalóide benzilisoquinolina do ópio que não é um narcótico, mas possui ação analgésica leve e é um potente espasmolítico; não provoca tolerância nem dependência; usado no tratamento da impotência masculina por injeção local. Também está disponível na forma de cloridrato de papaverina. [L. *papaver*, papoula]

pa·paw (pǎ-paw′). Mamão. VER papaya.

pa·pa·ya (pǎ-pī′yah, pǎ-pā′yah). Mamão; o fruto do mamoeiro, *Carica papaya* (família Caricaceae), uma árvore da América tropical; possui ação proteolítica e é a fonte da papaína. SIN carica. [Esp.]

pap·a·yo·tin (pap-ā′yō-tin). Papaína. SIN papain.

pa·per (pā′per). **1.** Papel; substância fabricada em folhas finas a partir da madeira, farrapos ou outros materiais. **2.** Papelote; quadrado de papel dobrado de modo a formar um envelope contendo uma dose de qualquer pó medicinal. **3.** Um pedaço de papel absorvente ou papel de filtro, impregnado com uma solução medicinal, seco e queimado; antigamente, a fumaça era inalada no tratamento da asma e de outras afecções respiratórias. [L. *papyrus;* G. *papyros*, tipo de junco do qual era feito o papel para escrita]
  articulating p., papel de articulação. SIN occluding p.
  chromatography p., papel de cromatografia; usado na cromatografia de papel. SIN high-quality filter p.
  Congo red p., papel impregnado com vermelho Congo; usado como indicador do pH, passando do azul-violeta em pH 3,0 para vermelho em pH 5,0.
  filter p., papel de filtro; papel hidrófilo usado em farmácia e química para filtragem de soluções; muitos tipos são usados para cromatografia em papel.
  high-quality filter p., p. de filtro de alta qualidade. SIN chromatography p.
  niter p., p. de nitro; papel impregnado com nitrato de potássio, sendo incendiado para produzir fumos, que são inalados como tratamento para asma. SIN potassium nitrate p., saltpeter p.
  occluding p., papel de oclusão; papel coberto com tinta ou borracha e interposto entre dentes naturais ou artificiais para determinar os contatos entre os dentes. SIN articulating p.
  potassium nitrate p., p. de nitrato de potássio. SIN niter p.
  saltpeter p., p. de salitre. SIN niter p.

Papez, James W., anatomista norte-americano, 1883–1958. VER P. *circuit*.

PAPILLA

pa·pil·la, pl. **pa·pil·lae** (pǎ-pil′ǎ, -pil′ē) [TA]. Papila; qualquer estrutura semelhante a um mamilo pequeno. SIN teat (3). [L. mamilo, dim. de *papula*, pápula]
  acoustic p., órgão espiral. SIN spiral organ.
  basilar p., p. basilar; o órgão da audição de aves, anfíbios e répteis; homólogo ao órgão de Corti em mamíferos.
  Bergmeister p., p. de Bergmeister; pequena massa de tecido glial que forma, durante a vida fetal, um revestimento cônico temporário da artéria hialóide em sua emergência na câmara vítrea; vestígios dessa massa podem persistir como uma membrana pré-papilar.
  bile p., p. maior do duodeno. SIN major duodenal p.
  p. of breat, mamilo. SIN nipple.
  circumvallate papillae, papilas circunvaladas. SIN vallate papillae.
  clavate papillae, papilas fungiformes. SIN fungiform papillae.
  conic papillae, papilas cônicas. SIN conical papillae.
  papil′lae con′icae, papilas cônicas. SIN conical papillae.
  conical papillae, papilas cônicas; numerosas projeções no dorso da língua, dispersas entre as papilas filiformes e semelhantes a estas, porém mais curtas. SIN conic papillae, papillae conicae.
  papil′lae co′rii, papilas do cório; *termo oficial alternativo para p. of dermis.

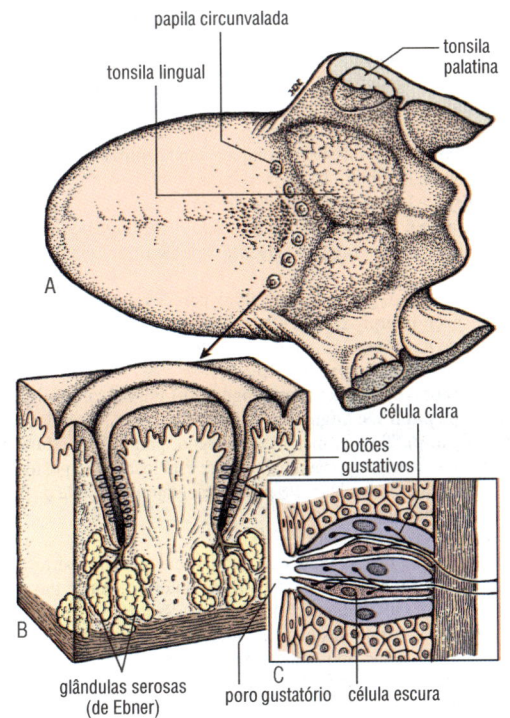

papila circunvalada da língua: (A) vista superior da língua, (B) papila circunvalada em detalhes, (C) botão gustativo em detalhe

papillae of corium, papilas do cório; *termo oficial alternativo para p. of dermis.
dental p. [TA], p. do dente; projeção do tecido mesenquimal da mandíbula em desenvolvimento para a escavação do órgão do esmalte; sua camada externa torna-se uma camada de células colunares especializadas, os odontoblastos, que formam a dentina. SIN p. dentis [TA], dentinal p.
dentinal p., p. do dente. SIN dental p.
p. den'tis [TA], p. do dente. SIN dental p.
dermal papillae, papilas dérmicas, papilas da derme. SIN p. of dermis.
papil'lae der'mis [TA], papilas da derme. SIN p. of dermis.
p. of dermis [TA], papilas da derme, papilas dérmicas; as projeções superficiais da derme (cório) que se interdigitam com os recessos na epiderme sobrejacente; contêm alças vasculares e terminações nervosas especializadas, e estão dispostas em linhas semelhantes a estrias, mais bem desenvolvidas na mão e no pé. SIN papillae dermis [TA], papillae corii*, papillae of corium*, dermal papillae.
p. ductus parotidei [TA], p. do ducto parotídeo. SIN p. of parotid gland.
p. duode'ni ma'jor [TA], p. maior do duodeno. SIN major duodenal p.
p. duode'ni mi'nor [TA], p. menor do duodeno. SIN minor duodenal p.
filiform papillae [TA], papilas filiformes; numerosas projeções queratinizadas cônicas e alongadas no dorso da língua. SIN papillae filiformes [TA].
papil'lae filifor'mes [TA], papilas filiformes. SIN filiform papillae.
papil'lae folia'tae [TA], papilas folhadas. SIN foliate papillae.
foliate papillae [TA], papilas folhadas; numerosas projeções dispostas em várias pregas transversas nas margens laterais da língua, logo na frente do músculo palatoglosso. SIN papillae foliatae [TA], folia linguae.
fungiform papillae [TA], papilas fungiformes; numerosas elevações diminutas no dorso da língua, com formato de cogumelo ornamental, sendo a extremidade mais larga que a base; o epitélio de muitas dessas papilas possui botões gustativos. SIN papillae fungiformes [TA], clavate papillae.
papil'lae fungifor'mes [TA], papilas fungiformes. SIN fungiform papillae.
gingival p. [TA], p. gengival; espessamento (observado como uma elevação) da gengiva que ocupa o espaço interproximal entre dois dentes adjacentes. SIN p. gingivalis [TA], interdental p.*, p. interdentalis*, gingival septum, interproximal p.
p. gingivalis [TA], p. gengival. SIN gingival p.
hair p., p. pilosa; entalhe semelhante a um botão, na base do folículo piloso, no qual o bulbo piloso se encaixa como um capuz; é derivado do cório e contém alças vasculares para a nutrição da raiz do pêlo. SIN p. pili.
ileal p. [TA], p. ileal; observada no cadáver como uma proeminência bilabial do íleo terminal, que se protrai para o intestino grosso na junção cecocólica; no indivíduo vivo, apresenta-se como um cone truncado com um orifício em forma de estrela. SIN p. ilealis [TA], valva ileocecalis [TA], Bauhin valve, ileocecal eminence, ileocecal valve, ileocolic valve, Tulp valve, Tulpius valve, valve of Varolius.
p. ilealis [TA], p. ileal. SIN ileal p.
p. incisi'va [TA], p. incisiva. SIN incisive p.
incisive p. [TA], p. incisiva; pequena elevação da mucosa na extremidade anterior da rafe do palato. SIN p. incisiva [TA], palatine p.
interdental p., p. gengival; * termo oficial alternativo para gingival p.
p. interdentalis, p. gengival; * termo oficial alternativo para gingival p.
interproximal p., p. gengival. SIN gingival p.
lacrimal p. [TA], p. lacrimal; pequena projeção da margem de cada pálpebra, localizada próximo da comissura medial, em cujo centro está o ponto lacrimal (abertura do ducto lacrimal). SIN p. lacrimalis [TA].
p. lacrima'lis [TA], p. lacrimal. SIN lacrimal p.
lenticular papillae, folículos da língua. SIN *folliculi* linguales, em *folliculus*.
lingual papillae, papilas linguais; **(1)** SIN papillae of tongue; **(2)** SIN lingual gingival p.
lingual gingival p., p. gengival lingual; as porções linguais da gengiva que ocupam o espaço interproximal entre dentes adjacentes; nas áreas molar e pré-molar, pode haver papilas interdentais bucais e linguais distintas. SIN lingual interdental p., lingual papillae (2).
lingual interdental p., p. interdental lingual. SIN lingual gingival p.
p. lingua'lis, pl. **papil'lae lingua'les,** papilas linguais. SIN papillae of tongue.
major duodenal p. [TA], p. maior do duodeno; ponto de abertura do ducto colédoco e ducto pancreático para o duodeno; está localizado posteriormente, na parte descendente do duodeno. SIN p. duodeni major [TA], bile p., p. of Vater, Santorini major caruncle.
p. mam'mae [TA], mamilo. SIN nipple.
minor duodenal p. [TA], p. menor do duodeno; o local de abertura do ducto pancreático acessório no duodeno, localizado anteriormente e um pouco acima da papila maior. SIN p. duodeni minor [TA], Santorini minor caruncle.
nerve p., p. nervosa; uma das papilas da derme que contêm um corpúsculo tátil ou outra forma de órgão final. SIN neurothele.
p. ner'vi op'tici, disco óptico. SIN optic *disk*.
optic p. (p), disco óptico. SIN optic *disk*.
palatine p., p. incisiva. SIN incisive p.
parotid p., p. do ducto parotídeo. SIN p. of parotid gland.
p. parotid'ea, p. do ducto parotídeo. SIN p. of parotid gland.
p. of parotid gland [TA], p. do ducto parotídeo; a projeção na abertura do ducto parotídeo para o vestíbulo da boca oposto ao colo do segundo dente molar superior. SIN p. ductus parotidei [TA], p. parotidea, parotid p.
p. pi'li, p. pilosa. SIN hair p.
renal p. [TA], p. renal; o ápice de uma pirâmide renal que se projeta para um cálice menor; cerca de 10–25 aberturas dos ductos papilares ocorrem em sua extremidade, formando a área cribriforme. SIN p. renalis [TA]
p. rena'lis, pl. **papil'lae rena'les** [TA], p. renal. SIN renal p.
retrocuspid p., p. retrocúspide; pequeno apêndice tecidual localizado na gengiva mandibular lingual aos dentes cuspidados; geralmente é bilateral, sendo mais comum em crianças e considerada uma estrutura anatômica normal.
tactile p., p. tátil; uma das papilas da derme que contêm uma célula ou corpúsculo tátil.
papillae of tongue [TA], papilas linguais; numerosas projeções de tamanhos variados da mucosa do dorso da língua; incluem as papilas filiformes, folhadas, fungiformes e circunvaladas. SIN lingual papillae (1), p. lingualis.
urethral p., p. urethra'lis, p. uretral; a pequena projeção freqüentemente presente no vestíbulo da vagina marcando o óstio uretral.
papillae valla'tae, pl. **papil'lae valla'tae** [TA], papila circunvalada. SIN vallate papillae.
vallate papillae [TA], papilas circunvaladas; uma dentre oito ou 10 projeções do dorso da língua, formando uma fileira anterior e paralela ao sulco terminal; cada papila é circundada por uma fossa circular que possui uma parede externa ligeiramente elevada (valo); nas laterais da papila circunvalada e na margem oposta do valo, há numerosos botões gustativos. SIN papillae vallatae [TA], circumvallate papillae.
vascular papillae, papilas vasculares; papilas dérmicas contendo alças vasculares.
p. of Vater, p. de Vater. SIN major duodenal p.

pap·il·lary, pap·il·late (pap'i - lār - ē, - i - lāt). Papilar; relativo a, semelhante a ou formado por papilas.
pap·il·lec·to·my (pap - i - lek'tō - mē). Papilectomia; remoção cirúrgica de qualquer papila. [papilla + G. *ektomē*, excisão]
pa·pil·le·de·ma (pa - pil - e - dē'mă). Papiledema; edema do disco óptico, freqüentemente devido a aumento da pressão intracraniana. SIN choked disk. [papilla + edema]
pap·il·lif·er·ous (pap - i - lif'er - ŭs). Papilífero; provido de papilas. [papilla + L. *fero*, carregar]
pa·pil·li·form (pă - pil'i - fōrm). Papiliforme; semelhante ou com o formato de uma papila.
pap·il·li·tis (pap - i - lī'tis). Papilite. **1.** Neurite óptica com edema do disco óptico. **2.** Inflamação da papila renal. [papilla + G. *-itis*, inflamação]
 foliate p., p. folhada; papilas folhadas vestigiais inflamadas na parte lateral posterior da língua.
 necrotizing p., p. necrotizante. SIN renal papillary *necrosis*.
papillo-. Papilo-; uma papila, papilar. [L. *papilla*]
pap·il·lo·ad·e·no·cys·to·ma (pap'i - lō - ad'ĕ - nō - sis - tō'mă). Papiloadenocistoma; neoplasia epitelial benigna caracterizada por glândulas ou estruturas glandulares, formação de cistos e projeções digitiformes, de células neoplásicas cobrindo um centro de tecido conjuntivo fibroso.
pap·il·lo·car·ci·no·ma (pap'i - lō - kar - si - nō'mă). Papilocarcinoma; carcinoma caracterizado por projeções digitiformes, papilares, de células neoplásicas associadas a centros de estroma fibroso como uma estrutura de sustentação. [papilla + G. *karkinōma*, câncer]
pap·il·lo·ma (pap - i - lō'mă). Papiloma; tumor epitelial benigno, circunscrito, que se projeta da superfície adjacente; mais precisamente, uma neoplasia epitelial benigna que consiste em crescimentos vilosos ou arborescentes de estroma fibrovascular coberto por células neoplásicas. SIN papillary tumor. [papilla + G. *-oma*, tumor]

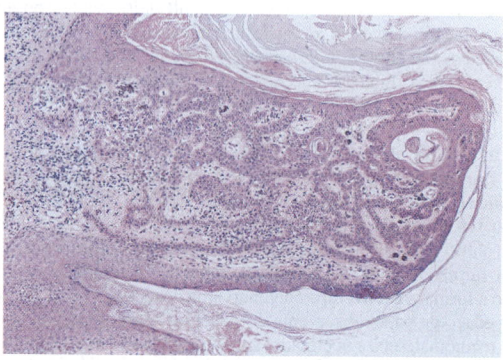

papiloma de células basais da pele: o tumor é composto de células semelhantes às da camada basal da epiderme; o tumor exofítico forma papilas que se projetam acima da superfície cutânea

papilloma

basal cell p., ceratose seborreica. SIN seborrheic *keratosis.*
p. canalic'ulum, p. canalicular; tumor benigno papilomatoso originado no ducto de uma glândula.
p. diffu'sum, p. difuso; ocorrência disseminada de papilomas.
duct p., p. ductal. SIN intraductal p.
p. du'rum, p. duro; uma verruga, calosidade ou corno cutâneo. SIN hard p.
hard p., p. duro. SIN p. durum.
Hopmann p., p. de Hopmann; supercrescimento papilomatoso da mucosa nasal. SIN Hopmann polyp.
p. inguina'le trop'icum, p. inguinal tropical; erupção cutânea, que ocorre na Colômbia, caracterizada por numerosas vegetações róseas delgadas na região inguinal.
intracystic p., p. intracístico; papiloma que cresce dentro de um adenoma cístico, preenchendo a cavidade com uma massa de processos epiteliais ramificados.
intraductal p., p. intraductal; papiloma benigno, pequeno, freqüentemente impalpável, que se origina em um ducto lactífero e freqüentemente causa hemorragia do mamilo. SIN duct p.
inverted p., p. invertido; tumor epitelial da bexiga ou da cavidade nasal na qual o epitélio proliferativo invagina-se sob a superfície e é mais suavemente arredondado que nos outros papilomas.
p. mol'le, p. mole. SIN skin *tag.*
Shope p., p. de Shope; crescimento papilomatoso encontrado em coelhos do gênero *Sylvilagus* selvagens, originalmente descrito por Shope, causado por um vírus da família Papovaviridae que pode ser transferido para coelhos domésticos, nos quais causará crescimentos semelhantes. Uma alta percentagem desses crescimentos pode tornar-se maligna.
soft p., p. mole. SIN skin *tag.*
transitional cell p., p. de células de transição. SIN urothelial p.
urothelial p., p. urotelial; tumor papilar benigno do urotélio. SIN transitional cell p.
villous p., p. viloso; papiloma composto de crescimentos digitiformes, delgados, que ocorrem na bexiga ou intestino grosso, ou do plexo coróide dos ventrículos cerebrais; o papiloma viloso do cólon geralmente é séssil e, freqüentemente, torna-se maligno. SIN villous tumor.
zymotic p., p. zimótico. SIN yaws.
pap·il·lo·ma·to·sis (pap′i-lō-mă-tō′sis). Papilomatose. **1.** O desenvolvimento de numerosos papilomas. **2.** Projeções papilares da epiderme, formando uma superfície ondulada.
confluent and reticulate p., p. confluente e reticulada; pápulas castanho-acinzentadas distintas e confluentes da região média anterior e posterior do tórax, disseminando-se gradualmente; a *Malassezia furfur* foi encontrada na camada de queratina. SIN Gougerot-Carteaud syndrome.
florid oral p., p. oral franca; envolvimento difuso dos lábios e da mucosa oral por papilomas escamosos benignos; microscopicamente, assemelha-se ao carcinoma verrucoso, mas não é invasivo ou localizado em uma área específica da mucosa oral.
juvenile p., p. juvenil; forma de doença fibrocística da mama em mulheres jovens, com adenose esclerosante franca que, microscopicamente, pode sugerir carcinoma.
laryngeal p., p. laríngea; múltiplos papilomas de células escamosas da laringe, mais comuns em crianças pequenas, geralmente causados por infecção pelo papilomavírus humano (HPV), que podem ser transmitidos ao nascimento pelos condilomas maternos; as recorrências são comuns, com remissão após vários anos. VER TAMBÉM recurrent respiratory p.
palatal p., p. palatina. SIN inflammatory papillary *hyperplasia.*
recurrent respiratory p., p. respiratória recorrente; doença das vias respiratórias causada pelo papilomavírus humano; caracterizada por rápida recorrência de papilomas após remoção cirúrgica, obstrução das vias aéreas e rouquidão, e mesmo afonia, quando há envolvimento da laringe. VER TAMBÉM laryngeal p.
subareolar duct p., p. ductal subareolar; tumor benigno por vezes semelhante, clinicamente, à doença de Paget, mas que é um crescimento papilar ou sólido de células colunares e mioepiteliais que produzem um padrão pseudo-infiltrativo franco. SIN adenoma of nipple, erosive adenomatosis of nipple.
pap·il·lo·ma·tous (pap-i-lō′mă-tŭs). Papilomatoso; relativo a um papiloma.
Pa·pil·lo·ma·vi·rus (pap-i-lō′mă-vī-rŭs). Gênero de vírus (família Papovaviridae) que contém DNA circular de duplo filamento (PM 5×10^6), possuindo vírions com aproximadamente 55 nm de diâmetro e incluindo os vírus do papiloma e da verruga de seres humanos e outros animais, alguns dos quais estão associados a induções de carcinoma. São conhecidos mais de 70 tipos que infectam seres humanos e são diferenciados por homologia do DNA. SIN papilloma virus.
Papillon, M.M., dermatologista francês do século XX. VER P.-Lefèvre *syndrome.*
Papillon-Léage, E., dentista francês do século XX. VER Papillon-Léage e Psaume *syndrome.*

pap·il·lo·ret·i·ni·tis (pap′i-lō-ret-i-nī′tis). Papilorretinite. SIN neuroretinitis.
pap·il·lot·o·my (pă-pi-lot′ō-mē). Papilotomia; uma incisão na papila; geralmente em referência à papila maior do duodeno. [papilla + G. *tome*, incisão]
pa·pil·lu·la, pl. **pa·pil·lu·lae** (pă-pil′ū-lă, -lē). Uma papila pequena. [L. mod. dim. do L. *papilla*]
Pa·po·va·vir·i·dae (pă-pō′vă-vir′i-dē). Família de vírus pequenos, antigenicamente distintos, que se replicam em núcleos de células infectadas; a maioria possui propriedades oncogênicas. Os vírions possuem 45–55 nm de diâmetro, não possuem envoltório e são resistentes ao éter; os capsídeos são icosaédricos, com 72 capsômeros, e contêm DNA circular de duplo filamento (PM $3–5 \times 10^6$). A família inclui 2 gêneros de Papillomavirus e Polyomavirus. [*pa*piloma + *po*lioma + *va*cuolizante]
pa·po·va·vi·rus (pă-pō′vă-vī′rŭs). Papovavírus; nome antigo de qualquer vírus da família Papovaviridae.
PAPP Abreviatura de *p*-aminopropiophenone (*p*-aminopropiofenona).
Pappenheim, Artur, médico alemão, 1870–1916. VER P. *stain;* Unna-P. *stain.*
Pap·pen·hei·mer, A.M., patologista norte-americano, 1878–1955. Seu trabalho em patologia experimental foi amplo e incluiu estudos do timo, identificação do papel da transmissão de piolhos na febre da trincheira (trench *fever*), desenvolvimento de um modelo experimental para raquitismo e avaliação de infecções virais em animais. VER Pappenheimer *bodies,* em *body.*
pap·pus (pap′ŭs). Os primeiros pêlos macios de barba. [G. *pappos,* lanugem]
PAPS Abreviatura de adenosine 3′-phosphate 5′-phosphosulfate (adenosina 3′-fosfato 5′-fosfossulfato); 3′-phosphoadenosine 5′- phosphosulfate (3′-fosfoadenosina 5′-fosfossulfato).
pap·u·lar (pap′ū-lăr). Papular; relativo a pápulas.
pap·ule (pap′ūl). Pápula; elevação sólida, circunscrita, com até 100 cm de diâmetro na pele. Uma pápula pode ser pediculada, séssil ou filiforme. [L. *papula,* pápula]
follicular p., p. folicular; lesão papular que se origina em torno de um folículo piloso; não é específica de qualquer condição.
moist p., mucous p., condiloma plano. SIN condyloma *latum.*
piezogenic pedal p., p. piezogênico do pé; pápulas do calcanhar induzidas por pressão, que provavelmente ocorrem em virtude de herniação do tecido adiposo.
pruritic urticarial p.'s and plaques of pregnancy (PUPPP), pápulas urticariformes pruriginosas e placas de gravidez; papulovesículas intensamente pruriginosas que começam no abdome no terceiro trimestre e disseminam-se para a periferia, resolvendo rapidamente após o parto, e não afetam o feto.
split p.'s, p. fendidas; pápulas nas comissuras labiais, observadas em alguns casos de sífilis secundária.
papulo-. Papulo-; pápula. [L. *papula,* pápula]
pap·u·lo·er·y·them·a·tous (pap′ū-lō-er-i-them′ă-tŭs, -thē′mă-tŭs). Papuloeritematoso; designa uma erupção de pápulas sobre uma superfície eritematosa.
pap·u·lo·pus·tu·lar (pap′ū-lō-pŭs′too-lăr). Papulopustular; designa uma erupção composta de pápulas e pústulas.
pap·u·lo·pus·tule (pap′ū-lō-pŭs′tŭl). Papulopústula; pequena elevação cutânea, semi-sólida, que rapidamente se transforma em uma pústula.
pa·pu·lo·sis (pap-ū-lō′sis). Papulose; a ocorrência de numerosas pápulas disseminadas.
bowenoid p., p. de Bowen; forma clinicamente benigna de neoplasia intraepitelial, microscopicamente semelhante à doença de Bowen ou carcinoma *in situ,* que ocorre em pessoas jovens, de ambos os sexos, na pele genital ou perianal, geralmente como múltiplas pápulas verrucosas pigmentadas bem demarcadas.
lymphomatoid p., p. linfomatóide; variante papular e ulcerativa crônica da pitiríase liquenóide e varioliforme aguda, caracterizada por infiltração perivascular por linfócitos T atípicos, sugestiva de linfoma; geralmente é benigna, mas já foi descrita transformação em linfoma.
malignant atrophic p., p. atrófica maligna; síndrome cutâneo-visceral, caracterizada por pápulas umbilicadas, branco-porcelana, patognomônicas, com bordas anulares telangiectáticas elevadas, seguida pelo desenvolvimento de úlceras intersticiais que perfuram, causando peritonite; as arteríolas nas lesões são ocluídas por trombose sem células inflamatórias, causando infarto, incapacidade neurológica progressiva e morte. SIN Degos disease, Degos syndrome.
pap·u·lo·squa·mous (pap′ū-lō-skwā′mŭs). Papuloescamoso; designa uma erupção composta de pápulas e escamas. [papulo- + L. *squamosus,* descamativo (escamoso)]
pap·u·lo·ves·i·cle (pap′ū-lō-ves′i-kl). Papulovesícula; pequena elevação cutânea que se transforma em uma vesícula.
pap·u·lo·ve·sic·u·lar (pap′ū-lō-ve-sik′ū-lăr). Papulovesicular; designa uma erupção composta de pápulas e vesículas.
PAPVR Abreviatura de partial anomalous pulmonary venous return (retorno venoso pulmonar anômalo parcial). VER anomalous pulmonary venous *connections,* total or partial, em *connection.*

pap·y·ra·ceous (pap-i-rā'shŭs). Papiráceo; semelhante a pergaminho ou papel. [L. *papyraceus*, feito de *papyrus*]

par. Par; especificamente um par de nervos cranianos, p. ex., p. nonum, nono par, glossofaríngeo; p. vagum, o nervo vago ou décimo par. [L. igual]

para (par'ă). Designa a mulher que deu à luz um ou mais fetos. *Para*, seguido por um algarismo romano ou precedido por um prefixo latino (primi-, secundi-, terti-, quadri-, etc.), designa o número de vezes que uma gravidez culminou em um parto único ou múltiplo; p. ex., **para I**, primípara, mulher que deu à luz pela primeira vez; **para II**, secundípara, mulher que deu à luz pela segunda vez a um ou mais lactentes. Cf. gravida. [L. *pario*, parir]

♲ **para-.** Para. **1.** Prefixo que designa uma divergência do normal. **2.** Prefixo que designa envolvimento de duas partes semelhantes ou um par. **3.** Prefixo que designa adjacente, paralelo, próximo, etc. **4.** (*p-*). Em química, um prefixo em itálico que designa duas substituições no anel benzeno dispostas simetricamente, isto é, ligadas aos átomos de carbono opostos no anel. Para palavras que começam com *para-* ou *p-*, ver o nome específico. [G. paralelo a, próximo]

para·ac·ti·no·my·co·sis (par-ă-ak'ti-nō-kō'sis). Para-actinomicose; infecção crônica, geralmente pulmonar, semelhante à actinomicose; comumente causada por nocardiose. SIN pseudoactinomycosis.

par·a·ami·no·ben·zo·ic ac·id (par'ă-mē'nō). Ácido para-aminobenzóico. SIN p-aminobenzoic acid.

para-ap·pen·di·ci·tis (par'ă-ă-pen-di-sī'tis) Para-apendicite. SIN periappendicitis.

par·a·ban·ic ac·id (par'ă-ban-ik). Ácido parabânico. SIN oxalylurea.

par·a·bi·o·sis (par-ă-bī-ō'sis). Parabiose. **1.** Fusão de ovos inteiros ou de embriões, como ocorre em algumas formas de gêmeos conjugados. **2.** União cirúrgica dos sistemas vasculares de dois organismos. [para- + G. *biōsis*, vida]

par·a·bi·ot·ic (par-ă-bī-ot'ik). Parabiótico; relativo a, ou caracterizado por, parabiose.

par·a·bu·lia (par-ă-boo'lē-ă). Parabulia; perversão da volição ou da vontade na qual um impulso é interrompido e substituído por outro. [para- + G. *boulē*, vontade]

par·ac·an·tho·ma (par'ak-an-thō'mă). Paracantoma; neoplasia originada de hiperplasia anormal da camada de células espinhosas da pele. [para- + G. *akantha*, espinho, + -*oma*, tumor]

par·ac·an·tho·sis (par'ak-an-thō'sis). Paracantose. **1.** O desenvolvimento de paracantomas. **2.** Uma divisão de tumores que inclui os epiteliomas cutâneos.

par·a·car·mine. Paracarmim. VER stain.

par·a·ca·se·in (par-ă-kā'sē-in). Paracaseína; a substância produzida pela ação da renina sobre a κ-caseína (que libera uma glicoproteína) e que se precita com íon cálcio sob a forma de um coalho insolúvel.

Paracelsus, Aureolus Theophrastus Bombastus von Hohenheim, médico suíço, 1493–1541. VER paracelsian *method*.

par·a·ce·nes·the·sia (par'ă-sē-nes-thē'zē-ă). Paracenestesia; deterioração da sensação de bem-estar corporal de uma pessoa, isto é, do funcionamento normal dos órgãos de uma pessoa. [para- + G. *koinos*, comum, + *aisthēsis*, sentimento]

par·a·cen·te·sis (par'ă-sen-tē'sis). Paracentese; a introdução, em uma cavidade, de um trocarte e cânula, agulha ou outro instrumento oco para fins de remover líquido; designada de acordo com a cavidade puncionada. SIN tapping (2). [G. *parakentēsis*, punção por causa de hidrópsia, de *para*, ao lado, + *kentēsis*, punção]

par·a·cen·tet·ic (par-ă-sen-tet'ik). Paracentésico; relativo à paracentese.

par·a·cen·tral (par-ă-sen'tral). Paracentral; próximo ou ao lado do centro ou de alguma estrutura designada "central".

par·a·cer·vi·cal (par-ă-ser'vi-kăl). Paracervical; tecido conjuntivo adjacente ao colo do útero.

par·a·cer·vix (par-ă-ser'viks) [TA]. Paracérvice; o tecido conjuntivo do assoalho pélvico, que se estende desde a camada subserosa fibrosa do colo do útero lateralmente, entre as camadas do ligamento largo.

par·ac·et·al·de·hyde (par-as-ē-tal'dē-hīd). Paracetaldeído. SIN paraldehyde.

par·a·cet·a·mol (par-ă-set'ă-mol). Paracetamol. SIN acetaminophen.

par·a·chlo·ro·phe·nol (par'ă-klōr-ō-fē'nol). Paraclorofenol; desinfetante efetivo contra a maioria dos organismos Gram-negativos; também disponível na forma de paraclorofenol canforado. SIN *p*-chlorophenol.

par·a·chol·e·ra (par-ă-kol'er-ă). Paracólera; doença clinicamente semelhante ao cólera asiático, mas causada por um vibrião especificamente diferente do *Vibrio cholerae*.

par·a·chor·dal (par-ă-kōr'dal). Paracordal; paralelo à porção anterior da notocorda no embrião; designa as barras cartilaginosas bilaterais que entram na formação da base do crânio. [para- + G. *chordē*, corda]

par·a·chro·ma (par-ă-krō'mă). Paracromia; coloração anormal da pele. [para- + G. *chrōma*, cor]

par·a·chy·mo·sin (par-ă-kī'mō-sin). Paraquimosina; enzima semelhante à quimosina.

par·a·ci·ne·sia, par·a·ci·ne·sis (par'ă-si-nē'zē-ă, -nē'sis). Paracinesia. SIN parakinesia.

par·ac·ma·sis (par-ak'mă-sis). Paracme. SIN paracme.

par·ac·mas·tic (par-ak-mas'tik). Paracmástico; relativo ao paracme.

par·ac·me (par-ak'mē). Paracme. **1.** O estágio de defervescência de uma febre. **2.** O período da vida após o apogeu; o declínio ou estágio de involução de um organismo. SIN paracmasis. [G. o ponto em que o apogeu já passou; de *para*, além, + *akmē*, ponto mais alto, apogeu]

Par·a·coc·cid·i·oi·des bra·sil·i·en·sis (par'ă-kok-sid-ē-oy'dēz bră-sil-ē-en'sis). Fungo dimórfico que causa paracoccidioidomicose. Em tecidos e em meio de cultura enriquecido a 37°C, brota como grandes células ovais ou esféricas que apresentam brotamentos únicos ou variados e geralmente é identificado por essa característica; em temperaturas menores, cresce lentamente como um mofo branco com esporulação mínima.

par·a·coc·cid·i·oi·din (par'ă-kok-sid-ē-oy'din). Paracoccidioidina; antígeno filtrado preparado a partir da forma filamentar do fungo patogênico *Paracoccidioides brasiliensis*; usado para demonstrar hipersensibilidade dérmica tardia em populações e útil na demonstração de áreas endêmicas em diferentes regiões geográficas.

par·a·coc·cid·i·oi·do·my·co·sis (par'ă-kok-sid-ē-oy'dō-mī-kō'sis). Paracoccidioidomicose; micose crônica caracterizada por lesões pulmonares primárias com disseminação para muitos órgãos viscerais, granulomas ulcerativos visíveis da mucosa bucal e nasal, com extensões para a pele, e linfangite generalizada; causada pelo *Paracoccidioides brasiliensis*. SIN Almeida disease, Lutz-Splendore-Almeida disease, paracoccidioidal granuloma, South American blastomycosis.

par·a·co·li·tis (par'ă-kō-lī'tis). Paracolite; inflamação da camada peritoneal do cólon.

par·a·col·pi·tis (par'ă-kol-pī'tis). Paracolpite. SIN paravaginitis. [para- + G. *kolpos*, vagina, + -*itis*, inflamação]

par·a·col·pi·um (par-ă-kol'pē-ŭm). Paracolpo; os tecidos ao longo da vagina. [para- + G. *kolpos*, vagina]

par·a·cone (par'ă-kōn). Paracone; a cúspide mesiobucal de um dente molar superior. [para- + G. *kōnos*, cone]

par·a·co·nid (par-ă-kon'id). Paracônide; a cúspide mesiobucal de um dente molar inferior.

par·a·cor·tex (par-ă-kōr'teks). Paracórtex; a área de um linfonodo entre o córtex subcapsular e os cordões medulares; contém principalmente os linfócitos de vida longa derivados do timo. SIN deep cortex, tertiary cortex, thymus-dependent zone.

par·a·cou·sis (par-ă-koo'sis). Paracusia. SIN paracusis.

par·a·crine (par'ă-krin). Parácrino; relativo a um tipo de função hormonal na qual os efeitos do hormônio são restritos ao ambiente local. Cf. endocrine. [para- + G. *krinō*, separar]

par·a·cu·sis, par·a·cu·sia (par'ă-koo'sis, -koo'sē-ă). Paracusia. **1.** Comprometimento da audição. **2.** Delírios ou alucinações auditivas. SIN paracousis. [para- + G. *akousis*, audição]

false p., p. falsa; o aparente aumento da audição de uma pessoa com surdez de condução ao conversar em locais barulhentos; deve-se ao fato de as outras pessoas falarem mais alto. SIN Willis p.

p. loci, p. de localização; perda ou diminuição da capacidade de determinar a direção do som.

Willis p., p. de Willis. SIN false p.

par·a·cy·e·sis (par-ă-sī-ē'sis). Paraciese. SIN ectopic *pregnancy*. [para- + G. *kyēsis*, gravidez]

par·a·cys·tic (par-ă-sis'tik). Paracístico; ao longo ou próximo de uma bexiga ou vesícula, especificamente da bexiga urinária. SIN paravesical. [para- + G. *kystis*, bexiga]

par·a·cys·ti·tis (par'ă-sis-tī'tis). Paracistite; inflamação do tecido conjuntivo e de outras estruturas ao redor da bexiga urinária. [para- + G. *kystis*, bexiga, + -*itis*, inflamação]

par·a·cys·ti·um (par-ă-sis'tē-ŭm). Paracístio; os tecidos adjacentes à bexiga. [para- + G. *kystis*, bexiga]

par·a·cy·tic (par-ă-sī'tik). Paracítico. **1.** Relativo às células diferentes daquelas normais no local onde são encontradas. **2.** Entre as células, mas independente delas. [para- + G. *kytos*, célula]

par·ad·e·ni·tis (par'ad'ē-nī'tis). Paradenite; inflamação dos tecidos adjacentes a uma glândula. [para- + G. *adēn*, glândula, + -*itis*, inflamação]

par·a·den·tal (par-ă-den'tăl). Paradental. SIN periodontal.

par·a·den·ti·um (par-ă-den'tē-oom). Periodonto. SIN periodontium.

par·a·did·y·mal (par-ă-did'i-măl). **1.** Referente ao paradídimo. **2.** Ao longo do testículo.

par·a·did·y·mis, pl. **par·a·did·y·mi·des** (par'ă-did'i-mis, -di-dim'i-dēz). [TA]. Paradídimo; pequeno corpo algumas vezes fixado à frente da parte inferior do cordão espermático acima da cabeça do epidídimo; os remanescentes dos túbulos do mesonefro. Seu equivalente na mulher é o paróforo. SIN parepididymis. [para- + G. *didymos*, gêmeo, no pl. *didymoi*, testículos]

par·a·dip·sia (par-ă-dip'sē-ă). Paradipsia; perversão do apetite para líquidos, ingeridos sem relação com as necessidades corporais. [para- + G. *dipsa*, sede]

par·a·dox (par´ă-doks). Paradoxo; aquilo que é aparentemente, embora na verdade não o seja, incompatível com ou contrário aos fatos conhecidos em qualquer caso. [G. *paradoxos*, inacreditável, além do que se pode crer, de *doxa*, crença]
  Weber p., p. de Weber; quando um músculo é sobrecarregado além de sua capacidade de contrair, ele pode alongar-se.
par·a·es·the·sia (par-es-thē´zē-ă). Parestesia. SIN paresthesia.
par·af·fin (par´ă-fin). Parafina. **1.** Uma das séries metano dos hidrocarbonetos acíclicos. **2.** SIN hard p. [L. *parum*, pouco, + *affinis*, próximo, afim, assim denominado devido à sua pequena tendência à reação química]
  chlorinated p., p. clorada; solvente da dicloramina-T.
  hard p., p. dura; mistura purificada de hidrocarbonetos sólidos derivados do petróleo. SIN paraffin (2).
  liquid p., p. líquida. SIN mineral oil.
  white soft p., vaselina branca. SIN white *petrolatum.*
  yellow soft p., vaselina. SIN petrolatum.
par·af·fi·no·ma (par´ă-fi-nō´mă). Parafinoma; tumefação, geralmente um granuloma, causada por prótese ou injeção terapêutica de parafina nos tecidos; algumas vezes usada em referência a lesões semelhantes resultantes da injeção de qualquer óleo, cera ou semelhantes. VER TAMBÉM lipogranuloma. SIN paraffin tumor.
Par·a fi·lar·ia mul·ti·pa·pil·lo·sa (par´ă-fi-lā´rē-ă mul´ti-pap-i-lō´să). Parasita filária comum que causa dermatorragia parasitária.
par·a·fla·gel·la (par´ă-fla-jel´ă). Paraflagelos; plural de paraflagellum.
par·a·flag·el·late (par-ă-flaj´e-lāt). Paraflagelado. **1.** Que possui um ou mais paraflagelos. **2.** SIN paramastigote.
par·a·fla·gel·lum, pl. **par·a·fla·gel·la** (par´ă-fla-jel´ŭm, -ă). Paraflagelo; pequeno flagelo acessório algumas vezes presente além do flagelo comum de alguns protozoários.
paraflocculus ventralis. Paraflóculo ventral. SIN ventral paraflocculus.
par·a·fol·lic·u·lar (par-ă-fo-lik´ū-lăr). Parafolicular; espacialmente associado a um folículo.
par·a·for·mal·de·hyde (par-ă-fōr-mal´dĕ-hīd). Paraformaldeído; polímero do formaldeído, usado como desinfetante. SIN trioxymethylene.
par·a·fuch·sin (par-ă-fuk´sin). Parafucsina. SIN pararosanilin.
par·a·gam·ma·cism (par´ă-gam´ă-sizm). Paragamacismo; substituição do som da letra g pelo som de outra letra. VER TAMBÉM gammacism. [para- + G. *gamma*, a letra g]
par·a·gan·glia (par´ă-gang´glē-ă). Paragânglios; plural de paraganglion.
par·a·gan·gli·o·ma (par´ă-gang-glē-ō´mă). Paraganglioma; neoplasia geralmente derivada do tecido cromorreceptor de um paragânglio, como o corpo carotídeo ou a medula da glândula supra-renal; esta última geralmente é denominada cromafinoma ou feocromocitoma.
  nonchromaffin p., p. não-cromafim. SIN chemodectoma.
par·a·gan·gli·on, pl. **par·a·gan·glia** (par-ă-gang´glē-on, -ă). Paragânglio; pequeno corpo arredondado contendo células cromafins; vários desses corpos podem ser encontrados no espaço retroperitoneal próximo da aorta e em órgãos como o rim, fígado, coração e gônadas. SIN chromaffin body.
par·a·gene (par´ă-jēn). Plasmídeo. SIN plasmid.
par·a·gen·i·tal (par-ă-jen´i-tal). Paragenital; ao longo das gônadas.
par·a·geu·sia (par-ă-gū´sē-ă, -joo´sē-ă). Parageusia. SIN dysgeusia. [para- + G. *geusis*, paladar]
par·a·geu·sic (par-ă-gū´sik). Parageúsico; relativo à parageusia.
pa·rag·na·thus (pa-rag´na-thŭs). Paragnato. **1.** Defeito do desenvolvimento que resulta em um indivíduo com uma mandíbula acessória. **2.** Um feto parasita ligado à mandíbula do autósito. [para- + G. *gnathos*, mandíbula]
par·ag·no·men (par-ag-nō´men). Reação inesperada. [para- + G. *gnōmen, gnōmē*, julgamento]
par·a·gon·i·mi·a·sis (par´ă-gon-i-mī´ă-sis). Paragonimíase; infecção por um verme do gênero *Paragonimus*, particularmente *P. westermani*. SIN pulmonary distomiasis.
Par·a·gon·i·mus (par-ă-gon´i-mŭs). Gênero de trematódeos pulmonares, parasitas de seres humanos e de uma grande variedade de mamíferos, que se alimentam de crustáceos portadores de metacercárias. [para- + G. *gonimos*, com capacidade geradora]
  P. kellicot´ti, espécie de trematódeo prevalente em alguns animais selvagens, como o guaxinim, e encontrado em cães, na região dos Grandes Lagos dos Estados Unidos; é morfologicamente semelhante ao *P. westermani*.
  P. rin´geri, SIN *P. westermani.*
  P. westerman´i, o trematódeo brônquico ou pulmonar; espécie que causa paragonimíase, encontrado principalmente no Japão, na Coréia, em Taiwan, na China, nas Filipinas e na Tailândia; os ovos são eliminados no escarro ou engolidos e eliminados nas fezes; os miracídios invadem caramujos *Melania* e produzem grandes números de cercárias de cauda curta que deixam o caramujo e invadem os músculos e as vísceras de camarões de água doce ou caranguejos e se encistam; em seres humanos, os vermes excistados invadem a parede intestinal e migram para os pulmões através do diafragma; os parasitas em desenvolvimento causam reação inflamatória intensa e, por fim, induzem nódulos de paredes fibrosas que, geralmente, contêm um par de vermes adultos, juntamente com exsudato, ovos e restos de hemácias; os nódulos fibroparasitários podem tornar-se contíguos e formam estruturas císticas multiloculadas; em alguns casos, os trematódeos invadem o encéfalo, fígado, peritônio, intestino ou pele. SIN *P. ringeri*.
par·a·gon·or·rhe·al (par´ă-gon-ō-rē´al). Paragonorreico; indiretamente relacionado ou conseqüente à gonorréia.
par·a·gram·ma·tism (par-ă-gram´ă-tizm). Paragramatismo; aliteração. SIN paraphasia.
par·a·graph·ia (par-ă-graf´ē-ă). Paragrafia. **1.** Perda da capacidade de escrever algo que está sendo ditado, embora as palavras sejam ouvidas e compreendidas. **2.** Escrever uma palavra quando se pretendia escrever outra. [para- + G. *graphō*, escrever]
par·a·he·pat·ic (par-ă-he-pat´ik). Para-hepático; adjacente ao fígado.
par·a·hi·dro·sis (par´ă-hi-drō´sis). Para-hidrose. SIN paridrosis.
par·a·hor·mone (par-ă-hōr´mōn). Para-hormônio; substância, produto do metabolismo comum, não produzida para um fim específico, que atua como um hormônio na modificação da atividade de algum órgão distante; p. ex., a ação do dióxido de carbono sobre o controle da respiração.
par·a·hy·poph·y·sis (par´ă-hī-pof´i-sis). Para-hipófise; pequena massa de tecido hipofisário, ou tecido com estrutura semelhante ao lobo anterior da hipófise, ocasionalmente encontrada na dura-máter que reveste a sela turca.
par·a·kap·pa·cism (par´ă-kap´ă-sizm). Paracapacismo; substituição do som da letra k por outra letra. VER TAMBÉM kappacism. [para- + G. *kappa*, a letra k]
par·a·ker·a·to·sis (par´ă-ker-ă-tō´sis). Paceratose; retenção de núcleos nas células do estrato córneo da epiderme, observada em muitas dermatoses descamativas como a psoríase e a dermatite subaguda ou crônica.
  p. pustulo´sa, p. pustulosa; ceratose subungueal idiopática com deformidade ou depressões das unhas e com alterações eczematosas pustulares ou descamativas bem demarcadas das pontas dos dedos; geralmente observada em meninas.
  p. scutula´ris, p. escutular; doença do couro cabeludo caracterizada pela formação de crostas que envolvem os fios de cabelo.
par·a·ki·ne·sia, par·a·ki·ne·sis (par´ă-ki-nē´zē-ă, -ki-nē´sis). Paracinesia; qualquer anormalidade motora. SIN paracinesia, paracinesis. [para- + G. *kinēsis*, movimento]
par·a·la·lia (par-ă-lā´lē-ă). Paralalia; qualquer defeito da fala; particularmente aquele no qual uma letra é habitualmente substituída por outra. [para- + G. *lalia*, fala]
  p. litera´lis, p. literal; gagueira. SIN stammering.
par·a·lamb·da·cism (par-ă-lam´dă-sizm). Paralambdacismo; erro de pronúncia da letra l, ou a substituição da letra l por outra. VER TAMBÉM lambdacism. [para- + G. *lambda*, letra l]
par·al·de·hyde (par-al´dĕ-hīd). Paraldeído; (CH$_3$CHO)$_3$; polímero cíclico do acetaldeído; potente sedativo hipnótico e anticonvulsivante adequado para administração oral, retal, intravenosa e intramuscular; o odor desagradável que apresenta limita seu uso; eficaz na supressão da abstinência da dependência de álcool. SIN paracetaldehyde.
par·a·lep·ro·sis (par-ă-lē-prō´sis). Paralepra; presença de determinadas alterações tróficas ou nervosas sugestivas de uma forma atenuada de hanseníase em regiões onde a doença predominou por muito tempo.
par·a·lep·sy (par´ă-lep-sē). Paralepsia. **1.** Termo raramente usado para designar uma crise temporária de inércia mental e desesperança. **2.** Uma mudança súbita de humor ou da tensão emocional. [para- + G. *lēpsis*, convulsão]
par·a·lex·ia (par-ă-lek´sē-ă). Paralexia; erro de compreensão das palavras escritas ou impressas, sendo substituídas por outras palavras sem sentido durante a leitura. [para- + G. *lexis*, fala]
par·al·ge·sia (par-al-jē´zē-ă). Paralgesia; parestesia dolorosa; qualquer distúrbio ou anormalidade na percepção da dor. [para- + G. *algēsis*, a percepção da dor]
par·al·gia (par-al´jē-ă). Paralgia; dor anormal ou incomum. [para- + G. *algos*, dor]
par·a·lip·o·pho·bia (par´ă-lip-ō-fō´bē-ă). Paralipofobia; medo mórbido de negligenciar obrigações. [G. *paraleipō*, omitir, negligenciar, + *phobos*, medo]
par·al·lac·tic (par-ă-lak´tik). Paráláctico; paralático; relativo a paralaxe.
par·al·lax (par´ă-laks). Paralaxe. **1.** O aparente deslocamento de um objeto após uma mudança na posição de observação. **2.** VER phi *phenomenon*. [G. alternadamente, de *par-allassō*, fazer alternar, de *allos*, outro]
  binocular p., p. binocular; a diferença nos ângulos formados pelas linhas de visão de dois objetos situados a distâncias diferentes dos olhos; um fator na percepção visual de profundidade. SIN stereoscopic p.
  heteronymous p., p. heterônima; o movimento aparente de um objeto em direção ao olho fechado; observada na exoforia.
  homonymous p., p. homônima; o movimento aparente de um objeto em direção ao olho aberto quando o outro está fechado; observada na esoforia.
  stereoscopic p., p. estereoscópica. SIN binocular p.

vertical p., p. vertical; o deslocamento vertical relativo da imagem quando cada olho é fechado de uma vez; observado na diplopia vertical ou heteroforia.

par·al·lel·ism (par′ă-lel-izm). Paralelismo. **1.** A condição de ser estruturalmente paralelo. **2.** Em psicologia, a doutrina mente–corpo que afirma que, para todo processo consciente, há um processo orgânico correspondente ou paralelo, sem afirmar uma inter-relação causal entre os dois. [para- + G. *allēlōn*, entre si, de *allos*, outro]

par·al·lel·om·e·ter (par′ă-lel-om′ĕ-ter). Paralelômetro; aparelho usado para igualar as conexões e limites para dentaduras parciais fixas ou móveis.

par·al·ler·gic (par-ă-ler′jik). Paralérgico; designa um estado alérgico no qual o corpo torna-se predisposto a estímulos inespecíficos após sensibilização original a um alérgeno específico.

par·a·lo·gia, pa·ral·o·gism, pa·ral·o·gy (par-ă-lō′jē-ă, pă-ral′ō-jizm, -ral′ō-jē). Paralogia, paralogismo; falso raciocínio, envolvendo a ilusão da própria pessoa. [G. *paralogia*, falácia, de *para*, ao lado de, + *logos*, razão]

thematic p., p. temático; raciocínio falso, principalmente em relação a um tema ou assunto, sobre o qual a mente divaga sem cessar.

pa·ral·y·sis, pl. **pa·ral·y·ses** (pă-ral′i-sis, -sēz). Paralisia. **1.** Perda da capacidade de movimentação voluntária de um músculo por lesão ou doença deste ou de seu suprimento nervoso. **2.** Perda de qualquer função, como sensibilidade, secreção ou capacidade mental. [G. de para- + *lysis*, afrouxamento]

acute ascending p., p. ascendente aguda; paralisia de evolução rápida que começa nas pernas e envolve progressivamente o tronco, braços e pescoço, culminando algumas vezes em morte em 1–3 semanas; geralmente causada por uma forma fulminante da síndrome de Guillain-Barré ou por uma mielopatia necrotizante ascendente. SIN ascending p.

p. ag'itans, p. agitante; designação obsoleta do parkinsonismo. [parkinsonism (1)]

ascending p., p. ascendente. SIN acute ascending p.

Brown-Séquard p., p. de Brown-Séquard. SIN Brown-Séquard *syndrome*.

bulbar p., p. bulbar. SIN progressive bulbar p.

central p., p. central; paralisia causada por lesão no encéfalo ou na medula espinal.

compression p., p. por compressão; paralisia causada por compressão externa de um nervo.

crossed p., p. cruzada. SIN alternating *hemiplegia*.

crutch p., p. por muleta; forma de paralisia compressiva que afeta o braço, causada por compressão do plexo braquial infraclavicular ou do nervo radial pela barra transversal de uma muleta. SIN crutch palsy.

diphtheritic p., p. diftérica. SIN postdiphtheritic p.

diver's p., p. do mergulhador; designação leiga da doença descompressiva (decompression *sickness*).

Duchenne-Erb p., p. de Duchenne-Erb. SIN Erb *palsy*.

Erb p., p. de Erb. SIN Erb *palsy*.

facial p., p. facial; paresia ou paralisia dos músculos da face, geralmente unilateral, causada por 1) uma lesão do núcleo ou do nervo facial periférico ao núcleo (paralisia facial periférica) ou por 2) uma lesão supranuclear no cérebro ou na parte superior do tronco cerebral (paralisia facial central); nesta última, a fraqueza facial geralmente é parcial e a parte superior da face é relativamente poupada, devido às conexões corticais bilaterais. SIN facial palsy, facioplegia, fallopian neuritis.

familial periodic p., p. periódica familiar; um dos distúrbios musculares hereditários que se manifestam como episódios recorrentes de fraqueza generalizada acentuada. VER hyperkalemic periodic p., hypokalemic periodic p., normokalemic periodic p.

faucial p., p. das fauces. SIN isthmoparalysis.

flaccid p., p. flácida; paralisia em que há perda do tônus muscular. Cf. spastic *diplegia*.

generalized p., p. generalizada. SIN global p.

ginger p., p. por gengibre. SIN jake p.

global p., p. global; paralisia de ambos os lados do corpo. SIN generalized p.

glossolabiolaryngeal p., glossolabiopharyngeal p., p. glossolabiolaríngea, p. glossolabiofaríngea. SIN progressive bulbar p.

glossopalatolabial p., p. glossopalatolabial. SIN progressive bulbar *palsy*.

glossopharyngeolabial p., p. glossofaringeolabial. SIN progressive bulbar *palsy*.

Gubler p., p. de Gubler. SIN Gubler *syndrome*.

hyperkalemic periodic p. [MIM*170500 tipo II], p. periódica hiperpotassêmica; forma de paralisia periódica na qual o nível sérico de potássio está elevado durante as crises; o início ocorre na lactância, as crises são freqüentes, mas relativamente leves, e freqüentemente há miotonia; herança autossômica dominante causada por mutação no gene do canal de sódio (SCN4A) no cromossoma 17q.

hypokalemic periodic p. [MIM*170400 tipo I], p. periódica hipopotassêmica; forma de paralisia periódica na qual o nível sérico de potássio é baixo durante as crises; o início geralmente ocorre entre 7 e 21 anos de idade; as crises podem ser precipitadas por exposição ao frio, refeições ricas em carboidratos ou álcool, podendo durar horas a dias e, também, causar paralisia respiratória; herança autossômica dominante causada por mutação na subunidade α-1 do canal de cálcio muscular sensível à diidropiridina (DHP) (CACNL1A3) no cromossoma 1q, ou herança ligada ao X.

hysterical p., p. histérica; dormência psicossomática de um membro que, algumas vezes, atinge o ponto de paralisia. VER hysteria.

immune p., p. imune; a indução de tolerância devida à injeção de grandes quantidades de antígeno. O antígeno é pouco metabolizado e a paralisia permanece apenas durante a persistência das condições supracitadas. VER immunologic *tolerance*. SIN immunologic p.

immunologic p., p. imunológica. SIN immune p.

jake p., p. por gengibre; polineuropatia causada pela ingestão de gengibre sintético jamaicano (nome popular *jake*) contendo triortocresilfosfato. SIN ginger p.

Klumpke p., p. de Klumpke. SIN Klumpke *palsy*.

Landry p., p. de Landry. SIN Guillain-Barré *syndrome*.

lead p., p. por chumbo. SIN lead *palsy*.

mimetic p., p. mimética; paralisia dos músculos faciais.

mixed p., p. mista; p. motora e sensorial combinada.

motor p., p. motora; perda da força de contração muscular.

musculospiral p., p. musculoespiral; paralisia dos músculos do antebraço devido à lesão do nervo radial (musculoespiral).

normokalemic periodic p. [type III MIM 170600], p. periódica normopotassêmica (tipo III); forma de paralisia periódica na qual o nível sérico de potássio está dentro dos limites normais durante a crise; o início geralmente se dá entre 2 e 5 anos de idade; freqüentemente há tetraplegia grave, que geralmente melhora com a administração de sais de sódio; herança autossômica dominante. SIN sodium-responsive periodic p.

obstetric p., p. obstétrica. SIN obstetric *palsy*.

ocular p., p. ocular; paralisia dos músculos extra-oculares e intra-oculares.

periodic p., p. periódica; termo para designar um grupo de doenças caracterizadas por episódios recorrentes de fraqueza muscular ou paralisia flácida sem perda da consciência, da fala ou da sensibilidade; as crises começam quando o paciente está em repouso, e entre elas, aparentemente há boa saúde. VER hyperkalemic periodic p., hypokalemic periodic p., normokalemic periodic p.

peripheral facial p., p. facial periférica. SIN Bell *palsy*.

postdiphtheritic p., p. pós-diftérica; paralisia que afeta mais amiúde a úvula, mas também qualquer outro músculo, causada por neurite tóxica; geralmente aparece na segunda ou terceira semana após o início da difteria. SIN diphtheritic p.

posti'cus p., p. dos músculos cricoaritenóideos posteriores.

Pott p., p. de Pott. SIN Pott *paraplegia*.

pressure p., p. por compressão; paralisia causada pela compressão de um nervo, tronco nervoso, plexo ou medula espinal. SIN pressure palsy.

progressive bulbar p., p. bulbar progressiva; fraqueza e atrofia progressivas dos músculos da língua, lábios, palato, faringe e laringe, que geralmente ocorre na velhice; na maioria das vezes é causada por doença do neurônio motor. SIN bulbar palsy, bulbar p., Erb disease, glossolabiolaryngeal p., glossolabiopharyngeal p.

pseudobulbar p., p. pseudobulbar; paralisia dos lábios e da língua, simulando paralisia bulbar progressiva, mas causada por lesões supranucleares com envolvimento bilateral dos neurônios motores superiores; caracterizada por dificuldades da fala e da deglutição, instabilidade emocional e risada deprimida, espasmódica.

sensory p., p. sensorial; perda da sensibilidade; anestesia.

sleep p., p. do sono; perda episódica breve do movimento voluntário que ocorre ao adormecer (paralisia do sono hipnagógica) ou ao acordar (paralisia do sono hipnopômpica). Uma das tétrades narcolépticas. SIN sleep dissociation.

sodium-responsive periodic p., p. periódica responsiva ao sódio. SIN normokalemic periodic p.

spastic spinal p., p. espinal espástica. SIN spastic *diplegia*.

spinal p., p. espinal; perda da capacidade motora causada por uma lesão da medula espinal. SIN myeloparalysis, myeloplegia, rachioplegia.

supranuclear p., p. supranuclear; paralisia causada por lesões acima dos neurônios motores primários.

tick p., p. por carrapatos; paralisia flácida ascendente causada pela presença contínua de fêmeas grávidas dos carrapatos *Dermacentor* e *Ixodes*; descritas na América do Norte e na Austrália; afeta seres humanos (principalmente crianças) e outros animais.

Todd p., p. de Todd; paralisia temporária (normalmente não dura mais que alguns dias) que acomete o membro ou membros envolvidos na epilepsia do tipo jacksoniana após a convulsão. SIN Todd postepileptic p.

Todd postepileptic p., p. pós-epiléptica de Todd. SIN Todd p.

vasomotor p., p. vasomotora. SIN vasoparesis.

Zenker p., p. de Zenker; parestesia e paralisia na área do nervo poplíteo externo.

pa·ra·lys·sa (par′ă-lis′ă). Forma paralítica de raiva, causada pela mordida do morcego vampiro (*Desmodus*). [paralysis + G. *lyssa*, loucura (raiva)]

par·a·lyt·ic (par-ă-lit´ik). Paralítico; relativo à paralisia ou que sofre de paralisia.

par·a·lyze (par´ă-līz). Paralisar; tornar incapaz de se movimentar.

par·a·mag·net·ic (par´ă-mag-net´ik). Paramagnético; que possui a propriedade de paramagnetismo; em ressonância magnética, os contrastes são escolhidos por suas propriedades paramagnéticas, que reduzem o tempo de relaxamento.

par·a·mag·ne·tism (par-ă-mag´ne-tizm). Paramagnetismo; a propriedade de possuir um forte momento magnético de um ou mais elétrons não-pareados, causando orientação em um campo magnético; são mais significativos na produção de imagens os íons de alguns metais de transição como o gadolínio, o ferro e o manganês, ou compostos orgânicos que são radicais livres estáveis; o oxigênio molecular também exibe paramagnetismo.

par·a·mas·ti·gote (par-ă-mas´ti-gōt). Paramastigota; mastigota que possui dois flagelos, um longo e um curto. SIN paraflagellate (2). [para- + G. *mastix*, flagelo]

par·a·mas·toid (par-ă-mas´toyd). Paramastóide; próximo ao processo mastóide.

Par·a·me·ci·um (par-ă-mē´shē-ŭm, -sē-ŭm). Gênero abundante de ciliados holotríquios de água doce que possuem formato característico de pantufas e, amiúde, são suficientemente grandes para serem vistos a olho nu; comumente usados para estudos genéticos e de outros tipos. [G. *paramēkēs*, bastante longos, de *mēkos*, comprimento]

par·a·me·di·an (par-ă-mē´dē-an). Paramediano; próximo à linha média. SIN paramesial.

par·a·med·ic (par-ă-med´ik). Paramédico; pessoa treinada e habilitada a prestar atendimento médico de emergência.

par·a·med·i·cal (par-ă-med´i-kăl). Paramédico. **1.** Relacionado à profissão médica de uma forma coadjuvante, p. ex., designando campos de saúde afins, como a fisioterapia, a patologia da fala, etc. **2.** Relativo a um paramédico.

par·a·me·nia (par-ă-mē´nē-ă). Paramenia; qualquer distúrbio ou irregularidade da menstruação. [para- + G. *mēn*, mês]

par·a·me·si·al (par´ă-sē-ăl). Paramesial; paramediano. SIN paramedian.

par·a·mes·o·neph·ric (par-ă-mes-ō-nef´rik). Paramesonéfrico; próximo ao, ou ao longo do, mesonefro embrionário. VER paramesonephric *duct*.

pa·ram·e·ter (pă-ram´e-ter). Parâmetro; uma das muitas dimensões ou formas de medir ou descrever um objeto ou de avaliar um assunto: **1.** Em uma expressão matemática, uma constante arbitrária que pode possuir diferentes valores, cada um definindo outras expressões, e pode determinar a forma específica, mas não a natureza geral da expressão; p. ex., na equação $y = a + bx$, a e b são parâmetros. **2.** Em estatística, termo usado para definir uma característica de uma população, ao contrário de uma amostra daquela população; p. ex., a média e o desvio padrão de uma população total. **3.** Em psicanálise, qualquer tática, além da interpretação, usada pelo analista para promover o progresso do paciente. [para- + G. *metron*, medida]

enzyme p.'s, parâmetros enzimáticos; aqueles fatores e constantes que controlam a velocidade de uma reação catalisada por enzimas, p. ex., $V_{máx}$ e K_m.

infection transmission p., p. de transmissão de infecção; a proporção de possíveis contatos totais entre casos infecciosos e susceptíveis que levam a novas infecções. VER TAMBÉM serial *interval*, mass action *principle*.

practice p.'s, parâmetros de prática. SIN practice *guidelines*, em *guideline*.

par·a·meth·a·di·one (par´ă-meth-ă-dī´ōn). Parametadiona; anticonvulsivante usado na epilepsia tipo pequeno mal.

par·a·meth·a·sone (par-ă-meth´ă-sōn). Parametasona; glicocorticóide com efeitos antiinflamatórios e tóxicos semelhantes aos da prednisona.

p. acetate, acetato de parametasona; éster acético da parametasona em C-21; glicocorticóide útil no tratamento da artrite reumatóide e de outras doenças do colágeno, condições alérgicas e alguns distúrbios hematológicos.

par·a·me·tri·al (par-ă-mē´trē-ăl). Parametrial; relativo ao paramétrio.

par·a·met·ric (par-ă-met´rik). Paramétrico; relativo ao paramétrio ou a estruturas imediatamente adjacentes ao útero.

par·a·me·trit·ic (par´ă-me-trit´ik). Parametrítico; relativo à parametrite.

par·a·me·tri·tis (par´ă-me-trī´tis). Parametrite; inflamação do tecido adjacente ao útero, particularmente no ligamento largo. SIN pelvic cellulitis. [parametrium + G. *-itis*, inflamação]

par·a·me·tri·um, pl. **par·a·me·tria** (par-ă-mē´trē-ŭm, -ă) [TA]. Paramétrio; o tecido conjuntivo do assoalho pélvico que se estende lateralmente da túnica subserosa fibrosa da porção supracervical do útero entre as camadas do ligamento largo. [para- + G. *mētra*, útero]

par·a·mim·ia (par-ă-mim´ē-ă). Paramimia; emprego de gestos inadequados para as palavras expressadas. [para- + G. *mimia*, imitação]

par·am·ne·sia (par-am-nē´zē-ă). Paramnésia; falsas lembranças, como as de eventos que nunca aconteceram ou esquecimento parcial de eventos que aconteceram. [para- + G. *amnēsia*, esquecimento]

Par·a·moe·ba (par´ă-mē´bă). Designação antiga de *Entamoeba*.

par·a·mo·lar (par-ă-mō´lăr). Paramolar; dente supranumerário situado entre os molares maxilares ou mandibulares, ou numa posição lingual ou bucal a estes.

par·a·mor·phine (par-ă-mōr´fen). Paramorfina. SIN thebaine.

Par·am·phis·to·mat·i·dae (par´am-fis-tō-mat´i-dē). Família de trematódeos parasitas caracterizada por grandes corpos carnosos com uma grande ventosa posterior; estão incluídos os gêneros *Paramphistomum*, *Gastrodiscoides* e *Watsonius*.

par·am·phis·to·mi·a·sis (par´am-fis-tō-mī´ă-sis). Paranfistomíase; infecção de animais e seres humanos por trematódeos da família Paramphistomatidae; a doença humana é por *Gastrodiscoides hominis*, na Ásia, e por *Watsonius watnosi*, na África.

Par·am·phis·to·mum (par-am-fis´tō-mŭm). O trematódeo de ruminantes, gênero de trematódeos digenéticos (família Paramphistomatidae) parasitas do rúmen ou pança bovina; as espécies incluem *P. microbothrioides*, *P. cervi* e *P. liorchis*. [para- + G. *amphistomos*, que possui uma boca dupla, de *amphi*, que tem dois lados, + *stoma*, boca]

par·a·mu·sia (par-ă-moo´zē-ă). Paramusia; perda da capacidade de ler ou de interpretar música corretamente. [para- + G. *mousa*, música, + -ia]

par·am·y·loi·do·sis (par-am´ī-loy-dō´sis). Paramiloidose. **1.** Deposição tecidual de uma proteína amiloidótica, semelhante às cadeias leves de imunoglobulinas na amiloidose primária ou (particularmente) na amiloidose atípica do mieloma múltiplo. **2.** Várias amiloidoses hereditárias (amiloidose portuguesa, amiloidose indiana) caracterizadas por polineurite hipertrófica progressiva com alterações sensoriais, ataxia, paresia e atrofia muscular, causadas por depósitos amilóides nos nervos periféricos e viscerais.

par·a·my·oc·lo·nus mul·ti·plex (par´ă-mī-ok´lō-nŭs). Paramioclônus múltiplo. SIN myoclonus multiplex. [para- + G. *mys*, músculo, + *klonos*, agitação]

par·a·my·o·to·nia (par´ă-mī-ō-tō´nē-ă). Paramiotonia; forma atípica de miotonia. SIN paramyotonus.

ataxic p., p. atáxica; distúrbio caracterizado por espasmo muscular tônico, ao tentar se movimentar, associado a discreta paresia e ataxia.

congenital p., p. congen'ita [MIM*168300], p. congênita; miotonia não-progressiva, induzida por exposição dos músculos ao frio; há episódios de paralisia flácida intermitente, mas não há atrofia nem hipertrofia dos músculos; herança autossômica dominante causada por mutação no gene do canal de sódio (SCN4A) no cromossoma 17q. Este é um distúrbio alélico à paralisia periódica hiperpotassêmica (hyperkalemic periodic *paralysis*). Há uma forma variante autossômica dominante [MIM*168350] na qual o frio não age como fator de provocação. SIN Eulenburg disease.

par·a·my·ot·o·nus (par-ă-mī-ot´ō-nŭs). Paramiotônus. SIN paramyotonia.

Par·a·myx·o·vir·i·dae (par´ă-mik´sō-vir´i-dē). Família de vírus que contêm RNA, apresentam aproximadamente o dobro do tamanho dos vírus influenza (Orthomyxoviridae), mas sua morfologia é semelhante a destes. Os vírions têm 150–300 nm de diâmetro, possuem envoltório, são sensíveis ao éter e contêm RNA polimerase RNA-dependente. Os nucleocapsídeos são helicoidais, consideravelmente maiores que os dos vírus influenza e contêm RNA monofilamentar não-segmentado. São conhecidos quatro gêneros: Paramyxovirus, Morbillivirus, Rubulavirus e Pneumovirus, todos os quais causam fusão celular e produzem inclusões eosinofílicas citoplasmáticas. As doenças associadas a esses vírus incluem crupe e outras infecções respiratórias altas, sarampo, caxumba e pneumonia.

Par·a·myx·o·vi·rus (par-ă-mik´sō-vi-rŭs). Gênero de vírus (família Paramyxoviridae) que inclui os vírus parainfluenza (tipos 1 e 3).

par·an·al·ge·sia (par-an-ăl-jē´zē-ă). Paranalgesia; analgesia da metade inferior do corpo. [para- + analgesia]

par·a·na·sal (par-ă-nā´săl). Paranasal; paralelo ao nariz.

par·a·ne·o·pla·sia (par´ă-nē-ō-plā´zē-ă). Paraneoplasia; distúrbios hormonais, neurológicos, hematológicos e outros distúrbios clínicos e bioquímicos associados a neoplasias malignas, mas não relacionados diretamente à invasão pelo tumor primário ou suas metástases.

par·a·ne·o·plas·tic (par´ă-nē-ō-plas´tik). Paraneoplásico; relativo a, ou característico de, paraneoplasia.

par·a·neph·ric (par-ă-nef´rik). Paranéfrico. **1.** Relativo ao paranefro. **2.** SIN pararenal.

par·a·neph·ros, pl. **par·a·neph·roi** (par-ă-nef´ros, -nef´roy). Glândula supra-renal. SIN suprarenal *gland*. [para- + G. *nephros*, rim]

par·an·es·the·sia (par-an-es-thē´zē-ă). Paranestesia; anestesia da metade inferior do corpo. [para- + anesthesia]

par·a·neu·rone (par-ă-noor´ōn). Paraneurônio; glândula ou conjunto de células contendo grânulos neurossecretores. SIN neuroendocrine cell (2).

pa·ran·gi (pă-rang´gē, -ran´jē). Doença semelhante à bouba que ocorre em Sri Lanka (antigo Ceilão).

par·a·noia (par-ă-noy´ă). Paranóia; transtorno mental grave, mas relativamente raro, caracterizado por delírios sistematizados, freqüentemente de caráter persecutório, no qual o indivíduo acredita estar sendo seguido, envenenado ou prejudicado por outros meios, sem outros distúrbios da personalidade. VER TAMBÉM paranoid *personality*. [G. perturbação, loucura, de para- + *noeō*, pensar]

acute hallucinatory p., p. alucinatória aguda; uma forma na qual ocorrem períodos de alucinação além dos delírios.

litigious p., p. litigiosa; forma de paranóia na qual uma pessoa é propensa a iniciar ações judiciais.

par·a·noi·ac (par-ă-noy′ak). Paranóico. **1.** Relativo a, ou afetado por, paranóia. **2.** Aquele que sofre de paranóia.

par·a·noid (par′ă-noyd). Paranóide. **1.** Relativo a, ou caracterizado por, paranóia. **2.** Que apresenta delírio persecutório.

par·a·no·mia (par-ă-nō′mē-ă). Paranomia; forma de afasia na qual os objetos são chamados por nomes errados. [para- + G. *onoma*, nome]

par·a·nu·cle·ar (par-ă-noo′klē-ăr). Paranuclear. **1.** SIN paranucleate. **2.** Do lado de fora, mas próximo do núcleo.

par·a·nu·cle·ate (par′ă-noo′klē-āt). Paranuclear; relativo a ou que possui um paranúcleo. SIN paranuclear (1).

par·a·nu·cle·o·lus (par′ă-noo-klē′ō-lŭs). Paranucléolo. VER sex *chromatin*.

par·a·nu·cle·us (par-ă-noo′klē-ŭs). Paranúcleo; núcleo acessório ou uma pequena massa de cromatina situada fora do núcleo, embora próxima dele.

par·a·om·phal·ic (par′ă-om-fal′ik). Paraonfálico. SIN paraumbilical. [para- + G. *omphalos*, umbigo]

par·a·op·er·a·tive (par-ă-op′er-ă-tiv). Perioperatório. SIN perioperative.

par·a·o·ral (par-ă-ō′ral). Paraoral; próximo ou adjacente à boca. [para- + L. *os* (*or*-), boca]

par·a·o·var·i·an (par′ă-ō-var′ē-an). Paraovariano. SIN parovarian (2).

par·a·ox·on (par-ă-ok′son). Paraoxon; inibidor da colinesterase organofosforado, usado em inseticidas; o paration é convertido em paraoxon no fígado.

par·a·pan·cre·at·ic (par′ă-pan-krē-at′ik). Parapancreático; próximo ou paralelo ao pâncreas.

par·a·pa·re·sis (par-ă-pă-rē′sis). Paraparesia; fraqueza que afeta os membros inferiores. [para- + paresis]

par·a·pa·ret·ic (par′ă-pă-ret′ik). Paraparético. **1.** Relativo à paraparesia. **2.** Uma pessoa com paraparesia.

par·a·pe·de·sis (par′ă-pē-dē′sis). Parapedese; excreção ou secreção através de um canal anormal [para- + G. *pedēsis*, curvatura, deflexão]

par·a·per·i·to·ne·al (par′ă-per′i-tō-nē′al). Paraperitoneal; fora do peritônio ou paralelo a ele.

par·a·pes·tis (par-ă-pes′tis). Parapeste. SIN ambulant *plague*. [para- + L. *pestis*, peste]

par·a·pha·sia (par-ă-fā′zē-ă). Parafasia; forma de afasia na qual uma pessoa perdeu a capacidade de falar corretamente, substituindo uma palavra por outra e confundindo palavras e sentenças de forma ininteligível. VER TAMBÉM jargon. SIN paragrammatism, paraphrasia, pseudoagrammatism. [para- + G. *phasis*, discurso]

thematic p., p. temática; discurso incoerente que se desvia do tema ou do assunto em discussão.

par·a·pha·sic (par-ă-fā′sik). Parafásico; relativo à parafasia.

pa·ra·phia (pa-rā′fē-ă). Parafia; qualquer distúrbio do sentido do tato. SIN pseudesthesia (1), pseudoesthesia (1). [para- + G. *haphē*, tato]

par·a·phil·ia (par-ă-fil′ē-ă). Parafilia. **1.** Condição, que acomete homens ou mulheres, de responsividade compulsiva e dependência obrigatória de estímulo externo inaceitável, do ponto de vista pessoal ou social, ou de fantasia interna para excitação sexual ou orgasmo. **2.** No discurso legal, uma perversão ou desvio. [para- + G. *philos*, afinidade]

par·a·phi·mo·sis (par′ă-fi-mō′sis). Parafimose. **1.** Constrição dolorosa da glande do pênis por um prepúcio fimótico, que foi retraído além da coroa. **2.** VER p. palpebrae. [para- + G. *phimosis*]

p. palpe'brae, p. palpebral; eversão espástica total das pálpebras superior e inferior.

par·a·pho·nia (par-ă-fō′nē-ă). Parafonia; qualquer distúrbio da voz, principalmente uma alteração de seu tom. [para- + G. *phōnē*, voz]

par·a·phra·sia (par-ă-frā′zē-ă). Parafrasia. SIN paraphasia. [para- + G. *phrasis*, discurso]

par·a·phys·i·al, par·a·phys·e·al (par-ă-fiz′ē-ăl). Parafisário; relativo à paráfise.

pa·raph·y·sis, pl. **pa·raph·y·ses** (pă-raf′i-sis, -sēz). Paráfise; órgão mediano que se desenvolve do teto do diencéfalo em determinados vertebrados inferiores. Presente no embrião humano e no feto por um curto período. SIN paraphysial body. [G. ramo]

par·a·pin·e·al (par-ă-pin′ē-ăl). Parapineal; ao lado da pineal; designa a porção visual ou fotorreceptora do corpo pineal presente, se não estiver funcionando, em alguns lagartos.

par·a·plasm (par′ă-plazm). Paraplasma. **1.** Designação obsoleta de hialoplasma. **2.** Tecido malformado ou anormal. [para- + G. *plasma*, algo formado]

par·a·plas·tic (par-ă-plas′tik). Paraplástico; relativo ao paraplasma.

par·a·ple·gia (par-ă-plē′jē-ă). Paraplegia; paralisia de ambos os membros inferiores e, geralmente, da parte inferior do tronco. [para- + *plēgē*, acesso]

ataxic p., p. atáxica; ataxia progressiva e paresia dos músculos da perna causadas por esclerose dos funículos lateral e posterior da medula espinal.

congenital spastic p., p. espástica congênita; paralisia espástica dos membros inferiores que ocorre no lactente. SIN infantile spastic p.

p. doloro'sa, p. dolorosa; paralisia dos membros inferiores na qual as partes afetadas, apesar da perda do movimento e da sensibilidade, são a fonte de dor excruciante; ocorre em alguns casos de câncer da medula espinal. SIN painful p.

p. in extension, p. em extensão; paralisia das pernas, mantidas em posição estendida por músculos extensores hipertônicos.

p. in flexion, p. em flexão; a fixação das pernas paralisadas em uma postura fletida; geralmente na transecção da medula espinal.

infantile spastic p., p. espástica do lactente. SIN congenital spastic p.

painful p., p. dolorosa. SIN p. dolorosa.

Pott p., p. de Pott; paralisia da parte inferior do corpo e dos membros, causada por compressão da medula espinal em virtude de espondilite tuberculosa. SIN Pott paralysis.

spastic p., p. espástica; paresia dos membros inferiores com aumento do tônus muscular e contração espasmódica dos músculos. SIN Erb-Charcot disease (2).

superior p., p. superior; paralisia de ambos os braços.

par·a·ple·gic (par-ă-plē′jik). Paraplégico; relativo a, ou que sofre de, paraplegia.

Par·a·pox·vi·rus (par-ă-poks′vī-rŭs). O gênero de vírus (família Poxviridae) que inclui os vírus do ectima contagioso dos ovinos, da estomatite pavular bovina e paravacínia. Eles possuem o antígeno da nucleoproteína comum a todos os vírus incluídos na família, mas diferem dos outros poxvírus em morfologia (p. ex., os víríons são menores e possuem revestimentos externos mais espessos) e por não se multiplicarem em ovos embrionados.

par·a·prax·ia (par-ă-prak′sē-ă). Parapraxia; uma condição análoga à parafasia e paragrafia, na qual há um distúrbio na realização de atos intencionais; p. ex., lapsos verbais ou colocação de objetos em locais errados. [para- + G. *praxis*, fazer]

par·a·proc·ti·tis (par′ă-prok-tī′tis). Paraproctite; inflamação do tecido celular adjacente ao reto. [para- + G. *prōktos*, ânus, + -*itis*, inflamação]

par·a·proc·ti·um, pl. **par·a·proc·tia** (par′ă-prok′shē-um, -tē-ŭm; -ă). O tecido celular adjacente ao reto. [para- + G. *proktos*, ânus]

par·a·pros·ta·ti·tis (par′ă-pros-ta-tī′tis). Paraprostatite; designação obsoleta da inflamação do tecido adjacente à próstata. [para- + L. *prostata*, próstata, + -*itis*, inflamação]

par·a·pro·tein (par-a-prō′tēn). Paraproteína. **1.** Uma imunoglobulina monoclonal do plasma sanguíneo, observada eletroforeticamente como uma faixa intensa nas regiões γ, β ou α, devido a um aumento isolado de um único tipo de imunoglobulina em virtude de um clone de plasmócitos originados da multiplicação rápida anormal de uma única célula. O achado de uma paraproteína no soro de um paciente indica a presença de um clone proliferativo de células produtoras de imunoglobulina, e pode ser observada em várias doenças malignas, benignas ou não-neoplásicas. **2.** SIN monoclonal *immunoglobulin*. [para- + proteína, do G. *protos*, primeiro]

par·a·pro·tein·e·mia (par′ă-prō-tēn-ē′mē-ă). Paraproteinemia; a presença de uma gamopatia monoclonal no sangue.

par·a·pso·ri·a·sis (par′ă-sō-rī′ă-sis). Parapsoríase; grupo heterogêneo de distúrbios cutâneos não relacionados à psoríase, incluindo pitiríase liquenóide e parapsoríase em placas pequenas e grandes.

p. en plaque, p. em placas; forma de parapsoríase em grandes placas que aparece na meia-idade e freqüentemente se transforma em micose fungóide. Afeta o tronco e a parte proximal dos membros, as lesões têm mais de 5 cm de diâmetro e freqüentemente são simétricas. A parapsoríase em pequenas placas é uma variante benigna, também denominada dermatose digitiforme.

p. gutta'ta, p. em gotas. SIN *pityriasis* lichenoides.

p. lichenoi'des, p. liquenóide. SIN *poikiloderma* atrophicans vasculare.

p. lichenoi'des et variolifor'mis acu'ta, p. liquenóide e varioliforme aguda. SIN *pityriasis* lichenoides et varioliformis acuta.

small plaque p., p. em pequenas placas. SIN digitate *dermatosis*.

p. variolifor'mis, p. varioliforme. SIN *pityriasis* lichenoides et varioliformis acuta.

par·a·psy·chol·o·gy (par′ă-sī-kol′ō-jē). Parapsicologia; o estudo da percepção extra-sensorial, como a transmissão de pensamento (telepatia) e clarividência.

par·a·quat (par′ă-kwaht). Paraquat; agente destruidor de ervas daninhas que produz efeitos tóxicos tardios no fígado, rins e pulmões quando ingerido; pode haver desenvolvimento de pneumonia intersticial progressiva com proliferação das células de revestimento alveolar.

par·a·ra·ma (par-ă-rā′mă). Parama; doença dolorosa ou incapacitante dos dedos das mãos, descrita pela primeira vez em seringueiros brasileiros, produzida por contato acidental com as cerdas das larvas da traça *Premolis semirufa*; prurido imediato, hiperemia e edema local podem ser seguidos por edema crônico e imobilidade, que podem levar à perda de um ou mais dedos das mãos, apresentando um quadro clínico correspondente à anquilose.

par·a·rec·tal (par-ă-rek′tăl). Pararretal; próximo do reto ou do músculo reto.

par·a·re·nal (par-ă-rē′năl). Pararrenal; próximo ou adjacente aos rins. SIN paranephric (2).

par·a·rho·ta·cism (par′ă-rō′tă-sizm). Pararrotacismo; substituição do fonema r por outro. VER TAMBÉM rhotacism. [para- + G. *rho*, letra r]

par·a·ro·san·i·lin (par´ă-rō-san´ĭ-lin) [C.I. 42500]. Pararrosanilina; cloridrato de tri(aminofenil)metano; importante corante biológico vermelho usado no reagente de Schiff para detectar DNA celular (corante de Feulgen), mucopolissacarídeos (coloração PAS) e proteínas (coloração de ninidrina-Schiff). SIN parafuchsin.

par·ar·rhyth·mia (par-ă-ridh´mē-ă). Pararritmia; arritmia cardíaca na qual coexistem dois ritmos independentes, mas não causada por bloqueio A–V; a pararritmia então inclui parassístole e dissociação A–V (2), mas não bloqueio A–V completo. [para- + G. *rhythmos*, ritmo]

par·a·sac·ral (par-ă-sā´kral). Parassacral; paralelo ao sacro.

par·a·sal·pin·gi·tis (par´ă-sal-pin-jī´tis). Parassalpingite; inflamação dos tecidos adjacentes à tuba uterina ou auditiva. [para- + salpinx + G. *-itis*, inflamação]

Par·as·ca·ris equo·rum (par-ras´ka-ris ē-kwō´rum). Um grande nematódeo ascarídeo, de corpo pesado, extremamente comum no intestino delgado de cavalos e outros eqüinos. As larvas podem desenvolver-se em seres humanos ou em camundongos, mas não chegam ao estágio adulto. SIN *Ascaris equorum*.

par·a·scar·la·ti·na (par´ă-skar-lă-tē´nă). Paraescarlatina. SIN Filatov-Dukes *disease.*

par·a·sex·u·al·i·ty (par´ă-sek-shŭ-al´ĭ-tē). Parassexualidade; anormalidade ou perversão da sexualidade.

par·a·sig·ma·tism (par-ă-sig´mă-tizm). Parassigmatismo. SIN lisping. [para- + G. *sigma*, a letra s]

par·a·si·noi·dal (par´ă-sī-noy´dal). Parassinusal; próximo de um seio, sobretudo um seio cerebral.

par·a·site (par´ă-sīt). Parasita. **1.** Organismo que vive sobre ou no interior de outro e dele retira sua nutrição. **2.** No caso de uma inclusão fetal ou gêmeos conjugados, o gêmeo geralmente incompleto que retira seu sustento do autósito mais próximo do normal. [G. *parasitos*, um hóspede, de *para*, ao lado de, + *sitos*, alimento]

  accidental p., p. acidental. SIN incidental p.
  autistic p., p. autóctone; parasita oriundo dos tecidos do hospedeiro. SIN autochthonous p.
  autochthonous p., p. autóctone. SIN autistic p.
  commensal p., p. comensal. VER commensal (2).
  euroxenous p., p. euroxeno; parasita com uma faixa de hospedeiros ampla ou inespecífica.
  facultative p., p. facultativo; organismo que pode levar uma existência independente ou viver como parasita, ao contrário do parasita obrigatório.
  heterogenetic p., p. heterogenético; parasita cujo ciclo vital envolve uma alternação de gerações.
  heteroxenous p., p. heteroxeno; parasita que possui mais de um hospedeiro obrigatório em seu ciclo vital.
  incidental p., p. incidental; parasita que normalmente vive em outro hospedeiro além de seu hospedeiro normal. SIN accidental p.
  inquiline p., p. inquilino. VER inquiline.
  malignant tertian malarial p., p. malárico terça maligno. SIN *Plasmodium falciparum.*
  obligate p., p. obrigatório; parasita que não consegue levar uma existência não-parasitária independente, ao contrário do parasita facultativo.
  quartan p., p. quartã. SIN *Plasmodium malariae.*
  specific p., p. específico; parasita que habitualmente vive em seu hospedeiro atual e está particularmente adaptado para a espécie do hospedeiro.
  spurious p., p. espúrio; organismos que parasitam outros hospedeiros que atravessam o intestino humano e são detectados nas fezes após a ingestão (p. ex., ovos de *Capillaria* sp. no fígado de animal).
  stenoxous p., p. estenoxeno; parasita com uma faixa de hospedeiros estreita ou específica.
  temporary p., p. temporário; organismo acidentalmente ingerido que sobrevive por um curto período no intestino.
  tertian p., p. terçã. SIN *Plasmodium vivax.*

par·a·si·te·mia (par´ă-si-tē´mē-ă). Parasitemia; a presença de parasitas no sangue circulante; usado particularmente em relação aos agentes da malária e a outros protozoários e microfilárias.

par·a·sit·ic (par-ă-sit´ik). Parasitário. **1.** Relativo a parasita ou que possui a mesma natureza deste. **2.** Designa organismos que normalmente crescem apenas no interior ou sobre o corpo vivo de um hospedeiro.

par·a·sit·i·ci·dal (par´ă-sit-i-sī´dăl). Parasiticida; destrutivo para os parasitas.

par·a·sit·i·cide (par-ă-sit´ĭ-sīd). Parasiticida; agente que destrói parasitas. [parasite + L. *caedo*, matar]

par·a·sit·ism (par´ă-si-tizm). Parasitismo; relação simbiótica na qual uma espécie (o parasita) beneficia-se à custa do outro (o hospedeiro). Cf. mutualism, commensalism, symbiosis, metabiosis.
  multiple p., p. múltiplo; condição na qual parasitas de diferentes espécies parasitam um único hospedeiro, ao contrário do superparasitismo (superparasitism) (2) ou hiperparasitismo (hyperparasitism).

par·a·si·tize (par´ă-si-tīz). Parasitar; invadir como parasita.

par·a·si·to·ce·nose (par-ă-sī´tō-sē-nōz). Parasitocenose; complexo de todas as espécies de parasitas e indivíduos associados a um hospedeiro específico. SIN parasite-host ecosystem. [parasite + G. *koinos*, comum, junto]

par·a·si·to·gen·e·sis (par´ă-sī-tō-jen´ĕ-sis). Parasitogênese; a evolução das relações entre parasita e hospedeiro.

par·a·si·to·gen·ic (par´-ă-sī-tō-jen´ik). Parasitogênico. **1.** Causado por determinados parasitas. **2.** Que favorece o parasitismo. [parasite + G. *-gen*, que produz]

par·a·si·toid (par-ă-sī´toyd). Parasitóide; designa uma relação alimentar intermediária entre a predação e o parasitismo, na qual o parasita acaba por destruir seu hospedeiro; refere-se particularmente a vespas parasitárias (ordem Hymenoptera), cujas larvas se alimentam de uma lagarta e acabam destruindo-a ou a outro hospedeiro artrópode picado pela vespa-mãe antes de pôr seu(s) ovo(s) no hospedeiro. [parasite + G. *eidos*, aparência]

par·a·si·tol·o·gist (par´ă-sī-tol´ō-jist). Parasitologista; aquele que se especializa na ciência da parasitologia.

par·a·si·tol·o·gy (par´ă-sī-tol´ō-jē). Parasitologia; ramo da biologia e da medicina que estuda todos os aspectos do parasitismo. [parasite + G. *logos*, estudo]

par·a·si·tome (par´ă-sī-tōm). Parasitoma; a massa ou o número total de indivíduos de todos os estágios de desenvolvimento de uma única espécie de parasita em um hospedeiro. [parasite + *-ome* (do G. *-ōma*), grupo, massa]

par·a·si·to·pho·bia (par´ă-sī-tō-fō´bē-ă). Parasitofobia; medo mórbido de parasitas. [parasite + G. *phobos*, medo]

par·a·sit·o·sis (par´ă-sī-tō´sis). Parasitose; infestação ou infecção por parasitas.

par·a·si·to·trop·ic (par´ă-sī-tō-trop´ik). Parasitotrópico; relativo a, ou caracterizado por, parasitotropismo.

par·a·si·tot·ro·pism (par´ă-sī-tot´rō-pizm). Parasitotropismo; a afinidade especial de determinados medicamentos ou outros agentes para parasitas e não para seus hospedeiros, incluindo microparasitas que infectam um parasita maior. Cf. organotropism. SIN parasitotropy. [parasite + G. *tropē*, uma volta]

par·a·si·tot·ro·py (par´ă-sī-tot´rō-pē). Parasitotropia. SIN parasitotropism.

par·a·som·nia (par-ă-som´nē-ă). Parassonia; qualquer disfunção associada ao sono, p. ex., sonambulismo, terror noturno, enurese ou convulsões noturnas.

par·a·sta·sis (par-ă-sta´sis). Parastasia; relação recíproca entre mecanismos causais que podem compensar ou mascarar defeitos um no outro; em genética, uma relação entre não-alelos (classificada por alguns como uma forma de epistasia). [G. ficar lado a lado]

par·a·ster·nal (par-ă-ster´năl). Paraesternal; paralelo ao esterno.

Par·a·stron·gy·lus (par´ă-stron´ji-lus). SIN Angiostrongylus.

parasubiculum. Parassubículo; região estreita do córtex localizada entre a área entorrinal (córtex) e o subículo.

par·a·sym·pa·thet·ic (par-ă-sim-pa-thet´ik). Parassimpático; relativo a uma divisão do sistema nervoso autônomo. VER autonomic *division* of nervous system.

par·a·sym·pa·tho·lyt·ic (par-ă-sim´pa-thō-lit´ik). Parassimpaticolítico; relativo a um agente que anula ou antagoniza os efeitos do sistema nervoso parassimpático; p. ex., atropina.

par·a·sym·pa·tho·mi·met·ic (par-ă-sim´pa-thō-mi-met´ik). Parassimpaticomimético; relativo a medicamentos ou substâncias químicas com ação semelhante àquela causada por estimulação do sistema nervoso parassimpático. VER TAMBÉM cholinomimetic. [para- + G. *sympatheia*, simpatia, + *mimētikos*, que imita]

par·a·sym·pa·tho·to·nia (par-ă-sim´pa-thō-tō´nē-ă). Parassimpaticotonia. SIN vagotonia.

par·a·sy·nap·sis (par´ă-si-nap´sis). Parassinapse; união de cromossomas lado a lado no processo de redução. [para- + G. *synapsis*, uma conexão, junção]

par·a·sy·no·vi·tis (par´ă-si-nō-vī´tis). Parassinovite; inflamação dos tecidos imediatamente adjacentes a uma articulação. [para- + synovitis]

par·a·syph·i·lis (par-ă-sif´ĭ-lis). Parassífilis; qualquer condição indiretamente causada por sífilis. SIN metasyphilis (2), parasyphilosis, quaternary syphilis.

par·a·syph·i·lit·ic (par´ă-sif-i-lit´ik). Parassifilítico; designa algumas doenças consideradas indiretamente causadas pela sífilis, mas que não apresentam nenhuma das lesões reconhecidas dessa infecção. SIN metaluetic (3). SIN metasyphilitic (3).

par·a·syph·i·lo·sis (par´ă-sif-i-lō´sis). Parassifilose. SIN parasyphilis.

par·a·sys·to·le (par-ă-sis´tō-lē). Parassístole; ritmo automático secundário simultâneo ao ritmo sinusal normal ou a outro ritmo dominante, sendo o centro parassistólico protegido dos impulsos do ritmo dominante, de forma que seu ritmo básico não é perturbado, embora possa se manifestar no ECG apenas em vários múltiplos de sua periodicidade básica. SIN parasystolic beat. [para- + G. *systolē*, uma contração]

par·a·tax·ia (par-ă-tak´sē-ă). Parataxia. SIN parataxis.

par·a·tax·ic (par-ă-tak'sik). Parataxico; relativo à parataxia.

par·a·tax·is (par-ă-tak'sis). Parataxia; designação antiga do estado psicológico ou repositório de atitudes, idéias e experiências acumuladas durante o desenvolvimento da personalidade que não são efetivamente assimilados ou integrados na massa em crescimento e no montante das outras atitudes, idéias e experiências da personalidade de um indivíduo. SIN parataxia. [para- + G. *taxis*, disposição ordenada]

par·a·te·ne·sis (par-ă-te-nē'sis). Paratênese; passagem de um agente infeccioso por um hospedeiro paratênico, ou por uma série deles, na qual o agente é transportado entre hospedeiros, mas não sofre desenvolvimento adicional. [parasite + L. *teneo*, segurar, manter]

par·a·ten·on (par-ă-ten'on). Paratendão; o tecido, adiposo ou sinovial, entre um tendão e sua bainha. [para- + G. *tenōn*, tendão]

par·a·ter·mi·nal (par-ă-ter'mi-nal). Paraterminal; próximo ou paralelo a qualquer terminação.

par·a·thi·on (par-ă-thī'on). Parathion; inseticida organofosforado, altamente tóxico para animais e seres humanos, que é um inibidor irreversível das colinesterases.

par·a·thor·mone (par-ă-thōr'mōn). Paratormônio. SIN parathyroid *hormone*.

par·a·thy·mia (par-ă-thī'mē-ă). Paratimia; má orientação das faculdades emocionais; transtorno do humor. [para- + G. *thymos*, alma, mente]

par·a·thy·rin (par-ă-thī'rin). Paratormônio. SIN parathyroid *hormone*.

par·a·thy·roid (par-ă-thī'royd). Paratireóide. 1. Adjacente à glândula tireóide. 2. SIN parathyroid *gland*.

par·a·thy·roid·ec·to·my (pa'ră-thī-roy-dek'to-mē). Paratireoidectomia; excisão das paratireóides. [parathyroid + G. *ektomē*, excisão]

par·a·thy·ro·tro·pic, par·a·thy·ro·tro·phic (par'ă-thī-rō-trop'ik-trof'ik). Paratireotrófico; que influencia o crescimento ou a atividade das glândulas paratireóides. [parathyroid + G. *trope*, uma volta; *trophē*, nutrição]

par·a·tope (par'ă-tōp). Paratopo; parte de uma molécula de anticorpo composta das regiões variáveis de cadeias leves e pesadas que se combinam ao antígeno. SIN antibody-combining site, antigen-binding site. [para- + -tope]

par·a·tri·cho·sis (par'ă-tri-kō'sis). Paratricose; qualquer distúrbio do crescimento dos pêlos, com particular referência à quantidade. [para- + G. *trichōsis*, tornar ou estar piloso, de *thrix* (*trich*-), pêlos]

par·a·trip·sis (par-ă-trip'sis). Paratripsia; fricção. [G. fricção, de *para*, ao lado de, + *tripsis*, esfregar]

par·a·tro·phic (par-ă-trof'ik). Paratrófico; que retira seu sustento de material orgânico vivo. VER TAMBÉM metatrophic, prototrophic. [para- + G. *trophē*, nutrição]

par·a·typh·li·tis (par'ă-tif-lī'tis). Paratiflite; inflamação do tecido conjuntivo adjacente ao ceco. [para- + G. *typhlon*, ceco, + *-itis*, inflamação]

par·a·ty·phoid (par-ă-tī'foyd). Febre paratifóide. SIN paratyphoid *fever*.

par·a·um·bil·i·cal (par'ă-ŭm-bil'i-kal). Paraumbilical; próximo do umbigo. SIN paraomphalic, paraumbilical.

par·a·u·re·thral (par'ă-ū-rē'thral). Parauretral; paralelo à uretra.

par·a·vac·cin·ia (par'ă-vak-sin'ē-ă). Paravacínia; nome antigo do vírus Pseudocowpox. SIN milkers' *nodules*, em *nodule*.

par·a·vag·i·nal (par-ă-vaj'i-nal). Paravaginal; paralelo à vagina.

par·a·vag·i·ni·tis (par'ă-vaj-i-nī'tis). Paravaginite; inflamação do tecido conjuntivo paralelo à vagina. SIN paracolpitis.

par·a·val·vu·lar (par-ă-val'vū-lăr). Paravalvular; paralelo ou adjacente a uma válvula.

par·a·ve·nous (par'ă-vē'nŭs). Paravenoso; ao lado de uma veia.

par·a·ver·te·bral (par-ă-ver'te-bral). Paravertebral; paralelo a uma vértebra ou à coluna vertebral.

par·a·ves·i·cal (par-ă-ves'i-kăl). Paravesical. SIN paracystic.

par·ax·i·al (par-ak'sē-ăl). Paraxial; ao lado do eixo de qualquer corpo ou parte.

par·ax·on (par-ak'son). Paraxônio; um ramo colateral de um axônio. [para- + G. *axōn*, eixo]

Par·a·zoa (par-ă-zō'ă). Sub-reino que inclui as esponjas (filo Porifera), considerado por muitos zoólogos intermediário entre os sub-reinos Protozoa e Metazoa.

par·a·zo·on (par-ă-zō'on). Parazoário. 1. Um animal parasita. 2. Um membro do sub-reino Parazoa. [para- + G. *zōon*, animal]

parch·ment crack·ling (parch'ment krak'ling). Crepitação de pergaminho; a sensação de crepitação de pergaminho ou de papel duro à palpação do crânio em casos de craniotabes.

Paré, Ambroïse, cirurgião francês, 1510–1590. VER P. *suture*.

par·e·gor·ic (par-ē-gōr'ik). Paregórico; tintura de ópio canforada, agente antiperistáltico contendo ópio em pó, óleo de erva-doce, ácido benzóico, cânfora, glicerina e álcool diluído. [G. *paregorikos*, calmante]

pa·rei·ra (pă-rā'-ră). Parreira-brava, erva-do-mato; a raiz de *Chondodendron tomentosum* e de outras espécies de *Chondodendron* (família Menispermaceae), videira da América tropical; uma das principais fontes de D-tubocurarina; possui propriedades diuréticas e anti-sépticas urinárias. [Pg. *parreira*, videira que cresce de encontro a uma parede]

par·e·lec·tro·nom·ic (par'ē-lek-trō-nom'ik). Pareletronômico; não sujeito às leis da eletricidade, isto é, não excitado por um estímulo elétrico. [para- + G. *ēlektron*, âmbar (eletricidade), + *nomos*, lei]

par·en·ce·pha·lia (par'en-se-fā'lē-ă). Parencefalia; defeito congênito do encéfalo. [para- + G. *enkephalos*, encéfalo]

par·en·ceph·a·li·tis (par'en-sef-ă-lī'tis). Parencefalite; inflamação do cerebelo. [parencephalon + G. *-itis*, inflamação]

par·en·ceph·a·lo·cele (par-en-sef'ă-lō-sēl). Parencefalocele; protrusão do cerebelo através de um defeito no crânio. [parencephalon + G. *kēlē*, hérnia]

par·en·ceph·a·lous (par-en-sef'ă-lŭs). Parencéfalo; relativo à parencefalia.

pa·ren·chy·ma (pă-reng'ki-mă) [TA]. Parênquima. 1. As células diferenciadas ou específicas de uma glândula ou órgão, contidas e sustentadas pela estrutura de tecido conjuntivo, ou estroma. 2. O endoplasma de um protozoário. [G. qualquer coisa derramada ao lado de, de *parencheō*, derramar ao lado de]

p. glandulae thyroideae [TA], p. da glândula tireóide. SIN p. of thyroid gland.

p. prostatae [TA], p. da próstata. SIN p. of prostate.

p. of prostate [TA], p. da próstata; o tecido celular básico (substância) que forma a próstata. SIN p. prostatae [TA].

p. tes'tis [TA], p. do testículo. SIN p. of testis.

p. of testis [TA], p. do testículo; a substância tecidual celular básica que forma o testículo, consistindo nos túbulos seminíferos e nas células intersticiais (células de Leydig e Sertoli) localizadas nos lóbulos. SIN p. testis [TA].

p. of thyroid gland [TA], p. da glândula tireóide; o tecido celular básico (substância) que forma a tireóide, organizado na forma de folículos. SIN p. glandulae thyroideae [TA].

pa·ren·chy·mal (pă-reng'ki-mal). Parenquimatoso. SIN parenchymatous.

pa·ren·chy·ma·ti·tis (pă-reng'ki-mă-tī'tis). Parenquimatite; inflamação do parênquima ou substância diferenciada de uma glândula ou órgão.

par·en·chym·a·tous (par'eng-kim'ă-tŭs). Parenquimatoso; relativo ao parênquima. SIN parenchymal.

par·ent (par'ent). Genitor; pai ou mãe. 1. Indivíduo que teve pelo menos um descendente através de reprodução sexuada. 2. Qualquer origem ou base, como para a elaboração de uma substância. [L. *parens*, de *pario*, produzir, parir]

par·en·ter·al (pă-ren'ter-ăl). Parenteral; por outra via que não seja o trato gastrointestinal; referindo-se sobretudo à introdução de substâncias em um organismo por injeção intravenosa, subcutânea, intramuscular ou intramedular. [para- + G. *enteron*, intestino]

Parenti, Gian Carlo, médico italiano. VER Parenti-Fraccaro *syndrome*.

par·ep·i·cele (par-ep'i-sēl). Parepicele; o recesso lateral do quarto ventrículo do encéfalo. [para- + G. *epi*, sobre, + *koilia*, cavidade]

par·ep·i·did·y·mis (par'ep'i-did'i-mis). Parepidídimo. SIN paradidymis.

par·ep·i·thy·mia (par'ep-i-thī'mē-ă). Parepitimia; designação antiga para um desejo mórbido; um desejo ou ânsia anormal. [para- + G. *epithymia*, desejo]

par·e·re·thi·sis (par-ĕ-rēth'i-sis). Pareretise; termo antigo para excitação anormal ou mórbida. [para- + G. *erethizō*, excitar]

pa·re·sis (pă-rē'sis, par'ĕ-sis). Paresia; paralisia parcial ou incompleta. [G. relaxamento, atonia, paralisia, de *pariēmi*, relaxar]

divergence p., p. divergente; esodesvio dos olhos maior a distância que para perto, e que pode ser um sinal de doença do sistema nervoso central ou de leve paralisia bilateral do VI nervo.

general p., p. geral. SIN paretic *neurosyphilis*.

par·es·the·sia (par-es-thē'zē-ă). Parestesia; sensação anormal, como de queimação, espetadelas, cócegas ou formigamento. SIN paraesthesia. [para- + G. *aisthēsis*, sensação]

par·es·thet·ic (par-es-thet'ik). Parestésico; relativo a, ou caracterizado por, parestesia; designa dormência e formigamento em um membro, geralmente ocorrendo quando há reinício do fluxo sanguíneo para um nervo após compressão temporária ou pequena lesão.

pa·ret·ic (pa-ret'ik). Parético; relativo a, ou que sofre de, paresia.

pa·reu·nia (par-ū'nē-ă). Coito; relação sexual. SIN coitus. [G. *pareunos*, deitado ao lado de, de *para*, ao lado de, + *eunē*, cama]

par·gy·line hy·dro·chlo·ride (par'ji-lēn). Cloridrato de pargilina; inibidor da monoamina oxidase não-hidrazínico, usado como anti-hipertensivo.

par·i·dro·sis (par-i-drō'sis). Paridrose; qualquer distúrbio da transpiração. SIN parahidrosis. [para- + G. *hidrōsis*, sudorese]

par·i·es, gen. **pa·ri·'e·tis**, pl. **pa·ri·e·tes** (par'i-ēz, pā'ri-ēz; pă-rī'ĕ-tēz). [TA]. Parede. SIN wall. [L. parede]

p. ante'rior gas'tris [TA], p. anterior do estômago. SIN anterior *wall* of stomach.

p. ante'rior vagi'nae [TA], p. anterior da vagina. SIN anterior *wall* of vagina.

p. carot'icus ca'vi tym'pani [TA], p. carótica da cavidade timpânica. SIN carotid *wall* of tympanic cavity.

p. exter'nus duc'tus cochlea'ris [TA], p. externa do ducto coclear. SIN external *surface* of cochlear duct.

p. infe'rior or'bitae [TA], p. inferior da órbita. SIN *floor* of orbit.

p. jugula'ris ca'vi tym'pani [TA], p. jugular da cavidade timpânica. SIN jugular wall of middle ear.
p. labyrin'thicus ca'vi tym'pani [TA], p. labiríntica da cavidade timpânica. SIN labyrinthine wall of tympanic cavity.
p. latera'lis or'bitae [TA], p. lateral da órbita. SIN lateral wall of orbit.
p. mastoi'deus ca'vi tym'pani [TA], p. mastóidea da cavidade timpânica. SIN mastoid wall of tympanic cavity.
p. media'lis or'bitae [TA], p. medial da órbita. SIN medial wall of orbit.
p. membrana'ceus ca'vi tym'pani [TA], p. membranácea da cavidade timpânica. SIN membranous wall of tympanic cavity.
p. membrana'ceus tra'cheae [TA], p. membranácea da traquéia. SIN membranous wall of trachea.
p. poste'rior gas'tris [TA], p. posterior do estômago. SIN posterior wall of stomach.
p. poste'rior vagi'nae [TA], p. posterior da vagina. SIN posterior wall of vagina.
p. supe'rior or'bitae [TA], p. superior da órbita. SIN roof of orbit.
p. tegmenta'lis ca'vi tym'pani [TA], p. tegmental da cavidade timpânica. SIN tegmental wall of tympanic cavity.
p. tympan'icus duc'tus cochlea'ris [TA], p. timpânica do ducto coclear. SIN tympanic surface of cochlear duct.
p. vestibula'ris duc'tus cochlea'ris [TA], p. vestibular do ducto coclear. SIN vestibular surface of cochlear duct.
pa·ri·e·tal (pă-rī′ĕ-tăl). Parietal. 1. Relativo à parede de qualquer cavidade. 2. SIN somatic (1). 3. SIN somatic (2). 4. Relativo ao osso parietal.
pa·ri·e·tes (pă-rī′ĕ-tēz). Paredes, plural de paries. [L.]
parieto-. Parieto-; uma parede (do corpo, p. ex., a parede abdominal); um osso parietal. [L. paries, parede]
pa·ri·e·to·fron·tal (pa-rī′ĕ-tō-frŏn′tăl). Parietofrontal; relativo aos ossos parietal e frontal ou às partes do córtex cerebral correspondentes.
pa·ri·e·tog·ra·phy (pa-rī′ĕ-tog′ră-fē). Parietografia; termo raramente usado para designar um exame radiográfico da parede do estômago utilizando uma combinação de pneumoperitônio e uso de ar e bário intraluminal. [parieto- + G. graphē, escrita]
pa·ri·e·to·mas·toid (pă-rī′ĕ-to-mas′toyd). Parietomastóide; relativo ao osso parietal e à porção mastóide do osso temporal.
pa·ri·e·to·oc·cip·i·tal (pă-rī′ĕ-tō-ok-sip′ĭ-tăl). Parietoocipital; parietoccipital; relativo aos ossos parietal e occipital ou às partes do córtex cerebral correspondentes.
pa·ri·e·to·sphe·noid (pă-rī′ĕ-tō-sfē′noyd). Parietoesfenóide; relativo aos ossos parietal e esfenóide.
pa·ri·e·to·splanch·nic (pă-rī′ĕ-tō-splangk′nik). Parietoesplâncnico. SIN parietovisceral.
pa·ri·e·to·squa·mo·sal (pă-rī′ĕ-tō-skwā-mō′săl). Parietoescamoso; relativo ao osso parietal e à porção escamosa do osso temporal.
pa·ri·e·to·tem·po·ral (pă-rī′ĕ-tō-tem′pŏ-răl). Parietotemporal; relativo aos ossos parietal e temporal.
pa·ri·e·to·vis·cer·al (pă-rī′ĕ-tō-vis′er-ăl). Parietovisceral; relativo à parede de uma cavidade e às vísceras contidas. SIN parietosplanchnic.
Parinaud, Henri, oftalmologista francês, 1844–1905. VER P. conjunctivitis, ophthalmoplegia, syndrome, oculoglandular syndrome.
Par·is green. Verde-Paris; acetoarsenito de cobre, usado como inseticida e como pigmento.
Par·is yel·low [C.I. 77600]. Amarelo-cromo. SIN chrome yellow.
par·i·ty (par′ĭ-tē). Paridade; a condição de ter dado à luz um feto ou fetos, vivos ou mortos; um parto múltiplo é considerado como uma única experiência de parto. [L. pario, dar à luz]
Park, Henry, cirurgião inglês, 1745–1831. VER P. aneurysm.
Park, William H., bacteriologista norte-americano, 1863–1939. VER P.-Williams fixative.
Parker, Edward Mason, cirurgião norte-americano, 1860–1941. VER P.-Kerr suture.
Parkinson, James, médico inglês, 1755–1824. VER parkinsonism (1); P. disease, facies.
Parkinson, Sir John, cardiologista inglês, 1885–1976. VER Wolff-P.-White syndrome.
par·kin·so·ni·an (par-kin-sō′nē-an). Parkinsoniano; relativo a, ou que sofre de, parkinsonismo (parkinsonism) (1).
par·kin·son·ism (par′kin-son-izm). Parkinsonismo, parquinsonismo. 1. Síndrome neurológica que, geralmente, resulta da deficiência do neurotransmissor dopamina em virtude de alterações degenerativas, vasculares ou inflamatórias nos núcleos da base; caracterizada por tremores musculares rítmicos, rigidez de movimento, festinação, postura abatida e fácies semelhante a uma máscara. SIN Parkinson disease, shaking palsy, trembling palsy. 2. Síndrome semelhante ao parkinsonismo que surge como efeito colateral de algumas drogas antipsicóticas. [J. Parkinson]
Parnas, Jakob Karol, químico e fisiologista polonês, 1884–1955. VER Embden-Meyerhof-P. pathway.

par·oc·cip·i·tal (par′ok-sip′ĭ-tăl). Paraoccipital; próximo ou ao lado do osso occipital ou occipúcio. [para- + occipital]
par·o·don·ti·tis (par′ō-don-tī′tis). Parodontite; termo obsoleto para periodontite.
pa·ro·don·ti·um (par-ō-don′shē-ŭm). Periodonto. SIN periodontium. [para- + G. odous, dente]
par·o·dyn·ia (par-ō-din′ē-ă). Parodinia. SIN labor pains, em pain. [L. pario, dar à luz, + G. odynē, dor]
pa·role (pă-rōl′). Palavra de honra; libertar sob palavra; em psiquiatria, termo para liberação condicional de um paciente formalmente confinado em um hospital psiquiátrico antes da alta formal, de forma que o paciente possa ser conduzido de volta ao hospital, se necessário, sem nova ação legal. [Fr., do L. parabola, discurso, do G. parabolē]
par·ol·fac·to·ry (par-ol-fak′tŏr-ē). Paraolfatório; associado ou relacionado ao sistema olfatório.
par·ol·i·vary (par-ol′ĭ-var-ē). Paraolivar; ao lado da oliva ou próximo desta. [para- + L. oliva, oliva]
par·o·mo·my·cin sul·fate (par′ō-mō-mī′sin). Sulfato de paromomicina; antibiótico de amplo espectro produzido pelo Streptomyces rimosus forma paromomycinus; usado no tratamento da enterite bacteriana e da amebíase, e na supressão pré-operatória de bactérias intestinais.
par·om·pha·lo·cele (par-om′fă-lō-sēl). Paraonfalocele. 1. Tumor próximo do umbigo. 2. Hérnia através de um defeito na parede abdominal próximo do umbigo. [para- + G. omphalos, umbigo, + kēlē, tumor, hérnia]
Parona, Francesco, cirurgião italiano do século XIX. VER P. space.
par·o·nych·ia (par-ō-nik′ē-ă). Paroníquia; inflamação supurativa da prega ungueal adjacente à lâmina ungueal; pode ser causada por bactérias ou fungos, na maioria das vezes estafilococos e estreptococos. [para- + G. onyx, unha]

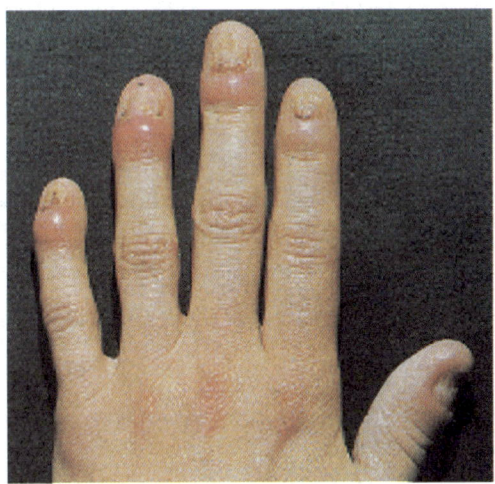

paroníquia: forma crônica

par·o·oph·o·ri·tis (par′ō-of′ō-rī′tis). Paraooforite; inflamação dos tecidos adjacentes aos ovários. [paroophoron + G. -itis, inflamação]
par·o·öph·o·ron (par-ō-of′or-on). [TA]. Paraoóforo; remanescentes dos túbulos e glomérulos da parte inferior do mesonefro que se apresenta como alguns túbulos dispersos no ligamento largo entre o epoóforo e o útero. Seu equivalente no homem é o paradídimo. SIN parovarium. [para- + oophoron, ovário]
par·or·chid·i·um (par-ōr-kid′ē-ŭm). Paraorquidia, ectopia testicular. SIN testis ectopia. [para- + G. orchis, testículo]
par·or·chis (par-ōr′kis). Parorquia. SIN epididymis. [para- + G. orchis, testículo]
par·o·rex·ia (par-ō-rek′sē-ă). Parorexia; anormalidade ou perturbação do apetite. [para- + G. orexis, apetite]
par·os·mia (par-oz′mē-ă). Parosmia. SIN dysosmia. [para + G. osmē, sentido do olfato]
par·os·phre·sia (par-os-frē′zē-ă). Parosfresia. SIN dysosmia. [para- + G. osphrēsis, olfato]
par·os·te·al (par-os′tē-ăl). Parosteal; relativo aos tecidos imediatamente adjacentes ao periósteo de um osso.
par·os·te·i·tis (păr-os-tē-ī′tis). Parosteíte; inflamação dos tecidos imediatamente adjacentes a um osso. SIN parostitis. [para- + G. osteon, osso, + -itis, inflamação]

par·os·te·o·sis, par·os·to·sis (par′os-tē-ō′sis, -os-tō′sis). Parosteose. **1.** Desenvolvimento de osso em um local incomum, como na pele. **2.** Ossificação anormal ou deficiente. [para- + G. *osteon*, osso, + *-osis*, condição]

par·os·ti·tis (par-os-tī′tis). Parosteíte; inflamação dos tecidos imediatamente adjacentes a um osso. SIN parosteitis. [para- + G. *osteon*, osso, + *-itis*, inflamação]

pa·rot·ic (pă-rot′ik). Parótico; próximo ou ao lado da orelha. [para- + G. *ous*, orelha]

pa·rot·id (pă-rot′id). Parótida; situado próximo da orelha; designa várias estruturas nessas adjacências. Geralmente refere-se à glândula salivar parótida. [G. *parōtis* (*parōtid-*), a glândula ao lado da orelha, de *para*, ao lado de, + *ous* (*ōt-*), orelha]

pa·rot·i·dec·to·my (pă-rot′i-dek′tō-mē). Parotidectomia; remoção cirúrgica da glândula parótida. [parotid + G. *ektomē*, excisão]

pa·rot·i·di·tis (pă-rot-i-dī′tis). Parotidite; inflamação da glândula parótida. SIN parotitis.
  epidemic p., p. epidêmica; caxumba. SIN mumps.
  postoperative p., p. pós-operatória; inflamação aguda da glândula parótida que ocorre no período pós-operatório, principalmente em pacientes debilitados ou desidratados; freqüentemente resulta em formação de abscesso e celulite que se dissemina rapidamente e pode ser fatal.
  punctate p., p. pontilhada; p. recorrente ou crônica com sialectasia terminal, que produz um padrão pontilhado à sialografia; associada a hiperplasia epitelial dos ductos intralobulares, atrofia dos ácinos e infiltração linfocítica, característica na doença de Sjögren (Sjögren *disease*).

pa·ro·ti·do·au·ri·cu·la·ris (pă-rot′i-dō-aw-rik-ū-la′ris). Parotidoauricular. **1.** Uma faixa ocasional de fibras musculares que seguem da superfície da glândula parótida até a orelha. **2.** Relativo à glândula parótida e à orelha externa.

par·o·tin (par′ō-tin). Parotina; globulina obtida de glândulas parótidas que causa hipocalcemia, tem efeitos sobre os tecidos mesenquimais, provoca primeiro leucopenia e, depois, leucocitose, e promove calcificação da dentina. SIN salivary gland hormone.

par·o·ti·tis (par-o-tī′tis). Parotidite. SIN parotiditis.

par·ous (par′us). Parido; relativo à paridade. [L. *pario*, dar à luz]

par·o·var·i·an (par-ō-var′ē-an). Parovárico. **1.** Relativo ao paroóforo. **2.** Ao lado de ou adjacente ao ovário. SIN paraovarian.

par·o·var·i·ot·o·my (par′ō-var-ē-ot′ō-mē). Parovariotomia; incisão ou remoção de um tumor do parovário. [parovarium + G. *tomē*, incisão]

par·o·va·ri·tis (par′ō-var-ī′tis). Parovarite; inflamação do parovário.

par·o·var·i·um (par-ō-var′ē-um). Parovário. SIN paraoöphoron. [para- + L. *ovarium*, ovário]

par·ox·y·pro·pi·one (par-ok-si-prō′pē-ōn). Paroxipropiona; inibidor do hormônio gonadotrófico hipofisário.

par·ox·ysm (par′ok-sizm). Paroxismo. **1.** Espasmo ou convulsão súbita. **2.** Início súbito de um sintoma ou de uma doença, sobretudo com manifestações recorrentes como os calafrios e os tremores da malária. [G. *paroxysmos*, de *paroxynō*, estimular, irritar, de *oxys*, agudo]

par·ox·ys·mal (par-ok-siz′mal). Paroxístico; relativo a, ou que ocorre, em paroxismos.

par·ri·cide (par′i-sīd). **1.** Parricídio; o assassinato de um dos genitores (patricídio ou matricídio). **2.** Parricida; aquele que comete tal ato. [L. *parricidium*, assassinato de um parente próximo]

Parrot, Jules, médico francês, 1829–1883. VER P. *disease*.

Parry, Caleb H., médico inglês, 1755–1822. VER P. *disease*.

PARS

pars, pl. **par·tes** (pars, par′tēz) [TA]. Parte. SIN part. [L. *pars* (*part-*) uma parte]
  p. abdomina'lis aor'tae [TA], p. abdominal da aorta. SIN abdominal *aorta*.
  p. abdomina'lis duc'tus thora'cici [TA], p. abdominal do ducto torácico. SIN abdominal *part* of thoracic duct.
  p. abdomina'lis esoph'agi [TA], p. abdominal do esôfago. SIN abdominal *part* of esophagus.
  p. abdominalis musculi pectorales majoris [TA], p. abdominal do músculo peitoral maior. SIN abdominal *part* of pectoralis major (muscle).
  p. abdominalis plexus visceralis et ganglii visceralis [TA], p. abdominal dos plexos viscerais e gânglios viscerais. SIN abdominal *part* of peripheral autonomic plexuses and ganglia.
  p. abdomina'lis ure'teris [TA], p. abdominal do ureter. SIN abdominal *part* of ureter.
  p. acromialis musculi deltoidei [TA], p. acromial do músculo deltóide. SIN acromial *part* of deltoid (muscle).
  p. ala'ris mus'culi nasa'lis [TA], p. alar do músculo nasal. SIN alar *part* of nasalis muscle. VER nasalis (*muscle*).
  p. alveola'ris mandib'ulae [TA], p. alveolar da mandíbula. SIN alveolar *part* of mandible.
  p. amor'pha, p. amorfa; a parte do nucléolo que ocupa espaços irregulares no nucleolonema e contém substância finamente filamentar. VER TAMBÉM p. granulosa.
  p. ante'rior [TA], p. anterior. SIN anterior *part*.
  p. ante'rior commissu'rae anterio'ris [TA], p. anterior da comissura anterior. SIN anterior *part* of anterior commissure of brain.
  p. ante'rior commissu'rae rostra'lis, p. anterior da comissura anterior. SIN anterior *part* of anterior commissure of brain.
  p. ante'rior facie'i diaphrag'matis hepa'tis [TA], p. anterior da face diafragmática do fígado. SIN anterior *part* of diaphragmatic surface of liver.
  p. ante'rior for'nicis vagi'nae [TA], p. anterior do fórnice da vagina. SIN anterior *part* of fornix of vagina.
  p. anterior linguae [TA], p. pré-sulcal da língua. SIN anterior *part* of tongue.
  p. anula'ris vagi'nae fibro'sae digitorum manus et pedis [TA], p. anular das bainhas fibrosas dos dedos da mão e do pé. SIN anular *part* of fibrous digital sheath of digits of hand and foot.
  p. aryepiglottica musculi arytenoidei obliqui [TA], p. ariepiglótica do músculo aritenóideo oblíquo. SIN aryepiglottic *part* of oblique arytenoid muscle.
  p. ascen'dens aor'tae [TA], p. ascendente da aorta. SIN ascending *aorta*.
  p. ascen'dens duode'ni [TA], p. ascendente do duodeno. SIN ascending *part* of duodenum.
  p. ascendens musculi trapezii [TA], p. ascendente do músculo trapézio. SIN ascending *part* of trapezius (muscle).
  p. atlantica arteriae vertebralis [TA], p. atlântica da artéria vertebral. SIN atlantic *part* of vertebral artery.
  p. autonom'ica systematis nervosi peripherici [TA], divisão autônoma do sistema nervoso. SIN autonomic *division* of nervous system.
  p. basalis [TA], p. basilar. SIN basal *part*.
  p. basalis arteriarum lobarium inferiorum pulmonis sinistri et dextri [TA], p. basilar das artérias lobares inferiores dos pulmões esquerdo e direito. SIN basal *part* of left and right inferior pulmonary arteries.
  p. basa'lis arte'riae pulmona'lis, p. basilar das artérias pulmonares. VER right pulmonary *artery*, left pulmonary *artery*.
  p. basilaris [TA], p. basilar. SIN basal *part*.
  p. basilaris pontis [TA], p. basilar da ponte. SIN basilar *part* of pons.
  p. basila'ris os'sis occipita'lis [TA], p. basilar do occipital. SIN basilar *part* of occipital bone.
  p. buccopharyn'gea mu'sculi constricto'ris phary'ngei superio'ris, p. bucofaríngea do músculo constritor superior da faringe. SIN buccopharyngeal *part* of superior pharyngeal constrictor. VER superior pharyngeal constrictor (*muscle*).
  p. canalis ner'vi op'tici [TA], p. do canal do nervo óptico. SIN *part* of optic nerve in canal.
  p. cardi'aca gas'tricae [TA], cárdia do estômago. SIN cardia.
  p. cardi'aca ventric'uli, cárdia. SIN cardia.
  p. cartilagin'ea sep'ti na'si, p. cartilagínea do septo nasal. SIN septal nasal *cartilage*.
  p. cartilaginea systema'tis skeleta'lis [TA], p. cartilagínea do sistema esquelético. SIN cartilaginous *part* of skeletal system.
  p. cartilagin'ea tu'bae auditi'vae [TA], p. cartilagínea da tuba auditiva. SIN cartilaginous *part* of pharyngotympanic (auditory) tube.
  p. cartilaginea tubae auditoriae, p. cartilagínea da tuba auditiva. SIN cartilaginous *part* of pharyngotympanic (auditory) tube.
  p. caverno'sa, p. esponjosa da uretra. SIN spongy *urethra*.
  p. caverno'sa arte'riae caro'tidis inter'nae [TA], p. cavernosa da artéria carótida interna. SIN cavernous *part* of internal carotid artery.
  p. ce'ca ret'inae, p. cega da retina; a parte anterior embriológica da retina que se transforma na parte ciliar da retina e na parte irídica da retina.
  p. centra'lis systematis nervosi [TA], p. central do sistema nervoso. SIN central nervous *system*.
  p. centra'lis ventric'uli latera'lis [TA], p. central do ventrículo lateral; o corpo do ventrículo lateral do encéfalo, que se estende do forame interventricular (de Monro) até o trígono colateral (isto é, a junção dos cornos posterior e inferior). SIN body of lateral ventricle, cella media, central part of lateral ventricle.
  p. ceratopharyn'gea mu'sculi constricto'ris phary'ngis me'dii [TA], p. ceratofaríngea do músculo constritor médio da faringe. SIN ceratopharyngeal *part* of middle constrictor muscle of pharynx. VER middle constrictor (*muscle*) of pharynx.
  p. cerebra'lis arte'riae caro'tidis inter'nae [TA], p. cerebral da artéria carótida interna. SIN cerebral *part* of internal carotid artery.
  p. cervica'lis arte'riae caro'tidis inter'nae [TA], p. cervical da artéria carótida interna. SIN cervical *part* of internal carotid artery.
  p. cervicalis arteriae vertebralis [TA], p. transversária da artéria vertebral. SIN cervical *part* of vertebral artery.

p. cervica'lis duc'tus thora'cici [TA], p. cervical do ducto torácico. SIN cervical *part* of thoracic duct.
p. cervica'lis esoph'agi [TA], p. cervical do esôfago. SIN cervical *part* of esophagus.
p. cervica'lis medul'lae spina'lis [TA], p. cervical da medula espinal. SIN cervical *part* of spinal cord.
p. chondropharyn'gea muscu'li constricto'ris pharyn'gei medi'i [TA], p. condrofaríngea do músculo constritor médio da faringe. SIN chondropharyngeal *part* of middle constrictor muscle of pharynx. VER middle constrictor (*muscle*) of pharynx.
p. cilia'ris ret'inae [TA], p. ciliar da retina. SIN ciliary *part* of retina. VER retina.
p. clavicularis musculi deltoidei [TA], p. clavicular do músculo deltóide. SIN clavicular *part* of deltoid (*muscle*).
p. clavicula'ris mus'culi pectoral'is major'is [TA], p. clavicular do músculo peitoral maior. SIN clavicular *head* of pectoralis major muscle. VER pectoralis major (*muscle*).
p. coccyg'ea medul'lae spina'lis [TA], p. coccígea da medula espinal. SIN coccygeal *part* of spinal cord.
p. cochlea'ris ner'vi vestibulocochlea'ris, p. coclear do nervo vestibulococlear. SIN cochlear *nerve*.
p. coeliacoduodenalis musculi (ligamenti) suspensorii duodeni [TA], p. celiacoduodenal do músculo suspensor do duodeno. SIN celiacoduodenal *part* of suspensory muscle (ligament) of duodenum.
p. convolu'ta lo'buli cortica'lis re'nis, p. convoluta dos lóbulos corticais renais. SIN convoluted *part* of kidney lobule.
p. corneosclera'lis reti'culi trabecula'ris sclerae [TA], p. corneoescleral do retículo trabecular da esclera. SIN corneoscleral *part* of trabecular tissue of sclera.
par'tes cor'poris huma'ni [TA], partes do corpo humano. SIN *parts* of human body, em *part*.
p. cortica'lis, p. cortical. SIN cortical *part*. VER middle cerebral *artery*, posterior cerebral *artery*.
p. cortica'lis arteri'ae cerebra'lis medi'ae, ramos terminais da artéria cerebral média. VER terminal *branches* of middle cerebral artery, em *branch*.
p. costa'lis disphrag'matis [TA], p. costal do diafragma. SIN costal *part* of diaphragm.
p. costalis pleurae parietalis [TA], p. costal da pleura parietal. SIN costal *part* of parietal pleura.
p. cranialis partis parasympathetici divisionis autonomici systematis nervosi [TA], p. craniana da parte parassimpática da divisão autônoma do sistema nervoso. SIN cranial *part* of parasympathetic part of autonomic division of nervous system.
p. craniocervicalis plexuum et gangliorum visceralium [TA], p. craniocervical dos plexos e gânglios viscerais. SIN craniocervical *part* of peripheral autonomic plexuses and ganglia.
p. cricopharyn'gea mus'culi constricto'ris pharyn'gis inferio'ris [TA], p. cricofaríngea do músculo constritor inferior da faringe. SIN cricopharyngeal *part* of inferior constrictor (muscle) of pharynx. VER inferior constrictor (*muscle*) of pharynx.
p. crucifor'mis vagi'nae fibro'sae [TA], p. cruciforme da bainha fibrosa. SIN cruciform *part* of fibrous digital sheath.
p. cuneiformis vomeris [TA], p. cuneiforme do vômer. SIN cuneiform *part* of vomer.
p. cupula'ris reces'sus epitympan'ici [TA], p. cupular do recesso epitimpânico. SIN cupular *part* of epitympanic recess.
p. cys'tica, p. cística; a divisão caudal menor do broto hepático embrionário primitivo, que se transforma na vesícula biliar e no ducto cístico.
p. descen'dens aor'tae [TA], p. descendente da aorta. SIN descending *aorta*.
p. descen'dens duode'ni [TA], p. descendente do duodeno. SIN descending *part* of duodenum. VER duodenum.
p. descendens ligamenti iliofemoralis [TA], p. descendente do ligamento iliofemoral. SIN descending *part* of iliofemoral ligament.
p. descendens musculi trapezii [TA], p. descendente do (músculo) trapézio. SIN descending *part* of trapezius (muscle).
p. dex'tra facie'i diaphragma'ticae hepa'tis [TA], p. direita da face diafragmática do fígado. SIN right *part* of diaphragmatic surface of liver.
p. diaphragmatica pleurae parietalis [TA], p. diafragmática da pleura parietal. SIN diaphragmatic *part* of parietal pleura.
p. dista'lis adenohypophyseos [TA], p. distal da adeno-hipófise. SIN distal *part* [TA] of anterior lobe of hypophysis.
p. distalis prostatae [TA], p. distal da próstata. SIN distal *part* of prostate.
p. distalis urethrae prostaticae [TA], p. distal da parte prostática da uretra masculina. SIN distal *part* of prostatic urethra.
partes dorsales musculorum intertransversariorum lateralium lumborum [TA], partes dorsais dos músculos intertransversários laterais do lombo. SIN dorsal *part* of intertransversarii laterales lumborum (muscles).
p. dorsa'lis pon'tis, p. dorsal da ponte. SIN dorsal *part* of pons.

p. duralis fili terminalis [TA], p. dural do filamento terminal. VER terminal *filum*.
p. endocri'na pancrea'tis [TA], p. endócrina do pâncreas. SIN endocrine *part* of pancreas. VER pancreas.
p. exocri'na pancrea'tis [TA], p. exócrina do pâncreas. SIN exocrine *part* of pancreas. VER pancreas.
p. extraocularis arteriae et venae centralis retinae [TA], p. extra-ocular da artéria e veia central da retina. SIN extraocular *part* of central retinal artery and vein.
p. feta'lis placen'tae, p. fetal da placenta. SIN fetal *placenta*.
p. flac'cida membra'nae tym'panae [TA], p. flácida da membrana timpânica. SIN flaccid *part* of tympanic membrane.
p. fronta'lis cor'poris callo'si, p. frontal do corpo caloso. SIN minor *forceps*.
p. funicularis ductus deferentis [TA], p. funicular do ducto deferente. SIN funicular *part* of ductus deferens.
par'tes genita'les femini'nae exter'nae, partes genitais femininas externas; termo obsoleto para external female genital *organs*, em *organ*.
par'tes genita'les masculi'nae exter'nae, partes genitais masculinas externas; termo obsoleto para external male genital *organs*, em *organ*.
p. glossopharyn'gea mus'culi constrictor'is pharyn'gis superior'is, p. glossofaríngea do músculo constritor superior da faringe. SIN glossopharyngeal *part* of superior pharyngeal constrictor. VER superior pharyngeal constrictor (*muscle*).
p. granulo'sa, p. granulosa; a parte granular e filamentar do nucleolonema do nucléolo.
p. hepat'ica, p. hepática; a maior divisão craniana do broto hepático embrionário primitivo, que se transforma no fígado propriamente dito.
p. hepatis dextra [TA], p. hepática direita. SIN right *liver*.
p. hepatis sinistra [TA], p. hepática esquerda. SIN left *liver*.
p. horizonta'lis duode'ni [TA], p. horizontal do duodeno. SIN inferior *part* of duodenum. VER duodenum.
p. iliaca fasciae iliopsoaticae [TA], p. ilíaca da fáscia iliopsoas. SIN iliac *fascia*.
p. infe'rior [TA], p. inferior. SIN inferior *part*.
p. inferior alae lobuli centralis [TA], p. inferior da asa do lóbulo central. SIN ala central *lobule*.
p. infe'rior duode'ni, p. inferior do duodeno;*termo oficial alternativo para inferior *part* of duodenum.
p. infe'rior gang'lii vestibula'ris [TA], p. inferior do nervo vestibular. SIN inferior *part* of vestibular ganglion.
p. infe'rior venae lingularis venae pulmonalis superioris sinistrae [TA], p. inferior da veia lingular (da veia pulmonar esquerda superior). SIN inferior *part* of lingular vein (of left superior pulmonary vein).
p. infraclavicula'ris plex'us brachia'lis [TA], p. infraclavicular do plexo braquial. SIN infraclavicular *part* of brachial plexus.
p. infraloba'ris venae posterio'ris ve'nae pulmona'lis superioris dex'trae [TA], p. infralobar da veia posterior (da veia pulmonar direita superior). SIN infralobar *part* of posterior vein (of right superior pulmonary vein).
p. infundibula'ris, p. tuberal. SIN *p. tuberalis*.
p. inguinalis ductus deferentis [TA], p. inguinal do ducto deferente. SIN inguinal *part* of ductus deferens.
p. insula'ris, lobo da ínsula. SIN *lobus* insula.
p. insularis arte'riae cerebri mediae [TA], p. insular da artéria cerebral média. SIN insular *part* of middle cerebral artery. VER middle cerebral *artery*.
p. interarticula'ris (in - ter - ar - tik'ū - lar - is), p. interarticular; o segmento de osso entre as faces articulares superior e inferior, principalmente na coluna lombar.
p. intercartilagin'ea ri'mae glot'tidis [TA], p. intercartilagínea da rima da glote. SIN intercartilaginous *part* of rima glottidis.
p. interme'dia [TA], p. intermédia. SIN intermediate *part*.
p. interme'dia adenohypophys'eos [TA], p. intermédia da adeno-hipófise. SIN intermediate *part* of adenohypophysis.
p. interme'dia commissurae bulbo'rum, comissura dos bulbos. SIN *commissure* of bulbs.
p. intermedia urethrae masculinae [TA], p. membranácea da uretra masculina. SIN intermediate *part* of male urethra.
p. intermembrana'cea ri'mae glot'tidis [TA], p. intermembranácea da rima da glote. SIN intermembranous *part* of rima glottidis.
partes intersegmenta'les venarum pulmonum [TA], partes intersegmentares das raízes das veias pulmonares. SIN intersegmental *vein*.
p. intracrania'lis arte'riae vertebra'lis [TA], p. intracraniana da artéria vertebral. SIN intracranial *part* of vertebral artery. VER vertebral *artery*.
p. intracrania'lis ner'vi op'tici [TA], p. intracraniana do nervo óptico. SIN intracranial *part* of optic nerve.
p. intralamina'ris ner'vi op'tici intraocularis [TA], p. intralaminar da parte intra-ocular do nervo óptico. SIN intralaminar *part* of intraocular part of optic nerve.
p. intraloba'ris (intersegmentalis) venae posterio'ris lobi superioris pulmonis dextri [TA], p. intralobar da veia posterior da veia pulmonar direita

superior. SIN intralobar *part* of the posterior vein (of the right superior pulmonary vein).
p. intramuralis urethrae masculinae [TA], p. intramural da uretra masculina. SIN intramural *part* of male urethra.
p. intraocula'ris ner'vi op'tici [TA], p. intra-ocular do nervo óptico. SIN intraocular *part* of optic nerve.
p. intrasegmenta'lis venae pulmonum [TA], p. intra-segmentar das raízes das veias pulmonares. SIN intrasegmental *part* of pulmonary veins.
p. irid'ica ret'inae [TA], p. irídica da retina. SIN iridial *part* of retina. VER retina.
p. labia'lis mus'culi orbicula'ris o'ris [TA], p. labial do músculo orbicular da boca. SIN labial *part* of orbicularis oris (muscle).
p. lacrima'lis mus'culi orbicula'ris oc'uli [TA], p. profunda do músculo orbicular do olho. SIN lacrimal *part* of orbicularis oculi muscle. VER orbicularis oculi (*muscle*).
p. laryn'gea pharyn'gis [TA], p. laríngea da faringe. SIN laryngopharynx.
p. latera'lis ar'cus pe'dis longitudina'lis [TA], p. lateral do arco longitudinal do pé. SIN lateral *part* of longitudinal arch of foot. VER longitudinal *arch* of foot.
p. lateralis compartimenti antebrachii posterioris (extensorum) [TA], p. lateral do compartimento posterior do antebraço. SIN lateral *part* of posterior (extensor) compartment of forearm.
p. latera'lis for'nicis vagi'nae [TA], p. lateral do fórnice da vagina. SIN lateral *part* of vaginal fornix. VER vaginal *fornix*.
p. latera'lis mus'culorum intertransversa'riorum posterio'rum cer'vicis [TA], p. lateral dos músculos intertransversários posteriores do pescoço. VER posterior cervical intertransversarii (*muscles*), em *muscle*.
p. lateralis nuclei accumbentis [TA], p. lateral do nucleus acumbens. VER *nucleus* accumbens.
p. latera'lis os'sis occipita'lis [TA], p. lateral do osso occipital. SIN lateral *part* of occipital bone.
p. latera'lis os'sis sa'cri [TA], p. lateral do sacro. SIN lateral *part* of sacrum.
p. latera'lis venae lo'bi medi'i ve'nae pulmona'lis dex'tri superi'oris, p. lateral da veia do lobo médio da veia pulmonar direita superior. SIN lateral *part* of middle lobe vein (of right superior pulmonary vein).
p. libera membri inferioris [TA], p. livre do membro inferior. SIN free *part* of lower limb.
p. libera membri superioris [TA], p. livre do membro superior. SIN free *part* of upper limb.
p. lumba'lis diaphrag'matis [TA], p. lombar do diafragma. SIN lumbar *part* of diaphragm.
p. lumba'lis medul'lae spina'lis [TA], p. lombar da medula espinal. SIN lumbar *part* of spinal cord.
p. margina'lis mus'culi orbicula'ris o'ris [TA], p. marginal do músculo orbicular da boca. SIN marginal *part* of orbicularis oris (muscle).
p. mastoi'dea os'sis tempora'lis, processo mastóide do osso temporal. SIN mastoid *process* of petrous part of temporal bone.
p. media'lis ar'cus pe'dis longitudina'lis [TA], p. medial do arco longitudinal do pé. SIN medial *part* of longitudinal arch of foot. VER longitudinal *arch* of foot.
p. media'lis mus'culorum intertransversa'riorum posterio'rum cer'vicis [TA], p. medial dos músculos intertransversários posteriores do pescoço. VER posterior cervical intertransversarii (*muscles*), em *muscle*.
p. medialis nuclei accumbentis [TA], p. medial do núcleo acumbens. VER *nucleus* accumbens.
p. media'lis venae lo'bi me'dii ve'nae pulmo'nis dex'tri superio'ris [TA], p. medial da veia do lobo médio da veia pulmonar direita superior. SIN medial *part* of middle lobe vein (of right superior pulmonary vein).
p. mediastinalis pleurae parietalis [TA], p. mediastinal da pleura parietal. SIN mediastinal *part* of parietal pleura.
p. mediastina'lis pulmo'nis, p. mediastinal do pulmão. SIN mediastinal *surface* of lung.
p. membrana'cea sep'ti interventricula'ris [TA], p. membránacea do septo. SIN membranous *part* of interventricular septum.
p. membrana'cea sep'ti na'si [TA], p. membránacea do septo nasal. SIN membranous *part* of nasal septum.
p. membrana'cea ure'thrae masculi'nae, p. membránacea da uretra masculina; *termo oficial alternativo para intermediate *part* of male urethra.
p. mo'bilis sep'ti na'si [TA], p. móvel do septo nasal. SIN mobile *part* of nasal septum.
p. muscula'ris sep'ti interventricula'ris (cor'dis) [TA], p. muscular do septo interventricular (do coração). SIN muscular *part* of interventricular septum (of heart).
p. mylopharyn'geus mus'culi constricto'ris pharyn'gis superio'ris [TA], p. milofaríngea do músculo constritor superior da faringe. SIN mylopharyngeal *part* of superior constrictor muscle of pharynx. VER superior pharyngeal constrictor (*muscle*).
p. nasa'lis os'sis fronta'lis [TA], p. nasal do (osso) frontal. SIN nasal *part* of frontal bone.

p. nasa'lis pharyn'gis [TA], p. nasal da faringe. SIN nasopharynx.
p. nervo'sa hypophys'eos, neuro-hipófise; *termo oficial alternativo para neurohypophysis.
p. nervo'sa ret'inae, p. nervosa da retina. SIN nervous *part* of retina. VER retina.
p. obli'qua mus'culi cricothyroi'dei [TA], p. oblíqua do músculo cricotireóideo. SIN oblique *part* of cricothyroid (muscle). VER cricothyroid *muscle*.
p. occipita'lis cor'poris callo'si, p. occipital do corpo caloso. SIN major *forceps*.
p. olfactoria tunicae mucosae [TA], p. olfatória da túnica mucosa. SIN olfactory *region* of nasal mucosa.
p. opercula'ris [TA], p. opercular. SIN opercular *part*.
p. op'tica ret'inae [TA], p. óptica da retina. SIN cerebral *layer* of retina. VER retina.
p. ora'lis pharyn'gis [TA], p. oral da faringe. SIN oropharynx.
p. orbitalis [TA], p. orbital. SIN orbital *part* [TA] of inferior frontal gyrus.
p. orbita'lis glan'dulae lacrima'lis [TA], p. orbital da glândula lacrimal. SIN orbital *part* of lacrimal gland. VER lacrimal *gland*.
p. orbita'lis mus'culi orbicula'ris oc'uli [TA], p. orbital do músculo orbicular do olho. SIN orbital part of orbicularis oculi (muscle) [TA]. VER orbicularis oculi (*muscle*).
p. orbita'lis ner'vi op'tici [TA], p. orbital do nervo óptico. SIN orbital *part* of optic nerve.
p. orbita'lis os'sis fronta'lis [TA], p. orbital do frontal. SIN orbital *part* of frontal bone.
p. os'sea sep'ti na'si [TA], p. óssea do septo nasal. SIN bony *part* of nasal septum.
p. os'sea syste'matis skeleta'lis [TA], p. óssea do sistema esquelético. SIN bony *part* of skeletal system.
p. os'sea tu'bae auditi'vae [TA], p. óssea da tuba auditiva. SIN bony *part* of pharyngotympanic (auditory) tube.
p. ossea tubae auditoriae, p. óssea da tuba auditiva. SIN bony *part* of pharyngotympanic (auditory) tube.
p. palpebra'lis glan'dulae lacrima'lis [TA], p. palpebral da glândula lacrimal. SIN palpebral *part* of lacrimal gland. VER lacrimal *gland*.
p. palpebra'lis mus'culi orbicula'ris oc'uli [TA], p. palpebral do músculo orbicular do olho. SIN palpebral *part* of orbicularis oculi (muscle). VER orbicularis oculi (*muscle*).
p. parasympath'ica divisionis automaticae systematis nervosi peripherici [TA], p. parassimpática da divisão autônoma do sistema nervoso. SIN parasympathetic *part* of autonomic division of peripheral nervous system.
p. patens arteriae umbilicalis [TA], p. patente da artéria umbilical. SIN patent *part* of umbilical artery.
p. pel'vica [TA], p. pélvica. SIN pelvic *part*.
p. pelvica ductus deferentes [TA], p. pélvica do ducto deferente. SIN pelvic *part* of ductus deferens.
p. pel'vica ure'teris [TA], p. pélvica do ureter. SIN pelvic *part* of ureter.
p. peripher'ica systematis nervosi [TA], p. periférica do sistema nervoso. SIN peripheral nervous *system*.
p. perpendicula'ris [TA], lâmina perpendicular. SIN perpendicular *plate*.
p. petro'sa arte'riae caro'tidis inter'nae [TA], p. petrosa da artéria carótida interna. SIN petrous *part* of internal carotid artery. VER internal carotid *artery*.
p. petro'sa os'sis tempora'lis [TA], p. petrosa do (osso) temporal. SIN petrous *part* of temporal bone. VER temporal *bone*.
p. phal'lica, p. fálica; a porção interior do seio urogenital relacionada à base do tubérculo genital.
p. pharyn'gea hypophys'eos, p. faríngea da hipófise. SIN pharyngeal *hypophysis*.
p. phrenicocoeliaca musculi (ligamenti) suspensorii duodeni [TA], p. frenicocelíaca do músculo suspensor do duodeno. SIN phrenicoceliac *part* of suspensory muscle (ligament) of duodenum.
p. pialis fili terminalis [TA], p. pial do filamento terminal. SIN pial *part* of filum terminale.
p. pigmento'sa, estrato pigmentoso da retina. SIN pigmented *part* of retina. VER retina.
p. pla'na, orbículo ciliar. SIN orbiculus ciliaris.
p. postcommunicalis arteriae cerebri anterioris [TA], p. pós-comunicante da artéria cerebral anterior. SIN post-communicating *part* of anterior cerebral artery.
p. posterior commissurae anterioris [TA], p. posterior da comissura anterior. SIN posterior *part* of anterior commissure of brain.
p. poste'rior facie'i diaphrag'matis hep'atis [TA], p. posterior da face diafragmática do fígado. SIN posterior *part* of the diaphragmatic surface of the liver.
p. posterior fornicis vaginae [TA], p. posterior do fórnice da vagina. SIN posterior *part* of vaginal fornix.
p. posterior linguae [TA], p. pós-sulcal. SIN posterior *part* of tongue.
p. postlamina'ris ner'vi op'tici intraocularis [TA], p. pós-laminar da parte intra-ocular do nervo óptico. SIN postlaminar *part* of intraocular part of optic nerve.

p. postsulcalis linguae, p. pós-sulcal da língua; *termo oficial alternativo para posterior *part* of tongue.
p. precommunica'lis arteri'ae cere'bri anterio'ris [TA], p. pré-comunicante da artéria cerebral anterior. SIN precommunicating *part* of anterior cerebral artery. VER anterior cerebral *artery*.
p. precommunica'lis arteri'ae cere'bri posterio'ris [TA], p. pré-comunicante da artéria cerebral posterior. SIN precommunicating *part* of posterior cerebral artery.
p. prelamina'ris ner'vi op'tici intraocularis [TA], p. pré-laminar da parte intra-ocular do nervo óptico. SIN prelaminar *part* of intraocular part of optic nerve.
p. preprostatica urethrae masculinae, p. intramural da uretra masculina; *termo oficial alternativo para intramural *part* of male urethra.
p. presulca'lis, p. pré-sulcal; *termo oficial alternativo para anterior *part* of tongue.
p. presulcalis linguae, p. pré-sulcal da língua; *termo oficial alternativo para anterior *part* of tongue.
p. prevertebralis arteriae prevertebralis [TA], p. pré-vertebral da artéria vertebral. SIN prevertebral *part* of vertebral artery. VER vertebral *artery*.
p. proximalis prostatae [TA], p. proximal da próstata. SIN proximal *part* of prostate.
p. prima duodeni, p. superior do duodeno. SIN superior *part* of duodenum.
p. profunda compartimenti antebrachii anterioris [TA], p. profunda do compartimento anterior do antebraço. SIN deep *part* of anterior compartment of forearm.
p. profunda compartimenti cruris posterioris [TA], p. profunda do compartimento posterior da perna. SIN deep *part* of posterior (flexor) compartment of leg.
p. profun'da glan'dulae parotid'eae, p. profunda da glândula parótida. VER parotid *gland*.
p. profunda glandulae parotidis [TA], p. profunda da glândula parótida. SIN deep *part* of parotid gland.
p. profun'da mus'culi masse'teri [TA], p. profunda do músculo masseter. SIN deep *part* of masseter (*muscle*).
p. profun'da mus'culi sphinc'teri a'ni exter'ni, p. profunda do músculo esfíncter externo do ânus. SIN deep *part* of external anal sphincter. VER external anal *sphincter*.
p. profunda partis palpebralis musculi orbicularis oculi [TA], p. profunda da parte palpebral do músculo orbicular do olho. SIN deep *part* of palpebral part of orbicularis oculi (muscle).
p. prostat'ica ure'thrae [TA], p. prostática da uretra. SIN prostatic *urethra.*
p. proximalis urethrae prostaticae [TA], p. proximal da parte prostática da uretra. SIN proximal *part* of prostatic urethra.
p. psoatica fasciae iliopsoaticae [TA], p. do psoas da fáscia iliopsoas. SIN psoatic *part* of iliopsoas fascia.
p. pterygopharyn'gea mus'culi constricto'ris pharyn'gis superio'ris, p. pterigofaríngea do músculo constritor superior da faringe. SIN pterygopharyngeal *part* of superior constrictor muscle of pharynx. VER superior pharyngeal constrictor (*muscle*).
p. pylo'rica gas'tris [TA], p. pilórica do estômago. SIN pyloric *part* of stomach.
p. pylo'rica ventric'uli, p. pilórica do estômago. SIN pyloric *part* of stomach.
p. quadra'ta hep'atis, parte anterior do segmento medial esquerdo do fígado. SIN anterior *portion* of left medial segment IV of liver.
p. radia'ta lo'buli cortica'lis re'nis, Raio medular. SIN medullary *ray*.
p. rec'ta mus'culi cricothyroi'dei, p. reta do músculo cricotireóideo. VER cricothyroid *muscle*.
p. respiratoria tunicae mucosae [TA], p. respiratória da túnica mucosa da cavidade nasal. SIN respiratory *region* of mucosa of nasal cavity.
p. retrolentifor'mis cap'sulae inter'nae [TA], p. retrolentiforme da cápsula interna. SIN retrolenticular *part* of internal capsule.
p. retrolentiformis cruris posterior [TA], p. retrolentiforme da cápsula interna. SIN retrolentiform *limb* of internal capsule.
p. sacra'lis medul'lae spina'lis [TA], p. sacral da medula espinal. SIN sacral *part* of spinal cord.
p. scrotalis ductus deferentis [TA], p. escrotal do ducto deferente. SIN scrotal *part* of ductus deferens.
p. secundum duodeni, parte descendente do duodeno. SIN descending *part* of duodenum.
p. sella'ris, sela turca. SIN *sella* turcica.
p. solealis compartimenti cruris posterioris [TA], p. profunda do compartimento posterior da perna. SIN soleal *part* of posterior (plantar flexor) compartment of leg.
p. sphenoida'lis arte'riae cerebra'lis me'diae [TA], p. esfenoidal da artéria cerebral média. SIN sphenoid *part* of middle cerebral artery. VER middle cerebral *artery*.
p. spinalis fili terminalis [TA], p. espinal do filamento terminal. SIN spinal *part* of filum terminale.

p. spinalis musculi deltoidei [TA], p. espinal do músculo deltóide. SIN spinal *part* of deltoid (*muscle*).
p. spina'lis ner'vi accesso'rii, raiz espinal do nervo acessório; *termo oficial alternativo para spinal *root* of accessory nerve.
p. spongio'sa ure'thrae masculi'nae [TA], p. esponjosa da uretra masculina. SIN spongy *urethra*.
p. squamo'sa os'sis tempora'lis [TA], p. escamosa do (osso) temporal. SIN squamous *part* of temporal bone.
p. sterna'lis diaphrag'matis [TA], p. esternal do diafragma. SIN sternal *part* of diaphragm.
p. sternocosta'lis mus'culi pectora'lis majo'ris [TA], p. esternocostal do músculo peitoral maior. SIN sternocostal *head* of pectoralis major (*muscle*).
p. subcuta'nae mus'culi sphinc'teri a'ni exter'ni [TA], p. subcutânea do músculo esfíncter externo do ânus. SIN subcutaneous *part* of external anal sphincter. VER external anal *sphincter*.
p. sublentifor'mis cap'sulae inter'nae [TA], p. sublentiforme da cápsula interna. SIN sublenticular *part* of internal capsule.
p. sublentiformis cruris posterioris [TA], p. sublentiforme da cápsula interna. SIN sublentiform *limb* of internal capsule.
p. superficialis compartimenti antebrachii anterioris [TA], p. superficial do compartimento anterior do antebraço. SIN superficial *part* of anterior (flexor) compartment of forearm.
p. superficialis compartimenti cruris posterioris [TA], p. superficial do compartimento posterior da perna. SIN superficial *part* of posterior (plantar flexor) compartment of leg.
p. superficia'lis glan'dulae parotid'eae [TA], p. superficial da glândula parótida. SIN superficial *part* of parotid gland. VER parotid *gland*.
p. superficia'lis mus'culi masse'teri [TA], p. superficial do músculo masseter. SIN superficial *part* of masseter muscle. VER masseter (*muscle*).
p. superficia'lis mus'culi sphinc'teri a'ni exter'ni [TA], p. superficial do músculo esfíncter externo do ânus. SIN superficial *part* of external anal sphincter. VER external anal *sphincter*.
p. superior ali lobuli centralis [TA], p. superior da asa do lóbulo central. SIN ala central *lobule*.
p. supe'rior duode'ni [TA], p. superior do duodeno. SIN superior *part* of duodenum.
p. supe'rior facie'i diaphrag'maticae hep'atis [TA], p. superior da face diafragmática do fígado. SIN superior *part* of diaphragmatic surface of liver.
p. supe'rior gan'glii vestibula'ris [TA], p. superior do nervo vestibular. SIN superior *part* of vestibular ganglion.
p. supe'rior venae lingula'ris ve'nae pulmo'nis superioris sin'istri [TA], p. superior da veia lingular da veia pulmonar esquerda superior. SIN superior *part* of lingular vein (of left superior pulmonary vein).
p. supraclavicula'ris plex'us brachia'lis [TA], p. supraclavicular do plexo braquial. SIN supraclavicular *part* of brachial plexus.
p. sympath'ica (divisionis autonomicae systematis nervosei peripherici) [TA], p. simpática (divisão autônoma do sistema nervoso). SIN sympathetic *part* of autonomic division of peripheral nervous system.
p. tec'ta, p. oculta; termo obsoleto; **p. tecta pancreatis,** parte oculta do pâncreas; parte do pâncreas coberta pela raiz do mesocolo transverso, a coalescência do mesocolo ascendente e a raiz do mesentério; **p. tecta renalis,** parte oculta do rim; parte do rim coberta pela raiz do mesocolo transverso; **p. tecta ureteralis,** parte oculta do ureter; parte do ureter direito recoberta (cruzada) pela raiz do mesentério, e do ureter esquerdo recoberta (cruzada) pela raiz do mesocolo sigmóide. SIN hidden part.
p. tec'ta duode'ni, p. oculta do duodeno. SIN hidden *part* of duodenum.
p. ten'sa membra'nae tym'pani [TA], p. tensa da membrana timpânica. SIN tense *part* of the tympanic membrane.
p. termina'lis, ramos terminais. VER middle cerebral *artery*, posterior cerebral *artery*. SIN terminal part.
p. terminalis ilei [TA], p. terminal do íleo. SIN terminal *ileus*.
p. thorac'ica aor'tae [TA], p. torácica da aorta. SIN thoracic *aorta*.
p. thorac'ica duc'tus thorac'ici [TA], p. torácica do ducto torácico. SIN thoracic *part* of thoracic duct. VER thoracic *duct*.
p. thorac'ica esoph'agi [TA], p. torácica do esôfago. SIN thoracic *part* of esophagus.
p. thorac'ica medul'lae spina'lis [TA], p. torácica da medula espinal. SIN thoracic *part* of spinal cord.
p. thoracica muscularis iliocostalis lumborum [TA], p. torácica do músculo iliocostal do lombo. SIN thoracic *part* of iliocostalis lumborum (muscle).
p. thoracica plexum et ganglionorum visceralium [TA], p. torácica dos plexos e gânglios viscerais. SIN thoracic *part* of peripheral autonomic plexuses and ganglia.
p. thoracica tracheae [TA], p. torácica da traquéia. SIN thoracic *part* of trachea.
p. thyroepiglottica musculi thyroarytenoidei [TA], p. tireoepiglótica do músculo tireoaritenóideo. SIN thyroepiglottic *part* of thyroarytenoid (muscle).
p. thyropharyn'gea mus'culi constricto'ris pharyn'gis inferio'ris [TA], p. tireofaríngea do músculo constritor inferior da faringe. SIN thyropharyngeal *part*

of inferior constrictor muscle of pharynx. VER inferior constrictor (*muscle*) of pharynx.

p. tibiocalcanea ligamenti deltoidei, p. tibiocalcânea do ligamento deltóideo (ligamento colateral medial) ; *termo oficial alternativo para tibiocalcaneal *part* of medial ligament of ankle joint.

p. tibiocalca'nea ligamen'ti collateralis media'lis articulationis talocruralis [TA], p. tibiocalcânea do ligamento colateral medial (deltóideo) da articulação talocrural. SIN tibiocalcaneal *part* of medial ligament of ankle joint.

p. tibionavicula'ris ligamen'ti collateralis media'lis articulationes talocruralis [TA]. SIN tibionavicular *part* of medial ligament of ankle joint.

p. tibiotala'ris ante'rior ligamen'ti collateralis media'lis articulationis talocruralis [TA], p. tibiotalar anterior do ligamento colateral medial (deltóideo) da articulação talocrural. SIN anterior tibiotalar *part* of medial ligament of ankle joint.

p. tibiotala'ris poste'rior ligamen'ti collateralis media'lis articulationis talocruralis [TA], p. tibiotalar posterior do ligamento colateral medial (deltóideo) da articulação talocrural. SIN tibiotalar *part* of medial ligament of ankle joint.

p. transversa ligamenti iliofemoralis [TA], p. transversa do ligamento iliofemoral. SIN transverse *part* of iliofemoral ligament.

p. transver'sa mus'culi nasa'lis [TA], p. transversa do músculo nasal. SIN transverse *part* of nasalis muscle. VER nasalis (*muscle*).

p. transversa musculi trapezii [TA], p. transversa do músculo trapézio. SIN transverse *part* of trapezius (muscle).

p. transver'sa ra'mi si'nistri ve'nae por'tae hepa'tis [TA], p. transversa do ramo esquerdo da veia porta do fígado. SIN transverse *part* of left branch of portal vein.

p. transversa'ria arte'riae vertebra'lis, p. transversária da artéria vertebral. VER vertebral *artery*.

p. triangula'ris [TA], p. triangular. SIN triangular *part*.

p. tricipitalis compartimenti cruris posterioris, p. superficial do compartimento posterior da perna; *termo oficial alternativo para superficial *part* of posterior (plantar flexor) compartment of leg.

p. tubera'lis [TA], p. tuberal da hipófise; a extensão superior do lobo anterior que envolve o pedículo infundibular; suas células, na maioria gonadotróficas, estão dispostas em cordões e grupos; é suprida pelas artérias hipofisárias superiores e contém o primeiro leito capilar e as vênulas de um sistema porta que transporta fatores neurossecretores do hipotálamo para um leito capilar secundário na adeno-hipófise, onde regulam a liberação de hormônios. VER TAMBÉM pituitary *gland*. SIN infundibular part, p. infundibularis.

p. tympan'ica os'sis tempora'lis [TA], p. timpânica do (osso) temporal. SIN tympanic *plate* of temporal bone.

p. umbilica'lis ra'mi si'nistri ve'nae por'tae hepa'tis [TA], p. umbilical do ramo esquerdo da veia porta do fígado. SIN umbilical *part* of left branch of portal vein.

p. uteri'na placen'tae, p. uterina da placenta; a parte da placenta derivada do tecido uterino. VER TAMBÉM placenta. SIN maternal placenta, placenta uterina.

p. uteri'na tu'bae uteri'nae [TA], p. uterina da tuba uterina. SIN uterine *part* of uterine tube.

p. uvea'lis reti'culi trabecula'ris sclerae [TA], p. uveal do retículo trabecular da esclera. SIN uveal *part* of trabecular tissue of sclera.

p. vaga'lis ner'vi accesso'rii, raiz craniana do nervo acessório; *termo oficial alternativo para cranial *root* of accessory nerve.

p. ventralis musculi intertransversarii lateralium lumborum [TA], p. ventral dos músculos intertransversários laterais do lombo. SIN ventral *part* of intertransversarii laterales lumborum (muscles).

p. ventralis pontis, p. basilar da ponte. SIN basilar *part* of pons.

p. vertebra'lis facie'i costa'lis pulmo'nis [TA], p. vertebral da face costal do pulmão. SIN vertebral *part* of the costal surface of the lungs.

p. vestibula'ris ner'vi vestibulocochlea'ris, p. vestibular do nervo vestibulococlear. SIN vestibular *nerve*.

pars-pla.ni.tis (parz′plā - nī′tis). Pars planitis; uma síndrome clínica que consiste em inflamação da retina periférica e/ou pars plana, exsudação para a base vítrea subjacente e edema do disco óptico e da retina adjacente.

part. Parte. SIN pars [TA].

abdominal p. of aorta, p. abdominal da aorta. SIN abdominal *aorta*.

abdominal p. of esophagus [TA], p. abdominal do esôfago; a parte do esôfago do ponto que atravessa o diafragma até o estômago. VER esophagus. SIN pars abdominalis esophagi [TA], epicardia.

abdominal p. of pectoralis major (muscle) [TA], p. abdominal do músculo peitoral maior; parte do músculo peitoral maior que se origina na bainha do reto. SIN pars abdominalis musculi pectorales majoris [TA].

abdominal p. of peripheral autonomic plexuses and ganglia [TA], p. abdominal dos plexos viscerais e gânglios viscerais; parte do sistema nervoso autônomo (redes compostas principalmente de fibras nervosas autônomas — mas que também incluem fibras aferentes viscerais — e gânglios associados aos vasos sanguíneos e órgãos) encontrada nos espaços retroperitoneal e intraperitoneal na cavidade abdominal. SIN pars abdominalis plexus visceralis et ganglii visceralis [TA].

abdominal p. of thoracic duct [TA], p. abdominal do ducto torácico; a parte do ducto torácico entre a cisterna do quilo e o hiato aórtico do diafragma. SIN pars abdominalis ductus thoracici [TA].

abdominal p. of ureter [TA], p. abdominal do ureter; a parte do ureter situada entre a pelve renal e a margem da pelve. SIN pars abdominalis ureteris [TA].

acromial p. of deltoid (muscle) [TA], p. acromial do músculo deltóide; parte do músculo deltóide que se origina no acrômio. SIN pars acromialis musculi deltoidei [TA].

alar p. of nasalis muscle [TA], p. alar do músculo nasal. VER nasalis (*muscle*). SIN pars alaris musculi nasalis [TA].

alveolar p. of mandible [TA], p. alveolar da mandíbula; a parte do corpo da mandíbula que circunda e sustenta os dentes inferiores. SIN pars alveolaris mandibulae [TA].

anterior p., [TA], p. anterior; a parte de uma estrutura em posição mais anterior, ou mais próxima da superfície anterior em relação a outras partes; em anatomia humana, a porção ventral de uma estrutura. VER anterior part of: anterior commissure of brain; guadrangular lobule of cerebellum; central lobule of cerebellum; culmen; lateral parabranchial nucleus; diaphragmatic surface of liver; tongue; fornix of vagina. SIN pars anterior [TA].

anterior p. of anterior commissure of brain [TA], p. anterior da comissura anterior do encéfalo; a parte anterior da comissura anterior ou rostral do encéfalo. SIN pars anterior commissurae anterioris [TA], pars anterior commissurae rostralis.

anterior p. of diaphragmatic surface of liver [TA], p. anterior da face diafragmática do fígado; a parte da face diafragmática do fígado situada profundamente aos arcos costais e ao processo xifóide. SIN pars anterior faciei diaphragmatis hepatis [TA].

anterior p. of fornix of vagina [TA], p. anterior do fórnice da vagina; a parte do fórnice da vagina anterior ao colo do útero. SIN pars anterior fornicis vaginae [TA].

anterior p. of pons, p. basilar da ponte. SIN basilar p. of pons.

anterior tibiotalar p. of deltoid ligament, p. tibiotalar anterior do ligamento deltóideo. SIN anterior tibiotalar p. of medial ligament of ankle joint.

anterior tibiotalar p. of medial ligament of ankle joint [TA], p. tibiotalar anterior do ligamento colateral medial da articulação talocrural; a parte do ligamento colateral medial ou deltóideo que se estende do maléolo medial até o colo do tálus. SIN pars tibiotalaris anterior ligamenti collateralis medialis articulationis talocruralis [TA], anterior talotibial ligament, anterior tibiotalar ligament, anterior tibiotalar p. of deltoid ligament, ligamentum mediale, ligamentum talotibiale anterius.

anterior p. of tongue [TA], p. pré-sulcal da língua; parte da língua (≈ 2/3) anterior ao sulco terminal, distinta da parte posterior em origem embriológica e inervação. SIN pars anterior linguae [TA], pars presulcalis linguae*, pars presulcalis*, presulcal p. of tongue*.

anular p. of fibrous digital sheath of digits of hand and foot [TA], p. anular da bainha fibrosa dos dedos da mão e do pé; uma das cinco faixas fibrosas circulares ou tróclas (A1-A5) das bainhas fibrosas dos dedos e das estruturas correspondentes dos dedos dos pés fixadas ao corpo das falanges proximal e média e das cápsulas articulares associadas. SIN pars anularis vaginae fibrosae digitorum manus et pedis [TA], anular pulley, anulus of fibrous sheath, ligamentum anulare digitorum.

aryepiglottic p. of oblique arytenoid muscle [TA], p. ariepiglótica do músculo aritenóideo oblíquo; fibras do músculo aritenóideo oblíquo que continuam após o ápice da cartilagem aritenóidea até a lateral da epiglote; *ação*, contrai a abertura laríngea de forma semelhante a um "cordão de bolsa". SIN pars aryepiglottica musculi arytenoidei obliqui [TA], aryepiglottic muscle, musculus aryepiglotticus.

ascending p. of aorta, p. ascendente da aorta. SIN ascending *aorta*.

ascending p. of duodenum [TA], p. ascendente do duodeno; a porção terminal, ou quarta parte do duodeno, que ascende da parte horizontal até o jejuno. SIN pars ascendens duodeni [TA].

ascending p. of trapezius (muscle) [TA], p. ascendente do músculo trapézio; terço inferior do trapézio que ascende para se inserir na espinha da escápula; age de forma independente de outras partes para abaixar a escápula (abaixar os ombros); age com outras partes para afastar e rodar a escápula. SIN pars ascendens musculi trapezii [TA], inferior p. of trapezius (muscle)*.

atlantic p. of vertebral artery [TA], p. atlântica da artéria vertebral; parte suboccipital da artéria vertebral. VER vertebral *artery*. SIN pars atlantica arteriae vertebralis [TA], suboccipital p. of vertebral artery.

autonomic p. of peripheral nervous system, divisão autônoma do sistema nervoso periférico; *termo oficial alternativo para autonomic *division* of nervous system.

basal p. [TA], p. basilar; parte de uma estrutura que forma sua base — a parte inferior ou parte oposta ao ápice da estrutura — ou um ramo que serve àquela parte da estrutura; p. ex., a base dos pulmões (formada pelos quatro segmentos basilares broncopulmonares de cada lado) irrigada pelas partes basilares das artérias pulmonares direita e esquerda. SIN basilar p.'s [TA], pars basalis [TA], pars basilaris [TA].

basal p. of left and right inferior pulmonary arteries [TA], p. basilar das artérias lobares inferiores pulmonares esquerda e direita. VER right pulmonary *artery*, left pulmonary *artery*. SIN pars basalis arteriarum lobarium inferiorum pulmonis sinistri et dextri [TA]. VER right pulmonary *artery*, left pulmonary *artery*.

basal p. of occipital bone, p. basilar do (osso) occipital. SIN basilar p. of occipital bone.

basilar p.'s [TA], partes basilares. SIN basal p.

basilar p. of occipital bone [TA], p. basilar do (osso) occipital; a parte cuneiforme do osso occipital (anterior ao forame magno) que se une ao corpo do osso esfenóide. SIN pars basilaris ossis occipitalis [TA], basal p. of occipital bone, basilar apophysis, basilar process of occipital bone, basilar process, basiociput.

basilar p. of pons [TA], p. basilar da ponte; a grande porção bulbar da ponte observada na porção ventral do tronco encefálico e ventral ao lemnisco medial em corte transversal: contém fibras orientadas longitudinalmente (corticospinais, corticopontinas, corticorreticulares e outras) e as fibras pontocerebelares orientadas transversalmente. SIN pars basilaris pontis [TA], pons basilaris pontis [TA], anterior p. of pons, pars ventralis pontis, ventral p. of pons.

bony p. of external acoustic meatus, p. óssea do meato acústico externo; os dois terços mediais do meato acústico externo, formados quando se desenvolve a parte timpânica do (osso) temporal; estende-se aproximadamente 16 mm desde sua junção com a parte cartilaginosa até a membrana timpânica.

bony p. of nasal septum [TA], p. óssea do septo nasal; a principal parte do septo nasal, incluindo o vômer (sustentada por este) e a lâmina perpendicular do etmóide. SIN pars ossea septi nasi [TA].

bony p. of pharyngotympanic (auditory) tube [TA], p. óssea da tuba auditiva; a parte da tuba auditiva (faringotimpânica) formada pela parte petrosa do osso temporal que segue da cavidade timpânica ântero-medialmente, através do semicanal da tuba auditiva. SIN pars ossea tubae auditivae [TA], pars ossea tubae auditoriae.

bony p. of skeletal system [TA], p. óssea do sistema esquelético; parte do esqueleto composta de osso cortical, compacto ou esponjoso. SIN pars ossea systematis skeletalis [TA], osseous p. of skeletal system.

buccopharyngeal p. of superior pharyngeal constrictor, p. bucofaríngeo do músculo constritor superior da faringe. VER superior pharyngeal constrictor (*muscle*). SIN pars buccopharyngea musculi constrictoris pharyngei superioris.

cardiac p. of stomach, cárdia. SIN cardia.

cardial p. of stomach, cárdia. SIN cardia.

cartilaginous p. of external acoustic meatus, p. cartilagínea do meato acústico externo; o terço lateral do meato acústico externo, contínuo com a cartilagem auricular e fixado à circunferência da parte óssea.

cartilaginous p. of nasal septum [TA], p. cartilagínea do septo nasal; parte do septo nasal sustentada por cartilagem (em vez de osso).

cartilaginous p. of pharyngotympanic (auditory) tube, p. cartilagínea da tuba auditiva; aquela parte da tuba auditiva sustentada por cartilagem; avança em sentido ântero-medial, a partir da parte óssea, para se abrir na nasofaringe. SIN pars cartilaginea tubae auditivae [TA], pars cartilaginea tubae auditoriae.

cartilaginous p. of skeletal system [TA], p. cartilagínea do sistema esquelético; a parte do esqueleto composta de cartilagem. SIN pars cartilaginea systematis skeletalis [TA].

cavernous p. of internal carotid artery [TA], p. cavernosa da artéria carótida interna; a parte mais tortuosa da artéria carótida interna que atravessa o seio cavernoso; possui muitos ramos pequenos. SIN pars cavernosa arteriae carotidis internae [TA].

celiacoduodenal p. of suspensory muscle (ligament) of duodenum [TA], p. celiacoduodenal do músculo suspensor do duodeno; faixa fibromuscular de músculo liso que sai da parte terminal do duodeno e da flexura duodenojejunal para terminar no tecido conjuntivo, nas adjacências do tronco celíaco. SIN pars coeliacoduodenalis musculi (ligament) suspensorii duodeni [TA].

central p. of lateral ventricle, p. central do ventrículo lateral. SIN *pars* centralis ventriculi lateralis.

ceratopharyngeal p. of middle constrictor muscle of pharynx [TA], p. ceratofaríngea do músculo constritor médio da faringe. VER middle constrictor (*muscle*) of pharynx. SIN pars ceratopharyngea musculi constrictoris pharyngei medii [TA], ceratopharyngeal p. of middle pharyngeal constrictor (muscle) of pharynx.

ceratopharyngeal p. of middle pharyngeal constrictor (muscle) of pharynx, p. ceratofaríngea do músculo constritor médio da faringe. SIN ceratopharyngeal p. of middle constrictor muscle of pharynx.

cerebral p. of arachnoid, p. encefálica da aracnóide-máter. SIN cranial *arachnoid* mater.

cerebral p. of dura mater, p. encefálica da dura-máter. SIN cranial *dura mater*.

cerebral p. of internal carotid artery [TA], p. cerebral da artéria carótida interna; a parte da artéria carótida interna que fica em contato com o encéfalo e o irriga diretamente; seus ramos são: hipofisária superior, do clivo, oftálmica, corióidea anterior, cerebral anterior e cerebral média. SIN pars cerebralis arteriae carotidis internae [TA].

cervical p. of esophagus [TA], p. cervical do esôfago; a parte do esôfago localizada no pescoço. VER esophagus. SIN pars cervicalis esophagi [TA].

cervical p. of internal carotid artery [TA], p. cervical da artéria carótida interna; a porção não ramificada localizada no pescoço. SIN pars cervicalis arteriae carotidis internae [TA].

cervical p. of spinal cord [TA], p. cervical da medula espinal; a parte da medula espinal localizada no pescoço, que consiste em oito segmentos cervicais [C1–C8] e dá origem aos primeiros oito pares de nervos espinais [C1–C8]. SIN pars cervicalis medullae spinalis [TA], segmenta cervicalia medullae spinalis [TA], segmenta medullae spinalis cervicalia C1–C8 [TA], cervical segments of spinal cord [C1–C8]*, segmenta cervicalia C1–C5.

cervical p. of thoracic duct [TA], p. cervical do ducto torácico; a parte do ducto torácico acima da primeira costela. SIN pars cervicalis ductus thoracici [TA].

cervical p. of vertebral artery [TA], p. transversária da artéria vertebral; parte da artéria vertebral que atravessa os forames transversos das vértebras cervicais C1–C6 e dá origem aos ramos espinais e musculares. SIN pars cervicalis arteriae vertebralis [TA], transversarial p. of vertebral artery [TA].

chondropharyngeal p. of middle constrictor muscle of pharynx [TA], p. condrofaríngea do músculo constritor médio da faringe. VER middle constrictor (*muscle*) of pharynx. SIN pars chondropharyngea musculi constrictoris pharyngei medii [TA], chondropharyngeal p. of middle pharyngeal constrictor (muscle) of pharynx.

chondropharyngeal p. of middle pharyngeal constrictor (muscle) of pharynx, p. condrofaríngea do músculo constritor médio da faringe. SIN chondropharyngeal p. of middle constrictor muscle of pharynx.

ciliary p. of retina [TA], p. ciliar da retina. VER retina. SIN pars ciliaris retinae [TA].

clavicular p. of deltoid (muscle) [TA], p. clavicular do músculo deltóide; porção anterior do músculo deltóide que se origina da clavícula; atua independentemente de outras partes para ajudar na flexão da articulação do ombro. SIN pars clavicularis musculi deltoidei [TA].

clavicular p. of pectoralis major (muscle), p. clavicular do músculo peitoral maior. SIN clavicular *head* of pectoralis major muscle. VER pectoralis major (*muscle*).

coccygeal p. of spinal cord [TA], p. coccígea da medula espinal; a p. terminal da medula espinal que consiste nos três segmentos coccígeos da medula espinal, do qual se originam os três pares de nervos coccígeos. SIN pars coccygea medullae spinalis [TA], segmenta coccygea medullae spinalis [TA].

cochlear p. of vestibulocochlear nerve, p. coclear do nervo vestibulococlear. SIN cochlear *nerve*.

convoluted p. of kidney lobule, p. convoluta do lóbulo renal; túbulos convolutos proximais e distais e os corpúsculos renais associados irrigados por ramos das artérias interlobulares. SIN labyrinthus, Ludwig labyrinth, pars convoluta lobuli corticalis renis, renal labyrinth.

corneoscleral p. of trabecular tissue of sclera [TA], p. corneoescleral do retículo trabecular da esclera; a p. anterior do retículo trabecular, localizada entre o seio venoso da esclera, o esporão da esclera e a membrana limitante posterior da córnea. SIN pars corneoscleralis reticuli trabecularis sclerae [TA].

cortical p., ramos terminais. SIN pars corticalis. VER middle cerebral *artery*, posterior cerebral *artery*.

cortical p. of middle cerebral artery, ramos terminais da artéria cerebral média. VER middle cerebral *artery*.

costal p. of diaphragm [TA], p. costal do diafragma; a p. do diafragma que se origina da face interna das seis cartilagens costais inferiores e das quatro costelas inferiores e se insere na parte ântero-lateral do tendão central. SIN pars costalis diaphragmatis [TA].

costal p. of parietal pleura [TA], p. costal da pleura parietal; p. da pleura parietal que reveste a face interna das costelas e músculos intercostais. SIN pars costalis pleurae parietalis [TA], costal pleura, pleura costalis.

cranial p. of parasympathetic part of autonomic division of nervous system [TA], p. craniana da parte parassimpática da divisão autônoma do sistema nervoso; as raízes e ramos dos gânglios parassimpáticos (ciliar, pterigopalatino, ótico e submandibular/sublingual) da cabeça. SIN pars cranialis partis parasympathetici divisionis autonomici systematis nervosi [TA].

craniocervical p. of peripheral autonomic plexuses and ganglia [TA], p. craniocervical dos plexos viscerais e gânglios viscerais; redes de fibras nervosas simpáticas pós-sinápticas que acompanham as artérias carótidas e seus ramos na cabeça e pescoço. SIN pars craniocervicalis plexuum et gangliorum visceralium [TA].

cricopharyngeal p. of inferior constrictor (muscle) of pharynx [TA], p. cricofaríngea do músculo constritor inferior da faringe. VER inferior constrictor (*muscle*) of pharynx. SIN pars cricopharyngea musculi constrictoris pharyngis inferioris [TA], cricopharyngeus muscle*.

cruciform p. of fibrous digital sheath [TA], p. cruciforme da bainha fibrosa dos dedos; as fibras da bainha fibrosa dos dedos da mão e do pé que constituem três trócleas em forma de X (C1–C3) sobre as falanges proximal e média. SIN pars cruciformis vaginae fibrosae [TA], crucial ligament (4), cruciform p. of fibrous sheath, cruciform pulley, ligamenta cruciata digitorum.

cruciform p. of fibrous sheath, p. cruciforme da bainha fibrosa. SIN cruciform p. of fibrous digital sheath.

cuneiform p. of vomer [TA], p. cuneiforme do vômer; a porção anterior fina cuneiforme do vômer. SIN pars cuneiformis vomeris [TA].

cupular p. of epitympanic recess [TA], p. cupular do recesso epitimpânico; a porção mais alta, em forma de cúpula, do recesso epitimpânico. SIN pars cupularis recessus epitympanici [TA].

deep p. of anterior compartment of forearm [TA], p. profunda do compartimento anterior do antebraço; p. do compartimento anterior (flexor) do antebraço que inclui os músculos flexor longo do polegar, flexor profundo dos dedos e pronador quadrado. SIN pars profunda compartimenti antebrachii anterioris [TA].

deep p. of external anal sphincter [TA], p. profunda do esfíncter externo do ânus. VER external anal *sphincter*. SIN pars profunda musculi sphincteri ani externi.

deep p. of flexor retinaculum, p. profunda do retináculo dos músculos flexores. SIN flexor *retinaculum*.

deep p. of masseter (muscle) [TA], p. profunda do músculo masseter. VER masseter (*muscle*). SIN pars profunda musculi masseteri [TA].

deep p. of palpebral part of orbicularis oculi (muscle) [TA], p. profunda da parte palpebral do músculo orbicular do olho; porção da parte palpebral do músculo orbicular do olho originada na face posterior do ligamento palpebral medial e no osso adjacente. SIN pars profunda partis palpebralis musculi orbicularis oculi [TA].

deep p. of parotid gland [TA], p. profunda da glândula parótida; a p. da glândula salivar localizada atrás da mandíbula e que ocupa o espaço entre o ramo da mandíbula e o processo mastóide, que se estende medialmente até a parede da faringe. SIN pars profunda glandulae parotidis [TA], processus retromandibularis glandulae parotidis, processus retromandibularis, retromandibular process of parotid gland. VER parotid *gland*.

deep p. of posterior (flexor) compartment of leg [TA], p. profunda do compartimento posterior da perna; p. do compartimento posterior (flexor) da perna, incluindo os músculos flexor longo dos dedos, flexor longo do hálux e tibial posterior. SIN pars profunda compartimenti cruris posterioris [TA].

descending p. of aorta, p. descendente da aorta. SIN descending *aorta*.

descending p. of duodenum [TA], p. descendente do duodeno. VER duodenum. SIN pars descendens duodeni [TA], pars secundum duodeni, second p. of duodenum.

descending p. of facial canal, p. descendente do canal facial; segunda porção do canal facial, após as partes horizontais, que começa na extremidade posterior do ramo lateral, onde o canal começa a descer. Segue verticalmente para baixo, terminando no forame estilomastóideo. Anteriormente, a p. descendente do canal facial comunica-se com a cavidade timpânica através do canalículo para o nervo até o músculo estapédio e o canalículo posterior da corda do tímpano. VER TAMBÉM facial *canal*.

descending p. of iliofemoral ligament [TA], p. descendente do ligamento iliofemoral; o mais vertical dos ramos do ligamento iliofemoral, tendo a forma de Y invertido (ao contrário da parte transversa, que é mais horizontal). SIN pars descendens ligamenti iliofemoralis [TA].

descending p. of trapezius (muscle) [TA], p. descendente do músculo trapézio; o terço superior do músculo trapézio que desce para se inserir na clavícula e no acrômio; agindo independentemente das outras partes, eleva a escápula (retrai os ombros). SIN pars descendens musculi trapezii [TA].

diaphragmatic p. of parietal pleura [TA], p. diafragmática da pleura parietal; p. da camada externa (parietal) da pleura que reveste a face superior do diafragma de cada lado do pericárdio. SIN pars diaphragmatica pleurae parietalis [TA], diaphragmatic pleura, phrenic pleura, pleura diaphragmatica, pleura phrenica.

distal p. of prostate [TA], p. distal da próstata; p. da próstata derivada do primórdio mais caudal; inclui os lobos direito, esquerdo e posterior da próstata. SIN pars distalis prostatae [TA].

distal p. of prostatic urethra [TA], p. distal da parte prostática da uretra masculina; p. da uretra prostática inferior à fusão das vias urinária e genital nas aberturas dos ductos ejaculatórios. SIN pars distalis urethrae prostaticae [TA].

distal p. [TA] of anterior lobe of hypophysis, p. distal da adeno-hipófise; a maior p. da adeno-hipófise, composta de cordões de células epiteliais individualmente especializadas para secretar vários hormônios trópicos que exercem seu efeito sobre vários órgãos-alvo do corpo. A atividade secretora dessas células é controlada por fatores liberadores ou inibidores produzidos por neurônios hipotalâmicos e transportados até a adeno-hipófise pelo sistema porta hipotalâmico-hipofisário. SIN pars distalis adenohypophyseos [TA].

dorsal p. of intertransversarii laterales lumborum (muscles) [TA], p. dorsal dos músculos intertransversários laterais do lombo; p. dos músculos intertransversários laterais da região lombar que une os processos acessórios de uma vértebra aos processos transversos da vértebra acima. SIN partes dorsales musculorum intertransversariorum lateralium lumborum [TA].

dorsal p. of pons, p. dorsal da ponte; a p. da ponte limitada, lateralmente, pelos pedúnculos cerebelares médios e, anteriormente, pela parte ventral da ponte; é contínua com o tegmento do mesencéfalo e contém longos tratos, como os lemniscos medial e lateral, núcleos dos nervos cranianos e formação reticular. SIN tegmentum of pons [TA], tegmentum pontis [TA], pars dorsalis pontis.

dural p. of filum terminale [TA], p. dural do filamento terminal; a terminação filiforme da dura-máter espinal que circunda o filamento terminal da medula espinal e está fundida a ele e fixada ao ligamento sacrococcígeo dorsal profundo; estende-se do nível vertebral S2–3 ao nível Co2. VER TAMBÉM terminal *filum*. SIN coccygeal ligament*, filum terminale externum*, filum durae matris spinalis, filum of spinal dura mater.

endocrine p. of pancreas [TA], p. endócrina do pâncreas. VER pancreas. SIN pars endocrina pancreatis [TA].

exocrine p. of pancreas [TA], p. exócrina do pâncreas. VER pancreas. SIN pars exocrina pancreatis [TA].

extraocular p. of central retinal artery and vein [TA], p. extra-ocular da artéria e veia centrais da retina; p. orbital da artéria e veia centrais da retina externa (posterior) ao bulbo do olho. SIN pars extraocularis arteriae et venae centralis retinae [TA].

first p. of duodenum, primeira p. do duodeno. SIN superior p. of duodenum.

flaccid p. of tympanic membrane [TA], p. flácida da membrana timpânica; p. frouxa triangular da membrana timpânica situada entre as pregas maleolares. SIN pars flaccida membranae tympanae [TA], flaccid membrane, membrana flaccida, Rivinus membrane, Shrapnell membrane.

free p. of lower limb [TA], p. livre do membro inferior; p. do esqueleto apendicular do membro inferior distal à articulação do quadril; o cíngulo do membro inferior está excluído. SIN pars libera membri inferioris [TA].

free p. of upper limb [TA], p. livre do membro superior; p. do esqueleto apendicular do membro superior distal à articulação do ombro; o cíngulo do membro superior não está incluído. SIN pars libera membri superioris [TA].

frontal p. of corpus callosum, p. frontal do corpo caloso. SIN minor *forceps*.

funicular p. of ductus deferens [TA], p. funicular do ducto deferente; p. do ducto deferente contida no cordão espermático. SIN pars funicularis ductus deferentis [TA].

glossopharyngeal p. of superior pharyngeal constrictor, p. glossofaríngea do músculo constritor superior da faringe. VER superior pharyngeal constrictor (*muscle*). SIN pars glossopharyngea musculi constrictoris pharyngis superioris.

hidden p., p. oculta. SIN pars tecta.

hidden p. of duodenum, p. oculta do duodeno; a p. do duodeno coberta pela raiz do mesocolo transverso, coalescência do mesocolo ascendente e raiz do mesentério. SIN pars tecta duodeni.

horizontal p. of duodenum, p. horizontal do duodeno; *termo oficial alternativo para inferior p. of duodenum. VER duodenum.

horizontal p. of facial canal, p. horizontal do canal do nervo facial; primeira p. do canal facial, situada entre o início do canal (no intróito do canal facial na extremidade do meato acústico interno) e o ponto no qual faz a volta para descer, começando a parte descendente (*descending part*). Há dois componentes (ramos) da parte horizontal: o ramo medial, orientado anteriormente e localizado medialmente, e o ramo lateral, orientado posteriormente e posicionado lateralmente, sendo os dois contínuos em uma curva aguda, o joelho do canal do nervo facial. Essa parte lateral é onde está localizado o gânglio geniculado, comunicando-se com a fossa média do crânio por meio do hiato do canal do nervo facial, através do qual passa o nervo petroso superficial maior.

p.'s of human body [TA], partes do corpo humano; cabeça, pescoço, tronco, membros e cavidades. SIN partes corporis humani [TA].

inferior p. [TA], p. inferior; a p. mais baixa de uma estrutura em relação às outras partes; a parte mais próxima das regiões plantares. VER inferior part of: duodenum, lingular branch of left pulmonary vein, and vestibular ganglion. SIN pars inferior [TA].

inferior p. of duodenum [TA], p. horizontal do duodeno; terceira p. do duodeno, inferior à cabeça do pâncreas, situada entre os vasos mesentéricos superiores, anteriormente, e a aorta e a veia cava inferior, posteriormente. SIN pars horizontalis duodeni [TA], horizontal p. of duodenum*, pars inferior duodeni*, third p. of duodenum.

inferior p. of lingular vein (of left superior pulmonary vein) [TA], p. inferior da veia lingular (da veia pulmonar esquerda superior); a veia que drena o segmento broncopulmonar lingular inferior do pulmão esquerdo. SIN pars inferior venae lingularis venae pulmonalis superioris sinistrae [TA].

inferior p. of trapezius (muscle), p. ascendente do músculo trapézio; *termo oficial alternativo para ascending p. of trapezius (muscle).

inferior p. of vestibular ganglion [TA], p. inferior do gânglio vestibular; a p. inferior do gânglio vestibular que recebe fibras da mácula do sáculo e da ampola do ducto semicircular posterior. SIN pars inferior ganglii vestibularis [TA].

inferior p. of vestibulocochlear nerve, p. inferior do nervo vestibulococlear. SIN cochlear *nerve*.

infraclavicular p. of brachial plexus [TA], p. infraclavicular do plexo braquial; a p. do plexo braquial que se estende do nível da clavícula para baixo até a axila; inclui os cordões do plexo e seus ramos. SIN pars infraclavicularis plexus brachialis [TA].

infralobar p. of posterior vein (of right superior pulmonary vein) [TA], p. infralobar da veia posterior (da veia pulmonar direita superior); a veia que drena o segmento posterior do pulmão direito que emerge inferior ao lobo superior; tributária do ramo posterior da veia pulmonar direita superior. SIN pars infralobaris venae posterioris venae pulmonalis superioris dextrae [TA].

infrasegmental p., p. infra-segmentar. SIN intersegmental *vein.*

infundibular p., p. infundibular. SIN *pars* tuberalis.

inguinal p. of ductus deferens [TA], p. inguinal do ducto deferente; p. do ducto deferente localizada no canal inguinal, isto é, entre os anéis inguinais superficial e profundo. SIN pars inguinalis ductus deferentis [TA].

insular p., lobo insular. SIN *lobus* insula.

insular p. of middle cerebral artery [TA], p. insular da artéria cerebral média. VER middle cerebral *artery.* SIN pars insularis arteriae cerebri mediae [TA].

intercartilaginous p. of glottic opening, p. intercartilagínea da rima da glote. SIN intercartilaginous p. of rima glottidis.

intercartilaginous p. of rima glottidis [TA], p. intercartilagínea da rima da glote; a abertura entre os processos vocais das cartilagens aritenóideas; essa parte fica aberta ao sussurrar e se fecha durante a fonação e a manobra de Valsalva. SIN pars intercartilaginea rimae glottidis [TA], glottis respiratoria, intercartilaginous p. of glottic opening.

intermediate p. [TA], p. intermédia; porção central; a porção localizada entre porções extremas de uma estrutura; uma parte interposta. VER intermediate p. of adenohypophysis, intermediate p. of male urethra. SIN pars intermedia [TA].

intermediate p. of adenohypophysis [TA], p. intermédia da adeno-hipófise; a p. da adeno-hipófise localizada entre a parte distal e a parte nervosa; pouco desenvolvida nos seres humanos. SIN pars intermedia adenohypophyseos [TA].

intermediate p. of male urethra [TA], p. membranácea da uretra masculina; a porção mais curta e mais estreita da uretra masculina, com cerca de 1 cm de comprimento, que se estende da próstata até o início da uretra no corpo esponjoso, logo após o bulbo. SIN pars intermedia urethrae masculinae [TA], membranous urethra*, pars membranacea urethrae masculinae*, membranous p. of male urethra.

intermediate p. of vestibular bulb, comissura dos bulbos. SIN *commissure* of bulbs.

intermembranous p. of glottic opening, p. intermembranácea da rima da glote. SIN intermembranous p. of rima glottidis.

intermembranous p. of rima glottidis [TA], p. intermembranácea da rima da glote; a p. da abertura anterior aos processos vocais das cartilagens aritenóideas limitados pelos ligamentos vocais; essa p. é fechada por contração do músculo cricoaritenóideo lateral apenas durante o sussurro. SIN pars intermembranacea rimae glottidis [TA], glottis vocalis, intermembranous p. of glottic opening.

intersegmental p. of pulmonary vein [TA], p. intersegmentar das raízes da veia pulmonar. SIN intersegmental *vein.*

intracranial p. of optic nerve [TA], p. intracraniana do nervo óptico; a p. do nervo óptico situada entre o canal óptico e o quiasma óptico. SIN pars intracranialis nervi optici [TA].

intracranial p. of vertebral artery [TA], p. intracraniana da artéria vertebral. VER vertebral *artery.* SIN pars intracranialis arteriae vertebralis [TA].

intralaminar p. of intraocular part of optic nerve [TA], p. intralaminar da p. intra-ocular do nervo óptico; a porção da parte intra-ocular do nervo óptico quando atravessa a lâmina cribriforme da esclera. SIN pars intralaminaris nervi optici intralocularis [TA].

intralobar p. of the posterior vein (of the right superior pulmonary vein) [TA], p. intralobar da veia posterior (da veia pulmonar direita superior); a veia que drena os segmentos apical e posterior do pulmão direito; tributária do ramo posterior da veia pulmonar direita superior. SIN pars intralobaris (intersegmentalis) venae posterioris lobi superioris pulmonis dextri [TA].

intramural p. of male urethra [TA], p. intramural da uretra masculina; porção inicial da uretra masculina que atravessa a parede (assoalho) da bexiga. SIN pars intramuralis urethrae masculinae [TA], pars preprostatica urethrae masculinae*, preprostatic p. of male urethra*.

intraocular p. of optic nerve [TA], p. intra-ocular do nervo óptico; a p. do nervo óptico situada dentro do bulbo do olho; é dividida em partes intralaminar, pós-laminar e pré-laminar. SIN pars intraocularis nervi optici [TA].

intrasegmental p. of pulmonary veins [TA], p. intra-segmentar das veias pulmonares; uma p. que emerge do segmento broncopulmonar que ela drena; tributária de um ramo de uma artéria pulmonar. SIN pars intrasegmentalis venae pulmonum [TA], intrasegmental veins.

iridial p. of retina [TA], p. irídica da retina. VER retina. SIN pars iridica retinae [TA].

labial p. of orbicularis oris (muscle) [TA], p. labial do músculo orbicular da boca; a maior p. do músculo orbicular da boca dentro do corpo dos lábios. SIN pars labialis musculi orbicularis oris [TA].

lacrimal p. of orbicularis oculi muscle [TA], p. profunda da p. palpebral do músculo orbicular do olho; p. do músculo orbicular do olho que se origina no osso lacrimal. VER orbicularis oculi (*muscle*). SIN pars lacrimalis musculi orbicularis oculi [TA], Duverney muscle, Horner muscle, musculus tensor tarsi.

laryngeal p. of pharynx, p. laríngea da faringe. SIN laryngopharynx.

lateral p. of longitudinal arch of foot [TA], p. lateral do arco longitudinal do pé; p. do arco longitudinal do pé formada pelo calcâneo, cubóide e pelos dois metatarsais laterais (N–V); situa-se em posição mais baixa e é menos móvel que a p. medial; atua na transmissão de peso, enquanto a p. medial do arco absorve o choque do pé durante a locomoção. SIN pars lateralis arcus pedis longitudinalis [TA].

lateral p. of middle lobe vein (of right superior pulmonary vein) [TA], p. lateral da veia do lobo médio (da veia pulmonar direita superior); a veia que drena o segmento broncopulmonar lateral do lobo médio do pulmão direito. SIN pars lateralis venae lobi medii venae pulmonalis dextri superioris.

lateral p. of occipital bone [TA], p. lateral do occipital; a p. do osso occipital situada de cada lado do forame magno. SIN pars lateralis ossis occipitalis [TA], exoccipital bone.

lateral p. of posterior cervical intertransversarii (muscles), p. lateral dos músculos intertransversários posteriores do pescoço. VER posterior cervical intertransversarii (*muscles*), em *muscle*.

lateral p. of posterior (extensor) compartment of forearm [TA], p. lateral do compartimento posterior do antebraço; p. do compartimento fascial posterior do antebraço que inclui os músculos de "enchimento laterais"; braquiorradial e extensor radial. SIN pars lateralis compartimenti antebrachii posterioris (extensorum) [TA], radial p. of posterior compartment of forearm*.

lateral p. of sacrum [TA], p. lateral do sacro; a massa do sacro lateral aos forames sacrais formada pelos elementos costais fundidos. SIN pars lateralis ossis sacri [TA].

lateral p. of vaginal fornix [TA], p. lateral do fórnice da vagina. VER vaginal *fornix.* SIN pars lateralis fornicis vaginae [TA].

left p. of liver, p. esquerda do fígado; *termo oficial alternativo para left *liver.*

lumbar p. of diaphragm [TA], p. lombar do diafragma; a p. do diafragma que se origina das vértebras lombares superiores e dos ligamentos arqueados medial e lateral. VER right *crus* of diaphragm, left *crus* of diaphragm, lateral arcuate *ligament*, medial arcuate *ligament.* SIN pars lumbalis diaphragmatis [TA], vertebral p. of diaphragm.

lumbar p. of spinal cord [TA], p. lombar da medula espinal; p. da medula espinal que consiste nos cinco segmentos lombares (L1–L5) e dos quais se originam cinco pares de nervos espinais lombares; no adulto está localizada na porção T10–L1 do canal vertebral, e está aumentada em relação às outras partes da medula espinal devido ao seu envolvimento na inervação do membro inferior. SIN pars lumbalis medullae spinalis [TA], lumbar segments L1–L5 of spinal cord, segmenta lumbalia L1–L5, segmenta lumbalia medullae spinalis.

marginal p. of orbicularis oris (muscle) [TA], p. marginal do músculo orbicular da boca; a p. do músculo orbicular da boca localizada na margem dos lábios, isto é, a área vermelha. SIN pars marginalis musculi orbicularis oris [TA].

mastoid p. of the temporal bone, p. mastóidea do osso temporal. SIN mastoid *process* of petrous part of temporal bone.

medial p. of longitudinal arch of foot [TA], p. medial do arco longitudinal do pé; p. do arco longitudinal do pé formada pelo calcâneo, tálus, navicular, cuneiformes e metatarsais mediais [I–III]. VER longitudinal *arch* of foot. SIN pars medialis arcus pedis longitudinalis [TA]. VER longitudinal *arch* of foot.

medial p. of middle lobe vein (of right superior pulmonary vein) [TA], p. medial da veia do lobo médio (da veia pulmonar direita superior); a veia que drena o segmento broncopulmonar medial do lobo médio do pulmão direito. SIN pars medialis venae lobi medii venae pulmonis dextri superioris [TA].

mediastinal p. of lung, p. mediastinal dos pulmões. SIN mediastinal *surface* of lung.

mediastinal p. of parietal pleura [TA], p. mediastinal da pleura parietal; a continuação da pleura costal e diafragmática de cada lado, que parte da coluna vertebral e do esterno, cobrindo as laterais do mediastino. SIN pars mediastinalis pleurae parietalis [TA], mediastinal pleura, pleura mediastinalis.

membranous p. of interventricular septum [TA], p. membranácea do septo interventricular; p. do esqueleto fibroso do coração observada como uma área não-muscular pequena, fina, redonda ou oval na extremidade superior do septo interventricular; situa-se imediatamente abaixo da porção do anel fibroso da valva aórtica que sustenta as válvulas anterior e posterior, sendo contínua com essa porção e com o trígono fibroso direito; o fascículo atrioventricular do tecido de condução segue ao longo de sua margem dorsal e bifurca-se, em sua margem inferior, nos ramos direito e esquerdo. SIN pars membranacea septi interventricularis [TA], membranous septum (2), septum membranaceum ventriculorum.

membranous p. of male urethra, p. membranácea da uretra masculina. SIN intermediate p. of male urethra.

membranous p. of nasal septum [TA], p. membranácea do septo nasal; a pequena porção do septo nasal anterior e inferior à porção sustentada pela cartilagem do septo nasal. SIN pars membranacea septi nasi [TA], membranous septum (1).

mobile p. of nasal septum [TA], p. móvel do septo nasal; a p. móvel ânteroinferior do septo nasal formada pela parte membranácea e pelo ramo medial da cartilagem alar maior de cada lado. SIN pars mobilis septi nasi [TA], septum mobile nasi.

muscular p. of interventricular septum (of heart) [TA], p. muscular do septo interventricular (do coração); a p. muscular espessa que forma a maior parte do septo interventricular do coração. SIN pars muscularis septi interventricularis (cordis) [TA], septum musculare ventriculorum.

mylopharyngeal p. of superior constrictor muscle of pharynx [TA], p. milofaríngea do (músculo) constritor superior da faringe. VER superior pharyngeal constrictor (*muscle*). SIN pars mylopharyngeus musculi constrictoris pharyngis superioris [TA], mylopharyngeal p. of superior pharyngeal constrictor (muscle) of pharynx.

mylopharyngeal p. of superior pharyngeal constrictor (muscle) of pharynx, p. milofaríngea do (músculo) constritor superior da faringe. SIN mylopharyngeal p. of superior constrictor muscle of pharynx.

nasal p. of frontal bone [TA], p. nasal do frontal; porção nasal do osso frontal situada entre as duas partes orbitais, anteriormente, e que forma parte do teto da cavidade nasal. SIN pars nasalis ossis frontalis [TA].

nasal p. of pharynx, p. nasal da faringe. SIN nasopharynx.

nervous p. of retina, p. óptica da retina. SIN optic p. of retina. SIN pars nervosa retinae.

neural p. of hypophysis, neuro-hipófise. SIN neurohypophysis.

oblique p. of cricothyroid (muscle), p. oblíqua do músculo cricotireóideo. VER cricothyroid *muscle*. SIN pars obliqua musculi cricothyroidei [TA].

occipital p. of corpus callosum, fórceps occipital.. SIN major *forceps*.

opercular p. [TA], p. opercular; um dos três pequenos giros corticais que, juntos, formam uma cobertura para a região insular. Os opérculos são frontal, temporal e parietal. SIN pars opercularis [TA].

p. of optic nerve in canal [TA], p. do canal do nervo óptico; a p. do nervo óptico situada no canal óptico. SIN pars canalis nervi optici [TA].

optic p. of retina [TA], p. óptica da retina. VER retina. SIN nervous p. of retina.

oral p. of pharynx, p. oral da faringe. SIN oropharynx.

orbital p. of frontal bone [TA], p. orbital do frontal; a p. do osso frontal que contribui para a formação das órbitas. SIN pars orbitalis ossis frontalis [TA].

orbital p. of lacrimal gland [TA], p. orbital da glândula lacrimal. VER lacrimal *gland*. SIN pars orbitalis glandulae lacrimalis [TA].

orbital p. of optic nerve [TA], p. orbital do nervo óptico; a p. do nervo óptico situada entre o bulbo do olho e o canal óptico, isto é, no interior da órbita. SIN pars orbitalis nervi optici [TA].

orbital p. of orbicularis oculi (muscle) [TA], p. orbital do músculo orbicular do olho. SIN *pars* orbitalis musculi orbicularis oculi. VER orbicularis oculi (*muscle*).

orbital p. [TA] of inferior frontal gyrus, p. orbital do giro frontal inferior; a porção rostral e algo ventral do giro frontal inferior. SIN pars orbitalis [TA].

osseous p. of skeletal system, p. óssea do sistema esquelético. SIN bony p. of skeletal system.

palpebral p. of lacrimal gland [TA], p. palpebral da glândula lacrimal. VER lacrimal *gland*. SIN pars palpebralis glandulae lacrimalis [TA].

palpebral p. of orbicularis oculi (muscle) [TA], p. palpebral do músculo orbicular do olho. VER orbicularis oculi (*muscle*). SIN pars palpebralis musculi orbicularis oculi [TA].

parasympathetic p. of autonomic division of peripheral nervous system [TA], p. parassimpática da divisão autônoma do sistema nervoso; os neurônios pré-sinápticos (pré-ganglionares) que possuem corpos celulares localizados no encéfalo, associados aos núcleos motores de alguns nervos cranianos [NC III, VII, IX e X], ou na substância cinzenta dos segmentos S2–S4 da medula espinal, e os neurônios pós-sinápticos com os quais as fibras pré-sinápticas fazem conexão (sinapse); na cabeça, há quatro gânglios parassimpáticos distintos: ciliar, pterigopalatino, ótico e submandibular/sublingual; no tronco, as células pós-sinápticas ocorrem como gânglios intrínsecos isolados. VER autonomic *division* of nervous system. SIN pars parasympathica divisionis automaticae systematis nervosi peripherici [TA], bulbosacral system, craniosacral division of autonomic nervous system, craniosacral nervous system.

patent p. of umbilical artery [TA], p. patente da artéria umbilical; p. da artéria umbilical entre sua origem como ramo da artéria ilíaca interna e sua oclusão pós-natal distal à origem das artérias vesicais superiores. SIN pars patens arteriae umbilicalis [TA].

pelvic p. [TA], p. pélvica; a p. de uma estrutura localizada dentro da pelve ou relacionada a ela. VER pelvic part of ductus deferens, of parasympathetic part of autonomic division of nervous system, and of ureter. SIN pars pelvica [TA].

pelvic p. of ductus deferens [TA], p. pélvica do ducto deferente; p. do ducto deferente que se estende entre o anel inguinal profundo e a ampola. SIN pars pelvica ductus deferentes [TA].

pelvic p. of peripheral autonomic plexuses and ganglia [TA], p. pélvica dos plexos viscerais e gânglios viscerais; p. dos plexos nervosos autônomos que se estende até a pelve menor e localiza-se em seu interior, isto é, inferior ao plano da abertura superior da pelve; estão incluídos os plexos hipogástricos superior e inferior, e os plexos das vísceras pélvicas: plexos retais médio e inferior, vesical, uterovaginal, prostático e deferencial; embora tecnicamente saiam da pelve e sigam no interior dos corpos eréteis do períneo, os nervos cavernosos do pênis e do clitóris também são incluídos. SIN pars pelvica plexus visceralis et ganglii visceralis [TA].

pelvic p. of ureter [TA], p. pélvica do ureter; a p. do ureter entre a margem da pelve e a bexiga. SIN pars pelvica ureteris [TA].

pelvic p. of the urogenital sinus, p. pélvica do seio urogenital; a porção pélvica superior do seio urogenital embriológico.

peripheral p. of nervous system, p. periférica do sistema nervoso. SIN peripheral nervous *system*.

petrous p. of internal carotid artery [TA], p. petrosa da artéria carótida interna; a p. da artéria carótida interna situada no canal carótico; seus ramos são as artérias caroticotimpânicas e a artéria do canal pterigóideo. SIN pars petrosa arteriae carotidis internae [TA], petrous bone.

petrous p. of temporal bone [TA], p. petrosa do temporal; a p. do osso temporal que contém as estruturas da orelha interna e a segunda parte da artéria carótida interna; na vida pré-natal, apresenta-se como um centro de ossificação distinto. SIN pars petrosa ossis temporalis [TA], periotic bone, petrosal bone, petrous pyramid.

phrenicoceliac p. of suspensory muscle (ligament) of duodenum [TA], p. frenicocelíaca do músculo suspensor do duodeno; tira de músculo esquelético, originada do pilar direito do diafragma, próxima do hiato esofágico e que se une à p. celiacoduodenal para se fixar ao duodeno terminal e à flexura duodenojejunal. SIN pars phrenicocoeliaca musculi (ligamenti) suspensorii duodeni [TA].

pial p. of filum terminale [TA], p. pial do filamento terminal; p. do filamento terminal dentro do saco dural; é composta de um prolongamento da pia-máter caudal à terminação da medula espinal na extremidade do cone medular. VER TAMBÉM terminal *filum*. SIN pars pialis fili terminalis [TA], filum terminale internum*, pial filament*.

pigmented p. of retina, estrato pigmentoso da p. óptica da retina. SIN pars pigmentosa. VER retina.

postcommunicating p. of anterior cerebral artery [TA], p. pós-comunicante da artéria cerebral anterior; p. da artéria cerebral anterior distal à artéria comunicante anterior. SIN pars postcommunicalis arteriae cerebri anterioris [TA], A2 segment of anterior cerebral artery*, segmentum A2 arteriae cerebri anterioris*.

postcommunicating p. of posterior cerebral artery [TA], p. pós-comunicante da artéria cerebral posterior; p. da artéria cerebral posterior distal à artéria comunicante posterior. SIN pars postcommunicalis arteriae cerebri posterioris [TA], P2 segment of posterior cerebral artery*.

posterior p. [TA], p. posterior; a porção posterior da comissura anterior do cérebro.

posterior p. of anterior commissure of brain [TA], p. posterior da comissura anterior do cérebro; parte importante, posterior, da conexão entre o par de bulbos olfatórios e as partes adjacentes do córtex dos lobos frontal e temporal. SIN pars posterior commissurae anterioris [TA].

posterior p. of the diaphragmatic surface of the liver [TA], p. posterior da face diafragmática do fígado; aquela p. da face diafragmática do fígado que inclui a área nua e o lobo caudado. SIN pars posterior faciei diaphragmatis hepatis [TA].

posterior p. of liver, p. posterior do fígado; *termo oficial alternativo para posterior hepatic *segment* I.

posterior tibiotalar p. of deltoid ligament, p. tibiotalar posterior do ligamento deltóideo. SIN tibiotalar p. of medial ligament of ankle joint.

posterior tibiotalar p. of medial ligament of ankle joint [TA], p. tibiotalar posterior do ligamento colateral medial da articulação talocrural. VER medial *ligament* of ankle joint.

posterior p. of tongue [TA], p. pós-sulcal da língua; p. (terço posterior) da língua posterior ao sulco terminal; é distinta da parte pré-sulcal (dois terços anteriores) da língua tanto em sua origem embriológica quanto em sua inervação. VER TAMBÉM *dorsum* of tongue. SIN pars posterior linguae [TA], pars postsulcalis linguae*, postsulcal p. of tongue*.

posterior p. of vaginal fornix [TA], p. posterior do fórnice vaginal. SIN pars posterior fornicis vaginae [TA].

postlaminar p. of intraocular part of optic nerve [TA], p. pós-laminar da parte intra-ocular do nervo óptico; a porção da p. intra-ocular do nervo óptico imediatamente posterior à lâmina cribriforme da esclera. SIN pars postlaminaris nervi optici intraocularis [TA].

postsulcal p. of tongue, p. pós-sulcal da língua; *termo oficial alternativo para posterior p. of tongue.

precommunicating p. of anterior cerebral artery [TA], p. pré-comunicante da artéria cerebral anterior; porção da artéria cerebral anterior proximal à artéria comunicante anterior. SIN pars precommunicalis arteriae cerebri anterioris [TA], A1 segment of anterior cerebral artery*, segmentum A1 arteriae cerebri anterioris*, precommunical segment of anterior cerebral artery.

precommunicating p. of posterior cerebral artery [TA], p. pré-comunicante da artéria cerebral posterior; porção da artéria cerebral posterior proximal à artéria comunicante posterior. SIN pars precommunicalis arteriae cerebri posterioris [TA], P1 segment of posterior cerebral artery, precommunical segment of posterior cerebral artery.
prelaminar p. of intraocular part of optic nerve [TA], p. pré-laminar da p. intra-ocular do nervo óptico; a porção da p. intra-ocular do nervo óptico imediatamente anterior à lâmina cribriforme da esclera. SIN pars prelaminaris nervi optici intraocularis [TA].
preprostatic p. of male urethra, p. intramural da uretra masculina; *termo oficial alternativo para intramural p. of male urethra.
presulcal p. of tongue, p. pré-sulcal da língua; *termo oficial alternativo para anterior p. of tongue.
prevertebral p. of vertebral artery [TA], p. pré-vertebral da artéria vertebral. VER vertebral *artery*. SIN pars prevertebralis arteriae prevertebralis [TA].
proximal p. of prostate [TA], p. proximal da próstata; porção da próstata derivada do primórdio mais rostral; inclui os lobos anterior e médio da próstata madura. SIN pars proximalis prostatae [TA].
proximal p. of prostatic urethra [TA], p. proximal da p. prostática da uretra; porção da uretra prostática superior à fusão das vias urinária e genital nas aberturas dos ductos ejaculatórios. SIN pars proximalis urethrae prostaticae [TA].
psoatic p. of iliopsoas fascia [TA], p. do psoas da fáscia iliopsoas; porção da fáscia sobrejacente ao músculo iliopsoas, com a porção específica diretamente relacionada à porção do psoas. SIN pars psoatica fasciae iliopsoaticae [TA].
pterygopharyngeal p. of superior constrictor muscle of pharynx [TA], p. pterigofaríngea do músculo constritor superior da faringe. VER superior pharyngeal constrictor (*muscle*). SIN pars pterygopharyngea musculi constrictoris pharyngis superioris.
pyloric p. of stomach [TA], p. pilórica do estômago; p. do estômago situada entre a incisura angular e o piloro; sua mucosa contém glândulas pilóricas. SIN pars pylorica gastris [TA], pars pylorica ventriculi.
quadrate p. of liver [TA], p. anterior do segmento medial esquerdo. SIN anterior *portion* of left medial segment IV of liver.
radial p. of posterior compartment of forearm, p. lateral do compartimento posterior do antebraço; *termo oficial alternativo para lateral p. of posterior (extensor) compartment of forearm.
retrolenticular p. of internal capsule, p. retrolentiforme da cápsula interna; a p. da cápsula caudal ao núcleo lentiforme e que contém fibras occipitopontinas [TA], fibras occipitotetais [TA], radiação óptica [TA] (fibras geniculocalcarinas), radiação talâmica posterior [TA] e outros sistemas de fibras. VER TAMBÉM retrolenticular *limb* of internal capsule. SIN pars retrolentiformis capsulae internae [TA].
right p. of diaphragmatic surface of liver [TA], p. direita da face diafragmática do fígado; a p. da face diafragmática do fígado situada profundamente aos corpos das costelas inferiores no lado direito. SIN pars dextra faciei diaphragmaticae hepatis [TA].
right p. of liver, p. direita do fígado; *termo oficial alternativo para right *liver*.
sacral p. of spinal cord [TA], p. sacral da medula espinal; a p. da medula espinal que inclui os cinco segmentos sacrais da medula espinal (S1–S5) e da qual se originam cinco pares de nervos sacrais. SIN pars sacralis medullae spinalis [TA], segmenta sacralia medullae spinalis [TA].
scrotal p. of ductus deferens [TA], p. escrotal do ducto deferente; p. inicial do ducto deferente, entre o epidídimo e o cordão espermático, quando o ducto segue paralelo ao epidídimo e ao testículo. SIN pars scrotalis ductus deferentis [TA].
second p. of duodenum, segunda p. do duodeno. SIN descending p. of duodenum.
soft p.'s, partes moles; as partes não-ósseas e não-cartilaginosas do corpo.
soleal p. of posterior (plantar flexor) compartment of leg [TA], p. profunda do compartimento posterior da perna; p. do compartimento osteofascial posterior da perna que inclui o músculo sóleo. SIN pars solealis compartimenti cruris posterioris [TA].
sphenoid p. of middle cerebral artery [TA], p. esfenoidal da artéria cerebral média. VER middle cerebral *artery*. SIN pars sphenoidalis arteriae cerebralis mediae [TA].
spinal p. of accessory nerve, p. espinal do nervo acessório; *termo oficial alternativo para spinal *root* of accessory nerve.
spinal p. of arachnoid, p. espinal da aracnóide-máter. SIN spinal *arachnoid mater*.
spinal p. of deltoid (muscle) [TA], p. espinal do músculo deltóide; p. do músculo deltóide que se origina na espinha da escápula. SIN pars spinalis musculi deltoidei [TA].
spinal p. of filum terminale [TA], p. espinal do filamento terminal; p. inicial (mais alta) do filamento terminal, na extremidade do cone medular, que ainda inclui um canal central. SIN pars spinalis fili terminalis [TA].
spongy p. of the male urethra, p. esponjosa da uretra masculina. SIN spongy *urethra*.

squamous p. of frontal bone [TA], escama frontal; a porção larga e curva do osso frontal que forma a fronte. SIN squama frontalis [TA].
squamous p. of occipital bone [TA], escama occipital; a porção laminar ou escamosa do osso occipital. SIN squama occipitalis, occipital squama [TA], frontal squama.
squamous p. of temporal bone [TA], p. escamosa do temporal; a porção larga, plana, fina (semelhante a uma escama), ântero-superior do osso temporal, que forma parte da parede lateral da abóbada craniana. SIN pars squamosa ossis temporalis [TA], squama temporalis, temporal squama.
sternal p. of diaphragm [TA], p. esternal do diafragma; a pequena tira de cada lado que se origina da superfície interna do processo xifóide e se insere no tendão central. SIN pars sternalis diaphragmatis [TA].
sternocostal p. of pectoralis major muscle, p. esternocostal do músculo peitoral maior. SIN sternocostal *head* of pectoralis major (*muscle*). VER pectoralis major (*muscle*).
straight p. of cricothyroid muscle [TA], p. reta do músculo cricotireóideo. VER cricothyroid *muscle*.
subcutaneous p. of external anal sphincter [TA], p. subcutânea do músculo esfíncter externo do ânus. VER external anal *sphincter*. SIN pars subcutanea musculi sphincteri ani externi [TA], subcutaneous portion of external anal sphincter.
sublenticular p. of internal capsule, p. sublentiforme da cápsula interna; a p. da cápsula interna, situada abaixo do terço caudal do núcleo lentiforme, que contém a radiação acústica [TA] (geniculotemporal fibers), fibras corticotetais [TA], fibras temporopontinas [TA] e fibras corticotalâmicas, bem como aquela parte da radiação óptica que representa a parte superior da metade contralateral do campo visual binocular. VER TAMBÉM sublentiform *limb* of internal capsule. SIN pars sublentiformis capsulae internae [TA].
suboccipital p. of vertebral artery, p. atlântica da artéria vertebral. SIN atlantic p. of vertebral artery.
superficial p. of anterior (flexor) compartment of forearm [TA], p. superficial do compartimento anterior do antebraço; p. do compartimento anterior (flexor) do antebraço, incluindo as camadas superficial e intermediária dos músculos pronadores e flexores: pronador redondo, flexor radial do carpo, palmar longo, flexor ulnar do carpo e flexor superficial dos dedos. SIN pars superficialis compartimenti antebrachii anterioris [TA].
superficial p. of external anal sphincter [TA], p. superficial do músculo esfíncter externo do ânus. VER external anal *sphincter*. SIN pars superficialis musculi sphincteri ani externi [TA].
superficial p. of masseter muscle [TA], p. superficial do músculo masseter. VER masseter (*muscle*). SIN pars superficialis musculi masseteri [TA].
superficial p. of parotid gland [TA], p. superficial da glândula parótida. VER parotid *gland*. SIN pars superficialis glandulae parotidae [TA].
superficial p. of posterior (plantar flexor) compartment of leg [TA], p. superficial do compartimento posterior da perna; p. do compartimento posterior (flexor plantar) da perna, incluindo os músculos gastrocnêmio e sóleo; é separada da parte profunda pelo septo intermuscular transverso da perna. SIN pars superficialis compartimenti cruris posterioris [TA], pars tricipitalis compartimenti cruris posterioris*.
superior p. of diaphragmatic surface of liver [TA], p. superior da face diafragmática do fígado; a porção superior convexa da face diafragmática do fígado. SIN pars superior faciei diaphragmaticae hepatis [TA].
superior p. of duodenum, p. superior do duodeno; p. inicial (primeira) do duodeno imediatamente distal ao piloro e proximal à parte descendente (segunda). VER duodenum. SIN pars superior duodeni [TA], first p. of duodenum, pars prima duodeni. VER duodenum.
superior p. of lingular vein (of left superior pulmonary vein) [TA], p. superior da veia lingular (da veia pulmonar esquerda superior); a veia que drena o segmento broncopulmonar lingular superior do pulmão esquerdo. SIN pars superior venae lingularis venae pulmonis superioris sinistri [TA].
superior p. of vestibular ganglion [TA], p. superior do gânglio vestibular; parte rostral, a p. superior do gânglio vestibular que recebe fibras das máculas do utrículo e do sáculo e da ampola dos ductos semicirculares anteriores e laterais. SIN pars superior ganglii vestibularis [TA].
superior p. of vestibulocochlear nerve, p. superior do nervo vestibulococlear. SIN vestibular *nerve*.
supraclavicular p. of brachial plexus [TA], p. supraclavicular do plexo braquial; a p. do plexo braquial acima da clavícula; inclui as raízes, troncos e divisões que dão origem aos nervos escapular dorsal, torácico longo, supra-escapular e subclávio. SIN pars supraclavicularis plexus brachialis [TA].
supravaginal p. of cervix [TA], porção supravaginal do colo; a p. do colo do útero situada acima da fixação da vagina. SIN portio supravaginalis cervicis [TA].
sympathetic p. of autonomic division of peripheral nervous system [TA], p. simpática da divisão autônoma do sistema nervoso; a p. simpática da divisão autônoma do sistema nervoso. VER TAMBÉM autonomic *division* of nervous system. SIN pars sympathica (divisionis autonomicae systematis nervosei peripherici) [TA], sympathetic nervous system, thoracolumbar nervous system.

tense p. of the tympanic membrane [TA], p. tensa da membrana timpânica; a maior porção da membrana timpânica que é tensa e firme, contrastando com a pequena parte flácida, triangular, da membrana timpânica. SIN pars tensa membranae tympani [TA], membrana tensa, membrana vibrans.

terminal p., ramos terminais. SIN *pars terminalis.* VER terminal *branches* of middle cerebral artery, em *branch*, posterior cerebral *artery*.

third p. of duodenum, terceira parte do duodeno. SIN inferior p. of duodenum.

thoracic p. of aorta, p. torácica da aorta. SIN thoracic *aorta*.

thoracic p. of esophagus [TA], p. torácica do esôfago; a p. do esôfago situada entre a abertura superior do tórax e o diafragma. SIN pars thoracica esophagi [TA].

thoracic p. of iliocostalis lumborum (muscle) [TA], p. torácica do músculo iliocostal do lombo; p. do músculo iliocostal que se estende para cima, a partir dos ângulos costais das seis costelas inferiores até os ângulos costais das seis costelas superiores e o processo transverso da vértebra C7, entre o músculo iliocostal do lombo, inferior e lateralmente, e o músculo iliocostal do pescoço, superior e medialmente. SIN pars thoracica muscularis iliocostalis lumborum [TA].

thoracic p. of peripheral autonomic plexuses and ganglia [TA], p. torácica dos plexos viscerais e gânglios viscerais; plexos autônomos das vísceras torácicas: coração/aorta, pulmões/brônquios e esôfago, e gânglios parassimpáticos associados. SIN pars thoracica plexuum et ganglionorum visceralium [TA].

thoracic p. of spinal cord [TA], p. torácica da medula espinal; a p. da medula espinal que consiste nos 12 segmentos torácicos [T1–T12] da medula espinal da qual se originam os 12 pares de nervos torácicos [T1–T12]. SIN pars thoracica medullae spinalis [TA], segmenta thoracica medullae spinalis [TA].

thoracic p. of thoracic duct [TA], p. torácica do ducto torácico; p. do ducto torácico situada dentro do tórax, do hiato aórtico até o nível da primeira vértebra torácica. SIN pars thoracica ductus thoracici [TA].

thoracic p. of trachea [TA], p. torácica da traquéia; a p. intratorácica da traquéia, isto é, a p. localizada entre o plano da abertura superior do tórax, acima, e a bifurcação da traquéia ao nível do ângulo esternal, abaixo. SIN pars thoracica tracheae [TA].

thyroepiglottic p. of thyroarytenoid (muscle) [TA], p. tireoepiglótica do músculo tireoaritenóideo; músculo intrínseco da laringe; *origem*, face interna da cartilagem tireóidea em comum com a parte tireoaritenóidea; *inserção*, prega ariepiglótica e margem da epiglote; *ação*, deprime a base da epiglote; *inervação*, laríngeo recorrente. SIN pars thyroepiglottica musculi thyroarytenoidei [TA], depressor muscle of epiglottis, musculus thyroepiglotticus, thyroepiglottic muscle, thyroepiglottidean muscle, ventricularis (2).

thyropharyngeal p. of inferior constrictor muscle of pharynx [TA], p. tireofaríngea do músculo constritor inferior da faringe. VER inferior constrictor (*muscle*) of pharynx. SIN pars thyropharyngea musculi constrictoris pharyngis inferioris [TA], thyropharyngeal p. of inferior pharyngeal constrictor (muscle) of pharynx.

thyropharyngeal p. of inferior pharyngeal constrictor (muscle) of pharynx, p. tireofaríngea do músculo constritor inferior da faringe. SIN thyropharyngeal p. of inferior constrictor muscle of pharynx.

tibiocalcaneal p. of deltoid ligament, p. tibiocalcânea do ligamento deltóideo; *termo oficial alternativo para tibiocalcaneal p. of medial ligament of ankle joint.

tibiocalcaneal p. of medial ligament of ankle joint [TA], p. tibiocalcânea do ligamento colateral medial da articulação talocrural; a p. do ligamento colateral medial ou deltóideo que se estende do maléolo medial até o sustentáculo do tálus do calcâneo. SIN pars tibiocalcanea ligamenti collateralis medialis articulationis talocruralis [TA], pars tibiocalcanea ligamenti deltoidei*, tibiocalcaneal p. of deltoid ligament*, calcaneotibial ligament, ligamentum calcaneotibiale, tibiocalcaneal ligament.

tibionavicular p. of deltoid ligament, p. tibionavicular do ligamento deltóideo. SIN tibionavicular p. of medial ligament of ankle joint.

tibionavicular p. of medial ligament of ankle joint [TA], p. tibionavicular do ligamento colateral medial da articulação talocrural; a p. do ligamento colateral medial (deltóideo) que se estende do maléolo medial até o osso navicular. VER TAMBÉM medial *ligament* of ankle joint. SIN pars tibionavicularis ligamenti collateralis medialis articulationis talocruralis [TA], ligamentum tibionaviculare, tibionavicular ligament, tibionavicular p. of deltoid ligament.

tibiotalar p. of medial ligament of ankle joint [TA], p. tibiotalar do ligamento colateral medial da articulação talocrural; a p. do ligamento colateral medial ou deltóideo que se estende do maléolo medial até o processo posterior do tálus. SIN pars tibiotalaris posterior ligamenti collateralis medialis articulationis talocruralis [TA], ligamentum talotibiale posterius, posterior talotibial ligament, posterior tibiotalar ligament, posterior tibiotalar p. of deltoid ligament.

transversarial p. of vertebral artery [TA], p. transversária da artéria vertebral. SIN cervical p. of vertebral artery.

transverse p. of iliofemoral ligament [TA], p. transversa do ligamento iliofemoral; o ramo mais horizontal do ligamento iliofemoral em forma de Y invertido. SIN pars transversa ligamenti iliofemoralis [TA].

transverse p. of left branch of portal vein [TA], p. transversa do ramo esquerdo da veia porta; a porção longa, não-ramificada, do ramo esquerdo da veia porta. SIN pars transversa rami sinistri venae portae hepatis [TA].

transverse p. of nasalis muscle [TA], p. transversa do músculo nasal. VER nasalis (*muscle*). SIN pars transversa musculi nasalis [TA].

transverse p. of trapezius (muscle) [TA], p. transversa do músculo trapézio; terço médio do músculo trapézio com fibras musculares que seguem transversalmente à espinha da escápula; atua retraindo as escápulas (ombros) na articulação escapulotorácica conceitual. SIN pars transversa musculi trapezii [TA].

triangular p. [TA], p. triangular; a p. média das três pequenas convoluções que, juntas, compõem o giro frontal inferior do córtex cerebral, sendo as outras duas a parte orbital e a parte opercular. SIN pars triangularis [TA].

tympanic p. of temporal bone, p. timpânica do temporal. SIN tympanic *plate* of temporal bone.

umbilical p. of left branch of portal vein [TA], p. umbilical do ramo esquerdo da veia porta do fígado; a p. bastante ramificada do ramo esquerdo da veia porta; os ligamentos redondo e venoso fixam-se a essa parte. SIN pars umbilicalis rami sinistri venae portae hepatis [TA].

uterine p. of uterine tube [TA], p. uterina da tuba uterina; a p. da tuba uterina localizada na parede do útero. SIN pars uterina tubae uterinae [TA].

uveal p. of trabecular reticulum, p. uveal do retículo trabecular da esclera. SIN uveal p. of trabecular tissue of sclera.

uveal p. of trabecular tissue of sclera [TA], p. uveal do retículo trabecular da esclera; a p. posterior do retículo trabecular, localizada entre o esporão da esclera, o corpo ciliar e a superfície anterior da íris. SIN pars uvealis reticuli trabecularis sclerae [TA], uveal p. of trabecular reticulum.

vagal p. of accessory nerve, raiz craniana do nervo acessório; *termo oficial alternativo para cranial *root* of accessory nerve. VER accessory *nerve* [NC XI].

vaginal p. of cervix [TA], porção vaginal do colo; a p. do colo do útero contida na vagina. SIN portio vaginalis cervicis [TA].

ventral p. of intertransversarii laterales lumborum (muscles) [TA], p. ventral dos músculos intertransversários do lombo; partes dos músculos intertransversários laterais da região lombar que unem os elementos costais dos processos transversos das vértebras lombares. SIN pars ventralis musculi intertransversarii lateralium lumborum [TA].

ventral p. of pons, p. basilar da ponte. SIN basilar p. of pons.

vertebral p. of the costal surface of the lungs [TA], p. vertebral da face costal do pulmão; a parte da face medial do pulmão que fica em contato com os corpos vertebrais. SIN pars vertebralis faciei costalis pulmonis [TA].

vertebral p. of diaphragm, p. lombar do diafragma. SIN lumbar p. of diaphragm.

vestibular p. of vestibulocochlear nerve, p. vestibular do nervo vestibulococlear. SIN vestibular *nerve*.

part. aeq. Abreviatura do L. *partes aequales*, em partes (quantidades) iguais.

par·tes (par'tēz). Partes; plural de pars.

par·the·no·gen·e·sis (par'the-nō-jen'ĕ-sis). Partenogênese; uma forma de reprodução assexuada, ou agamogênese, em que a fêmea se reproduz sem fecundação pelo macho. SIN apogamia, apogamy, apomixia, virgin generation. [G. *parthenos*, virgem, + *genesis*, produto]

par·the·no·pho·bia (par'the-nō-fō'bē-ă). Partenofobia; medo mórbido de meninas. [G. *parthenos*, virgem, + *phobos*, medo]

par·ti·cle (par'ti-kl). Partícula. **1.** Um pedaço ou uma porção muito pequena de qualquer coisa. **2.** Uma parte elementar, como um próton ou elétron. [L. *particula*, dim. de *pars*, parte]

alpha p. (α), p. alfa; uma p. que consiste em dois nêutrons e dois prótons, com uma carga elétrica positiva (2e$^+$); emitida energeticamente dos núcleos de isótopos instáveis de alto número atômico (elementos com número de massa a partir de 82); idêntica ao núcleo do hélio. SIN alpha ray.

beta p., p. beta; um elétron, com carga elétrica positiva (positron, β$^+$) ou negativa (negatron, β$^-$), emitido durante o decaimento beta de um radionuclídeo. VER TAMBÉM cathode *rays*, em *ray*. SIN beta ray.

chromatin p.'s, partículas de cromatina; pontos azulados finos que parecem representar remanescentes do núcleo, ocasionalmente observados em eritrócitos corados.

core p., p. nuclear; partícula liberada por digestão enzimática parcial da cromatina.

Dane p.'s, partículas de Dane; as formas esféricas maiores de antígenos associados à hepatite; formam o vírion do vírus da hepatite B, contendo um "cerne" de 27 nm no qual foram encontrados DNA polimerase DNA-dependente e DNA de duplo filamento circular.

defective interfering p., vírus incompleto incapaz de se replicar e que interfere com a replicação de um vírus infeccioso.

D.I. p., abreviatura de defective interfering p.

electron transport p.'s (ETP), partículas de transporte de elétrons; fragmentos de mitocôndrias ainda capazes de transportar elétrons. SIN submitochondrial p.'s.

elementary p., (1) Plaqueta. SIN platelet; **(2)** p. elementar; uma das unidades presentes na superfície matricial das cristas mitocondriais; a cabeça da partícula, com cerca de 9 nm, fixa-se à membrana da crista por um pedículo com 5 nm de comprimento; as partículas estariam envolvidas no sistema de transporte de elétrons.

kappa p.'s, partículas capa; simbiontes citoplasmáticos hereditários, antigamente considerados partículas constituídas, principal ou exclusivamente, por DNA, ocorrendo em algumas cepas de *Paramecium*; capazes de produzir um produto letal para outras cepas.
signal recognition p. (SRP), p. de reconhecimento de sinal; pequeno complexo de RNA-proteína que interage com a seqüência de sinais de proteínas secretoras nascentes. A união da proteína de reconhecimento do sinal resulta em interrupção da tradução até a interação com a proteína de atracamento, uma parte integrante da membrana do retículo endoplasmático.
submitochondrial p.'s, partículas submitocondriais. SIN electron transport p.'s.
Zimmermann elementary p., p. elementar de Zimmermann; termo obsoleto para plaqueta.
par·tic·u·late (par - tik′ū - lāt). Particulado; relativo a, ou que ocorre em forma de, partículas finas.
par·tic·u·lates (par - tik′ū - lats). Particulados; elementos formados, corpos bem definidos, ao contrário do material líquido ou semilíquido adjacente; p. ex., grânulos ou mitocôndrias nas células.
par·to·gram (par′tō - gram). Partograma; gráfico dos parâmetros de tempo e dilatação no trabalho de parto, com linhas de alerta e ação para dar o sinal para intervenção se a curva desviar-se do esperado. SIN Friedman curve, labor curve. [L. *partus*, parto, + -gram]

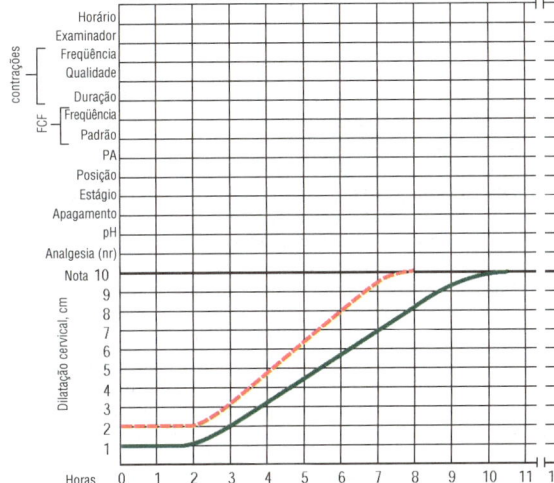

partograma: fluxograma para representação gráfica do progresso do trabalho de parto; FCF = freqüência cardíaca fetal

par·tu·ri·ent (par - too′rē - ent). Parturiente; relacionado com o ou no processo de parto. [L. *parturio*, estar em trabalho de parto]
par·tu·ri·fa·cient (par - toor - ē - fā′shent). Parturifaciente. **1.** Que induz ou acelera o trabalho de parto. **2.** Agente que induz ou acelera o trabalho de parto. SIN oxytocic (2). [L. *parturio*, estar em trabalho de parto, + *facio*, fazer]
par·tu·ri·tion (par - toor - ish′ŭn). Parto. SIN childbirth. [L. *parturitio*, de *parturio*, estar em trabalho de parto]
part. vic. Abreviatura do L. *partes vicibus*, em doses divididas.
pa·ru·lis, pl. **pa·ru·li·des** (pă - roo′lis, - li - dēz). Parúlia; parúlide. SIN gingival abscess. [G. *paroulis*, abscesso da gengiva, de *para*, ao lado de, + *oulon*, gengiva]
par·um·bil·i·cal (par′ŭm - bil′i - kăl). Paraumbilical. SIN paraumbilical.
par·u·re·sis (par - ū - rē′sis). Parurese; inibição da micção, principalmente na presença de estranhos. [para- + G. *ourēsis*, micção]
par·val·bu·min (par - val - bū′min). Parvalbumina; qualquer dentre um grupo de pequenas proteínas hidrossolúveis, ligadas ao cálcio, distintas da calmodulina e de outras proteínas de ligação do cálcio; encontrada no cérebro, músculo esquelético e retina, mas não no coração, fígado ou baço de várias espécies. [L. *parvus*, pequeno + albumina]
Par·vo·bac·te·ri·a·ce·ae (par′vō - bak - tēr - ē - ā′sē - ē). Denominação de família tida como antecessora da família de bactérias Brucellaceae. Nenhum gênero típico jamais foi proposto para essa família.
par·vo·cel·lu·lar (par - vō - sel′ū - lăr). Parvocelular; relacionado a, ou composto por, células pequenas. [L. *parvus*, pequeno, + L. mod. *cellularis*, celular]
par·vo·line (par′vō - lēn). Parvolina; uma ptomaína, $C_9H_{13}N$, resultante da decomposição de peixes.
Par·vo·vir·i·dae (par - vō - vir′i - dē). Família de pequenos vírus contendo DNA de filamento único. Os vírions possuem 18–26 nm de diâmetro, não possuem envoltório e são resistentes ao éter. Os capsídeos possuem simetria cúbica, com 32 capsômeros. A replicação e o agrupamento ocorrem no núcleo de células infectadas. São reconhecidos três gêneros na subfamília Parvovirinae: Parvovirus, Erythrovirus e Dependovirus, que inclui o vírus adeno-associado. Uma segunda subfamília, Densovirinae, tem 3 outros gêneros e todos infectam artrópodes.
Par·vo·vi·rus (par′vō - vi - rŭs). Gênero de vírus (família Parvoviridae) que se replicam de forma autônoma em células adequadas. A cepa B19 infecta seres humanos, causando eritema infeccioso e crise aplásica na anemia hemolítica. [L. *parvus*, pequeno, + virus]

Par·vo·vi·rus B19. Vírus de DNA de filamento único pertencente à família Parvoviridae; a causa do eritema infeccioso (quinta doença) e de crises aplásicas.

O parvovírus B19 (B19V) foi isolado pela primeira vez em 1975, de uma amostra de sangue de doador saudável. Em 1983 foi relacionado ao eritema infeccioso, também denominado quinta doença da infância, um exantema febril de crianças geralmente benigno. A infecção por B19V ocorre em todo o mundo e pode atacar pessoas de qualquer idade. Na maioria das vezes é contraída na infância; 30–60% dos adultos possuem anticorpos IgG protetores contra o vírus. A infecção é assintomática em 20–50% das pessoas que a adquirem. A transmissão geralmente se dá pelas secreções respiratórias. O vírus replica-se na medula óssea. O eritema infeccioso clássico ocorre tipicamente em crianças de 4–15 anos de idade. Surtos esporádicos são comuns, e a incidência máxima ocorre no inverno e na primavera. Após um período de incubação de 4–14 dias, a criança desenvolve sinais e sintomas prodrômicos, geralmente leves, que consistem em cefaléia, febre, calafrios, dores articulares e mal-estar. Cerca de 1 semana depois, surge uma erupção facial de tom vermelho-vivo semelhante à "face esbofeteada" e, nos 3–4 dias subseqüentes, a erupção dissemina-se para o restante do corpo (partes proximais dos membros, depois o tronco e as partes distais, incluindo as regiões palmares e plantares), onde seu aspecto é reticular ou maculopapular. Se houver prurido, este é leve. A erupção cutânea é uma resposta imune, que anuncia o surgimento de anticorpo IgM e o fim do período contagioso. A doença tipicamente tem uma evolução benigna, e o tratamento é apenas sintomático. (Como alguns outros vírus, o B19V por vezes também causa um exantema benigno conhecido como síndrome de luvas e meias papulares purpúricas.) A infecção em adultos segue um padrão diferente: não é observada a "face esbofeteada", e a erupção cutânea no tronco e nos membros tende a ser mais leve e mais sutil, mas 15–20% dos pacientes adultos, praticamente todos do sexo feminino, apresentam envolvimento articular significativo. A deposição de imunocomplexos nas membranas articulares causa início súbito de poliartrite simétrica, afetando sobretudo as articulações metacarpofalângicas e interfalângicas proximais, os punhos e os joelhos. Pode ou não haver edema. A dor e a incapacidade podem ser intensas, e os sintomas podem persistir por semanas ou meses, embora a resolução espontânea final seja a regra. Como o B19V infecta a medula óssea, a maioria dos pacientes apresenta diminuição transitória do número de hemácias, leucócitos e plaquetas. Geralmente isso não tem conseqüências, mas algumas vezes evolui para uma crise aplásica transitória (CAT), na qual a produção de hemácias praticamente cessa e o número de hemácias diminui rapidamente. O risco dessa complicação é muito maior na anemia falciforme, em anemias hemolíticas auto-imunes, imunodeficiência e gravidez. Com a formação de anticorpos IgG pelo sistema imune, a formação de hemácias é reiniciada e a anemia resolve. Entretanto, em pacientes com imunodeficiência congênita ou adquirida, a ausência de formação de anticorpos pode levar a anemia prolongada. A infecção em uma mulher grávida tem aproximadamente 1 chance em 3 de ser transmitida para o feto e induzir uma crise aplásica fetal. Isso, por sua vez, pode resultar em insuficiência cardíaca congestiva e hidropisia fetal. A recuperação espontânea é típica, mas há morte fetal em até 10% dos casos. A infecção fetal por B19V aparentemente não causa anomalias congênitas. A infecção aguda por B19V pode ser confirmada por um rápido aumento e diminuição dos anticorpos IgM. O diagnóstico também pode ser estabelecido por cultura do vírus em material da medula óssea ou por detecção ELISA do antígeno no soro. O tratamento de todas as formas de infecção por B19V é puramente sintomático e de suporte, pois não há tratamento antiviral específico disponível. Os pacientes hospitalizados com B19V são isolados, e as funcionárias grávidas são aconselhadas a evitar contato com eles. A anemia grave pode exigir transfusões sanguíneas. Quando a anemia prolongada resulta da incapacidade de formar anticorpo IgM, o uso de imunoglobulina intravenosa pode ser útil.

par·vule (par′vool). Párvulo; um comprimido muito pequeno. [L. *parvulus*, muito pequeno, de *parvus*, pequeno]
par·vus (par′vŭs). Pequeno. [L.]

PAS Abreviatura de *p*-aminosalicylic acid (ácido *p*-aminossalicílico); periodic acid-Schiff *stain* (coloração com ácido periódico de Schiff).
PASA Abreviatura de *p*-aminosalicylic acid (ácido *p*-aminossalicílico).
Pascal, Blaise, cientista francês, 1623–1662. VER pascal; P. *law.*
pas·cal (Pa) (pas′kăl). Pascal; unidade derivada de pressão ou tensão no sistema SI, expresso em newtons por metro quadrado; igual a 10^{-5} bar ou $7,50062 \times 10^{-3}$ torr. [B. *Pascal*]
Pascheff (Pashev), Konstantin M., oftalmologista búlgaro. 1873–1961. VER P. *conjunctivitis.*
Paschen, Enrique, patologista alemão, 1860–1936. VER P. *bodies,* em *body.*
Pashev. VER Pascheff.
Pasini, Augustine, dermatologista argentino do século XX. VER *atrophoderma* of P. and Pierini.
pas·pal·ism (pas′păl-izm). Paspalismo; envenenamento por sementes de uma espécie de grama, *Paspalum scrobiculatum.* [G. *paspalos,* tipo de milho miúdo, de *pas,* todo, + *palē,* alimento]
pas·sage (pas′ij). **1.** Passagem; o ato de passar. **2.** Excremento, como do intestino ou de urina. **3.** Inoculação de uma série de animais com a mesma cepa de um microrganismo patogênico cuja virulência geralmente é aumentada, mas algumas vezes é diminuída. **4.** Um canal, ducto, poro ou abertura. [L. mediev. *passo,* passar]
blind p., passagem às cegas; transferência sucessiva de um agente através de culturas ou de animais sem aparente replicação ou doença.
nasopharyngeal p., meato nasofaríngeo. SIN nasopharyngeal *meatus.*
oropharyngeal p., fauces. SIN fauces.
serial p., passagem seriada; transferência sucessiva de um agente infeccioso através de uma série de culturas ou animais experimentais, geralmente com patogenicidade atenuada.
Pas·sal·u·rus am·big·u·us (pa-sal′ū-rŭs am-big′ū-ŭs). O oxiúro do coelho, um nematódeo oxiurídeo encontrado em abundância no ceco e no intestino grosso de coelhos.
Passavant, Philippas G., médico alemão, 1815–1893. VER P. *bar, cushion, pad, ridge.*
Passey, R.D., patologista inglês do século XX. VER Harding-P. *melanoma.*
pas·si·flo·ra (pas-i-flō′ră). Passiflora; o maracujá, *Passiflora incarnata* (família Passifloraceae), erva trepadeira do sul dos Estados Unidos; as flores secas e os frutos foram usados no tratamento da neuralgia, dismenorréia e insônia, e como aplicação nas hemorróidas e queimaduras. [L. *passio,* paixão, + *flos* (*flor*-), flor]
pas·sion (pash′ŭn). **1.** Paixão; emoção intensa. **2.** Termo obsoleto para sofrimento ou dor. [L. *passio,* de *patior,* pp. *passus,* sofrer]
pas·sive (pas′iv). Passivo; não ativo; submisso, inerte. [L. *passivus,* de *patior,* resistir]
pas·siv·ism (pas′iv-izm). Passividade. **1.** Atitude de submissão. **2.** Prática sexual na qual a pessoa se submete à vontade do parceiro em comportamento que geralmente exige o consentimento de ambos os participantes (p. ex., sexo anal). VER TAMBÉM pathic. [ver passive]
pas·siv·i·ty (pas-iv′i-tē). Passividade. **1.** A condição de um metal que formou uma camada protetora de óxido; p. ex., metais inoxidáveis e o alumínio tornam-se passivos (inertes) no ar. **2.** Em odontologia, a qualidade ou condição de inatividade (inércia) ou repouso adotada pelos dentes, tecidos e dentadura quando uma dentadura parcial removível está no lugar, mas não sob pressão mastigatória.
pas·ta, gen. and pl. **pas·tae** (pas′tă, -tē). Pasta. SIN paste. [L.]
paste (pāst). Pasta; material semi-sólido de consistência mais firme que a da papa, mas ainda suficientemente mole para fluir lentamente e não manter seu formato. SIN pasta. [L. *pasta*]
dermatologic p., p. dermatológica; classe de preparações que consistem em amido, dextrina, enxofre, carbonato de cálcio ou óxido de zinco transformados em pasta com glicerina, sabão líquido, vaselina ou alguma gordura, à qual é incorporada alguma substância medicinal.
desensitizing p., p. dessensibilizante; ungüento, geralmente cáustico, coagulante ou citotóxico, formulado para ser aplicado ao colo de um dente a fim de aliviar a dor decorrente da exposição do cemento ou dentina sensíveis.
past·er (pā′ster). O segmento responsável pela visão de perto das lentes bifocais.
Pasteur, Louis, químico e bacteriologista francês, 1822–1895. VER P. *vaccine, effect, pipette.*
Pas·teu·rel·la (pas-ter-el′ă). Gênero de bactérias aeróbicas ou anaeróbicas facultativas, imóveis (família Brucellaceae), contendo cocos Gram-negativos muito pequenos ou bacilos elipsóides a alongados que, com métodos especiais, podem exibir coloração bipolar. Esses microrganismos são parasitas de seres humanos e de outros animais, incluindo aves. A espécie típica é *P. multocida.* [L. *Pasteur*]
P. aerogenes, espécie encontrada em suínos que pode causar infecção de feridas no homem após ser mordido por um porco.
P. multoci·da, espécie de bactéria causadora de cólera em aves domésticas e de septicemia hemorrágica em animais homeotérmicos, pode infectar mordidas ou arranhaduras de cães e gatos e causar celulite e septicemia nos seres humanos com doença crônica. Patógeno mais comum associado a mordidas de cães e gatos. Causadora da pasteurelose. É a espécie típica do gênero P.
P. pes′tis. SIN *Yersinia pestis.*
P. pseudotuberculo′sis. SIN *Yersinia pseudotuberculosis.*
P. "SP", microrganismo raramente encontrado, de taxonomia problemática, que pode causar infecções após uma mordida de cobaia; as infecções humanas são muito raras, provavelmente porque a bactéria não é disseminada e tem baixa virulência.
P. tularen′sis. SIN *Francisella tularensis.*
pas·teu·rel·la, pl. **pas·teu·rel·lae** (pas-ter-el′ă, pas-ter-el′ē). Pasteurela; termo usado para se referir a qualquer membro do gênero *Pasteurella.*
pas·teur·el·lo·sis (pas′ter-ě-lō′sis). Pasteurelose; infecção por bactérias do gênero *Pasteurella.*
pas·teur·i·za·tion (pas′ter-i-zā′shŭn). Pasteurização; o aquecimento do leite, vinhos, sucos de frutas, etc., a 68°C (154,4°F) por cerca de 30 minutos, com destruição das bactérias vivas e preservação do sabor ou buquê; os esporos não são afetados, mas ficam impedidos de se desenvolverem por resfriamento imediato do líquido a 10°C (50°F) ou menos. VER TAMBÉM sterilization. [L. *Pasteur*]
pas·teur·ize (pas′ter-īz). Pausterizar; tratar por pasteurização.
pas·teur·iz·er (pas′ter-ī-zer). Pasteurizador; aparelho usado em pasteurização.
Pastia, Constantin C., médico romeno, 1883–1926. VER P. *sign.*
pas·til, pas·tille (pas′til, pas-tēl). Pastilha. **1.** Pequena massa de benzoína e outras substâncias aromáticas para ser queimada para fumigação. **2.** SIN troche. [Fr. *pastille;* L. *pastillus,* um rolo (de pão), dim. de *panis,* pão]
Sabouraud p.'s, pastilhas de Sabouraud; discos contendo platinocianeto de bário que sofrem alteração da cor quando expostos aos raios X; usadas antigamente para indicar a dose administrada.
past·point·ing (past′poynt′ing). Teste do indicador; um teste da integridade do sistema vestibular: o indivíduo, sentado em uma cadeira giratória, é rodado para a direita 10 vezes, com os olhos fechados; depois, com o braço mantido na posição horizontal, o dedo indicador direito é encostado na ponta do dedo do examinador; a seguir, o braço é levantado verticalmente e o indivíduo é instruído a tocar o dedo do examinador ao trazer o braço de volta para a posição horizontal; se o aparelho vestibular estiver normal, o dedo será posicionado vários centímetros à direita do dedo do examinador; quando a rotação é feita para a esquerda, ocorre o inverso. Na doença cerebelar, um paciente que tente tocar um ponto com o dedo irá ultrapassá-lo. O teste também é usado em conjunto com a estimulação calórica. Em alguns distúrbios vestibulares, a prova do indicador é positiva sem rotação ou estimulação calórica.
pa·ta·gi·um, pl. **pa·ta·gia** (pă-tā′jē-ŭm, -ă). Patágio; membrana semelhante a uma asa. [L. orla de ouro em um vestido feminino]
Patau, Klaus, citogeneticista norte-americano do século XX. VER P. *syndrome.*
patch. 1. Mancha; pequena área circunscrita que difere em cor ou estrutura da superfície adjacente. **2.** Em dermatologia, uma área plana maior que 1,0 cm de diâmetro. **3.** Um estágio intermediário na formação de uma cobertura sobre a superfície de uma célula.
butterfly p., placa em forma de borboleta. SIN butterfly (2).
p. clamping, técnica usada no estudo de canais iônicos na qual é medido o movimento de íons através de um pequeno pedaço de membrana isolado quando a membrana é eletricamente polarizada ou hiperpolarizada e mantida nesse potencial. SIN patch clamp.
cotton-wool p.'s, manchas algodonosas; áreas brancas, irregulares, na superfície da retina (acúmulos de organelas celulares) causadas por lesão (geralmente infarto) da camada de fibras nervosas da retina. SIN cotton-wool spots.
herald p., mancha precursora; a lesão inicial papuloescamosa vermelha, oval, que aumenta rapidamente, geralmente localizada no tronco, prenunciando a erupção disseminada de pitiríase rósea, à qual precede de 7–14 dias.
Hutchinson p., mancha de Hutchinson. SIN salmon p.
mucous p., p. mucosa; uma ou mais lesões ovais ou redondas, amarelo-acinzentadas ou brancas, cobertas por membrana, encontradas nas mucosas; geralmente é observada na sífilis secundária.
Peyer p.'s, placas de Peyer. SIN aggregated lymphoid *nodules* of small intestine, em *nodule.*
salmon p., (1) hemorragia intra-retiniana observada na retinopatia falciforme (sickle cell *retinopathy*); **(2)** o aspecto de um tumor linfóide orbital observado no espaço subconjuntival; **(3)** uma malformação vascular macular comum, rosa-alaranjado ou vermelha, presente na cabeça e pescoço, ao nascimento ou logo depois, que involui durante a infância. SIN Hutchinson p.
shagreen p., p. chagrém. SIN shagreen *skin.*
smoker's p.'s, leucoplaquia. SIN leukoplakia.
soldier's p.'s, manchas lácteas. SIN milk *spots* (1), em *spot.*
Patein, G., médico francês, 1857–1928. VER P. *albumin.*
pa.tel.la, gen. e pl. **pa.tel.lae** (pa-tel′ă, -ē). [TA]. Patela; o grande osso sesamóide, no tendão combinado dos extensores da perna, que cobre a superfície anterior do joelho. SIN kneecap. [L. uma pequena placa, a rótula, dim. de *patina,* um disco raso, de *pateo,* ficar aberto]

p. alta, p. alta; termo usado para descrever a posição um pouco mais proximal da patela que o previsto quando é visualizada em uma radiografia lateral do joelho. [patella + L. *alta,* alta]

p. baja, p. baixa; termo usado para descrever uma posição um pouco mais distal da patela que o previsto quando é visualizada em uma radiografia lateral do joelho. [patella + Esp. *baja,* baixa]

floating p., p. flutuante; patela elevada em decorrência de derrame na articulação do joelho.

slipping p., p. deslizante; luxação espontânea ou facilmente provocada da patela.

pa·tel·lar (pa-tel′ar). Patelar; relativo à patela.

pat·el·lec·to·my (pat′e-lek′to-me). Patelectomia; excisão da patela. [patella + G. *ektome,* excisão]

pa·tel·li·form (pa-tel′i-form). Pateliforme; que possui o formato da patela.

pa·ten·cy (pa′ten-se). Desobstrução; desimpedimento; o estado de estar livremente aberto ou exposto.

probe p., desobstrução do forame oval à sondagem; termo introduzido por B.M. Patten para designar a adesão fibrosa incompleta de uma válvula do forame oval no fechamento pós-natal desse forame.

pa·tent (pa′tent, pat′ent). Permeável; desobstruído; pérvio; aberto ou exposto. SIN patulous. [L. *patens,* part. pres. de *pateo,* ficar aberto]

pa·tent blue V. Azul patente V. SIN leuco patent blue.

Paterson, Donald R., otorrinolaringologista inglês, 1863–1939. VER P.-Kelly *syndrome;* Paterson-Brown-Kelly *syndrome.*

path. Trajeto, via, trajetória; o curso seguido por uma corrente elétrica ou por impulsos nervosos. VER TAMBÉM pathway. [A.S. *paeth*]

clinical p., mapa clínico; mapa que define todo o curso ou trajetória que se espera que um paciente siga durante o tratamento e depois.

condyle p., trajeto condilar; o trajeto percorrido pelo processo condilar da mandíbula, na articulação temporomandibular, durante os vários movimentos da mandíbula.

generated occlusal p., trajeto oclusal gerado; um registro dos trajetos de movimento das superfícies oclusais dos dentes mandibulares sobre uma superfície plástica ou abrasiva fixada ao arco maxilar. VER TAMBÉM functional chewin *record.*

incisal p., trajeto incisal. SIN incisal *guidance.*

p. of insertion, trajeto de inserção; a direção em que uma prótese dentária é colocada nos tecidos de sustentação ou nos dentes adjacentes ou deles retirada.

milled-in p.'s, curvas de articulação; (1) contornos esculpidos por vários movimentos mandibulares, na superfície oclusal de uma borda de oclusão, pelos dentes ou tachões colocados na borda de oclusão oposta; as curvas ou contornos podem ser esculpidos em cera, plástico de modelagem ou gesso; (2) as curvas de oclusão desenvolvidas por movimentos de mastigação ou deslizamento nas bordas de oclusão, compostas de materiais incluindo abrasivos. VER TAMBÉM functional chew-in *Record.* SIN milled-in curves.

occlusal p., trajeto oclusal; (1) um contato oclusal deslizante; (2) o trajeto de movimento de uma superfície oclusal.

path-, -pathy, patho-, path·ic. Pat-, pato-, -pático; doença. [G. *pathos,* sentimento, sofrimento, doença]

pa·the·ma (pa-the′ma). Pátema; termo obsoleto para designar uma doença ou condição mórbida. [G. *pathema,* sofrimento]

path·er·gy (path′er-je). Patergia; aquelas reações resultantes de um estado de atividade alterada, tanto alérgicas (imunes) quanto não-alérgicas. [G. *pathos,* doença, + *ergon,* trabalho]

pa·thet·ic (pa-thet′ik). 1. Designa o quarto nervo craniano (outrora nervo patético), o nervo troclear. 2. Patético; designa o que desperta compaixão ou piedade. [G. *pathetikos,* relativo aos sentimentos]

path·find·er (path′fin-der). Guia; sonda filiforme que é introduzida através de uma extremidade estreita para servir como guia para a passagem de uma sonda ou cateter maior.

path·ic (path′ik). Pessoa que assume o papel passivo em práticas sexuais menos comuns. VER TAMBÉM passivism (2). [G. *pathikos,* que permanece passivo]

patho-. Pato. VER path-.

path·o·am·ine (path-o-am′en). Patoamina; uma ptomaína; amina tóxica que causa doença ou resultante de um processo patológico.

path·o·bi·ol·o·gy (path′o-bi-ol′o-je). Biopatologia; patologia com maior ênfase nos aspectos biológicos que nos aspectos médicos.

path·o·ci·din (path-o-si′din). Patocidina; 8-azaguanina.

path·o·cli·sis (path-o-klis′is). Patóclise; tendência específica à sensibilidade a toxinas especiais; uma tendência das toxinas de atacar determinados órgãos. [patho- + G. *klisis,* inclinação, propensão]

path·o·crin·ia (path-o-krin′e-a). Patocrinia; termo obsoleto para designar qualquer distúrbio das glândulas endócrinas. [patho- + G. *krino,* separar]

path·o·don·tia (path-o-don′she-a). Patodontia; a ciência que estuda as doenças dos dentes. [patho- + G. *odous,* dente]

path·o·for·mic (path-o-for′mik). Patofórmico; relativo ao início da doença; designa principalmente alguns sintomas que ocorrem no período de transição entre um estado normal e de doença. [patho- + L. *formo,* formar]

path·o·gen (path′o-jen). Patógeno; qualquer vírus, microrganismo ou outra substância que cause doença. [patho- + G. *-gen,* produzir]

behavioral p., p. comportamental; os hábitos pessoais e o estilo de vida de um indivíduo associados a um aumento do risco de doença e disfunção física. VER TAMBÉM risk *factor.*

opportunistic p., p. oportunista; organismo capaz de causar doença apenas quando a resistência do hospedeiro está diminuída, p. ex., por outras doenças ou drogas.

path·o·gen·e·sis (path-o-jen′e-sis). Patogenia; patogênese; o mecanismo patológico, fisiológico ou bioquímico que resulta no desenvolvimento de uma doença ou processo mórbido. Cf. etiology. [patho- + G. *genesis,* produção]

drug p., p. medicamentosa; a produção de sinais e sintomas mórbidos por drogas.

path·o·gen·ic, path·o·ge·net·ic (path-o-jen′ik, -je-net′ik). Patogênico; que causa doença ou anormalidade. SIN morbific, morbigenous, nosogenic, nosopoietic.

path·o·ge·nic·i·ty (path′o-je-nis′i-te). Patogenicidade; a condição ou qualidade de ser patogênico, ou a capacidade de causar doença.

pa·thog·e·ny (pa-thoj′e-ne). Patogenia; sinônimo de *pathogenesis* raramente usado.

path·og·no·mon·ic (path′og-no-mon′ik). Patognomônico; característico ou indicativo de uma doença; designa principalmente um ou mais sintomas ou achados típicos, ou um padrão de anormalidades específicas de determinada doença e não encontrado em qualquer outro distúrbio. [ver pathognomy]

path·og·no·my (pa-thog′no-me). Patognomia; termo raramente usado para diagnóstico por meio de um estudo dos sinais e sintomas típicos de uma doença, ou das sensações subjetivas do paciente. [patho- + G. *gnome,* uma marca, um sinal]

path·og·nos·tic (path-og-nos′tik). Patognóstico; sinônimo raramente usado de pathognomonic (patognomônico). [patho- + G. *gnostikos,* relativo ao conhecimento]

path·o·log·ic, path·o·log·i·cal (path-o-loj′ik, -i-kal). Patológico. 1. Relativo à patologia. 2. Mórbido ou doente; resultante de doença.

pa·thol·o·gist (pa-thol′o-jist). Patologista; um especialista em patologia; um médico que realiza, avalia ou supervisiona testes diagnósticos, utilizando materiais removidos de pacientes vivos ou mortos, e atua como um consultor laboratorial dos médicos, ou que realiza experiências ou outras investigações para determinar as causas ou a natureza das alterações patológicas.

speech-language p., terapeuta da fala; profissional envolvido no diagnóstico e reabilitação de pessoas com transtornos da voz, fala e linguagem.

pa·thol·o·gy (pa-thol′o-je). Patologia; a ciência médica e a especialidade relacionada com todos os aspectos da doença, mas com especial referência à natureza essencial, causas e desenvolvimento de condições anormais, bem como às alterações estruturais e funcionais resultantes dos processos patológicos. [patho- + G. *logos,* estudo, tratado]

anatomic p., anatomia patológica; a subespecialidade da p. que diz respeito ao estudo macroscópico e microscópico de órgãos ou tecidos removidos por biopsia ou durante exame *postmortem,* e também à interpretação dos resultados desse estudo. SIN pathological anatomy.

cellular p., p. celular; (1) a interpretação de doenças em termos de alterações celulares, isto é, as formas pelas quais as células não conseguem manter a homeostasia; (2) algumas vezes usado como sinônimo de citopatologia (cytopathology) (1).

clinical p., p. clínica; (1) qualquer parte da prática médica da patologia relativa ao tratamento de pacientes; (2) a subespecialidade da p. que diz respeito aos aspectos teóricos e técnicos (isto é, os métodos ou procedimentos) da química, imuno-hematologia, microbiologia, parasitologia, imunologia, hematologia e outros campos no que se refere ao diagnóstico de doenças e ao tratamento de pacientes, bem como à prevenção de doenças.

comparative p., p. comparativa; a p. das doenças de animais, principalmente em relação à patologia humana.

dental p., p. dental. SIN oral p.

functional p., p. funcional; p. relativa às anormalidades da função de um tecido, órgão ou parte, com ou sem alterações associadas da estrutura.

humoral p., p. humoral; a tese que afirma que distúrbios nos líquidos do corpo, principalmente no sangue, são os fatores básicos na doença.

medical p., p. clínica; p. relativa às várias doenças que não devem receber tratamento cirúrgico.

molecular p., p. molecular; o estudo dos mecanismos celulares bioquímicos e biofísicos como os fatores básicos na doença.

oral p., p. oral; o ramo da odontologia que estuda a etiologia, a patogenia e os aspectos clínicos, macroscópicos e microscópicos da doença oral e paraoral, incluindo os tecidos moles da boca, os dentes, a mandíbula e maxila e as glândulas salivares. SIN dental p.

speech p., p. da fala; a ciência que estuda os defeitos e distúrbios funcionais e orgânicos da fala. SIN speech-language p.

speech-language p., p. da fala. SIN speech p.

surgical p., p. cirúrgica; um campo da p. anatômica relacionado ao exame de tecidos removidos de pacientes vivos para diagnóstico de doença e orientação no tratamento dos pacientes.

path·o·met·ric (path-ō-met′rik). Patométrico; relativo à patometria.

pa·thom·e·try (pă-thom′e-trē). Patometria; termo raramente usado para a determinação do número proporcional de indivíduos afetados por determinada doença em determinado período, e das condições que causam aumento ou diminuição desse número. [patho- + G. *metron*, medida]

path·o·mi·me·sis (path′ō-mi-mē′sis). Patomimese; simulação de uma doença ou disfunção, seja intencional ou inconsciente. SIN pathomimicry. [patho- + G. *mimēsis*, imitação]

path·o·mim·ic·ry (path-ō-mim′i-krē). Patomimese. SIN pathomimesis.

path·o·mi·o·sis (path-ō-mi-ō′sis). Patomiose; a atitude que leva um paciente a minimizar sua doença. [patho- + G. *meiōsis*, diminuição]

path·o·mor·phism (path-ō-mōr′fizm). Patomorfismo; morfologia anormal.

path·o·no·mia, pa·thon·o·my (path-ō-nō′mē-ă, pă-thon′ō-mē). Patonomia; a ciência das leis das alterações mórbidas. [patho- + G. *nomos*, lei]

path·o·pho·bia (path-ō-fō′bē-ă). Patofobia. SIN nosophobia. [patho- + G. *phobos*, medo]

path·o·phys·i·ol·o·gy (path′ō-fiz-ē-ol′ō-jē). Fisiopatologia; distúrbio da função observado na doença; alteração da função distinta de defeitos estruturais.

path·o·poi·e·sis (path′ō-poy-ē′sis). Patopoese; termo raramente usado para designar a forma de produção de doença. [patho- + G. *poiēsis*, produção]

pa·tho·sis (pă-thō′sis). Patose; termo raramente usado para designar um estado mórbido, condição patológica ou entidade mórbida. [patho- + G. *-osis*, condição]

pa·thot·ro·pism (pa-thot′rō-pizm). Patotropismo; atração dos fármacos por estruturas patológicas. [patho- + G. *tropos*, uma volta]

path·way (path′wā). Via; trajeto. **1.** Um conjunto de axônios que estabelecem uma via de condução para impulsos nervosos de um grupo de células nervosas para outro grupo ou para um órgão efetor composto de células musculares ou glandulares. **2.** Qualquer seqüência de reações químicas que levam de um composto a outro; se ocorre em tecido vivo, geralmente é denominado **biochemical p.** (via bioquímica).

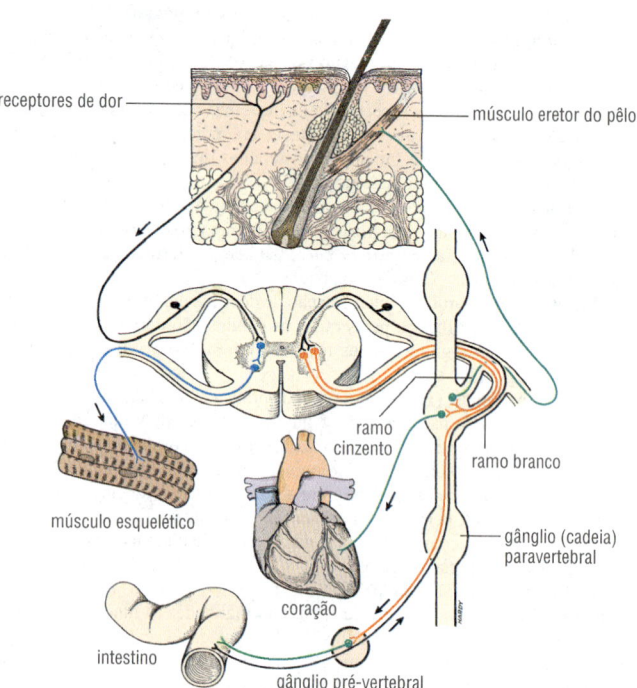

vias reflexas somáticas e viscerais: representação em diagrama; as setas indicam a direção da transmissão do impulso; os neurônios aferentes viscerais, mostrados à direita, são pré-ganglionares (linhas vermelhas) e pós-ganglionares (linhas verdes); as sinapses ocorrem nos gânglios paravertebrais ou nos gânglios pré-vertebrais

4-aminobutyrate p., via do 4-aminobutirato; a via que faz a conversão final de 4-aminobutirato em succinato; o succinato então é convertido em α-cetoglutarato, através do ciclo do ácido tricarboxílico, que então sofre a ação da glutamato desidrogenase; o glutamato então é descarboxilado para formar novamente o 4-aminobutirato; uma via importante para as células que produzem essa molécula neuroativa. SIN GABA p.

auditory p., via auditiva; vias e conexões neurais no sistema nervoso central, começando com as células ciliadas do órgão de Corti, continuando ao longo do oitavo nervo e terminando no córtex auditivo.

critical p., via crítica; resumo ou diagrama que documenta o processo de diagnóstico ou tratamento considerado apropriado para uma condição baseada em orientações práticas.

Embden-Meyerhof p., via de Embden-Meyerhof; a via glicolítica anaeróbica pela qual a D-glicose (mais notavelmente no músculo) é convertida em ácido lático. Cf. glycolysis. SIN Embden-Meyerhof-Parnas p.

Embden-Meyerhof-Parnas p., via de Embden-Meyerhof-Parnas. SIN Embden-Meyerhof p.

Entner-Douderoff p., via de Entner-Douderoff; uma via degradativa para carboidratos em alguns microrganismos (p. ex., *Pseudomonas* sp.) que não possuem hexocinase, fosfofrutocinase e gliceraldeído-3-fosfato desidrogenase.

GABA p., via do GABA. SIN 4-aminobutyrate p.

hexose monophosphate p., via da hexose monofosfato. SIN pentose phosphate p.

lacrimal p. [TA], rego lacrimal; espaço entre as pálpebras fechadas e o bulbo do olho através do qual as lágrimas fluem para o ponto lacrimal. SIN rivus lacrimalis [TA], Ferrein canal.

mercapturic acid p., via do ácido mercaptúrico; uma via glutatião-dependente para a detoxificação de várias substâncias, incluindo óxidos arena; é formado um glutatião com substituição do *S*, que, finalmente, é convertido em um ácido mercaptúrico (uma L-cisteína *N*-acetilada *S*-substituída), que é excretado; acredita-se que os leucotrienos sejam degradados através dessa via.

pentose phosphate p., via da pentose fosfato; uma via secundária para a oxidação da D-glicose (que não ocorre no músculo esquelético), gerando uma força redutora (NADPH) no citoplasma fora das mitocôndrias e sintetizando pentoses e alguns outros açúcares. Também proporciona um meio de converter pentoses e alguns outros açúcares em intermediários da via glicolítica. Prossegue da D-glicose 6-fosfato para D-ribulose fosfato e D-ribose fosfato, daí (com D-xilulose-5-fosfato) para D-sedoeptulose 7-fosfato e D-gliceraldeído 3-fosfato; dióxido de carbono é liberado na etapa da gluconato-ribulose. Em vegetais, participa da formação da D-glicose a partir do dióxido de carbono nas reações de fotossíntese no escuro. Essa via é deficiente em algumas doenças hereditárias, p. ex., deficiência de glicose-6-fosfato desidrogenase. SIN Dickens shunt, hexose monophosphate p., hexose monophosphate shunt, pentose monophosphate shunt, pentose phosphate cycle, phosphogluconate p., Warburg-Dickens-Horecker shunt, Warburg-Lipmann-Dickens-Horecker shunt.

phosphogluconate p., via do fosfogluconato. SIN pentose phosphate p.

polyol p., via do poliol. SIN sorbitol p.

salvage p., via de recuperação; a utilização de bases purina e pirimidina pré-formadas para sintetizar nucleotídeos.

sorbitol p., via do sorbitol; via responsável pela formação da D-frutose a partir do sorbitol; sua atividade aumenta quando a concentração de glicose aumenta no diabetes. SIN polyol p.

ubiquitin-protease p., via da ubiquitina-protease; via na qual um pequeno cofator proteico, a ubiquitina, acopla-se ao substrato protéico para catalisar a destruição proteolítica por proteases; essa via é extremamente seletiva e estritamente regulada, e é responsável pela degradação proteica observada em doenças consuntivas musculares.

visual p., via visual; vias e conexões neurais no sistema nervoso central, começando com a retina e terminando no córtex occipital.

-pathy. VER path-.

pa·tient (pā′shent). Paciente; aquele que sofre de qualquer doença ou transtorno do comportamento e está em tratamento. Cf. case (1). [L. *patiens*, part. pres. de *patior*, sofrer]

target p., p.-alvo; em terapia de grupo, o paciente que está sendo analisado por outro paciente do grupo.

pat·ri·cide (pat′ri-sīd). Patricida. **1.** Aquele que mata o próprio pai. **2.** Aquele que comete tal ato. VER parricide. Cf. matricide. [L. *pater*, pai, + *caedō*, matar]

Patrick, Hugh T., neurologista norte-americano, 1860–1938. VER P. test.

pat·ri·lin·e·al (pat-ri-lin′ē-ăl). Patrilinear; relativo à descendência através da linhagem masculina; a herança do cromossoma Y é exclusivamente patrilinear. [L. *pater*, pai, + *linea*, linha]

pat·tern (pat′ern). **1.** Padrão; configuração; freqüentemente refere-se a achados nas radiografias de tórax. **2.** Matriz; em odontologia, uma forma usada para fazer um molde, como para uma obturação ou estrutura de dentadura parcial.

airspace-filling p., p. alveolar. SIN alveolar p.

airway p., p. das vias aéreas; imagem à radiografia de tórax de paredes brônquicas espessadas, bronquiectasia, bronquiolite ou consolidação acinar.

alveolar p., p. alveolar; imagens nebulosas a densas, encobrindo a trama vascular, nas radiografias do tórax. SIN airspace-filling p.

ballerina-foot p., p. em pé de bailarina; contração póstero-medial vigorosa do ventrículo esquerdo associada à convexidade, anteriormente, que algumas vezes resulta da contração deficiente da parede anterior oposta; é a dissinergia mais freqüentemente observada na síndrome do prolapso da valva mitral (mesmo com uma parede anterior normal) e produz uma configuração de contraste angiográfico na incidência oblíqua anterior direita, semelhante a um pé de bailarina; algumas vezes é denominada malformação em pé de dançarina.

butterfly p., p. em asa de borboleta; imagens opacas alveolares pulmonares, simétricas, bilaterais, que poupam a periferia, em radiografias do tórax; geralmente causadas por edema pulmonar.

ground-glass p., p. em vidro fosco; imagem hipotransparente mal definida nas radiografias ou na TC que não encobre a trama vascular pulmonar.

honeycomb p., p. em favo de mel; imagens circulares, ligeiramente irregulares, densas, mais comuns próximo a pleura na base pulmonar, em radiografias ou TC do tórax; causado por fibrose intersticial crônica de causas diversas.

hourglass p., p. em ampulheta; contração anular vigorosa, observada à angiografia no ventrículo esquerdo, na incidência oblíqua anterior direita, semelhante a uma ampulheta; é observada na síndrome de prolapso da valva mitral.

interstitial p., p. intersticial; um dos vários padrões à radiografia de tórax associados a infiltração ou espessamento intersticial, incluindo p. em favo de mel, p. miliar, p. reticulonodular ou linhas septais.

juvenile p., p. juvenil; inversão da onda T precordial, algumas vezes com elevações de J-ST em um eletrocardiograma, semelhante à observada em crianças normais, que ocorre como uma variante normal em alguns adultos, sobretudo negros, e principalmente nas derivações V_1, V_2 e V_3.

miliary p., p. miliar; imagens finas e arredondadas observadas na radiografia de tórax, típicas da disseminação hematogênica da tuberculose; o tamanho tem alguma relação com o de uma semente de milhete.

mosaic p., p. de mosaico; na TC de alta resolução dos pulmões, um p. de regiões mais brilhantes e mais escuras que correspondem a diferenças na perfusão ou ventilação; encontrado em alguns casos de tromboembolismo crônico ou de bronquiolite obliterante. Cf. oligemia.

occlusal p., p. oclusal. SIN occlusal form.

reticulonodular p. (re-tik′u-lo-nod′u-lar), p. reticulonodular; um p. algo reticular à radiografia do tórax, com espessamento nodular nas intersecções das linhas; um p. intersticial inespecífico.

wax p., forma de cera; uma matriz de cera que, quando revestida e queimada, ou eliminada de outra forma, produzirá um molde no qual se pode fazer uma peça moldada. SIN wax form.

pat·u·lin (pat′u-lin). Patulina; antibiótico derivado de metabólitos de fungos, como espécies de *Aspergillus, Penicillium* e *Gymnoascus*; tem atividade carcinogênica.

pat·u·lous (pat′u-lus). Aberto; dilatado. SIN patent. [L. *patulus*, de *pateo*, ficar aberto]

pau·ci·ar·ti·cu·lar (paw-se-ar-tik′u-lar). Pauciarticular; uma condição na qual são acometidas apenas algumas (> 1, < 5) articulações. [L. *pauci*, poucos, + articular]

pau·ci·bac·il·lary (paw-se-bas′i-lar-e). Paucibacilar; constituído ou que designa a presença de poucos bacilos.

pau·ci·sy·nap·tic (paw′se-si-nap′tik). Paucissináptico. SIN oligosynaptic. [L. *paucus*, poucos, + synapse]

Paul, Gustav, médico austríaco, 1859–1935. VER P. *reaction, test*; P.-Bunnell *test*.

Pauli, Wolfgang, físico austríaco-norte-americano e Prêmio Nobel, 1900–1958. VER P. exclusion *principle*.

Pauling, Linus C., químico norte-americano e Prêmio Nobel, 1901–1994. VER P. *theory*; P.-Corey *helix*.

pause (pawz). Pausa; parada temporária. [G. *pausis*, cessação]

apneic p., p. apnéica; interrupção do fluxo de ar por mais de 10 segundos. VER sleep *apnea*.

compensatory p., p. compensatória; a p. após uma extra-sístole, quando a p. é suficientemente longa para compensar a prematuridade da extra-sístole; o ciclo curto que termina com a extra-sístole e a pausa após a extra-sístole são iguais a dois ciclos regulares.

postextrasystolic p., p. pós-extra-sistólica; o ciclo um pouco prolongado imediatamente após uma extra-sístole.

preautomatic p., p. pré-automática; uma p. temporária na atividade cardíaca antes do escape de um marcapasso automático. VER TAMBÉM escape.

respiratory p., p. respiratória; cessação do fluxo de ar por menos de 10 segundos. VER sleep *apnea*.

sinus p., p. sinusal; interrupção espontânea do ritmo sinusal regular, a p. que dura por um período que não é um múltiplo exato do ciclo sinusal. VER TAMBÉM sinus *arrest*, sinus *standstill*.

Pautrier, Lucien M.A., dermatologista francês, 1876–1959. VER P. *abscess, microabscess*.

Pauzat, Jean E., médico francês do século XIX.

Pavlov, Ivan P., fisiologista russo e Prêmio Nobel, 1849–1936. VER pavlovian *conditioning*; P. *method, pouch, stomach, reflex*.

pav·or noc·tur·nus (pā′vor nok-ter′nŭs). Terror noturno. SIN night terrors. [L.]

Pavy, Frederick W., médico inglês, 1829–1911. VER P. *disease*.

paw·paw. Mamão. VER papaya.

Payne, J. Howard, cirurgião norte-americano, *1916. VER P. *operation*.

Payr, Erwin, cirurgião alemão, 1871–1946. VER P. *clamp, membrane, sign*.

Pb Símbolo de plumbum (chumbo).

PBG Abreviatura de porphobilinogen (porfobilinogênio).

PBI Abreviatura de protein-bound *iodine* (iodo ligado a proteína).

p.c. Abreviatura do L. *post cibum*, após uma refeição.

PCA Abreviatura de passive cutaneous *anaphylaxis* (anafilaxia cutânea passiva); patient-controlled *analgesia* (analgesia controlada pelo paciente); patient-controlled *anesthesia* (anestesia controlada pelo paciente).

pCa Forma de relatar os níveis de íon cálcio; igual ao logaritmo decádico negativo da concentração de íon cálcio.

PCB Abreviatura de polychlorinated *biphenyl* (bifenilpoliclorado).

PCIS Abreviatura de patient care information system (sistema de informações do tratamento do paciente), o sistema computadorizado interativo usado para armazenar prontuários médicos em um hospital.

PCMB, *p*CMB Abreviatura de *p*-chloromercuribenzoate (*p*-cloromercuribenzoato).

P con·gen·i·ta·le (kon-jen-i-tā′le). P congênita; o padrão de onda P no eletrocardiograma, observado em alguns casos de cardiopatia congênita, que consiste em ondas P apiculadas altas nas derivações I, II, aVF e aVL (geralmente maiores em DII) com positividade predominante de ondas difásicas em V1-2.

PCP Abreviatura de phencyclidine (fenciclidina); *Pneumocystis carinii* pneumonia (pneumonia por *Pneumocystis carinii*).

PCR Abreviatura de polymerase chain *reaction* (reação da cadeia da polimerase).

PCT 1. Abreviatura de *porphyria* cutanea tarda (porfiria cutânea tardia). 2. Abreviatura de patient care technician (técnico de saúde).

PCWP Abreviatura de pulmonary capillary wedge *pressure* (pressão capilar pulmonar).

PD Abreviatura de phenyldichloroarsine (fenildicloroarsina).

Pd Símbolo do palladium (paládio).

p.d. Abreviatura de prism *diopter* (dioptria do prisma).

P-dex·tro·car·di·a·le (deks′tro-kar-de-ā′le). P-dextrocardíaco; síndrome eletrocardiográfica característica da sobrecarga do átrio direito, amiúde é erroneamente denominado P-pulmonale porque a síndrome pode resultar de qualquer sobrecarga do átrio direito (p. ex., estenose tricúspide) e independentemente do cor pulmonale.

PDGF Abreviatura de platelet-derived growth *factor* (fator de crescimento derivado de plaquetas).

PDI Abreviatura de Periodontal Disease Index.

PDL. Abreviatura de pulsed dye *laser* (laser de corante pulsado).

PEA Abreviatura de pulseless electrical *activity* (atividade elétrica sem pulso).

peach ker·nel oil (pēch ker′nel). Óleo de semente de pêssego. VER persic oil.

peak (pēk). Pico; o topo ou limite superior de um traçado gráfico ou de qualquer variável. [I.m. *peke, pike*, do Esp. *pico*, pico, do L. *picus*, pega]

biclonal p., p. biclonal; duas faixas eletroforéticas estreitas consideradas representantes das imunoglobulinas de duas linhagens celulares.

juxtaphrenic p. (jŭks-tă-fren′ik pēk), p. justafrênico; à radiografia do tórax, uma imagem densa triangular, no topo do hemidiafragma direito, provavelmente causada por tensão do nervo frênico na pleura sobre o diafragma.

monoclonal p., p. monoclonal; uma faixa estreita visível à eletroforese ou uma faixa anormal são observadas à imunoeletroforese, consideradas representantes da imunoglobulina de um clone celular.

pea·nut oil (pē′nŭt). Óleo de amendoim; óleo extraído das sementes de um ou mais tipos cultivados de *Arachis hypogaea* (família Leguminosae); usado como solvente para injeções intramusculares e no preparo de alimentos. SIN arachis oil.

Pearl, Raymond, biólogo norte-americano, 1879–1940. VER P. *index*.

pearl (perl). Pérola. 1. Uma concreção formada em torno de um grão de areia ou de outro corpo estranho no interior da concha de alguns moluscos. 2. Uma dentre várias massas pequenas resistentes, tais como o muco que ocorre no escarro na asma. 3. Pérola de queratina. SIN keratin p.

Elschnig p.'s, pérolas de Elschnig; retenção focal de fibras da lente que sofreram alterações proliferativas e degenerativas circundadas por fragmentos capsulares da lente observada após extração de catarata extracapsular.

enamel p., p. de esmalte. SIN enameloma.

epithelial p., p. epitelial. SIN keratin p.

Epstein p.'s, pérolas de Epstein; múltiplos e pequenos cistos de inclusão epitelial, brancos, encontrados na linha média do palato em recém-nascidos.

gouty p., tofo. SIN tophus.

keratin p., p. de queratina; foco de queratinização central dentro de camadas concêntricas de células escamosas anormais; observada no carcinoma de células escamosas. SIN epithelial nest, epithelial p., pearl (3), squamous p.

Laënnec p.'s, pérolas de Laënnec; designação obsoleta de corpos pequenos, redondos, translúcidos, de consistência viscosa, no escarro de algumas pessoas com asma; quando colocados na água para flutuar, eles se desenrolam e são então denominados espirais de Curschmann.

squamous p., p. de queratina. SIN keratin p.

pearl-ash. Perlasso. SIN potash.

Pearson, Karl, matemático inglês, 1857–1936. VER Poisson-P. *formula*; McArdle-Schmid-P. *disease*.

peau d'orange (pō - dō - rahnj'). Casca de laranja; superfície cutânea com edema depressível, superposta ao carcinoma de mama, em que há infiltração do estroma e obstrução linfática com edema. [Fr. casca de laranja]

pec·cant (pek'ant). Insalubre; que produz doença. [L. *peccans* (*-ant-*), part. pres. de *pecco*, pecar]

pec·ca·ti·pho·bia (pek'kă - ti - fō'bē - ă). Pecatifobia; medo mórbido de pecar. [L. *peccatum*, pecado, + G. *phobos*, medo]

pecilo-. Pecilo-. VER poikilo-.

pe·cil·o·cin (pē - sil'ō - sin). Pecilocina; um agente antifúngico.

Pecquet, Jean, anatomista francês, 1622–1674. VER P. *cistern, duct; receptaculum pecqueti*; P. *reservoir*.

pec·tase (pek'tās). Pectase; enzima que converte a pectina em ácido D-galacturônico (ácido péctico); usada no tratamento de alguns alimentos. SIN pectinesterase.

pec·ten (pek'ten). 1. [NA] Pécten; estrutura com prolongamentos ou projeções semelhantes a um pente. 2. SIN anal p. [L. pente]

anal p. [TA], p. anal; o terço médio do canal anal cirúrgico; a metade superior do canal anatômico estende-se entre a linha pectinada e o sulco interesfinctérico, e é revestida por anoderme. SIN p. analis [TA], pecten (2).

p. ana'lis [TA], p. anal. SIN anal p.

p. os'sis pu'bis [TA], SIN p. pubis.

p. pu'bis [TA], linha pectínea do púbis; a continuação da linha terminal no ramo superior do púbis, formando uma crista aguda. SIN p. ossis pubis [TA], pectineal line of pubis.

pec·ten·i·tis (pek - ten - ī'tis). Pectenite; inflamação do esfíncter anal. [L. *pecten*, pente, + G. *-itis*, inflamação]

pec·ten·o·sis (pek - ten - ō'sis). Pectenose; aumento exagerado da faixa do pécten.

pec·tic (pek'tik). Péctico; relativo a qualquer uma das substâncias ou materiais atualmente conhecidos como pectina. [G. *pēktos* denso, coagulado]

pec·tic ac·id. Ácido péctico. SIN D-galacturonic acid.

pec·tin (pek'tin). Pectina. 1. Termo genérico amplo pelo qual são conhecidas atualmente as substâncias ou materiais pécticos; especificamente, uma substância gelatinosa, que consiste, principalmente, em cadeias longas constituídas sobretudo por unidades de ácido D-galacturônico (tipicamente ligações α-1,4 e algumas vezes presentes como ésteres metil), extraída de frutas, onde se presume que exista como protopectina (pectose). 2. As pectinas comerciais, algumas vezes denominadas ácido pectínico, são pós solúveis, esbranquiçados, preparados a partir da casca de frutas cítricas. São usadas no preparo de geléias, gelatinas e alimentos semelhantes, cuja viscosidade aumentam; terapeuticamente, são usadas no controle da diarréia (geralmente associadas a outros agentes), como expansor plasmático e como protetor; as pectinas ligam-se aos íons cálcio e são altamente hidratadas.

p. lyase, p. liase; enzima que catalisa a eliminação de resíduos 6-metil-Δ-4,5-D-galacturonato da pectina; assim, desencadeia despolimerização; não atua sobre a pectina desesterificada; é usada no tratamento de alguns alimentos.

pec·tin·ase (pek'tin - ās). Pectinase. SIN polygalacturonase.

pec·ti·nate (pek'ti - nāt). Pectinado. 1. Pectiniforme; em forma de pente. SIN pectiniform. 2. Em fungos, é usado para descrever um tipo específico de hifas ramificadas em culturas de dermatófitos.

pec·tin·e·al (pek - tin'ē - al). Pectíneo; sulcado; estriado; relativo ao osso púbis ou a qualquer estrutura semelhante a um pente. SIN pectineus (1).

pec·tin·es·ter·ase (pek - tin - es'ter - ās). Pectinesterase. SIN pectase.

pec·ti·ne·us (pek'ti - nē'ŭs). Pectíneo. 1. SIN pectineal. 2. VER pectineus (*muscle*). [L.]

pec·tin·ic ac·ids (pek - tin'ik). Ácidos pectínicos; termo usado algumas vezes para pectinas comerciais.

pec·tin·i·form (pek - tin'i - fōrm). Pectiniforme. SIN pectinate (1).

pec·ti·za·tion (pek - ti - zā'shŭn). Pectização; em química coloidal, coagulação. [G. *pēktikos*, coagulação]

pec·to·ral (pek'tō - răl). Peitoral; relativo ao tórax. [L. *pectoralis*; de *pectus*, osso do peito]

pec·to·ral·gia (pek - tō - ral'jē - ă). Pectoralgia; dor no tórax. [L. *pectus* (*pector-*), tórax, + G. *algos*, dor]

pec·to·ril·o·quy (pek - tō - ril'ō - kwē). Pectorilóquia; aumento da transmissão do som vocal através das estruturas pulmonares, de forma que seja claramente audível à ausculta do tórax; geralmente indica consolidação do parênquima pulmonar subjacente. SIN pectorophony. [L. *pectus*, tórax, + *loquor*, falar]

aphonic p., p. afônico. SIN Baccelli sign.

whispered p., whispering p., p. sussurrada; broncofonia sussurrada; pectorilóquia de sons sussurrados da mesma forma que os sons vocais. SIN whispered bronchophony.

pec·to·roph·o·ny (pek - tō - rof'ō - nē). Pectorofonia. SIN pectoriloquy. [L. *pectus*, tórax, + G. *phōnē*, voz]

pec·tose (pek'tōs). Pectose. VER pectin, protopectin.

pec·tous (pek'tŭs). Pectinoso. 1. Relativo a, ou que consiste em, pectina ou pectose. 2. Designa uma condição coagulada firme algumas vezes assumida por um gel, que é permanente porque a substância não consegue voltar à forma de gel.

pec·tus, gen. **pec·to·ris,** pl. **pec·to·ra** (pek'tŭs, pek'tō - ris, pek'tō - ră). Peito; tórax. SIN chest. [L.]

p. carina'tum, peito (tórax) de pombo; tórax quereniforme; achatamento do hemitórax direito e/ou esquerdo com projeção do esterno para a frente, semelhante à quilha de um barco. SIN chicken breast, keeled chest, pigeon breast, pigeon chest.

p. excava'tum, peito (tórax) escavado; depressão na parte inferior do tórax causada por deslocamento da cartilagem xifóide para trás. SIN foveated chest, funnel chest, funnel breast, koilosternia, p. recurvatum, trichterbrust.

p. recurva'tum, SIN p. excavatum.

ped-, pedi-, pedo-. Ped-, pedi-, pedo-. 1. Criança. [G. *pais*, criança] 2. Pé, pés. [L. *pes*, pé]

ped·al (ped'ăl). Pedal; podálico; relativo aos pés ou a qualquer estrutura denominada pé (pes). [L. *pedalis*, de *pes* (*ped-*), pé]

pe·da·tro·phia, pe·dat·ro·phy (ped - ă - trō'fē - ă, - at'rō - fē). Pedatrofia. SIN marasmus. [G. *pais* (*paid-*), criança, + atrophy]

ped·er·ast (ped'er - ast). Pederasta; aquele que pratica pederastia.

ped·er·as·ty (ped'er - as - tē). Pederastia; coito anal homossexual, principalmente quando praticada em meninos. [G. *paiderastia*; de *pais* (*paid-*), menino, + *eraō*, ansiar]

Pedersen spec·u·lum. Espéculo de Pedersen. Ver em speculum.

pe·de·sis (pē - dē'sis). Pedese. SIN brownian movement. [G. *pēdēsis*, salto]

pedi-. VER ped-.

pe·di·at·ric (pē - dē - at'rik). Pediátrico; relativo à pediatria. [G. *pais* (*paid-*), criança, + *iatrikos*, relativo à medicina]

pe·di·a·tri·cian (pē'dē - ă - trish'ăn). Pediatra; um especialista em pediatria. SIN pediatrist.

pe·di·at·rics (pē - dē - at'riks). Pediatria; a especialidade médica que diz respeito ao estudo e tratamento de crianças saudáveis e doentes, durante o desenvolvimento, desde o nascimento até a adolescência. [G. *pais*, (*paid-*), criança, + *iatreia*, tratamento médico]

pe·di·a·trist (pē'dē - at'rist). Pediatra. SIN pediatrician.

ped·i·a·try (pē'dē - at - rē, pē - dī'ă - trē). Pediatria; termo raramente usado.

ped·i·cel (ped'i - sel). Pedicelo; o prolongamento secundário de um podócito, que ajuda a formar a cápsula visceral de um corpúsculo renal. SIN footplate (2), foot-plate*, foot process. [L. mod. *pedicellus*, dim. do L. *pes*, pé]

ped·i·cel·late (ped'i - sel - lāt). Pediculado. SIN pediculate.

ped·i·cel·la·tion (ped'i - sē - lā'shŭn). Pedicelação; formação de um pedículo ou pedúnculo.

ped·i·cle (ped'ī - kl). [TA]. Pedículo; pedúnculo. 1. Uma porção estreita ou talo. SIN pediculus (1) [TA]. 2. Um talo pelo qual um tumor não-séssil está fixado ao tecido normal. SIN pedunculus [TA], peduncle (2). 3. Um talo através do qual um retalho de tecido é vascularizado, permitindo transferência para outro local. [L. *pediculus*, dim. de *pes*, pé]

p. of arch of vertebra [TA], p. do arco vertebral; a porção estreitada do arco de cada lado, que se estende do corpo até a lâmina; limitado pelos forames intervertebrais, superior e inferiormente. SIN pediculus arcus vertebrae [TA], radix arcus vertebrae.

vascular p., p. vascular; os tecidos contendo artérias e veias de um órgão; especificamente em radiologia do tórax, o mediastino (sua largura) ao nível do arco da aorta e da veia cava superior.

pe·dic·u·lar (pē - dik'ū - lăr). Pedicular; relativo aos piolhos. [L. *pedicularis*]

pe·dic·u·late (pē - dik'ū - lāt). Pediculado; não-séssil, que possui um pedículo ou pedúnculo. SIN pedicellate, pedunculate. [L. *pediculatus*]

pe·dic·u·li (pē - dik'ū - lī). Pedículos; plural de pediculus. [L.]

pe·dic·u·li·cide (pē - dik'ū - li - sīd). Pediculicida; agente usado para matar piolhos. [L. *pediculus*, piolho, + *caedo*, matar]

Pe·dic·u·loi·des ven·tri·co·sus (pē - dik - ū - loy'dez ven - tri - kō'sŭs). SIN *Pyemotes tritici.* [L. mod., do L. *pediculus*, piolho, + *venter*, ventre]

pe·dic·u·lo·pho·bia (pē - dik'ū - lō - fō'bē - ă). Pediculofobia; medo mórbido de infestação por piolhos. SIN phthiriophobia. [L. *pediculus*, piolho, + G. *phobos*, medo]

pe·dic·u·lo·sis (pē - dik'ū - lō'sis). Pediculose; o estado de estar infestado por piolhos. [L. *pediculus*, piolho, + G. *-osis*, condição]

p. cap'itis, p. da cabeça; a presença de piolhos no couro cabeludo, principalmente em crianças, com lêndeas presas aos fios de cabelo.

p. cor'poris, p. do corpo; a presença de piolhos do corpo, que vivem nas costuras das roupas. Suas picadas causam prurido e escoriações.

p. palpebra'rum, p. palpebral; a presença de piolhos nos cílios.

p. pu'bis, p. do púbis; infestação pelo piolho do púbis, *Pthirus pubis*, principalmente nos pêlos pubianos, causando prurido e máculas cerúleas.

pe·dic·u·lous (pē-dik′ū-lŭs). Pediculoso; infestado por piolhos. SIN lousy.

Pe·dic·u·lus (pē-dik′ū-lŭs). Gênero de piolhos parasitas (família Pediculidae) que vivem no cabelo e alimentam-se periodicamente de sangue. As espécies importantes incluem *P. humanus*, a espécie de piolho que infecta seres humanos; *P. humanus* var. *capitis*, o piolho da cabeça de seres humanos; *P. humanus* var. *corporis* (também denominado *P. vestimenti* ou *P. corporis*), o piolho do corpo ou das roupas, que vive e põe ovos (lêndeas) nas roupas e alimenta-se no corpo humano; e *P. pubis*. [L.]

pe·dic·u·lus, pl. **pe·dic·u·li** (pē-dik′ū-lŭs, -lī) [TA]. Pedículo. **1.** SIN pedicle (1). [L. pedículo] **2.** Um piolho. VER *Pediculus*. [L.]
  p. ar′cus ver′tebrae [TA], pedículo do arco vertebral. SIN pedicle of arch of vertebra.

ped·i·cure (ped′i-kūr). Pedicuro; cuidado e tratamento dos pés. [L. *pes* (*ped-*), pé, + *cura*, tratamento]

ped·i·gree (ped′i-grē). Árvore genealógica; heredograma; linha ancestral de descendência, principalmente a representada em um gráfico para mostrar a história ancestral; usada em genética para analisar a herança. [I.m. *pedegra* do Fr. ant. *pie de grue*, pé de grua]

pe·di·o·pho·bia (pē-dē-o-fō′bē-ă). Pediofobia; medo mórbido despertado pela visão de uma criança ou de uma boneca. [G. *paidion*, uma criança pequena, + *phobos*, medo]

ped·i·pha·lanx (ped′i-fā′langks). Uma falange do pé, distinta da falange da mão (maniphalanx). [L. *pes* (*ped-*), pé, + *phalanx*]

pedo-. VER ped-.

pe·do·don·tia (pē-dō-don′shē-ă). Pedodontia; odontopediatria. SIN pedodontics.

pe·do·don·tics (pē-dō-don′tiks). Pedodontia; odontopediatria; o ramo da odontologia relacionado com os cuidados e tratamento dentário de crianças. SIN pediatric dentistry, pedodontia. [G. *pais*, criança, + *odous*, dente]

pe·do·don·tist (pē-dō-don′tist). Pedodontista; odontopediatra; dentista que pratica pedodontia.

ped·o·dy·na·mom·e·ter (ped′ō-dī-nă-mom′ē-ter). Pedodinamômetro; instrumento para medir a força dos músculos da perna. [L. *pes* (*ped-*), pé, + G. *dynamis*, força, + G. *metron*, medida]

pe·do·gen·e·sis (pē-dō-jen′ē-sis). Pedogênese; estágio larval permanente com desenvolvimento sexual, como em determinados mosquitos (gênero *Miastor*). Cf. neoteny. [G. *pais* (*paid-*), criança, + *genesis*, origem]

ped·o·gram (ped′ō-gram). Pedograma; registro feito pelo pedógrafo.

ped·o·graph (ped′ō-graf). Pedógrafo; instrumento para registrar e estudar a marcha. [L. *pes* (*ped-*), pé, + G. *graphō*, escrever]

pe·dog·ra·phy (pē-dog′ră-fē). Pedografia; produção de um registro feito por um pedógrafo.

pe·dom·e·ter (pē-dom′ē-ter). Pedômetro; instrumento para medir a distância percorrida ao caminhar. SIN podometer. [L. *pes* (*ped-*), pé]

pe·do·mor·phism (pē-dō-mōr′fizm). Pedomorfismo; descrição do comportamento adulto em termos apropriados para o comportamento da criança. [G. *pais* (*paid*), criança, + *morphē*, forma]

pe·do·phil·ia (pē-dō-fil′ē-ă). Pedofilia; em psiquiatria, uma atração anormal de um adulto por crianças para fins sexuais. [G. *pais*, criança, + *philos*, amigo]

pe·do·phil·ic (pē-dō-fil′ik). Pedófilo; relativo a ou que exibe pedofilia.

pe·dun·cle (pe-dŭng′kl, pē′dŭng-kl). Pedúnculo. **1.** Em neuroanatomia, termo livremente aplicado a várias estruturas de conexão semelhantes a pedículos no encéfalo, compostas exclusivamente de substância branca (p. ex., pedúnculo cerebelar) ou de substância branca e cinzenta (p. ex., pedúnculo cerebral). **2.** SIN pedicle (2). [L. mod. *pedunculus*, dim. de *pes*, pé]
  cerebral p. [TA], p. cerebral; originalmente designa uma das duas metades do mesencéfalo (um "colo" relativamente estreito une o prosencéfalo ao telencéfalo); esse termo tem sido usado variavelmente para designar apenas aqueles grandes feixes de fibras corticífugas que formam os pilares do cérebro ou para designar os pilares do cérebro mais o tegmento do mesencéfalo; este último uso, mais inclusivo (pilares do cérebro e tegmento do mesencéfalo), é preferido; a substância negra, uma parte da base do pedúnculo, é considerada uma estrutura que separa o tegmento do mesencéfalo dos pilares do cérebro. VER TAMBÉM *crus* cerebri. SIN pedunculus cerebri [TA].
  p. of corpus callosum, área subcalosa. SIN subcallosal *gyrus*.
  p. of flocculus [TA], p. do flóculo; o feixe de fibras nervosas aferentes e eferentes que ligam o flóculo e o nódulo do cerebelo; parte de seu trajeto se dá no véu medular inferior. SIN pedunculus flocculi [TA].
  inferior cerebellar p., p. cerebelar inferior; par de grandes feixes de fibras nervosas que se desenvolvem nas superfícies dorsolaterais da parte superior do bulbo, estendem-se sob os recessos laterais da fossa rombóide e curvam-se dorsalmente até o cerebelo, caudomedial ao pedúnculo cerebelar médio; composto pelo feixe maior (lateral), pelo corpo restiforme [TA] e por um pequeno feixe (medial), o corpo justarrestiforme [TA]. As fibras que formam esse feixe composto originam-se dos neurônios espinais e dos núcleos de liberação bulbares. O maior constituinte (corpo restiforme) contém fibras cruzadas da oliva inferior; também contém o trato espinocerebelar dorsal e as projeções cerebelares do núcleo reticular lateral, o núcleo cuneiforme acessório, os núcleos reticulares paramedianos, os núcleos peri-hipoglossais e outros núcleos. As fibras vestibulocerebelares são posicionadas medialmente, no pedúnculo cerebelar inferior, e identificadas separadamente como corpo justarrestiforme. SIN pedunculus cerebellaris inferior [TA].
  inferior thalamic p., radiação inferior do tálamo; um grande feixe de fibras que emerge da parte anterior do tálamo na direção ventral, em parte unindo-se às fibras mediais da cápsula interna, em outra parte curvando-se lateralmente ao redor da margem medial da cápsula até a substância inominada. Muitas dessas fibras estabelecem uma conexão recíproca do núcleo mediodorsal do tálamo com os giros orbitais do lobo frontal, mas muitas outras formam um sistema de condução da amígdala e do córtex olfatório até o núcleo mediodorsal. VER TAMBÉM *ansa* peduncularis. SIN inferior thalamic radiation [TA], radiatio inferior thalami [TA], pedunculus thalami inferior.
  lateral thalamic p., radiação central do tálamo; o grande grupo de fibras que emerge da face látero-dorsal do tálamo para se unir à coroa radiada; une reciprocamente o núcleo lateral e os corpos geniculados do tálamo com as regiões correspondentes do córtex cerebral. VER TAMBÉM central thalamic *radiation*. SIN pedunculus thalami lateralis.
  p. of mammillary body, fascículo pedunculomamilar; um fascículo de fibras nervosas que seguem até o corpo mamilar ao longo da superfície ventral do mesencéfalo; consiste em fibras que se originam dos núcleos tegmentais posteriores e anteriores. SIN fasciculus pedunculomammillaris, pedunculomammillary fasciculus, pedunculus corporis mammillaris.
  middle cerebellar p. [TA], p. cerebelar médio; o maior dos três pares de pedúnculos cerebelares, composto principalmente de fibras que se originam nos núcleos pontinos, atravessam a linha média na ponte basilar e emergem, do lado oposto, como um grande feixe que se curva dorsalmente ao longo da face lateral do tegmento da ponte até o cerebelo; há algumas fibras pontocerebelares não cruzadas nesse pedúnculo; suas fibras são distribuídas principalmente para o córtex do hemisfério cerebelar, com algumas fibras colaterais que seguem até os núcleos cerebelares. SIN pedunculus cerebellaris medius [TA], brachium pontis.
  olfactory p., p. olfatório. SIN olfactory *tract*.
  superior cerebellar p. [TA], p. cerebelar superior; um grande feixe (fascículo) de fibras nervosas que se origina dos núcleos denteado, globoso e emboliforme e emerge do cerebelo na direção rostral, ao longo da parede lateral do quarto ventrículo. O fascículo submerge da superfície dorsal do tronco cerebral no tegmento do mesencéfalo, onde a maioria de suas fibras cruza na grande decussação dos pedúnculos cerebelares superiores. Parte do fascículo termina no núcleo rubro contralateral; a maioria das fibras continua rostralmente até partes do núcleo intermédio ventral do tálamo, núcleo póstero-lateral ventral do tálamo e núcleo lateral central do tálamo. SIN pedunculus cerebellaris superior [TA], brachium conjunctivum cerebelli.
  ventral thalamic p., radiação posterior do tálamo; o grande sistema de feixes de fibras que emergem através das bordas ventral, lateral e anterior do tálamo para se unirem à cápsula interna e a partes da coroa radiada; contém as fibras que unem reciprocamente os núcleos talâmicos ventrais aos giros pré-central e pós-central do córtex cerebral. SIN pedunculus thalami ventralis.

pe·dun·cu·lar (pē-dŭng′kū-lăr). Peduncular; relativo a um pedículo ou pedúnculo.

pe·dun·cu·late (pē-dŭng′kū-lăt). Pediculado. SIN pediculate.

pe·dun·cu·lot·o·my (pe-dŭng′kū-lot′ō-mē). Pedunculotomia. **1.** Secção total ou parcial de um pedúnculo cerebral. **2.** Tratotomia piramidal mesencefálica. [peduncle + G. *tomē*, incisão]

pe·dun·cu·lus, pl. **pe·dun·cu·li** (pe-dŭng′kū-lŭs, -kū-lī) [TA]. Pedúnculo; pedículo. SIN pedicle (2). [L. mod. dim. de *pes*, pé]
  p. cerebella′ris infe′rior [TA], p. cerebelar inferior. SIN inferior cerebellar *peduncle*.
  p. cerebella′ris me′dius [TA], p. cerebelar médio. SIN middle cerebellar *peduncle*.
  p. cerebella′ris supe′rior [TA], p. cerebelar superior. SIN superior cerebellar *peduncle*.
  p. cer′ebri [TA], p. cerebral. SIN cerebral *peduncle*.
  p. cor′poris callo′si, área subcalosa. SIN subcallosal *gyrus*.
  p. cor′poris mammilla′ris, fascículo pedunculomamilar. SIN *peduncle* of mammillary body.
  p. floc′culi [TA], p. do flóculo. SIN *peduncle* of flocculus.
  p. of pineal body, p. do corpo pineal. VER habenula (2).
  p. thal′ami infe′rior, radiação inferior do tálamo. SIN inferior thalamic *peduncle*.
  p. thal′ami latera′lis, radiação lateral do tálamo. SIN lateral thalamic *peduncle*.
  p. thal′ami ventra′lis, radiação posterior do tálamo. SIN ventral thalamic *peduncle*.
  p. vitelli′nus, p. vitelino; termo obsoleto para yolk *stalk*.

peel. Descascar; descorticar; remover a camada externa.
  face p., retirada de marcas da pele como rugas, efélides ou cicatrizes de acne por agentes químicos que produzem lesão (ácido tricloroacético, fenol ou outros ácidos orgânicos) ou dióxido de carbono sólido.

peel·ing (pēl'ing). *Peeling*; descamação; retirada ou perda da epiderme, como na queimadura solar. [I.m. *pelen*]
  chemical p., *peeling* químico. SIN chemexfoliation.
pee·nash (pē'nash). Rinite causada por larvas de insetos nas vias nasais. [leste da Índia]
PEEP Abreviatura de positive end-expiratory *pressure* (pressão expiratória final positiva).
peer re·view. Revisão por pares; processo de revisão por colegas de propostas de pesquisa, manuscritos apresentados para publicação e sumários apresentados para publicação em um encontro científico, no qual são avaliados os méritos técnicos e científicos por outros cientistas do mesmo campo.
peg. Uma projeção cilíndrica.
  rete p.'s, cristas interpapilares. SIN rete *ridge*.
PEGs Abreviatura de polyethylene glycols (polietileno glicóis).
Peiffer, J., médico alemão, *1922. VER Hirsch-P. *stain*.
pe·jor·ism (pē'jōr-izm). Uma atitude pessimista. [L. *pejor*, pior]
PEL. Abreviatura de permissible exposure *limit* (limite de exposição permissível).
Pel, Pieter K., médico holandês, 1852–1919. VER P.-Ebstein *disease, fever*.
pe·lade (pē-lad', -lahd'). Pelada. SIN alopecia. [Fr. *peler*, remover o cabelo de um couro].
pel·ar·gon·ic ac·id (pel-ar-gon'ik). Ácido pelargônico; usado na fabricação de vernizes e plásticos; produzido na clivagem oxidativa do ácido oléico. SIN *n-nonanoic acid*.
Pelger, Karel, médico holandês, 1885–1931. VER P.-Huët nuclear *anomaly*.
pe·li·o·sis (pē-lē-ō'sis, pel-). Peliose. SIN purpura. [G. *peliōsis*, uma mancha lívida, lividez]
  bacterial p., p. bacteriana; infecção bacteriana de cistos hemorrágicos do fígado, baço ou linfonodos, observada em pessoas imunodeprimidas, causada por *Rochalimaea henselae*.
  p. hep'atis, p. hepática; a presença, em todo o fígado, de cavidades cheias de sangue que podem ser revestidas por endotélio ou tornar-se organizadas.
Pelizaeus, Friedrich, neurologista alemão, 1850–1917. VER Merzbacher-P. *disease*; P.-Merzbacher *disease*.
pel·lag·ra (pē-lag'ră, pē-lā'gră). Pelagra; afecção caracterizada por distúrbios gastrointestinais, eritema (sobretudo em áreas expostas) seguido por descamação e transtornos nervosos e mentais; pode dever-se a dieta insatisfatória, alcoolismo ou a alguma outra doença que cause comprometimento nutricional; comumente observada quando o milho é o principal nutriente na dieta, resultando em deficiência de niacina. SIN Alpine scurvy, maidism, mal de la rosa, mal rosso, mayidism, psychoneurosis maidica, Saint Ignatius itch. [It. *pelle*, pele, + *agra*, áspero]
  infantile p., p. do lactente. SIN kwashiorkor.
  secondary p., p. secundária; pelagra resultante de qualquer condição mórbida que comprometa a nutrição por aumento da necessidade ou redução do suprimento de vitaminas disponível.
  p. si'ne p., p. sem pelagra; pelagra sem as lesões cutâneas características.
pel·lag·roid (pē-lag'royd). Pelagróide; semelhante à pelagra.
pel·lag·rous (pē-lag'rŭs). Pelagroso; relativo à pelagra ou que sofre dessa afecção.
Pellegrini, Augusto, cirurgião italiano, *1877. VER P. *disease*; P.-Stieda *disease*.
pel·let (pel'et). *Pellet*. 1. Uma pílula muito pequena. 2. Uma formulação farmacêutica cilíndrica ou ovóide, pequena, estéril e composta essencialmente de hormônios esteróides puros na forma comprimida, para implantação subcutânea nos tecidos do corpo; serve como depósito, com liberação lenta do hormônio durante um longo período. [Fr. *pelote*; L. *pila*, uma bola]
pel·li·cle (pel'i-kl). Película. 1. Literal e inespecificamente, uma pele fina. 2. Uma película ou espuma sobre a superfície de um líquido. 3. Limite celular de esporozoítas e merozoítas entre membros do subfilo protozoário Apicomplexa (Sporozoa), que consiste em uma unidade de membrana externa e uma camada interna com duas unidades de membrana. [L. *pellicula*, dim. de *pellis*, pele]
  acquired p., p. adquirida; uma película fina (cerca de 1 μ), derivada principalmente das glicoproteínas salivares, que se forma sobre a superfície de uma coroa dentária limpa quando é exposta à saliva. SIN acquired cuticle, acquired enamel cuticle, brown p., posteruption cuticle.
  brown p., p. castanha. SIN acquired p.
pel·lic·u·lar, pel·lic·u·lous (pe-lik'ū-lăr, -lŭs). Pelicular; relativo a uma película.
Pellizzari, Pietro, dermatologista italiano, 1823–1892. VER Jadassohn-P. *anetoderma*.
Pellizzi, G.B., médico italiano dos séculos XIX–XX. VER P. *syndrome*.
pe·llo·te (pā-yō'tā). Peiote. SIN peyote. [Asteca, *peyotl*]
pel·lu·cid (pe-loo'sid). Pelúcido; translúcido; que permite a passagem de luz. [L. *pellucidus*]
pel·ma (pel'mă). Planta, sola. SIN sole. [G.]
pel·mat·ic (pel-mat'ik). Pelma; relativo à planta do pé. [G. *pelma*, planta do pé]

pel·mat·o·gram (pel-mat'ō-gram). Pelmatograma; impressão da planta do pé, que pode ser feita pelo repouso do pé pintado sobre uma folha de papel ou pela compressão do pé engordurado sobre gesso em pasta. [G. *pelma* (*pelmat-*), planta do pé, + *gramma*, figura]
pe·lop·a·thy (pē-lop'ă-thē). Peloterapia. SIN pelotherapy. [G. *pēlos*, barro, + *pathos*, sofrimento]
pel·o·ther·a·py (pē'lō-thār-ă-pē). Peloterapia; aplicação de pelóides, como lama, turfa ou argila, a uma parte do corpo ou a todo ele. SIN pelopathy. [G. *pēlos*, lama, barro, + *therapeia*, tratamento]
pel·ta (pel'tă). Pelta; pequeno escudo; uma organela membranácea, em forma de crescente, que se cora com a prata, localizada anteriormente, próximo à base dos flagelos em determinados protozoários flagelados, como no *Trichomonas*. [L. um escudo]
pel·ta·tion (pel-tā'shŭn). Peltação; proteção produzida pela inoculação de um anti-soro ou de uma vacina. [L. *pelta*, um pequeno escudo, do G. *peltē*]
♻ **pelvi-, pelvio-, pelvo-.** A pelve. Cf. pyelo-, pelyco-. [L. *pelvis*, bacia (pelve)]
pel·vic (pel'vik). Pélvico; relativo à pelve.
pel·vic di·rec·tion (pel'vik dī-rek'shŭn). Direção pélvica; a direção do eixo da pelve.
pel·vi·ceph·a·log·ra·phy (pel'vi-sef-ă-log'ră-fē). Pelvicefalografia. SIN cephalopelvimetry. [pelvi- + G. *kephalē*, cabeça, + *graphō*, escrever]
pel·vi·ceph·a·lom·e·try (pel'vi-sef-ă-lom'ĕ-trē). Pelvicefalometria; medida dos diâmetros pélvicos femininos em relação aos diâmetros da cabeça fetal. [pelvi- + G. *kephalē*, cabeça, + *metron*, medida]
pel·vi·fix·a·tion (pel-vi-fik-sā'shŭn). Pelvifixação; fixação cirúrgica de um órgão pélvico flutuante à parede da cavidade pélvica.
pel·vi·li·thot·o·my (pel'vi-li-thot'ō-mē). Pelvilitotomia. SIN pyelolithotomy. [pelvi- + G. *lithos*, pedra, + *tomē*, incisão]
pel·vim·e·try (pel-vim'ĕ-trē). Pelvimetria; medida dos diâmetros da pelve. SIN radiocephalpelvimetry. [pelvi- + G. *metron*, medida]
  CT p., p. por TC; procedimento para medida da pelve óssea e da cabeça fetal por meio de imagens de TC; atualmente é a técnica mais acurada de diagnóstico por imagens.
  manual p., p. manual; medida dos diâmetros essenciais da pelve óssea utilizando as mãos.
  radiographic p., p. radiográfica; procedimento para medida da pelve óssea e da cabeça fetal utilizando incidências ântero-posteriores e laterais, com um dispositivo para correção da ampliação.
♻ **pelvio-.** VER pelvi-.
pel·vi·o·li·thot·o·my (pel-vē-ō-li-thot'ō-mē). Pielolitotomia. SIN pyelolithotomy.
pel·vi·o·per·i·to·ni·tis (pel'vē-ō-per-i-tō-nī'tis). Pelviperitonite. SIN pelvic *peritonitis*.
pel·vi·o·plas·ty (pel'vē-ō-plas-tē). Pelviplastia; pieloplastia. SIN pyeloplasty. [pelvio- + G. *plastos*, formado]
pel·vi·os·co·py (pel-vē-os'kŏ-pē). Pelvioscopia; pelviscopia; exame da pelve para qualquer fim, geralmente por endoscopia. SIN pelvoscopy. [pelvio- + G. *skopeō*, ver]
pel·vi·per·i·to·ni·tis (pel-vē-per-i-tō-nī'tis). Pelviperitonite. SIN pelvic *peritonitis*.

PELVIS

pel·vis, pl. **pel·ves** (pel'vis, pel'vēz) [TA]. Pelve. 1. [NA]. O grande anel ósseo caliciforme, com seus ligamentos, na extremidade inferior do tronco, formado pelo osso do quadril (púbis, ílio e ísquio), de cada lado e na frente, e pelo sacro e cóccix, posteriormente. 2. Qualquer cavidade semelhante a uma bacia ou caliciforme, como a pelve renal. [L. bacia]
  android p., p. andróide; uma p. masculina ou afunilada.
  anthropoid p., p. antropóide; p. com um grande diâmetro ântero-posterior e um pequeno diâmetro transverso.
  assimilation p., p. de assimilação; deformidade em que os processos transversos da última vértebra lombar estão fundidos ao sacro, ou os da última vértebra sacral com o primeiro corpo coccígeo.
  beaked p., p. em bico; p. rostriforme. SIN osteomalacic p.
  brachypellic p., p. braquipélica; p. na qual o diâmetro transverso é mais de 1 cm e menos de 3 cm maior que o diâmetro ântero-posterior. SIN transverse oval p.
  caoutchouc p., p. de borracha; na osteomalacia, uma p. na qual os ossos ainda são moles. SIN rubber p.
  contracted p., p. contraída; p. com medidas menores que o normal em qualquer diâmetro.
  cordate p., cordiform p., p. em forma de coração; p. com o sacro projetado para a frente entre os ílios, dando à borda o formato de coração. SIN heart-shaped p.

Deventer p., p. de Deventer; p. com diâmetro ântero-posterior reduzido.
dolichopellic p., p. dolicopélica; p. na qual o diâmetro ântero-posterior é maior que o transverso. SIN longitudinal oval p.
dwarf p., p. anã; p. muito pequena, na qual os vários ossos estão unidos por cartilagem, como no lactente. SIN nana.
false p., p. falsa; p. maior. SIN greater p.
flat p., p. plana; p. em que o diâmetro ântero-posterior está uniformemente contraído e o sacro é deslocado para a frente, entre os ossos ilíacos. SIN p. plana.
frozen p., p. congelada; condição na qual a p. verdadeira está completamente endurecida, principalmente por carcinoma. SIN hardened p.
funnel-shaped p., f. afunilada; p. na qual as dimensões da entrada da p. são normais, mas a saída está contraída no diâmetro transverso ou em ambos os diâmetros, transverso e ântero-posterior.
p. of gallbladder, bolsa da vesícula biliar. SIN Hartmann *pouch.*
greater p. [TA], p. maior; a porção expandida da p. acima da borda. SIN p. major [TA], false p., large p., p. spuria.
gynecoid p., p. ginecóide; a p. feminina normal.
hardened p., p. congelada. SIN frozen p.
heart-shaped p., p. em forma de coração. SIN cordate p.
inverted p., p. invertida; p. dividida com separação no púbis.
p. jus'to ma'jor, p. simétrica com medidas maiores que o normal em todos os diâmetros.
p. jus'to mi'nor, p. do tipo feminino, mas que possui todos os seus diâmetros menores que o normal.
juvenile p., p. juvenil; p. *justo minor* na qual os ossos são finos.
kyphoscoliotic p., p. cifoescoliótica; p. com acentuada curvatura ântero-posterior da coluna, associada à curvatura lateral da coluna, geralmente causada por raquitismo grave.
kyphotic p., p. cifótica; p. deformada associada a uma deformidade cifótica da coluna vertebral.
large p., p. maior. SIN greater p.
lesser p. [TA], p. menor; a cavidade da p. abaixo da borda ou da abertura superior. SIN p. minor [TA], p. vera, small p., true p.
longitudinal oval p., p. dolicopélica. SIN dolichopellic p.
lordotic p., p. lordótica; p. deformada associada a curvatura lordótica da coluna vertebral.
p. ma'jor [TA], p. maior. SIN greater p.
masculine p., p. masculina; **(1)** uma p. *justo minor* na qual os ossos são grandes e pesados; **(2)** um pequeno grau de afunilamento da p. na mulher, no qual o formato aproxima-se do formato da pelve masculina.
mesatipellic p., p. mesatipélica; termo obsoleto para a p. na qual os diâmetros ântero-posterior e transverso são iguais ou o diâmetro transverso não é mais que 1 cm maior que o diâmetro ântero-posterior. SIN round p.
p. mi'nor [TA], p. menor. SIN lesser p.
Nägele p., p. de Nägele; p. sinostótica contraída unilateral ou p. caracterizada por interrupção do desenvolvimento da metade lateral do sacro, geralmente anquilose da articulação sacroilíaca daquele lado, rotação do sacro para o mesmo lado e desvio da sínfise púbica para o lado oposto.
p. na'na, p. anã. SIN dwarf p.
p. obtec'ta, p. obtecta; forma de p. cifótica na qual a curvatura angular da coluna vertebral é baixa e extrema, de forma que a coluna vertebral projeta-se horizontalmente através da entrada da pelve.
osteomalacic p., p. osteomalácica; deformidade pélvica na osteomalacia; a pressão do tronco sobre o sacro e a pressão lateral das cabeças dos fêmures produzem uma abertura pélvica com três ângulos ou em forma de coração ou trevo, enquanto o osso púbis adquire um formato de bico. SIN beaked p., rostrate p.
Otto p., p. de Otto. SIN Otto *disease.*
p. pla'na, p. plana. SIN flat p.
platypellic p., p. platipélica; p. oval plana na qual o diâmetro transverso é mais de 3 cm maior que o diâmetro ântero-posterior.
platypelloid p., p. platipelóide; p. plana simples.
Prague p., p. de Prague. SIN spondylolisthetic p.
pseudoosteomalacic p., p. pseudo-osteomalácica; grau extremo de pelve raquítica, semelhante à pelve osteomalácica puerperal, na qual o canal pélvico é obstruído pela projeção para a frente do sacro e por uma aproximação dos acetábulos.
rachitic p., p. raquítica; p. contraída e deformada; mais comumente, uma p. plana que decorre do amolecimento raquítico dos ossos no início da vida.
renal p. [TA], p. renal; uma expansão afunilada achatada da extremidade superior do ureter que recebe os cálices, sendo o ápice contínuo com o ureter. SIN p. renalis [TA], ureteric p.
p. rena'lis [TA], p. renal. SIN renal p.
reniform p., p. reniforme; pelve em forma de coração modificado, com um longo diâmetro transverso, conferindo à borda um formato de rim.
Robert p., p. de Robert; termo obsoleto para designar uma p. estreitada transversalmente, em consequência da ausência quase completa das asas do sacro.

Rokitansky p., p. de Rokitansky. SIN spondylolisthetic p.
rostrate p., p. rostriforme. SIN osteomalacic p.
round p., p. redonda. SIN mesatipellic p.
rubber p., p. de borracha. SIN caoutchouc p.
scoliotic p., p. escoliótica; p. deformada associada a curvatura lateral da coluna vertebral.
small p., p. menor. SIN lesser p.
spider p., p. aracneiforme; cálices estreitos da pelve renal.
split p., p. fendida; p. na qual não há sínfise púbica, estando os ossos pélvicos bem separados; geralmente associada à extrofia da bexiga.
spondylolisthetic p., p. espondilolistética; p. cuja borda está mais ou menos ocluída pelo deslocamento para a frente do corpo da vértebra lombar inferior. SIN Prague p., Rokitansky p.
p. spu'ria, p. falsa. SIN greater p.
transverse oval p., p. braquipélica. SIN brachypellic p.
true p., p. verdadeira. SIN lesser p.
ureteric p., p. renal. SIN renal p.
p. ve'ra, p. verdadeira. SIN lesser p.

---

pel·vi·sa·cral (pel - vi - sā′kral). Pelvissacra; relativo à pelve, ou ossos do quadril, e ao sacro.
pel·vi·scope (pel′vi - skōp). Pelviscópio; instrumento endoscópico para examinar o interior da pelve. [pelvi- + G. *skopeō*, ver]
pel·vi·therm (pel′vi - therm). Pelvitermo; instrumento para aplicar calor aos órgãos pélvicos. [pelvi- + G. *thermē*, calor]
pel·vi·u·re·ter·og·ra·phy (pel - vi - ū - rē - ter - og′rā - fē). Pelviureterografia; pielografia. SIN pyelography.
△ **pelvo-.** VER pelvi-.
pel·vo·ca·li·ec·ta·sis (pel′vō - kal - ē - ek - tā′sis). Hidronefrose. SIN hydronephrosis.
pel·vo·ceph·a·log·ra·phy (pel′vō - sef - ă - log′rā - fē). Pelvicefalografia. SIN cephalopelvimetry.
pel·vos·co·py (pel - vos′cō - pē). Pelviscopia. SIN pelvioscopy.
pel·vo·spon·dy·li·tis os·sif·i·cans (pel′vō - spon - di - lī′tis os - if′i - kanz). Pelviespondilite ossificante; depósitos de substância óssea entre as vértebras do sacro. [L. *pelvis*, bacia, + G. *spondylos*, vértebra, + *-itis*; L. *os*, osso, + *facio*, fazer]
△ **pelyco-.** A pelve. VER pelvi-. [G. *pelyx*, concavidade (pelve)]
pem·o·line (pem′ō - lēn). Pemolina; psicoestimulante usado no tratamento do distúrbio de déficit de atenção (hiperatividade) em crianças.
pem·phi·goid (pem′fi - goyd). Penfigóide. **1.** Semelhante ao pênfigo. **2.** Doença semelhante ao pênfigo, mas bastante diferente histológica (não-acantolítica) e clinicamente (a evolução geralmente é benigna). [G. *pemphix*, bolha, + *eidos*, semelhança]
benign mucosal p., p. benigno da mucosa. SIN ocular cicatricial p.
bullous p., p. bolhoso; doença crônica, geralmente benigna, mais comum em idosos, caracterizada por bolhas tensas e não-acantolíticas nas quais os anticorpos séricos estão localizados em componentes hemidesmossômicos da membrana basal epidérmica, causando separação da epiderme em toda a sua espessura.
localized p. of Brunsting-Perry, p. localizado de Brunsting-Perry; variante do p., basicamente no couro cabeludo e na face, com alguma formação de cicatriz (fibrose).
ocular p., p. cicatricial ocular. SIN ocular cicatricial p.
ocular cicatricial p., p. cicatricial ocular; doença crônica que produz aderências com fibrose e retração progressivas das mucosas conjuntival, oral e vaginal. SIN benign mucosal p., ocular p.
pem·phi·gus (pem′fi - gŭs). Pênfigo. **1.** Doenças bolhosas auto-imunes com acantólise: p. vulgar, p. foliáceo, p. eritematoso ou p. vegetante. **2.** Termo inespecífico para designar doenças cutâneas bolhosas. [G. *pemphix*, bolha]
benign familial chronic p. [MIM*169600], p. crônico familiar benigno; erupção recorrente de vesículas e bolhas que se tornam lesões descamativas e crostosas com bordas vesiculares, predominantemente no pescoço, na região inguinal e nas regiões axilares; herança autossômica dominante, apresentando-se no final da adolescência ou no início da vida adulta. SIN Hailey-Hailey disease.
Brazilian p., p. brasileiro. SIN fogo selvagem.
p. erythemato'sus, p. eritematoso; erupção que envolve a pele exposta ao sol, principalmente a face; as lesões são máculas eritematosas descamativas e bolhas, combinando as manifestações clínicas do lúpus eritematoso e do pênfigo vulgar; as bolhas são subcórneas; provavelmente é uma variante do p. foliáceo, algumas vezes induzido por penicilamina. SIN Senear-Usher disease, Senear-Usher syndrome
p. folia'ceus, p. foliáceo; forma geralmente crônica de p., que raramente afeta as mucosas, na qual pode haver dermatite esfoliativa extensa, sem formação perceptível de bolhas, associada às bolhas; os auto-anticorpos séricos induzem bolhas e lesões epidérmicas superficiais acantolíticas crostosas.

p. gangreno'sus, p. gangrenoso; **(1)** SIN *dermatitis* gangrenosa infantum; **(2)** SIN bullous *impetigo* of newborn.
paraneoplastic p., p. paraneoplásico; erosões dolorosas da mucosa e erupções cutâneas polimórficas com achados à biopsia semelhantes aos do p. vulgar, associadas a neoplasia e a anticorpos séricos que reagem com a substância intercelular de todos os epitélios; em geral é rapidamente fatal.
p. veg'etans, p. vegetante; **(1)** forma rara, verrucosa, do p. vulgar na qual surgem vegetações nas superfícies erodidas deixadas pela ruptura das bolhas; novas bolhas continuam a se formar. SIN Neumann disease. **(2)** Forma vegetante benigna crônica de p., com lesões comumente nas axilas e no períneo; ocorrem remissões espontâneas e, ocasionalmente, cura permanente. SIN Hallopeau disease.
p. vulga'ris, p. vulgar; forma grave de p., que ocorre na meia-idade, na qual bolhas cutâneas suprabasais acantolíticas flácidas e erosões da mucosa oral podem permanecer localizadas alguns meses antes de se tornarem generalizadas; as bolhas rompem-se facilmente e cicatrizam lentamente; resulta da ação de anticorpos auto-imunes localizados no espaço intercelular do epitélio escamoso estratificado.

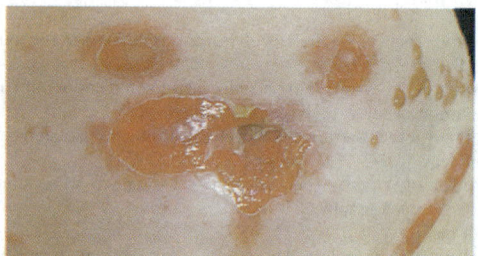

pênfigo vulgar

pem·pi·dine (pem'pi-dēn). Pempidina; amina secundária do grupo mecamilamina, efetiva como agente bloqueador ganglionar; também disponível na forma de tartarato de pempidina, com os mesmos empregos.
pen·del·luft (pen-del-lŭft'). Movimento transitório de saída de gás de alguns alvéolos e entrada em outros quando o fluxo acabou de cessar no fim da inspiração, ou esse movimento na direção oposta logo no fim da expiração; ocorre quando regiões do pulmão diferem em complacência, resistência das vias aéreas ou inércia de tal forma que as constantes de tempo de seu enchimento (ou esvaziamento) em resposta a uma alteração da pressão transpulmonar não são iguais. [Al. *Pendel*, pêndulo, + *Luft*, ar]
Pendred, Vaughan, cirurgião inglês, 1869–1946. VER P. *syndrome*.
pe·nec·to·my (pē-nek'tō-mē). Penectomia. SIN phallectomy. [L. *penis* + G. *ektomē*, excisão]
pe·nes. Plural de penis, como no dífalo (*diphallus*).
pen·e·trance (pen'ĕ-trans). Penetrância; a freqüência, expressa como fração ou percentagem, de indivíduos fenotipicamente afetados, entre pessoas de um genótipo apropriado (isto é, homozigotos ou hemizigotos para recessivos, heterozigotos ou hemizigotos para dominantes); para um distúrbio autossômico dominante, se apenas uma parte dos indivíduos que possuem o alelo mutante exibe o fenótipo anormal, diz-se que o traço possui penetrância incompleta. Se todos que possuem o alelo mutante exibem o fenótipo anormal, diz-se que o traço tem penetrância completa. VER penetration.
genetic p. (pen'ĕ-trans), p. genética; o quanto uma condição geneticamente determinada é expressa em um indivíduo.
pen·e·trate (pen'ĕ-trāt). Penetrar; perfurar; entrar nos tecidos mais profundos ou em uma cavidade.
pen·e·tra·tion (pen-ĕ-trā'shŭn). Penetração. **1.** Uma perfuração ou entrada. **2.** Acuidade mental. **3.** SIN focal *depth*. [L. *penetratio*, de *penetro*, pp. *-atus*, entrar]
pen·e·trom·e·ter (pen-ĕ-trom'ĕ-ter). Penetrômetro; instrumento obsoleto usado para medir a capacidade de penetração de raios X de qualquer fonte. [penetration + G. *metron*, medida]
-penia. -penia; deficiência. [G. *penia*, escassez]
pe·ni·al (pē'nē-ăl). Peniano. SIN penile.
pe·ni·a·pho·bia (pē'nē-ă-fō'bē-ă). Peniafobia; medo mórbido da pobreza. [G. *penia*, pobreza, + *phobos*, medo]
pen·i·cil·la·mine (pen-i-sil'ă-mēn). Penicilamina; produto da degradação da penicilina; agente quelante usado no tratamento da intoxicação por chumbo, degeneração hepatolenticular e cistinúria, e na remoção do excesso de cobre na doença de Wilson; também disponível como cloridrato de penicilamina. SIN β,β-dimethylcysteine.
pen·i·cil·la·nate (pen-i-sil'ă-nāt). Penicilanato; um sal do ácido penicilânico.
pen·i·cil·lan·ic ac·id (pen-i-si-lan'ik). Ácido penicilânico; uma penicilina sem o grupamento R característico (com H– substituindo ROONH–) da penicilina.

pen·i·cil·lar·y (pen-i-sil'ă-rē). Penicilar; designa um penicílio (1).
pen·i·cil·late (pen-i-sil'āt). Penicilato. **1.** Relativo a um penicílio. **2.** Que possui estrutura semelhante a um tufo.
pen·i·cil·lic ac·id (pen-i-sil'ik). Ácido penicílico; antibiótico produzido por *Penicillium puberulum*, fungo encontrado no milho, e do *P. cyclopium*; ativo contra bactérias Gram-positivas e Gram-negativas, mas tóxico para tecidos animais.
pen·i·cil·in (pen-i-sil'in). Penicilina. **1.** Originalmente, um antibiótico obtido de culturas dos fungos *Penicillium notatum* ou *P. chrysogenum;* interfere com a síntese da parede celular em bactérias. **2.** Pertencente a uma família de variantes naturais ou sintéticas do ácido penicílico. As penicilinas possuem ação principalmente bactericida, são particularmente ativas contra microrganismos Gram-positivos e, com exceção das reações de hipersensibilidade, exibem uma ação tóxica particularmente baixa sobre o tecido animal. [ver penicillus]
aluminum p., p. alumínio; o sal de alumínio trivalente de um ou mais antibióticos produzidos pelo crescimento dos fungos *Penicillium notatum* ou *P. chrysogenum;* uso oral ou sublingual.
p. amidase, p. amidase; enzima que catalisa a hidrólise da ligação amida nas penicilinas, produzindo um ânion do ácido carboxílico e penicina; a penicina é o precursor de muitas penicilinas sintéticas.
p. B, p. B. SIN phenethicillin potassium.
benzyl p., benzilpenicilina, p. G. SIN p. G.
buffered crystalline p. G, p. G cristalina tamponada; p. G potássica cristalina ou p. G sódica cristalina com não menos de 4% e não mais de 5% de citrato de sódio.
chloroprocaine p. O, p. O cloroprocaína; sal cristalino de 2-cloroprocaína e p. O, insolúvel em água; o nível do antibiótico no sangue persiste por 24 horas; sua atividade antibacteriana é semelhante à das penicilinas O e G.
p. G, p. G; p. comumente usada; constitui 85% dos sais de p.: sódio, potássio, alumínio e procaína, com este último exercendo ação prolongada quando da injeção intramuscular, devido à limitada solubilidade. Um antibiótico obtido do fungo *Penicillium chrysogenum* usado por via oral e parenteral; ativo basicamente contra estreptococos e estafilococos Gram-positivos; destruído por β-lactamase bacteriana. SIN benzyl p., benzylpenicillin.
p. G benzathine, p. G benzatina; preparado relativamente insolúvel que pode permanecer no corpo por 1–2 semanas.
p. G. hydrabamine, p. G hidrabamina; uma dipenicilina, mistura de sais de p. G que consiste principalmente no sal da base diacídica *N,N'*-bis-(desidroabietil)etilenodiamina.
p. G potassium, p. G potássica; o sal potássico da p. G, que contém 85–90% de p. G.
p. G procaine, p. G procaína; o sal procaína da p. G; tem ação mais prolongada que a p. G.
p. G sodium, p. G sódica; o sal sódico de p. G, que contém não menos que 85% de p. G.
p. N, p. N. SIN cephalosporin N.
p. O, p. O; produzida pelo crescimento do fungo em um meio contendo ácido alilmercaptometilacético; também disponível como sais potássico e sódico. SIN allylmercaptomethylpenicillin.
p. phenoxymethyl, p. fenoximetílica. SIN p. V.
p. V, p. V; derivado da p. contendo um grupamento fenoxiacetil; obtida do *Penicillium chrysogenum* Q 176; ácido não-hidroscópico cristalino, muito estável mesmo em condições de alta umidade; resiste à destruição pelo suco gástrico; o sal potássico é usado por via oral; precursor para a síntese de análogos da cefalosporina C. SIN p. phenoxymethyl, phenoxymethylpenicillin.
p. V benzathine, p. V benzatina; p. para uso oral.
p. V hydrabamine, p. V hidrabamina; composto com preparo e usos análogos aos da p. G hidrabamina.
pen·i·cil·li·nase (pen-i-sil'i-nās). Penicilinase. **1.** SIN β-lactamase. **2.** Preparado de enzima purificado obtido de culturas de uma cepa de *Bacillus cereus*; antigamente usado no tratamento de reações à penicilina tardias ou que se desenvolvem lentamente. Usada por bactérias para desenvolver resistência à penicilina.
pen·i·cil·li·nate (pen-i-sil'i-nāt). Penicilinato; um sal de um ácido penicílico (isto é, de uma penicilina).
penicilliosis. Peniciliose; infecção invasiva por uma espécie de *Penicillium*.
Pen·i·cil·li·um (pen-i-sil'ē-ŭm). Gênero de fungos (classe Ascomycetes, ordem Aspergillales), cujas espécies fornecem várias substâncias antibióticas e biológicas; p. ex., *P. citrinum* produz citrinina; *P. claviforme*, *P. expansum* e *P. patulum* produzem patulina; *P. chrysogenum* produz penicilina; *P. griseofulvum* produz griseofulvina; *P. notatum* produz penicilina e notatina; *P. cyclopium* e *P. puberulum* produzem ácido penicílico; *P. purpurogenum* e *P. rubrum* produzem rubratoxina. *P. marneffei* é um patógeno verdadeiro no Sudeste Asiático e em ratos do bambu. [ver penicillus]
P. lilacinum. SIN *Paecilomyces lilacinus*.
pen·i·cil·lo·ic ac·id (pen'i-si-lō'ik). Ácido peniciloico; produto alcalino e da degradação bacteriana de uma penicilina, resultante da hidrólise da ligação 1,7.
pen·i·cil·loyl pol·y·ly·sine (pen-i-sil'ō-il). Peniciloil polilisina; preparado de polilisina e um ácido penicílico, usado por via intradérmica no diagnóstico da sensibilidade à penicilina; pessoas sensíveis podem apresentar reações sistêmicas, incluindo erupções cutâneas generalizadas.

pen·i·cil·lus, pl. **pe·ni·cil·li** (pen-i-sil′ŭs, -sil′ī) [TA]. Penicilo. **1** [NA]. Um dos tufos formados pela subdivisão repetida das pequenas ramificações arteriais no baço. **2.** Em fungos, um dos conidióforos ramificados que possuem cadeias de conídios em espécies de *Penicillium*. [L. pincel]

pen·i·cin (pen′i-sin). Penicina. SIN 6-aminopenicillanic acid.

pe·nile (pē′nīl). Peniano; relativo ao pênis. SIN penial.

pe·nil·lic ac·ids (pe-nil′ik). Ácidos penílicos; produtos da degradação ácida das penicilinas, produzidos pela clivagem da ligação 1,7, formando ácido penicilóico, e a formação de uma ligação entre o carbono carbonila exocíclico e N-1, com eliminação de H_2O desses dois e do NH exocíclico.

pen·in (pen′in). Penina; ácido 6-aminopenicilânico; um intermediário na síntese de penicilinas.

pe·nis, pl. **pe·nes** (pē′nis) [TA]. Pênis; o órgão de cópula e micção no homem; é formado por três colunas de tecido erétil, duas dispostas lateralmente, no dorso (corpos cavernosos do pênis), e uma mediana, abaixo (corpo esponjoso); a uretra atravessa esta última; a extremidade (glande do pênis) é formada por uma expansão do corpo esponjoso, sendo mais ou menos completamente coberta por uma prega livre de pele (prepúcio). SIN intromittent organ, membrum virile, phallus, priapus, virga. [L. cauda]

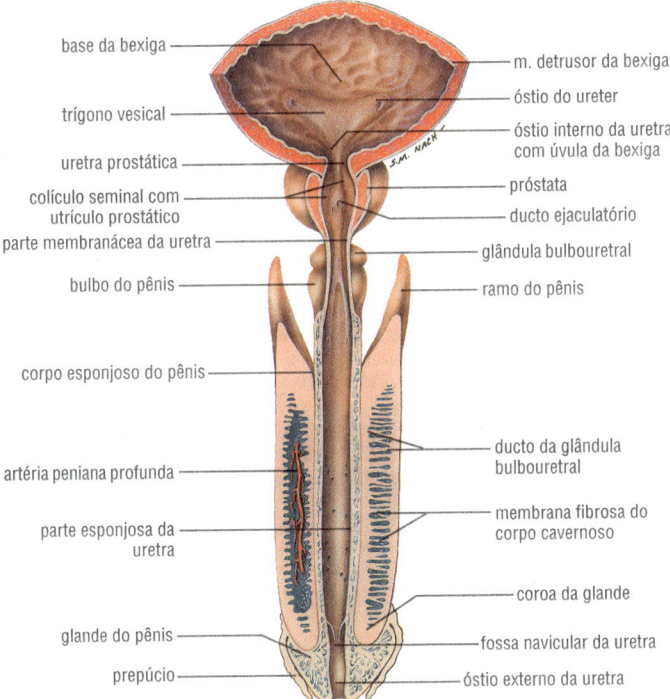

pênis, base da bexiga e uretra: corte longitudinal (a pele do pênis foi removida até o prepúcio)

bifid p., p. bífido. SIN diphallus.
buried p., p. encoberto; p. normal encoberto por gordura suprapúbica.
clubbed p., p. em clava; deformidade do p. ereto, caracterizada por uma curva para um lado ou em direção ao escroto.
concealed p., p. oculto; geralmente uma complicação da circuncisão na qual a linha anastomótica entre a pele do corpo e o colar do prepúcio fecha-se como uma íris ou cicatriz sobre a glande (alguns consideram este igual ao pênis encoberto).
p. femin'eus, termo obsoleto para clítoris.
gryposis p., corda venérea. SIN chordee (1).
p. mulie'bris, termo obsoleto para clítoris.
webbed p., p. membranoso; deficiência da pele do corpo ventral do p. que fica encoberto no escroto ou preso à linha média deste último por uma prega ou membrana de pele. A uretra e os corpos eréteis geralmente são normais.

pe·nis·chi·sis (pē-nis′ki-sis). Penisquise; uma fissura do pênis que resulta em abertura anormal para a uretra, seja em cima (epispádia), embaixo (hipospádia) ou em um lado (paraspádia). [L. *penis* + G. *schisis*, fissura]

pen·nate (pen′āt). Peniforme; emplumado; semelhante a uma pena. SIN penniform. [L. *pennatus*, de *penna*, pena]

pen·ni·form (pen′i-fōrm). Peniforme. SIN pennate. [L. *penna*, pena, + *forma*, forma]

pen·ny·roy·al (pen′ē-roy-ăl). Nome popular dado à *Mentha pulegium* (poejo) (aromática), ou à *Hedeoma pulegeoides* (poejo americano) (família Labiatae); estimulante aromático usado antigamente como emenagogo.

pe·no·scro·tal (pē′nō-skrō′tăl). Penoescrotal; relativo ao pênis e ao escroto.

pe·not·o·my (pē-not′o-mē). Penotomia. SIN phallotomy. [L. *penis* + G. *tomē*, corte]

Penrose, Charles B., ginecologista norte-americano, 1862–1925. VER P. *drain*.

penta-. Penta-; forma combinante que significa cinco. [G. *pente*, cinco]

pen·ta·ba·sic (pen-tă-bā′sik). Pentabásico; indica um ácido que possui cinco átomos de hidrogênio substituíveis. [penta- + G. *basis*, base]

pen·ta·chlo·ro·phe·nol (pen-tă-klōr-ō-fēn′ol). Pentaclorofenol; inseticida para controle de cupins; desfolhante pré-colheita; herbicida geral. Tem sido muito usado na preservação de madeira, produtos de madeira, amidos, dextrinas, colas. Não está mais disponível para o consumidor; um potente irritante.

pen·tad. Grupo de cinco. **1.** Um conjunto de cinco coisas relacionadas de alguma forma. **2.** Em química, um elemento pentavalente. [G. *pentas*, o número cinco]
Reynolds p., dor abdominal, febre, icterícia, choque e depressão da função do sistema nervoso central; geralmente indica colangite supurativa aguda.

pen·ta·dac·tyl, pen·ta·dac·tyle (pen-tă-dak′til). Pentadáctilo; que tem cinco dedos em cada mão ou pé. SIN quinquedigitate. [penta- + G. *daktylos*, dedo]

pen·ta·e·ryth·ri·tol (pen-tă-ē-rith′ri-tol). Pentaeritritol; o tetranitrato é um vasodilatador coronariano com ação semelhante à dos outros nitratos orgânicos de ação lenta.

pen·ta·e·ryth·ri·tol tet·ra·ni·trate. Tetranitrato de pentaeritritol; nitrato orgânico usado como vasodilatador no tratamento da angina de peito; sua ação é mais prolongada que a da nitroglicerina; atua através da conversão em ácido nítrico.

pen·ta·gas·trin (pen-tă-gas′trin). Pentagastrina; o pentapeptídeo substituído, BOC-β-Ala-Trp-Met-Asp-Phe(NH_2); um estimulante do ácido gástrico.

pen·tal·o·gy (pen-tal′o-jē). Pentalogia; termo raramente usado para uma combinação de cinco elementos, como cinco sintomas concomitantes. [penta- + G. *logos*, tratado, palavra]
p. of Cantrell, p. de Cantrell; defeito congênito que envolve uma fenda na parte inferior do esterno, um defeito diafragmático anterior, ausência do pericárdio parietal, uma onfalocele associada ou distinta, e uma grande anomalia cardíaca, na maioria das vezes tetralogia de Fallot (*tetralogy* of Fallot) e divertículo ventricular esquerdo. SIN thoracoabdominal ectopia cordis.
p. of Fallot, p. de Fallot; tetralogia de Fallot associada à persistência do forame oval ou à comunicação interatrial.

pen·ta·mer (pen′tă-mer). Pentâmero. VER virion. [penta- + G. *meros*, parte]

pen·tam·i·dine is·e·thi·o·nate (pen-tam′i-dēn). Isetionato de pentamidina; fármaco tóxico, mas efetivo, na profilaxia e no tratamento dos estágios iniciais de ambos os tipos de doença do sono africana (tripanossomíase gambiense e rodesiana). Não atravessa a barreira hematoencefálica e não é efetivo no tratamento do estágio avançado (neurológico) da doença. Também é usado no tratamento da leishmaniose que não responde aos antimoniais pentavalentes e no tratamento da pneumonia causada por *Pneumocystis carinii*.

pen·ta·no·ic ac·id (pen-tă-nō′ik). Ácido pentanóico. SIN valeric acid.

pen·ta·pep·tide (pen′tă-pep′tid). Pentapeptídeo; composto que contém cinco resíduos aminoácidos unidos por ligações peptídicas.

pen·ta·pip·er·ide fu·ma·rate (pen-tă-pip′er-īd). Fumarato de pentapiperida; antiespasmódico intestinal.

pen·ta·pi·per·i·um meth·yl·sul·fate (pen′tă-pī-per′ē-ŭm). Metilsulfato de pentapipério; um agente anticolinérgico.

pen·ta·quine (pen′tă-kwīn). Pentaquina; agente antimalárico que possui íntima relação química com a pamaquina, porém é menos tóxico e mais efetivo; é administrado com a quinina, e os dois fármacos agem sinergicamente; é ativa contra infecções por *Plasmodium vivax*.

Pen·tas·to·ma (pen-tas′tō-mă). Nome antigo de um gênero de Pentastomida, agora denominado *Linguatula*. Foi comprovado que a espécie descrita como *P. denticulatum* era a larva da *Linguatula rhinaria*, que algumas vezes parasita o nariz do homem e de outros mamíferos; os adultos são encontrados nos pulmões de répteis. [penta- + G. *stoma*, boca]

pen·ta·sto·mi·a·sis (pen′tă-stō-mī′ă-sis). Pentastomíase; infecção de animais herbívoros, suínos e seres humanos por pentastomídeos; as lesões ocorrem principalmente nos linfonodos do trato digestivo, onde freqüentemente assemelham-se às lesões da tuberculose.

Pen·ta·stom·i·da (pen-tă-stom′i-dă). Vermes com corpo em forma de língua, um grupo de animais parasitas, vermiformes, considerados formadores de um filo separado, descendentes dos artrópodes primitivos, contudo modificados pelo parasitismo para formar organismos alongados, pseudo-segmentados, vermiformes, com dois a três pares de membros degenerados, germiformes na larva, e ganchos, semelhantes a presas, ocos, anteriores no adulto. Os adultos geralmente parasitam os pulmões ou as vias respiratórias de vertebrados, geralmente cobras e outros répteis, embora um grupo parasite os sacos aéreos de aves e uma família (Linguatulidae) tenha se adaptado aos pulmões de mamíferos carnívoros (famílias Felidae e Canidae). As larvas são encontradas nas vísceras de muitos hospedeiros que servem como presas dos hospedeiros definitivos (insetos, peixes, anfíbios, principalmente rãs, e mamíferos, principalmente roedores). Os cães podem desenvolver *Linguatula serrata* adulta nas vias nasais a partir das larvas infecciosas (ninfas) encontradas nas vísceras de carneiros, bois ou coelhos, que foram infestados pela água ou vegetação contaminada por ovos eliminados por cães infectados; o homem também pode desenvolver uma infecção larvar por essa fonte. Já foi descrita infecção humana do fígado, baço e pulmões, na África, pelo *Armillifer armillatus* e, na China, pelo *A. moniliformis* provenientes da água ou vegetação contaminada ou pelo manuseio de cobras infectadas. [ver *Pentastoma*]

pent·a·tom·ic (pent′a-tom-ik). Pentatômico; indica cinco átomos por molécula. [penta- + atomic]

Pen·ta·trich·o·mon·as (pen′ta-trik-o-mō′nas, pen′ta-tri-kom′o-nas). Gênero de flagelados protozoários parasitas, antigamente considerados parte do gênero *Trichomonas*, mas agora separados como um gênero distinto pela presença de cinco flagelos anteriores e um corpo parabasal granular. A espécie *Pentatrichomonas hominis* vive como um comensal no colo de seres humanos e outros primatas, cães, gatos, bois e vários roedores. [penta- + *Trichomonas*]

pen·ta·va·lent (pen-ta-vā′lent, pen-tav′a-lent). Pentavalente; que possui uma capacidade de combinação (valência) igual a cinco. SIN quinquevalent.

pen·taz·o·cine (pen-taz′o-sen). Pentazocina; um agonista/antagonista opióide analgésico, com alguma probabilidade de causar dependência, mas apenas raramente causa síndrome de abstinência e tolerância; muito irritante para os tecidos em injeções locais; encontrado na forma de cloridrato e sais de lactato.

pen·te·tate tri·so·di·um cal·ci·um (pen′te-tat). Pentetato trissódico de cálcio; o sal trissódico de cálcio do ácido pentético. SIN calcium trisodium pentetate.

pen·tet·ic ac·id (pen-tet′ik). Ácido pentético; ácido pentaacético triaminado com afinidade por metais pesados; usado como quelato sódico de cálcio no tratamento da doença por depósito de ferro e intoxicação por metais pesados e metais radioativos. VER TAMBÉM ethylenediaminetetraacetic acid.

pen·thi·e·nate bro·mide (pen-thi′e-nat). Brometo de pentionato; agente anticolinérgico.

pen·tif·yl·line (pen-tif′i-len). Pentifilina; vasodilatador; possui maior lipossolubilidade que a teobromina.

pen·ti·tol (pen′ti-tol). Pentitol; uma pentose reduzida; p. ex., ribitol, lixitol, xilitol.

pen·to·bar·bi·tal (pen-tō-bar′bi-tahl). Pentobarbital; sedativo oral e intravenoso e barbitúrico hipnótico de ação curta; amplamente substituído pelos benzodiazepínicos.

pen·to·lin·i·um tar·trate (pen-tō-lin′e-um). Tartarato de pentolínio; composto de amônio quaternário com potente ação bloqueadora ganglionar; usado no tratamento da hipertensão grave e maligna e das doenças vasoespásticas periféricas.

pen·ton (pen′ton). Penton; o capsômero pentagonal (base penton) juntamente com a fibra protrusa em cada um dos 12 vértices do capsídio do adenovírus; antigenicamente, a base penton difere da fibra, e ambos diferem dos outros capsômeros (hexagonais).

pen·to·san (pen′to-san). Pentosana; poli- ou oligossacarídeo de uma pentose; p. ex., arabanas, xilanas.

pen·tose (pen′tos). Pentose; monossacarídeo que contém cinco átomos de carbono na molécula; p. ex., arabinose, lixose, xilose, xilulose.

p. nucleotide, nucleotídeo pentose; nucleotídeo que possui uma pentose como o componente açúcar.

pen·to·sta·tin (pen′to-stat′in). Pentostatina; antineoplásico; potente inibidor da adenosina desaminase; interfere com a síntese do dinucleotídeo nicotinamida adenina. SIN 2-deoxycoformycin.

pen·to·su·ria (pen′to-soo′re-a). Pentosúria; a excreção de uma ou mais pentoses em quantidades elevadas de urina.

alimentary p., p. alimentar; a excreção urinária de L-arabinose e L-xilose, em virtude da ingestão excessiva de frutas contendo essas pentoses.

essential p. [MIM*260800], p. essencial; distúrbio hereditário benigno no qual o débito urinário de L-xilulose é de 1–4 g/24 h; ocorre principalmente em judeus asquenazim; herança autossômica recessiva. SIN L-xylulosuria, primary p.

primary p., p. primária. SIN essential p.

pen·tox·ide (pen-tok′sid). Pentóxido; um óxido que contém cinco átomos de oxigênio; p. ex., p. de fósforo, P_2O_5.

pen·tox·if·yl·line (pen-toks-if′i-len). Pentoxifilina; um derivado da dimetilxantina que diminui a viscosidade sanguínea e aumenta o fluxo sanguíneo; usada no tratamento da claudicação intermitente.

pen·tu·lose (pen′tu-los). Pentulose; uma cetopentose; p. ex., ribulose, xilulose.

pen·tyl (pen′til). Pentil. **1.** SIN amyl. **2.** A porção $CH_3(CH_2)_3CH_2-$.

pen·ty·lene·tet·ra·zol (pen′ti-len-tet′ra-zol). Pentilenotetrazol; um potente estimulante do sistema nervoso central; foi usado para causar convulsão generalizada no tratamento de choque de estados emocionais e como estimulante respiratório; usado principalmente em estudos experimentais dos mecanismos de convulsão e na pesquisa de fármacos anticonvulsivantes.

pe·num·bra (pe-num′bra). Penumbra; a região de iluminação ou radiação parcial causada por luz ou raios X não originados de uma fonte pontual; também denominada borramento geométrico. [L. mod., do L. *paene*, quase, + *umbra*, sombra]

pep·lo·mer (pep′lo-mer). Peplômero; uma parte ou subunidade, semelhante a um botão, do peplo de um vírion, cujo conjunto produz um peplo completo; freqüentemente, uma glicoproteína de superfície sobre revestimento lipoproteico. [ver peplos]

pep·los (pep′los). Peplo; o revestimento ou envoltório de material lipoproteico que circunda determinados vírions. [G. uma vestimenta externa usada por mulheres]

Pepper, William, Jr., médico norte-americano, 1874–1947. VER P. *syndrome*.

pep·per·mint (pep′er-mint). Hortelã-pimenta; as folhas secas e flores da *Mentha piperita* (família Labiatae); carminativo e antiemético.

p. camphor, mentol. SIN menthol.

p. oil, óleo de hortelã-pimenta; o óleo volátil destilado com vapor das partes frescas, excluindo a raiz, da planta florida da *Mentha piperita*, retificado por destilação e nem parcial nem completamente desmentolizado; um aromatizante.

pep·sic (pep′sik). Péptico. SIN peptic.

pep·sin (pep′sin). Pepsina; um grupo de proteinases aspárticas intimamente relacionadas. A pepsina A é a principal enzima digestiva do suco gástrico, formada a partir do pepsinogênio; hidrolisa ligações peptídicas em baixos valores de pH (é lábil em ambiente alcalino), preferencialmente adjacente aos resíduos fenilalanil e leucil, assim reduzindo as proteínas a moléculas menores (denominadas proteoses e peptonas); a pepsina B (gelatinase) é semelhante à pepsina A, mas é formada a partir do pepsinogênio B suíno e tem uma especificidade mais restrita; a pepsina C (gastricsina é a pepsina C humana) também é semelhante à pepsina A e estruturalmente relacionada a ela, possuindo uma especificidade mais restrita. [G. *pepsis*, digestão]

pep·si·nate (pep′si-nat). Pepsinar; misturar com pepsina.

pep·si·nif·er·ous (pep-si-nif′er-us). Pepsinífero. SIN pepsinogenous.

pep·sin·o·gen (pep-sin′o-jen). Pepsinogênio; uma pró-enzima ou zimogênio formado e secretado pelas células principais da mucosa gástrica; a acidez do suco gástrico e da própria pepsina remove 44 resíduos aminoacil da pepsina para formar pepsina ativa. SIN propepsin. [pepsin + G. *-gen*, que produz]

pep·sin·og·e·nous (pep-sin-oj′e-nus). Pepsinogênico; que produz pepsina. SIN pepsiniferous.

pep·si·nu·ria (pep-si-noo′re-a). Pepsinúria; excreção de pepsina na urina. [pepsin + G. *ouron*, urina]

pep·sta·tin (pep-sta′tin). Pepstatina; peptídeo inibidor de actinomicetos que inibe a pepsina e a catepsina D.

pep·tic (pep′tik). Péptico; relativo ao estômago, à digestão gástrica ou à pepsina A. SIN pepsic. [G. *peptikos*, de *pepto*, digerir]

pep·ti·dase (pep′ti-das). Peptidase; enzima capaz de hidrolisar uma ligação peptídica de um peptídeo; p. ex., carboxipeptidases, aminopeptidases. SIN peptide hydrolase.

p. D, p. D. SIN *proline* dipeptidase.

p. P, p. P. SIN peptidyl dipeptidase A.

pep·tide (pep′tid). Peptídeo; composto de dois ou mais aminoácidos no qual um grupamento carboxila de um se une a um grupo amino do outro, com a eliminação de uma molécula de água, assim formando uma ligação peptídica, –CO–NH–; isto é, uma amida substituída. Cf. eupeptide *bond*, isopeptide *bond*.

adrenocorticotropic p., p. adrenocorticotrópico; p. com atividade ACTH, isolado de extratos hipofisários.

anionic neutrophil-activating p. (ANAP), p. ativador de neutrófilos aniônico. SIN interleukin-8.

antigen p.'s, peptídeos antigênicos; os fragmentos de proteína que se ligam às moléculas do MHC (CPH).

atrial natriuretic p. (ANP) (na′tre-oo-ret′ik). p. natriurético atrial (PNA); um p. com 28 aminoácidos (α-PNA), derivado dos átrios cardíacos, vários fragmentos menores e α-PNA, e um dímero de α-PNA com 56 aminoácidos (β-PNA) que estão presentes no plasma na insuficiência cardíaca. As ações do PNA incluem filtração capilar crescente e excreção renal de sódio e água, bem como diminuição da pressão arterial e da secreção de renina, angiotensina, aldosterona e hormônio antidiurético. SIN atriopeptin, cardionatrin.

bitter p.'s, peptídeos amargos; peptídeos de sabor amargo e que podem estragar alguns alimentos; freqüentemente contêm grandes proporções de leucil, valil e resíduos aminoacil aromatizantes.

bradykinin-potentiating p., p. potencializador da bradicinina. SIN teprotide.

calcitonin gene-related p. (CGRP), p. relacionado ao gene da calcitonina (PRGC); um segundo produto transcrito do gene da calcitonina. O PRGC é encontrado em vários tecidos, incluindo o tecido nervoso. É um vasodilatador que pode participar da resposta tripla cutânea.

cyclic p., p. cíclico; p. que forma uma estrutura em anel; p. ex., a tirocidina A, um antibiótico, é um decapeptídeo cíclico; a valinomicina é um depsipeptídeo cíclico.

gastric inhibitory p. (GIP), p. inibitório gástrico. SIN gastric inhibitory polypeptide.
glucagonlike p., p. semelhante ao glucagon; hormônio intestinal que lentifica o esvaziamento gástrico e estimula a secreção de insulina. No futuro pode ser útil no tratamento do diabetes melito não-insulino-dependente, talvez administrado por adesivo, inalador ou pílula oral.
glucagonlike insulinotropic p., p. insulinotrópico glucagon-símile; substância insulinotrópica originada no trato gastrointestinal e liberada para a circulação após a ingestão de uma refeição contendo glicose.
heterodetic p., p. heterodético; p. que contém ligações peptídicas, bem como ligações covalentes entre determinados resíduos aminoacil que não são ligações peptídicas; p. ex., valinomicina, ocitocina. [hetero- + G. *detos*, ligado, de *deō*, ligar, + -ic]
heteromeric p., p. heteromérico; p. que, à hidrólise, produz outras substâncias diferentes dos aminoácidos, além destes; p. ex., ácido pteroilglutâmico.
homodetic p., p. homodético; p. no qual todas as ligações covalentes entre os aminoácidos constituintes são ligações peptídicas; p. ex., bradicinina. [homo- + G. *detos*, ligado, de *deō*, ligar, + -ic]
homomeric p., p. homomérico; **(1)** p. que, à hidrólise, produz apenas aminoácidos; p. ex., glutationa; **(2)** peptídeo que consiste apenas em um aminoácido específico; p. ex., alanilalanilalanina.
p. hydrolase [EC subclasse 3,4], p. hidrolase. SIN peptidase.
parathyroid hormone-related p., p. relacionado ao paratormônio; hormônio que pode ser produzido por tumores, principalmente do tipo de células escamosas; a grande superprodução pode causar hipercalcemia e outras manifestações de hiperparatireoidismo. O PTHrP exerce uma ação biológica semelhante à ação do paratormônio (PTH), agindo através do mesmo receptor, sendo expresso em muitos tecidos, porém é mais abundante no rim, no osso e na cartilagem da placa de crescimento. Aparentemente não tem ações significativas durante o desenvolvimento, mas não se sabe ao certo se o PTHrP realmente circula ou se tem qualquer função em seres humanos adultos normais. A estrutura do gene para o PTHrP humano é mais complexa que a do PTH, e existem várias formas moleculares, incluindo proteínas com 141, 139 e 173 aminoácidos, que compartilham uma homologia significativa com o paratormônio.
phenylthiocarbamoyl p., PTC p., p. feniltiocarbamoil; o peptídeo formado por combinação do fenilisotiocianato e um grupamento α-amino de um peptídeo. VER TAMBÉM phenylthiohydantoin.
S p., p. S. VER S *protein*.
sigma p., p. sigma; p. com uma extremidade ligada a um ponto dentro da cadeia, geralmente por meio do grupamento dissulfeto de um resíduo cistina, de forma que apenas uma extremidade do p. é livre; assim denominado porque a cadeia peptídica apresenta então formato semelhante ao da letra grega sigma; p. ex., ocitocina.
p. synthetase [EC 6.3.2.x], p. sintetase; qualquer enzima que catalisa a síntese de ligações peptídicas, com a hidrólise concomitante de um nucleosídeo trifosfato.
vasoactive intestinal p., p. intestinal vasoativo. SIN vasoactive intestinal polypeptide.
pep·ti·der·gic (pep-ti-der′jik). Peptidérgico; referente às células ou fibras nervosas que, supostamente, empregam pequenas moléculas peptídicas como neurotransmissor. [peptide + G. *ergon*, trabalho]
pep·ti·do·gly·can (pep′ti-dō-glī′kan). Peptidoglicano; composto contendo aminoácidos (ou peptídeos) ligados a açúcares, com predomínio destes últimos. Cf. glycopeptide. SIN mucopeptide (2).
pep·ti·doid (pep′ti-doyd). Peptidóide; um produto da condensação de dois aminoácidos envolvendo pelo menos um grupo de condensação diferente dos grupos α-carboxila ou α-amino, p. ex., glutationa.
pep·ti·do·lyt·ic (pep′ti-dō-lit′ik). Peptidolítico; que causa a clivagem ou digestão de peptídeos. [peptide + G. *lytikos*, solvente]
pep·ti·dyl di·pep·ti·dase A (pep′ti-dil). Peptidil dipeptidase A; hidrolase contendo zinco que cliva os dipeptídeos C-terminais de vários substratos, incluindo angiotensina I, que é convertida em angiotensina II e histidil-leucina (uma etapa importante no metabolismo de alguns agentes vasopressores). Fármacos que a inibem são usados no tratamento da hipertensão e da insuficiência cardíaca congestiva. SIN angiotensin-converting enzyme, carboxycathepsin, dipeptidyl carboxypeptidase, kinase II, peptidase P.
pep·ti·dyl·trans·fer·ase (pep-tī′dil-trans′fer-ās). Peptidiltransferase; a enzima responsável pela formação da ligação peptídica no ribossoma durante a biossíntese proteica, peptidyl-RNAt¹ + aminoacil-RNAt² → RNAt¹ + peptidilaminoacil-RNAt².
pep·ti·za·tion (pep-ti-zā′shŭn). Peptização; em química coloidal, um aumento do grau de dispersão, que tende a uma distribuição uniforme da fase dispersa.
Pep·to·coc·ca·ce·ae (pep′tō-kok-ā′sē-ē). Família de bactérias anaeróbicas, não-formadoras de esporos, imóveis (ordem Eubacteriales), contendo cocos Gram-positivos (a coloração pode ser questionável), com 0,5–1,6 μm de diâmetro, que ocorrem isoladamente, em pares, cadeias, tétrades e massas irregulares, mas não em grupos cúbicos tridimensionais. Esses microrganismos são quimiorganotróficos e têm exigências nutricionais complexas. Os carboidratos podem ou não ser fermentados por esses microrganismos, que produzem gás, principalmente CO_2 e geralmente H_2, a partir de aminoácidos e/ou carboidratos. São encontrados na boca e nas vias intestinais e respiratórias dos seres humanos e de outros animais; são freqüentemente encontrados nas vias urogenitais femininas humanas normais e doentes.

Pep·to·coc·cus (pep′tō-kok′ŭs). Gênero de bactérias quimiorganotróficas, anaeróbicas, imóveis (família Peptococcaceae), contendo células esféricas, Gram-positivas, que ocorrem isoladamente, em pares, tétrades ou massas irregulares, e, raramente, em cadeias curtas. São encontradas freqüentemente em associação a condições patológicas. A espécie típica é *P. niger*. [G. *peptō*, digerir, + *kokkos*, coco]
P. aero′genes, nome antigo do *Peptostreptococcus asaccharolyticus*.
P. constellatus, espécie de bactéria encontrada nas amígdalas, na pleurisia purulenta, no apêndice, no nariz, na orofaringe e nas gengivas, bem como, raramente, na pele e na vagina.
P. ni′ger, espécie de bactéria encontrada uma vez na urina de uma mulher idosa; a espécie típica do gênero *P*.
pep·to·crin·ine (pep-tō-krin′en). Peptocrinina; um extrato da mucosa intestinal semelhante à secretina.
pep·to·gen·ic, pep·tog·e·nous (pep-tō-jen′ik, pep-toj′e-nŭs). Peptogênico. **1.** Que produz peptonas. **2.** Que promove digestão.
pep·toid (pep′toyd). Peptóide; peptídeo com um ou mais grupos não-aminoacil (p. ex., açúcar, lipídios, etc.) ligados de forma covalente ao peptídeo.
pep·to·lide (pep′tō-līd). Peptolídeo. **1.** Um depsipeptídeo cíclico; p. ex., valinomicina. **2.** Um depsipeptídeo heteromérico.
pep·tol·y·sis (pep-tol′i-sis). Peptólise; a hidrólise de peptonas.
pep·to·lyt·ic (pep-tō-lit′ik). Peptolítico. **1.** Relativo à peptólise. **2.** Designa uma enzima ou outro agente que hidrolisa peptonas.
pep·tone (pep′tōn). Peptona; termo descritivo aplicado a produtos polipeptídicos intermediários, formados na hidrólise parcial de proteínas, que são solúveis em água, difusíveis e não-coaguláveis pelo calor; usada em meios de cultura para bactérias.
pep·ton·ic (pep-ton′ik). Peptônico; relativo à peptona ou que a contém.
pep·to·ni·za·tion (pep′ton-i-zā′shŭn). Peptonização; conversão, por ação enzimática, de proteína nativa em peptona solúvel.
Pep·to·strep·to·coc·cus (pep′tō-strep-tō-kok′ŭs). Gênero de bactérias quimiorganotróficas, anaeróbicas, imóveis (família Peptococcaceae), compreendendo células esféricas ou ovóides, Gram-positivas, que ocorrem em pares e cadeias curtas ou longas. Esses microrganismos são encontrados no trato genital feminino normal ou doente e no sangue na febre puerperal, nas vias respiratórias e intestinais de seres humanos e outros animais normais, na cavidade oral e em infecções piogênicas, feridas de guerra putrefatas e na apendicite; podem ser patogênicos. A espécie típica é o *P. anaerobius*. [G. *peptō*, digerir, + *streptos*, curvo, + *kokkos*, coco]
P. anaero′bius, espécie de bactéria encontrada na boca, nas vias intestinal e respiratória, e nas cavidades, principalmente a vagina, de seres humanos e outros animais; pode ser patogênica; é a espécie típica do gênero *P*.
P. asaccharoly′ticus, espécie de bactéria encontrada no intestino grosso, na cavidade bucal, na pleura, no útero e na vagina humanos; também é encontrada em casos de febre puerperal; caracterizada por sua incapacidade de metabolizar açúcares.
P. evolu′tus, espécie de bactéria encontrada na via respiratória, na boca e na vagina de seres humanos.
P. foe′tidus, espécie de bactéria encontrada em abscessos, no sangue, no trato intestinal, na vagina e na boca do homem e de outros animais; algumas vezes é fatal.
P. interme′dius. SIN *Streptococcus intermedius*.
P. mag′nus, espécie de bactéria encontrada na carne de açougue em putrefação e em um caso de apendicite.
P. mi′cros, espécie de bactéria encontrada em cavidades naturais dos seres humanos e de outros animais; tem sido isolada em várias condições patológicas.
P. morbillo′rum, espécie de bactéria encontrada no nariz, na orofaringe, nos olhos, nas orelhas, nas secreções mucosas e no sangue em casos de sarampo, sendo, porém, irrelevante para a etiologia do sarampo; provavelmente está presente em condições normais e desenvolve-se como um invasor secundário. SIN *Streptococcus morbillorum*.
P. paleopneumo′niae, espécie de bactéria encontrada na cavidade orofaríngea e nas vias respiratórias superiores dos seres humanos.
P. par′vulus, nome antigo de *Atopobium parvulus*.
P. plagarumbel′li, espécie de bactéria comumente encontrada em feridas de guerra sépticas.
P. produc′tus, nome antigo de *Ruminococcus productus*.
P. pu′tridus, espécie de bactéria encontrada na boca e no trato intestinal dos seres humanos, mas principalmente na vagina.
per-. Per-. **1.** Através, que indica intensidade. **2.** Em química, um prefixo que designa 1) mais ou máximo, em relação à quantidade de determinado elemento (geralmente oxigênio, como no ácido perclórico) ou radical contido em uma substância, ou 2) o grau de substituição de hidrogênio, como em peróxidos,

ácidos peroxi (p. ex., peróxido de hidrogênio, ácido peroxifórmico). VER TAMBÉM peroxy-. [L. através, extremamente]

per·a·ceph·a·lus (per-ă-sef'ă-lŭs). Peracéfalo; onfalósito que não possui cabeça nem braços, apresentando tórax defeituoso; tipicamente, o corpo consiste em pouco mais do que pelve e pernas. [per- + G. *a-* priv. + *kephalē*, cabeça]

per·ac·id (per-as'id). Perácido; um ácido que contém um grupamento peróxido (–O–OH); p. ex., ácido peracético. SIN peroxy acid.

per·a·cute (per-ă-kyut'). Peragudo; muito agudo; diz-se de uma doença. [L. *peracutus*, muito agudo]

per an·um (per ā'nŭm). Pelo ânus ou através dele. [L.]

per·ar·tic·u·la·tion (per'ar-tik'ū-lā'shŭn). Articulação sinovial. SIN synovial joint. [per- + L. *articulatio*, articulação]

per·a·to·dyn·ia (per'ă-tō-din'ē-ă). Peratodinia; termo obsoleto para pirose. [G. *peratos*, do lado oposto, + *odynē*, dor]

per·ax·il·lary (per-ak'si-lār-ē). Peraxilar; através da axila.

per·a·zine (per'ă-zēn). Perazina; um antipsicótico.

per·cen·tile (per-sen'tīl). Percentil; a posição relativa de um indivíduo em uma ordem seriada de dados, estabelecida em termos de que percentagem do grupo ele iguala ou excede.

per·cept (per'sept). Percepto. **1.** O que é percebido; a imagem mental completa, formada pelo processo de percepção, de um objeto ou idéia. **2.** Em psicologia clínica, uma única unidade de relato da percepção, tal como uma das respostas a um borrão de tinta no teste de Rorschach. [L. *perceptum*, algo percebido]

per·cep·tion (per-sep'shun). Percepção; o processo mental de tomada de consciência ou de reconhecimento de um objeto ou idéia; basicamente cognitivo, em vez de afetivo ou conativo, embora todos os três aspectos se manifestem. SIN esthesia (1).

depth p., p. de profundidade; a capacidade visual de julgar profundidade ou distância.

extrasensory p. (ESP), p. extra-sensorial; p. por outro meio além dos sentidos comuns; p. ex., telepatia, clarividência, precognição.

simultaneous p., p. simultânea; uma combinação de duas imagens ligeiramente diferentes em uma única imagem.

per·cep·tive (per-sep'tiv). Perceptivo; relativo a ou que possui uma capacidade de percepção maior que o normal.

per·cep·tiv·i·ty (per-sep-tiv'i-tē). Perceptividade; a capacidade de percepção.

per·cep·to·ri·um (per-sep-tōr'ē-ŭm). Perceptório. SIN sensorium (2).

per·co·la·tion (per-kō-lā'shŭn). Percolação. **1.** SIN filtration. **2.** Extração da parte solúvel de uma mistura sólida pela passagem de um solvente líquido através dela. **3.** Entrada de saliva ou de outros líquidos na interface entre a estrutura e a restauração do dente; algumas vezes é induzida por alterações térmicas. [L. *percolatio*, de *per-* + *colare*, coar]

per·co·la·tor (per'kō-lā-ter). Percolador; recipiente em forma de funil usado no processo de percolação em farmácia.

per·co·morph oil (per-kō-morf). Óleo de percomorfo; óleo de fígado de peixe da ordem Percomorphi, com uma quantidade padronizada de vitaminas A e D.

per con·tig·u·um (per-kon-tig'ū-ŭm). Por contigüidade; em contigüidade; designa o modo pelo qual uma reação inflamatória ou outro processo mórbido dissemina-se para uma estrutura contígua adjacente. [per- + L. *contiguus*, que toca, de *tango*, tocar]

per con·tin·u·um (per kon-tin'ū-ŭm). Por continuidade; em continuidade; contínuo; designa o modo pelo qual uma inflamação ou outro processo mórbido dissemina-se de uma parte para outra através de tecido contínuo. [per- + L. *continuus*, que mantém junto, contínuo, de *teneo*, segurar]

per·cuss (per-kŭs'). Percutir; realizar percussão.

per·cus·sion (per-kŭsh'ŭn). Percussão. **1.** Procedimento diagnóstico destinado a determinar a densidade de uma parte do corpo pelo som produzido golpeando-se levemente a superfície com o dedo ou percussor; realizado basicamente sobre o tórax, para determinar a presença de conteúdo normal de ar nos pulmões, e sobre o abdome, para avaliar se existe ar nas alças intestinais e o tamanho de órgãos sólidos como o fígado e o baço. **2.** Uma forma de massagem que consiste em repetidos golpes ou pancadas de força variável. [L. *percussio*, de *per-cutio*, pp. *-cussus*, bater, de *quatio*, agitar, bater]

auscultatory p., p. auscultatória; ausculta do tórax ou de outra parte ao mesmo tempo que se faz a p., para ajudar a ouvir o som produzido pela p.

bimanual p., p. bimanual; p. imediata na qual o dedo de uma mão golpeia a outra mão; uma forma de p. indireta.

clavicular p., p. clavicular; p., geralmente direta, ao longo de toda a clavícula, para demonstrar macicez, sobretudo na tuberculose pulmonar atípica.

deep p., p. profunda; p. forte para obter informações sobre órgãos ou estruturas profundas.

direct p., p. direta. SIN immediate p.

finger p., p. digital; p. na qual um dedo de uma mão é usado como plessímetro e o da outra mão usado como percussor.

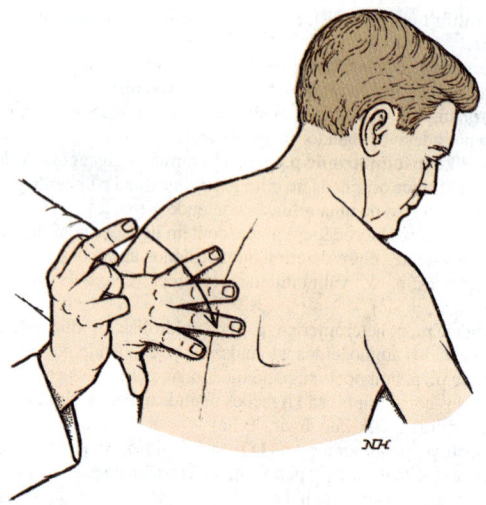

percussão bimanual: a falange distal do dedo médio esquerdo é pressionada firmemente contra a parede torácica paralela às costelas; é aplicado um golpe curto e rápido na base da falange distal do dedo médio com a ponta do dedo médio da mão direita

immediate p., p. imediata; p. direta; o golpeamento da parte examinada diretamente com o dedo ou um percussor, sem a intervenção de outro dedo ou plessímetro. SIN direct p.

mediate p., p. indireta; p. realizada pela intervenção de um dedo ou plessímetro entre o dedo ou percussor que golpeia e a parte percutida.

Murphy p., p. de Murphy; pesquisa de macicez golpeando-se a parede torácica diretamente com as pontas dos dedos de uma mão sucessivamente, começando com o quinto dedo. SIN piano p.

palpatory p., p. palpatória; p. digital na qual a atenção se concentra na resistência e na reverberação dos tecidos sob o dedo da mão, bem como no som produzido. SIN plessesthesia.

piano p., p. de Murphy. SIN Murphy p.

threshold p., p. limiar; p. realizada por meio de um bastão de vidro usado como plessímetro, estando o bastão inclinado para a parede do tórax ou do abdome, tocando-a apenas com uma extremidade.

per·cus·sor (per-kŭs'er). Percussor. SIN plessor.

per·cu·ta·ne·ous (per-kū-tā'nē-ŭs). Percutâneo; indica a passagem de substâncias através da pele intata, como na absorção por unção; também a passagem através da pele por perfuração com agulha, incluindo a introdução de fios e cateteres pela técnica de Seldinger (Seldinger *technique*). SIN transcutaneous, transdermic.

per·en·ceph·a·ly (per-en-sef'ă-lē). Perencefalia; condição caracterizada por um ou mais cistos cerebrais. [G. *pēra*, bolsa, estojo, + *enkephalos*, encéfalo]

Perez, Bernard, médico francês, 1836–1903. VER P. *reflex*.

Perez, George V., médico espanhol, †1920. VER P. *sign*.

per·fec·tion·ism (per-fek'shŭn-izm). Perfeccionismo; tendência a estabelecer rigorosos e elevados padrões de desempenho para si próprio.

per·fla·tion (per-flā'shŭn). Perflação; ato de forçar a entrada ou passagem de ar em uma cavidade ou canal a fim de causar o afastamento de suas paredes ou para expelir qualquer material nele contido. [L. *per-flo*, pp., *-flatus*, soprar]

per·flu·bron (per-floo'bron). Perflubron; nome genérico do bromuro de perfluorooctil.

per·flu·o·ro·octyl bro·mide (PFOB) (per-floo'rō-ok-til brō'mid). Brometo de perfluorooctil; fluorocarbono bromo-substituído, preparado como uma emulsão de partículas, usado como contraste para TC, RM e ultra-sonografia.

per·fo·rans (per'fō-rans). Perfurante; termo aplicado a vários músculos e nervos que, em seu trajeto, perfuram outras estruturas. [L. *perfurante*]

per·fo·rat·ed (per'fō-rāt-ed). Perfurado; com uma ou mais perfurações. [L. *perforatus*, de *per-foro*, pp. *-atus*, perfurar]

per·fo·ra·tion (per-fō-rā'shŭn). Perfuração; abertura anormal em um órgão ou víscera oca. SIN tresis [ver perforated]

per·fo·ra·tor (per'fōr-ā-ter). Perfurador; instrumento para fazer uma abertura óssea através do crânio. SIN trephine (1).

per·fo·rin (per'fōr-in). Perforina; proteína encontrada nos grânulos citoplasmáticos dos linfócitos T citotóxicos e das células exterminadoras naturais (natural Killer cells). Essa proteína está envolvida na lise de células-alvo pelas células NK. [L. *per-foro*, perfurar, + *-in*]

per·for·mic ac·id (per-fōr'mik). Ácido perfórmico; perácido orgânico usado na clivagem de ligações dissulfeto em peptídeos por oxidação de resíduos cistinil em ácido cisteico. SIN peroxyformic acid.

per·frig·er·a·tion (per-frij-er-ā'shŭn). Perfrigeração; leve grau de geladura. [L. *per-frigero*, pp. *-atus*, tornar frio, de *frigus*, frio]

per·fus·ate (per'fū-sāt). Perfusado; o líquido usado para perfusão; algumas vezes aplicado de forma mais ampla ao líquido que sofreu passagem forçada através de qualquer membrana ou material mais ou menos poroso. [ver perfuse]

per·fuse (per-fyūs'). Perfundir; forçar o fluxo de sangue ou outro líquido da artéria através do leito vascular de um tecido ou através da luz de uma estrutura oca (p. ex., um túbulo renal isolado). Cf. perifuse, superfuse. [L. *perfusio*, de per- + *fusio*, derramar]

per·fu·sion (per-fū'zhŭn). Perfusão. **1.** O ato de perfundir. **2.** O fluxo de sangue ou de outro perfusado por unidade de volume de tecido, como na razão ventilação/perfusão.
  regional p., p. regional; perfusão de parte do corpo, principalmente um membro, e particularmente com agentes quimioterápicos, para tratamento de um tumor maligno, primário, recorrente ou metastático.

per·go·lide mes·y·late (per'go-līd). Mesilato de pergolida; derivado do esporão do centeio com propriedades dopaminérgicas; usado no parkinsonismo.

per·hex·il·ine ma·le·ate (per-hek'si-lēn). Maleato de perexilina; vasodilatador coronariano e diurético.

per·hy·dro·cy·clo·pen·ta[a]phen·an·threne. Peridrociclopenta[a]fenantreno. SIN tetracyclic steroid *nucleus.*

peri-. Peri-; ao redor, em torno, próximo. Cf. circum-. [G. ao redor]

per·i·ac·cre·tio pe·ri·car·dii (per'i-ă-krē'shē-ō per-i-kar'dē-ī). Aderência do periaccretio pericardii ou de parte dele à superfície cardíaca devido a inflamação prévia.

per·i·ac·i·nal, per·i·ac·i·nous (per-ē-as'i-năl, -i-nŭs). Periacinoso; que circunda um ácino.

per·i·ad·e·ni·tis (per'ē-ad-ē-nī'tis). Periadenite; inflamação dos tecidos que circundam uma glândula. [peri- + G. *aden*, glândula, + *-itis*, inflamação]
  p. muco'sa necrot'ica recur'rens, p. mucosa necrótica recorrente. SIN *aphthae major*, em *aphtha.*

per·i·a·nal (per-ē-ā'năl). Perianal. SIN circumanal.

per·i·an·gi·o·cho·li·tis (per'ē-an'jē-ō-kō-lī'tis). Periangiocolite. SIN pericholangitis. [peri- + G. *angeion*, vaso, + *cholē*, bile, + *-itis*, inflamação]

per·i·an·gi·tis (per'ē-an-jī'tis). Periangeíte; periangiite; inflamação da adventícia de um vaso sanguíneo ou dos tecidos que o circundam ou de um vaso linfático. VER TAMBÉM periarteritis, periphlebitis, perilymphangitis. SIN perivasculitis. [peri- + G. *angeion*, um vaso, + *-itis*, inflamação]

per·i·a·or·tic (per'ē-ā-ōr'tik). Periaórtico; que circunda a aorta ou adjacente a ela.

per·i·a·or·ti·tis (per'ē-ā-ōr-tī'tis). Periaortite; inflamação da adventícia da aorta e dos tecidos que a circundam.

per·i·a·pex (per'ē-ā'peks). Periápice; as estruturas periapicais, particularmente a membrana periodontal e o osso adjacente. [peri- L. *apex*, ápice]

per·i·ap·i·cal (per-ē-ap'i-kăl). Periapical. **1.** No ápice da raiz de um dente ou ao seu redor. **2.** Designa o periápice.

per·i·ap·pen·di·ci·tis (per'ē-ă-pen-di-sī'tis). Periapendicite; inflamação do tecido que circunda o apêndice vermiforme. SIN para-appendicitis.
  p. decidua'lis, p. decidual; a presença de células deciduais no peritônio do apêndice vermiforme em casos de gravidez tubária direita com aderências entre a tuba de Falópio (tuba uterina) e o apêndice.

per·i·ap·pen·dic·u·lar (per'ē-ap-en-dik'ū-lăr). Periapendicular; que circunda um apêndice, principalmente o apêndice vermiforme.

per·i·ar·te·ri·al (per'ē-ar-tē'rē-ăl). Periarterial; que circunda uma artéria.

per·i·ar·te·ri·tis (per'ē-ar-ter-ī'tis). Periarterite; inflamação da adventícia de uma artéria. SIN exarteritis.
  p. nodo'sa, p. nodosa. SIN polyarteritis nodosa.

per·i·ar·thric (per'ē-ar'thrik). Periártrico. SIN circumarticular.

per·i·ar·thri·tis (per'ē-ar-thrī'tis). Periartrite; inflamação das partes que circundam uma articulação. [peri- + *arthritis*]

per·i·ar·tic·u·lar (per'ē-ar-tik'ū-lăr). Periarticular. SIN circumarticular.

per·i·a·tri·al (per'ē-ā'trē-ăl). Periatrial; que circunda o átrio do coração. SIN periauricular (1).

per·i·au·ric·u·lar (per'ē-aw-rik'ū-lăr). Periauricular. **1.** SIN periatrial. **2.** SIN periconchal. **3.** Ao redor da orelha externa.

per·i·ax·i·al (per'ē-ak'sē-ăl). Periaxial; que circunda um eixo.

per·i·ax·il·lary (per'ē-ak'sē-lār-ē). Periaxilar. SIN circumaxillary.

per·i·ax·o·nal (per'ē-ak'sō-năl). Periaxonal; que circunda o axônio de um nervo. [peri- + G. *axon*, eixo]

per·i·blast (per'i-blast). Periblasto; região especializada da superfície vitelina imediatamente periférica ao blastoderma em ovos telolécitos. [peri- + G. *blastos*, germe]

per·i·bron·chi·al (per-i-brong'kē-ăl). Peribrônquico; que circunda um brônquio ou os brônquios.

per·i·bron·chi·o·lar (per-i-brong'kē-ō'lăr). Peribronquiolar; que circunda os bronquíolos.

per·i·bron·chi·o·li·tis (per'i-brong'kē-ō-lī'tis). Peribronquiolite; inflamação dos tecidos que circundam os bronquíolos.

per·i·bron·chi·tis (per'i-brong-kī'tis). Peribronquite; inflamação dos tecidos que circundam os brônquios ou tubos brônquicos.

per·i·buc·cal (per'i-bŭk'al). Peribucal; que circunda a bochecha.

per·i·bul·bar (per-i-bŭl'bar). Peribulbar; que circunda qualquer bulbo, principalmente o bulbo do olho ou o bulbo da uretra. SIN circumbulbar.

per·i·bur·sal (per-i-ber'săl). Que circunda uma bolsa.

per·i·can·a·lic·u·lar (per'i-kan-ă-lik'oo-lăr). Pericanalicular; que circunda um canalículo.

per·i·car·dec·to·my (per'i-kar-dek'tō-mē). Pericardectomia. SIN pericardiectomy.

per·i·car·di·a (per-i-kar'dē-ă). Pericárdios; plural de pericardium.

per·i·car·di·ac, per·i·car·di·al (per-i-kar'dē-ak, -dē-ăl). Pericárdico. **1.** Que circunda o coração. **2.** Relativo ao pericárdio.

per·i·car·di·cen·te·sis (per-i-kar'dē-sen-tē'sis). Pericardiocentese. SIN pericardiocentesis.

per·i·car·di·ec·to·my (per'i-kar-dē-ek'tō-mē). Pericardiectomia; excisão de uma parte do pericárdio. SIN pericardectomy. [pericardium + G. *ektomē*, excisão]
  radical p., p. radical; excisão de quase todo o pericárdio.

per·i·car·di·o·cen·te·sis (per-i-kar'dē-ō-sen-tē'sis). Pericardiocentese; drenagem do pericárdio por agulha ou cateter. SIN pericardial tap, pericardicentesis. [peri- + G. *kardia*, coração, + *kentēsis*, punção]

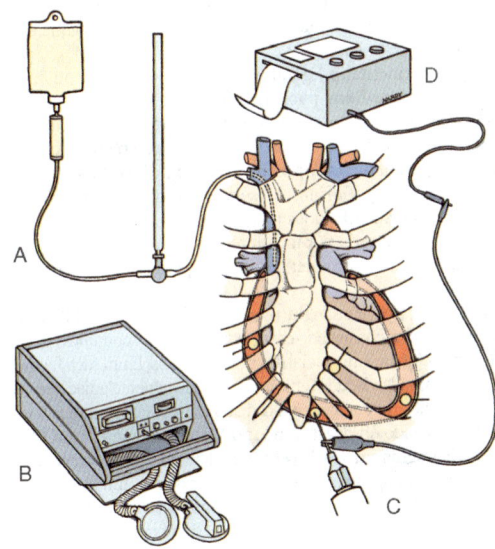

pericardiocentese: suporte para pacientes; (A) acesso IV para monitorização da pressão venosa central aberto para fármacos de emergência, (B) desfibrilador e equipamento de reanimação preparados, (C) pericardiocentese, com seringa e agulha à qual foi acoplado cabo de ECG, (D) monitorização ECG (os pequenos círculos indicam locais de aspiração pericárdica)

per·i·car·di·ol·ogy (per-ē-kar-dē-ol'ō-jē). Pericardiologia; a ciência ou o estudo do pericárdio, sua fisiologia e doenças.

per·i·car·di·o·per·i·to·ne·al (per-i-kar'dē-ō-per-i-tō-nē'al). Pericardioperitoneal; relativo às cavidades pericárdica e peritoneal.

per·i·car·di·o·phren·ic (per-i-kar'dē-ō-fren'ik). Pericardiofrênico; relativo ao pericárdio e ao diafragma. [pericardium + G. *phrēn*, diafragma]

per·i·car·di·o·pleur·al (per-i-kar'dē-ō-ploor'ăl). Pericardiopleural; relativo às cavidades pericárdica e pleural.

per·i·car·di·or·rha·phy (per'i-kar-dē-ōr'ă-fē). Pericardiorrafia; sutura do pericárdio. [pericardium + G. *rhaphē*, sutura]

per·i·car·di·os·to·my (per'i-kar-dē-os'tō-mē). Pericardiostomia; estabelecimento de uma abertura no pericárdio. [pericardium + G. *stoma*, boca]

per·i·car·di·ot·o·my (per'i-kar-dē-ot'ō-mē). Pericardiotomia; incisão do pericárdio. SIN pericardotomy. [pericardium + G. *tomē*, incisão]

per·i·car·dit·ic (per'i-kar-dit'ik). Pericardítico; relativo à pericardite.

per·i·car·di·tis (per'i-kar-dī'tis). Pericardite; inflamação do pericárdio.
  acute fibrinous p., p. fibrinosa aguda; a lesão habitual da p. aguda na qual a inflamação produz grandes quantidades de fibrina.
  adhesive p., p. adesiva; p. com aderências entre as duas camadas pericárdicas, entre o pericárdio e o coração, ou entre o pericárdio e estruturas vizinhas. SIN adherent pericardium.
  bacterial p., p. bacteriana; p. produzida por infecção bacteriana.
  p. calculosa, p. calculosa; calcificação pericárdica devida à pericardite prévia.
  carcinomatous p., p. carcinomatosa; p. causada por infiltração de células carcinomatosas, geralmente provenientes de estruturas adjacentes.

chronic constrictive p., p. constritiva crônica; fibrose do pericárdio com espessamento da membrana e constrição prolongada das câmaras cardíacas.
constrictive p., p. constritiva; espessamento e fibrose pós-inflamatória da membrana, produzindo constrição das câmaras cardíacas; pode ser aguda, subaguda ou crônica. Antigamente denominada pericardite constritiva crônica.
dry p., p. seca; inflamação pericárdica na ausência de derrame pericárdico demonstrável.
epistenocardiac p., p. epistenocardíaca; p. associada a infarto do miocárdio transmural e limitada à área sobre o infarto. SIN p. epistenocardica.
p. epistenocardica, p. epistenocardíaca. SIN epistenocardiac p.
fibrinous p., p. fibrinosa; p. aguda com exsudato fibrinoso. VER TAMBÉM bread-and-butter *pericardium*. SIN hairy heart, p. villosa, shaggy pericardium.
fibrous p., p. fibrosa; fibrose, geralmente com aderências, de todo o pericárdio ou de sua maior parte.
hemorrhagic p., p. hemorrágica; p. com derrame tinto de sangue.
internal adhesive p., p. adesiva interna. SIN concretio cordis.
p. oblit'erans, p. obliterante; inflamação do pericárdio que leva à aderência das duas camadas, obliterando o saco. VER TAMBÉM adhesive p.
obliterative p., p. obliterativa; obliteração completa por aderências pós-inflamatórias da cavidade pericárdica.
postmyocardial infarction p., p. pós-infarto do miocárdio; forma aguda de p. que geralmente se desenvolve uma semana após um infarto do miocárdio.
postpericardiotomy p., p. pós-pericardiotomia; síndrome caracterizada por febre, dor torácica subesternal e atrito pericárdico após cirurgia pericárdica.
posttraumatic p., p. pós-traumática; inflamação pericárdica que se desenvolve após traumatismo torácico.
purulent p., p. purulenta; p., geralmente bacteriana, com pus no saco. SIN empyema of the pericardium, pyopericardium.
rheumatic p., p. reumática; p. fibrinosa que ocorre na febre reumática aguda.
p. sic'ca, p. seca; p. fibrinosa sem derrame pericárdico significativo.
tuberculous p., p. tuberculosa; p. causada por infecção tuberculosa.
uremic p., p. urêmica; p. fibrinosa observada na insuficiência renal crônica.
p. villo'sa, p. vilosa. SIN fibrinous p.
viral p., p. viral; p. causada por uma infecção viral.
p. with effusion, p. com derrame; inflamação pericárdica que produz excesso de líquido pericárdico.

per·i·car·di·um, pl. **per·i·car·dia** (per-i-kar'dē-ŭm, -ă) [TA]. Pericárdio; a membrana fibrosserosa, consistindo em mesotélio e tecido conjuntivo submesotelial, que recobre o coração e a parte inicial dos grandes vasos. É um saco fechado que tem duas camadas: a camada visceral (epicárdio), imediatamente adjacente e superposta a todas as superfícies do coração, e a camada parietal externa, que forma o saco, composta de forte tecido fibroso revestido por uma membrana serosa. O nervo frênico segue até o diafragma através do pericárdio anterior e divide o pericárdio em porções antefrênica e retrofrênica; o hilo pulmonar divide ambas essas porções em porções supra-hilar, hilar e infra-hilar. SIN capsula cordis, heart sac, membrana cordis, theca cordis. [L. do G. *pericardion*, a membrana ao redor do coração]
adherent p., pericardite adesiva. SIN adhesive *pericarditis*.
bread-and-butter p., tipo pão com manteiga; p. fibrinosa na qual as superfícies visceral e parietal do pericárdio assemelham-se às superfícies de dois pedaços de pão com manteiga que foram encostados e depois afastados, quando são separadas durante cirurgia ou necropsia.
p. fibro'sum [TA], p. fibroso. SIN fibrous p.
fibrous p. [TA], p. fibroso. VER pericardium. SIN p. fibrosum [TA].
p. sero'sum, p. seroso. SIN serous p.
serous p. [TA], p. seroso. VER pericardium. SIN p. serosum.
shaggy p., pericardite fibrinosa. SIN fibrinous *pericarditis*.
visceral p., p. visceral; a camada do saco pericárdico na superfície epicárdica do coração. É composto principalmente de uma única camada de mesotélio.

per·i·car·dot·o·my (per-i-kar-dot'ō-mē). Pericardiotomia. SIN pericardiotomy.
per·i·ce·cal (per'i-sē'kăl). Pericecal; que circunda o ceco. SIN perityphlic.
per·i·cel·lu·lar (per'i-sel'ū-lăr). Pericelular; que circunda uma célula. SIN pericytial.
per·i·ce·men·tal (per'i-sē-men'tăl). Pericemental. SIN periodontal.
per·i·cen·tral (per-i-sen'trăl). Pericentral; que circunda o centro.
per·i·cho·lan·gi·tis (per'i-kō-lan'jī'tis). Pericolangite; inflamação dos tecidos ao redor dos ductos biliares. SIN periangiocholitis. [peri- + G. *cholē*, bile, + *angeion*, vaso, + -*itis*, inflamação]
per·i·chon·dral, per·i·chon·dri·al (per-i-kon'drăl, -kon'drē-ăl). Pericondral; relativo ao pericôndrio.
per·i·chon·dri·tis (per'i-kon-drī'tis). Pericondrite; inflamação do pericôndrio.
peristernal p., p. periesternal. SIN Tietze *syndrome*.
relapsing p., p. recidivante. SIN relapsing *polychondritis*.
per·i·chon·dri·um (per-i-kon'drē-ŭm). [TA]. Pericôndrio; a membrana de tecido conjuntivo irregular denso ao redor da cartilagem. [peri- + G. *chondros*, cartilagem]
per·i·chord (per'i-kōrd). Pericórdio; bainha do notocórdio.
per·i·chor·dal (per-i-kōr'dăl). Relativo ao pericórdio.

per·i·cho·roi·dal (per-i-kō-roy'dăl). Pericoroidal; que envolve a corióide do olho.
per·i·chrome (per'i-krōm). Pericromo; indica uma célula nervosa na qual a substância cromófila, ou material corável, está dispersa em todo o citoplasma. [peri- + G. *chrōma*, cor]
per·i·col·ic (per'i-kol'ik). Pericólico; que envolve ou circunda o colo.
per·i·co·li·tis (per'i-kō-lī'tis). Pericolite; inflamação do tecido conjuntivo ou peritônio que circunda o colo. SIN pericolonitis, serocolitis.
p. dex'tra, p. direita; pericolite que envolve o colo ascendente.
p. sinis'tra, p. esquerda. SIN perisigmoiditis.
per·i·co·lon·i·tis (per'i-kō-lon-ī'tis). Pericolite. SIN pericolitis.
per·i·col·pi·tis (per'i-kol-pī'tis). Pericolpite. SIN perivaginitis. [peri- + G. *kolpos*, vagina, + -*itis*, inflamação]
per·i·con·chal (per'i-kong'kăl). Periauricular; que circunda a concha da orelha. SIN periauricular (2).
per·i·cor·ne·al (per-i-kōr'nē-ăl). Pericórneo; que circunda a córnea. SIN circumcorneal, perikeratic.
per·i·cor·o·nal (per-i-kōr'ō-năl). Pericoronal; ao redor da coroa de um dente.
per·i·cor·o·ni·tis (per-i-kōr-ō-nī'tis). Pericoronite; inflamação ao redor da coroa de um dente, em geral que está incompletamente irrompido na cavidade oral. [peri- + L. *corona*, coroa, + G. -*itis*, inflamação]
per·i·cra·ni·al (per'i-krā'nē-ăl). Pericranial; relativo ao pericrânio; que circunda o crânio.
per·i·cra·ni·tis (per'i-krā-nī'tis). Pericranite; inflamação do pericrânio.
per·i·cra·ni·um (per'i-krā'nē-ŭm) [TA]. Pericrânio; o periósteo do crânio. SIN periosteum cranii [TA]. [peri- + G. *kranion*, crânio]
per·i·cy·a·zine (per-i-sī'ă-zēn). Periciazina; antipsicótico.
per·i·cys·tic (per'i-sis'tik). Pericístico. 1. Que circunda a bexiga. 2. Que circunda a vesícula biliar. 3. Que circunda um cisto. SIN perivesical. [peri- + G. *kystis*, vesícula]
per·i·cys·ti·tis (per'i-sis-tī'tis). Pericistite; inflamação dos tecidos ao redor de uma bexiga ou vesícula, particularmente a bexiga urinária.
per·i·cys·ti·um (per-i-sis'tē-ŭm). Pericisto. 1. Os tecidos que circundam a bexiga ou a vesícula biliar. 2. O revestimento vascular de um tumor cístico. [peri- + G. *kystis*, bexiga, cisto]
per·i·cyte (per'i-sīt). Pericito; uma das delgadas células semelhantes às mesenquimais, encontradas em íntima associação com a parede externa das vênulas pós-capilares; é relativamente indiferenciado e pode tornar-se um fibroblasto, macrófago ou célula muscular lisa. SIN adventitial cell, pericapillary cell, perithelial cell. [peri- + G. *kytos*, célula]
per·i·cy·ti·al (per'i-sish'ē-ăl, -sit'ē-ăl). Pericelular. SIN pericellular.
per·i·dens (per'i-denz). Peridente; um dente supranumerário que aparece em qualquer outro lugar além da linha média do arco dental. [peri- + L. *dens*, dente]
per·i·den·tal (per-i-den'tăl). Peridental. SIN periodontal.
per·i·den·ti·tis (per'i-den-tī'tis). Peridentite; termo obsoleto para periodontite.
per·i·den·ti·um (per'i-den'tē-ŭm). Periodonto. SIN periodontium.
per·i·derm, per·i·der·ma (per'i-derm, -i-der'mă). Periderme; a camada mais externa da epiderme do embrião e do feto até o sexto mês de vida intrauterina; as células peridérmicas descamadas são um componente considerável do verniz caseoso. SIN epitrichium. [peri- + G. *derma*, pele]
per·i·der·mal, per·i·der·mic (per-i-der'măl, -mik). Peridérmico; relativo à periderme.
per·i·des·mic (per-i-dez'mik). Peridésmico. 1. Que circunda um ligamento. 2. Relativo ao peridesmo. SIN periligamentous.
per·i·des·mi·tis (per'i-dez-mī'tis). Peridesmite; inflamação do tecido conjuntivo que circunda um ligamento. [peri- + G. *desmos*, faixa, + -*itis*, inflamação]
per·i·des·mi·um (per-i-dez'mē-ŭm). Peridesmo; a membrana de tecido conjuntivo que circunda um ligamento. [peri- + G. *desmion* (*desmos*), faixa]
per·i·did·y·mis (per-i-did'i-mis). Túnica albugínea do testículo. SIN tunica albuginea of testis. [G. *didymos*, gêmeo, pl. *didymoi*, testículos]
per·i·did·y·mi·tis (per'i-did-i-mī'tis). Perididimite; inflamação do perididimo.
pe·rid·i·um (pe-rid'ē-ŭm). Perídio; em fungos, a estrutura de hifas que circunda os ascos. [G. *pēridion*, dim. de *pēra*, bolsa de couro]
per·i·di·ver·tic·u·li·tis (per'i-dī'ver-tik'ū-lī'tis). Peridiverticulite; inflamação ao redor do divertículo.
per·i·duo·de·ni·tis (per'i-doo'ō-dē-nī'tis). Periduodenite; inflamação em torno do duodeno.
per·i·du·ral (per-i-doo'răl). Peridural. SIN epidural.
per·i·en·ceph·a·li·tis (per'ē-en-sef-ă-lī'tis). Periencefalite; inflamação das membranas cerebrais, sobretudo das leptomeninges, ou inflamação da pia-máter com envolvimento do córtex subjacente. [peri- + G. *enkephalos*, encéfalo]
per·i·en·ter·ic (per-ē-en-ter'ik). Perientérico; que circunda o intestino. SIN circumintestinal.
per·i·en·ter·i·tis (per'ē-en-ter-ī'tis). Perienterite; inflamação do revestimento peritoneal do intestino. SIN seroenteritis.
per·i·e·pen·dy·mal (per'ē-e-pen'di-măl). Periependimário; que circunda o epêndima.

per·i·e·soph·a·ge·al (per′ē-e-sof′ă-jē′ăl). Periesofágico; que circunda o esôfago.

per·i·e·soph·a·gi·tis (per′ē-e-sof′ă-jī′tis). Periesofagite; inflamação dos tecidos ao redor do esôfago.

per·i·fo·cal (per-i-fō′kal). Perifocal; que circunda um foco; designa tecidos, ou o sangue que eles contêm, na vizinhança de um foco infeccioso.

per·i·fol·lic·u·lar (per′i-fō-lik′ū-lăr). Perifolicular; que circunda um folículo piloso; geralmente usado para descrever o aspecto histopatológico do infiltrado que circunda um folículo piloso.

per·i·fol·lic·u·li·tis (per′i-fō-lik′ū-lī′tis). Perifoliculite; a presença de um infiltrado inflamatório circundando os folículos pilosos; freqüentemente ocorre em conjunto com a foliculite.
 p. absce′dens et suffo′diens, p. abscedante da cabeça; foliculite dissecante crônica do couro cabeludo. SIN dissecting cellulitis.

per·i·fuse (per′i-fūs). Enxaguar; lavar com um jato de um líquido de embebição fresco todas as superfícies externas de um pequeno pedaço de tecido nele imerso. Cf. perfuse, superfuse. [peri- + L. *fusio*, derrame]

per·i·fu·sion (per-i-fū′shŭn). O ato de enxaguar.

per·i·gan·gli·on·ic (per′i-gang-glē-on′ik). Periganglionar; que circunda um gânglio, principalmente um gânglio nervoso.

per·i·gas·tric (per-i-gas′trik). Perigástrico; que circunda o estômago. [peri- + G. *gaster*, ventre, estômago]

per·i·gas·tri·tis (per′i-gas-trī′tis). Perigastrite; inflamação do revestimento peritoneal do estômago.

per·i·gem·mal (per′i-jem′ăl). Perigemal. SIN circumgemmal. [peri- + L. *gemma*, broto]

per·i·glan·du·li·tis (per′i-glan-doo-lī′tis). Periglandulite; inflamação dos tecidos que circundam uma glândula.

per·i·glot·tic (per-i-glot′ik). Periglótico; ao redor da língua, principalmente ao redor da base da língua e da epiglote, ou ao redor da glote (laringe), a rima da glote. [peri- + G. *glōssa* ou *glōtta*, língua]

per·i·glot·tis (per-i-glot′is). Periglote; a mucosa da língua. [G. *periglōttis*, que cobre a língua]

per·i·he·pat·ic (per-i-he-pat′ik). Periepático; que circunda o fígado. [peri- + G. *hēpar*, fígado]

per·i·hep·a·ti·tis (per′i-hep-ă-tī′tis). Periepatite; inflamação do revestimento seroso, ou peritoneal, do fígado. SIN hepatic capsulitis, hepatitis externa, hepatoperitonitis. [peri- + G. *hēpar*, fígado, + *-itis*, inflamação]

per·i·her·ni·al (per-i-her′nē-ăl). Perierniário; que circunda uma hérnia.

peri-im·plan·to·cla·sia (per′ē-im-plan′tō-klă-zē-ă). Perimplantoclasia; em odontologia, termo genérico para designar a doença do osso de sustentação que envolve um implante; a doença pode ser de natureza esfoliativa, reabsortiva, traumática ou ulcerativa. [peri- + L. *im*, em, + *planto*, plantar, + G. *klasis*, ruptura]

per·i·je·ju·ni·tis (per′i-jē-joo-nī′tis). Perijejunite; inflamação ao redor do jejuno.

per·i·kar·y·on, pl. **per·i·kar·ya** (per-i-kar′ē-on, -ă). Pericário. **1.** O citoplasma ao redor do núcleo, como o observado no corpo celular das células nervosas. **2.** O corpo do odontoblasto, excluindo a fibra da dentina. **3.** O corpo celular da célula nervosa, distinto de seu axônio e dendritos. [peri- + G. *karyon*, núcleo]

per·i·ker·at·ic (per-i-ke-rat′ik). Pericerático. SIN pericorneal. [peri- + G. *keras*, corno]

per·i·ky·ma·ta, sing. **per·i·ky·ma** (per-i-kī′mă-tă, -kī′mă). Pericimo; as cristas e sulcos transversos na superfície do esmalte dental. [peri- + G. *kyma*, onda]

per·i·lab·y·rin·thi·tis (per′i-lab′ĭ-rin-thī′tis). Perilabirintite; inflamação das partes ao redor do labirinto.

per·i·la·ryn·ge·al (per′i-lă-rin′jē-ăl). Perilaríngeo; que circunda a laringe.

per·i·len·tic·u·lar (per-i-len-tik′ū-lăr). Perilenticular; que circunda a lente do olho. SIN circumlental.

per·i·lig·a·men·tous (per′i-lig-ă-men′tŭs). Periligamentar. SIN peridesmic.

per·i·lymph (per′i-limf) [TA]. Perilinfa; o líquido contido no labirinto ósseo, que circunda e protege o labirinto membranáceo; a perilinfa tem composição semelhante à do líquido extracelular (os sais de sódio são o eletrólito positivo predominante) e, através do ducto perilinfático, está em continuidade com o líquido cerebroespinal. SIN perilympha [TA], Cotunnius liquid, liquor cotunnii.

per·i·lym·pha (per′i-limf′ă) [TA]. Perilinfa. SIN perilymph. [peri- + L. *lympha*, um líquido claro (linfa)]

per·i·lym·phan·gi·al (per′i-lim-fan′jē-ăl). Perilinfangial; que circunda um vaso linfático.

per·i·lym·phan·gi·tis (per′i-lim-fan-jī′tis). Perilinfangite; inflamação dos tecidos que circundam um vaso linfático.

per·i·lym·phat·ic (per′i-lim-fat′ik). Perilinfático. **1.** Que circunda uma estrutura linfática (nodo ou vaso). **2.** Os espaços e tecidos que circundam o labirinto membranáceo da orelha interna.

per·i·men·in·gi·tis (per′i-men-in-jī′tis). Perimeningite. SIN pachymeningitis.

per·i·men·o·pause (per′i-men′ō-paws). Perimenopausa; o período de 3–5 anos que precede a menopausa, durante o qual os níveis de estrogênio começam a cair.

pe·rim·e·ter (pe-rim′e-ter). Perímetro. **1.** Uma circunferência, margem ou borda. **2.** Um instrumento, geralmente metade de um círculo ou esfera, usado para medir o campo de visão. [G. *perimetros*, circunferência, de *peri*, ao redor, + *metron*, medida]
 arc p., p. do arco; perímetro que consiste em uma estrutura semicircular para o centro da qual o paciente olha enquanto um objeto branco se move ao longo do arco, sendo observado e registrado em um cartão o ponto exato onde se torna visível ou invisível.
 Goldmann p., p. de Goldmann; p. de projeção que aumenta a precisão por controle da iluminação do ambiente.
 projection p., p. de projeção; p. utilizando como alvo um ponto de luz que pode ser ajustado rapidamente quanto ao tamanho, brilho e cor, e move-se silenciosamente em qualquer velocidade desejada.
 Tübinger p., p. de Tübinger; uma projeção curva na qual um estímulo estático foi aumentado em intensidade até ser detectado. [*Tübingen*, cidade alemã]

per·i·met·ric (per-i-met′rik). Perimétrico. **1.** Que circunda o útero; relativo ao perimétrio. SIN periuterine. [G. *peri*, ao redor, + *metra*, útero] **2.** Relativo à circunferência de qualquer parte ou área. [G. *perimetros*, circunferência] **3.** Relativo à perimetria.

per·i·me·trit·ic (per-i-me-trit′ik). Perimetrítico; relativo a, ou caracterizado por, perimetrite.

per·i·me·tri·tis (per′i-me-trī′tis). Perimetrite; inflamação do útero envolvendo o perimétrio. SIN metroperitonitis. [perimetrium + G. -*itis*, inflamação].

per·i·me·tri·um, pl. **per·i·me·tria** (per-i-mē′trē-ŭm, -ă). Perimétrio; o revestimento seroso (peritoneal) do útero. SIN tunica serosa uteri [TA]. [peri- + G. *mētra*, útero]

pe·rim·e·try (pe-rim′ē-trē). Perimetria. **1.** A determinação dos limites do campo visual. **2.** O mapeamento dos contornos de sensibilidade do campo visual. [G. *perimetros*, circunferência]
 computed p., p. computadorizada; determinação do campo visual por meio de uma rotina programada de estímulos estáticos.
 flicker p., p. de cintilação; técnica de p. que utiliza o critério da freqüência de fusão crítica. SIN flicker fusion frequency technique.
 kinetic p., p. cinética; mapeamento do campo visual pelo uso de um objeto de teste móvel, e não estático.
 mesopic p., p. mesópica; exploração do campo visual com pouca iluminação.
 objective p., p. objetiva; determinação do campo visual por constrição pupilar, eletroencefalografia ou movimentos oculares.
 quantitative p., p. quantitativa; representação do campo visual em isópteros de igual sensibilidade retiniana.
 scotopic p., p. escotópica; projeção de um olho adaptado à escuridão.
 static p., p. estática; determinação do campo visual pelo uso de objetos de teste em posições fixas e aumento crescente da luminância até o limiar de visibilidade.

per·i·mol·y·sis (per-ē-mol′i-sis). Perimilólise; descalcificação dos dentes por exposição ao ácido gástrico em pessoas que apresentam vômito crônico. [=perimylolysis, de peri- + G. *mylos*, molar, + *lysis*, afrouxamento, dissolução, de *luō*, afrouxar]

per·i·my·e·lis (per-i-mī′ē-lis). Perimielo; endósteo. SIN endosteum. [peri- + G. *myelos*, medula óssea]

per·i·my·e·li·tis (per-i-mī-e-lī′tis). Perimielite. SIN endosteitis.

per·i·my·o·car·di·tis (per-i-mī′ō-kar-dī-tis). Perimiocardite; pericardite e miocardite simultâneas, geralmente causadas pelo mesmo agente etiológico.

per·i·my·o·si·tis (per′i-mī-ō-sī′tis). Perimiosite; inflamação do tecido celular frouxo que circunda um músculo. SIN perimysiitis (2), perimysitis.

per·i·my·si·al (per-i-mis′ē-ăl, -miz′ē-ăl). Perimisial; relativo ao perimísio; que circunda um músculo.

per·i·my·si·i·tis, per·i·my·si·tis (per′i-mis-ē-ī′tis, -mī-sī′tis). Perimisiite. **1.** Inflamação do perimísio. **2.** SIN perimyositis.

per·i·my·si·um, pl. **per·i·my·sia** (per-i-mis′ē-ŭm, -miz′ē-ŭm -ē-ă). [TA]. Perimísio; o envoltório fibroso de cada um dos fascículos das fibras musculares esqueléticas. [peri- + G. *mys*, músculo]
 p. exter′num, epimísio. SIN epimysium.
 p. inter′num, p. interno; na literatura antiga, um termo que se refere ao tecido conjuntivo que envolve os fascículos secundários e terciários e as fibras individuais, e também à estrutura de sustentação do miocárdio.

per·i·na·tal (per-i-nā′tăl). Perinatal; que ocorre durante o nascimento, ou é relativo aos períodos antes, no decorrer ou depois do nascimento; isto é, a partir da 22.ª semana de gestação até os primeiros 28 dias após o parto. [peri- + L. *natus*, pp. de *nascor*, nascer]

per·i·nate (per′i-nāt). Perinato; um lactente no período neonatal.

per·i·na·tol·o·gist (per-i-nā-tol′ō-jist). Perinatologista; um obstetra subespecializado em perinatologia.

per·i·na·tol·o·gy (per-i-nā-tol′ō-jē). Perinatologia; subespecialidade da obstetrícia que cuida da mãe e do feto durante a gravidez, o trabalho de parto e o parto, sobretudo quando a mãe e/ou o feto correm alto risco de apresentar complicações. SIN perinatal medicine.

per·i·ne·al (per′i-nē′ăl). Perineal; relativo ao períneo.

perineo-. Perineo-; o períneo. [L. do G. *perineos, perinaion*]

perineocele

per·i·ne·o·cele (per-i-nē´ō-sēl). Perineocele; uma hérnia na região perineal, seja entre o reto e a vagina ou entre o reto e a bexiga, ou paralela ao reto. [perineo- + G. *kēlē*, hérnia]

per·i·ne·om·e·ter (per'i-nē-om´ē-ter). Perineômetro; instrumento usado para medir a força de contrações musculares voluntárias do períneo. [perineo- + G. *metron*, medida]

per·i·ne·o·plas·ty (per-i-nē´ō-plas-tē). Perineoplastia; cirurgia plástica do períneo. [perineum + G. *plastos*, formado]

per·i·ne·or·rha·phy (per-i-nē-ōr´a-fē). Perineorrafia; sutura do períneo, realizada na perineoplastia. [perineum + G. *rhaphē*, sutura]

per·i·ne·o·scro·tal (per-i-nē´ō-skrō´tal). Perineoescrotal; relativo ao períneo e ao escroto.

per·i·ne·os·to·my (per-i-nē-os´tō-mē). Perineostomia; uretrostomia através do períneo. [perineo- + G. *stoma*, boca]

per·i·ne·o·syn·the·sis (per'i-nē-ō-sin´thē-sis). Perineossíntese; termo raramente usado para perineoplastia em um caso de extensa laceração do períneo.

per·i·ne·ot·o·my (per-i-nē-ot´ō-mē). Perineotomia; incisão do períneo para facilitar o parto. VER TAMBÉM episiotomy.

per·i·ne·o·vag·i·nal (per-i-nē´ō-vaj'i-nal). Perineovaginal; relativo ao períneo e à vagina.

per·i·neph·ri·al (per'i-nef´rē-al). Perinéfrico; relativo ao perinefro.

per·i·neph·ric (per'i-nef´rik). Perinéfrico; que circunda o rim no todo ou em parte. SIN circumrenal, perirenal.

per·i·neph·ri·tis (per'i-ne-frī´tis). Perinefrite; inflamação do tecido perinéfrico.

per·i·neph·ri·um, pl. **per·i·neph·ria** (per'i-nef´rē-um, -nef´rē-a). Perinefro; o tecido conjuntivo e a gordura que circundam o rim. [peri- + G. *nephros*, rim]

per·i·ne·um, pl. **per·i·nea** (per'i-nē´um, -nē´a). [TA]. Períneo. **1.** [NA]. A área situada entre as coxas, que se estende do cóccix até o púbis e está abaixo do diafragma pélvico. **2.** A superfície externa do tendão central do períneo, situada entre a vulva e o ânus, na mulher, e entre o escroto e o ânus, no homem. [L. do G. *perineon, perinaion*]
  watering-can p., p. em regador; períneo crivado de fístulas resultantes de estenose uretral.

per·i·neu·ral (per'i-noo´ral). Perineural; que circunda um nervo. [peri- + G. *neuron*, nervo]

per·i·neu·ri·al (per'i-noo´rē-al). Perineural; relativo ao perineuro.

per·i·neu·ri·tis (per'i-noo-rī´tis). Perineurite; inflamação do perineuro. VER TAMBÉM adventitial *neuritis*.

per·i·neu·ri·um, pl. **per·i·neu·ria** (per-i-noo´rē-um, -rē-a). Perineuro; uma das estruturas de sustentação dos troncos nervosos periféricos, consistindo em camadas de células achatadas e tecido conjuntivo colágeno, que circundam os fascículos nervosos e formam a principal barreira à difusão no nervo; juntamente com o endoneuro e o epineuro, forma o estroma do nervo periférico. [L. de peri- + G. *neuron*, nervo]

per·i·nu·cle·ar (per-i-noo´klē-ar). Perinuclear; que circunda um núcleo. SIN circumnuclear.

per·i·oc·u·lar (per-i-ok´u-lar). Periocular. SIN circumocular.

pe·ri·od (pēr´ē-od). Período. **1.** Determinada duração ou divisão do tempo. **2.** Um dos estágios de uma doença, p. ex., período de incubação, período de convalescença. VER TAMBÉM stage, phase. **3.** Termo coloquial para menstruação. **4.** Qualquer uma das linhas horizontais dos elementos químicos na tabela periódica. [G. *periodos*, um caminho circular, um ciclo, de *peri*, ao redor, + *hodos*, caminho]
  absolute refractory p., p. refratário absoluto; o p. após a excitação quando nenhuma resposta é possível, independentemente da intensidade do estímulo.
  amblyogenic p., p. ambliogênico; p. durante o início do desenvolvimento visual, quando o sistema neurossensorial visual é vulnerável a desenvolver ambliopia por formação de imagem borrada na retina e/ou supressão cortical bilateral (como na ambliopia estrábica, strabismic *amblyopia*). SIN critical p. (3).
  critical p., p. crítico; **(1)** nas primeiras horas após o nascimento, o p. de máxima capacidade de gravação na memória; o p. antes e depois do qual é difícil ou impossível gravar na memória; **(2)** em animais, um p. após o nascimento no qual os processos subjacentes à capacidade de socialização são ativados ou gravados; **(3)** p. ambliogênico. SIN amblyogenic p.
  eclipse p., p. de eclipse; o tempo entre a infecção por (ou indução de) um bacteriófago, ou outro vírus, e o surgimento de um vírus maduro dentro da célula; um p. de tempo durante o qual a infectividade viral não pode ser recuperada. SIN eclipse phase.
  effective refractory p., p. refratário efetivo; o p. durante o qual pode haver impulsos, mas eles são demasiado fracos para serem conduzidos; o maior intervalo entre estímulos adequados, terminando imediatamente antes do tempo necessário para permitir que uma resposta propagada seja evocada em um tecido pelo segundo estímulo; diferente do p. refratário funcional porque é uma medida do intervalo de estímulo, e não do intervalo de resposta.
  ejection p., p. de ejeção. SIN sphygmic *interval*.
  extrinsic incubation p. (eks-trin´sik). p. de incubação extrínseco; tempo necessário para o desenvolvimento de um agente patológico em um vetor, desde

period

o momento da aquisição do agente até o momento em que o vetor torna-se capaz de transmiti-lo.
  fertile p., p. fértil; o período em um ciclo menstrual regular durante o qual a concepção é mais provável.
  functional refractory p., p. refratário funcional; o mínimo intervalo possível entre respostas sucessivas à estimulação de um tecido.
  gap$_1$ p., p. de intervalo 1; o p. do ciclo celular após a divisão celular, em que há síntese de RNA e proteína; pode durar algumas horas em um tecido que cresce rapidamente, ou toda a vida em células que não se renovam, como as células nervosas. SIN gap$_1$ phase, postmitotic phase.
  gap$_2$ p., p. de intervalo 2; o p. no ciclo celular em que a síntese de DNA é concluída, mas antes de começar a mitose. SIN gap$_2$ phase, premitotic phase.
  gap$_0$ p., p. de intervalo 0; fase de uma célula que não está mais no ciclo celular e, portanto, é, ao menos temporariamente, incapaz de se dividir. SIN gap$_0$ phase.
  incubation p., p. de incubação; **(1)** intervalo de tempo entre a invasão do corpo por um organismo infectante e o surgimento do primeiro sinal ou sintoma que causa. SIN incubative stage, latent p. (2), latent stage, stage of invasion. **(2)** No vetor de uma doença, o p. entre a entrada do organismo da doença e o momento em que o vetor é capaz de transmitir a doença para outro hospedeiro humano.
  induction p., p. de indução; o p. necessário para que um agente específico produza uma doença; o intervalo entre a ação causal de um fator e o início da doença, p. ex., o intervalo entre a exposição à radiação e o início da leucemia; o intervalo entre uma injeção inicial de antígeno e o surgimento de anticorpos demonstráveis no sangue.
  intrapartum p., p. intraparto; em obstetrícia, o período decorrido desde o início do trabalho de parto até o fim do terceiro estágio do trabalho de parto.
  isoelectric p., p. isoelétrico; período anormal que ocorre no eletrocardiograma, entre o fim da onda S e o início da onda T, durante o qual as forças elétricas estão agindo em direções que neutralizam uma a outra, de forma que não há diferença no potencial sob os eletrodos. SIN abnormal ST segment.
  isometric p. of cardiac cycle, p. isométrico do ciclo cardíaco; aquele p. no qual as fibras musculares não se encurtam, embora o músculo cardíaco seja excitado e a pressão nos ventrículos aumente, estendendo-se do fechamento das valvas atrioventriculares até a abertura das valvas semilunares (constrição isovolumétrica) ou o inverso (relaxamento isovolumétrico). SIN isovolumic p.
  isometric contraction p., p. de contração isométrica; o tempo entre o fechamento das valvas atrioventriculares e a abertura das valvas semilunares.
  isometric relaxation p., p. de relaxamento isométrico; diástole ventricular inicial que começa com o fechamento das valvas aórtica e pulmonar e precede a abertura das valvas atrioventriculares.
  isovolumic p., p. isovolumétrico. SIN isometric p. of cardiac cycle.
  latency p., p. de latência. SIN latency *phase*.
  latent p., p. latente; **(1)** o p. decorrido entre a aplicação de um estímulo e a resposta, p. ex., contração de um músculo; **(2)** período de incubação. SIN incubation p. (1).
  masticatory silent p., p. de silêncio mastigatório; uma pausa nos padrões eletromiográficos associada aos contatos dentários durante a mastigação e a mordida; uma parte do complexo mecanismo de retroalimentação do controle mandibular envolvendo receptores no ligamento periodontal e nos músculos.
  menstrual p., p. menstrual. SIN menses.
  missed p., a ausência de menstruação no período previsto em qualquer mês.
  mitotic p., p. mitótico; o p. do ciclo celular no qual ocorrem todas as fases da mitose. SIN M phase.
  oedipal p., fase edipiana. SIN oedipal *phase*.
  preejection p., p. pré-ejeção; o intervalo entre o início do complexo QRS e a ejeção cardíaca; a sístole eletromecânica menos o tempo de ejeção.
  prepatent p., p. pré-patente; em parasitologia, o período equivalente ao período de incubação das infecções microbianas; entretanto, é biologicamente diferente porque o parasita está passando por estágios do desenvolvimento no hospedeiro.
  prodromal p., p. prodrômico; o intervalo de tempo durante o qual um processo patológico se iniciou, mas ainda não é clinicamente evidente.
  puerperal p., p. puerperal; o p. entre o fim do trabalho de parto e o retorno do aparelho reprodutor à sua condição normal; as 6 semanas após o fim do trabalho de parto.
  pulse p., p. de pulso; a recíproca do índice de repetição; p. ex., o intervalo entre os inícios de pulsos sucessivos.
  quarantine p., p. de quarentena; o p. durante o qual um indivíduo ou uma área infectada é mantida em isolamento, evitando contato com indivíduos não-infectados; pode ser qualquer p. especificado, variando com a doença em questão. O termo é derivado da palavra italiana para 40, pois o p. de isolamento das pessoas com suspeita de peste na Idade Média era de 40 dias.
  refractory p., p. refratário; **(1)** o período, após estimulação efetiva, durante o qual um tecido excitável, como o músculo cardíaco e o nervo, não responde a um estímulo de intensidade limiar (isto é, a excitabilidade é deprimida); **(2)** um período de resistência psicofisiológica temporária para estimulação sexual adicional que ocorre imediatamente após o orgasmo.
  refractory p. of electronic pacemaker, p. refratário do marcapasso eletrônico; o tempo necessário para o restabelecimento da completa sensibilidade após a detecção de atividade cardíaca ou aplicação de um impulso.

relative refractory p., p. refratário relativo; o período entre o p. refratário efetivo e o fim do p. refratário; as fibras então respondem apenas a estímulos de alta intensidade e os impulsos são conduzidos mais lentamente que o normal.

silent p., p. silencioso; (**1**) o período durante o qual não há atividade elétrica em um músculo após sua rápida descarga; (**2**) qualquer pausa em uma série contínua de eventos eletrofisiológicos.

synthesis p., p. de síntese; o p. do ciclo celular em que há síntese de DNA e histona; ocorre entre Gap_1 e Gap_2. SIN S phase.

total refractory p., p. refratário total; o p. refratário absoluto somado ao p. refratário relativo.

vulnerable p., vulnerable p. of heart, p. vulnerável, p. vulnerável do coração; um breve p., durante o ciclo cardíaco, quando é particularmente provável que os estímulos induzam atividade repetitiva, como taquicardia, *flutter* ou fibrilação, que persiste após cessar o estímulo; para o ventrículo, ocorre durante a última parte da sístole, durante o p. refratário relativo coincidente com a inscrição da última metade da onda T do eletrocardiograma.

Wenckebach p., p. de Wenckebach; uma seqüência de ciclos cardíacos no eletrocardiograma, que termina em um batimento "perdido" devido ao bloqueio AV, com os ciclos precedentes exibindo aumento progressivo dos intervalos PR; o intervalo PR, após o batimento "perdido", é novamente curto.

per·i·o·date (per-ī′-ō-dāt) Periodato; um sal do ácido periódico.

pe·ri·od·ic (pēr-ē-od′ik). Periódico. **1.** Que ocorre a intervalos regulares. **2.** Designa uma doença com exacerbações ou paroxismos que recorrem regularmente. **3.** Designa qualquer um dos vários oxiácidos do iodo.

pe·ri·od·ic ac·id (per-ī′ō-dik). Ácido periódico. **1.** HIO_4, porém encontrado em solução geralmente na forma hidratada; usado na detecção e análise de carboidratos. SIN metaperiodic acid. **2.** Qualquer um dos vários ácidos iódicos (VII) formados pela combinação de heptóxido de iodo, I_2O_7, com água.

per·i·o·dic·i·ty (pēr̄-ē-ō-dis′i-tē). Periodicidade; tendência à recorrência a intervalos regulares.

diurnal p., p. diurna; ritmo circadiano com expressão primária da periodicidade durante o dia, como na liberação de microfilárias de *Loa loa* para o sangue periférico durante o dia, com liberação muito menor à noite; associado aos hábitos diurnos do vetor, do gênero *Chrysops*.

filarial p., p. filarial; o ritmo circadiano observado no surgimento de microfilárias no sangue periférico. VER TAMBÉM diurnal p., nocturnal p.

lunar p., p. lunar; qualquer fenômeno rítmico que siga um ciclo lunar ou mensal.

malarial p., p. malarial; uma ritmicidade clínica refletida em febres periódicas e calafrios que recorrem a intervalos de aproximadamente 48 horas na malária terçã (*Plasmodium vivax* ou *P. ovale*) ou a intervalos de 72 horas na malária quartã (*P. malariae*); o ritmo dos ciclos de terçã ou de 48 horas é freqüentemente modificado na malária terçã maligna ou falcípara (*P. falciparum*); associada à liberação de merozoítas das hemácias durante esquizogonia eritrocitária, embora o mecanismo de controle para a liberação sincrônica não seja conhecido.

nocturnal p., p. noturna; ritmo circadiano com a periodicidade expressa durante a noite, como na liberação noturna de microfilárias da filária humana *Wuchereria brancrofti* para o sangue periférico; esse tipo de periodicidade é encontrado em regiões onde o mosquito vetor é uma espécie que pica à noite.

subperiodic p., p. subperiódica; um ritmo circadiano modificado no qual a periodicidade não é nítida, como em determinadas cepas não-zoonóticas de filariose malaia causada por *Brugia malayi*; como em exemplos de periodicidade filarial estrita, essa resposta está correlacionada aos hábitos de alimentação do inseto vetor (mosquito), embora o mecanismo preciso que induz essa resposta das microfilárias não esteja claramente estabelecido.

per·i·o·don·tal (per′ē-ō-don′tăl). Periodontal; ao redor de um dente. SIN paradental, pericemental, perideral. [peri- + G. *odous*, dente]

Per·i·o·don·tal Dis·ease In·dex (PDI). Índice de Doença Periodontal (IDP); índice usado para estimar o grau de doença periodontal com base na avaliação de seis dentes representativos quanto à inflamação gengival, profundidade da bolsa periodontal, cálculo e placa, atrito, mobilidade e falta de contato.

Per·i·o·don·tal In·dex (PI). Índice Periodontal; índice usado para a classificação epidemiológica da doença periodontal.

per·i·o·don·tia (per′ē-ō-don′shē-ă). **1.** Periodontos; plural de periodontium. **2.** Periodontia. SIN periodontics.

per·i·o·don·tics (per′ē-ō-don′tiks). Periodontia; periodontologia; o ramo da odontologia que estuda os tecidos normais e o tratamento de condições anormais dos tecidos imediatamente ao redor dos dentes. SIN periodontia (2). [peri- + G. *odous*, dente]

per·i·o·don·tist (per′ē-ō-don′tist). Periodontista; um dentista especializado em periodontologia.

per·i·o·don·ti·tis (per′ē-ō-don-tī′tis). Periodontite. **1.** Inflamação do periodonto. **2.** Doença inflamatória crônica do periodonto que ocorre em resposta à placa bacteriana nos dentes adjacentes; caracterizada por gengivite, destruição do osso alveolar e do ligamento periodontal, migração apical da fixação epitelial resultando na formação de bolsas periodontais e, finalmente, afrouxamento e esfoliação dos dentes. [periodontium + G. *-itis*, inflamação]

apical p., p. apical; inflamação do ligamento periodontal que circunda o ápice da raiz de um dente; geralmente é uma consequência da inflamação pulpar ou necrose.

p. com′plex, p. complexa; reabsorção vertical do processo alveolar com bolsas de profundidade desigual em dentes adjacentes, e com oclusão traumática como um fator.

juvenile p., p. juvenil; doença periodontal degenerativa de adolescentes na qual a destruição periodontal é desproporcional aos fatores irritantes locais encontrados nos dentes adjacentes; as alterações inflamatórias são superpostas, e são observadas perda óssea, migração e extrusão. São reconhecidas duas formas: 1) localizada, na qual a destruição é limitada aos incisivos e primeiros molares; e 2) generalizada, envolvendo todos os dentes. SIN periodontosis.

p. sim′plex, p. simples; reabsorção horizontal do processo alveolar com bolsas de profundidade uniforme nos dentes adjacentes; a oclusão traumática não é um fator.

suppurative p., p. supurativa; p. acompanhada por exsudato purulento.

per·i·o·don·ti·um, pl. **per·i·o·don·tia** (per′ē-ō-don′shē-ŭm, -shē-ă) [TA]. Periodonto; o tecido conjuntivo que circunda a raiz do dente e fixa-se ao seu alvéolo dental; consiste em fibras fixadas no cemento e que se estendem até o osso alveolar; os tecidos que circundam e sustentam os dentes, incluindo as gengivas, cemento, desmodonto, fibras periodontais e osso alveolar e de sustentação. SIN periodontal ligament [TA], periodontal membrane*, alveolar periosteum, periosteum alveolare, alveolodental ligament, alveolodental membrane, gingivodental ligament, paradentium, parodontium, peridental ligament, peridental membrane, peridentium, tapetum alveoli. [L. de peri- + G. *odous*, dente]

per·i·o·don·to·cla·sia (per′ē-ō-don-tō-klā′zē-ă). Periodontoclasia; destruição dos tecidos periodontais, gengiva, pericemento, osso alveolar e cemento. SIN periodontolysis. [periodontium + *klasis*, ruptura]

per·i·o·don·tol·y·sis (par′ē-ō-don-tol′i-sis). Periodontólise. SIN periodontoclasia. [periodontium + G. *lysis*, dissolução]

per·i·o·don·to·sis (per′ē-ō-don-tō′sis). Periodontose. SIN juvenile periodontitis. [periodontium + G. *-osis*, condição]

per·i·om·phal·ic (per′ē-om-fal′ik). Perionfálico. SIN periumbilical. [peri- + G. *omphalos*, umbigo)

per·i·o·nych·ia (per-ē-ō-nik′ē-ă). **1.** Paroníquia; panarício; inflamação do perioníquio. **2.** Perioníquios; plural de perionychium.

per·i·o·nych·i·um, pl. **per·i·o·nych·ia** (per-ē-ō-nik′ē-ŭm, -nik′ē-ă). Perioníquio. SIN eponychium (2). [peri- + G. *onyx*, unha]

per·i·on·yx (per-ē-on′iks). [TA]. Perioníquio; remanescente do eponíquio que permanece na prega estreita superposta à parte proximal da lúnula, surgindo no oitavo mês de gravidez e permanecendo durante toda a vida. [peri- + G. *onyx*, unha]

per·i·o·o·pho·ri·tis (per′ē-ō-of′ō-rī′tis). Periooforite; inflamação do revestimento peritoneal do ovário. SIN periovaritis. [peri- + L. mod. *oophoron*, ovário, + *-itis*, inflamação]

per·i·o·o·pho·ro·sal·pin·gi·tis (per′ē-ō-of′ō-rō-sal-pin-jī′tis). Periooforossalpingite; inflamação do peritônio e de outros tecidos ao redor do ovário e do oviduto. SIN perisalpingoovaritis. [peri- + L. mod. *oophoron*, ovário, + *salpinx*, trompa, + *-itis*, inflamação]

per·i·op·er·a·tive (per-ē-op′er-ă-tiv). Perioperatório; por volta do momento da cirurgia. SIN paraoperative.

per·i·oph·thal·mic (per′ē-of-thal′mik). Perioftálmico. SIN circumocular. [peri- + G. *ophthalmos*, olho]

per·i·oph·thal·mi·tis (per′ē-of-thal-mī′tis). Perioftalmite; inflamação dos tecidos ao redor do olho.

per·i·o·ral (per-ē-ō′răl). Perioral; ao redor da boca. SIN circumoral, peristomal, peristomatous.

per·i·or·bit (per-ē-ōr′bit). Periórbita. SIN periorbita.

pe·ri·or·bi·ta (per′ē-ōr′bi-tă). [TA]. Periórbita; o periósteo da órbita. SIN periorbit, periorbital membrane. [peri- + L. *orbita*, órbita]

per·i·or·bi·tal (per-ē-ōr′bi-tăl). Periorbital. **1.** Relativo à periórbita. **2.** SIN circumorbital.

per·i·or·chi·tis (per′ē-ōr-kī′tis). Periorquite; inflamação da túnica vaginal do testículo. [peri- + G. *orchis*, testículo, + *-itis*, inflamação]

p. hemorrha′gica, p. hemorrágica; hematocele crônica da túnica vaginal do testículo.

per·i·ost (per′ē-ost). Periósteo. SIN periosteum.

pe·ri·os·tea (per-ē-os′tē-ă). Periósteos; plural de periosteum.

per·i·os·te·al (per-ē-os′tē-ăl). Periosteal; relativo ao periósteo. SIN periosteous.

per·i·os·te·i·tis (per′ē-oste-ī′tis). Periosteíte. SIN periostitis.

periosteo-. Periósteo-; o periósteo. [L. mod. *periosteum*]

per·i·os·te·o·ma (per′ē-os′tē-ō′mă). Periosteoma; uma neoplasia derivada do periósteo. SIN periosteophyte, periostoma.

per·i·os·te·o·med·ul·li·tis (per-ē-os′tē-ō-med-ŭ-lī′tis). Periosteomedulite. SIN periosteomyelitis. [periosteo- + L. *medulla*, medula óssea, + G. *-itis*, inflamação]

per·i·os·te·o·my·e·li·tis (per-ē-os′tē-ō-mī-ĕ-lī′tis). Periosteomielite; inflamação de todo o osso, com o periósteo e a medula óssea. SIN periosteomedullitis. [periosteo- + G. *myelos*, medula óssea, + *-itis*, inflamação]

per·i·os·te·op·a·thy (par′ē-os-tē-op′ă-thē). Periosteopatia; qualquer doença do periósteo.

per·i·os·te·o·phyte (per-ē-os′tē-ō-fit). Periosteófito. SIN periosteoma. [periosteo- + G. *phyton*, crescimento]

per·i·os·te·o·sis (per′ē-os-tē-ō′sis). Periosteose; a formação de um periosteoma. SIN periostosis.
per·i·os·te·o·tome (per′ē-os′tē-ō-tōm). Periosteótomo; lâmina forte, em forma de bisturi, para cortar o periósteo. SIN periostotome.
per·i·os·te·ot·o·my (per′ē-os-tē-ot′ō-mē). Periosteotomia; a incisão através do periósteo até o osso. SIN periostotomy. [periosteo- + G. *tomē*, incisão]
per·i·os·te·ous (per-ē-os′tē-us). Periósteo. SIN periosteal.
per·i·os·te·um, pl. **per·i·os·tea** (per-ē-os′tē-um, -ă) [TA]. Periósteo; a membrana fibrosa espessa que cobre toda a superfície de um osso, exceto sua cartilagem articular. Em ossos jovens, consiste em duas camadas: uma camada celular interna osteogênica, que forma novo tecido ósseo, e uma camada de tecido conjuntivo fibroso externa, que conduz os vasos sanguíneos e os nervos que suprem o osso; em ossos mais velhos, a camada osteogênica está reduzida. VER TAMBÉM perichondral *bone*. SIN periost. [L. mod. do G. *periosteon*, neutro de adj. *periosteos*, ao redor dos ossos, de *peri*, ao redor, + *osteon*, osso]

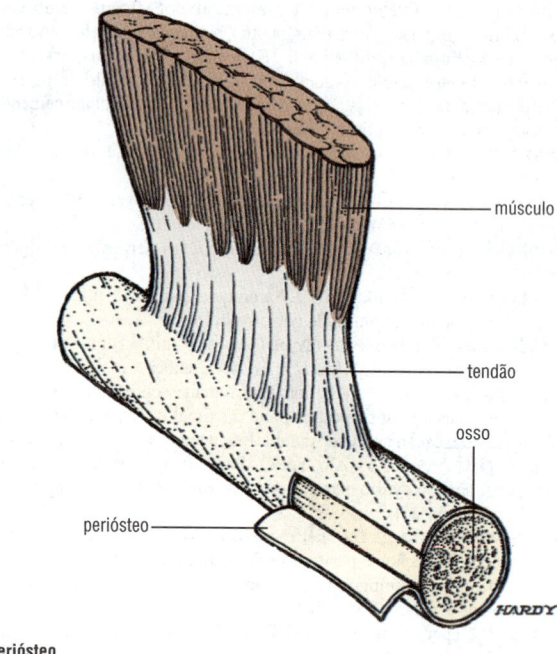

periósteo

alveolar p., p. alveola're, periodonto. SIN periodontium.
p. cra'nii [TA], pericrânio. SIN pericranium.
per·i·os·ti·tis (per′ē-os-tī′tis). Periostite; inflamação do periósteo. SIN periosteitis.
per·i·os·to·ma (per′ē-os-tō′mă). Periostoma. SIN periosteoma.
per·i·os·to·sis, pl. **per·i·os·to·ses** (per′ē-os-tō′sis, -sēz). Periostose. SIN periosteosis.
per·i·os·tos·te·i·tis (per-ē-os′tos-tē-ī′tis). Periosteosteíte; inflamação de um osso com envolvimento do periósteo. [periosteum + G. *osteon*, osso, + *-itis*, inflamação]
per·i·os·to·tome (per-ē-os′tō-tōm). Periostótomo. SIN periosteotome.
per·i·os·tot·o·my (per-ē-os-tot′ō-mē). Periosteotomia. SIN periosteotomy.
per·i·ot·ic (per′ē-ō′tik, -ot′ik). Periótico; que circunda a orelha interna; referente à porção petrosa do osso temporal, ou aos espaços e tecidos no labirinto ósseo que circundam o labirinto membranáceo. [peri- + G. *ous*, ouvido]
per·i·o·va·ri·tis (per′ē-ō-vă-rī′tis). Periovarite. SIN perioophoritis.
per·i·o·vu·lar (per′ē-ō′vū-lăr). Periovular; que circunda o óvulo.
per·i·pach·y·men·in·gi·tis (per′i-pak′ē-men-in-jī′tis). Peripaquimeningite; inflamação da área entre a dura-máter e o revestimento ósseo do sistema nervoso central. [peri- + *pachymeninx* (dura-máter) + G. *-itis*, inflamação]
per·i·pan·cre·a·ti·tis (per′i-pan′krē-ă-tī′tis). Peripancreatite; inflamação do revestimento peritoneal do pâncreas.
per·i·pap·il·lary (per-i-pap′i-lār-ē). Peripapilar; que circunda uma papila.
per·i·pa·tet·ic (per′i-pă-tet′ik). Peripatético; perambulando; passeando; usado antigamente para descrever um paciente com febre tifóide leve. [G. *peripatēsis*, passear]
per·i·pe·ni·al (per-i-pē′nē-ăl). Peripeniano; que circunda o pênis.
per·i·pha·ryn·ge·al (per′i-fă-rin′jē-ăl). Perifaríngeo; que circunda a faringe.
pe·riph·er·ad (pĕ-rif′ĕ-rad). Em direção à periferia. [G. *periphereia*, periferia, + L. *ad*, para]
pe·riph·e·ral (pĕ-rif′ĕ-răl) [TA]. Periférico. **1.** Relativo a, ou situado na periferia. **2.** Situado mais próximo da periferia de um órgão ou parte do corpo em relação a um ponto de referência específico; oposto de central. SIN peripheralis [TA], eccentric (3).
pe·riph·e·ra·lis (pĕ-rif-ē-ră′lis). [TA]. Periférico. SIN peripheral.
pe·riph·e·rin (pĕri-fer-in). Periferina; uma glicoproteína que, aparentemente, é necessária para manter o formato das membranas do disco do segmento externo de bastonetes e cones; muitos pesquisadores acreditam que um defeito na periferina está associado a determinados tipos de cegueira.
pe·riph·e·ro·cen·tral (pĕ-rif′ē-rō-sen′trăl). Periferocentral; relativo à periferia e ao centro do corpo ou de qualquer parte.
pe·riph·e·ry (pĕ-rif′ĕ-rē). Periferia. **1.** A parte de um corpo distante do centro; a parte ou superfície externa. **2.** SIN denture *border*. [G. *periphereia*, de *peri*, ao redor, + *pherō*, conduzir]
per·i·phle·bit·ic (per′i-fle-bit′ik). Periflebítico; relativo à periflebite.
per·i·phle·bi·tis (per′i-fle-bī′tis). Periflebite; inflamação da camada externa de uma veia ou dos tecidos que a circundam. [peri- + G. *phleps*, veia, + *-itis*, inflamação]
Per·i·pla·ne·ta (per-i-pla-nē′tă). Gênero de baratas grandes que inclui diversas pragas domésticas encontradas em qualquer lugar onde haja alimento disponível, principalmente em áreas úmidas protegidas. *P. americana* (barata-americana), uma espécie muito grande que tem o peito marrom, com 30–40 mm de comprimento, provavelmente nativa da África, mas agora de distribuição mundial; a *P. fuliginosa* (a barata castanho-enegrecida) é uma praga doméstica comum no leste e no sudeste dos Estados Unidos. [peri- + G. *planētēs*, nômade]
per·i·plasm (per′i-plazm). Periplasma; o espaço entre as membranas celulares e a parede celular, em bactérias Gram-negativas; contém proteínas secretadas pela célula.
pe·rip·lo·cin (pe-rip′lō-sin). Periplocina; glicosídeo cardiotônico obtido da casca e caule da *Periploca graeca* (família Asclepiadaceae), uma planta do sul da Europa. [G. *peri-plokē*, enrolado ao redor de, de *plekō*, entrelaçar, dobrar]
per·i·po·lar (per-i-pō′lăr). Peripolar; que circunda o pólo ou os pólos de qualquer corpo, ou quaisquer pólos elétricos ou magnéticos.
per·i·po·le·sis (per′i-pō-lē′sis). Peripoese; penetração de células em migração entre células teciduais fixas que, normalmente, se encontram em contato íntimo. [peri- + G. *poleomai*, perambular]
per·i·po·ri·tis (per′i-pŏ-rī′tis). Periporite; pápulas e papulovesículas miliares com infecção estafilocócica; na maioria das vezes ocorre na face e em lactentes. [peri- + G. *poros*, poro, + *-itis*, inflamação]
per·i·por·tal (per-i-pōr′tăl). Periporta; que circunda a veia porta. SIN peripylic.
per·i·proc·tic (per′ē-prok′tik). Periprócico. SIN circumanal. [peri- + G. *prōktos*, ânus]
per·i·proc·ti·tis (per′i-prok-tī′tis). Periproctite; inflamação do tecido areolar ao redor do reto. SIN perirectitis.
per·i·pros·tat·ic (per′i-pros-tat′ik). Periprostático; que circunda a próstata.
per·i·pros·ta·ti·tis (per′i-pros-tă-tī′tis). Periprostatite; designação obsoleta da inflamação dos tecidos que circundam a próstata.
per·i·py·le·phle·bi·tis (per′i-pī′lē-fle-bī′tis). Peripileflebite; inflamação dos tecidos ao redor da veia porta. [peri- + G. *pylē*, portão, + *phleps*, veia, + *-itis*, inflamação]
per·i·py·lic (per′i-pī′lik). Peripílico. SIN periportal. [peri- + G. *pylē*, portal, portão]
per·i·py·lor·ic (per′i-pī-lōr′ik, -pĕ-lōr′ik). Peripilórico; que circunda o piloro.
per·i·rec·tal (per′i-rek′tăl). Perirretal; que circunda o reto.
per·i·rec·ti·tis (per′i-rek-tī′tis). Perirretite. SIN periproctitis.
per·i·re·nal (per′i-rē′năl). Perirrenal. SIN perinephric. [peri- + L. *ren*, rim]
per·i·rhi·nal (per′i-rī′năl). Perirrinal; ao redor do nariz ou da cavidade nasal. [peri- + G. *rhis*, nariz]
per·i·rhi·zo·cla·sia (per′ē-rī-zō-klā′zē-ă). Perirrizoclasia; destruição inflamatória dos tecidos situados imediatamente ao redor da raiz de um dente, isto é, pericemento, cemento e camadas próximas do osso alveolar. [peri- + G. *rhiza*, raiz, + *klasis*, destruição]
per·i·sal·pin·gi·tis (per′i-sal-pin-jī′tis). Perissalpingite; inflamação do revestimento peritoneal da tuba uterina. [peri- + G. *salpinx*, trompa, + *-itis*, inflamação]
per·i·sal·pin·go·o·va·ri·tis (per′i-sal-ping′gō-ō-vă-rī′tis). Perissalpingoovarite. SIN perioophorosalpingitis. [peri- + G. *salpinx*, trompa, + ovário + G. *-itis*, inflamação]
per·i·sal·pinx (per′i-sal′pingks). Perissalpinge; o revestimento peritoneal da tuba uterina. [peri- + G. *salpinx* (*salping*-), trompa]
per·i·scop·ic (per′i-skop′ik). Periscópico; designa aquilo que permite ver objetos de um lado e, também, no eixo direto de visão. [peri- + G. *skopeō*, ver]

per·i·sig·moi·di·tis (per′i-sig-moy-di′tis). Perissigmoidite; inflamação dos tecidos conjuntivos que circundam a flexura sigmóide, causando sinais e sintomas referidos na fossa ilíaca esquerda, semelhantes aos da peritiflite na fossa ilíaca direita. SIN pericolitis sinistra.

per·i·sin·u·ous (per′i-sin′u-ŭs). Perissinusal; que circunda um seio, principalmente um seio da dura-máter.

per·i·sper·ma·ti·tis (per′i-sper-mă-ti′tis). Periespermatite; inflamação dos tecidos ao redor do cordão espermático.
  p. sero'sa, p. serosa; hidrocele do cordão espermático.

per·i·splanch·nic (per′i-splangk′nik). Perisplâncnico; que circunda qualquer víscera. SIN perivisceral. [peri- + G. *splanchna*, víscera]

per·i·splanch·ni·tis (per′i-splangk-ni′tis). Perisplancnite; inflamação adjacente a qualquer víscera. [peri- + G. *splanchna*, víscera, + *-itis*, inflamação]

per·i·splen·ic (per-i-splen′ik). Perisplênico; ao redor do baço.

per·i·sple·ni·tis (per′i-sple-ni′tis). Perisplenite; inflamação do peritônio que recobre o baço.

per·i·spon·dyl·ic (per-i-spon-dil′ik). Perispondílico. SIN perivertebral. [peri- + G. *spondylos*, vértebra]

per·i·spon·dy·li·tis (per-i-spon-di-li′tis). Perispondilite; inflamação dos tecidos ao redor de uma vértebra. [peri- + G. *spondylos*, vértebra, + *-itis*, inflamação]

per·i·stal·sis (per-i-stal′sis). Peristalse; o movimento do intestino ou de outra estrutura tubular, caracterizado por ondas alternadas de contração circular e relaxamento do tubo que propelem o conteúdo. SIN vermicular movement. [peri- + G. *stalsis*, constrição]
  mass p., p. de massa; movimentos peristálticos forçados de curta duração, que ocorrem apenas três ou quatro vezes ao dia e que deslocam o conteúdo do intestino grosso de uma divisão para a seguinte, como do colo ascendente para o colo transverso. SIN mass movement.
  reversed p., p. inversa; onda de contração intestinal em uma direção inversa ao normal, pela qual o conteúdo intestinal é forçado para trás. SIN antiperistalsis.

per·i·stal·tic (per-i-stal′tik). Peristáltico; relativo à peristalse.

pe·ris·ta·sis (pĕ-ris′tă-sis). Peristasia; fases de inatividade de vasoconstrição na inflamação. SIN peristatic hyperemia. [peri- + G. *stasis*, permanecer imóvel]

pe·ris·to·le (pĕ-ris′tō-lē). Perístole; a atividade tônica das paredes do estômago pela qual o órgão se contrai em torno de seu conteúdo; contrasta com as ondas peristálticas que seguem do cárdia para o piloro (peristalse). [peri- + G. *stellō*, contrair]

per·i·stol·ic (per-i-stol′ik). Peristólico; relativo à perístole.

pe·ris·to·ma (per-ris′tō-mă, per-i-stō′mă). Perístoma. SIN peristome.

per·i·sto·mal, per·i·sto·ma·tous (per′i-stō′mal, -stō′mă-tŭs). Peristomático. SIN perioral.

per·i·stome (per′i-stōm). Perístoma; sulco que parte do cistostoma no ciliado e em algumas outras formas de protozoários. SIN peristoma. [peri- + G. *stoma*, boca]

per·i·stru·mous (per′i-stroo′mŭs). Peristrumoso; situado ao redor ou próximo de um bócio. [peri- + L. *struma*, bócio]

per·i·syn·o·vi·al (per′i-si-nō′vē-al). Perissinovial; ao redor de uma membrana sinovial.

per·i·sys·tol·ic (per-i-sis-tol′ik). Perissistólico; descritivo de eventos que ocorrem antes e depois da sístole ventricular.

per·i·tec·to·my (per′i-tek′tō-mē). Peritectomia. 1. A remoção de uma fita paracorneana da conjuntiva para alívio de doença da córnea. 2. SIN circumcision (2). [peri- + G. *ektomē*, excisão]

pe·ri·ten·di·ne·um, pl. **pe·ri·ten·di·nea** (per-i-ten-din′ē-ŭm, -ē-ŭ). Peritendíneo; uma das bainhas fibrosas que circundam os feixes primários de fibras em um tendão. [L. de peri- + G. *tenōn*, tendão]

per·i·ten·di·ni·tis (per′i-ten-di-ni′tis). Peritendinite; inflamação da bainha de um tendão. SIN peritenonitis, peritenontitis.
  p. calca'rea, p. calcária; depósito de cálcio (cretáceo) em torno de um tendão.
  p. sero'sa, p. serosa. SIN ganglion (2).

per·i·ten·on (per′i-ten-on). Peritendão. SIN tendinous sheath of extensor carpi ulnaris muscle. [peri- + G. *tenōn*, tendão]

per·i·ten·on·ti·tis (per′i-ten-on-ti′tis). Peritendinite. SIN peritendinitis.

per·i·the·ci·um, pl. **per·i·the·cia** (per-i-thē′sē-ŭm, -sē-ă). Peritécio; em fungos, um ascocarpo em forma de cantil, um dos muitos formatos de estruturas que contêm ascos e ascosporos; útil como auxiliar na identificação de um fungo. [peri- + G. *thēkē*, cantil]

per·i·the·li·um, pl. **per·i·the·lia** (per-i-thē′lē-ŭm, -ă). Peritélio; o tecido conjuntivo que circunda vasos menores e capilares. [peri- + G. *thēlē*, mamilo]
  Eberth p., p. de Eberth; uma camada incompleta de células de tecido conjuntivo que encerra os capilares sanguíneos.

per·i·tho·rac·ic (per-i-thō-ras′ik). Peritorácico; que circunda ou envolve o tórax.

per·i·thy·roi·di·tis (per′i-thi-roy-di′tis). Peritireoidite; inflamação da cápsula ou dos tecidos que circundam a tireóide.

pe·rit·o·mist (pe-rit′ō-mist). Peritomista; aquele que realiza circuncisão.

pe·rit·o·my (pe-rit′ō-mē). Peritomia; incisão ao redor da córnea através da conjuntiva. [G. *peritomē*, de peri, ao redor, + *tomē*, incisão]

per·i·to·ne·al (per′i-tō-nē′al). Peritoneal; relativo ao peritônio.

per·i·to·ne·al·gia (per′i-tō-nē-al′jē-ă). Peritonealgia; termo raramente usado para designar a dor no peritônio. [peritoneum + G. *algos*, dor]

△ **peritoneo-**. Peritoneo-; o peritônio. [L. *peritoneum*]

per·i·to·ne·o·cen·te·sis (per′i-tō-nē′ō-sen-tē′sis). Peritoneocentese; paracentese do abdome. [peritoneum + G. *kentēsis*, punção]

per·i·to·ne·oc·ly·sis (per′i-tō-nē-ok′li-sis). Peritoneoclise; irrigação da cavidade abdominal. [peritoneum, + G. *klysis*, lavagem]

per·i·to·ne·op·a·thy (per′i-tō-nē-op′a-thē). Peritoneopatia; termo raramente usado para designar inflamação ou outra doença do peritônio. [peritoneum, + *pathos*, que sofre]

per·i·to·ne·o·per·i·car·di·al (per′i-tō-nē′ō-per′i-kar′dē-al). Peritoneopericárdico; relativo ao peritônio e ao pericárdio.

per·i·to·ne·o·pexy (per′i-tō-nē-ō-pek-sē). Peritoneopexia; uma suspensão ou fixação do peritônio. [peritoneum + G. *pēxis*, fixação]

per·i·to·ne·o·plas·ty (per′i-tō-nē′ō-plas-tē). Peritoneoplastia; desprendimento de aderências e revestimento das superfícies desnudas com peritônio para evitar a formação de novas aderências. [peritoneum + G. *plastos*, formado]

per·i·to·ne·o·scope (per′i-tō-nē′ō-skōp). Peritoneoscópio. SIN laparoscope. [peritoneum + G. *skopeō*, ver]

per·i·to·ne·os·co·py (per′i-tō-nē-os′kō-pē). Peritoneoscopia; exame do conteúdo do peritônio com um peritoneoscópio introduzido através da parede abdominal. VER laparoscopy. SIN celioscopy, ventroscopy.

per·i·to·ne·ot·o·my (per′i-tō-nē-ot′ō-mē). Peritoneotomia; incisão do peritônio. [peritoneum + G. *tomē*, incisão]

per·i·to·ne·um, pl. **pe·ri·to·nea** (per′i-tō-nē′ŭm, -ă). [TA]. Peritônio; o saco seroso, consistindo em mesotélio e em uma camada fina de tecido conjuntivo irregular, reveste a cavidade abdominal e cobre a maioria das vísceras nela contidas; forma dois sacos: o saco peritoneal (ou maior) e a bolsa omental (saco menor) unidos pelo forame epiplóico. SIN membrana abdominis. [L. mod. do G. *peritonaion*, de *periteinō*, estender sobre]
  parietal p. [TA], p. parietal; a camada de p. que reveste as paredes abdominais. SIN p. parietale [TA].
  p. parieta'le [TA], p. parietal. SIN parietal p.
  urogenital p. [TA], p. urogenital; p. da cavidade pélvica, incluindo as pregas e fossas formadas por ele. SIN p. urogenitale [TA].
  p. urogenitale [TA], p. urogenital. SIN urogenital p.
  visceral p. [TA], p. visceral; a camada de p. que reveste os órgãos abdominais. SIN p. viscerale [TA].
  p. viscera'le [TA], p. visceral. SIN visceral p.

per·i·to·ni·tis (per′i-tō-ni′tis). Peritonite; inflamação do peritônio.
  adhesive p., p. adesiva; forma de p. na qual ocorre um exsudato fibrinoso, provocando aderência entre o intestino e vários outros órgãos.
  benign paroxysmal p., p. paroxística benigna. SIN familial paroxysmal polyserositis.
  bile p., p. biliar; inflamação do peritônio causada pelo extravasamento de bile para a cavidade peritoneal. SIN choleperitonitis.
  chemical p., p. química; p. causada pelo extravasamento de bile, do conteúdo do trato gastrointestinal ou do suco pancreático para a cavidade peritoneal; o conteúdo do líquido causa lesão química, choque e exsudação peritoneal antes da ocorrência de qualquer infecção associada.
  chyle p., p. quilosa; p. causada por quilo livre na cavidade peritoneal.
  circumscribed p., p. circunscrita. SIN localized p.
  p. defor'mans, p. deformante; p. crônica na qual o espessamento da membrana e as aderências retráteis causam encurtamento do mesentério e torção e retração do intestino.
  diaphragmatic p., p. diafragmática; p. que afeta principalmente a superfície peritoneal do diafragma.
  diffuse p., p. difusa. SIN general p.
  p. encap'sulans, p. encapsulante; p. fibrosa ou adesiva localizada que permanece após uma p. generalizada quase ter desaparecido; é caracterizada por dor, constipação e um tumor palpável.
  fibrocaseous p., p. fibrocaseosa; p. caracterizada por caseificação e fibrose, geralmente causada pelo bacilo da tuberculose.
  gas p., p. gasosa; inflamação do peritônio acompanhada por acúmulo intraperitoneal de gás.
  general p., p. geral; p. em toda a cavidade peritoneal. SIN diffuse p.
  localized p., p. localizada; p. limitada a uma região demarcada da cavidade peritoneal. SIN circumscribed p.
  meconium p., p. meconial; p. causada por perfuração intestinal no feto ou no recém-nascido; associada à obstrução congênita ou causada por fibrose cística.
  pelvic p., p. pélvica; inflamação generalizada do peritônio circundando o útero e as tubas de Falópio. SIN pelvioperitonitis, pelviperitonitis.

periodic p., p. periódica. SIN familial paroxysmal *polyserositis*.
productive p., p. produtiva. SIN pachyperitonitis.
tuberculous p., p. tuberculosa; p. causada pelo bacilo da tuberculose.
per·i·ton·sil·lar (per'i-ton'si-lar). Peritonsilar; ao redor de uma tonsila ou das tonsilas.
per·i·ton·sil·li·tis (per'i-ton'si-lī'tis). Peritonsilite; inflamação do tecido conjuntivo acima e atrás da tonsila.
per·i·tra·che·al (per-i-trā'kē-al). Peritraqueal; ao redor da traquéia.
pe·rit·ri·chal, pe·rit·ri·chate, per·i·trich·ic (pe-rit'ri-kal, -rit'ri-kāt, per-i-trik'ik). Peritríquio. SIN peritrichous (2).
Per·i·trich·i·da (per-i-trik'i-da). Ordem de ciliados (subclasse Peritrichia, filo Ciliophora) caracterizada por um formato cilíndrico, com os cílios geralmente limitados à zona que circunda a abertura da boca; inclui a subordem Mobilina, cujos membros são todos ecto- ou endoparasitas de invertebrados e vertebrados aquáticos, cujo gênero *Trichodina* inclui parasitas das guelras de peixes economicamente importantes. [peri- + G. *thrix*, pêlo]
pe·rit·ri·chous (pe-rit'ri-kŭs). Peritríquio. **1.** Relativo aos cílios ou outros órgãos apendiculares que se projetam da periferia de uma célula. **2.** Que possui flagelos uniformemente distribuídos sobre uma célula; usado particularmente em relação a bactérias. SIN peritrichal, peritrichate, peritrichic. [peri- + G. *thrix*, pêlo]
per·i·tro·chan·ter·ic (per'i-trō'kan-ter'ik). Peritrocantérico; ao redor de um trocânter.
per·i·typh·lic (per'i-tif'lik). Peritíflico. SIN pericecal. [peri- + G. *typhlon*, ceco]
per·i·typh·li·tis (per'ī-tif-lī'tis). Peritiflite; inflamação do peritônio que circunda o ceco.
perityphlitis actinomyco'tica (per'ī-tif-lī-tis ak'ti-nō-mī-kot-i-ka), p. actinomicótica, infecção abdominal, predominantemente ao redor do ceco, por Actinomycetes, geralmente *Actinomyces israelii*.
per·i·um·bil·i·cal (per'i-ŭm-bil'i-kal). Periumbilical; ao redor ou próximo do umbigo. SIN periomphalic.
per·i·un·gual (per'i-ŭng'gwal). Periungueal; que circunda uma unha; que envolve as pregas ungueais. [peri- + L. *unguis*, unha]
per·i·u·re·ter·al, per·i·u·re·ter·ic (per'i-ū-rē'ter-al, -ū're-ter'ik). Periureteral; que circunda um ou ambos os ureteres.
per·i·u·re·ter·i·tis (per'i-ū-rē'ter-ī'tis). Periureterite; inflamação dos tecidos ao redor de um ureter. [peri- + ureter + G. *-itis*, inflamação]
p. plas'tica, p. plástica. SIN retroperitoneal *fibrosis*.
per·i·u·re·thral (per'i-ū-rē'thral). Periuretral; que circunda a uretra.
per·i·u·re·thri·tis (per'i-ū-rē-thrī'tis). Periuretrite; inflamação dos tecidos ao redor da uretra. [peri- + urethra + G. *-itis*, inflamação]
per·i·u·ter·ine (per'i-ū'ter-in). Periuterino. SIN perimetric (1).
per·i·u·vu·lar (per'i-ū'vū-lar). Periuvular; ao redor da úvula.
per·i·vag·i·ni·tis (per'i-vaj-i-nī'tis). Perivaginite; inflamação do tecido conjuntivo ao redor da vagina. SIN pericolpitis.
per·i·vas·cu·lar (per'i-vas'kū-lar). Perivascular; que circunda um vaso sanguíneo ou linfático. SIN circumvascular. [peri- + L. *vasculum*, vaso]
per·i·vas·cu·li·tis (per'i-vas-koo-lī'tis). Perivasculite. SIN periangitis.
per·i·ve·nous (per-i-vē'nŭs). Perivenoso; que circunda uma veia.
per·i·ver·te·bral (per-i-ver'te-bral). Perivertebral; ao redor de uma vértebra ou vértebras. SIN perispondylic.
per·i·ves·i·cal (per-i-ves'i-kal). Perivesical. SIN pericystic. [peri- + L. *vesica*, bexiga]
per·i·vis·cer·al (per-ivis'er-al). Perivisceral. SIN perisplanchnic.
per·i·vis·cer·i·tis (per'i-vis-er-ī'tis). Periviscerite; inflamação ao redor de qualquer víscera. [peri- + L. *viscera*, órgãos internos, + G. *-itis*, inflamação]
per·i·vi·tel·line (per'i-vi-tel'in, -īn). Perivitelino; que circunda o vitelo. [peri- + L. *vitellus*, vitelo]
per·i·win·kle (per'i-wing-kl). *Vinca rosea*. SIN *Vinca rosea*.
per·kin·ism (per'kin-izm). Perkinismo; forma de charlatanismo que se propõe a tratar doenças pela aplicação de metais com propriedades magnéticas e mágicas.
Perkins, Elisha, médico norte-americano, 1741–1799. VER perkinism.
per·lèche (per-lesh'). Perlèche. SIN angular *cheilitis*. [Fr. *per*, intensivo, + *lécher*, lamber]
Perlia, Richard, oftalmologista alemão do século XIX. VER P. *nucleus*; convergence *nucleus* of P.
per·lin·gual (per-ling'gwal). Perlingual; através ou por meio da língua, designando um método de medicação. [L. *per*, através, + *lingua*, língua]
Perls, Max, patologista alemão, 1843–1881. VER P. Prussian blue *stain, test*.
per·man·ga·nate (per-mang'ga-nāt). Permanganato; um sal do ácido permangânico. Usado antigamente em tentativas (provavelmente malsucedidas) de oxidar e, assim, detoxificar venenos alcalóides.
per·man·gan·ic ac·id (per-mang-gan'ik). Ácido permangânico; um ácido, HMnO₄, derivado do manganês, que forma permanganatos com bases. VER TAMBÉM *potassium* permanganate.
per·me·a·bil·i·ty (per'mē-a-bil'i-tē). Permeabilidade; a propriedade de ser permeável.

per·me·a·ble (per'mē-a-bl). Permeável; que permite a passagem de substâncias (p. ex., líquidos, gases, calor), como através de uma membrana ou de outra estrutura. SIN pervious. [L. *permeabilis* (ver permeate)]
per·me·ant (per'mē-ant). Capaz de atravessar determinada membrana semipermeável. [L. *permeabilis* (ver permeate)]
per·me·ase (per'mē-ās). Permease; qualquer um de um grupo de portadores ligados à membrana (enzimas) que realiza o transporte de soluto através de uma membrana semipermeável; esse termo não é tipicamente usado com eucariotas.
per·me·ate (per'mē-āt). Permear. **1.** Atravessar uma membrana ou outra estrutura, tipicamente por difusão. **2.** Aquele que pode atravessar dessa forma. [L. *permeo*, atravessar]
per·me·a·tion (per-mē-ā'shŭn). Permeação; o processo de se disseminar através ou penetrar, como a extensão de uma neoplasia maligna por proliferação das células continuamente ao longo dos vasos sanguíneos ou linfáticos. [L. *per-meo*, pp. *-meatus*, atravessar]
per·nic·i·o·si·form (per-nish'ē-o'si-fōrm). Perniciosiforme; termo raramente usado que significa aparentemente pernicioso, designando uma condição ou doença que parece ser perniciosa ou maligna.
per·ni·cious (per-nish'ŭs). Pernicioso; destrutivo; prejudicial; designa uma doença de caráter grave e geralmente fatal, sem tratamento apropriado. [L. *perniciosus*, destrutivo, de *pernicies*, destruição]
per·ni·o·sis (per-nē-ō'sis). Perniose. SIN chilblain. [L. *pernio*, frieira, + G. *-osis*, condição]
△ **pero-**. Mutilado, malformado. [G. *pēros*]
pe·ro·bra·chi·us (pē-rō-brā'kē-ŭs). Perobráquio; indivíduo com uma malformação congênita de uma ou ambas as mãos e antebraços. [pero- + G. *brachiōn*, braço]
pe·ro·ceph·a·lus (pē-rō-sef'a-lŭs). Perocéfalo; um indivíduo com defeito congênito da face e da cabeça. [pero- + G. *kephalē*, cabeça]
pe·ro·chi·rus (pē-rō-kī'rus). Peroquiro; indivíduo com uma malformação congênita de uma ou de ambas as mãos. [pero- + G. *cheir*, mão]
pe·ro·dac·ty·ly, pe·ro·dac·tyl·ia (pē-rō-dak'ti-lē, -dak-til'ē-a). Perodactilia; malformação congênita dos dedos das mãos ou dos pés. [pero- + G. *daktylos*, dedo da mão ou do pé]
per·o·gen (per'ō-jen). Perogênio; uma preparação de perborato de sódio que, quando misturado ao catalisador associado, libera 10% do oxigênio no sal.
pe·ro·me·lia, pe·rom·e·ly (pē-rō-mē'lē-a, pĕ-rom'e-lē). Peromelia; malformações congênitas graves dos membros, incluindo ausência da mão ou do pé. [pero- + G. *melos*, membro]
per·o·ne (per-ō'nē). Fíbula. SIN fibula. [G. *peronē*, broche, o pequeno osso do braço ou da perna, a fíbula, de *peirō*, perfurar]
per·o·ne·al (per-ō-nē'al). Fibular. SIN fibular. [L. *peroneus*, do G. *peronē*, fíbula]
per·o·ne·o·tib·i·al (per'ō-nē'ō-tib'ē-al). Tibiofibular. SIN tibiofibular.
pe·ro·pus (pē'rō-pŭs). Perópode; pessoa com malformação congênita de um ou de ambos os pés. [pero- + G. *pous*, pé]
per·o·ral (per-ō'ral). Peroral; através da boca, designa um método de medicação ou uma abordagem. [L. *per*, através, + *os* (*or-*), boca]
per os (PO). Por via oral; por meio ou através da boca, designando um método de medicação. [L.]
pe·ro·splanch·nia (pē-rō-splank'nē-a). Perosplancnia; malformação congênita das vísceras. [pero- + G. *splanchnon*, víscera]
per·os·se·ous (per-os'ē-ŭs). Perósseo; através do osso. [L. *per*, através, + *os*, osso]
△ **peroxi-**. Peroxi-. VER peroxy-.
per·ox·i·das·es (per-ok'si-dās-ez) [EC subclasse 1,11]. Peroxidases; oxidorredutases que reduzem o peróxido de hidrogênio; enzimas presentes nos tecidos animais e vegetais que catalisam a desidrogenação (oxidação) de várias substâncias na presença de peróxido de hidrogênio, o qual atua como aceptor de hidrogênio, sendo convertido em água no processo.
horseradish p., p. da raiz-forte; uma peroxidase isolada da raiz-forte, que é usada em imuno-histoquímica para marcar o complexo antígeno-anticorpo.
per·ox·ide (per-ok'sīd). Peróxido. **1.** O óxido de uma série que contém o maior número de átomos de oxigênio; aplicado de forma mais correta a substâncias que contêm uma ligação –O–O–, como no peróxido de hidrogênio (H–O–O–h); um hidroperóxido é R–O–O–H. **2.** O íon O_2^{2-}. **3.** Qualquer membro de uma classe de óxidos metálicos que contêm o íon peróxido.
per·ox·i·some (per-ok'si-sōm). Peroxissoma; uma organela ligada à membrana que ocorre em muitas células eucarióticas e, freqüentemente, tem uma inclusão cristalina elétron-densa contendo catalase, urato oxidase e outras enzimas oxidativas relacionadas com a formação e degradação de H_2O_2; considerada importante na detoxificação de várias moléculas e na catálise da decomposição de ácidos graxos em acetil-CoA; os indivíduos com a síndrome de Zellweger não têm peroxissomas. [peroxide + G. *sōma*, corpo]
△ **peroxy-**. Peroxi-; prefixo que designa a presença de um átomo adicional de O, como em peróxidos, ácidos peroxi (p. ex., peróxido de hidrogênio, ácido peroxifórmico). Freqüentemente é abreviado para per-.

per·ox·y·a·ce·tyl ni·trate (per-ok-sē-ă-sē′til). Nitrato de peroxiacetil; o principal poluente responsável pela irritação ocular e nasal na mistura de nevoeiro e fumaça.

per·oxy ac·id (per-ok′sē). Ácido peroxi. SIN peracid.

per·ox·y·for·mic ac·id (per-ok′sē-fōr′mik). Ácido peroxifórmico. SIN performic acid.

per·ox·yl (per-ok′sil). Peroxila; H–O–O; um dos radicais livres presumidamente formados em virtude do bombardeio do tecido por radiação de alta energia.

per·phe·na·zine (per-fen′ă-zēn). Perfenazina; antipsicótico do tipo fenotiazina.

per pri·mam (per prī′mam in-ten-shē-ō′nem). Por primeira intenção. VER *healing* by first intention. [L.]

per rec·tum (per rek′tŭm). Por via retal; por meio ou através do reto, designando um método de medicação. [L.]

per·salt (per′sawlt). Persal; em química, qualquer sal que contenha a maior quantidade possível do radical ácido.

per sal·tum (per sal′tŭm). Em um salto; em um pulo; que não ocorre gradualmente ou através de diferentes estágios. [L.]

per·sev·er·a·tion (per-sev-er-ā′shun). Perseveração. **1.** A repetição constante de uma palavra ou frase sem significado. **2.** A duração de uma impressão mental, medida pela rapidez com que uma impressão segue outra, determinada pela rotação de um disco de duas cores. **3.** Em psicologia clínica, a repetição incontrolável de uma resposta previamente apropriada ou correta, embora a resposta repetida tenha se tornado inadequada ou errada. [L. *persevero*, persistir]

per·sic oil (per′sik). Óleo pérsico; o óleo fixo espremido das sementes de variedades de *Prunus armeniaca* (óleo de semente de damasco) ou *Prunus persica* (óleo de semente de pêssego); usado como veículo.

per·sis·tence (per-sis′tens). Persistência; continuação obstinada de comportamento característico, ou de existência apesar de tratamento ou de condições ambientais adversas. [L. *persisto*, permanecer, ficar firme]

  lactase p., p. de lactase; uma característica hereditária (autossômica dominante) em que os níveis de lactase não diminuem após o desmame. Cf. lactase restriction.

  microbial p., p. microbiana; o fenômeno de sobrevida, em alta concentração de uma substância antimicrobiana, de micróbios que não parecem ser formas resistentes (mutantes), pois sua prole é totalmente susceptível.

per·sist·er (per-sis′ter). Persistente; aquele que é capaz de persistir; principalmente uma bactéria que exibe persistência microbiana.

per·so·na (per-sō′nă). *Persona*; termo que corporifica a totalidade do indivíduo, o conjunto total das características físicas, psicológicas e comportamentais de cada indivíduo único; na psicologia junguiana, o aspecto externo do caráter, ao contrário do anima (2); a personalidade adotada para mascarar a verdadeira. [L. *per*, através, + *sonare*, soar: originário do pequeno megafone usado nas antigas máscaras de teatro para ajudar a projetar a voz do ator]

per·son·al·i·ty (per-sŏn-al′i-tē). Personalidade. **1.** O eu único; o sistema organizado de atitudes e predisposições de comportamento através do qual uma pessoa sente, pensa e imprime e estabelece relações com outras. **2.** Um indivíduo com um padrão de personalidade específico.

  affective p., p. afetiva; padrão de comportamento crônico em um transtorno permanente dos sentimentos ou do humor, expresso como uma forma de depressão e aspectos emocionais correlatos que afetam toda a vida psíquica.

  antisocial p., p. anti-social. VER psychopath, sociopath, antisocial personality *disorder*. SIN psychopathic p.

  asthenic p., p. astênica; termo outrora utilizado para designar um tipo de personalidade caracterizada por baixo nível de energia, fácil fatigabilidade, incapacidade de se divertir, ausência de entusiasmo e hipersensibilidade ao estresse físico e emocional. SIN asthenic personality disorder.

  authoritarian p., p. autoritária; grupo de traços da personalidade que refletem um desejo de segurança e ordem, p. ex., rigidez, ponto de vista extremamente convencional, obediência sem questionamentos, procura de bodes expiatórios, desejo de linhas estruturadas de autoridade.

  avoidant p., p. esquiva. SIN avoidant personality *disorder*.

  basic p., p. básica. VER basic personality *type*.

  borderline p., p. limítrofe. VER borderline personality *disorder*.

  compulsive p., p. compulsiva. SIN obsessive-compulsive personality *disorder*.

  cyclothymic p., p. ciclotímica; transtorno da p. no qual uma pessoa apresenta períodos rapidamente alternantes de entusiasmo e depressão, menos intenso que o observado no distúrbio bipolar, geralmente não relacionado a circunstâncias externas. SIN cyclothymic personality disorder.

  dependent p., p. dependente. SIN dependent personality *disorder*.

  dual p., p. dupla; termo outrora utilizado para designar transtornos mentais nos quais uma pessoa adota alternantemente duas identidades diferentes sem que uma personalidade esteja consciente da outra. VER TAMBÉM multiple p.

  hysterical p., p. histérica. SIN histrionic personality *disorder*.

  inadequate p., p. inadequada; transtorno da p. caracterizado por inaptidão pessoal e social mais instabilidade emocional e física, que tornam o indivíduo incapaz de enfrentar as vicissitudes da vida.

  masochistic p., p. masoquista; transtorno da p. no qual o indivíduo aceita ser explorado e sacrifica seu próprio interesse enquanto, ao mesmo tempo, sente-se moralmente superior ou aparenta superioridade moral, tentando obter simpatia e induzir culpa nos outros.

  multiple p., p. múltipla. SIN dissociative identity *disorder*.

  neurasthenic p., p. neurastênica; termo obsoleto que designa uma condição caracterizada por algumas das seguintes características: perda de apetite ou ingestão excessiva de alimentos, insônia ou hipersonia, baixa energia ou fadiga, baixa auto-estima, má concentração ou dificuldade em tomar decisões e sentimentos de desesperança. Em sua forma mais grave, pode tornar-se um transtorno crônico do humor denominado distimia (neurose depressiva), no qual um humor depressivo acompanha as características já citadas.

  obsessive p., p. obsessiva. SIN obsessive-compulsive personality *disorder*. VER obsessive-compulsive p., obsessive-compulsive *disorder*.

  obsessive-compulsive p., p. obsessivo-compulsiva. SIN obsessive-compulsive personality *disorder*.

  paranoid p., p. paranóide. SIN paranoid personality *disorder*.

  passive-agressive p., p. passivo-agressiva; transtorno da p. caracterizado por um padrão difuso e duradouro de comportamento no qual sentimentos agressivos manifestam-se de forma passiva, principalmente através de leve obstrucionismo e resistência.

  perfectionistic p., p. perfeccionista; p. caracterizada por rigidez, inibição extrema e preocupação excessiva com a conformidade e a obediência a padrões que, freqüentemente, são únicos.

  psychopathic p., p. psicopática. SIN antisocial p.

  schizoid p., p. esquizóide. SIN schizoid personality *disorder*.

  schizotypal p., p. esquisotípica. SIN schizotypal personality *disorder*.

  shut-in p., p. confinada; termo usado raramente para designar uma pessoa que responde inadequadamente a contatos com outras pessoas.

  syntonic p., p. sintônica; termo raramente usado para designar uma p. estável, caracterizada por temperamento constante.

  type A p., type B p., p. tipo A, p. tipo B. VER type A *behavior*, type B *behavior*.

per·son-years. Pessoas-ano; o produto do número de anos multiplicado pelo número de membros de uma população afetados por determinada condição; p. ex., anos de tratamento com determinado fármaco.

pers·pi·ra·tion (pers-pi-rā′shŭn). Transpiração. **1.** A excreção de líquido pelas glândulas sudoríparas da pele. SIN diaphoresis, sudation, sweating. VER TAMBÉM sweat. **2.** Toda a perda de líquido através da pele normal, seja por secreção das glândulas sudoríparas, seja por difusão através de outras estruturas cutâneas. **3.** O líquido hipotônico excretado pelas glândulas sudoríparas; consiste em água contendo cloreto de sódio e fosfato, uréia, amônia, sulfatos etéreos, creatinina, gorduras e outros resíduos; a quantidade diária média é estimada em aproximadamente 1.500 g. SIN sudor. VER TAMBÉM sweat (1). [L. *per-spiro*, pp. -*atus*, respirar em toda parte]

  insensible p., t. insensível; t. que evapora antes de ser percebida como umidade sobre a pele; o termo algumas vezes inclui evaporação dos pulmões.

  sensible p., t. sensível; a t. exagerada, ou quando há muita umidade na atmosfera, de forma que se apresenta como umidade (suor) sobre a pele.

per·stil·la·tion (per-sti-lā′shŭn). Pervaporação. VER pervaporation. [L. *per*, através, + *stillo*, gotejar, destilar]

per·sua·sion (per-swā′zhŭn). Persuasão; o ato de influenciar a mente de outra pessoa por autoridade, argumento, razão ou discernimento pessoal; um elemento importante na maioria dos tipos de psicoterapia. [L. *persuasio*, de *persuadeo*, persuadir]

per·sul·fate (per-sŭl′fāt). Persulfato; um sal do ácido persulfúrico.

per·sul·fide (per-sŭl′fīd). Persulfeto. **1.** O composto de uma série de sulfetos que contêm mais átomos de enxofre que outro. **2.** O análogo sulfúrico de um peróxido.

per·sul·fu·ric ac·id (per-sŭl-fūr′ik). Ácido persulfúrico; H_2SO_5; ácido peroximonossulfúrico; um agente oxidante.

pertactin (per-tak′tin). Pertactina; material antigênico produzido por *Bordetella pertussis* usado para melhorar a efetividade das vacinas contra coqueluche. [*per*tussis + *act* + *-in*]

per·tech·ne·tate (per-tek-ne-tāt). Pertecnetato; forma aniônica de tecnécio usada amplamente na cintigrafia nuclear; TcO_4^{99m}.

Perthes, Georg C., cirurgião alemão, 1869–1927. VER P. *disease, test;* Calvé-P. *disease;* Legg-Calvé-P. *disease*.

perthio-. Prefixo que designa a substituição por enxofre de cada oxigênio em uma substância; p. ex., ácido pertiocarbônico, H_2CS_3.

Pertik, Otto, patologista húngaro, 1852–1913. VER P. *diverticulum*.

per tu·bam (per-too′bam). Através de um tubo. [L.]

per·tus·sis (per-tŭs′is). Coqueluche; inflamação aguda infecciosa da laringe, traquéia e brônquios causada por *Bordetella pertussis*; caracterizada por crises recorrentes de tosse espasmódica que continua até a exaustão respiratória, terminando então em um estridor inspiratório ruidoso (o "grito") causado por espasmo laríngeo. SIN pertussis syndrome, whooping cough. [L. *per*, muito (intenso), + *tussis*, tosse]

Pe·ru·vi·an bark. Cinchona. SIN cinchona.

per·vap·o·ra·tion (per′vap-ōr-ā′shŭn). Pervaporação; o aquecimento de um líquido em uma bolsa de diálise suspensa sobre uma chapa quente, com a evaporação ocorrendo rapidamente através da membrana; quaisquer colóides em solução permanecem dentro da bolsa, enquanto os cristalóides difundem-se para fora e cristalizam na superfície externa da bolsa. [L. *per*, através, + *vapor*, vapor]

per·ver·sion (per-ver′zhŭn). Perversão; um desvio do padrão, principalmente no que se refere aos interesses ou ao comportamento sexual. [L. *perversio*, de *per-verto*, pp. *-versus*, voltar-se]

  polymorphous p., p. polimórfica; (1) em teoria psicanalítica, as atividades e os interesses sexuais variados de uma criança; (2) em geral, as perversões múltiplas apresentadas por um adulto.

  sexual p., p. sexual. SIN sexual deviation.

per·vert (per′vert). Pervertido; aquele que pratica perversões. VER TAMBÉM deviant (2).

per·vert·ed (per-ver′ted). Pervertido; anormal, desviado ou perturbado.

per vi·as na·tu·ra·les (per vī′as nach′er-ā′lez). Por vias naturais; através das vias naturais; p. ex., designa um parto vaginal, ao contrário da cesariana, ou a eliminação de um corpo estranho nas fezes, em vez de sua remoção cirúrgica. [L.]

per·vi·ous (per′vē-ŭs). Pérvio. SIN permeable. [L. *pervius*, de *per*, através, + *via*, caminho]

pes, gen. **pe·dis**, pl. **pe·des** (pes, pē′dis, -dēz). Pé. **1** [TA]. SIN foot (1). **2.** Qualquer estrutura ou parte basal semelhante a um pé. **3.** Talipe. Nesse sentido, o pé é sempre qualificado por uma palavra que expressa o tipo específico. [L.]

  p. abduc′tus, pé abduzido. SIN talipes valgus.
  p. adduc′tus, pé aduzido. SIN talipes varus.
  p. anseri′nus, pé anserino; (1) SIN parotid plexus of facial nerve; (2) as expansões tendíneas combinadas dos músculos sartório, grácil e semitendíneo na borda medial da tuberosidade da tíbia.
  p. ca′vus, pé cavo. SIN talipes cavus.
  p. equi′noval′gus, pé eqüinovalgo. SIN talipes equinovalgus.
  p. equi′nova′rus, pé eqüinovaro. SIN talipes equinovarus.
  p. gi′gas, pé gigante. SIN macropodia.
  p. hippocam′pi [TA], pé do hipocampo. SIN foot of hippocampus.
  p. pla′nus, pé plano; uma condição na qual o arco longitudinal se rompe, com toda a planta tocando o chão. SIN flatfoot, talipes planus.
  p. prona′tus, pé pronado. SIN talipes valgus.
  p. val′gus, pé valgo. SIN talipes valgus.
  p. va′rus, pé varo. SIN talipes varus.

pes·co·veg·e·tar·i·an. Pescovegetariano; um vegetariano que consome laticínios, ovos e peixe, mas não consome carne de outros animais.

pes·sa·ry (pes′ā-rē). Pessário. **1.** Dispositivo de formato variado, introduzido na vagina para dar suporte ao útero ou para corrigir qualquer deslocamento. **2.** Medicamento na forma de supositório vaginal. [L. *pessarium*, do G. *pessos*, uma pedra oval usada em alguns jogos]

  cube p., p. cúbico; pessário de plástico ou borracha de formato cúbico, particularmente adequado para mulheres idosas com prolapso uterino.
  diaphragm p., p. em diafragma; anel com abertura coberta, usado como plataforma para dar suporte ao útero, à bexiga ou ao reto.
  doughnut p., p. anular. SIN ring p.
  Dumontpallier p., p. de Dumontpallier; pessário anular elástico. SIN Mayer p.
  Gariel p., p. de Gariel; pessário de borracha oco, inflável, com o formato de um anel ou pêra.
  Hodge p., p. de Hodge; pessário oblongo, de curvatura dupla, empregado para correção de retrodesvios do útero.
  Mayer p., p. de Mayer. SIN Dumontpallier p.
  Menge p., p. de Menge; pessário anular com uma barra horizontal central na qual é introduzido um cabo destacável.
  ring p., p. anular; anel de borracha, plástico ou metal em que se apóia o colo do útero; elaborado para dar suporte ao útero e para corrigir o prolapso uterino. SIN doughnut p.

pes·si·mism (pes′i-mizm). Pessimismo; tendência a ver ou prever o pior. [L. *pessimus*, pior, superl. irreg. de *malus*, mau]

  therapeutic p., p. terapêutico; descrença nas virtudes curativas dos remédios em geral e principalmente dos fármacos.

pest. Peste. SIN plague (2). [L. *pestis*]

pes·ti·ce·mia (pes-ti-sē′mē-ā). Pesticemia; bacteriemia por *Yersinia pestis*. [L. *pestis*, peste, + G. *haima*, sangue]

pes·ti·cide (pes′ti-sīd). Pesticida; termo genérico para um agente que destrói fungos, insetos, roedores ou qualquer outra peste.

pes·tif·er·ous (pes-tif′e-rŭs). Pestífero. SIN pestilential.

pes·ti·lence (pes′ti-lens). **1.** Peste. SIN plague (2). **2.** Pestilência; deflagração virulenta de qualquer doença. [L. *pestilentia*]

pes·ti·len·tial (pes-ti-len′shăl). Pestilencial; relativo a, ou que tende a provocar pestilência. SIN pestiferous.

pes·tis. Peste. SIN plague (2). [L.]

  p. am′bulans, p. ambulante. SIN ambulant *plague*.
  p. bubonica (pes′tis boo′bon′ik-ā), p. bubônica. SIN bubonic *plague*.
  p. ful′minans, peste bubônica. SIN bubonic *plague*.
  p. ma′jor, peste bubônica. SIN bubonic *plague*.
  p. mi′nor, p. ambulante. SIN ambulant *plague*.
  p. sid′erans, p. septicêmica. SIN septicemic *plague*.

Pes·ti·vi·rus (pes′ti-vī′rŭs). Gênero de vírus (família Flaviviridae) composto pelo vírus da cólera suína e vírus correlatos. [L. *pestis*, peste, + vírus]

pes·tle (pes′l). Pilão; instrumento em forma de um bastão com uma extremidade arredondada e pesada, usado para amassar, quebrar, moer e misturar substâncias em um almofariz. [L. *pistillum*, de *pinso*, ou *piso*, triturar]

PET Abreviatura de positron emission *tomography* (tomografia com emissão de positrons).

peta- (**P**). Peta-; prefixo usado nos sistemas SI e métrico para designar múltiplos de um quadrilhão (10^{15}).

-petal. -peta; que busca; movimento em direção à parte indicada pela porção principal da palavra. [L. *peto*, buscar, lutar por]

pe·te·chi·ae, sing. **pe·te·chia** (pe-tē′kē-ē, pē-tek′-; pe-tē′kē-ā). Petéquia; diminutos pontos hemorrágicos na pele, puntiformes ou do tamanho da cabeça de um alfinete, que não empalidecem quando comprimidos. [L. mod. forma do It. *petecchie*]

  calcaneal p., p. no calcâneo; hemorragia traumática para o estrato córneo do calcanhar que pode persistir por várias semanas como pontos pretos confluentes centralmente. SIN black heel.
  Tardieu petechiae, petéquias de Tardieu. SIN Tardieu *ecchymoses*, em *ecchymosis*.

pe·te·chi·al (pē-tē′kē-al, pē-tek′-). Petequial; relativo a, ou acompanhado ou caracterizado por petéquias.

Peters, Albert, médico alemão, 1862–1938. VER P. *anomaly*.

Peters, Hubert, obstetra austríaco, 1859–1934. VER P. *ovum*.

Petersen, C.F., cirurgião alemão, 1845–1908.

peth·i·dine (peth′ī-dēn). Petidina. SIN meperidine hydrochloride.

pet·i·o·late, pet·i·o·lat·ed (pet′ē-ō-lāt, -lāt-ed). Peciolado; que possui um pecíolo ou pedículo. SIN petioled. [L. *petiolus*]

pet·i·ole (pet′ē-ōl). Pecíolo. SIN petiolus.

pet·i·oled (pet′ē-ōld). Peciolado. SIN petiolate.

pe·ti·o·lus (pe-tī′ō-lŭs). Pecíolo; uma haste ou pedículo. SIN petiole. [L. dim. de *pes* (pé), a haste de uma fruta]

  p. epiglot′tidis, pecíolo epiglótico. SIN stalk of epiglottis.

Petit, Alexis T., físico francês, 1791–1820. VER Dulong-P. *law*.

Petit, François du, cirurgião e anatomista francês, 1664–1741, VER P. *canals*, em *canal, sinus*.

Petit, Jean L., cirurgião parisiense, 1674–1750. VER P. *hernia herniotomy*, lumbar *triangle*.

Petit, Paul, anatomista francês, *1889. VER P. *aponeurosis*.

Petri, Julius, bacteriologista alemão, 1852–1921. VER P. *dish*; Petri dish *culture*.

pet·ri·fac·tion (pet-ri-fak′shŭn). Petrificação; fossilização, como na conversão em pedra. [L. *petra*, pedra + *facio*, fazer]

pé·tris·sage (pā-trē-sazh′). Amassamento; manipulação em massagem, que consiste em amassamento dos músculos. [Fr. amassamento]

petro-. Petro-; pedra; dureza semelhante à da pedra. [L. *petra*, rocha; G. *petros*, pedra]

pet·roc·cip·i·tal (pet′rok-sip′i-tăl). Petroccipital. SIN petrooccipital.

pe·tro·la·tum (pet-rō-lā′tum). Petrolato; vaselina; mistura amarelada dos outros membros da parafina ou da série metano de hidrocarbonetos, obtida do petróleo como um produto intermediário em sua destilação; usada como aplicação suavizante para queimaduras e escoriações da pele e como base para pomadas. SIN petroleum jelly, yellow soft paraffin.

  heavy liquid p., óleo mineral. SIN mineral oil.
  hydrophilic p., vaselina hidrofílica; vaselina composta de 30 g de colesterol, 30 g de álcool esteárilico; 80 g de cera branca e 860 g de vaselina branca, para compor 1.000 g.
  light liquid p., óleo mineral leve.
  white p., vaselina branca; possui a mesma composição da vaselina, exceto por ser descorada pelo tratamento com carvão ativado; usada para os mesmos fins que a vaselina. SIN white soft paraffin.

pe·tro·le·um (pē-trō′lē-ŭm). Petróleo; mistura de hidrocarbonetos líquidos encontrados na terra em várias partes do mundo e supostamente derivados de resíduos animais e vegetais fossilizados; a fonte da vaselina, além de seu uso para fins de iluminação e aquecimento. SIN coal oil, rock oil. [L. *petra*, rocha, + *oleum*, óleo]

  p. benzin, benzina de petróleo; frações purificadas com baixo ponto de ebulição, destiladas a partir do petróleo, que consistem em hidrocarbonetos, principalmente da série metano; é extremamente inflamável, e seus vapores, quando misturados com ar e inflamados, podem explodir; usada como solvente. SIN benzin, benzine, naphtha, p. ether.

p. ether, éter de petróleo. SIN p. benzin.
liquid p., óleo mineral. SIN mineral oil.

pe·tro·le·um jel·ly. Vaselina; petrolato. SIN petrolatum.

pet·ro·mas·toid (pet′rō-mas′toyd). Petromastóide; relativo às partes petrosa e escamosa do osso temporal, que geralmente estão unidas ao nascimento pela sutura petroescamosa. SIN petrosomastoid.

pet·ro·oc·cip·i·tal (pet′rō-ok-sip′i-tāl). Petroccipital; designa a sutura craniana entre o osso occipital e a parte petrosa do temporal. SIN petroccipital.

pet·ro·pha·ryn·ge·us. Petrofaríngeo. VER *musculus* petropharyngeus.

pe·tro·sa, pl. **pe·tro·sae** (pe-trō′sǎ, -sē). Petrosa; a parte petrosa do osso temporal. [L. de *petra*, rocha]

pe·tro·sal (pe-trō′sǎl). Petroso; relativo à parte petrosa. SIN petrous (2).

pe·tro·sal·pin·go·sta·phy·li·nus (pet′rō-sal′pin-gō-staf-i-lī′nŭs). Petrossalpingoestafilino; termo obsoleto para designar o músculo levantador do véu palatino. [petrosa + G. *salpinx*, trompa, + *staphylē*, úvula]

pet·ro·si·tis (pet-rō-sī′tis). Petrosite; inflamação que envolve a parte petrosa do osso temporal e suas células aéreas. SIN petrousitis.

pet·ro·so·mas·toid (pet-rō′sō-mas′toyd). Petrosomastóide. SIN petromastoid.

pet·ro·sphe·noid (pet′rō-sfē′noyd). Petroesfenóide; relativo à porção petrosa do osso temporal e ao osso esfenóide.

pet·ro·squa·mo·sal, pet·ro·squa·mous (pet′rō-skwa-mō′sǎl, -skwa′mŭs). Petroescamoso; relativo às partes petrosa e escamosa do osso temporal. SIN squamopetrosal.

pe·tro·sta·phy·li·nus (pet′rō-staf-i-lī′nŭs). Petroestafilino; designação obsoleta do músculo levantador do véu palatino (levator veli palatini (muscle)). [G. *petra*, pedra, + *staphylē*, úvula]

pet·rous (pet′rŭs, pē′trŭs). Petroso. **1.** De consistência pétrea. **2.** SIN petrosal. [L. *petrosus*, de *petra*, uma rocha]

pet·rou·si·tis (pet-roo-sī′tis). Petrosite. SIN petrositis.

Pette, H.H., neuropatologista alemão, 1887–1964. VER P.-Döring *disease*.

Pettit, Auguste, médico francês, 1869–1939. VER Bachman-P. *test*.

Peutz, J.L.A., médico holandês. VER P.-Jeghers *syndrome*; Jeghers-P. *syndrome*.

pex·in (pek′sin). Pexina. SIN chymosin.

pex·in·o·gen (pek-sin′ō-jen). Pexinogênio. SIN prochymosin.

pex·is (pek′sis). Pexia; fixação de substâncias nos tecidos. [G. *pēxis*, fixação]

-pexy. -Pexia; fixação, geralmente cirúrgica. [G. *pēxis*, fixação]

Peyer, Johann K., anatomista suíço, 1653–1712. VER P. *glands*, em *gland*; aggregated lymphoid *nodules* of small intestine, em *nodule*.

pe·yo·te, pe·yo·tl (pā-yō′tē, pā-yō′tl). Peiote; mescal; nome asteca para *Lophophora williamsii*, um pequeno cacto nativo do México e do sudoeste dos Estados Unidos, e usado em cerimônias tribais de nativos americanos, onde produz transe e alucinações: o principal componente ativo do peiote é a mescalina. SIN pellote. [Esp.]

Peyronie, Francois de la, cirurgião francês, 1678–1747. VER P. *disease*.

Peyrot, Jean J., cirurgião francês, 1843–1918. VER P. *thorax*.

Pezzer, O. de. VER de Pezzer.

Pfannenstiel, Hermann Johann, ginecologista alemão, 1862–1909. VER P. *incision*.

Pfaundler, Meinhard von, médico alemão, 1872–1947. VER P.-Hurler *syndrome*.

Pfeiffer, Richard F.J., médico alemão, 1858–1945. VER *Pfeifferella*; P. *phenomenon, syndrome*.

Pfeif·fer·el·la (fī-fer-el′lǎ). Gênero obsoleto de bactérias cuja espécie típica, *P. mallei*, outrora era posicionada no gênero *Actinobacillus* e, atualmente, no gênero *Pseudomonas*. [R.F.J. *Pfeiffer*]

PFFD Abreviatura de proximal femoral focal *deficiency* (deficiência).

Pflüger, Eduard F.W., anatomista e fisiologista alemão, 1829–1910. VER P. *law*.

PFOB Abreviatura de perfluorooctyl bromide (brometo de perfluorooctil).

Pfuhl, Eduard, médico alemão, 1852–1905. VER P. *sign*.

PG Abreviatura de prostaglandin (prostaglandina).

pg Símbolo de picogram (picograma).

PGA, PGB, PGC, PGD Abreviaturas, com subscritos numéricos de acordo com a estrutura, freqüentemente usados para prostaglandinas. As letras A, B, etc. indicam a natureza do anel ciclopentano (substituintes, ligações duplas, orientação); os subscritos numéricos indicam o número de ligações duplas nas cadeias alquil.

P-glycoprotein (glī-kō-prō′tēn). P-glicoproteína; proteína associada à resistência do tumor a múltiplas drogas; atua como bomba de efluxo que exige energia para muitas classes de produtos naturais e quimioterápicos. SIN P-170.

PGR Abreviatura de psychogalvanic *response* (resposta psicogalvânica).

P₂Gri Símbolo de diphosphoglycerate (difosfoglicerato).

1,3-P₂Gri Símbolo de 1,3-bisphosphoglycerate (1,3-bisfosfoglicerato).

2,3-P₂Gri Símbolo de 2,3-bisphosphoglycerate (2,3-bisfosfoglicerato).

Ph Símbolo de phenyl (fenil).

Ph1. Abreviatura de Philadelphia *chromosome* (cromossoma Philadelphia).

pH Símbolo do logaritmo decádico negativo da concentração de íon H⁺ (medida em moles por litro); uma solução com pH 7,00 (1×10^{-7} g peso molecular de hidrogênio por litro) é neutra a 22°C (isto é, [H⁺] = [OH⁻]), com pH > 7,00 é alcalina e, com pH < 7,00, é ácida. A uma temperatura de 37°C, a neutralidade ocorre em um pH de 6,80. Cf. dissociation *constant* of water. [p (potência) de [H⁺]]

blood pH, pH sanguíneo; pH do sangue arterial; o normal é 7,4 (faixa normal 7,36–7,44).

critical pH, pH crítico; a faixa de pH, aproximadamente 5,5, na qual a saliva deixa de ser saturada em relação ao cálcio e ao fosfato, e abaixo da qual o mineral do dente se dissolverá.

optimum pH, pH ideal; o pH no qual uma reação enzimática ou qualquer outra reação ou processo é mais efetivo em determinado conjunto de condições.

PHA Abreviatura de phytohemagglutinin (fitoemaglutinina).

phaco-. Faco-. **1.** Que tem o formato de uma lente, relativo a uma lente. **2.** Sinal de nascença; como na facomatose. [G. *phakos*, lentilha (lente), qualquer coisa com o formato de uma lentilha]

phac·o·an·a·phy·lax·is (fak′ō-an-ǎ-fi-lak′sis). Facoanafilaxia; hipersensibilidade à proteína da lente do olho.

phac·o·cele (fak′ō-sēl). Facocele; hérnia da lente do olho através da esclera. [phaco- + G. *kēlē*, hérnia]

phac·o·cyst (fak′ō-sist). Cápsula da lente. SIN capsule of lens. [phaco- + G. *kystis*, bexiga]

phac·o·cys·tec·to·my (fak′ō-sis-tek′tō-mē). Facocistectomia; termo raramente usado para remoção cirúrgica de uma parte da cápsula da lente do olho. [phaco- + G. *kystis*, bexiga, + *ektomē*, excisão]

phac·o·don·e·sis (fak′ō-don-ē′sis). Facodonese; tremor da lente do olho. [phaco- + G. *doneō*, balançar para frente e para trás]

phac·o·e·mul·si·fi·ca·tion (fak′ō-ē-mŭl-si-fi-kā′shŭn). Facoemulsificação; método de emulsificação e aspiração de uma catarata com uma agulha ultrasônica de baixa freqüência.

phac·o·er·y·sis (fak-ō-er′i-sis). Facoérise; extração da lente do olho por meio de uma ventosa. [phaco- + G. *erysis*, tração, retirada]

phac·o·frag·men·ta·tion (fak′ō-frag′men-tā′shŭn). Facofragmentação; ruptura e aspiração da lente.

pha·coid (fak′oyd). Facóide; que possui o formato de lentilha. [phaco- + G. *eidos*, semelhança]

pha·col·y·sis (fa-kol′i-sis). Facólise; divisão cirúrgica e remoção da lente. [phaco- + G. *lysis*, dissolução]

pha·co·lyt·ic (fak-ō-lit′ik). Facolítico; caracterizado por, ou que se refere à facólise.

pha·co·ma (fa-kō′mǎ). Facoma; hamartoma encontrado na facomatose; freqüentemente, refere-se a um hamartoma da retina na esclerose tuberosa. SIN phakoma. [phaco- + G. *-oma*, tumor]

phac·o·ma·la·cia (fak′ō-mǎ-lā′shē-ǎ). Facomalacia; amolecimento da lente, como pode ocorrer na catarata hipermadura. [phaco- + G. *malakia*, amolecimento]

phac·o·ma·to·sis (fak′ō-mǎ-tō′sis). Facomatose; termo genérico para designar um grupo de doenças hereditárias caracterizadas por hamartomas que envolvem múltiplos tecidos; p. ex., doença de von Hippel-Lindau, neurofibromatosis, Sturge-Weber syndrome, tuberous sclerosis. SIN phakomatosis. [Van der Hoeve's coinage do G. *phakos*, mancha-mãe]

phac·o·scope (fak′ō-skōp). Facoscópio; instrumento na forma de uma câmara escura para observar as alterações na lente durante a acomodação. [phaco- + G. *skopeō*, ver]

Phae·ni·cia ser·i·ca·ta (fen-ī′sē-ǎ ser-i-kā′tǎ). Uma espécie comum de mosca varejeira verde-amarelada ou metálica (família Calliphoridae, ordem Diptera); inseto abundante, que se alimenta de substâncias putrefeitas ou excrementos, e implicado no acometimento de ovelhas e em outras formas de miíase. SIN *Lucilia sericata*.

phaeo-. VER pheo-.

phae·o·hy·pho·my·co·sis (fē′ō-hī′fō-mī-kō′sis). Feoifomicose; grupo de infecções superficiais e profundas causadas por fungos que formam hifas pigmentadas e células semelhantes a leveduras nos tecidos, isto é, outras infecções fúngicas dematiáceas além da cromoblastomicose e dos micetomas. Em seres humanos, gatos e cavalos, a feoifomicose é causada por muitas espécies. [G. *phaios*, escuro, + *hyphē*, teia, + *mycosis*]

phage (fāj). Fago. SIN bacteriophage.

β p., f. β. SIN β *corynebacteriophage*.

defective p., f. defeituoso. SIN defective *bacteriophage*.

lambda p., f. lambda; bacteriófago amplamente usado em sistemas experimentais.

-phage, -phagia, -phagy. -Fago, -fagia; que come, que devora. [G. *phagō*, comer]

phag·e·de·na (faj-e-dē′nǎ). Fagedena; termo obsoleto para designar uma úlcera que se dissemina rapidamente para a periferia, destruindo os tecidos à medida que aumenta de tamanho. [G. *phagedaina*, cancro]

p. gangreno·sa, f. gangrenosa; gangrena grave com descamação.

p. nosocomia·lis, f. nosocomial; gangrena que surge no hospital por infecção cruzada.

phagedena 1208 **phalanx**

p. trop'ica, f. tropical; a úlcera tropical da leishmaniose cutânea do Velho Mundo.
phag·e·den·ic (faj-ĕ-den'ik). Fagedênico; termo obsoleto para designar o que tem relação com fagedena ou apresenta as características deste.
phago-. Fago-; que come, que devora. [G. *phagō*, comer]
phag·o·cyte (fag'ō-sīt). Fagócito; uma célula que possui a propriedade de fagocitar bactérias, partículas estranhas e outras células. Os fagócitos são divididos em duas classes gerais: 1) micrófagos, leucócitos polimorfonucleares que ingerem principalmente bactérias; 2) macrófagos, células mononucleadas (histiócitos e monócitos) que são basicamente "lixeiros", fagocitando tecido morto e células degeneradas. SIN carrier cell, scavenger cell. [phago- + G. *kytos*, célula]
phag·o·cyt·ic (fag-ō-sit'ik). Fagocítico; relativo a fagócitos ou à fagocitose.
phag·o·cy·tin (fag-ō-sī'tin). Fagocitina; substância bactericida muito lábil que pode ser isolada dos leucócitos polimorfonucleares.
phag·o·cy·tize (fag'ō-si-tīz). Fagocitar. SIN phagocytose.
phag·o·cy·to·blast (fag-ō-sī'tō-blast). Fagocitoblasto; uma célula primitiva que se transforma em um fagócito. [phagocyte + G. *blastos*, germe]
phag·o·cy·tol·y·sis (fag'ō-sī-tol'ĭ-sis). Fagocitólise. **1.** Destruição de fagócitos, ou leucócitos, que ocorre no processo da coagulação sanguínea ou em virtude da introdução de algumas substâncias estranhas antagonistas no corpo. SIN phagolysis. **2.** Decomposição espontânea dos fagócitos, preliminar (de acordo com Metchnikoff) à liberação de citase, ou complemento. [phagocyte + G. *lysis*, dissolução]
phag·o·cy·to·lyt·ic (fag'ō-sī-tō-lit'ik). Fagocitolítico; relativo à fagocitólise. SIN phagolytic.
phag·o·cy·tose (fag'ō-si-tōz). Fagocitar; realizar fagocitose, designando a ação das células fagocíticas. SIN phagocytize.
phag·o·cy·to·sis (fag-ō-sī-tō'sis). Fagocitose; o processo de "ingestão" e digestão celular de substâncias sólidas, p. ex., outras células, bactérias, fragmentos de tecido necrosado, partículas estranhas. VER TAMBÉM endocytosis. [phagocyte + G. *-osis*, condição]

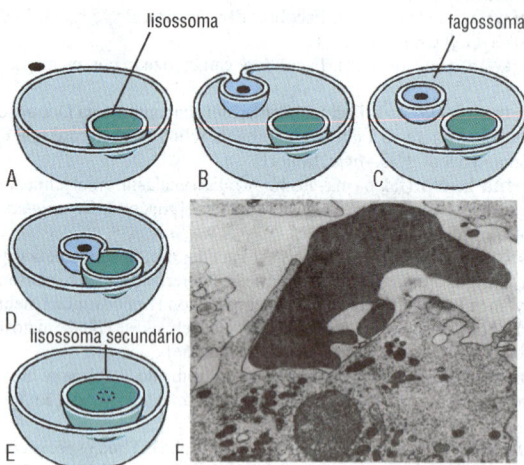

fagocitose: (A) célula e partícula estranha convergindo; (B) partícula endocitada; (C) fagossoma aproximando-se do lisossoma; (D) fagossoma e lisossoma fundidos; (E) partícula digerida no lisossoma secundário; (F) estágio inicial da fagocitose do eritrócito por granulócito neutrófilo (cobaia)

induced p., f. induzida; f. que ocorre quando as bactérias estão sujeitas à ação das opsoninas no sangue e, depois, são colocadas em contato com os leucócitos.
spontaneous p., f. espontânea; f. que ocorre quando uma cultura de bactérias é colocada em contato com leucócitos lavados em um meio indiferente, como uma solução salina fisiológica.
phag·o·dy·na·mom·e·ter (fag'ō-dī-nă-mom'ĕ-ter). Fagodinamômetro; dispositivo para medir a força necessária para mastigar vários alimentos. [phago- + G. *dynamis*, força, + *metron*, medida]
pha·gol·y·sis (fa-gol'ĭ-sis). Fagólise. SIN phagocytolysis (1).
phag·o·ly·so·some (fag-ō-lī'sō-sōm). Fagolisossoma; corpúsculo formado pela união de um fagossoma ou partícula ingerida com um lisossoma, que possui enzimas hidrolíticas.
phag·o·lyt·ic (fag-ō-lit'ik). Fagolítico. SIN phagocytolytic.
phag·o·pho·bia (fag-ō-fō'bē-ă). Fagofobia; medo mórbido de comer. [phago- + G. *phobos*, medo]

phag·o·some (fag'ō-sōm). Fagossoma; uma vesícula que se forma ao redor de uma partícula (bacteriana ou de outro tipo) dentro do fagócito que a fagocitou, separa-se da membrana celular e, depois, funde-se aos grânulos citoplasmáticos (lisossomas) e recebe seu conteúdo, assim formando um fagolisossoma, no qual ocorre digestão da partícula engolfada. [phago- + G. *sōma*, corpo]
phag·o·type (fag'ō-tīp). Fagotipo; em microbiologia, subdivisão de uma espécie distinta das outras cepas pela sensibilidade a determinado bacteriófago ou conjunto de bacteriófagos. [phago- + G. *typos*, tipo]
-phagy. VER -phage.
phako-. Faco-; quanto às palavras que começam assim e não estejam relacionadas aqui, ver phaco-.
pha·ko·ma (fa-kō'mă). Facoma. SIN phacoma.
phak·o·ma·to·sis (fak'ō-mă-tō'sis). Facomatose. SIN phacomatosis.
pha·lan·ge·al (fă-lan'jē-ăl). Falângico; relativo a uma falange.
phal·an·gec·to·my (fal-an-jek'tō-mē). Falangectomia; excisão de uma ou mais falanges da mão ou do pé. [phalang- + G. *ektomē*, excisão]
pha·lan·ges (fă-lan'jēz). Falanges; plural de phalanx. [L.]
pha·lanx, gen. **pha·lan·gis,** pl. **pha·lan·ges** (fa'langks, fă-langks'; fă-lan'jis; -jēz). [TA]. Falange. **1.** [NA]. Um dos ossos longos dos dedos; há 14 falanges em cada mão ou pé, duas no polegar ou no hálux e três em cada um dos outros dedos; designadas como proximal, média e distal, a partir do metacarpo. **2.** Uma dentre várias lâminas cuticulares, dispostas em várias fileiras, sobre a superfície do órgão espiral (de Corti), que são as cabeças da fileira externa das células pilares e das células falângicas; entre elas estão as extremidades livres das células ciliadas. [L. do G. *phalanx* (*-ang-*), linha de soldados, osso entre duas articulações dos dedos das mãos e dos pés]

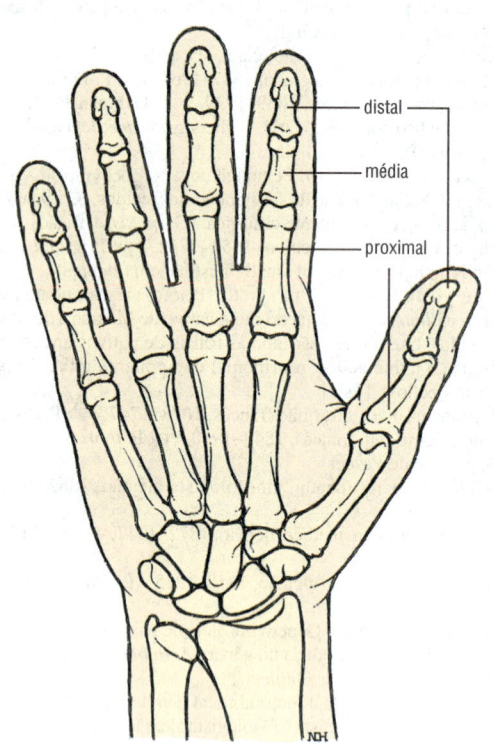

falanges dos dedos da mão

distal p. of foot [TA], f. distal do pé; cada um dos pequenos ossos, relativamente planos, dos dedos dos pés subjacentes ao leito ungueal, possuindo uma tuberosidade em sua face plantar distal, a partir da qual se irradiam filamentos de tecido conjuntivo (ligamentos cutâneos) através da polpa; as bases das falanges dos quatro dedos laterais do pé articulam-se proximalmente com as cabeças das falanges médias, enquanto a do hálux articula-se com uma falange proximal. SIN p. distalis pedis [TA].
distal p. of hand [TA], f. distal da mão; cada um dos pequenos ossos em forma de pá nas extremidades dos dedos das mãos subjacentes ao leito ungueal, possuindo uma tuberosidade em sua face palmar distal, a partir da qual se irradiam filamentos de tecido conjuntivo (ligamentos cutâneos) através da polpa; as bases das falanges dos quatro dedos mediais articulam-se proximalmente com as cabeças das falanges médias; a do polegar articula-se com uma falange proximal. SIN p. distalis manus [TA]
p. distalis manus [TA], f. distal da mão. SIN distal p. of hand.

p. distalis pedis [TA], f. distal do pé. SIN distal p. of foot.
p. media pedis et manus [TA], f. média do pé e da mão. SIN middle phalanges of foot and hand.
middle phalanges of foot and hand [TA], falanges médias do pé e da mão; o osso longo, pequeno, situado no meio dos quatro dedos laterais e quatro dedos mediais, posicionado entre uma falange distal e uma falange proximal e articulando-se com elas. SIN p. media pedis et manus [TA].
proximal p. of foot [TA], f. proximal do pé; o osso relativamente maior dos dedos do pé que se articula proximalmente com a cabeça de um metatarsal; aqueles dos quatro dedos laterais do pé articulam-se distalmente com uma falange média; a do hálux articula-se distalmente com uma falange distal. SIN p. proximalis pedis [TA].
proximal p. of hand [TA], f. proximal da mão; o osso relativamente maior dos dedos que se articula proximalmente com a cabeça de um metacarpal; aqueles dos quatro dedos mediais articulam-se distalmente com uma falange média; aquele do polegar articula-se distalmente com uma falange distal. SIN p. proximalis manus [TA].
p. proximalis manus [TA], f. proximal da mão. SIN proximal p. of hand.
p. proximalis pedis [TA], f. proximal do pé. SIN proximal p. of foot.
tufted p., f. em tufo; uma das falanges terminais dos dedos das mãos na acromegalia; possui uma extremidade expandida semelhante a um feixe de trigo.
ungual p., f. ungueal; a falange distal de cada dedo; assim denominada devido à tuberosidade achatada em sua terminação que sustenta a unha.

phall-, phalli-, phallo-. Fal-, falo-; o pênis. [G. *phallos*]
phal·lal·gia (fal-al′jē-ă). Falalgia. SIN phallodynia. [phall- + G. *algos*, dor]
phal·lec·to·my (fal-ek′tō-mē). Falectomia; remoção cirúrgica do pênis. SIN penectomy. [phall- + G. *ektomē*, excisão]
phal·lic (fal′ik). Fálico. 1. Relativo ao pênis. 2. Em psicanálise, relativo ao pênis, principalmente durante as fases da psicossexualidade infantil. VER TAMBÉM phallic *phase*. [G. *phallos*, pênis]
phal·li·cism (fal′i-sizm). Falicismo; o culto da genitália masculina. SIN phallism.
phal·li·form (fal′i-fōrm). Faliforme. SIN phalloid.
phal·lism (fal′izm). Falismo. SIN phallicism.
phallo-. VER phall-.
phal·lo·camp·sis (fal-ō-kamp′sis). Falocampse; curvatura do pênis ereto. VER TAMBÉM chordee. [phallo- + G. *kampsis*, curvatura]
phal·lo·cryp·sis (fal-ō-krip′sis). Falocripsia; deslocamento e retração do pênis. [phallo- + G. *krypsis*, ocultação]
phal·lo·dyn·ia (fal-ō-din′ē-ă). Falodinia; dor no pênis. SIN phallalgia. [phallo- + G. *odynē*, dor]
phal·loid (fal′oyd). Falóide; de formato semelhante ao do pênis. SIN phalliform. [phallo- + G. *eidos*, semelhança]
phal·loi·din (fă-loy′din). Faloidina; o mais conhecido dos peptídeos cíclicos tóxicos produzidos pelo cogumelo venenoso *Amanita phalloides*; intimamente relacionado à amanitina.
phal·lol·y·sin (fă-lol′i-sin). Falolisina; uma glicoproteína que é a toxina termossensível (destruída pelo cozimento) do cogumelo *Amanita phalloides*.
phal·lon·cus (fal-ong′kŭs). Faloncose; tumor ou tumefação do pênis. [phallo- + G. *onkos*, massa]
phal·lo·plas·ty (fal′ō-plas-tē). Faloplastia; reconstrução cirúrgica do pênis. [phallo- + G. *plastos*, formado]
phal·lot·o·my (fal-ot′ō-mē). Falotomia; incisão cirúrgica do pênis. SIN penotomy. [phallo- + G. *tomē*, corte]
phal·lo·tox·ins (fal′ō-toks′ins). Falotoxinas; classe de heptapeptídeos cíclicos heterodéticos presentes na *Amanita phalloides*; juntamente com as amatoxinas, os principais componentes tóxicos desse fungo.
phal·lus, pl. **phalli** (fal′ŭs, fal′ī). Falo, pênis. SIN penis. [L.; G. *phallos*]

phanero-. Fanero-; visível, óbvio. [G. *phaneros*]
phan·er·o·gen·ic (fan′er-ō-jen′ik). Fanerogênico; indica uma doença cuja etiologia é evidente. Cf. cryptogenic. [phanero- + G. *genesis*, origem]
phan·er·o·ma·nia (fan′er-ō-mā′nē-ă). Faneromania; termo obsoleto para designar a preocupação constante com alguma parte externa, como arrancar fios da barba, puxar o lobo da orelha, ficar mexendo em uma espinha, etc. [phanero- + G. *mania*, mania]
phan·er·o·scope (fan′er-ō-skōp). Faneroscópio; lente usada para concentrar a luz de uma lâmpada sobre a pele, facilitando o exame de lesões da pele e dos tecidos subcutâneos. [phanero- + G. *skopeō*, ver]
phan·er·o·sis (fan-er-ō′sis). Fanerose; o ato ou o processo de tornar-se visível. [phanero- + G. *osis*, condição]
fatty p., f. gordurosa; revelação presumida de gordura previamente invisível no citoplasma celular; a metamorfose gordurosa acentuada está associada a um aumento absoluto no conteúdo de gordura das células, de forma que a ocorrência de fanerose é questionada.

phan·er·o·zo·ite (fan′er-ō-zō′īt). Fanerozoíto; estágio tecidual exoeritrocítico da malária, além dos estágios exoeritrocíticos primários (gerações de criptozoíto e metacriptozoíto); consiste principalmente em reinfecção do fígado por merozoítos produzidos por uma infecção sanguínea (não encontrada na malária falcípara). [phanero- + G. *zōon*, animal]
phan·quone (fan′kwōn). Fanquona; um amebicida.
phan·ta·sia (fan-tā′zē-ă). Fantasia. SIN fantasy. [G. aparição]
phan·tasm (fan′tazm). Fantasma; a imagem mental produzida por fantasia. SIN phantom (1). [G. *phantasma*, uma aparição]
phan·tas·ma·go·ria (fan-taz-mă-gōr′ē-ă). Fantasmagoria; uma seqüência fantástica de imagens casualmente associativas.
phan·tas·mol·o·gy (fan-tas-mol′ō-jē). Fantasmologia; o estudo de manifestações espirituais e de aparições. [G. *phantasma*, uma aparição, + -*logos*, estudo]
phan·tas·mo·sco·pia, phan·tas·mos·co·py (fan-taz-mō-skō′pē-ă, -mos′kō-pē). Fantasmoscopia; termo raramente usado para designar o delírio de ver fantasmas. [G. *phantasma*, uma aparição, + *skopeō*, ver]
phan·tom (fan′tŏm). 1. Fantasma. SIN phantasm. 2. Um modelo, principalmente transparente, do corpo humano ou de qualquer uma de suas partes. VER TAMBÉM manikin. 3. Em radiologia, um modelo mecânico ou feito em computador para prever a dosagem de radiação nas partes profundas do corpo. [G. *phantasma*, uma aparição]
Schultze p., modelo de Schultze; modelo de uma pelve feminina usado para demonstrar o mecanismo de parto e a aplicação de fórceps.
sensory p., sensação percebida sem relação com, ou distinta de, qualquer estímulo real, podendo ocorrer em qualquer um dos sentidos.
phan·tom·ize (fan′tŏm-īz). Fantasiar; em psiquiatria, criar imagens mentais por fantasia.

phar·ma·cal (far′mă-kăl). Farmacêutico. SIN pharmaceutic.
phar·ma·ceu·tic, phar·ma·ceu·ti·cal (far-mă-soo′tik, soo′ti-kăl). Farmacêutico; relativo à farmácia. SIN pharmacal. [G. *pharmakeutikos*, relativo a drogas]
phar·ma·ceu·tics (far-mă-soo′tiks). Farmácia. 1. SIN pharmacy (1). 2. A ciência dos sistemas farmacêuticos, isto é, preparações, apresentações, etc.
phar·ma·ceu·tist (far-mă-soo′tist). Farmacêutico. SIN pharmacist.
phar·ma·cist (far′mă-sist). Farmacêutico; aquele que está licenciado para preparar e dispensar fármacos e substâncias, e que conhece suas propriedades. SIN pharmaceutist. [G. *pharmakon*, um fármaco]
pharmaco-. Farmaco-; medicamentos. [G. *pharmakon*, medicamento]
phar·ma·co·chem·is·try (far′mă-kō-kem′is-trē). Farmacoquímica. SIN pharmaceutical *chemistry*.
phar·ma·co·di·ag·no·sis (far′mă-kō-dī-ag-nō′sis). Farmacodiagnóstico; uso de fármacos no diagnóstico.
phar·ma·co·dy·nam·ic (far′mă-kō-dī-nam′ik). Farmacodinâmico; relativo à ação dos fármacos.
phar·ma·co·dy·nam·ics (far′mă-kō-dī-nam′iks). Farmacodinâmica; o estudo da absorção, do movimento, da ligação e das interações de moléculas farmacologicamente ativas em seus locais teciduais de ação. [pharmaco- + G. *dynamis*, força]
phar·ma·co·en·do·cri·nol·o·gy (far′mă-kō-en′dō-krin-ol′ō-jē). Farmacoendocrinologia; a farmacologia da função endócrina.
phar·ma·co·ep·i·dem·i·ol·o·gy (far′mă-kō-ep-i-dē-mē-ol′ō-jē). Farmacoepidemiologia; o estudo da distribuição e dos determinantes de eventos relacionados a fármacos nas populações, e a aplicação desse estudo à farmacoterapia eficaz.
phar·ma·co·ge·net·ics (far′mă-kō-jē-net′iks). Farmacogenética; o estudo de variações determinadas geneticamente em resposta a fármacos em seres humanos ou em organismos de laboratório. SIN pharmacogenomics.
pharmacogenomics (far′mă-kō-jēn-om′iks). Farmacogenética. SIN pharmacogenetics.
phar·ma·cog·no·sist (far-mă-kog′nō-sist). Farmacognosista; uma pessoa habilitada em farmacognosia.
phar·ma·cog·no·sy (far-mă-kog′nō-sē). Farmacognosia; ramo da farmacologia que trata das características físicas e das fontes botânicas e animais dos fármacos em estado natural. SIN pharmaceutical biology. [pharmaco- + G. *gnōsis*, conhecimento]
phar·ma·cog·ra·phy (far-mă-kog′ră-fē). Farmacografia; um tratado (ou descrição) sobre fármacos. [pharmaco- + G. *graphē*, descrição]
phar·ma·co·ki·net·ic (far′mă-kō-ki-net′ik). Farmacocinético; relativo ao movimento dos fármacos no corpo (isto é, sua absorção, distribuição, metabolismo e eliminação).
phar·ma·co·ki·net·ics (far′mă-kō-ki-net′iks). Farmacocinética; movimentos dos fármacos nos sistemas biológicos, afetados pela captação, distribuição, ligação, eliminação e biotransformação, particularmente pelas velocidades desses movimentos. [pharmaco- + G. *kinēsis*, movimento]
phar·ma·co·log·ic, phar·ma·co·log·i·cal (far′mă-kō-loj′ik, -loj′i-kăl). Farmacológico. 1. Relativo à farmacologia ou à composição, propriedades e ações dos fármacos. 2. Algumas vezes usado em fisiologia para designar uma dose (de um agente químico que é ou imita um hormônio, neurotransmissor ou outro agente natural), bem maior ou mais potente do que seria natural, a ponto de ter efeitos qualitativamente diferentes. Cf. homeopathic (2), physiologic (4), supraphysiologic.

phar·ma·col·o·gist (far-mă-kol'ō-jist). Farmacologista; um especialista em farmacologia.
  clinical p., f. clínico; farmacologista que recebeu treinamento em farmacologia básica, farmacologia clínica e em uma das várias especialidades da prática médica.

phar·ma·col·o·gy (far-mă-kol'ō-jē). Farmacologia; a ciência que estuda os fármacos, suas origens, aparência, química, ações e empregos. [pharmaco- + G. *logos*, estudo]
  biochemical p., f. bioquímica; ramo da farmacologia que estuda os mecanismos bioquímicos responsáveis pelas ações dos fármacos.
  clinical p., f. clínica; o ramo da farmacologia que estuda a farmacologia dos agentes terapêuticos na prevenção, tratamento e controle das doenças nos seres humanos.
  marine p., f. marinha; ramo da farmacologia que estuda substâncias farmacologicamente ativas presentes em plantas e animais aquáticos; seu objetivo é encontrar e desenvolver novos agentes terapêuticos.

phar·ma·co·ma·nia (far'mă-kō-mā'nē-ă). Farmacomania; impulso mórbido de tomar medicamentos. [pharmaco- + G. *mania*, mania]

Phar·ma·co·pe·ia, Phar·ma·co·poe·ia (far'mă-kō-pē'ă). Farmacopéia; trabalho que contém monografias de agentes terapêuticos, parâmetros de concentração e pureza, e suas fórmulas. As várias farmacopéias nacionais são designadas por abreviaturas, sendo as seguintes as mais freqüentemente encontradas: *USP*, a Farmacopéia dos Estados Unidos da América (United States Pharmacopeia); *BP*, Farmacopéia Inglesa (British Pharmacopeia); *Codex medicamentarius*, a Farmacopéia Francesa; *I. C. Add.* (ou *BA*), o Adendo Indiano e Colonial à BP; *IP*, Farmacopéia Internacional (International Pharmacopeia); *Pharmacopeia Austr.*, a Farmacopéia Austríaca; *Ph.G.*, a Farmacopéia Alemã (D.A.B.); *Pharmacopeia Helv.*, a Farmacopéia Suíça. A primeira edição da USP foi compilada em 1820 e tornou-se um parâmetro legal pelos termos do *National Food and Drugs Act* em janeiro de 1907. [G. *pharmakopoiia*, de *pharmakon*, um medicamento, + *poieo*, fazer]

phar·ma·co·pe·ial (far'mă-kō-pē'ăl). Farmacopeico; relativo à Farmacopéia; designa uma droga na lista da Farmacopéia. VER TAMBÉM official.

phar·ma·co·phi·lia (far'mă-kō-fil'ē-ă). Farmacofilia; gosto mórbido por tomar medicamentos. [pharmaco- + G. *phileo*, amar]

phar·ma·co·pho·bia (far'mă-kō-fō'bē-ă). Farmacofobia; medo mórbido de tomar medicamentos. [pharmaco- + G. *phobos*, medo]

phar·ma·co·psy·cho·sis (far'mă-kō-sī-kō'sis). Farmacopsicose; termo raramente usado para designar uma psicose que tem relação etiológica com um fármaco. [pharmaco- + psychosis]

phar·ma·co·ther·a·py (far'mă-kō-thar'ă-pē). Farmacoterapia; tratamento de doença por meio de fármacos. VER TAMBÉM chemotherapy. [pharmaco- + G. *therapeia*, terapia]

phar·ma·cy (far'mă-sē). Farmácia. **1.** A prática de preparar e dispensar fármacos. SIN pharmaceutics (1). **2.** Uma drogaria. [G. *pharmakon*, fármaco]
  clinical p., f. clínica; ramo da prática de farmácia que dá ênfase ao uso terapêutico dos fármacos e não ao seu preparo e sua distribuição.

Pharm. D. Abreviatura de Doctor of Pharmacy (Doutor em Farmácia).

pharyng-. VER pharyngo-.

pha·ryn·ge·al (fă-rin'jē-ăl). Faríngeo; relativo à faringe. SIN pharyngeus. [L. mod. *pharyngeus*]

phar·yn·gec·to·my (far'in-jek'tō-mē). Faringectomia; ressecção da faringe. [pharyng- + G. *ektome*, excisão]

phar·yn·gei (far-in'jē-ī). Ramos faríngeos. SIN pharyngeal branches, em branch.

pha·ryn·ges (fă-rin'jēz). Faringes; plural de pharynx.

pha·ryn·ge·us (far'in-jē'us). Faríngeo. SIN pharyngeal. [L. mod.]

phar·yn·gis·mus (far-in-jiz'mŭs). Faringismo; espasmo dos músculos da faringe. SIN pharyngospasm.

phar·yn·git·ic (far-in-jit'ik). Faringítico; relativo à faringite.

phar·yn·gi·tis (far-in-jī'tis). Faringite; inflamação da mucosa e das partes subjacentes da faringe. [pharyng- + G. *-itis*, inflamação]
  atrophic p., f. atrófica; f. crônica acompanhada por atrofia variável das glândulas mucosas e ausência de secreção. SIN p. sicca.
  gangrenous p., f. gangrenosa; inflamação gangrenosa da mucosa faríngea.
  membranous p., f. membranosa; inflamação acompanhada por exsudato fibrinoso, formando uma falsa membrana não-diftérica.
  p. sic'ca, f. seca, f. atrófica. SIN atrophic p.
  ulcerative p., f. ulcerativa; inflamação da faringe caracterizada por ulceração da mucosa; pode ter uma etiologia viral.
  ulceromembranous p., f. ulceromembranosa; inflamação da mucosa faríngea com resíduos membranosos sobre as lesões ulcerativas.

pharyngo-, pharyng-. Faringo-, faring-; a faringe. [L. mod. do G. *pharynx*]

pha·ryn·go·cele (fă-ring'gō-sēl). Faringocele; um divertículo da faringe. [pharyngo- + G. *kele*, hérnia]

pha·ryn·go·ep·i·glot·tic, pha·ryn·go·ep·i·glot·tid·e·an (fă-ring'gō-ep'i-glot'ik, -glo-tid'ē-an). Faringoepiglótico; relativo à faringe e à epiglote.

pha·ryn·go·e·soph·a·ge·al (fă-ring'gō-ē-sof'ă-jē'ăl). Faringoesofágico; relativo à faringe e ao esôfago.

pha·ryn·go·e·soph·a·go·plas·ty (fă-ring'gō-ē-sof'ă-gō-plas-tē). Faringoesofagoplastia; cirurgia plástica da faringe e do esôfago. [pharyngo- + esophago- + G. *plastos*, formado]

pha·ryn·go·glos·sal (fă-ring'gō-glos'ăl). Faringoglosso; relativo à faringe e à língua.

pha·ryn·go·glos·sus (fă-ring-gō-glos'us). Músculo constritor superior da faringe. VER superior pharyngeal constrictor (*muscle*).

pha·ryn·go·la·ryn·ge·al (fă-ring'gō-lă-rin'jē-ăl). Faringolaríngeo; relativo à faringe e à laringe.

pha·ryn·go·lar·yn·gi·tis (fă-ring'gō-lar-in-jī'tis). Faringolaringite; inflamação da faringe e da laringe.

pha·ryn·go·lith (fă-ring'gō-lith). Faringólito; uma concreção na faringe. SIN pharyngeal calculus. [pharyngo- + G. *lithos*, pedra]

pha·ryn·go·max·il·lary (fă-ring'gō-mak-si-lār-ē). Faringomaxilar; relativo à faringe e à maxila.

pha·ryn·go·na·sal (fă-ring'gō-nā'săl). Faringonasal; relativo à faringe e à cavidade nasal.

pha·ryn·go-oral (fă-ring'gō-ō'răl). Orofaríngeo; relativo à faringe e à boca. [pharyngo- + L. *os* (*or-*), boca]

pha·ryn·go·pal·a·tine (fă-ring'gō-pal'ă-tīn). Faringopalatino; relativo à faringe e ao palato.

pha·ryn·go·pa·la·ti·nus (fă-ring'gō-pal-ă-tī'nus). Músculo palatofaríngeo. SIN palatopharyngeus (*muscle*). [L.]

pha·ryn·go·plas·ty (fă-ring'gō-plas-tē). Faringoplastia; cirurgia plástica da faringe; procedimento que visa corrigir disfunção velofaríngea. [pharyngo- + G. *plastos*, formado]

pha·ryn·go·ple·gia (fă-ring'gō-plē'jē-ă). Faringoplegia; paralisia dos músculos da faringe. [pharyngo- + G. *plege*, golpe]

pha·ryn·go·rhi·nos·co·py (fă-ring'gō-rī-nos'kō-pē). Faringorrinoscopia; inspeção da nasofaringe e da parte posterior das narinas por meio do espelho rinoscópico. [pharyngo- + G. *rhis*, nariz + *skopeo*, ver]

pha·ryn·go·scope (fă-ring'gō-skōp). Faringoscópio; instrumento semelhante a um laringoscópio, usado para inspeção da faringe. [pharyngo- + G. *skopeo*, ver]

phar·yn·gos·co·py (far'ing-gos'kō-pē). Faringoscopia; inspeção e exame da faringe. [pharyngo- + G. *skopeo*, ver]

pha·ryn·go·spasm (fă-ring'gō-spazm). Faringospasmo. SIN pharyngismus.

pha·ryn·go·sta·phy·li·nus (fă-ring'gō-staf-i-lī'nus). Músculo palatofaríngeo. SIN palatopharyngeus (*muscle*). [L. de pharyngo- + G. *staphyle*, úvula]

pha·ryn·go·ste·no·sis (fă-ring'gō-ste-nō'sis). Faringostenose; estreitamento da faringe. [pharyngo- + G. *stenosis*, estreitamento]

phar·yn·got·o·my (far'ing-got'ō-mē). Faringotomia; qualquer cirurgia de corte da faringe por fora ou por dentro. [pharyngo- + G. *tome*, incisão]

pha·ryn·go·ton·sil·li·tis (fă-ring'gō-ton-si-lī'tis). Faringotonsilite; inflamação da faringe e das tonsilas. [pharyngo- + tonsillitis]

phar·ynx, gen. **pha·ryn·gis,** pl. **pha·ryn·ges** (far'ingks, fă-rin'jis, fă-rin'jēz) [TA]. Faringe; a porção superior expandida do tubo digestivo, entre o esôfago, abaixo, e a boca e cavidades nasais, acima e na frente; é distinta do restante do tubo digestivo porque é composta exclusivamente de músculo esquelético (voluntário) disposto em camadas circular externa e longitudinal interna. [L. mod. do G. *pharynx* (*pharyng-*), garganta, a abertura conjunta da garganta e da traquéia]
  laryngeal p., parte laríngea da faringe. SIN laryngopharinx.
  nasal p., parte nasal da faringe. SIN nasopharynx.
  oral p., parte oral da faringe. SIN oropharynx.

phase (fāz). Fase. **1.** Um estágio no decorrer da alteração ou do desenvolvimento. **2.** Uma porção homogênea, fisicamente distinta e separável de um sistema heterogêneo; p. ex., óleo, goma e água são três fases de uma emulsão. **3.** A relação temporal entre dois ou mais eventos. **4.** Determinada parte de um padrão recorrente de tempo ou onda. VER TAMBÉM stage, period. [G. *phasis*, aparência]
  anal p., f. anal; na teoria psicanalítica da personalidade, o estágio de desenvolvimento psicossexual, que ocorre quando uma criança tem entre 1 e 3 anos de idade, durante o qual as atividades, interesses e preocupações concentram-se ao redor da região anal.
  aqueous p., f. aquosa; a porção aquosa de um sistema que consiste em duas fases líquidas, sendo uma principalmente água, e a outra, um líquido imiscível com água (p. ex., benzeno, éter).
  cis p., f. cis. VER coupling p.
  continuous p., f. contínua. SIN external p.
  coupling p., f. de acoplamento; a relação física entre dois genes sintênicos. Caso estejam no mesmo cromossoma, diz-se que estão "em acoplamento" ou "na fase cis"; caso estejam em membros opostos de um par de cromossomas, "em repulsão" ou "na fase trans".
  discontinuous p., f. descontínua. SIN internal p.

dispersed p., f. dispersa. SIN internal p.
dispersion p., f. de dispersão. SIN external p.
eclipse p., f. de eclipse. SIN eclipse period.
p. encoding, codificação de fase; em ressonância magnética, a técnica de induzir um gradiente no campo magnético, no eixo x ou no y, para induzir diferenças de fase com localização. SIN gradient encoding.
eruptive p., f. eruptiva; período na formação do dente que inclui o desenvolvimento das raízes, do ligamento periodontal e da junção dentogengival do dente.
external p., f. externa; o meio ou líquido no qual um elemento disperso está suspenso. SIN continuous p., dispersion medium, dispersion p., external medium.
gap$_1$ p., período de intervalo 1. SIN gap$_1$ period.
gap$_2$ p., período de intervalo 2. SIN gap$_2$ period.
gap$_0$ p., período de intervalo 0. SIN gap$_0$ period.
genital p., f. genital; na teoria psicanalítica da personalidade, o estágio final do desenvolvimento psicossexual, que ocorre durante a puberdade, no qual o desenvolvimento psicossexual do indivíduo é organizado de forma que possa ser obtido prazer sexual por contato genitogenital, e exista a capacidade de um relacionamento afetivo com um indivíduo do sexo oposto. VER phallic p.
horizontal growth p., f. de crescimento horizontal; um estágio inicial do desenvolvimento do melanoma cutâneo por disseminação intra-epidérmica de melanócitos atípicos.
internal p., f. interna; as partículas contidas em uma solução colóide. SIN discontinuous p., dispersed p.
lag p., f. de retardo; breve período no decorrer do crescimento de uma cultura bacteriana, principalmente no início, durante o qual o crescimento é muito lento ou praticamente imperceptível.
latency p., f. de latência; na teoria psicanalítica da personalidade, o período de desenvolvimento psicossexual, em crianças, que se estende desde aproximadamente os 5 anos de idade até o início da adolescência, aos 12 anos, durante o qual a aparente cessação da preocupação sexual provém de um bloqueio forte e agressivo dos impulsos libidinosos e sexuais em uma tentativa de evitar relações edipianas; durante esse período, meninos e meninas tendem a escolher amigos e aderir a grupos do mesmo sexo. SIN latency period.
logarithmic p., f. logarítmica, exponencial; período durante o crescimento de uma cultura bacteriana no qual está havendo multiplicação máxima por progressão geométrica; assim, se os logaritmos de seus números forem extrapolados em relação ao tempo, eles formarão uma linha reta ascendente.
luteal p., f. lútea; aquela parte do ciclo menstrual que vai do momento da formação do corpo lúteo até o início da menstruação, geralmente durando 14 dias;
short luteal p., f. lútea curta; período de 10 dias ou menos entre a ovulação e o início da menstruação, freqüentemente associado à infertilidade.
M p., f. M. SIN mitotic period.
meiotic p., f. meiótica; o estágio de alterações nucleares nas células sexuadas durante o qual ocorre redução do número de cromossomos; compreende as gerações celulares dos espermatócitos e ovócitos. SIN reduction p.
negative p., f. negativa; período durante o qual o índice opsônico é reduzido após a injeção de uma vacina.
oedipal p., f. edipiana; em psicanálise, um estágio do desenvolvimento psicossexual da criança caracterizado por fixação erótica no genitor do sexo oposto, sendo reprimido devido ao medo do genitor do mesmo sexo; geralmente ocorre entre 3 e 6 anos de idade. SIN oedipal period.
oral p., f. oral; na teoria psicanalítica da personalidade, o primeiro estágio do desenvolvimento psicossexual, que persiste durante os primeiros 18 meses de vida e durante o qual a zona oral é o centro das necessidades, expressão, gratificação e experiência erótica agradável do lactente; tem uma forte influência sobre a organização e o desenvolvimento da psique da criança.
phallic p., f. fálica; na teoria psicanalítica da personalidade, o estágio do desenvolvimento psicossexual que ocorre quando em criança, entre os 2 e os 6 anos de idade, durante o qual o interesse, a curiosidade e as experiências prazerosas concentram-se no pênis, em meninos, e no clitóris, em meninas. VER genital p.
positive p., f. positiva; o período posterior à fase negativa, durante o qual o índice opsônico aumenta.
postmeiotic p., f. pós-meiótica; o estágio posterior àquele de redução dos cromossomas nas células sexuais, representando as formas maduras dessas células, terminando com a conjugação dos núcleos no óvulo impregnado. SIN postreduction p.
postmitotic p., período de intervalo 1. SIN gap$_1$ period.
postreduction p., f. pós-meiótica. SIN postmeiotic p.
poststationary p., f. pós-estacionária; o período do crescimento de uma cultura bacteriana no qual o crescimento está diminuindo.
pregenital p., f. pré-genital; em psicanálise, a fase do desenvolvimento psicossexual coletivo que precede a fase genital.
premeiotic p., f. pré-meiótica; o estágio de alterações nucleares nas células sexuais antes da redução dos cromossomas, compreendendo as gerações celulares até a geração das espermatogônias e ovogônias. SIN prereduction p.
premitotic p., f. pré-mitótica. SIN gap$_2$ period.
pre-oedipal p., f. pré-edipiana; em psicanálise, o conjunto das fases do desenvolvimento psicossexual que precedem a fase edipiana.
prereduction p., f. pré-meiótica. SIN premeiotic p.
radial growth p., f. de crescimento radial, o padrão inicial do crescimento do melanoma maligno cutâneo, no qual as células tumorais se propagam lateralmente na epiderme.
reduction p., f. meiótica. SIN meiotic p.
S p., f. S. SIN synthesis period.
stationary p., f. estacionária; (1) o período do crescimento de uma cultura bacteriana durante o qual a multiplicação dos microrganismos torna-se gradualmente menor e as bactérias que se dividem estão em equilíbrio com aquelas que morrem; (2) refere-se ao componente imóvel, geralmente sólido na cromatografia de partição.
supernormal recovery p., f. de recuperação supernormal; breve período, durante a recuperação do músculo cardíaco após excitação, quando o músculo doente é mais (isto é, menos anormalmente) excitável; corresponde ao fim da onda T no ECG.
synaptic p., f. sináptica. SIN synapsis.
trans p., f. trans. VER coupling p.
vertical growth p., f. de crescimento vertical; período de disseminação de células de melanoma da epiderme para a derme e, depois, para o tecido subcutâneo, durante o qual podem ocorrer metástases.
vulnerable p., f. vulnerável; período no ciclo cardíaco durante o qual um impulso ectópico pode levar a atividade repetitiva, como *flutter* ou fibrilação da câmara afetada.

phas·mid (faz′mid). Fasmídeo. 1. Um dos componentes de um par de quimiorreceptores caudais observados em nematódeos da classe Secernentasida (Phasmidia). 2. Designação comum de um membro da classe Phasmidia, agora Secernentasida.

Phas·mid·ia (faz - mid′ē - ă). SIN Secernentasida. [G. *phasma*, aparência]

phas·mo·pho·bia (fas - mō - fō′bē - ă). Fasmofobia; medo mórbido de fantasmas. [G. *phasma*, aparição, + *phobos*, medo]

phat·nor·rha·gia (fat - nō - rā′jē - ă). Hemorragia de um alvéolo dental. [G. *phatnōma*, manjedoura (alvéolo), + G. *rhēgnymi*, irromper]

Ph.D. Abreviatura de Doctor of Philosophy (Doutor em Filosofia).

Phe Símbolo de phenylalanine (fenilalanina) ou phenylalanyl (fenilalanil).

Phemister, Dallas B., cirurgião americano, 1882–1951.

△ **phen-, pheno-.** Fen-, feno-. 1. Forma combinante que significa aparência. 2. Em química, forma combinante que designa derivação do benzeno (fenil-). [do G. *phainō*, aparecer, mostrar]

phen·a·caine hy·dro·chlo·ride (fen′ă - kān). Cloridrato de fenacaína; potente anestésico local de superfície usado em oftalmologia.

phen·ac·e·mide (fe - nas′ē - mīd). Fenacemida; anticonvulsivante usado no tratamento da epilepsia. SIN phenylacetylurea.

phen·ac·e·tin (APC) (fe - nas′e - tin). Fenacetina; analgésico e antipirético; o "P" no APC, uma combinação analgésica que também contém ácido acetilsalicílico e cafeína; biotransformado em acetaminofeno. SIN acetophenetidin.

phen·ac·e·to·lin (fen′ă - set′ō - lin). Fenacetolina; um pó vermelho, $(C_{16}H_{12})_2$, usado como indicador. Tem uma faixa de pH de 5 a 6, sendo amarelo em pH 5 e vermelho em pH 6.

phen·ac·e·tur·ic ac·id (fē - nas - ē - toor′ik). Ácido fenacetúrico; um produto final do metabolismo dos ácidos graxos fenilados com números pares de átomos de carbono. SIN phenylaceturic acid.

phen·ac·ri·dane chlo·ride (fe - nas′ri - dān). Cloreto de fenacridana; antiséptico tópico.

phen·a·cy·cla·mine (fen - ă - sī′klă - mēn). Fenaciclamina. SIN phenetamine.

phen·a·gly·co·dol (fen - ă - glī′kō - dol). Fenaglicodol; depressor do sistema nervoso central usado no tratamento da ansiedade e de neuroses simples.

phen·an·threne (fē - nan′thrēn). Fenantreno; composto isomérico com antraceno, derivado do alcatrão; um importante componente de esteróides, como o ciclopenta[α]fenantreno. Usado como base para a síntese de vários corantes e drogas.

phen·ar·sen·a·mine (fen - ar - sen - am′ēn). Fenarsenamina. SIN arsphenamine.

phen·ar·sone sulf·ox·y·late (fen - ar′sōn sŭl - fok′si - lāt). Sulfoxilato de fenarsona; um arsenical pentavalente usado na vaginite por tricômonas.

phe·nate (fē′nāt). Fenato; sal ou éster do fenol (ácido carbólico). SIN carbolate (1).

phe·naz·o·cine (fen - ā′zō - sēn). Fenazocina; potente analgésico, quando administrado por via intramuscular ou intravenosa, sendo menos efetivo por via oral.

phen·az·o·line hy·dro·chlo·ride (fen - az′ō - lēn). Cloridrato de fenazolina. SIN antazoline hydrochloride.

phen·az·o·pyr·i·dine hy·dro·chlo·ride (fen - ă - zō - pēr′i - dēn). Cloridrato de fenazopiridina; analgésico das vias urinárias administrado por via oral.

phen·cy·cli·dine (PCP) (fen - sī′kli - dēn). Fenciclidina; substância de abuso, usada por suas propriedades alucinógenas, que pode provocar profundos distúrbios psicológicos e comportamentais; o cloridrato possui propriedades analgésicas e anestésicas.

phen·di·me·tra·zine tar·trate (fen-di-met′ră-zēn). Tartarato de fendimetrazina; agente anoréxico.
phen·el·zine sul·fate (fen′el-zēn). Sulfato de fenelzina; inibidor da monoamina oxidase usado como antidepressivo.
phe·net·a·mine (fĕ-net′a-mēn). Fenetamina; antiespasmódico intestinal. SIN phenacyclamine.
phe·neth·i·cil·lin po·tas·si·um (fĕ-neth-i-sil′in) Feneticilina potássica; preparação de penicilina estável em ácido gástrico e que é absorvida rapidamente, porém apenas parcialmente pelo trato gastrointestinal. SIN α-phenoxyethylpenicillin potassium, penicillin B.
phen·eth·yl al·co·hol (fĕ-neth′il). Álcool fenetílico. SIN phenylethyl alcohol.
phe·net·sal (fĕ-net′sal). Acetaminossalol. SIN acetaminosalol.
phe·net·u·ride (fĕ-net′ū-rīd). Feneturida; antiepiléptico com ação semelhante à fenacemida.
phen·for·min hy·dro·chlo·ride (fen-fōr′min). Cloridrato de fenformina; agente hipoglicemiante oral que não é mais usado nos Estados Unidos devido à alta incidência de acidose lática fatal associada a seu uso. A metformina, um agente quimicamente relacionado, é usada atualmente.
phen·glu·tar·i·mide hy·dro·chlo·ride (fen-gloo-tar′i-mīd). Cloridrato de fenglutarimida; o cloridrato da α-2-dietilaminoetil-α-fenil-glutarimida; anti-histamínico usado para reduzir ou evitar a cinetose, assim como para controlar a doença de Ménière e o vômito.
phen·go·pho·bia (fen-gō-fō′bē-ă). Fengofobia; medo mórbido da luz do dia. [G. *phengos*, luz do dia, + *phobos*, medo]
phen·i·car·ba·zide (fen-i-kar′ba-zīd). Fenicarbazida; um antipirético.
phe·nin·da·mine tar·trate (fĕ-nin′dă-mēn). Tartarato de fenindamina; um anti-histamínico.
phen·in·di·one (fĕ-nin-dī′ōn). Fenindiona; 2-fenil-1,3-indanediona; anticoagulante sintético com ação e empregos semelhantes aos da bisidroxicumarina. SIN phenylindanedione.
phen·ir·a·mine ma·le·ate (fĕ-nir′a-mēn, -min). Maleato de feniramina; um anti-histamínico H$_1$. SIN prophenpyridamine maleate.
phen·meth·y·lol (fen-meth′il-ol). Fenmetilol. SIN benzyl alcohol.
phen·met·ra·zine hy·dro·chlo·ride (fen-met′ră-zēn). Cloridrato de fenmetrazina; agente anoréxico com propriedades simpaticomiméticas.
♻ **pheno-.** VER phen-.
phe·no·bar·bi·tal (fē-nō-bar′bi-tahl). Fenobarbital; sedativo oral ou parenteral de ação prolongada, anticonvulsivante e hipnótico; também disponível como um sal de sódio solúvel; também usado no tratamento da epilepsia e na indução de enzimas microssomais hepáticas. SIN phenylethylbarbituric acid, phenylethylmalonylurea.
phe·no·bu·ti·o·dil (fen′ō-bū-tī′ō-dil). Fenobutiodil; um contraste radiográfico usado antigamente para colecistografia.
phe·no·copy (fē′nō-kop′ē). Fenocópia; imitação de uma doença ambientalmente induzida, que é caracteristicamente produzida por um gene específico. [G. *phainō*, exibir, + copy]
phe·no·din (fē′nō-din). Fenodina. SIN hematin.
phe·nol (fē′nol). Fenol; hidroxibenzeno; anti-séptico, anestésico e desinfetante; localmente escarótico na forma concentrada e neurolítico em soluções de 3–4%; internamente, um poderoso veneno escarótico. SIN carbolic acid, phenyl alcohol.
   camphorated p., f. canforado; ácido carbólico canforado, que consiste em fenol, cânfora e vaselina líquida; usado como anestésico local e para alívio da dor de dente.
   liquefied p., f. liquefeito; ácido carbólico liquefeito, fenol liquefeito pela adição de 10% de água.
   p. oxidase, f. oxidase. SIN laccase.
phe·no·lase (fē′nō-lās). Fenolase. SIN laccase.
phe·no·lat·ed (fē′nō-lāt-ed). Fenolado; impregnado ou misturado com fenol. SIN carbolated.
phe·nol·e·mia (fē-nol-ē-mē-ă). Fenolemia; a presença de fenóis no sangue. [phenol + G. *haima*, sangue]
phe·nol·o·gy (fe-nol′ō-jē). Fenologia; o estudo dos ritmos biológicos de plantas e animais, sobretudo aqueles que exibem variação sazonal. [G. *phainō*, aparecer, + *logos*, estudo]
phe·nol·phtha·le·in (fē-nol-thal′ē-in, -thal′ēn). Fenolftaleína; obtida pela ação do fenol sobre o anidrido ftálico; usado como indicador do íon hidrogênio e usado antigamente como laxante.
phe·nol red. Vermelho fenol. SIN phenolsulfonphthalein.
phe·nol·sul·fon·phthal·e·in (PSP) (fē′nol-sŭl-fon-thal′ē-in, -thal′ēn) Fenolsulfonftaleína; ocorre como um pó cristalino vermelho-brilhante ou escuro; usado como indicador em meios de cultura tecidual (amarelo em pH 6,8; vermelho em pH 8,4); no passado era administrado por injeção parenteral para testar a função renal. SIN phenol red.
phe·nol·u·ria (fē-nol-ū′rē-ă). Fenolúria; a excreção de fenóis na urina.
phe·nom·e·nol·o·gy (fē-nom-ē-nol′ō-jē). Fenomenologia. **1.** A descrição e classificação sistemáticas de fenômenos sem tentar explicar ou interpretar. **2.** O estudo de experiências humanas, independentemente de distinções objetivo-subjetivas. VER TAMBÉM existential *psychology*. [phenomenon, + G. *logos*, estudo]

PHENOMENON

phe·nom·e·non, pl. **phe·nom·e·na** (fĕ-nom′ē-non, -nă). Fenômeno. **1.** Uma manifestação; uma ocorrência de qualquer tipo, seja ordinária ou extraordinária, em relação a uma doença. **2.** Qualquer fato ou ocorrência incomum. [G. *phainomenon*, de *phainō*, fazer surgir]
   adhesion p., f. de aderência; f. secundário à aderência do complexo antígeno-anticorpo-complemento a "células indicadoras" (microrganismos, plaquetas, leucócitos ou eritrócitos), sendo a reação sensível e específica para o antígeno e anticorpo no complexo. SIN erythrocyte adherence p., immune adherence p., red cell adherence p.
   AFORMED p., acrônimo de *a*lternating, *f*ailure *o*f *r*esponse, *m*echanical, to *e*lectrical *d*epolarization, (falha alternante da resposta mecânica às despolarizações elétricas); à medida que o pulso alternante induzido evolui, desenvolve-se um estado no qual despolarizações cardíacas alternadas não resultam em ejeção de sangue, assim permitindo um enchimento diastólico mais prolongado; o batimento subseqüente consegue produzir uma ejeção significativa; em freqüências elevadas, o volume-minuto cardíaco e a pressão arterial podem parecer normais.
   Anrep p., f. de Anrep; auto-regulação homeométrica do coração pela qual o desempenho cardíaco melhora à medida que aumenta a pós-carga (estresse da parede sistólica).
   aqueous influx p., f. de influxo aquoso; o enchimento da veia aquosa (que normalmente leva sangue e líquido aquoso) com líquido aquoso, quando a junção da veia aquosa com a veia receptora é parcialmente ocluída. SIN Ascher aqueous influx p.
   Arias-Stella p., f. de Arias-Stella; alterações deciduais, incomuns, focais no epitélio endometrial, que consistem em brotamento intraluminal e aumento nuclear e hipercromatismo com tumefação citoplasmática e vacuolação; pode estar associado a gravidez ectópica ou uterina. SIN Arias-Stella effect, Arias-Stella reaction.
   arm p., f. de Pool. SIN Pool p. (2).
   Arthus p., f. de Arthus; forma de hipersensibilidade imediata que resulta em eritema, edema, hemorragia e necrose observadas em coelhos após injeção de antígeno ao qual o animal já foi sensibilizado e contra o qual possui anticorpos IgG específicos. A reação é causada pela inflamação resultante da deposição de complexos antígeno-anticorpo nos espaços teciduais e nas paredes dos vasos sanguíneos que ativam o complemento; a maior parte da lesão aparentemente é causada por leucócitos polimorfonucleares que fagocitam os depósitos e liberam enzimas lisossômicas. O fenômeno, descrito por Arthus, foi observado em coelhos, mas são observadas reações semelhantes (reações tipo Arthus) em cobaias, ratos e cães, bem como em seres humanos. VER TAMBÉM Arthus *reaction* (2). SIN Arthus reaction (1).
   Ascher aqueous influx p., f. do influxo aquoso de Ascher. SIN aqueous influx p.
   Aschner p., f. de Aschner. SIN oculocardiac *reflex*.
   Ashman p., f. de Ashman; condução ventricular aberrante de um batimento que encerra um ciclo curto precedido por um ciclo mais longo, na maioria das vezes durante fibrilação atrial.
   Aubert p., f. de Aubert; f. no qual uma linha perpendicular brilhante parece inclinar-se para um lado quando o observador vira a cabeça para o lado oposto em um quarto escuro.
   Austin Flint p., f. de Austin Flint; o sopro da estenose mitral relativa durante regurgitação aórtica significativa causado por estreitamento do orifício mitral por pressão do fluxo regurgitante aórtico no folheto mitral anterior. SIN Austin Flint murmur.
   autoscopic p., f. autoscópico; o encontro de uma imagem de si próprio, sendo a imagem uma ilusão, uma alucinação ou uma fantasia vívida.
   Babinski p., f. de Babinski. SIN Babinski *sign* (1).
   Bell p., f. de Bell; desvio reflexo do olho para cima ao tentar fechar o olho; observado em vários distúrbios, incluindo mononeuropatias faciais, síndrome de Guillain-Barré e miastenia gravis.
   Bombay p., f. de Bombay; um traço recessivo raro em um *locus* que, comumente, fabrica substância H, o precursor a partir do qual são produzidos os fenótipos A e B; a forma mutante causa ausência de produção da substância H e, não importa qual seja o genótipo no *locus* ABO, o fenótipo é O. O fenótipo de Bombay é epistático em relação ao *locus* ABO. [*Bombay*, Índia, onde foi descrito pela primeira vez]
   Bordet-Gengou p., f. de Bordet-Gengou; o f. de fixação do complemento; quando soro contendo complemento é adicionado a uma mistura de bactérias e anticorpo específico, o complemento é removido (fixado) e não está disponí-

vel para lisar eritrócitos adicionados subseqüentemente sensibilizados com anticorpo específico. VER TAMBÉM Gengou p.

breakoff p., breakaway p., f. de rompimento; a ocorrência, durante vôos em grandes altitudes, de uma sensação de estar totalmente desligado da terra e das outras pessoas.

Brücke-Bartley p., f. de Brücke-Bartley; a sensação de ofuscamento em resposta a estímulos sucessivos em freqüências logo abaixo do ponto de fusão.

Capgras p., f. de Capgras. SIN Capgras *syndrome*.

centralization p., f. de centralização; a alteração relativamente rápida na localização percebida da dor, variando de mais periférica, ou distal, a uma localização mais proximal, ou central; comumente ocorre durante a avaliação inicial de pacientes com dor lombar e dor que se irradia para o membro; útil para determinar o tipo e o prognóstico da fisioterapia.

cervicolumbar p., f. cervicolombar; sensação de fraqueza nos membros inferiores ao movimento do pescoço quando há uma lesão na parte superior da medula espinal; ou sensações referidas no pescoço quando existe uma lesão na parte inferior da medula espinal.

cogwheel p., f. de roda dentada; interrupção súbita e breve da respiração geralmente tranqüila ou em outra atividade motora. SIN Negro p.

constancy p., f. de constância; na percepção, a tendência do brilho, cor, tamanho ou formato permanecerem relativamente constantes, no que se refere à percepção, apesar de alterações reais na cor, tamanho, formato ou outras condições de observação.

crowding p., f. de aglomeração; uma característica da visão ambliópica na qual a visão é melhor para a apresentação de um optótipo único que para a apresentação simultânea de múltiplos optótipos.

Cushing p., f. de Cushing; aumento da pressão arterial sistêmica quando a pressão intracraniana aumenta agudamente, em geral acima de 50% da pressão arterial sistólica. SIN Cushing effect, Cushing response.

Danysz p., f. de Danysz; redução do efeito neutralizador de uma antitoxina quando a toxina é misturada a ela em partes divididas, em vez de acrescentar a mesma quantidade total de toxina em uma etapa.

dawn p., f. do amanhecer; aumentos súbitos dos níveis plasmáticos de glicose em jejum entre 5 e 9 horas da manhã, na ausência de hipoglicemia prévia; ocorre em pacientes diabéticos que recebem insulinoterapia.

Debré p., f. de Debré; no sarampo, a ausência de desenvolvimento de erupção cutânea no lugar da injeção de soro imune.

declamping p., f. de desclampeamento; choque ou hipotensão após súbita retirada de clampes de uma grande porção do leito vascular, como da aorta; aparentemente causado por acúmulo transitório de sangue em uma área previamente isquêmica. SIN declamping shock.

déjà vu p., f. de déjà vu; a impressão mental de que uma nova experiência (p. ex., uma situação, uma visão, um som ou uma ação) já aconteceu antes; fenômeno comum em algumas pessoas que pode ser mais freqüente ou contínuo em determinados distúrbios emocionais ou orgânicos. Também denominado déjà entendu, déjà éprouvé, déjà fait, déjà pensé, déjà raconté, déjà vécu ou déjà voulu, dependendo da experiência ou do sentido evocado.

Dejerine hand p., f. da mão de Dejerine; contrações clônicas dos flexores da mão (punho) ao se golpear levemente o dorso da mão ou a face volar do antebraço próximo ao punho; ocorre em pessoas normais, mas é exagerada nas lesões do trato piramidal. SIN Dejerine reflex.

Denys-Leclef p., f. de Denys-Leclef; aumento da fagocitose de microrganismos por leucócitos, na presença de soro imune.

d'Herelle p., f. d'Herelle. SIN Twort-d'Herelle p.

dip p., f. de depressão; desaparecimento completo da excitabilidade ventricular seguido por recuperação progressiva em alguns microssegundos ao fim da excitação; o músculo como um todo repolariza de forma um pouco heterogênea, de modo que esse período é muito sensível a estímulos exógenos ou endógenos e à reentrada.

Donath-Landsteiner p., f. de Donath-Landsteiner; a hemólise que ocorre na amostra de sangue de um indivíduo com hemoglobinúria paroxística quando a amostra é resfriada a cerca de 5°C e, depois, novamente aquecida.

Doppler p., f. Doppler. SIN Doppler *effect*.

Duckworth p., f. de Duckworth; parada respiratória antes da parada cardíaca em virtude de doença intracraniana.

Ehret p., f. de Ehret; pulsação súbita palpada pelo dedo da mão sobre a artéria braquial, à medida que a pressão no esfigmomanômetro cai durante uma medida da pressão arterial; diz-se que indica a pressão diastólica com razoável acurácia.

Ehrlich p., f. de Ehrlich; a diferença entre a quantidade de toxina diftérica que neutralizará exatamente uma unidade de antitoxina e a quantidade que, adicionada a uma unidade de antitoxina, deixará uma dose letal livre, é maior que uma dose letal de toxina; isto é, é necessário acrescentar mais de uma dose letal de toxina a uma mistura neutra de toxina e antitoxina para tornar a mistura letal (a base da dose L$_+$).

erythrocyte adherence p., f. de aderência eritrocitária. SIN adhesion p.

escape p., f. de escape; incapacidade da pupila de um olho com neurite óptica de manter a constrição quando ambos os olhos são estimulados alternadamente com luz.

facialis p., f. facial; espasmo facial produzido pela leve fricção da pele ou por um leve golpe sobre o zigoma; algumas vezes, a percussão acima do zigoma causa contração apenas do lábio; observado na tetania e, algumas vezes, no bócio exoftálmico.

finger p., f. do dedo; sinal de hemiplegia orgânica; com o cotovelo do paciente apoiado sobre uma mesa, a mão do examinador segura o punho do paciente, usando o polegar para exercer pressão sobre a face radial do osso pisiforme do paciente; se a hemiplegia for orgânica, alguns dedos da mão do paciente, ou todos eles, estendem-se e afastam-se como um leque. SIN Gordon sign.

Flynn p., f. de Flynn. SIN paradoxical pupillary *reflex*.

Friedreich p., f. de Friedreich; o som produzido à percussão timpânica de uma cavidade pulmonar é um pouco mais agudo à inspiração profunda.

Galassi pupillary p., f. pupilar de Galassi. SIN eye-closure pupil *reaction*.

Gallavardin p., f. de Gallavardin; dissociação entre os elementos ruidosos e musicais do sopro de ejeção da estenose aórtica, sendo o elemento musical mais bem auscultado na borda esternal esquerda e no ápice cardíaco, enquanto o elemento ruidoso é mais bem ouvido no foco aórtico; projeção do sopro da estenose aórtica para a borda esternal esquerda baixa.

gap p., f. de intervalo; um curto período, no ciclo da condução atrioventricular ou intraventricular, que permite a passagem de um impulso que, em outros momentos, teria seu trânsito bloqueado. SIN excitable gap.

Gärtner vein p., f. venoso de Gärtner; repleção das veias do braço e da mão abaixo do nível do coração e colapso a uma determinada distância variável acima desse nível. Um teste não-fidedigno da pressão venosa.

generalized Shwartzman p., f. de Shwartzman generalizado; quando tanto a injeção primária de filtrado contendo endotoxina quanto a injeção secundária são administradas por via intravenosa com um intervalo de 24 horas, o animal geralmente morre nas primeiras 24 horas após a segunda inoculação; as lesões características no coelho incluem hemorragias disseminadas no pulmão, fígado e em outros órgãos, bem como necrose cortical bilateral do rim. Essa reação não tem base imunológica. SIN Sanarelli p., Sanarelli-Shwartzman p.

Gengou p., f. de Gengou; uma extensão do fenômeno de Bordet-Gengou; antígenos acelulares, quando misturados com anticorpo específico, também fixam o complemento.

gestalt p., VER gestalt.

Glover p., f. de Glover; variação não-aleatória (isto é, casual) entre comunidades nas taxas de realização de procedimentos eletivos comuns, como tonsilectomia, histerectomia, atribuível a variações locais nas práticas clínicas e cirúrgicas.

Grasset p., f. de Grasset; na paralisia orgânica do membro inferior, o paciente em decúbito dorsal pode elevar cada membro separadamente, mas não os dois juntos. SIN Grasset-Gaussel p.

Grasset-Gaussel p., f. de Grasset-Gaussel. SIN Grasset p.

Gunn p., f. de Gunn. SIN jaw-winking *syndrome*.

Hamburger p., f. de Hamburger. SIN chloride *shift*.

Hill p., f. de Hill. SIN Hill *sign*.

hip p., f. do quadril. SIN Joffroy *reflex*.

hip-flexion p., f. de flexão do quadril; quando um hemiplégico tenta levantar-se de uma postura deitada, o quadril do lado paralisado é fletido primeiro; o mesmo movimento é feito ao deitar.

Hoffmann p., f. de Hoffmann; irritabilidade excessiva dos nervos sensoriais a estímulos elétricos ou mecânicos na tetania.

Houssay p., f. de Houssay. VER Houssay *animal*.

Hunt paradoxic p., f. paradoxal de Hunt; na distonia muscular deformante, se for feita uma tentativa de flexão plantar do pé quando está em espasmo dorsal, a única resposta é um aumento do espasmo extensor ou dorsal; entretanto, se o paciente é instruído a estender o pé que já está em um estado de forte flexão dorsal, haverá um súbito movimento de flexão plantar; o mesmo fenômeno, *mutatis mutandis*, é observado quando há forte flexão plantar.

immune adherence p., f. de aderência imune. SIN adhesion p.

jaw-winking p., f. da mandíbula-piscadela. SIN jaw-winking *syndrome*.

Jod-Basedow p., f. de Jod-Basedow; indução de tireotoxicose em um indivíduo previamente eutireóideo por exposição a grandes quantidades de iodo; é mais freqüente em áreas de bócio endêmico por deficiência de iodo e em pacientes com bócio multinodular; também pode se desenvolver após o uso de agentes contendo iodo para fins diagnósticos. SIN iodine-induced hyperthyroidism.

Köbner p., f. de Köbner. SIN isomorphic *response*.

Koch p., f. de Koch; **(1)** o fenômeno de imunidade à infecção; os bacilos da tuberculose (*Mycobacterium tuberculosis*) vivos não causam reinfecção quando inoculados em cobaias tuberculosas (isto é, os animais são "imunes" à reinfecção), embora as infecções originais continuem a se desenvolver e acabem matando os animais; **(2)** aumento da temperatura e aumento da lesão local, em um indivíduo tuberculoso, após uma injeção de tuberculina.

Kohnstamm p., f. de Kohnstamm. SIN aftermovement.

Kühne p., f. de Kühne; quando uma corrente constante é passada através de um músculo, é observada uma ondulação que segue do pólo positivo para o negativo.

LE p., f. LE; a formação de células LE na medula óssea ou no sangue ao acrescentar soro de pacientes com lúpus eritematoso disseminado.

Leede-Rumpel p., f. de Leede-Rumpel. Rumpel-Leede p. (q.v.).

leg p., f. da perna. SIN Pool p. (1).

Lucio leprosy p., f. da hanseníase de Lucio. SIN Lucio *leprosy*.

Marcus Gunn p., f. de Marcus Gunn. SIN jaw-winking *syndrome*.

misdirection p., regeneração aberrante. SIN aberrant *regeneration*.

Mitsuo p., f. de Mitsuo; restauração da cor normal do fundo de olho com adaptação ao escuro na doença de Oguchi.

Negro p., f. de Negro. SIN cogwheel p.

no reflow p., f. de ausência de refluxo; ausência de fluxo sanguíneo, ao nível da microcirculação, em uma área lesada do encéfalo após reperfusão.

on-off p., f. de intermitência; um estado, no tratamento da doença de Parkinson com L-dopa, no qual há uma rápida flutuação de movimentos acinéticos (desligados) e coreoatetóticos (ligados).

orbicularis p., f. orbicular. SIN eye-closure pupil *reaction*.

paradoxical diaphragm p., f. do diafragma paradoxal; no piopneumotórax, hidropneumotórax e alguns casos de lesão, o diafragma do lado afetado eleva-se durante a inspiração e abaixa durante a expiração.

paradoxical pupillary p., f. pupilar paradoxal. SIN paradoxical pupillary *reflex*.

peroneal p., f. peroneal; a leve percussão do nervo fibular abaixo da cabeça da fíbula causa dorsiflexão e abdução do pé.

Pfeiffer p., f. de Pfeiffer; alteração e desintegração completa dos vibriões do cólera quando introduzidos na cavidade peritoneal de uma cobaia imunizada, ou na cavidade peritoneal de uma cobaia normal se for injetado soro imune ao mesmo tempo; ampliado para incluir a bacteriólise em geral.

phi p., f. fi; uma ilusão de movimento, que ocorre por meio de impressões visuais sucessivas a intervalos de 1/15 a 1/20 s; quando se passa um oclusor de um olho para o outro, enquanto se observa uma luz distante, a luz parece mover-se com o oclusor quando há exoforia, mas, na direção oposta, quando há esoforia.

Pool p., f. de Pool; **(1)** na tetania, espasmo dos músculos do quadríceps e da panturrilha quando a perna estendida é fletida no quadril. SIN leg p., Pool-Schlesinger sign, Schlesinger sign; **(2)** na tetania, contração dos músculos do braço após o estiramento do plexo braquial por elevação do braço acima da cabeça com o antebraço estendido, assemelhando-se à contração resultante da estimulação do nervo ulnar. SIN arm p.

pseudo-Graefe p., pseudofenômeno de Graefe; retração da pálpebra superior ao movimentar os olhos para baixo.

psi p., f. psi; f. que inclui psicocinese e percepção extra-sensorial; os processos mentais extra-sensoriais envolvidos na suposta capacidade de enviar ou receber mensagens telepáticas.

Pulfrich p., f. de Pulfrich; a percepção binocular de que um pequeno alvo oscilante no plano frontal está se movendo em um trajeto elíptico observado quando um olho é coberto por um filtro ou na presença de uma neuropatia óptica unilateral.

Purkinje p., f. de Purkinje; no olho adaptado à luz, a região de máximo brilho está no amarelo; no olho adaptado ao escuro, a região de máximo brilho está no verde. SIN Purkinje effect, Purkinje shift.

quellung p., intumescimento capsular de Neufeld. SIN Neufeld capsular *swelling*.

radial p., f. radial; flexão dorsal da mão que ocorre involuntariamente com a flexão palmar dos dedos.

Raynaud p., f. de Raynaud; espasmo das artérias digitais, com palidez e dormência ou dor dos dedos, freqüentemente precipitados pelo frio. Os dedos apresentam-se variavelmente vermelhos, brancos e azuis.

rebound p., f. de rebote; **(1)** SIN Stewart-Holmes *sign*; **(2)** genericamente, qualquer fenômeno no qual uma variável que foi deslocada de seu estado normal por uma influência perturbadora desvia-se temporariamente do normal na direção oposta, quando a influência é subitamente interrompida, antes de, finalmente, estabilizar-se em seu estado normal, isto é, um fenômeno que envolve subultrapassagem; p. ex., a hipoglicemia subseqüente que pode suceder a injeção de glicose, porque a hiperglicemia inicial causou secreção excessiva de insulina.

reclotting p., f. de recoagulação. SIN thixotropy.

red cell adherence p., f. de aderência eritrocitária. SIN adhesion p.

reentry p., f. de reentrada. VER reentry.

release p., f. de liberação; o aumento do tônus e a hiperirritabilidade dos reflexos de estiramento muscular que ocorrem após lesão das partes superiores do sistema extrapiramidal.

Riddoch p., f. de Riddoch; capacidade de observar um pequeno objeto em movimento em uma área do campo visual cega para objetos estáticos; associado sobretudo a lesões do lobo occipital.

Ritter-Rollet p., f. de Ritter-Rollet; à estimulação elétrica igual dos troncos de nervos motores, os grupos musculares flexores e abdutores reagem mais facilmente que os extensores e adutores.

R-on-T p., f. R sobre T; um complexo ventricular (QRS) prematuro, no eletrocardiograma, que interrompe a onda T do batimento precedente; freqüentemente predispõe a arritmias ventriculares graves.

Rumpel-Leede p., f. de Rumpel-Leede; surgimento de petéquias em uma área conseqüente à aplicação de constrição vascular, como por um torniquete, geralmente após 10 minutos, mas pode surgir após um período menor, como depois da aplicação de torniquete para colher amostras de sangue ou do uso do esfigmomanômetro; é decorrente de fragilidade capilar ou de anormalidade do número (p. ex., trombocitopenia) ou da função das plaquetas.

Rust p., f. de Rust; no câncer ou na destruição das vértebras cervicais superiores, o paciente sempre sustentará a cabeça com as mãos ao passar do decúbito para a posição sentada, ou o inverso.

Sanarelli p., f. de Sanarelli. SIN generalized Shwartzman p.

Sanarelli-Shwartzman p., f. de Sanarelli-Shwartzman. SIN generalized Shwartzman p.

Schellong-Strisower p., f. de Schellong-Strisower; redução da pressão arterial sistólica, acompanhada algumas vezes por vertigem, ao passar da posição horizontal para a ortostática.

Schiff-Sherrington p., f. de Schiff-Sherrington; quando a medula espinal é transeccionada na região torácica média ou um pouco abaixo, o reflexo de estiramento e outros reflexos posturais do membro superior são exagerados; se a transecção é feita na medula sacral, observa-se um efeito semelhante nos membros inferiores. O efeito é considerado um fenômeno de liberação, isto é, liberação de uma influência inibitória normalmente exercida pelos segmentos espinais abaixo da transecção.

Schüller p., f. de Schüller; quando pacientes com hemiplegia caminham, se o distúrbio for funcional eles viram-se para o lado não afetado; se for orgânico, eles viram-se para o lado afetado.

Schultz-Charlton p., f. de Schultz-Charlton. SIN Schultz-Charlton *reaction*.

Sherrington p., f. de Sherrington; após os músculos da perna terem sido privados de sua inervação motora por secção das raízes ventrais que contêm fibras para o nervo ciático, e dando-se tempo para que haja degeneração das fibras, a estimulação do nervo ciático causa contração lenta dos músculos.

shot-silk p., f. de seda molhada. SIN shot-silk *retina*.

Shwartzman p., f. de Shwartzman; um coelho recebe injeção intradérmica de pequena dose de lipopolissacarídeo (endotoxina) seguida por uma segunda injeção intravenosa 24 horas depois, e desenvolverá uma lesão hemorrágica e necrótica no local da primeira injeção. VER TAMBÉM generalized Shwartzman p. SIN Shwartzman reaction.

Somogyi p., f. de Somogyi; f. de rebote de hiperglicemia reativa após um período de hipoglicemia relativa, que pode ser subclínica e difícil de detectar; a hiperglicemia induz o uso de mais insulina, assim agravando o problema. SIN posthypoglycemic hyperglycemia.

Soret p., f. de Soret; em uma solução mantida em um tubo longo, vertical, à temperatura ambiente, a parte superior, sendo a mais quente, também é a mais concentrada.

sparing p., f. poupador. SIN sparing *action*.

Splendore-Hoeppli p., f. de Splendore-Hoeppli; depósitos eosinofílicos irradiados ou anulares de materiais provenientes do hospedeiro, bem como, possivelmente, de antígenos do parasita, que se formam ao redor de fungos, helmintos ou colônias de bactérias no tecido.

staircase p., f. da escada. SIN treppe.

Staub-Traugott p., f. de Staub-Traugott; o aumento da taxa de remoção da glicose administrada logo após uma dose grande inicial de glicose.

steal p., f. de seqüestro. VER steal.

Strümpell p., f. de Strümpell; flexão dorsal do hálux, algumas vezes de todo o pé, em um membro paralisado quando a extremidade é erguida contra o corpo, fletindo o joelho e o quadril. SIN tibial p.

symbiotic fermentation p., f. de fermentação simbiótica; "dois organismos, nenhum dos quais, isoladamente, produz fermentação gasosa em determinados carboidratos, podem fazê-lo quando vivem em simbiose ou quando misturados artificialmente" (Castellani).

Theobald Smith p., f. de Theobald Smith; fenômeno observado em cobaias que sobreviveram ao uso para padronização da antitoxina diftérica, tendo os animais se tornado altamente suscepíveis à inoculação subseqüente de soro eqüino.

tibial p., f. tibial. SIN Strümpell p.

toe p., f. do artelho. SIN Babinski *sign* (1).

tongue p., f. da língua. SIN Schultze *sign*.

Tournay p., f. de Tournay; dilatação da pupila no olho abduzido no olhar lateral extremo. Ocorre apenas em uma pequena percentagem da população normal e não tem associação conhecida com doença. SIN Tournay sign.

Tullio p., f. de Tullio; vertigem momentânea causada por qualquer som alto, que ocorre notavelmente em casos de fístula labirintina ativa.

two-dimension–three-dimension p., f. bidimensional-tridimensional; uma experiência em endoscopia telescópica na qual uma imagem bidimensional parece ser tridimensional devido ao movimento do endoscópio dentro e fora da vista do objeto.

Twort p., f. de Twort. SIN Twort-d'Herelle p.
Twort-d'Herelle p., f. de Twort-d'Herelle; a lise de bactérias por bacteriófagos. SIN d'Herelle p., Twort p.
Tyndall p., f. de Tyndall; a visibilidade de partículas flutuantes em gases ou líquidos quando iluminados por um raio de luz solar e vistos formando ângulos retos com esse raio. SIN Tyndall effect.
vacuum disk p., f. do disco com vácuo; o surgimento de uma faixa radiotransparente em um disco intervertebral, uma manifestação de degeneração do disco; um nome errado, pois há gás.
warmup p., f. de aquecimento; diminuição progressiva da resposta miotônica de um músculo durante contração repetida do músculo.
Wenckebach p., f. de Wenckebach; aumento progressivo do tempo de condução em qualquer tecido cardíaco (na maioria das vezes, o nó ou junção AV) até que, finalmente, há perda de um batimento (Wenckebach AV) ou reversão para o tempo de condução inicial (como no Wenckebach QRS).
Westphal-Piltz p., f. de Westphal-Piltz. SIN eye-closure pupil *reaction.*
Wever-Bray p., f. de Wever-Bray. SIN cochlear microphonic.

---

phe·no·per·i·dine (fē - nō - per′i - dēn). Fenoperidina; um analgésico.
phe·no·thi·a·zine (fē - nō - thī′a - zēn). Fenotiazina; composto muito usado antigamente para o tratamento de nematódeos intestinais em animais; sem atividade depressora do sistema nervoso central por si só, serve como o composto original para síntese de um grande número de compostos antipsicóticos, incluindo a clorpromazina, a tioridazina, a perfenazina e a flufenazina. SIN dibenzothiazine, thiodiphenylamine.
phe·no·type (fē′nō - tīp). Fenótipo; as características observáveis, a nível físico, morfológico ou bioquímico, de um indivíduo, determinadas pelo genótipo e pelo ambiente. [G. *phaino*, exibir, + *typos*, modelo]
phe·no·typ·ic (fē′nō - tip′ik, fen - ō-). Fenotípico; relativo ao fenótipo.
phen·ox·a·zine (fe - nok′sa - zēn). Fenoxazina; fenotiazina na qual S é substituído por O; como o derivado 3-oxo (fenoxazona), a fenoxazina é o cromóforo das actinomicinas.
phen·ox·a·zone (fe - nok′sa - zōn). Fenoxazona. VER phenoxazine.
phe·nox·y·ben·za·mine hy·dro·chlo·ride (fe - nok′si - ben′za - mēn). Cloridrato de fenoxibenzamina; potente bloqueador adrenérgico não-seletivo (receptor α) das β-haloalquilaminas; bloqueia a resposta excitatória do músculo liso e glândulas exócrinas à adrenalina; usado no tratamento de doenças vasculares periféricas e do feocromocitoma.
2-phe·nox·y·eth·a·nol (fē - nok - si - eth′a - nol). 2-Fenoxietanol; agente antibacteriano usado no tratamento tópico de infecções de feridas; é ativo contra bactérias Gram-negativas resistentes à maioria dos outros anti-sépticos.
α-phe·nox·y·eth·yl·pen·i·cil·lin po·tas·si·um (fē - nok′sē - eth′il - pen - i - sil′in). α-Fenoxietilpenicilina potássica. SIN phenethicillin potassium.
phe·nox·y·meth·yl·pen·i·cil·lin (fe - nok′si - meth′il - pen - i - sil′in). Fenoximetilpenicilina. SIN *penicillin* V.
α-phe·nox·y·pro·pyl·pen·i·cil·lin potassium (fē′nok - sē - prō′pil - pen - i - sil′in). α-Fenoxipropilpenicilina potássica. SIN propicillin.
phe·no·zy·gous (fē′nō - zī′gus, fe - noz′i - gŭs). Fenózigo; que possui um crânio estreito em comparação com a largura da face, de forma que, quando o crânio é visto de cima, os arcos zigomáticos são visíveis. [G. *phaino*, mostrar, + *zygon*, gema]
phen·pen·ter·mine tar·trate (fen - pen′ter - mēn). Tartarato de fempentermina; um agente anorexígeno.
phen·pro·ba·mate (fen - prō′ba - māt). Femprobamato; um relaxante da musculatura esquelética com ação ansiolítica semelhante à do meprobamato. SIN proformiphen.
phen·pro·cou·mon (fen - prō - koo′mon). Fenoprocumona; um anticoagulante efetivo por via oral, de ação prolongada.
phen·pro·pi·o·nate (fen - prō′pē - ō - nāt). Fempropionato; contração para 3-fenilpropionato aprovada pela USAN.
phen·sux·i·mide (fen - sŭk′si - mīd). Fensuximida; anticonvulsivante usado no tratamento da crise de ausência (epilepsia tipo pequeno mal).
phen·ter·mine (fen′ter - mēn). Fentermina; agente anorexígeno semelhante à anfetamina; também disponível na forma de cloridrato.
phen·tol·a·mine hy·dro·chlo·ride (fen - tol′a - mēn). Cloridrato de fentolamina; um agente bloqueador adrenérgico (receptor α) não-seletivo.
phen·tol·a·mine mes·y·late. Mesilato de fentolamina; as mesmas ações do cloridrato de fentolamina, apenas para uso intravenoso.
phen·yl (Ph, Φ) (fen′il). Fenil; a porção univalente, C_6H_5-, do benzeno.
   p. alcohol, fenol. SIN phenol.
   p. aminosalicylate, aminossalicilato de fenil; medicamento antituberculoso de segunda linha com alta incidência de reações de hipersensibilidade e perturbação gastrointestinal.
   p. salicylate, salicilato de fenil; o éster salicílico do fenol; o éster fenílico do ácido salicílico; analgésico intestinal e antipirético; tem sido usado no tratamento do reumatismo, da diarréia e da faringite, como revestimento entérico de comprimidos, e em cremes para prevenção de queimadura solar. SIN salol.

phen·yl·a·ce·tic ac·id (fen′il - ă - sē′tik). Ácido fenilacético; um produto anormal do catabolismo da fenilalanina, que aparece na urina de indivíduos com fenilcetonúria.
phen·yl·a·ce·tur·ic ac·id (fen′il - as - ē - toor′ik). Ácido fenilacetúrico. SIN phenaceturic acid.
phen·yl·a·ce·tyl·u·rea (fen - il - as′ē - til - ū - rē′a). Fenilacetiluréia. SIN phenacemide.
phen·yl·a·cryl·ic ac·id (fen′il - ă - kril′ik). Ácido fenilacrílico. SIN cinnamic acid.
phen·yl·al·a·nin·ase (fen - il - al′ă - nin - ās). Fenilalaninase; fenilalanina 4-monoxigenase.
phen·yl·al·a·nine (Phe, F) (fen - il - al′ă - nēn). Fenilalanina; ácido 2-amino-3-fenilpropiônico; o L-isômero dos aminoácidos comuns em proteínas, um aminoácido nutricionalmente essencial.
   p. ammonia-lyase, f. amônia-liase; uma enzima, não encontrada em mamíferos, que catalisa a conversão de L-fenilalanina em *trans*-cinamato e amônia; tem sido usada no tratamento da fenilcetonúria.
   p. 4-hydroxylase, f. 4-hidroxilase. SIN p. 4-monooxygenase.
   p. 4-monooxygenase, f. 4-monooxigenase; enzima que catalisa a oxidação da L-fenilalanina em L-tirosina com O_2 e tetraidrobiopterina (esta última formando o derivado diidro), que, por sua vez, é reduzida para a forma ativa pelo NADPH e por uma redutase; a deficiência de qualquer dessas enzimas resultará em fenilcetonúria. SIN p. 4-hydroxylase.
phen·yl·a·mine (fe - nil′ă - mēn). Fenilamina. SIN aniline.
phen·yl·ben·zene (fen - il - ben′zēn). Fenilbenzeno. SIN diphenyl.
phen·yl·bu·ta·zone (fen - il - bū′ta - zōn). Fenilbutazona; agente analgésico, antipirético, antiinflamatório e uricosúrico.
phen·yl·car·bi·nol (fen - il - kar′bi - nol). Fenilcarbinol. SIN *benzyl* alcohol.
phen·yl·di·chlo·ro·ar·sine (PD) (fen′il - dī - klōr - ō - ar′sēn). Fenildicloroarsina; líquido tóxico que tem sido usado como agente vesicante e causador de vômito por algumas organizações militares e policiais; foi usado pela primeira vez de forma limitada na I Guerra Mundial.
phen·yl·eph·rine hy·dro·chlo·ride (fen - il - ef′rin). Cloridrato de fenilefrina; potente vasoconstritor, usado como descongestionante nasal e midriático.
phen·yl·eth·a·no·la·mine *N*-meth·yl·trans·fer·ase (PNMT) (fē′nil - eth - an - ol′a - mēn). Feniletanolamina *N*-metiltransferase; enzima fundamental na biossíntese das catecolaminas que catalisa a conversão de norepinefrina em epinefrina, utilizando S-adenosil-L-metionina; encontrada na medula da supra-renal e em alguns neurônios; a biossíntese dessa enzima é induzida por cortisol.
phen·yl·eth·yl al·co·hol (fen - il - eth′il). Álcool feniletílico; um constituinte natural de alguns óleos essenciais (rosa, gerânio, nerol); usado como agente antibacteriano em soluções oftálmicas. SIN benzyl carbinol, phenethyl alcohol.
phen·yl·eth·yl·bar·bi·tur·ic ac·id (fen′il - eth′il - bar - bi - tūr′ik). Ácido feniletilbarbitúrico. SIN phenobarbital.
phen·yl·eth·yl·ma·lo·na·mide (fen′il - eth′il - mal - on - ă - mīd). Feniletilmalonamida; metabólito da primidona, agente antiepiléptico. A feniletilmalonamida tem atividade anticonvulsivante em animais, mas não foi avaliada como agente antiepiléptico em seres humanos.
phen·yl·eth·yl·mal·o·nyl·u·rea (fen′il - eth′il - mal′ō - nil - ū - rē′a). Feniltilmaloniluréia. SIN phenobarbital.
phen·yl·gly·col·ic ac·id (fen′il - glī - kol′ik). Ácido fenilglicólico. SIN mandelic acid.
phen·yl·in·dane·di·one (fen′il - in - dān′dī - ōn). Fenilindanediona. SIN phenindione.
phen·yl·i·so·thi·o·cy·a·nate (PITC, PhNCS) (fen′il - ī′sō - thī - ō - sī′ă - nāt). Fenilisotiocianato; reagente que se liga ao grupamento amino N-terminal livre de uma cadeia peptídica para formar uma feniltioidantoína no método Edman para identificação de aminoácidos N-terminais. SIN Edman reagent.
phen·yl·ke·to·nu·ri·a (PKU) (fen′il - kē′tō - noo′rē - ă). Fenilcetonúria; erro congênito do metabolismo da fenilalanina, com herança autossômica recessiva, caracterizado por deficiência de 1) fenilalanina hidroxilase [MIM*261600] causada por mutação no gene da fenilalanina hidroxilase (PAH) em 12q; 2) ocasionalmente, diidropteridina redutase [MIM*261630], causada por mutação no gene da diidropteridina redutase (DHPR) em 4p; 3) raramente, diidrobiopterina sintetase [MIM*261640], causada por mutação no gene da piruvoil tetraidropterina sintase (PTS) em 11q; ou 4) ainda mais raramente, guanidina trifosfato cicloidrolase 1 [MIM*233910]. O distúrbio é caracterizado por formação inadequada de L-tirosina, elevação da L-fenilalanina sérica, excreção urinária de ácido fenilpirúvico e de outros derivados, e acúmulo de fenilalanina e seus metabólitos, que pode produzir lesão cerebral, resultando em grave retardo mental, freqüentemente com convulsões, outras anormalidades neurológicas, com retardo da mielinização e deficiência da formação de melanina, levando à hipopigmentação da pele e eczema. Cf. hyperphenilalaninemia. SIN Folling disease, phenylpyruvate oligophrenia. [phenyl + ketone + G. *ouron*, urina]

nonclassical p., f. não-clássica. SIN malignant *hyperphenylalaninemia.*
phen·yl·lac·tic ac·id (fen - il - lak'tik). Ácido fenilático; produto do catabolismo da fenilalanina, surgindo de forma proeminente na urina de indivíduos com fenilcetonúria.
phen·yl·mer·cu·ric ac·e·tate (fen'il - mer - kū'rik). Acetato fenilmercúrico; conservante bacteriostático, fungicida e herbicida (especialmente para capim-das-hortas).
phen·yl·mer·cu·ric ni·trate. Nitrato fenilmercúrico; uma mistura de nitrato fenilmercúrico e hidróxido fenilmercúrico; um anti-séptico usado para a desinfecção profilática da pele intacta ou de pequenas feridas.
phen·yl·pro·pa·nol·a·mine (fen'il - prō - pā - nol'ā - mēn). Fenilpropanolamina; uma amina simpaticomimética, usada como descongestionante nasal, broncodilatador e supressor do apetite.
phe·nyl·py·ru·vic ac·id (fen'il - pī - roo'vik). Ácido fenilpirúvico; o produto transaminado da ação da fenilalanina aminotransferase; elevada na urina de indivíduos com fenilcetonúria.
phen·yl·thi·o·car·ba·mide (fen'yl - thī - ō - kar'bā - mīd). Feniltiocarbamida. SIN phenylthiourea.
phen·yl·thi·o·car·bam·o·yl (PTC). Feniltiocarbamoil. VER phenylthiocarbamoyl *peptide.*
phen·yl·thi·o·hy·dan·to·in (PTH) (fen'il - thī'ō - hī - dan'tō - in). Feniltioidantoína; o composto formado a partir de um aminoácido no método Edman de degradação de proteínas, no qual o fenilisotiocianato reage com a porção amino do aminoácido N-terminal para formar um peptídeo ou proteína feniltiocarbamoil, sobre os quais os ácidos fracos agem para liberar a feniltioidantoína que contém o aminoácido N-terminal.
phen·yl·thi·o·u·rea (fen'il - thī'ō - ū - rē'a) [MIM*171200]. Feniltiouréia; uma substância que tem sabor amargo para algumas pessoas, mas é insípida para outras. Acredita-se que a capacidade de perceber o gosto seja uma característica autossômica dominante. A feniltiouréia contém o grupamento N–C≠ S do qual, aparentemente, depende a peculiaridade do sabor; substâncias bociogênicas ou antitireóideas (p. ex., tiouréia e tiouracil), que também contêm esse grupamento, possuem a mesma propriedade em relação ao sabor. SIN phenylthiocarbamide.
phen·yl·to·lox·a·mine (fen'il - tol - ok'sā - mēn). Feniltoloxamina; um anti-histamínico.
phen·yl·tri·meth·yl·am·mo·ni·um (PTMA) (fen'il - trī - meth'il - ā - mō'nē - ūm). Feniltrimetilamônio; estimulante extremamente seletivo das placas terminais motoras do músculo esquelético.
phen·y·ram·i·dol hy·dro·chlo·ride (fen - i - ram'i - dol). Cloridrato de feniramidol; analgésico e relaxante muscular.
phen·yt·o·in (fen'i - tō - in). Fenitoína; anticonvulsivante usado no tratamento da epilepsia tônico-clônica generalizada e da epilepsia parcial complexa. Também disponível na forma de fenitoína sódica, com os mesmos empregos que a fenitoína. SIN 5,5-diphenylhydantoin.
♻ **pheo-.** Feo-. **1.** Prefixo que designa os mesmos substituintes em um resíduo forbina ou forbida (porfirina) presentes na clorofila, excluindo quaisquer resíduos éster e Mg. **2.** Forma combinante que significa cinza, escuro. [G. *phaios,* pardo]
phe·o·chrome (fē'ō - krōm). Feocromo. **1.** SIN chromaffin. **2.** Que adquire coloração escura com sais crômicos. [G. *phaios,* pardo, + *chrōma,* cor]
phe·o·chro·mo·blast (fē - ō - krō'mō - blast). Feocromoblasto; célula cromafin primitiva que, com simpatetoblastos, entra na formação da glândula supra-renal. [G. *phaios,* pardo, + *chrōma,* cor, + *blastos,* germe]
phe·o·chro·mo·cyte (fē - ō - krō'mō - sīt). Feocromócito; célula cromafin de um paragânglio simpático, medula de uma glândula supra-renal ou feocromocitoma. [pheochrome + G. *kytos,* célula]
phe·o·chro·mo·cy·to·ma (fē'ō - krō'mō - sī - tō'mă). Feocromocitoma; cromafinoma funcional, geralmente benigno, derivado de células do tecido medular supra-renal e caracterizado pela secreção de catecolaminas, resultando em hipertensão arterial, que pode ser paroxística e associada a episódios de palpitação, cefaléia, náuseas, dispnéia, ansiedade, palidez e sudorese profusa. O feocromocitoma freqüentemente é hereditário, não apenas em facomas como a doença de Hippel-Lindau, neurofibromatose e neoplasia endócrina familiar, mas também como um defeito isolado [MIM*171300] como um traço autossômico dominante. VER TAMBÉM paraganglioma.
phe·o·mel·a·nin (fē - ō - mel'ā - nin). Feomelanina; tipo de melanina encontrada no cabelo ruivo; contém enxofre e é solúvel em álcalis; são encontrados níveis elevados no tipo ruivo de albinismo oculocutâneo. Cf. eumelanin. [G. *phaios,* pardo, + *melos* (*melan-*), preto]
phe·o·mel·a·no·gen·e·sis (fē'ō - mel'ā - nō - jen'ē - sis). Feomelanogênese; a produção de feomelanina por células vivas.
phe·o·mel·a·no·some (fē - ō - mel'ā - nō - sōm). Feomelanossoma; melanossoma esférico de feomelanina no cabelo ruivo.
phe·re·sis (fe - rē'sis). Ferese; procedimento pelo qual o sangue é removido de um doador, separado, sendo uma parte retida, e o restante devolvido ao doador. VER TAMBÉM leukapheresis, plateletpheresis, plasmapheresis. [G. *aphairesis,* retirada]

pher·o·mones (fer'ō - mōnz). Feromônios; ferormônios; feromonas; tipo de ectormônio secretado por um indivíduo e percebido por um segundo indivíduo da mesma espécie ou de espécie semelhante, assim produzindo uma alteração do comportamento social ou sexual desse segundo indivíduo. Cf. allelochemicals, allomones, kairomones. [G. *pherō,* carregar, + *hormaō,* excitar, estimular]
Ph.G. 1. Abreviatura de *Pharmacopoeia Germanica* (Farmacopéia Alemã). **2.** Abreviatura de Graduate in Pharmacy (Graduado em Farmácia), um grau que não é mais oferecido nos Estados Unidos.
phi (φ, Φ) (fī). **1.** A 21.ª letra do alfabeto grego. **2.** (Φ) Símbolo de phenyl (fenil); potencial energy (energia potencial); magnetic flux (fluxo magnético). **3.** (φ) Símbolo do plane angle (ângulo plano); volume fraction (fração de volume); quantum yield (rendimento quântico); o ângulo diédrico de rotação em torno da ligação N–C$_\alpha$ associada a uma ligação peptídica.
phi·al (fī'al). Pequeno frasco. SIN vial. [G. *phialē,* um recipiente largo e plano]
phi·a·lide (fī'ā - līd). Fiálide; célula conidiógena na qual a extremidade meristemática permanece inalterada enquanto sucessivos conídios são expulsos para formar cadeias. [G. *phialē,* um recipiente plano e largo]
phi·a·lo·con·id·i·um, pl. **phi·a·lo·co·nid·ia** (fī'ā - lō - ko - nid'ē - ūm, fī'ā - lō - kō - nid'ē - ā). Fialoconídio; conídio produzido por uma fiálide.
Phi·a·loph·o·ra (fī - ā - lof'ō - ră). Gênero de fungos do qual pelo menos duas espécies, *P. verrucosa* e *P. dermatitidis* (*Exophiala dermatidites*), causam cromoblastomicose. [G. *phialē,* um recipiente largo e plano, + *phoreō,* carregar]
♻ **-phil, -phile, -philic, -philia.** -fil, -filo, -fílico, -filia; afinidade por, atração por. VER TAMBÉM philo-. [G. *philos,* amigo, amante; *phileō,* amar]
phil·i·a·ter (fil'ē - ā'ter, fi - lī'ā - ter). Filiatra; termo raramente usado para designar aquele interessado no estudo da medicina. [G. *philos,* amigo, + *iatreia,* prática da medicina]
Philip, Sir Robert W., médico escocês, 1857–1939. VER P. *glands,* em gland.
Philippe, Claudien, patologista francês, 1866–1903. VER P. *triangle.*
Philipps, Charles, urologista francês, 1809–1871. VER P. *catheter.*
Phillipson re·flex. Reflexo de Phillipson. Ver em reflex.
♻ **philo-.** VER -phil. [G. *philos,* amigo, amante; *phileō,* amar]
phi·lo·mi·me·sia (fil'ō - mī - mē'sē - ā). Filomimesia; termo raramente usado para designar um impulso mórbido de imitar ou simular. [philo- + G. *mimēsis,* imitação]
Phil·o·pia ca·sei (fil - ō'pē - ā kā'sē - ī). Espécie que pode causar míiase intestinal temporária. SIN cheese maggot.
phil·o·pro·gen·i·tive (fil'ō - prō - jen'i - tiv). Filoprogenitivo. **1.** Procriativo, que produz descendência. **2.** Em psiquiatria, termo obsoleto para designar pedofilia. [philo- + L. *progenies,* descendência, prole]
phil·trum, pl. **phil·tra** (fil'trum, - tră). [TA] Filtro. **1.** Um filtro ou poção do amor. **2** [NA]. A depressão infranasal; o sulco na linha média do lábio superior. [L., do G. *philtron,* feitiço de amor, depressão no lábio superior, de *phileō,* amar]
phi·mo·sis, pl. **phi·mo·ses** (fī - mō'sis, - sēz). Fimose; estreitamento da abertura do prepúcio, impedindo que seja retraído sobre a glande. [G. amordaçamento, de *phimos,* mordaça]
p. clitor'idis, f. do clitóris; aglutinação das pregas do clitóris.
p. vagina'lis, p. vaginal; estreitamento da vagina.
phi·mot·ic (fī - mot'ik). Fimótico; relativo à fimose.
♻ **phleb-.** VER phlebo-.
phle·bal·gia (flē - bal'jē - ă). Flebalgia; dor que se origina em uma veia. [phlebo- + G. *algos,* dor]
phleb·ec·ta·sia (fleb - ek - tā'zē - ă). Flebectasia; vasodilatação das veias. SIN venectasia. [phlebo- + G. *ektasis,* estiramento]
phle·bec·to·my (fle - bek'tō - mē). Flebectomia; excisão de um segmento de uma veia, algumas vezes realizada para a cura de veias varicosas. VER TAMBÉM strip (2). SIN venectomy. [phlebo- + G. *ektomē,* excisão]
phleb·eu·rysm (fleb'ū - rizm). Fleborismo; dilatação patológica (variz) de uma veia. [phlebo- + G. *eurys,* largo]
phle·bit·ic (fle - bit'ik). Flebítico; relativo à flebite.
phle·bi·tis (fle - bī'tis). Flebite; inflamação de uma veia. [phlebo- + G. *-itis,* inflamação]
adhesive p., f. adesiva; forma de f. na qual as paredes se aderem, levando à obliteração do vaso.
p. nodula'ris necroti'sans, f. nodular necrotizante; termo obsoleto para designar f. na qual se formam nódulos tuberculosos na pele; as lesões disseminam-se perifericamente e sofrem necrose central.
septic p., f. séptica; inflamação de uma veia devido a infecção.
♻ **phlebo-, phleb-.** Flebo-, fleb-; veia. [G. *phleps*]
phleb·o·cly·sis (flē - bok'li - sis). Fleboclise; injeção intravenosa de um volume grande de uma solução isotônica de glicose ou outras substâncias. SIN venoclysis. [phlebo- + G. *klysis,* lavagem]
drip p., f. por gotejamento; injeção intravenosa de um líquido gota a gota, pelo método de gotejamento.

phleb·o·dy·nam·ics (fleb′o-di-nam′iks). Flebodinâmica; leis e princípios que governam as pressões arteriais e o fluxo na circulação venosa. [phlebo- + G. *dynamis*, força]

phleb·o·gram (fleb′o-gram). Flebograma; um traçado do pulso jugular ou de outro pulso venoso. SIN venogram (2). [phlebo- + G. *gramma*, algo escrito]

phleb·o·graph (fleb′o-graf). Flebógrafo; esfigmógrafo venoso; aparelho para fazer um traçado do pulso venoso. [phlebo- + G. *graphō*, escrever]

phle·bog·ra·phy (fle-bog′ra-fe). Flebografia. 1. O registro do pulso venoso. 2. SIN venography. [phlebo- + G. *graphē*, escrita]

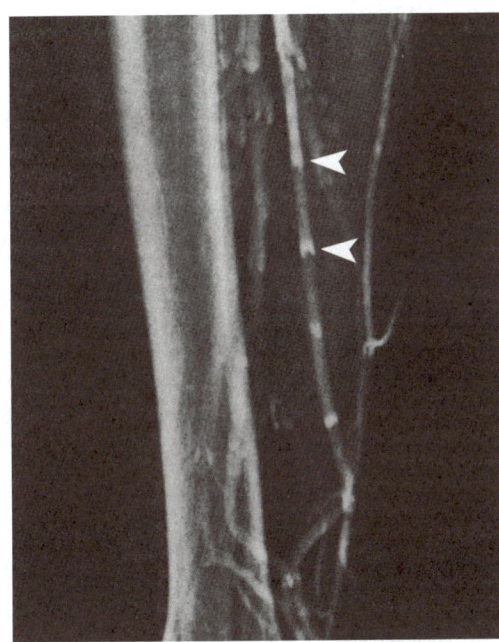

flebografia: vista lateral da perna esquerda; as valvas venosas são claramente visíveis (setas)

phleb·oid (fleb′oyd). Flebóide. 1. Semelhante a uma veia. 2. SIN venous. 3. Que contém muitas veias. [phlebo- + G. *eidos*, semelhança]

phleb·o·lite (fleb′o-lit). Flebólito. SIN phlebolith.

phleb·o·lith (fleb′o-lith). Flebólito; depósito calcificado em uma parede venosa ou trombo; comumente observado em radiografias abdominais na região pélvica inferior. SIN phlebolite, vein stone. [phlebo- + G. *lithos*, cálculo]

phleb·o·li·thi·a·sis (fleb′o-li-thi′a-sis). Flebolitíase; a formação de flebólitos.

phle·bol·o·gy (fle-bol′o-je). Flebologia; o ramo da ciência médica que estuda a anatomia e as doenças das veias. [phlebo- + G. *logos*, estudo]

phle·bo·ma·nom·e·ter (fleb′o-ma-nom′e-ter). Flebomanômetro; manômetro para medir a pressão venosa.

phleb·o·me·tri·tis (fleb′o-me-tri′tis). Flebometrite; inflamação das veias uterinas. [phlebo- + G. *metra*, útero, + -itis, inflamação]

phleb·o·my·o·ma·to·sis (fleb′o-mi-o-ma-to′sis). Flebomiomatose; espessamento das paredes de uma veia por supercrescimento das fibras musculares dispostas irregularmente, entrecruzando-se sem qualquer relação definida com o eixo do vaso. [phlebo- + myoma + G. -osis, condição]

phleb·o·phle·bos·to·my (fleb′o-fle-bos′to-me). Fleboflebostomia. SIN venovenostomy.

phleb·o·plas·ty (fleb′o-plas-te). Fleboplastia; reparo de uma veia. [phlebo- + G. *plastos*, formado]

phle·bor·rha·phy (fle-bor′a-fe). Fleborrafia; sutura de uma veia. [phlebo- + G. *rhaphē*, sutura]

phleb·o·scle·ro·sis (fleb′o-skle-ro′sis). Flebosclerose; endurecimento fibroso das paredes das veias. SIN venofibrosis, venosclerosis. [phlebo- + G. *sklērōsis*, endurecimento]

phle·bos·ta·sis (fle-bos′ta-sis). Flebostase. 1. Movimento anormalmente lento do sangue nas veias, em geral com distensão venosa. 2. Tratamento de insuficiência cardíaca congestiva por compressão das veias proximais dos membros com torniquetes. SIN bloodless phlebotomy. SIN venostasis. [phlebo- + G. *stasis*, estase]

phleb·o·ste·no·sis (fleb′o-ste-no′sis). Flebostenose; estreitamento da luz de uma veia por qualquer causa. [phlebo- + G. *stenōsis*, estreitamento]

phleb·o·throm·bo·sis (fleb′o-throm-bo′sis). Flebotrombose; trombose, ou coagulação, em uma veia sem inflamação primária. [phlebo- + thrombosis]

phle·bot·o·mine (fle-bot′o-men). Flebotomíneo; relativo aos mosquitos do gênero *Phlebotomus*.

phle·bot·o·mist (fle-bot′o-mist). Flebotomista; indivíduo treinado e hábil em flebotomia.

phle·bot·o·mize (fle-bot′o-miz). Flebotomizar. 1. Retirar sangue de. 2. Obter redução da sobrecarga de ferro por repetidas retiradas de sangue, como na hemocromatose.

Phle·bot·o·mus (fle-bot′o-mus). Gênero de mosquitos hematófagos muito pequenos da subfamília Phlebotominae, família Psychodidae. [phlebo- + G. *tomos*, cortante]

P. argen′tipes, o vetor do calazar na Índia.
P. chinen′sis, o vetor do calazar na China.
P. flaviscutel′latus. SIN *Lytzomyia flaviscutellata.*
P. longipal′pis, um vetor do calazar na América do Sul. SIN *Lutzomyia longipalpis.*
P. ma′jor, um vetor do calazar na região do Mediterrâneo.
P. nogu′chi, o transmissor de *Bartonella*, o agente causador da febre de Oroya.
P. orienta′lis, um vetor do calazar no Sudão.
p. papata′sii, transmissor do vírus da febre hemorrágica; também é um vetor da *Leishmania tropica* na região do Mediterrâneo.
P. pernicio′sus, um vetor do calazar na região do Mediterrâneo.
P. sergen′ti, um vetor da *Leishmania tropica*, a causa da leishmaniose cutânea antroponótica.
P. verruca′rum, uma forma encontrada no Peru que transmite *Bartonella*, o agente causador da febre de Oroya.

phle·bot·o·my (fle-bot′o-me). Flebotomia; incisão ou punção por agulha de uma veia para colher sangue. SIN venesection, venotomy. [phlebo- + G. *tomē*, incisão]

bloodless p., f. exangue. SIN phlebostasis (2).

Phleb·o·vi·rus (fleb′o-vi-rus). Gênero da família Bunyaviridae com mais de 40 vírus que reagem de forma cruzada; transmitido por artrópodes basicamente do gênero *Phlebotomus*; causa febre hemorrágica e febre do Vale Rift.

phlegm (flem). Flegma; fleuma. 1. Quantidade anormal de muco, principalmente expectorado pela boca. 2. Um dos quatro humores do corpo, de acordo com a doutrina humoral (humoral *doctrine*) da Grécia antiga. [G. *phlegma*, inflamação]

phleg·ma·sia (fleg-ma′ze-a). Flegmasia; termo obsoleto para designar inflamação, principalmente quando aguda e grave. [G. de *phlegma*, inflamação]

p. ceru′lea do′lens, trombose das veias de um membro acompanhada de dor súbita e forte com edema, cianose e edema da parte, seguida por colapso circulatório e choque.

phleg·mat·ic (fleg-mat′ik). Flegmático; fleumático; relativo ao mais pesado dos quatro humores da Grécia antiga (ver phlegm) e, portanto, calmo, impassível, inexcitável. [G. *phlegmatikos*, relativo à fleuma]

phleg·mon·ous (fleg′mon-us). Flegmonoso; fleimonoso; designa o fleimão.

phlo·gis·ton (flo-jis′ton). Flogisto; flogístico; substância hipotética de massa negativa que, de acordo com a teoria de G.E. Stahl, desprendia-se de uma substância quando esta sofria combustão, assim causando diminuição da massa de cinzas em relação à substância original; abandonado após as descobertas de Priestley e Lavoisier acerca do oxigênio. [G. *phlogistos*, inflamável]

phlo·go·sin (flo′go-sin). Flogosina; substância isolada de culturas de cocos produtores de pus, e injeções de soluções esterilizadas dessa substância causarão supuração. [G. *phlogōsis*, inflamação]

phlo·go·ther·a·py (flo′go-thar′a-pe). Flogoterapia. SIN nonspecific therapy. [G. *phlogōsis*, inflamação, + therapy]

phlo·rid·zin. Floridizina; diidrocalcona encontrada em muitas partes da macieira; usada experimentalmente para produzir glicosúria em animais. SIN phlorizin.

phlo·ri·zin. Florizina. SIN phloridzin.

phlor·o·glu·cin, phlor·o·glu·cin·ol, phlor·o·glu·col (flor-o-gloo′sin, -gloo′sin-ol, -gloo′kol). Floroglucina, foroglucinol, floroglucol; isômero do pirogalol, obtido a partir do resorcinol por fusão com soda cáustica; usado como reagente com a vanilina, como descalcificador de amostras de osso e como antiespasmódico. [phloridizin + G. *glykys*, doce, + -in]

phlox·ine (flok-sen, -sin). [I.C. 45405]. Floxina; corante ácido vermelho usado como corante citoplasmático em histologia.

phlyc·ten·u·la, pl. **phlyc·ten·u·lae** (flik-ten′u-la). Flictênula; pequeno nódulo vermelho de células linfóides, com ápice ulcerado, que ocorre na conjuntiva. SIN phlyctenule. [L. mod. dim. do G. *phlyktaina*, vesícula]

phlyc·ten·u·lar (flik-ten′u-lar). Flictenular; relativo a uma flictênula.

phlyc·ten·ule (flik′ten-ul). Flictênula. SIN phlyctenula.

phlyc·ten·u·lo·sis (flik-ten′u-lo′sis). Flictenulose; afecção nodular hipersensível do epitélio da córnea e da conjuntiva causada por toxina endógena.

PhNCS Símbolo de phenylisothiocyanate (fenilisotiocianato).

PHOBIA

pho·bia (fō′bē-ă). Fobia; qualquer medo ou temor mórbido objetivamente infundado que causa um estado de pânico. A palavra é usada como uma forma combinante em muitos termos que expressam o objeto que inspira o medo. [G. *phobos*, medo]
alcoholism (alcoolismo), alcoolofobia.
animals (animais), zoofobia.
bees (abelhas), apifobia, melissofobia.
being beaten (de ser mordido), rabdofobia.
being buried alive (de ser sepultado vivo), tafofobia.
being dirty (de estar sujo), automisofobia.
being locked in (de ficar trancado), clitrofobia.
being stared at (de ser visto), escopofobia.
birth of malformed fetus (do nascimento de um feto malformado), teratofobia.
blood (sangue), hemofobia.
blushing (de enrubescer), ereutofobia.
cancer (câncer), cancerofobia, carcinofobia.
cats (gatos), ailurofobia.
childbirth (de parir), tocofobia.
children (crianças), pedofobia.
choking (de asfixia), pnigofobia.
climbing (de subir escadas), climacofobia.
cold (frio), psicrofobia.
colors (cores), cromatofobia, cromofobia.
confinement (confinamento), claustrofobia.
corpses (cadáveres), necrofobia.
crossing a bridge (de atravessar uma ponte), gefirofobia.
crowds (multidão), oclofobia.
dampness (umidade), higrofobia.
darkness (escuridão), nictofobia, escotofobia.
dawn (alvorada), eosofobia.
daylight (luz do dia), fengofobia.
death (morte), tanatofobia.
deep places (lugares profundos), batofobia.
deserted places (lugares desertos), eremofobia.
dirt (sujeira), misofobia, ripofobia.
disease (doença), nosofobia, patofobia.
disorder (desordem), ataxiofobia.
dogs (cães), cinofobia.
dolls (bonecas), pediofobia.
drafts (correntes de ar), aerofobia, anemofobia.
drugs (fármacos), farmacofobia.
eating (de alimentar-se), fagofobia.
electricity (eletricidade), eletrofobia.
enclosed space (espaços fechados), claustrofobia.
error (erro), hamartofobia.
everything (tudo), panfobia.
excrement (excremento), coprofobia.
fatigue (fadiga), ponofobia, copofobia.
fever (febre), pirexiofobia.
filth (sujeira, imundície), ripofobia.
fire (fogo), pirofobia.
fish (peixe), ictiofobia.
food (alimento), cibofobia.
forests (florestas), hilefobia.
fur (pele de animais), dorafobia.
germs (germes), microfobia.
ghosts (fantasmas), fasmofobia.
girls (meninas), partenofobia.
glare of light (ofuscamento por luz), fotaugiafobia
glass (vidro), cristalofobia, hialofobia.
God (Deus), teofobia.
hair (cabelo), tricofobia, tricopatofobia.
heart disease (cardiopatia), cardiofobia.
heat (calor), termofobia.
heights (altura), acrofobia.
home, returning to (de voltar para a casa), nostofobia.
human companionship (companhia humana), antropofobia, misantropia.
ideas (idéias), ideofobia.
infection (infecção), molismofobia.
insects (insetos), entomofobia.
itching (prurido), acarofobia.
jealousy (ciúme), zelofobia.
lice (piolhos), pediculofobia, ftiriofobia.
light (luz), fotofobia.
lightning (relâmpago), astrapofobia, ceraunofobia.
machinery (máquina), mecanofobia.
malignancy (câncer), cancerofobia, carcinofobia.
many things (muitas coisas), polifobia.
marriage (casamento), gamofobia.
men (homens), androfobia.
metal objects (objetos metálicos), metalofobia.
microorganisms (microrganismos), microfobia.
minute objects (objetos pequenos), microfobia.
mirrors (espelhos), espectrofobia.
missiles (projéteis), balistofobia.
moisture (umidade), higrofobia.
movements (movimentos), cinesiofobia.
nakedness (nudez), gimnofobia.
names (nomes), nomatofobia, onomatofobia.
neglect of duty, omission of duty (negligência do dever, omissão do dever), paralipofobia.
night (noite), nictofobia.
novelty (novidade), neofobia.
odors (odores), olfatofobia, osmofobia, osfresiofobia, bromidosifobia.
open spaces (espaços abertos), agorafobia.
pain (dor), algofobia.
parasites (parasitas), parasitofobia.
phobias (fobias), fobofobia.
places (lugares), topofobia.
pleasure (prazer), hedonofobia.
pointed objects (objetos pontiagudos), aicmofobia.
poisoning (envenenamento), toxicofobia, iofobia.
poverty (pobreza), peniafobia.
precipices (precipícios), cremnofobia.
pregnancy (gravidez), maieusiofobia.
radiation (radiação), radiofobia.
rain (chuva), ombrofobia.
rectal disease (doença retal), proctofobia, retofobia.
religious objects, sacred objects (objetos religiosos, objetos sagrados), hierofobia.
responsibility (responsabilidade), hipengiofobia.
rivers (rios), potamofobia.
robbers (ladrões), harpaxofobia.
school p., (fobia à escola), súbita aversão ou medo de uma criança pequena de ir à escola; geralmente considerada uma manifestação de ansiedade de separação.
sea (mar), talassofobia.
self (de si próprio), autofobia.
semen, loss of (perda de sêmen), espermatofobia.
sexual intercourse (relações sexuais), coitofobia, cipridofobia.
sexual love (amor sexual), erotofobia.
sharp objects (objetos pontiagudos), belonefobia.
simple p. (fobia simples). SIN specific p.
sin (pecado), hamartofobia.
sinning (de pecar), pecatifobia.
skin of animals (pele de animais), dorafobia.
skin diseases (doenças cutâneas), dermatofobia.
sleep (sono), hipnofobia.
snakes (cobras), ofidiofobia.
social p. (fobia social); (1) padrão persistente de medo significativo de uma situação social ou de desempenho, que se manifesta por ansiedade ou pânico quando exposto à situação ou ao prevê-la, que a pessoa percebe como irracional ou excessivo e interfere significativamente na sua vida; (2) um diagnóstico DSM estabelecido quando são atendidos critérios específicos.
solitude (solidão), eremofobia, autofobia, monofobia.
sounds (sons), acusticofobia, fonofobia.
speaking (de falar), laliofobia.
specific p. (fobia específica), (1) um padrão persistente de medo significativo de objetos ou situações específicas, que se manifesta por ansiedade ou pânico durante a exposição ao objeto ou à situação ou ao prevê-los, que a pessoa percebe como irracional ou excessivo e interfere significativamente na sua vida; (2) um diagnóstico DSM estabelecido quando são atendidos os critérios específicos. SIN simple p.
spiders (aranhas), aracnofobia.
stairs (escadas), climacofobia.
stealing (de roubar), cleptofobia.
strangers (estranhos), xenofobia.
stuttering (de gaguejar), laliofobia.
sun (sol), heliofobia.
teeth (dentes), odontofobia.
thirteen (treze), triscaidecafobia.

thunder (trovão), ceraunofobia, tonitrofobia, brontofobia.
time (tempo), cronofobia.
touching, being touched (tocar, ser tocado), afefobia, hafefobia.
traveling (de viajar), hodofobia.
trembling (de tremor), tremofobia.
uncleanliness (sujeira), automisofobia.
vaccination (vacinação), vacinofobia.
vehicles (veículos), amaxofobia, hamaxofobia.
venereal disease (doença venérea), cipridofobia, venereofobia.
voices (vozes), fonofobia.
walking (de andar), basifobia.
water (água), hidrofobia.
wind (vento), anemofobia.
women (mulheres), ginefobia.
work (trabalho), ergasiofobia.
worms (vermes), helmintofobia.
writing (de escrever), grafofobia.

pho·bic (fō′bik). Fóbico; relativo a, ou caracterizado por, fobia.
pho·bo·pho·bia (fō-bō-fō′bē-ă). Fobofobia; medo mórbido de desenvolver alguma fobia. [G. *phobos*, medo]
pho·co·me·lia, pho·com·e·ly (fō-kō-mē′lē-ă, fō-kom′e-lē). Focomelia; defeito do desenvolvimento dos braços e/ou das pernas, de forma que as mãos e os pés ficam próximos do corpo, semelhante às nadadeiras de uma foca. [G. *phōkē*, foca, + *melos*, extremidade]
phol·co·dine (fol′kō-dēn). Folcodina; narcótico com pequena ou nenhuma atividade analgésica ou euforigênica, usado principalmente como antitussígeno.
phol·e·drine (fōl′e-drēn). Foledrina; agente simpaticomimético para tratamento do choque; também um adrenérgico e vasopressor.
Pho·ma (fō′mă). Gênero de fungos de crescimento rápido, contaminantes comuns de laboratório e patógenos vegetais comuns; causa rara de infecção em pacientes imunodeprimidos.
phon (fōn). Fon; unidade de intensidade do som.
phon-. VER phono-.
pho·nac·o·scope (fō-nak′ō-skōp). Fonacoscópio; instrumento para aumentar a intensidade da nota de percussão ou dos sons da voz, sendo o ouvido do examinador ou o estetoscópio colocado do lado oposto do tórax. [phon- + G. *akouō*, ouvir, + *skopeō*, ver]
pho·na·cos·co·py (fō-nă-kos′kŏ-pē). Fonacoscopia; exame do tórax por meio do fonacoscópio.
pho·nal (fō′năl). Fônico; relativo à voz ou ao som. [G. *phōnē*, voz]
pho·nar·te·ri·o·gram (fōn-ar-tēr′ē-ō-gram). Fonarteriograma; técnica obsoleta para registrar o som produzido nas artérias.
pho·nar·te·ri·og·ra·phy (fōn-ar-tēr′ē-og′ră-fē). Fonarteriografia; o procedimento de obtenção de um fonarteriograma.
phon·as·the·nia (fō-nas-thē′nē-ă). Fonastenia; voz cansada, que pode ser devida à fadiga. SIN functional vocal fatigue. [phon- + G. *astheneia*, fraqueza]
pho·na·tion (fō-nā′shŭn). Fonação; a produção de sons por vibração das pregas vocais. [G. *phōnē*, voz]
pho·na·tory (fō′nă-tōr-ē). Fonatório; relativo à fonação.
pho·neme (fō′nēm). Fonema; a menor unidade de som da fala que proporciona significado. [G. *phōnēma*, uma voz]
pho·ne·mic (fō-nē′mik). Fonêmico; relativo a, ou que possui as características de, um fonema.
pho·nen·do·scope (fō-nen′dō-skōp). Fonendoscópio; um estetoscópio que intensifica os sons auscultatórios por meio de duas placas ressonantes paralelas, uma apoiada sobre o tórax do paciente ou fixada ao tubo de um estetoscópio, a outra vibrando em uníssono com ela. [phon- + G. *endon*, dentro, + *skopeō*, ver]
pho·net·ic (fō-net′ik). Fonético; relativo à fala ou à voz. VER TAMBÉM phonic. [G. *phōnetikos*]
pho·net·ics (fō-net′iks). Fonética; a ciência da fala e da pronúncia. SIN phonology.
pho·ni·at·rics (fō-nē-at′riks). Foniatria; o estudo da fala; a ciência da fala. [phon- + G. *iatrikos*, da arte de curar]
phon·ic (fon′ik, fō′nik). Fônico; relativo à voz ou ao som. VER TAMBÉM phonetic.
phono-, phon-. Fono-, fon-; som, fala ou sons vocais. [G. *phōnē*]
pho·no·an·gi·og·ra·phy (fō′nō-an-jē-og′ră-fē). Fonoangiografia; registro e análise dos componentes de freqüência—intensidade do ruído do fluxo sanguíneo arterial turbulento através de uma lesão estenótica. [phono- + G. *angeion*, vaso, + *graphō*, escrever]
pho·no·car·di·o·gram (fō′nō-kar′dē-ō-gram). Fonocardiograma; um registro dos sons cardíacos produzidos por meio de um fonocardiógrafo.
pho·no·car·di·o·graph (fō-nō-kar′dē-ō-graf). Fonocardiógrafo; aparelho, utilizando microfones, amplificadores e filtros, para registrar graficamente os sons cardíacos, exibidos em um osciloscópio ou traçado analógico.

linear p., f. linear; f. que registra todas as vibrações da parede torácica resultantes da atividade cardíaca, com ênfase em vibrações de baixa freqüência devido a suas características de filtro.
logarithmic p., f. logarítmico; f. que registra apenas vibrações teoricamente audíveis com ênfase nas maiores freqüências devido às características de filtro designadas para imitar a resposta de freqüência–intensidade logarítmica do aparelho auditivo humano.
spectral p., f. espectral; aparelho para registrar os sons cardíacos no qual as alterações elétricas criadas por este partem de um microfone e atravessam uma série de filtros, cada um sintonizado em determinada faixa de freqüência; a saída de cada filtro ativa uma lâmpada separada, de brilho proporcional à intensidade do som transmitido através do filtro correspondente; as luzes são dispostas verticalmente em ordem decrescente de freqüência. É obtido um registro fotografando-se a fileira vertical de luzes.
stethoscopic p., f. estetoscópico; fonocardiógrafo que registra todas as vibrações sonoras, audíveis e inaudíveis, conduzidas pelo estetoscópio; entretanto, vibrações de freqüência muito baixa (na amplitude dos movimentos corporais) são filtradas.

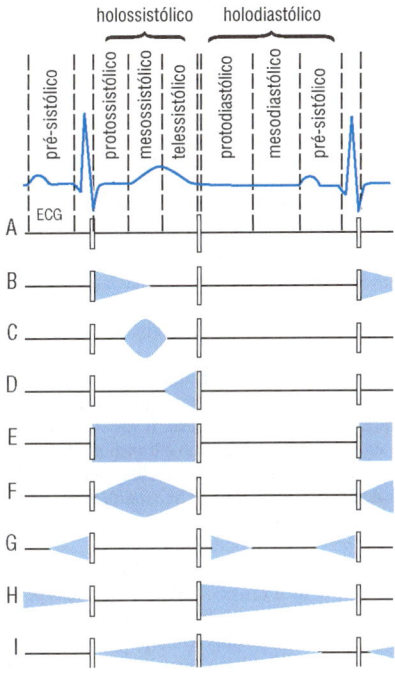

fonocardiografia (mostrando o momento e a intensidade de vários sopros cardíacos): (A) seqüência temporal da primeira e segunda bulhas; (B) sopro protossistólico em decrescendo (p. ex., na insuficiência mitral e tricúspide); (C) sopro mesossistólico em fuso (p. ex., na estenose aórtica); (D) sopro telessistólico em crescendo (p. ex., atrito pericárdico vestigial; na insuficiência mitral); (E) sopro holossistólico em faixa (p. ex., na comunicação interventricular, insuficiência mitral); (F) sopro holossistólico em diamante (p. ex., na estenose pulmonar); (G) sopros em crescendo pré-sistólico e protodiastólico em decrescendo — este último é separado da segunda bulha por um breve intervalo (sopro de Flint na estenose mitral); (H) sopro holodiastólico em decrescendo que começa imediatamente após a segunda bulha (como na insuficiência aórtica); (I) sopro contínuo (p. ex., na persistência do canal arterial ou no aneurisma atrioventricular)

pho·no·car·di·og·ra·phy (fō′nō-kar-dē-og′ră-fē). Fonocardiografia. **1.** Registro dos sons cardíacos com um fonocardiógrafo. **2.** A ciência de interpretar fonocardiogramas. [phono- + G. *kardia*, coração, + *graphō*, registrar]
pho·no·cath·e·ter (fō-nō-kath′e-ter). Fonocateter; cateter cardíaco com um pequeno microfone em sua extremidade, para registrar sons e sopros no interior do coração e dos grandes vasos.
pho·no·gram (fō′nō-gram). Fonograma; curva gráfica que representa a duração e a intensidade de um som. [phono- + G. *gramma*, diagrama]
pho·nol·o·gy (fō-nol′ō-jē). Fonologia. SIN phonetics. [phono- + G. *logos*, estudo]
pho·no·ma·nia (fō-nō-mā′nē-ă). Fonomania; termo raramente usado para uma mania homicida. [G. *phonos*, assassino, + *mania*, mania]
pho·nom·e·ter (fō-nom′e-ter). Fonômetro; aparelho para medir a freqüência e a intensidade dos sons. [phono- + G. *metron*, medida]

pho·no·my·oc·lo·nus (fō'nō - mī - ok'lō - nŭs). Fonomioclônus; espasmos clônicos dos músculos em resposta a estímulos aurais. [phono- + G. *mys*, músculo, + *klonos*, tumulto]

pho·no·my·og·ra·phy (fō'nō - mī - og'ră - fē). Fonomiografia; o registro dos vários sons produzidos pela contração do tecido muscular. [phono- + G. *mys*, músculo, + *grephē*, desenho]

pho·nop·a·thy (fō - nop'ă - thē). Fonopatia; qualquer doença do sistema vocal que afeta a fala. [phono- + G. *pathos*, que sofre]

pho·no·pho·bia (fō - nō - fō'bē - ă). Fonofobia; medo mórbido da própria voz, ou de qualquer som. [phono- + G. *phobos*, medo]

pho·no·phore (fō'nō - fōr). Fonóforo; forma de estetoscópio biauricular com a parte torácica em forma de sino, para o interior da qual se projetam as extremidades curvas dos tubos de som. [phono- + G. *phoros*, que conduz]

pho·no·pho·tog·ra·phy (fō'nō - fō - tog'ră - fē). Fonofotografia; o registro em uma placa fotográfica móvel dos movimentos conferidos a um diafragma por ondas sonoras. [phono- + photography]

pho·nop·sia (fō - nop'sē - ă). Fonopsia; condição na qual a audição de determinados sons dá origem a uma sensação subjetiva de cor. [phono- + G. *opsis*, visão]

pho·no·re·cep·tor (fō'nō - rē - sep'ter). Fonorreceptor; um receptor para estímulos sonoros.

pho·no·scope (fō'nō - skōp). Fonoscópio; designação obsoleta de um aparelho para registrar a percussão auscultatória; originalmente usado para registro fotográfico dos sons cardíacos. [phono- + G. *skopeō*, ver]

pho·nos·co·py (fō - nos'kō - pē). Fonoscopia; o registro feito por um fonoscópio.

pho·no·sur·gery (fō'nō - ser'jer - ē). Fonocirurgia; grupo de operações designadas para melhorar ou alterar a voz.

⚠ **phor-**. VER phoro-.

phor·bin (fōr'bin). Forbina; o hidrocarboneto que dá origem à clorofila; difere da porfina (porfirina) pela presença de um anel isocíclico formado pela adição de um grupamento de dois carbonos que une as posições 13 e 15 da porfina (porfirina) e por saturação da ligação dupla 17–18 (com realinhamento das ligações duplas conjugadas). O acréscimo de cadeias laterais de hidrocarbonetos em localizações específicas produz forbinas caracterizadas por prefixos; p. ex., fenoforbina.

phor·bol (fōr'bol). Forbol; o álcool original dos cocarcinógenos, que são 12,13(9,9a) diésteres do forbol encontrados no óleo de cróton; o esqueleto do hidrocarboneto é um ciclopropabenzazuleno; os ésteres de forbol imitam o 1,2-diacilglicerol como ativadores da proteinoquinase C.

pho·re·sis (fō'rē - sis, fō - rē'sis). Forese. **1.** SIN electrophoresis. **2.** Uma associação biológica na qual um organismo é transportado por outro, como na fixação dos ovos de *Dermatobia hominis*, a mosca-do-berne humana e de bovinos, às pernas de um mosquito, que os transporta até o homem, o boi ou outro hospedeiro no qual os bernes se desenvolvem. SIN epizoic commensalism, phoresy. [G. *phorēsis*, que é conduzido]

phor·e·sy (for'ē - sē). Forese. SIN phoresis (2).

phor·ia (fōr'ē - ă). Foria; as direções relativas adotadas pelos olhos durante a fixação binocular de determinado objeto na ausência de um estímulo de fusão adequado. VER cyclophoria, esophoria, exophoria, heterophoria, hyperphoria, hypophoria, orthophoria. [G. *phora*, transporte, movimento]

Phor·mia re·gi·na (fōr'mē - ă re - jī'nă). A mosca preta, cujas larvas eram usadas antigamente no tratamento de feridas sépticas porque secretam uma enzima proteolítica que ajuda na remoção de tecido morto; é uma causa frequente de infestação de carneiros por larvas, depositando ovos na lã; é uma espécie do clima frio, com ampla distribuição, que deposita seus ovos em tecidos mortos em deterioração.

⚠ **phoro-, phor-**. Foro-, for-; que transporta, conduz; um carregador, um transportador; fobia. [G. *phoros*, que transporta, que conduz]

Pho·rop·tor (fō - rop'ter). Foróptero; aparelho que contém diferentes lentes, usado para refração do olho.

phor·o·zo·on (fōr - ō - zō'on). Forozoário; o estágio assexuado na história da vida de um animal que atravessa várias fases em seu ciclo vital. [phoro- + G. *zōon*, animal]

⚠ **phos-**. Fos-; luz. [G. *phōs*]

phos·gene (CG) (fos'jēn). Fosgênio; cloreto de carbonila; um líquido incolor abaixo de 8,2°C, mas um gás extremamente venenoso em temperaturas comuns; é um gás insidioso, pois não causa irritação imediata, mesmo quando são inaladas concentrações fatais; mais de 80% das mortes causadas por agentes químicos na I Guerra Mundial foram devidas ao fosgênio.

p. oxime (CX), fosgênio oxima; agente vesicante armazenado pelos militares de alguns governos; um potente irritante que causa dor imediata. SIN dichloroformoxime.

⚠ **phosph-, phospho-, phosphor-, phosphoro-**. Fosf-, fosfo-, fosfor-, fosforo-; prefixos que indicam a presença de fósforo em um composto. Ver phospho- para o uso específico desse prefixo. [G. *phōs*, luz, *phoros*, que conduz]

phos·pha·gen (fos'fă - jen). Fosfagênio; fosfato de guanidínio ou amidina rico em energia, que serve como reservatório de energia no músculo e no encéfalo;

p. ex., fosfocreatina em mamíferos e fosfoarginina em invertebrados. Outros fosfagênios incluem fosfoagmatina, fosfoglicociamina e fosfolombricina.

phos·pha·gen·ic (fos - fă - jen'ik). Fosfagênico; que produz fosfato.

phos·pham·ic ac·id (fos - fam'ik). Ácido fosfâmico; R–NH–PO$_3$H$_2$, um dos três tipos de fosfatos de alta energia (sendo os outros ácidos fosfofosfóricos e ácidos fosfossulfúricos).

phos·pham·i·dase (fos - fam'i - dās). Fosfamidase. SIN phosphoamidase.

phos·pha·stat (fos'fă - stat). Mecanismo conceitual pelo qual o paratormônio está aumentado quando os níveis de fósforo aumentam até um nível acima do normal; ainda não há evidências satisfatórias de sua existência. [phosphate + L. *status*, situação]

phos·pha·tase (fos'fă - tās). Fosfatase; qualquer uma dentre um grupo de enzimas [EC 3.1.3.x] que liberam ortofosfato dos ésteres fosfóricos. VER TAMBÉM phosphohydrolases.

acid p., f. ácida; f. com um pH ideal < 7,0 (para várias isozimas, é de 5,4), notavelmente presente na próstata; demonstrável em lisossomas com coloração para f. ácida inespecífica de Gomori; hidrolisa muitos monoésteres ortofosfóricos.

alkaline p., f. alcalina; f. com um pH ideal > 7,0 (p. ex., 8,6), onipresente; localizada quimicamente em membranas por modificações da coloração para f. alcalina inespecífica de Gomori; hidrolisa muitos monoésteres ortofosfóricos; baixos níveis dessa enzima são observados em casos de hipofosfatasia.

phos·phate (fos'fāt). Fosfato. **1.** Um sal ou éster do ácido fosfórico. Para fosfatos individuais não apresentados aqui, ver o nome da base. **2.** O íon trivalente, PO$_4^{3-}$.

bone p., f. ósseo. SIN tribasic *calcium* phosphate.

codeine p., f. de codeína; um sal hidrossolúvel de codeína frequentemente usado na preparação farmacêutica de medicamentos líquidos que contêm codeína.

cyclic p., f. cíclico. SIN adenosine 3',5'-cyclic monophosphate.

dihydrogen p., f. de diidrogênio; ácido fosfórico com um terço neutralizado; p. ex., NaH$_2$PO$_4$, KH$_2$PO$_4$.

disodium p., f. dissódico; Na$_2$HPO$_4$.

energy-rich p., fosfatos ricos em energia. SIN high-energy p.'s.

high-energy p.'s, fosfatos de alta energia; aqueles ésteres de fosfato e fosfoanidridos que, à hidrólise, produzem uma quantidade incomumente grande de energia; p. ex., nucleotídeo fosfatases como ATP, fosfatos de enol como fosfoenolpiruvato (phosphoenol pyruvate). VER TAMBÉM high-energy *compounds*, em *compound*. SIN energy-rich p.'s.

inorganic p. (Pi), f. inorgânico. SIN inorganic *orthophosphate*.

monopotassium p., f. monopotássico; KH$_2$PO$_4$; um f. diidrogênio usado como reagente; comumente usado em tampões.

monosodium p., f. monossódico; NaH$_2$PO$_4$; um f. diidrogênio usado como reagente; comumente usado em tampões.

normal p., f. normal; um sal do ácido fosfórico ou ácido pirofosfórico no qual todos os átomos de hidrogênio estão deslocados; p. ex., Na$_3$PO$_4$, Na$_4$P$_2$O$_7$.

organic p., f. orgânico; um éster do ácido fosfórico; p. ex., fosfato de glicerol, fosfato de adenosina, fosfato de hexose.

triple p., f. triplo; **(1)** fosfato de amônio magnesiano; MgNH$_4$PO$_4$; **(2)** fosfato bruto fertilizante, produto da rocha fosfática e ácido fosfórico.

trisodium p., f. trissódico; Na$_3$PO$_4$; usado para emulsificar gorduras, óleo e graxa; um irritante.

phos·phate ace·tyl·trans·fer·ase. Fosfato acetiltransferase; transferência, catalisada por enzima, de uma porção acetil da acetil-CoA para o ortofosfato, formando acetil fosfato e coenzima A. SIN phosphoacylase, phosphotransacetylase.

phos·phat·ed (fos'fāt - ed). Fosfatado; que contém fosfatos.

phos·pha·te·mia (fos - fă - tē'mē - ă). Fosfatemia; uma concentração anormalmente alta de fosfatos inorgânicos no sangue. [phosphate + G. *haima*, sangue]

phos·phat·ic (fos - fat'ik). Fosfático; relativo a ou que contém fosfatos.

phos·pha·ti·dal (fos - fă - tī'dăl). Fosfatidal; nome trivial antigo para alc-1-enil-glicerofosfolipídio; plasmalógeno.

phos·pha·ti·dase (fos - fă - tī'dās). Fosfatidase. SIN phospholipase A$_2$.

phos·pha·ti·date (fos - fă - tī'dāt). Fosfatidato; um sal ou éster de um ácido fosfatídico.

p. phosphatase, f. fosfatase; enzima que catalisa a hidrólise do fosfatidato, produzindo ortofosfato e 1,2-diacilglicerol; essa enzima participa do metabolismo dos fosfolipídios e triacilglicerol.

phos·pha·tide (fos'fă - tīd). Fosfatídeo; designação antiga de 1) ácido fosfatídico e 2) fosfatidato.

phos·pha·tid·ic ac·id (fos'fă - tid'ik). Ácido fosfatídico; fosfato de 1,2-diacilglicerol; um derivado do ácido glicerofosfórico no qual os dois grupos hidroxila remanescentes do glicerol são esterificados com ácidos graxos; p. ex., ácidos fosfatídicos fixados à colina são fosfatidilcolinas (lecitinas).

phos·pha·ti·do·lip·ase (fos'fă - tī - dō - lip'ās). Fosfatidolipase. SIN *phospholipase* A$_2$.

phos·pha·ti·dyl (Ptd) (fos - fă - tī'dĭl). Fosfatidil; o radical de um ácido fosfatídico; p. ex., fosfatidilcolina.

phos·pha·ti·dyl·cho·line (PtdCho) (fos-fă-tĭ′dĭl-kō′lēn). Fosfatidilcolina. VER lecithin.

phos·pha·ti·dyl·eth·a·nol·a·mine (PtdEth) (fos-fă-tĭ′dĭl-eth-ă-nol′ă-mēn). Fosfatidiletanolamina; o produto da condensação de um ácido fosfatídico e etanolamina; encontrada em biomembranas. VER TAMBÉM cephalin.
  p. cytidylyltransferase, p. citidiltransferase; uma enzima fundamental na biossíntese da cefalina; catalisa a reação da fosfoetanolamina e CTP para formar CDP-etanolamina e pirofosfato.

phos·phat·i·dyl·glyc·er·ol (fos-fă-tĭ′dĭl-glis′er-ol). Fosfatidilglicerol; um ácido fosfatídico no qual uma segunda molécula de glicerol substitui a colina habitual, ou etanolamina ou serina; um constituinte do líquido amniótico humano que indica maturidade pulmonar fetal quando presente no último trimestre.

phos·pha·ti·dyl·in·o·si·tol (PtdIns) (fos-fă-tĭ′dĭl-in-ō′si-tol). Fosfatidilinositol; um ácido fosfatídico combinado ao inositol encontrado em biomembranas e um precursor de determinados sinais celulares. Algumas vezes denominado inositídeo. SIN phosphoinositide.
  p. 4,5-bisphosphate (PIP$_2$, PtdIns(4,5)P$_2$), 4,5-bifosfato de f.; fosfato com dois locais adicionais de fosforilação; um importante constituinte dos fosfolipídios da membrana celular e precursor dos mensageiros secundários, o diacilglicerol e o 1,4,5-trifosfato de inositol.
  p. 4-phosphate, 4-fosfato de f.; o intermediário na biossíntese do 4,5-bifosfato de fosfatidilinositol a partir do fosfatidilinositol.
  p. synthase, f. sintase; enzima que catalisa a reação do CDP-diacilglicerol com inositol para formar CMP e fosfatidilinositol; encontrada no retículo endoplasmático.

phos·pha·ti·dyl·ser·ine (PtdSer) (fos-fă-tĭ′dĭl-ser′ēn). Fosfatidilserina; o produto da condensação do ácido fosfatícido e da serina; encontrada em biomembranas. VER TAMBÉM cephalin.

phos·pha·tu·ria (fos-fă-too′rē-ă). Fosfatúria; excreção excessiva de fosfatos na urina. SIN phosphoruria, phosphuria. [phosphate + G. *ouron*, urina]

phos·phene (fos′fēn). Fosfeno; sensação de luz produzida por estimulação mecânica ou elétrica da via óptica periférica ou central do sistema nervoso. [G. *phōs*, luz, + *phainō*, mostrar]
  accommodation p., f. de acomodação; fosfeno que ocorre durante a acomodação, causado por súbito relaxamento do músculo ciliar.

phos·phide (fos′fīd). Fosfeto; fosforeto; composto de fósforo com valência −3; p. ex., fosfeto de sódio, Na$_3$P.

phos·phine (fos′fēn, -fin). Fosfina; gás de guerra venenoso incolor com um odor característico semelhante ao do olho; também o agente ativo em alguns rodenticidas; formado em pequenas quantidades na putrefação da matéria orgânica que contém fósforo. SIN hydrogen phosphide, phosphureted hydrogen.

⚠ **phosphinico-.** Fosfínico-; em química, ácido fosfínico duplamente substituído simetricamente, R$_2$P(O)OH.

phos·phite (fos′fīt). Fosfito; um sal do ácido fosforoso.

⚠ **phospho-.** Fosfo-; prefixo para *O*-fosfono-, que pode substituir o sufixo fosfato; p. ex., o fosfato de glicose é *O*-fosfonoglicose ou fosfoglicose. VER TAMBÉM phosph-, phosphoryl-.

phos·pho·ac·y·lase (fos-fō-as′i-lās). Fosfoacilase. SIN phosphate acetyltransferase.

3′-phos·pho·aden·o·sine 5′-phos·phate (PAP) (fos′fō-a-den′ō-sēn). 3′-fosfoadenosina 5′-fosfato; um produto nas reações de transferência sulfuril.

3′-phos·pho·aden·o·sine 5′-phos·pho·sul·fate (PAPS). 3′-fosfoadenosina 5′-fosfossulfato. VER adenosine 3′-phosphate 5′-phosphosulfate.

phos·pho·am·i·dase (fos-fō-am′i-dās). Fosfoamidase; enzima que catalisa a hidrólise de ligações fósforo–nitrogênio, notavelmente a hidrólise de *N*-fosfocreatina em creatina e ortofosfato. SIN phosphamidase.

phos·pho·am·ides (fos-fō′am′ĭdz). Fosfoamidas; amidas do ácido fosfórico (ácidos fosforamídicos) e seus sais ou ésteres (fosforamidatos), da fórmula geral (HO)$_2$P(O)–NH$_2$; p. ex., fosfato de creatina.

phos·pho·ar·gi·nine (fos-fō-ar′gi′nēn). Fosfoarginina; um composto (em particular, um fosfagênio) da L-arginina com ácido fosfórico contendo a ligação fosfoamida; uma fonte de energia, na contração do músculo em invertebrados, que corresponde à fosfocreatina nos músculos dos vertebrados. Cf. phosphocreatine. SIN arginine phosphate.

phos·pho·cho·line (fos-fō-kō′lēn). Fosfocolina; colina *O*-fosfato; importante no metabolismo da colina, p. ex., na biossíntese das lecitinas. SIN phosphorylcholine.
  p. cytidylyltransferase, f. citidiltransferase; enzima que catalisa a reação da fosfocolina com CTP para formar pirofosfato e CDP-colina; a etapa limitadora de velocidade da biossíntese da lecitina; a forma citossólica da enzima é inativa (uma forma fosforilada da enzima).
  p. diacylglycerol transferase, f. diacilglicerol transferase; enzima na biossíntese da lecitina que catalisa a reação do 1,2-diacilglicerol com CDP-colina para formar CMP e fosfatidilcolina.

phos·pho·cre·a·tine (fos-fō-krē′ă-tēn). Fosfocreatina; um fosfagênio; um composto da creatina (através de seu grupamento NH$_2$) com ácido fosfórico; uma fonte de energia na contração do músculo vertebrado, e sua degradação fornece fosfato para a ressíntese de ATP a partir do ADP pela creatinoquinase. Cf. phosphoarginine. SIN creatine phosphate, N.°-phosphonocreatine.

phos·pho·di·es·ter (fos′fō-dī-es′ter). Fosfodiéster; um ácido ortofosfórico diesterificado, RO–(PO$_2$H)–OR′, como nos ácidos nucleicos.
  p. hydrolases, f. hidrolases. SIN phosphodiesterases.

phos·pho·di·es·ter·as·es (fos′fō-dī-es′ter-ās-ez). Fosfodiesterases; enzimas (EC 3.1.4.x) que clivam ligações fosfodiéster, como aquelas existentes no AMPc ou entre nucleotídeos nos ácidos nucleicos, liberando menores unidades de poli- ou oligonucleotídeos ou mononucleotídeos, mas não ortofosfato. SIN phosphodiester hydrolases.
  spleen p., f. esplênicas. SIN micrococcal endonuclease.

phos·pho·dis·mu·tase (fos-fō-dis′mū-tās). Fosfodismutase. SIN phosphomutase.

phos·pho*enol*py·ru·vate car·box·y·kin·ase. Fosfo*enol*piruvato carboxiquinase. SIN *phosphoenolpyruvic acid* carboxykinase.

phos·pho·e·*nol*·pyr·u·vic ac·id (fos′fō-ē′nol-pī-roo′vik). Ácido fosfoenolpirúvico; o éster fosfórico do ácido pirúvico na forma enol deste último; um intermediário na conversão da D-glicose em ácido pirúvico e um exemplo de um éster fosfato de alta energia.
  p.a. carboxykinase, carboxiquinase do ácido fosfoenolpirúvico; enzima que catalisa a reação de oxaloacetato e GTP para formar ácido fosfoenolpirúvico, CO$_2$ e GDP; uma enzima fundamental na gliconeogênese; a biossíntese dessa enzima é diminuída pela insulina. SIN phospho*enol*pyruvate carboxykinase.

phos·pho·eth·a·no·la·mine (fos′fō-eth-an-ol′a-mēn). Fosfoetanolamina; um intermediário fundamental na formação das cefalinas; produzido no fígado e no encéfalo por fosforilação de etanolamina.
  p. cytidylyltransferase, f. citidililtransferase; enzima fundamental na biossíntese das cefalinas; catalisa a reação da fosfoetanolamina e CTP para formar CDP-etanolamina e pirofosfato.

1-phos·pho·fruc·tal·do·lase (fos′-fō-frŭk-tal′dō-lās). 1-Fosfofrutaldolase. SIN fructose-bisphosphate aldolase.

1-phos·pho·fruc·to·ki·nase (fos′fō-frŭk-tō-kī′nās). 1-Fosfofrutocinase; frutose-1-fosfato cinase; enzima que catalisa a fosforilação de D-frutose 1-fosfato pelo ATP (ou outro NTP) em D-frutose 1,6-bifosfato e ADP (ou outro NDP); uma etapa fundamental no metabolismo da D-frutose; deficiência da enzima do músculo pode resultar em doença do armazenamento de glicogênio tipo VII.

6-phos·pho·fruc·to·ki·nase. 6-Fosfofrutocinase; fosfofrutocinase I; enzima que catalisa a fosforilação da D-frutose 6-fosfato pelo ATP (ou outro NTP) em frutose 1,6-bifosfato e ADP (ou outro NDP); essa enzima catalisa uma etapa na glicólise; é inibida por níveis elevados de ATP ou citrato; a deficiência dessa enzima pode causar anemia hemolítica. SIN phosphohexokinase.

phos·pho·ga·lac·to·i·som·er·ase (fos′fō-gă-lak′tō-ī-som′er-ās). Fosfogalactoisomerase. SIN UDPglucose-hexose-1-phosphate uridylyltransferase.

phos·pho·glu·co·ki·nase (fos′fō-gloo-kō-kī′nās). Fosfoglucoquinase; uma enzima que, na presença de ATP, catalisa a fosforilação da D-glicose 1-fosfato para formar D-glicose 1,6-bifosfato e ADP; encontrada na levedura e no músculo; a D-glicose 1,6-bifosfato é um co-fator necessário de uma das enzimas da glicogenólise. SIN glucose-1-phosphate kinase.

phos·pho·glu·co·mu·tase (fos′fō-gloo-kō-mū′tās). Fosfoglucomutase; enzima que catalisa a reação reversível, α-D-glicose 1-fosfato ⇌ α-D-glicose 6-fosfato, sendo a glicose 1,6-bifosfato um co-fator necessário; uma das etapas na glicogenólise. SIN glucose phosphomutase.

phos·pho·glu·co·nate de·hy·dro·gen·ase (fos-fō-gloo′kō-nāt). Fosfogluconato desidrogenase; 6-fosfoglucônico desidrogenase; enzima que catalisa a reação do 6-fosfo-D-gluconato e NAD(P)$^+$ para formar 6-fosfo-2-ceto-D-gluconato e NAD(P)H; já foi descrita uma deficiência dessa enzima, mas não foi observada ruptura celular.

phos·pho·glu·co·nate de·hy·dro·gen·ase (de·car·box·y·lat·ing). Fosfogluconato desidrogenase (descarboxilante); enzima, parte da via da pentosefosfato, que catalisa a reação do 6-fosfo-D-gluconato e NADP$^+$ para produzir CO$_2$, NADPH e D-ribulose 5-fosfato.

6-phos·pho·glu·co·no·lac·to·nase (fos′fō-gloo′kō-nō-lak′tō-nās). 6-Fosfogluconolactonase; hidrolase que catalisa a hidrólise de 6-fosfo-D-glucono δ-lactona em 6-fosfo-D-gluconato; essa enzima é uma parte da via da pentosefosfato.

6-phos·pho-D-glu·co·no-δ-lac·tone. 6-Fosfo-D-glucono-δ-lactona; intermediário na via da pentosefosfato sintetizado a partir da D-glicose 6-fosfato.

phos·pho·glyc·er·ac·e·tals (fos′fō-glis-er-as′ē-tālz). Plasmalógenos. SIN plasmalogens.

phos·pho·glyc·er·ate ki·nase (fos-fō-glis′er-āt). Fosfoglicerato quinase; enzima que catalisa a formação de 3-fosfo-D-glicerol fosfato e ADP a partir do 3-fosfo-D-glicerato e ATP; essa enzima é uma parte da via glicolítica; a deficiência de fosfoglicerato quinase (uma doença ligada ao X) resulta em comprometimento da glicólise na maioria das células.

phos·pho·glyc·er·ic ac·id (fos′fō-gli-ser′ik, -glis′er-ik). Ácido fosfoglicérico. **1.** Ácido gliceroil fosfórico; gliceroil fosfato; um anidrido ácido entre o ácido glicérico e o ácido fosfórico. **2.** Ácido 2-fosfoglicérico; a forma desprotonada, 2-fosfoglicerato, é um intermediário na glicólise. **3.** Ácido 3-fosfoglicérico; a forma desprotonada, 3-fosfoglicerato, é um intermediário na glicólise.

phos·pho·glyc·er·ides (fos-fō-glis'er-īdz). Fosfoglicerídeos; fosfatos acilglicerol e diacilglicerol; constituintes do tecido nervoso e envolvidos no transporte e no armazenamento de gordura.

phos·pho·glyc·er·o·mu·tase (fos'fō-glis'er-ō-mū'tās). Fosfogliceromutase; enzima isomerizante que catalisa a interconversão reversível do 2-fosfoglicerato e 3-fosfoglicerato com 2,3-bifosfoglicerato presente como um co-fator; a deficiência dessa enzima, que desempenha um papel na glicólise, é um distúrbio hereditário que resulta em intolerância ao exercício vigoroso.

phos·pho·hex·o·ki·nase (fos'fō-hek-sō-kī'nās). Fosfoexoquinase. SIN 6-phosphofructokinase.

phos·pho·hex·o·mu·tase (fos'fō-hek-sō-mū'tās). Fosfoexomutase. SIN glucose-phosphate isomerase.

phos·pho·hex·ose isom·er·ase (fos-fō-hek'sōs). Fosfoexose isomerase. SIN glucose-phosphate isomerase.

phos·pho·hy·dro·las·es (fos-fo-hī'drō-lās-ez). Fosfoidrolases; monoéster fosfórico hidrolases; enzimas (EC 3.1.3.x) que clivam o ácido fosfórico (na forma de ortofosfato) a partir de seus ésteres; os nomes populares geralmente terminam em fosfato.

phos·pho·in·o·si·tide (fos'fō-in-ō'si-tīd). Fosfoinositídeo. SIN phosphatidylinositol.

phos·pho·ki·nase (fos'fō-kī'nās). Fosfoquinase; uma fosfotransferase ou uma quinase.

phos·pho·li·pase (fos-fō-lip'ās). Fosfolipase; enzima que catalisa a hidrólise de um fosfolipídio. SIN lecithinase.

p. A$_1$, f. A$_1$; enzima que hidrolisa uma lecitina (1,2-diacilglicerofosfocolina) em uma 2-acilglicerofosfocolina e um ânion de ácido graxo.

p. A$_2$, f. A$_2$; enzima que catalisa a hidrólise de uma lecitina em uma lisolecitina pela remoção do grupamento 2-acil; também atua sobre outros fosfolipídios pela remoção de um ácido graxo da posição 2; essa enzima é importante na biossíntese de prostaglandina e leucotrieno. SIN lecithinase A, phosphatidase, phosphatidolipase.

p. B, f. B; (1) SIN lysophospholipase; (2) uma mistura de f. A$_1$ e f. A$_2$.

p. C, f. C; α-toxina do *Clostridium welchii*; β e γ-toxinas de *Clostridium oedematiens*; uma enzima que catalisa a hidrólise da fosfatidilcolina (e, talvez, de outros fosfolipídios) para produzir colina fosfato e 1,2-diacilglicerol; também atua na esfingomielina; uma enzima fundamental na formação de inositol 1,4,5-trifosfato. SIN lecithinase C, lipophosphodiesterase I.

p. D, f. D; enzima que hidrolisa a fosfatidilcolina para produzir colina e um fosfatidato; também atua em outros ésteres fosfatidil. SIN choline phosphatase, lecithinase D, lipophosphodiesterase II.

phos·pho·lip·id (fos-fō-lip'id). Fosfolipídio; lipídio que contém fósforo, assim incluindo as lecitinas e outros derivados fosfatidil, esfingomielina e plasmalogênios; os constituintes básicos das biomembranas.

phos·pho·mu·tase (fos-fō-mū'tās). Fosfomutase; uma dentre várias enzimas (mutases) (EC 5.4.2.x) que, aparentemente, catalisam a transferência intramolecular porque o doador é regenerado (p. ex., fosfogliceromutase, fosfoglucomutase). SIN phosphodismutase.

phos·pho·ne·cro·sis (fos-fō-ne-krō'sis). Fosfonecrose; necrose do osso da mandíbula, resultante da intoxicação por inalação de fumos de fósforo, ocorrendo principalmente em pessoas que trabalham com esse elemento. [phosphorus + G. *nekrōsis*, morte (necrose)]

phos·pho·ni·um (fos-fō'nē-ŭm). Fosfônio; o radical, (PR$_4$)$^+$.

⚠ **O-phosphono-.** *O*-fosfono-; prefixo que indica um radical ácido fosfônico (-PO$_3$H$_2$) fixado através de um átomo de oxigênio, portanto um éster fosfórico. VER TAMBÉM phospho-.

N$^\omega$-**phosphonocreatine.** *N*$^\omega$-fosfonocreatina. SIN phosphocreatine.

4'-phos·pho·pan·te·the·ine (fos'fō-pan-tē-thē'in). 4'-Fosfopanteteína; o grupo protético da proteína carreadora acil no complexo da ácido graxo sintase. SIN pantetheine 4'-phosphate.

phos·pho·pen·ia (fos'fō-pē'nē-ă). Fosfopenia; baixos níveis séricos de fosfato. SIN phosphorpenia. [phospho- + G. *penia*, escassez]

phos·pho·pen·tose ep·i·mer·ase (fos-fō-pen'tōs ē-pim-er-ās). Fosfopentose epimerase; enzima que catalisa a epimerização reversível de vários açúcares de cinco carbonos, fosforilados; mais notavelmente ribulose 5-fosfato em xilulose 5-fosfato na via da pentose fosfato.

phos·pho·pen·tose isom·er·ase (fos-fō-pen'tōs). Fosfopentose isomerase. SIN ribose 5-phosphate isomerase.

phos·pho·pho·rin (fos-fō-fōr'in). Fosfoforina; uma proteína (PM = 155.000) encontrada na dentina que parece atuar na mineralização.

phos·pho·pro·tein (fos-fō-prō'tēn). Fosfoproteína; uma proteína que contém grupamentos fosforil fixados diretamente às cadeias laterais de alguns de seus aminoácidos constituintes, geralmente ao grupo hidroxila de um resíduo L-seril ou L-treonil; p. ex., caseína, vitelina, ovalbumina.

phos·pho·py·ru·vate hy·dra·tase (fos-fō-pī'roo-vāt). Fosfopiruvato hidratase. SIN enolase.

⚠ **phos·phor** (fos'fōr). Fósforo. **1.** Substância química que transforma a energia eletromagnética ou radioativa incidente em luz, como nas determinações de radioatividade por cintilação ou *écrans* de intensificação radiológica ou amplificadores de imagem. **2.** Qualquer substância capaz de exibir fosforescência. [G. *phōs*, luz, + *phoros*, que conduz]

photostimulable p., f. foto-estimulável; o revestimento químico da placa de fósforo em um sistema radiográfico digital; a imagem latente é lida por varredura com laser.

⚠ **phosphor-, phosphoro-.** Fosfor-, fósforo-. VER phosph-.

phos·phor·at·ed (fos'fōr-āt-ed). Fosforado; que forma um composto com o fósforo.

phos·pho·res·cence (fos-fo-res'ens). Fosforescência; a qualidade ou propriedade de emitir luz sem combustão ativa ou produção de calor, geralmente em virtude de exposição prévia à radiação, que persiste após ser removida a causa incitante. [G. *phōs*, luz, + *phoros*, que conduz]

phos·pho·res·cent (fos'fō-res'ent). Fosforescente; que possui a propriedade de fosforescência.

phos·phor·hi·dro·sis (fos'fōr-hī-drō'sis). Fosforidrose; a excreção de suor luminoso. SIN phosphoridrosis. [G. *phōs*, luz, + *phoros*, que conduz, + *hidrōsis*, sudorese]

phos·pho·ri·bo·i·som·er·ase (fos'fō-rī-bō-ī-som'er-ās). Fosforriboisomerase. SIN ribose 5-phosphate isomerase.

5-phos·pho·ri·bose 1-di·phos·phate. 5-Fosforribose 1-difosfato. SIN 5-phospho-α-D-ribosyl-1-pyrophosphate.

5-phos·pho·ri·bo·syl·am·ine (fos'fō-rī-bō-sil-a-mēn). 5-Fosforribosilamina; um intermediário na biossíntese da purina.

phos·pho·ri·bo·syl·gly·cine·a·mide syn·the·tase (fos'fō-rī'bō-sil-gli-sīn'ă-mīd). Fosforribosilglicinamida sintetase; glicinamida ribonucleotídeo sintetase; enzima que causa reação da glicina com a ribosilamina 5-fosfato e ATP para formar ADP, ortofosfato e fosforribosilglicinamida no decorrer da biossíntese da purina.

5-phos·pho-α-D-ri·bo·syl-1-py·ro·phos·phate (PPRibp, PPRP, PRPP). 5-fosfo-α-D-ribosil-1-pirofosfato; 5-fosforribosil 1-difosfato; D-ribose que transporta um grupamento fosfato no carbono 5 da ribose e um grupo pirofosfato no carbono 1 da ribose; um intermediário na formação dos nucleotídeos pirimidina e purina e, também, do NAD$^+$. SIN 5-phosphoribose 1-diphosphate.

phos·pho·ri·bo·syl·trans·fer·ase (fos'fō-rī'bō-sil-trans'fer-ās). Fosforribosiltransferase; enzima pertencente a um grupo (EC 2.3.2.x, pentosiltransferases) que transfere D-ribose 5-fosfato do 5-fosfo-α-D-ribosil pirofosfato para um aceptor de purina, pirimidina ou piridina, formando um 5'-nucleotídeo e pirofosfato, ou D-ribose do D-ribosil fosfato para uma base, formando um nucleosídeo, ou transferências semelhantes de pentose; importante na biossíntese de nucleotídeos. As fosforribosiltransferases específicas são precedidas pelo nome da base aceptora, p. ex., uracil fosforribosiltransferase (isto é, uracil + PRPP ⚠ UMP + pyrophosphate).

phos·pho·ri·bu·lo·ki·nase (fos'fō-rī'bū-lō-kī'nās). Fosforribuloquinase; enzima que, na presença de ATP, catalisa a fosforilação de D-ribulose 5-fosfato em D-ribulose 1,5-bifosfato e ADP, uma reação importante no ciclo de fixação do dióxido de carbono da fotossíntese.

phos·pho·ri·bu·lose ep·i·mer·ase (fos-fō-rī'bū-lōs). Fosforribulose epimerase. SIN ribulose-phosphate 3-epimerase.

phos·phor·ic ac·id (fos-fōr'ik). Ácido fosfórico; ácido ortofosfórico; um ácido forte de importância industrial; ponto de fusão 42,35°C; soluções diluídas foram usadas como acidificantes urinários e como curativos para remover resíduos necróticos. Em odontologia, constitui cerca de 60% do líquido usado nos cimentos de fosfato de zinco e silicato; são usadas soluções em concentrações variáveis para condicionamento ácido das superfícies do esmalte e da dentina antes da aplicação de vários tipos de resinas.

cyclic p. a., a.f. cíclico; **(1)** em geral, um polímero linear de resíduos do ácido fosfórico em ligação pirofosfato no qual os resíduos α e ω são ligados de forma semelhante para produzir um composto com alça contínua ou cíclico; **(2)** especificamente, um termo genérico aplicado a compostos nos quais um resíduo do ácido fosfórico é esterificado em dois grupamentos hidroxila de uma única cadeia de carbono, como na adenosina ácido 3',5'-fosfórico, adenosina ácido 2',3'-fosfórico, etc.

dilute p.a., a.f. diluído; solvente contendo 10% de H$_3$PO$_4$.

glacial p.a., a.f. glacial; um anidrido do ácido fosfórico usado como reagente e na fabricação de cimento de oxifosfato de zinco para odontologia. SIN metaphosphoric acid.

phos·phor·i·dro·sis (fos'fōr-i-drō'sis). Fosforidrose. SIN phosphorhidrosis.

phos·phor·ism (fos'fōr-izm). Fosforismo; intoxicação crônica por fósforo.

phos·phor·ized (fos'fōr-īzd). Fosforizado; que contém fósforo.

phos·pho·rol·y·sis (fos-fō-rol'i-sis). Fosforólise; reação análoga à hidrólise, exceto pelo fato de serem acrescentados elementos do ácido fosfórico, e não da água, no transcurso da divisão de uma ligação; p. ex., a formação de glicose 1-fosfato a partir do glicogênio. SIN phosphoroclastic cleavage.

phos·pho·rous (fos'for-ŭs, fos-for'ŭs). Fósforo. **1.** Relativo ao fósforo ou que contém ou se assemelha a esse elemento. **2.** Referente ao fósforo em seu menor estado de valência (+3).

phos·pho·rous ac·id. Ácido fosforoso; H_3PO_3; seus sais são fosfitos.

phos·phor·pen·ia (fos'for-pē'nē-ă). Fosfopenia. SIN phosphopenia.

phos·phor·u·ria (fos-fō-roo'rē-ă). Fosfatúria. SIN phosphaturia.

phos·pho·rus (P) (fos'fōr-ŭs). Fósforo; elemento químico não-metálico, de n.° atômico 15, peso atômico 30,973762, abundante na natureza, sempre em combinação, como fosfatos, fosfitos, etc., e na forma de fosfato em toda célula viva; a forma elementar é extremamente venenosa, causando inflamação intensa e degeneração gordurosa; a inalação repetida de fumos do fósforo pode causar necrose da mandíbula (fosfonecrose); a dose fatal aproximada é de 50–100 mg. [G. *phosphoros*, de *phōs*, luz, + *phoros*, que carrega]
  amorphous p., red p., f. amorfo, f. vermelho; forma alotrópica de f. produzida por aquecimento do fósforo comum, na ausência de oxigênio, a 260°C; ocorre como uma massa ou pó vermelho-escuro amorfo, não-venenoso, e muito menos inflamável que o f. comum; pode ser reconvertido neste último por aquecimento a 454,4°C em gás nitrogênio.
  p. pentoxide, pentóxido de fósforo; o anidrido final do ácido ortofosfórico; um agente secante e desidratante; corrosivo.

phos·pho·rus-32 (^{32}P). Fósforo-32; isótopo do fósforo radioativo; emissor beta com meia-vida de 14,28 dias; usado como marcador em estudos metabólicos e no tratamento de algumas doenças dos sistemas ósseo e hematopoético.

phos·pho·rus-33 (^{33}P). Fósforo-33; um isótopo radioativo do fósforo com uma meia-vida de 25,3 dias; usado como marcador em estudos metabólicos.

phos·pho·ryl (fos'fō-ril). Fosforila; o radical, O≠P–, como no cloreto de fosforila, $POCl_3$.

⚠ **phosphoryl-**. Fosforil-; prefixo usado incorretamente para indicar um fosfato (p. ex., fosforilcolina) no lugar do prefixo correto *O-*fosfono- ou fosfo-.

phos·pho·ryl·ase (fos-fōr'i-lās). Fosforilase; enzima fosforilada que cliva poli(1,4-α-D-glucosil)$_n$ com ortofosfato para formar poli(1,4-α-D-glicosil)$_{n-1}$ e α-D-glicose 1-fosfato. SIN α-glucan phosphorylase, glycogen phosphorylase, P enzyme, p. *a*, polyphosphorylase.
  p. *a*. f. *a*. SIN phosphorylase.
  p. *b*. f. *b*; f. *a* desfosforilada. Na maioria das vezes, a forma inativa de fosforilase; ativa na presença de AMP. VER p. phosphatase.
  p. kinase, f. quinase; enzima que usa ATP para fosforilar a fosforilase *b* e, assim, formar novamente a fosforilase *a*, a forma ativa da fosforilase; a forma ativa da fosforilase quinase é uma proteína fosforilada; quando há desfosforilação da fosforilase quinase, a enzima é inativada; ela pode ser refosforilada com uma proteinoquinase AMPc-dependente; a fosforilase quinase é deficiente em alguns tipos de doença de armazenamento de glicogênio.
  p. phosphatase, f. fosfatase; enzima que catalisa a conversão de uma fosforilase *a* em duas fosforilases *b*, com liberação de quatro ortofosfatos. SIN phosphorylase-rupturing enzyme.

phos·pho·ryl·as·es (fos-fōr'i-lās-ez). Fosforilases. **1.** Termo genérico para designar enzimas que transferem um grupamento fosforila para algum aceptor orgânico, portanto pertencente às transferases. **2.** Especificamente, enzimas que liberam um único resíduo glucosil de uma poliglicose como D-glicose 1-fosfato, sendo o fosfato proveniente do ortofosfato; p. ex., fosfoforilase, sacarose fosforilase, celobiose fosforilase.
  nucleoside p., nucleosídeo fosforilase; enzimas que catalisam a fosforólise de um nucleosídeo, formando a purina ou pirimidina livre mais ribose (ou desoxirribose 1-fosfato); p. ex., purina-nucleosídeo fosforilases.

phos·pho·ryl·a·tion (fos-fōr-i-lā'shŭn). Fosforilação; adição de fosfato a um composto orgânico, como a glicose, para produzir glicose monofosfato através da ação de uma fosfotransferase (fosforilase) ou quinase.
  oxidative p., f. oxidativa; formação de ligações fosfóricas de alta energia (p. ex., em pirofosfatos) a partir da energia liberada pelo fluxo de elétrons para O_2 e a desidrogenação (isto é, oxidação) de vários substratos, mais notavelmente ácido isocítrico, α-cetoglutárico, ácido succínico e ácido málico no ciclo do ácido tricarboxílico.
  substrate-level p., f. ao nível do substrato; a síntese de ATP (ou outro NTP), não envolvendo o transporte de elétrons, associada à fosforilação oxidativa ou à fotofosforilação.

phos·pho·ryl·cho·line (fos'fōr-il-kō'lēn). Fosforilcolina. SIN phosphocholine.

phos·pho·ryl·eth·a·nol·a·mine glyc·er·ide·trans·fer·ase (fos'fōr-il-eth-ă-nol'ă-mēn). Fosforiletanolamina gliceridotransferase; etanolaminofosfotransferase. SIN ethanolaminephosphotransferase.

***O*-phos·pho·ser·ine** (fos-fō-ser'ēn). *O*-fosfosserina; o éster fosfórico da serina; encontrado como constituinte em muitas proteínas (p. ex., fosforilase *a* e fosvitina).

phos·pho·sphin·go·sides (fos-fō-sfing'gō-sīdz). Fosfoesfingosídeos. SIN sphingomyelins.

phos·pho·sug·ar (fos-fō-shug'er). Fosfoaçúcar; sacarídeo fosforilado; qualquer açúcar que contenha um grupo alcoólico esterificado com ácido fosfórico.

phos·pho·trans·a·cet·y·lase (fos'fō-trans-ă-set'i-lās). Fosfotransacetilase. SIN phosphate acetyltransferase.

phos·pho·trans·fer·as·es (fos-fō-trans'fer-ās-ez). Fosfotransferases; uma subclasse de transferases (EC subclasse 2.7) que transfere grupamentos contendo fósforo. As fosfotransferases incluem as "quinases" (2.7.1) que transferem fosfato para os álcoois, para grupamentos carboxila (2.7.2), para grupamentos nitrogenados (2.7.3) ou para outro grupamento fosfato (2.7.4). As fosfomutases (5.4.2) catalisam aparentes transferências intramoleculares; as pirofosfoquinases (2.7.6) catalisam a transferência do grupamento pirofosfato; as nucleotidiltransferases (2.7.7) catalisam a transferência dos grupamentos nucleotídeos (nucleotidil) (incluindo a polirribonucleotídeo nucleotidiltransferase) e outros grupamentos semelhantes (2.7.8). SIN transphosphatases.

phos·pho·tri·ose isom·er·ase (fos-fō-trī'ōs). Fosfotriose isomerase. SIN triosephosphatase isomerase.

phos·pho·tung·stic ac·id (PTA) (fos-fō-tŭng'stik). Ácido fosfotúngstico; mistura de ácidos fosfórico e túngstico; precipitante de proteínas e reagente para arginina, lisina, histidina e cistina; usado com hematoxilina para coloração nuclear e muscular; também é usado em microscopia eletrônica como corante para colágeno e como corante negativo.

phos·pho·vi·tin. Fosfovitina. SIN phosvitin.

phos·phu·re·sis (fos'foo-rē'sis). Fosfurese; excreção de quantidades excessivas de fosfato na urina. [phospho- + G. *ourēsis*, micção]

phos·phu·ria (fos-foo'rē-ă). Fosfatúria. SIN phosphaturia.

phos·vi·tin (fos-vī'tin). Fosvitina; uma proteína fosfatada que forma cerca de 7% da proteína da gema do ovo; consiste em cerca de 60% de serina, principalmente como *O*-fosfosserina, e tem propriedades anticoagulantes; um anticoagulante. SIN phosphovitin.

phot (fōt). Fot; unidade de iluminação; 1 fot é igual a 1 lúmen/cm^2 de superfície. [G. *phōs* (*phōt-*), luz]

⚠ **phot-**. VER photo-.

pho·tal·gia (fō-tal'jē-ă). Fotalgia; dor induzida pela luz, principalmente dos olhos; p. ex., na uveíte, o movimento da íris induzido pela luz pode ser doloroso. SIN photodynia, photophobia. [phot- + G. *algos*, dor]

pho·tau·gi·a·pho·bia (fō-taw'jē-ă-fō'bē-ă). Fotaugiafobia; medo mórbido ou reação excessiva a um brilho de luz. [G. *phōtaugeia*, brilho de luz, + *phobos*, medo]

pho·tes·the·sia (fō-tes-thē'zē-ă). Fotestesia; percepção da luz. [photo- + G. *aisthēsis*, sensação]

pho·tic (fō'tik). Fótico; relativo à luz.

pho·tism (fō'tizm). Fotismo; produção de uma sensação de luz ou cor por um estímulo em outro órgão do sentido, como de audição, paladar ou tato. SIN pseudophotesthesia.

⚠ **photo-, phot-**. Foto-, fot-; luz. [G. *phōs* (*phōt-*)]

pho·to·ab·la·tion (fō'tō-ab-lā'shŭn). Fotoablação; o processo de decomposição fotoablativa do tecido por laser, p. ex., na ceratectomia fotorrefrativa.

pho·to·ac·tin·ic (fō'tō-ak-tin'ik). Fotoactínico; designa a radiação que produz efeitos luminosos e químicos. [photo- + G. *aktis*, raio]

photoaging (fō'tō-āj'ing). Fotoenvelhecimento; lesão causada por anos de exposição ao sol, sobretudo enrugamento da pele. [photo- + aging]

pho·to·al·ler·gy (fō'tō-al'er-jē). Fotoalergia. VER photosensitization.

pho·to·au·to·troph (fō'tō-aw'tō-trōf). Fotoautótrofo; organismo que depende apenas da luz para obter energia e principalmente do dióxido de carbono para obter seu carbono. Cf. photoheterotroph, photolithotroph, phototroph. [photo- + G. *autos*, auto, + *trophē*, nutrição]

pho·to·au·to·tro·phic (fō-tō-aw'tō-trōf'ik). Fotoautotrófico; relativo a um fotoautótrofo.

pho·to·bac·te·ria (fō'tō-bak-tēr'ē-ă). Fotobactérias; plural de photobacterium.

Pho·to·bac·te·ri·um (fō'tō-bak-tēr'ē-ŭm). Gênero de bactérias móveis e imóveis, aeróbicas ou facultativamente anaeróbicas (família Pseudomonadaceae) que compreende cocobacilos Gram-negativos e alguns bacilos; em condições adversas, freqüentemente ocorrem formas pleomórficas. As células móveis possuem flagelos polares. O metabolismo desses microrganismos é fermentativo. Geralmente são luminescentes e ocorrem simbioticamente em tecidos de órgãos luminosos de cefalópodes e peixes das profundezas marinhas, assim como na pele e no intestino de alguns peixes marinhos. A espécie típica é *P. phosphoreum*.
  ***P. phospho'reum*,** espécie luminescente encontrada em peixes mortos e na água do mar; é a espécie típica do gênero *P*.

pho·to·bac·te·ri·um, pl. **pho·to·bac·te·ria** (fō'tō-bak-tēr'ē-ŭm, -bak-tēr'ē-ă). Fotobactéria; termo vernacular usado para se referir a qualquer membro do gênero *Photobacterium*.

pho·to·bi·ol·o·gy (fō'tō-bī-ol'ō-jē). Fotobiologia; o estudo dos efeitos da luz sobre plantas e animais.

pho·to·bi·ot·ic (fō'tō-bī-ot'ik). Fotobiótico; que vive ou floresce apenas na luz. [photo- + G. *bios*, vida]

pho·to·bleach (fō'tō-blēch). Fotoclareamento; perder cor ou tornar branco pela ação da luz; p. ex., o uso de um laser para clarear um corante fluorescente ligado a uma macromolécula de forma covalente.

pho·to·cat·a·lyst (fō-tō-kat′a-list). Fotocatalisador; substância que ajuda a produzir uma reação catalisada pela luz; p. ex., clorofila. [photo- + G. *katalysis*, dissolução (catálise)]

pho·to·cep·tor (fō′tō-sep′ter, -tōr). Fotorreceptor. SIN photoreceptor.

pho·to·chem·i·cal (fō-tō-kem′i-kal). Fotoquímico; designa alterações químicas causadas pela luz ou que envolvem a luz.

pho·to·chem·is·try (fō-tō-kem′is-trē). Fotoquímica; o ramo da química que estuda as alterações químicas causadas pela luz ou que envolvem a luz.

pho·to·che·mo·ther·a·py (fō′tō-kem-ō-thār′a-pē, -kē-mō-). Fotoquimioterapia. SIN photoradiation.

pho·to·chro·mo·gens (fō′tō-krō′mō-jenz). Fotocromógenos. SIN Runyon group I *mycobacteria*. [photo- + G. *chrōma*, cor, + *-gen*, que produz]

pho·to·co·ag·u·la·tion (fō′tō-kō-ag′ū-lā′shŭn). Fotocoagulação; método pelo qual um feixe de energia eletromagnética é direcionado para um tecido desejado sob controle visual; a coagulação localizada resulta da absorção de energia luminosa e sua conversão em calor ou conversão de tecido em plasma (átomos desprovidos de elétrons). [photo- + L. *coagulo*, pp. *-atus*, coagular]

pho·to·co·ag·u·la·tor (fō′tō-kō-ag′ū-lā′ter, tōr). Fotocoagulador; o aparelho usado na fotocoagulação.

 laser p., f. a laser; fonte de radiação eletromagnética de alta energia. VER laser.

 xenon-arc p., f. de arco de xenônio; fotocoagulador no qual uma lâmpada de arco de xenônio aplica radiação do espectro visível e próximo do infravermelho.

pho·to·der·ma·ti·tis (fō′tō-der-mă-tī′tis). Fotodermatite; dermatite causada ou desencadeada por exposição à luz solar; pode ser fototóxica ou fotoalérgica, bem como resultar de aplicação tópica, ingestão, inalação ou injeção de material fototóxico ou fotoalérgico de mediação. VER TAMBÉM photosensitization. SIN actinic dermatitis. [photo- + G. *derma*, pele, + *-itis*, inflamação]

pho·to·dis·tri·bu·tion (fō′tō-dis-tri-bū′shŭn). Fotodistribuição; áreas na pele que recebem a maior exposição à luz solar e que estão envolvidas em erupções devidas à fotossensibilidade.

pho·tod·ro·my (fō-tod′rō-mē). Fotodromia; na clarificação induzida ou espontânea de algumas suspensões, a sedimentação de partículas no lado mais próximo da luz (**fotodromia positiva**) ou no lado escuro (**fotodromia negativa**). [photo- + G. *dromos*, corrida]

pho·to·dy·nam·ic (fō′tō-dī-nam′ik). Fotodinâmico; relativo à energia ou força exercida pela luz. [photo- + G. *dynamis*, força]

pho·to·dyn·ia (fō-tō-din′ē-ă). Fotodinia. SIN photalgia. [photo- + G. *odynē*, dor]

pho·to·dys·pho·ria (fō′tō-dis-fōr′ē-ă). Fotodisforia; fotofobia extrema. [photo- + G. *dysphoria*, desconforto extremo]

pho·to·e·lec·tric (fō′tō-ēlek′trik). Fotoelétrico; designa efeitos eletrônicos ou elétricos produzidos pela ação da luz. VER photoelectric *effect*, photoelectric *absorption*.

pho·to·e·lec·trom·e·ter (fō′tō-ē-lek-trom′ē-ter). Fotoeletrômetro; dispositivo que emprega uma célula fotoelétrica para medir a concentração de substâncias em solução.

pho·to·e·lec·tron (fō′tō-ē-lek′tron). Fotoelétron; um elétron liberado pela ação da luz.

pho·to·er·y·the·ma (fō′tō-er-i-thē′mă). Fotoeritema; eritema causado por exposição à luz. [photo- + G. *erythema*, rubor]

pho·to·es·thet·ic (fō′tō-es-thet′ik). Fotoestético; sensível à luz. [photo- + G. *aisthēsis*, sensação]

pho·to·flu·o·rog·ra·phy (fō′tō-flor-og′ra-fē). Fotofluorografia; radiografias em miniatura realizadas por fotografia de contato de uma tela fluoroscópica, usada antigamente no exame radiográfico em massa dos pulmões. SIN fluorography, fluororoentgenography. [photo- + L. *fluor*, fluxo, + G. *graphē*, escrita]

pho·to·gas·tro·scope (fō′tō-gas′trō-skōp). Fotogastroscópio; instrumento para fazer fotografias do interior do estômago. [photo- + G. *gaster*, estômago, + *skopeō*, ver]

pho·to·gen (fō′tō-jen). Fotógeno; microrganismo que produz luminescência. [photo- + G. *gen-*, que produz]

pho·to·gen·e·sis (fō-tō-jen′ē-sis). Fotogênese; produção de luz, como por bactérias, insetos ou fosforescência. [photo- + G. *genesis*, produção]

pho·to·gen·ic, pho·tog·e·nous (fō-tō-jen′ik, fō-toj′ē-nŭs). Fotogênico; designa o que é capaz de fotografar.

pho·to·he·mo·ta·chom·e·ter (fō′tō-hē′mō-tă-kom′ē-ter). Foto-hemotacômetro; aparelho para registrar fotograficamente a velocidade da corrente sanguínea. [photo- + G. *haima*, sangue, + *tachos*, velocidade, + *metron*, medida]

pho·to·het·er·o·troph (fō′tō-het′er-ō-trof, -trōf). Fotoeterótrofo; organismo que depende da luz para obter a maior parte de sua energia e principalmente de compostos orgânicos para obter seu carbono. Cf. photoautotroph, photolithotroph, phototroph. [photo- + G. *heteros*, outro, + *trophē*, nutrição]

pho·to·het·er·o·tro·phic (fō-tō-het′er-ō-trof′ik). Fotoeterotrófico; relativo a um foto-heterótrofo.

pho·to·in·ac·ti·va·tion (fō′tō-in-ak-ti-vā′shŭn). Fotoinativação; inativação pela luz; p. ex., como no tratamento do herpes simples por aplicação local de um corante fotoativo seguida por exposição a uma lâmpada fluorescente.

pho·to·ker·a·to·scope (fō′tō-ker′ah-tō-skōp). Fotoceratoscópio; ceratoscópio adaptado a uma câmara de filmagem fixa.

pho·to·ki·ne·sis (fō′tō-ki-nē′sis). Fotocinesia; alteração de movimentos aleatórios de organismos móveis em resposta à luz. [photo- + G. *kinēsis*, movimento]

pho·to·ki·net·ic (fō′tō-ki-net′ik). Fotocinético. **1.** Relativo à fotocinesia. **2.** Relativo à fotocinética.

pho·to·ki·net·ics (fō′tō-ki-net′iks). Fotocinética; as alterações na velocidade de uma reação química em resposta à luz. [photo- + G. *kinētikos*, relativo ao movimento]

pho·to·ky·mo·graph (fō-tō-kī′mō-graf). Fotocimógrafo; dispositivo para movimentar o filme a uma velocidade constante de forma que possa ser obtido um registro contínuo de um evento fisiológico, como por um feixe de luz incidindo sobre o filme. [photo- + G. *kyma*, onda, + *graphō*, registrar]

pho·to·lith·o·troph (fō′tō-lith′ō-trof). Fotolitótrofo; organismo que precisa de compostos inorgânicos e que usa a luz para atender à maior parte de suas necessidades de energia. Cf. photoautotroph, photoheterotroph, phototroph. [photo- + G. *lithos*, cálculo, mineral, + *trophē*, nutrição]

pho·to·lu·mi·nes·cent (fō′tō-loo-mi-nes′ent). Fotoluminescente; que tem a capacidade de tornar-se luminescente quando exposto à luz visível. [photo- + L. *lumen*, luz]

pho·to·ly·ase (fō-tō-lī′ās). Fotoliase. VER deoxyribodipyrimidine photolyase. [photo- + G. *lyo*, afrouxar, + *-ase*]

pho·tol·y·sis (fō-tol′i-sis). Fotólise; decomposição de uma substância química ou clivagem de uma ligação química pela ação da luz. [photo- + G. *lysis*, dissolução]

pho·to·lyte (fō′tō-līt). Fotólito; qualquer produto da decomposição pela luz.

pho·to·lyt·ic (fō-tō-lit′ik). Fotolítico; relativo à fotólise.

pho·to·mac·rog·ra·phy (fō′tō-mă-krog′ra-fē). Fotomacrografia; técnica para investigar e registrar condições e procedimentos envolvendo pequenos objetos que comumente seriam examinados com uma lupa, e não com um microscópio. [photo- + G. *makros*, grande, + *graphō*, escrever]

pho·to·ma·nia (fō-tō-mā′nē-ă). Fotomania; desejo mórbido ou exagerado de luz. [photo- + G. *mania*, mania]

pho·tom·e·ter (fō-tom′ē-ter). Fotômetro; instrumento designado para medir a intensidade da luz ou determinar o limiar luminoso. [photo- + G. *metron*, medida]

 flame p., f. de chama; instrumento que usa espectrofotometria com emissão de chama para medir a intensidade e outras propriedades da luz.

 flicker p., aparelho que compara dois estímulos visuais variáveis através do controle da freqüência de uma luz oscilante.

pho·tom·e·try (fō-tom′ē-trē). Fotometria; a medida da intensidade da luz.

pho·to·mi·cro·graph (fō′tō-mī′krō-graf). Fotomicrografia; uma fotografia ampliada de um objeto visto ao microscópio; diferente da microfotografia. SIN micrograph (2). [photo- + G. *mikros*, pequeno, + *graphē*, registro]

pho·to·mi·crog·ra·phy (fō′tō-mī′krog′ra-fē). Fotomicrografar; a produção de uma fotomicrografia. SIN micrography (3).

pho·to·my·oc·lo·nus (fō′tō-mī-ok′lō-nŭs). Fotomioclônus; espasmos clônicos dos músculos em resposta a estímulos visuais. [photo- + G. *mys*, músculo, + *klonos*, movimento confuso]

 hereditary p. [MIM*172500], f. hereditário; f. associado a diabetes melito, surdez, nefropatia e disfunção cerebral; herança autossômica dominante.

pho·ton (hν, γ) (fō′ton). Fóton; em física, um corpúsculo de energia ou partícula de luz; um quantum de luz ou outra radiação eletromagnética.

pho·top·a·thy (fō-top′ă-thē). Fotopatia; qualquer doença causada por exposição à luz. [photo- + G. *pathos*, que sofre]

pho·to·peak (fō′tō-pēk). Fotópico; as energias características de fótons emitidos por um radionuclídeo, usadas para estabelecer os parâmetros de varredura.

pho·to·per·cep·tive (fō′tō-per-sep′tiv). Fotoperceptivo; capaz de receber e perceber a luz.

pho·to·pe·ri·od·ism (fō′tō-pēr′ē-ō-dizm). Fotoperiodismo; as atividades, comportamento ou alterações periódicas (sazonais ou diurnas) em vegetais ou animais produzidas pela ação da luz.

pho·to·pho·bia (fō-tō-fō′bē-ă). Fotofobia. SIN photalgia. [photo- + G. *phobos*, medo]

pho·to·pho·bic (fō-tō-fō′bik). Fotofóbico; relativo a, ou que sofre de, fotofobia.

pho·to·phore (fō′tō-fōr). Fotóforo; em bacteriologia, o órgão que produz bioluminescências intracelulares em alguns organismos. [photo- + G. *phoros*, que conduz]

pho·to·pho·re·sis. Fotoforese. VER extracorporeal p.

 extracorporeal p., f. extracórpórea; destruição de células separadas do sangue em um sistema de fluxo extracórpóreo por ativação de agentes quimioterápicos (p. ex., psoralenos) com luz ultravioleta.

pho·to·phos·pho·ry·la·tion (fō-tō-fos′fōr-i-lā′shŭn). Fotofosforilação; formação de ATP em virtude de absorção de luz.

pho·toph·thal·mia (fō′tof-thal′mē-ă). Fotoftalmia; ceratoconjuntivite causada por energia ultravioleta, como na cegueira pela neve, exposição a uma lâmpada ultravioleta, arco de solda ou o curto-circuito de uma corrente elétrica de alta tensão. VER TAMBÉM photoretinopathy. [photo- + G. *ophthalmos*, olho]

pho·to·pia (fō-tō′pē-ă). Fotopia. SIN photopic vision. [photo- + G. *opsis*, visão]

pho·top·ic (fō-top′ik). Fotópico; relativo à visão fotópica.

pho·top·sia (fō-top′sē-ă). Fotopsia; sensação subjetiva de luzes, centelhas ou cores causada por estimulação elétrica ou mecânica do sistema ocular. VER TAMBÉM Moore lightning *streaks*, em *streak*. SIN photopsy. [photo- + G. *opsis*, visão]

pho·top·sin (fō-top′sin). Fotopsina; a porção proteína (opsina) do pigmento (iodopsina) nos cones da retina.

pho·top·sy (fō-top′sē). Fotopsia. SIN photopsia.

pho·to·ptar·mo·sis (fō′tō-tar-mō′sis). Reflexo fótico de espirro; o ato de espirrar ao olhar diretamente para uma luz, principalmente uma luz brilhante (p. ex., a luz do sol), um reflexo cujas vias neuroanatômicas são discutidas; transmissão autossômica dominante. SIN photic-sneeze reflex. [photo- + G. *ptarmos*, espirro, + *-osis*, condição]

pho·to·ra·di·a·tion (fō′tō-rā-dē-ā′shŭn). Fotorradiação; tratamento de câncer por injeção intravenosa de um agente fotossensibilizante, como hematoporfirina, seguida por exposição de tumores superficiais ou de tumores profundos a luz visível (por uma sonda de fibra óptica). SIN photochemotherapy, photodynamic therapy, photoradiation therapy.

pho·to·re·ac·tion (fō′tō-rē-ak′shŭn). Fotorreação; reação causada ou afetada pela luz; p. ex., uma reação fotoquímica, fotólise, fotossíntese, fototropismo, formação de dímero de timina.

pho·to·re·ac·ti·va·tion (fō′tō-rē-ak-ti-vā′shŭn). Fotorreativação; ativação pela luz de alguma coisa ou de algum processo previamente inativo ou inativado; p. ex., dímeros de pirimidina, formados em ácidos polinucleicos pela ação da luz UV, podem ser monitorizados por luz UV de um comprimento de onda diferente através da DNA fotoliase.

pho·to·re·cep·tive (fō′tō-rē-sep′tiv). Fotorreceptivo; que funciona como um fotorreceptor.

pho·to·re·cep·tor (fō′tō-rē-sep′ter, tōr). Fotorreceptor; receptor sensível à luz, p. ex., um bastonete ou cone retiniano. SIN photoceptor. [photo- + L. *recipio*, pp. *-ceptus*, receber, de *capio*, tomar]

pho·to·res·pi·ra·tion (fō′tō-res-pi-rā′shŭn). Fotorrespiração; respiração estimulada pela luz em organismos que realizam fotossíntese; isto é, a luz aumenta a utilização de O₂.

pho·to·ret·i·ni·tis (fō′tō-ret′i-nī′tis). Fotorretinite. VER photoretinopathy.

pho·to·ret·i·nop·a·thy (fō′tō-ret′i-nop′ă-thē). Fotorretinopatia; queimadura macular decorrente da exposição excessiva à luz solar ou a outra luz intensa (p. ex., o clarão de um curto-circuito); caracterizada subjetivamente por redução da acuidade visual. VER TAMBÉM solar *maculopathy*. SIN electric retinopathy, solar retinopathy. [photo- + retina, + G. *pathos*, que sofre]

pho·to·scan (fō′tō-skan). Fotocintilografia. SIN scintiscan.

pho·to·sen·si·tive (fō-tō-sen′si-tiv). Fotossensível. **1.** Aumento anormal da reatividade da pele à luz do sol. **2.** Que responde à luz, p. ex., como por uma fotocélula. [photo + L. *sensus*, uma sensibilidade, de *sentio*, sentir]

pho·to·sen·si·tiv·i·ty (fō′tō-sen-si-tiv′i-tē). Fotossensibilidade; sensibilidade anormal à luz, principalmente dos olhos. Por exemplo, a luz pode irritar as pálpebras, a conjuntiva, a córnea ou, em excesso, a retina; quando dispersa por uma lente acometida por catarata, a luz pode produzir ofuscação; pode causar enxaqueca ou exotropia temporária. VER photophobia, photalgia, photesthesia.

pho·to·sen·si·ti·za·tion (fō′tō-sen-si-ti-zā′shŭn). Fotossensibilização. **1.** Sensibilização da pele à luz, geralmente causada pela ação de alguns fármacos, vegetais ou outras substâncias; pode ocorrer logo após a administração do fármaco (sensibilidade fototóxica), ou somente após um período latente de dias a meses (sensibilidade fotoalérgica, ou fotoalergia). **2.** SIN photodynamic sensitization.

pho·to·sen·sor (fō′tō-sen′ser, sōr). Fotossensor; dispositivo que responde à luz e transmite os impulsos resultantes para interpretação, movimento ou controle operacional. VER sensor.

pho·to·sta·ble (fō′tō-stā-bl). Fotoestável; não sujeito a alteração após exposição à luz.

pho·to·steth·o·scope (fō-tō-steth′ō-skōp). Fotoestetoscópio; aparelho que converte o som em clarões de luz; usado para observação contínua do coração fetal.

pho·to·stress (fō′tō-stres). Fotoestresse; exposição à iluminação intensa. VER TAMBÉM photostress *test*.

pho·to·syn·the·sis (fō-tō-sin′thĕ-sis). Fotossíntese. **1.** A composição ou acúmulo de substâncias químicas sob a influência da luz. **2.** O processo pelo qual as plantas verdes, utilizando clorofila e a energia da luz solar, produzem carboidratos a partir da água e do dióxido de carbono, liberando oxigênio molecular no processo. [photo- + G. *synthesis*, reunião]

bacterial p., f. bacteriana; forma primitiva de f. observada em algumas bactérias utilizando apenas um fotossistema e algum outro agente redutor além da água.

pho·to·tax·is (fō-tō-tak′sis). Fototaxia; reação de protoplasma vivo ao estímulo luminoso, envolvendo o movimento corporal do organismo como um todo aproximando-se (**fototaxia positiva**) ou afastando-se (**fototaxia negativa**) do estímulo. Cf. phototropism. [photo- + G. *taxis*, arranjo ordenado]

pho·to·ther·a·py (fō-tō-thar′ă-pē). Fototerapia; tratamento de doença por meio de raios luminosos. SIN light treatment.

pho·to·ther·mal (fō-tō-ther′măl). Fototérmico; relativo ao calor radiante. [photo- + G. *therme*, calor]

pho·to·tim·er (fō-tō-tim′er). Fototemporizador; dispositivo eletrônico em radiografia que mede a radiação que atravessou o paciente e interrompe a exposição aos raios X quando esta é suficiente para formar uma imagem.

pho·to·tox·ic (fō-tō-tok′sik). Fototóxico; relativo a, caracterizado por ou que causa fototoxicidade.

pho·to·tox·ic·i·ty (fō-tō-tok-sis′i-tē). Fototoxicidade; a condição resultante da superexposição à luz ultravioleta, ou da combinação de exposição a determinados comprimentos de onda de luz e a uma substância fototóxica. VER TAMBÉM photosensitization. [photo- + G. *toxikon*, tóxico]

pho·to·troph (fō′tō-trōf). Fotótrofo; organismo que usa luz para satisfazer as suas necessidades de energia. Cf. photoautotroph, photoheterotroph, photolithotroph.

pho·tot·ro·pism (fō-to′trō-pizm). Fototropismo; movimento de uma parte de um organismo aproximando-se (**fototropismo positivo**) ou afastando-se (**fototropismo negativo**) do estímulo luminoso. Cf. phototaxis. [photo- + G. *trope*, uma volta]

pho·tu·ria (fō-too′rē-ă). Fotúria; a eliminação de urina fosforescente. [photo- + G. *ouron*, urina]

PHP Abreviatura de panhypopituitarism (pan-hipopituitarismo).

phrag·mo·plast (frag′mō-plast). Fragmoplasto; aumento em forma de barril do fuso associado à formação da nova membrana celular durante a telófase em células vegetais. [G. *phragma*, barreira, cercado, + *plasso*, formar]

phren (fren). **1.** Diafragma. SIN diaphragm (1). **2.** A mente. [G. *phren*, o diafragma, mente, coração (como sede das emoções)]

phren-. VER phreno-.

phre·nal·gia (fre-nal′jē-ă). Frenalgia. **1.** SIN psychalgia (1). **2.** Dor no diafragma. [phren- + G. *algos*, dor]

phre·nec·to·my (fre-nek′tō-mē). Frenectomia. SIN phrenicectomy.

phren·em·phrax·is (fren′em-frak′sis). Freniclasia. SIN phreniclasia. [phren- + G. *emphraxis*, interrupção]

phre·net·ic (fre-net′ik). Frenético. **1.** Maníaco. **2.** Indivíduo que exibe esse comportamento. [G. *phrenitikos*, arrebatado]

phreni-. VER phreno-.

-phrenia. -Frenia. **1.** O diafragma. **2.** A mente. VER phreno-. [G. *phren*, o diafragma, a mente, o coração (como sede das emoções)]

phren·ic (fren′ik). Frênico. **1.** Diafragmático. SIN diaphragmatic. **2.** Relativo à mente.

phren·i·cec·to·my (fren-i-sek′tō-mē). Frenicectomia; excisão de uma parte do nervo frênico, para evitar reunião como a que pode ocorrer após frenicotomia. SIN phrenectomy, phrenicoexeresis, phreniconeurectomy. [phreni- + G. *ektome*, excisão]

phren·i·cla·sia (fren-i-klā′zē-ă). Frenicoclasia; esmagamento de uma parte do nervo frênico para provocar paralisia temporária do diafragma. SIN phrenemphraxis, phrenicotripsy. [phreni- + G. *klasis*, ruptura]

phren·i·co·col·ic (fren′i-kō-kol′ik). Frenicocólico; relativo ao diafragma e ao colo. SIN phrenocolic.

phren·i·co·ex·er·e·sis (fren′i-kō-ek-ser′ē-sis). Frenicoexérese. SIN phrenicectomy. [phrenico- + G. *exairesis*, tirar, de *haireo*, tomar, agarrar]

phren·i·co·gas·tric (fren′i-kō-gas′trik). Frenicogástrico; relativo ao diafragma e ao estômago. SIN phrenogastric.

phren·i·co·glot·tic (fren′i-kō-glot′ik). Frenicoglótico; relativo ao diafragma e à glote; designa o espasmo que envolve o diafragma e as pregas vocais.

phren·i·co·he·pat·ic (fren′i-kō-he-pa′tik). Frenoepático; relativo ao diafragma e ao fígado. SIN phrenohepatic.

phren·i·co·neu·rec·to·my (fren′i-kō-noo-rek′tō-mē). Freniconeurectomia. SIN phrenicectomy.

phren·i·co·splen·ic (fren′i-kō-splen′ik). Frenicoesplênico; relativo ao diafragma e ao baço.

phren·i·cot·o·my (fren-i-kot′ō-mē). Frenicotomia; corte do nervo frênico a fim de induzir paralisia unilateral do diafragma, que é então empurrado para cima pelas vísceras abdominais e comprime um pulmão doente. [phrenico- + G. *tome*, incisão]

phren·i·co·trip·sy (fren′i-kō-trip′sē). Frenicotripsia. SIN phreniclasia. [phrenico- + G. *tripsis*, fricção, esmagamento]

phreno-, phren-, phreni-, phrenico-. Freno-, fren-, freni-, frenico. **1.** O diafragma. **2.** A mente. **3.** O nervo frênico. [G. *phrēn*, diafragma, mente, coração (como a sede das emoções)]

phren·o·car·di·a (fren-ō-kar'dē-ă). Frenocardia; dor precordial e dispnéia de origem psicogênica, freqüentemente um sintoma de neurose de ansiedade. VER cardiac *neurosis*. SIN cardiophrenia. [phreno- + G. *kardia*, coração]

phren·o·col·ic (fren'ō-kol'ik). Frenocólico. SIN phrenicocolic. [phreno- + G. *kolon*, colo]

phren·o·gas·tric (fren-ō-gas'trik). Frenogástrico. SIN phrenicogastric. [phreno- + G. *gastēr*, estômago]

phren·o·graph (fren'ō-graf). Frenógrafo; instrumento para realizar o registro gráfico dos movimentos do diafragma. [phreno- + G. *graphō*, registrar]

phren·o·he·pat·ic (fren'ō-hĕ-pat'ik). Frenoepático; frenepático. SIN phrenicohepatic. [phreno- + G. *hepar*, fígado]

phre·nol·o·gist (frĕ-nol'ō-jist). Frenologista; aquele que afirma ser capaz de diagnosticar características mentais e comportamentais por um estudo da configuração externa do crânio. [ver phrenology]

phre·nol·o·gy (frĕ-nol'ō-jē). Frenologia; doutrina obsoleta que afirma que cada uma das faculdades mentais está localizada em uma parte definida do córtex cerebral, e o tamanho de cada parte é diretamente proporcional ao desenvolvimento e à capacidade da faculdade correspondente, sendo esse tamanho indicado pela configuração externa do crânio. SIN craniognomy. [phreno- + G. *logos*, estudo]

phren·o·ple·gia (fren-ō-plē'jē-ă). Frenoplegia; paralisia do diafragma. [phreno- + G. *plēgē*, ataque]

phren·op·to·sia (fren-op-tō'sē-ă). Frenoptose; descida anormal do diafragma. [phreno- + G. *ptōsis*, queda]

phren·o·sin (fren'ō-sin). Frenosina; um cerebrosídeo abundante na substância branca do encéfalo, composto de ácido cerebrônico, D-galactose e esfingosina. SIN cerebron.

phren·o·sin·ic ac·id (fren-ō-sin'ik). Ácido frenosínico. SIN cerebronic acid.

phren·o·spasm (fren'ō-spazm). Frenospasmo; espasmo do diafragma, como no soluço. [phreno- + G. *spasmos*, espasmo]

phren·o·tro·pic (fren-ō-trop'ik). Frenotrópico; que afeta ou atua através da mente ou do encéfalo. [phreno- + G. *tropē*, uma volta]

phryn·o·der·ma (frin-ō-der'mă). Frinoderma; erupção hiperceratótica folicular supostamente causada por deficiência de vitamina A. SIN toad skin. [G. *phrynos*, sapo, + *derma*, pele]

phry·nol·y·sin (frī-nol'ī-sin). Frinolisina; o veneno do sapo do fogo (*Bombinator igneus*). [G. *phrynos*, sapo, + *lysis*, solução]

PHS Abreviatura de Public Health Service (Serviço de Saúde Pública).

pH-stat. Um dispositivo para determinar continuamente o pH de uma solução e automaticamente acrescentar ácidos ou álcalis quando necessário para manter o pH constante; usado para acompanhar o curso de reações que liberam um ácido ou álcali.

o-**phtha·lal·de·hyde** (thal-al'dĕ-hīd). *o*-ftalaldeído; reagente usado na identificação e na detecção de aminoácidos.

phthal·ein (thal'ē-in). Ftaleína; membro de um grupo de compostos altamente coloridos que têm como base a trifenilmetila; p. ex., fenolftaleína.

phthal·ic ac·id (thal'ik). Ácido ftálico; ácido *o*-benzenodicarboxílico.

phthal·o·yl (thal'ō-il). Ftaloíla; o radical diacil do ácido ftálico.

phthal·yl (thal'il). Ftalil; o radical monoacil do ácido ftálico.

phthal·yl·sul·fa·cet·a·mide (thal'il-sŭl-fă-set'ă-mīd). Ftalilsulfacetamida; N^1-acetil-N^4-ftalilsulfanilamida; sulfonamida usada no tratamento de infecções entéricas.

phthal·yl·sul·fa·thi·a·zole (thal'il-sŭl-fă-thī'ă-zōl). Ftalilsulfatiazol; sulfonamida usada no tratamento de infecções entéricas.

phthi·ri·o·pho·bia (thī'rē-ō-fō'bē-ă). Pediculofobia. SIN pediculophobia. [G. *phtheir*, piolho, + *phobos*, medo]

Phthi·rus (thī'rus). VER *Pthirus*. [L. *phthir*; G. *phtheir*, piolho]

phthisio-. Tisio-; tísica (tuberculose). [G. *phthisis*, desgaste]

phthis·i·ol·o·gist (thī-zē-ol'ō-jist). Tisiologista; termo obsoleto para especialista em tuberculose.

phyco-. Fico-; alga marinha. [G. *phykos*]

Phy·co·my·ce·tes (fī'kō-mi-sē'tēz). SIN Zygomycetes. [phyco- + G. *mykēs*, fungo]

phy·co·my·ce·to·sis (fī'kō-mī-sē-tō'sis). Ficomicetose. SIN zygomycosis.

phy·co·my·co·sis (fī'kō-mī'kō-sis). Ficomicose. SIN zygomycosis.
subcutaneous p., f. subcutânea. SIN entomophthoramycosis basidiobolae.

phy·lac·a·gog·ic (fī-lak-ă-goj'ik). Filacagógico; que estimula a produção de anticorpos protetores. [G. *phylaxis*, guarda, proteção, + *agogos*, que leva]

phy·lax·is (fī-lak'sis). Filaxia; proteção contra infecção. [G. guarda, proteção]

phy·let·ic (fī-let'ik). Filético; designa a evolução de alterações seqüenciais em uma linha de descendência pela qual uma espécie é transformada em uma nova espécie. [G. *phyletikos*, tribal, de *phylē*, tribo]

phyllo-. Filo-; uma folha; semelhante a uma folha; clorofila. [G. *phyllon*, folhagem]

phyl·lode (fil'ōd). Filódio; pecíolo achatado, semelhante a uma folha; termo aplicado a qualquer estrutura semelhante a uma folha, principalmente a um corte transversal de uma neoplasia com uma estrutura foliada, como o cistossarcoma filóide. [G. *phyllōdēs*, semelhante a folhas, de *phyllon*, folha, + *eidos*, semelhança]

phyl·lo·qui·none (K), phyl·lo·qui·none K (fil-ō-kwin'ōn, -kwī'nōn). Filoquinona; isolado da alfafa; também preparado sinteticamente; principal forma de vitamina K encontrada em vegetais. SIN phytomenadione, phytonadione, vitamin K_1, vitamin K_1 (20).
p. reductase, f. redutase. SIN NADPH dehydrogenase (quinone).

phylo-. Filo-; tribo, raça; um filo taxonômico. [G. *phylon*, tribo]

phy·lo·a·nal·y·sis (fī'lō-ă-nal'i-sis). Filoanálise. **1.** O estudo das origens biorraciais. **2.** Termo raramente usado para designar um método de investigação de distúrbios comportamentais individuais e coletivos supostamente causados por comprometimento dos processos tensionais. [phylo- + analysis]

phy·lo·gen·e·sis (fī-lō-jen'ĕ-sis). Filogênese. SIN phylogeny. [phylo- + G. *genesis*, origem]

phy·lo·ge·net·ic, phy·lo·gen·ic (fī'lō-jĕ-net'ik, -jen'ik). Filogenético, filogênico; relativo à filogênese.

phy·log·e·ny (fī-loj'ĕ-nē). Filogenia; o desenvolvimento evolutivo das espécies, distinto da ontogenia, desenvolvimento do indivíduo. SIN phylogenesis.

phy·lum, pl. **phy·la** (fī'lŭm, fī'lă). Filo; divisão taxonômica abaixo do reino e acima da classe. [L. mod. do G. *phylon*, tribo]

phy·ma·toid (fī'mă-toyd). Fimatóide; semelhante a uma neoplasia. [G. *phyma*, um tumor, + *eidos*, semelhança]

phy·ma·tor·rhy·sin (fī'mă-tōr'i-sin). Fimatorrisina; variedade de melanina obtida de algumas neoplasias melanóticas e dos pêlos e de outras partes intensamente pigmentadas. [G. *phyma* (*phymat*-), tumor, + *rhysis*, fluxo]

Phy·sa (fī'să). Gênero típico dos caramujos pulmonados de água doce (família Physidae) que inclui várias espécies americanas comuns como *P. parkeri*, *P. gyrina* e *P. integra*; são hospedeiros intermediários de vários trematódeos de aves e animais, incluindo vários que causam dermatite por esquistossoma em seres humanos. [G. um par de foles; uma bolha de ar; bexiga]

Physalia. Gênero do filo invertebrado Cnidaria, que inclui a caravela.
P. physalis, a caravela, um animal gelatinoso que consiste em uma colônia complexa cujos membros podem infligir picadas extremamente dolorosas. SIN Portuguese man-of-war.

phys·a·lif·er·ous (fis-ă-lif'er-ŭs). Fisalíforo. SIN physaliphorous.

phys·a·li·form (fi-sal'i-fōrm). Fisaliforme; semelhante a uma bolha ou pequena vesícula. [G. *physallis*, bexiga, bolha, + L. *forma*, forma]

phys·a·li·phore (fi-sal'i-fōr). Fisalíforo; uma célula-mãe ou célula gigante que contém um grande vacúolo, em um tumor maligno. [G. *physallis*, bexiga, bolha, + *phoros*, que conduz]

phys·a·liph·or·ous (fis-ă-lif'or-ŭs). Fisalíforo; que possui bolhas ou vacúolos. SIN physaliferous. [G. *physallis*, bexiga, bolha, + *phoros*, que conduz]

phys·a·lis (fis'ă-lis). Fisálide; vacúolo em uma célula gigante encontrado em determinadas neoplasias malignas, como o cordoma. [G. *physallis*, bexiga]

Phy·sa·lop·te·ra (fī'să-lop'ter-ă, fis-). Grande gênero de nematódeos espirúroides parasitas do estômago e do duodeno de vertebrados, principalmente de aves e mamíferos; são transmitidos por insetos e anelídeos, hospedeiros intermediários, sendo freqüentemente patogênicos, causando erosões e gastrite catarral. *P. caucasica* é uma espécie descrita em seres humanos no sul da antiga União Soviética; *P. mordens* é uma espécie da África tropical encontrada apenas raramente no esôfago, estômago e intestino de seres humanos (provavelmente, casos de infecção temporária por ingestão de insetos infectados). [G. *physallis*, bexiga, + *pteron*, asa]

phy·sa·lop·ter·i·a·sis (fī'să-lop-ter-ī'ă-sis). Fisalopteríase; infecção de animais e seres humanos por nematódeos do gênero *Physaloptera*.

phys·e·al (fiz'ē-ăl). Fisário(a); relativo à fise, ou área da cartilagem de crescimento, que separa a metáfise e a epífise em ossos esqueleticamente imaturos.

physi-. Fisi-. VER physio-.

phys·i·at·ri·cian (fiz'ē-ă-trish'ŭn). Fisiatra; médico que se especializa em fisiatria (medicina de reabilitação).

phys·i·at·rics (fiz-ē-at'riks). Fisiatria. **1.** Designação antiga de physical *therapy* (fisioterapia). **2.** Terapia de reabilitação. [G. *physis*, natureza, + *iatrikos*, cura]

phys·i·a·trist (fiz-ī'ă-trist). Fisiatra; médico especializado em fisiatria.

phys·i·a·try (fi-zī'ă-trē; fiz-ē-at'rē). Fisiatria. SIN physical *medicine*.

phys·ic (fiz'ik). **1.** Medicina; a arte da medicina. **2.** Remédio; medicamento; freqüentemente um termo usado por leigo para catártico. [G. *physikos*, natural, físico]

phys·i·cal (fiz'i-kăl). Físico; relativo ao corpo, distinto da mente. [L. mod. *physicalis*, do G. *physikos*]

phy·si·cian (fi-zish'ŭn). Médico. **1.** Pessoa que foi educada, treinada e licenciada para praticar a arte e a ciência da medicina. **2.** Um clínico, em contraste com um cirurgião. [Fr. *physicien*, um filósofo natural]
attending p., (1) médico assistente; médico responsável pelo tratamento de um paciente; (2) médico que supervisiona o tratamento de pacientes por internos,

residentes e/ou estudantes de medicina. (3) médico que completou o internato e a residência.
family p., médico de família; médico especializado em medicina de família.
hospital-based p., hospitalista. SIN hospitalist (1).
osteopathic p., médico osteopata; médico que pratica a osteopatia. SIN osteopath.
resident p., médico residente. SIN resident.

phy·si·cian as·sis·tant (P.A.). Auxiliar médico; pessoa treinada, certificada e licenciada para realizar anamnese, exame físico, diagnóstico e tratamento de problemas clínicos comuns, e algumas manobras técnicas, sob a supervisão de um médico licenciado, e que, portanto, amplia a capacidade do médico de prestar assistência. Existem muitos subespecialistas, como auxiliar de ortopedia, auxiliar em lesões esportivas, auxiliar de pediatria, etc.

Physick, Philip Syng, cirurgião norte-americano, 1768–1837. VER P. *pouches*, em *pouch*.

phys·i·co·chem·i·cal (fiz'i-kō-kem'i-kal). Físico-químico; relativo ao campo da físico-química.

phys·ics (fiz'iks). Física; o ramo da ciência que estuda os fenômenos da matéria e energia e suas interações. VER physic.
radiation p., f. nuclear; a disciplina científica da aplicação da f. ao uso da radiação ionizante no tratamento e na radiologia diagnóstica; incluindo, por extensão, aplicações de medicina nuclear, ultra-sonografia e ressonância magnética.

physio-, physi-. Fisio-, fisi-. **1.** Físico, fisiológico. **2.** Natural, relativo à física. [G. *physis*, natureza]

phys·i·o·gen·ic (fiz'ē-ō-jen'ik). Fisiogênico; relativo a, ou causado por, atividade fisiológica. [physio- + G. *genesis*, origem]

phys·i·og·no·my (fiz-ē-og'nō-mē). Fisiognomonia. **1.** A aparência física da face, fisionomia ou biotipo de uma pessoa, particularmente considerada como uma indicação do caráter. **2.** Estimativa do caráter e das qualidades mentais de uma pessoa por um estudo da face e de outras características corporais externas. [physio- + G. *gnōmon*, julgamento]

phys·i·og·no·sis (fiz-ē-og-nō'sis). Fisiognose; diagnóstico de doenças baseado em um estudo da aparência facial ou do biotipo. [physio- + G. *gnōsis*, conhecimento]

phys·i·o·log·ic, phys·i·o·log·i·cal (fiz-ē-ō-loj'ik, -loj'i-kal). Fisiológico. **1.** Relativo à fisiologia. **2.** Normal, ao contrário do patológico; designa os vários processos vitais. **3.** Designa algo que é aparente por seus efeitos funcionais, e não por sua estrutura anatômica; p. ex., um esfíncter fisiológico. **4.** Designa uma dose ou os efeitos desta dose (de um agente químico que é ou imita um hormônio, neurotransmissor ou outro agente de ocorrência natural) dentro da faixa de concentrações ou potências que ocorreriam naturalmente. Cf. homeopathic (2), pharmacologic (2), supraphysiologic.

phys·i·o·log·i·co·an·a·tom·i·cal (fiz'ē-ō-loj'i-kō-an-ă-tom'i-kal). Fisiológico-anatômico; relativo à fisiologia e à anatomia.

phys·i·ol·o·gist (fiz-ē-ol'ō-jist). Fisiologista; um especialista em fisiologia.

phys·i·ol·o·gy (fiz-ē-ol'ō-jē). Fisiologia; a ciência que estuda os processos vitais normais de organismos animais e vegetais, principalmente no que se refere à forma como as coisas funcionam normalmente no organismo vivo, e não à sua estrutura anatômica, sua composição bioquímica, ou à forma como são afetadas por fármacos ou doenças. [L. ou G. *physiologia*, do G. *physis*, natureza, + *logos*, estudo]
comparative p., f. comparativa; a ciência que estuda as diferenças nos processos vitais em diferentes espécies de organismos, visando sobretudo a adaptação dos processos às necessidades específicas da espécie, a elucidação das relações evolucionárias entre diferentes espécies, ou o estabelecimento de outras generalizações e relações entre espécies.
general p., f. geral; a ciência das funções ou dos processos vitais comuns a quase todos os seres vivos, sejam animais ou vegetais, ao contrário dos aspectos da fisiologia peculiares a determinados tipos de animais ou vegetais, ou a aplicação da fisiologia às ciências aplicadas como medicina e agricultura.
hominal p., f. humana; fisiologia aplicada ao esclarecimento das funções normais do ser humano.
pathologic p., fisiopatologia; parte da ciência que estuda a perturbação da função, distinta das lesões anatômicas. SIN physiopathology.

phys·i·o·path·o·log·ic (fiz'ē-ō-path-ō-loj'ik). Fisiopatológico; relativo à fisiopatologia.

phys·i·o·pa·thol·o·gy (fiz'ē-ō-pă-thol'ō-jē). Fisiopatologia. SIN pathologic *physiology*.

phys·i·o·psy·chic (fiz'ē-ō-sī'kik). Fisiopsíquico; relativo à mente e ao corpo.

phys·i·o·py·rex·ia (fiz'ē-ō-pī-rek'sē-ă). Fisiopirexia; febre produzida por um agente físico. [physio- + G. *pyrexis*, febre]

phys·i·o·ther·a·peu·tic (fiz'ē-ō-thār-ă-pū'tik). Fisioterapêutico; relativo à fisioterapia. SIN physical *therapy*.

phys·i·o·ther·a·pist (fiz'ē-ō-thār'ă-pist). Fisioterapeuta. VER physical *therapy* (2).

phys·i·o·ther·a·py (fiz'ē-ō-thār'ă-pē). Fisioterapia. SIN physical *therapy* (1). [physio- + G. *therapeia*, tratamento]
oral p., f. oral; o uso de uma escova de dentes, estimulador interdental, fio dental, dispositivo de irrigação ou outro auxiliar para manter a saúde oral.

phy·sique (fi-zēk'). Físico; tipo constitucional; a estrutura física ou corporal; a "constituição". [Fr.]

phy·sis (fi'sis). Fise; termo usado algumas vezes para se referir à cartilagem epifisária. [G. crescimento]

physo-. Fiso-. **1.** Tendência a inchar ou inflar. **2.** Relação com ar ou gás. [G. *physaō*, inflar, distender]

phy·so·cele (fi'sō-sēl). Fisocele. **1.** Tumefação circunscrita causada pela presença de gás. **2.** Saco herniário distendido com gás. [physo- + G. *kēlē*, tumor, hérnia]

Phy·so·ceph·a·lus sex·a·la·tus (fī'sō-sef'ă-lŭs sek'să-lā'tŭs). Uma pequena espécie de nematódeos espiruróides (família Spiruridae) encontrada no estômago de porcos, cavalos, camelos, coelhos e éguas; tem distribuição mundial, sendo particularmente prevalente em porcos. [G. *physa*, fole, + *kephalē*, cabeça]

phy·so·ceph·a·ly (fī-sō-sef'ă-lē). Fisocefalia; tumefação da cabeça resultante da introdução de ar nos tecidos subcutâneos. [physo- + G. *kephalē*, cabeça]

phy·so·me·tra (fī-sō-mē'tră). Fisometria; distensão da cavidade uterina por ar ou gás. SIN uterine tympanites. [physo- + G. *mētra*, útero]

Phy·sop·sis (fī-sop'sis). Subgênero do gênero *Bulinus*, cuja maioria das espécies transmite o trematódeo sanguíneo humano, *Schistosoma haematobium*, e alguns esquistossomas animais na África, ao sul do Saara. [G. *physis*, crescimento, + *opsis*, aspecto, aparência]

phy·so·py·o·sal·pinx (fī'sō-pī-ō-sal'pingks). Fisopiossalpinge; piossalpinge acompanhada por formação de gás em uma tuba uterina. [physo- + G. *pyon*, pus, + *salpinx*, trompa]

phy·so·stig·ma (fī-sō-stig'mă). Fisostigma; a semente seca da *Pysostigma venenosum* (família Leguminosae), uma trepadeira do oeste da África; contém os alcalóides fisostigmina (eserina), eseramina, eseridina (geneserina) e fisovenina; em doses tóxicas causa vômitos, cólica, salivação, diarréia, convulsões, sudorese, dispnéia, vertigem, pulso lento e prostração extrema. SIN Calabar bean, ordeal bean. [G. *physa*, fole, + *stigma*, uma marca, mancha; assim denominada devido ao formato do estigma]

phy·so·stig·mine (fī-sō-stig'mēn, -min). Fisostigmina; um alcalóide da fisostigmina; é um inibidor reversível das colinesterases e impede a destruição da acetilcolina; usada como agente colinérgico e, experimentalmente, para estimular a ação da acetilcolina em qualquer um de seus locais de liberação. SIN eserine.
p. salicylate, salicilato de fisostigmina; usado por instilação conjuntival para reduzir a tensão no glaucoma, no tratamento da atonia intestinal pós-operatória e da retenção urinária, no tratamento da miastenia grave e para neutralizar doses excessivas de tubocurarina; também disponível na forma de sulfato de f., com os mesmos empregos. SIN eserine salicylate.

phyt-. VER phyto-.

phy·tan·ate (fī'tan-āt). Fitanato; o ânion do ácido fitânico.
p. α-oxidase, f. α-oxidase; enzima que oxida o ácido fitânico, removendo o grupamento carboxila.

phy·tan·ic ac·id (fī-tan'ik). Ácido fitânico; um ácido graxo de cadeia ramificada que se acumula no soro e nos tecidos na doença de Refsum e atribuído à ausência hereditária de fitanato α-oxidase; origina-se do fitol e atua como inibidor da α-oxidação do ácido palmítico (hexadecanóico); também se acumula em vários outros distúrbios, notavelmente em distúrbios do peroxissoma.

6-phy·tase (fī'tās). 6-Fitase; fitato-6-fosfato; enzima que hidrolisa o ácido fítico, removendo o grupamento 6-fosfórico, assim produzindo ortofosfato e 1L-*mio*-1,2,3,4,5-pentacisfosfato.

phy·tate (fī'tāt). Fitato; um sal ou éster do ácido fítico.

phy·tic ac·id (fī'tik). Ácido fítico; o éster hexacisfosfórico do mio-inositol (*myo*-inositol); o sal misto com magnésio e cálcio é a fitina.

phy·tin (fī'tin). Fitina; o sal de magnésio e cálcio do ácido fítico; um suplemento alimentar usado para fornecer cálcio, fósforo orgânico e mio-inositol (*myo*-inositol).

phyto-, phyt-. Fito-, fit-; plantas. [G. *phyton*, uma planta]

phy·to·ag·glu·ti·nin (fī'tō-ă-gloo'ti-nin). Fitoaglutinina; lectina que causa a aglutinação de eritrócitos ou de leucócitos.

phy·to·be·zoar (fī-tō-bē'zor). Fitobezoar; concreção gástrica formada por fibras vegetais, com as sementes e cascas de frutas, e, algumas vezes, grânulos de amido e glóbulos de gordura. SIN food ball. [phyto- + bezoar]

phy·to·chem·is·try (fī-tō-kem'is-trē). Fitoquímica; o estudo bioquímico dos vegetais; relacionado à identificação, biossíntese e metabolismo dos constituintes químicos dos vegetais; usado particularmente em relação a produtos naturais.

phy·to·der·ma·ti·tis (fī'tō-der-mă-ti'tis). Fitodermatite; dermatite causada por vários mecanismos, incluindo lesão mecânica e química, alergia ou fotossensibilização (fitofotodermatite) em locais cutâneos previamente expostos a vegetais.

Phy·to·fla·gel·la·ta (fi'tō - flaj - ĕ - lā'tă). Subclasse de Phytomastigophorea, cujos membros possuem cromatóforos amarelos ou verdes. [phyto- + L. *flagellum*, flagelo]

phy·to·hem·ag·glu·ti·nin (PHA) (fi'tō - hēm - ă - glooʹti - nin). Fitoemaglutinina; um fitomitógeno proveniente de vegetais que aglutina hemácias. O termo é comumente usado especificamente para se referir à lectina obtida do feijão (*Phaseolus vulgaris*), que também é um mitógeno que estimula mais vigorosamente os linfócitos T que os linfócitos B. SIN phytolectin.

phy·toid (fi'toyd). Fitóide; semelhante a um vegetal; designa um animal que possui muitas das características biológicas de um vegetal. [G. *phytōdēs*, de *phyton*, vegetal, + *eidos*, semelhança]

phy·tol (fi'tol). Fitol; álcool primário insaturado derivado da hidrólise da clorofila; um constituinte das vitaminas E e K_1. SIN phytyl alcohol.

phy·to·lec·tin (fī - tō - lek'tin). Fitolectina. SIN phytohemagglutinin.

Phy·to·mas·ti·gi·na (fi'tō - mas - ti - jī'nă). Designação antiga de flagelados semelhantes a vegetais, originalmente classificados como uma subordem ou ordem, elevados à classe Phytomastigophorea (Phytomastigophorasida) em classificações recentes. [phyto- + G. *mastix*, flagelo]

Phy·to·mas·ti·go·pho·ras·i·da (fi'tō - masʹti - gō - fō - rasʹi - dă). SIN Phytomastigophorea.

Phy·to·mas·ti·goph·o·rea (fi'tō - masʹti - gof - ō - rē'ă). Classe do subfilo Mastigophora (flagelados) no filo Sarcomastigophora (protozoários flagelados e amebóides), consistindo principalmente em flagelados de vida livre, semelhantes a vegetais, com ou sem cloroplastos, e geralmente com um ou dois flagelos. Cf. Zoomastigophorea. SIN Phytomastigophorasida. [phyto- + G. *mastix*, flagelo, + *phoros*, que conduz]

phy·to·men·a·di·one (fī'tō - men - ă - dī'ōn). Fitomenadiona. SIN phylloquinone.

phy·to·mi·to·gen (fī - tō - mī'tō - jen). Fitomitógeno; lectina mitogênica que causa transformação de linfócitos acompanhada por proliferação mitótica das células blásticas resultantes idêntica àquela produzida por estimulação antigênica; p. ex., fitoemaglutinina, concanavalina A.

phy·to·na·di·one (fī'tō - nă - dī'ōn). Fitonadiona. SIN phylloquinone.

phy·toph·a·gous (fī - tofʹă - gŭs). Fitófago; que come vegetais; vegetariano. [phyto- + G. *phagō*, comer]

phy·to·pho·to·der·ma·ti·tis (fī'tō - fō'tō - der - mă - tī'tis). Fotofitodermatite; fitodermatite resultante da fotossensibilização.

phy·to·pneu·mo·co·ni·o·sis (fī'tō - nooʹmō - kō - nē - ō'sis). Fitopneumoconiose; reação fibrosa crônica nos pulmões causada por inalação de partículas de origem vegetal. [phyto- + pneumoconiosis]

phy·to·por·phy·rin (fī - tō - pōrʹfī - rin). Fitoporfirina. 1. Uma porfirina semelhante à feoforbida das clorofinas, mas com o grupamento vinila substituído por um grupamento etila, sem grupamento metoxicarbonila, e menos dois átomos de hidrogênio, produzindo uma ou mais ligações duplas no anel D. 2. Qualquer porfirina vegetal.

phy·to·sis (fī - tō - sis). Fitose; processo patológico causado por infecção por um organismo vegetal, como um fungo.

phy·to·sphin·go·sine (fī - tō - sfingʹgō - sēn, - sin) Fitoesfingosina; um derivado da esfingosina isolado de vários vegetais.

phy·to·ste·rol (fī - tō - stērʹol). Fitosterol; termo genérico para designar os esteróis dos vegetais.

phy·to·ste·ro·lem·i·a (fī - tō - stērʹol - ē - mē - ă). Fitosterolemia; distúrbio hereditário no qual há hiperabsorção de fitosteróis e esteróis de crustáceos, resultando em xantomas tendinosos e tuberosos. SIN sitosterolemia.

phy·to·tox·ic (fī - tō - tokʹsik). Fitotóxico. 1. Venenoso para a vida vegetal. 2. Relativo a uma fitotoxina.

phy·to·tox·in (fī - tō - tokʹsin). Fitotoxina; substância tóxica de origem vegetal. SIN plant toxin. [phyto- + G. *toxikon*, veneno]

phy·to·trich·o·be·zoar (fī'tō - trikʹō - bēʹzōr). Fitotricobezoar. SIN trichophytobezoar.

phy·tyl (fī'til). Fitil; o radical encontrado na filoquinona (vitamina K_1); um radical tetraprenila, reduzido em 3 dos 4 grupamentos prenila.

phy·tyl al·co·hol. Álcool fitílico. SIN phytol.

PI Abreviatura de Periodontal Index (Índice Periodontal).

Pi Abreviatura de inorganic *phosphate* (fosfato inorgânico).

p*I* O valor do pH para o ponto isoelétrico (isoeletric *point*) de determinada substância.

pi (π, Π) (pī). 1. Pi; a 16.ª letra do alfabeto grego. 2. (Π). Símbolo de pressão osmótica; em matemática, símbolo do produto de uma série. 3. (π). Símbolo da razão entre a circunferência de um círculo e seu diâmetro (aproximadamente 3,14159). 4. Símbolo de *pros*.

pia (pīʹă, pēʹă). Pia-máter. VER pia mater. [L. fem. de *pius*, sensível]

pia-a·rach·ni·tis (pīʹă - ă - rak - nīʹtis). Pia-aracnite. SIN leptomeningitis.

pia-a·rach·noid (pīʹă - ă - rakʹnoyd, pēʹă). Pia-aracnóide. SIN leptomeninx.

pi·al (pīʹal, pēʹal). Pial; relativo à pia-máter.

pia mat·er (pīʹă māʹter, pēʹă mahʹter) [TA]. Pia-máter; uma delicada membrana fibrosa vascularizada firmemente aderida à cápsula glial do encéfalo (parte encefálica da p.m.) e à medula espinal (parte espinal da p. m. ou membrana limitante da glia); seguindo exatamente as impressões externas do cérebro e, também, a circunferência do revestimento ependimal das membranas e plexo corióides, reveste o cerebelo, mas não de forma tão íntima como reveste o cérebro, não se aprofundando nos sulcos menores. A pia-máter e a aracnóide são coletivamente denominadas aracnóide-máter [TA], distinta da dura-máter ou paquimeninge. SIN pia. [L. mãe afetuosa, sensível]

pi·an (pē - anʹ, pīʹan). Bouba. SIN yaws.
  p. bois, forma de leishmaniose cutânea do Novo Mundo causada por *Leishmania braziliensis guyanensis* no delta do rio Amazonas; acredita-se que uma pequena fração dos casos metastatize para a mucosa nasal, com envolvimento semelhante ao da espúndia. SIN bosch yaws, bush yaws.

pi·a·rach·noid (pīʹă - rakʹnoyd). Pia-aracnóide. SIN leptomeninx.

pi·blok·to, pi·blok·tog (pib - lokʹtō). Estado dissociativo histérico, que geralmente ocorre em mulheres esquimós, no qual a pessoa grita, rasga a roupa e corre para a neve, sem que se lembre do episódio depois. [Nativo]

pi·ca (pīʹkă, pēʹkă). Pica; perversão do apetite para substâncias inadequadas como alimento ou sem valor nutricional; p. ex., barro, tinta seca, amido, gelo. [L. *pica*, pega]

Picchini. Luigi, médico italiano do final do século XIX. VER Picchini *syndrome*.

Pick, Arnold, psiquiatra tchecoslovaco, 1851–1924. VER P. *atrophy, bundle, disease*.

Pick, Friedel, médico alemão, 1867–1926. VER P. *bodies*, em *body, disease, syndrome*.

Pick, Ludwig, médico alemão, 1868–1935. VER P. *cell*; Niemann-P. *cell, disease*.

Pickles, William, clínico geral inglês, pesquisador da transmissão de infecções em comunidades isoladas, 1885–1969. VER P. *chart*.

pick·ling (pikʹling). Decapagem; em odontologia, o processo de limpeza das superfícies metálicas dos produtos de oxidação e outras impurezas por imersão em ácido.

Pickworth, Frederick A., *1889. VER Lepehne-P. *stain*.

♻ **pico-**. Pico-. 1. Forma combinante que significa pequeno. 2 (**p**). Prefixo usado no SI e no sistema métrico para designar submúltiplos de um trilionésimo (10^{-12}). SIN bicro-. [It. *piccolo*]

pi·co·gram (pg) (pīʹkō - gram, pēʹkō - gram). Picograma; um trilionésimo de um grama.

pi·co·ka·tal (pkat) (pīʹkō - katʹal; pēʹko - katʹal). Picokatal; um trilionésimo de um katal (10^{-12} katal).

pi·co·lin·ic ac·id (pik - ō - linʹik). Ácido picolínico; ácido piridina-4-carboxílico; um isômero do ácido nicotínico.

pi·co·li·nur·ic ac·id (pik - ō - li - noorʹik). Ácido picolinúrico; *N*-picolinoilglicina; a amida, com glicina, do ácido picolínico; um análogo do ácido hipúrico no qual o ácido picolínico, em vez do ácido benzóico, é conjugado com a glicina e excretado.

pi·com·e·ter (pm) (pīʹkō - mē - ter). Picômetro; um trilionésimo de um metro. SIN bicron.

pi·co·mole (pmol) (pēʹkō - mōl; pīʹkō - mōl). Picomol; um trilionésimo de um mol (10^{-12} mol).

Pi·cor·na·vir·i·dae (pi - kōr - nă - virʹi - dē). Família de vírus muito pequenos (20–30 nm), resistentes ao éter, sem envoltório, que possuem um cerne de RNA infeccioso monofilamentar de sentido positivo, encerrado em um capsídeo de simetria icosaédrica com 60 capsômeros. Muitas espécies (incluindo poliovírus, vírus coxsackie e ECHO) estão incluídas na família. Há cinco gêneros aceitos: Enterovirus, Rhinovirus, Hepatovirus, Cardiovirus e Aphthovirus. [It. *piccolo*, muito pequeno, + RNA + -viridae]

pi·cor·na·vi·rus (pi - kōr - nă - vīʹrŭs). Picornavírus; vírus da família Picornaviridae.

pic·ram·ic ac·id (pī - kramʹik). Ácido picrâmico; cristais vermelhos algumas vezes encontrados no sangue de pessoas envenenadas por ácido pícrico; os cristais são formados em virtude de redução parcial do ácido pícrico.

Pic·ras·ma (pi - krazʹmă). Quássia, pau-amargo. VER quassia. [L., do G. *pikrasmos*, amargor]

pic·rate (pikʹrāt). Picrato; um sal do ácido pícrico.

pic·ric ac·id (pikʹrik). Ácido pícrico; tem sido aplicado em queimaduras, eczema, erisipela e prurido. SIN carbazotic acid, nitroxanthic acid. [G. *pikros*, amargo]

pic·ro·car·mine (pik - rō - karʹmin, - mēn). Picrocarmim. VER picrocarmine *stain*.

pic·ro·for·mol (pikʹrō - fōrʹmol). Picroformol. VER picroformol *fixative*.

pic·ro·ni·gro·sin (pikʹrō - nīʹgrō - sin). Picronigrosina. VER picronigrosin *stain*.

pic·ro·tox·in (pikʹrō - tokʹsin). Picrotoxina; princípio neutro muito amargo, derivado do fruto da *Anamirta cocculus* (família Menispermaceae); estimulante do sistema nervoso central, usado como antídoto para envenenamento por barbitúricos e alguns outros fármacos depressores do SNC; convulsivante e antagonista do GABA amplamente usado em procedimentos experimentais que estudam mecanismos convulsivos. SIN cocculin. [G. *pikros*, amargo, + *toxicon*, veneno]

pic·ro·tox·in·in (pik-rō-tok'si-nin). Picrotoxinina; produto da decomposição da lactona; as propriedades farmacológicas assemelham-se às da picrotoxina.

pic·ryl (pik'ril). Picrilo; o radical orgânico derivado do ácido pícrico por remoção do grupamento hidroxila.

pic·to·graph (pik'tō-graf). Pictografia; tabela de exame visual para analfabetos.

PID Abreviatura de pelvic inflammatory *disease* (doença inflamatória pélvica).

Pidgin Sign English (PSE) (pij'in). Sistema de comunicação que é uma representação manual do inglês no qual são usados os sinais da Linguagem de Sinais Americana (American Sign Language) na ordem de palavras inglesa; não há sinais de inflexão, e os nomes próprios são soletrados com os dedos.

pie·bald·ism (pī'bawld-izm) [MIM*172800]. Piebaldismo; ausência segmentar da pigmentação no cabelo, produzindo um aspecto listrado; pode haver manchas de vitiligo em outras áreas devido à ausência de melanócitos; freqüentemente transmitido como uma característica autossômica dominante causada por mutação no proto-oncogene KIT em 4q, podendo estar associado a defeitos neurológicos [MIM*172850] ou alterações oculares [MIM*172870]. Cf. Waardenburg *syndrome*. SIN cutaneous albinism, piebald skin, piebaldness.

pie·bald·ness (pī'bawld-ness). Piebaldismo. SIN piebaldism.

piece (pēs). Parte, fragmento, porção.
  end p., parte terminal; uma parte do espermatozóide consistindo em um axonema circundado apenas pela membrana flagelar.
  Fab p., porção Fab. SIN Fab *fragment.*
  Fc p., porção Fc. SIN Fc *fragment.*
  middle p., parte média; parte do espermatozóide caracterizada por um axonema e por uma bainha de mitocôndrias dispostas em uma hélice apertada.
  principal p., parte principal; a principal parte do espermatozóide, que tem cerca de 45 μm de comprimento e apresenta uma bainha fibrosa característica circundando o axonema.

pie·dra (pē-ā'drä). Piedra; doença fúngica do cabelo, caracterizada pela formação de muitas massas nodulares, pequenas, firmes e céreas no fio de cabelo. VER TAMBÉM trichosporosis. [Esp. uma pedra]
  black p., p. negra; piedra que envolve o cabelo, causada por *Piedraia hortae* e caracterizada por nódulos arenosos, duros, pretos, firmemente aderidos, compostos de uma massa organizada, firmemente cimentada, de células fúngicas; o crescimento fúngico está sempre localizado acima do nível dos folículos pilosos; a doença ocorre em áreas tropicais úmidas das Américas, África e Ásia, acometendo chimpanzés e outros primatas, bem como os seres humanos.
  p. nos'tras, condição semelhante à piedra, mas que afeta os pêlos da barba.
  white p., p. branca; piedra da barba, do bigode e das áreas genitais, e também do couro cabeludo, causada por *Trichosporon beigelii* e encontrada na América do Sul, na Europa e no Japão; caracterizada por nódulos de consistência mole, mucilaginosos, de cor branca a castanho-clara, tanto dentro como em cima dos fios.

Pi·e·dra·ia (pī'ē-drī'ä). Gênero de fungos, baseado na *P. hortae*, que provavelmente é a única espécie e que causa a piedra negra. [ver piedra]

pieds ter·mi·naux (pē-e'ter-mē-nō'). Terminações axônicas. SIN axon *terminals,* em *terminal.* [Fr., pés terminais]

Pierini, Luigi, dermatologista argentino do século XX. VER *atrophoderma* of Pasini and P.

Pierre Robin. VER Robin.

pi·e·sim·e·ter, pi·e·som·e·ter (pī-ē-sim'ē-ter, pī-ē-som'ē-ter). Piezômetro; instrumento para medir a pressão de um gás ou líquido. SIN piezometer. [G. *piesis*, pressão]
  Hales p., p. de Hales; tubo de vidro introduzido em uma artéria em ângulos retos com seu eixo, sendo a pressão demonstrada pela altura de ascensão do sangue no tubo.

pi·e·sis (pī'ē-sis). Pressão sanguínea. SIN blood *pressure.* [G. pressão]

pi·e·zo·chem·is·try (pī-ē-zō-kem'is-trē). Piezoquímica; o estudo do efeito de pressões muito altas em reações químicas.

pi·e·zo·e·lec·tric (pī'ē-zō-ē-lek'trik). Piezoelétrico; piezelétrico; relativo à piezoeletricidade.

pi·e·zo·e·lec·tric·i·ty (pī'ē-zō-ē-lek-tris'i-tē). Piezoeletricidade; correntes elétricas geradas por pressão sobre determinados cristais, p. ex., quartzo, mica, calcita. [G. *piezo*, pressionar, comprimir, + electricity]

pi·e·zo·gen·ic (pī'ē-zō-jen'ik). Piezogênico; resultante de pressão. [G. *piezo*, pressionar, comprimir, + *genesis*, origem]

pi·e·zom·e·ter (pī-ē-zom'ē-ter). Piezômetro. SIN piesimeter.

pig. Transportador e protetor de seringas e frascos; recipiente, geralmente feito de chumbo, usado para proteger frascos ou seringas contendo material radioativo. [jargão]

pig·bel. Um tipo de enterite necrotizante endêmica nas regiões montanhosas da Papua Nova Guiné, causado pela toxina B do *Clostridium perfringens* tipo C; ocorre predominantemente em crianças devido à baixa imunidade contra a toxina B e a um baixo nível de proteases intestinais resultantes de uma dieta pobre em proteínas e rica em batatas-doces.

pig·ment. Pigmento. **1.** Qualquer substância corante, como as hemácias, do cabelo, da íris, etc., ou os corantes usados em trabalhos histológicos ou bacteriológicos, ou em pinturas. **2.** Preparação medicinal para uso externo, aplicada à pele, como tinta ou agentes corantes usados em tintas. [L. *pigmentum*, tinta]
  bile p.'s, pigmentos biliares; substância corante na bile derivada das porfirinas por ruptura de uma ponte metano; p. ex., bilirrubina, biliverdina.
  chymotropic p., p. quimiotrópico; p. dissolvido no vacúolo de uma célula vegetal. [G. *chymos*, suco, + *tropē*, volta, inclinação, + -ic]
  formalin p., p. de formol; p. formado quando soluções aquosas ácidas de formaldeído atuam sobre tecidos ricos em sangue; caracterizado por rotação do plano de luz polarizada, resistindo à extração em solventes aquosos e lipídicos, sendo alvejado em ácidos e peróxido de hidrogênio; não é formado quando o tecido é fixado com formaldeído tamponado em níveis de pH acima de 6.
  hematogenous p., p. hematogênico; p. derivado da hemoglobina das hemácias.
  hepatogenous p., p. hepatogênico; p. biliar derivado da destruição da hemoglobina no fígado.
  malarial p., p. malárico; p. granular castanho-escuro que roda o plano de luz polarizada e tem outras propriedades semelhantes às do pigmento de formol; encontrado em parasitas, como o *Plasmodium malariae*, ao redor dos capilares encefálicos, e em macrófagos fixos do baço, fígado, medula óssea e linfonodos; composto de proteína em excesso, uma ferro-porfirina e hematina deixadas do metabolismo da hemoglobina pelo parasita malárico na hemácia. VER malarial pigment *stain.*
  melanotic p., melanina. SIN melanin.
  natural p., p. natural; substância colorida natural; absorve a luz na faixa visível do espectro eletromagnético. Cf. structural *color.* SIN biochrome.
  respiratory p.'s, pigmentos respiratórios; as substâncias transportadoras de oxigênio (coloridas) no sangue e nos tecidos (hemoglobina, mioglobina, hemocianina, etc.)
  visual p.'s, pigmentos visuais; os fotopigmentos nos cones e bastonetes da retina que absorvem luz e iniciam o processo visual.
  wear-and-tear p., p. de desgaste; p. de envelhecimento; lipofuscina que se acumula em células em envelhecimento ou atróficas na forma de um resíduo de digestão lisossômica.

pig·men·tary (pig'men-tār-ē). Pigmentar; relativo a um pigmento.

pig·men·ta·tion (pig-men-tā'shun). Pigmentação; coloração, seja normal ou patológica, da pele ou tecidos resultante de um depósito de pigmento.
  arsenic p., p. arsenical; aumento generalizado, mas irregular, da pigmentação cutânea por melanina no envenenamento crônico por arsênico.
  exogenous p., p. exógena; coloração da pele ou dos tecidos por um pigmento introduzido de fora.

pig·ment·ed (pig'men-ted). Pigmentado; colorido em virtude de um depósito de pigmento.

pig·men·to·ly·sin (pig-men-tol'i-sin). Pigmentolisina; anticorpo que causa destruição de pigmento. [L. *pigmentum*, pigmento, + G. *lysis*, afrouxamento]

pig·men·tum ni·grum (pig-men'tum nī'grum). Pigmento negro; melanina da corióide do olho.

pig·my (pig'mē). Pigmeu. SIN pygmy.

Pignet, Maurice-C.J., cirurgião francês, *1871. VER P. *formula.*

pi·lar, pi·la·ry (pī'lar, pil'ä-rē). Piloso. SIN hairy. [L. *pilus*, pêlo]

pile (pīl). **1.** Pilha; uma série de placas de dois metais diferentes impostas alternadamente uma sobre a outra, separadas por uma lâmina de material umedecido com uma solução ácida diluída, usada para produzir uma corrente elétrica. [L. *pīla*, pilar.] **2.** Um tumor hemorroidário individual. VER hemorrhoids. [L. *pīla*, bola]
  sentinel p., espessamento circunscrito da mucosa na extremidade inferior de uma fissura do ânus.
  thermoelectric p., pilha termoelétrica. SIN thermopile.

piles (pīlz). Hemorróidas. SIN hemorrhoids. [L. *pila*, bola]

pi·le·us (pī'lē-us). Omento maior. SIN greater *omentum.* [L. *pileum* ou *pileus*, um capuz de feltro]

pi·li (pī'lī). Pêlos; plural de pilus. [L.]

pi·li·mic·tion (pī-li-mik'shun). Pilimicção; eliminação de pêlos na urina, como em casos de tumores desmóides, ou de filamentos de muco na urina. [L. *pilus*, pêlo, + *mictio*, micção]

pil·in (pi'lin). Pilina; o componente proteico dos apêndices adesivos bacterianos que ajudam a bactéria a aderir às superfícies de um tecido ou recipiente, freqüentemente as glicoproteínas na superfície das células eucarióticas. [pilus 2, + -in]

pill. Pílula. **1.** Pequena massa globular de alguma substância coesa, mas solúvel, contendo uma substância medicinal a ser engolida. VER TAMBÉM tablet. **2.** A Pílula; termo coloquial para contraceptivos orais. [L. *pilula*; dim. de *pila*, bola]
  bread p., p. de pão; placebo feito de miolo de pão ou de outras substâncias inativas.
  morning after p., p. da manhã seguinte; medicamento oral que, quando tomado por uma mulher nas 48 a 72 horas após a relação sexual, reduz a probabilidade de gravidez. SIN emergency hormonal contraception.

Geralmente, o termo refere-se a contraceptivos orais (pílulas anticoncepcionais) tomados por um curto período em dose maior que a habitual. O uso de contraceptivos orais foi aprovado pelo órgão norte-americano *Food and Drug Administration* como forma de "contracepção de emergência" após estupro ou relação sexual não planejada e sem proteção, mas não como forma regular de evitar a gravidez. O protocolo de Yupze consiste em uma combinação de progestogênio (0,25 mg de levonorgestrel ou 0,5 mg de norgestrel) e estrogênio (0,05 mg de etinilestradiol) tomados juntos e repetidos em 12 horas. Dependendo do produto usado, esse protocolo exige o uso de 2–4 comprimidos de um contraceptivo oral padrão. A primeira dose deve ser tomada de preferência 24 horas após a relação sexual, e não mais de 72 horas depois. O método reduz a probabilidade de gravidez em aproximadamente 75%. Cerca de 50% das mulheres apresentam sangramento uterino dentro de 1 semana, e a maioria das outras em 3 semanas, exceto se houve concepção. Se forem tomados suficientemente cedo, os hormônios impediriam a fertilização por alterarem a função tubária ou serem tóxicos para o óvulo. Provavelmente, entretanto, eles geralmente atuam impedindo a implantação de um óvulo fertilizado. Nessa dosagem hormonal, a incidência de náuseas é de aproximadamente 50% e de vômitos, de aproximadamente 20%; também pode haver cefaléia, retenção hídrica e dor à palpação da mama. (Foi descrito que o levonorgestrel administrado isoladamente causa menos náuseas que em associação e produz proteção comparável ou melhor contra gravidez.) Esse procedimento é contra-indicado em mulheres para as quais os contraceptivos orais são contra-indicados, como aquelas com hipertensão ou história pregressa de acidente vascular cerebral ou doença tromboembólica. O breve curso de hormônios em doses altas provavelmente não interrompe uma gravidez após a implantação, e não há evidências de danos fetais quando tal gravidez continua até o termo. Entretanto, o uso de hormônios é contra-indicado na gravidez conhecida ou se a mulher manteve relações sexuais sem proteção nos 3–10 dias anteriores.

pep. p.'s, estimulante; bolinha; designação coloquial de comprimidos contendo um estimulante do sistema nervoso central, principalmente anfetamina.

pil·lar (pil'ăr). Pilar; estrutura ou parte semelhante a uma coluna ou pilar. [L. *pila*]

anterior p. of fauces, arco palatoglosso; *termo oficial alternativo para palatoglossal *arch*.

anterior p. of fornix, coluna do fórnice. SIN *column* of fornix.

Corti p.'s, pilares de Corti. SIN *pillar cells*, em *cell*.

p.'s of fauces, arcos das fauces. VER palatoglossal *arch*, palatopharyngeal *arch*.

p.'s of fornix, a coluna do fórnice [TA] e o pilar do fórnice [TA].

p. of iris, retículo trabecular da íris. SIN *trabecular tissue* of *sclera*.

posterior p. of fauces, arco palatofaríngeo; *termo oficial alternativo para palatopharyngeal *arch*.

posterior p. of fornix, pilar do fórnice. SIN *crus fornicis*.

pil·let (pil'et). Uma pílula pequena.

pill mass. Massa pilular. SIN *pilular mass*.

pill-roll·ing (pil'rōl'ing). Enrolamento de pílula; movimento circular das extremidades opostas do polegar e do indicador que aparece como uma forma de tremor na paralisia agitante.

⚠ **pilo-.** Pilo-; pêlo. [L. *pilus*]

pi·lo·car·pine (pī-lō-kar'pēn). Pilocarpina; alcalóide obtido das folhas do *Pilocarpus; Microphyllus* ou *P. jaborandi* (família Rutaceae), arbustos das Índias Ocidentais e da região tropical da América; agente parassimpaticomimético usado como diaforético, sialagogo e estimulante da motilidade intestinal, e, externamente, como miótico e no tratamento do glaucoma; usado na forma de cloridrato e sais nitrato. [G. *pilos*, um chapéu de feltro, + *karpos*, fruta]

pi·lo·car·pus (pil'ō-kar-pŭs). Pilocarpo; gênero de árvores e arbustos encontrados na América Central e na América do Sul e nas Índias Ocidentais. Constitui a origem botânica da pilocarpina, um alcalóide que ativa receptores muscarínicos colinérgicos. A pilocarpina é usada no tratamento do glaucoma, no qual é instilada nos olhos. Sudorífico; miótico. SIN Jaborandi.

pi·lo·cys·tic (pī'lō-sis'tik). Pilocístico; designa um cisto dermóide que contém pêlos. [pilo- + G. *kystis*, bexiga]

pi·lo·e·rec·tion (pī'lō-ē-rek'shŭn). Piloereção; ereção dos pêlos devido à ação dos músculos eretores dos pêlos.

pi·loid (pī'loyd). Semelhante a pêlo. [pilo- + G. *eidos*, semelhança]

pi·lo·ma·trix·o·ma (pī'lō-mă-trik-sō'mă). Pilomatrixoma; tumor benigno do folículo piloso solitário, freqüentemente surgindo na segunda infância, que contém células semelhantes às do carcinoma de células basais e áreas de necrose epitelial, formando células-fantasma eosinofílicas com calcificação variável e reação de células gigantes do tipo corpo estranho no estroma fibroso. SIN Malherbe calcifying epithelioma. [pilo- + matrix + G. *-oma*, tumor]

pi·lo·mo·tor (pī'lō-mō'ter). Pilomotor; que move o pêlo; designa os músculos eretores dos pêlos da pele e as fibras nervosas simpáticas pós-ganglionares que inervam esses pequenos músculos lisos. [pilo- + L. *motor*, motor]

pi·lo·ni·dal (pī-lō-nī'dăl). Pilonidal; designa a presença de pêlos em um cisto dermóide ou em um seio que se abre na pele. [pilo- + L. *nidus*, ninho]

pi·lose (pī'lōs). Piloso. SIN hairy. [L. *pilosus*]

pi·lo·se·ba·ceous (pī'lō-sē-bā'shŭs). Pilossebáceo; relativo aos folículos pilosos e às glândulas sebáceas. [pilo- + L. *sebum*, sebo]

pi·lo·sis (pī-lō'sis). Pilose. SIN hirsutism. [pilo- + G. *-osis*, condição]

Piltz, Jan, neurologista polonês, 1870–1931. VER P. *sign*; Westphal-P. *phenomenon*.

pil·u·la, gen. e pl. **pil·u·lae** (pil'ū-lă, -lē). Pílula. [L. dim. de *pila*, uma bola]

pil·u·lar (pil'ū-lar). Pilular; relativo a uma pílula.

pil·ule (pil'ūl). Uma pílula pequena. [L. *pilula*]

pi·lus, pl. **pi·li** (pī'lŭs, pī'lī) [TA]. Pêlo. SIN hair (1). **2.** Um apêndice filamentoso fino, algo análogo ao flagelo, presente em algumas bactérias. Os pili consistem apenas em proteínas e são mais curtos, mais retos e muito mais numerosos, podendo ser quimicamente semelhantes aos flagelos; pili especializados (pili F, pili I e outros pili de conjugação) parecem mediar a conjugação bacteriana. SIN fimbria (2). VER TAMBÉM conjugative *plasmid*. [L.]

pi'li annula'ti, cabelo com anéis. SIN ringed *hair*.

F pili, pili F. VER pilus (2).

F p., estrutura responsável pela fixação de bactérias masculinas (F⁺) a femininas (F⁻) individuais, formando pares conjugados.

I pili, pili I. VER pilus (2).

pi'li multigem'ini, a presença de vários pêlos em um único folículo.

R pili, pili R; pili especializados encontrados em células bacterianas, semelhantes aos pili F e associados aos plasmídeos R.

pi'li tor'ti, condição na qual muitos fios de cabelo são torcidos no eixo longitudinal, podendo ser congênita ou adquirida em virtude de distorção dos folículos por um processo inflamatório fibrosante, estresse mecânico ou alopecia cicatrizante; as hastes dos pêlos assemelham-se a lantejoulas na luz refletida, são quebradiças e quebram-se em comprimentos variáveis, com muitas áreas parecendo calvas com um restolho escuro; como um defeito congênito, pode manifestar-se em síndromes tais como Bjornstad, Crandall e Menkes. SIN twisted hairs.

pi·mar·i·cin (pi-mar'i-sin). Pimaricina; antibiótico antifúngico para uso tópico, produzido pelo *Streptomyces natalensis*; efetiva contra os gêneros *Aspergillus, Candida* e *Mucor*. SIN natamycin.

pi·mel·ic ac·id (pī-mel'ik). Ácido pimélico; ácido heptanedióico; um intermediário na oxidação do ácido oleico em alguns microrganismos; um precursor da biotina.

⚠ **pimelo-.** Pimelo-; gordura, gorduroso. [G. *pimelē*, gordura flácida, banha de porco, de *piar*, gordura]

pim·e·lor·rhea (pim'ē-lō-rē'ă). Pimelorréia. SIN fatty *diarrhea*. [pimelo- + G. *rhoia*, um fluxo]

pim·e·lor·thop·nea (pim'ē-lōr-thop'nē-ă, -nē'ă). Pimelortopnéia; ortopnéia; dificuldade respiratória em qualquer posição, exceto a ortostática, devido à obesidade. SIN piorthopnea. [pimelo- + G. *orthos*, reto, + *pnoē*, respiração]

pi·men·ta, pi·men·to (pi-men'tă, -tō). Pimenta; o fruto seco da *Pimenta officinalis* (família Myrtaceae), uma árvore nativa da Jamaica e de outras partes da América tropical, usado como carminativo e condimento aromático; o óleo de pimenta representa 3 a 4% do fruto seco. [Esp. do L. *pigmentum*, tinta [L. mediev. tempero]

p. oil, óleo de pimenta; representa 3–4,5% do fruto seco. SIN allspice oil.

pim·o·zide (pim'ō-zīd). Pimozida; um antipsicótico tranqüilizante.

pim·ple (pim'pl). Uma pápula ou pequena pústula; geralmente designa uma lesão inflamatória da acne.

PIN Abreviatura de prostatic intraepithelial *neoplasia* (neoplasia intra-epitelial prostática).

pin. Pino; implante metálico usado no tratamento cirúrgico de fraturas ósseas. VER TAMBÉM nail. [I. ant. *pinn*, do L. *pinna*, pena]

Steinmann p., p. de Steinmann; pino usado para transfixar o osso para tração ou fixação.

pin·a·cy·a·nol (pin-ă-sī'ă-nol) [antigo I.C. 808]. Pinacianol; corante básico, usado como sensibilizador para cor (vermelho-violeta na água, azul no álcool) em fotografia e para coloração vital dos leucócitos.

Pinard, Adolphe, obstetra francês, 1844–1934. VER P. *maneuver*.

pince·ment (pans-mon'). Pinçamento; manipulação por pinçamento na massagem. [Fr. pinçamento]

ℹ **pinch.** Pinçar; preensão entre dedos das mãos nas articulações mais distais (técnica usada em terapia ocupacional).

Pindborg, Jens J., patologista oral dinamarquês, 1921–1995. VER P. *tumor*.

pin·do·lol (pin'dō-lol). Pindolol; um bloqueador β-adrenérgico usado no tratamento da hipertensão; também possui atividade simpaticomimética intrínseca.

pine (pīn). Pinheiro; árvore conífera perene do gênero *Pinus* (família Pinaceae), do qual várias espécies fornecem alcatrão, terebentina, resina e óleos voláteis. [L. *pinus*, pinheiro]

p.-needle oil, óleo de agulha de pinho; óleo volátil destilado com vapor da folha fresca do *Pinus mugo*; foi usado por inalação e *spray* em afecções catarrais das

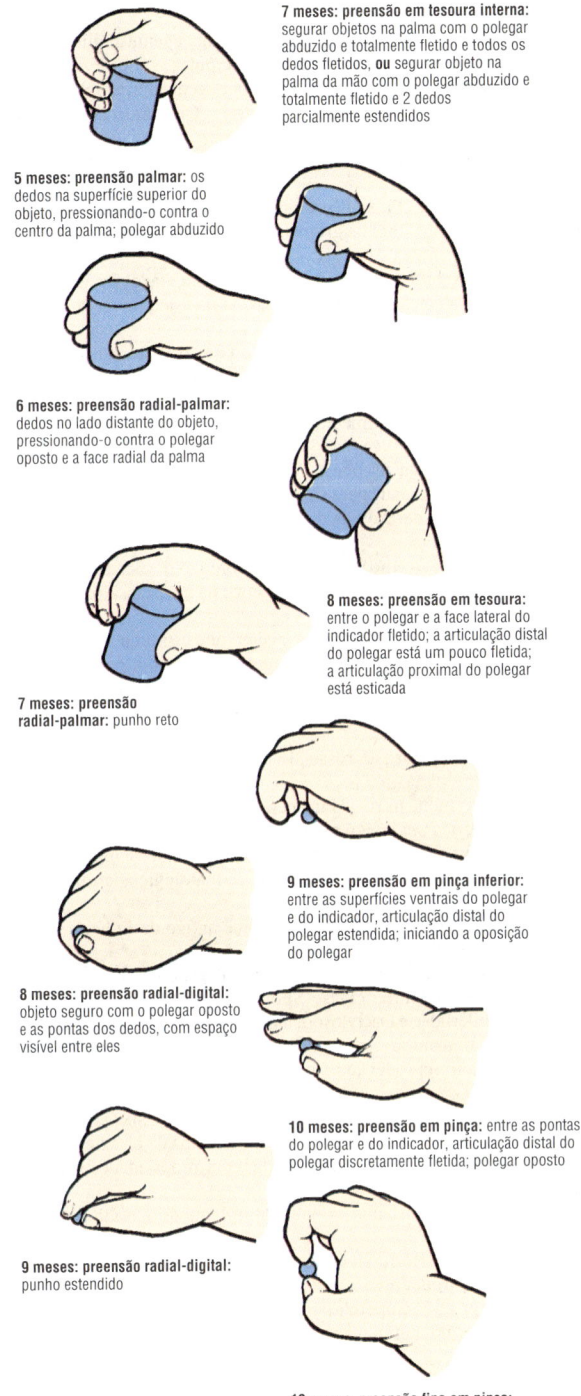

padrões de pinçamento e preensão

vias aéreas, bem como localmente no reumatismo; também usado como flavorizante e em perfumaria.
 p. oil, óleo de pinho; o óleo volátil da madeira de *Pinus palustris* e outras espécies de *Pinus*; usado como desodorante e desinfetante.
 p. tar, alcatrão de pinheiro; obtido pela destilação destrutiva da madeira do *Pinus palustris* e de outras espécies de *Pinus*; prescrito internamente como expectorante e externamente para doenças cutâneas. SIN liquid pitch.
 white p., p. branco; a casca interna seca do *Pinus strobus*, usado como ingrediente em xaropes para tosse.
pin·e·al (pĭn′ē-ăl). Pineal. **1.** Que tem o formato de uma pinha. SIN piniform. **2.** Relativo à glândula pineal. [L. *pineus*, relativo a pinha, *pinus*]
pin·e·al·ec·to·my (pĭn′ē-ă-lĕk-tō′mē). Pinealectomia; remoção da glândula pineal. [pineal + G. *ektomē*, excisão]

pin·e·a·lo·cyte (pĭn-ē′ăl-ō-sīt). Pinealócito; uma célula da glândula pineal com longos prolongamentos que terminam em expansões bulbosas. Os pinealócitos recebem inervação direta de neurônios simpáticos que formam sinapses reconhecíveis. As terminações claviformes dos prolongamentos do pinealócito terminam nos espaços perivasculares que circundam os capilares. SIN chief cell of corpus pineale, parenchymatous cell of corpus pineale. [pineal + G. *kytos*, célula]
pin·e·a·lo·ma (pĭn′ē-ă-lō′mă). Pinealoma; termo que foi variavelmente usado para designar tumores das células germinativas, pineocitomas e pineoblastomas da glândula pineal. [pineal + G. *-oma*, tumor]
 ectopic p., p. ectópico; termo obsoleto para uma neoplasia indiferenciada semelhante a um pinealoma, geralmente encontrada próximo da hipófise; considerado por alguns um teratoma indiferenciado.
 extrapineal p., p. extrapineal; termo obsoleto para pinealoma ectópico.
pin·e·a·lop·a·thy (pĭn′ē-ă-lŏp′ă-thē). Pinealopatia; doença da glândula pineal. [pineal + G. *pathos*, doença]
pine·ap·ple (pīn′ăp-ĕl). Abacaxi; o fruto do *Ananas sativa* ou *Bromelia ananas* (família Bromeliaceae); contém uma enzima proteolítica e que coagula o leite, a bromelina.
Pinel, Philippe, psiquiatra francês, 1745–1826. VER P. *system*.
pin·e·o·blas·to·ma (pĭn′ē-ō-blăs-tō′mă). Pineoblastoma; tumor mal diferenciado da glândula pineal, mais freqüente nas primeiras três décadas de vida, que consiste em pequenas células com citoplasma escasso e freqüentemente formando pseudo-rosetas; histologicamente, assemelha-se a um meduloblastoma; um tipo de tumor primitivo do neuroectoderma. [pineal + G. *blastos*, germe, + *-oma*, tumor]
pin·e·o·cy·to·ma (pĭn′ē-ō-cī′tō′mă). Pineocitoma; tumor originado na glândula pineal que se assemelha ao parênquima pineal normal.
ping-pong (pĭng′pŏng). Pingue-pongue. VER ping-pong *mechanism*. [Ping-Pong, marca registrada do tênis de mesa]
pin·guec·u·la, pin·guic·u·la (pĭng-gwĕk′ū-lă, pĭng-gwĭk′ū-lă). Pinguécula; acúmulo amarelado de tecido conjuntivo que espessa a conjuntiva; ocorre em idosos. [L. *pinguiculus*, gorduroso, de *pinguis*, gordura]
pin·i·form (pĭn′ĭ-fōrm, pī′nĭ-). Piniforme. SIN pineal (1). [L. *pinus*, pinha, + *forma*, forma]
pink·eye (pĭnk′ī). Conjuntivite contagiosa aguda. SIN acute contagious *conjunctivitis*.
pin·ledge (pĭn′lĕdj). Restauração dental metálica ou técnica que emprega pinos paralelos como parte do modelo para aumentar a retenção da restauração.
pin·na, pl. **pin·nae** (pĭn′ă, pĭn′ē). **1.** Orelha. SIN auricle (1). **2.** Uma pena, asa ou barbatana. [L. *pinna* ou *penna*, pena, no pl. asa]
 p. na′si, asa do nariz. SIN ala of nose.
pin·nal (pĭn′ăl). Relativo à orelha.
pin·ni·ped (pĭn′ĭ-pĕd). Pinípede; membro da subordem Pinnipedia, mamíferos carnívoros aquáticos com os quatro membros modificados em nadadeiras (p. ex., foca, morsa). [L. *pinna*, pena (asa) + *pes* (*ped*-), pé]
pin·o·cyte (pĭn′ō-sīt, pī′nō-). Pinócito; célula que exibe pinocitose. [G. *pineō*, beber, + *kytos*, célula]
pin·o·cy·to·sis (pĭn′ō-sī-tō′sĭs, pī′nō-). Pinocitose; o processo celular de engolfar líquido ativamente, um fenômeno no qual se formam diminutas invaginações na superfície da membrana celular, que se fecham para formar vesículas cheias de líquido; assemelha-se à fagocitose. [pinocyte + G. *-osis*, condição]
pin·o·some (pĭn′ō-sōm, pī′nō-). Pinossoma; vacúolo cheio de líquido formado por pinocitose. [G. *pineō*, beber, + *sōma*, corpo]
Pins, Emil, médico austríaco, 1845–1913. VER P. *sign*, *syndrome*.
pint (pīnt). Pinta; medida de quantidade líquida norte-americana que contém 16 onças líquidas, 28,875 polegadas cúbicas; 473,1765 cm³. Uma pinta imperial contém 20 onças britânicas, 34,67743 polegadas cúbicas; 568,2615 cm³.
pin·ta (pĭn′tă, pēn′tă). Pinta; doença causada por um espiroqueta, *Treponema carateum*, endêmica no México e na América Central, é caracterizada por uma pequena pápula primária seguida por uma placa crescente e máculas secundárias disseminadas de cor variável, denominadas píntides, que acabam tornando-se brancas. VER TAMBÉM nonvenereal *syphilis*. SIN azul, carate, mal del pinto. [Esp. pintado]
pin·tids; Píntides; lesões semelhantes a placas na fase secundária da pinta; as lesões, que variam em cor (hipocrômicas, hipercrômicas e eritematoescamosas), resultam em despigmentação. [pinta + -id(1)]
pi·nus (pī′nŭs). Glândula pineal. SIN pineal *body*. [L. pinheiro]
pin·worm (pĭn′wĕrm). Oxiúro; membro do gênero *Enterobius* ou gêneros correlatos de nematódeos na família Oxyuridae, abundante em uma grande variedade de vertebrados, incluindo espécies como *Oxyuris equi* (o oxiúro eqüino), *Enterobius vermicularis* (o oxiúro humano), os gêneros *Syphacia* e *Aspiculuris* (o oxiúro do camundongo), *Passalurus ambiguus* (o oxiúro do coelho) e *Syphacia muris* (o oxiúro do rato). SIN seatworm.
Pi·oph·i·la ca·sei (pī-ŏf′ĭ-lă kā′sē-ī). A mosca do queijo, uma espécie de insetos muscóides cujos ovos são depositados sobre o queijo, carnes curadas e outros alimentos expostos, e assim são ingeridos, algumas vezes causando

miíase intestinal temporária, com diarréia, cólica e vômitos. [l., do G. *piôn*, gordura, + *philos*, amigo; L. *caseus*, queijo]

pi·or·thop·nea (pi-or-thop'ne-, -ne'a). Piortopnéia. SIN pimelorthopnea. [G. *piôn*, gordura, + *orthos*, reto, + *pnoe*, respiração]

PIP$_2$ Abreviatura de *phosphatidylinositol* 4,5-bisphosphate (fosfatidilinositol 4,5-bisfosfato).

pi·pam·a·zine (pi-pam'a-zen). Pipamazina; análogo da fenotiazina com propriedades antieméticas e tranqüilizantes.

pi·pam·per·one (pi-pam'per-on). Pipamperona; tranqüilizante antipsicótico.

pi·paz·e·thate (pi-paz'e-that). Pipazetato; agente antitussígeno.

pip·e·co·lic ac·id (pip'e-ko'lik, -kol'ik). Ácido pipecólico; diidrobaiquianina; ácido 2-piperidinocarboxílico; ácido picolínico saturado; os L-isômeros dos ácidos Δ^1- e Δ^6-desidroepicólico são intermediários no catabolismo da L-lisina; o ácido pipecólico acumula-se em distúrbios dos peroxissomas. SIN homoproline, pipecolinic acid.

pip·e·co·lin·ic ac·id (pip-e-ko-lin'ik, -kol'i-nik). Ácido pipecolínico. SIN pipecolic acid.

pip·e·cur·o·ni·um (pip'e-kur-o'ne-um). Pipecurônio; relaxante muscular esteróide não-despolarizante, estruturalmente relacionado ao pancurônio e caracterizado por ação prolongada.

pip·e·cu·ron·i·um bro·mide (pi-pe-kur-o'ne-um bro'mid). Brometo de pipecurônio; bloqueador neuromuscular com propriedades não-despolarizantes, portanto semelhante à D-tubocurarina, mas com ação paralítica mais breve.

pip·pen·zo·late meth·yl·bro·mide (pi-pen'zo-lat). Metilbrometo de pipenzolato; fármaco anticolinérgico.

Piper, E.B., ginecologista-obstetra norte-americano, 1881–1935. VER P. *forceps*.

pip·er (pi'per). Pimenta negra; o fruto verde e seco da *Piper nigrum* (família Piperaceae), uma planta trepadeira da Índia Oriental; usada como condimento, diaforético, estimulante e carminativo, e localmente como contra-irritante. [L. pimenta]

pi·per·a·cil·lin so·di·um (pi-per'a-sil'in). Piperacilina sódica; penicilina semi-sintética, de amplo espectro, ativa contra várias bactérias Gram-positivas e Gram-negativas.

pi·per·a·zine (pi-per'a-zen, -zin). Piperazina; seu uso antigamente no tratamento da gota baseava-se em sua propriedade de dissolver o ácido úrico *in vitro*, mas não aumenta efetivamente a excreção de ácido úrico; seus compostos agora são usados como anti-helmínticos na oxiuríase e na ascaridíase. SIN diethylenediamine.

p. adipate, adipato de p.; anti-helmíntico e filaricida veterinário.

p. calcium edetate, edetato cálcico de p.; um anti-helmíntico.

p. citrate, citrato de p.; vermífugo para oxiúros e nematódeos.

p. estrone sulfate, sulfato de estrona de p.; preparação purificada de sulfato de estrona natural; a piperazina atua como tampão para aumentar a estabilidade do sulfato de estrona.

p. tartrate, tartarato de p., anti-helmíntico útil no tratamento da infestação por nematódeos.

pi·per·a·zine di·eth·ane·sul·fon·ic ac·id (PIPES). Ácido dietanossulfônico de piperazina; um dos vários ácidos aminossulfônicos (como os HEPES) usados em tampões biológicos; faixa de atividade, 6,0–8,5.

pi·per·i·dine (pi'per-i-den). Piperidina. **1.** Hexaidropiridina; composto do qual são derivados antipsicóticos fenotiazínicos, como o cloridrato de tioridazina e besilato de mesoridazina. **2.** Pertencente a uma classe de alcalóides que contém uma porção piperidina (1).

pi·per·i·do·late hy·dro·chlo·ride (pi-per'i-do-lat). Cloridrato de piperidolato; agente anticolinérgico.

pi·per·o·caine hy·dro·chlo·ride (pip'er-o-kan, pi'per-). Cloridrato de piperocaína; anestésico local de ação rápida para infiltração e bloqueios de nervos.

pi·per·ox·an hy·dro·chlo·ride (pip-er-ok'san). Cloridrato de piperoxano; adrenérgico (agente bloqueador de α-receptor da série de Fourneau dos benzodioxanos); usado como teste diagnóstico para feocromocitoma. SIN Fourneau 933.

PIPES Abreviatura de piperazine diethanesulfonic acid (ácido dietanossulfônico de piperazina).

pi·pette, pi·pet (pi-pet', pi-pet'). Pipeta; tubo graduado (com marcação em mL) usado para transportar um volume definido de um gás ou líquido em laboratórios. [Fr. dim. de *pipe*, pipa]

blowout p., pipeta calibrada para liberar seu valor nominal, permitindo primeiro a drenagem e, depois, soprando a última gota presa na ponta.

graduated p., p. graduada; pipeta com um tubo simples, estreito, alongado até uma ponta e graduado uniformemente ao longo de seu comprimento. As marcas de calibração podem ser limitadas à haste (p. de Mohr) ou estender-se até a extremidade (p. sorológica).

Mohr p., p. de Mohr. VER graduated p.

Pasteur p., p. de Pasteur; tubo de vidro, com tampão de algodão, que se estende até uma ponta fina, usado para a transferência estéril de pequenos volumes de líquido.

serologic p., p. sorológica. VER graduated p.

pip·o·bro·man (pip-o-bro'man). Pipobromano; agente alquilante usado na policitemia vera e na leucemia granulocítica crônica.

pi·po·sul·fan (pi-po-sul'fan). Pipossulfano; agente antineoplásico.

pi·pra·drol hy·dro·chlo·ride (pip'ra-drol). Cloridrato de pipradrol; um estimulante do sistema nervoso central.

pi·prin·hy·dri·nate (pip-rin-hi'dri-nat). Piprinidrinato; anti-histamínico e antiemético.

pip·syl (Ips) (pip'sil). Pipsila; *p*-iodofenilsulfonil, o radical do cloreto de pipsila que se combina com os grupamentos amino de aminoácidos e proteínas.

pir·bu·ter·ol (pir-bu'ter-ol). Pirbuterol; broncodilatador β_2-adrenérgico seletivo usado no tratamento do broncoespasmo na asma ou na doença pulmonar obstrutiva crônica.

Pi·re·nel·la (pir-e-nel'a). Gênero de caramujos operculados da água marinha e salobra (prosobrânquios). *P. conica* é o hospedeiro intermediário do *Heterophyes heterophyes*, o trematódeo de peixes que parasita seres humanos e aves e mamíferos que se alimentam de peixes na costa do Mediterrâneo e do Mar Vermelho.

pi·ren·zep·ine (pi-ren'ze-pen). Pirenzepina; agente anticolinérgico que exibe relativa especificidade para supressão da secreção gástrica de ácido clorídrico; relativamente desprovida de efeitos colaterais anticolinérgicos; usada no tratamento da úlcera.

pi·ret·a·nide (pi-ret'a-nid). Piretanida; diurético de alça semelhante à bumetanida e à furosemida; usado como diurético na hipertensão e na insuficiência cardíaca congestiva.

pi·rib·ed·il (pi-rib'e-dil). Piribedil; agente que estimula receptores da dopamina no encéfalo e também exerce efeito vasodilatador periférico.

Pirie, George A., radiologista escocês, 1864–1929. VER P. *bone*.

pir·i·form (pir'i-form, pi're-). Piriforme; em forma de pêra. SIN pyriform. [L. *pirum*, pra, + *forma*, forma]

Pirogoff, Nikolai I., cirurgião russo, 1810–1881. VER P. *amputation, angle, triangle*.

pir·o·men (pir'o-men, pi'ro-). Piromena; extrato estéril, não-proteico, não-anafilactogênico, de *Pseudomonas aeruginosa* e *Proteus vulgaris*. Os componentes ativos são polissacarídeos bacterianos de baixa toxicidade; usado no tratamento de alguns distúrbios alérgicos, dermatológicos e oftálmicos. SIN pyromen.

Pi·ro·plas·ma (pir'o-plaz'ma, pi'ro-). Nome antigo da *Babesia*. [L. *pirum*, pêra, + G. *plasma*, algo formado]

Pi·ro·plas·mi·da (pi'ro-plaz-mi'da). Ordem de protozoários esporozoários (subclasse Piroplasmia, classe Sporozoea) que consiste nas famílias Habesiidae, Theileriidae e Dactylosomatidae; inclui hemoparasitas heteroxenos de vertebrados, transmitidos por carrapatos, com complexo apical reduzido, sem esporos, e com reprodução assexuada por divisão binária ou esquizogonia.

pir·o·plas·mo·sis (pir'o-plas-mo'sis). Piroplasmose. SIN babesiosis.

pir·ox·i·cam ol·a·mine (pir-oks'i-kam). Olamina de piroxicam; antiinflamatório não-esteróide de ação prolongada, com propriedades analgésicas e antipiréticas.

pir·pro·fen (pir-pro'fen). Pirprofeno; antiinflamatório usado no tratamento da artrite reumatóide.

Pirquet von Cesenatico, Clemens P., médico austríaco, 1874–1929. VER Pirquet *reaction*; Pirquet *test*.

Pis·ces (pis'ez, pi'sez). Superclasse de vertebrados, geralmente conhecidos como peixes; o termo algumas vezes é limitado aos peixes ósseos. [L. pl. de *piscis*, um peixe]

pis·i·form (pis'i-form). [TA]. Pisiforme; do tamanho ou da forma da ervilha. [L. *pisum*, ervilha, + *forma*, aparência]

pit. 1. Depressão; fóvea. SIN fovea. **2.** Uma das cicatrizes deprimidas, do tamanho de uma cabeça de alfinete, que sucedem a pústula da acne, da varicela ou da varíola (marca de bexiga). **3.** Fóssula; depressão pontiaguda na superfície do esmalte de um dente, causada por calcificação deficiente ou incompleta ou formada no ponto de confluência de dois ou mais lobos de esmalte. **4.** Cacifo; indentar, como por pressão do dedo da mão sobre a pele edemaciada; apresentar cacifo, diz-se dos tecidos edemaciados quando é aplicada compressão com a ponta do dedo.

anal p., proctódio. SIN proctodeum (1).

articular p. of head of radius, fóvea articular da cabeça do rádio. SIN articular facet of radial head.

p. of atlas for dens, fóvea do dente. SIN facet (of atlas) for dens.

auditory p.'s, depressões auditivas. SIN otic p.'s.

buccal p., fóssula vestibular; depressão estrutural encontrada no esmalte bucal dos molares.

central p., fóvea central. SIN central retinal fovea.

coated p., depressão revestida; depressões especializadas na superfície celular envolvidas na endocitose mediada por receptor; a camada proteinácea visível na face citossólica da depressão confere o aspecto de revestimento.

commisural p.'s, depressões comissurais; semelhantes às depressões labiais, mas são encontradas nas comissuras dos lábios.

costal p. of transverse process, face costal do processo transverso. SIN transverse costal *facet*.

gastric p. [TA], fovéola gástrica; uma das muitas pequenas depressões na mucosa gástrica que são as aberturas das glândulas gástricas. SIN foveola gastrica [TA].

granular p.'s, fovéolas granulares. SIN granular *foveolae*, em *foveola*.

p. of head of femur, fóvea da cabeça do fêmur. SIN *fovea* for ligament of head of femur.

inferior articular p. of atlas, face articular inferior do atlas. SIN inferior articular *surface* of atlas.

inferior costal p., face costal inferior. SIN inferior costal *facet*.

iris p.'s, depressões da íris; colobomas que afetam o estroma da íris com epitélio pigmentar intacto.

lens p.'s, depressões da lente; as depressões pares formadas no ectoderma superficial da cabeça do embrião quando os placóides da lente afundam no cálice óptico; as aberturas externas das depressões são fechadas quando as vesículas da lente se formam.

lip p.'s, depressões labiais; malformações do lábio observadas em depressões ou fístulas uni ou bilaterais. Podem ser hereditárias ou associadas a fenda labial e/ou palatina.

Mantoux p., depressão de Mantoux; depressões superficiais de 2-3 mm nas regiões palmar e plantar na síndrome do nevo basocelular.

nail p.'s, depressões da unha; pequenas depressões pontilhadas, na superfície da placa ungueal, causadas por defeito na formação da unha; observadas na psoríase e em outros distúrbios. VER TAMBÉM geographic *stippling* of nails.

nasal p.'s, depressões nasais; as depressões pares formadas quando os placóides nasais situam-se abaixo do contorno externo geral da face em desenvolvimento em virtude do rápido crescimento das elevações nasais adjacentes; as depressões são os primórdios das porções rostrais das câmaras nasais. SIN olfactory p.'s.

oblong p. of arytenoid cartilage, fóvea oblonga da cartilagem aritenóidea. SIN oblong *fovea* of arytenoid cartilage.

olfactory p.'s, depressões olfatórias. SIN nasal p.'s.

optic p., depressão óptica; anomalia congênita caracterizada por uma depressão focal da parte temporal do disco óptico.

otic p.'s, depressões óticas; par de depressões, uma de cada lado da cabeça do embrião, marcando a localização das futuras vesículas auditivas. SIN auditory p.'s.

preauricular p., seio pré-auricular. SIN preauricular *sinus*.

primitive p., depressão primitiva; a depressão no nodo primitivo que serve para unir o canal notocórdico ao ectoderma de superfície.

pterygoid p., fóvea pterigóidea. SIN pterygoid *fovea*.

p. of stomach, fossa epigástrica. SIN epigastric *fossa*.

sublingual p., fóvea sublingual. SIN sublingual *fossa*.

superior articular p. of atlas, face articular superior do atlas. SIN superior articular *surface* of atlas.

superior costal p., face costal superior. SIN superior costal *facet*.

surpameatal p., fovéola suprameática. SIN suprameatal *triangle*.

triangular p. of arytenoid cartilage, fóvea triangular da cartilagem aritenóidea. SIN triangular *fovea* of arytenoid cartilage.

trochlear p., fóvea troclear. SIN trochlear *fovea*.

pit-1. Fator de transcrição de ligação nuclear encontrado em muitas células na hipófise humana normal e expresso em uma grande percentagem de adenomas hipofisários, em particular aqueles positivos para hormônio do crescimento ou tireotrofina.

PITC Abreviatura de phenylisothiocyanate (fenilisotiocianato).

pitch (pich). Piche; substância resinosa obtida do alcatrão após expelidas as substâncias voláteis por ebulição. SIN pix. [L. *pix*]

Burgundy p., p. da Borgonha; resina obtida do abeto ou da espruce da Noruega, *Picea excelsa*; foi usado como contra-irritante na forma de emplastro. SIN white p.

liquid p., p. líquido. SIN pine tar.

white p., p. branco. SIN Burgundy p.

pitch·blende (pich'blend). Pechblenda; uraninita; mineral de aspecto semelhante ao do piche, principalmente o dióxido de urânio, a principal fonte de urânio e elementos, como o rádio, produzidos pela desintegração radioativa daquele elemento. SIN uraninite.

pith. 1. Medula; o centro de um pêlo. 2. A medula espinal e o bulbo. 3. Perfurar o bulbo de um animal com um instrumento pontiagudo introduzido na base do crânio. [A.S. *pitha*]

pith·e·coid (pith'ē-koyd). Pitecóide; semelhante a um macaco. [G. *pithēkos*, macaco, + *eidos*, semelhança]

pith·ode (pith'ōd). O fuso nuclear na cariocinese. [G. *pithōdēs*, como uma jarra, de *pithos*, jarra de vinho feita de louça, + *eidos*, semelhança]

Pitot, Henri, engenheiro francês, 1695–1771. VER P. *tube*.

Pitres, Jean A., médico francês, 1848–1927. VER P. *area, sign*.

Pi·tressin (pi-tres'in). Nome comercial norte-americano da vasopressina. SIN vasopressin.

pit·ting. Em odontologia, a formação de depressões relativamente profundas, bem definidas em uma superfície; termo geralmente usado para descrever defeitos nas superfícies (freqüentemente de ouro, solda ou amálgama). Pode ter várias causas, embora a ocorrência clínica freqüentemente esteja associada a corrosão. VER TAMBÉM pitting *edema*, nail *pits*, em *pit*.

pi·tu·i·cyte (pi-too'i-sit). Pituícito; a célula primária do lobo posterior da hipófise, uma célula fusiforme intimamente relacionada à neuróglia. [pituitary + G. *kytos*, célula]

pi·tu·i·cy·to·ma (pi-too'i-sī-tō'mă). Pituicitoma; uma neoplasia gliogenosa rara derivada de pituícitos, encontrada no lobo posterior da hipófise e caracterizada por células com núcleos redondos ou ovais, relativamente pequenos, e longos prolongamentos ramificados que formam uma rede complexa de material citoplasmático, no qual podem ser demonstradas numerosas gotículas de gordura. [pituicyte + G. *-oma*, tumor]

pi·tu·i·ta (pi-too'i-tă). Pituíta; secreção nasal espessa. SIN glairy mucus. [L. fleuma ou secreção mucosa espessa]

pi·tu·i·ta·rism (pi-too'i-tār-izm). Pituitarismo; disfunção hipofisária. VER hyperpituitarism, hypopituitarism.

pi·tu·i·ta·ri·um (pi-too-i-tā'rē-ŭm). Pituitária. SIN pituitary. [L. mod.]

pi·tu·i·tary (pi-too'i-tār-ē). Pituitária; relativo à pituitária (hipófise). SIN pituitarium. [L. *pituita*, fleuma]

anterior p., hipófise anterior; o lobo anterior seco, parcialmente desengordurado e pulverizado da glândula hipófise de bovinos, ovinos ou suínos; agora raramente é usada terapeuticamente.

desiccated p., h. dessecada. SIN posterior p.

pharyngeal p., h. faríngea; o remanescente embrionário da extremidade oral da bolsa de Rathke, que é separado da adeno-hipófise pelo osso esfenóide em desenvolvimento; composto principalmente de cromófobos e, em condições normais, considerado fisiologicamente inativo. VER pituitary *gland*.

posterior p., h. posterior; o lobo posterior limpo, seco e pulverizado obtido do corpo da hipófise de animais domésticos usado como alimento pelo homem; ocitócico, vasoconstritor, antidiurético e estimulante da motilidade intestinal. SIN desiccated p., hypophysis sicca.

pi·tu·i·tous (pi-too'i-tŭs). Pituitoso; relativo à pituíta.

pit·y·ri·a·sis (pit-i-rī'ă-sis). Pitiríase; dermatose caracterizada por descamação furfurácea. [G. de *pityron*, farelo, caspa]

p. al'ba, p. alba; hipopigmentação segmentar da pele resultante de dermatite leve.

p. al'ba atroph'icans, p. alba atrófica; condição descamativa da pele seguida por atrofia.

p. cap'itis, p. da cabeça. SIN dandruff.

p. circina'ta, p. circinada. SIN p. rosea.

p. lichenoi'des, p. liquenóide; distúrbio cutâneo autolimitado de crianças e adultos, geralmente dividido em pitiríase liquenóide varioliforme aguda e pitiríase liquenóide crônica. SIN parapsoriasis guttata.

p. lichenoi'des et variolifor'mis acu'ta (PLEVA), p. liquenóide e varioliforme aguda; dermatite aguda que afeta crianças e adultos jovens, tem evolução relativamente leve e é autolimitada, embora a persistência de lesões e a recorrência de ataques não sejam raras; vesículas, pápulas e lesões crostosas acabam por produzir cicatrizes semelhantes às da varíola. SIN Mucha-Habermann disease, parapsoriasis lichenoides et varioliformis acuta, parapsoriasis varioliformis.

p. linguae, língua geográfica. SIN geographic *tongue*.

p. macula'ta, p. rósea. SIN p. rosea.

p. ni'gra, p. negra. SIN tinea nigra.

p. ro'sea, p. rósea; erupção autolimitada de máculas ou pápulas envolvendo o tronco e, menos freqüentemente, os membros, o couro cabeludo e a face; as lesões geralmente são ovais e seguem as linhas de tensão da pele; é mais comum em crianças e adultos jovens e freqüentemente é precedida por uma única lesão descamativa maior conhecida como lesão-mãe. SIN p. circinata, p. maculata.

p. ru'bra pila'ris, p. rubra pilosa; erupção pruriginosa crônica incomum dos folículos pilosos, que se tornam firmes, vermelhos, encimados por um tampão córneo e freqüentemente confluentes para formar placas descamativas; é observada mais visivelmente nos dorsos dos dedos das mãos e nos cotovelos e joelhos, e está associada a eritema, espessamento das regiões palmares e plantares e a espessamento opaco das unhas.

p. versic'olor, p. versicolor. SIN tinea versicolor.

pit·y·ri·a·sis li·che·noi·des chron·i·ca (līk'en-noyd'ēz kron'ik-ā). Pitiríase liquenóide crônica; erupção, com duração de até alguns anos, de pápulas castanho-avermelhadas com descamação central; desaparece sem cicatriz. [lichenoides L. mod., do G. *leichēn*, líquen, uma erupção semelhante a líquen, + *eidos*, semelhança; chronica L. mod. crônico, do G. *chronikos*, relativo ao tempo; de *chronos*, tempo]

pit·y·roid (pit'i-royd). Furfuráceo. SIN furfuraceous. [G. *pityrōdēs*, fareláceo, de *pityron*, farelo, + *eidos*, semelhança]

Pit·y·ro·spo·rum (pit-i-ros′pō-rŭm, pit′i-rō-spō′rŭm). Gênero de fungos cuja patogenicidade é discutível, sendo encontrado na caspa e na dermatite seborreica. [G. *pityron*, farelo, + *sporos*, semente]
   P. orbicula're, SIN *Malassezia furfur.*
   P. ova'le, SIN *Malassezia furfur.*

piv·a·late (piv′ă-lāt). Pivalato; contração para trimetilacetato $(CH_3)_3C-CO_2^-$ aprovada pela USAN.

piv·ot (piv′ŏt). Pivô; pilar no qual alguma coisa se articula ou gira.
   adjustable occlusal p., p. oclusal ajustável; um pivô oclusal que pode ser ajustado verticalmente por meio de um parafuso ou por outro meio.
   occlusal p., p. oclusal; elevação produzida na superfície oclusal, geralmente na região molar, destinada a atuar como fulcro e a induzir rotação mandibular sagital.

pix, gen. **pi·cis** (piks, pī′sis). SIN pitch. [L.]

pix·el (pik′sel). Pixel; contração de picture element (elemento de imagem), representação bidimensional de um elemento de volume (voxel) na exibição da imagens de TC ou RM, geralmente 512 × 512 ou 256 × 256 pixels, respectivamente.

PK Abreviatura de *pyruvate* kinase (piruvatoquinase, piruvatocinase).

pK_a, O logaritmo na base 10 negativo da constante de ionização (K_a) de um ácido; é igual ao valor do pH no qual estão presentes concentrações iguais das formas ácida e base conjugada de uma substância (freqüentemente um tampão).

pkat Abreviatura de picokatal.

PKU Abreviatura de phenylketonuria (fenilcetonúria).

pkV kVp; abreviatura de peak kilovoltage (quilovoltagem de pico), a voltagem nominal percebida pelo aparelho de raios X.

PL Abreviatura de placental lactogen (lactogênio placentário).

pla·ce·bo (plă-sē′bō). Placebo. **1.** Substância inerte administrada como medicamento por seu efeito sugestivo. **2.** Um composto inerte com aspecto idêntico ao material testado em pesquisa experimental, que pode ou não ser conhecido pelo médico e/ou paciente, administrado para distinguir entre a ação do fármaco e o efeito sugestivo do material em estudo. SIN active p. [L. agradarei, futuro de *placeo*]
   active p., p. ativo. SIN placebo.

PLACENTA

pla·cen·ta (plă-sen′tă). Placenta; órgão de troca metabólica entre o feto e a mãe. Possui uma parte de origem embrionária, derivada de uma área altamente desenvolvida da membrana embrionária mais externa (cório frondoso) e uma parte materna formada por uma modificação da parte da mucosa uterina (decídua basal) na qual a vesícula coriônica é implantada. Dentro da placenta, as vilosidades coriônicas, com seus capilares contidos que transportam sangue da circulação embrionária, são expostas ao sangue materno nos espaços intervilosos nos quais se situam as vilosidades; não ocorre mistura direta do sangue fetal e materno, mas o tecido interposto (a membrana placentária) é suficientemente fino para permitir a passagem de nutrientes, oxigênio e algumas substâncias nocivas, como vírus, para o sangue fetal e a liberação de dióxido de carbono e escórias nitrogenadas dele. A termo, a placenta humana tem formato de disco, cerca de 4 cm de espessura e 18 cm de diâmetro, pesando, em média, 1/6 a 1/7 do peso do feto; sua superfície fetal é lisa, sendo formada pelo âmnio aderente, com o cordão umbilical normalmente fixado próximo de seu centro; a superfície materna de uma placenta descolada é rugosa, devido ao tecido decidual lacerado aderido ao cório, e exibe elevações lobulares denominadas cotilédones ou lobos. [L. um bolo]
   accessory p., p. acessória; massa de tecido placentário distinta da p. principal. SIN succenturiate p., supernumerary p.
   p. accre'ta, p. acreta; a aderência anormal das vilosidades coriônicas ao miométrio, associada à ausência parcial ou completa da decídua basal e, em particular, do estrato esponjoso. VER TAMBÉM p. percreta.
   p. accre'ta ve'ra, p. acreta verdadeira; termo empregado quando as vilosidades estão justapostas ao miométrio.
   adherent p., p. aderida; p. que não se separa facilmente do útero após o parto.
   anular p., p. anular; p. na forma de uma faixa circundando o interior do útero. SIN ring-shaped p., zonary p.
   battledore p., p. em raquete; p. na qual o cordão umbilical está inserido na margem; assim denominada devido a uma suposta semelhança com a raquete usada no jogo de *battledore* (tamborete e peteca), um precursor do *badminton*.
   bidiscoidal p., p. bidiscóide; p. com duas porções distintas, em forma de disco, fixadas às paredes opostas do útero; normal em determinados macacos e em musaranhos, sendo ocasionalmente encontrada em seres humanos.
   p. bilo'ba, p. bilobada; p. dupla na qual as duas partes estão separadas por uma constrição. SIN p. bipartita.
   p. biparti'ta, p. bipartida. SIN p. biloba.
   central p. pre'via, p. prévia central. SIN p. previa centralis.
   chorioallantoic p., p. corioalantóica; placenta (como a de primatas) na qual o córion é formado pela fusão do mesoderma e vasos alantóicos até a face interna da serosa.
   chorioamnionic p., p. corioamniótica; forma de placentação na qual o âmnion está fundido à face interna do córion, assim permitindo a troca de água e eletrólitos entre a mãe e o feto.
   p. circumvalla'ta, p. circumvalada; p. caliciforme com bordas elevadas, que possuem um anel espesso, redondo, branco, opaco ao redor de sua periferia; uma parte da decídua separa a margem da p. de sua placa coriônica; o restante da superfície coriônica tem aspecto normal, mas os vasos fetais são limitados em seu trajeto através da p. pelo anel. VER TAMBÉM p. marginata, p. reflexa.
   cotyledonary p., p. cotiledonária; p. na qual a substância é dividida em lobos ou cotilédones.
   deciduate p., p. deciduada; p. na qual a substância é expulsa com a placenta fetal.
   dichorionic diamnionic p., p. diamniótica dicoriônica. VER twin p.
   p. diffu'sa, p. difusa. SIN p. membranacea.
   p. dimidia'ta, p. dimidiada. SIN p. duplex.
   disperse p., p. dispersa; p. na qual as artérias umbilicais dividem-se dicotomicamente antes de entrarem na substância placentária.
   Duncan p., p. de Duncan; p. separada que se apresenta na vulva com a superfície coriônica exteriorizada.
   p. du'plex, p. dupla; p. que consiste em duas partes, quase totalmente separada, estando unida apenas no ponto de fixação do cordão umbilical. VER p. biloba. SIN p. dimidiata.
   endotheliochorial p., p. endoteliocorial; p. na qual o tecido coriônico penetra no endotélio dos vasos sanguíneos maternos.
   endothelio-endothelial p., p. endotelioendotelial; p. na qual o endotélio dos vasos maternos entra em contato direto com o endotélio dos vasos fetais para formar a barreira placentária.
   epitheliochorial p., p. epiteliocorial; p. na qual o córion está apenas em contato com o endométrio, e não causa erosão.
   p. extrachora'les, p. extracorial; p. na qual a placa coriônica é limitada por uma fina prega membranácea na margem.
   p. fenestra'ta, p. fenestrada; p. na qual há áreas de adelgaçamento, algumas vezes estendendo-se até a total ausência de tecido placentário.
   fetal p., p. feta'lis, p. fetal; a porção coriônica da p. que contém os vasos sanguíneos fetais, da qual se desenvolve o cordão umbilical; especificamente, em seres humanos, desenvolve-se do córion frondoso. SIN pars fetalis placentae.
   hemochorial p., p. hemocorial; o tipo de p., como em seres humanos e em alguns roedores, no qual o sangue materno está em contato direto com o córion.
   hemoendothelial p., p. hemoendotelial; o tipo de p., como em coelhos, no qual o trofoblasto torna-se tão adelgaçado que, à microscopia óptica, o sangue materno parece estar separado do sangue fetal apenas pelo endotélio dos capilares coriônicos.
   horseshoe p., p. em ferradura; p. exagerada, reniforme e curva, lembrando a forma de uma ferradura; presente em algumas gestações gemelares.
   incarcerated p., p. encarcerada. SIN retained p.
   p. incre'ta, p. increta; forma de p. acreta na qual as vilosidades coriônicas invadem o miométrio.

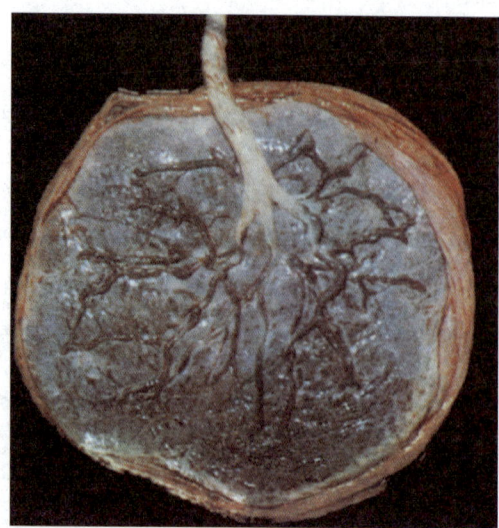

placenta: superfície amniótica, com cordão umbilical

labyrinthine p., p. labiríntica; p. na qual o sangue materno circula através de canais no sinciciotrofoblasto fetal.
p. margina'ta, p. marginal; p. com margens elevadas, menos acentuada que a p. circunvalada. VER TAMBÉM p. reflexa.
maternal p., p. materna. SIN *pars uterina placentae.*
p. membrana'cea, p. membranácea; p. anormalmente fina que cobre uma área incomumente grande do revestimento uterino. SIN p. diffusa.
monochorionic diamnionic p., p. diamniótica monocoriônica. VER twin p.
monochorionic monoamnionic p., p. monoamniótica monocoriônica. VER twin p.
p. multilo'ba, p. multilobada; p. com mais de três lobos separados entre si por constrições simples, sendo o feto único. SIN p. multipartita.
p. multiparti'ta, p. multipartida. SIN p. multiloba.
nondeciduous p., p. não-decídua; p. na qual a parte fetal é expelida, deixando a mucosa uterina intacta (p. ex., uma p. epiteliocorial).
p. pandurafor'mis, p. panduriforme; forma de p. dimidiada com as duas metades colocadas lado a lado, com o formato sugestivo de um instrumento musical semelhante ao alaúde (pandora).
p. percre'ta, p. percreta; o termo aplicado quando as vilosidades invadem toda a espessura do miométrio chegando até a serosa do útero ou atravessando-a, causando ruptura uterina incompleta ou completa, respectivamente. VER TAMBÉM p. accreta.
p. pre'via, p. prévia; a condição na qual a p. está implantada no segmento inferior do útero, estendendo-se até a margem do óstio interno do colo uterino ou causando obstrução parcial ou completa do óstio. SIN placental presentation.

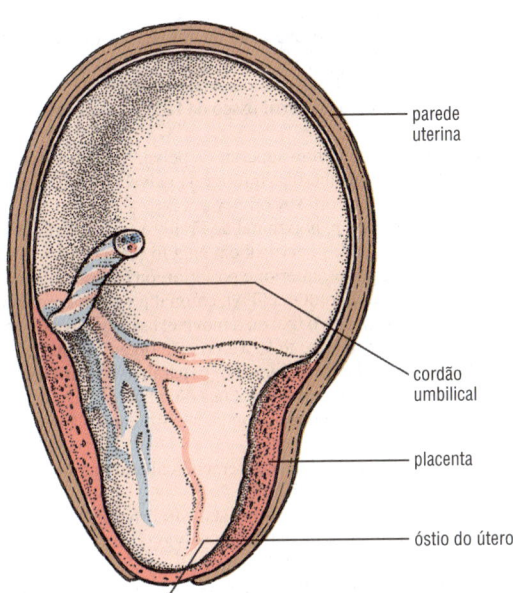

placenta prévia central: a placenta cobre totalmente o óstio interno do útero; o feto não é mostrado

p. pre'via centra'lis, p. prévia central; p. prévia na qual a p. cobre totalmente o óstio interno do colo do útero. SIN central p. previa, total p. previa.
p. pre'via margina'lis, p. prévia marginal; p. prévia na qual a p. chega até a margem do óstio interno do colo do útero, mas não o oclui.
p. pre'via partia'lis, p. prévia parcial; p. prévia na qual o óstio interno do colo do útero é parcialmente coberto por tecido placentário.
p. reflex'a, p. reflexa; anomalia da p. na qual a margem está espessada a ponto de parecer voltada sobre si própria. VER TAMBÉM p. circumvallata, p. marginata.
p. renifor'mis, p. reniforme; uma placenta em forma de rim.
retained p., p. retida; separação incompleta da placenta e sua incapacidade de ser expelida no tempo normal após o nascimento da criança. SIN incarcerated p.
ring-shaped p., p. anular. SIN anular p.
Schultze p., p. de Schultze; p. que aparece na vulva mostrando a superfície fetal brilhante (âmnio).
p. spu'ria, p. espúria; massa de tecido placentário sem conexões vasculares com a p. principal.
succenturiate p., p. sucenturiada. SIN accessory p.
supernumerary p., p. supranumerária. SIN accessory p.
total p. pre'via, p. prévia total. SIN p. previa centralis.
p. tri'loba, p. trilobada. SIN p. tripartita.

p. triparti'ta, p. tripartida; p. que consiste em três partes quase totalmente separadas, sendo unidas apenas pelos vasos sanguíneos do cordão umbilical; o feto é único. SIN p. triloba, p. triplex.
p. tri'plex, p. tripla. SIN p. tripartita.
twin p., p. gemelar; a(s) placenta(s) de uma gravidez gemelar; se dizigóticas, as placentas podem ser separadas ou fundidas, e estas últimas preservam dois sacos amnióticos e dois sacos coriônicos (placenta diamniótica dicoriônica); se monozigótica, a p. pode ser **monoamniótica monocoriônica** ou **monocoriônica diamniótica**, dependendo do estágio no qual ocorreu a gemelaridade; se a gemelaridade ocorre precocemente, pode haver uma p. fundida com duas membranas coriônicas e duas membranas amnióticas.
p. uteri'na, p. uterina. SIN *pars uterina placentae.*
p. velamento'sa, p. velamentosa; p. na qual o cordão umbilical está fixado às membranas adjacentes, com os vasos umbilicais espalhados e entrando na p. independentemente.
villous p., p. vilosa; p. na qual o córion forma vilosidades.
zonary p., p. zonária. SIN anular p.

pla·cen·ta·go·nad·o·trop·in. Gonadotrofina placentária; gonadotrofina coriônica. SIN chorionic gonadotropin.
pla·cen·tal (pla-sen'tal). Placentário; relativo à placenta.
pla·cen·tal dys·ma·ture. Desenvolvimento imaturo da placenta de forma que esta não funciona normalmente.
Pla·cen·ta·lia (plas-en-tā'lē-ă). VER Eutheria. [L. *placenta*]
plac·en·ta·tion (plas-en-tā'shŭn). Placentação; a organização estrutural e a forma de fixação dos tecidos fetais aos tecidos maternos na formação da placenta. Os tipos de placenta são definidos sob o verbete placenta.
plac·en·ti·tis (plas-en-tī'tis). Placentite; inflamação da placenta.
plac·en·to·ma (plas-en-tō'mă). Placentoma. SIN deciduoma.
pla·cen·to·ther·a·py (plă-sen'tō-thar'ă-pē). Placentoterapia; uso terapêutico de um extrato do tecido placentário.
Placido da Costa, Antonio, oftalmologista português, 1848–1916. VER P. da C. *disk.*
plac·ode (plak'ōd). Placóide; espessamento local no ectoderma embrionário; as células do placóide habitualmente constituem um grupo primordial do qual se desenvolve um órgão do sentido ou gânglio. [G. *plakōdēs*, de *plax*, qualquer coisa plana ou larga, + *eidos*, semelhante]
auditory p.'s, placóides auditivos. SIN otic p.'s.
epibranchial p.'s, placóides epibranquiais; espessamentos ectodérmicos associados às partes mais dorsais dos arcos branquiais embrionários; suas células contribuem para a formação dos gânglios cranianos, incluindo os dos nervos V, VII, IX e X.
lens p.'s, placóides da lente; par de placóides ectodérmicos que se invaginam para formar as vesículas da lente embrionária.
nasal p.'s, placóides nasais. SIN olfactory p.'s.
olfactory p.'s, placóides olfatórios; par de placóides ectodérmicos que passam a se localizar no fundo das fossas nasais à medida que as fossas se aprofundam pelo crescimento das proeminências nasais medial e lateral adjacentes. SIN nasal p.'s.
optic p.'s, placóides ópticos. SIN lens p.'s.
otic p.'s, placóides óticos; par de placóides ectodérmicos que afundam abaixo do nível geral do ectoderma superficial para formar as vesículas óticas. SIN auditory p.'s.
pla·fond (plă-fon'd). Teto; um teto, principalmente o teto da articulação do tornozelo, isto é, a superfície articular da extremidade distal da tíbia. [Fr. teto]
plagio-. Plagio-; oblíquo, inclinado. [G. *plagios*]
pla·gi·o·ce·phal·ic (plā'jē-ō-se-fal'ik). Plagiocefálico; relativo a, ou caracterizado por, plagiocefalia. SIN plagiocephalous.
pla·gi·o·ceph·a·lism (plā'jē-ō-sef'ă-lizm). Plagiocefalia. SIN plagiocephaly.
pla·gi·o·ceph·a·lous (plā'jē-ō-sef'ă-lŭs). Plagiocefálico. SIN plagiocephalic.
pla·gi·o·ceph·a·ly (plā'jē-ō-sef'ă-lē). Plagiocefalia; cranioestenose assimétrica causada por fechamento prematuro das suturas lambdóide e coronal de um lado; caracterizada por deformidade oblíqua do crânio. SIN asynclitism of the skull, plagiocephalism. [G. *plagios*, oblíquo, + *kephalē*, cabeça]
plague (plāg). Peste. **1.** Qualquer doença de prevalência significativa ou de mortalidade excessiva. **2.** Doença infecciosa aguda causada pela bactéria *Yersinia pestis* e caracterizada clinicamente por febre alta, toxemia, prostração, erupção petequial, linfadenopatia e pneumonia, ou hemorragia das mucosas; basicamente é uma doença de roedores, transmitida aos seres humanos por pulgas que picaram animais infectados. Nos seres humanos, a doença pode assumir quatro formas clínicas: p. bubônica, p. septicêmica, p. pneumônica ou p. menor. SIN pest, pestilence (1), pestis. [L. *plaga*, um choque, lesão]
ambulant p., ambulatory p., p. menor; forma leve de p. bubônica caracterizada por manifestações como febre leve e linfadenite. SIN larval p., parapestis, pestis ambulans, pestis minor.

black p., p. negra. VER black *death*.
bubonic p., p. bubônica; a forma habitual de p. cujas manifestações incluem linfadenopatia inflamatória na região inguinal, axilas ou outras partes. SIN glandular p., pestis bubonica, pestis fulminans, pestis major, polyadenitis maligna.
glandular p., p. bubônica. SIN bubonic p.
hemorrhagic p., p. hemorrágica; a forma hemorrágica da p. bubônica.
larval p., p. menor. SIN ambulant p.
Pahvant Valley p., p. do Vale Pahvant, tularemia. SIN tularemia.
pneumonic p., p. pneumônica; forma rapidamente progressiva e freqüentemente fatal de p. na qual há áreas de consolidação pulmonar, com calafrios, dor na parte lateral do corpo, expectoração com sangue, febre alta e possível transmissão entre seres humanos. SIN plague pneumonia, pulmonic p.
pulmonic p., p. pneumônica. SIN pneumonic p.
septicemic p., p. septicêmica; forma geralmente fatal de p. na qual há bacteriemia intensa, com sinais e sintomas de toxemia profunda. SIN pestis siderans.
sylvatic p., p. silvestre; p. bubônica em ratos e outros animais selvagens.
plak·al·bu·min (plak-al-bū′min). Placalbumina; o produto da ação da subtilisina sobre a albumina do ovo, removendo um hexapeptídeo.
pla·kins (plā′kinz). Plaquinas; substâncias bactericidas semelhantes às leucinas extraídas das plaquetas do sangue. [G. *plax, plakos*, qualquer coisa plana, + -in]
plan-. VER plano-.
pla·na (plā′nă). Planos; plural de planum. [L.]
plan·chet (plan′shet). Prancheta; uma pequena placa ou disco plano usado como suporte de uma amostra para determinação da radioatividade; a amostra geralmente é evaporada na prancheta. [Fr. *planchette*, dim. de *planche*, prancha]
Planck, Max, físico alemão e ganhador do Prêmio Nobel, 1858–1947. VER P. *constant, theory.*

PLANE

plane (plān) [TA]. **1.** Plano; uma superfície plana bidimensional. VER planum. **2.** Uma superfície imaginária formada por extensão de um ponto através de qualquer eixo ou dois pontos definidos, em referência principalmente à craniometria e à pelvimetria. SIN planum. [L. *planus*, plano]
Addison clinical p.'s, planos clínicos de Addison; uma série de planos usados como pontos de reparo em topografia toracoabdominal; o tronco é dividido verticalmente por um *p. mediano* desde a borda superior do manúbrio do esterno até a sínfise púbica, por um *p. lateral* traçado verticalmente de cada lado através de um ponto a meio caminho entre a espinha ilíaca ântero-superior e o p. mediano no p. interespinal, e por um *p. interespinal* que segue verticalmente através da espinha ilíaca ântero-superior de cada lado; transversalmente, o tronco é dividido por um *p. transtorácico* que atravessa o tórax 3,2 cm acima da borda inferior do corpo do esterno, por um *p. transpilórico* a meio caminho entre a incisura jugular do esterno e a sínfise púbica, correspondente ao disco entre a primeira e a segunda vértebras lombares, e por um *p. intertubercular* que atravessa os tubérculos ilíacos e, geralmente, corta a quinta vértebra lombar; os planos formados por essas linhas, bem como os planos transversos que cortam a borda superior do manúbrio e a borda superior da sínfise púbica, constituem os planos clínicos de Addison.
Aeby p., p. de Aeby; em craniometria, um p. perpendicular ao plano mediano do crânio, cortando o násio e o básio.
auriculoinfraorbital p., p. auriculoinfra-orbital. SIN orbitomeatal p.
axial p., p. axial; p. transversal que forma ângulos retos com o eixo longitudinal do corpo, como na TC. SIN transaxial p.
axiolabiolingual p., p. axiolabiolingual; p. paralelo ao eixo longitudinal de um dente e que se estende na direção labiolingual.
axiomesiodistal p., p. axiomesiodistal; p. paralelo aos eixos longitudinais dos dentes e que se estende em direção mesiodistal.
bite p., p. de mordida. SIN occlusal p.
Broca visual p., p. visual de Broca; p. traçado através dos eixos visuais de cada olho.
Camper p., p. de Camper; p. que segue da extremidade da espinha nasal anterior (acântio) até o centro do meato acústico externo ósseo dos lados direito e esquerdo.
canthomeatal p., p. cantomeatal; p. que atravessa os dois ângulos laterais do olho e o centro do meato acústico externo; esse p. situa-se aproximadamente a meio caminho entre os planos de Frankfort e o plano supra-orbitomeatal.
coronal p., p. coronal. SIN frontal p.
cove p., descrição clássica de inversão terminal da onda T do eletrocardiograma com a porção inicial curva acima da linha de base e a porção terminal abaixo dela, sendo a primeira arredondada e a última pontiaguda.
datum p., p. de dados; p. arbitrário usado como base a partir da qual se fazem medidas craniométricas.
Daubenton p., p. de Daubenton; o p. do forame magno. VER TAMBÉM Daubenton *angle*, Daubenton *line*.
equatorial p., p. equatorial; na metáfase da mitose, o p. que toca todos os centrômeros e suas fixações em fuso.
eye-ear p., p. orbitomeatal. SIN orbitomeatal p.
facial p., p. facial; medida do perfil ósseo da face. SIN nasion-pogonion measurement.
first parallel pelvic p., abertura superior da pelve. SIN pelvic *inlet*.
fourth parallel pelvic p., abertura inferior da pelve. SIN pelvic *outlet*.
Frankfort p., p. de Frankfort. SIN orbitomeatal p.
Frankfort horizontal p., p. horizontal de Frankfort. SIN orbitomeatal p.
frontal p. [TA], p. frontal; p. vertical em ângulo reto com um plano sagital, dividindo o corpo nas partes anterior e posterior, ou qualquer p. paralelo ao p. coronal central. SIN plana frontalia [TA], coronal p., plana coronalia.
guide p., p. de guia; dispositivo fixo ou removível usado para deslocar um único dente, um segmento do arco ou todo o arco para obter uma melhor relação.
horizontal p.'s [TA], planos horizontais; p. paralelo e relativo ao horizonte; na posição anatômica, os planos horizontais são planos transversais; em decúbito dorsal ou ventral, os planos horizontais são frontais (planos coronais). SIN plana horizontalia [TA].
p. of incidence, p. de incidência; o p. perpendicular a uma superfície da lente que contém o raio luminoso incidente.
infraorbitomeatal p., p. infra-orbitomeatal. SIN orbitomeatal p.
p. of inlet, abertura superior da pelve. SIN pelvic *inlet*.
interspinal p., p. interespinal. SIN interspinous p.
interspinous p. [TA], p. interespinal; p. que atravessa as espinhas ilíacas ântero-superiores; marca o limite entre as regiões lateral e umbilical, superiormente, e as regiões inguinal e púbica, inferiormente. SIN planum interspinale [TA], interspinal p., Lanz line.
intertubercular p. [TA], p. intertubercular; p. que atravessa os tubérculos ilíacos. SIN planum intertuberculare [TA].
labiolingual p., p. labiolingual; p. paralelo às superfícies labial e lingual dos dentes.
p. of least pelvic dimensions, p. das menores dimensões pélvicas. SIN pelvic p. of least dimensions.
mean foundation p., a média das várias irregularidades na forma e inclinação da sede basal; a condição ideal para estabilidade da dentadura se dá quando esse p. está quase em ângulo reto com a direção da força.
Meckel p., p. de Meckel; p. craniométrico que corta os pontos alveolar e auricular.
median p. [TA], p. mediano; p. vertical, na posição anatômica, que atravessa a linha média do corpo, dividindo-o nas metades direita e esquerda. VER TAMBÉM Addison clinical p.'s. SIN planum medianum [TA].
p. of midpelvis, p. mesopélvico. SIN pelvic p. of least dimensions.
midsagittal p., p. sagital mediano; termo obsoleto para p. mediano.
Morton p., p. de Morton; p. que atravessa os ápices das protuberâncias parietal e occipital.
nasion-postcondylar p., p. násio-pós-condilar; p. que atravessa o násio anteriormente e até um ponto imediatamente atrás de cada processo condilar da mandíbula, posteriormente.
nodal p., p. nodal; o p. que corresponde ao centro óptico de uma lente simples. VER nodal *point*.

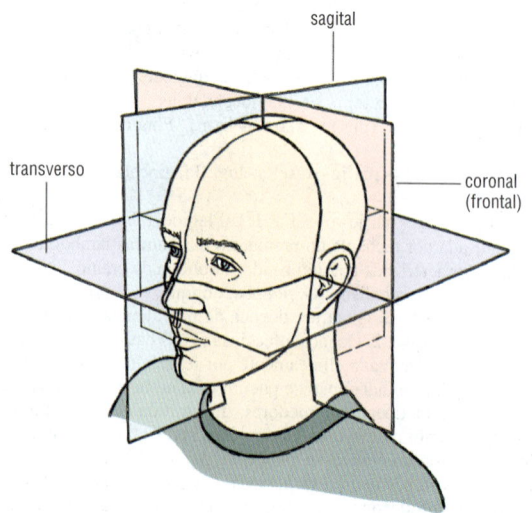

planos do corpo

nuchal p., p. nucal; a superfície externa da parte escamosa do osso occipital abaixo da linha nucal superior, dando fixação aos músculos do dorso do pescoço.

occipital p. [TA], p. occipital; a superfície externa do osso occipital acima da linha nucal superior. SIN planum occipitale [TA].

occlusal p., p. of occlusion, p. oclusal, p. de oclusão; uma superfície imaginária relacionada anatomicamente ao crânio e que, teoricamente, toca as margens incisais dos dentes incisivos e as extremidades das superfícies oclusais dos dentes posteriores; não é um p. no sentido real da palavra, mas representa a média da curvatura da superfície. VER TAMBÉM *curve* of occlusion. SIN bite p.

orbital p., p. orbital; a superfície orbital da maxila, situada perpendicular ao p. orbitomeatal na órbita. SIN planum orbitale.

orbitomeatal p., p. orbitomeatal; (1) uma linha que se aproxima da base do crânio, que segue da crista infra-orbital até a linha média do occipúcio, cruzando a margem superior do meato acústico externo; o crânio está na posição anatômica quando a linha basal se situa no plano horizontal e os lados direito e esquerdo estão no mesmo nível. (2) um p. de referência craniométrico padrão que atravessa as porções direita e esquerda e a órbita esquerda; desenhado na radiografia ou fotografia de perfil desde a margem superior do meato acústico até à órbita. SIN auriculoinfraorbital p., eye-ear p., Frankfort horizontal p., Frankfort p., infraorbitomeatal p.

p. of outlet, abertura inferior da pelve. SIN pelvic *outlet*.

parasagittal p., p. parassagital; termo obsoleto para p. sagital.

p. of pelvic canal, p. do canal pélvico. SIN *axis* of pelvis.

pelvic p. of greatest dimensions, p. das maiores dimensões pélvicas, o p. que se estende do meio da superfície posterior da sínfise púbica até a junção da segunda e terceira vértebras sacrais, seguindo lateralmente através dos ossos ísquios pelo meio do acetábulo. SIN second parallel pelvic p., wide p.

pelvic p. of inlet, abertura superior da pelve. SIN pelvic *inlet*.

pelvic p. of least dimensions, p. de menores dimensões pélvicas, o p. que se estende da extremidade do sacro até a borda inferior da sínfise púbica; é limitado posteriormente pela extremidade do sacro, lateralmente pelas espinhas isquiáticas e anteriormente pela borda inferior da sínfise púbica. SIN midplane, p. of least pelvic dimensions, p. of midpelvis, third parallel pelvic p.

pelvic p. of outlet, abertura inferior da pelve. SIN pelvic *outlet*.

popliteal p. of femur, p. poplíteo do fêmur. SIN popliteal *surface* of femur.

principal p., p. principal; o p. teórico de um sistema de lente composto. VER principal *point*.

p.'s of reference, planos de referência; planos que atuam como orientação para a localização de outros planos.

p. of regard, p. de observação; p. imaginário no qual o ponto de observação se move quando os olhos se voltam de um lado para outro.

sagittal p. [TA], p. sagital; p. paralelo ao p. mediano; os planos sagitais são planos verticais na posição anatômica. SIN plana sagittalia [TA].

second parallel pelvic p., p. de maiores dimensões pélvicas. SIN pelvic p. of greatest dimensions.

spectacle p., p. de óculos; p. no qual são usados óculos.

sternal p., p. esternal; p. indicado pela superfície frontal do esterno. SIN planum sternale.

subcostal p. [TA], p. subcostal; p. que atravessa os limites inferiores da margem costal, isto é, as décimas cartilagens costais; marca o limite entre as regiões do hipocôndrio e epigástrio superiormente, e as regiões lateral e umbilical, inferiormente. SIN planum subcostale [TA], infracostal line.

supracrestal p., p. supracristal. SIN supracristal p.

supracristal p. [TA], p. supracristal; p. que atravessa os ápices das cristas ilíacas; geralmente atravessa o quarto processo espinhoso lombar. SIN planum supracristale [TA], supracrestal p.

supraorbitomeatal p., p. supra-orbitomeatal; p. que passa pelas margens orbitais superiores e pela margem superior dos meatos acústicos externos; faz um ângulo de aproximadamente 25°–30° com o p. de Frankfort; imagens de TC de rotina do encéfalo são feitas paralelas a esse p. para limitar a exposição do bulbo do olho à radiação ionizante.

suprasternal p., p. supra-esternal; p. que atravessa o corpo ao nível da margem superior do manúbrio do esterno.

temporal p. [TA], p. temporal; área algo deprimida na lateral do crânio, abaixo da linha temporal inferior, formada pelos ossos temporal e parietal, pela asa maior do esfenóide e por uma parte do osso frontal. SIN planum temporale [TA].

third parallel pelvic p., p. de menores dimensões pélvicas. SIN pelvic p. of least dimensions.

tooth p., p. dental; qualquer um dos planos imaginários de secção de um dente, como o axial, o horizontal ou o vertical.

transaxial p., p. transaxial. SIN axial p.

transpyloric p. [TA], p. transpilórico; p. transverso a meio caminho entre as margens superiores do manúbrio do esterno e a sínfise púbica; o piloro pode estar localizado nesse p. em decúbito dorsal ou ventral, mas, na posição ortostática (anatômica), desce para um nível mais baixo. SIN planum transpyloricum [TA]

transverse p. [TA], p. transverso; p. que atravessa o corpo formando ângulos retos com os planos coronal e sagital; os planos transversos são perpendiculares ao eixo longitudinal do corpo ou dos membros, independentemente da posição do corpo ou do membro; na posição anatômica, os planos transversos são planos horizontais; em outra situação os dois termos não são sinônimos. SIN plana transversalia [TA].

wide p., p. de maiores dimensões pélvicas. SIN pelvic p. of greatest dimensions.

△ **plani-**. VER plano-.

pla·nig·ra·phy (pla-nig′ra-fē). Planigrafia. SIN tomography. [L. *planum*, plano, + G. *graphē*, escrita]

pla·nim·e·ter (pla-nim′e-ter). Planímetro; instrumento formado de alavancas articuladas com um indicador de registro, usado para medir a área de qualquer superfície pelo traçado de seus limites. [L. *planum*, plano, + G. *metron*, medida]

pla·nim·e·try (pla-nim′e-trē). Planimetria; a medida das áreas de superfície e perímetros pelo traçado dos limites. A planimetria em fotomicrografias ou imagens projetadas pode ser usada para avaliar o tamanho das células.

plan·i·tho·rax (plan′i-thō′raks). Planitórax; diagrama do tórax mostrando a frente e o dorso em projeção plana, de acordo com a projeção de Mercator da superfície terrestre.

plank·ter (plangk′ter). Qualquer tipo de plâncton.

plank·ton (plangk′ton). Plâncton; termo geral para muitas formas marinhas flutuantes, em sua maioria de tamanho microscópico ou pequeno, que são deslocadas passivamente por ventos, ondas, marés ou correntes; inclui diatomáceas, algas, copépodes e muitos protozoários, crustáceos, moluscos e vermes. [G. *planktos*, errante]

plank·ton·ic (plangk-ton′ik). Plactônico; relativo ao plâncton; semelhante ao plâncton.

△ **plano-, plan-, plani-**. Plano-, plan-, plani-. 1. Um plano; achatado, liso. [L. *planum*, plano; *planus*, plano] 2. Errante. [G. *planos*, ação de vagar]

pla·no·cel·lu·lar (plā-nō-sel′u-lar). Planocelular; relativo a, ou composto de, células planas. [L. *planus*, plano, + celular]

pla·no·con·cave (plā′nō-kon-kāv′). Planocôncavo; plano de um lado e côncavo do outro; designa uma lente com esse formato.

pla·no·con·vex (plā′nō-kon-veks′). Planoconvexo; plano de um lado e convexo do outro; designa uma lente com esse formato.

pla·nog·ra·phy (pla-nog′ra-fē). Planografia. SIN tomography.

plan·o·ma·nia (plan-ō-mā′nē-a). Planomania; termo raramente usado para designar o impulso mórbido de deixar o lar e desprezar limites sociais. [G. *planos*, ação de vagar, + *mania*, mania]

Pla·nor·bis (plan-ōr′bis). Gênero europeu e norte-africano de caramujos da água doce (família Planorbidae), incluindo *P. planorbis*, hospedeiro intermediário do trematódeo de ovinos e bovinos, *Paramphistoma cervi*. [G. *planos*, ação de vagar, + L. *orbis*, círculo, anel]

pla·no·val·gus (plā-nō-val′gus). Planovalgo; uma condição na qual o arco longitudinal do pé está retificado e a parte posterior do pé está evertida. [plano- + L. *valgus*, voltado para fora]

plan·ta, gen. e pl. **plan·tae** (plan′ta, plan′tē) [TA]. Planta. SIN sole. [L.]

p. pe′dis [TA], planta do pé. SIN *sole* of foot.

plan·ta·go (plan-tā′gō). Tanchagem; a raiz e as folhas da tanchagem comum ou de folhas grandes, *Plantago major* (família Plantaginaceae). [L. tanchagem]

p. ovata coating, película de plantago ovata; as lâminas mucilaginosas externas separadas das sementes de *Plantago ovata*; usada na constipação simples associada à ausência de volume suficiente.

p. seed, semente de tanchagem; semente de psílio. SIN psyllium seed.

plan·tain seed. Semente de tanchagem. SIN psyllium seed.

plan·tal·gia (plan-tal′jē-a). Dor na superfície plantar do pé sobre a fáscia plantar. [L. *planta*, planta do pé, + G. *algos*, dor]

plan·tar (plan′tar) [TA]. Plantar; relativo à planta do pé. SIN plantaris [TA]. [L. *plantaris*].

plan·tar·is (plan-tār′is) [TA]. Plantar. SIN plantar [L.]

plan·ti·grade (plan′ti-grād). Plantígrado; que caminha com toda a planta do pé e o calcanhar no chão, como o homem e o urso. [L. *planta*, planta, + *gradior*, caminhar]

plan·u·la, pl. **plan·u·lae** (plan′u-lā, -lē). Plânula; nome dado por Lankester a um embrião de celenterado quando este consiste apenas em duas camadas germinativas primárias, o ectoderma e o endoderma. [L. dim. de *planum*, superfície plana]

invaginate p., p. invaginada. SIN gastrula.

pla·num, pl. **pla·na** (plā′num, plā′na). Plano. SIN plane. [L. plane]

plana coronalia, planos frontais. SIN frontal *plane*.

plana frontalia, p. frontal. SIN frontal *plane*.

horizontal planes [TA], planos horizontais; p. paralelo e relativo ao horizonte; na posição anatômica, os planos horizontais são planos transversos; no decúbito dorsal ou ventral, os planos horizontais são frontais (planos coronais). SIN plana horizontalia [TA].

plana horizontalia [TA], planos horizontais. SIN horizontal planes.

p. interspina'le [TA], p. interespinal. SIN interspinous *plane*. VER TAMBÉM Addison clinical *planes*, em *plane*.
p. intertubercula're [TA], SIN intertubercular plane. VER TAMBÉM Addison clinical *planes*, em *plane*.
p. medianum [TA], p. mediano. SIN median *plane*.
p. occipita'le [TA], p. occipital. SIN occipital *plane*.
p. orbita'le, p. orbital. SIN orbital *plane*.
p. poplit'eum, p. poplíteo. SIN popliteal *surface* of femur.
plana sagittalia [TA], planos sagitais. SIN sagittal *plane*.
p. semiluna'tum, p. semilunar; a área do epitélio que limita a área sensorial da crista ampular.
p. sphenoida'le [TA], jugo esfenoidal. SIN jugum sphenoidale.
p. sterna'le, p. esternal. SIN sternal *plane*.
p. subcosta'le, p. subcostal. SIN subcostal *plane*.
p. supracrista'le [TA], p. supracristal. SIN supracristal *plane*.
p. tempora'le [TA], p. temporal. SIN temporal *plane*.
p. transpylo'ricum [TA], p. transpilórico. SIN transpyloric *plane*. VER Addison clinical *planes*, em *plane*.
plana transversalia [TA], planos transversos. SIN transverse *plane*.
pla·nu·ria (plă-noo′rē-ă). Planúria. **1.** Extravasamento de urina. **2.** A eliminação de urina por uma abertura anormal. [G. *planos*, errante, + *ouron*, urina]
plaque (plak). Placa. **1.** Uma mancha ou pequena área diferenciada na superfície de um corpo (p. ex., pele, mucosa ou endotélio arterial) ou na superfície de corte de um órgão como o encéfalo; na pele, uma área circunscrita, elevada, superficial e sólida com mais de 1,0 cm de diâmetro. **2.** Área de clareamento em um crescimento confluente plano de bactérias ou células teciduais, como aquela causada pela ação lítica de bacteriófagos em uma cultura de bactérias em placa de ágar, pelo efeito citopático de determinados vírus animais em uma lâmina de células teciduais cultivadas, ou por anticorpo (hemolisina) produzido por linfócitos cultivados na presença de eritrócitos e aos quais foi acrescentado complemento. **3.** Uma zona bem definida de desmielinização característica de esclerose múltipla. **4.** VER dental p. [Fr. uma placa]
atheromatous p., p. ateromatosa; uma área amarela ou tumefação bem demarcada na superfície íntima de uma artéria; produzida por depósito de lipídios na íntima.
bacterial p., p. bacteriana; em odontologia, uma massa de microrganismos filamentosos e uma grande variedade de formas menores fixadas à superfície de um dente que, dependendo da atividade bacteriana e de fatores ambientais, pode dar origem a cáries, tártaro ou alterações inflamatórias no tecido adjacente. SIN dental p. (2), mucous p., mucinous p.
bacteriophage p., p. de bacteriófago; uma zona circular clara em um crescimento de bactérias confluente em uma superfície de ágar, resultante da lise de bactérias por vírus bacterianos.
dental p., p. dentária; **(1)** o acúmulo não-calcificado, principalmente de microrganismos orais e seus produtos, que adere firmemente aos dentes e não é facilmente removido; **(2)** SIN bacterial p.
Hollenhorst p.'s, placas de Hollenhorst; êmbolos ateromatosos, laranja-amarelado, brilhantes nas arteríolas retinianas, que contêm cristais de colesterol e originam-se na artéria carótida ou nos grandes vasos.
mucous p., mucinous p., p. mucosa. SIN bacterial p.
neuritic p., p. neurítica. SIN senile p.
pleural p., p. pleural; espessamento fibroso da pleura parietal, caracteristicamente causado por exposição inalatória ao asbesto; é comum haver calcificação microscópica e macroscópica nessa lesão.
Randall p.'s, placas de Randall; concentrações de minerais nas papilas renais.
senile p., p. senil; uma massa esférica composta basicamente de fibrilas amilóides e processos neuronais entrelaçados, freqüentemente, embora não exclusivamente, observada na doença de Alzheimer. SIN neuritic p.
Plaque In·dex. Índice de Placa; índice para estimar o estado de higiene oral medindo-se a placa dental que ocorre nas áreas adjacentes à margem gengival.
-plasia. -Plasia; formação (principalmente de células). VER plasma-. [G. *plassō*, formar]
plasm (plazm). Plasma. SIN plasma.
plas·ma (plaz′mă). Plasma. **1.** A porção líquida proteinácea (acelular) do sangue circulante, distinta do soro obtido após coagulação. SIN blood p. **2.** A porção líquida da linfa. **3.** O líquido no qual as gotículas de gordura do leite estão suspensas. **4.** Um "quarto estado da matéria" no qual, devido à temperatura elevada, os átomos se romperam para formar elétrons livres e núcleos mais ou menos despojados; produzido no laboratório em conjunto com a pesquisa de fusão de hidrogênio (termonuclear). SIN plasm. [G. algo formado]
antihemophilic p., p. anti-hemofílico; p. humano no qual o componente globulina anti-hemofílica lábil, presente no p. fresco, foi preservado; é usado para aliviar temporariamente a disfunção do mecanismo hemostático na hemofilia.
blood p., p. sanguíneo. SIN plasma (1).
p. expander (plaz′mă eks-pan′der). Expansor plasmático. SIN plasma substitute.
fresh frozen p. (FFP), p. fresco congelado; p. separado; congelado nas 6 horas seguintes à coleta, usado na hipovolemia e na deficiência de fator da coagulação.

plasma sanguíneo		
componentes selecionados do plasma ou soro: faixas normais		
ácido úrico (enzimático)	♂ 155–404 ♀ 119–375	μmol/l
ácidos graxos, livres	200–900	μmol/l
bicarbonato	21–25	mmol/l
bilirrubina (direta)	até 6,8	μmol/l
bilirrubina (total)	5,1–18,8	μmol/l
cálcio	2,2–2,7	mmol/l
capacidade de ligação do ferro		
-total	♂ 53,7–71,6 ♀ 44,8–62,7	μmol/l
-livre	♂ 35,8–53,7 ♀ 26,9–44,8	μmol/l
chumbo (sangue total)	até 2,0	μmol/l
cloreto	94–111	mmol/l
cobre	♂ 11,0–22,0 ♀ 13,4–24,4	μmol/l
colesterol	3,36–5,20*	mmol/l
creatina	♂ 23–61 ♀ 23–92	μmol/l
creatinina	♂ 62–106 ♀ 44–88	μmol/l
ferro	♂ 16,1–25,1 ♀ 14,3–21,5	μmol/l
fósforo, inorgânico	0,81–1,55	mmol/l
frutose	até 0,55	mmol/l
galactose	até 0,24	mmol/l
glicose	3,33–5,55*	mmol/l
gordura, total	3,6–8,2*	g/l
lactato	1,00–1,78	mmol/l
LDL-colesterol		
lítio	0,4–6,3	μmol/l
magnésio	0,66–0,90	mmol/l
nitrogênio amoniacal (sangue total)	53–143	μmol/l
potássio	4,1–5,6	mmol/l
proteínas totais	67–87	g/l
sódio	137–148	mmol/l
tiroxina	66–187	nmol/l
triglicerídeos	0,4–15	g/l
uréia	3,33–6,66	mmol/l

*dependente da idade

p. hydrolysate, hidrolisado de p.; condensado artificial de proteínas derivadas do p. sanguíneo bovino, preparado por um método de hidrólise suficiente para fornecer mais da metade do nitrogênio total presente na forma de α-amino nitrogênio; usado quando está indicado aporte proteico elevado que não pode ser obtido através de alimentos comuns. VER TAMBÉM protein hydrolysate.
p. mari'num, p. marinho; água do mar diluída para torná-la isotônica em relação ao plasma.
muscle p., p. muscular; líquido alcalino no músculo que se coagula espontaneamente, separando-se em miosina e soro muscular.
normal human p., p. humano normal; p. estéril obtido por reunião de quantidades aproximadamente iguais da porção líquida do sangue total citratado de oito ou mais seres humanos adultos sem qualquer doença transmissível por transfusão, e tratado com radiação ultravioleta para destruir possíveis contaminantes bacterianos e virais.
salted p., p. salgado; a porção líquida de sangue retirada dos vasos, cuja coagulação é impedida por colocação em uma solução de sulfato de sódio ou de magnésio. SIN salted serum.
plasma-, plasmat-, plasmato-, plasmo-. Plasma-, plasmat-, plasmato-, plasmo-; formador, organizado; plasma. [G. *plasma*, algo formado]
plas·ma·blast (plaz′mă-blast). Plasmoblasto; precursor do plasmócito. SIN plasmacytoblast. [plasma + G. *blastos*, germe]
plas·ma cell dys·cra·sia. Discrasia de plasmócitos; grupo diverso de doenças caracterizado pela proliferação de um único clone de células que produz

uma imunoglobulina monoclonal ou fragmento de imunoglobulina (um componente M sérico). As células geralmente possuem morfologia de plasmócitos, mas podem ter morfologia linfocítica ou linfoplasmacítica. Esse grupo inclui mieloma múltiplo, macroglobulinemia de Waldenström, doença da cadeia pesada, gamopatia monoclonal benigna e amiloidose imunocítica.

plas·ma·crit (plaz′mă-krit). Plasmácrito; medida da percentagem do volume de sangue ocupado por plasma, em contraste com um hematócrito. [plasma + G. *krino*, separar]

plas·ma·cyte (plaz′mă-sīt). Plasmócito. SIN plasma cell.

plas·ma·cy·to·blast (plas-mă-sī′tō-blast). Plasmacitoblasto. SIN plasmablast.

plas·ma·cy·to·ma (plaz′mă-sī-tō′mă). Plasmacitoma; massa distinta, provavelmente solitária, de plasmócitos neoplásicos no osso ou em um dos vários locais extramedulares; em seres humanos, essas lesões provavelmente são a fase inicial do mieloma de plasmócitos em desenvolvimento. [plasmacyte + G. *-oma*, tumor]

plas·ma·cy·to·sis (plaz′mă-sī-tō′sis). Plasmocitose. **1.** Presença de plasmócitos no sangue circulante. **2.** Presença de proporções incomumente grandes de plasmócitos nos tecidos ou exsudatos. [plasmacyte + G. *-osis*, condição]

plas·ma·gene (plaz′mă-jēn). Plasmagene; determinante de uma característica hereditária localizado no citoplasma. SIN cytogene. [plasma + gene]

plas·ma·ki·nins (plaz′mă-kī′ninz). Plasmacininas; grupo de oligopeptídeos altamente ativos encontrados em soros que atuam sobre o músculo liso de vasos sanguíneos, útero, brônquios, etc.; p. ex., bradicinina, calidina.

plas·ma·lem·ma (plaz-mă-lem′ă). Plasmalema, membrana celular. SIN cell membrane. [plasma + G. *lemma*, casca]

plas·mal·o·gens (plaz-mal′ō-jenz). Plasmalogênios; termo genérico para glicerofosfolipídios nos quais a porção glicerol possui um grupamento 1-alquenil éter (em ocasiões mais raras, um grupamento 1-alquil éter); p. ex., alqui-1-enilglicerofosfolipídio; a síntese de plasmalogênios está reduzida em distúrbios do peroxissoma. SIN phosphoglyceracetals.

plas·mals (plaz′mălz). Plasmais; aldeídos de cadeia longa que ocorrem em plasmalogênios; p. ex., estearaldeído, palmitaldeído.

plas·ma·phe·re·sis (plaz′mă-fĕ-rē′sis). Plasmaférese; remoção de todo o sangue do corpo, separação de seus elementos celulares por centrifugação e reinfusão deles suspensos em solução salina ou algum outro substituto do plasma, assim causando depleção do plasma corporal sem que haja depleção de suas células. [plasma + G. *aphairesis*, retirada]

plas·ma·phe·ret·ic (plaz′mă-fĕ-ret′ik). Plasmaferético; relativo à plasmaférese.

plasmat-. VER plasma-.

plas·mat·ic (plaz-mat′ik). Plasmático; relativo ao plasma. SIN plasmic.

plas·ma·tog·a·my (plaz-mă-tog′ă-mē). Plasmatogamia. SIN plasmogamy.

plas·men·ic ac·id (plaz′men-ik). Ácido plasmênico; nome proposto para fosfatidatos como 2-acil-1-alqui-enilglicerol 3-fosfato.

plas·mic (plaz′mik). Plásmico. SIN plasmatic.

plas·mid (plaz′mid). Plasmídeo; partícula genética fisicamente separada do cromossoma da célula hospedeira (principalmente bacteriana) que consegue funcionar de forma estável e replicar-se, geralmente, conferindo alguma vantagem à célula hospedeira; não-essencial para o funcionamento básico da célula. SIN extrachromosomal element, extrachromosomal genetic element, paragene. [cyto*plasm*, + -id]

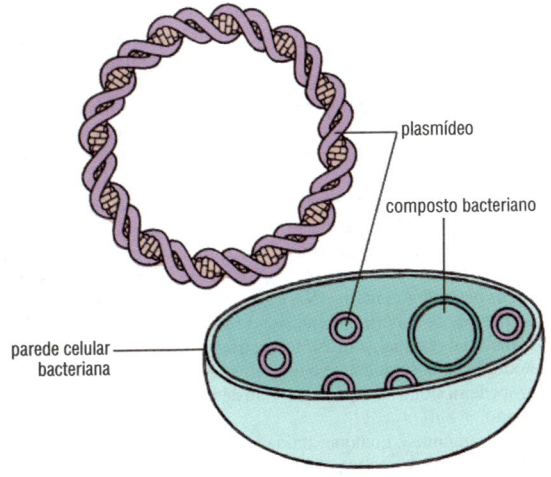

plasmídeo

bacteriocinogenic p.'s, plasmídeos bacteriocinogênicos; plasmídeos bacterianos responsáveis pela produção de bacteriocinas. SIN bacteriocin factors, bacteriocinogens.

conjugative p., p. conjugativo; p. que pode realizar sua própria transferência intercelular por meio de conjugação; essa transferência é realizada pela transformação de uma bactéria em doador, geralmente com *pili* especializados. SIN infectious p., transmissible p.

F p., p. F; o protótipo conjugativo associado à conjugação na cepa K-12 da *Escherichia coli.* SIN fertility factor, sex factor.

infectious p., p. infeccioso. SIN conjugative p.

nonconjugative p., p. não-conjugativo; p. que não pode realizar conjugação e autotransferência para outra bactéria (cepa bacteriana); a transferência depende da mediação de outro p. (conjugativo).

R p.'s, plasmídeos R. SIN resistance p.'s.

resistance p.'s, plasmídeos de resistência; plasmídeos que transportam genes responsáveis pela resistência a antibióticos (ou fármaco antibacteriano) entre bactérias (notavelmente Enterobacteriaceae); podem ser plasmídeos conjugativos ou não-conjugativos, com o primeiro possuindo genes de transferência (fator de transferência de resistência) ausentes no último. SIN R factors, R p.'s, resistance factors, resistance-transferring episomes.

transmissible p., p. transmissível. SIN conjugative p.

plas·min (plaz′min). Plasmina; proteinase sérica que hidrolisa peptídeos e ésteres da L-arginina e L-lisina e converte a fibrina em produtos solúveis; encontrada no plasma na forma do precursor plasminogênio (pró-fibrinolisina) e é ativada em plasmina por solventes orgânicos, que removem um inibidor, e pela estreptocinase, tripsina e ativador do plasminogênio, todos clivando uma única ligação arginil-valil; a plasmina é responsável pela dissolução de coágulos sanguíneos. SIN fibrinase (2), fibrinolysin.

plas·min·o·gen (plaz-min′ō-jen). Plasminogênio; um precursor da plasmina. Há deficiência autossômica dominante de plasmina [MIM*173350] que pode promover trombose. VER plasmin.

plas·min·o·ki·nase (plaz′min-ō-kī′nās). Plasminocinase, estreptoquinase. SIN streptokinase.

plas·min·o·plas·tin (plaz′min-ō-plas′tin). Plasminoplastina; termo proposto para agentes ativadores que produzem plasmina por ação direta sobre o plasminogênio; p. ex., estafilocinase, ativador do plasminogênio.

plasmo-. VER plasma-.

plas·mo·dia (plaz-mō′dē-ă). Plasmódios; plural de plasmodium. [L.]

plas·mo·di·al (plaz-mō′dē-ăl). Plasmodial. **1.** Relativo a um plasmódio. **2.** Relativo a qualquer espécie do gênero *Plasmodium.*

plas·mo·di·o·tro·pho·blast (plaz-mō′dē-ō-trō′fō-blast). Plasmodiotrofoblasto. SIN syncytiotrophoblast. [plasmodium + G. *trophē*, nutrição, + *blastos*, germe]

Plas·mo·di·um (plaz-mō′dē-ŭm). Gênero da família de protozoários Plasmodiidae (subordem Haemosporina, subclasse Coccidia), parasitas sanguíneos de vertebrados, caracterizados por microgametas e macrogametas distintos, um oocineto móvel, esporogonia no hospedeiro invertebrado e merogonia (esquizogonia) no hospedeiro vertebrado; inclui os agentes causadores da malária nos seres humanos e em outros animais, com um ciclo assexuado ocorrendo no fígado e nas hemácias de vertebrados e um ciclo sexuado em mosquitos, com este último ciclo resultando na produção de numerosos esporozoítas infecciosos nas glândulas salivares do vetor, que são transmitidos quando o mosquito pica e retira sangue. A malária dos primatas é transmitida por várias espécies de mosquitos *Anopheles*, e a malária das aves, por espécies de *Aedes, Culex, Anopheles* e *Culiseta.* [L. mod. do G. *plasma*, algo formado, + *eidos*, aparência]

P. aethio′picum. SIN *P. falciparum.*

P. ber′ghei, espécie de protozoário que é o agente etiológico da malária de roedores da África central; uma fonte importante de malária experimental em mamíferos não-primatas.

P. brazilian′um, espécie de protozoário encontrada em macacos do Novo Mundo da família Cebidae no norte da América do Sul e no Panamá, que pode causar malária leve no homem.

P. cynomol′gi, espécie de protozoário semelhante ao *P. vivax* que ocorre naturalmente no macaco, mas que infecta seres humanos de forma acidental e experimental; provoca um tipo de malária semelhante à causada pelo *P. -vivax.*

P. falcip′arum, *Laverania falciparum*, espécie causadora da malária falcípara (terçã maligna); um trofozoíta jovem tem cerca de um quinto do tamanho de um eritrócito, mas raramente são observados estágios eritrocíticos no sangue circulante, pois tornam as células infectadas aderentes e causam sua concentração em capilares nos órgãos vitais, particularmente o encéfalo e o coração; um esquizonte ocupa cerca de metade a dois terços da hemácia e tem grânulos finos, esparsos (observados apenas no sangue periférico de pacientes moribundos); os eritrócitos infectados são de tamanho normal ou pequenos e, provavelmente, contêm grânulos basófilos e pontos vermelhos (fendas ou pontos de Maurer); a infecção múltipla é extremamente freqüente e causa episódios de febre algo irregulares, pois os ciclos de multiplicação do parasita geralmente são assincrônicos. SIN malignant tertian malarial parasite, *P. aethiopicum.*

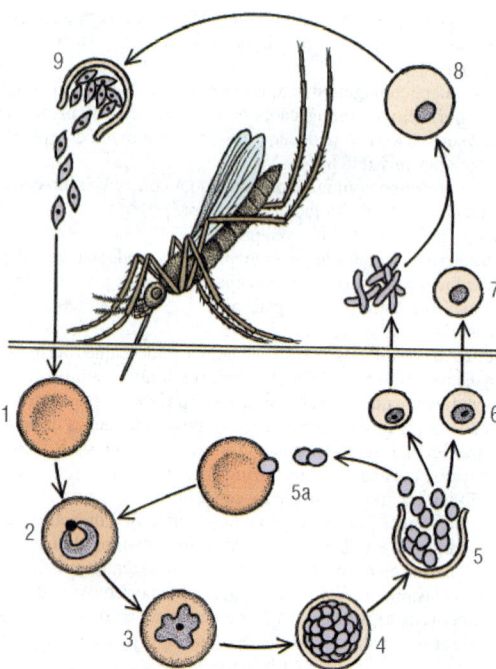

plasmódio: ciclo vital; (1) esporozoíta invadindo a hemácia; (2) estágio "anular" do desenvolvimento; (3) estágio amebóide do desenvolvimento; (4) divisão assexuada; (5) ruptura celular com liberação de esporo; (5a) reinfecção de hemácias por alguns esporos; (6) desenvolvimento de outros esporos em formas sexuadas; (7) desenvolvimento em óvulo e espermatozóide após serem sugados pelo mosquito; (8) transformação de célula fertilizada em cisto; (9) ruptura do cisto com liberação de esporozoítas

P. knowles'i, espécie de protozoário do Sudeste Asiático que causa malária do macaco com um ciclo febril cotidiano; altamente fatal em macacos rhesus; naturalmente adquirido por um ser humano na Malásia, sendo também transmitido experimentalmente aos seres humanos.

P. ko'chi, espécie de *P.* agora reconhecida como *Hepatocystis kochi.*

P. mala'riae, espécie de protozoário causadora da malária quartã; um trofozoíta no estágio anular é triangular, ovóide ou ligeiramente reniforme, com grânulos pretos, finos ou grosseiros, e aproximadamente um terço do tamanho de um eritrócito; o esquizonte é oval ou arredondado e ocupa quase toda a hemácia; os eritrócitos infectados têm tamanho normal ou ligeiramente reduzido, geralmente sem pontilhado (as duas características mais importantes que os distinguem do *P. vivax*), embora possam ser observados pontos de Ziemann extremamente finos; a infecção múltipla é extremamente rara; assim, os episódios de febre ocorrem regularmente a intervalos de 72 horas; a parasitemia assintomática prolongada é característica da espécie, e pode haver recrudescência da febre 10 anos ou mais após o episódio inicial. SIN quartan parasite.

P. ova'le, espécie de protozoário que é o agente da forma menos comum de malária humana; assemelha-se ao *P. vivax* em seus estágios anteriores, mas freqüentemente modifica a membrana celular, causando a formação de um contorno fimbriado, e, freqüentemente, assume um formato oval; os pontos de Schüffner são abundantes e surgem cedo, as células hospedeiras são normais ou apenas ligeiramente aumentadas, e são produzidos apenas cerca de 8–10 merozoítos semelhantes a uvas; a febre é terçã (a cada 48 horas) e as recidivas são pouco freqüentes.

P. vi'vax, espécie de protozoário que é o parasita mais comum da malária nos seres humanos (exceto no oeste da África, onde a forma do antígeno Duffy (FyFy) protege a maioria das populações residentes, o que permitiu que o *P. ovale* substituísse o *P. vivax*); o trofozoíta inicial é irregular e amebóide, um quarto a um terço do tamanho de uma hemácia, e contém vários grânulos finos; o esquizonte tem formato irregular, ocupa o eritrócito aumentado e contém numerosos grânulos de pigmentos amarelo-acastanhados; as hemácias afetadas são pálidas, aumentadas e contêm pontos de Schüffner nos estágios avançados de crescimento; caracteristicamente, causa episódios de febre bastante regulares a intervalos de 48 horas, mas é comum haver infecção múltipla, causando padrões irregulares de febre. SIN tertian parasite.

plas·mo·di·um, pl. **plas·mo·dia** (plaz-mō′dē-ŭm, -dē-ă). Plasmódio; massa protoplasmática que contém vários núcleos, resultante da multiplicação do núcleo com divisão celular. [L. mod. do G. *plasma,* algo formado, + *eidos,* aparência]

placental p., sinciciotrofoblasto. SIN syncytiotrophoblast.

Plas·mo·dro·ma·ta (plaz-mō-drō′ma-tă). Categoria taxonômica antiga que incluía Protozoa amebóides e flagelados nos quais o núcleo não é separa-do em porções reprodutiva (micro) e vegetativa (macro); equivalente ao atual filo Sarcomastigophora. [plasmo- + G. *dromos,* deslocamento, curso]

plas·mog·a·my (plaz-mog′ă-mē). Plasmogamia; união de duas ou mais células com preservação dos núcleos individuais; formação de um plasmódio. SIN plasmatogamy, plastogamy. [plasmo- + G. *gamos,* casamento]

plas·mo·gen (plaz-mō-jen). Plasmogênio, protoplasma. SIN protoplasm. [plasmo- + G. *-gen,* que produz]

plas·mo·ki·nin (plaz-mō-kī′nin). Plasmocinina; termo obsoleto para designar o fator VIII (*factor* VIII).

plas·mo·lem·ma (plaz-mō-lem′ă). Plasmolema. SIN cell membrane.

plas·mol·y·sis (plaz-mol′i-sis). Plasmólise; retração de células vegetais por perda osmótica de água citoplasmática. SIN protoplasmolysis. [plasmo- + G. *lysis,* dissolução]

plas·mo·lyt·ic (plaz-mō-lit′ik). Plasmolítico; relativo à plasmólise.

plas·mo·lyze (plaz′mō-līz). Plasmolisar; submeter a plasmólise.

plas·mon (plaz′mon). Plasmônio; o total dos determinantes genéticos extra-cromossômicos do citoplasma da célula eucariótica. SIN plasmotype. [cyto*plasm* + -on]

plas·mor·rhex·is (plaz-mō-rek′sis). Plasmorrexe; a abertura violenta de uma célula por pressão do protoplasma.

plas·mos·chi·sis (plaz-mos′ki-sis). Plasmosquise; a divisão do protoplasma em fragmentos. [plasmo- + G. *schisis,* clivagem]

plas·mo·sin (plaz′mō-sin). Plasmosina; substância altamente viscosa no citoplasma que contém fibras distintas de comprimento considerável; uma nucleoproteína considerada como a base estrutural da célula.

plas·mot·o·my (plaz-mot′ō-mē). Plasmotomia; forma de mitose em células de protozoários multinucleados na qual o citoplasma divide-se em duas massas ou mais, depois se reproduzindo, em alguns casos por esporulação. [plasmo- + G. *tome,* incisão]

plas·mo·tro·pic (plaz-mō-trop′ik). Plasmotrópico; relativo a ou que exibe plasmotropismo.

plas·mot·ro·pism (plaz-mot′rō-pizm). Plasmotropismo; condição na qual a medula óssea, o baço e o fígado são locais para a destruição dos eritrócitos, ao contrário da destruição no sangue circulante. [plasmo- + G. *trope,* volta]

plas·mo·type (plaz′mō-tip). Plasmótipo. SIN plasmon.

plas·mo·zyme (plaz′mō-zīm). Plasmozima; designação obsoleta de protrombina. [plasmo- + G. *zyme,* levedura]

plas·tein (plas′tē-in). Plasteína. **1.** Polipeptídeo insolúvel formado pela condensação aleatória de aminoácidos ou peptídeos sob a influência catalítica de uma quimiotripsina semelhante a uma proteinase; são descritos pesos moleculares de até 500.000. **2.** Gel formado ao se tratar um hidrolisado parcial de uma proteína com uma endopeptidase.

plas·ter. 1. Emplastro; preparação sólida que pode ser espalhada quando aquecida e que se torna aderente à temperatura do corpo; usada para manter as bordas de uma ferida em aposição, para proteger superfícies desnudas e, quando medicado, para enrubescer ou formar vesículas na pele, como no emplastro de mostarda, ou para aplicar medicamentos à superfície a fim de obter seus efeitos sistêmicos. **2.** Em odontologia, coloquialismo para gesso. [L. *emplastrum;* G. *emplastron,* gesso ou molde]

p. of Paris, gesso; sulfato de cálcio dessecado do qual foi expelida a água de cristalização por calor, mas que, quando misturado com água, formará uma pasta que depois endurece.

plas·tic (plas′tik). Plástico. **1.** Capaz de ser formado ou moldado. **2.** Material que pode ser moldado por pressão ou calor na forma de uma cavidade ou molde. [G. *plastikos,* relativo à moldagem]

Bingham p., p. de Bingham; material que, em situação ideal, não flui até que seja ultrapassada uma tensão crítica (tensão de escoamento), fluindo então a uma velocidade proporcional ao excesso de tensão acima da tensão de escoamento; os materiais reais provavelmente apenas se aproximam deste modelo ideal.

modeling p., p. de modelagem; material termoplástico geralmente composto de goma de damar e greda preparada, usado particularmente para fazer impressões dentais. SIN impression compound, modeling composition, modeling compound.

plas·tic·i·ty (plas-tis′i-tē). Plasticidade; a capacidade de ser formado ou moldado; a qualidade de ser plástico.

plas·tid (plas′tid). Plastídio. **1.** Uma das estruturas diferenciadas no citoplasma de células vegetais, onde são realizados a fotossíntese ou outros processos celulares; os plastídios contêm DNA e são auto-replicantes. SIN trophoblast. **2.** Um dos grânulos de matéria estranha ou diferenciada, partículas de alimentos, gordura, material residual, cromatóforos, tricocistos, etc., nas células. **3.** Partícula autoduplicante, semelhante a um vírus, que se multiplica dentro de uma célula hospedeira, como as partículas κ em determinados paramécios. [G. *plastos,* formado, + -id]

blood p., p. sanguíneo; qualquer unidade morfológica básica na composição biológica do sangue, p. ex., um eritrócito.

plas·to·chro·man·ol-3, plas·to·chro·ma·nol E$_3$ (plas-tō-krō′man-ol). Plastocromanol-3, plastocromanol E$_3$; um γ-tocotrienol. VER tocotrienol.

plas·to·chro·men·ol-8 (plas-tō-krō′men-ol). Plastocromenol-8; a forma cromenol (isomérica) da plastoquinona-9. SIN solanochromene.

plas·tog·a·my (plas-tog′a-mē). Plastogamia. SIN plasmogamy.

plas·to·quin·one (PQ) (plas-tō-kwin′ōn, -kwi′nōn). Plastoquinona; 2,3-dimetil-1,4-benzoquinona com uma cadeia lateral multiprenil; nome trivial usado algumas vezes para plastoquinona-9.

plas·to·quin·one-9 (PQ-9), plas·to·quin·one E$_9$. Plastoquinona-9, plastoquinona E$_9$; 2,3-dimetil-6-nonaprenil-1,4-benzoquinona; pertencente a um grupo de vitaminas E e K e coenzimas Q; a forma isomérica é o plastocromenol-8; um participante do transporte de elétrons na fotossíntese.

plas·tron. Plastrom; plastrão; o esterno com as cartilagens costais a ele fixadas. [Fr. plastrom]

-plasty. -Plastia; moldagem ou o resultado desta; procedimento cirúrgico para reparo de um defeito ou restauração de uma forma e/ou função de uma parte. [G. *plastos*, formado]

plate (plāt). **1** [TA]. Lâmina; em anatomia, uma estrutura fina, relativamente plana. SIN lamina [TA]. **2.** Placa óssea; uma placa de metal com perfurações destinadas à penetração de parafusos, aplicada a um osso fraturado a fim de manter as extremidades em aposição. **3.** A camada de ágar em uma placa de Petri ou recipiente semelhante. **4.** Semear; formar uma camada muito fina de uma cultura bacteriana pelo método de estriação da superfície de uma placa de ágar (geralmente em uma placa de Petri) para isolar microrganismos individuais a partir dos quais se desenvolverá uma colônia de clones. **5.** Qualquer uma das placas perfuradas horizontais que formam o componente de fracionamento de uma coluna na destilação fracionada (ou o equivalente teórico dessa placa). [Fr. ant. *plat*, um objeto plano, do G. *platys*, plano, largo]

alar p. of neural tube, placa alar do tubo neural. SIN alar *lamina* of neural tube.
amorphous selenium p., placa de selênio amorfo. SIN selenium p.
anal p., placa anal; a porção anal da placa cloacal.
axial p., placa axial; a crista primitiva de um embrião.
basal p. of neural tube, lâmina basal do tubo neural. SIN basal *lamina* of neural tube.
base p., placa basal. VER baseplate.
blood p., termo obsoleto para plaqueta (*platelet*).
bone p., placa de metal com perfurações para a inserção de parafusos; usada para imobilizar segmentos fraturados.
buttress p., placa de apoio; placa de metal usada para manter a fixação interna de uma fratura e evitar deslocamento.
cardiogenic p., placa cardiogênica; a camada espessa de mesoderma esplâncnico da qual são derivados os primórdios cardiopericárdicos de embriões muito jovens.
cell p., placa celular; estrutura não constituída de celulose, que é a precursora da parede celular; forma-se entre núcleos-filhos durante a mitose.
chorionic p., p. coriônica; aquela parte da parede coriônica situada na região de sua fixação uterina; consiste no mesoderma que reveste a vesícula coriônica e, do lado materno, no trofoblasto que reveste os espaços intervilosos; na última metade da gestação, o tecido conjuntivo mesodérmico é quase todo substituído por material fibrinóide, e a membrana amniótica está aderida ao lado fetal da placa.
cloacal p., p. cloacal; placa, composta de uma camada de endoderma cloacal em contato com uma camada de ectoderma do proctódio, que depois se torna a membrana cloacal e se rompe, formando as aberturas anal e urogenital do embrião.
compression p., p. de compressão; placa para fixação interna de fratura com orifícios para introdução de parafusos, projetados de forma que a inserção dos parafusos una os fragmentos ósseos de forma mais firme.
cribriform p. of ethmoid bone [TA], lâmina cribriforme do etmóide; lâmina horizontal da qual estão suspensos o labirinto, de cada lado, e a lâmina perpendicular, no centro; encaixa-se na incisura etmoidal do osso frontal e sustenta os lobos olfatórios do cérebro, apresentando numerosas perfurações para a passagem dos nervos olfatórios. SIN lamina cribrosa ossis ethmoidalis [TA], cribrum, sieve bone, sieve p.
cutis p., dermátomo. SIN dermatome (2).
dorsal p. of neural tube, placa dorsal do tubo neural. SIN roof p.
dorsolateral p. of neural tube, placa dorsolateral do tubo neural. SIN alar *lamina* of neural tube.
end p., p. terminal. VER endplate.
epiphysial p. [TA], lâmina epifisial; o disco de cartilagem situado entre a metáfise e o epidídimo de um osso longo imaturo, permitindo crescimento em comprimento. SIN lamina epiphysialis [TA], growth p.
equatorial p., p. equatorial; a reunião dos cromossomas na mitose.
ethmovomerine p., p. etmovomerina; a porção central do osso etmóide, que forma um elemento distinto ao nascimento.
flat p., jargão para radiografia simples (plain *film*).
floor p., placa do assoalho; placa ventral; adelgaçamento ventral na linha média do tubo neural em desenvolvimento, uma continuidade entre as lâminas basais de cada lado; oposta à placa do teto. SIN ventral p.
foot p., p. do pé. VER footplate.
frontal p., p. frontal; no feto, uma placa de cartilagem entre as partes laterais da cartilagem etmóide e o osso esfenóide em desenvolvimento.
growth p., p. de crescimento. SIN epiphysial p.
horizontal p. of palatine bone [TA], lâmina horizontal do palatino; a parte do palatino que forma a porção posterior (aproximadamente um terço) do palato ósseo. SIN lamina horizontalis ossis palatini [TA].
Kühne p., p. de Kühne; a placa terminal de uma fibra nervosa motora em um fuso muscular.
lateral p., p. lateral; uma massa não-segmentada de mesoderma na periferia lateral do disco embrionário; forma o mesoderma somatopleural (parietal) e esplancnopleural (visceral).
lateral cartilaginous p., lâmina lateral da cartilagem da tuba auditiva. SIN lateral *lamina* of cartilage of pharyngotympanic (auditory) tube.
lateral p. of cartilaginous auditory tube, lâmina lateral da cartilagem da tuba auditiva. SIN lateral *lamina* of cartilage of pharyngotympanic (auditory) tube.
lateral pterygoid p. [TA], lâmina lateral do processo pterigóide; a maior e mais lateral das duas lâminas ósseas que descem a partir do ponto de união do corpo e da asa maior do osso esfenóide de cada lado; forma a parede medial da fossa infratemporal e dá origem aos músculos pterigóideos. SIN lamina lateralis processus pterygoidei [TA], lateral p. of pterygoid process.
lateral p. of pterygoid process, lâmina lateral do processo pterigóide. SIN lateral pterygoid p.
lingual p., placa lingual. SIN linguoplate.
medial cartilaginous p., lâmina medial da cartilagem da tuba auditiva. SIN medial *lamina* of cartilage of pharyngotympanic (auditory) tube.
medial p. of cartilaginous auditory tube, lâmina medial da cartilagem da tuba auditiva. SIN medial *lamina* of cartilage of pharyngotympanic (auditory) tube.
medial pterygoid p. [TA], lâmina medial do processo pterigóide; a menor e mais medial das duas lâminas ósseas que se estendem para baixo a partir do ponto de união do corpo e da asa maior do esfenóide de cada lado, terminando inferiormente no hâmulo pterigóideo. SIN lamina medialis processus pterygoidei [TA], medial p. of pterygoid process.
medial p. of pterygoid process, lâmina medial do processo pterigóide. SIN medial pterygoid p.
medullary p., placa neural. SIN neural p.
p. of modiolus, lâmina do modíolo. SIN lamina of modiolus of cochlea.
motor p., placa motora; uma placa terminal motora.
muscle p., placa muscular. SIN myotome (2).
nail p., placa ungueal. SIN nail (1).
neural p., placa neural; a região neuroectodérmica da superfície dorsal do embrião inicial que mais tarde é transformada no tubo neural e crista neural. SIN medullary p.
neutralization p., placa de neutralização; placa metálica usada para fixação interna de uma fratura óssea para neutralizar as forças que produzem deslocamento.
notochordal p., placa da notocorda; a lâmina de células da notocorda intercalada no teto endodérmico do saco vitelino primitivo. VER TAMBÉM head *process*.
oral p., placa oral; área circunscrita de fusão do endoderma do intestino anterior e do ectoderma do estomódio no embrião, rompendo-se no início do desenvolvimento para estabelecer a abertura da boca. VER TAMBÉM buccopharyngeal *membrane*.
orbital p., lâmina orbital. SIN orbital p. of ethmoid bone.
orbital p. of ethmoid bone [TA], lâmina orbital do etmóide; uma fina lâmina do osso etmóide que forma parte da parede medial da órbita e a parede lateral do labirinto etmoidal. SIN lamina orbitalis ossis ethmoidalis [TA], lamina papyracea, orbital lamina of ethmoid bone, orbital layer of ethmoid bone, orbital p., paper p., papyraceous p.
palatal p., placa palatina; conector principal de dentadura parcial cuja largura ântero-posterior é maior que a dos dois pré-molares maxilares.
palmar p.'s, placas palmares. SIN palmar *ligaments* of metacarpophalangeal joints, em *ligament*.
paper p., papyraceous p., lâmina papirácea. SIN orbital p. of ethmoid bone.
parachordal p., p. paracordal; os primórdios cartilaginosos da base do crânio situados de cada lado da parte cefálica da notocorda.
parietal p., lâmina parietal; **(1)** a mais externa das duas camadas do mesoderma da lâmina lateral, que é associada ao ectoderma; o ectoderma e o mesoderma da lâmina parietal juntos formam a somatopleura; **(2)** a lâmina do osso etmóide que forma parte do septo nasal.
perpendicular p. [TA], lâmina perpendicular; porção plana de um osso situada em um plano vertical ou que se aproxima muito dele. VER perpendicular p. of ethmoid bone, perpendicular p. of palatine bone. SIN lamina perpendicularis [TA], pars perpendicularis, vertical p.
perpendicular p. of ethmoid bone [TA], lâmina perpendicular do etmóide; uma lâmina fina de osso que se projeta para baixo a partir da crista etmoidal; forma parte do septo nasal. SIN lamina perpendicularis ossis ethmoidalis [TA].
perpendicular p. of palatine bone [TA], lâmina perpendicular do palatino que se estende verticalmente para cima a partir da lâmina horizontal; forma parte da parede lateral da cavidade nasal. SIN lamina perpendicularis ossis palatini. [TA].

phosphor p., placa de fósforo; a placa revestida usada no lugar de um chassi radiológico em um sistema radiológico computadorizado. VER TAMBÉM selenium p., amorphous *silicon*.
polar p.'s, placas polares; corpos semelhantes a placas condensados nas extremidades do fuso durante a mitose de alguns tipos de células.
prechordal p., placa pré-cordal. SIN prochordal p.
prochordal p., placa pré-cordal; uma pequena área imediatamente rostral à extremidade cefálica da notocorda onde o ectoderma e o endoderma estão em contato; quando voltada sob a cabeça em crescimento, forma a membrana buceofaríngea. VER TAMBÉM oral p. SIN prechordal p.
pterygoid p.'s, lâminas pterigóides. VER lateral pterygoid p., medial pterygoid p.
quadrigeminal p., lâmina do teto do mesencéfalo. SIN lamina of mesencephalic tectum.
roof p., lâmina do teto; a camada fina do tubo neural embrionário que une as lâminas alares dorsalmente. SIN dorsal p. of neural tube.
secondary spiral p., lâmina espiral secundária. SIN secondary spiral *lamina*.
segmental p., placa segmentar. SIN segmental *zone*.
selenium p., placa de selênio; material radiossensível usado em radiografia digital dirigida (directed digital *radiography*). VER TAMBÉM digital *radiography*. SIN amorphous selenium p.
sieve p., lâmina cribriforme do etmóide. SIN cribriform p. of ethmoid bone.
spiral p., lâmina espiral. SIN osseous spiral *lamina*.
stigmal p.'s, placas do estigma; área nas larvas de artrópodes onde o sistema traqueal se abre para o exterior; a morfologia dessa área é usada para identificar várias larvas de artrópodes. VER TAMBÉM spiracle.
suction p., placa de sucção; em odontologia, uma placa mantida no lugar pela pressão atmosférica.
tarsal p.'s, placas tarsais. VER superior *tarsus*, inferior *tarsus*.
tectal p. [TA], lâmina do teto do mesencéfalo. SIN lamina of mesencephalic tectum.
terminal p., lâmina terminal. SIN lamina terminalis of cerebrum.
tympanic p. of temporal bone [TA], parte timpânica do osso temporal; a parte óssea que forma a maior parte da parede anterior da parte óssea do meato acústico externo e da cavidade timpânica, assim como a parede posterior da fossa mandibular. SIN pars tympanica ossis temporalis [TA], tympanic part of temporal bone.
urethral p., placa uretral; o revestimento endodérmico do sulco uretral que forma o revestimento da uretra peniana.
ventral p., placa ventral. SIN floor p.
ventral p. of neural tube, p. ventral do tubo neural. SIN basal *lamina* of neural tube
vertical p., lâmina vertical. SIN perpendicular p.
visceral p., placa visceral; a camada interna das duas camadas do mesoderma lateral; o mesoderma esplâncnico que se associa ao endoderma e, juntamente com este, forma a esplancnopleura.
wing p., lâmina alar. SIN alar *lamina* of neural tube.
Plateau, Joseph Antoine Ferdinand, físico belga, 1801–1883. VER P.-Talbot *law*.
pla·teau (plă-tō). Platô; segmento plano elevado de um registro gráfico. [Fr.]
ventricular p. p. ventricular; uma porção diastólica plana da curva de pressão intraventricular, representando graficamente um equilíbrio ou estado final de enchimento.
plate·let (plāt′let). Plaqueta; um fragmento citoplasmático discóide, de formato irregular, de um megacariócito, eliminado no seio da medula óssea e subseqüentemente encontrado no sangue periférico, onde atua na coagulação. Uma plaqueta contém grânulos na parte central (granulômero) e, perifericamente, protoplasma claro (hialômero), mas sem núcleo definido; tem aproximadamente um terço a metade do tamanho de um eritrócito e não contém hemoglobina. SIN Bizzozero corpuscle, blood disk, elementary bodies (2), elementary particle (1), third corpuscle, thrombocyte, thromboplastid (1), Zimmermann corpuscle. [ver plate]
plate·let·phe·re·sis (plāt′let-fĕ-rē′sis). Plaquetoférese; remoção de sangue de um doador com reposição de todos os componentes do sangue, exceto as plaquetas. [platelet + G. *aphairesis*, retirada]
plat·ing (plāt′ing). 1. Plaqueamento; semeadura de bactérias em meio sólido em uma placa de Petri ou recipiente semelhante; a confecção de uma cultura em placa. 2. Aplicação de uma placa de metal para manter as extremidades de um osso fraturado em aposição. 3. Deposição eletrolítica de um metal.
compression p., técnica para fixação interna que utiliza uma placa de compressão.
replica p., plaqueamento de réplicas; procedimento para produzir uma cópia precisa de colônias bacterianas de uma placa de ágar para outra.
pla·tin·ic (pla-tin′ik). Platínico; relativo à platina; designa um composto que contém platina em sua maior valência.
plat·i·nous (plat′i-nŭs). Platinoso; relativo à platina; designa um composto que contém platina em sua menor valência.
plat·i·num (Pt) (plat′i-nŭm). Platina; elemento metálico, n.° atômico 78, peso atômico 195,08, usado para a confecção de pequenas partes de aparelhos químicos devido à sua resistência aos ácidos; na forma de pó (**platina preta**), é importante catalisador na hidrogenação. Alguns de seus sais foram usados no tratamento da sífilis. Um derivado da platina, a cisplatina, é usado como agente antineoplásico. [L. mod., originalmente *platina*, do Esp. *plata*, prata]
plat·i·num foil. Folha de platina; platina pura enrolada em folhas extremamente finas; seu alto ponto de fusão torna-a adequada como matriz para vários procedimentos de soldagem em odontologia, bem como para proporcionar forma interna para restaurações de porcelana durante sua fabricação.
plat·i·num group. Grupo da platina; grupo de seis elementos anfotéricos: irídio, ósmio, paládio, platina, ródio e rutênio.
Platt, Sir Harry, cirurgião inglês, *1886. VER Putti-P. *operation*, *procedure*.
platy-. Plati-; largura; qualidade de plano. [G. *platys*, plano, largo]
plat·y·ba·sia (plat-i-bā′sē-ă). Platibasia; uma anomalia do desenvolvimento do crânio ou um amolecimento adquirido dos ossos deste, de forma que o assoalho da sua fossa posterior salienta-se para cima, na região em torno do forame magno. SIN basilar invagination. [platy- + G. *basis*, base]
plat·y·ceph·a·ly (plat′i-sef′ă-lē). Platicefalia; achatamento do crânio, condição na qual o índice craniano vertical é menor que 70. SIN platycrania. [platy- + G. *kephalē*, cabeça]
plat·yc·ne·mia (plat′ik-nē′mē-ă). Platicnemia; condição na qual a tíbia é anormalmente larga e plana. SIN platycnemism. [platy- + G. *knēmē*, perna]
plat·yc·ne·mic (plat′ik-nē′mik). Platicnêmico; relativo a, ou caracterizado por, plactinemia.
plat·yc·ne·mism (plat′ik-nē′mizm). Platicnemia. SIN platycnemia.
plat·y·cra·nia (plat′i-krā′nē-ă). Platicrânia. SIN platycephaly. [platy- + G. *kranion*, crânio]
plat·y·cyte (plat′i-sīt). Termo obsoleto para designar uma célula gigante relativamente pequena, formada algumas vezes em tubérculos. [platy- + G. *kytos*, célula]
plat·y·glos·sal (plat′i-glos′ăl). Platiglosso; que possui uma língua larga e achatada. [platy- + G. *glōssa*, língua]
plat·y·hel·minth (plat-i-hel′minth). Platelminto; designação comum de qualquer verme achatado do filo Platyhelminthes; qualquer cestódeo (tênia) ou trematódeo. [platy- + G. *helmins*, verme]
Plat·y·hel·min·thes (plat′i-hel-min′thēz). Filo de vermes planos, bilateralmente simétricos, achatados e acelomados. Alguns platelmintos (Cestoda) não possuem trato digestivo, ou o intestino pode ser incompleto (sem ânus), como nos Trematoda; a maioria das formas é hermafrodita. Há três classes principais, mas as espécies parasitas que têm importância médica e veterinária estão na subclasse Cestoda (as verdadeiras tênias) da classe Cestoidea, e na subclasse Digenea (os trematódeos digenéticos) da classe Trematoda.
plat·y·hi·er·ic (plat-i-hī-er′ik). Platiiérico; que possui um sacro largo. [platy- + G. *heiron*, sacro]
plat·y·mer·ic (plat-i-mē′rik, -mer′ik). Platimérico; que possui um fêmur largo. [platy- + G. *mēros*, coxa]
plat·y·mor·phia (plat′i-mōr′fē-ă). Platimorfia; que possui um formato plano; termo que designa um olho com um eixo ântero-posterior curto. [platy- + G. *morphē*, formato]
plat·y·o·pia (plat′i-ō′pē-ă). Platiopia; face larga; designa uma condição na qual o índice orbitonasal é menor que 107,5. [platy- + G. *ōps*, olho, face]
plat·y·op·ic (plat′i-op′ik, -ō′pik). Platiópico; relativo a, ou caracterizado por, platiopia.
plat·y·pel·lic (plat-i-pel′ik). Platipélico; que possui uma pelve larga, com um índice menor que 90°. VER platypellic *pelvis*. SIN platypelloid. [platy- + G. *pellis*, pelve]
plat·y·pel·loid (plat-ē-pel′oyd). Platipelóide. SIN platypellic.
pla·typ·nea (pla-tip′nē-ă). Platipnéia; dificuldade respiratória em posição ortostática, aliviada em decúbito. Cf. orthopnea. [platy- + G. *pnoē*, respiração]
plat·yr·rhine (plat′i-rīn). Platirrino. 1. Caracterizado por um nariz muito largo em relação ao seu comprimento. 2. Designa um crânio com um índice nasal entre 53 e 58. [platy- + G. *rhis*, nariz]
plat·yr·rhi·ny (plat′i-ri-nē). Platirrinia; condição na qual o nariz é largo em relação ao comprimento.
pla·tys·ma, pl. **pla·tys·mas, pla·tys·ma·ta** (plă-tiz′mă, -tiz′mă-tă) [TA]. Platisma. SIN platysma (*muscle*). [G. *platysma*, uma placa plana]
plat·y·spon·dyl·ia, plat·y·spon·dyl·i·sis (plat-i-spon-dil′ē-ă, plat′i-spon-dil′i-sis). Platispondilia; achatamento dos corpos vertebrais. [platy- + G. *spondylos*, vértebra]
pla·tys·ten·ceph·a·ly (plă-tis′ten-sef′ă-lē). Platistencefalia; largura extrema do crânio na região occipital, com estreitamento anterior e prognatismo. [G. *platystos*, mais largo, superl. de *platys*, largo, + *enkephalē*, encéfalo]
Pleasure, Max A., dentista norte-americano, 1903–1965. VER P. *curve*.
plec·trid·i·um (plek-trid′ē-ŭm). Plectrídio; célula bacteriana em forma de bastonete que contém um esporo em uma extremidade, conferindo-lhe um formato de baqueta, como as células que contêm esporos no microrganismo causador do tétano, *Clostridium tetani*. [L. mod. dim. do G. *plēktron*, um instrumento para golpear]

pled·get (plej'et). Compressa; um tufo de lã, algodão ou linho.
-plegia. -Plegia; paralisia. [G. *plēgē*, acesso]
pleio-. Pleio-; grafia alternativa raramente usada para pleo-.
plei·o·tro·pic (plī-ō-trop'ik). Pleiotrópico; que designa, ou caracterizado por, pleiotropia. SIN polyphenic.
plei·ot·ro·py, plei·o·tro·pia (plī-ot'rō-pē, plī-ō-trō'pē-ă). Pleiotropia; pliotropia; produção por um único gene mutante de efeitos múltiplos, aparentemente não relacionados, em nível clínico ou fenotípico. [pleio- + G. *tropos*, volta]
  functional p., p. funcional; p. causada pela participação da mesma alteração alélica em múltiplos processos distintos; p. ex., a heparina é ativa em muitas reações corporais, incluindo coagulação e o metabolismo de gordura.
  structural p., p. estrutural; p. que ocorre quando duas ou mais regiões de um polipeptídeo podem ter funções biológicas distintas e não-correlatas, sem nada em comum, exceto por serem transcritas e traduzidas ao mesmo tempo.
Pleis·to·pho·ra (plis-tof'er-ah). Gênero de microsporídios no filo de protozoários Microspora, comumente encontrado em peixes e insetos, com esporos mononucleados, de paredes espessas, em grupos de mais de oito. Uma espécie não descrita, mas distinta de *Pleistophora* foi implicada como causa de uma miosite microsporidiana disseminada em um homem imunodeprimido.
pleo-. Pleo-; mais numeroso. [G. *pleiōn*]
ple·o·chro·ic (plē-ō-krō'ik). Pleocrômico. SIN pleochromatic. [pleo- + G. *chroa*, cor]
ple·och·ro·ism (plē-ok'rō-izm). Pleocromia. SIN pleochromatism.
ple·o·chro·mat·ic (plē-ō-krō-mat'ik). Pleocrômico; relativo a pliocromia. SIN pleochroic.
ple·o·chro·ma·tism (plē-ō-krō'mă-tizm). Pleocromia; propriedade de exibir alterações de cor quando iluminado ao longo de diferentes eixos, como determinados cristais ou líquidos. SIN pleochroism. [pleo- + G. *chrōma*, cor]
ple·o·cy·to·sis (plē'ō-sī-tō'sis). Pleocitose; presença de mais células que o normal, freqüentemente designando leucocitose e, principalmente, linfocitose ou infiltração por células redondas; originalmente aplicado à linfocitose do líquido cerebrospinal presente na sífilis do sistema nervoso central. [pleo- + G. *kytos*, célula, + *-osis*, condição]
ple·o·mas·tia, ple·o·ma·zia (plē-ō-mas'tē-ă, mā'zē-ă). Pleomastia, pleomazia. SIN polymastia. [pleo- + G. *mastos*, mama]
ple·o·mor·phic (plē-ō-mōr'fik). Pleomorfo. **1.** SIN polymorphic. **2.** Entre fungos, que possui duas ou mais formas de esporos; também usado para descrever um dermatófito mutante estéril resultante de alterações degenerativas em cultura.
ple·o·mor·phism (plē-ō-mōr'fizm). Pleomorfismo. SIN polymorphism. [pleo- + G. *morphē*, forma]
ple·o·mor·phous (plē-ō-mōr'fŭs). Pleomorfo. SIN polymorphic.
ple·o·nasm (plē'ō-nazm). Pleonasmo; excesso em número ou tamanho das partes. [G. *pleonasmos*, exagero, excessivo, de *pleiōn*, mais]
ple·on·os·te·o·sis (plē'on-os-tē-ō'sis). Pleonosteose; superabundância de formação óssea. [pleo- + G. *osteon*, osso, + *-osis*, condição]
  Leri' p., p. de Leri. SIN dyschondrosteosis.
ple·op·tics (plē-op'tiks). Pleóptica; termo introduzido por Bangerter para incluir todas as formas de tratamento para ambliopia, particularmente aquela associada à fixação excêntrica. [pleo- + optics]
ple·op·to·phor (plē-op'tō-fōr). Pleoptóforo; instrumento para tratamento da ambliopia. [pleo- + G. *optos*, visível, + *phoros*, que conduz]
ple·ro·cer·coid (plē-rō-ser'koyd). Plerocercóide; estágio no desenvolvimento de uma tênia após a fase de procercóide, que se desenvolve em um animal que serve como segundo hospedeiro intermediário ou subseqüente; uma larva não-segmentada, semelhante a um verme, com um escólex em uma extremidade, geralmente não-encistado na carne de vários peixes, répteis ou anfíbios, cuja ingestão transmite o parasita para o hospedeiro final. VER TAMBÉM *Diphyllobothrium latum*. [G. *plērēs*, cheio, completo, + *kerkos*, cauda]
plesio-. Proximidade, semelhança. [G. *plēsios*, perto, próximo]
Ples·i·o·mo·nas. Gênero de bactérias Gram-negativas, facultativamente anaeróbicas, quimioorganotróficas, em forma de bastonetes, móveis. Possui o antígeno enterobacteriano comum. Esse gênero é encontrado em peixes e outros animais aquáticos e em alguns outros animais. Associado à diarréia e à infecção oportunista ocasional em seres humanos.
  P. shigelloides, espécie que é um patógeno entérico e um agente etiológico de várias infecções extra-intestinais transmitidas aos seres humanos por alimento ou água contaminados ou como colonizador de vários animais. Esta é a única espécie do gênero e também foi denominada *Pseudomonas s., Aeromonas s.,* C57 e *Vibrio s.*
ple·si·o·mor·phic (plē'sē-ō-mōr'fik). Plesiomórfico; semelhante na forma. SIN plesiomorphous.
ple·si·o·mor·phism (plē'sē-ō-mōr'fizm). Plesiomorfismo; semelhança na forma. [plesio- + G. *morphē*, forma]
ple·si·o·mor·phous (plē'sē-ō-mōr'fŭs). Plesiomorfo. SIN plesiomorphic.
pless-, plessi-. Pless-, plessi-, plesso-; um golpe, principalmente percussão. [G. *plēssō*, bater]

ples·ses·the·sia (ples-es-thē'zē-ă). Plessestesia. SIN palpatory percussion. [G. *plēsso*, bater, + *aisthēsis*, sensação]
ples·sim·e·ter (ple-sim'e-ter). Plessímetro; placa flexível e oblonga usada na percussão mediata, sendo colocada contra a superfície e golpeada com o plessor. SIN pleximeter, plexometer. [G. *plēssō*, bater, + *metron*, medida]
ples·si·met·ric (ples-i-met'rik). Plessimétrico; relativo a um plessímetro.
ples·sor (ples'er). Plessor; pequeno martelo, geralmente com cabeça de borracha macia, usado para percutir diretamente, ou com um plessímetro, o tórax ou outra parte. SIN percussor, plexor. [G. *plēssō*, bater]
pleth·o·ra (pleth'ō-ră). Pletora. **1.** SIN hypervolemia. **2.** Excesso de qualquer um dos líquidos corporais. [G. *plēthōrē*, plenitude, de *plēthō*, tornar-se cheio]
pleth·or·ic (ple-thor'ik, pleth'ō-rik). Pletórico; relativo à pletora. SIN sanguine (1), sanguineous (2).
ple·thys·mo·graph (ple-thiz'mō-graf). Pletismógrafo; aparelho para medir e registrar alterações no volume de uma parte, órgão ou de todo o corpo. [G. *plēthysmos*, aumento, + *graphō*, escrever]
  body p., p. corporal; aparelho de câmara que circunda todo o corpo, comumente usado em estudos da função respiratória.
  digital p., p. digital; p. aplicado a um dedo da mão ou do pé para medir o fluxo sangüíneo cutâneo.
  pressure p., p. de pressão; **(1)** p. aplicado a uma parte do corpo, p. ex., um segmento do membro, e disposto de forma que o volume seja medido durante aplicação temporária de pressão suficiente a essa parte para esvaziar seus vasos sangüíneos; **(2)** um p. corporal no qual as alterações do volume corporal são medidas em termos das alterações conseqüentes na pressão do ar no p. corporal.
  volume-displacement p., p. de deslocamento de volume; um p., geralmente um p. corporal, no qual alterações de volume deslocam um volume correspondente para dentro ou para fora de um dispositivo de medida muito complacente, como um espirômetro de Krogh ou fluxômetro de integração.
pleth·ys·mog·ra·phy (pleth-iz-mog'ră-fē). Pletismografia; medida e registro de alterações no volume de um órgão ou outra parte do corpo por um pletismógrafo. [G. *plēthysmos*, aumento, + *graphē*, uma escrita]
  impedance p., p. de impedância; registro de alterações na impedância elétrica entre eletrodos colocados em lados opostos de uma parte do corpo, como uma medida de alterações de volume no trajeto da corrente. SIN dielectrography.
  venous occlusion p., p. de oclusão venosa; medida da taxa de influxo arterial em um órgão ou segmento de um membro através da medida de sua velocidade inicial de aumento do volume quando seu efluxo venoso é subitamente ocluído.
pleth·ys·mom·e·try (pleth-iz-mom'e-trē). Pletismometria; medida da repleção de um órgão oco ou vaso, como do pulso. [G. *plēthysmos*, aumento, + *metron*, medida]
pleur-, pleura-, pleuro-. Pleur-, pleura-, pleuro-; costela, lado, pleura. [G. *pleura*; uma costela, a lado]
pleu·ra, gen. e pl. **pleu·rae** (ploor'ă, ploor'ē). [TA]. Pleura; a membrana serosa que envolve os pulmões e reveste as paredes da cavidade pleural. SIN membrana succingens. [G. *pleura*, uma costela, pl. a lateral]
  cervical p. [TA], cúpula da pleura; o teto abobadado da cavidade pleural que se estende para cima, através da abertura superior do tórax. SIN cupula pleurae [TA], dome of pleura*, pleural cupula*.
  costal p., parte costal da pleura parietal. SIN costal part of parietal pleura.
  p. costa'lis, parte costal da pleura parietal. SIN costal part of parietal pleura.
  diaphragmatic p., parte diafragmática da pleura parietal. SIN diaphragmatic part of parietal pleura.
  p. diaphragmat'ica, parte diafragmática da pleura parietal. SIN diaphragmatic part of parietal pleura.
  mediastinal p., parte mediastinal da pleura parietal. SIN mediastinal part of parietal pleura.
  p. mediastina'lis, parte mediastinal da pleura parietal. SIN mediastinal part of parietal pleura.
  parietal p. [TA], p. parietal; aquela que reveste as diferentes partes da parede da cavidade pleural; denominada costal, diafragmática e mediastinal, de acordo com as partes revestidas. SIN p. parietalis [TA].
  p. parieta'lis [TA], p. parietal. SIN parietal p.
  p. pericardi'aca, pericardial p., p. pericárdica; a porção da parte mediastinal da pleura parietal que está fundida com o pericárdio.
  phrenic p., parte diafragmática da pleura parietal. SIN diaphragmatic part of parietal pleura.
  p. phren'ica, parte diafragmática da pleura parietal. SIN diaphragmatic part of parietal pleura.
  p. pulmona'lis, p. visceral; *termo oficial alternativo para visceral p.
  pulmonary p., p. visceral; *termo oficial alternativo para visceral p.
  visceral p. [TA], p. visceral; a camada que reveste os pulmões e mergulha nas fissuras entre os vários lobos. SIN p. visceralis [TA], p. pulmonalis*, pulmonary p*.
  p. viscera'lis [TA], p. visceral. SIN visceral p.

pleu·ra·cen·te·sis (ploor'ă-sen-tē'sis). Pleurocentese; toracocentese. SIN thoracentesis.

pleu·ral (ploor'ăl). Pleural; relativo à pleura.

pleu·ral crac·kles (krăk'lz). Crepitações pleurais; sons auscultados em virtude de inflamação da pleura associada a exsudato fibrinoso.

pleu·ral·gia (ploo-ral'jē-ă). Pleuralgia; sinônimo raramente usado para pleurodinia (2). [pleur- + G. *algos*, dor]

pleur·a·poph·y·sis (ploor'ă-pof'i-sis). Pleurapófise; uma costela, ou o processo em uma vértebra cervical ou lombar correspondente a ela. Cf. superior articular *process*. [pleur- + G. *apophysis*, processo, ramo]

pleur·ec·to·my (ploo-rek'tō-mē). Pleurectomia; excisão da pleura, geralmente parietal. [pleur- + G. *ektomē*, excisão]

pleu·ri·sy (ploor'i-sē). Pleurisia; inflamação da pleura. SIN pleuritis. [L. *pleurisis*, do G. *pleuritis*]

   adhesive p., pleurisia adesiva. SIN dry p.
   benign dry p., p. seca benigna. SIN epidemic *pleurodynia*.
   bilateral p., p. bilateral; inflamação da pleura dos dois lados do tórax. SIN double p.
   chronic p., p. crônica; termo vago ou indefinido para inflamação crônica da pleura de qualquer etiologia (p. ex., tuberculose).
   costal p., p. costal; inflamação da pleura que reveste as paredes torácicas.
   diaphragmatic p., p. diafragmática. SIN epidemic *pleurodynia*.
   double p., p. dupla. SIN bilateral p.
   dry p., p. seca; p. com exsudação fibrinosa, sem derrame de soro, resultando em adesão das superfícies opostas da pleura. SIN adhesive p., fibrinous p., plastic p.
   encysted p., p. encistada; forma de p. serofibrinosa, na qual ocorrem aderências em vários pontos, circunscrevendo o derrame seroso.
   epidemic benign dry p., p. seca benigna epidêmica. SIN epidemic *pleurodynia*.
   epidemic diaphragmatic p., p. diafragmática epidêmica. SIN epidemic *pleurodynia*.
   fibrinous p., p. fibrinosa. SIN dry p.
   hemorrhagic p., p. hemorrágica; p. com derrame de soro tinto de sangue.
   interlobular p., p. interlobular; inflamação limitada à pleura nos sulcos entre os lobos pulmonares.
   mediastinal p., p. mediastinal; inflamação da parte da pleura que reveste a superfície mediastinal do pulmão.
   plastic p., p. plástica. SIN dry p.
   productive p., p. produtiva. SIN pachypleuritis.
   proliferating p., p. proliferativa; p. com tendência à proliferação de exsudato inflamatório.
   pulmonary p., p. pulmonar; inflamação da pleura que reveste os pulmões. SIN visceral p.
   purulent p., p. purulenta; p. com empiema. SIN suppurative p.
   sacculated p., p. saculada; p. com o exsudato inflamatório dividido em regiões distintas por aderências ou alterações inflamatórias.
   serofibrinous p., p. serofibrinosa; a forma mais comum de p., caracterizada por exsudato fibrinoso na superfície da pleura e derrame de líquido seroso substancial para a cavidade pleural.
   serous p., p. serosa. SIN p. with effusion.
   suppurative p., p. supurativa. SIN purulent p.
   typhoid p., p. tifóide; termo obsoleto para p. aguda ou subaguda com sintomas tifóides (confusão ou demência).
   visceral p., p. visceral. SIN pulmonary p.
   wet p., p. úmida. SIN p. with effusion.
   p. with effusion, p. com derrame; p. acompanhada por exsudação serosa. SIN serous p., wet p.

pleu·rit·ic (ploo-rit'ik). Pleurítico; relativo à pleurisia.

pleu·ri·tis (ploo-rī'tis). Pleurite. SIN pleurisy. [G. de *pleura*, lado, + *-itis*, inflamação]

pleur·i·tog·e·nous (ploor-i-toj'ē-nŭs). Pleuritogênico; que tende a produzir pleurisia. [G. *pleuritis*, pleurisia, + *genesis*, origem]

⚠ **pleuro-**. VER pleur-.

pleu·ro·cele (ploor'ō-sēl). Pleurocele. SIN pneumocele. [pleuro- + G. *kēlē*, hérnia]

pleu·ro·cen·te·sis (ploor'ō-sen-tē'sis). Pleurocentese. SIN thoracentesis. [pleuro- + G. *kentēsis*, punção]

pleu·ro·cen·trum (ploor'ō-sen'trŭm). Pleurocentro; uma das metades laterais do corpo de uma vértebra. [pleuro- + G. *kentron*, centro]

pleu·roc·ly·sis (ploor-ok'li-sis). Pleuróclise; lavagem da cavidade pleural. [pleuro- + G. *klysis*, lavagem]

pleu·rod·e·sis (ploo-od'ē-sis). Pleurodese; a criação de aderência fibrosa entre as camadas visceral e parietal da pleura, assim obliterando a cavidade pleural; é realizada cirurgicamente por abrasão da pleura ou por introdução de um irritante estéril no espaço pleural, e aplicada como tratamento em casos de derrame pleural maligno, pneumotórax espontâneo recorrente e quilotórax. [pleuro- + G. *desis*, união]

pleu·ro·dyn·ia (ploor-ō-din'ē-ă). Pleurodinia. **1.** Dor pleurítica no tórax. **2.** Afecção dolorosa das inserções tendíneas dos músculos torácicos, em geral apenas de um lado. SIN costalgia. [pleuro- + G. *odynē*, dor]

   epidemic p., p. epidêmica; doença infecciosa aguda que geralmente ocorre na forma epidêmica, caracterizada por paroxismos de dor, geralmente torácica, e associada a cepas de enterovírus coxsackie tipo B. SIN benign dry pleurisy, Bornholm disease, Daae disease, devil grip, diaphragmatic pleurisy, epidemic benign dry pleurisy, epidemic diaphragmatic pleurisy, epidemic myalgia, epidemic myositis, myositis epidemica acuta, epidemic transient diaphragmatic spasm, Sylvest disease.

pleu·ro·gen·ic (ploor-ō-jen'ik). Pleurogênico; de origem pleural; que começa na pleura. SIN pleurogenous (1). [pleuro- + G. *-gen*, que produz]

pleu·rog·e·nous (ploor-oj'ē-nŭs). Pleurogênico. **1.** SIN pleurogenic. **2.** Em fungos, designa esporos ou conídios desenvolvidos nas laterais de um conidióforo ou hifa.

pleu·rog·ra·phy (ploor-og'ră-fē). Pleurografia; radiografia da cavidade pleural após injeção de contraste. [pleuro- + G. *graphō*, escrever]

pleu·ro·hep·a·ti·tis (ploor'ō-hep-ă-tī'tis). Pleuro-hepatite; hepatite com extensão da inflamação para a porção adjacente da pleura. [pleuro- + G. *hēpar*, fígado, + *-itis*, inflamação]

pleu·ro·lith (ploor'ō-lith). Pleurólito; concreção na cavidade pleural. SIN pleural calculus. [pleuro- + G. *lithos*, cálculo]

pleu·rol·y·sis (ploor-ol'i-sis). Pleurólise; localização de aderências pleurais com a ajuda de um endoscópio seguida por sua divisão com o cautério elétrico. [pleuro- + G. *lysis*, dissolução]

pleu·ro·per·i·car·di·al (ploor'ō-per-i-kar'dē-ăl). Pleuropericárdico; relativo à pleura e ao pericárdio.

pleu·ro·per·i·car·di·tis (ploor'ō-per-i-kar-dī'tis). Pleuropericardite; inflamação combinada do pericárdio e da pleura. [pleuro- + pericardium + G. *-itis*, inflamação]

pleu·ro·per·i·to·ne·al (ploor'ō-per-i-tō-nē'ăl). Pleuroperitoneal; relativo à pleura e ao peritônio.

pleuropneumonectomy. Pleuropneumectomia; ressecção cirúrgica de um pulmão inteiro juntamente com a pleura parietal; antigamente era usado sobretudo no pulmão destruído por tuberculose; atualmente é um método de tratamento do mesotelioma maligno.

pleu·ro·pul·mo·nary (ploor-ō-pul'mō-ner-ē). Pleuropulmonar; relativo à pleura e aos pulmões.

pleu·ros·co·py (ploor-os'kō-pē). Pleuroscopia. SIN thoracoscopy. [pleuro- + G. *skopeō*, inspecionar]

pleu·rot·o·my (ploo-rot'ō-mē). Pleurotomia. SIN thoracotomy. [pleuro- + G. *tomē*, incisão]

pleu·ro·ty·phoid (plur-ō-tī'foyd). Pleurotifóide; febre tifóide na qual o estágio inicial é mascarado pelos sinais físicos de pleurisia.

pleu·ro·vis·cer·al (ploor'ō-vis'er-ăl). Pleurovisceral. SIN visceropleural.

PLEVA. Acrônimo para *pityriasis* lichenoides et varioliformis acuta (pitiríase liquenóide e varioliforme aguda).

plex·al (plek'săl). Relativo a um plexo.

plex·ec·to·my (plek-sek'tō-mē). Plexectomia; excisão cirúrgica de um plexo. [plexus + G. *ektomē*, excisão]

plex·i·form (plek'si-fōrm). Plexiforme; semelhante a uma rede ou a um plexo, ou que o forma. [plexus + L. *forma*, forma]

plex·im·e·ter (plek-sim'i-ter). Pleximetro. SIN plessimeter. [G. *plēxis*, golpe]

plex·i·tis (plek-sī'tis). Plexite; inflamação de um plexo.
   brachial p., amiotrofia neurálgica. SIN neuralgic *amyotrophy*.

plex·o·gen·ic (plek-sō-jen-ik). Plexogênico; que dá origem a estruturas semelhantes a membranas ou plexiformes. [plexus + G. *-gen*, que produz]

plex·om·e·ter (plek-som'ē-ter). Plexômetro. SIN plessimeter.

plex·o·path·y (pleks-op'ă-thē). Plexopatia; distúrbio que envolve um dos principais plexos neurais periféricos: cervical, braquial ou lombossacro. [plexus + G. *pathos*, doença]

plex·or (plek'ser). Plexor. SIN plessor. [G. *plēxis*, um golpe]

PLEXUS

plex·us, pl. **plex·us**, **plex·us·es** (plek'sŭs, -sŭs-ez). [TA]. Plexo; uma rede ou interconexão de nervos e vasos sanguíneos ou de vasos linfáticos. [L. trança]

   abdominal aortic (nervous) p. [TA], p. aórtico abdominal; p. autônomo que circunda a aorta abdominal, diretamente contínuo com o p. aórtico torácico superiormente, continuando inferiormente até a bifurcação da aorta como o p. hipogástrico superior. SIN p. nervosus aorticus abdominalis [TA]
   acromial p., anastomose acromial da artéria toracoacromial. SIN acromial *anastomosis* of the thoracoacromial artery.
   p. annula'ris, p. anular. SIN anular p.
   anterior coronary periarterial p., p. periarterial coronariano anterior; a parte do p. cardíaco que acompanha as artérias coronárias na face anterior do coração.

anular p., p. anular; p. nervoso próximo da junção corneoescleral a partir do qual nervos mielinizados e não-mielinizados seguem até a córnea. SIN p. annularis.

aortic lymphatic p., p. linfático aórtico; p. de linfonodos e vasos de união situados ao longo da porção inferior da aorta abdominal. SIN p. aorticus.

p. aor'ticus, p. linfático aórtico. SIN aortic lymphatic p.

areolar venous p. [TA], p. venoso areolar; p. venoso na aréola que circunda o mamilo, formado pelas veias mamárias, e que envia seu sangue para a veia torácica lateral; o tecido erétil da aréola do mamilo. SIN p. venosus areolaris [TA], circulus venosus halleri, Haller circle (2), vascular circle (2), venous circle of mammary gland.

p. arte'riae choroi'deae, p. periarterial da artéria corióidea. SIN periarterial p. of choroid artery.

arterial p. [TA], p. arterial; rede vascular formada por anastomoses entre pequenas artérias logo antes de se tornarem capilares. SIN rete arteriosum [TA], arteriolar network.

articular vascular p. [TA], p. vascular articular; rede vascular na adjacência de uma articulação, onde esses arranjos são comuns, permitindo uma circulação colateral pela qual o sangue será suprido distal à articulação independentemente das acomodações resultantes da posição articular. SIN rete vasculosum articulare [TA], articular network, articular vascular circle, articular vascular network, circulus articularis vasculosus.

ascending pharyngeal p., p. periarterial da artéria faríngea ascendente. SIN periarterial p. of ascending pharyngeal artery.

Auerbach p., p. de Auerbach. SIN myenteric (nervous) p.

autonomic plexuses [TA], plexos autônomos; plexos nervosos em relação aos vasos sanguíneos e vísceras, cujas fibras componentes são simpáticas, parassimpáticas e sensoriais. SIN plexus viscerales.

p. autonomicus brachialis [TA], p. autônomo braquial. SIN brachial autonomic p.

axillary p., p. linfático axilar. SIN axillary lymphatic p.

axillary lymphatic p., p. linfático axilar; p. linfático formado por linfonodos, com seus vasos aferentes e eferentes, na axila. SIN axillary p., p. lymphaticus axillaris.

basilar venous p. [TA], p. venoso basilar; p. venoso sobre o clivo, unido aos seios cavernoso e petroso e ao plexo venoso vertebral interno (epidural). SIN p. venosus basilaris [TA], basilar sinus.

Batson p., p. de Batson. SIN vertebral venous system.

brachial p., [TA], p. braquial; principal p. nervoso formado pelos ramos primários ventrais desde o quinto nervo espinal cervical até o primeiro nervo torácico para inervação do membro superior. Os ramos primários ventrais que entram na formação do p. constituem as suas raízes; as raízes estão localizadas no triângulo posterior do pescoço; convergindo para emergir dos músculos escalenos anterior e médio. Quando emergem do hiato escaleno, as raízes de C5 e C6 juntam-se para formar o tronco superior, a raiz de C7 permanece isolada como tronco médio, e as raízes de C8 e T1 combinam-se para formar o tronco inferior do p. Os troncos passam sob a clavícula, seguindo do pescoço até a axila através do canal cervicoaxilar. Quando cruzam a primeira costela, os três troncos separam-se, formando as divisões anterior e posterior do p. As fibras nervosas contidas nas divisões anteriores são destinadas à face anterior do membro; aquelas contidas nas divisões posteriores são destinadas à face posterior do membro. Na axila, as divisões anteriores dos troncos superior e médio fundem-se para formar o cordão lateral do p.; a divisão anterior do tronco inferior torna-se o cordão medial do p.; e as divisões posteriores de todos os três troncos tornam-se o cordão posterior, sendo os cordões denominados de acordo com sua posição em relação à artéria axilar, à qual seguem paralelos e a circundam. Os cordões do p. braquial dão origem à maioria dos nervos periféricos mencionados, que são os produtos da formação do p. Os principais nervos do cordão lateral são o nervo musculocutâneo e a raiz lateral do nervo mediano. O cordão medial dá origem à raiz ulnar e medial do nervo mediano. As raízes lateral e medial do nervo mediano fundem-se para formar o nervo medial. O cordão posterior do plexo emite os nervos radial e axilar. SIN p. brachialis [TA].

brachial autonomic p. [TA], p. autônomo braquial; p. autônomo periarterial da artéria braquial. SIN p. autonomicus brachialis [TA].

p. brachia'lis [TA], p. braquial. SIN brachial p.

cardiac (nervous) p. [TA], p. cardíaco; uma ampla rede formada por nervos cardiopulmonares e esplâncnicos anastomosados que conduzem fibras nervosas aferentes e autônomas (simpáticas e parassimpáticas), que circundam o arco da aorta, a artéria pulmonar e seguem até os átrios, ventrículos e vasos coronários. SIN p. nervosus cardiacus [TA].

p. cardi'acus profun'dus, p. cardíaco profundo. SIN deep cardiac p.

p. carot'icus inter'nus, p. carótico comum interno. SIN internal carotid venous p.

cavernous p. of clitoris, nervos cavernosos do clitóris. SIN cavernous nerves of clitoris, em nerve.

cavernous nervous p. [TA], p. cavernoso; a porção do p. carótico interno no seio cavernoso. SIN p. nervosus cavernosus [TA], intracavernous p., Walther p.

cavernous p. of penis, nervos cavernosos do pênis. SIN cavernous nerves of penis, em nerve.

cavernous (vascular) p. of conchae [TA], p. cavernoso das conchas; tecido erétil na mucosa que cobre as conchas da cavidade nasal. SIN p. vascularis cavernosus conchae [TA], corpus cavernosum conchae.

celiac p., p. celíaco; rede relacionada ao tronco celíaco. VER celiac (nervous) p., celiac (lymphatic) p.

celiac (lymphatic) p., p. (linfático) celíaco; rede formada pelos vasos linfáticos eferentes e aferentes dos linfonodos celíacos e relacionada ao tronco celíaco; os vasos linfáticos aferentes trazem linfa basicamente das estruturas servidas pela artéria celíaca (estômago, duodeno, pâncreas e face visceral do fígado); os vasos eferentes drenam para a cisterna do quilo/ducto torácico através dos troncos linfáticos intestinais.

celiac (nervous) p. [TA], p. celíaco; a porção superior e mais substancial do p. aórtico abdominal situada anterior à aorta, ao nível de origem do tronco celíaco (nível vertebral T-12); os gânglios celíacos situam-se no p.; é formado por contribuições dos nervos esplâncnico maior e vago (principalmente o vago posterior ou direito) e por ramos comunicantes que entram nos gânglios e plexos mesentérico superior e renal e os deixam; a maioria das fibras aferentes simpáticas, parassimpáticas e viscerais que servem às vísceras abdominais atravessam esse plexo. SIN plexus coeliacus [TA], p. nervosus celiacus [TA], solar p.

cervical p., p. cervical; formado por alças que unem os ramos primários ventrais adjacentes dos quatro primeiros nervos cervicais e recebem ramos comunicantes cinzentos do gânglio cervical superior; situa-se profundamente ao músculo esternocleidomastóideo e envia numerosos ramos cutâneos, musculares e comunicantes. SIN p. cervicalis.

p. cervica'lis, p. cervical. SIN cervical p.

choroid p. [TA], p. corióideo; proliferação vascular ou franja da tela corióidea no terceiro e quarto ventrículos e no ventrículo lateral; secreta líquido cerebrospinal, assim regulando parcialmente a pressão intraventricular. SIN p. choroideus [TA], tela vasculosa.

p. choroi'deus [TA], p. corióideo. SIN choroid p.

p. choroi'deus ventric'uli latera'lis [TA], p. corióideo do ventrículo lateral. SIN choroid p. of lateral ventricle.

p. choroi'deus ventric'uli quar'ti [TA], p. corióideo do quarto ventrículo. SIN choroid p. of fourth ventricle.

p. choroi'deus ventric'uli ter'tii [TA], p. corióideo do terceiro ventrículo. SIN choroid p. of third ventricle.

choroid p. of fourth ventricle [TA], p. corióideo do quarto ventrículo; uma dentre duas franjas vasculares de pia-máter que se projetam de cada lado da parte inferior do teto do quarto ventrículo cerebral. SIN p. choroideus ventriculi quarti [TA].

choroid p. of lateral ventricle [TA], p. corióideo do ventrículo lateral; a franja vascular que se projeta da fissura corióidea para cada ventrículo lateral. SIN p. choroideus ventriculi lateralis [TA].

choroid p. of third ventricle [TA], p. corióideo do terceiro ventrículo; a dupla fileira de projeções vasculares da superfície inferior da tela corióidea, onde cobre o terceiro ventrículo. SIN p. choroideus ventriculi tertii [TA].

ciliary ganglionic p., p. ganglionar ciliar; p. autônomo situado sobre o músculo ciliar, derivado do oculomotor, trigêmeo e simpático. SIN p. gangliosus ciliaris.

coccygeal p. [TA], p. coccígeo; pequeno p. formado pelo quinto nervo sacral e pelos nervos coccígeos; dá origem aos nervos anococcígeos. SIN p. coccygeus [TA].

p. coccyg'eus [TA], p. coccígeo. SIN coccygeal p.

common carotid p., p. carótico comum. SIN common carotid nervous p.

common carotid nervous p. [TA], p. carótico comum; p. autônomo que acompanha a artéria de mesmo nome, formado por fibras do gânglio cervical médio. SIN p. nervosus caroticus communis [TA], common carotid p.

p. corona'rii cor'dis, plexos periarteriais das artérias coronárias. SIN periarterial plexuses of coronary arteries.

coronary p., plexos periarteriais das artérias coronárias. SIN periarterial plexuses of coronary arteries.

Cruveilhier p., p. de Cruveilhier; p. nervoso formado por comunicação entre os ramos primários dorsais dos três primeiros nervos cervicais; situa-se profundamente ao músculo semi-espinal da cabeça.

deep cardiac p., p. cardíaco profundo; a parte mais profunda do p. cardíaco inferior ao arco da aorta. SIN p. cardiacus profundus.

deferential (nervous) p. [TA], p. deferencial; p. autônomo na vesícula seminal e ampola do ducto deferente de cada lado, derivado do p. hipogástrico inferior. SIN p. nervosus deferentialis [TA], p. of ductus deferens.

p. of ductus deferens, p. deferencial. SIN deferential (nervous) p.

enteric (nervous) p. [TA], p. entérico; o p. autônomo na parede do intestino; consiste em três partes, submucosa, mioentérica e subserosa; as células ganglionares encontram-se dispersas através dos plexos mioentérico e submucoso. SIN p. nervosus entericus [TA].

esophageal (nervous) p. [TA], p. esofágico; um dentre dois plexos nervosos, posterior e anterior, nas paredes do esôfago; o primeiro é formado por ramos dos nervos vago direito e recorrente esquerdo, e o segundo pela anastomose dos troncos do nervo vago após sair dos plexos pulmonares; os ramos suprem as túnicas mucosa e muscular do esôfago. SIN p. nervosus esophageus [TA], p. gulae.

Exner p., p. de Exner; p. formado por fibras nervosas tangenciais na camada plexiforme ou molecular superficial do córtex cerebral.

external carotid (nervous) p. [TA], p. carótico externo; p. autônomo formado pelos nervos caróticos externos que circundam a artéria de mesmo nome e dão origem a vários plexos secundários ao longo dos ramos dessa artéria e a ramos para o corpo carótico. SIN p. nervosus caroticus externus [TA].

external iliac lymphatic p., p. linfático ilíaco externo; p. linfático formado pelos linfonodos ao longo da artéria ilíaca externa, de cada lado, e seus vasos aferentes e eferentes. SIN p. lymphaticus iliacus externus.

external maxillary p., p. periarterial da artéria facial. SIN periarterial p. of facial artery.

facial p., p. periarterial da artéria facial. SIN periarterial p. of facial artery.

femoral (nervous) p. [TA], p. femoral; p. autônomo que circunda a artéria femoral, derivado do p. ilíaco. SIN p. nervosus femoralis [TA].

p. ganglio'sus cilia'ris, p. ganglionar ciliar. SIN ciliary ganglionic p.

gastric plexuses of autonomic system, plexos gástricos do sistema autônomo. SIN gastric nervous plexuses.

p. gas'trici syste'matis autono'mici, p. gástrico do sistema autônomo. SIN gastric nervous plexuses.

gastric nervous plexuses [TA], plexos gástricos; os plexos ao longo das curvaturas maior e menor do estômago derivados do p. celíaco; também conhecidos como plexos inferior e superior. SIN p. nervorum gastricorum [TA], gastric plexuses of autonomic system, p. gastrici systematis autonomici.

p. gu'lae, p. esofágico. SIN esophageal (nervous) p.

Haller p., p. de Haller; p. nervoso de filamentos simpáticos e ramos do nervo laríngeo externo na superfície do músculo constritor inferior da faringe.

Heller p., p. de Heller; p. de pequenas artérias na parede do intestino.

hemorrhoidal p., p. venoso retal. SIN rectal venous p. VER TAMBÉM inferior rectal (nervous) p., middle rectal (nervous) p., superior rectal (nervous) p.

hepatic (nervous) p. [TA], p. nervoso hepático; p. autônomo ímpar situado na artéria hepática e seus ramos no fígado. SIN p. nervosus hepaticus [TA].

iliac (nervous) p. [TA], p. ilíaco; o p. autônomo situado nas artérias ilíacas, derivado do p. aórtico. SIN p. nervosus iliacus [TA].

inferior dental (nervous) p. [TA], p. dental inferior; formado por ramos do nervo alveolar inferior entrelaçados antes de suprirem os dentes; emite ramos dentais interiores para os dentes e ramos gengivais inferiores para as gengivas. SIN p. nervosus dentalis inferior [TA].

inferior hemorrhoidal plexuses, plexos retais inferiores. SIN inferior rectal (nervous) p.

inferior hypogastric (nervous) p., p. hipogástrico inferior; um dos plexos autônomos bilaterais na pelve distribuídos para as vísceras pélvicas; recebe os nervos hipogástricos e esplâncnicos pélvicos. SIN p. nervosus hypogastricus inferior [TA], pelvic (nervous) p*., p. nervosus pelvicus*.

inferior mesenteric (nervous) p. [TA], p. mesentérico inferior; p. autônomo, derivado do p. aórtico abdominal, que circunda a artéria mesentérica inferior e envia ramos para o colo descendente, colo sigmóide e reto. SIN p. nervosus mesentericus inferior [TA].

inferior rectal (nervous) p. [TA], p. retal inferior; os plexos autônomos ao longo do ânus derivados do plexo hipogástrico inferior. SIN p. nervosus rectalis inferiores [TA], inferior hemorrhoidal plexuses.

inferior thyroid p., p. periarterial da artéria tireóidea inferior. SIN periarterial p. of inferior thyroid artery.

inferior vesical venous p., p. venoso vesical inferior; p. venoso na mulher que corresponde ao p. venoso prostático no homem. SIN p. venosus vesicalis inferior.

inguinal lymphatic p., p. linfático inguinal; p. linfático formado por 10–15 linfonodos com seus vasos de união situados superficialmente próximo ao fim da veia safena magna e mais profundamente ao longo da artéria e veia femorais. VER superficial inguinal *lymph nodes*, em *lymph node*. SIN p. lymphaticus inguinalis.

intermesenteric (nervous) p. [TA], p. intermesentérico; a parte do p. aórtico abdominal situada entre os plexos mesentéricos superior e inferior. SIN p. nervosus intermesentericus [TA].

internal carotid (nervous) p. [TA], p. carótico interno; p. nervoso autônomo que circunda a artéria carótida interna no canal carótico e seio cavernoso, enviando ramos para o p. timpânico, gânglio esfenopalatino, nervos abducente e oculomotor, vasos cerebrais e gânglio ciliar. SIN p. nervosus arteriae carotidis internae.

internal carotid venous p., p. venoso carótico interno; rede venosa ao redor da artéria carótida interna, no canal carótico do osso temporal, que se une ao seio cavernoso e à veia jugular interna. SIN p. caroticus internus, p. venosus caroticus internus.

internal mammary p., p. mamário interno. SIN periarterial p. of internal thoracic artery.

internal maxillary p., p. maxilar interno. SIN periarterial p. of maxillary artery.

internal thoracic p., p. periarterial da artéria torácica interna. SIN periarterial p. of internal thoracic artery.

internal thoracic lymphatic p., p. linfático torácico interno; p. linfático, que inclui os linfonodos paraesternais (torácicos internos) com seus vasos, paralelo ao trajeto das veias torácicas internas. SIN mammary p., p. mammarius.

intracavernous p., p. intracavernoso. SIN cavernous nervous p.

p. intraparoti'deus nervi facialis, p. intraparotídeo do nervo facial. SIN parotide p. of facial nerve.

intraparotid p. of facial nerve, p. intraparotídeo do nervo facial. SIN parotid p. of facial nerve.

ischiadic p., p. isquiático. SIN sacral p.

Jacobson p., p. de Jacobson. SIN tympanic (nervous) p.

Jacques p., p. de Jacques; p. nervoso na túnica muscular da tuba uterina (de Falópio).

jugular lymphatic p., p. linfático jugular; p. linfático que inclui o grupo cervical profundo dos linfonodos, com seus vasos aferentes e eferentes, estendendo-se ao longo da veia jugular interna (bainha carótica). SIN p. lymphaticus jugularis.

Leber p., p. de Leber; pequeno p. venoso no olho entre os seios venosos da esclera (de Schlemm) e os espaços do ângulo iridocorneal (de Fontana).

lingual p., p. periarterial da artéria lingual. SIN periarterial p. of lingual artery.

lumbar lymphatic p., p. linfático lombar; p. linfático formado por aproximadamente 20 linfonodos e vasos de união situados ao longo da porção inferior da aorta e dos vasos ilíacos comuns. SIN p. lymphaticus lumbalis.

lumbar (nervous) p., p. lombar; p. nervoso, formado pelos ramos ventrais dos quatro primeiros nervos lombares; situa-se na substância do músculo psoas. SIN p. nervorum lumbalium.

lumbosacral (nervous) p. [TA], p. lombossacral; formado pela união dos ramos anteriores dos nervos lombar e sacral; é dividido em plexos lombar e sacral. SIN p. nervosus lumbosacralis [TA].

lymphatic p., p. linfático; p. de capilares linfáticos, geralmente sem válvulas, que se abre para um ou mais vasos linfáticos maiores. SIN p. lymphaticus.

p. lymph'aticus, p. linfático. SIN lymphatic p.

p. lymphaticus axilla'ris, p. linfático axilar. SIN axillary lymphatic p.

p. lymphaticus ili'acus exter'nus, p. linfático ilíaco externo. SIN external iliac lymphatic p.

p. lymphaticus inguina'lis, p. linfático inguinal. SIN inguinal lymphatic p.

p. lymphaticus jugula'ris, p. linfático jugular. SIN jugular lymphatic p.

p. lymphaticus lumbalis, p. linfático lombar. SIN lumbar lymphatic p.

plexo lombossacral e **plexo ciático**

p. lymphaticus sacra'lis me'dius, p. linfático sacral médio. SIN middle sacral lymphatic p.
p. mamma'rius, p. linfático torácico interno. SIN internal thoracic lymphatic p.
p. mamma'rius inter'nus, p. periarterial da artéria torácica interna. SIN periarterial p. of internal thoracic artery.
mammary p., p. linfático torácico interno. SIN internal thoracic lymphatic p.
p. maxilla'ris exter'nus, p. periarterial da artéria facial. SIN periarterial p. of facial artery.
p. maxilla'ris inter'nus, p. periarterial da artéria maxilar. SIN periarterial p. of maxillary artery.
maxillary p., p. periarterial da artéria maxilar. SIN periarterial p. of maxillary artery.
Meissner p., p. de Meissner. SIN submucosal (nervous) p.
meningeal p., p. meníngeo; p. nervoso nas meninges cerebrais, derivado do p. carótico externo. SIN p. meningeus.
p. menin'geus, p. meníngeo. SIN meningeal p.
middle hemorrhoidal plexuses, plexos retais médios. SIN middle rectal (nervous) p.
middle rectal (nervous) p. [TA], p. retal médio; os plexos autônomos ao longo do reto derivados do p. hipogástrico inferior. SIN middle hemorrhoidal plexuses, p. nervosus rectalis medius.
middle sacral lymphatic p., p. linfático sacral médio; p. linfático formado de linfonodos e vasos de união, situados principalmente no mesorreto, anteriores e inferiores ao promontório sacral. SIN p. lymphaticus sacralis medius.
myenteric (nervous) p. [TA], p. mioentérico; p. de fibras não-mielinizadas e corpos de células autônomas pós-ganglionares situados na túnica muscular do esôfago, estômago e intestino; comunica-se com os plexos subseroso e submucoso, todos subdivisões do p. entérico. SIN p. (nervosus) myentericus [TA], Auerbach p.
nerve p. [TA], p. nervoso; p. formado pelo entrelaçamento de nervos ou fibras nervosas por meio de numerosos ramos ou fibras que se comunicam. SIN p. nervosus [TA].
p. nervorum gastricorum [TA], p. gástrico. SIN gastric nervous plexuses.
p. nervorum lumba'lium [TA], p. lombar. SIN lumbar (nervous) p.
p. nervo'rum spina'lium [TA], p. nervoso espinal. SIN spinal nerve p.
p. nervo'sus [TA], p. nervoso. SIN nerve p.
p. nervosus aor'ticus abdomina'lis [TA], p. aórtico abdominal. SIN abdominal aortic (nervous) p.
p. (nervosus) aor'ticus thora'cicus [TA], p. aórtico torácico. SIN thoracic aortic (nervous) p.
p. nervosus arteriae carotidis internae, p. carótico interno. SIN internal carotid (nervous) p.
p. nervosus cardi'acus [TA], p. cardíaco. SIN cardiac (nervous) p.
p. (nervosus) cardi'acus superficia'lis [TA], p. cardíaco. SIN superficial cardiac (nervous) p.
p. nervosus carot'icus commu'nis [TA], p. carótico comum. SIN common carotid nervous p.
p. nervosus carot'icus exter'nus [TA], p. carótico externo. SIN external carotid (nervous) p.
p. nervosus caverno'sus [TA], p. cavernoso. SIN cavernous nervous p.
p. nervosus celi'acus [TA], p. celíaco. SIN celiac (nervous) p.
p. nervosus cervicalis posterior [TA], p. cervical posterior. SIN posterior cervical (nervous) p.
p. nervosus deferentia'lis [TA], p. deferencial. SIN deferential (nervous) p.
p. nervosus denta'lis infe'rior [TA], p. dental inferior. SIN inferior dental (nervous) p.
p. (nervosus) denta'lis supe'rior [TA], p. dental superior. SIN superior dental (nervous) p.
p. nervosus enter'icus [TA], p. entérico. SIN enteric (nervous) p.
p. nervosus esopha'geus [TA], p. esofágico. SIN esophageal (nervous) p.
p. nervosus femora'lis [TA], p. femoral. SIN femoral (nervous) p.
p. nervosus hepat'icus [TA], p. hepático. SIN hepatic (nervous) p.
p. nervosus hypogas'tricus infe'rior [TA], p. hipogástrico inferior. SIN inferior hypogastric (nervous) p.
p. (nervosus) hypogas'tricus supe'rior [TA], p. hipogástrico superior. SIN superior hypogastric (nervous) p.
p. nervosus ili'acus [TA], p. ilíaco. SIN iliac (nervous) p.
p. nervosus intermesenter'icus [TA], p. intermesentérico. SIN intermesenteric (nervous) p.
p. (nervosus) liena'lis, p. esplênico; *termo oficial alternativo para splenic (nervous) p.
p. nervosus lumbosacra'lis [TA], p. lombossacral. SIN lumbossacral (nervous) p.
p. nervosus mesenter'icus infe'rior [TA], p. mesentérico inferior. SIN inferior mesenteric (nervous) p.
p. (nervosus) mesenter'icus supe'rior [TA], p. mesentérico superior. SIN superior mesenteric (nervous) p.

p. (nervosus) myenter'icus [TA], p. mioentérico. SIN myenteric (nervous) p.
p. (nervosus) ova'ricus [TA], p. ovárico. SIN ovarian (nervous) p.
p. (nervosus) pancreat'icus [TA], p. pancreático. SIN pancreatic (nervous) p.
p. nervosus pel'vicus, p. hipogástrico inferior; *termo oficial alternativo para inferior hypogastric (nervous) p.
p. nervosus pharyn'geus [TA], p. faríngeo. SIN pharyngeal (nervous) p.
p. nervosus prostat'icus [TA], p. prostático. SIN prostatic (nervous) p.
p. (nervosus) pulmona'lis [TA], p. pulmonar. SIN pulmonary (nervous) p.
p. nervosus recta'lis inferio'res [TA], p. retal inferior. SIN inferior rectal (nervous) p.
p. nervosus recta'lis me'dius, p. retal médio. SIN middle rectal (nervous) p.
p. (nervosus) recta'lis supe'rior [TA], p. retal superior. SIN superior rectal (nervous) p.
p. (nervosus) rena'lis [TA], p. renal. SIN renal (nervous) p.
p. (nervosus) sple'nicus [TA], p. esplênico. SIN splenic (nervous) p.
p. (nervosus) submuco'sus [TA], p. submucoso. SIN submucosal (nervous) p.
p. (nervosus) subsero'sus [TA], p. subseroso. SIN subserous (nervous) p.
p. (nervosus) suprarena'lis [TA], p. supra-renal. SIN suprarenal (nervous) p.
p. (nervosus) tympan'icus [TA], p. timpânico. SIN tympanic (nervous) p.
p. (nervosus) ureter'icus [TA], p. (nervoso) ureteral. SIN ureteric (nervous) p.
p. (nervosus) uterovagina'lis [TA], p. uterovaginal. SIN uterovaginal (nervous) p.
p. vesica'lis [TA], p. vesical. SIN vesical (nervous) p.
plexus viscerales, plexos viscerais. SIN autonomic plexuses.
occipital p., p. periarterial da artéria occipital. SIN periarterial p. of occipital artery.
ovarian (nervous) p. [TA], p. ovárico; p. autônomo derivado do p. aórtico e que acompanha a artéria ovárica até o ovário, ligamento largo e tuba uterina. SIN p. (nervosus) ovaricus [TA].
pampiniform venous p., p. venoso pampiniforme; p. formado, no homem, por veias oriundas do testículo e epidídimo, que consiste em 8 ou 10 veias situadas na frente do ducto deferente e que forma parte do cordão espermático; na mulher as veias ováricas formam esse p. entre as camadas do ligamento largo; no homem é parte do sistema termorregulador do testículo, ajudando a manter o testículo a uma temperatura constante (um pouco menor que a temperatura corporal). SIN p. venosus pampiniformis [TA].
pancreatic (nervous) p. [TA], p. pancreático; o p. autônomo que acompanha as artérias pancreáticas. SIN p. (nervosus) pancreaticus [TA].
parotid p. of facial nerve [TA], p. intraparotídeo; os ramos divergentes do nervo facial que atravessam a substância da glândula parótida, unidos por muitas anastomoses em alça. SIN intraparotid p. of facial nerve, pes anserinus (1), p. intraparotideus nervi facialis.
pelvic (nervous) p., p. hipogástrico inferior; *termo oficial alternativo para inferior hypogastric (nervous) p.
periarterial p. [TA], p. periarterial; p. autônomo que acompanha uma artéria, circundando-a em uma rede de fibras nervosas autônomas. SIN p. periarterialis [TA].
periarterial p. of anterior cerebral artery, p. periarterial da artéria cerebral anterior; p. autônomo que acompanha a artéria cerebral anterior, derivado do p. carótico interno. SIN p. periarterialis arteriae cerebri anterioris.
periarterial p. of ascending pharyngeal artery, p. periarterial da artéria faríngea ascendente; p. autônomo sobre a artéria faríngea ascendente, formado por fibras do gânglio cervical superior. SIN ascending pharyngeal p., p. periarterialis arteriae pharyngeae ascendentis.
periarterial p. of choroid artery, p. periarterial da artéria corióidea; p. autônomo que acompanha a artéria de mesmo nome, derivada do p. carótico interno. SIN p. arteriae choroideae, p. periarterialis arteriae choroideae.
periarterial plexuses of coronary arteries, plexos periarteriais das artérias coronárias; a continuação do p. cardíaco sobre as artérias coronárias. SIN coronary p., p. coronarii cordis.
periarterial p. of facial artery, p. periarterial da artéria facial; p. autônomo sobre a artéria facial derivada do p. carótico externo; emite um ramo para o gânglio submandibular. SIN external maxillary p., facial p., p. maxillaris externus, p. periarterialis arteriae facialis.
periarterial p. of inferior phrenic artery, p. periarterial da artéria frênica inferior; p. autônomo que circunda a artéria frênica inferior. SIN phrenic p., p. phrenicus, p. periarterialis arteriae phrenicae inferioris.
periarterial p. of inferior thyroid artery, p. periarterial da artéria tireóidea inferior; p. autônomo sobre a artéria tireóidea inferior derivado do p. subclávio. SIN inferior thyroid p., p. thyroideus inferior.
periarterial p. of internal thoracic artery, p. periarterial da artéria torácica interna; p. autônomo sobre a artéria torácica interna, derivado do p. subclávio. SIN internal mammary p., internal thoracic p., p. mammarius internus, p. periarterialis arteriae thoracicae internae.
p. periarteria'lis [TA], p. periarterial. SIN periarterial p.
p. periarterialis arteriae auricula'ris poste'rioris, p. periarterial da artéria auricular posterior. SIN periarterial p. of posterior auricular artery.
p. periarterialis arte'riae cer'ebri anterio'ris, p. periarterial da artéria cerebral anterior. SIN periarterial p. of anterior cerebral artery.

p. periarterialis arte'riae cer'ebri me'diae, p. periarterial da artéria cerebral média. SIN periarterial p. of middle cerebral artery.
p. periarterialis arteriae choroideae, p. periarterial da artéria corióidea. SIN periarterial p. of choroid artery.
p. periarterialis arteriae facialis, p. periarterial da artéria facial. SIN periarterial p. of facial artery.
p. periarterialis arteriae lingualis, p. periarterial da artéria lingual. SIN periarterial p. of lingual artery.
p. periarterialis arteriae maxillaris, p. periarterial da artéria maxilar. SIN periarterial p. of maxillary artery.
p. periarterialis arteriae occipita'lis, p. periarterial da artéria occipital. SIN periarterial p. of occipital artery.
p. periarterialis arteriae ophthal'micae, p. periarterial da artéria oftálmica. SIN periarterial p. of ophthalmic artery.
p. periarterialis arteriae pharyn'geae ascen'dentis, p. periarterial da artéria faríngea ascendente. SIN periarterial p. of ascending pharyngeal artery.
p. periarterialis arteriae phrenicae inferioris, p. periarterial da artéria frênica inferior. SIN periarterial p. of inferior phrenic artery.
p. periarterialis arteriae popliteae, p. periarterial da artéria poplítea. SIN periarterial p. of popliteal artery.
p. periarterialis arteriae subcla'viae [TA], p. periarterial da artéria subclávia. SIN periarterial p. of subclavian artery.
p. periarterialis arteriae tempora'lis superficia'lis, p. periarterial da artéria temporal superficial. SIN periarterial p. of superficial temporal artery.
p. periarterialis arteriae testicula'ris, p. periarterial da artéria testicular. SIN periarterial p. of testicular artery.
p. periarterialis arteriae thoracicae internae, p. periarterial da artéria torácica interna. SIN periarterial p. of internal thoracic artery.
p. periarterialis arteriae thyroi'deae superio'ris, p. periarterial da artéria tireóidea superior. SIN periarterial p. of superior thyroid artery.
p. periarterialis arteriae vertebralis, p. periarterial da artéria vertebral. SIN periarterial p. of vertebral artery.
periarterial p. of lingual artery, p. periarterial da artéria lingual; p. autônomo sobre a artéria lingual, derivado do p. carótico externo. SIN lingual p., p. periarterialis arteriae lingualis.
periarterial p. of maxillary artery, p. periarterial da artéria maxilar; p. autônomo sobre a artéria maxilar derivado do p. carótico externo. SIN internal maxillary p., maxillary p., p. maxillaris internus, p. periarterialis arteriae maxillaris.
periarterial p. of middle cerebral artery, p. periarterial da artéria cerebral média; p. autônomo que acompanha a artéria cerebral média, derivado do p. carótico interno. SIN p. periarterialis arteriae cerebri mediae.
periarterial p. of occipital artery, p. periarterial da artéria occipital; p. autônomo sobre a artéria occipital derivado do p. carótico externo. SIN occipital p., p. periarterialis arteriae occipitalis.
periarterial p. of ophthalmic artery, p. periarterial da artéria oftálmica; p. autônomo que entra na órbita juntamente com a artéria oftálmica, derivado do p. carótico interno. SIN p. periarterialis arteriae ophthalmicae.
periarterial p. of popliteal artery, p. periarterial da artéria poplítea; p. nervoso que circunda a artéria poplítea, derivado do p. femoral. SIN p. periarterialis arteriae popliteae, popliteal p., p. popliteus.
periarterial p. of posterior auricular artery, p. periarterial da artéria auricular posterior; p. autônomo sobre a artéria auricular posterior, derivado do p. carótico externo. SIN p. periarterialis arteriae auricularis posterioris, posterior auricular p.
periarterial p. of subclavian artery [TA], p. periarterial da artéria subclávia; o p. autônomo acompanhando a artéria que tem esse nome, formado por fibras do gânglio estrelado, e que emite plexos secundários ao longo dos ramos da artéria subclávia. SIN p. periarterialis arteriae subclaviae [TA], subclavian p.
periarterial p. of superficial temporal artery, p. periarterial da artéria temporal superficial; p. autônomo de nervos sobre a artéria que tem esse nome, derivado do p. carótico externo. SIN p. periarterialis arteriae temporalis superficialis, superficial temporal p.
periarterial p. of superior thyroid artery, p. periarterial da artéria tireóidea superior; p. autônomo sobre a artéria tireóidea superior, derivado do p. carótico externo. SIN p. periarterialis arteriae thyroideae superioris, superior thyroid p.
periarterial p. of testicular artery, p. periarterial da artéria testicular; o p. autônomo derivado do p. aórtico e que acompanha a artéria testicular. SIN p. periarterialis arteriae testicularis, spermatic p., testicular p.
periarterial p. of thyroid artery, p. periarterial da artéria tireóidea; p. autônomo sobre a artéria tireóidea, derivado do p. subclávio.
periarterial p. of vertebral artery, p. periarterial da artéria vertebral; p. de nervos autônomos sobre a artéria vertebral, proveniente do p. subclávio. SIN p. periarterialis arteriae vertebralis, p. vertebralis, vertebral p.
pharyngeal (nervous) p., p. faríngeo; **(1)** o p. de nervos, incluindo ramos dos nervos glossofaríngeo, vago e acessório (raiz cranial), situado ao longo da parede posterior da faringe; **(2)** [TA] p. venoso nas paredes póstero-laterais da faringe, que se esvazia através das veias faríngeas na veia jugular interna. SIN p. nervosus pharyngeus [TA].
phrenic p., p. phren'icus, p. periarterial da artéria frênica inferior. SIN periarterial p. of inferior phrenic artery.
popliteal p., p. poplit'eus, p. poplíteo. SIN periarterial p. of popliteal artery.
posterior auricular p., p. auricular posterior. SIN periarterial p. of posterior auricular artery.
posterior cervical (nervous) p. [TA], p. cervical posterior; esse p. não é tradicionalmente descrito com os principais plexos nervosos, todos formados por ramos ventrais, e refere-se aos ramos dorsais dos nervos espinais cervicais superiores e aos ramos comunicantes relativamente pequenos que se estendem entre eles. SIN p. nervosus cervicalis posterior [TA].
posterior coronary p., p. coronário posterior; a porção do p. cardíaco que acompanha ramos das artérias coronárias na superfície póstero-inferior do coração.
prostatic (nervous) p. [TA], p. prostático; p. autônomo de nervos intimamente associado à cápsula da próstata, derivado do p. hipogástrico inferior e dando origem aos nervos cavernosos para o tecido erétil do pênis; a lesão cirúrgica desse p. freqüentemente resulta em impotência. SIN p. nervosus prostaticus [TA].
prostaticovesical venous p., p. venoso prostaticovesical; plexo venoso que inclui o plexo venoso prostático ao redor da próstata e do colo da bexiga; comunica-se com os plexos vesical e pudendo, recebe a veia dorsal profunda do pênis, e esvazia-se, por um ou mais vasos eferentes, na veia ilíaca interna (hipogástrica); corresponde ao p. vesical inferior na mulher. SIN p. venosus prostaticovesicalis.
prostatic venous p. [TA], p. venoso prostático; p. venoso, originado principalmente na veia dorsal do pênis, situado abaixo da base da bexiga nas laterais da próstata. VER TAMBÉM prostaticovesical venous p. SIN p. venosus prostaticus [TA], p. pudendalis, Santorini labyrinth.
pterygoid venous p. [TA], p. pterigóideo; p. venoso que ocupa a fossa infratemporal, recebendo veias que acompanham os ramos da artéria maxilar e terminando posteriormente na veia maxilar; anteriormente, o p. pterigóideo drena através da veia facial profunda para a veia facial. SIN p. venosus pterygoideus.
p. pudenda'lis, p. pudendo. SIN prostatic venous p.
p. puden'dus nervo'sus, p. nervoso pudendo. SIN pudendal nerve.
pulmonary (nervous) p. [TA], p. pulmonar; um dentre dois plexos anatômicos, anterior e posterior, no hilo de cada pulmão, formado por nervos esplâncnicos cardiopulmonares do tronco simpático e por ramos brônquicos do nervo vago; a partir deles, vários ramos acompanham os brônquios e artérias até o pulmão. SIN p. (nervosus) pulmonalis [TA].
Quénu hemorrhoidal p., p. hemorroidário de Quénu; plexos linfáticos na pele ao redor do ânus.
Ranvier p., p. de Ranvier; p. do estroma sub-basal da córnea. VER stroma p.
rectal plexuses, plexos retais. VER inferior rectal (nervous) p., middle rectal (nervous) p., superior rectal (nervous) p.
rectal venous p. [TA], p. venoso retal; um p. venoso que se apóia nas paredes posterior e lateral do reto; drena para a veia renal superior e, daí, para a veia porta, com as veias retais médias drenando para a veia ilíaca interna, e as veias retais inferiores, para a veia pudenda interna. SIN p. venosus rectalis [TA], hemorrhoidal p.
Remak p., p. de Remak. SIN submucosal (nervous) p.
renal (nervous) p. [TA], p. renal; o p. autônomo que circunda a artéria renal e estende-se com ela para a substância do rim. SIN p. (nervosus) renalis [TA].
sacral p. [TA], p. sacral; p. formado pelo quarto e quinto nervos lombares (tronco lombossacral) e pelo primeiro, segundo e terceiro nervos sacrais; situa-se na superfície interna da parede posterior da pelve, geralmente incrustado no músculo piriforme; seus nervos suprem os membros inferiores, sendo seu principal produto o nervo ciático. SIN p. sacralis [TA], ischiadic p., sciatic p.
p. sacra'lis [TA], p. sacral. SIN sacral p.
sacral venous p., p. venoso sacral; um p. venoso na superfície pélvica do sacro, formado por tributárias das veias sacrais laterais. SIN p. venosus sacralis.
Santorini p., p. de Santorini; p. venoso nas superfícies prostáticas ventral e lateral.
Sappey p., p. de Sappey; uma rede de linfáticos na aréola do mamilo.
sciatic p., p. ciático. SIN sacral p.
solar p., p. solar. SIN celiac (nervous) p.
spermatic p., p. espermático. SIN periarterial p. of testicular artery.
spinal nerve p. [TA], p. nervoso espinal; um entrelaçado de fascículos de fibras provenientes dos nervos espinais adjacentes para formar uma rede; os principais plexos são o cervical, o braquial e o lombossacral. SIN p. nervorum spinalium [TA], p. of spinal nerves [TA].
p. of spinal nerves [TA], p. nervoso espinal. SIN spinal nerve p.
splenic (nervous) p. [TA], p. esplênico; o p. de nervos autônomos ao longo da artéria esplênica. SIN p. (nervosus) splenicus [TA], p. (nervosus) lienalis*.
Stensen p., p. de Stensen; a rede venosa que circunda o ducto parotídeo (de Stensen).
stroma p., p. do estroma; p. de nervos no parênquima da córnea que consiste no p. primário ou profundo, na substância da córnea e no p. sub-basal ou superficial imediatamente subjacente à membrana limitante anterior.

subclavian p., p. subclávio. SIN periarterial p. of subclavian artery.
submucosal (nervous) p. [TA], p. submucoso; p. ganglionar de fibras nervosas não-mielinizadas, derivado principalmente do p. mesentérico superior, ramificando-se na submucosa intestinal. SIN p. (nervosus) submucosus [TA], Meissner p., Remak p.
suboccipital venous p. [TA], p. venoso suboccipital; o extenso p. de veias na região suboccipital. SIN p. venosus suboccipitalis [TA].
subserous (nervous) p. [TA], p. subseroso; a parte subserosa do p. entérico de nervos autônomos. SIN p. (nervosus) subserosus [TA].
superficial cardiac (nervous) p. [TA], p. cardíaco superficial; a subdivisão superficial e menor do p. cardíaco, formada pelos ramos cardíacos cervicais superiores do nervo vago esquerdo e pelo tronco simpático cervical; é encontrado sob o arco da aorta, entre o arco e a bifurcação do tronco pulmonar. SIN p. (nervosus) cardiacus superficialis [TA].
superficial temporal p., p. temporal superficial. SIN periarterial p. of superficial temporal artery.
superior dental (nervous) p. [TA], p. dental superior; formado por ramos do nervo infra-orbital, emite os ramos dentais superiores para a parte superior e os ramos gengivais superiores para a gengiva. SIN p. (nervosus) dentalis superior [TA].
superior hemorrhoidal p., p. hemorroidário superior. SIN superior rectal (nervous) p.
superior hypogastric (nervous) p. [TA], p. hipogástrico superior; a continuação do plexo aórtico abaixo da bifurcação da aorta ao nível da quinta vértebra lombar e entrando na pelve, onde se divide em dois nervos hipogástricos ao lado do reto; estes se unem aos nervos esplâncnicos pélvicos para formar o plexo hipogástrico inferior, que supre as vísceras pélvicas. SIN p. (nervosus) hypogastricus superior [TA], nervus presacralis*, presacral nerve*, Latarget nerve (1).
superior mesenteric (nervous) p. [TA], p. mesentérico superior; um plexo autônomo, continuação do plexo aórtico abdominal, que envia nervos para o intestino e forma com o vago os plexos subseroso, mioentérico e submucoso; esse plexo periarterial é tão denso que forma um "colar" perivascular característico, distinguindo a artéria mesentérica superior da veia mesentérica superior em várias modalidades de estudo por imagens, como por ultra-som. SIN p. (nervosus) mesentericus superior [TA].
superior rectal (nervous) p. [TA], p. retal superior; o plexo autônomo que se origina como uma continuação do plexo mesentérico inferior que acompanha a artéria retal superior. SIN p. (nervosus) rectalis superior [TA], superior hemorrhoidal p.
superior thyroid p., p. tireóideo superior. SIN periarterial p. of superior thyroid artery.
suprarenal (nervous) p. [TA], p. supra-renal; plexo autônomo formado principalmente por ramos do gânglio celíaco, situado no hilo da glândula suprarenal. SIN p. (nervosus) suprarenalis [TA].
sympathetic plexuses [TA], plexos simpáticos; plexos autônomos, nos quais há predomínio de fibras nervosas simpáticas pós-sinápticas.
testicular p., p. testicular. SIN periarterial p. of testicular artery.
thoracic aortic (nervous) p. [TA], p. aórtico torácico; plexo autônomo que circunda a aorta torácica e segue com ela através da abertura aórtica no diafragma para tornar-se contínuo com o plexo aórtico abdominal. SIN p. (nervosus) aorticus thoracicus [TA].
p. thyroi'deus infe'rior, p. tireóideo inferior. SIN periarterial p. of inferior thyroid artery.
tympanic (nervous) p. [TA], p. timpânico; um plexo situado sobre o promontório da parede labiríntica da cavidade timpânica, formado pelo nervo timpânico, um ramo anastomótico do nervo facial e por ramos simpáticos do plexo carótico interno; supre a mucosa da orelha média, as células mastóideas e a tuba auditiva (de Eustáquio), emitindo o nervo petroso superficial menor para o gânglio ótico. SIN p. (nervosus) tympanicus [TA], Jacobson p.
unpaired thyroid venous p. [TA], p. tireóideo ímpar; um plexo venoso situado na frente da porção inferior da traquéia, formado por anastomoses entre as veias laríngeas inferiores e as veias que emergem da borda caudal da tireóide; termina na veia tireóidea inferior ímpar. SIN p. venosus thyroideus impar.
ureteric (nervous) p. [TA], p. uretérico; o plexo autônomo derivado do plexo celíaco que acompanha o ureter. SIN p. (nervosus) uretericus [TA].
uterine venous p. [TA], p. uterino; as veias plexiformes situadas ao lado do útero no ligamento largo. SIN p. venosus uterinus [TA].
uterovaginal (nervous) p. [TA], p. uterovaginal; plexo autônomo ganglionar situado de cada lado do colo do útero, derivado do plexo hipogástrico inferior. SIN p. (nervosus) uterovaginalis [TA], Frankenhäuser ganglion, Lee ganglion.
vaginal venous p. [TA], p. venoso vaginal; o p. venoso que circunda a vagina. SIN p. venosus vaginalis [TA].
vascular p. [TA], p. vascular; rede vascular formada por anastomoses freqüentes entre os vasos sanguíneos (artérias ou veias) de uma parte. SIN p. vasculosus [TA].
p. vascularis cavernosus conchae [TA], p. cavernoso das conchas. SIN cavernous (vascular) p. of conchae.
p. vasculo'sus [TA], p. vascular. SIN vascular p.
p. veno'sus [TA], p. venoso. SIN venous p.
p. veno'sus areola'ris [TA], p. venoso areolar. SIN areolar venous p.
p. venosus basila'ris [TA], p. basilar. SIN basilar venous p.
p. veno'sus cana'lis hypoglos'si [TA], p. venoso do canal do nervo hipoglosso. SIN venous p. of canal of hypoglossal nerve.
p. veno'sus carot'icus inter'nus, p. venoso carótico interno. SIN internal carotid venous p.
p. veno'sus foram'inis ova'lis [TA], p. venoso do forame oval. SIN venous p. of foramen ovale.
p. venosus pampinifor'mis [TA], p. pampiniforme. SIN pampiniform venous p.
p. venosus prostaticovesica'lis, p. venoso prostaticovesical. SIN prostaticovesical venous p.
p. veno'sus prostat'icus [TA], p. venoso prostático. SIN prostatic venous p.
p. venosus pterygoi'deus, p. pterigóideo. SIN pterygoid venous p.
p. veno'sus recta'lis [TA], p. venoso retal. SIN rectal venous p.
p. veno'sus sacra'lis, p. venoso sacral. SIN sacral venous p.
p. veno'sus suboccipita'lis [TA], p. venoso suboccipital. SIN suboccipital venous p.
p. venosus thyroi'deus im'par, p. venoso tireóideo ímpar. SIN unpaired thyroid venous p.
p. veno'sus uteri'nus [TA], p. venoso uterino. SIN uterine venous p.
p. veno'sus vagina'lis [TA], p. venoso vaginal. SIN vaginal venous p.
p. veno'sus vertebra'lis, p. venoso vertebral. SIN vertebral venous *system*.
p. veno'sus vesica'lis [TA], p. venoso vesical. SIN vesicular venous p.
p. venosus vesica'lis infe'rior, p. venoso vesical inferior. SIN inferior vesical venous p.
venous p. [TA], p. venoso; rede vascular formada por numerosas anastomoses entre veias. SIN p. venosus [TA].
venous p. of bladder, p. venoso vesical. SIN vesicular vernous p.
venous p. of canal of hypoglossal nerve [TA], p. venoso do canal do nervo hipogloso; pequena rede venosa em torno do nervo hipoglosso, que se une ao seio occipital, seio petroso inferior e veia jugular interna. SIN venous canalis hypoglossi [TA], circellus venosus hypoglossi, rete canalis hypoglossi.
venous p. of foramen ovale [TA], p. venoso do forame oval; uma rede venosa ao redor do nervo mandibular que une o seio cavernoso e o p. pterigóideo. SIN p. venosus foraminis ovalis [TA], rete foraminis ovalis.
vertebral p., p. vertebral. SIN periarterial p. of vertebral artery.
p. vertebra'lis, p. vertebral. SIN periarterial p. of vertebral artery.
vertebral venous p., p. venoso vertebral. SIN vertebral venous *system*.
vesical (nervous) p. [TA], p. vesical; p. autônomo sobre a bexiga, derivado do plexo hipogástrico inferior. SIN p. vesicalis [TA].
vesicular venous p. [TA], p. venoso vesical; plexo de veias ao redor do fundo e das laterais da bexiga. SIN p. venosus vesicalis [TA], venous p. of bladder.
Walther p., p. de Walther. SIN cavernous nervous p.

PLICA

pli·ca, gen. e pl. **pli·cae** (plī'kă, plī'sē). [TA] Prega. SIN fold (1). [L. mod. dobra ou prega]
pli'cae adipo'sae pleurae, pregas adiposas da pleura. SIN fatty *folds* of pleura, em *fold*.
pli'cae ala'res plicae synovialis infrapatellaris, pregas alares da prega sinovial infrapatelar. SIN alar *folds* of infrapatellar synovial fold, em *fold*.
pli'cae ampulla'res tu'bae uteri'nae, pregas ampulares da tuba uterina. SIN ampullary *folds* of uterine tube, em *fold*.
p. anterior faucium, prega anterior das fauces; arco palatoglosso; *termo oficial alternativo para palatoglossal *arch*.
p. aryepiglot'tica [TA], p. ariepiglótica. SIN aryepiglottic *fold*.
p. axilla'ris, p. axilar. SIN axillary *fold*.
pli'cae ceca'les [TA], pregas cecais. SIN cecal *folds*, em *fold*.
p. ceca'lis vascula'ris [TA], p. cecal vascular. SIN vascular *fold* of the cecum.
p. chor'dae tym'pani [TA], p. da corda do tímpano. SIN *fold* of chorda tympani.
p. choroi'dea, p. corióidea; no embrião, uma invaginação da pia-máter a partir da qual se desenvolve o plexo corióide.
pli'cae cilia'res [TA], pregas ciliares. SIN ciliary *folds*, em *fold*.
pli'cae circula'res intestini tenuis [TA], pregas circulares do intestino delgado. SIN circular *folds* of small intestine, em *fold*.
p. duodena'lis infe'rior [TA], p. duodenal inferior. SIN inferior duodenal *fold*.
p. duodena'lis supe'rior [TA], p. duodenal superior. SIN superior duodenal *fold*.
p. duodenojejuna'lis, p. duodenojejunal; *termo oficial alternativo para superior duodenal *fold*.

p. duodenomesocol'ica, p. duodenomesocólica; *termo oficial alternativo para inferior duodenal fold.
p. epigas'trica, p. epigástrica. SIN lateral umbilical fold.
pli'cae epiglot'ticae, pregas epiglóticas. SIN epiglottic folds, em fold.
p. fimbria'ta faciei inferioris linguae [TA], prega franjada da face inferior da língua. SIN fimbriated fold of inferior surface of tongue.
pli'cae gas'tricae [TA], pregas gástricas. SIN gastric folds, em fold.
pli'cae gastropancreat'icae [TA], pregas gastropancreáticas. SIN gastropancreatic folds, em fold.
p. glossoepiglot'tica latera'lis [TA], p. glossoepiglótica lateral. SIN lateral glossoepiglottic fold.
p. glossoepiglot'tica media'na [TA], p. glossoepiglótica mediana. SIN median glossoepiglottic fold.
p. guberna'trix, ligamento genitoinguinal. SIN genitoinguinal ligament.
p. hypogas'trica, p. hipogástrica. SIN medial umbilical fold.
p. ilioceca'lis [TA], p. iliocecal. SIN ileocecal fold.
p. incu'dis, p. da bigorna. SIN incudal fold.
p. inguina'lis, p. inguinal; um espessamento mesodérmico embrionário que une a extremidade caudal da crista urogenital à parede anterior do abdome; o gubernáculo do testículo nele se desenvolve. SIN inguinal fold.
p. interdigita'lis, p. interdigital. SIN web of fingers/toes.
p. interureter'ica [TA], p. interuretérica. SIN interureteric crest.
pli'cae ir'idis [TA], pregas da íris. SIN folds of iris, em fold.
p. lacrima'lis [TA], p. lacrimal. SIN lacrimal fold.
p. longitudina'lis duode'ni [TA], p. longitudinal do duodeno. SIN longitudinal fold of duodenum.
p. luna'ta, p. semilunar. SIN p. semilunaris of conjunctiva.
plicae mallea'res (anterior et posterior) [TA], pregas maleares (anterior e posterior). SIN mallear folds, em fold.
p. membra'nae tym'pani, p. da membrana timpânica. SIN mallear folds, em fold.
pli'cae muco'sae vesi'cae biliaris [TA], pregas da mucosa da vesícula biliar. SIN mucosal folds of gallbladder, em fold.
p. ner'vi laryn'gei superioris [TA], p. do nervo laríngeo superior. SIN fold of superior laryngeal nerve.
p. palati'na transver'sa [TA], prega palatina transversa. SIN transverse palatine fold.
pli'cae palma'tae canalis cervicis uteri [TA], pregas palmadas do canal do colo do útero. SIN palmate folds of cervical canal, em fold.
p. palpebronasa'lis [TA], p. palpebronasal. SIN palpebronasal fold.
p. paraduodena'lis [TA], p. paraduodenal. SIN paraduodenal fold.
p. posterior faucium, p. posterior das fauces; arco palatofaríngeo; *termo oficial alternativo para palatopharyngeal arch.
pli'cae rec'ti, pregas retais. SIN transverse folds of rectum, em fold.
p. rectouteri'na [TA], p. retouterina. SIN rectouterine fold.
p. rectovagina'lis, p. retovaginal. SIN sacrovaginal fold.
p. salpingopalatin'a [TA], p. salpingopalatina. SIN salpingopalatine fold.
p. salpingopharyn'gea [TA], p. salpingofaríngea. SIN salpingopharyngeal fold.
plicae semilunares coli [TA], pregas semilunares do colo. SIN semilunar folds of colon, em fold.
plicae semiluna'res of colon, pregas semilunares do colo. SIN semilunar folds of colon, em fold.
p. semiluna'ris [TA], p. semilunar. SIN semilunar fold.
p. semiluna'ris of conjuncti'va [TA], p. semilunar da túnica conjuntiva; (1) [NA], a prega semilunar formada pela conjuntiva palpebral no ângulo medial do olho; (2) uma prega da túnica mucosa conjuntival encontrada em muitos animais; normalmente está parcialmente oculta no canto medial do olho, quando em repouso, mas pode ser estendida para cobrir parte da córnea ou toda ela, em uma ação semelhante ao piscar para limpar a córnea, como nas aves. SIN membrana nictitans, nictitating membrane, palpebra III, palpebra tertia, third eyelid. SIN p. semilunaris conjunctivae [TA], p. lunata, p. semilunaris of eye, semilunar conjunctival fold.
p. semilunaris conjunctivae [TA], p. semilunar da túnica conjuntiva. SIN p. semilunaris of conjunctiva.
p. semilunaris of eye, p. semilunar do olho. SIN p. semilunaris of conjunctiva.
p. spira'lis duc'tus cys'tici [TA], p. espiral do ducto cístico. SIN spiral fold of cystic duct.
p. stapedialis, p. estapedial. SIN fold of stapes.
p. sublingua'lis [TA], p. sublingual. SIN sublingual fold.
p. synovia'lis, p. sinovial. SIN synovial fold.
p. synovia'lis infrapatella'ris [TA], p. sinovial infrapatelar. SIN infrapatellar synovial fold.
p. synovia'lis patella'ris, p. sinovial patelar. SIN infrapatellar synovial fold.
pli'cae transversa'les rec'ti [TA], pregas transversas do reto. SIN transverse folds of rectum, em fold.
p. triangula'ris [TA], p. triangular. SIN triangular fold.
pli'cae tuba'riae tu'bae uteri'nae [TA], pregas tubárias da tuba uterina. SIN folds of uterine tubes, em fold.
p. tubopalati'na, p. tubopalatina. SIN salpingopalatine fold.
p. umbilica'lis latera'lis [TA], p. umbilical lateral. SIN lateral umbilical fold.
p. umbilica'lis media'lis [TA], p. umbilical medial. SIN medial umbilical fold.
p. ura'chi, p. do úraco. SIN median umbilical fold.
p. ureter'ica, p. uretérica. SIN interureteric crest.
p. uterovesica'lis, p. uterovesical. SIN uterovesical ligament.
p. ve'nae ca'vae sinis'trae [TA], p. da veia cava esquerda. SIN fold of left vena cava.
p. ventricula'ris, p. ventricular. SIN vestibular fold.
p. vesica'lis transver'sa, p. vesical transversa. SIN transverse vesical fold.
p. vesicouteri'na, p. vesicouterina. SIN uterovesical ligament.
p. vestibula'ris [TA], p. vestibular. SIN vestibular fold.
p. vestib'uli, p. do vestíbulo; uma prega de mucosa que forma uma crista no septo do nariz.
p. villo'sa, p. vilosa; uma das cristas da mucosa do estômago na região do piloro.
p. voca'lis [TA], p. vocal. SIN vocal fold.

pli·cate (pli′kāt). Pregueado; dobrado; franzido.
pli·ca·tion (plī-kā′shun, pli-). Plicatura; pregueamento ou reunião em pregas; especificamente, uma operação para reduzir o tamanho de uma víscera oca fazendo-se pregas ou dobras em suas paredes. [L. *plico*, pp. *-atus*, preguear]
pli·cot·o·my (plī-kot′ō-mē). Plicotomia; divisão da prega maleolar posterior. [plica + G. *tomē*, incisão]
-ploid. -Plóide; múltiplo em forma; suas combinações são usadas na forma de adjetivo e substantivo de um múltiplo (específico) de cromossomas. [G. *-plo-*, *-prega*, + *-ides*, em forma; L. *-ploïdeus*]
ploi·dy (ploy′dē). Ploidia; o número de conjuntos haplóides em uma célula. Os gametas normalmente contêm um; as células somáticas, dois. VER TAMBÉM polyploidy. [-ploid + -y, condição]
plom·bage (plom-bahzh′). Plumbagem; antigamente, o uso de um material inerte no colapso pulmonar no tratamento cirúrgico da tuberculose pulmonar. [Fr. lit. trabalho com chumbo]
plo·sive (plō′siv). Plosivo; som da fala produzido prendendo-se o fluxo de ar por um momento e, depois, liberando-o subitamente.
plot (plot). Gráfico; uma representação gráfica.
  double-reciprocal p., gráfico do duplo-recíproco; uma representação gráfica de dados cinéticos enzimáticos na qual $1/v$ (no eixo vertical), onde v é a velocidade inicial, é representado como uma função da recíproca da concentração de substrato $(1/[S])$. SIN Lineweaver-Burk p. Woolf-Lineweaver-Burk p.
  Eadie-Hofstee p., gráfico de Eadie-Hofstee; representação gráfica de dados cinéticos enzimáticos na qual as velocidades, v, são representadas no eixo vertical como uma função da razão $v/[S]$ no eixo horizontal. Ocasionalmente, esses eixos são invertidos. Algumas vezes é denominado gráfico de Eadie-Augustinsson ou gráfico de Woolf-Eadie-Augustinsson-Hofstee.
  funnel p., gráfico do funil; método gráfico para detecção de viés de publicação. A estimativa de risco derivada de um conjunto de estudos epidemiológicos usados em uma metaanálise é representada contra o tamanho da amostra. Se não houver viés de publicação, o gráfico tem o formato de um funil; se for mais provável a publicação de estudos com resultados significativos que de estudos negativos, o gráfico é assimétrico. VER TAMBÉM metaanalysis.
  Hanes p., gráfico de Hanes; representação gráfica de dados cinéticos enzimáticos na qual a concentração de substrato dividida pela velocidade (isto é, a razão $[S]/v$) é representada no eixo vertical como uma função de $[S]$. Algumas vezes é denominado gráfico de Hanes-Wilkinson.
  Hill p., gráfico de Hill; representação gráfica de dados cinéticos enzimáticos ou de fenômenos de ligação para avaliar o grau de cooperatividade de um sistema; o eixo vertical em um gráfico de Hill é log $[Y/(1-Y)]$, no qual Y é o grau de saturação (para enzimas, o eixo vertical é log $[v/(V_{máx} - v)]$, onde v é a velocidade inicial e $V_{máx}$ é a velocidade máxima, e o eixo horizontal é o logaritmo da concentração de ligante.
  Lineweaver-Burk p., gráfico de Lineweaver-Burk. SIN double-reciprocal p.
  Ramachandran p., gráfico de Ramachandran; representação gráfica na qual o ângulo diédrico de rotação em torno da ligação α-carbono-carbonil em polipeptídeos é representada em relação ao ângulo diédrico de rotação em torno da ligação α-carbono-nitrogênio. SIN conformational map.
  Scatchard p., gráfico de Scatchard; (1) uma representação gráfica usada na análise de fenômenos de ligação na qual a concentração de ligante unido dividida pela concentração de ligante livre é representada contra a concentração de ligante unido; (2) semelhante a (1), exceto pelo fato de a concentração de ligante unido estar no eixo vertical.
  Woolf-Lineweaver-Burk p., gráfico de Woolf-Lineweaver-Burk. SIN double-reciprocal p.
PLP Abreviatura de *pyridoxal* 5-phosphate (piridoxal 5-fosfato); parathyroid hormonelike *protein* (proteína semelhante ao paratormônio).
plug (plŭg). Tampão; qualquer massa que enche uma cavidade ou fecha um orifício.

Dittrich p.'s, tampões de Dittrich; pequenas massas de coloração cinza-escuro, fétidas, de bactérias e cristais de ácidos graxos no escarro na gangrena pulmonar e na bronquite fética. SIN Traube p.'s.

epithelial p., t, epitelial; massa de células epiteliais que oclui temporariamente uma abertura embrionária; o termo é mais usado em relação às narinas externas.

laminated epithelial p., ceratose obliterante. SIN keratosis obturans.

meconium p., tampão meconial; tampão de mecônio espesso, viscoso, que pode causar obstrução intestinal.

mucous p., tampão mucoso; massa de muco e células que enche o canal cervical entre os períodos menstruais ou durante a gravidez; uma massa de muco que oclui um brônquio principal ou lobar.

Traube p.'s, tampões de Traube. SIN Dittrich p.'s.

plug·ger. Obturador; instrumento dental usado para condensar ouro (em folha), amálgama ou qualquer material plástico em uma cavidade; operado por meios manuais ou mecânicos. SIN packer (2), plugging instrument.

automatic p., obturador automático; dispositivo ativado mecânica ou eletricamente, usado para produzir pressão de condensação na colocação de amálgama ou de folha de ouro na preparação de uma cavidade. SIN automatic condenser.

back-action p., obturador de ação retrógrada; instrumento para condensar folha de ouro ou amálgama em áreas que não podem ser diretamente alcançadas.

foot p., obturador de pé; um obturador, cujo formato se assemelha ao de um pé, usado para condensar folha de ouro; a superfície de trabalho pode ser plana ou curva na direção calcanhar–dedo.

root canal p., obturador do canal radicular; instrumento para um canal radicular bem afilado, de ponta romba, usado para comprimir ou forçar um cone de guta-percha no canal radicular.

plum·ba·go (plŭm-bā′gō). Grafite. SIN graphite. [L. *plumbago*, grafite]

plum·bic (plŭm′bik). Plúmbico. 1. Relativo ao chumbo ou que o contém. 2. Designa a maior valência do íon chumbo, Pb^{4+}. [L. *plumbum*, chumbo]

plum·bism (plŭm′bizm). Plumbismo. SIN lead poisoning. [L. *plumbum*, chumbo]

plum·bum (plŭm′bŭm). Chumbo. SIN lead. [L.]

Plummer, Henry S., médico norte-americano, 1874–1937. VER P. *disease*; P.-Vinson *syndrome*.

plu·mose (ploo′mōs). Plumoso. [L. *pluma*, pena]

pluri-. Pluri-; muitos, vários. VER TAMBÉM multi-, poly-. [L. *plus, pluris*]

plu·ri·cau·sal (ploor-i-kaw′zăl). Pluricausal; que tem duas ou mais causas; usado em referência à etiologia de uma doença; freqüentemente indica que determinada doença desenvolve-se apenas quando dois ou mais fatores causadores operam simultaneamente.

plu·ri·glan·du·lar (ploo-ri-glan′doo-lăr). Pluriglandular; designa várias glândulas ou suas secreções. SIN multiglandular, polyglandular.

plu·ri·loc·u·lar (ploo-ri-lok′u-lăr). Plurilocular. SIN multilocular.

plu·ri·nu·cle·ar (ploo-ri-noo′klē-ăr). Plurinuclear. SIN multinuclear.

plu·rip·o·tent, plu·ri·po·ten·tial (ploo-rip′ō-tent, ploo′rē-pō-ten′shăl). Pluripotente, pluripotencial. 1. Que tem a capacidade de afetar mais de um órgão ou tecido. 2. Não fixo quanto ao potencial de desenvolvimento. VER TAMBÉM pluripotent *cells*, em *cell*.

plu·ri·re·sis·tant (ploo′ri-rē-sis′tănt). Plurirresistente; que possui múltiplos aspectos de resistência.

plu·to·ma·nia (ploo-tō-mā′nē-ă). Plutomania; delírio de um indivíduo de que tem grande riqueza. [G. *ploutos*, riqueza, + *mania*, mania]

plu·to·nism (ploo-ton-izm). Plutonismo; efeitos produzidos, conforme demonstrado em animais experimentais, por meio de exposição ao elemento radioativo plutônio presente em reatores atômicos; consistem em lesão hepática, alterações ósseas e encanecimento do cabelo.

plu·to·ni·um (Pu) (ploo′tō′nē-ŭm). Plutônio; um elemento radioativo artificial transurânico, de n.º atômico 94, peso atômico 244,064. O isótopo emissor α mais conhecido é o Pu^{239} (meia-vida de 24.110 anos) que, como o U^{235}, é físsil e pode ser usado em bombas atômicas e nas usinas nucleares; Pu^{238} (meia-vida 87,74 anos) é usado como fonte de energia em marcapassos. Os íons do Pu buscam o osso; a ingestão leva a risco de radiação, como ocorre com o rádio e o radioestrôncio. [planeta, *Plutão*]

Pm Símbolo de promethium (promécio).

pM Abreviatura de picomolar (10^{-12} M).

pm Símbolo de picometer (picômetro).

P mit·ra·le (mī-trā′lē). P mitral; ondas P largas, entalhadas em algumas ou muitas derivações do eletrocardiograma com um proeminente componente negativo tardio da onda P em V_1, considerada característica de doença valvular mitral. (Embora esse termo seja amplamente usado em literatura eletrocardiográfica, é, na verdade, um nome inadequado e seria mais apropriadamente denominado P-sinistrocárdico, pois resulta de sobrecarga do átrio esquerdo a despeito da causa e pode ocorrer independentemente de doença da valva mitral.)

PML Abreviatura de progressive multifocal *leukoencephalopathy* (leucoencefalopatia multifocal progressiva).

pmol Abreviatura de picomole (picomol).

PMR Abreviatura de proportional mortality ratio (razão de mortalidade proporcional).

PMS Abreviatura de premenstrual *syndrome* (síndrome pré-menstrual).

-pnea. -Pnéia; respiração. [G. *pneō*, respirar]

pneo-. Forma combinante que significa respiração. VER TAMBÉM pneum-, pneumo-. [G. *pneō*, respirar]

pneum-, pneuma-, pneumat-, pneumato-. Pneum-, pneuma-, pneumat-, pneumato-; presença de ar ou gás, os pulmões, ou a respiração. VER TAMBÉM pneo-, pneumo-. [G. *pneuma, pneumatos*, ar, respiração]

pneu·ma (noo′mă). Na filosofia e na medicina da Grécia antiga: 1. Ar ou uma essência flamejante impregnante no ar (que hoje seria identificada com o oxigênio), que era o espírito criativo e animador do universo; introduzida no corpo através dos pulmões, essa essência gerava e mantinha o calor inato no ventrículo esquerdo e era distribuída pelas artérias para o cérebro e para todas as partes do corpo. 2. Alma ou psique. [G. *pneuma*, ar, respiração]

pneu·marth·ro·gram (noo-marth′rō-gram). Pneumartrograma; registros de pneumartrografia em filme.

pneu·marth·rog·ra·phy (noo-marth-rog′ră-fē). Pneumartrografia; exame radiológico de uma articulação após a introdução de ar, com ou sem outro meio de contraste.

pneu·mar·thro·sis (noo-mar-thrō′sis). Pneumartrose; presença de ar em uma articulação. [G. *pneumo*, ar, + *arthron*, articulação, + *-osis*, condição]

pneu·mat·ic (noo-mat′ik). Pneumático. 1. Relativo a ar ou gás, ou a uma estrutura cheia de ar. 2. Relativo à respiração. [G. *pneumatikos*]

pneu·mat·ic an·ti·shock gar·ment. Veste pneumática antichoque; veste inflável usada para comprimir a circulação periférica, assim reduzindo o fluxo sanguíneo e a exsudação de líquido para os tecidos, a fim de manter o fluxo sanguíneo central na presença de choque. SIN military antishock trousers.

pneu·mat·ics (noo′mat′iks). Pneumática; ciência que estuda as propriedades físicas do ar e dos outros gases. [G. *pneuma*, ar ou gás]

pneu·ma·tism (noo′mă-tizm). Pneumatismo; a doutrina dos pneumatistas.

pneu·ma·tists (noo′mă-tists). Pneumatistas; os seguidores da escola cuja fisiologia centralizava-se no pneuma e que concebia as causas de doenças como distúrbios desse princípio vital.

pneu·ma·ti·za·tion (noo′mă-ti-zā′shŭn). Pneumatização; o desenvolvimento de células aéreas como aquelas dos ossos mastóide e etmóide. [G. *pneuma*, ar]

pneu·ma·tized (noo′mă-tīzd). Pneumatizado; que contém ar.

pneumato-. Pneumato-. VER pneum-.

pneu·ma·to·car·dia (noo′mă-tō-kar′dē-ă). Pneumatocardia; presença de bolhas de ar ou gás no sangue do coração; produzida por embolia aérea.

pneu·ma·to·cele (noo′mat′o-sēl). Pneumatocele. 1. Edema enfisematoso ou gasoso. 2. SIN pneumocele. 3. Uma cavidade de paredes finas no pulmão, uma das seqüelas características da pneumonia estafilocócica e da pneumonia por *Pneumocystis carinii*. [G. *pneuma*, ar, + *kēlē*, tumor, hérnia]

extracranial p., p. extracraniana; coleção de gás sob a gálea aponeurótica, geralmente devido a fratura nos seios paranasais. SIN extracranial pneumocele.

intracranial p., p. intracraniana; coleção de gás no crânio, no encéfalo ou nas meninges. SIN intracranial pneumocele.

pneu·ma·to·en·ter·ic. Pneumatoentérico. SIN celomic bay.

pneu·ma·to·he·mia (noo′mă-tō-hē′mē-ă). Pneumatemia. SIN pneumohemia.

pneu·ma·tom·e·ter (noo-mă-tom′e-ter). Pneumatômetro; termo obsoleto para espirômetro.

pneu·ma·tor·rha·chis (noo-mă-tōr′ă-kis). Pneumatórraque. SIN pneumatorrhachis. [G. *pneuma*, ar, + *rhachis*, espinha]

pneu·ma·to·scope (noo′mă-tō-skōp, noo-mat′ō-skōp). Pneumatoscópio. 1. Termo obsoleto para designar um instrumento para medida da extensão das incursões respiratórias do tórax. 2. Termo obsoleto para designar um instrumento para uso em percussão auscultatória, sendo os sons da percussão do tórax ouvidos na boca. SIN pneumoscope. [G. *pneuma*, ar, + *skopeō*, examinar]

pneu·ma·to·sis (noo-mă-tō′sis). Pneumatose; acúmulo anormal de gás em qualquer tecido ou parte do corpo. [G. uma explosão]

p. coli, p. colônica; condição geralmente benigna na qual se observa radiologicamente a presença de gás na parede do colo; algumas vezes está associada a doença pulmonar obstrutiva.

p. cystoi'des intestina'lis, p. cistóide intestinal; condição de causa desconhecida caracterizada pela ocorrência de cistos de gás na mucosa intestinal; pode causar obstrução intestinal. SIN intestinal emphysema.

pneu·ma·tu·ria (noo-mă-too′rē-ă). Pneumatúria; a eliminação de gás ou ar pela uretra durante ou após a micção, resultante de urina infectada ou, na maioria das vezes, de uma fístula intestinal. [G. *pneuma*, ar, + *ouron*, urina]

pneu·ma·type (noo′mă-tīp). Pneumótipo; aparelho para determinar a pervidade das fossas nasais pela expiração através do nariz contra uma lâmina de vidro resfriada. [G. *pneuma*, respiração, + *typos*, tipo]

pneumo-, pneumon-, pneumono-. Pneumo-, pneumon-, pneumono-; os pulmões, ar ou gás, respiração ou pneumonia. VER TAMBÉM aer-, pneo-, pneum-. [G. *pneumōn, pneumonos*, pulmão]

pneumoarthrography / pneumology

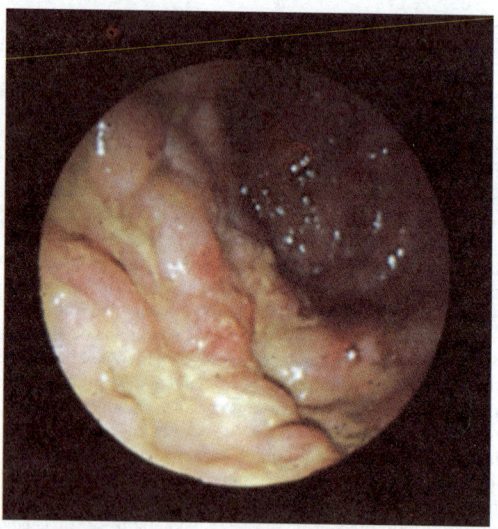

pneumatose cistóide intestinal: imagem endoscópica de cistos de gás

pneu·mo·ar·throg·ra·phy (noo′mō-ar-throg′ra-fē). Pneumartrografia; radiografia de uma articulação após injeção de ar e geralmente um contraste hidrossolúvel. [G. *pneuma*, ar, + *arthron*, articulação, + *graphō*, escrever]

pneu·mo·ba·cil·lus (noo′mō-ba-sil′us). SIN *Klebsiella pneumoniae.*

pneu·mo·bul·bar (noo-mō-bul′bar). Pneumobulbar; relativo aos pulmões e à sua conexão com o bulbo através do nervo vago. [G. *pneumōn*, pulmão, + L. *bulbus*, bulbo]

pneu·mo·car·di·al (noo′mō-kar′dē-al). Cardiopulmonar. SIN cardiopulmonary.

pneu·mo·cele (noo′mō-sēl). Pneumocele. SIN pneumonocele.
  extracranial p., p. extracraniana. SIN extracranial *pneumatocele.*
  intracranial p., p. intracraniana. SIN intracranial *pneumatocele.*

pneu·mo·cen·te·sis (noo-mō-sen-tē′sis). Pneumocentese. SIN pneumonocentesis.

pneu·mo·ceph·a·lus (noo-mō-sef′a-lus). Pneumocéfalo; presença de ar ou gás na cavidade craniana. [G. *pneuma*, ar, + *kephalē*, cabeça]

pneu·mo·cho·le·cys·ti·tis (noo′mō-kō′lē-sis-tī′tis). Pneumocolecistite; colecistite causada por microrganismos formadores de gás que produzem gás na vesícula biliar.

pneu·mo·coc·cal (noo-mō-kok′al). Pneumocócico; relativo a pneumococo ou que o contém.

pneu·mo·coc·ce·mia (noo′mō-kok-sē′mē-a). Pneumococcemia; a presença de pneumococcus no sangue. [pneumococcus + G. *haima*, sangue]

pneu·mo·coc·ci·dal (noo′mō-kok-si′dal). Pneumococcida; destrutivo para pneumococcus. [pneumococcus + L. *caedo*, matar]

pneu·mo·coc·col·y·sis (noo′mō-kok-ol′i-sis). Pneumocólise; lise ou destruição de pneumococcus. [pneumococcus + G. *lysis*, dissolução]

pneu·mo·coc·co·sis (noo′mō-kok-ō′sis). Pneumococose; termo raramente usado para infecção por pneumococcus.

pneu·mo·coc·co·su·ri·a (noo′mō-kok-o-soo′rē-a). Pneumococosúria; a presença de pneumococcus ou de sua substância capsular específica na urina. [pneumococcus + G. *ouron*, urina]

pneu·mo·coc·cus, pl. **pneu·mo·coc·ci** (noo-mō-kok′us, -kok′sī). Pneumococo. SIN *Streptococcus pneumoniae.* [G. *pneumōn*, pulmão, + *kokkos*, coco]
  Fraenkel p., p. de Fraenkel. SIN *Streptococcus pneumoniae.*

pneu·mo·co·lon (noo-mō-kō′lon). Pneumocolo; gás no colo ou gás intersticial na parede do colo. [G. *pneuma*, ar, + *kolon*, colo]

pneu·mo·co·ni·o·sis, pneu·mo·ko·ni·o·sis, pl. **pneu·mo·co·ni·o·ses** (noo′mō-kō-nē-ō-sis, -sēz). Pneumoconiose; inflamação que comumente leva a fibrose dos pulmões causada pela inalação de poeira incidente em diversas ocupações; caracterizada por dor torácica, tosse com pouca ou nenhuma expectoração, dispnéia, redução da excursão torácica, algumas vezes cianose e fadiga após pequeno esforço; o grau de incapacidade depende dos tipos de partículas inaladas, bem como do nível de exposição a elas. SIN anthracotic tuberculosis, pneumonoconiosis, pneumonokoniosis. [G. *pneumōn*, pulmão, + *konis*, poeira, + *-osis*, condição]
  bauxite p., p. por bauxita; condição causada pela inalação ocupacional de fumos de bauxita emitidos durante a fabricação de abrasivos de alumina; caracterizada por tosse, dispnéia, um padrão respiratório obstrutivo e restritivo combinado e comprometimento da capacidade de difusão. SIN Shaver disease.
  coal worker's p., p. dos mineiros de carvão. SIN anthracosilicosis.
  collagenous p., p. colagenosa; doença dos pulmões, caracterizada por fibrose intersticial, causada por inalação de poeiras ou toxinas no local de trabalho.
  p. siderotica (sid-er-ot′i-ka). Siderose; pneumonia causada por inalação da poeira de ferro. SIN pulmonary siderosis.

pneu·mo·cra·ni·um (noo-mō-krā′nē-um). Pneumocrânio; presença de ar entre o crânio e a dura-máter; o termo é comumente usado para indicar ar extradural ou subdural. [G. *pneuma*, ar, + *kranion*, crânio]

ℹ️ ***Pneu·mo·cys·tis ca·ri·nii*** (noo-mō-sis′tis ka-rī′nē-ī). O microrganismo eucariótico responsável pela pneumonia intersticial em pacientes imunodeprimidos. A posição taxonômica exata permanece obscura, pois o organismo tem semelhanças morfológicas com protozoários, mas compartilha substancial RNA ribossômico 16S e DNA mitocondrial com algumas espécies dos Ascomycetes. *P. carinii* não cresce em meios de cultura fúngica, mas é corado por métodos para fungos, e as infecções causadas por ele respondem a fármacos antiprotozoários e também a alguns antifúngicos. [G. *pneuma*, ar, respiração, + *kystis*, bexiga, bolsa]

pneu·mo·cys·tog·ra·phy (noo′mō-sis-tog′ra-fē). Pneumocistografia; radiografia da bexiga após injeção de ar. [G. *pneuma*, ar, + *kystis*, bexiga, + *graphō*, escrever]

pneu·mo·cys·to·sis (noo′mō-sis-tō′sis). Pneumocistose. SIN *Pneumocystis carinii pneumonia.*

pneu·mo·cyte (noo′mō-sīt). Pneumócito. SIN alveolar cell. [pneumo- + G. *kytos*, célula]

pneu·mo·der·ma (noo-mō-der′ma). Pneumoderma. SIN subcutaneous *emphysema.* [G. *pneuma*, ar, + *derma*, pele]

pneu·mo·dy·nam·ics (noo′mō-di-nam′iks). Pneumodinâmica; a mecânica da respiração. [G. *pneuma*, respiração, + *dynamis*, força]

pneu·mo·em·py·e·ma (noo′mō-em′pī-ē′ma). Pneumoempiema; termo raramente usado para piopneumotórax.

pneu·mo·en·ceph·a·lo·gram (noo′mō-en-sef′a-lō-gram). Pneumoencefalograma; radiografias obtidas por pneumoencefalografia.

pneu·mo·en·ceph·a·log·ra·phy (noo′mō-en-sef′a-log′ra-fē). Pneumoencefalografia; visualização radiográfica dos ventrículos cerebrais e dos espaços subaracnóides pelo uso de gás como ar; não é mais usada devido à TC e à RM. [G. *pneuma*, ar, + *enkephalos*, encéfalo, + *graphō*, escrever]

pneu·mo·gas·tric (noo-mō-gas′trik). Pneumogástrico. 1. Relativo aos pulmões e ao estômago. 2. Designação obsoleta do nervo vago. SIN gastropneumonic, gastropulmonary. [G. *pneumōn*, pulmão, + *gastēr*, estômago]

pneu·mo·gas·trog·ra·phy (noo′mō-gas-trog′ra-fē). Pneumogastrografia; estudo radiográfico do estômago após injeção de ar, sendo raramente usado. [G. *pneuma*, ar, + *gastēr*, estômago, + *graphō*, escrever]

pneu·mo·gram (noo′mō-gram). Pneumograma. 1. O registro ou traçado feito por um pneumógrafo. 2. Registro radiográfico de pneumografia. [G. *pneumōn*, pulmão, + *gramma*, desenho]

pneu·mo·graph (noo′mō-graf). Pneumógrafo; termo genérico usado para qualquer dispositivo que registre as excursões respiratórias por movimentos da superfície corporal; p. ex., um pneumógrafo de impedância, que aplica os princípios da pletismografia de impedância ao tórax. [G. *pneumōn*, pulmão, + *graphō*, escrever]

pneu·mog·ra·phy (noo-mog′ra-fē). Pneumografia. 1. Exame com um pneumógrafo. 2. Termo geral que indica radiografia após injeção de ar. SIN pneumoradiography, pneumoroentgenography. [G. *pneumōn*, pulmão, + *graphō*, escrever]

pneu·mo·he·mia (noo-mō-hē′mē-a). Pneumoemia; pneumemia; presença de ar nos vasos sanguíneos. VER TAMBÉM air *embolism.* SIN pneumatohemia. [G. *pneuma*, ar, + *haima*, sangue]

pneu·mo·he·mo·per·i·car·di·um (noo′mō-hē-mō-per-i-kar′dē-um). Hemopneumopericárdio. SIN hemopneumopericardium.

pneu·mo·he·mo·tho·rax (noo′mō-hē-mō-thōr′aks). Pneumoemotórax; pneumemotórax; hemopneumotórax. SIN hemopneumothorax.

pneu·mo·hy·dro·me·tra (noo′mō-hī-drō-mē′tra). Pneumoidrometria; presença de gás e soro na cavidade uterina. [G. *pneuma*, ar, + *hydōr* (hydr-), água, + *mētra*, útero]

pneu·mo·hy·dro·per·i·car·di·um (noo′mō-hī′drō-par-i-kar′dē-um). Pneumoidropericárdio. SIN hydropneumopericardium.

pneu·mo·hy·dro·per·i·to·ne·um (noo′mō-hī-drō-per-i-tō-nē′um). Pneumoidroperitônio. SIN hydropneumoperitoneum.

pneu·mo·hy·dro·tho·rax (noo-mō-hī-drō-thōr′aks). Pneumoidrotórax. SIN hydropneumothorax.

pneu·mo·hy·po·der·ma (noo′mō-hī-pō-der′ma). Pneumoipodermia. SIN subcutaneous *emphysema.* [G. *pneuma*, ar, + *hypo*, sob, + *derma*, pele]

pneu·mo·ko·ni·o·sis. VER pneumoconiosis.

pneu·mo·lith (noo′mō-lith). Pneumólito; um cálculo no pulmão. SIN pulmolith. [G. *pneumōn*, pulmão, + *lithos*, cálculo]

pneu·mo·li·thi·a·sis (noo-mō-li-thī′a-sis). Pneumolitíase; formação de cálculos nos pulmões.

pneu·mol·o·gy (noo-mol′o-jē). Pneumologia; termo raramente usado para o estudo de doenças do pulmão e das vias aéreas. [G. *pneumōn*, pulmão, + *logos*, estudo]

pneu·mol·y·sis (noo - mol′i - sis). Pneumólise; separação cirúrgica do pulmão e da pleura costal desde a fáscia endotorácica; usado antigamente na terapia de colapso para tuberculose. [G. *pneumōn*, pulmão, + *lysis*, afrouxamento]

pneu·mo·ma·la·cia (noo - mō - ma - lā′shē - a). Pneumomalacia; amolecimento do tecido pulmonar. [G. *pneumōn*, pulmão, + *malakia*, amolecimento]

pneu·mo·mas·sage (noo′mō - ma - sahzh′). Pneumomassagem; compressão e rarefação do ar no meato auditivo externo, causando movimento de uma membrana timpânica íntegra. [G. *pneuma*, ar, + *massage*]

pneu·mo·me·di·as·ti·num (noo′mō - mē·dē - a - sti′num). Pneumomediastino; presença anormal de ar nos tecidos mediastinais; múltiplas causas incluem enfisema pulmonar intersticial, ruptura de bolha, perfuração do esôfago cervical ou torácico ou das vias aéreas, infecção cervicomediastinal e víscera abdominal perfurada. SIN mediastinal emphysema. [G. *pneuma*, ar, + *mediastinum*]

pneu·mo·mel·a·no·sis (noo′mō - mel - ā - nō′sis). Pneumomelanose; enegrecimento do tecido pulmonar por inalação de poeira de carvão ou de outras partículas negras. VER TAMBÉM anthracosis. SIN pneumonomelanosis. [G. *pneumōn*, pulmão, + *melanosis*, tornar-se preto]

pneu·mo·my·co·sis (noo′mō - mī - kō′sis). Pneumomicose; termo obsoleto para designar qualquer doença pulmonar causada pela presença de fungos. [G. *pneumōn*, pulmão, + *mykēs*, fungo]

pneu·mo·my·e·log·ra·phy (noo′mō - mī′ē - log′ra - fē). Pneumomielografia; exame radiográfico do canal central da medula espinal após injeção de ar ou gás no espaço subaracnóide, sendo raramente usado. [G. *pneuma*, ar, + *myelos*, medula óssea, + *graphō*, escrever]

pneumon-. VER pneumo-.

pneu·mo·nec·to·my (noo′mō - nek′tō - mē). Pneumonectomia; remoção de um pulmão inteiro. SIN pulmonectomy. [G. *pneumōn*, pulmão, + *ektomē*, excisão]

pneu·mo·nia (noo - mō′nē - a). Pneumonia; inflamação do parênquima pulmonar caracterizada por consolidação da parte afetada, ficando os espaços aéreos alveolares cheios de exsudato, células inflamatórias e fibrina. A maioria dos casos é causada por infecção por bactérias ou vírus, alguns por inalação de substâncias químicas ou traumatismo da parede torácica, e uma pequena minoria por riquétsias, fungos e leveduras. A distribuição pode ser lobar, segmentar ou lobular; quando lobular e associada a bronquite, é denominada broncopneumonia. VER TAMBÉM pneumonitis. [G. de *pneumōn*, pulmão, + *-ia*, condição]

acute interstitial p., p. intersticial aguda; forma grave e geralmente fatal de p. que ocorre basicamente em lactentes; geralmente é considerada uma forma de pneumonite por hipersensibilidade (hypersensitivity *pneumonitis*).

alcoholic p., p. alcoólica; p. que ocorre em paciente com alcoolismo, geralmente após um período de intoxicação com torpor, resultando em aspiração.

anaerobic p., p. anaeróbica; p. causada por bactérias geralmente originada na boca, principalmente na presença de doença periodontal; a cavitação é comum.

apex p., apical p., p. apical; p. do ápice ou dos ápices.

aspiration p., p. por aspiração; broncopneumonia resultante da inalação de material estranho, geralmente partículas alimentares ou vômito, para os brônquios; p. secundária à presença de líquido, sangue, saliva ou conteúdo gástrico nas vias aéreas. SIN deglutition p.

atypical p., p. atípica; p. causada por um patógeno não-bacteriano, classicamente causada por *Mycoplasma pneumoniae*, mas geralmente esse termo é usado em referência a qualquer pneumonia não-bacteriana com sintomas sistêmicos leves, incluindo virais. VER primary atypical p.

bacterial p., p. bacteriana; infecção pulmonar por qualquer uma dentre uma grande variedade de bactérias, principalmente *Streptococcus pneumoniae* (pneumococo).

bilious p., p. biliosa; p. após aspiração de conteúdo gástrico contendo bile.

bronchial p., p. brônquica. SIN bronchopneumonia.

caseous p., p. caseosa; forma de tuberculose pulmonar grave na qual não há tubérculos proeminentes, mas com infiltração celular extensa e difusa que sofre caseificação, afetando grandes áreas de pulmão.

central p., p. central; forma de p. na qual a exsudação é limitada por um tempo à porção central de um lobo ou à região hilar. SIN core p.

chemical p., p. química; p. causada por inalação de gás tóxico, como os gases de guerra fosgênio ou clorino; a exsudação para os alvéolos causa edema e hemorragia pulmonar; grandes quantidades de líquido que enchem as vias aéreas bloqueiam a troca gasosa; ocorre recuperação, a lesão permanente dos pulmões permanece e é comum haver infecções pulmonares recorrentes.

chronic p., p. crônica; designação vaga ou indefinida de inflamação prolongada do tecido pulmonar de qualquer etiologia.

chronic eosinophilic p., p. eosinofílica crônica; doença caracterizada por sudorese noturna, dispnéia aos esforços, sibilos ocasionais e eosinofilia periférica. As radiografias mostram infiltrados pulmonares não-segmentares, periféricos, que podem ser nodulares com cavitação. Responde ao tratamento com corticosteróides. SIN Carrington disease.

community-acquired p., p. comunitária; p. causada por qualquer microrganismo encontrado regularmente fora do hospital; os microrganismos comuns incluem *Streptococcus pneumoniae*, *Haemophilus influenzae*, *Mycoplasma*, ao contrário da pneumonia hospitalar ou nosocomial.

congenital p., p. congênita; p. no recém-nascido, sendo a infecção contraída no período pré-natal.

core p., p. central. SIN central p.

deglutition p., p. por aspiração. SIN aspiration p.

desquamative p., p. descamativa; forma relativamente rara de p. com enchimento homogêneo dos espaços aéreos alveolares com macrófagos e algumas células de revestimento epitelial tipo II, alguma infiltração septal alveolar com células teciduais inflamatórias e conjuntivas; geralmente é idiopática, mas foram descritos alguns casos associados a fármacos ou a doença do tecido conjuntivo sistêmica subjacente; raramente evolui para doença pulmonar em estágio terminal.

desquamative interstitial p. (D.I.P.), p. intersticial descamativa; proliferação difusa de células epiteliais alveolares, que descamam para os sacos aéreos e tornam-se líquidas com macrófagos, acompanhada por infiltração celular intersticial e fibrose; há início gradual de dispnéia e tosse improdutiva.

p. dis'secans, p. dissecante. SIN p. interlobularis purulenta.

double p., p. dupla; p. lobar envolvendo ambos os pulmões.

embolic p., p. embólica; infarto após embolização de uma artéria ou artérias pulmonares.

eosinophilic p., p. eosinofílica. SIN Loeffler *syndrome* I. SIN eosinophilic pneumonopathy.

fibrous p., p. fibrosa; processo que afeta o tecido pulmonar e causa deposição de colágeno, seja intersticialmente ou nos sacos alveolares.

Friedländer p., p. de Friedländer; forma de p. causada por infecção por *Klebsiella pneumoniae* (bacilo de Friedländer), caracteristicamente grave e de distribuição lobar.

Friedländer bacillus p., p. por bacilo de Friedländer; p. causada por *Klebsiella pneumoniae*, o bacilo de Friedländer.

gangrenous p., p. gangrenosa; gangrena dos pulmões.

giant cell p., p. de células gigantes; uma complicação rara do sarampo, com o achado *postmortem* de células gigantes multinucleadas revestindo os alvéolos. SIN Hecht p., interstitial p.

Hecht p., p. de Hecht. SIN giant cell p.

hospital-acquired p., p. hospitalar; p. em um paciente em um hospital, ou ambiente do tipo hospitalar, como uma unidade de reabilitação. Freqüentemente causada por microrganismos Gram-negativos ou estafilocócicos. SIN nosocomial p.

hypostatic p., p. hipostática; p. resultante de infecção que se desenvolve nas porções inferiores dos pulmões causada por diminuição da ventilação dessas áreas, com conseqüente falha da drenagem de secreções brônquicas; ocorre basicamente nas pessoas idosas ou debilitadas por doença que permanecem na mesma posição por longos períodos.

influenza p., p. da *influenza*; p. que complica a *influenza*.

influenzal virus p., p. pelo vírus *influenza*; forma grave, freqüentemente fatal, de p. causada por um vírus do tipo *influenza*; ocorre em epidemias e pandemias.

p. interlobula'ris purulen'ta, p. interlobular purulenta; p. na qual os lóbulos pulmonares são separados por coleções de exsudato purulento. SIN p. dissecans.

interstitial p., p. intersticial. SIN giant cell p.

interstitial plasma cell p., p. intersticial por plasmócitos. SIN *Pneumocystis carinii* p.

intrauterine p., p. intra-uterina; p. fetal contraída *in utero* e que se manifesta no início do período neonatal.

lipid p., lipoid p., p. lipídica; p. lipóide; condição pulmonar caracterizada por alterações inflamatórias e fibróticas nos pulmões causada por inalação de várias substâncias oleosas ou gordurosas, particularmente vaselina líquida, ou resultante do acúmulo de material lipídico endógeno nos pulmões, seja colesterol por pneumonite obstrutiva ou após fratura de um osso; geralmente há fagócitos contendo lipídios. SIN oil p.

lobar p., p. lobar; p. que afeta um ou mais lobos do pulmão, ou parte de um lobo, na qual a consolidação é praticamente homogênea; freqüentemente causada por infecção por *Streptococcus pneumoniae*; o escarro é escasso e, em geral, tem coloração ferruginosa devido ao sangue modificado.

lymphocytic interstitial p. (LIP), p. intersticial linfocítica. SIN lymphocytic interstitial *pneumonitis*.

lymphoid interstitial p. (LIP), p. intersticial linfóide. SIN lymphocytic interstitial *pneumonitis*.

p. malleosa (ma - lē′o - sa). p. associada a mormos.

metastatic p., p. metastática; inflamação purulenta nos pulmões causada por êmbolos infectados.

migratory p., p. migratória; forma de p. na qual são afetadas áreas sucessivas do pulmão; pode ocorrer na aspergilose broncopulmonar. SIN wandering p.

nosocomial p., p. nosocomial. SIN hospital-acquired p.

obstructive p., p. obstrutiva; infecção pulmonar devida à obstrução das vias aéreas por estreitamento resultante de processo patológico persistente, broncoespasmo persistente ou secreções espessas, ou por aspiração de um corpo estranho.

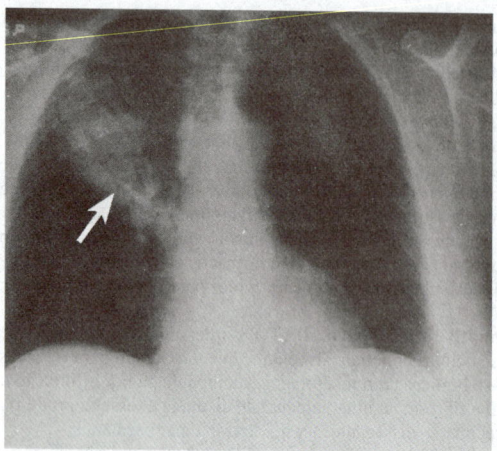

pneumonia lobar: radiografia do tórax exibindo infiltrados pulmonares (seta) no lobo superior do pulmão direito

oil p., p. lipídica. SIN lipid p.
Pittsburgh p., p. de Pittsburgh; uma variante da doença dos Legionários causada por *Legionella micdadei*.
plague p., peste pneumônica. SIN pneumonic plague.
pleuritic p., p. pleurítica; p. associada a inflamação da pleura sobrejacente. SIN pneumonopleuritis.
***Pneumocystis carinii* p. (PCP)**, p. por *Pneumocystis carinii*; p. resultante de infecção por *Pneumocystis carinii*, freqüentemente observada em pacientes imunologicamente comprometidos, como as pessoas com AIDS/SIDA, ou indivíduos tratados com esteróides, idosos ou bebês prematuros ou debilitados durante os 3 primeiros meses de vida. Em pacientes com AIDS/SIDA, a lesão tecidual geralmente é restrita ao parênquima pulmonar, enquanto, na forma infantil da doença, os alvéolos estão cheios de uma rede espumosa ou semelhante a um favo de mel de material acidófilo, que aparentemente não é fibrina nem se cora pela prata, dentro da qual os microrganismos, individualmente ou em grupos, estão emaranhados; nas paredes alveolares e septos pulmonares, há infiltração difusa de células inflamatórias mononucleares, principalmente plasmócitos e macrófagos, bem como alguns linfócitos. Os pacientes podem apresentar-se apenas levemente febris (ou mesmo afebris), mas tendem a exibir fraqueza extrema, dispnéia e cianose. Esta é uma importante causa de morbidade em pacientes com AIDS/SIDA. SIN interstitial plasma cell p., pneumocystosis.
postobstructive p., p. pós-obstrutiva; p. que ocorre distalmente a uma obstrução brônquica.
primary atypical p., p. atípica primária; termo antigo que se refere a uma doença sistêmica aguda com envolvimento dos pulmões, geralmente causada por *Mycoplasma pneumoniae* e caracterizada por febre, tosse, relativamente poucos sinais físicos e densidades dispersas em radiografias; geralmente está associada ao desenvolvimento de crioaglutininas e anticorpos contra o agente infeccioso.
purulent p., p. purulenta; p. causada por um microrganismo que produz pus, indicando que pode haver destruição do tecido pulmonar com alterações permanentes; geralmente o escarro contém pus. Estafilococos (*Staphylococci*), estreptococos hemolíticos (hemolytic *streptococci*, em *streptococcus*) e bacilo de Friedländer (Friedländer *bacillus*) são causas típicas, ao contrário do *Streptococcus pneumoniae*, que raramente causa p. purulenta.
rheumatic p., p. reumática; p. que ocorre raramente na febre reumática aguda, mesmo quando a doença era comum; ocorre consolidação, e os pulmões apresentam uma consistência elástica, com exsudato de fibrina e pequenas hemorragias, bem como edema por insuficiência ventricular esquerda.
septic p., p. séptica. SIN suppurative p.
staphylococcal p., p. estafilocócica; p., em geral causada por *Staphylococcus aureus*, e que quase sempre causa supuração e destruição do tecido pulmonar.
streptococcal p., p. estreptocócica; p. causada por *Streptococcus pyogenes*.
suppurative p., p. supurativa; qualquer p. associada a formação de pus e destruição do tecido pulmonar; pode haver formação de abscesso. SIN septic p.
terminal p., p. terminal; p. que ocorre no decorrer de alguma outra doença próxima ao seu término fatal.
tularemic p., p. tularêmica; tularemia com lesões pulmonares.
typhoid p., p. tifóide; p. que complica a febre tifóide.
unresolved p., p. não-resolvida; p. na qual o exsudato alveolar persiste e acaba por sofrer fibrose.
uremic p., p. urêmica; **(1)** SIN uremic lung; **(2)** pneumonia infecciosa terminal que ocorre em um paciente com uremia.

usual interstitial p. of Liebow (UIP), p. intersticial habitual de Liebow; distúrbio inflamatório progressivo que começa com lesão alveolar difusa e resulta em fibrose e formação de um padrão em favo de mel durante um período variável; também é uma característica comum as colagenoses.
wandering p., p. migratória. SIN migratory p.
woolsorter's p., p. dos tosquiadores. SIN pulmonary anthrax.
pneu·mon·ic (noo-mon'ik). Pneumônico. **1.** SIN pulmonary. **2.** Relativo à pneumonia.
pneu·mo·ni·tis (noo-mō-nī'tis). Pneumonite; inflamação dos pulmões. VER TAMBÉM pneumonia. SIN pulmonitis. [G. *pneumōn*, pulmão, + *-itis*, inflamação]
  acute interstitial p., p. intersticial aguda; geralmente considerada uma forma de pneumonia por hipersensibilidade.
  hypersensitivity p., p. por hipersensibilidade; forma progressiva crônica de pneumonia com sibilos, dispnéia, infiltrados difusos observados em radiografias; ocorre após exposição a um dentre vários antígenos, algumas vezes é ocupacional e muitos nomes são dados a casos com tipos conhecidos de exposição (como pulmão de fazendeiro, pulmão dos cortadores de casca do bordo, pulmão dos criadores de pássaros, bagaçose, bissinose e doença pulmonar devida aos sistemas de ar condicionado e de umidificação do ar); os achados à biopsia geralmente mostram infiltração segmentar das paredes alveolares com linfócitos, plasmócitos e outras células inflamatórias; pode evoluir para doença fibrótica intersticial irreversível com padrão restritivo à função pulmonar, mas, na doença inicial, a maioria das manifestações é reversível se o antígeno agressor for identificado e removido do ambiente.
  lymphocytic interstitial p., p. intersticial linfocítica; doença rara caracterizada por acúmulo intersticial de linfócitos nos pulmões e fibrose tardia; geralmente resulta de um linfoma, ocasionalmente observada na AIDS/SIDA, principalmente em crianças; algumas vezes é observada como um distúrbio auto-imune. SIN lymphocytic interstitial pneumonia, lymphoid interstitial pneumonia.
  radiation p., p. por radiação; a pneumonia intersticial e fibrose que sucede a irradiação pulmonar em doses radioterapêuticas.
  uremic p., p. urêmica. SIN uremic lung.
♻ **pneumono-.** VER pneumo-.
pneu·mo·no·cele (noo-mōn'ō-sēl). Pneumonocele; protrusão de uma parte do pulmão através de um defeito na parede torácica. SIN pleurocele, pneumatocele (2), pneumocele.
pneu·mo·no·cen·te·sis (noo'mō-nō-sen-tē'sis). Pneumocentese; termo raramente usado para designar paracentese do pulmão. SIN pneumocentesis. [G. *pneumōn*, pulmão, + *kentēsis*, punção]
pneu·mo·no·coc·cal (noo'mō-nō-kok'ăl). Pneumocócico; relativo ou associado ao *Streptococcus pneumoniae*.
pneu·mo·no·coc·cus (noo'mō-nō-kok'ŭs). Pneumococo. SIN *Streptococcus pneumoniae*.
pneu·mo·no·co·ni·o·sis, pneu·mo·no·ko·ni·o·sis (noo'mō-nō-kō-nē-ō'sis). Pneumoconiose. SIN pneumoconiosis.
pneu·mo·no·cyte (noo'mō-nō-sīt). Pneumócito; termo inespecífico referente às células que revestem os alvéolos na parte respiratória do pulmão. [G. *pneumōn*, pulmão, + *kytos*, célula]
  granular p.'s, pneumócitos granulares. SIN great alveolar cells, em cell.
  phagocytic p., p. fagocítico; fagócito alveolar que contém hemossiderina, carbono ou outras partículas estranhas.
pneu·mo·no·ko·ni·o·sis. Pneumoconiose. VER pneumonoconiosis.
pneu·mo·no·mel·a·no·sis (noo'mō-nō-mel-ă-nō'sis). Pneumomelanose. SIN pneumomelanosis.
pneu·mo·nop·a·thy (noo'mō-nop'ă-thē). Pneumopatia; doença do pulmão.
  eosinophilic p., p. eosinofílica. SIN eosinophilic pneumonia.
pneu·mo·no·pexy (noo'mō-nō-pek-sē). Pneumopexia; fixação do pulmão por sutura das pleuras parietal e visceral, ou causando-se adesão dessas duas camadas. SIN pneumopexy. [G. *pneumōn*, pulmão, + *pēxis*, fixação]
pneu·mo·no·pleu·ri·tis (noo'mō'nō-ploo-rī'tis). Pneumopleurite. SIN pleuritic pneumonia.
pneu·mo·nor·rha·phy (noo-mō-nōr'ă-fē). Pneumorrafia; sutura do pulmão. [G. *pneumōn*, pulmão, + *rhaphē*, sutura]
pneu·mo·not·o·my (noo-mō-not'ō-mē). Pneumotomia; incisão do pulmão. SIN pneumotomy. [G. *pneumōn*, pulmão, + *tomē*, incisão]
pneu·mo·or·bi·tog·ra·phy (noo'mō-ōr'bi-tog'ră-fē). Pneumo-orbitografia; visualização radiográfica do conteúdo orbital após injeção de um gás, geralmente ar.
pneu·mo·per·i·car·di·um (noo'mō-per-i-kar'dē-ŭm). Pneumopericárdio; presença de gás (geralmente ar) no saco pericárdico. [G. *pneuma*, ar, + *pericardium*, pericárdio]
  tension p., p. hipertensivo; a presença de ar sob pressão no espaço pericárdico, com a possibilidade de haver tamponamento cardíaco.
pneu·mo·per·i·to·ne·um (noo'mō-per-i-tō-nē'ŭm). Pneumoperitônio; presença de ar ou gás na cavidade peritoneal em virtude de doença, ou produzida artificialmente no abdome para obter exposição durante cirurgia laparoscópica. [G. *pneuma*, ar, + *peritoneum*]

pneu·mo·per·i·to·ni·tis (noo′mō - per - i - tō - nī′tis). Pneumoperitonite; inflamação do peritônio com acúmulo de gás na cavidade peritoneal. [G. *pneuma*, ar, + peritonitis]
pneu·mo·pexy (noo′mō - pek - sē). Pneumopexia. SIN pneumonopexy.
pneu·mo·pha·gia (noo - mō - fā′jē - ā). Pneumofagia. SIN aerophagia.
pneu·mo·pleu·ri·tis (noo′mō - ploo - rī′tis). Pneumopleurite; pleurite com ar ou gás na cavidade pleural. [G. *pneuma*, ar, + pleur- + *-itis*, inflamação]
pneu·mo·py·e·log·ra·phy (noo′mō - pī - ē - log′rā - fē). Pneumopielografia; radiografia do rim após a injeção de ar ou gás na pelve renal. [G. *pneuma*, ar, + *pyelos*, pelve, + *graphō*, escrever]
pneu·mo·ra·di·og·ra·phy (nu′mo - ra - dī - og′rā - fī). Pneumorradiografia. SIN pneumography (2).
pneu·mo·re·sec·tion (noo′mō - rē - sek′shŭn). Pneumorressecção; excisão de parte de um pulmão. [G. *pneumōn*, pulmão, + resection]
pneu·mo·ret·ro·per·i·to·ne·um (noo′mō - ret′rō - per - i - tō - nē′ŭm). Pneumorretroperitônio; presença patológica de ar nos tecidos retroperitoneais.
pneu·mo·roent·gen·og·ra·phy (noo′mō - rent′gē - nog′rā - fē). Pneumorradiografia. SIN pneumography (2).
pneu·mor·rha·chis (noo - mō - rā′kis, noo - mōr′ā - kis). Pneumorraque; a presença de gás no canal central da medula espinal. SIN pneumatorrhachis. [G. *pneuma*, ar, + *rhachis*, coluna vertebral]
pneu·mo·scope (noo′mō - skōp). Pneumoscópio. SIN pneumatoscope.
pneu·mo·ser·o·tho·rax (noo′mō - sēr - ō - thōr′aks). Hidropneumotórax. SIN hydropneumothorax.
pneu·mo·sil·i·co·sis (noo′mō - sil′i - kō′sis). Silicose. SIN silicosis.
pneu·mo·tach·o·gram (noo - mō - tak′ō - gram). Pneumotacograma; registro do fluxo de gás respirado em função do tempo, produzido por um pneumotacógrafo. [G. *pneuma*, ar, + *tachys*, rápido, + *gramma*, algo escrito]
pneu·mo·tach·o·graph (noo - mō - tak′ō - graf). Pneumotacógrafo; instrumento para medir o fluxo instantâneo dos gases respiratórios. SIN pneumotachometer.
  Fleisch p., p. de Fleisch; p. que mede o fluxo em termos da queda de pressão proporcional ao atravessar uma resistência que consiste em numerosos tubos capilares paralelos.
  Silverman-Lilly p., p. de Silverman-Lilly; p. que mede o fluxo em termos da queda de pressão proporcional ao atravessar uma resistência que consiste em uma tela muito fina.
pneu·mo·ta·chom·e·ter (noo′mō - tă - kom′ē - ter). Pneumotacômetro, pneumotacógrafo. SIN pneumotachograph. [G. *pneuma*, ar, + *tachys*, rápido, + *metron*, medida]
pneu·mo·ther·mo·mas·sage (noo - mō - ther′mō - mă - sahzh′). Pneumotermomassagem; aplicação corporal de ar quente sob vários graus de pressão. [G. *pneuma*, ar, + *thermē*, calor, + Fr. *massage*]
pneu·mo·tho·rax (noo - mō - thōr′aks). Pneumotórax; a presença de ar ou gás livre na cavidade pleural. [G. *pneuma*, ar, + thorax]

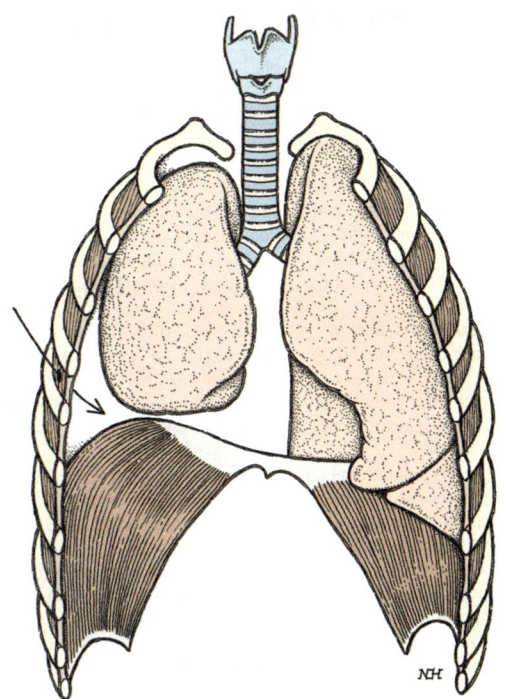

pneumotórax: causado por ferida perfurante da parede torácica

  artificial p., p. artificial; p. produzido pela injeção de ar, ou de um gás absorvido mais lentamente como o nitrogênio, no saco pleural; antigamente era usado na colapsoterapia da tuberculose. SIN therapeutic p.
  catamenial p., p. catamenial; p. que ocorre em mulheres jovens durante a menstruação, geralmente do lado direito.
  extrapleural p., p. extrapleural; a presença de gás entre a camada pleural-fáscia endotorácica e a parede torácica adjacente.
  iatrogenic p., p. iatrogênico; p. causado por um procedimento médico, na maioria das vezes inserção de um cateter venoso central (central venous *catheter*), toracocentese ou biopsia pulmonar transbrônquica e transtorácica.
  open p., p. aberto; uma comunicação livre entre a atmosfera e o espaço pleural através do pulmão ou da parede torácica. SIN sucking chest wound.
  pressure p., p. hipertensivo. SIN tension p.
  p. sim′plex, p. simples; p., sem causa conhecida, em uma pessoa saudável.
  spontaneous p., p. espontâneo; p. que ocorre sem traumatismo iatrogênico ou de outro tipo; o p. espontâneo primário geralmente ocorre em pessoas jovens com bolhas apicais, mas com pulmões normais nos demais aspectos; o p. espontâneo secundário ocorre em pessoas com doença pulmonar subjacente, na maioria das vezes doença pulmonar obstrutiva crônica e, com menor freqüência, doença pulmonar intersticial, pneumonia, abscesso pulmonar e tumores pulmonares.
  tension p., p. hipertensivo; p. no qual o ar entra na cavidade pleural e é retido durante a expiração; a pressão intratorácica aumenta até níveis acima da pressão atmosférica, comprime o pulmão e pode deslocar o mediastino e suas estruturas em direção ao lado oposto, com conseqüente comprometimento cardiopulmonar. SIN pressure p.
  therapeutic p., p. terapêutico. SIN artificial p.
  traumatic p., p. traumático; p. causado por lesão torácica penetrante ou não-penetrante.
pneu·mot·o·my (noo - mot′ō - mē). Pneumotomia. SIN pneumonotomy.
pneu·mo·ven·tri·cle (noo - mō - ven′tri - kl). Pneumoventrículo; ar no sistema ventricular do encéfalo; ocorre como complicação de uma fratura do crânio que atravessa os seios nasais acessórios.
Pneu·mo·vi·rus (noo′mō - vī′rŭs). Gênero de vírus (família Paramyxoviridae) que inclui o vírus sincicial respiratório, causando doença grave das vias respiratórias inferiores em lactentes. Os nucleocapsídeos possuem 14–15 nm de diâmetro e, assim, são intermediários em tamanho entre outros Paramyxoviridae e os Orthomyxoviridae; as inclusões citoplasmáticas são consideravelmente mais densas que as de outros vírus da família.
pneu·sis (noo′sis). Respiração. SIN breathing. [G. *pneō*, respirar]
pni·go·pho·bia (nī - gō - fō′bē - ā). Pnigofobia; medo mórbido de sufocação. [G. *pnigos*, sufocação, + *phobos*, medo]
PNMT Abreviatura de phenylethanolamine *N*-methyltransferase (feniletanolamina *N*-metiltransferase).
PNP Abreviatura de psychogenic nocturnal *polydipsia* (polidipsia noturna psicogênica).
PNPB Abreviatura de positive-negative pressure *breathing* (respiração sob pressão positivo-negativa).
PO Abreviatura de per os (por via oral).
Po Símbolo de polonium (polônio).
pock (pok). Pústula; a lesão cutânea pustular específica da varíola. [A.S. *poc*, uma pústula]
pock·et (pok′et). Bolsa. **1.** Um fundo-de-saco ou cavidade semelhante a uma bolsa. **2.** Uma fixação gengival doente; um espaço entre a gengiva inflamada e a superfície de um dente, limitado apicalmente por uma fixação epitelial. **3.** Encerrar em um espaço limitado, como o coto do pedículo de um tumor de ovário ou outro tumor abdominal entre os lábios da ferida externa. **4.** Uma coleção de pus em um saco quase fechado. **5.** Aproximar-se da superfície em um ponto localizado, como na parede adelgaçada de um abscesso que está prestes a romper. [Fr. *pochette*]
  gingival p., bolsa gengival; uma fixação gengival doente na qual o aumento da profundidade do sulco é causado por aumento no volume de sua parede gengival.
  infrabony p., intrabony p., bolsa infra-óssea; bolsa intra-óssea. SIN subcrestal p.
  periodontal p., bolsa periodontal; aprofundamento patológico do sulco gengival resultante de separação da gengiva do dente.
  Rathke p., bolsa de Rathke. SIN pituitary *diverticulum*.
  retraction p.'s, bolsas de retração; pequenas áreas de retração da membrana timpânica, causadas por pressão negativa crônica na orelha média, que podem levar à formação de colesteatoma.
  rheumatoid p., epítopo reumatóide. SIN susceptibility *cassette*.
  Seessel p., bolsa de Seessel; a parte do intestino anterior embrionário que se estende cefalicamente até o nível da lâmina oral e caudal ao divertículo hipofisário (bolsa de Rathke). SIN preoral gut.
  subcrestal p., bolsa que se estende em sentido apical abaixo do nível da crista alveolar adjacente. SIN infrabony p., intrabony p.
  Tröltsch p.'s, bolsas de Tröltsch. SIN anterior *recess* of tympanic membrane, posterior *recess* of tympanic membrane.

pock·mark (pok′mark). A pequena cicatriz deprimida deixada após a cicatrização da pústula da varíola.

po·cu·lum (pok′u-lŭm). Taça. SIN cup (1). [L.]
 p. diog'enis, taça de Diógenes. SIN cup of palm.

♻ **pod-, podo-.** Pé, em forma de pé. Cf. ped-. [G. *pous, podos*]

po·dag·ra (po-dag′ra). Podagra; dor forte no pé, principalmente aquela da gota típica no hálux. [G. de *pous*, pé, + *agra*, uma convulsão]

po·dag·ral, po·dag·ric, po·dag·rous (pod′a-gral, po-dag′rik, pod′a-grŭs). Relativo a, ou caracterizado por, podagra.

po·dal·gia (po-dal′je-a). Podalgia; dor no pé. SIN pododynia, tarsalgia. [pod- + G. *algos*, dor]

po·dal·ic (po-dal′ik). Podálico; relativo ao pé. [G. *pous* (pod-), pé]

pod·ar·thri·tis (pod-ar-thri′tis). Podartrite; inflamação de qualquer uma das articulações do tarso ou metatarso. [pod- + arthritis]

pod·e·de·ma (pod-e-de′ma). Podedema; edema dos pés e tornozelos.

po·di·a·tric (po-di′a-trik). Podiátrico; relativo à podiatria.

po·di·a·trist (po-di′a-trist). Podiatra; profissional de podiatria. SIN chiropodist, podologist. [pod- + G. *iatros*, médico]

po·di·a·try (po-di′a-tre). Podiatria; a especialidade relacionada ao diagnóstico e/ou tratamento clínico, cirúrgico, mecânico, físico e auxiliar das doenças, lesões e defeitos do pé humano. SIN chiropody, podiatric medicine, podology. [pod- + G. *iatreia*, tratamento clínico]

po·dis·mus (po-diz′mŭs). Podismo. SIN podospasm.

po·di·tis (po-di′tis). Podite; distúrbio inflamatório do pé. [pod- + G. *-itis*, inflamação]
 tourniquet p., p. por torniquete; edema inflamatório agudo pós-isquêmico no pé (ou pata), em virtude de obstrução completa da circulação para esse membro por uso de um torniquete; produzida experimentalmente em animais como uma forma de avaliar a eficácia antiinflamatória dos fármacos.

♻ **podo-.** VER pod-.

pod·o·bro·mi·dro·sis (pod′o-bro-mi-dro′sis). Podobromidrose; transpiração fétida dos pés. [podo- + G. *bromos*, um odor fétido, + *hidros*, suor]

pod·o·cyte (pod′o-sit). Podócito; célula epitelial da camada visceral da cápsula de Bowman no corpúsculo renal, fixada à superfície externa da membrana basal capilar glomerular por prolongamentos podálicos citoplasmáticos (pedicelos); acredita-se que represente um papel na ultrafiltração do sangue. [podo- + G. *kytos*, uma cavidade (célula)]

pod·o·dy·na·mom·e·ter (pod′o-di′na-mom′e-ter). Pododinamômetro; instrumento para medir a força dos músculos do pé ou da perna. [podo- + G. *dynamis*, força, + *metron*, medida]

pod·o·dyn·ia (pod-o-din′e-a). Pododinia. SIN podalgia. [podo- + G. *odyne*, dor]

podofilox (po-dof′il-oks). Podofilox; agente antimitótico derivado de espécies de *Juniperus* e *Podophyllum*; usado no tratamento de verrugas genitais externas e perianais.

pod·o·gram (pod′o-gram). Podograma; impressão da planta do pé, exibindo o contorno e a condição do arco, ou um traçado do contorno. [podo- + G. *gramma*, escrito]

pod·o·graph (pod′o-graf). Podógrafo; aparelho para fazer um esboço do pé e uma impressão da sua planta. [podo- + G. *grapho*, escrever]

pod·o·lite (pod′o-lit). Podólito. SIN dahllite.

po·dol·o·gist (po-dol′o-jist). Podólogo. SIN podiatrist.

po·dol·o·gy (po-dol′o-je). Podologia. SIN podiatry. [podo- + G. *logos*, estudo]

pod·o·mech·a·no·ther·a·py (pod-o-mek′a-no-thar′a-pe). Podomecanoterapia; tratamento de distúrbios do pé com aparelhos mecânicos; p. ex., suportes de arco, órteses.

po·dom·e·ter (po-dom′e-ter). Podômetro. SIN pedometer. [podo- + G. *metron*, medida]

pod·o·phyl·lin (pod-o-fil′in). Podofilina. SIN podophyllum resin.

pod·o·phyl·lo·tox·in (pod′o-fil-o-tok′sin). Podofilotoxina; substância policíclica tóxica, $C_{22}H_{22}O_8$, com propriedades catárticas, presente no podofilo; tem ação antineoplásica.

pod·o·phyl·lum (pod-o-fil′ŭm). Podofilo; o rizoma do *Podophyllum peltatum* (família Berberidaceae), usado como potente laxante. SIN May apple, vegetable calomel.
 Indian p., p. indiano; o rizoma e as raízes secas de *P. emodi*, uma planta do Himalaia; um colagogo e catártico.

pod·o·spasm, pod·o·spas·mus (pod′o-spazm, -spaz-mŭs). Podospasmo; espasmo do pé. SIN podismus. [podo- + G. *spasmos*, espasmo]

Po·do·vir·i·dae (po-do-vir′i-de). Nome de uma família de vírus bacterianos com caudas curtas e genomas de DNA de duplo filamento (PM 12–73 × 10^6); as cabeças podem ser isométricas ou alongadas. A família inclui o grupo fago T-7 e, provavelmente, outros gêneros.

POEMS Acrônimo para *p*olineuropatia, *o*rganomegalia, *e*ndocrinopatia, gamopatia *m*onoclonal e alterações cutâneas (*s*kin changes). VER POEMS syndrome. SIN Crow-Fukase syndrome.

po·go·ni·a·sis (po-go-ni′a-sis). Pogoníase; termo usado raramente para designar o crescimento de barba em uma mulher, ou o excesso de pêlos na face em homens. VER TAMBÉM hirsutism. [G. *pogon*, barba, + *-iasis*, condição]

po·go·ni·on (po-go′ni-on). Pogônio; em craniometria, o ponto mais anterior na mandíbula na linha média; o ponto proeminente, mais anterior no queixo. SIN mental point. [G. dim. de *pogon*, barba]

Po·go·no·myr·mex (po-go-no-mir′meks, -mer′meks). Gênero de formigas que atacam seres humanos e pequenos animais. SIN harvester ant. [G. *pogon*, barba, + *myrmex*, formiga]

pOH. O logaritmo decádico negativo da concentração de OH^- (em moles por litro).

♻ **-poiesis.** -Poese; produção; que produz. [G. *poiesis*, uma produção]

poi·e·tin. -Poetina; sufixo usado com palavras para indicar um agente com efeito estimulante sobre o crescimento ou a multiplicação de células, como a eritropoetina e outros. [G. *poietes*, que produz, + -in]

♻ **poikilo-.** Poiquilo-; irregular, variado. [G. *poikilos*, de muitas cores, variado]

poi·ki·lo·blast (poy′ki-lo-blast). Poiquiloblasto; uma hemácia nucleada de formato irregular. [poikilo- + G. *blastos*, germe]

ℹ **poi·ki·lo·cyte** (poy′ki-lo-sit). Poiquilócito; hemácia de formato irregular. [poikilo- + G. *kytos*, célula]

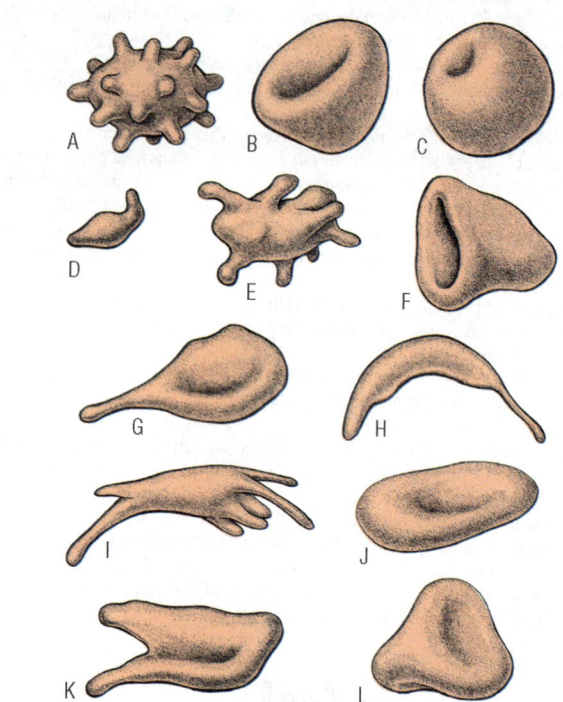

poiquilócitos: (A) equinócito, (B) estomatócito, (C) esferócito, (D) esquistócito, (E) acantócito, (F) codócito (célula em alvo), (G) dacriócito (lágrima), (H) drepanócito (foice), (I) drepanócito (folha de azevinho), (J) eliptócito, (K) ceratócito (célula em capacete), (L) cnizócito

poi·ki·lo·cy·the·mia (poy′ki-lo-si-the′me-a). Poiquilocitose. SIN poikilocytosis. [poikilocyte + G. *haima*, sangue]

ℹ **poi·ki·lo·cy·to·sis** (poy′ki-lo-si-to′sis). Poiquilocitose; a presença de poiquilócitos no sangue periférico. SIN poikilocythemia. [poikilocyte + G. *-osis*, condição]

poi·ki·lo·den·to·sis (poy′ki-lo-den-to′sis). Poiquilodentose; defeitos hipoplásicos ou mosqueamento do esmalte devido ao excesso de flúor na água. [poikilo- + L. *dens*, dente, + G. *-osis*, condição]

poi·ki·lo·der·ma (poy′ki-lo-der′ma). Poiquilodermia; hiperpigmentação variegada e telangiectasia cutânea, seguida por atrofia. [poikilo- + G. *derma*, pele]
 p. atroph'icans and cataract, p. atrófica e catarata. SIN Rothmund syndrome.
 p. atroph'icans vascula're, p. atrófica vascular; condição rara que simula a radiodermatite crônica em aparência; pode resultar em micose fungóide. SIN parapsoriasis lichenoides.
 p. of Civatte, p. de Civatte; pigmentação reticulada e telangiectasia das laterais das bochechas e do pescoço; comum em mulheres de meia-idade.
 p. congenita'le, p. congênita. SIN Rothmund syndrome.

poi·ki·lo·therm (poy′ki-lo-therm). Poiquilotermo; pecilotermo; um animal pecilotérmico. SIN allotherm, cold-blooded animal.

poi·ki·lo·ther·mic, poi·ki·lo·ther·mal, poi·ki·lo·ther·mous (poy′ki-lo-ther′mic, -mal, -mŭs). Poiquilotérmico; pecilotérmico. **1.** Aquele cuja temperatura varia de acordo com a temperatura no meio ambiente; designa os denominados animais de sangue frio, como os répteis e anfíbios, e as plantas. **2.** Capaz de viver e crescer em meios de várias temperaturas. Cf. heterothermic, homeothermic. **3.** Que causa uma ruptura da função termorreguladora hipotalâmica normal, observada com fármacos como as fenotiazinas. SIN cold-blooded, hematocryal. [poikilo- + G. *thermē*, calor]

poi·ki·lo·ther·my, poi·ki·lo·ther·mism (poy′ki-lō-ther′mē, -therm′izm). Poiquilotermia; pecilotermia; a condição de plantas e animais de sangue frio, cuja temperatura varia com as alterações na temperatura do meio ambiente. [poikilo- + G. *thermē*, calor]

poi·ki·lo·throm·bo·cyte (poy′ki-lō-throm′bō-sit). Poiquilotrombócito; uma plaqueta sanguínea de formato anormal. [poikilo- + G. *thrombos*, coágulo, + *kytos*, célula]

poi·ki·lo·thy·mia (poy′ki-lō-thī′mē-ă). Poiquilotimia; termo raramente usado para designar um estado mental caracterizado por variações anormais do humor. [poikilo- + G. *thymos*, mente]

POINT

point (poynt). **1.** Ponto. SIN punctum. **2.** Ponta; uma extremidade ou ápice pontiagudo. **3.** Uma pequena projeção. **4.** Um estágio ou condição atingida, como o ponto de fervura. **5.** Apontar; estar pronto para abrir, como em relação a um abscesso ou furúnculo cuja parede está se adelgaçando e prestes a se romper. **6.** Em matemática, um elemento geométrico sem dimensão. **7.** Uma localização ou posição em um gráfico, representação ou diagrama. **8.** Ponto decimal. [Fr.; L. *punctum*, de *pungo*, pp. *punctus*, perfurar]

p. A, p. A. SIN subspinale.
absorbent p.'s, pontos absorventes; cones de papel ou produtos de papel usados para secar ou manter medicamentos durante a terapia do canal radicular.
alveolar p., p. alveolar. SIN prosthion.
anterior focal p., p. focal anterior; o ponto onde são focalizados os raios paralelos da retina.
apophysary p., apophysial p., p. apofisário; **(1)** SIN subnasal p; **(2)** SIN Trousseau p.
auricular p., p. auricular. SIN auriculare.
axial p., p. axial. SIN nodal p.
p. B, p. B. SIN supramentale.
boiling p. (b.p.), p. de fervura; a temperatura em que a pressão do vapor de um líquido é igual à pressão atmosférica ambiente.
Cannon p., p. de Cannon; a localização na porção média do colo transverso em que a inervação por plexos mesentéricos superior e inferior superpõe-se na junção dos intestinos médio e posterior primitivos, freqüentemente resultando em estreitamento evidente ao enema baritado. VER Cannon *ring.* SIN Cannon ring.
Capuron p.'s, pontos de Capuron; as eminências iliopubianas e as articulações sacroilíacas, que formam quatro pontos fixos na abertura superior da pelve.
cardinal p.'s, pontos cardinais; **(1)** os quatro pontos na abertura superior da pelve, estando o occipúcio do bebê geralmente voltado para um deles no caso de apresentação cefálica: duas articulações sacroilíacas e as duas eminências iliopectíneas correspondentes aos acetábulos; **(2)** seis pontos de um sistema óptico composto: o ponto focal anterior, o ponto focal posterior, os dois pontos principais e os dois pontos nodais.
central-bearing p., p. de apoio central; o ponto de contato de um aparelho com apoio central.
Clado p., p. de Clado; ponto na junção das linhas interespinal e semilunar direita, na borda lateral do músculo reto do abdome, onde há dor à compressão em alguns casos de apendicite.
clinical end p., p. final clínico; medidas clínicas tradicionais de impacto diagnóstico ou terapêutico que podem ou não ser percebidas pelo paciente.
cold-rigor p., p. de rigor pelo frio; o grau de temperatura reduzida no qual a atividade de uma célula cessa e a célula entra em estado de narcose ou hibernação.
congruent p.'s, pontos congruentes; o p. em cada retina referente ao mesmo estímulo externo.
conjugate p., p. conjugado; um ponto tão relacionado a outro que um objeto em um deles tem sua imagem formada em outro.
contact p., p. de contato. SIN contact *area.*
p.'s of convergence, pontos de convergência. VER convergence.
craniometric p.'s, pontos craniométricos; pontos fixos sobre o crânio usados como pontos de reparo em craniometria.
critical p., p. crítico; ponto em que duas fases tornam-se idênticas; assim, em dada temperatura e pressão críticas, os estados líquido e gasoso de determinada substância não podem mais ser diferenciados.
dew p., p. de orvalho; a temperatura na qual e abaixo da qual a umidade se condensará para uma umidade específica.

p. of elbow, olécrano. SIN olecranon.
end p., p. terminal; a conclusão de uma reação; geralmente evidenciada pela primeira alteração perceptível da cor de um indicador adicionado.
equivalence p., p. de equivalência. SIN equivalence *zone.*
far p., p. distante; aquele ponto no foco conjugado com a retina quando o olho não está se acomodando. SIN punctum remotum.
p. of fixation, p. de fixação; o ponto na retina em que são focalizados os raios provenientes de um objeto fitado diretamente. SIN p. of regard.
flash p., p. de ignição; a menor temperatura em que vapores de um líquido podem ser inflamados por uma chama.
focal p., p. focal. VER anterior focal p., posterior focal p.
freezing p., p. de congelamento; a temperatura em que um líquido se solidifica.
fusing p., p. de fusão. VER fusion *temperature* (wire method).
Guéneau de Mussy p., p. de Guéneau de Mussy; ponto doloroso à compressão, na junção de uma linha que prolonga a borda esquerda do esterno e uma linha horizontal ao nível da extremidade da porção óssea da décima costela; é encontrado em casos de pleurite diafragmática.
gutta-percha p.'s, pontos de guta-percha; cones de um composto de gutapercha usado para preencher canais radiculares em conjunto com um cemento, pasta ou plástico.
Hallé p., p. de Hallé; um ponto na intersecção de uma linha horizontal que toca a espinha ântero-superior do ílio e uma linha perpendicular desenhada a partir da espinha do púbis; aqui o ureter pode ser palpado mais facilmente.
heat-rigor p., p. de rigor pelo calor; o grau de temperatura elevada em que ocorre coagulação do protoplasma com morte da célula.
incident p., p. de incidência; o ponto no qual um raio de luz entra em um sistema óptico.
incisal p., p. incisal; o ponto localizado entre as margens incisais dos incisivos centrais inferiores; a projeção gráfica das excursões do ponto incisal em alguns planos geralmente é usada para ilustrar a amplitude do movimento mandibular.
isoelectric p. (p*l***, IEP, I.P., i.p.),** p. isoelétrico; o pH em que uma substância anfotérica, como uma proteína ou um aminoácido, é eletricamente neutra.
isoionic p., p. isoiônico; o pH em que um zwitteríon tem um número igual de cargas elétricas positivas e negativas; na água e na ausência de outros solutos, esse é o ponto isoelétrico.
isosbestic p., p. isosbéstico; em espectroscopia aplicada, um comprimento de onda no qual a absorbância de duas substâncias, uma das quais pode ser convertida na outra, é igual.
J p., p. J; o ponto que marca o fim do complexo QRS e o início da onda S ou T no eletrocardiograma. SIN ST junction.
jugal p., p. jugal. SIN jugale.
lower alveolar p., p. alveolar inferior. SIN infradentale.
malar p., p. malar; ápice da tuberosidade do osso zigomático (malar).
p. of maximal impulse, p. de impulso máximo; o ponto, na parede torácica em que se vê ou sente o impulso cardíaco máximo.
maximum occipital p., p. occipital máximo; o ponto, na escama do osso occipital, mais distante da glabela.
Mayo-Robson p., p. de Mayo-Robson; um ponto situado logo acima e à direita do umbigo, onde há dor à compressão na doença do pâncreas.
McBurney p., p. de McBurney; ponto entre 3,84 e 5,12 cm súpero-medial à espinha ilíaca ântero-superior, sobre uma linha que une esse processo e o umbigo, onde a compressão causa dor na apendicite aguda.
median mandibular p., p. mandibular mediano; ponto no centro ântero-posterior da crista mandibular, no plano sagital mediano.
melting p. (m.p., T_m**),** p. de fusão; **(1)** a temperatura na qual um sólido torna-se líquido; **(2)** a temperatura em que 50% de uma macromolécula torna-se desnaturada.
mental p., pogônio. SIN pogonion.
metopic p., metópio. SIN metopion.
motor p., p. motor; ponto na pele sobre as placas terminais de um músculo subjacente; a aplicação de um estímulo elétrico, através de um eletrodo, causará contração do músculo.
Munro p., p. de Munro; um ponto na margem direita do músculo reto do abdome, entre o umbigo e a espinha ilíaca ântero-superior, onde a pressão causa dor à palpação na apendicite.
nasal p., násio. SIN nasion.
near p., p. próximo; aquele ponto no foco conjugado com a retina quando o olho exerce acomodação máxima. SIN punctum proximum.
neutral p., p. neutro; um ponto no qual uma solução não é ácida nem alcalina (pH 7 a 22°C para soluções aquosas).
nodal p., p. nodal; um dentre dois pontos em um sistema óptico composto tão relacionados que um raio direcionado para o primeiro ponto parecerá ter atravessado o segundo ponto paralelo à sua direção original. SIN axial p.
occipital p., p. occipital; o ponto posterior mais proeminente no osso occipital acima do ínio.
p. of ossification, centro de ossificação. SIN ossification *center.*

painful p., p. doloroso. VER Valleix p.'s.
posterior focal p., p. focal posterior; o ponto de um sistema óptico composto onde são focalizados raios paralelos entrando no sistema.
power p., em odontologia, a dimensão vertical na qual pode ser registrada a força mastigatória máxima.
preauricular p., p. pré-auricular; um ponto da raiz posterior do arco zigomático situado imediatamente na frente da extremidade superior do trago.
pressure p., p. de pressão; um local na pele apresentando elementos sensíveis à pressão que, quando comprimidos, produzem uma sensação de pressão.
primary p. of ossification, centro primário de ossificação. SIN primary ossification center.
principal p., p. principal; um dentre dois pontos sobre um eixo óptico tão relacionados que um objeto situado em um ponto tem sua imagem exata formada no outro sem ampliação, redução ou inversão.
p. of proximal contact, p. de contato proximal. SIN contact area.
p. of regard, p. de atenção. SIN p. of fixation.
retention p., p. de retenção; preparação feita dentro de uma cavidade dental para manter no lugar os primeiros pedaços de ouro ao se fazer uma restauração de ouro direta.
secondary p. of ossification, centro secundário de ossificação. SIN secondary ossification center.
silver p., p. de prata; um cone central sólido de prata usado no enchimento de canais radiculares em conjunto com um cimento ou pasta.
spinal p., p. subnasal. SIN subnasal p.
subnasal p., p. subnasal; o centro da raiz da espinha nasal anterior. SIN apophysary p. (1), apophysial p., spinal p.
Sudeck critical p., p. crítico de Sudeck; região no colo entre o suprimento das artérias sigmóideas e o da artéria retal superior.
supra-auricular p., p. supra-auricular; ponto craniométrico sobre a raiz posterior do processo zigomático do osso temporal, diretamente acima do ponto auricular.
supranasal p., ófrio. SIN ophryon.
supraorbital p., ófrio. SIN ophryon.
sylvian p., p. de Sylvius; o ponto mais próximo, no crânio, da fissura lateral (de Sylvius), cerca de 30 mm atrás do processo zigomático do osso frontal.
tender p.'s, pontos dolorosos. SIN Valleix p.'s.
trigger p., p. gatilho; p. desencadeante; um ponto ou uma área específica na qual a estimulação por toque, dor ou pressão induz uma resposta dolorosa. SIN dolorogenic zone, trigger area, trigger zone.
triple p., p. triplo; a temperatura em que todas as três fases (isto é, sólida, líquida e gasosa) estão em equilíbrio; o ponto triplo da água (273,16 K) é um ponto fixo fundamental nas escalas de temperatura.
Trousseau p., p. de Trousseau; um ponto doloroso, na neuralgia, no processo espinhoso da vértebra abaixo da qual se origina o nervo agressor. SIN apophysary p. (2), apophysial p.
Valleix p.'s, pontos de Valleix; vários pontos no trajeto de um nervo, cuja compressão é dolorosa em casos de neuralgia; esses pontos são: 1) onde o nervo emerge do canal ósseo; 2) onde perfura um músculo ou aponeurose para chegar à pele; 3) onde um nervo superficial apóia-se sobre uma superfície resistente em que é facilmente comprimido; 4) onde o nervo emite um ou mais ramos; e 5) onde o nervo termina na pele. SIN tender p.'s.
Weber p., p. de Weber; ponto situado 1 cm abaixo do promontório do sacro; Weber acreditava que representasse o centro de gravidade do corpo.
zygomaxillary p., p. zigomaxilar. SIN zygomaxillare.

poin·til·lage (pwan-tē-yazh'). Uma manipulação por massagem com as pontas dos dedos das mãos. [Fr. pontilhado]
point·ing (poynt'ing). Apontando; preparando-se para abrir espontaneamente, em relação a um abscesso ou furúnculo.
point source. Fonte pontual; em fotometria; uma fonte luminosa muito pequena, considerada como um ponto geométrico do qual a luz emana em linhas retas em todas as direções.
Poirier, Paul J., cirurgião francês, 1853–1907. VER P. gland, line.
poise (P) (poyz, pwahz). Poise; no sistema CGS, a unidade de viscosidade igual a 1 dina-segundo por centímetro quadrado e a 0,1 pascal-segundo. [J.-L. M. Poiseuille]
Poiseuille, Jean Léonard Marie, fisiologista e físico francês, 1799–1869. VER poise; P. viscosity coefficient, law, space.
poi·son (poy'zŭn). Veneno; qualquer substância, seja tomada internamente ou aplicada externamente, que é prejudicial para a saúde ou perigosa para a vida. [Fr., do L. potio, poção, dose]
acrid p., v. corrosivo; veneno que provoca irritação local destrutiva, bem como efeitos sistêmicos.
arrow p., v. de flecha; **(1)** Curare. SIN curare; **(2)** qualquer toxina natural usada para revestir flechas, lanças e dardos (p. ex., extratos contendo aconitina, ouabaína, glicosídeos cardíacos, batracotoxina, curare).
fish p., veneno de peixe; ictiotoxina; **(1)** SIN ichthyotoxicon; **(2)** SIN fugu p.
fugu p. (foo'goo), um veneno na ova e em outras partes de várias espécies de Diodon, Triodon e Tetradon, peixes das águas asiáticas orientais. SIN fish p. (2). [Jap. fugu, um peixe venenoso]
respiratory p., veneno respiratório. SIN respiratory inhibitor.

poi·son·ing (poy'zŏn-ing). Envenenamento; intoxicação. **1.** A administração de veneno. **2.** O estado de estar envenenado. SIN intoxication (1).
ackee p., envenenamento por ackee (fruto da Jamaica); doença emética aguda e freqüentemente fatal, associada a sinais e sintomas referentes ao sistema nervoso central e à hipoglicemia acentuada, causado pela ingestão do fruto verde da Blighia spaida, uma árvore comum na Jamaica. SIN Jamaican vomiting sickness.
bacterial food p., intoxicação alimentar bacteriana; termo comumente usado para referir-se a condições limitadas à enterite ou gastroenterite (excluindo as febres entéricas e as disenterias) causada pela própria multiplicação bacteriana ou por uma exotoxina bacteriana solúvel.
blood p., septicemia. VER septicemia, pyemia.
carbon disulfide p., intoxicação por dissulfeto de carbono; intoxicação aguda ou crônica por CS_2, doença ocupacional encontrada em trabalhadores na indústria de borracha e na fabricação de seda artificial (raion) pelo processo da viscose; caracterizada por insônia, desatenção e irritabilidade, seguidas por paralisias, comprometimento da visão, úlcera péptica e psicoses.
carbon monoxide p., intoxicação por monóxido de carbono; intoxicação aguda ou crônica, potencialmente fatal, causada por inalação do gás monóxido de carbono, que tem uma afinidade 210 vezes maior que a do oxigênio pela ligação com a hemoglobina (carboxiemoglobina) e, assim, interfere com o transporte de oxigênio e dióxido de carbono pelo sangue.
crotalaria p., intoxicação por crotalária; intoxicação de seres humanos e animais com alcalóides dos vegetais Senecio (senécio), Crotalaria (crotalária) e Heliotropum; provoca uma doença venooclusiva do fígado semelhante à doença de Chiari. SIN crotalism.
cyanide p., intoxicação por cianeto; uma doença bastante comum de animais herbívoros, causada pela ingestão de vegetais cianogênicos contendo glucosídeos que são hidrolisados, produzindo ácido hidrociânico; alguns produtos químicos usados no meio rural, como fungicidas ou inseticidas, podem ser causas de intoxicação por cianeto; o cianeto de hidrogênio e seus sais são extremamente venenosos para os seres humanos, seja por inalação ou por ingestão.
Datura p., intoxicação por Datura; intoxicação resultante da ingestão de plantas do gênero Datura; os sinais e sintomas são de natureza parassimpaticolítica e, na intoxicação grave, incluem depressão do sistema nervoso central, insuficiência circulatória e depressão respiratória.
djenkol p., intoxicação por djenkol; intoxicação considerada resultante da ingestão exagerada de um feijão, Pitecolobium lobatum; os sintomas são dor na região renal, disúria e, posteriormente, anúria; o djenkol tem um alto conteúdo de vitamina B e é usado na alimentação, apesar de seus efeitos tóxicos.
ergot p., intoxicação pelo esporão do centeio; uma síndrome produzida pelo consumo de pão (notavelmente de centeio) contaminado pelo fungo Claviceps purpurea (ferrugem do centeio), a fonte de muitos alcalóides do esporão do centeio. Os efeitos observados incluem vasoconstrição periférica levando a gangrena, paralisia parcial com dormência, formigamento e queimação nos membros, pulso fraco, agitação, torpor ou delírio; pode ser fatal.
food p., intoxicação alimentar; intoxicação na qual o agente ativo está contido no alimento ingerido.
lead p., intoxicação por chumbo; intoxicação aguda ou crônica por chumbo ou qualquer um de seus sais; as manifestações de **i. aguda por chumbo** geralmente são aquelas de gastroenterite aguda em adultos ou encefalopatia em crianças; a **i. crônica por chumbo** manifesta-se principalmente por anemia, constipação, cólica abdominal, neuropatia com paralisia e queda do punho envolvendo os músculos extensores do antebraço, linha de chumbo azulada na gengiva e nefrite intersticial; podem ocorrer gota saturnina, convulsões e coma. SIN plumbism, saturnism.
mercury p., intoxicação por mercúrio; doença geralmente causada pela ingestão ou inalação de mercúrio ou de compostos mercuriais, que são tóxicos por causa de sua capacidade de produzir íons mercúricos; em geral, a **i. aguda por mercúrio** está associada a ulcerações da boca (incluindo amolecimento dos dentes), estômago e intestino e alterações tóxicas nos túbulos renais; pode haver anúria e anemia; a inalação pode ser seguida por angústia respiratória e pneumonia; geralmente a **i. crônica por mercúrio** é conseqüente a intoxicação ocupacional e causa malformações gastrointestinais ou do sistema nervoso central, incluindo estomatite, diarréia, cefaléias, ataxia, tremor, hiper-reflexia, comprometimento neurossensorial, instabilidade emocional e, algumas vezes, delírio (síndrome do Chapeleiro Louco). SIN hydrargyria, hydrargyrism, mercurialism.
mushroom p., envenenamento por cogumelos. VER mycetism.
oxygen p., intoxicação por oxigênio. SIN oxygen toxicity.
radiation p., intoxicação por radiação. SIN radiation sickness.
Salmonella food p., intoxicação alimentar por Salmonella; gastroenterite causada por várias cepas de Salmonella que se multiplicam livremente no trato

gastrointestinal, mas não provocam septicemia; os sintomas geralmente começam em 8–24 horas e incluem febre, cefaléia, náuseas, vômitos, diarréia e dor abdominal.

scombroid p., intoxicação por escombróide; intoxicação pela ingestão das toxinas termoestáveis produzidas por ação bacteriana sobre peixes de carne escura inadequadamente preservados da ordem Scombroidea (atum, bonito, cavalinha, albacora, peixe-serra); caracterizada por dor epigástrica, náuseas e vômitos, cefaléia, sede, dificuldade à deglutição e urticária.

silver p., intoxicação por prata. SIN argyria.

Staphylococ'cus food p., intoxicação alimentar por *Staphylococcus*; episódios comumente causados pela enterotoxina estafilocócica e caracterizados por início abrupto de gastroenterite algumas horas após a ingestão do alimento contaminado com a exotoxina pré-formada; o vômito geralmente é mais intenso e a diarréia menos intensa que nas formas infecciosas de intoxicação alimentar bacteriana.

systemic p., intoxicação sistêmica. SIN toxicosis.

tetraethyl p., i. por chumbo tetraetila. VER tetraethyllead.

thallium p., i. por tálio; condição caracterizada por vômitos, diarréia, dor nas pernas e polineuropatia sensorimotora grave; cerca de 3 semanas após a intoxicação, tipicamente ocorre extensa queda de cabelo temporária; geralmente ocorre após a ingestão acidental de um rodenticida.

turpentine p., intoxicação por terebintina; intoxicação por óleo de terebintina; os sinais e sintomas incluem hematúria, albuminúria e coma; a urina pode ter um odor de violetas. SIN terebinthinism.

poi·son ivy, poi·son oak, poi·son su·mac. Hera venenosa, carvalho venenoso, sumagre venenoso. **1.** VER *Toxicodendron.* **2.** Nome comum da erupção cutânea (dermatite por *rhus*) causada por contato com essas espécies de *Toxicodendron.*

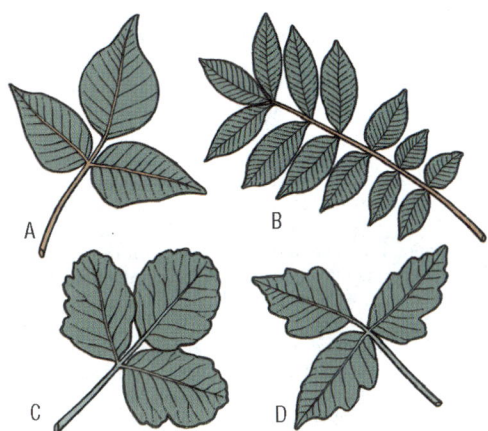

Toxicodendron: (A) hera venenosa, (B) sumagre venenoso, (C) carvalho venenoso (Ocidente), (D) carvalho venenoso (Oriente)

poi·son·ous (poy'zŭn - ŭs). Venenoso; caracterizado por, que possui a característica de, ou que contém um veneno. SIN toxic (1), toxicant (1), toxiferous, venenous.

Poisson, Siméon Denis, matemático francês, 1781–1840. VER P. *distribution.* P.-Pearson *formula.*

po·lar (pō'lăr). Polar. **1.** Relativo a um pólo. **2.** Que tem pólos, diz-se de algumas células nervosas que possuem um ou mais prolongamentos. [L. mod. *polaris*, de *polus*, pólo]

po·lar·im·e·ter (pō'lăr - im'ĕ - ter). Polarímetro; instrumento para medir o ângulo de rotação em polarização ou a quantidade de luz polarizada. [L. mod. *polaris*, polar, + G. *metron*, medida]

po·lar·im·e·try (pō'lăr - im'ĕ - trē). Polarimetria; medida por polarímetro.

po·lar·i·scope (pō - lăr'i - skōp). Polariscópio; instrumento para estudar os fenômenos de polarização da luz. [L. mod. *polaris*, polar, + G. *skopeō*, examinar]

po·lar·i·scop·ic (pō - lăr - i - skop'ik). Polariscópico; relativo ao polariscópio ou à polariscopia.

po·lar·is·co·py (pō'lă - ris'kŏ - pē). Polariscopia; uso do polariscópio no estudo das propriedades da luz polarizada.

po·lar·i·ty (pō - lăr'i - tē). Polaridade. **1.** A propriedade de ter dois pólos opostos, como os possuídos por um magneto. **2.** A posse de propriedades ou características opostas. **3.** A direção ou orientação da positividade em relação à negatividade. **4.** A direção ao longo de uma cadeia de polinucleotídeos, ou qualquer biopolímero ou macroestrutura (p. ex., microtúbulos). **5.** Em relação aos solventes, a capacidade ionizante. **6.** A tendência de um organismo de se desenvolver diferencialmente ao longo de um eixo. [L. mod. *polaris*, polar]

po·lar·i·za·tion (pō'lăr - i - zā'shŭn). Polarização. **1.** Em eletricidade, o revestimento de um eletrodo com uma camada espessa de bolhas de hidrogênio, resultando no enfraquecimento ou na interrupção do fluxo de corrente. **2.** Alteração efetuada em um raio de luz que atravessa determinados meios, na qual as vibrações transversas ocorrem apenas em um plano, e não em todos os planos como em um raio luminoso comum. **3.** Desenvolvimento de diferenças no potencial entre dois pontos em tecidos vivos, como entre o interior e o exterior de uma parede celular.

po·lar·ize (pō'lăr - īz). Polarizar; colocar em um estado de polarização.

po·lar·iz·er (pō'lă - rīz'er). Polarizador; o primeiro elemento de um polariscópio que polariza a luz, distinto do analisador, o segundo elemento polarizante.

po·lar·og·ra·phy (pō'lă - rog'ră - fē). Polarografia; ramo da eletroquímica que estuda a variação no fluxo de corrente através de uma solução enquanto a voltagem varia; esta variará com a concentração iônica de substâncias redutíveis, de forma que a polarografia possa ser usada em análise química. A polarografia é comumente empregada na forma de redução em um eletrodo gotejante de mercúrio. [L. mod. *polaris*, polar, + G. *graphō*, escrever]

pol·dine meth·yl·sul·fate (pōl'dēn). Metilsulfato de poldina; um agente anticolinérgico.

pole (pōl). [TA]. Pólo. **1.** Um dos dois pontos nas extremidades do eixo de qualquer órgão ou corpo. **2.** Um dos dois pontos sobre uma esfera na maior distância do equador. **3.** Um dos dois pontos em um magneto ou em uma bateria ou célula elétrica que possui extremos de propriedades opostas; o pólo negativo é um catodo e o pólo positivo, um anodo. **4.** Uma das extremidades de um fuso. **5.** Uma das zonas diferenciadas nas extremidades opostas de um eixo em uma célula, órgão ou organismo. SIN polus [TA]. [L. *polus*, a extremidade de um eixo, pólo, do G. *polos*]

abapical p., p. abapical; em um óvulo, o pólo oposto ao pólo animal (isto é, o pólo vegetal).

animal p., p. animal; o ponto em um ovo telolécito oposto ao vitelo, onde está concentrada a maior parte do protoplasma e localizado o núcleo; a partir dessa região, os corpos polares são expulsos durante a maturação. SIN germinal p.

anterior p. of eyeball [TA], p. anterior do bulbo do olho; o centro da curvatura corneal do olho. SIN polus anterior bulbi oculi [TA].

anterior p. of lens [TA], p. anterior da lente; o ponto central na superfície anterior da lente do olho. SIN polus anterior lentis [TA].

cephalic p., p. cefálico; a extremidade da cabeça do feto.

frontal p. [TA], p. frontal. SIN frontal p. [TA] of cerebrum.

frontal p. [TA] of cerebrum, p. frontal [TA] do cérebro; o promontório mais anterior de cada hemisfério cerebral. SIN frontal p. [TA], polus frontalis [TA].

germinal p., p. germinal. SIN animal p.

inferior p. [TA], p. inferior; em uma estrutura que possui um eixo longitudinal orientado verticalmente, o ponto situado na extremidade inferior do eixo, mais próximo das plantas dos pés; o ponto mais baixo na superfície de uma estrutura. VER inferior p. of kidney, lower p. of testis. SIN extremitas inferior [TA], lower p. [TA], inferior extremity (1)*, polus inferior*.

inferior p. of kidney [TA], p. inferior do rim; a extremidade inferior do rim. SIN extremitas inferior renis [TA], inferior extremity of kidney*, polus inferior renis*.

inferior p. of testis, p. inferior do testículo; *termo oficial alternativo para lower p. of testis.

lateral p., p. lateral. SIN tubal extremity of ovary.

lower p. [TA], p. inferior. SIN inferior p.

lower p. of testis [TA], p. inferior do testículo; a extremidade inferior do testículo. SIN extremitas inferior testis [TA], inferior p. of testis*, polus inferior testis*.

medial p. of ovary, p. medial do ovário. SIN uterine extremity of ovary.

occipital p. [TA], p. occipital. SIN occipital p. [TA] of cerebrum.

occipital p. [TA] of cerebrum, p. occipital [TA] do cérebro; o promontório mais posterior de cada hemisfério cerebral; o ápice do lobo occipital. SIN occipital p. [TA], polus occipitalis [TA].

pelvic p., p. pélvico; a extremidade pélvica do feto.

posterior p. of eyeball [TA], p. posterior do bulbo do olho; o centro da curvatura posterior do olho. SIN polus posterior bulbi oculi [TA].

posterior p. of lens [TA], p. posterior da lente; o ponto central na superfície posterior da lente do olho. SIN polus posterior lentis [TA].

superior p. [TA], p. superior; em uma estrutura que possui um eixo longitudinal vertical, o ponto, na extremidade superior do eixo, mais distante da extremidade inferior, o ponto mais alto da superfície de uma estrutura. VER superior p. of kidney, upper p. of testis. SIN extremitas superior [TA], upper p. [TA], polus superior*, superior extremity (1)*.

superior p. of kidney [TA], p. superior do rim; a extremidade superior do rim. SIN extremitas superior renis [TA], polus superior renis*, superior extremity of kidney*.

superior p. of testis, p. superior do testículo; *termo oficial alternativo para upper p. of testis.

temporal p. [TA], p. temporal. SIN temporal p. [TA] of cerebrum.
temporal p. [TA] of cerebrum, p. temporal [TA] do cérebro; a parte mais proeminente da extremidade anterior do lobo temporal de cada hemisfério cerebral, uma pequena distância abaixo da fissura de Sylvius. SIN polus temporalis [TA], temporal p. [TA].
upper p. [TA], p. superior. SIN superior p.
upper p. of testis [TA], p. superior do testículo; a extremidade superior do testículo. SIN extremitas superior testis☆ [TA], polus superior testis, superior p. of testis☆.
vegetal p., vegetative p., p. vegetal, p. vegetativo; a parte de um ovo telolécito em que está situada a maior parte do vitelo.
vitelline p., p. vitelino; o pólo vegetativo de um óvulo.
Polenské num·ber. Número de Polenské. Ver em number.
po·lice·man (po-les'man). Um instrumento, geralmente um bastão com ponta de borracha, para remover partículas sólidas de um recipiente, particularmente das paredes do recipiente.
po·li·o (po'le-o). Pólio; abreviação de poliomielite.
polio-. Cinzento; substância cinzenta. [G. *polios*]
po·li·o·clas·tic (po'le-o-klas'tik). Polioclástico; destrutivo para a substância cinzenta do sistema nervoso. [polio- + G. *klastos*, quebrado]
po·li·o·dys·tro·phia (po'le-o-dis-tro'fe-a). Poliodistrofia. SIN poliodystrophy.
 p. cer'ebri progressi'va infan'tilis [MIM*203700], p. cerebral progressiva do lactente; paresia espástica progressiva hereditária autossômica recessiva dos membros, com deterioração mental progressiva, desenvolvimento de convulsões, cegueira e surdez, começando durante o primeiro ano de vida, e destruição e desorganização das células nervosas do córtex cerebral. SIN Alpers disease, Christensen-Krabbe disease, progressive cerebral poliodystrophy.
po·li·o·dys·tro·phy (po'le-o-dis'tro-fe). Poliodistrofia; desgaste da substância cinzenta do sistema nervoso. SIN poliodystrophia. [polio- + G. *dys*-, mau, + *trophe*, nutrição]
 progressive cerebral p., p. cerebral progressiva. SIN poliodystrophia cerebri progressiva infantilis.
po·li·o·en·ceph·a·li·tis (po'le-o-en-sef'a-li'tis). Polioencefalite; inflamação da substância cinzenta do cérebro, seja do córtex ou dos núcleos centrais; ao contrário da inflamação da substância branca. [polio- + G. *enkephalos*, encéfalo, + *-itis*, inflamação]
 p. infecti'va, p. infecciosa. SIN von Economo disease.
 inferior p., p. inferior; p. com predomínio de paralisia bulbar.
 superior p., p. superior; p. com oftalmoplegia.
 superior hemorrhagic p., p. hemorrágica superior. SIN Wernicke syndrome.
po·li·o·en·ceph·a·lo·me·nin·go·my·e·li·tis (po'le-o-en-sef'a-lo-mening'go-mi-e-li'tis). Polioencefalomeningomielite; inflamação da substância cinzenta do encéfalo e da medula espinal e do revestimento meníngeo das partes. [polio- + G. *enkephalos*, encéfalo, + *meninx*, membrana, + *myelon*, medula óssea, + *-itis*, inflamação]
po·li·o·en·ceph·a·lo·my·e·li·tis (po'le-o-en-sef'a-lo-mi'e-li'tis). Polioencefalomielite; inflamação da substância cinzenta do encéfalo e da medula espinal.
po·li·o·en·ceph·a·lop·a·thy (po'le-o-en-sef'a-lop'a-the). Polioencefalopatia; qualquer doença da substância cinzenta do encéfalo. [polio- + G. *enkephalos*, encéfalo, + *pathos*, que sofre]
po·li·o·my·e·li·tis (po'le-o-mi'e-li'tis). Poliomielite; um processo inflamatório que envolve a substância cinzenta da medula. [polio- + G. *myelos*, medula óssea, + *-itis*, inflamação]
 acute anterior p., p. anterior aguda; doença que resulta em morte ou lesão irreversível das células motoras no cérebro, tronco cerebral e medula espinal, causada por infecção por pequenos enterovírus RNA do grupo Picornaviridae; antigamente era causada quase somente por um dentre três tipos de vírus pólio, mas agora é causada, na maioria das vezes, por vírus Coxsackie A e B, ou por vírus ECHO.
 acute bulbar p., p. bulbar aguda; infecção pelo vírus da poliomielite que afeta células nervosas no bulbo e produz paralisia dos nervos cranianos motores inferiores.
 chronic anterior p., p. anterior crônica; atrofia muscular dos membros superiores e do pescoço, na qual há longos intervalos de quiescência ou melhora; não deve ser confundida com infecções pelo vírus da poliomielite.
po·li·o·my·e·lo·en·ceph·a·li·tis (po'le-o-mi'e-lo-en-sef'a-li'tis). Poliomieloencefalite; poliomielite anterior aguda com acentuados sinais cerebrais. [polio- + G. *myelon*, meo, + *enkephalos*, encéfalo, + *-itis*, inflamação]
po·li·o·my·e·lop·a·thy (po'le-o-mi'e-lop'a-the). Poliomielopatia; qualquer doença da substância cinzenta da medula espinal. [polio- + G. *myelon*, medula óssea, + *pathos*, que sofre]
po·li·o·sis (po-le-o'sis). Poliose; ausência segmentar ou diminuição da melanina nos fios de cabelo, das sobrancelhas ou dos cílios, causada por ausência do pigmento na epiderme; ocorre em várias síndromes hereditárias, mas pode ser causada por inflamação, irradiação ou infecção como herpes zoster. SIN trichopoliosis. [G. de *polios*, cinza]
 ciliary p., p. ciliar. SIN piebald eyelash.

po·li·o·vi·rus. Poliovírus; um enterovírus da família Picornaviridae. Há 3 sorotipos distintos, sendo o tipo 1 responsável por 85% dos casos de pólio paralítica e pela maioria das epidemias.
po·li·o·vi·rus hom·i·nis (po'le-o-vi'rus hom'i-nis). Vírus da poliomielite. SIN poliomyelitis virus.
pol·ish·ing. Polimento; em odontologia, o ato ou processo de tornar uma restauração lisa e brilhante.
Politzer, Adam, otologista austríaco, 1835–1920. VER P. *bag, method,* luminous *cone.*
pol·itz·er·i·za·tion (pol'it-zer-i-za'shŭn). Ducha de ar de Politzer; insuflação da tuba de Eustáquio e da orelha média pelo método de Politzer.
 negative p., ducha de ar de Politzer negativa; retirada de secreções de uma cavidade por sucção, realizada fixando-se uma bolsa de Politzer comprimida, ou uma pêra de borracha, a um tubo introduzido na cavidade.
pol·kis·sen of Zimmermann (pol'kis-en). Mesângio extraglomerular. SIN extraglomerular *mesangium.* [Al. *Polkissen,* pólo + coxim]
pol·la·ki·dip·sia (pol'a-ki-dip'se-a). Polacidipsia; termo raramente usado para a sede freqüente demais. [G. *pollakis,* freqüentemente, + *dipsa,* sede]
pol·la·ki·u·ria (pol'a-ke-u-re-a). Polaciúria; termo raramente usado para designar a freqüência urinária muito alta.
pol·len (pol'en). Pólen; microsporos de sementes de vegetais levados pelo vento ou por insetos antes da fertilização; importante na etiologia da febre do feno e de outras alergias. [L. poeira fina, farinha fina]
pol·le·no·sis (pol-e-no'sis). Polenose. SIN pollinosis.
pol·lex, gen. **pol·li·cis,** pl. **pol·li·ces** (pol'eks, pol'i-sis, -sez) [TA]. Polegar. SIN thumb. [L.]
 p. pe'dis, hálux. SIN great *toe* I.
pol·li·ci·za·tion (pol'i-si-za'shŭn). Policização; construção de um polegar substituto. [L. *pollex,* polegar, + *-ize,* fazer semelhante, + *-ation,* estado]
pol·li·no·sis (pol-i-no'sis). Polenose; febre do feno excitada pelo pólen de várias plantas. SIN pollenosis. [L. *pollen,* pólen, + G. *-osis,* condição]
pol·lu·tant (po-loo'tănt). Poluente; um contaminante indesejado que resulta em poluição.
pol·lu·tion (po-loo'shŭn). Poluição; tornar sujo ou inadequado por contato ou mistura com um contaminante indesejado. [L. *pollutio,* de *pol-luo,* pp. *-lutus,* sujar]
 air p., p. atmosférica; contaminação do ar por fumaça e gases prejudiciais, principalmente óxidos de carbono, enxofre e nitrogênio, como de escapamentos de automóveis, despejos industriais ou resíduos de combustão. VER TAMBÉM smog.
 noise p., p. sonora; níveis de ruído ambiental perturbadores ou prejudiciais, como de motores de automóveis, máquinas industriais ou música amplificada.
po·lo·cyte (po'lo-sit). Polócito. SIN polar *body.* [G. *polos,* pólo, + *kytos,* célula]
po·lo·ni·um (Po) (po-lo'ne-ŭm). Polônio; um elemento radioativo, de n.º atômico 84, isolado da uraninita; o isótopo de vida mais longa é o Po^{209} (meia-vida 102 anos); o Po^{210} é o rádio F (meia-vida de 138,38 dias), o único isótopo facilmente acessível. [L. de *Polonia,* Polônia, país onde nasceu Mme. M.S. Curie que, com seu marido, P. Curie, descobriu a substância]
pol·ox·a·lene (pol-ok-sa-len). Poloxaleno; um polímero oxialquileno, agente tensoativo aniônico, com ações e empregos semelhantes aos do dioctil sulfossuccinato de sódio; usado na constipação causada por fezes secas e de consistência dura. SIN poloxalkol.
pol·ox·al·kol (pol-ok'sal-kol). Poloxalcol. SIN poloxalene.
pol·ster (pol'ster). Uma saliência de células musculares lisas, como nas artérias e veias penianas, antigamente considerada capaz de regular o fluxo sanguíneo. [G. coxim, suporte]
po·lus, pl. **po·li** (po'lus, -li) [TA]. Pólo. SIN pole. [L. pole]
 p. ante'rior bul'bi oc'uli [TA], p. anterior do bulbo do olho. SIN anterior *pole* of eyeball.
 p. ante'rior len'tis [TA], p. anterior da lente. SIN anterior *pole* of lens.
 p. fronta'lis [TA], p. frontal. SIN frontal *pole* [TA] of cerebrum.
 p. inferior, p. inferior; *termo oficial alternativo para inferior *pole.*
 p. inferior renis, p. inferior do rim; *termo oficial alternativo para inferior *pole* of kidney.
 p. inferior testis, p. inferior do testículo; *termo oficial alternativo para lower *pole* of testis.
 po'li liena'lis infe'rior et supe'rior, pólos inferior e superior do baço. VER anterior *extremity* of spleen, posterior *extremity* of spleen.
 p. occipita'lis [TA], p. occipital. SIN occipital *pole* [TA] of cerebrum.
 p. poste'rior bul'bi oc'uli [TA], p. posterior do bulbo do olho. SIN posterior *pole* of eyeball.
 p. poste'rior len'tis [TA], p. posterior da lente. SIN posterior *pole* of lens.
 poli rena'les infe'rior et supe'rior, pólos inferior e superior do rim. VER superior *pole* of kidney, inferior *pole* of kidney.
 p. superior, p. superior; *termo oficial alternativo para superior *pole.*
 p. superior renis, p. superior do rim; *termo oficial alternativo para superior *pole* of kidney.

p. superior testis, p. superior do testículo; *termo oficial alternativo para upper pole of testis.
p. tempora'lis [TA], p. temporal. SIN temporal *pole* [TA] of cerebrum.
poly (pol'ē). Forma abreviada e coloquialismo de polymorphonuclear *leukocyte* (leucócito polimorfonuclear).
poly-. Poli-. **1.** Prefixo que designa muitos; multiplicidade. Cf. multi-, pluri-. **2.** Em química, prefixo que significa "polímero de", como em polipeptídeo, polissacarídeo, polinucleotídeo; freqüentemente usado com símbolos, como em poli(A) para ácido poliadenílico, poli(Lys) para poli(L-lisina). [G. *polys*, muito, muitos]
Pólya, Jenö (Eugene), cirurgião húngaro, 1876–1944. VER Pólya *gastrectomy*; P. *operation*; Reichel-P. stomach *procedure*.
pol.y.(A) 1. Abreviatura de polyadenylic acid (ácido poliadenílico). **2.** Alcalóide de indol iridóide isolado da *Vinca* sp.; pode ter aplicações farmacológicas; pertencem a essa classe a vimblastina e a vincristina. **3.** Excreção de ácido D-glicérico na urina; encontrada em cálculos renais. **4.** Erro congênito do metabolismo, resultando em acidúria D-glicérica (1). **5.** Uma classe de peptídeos antibióticos básicos, encontrada em neutrófilos, que aparentemente destrói bactérias causando lesão da membrana.
poly(a) polymerase, poli(a) polimerase; enzima que catalisa a formação de uma seqüência de ácido poliadenílico.
pol·y·ac·id (pol-ē-as'id). Poliácido; ácido capaz de liberar mais de um íon hidrogênio por molécula; p. ex., H_2SO_4, ácido cítrico. [G. *polys*, muito, muitos + ácido]
pol·y·ac·ry·la·mide (pol-ē-a-kril-a-mīd). Poliacrilamida; polímero ramificado da acrilamida ($H_2C \neq CHCONH_2$) usado na eletroforese em gel; p. ex., R–CH_2–CH($CONH_2$)–CH($CONHR$)CH($CONHR'$)–R".
pol·y·ad·e·ni·tis (pol'ē-ad-ē-nī'tis). Poliadenite; inflamação de muitos linfonodos, principalmente em relação ao grupo cervical.
p. malig'na, peste bubônica SIN bubonic *plague.*
pol·y·ad·e·nop·a·thy (pol'ē-ad-ē-nop'a-thē). Poliadenopatia; quando muitos linfonodos são afetados. SIN polyadenosis.
pol·y·ad·e·no·sis (pol'ē-ad-ē-nō'sis). Poliadenose. SIN polyadenopathy.
pol·y·ad·e·nous (pol-ē-ad'ē-nŭs). Poliadenoso; relativo a ou que envolve muitos linfonodos.
pol·y·ad·e·nyl·a·tion. Poliadenilação. **1.** O processo de formação de ácido poliadenílico. **2.** A modificação covalente de uma macromolécula (p. ex., RNAm) pela formação de uma porção poliadenilil ligada de forma covalente à macromolécula.
pol·y·(ad·en·yl·ic ac·id) (pol·y·(A)) (pol-ē-ă-dē-nil'ik). Ácido poliadenílico (poli(A)); homopolímero do ácido adenílico; freqüentemente observado na extremidade 3′ de muitos RNAms eucarióticos.
pol·y·al·co·hol (pol-ē-al'kō-hol). Poliálcool; molécula alifática ou alicíclica caracterizada por dois ou mais grupamentos hidroxila; p. ex., glicerol, inositol. [G. *polys*, muito, muitos, + alcohol]
pol·y·al·lel·ism (pol'ē-ă-lēl'izm). Polialelismo; a existência de múltiplos alelos em um *locus* genético.
pol·y·a·mine (pol-ē-am'ēn). Poliamina; nome de classe das substâncias de fórmula geral $H_2N(CH_2)_nNH_2$, $H_2N(CH_2)_nNH(CH_2)_nNH_2$, $H_2N(CH_2)_n$-$NH(CH_2)_nNH(CH_2)_nNH_2$, onde $n = 3$, 4 ou 5. Muitas poliaminas originam-se por ação bacteriana sobre as proteínas; muitas são constituintes corporais normais de ampla distribuição ou são fatores de crescimento essenciais para microrganismos. [G. *polys*, muito, muitos + amine]
p. oxidase, p. oxidase; enzima dos peroxissomos hepáticos que usa oxigênio molecular para oxidar espermina em espermidina e espermidina em putrescina, em ambos os casos produzindo também H_2O_2 e β-aminopropionaldeído; uma parte da via catabólica das poliaminas.
pol·y(ami·no ac·ids). Poli(aminoácidos); polipeptídeos que são polímeros de grupamentos aminoacil, isto é, de –NH-CHR–CO–; tipicamente, um termo usado com homopolímeros. VER poly- (2).
pol·y·an·gi·i·tis (pol'ē-an-jē-ī'tis). Poliangeíte; inflamação de múltiplos vasos sanguíneos envolvendo mais de um tipo de vaso, p. ex., artérias e veias, ou arteríolas e capilares.
microscopic p., p. microscópica; inflamação de pequenos vasos não-granulomatosa, sistêmica, associada a glomerulonefrite, capilarite pulmonar, púrpura palpável e auto-anticorpos citoplasmáticos antineutrofílicos.
pol·y·an·i·on (pol-ē-an'ī-on). Poliânion; sítios aniônicos em proteoglicanas nos glomérulos renais que restringem a filtração de moléculas aniônicas e facilitam a infiltração de proteínas catiônicas; a perda de poliânions pode causar albuminúria na nefrose lipóide.
pol·y·ar·ter·i·tis (pol'ē-ar-ter-ī'tis). Poliarterite; inflamação simultânea de várias artérias.
p. nodo'sa, p. nodosa; inflamação segmentar, com infiltração por eosinófilos e necrose de artérias pequenas ou médias, mais comum em homens, com vários sinais e sintomas relacionados ao envolvimento das artérias nos rins, músculos, trato gastrointestinal e coração. SIN arteritis nodosa, Kussmaul disease, periarteritis nodosa.
pol·y·ar·thric (pol-ē-ar'thrik). Poliarticular. SIN multiarticular.

pol·y·ar·thri·tis (pol'ē-ar-thrī'tis). Poliartrite; inflamação simultânea de várias articulações. [poly- + G. *arthron*, articulação, + *-itis*, inflamação]
p. chron'ica, p. crônica; termo obsoleto para designar artrite reumatóide (rheumatoid *arthritis*).
p. chron'ica villo'sa, p. crônica vilosa; inflamação crônica limitada à membrana sinovial, envolvendo diversas articulações; ocorre em mulheres na menopausa e em crianças.
epidemic p., p. epidêmica; doença febril leve de seres humanos na Austrália, caracterizada por poliartralgia e exantema, causada pelo vírus do rio Ross, um membro da família Togaviridae, e transmitida por mosquitos. SIN epidemic exanthema, Murray Valley rash, Ross River fever.
p. rheumat'ica acu'ta, p. reumática aguda; termo obsoleto para designar poliartrite associada a febre reumática.
vertebral p., p. vertebral; inflamação de vários discos intervertebrais sem envolvimento dos corpos vertebrais.
pol·y·ar·tic·u·lar (pol-ē-ar-tik'ū-lar). Poliarticular. SIN multiarticular. [poly- + L. *articulus*, articulação]
pol·y·a·sple·nia. Polisplenia. SIN polysplenia. [fusão de *polysplenia* e *asplenia*]
pol·y·aux·o·troph (pol-ē-awks'ō-trof). Poliauxotrófico; organismo mutante que requer vários nutrientes não requeridos pelo organismo do tipo selvagem. Cf. auxotroph, monoauxotroph.
pol·y·a·vi·ta·min·o·sis (pol'ē-ā'vī-tă-mi-nō'sis). Poliavitaminose; deficiências de múltiplas vitaminas.
pol·y·ba·sic (pol-ē-bās'ik). Polibásico; que tem mais de um átomo de hidrogênio substituível, designando um ácido com uma basicidade maior que 1.
pol·y·blen·nia (pol-ē-blen'ē-ă). Poliblenia; produção excessiva de muco. [poly- + G. *blennos*, muco]
pol·y·car·bo·phil (pol-ē-kar'bō-fil). Policarbófilo; um ácido poliacrílico com ligação cruzada com o divinil glicol; usado como absorvente gastrointestinal.
pol·y·car·dia (pol-ē-kar'dē-ă). Taquicardia. SIN tachycardia.
pol·y·cen·tric (pol-ē-sen'trik). Policêntrico; que tem vários centros.
pol·y·chei·ria, pol·y·chi·ria (pol-ē-kī'rē-ă). Poliquiria; presença de mãos supranumerárias. [poly- + G. *cheir*, mão]
pol·y·chon·dri·tis (pol'ē-kon-drī'tis). Policondrite; inflamação de cartilagem. [poly- + G. *chondros*, cartilagem, + *-itis*, inflamação]
chronic atrophic p., p. atrófica crônica. SIN relapsing p.
relapsing p., p. recidivante; doença degenerativa da cartilagem que produz uma forma bizarra de artrite, com colapso das orelhas, da porção cartilaginosa do nariz e da árvore traqueobrônquica; pode haver morte por infecção crônica ou sufocação devido à perda da estabilidade na árvore traqueobrônquica; de origem autossômica. SIN chronic atrophic p., generalized chondromalacia, Meyenburg disease, Meyenburg-Altherr-Uehlinger syndrome, relapsing perichondritis, systemic chondromalacia.
pol·y·chro·ma·sia (pol'ē-krō-mā'zē-ă). Policromasia. SIN polychromatophilia.
pol·y·chro·mat·ic (pol-ē-krō-mat'ik). Policromático; multicolorido.
pol·y·chro·mat·o·cyte (pol'ē-krō-mat'ō-sīt). Policromatócito. SIN polychromatophil (2).
pol·y·chro·ma·to·phil, pol·y·chro·ma·to·phile (pol-ē-krō'mă-tō-fil, -fil). Policromatófilo. **1.** Que se cora facilmente por corantes ácidos, neutros e básicos; designa determinadas células, principalmente algumas hemácias. SIN polychromatophilic. **2.** Eritrócito jovem ou em degeneração que apresenta afinidade por corantes ácidos e básicos. SIN polychromatocyte. SIN polychromophil. [poly- + G. *chrōma*, cor, + *phileō*, amar]
pol·y·chro·ma·to·phil·ia (pol-ē-krō'mă-tō-fil'ē-ă). Policromatofilia. **1.** A tendência de algumas células, como as hemácias na anemia perniciosa, de serem coradas por corantes básicos e também ácidos. **2.** Condição caracterizada por muitas hemácias com afinidade por corantes ácidos, básicos ou neutros. SIN polychromasia, polychromatosis, polychromophilia.
pol·y·chro·ma·to·phil·ic (pol-ē-krō'mă-tō-fil'ik). Policromatófilo. SIN polychromatophil (1).
pol·y·chro·ma·to·sis (pol'ē-krō-mă-tō'sis). Policromatose. SIN polychromatophilia.
pol·y·chro·me·mia (pol-ē-krō-mē'mē-ă). Policromemia; aumento da quantidade total de hemoglobina no sangue.
pol·y·chro·mia (pol-ē-krō'mē-ă). Policromia; aumento da pigmentação em qualquer parte.
pol·y·chro·mo·phil (pol-ē-krō'mō-fil). Policromatófilo. SIN polychromatophil.
pol·y·chro·mo·phil·ia (pol-ē-krō-mō-fil'ē-ă). Policromatofilia. SIN polychromatophilia.
pol·y·chy·lia (pol-ē-kī'lē-ă). Poliquilia; aumento da produção de quilo. [poly- + G. *chylos*, quilo, + *-ia*, condição]
pol·y·cis·tron·ic (pol-ē-sis-tron'ik). Policistrônico; relativo ao RNAm que transporta informações para síntese de mais de uma proteína.
pol·y·clin·ic (pol-ē-klin'ik). Policlínico; dispensário para o tratamento e estudo de doenças de todos os tipos. [poly- + G. *klinē*, cama]

pol·y·clo·nal (pol-ē-klō′năl). Policlonal; em imunoquímica, relativo a proteínas (isto é, anticorpos) de mais de um único clone de células, ao contrário do monoclonal.

pol·y·clo·nia (pol′ē-klō′nē-ă). Mioclônus múltiplo. SIN *myoclonus multiplex.* [poly- + G. *klonos*, tumulto]

pol·y·co·ria (pol-ē-krō′rē-ă). Policoria; a presença de duas ou mais pupilas em uma íris. [poly- + G. *korē*, pupila]

pol·y·crot·ic (pol-ē-krot′ik). Policrótico; relativo a, ou caracterizado por, policrotismo.

po·lyc·ro·tism (pol-ik′rō-tizm). Policrotismo; condição na qual o traçado esfigmográfico mostra várias quebras ascendentes na onda descendente. [poly- + G. *krotos*, batimento]

pol·y·cy·e·sis (pol-ē-sī-ē′sis). Policiese, gravidez múltipla. SIN multiple pregnancy. [poly- + G. *kyēsis*, gravidez]

pol·y·cys·tic (pol-ē-sis′tik). Policístico; composto de muitos cistos.

pol·y·cy·the·mia (pol-ē-sī-thē′mē-ă). Policitemia; aumento acima do normal no número de hemácias no sangue. SIN erythrocythemia. [poly- + G. *kytos*, célula, + *haima*, sangue]

compensatory p., p. compensatória; p. secundária resultante de anoxia, p. ex., na cardiopatia congênita, enfisema pulmonar ou residência prolongada em grande altitude.

p. hyperton'ica, p. hipertônica; p. associada a hipertensão, mas sem esplenomegalia. SIN Gaisböck syndrome.

relative p., p. relativa; aumento relativo do número de hemácias em virtude de perda da porção líquida do sangue.

p. ru'bra, p. vera. SIN p. vera.

p. ru'bra ve'ra, p. vera. SIN p. vera.

p. ve'ra, p. vera; forma crônica de p. de causa desconhecida; caracterizada por hiperplasia da medula óssea, aumento do volume sanguíneo e também do número de hemácias, vermelhidão ou cianose da pele e esplenomegalia. SIN erythremia, Osler disease, Osler-Vaquez disease, p. rubra vera, p. rubra, Vaquez disease.

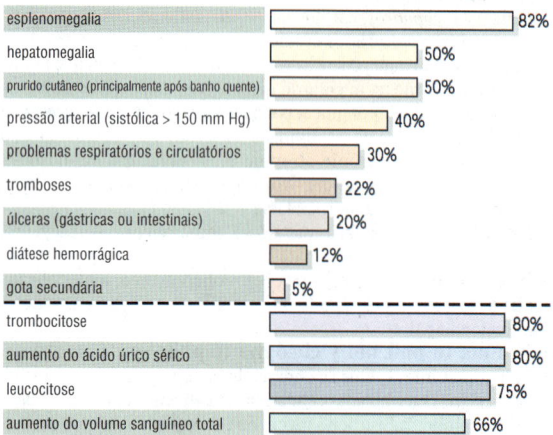

policitemia vera: freqüência relativa dos principais sintomas

pol·y·dac·tyl·ism (pol-ē-dak′ti-lizm). Polidactilia. SIN polydactyly.

pol·y·dac·tyl·ous (pol-ē-dak′til-ŭs). Polidáctilo; relativo à polidactilia.

pol·y·dac·ty·ly (pol-ē-dak′ti-lē). Polidactilia; presença de mais cinco dedos na mão ou no pé. SIN polydactylism. [poly- + G. *daktylos*, dedo]

pol·y·den·tia (pol-ē-den′shē-ă). Polidontia. SIN polyodontia. [poly- + L. *dens*, dente]

pol·y·dip·sia (pol-ē-dip′sē-ă). Polidipsia; sede excessiva e relativamente prolongada. [poly- + G. *dipsa*, sede]

hysterical p., p. histérica. SIN psychogenic p.

psychogenic p., p. psicogênica; consumo excessivo de líquido resultante de distúrbio da personalidade, sem lesão orgânica demonstrável. SIN hysterical p.

psychogenic nocturnal p. (PNP), p. noturna psicogênica. VER psychogenic nocturnal polydipsia *syndrome.*

pol·y·dis·per·soid (pol′ē-dis-per′soyd). Polidispersóide; sistema colóide no qual a fase dispersa é composta de partículas que apresentam diferentes graus de dispersão.

pol·y·dys·pla·sia (pol′ē-dis-plā′zē-ă). Polidisplasia; desenvolvimento tecidual anormal em vários aspectos. [poly- + G. *dys-*, mau, + *plasis*, moldagem]

pol·y·dys·tro·phic (pol′ē-dis-trof′ik). Polidistrófico; relativo à polidistrofia.

pol·y·dys·tro·phy (pol-ē-dis′trō-fē). Polidistrofia; condição caracterizada por muitas anomalias congênitas. [poly- + dystrophy]

pseudo-Hurler p., pseudodistrofia de Hurler. SIN *mucolipidosis* III.

pol·y·em·bry·o·ny (pol-ē-em-brē′ō-nē). Poliembrionia; condição de um zigoto dar origem a dois ou mais embriões. [poly- + G. *embryon*, embrião]

poly·en·do·crin·op·athy (pol′ē-en′dō-kri-nop′a-thē). Poliendocrinopatia; doença geralmente causada por insuficiência de múltiplas glândulas endócrinas. VER multiple endocrine deficiency *syndrome.*

pol·y·ene (pol-ē-ēn′). Polieno; um composto químico que possui uma série de ligações duplas conjugadas (alternadas); p. ex., os carotenóides.

pol·y·e·nic ac·ids (pol-ē-ē′nik). Ácidos poliênicos. SIN polyenoic acids.

pol·y·e·no·ic ac·ids (pol-ē-en′ik). Ácidos polienóicos; ácidos graxos com mais de uma ligação dupla na cadeia de carbono; p. ex., ácidos linoleico, linolênico e araquidônico. SIN polyenic acids.

pol·y·er·gic (pol-ē-er′jik). Poliérgico; capaz de atuar de várias formas diferentes. [poly- + G. *ergon*, trabalho]

pol·y·es·the·sia (pol-ē-es-thē′zē-ă). Poliestesia; distúrbio da sensibilidade no qual um único toque ou outro estímulo é percebido como vários estímulos. [poly- + G. *aisthēsis*, sensação]

pol·y·es·tra·di·ol phos·phate (pol′ē-es-tră-dī′ol). Fosfato de poliestradiol; polímero do fosfato de estradiol, usado como estrogênio de ação prolongada no tratamento do carcinoma da próstata.

pol·y·es·trous (pol-ē-es′trŭs). Poliestro; que tem dois ou mais ciclos estrais em um período de acasalamento.

pol·y·eth·y·lene gly·cols (PEGs) (pol-ē-eth′i-lēn). Polietilenoglicóis; polímeros da condensação do óxido de etileno e da água, da fórmula geral $HO(CH_2CH_2O)_nH$, onde *n* é igual ao número médio de grupamentos oxietileno (300-6.000); eles variam em consistência de acordo com o tamanho molecular; PEG 300 é um líquido viscoso; PEG 6.000 é um sólido semelhante a cera; os PEGs são solúveis em água e são usados como auxílios farmacêuticos.

pol·y·fruc·tose (pol-ē-fruk′tōs). Polifrutose. SIN fructosan (1).

pol·y·ga·lac·tia (pol′ē-gă-lak′tē-ă, -shē-ă). Poligalactia; secreção mamária excessiva de leite, principalmente no período de desmame. [poly- + G. *gala*, leite]

pol·y·ga·lac·tu·ro·nase (pol′ē-gă-lak′too-ron-ās). Poligalacturonase; pectina polimerase; enzima que catalisa a hidrólise aleatória de ligações 1,4-α-D-galactosidurônicas no pectato e em outros galacturonanos. SIN pectinase.

pol·y·gan·gli·on·ic (pol′ē-gang-glē-on′ik). Poliganglionar; que contém ou envolve muitos gânglios.

pol·y·gene (pol′ē-jēn). Poligene; um de muitos genes que contribuem para o valor fenotípico de um fenótipo mensurável.

pol·y·gen·ic (pol-ē-jen′ik). Poligênico; relativo a uma doença hereditária ou característica normal controlada pelos efeitos adicionados de genes em múltiplos *loci.*

polyglactin 910 (pol′ē-glak′tin). Poliglactina 910; fio de sutura absorvível sintético para sustentação de ferida de aproximação superficial da pele e mucosa.

pol·y·glan·du·lar (pol-ē-glan′doo-lăr). Poliglandular. SIN pluriglandular.

poly-β-glu·co·sa·min·i·dase. Poli-β-glucosaminidase. SIN chitinase.

pol·y·glu·ta·mate (pol-ē-gloo′tă-māt). Poliglutamato. SIN poly(glutamic acid).

pol·y(glu·tam·ic ac·id) (pol′ē-gloo-tam′ik). Ácido poliglutâmico; polímero de resíduos ácido glutâmico na ligação peptídica habitual (α-carboxil para α-amino). VER poly- (2). VER TAMBÉM poly(γ-glutamic acid). SIN polyglutamate.

pol·y(γ-glu·tam·ic ac·id). Ácido γ-poliglutâmico; polipeptídeo formado de resíduos ácido glutâmico, sendo o grupamento γ-carboxila de um ácido glutâmico condensado no grupo amino de seu vizinho; ocorre naturalmente na cápsula do bacilo do antraz.

poly(gly·col·ic ac·id) (pol′ē-glī-kol′ik). Ácido poliglicólico; polímero do ácido glicólico, usado em fios de sutura cirúrgicos absorvíveis. [ver poly- (2)]

pol·y·gna·thus (pol-ē-nath′ŭs, pō-lig′na-thŭs). Polignato; gêmeos conjugados desiguais em que o parasita está fixado à mandíbula do autósito. VER conjoined *twins,* em *twin.* [poly- + G. *gnathos*, mandíbula]

pol·y·graph (pol′ē-graf). Polígrafo. **1.** Instrumento para obter traçados simultâneos de várias fontes diferentes; p. ex., pulso radial e jugular, batimento cardíaco apical, fonocardiograma, eletrocardiograma. Quase sempre é incluído o ECG para controle. **2.** Instrumento para registrar alterações na respiração, pressão arterial, resposta cutânea galvânica e outras alterações fisiológicas, enquanto a pessoa é questionada sobre algum assunto ou solicitada a fazer associações com palavras relevantes e irrelevantes; presume-se que as alterações fisiológicas sejam indicadores de reações emocionais, indicando assim se a pessoa está falando a verdade. SIN lie detector. [poly- + G. *graphō*, escrever]

Mackenzie p., p. de Mackenzie; instrumento que consiste em um sistema de tambores e um marcador de tempo para registrar simultaneamente os pulsos jugular e arterial e o batimento apical; usado antigamente na investigação clínica de arritmias cardíacas.

pol·y·gy·ria (pol-ē-jī′rē-ă). Poligiria; condição na qual o encéfalo tem um número excessivo de convoluções. [poly- + G. *gyros*, círculo, giro]

pol·y·he·dral (pol-ē-hē′drăl). Poliédrico; que tem muitos lados ou faces. [G. *polyedros*, de muitos lados, de poly- + G. *hedra*, sítio, face]

pol·y·hex·os·es (pol-ē-heks′ōs-ez). Poliexoses. SIN hexosans.

pol·y·hi·dro·sis (pol′ē-hi-drō′sis). Poliidrose. SIN hyperhidrosis.

pol·y·hy·brid (pol-ē-hi′brid). Poliíbrido; a prole de pais diferentes entre si em mais de três características.

pol·y·hy·dram·ni·os (pol′ē-hi-dram′nē-os). Poliidrâmnio. SIN hydramnios.

pol·y·hy·dric (pol-ē-hi′drik). Poliídrico; que contém mais de um grupamento hidroxila, como em álcoois poliídricos (glicerol, $C_3H_5(OH)_3$) ou ácidos poliídricos (ácido o-fosfórico, $OP(OH)_3$).

pol·y·hy·per·men·or·rhea (pol-ē-hi′per-men-ō-rē′ă). Poliipermenorréia; menstruação freqüente e excessiva. [poly- + G. *hyper*, acima, + *mēn*, mês, + *rhoia*, fluxo]

pol·y·hy·po·men·or·rhea (pol-ē-hi′pō-men-ō-rē′ă). Poliipomenorréia; menstruação freqüente, mas escassa. [poly- + G. *hypo*, abaixo, + *mēn*, mês, + *rhoia*, fluxo]

pol·y·iso·pre·nes (pol-ē-i′sō-prēnz). Poliisoprenos. SIN polyterpenes.

pol·y·iso·pre·noids (pol-ē-i-sō-prē-noydz). Poliisoprenóides. SIN polyterpenes.

pol·y·kar·y·o·cyte (pol-ē-kar′ē-ō-sit). Policariócito; célula que contém muitos núcleos, como o osteoclasto. [poly- + G. *karyon*, núcleo, + *kytos*, célula]

pol·y·lac·to·sa·mines (pol-ē-lak-tōs′ă-mēnz). Polilactosaminas; classe de glicoproteínas que contém unidades lactosamina repetidas em seus componentes oligossacarídeos; as substâncias do grupo sanguíneo I/i pertencem a essa classe.

pol·y·lep·tic (pol-ē-lep′tik). Poliléptico; designa uma doença que ocorre em muitos paroxismos, p. ex., malária, epilepsia. [poly- + G. *lēpsis*, acesso]

pol·y·link·er (pol-ē-link′er). Sítio de policlonagem; seqüência de DNA inserida em vetores de DNA recombinante que consiste em um grupo de numerosos sítios de endonuclease de restrição únicos no plasmídeo; também denominado *restriction site bank* e *polycloning site*.

pol·y·lo·gia (pol-ē-lō′jē-ă). Polilogia; fala contínua e freqüentemente incoerente. [poly- + G. *logos*, palavra]

pol·y·mas·tia (pol-ē-mas′tē-ă). Polimastia; em seres humanos, uma condição na qual há mais de duas mamas. SIN hypermastia (1), multimammae, pleomastia, pleomazia. [poly- + G. *mastos*, mama]

pol·y·mas·ti·gote (pol-ē-mas′ti-gōt). Polimastigota; mastigota com vários flagelos agrupados. [poly- + G. *mastix*, chicote]

pol·y·meg·eth·ism (pol′ē-meg′ĕ-thism). Polimegetismo; variação maior que o normal no tamanho das células endoteliais da córnea humana.

pol·y·me·lia (pol-ē-mē′lē-ă). Polimelia; defeito do desenvolvimento no qual há membros ou partes de membros supranumerários. [poly- + G. *melos*, membro]

pol·y·men·or·rhea (pol-ē-men-ō-rē′ă). Polimenorréia; ocorrência de ciclos menstruais de freqüência maior que a habitual. [poly- + G. *mēn*, mês, + *rhoia*, fluxo]

pol·y·mer (pol′i-mer). Polímero; substância de alto peso molecular formada por uma cadeia de unidades repetidas, algumas vezes denominadas "meros". VER TAMBÉM biopolymer. [ver -mer (1)]

cross-linked p., p. de ligação cruzada; polímero no qual moléculas de cadeia longa são unidas entre si, formando uma rede bi ou tridimensional. SIN cross-linked resin.

pol·y·mer·ase (po-lim′er-ās). Polimerase; termo geral para designar qualquer enzima que catalisa uma polimerização, como a de nucleotídeos em polinucleotídeos, assim pertencendo à EC classe 2, as transferases.

p. alpha, p. alfa; uma classe de DNA polimerases de mamíferos, encontradas no núcleo, que atuam na replicação do cromossoma. SIN polymerase α.

p. beta, p. beta; classe de DNA polimerases de mamíferos, situadas no núcleo, que não participam da replicação, mas podem participar do reparo do DNA. SIN polymerase β.

p. gamma, p. gama; classe de DNA polimerases de mamíferos, situada nas mitocôndrias, responsável pela replicação do genoma mitocondrial. SIN polymerase γ.

Taq p., Taq p.; DNA polimerase termorresistente, isolada do *Thermus aquaticus*, que pode ampliar iniciadores em altas temperaturas; usada na reação da cadeia da polimerase.

pol·y·mer·ase γ. Polimerase γ. SIN *polymerase* gamma.

pol·y·mer·ase α. Polimerase α. SIN *polymerase* alpha.

pol·y·mer·ase β. Polimerase β. SIN *polymerase* beta.

pol·y·mer·ia (pol-ē-mēr′ē-ă). Polimeria; condição caracterizada por um número excessivo de partes, membros ou órgãos do corpo. [poly- + G. *meros*, parte]

pol·y·mer·ic (pol-i-mer′ik). Polimérico. **1.** Que possui as propriedades de um polímero. **2.** Relativo a, ou caracterizado por, polimeria. **3.** Sinônimo raramente usado de poligênico.

po·lym·er·i·za·tion (po-lim′er-i-za′shŭn). Polimerização; uma reação na qual um produto de alto peso molecular é produzido por sucessivas adições ou condensações de um composto mais simples; p. ex., o poliestireno pode ser produzido a partir do estireno, ou a borracha a partir do isopreno, ou um polinucleotídeo a partir de mononucleotídeos, ou microtúbulos a partir da tubulina.

po·lym·er·ize (pol′i-mer-iz, po-lim′er-iz). Polimerizar; produzir polimerização.

pol·y·met·a·car·pa·lia, pol·y·met·a·car·pa·lism (pol′ē-met-ă-kar-pā′lē-ă, -kar′pă-lizm). Polimetacarpalismo; anomalia congênita caracterizada por ossos metacarpais supranumerários.

pol·y·met·a·tar·sa·lia, pol·y·met·a·tar·sa·lism (pol′ē-met-ă-tar-sā′lē-ă, -tar′să-lizm). Polimetatarsalismo; anomalia congênita caracterizada pela presença de ossos metatarsais supranumerários.

pol·y·mi·cro·lip·o·ma·to·sis (pol-ē-mi′krō-lip′ō-mă-tō′sis). Polimicrolipomatose; a ocorrência de múltiplas e pequenas massas nodulares, bem distintas, de lipídios, no tecido conjuntivo subcutâneo. [poly- + G. *mikros*, pequeno, + lipoma + G. -*osis*, condição]

po·lym·i·tus (pō-lim′i-tŭs). Exflagelação. SIN exflagellation. [poly- + G. *mitos*, fio]

pol·y·morph (pol′ē-morf). Polimorfo; termo coloquial para leucócito polimorfonuclear (polymorphonuclear *leukocyte*).

pol·y·mor·phic (pol-ē-mor′fik). Polimórfico; que ocorre em mais de uma forma morfológica. SIN multiform, pleomorphic (1), pleomorphous, polymorphous. [G. *polymorphos*, multiforme]

pol·y·mor·phism (pol-ē-mor′fizm). Polimorfismo; ocorrência em mais de uma forma; existência, na mesma espécie ou em outro grupo natural, de mais de um tipo morfológico. SIN pleomorphism.

balanced p., p. balanceado; traço unilocal no qual dois alelos são mantidos em freqüências estáveis porque o heterozigoto está mais adaptado que qualquer um dos homozigotos. VER TAMBÉM overdominance.

corneal endothelial p., p. endotelial corneano; variação maior que o normal no formato das células.

DNA p., p. do DNA; condição na qual uma dentre duas seqüências de nucleotídeos normais, porém diferentes, pode existir em um local específico no DNA.

genetic p., p. genético; a ocorrência, na mesma população, de múltiplos estados alélicos distintos, dos quais pelo menos dois têm alta freqüência (convencionalmente de 1% ou mais).

lipoprotein p., p. de lipoproteína; variações hereditárias nas β-lipoproteínas de baixa densidade; as lipoproteínas variantes exibem diferentes propriedades antigênicas e químicas quando comparadas às lipoproteínas normais.

restriction fragment length p. (RFLP), p. do comprimento do fragmento de restrição; usado na análise genética de populações ou de relações individuais. Em regiões do genoma humano que não codificam proteínas, freqüentemente há uma grande variedade de seqüência entre indivíduos que pode ser medida; na verdade, a distância (em nucleotídeos no cromossoma) pode ser diferente, geralmente devido a padrões de bases repetidos.

restriction length p., fragment length p., p. do comprimento do fragmento, a existência de formas alélicas reconhecíveis pelo comprimento dos fragmentos resultantes do tratamento da cadeia de nucleotídios com uma enzima de restrição específica que retira uma determinada seqüência de nucleotídios sempre que esta ocorre. Uma mutação nessa seqüência modifica a clivagem e, portanto, o número de fragmentos.

restriction-site p., p. de sítio de restrição; p. do DNA no qual a seqüência de uma forma do p. contém um sítio de reconhecimento para determinada endonuclease, mas a seqüência da outra forma não possui esse sítio.

pol·y·mor·pho·cel·lu·lar (pol-ē-mor′fō-sel′ŭ-lăr). Polimorfocelular; relativo a, ou formado por células de vários tipos diferentes. [G. *polymorphos*, multiforme, + L. *cellula*, célula]

pol·y·mor·pho·nu·cle·ar (pol′ē-mor-fō-noo′klē-ăr). Polimorfonuclear; que possui núcleos de várias formas; designa um tipo de leucócito. [G. *polymorphos*, multiforme, + L. *nucleus*, núcleo]

pol·y·mor·phous (pol-ē-mor′fŭs). Polimorfo. SIN polymorphic.

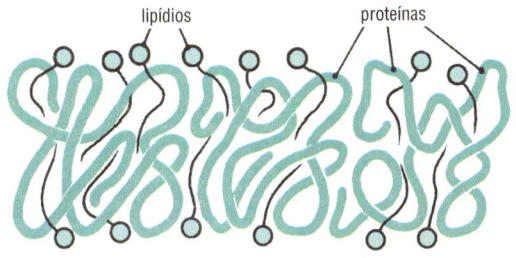

membrana de polímero (estrutura)

pol·y·my·al·gia (pol'ē-mī-al'jē-ă). Polimialgia; dor em vários grupos musculares. [poly- + G. *mys*, músculo, + *algos*, dor]
  p. arterit'ica, p. arterítica; p. reumática resultante de arterite, principalmente de arterite de célula gigante disseminada.
  p. rheumat'ica, p. reumática; síndrome pertencente ao grupo das doenças do colágeno diferente da espondilartrite ou da periartrite escapular umeral pela velocidade de hemossedimentação elevada; muito mais comum em mulheres que em homens.
pol·y·my·oc·lo·nus (pol'ē-mī-ok'lō-nŭs). Polimioclônus. SIN *myoclonus multiplex.*
pol·y·my·o·si·tis (pol'ē-mī-ō-sī'tis). Polimiosite; inflamação de vários músculos voluntários simultaneamente. [poly- + G. *mys*, músculo, + *-itis*, inflamação]
pol·y·myx·in (pol-ē-mik'sin). Polimixina; uma mistura de substâncias antibióticas obtidas de culturas de *Bacillus polymyxa* (*B. serosporus*), microrganismo encontrado na água e no solo e que pode ser obtido como um cloridrato cristalino; todos são polipeptídeos contendo vários aminoácidos e um ácido graxo de cadeia ramificada, geralmente o ácido (+)-6-metiloctanóico. Existem várias polimixinas (p. ex., designadas A, B$_1$, C, D, E, M, T), que têm efetividade aproximadamente igual contra bactérias Gram-negativas, mas que diferem em toxicidade, sendo a polimixina E (colistina) e a polimixina B as menos tóxicas. VER TAMBÉM *colistin* sulfate, colistimethate sodium.
  p. B sulfate, sulfato de p. B; antibacteriano efetivo na tularemia, brucelose, infecções por *Pseudomonas* e infecções urinárias, mas que só é usado sistemicamente nas infecções graves que não respondem a agentes menos tóxicos; também é usado localmente. A p. B é uma mistura de p. B$_1$ e p. B$_2$.
pol·y·ne·sic (pol-i-nē'sik). Polinésico; que ocorre em muitos focos distintos; designando algumas formas de inflamação ou infecção. [poly- + G. *nēsos*, ilha]
pol·y·neu·ral (pol-ē-noo'răl). Polineural; relativo a, suprido por ou que afeta vários nervos. [poly- + G. *neuron*, nervo]
pol·y·neu·ral·gia (pol'ē-noo-ral'jē-ă). Polineuralgia; neuralgia de vários nervos simultaneamente.
pol·y·neu·ri·tis (pol'ē-noo-rī'tis). Polineurite. SIN *polyneuropathy* (2).
  acute idiopathic p., p. idiopática aguda. SIN *Guillain-Barré syndrome.*
  chronic familial p., p. familiar crônica; inflamação dos nervos relacionada à infiltração por amilóide.
  infectious p., p. infecciosa. SIN *Guillain-Barré syndrome.*
  postinfectious p., p. pós-infecciosa. SIN *Guillain-Barré syndrome.*
pol·y·neu·ro·ni·tis (pol'ē-noo-rō-nī'tis). Polineuronite; inflamação de vários grupos de células nervosas.
pol·y·neu·rop·a·thy (pol'ē-noo-rop'ă-thē). Polineuropatia. **1.** Processo mórbido que envolve vários nervos periféricos (sentido literal). **2.** Distúrbio generalizado atraumático dos nervos periféricos que afeta mais intensamente as fibras distais, com atenuação proximal (p. ex., os pés são afetados mais cedo ou mais intensamente que as mãos) e, tipicamente, de forma simétrica; na maioria das vezes, afeta fibras motoras e sensitivas quase igualmente, mas pode envolver apenas um tipo de fibra ou o acometimento pode ser muito desproporcional; classificada como causadora de degeneração axonal ou desmielinizante; tem muitas causas, particularmente metabólicas e tóxicas; é de natureza familiar ou esporádica. SIN *polyneuritis.* SIN multiple neuritis, symmetric distal neuropathy. [poly- + G. *neuron*, nervo, + *pathos*, doença]
  acute inflammatory p., p. inflamatória aguda. SIN *Guillain-Barré syndrome.*
  alcoholic p., p. alcoólica; p. axonal nutricional associada ao alcoolismo crônico.
  arsenical p., p. arsenical; p. axonal que resulta de envenenamento subagudo ou crônico por arsênico; quase sempre é precedida por sinais e sintomas gastrointestinais; uma das neuropatias por metais pesados.
  axonal p., p. por perda axonal. SIN *axon loss p.*
  axon loss p., p. por perda axonal; tipo de p. no qual a degeneração axonal é o fator único/predominante; tem muitas etiologias, particularmente tóxicas e metabólicas; em estudos da condução nervosa, afeta as amplitudes das respostas, mas não causa lentificação nem bloqueio da condução. SIN axonal p.
  buckthorn p., p. por *Karwinskia humboldtiana*; p. ascendente resultante da ingestão do fruto da *Karwinskia humboldtiana*.
  chronic inflammatory demyelinating p. (CIDP), p. desmielinizante inflamatória crônica; p. sensorimotora desmielinizante, adquirida, incomum, clinicamente caracterizada por início insidioso, evolução lenta (seja progressão contínua ou gradual) e crônica; a fraqueza muscular simétrica é predominante, freqüentemente envolvendo os músculos proximais da perna, acompanhada por parestesias, mas não por dor; o exame do líquido cerebrospinal mostra elevação da proteína, enquanto estudos eletrodiagnósticos revelam evidências de um processo desmielinizante, basicamente de lentificação da condução, e não de bloqueio; algumas vezes responde à prednisona.
  critical ilness p., p. por doença grave; p. sensorimotor axonal difusa, observada em pacientes em estado grave, em geral na unidade de terapia intensiva; a maioria dos pacientes usam múltiplos medicamentos e não podem ser retirados do suporte ventilatório; estudos eletrodiagnósticos mostram evidências de polineuropatia axonal, predominantemente motora; de etiologia desconhecida.
  demyelinating p., p. desmielinizante; um tipo de p. no qual é afetada quase somente a mielina dos nervos periféricos; pode ser familiar (p. ex., doença de Charcot-Marie-Tooth, tipo 1) ou adquirida (p. ex., síndrome de Guillain-Barré); em estudos da condução nervosa motora, apresenta-se como lentificação ou bloqueio da condução. SIN segmental demyelinating p.
  diabetic p., p. diabética; p. distal, simétrica, em geral sensorimotora, que é uma complicação freqüente do diabetes melito.
  isoniazid p., p. por isoniazida; p. axonal observada em alguns pacientes tratados com isoniazida.
  nitrofurantoin p., p. por nitrofurantoína; p. axonal, freqüentemente grave, observada em alguns pacientes tratados com nitrofurantoína, sobretudo quando têm insuficiência renal crônica.
  nutritional p., p. nutricional; p. axonal observada no beribéri, no alcoolismo crônico e em outros estados clínicos, resultante da deficiência de tiamina.
  progressive hypertrophic p., p. hipertrófica progressiva. SIN *Dejerine-Sottas disease.*
  segmental demyelinating p., p. desmielinizante segmentar. SIN *demyelinating p.*
  uremic p., p. urêmica; p. sensorial e motora distal, sem inflamação visível e atribuída aos efeitos metabólicos da insuficiência renal crônica.
pol·y·nox·y·lin (pol-ē-nok'si-lin). Polinoxilina; poli {metilenobis[*N*,*N*'-di(hidroximetil)uréia]}; um polímero da uréia com formaldeído, usado como anti-séptico tópico.
pol·y·nu·cle·ar, pol·y·nu·cle·ate (pol-ē-noo'klē-ăr, -klē-āt). Polinuclear, polinucleado. SIN *multinuclear.*
pol·y·nu·cle·o·sis (pol'ē-noo-klē-ō'sis). Polinucleose; a presença de células polinucleares ou multinucleares no sangue periférico. SIN multinucleosis.
pol·y·nu·cle·o·ti·das·es (pol'ē-noo'klē-ō-tī'dās-ez). Polinucleotidases. **1.** Enzimas que catalisam a hidrólise de polinucleotídeos em oligonucleotídeos ou em mononucleotídeos; p. ex., fosfodiesterases, nucleases. **2.** Termo antigamente aplicado às duas polinucleotideofosfatases, 2'(3')- e 5'-, que não clivam ligações internucleotídeos.
pol·y·nu·cle·o·tide (pol-ē-noo'klē-ō-tīd). Polinucleotídeo; um polímero linear contendo um número indefinido (geralmente grande) de nucleotídeos, ligados de uma ribose (ou desoxirribose) a outra através de resíduos fosfóricos. Cf. oligonucleotide.
  p. methyltransferases, p. metiltransferases; enzimas que catalisam a metilação de bases purina e/ou pirimidina de polinucleotídeos ou dos açúcares dos polinucleotídeos. SIN polynucleotide methylases.
  p. phosphorylase, p. fosforilase. SIN *polyribonucleotide nucleotidyltransferase.*
  p. thioltransferases, p. tioltransferases; enzimas que catalisam a reação específica de tiolação de bases purina e/ou pirimidina em polinucleotídeos.
pol·y·nu·cle·o·tide meth·yl·ases. Polinucleotídeo metilases. SIN *polynucleotide* methyltransferases.
pol·y·o·don·tia (pol'ē-ō-don'shē-ă). Polidontia; presença de dentes supranumerários. SIN polydentia. [poly- + G. *odous*, dente]
pol·y·ol (pol'ē-ol). Poliol; álcool poliidroxi; um açúcar que contém muitos grupamentos –OH (-ol), como os álcoois e inositóis de açúcar.
  p. dehydrogenases, p. desidrogenases; enzimas oxidantes que catalisam a desidrogenação de álcoois de açúcar em monossacarídeos (na EC classe 1.1), p. ex., L-iditol desidrogenase e aldose redutase.
Pol·y·o·ma·vi·rus (pol-ē-ō'mă-vī'rŭs). Gênero de vírus (família Papovaviridae) contendo DNA (PM 3 × 10⁶), que possui vírions com aproximadamente 45 nm de diâmetro, incluindo vírus oncogênicos para animais; inclui o vírus polioma de roedores, vírus vacuolantes (SV40) de primatas e os vírus BK e JC dos seres humanos. [poly- + G. *-ōma*, tumor]
pol·y·on·co·sis, pol·y·on·cho·sis (pol'ē-ong-kō'sis). Polioncose; formação de múltiplos tumores. [poly- + G. *onkos*, tumor, + *-osis*, condição]
pol·y·o·nych·ia (pol-ē-ō-nik'ē-ă). Polioníquia; presença de unhas supranumerárias nos dedos das mãos ou dos pés. SIN polyunguia. [poly- + G. *onyx*, unha]
pol·y·o·pia, pol·y·op·sia (pol'ē-ō'pē-ă, -op'sē-ă). Poliopia; poliopsia; a percepção de várias imagens do mesmo objeto. SIN multiple vision. [poly- + G. *ōps*, olho]
pol·y·or·chism, pol·y·or·chid·ism (pol-ē-ōr'kizm, -ōr'kid-izm). Poliorquia; poliorquidismo; a presença de um ou mais testículos supranumerários. [poly- + G. *orchis*, testículo]
pol·y·os·tot·ic (pol'ē-os-tot'ik). Poliostótico; que envolve mais de um osso. [poly- + G. *osteon*, osso]
pol·y·o·tia (pol-ē-ō'shē-ă). Poliotia; presença de uma orelha supranumerária em um ou ambos os lados da cabeça. [poly- + G. *ous*, orelha]
pol·y·ov·u·lar (pol-ē-ō'vū-lăr). Poliovular; que contém mais de um óvulo.
pol·y·ov·u·la·to·ry (pol-ē-ō'vū-lă-tōr-ē). Poliovulatório; que libera vários óvulos em um ciclo ovulatório. SIN polyzygotic.
pol·y·ox·yl 40 ste·a·rate (pol-ē-ok'sil). Estearato de polioxil 40; uma mistura dos ésteres monoestearato e diestearato de um polímero de condensa-

ção, H(OCH$_2$CH$_2$)$_n$·OCOC$_{16}$H$_{32}$CH$_3$ (*n* é aproximadamente 40); é um agente tensoativo aniônico usado como emulsificante em pomadas hidrofílicas e outras emulsões.

pol·yp (pol'ip). Pólipo; termo descritivo geral usado em relação a qualquer massa de tecido que se saliente ou projete para fora ou para cima em relação ao nível normal da superfície, assim sendo macroscopicamente visível como uma estrutura hemisferóide, esferóide ou com a forma irregular semelhante a um monte que cresce a partir de uma base relativamente larga ou de um pedículo fino; os pólipos podem ser neoplasias, focos de inflamação, lesões degenerativas ou malformações. SIN polypus. [L. *polypus*; G. *polypous*, contr. do G. *polys*, muitos, + *pous*, pé]

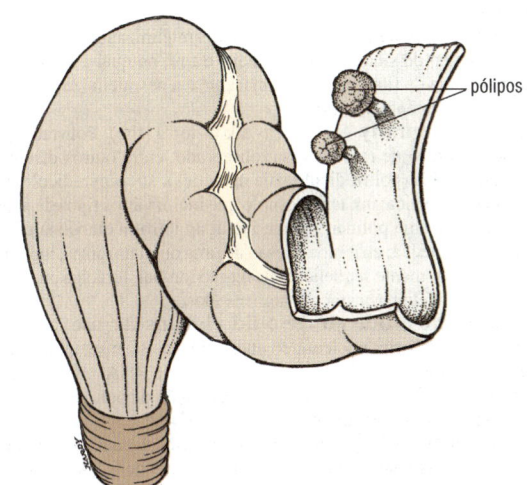

pólipos: na região sigmóide do intestino grosso

 adenomatous p., p. adenomatoso; p. que consiste em tecido neoplásico benigno derivado do epitélio glandular. SIN cellular p., polypoid adenoma.
 bleeding p., p. hemorrágico. SIN vascular p.
 bronchial p., p. brônquico; p. que cresce a partir da mucosa brônquica.
 cardiac p., p. cardíaco; geralmente um trombo arredondado preso ao endocárdio.
 cellular p., p. celular. SIN adenomatous p.
 choanal p., p. coanal; p. antrocoanal que se estende até a nasofaringe; origina-se no seio maxilar.
 cystic p., p. cístico; um cisto pediculado. SIN hydatid p.
 dental p., p. dental. SIN hyperplastic *pulpitis.*
 fibroepithelial p. (fi'brō-ep-the'lē-al), p. fibroepitelial. SIN skin *tag.*
 fibrous p., p. fibroso; p. que consiste principalmente em tecido fibroso celular, freqüentemente com focos de material colágeno ou hialino muito denso (ou ambos).
 fleshy p., p. miomatoso. SIN myomatous p.
 gelatinous p., p. gelatinoso; **(1)** p. que consiste em tecido conjuntivo edematoso, frouxo, delicado; **(2)** um mixoma polipóide.
 Hopmann p., p. de Hopmann. SIN Hopmann *papilloma.*
 hydatid p., p. hidático. SIN cystic p.
 hyperplastic p., p. hiperplásico; p. séssil, pequeno e benigno do intestino grosso, exibindo alongamento e dilatação cística das glândulas mucosas; também aplicado aos pólipos não-neoplásicos da mucosa gástrica. SIN metaplastic p.
 inflammatory p., p. inflamatório. SIN pseudopolyp.
 juvenile p., p. juvenil; hamartoma da mucosa do intestino grosso, suavemente arredondado, que pode ser múltiplo e causar hemorragia retal, principalmente na primeira década de vida; não é pré-canceroso. SIN retention p.
 laryngeal p., p. laríngeo; p. que se projeta da superfície de uma das pregas vocais.
 lipomatous p., p. lipomatoso; **(1)** p. que consiste principalmente em tecido adiposo; **(2)** lipoma que se projeta da superfície ou está preso por meio de um pedículo.
 lymphoid p., p. linfóide; p. benigno que consiste em agregados de linfócitos no reto.
 metaplastic p., p. metaplásico. SIN hyperplastic p.
 mucous p., p. mucoso; **(1)** p. adenomatoso no qual são formadas notáveis quantidades de mucina; **(2)** um cisto polipóide que contém muco.
 myomatous p., p. miomatoso; p. que consiste em tecido neoplásico benigno derivado do músculo não-estriado (liso). SIN fleshy p.
 nasal p., p. nasal; p. inflamatório ou alérgico, originário do óstio ou cavidade de um dos seios paranasais, que se projeta para a cavidade nasal.
 osseous p., p. ósseo; p. formado parcialmente por tecido ósseo.
 pedunculated p., p. pediculado; qualquer forma de p. fixada ao tecido basal por meio de um fino pedículo.
 placental p., p. placentário; p. desenvolvido a partir de um pedaço de placenta retida.
 pulp p., p. pulpar. SIN hyperplastic *pulpitis.*
 regenerative p., p. regenerativo; p. hiperplásico da mucosa gástrica.
 retention p., p. de retenção. SIN juvenile p.
 sessile p., p. séssil; qualquer forma de p. que tenha uma base relativamente larga.
 tooth p., p. dental. SIN hyperplastic *pulpitis.*
 vascular p., p. vascular; um angioma saliente ou protruso da mucosa nasal. SIN bleeding p.

pol·y·pap·il·lo·ma (pol'ē-pap-i-lō'mă). Polipapiloma; papilomas múltiplos.

pol·y·path·ia (pol-ē-path'ē-ă). Polipatia; multiplicidade de doenças ou distúrbios. [poly- + G. *pathos*, doença]

pol·y·pec·to·my (pol-i-pek'tō-me). Polipectomia; excisão de um pólipo. [polyp + G. *ektomē*, excisão]
 p. snare, alça de polipectomia; dispositivo em forma de alça destinado a deslizar sobre um pólipo e, ao ser fechado, resultar na transecção do pedículo do pólipo.

pol·y·pep·tide (pol-ē-pep'tīd). Polipeptídeo; peptídeo formado pela união de um número indefinido (incomumente grande) de aminoácidos por ligações peptídicas (–NH–CO–).
 gastric inhibitory p. (GIP), p. inibitório gástrico; hormônio peptídico secretado pelo estômago; o PIG inibe a secreção de ácidos e de pepsina e estimula a liberação de insulina como parte do processo digestivo. SIN gastric inhibitory peptide.
 glucose-dependent insulinotropic p., p. insulinotrópico glicose-dependente; substância insulinotrópica que se origina no trato gastrointestinal e é liberada para a circulação após a ingestão de uma refeição contendo glicose.
 pancreatic p., p. pancreático; **(1)** peptídeo com 36 aminoácidos, secretado pelas células das ilhotas do pâncreas em resposta a uma refeição e cuja função fisiológica é incerta; **(2)** uma família de peptídeos gastrointestinais, incluindo o polipeptídeo pancreático, o neuropeptídeo Y e peptídeo YY.
 trefoil p., p. em trevo; grupo de p. que compartilham a porção em trevo de uma estrutura em três alças altamente estável mantida unida por ligações dissulfeto baseadas em resíduos cisteína; são amplamente expressos em tecidos gastrointestinais e secretados por células mucosas; suas funções ainda são desconhecidas.
 vasoactive intestinal p. (VIP), p. intestinal vasoativo; hormônio peptídico secretado mais comumente por tumores de células das ilhotas não-β do pâncreas; aumenta a taxa de glicogenólise e estimula a secreção pancreática de bicarbonato; a produção excessiva causa diarréia aquosa abundante e perda fecal de eletrólitos, com hipopotassemia e hipocloridria. SIN vasoactive intestinal peptide.

pol·y·pha·gia (pol-ē-fā'jē-ă). Polifagia; ingestão excessiva de alimentos; glutonaria. [poly- + G. *phago*, comer]

pol·y·pha·lan·gism (pol'ē-fā-lan'jizm). Hiperfalangismo. SIN hyperphalangism.

pol·y·phal·lic (pol-ē-fal'ik). Polifálico; relativo à fantasia de possuir múltiplos pênis.

pol·y·phar·ma·cy (pol-ē-far'mă-sē). Polifarmácia; a administração simultânea de muitos fármacos. VER TAMBÉM shotgun *prescription.*

pol·y·phen·ic (pol-ē-phēn'ik). Pleotrópico. SIN pleiotropic. [poly- + G. *phainō*, exibir]

pol·y·phe·nol ox·i·dase (pol-ē-fē'nol). Polifenol oxidase. SIN laccase.

pol·y·pho·bia (pol-ē-fō'bē-ă). Polifobia; medo mórbido de muitas coisas; condição caracterizada por muitas fobias. [poly- + G. *phobos*, medo]

pol·y·phos·phor·y·lase (pol'ē-fos-fōr'i-lās). Polifosforilase. SIN phosphorylase.

pol·y·phra·sia (pol-ē-frā'zē-ă). Logorréia; hábito de falar em excesso. VER logorrhea. [poly- + G. *phrasis*, fala]

pol·y·phy·let·ic (pol'ē-fi-let'ik). Polifilético. **1.** Originado de mais de uma fonte, ou que possui várias linhas de descendência, ao contrário de monofilético. **2.** Em hematologia, relativo a polifiletismo.

pol·y·phy·le·tism (pol-ē-fī'lĕ-tizm). Polifiletismo; em hematologia, a teoria de que as células do sangue são derivadas de várias células-tronco diferentes, dependendo do tipo celular específico. SIN polyphyletic theory. [poly- + G. *phylē*, tribo]

pol·y·phy·o·dont (pol-ē-fī'ō-dont). Polifiodonte; que tem vários conjuntos de dentes formados em sucessão durante toda a vida. [poly- + G. *phyō*, produzir, + *odous* (*odont-*), dente]

po·ly·pi (pol'i-pī). Pólipos; plural de polypus.

pol·yp·i·form (po-lip'i-form). Polipiforme. SIN polypoid.

pol·y·plas·mia (pol-ē-plaz′mē-ă). Hidremia. SIN hydremia.
pol·y·plas·tic (pol-ē-plas′tik). Poliplásico. **1.** Formado por várias estruturas diferentes. **2.** Capaz de assumir várias formas. [poly- + G. *plastikos*, plástico]
Pol·y·plax (pol′ē-plaks). Um piolho sugador (ordem Anoplura) de ratos e camundongos. Foi demonstrado experimentalmente que a espécie *P. serratus* (o piolho do camundongo) é capaz de transmitir tularemia e também pode ser um vetor do tifo murino e do *Trypanosoma lewisi*. [poly- + G. *plax*, placa]
pol·yp·loid (pol′ē-ployd). Poliplóide; caracterizado por, ou relativo à, poliploidia.
pol·y·ploi·dy (pol′ē-ploy′dē). Poliploidia; o estado de um núcleo celular que contém três ou mais conjuntos haplóides. As células que contêm três, quatro, cinco ou seis múltiplos são denominadas, respectivamente, triplóides, tetraplóides, pentaplóides ou hexaplóides. [poly- + G. *ploidēs*, em forma]
pol·yp·nea (pol-ip-nē′ă). Polipnéia. SIN tachypnea. [poly- + G. *pnoia*, respiração]
pol·y·po·dia (pol-i-pō′dē-ă). Polipodia; presença de pés supranumerários.
pol·yp·oid (pol′i-poyd). Polipóide; semelhante a um pólipo nas características macroscópicas. SIN polypiform. [polyp + G. *eidos*, semelhança]
po·lyp·or·ous (pol-ip′or-ŭs). Cribriforme. SIN cribriform. [poly- + G. *poros*, poro]
Pol·y·po·rus (pol-lip′ō-rŭs). Gênero de cogumelos. VER agaric. [poly- + G. *poros*, poro]
pol·y·po·sia (pol-ē-pō′zē-ă). Poliposia; termo raramente usado para designar o consumo excessivo e constante de líquidos. [poly- + G. *posis*, bebida]
pol·y·po·sis (pol′i-pō′sis). Polipose; presença de vários pólipos. [polyp + G. -*osis*, condição]
   adenomatous p. coli, p. adenomatosa do colo. SIN familial adenomatous p.
   familial adenomatous p. (FAP) [MIM*175100], p. adenomatosa familiar; polipose que geralmente começa na infância; os pólipos aumentam em número, causando sinais e sintomas de colite crônica; freqüentemente são encontradas lesões pigmentadas da retina; o carcinoma do colo quase invariavelmente se desenvolve em casos não-tratados; herança autossômica dominante, causada por mutação no gene da polipose adenomatosa do colo (PAC) em 5q. Na síndrome de Gardner, que é alélica para PAF, há alterações extracolônicas (tumores desmóides, osteomas, cistos mandibulares). SIN adenomatous p. coli, familial p. coli, multiple intestinal p. (1).
   familial p. coli, p. colônica familiar. SIN familial adenomatous p.
   lymphomatoid p., p. linfomatóide; linfoma multifocal de células do manto, que produz numerosos pólipos linfóides nos intestinos.
   multiple intestinal p. [MIM*175100], p. intestinal múltipla; **(1)** SIN familial adenomatous p; **(2)** p. hamartomatosa do intestino delgado ou grosso, síndrome de Peutz-Jeghers [MIM*175200] com manchas de melanina nos lábios, menos comum.

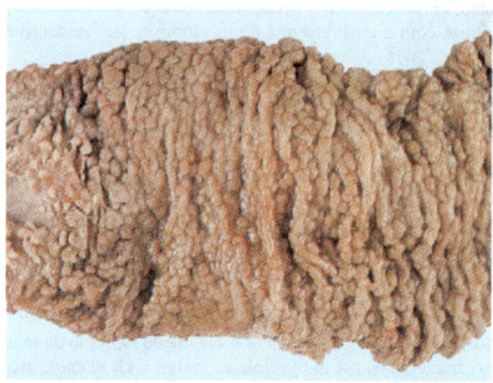

polipose (intestinal múltipla)

po·lyp·o·tome (po-lip′ō-tōm). Polipótomo; instrumento usado para seccionar um pólipo. [polyp + G. *tomos*, que corta]
pol·yp·o·trite (pol-ip′ō-trīt). Polipótrito; instrumento para triturar pólipos. [polyp + L. *tero*, pp. *tritus*, esfregar]
pol·y·pous (pol′i-pŭs). Poliposo; relativo a, que manifesta as características macroscópicas de, ou caracterizado por um pólipo ou pólipos.
pol·y·prag·ma·sy (pol-ē-prag′mă-sē). Polipragmasia; administração de muitos remédios diferentes ao mesmo tempo. [poly- + G. *pragma*, uma coisa]
pol·y·pre·nols (pol-ē-prēn-olz). Poliprenóis; álcoois poliisopreno acíclicos.
pol·yp·tych·i·al (pol-ē-tik′ē-ăl). Pregueado ou disposto formando mais de uma camada. [G. *polyptychos*, que tem muitas pregas ou camadas, de poly- + *ptychē*, prega ou camada]

pol·y·pus, pl. **po·ly·pi** (pol′i-pŭs, -pī). Pólipo. SIN polyp. [L.]
pol·y·ra·dic·u·li·tis (pol′ē-ra-dik′ū-lī′tis). Polirradiculite. SIN polyradiculopathy.
pol·y·ra·dic·u·lo·my·op·a·thy (pol′ē-ra-dik′ū-lō-mī-op′ă-thē). Polirradiculomiopatia; polirradiculopatia e miopatia coexistente.
pol·y·ra·dic·u·lo·neu·rop·a·thy (pol-ē-ra-dik′ū-lō-noo-rop′ă-thē). Polirradiculoneuropatia. **1.** Literalmente, um processo patológico que afeta as raízes e os nervos periféricos. **2.** Um distúrbio generalizado atraumático, na maioria dos casos esporádico, das raízes nervosas e dos nervos periféricos, que pode afetar as fibras motoras ou sensitivas, mas geralmente afeta ambas, embora freqüentemente não no mesmo grau; classificado como degenerativo axonal ou desmielinizante. Esse distúrbio tem muitas causas, basicamente mediadas pelo sistema imune, e inclui a síndrome de Guillain-Barré e a polineuropatia inflamatória crônica.
   acute inflammatory demyelinating p., p. desmielinizante inflamatória aguda; o tipo clássico de síndrome de Guillain-Barré, no qual a forma predominante de patologia da fibra nervosa subjacente é a desmielinização. VER TAMBÉM acute motor axonal *neuropathy*.
pol·y·ra·dic·u·lop·a·thy (pol-ē-ra-dik′ū-lop′ă-thē). Polirradiculopatia; envolvimento difuso de raiz nervosa; observado, entre outros distúrbios, na neuropatia diabética (polirradiculopatia diabética). SIN polyradiculitis.
   diabetic p., p. diabética; um termo amplo que inclui vários tipos de neuropatia diabética além de uma polineuropatia; inclui amiotrofia diabética e radiculopatia torácica diabética; atribuída à lesão de uma ou mais raízes, induzida pelo diabetes, freqüentemente seqüencial, na região lombar, torácica ou, ocasionalmente, cervical; afeta basicamente homens idosos.
pol·y·ri·bo·nu·cle·o·tide nu·cle·o·tid·yl trans·fer·ase (pol′ē-rī-bō-noo′klē-ō-tīd). Polirribonucleotídeo nucleotidiltransferase; uma enzima que catalisa a fosforólise de polirribonucleotídeos ou de RNA, que produz nucleosídeo difosfato (ou o inverso, a primeira formação de polinucleotídeo artificial descoberta). SIN polynucleotide phosphorylase.
pol·y·ri·bo·somes (pol-ē-rī′bō-sōmz). Polirribossomas; conceitualmente, dois ou mais ribossomas ligados por uma molécula de RNA mensageiro; as estruturas que satisfazem esse conceito podem ser observadas em micrografias eletrônicas e sedimentadas em taxas compatíveis com agregados de ribossomas (motivo pelo qual é freqüentemente, algumas vezes erradamente, suposto que agregados contendo ribossomas são polirribossomas verdadeiros); os polirribossomas são ativos na síntese proteica. SIN polysomes.
pol·yr·rhea (pol-i-rē′ă). Polirréia; eliminação abundante de líquido seroso ou de outro tipo. [poly- + G. *rhoia*, fluxo]
pol·y·sac·char·ide (pol-ē-sak′ă-rīd). Polissacarídeo; carboidrato que contém um grande número de grupamentos sacarídeos; p. ex., amido. Cf. oligosaccharide. SIN glycan.
   pneumococcal p., p. pneumocócico. SIN specific capsular *substance*.
   specific soluble p., p. solúvel específico. SIN specific capsular *substance*.
pol·y·sce·lia (pol-ē-sē′lē-ă). Poliscelia; forma de polimelia envolvendo a presença de mais de duas pernas. [poly- + G. *skelos*, perna]
pol·y·scope (pol′ē-skōp). Poliscópio. SIN diaphanoscope.
pol·y·ser·o·si·tis (pol′ē-ser-ō-sī′tis). Polisserosite; inflamação crônica com derrames em várias cavidades serosas; pode resultar em espessamento fibroso da serosa, incluindo pericardite constritiva. SIN Bamberger disease (2), Concato disease, multiple serositis. [poly- + L. *serum*, soro, + G. -*itis*, inflamação]
   familial paroxysmal p. [MIM*249100], p. paroxística familiar; ataques recorrentes transitórios de dor abdominal, febre, pleurite, artrite e exantema; a condição é assintomática entre as crises; herança autossômica recessiva, causada por mutação no gene marenostrina em 16p. Há uma forma autossômica dominante [MIM*134610] na qual a amiloidose é comum. SIN benign paroxysmal peritonitis, familial Mediterranean fever, familial recurrent p., Mediterranean fever (2), periodic peritonitis, periodic p.
   familial recurrent p., p. recorrente familiar. SIN familial paroxysmal p.
   periodic p., p. periódica. SIN familial paroxysmal p.
   recurrent p., p. recorrente; febre familiar do Mediterrâneo (familial Mediterranean *fever*).
pol·y·si·nu·si·tis (pol′ē-sī-nŭ-sī′tis). Polissinusite; inflamação simultânea de dois seios da face ou mais.
pol·y·somes (pol′ē-sōmz). Polissomas. SIN polyribosomes.
pol·y·so·mia (pol-ē-sō′mē-ă). Polissomia; malformação fetal envolvendo dois ou mais corpos imperfeitos e parcialmente fundidos. [poly- + G. *sōma*, corpo]
pol·y·so·mic (pol-ē-sō′mik). Polissômico; relativo a, ou caracterizado por, polissomia.
pol·y·som·no·gram (pol-ē-som′nō-gram). Polissonograma; a função (ou funções) fisiológica registrada obtida em polissonografia. [poly- + L. *somnus*, sono, + G. *gramma*, diagrama]
pol·y·som·nog·ra·phy (pol′ē-som-nog′ră-fē). Polissonografia; monitorização simultânea e contínua de atividade fisiológica normal e anormal relevante durante o sono. [poly- + L. *somnus*, sono, + G. *graphō*, escrever]

pol·y·so·my (pol - ē - sō′mē). Polissomia; estado de um núcleo celular no qual um cromossoma específico é representado mais de duas vezes. Células contendo três, quatro ou cinco cromossomas homólogos são denominadas, respectivamente, trissômicas, tetrassômicas ou pentassômicas. Cf. polyploidy. [poly- + G. *sōma*, corpo (cromossoma)]

pol·y·sor·bate 80 (pol - ē - sōr′bat). Polissorbato 80; uma mistura de éteres de polioxetileno de ésteres oleicos parciais mistos de anidridos do sorbitol; usado como emulsificante, como no preparo de produtos farmacológicos.

pol·y·sper·mia, pol·y·sper·mism (pol - ē - sper′mē - ă, - sper′mizm). Poliespermia; polispermia. **1.** SIN polyspermy. **2.** Uma secreção espermática anormalmente abundante.

pol·y·sper·my (pol′ē - sper - mē). Polispermia; a penetração de mais de um espermatozóide no ovo. SIN polyspermia (1). polyspermism.

pol·y·sple·nia (pol - ē - sple′nē - ă) [MIM*208530]. Polisplenia; condição na qual o tecido esplênico é dividido em massas quase iguais ou está totalmente ausente; é comum haver cardiopatia congênita e mau posicionamento e mau desenvolvimento de órgãos abdominais; pode estar relacionada ao *situs inversus*. A maioria dos casos é esporádica, embora alguns sugiram herança autossômica recessiva. VER TAMBÉM bilateral *left-sidedness*. SIN asplenia with cardiovascular anomalies, Ivemark syndrome, polyasplenia. [poly- + G. *splēn*, baço]

pol·y·ster·ax·ic (pol′ē - ster - ak′sik). Termo raramente usado para designar comportamento caracterizado por sua qualidade socialmente provocadora.

pol·y·stich·ia (pol - ē - stik′ē - ă). Polistiquia; arranjo dos cílios em duas ou mais fileiras. [poly- + G. *stichos*, fileira]

pol·y·sul·fide rub·ber (pol - ē - sul′fid). Borracha de polissulfeto; borracha sintética usada como material para impressão dental.

pol·y·sus·pen·soid (pol′ē - sŭs - pen′soyd). Polissuspensóide; sistema colóide de fases sólidas que possuem diferentes graus de dispersão.

pol·y·sym·brach·y·dac·ty·ly (pol′ē - sim - brak - ē - dak′ti - lē). Polissimbraquidactilia; malformação da mão ou do pé na qual os dedos encurtados são sindácticos e polidácticos. [poly- + symbrachydactyly]

pol·y·syn·ap·tic (pol′ē - si - nap′tik). Polissináptico; referente às vias neurais formadas por uma cadeia de um grande número de células nervosas conectadas sinapticamente, diferente dos sistemas de condução oligossinápticos. SIN multisynaptic.

pol·y·syn·dac·ty·ly (pol′ē - sin - dak′ti - lē). Polissindactilia; sindactilia de vários dedos das mãos ou dos pés. Há várias formas: uma simples [MIM*174700] e uma com formato anormal do crânio, síndrome de cefalopolissindactilia de Grieg [MIM*175700], ambas herdadas de forma autossômica dominante; uma forma recessiva está associada a defeitos cardíacos [MIM*263630].

pol·y·ten·di·ni·tis (pol′ē - ten - di - nī′tis). Politendinite; inflamação de vários tendões.

pol·y·tene (pol′i - tēn). Politeno; que consiste em muitos filamentos de cromatina em virtude da divisão repetida do cronomena sem separação de filamentos.

pol·y·ten·i·za·tion (pol′ē - ten - i - zā′shŭn). Politenização; o processo de formação do politeno sem separação.

pol·y·ter·penes (pol - ē - ter′penz). Politerpenos; polímeros acíclicos que contêm um grande número de subunidades isopreno, geralmente insaturados. SIN polyisoprenes, polyisoprenoids.

pol·y·the·lia (pol - ē - thē′lē - ă). Politelia; presença de mamilos supranumerários, seja na mama ou em outra parte do corpo. SIN hyperthelia. [poly- + G. *thēlē*, mamilo]

pol·y·thi·a·zide (pol - ē - thī′ă - zīd). Politiazida; diurético e anti-hipertensivo do grupo da benzotiadiazina.

po·lyt·o·cous (pō - lit′ō - kŭs). Polítoco; que tem muitos filhos em um parto. [poly- + G. *tokos*, nascimento]

pol·y·to·mog·ra·phy (pol - i - tō - mog′ră - fē). Politomografia; radiografia seccional do corpo que utiliza um aparelho destinado a realizar um movimento hipociclóide completo; produz uma imagem de um plano tecidual mais fino que a tomografia linear simples ou circular.

pol·y·trich·ia (pol - ē - trik′ē - ă). Politriquia; excesso de pêlos. SIN polytrichosis. [poly- + G. *thrix* (*trich*-), pêlo]

pol·y·tri·cho·sis (pol′ē - tri - kō′sis). Politricose. SIN polytrichia.

pol·y·tro·phic (pol′ē - trō - fik). Politrópico; que exibe uma atração, tropismo, por múltiplos órgãos; geralmente usado para designar um vírus que afeta múltiplos sistemas orgânicos.

pol·y.(U) Poli(U); abreviatura de (poly)uridylic acid (ácido poliuridílico).

pol·y·un·guia (pol - ē - ŭng′gwē - ă). Polioníquia. SIN polyonychia. [poly- + L. *unguis*, unha]

pol·y·u·ria (pol - ē - ū′rē - ă). Poliúria; excreção excessiva de urina, resultando em micção abundante e freqüente. [poly- + G. *ouron*, urina]

pol·y·(uri·dyl·ic ac·id) (pol·y·(U)). Ácido poliuridílico (poli(U)); um homopolímero dos ácidos uridílicos.

pol·y·uro·nides (pol - ē - ūr′ō - nīdz). Poliuronidas; polímeros dos ácidos urônicos (p. ex., ácido glucurônico, ácido galacturônico); as pectinas são poliuronidas.

pol·y·va·lent (pol - ē - vā′lent). Polivalente. **1.** SIN multivalent. **2.** Relativo a um anti-soro polivalente.

pol·y·vi·done (pol - ē - vī′don). Polividona. SIN povidone.

pol·y·vi·nyl (pol - ē - vī′nal). Polivinil; refere-se a um composto que contém vários grupamentos vinila na forma polimerizada.

pol·y·vi·nyl al·co·hol. Álcool polivinílico; um composto, $CH_2(CHOH)_n$, solúvel em água; um adesivo e emulsificante.

pol·y·vi·nyl chlo·ride (PVC). Cloreto polivinílico; substância usada como substituto da borracha em muitas aplicações industriais e suspeita de ser carcinogênica em seres humanos. SIN chlorethene homopolymer.

pol·y·vi·nyl·pyr·rol·i·done (PVP) (pol - ē - vī′nil - pi - rol′i - dōn). Polivinilpirrolidona. SIN povidone.

pol·y·vi·nyl·pyr·rol·i·done-io·dine com·plex. Complexo polivinilpirrolidona-iodo. SIN povidone *iodine.*

pol·y·zo·ic (pol - ē - zō′ik). Polizóico; forma corporal segmentada, como nas tênias superiores, subclasse Cestoda. VER TAMBÉM strobila, monozoic.

pol·y·zy·got·ic (pol - ē - zī - got′ik). Polizigótico. SIN polyovulatory. [poly- + G. *zygōtos*, unido]

po·made (pō - mād′, pō - mahd′). Pomada; ungüento ou creme que contém medicamentos; geralmente usada no cabelo. SIN pomatum. [Fr. *pomade*, do L. *pomum*, maçã]

po·ma·tum (pō - mā′tŭm). Pomada. SIN pomade. [L. mod.]

POMC Abreviatura de proopiomelanocortin (propiomelanocortina).

pome·gran·ate (pom′gran - at). Romã; o fruto da *Punica granatum* (família Punicaceae), um fruto amarelo-avermelhado, do tamanho de uma laranja, que contém muitas sementes em uma polpa ácida avermelhada; usada na diarréia por suas propriedades adstringentes; a casca da árvore e a raiz contêm peletierina e outros alcalóides; foi usada como tenicida. SIN granatum. [L. *pomum*, maçã, + *granatus*, de muitas sementes, de *granum*, grão ou semente]

Pomeroy, Ralph H., obstetra-ginecologista norte-americano, 1867–1925. VER P. *operation*.

POMP Abreviatura de Purinethol® (6-mercaptopurina), Oncovin® (sulfato de vincristina), metotrexato e prednisona, um esquema quimioterápico para câncer.

Pompe, J.C., médico holandês do século XX. VER P. *disease*.

pom·pho·lyx (pom′fō - liks). Ponfólige. SIN dyshidrosis. [G. uma bolha, de *pomphos*, vesícula]

pon·ceau de xy·li·dine (pon - sō′ dĕ zī′li - dēn) [I.C.-16151]. Vermelho de xilidina; corante ácido monoazo originalmente empregado como um contracorante histológico vermelho na coloração tricrômica de Masson.

Ponfick, Emil, patologista alemão, 1844–1913. VER P. *shadow*.

△ **pono-.** Pono-; esforço corporal, fadiga, trabalho excessivo, dor. [G. *ponos*, trabalho difícil, fadiga, dor]

po·no·graph (pō′nō - graf). Ponógrafo; instrumento para registro gráfico da fadiga progressiva de um músculo em contração. [pono- + G. *graphō*, escrever]

po·no·pal·mo·sis (pō′nō - pal - mō′sis). Termo raramente usado para designar uma condição de coração irritável no qual um pequeno esforço provoca palpitação. [pono- + G. *palmos*, palpitação]

po·no·pho·bia (pō - nō - fō′bē - ă). Ponofobia; medo mórbido de trabalho excessivo ou de ficar cansado. [pono- + G. *phobos*, medo]

po·nos (pō′nos). Ponose; doença que ocorre em crianças pequenas em algumas ilhas da Grécia, caracterizada por aumento do baço, hemorragias, febre e caquexia; possivelmente a forma infantil da leishmaniose visceral. [G. trabalho difícil, fadiga, dor]

pons, pl. **pon·tes** (ponz, pon′tēz). **1** [TA] Ponte; em neuroanatomia, a ponte de Varólio ou ponte do cerebelo; aquela parte do tronco cerebral entre o bulbo, caudalmente, e o mesencéfalo, rostralmente, composta da parte basilar da ponte e do tegmento da ponte. Na superfície ventral do encéfalo, a parte basilar da ponte, a protuberância pontina branca, é demarcada do bulbo e do mesencéfalo por sulcos transversos distintos. SIN p. cerebelli, p. varolii. **2.** Qualquer formação semelhante a uma ponte que une duas partes mais ou menos desunidas da mesma estrutura ou órgão. [L. ponte]

p. basilaris pontis [TA], parte basilar da ponte. SIN basilar *part* of pons.
p. cerebel′li, ponte do cerebelo. SIN pons (1).
pontes grisei caudolenticulares [TA], pontes cinzentas caudolenticulares. SIN caudolenticular gray *bridges*, em *bridge*.
p. hep′atis, p. do fígado; uma ponte de tecido hepático que, algumas vezes, se superpõe à fossa da veia cava inferior, convertendo-a em um canal. SIN ponticulus hepatis.
p. varo′lii, ponte do cerebelo. SIN pons (1).

pon.tes (pon′tēz). Pontes; plural de pons. [L.]

pon.tic (pon′tik). Pôntico; um dente artificial em uma dentadura parcial fixa; substitui o dente natural perdido, restabelece suas funções e geralmente ocupa o espaço previamente ocupado pela coroa natural. SIN dummy.

pon·ti·cu·lus (pon - tik′ū - lŭs). Pontículo; uma crista vertical sobre a eminência da concha que dá inserção para o músculo auricular posterior. [L. dim. de *pons*, ponte]

p. hep'atis, ponte do fígado. SIN *pons hepatis.*
p. na'si, ponte do nariz.
p. promonto'rii, subículo do promontório. SIN *subiculum promontorii.*
pon·tile, pon·tine (pon'tīl, -tin; -tēn). Pontino; relativo a uma ponte.
pontocerebellum. Pontocerebelo; as áreas do córtex cerebelar que recebem impulsos das células dos núcleos pontinos basilares; inclui todas as regiões corticais; projeções para o hemisfério maiores que para o verme; as fibras pontocerebelares enviam colaterais para os núcleos cerebelares no trajeto para o córtex sobrejacente.
Pool, Eugene H., cirurgião norte-americano, 1874–1949. VER P. *phenomenon;* P.-Schlesinger *sign.*
pool (pool). **1.** Uma coleção de sangue ou outro líquido em qualquer região do corpo; a coleção de sangue resulta de dilatação e retardo da circulação nos capilares e veias da região. **2.** Uma combinação de recursos. [A.S. *pōl*]
abdominal p., coleção abdominal; o volume de sangue no abdome.
gene p., capital genético; o conjunto dos genes disponíveis para herança em uma população específica em acasalamento.
metabolic p., reserva metabólica; a quantidade de determinado composto químico ou grupo de compostos relacionados que participam de reações metabólicas; pode constituir apenas uma parte do conteúdo corporal total desses compostos.
vaginal p., as secreções e o material que se acumulam no fórnice posterior da vagina; usado para amostragem, principalmente para avaliação após ruptura prematura das membranas.
pop·les (pop'lēz). Fossa poplítea. SIN popliteal *fossa.* VER TAMBÉM popliteal *fossa.* [L. o jarrete do joelho].
pop·lit·e·al (pop-lit'ē-ăl). Poplíteo; relativo à fossa poplítea. SIN popliteus (1).
pop·li·te·us (pop-li-tē'ŭs). Poplíteo. **1.** SIN popliteal. **2.** SIN popliteal *fossa.* **3.** SIN popliteus (muscle) [L.].
POPOP Abreviatura de 1,4-bis(5-fenilоxazol-2-il)benzeno, um cintilador líquido.
pop·py (pop'ē). Papoula. SIN Papaver.
p. oil, óleo de p.; um óleo fixo (secante) extraído da semente da *Papaver somniferum;* usado algumas vezes no preparo de linimentos e como solvente do iodo em óleo iodado.
pop·u·la·tion (pop-ū-lā'shŭn). População; termo estatístico que designa todos os objetos, eventos ou indivíduos de determinada classe. Cf. sample. [L. *populus,* um povo, nação]
POR Abreviatura de problem-oriented *record* (prontuário orientado ao problema).
por-. VER poro-.
por·ce·lain (pōr'sĕ-lin). Porcelana; pó composto de argila, sílica e um fluxo que, quando misturado com água, forma uma pasta moldada para confeccionar dentes artificiais, restaurações *inlay,* coroas de jaqueta e dentaduras. Quando aquecido, o material funde-se para formar uma cerâmica.
por·cine (pōr'sīn, -sin). Suíno; relativo a porcos. [L. *porcinus,* de *porcus,* um porco]
pore (pōr) [TA]. Poro. **1.** Abertura, orifício, perfuração ou forame. Um poro, meato ou forame. VER TAMBÉM opening. **2.** Poro sudorífero. SIN sweat p. VER TAMBÉM opening, meatus, foramen. [G. *poros,* passagem]
alveolar p.'s, poros alveolares; aberturas nos septos interalveolares do pulmão que permitem o fluxo de ar entre alvéolos adjacentes.
dilated p., p. dilatado; abertura folicular aumentada da pele, com um tampão de queratina e, algumas vezes, lanugo ou pêlos maduros.
external acoustic p., external auditory p. [TA], poro acústico externo; o orifício do meato acústico externo na porção timpânica do osso temporal. SIN porus acusticus externus [TA], external acoustic aperture*, external acoustic foramen, external auditory foramen, opening of external acoustic meatus, orifice of external acoustic meatus.
gustatory p., p. gustatório. SIN taste p.
interalveolar p.'s, poros interalveolares; aberturas nos septos interalveolares do pulmão. SIN Kohn p.'s.
internal acoustic p., auditory p., poro acústico interno, poro auditivo; a abertura interna do meato acústico interno na superfície posterior da parte petrosa do osso temporal. SIN internal acoustic opening [TA], internal acoustic foramen, internal auditory foramen, opening of internal acoustic meatus, orifice of internal acoustic meatus, porus acusticus internus.
Kohn p.'s, poros de Kohn. SIN interalveolar p.'s.
nuclear p., p. nuclear; abertura octagonal, com cerca de 70 nm de diâmetro transversal, onde as membranas interna e externa do envoltório nuclear são contínuas.
skin p., p. cutâneo. SIN sweat p.
slit p.'s, poros de filtração; as fendas intercelulares entre os pedicelos interdigitados dos podócitos; eles são parte da barreira de filtração dos corpúsculos renais. SIN filtration slits.
sweat p. [TA], poro sudorífero; a abertura superficial do ducto de uma glândula sudorípara. SIN pore (2) [TA], porus sudiferus, porus, skin p.

taste p. [TA], poro gustatório; a pequena abertura de uma papila gustatória, na superfície da mucosa oral, através da qual se projetam os pêlos gustatórios das células gustatórias neuroepiteliais especializadas. SIN porus gustatorius [TA], gustatory p.
por·en·ce·pha·lia (pōr'en-se-fā'lē-ă). Porencefalia. SIN porencephaly.
por·en·ce·phal·ic (pōr'en-se-fal'ik). Porencefálico; relativo a, ou caracterizado por, porencefalia. SIN porencephalous.
por·en·ceph·a·li·tis (pōr'en-sef-ă-lī'tis). Porencefalite; inflamação crônica do encéfalo com a formação de cavidades na substância do órgão. [G. *poros,* poro, + *enkephalos,* encéfalo, + *-itis,* inflamação]
por·en·ceph·a·lous (pōr-en-sef'ă-lŭs). Porencefálico. SIN porencephalic.
por·en·ceph·a·ly (pōr-en-sef'ă-lē). Porencefalia; a ocorrência de cavidade, na substância encefálica, que geralmente se comunica com os ventrículos laterais. SIN porencephalia, splencephaly. [G. *poros,* poro, + *enkephalos,* encéfalo]
Porges, Otto, bacteriologista austríaco, 1879–1968. VER P. *method;* P.-Meier *test.*
po·ri (pō'rī). Poros; plural de porus.
po·ria (pōr'ē-ă). Pórios; plural de porion.
Po·rif·era (pō-rif'er-ă). As esponjas; um filo do Metazoa, constituindo um grupo de animais aquáticos, sésseis, que possuem um endoesqueleto e muitos canais ramificados, revestidos por coanócitos flagelados; a comunicação dos canais com a superfície é feita através de muitos poros ou através de aberturas maiores e ósculos. VER TAMBÉM Parazoa. [L. *porus,* poro, + *fero,* conduzir]
po·rins (pōr'inz). Porinas; proteínas encontradas na membrana externa de uma dupla membrana permeável à maioria das moléculas pequenas. [G. *poros,* passagem, + *-in*]
por·i·o·ma·nia (pōr'ē-ō-mā'nē-ă). Poriomania; impulso mórbido de vagar ou sair de casa. [G. *poreia,* uma jornada, + *mania,* mania]
por·i·on, pl. **po·ria** (pōr'ē-on, -ē-ă). Pório; o ponto central na margem superior do meato acústico externo; como um ponto de reparo cefalométrico, está localizado no meio dos bastões metálicos do cefalômetro. [G. *poros,* passagem]
PORN Acrônimo para progressive outer retinal *necrosis* (necrose externa progressiva da retina).
por·no·lag·nia (pōr-nō-lag'nē-ă). Pornolagnia; termo raramente usado para designar a atração sexual por prostitutas. [G. *pornē,* prostituta, + *lagneia,* prazer]
poro-, por-. Poro-, por-. **1.** Um poro, um ducto, uma abertura. [G. *poros* (L. *porus),* passagem] **2.** Uma passagem. [G. *poreia,* uma jornada, passagem] **3.** Um calo; um endurecimento. [G. *poros,* um tipo de mármore, uma pedra]
po·ro·ceph·a·li·a·sis (pō'rō-sef-ă-lī'ă-sis). Porocefalíase; infecção por uma espécie dos vermes *Porocephalus.* SIN porocephalosis.
Po·ro·ce·phal·i·dae (pō'rō-se-fal'i-dē). Família de vermes pentastomídeos (ordem Porocephalida, filo Pentastomida) caracterizada por quatro ganchos dispostos em uma linha curva de cada lado da boca. Os adultos são encontrados nos pulmões de répteis, e larvas ou ninfas são encontradas nos tecidos de uma grande variedade de vertebrados, incluindo seres humanos. VER TAMBÉM Linguatulidae, *Armillifer, Linguatula.* [G. *poros,* poro, + *kephalē,* cabeça]
po·ro·ceph·a·lo·sis (pō'rō-sef-ă-lō'sis). Porocefalose. SIN porocephaliasis.
Po·ro·ceph·a·lus (pō-rō-sef'ă-lŭs). Gênero de pentastomídeos da família Porocephalidae, cujos vermes adultos ou larvas causam porocefalíase em várias espécies de animais, incluindo seres humanos. [G. *poros,* poro, + *kephalē,* cabeça]
P. armilla'tus. SIN *Armillifer armillatus.*
po·ro·co·nid·i·um (pōr'ō-kō-nid'ē-ŭm). Poroconídio; em fungos, um conídio produzido através do poro microscópico do conidióforo. SIN porospore.
po·ro·ker·a·to·sis (pō'rō-ker-ă-tō'sis). Poroceratose; dermatose rara na qual há espessamento do estrato córneo com uma margem ceratótica anular ou lamela cornóide que circunda uma área de atrofia centrífuga progressiva; foi descrito que o carcinoma cutâneo origina-se nas lesões. SIN Mibelli disease. [G. *poros,* poro, + *keratosis*]
actinic p., p. actínica; lesão que ocorre basicamente nas áreas expostas dos membros; tem uma semelhança com a ceratose actínica, mas as características histológicas são de poroceratose.
po·ro·ma (pō-rō'ma). Poroma. **1.** Calosidade. SIN callosity. **2.** Exostose. SIN exostosis. **3.** Endurecimento após um fleimão. **4.** Um tumor de células que revestem as aberturas cutâneas das glândulas sudoríferas. [G. *pōrōma,* calo, de *pōros,* pedra]
eccrine p., p. écrino; um poroma ou acrospiroma das glândulas sudoríferas écrinas, que geralmente ocorrem na planta do pé, como um nódulo avermelhado de consistência mole composto de células basalóides e tecido fibrovascular.
po·ro·sis, pl. **po·ro·ses** (pō-rō'sis, -sēz). Porosidade; condição porosa. SIN porosity (1). [L. *porosus,* poroso]
cerebral p·, p. cerebral; uma condição porosa do encéfalo causada por crescimento *postmortem* de *Clostridium perfringens* ou de outros organismos produtores de gás no tecido.

po·ros·i·ty (pō-rosʹi-tē). Porosidade. **1.** SIN porosis. **2.** Uma perfuração. [G. *poros*, poro]

por·o·spore (porʹō-spor). Porosporo. SIN poroconidium.

po·rot·ic (pō-rotʹik). Poroso, como em osteoporótico.

po·rous (poʹrus). Poroso; que possui aberturas para atravessar direta ou indiretamente a substância.

por·phin, por·phine (porʹfin). Porfina; o núcleo tetrapirrol cíclico não substituído que é a base das porfirinas. VER TAMBÉM porphyrins. Cf. chlorin, phorbin, corrin. SIN porphyrin.

por·pho·bi·lin (porʹfō-bīʹlin). Porfobilina; termo geral que designa intermediários entre o monopirrol, porfobilinogênio e o tetrapirrol cíclico do heme (um derivado da porfina). VER TAMBÉM bilin.

por·pho·bi·lin·o·gen (PBG) (porʹfō-bī-linʹō-jen). Porfobilinogênio; porfirina precursora dos porfirinogênios, porfirinas e heme; encontrado em grandes quantidades na urina em casos de porfiria aguda ou congênita.
  p. synthase, p. sintase; enzima hepática que catalisa a formação de porfobilinogênio e água a partir de duas moléculas de δ-aminolevulinato, uma importante reação na biossíntese da porfirina; inibida pelo chumbo em casos de intoxicação por chumbo; a deficiência dessa enzima resulta em níveis elevados de δ-aminolevulinato e distúrbios neurológicos. SIN δ-aminolevulinate dehydratase.

por·phyr·ia (por-firʹē-ā). Porfiria; grupo de distúrbios envolvendo a biossíntese do heme, caracterizado pela excreção excessiva de porfirinas ou seus precursores; pode ser hereditária ou adquirida, como decorrente dos efeitos de determinados agentes químicos (p. ex., hexaclorobenzeno).
  acute intermittent p., acute p., p. intermitente aguda, p. aguda. SIN intermittent acute p.
  δ-aminolevulinate dehydratase p., p. por δ-aminolevulinato desidratase; distúrbio hereditário no qual há deficiência de porfobilinogênio sintetase; os níveis de δ-aminolevulinato estão elevados, causando distúrbios neurológicos. SIN porphobilinogen synthase p.
  congenital erythropoietic p. [MIM*263700], p. eritropoética congênita; aumento da formação de porfirina pelas células eritróides na medula óssea, causando porfirinúria grave, freqüentemente combinado com anemia hemolítica e fotossensibilidade cutânea persistente; causada por deficiência de uroporfirinogênio III co-sintetase; herança autossômica recessiva, causada por mutação no gene da uroporfirinogênio III sintetase (UROS) no cromossoma 10q; há superprodução de isômeros da porfirina tipo I.
  p. cuta'nea tar'da (PCT) [MIM*176090, MIM*176100], p. cutânea tardia; p. familiar ou esporádica, caracterizada por disfunção hepática e lesões cutâneas fotossensíveis, com bolhas, hiperpigmentação e alterações cutâneas semelhantes às encontradas na esclerodermia e aumento da excreção de uroporfirina; causada por uma deficiência de uroporfirinogênio descarboxilase induzida em casos esporádicos por alcoolismo crônico; herança autossômica dominante em casos familiares. SIN symptomatic p.
  p. cuta'nea tar'da heredita'ria, p. cutânea tardia hereditária. SIN p. cutanea tarda.
  p. cuta'nea tar'da symptoma'tica, p. cutânea tardia sintomática. VER p. cutanea tarda.
  erythropoietic p., p. eritropoética; classificação de p. que inclui a p. eritropoética e a protoporfiria eritropoética.
  hepatic p. [MIM*176100.0002], p. hepática; categoria de p. que inclui a p. cutânea tardia, a p. variegada e a coproporfiria. SIN p. hepatica.
  p. hepatica (he-patʹī-kă), p. hepática. SIN hepatic p.
  hepatoerythropoietic p., p. hepatoeritropoética; distúrbio autossômico recessivo no qual há deficiência ou ausência de uroporfirinogênio descarboxilase; resulta em fotossensibilidade e produção hepática excessiva de 8- e 7-carboxilato porfirinas.
  intermittent acute p. (IAP) [MIM*176000], p. aguda intermitente; p. causada por superprodução hepática de ácido δ-aminolevulínico, com grande aumento da excreção urinária deste e de porfobilinogênio, e algum aumento de uroporfirina, causada por deficiência de porfobilinogênio desaminase; caracterizada por crises agudas intermitentes de hipertensão, cólica abdominal, psicose e polineuropatia, mas sem fotossensibilidade; herança autossômica dominante, causada por mutação no gene da porfobilinogênio desaminase humana em 11q24; a exacerbação é causada pela ingestão de alguns fármacos (p. ex., barbitúricos). SIN acute intermittent p., acute p.
  ovulocyclic p., p. ovulocíclica; exacerbações episódicas agudas de porfiria que ocorrem no período pré-menstrual.
  porphobilinogen synthase p., p. por porfobilinogênio sintetase. SIN δ-aminolevulinate dehydratase p.
  South African type p., p. do tipo sul-africana. SIN variegate p.
  symptomatic p., p. sintomática. SIN p. cutanea tarda.
  variegate p. (VP) [MIM*176200], p. variegada; p. caracterizada por dor abdominal e anormalidades neuropsiquiátricas, por sensibilidade dérmica à luz e ao traumatismo mecânico, aumento da excreção fecal de proto e coproporfirina, e por aumento da excreção urinária de ácido δ-aminolevulínico, porfobilinogênio e porfirinas; causada por deficiência de protoporfirinogênio oxidase; herança autossômica dominante, causada por mutação no gene da protoporfirinogênio oxidase (PPOX) no cromossoma 1q. SIN protocoproporphyria hereditária, South African type p.

por·phy·rin (porʹfi-rin). Porfirina. SIN porphin.

por·phy·rin·o·gens (por-fi-rinʹō-jenz). Porfirinogênios; intermediários na biossíntese do heme, da seguinte forma: quatro porfobilinogênios condensam-se para formar uroporfirinogênios I e III (originando os produtos laterais uroporfirinas I e III), que são descarboxilados para formar coproporfirinogênios I e III (dando origem aos produtos laterais coproporfirinas I e III); o coproporfirinogênio III é oxidado em protoporfirinogênio III (IX) que, a seguir, é oxidado para formar a protoporfirina III (IX) (este último intermediário acrescenta ferro ferroso para produzir heme); alguns porfirinogênios estão elevados em algumas porfirias.

por·phy·ri·nop·a·thy (porʹfir-in-opʹa-thē). Porfirinopatia; síndrome resultante do metabolismo anormal da porfirina como porfiria aguda. SIN porphyrism. [porphyrin + G. *pathos*, doença]

por·phy·rins (porʹfi-rinz). Porfirinas; pigmentos amplamente distribuídos na natureza (p. ex., heme, pigmentos biliares, citocromos) que consistem em quatro pirróis unidos em uma estrutura em anel porfina. São produtos de substituição da porfina (porfirina) e constituem diversos tipos, diferindo na maior parte nas cadeias laterais (metil, etil, vinil, formil, carboxietil, carboximetil, etc.) presente nas oito posições disponíveis nos anéis pirróis. Dependendo da natureza das cadeias laterais, os prefixos dentero-, etio-, meso-, proto-, etc., são acrescentados à porfirina; a distribuição dentro de cada classe é dada pelo tipo I, II, III e IV. As porfirinas combinam-se com vários metais (ferro, cobre, magnésio, etc.) para formar metaloporfirinas, e com substâncias nitrogenadas.

por·phy·ri·nu·ria (porʹfir-i-nooʹrē-ā). Porfirinúria; excreção de porfirinas e compostos correlatos na urina. SIN porphyruria, purpurinuria.

por·phy·rism. Porfirismo. SIN porphyrinopathy.

por·phy·ri·za·tion (porʹfi-ri-zāʹshun). Porfirização; pulverização em um almofariz (antigamente sobre uma placa de pórfiro).

Por·phy·ro·mo·nas (porʹfir-ō-mōnʹas). Gênero de pequenos cocos imóveis Gram-negativos, anaeróbicos e geralmente bastões curtos, que produzem colônias lisas, pigmentadas cinza ou pretas, cujo tamanho varia com a espécie. Em seres humanos, são encontrados como parte da flora normal na orofaringe, incluindo os sulcos gengivais, e nos tratos vaginal e intestinal. A espécie típica é *P. asaccharolytica*.
  P. asaccharolytica, espécie que raramente causa infecções independentemente, mas é um componente importante de infecções mistas associadas a abscessos orais, genitourinários e intra-abdominais, bem como de infecções associadas a comprometimento da circulação e gangrena diabética.

por·phy·ru·ria (por-fi-rooʹrē-ā). Porfirúria. SIN porphyrinuria.

Porro, Edoardo, obstetra italiano, 1842–1902. VER P. *hysterectomy*.

port (port). Porta. SIN portal.
  ancillary p.'s, portas auxiliares; durante cirurgia endoscópica, a instituição de mais de um local de entrada para permitir a introdução de outros instrumentos além do endoscópio.

por·ta, pl. **por·tae** (porʹtă, -tē). Porta. **1.** SIN hilum (1). **2.** SIN interventricular *foramen*. [L. portão]
  p. hepʹatis [TA], p. do fígado; fissura transversal na superfície visceral do fígado, entre os lobos caudado e quadrado, que aloja a veia porta, artéria hepática, plexo nervoso hepático, ductos hepáticos e vasos linfáticos. SIN caudal transverse fissure, portal fissure.
  p. lieʹnis, hilo esplênico. SIN splenic *hilum*.
  p. pulmoʹnis, hilo do pulmão. SIN *hilum* of lung.
  p. reʹnis, hilo renal. SIN *hilum* of kidney.

Port-a-Cath (portʹā-kath). Cateter venoso central de uso prolongado com abertura(s) subcutânea(s). [nome comercial]

por·ta·ca·val (porʹtă-kāʹval). Portocava; relativo à veia porta e à veia cava inferior.

por·tal (porʹtăl). Portal. **1.** Relativo a qualquer porta ou hilo, especificamente à porta do fígado e à veia porta. **2.** O ponto de entrada no corpo de um microrganismo patogênico. SIN port. [L. *portalis*, relativo a uma porta (portão)]
  anterior intestinal p., porta intestinal anterior. SIN *fovea cardiaca*.
  posterior intestinal p., porta intestinal posterior; em embriões jovens, as comunicações entre o intestino médio e o intestino posterior.

Porter, Curt C., bioquímico norte-americano, *1914. VER P.-Silver *chromogens*, em *chromogen*, *reaction*, chromogens *test*.

Porter, Thomas C., cientista inglês, 1860–1933. VER Ferry-P. *law*.

Porter, William H., cirurgião irlandês, 1790–1861. VER P. *fascia*.

por·tio, pl. **por·ti·o·nes** (porʹshē-ō, -ōʹnez). Porção; uma parte. [L. porção]
  p. interme'dia, nervo intermédio. SIN intermediate *nerve*.
  p. ma'jor ner'vi trigem'ini, raiz sensitiva do nervo trigêmeo. SIN sensory *root* of trigeminal nerve.
  p. mi'nor ner'vi trigem'ini, raiz motora do nervo trigêmeo. SIN motor *root* of trigeminal nerve.

p. supravagina'lis cervicis [TA], porção supravaginal do colo do útero. SIN supravaginal *part* of cervix.
p. vagina'lis cervicis [TA], porção vaginal do colo do útero. SIN vaginal *part* of cervix.

por·tion (pōr'shun). Porção; parte ou divisão.
accessory p. of spinal accessory nerve, raiz craniana do nervo acessório espinal. SIN cranial *root* of accessory nerve.
anterior p. of left medial segment IV of liver [TA], parte anterior do segmento medial esquerdo do fígado que inclui o lobo quadrado. SIN quadrate part of liver [TA], pars quadrata hepatis.
mesenteric p. of small intestine, porção mesentérica do intestino delgado; a porção livremente móvel do intestino delgado suprida por um mesentério, que forma o jejuno e o íleo. SIN intestinum tenue mesenteriale.
subcutaneous p. of external anal sphincter, porção subcutânea do esfíncter externo do ânus. SIN subcutaneous *part* of external anal sphincter. VER external anal *sphincter*.

por·ti·plex·us (pōr-ti-plek'sŭs). Portiplexo; a união do plexo coróide do ventrículo lateral com o do terceiro ventrículo no forame interventricular (de Monro).

♲ **porto-.** Porto-; portal. [L. *porta*, portão]

por·to·bil·i·o·ar·te·ri·al (pōr'tō-bil'ē-ō-ar-tēr'ē-ăl). Portobilioarterial; relativo à veia porta, aos ductos biliares e à artéria hepática, que têm distribuições semelhantes. VER TAMBÉM portal *triad*.

por·to·en·ter·os·to·my (pōr'tō-en-ter-os'tō-mē). Portoenterostomia; operação para atresia biliar na qual uma alça de jejuno em Y de Roux é anastomosada à extremidade hepática das estruturas portais extravasculares divididas, incluindo ductos biliares rudimentares. SIN Kasai operation.

por·to·gram (pōr'tō-gram). Portograma; registro radiográfico da portografia. [porto- + G. *gramma*, escrito]

por·tog·ra·phy (pōr-tog'ră-fē). Portografia; delineação da circulação porta por radiografia, utilizando material radiopaco, geralmente introduzido no baço ou na veia porta durante cirurgia. SIN portovenography. [porto- + G. *graphō*, escrever]

por·to·sys·tem·ic (pōr'tō-sis-tem'ik). Portossistêmico; relativo a conexões entre os sistemas venosos porta e sistêmico.

por·to·ve·nog·ra·phy (pōr'tō-vē-nog'ră-fē). Portovenografia. SIN portography.

po·rus, pl. **po·ri** (pō'rŭs, -rī). Poro. SIN sweat *pore*. VER TAMBÉM opening. [L. do G. *poros*, passagem]
p. acus'ticus exter'nus [TA], p. acústico externo. SIN external acoustic *pore*.
p. acus'ticus inter'nus, p. acústico interno. SIN internal acoustic *pore*.
p. crotaphy'tico-buccinato'rius, p. crotafítico-bucinatório; um forame ocasional no osso esfenóide através do qual passa a porção motora do nervo trigêmeo; é formado por ossificação de um ligamento ínfero-lateral ao forame oval. SIN Hyrtl foramen.
p. gustato'rius [TA], poro gustatório. SIN taste *pore*.
p. op'ticus, p. óptico. SIN optic *disk*.
p. sudorif'erus, p. sudorífero. SIN sweat *pore*.

Posadas, Alejandro, patologista argentino, 1870–1902. VER P. *disease*.

POSITION

ℹ **po·si·tion** (pŏ-zish'ŭn). Posição. **1.** Uma atitude, postura ou lugar ocupado. **2.** Postura ou atitude assumida por um paciente para obter conforto e para facilitar a realização de procedimentos diagnósticos, cirúrgicos ou terapêuticos. **3.** Em obstetrícia, a relação entre uma parte arbitrariamente escolhida do feto e o lado direito ou esquerdo da mãe; para cada apresentação pode haver uma posição direita ou esquerda; o occipúcio, o queixo e o sacro do feto são os pontos determinantes de posição nas apresentações de vértice, face e pélvica, respectivamente. Cf. presentation. [L. *positio*, uma posição, de *pono*, colocar]

ℹ **anatomic p.,** p. anatômica; a p. ereta do corpo com a face voltada para a frente (crânio alinhado no plano orbitomeatal ou de Frankfort), os braços ao lado do corpo e as palmas das mãos voltadas para a frente; os termos posterior, anterior, lateral, medial, etc., são aplicados às partes de acordo com sua relação entre si e com o eixo do corpo quando nessa posição.
Bozeman p., p. de Bozeman; posição genocubital, estando o paciente preso a apoios.
Casselberry p., p. de Casselberry; posição de decúbito ventral que permite a um paciente intubado ingerir líquidos sem risco de penetração no tubo.
centric p., p. cêntrica; a posição da mandíbula em sua relação livre mais retraída com o maxilar. VER TAMBÉM centric jaw *relation*.
condylar hinge p., p. do gínglimo condilar; **(1)** a posição dos côndilos nas articulações temporomandibulares a partir da qual é possível um movimento tipo gínglimo; **(2)** a relação maxilomandibular a partir da qual pode ser executado um movimento de gínglimo verdadeiro estimulado conscientemente.
dorsal p., p. dorsal. SIN supine p.
dorsosacral p., p. dorso-sacral. SIN lithotomy p.
eccentric p., p. excêntrica. SIN eccentric *relation*.
electrical heart p., p. elétrica do coração; descrição do eixo elétrico do coração baseada na forma dos complexos QRS nas derivações aVL, aVF, V_1 e V_6. Algumas vezes usado de forma livre (e imprecisa) para descrever o eixo elétrico do plano frontal. SIN heart p.
Elliot p., posição de Elliot; p. de decúbito dorsal sobre um plano inclinado duplo ou sobre um plano inclinado único, com uma almofada sob as costas ao nível do fígado; usada para facilitar a secção abdominal.
English p., p. inglesa. SIN Sims p.
flank p., p. de flanco; p. de decúbito lateral, com a perna de baixo fletida, a perna de cima estendida e extensão convexa do lado superior do corpo; usada para nefrectomia.
Fowler p., p. de Fowler; p. inclinada obtida elevando-se a cabeceira do leito cerca de 50 a 76 cm para promover a coleta de líquido intra-abdominal na parte inferior do abdome.
frog leg p., p. de rã; decúbito dorsal com as plantas dos pés juntas e os joelhos afastados para expor o períneo.
frontoanterior p., p. frontoanterior; apresentação cefálica do feto com a fronte voltada para a direita (**frontoanterior direita**, FAD) ou para a esquerda (**frontoanterior esquerda**, FAE) do acetábulo da mãe.
frontoposterior p., p. frontoposterior; apresentação cefálica do feto com sua fronte voltada para a articulação sacroilíaca direita (**frontoposterior direita**, FPD) ou esquerda (**frontoposterior esquerda**, FPE) da mãe.
frontotransverse p., p. frontotransversa; apresentação cefálica do feto com sua fronte voltada para a fossa ilíaca direita (**frontotransversa direita**, FTD) ou esquerda (**frontotransversa esquerda**, FTE) da mãe.
genucubital p., p. genunlar. SIN knee-elbow p.
genupectoral p., p. genupeitoral. SIN knee-chest p.
heart p., p. cardíaca. SIN electrical heart p.
hinge p., p. em dobradiça; em odontologia, a orientação de partes de uma forma que permita movimento em dobradiça entre elas.
intercuspal p., p. intercuspidal; a p. da mandíbula quando as cúspides e sulcos dos dentes maxilares e mandibulares estão em seu maior contato e a mandíbula está em sua posição mais fechada.
knee-chest p., p. genupeitoral; p. em decúbito ventral apoiada sobre os joelhos e a parte superior do tórax, adotada para exame ginecológico ou retal. SIN genupectoral p.
knee-elbow p., p. genucubital; p. em decúbito ventral apoiada sobre os joelhos e os cotovelos, adotada para exame ou cirurgia ginecológica ou retal. SIN genucubital p.
lateral recumbent p., p. de Sims. SIN Sims p.
leapfrog p., p. de pular carniça; posição de inclinação, como aquela adotada por crianças ao pular carniça, adotada para exame retal.
lithotomy p., p. de litotomia; posição de decúbito dorsal com as nádegas na extremidade da mesa de cirurgia, os quadris e os joelhos estando completamente fletidos com os pés presos na posição. SIN dorsosacral p.
mandibular hinge p., p. da dobradiça mandibular; qualquer p. da mandíbula que existe quando os côndilos estão situados nas articulações temporomandibulares de forma que possam ser feitos movimentos de abertura ou fechamento no eixo da dobradiça.
Mayo-Robson p., p. de Mayo-Robson; p. de decúbito dorsal com uma almofada espessa sob a região lombar, causando lordose acentuada nessa região; usada em cirurgias da vesícula biliar.
mentoanterior p. (MA), p. mentoanterior; apresentação cefálica do feto com seu queixo apontando para a sínfise ou rodado para o acetábulo direito (**mentoanterior direita**, MAD) ou esquerdo (**mentoanterior esquerda**, MAE) da mãe.
mentoposterior p. (MP), p. mentoposterior; apresentação cefálica do feto com seu queixo apontando para o sacro ou rodado para a articulação sacroilíaca direita (**mentoposterior direita**, MPD) ou esquerda (**mentoposterior esquerda**, MPE) da mãe.
mentotransverse p., p. mentotransversa; apresentação cefálica do feto com seu queixo apontando para a fossa ilíaca direita (**mentotransversa direita**, MTD) ou esquerda (**mentotransversa esquerda**, MTE) da mãe.
Noble p., p. de Noble; paciente de pé e discretamente inclinado para a frente; útil para inspeção de edema da região lombar que pode ocorrer na pielonefrite.
obstetric p., p. obstétrica; a p. adotada pela parturiente, seja de decúbito dorsal ou de decúbito lateral.
occipitoanterior p. (OA), p. occipitoanterior; apresentação cefálica do feto com seu occipúcio sob a sínfise ou rodado para o acetábulo direito (**occipitoanterior direita**, OAD) ou esquerdo (**occipitoanterior esquerda**, OAE) da mãe.
occipitoposterior p. (OP), p. occipitoposterior; apresentação cefálica do feto com seu occipúcio voltado para o sacro ou rodado para a articulação sacroilíaca direita (**occipitoposterior direita**, OPD) ou esquerda (**occipitoposterior esquerda**, OPE) da mãe.

occipitotransverse p., p. occipitotransversa; apresentação cefálica do feto com seu occipúcio voltado para a fossa ilíaca direita (**occipitotransversa direita**, OTD) ou esquerda (**occipitotransversa esquerda**, OTE) da mãe.
occlusal p., p. oclusal; a relação entre a mandíbula e a maxila quando estão fechadas e os dentes estão em contato; pode ou não coincidir com a oclusão cêntrica.
orthopnea p., p. ortopneica. SIN orthopneic p.
orthopneic p., p. ortopneica; a posição adotada por paciente com ortopnéia, sentado na cama levantado por vários travesseiros. SIN orthopnea p.
physiologic rest p., p. de repouso fisiológico; a p. habitual da mandíbula quando o paciente está repousando confortavelmente na posição vertical e os côndilos estão em uma posição neutra sem esforço nas fossas glenóides. VER TAMBÉM rest *relation*. SIN postural p., postural resting p., rest p.
postural p., postural resting p., p. postural, p. de repouso postural. SIN physiologic rest p.
prone p., p. de decúbito ventral; voltado com o rosto para baixo.
protrusive p., p. protrusiva; uma posição para frente da mandíbula produzida por esforço muscular.
rest p., p. de repouso. SIN physiologic rest p.
reverse Trendelenburg p., p. de Trendelenburg inversa; posição de decúbito dorsal, sem fletir ou estender, na qual a cabeça fica mais alta que os pés.
Rose p., p. de Rose; p. de decúbito dorsal com a cabeça fora da extremidade da mesa, o pescoço em extensão; usada em cirurgias na boca ou faringe.
sacroanterior p. (SA), p. sacroanterior; apresentação pélvica do feto com o sacro sob a sínfise ou rodado para o acetábulo direito (**sacroanterior direita**, SAD) ou esquerdo (**sacroanterior esquerda**, SAE) da mãe.
sacroposterior p. (SP), p. sacroposterior; apresentação pélvica do feto com o sacro próximo ao sacro materno ou rodado apontando para a articulação sacroilíaca direita (**sacroposterior direita**, SPD) ou esquerda (**sacroposterior esquerda**, SPE) da mãe.
sacrotransverse p., p. sacrotransversa; apresentação pélvica do feto com seu sacro apontando para a articulação sacroilíaca direita (**sacrotransversa direita**, STD) ou esquerda (**sacrotransversa esquerda**, STE) da mãe.
Scultetus p., p. de Scultetus; posição de decúbito dorsal sobre um plano inclinado com cabeça baixa, recomendado por Scultetus para herniotomia e castração.
semi-Fowler p., p. de semi-Fowler; posição inclinada obtida elevando-se a cabeceira do leito 25 a 37 cm, fletindo os quadris e colocando um apoio sob os joelhos de forma que fiquem curvos a aproximadamente 90°, assim permitindo que o líquido na cavidade abdominal acumule-se na pelve.
semiprone p., p. de semidecúbito ventral. SIN Sims p.
Simon p., p. de Simon; p. para exame vaginal; posição de decúbito dorsal com quadris elevados, coxas e pernas fletidas e coxas amplamente separadas.
Sims p., p. de Sims; p. para facilitar o exame vaginal, com a paciente em decúbito lateral com o braço de baixo atrás das costas, as coxas fletidas, a coxa de cima mais que a de baixo. SIN English p., lateral recumbent p., semiprone p.
supine p., p. de decúbito dorsal; deitado sobre as costas. SIN dorsal p.
terminal hinge p., p. em dobradiça terminal; a posição de dobradiça mandibular a partir da qual a abertura adicional da mandíbula produziria movimento de translação, e não de dobradiça.
Trendelenburg p., p. de Trendelenburg; posição de decúbito dorsal sobre a mesa de cirurgia, que é inclinada em vários ângulos de forma que a pelve fica mais alta que a cabeça; usada durante e após cirurgias na pelve ou no choque.
Valentine p., p. de Valentine; posição de decúbito dorsal sobre uma mesa com plano inclinado duplo de forma a causar flexão nos quadris; usada para facilitar a irrigação uretral.
Walcher p., p. de Walcher; termo obsoleto para designar uma p. de decúbito dorsal da parturiente com os membros inferiores pendentes sobre a borda da mesa.

po·si·tion·er (pō - zish′un - er). Posicionador; um aparelho elastoplástico ou de borracha elástico ajustado sobre a superfície oclusal dos dentes, para obter movimento limitado e/ou estabilização, geralmente usado no fim do tratamento ortodôntico.
pos·i·tive (poz′i - tiv). Positivo. **1.** Afirmativo; definido; não-negativo. **2.** Designa uma resposta, a ocorrência de uma reação, ou a existência da entidade ou condição em questão. **3.** Que tem um valor maior que zero. [L. *positivus*, estabelecido por consenso arbitrário, de *pono*, pp. *positus*, estabelecer, colocar]
pos·i·tive G. G positivo; gravidade ou aceleração na direção da cabeça para o pé habitual ao voar ou na posição de pé; o inverso de G negativo.
pos·i·tron (β^+) (poz′i - tron). Pósitron; uma partícula subatômica de massa e carga elétrica igual ao elétron, mas de carga oposta (isto é, positiva). SIN positive electron.
po·so·log·ic (pō - sō - loj′ik). Posológico; relativo à posologia.
po·sol·o·gy (pō - sol′ō - jē). Posologia; o ramo da farmacologia e terapêutica relacionado com uma determinação das doses de remédios; a ciência da dosagem. [G. *posos*, quanto, + *logos*, estudo]
post (pōst). Em odontologia, um pino introduzido no canal radicular de um dente natural como uma fixação para uma coroa artificial.
post-. pós-, posterior a.; oposto de anti-. Cf. meta-. [L. *post*]
post·ac·e·tab·u·lar (pōst′as - e - tab′u - lar). Pós-acetabular; posterior à cavidade acetabular.
post·ad·o·les·cence (pōst - ad - ō - les′ens). Pós-adolescência; o período após a adolescência ou puberdade.
post·a·nal (pōst - a′nal). Pós-anal; posterior ao ânus.
post·an·es·thet·ic (pōst′an - es - thet′ik). Pós-anestésico; que ocorre após anestesia.
post·ap·o·plec·tic (pōst′ap - ō - plek′tik). Pós-apoplético; que ocorre após um ataque de apoplexia.
post·ax·i·al (pōst - ak′sē - al). Pós-axial. **1.** Posterior ao eixo do corpo ou de qualquer membro, estando este último na posição anatômica. **2.** Designa a parte do broto do membro situada caudal ao eixo do membro; a face ulnar do membro superior e a face fibular do membro inferior.
post·bra·chi·al (pōst′brā′kē - al). Pós-braquial; sobre o braço ou na parte posterior deste.
post·car·di·nal (pōst′kar′di - nal). Pós-cardinal; relativo às veias cardinais posteriores.
post·ca·va (pōst′kā′vă). Veia cava inferior. SIN inferior *vena* cava.
post·ca·val (pōst′kā′val). Relativo à veia cava inferior.
post·cen·tral (pōst - sen′tral). Pós-central; referente à convolução cerebral que forma a borda posterior do sulco central: o giro pós-central.
post·chrom·ing (pōst′krōm′ing). Pós-cromação. SIN afterchroming.
post·ci·bal (pōst - sī′bal). Após uma refeição ou depois de ingerir o alimento. [L. *cibum*, alimento]
post·cla·vic·u·lar (pōst′kla - vik′u - lar). Pós-clavicular; posterior à clavícula.
post·co·i·tal (pōst - kō′i - tal). Pós-coital; depois do coito.
post·co·i·tus (pōst - kō′i - tus). Pós-coito; o momento imediatamente após o coito.
post·cor·di·al (pōst′kor′jal). Pós-cordial; posterior ao coração. [L. *cor* (*cord*-), coração]
post·cos·tal (pōst - kos′tal). Pós-costal; atrás das costelas.
post·crown. Pós-coroa; uma coroa, para substituir a coroa natural, que é retida no coto da raiz de um dente do qual foi removida a polpa, por um pino integrado na coroa e fechado no canal radicular tratado com um cimento.
post·cu·bi·tal (pōst′kū′bi - tal). Pós-ulnar; situado sobre o antebraço ou na parte posterior ou dorsal deste.

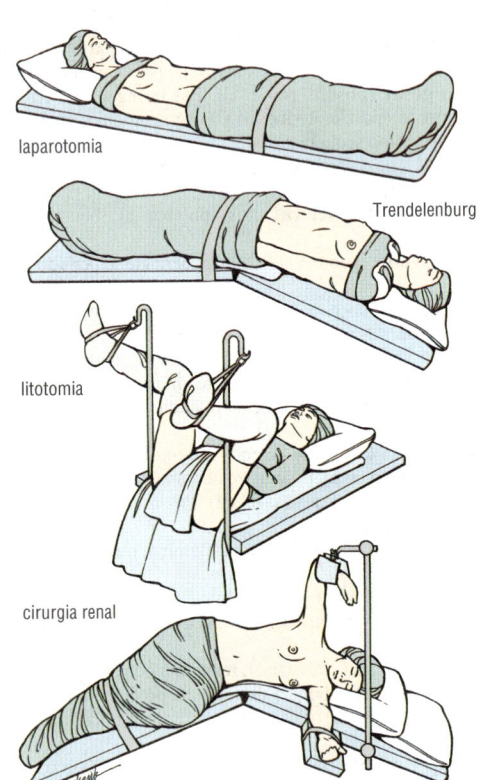

posições na mesa de cirurgia

post·dam. Dique posterior. SIN posterior palatal *seal.*
post·di·a·stol·ic (pōst'dī-ă-stol'ik). Pós-diastólico; que sucede a diástole.
post·di·crot·ic (pōst-dī-krot'ik). Pós-dicrótico; que sucede a onda dicrótica em um esfigmograma; designa uma variação adicional na linha descendente do traçado de pulso.
post·diph·the·rit·ic (pōst'dif-the-rit'ik). Pós-difterítico; que sucede ou ocorre como seqüela de difteria.
post·dor·mi·tal (pōst-dōr'mi-tăl). Pós-dormital; relativo ao período pós-dórmito.
post·dor·mi·tum (pōst-dōr'mi-tŭm). Pós-dórmito; o período de consciência crescente entre o sono e o despertar. [L. *dormio,* dormir]
post·duc·tal (pōst-dŭk'tal). Pós-ductal; relativo à parte da aorta distal à abertura aórtica do canal arterial.
post·en·ceph·a·lit·ic (pōst-en-sef'ă-lit'ik). Pós-encefalítico; que sucede a encefalite.
post·ep·i·lep·tic (pōst'ep-i-lep'tik). Pós-epiléptico; que sucede uma convulsão epiléptica.
pos·te·ri·or (pos-tēr'ē-ŏr). [TA]. Posterior. **1.** Após, em relação ao tempo ou espaço. **2** [NA]. Em anatomia humana, designa a superfície posterior do corpo. Freqüentemente usado para indicar a posição de uma estrutura em relação a outra, isto é, mais próxima do dorso do corpo. SIN dorsal (2) [TA], dorsalis [TA], posticus. **3.** Próximo da cauda ou da extremidade caudal de determinados embriões. **4.** Um substituto indesejável e confuso para caudal em quadrúpedes; em anatomia veterinária, o termo posterior é usado apenas para designar algumas estruturas da cabeça. [L. comparativo de *posterus,* subseqüente]
pos·te·ri·us (pos-tēr'ē-ŭs). Neutro de posterior. [L.]
postero-. Posterior; no dorso de. [L. *posterior*]
pos·ter·o·an·te·ri·or (pos'ter-ō-an-tēr'ē-ŏr). Póstero-anterior; termo que designa a direção de imagem ou progressão, póstero-anterior, através de uma parte.
pos·ter·o·clu·sion (pos'ter-ō-kloo'shŭn). Póstero-oclusão. SIN posterior *occlusion.*
pos·ter·o·ex·ter·nal (pos'ter-ō-ek-ster'nal). Póstero-externo. SIN posterolateral.
pos·ter·o·in·ter·nal (pos'ter-ō-in-ter'nal). Póstero-interno. SIN posteromedial.
pos·ter·o·lat·er·al (pos'ter-ō-lat'ē-răl). Póstero-lateral; por trás e de um lado, especificamente do lado externo. SIN posteroexternal.
pos·ter·o·me·di·al (pos'ter-ō-mē'dē-ăl). Póstero-medial; por trás e do lado interno. SIN posterointernal.
pos·ter·o·me·di·an (pos'ter-ō-mē'dē-an). Póstero-mediano; que ocupa uma posição central posteriormente.
pos·ter·o·pa·ri·e·tal (pos'ter-ō-pa-rī'ē-tăl). Póstero-parietal; relativo à porção posterior do lobo parietal do cérebro.
pos·ter·o·su·pe·ri·or (pos'ter-ō-soo-pē'rē-ŏr). Póstero-superior; situado atrás e na parte superior.
pos·ter·o·tem·po·ral (pos'ter-ō-tem'po-răl). Póstero-temporal; relativo ao, ou situado na porção posterior do, lobo temporal do cérebro.
post·e·soph·a·ge·al (pōst'ē-sof'ă-jē'ăl, ē-sŏ-faj'ē-ăl). Pós-esofágico; atrás do esôfago.
post·es·trus, post·es·trum (pōst-es'trŭs, -trŭm). Pós-estro; o período no ciclo estral após o estro; caracterizado pelo crescimento do corpo lúteo e por alterações fisiológicas relacionadas à produção de progesterona.
post·feb·rile (pōst-fē'bril). Pós-febril; que ocorre após uma febre. SIN metapyretic.
post·gan·gli·on·ic (pōst'gang-glē-on'ik). Pós-ganglionar; situado distal a ou além de um gânglio; refere-se às fibras nervosas desmielinizadas que se originam de células em um gânglio autônomo. SIN neurofibrae postganglionicae.
post·hem·i·ple·gic (pōst'hem-i-plē'jik). Pós-hemiplégico; após hemiplegia.
post·hem·or·rha·gic (pōst-hem-ŏ-raj'ik). Pós-hemorrágico; após uma hemorragia.
post·he·pat·ic (pōst-he-pat'ik). Pós-hepático; atrás do fígado.
pos·thet·o·my (pos-thet'ō-mē). Postetomia; abertura dorsal do prepúcio. [G. *posthē,* prepúcio, + *tomē,* incisão]
pos·thi·o·plas·ty (pos'thē-ō-plas-tē). Postioplastia; reconstrução cirúrgica do prepúcio. [G. *posthion,* forma dim. de *posthē,* prepúcio, + *plastos,* formado]
pos·thi·tis (pos-thī'tis). Postite; inflamação do prepúcio. [G. *posthē,* prepúcio, + *-itis,* inflamação]
pos·tho·lith (pos'thō-lith). Postólito. SIN preputial *calculus.* [G. *posthē,* prepúcio, + *lithos,* cálculo]
post·hy·oid (pōst-hī'oyd). Pós-hióide; atrás do osso hióide.
post·hyp·not·ic (pōst-hip-not'ik). Pós-hipnótico; após hipnose; designa um ato sugerido durante a hipnose que deve ser realizado em algum momento após o indivíduo hipnotizado despertar.
post·ic·tal (pōst-ik'tăl). Pós-ictal; após uma convulsão, p. ex., epiléptico.

pos·ti·cus (pos-tī'kŭs). SIN posterior (2). [L. de *post,* após]
post·in·flu·en·zal (post'in-floo-en'zăl). Pós-influenza; que ocorre como uma seqüela da influenza.
post·is·chi·al (pōst-is'kē-ăl). Pós-isquiático; posterior ao ísquio.
post·ma·lar·i·al (pōst-mă-lār'ē-ăl). Pós-malárico; que ocorre como uma seqüela da influenza.
post·mas·toid (pōst'mas'toyd). Pós-mastóide; posterior ao processo mastóide.
post·ma·ture (pōst-mă-toor', mă-tūr'). Pós-maduro; referente a um feto que permanece no útero por tempo maior que o período gestacional normal; isto é, mais de 42 semanas (288 dias) em seres humanos.
post·me·di·an (pōst'mē'dē-an). Pós-mediano; posterior ao plano mediano.
post·me·di·as·ti·nal (pōst'mē-dē-as'ti-năl, -mē'dē-ă-stī'năl). Pós-mediastinal. **1.** Posterior ao mediastino. **2.** Relativo ao mediastino posterior.
post·me·di·as·ti·num (pōst'mē'dē-ă-stī'nŭm). Pós-mediastino. SIN posterior *mediastinum.*
post·men·o·pau·sal (pōst-men-ō-paw'săl). Pós-menopausa; relativo ao período após a menopausa.
post·min·i·mus (pōst-min'i-mŭs). Pós-mínimo; um pequeno apêndice acessório fixado à lateral do quinto dedo da mão ou do pé; pode assemelhar-se a um dedo normal ou ser apenas uma massa carnosa. [post- + L. *minimus,* mínimo (dedo)]
post·mor·tem (pōst-mōr'tem). **1.** Relativo ao período após a morte ou que ocorre durante esse período. **2.** Coloquialismo para autopsia (1). [post- + L. acusativo de caso de *mors* (*mort-*), morte]
post·na·ri·al (pōst'nā'rē-ăl). Relativo às narinas posteriores ou coanas.
post·na·ris (pōst'nā'ris). Coana. SIN choanae.
post·na·sal (pōst'nā'săl). Pós-nasal. **1.** Posterior à cavidade nasal. **2.** Relativo à parte posterior da cavidade nasal.
post·na·tal (pōst-nā'tăl). Pós-natal; que ocorre após o nascimento. [L. *natus,* nascimento]
post·ne·crot·ic (post-ne-krot'ik). Pós-necrótico; subseqüente à morte de um tecido ou parte do corpo.
post·neu·rit·ic (pōst-noo-rit'ik). Pós-neurítico; subseqüente à neurite.
post·oc·u·lar (pōst'ok'ū-lăr). Pós-ocular; posterior ao bulbo do olho. [L. *oculus,* olho]
post·op·er·a·tive (pōst-op'er-ă-tiv). Pós-operatório; após uma operação.
post·o·ral (pos-tō'răl). Pós-oral; na parte posterior da boca, ou posterior a ela. [L. *os* (*or-*), boca]
post·or·bi·tal (pōst'ōr'bi-tăl). Pós-orbital; posterior à órbita.
post·pal·a·tine (pōst'pal'ă-tīn). Pós-palatino; posterior aos ossos palatinos. Geralmente usado em referência ao palato mole.
post·par·a·lyt·ic (pōst'par-ă-lit'ik). Pós-paralítico; que ocorre após paralisia ou conseqüente a esta.
post·par·tum (pōst-par'tŭm). Pós-parto; após o parto. Cf. antepartum, intrapartum. [L. *partus,* parto (substantivo), de *pario,* pp. *partus,* dar à luz]
post·pha·ryn·ge·al (pōst'fă-rin'jē-ăl). Pós-faríngeo; posterior à faringe.
post·pneu·mon·ic (post-noo-mon'ik). Pós-pneumônico; que sucede a pneumonia ou ocorre como seqüela desta.
post·pran·di·al (pōst-pran'dē-ăl). Pós-prandial; após uma refeição. [L. *prandium,* desjejum]
post·pu·ber·al, post·pu·ber·tal (pōst-poo'ber-ăl, -ber-tăl). Pós-puberal. SIN postpubescent.
post·pu·ber·ty (pōst-poo'ber-tē). Pós-puberdade; o período após a puberdade.
post·pu·bes·cent (pōst-poo-bes'ent). Pós-pubescente; subseqüente ao período da puberdade. SIN postpuberal, postpubertal.
post·pyk·not·ic (pōst-pik-not'ik). Pós-picnótico; após o estágio de picnose em uma hemácia, designando o desaparecimento do núcleo (cromatólise).
post·ro·lan·dic (pos'trō-lan'dik). Pós-rolândico; atrás da fissura de Rolando, ou sulco central. VER postcentral.
post·sa·cral (pōst'sā'krăl). Pós-sacral; referente ao cóccix.
post·scap·u·lar (pōst-skap'ū-lăr). Pós-escapular; posterior à escápula.
post·scar·la·ti·nal (pōst'skar-lă-tē'năl). Pós-escarlatina; que ocorre como uma seqüela da escarlatina.
post·sphyg·mic (pōst-sifg'mik). Pós-esfígmico; que ocorre após a onda de pulso. [G. *sphygmos,* pulso]
post·splen·ic (pōst'splen'ik). Pós-esplênico; posterior ao baço.
post·syn·ap·tic (pōst-si-nap'tik). Pós-sináptico; relativo à área na face distal de uma fenda sináptica.
post·tar·sal (pōst'tar'săl). Pós-tarsal; relativo à porção posterior do tarso.
post·tec·ta (pōst'tek'tă). Aboral à parte oculta do duodeno.
post·tib·i·al (pōst'tib'ē-ăl). Pós-tibial; posterior à tíbia; situado na porção posterior da perna.
post·trans·crip·tion·al (pōst-tran-skrip'shŭn-al). Pós-transcricional; referente aos eventos que ocorrem após a transcrição.
post·trans·la·tion·al (pōst-trans-lā'shŭn-al). Pós-tradução; referente aos eventos que ocorrem após a tradução.

post·trans·verse (pōst-tranz′vers). Pós-transverso; atrás de um processo transverso.

post·trau·mat·ic (pōst-traw-mat′ik). Pós-traumático; que ocorre após traumatismo e, por implicação, causado por ele.

post·tre·mat·ic (pōst-trē-mat′ik). Relativo à superfície caudal de uma fenda branquial. [post- + G. *trēma*, perfuração]

post·tus·sis (pōst-tūs′is). Após a tosse; geralmente refere-se a determinados ruídos auscultados. [L. *tussis*, tosse]

post·ty·phoid (pōst-tī′foyd). Pós-tifóide; que ocorre como uma seqüela da febre tifóide.

pos·tu·late (pos′tū-lāt). Postulado; uma proposição tida como auto-evidente ou suposta sem comprovação como base para análise adicional. VER TAMBÉM hypothesis, theory. [L. *postulo*, pp. *-atus*, demandar]
 Ampère p., p. de Ampère. SIN Avogadro *law.*
 Avogadro p., p. de Avogadro. SIN Avogadro *law.*
 Ehrlich p., p. de Ehrlich. SIN side-chain *theory.*
 Koch p.'s, postulados de Koch; para estabelecer a especificidade de um microrganismo patogênico, este deve estar presente em todos os casos da doença, inoculações de suas culturas puras devem produzir doença em animais e, destes, deve ser novamente obtido e propagado em culturas puras. SIN Koch law.

pos·tur·al (pos′tū-rāl, pos′cher-al). Postural; relativo à postura ou por ela afetado.

pos·ture (pos′choor, pos′cher). Postura; a posição dos membros ou do corpo como um todo. [L. *positura*, de *pono*, pp. *positus*, colocar]
 Stern p., p. de Stern; posição de decúbito dorsal com a cabeça estendida e pendente sobre a extremidade da mesa, na qual surge ou torna-se mais distinto o sopro em casos de insuficiência tricúspide.

pos·tur·og·ra·phy (pos-tyur-og′ra-fē). Posturografia. SIN dynamic p. [posture + G. *graphō*, escrever]
 dynamic p., p. dinâmica; medida da estabilidade postural com estímulos visuais e proprioceptivos variados. SIN posturography.

post·u·ter·ine (pōst-ū′ter-in). Pós-uterino; posterior ao útero.

post·vac·ci·nal (pōst-vak′si-nāl). Pós-vacinal; após a vacinação.

post·val·var, post·val·vu·lar (pōst-val′var, -val′vū-lar). Pós-valvar, pós-valvular; relativo a uma posição distal à valva pulmonar ou aórtica.

po·ta·ble (pō′ta-bl). Potável; que se pode beber. [L. *potabilis*, de *poto*, beber]

Potain, Pierre C.E., médico francês, 1825–1901. VER P. sign.

pot·a·mo·pho·bia (pot′ă-mō-fō′bē-ă). Potamofobia; medo mórbido provocado pela visão e, algumas vezes, pelo pensamento de um rio ou de qualquer fluxo de água. [G. *potamos*, rio, + *phobos*, medo]

pot·ash. Potassa; carbonato de potássio impuro. SIN pearl-ash. [E. pot-ashes]
 caustic p., p. cáustica. SIN potassium hydroxide.
 sulfurated p., p. sulfurada; mistura composta principalmente de polissulfetos de potássio e tiossulfato de potássio; usada externamente na escaviose, acne e psoríase; usada na fabricação de "loção branca". SIN liver of sulfur.

po·tas·sic (pō-tas′ik). Potássico; relativo a ou que contém potássio.

po·tas·si·um (K) (pō-tas′ē-ŭm). Potássio; elemento metálico alcalino, n.º atômico 19, peso atômico 39,0983, abundante na natureza, mas sempre em combinação; seus sais são usados com fins medicinais. No caso de sais de potássio orgânicos, não relacionados a seguir, ver o nome do ânion. SIN kalium. [L. mod., do inglês potash (de pot + ashes), + *-ium*]
 p. acetate, acetato de potássio; diurético, diaforético e alcalinizante sistêmico e urinário. SIN sal diureticum.
 p. acid tartrate, tartarato ácido de potássio. SIN p. bitartrate.
 p. alum, alume de potássio. SIN aluminum potassium sulfate.
 p. aminosalicylate, aminossalicilato de potássio. VER *p*-aminosalicylic acid.
 p. antimonyltartrate, antimoniotartarato de potássio. SIN antimony potassium tartrate.
 p. atractylate, atractilato de potássio; o sal de potássio do ácido atractílico, a fonte natural deste último.
 p. bicarbonate, bicarbonato de potássio; usado como diurético para reduzir a acidez da urina e como repositor de eletrólitos.
 p. bitartrate, bitartarato de potássio; diurético e laxante. SIN cream of tartar, p. acid tartrate.
 p. bromide, brometo de potássio; KBr; sedativo e hipnótico obsoleto (geralmente é preferido o brometo de sódio).
 p. chlorate, clorato de potássio; clorato de potassa, $KClO_3$, usado como colutório e gargarejo na estomatite e na faringite folicular; é incompatível no estado seco com todas as substâncias facilmente oxidáveis.
 p. chloride, cloreto de potássio; usado para corrigir a deficiência de potássio.
 p. citrate, citrato de potássio; pó deliqüescente, solúvel em água; usado como diurético, diaforético, expectorante e alcalinizante sistêmico e urinário. SIN Rivière salt.
 p. cyanide, cianeto de potássio; fumegante comercial.
 dibasic p. phosphate, fosfato de potássio dibásico. SIN p. phosphate.
 p. dichromate, p. bichromate, dicromato de potássio; usado externamente como adstringente, anti-séptico e cáustico; forte agente oxidante que deve ser manuseado com cuidado.
 effervescent p. citrate, citrato de potássio efervescente; uma mistura de citrato de potássio, ácido cítrico, bicarbonato de sódio e ácido tartárico; usado como antiácido gástrico e alcalinizante da urina.
 p. ferrocyanide, ferrocianeto de potássio; prussiato de potassa amarelo, usado no preparo de vários cianetos e na medicina como antídoto do sulfato de cobre.
 p. gluconate, gluconato de potássio; sal potássico do ácido glucônico, usado na hipopotassemia para fins de reposição.
 p. guaiacolsulfonate, guaiacolsulfonato de potássio; usado como expectorante.
 p. hydroxide, hidróxido de potássio; KOH; um cáustico forte e penetrante. SIN caustic potash.
 p. hypophosphite, hipofosfito de potássio; antigamente considerado como tendo um efeito tônico sobre o sistema nervoso; pode ser explosivo se triturado ou aquecido com agentes oxidantes.
 p. iodate, iodato de potássio; agente oxidante e desinfetante.
 p. iodide, iodeto de potássio; KI; usado como restaurador da saúde e expectorante e em determinadas micoses.
 p. metaphosphate, metafosfato de potássio; um auxiliar farmacêutico (tampão).
 monobasic p. phosphate, fosfato monobásico de potássio; usado como acidificante e tampão urinário.
 p. nitrate, nitrato de potássio; algumas vezes usado como diurético e diaforético; antigamente era incluído em pós para tratamento da asma contendo folhas de estramônio. SIN niter, salpeter.
 penicillin G p., penicilina G potássica. VER *penicillin* G potassium.
 p. perchlorate, perclorato de potássio; ocasionalmente usado, como alternativa a um derivado tiouracil, no controle do hipertireoidismo.
 p. permanganate, permanganato de potássio; forte agente oxidante, usado em solução como anti-séptico e desodorizante em lesões fétidas, sendo antigamente usado como lavagem gástrica no envenenamento por morfina, estricnina, aconita e picrotoxina; à microscopia eletrônica, cora bem as membranas citoplasmáticas e oferece resultados semelhantes aos da coloração por hidróxido de chumbo; também é usado como fixador (Luft).
 p. phosphate, fosfato de potássio; um diurético e catártico salino leve. SIN dibasic p. phosphate, dipotassium phosphate.
 p. rhodanate, rodanato de potássio. SIN p. thiocyanate.
 p. sodium tartrate, tartarato sódico de potássio; catártico salino leve, usado como ingrediente em pós efervescentes compostos. SIN Rochelle salt, Seignette salt, sodium potassium tartrate.
 p. sorbate, sorbato de potássio; sal potássico do ácido 2,3-hexadienóico; um inibidor de fungos e leveduras, usado como preservativo.
 p. succinate, succinato de potássio; pó deliqüescente usado como hemostático.
 p. sulfate, sulfato de potássio; laxante obsoleto.
 p. sulfocyanate, sulfocianato de potássio. SIN p. thiocyanate.
 p. tartrate, tartarato de potássio; purgante leve e diurético. SIN soluble tartar.
 p. thiocyanate, tiocianato de potássio; usado antigamente no tratamento da hipertensão essencial e como reagente na detecção de cobre, ferro e prata. SIN p. rhodanate, p. sulfocyanate.

potassium-39 (^{39}K). Potássio-39; o isótopo não-radioativo mais abundante do potássio; representa 93,1% do potássio natural.

po·tas·si·um-40 (^{40}K). Potássio-40; isótopo radioativo natural (0,0117%) do potássio; emissor beta com meia-vida de 1,26 bilhão de anos; principal fonte de radioatividade natural do tecido vivo.

po·tas·si·um-42 (^{42}K). Potássio-42; isótopo artificial do potássio; emissor beta com meia-vida de 12,36 h, usado como marcador em estudos da distribuição do potássio nos compartimentos de líquido corporal e na localização de tumores cerebrais.

po·tas·si·um-43 (^{43}K). Potássio-43; isótopo artificial do potássio; um emissor beta com meia-vida de 22,3 h, usado como marcador em estudos de perfusão miocárdica.

po·ten·cy (pō′ten-sē). Potência. **1.** Energia, força ou poder; a condição ou qualidade de ser potente. **2.** Especificamente, potência sexual. **3.** Em terapêutica, a atividade farmacológica relativa de uma dose de uma substância em comparação a dose de um outro agente que tem os mesmos efeitos; p. ex., aspirina e acetaminofeno têm igual potência no alívio da cefaléia (é necessária a mesma dose), mas o cetorolac exibe maior potência que o ibuprofeno, pois 20 mg do primeiro têm a mesma eficácia que 400 mg do último. [L. *potentia*, potência]
 sexual p., p. sexual; a capacidade de realizar e consumar uma relação sexual, geralmente referindo-se ao homem.

po·tent (pō′tent). Potente. **1.** Que tem força, poder, vigor. **2.** Indica a capacidade de diferenciação de uma célula primitiva. VER TAMBÉM totipotent, pluripotent, unipotent. **3.** Em psiquiatria, que tem potência sexual.

po·ten·tial (pō-ten′shăl). Potencial. **1.** Capaz de fazer ou ser, embora ainda não esteja fazendo ou sendo; possível, mas não real. **2.** Um estado de tensão em uma fonte elétrica que permite trabalhar em condições adequadas; em relação à eletricidade, o potencial é análogo à temperatura em relação ao calor. [L. *potentia*, energia, potência]

action p., p. de ação; a alteração no potencial de membrana que ocorre no nervo, músculo ou outro tecido excitável quando há excitação.

after-p., pós-p. VER afterpotential.

bioelectric p., p. bioelétrico; potenciais elétricos que ocorrem em organismos vivos.

biotic p., p. biótico; uma medida teórica da capacidade de uma espécie de sobreviver ou competir com sucesso.

brain p., p. cerebral; a carga elétrica do cérebro em comparação com um ponto no corpo; o potencial pode ser contínuo (p. DC) ou pode flutuar em freqüências específicas quando registrado em relação ao tempo, dando origem ao eletroencefalograma.

brainstem auditory evoked p., p. evocado auditivo do tronco encefálico; respostas deflagradas por estímulos sonoros (estalos), gerados no nervo acústico e nas vias auditivas do tronco encefálico; registrado sobre o couro cabeludo.

chemical p. (μ), p. químico; uma medida da forma como a energia livre de Gibbs de uma fase depende de qualquer alteração na composição dessa fase.

cochlear p., p. coclear. SIN cochlear microphonic.

compound action p., p. de ação composto; os potenciais combinados resultantes da ativação da divisão auditiva do oitavo nervo craniano.

demarcation p., p. de demarcação; a diferença de potencial registrada quando um eletrodo é colocado sobre fibras nervosas ou fibras musculares intactas e o outro eletrodo é colocado sobre as extremidades lesadas das mesmas fibras; a porção intacta é positiva em relação à porção lesada. SIN injury p.

early receptor p. (ERP), p. receptor precoce; uma voltagem que se origina através do olho por um deslocamento de carga no pigmento fotorreceptor em resposta a um forte clarão de luz.

endocochlear p., p. endococlear; o potencial de corrente contínua permanente na endolinfa em relação à perilinfa, medindo 80 mV positivo.

evoked p., p. evocado; potencial relacionado a um evento, produzido por um estímulo e temporário. VER TAMBÉM evoked *response*.

excitatory junction p. (EJP), p. de junção excitatório; despolarização parcial distinta do músculo liso produzida por estimulação de nervos excitatórios; semelhante aos pequenos potenciais da placa terminal somados a estímulos repetidos.

excitatory postsynaptic p. (EPSP), p. pós-sináptico excitatório; a alteração no potencial produzida na membrana do próximo neurônio quando um impulso que tem uma influência excitatória chega na sinapse; é uma alteração local na direção da despolarização; a soma desses potenciais pode levar à liberação de um impulso pelo neurônio.

generator p., p. gerador; despolarização local do potencial de membrana na extremidade de um neurônio sensorial em resposta graduada à intensidade de um estímulo aplicado ao órgão receptor associado, p. ex., um corpúsculo de Pacini; se o potencial gerador tornar-se suficientemente grande (porque o estímulo tem o mínimo intensidade limiar), causa excitação no nodo de Ranvier mais próximo e um potencial de ação propagado.

inhibitory juncion p. (IJP), p. de junção inibitório; hiperpolarização do músculo liso produzida por estimulação de nervos inibitórios.

inhibitory postsynaptic p. (IPSP), p. pós-sináptico inibitório; a alteração no potencial produzida na membrana do próximo neurônio quando um impulso que tem influência inibitória chega na sinapse; é uma alteração local na direção da hiperpolarização; a freqüência de descarga de um dado neurônio é determinada pela extensão com que os impulsos que podem levar a potenciais pós-sinápticos excitatórios predominam sobre aqueles que causam potenciais pós-sinápticos inibitórios.

injury p., p. de lesão. SIN demarcation p.

membrane p., p. de membrana; o potencial no interior de uma membrana celular, medido em relação ao líquido imediatamente fora; é negativo em condições de repouso e torna-se positivo durante um potencial de ação. SIN transmembrane p.

myogenic p., p. miogênico; potencial de ação do músculo.

oscillatory p., p. oscilatório; a voltagem variável na deflexão positiva do eletrorretinograma (onda β) do olho adaptado ao escuro, originada nas células amácrinas.

Ottoson p., p. de Ottoson. SIN electroolfactogram.

oxidation-reduction p. (E_0^+), p. de oxidação-redução, p. de oxirredução; o potencial, em volts, de um eletrodo metálico inerte, medido em um sistema com uma razão entre [oxidante] e [redutor] escolhida arbitrariamente e referido ao eletrodo de hidrogênio normal em temperatura absoluta; é calculado a partir da seguinte equação:

$$E_0^+ = E_0 + \frac{RT}{nF} \ln \frac{[\text{oxidante}]}{[\text{redutor}]},$$

na qual R é a constante de gás expressa em unidades elétricas, T é a temperatura absoluta (Kelvin), n é o número de elétrons transferidos, F é o faraday, ln é o logaritmo natural e E_0 é o símbolo normal do potencial do sistema em pH 0; para sistemas biológicos, E_0' é freqüentemente usado (no qual o pH = 7). Cf. Nernst *equation*. SIN redox p.

pacemaker p., p. do marca-passo; a voltagem inscrita por impulsos de um marca-passo eletrônico artificial.

redox p., p. redox. SIN oxidation-reduction p.

S p., p. S; respostas prolongadas, lentas, despolarizantes ou hiperpolarizantes à iluminação; iniciada entre as camadas de células fotorreceptoras e ganglionares da retina.

somatosensory evoked p., p. evocado somatossensorial; as respostas corticais e subcorticais, com média calculada por computador, à estimulação repetitiva de fibras sensitivas dos nervos periféricos.

spike p., p. em ponta; a principal onda no potencial de ação de um nervo; é seguida por pós-potenciais negativos e positivos.

summating p.'s, potenciais de soma; respostas às correntes alternadas do órgão de Corti à estimulação acústica.

thermodynamic p., p. termodinâmico. VER free *energy*.

transmembrane p., p. transmembrana. SIN membrane p.

ventricular late p., p. ventricular tardio; sinais eletrocardiográficos de microvoltagem de alta freqüência ao fim do complexo QRS.

visual evoked p., p. evocado visual; flutuações de voltagem que podem ser registradas na área occipital do couro cabeludo em virtude de estimulação da retina por uma luz piscando a intervalos de 1/4 s; comumente somadas e com a média calculada por computador.

zeta p., p. zeta; o grau de carga negativa na superfície de uma hemácia; isto é, a diferença de potencial entre as cargas negativas sobre a hemácia e o cátion na porção líquida do sangue.

zoonotic p., p. zoonótico; o potencial de infecções de animais subumanos de serem transmissíveis para seres humanos.

po·ten·ti·a·tion (po-ten′she-a′shun). Potencialização; interação entre dois ou mais fármacos ou agentes que resulta em uma resposta farmacológica maior que a soma das respostas individuais a cada fármaco ou agente.

po·ten·ti·a·tor (po-ten′she-a-ter, -tor). Potencializador; em quimioterapia, um fármaco usado em conjunto com outros fármacos para produzir potencialização deliberada.

po·ten·ti·om·e·ter (po-ten-she-om′e-ter). Potenciômetro. **1.** Instrumento usado para medir pequenas diferenças de potencial elétrico. **2.** Resistor elétrico com resistência total fixa entre dois terminais, mas com um terceiro terminal fixado a um cursor que pode estabelecer contato em qualquer ponto desejado ao longo da resistência. [L. *potentia*, potência, + G. *metron*, medida]

po·tion (po′shun). Poção; um gole ou uma grande dose de medicamento líquido. [L. *potio, potus*, de *poto*, beber]

Pott, Sir Percivall, cirurgião inglês, 1714–1788. VER P. *abscess, aneurysm, curvature, disease, fracture, paralysis, paraplegia*.

Potter, Edith L., patologista perinatal norte-americano, *1901. VER P. *disease, facies, syndrome*.

Potter, Irving White, obstetra norte-americano, 1868–1956. VER P. *version*.

Potts, Willis J., cirurgião pediátrico norte-americano, 1895–1968. VER P. *anastomosis, clamp, operation*.

pouch (powch). Bolsa; fundo-de-saco. VER TAMBÉM fossa, recess, sac.

antral p., b. antral; uma bolsa feita no antro do estômago de animais experimentais.

branchial p.'s, bolsas branquiais. SIN pharyngeal p.'s.

Broca p., b. de Broca. SIN pudendal *sac*.

deep perineal p., b. perineal profunda. SIN deep perineal *space*.

Denis Browne p., b. de Denis Browne; bolsa formada entre a fáscia de Scarpa e a fáscia oblíqua externa adjacente ao anel inguinal externo; um local de alojamento comum dos testículos não-descidos (como no criptorquidismo). SIN superficial inguinal p.

p. of Douglas, b. de Douglas; fundo-de-saco de Douglas. SIN rectouterine p.

Douglas p., b. de Douglas. SIN rectouterine p.

endodermal p.'s, bolsas endodérmicas. SIN pharyngeal p.'s.

Hartmann p., b. de Hartmann; bolsa esferóide ou cônica na junção do colo da vesícula biliar e do ducto cístico. SIN ampulla of gallbladder, fossa provesicalis, pelvis of gallbladder.

Heidenhain p., b. de Heidenhain; um pequeno saco (bolsa) do estômago, desnervado do vago e isolado da cavidade principal, mas com uma abertura através da parede abdominal, feita para obter suco gástrico e para estudar a secreção gástrica em experiências fisiológicas.

hepatorenal p., b. hepatorrenal. SIN hepatorenal *recess* of subhepatic space.

hypophyseal p., b. hipofisária. SIN pituitary *diverticulum*.

ileoanal p. (il′e-o-a′nal), b. ileoanal; bolsa construída a partir do íleo e anastomosada à parte proximal do ânus para restauração da continência após proctocolectomia.

Kock p., b. de Kock; ileostomia continente com um reservatório e abertura provida de válvula, criada a partir de alças duplas de íleo. SIN Kock ileostomy.

laryngeal p., b. laríngea. SIN laryngeal *saccule*.

Morison p., b. de Morison. SIN hepatorenal *recess* of subhepatic space.

paracystic p., b. paracística. SIN paravesical *fossa*.

pararectal p., b. pararretal. SIN pararectal *fossa*.

paravesical p., b. paravesical. SIN paravesical *fossa*.

Pavlov p., b. de Pavlov; secção do estômago de um cão, preservando sua inervação vagal, mas isolada de toda comunicação com a parte principal do órgão e conectada ao exterior por uma fístula; usada em estudos das secreções gástricas. SIN miniature stomach, Pavlov stomach.

pharyngeal p.'s, bolsas faríngeas; evaginações pares do endoderma faríngeo embrionário, entre os arcos branquiais, estendendo-se em direção aos sulcos branquiais correspondentes revestidos de ectoderma; durante o desenvolvimento transformam-se em tecidos e órgãos epiteliais, como o timo e as glândulas tireóides. SIN branchial p.'s, endodermal p.'s.

Physick p.'s, bolsas de Physick; proctite com secreção mucosa e dor em queimação, envolvendo principalmente as saculações entre as válvulas retais.

Prussak p., b. de Prussak. SIN superior recess of tympanic membrane.

Rathke p., b. de Rathke. SIN pituitary *diverticulum*.

rectouterine p. [TA], escavação retouterina; bolsa formada pela deflexão do peritônio do reto para o útero. SIN excavatio rectouterina [TA], cavum douglasi, cul-de-sac (2), Douglas cul-de-sac, Douglas p., p. of Douglas, rectovaginouterine p.

rectovaginouterine p., b. retovaginouterina. SIN rectouterine p.

rectovesical p. [TA], escavação retovesical; bolsa formada pela deflexão do peritônio do reto para a bexiga no homem. SIN excavatio rectovesicalis [TA], Proust space.

Seessel p., b. de Seessel. VER Seessel *pocket*.

superficial inguinal p., b. inguinal superficial. SIN Denis Browne p.

superficial perineal p., b. perineal superficial. SIN superficial perineal *space*.

ultimobranchial p., b. ultimobranquial; quinta bolsa faríngea transitória; agora é considerada incorporada ao complexo faríngeo caudal, cujas células tornam-se as células parafoliculares (células C) da tireóide.

uterovesical p., b. uterovesical. SIN vesicouterine p.

vesicouterine p. [TA], escavação vesicouterina; bolsa formada pela deflexão do peritônio da bexiga para o corpo do útero na mulher. SIN excavatio vesicouterina [TA], cavum vesicouterinum, uterovesical p.

Willis p., b. de Willis; termo obsoleto para omento menor (lesser *omentum*).

pouch·i·tis (pow-chī'tis). Bolsite; inflamação aguda da mucosa de um reservatório ou bolsa ileal criado cirurgicamente, em geral após colectomia total para tratamento de doença inflamatória intestinal ou de polipose múltipla. [pouch + *-itis*, inflamação]

pou·drage (poo-drahzh′). **1.** Pulverização. **2.** SIN talc *operation*. [F.]

pleural p., pulverização pleural; cobertura das superfícies pleurais opostas com um pó ligeiramente irritante a fim de assegurar aderência.

poul·tice (pōl'tis). Cataplasma; emulsão mole ou papa preparada umedecendo-se vários pós ou outras substâncias absorventes com líquidos oleosos ou aquosos, algumas vezes medicinais, e geralmente aplicada quente à superfície; exerce efeito emoliente, relaxante ou estimulante, contra-irritante sobre a pele e os tecidos subjacentes. SIN cataplasm. [L. *puls* (*pult-*), uma papa espessa; G. *poltos*]

pound (pownd). Libra; uma unidade de peso, que contém 12 onças no sistema apotecário, ou 16 onças no sistema avoirdupois. [A.S. *pund*; L. *pondus*, peso]

pound·al (pownd'ăl). Poundal; a força necessária para dar a uma massa de 1 libra uma aceleração de 1 pé/s^2; igual a 0,138255 N.

Poupart, François, anatomista francês, 1616–1708. VER P. *ligament, line*.

po·vi·done (pō'vi-dōn). Povidona; polímero sintético que consiste principalmente em grupos 1-vinil-2-pirrolidona lineares, com pesos moleculares médios que variam de 10.000 a 70.000; usado como agente dispersante e suspensor; a povidona com peso molecular entre 20.000 e 40.000 foi usada como extensor plasmático. Não é metabolizada, mas é excretada de forma inalterada pelo rim. SIN polyvidone, polyvinylpyrrolidone.

po·vi·done-io·dine. Povidona-iodo. SIN povidone *iodine*.

pow·der. Pó. **1.** Uma massa seca de pequenas partículas separadas de qualquer substância. **2.** Em farmácia, uma dispersão homogênea de partículas relativamente secas, finamente divididas, que consiste em uma ou mais substâncias; o grau de divisão de um pó está relacionado à passagem do material através de peneiras padronizadas. **3.** Uma única dose de um fármaco pulverizado, contida em um envelope de papel. **4.** Pulverizar; reduzir uma substância sólida a um estado de divisão muito fina. [Fr. *poudre*; L. *pulvis*]

bleaching p., cal clorada. SIN chlorinated *lime*.

pow·er (pow'er). Potência. **1.** Em óptica, a vergência refrativa de uma lente. **2.** Em física e em engenharia, a velocidade de execução de um trabalho. **3.** O expoente de um número ou expressão que determina o número de vezes que esse número deve ser multiplicado por si mesmo.

back vertex p., p. de vértice posterior; a potência efetiva de uma lente medida a partir de uma superfície em direção ao olho; um padrão para medida das lentes oftálmicas.

carbon dioxide combining p., p. de combinação do dióxido de carbono; uma medida do CO_2 total que pode ser ligado como HCO_2 em uma PCO_2 de 40 mm Hg a 25°C pelo soro, plasma ou sangue total.

equivalent p., p. equivalente; a potência igual a uma lente infinitamente fina, medida sobre um banco óptico.

resolving p., p. de resolução; **(1)** definição de uma lente; em uma lente objetiva microscópica, é calculada dividindo-se o comprimento de onda da luz usada pelo dobro da abertura numérica da objetiva. VER TAMBÉM definition; **(2)** analogias a outras modalidades, p. ex., a discriminação entre dois pontos em um exame neurológico. Comumente é erroneamente interpretada como erro aleatório, embora não apresente nenhuma de suas propriedades. **(3)** SIN resolution (2).

statistical p., p. estatística; no teste da hipótese de Neyman-Pearson, a probabilidade de rejeição da hipótese nula quando é falsa; o complemento de um erro (*error*) do segundo tipo.

pox (poks). **1.** Uma doença eruptiva, geralmente qualificada por um prefixo descritivo; p. ex., smallpox (varíola), cowpox (vacínia), chickenpox (varicela). Ver o termo específico. **2.** Termo arcaico ou coloquial para sífilis. [var. do pl. *pocks*]

Kaffir p., alastrim. SIN alastrim.

Pox·vir·i·dae (poks-vir'i-dē). Família de grandes vírus complexos, com grande afinidade pelo tecido cutâneo, patogênicos para os seres humanos e outros animais. Os vírions são grandes, com até 250 × 400 nm, e possuem envoltório (membranas duplas). A replicação ocorre totalmente no citoplasma de células infectadas. Os capsídeos têm simetria complexa e contêm DNA de duplo filamento (PM 160 × 10^6), sendo o antígeno nucleoproteico comum a todos os membros da família. São reconhecidos vários gêneros, incluindo: Orthopoxvirus, Avipoxvirus, Capripoxvirus, Leporipoxvirus e Parapoxvirus.

pox·vi·rus (poks'vī-rŭs). Poxvírus; qualquer vírus da família Poxviridae.

p. officina'lis. SIN vaccinia *virus*.

Pozzi, Samuel J., ginecologista e anatomista francês, 1846–1918. VER P. *muscle*.

PP Abreviatura de pyrophosphate (pirofosfato).

PP$_1$ Abreviatura de inorganic *pyrophosphate* (diphosphate).

P.p. Abreviatura de *punctum* proximum.

ppb Abreviatura de partes por bilhão (parts per billion).

PPCA Abreviatura de proserum prothrombin conversion *accelerator* (acelerador da conversão da protrombina).

PPCF Abreviatura de plasmin prothrombin conversion *factor* (fator V).

PPD Abreviatura de purified protein derivative of *tuberculin* (derivado proteico purificado de tuberculina).

PPLO Abreviatura de pleuropneumonia-like *organisms* (microrganismos semelhantes aos causadores de pleuropneumonia) em *organism*.

ppm Abreviatura de partes por milhão (parts per million).

PPO Abreviatura de 2,5-diphenyloxazole (2,5-difeniloxazol), um cintilador líquido; preferred provider *organization*.

PPPPPP Um mnemônico de 6 "P", designando o complexo de sintomas da oclusão arterial aguda. [dor (*pain*), palidez, parestesia, ausência de pulso, paralisia, prostração]

PPRibp, PPRP Abreviatura de 5-fosfo-α-D-ribosil-1-pirofosfato (5-phospho-α-D-ribosyl-1-pyrophosphate).

P pul·mo·na·le (pul-mō-nā'lā). P *pulmonale*; ondas P apiculadas, altas, estreitas nas derivações eletrocardiográficas II, III e aVF, e muitas vezes um componente de onda P positiva inicial proeminente em V$_1$, presumidamente característica de *cor pulmonale*. (Embora esse termo seja amplamente usado na literatura eletrocardiográfica, na verdade é inadequado e teria sido mais apropriadamente substituído por P-*dextrocardiale*, pois essas ondas resultam da sobrecarga do átrio direito, independentemente da causa, como na estenose tricúspide, e podem ocorrer independentemente do *cor pulmonale*.) Na doença pulmonar, a P *pulmonale* geralmente é transitória, ocorrendo durante exacerbações, geralmente asmáticas.

PQ Abreviatura de plastoquinone (plastoquinona).

PQ-9 Abreviatura de plastoquinone-9 (plastoquinona-9).

P.r. abreviatura de *punctum* remotum.

Pr 1. Abreviatura de presbiopia. **2.** Símbolo de praseodímio; propil.

PRA Abreviatura de plasma renin *activity*; fosforribosilamina (phosphoribosylamine).

prac·tice (prak'tis). Prática; o exercício da profissão médica ou de uma das profissões da área de saúde relacionadas. [L. mediev. *practica*, negócio, G. *praktikos*, relativo à ação]

extramural p., medicina extramuros; prestação de serviços de assistência à saúde por equipes de universidades ou hospitalares em tempo integral às pessoas, além dos limites físicos de seus respectivos centros médicos.

family p., medicina de família; uma especialidade da medicina na qual o médico assume a responsabilidade pela saúde e pelo tratamento médico de todos os membros de um grupo familiar, independentemente da idade ou sexo, mas geralmente exerce de forma limitada a obstetrícia e a cirurgia.

general p., medicina geral; termo relativamente obsoleto para designar médicos que cuidam de todos os tipos de problemas médicos, incluindo doenças internas, pediátricas, obstétricas e cirúrgicas. O treinamento de pós-graduação para clínicos era limitado e não havia certificação de especialidade; o campo foi substituído por profissionais de família que recebem treinamento mais amplo.

group p., medicina de grupo; a prática cooperativa da medicina por um grupo de médicos, em geral tendo um especialista em determinado campo; esse grupo freqüentemente compartilha um conjunto comum de consultórios, laboratórios, equipe, equipamento, etc.

intramural p., medicina intramuros; prestação de serviços de assistência à saúde por equipes de universidades ou hospitalares em tempo integral realizada dentro dos limites físicos de seus respectivos centros médicos.

prac·ti·tion·er (prak - tish′ŭn - er). Profissional; indivíduo que exerce a medicina ou uma das profissões da área de saúde relacionadas.

Prader, Andrea, pediatra suíço, *1919. VER P.-Willi *syndrome.*

prae-. VER pre-.

prag·mat·ics (prag - mat′iks). Pragmática; ramo da semiologia; a teoria que lida com a relação entre os signos e seus usuários, tanto transmissores quanto receptores. [G. *pragmatikos,* de *pragma,* algo feito]

prag·ma·tism (prag′mă - tizm). Pragmatismo; filosofia que enfatiza as aplicações práticas e as conseqüências das crenças e teorias, sustentando que o significado das idéias ou das coisas é determinado pela testabilidade da idéia na vida real. [G. *pragma* (*pragmat-*), algo realizado]

2-pra·li·dox·ime (2-PAM). 2-Pralidoxima; uma dentre várias oximas eficazes na reversão da inibição da colinesterase por organofosfatos. A 2-PAM facilita a hidrólise da enzima fosforilada de forma a regenerar a colinesterase ativa.

pral·i·dox·ime chlo·ride (pral - i - dok′sēm, prā - li -). Cloreto de pralidoxima; usado para restaurar a atividade da colinesterase inativada, resultante de intoxicação por organofosforado; tem utilidade um pouco limitada como antagonista do tipo carbamato de inibidores da colinesterase usados no tratamento da miastenia gravis. Pode haver tonteira, borramento visual, sonolência, náuseas, taquicardia e fraqueza muscular.

pra·mox·ine hy·dro·chlo·ride (prā - mok′sēn, - sin). Cloridrato de pramoxina; anestésico local não-éster, não-amida para uso dérmico e retal.

pran·di·al (pran′dē - ăl). Prandial; relativo a uma refeição. [L. *prandium,* desjejum]

pra·se·o·dym·i·um (Pr) (prā - sē - ō - dim′ē - ŭm). Praseodímio; um elemento do grupo dos lantanídeos ou "terras raras"; n.º atômico 59, peso atômico 140,90765. [G. *prasios,* verde-claro, de *prason,* alho-poró, + *didymos,* gêmeo]

Pratt, Joseph H., médico norte-americano, 1872–1956. VER P. *symptom.*

Prausnitz, Otto Carl, higienista alemão, 1876–1963. VER P.-Küstner *antibody, reaction;* reversed P. *reaction.*

prav·a·sta·tin. Pravastatina; um inibidor da enzima 3-hidroxi-3-metilglutaril coenzima A (HMG-CoA), a enzima limitadora de velocidade na biossíntese do colesterol; usada no tratamento da hipercolesterolemia; semelhante à lovastatina e sinvastatina.

prax·i·ol·o·gy (prak - sē - ol′ō - jē). Praxiologia; a ciência ou estudo do comportamento; exclui o estudo da consciência e de conceitos metafísicos não-objetivos semelhantes. [G. *praxis,* ação, + *logos,* estudo]

prax·is (prak′sis). Práxis; a realização de uma ação. [G. *praxis,* ação]

pra·ze·pam (prā′zē - pam). Prazepam; agente ansiolítico da classe dos benzodiazepínicos; uma pró-droga do nordiazepam.

pra·zi·quan·tel (prā - zi - kwahn′tel). Praziquantel; um derivado da pirazinoisoquinolina; um agente anti-helmíntico de amplo espectro, heterocíclico, sintético, eficaz contra todas as espécies de esquistossoma que parasitam os seres humanos, bem como contra a maioria dos outros trematódeos e cestódeos adultos.

pra·zo·sin hy·dro·chlo·ride (prā′zō - sin). Cloridrato de prazosin; um agente anti-hipertensivo, que é um bloqueador adrenérgico α₁-específico.

pre-. Pré-; anterior; antes (no tempo ou no espaço). VER TAMBÉM ante-, pro- (1). [L. *prae*]

pre·ag·o·nal (prē - ag′ō - năl). Pré-agônico; que precede imediatamente a morte. [pre- + G. *agōn,* luta (agonia)]

pre·al·bu·min (prē - al - bū′min). Pré-albumina. **1.** Um componente proteico do plasma que possui um peso molecular de aproximadamente 55.000 e contém 1,3% de carboidratos; a concentração plasmática estimada é de 0,3 g/100 ml; são encontrados níveis anormais de pré-albumina em casos de amiloidose familiar. SIN transthyretin. **2.** A zona contendo proteínas observada na eletroforese zonal do soro que migra mais rapidamente que a albumina sérica.

thyroxine-binding p. (TBPA), p. de ligação da tiroxina; proteína localizada na zona da "pré-albumina" à análise eletroforética das proteínas plasmáticas; sua afinidade pela ligação à tiroxina é menor que a da globulina de ligação à tiroxina, porém maior que a da albumina. SIN thyroxine-binding protein (2).

pre·a·nal (prē - ā′nal). Pré-anal; anterior ao ânus.

pre·an·es·thet·ic (prē - an - es - thet′ik). Pré-anestésico; antes da anestesia.

pre·an·ti·sep·tic (prē′an - ti - sep′tik). Pré-anti-séptico; designa o período, principalmente em relação à cirurgia, antes da adoção dos princípios de anti-sepsia.

pre·a·or·tic (prē′ā - ōr′tik). Pré-aórtico; anterior à aorta; designa alguns linfonodos assim situados.

pre·a·sep·tic (prē - ā - sep′tik). Pré-asséptico; designa o período, principalmente o período anti-séptico inicial em relação à cirurgia, antes que fossem conhecidos ou adotados os princípios de assepsia.

pre·au·ric·u·lar (prē - aw - rik′ū - lăr). Pré-auricular; anterior à orelha; designa linfonodos assim situados.

pre·ax·i·al (prē - ak′sē - ăl). Pré-axial. **1.** Anterior ao eixo do corpo ou de um membro, estando este último em posição anatômica. **2.** Designa a parte do broto de um membro situada cranial ao eixo do membro; a face radial do membro superior e a face tibial do membro inferior.

pre·cal·cif·er·ol (prē - kal - si′fer - ol). Pré-calciferol; o precursor imediato do ergocalciferol e do lumisterol.

pre·can·cer (prē - kan′ser). Pré-câncer; uma lesão a partir da qual se atribui o desenvolvimento de uma neoplasia maligna em um grande número de casos, e que pode ou não ser reconhecível clinicamente ou por alterações microscópicas no tecido afetado.

pré-cânceres		
órgão ou tecido	pré-neoplasia	neoplasia maligna posterior
A) irritação crônica		
pele	fotodermatite	"câncer solar"
	dermatite por raios X	câncer por raios X
	dermatite por alcatrão	câncer dos trabalhadores com carvão
	dermatite por arsênico	câncer por arsênico
	dermatite lúpica	câncer lúpico
	ceratose senil doença de Paget condiloma	câncer de pele
cicatrizes	cicatriz de queimadura cicatriz sifilítica cicatriz de fístula cicatriz de úlcera de perna	câncer cicatricial
úlceras	úlcera crônica úlcera varicosa	câncer ulcerado
	fístula óssea fístula retal	câncer de fístula
esôfago	esôfago de Barrett	metaplasia escamosa
estômago	úlcera gástrica gastrite	carcinoma *ex ulcere*
fígado, vesícula biliar	colelitíase	adenocarcinoma, carcinoma cirroso, carcinoma da vesícula biliar
vagina	craurose vulvar	carcinoma vulvar
B) doenças sistêmicas, deformidades teciduais, neoplasias benignas		
pele	nevo pigmentado	melanoma maligno
	dermatose bowenóide xeroderma pigmentoso eritroplasia	carcinomas e sarcomas da pele
mucosa	leucoplasia	câncer da língua câncer da face câncer do palato câncer de pênis
ossos	doença de Paget do osso exostoses	osteossarcoma condrossarcoma
	encondroma	
	osteíte fibrosa leontíase óssea	osteossarcoma osteossarcoma
sistema nervoso	neurofibromatose	fibrossarcoma
estômago/intestino	polipose	adenocarcinoma
útero	mola hidatiforme	epitelioma coriônico
	hiperplasia adenomatosa carcinoma *in situ*	cânceres do útero e do colo do útero
tireóide	nódulo	câncer da tireóide

pre·can·cer·ous (prē - kan′ser - ŭs). Pré-canceroso; relativo a qualquer lesão interpretada como pré-câncer. SIN premalignant.

pre·cap·il·lary (prē - kap′i - lār - ē). Pré-capilar; que precede um capilar; uma arteríola ou vênula.

pre·car·di·ac (prē - kar′dē - ak). Pré-cardíaco; anterior ao coração.

pre·car·di·nal (prē - kar′di - nal). Pré-cardinal; relativo às veias cardinais anteriores.

pre·car·ti·lage (prē-kar′ti-lij). Pré-cartilagem; agregado compacto de células mesenquimais imediatamente antes de sua diferenciação em cartilagem embrionária.

precautions. Precauções. VER Universal Precautions.

pre·ca·va (prē-kā′va). Veia cava superior. SIN superior vena cava.

pre·cen·tral (prē-sen′tral). Pré-central; referente à convolução cerebral imediatamente anterior ao sulco central; giro pré-central.

pre·chor·dal (prē-kōr′dal). Pré-cordal. SIN prochordal.

pre·chrom·ing (prē-krōm′ing). Pré-cromagem; tratamento de um tecido primeiramente com um mordente metálico, seguido por um corante.

pre·cip·i·ta·ble (prē-sip′i-tă-bl). Precipitável; capaz de precipitar.

pre·cip·i·tant (prē-sip′i-tant). Precipitante; qualquer coisa que cause precipitação de uma solução.

pre·cip·i·tate (prē-sip′i-tāt). **1.** Precipitar; fazer com que uma substância em solução separe-se como um sólido. **2.** Precipitado; um sólido separado de uma solução ou suspensão; um floco ou grumo, como aquele resultante da mistura de um antígeno específico e seu anticorpo. **3.** Acúmulo de células inflamatórias no endotélio corneano na uveíte (precipitados ceráticos). [L. *praecipito*, pp. -*atus*, lanças de cabeça para baixo]
   keratic p.'s, precipitados ceráticos; células inflamatórias no endotélio da córnea. SIN punctate keratitis, keratitis punctata.
   mutton-fat keratic p.'s, precipitados ceráticos de gordura de carneiro; precipitados coalescentes que formam pequenas placas que se tornam gradualmente mais translúcidas.
   pigmented keratic p.'s, precipitados ceráticos pigmentados; precipitados que ocorrem em olhos com íris castanha ou após inflamação prolongada.
   red p., precipitado vermelho. SIN mercuric oxide, red.
   sweet p., calomel. SIN calomel.
   white mercuric p., precipitado mercúrico branco. SIN ammoniated mercury.
   yellow p., precipitado amarelo. SIN mercuric oxide, yellow.

pre·cip·i·ta·tion (prē-sip-i-tā′shŭn). Precipitação. **1.** O processo de formação de um sólido previamente mantido em solução ou suspensão em um líquido. **2.** O fenômeno de aglomeração de proteínas no soro produzido pela adição de uma precipitina específica. [ver precipitate]
   double antibody p., p. de anticorpo duplo; método de separação de antígeno ligado ao anticorpo (p. ex., insulina) do antígeno livre pela precipitação do primeiro com anticorpo específico para imunoglobulina. SIN double antibody immunoassay, double antibody method.
   immune p., imunoprecipitação. SIN immunoprecipitation.

pre·cip·i·tin (prē-sip′i-tin). Precipitina; anticorpo que, em condições adequadas, combina-se ao seu antígeno específico e solúvel e causa sua precipitação da solução. SIN precipitating antibody.

pre·cip·i·tin·o·gen (prē-sip-i-tin′ō-jen). Precipitinogênio. **1.** Antígeno que estimula a formação de precipitina específica quando injetado no corpo de um animal. **2.** Um antígeno solúvel precipitável. SIN precipitogen. [precipitin + G. -*gen*, que produz]

pre·cip·i·tin·o·ge·noid (prē-sip-i-tin′ō-jĕ-noyd). Precipitinogenóide; precipitinogênio alterado por meio de aquecimento, assim resultando em uma substância que se combina à precipitina específica, mas não leva à formação de um precipitado.

pre·cip·i·to·gen (prē-sip′i-tō-jen). Precipitinogênio. SIN precipitinogen.

pre·cip·i·toid (prē-sip′i-toyd). Precipitóide; precipitina tratada com calor que, quando misturada ao precipitinogênio específico, não causa um precipitado e ainda interfere com o efeito precipitante da precipitina não-aquecida adicional. [precipitin + G. *eidos*, semelhança]

pre·cip·i·to·phore (prē-sip′i-tō-fōr). Precipitóforo; na teoria da cadeia lateral de Ehrlich, a porção de uma molécula de precipitina necessária na formação de um precipitado, distinta do grupo haptóforo. [precipitin + G. *phoros*, que conduz]

pre·ci·sion (prē-sĭ′zhun). Precisão. **1.** A qualidade de ser bem definido ou declarado; uma medida de precisão é o número de alternativas distinguíveis a uma medida. **2.** Em estatística, o inverso da variação de uma medida ou estimativa. **3.** Reprodutibilidade de um resultado quantificável; uma indicação do erro aleatório.

pre·clin·i·cal (prē-klin′i-kăl). Pré-clínico. **1.** Antes do início da doença. **2.** Um período na educação médica antes de o estudante se envolver com pacientes e trabalho clínico.

pre·co·cious (prē-kō′shŭs). Precoce; que se desenvolve cedo ou rápido demais. [L. *praecox*, prematuro]

pre·coc·i·ty (prē-kos′i-tē). Precocidade; desenvolvimento incomumente cedo ou rápido de características mentais ou físicas. [ver precocious]

pre·cog·ni·tion (prē-kog-nish′un). Precognição; conhecimento prévio, por outros meios além dos sentidos normais, de um evento futuro; uma forma de percepção extra-sensorial. [L. *praecogito*, considerar antes]

pre·con·scious (prē-kon′shŭs). Pré-consciente; em psicanálise, uma das três divisões da psique de acordo com a psicologia topográfica de Freud, sendo as outras duas o consciente e o inconsciente; inclui todas as idéias, pensamentos, experiências passadas e outras impressões da memória que, com esforço, podem ser relembradas conscientemente. Cf. foreconscious.

pre·con·vul·sive (prē-kon-vŭl′siv). Pré-convulsivo; designa o estágio em um paroxismo epiléptico que precede convulsões (p. ex., aura).

pre·cor·dia (prē-kōr′dē-ă). Precórdios; o epigástrio e a superfície anterior da parte inferior do tórax. SIN antecardium. [L. *praecordia* (apenas pl. neutro), o diafragma, as entranhas, de *prae*, antes, + *cor*, (*cord*-), coração]

pre·cor·di·al (prē-kōr′dē-ăl). Precordial; relativo ao precórdio.

pre·cor·di·al·gia (prē′kōr-dē-al′jē-ă). Precordialgia; dor na região precordial. [precordia + G. *algos*, dor]

pre·cor·di·um (prē-kōr′dē-ŭm). Precórdio; singular de precordia.

pre·cos·tal (prē-kos′tal). Pré-costal; anterior às costelas. [pre- + L. *costa*, costela]

pre·crit·i·cal (prē-krit′i-kăl). Pré-crítico; relativo à fase antes de uma crise.

pre·cu·ne·al (prē-koo′nē-ăl). Pré-cuneal; anterior ao cúneo.

pre·cu·ne·ate (prē-koo′nē-āt). Relativo ao pré-cúneo.

pre·cu·ne·us (prē-koo′nē-ŭs) [TA]. Pré-cúneo; divisão da superfície medial de cada hemisfério cerebral entre o cúneo e o lóbulo paracentral; situa-se acima do sulco subparietal e é limitada, anteriormente, pelo ramo marginal do sulco do cíngulo e, posteriormente, pelo sulco parietooccipital. SIN lobulus quadratus (2), quadrate lobe (3), quadrate lobule (2). [pre- + L. *cuneus*, cunha]

pre·cur·sor (prē-ker′ser). Precursor; aquilo que precede outro ou do qual outro é derivado, aplicado especificamente a uma substância fisiologicamente inativa que é convertida em uma enzima ativa, vitamina, hormônio, etc., ou em uma substância química que é transformada em uma estrutura maior no decorrer da síntese desta última. [L. *praecursor*, de *prae*-, pré-, + *curro*, correr]

pre·den·tin (prē-den′tin). Pré-dentina; a matriz fibrilar orgânica da dentina antes de sua calcificação.

pre·di·a·be·tes (prē′dī-ă-bē′tēz). Pré-diabetes; estado de diabetes melito potencial, com tolerância normal à glicose, mas com maior risco de desenvolver diabetes (p. ex., história familiar). Termo declarado obsoleto pela *American Diabetes Association*.

pre·di·as·to·le (prē-dī-as′tō-lē). Pré-diástole; o intervalo no ritmo cardíaco imediatamente anterior à diástole. SIN late systole.

pre·di·a·stol·ic (prē-dī-ă-stol′ik). Pré-diastólico; sistólico tardio (telessistólico), relativo ao intervalo que precede a diástole cardíaca.

pre·di·crot·ic (prē-dī-krot′ik). Pré-dicrótico; que precede a incisura dicrótica.

pre·di·ges·tion (prē-dī-jes′chun). Pré-digestão; o início artificial da digestão de proteínas (proteólise) e amidos (amilólise) antes de serem ingeridos.

pre·dis·pose (prē′dis-pōz). Predispor; tornar suscetível.

pre·dis·po·si·tion (prē′dis-pō-zish′un). Predisposição; uma condição de suscetibilidade especial a uma doença.

pred·nis·o·lone (pred-nis′ō-lōn). Prednisolona; análogo desidrogenado do cortisol com as mesmas ações e empregos do cortisol; um potente glicocorticóide.
   p. acetate, acetato de p.; mesmos empregos que a p.; adequado para administração intramuscular.
   p. butylacetate, butilacetato de p.. SIN p. tebutate.
   p. sodium phospate, fosfato sódico de p.; mais solúvel que a p. e os outros ésteres da p. e útil quando se deseja uma ação com início rápido ou de curta duração; adequado para administração intra-sinovial, parenteral e tópica.
   p. succinate, succinato de p.; composto de p. adequado para administração intramuscular, intravenosa ou retal.
   p. tebutate, tebutato de p.; mesmas ações e empregos que a p., mas com maior duração da ação e adequado para injeção intra-sinovial e nos tecidos moles. SIN p. butylacetate.

pred·ni·sone (pred′ni-sōn). Prednisona; um análogo desidrogenado da cortisona, com as mesmas ações e empregos; deve ser convertida em prednisolona antes de tornar-se ativa; inibe a proliferação de linfócitos.

pred·nyl·i·dene (pred-nil′i-dēn). Prednilideno; um glicocorticóide.

pre·dor·mi·tal (prē-dōr′mi-tăl). Relativo ao *predormitum*.

pre·dor·mi·tum (prē-dōr′mi-tŭm). O estágio de semi-inconsciência que precede o sono. [pre- + L. *dormio*, dormir]

pre·duc·tal (prē-dŭk′tal). Pré-ductal; relativo à parte da aorta proximal à abertura aórtica do canal arterial.

pre-e·clamp·sia (prē-ē-klamp′sē-ă). Pré-eclâmpsia; desenvolvimento de hipertensão arterial com proteinúria e/ou edema, devido à gravidez ou à influência de uma gravidez recente; geralmente ocorre após a 20.ª semana de gestação, mas pode se desenvolver antes desse período na presença de doença trofoblástica. [pre- + G. *eklampsis*, brilho vivo (eclâmpsia)]
   superimposed p., p. superposta; o desenvolvimento de pré-eclâmpsia em um paciente com doença vascular ou renal hipertensiva crônica; quando a hipertensão arterial precede a gravidez conforme estabelecido por registros prévios da pressão arterial, é necessário que haja aumento da pressão sistólica de 30 mm Hg ou aumento da pressão diastólica de 15 mm Hg e o desenvolvimento de proteinúria e/ou edema, durante a gravidez, para estabelecer o diagnóstico.

pre·ep·i·glot·tic (prē′ep-i-glot′ik). Pré-epiglótico; anterior à epiglote.

pre·e·rup·tive (prē-e-rŭp′tiv). Pré-eruptivo; indica a fase de uma doença exantematosa que precede a erupção.
pre·ex·ci·ta·tion (prē′ek-sī-tā′shŭn). Pré-excitação; ativação prematura de parte do miocárdio ventricular por um impulso que segue por uma via anômala e, assim, evita retardo fisiológico na junção atrioventricular; uma parte intrínseca da síndrome de Wolff-Parkinson-White.
  ventricular p., p. ventricular. VER Wolff-Parkinson-White *syndrome*.
pre·for·ma·tion. Pré-formação. VER preformation *theory*.
pre·fron·tal (prē-fron′tăl). Pré-frontal. **1.** Designa a porção anterior do lobo frontal do cérebro. **2.** Designa o córtex frontal granular rostral à área pré-motora.
pre·gan·gli·on·ic (prē′gang-glē-on′ik). Pré-ganglionar; situado proximal a ou precedendo um gânglio; referente especificamente aos neurônios motores pré-ganglionares do sistema nervoso autônomo (localizados na medula espinal e no tronco cerebral) e às fibras nervosas mielinizadas, pré-ganglionares, pelas quais estão unidos aos gânglios autônomos.
preg·nan·cy (preg′nan-sē). Gravidez; o estado de uma mulher após a concepção e até o fim da gestação. SIN fetation, gestation, gravidism, graviditas. [L. *praegnans* (*praegnant-*), grávida, de *prae*, antes, + *gnascor*, pp. *natus*, nascer]

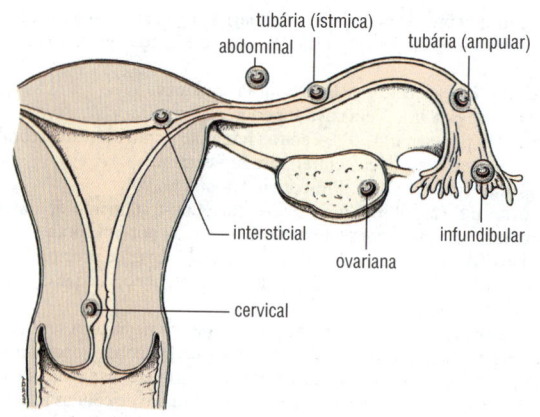

locais de gravidez ectópica

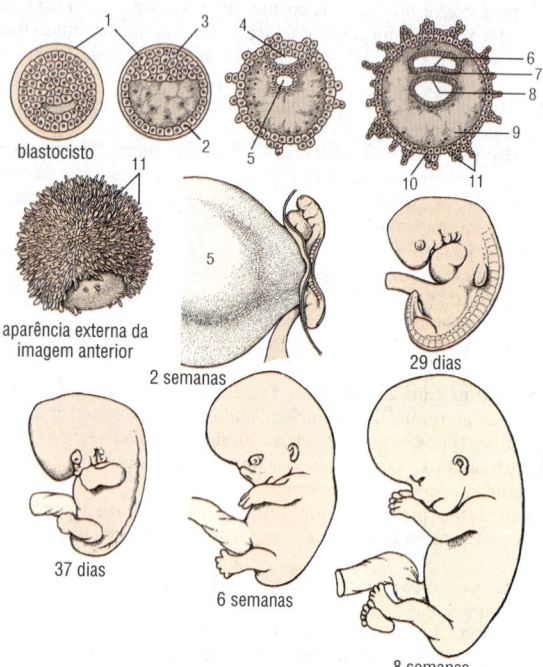

desenvolvimento: do blastocisto ao feto; (1) zona pelúcida, (2) trofectoderma, (3) massa celular interna, (4) cavidade amniótica, (5) saco vitelino, (6) ectoderma, (7) mesoderma, (8) endoderma, (9) mesoderma, (10) trofectoderma, (11) vilosidades coriônicas

abdominal p., g. abdominal; a implantação e o desenvolvimento do ovo na cavidade peritoneal, geralmente secundário a uma ruptura precoce de uma prenhez tubária; muito raramente, pode haver implantação primária na cavidade peritoneal. SIN abdominocyesis (1), intraperitoneal p.
aborted ectopic p., g. ectópica abortada. SIN tubal *abortion*.
ampullar p., g. ampular; g. tubária situada próximo da porção média do oviduto.
cervical p., g. cervical; a implantação e o desenvolvimento do óvulo impregnado no canal cervical.
chemical p., g. química; pequeno aumento, não-mantido, dos níveis de HCG.
combined p., g. combinada; g. uterina e ectópica coexistente.
compound p., g. composta; desenvolvimento de g. uterina além de uma g. ectópica previamente existente (geralmente um litopédio).
cornual p., g. cornual; a implantação e o desenvolvimento do óvulo fecundado em um dos cornos do útero.
ectopic p., g. ectópica; o desenvolvimento de um óvulo fecundado fora da cavidade uterina. SIN eccyesis, extrauterine p., heterotopic p., paracyesis.
extraamniotic p., g. extra-amniótica; g. na qual o córion está intacto, mas o âmnion sofreu ruptura e retração. SIN graviditas examnialis.
extrachorial p., g. extracorial; g. na qual as membranas se rompem e se retraem, causando o desenvolvimento do feto fora do saco coriônico, porém dentro do útero. SIN graviditas exochorialis.
extramembranous p., g. extramembranosa; g. na qual, durante a gestação, o feto rompeu seus envoltórios, entrando em contato direto com as paredes uterinas.
extrauterine p., g. extra-uterina. SIN ectopic p.
fallopian p., g. tubária. SIN tubal p.
false p., falsa g.; condição na qual alguns sinais e sintomas sugerem g., embora a mulher não esteja grávida. SIN hysterical p., pseudocyesis, pseudopregnancy (1), spurious p.
heterotopic p., g. heterotópica. SIN ectopic p.
heterotropic p.'s, gravidezes heterotrópicas; gravidezes que ocorrem simultaneamente em diferentes locais, p. ex., intra-uterina e ampular.
higher order p., g. de maior ordem; g. que possui três fetos (trigêmeos) ou mais.
hydatid p., g. hidática; a presença de uma mola hidatiforme no útero grávido.
hysterical p., g. histérica. SIN false p.
interstitial p., g. intersticial. SIN intramural p.
intraligamentary p., g. intraligamentar; gravidez no ligamento largo.
intramural p., g. intramural; desenvolvimento do óvulo fertilizado na porção uterina da tuba de Falópio. SIN interstitial p., tubouterine p.
intraperitoneal p., g. intraperitoneal. SIN abdominal p.
molar p., g. molar; g. caracterizada por uma neoplasia no interior do útero, na qual parte das vilosidades coriônicas ou todas elas são convertidas em uma massa de vesículas transparentes.
multiple p., g. múltipla; g. de dois ou mais fetos simultaneamente. SIN polycyesis.
mural p., g. mural; g. na parede muscular uterina.
ovarian p., g. ovariana; desenvolvimento de um óvulo fecundado em um folículo ovariano. VER TAMBÉM Spiegelberg *criteria*, em *criterion*. SIN oocyesis, ovariocyesis.
ovarioabdominal p., g. ovarioabdominal; g. ovariana que, em virtude do crescimento do embrião, torna-se abdominal.
persistent ectopic p., g. ectópica persistente; g. ectópica que possui tecido viável persistente, secretando hCG após cirurgia conservadora.
postdate p., g. pós-data; g. de mais de 294 dias ou 42 semanas completas. SIN prolonged p.
prolonged p., g. prolongada. SIN postdate p.
secondary abdominal p., g. abdominal secundária; uma condição na qual o embrião ou feto continua a crescer na cavidade abdominal após sua expulsão da tuba de Falópio ou outro local de seu desenvolvimento primário. SIN abdominocyesis (2).
spurious p., falsa g. SIN false p.
tubal p., g. tubária; desenvolvimento de um óvulo fecundado na tuba de Falópio. SIN fallopian p., salpingocyesis.
tuboabdominal p., g. tuboabdominal; desenvolvimento de g. ectópica parcialmente na tuba de Falópio e parcialmente na cavidade abdominal.
tuboovarian p., g. tubovariana; desenvolvimento do óvulo na extremidade fimbriada da tuba de Falópio e envolvendo o ovário.
tubouterine p., g. tubouterina. SIN intramural p.
twin p., g. gemelar; g. que pode resultar da fertilização de dois óvulos distintos ou de um único óvulo. VER TAMBÉM twin.
uterine p., g. uterina; desenvolvimento do feto no útero.
uteroabdominal p., g. uteroabdominal; desenvolvimento do ovo basicamente no útero e, depois, em virtude da ruptura do útero, na cavidade abdominal.
preg·nane (preg′nān). Pregnano; hidrocarboneto que dá origem a duas séries de esteróides provenientes do 5α-pregnano (originalmente alopregnano) e 5β-pregnano (17β-etiletiocolano). O 5β-pregnano dá origem às progesteronas, álcoois pregnanos, cetonas e vários hormônios adrenocorticais, e é encontrado

principalmente na urina como um produto metabólico dos compostos 5β-pregnano. Quanto à estrutura, ver steroids.

preg·nane·di·ol (preg-nan-dī′ol). Pregnanediol; 5β-pregnano-3α,20α-diol; o principal metabólito esteróide da progesterona, biologicamente inativo e presente como glucuronato de pregnanediol na urina.

preg·nane·di·one (preg-nan-dī′ōn). Pregnanediona; 5β-pregnano-3,20-diona; um metabólito da progesterona, formado em quantidades relativamente pequenas, que ocorre nas formas isoméricas 5α e 5β.

preg·nane·tri·ol (preg-nan-trī′ol). Pregnanetriol; 5β-pregnano-3α,17α,20α-triol; um metabólito urinário da 17-hidroxiprogesterona e um precursor da biossíntese do cortisol; sua excreção está aumentada em algumas doenças do córtex supra-renal e após administração de corticotropina.

preg·nant. Grávida; indica uma fêmea grávida. SIN gravid. [ver pregnancy]

preg·nene (preg′nēn). Pregneno; um esteróide insaturado que tem importância basicamente terminológica; utilizado na nomenclatura sistêmica de esteróides apropriados de 21 carbonos.

preg·nen·in·o·lone (preg-nen-in′ō-lōn, preg-nen′in-). Pregneninolona. SIN ethisterone.

preg·nen·o·lone (preg-nen′ō-lōn). Pregnenolona; 3β-hidroxi-5-pregneno-20-ona; esteróide que serve como intermediário na biossíntese de numerosos hormônios, incluindo a progesterona.
  p. succinate, succinato de p.; corticosteróide usado no tratamento da artrite reumatóide.

pre·hal·lux (prē-hal′uks). Pré-hálux; dedo supranumerário, geralmente apenas parcial, fixado à borda medial do hálux. [pre- + L. mod. *hallux*, hálux]

pre·hel·i·cine (prē-hel′i-sēn). Pré-helicino; na frente da hélice da orelha.

pre·he·ma·tam·in·ic ac·id (prē′hem-ta-min′ik). Ácido pré-hematamínico. SIN neuraminic acid.

pre·hen·sile (prē-hen′sil). Preênsil; adaptado para segurar ou agarrar. [L. *prehendo*, pp. -*hensus*, agarrar, apreender]

pre·hen·sion (prē-hen′shŭn). Preensão; o ato de apreender ou agarrar.

pre·hor·mone (prē-hor′mōn). Pré-hormônio; um produto secretor glandular, que tem pequena ou nenhuma potência biológica inerente, convertido perifericamente em um hormônio ativo. Cf. prohormone (1).

pre·hy·oid (prē-hī′oyd). Pré-hióide; anterior ou superior ao osso hióide; designa algumas glândulas tireóides acessórias situadas acima do músculo milohióideo.

pre·ic·tal (prē-ik′tal). Pré-ictal; que ocorre antes de uma convulsão ou acidente vascular cerebral. [pre- + L. *ictus*, golpe]

pre·in·duc·tion (prē-in-dŭk′shŭn). Pré-indução; um efeito na terceira geração resultante da ação do ambiente sobre as células germinativas dos avós. [L. *prae*, antes, + *inductio*, indução, de *induco*, induzir]

Preisz, Hugo von, bacteriologista húngaro, 1860–1940.

pre·kal·li·krein (prē-kal-i-krē′in). Pré-calicreína; glicoproteína plasmática que, associada ao cininogênio, serve como co-fator na ativação do fator XII. A pré-calicreína também serve como a pró-enzima para a calicreína plasmática. SIN Fletcher factor.

pre·lac·ri·mal (prē-lak′ri-mal). Pré-lacrimal; anterior ao saco lacrimal.

pre·la·ryn·ge·al (prē-la-rin′jē-al). Pré-laríngeo; anterior à laringe; designa particularmente um ou dois pequenos linfonodos.

pre·lep·to·tene (prē-lep′tō-tēn). Pré-leptóteno; o estágio inicial da prófase na meiose, caracterizado por alterações físico-químicas no citoplasma e no carioplasma e pela contração inicial dos cromossomas. [pre- + leptotene, do G. *leptos*, delgado, + *tainia*, faixa]

pre·leu·ke·mia (prē-loo-kē′mē-a). Pré-leucemia; uma síndrome que, com o tempo, pode transformar-se em leucemia manifesta. É caracterizada por disfunção da medula óssea, que se manifesta por anemia, neutropenia e trombocitopenia. SIN myelodysplastic syndrome.

pre·lim·bic (prē-lim′bik). Pré-límbico; anterior ao limbo da fossa oval.

pre·load (prē′lōd). Pré-carga. **1.** A carga a que um músculo é submetido antes do encurtamento. **2.** SIN ventricular p.
  ventricular p., p. ventricular; antigamente, a pressão diastólica final que distende as paredes ventriculares, determinando o comprimento diastólico final da fibra no início da contração ventricular, ou alguma outra medida dessa carga sobre as fibras musculares antes da contração; hoje é expressa com mais rigor, em termos da tensão na parede nesse momento, relacionada à tensão por unidade de área de secção transversal nas fibras musculares ventriculares (calculada pela lei de Laplace a partir do raio interno e da pressão modificada pela espessura da parede) que equilibra essa pressão transmural imediatamente antes do início da contração. SIN preload (2).

pre·ma·lig·nant (prē-ma-lig′nant). Pré-maligno. SIN precancerous.

pre·ma·ni·a·cal (prē-ma-nī′a-kal). Pré-maníaco; que precede um ataque de mania.

pre·ma·ture (prē-ma-toor′, -choor). Prematuro. **1.** Que ocorre antes do momento habitual ou esperado. **2.** Designa um lactente nascido em uma idade gestacional inferior a 37 semanas; o peso ao nascimento não é mais considerado um critério crítico para uso dessa designação. [L. *praematurus*, muito cedo, de *prae*-, pre- + *maturus*, maduro]

pre·ma·tu·ri·ty (prē-ma-toor′i-tē, -choor′i-tē). Prematuridade. **1.** O estado de ser prematuro. **2.** Em odontologia, contato oclusal deflectivo (deflective occlusal *contact*).

pre·max·il·la (prē-mak-sil′a). Pré-maxila; osso incisivo. **1.** *Termo oficial alternativo para incisive *bone*. **2.** A parte óssea isolada central em uma fenda bilateral completa do lábio. [pre- + L. *maxilla*, maxila]

pre·max·il·lary (prē-mak′si-lār-ē). Pré-maxilar. **1.** Anterior à maxila. **2.** Designa a pré-maxila.

pre·med·i·ca·tion (prē′med-i-ka′shŭn). Pré-medicação. **1.** Administração de fármacos antes da anestesia para aliviar a apreensão, produzir sedação e facilitar a administração de anestesia. **2.** Fármacos usados para esses fins.

pre·mel·a·no·some (prē-mel′a-nō-sōm). Pré-melanossoma; uma vesícula não-pigmentada, ligada à membrana, em um melanócito que contém tirosina e amadurece, transformando-se no melanossoma cheio de melanina; proeminente em melanócitos de albinos.

pre·men·stru·al (prē-men′stroo-al). Pré-menstrual; relativo ao período que precede a menstruação.

pre·men·stru·um (prē-men′stroo-ŭm). O período de poucos dias que precedem a menstruação. [pre- + L. *menstruum*, ntr. *menstrus*, uma vez ao mês, referente a menstruação].

pre·mi·to·chon·dria (prē-mī-tō-kon′drē-a). Pré-mitocôndria. SIN promitochondria.

pre·mo·lar (prē-mō′lar). Pré-molar. **1.** Anterior a um dente molar. **2.** Um dente bicúspide.

pre·mon·o·cyte (prē-mon′ō-sīt). Pré-monócito; um monócito imaturo que não é observado normalmente no sangue circulante. SIN promonocyte.

pre·mor·bid (prē-mor′bid). Pré-mórbido; que precede a ocorrência de uma doença. [pre- + L. *morbidus*, mórbido, de *morbus*, doença]

pre·mu·ni·tion (prē-moo-nish′ŭn). Premunição; um estado de resistência de um hospedeiro à infecção ou reinfecção por um parasita; usado especialmente na epidemiologia da malária. [L. *praemunitio*, fortificação antecipada, de *prae*-, + *munio*, fortificar]

pre·mu·ni·tive (prē-moo′ni-tiv). Premunitivo; relativo à premunição.

pre·my·e·lo·blast (prē-mī′e-lō-blast). Pré-mieloblasto; o primeiro precursor reconhecível do mieloblasto.

pre·my·e·lo·cyte (prē-mī′e-lō-sīt). Pré-mielócito. SIN promyelocyte.

pre·na·ris, pl. **pre·na·res** (prē-nā′ris, nā′rēz). Pré-narina. SIN naris.

pre·na·tal (prē-nā′tal). Pré-natal; que precede o nascimento. SIN antenatal. [pre- + L. *natus*, nascido]

pre·ne·o·plas·tic (prē′nē-ō-plas′tik). Pré-neoplásico; que precede a formação de qualquer neoplasia, benigna ou maligna; uma condição pré-neoplásica nem sempre é pré-cancerosa, embora o termo freqüentemente seja usado de forma errada nesse sentido. [pre- + G. *neos*, novo, + *plastikos*, formador]

Prentice, Charles F., óptico norte-americano, 1854–1946. VER P. *rule*.

pren·yl (pren′il). Prenil; resíduos poli ou multiprenil ou derivados dele, aparentemente formados por polimerização término-terminal de moléculas de isopreno; encontrado nos isoprenóides na natureza.

pre·nyl·a·mine (pre-nil′a-mēn). Prenilamina; um agente antianginoso.

pre·nyl·a·tion (pren′il-a′shŭn). Prenilação; a adição covalente de resíduos prenil e multiprenil a uma macromolécula.

pre·op·er·a·tive (prē-op′er-a-tiv). Pré-operatório; que precede uma operação.

pre·op·tic (prē-op′tik). Pré-óptico; referente à região pré-óptica (preoptic *region*).

pre·o·ral (prē-o′ral). Pré-oral; na frente da boca. [pre- + L. *os* (or-), boca]

pre·os·te·o·blast (prē-os′tē-ō-blast). Pré-osteoblasto. SIN osteoprogenitor cell.

pre·ox·y·gen·a·tion (prē′ok-sē-je-nā′shŭn). Pré-oxigenação; desnitrogenação com oxigênio a 100% antes da indução de anestesia geral.

prep (prep). Preparar a pele ou outra superfície corporal para um procedimento cirúrgico, geralmente por limpeza e aplicação de soluções anti-sépticas. [gíria para preparo]

pre·pal·a·tal (prē-pal′a-tal). Pré-palatino; relativo à parte anterior do palato, ou anterior ao osso palatino.

prep·a·ra·tion (prep-a-ra′shŭn). Preparo. **1.** Ato de aprontar. **2.** Algo aprontado, como uma mistura medicinal ou de outro tipo, ou uma amostra histológica. [L. *praeparatio*, de *prae*, antes, + *paro*, pp. -*atus*, aprontar]
  cavity p., p. da cavidade; **(1)** remoção de cáries dentárias e preparo cirúrgico da estrutura remanescente do dente para receber uma restauração dentária; **(2)** a forma final de uma escavação em um dente resultante desse preparo.
  corrosion p., p. por corrosão; p. no qual as partes ocas, como ductos, vasos ou alvéolos pulmonares, são preenchidas por uma substância que endurece e persiste após dissolver os tecidos por digestão.
  cytologic filter p., p. de filtro citológico; uma amostra citológica feita por deposição de uma amostra aquosa (obtida por vários métodos de muitos locais do corpo) sobre um filtro com poros de tamanho uniforme, menores que o material celular a ser concentrado; isso é seguido por fixação e coloração, geralmente com álcool etílico a 95% e coloração por Papanicolaou.

heart-lung p., p. cardiopulmonar; um preparo animal no qual o sangue (tornado incoagulável) circula através do coração e pulmões e através de um sistema artificial de vasos que representa a circulação sistêmica; este último é conectado à aorta dividida de um lado e à veia cava superior do outro; usado em estudos fisiológicos do coração e da circulação.

pre·par·tu·ri·ent (prē-par-too′rē-ent). Pré-parturiente; relativo ao período antes do nascimento.

pre·pa·tel·lar (prē-pă-tel′ăr). Pré-patelar; anterior à patela.

pre·per·i·to·ne·al (prē′per-i-tō-nē′ăl). Pré-peritoneal; designa uma camada adiposa entre o peritônio e a fáscia transversal na parede abdominal ânteroinferior.

pre·phe·nic ac·id (prē-fē′nik, -fen′ik). Ácido prefênico; intermediário na conversão microbiana do ácido xiquímico em L-fenilalanina e L-tirosina.

pre·pla·cen·tal (prē-pla-sen′tăl). Pré-placentário; antes da formação de uma placenta.

preponderance (prē-pon′der-ans). Preponderância; qualidade de supremacia, ou que excede em extensão ou importância.

   directional p., p. direcional; um predomínio direito ou esquerdo do nistagmo, calculado a partir das respostas ao teste calórico biaural, bitérmico.

pre·po·ten·tial (prē-pō-ten′shăl). Pré-potencial; um aumento gradual do potencial entre potenciais de ação como uma oscilação fásica na atividade elétrica da membrana celular, que estabelece sua freqüência de atividade automática, como no ureter ou no marcapasso cardíaco.

pre·pro·col·la·gen (prē-prō-kol-ō-jen). Pré-pró-colágeno; o precursor do colágeno sintetizado nos ribossomas; pró-colágeno com uma seqüência condutora ou sinalizadora que direciona a cadeia polipeptídica para o espaço vesicular do retículo endoplasmático.

pre·pro·in·su·lin (prē-prō-in′soo-lin). Pré-pró-insulina; a proteína precursora da pró-insulina. VER preprotein.

pre·pro·pro·tein (prē-prō-prō′tēn). Pré-pró-proteína; um precursor de uma pró-proteína secretora inativa.

pre·pro·tein (prē-prō′tēn). Pré-proteína; uma proteína secretora com uma região peptídica sinalizadora fixada.

pre·psy·chot·ic (prē-sī-kot′ik). Pré-psicótico. 1. Relativo ao período que precede o início da psicose. 2. Designa a possibilidade de sofrer um episódio psicótico, que parece iminente sob estresse contínuo.

pre·pu·ber·al, pre·pu·ber·tal (prē-pū′ber-ăl, -ber-tăl). Pré-púbere; antes da puberdade.

pre·pu·bes·cent (prē-pū-bes′ent). Pré-pubescente; imediatamente anterior ao início da puberdade.

pre·puce (prē′poos) [TA]. Prepúcio; uma prega cutânea livre que cobre. SIN preputium [TA], foreskin*. [L. praeputium, prepúcio]

   p. of clitoris [TA], p. do clitóris; a prega externa dos lábios menores, que forma um capuz sobre o clitóris. SIN preputium clitoridis.

   hooded p., p. coberto; formação circunferencial incompleta de prepúcio com um componente dorsal (o capuz dorsal), mas com uma porção ventral ausente ou incompleta. Tipicamente observado em meninos com hipospádias ou encurvamento distal isolado. Na condição rara de epispádia, a porção incompleta pode ser ventral.

   p. of penis [TA], p. do pênis; a prega cutânea livre que cobre, de forma mais ou menos completa, a glande do pênis. SIN foreskin of penis [TA], preputium penis [TA].

   ventral apron p., p. em avental ventral; o prepúcio incompleto observado em pacientes com epispádia, tipicamente de forma que permanece um avental ventral.

pre·pu·ti·al (pre-pū′shē-ăl). Prepucial; relativo ao prepúcio.

pre·pu·ti·ot·o·my (prē-pū′shē-ot′ō-mē). Prepuciotomia; incisão do prepúcio. [preputium + G. tomē, incisão]

pre·pu·ti·um, pl. **pre·pu·tia** (prē-pū′shē-ŭm, shē-ă) [TA]. Prepúcio. SIN prepuce. [L. praeputium]

   p. clitor′idis, p. do clitóris. SIN *prepuce* of clitoris.

   p. penis [TA], p. do pênis. SIN *prepuce* of penis.

pre·py·lor·ic (prē-pī-lōr′ik). Pré-pilórico; anterior ao piloro ou que o precede; designa a constrição temporária da parede do estômago que separa o fundo do antro durante a digestão.

pre·rec·tal (prē-rek′tăl). Pré-retal; anterior ao reto ou que o precede.

pre·re·duced (prē-rē-doosd′). Pré-reduzido; relativo a meios bacteriológicos que são fervidos, colocados em tubo sob gás sem oxigênio, com agentes redutores químicos e indicador colorimétrico redox em tubos ou frascos tampados, sendo depois esterilizados.

pre·re·nal (prē-rē′năl). Pré-renal; anterior a um rim. [L. ren, rim]

pre·ret·i·nal (prē-ret′i-năl). Pré-retiniano; anterior à retina.

pre·sa·cral (prē-sā′krăl). Pré-sacral; anterior ao sacro ou que o precede.

△ **presby-, presbyo-.** Presbi-, presbio-; idade avançada. VER TAMBÉM gero-. [G. *presbys,* homem idoso]

pres·by·a·cou·sia (prez-bē-ă-koo′sē-ă). Presbiacusia. SIN *presbyacusis.*

pres·by·a·cu·sis, pres·by·a·cu·sia (prez′bē-ă-koo′sis). Presbiacusia; perda da capacidade de perceber ou discriminar sons associada ao envelhecimento; o padrão e a idade de início variam. SIN presbyacousia, presbycusis. [presby- + G. *akousis,* audição]

pres·by·a·sta·sis (prez′bī-ă-stā′sis). Presbiastasia; comprometimento da função vestibular associado ao envelhecimento. [presby- + G. *a-* priv. + *stasis,* parado]

pres·by·at·rics (prez-bē-at′riks). Presbiatria; termo raramente usado para geriatria. [presby- + G. *iatreia,* tratamento médico]

pres·by·cu·sis (prez-bē-koo′sis). Presbiacusia. SIN *presbyacusis.*

pres·by·o·pia (Pr) (prez-bē-ō′pē-ă). Presbiopia; a perda fisiológica da acomodação dos olhos na idade avançada, diz-se que começa quando o ponto próximo se afastou além de 22 cm. [presby- + G. *ōps,* olho]

pres·by·op·ic (prez′bē-op′ik, -ō′pik). Presbiópico; relativo a ou que sofre de presbiopia.

pre·scribe (prē-skrīb). Prescrever; dar orientações, orais ou por escrito, para o preparo e a administração de um remédio a ser usado no tratamento de qualquer doença. [L. *prae-scribo,* pp. *-scriptus,* escrever antes]

pre·scrip·tion (prē-skrip′shun). Prescrição. **1.** Uma fórmula escrita para preparo e administração de qualquer remédio. **2.** Uma preparação medicinal composta de acordo com as orientações formuladas, que consistem em quatro partes: 1) *superescrição* (cabeçalho), consiste na palavra *receita* (*recipe*), tome ou em seu sinal, R; 2) *inscrição*, a parte principal da prescrição, que contém os nomes e as quantidades dos fármacos prescritos; 3) *subscrição*, orientações para misturar os ingredientes e designação da forma (comprimido, pó, solução, etc.) na qual o fármaco deve ser apresentado, geralmente começando com a palavra *misce*, misturar, ou sua abreviatura, M; 4) *signatura*, orientações para o paciente acerca da dose e do número de vezes que deve tomar o remédio, precedida pela palavra *signa*, designar, ou sua abreviatura, S. ou Sig. [L. *praescriptio;* ver prescribe]

   shotgun p.' uma prescrição contendo muitos ingredientes, alguns dos quais podem ser inúteis, em uma tentativa de cobrir todos os tipos possíveis de tratamento que podem ser necessários; um termo pejorativo.

pre·se·nile (prē-sē′nīl). Pré-senil; antes do início habitual da senilidade, como na demência pré-senil (presenile *dementia*), que é mais leve.

pre·se·nil·i·ty (prē-se-nil′i-tē). Pré-senilidade; idade avançada prematura; a condição de um indivíduo que não tem idade avançada, mas que exibe as características físicas e mentais da idade avançada, mas não ao ponto da senilidade. [pre- + L. *senilis,* senil]

pre·se·ni·um (prē-sē′nē-ŭm). O período que precede a idade avançada.

pre·sent (prē-zent′). **1.** Apresentar-se; preceder ou aparecer primeiro no óstio do útero, tratando-se da parte do feto que se palpa primeiro durante o exame. **2.** Apresentar-se para exame, tratamento, etc., tratando-se de um paciente. [L. *praesens* (*-sent-*), p. pres. de *prae-sum,* estar antes de, estar à mão]

ℹ **pre·sen·ta·tion** (prē′zen-tā′shun, prez′). Apresentação; a parte do feto que se apresenta no estreito superior da pelve materna; o occipúcio, o queixo e o sacro são, respectivamente, os pontos determinantes na apresentação de vértice, de face e pélvica. VER TAMBÉM position (3). Ver também entradas em position. [ver present]

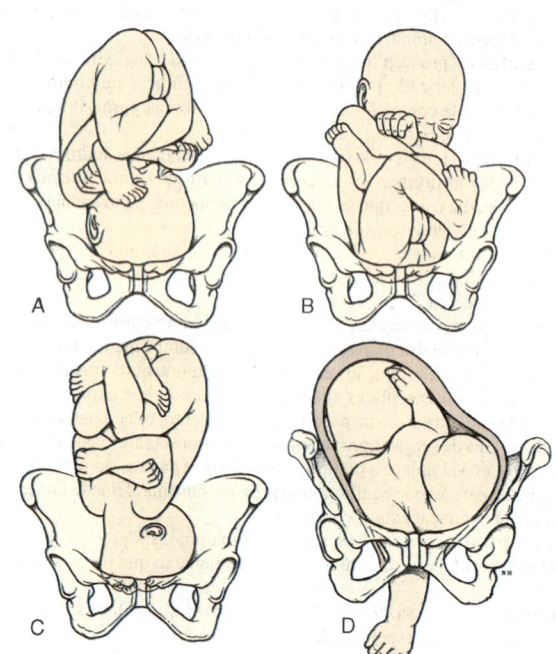

apresentações fetais: (A) cefálica, (B) pélvica, (C) face, (D) transversal

acromion p., a. de acrômio. SIN shoulder p.
breech p., a. pélvica; apresentação de qualquer parte da extremidade pélvica do feto, as nádegas, os joelhos ou os pés; mais apropriadamente, apenas as nádegas; a apresentação pélvica franca ocorre quando o feto se apresenta pela extremidade pélvica; as coxas podem estar fletidas e as pernas estendidas sobre as superfícies anteriores do corpo; na **apresentação pélvica completa,** as coxas podem estar fletidas sobre o abdome e as pernas sobre as coxas; e, na **apresentação podálica,** os pés podem ser a parte mais baixa; na **apresentação pélvica incompleta (modo de pé), apresentação pélvica incompleta (modo de joelho),** uma perna pode manter a posição que é típica de uma das apresentações mencionadas antes, enquanto o outro pé ou joelho pode se apresentar. SIN pelvic p.
brow p., a. de fronte. VER cephalic p.
cephalic p., a. cefálica; apresentação de qualquer parte da cabeça fetal, geralmente as partes superior e posterior, em virtude de flexão, de forma que o queixo fique em contato com o tórax na apresentação de vértice; pode haver graus de flexão de forma que a parte de apresentação é a grande fontanela na apresentação sincipital, a fronte na apresentação de fronte, ou a face na apresentação de face. SIN head p.
compound p., a. composta; prolapso de uma extremidade, geralmente a mão, ao longo da parte de apresentação, com ambos na pelve simultaneamente.
face p., a. de face. VER cephalic p.
footling p., a. podálica. VER breech p.
frank breech p., a. pélvica franca. VER breech p.
head p., a. cefálica. SIN cephalic p.
incomplete foot p., a. podálica incompleta. VER breech p.
knee p., a. de joelho. VER breech p.
pelvic p., a. pélvica. SIN breech p.
placental p., a. placentária. SIN placenta previa.
polar p., a. polar; a apresentação de um dos pólos do ovóide fetal; pode ser uma apresentação cefálica ou pélvica, ou uma situação longitudinal.
shoulder p., a. de ombro; apresentação córmica, nem cefálica nem pélvica, na qual o feto situa-se transversalmente no útero através do eixo do canal de parto. SIN acromion p.
sincipital p., a. de sincipício. VER cephalic. p.
transverse p., a. transversa, a. anormal, que não a cefálica ou a pélvica, na qual o feto está numa posição transversa em relação ao eixo do canal de nascimento.
vertex p., a. de vértice. VER cephalic p.
pre·ser·va·tive (prē-zer′vă-tiv). Conservante; substância adicionada a alimentos ou a uma solução orgânica para evitar alteração química ou ação bacteriana.
pre·so·mite (prē-sō′mīt). Pré-somito; relativo ao estágio embrionário antes do surgimento de somitos (antes do 19.º dia no ser humano).
pre·sphe·noid (prē-sfē′noyd). Pré-esfenóide; na frente do osso ou cartilagem esfenóide.
pre·sphyg·mic (prē-sfig′mik). Pré-esfígmico; que precede o batimento do pulso; designa um breve intervalo após o enchimento dos ventrículos com sangue antes que sua contração force a abertura das válvulas semilunares, correspondendo ao período de contração isovolumétrico. [pre- + G. *sphygmos,* pulso]
pre·spi·nal (prē-spī′năl). Pré-espinal; anterior à coluna vertebral.
pre·spon·dy·lo·lis·the·sis (prē-spon-di-lō-lis′thē-sis). Pré-espondilolistese; uma condição que predispõe à espondilolistese, consistindo em um defeito nas lâminas de uma vértebra lombar antes do desenvolvimento de qualquer deslocamento do corpo vertebral. VER spondylolysis.
pres·sor (pres′er, -ōr). Pressor; que excita a atividade vasomotora; que produz aumento da pressão arterial; designa fibras nervosas aferentes que, quando estimuladas, excitam vasoconstritores, que aumentam a resistência periférica. SIN hypertensor. [L. *premo,* pp. *pressus,* pressionar]
pres·so·re·cep·tive (pres′ō-rē-sep′tiv). Pressorreceptivo; capaz de receber como estímulos alterações da pressão, principalmente alterações da pressão arterial. SIN pressosensitive.
pres·so·re·cep·tor (pres′ō-rē-sep′ter, -tōr). Pressorreceptor. SIN baroreceptor.
pres·so·sen·si·tive (pres-ō-sen′si-tiv). Pressorreceptivo. SIN pressoreceptive.
pres·so·sen·si·tiv·i·ty (pres′ō-sen-si-tiv′i-tē). Pressossensibilidade; o estado de ser capaz de perceber alterações da pressão. VER TAMBÉM pressoreceptive.
reflexogenic p., p. reflexogênica; pressossensibilidade capaz de iniciar a regulação da freqüência cardíaca, do tônus vascular e da pressão arterial.
pres·sure (P, *P***)** (presh′ŭr). Pressão. **1.** Uma tensão ou força que atua em qualquer direção contra resistência. **2.** (*P,* freqüentemente seguido por um subscrito indicando a localização.) Em física e fisiologia, a força por unidade de área exercida por um gás ou líquido contra as paredes de seu recipiente ou que seria exercida sobre uma parede imersa naquele ponto no meio de um corpo líquido.

$$p = \frac{\text{força}}{\text{unidade de área}}$$

A pressão pode ser considerada em relação a alguma pressão de referência, como aquela da atmosfera ambiente (supostamente no outro lado da parede), ou em termos absolutos (em relação a um vácuo perfeito). [L. *pressura,* de *premo,* pp. *pressus,* pressionar]

pressão: várias unidades expressas em pascals (Pa)			
libras por polegada quadrada	lb/pol^2	=	6.894,76 Pa
atmosfera (padrão)	1 atm	=	101.325,0 Pa
atmosfera (técnico)	1 kg/cm^2	=	98.066,5 Pa
coluna de água	1 pol H$_2$O (60°F)	=	248,84 Pa
coluna de mercúrio	1 mm Hg (0°C)	=	133,32 Pa
torr	1 torr	=	133,32 Pa
bar	1 bar	=	100.000 Pa
dinas por centímetro quadrado	1 dina/cm^2	=	0,10 Pa

abdominal p., p. abdominal; p. que circunda a bexiga; estimada a partir da p. retal, gástrica ou intraperitoneal.
absolute p., p. absoluta; p. medida em relação à pressão zero. Cf. gauge p.
acoustic p., p. acústica; em ultra-sonografia, o valor instantâneo da pressão total menos a pressão ambiente; a unidade é o pascal (Pa).
atmospheric p., p. atmosférica. SIN barometric p.
back p., p. retrógrada; p. exercida a montante na circulação em virtude de obstrução ao fluxo, como ocorre quando a congestão na circulação pulmonar resulta de estenose da valva mitral ou de insuficiência ventricular esquerda.
barometric p. (P_B), p. barométrica; a pressão absoluta da atmosfera ambiente, que varia com o clima, a altitude, etc.; expressa em milibars (meteorologia) ou mm Hg ou torr (fisiologia respiratória); ao nível do mar, uma atmosfera (atm, 760 mm Hg ou torr) é equivalente a: 14,69595 lb/pol^2, 1.013,25 milibars, 1.013,25 × 10^6 dinas/cm^2; e, em unidades SI, 101.325 pascals (Pa). SIN atmospheric p.
biting p., p. de mordida. SIN occlusal p.
blood p. (BP), p. arterial; a p. ou tensão do sangue nas artérias sistêmicas, mantida pela contração do ventrículo esquerdo, resistência das arteríolas e capilares, elasticidade das paredes arteriais, bem como pela viscosidade e volume do sangue; expressa como relativa à pressão atmosférica ambiente. SIN piesis.
central venous p. (CVP), p. venosa central; a p. do sangue no sistema venoso na veia cava superior e na porção da veia cava inferior cefálica ao diafragma, normalmente entre 4 e 10 cm de água; está deprimida no choque circulatório e nas deficiências do volume sanguíneo circulante, e aumentada na insuficiência cardíaca e na congestão da circulação venosa.
cerebrospinal p., p. cerebrospinal; a p. do líquido cerebrospinal, normalmente 100–150 mm de água, em relação à pressão atmosférica ambiente.
continuous positive airway p. (CPAP), p. positiva contínua nas vias aéreas; uma técnica de terapia respiratória, usada em pacientes que respiram espontaneamente ou ventilados mecanicamente, na qual a pressão nas vias aéreas é mantida acima da pressão atmosférica durante todo o ciclo respiratório por pressurização do circuito ventilatório.
coronary perfusion p., p. de perfusão coronariana; a pressão na qual o sangue prossegue através da circulação coronariana, principalmente na diástole.
critical p., p. crítica; a pressão mínima necessária para liquefazer um gás na temperatura crítica.
detrusor p., p. do detrusor; o componente da pressão intravesical criado pela tensão (ativa e passiva) exercida pela parede vesical; a pressão transmural através da parede vesical, estimada subtraindo-se a pressão abdominal da pressão intravesical.
diastolic p., p. diastólica; a pressão intracardíaca durante o relaxamento diastólico ou resultante dele; a menor pressão arterial atingida durante qualquer ciclo ventricular.
differential blood p., p. sanguínea diferencial; a pressão arterial em pontos correspondentes nos dois lados do corpo.
Donders p., p. de Donders; aumento de aproximadamente 6 mm Hg mostrado por um manômetro conectado à traquéia quando se abre o tórax de um corpo morto; é causada pelo colapso dos pulmões quando há entrada de ar no tórax.
effective osmotic p., p. osmótica efetiva; a parte da pressão osmótica total de uma solução que orienta a tendência de seu solvente para atravessar um limite, geralmente uma membrana semipermeável; comumente é representada pelo produto da pressão osmótica total da solução e pela razão (corrigida para atividades) do número de partículas dissolvidas que não atravessam a membrana limitante até o número total de partículas na solução; equivalente, em signifi-

cado, à tonicidade; comumente expressa em unidades equivalentes de osmolalidade, e não como pressão em si.

gauge p., p. manométrica; p. medida em relação à pressão atmosférica ambiente; ao nível do mar, é pelo menos 1 atm menor que a pressão na atmosfera. Cf. absolute p.

hydrostatic p., p. hidrostática; a p. exercida por um líquido em virtude de sua energia potencial, ignorando sua energia cinética; freqüentemente usada para distinguir uma p. verdadeira de uma p. osmótica ou para enfatizar a variação de p. em uma coluna de líquido devido ao efeito da gravidade.

intracranial p. (ICP), p. intracraniana; p. na cavidade craniana.

intraocular p., p. intra-ocular; a p. (geralmente medida em milímetros de mercúrio) do líquido intra-ocular no olho, medida por meio de um manômetro.

leak point p., p. de perda; p. de armazenamento na bexiga em que ocorre extravasamento passivo, geralmente em pacientes com bexiga neuropática.

negative p., p. negativa; p. menor que a da atmosfera ambiente.

negative end-expiratory p. (NEEP), p. expiratória final negativa; p. subatmosférica nas vias aéreas ao fim da expiração.

occlusal p., p. oclusal; qualquer força exercida sobre as superfícies oclusais dos dentes. SIN biting p.

oncotic p., p. oncótica; p. osmótica exercida por colóides em solução.

osmotic p. (Π), p. osmótica; a p. que deve ser aplicada a uma solução para impedir a entrada nela de solvente quando a solução e o solvente puro são separados por uma membrana permeável apenas ao solvente (algumas vezes vista de forma menos correta como a força com que a solução atrai solvente através da membrana semipermeável).

partial p. (P), p. parcial; a p. exercida por um único componente de uma mistura de gases, comumente expressa em mm Hg ou torr; para um gás dissolvido em um líquido, a p. parcial é aquela em que um gás estaria em equilíbrio com o gás dissolvido. Antigamente, simbolizada por *p*, seguido pelo símbolo químico em letras maiúsculas (p. ex., pCO_2, pO_2); agora, em fisiologia respiratória, P, seguida por subscritos que indicam a localização e/ou a espécie química (p. ex., P_{CO_2}, P_{O_2}, Pa_{CO_2}).

pleural p., p. pleural; a pressão no espaço pleural entre as pleuras visceral e parietal.

positive end-expiratory p. (PEEP), p. expiratória final positiva (PEFP); técnica usada em terapia respiratória na qual se alcança pressão nas vias aéreas maior que a p. atmosférica ao fim da expiração, por introdução de uma impedância mecânica à expiração. A denominada "auto-PEFP" ocorre quando é necessário aumento do tempo de expiração durante ventilação mecânica e a próxima respiração é realizada antes de a pressão no sistema ter chegado a zero; este pode ser um fenômeno perigoso, que pode causar barotrauma e hipotensão.

pulmonary p., p. pulmonar; a pressão sanguínea na artéria pulmonar.

pulmonary capillary wedge p. (PCWP), p. de encunhamento capilar pulmonar (PECP); a pressão obtida pela introdução de um cateter no lado direito do coração até a artéria pulmonar, que é "encunhado" em uma artéria terminal. A PECP é medida deixando-se o fluxo sanguíneo pulmonar guiar a entrada de um cateter-balão flutuante em uma pequena artéria terminal pulmonar. A pressão distal ao cateter encunhado é uma aproximação da pressão diastólica final ventricular esquerda. A pressão registrada com o balão desinsuflado é a pressão na artéria pulmonar.

pulp p., p. da polpa; a pressão na cavidade pulpar dental associada à pressão no líquido extracelular, mas que exibe variações pulsáteis durante o ciclo cardíaco devido ao encerramento da polpa no dente.

pulse p., p. de pulso; a variação na pressão sanguínea que ocorre em uma artéria durante o ciclo cardíaco; é a diferença entre a pressão sistólica ou máxima e a pressão diastólica ou mínima.

selection p., p. de seleção; impacto da reprodução efetiva devido ao impacto ambiental sobre o fenótipo.

solution p., p. da solução; a força que leva átomos ou moléculas a deixar uma partícula sólida e entrar em uma solução (isto é, dissolver).

standard p., p. padrão; a pressão absoluta a que os gases são submetidos em condições padrões (STPD), isto é, 760 mm Hg, 760 torr ou 101.325 N/m² (isto é, 101.325 Pa).

systolic p., p. sistólica; a pressão intracardíaca durante a contração sistólica de uma câmara cardíaca, ou resultante dela; a maior pressão arterial alcançada durante qualquer ciclo ventricular.

transmural p., p. transmural; p. através da parede de uma câmara cardíaca ou de um vaso sanguíneo. No coração, a pressão transmural é o resultado da pressão intracavitária menos a pressão extracavitária (isto é, pericárdica) e é a pressão distensora, isto é, de enchimento verdadeiro da câmara cardíaca, medida quando realizada durante a diástole. Como a pressão pericárdica normalmente se aproxima de zero, a pressão de enchimento geralmente é igual à pressão ventricular diastólica média, evitando as complexidades de medir a pressão pericárdica.

transpulmonary p., p. transmural; a diferença entre a pressão do gás respirado na boca e a pressão pleural ao redor dos pulmões, medida quando as vias aéreas estão abertas; assim, inclui não apenas a pressão transmural do pulmão, mas também qualquer diminuição da pressão ao longo da árvore traqueobrônquica durante o fluxo.

transthoracic p., p. transtorácica; a pressão no espaço pleural medida em relação à pressão da atmosfera ambiente fora do tórax; a pressão transmural através da parede torácica.

vapor p., p. do vapor; a pressão parcial exercida pela fase de vapor de um líquido.

ventricular filling p., p. de enchimento ventricular; a pressão ventricular quando o ventrículo está cheio de sangue, comumente equivalente à pressão atrial média quando não há gradiente valvular AV. A pressão atrial pode ser usada no lugar da pressão transmural porque a pressão pericárdica geralmente varia entre −2 e +2 mm Hg e, portanto, é desprezível. Durante o tamponamento cardíaco, as pressões pericárdica e atrial equilibram-se de forma que a pressão transmural seja igual a zero e as altas pressões atriais não possam ser pressões de "enchimento".

wedge p., p. de encunhamento; a pressão intravascular obtida quando um cateter fino é introduzido até ocluir completamente um pequeno vaso sanguíneo ou é fixado no lugar por insuflação de um pequeno balão; comumente medida no pulmão (artéria pulmonar) para estimar a pressão atrial esquerda.

zero end-expiratory p. (ZEEP), p. expiratória final zero; pressão das vias aéreas que, ao fim da expiração, é igual à pressão atmosférica.

pre·ster·num (prē′ster′nŭm). Pré-esterno. SIN *manubrium* of sternum.

pre·sup·pu·ra·tive (prē-sŭp′u-rā′tiv). Pré-supurativo; designa um estágio inicial em uma inflamação antes da formação de pus.

pre·syn·ap·tic (prē′si-nap′tik). Pré-sináptico; relativo à área no lado proximal de uma fenda sináptica.

pre·sys·to·le (prē-sis′tō-lē). Pré-sístole; a parte da diástole imediatamente anterior à sístole. SIN late diastole.

pre·sys·tol·ic (prē-sis-tol′ik). Pré-sistólico; diastólico final, relativo ao intervalo imediatamente anterior à sístole.

pre·tar·sal (prē-tar′săl). Pré-tarsal; designa a porção anterior, ou inferior, do tarso.

pre·tec·ta (prē-tek′tă). Pré-tectal; oral à parte oculta do duodeno.

pre·tec·tum (prē-tek′tŭm). Pré-teto. SIN pretectal *area.*

pre·thy·roid, pre·thy·roi·de·al, pre·thy·roi·de·an (prē-thī′royd, -thī-roy′dē-ăl, -thī-roy′dē-an). Pré-tireóideo; anterior à ou que precede a glândula ou cartilagem tireóide.

pre·tib·i·al (prē-tib′ē-ăl). Pré-tibial; relativo à porção anterior da perna; designa particularmente alguns músculos.

pre·tra·che·al (prē-trā′kē-al). Pré-traqueal; anterior à traquéia; designa particularmente a camada média da fáscia cervical profunda.

pre·tre·mat·ic (prē-trē-mat′ik). Pré-tremático; relativo à superfície cranial de uma fenda branquial. [pre- + G. *trēma,* perfuração]

pre·tym·pan·ic (prē-tim-pan′ik). Pré-timpânico; anterior ao tímpano.

prev·a·lence (prev′ă-lens). Prevalência; o número de casos de uma doença existente em determinada população em um período específico (*p. no período*) ou em determinado momento (*p. pontual*).

pre·ven·tive (prē-ven′tiv). Preventivo. SIN prophylactic (1). [L. *prae-venio,* pp. *-ventus,* vir antes, evitar]

pre·ver·te·bral (prē-ver′tē-brăl). Pré-vertebral; anterior ao corpo de uma vértebra ou à coluna vertebral; designa particularmente a camada mais profunda da fáscia cervical profunda e os músculos na face anterior da coluna vertebral.

pre·ves·i·cal (prē-ves′i-kăl). Pré-vesical; anterior à bexiga; designa particularmente o espaço retropúbico. [pre- + L. *vesica,* bexiga]

Pre·vo·tel·la (prev′ō-tel′ah). Gênero de bacilos Gram-negativos, imóveis, não-formadores de esporos, obrigatoriamente anaeróbicos, quimio-organotróficos e pleomórficos; contém muitas espécies previamente classificadas no gênero Bacteroides.

pressão intracardíaca (mm Hg)

	onda A	colapso X	onda V	colapso Y	média
átrio direito	até 5	0	até 5	0	até 4
átrio esquerdo	cerca de 8	0	cerca de 10	0	cerca de 6–8
	sistólica		diastólica inicial		diastólica final
ventrículo direito	20–30		0		até 5
ventrículo esquerdo	cerca de 120		0		cerca de 7–10

P. bivia, a espécie de *Prevotella* existente em maior concentração no trato vaginal humano.
P. denticola, uma espécie de bactéria encontrada na boca do ser humano; uma causa de infecções da cavidade oral e das estruturas adjacentes.
P. di'siens, espécie de bactéria associada a infecções humanas, basicamente do aparelho genital feminino. SIN *Bacteroides disiens*.
P. heparinolytica, espécie de bactéria associada a doença periodontal humana.
P. intermedia, espécie encontrada nas fendas gengivais, particularmente associada a gengivite e a outras infecções orais.
P. melani'noge'nica, espécie encontrada na boca, nas fezes, em infecções da boca, tecidos moles, vias respiratórias, trato urogenital e trato intestinal; implicada na doença periodontal; observada na aspiração. A espécie típica de *Pretovella*. SIN *Bacteroides melaninogenicus*.
P. ora'lis, espécie de bactéria encontrada na fenda gengival de seres humanos, bem como em infecções da cavidade oral, das vias respiratórias superiores e do aparelho genital.
P. o'ris, espécie de bactéria isolada na fenda gengival, em infecções sistêmicas, em abscessos da face, pescoço e tórax, em drenagens de ferida, no sangue e em vários líquidos corporais.
pre·zone (pre'zōn). Pré-zona. SIN prozone.
pri·a·pism (prī'a - pizm). Priapismo; ereção persistente do pênis, acompanhada por dor e dor à palpação, resultante de uma condição patológica, e não de desejo sexual; termo livremente usado como sinônimo de satiríase. [ver priapus]
pri·a·pus (prī'a - pŭs). Príapo; pênis. SIN penis. [L. de *Priapus* (G. *Priapos*), deus da procriação]
Prib·now (prib'now). David, biólogo molecular norte-americano do século XX. VER Pribnow *box*.
Price, Ernest Arthur, bioquímico inglês, *1882. VER Carr-P. *reaction*.
Price-Jones, Cecil, hematologista inglês, 1863–1943. VER Price-Jones *curve*.
Priestley, John Gillies, fisiologista britânico, 1880–1941. VER Haldane-P. *sample*.
pril·o·caine hy·dro·chlo·ride (pril'ō - kān). Cloridrato de prilocaína; anestésico local do tipo amida, química e farmacologicamente relacionado com o cloridrato de lidocaína; usado para bloqueios peridurais, caudais e nervos, e para anestesia regional e por infiltração. SIN propitocaine hydrochloride.
pri·ma·cy (prī'ma - sē). Primazia; o estado de ser primário, ou o primeiro em ordem ou importância. [ver primary]
  genital p., p. genital; em psicanálise, a característica primária da fase genital do desenvolvimento psicossexual, isto é, a libido torna-se preponderantemente no pênis.
  oral p., p. oral; em psicanálise, a característica primária da fase oral do desenvolvimento psicossexual, isto é, a libido está concentrada basicamente na zona oral.
pri·mal (prī'măl). Primário. 1. Primeiro ou primário. 2. SIN primordial (2).
pri·ma·quine phos·phate (prī'ma - kwin). Fosfato de primaquina; agente antimalárico particularmente efetivo contra *Plasmodium vivax*, interrompendo a malária vivax recidivante; geralmente administrado com cloroquina.
  p. p. sensitivity, sensibilidade ao fosfato de primaquina; uma sensibilidade ao fosfato de primaquina observada em indivíduos com deficiência de glicose-6-fosfato desidrogenase.
pri·mary (prī'mār - ē). Primário. 1. O primeiro ou em primeiro lugar, como uma doença ou sintomas aos quais outros podem ser secundários ou ocorrer como complicações. 2. Relativo ao primeiro estágio de crescimento ou desenvolvimento. VER primordial. [L. *primarius*, de *primus*, primeiro]
pri·mary re·nin·ism (ren'in - izm). Reninismo primário; superprodução de renina por células justaglomerulares na ausência de um estímulo (como diminuição da perfusão renal); leva ao hiperaldosteronismo, hipertensão, hipocalemia e edema.
pri·mase (prī'māz). Primase; polimerase que atua sobre um filamento modelo de DNA para produzir RNA, resultando na formação de um RNA iniciador necessário na replicação do RNA. SIN dnaG. [primer + -ase]
pri·mate (prī'māt). Primata; um indivíduo da ordem Primates. [L. *primus*, primeiro]
Pri·ma·tes (prī - ma'tēz). A ordem mais elevada dos mamíferos, incluindo os seres humanos, os macacos e os lêmures. [L. *primus*, primeiro]
prim·er (prī'mer). Iniciador. 1. Uma molécula (que pode ser um pequeno polímero) que inicia a síntese de uma estrutura maior. SIN starter. 2. Um feromônio que causa uma alteração fisiológica em longo prazo.
pri·mer·ite (prī'mer - rīt) Protomérito. SIN protomerite. [L. *primus*, primeiro, + G. *meros*, parte]
pri·mi·done (prī'mi - dōn). Primidona; um anticonvulsivante usado no tratamento da epilepsia tônico-clônica generalizada e parcial completa.
pri·mi·grav·i·da (prī - mi - grav'i - dă). Primigrávida. VER gravida. [L. de *primus*, primeiro, + *gravida*, uma mulher grávida]
  elderly p., p. idosa; termo obsoleto referente a uma mulher com mais de 35 anos grávida pela primeira vez.
pri·mip·a·ra (prī - mip'a - ră). Primípara. VER para. [L. de *primus*, primeiro, + *pario*, parir]

pri·mi·par·i·ty (prī - mi - par'i - tē). Primiparidade; condição de ser uma primípara.
pri·mip·a·rous (prī - mip'a - rŭs). Primípara; designa uma primípara.
pri·mite (prī'mit). Primito; o membro anterior de um par de gamontes gregarinos em sizígia.
prim·i·tive (prim'i - tiv). Primitivo. SIN primordial (2). [L. *primitivus*, de *primus*, primeiro]
pri·mor·dia (prī - mōr'dē - ă). Plural de primordium.
pri·mor·di·al (prī - mōr'dē - ăl). Primordial. 1. Relativo a um primórdio. 2. Relativo a uma estrutura em seu primeiro estágio ou no estágio inicial de desenvolvimento. SIN primal (2), primitive.
pri·mor·di·um (prī - mōr' - dē - ŭm). Primórdio; um conjunto de células no embrião, indicando o primeiro traço de um órgão ou estrutura. SIN anlage (1). [L. origem, de *primus*, primeiro, + *ordior*, começar]
  genital p., p. genital; aglomeração ovóide de células observada nas larvas rabditiformes do *Strongyloides stercoralis* e ancilóstomos, que se torna o sistema reprodutivo.
prim·o·some (prī - mō - sōm). Primossoma; complexo de proteínas que se ligam à primase em seqüências específicas de DNA que servem como locais para a formação de RNA iniciadores; uma parte do replissoma. [primer + -some]
prim·u·la (prim'ū - lă). Prímula; o rizoma e as raízes de várias espécies de *Primula* (família Primulaceae), prímula ou primavera; foi usada como expectorante, diurético e anti-helmíntico. Em algumas pessoas sensíveis, o contato com a planta causa um exantema. [L. mediev. prímula, fem. do L. *primulus*, primeiro]
pri·mu·lin (prī'mū - lin). [I.C. 49000]. Primulina; corante ácido do tiazol amarelo, usado como corante vital fluorescente.
pri·mus (prī'mŭs). Primeiro; designa a primeira de uma série de estruturas semelhantes. [L.]
prin·ceps, pl. **prin·ci·pes** (prin'seps, -si - pēz). Principal; em anatomia, termo usado para distinguir a maior e mais importante de várias artérias. [L. principal, de *primus*, primeiro, + *capio*, tomar, escolher]
  p. cervi'cis, artéria principal cervical. SIN descending branch of occipital artery.
  p. pol'licis, artéria principal do polegar. SIN princeps pollicis artery.
Princeteau, L.R., médico francês, *1884. VER P. *tubercle*.
prin·ci·ple (prin'si - pl). Princípio. 1. Uma doutrina ou dogma geral ou fundamental. VER TAMBÉM law, rule, theorem. 2. O ingrediente essencial de uma substância, particularmente aquele que confere sua qualidade ou efeito. [L. *principium*, princípio, de *princeps*, principal]
  active p., p. ativo; um constituinte de um fármaco, geralmente um alcalóide ou glicosídeo, de cuja presença depende amplamente a ação terapêutica característica da substância.
  antianemic p., p. antianêmico; o material no fígado (e alguns outros tecidos) que estimula a hematopoese na anemia perniciosa; para fins práticos, o efeito antianêmico de extratos desses tecidos é aproximadamente equivalente ao conteúdo de vitamina B_{12}.
  Bernoulli p., p. de Bernoulli. SIN Bernoulli law.
  bitter p.'s, princípios amargos; classe de substâncias vegetais com um gosto amargo que produzem um aumento reflexo da secreção de saliva, bem como a secreção de sucos digestivos.
  closure p., p. de fechamento; em psicologia, o princípio segundo o qual, quando se vêem estímulos fragmentários formando uma figura quase completa (p. ex., um retângulo incompleto), tende-se a ignorar as partes ausentes e perceber a figura como um todo. VER gestalt.
  consistency p., p. da constância; em psicologia, o desejo do ser humano de ser constante, principalmente em suas atitudes e crenças; teorias de formação do comportamento e das mudanças baseadas no princípio da constância incluem a teoria do equilíbrio, segundo a qual o indivíduo procura evitar incongruências em suas diversas atitudes. VER TAMBÉM cognitive dissonance *theory*.
  Fick p., p. de Fick. SIN Fick method.
  follicle-stimulating p., p. folículo-estimulante. SIN follitropin.
  founder p., p. fundador; as probabilidades condicionais das freqüências de um conjunto de genes em qualquer data futura dependem da composição inicial dos fundadores da população e, em geral, não tendem a retornar para a composição da população da qual se originaram os próprios fundadores.
  hematinic p., p. hematínico; o princípio previamente considerado produzido pela ação do fator intrínseco de Castle sobre um fator extrínseco no alimento, agora reconhecido como vitamina B_{12}.
  Huygens p., p. de Huygens; usado em tecnologia de ultra-som; o princípio que afirma que qualquer fenômeno de onda pode ser analisado como a soma de muitas fontes simples apropriadamente escolhidas considerando-se a fase e a amplitude.
  p. of inertia, p. da inércia. SIN repetition-compulsion p.
  Le Chatelier p., p. de Le Chatelier. SIN Le Chatelier law.
  luteinizing p., p. luteinizante. SIN lutropin.
  mass action p., p. de ação de massa; o princípio fundamental na teoria epidêmica: a incidência de uma doença infecciosa é determinada pelo produto da

prevalência atual pelo número de indivíduos suscetíveis na população. VER TAMBÉM serial *interval*, infection transmission *parameter*.

melanophore-expanding p., p. expansor do melanóforo. SIN melanotropin.
Mitrofanoff p., p. de Mitrofanoff; uso de um canal cateterizável (apêndice, intestino, ureter) para drenar a bexiga como uma alternativa à uretra. VER TAMBÉM appendicovesicostomy.
nirvana p., p. do nirvana; em psicanálise, o princípio que expressa a tendência a atingir um estado de ausência de dor ou preocupação, sem conflito.
organic p., p. orgânico. SIN proximate p.
pain-pleasure p., p. da dor-prazer; um conceito psicanalítico que afirma que, na função psíquica do homem, a pessoa tende a buscar prazer e evitar a dor; um termo que a psicologia experimental tomou emprestado para designar a mesma tendência de um animal em uma situação de aprendizado. SIN pleasure p.
Pauli exclusion p., p. de exclusão de Pauli; a teoria que limita o número de elétrons na órbita ou periferia de um átomo; que não é possível para quaisquer dois elétrons ter todos os quatro números de quantum idênticos.
pleasure p., p. do prazer. SIN pain-pleasure p.
proximate p., p. da aproximação; em química, um composto orgânico que pode existir já formado como parte de alguma outra substância mais complexa (p. ex., vários açúcares, amidos e albuminas). SIN organic p.
reality p., p. da realidade; o conceito de que o princípio do prazer no desenvolvimento da personalidade é modificado pelas demandas da realidade externa; o princípio ou força que impele a criança em crescimento a adaptar-se às demandas da realidade externa.
repetition-compulsion p., p. da repetição-compulsão; em psicanálise, o impulso de redramatizar ou representar novamente experiências ou situações emocionais anteriores. SIN p. of inertia.
ultimate p., um dos elementos químicos.

Pringle, John J. dermatologista inglês, 1855–1922. VER P. *disease*; Bourneville-Pringle *disease*.
Prinzmetal, Myron, cardiologista norte-americano, 1908–1994. VER P. *angina*.

pri·on (prī'on). Príon; pequena partícula proteinácea infecciosa, sem ácido nucleico em sua composição, devido à sua resistência às nucleases; o agente causador, em uma base esporádica, genética ou infecciosa, de seis doenças neurodegenerativas em animais, e quatro em seres humanos; estas últimas são as encefalopatias espongiformes do kuru, doença de Creutzfeldt-Jakob, síndrome de Gerstmann-Straussler-Scheinker e insônia familiar fatal. O gene que codifica o PrP é encontrado no cromossoma 20. SIN prion protein. [proteinaceous infectious particle]

> Stanley B. Prusiner ganhou o Prêmio Nobel em Fisiologia ou Medicina em 1997 pela descoberta dos príons. Prusiner começou sua pesquisa em 1972, para identificar o agente infeccioso da doença de Creutzfeldt-Jakob. Em 1982, ele e seus colegas isolaram uma proteína capaz de transmitir infecção, mas que, ao contrário de outros patógenos conhecidos, não continha DNA nem RNA. O termo de Prusiner para essa proteína, *príon*, foi derivado da expressão *partícula infecciosa proteinácea*. Um gene que codifica essa proteína foi encontrado em todos os animais testados, incluindo seres humanos. A proteína do príon pode exibir 2 conformações estruturais, uma que é normal (mas de função desconhecida), designada PrPc, e uma que resulta em doença, denominada PrPSc. A proteína do príon normal é um componente de linfócitos e outras células, sendo particularmente abundante nas membranas celulares de neurônios do SNC. A proteína do príon PrPSc é extremamente estável e resistente à proteólise, a solventes orgânicos e a altas temperaturas. Uma vez produzida ou adquirida por um hospedeiro adequado, pode iniciar uma reação em cadeia na qual a proteína PrPc normal é convertida na forma PrPSc, mais estável. Após um longo período de incubação assintomático, o PrPSc causador de doença acumula-se para alcançar níveis neurotóxicos. Os sintomas das doenças por príon variam com as partes do encéfalo afetadas. Todas as doenças conhecidas causadas por príon levam à morte dos que são afetados. As doenças por príons são denominadas encefalopatias espongiformes devido ao aspecto histológico do córtex cerebral e do cerebelo afetados, que exibem grandes vacúolos. Provavelmente a maioria das espécies de mamíferos desenvolve essas doenças. Os príons não são vivos, são menores que os vírus e não produzem uma resposta imune em sua forma normal nem em sua forma causadora de doença. Dentre as doenças por príons, além da de Creutzfeldt-Jakob, incluem-se kuru (prevalente antigamente entre o povo Fore da Nova Guiné, que praticava canibalismo ritual), encefalopatia espongiforme bovina (EEB, doença da vaca louca) e scrapie, uma doença de ovinos. Uma nova variante da DCJ pode ter surgido através da transmissão de príons para seres humanos de gado bovino infectado por EEB. As doenças por príons são únicas por serem infecciosas e hereditárias. As formas hereditárias são causadas por mutações transmitidas no gene do príon, localizado no cromossoma 20 em seres humanos. A doença de Gerstmann-Sträussler-Scheinker (GSS) é uma demência hereditária resultante de uma mutação nesse gene. Foram identificadas aproximadamente 50 famílias com mutações GSS. Cerca de 10–15% dos casos de DCJ são causados por mutações hereditárias no gene da proteína do príon. Cepas de camundongos nas quais esse gene foi abolido são imunes à doença causada por príons. Ver Creutzfeldt-Jakob disease, bovine spongiform encephalopathy.

prism (prizm). Prisma; um sólido transparente, com lados convergindo em um ângulo, que deflete um raio luminoso em direção à parte mais grossa (a base) e divide a luz branca em suas cores componentes; em óculos, um prisma corrige o desequilíbrio dos músculos oculares. [G. *prisma*]
enamel p.'s, prismas de esmalte. SIN *prismata* adamantina, em *prisma*.
Fresnel p., p. de Fresnel; p. composto de anéis concêntricos.
Nicol p., p. de Nicol; p. que transmite apenas luz polarizada.
Risley rotary p., p. giratório de Risley; p. com uma base circular que é girada em uma estrutura metálica marcada com uma escala; usado no exame do desequilíbrio dos músculos oculares.

pris·ma, pl. **pris·ma·ta** (priz'mă, priz'mah - tă). Prisma; estrutura semelhante a um prisma. [G. algo serrado, um prisma]
pris'mata adamanti'na, prismas adamantinos; bastões microscópicos, calcificados, que se irradiam da superfície da dentina, formando a substância do esmalte de um dente. SIN enamel fibers, enamel prisms, enamel rods.

pris·mat·ic (priz - mat'ik). Prismático; relativo ou que se assemelha a um prisma.

pri·va·cy (prī'vă - sē). **1.** Privacidade; que está afastado de outros; isolamento; intimidade. **2.** Sigilo; particularmente em psiquiatria e psicologia clínica, respeito pela natureza confidencial da relação terapeuta–paciente.

PRK Acrônimo para photorefractive *keratectomy* (ceratectomia fotorrefrativa).
PRL Abreviatura de prolactin (prolactina).
p·r·n· Abreviatura do L. *pro re nata*, quando surgir a ocasião; quando necessário.
Pro Símbolo de prolina ou prolil.
pro-. 1. Prefixo que designa antes, para diante. VER TAMBÉM ante-, pre-. **2.** Em química, prefixo que indica precursor de. VER TAMBÉM -gen. [L. e G. *pro*]
pro·ac·cel·er·in (prō - ak - sel'er - in). Pró-acelerina. SIN *factor* V.
pro·ac·ro·sin (prō - ak'rō - sin). Pró-acrosina; uma proteína precursora da acrosina.
pro·ac·ro·so·mal (prō - ak - rō - sō'mǎl). Pró-acrossômico; relativo a um estágio inicial no desenvolvimento do acrossoma.
pro·ac·tin·i·um (prō - ak - tin'ē - ŭm). Protactínio. SIN protactinium.
pro·ac·ti·va·tor (prō - ak'ti - vā - ter). Pró-ativador; uma substância que, quando quimicamente dividida, produz um fragmento (ativador) capaz de tornar outra substância enzimaticamente ativa.
pro·al (prō - ǎl). Proal; relativo a um movimento para diante.
pro·am·ni·on (prō - am'nē - on). Pró-âmnion; uma área das membranas extra-embrionárias situada sob e na frente da cabeça em desenvolvimento de um embrião jovem que permanece sem mesoderma por algum tempo.
prob·a·bil·i·ty (P) (pro - bă - bil'ĭ - tē). Probabilidade. **1.** Uma medida, que varia de 0 a 1, da probabilidade de uma hipótese ou declaração ser verdadeira. **2.** O limite da freqüência relativa de um evento em uma seqüência de N provas aleatórias à medida que N se aproxima do infinito.
conditional p., p. condicional; probabilidade citada quando a variedade de escolhas admitidas é restrita, isto é, condicional; assim, a probabilidade de o filho de um homem cego para cores herdar o gene é de 1/2, se a criança for do sexo feminino, e de quase 0, se a criança for do sexo masculino.
joint p., p. conjunta; a probabilidade de que dois ou mais eventos ocorram juntos.
objective p., p. objetiva; probabilidade de um evento baseada em teoria incontestável ou em ampla experiência empírica com, exatamente, a mesma combinação de circunstâncias; a noção também implica que a realização envolvida não foi efetuada e, portanto, mesmo em princípio não é conhecida com certeza.
personal p., p. pessoal; um julgamento idiossincrásico sobre o resultado de um evento; pode incluir evidências muito sutis para serem usadas em uma probabilidade subjetiva.
posterior p., p. posterior; a melhor avaliação racional da probabilidade de um resultado com base em conhecimento estabelecido modificado e atualizado. VER TAMBÉM prior p., Bayes *theorem*. Cf. Bayes *theorem*.
prior p., p. prévia; a melhor avaliação racional da probabilidade de um resultado com base no conhecimento estabelecido antes da realização da experiência atual. Por exemplo, a probabilidade prévia de a filha de um portador de hemofilia ser uma portadora de hemofilia é de 1/2. Mas, se a filha já tem um filho afetado, a probabilidade posterior de ser uma portadora é igual à unidade, enquanto, se ela tem um filho normal, a probabilidade posterior de ela ser portadora é de 1/3. VER Bayes *theorem*.
subjective p., p. subjetiva; uma declaração razoável das chances que uma pessoa racional, bem informada, faria em relação ao resultado de uma experiência. A experiência pode ser única e não compreendida racionalmente (impe-

dindo tanto a previsão teoricamente fundamentada quanto a experiência empírica). A formulação é aplicável a experiências que foram realizadas, mas o resultado é desconhecido. (P. ex., é feita certa declaração sobre o sexo do feto no início da gravidez, mas talvez não seja acessível até que possa ser realizada a amniocentese.) Ao contrário da probabilidade pessoal, a probabilidade subjetiva deve ser igual para todos os conselheiros competentes que possuem as mesmas evidências.

pro·bac·te·ri·o·phage (prō - bak - tēr′ē - ō - fāj). Pró-bacteriófago; o estágio de um bacteriófago temperado no qual o genoma é incorporado ao aparelho genético do hospedeiro da bactéria. SIN prophage.

defective p., VER defective *bacteriophage*.

pro·band (prō′band). Probando; em genética humana, o paciente ou membro da família que coloca uma família em estudo. SIN index case. [L. *probo*, testar, provar]

pro·bang (prō - bang′). Bastão flexível com material de consistência macia na extremidade distal, usado de forma insensata para tentar avançar ou retirar corpos estranhos do esôfago; uma prática a ser condenada como perigosa. [alteração de *provang* (um termo de etimologia desconhecida cunhado pelo inventor, Walter Rumsey), sob a influência de *probe* (sonda)]

probe (prōb). Sonda. **1.** Um bastão delgado de material rígido ou flexível, com uma extremidade bulbar roma, usado para explorar seios, fístulas, outras cavidades ou feridas. **2.** Dispositivo ou agente usado para detectar ou explorar uma substância; p. ex., uma molécula usada para detectar a presença de um fragmento específico de DNA ou RNA ou de uma colônia bacteriana específica. **3.** Sondar; entrar e explorar, como se faz com uma sonda. [L. *probo*, testar]

> As sondas são instrumentos essenciais para análise do DNA. Cada molécula de DNA possui algumas seqüências de nucleotídeos únicas, o que a diferencia de todas as outras. Uma sonda é um fragmento de DNA fabricado, relativamente curto, que se encaixa, como uma chave na fechadura, em uma seqüência de nucleotídeos exclusiva do material que está sendo pesquisado. As sondas são usadas para "buscar" genes clonados em colônias de bactérias ou leveduras, de seqüências de nucleotídeos específicas em amostras de DNA, ou de genes específicos em cromossomas.

Bowman p., s. de Bowman; uma sonda de extremidade dupla para o canal lacrimal.

nucleic acid p., s. de ácido nucleico; um fragmento de ácido nucleico, marcado por um radioisótopo, biotina, etc., que é complementar a uma seqüência em outro ácido nucleico (fragmento) e que irá, por ligação do hidrogênio a este último, localizá-lo ou identificá-lo e ser detectado; uma técnica de diagnóstico baseada no fato de que cada espécie de micróbio possui algumas seqüências de ácidos nucleicos exclusivas, as quais a diferenciam de todas as outras, e assim podem ser usadas como marcadores de identificação ou "impressões digitais".

periodontal p., s. periodontal; instrumento calibrado usado para medir a profundidade e a topografia das bolsas periodontais.

radioactive p., s. radioativa. VER nucleic acid p.

vertebrated p., s. vertebrada; sonda constituída de uma série de secções curtas, articuladas juntas para flexibilidade na penetração de tratos convolutos.

viral p., s. viral. VER nucleic acid p.

pro·ben·e·cid (prō - ben′ē - sid). Probenecida; um inibidor competitivo da secreção de penicilina ou *p*-aminoipurato pelos túbulos renais; um agente uricosúrico usado na artrite gotosa crônica.

pro·bil·i·fus·cins (prō - bil′i - fŭs′in). Probilifuscinas. VER bilirubinoids.

pro·bi·o·sis (prō - bī - ō′sis). Probiose; associação de dois organismos que estimula os processos vitais de ambos. Cf. antibiosis (1), symbiosis, mutualism. [pro- + G. *biōsis*, vida]

pro·bi·ot·ic (prō - bī - ot′ik). Probiótico; relativo à probiose.

prob·lem. Problema; nas profissões que lidam com a saúde mental, termo freqüentemente usado para designar problemas da vida (as dificuldades ou desafios da vida); algumas vezes usado em preferência aos termos doença mental ou distúrbio mental. [G. *problēma*, proposição, tópico, de *proballo*, colocar para frente]

pro·bos·cis, pl. **pro·bos·ci·des, pro·bos·ci·ses** (prō - bos′is, prō - bos′i - dēz, - sēz). Probóscide. **1.** Longa tromba flexível, como a de um tapir ou de um elefante. **2.** Em teratologia, uma protuberância cilíndrica da face que, na ciclopia ou etmocefalia, representa o nariz. [G. *proboskis*, uma forma de fornecer alimento, de pro- + *boskein*, alimentar]

Prob·sty·may·ria vi·vip·a·ra (prob - sti - mā′rē - ă vi - vip′a - ră). Um nematódeo (família Atractidae) intimamente relacionado aos oxiúros verdadeiros (família Oxyuridae) e ainda comumente considerado o oxiúro do cavalo; está distribuído em todo o mundo, sendo freqüentemente encontrado em grandes números, devido à auto-reinfecção interna, no colo de cavalos e outros eqüinos.

pro·bu·col (prō′bū - kōl). Probucol; agente anti-hiperlipoproteinêmico.

pro·cain·a·mide hy·dro·chlo·ride (pro - kān′ă - mīd, pro′kăn - am′īd, - id). Cloridrato de procainamida; difere quimicamente da procaína por conter o grupo amida (CONH) em vez do grupo éster (COO). Deprime a irritabilidade dos músculos cardíacos, possuindo uma ação sobre o coração semelhante à da quinidina, e é usado em arritmias ventriculares.

pro·caine hy·dro·chlo·ride (prō′kān). Cloridrato de procaína; anestésico local para infiltração e anestesia raquidiana; já foi muito usado, mas agora raramente é empregado.

pro·cap·sid (prō - kap′sid). Procapsídeo; revestimento proteico que não possui um genoma viral.

pro·car·ba·zine hy·dro·chlo·ride (prō - kar′bă - zēn). Cloridrato de procarbazina; agente antineoplásico.

pro·car·box·y·pep·ti·dase (prō′kar - bok - sē - pep′ti - dās). Procarboxipeptidase; precursor inativo de uma carboxipeptidase.

pro·car·cin·o·gens (prō - kar - sin′ō - jens). Pró-carcinógenos; xenobióticos inativos que são convertidos em carcinógenos no organismo.

Pro·car·y·o·tae (pro - kar - ē - ō′tē). SIN Prokaryotae. [pro- + G. *karyon*, cerne, núcleo]

pro·car·y·ote (pro - kar′ē - ōt). Procariota. SIN prokaryote. [pro- + G. *karyon*, cerne, núcleo]

pro·car·y·ot·ic (prō′kar - ē - ot′ik). Procariótico. SIN prokaryotic.

pro·cat·arc·tic (prō - kă - tark′tik). Procatártico; termo raramente usado para designar a causa excitante de uma doença. [G. *prokatarktikos*, que começa antes]

pro·cat·arx·is (prō - kă - tark′sis). Procatarse. **1.** SIN exciting *cause*. **2.** O início de uma doença sob a influência da causa excitante, uma causa predisponente já existente. [G. um início de antemão, de *prokatararchomi*, começar primeiro, de *pro*, antes, + *kata*, sobre, + *archō*, começar]

pro·ce·dure (prō - sē′jŭr). Procedimento; ato ou conduta de diagnóstico, tratamento ou operação. VER TAMBÉM method, operation, technique.

back table p., procedimento realizado em um órgão removido de um paciente antes de ser substituído.

Batista p., p. de Batista; redução cirúrgica de um ou de ambos os ventrículos quando estão excessivamente dilatados; investigado incompletamente em 1999. SIN ventricular reduction surgery.

Belsey p., p. de Belsey. SIN Belsey *fundoplication*.

Chamberlain p., p. de Chamberlain; toracostomia anterior esquerda limitada para biopsia dos linfonodos mediastinais fora de alcance por mediastinoscopia cervical. VER TAMBÉM anterior *mediastinoscopy*. SIN anterior mediastinotomy.

Clagett p. for empyema, p. de Claggett para empiema; um procedimento cirúrgico em dois estágios para tratamento de empiema pós-pneumonectomia sem fístula broncopleural.

Collis-Belsey p., p. de Collis-Belsey. SIN Collis-Nissen *fundoplication*.

commando p., operação para tumores malignos do assoalho da cavidade oral, envolvendo a ressecção de partes da mandíbula em continuidade com a lesão oral e dissecção cervical radical. SIN commando operation.

Damus-Kaye-Stancel p., p. de Damus-Kaye-Stancel; p. para estenose subaórtica, permite a criação de uma anastomose término-lateral do tronco pulmonar/aorta, realizada juntamente com um procedimento de Fontan, sobretudo em pacientes com uma dupla entrada do ventrículo esquerdo. SIN Damus-Stancel-Kaye anastomosis.

dideoxy p., (di′dē - ōks - ē), p. didesoxi; procedimento enzimático para seqüenciamento de DNA empregando nucleotídeos didesoxi como interruptores da cadeia. VER Sanger *method*.

Dor p., p. de Dor. SIN Jatene p.

Eloesser p., p. de Eloesser; transposição de um retalho cutâneo pediculado, lingüiforme, desde a parede torácica até a parte profunda de uma incisão que se comunica com um empiema ou abscesso pulmonar periférico; usado para evitar o fechamento cicatricial do trajeto a fim de assegurar drenagem gravitacional obrigatória prolongada. VER TAMBÉM Eloesser *flap*.

endorectal pull-through p., remoção de mucosa retal doente juntamente com ressecção da porção inferior do intestino, seguida por anastomose do coto proximal ao ânus, para preservar a função do ânus.

Ewart p., p. de Ewart; elevação da laringe entre o polegar e o indicador para incitar repuxamento da traquéia.

Fontan p., p. de Fontan; colocação de um conduto (geralmente com valvas) do átrio direito para a artéria pulmonar principal como derivação para um ventrículo direito hipoplásico, p. ex., na atresia tricúspide. SIN Fontan operation.

Girdlestone p., p. de Girdlestone; ressecção ou excisão completa da cabeça e do colo do fêmur.

Harada-Ito p., p. de Harada-Ito; p. destinado a corrigir extorsão ocular causada por paralisia do IV nervo por retesamento seletivo das fibras anteriores do tendão oblíquo superior.

Hummelsheim p., p. de Hummelsheim; p. cirúrgico para corrigir um desvio ocular devido à paralisia do VI nervo no qual os tendões dos músculos retos superior e inferior são divididos e transferidos lateralmente.

Jatene p., p. de Jatene; método de reparo de estenose subaórtica congênita em túnel e estreitamento da junção ventrículo esquerdo-aorta por atrioventriculoplastia e substituição por prótese valvar. SIN Dor p.

Kestenbaum p., p. de Kestenbaum; p. cirúrgico nos músculos extra-oculares (extraocular *muscles*, em *muscle*), indicado em pacientes com torcicolo associado a nistagmo.

Konno p., p. de Konno; método de reparo de estenose subaórtica congênita em túnel e estreitamento da junção ventrículo esquerdo-aorta por atrioventriculoplastia e substituição por prótese valvar.

Konno-Rastan p., p. de Konno-Rastan; aortoventriculoplastia para dilatar o anel aórtico, principalmente quando há estenose fibromuscular subaórtica.

lateral tarsal strip p., correção cirúrgica de má posição da pálpebra inferior devido à frouxidão horizontal da pálpebra por encurtamento da pálpebra na extremidade do ângulo lateral.

loop electrocautery excision p. (LEEP), p. de excisão com eletrocautério em alça; biopsia excisional por eletrocautério de tecido cervical anormal.

loop electrosurgical excision p. (LEEP), p. de excisão eletrocirúrgica com alça. SIN loop *excision*.

McCall culdoplasty p., p. de culdoplastia de McCall; método de sustentação do fundo-de-saco vaginal, durante uma histerectomia vaginal, por fixação dos ligamentos útero-sacrais e cardinais à superfície peritoneal com fio de sutura que, quando amarrado, exerce tração para a linha média, ajudando a fechar o fundo-de-saco.

Mitchell p., p. de Mitchell; p. cirúrgico para corrigir um hálux valgo por combinação de excisão de joanete e correção dos tecidos moles da primeira articulação metatarsofalângica com osteotomia da porção proximal do primeiro metatarsal.

Mustard p., p. de Mustard. SIN Mustard *operation*.

Nick p., p. de Nick; dilata o anel aórtico por incisão do seio não-coronário e do teto do átrio esquerdo.

Noble-Collip p., p. de Noble-Collip; p. obsoleto no qual é induzido choque em ratos por rotação deles em um tambor.

Norwood p., p. de Norwood; p. complexo para tratar a atresia aórtica associada à síndrome de hipoplasia do coração esquerdo; algumas vezes realizado em dois estágios.

Puestow p., p. de Puestow; pancreatojejunostomia longitudinal para tratamento da pancreatite crônica.

push-back p., manobra cirúrgica destinada a reposicionar o palato mole posteriormente a fim de restabelecer a competência velofaríngea.

Putti-Platt p., p. de Putti-Platt. SIN Putti-Platt *operation*.

Reichel-Pólya stomach p., p. gástrico de Reichel-Pólya; anastomose retrocólica de toda a circunferência do estômago aberto até o jejuno.

Rittenhouse-Manogian p., p. de Rittenhouse-Manogian; dilata o anel aórtico mediante incisão da comissura coronária esquerda–não-coronária até o folheto anterior da valva mitral.

Ross p., p. de Ross; p. usado na estenose ou regurgitação aórtica, no qual a valva aórtica é substituída pela valva pulmonar do próprio paciente (auto-enxerto) e a valva pulmonar, por sua vez, é substituída por homoenxerto.

sacrocolpopexy p., p. de sacrocolpopexia; sustentação da abóbada vaginal por sua fixação ao periósteo do sacro após histerectomia. [sacro- + colpo- + -pexy]

sacrospinous vaginal vault suspension p., p. de suspensão sacroespinal da abóbada vaginal; reparo cirúrgico da abóbada vaginal prolapsada, suturando-a ao ligamento sacroespinal; realizada por via vaginal ou abdominal.

shelf p., inserção de um enxerto do ílio no teto do acetábulo para tratamento da luxação congênita do quadril.

Sugiura p., p. de Sugiura; transecção esofágica com desvascularização para-esofágica, no tratamento de varizes esofágicas.

Thal p., p. de Thal; correção de estenose benigna da parte inferior do esôfago na qual a área estreitada é aberta longitudinalmente e a parede gástrica externa adjacente é suturada sobre esse defeito.

Vineberg p., p. de Vineberg; cirurgia obsoleta para tratamento de isquemia do miocárdio na qual a artéria torácica interna é implantada no miocárdio a fim de melhorar o fluxo sanguíneo para o coração.

Walsh p., p. de Walsh; prostatectomia retropúbica radical anatômica (com preservação dos nervos).

pro·ce·lia (pro-sē'lē-ȧ). Um ventrículo lateral do encéfalo; a cavidade do prosencéfalo. [pro- + G. *koilia*, cavidade]

pro·ce·lous (prō-sē'lŭs). Procélico; côncavo anteriormente. [pro- + G. *koilos*, oco]

pro·cen·tri·ole (prō-sen'trē-ōl). Procentríolo; a fase inicial no desenvolvimento *de novo* de centríolos ou corpos basais da centrosfera; os procentríolos se formam em relação aos deuterossomas (organizadores do procentríolo).

pro·ce·phal·ic (prō-se-fal'ik). Procefálico; relativo à parte anterior da cabeça. [pro- + G. *kephalē*, cabeça]

pro·cer·coid (prō-ser'koyd). Procercóide; o primeiro estágio no ciclo vital aquático de alguns cestódeos, como os pseudofilídeos (família Diphyllobothriidae), após a ingestão de larvas recém-eclodidas (coracídio) por um copépode (pulga d'água). O procercóide transforma-se em uma larva caudada na cavidade corporal do crustáceo, que é o primeiro hospedeiro intermediário; quando o procercóide e seu hospedeiro são ingeridos por um peixe, o procercóide penetra nos novos tecidos do hospedeiro e torna-se um plerocercóide. VER TAMBÉM *Diphyllobothrium latum*, Pseudophyllidea. [pro- + G. *kerkos*, cauda, + *eidos*, semelhança]

pro·ce·rus (prō-sē'rŭs). Músculo prócero. SIN procerus (*muscle*). [L. longo, esticado]

PROCESS

pro·cess (pros'es, prō'ses) [TA]. Processo. **1.** Em anatomia, uma projeção ou crescimento. SIN processus [TA]. **2.** Um método ou forma de ação usado para alcançar determinado resultado. **3.** Um avanço, progresso ou método, como o de uma doença. VER processus. **4.** Uma condição patológica ou doença. **5.** Em odontologia, uma série de operações que convertem um molde de cera, como o da base de uma dentadura, em uma base de dentadura sólida ou outro material. VER dental *curing*. [L. *processus*, um avanço, progresso, process, de *procedo*, pp. *-cessus*, ir adiante]

A·B·C p., p. A.B.C.; purificação de água ou desodorização de esgoto por uma mistura de alume, sangue e carvão (*alum*, *blood*, *charcoal*).

accessory p. of lumbar vertebra [TA], p. acessório de vértebra lombar; uma pequena apófise na parte posterior da base do processo transverso de cada uma das vértebras lombares. SIN processus accessorius vertebrae lumbalis [TA], accessory tubercle.

acromial p., acrômio. SIN acromion.

agene p., p. agênico; branqueamento da farinha de trigo com tricloreto de nitrogênio (proibido nos Estados Unidos).

alar p., asa da crista etmoidal. SIN ala of crista galli.

alveolar p. of maxilla [TA], p. alveolar da maxila; a crista proeminente, na superfície inferior do corpo da maxila, que contém os alvéolos dentários; o termo também é aplicado à face superior do corpo da mandíbula, que também contém alvéolos dentários. SIN alveolar body, alveolar bone (1), alveolar border (2), alveolar ridge, basal ridge (1), dental p., processus alveolaris maxillae.

anterior clinoid p. [TA], p. clinóide anterior; a projeção direcionada para trás, que é a extremidade medial da crista esfenoidal (asa menor do esfenóide); dá fixação à borda livre da tenda do cerebelo. SIN processus clinoideus anterior [TA].

anterior p. of malleus [TA], p. anterior do martelo; esporão fino que segue para frente, a partir do colo do martelo, em direção à fissura petrotimpânica. SIN processus anterior mallei [TA], Folli p., follian p., long p. of malleus, processus gracilis, processus ravii, Rau p., Ravius p., slender p. of malleus.

apical p., dendrito apical; o prolongamento dendrítico que se estende do ápice de uma célula piramidal do córtex cerebral em direção à superfície. SIN apical dendrite.

articular p. [TA], p. articular; uma das pequenas projeções planas bilaterais nas superfícies dos arcos das vértebras, no ponto onde os pedículos e lâminas se unem, formando as superfícies das articulações dos processos articulares. SIN processus articularis [TA], zygapophysis.

ascending p., p. ascendente. SIN *processus* ascendens.

auditory p., parte timpânica; a borda áspera da placa timpânica onde se fixa a porção cartilagínea do meato acústico externo.

basilar p., parte basilar do osso occipital. SIN basilar *part* of occipital bone.

basilar p. of occipital bone, parte basilar do osso occipital. SIN basilar *part* of occipital bone.

binary p., p. binário; um evento aleatório com dois resultados exaustivos e mutuamente exclusivos; um processo de Bernoulli.

Budde p., p. de Budde; método de esterilização do leite; adiciona-se peróxido de hidrogênio ao leite fresco na proporção de 15 ml de uma solução a 3% para 1 litro de leite, e a mistura é aquecida a 51° ou 52°C (124°F) por 3 horas, quando o peróxido é decomposto e o oxigênio produzido atua como um eficiente germicida; o leite, então, é rapidamente resfriado e colocado em frascos fechados.

Burns falciform p., p. falciforme de Burns. SIN superior *horn* of falciform margin of saphenous opening.

calcaneal p. of cuboid [TA], p. calcâneo do cubóide; o processo que se projeta posteriormente a partir da superfície plantar do cubóide; sustenta a extremidade anterior do calcâneo. SIN processus calcaneus ossis cuboidei [TA].

caudate p. [TA], p. caudado do fígado; uma faixa estreita de tecido hepático que une os lobos caudado e direito do fígado posterior à porta do fígado. SIN processus caudatus [TA].

ciliary p. [TA], p. ciliar; uma das cristas pigmentadas radiadas, geralmente em número de 70, na superfície interna do corpo ciliar, aumentando em espessura à medida que avançam do orbículo ciliar até a margem externa da íris; estas, juntamente com as pregas nos sulcos entre elas, formam a coroa ciliar. SIN processus ciliaris [TA].

Civinini p., p. de Civinini. SIN pterygospinous p.

clinoid p. [TA], p. clinóide; um dos três pares de projeções ósseas do osso esfenóide, com os pares anterior e posterior circundando a fossa hipofisária como pés de cama. SIN processus clinoideus [TA], clinoid (2).
cochleariform p., p. cocleariforme. SIN *processus cochleariformis.*
complex learning p.'s, processos de aprendizado complexos; aqueles processos que exigem o uso de manipulações simbólicas, como no raciocínio.
condylar p. of mandible [TA], p. condilar da mandíbula; o processo articular do ramo da mandíbula; inclui a cabeça da mandíbula, o colo da mandíbula e a fóvea pterigóidea. SIN processus condylaris mandibulae [TA], condyloid p., mandibular condyle.
condyloid p., p. condilar da mandíbula. SIN condylar p. of mandible.
conoid p., tubérculo conóide (da clavícula). SIN conoid *tubercle* (of clavicle).
coracoid p. [TA], p. coracóide; uma projeção curva, longa, semelhante a um dedo fletido originando-se do colo da escápula e projetando-se sobre a cavidade glenóide; local de fixação da cabeça curta do músculo bíceps e dos músculos coracobraquial e peitoral menor, bem como dos ligamentos coronóide e coracoacromial. SIN processus coracoideus [TA].
coronoid p., p. coronóide; uma projeção triangular aguda de um osso. SIN processus coronoideus.
coronoid p. of the mandible [TA], p. coronóide da mandíbula; o processo anterior triangular do ramo da mandíbula, onde se fixa o músculo temporal. SIN processus coronoideus mandibulae [TA].
coronoid p. of the ulna [TA], p. coronóide da ulna; uma projeção, semelhante a um colchete, da porção anterior da extremidade proximal da ulna; sua superfície anterior é o local de fixação do músculo braquial, e sua superfície proximal entra na formação da incisura troclear. SIN processus coronoideus ulnae [TA].
costal p. [TA], p. costiforme da vértebra lombar; uma apófise que se estende lateralmente a partir do processo transverso de uma vértebra lombar; é o homólogo da costela. SIN processus costalis [TA].
dendritic p., dendrito. SIN dendrite (1).
dental p., p. alveolar da maxila. SIN alveolar p. of maxilla.
ensiform p., p. xifóide. SIN xiphoid p.
ethmoidal p. of inferior nasal concha [TA], p. etmoidal da concha nasal inferior; uma projeção da concha inferior, situada atrás do processo lacrimal e que se articula com o processo uncinado do etmóide. SIN processus ethmoidalis conchae nasalis inferioris [TA].
falciform p. of sacrotuberous ligament [TA], p. falciforme do ligamento sacrotuberal; uma continuação da borda interna do ligamento sacrotuberal para cima e para frente, sobre a face interna do ramo do ísquio. SIN processus falciformis ligamenti sacrotuberalis [TA], falciform ligament, ligamentum falciforme.
Folli p., p. de Folli. SIN anterior p. of malleus.
follian p., p. anterior do martelo. SIN anterior p. of malleus.
foot p., pedicelo. SIN pedicel.
frontal p. of maxilla [TA], p. frontal da maxila; a extensão superior do corpo da maxila, que se articula com o osso frontal. SIN processus frontalis maxillae [TA], nasal p.
frontal p. of zygomatic bone [TA], p. frontal do osso zigomático; o processo do osso zigomático que se estende para cima, para formar a margem lateral da órbita, articulando-se com o osso frontal e com a asa maior do osso esfenóide. SIN processus frontalis ossis zygomatici [TA], frontosphenoidal p.
frontonasal p., proeminência frontonasal. SIN frontonasal *prominence.*
frontosphenoidal p., p. frontal do osso zigomático. SIN frontal p. of zygomatic bone.
funicular p., p. funicular; a túnica vaginal que envolve o cordão espermático.
globular p., termo obsoleto para segmento intermaxilar (intermaxillary *segment*).
hamular p. of lacrimal bone, hâmulo lacrimal. SIN lacrimal *hamulus.*
hamular p. of sphenoid bone, p. hâmulo pterigóideo. SIN pterygoid *hamulus.*
head p., p. cefálico; o primórdio para o notocórdio. VER TAMBÉM notochordal p.
inferior articular p. [TA], p. articular inferior; um dos processos articulares na superfície inferior do arco vertebral. SIN zygapophysis inferior [TA].
Ingrassia p., p. de Ingrassia. SIN lesser *wing* of sphenoid (bone).
intrajugular p. [TA], p. intrajugular; pequeno p. pontiagudo de osso estendendo-se do meio da incisura jugular nos ossos occipital e temporal, os dois sendo unidos por um ligamento e dividindo o forame jugular em duas porções. SIN processus intrajugularis [TA].
jugular p. of occipital bone [TA], p. jugular do osso occipital; um processo curto que se projeta da parte posterior do côndilo do occipital, com sua borda anterior formando o limite posterior do forame jugular. SIN processus jugularis ossis occipitalis [TA].
lacrimal p. of inferior nasal concha [TA], p. lacrimal da concha nasal inferior; projeção da margem anterior da concha inferior que se articula com a margem inferior do osso lacrimal. SIN processus lacrimalis conchae nasalis inferioris [TA].

lateral p. of calcaneal tuberosity [TA], p. lateral da tuberosidade do calcâneo; a projeção lateral da parte posterior do calcâneo. SIN processus lateralis tuberis calcanei [TA].
lateral p. of malleus [TA], p. lateral do martelo; uma projeção curta da base do manúbrio do martelo, firmemente fixado ao tímpano. SIN processus lateralis mallei [TA], processus brevis, short p. of malleus, tuberculum mallei.
lateral nasal p., proeminência nasal lateral. SIN lateral nasal *prominence.*
lateral p. of septal nasal cartilage [TA], p. lateral da cartilagem do septo nasal; o processo plano da cartilagem do septo nasal localizado na parede lateral do nariz acima da cartilagem alar. SIN cartilago nasi lateralis, lateral cartilage of nose.
lateral p. of talus [TA], p. lateral do tálus; projeção na face lateral do tálus abaixo da superfície articular maleolar. SIN processus lateralis tali [TA].
Lenhossék p.'s, prolongamentos de Lenhossék; prolongamentos curtos ("axônios atrofiados") apresentados por algumas células ganglionares.
lenticular p. of incus [TA], p. lenticular da bigorna; saliência na extremidade do ramo longo da bigorna que se articula com o estribo. SIN processus lenticularis incudis [TA], lenticular apophysis, lenticular bone, orbicular bone, orbicular p., orbiculare, os orbiculare, os sylvii.
long p. of malleus, p. anterior do martelo. SIN anterior p. of malleus.
malar p., p. zigomático da maxila. SIN zygomatic p. of maxilla.
mammillary p. of lumbar vertebra [TA], p. mamilar da vértebra lombar; pequena apófise ou tubérculo na margem dorsal do processo articular superior de cada vértebra lombar e geralmente da décima segunda vértebra torácica. SIN processus mammillaris vertebrae lumbalis [TA], mammillary tubercle, metapophysis.
mandibular p., arco mandibular. SIN mandibular *arch.*
Markov p., p. de Markov; um processo estocástico de forma que a distribuição de probabilidade condicional para o estado em qualquer momento futuro, dado o estado atual, não é afetada por qualquer conhecimento adicional da história passada do sistema.
mastoid p. [TA], p. mastóide; a projeção mamilar da parte petrosa do osso temporal. SIN processus mastoideus [TA], mastoid bone, temporal apophysis.
mastoid p. of petrous part of temporal bone [TA], p. mastóide da parte petrosa do osso temporal; a porção da parte petrosa do osso temporal que contém o p. mastóide. SIN processus mastoideus partis petrosae ossis temporalis [TA], mastoid part of the temoral bone, pars mastoidea ossis temporalis.
maxillary p. of embryo, p. maxilar do embrião; a parte proximal do primeiro arco faríngeo que se desenvolve na maior parte da maxila.
maxillary p. of inferior nasal concha [TA], p. maxilar da concha nasal inferior; uma lâmina fina, de formato irregular, que se projeta do meio da borda superior da concha inferior, articulando-se com a maxila e fechando parcialmente o orifício do seio maxilar. SIN processus maxillaris conchae nasalis inferioris [TA].
medial p. of calcaneal tuberosity [TA], p. medial da tuberosidade do calcâneo; a projeção medial da parte posterior do calcâneo. SIN processus medialis tuberis calcanei [TA].
medial nasal p., proeminência nasal medial. SIN medial nasal *prominence.*
mental p., protuberância mentual. SIN mental *protuberance.*
middle clinoid p. [TA], p. clinóide médio; esporão ósseo pequeno, inconstante no corpo do esfenóide, póstero-lateral e, ocasionalmente, contínuo com o tubérculo da sela; é ao redor desse ponto que a artéria carótida interna faz uma volta de 180°, mudando a direção de anterior para posterior a fim de se unir ao círculo arterial cerebral. SIN processus clinoideus medius [TA].
muscular p. of arytenoid cartilage [TA], p. muscular da cartilagem aritenóidea; a projeção lateral romba da cartilagem aritenóidea onde se fixam os músculos cricoaritenóideos lateral e posterior da laringe. SIN processus muscularis cartilaginis arytenoideae [TA].
nasal p., p. frontal da maxila. SIN frontal p. of maxilla.
notochordal p., p. notocórdico; no embrião, uma coluna de células na linha média situadas rostrais ao linfonodo primitivo e que formam o notocórdio. VER TAMBÉM head p.
odontoblastic p., p. odontoblástico; a extensão do odontoblasto situada dentro do túbulo dentinário; a aplicação de estímulos à dentina pode causar aspiração do conteúdo do odontoblasto para o processo.
odontoid p., dente do áxis. SIN dens (2).
odontoid p. of epistropheus, dente do áxis. SIN dens (2).
olecranon p., olécrano. SIN olecranon.
orbicular p., p. lenticular da bigorna. SIN lenticular p. of incus.
orbital p. of palatine bone [TA], p. orbital do palatino; o anterior e maior dos dois processos da extremidade superior da lâmina perpendicular do palatino, articulando-se com a maxila, etmóide e esfenóide. SIN processus orbitalis ossis palatini [TA].
packing p., p. de inclusão; o método de colocação do material básico da dentadura em uma mufla para processamento.
palatine p. of maxilla [TA], p. palatino da maxila; prateleiras voltadas medialmente, a partir da maxila, que, com a lâmina horizontal do palatino, formam o palato ósseo. SIN processus palatinus ossis maxillae [TA].

papillary p. of caudate lobe of liver [TA], p. papilar do lobo caudado do fígado; o ângulo inferior esquerdo do lobo caudado do fígado, oposto ao processo caudado. SIN processus papillaris lobi caudati hepatis [TA].
paramastoid p. [TA], p. paramastóideo; um processo ocasional de osso que se estende para baixo, a partir do processo jugular do osso occipital em seres humanos. SIN processus paramastoideus [TA], paroccipital p.
paroccipital p., p. paramastóideo. SIN paramastoid p.
posterior clinoid p. [TA], p. clinóide posterior; os ângulos súpero-laterais agudos do dorso da sela, onde se fixam as fibras de tecido conjuntivo que irradiam da tenda do cerebelo. SIN processus clinoideus posterior [TA].
posterior p. of septal cartilage [TA], p. posterior da cartilagem do septo nasal; a extensão afilada da cartilagem septal situada entre a lâmina vertical do etmóide e o vômer. SIN processus posterior cartilaginis septi nasi [TA], sphenoid p. of septal nasal cartilage [TA], processus sphenoidalis cartilaginis septi nasi*.
posterior p. of talus [TA], p. posterior do tálus; uma projeção do tálus que possui tubérculos medial e lateral; situa-se posterior e inferior à tróclea. SIN processus posterior tali [TA], Stieda p.
primary p., p. primário; em psicanálise, o processo mental diretamente relacionado às funções das forças vitais primitivas associadas ao id e característico da atividade mental inconsciente; caracterizado por raciocínio desorganizado, ilógico, e pela tendência a buscar a imediata obtenção e satisfação das necessidades instintivas. Cf. secondary p.
progressive p.'s, processos progressivos; processos que persistem após não atenderem mais às necessidades do organismo, e após cessar o estímulo que os despertou.
pterygoid p. of sphenoid bone [TA], p. pterigóide do esfenóide; um p. longo que se estende para baixo a partir da junção do corpo e da asa maior do esfenóide de cada lado; é formado por duas lâminas (lateral e medial), unidas anteriormente, mas separadas abaixo para formar a incisura pterigóidea; a fossa pterigóidea é formada pela divergência dessas duas lâminas posteriormente. SIN processus pterygoideus ossis sphenoidalis [TA], os pterygoideum.
pterygospinous p. [TA], p. pterigoespinhoso; uma projeção pontiaguda da lâmina pterigóide lateral do esfenóide. SIN processus pterygospinosus [TA], Civinini p.
pyramidal p. of palatine bone [TA], p. piramidal do palatino; a porção do palatino que passa lateral e posterior, a partir do ângulo formado pelas lâminas perpendicular e horizontal. SIN processus pyramidalis ossis palatini [TA].
Rau p., p. de Rau. SIN anterior p. of malleus.
Ravius p., p. de Ravius. SIN anterior p. of malleus.
retromandibular p. of parotid gland, parte profunda da glândula parótida. SIN deep part of parotid gland.
secondary p., p. secundário; em psicanálise, o processo mental diretamente relacionado às funções aprendidas e adquiridas do ego e característico de atividades mentais conscientes e pré-conscientes; caracterizado por raciocínio lógico e pela tendência a retardar a gratificação por regulação da satisfação de exigências instintivas. Cf. primary p.
sheath p. of sphenoid bone, p. vaginal do esfenóide. SIN vaginal p. of sphenoid bone.
short p. of malleus, p. lateral do martelo. SIN lateral p. of malleus.
slender p. of malleus, p. anterior do martelo. SIN anterior p. of malleus.
sphenoid p., p. esfenóide. SIN sphenoidal p. of palatine bone.
sphenoidal p. of palatine bone [TA], p. esfenoidal do palatino; o posterior e menor dos dois processos na extremidade da lâmina perpendicular do palatino. SIN processus sphenoidalis ossis palatini [TA], sphenoid p.
sphenoid p. of septal nasal cartilage [TA], p. posterior da cartilagem do septo nasal. SIN posterior p. of septal cartilage.
spinous p. of sphenoid, espinha do esfenóide. SIN spine of sphenoid bone.
spinous p. of tibia, eminência intercondilar. SIN intercondylar eminence.
spinous p. of vertebra [TA], p. espinhoso da vértebra; a projeção dorsal do centro de um arco vertebral. SIN processus spinosus vertebrae [TA].
Stieda p., p. de Stieda. SIN posterior p. of talus.
stochastic p., p. estocástico; p. que incorpora algum elemento de aleatoriedade. [G. *stochastikos*, relativo à adivinhação, de *stochazomai*, adivinhar]
styloid p. of fibula, ápice da cabeça da fíbula. SIN apex of head of fibula.
styloid p. of radius [TA], p. estilóide do rádio; uma projeção grossa, pontiaguda, palpável na face lateral da extremidade distal do rádio. SIN processus styloideus radii [TA].
styloid p. of temporal bone [TA], p. estilóide do temporal; uma projeção pontiaguda, delgada, semelhante a uma agulha, que segue para baixo e ligeiramente para frente a partir da base da superfície inferior da porção petrosa do osso temporal, onde se une à porção timpânica; dá inserção aos músculos estiloglosso, estilo-hióideo e estilofaríngeo e aos ligamentos estilo-hióideo e estilomandibular. SIN processus styloideus ossis temporalis [TA].
styloid p. of third metacarpal bone [TA], p. estilóide do terceiro metacarpal; projeção pontiaguda do ângulo dorsolateral da base do terceiro metacarpal; algumas vezes existe como um ossículo distinto. SIN processus styloideus ossis metacarpalis III [TA].
styloid p. of ulna [TA], p. estilóide da ulna; projeção cilíndrica, pontiaguda, palpável nas faces medial e posterior da cabeça da ulna, em cuja extremidade está fixado o ligamento colateral ulnar do punho. SIN processus styloideus ulnae [TA].
superior articular p. [TA], p. articular superior da vértebra; um dos processos articulares na superfície superior do arco vertebral. SIN zygapophysis superior [TA], diapophysis.
superior articular p. of sacrum [TA], p. articular superior da vértebra da base do sacro; o grande processo de cada lado do sacro posteriormente, que se articula com o processo articular inferior correspondente da quinta vértebra lombar. SIN processus articularis superior ossis sacri [TA].
supracondylar p. of humerus [TA], processo supracondilar do úmero; a espinha ocasional que se projeta da superfície ântero-medial do úmero cerca de 5 cm acima do epicôndilo medial, ao qual é fixada por uma faixa fibrosa. O forame supracondilar assim formado dá passagem à artéria braquial e ao nervo mediano. SIN processus supraepicondylaris humeri [TA], supraepicondylar p.
supraepicondylar p., p. supracondilar. SIN supracondylar p. of humerus.
temporal p. of zygomatic bone [TA], p. temporal do zigomático que se articula com o processo zigomático do osso temporal para formar o arco zigomático. SIN processus temporalis ossis zygomatici [TA].
Tomes p.'s, processos de Tomes; processos apicais dos ameloblastos.
transverse p. of vertebra [TA], p. transverso da vértebra; uma protrusão óssea de cada lado do arco de uma vértebra, a partir da junção da lâmina ao pedículo, que funciona como uma alavanca para os músculos fixados. SIN processus transversus vertebrae [TA].
trochlear p., tróclea fibular do calcâneo. SIN fibular *trochlea* of calcaneus.
uncinate p. of cervical vertebra [TA], unco do corpo da vértebra cervical; margens laterais elevadas da superfície superior das vértebras cervicais; com o envelhecimento, eles em geral se estendem para cima o suficiente para tocar a vértebra superior, formando uma articulação uncovertebral. SIN processus uncinatus vertebrae cervicalis [TA].
uncinate p. of ethmoid bone [TA], p. uncinado do etmóide; processo falciforme de osso na parede medial do labirinto etmoidal abaixo da concha média; articula-se com o processo etmoidal da concha inferior e fecha parcialmente o orifício do seio maxilar. SIN processus uncinatus ossis ethmoidalis [TA].
uncinate p. of first thoracic vertebra [TA], unco do corpo da primeira vértebra torácica; borda lateral elevada da superfície superior. VER TAMBÉM uncinate p. of cervical vertebra. SIN processus uncinatus vertebrae thoracicae primae [TA].
uncinate p. of pancreas [TA], p. uncinado do pâncreas; parte da cabeça do pâncreas que se curva ao redor da parte posterior dos vasos mesentéricos superiores, algumas vezes entrando no "quebra-nozes" formado pela artéria mesentérica superior e pela aorta abdominal. SIN processus uncinatus pancreatis [TA], lesser pancreas, pancreas minus, small pancreas, uncinate pancreas, unciforme pancreas, Willis pancreas, Winslow pancreas.
vaginal p., bainha. SIN *sheath* of styloid process.
vaginal p. of peritoneum, túnica vaginal do peritônio. SIN *processus* vaginalis of peritoneum.
vaginal p. of sphenoid bone [TA], p. vaginal do esfenóide; uma fina lâmina de osso que se estende medialmente sob o corpo do esfenóide a partir da lâmina medial do processo pterigóide; articula-se com o vômer e com o palatino. SIN processus vaginalis ossis sphenoidalis [TA], sheath p. of sphenoid bone.
vaginal p. of testis, túnica vaginal do testículo. SIN tunica vaginalis testis.
vermiform p., apêndice vermiforme. SIN appendix (2).
vocal p., p. vocal da cartilagem aritenóidea. SIN vocal p. of arytenoid cartilage.

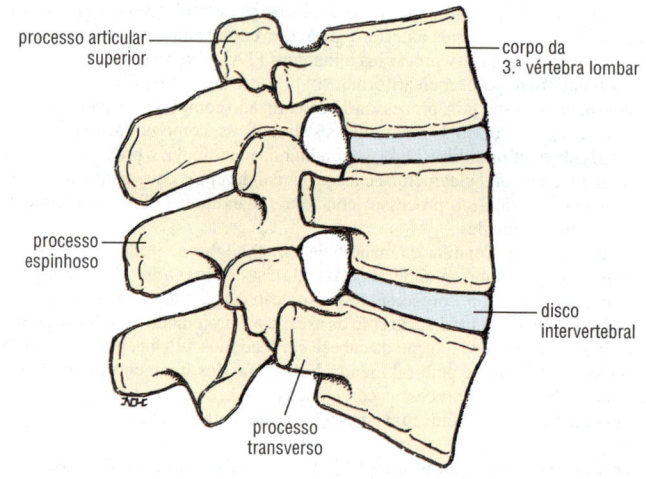

processos vertebrais em três vértebras lombares

vocal p. of arytenoid cartilage [TA], p. vocal da cartilagem aritenóidea; a extremidade inferior da margem anterior da cartilagem aritenóidea, à qual se fixa a prega vocal. SIN processus vocalis cartilaginis arytenoideae [TA], vocal p.

xiphoid p. [TA], p. xifóide; a cartilagem na extremidade inferior do esterno. SIN processus xiphoideus [TA], ensiform p., ensisternum, metasternum, mucro sterni, xiphisternum, xiphoid cartilage.

zygomatic p. of frontal bone [TA], p. zigomático do frontal; a grande projeção do osso frontal que une o osso zigomático para formar a margem lateral da órbita. SIN processus zygomaticus ossis frontalis [TA].

zygomatic p. of maxilla [TA], p. zigomático da maxila; a projeção grosseira da maxila que se articula com o osso zigomático. SIN processus zygomaticus maxillae [TA], malar p.

zygomatic p. of temporal bone [TA], p. zigomático do temporal; o p. anterior do osso temporal que se articula com o processo temporal do osso zigomático para formar o arco zigomático. SIN processus zygomaticus ossis temporalis [TA].

---

pro·cess·ing (pros′es-ing). Processamento. **1.** Modificação pós-tradução de proteínas, sobretudo proteínas secretoras e proteínas direcionadas para membranas ou localizações celulares específicas. SIN trafficking. **2.** Modificação pós-transcricional de ácidos polinucleicos.

pro·ces·sor (pro′ses-sōr). Processador; dispositivo que converte uma forma de energia em outra forma de energia, ou uma forma de material em outra forma de material.

speech p., p. da fala; a parte de um implante coclear que converte a fala em impulsos elétricos usados para estimular os neurônios da divisão auditiva do oitavo nervo craniano.

PROCESSUS

pro·ces·sus, pl. **pro·ces·sus** (prō-ses′ŭs). [TA]. Processo. SIN process (1). [L. ver process]

p. accesso′rius vertebrae lumbalis [TA], p. acessório da vértebra lombar. SIN accessory process of lumbar vertebra.

p. alveola′ris maxillae, p. alveolar da maxila. SIN alveolar process of maxilla. VER TAMBÉM alveolar bone (2).

p. ante′rior mal′lei [TA], p. anterior do martelo. SIN anterior process of malleus.

p. articula′ris [TA], p. articular. SIN articular process.

p. articula′ris supe′rior os′sis sa′cri [TA], p. articular superior da base do sacro. SIN superior articular process of sacrum.

p. ascen′dens, p. ascendente; uma extensão superior da cartilagem pterigoquadrada embrionária; transforma-se na asa maior do esfenóide. SIN ascending process.

p. bre′vis, processo lateral do martelo. SIN lateral process of malleus.

p. calca′neus os′sis cuboi′dei [TA], p. calcâneo do cubóide. SIN calcaneal process of cuboid.

p. cauda′tus [TA], p. caudado do fígado. SIN caudate process.

p. cilia′ris [TA], p. ciliar. SIN ciliary process.

p. clinoi′deus [TA], p. clinóide. SIN clinoid process.

p. clinoideus anterior [TA], p. clinóide anterior. SIN anterior clinoid process.

p. clinoideus medius [TA], p. clinóide médio. SIN middle clinoid process.

p. clinoideus posterior [TA], p. clinóide posterior. SIN posterior clinoid process.

p. cochlearifor′mis [TA], p. cocleariforme; processo angular ósseo (o fim do septo na tuba auditiva) acima da extremidade anterior da janela do vestíbulo, formando uma polia sobre a qual passa o tendão do músculo tensor do tímpano. SIN cochleariform process, p. trochleariformis.

p. condyla′ris mandibulae [TA], p. condilar da mandíbula. SIN condylar process of mandible.

p. coracoi′deus [TA], p. coracóide da escápula. SIN coracoid process.

p. coronoi′deus, p. coronóide. SIN coronoid process.

p. coronoideus mandibulae [TA], p. coronóide da mandíbula. SIN coronoid process of the mandible.

p. coronoideus ulnae [TA], p. coronóide da ulna. SIN coronoid process of the ulna.

p. costa′lis [TA], p. costiforme da vértebra lombar. SIN costal process.

p. ethmoida′lis conchae nasalis inferioris [TA], p. etmoidal da concha nasal inferior. SIN ethmoidal process of inferior nasal concha.

p. falcifor′mis ligamenti sacrotuberalis [TA], p. falciforme do ligamento sacrotuberal. SIN falciform process of sacrotuberous ligament.

p. ferrei′ni, raios medulares. SIN medullary ray.

p. fronta′lis maxil′lae [TA], p. frontal da maxila. SIN frontal process of maxilla.

p. fronta′lis os′sis zygomat′ici [TA], p. frontal do zigomático. SIN frontal process of zygomatic bone.

p. grac′ilis, p. anterior do martelo. SIN anterior process of malleus.

p. intrajugula′ris [TA], p. intrajugular. SIN intrajugular process.

p. jugula′ris ossis occipitalis [TA], p. jugular do occipital. SIN jugular process of occipital bone.

p. lacrima′lis conchae nasalis inferioris [TA], p. lacrimal da concha nasal inferior. SIN lacrimal process of inferior nasal concha.

p. latera′lis mal′lei [TA], p. lateral do martelo. SIN lateral process of malleus.

p. latera′lis ta′li [TA], p. lateral do tálus. SIN lateral process of talus.

p. latera′lis tu′beris calca′nei [TA], p. lateral da tuberosidade do calcâneo. SIN lateral process of calcaneal tuberosity.

p. lenticula′ris incu′dis [TA], p. lenticular da bigorna. SIN lenticular process of incus.

p. mammilla′ris vertebrae lumbalis [TA], p. mamilar da vértebra lombar. SIN mammillary process of lumbar vertebra.

p. mastoi′deus [TA], p. mastóide. SIN mastoid process.

p. mastoideus partis petrosae ossis temporalis [TA], p. mastóide da parte petrosa do osso temporal. SIN mastoid process of petrous part of temporal bone.

p. maxilla′ris conchae nasalis inferioris [TA], p. maxilar da concha nasal inferior. SIN maxillary process of inferior nasal concha.

p. media′lis tu′beris calca′nei [TA], p. medial da tuberosidade do calcâneo. SIN medial process of calcaneal tuberosity.

p. muscula′ris cartila′ginis arytenoi′deae [TA], p. muscular da cartilagem aritenóidea. SIN muscular process of arytenoid cartilage.

p. orbita′lis ossis palatini [TA], p. orbital do palatino. SIN orbital process of palatine bone.

p. palati′nus ossis maxillae [TA], p. palatino da maxila. SIN palatine process of maxilla.

p. papilla′ris lobi caudati hepatis [TA], p. papilar do lobo caudado do fígado. SIN papillary process of caudate lobe of liver.

p. paramastoi′deus [TA], p. paramastóideo. SIN paramastoid process.

p. poste′rior cartila′ginis sep′ti na′si [TA], p. posterior da cartilagem do septo nasal. SIN posterior process of septal cartilage.

p. poste′rior ta′li [TA], p. posterior do tálus. SIN posterior process of talus.

p. pterygoi′deus ossis sphenoidalis [TA], p. pterigóide do osso esfenoidal. SIN pterygoid process of sphenoid bone.

p. pterygospino′sus [TA] p. pterigoespinhoso. SIN pterygospinous process.

p. pyramida′lis ossis palatini [TA], p. pterigóide do palatino. SIN pyramidal process of palatine bone.

p. ra′vii, processo anterior do martelo. SIN anterior process of malleus.

p. retromandibula′ris, parte profunda da glândula parótida. SIN deep part of parotid gland.

p. retromandibula′ris glan′dulae paro′tidis, parte profunda da glândula parótida. SIN deep part of parotid gland.

p. sphenoida′lis cartila′ginis sep′ti na′si, processo posterior da cartilagem do septo nasal; *termo oficial alternativo para posterior process of septal cartilage.

p. sphenoida′lis ossis palatini [TA], p. esfenoidal do palatino. SIN sphenoidal process of palatine bone.

p. spino′sus [TA], espinha do esfenóide. SIN spine of sphenoid bone.

p. spinosus vertebrae [TA], p. espinhoso da vértebra. SIN spinous process of vertebra.

p. styloi′deus os′sis metacarpa′lis III [TA], p. estilóide do metacarpal terceiro. SIN styloid process of third metacarpal bone.

p. styloi′deus os′sis tempora′lis [TA], p. estilóide do temporal. SIN styloid process of temporal bone.

p. styloi′deus ra′dii [TA], p. estilóide do rádio. SIN styloid process of radius.

p. styloi′deus ul′nae [TA], p. estilóide da ulna. SIN styloid process of ulna.

p. supraepicondyla′ris hu′meri [TA], p. supracondilar do úmero. SIN supracondylar process of humerus.

p. tempora′lis ossis zygomatici [TA], p. temporal do osso zigomático. SIN temporal process of zygomatic bone.

p. transver′sus vertebrae [TA], p. transverso da vértebra. SIN transverse process of vertebra.

p. trochleariform′is, p. cocleariforme. SIN p. cochleariformis.

p. trochlea′ris, tróclea fibular do calcâneo. SIN fibular trochlea of calcaneus.

p. uncina′tus os′sis ethmoida′lis [TA], p. uncinado do etmóide. SIN uncinate process of ethmoid bone.

p. uncina′tus pancrea′tis [TA], p. uncinado do pâncreas. SIN uncinate process of pancreas.

p. uncinatus vertebrae cervicalis [TA], unco do corpo da vértebra cervical. SIN uncinate process of cervical vertebra.

p. uncinatus vertebrae thoracicae primae [TA], unco do corpo da primeira vértebra torácica. SIN uncinate process of first thoracic vertebra.

p. vagina′lis os′sis sphenoida′lis [TA], p. vaginal do esfenóide. SIN vaginal process of sphenoid bone.

p. vagina'lis peritone'i, p. vaginal do peritônio. SIN p. vaginalis of peritoneum.
p. vaginalis of peritoneum, túnica vaginal do peritônio; um divertículo peritoneal na parede abdominal ântero-inferior do embrião que atravessa o canal inguinal; no homem, forma a túnica vaginal do testículo e, normalmente, perde sua conexão com a cavidade peritoneal; um processo vaginal persistente na mulher é conhecido como canal de Nuck. SIN Nuck diverticulum, p. vaginalis peritonei, vaginal process of peritoneum, vaginal process of testis.
p. vermifor'mis, apêndice vermiforme. SIN appendix (2).
p. voca'lis cartila'ginis arytenoi'deae [TA], p. vocal da cartilagem aritenóidea. SIN vocal process of arytenoid cartilage.
p. xiphoi'deus [TA], p. xifóide. SIN xiphoid process.
p. zygomat'icus maxil'lae [TA], p. zigomático da maxila. SIN zygomatic process of maxilla.
p. zygomat'icus os'sis fronta'lis [TA], p. zigomático do frontal. SIN zygomatic process of frontal bone.
p. zygomat'icus os'sis tempora'lis [TA], p. zigomático do temporal. SIN zygomatic process of temporal bone.

pro·chei·lia, pro·chi·lia (prō - kī'lē - ă). Proquilia; lábios protrusos. [pro- + G. *cheilos*, lábio]
pro·chei·lon, pro·chi·lon (prō - kī'lon). Tubérculo do lábio superior. SIN tubercle of upper lip.
pro·chi·ral (prō - kī'ral). Proquiral; refere-se a um átomo em uma molécula (geralmente um átomo de carbono) que se tornaria quiral se um dentre dois substituintes idênticos fosse substituído por um novo ligante; isto é, um átomo que tem dois grupos enantiotópicos ligados a ele. Por exemplo, o carbono 1 do etanol é um carbono proquiral.
pro·chi·ral·i·ty (prō - ki - ral'i - tē). Proquiralidade; a propriedade de ser proquiral.
pro·chlor·per·a·zine (prō - klōr - per'ă - zēn). Proclorperazina; um composto fenotiazina com estrutura, ações e empregos semelhantes aos da clorpromazina; usado como tranqüilizante e antiemético; disponível na forma de edisilato, para administração oral e intramuscular, e de maleato para administração oral.
pro·chon·dral (prō - kon'drăl). Procondral; designa um estágio do desenvolvimento anterior à formação de cartilagem. [pro- + G. *chondros*, cartilagem]
pro·chor·dal (prō - kōr'dăl). Procordal; localizado cefálico ao notocórdio. SIN prechordal.
pro·chy·mo·sin (prō - kī'mō - sin). Proquimosina; o precursor da quimosina. SIN chymosinogen, pexinogen, prorennin, renninogen, rennogen.
pro·ci·den·tia (pros - i - den'shē - ă, prō'si-). Procidência; prolapso; queda ou prolapso de qualquer órgão ou parte; geralmente relacionado ao prolapso do útero. [L. queda, de *procido*, cair para frente]
p. u'teri, p. do útero. VER *prolapse* of the uterus.
pro·col·la·gen (prō - kol'ă - jen). Pró-colágeno; precursor solúvel do colágeno formado por fibroblastos e outras células no processo da síntese de colágeno; o pró-colágeno instável tipo III está associado à síndrome de Ehlers-Danlos tipo IV.
p. aminoproteinase, p. aminoproteinase; enzima extracelular que participa do processamento de colágeno, removendo a extensão peptídica na extremidade amino-terminal do pró-colágeno.
p. carboxyproteinase, p. carboxiproteinase; enzima extracelular que participa do processamento de colágeno, removendo a extensão peptídica na extremidade carboxi-terminal do pró-colágeno.
pro·con·ver·tin (prō - kon - ver'tin). Pró-convertina. SIN *factor VII*.
pro·cre·ate (prō'krē - āt). Procriar; gerar; produzir por ato sexual; diz-se geralmente do pai. [L. *pro-creo*, pp. *-creatus*, procriar]
pro·cre·a·tion (prō - krē - ă - shŭn). Procriação. SIN reproduction (1).
pro·cre·a·tive (prō'krē - ă - tiv). Procriador; que tem a capacidade de gerar ou procriar.
△ **proct-.** VER procto-.
proc·tal·gia (prok - tal'jē - ă). Proctalgia; dor no ânus ou no reto. SIN proctodynia, rectalgia. [proct- + G. *algos*, dor]
p. fu'gax, p. fugaz; espasmo doloroso do músculo ao redor do ânus sem causa conhecida; provavelmente uma neurose. SIN anorectal spasm.
proc·ta·tre·sia (prok - tă - trē'zē - ă). Proctatresia. SIN anal atresia. [proct- + G. *a-* priv. + *tresis*, perfuração]
proc·tec·ta·sia (prok - tek - tā'ze'ă). Proctectasia; termo obsoleto para dilatação do reto ou do ânus. [proct- + G. *ektasis*, extensão]
proc·tec·to·my (prok - tekt'tō - mē). Proctectomia; ressecção cirúrgica do reto. SIN rectectomy. [proct- + G. *ektomē*, excisão]
proc·ti·tis (prok - tī'tis). Proctite; inflamação da mucosa do reto. SIN rectitis. [proct- + G. *-itis*, inflamação]
chronic ulcerative p., p. ulcerativa crônica. SIN idiopathic p.
epidemic gangrenous p., p. gangrenosa epidêmica; doença geralmente fatal que afeta principalmente crianças nos trópicos, caracterizada por ulceração gangrenosa do reto e ânus, acompanhada por fezes aquosas freqüentes e tenesmo. SIN bicho, caribi, Indian sickness.

idiopathic p., p. idiopática; provavelmente uma forma de colite ulcerativa que envolve o reto; alguns casos evoluem para envolver o restante do colo também. SIN chronic ulcerative p.
△ **procto-, proct-.** Procto-; ânus; (na maioria das vezes) reto. Cf. recto-. [G. *prōktos*].
proc·to·cele (prok'tō - sēl). Proctocele; prolapso ou hérnia do reto. SIN rectocele. [procto- + G. *kēlē*, tumor]
proc·to·cly·sis (prok - tok'li - sis). Proctoclise; administração contínua lenta de solução salina por instilação no reto e no colo sigmóide. SIN Murphy drip, rectoclysis. [procto- + G. *klysis*, lavagem]
proc·to·coc·cy·pexy (prok - tō-kok'si - pek - sē). Proctococcipexia; sutura de um reto prolapsado aos tecidos anteriores ao cóccix. SIN rectococcypexy. [procto- + G. *kokkyx*, cóccix, + *pēxis*, fixação]
proc·to·co·lec·to·my (prok'tō - kō - lek'tō - mē). Proctocolectomia; remoção cirúrgica do reto juntamente com parte do colo ou todo ele. [procto- + G. *kolon*, cólon, + *ektomē*, excisão]
proc·to·co·li·tis (prok'tō - kō - lī'tis). Proctocolite. SIN coloproctitis.
proc·to·co·lo·nos·co·py (prok'tō - kō'lō - nos'kō - pē). Proctocolonoscopia; inspeção do interior do reto e colo. [procto- + G. *kolon*, cólon, + *skopeō*, ver]
proc·to·col·po·plas·ty (prok'tō - kol'pō - plas - tē). Proctocolpoplastia; fechamento cirúrgico de uma fístula retovaginal. [procto- + G. *kolpos*, vagina, + *plastos*, formado]
proc·to·cys·to·cele (prok'tō - sis'tō - sēl). Proctocistocele; herniação da bexiga para o reto. [procto- + G. *kystis*, bexiga, + *kēlē*, hérnia]
proc·to·cys·to·plas·ty (prok'tō - sis'tō - plas - tē). Proctocistoplastia; fechamento cirúrgico de uma fístula retovesical. [procto- + G. *kystis*, bexiga, + *plastos*, formado]
proc·to·cys·tot·o·my (prok'tō - sis - tot'o - mē). Proctocistotomia; incisão da bexiga a partir do reto. [procto- + G. *kystis*, bexiga, + *tomē*, incisão]
proc·to·de·al (prok'tō - dē - ăl). Proctodeal; relativo ao proctódio.
proc·to·de·um, pl. **proc·to·dea** (prok - tō - dē'um, - dē'ă). Proctódio. 1. Uma depressão revestida por ectoderma sob a raiz da cauda, adjacente à parte terminal do intestino posterior embrionário, em seu fundo, ectoderma proctodeal e endoderma cloacal formam a placa cloacal. Quando essa placa epitelial se rompe, são estabelecidos os orifícios anal e urogenital externos. SIN anal pit. 2. Porção terminal do canal alimentar do inseto, que se estende do piloro (área de fixação do túbulo de Malpighi) até a abertura anal; em determinados dípteros (moscas) e outros insetos, o proctódio é dividido em um intestino anterior tubular e um intestino posterior dilatado, ou reto, terminando no ânus. [L. do G. *prōktos*, ânus, + *hodaios*, no caminho, de *hodos*, um caminho]
proc·to·dyn·ia (prok'tō - din'ē - ă). Proctodinia. SIN proctalgia. [procto- + G. *odynē*, dor]
proc·to·log·ic (prok - tō - loj'ik). Proctológico; relativo à proctologia.
proc·tol·o·gist (prok - tol'ō - jist). Proctologista; um especialista em proctologia.
proc·tol·o·gy (prok - tol'ō - jē). Proctologia; especialidade cirúrgica que estuda o ânus e o reto e suas doenças. [procto- + G. *logos*, estudo]
proc·to·pa·ral·y·sis (prok'tō - pa - ral'i - sis). Proctoparalisia; paralisia do ânus, causando incontinência fecal.
proc·to·per·i·ne·o·plas·ty (prok'tō - per - i - nē'ō - plas - tē). Proctoperineoplastias; cirurgia plástica do ânus e do períneo. SIN rectoperineorraphy. [procto- + *perineum*, + G. *plastos*, formado]
proc·to·pexy (prok'tō - pek - sē). Proctopexia; fixação cirúrgica de um reto prolapsado. SIN rectopexy. [procto- + G. *pēxis*, fixação]
proc·to·pho·bia (prok - tō - fō'bē - ă). Proctofobia; medo mórbido de doença retal. SIN rectophobia. [procto- + G. *phobos*, medo]
proc·to·plas·ty (prok'tō - plas - tē). Proctoplastia; cirurgia plástica do ânus ou reto. SIN rectoplasty. [procto- + G. *plastos*, formado]
proc·to·ple·gia (prok - tō - plē'jē - ă). Proctoplegia; paralisia do ânus e reto que ocorre na paraplegia. [procto- + G. *plēgē*, ataque]
proc·to·pol·y·pus (prok - tō - pol'i - pŭs). Proctopólipo; pólipo do reto.
proc·top·to·sia, proc·top·to·sis (prok - top - tō'sē - ă, - tō'sis). Proctoptose; prolapso do reto e ânus. [procto- + G. *ptōsis*, queda]
proc·tor·rha·gia (prok - tō - rā'jē - ă). Proctorragia; estado caracterizado por secreção sanguinolenta pelo ânus. [procto- + G. *rhēgnymi*, explodir]
proc·tor·rha·phy (prok - tōr'ă - fē). Proctorrafia; reparo por sutura de laceração do reto ou ânus. SIN rectorrhaphy. [procto- + G. *rhaphē*, sutura]
proc·tor·rhea (prok - tō - rē'ă). Proctorréia; secreção mucosserosa do reto. [procto- + G. *rhoia*, fluxo]
proc·to·scope (prok'tō - skōp). Proctoscópio; espéculo retal. SIN rectoscope. [procto- + G. *skopeō*, ver]
Tuttle p., p. de Tuttle; espéculo retal tubular iluminado em sua extremidade distal; após a introdução, o obturador é retirado e uma janela de vidro é inserida na extremidade proximal; então, por meio de um bulbo e um tubo de borracha, conectados ao proctoscópio, a ampola retal pode ser insuflada.
proc·tos·co·py (prok - tos'kō - pē). Proctoscopia; exame visual do reto e do ânus, como por um proctoscópio. SIN rectoscopy.

proc·to·sig·moid (prok′tō - sig′moyd). Proctossigmóide; a área do canal anal e do colo sigmóide, geralmente usada para descrever a região visualizada por retossigmoidoscopia.

proc·to·sig·moi·dec·to·my (prok′tō - sig - moy - dek′tō - mē). Proctossigmoidectomia, retossigmoidectomia; excisão do reto e do colo sigmóide. [procto- + sigmoid, + G. *ektomē*, excisão]

proc·to·sig·moi·di·tis (prok′tō - sig - moy - dī′tis). Proctossigmoidite; inflamação do colo sigmóide e do reto. [procto- + sigmoid + G. *-itis*, inflamação]

proc·to·sig·moi·do·scope (prok′- tō - sig - moid′ō - skōp). Proctossigmoidoscópio, retossigmoidoscópio; aparelho usado no exame do colo sigmóide do reto.

proc·to·sig·moi·dos·co·py (prok′tō - sig - moy - dos′kō - pē). Proctossigmoidoscopia, retossigmoidoscopia; inspeção direta do reto e do colo sigmóide através de um retossigmoidoscópio. [procto- + sigmoid + G. *skopeō*, ver]

proc·to·spasm (prok′tō - spazm). Proctoespasmo. **1.** Contração espasmódica do ânus. **2.** Contração espasmódica do reto. [procto- + G. *spasmos*, espasmo]

proc·tos·ta·sis (prok - tos′tă - sis). Proctostasia; constipação com estase no reto. [procto- + G. *stasis*, estase]

proc·to·stat (prok′tō - stat). Proctostato; um tubo que contém rádio para inserção através do ânus no tratamento do câncer retal; obsoleto. [procto- + G. *statos*, estase]

proc·to·ste·no·sis (prok′tō - stĕ - nō′sis). Proctoestenose; estreitamento do reto ou do ânus. SIN rectostenosis. [procto- + G. *stenōsis*, estreitamento]

proc·tos·to·my (prok - tos′tō - mē). Proctostomia; a formação de uma abertura artificial para o reto. SIN rectostomy. [procto- + G. *stoma*, boca]

proc·to·tome (prok′tō - tōm). Proctótomo; instrumento para uso em proctotomia. SIN rectotome.

proc·tot·o·my (prok - tot′ō - mē). Proctotomia; incisão do reto. SIN rectotomy. [procto- + G. *tomē*, incisão]

proc·to·tre·sia (prok - tō - trē′zē - ă). Proctotresia; operação para correção de ânus imperfurado. [procto- + G. *trēsis*, perfuração]

proc·to·val·vot·o·my (prok′tō - val - vot′ō - mē). Proctovalvotomia; incisão das valvas retais.

pro·cum·bent (prō - kŭm′bent). Procumbente; termo raramente usado que significa decúbito ventral; deitado com a face para baixo. [L. *procumbens*, caído ou inclinado para frente]

pro·cur·va·tion (prō - ker - vā′shŭn). Procurvação; termo raramente usado para designar uma posição curvada para frente. [L. *pro-curvo*, curvo para frente]

pro·cy·cli·dine hy·dro·chlo·ride (prō - sī′kli - dēn). Cloridrato de prociclidina; agente anticolinérgico usado no tratamento da paralisia agitante e do parkinsonismo fármaco-induzido.

pro·cy·cli·dine meth·o·chlo·ride. Metocloreto de prociclidina; medicamento anticolinérgico usado no tratamento do espasmo gastrointestinal funcional. SIN tricyclamol chloride.

pro·dig·i·os·in (prō - dij′ē - ō - sin). Prodigiosina; pigmento vermelho sintetizado pela bactéria *Serratia marcescens*; agente antifúngico.

α**-pro·dine hy·dro·chlo·ride.** Cloridrato de α-prodina. VER alphaprodine.

pro·dro·mal (prō - drō′măl, prod′rō′măl). Prodromal; relativo a um pródromo. SIN prodromic, prodromous, proemial.

pro·drome (prō′drōm). Pródromo; um sinal ou sintoma inicial ou premonitório de uma doença. SIN prodromus. [G. *prodromos*, que ocorre antes, de pro- + *dromos*, um curso]

pro·dro·mic, pro·dro·mous (prō - drō′ - mik, prod′rō -; - mŭs). Prodrômico. SIN prodromal.

prod·ro·mus, pl. **prod·ro·mi** (prod′rō - mŭs, - mī). Pródromo. SIN prodrome.

pro·drug (prō′drŭg). Pró-droga; pró-medicamento; classe de fármacos cuja ação farmacológica resulta da conversão por processos metabólicos no corpo (biotransformação).

pro·duct (prod′ŭkt). Produto. **1.** Qualquer coisa produzida ou feita, seja natural ou artificialmente. **2.** Em matemática, o resultado da multiplicação. [L. *productus*, de *pro-duco*, pp. *-ductus*, levar adiante]

cleavage p., p. de clivagem; substância resultante da divisão de uma molécula em duas ou mais moléculas mais simples.

double p., p. duplo; o p. da pressão sistólica multiplicado pela freqüência cardíaca; uma medida da carga de trabalho cardíaco. VER Robinson *index*.

end p., p. final; o p. final em uma via metabólica.

fibrin/fibrinogen degradation p.'s (FDP), produtos da degradação da fibrina/fibrinogênio; diversos pequenos peptídeos, mal caracterizados, designados X, Y, D e E, resultantes da ação da plasmina sobre o fibrinogênio e a fibrina no processo fibrinolítico.

fission p., p. de fissão; uma espécie atômica produzida durante a fissão de um átomo maior como o U^{235}.

natural p.'s, produtos naturais; compostos naturais que são produtos finais do metabolismo secundário; freqüentemente, são compostos únicos de determinados organismos ou classes de organismos.

orphan p.'s, produtos-órfãos; fármacos, produtos biológicos e aparelhos médicos (incluindo testes diagnósticos *in vitro*) que podem ser úteis em doenças comuns ou raras, mas que não são considerados comercialmente viáveis. SIN orphan drugs.

spallation p., p. de fragmentação; espécie atômica produzida durante a fragmentação de qualquer átomo.

substitution p., p. de substituição; p. obtido substituindo-se um átomo ou grupamento em uma molécula por outro átomo ou grupamento.

pro·duc·tive (prō - dŭk′tiv). Produtivo; que produz ou é capaz de produzir; designa especialmente a inflamação que leva à produção de novo tecido com ou sem exsudato. [ver product]

pro·elas·tase (prō - ē - las′tās). Pró-elastase; a proteína precursora da elastase; formada no pâncreas (em vertebrados) e convertida em elastase pela ação da tripsina.

pro·e·mi·al (prō - ē′mē - ăl). Prodrômico. SIN prodromal. [L. *prooemium*, do G. *prooimion*, prelúdio]

pro·en·ceph·a·lon (prō - en - sef′ă - lon). Prosencéfalo. SIN prosencephalon.

pro·en·keph·a·lin (prō - en - kef′ă - lin). Proencefalina; proteína precursora que contém várias seqüências de encefalina. Cf. propiocortin.

pro·en·zyme (prō - en′zīm). Proenzima; o precursor de uma enzima, exigindo alguma alteração (geralmente a hidrólise de um fragmento inibidor que mascara um grupamento ativo) para torná-lo ativo; p. ex., pepsinogênio, tripsinogênio, pró-fibrinolisina. SIN zymogen.

pro·e·ryth·ro·blast (prō - ē - rith′rō - blast). Proeritroblasto. SIN pronormoblast.

pro·e·ryth·ro·cyte (prō - ē - rith′rō - sīt). Proeritrócito; o precursor de um eritrócito; hemácia imatura com núcleo.

pro·es·tro·gen (prō - es′trō - jen). Proestrogênio; substância que só atua como estrogênio após ser metabolizada no corpo em uma substância ativa.

pro·es·trum (prō - es′trŭm). Proestro. SIN proestrus.

pro·es·trus (prō - es′trŭs). Proestro; o período no ciclo estral que precede o estro, caracterizado pelo crescimento dos folículos de Graaf e alterações fisiológicas relacionadas à produção de estrogênio. SIN proestrum.

pro·fen·a·mine hy·dro·chlo·ride (pro - fen′ă - men). Cloridrato de profenamina. SIN ethopropazine hydrochloride.

Profeta, Giuseppe, dermatologista italiano, 1840–1910. VER P. *law*.

pro·fi·bri·nol·y·sin (prō′fī - bri - nol′i - sin). Pró-fibrinolisina. VER plasmin.

pro·fi·lac·tin (prō - fil - ak′tin). Profilactina; um complexo de actina e profilina. Cf. profilin.

pro·file (prō′fīl). Perfil. **1.** Um esboço ou contorno, principalmente o que representa uma vista lateral da cabeça humana. SIN norma (2). **2.** Um resumo, breve relato ou registro. [It. *profilo*, do L. *pro*, para frente, + *filum*, filamento, linha (contorno)]

biochemical p., p. bioquímico. SIN test p.

biophysical p., p. biofísico; técnica para avaliar o estado fetal utilizando monitorização da freqüência cardíaca fetal e avaliação ultra-sonográfica do volume de líquido amniótico, movimento fetal e movimento respiratório fetal.

facial p., p. facial; **(1)** o contorno da face a partir de uma vista lateral; **(2)** o contorno sagital da face.

personality p., p. de personalidade; **(1)** método pelo qual os resultados de teste psicológico são apresentados na forma gráfica; **(2)** um esboço ou breve descrição da personalidade.

test p., p. de teste; combinação de testes laboratoriais geralmente realizados por métodos automatizados e destinados a avaliar sistemas orgânicos de pacientes após internação em um hospital ou clínica. SIN biochemical p.

urethral pressure p., p. da pressão uretral; o registro contínuo da pressão através de um orifício na lateral de um pequeno cateter à medida que este é puxado (a uma velocidade constante, com infusão de água ou gás através do orifício) de um ponto dentro da bexiga, passando pelo colo vesical e por toda a uretra; forma de medida da resistência que fornece um traçado indicativo do comprimento funcional da uretra e dos pontos de máxima resistência uretral.

pro·fi·lin (prō - fil′in). Profilina; uma pequena proteína que se liga à actina monomérica (assim tornando-se profilactina), impedindo a polimerização prematura da actina. Também participa na inibição de uma isoforma de fosfolipase C.

pro·fi·lom·e·ter (prō′fī - lom′ē - ter). Profilômetro; instrumento para medir a rugosidade de uma superfície, p. ex., dos dentes.

pro·fla·vine (hem·i)sul·fate (prō - flā′vin - vēn). Hemissulfato de proflavina; o sulfato neutro do 3,6-diaminoacridina; um composto intimamente associado à acriflavina, que tem propriedades anti-sépticas semelhantes.

pro·for·mi·phen (prō - fōr′mi - fen). Proformifeno. SIN phenprobamate.

pro·fun·da (prō - fŭn′dă). Profunda; termo aplicado a estruturas (músculos, nervos, veias e artérias, etc.) situados profundamente nos tecidos, principalmente quando comparados a uma estrutura semelhante, mais superficial (sublimis). [L. fem. de *profundus*, profundo]

pro·fun·dus (prō - fŭn′dŭs) [TA]. Profundo. SIN deep. [L.]

pro·fu·sion (prō - fū′zhŭn). Profusão; um escore que reflete o número de lesões visíveis em uma região em radiografias do tórax de indivíduos com pneumoconiose. VER International Labour Organization *Classification*. [L. *profusio*, despejo em grande quantidade, de *profundo*, descarregar em grande quantidade]

pro·ga·bide (prō'gă-bīd). Progabida; anticonvulsivante que é um derivado lipossolúvel da forma amidada do ácido γ-aminobutírico (GABAmida) que, ao contrário do próprio ácido γ-aminobutírico (GABA), consegue atravessar a barreira hematoencefálica. Ao penetrar no encéfalo, o fármaco é convertido em vários metabólitos, alguns dos quais são formas ativas de GABA ou compostos relacionados que atuam sobre os receptores do GABA para aumentar a inibição no encéfalo.

pro·gas·trin (prō-gas'trin). Progastrina; precursor da secreção gástrica na mucosa do estômago.

pro·ge·nia (prō-jē'nē-ă). Prognatia; prognatismo. SIN prognathism. [pro- + L. *gena*, face]

pro·ge·ni·ta·lis (prō-jen-i-tā'lis). Progenital; sobre qualquer uma das superfícies expostas da genitália. [L. prefixo *pro-*, antes, na frente de, + *genitalis*, relativo aos órgãos reprodutivos, de *gigno*, gerar]

pro·gen·i·tor (prō-jen'i-ter,-tōr). Progenitor; um precursor, ancestral; aquele que gera. [L.]

prog·e·ny (proj'ē-nē). Progênie; prole; descendentes. [L. *progenies*, de *progigno*, gerar]

pro·ge·ria (prō-jēr'ē-ă) [MIM*176670]. Progeria; condição de envelhecimento precoce que começa ao nascimento ou no início da infância; caracterizada por retardo do crescimento, aspecto senil com pele seca e enrugada, alopecia total e face de passarinho; ocorrência precoce de aterosclerose nos vasos sanguíneos e morte prematura por doença coronariana; a genética é obscura. SIN Hutchinson-Gilford disease, Hutchinson-Gilford syndrome, premature senility syndrome. [pro- + G. *gēras*, idade avançada]
  p. with cataract, p. with microphthalmia, p. com catarata, p. com microftalmia. SIN dyscephalia mandibulo-oculofacialis.

pro·ges·ta·tion·al (prō'jes-tā'shŭn-ăl). Progestacional. **1.** Que favorece a gravidez; que conduz à gestação; capaz de estimular as alterações uterinas essenciais para implantação e crescimento de um óvulo fertilizado. **2.** Referente a progesterona ou a um fármaco com propriedades semelhantes às da progesterona.

pro·ges·ter·one (prō-jes'ter-ōn). Progesterona; esteróide antiestrogênico, considerado o princípio ativo do corpo lúteo, isolado do corpo lúteo e da placenta ou preparado sinteticamente; usado para corrigir anormalidades do ciclo menstrual e como contraceptivo e para controlar o abortamento habitual. SIN luteohormone, pregnancy hormone, progestational hormone.

pro·ges·tin (prō-jes'tin). Progestina. **1.** Um hormônio do corpo lúteo. **2.** Termo genérico para designar qualquer substância, natural ou sintética, que realiza algumas das alterações biológicas produzidas pela progesterona ou todas elas. **3.** SIN gestagen. [pro- + gestation + -in]

pro·ges·to·gen (prō-jes'tō-jen). Progestógeno. **1.** Qualquer agente capaz de produzir efeitos biológicos semelhantes àqueles da progesterona; a maioria dos progestógenos é composta por esteróides semelhantes aos hormônios naturais. **2.** Um derivado sintético da testosterona que exibe parte da atividade fisiológica e dos efeitos farmacológicos da progesterona; a progesterona é antiestrogênica, enquanto alguns progestógenos apresentam propriedades estrogênicas ou androgênicas além da atividade progestacional. [pro- + gestation + G. *-gen*, que produz]

pro·glos·sis (prō-glos'is). A porção anterior, ou extremidade, da língua. [+ G. *glōssa*, língua]

pro·glot·tid (prō-glot'id). Proglote; um dos segmentos de uma tênia, contendo os órgãos reprodutivos. SIN proglottis. [pro- + G. *glōssa*, língua]

pro·glot·tis, pl. **pro·glot·ti·des** (prō-glot'is, -i-dēz). Proglote. SIN proglottid.

prog·nath·ic (prog-nath'ik, -nā'thik). Prognático. **1.** Que possui uma mandíbula projetada para a frente; que tem um índice gnático acima de 103. **2.** Designa uma projeção anterior de uma ou de ambas as mandíbulas em relação ao esqueleto craniofacial. SIN prognathous. [pro- + G. *gnathos*, mandíbula]

prog·na·thism (prog'nă-thizm). Prognatismo; a condição de ser prognático; projeção para a frente anormal da maxila ou da mandíbula além da relação normal estabelecida com a base do crânio; os côndilos mandibulares estão em sua relação de repouso normal com as articulações temporomandibulares. SIN progenia.
  basilar p., p. basilar; o perfil facial côncavo ou posição do queixo para a frente, semelhante ao prognatismo mandibular, criado pela proeminência do osso da mandíbula no queixo ou mento.

prog·na·thous (prog'nă-thŭs). Prognático. SIN prognathic.

prog·nose (prog-nōs', -nōz'). Prognosticar. SIN prognosticate.

prog·no·sis (prog-nō'sis). Prognóstico; previsão da provável evolução e/ou resultado de uma doença. [G. *prognōsis*, de *pro*, antes, + *gignōskō*, conhecer]
  denture p., p. da prótese; opinião ou julgamento, feito antes do tratamento, das perspectivas de êxito na construção e utilidade de uma dentadura ou restauração.

prog·nos·tic (prog-nos'tik). Prognóstico. **1.** Relativo ao prognóstico. **2.** Um sinal ou sintoma no qual se baseia um prognóstico, ou indicativo da provável evolução. [G. *prognōstikos*]

prog·nos·ti·cate (prog-nos'ti-kāt). Prognosticar; fazer um prognóstico. SIN prognose.

prog·nos·ti·cian (prog-nos-tish'ŭn). Prognosticador; aquele hábil em fazer prognósticos.

pro·gon·o·ma (prō-gon-ō'mă). Progonoma; um nódulo ou massa resultante do deslocamento de tecido quando há atavismo no desenvolvimento embrionário; representa uma reversão à estrutura que não ocorre normalmente nos indivíduos de uma espécie, mas é observada em uma forma ancestral dessa espécie. [pro- + G. *gonos*, prole, + *-oma*, tumor]
  p. of jaw, p. da mandíbula. SIN melanotic neuroectodermal *tumor* of infancy.
  melanotic p., p. melanótico; um nevo piloso pigmentado.

pro·grade. Prógrado; na direção normal de fluxo.

pro·gram. Programa. **1.** Um conjunto formal de procedimentos para orientar uma atividade. **2.** Uma lista ordenada de instruções orientando um computador a realizar uma seqüência desejada de operações necessárias para resolver um problema.

pro·gram·ming (prō'gram-ing). Programação; método de treinamento em segmentos distintos.
  neurolinguistic p., p. neurolingüística; um ramo da psicologia cognitivo-comportamental que emprega técnicas específicas, usando a linguagem para acessar o inconsciente a fim de modificar os estados internos ou comportamentos externos de um cliente.

pro·gran·u·lo·cyte (prō-gran'ū-lō-sīt). Progranulócito. SIN promyelocyte.

pro·gress. 1. (prog'res). Progresso; um avanço; a evolução de uma doença. **2.** (prō-gres'). Progredir; avançar; evoluir; diz-se de uma doença, principalmente quando não-qualificada, que apresenta uma evolução desfavorável. [L. *progredior*, pp. *-gressus*, ir adiante, de *gradior*, andar, ir, de *gradus*, um passo]

pro·gress·ive (prō-gres'iv). Progressivo; que vai para frente; que avança; designa a evolução de uma doença, principalmente quando não-qualificada, uma evolução desfavorável.

pro·gua·nil hy·dro·chlo·ride (prō-gwah'nil). Cloridrato de proguanila. SIN chloroguanide hydrochloride.

pro·hor·mone (prō-hōr'mōn). Pró-hormônio. **1.** Um precursor intraglandular de um hormônio; p. ex., pró-insulina. Cf. prehormone. **2.** Termo obsoleto usado antigamente para designar uma substância desenvolvida no soro que antagoniza um anti-hormônio específico e, assim, potencializa a ação do hormônio correspondente.

pro·in·su·lin (prō-in'sŭ-lin). Pró-insulina; precursor da insulina com uma única cadeia.

pro·jec·tion (prō-jek'shŭn). **1.** Projeção; uma saliência; uma excrescência ou protuberância. **2.** A associação entre uma sensação e o objeto que a produz. **3.** Projeção; mecanismo de defesa pelo qual um complexo reprimido no indivíduo é negado e concebido como pertencendo a outra pessoa, como ocorre quando os erros que a pessoa tende a cometer são percebidos ou atribuídos a outras pessoas. **4.** Projeção; concepção pela consciência de uma ocorrência mental pertencente ao indivíduo como sendo de origem externa. **5.** Projeção; localização de impressões visuais no espaço. **6.** Em neuroanatomia, o sistema ou sistemas de fibras nervosas pelo qual um grupo de células nervosas libera seus impulsos nervosos ("projeta") para um ou mais diferentes grupos celulares. **7.** Projeção; a imagem de um objeto tridimensional sobre um plano, como em uma radiografia. **8.** Incidência; em radiografia, imagens padronizadas de partes do corpo, descritas pela posição da parte do corpo, direção do feixe de raios X através da parte do corpo, ou por epônimo. SIN norma (3), salient (1), view. [L. *projectio*; de *pro- jicio*, pp. *-jectus*, lançar antes]
  anteroposterior p., incidência ântero-posterior. SIN AP p.
  AP p., incidência AP; a incidência radiográfica frontal alternativa, usada principalmente em radiografia no leito ou com aparelho portátil. SIN anteroposterior p.
  apical lordotic p., incidência ápico-lordótica. SIN backprojection.
  axial p., incidência axial; incidência radiográfica destinada a obter visualização direta da base do crânio. SIN axial view, base p., submental vertex p., submentovertical p., verticosubmental view.
  base p., incidência axial. SIN axial p.
  Caldwell p., incidência de Caldwell; incidência radiográfica PA inclinada para permitir a visualização de estruturas da órbita não obstruídas pelas cristas petrosas. SIN Caldwell view.
  cross-table lateral p., incidência lateral transversal à mesa; radiografia em incidência lateral de um objeto em supinação utilizando um feixe de raios X horizontal.
  enamel p., projeção do esmalte; extensão do esmalte para a área de bifurcação.
  erroneous p., p. falsa. SIN false p.
  false p., p. falsa; a sensação visual errônea que se origina secundariamente à hipoatividade de um músculo ocular. SIN erroneous p.
  Fischer p., VER sugars.
  frog-leg lateral p., incidência lateral "em perna de rã"; uma incidência lateral do colo do fêmur feita com a coxa em abdução máxima.
  Granger p., incidência de Granger; incidência de Towne invertida; incidência PA do crânio raramente usada.

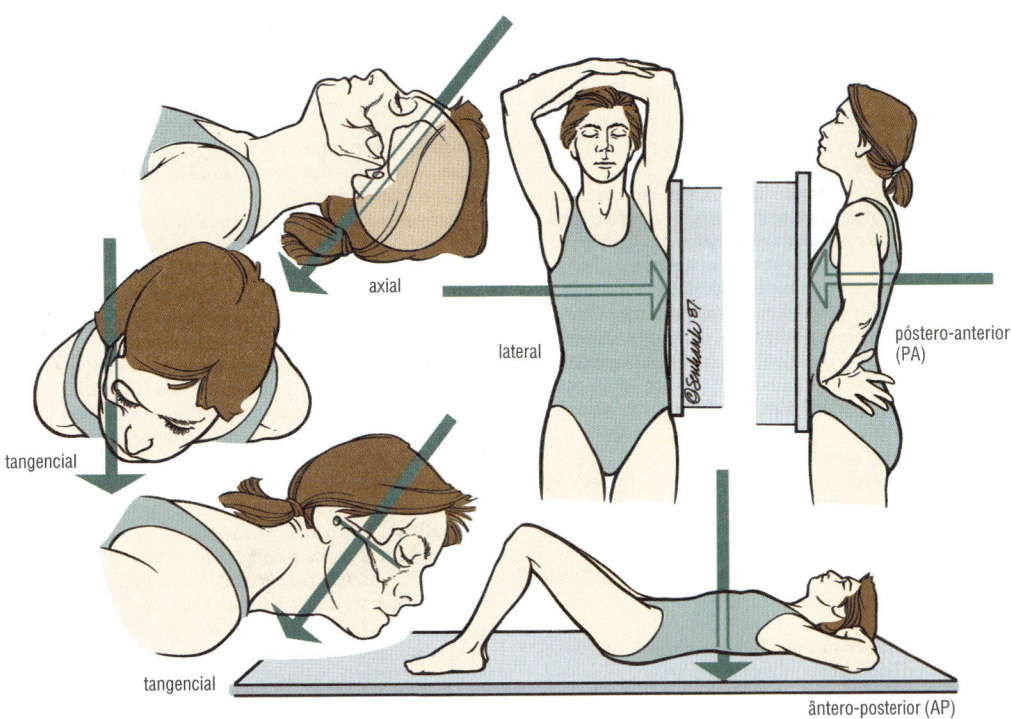

incidências radiográficas

half-axial p., incidência de Towne. SIN Towne p.
Haworth p., projeção de Haworth. VER sugars.
lateral p., incidência lateral; incidência radiográfica com o feixe de raios X em um plano coronal.
maximum intensity p. (MIP), projeção em intensidade máxima; um método de exibição de imagem computadorizada, usada em angiorressonância magnética e tomografia computadorizada helicoidal; uma série de cortes é combinada com exibição do pixel mais brilhante em qualquer corte, em cada localização, e supressão do fundo; simula uma angiografia por projeção (projection *angiogram*).
oblique p., incidência oblíqua; qualquer incidência radiográfica entre frontal e lateral.
occipitomental p., incidência occipitomental. SIN Waters p.
PA p., incidência PA; a incidência radiográfica frontal padrão; incidência radiográfica do crânio com a crista petrosa superposta nas órbitas. SIN posteroanterior p.
posteroanterior p., incidência póstero-anterior. SIN PA p.
Rhese p., incidência de Rhese; incidência radiográfica oblíqua do crânio para exibir o forame óptico.
Stenvers p., incidência de Stenvers; incidência radiográfica oblíqua do crânio destinada a permitir uma incidência não-obstruída do osso petroso, labirinto ósseo, canal auditivo interno e meato. SIN Stenvers view.
submental vertex p., incidência de vértice submental. SIN axial p.
submentovertical p., incidência submentovertical. SIN axial p.
Towne p., incidência de Towne; incidência radiográfica AP inclinada invertida destinada a permitir a demonstração de todo o osso occipital, forame magno e dorso da sela, bem como das cristas petrosas. SIN half axial view, half-axial p., Towne view.
visual p., projeção visual; uma síntese da percepção que envolve os mecanismos visuais.
Waters p., incidência de Waters; uma incidência radiográfica PA do crânio, feita com a linha orbitomeatal formando um ângulo de 37° com o plano do filme, para mostrar as órbitas e os seios maxilares. SIN occipitomental p., Waters view.
Pro·kar·y·o·tae (pro - kar - ē - ō'tē). Super-reino de organismos celulares que inclui o reino Monera (bactérias e algas azul-verdes) e é caracterizado pela condição procariótica, tamanho pequeno (0,2–10 μm para bactérias) e ausência da organização nuclear, capacidades mitóticas e organelas complexas que caracterizam o super-reino Eukaryotae. SIN Procaryotae.
pro·car·y·ote (prō-kar′ē-ōt). Procariota; membro do super-reino Prokaryotae; uma unidade organísmica que consiste em uma única e presumivelmente primitiva célula monérica, ou um microrganismo pré-celular, que não possui uma membrana nuclear, com cromossomas organizados aos pares, um mecanismo mitótico para divisão celular, microtúbulos e mitocôndrias. VER TAMBÉM Prokaryotae, Monera, eukaryote. SIN procaryote.

pro·kar·y·ot·ic (prō′kar-ē-ot′ik). Procariótico; relativo a, ou característico de, um procariota. SIN procaryotic.
pro·la·bi·al (prō-lā′bē-ăl). Prolabial; designa o segmento de tecidos moles central isolado do lábio superior no estado embrionário e em uma fenda palatina bilateral não-reparada.
pro·la·bi·um (prō-lā′bē-ŭm). Prolábio. **1.** A margem carmim exposta do lábio. **2.** O segmento de tecidos moles central isolado do lábio superior no estado embrionário e em uma fenda palatina bilateral não-reparada. [pro- + L. *labium*, lábio]
pro·lac·tin (PRL) (prō-lak′tin). Prolactina; hormônio proteico do lobo anterior da hipófise que estimula a secreção de leite e possivelmente, durante a gravidez, o crescimento mamário. SIN galactopoietic hormone, lactation hormone, lactogenic hormone, lactotropin, mammotropic factor, mammotropic hormone. [pro- + L. *lac, lact*-, leite, + -in]
pro·lac·ti·no·ma (prō-lak-ti-nō′mă). Prolactinoma. SIN prolactin-producing *adenoma.*
pro·lam·ines (prō-lam′ēnz, prō′lă-mēnz, -minz). Prolaminas; proteínas insolúveis em água ou soluções salinas neutras, solúveis em ácidos ou álcalis diluídos, e em álcool a 50–90%; p. ex., gliadina, zeína, hordeína; todos possuem conteúdo de prolina relativamente alto.
pro·lapse (prō-laps′). **1.** Prolapsar; queda, diz-se de um órgão ou outra parte. **2.** Prolapso; queda de um órgão ou outra parte, principalmente seu aparecimento em um orifício natural ou artificial. VER TAMBÉM procidentia, ptosis. [L. *prolapsus*, queda]
p. of the corpus luteum, p. do corpo lúteo; ectrópio do corpo lúteo, devido à eversão da membrana granulosa através da abertura no folículo roto; isso ocorre normalmente em alguns animais.
mitral valve p., p. da valva mitral; movimento retrógrado excessivo de um ou de ambos os folhetos da valva mitral para o átrio esquerdo durante a sístole ventricular esquerda, freqüentemente permitindo regurgitação mitral; responsável pelo clique-sopro da síndrome de Barlow e, raramente, é causado por cardite reumática, um distúrbio do tecido conjuntivo como a síndrome de Marfan, ou ruptura das cordas tendíneas ("folheto mitral plano").
Morgagni p., p. de Morgagni; inflamação crônica do ventrículo de Morgagni.
p. of umbilical cord, p. do cordão umbilical; apresentação de parte do cordão umbilical à frente do feto; pode causar morte fetal devido à compressão do cordão entre a parte de apresentação do feto e a pelve materna.
p. of the uterus, p. uterino; movimento descendente do útero devido à frouxidão e atonia das estruturas musculares e fasciais do assoalho pélvico, geralmente causada por lesões no parto ou pela idade avançada; o p. ocorre em três formas: **p. de primeiro grau,** o colo do útero prolapsado está bem dentro do óstio vaginal; **p. de segundo grau,** o colo está no intróito ou próximo dele; **p. de terceiro grau** (procidência uterina), o colo protrai-se além do óstio vaginal. SIN descensus uteri, falling of the womb.

valvular p., p. valvar; p. que pode envolver qualquer valva ou combinação de valvas, mas geralmente a valva mitral. O p. da valva pulmonar é extremamente raro.

pro·lec·tive (prō-lek-tiv). Prolectivo; relativo a dados colhidos por planejamento antecipado da razão de mortalidade proporcional. O número de mortes por determinada causa, em um período específico, por 100 ou por 1.000 mortes. [pro- + L. *lego*, pp. *lectum*, reunir]

pro·lep·sis (prō-lep'sis). Prolepse; recorrência do paroxismo de uma doença periódica a intervalos que diminuem regularmente. [G. *prolēpsis*, antecipação]

pro·lep·tic (prō-lep'tik). Proléptico; relativo a prolepse. SIN subintrant.

pro·leu·ko·cyte (prō-loo'kō-sīt). Proleucócito. SIN leukoblast.

pro·li·dase (prō'li-dās). Prolidase. SIN *proline* dipeptidase.

pro·lif·er·ate (prō-lif'ĕ-rāt). Proliferar; crescer e aumentar em número por meio de reprodução de formas semelhantes. [L. *proles*, prole, + *fero*, levar]

pro·lif·er·a·tion (prō-lif-ĕ-rā'shŭn). Proliferação; crescimento e reprodução de células semelhantes.
  diffuse mesangial p., glomerulonefrite proliferativa difusa. SIN mesangial proliferative *glomerulonephritis*.
  gingival p., hiperplasia gengival. SIN gingival *hyperplasia*.

pro·lif·er·a·tive, pro·lif·er·ous (prō-lif'er-ā-tiv, -er-ŭs). Proliferativo; que aumenta o número de formas semelhantes.

pro·lif·ic (prō-lif'ik). Prolífico; frutífero; que tem muitos filhos. [L. *proles*, prole, + *facio*, fazer]

pro·lig·er·ous (prō-lij'er-ŭs). Prolígero; que germina; que produz prole. [L. *proles*, prole, + *gero*, gerar]

pro·li·nase (prō'li-nās). Prolinase. SIN *prolyl* dipeptidase.

pro·line (Pro) (prō'lēn). Prolina; ácido pirrolidina-2-carboxílico; o L-isômero é encontrado em proteínas, principalmente os colágenos. SIN pyrrolidine-2-carboxylate.
  p. aminopeptidase, p. aminopeptidase. SIN p. iminopeptidase.
  p. dehydrogenase, p. desidrogenase. SIN pyrroline-2-carboxylate reductase, pyrroline-5-carboxylate reductase.
  p. dipeptidase, p. dipeptidase; enzima que cliva ligações aminoacil-L-prolina em dipeptídeos que contêm um resíduo prolina C-terminal; uma deficiência dessa enzima resulta em hiperimidodipeptidúria. SIN imidodipeptidase, peptidase D, prolidase.
  p. iminopeptidase, p. iminopeptidase; hidrolase que cliva resíduos L-prolil da posição N-terminal em peptídeos. SIN p. aminopeptidase.
  p. oxidase, p. oxidase. SIN pyrroline-2-carboxylate reductase, pyrroline-5-carboxylate reductase.
  p. racemase, p. racemase; enzima que converte reversivelmente D-prolina em L-prolina.
  D-p. reductase, D-p. redutase; oxidorredutase que causa reação reversível entre a D-prolina e o NADH para produzir 5-aminovalerato e NAD$^+$.

pro·lyl (Pro, pro·lyl) (prō'lil). Prolil; o radical acil da prolina.
  p. dipeptidase, p. dipeptidase; enzima que cliva ligações L-prolil-aminoácido em dipeptídeos contendo resíduos prolil N-terminais. SIN iminodipeptidase, prolinase, prolylglycine dipeptidase.
  p. hydroxilase, p. hidroxilase; enzima que catalisa a hidroxilação de alguns resíduos prolil em precursores do colágeno, utilizando oxigênio molecular, íon ferroso, ácido ascórbico e α-cetoglutarato; a deficiência de vitamina C afeta diretamente a atividade dessa enzima; uma forma dessa enzima (p. 4-hidroxilase) sintetiza resíduos 4-hidroxiprolil, enquanto outra produz resíduos 3-hidroxiprolil.

pro·lyl·gly·cine di·pep·ti·dase (prō'lil-glī'sēn). Prolilglicina dipeptidase. SIN *prolyl* dipeptidase.

pro·mas·ti·gote (prō-mas'ti-gōt). Promastigota; termo que agora geralmente é usado em substituição a "leptomônado" ou "estágio leptomônado", para evitar confusão com o gênero de flagelado *Leptomonas*. Designa o estágio flagelado de um protozoário tripanossomídeo no qual o flagelo origina-se de um cinetoplasto na frente do núcleo e emerge da extremidade anterior do microrganismo; geralmente é uma fase extracelular, como no inseto que é hospedeiro intermediário (ou em cultura) de parasitas *Leishmania*. [pro- + G. *mastix*, flagelo]

pro·meg·a·lo·blast (prō-meg'a-lō-blast). Promegaloblasto; o primeiro dos quatro estágios de maturação do megaloblasto. VER erythroblast. SIN pernicious anemia type rubriblast.

pro·met·a·phase (prō-met'ā-fāz). Prometáfase; o estágio de mitose ou meiose no qual a membrana nuclear desintegra-se e os centríolos chegam aos pólos da célula, enquanto os cromossomas continuam a se contrair.

pro·meth·a·zine hy·dro·chlo·ride (prō-meth'a-zēn). Cloridrato de prometazina; anti-histamínico com propriedades antieméticas, freqüentemente usado para aumentar a eficácia de narcóticos.

pro·meth·a·zine the·o·clate (prō-meth'a-zēn). Teoclato de prometazina; sal prometiazínico da 8-clorotofilina; um fármaco anti-histamínico usado para a cinetose.

pro·meth·es·trol di·pro·pi·o·nate (prō-meth'es-trol, dī-prō'pē-ō-nāt). Dipropionato de prometestrol; estrogênio sintético derivado a partir do estilbeno.

pro·me·thi·um (Pm) (prō-mē'thē-ŭm). Promécio; elemento radioativo da série terras raras, de número atômico 61; identificado quimicamente pela primeira vez em 1945; o Pm[145] tem a maior meia-vida conhecida (17,7 anos). [*Prometheus*, um Titã da mitologia grega que roubou o fogo para dar aos mortais]

prom·i·nence (prom'i-nens) [TA]. Proeminência, eminência; em anatomia, tecidos ou partes que se projetam além de uma superfície. SIN prominentia [TA]. [L. *prominentia*]
  Ammon p., p. de Ammon; uma proeminência externa no pólo posterior do bulbo do olho durante o início da embriogênese.
  canine p., eminência canina. SIN canine *eminence*.
  cardiac p., p. cardíaca; a saliência externa visível que aparece sobre a face ventral do embrião humano já na quarta semana, indicativo do desenvolvimento precoce do coração.
  p. of facial canal [TA], p. do canal do facial; a proeminência na parede medial da cavidade timpânica, acima da janela vestibular (oval), produzida pela presença do canal do facial. SIN prominentia canalis facialis [TA].
  forebrain p., p. frontonasal. SIN frontonasal p.
  frontonasal p., p. frontonasal; a proeminência embrionária ímpar formada pelos tecidos que circundam a vesícula do prosencéfalo. SIN forebrain eminence, forebrain p., frontonasal process.
  hepatic p., p. hepática; a saliência externa visível que aparece dorsocaudal à proeminência cardíaca sobre o dorso do embrião humano por volta da quarta semana, indicando o desenvolvimento precoce do fígado.
  hypothenar p., eminência hipotenar. SIN hypothenar *eminence*.
  laryngeal p. [TA], p. laríngea; a projeção na porção anterior do colo, formada pela cartilagem tireóidea da laringe; serve como indicação externa do nível da quinta vértebra cervical. SIN prominentia laryngea [TA], Adam's apple, protuberantia laryngea, thyroid eminence.
  lateral nasal p., p. nasal lateral; tumefação mesenquimal coberta por ectoderma que separa a depressão olfatória embrionária do olho em desenvolvimento; as asas do nariz desenvolvem-se a partir dele. SIN lateral nasal fold, lateral nasal process.
  p. of lateral semicircular canal [TA], p. do canal semicircular lateral; a pequena saliência na parede medial do recesso epitimpânico causada pela proximidade do canal semicircular lateral. SIN prominentia canalis semicircularis lateralis [TA].
  mallear p. [TA], p. malear da membrana timpânica; pequena proeminência na extremidade superior da estria malear produzida pelo processo lateral do martelo. SIN prominentia mallearis [TA].
  medial nasal p., p. nasal medial; tumefação mesenquimal coberta de ectoderma, situada medial ao placódio ou depressão olfatória no embrião; a extremidade nasal e o filtro do lábio desenvolvem-se a partir dele. SIN medial nasal fold, medial nasal process.
  spiral p. of cochlear duct [TA], p. espiral do ducto coclear; uma porção que se projeta do ligamento espiral da cóclea, limitando a margem inferior da estria vascular e contendo um vaso sanguíneo, o vaso proeminente. SIN prominentia spiralis ductus cochlearis [TA].
  styloid p. [TA], p. estilóide; eminência arredondada na parede posterior (mastóide) da cavidade timpânica correspondendo à base do processo estilóide. SIN prominentia styloidea [TA].
  thenar p., eminência tenar. SIN thenar *eminence*.
  tubal p., toro tubário. SIN *torus* tubarius.
  p. of venous valvular sinus, p. do seio valvular venoso; uma pequena eminência na parede externa de uma veia que se correlaciona com o seio valvular imediatamente proximal aos folhetos da válvula venosa. SIN agger valvae venae.

pro·mi·nens (prom'i-nens). Proeminente; em anatomia, designa uma proeminência. [L.]

prom·i·nen·tia, pl. prom·i·nen·ti·ae (prom-i-nen'shē-ā, -shē-ē) [TA]. Proeminência. SIN prominence. [L. de *promineo*, projetar-se, ser proeminente]
  p. cana'lis facia'lis [TA], p. do canal facial. SIN *prominence* of facial canial.
  p. cana'lis semicircula'ris latera'lis [TA], p. do canal semicircular lateral. SIN *prominence* of lateral semicircular canal.
  p. laryn'gea [TA], p. laríngea. SIN laryngeal *prominence*.
  p. mallea'ris [TA], p malear. SIN mallear *prominence*.
  p. spira'lis ductus cochlearis [TA], p. espiral do ducto coclear. SIN spiral *prominence* of cochlear duct.
  p. styloi'dea [TA], p. estilóide. SIN styloid *prominence*.

pro·mi·to·chon·dria (prō-mī-tō-kon'drē-ā). Promitocôndria; precursores das mitocôndrias que possuem estrutura interna pequena (p. ex., não há cristas) e não possuem proteínas para transporte de elétrons. SIN premitochondria.

PROMM Acrônimo para proximal myotonic *myopathy* (miopatia miotônica proximal).

pro·mon·o·cyte (prō-mon'ō-sīt). Promonócito. SIN premonocyte.

prom·on·to·ri·um, pl. prom·on·to·ria (prom'on-tō'rē-ŭm, -rē-ā) [TA]. Promontório. SIN promontory. [L. o cume de uma montanha, promontório, de *promineo*, projetar-se]

promontorium 1295 **propicillin**

p. ca'vi tym'pani [TA], p. da cavidade timpânica. SIN *promontory of tympanic cavity.*
p. os'sis sa'cri [TA], p. da base do sacro. SIN sacral *promontory.*
prom·on·to·ry (prom'on-tō-rē) [TA]. Promontório; eminência ou projeção; projeção de uma parte. SIN promontorium [TA]. [L. *promontorium*]
  pelvic p., p. da base do sacro. SIN sacral p.
  sacral p. [TA], p. da base do sacro; a projeção anterior mais proeminente da base do sacro. SIN promontorium ossis sacri [TA], pelvic p., p. of the sacrum.
  p. of the sacrum, p. da base do sacro. SIN sacral p.
  tympanic p., p. da cavidade timpânica. SIN p. of tympanic cavity.
  p. of tympanic cavity [TA], p. da cavidade timpânica; eminência arredondada sobre a parede labiríntica da orelha média, produzida pela primeira espiral da cóclea. SIN promontorium cavi tympani [TA], tuber cochleae, tympanic p.
pro·mot·er (prō-mō'ter). Promotor. **1.** Em química, uma substância que aumenta a atividade de um catalisador. **2.** Em biologia molecular, uma seqüência de DNA à qual a RNA polimerase se une e dá início à transcrição.
pro·mo·tion (prō-mō'shun). Promoção; estimulação de indução tumoral, após seu início, por um agente promotor que pode não ser carcinogênico.
  health p., p. da saúde; de acordo com a *Organização Mundial de Saúde,* o processo de permitir às pessoas ter maior controle de sua saúde e melhorá-la; envolve a população como um todo no seu cotidiano, em vez de concentrar-se em pessoas sob risco de apresentar doenças específicas, e está voltada para a atuação sobre os determinantes ou causas da saúde.
pro·my·e·lo·cyte (prō-mī'e-lō-sīt). Promielócito. **1.** O estágio de desenvolvimento de um leucócito granulócito entre o mieloblasto e o mielócito, quando surgem alguns grânulos específicos além dos azurófilos. **2.** Uma grande célula uninuclear observada no sangue circulante de pessoas com leucemia mielocítica. SIN premyelocyte, progranulocyte. [pro- + G. *myelos,* medula óssea, + *kytos,* célula]
pro·na·si·on (prō-nā'zē-on). A ponta do ângulo entre o septo do nariz e a superfície do lábio superior, situada no ponto onde uma tangente que passa pelo septo nasal encontra o lábio superior. [pro- + L. *nasus,* nariz]
pro·nate (prō'nāt). Pronar. **1.** Realizar pronação do antebraço ou do pé. **2.** Adotar, ou ser colocado em, uma posição de pronação. [L. *pronatus,* de *prono,* pp. -*atus,* curvar-se para frente, de *pronus,* curvo para frente]
pro·na·tion (prō-nā'shun) [TA]. Pronação; a condição de ser pronado; o ato de adotar uma posição de pronação ou ser colocado nessa posição; um movimento específico de rotação do antebraço que faz a palma da mão girar para trás; um movimento específico de rotação do pé em que a superfície plantar é girada para fora.
  p. of foot, p. do pé; eversão e abdução do pé, elevando a borda lateral.
  p. of forearm, p. do antebraço; rotação do antebraço de forma que a palma da mão fica voltada para trás, quando o braço está em posição anatômica, ou para baixo, quando o braço está estendido, formando um ângulo reto com o corpo.
pro·na·tor (prō-nā'ter, tōr) [TA]. Pronador; músculo que coloca uma parte do corpo em pronação. VER muscle. [L.]
prone (prōn). Prono; designa: **1.** O corpo quando deitado com a face voltada para baixo. **2.** Pronação do antebraço ou do pé. [L. *pronus,* dobrado para baixo ou para diante]
pro·neph·ros, pl. **pro·neph·roi** (prō-nef'ros, -roy). Pronefro. **1.** O órgão excretor definitivo dos peixes primitivos. SIN head kidney. **2.** Nos embriões de vertebrados superiores, uma estrutura vestigial consistindo em uma série de túbulos tortuosos que se esvaziam na cloaca através do ducto néfrico primário; no embrião humano, o pronefro é uma estrutura muito rudimentar e temporária, seguida pelo mesonefro e, depois, pelo metanefro. SIN forekidney, primordial kidney. [pro- + G. *nephros,* rim]
pro·no·grade (prō'nō-grād). Pronógrado; que caminha ou repousa com o corpo em posição horizontal, designando a postura dos quadrúpedes; o contrário de ortógrado. [L. *pronus,* inclinado para diante, + *gradior,* caminhar]
pro·nom·e·ter (prō-nom'e-ter). Pronômetro. SIN goniometer (3).
pro·nor·mo·blast (prō-nōr'mō-blast). Pronormoblasto; o primeiro dos quatro estágios no desenvolvimento do normoblasto. VER TAMBÉM erythroblast. SIN proerythroblast, rubriblast.
pro·nu·cle·us, pl. **pro·nu·clei** (prō-noo'klē-ūs, -klē-ī). Pronúcleo. **1.** Um dos dois núcleos que se fundem na cariogamia. **2.** Em embriologia, o material nuclear da cabeça do espermatozóide (**pronúcleo masculino**) ou do óvulo (**pronúcleo feminino**), após a penetração do espermatozóide no óvulo; cada pronúcleo normalmente possui um número haplóide de cromossomas, de forma que a fusão dos pronúcleos na fertilização restabelece o número diplóide.
proof·read·ing (pruf'rēd-ing). Revisão; a propriedade de algumas polimerases, p. ex., DNA polimerase, de usar sua atividade de exonuclease para remover bases introduzidas erradamente e substituí-las pelas bases corretas.
pro·opi·o·mel·a·no·cor·tin (POMC) (prō-ō'pē-ō-mel'ă-nō-kōr'tin). Pró-opiomelanocortina; uma grande molécula encontrada nos lobos anterior e intermédio da hipófise, no hipotálamo e em outras partes do encéfalo, bem como nos pulmões, no trato gastrointestinal e na placenta; precursora do ACTH, CLIP, β-LPH, γ-MSH, β-endorfina e met-encefalina.
pro·ot·ic (prō-ō'tik). Pró-ótico; na frente da orelha. [pro- + G. *ous,* orelha]

pro-ox·i·dants (prō-oks'i-dănts). Pró-oxidantes; compostos ou agentes capazes de gerar espécies tóxicas de oxigênio. Cf. antioxidant.
pro·pa·fen·one (prō-paf'ĕ-nōn). Propafenona; agente antiarrítmico classificado como classe I_c, assemelhando-se à flecainida e encainida. Bloqueia os canais rápidos de sódio e foi usada no tratamento de arritmias cardíacas ventriculares.
prop·a·gate (prop'ă-gāt). Propagar. **1.** Reproduzir; gerar. **2.** Mover ao longo de uma fibra, p. ex., propagação do impulso nervoso. [L. *propago,* pp. *-atus,* gerar, reproduzir]
prop·a·ga·tion (prop-ă-gā'shun). Propagação; o ato de propagar.
prop·a·ga·tive (prop-ă-gā'tiv). Propagativo; propagador; relativo ou que diz respeito à propagação; designando a parte sexual de um animal ou vegetal distinta do corpo.
pro·pal·i·nal (prō-pal'i-năl). Propalinal; para trás e para frente; designa um movimento anterior e posterior. [pro- + G. *palin,* para trás]
pro·pam·i·dine (prō-pam'i-dēn). Propamidina; ativa contra infecções por *Trypanosoma gambiense;* também significativamente bacteriostática; usada como agente antiinfeccioso local em solução aquosa a 0,1% e contra infecções fúngicas sistêmicas como blastomicose; também usada no tratamento da ceratite por *Acanthamoeba.*
pro·pane (prō'pān). Propano; uma das séries alcano de hidrocarbonetos.
pro·pane·di·o·ic ac·id (prō-pān-dī'ō-ik). Ácido propanodióico. SIN malonic acid.
1,2,3-pro·pane·tri·ol (prō-pān-trī'ol). 1,2,3-propanotriol, glicerol. SIN glycerol.
pro·pan·i·did (prō-pan'i-did). Propanidida; um eugenol de ação curta usado por via intravenosa para indução de anestesia geral.
pro·pa·no·ic ac·id (prō-pă-nō'ik). Ácido propanóico. SIN propionic acid.
pro·pa·nol (prō'pă-nol). Propanol. SIN propyl alcohol.
pro·pa·no·yl (prō'pă-nō-il). Propanoíla. SIN propionyl.
pro·pan·the·line bro·mide (prō-pan'the-lēn brō-mīd); o análogo isopropílico do brometo de metantelina; agente anticolinérgico.
pro·par·a·caine hy·dro·chlo·ride (prō-par'ă-kān). Cloridrato de proparacaína; agente anestésico de superfície usado em oftalmologia. SIN proxymetacaine hydrochloride.
pro·pa·tyl ni·trate (prō'pă-til). Nitrato de propatila; dilatador coronariano.
pro·pene (prō'pēn). . Propeno, propileno. SIN propylene.
pro·pent·dy·o·pents (prō-pent-dī'ō-pentz). VER bilirubinoids.
pro·pe·nyl (prō'pē-nil). Propenil; o radical, –CH₂≠CH–CH₃.
pro·pep·sin (prō-pep'sin). Propepsina, pepsinogênio. SIN pepsinogen.
pro·pep·tone (prō-pep'tōn). Propeptona; uma mistura não-descrita de produtos intermediários na conversão da proteína nativa em peptona.
pro·per·din (prō-per'din). Properdina; uma globulina do soro normal envolvida na resistência à infecção, que participa, juntamente com outros fatores, de uma via alternativa para a ativação dos componentes terminais do complemento; a deficiência de properdina impede a estabilização da enzima alternativa C3-convertase (um distúrbio recessivo ligado ao X). VER TAMBÉM properdin *system, component* of complement, *factor* P. [pro- + L. *perdo,* destruir]
pro·per·i·to·ne·al (prō'per-i-tō-nē'ăl). Properitoneal; na frente do peritônio.
pro·phage (prō'fāj). Profago. SIN probacteriophage.
  defective p., p. defeituoso. VER defective *bacteriophage.*
pro·phase (prō'fāz). Prófase; a primeira fase da mitose ou meiose, que consiste em contração linear e aumento da espessura dos cromossomas (cada um formado por duas cromátides) acompanhada por migração dos dois centríolos-filhos e seus ásteres em direção aos pólos da célula. Na meiose, a prófase é complexa e pode ser subdividida em estágios: preleptóteno, leptóteno, zigóteno, paquíteno, diplóteno e diacinese. [G. *prophasis,* de *prophainō,* prenunciar]
pro·phen·py·rid·a·mine ma·le·ate (prō'fen-pi-rid'ă-mēn). Maleato de profempiridamina. SIN pheniramine maleate.
pro·phy·lac·tic (prō-fi-lak'tik). Profilático. **1.** Que evita doenças; relativo à profilaxia. SIN preventive. **2.** Um agente que atua prevenindo uma doença. [G. *prophylaktikos;* ver prophylaxis]
pro·phy·lax·is, pl. **pro·phy·lax·es** (prō-fi-lak'sis, -sēz). Profilaxia; prevenção de doença ou de um processo que pode levar a doença. [L. mod. do G. *pro-phylassō,* guardar, tomar precaução]
  active p., p. ativa; uso de um agente antigênico (imunogênico) para estimular ativamente o mecanismo imunológico.
  chemical p., p. química; a administração de substâncias químicas ou fármacos a membros de uma comunidade a fim de reduzir o número de portadores de uma doença e evitar que outros a contraiam.
  dental p., p. dental; série de procedimentos nos quais são removidos tártaro, manchas e outros materiais das coroas clínicas dos dentes e polidas as superfícies do esmalte.
  passive p., p. passiva; uso de um anti-soro de outra pessoa ou animal para obter proteção temporária contra um agente infeccioso ou tóxico específico.
pro·pi·cil·lin (prō-pi-sil'in). Propicilina; penicilina semi-sintética, estável em meio ácido, que pode ser mais efetiva que a penicilina G. SIN α-phenoxypropylpenicillin potassium.

pro·pi·o·cor·tin (pro-pe-o-kor'ten). Propiocortina; polipeptídeo endógeno que poderia ser um precursor das encefalinas. Cf. proenkephalin.

pro·pi·o·lac·tone (pro-pe-o-lak'ton). Propiolactona; usada para esterilizar plasma, vacinas e enxertos teciduais.

pro·pi·o·nate (pro'pe-o-nat). Propionato; um sal ou éster do ácido propiônico.

Pro·pi·on·i·bac·te·ri·um (pro-pe-on-i-bak-ter'e-um). Gênero de bactérias imóveis, não-formadoras de esporos, anaeróbicas ou aerotolerantes (família Propionibacteriaceae) contendo bacilos Gram-positivos, geralmente pleomórficos, difteróides ou claviformes, com uma extremidade arredondada, a outra afilada ou pontiaguda. Algumas células podem ser cocóides, alongadas ou bífidas, ou até mesmo ramificadas. As células geralmente são observadas isoladamente, em pares, em configurações em V e Y, cadeias curtas ou grupos arrumados como "ideogramas chineses". O metabolismo desses microrganismos é fermentativo, e os produtos da fermentação incluem combinações de ácidos propiônico e acético. Esses microrganismos são encontrados em laticínios, na pele humana e no trato intestinal dos seres humanos e de outros animais. Podem ser patogênicos. A espécie típica é *P. freudenreichii*.

P. ac'nes, espécie de bactéria comumente encontrada nas pústulas da acne, embora seja encontrada em outros tipos de lesões nos seres humanos, e até mesmo como um sapráfita no intestino, na pele, nos folículos pilosos e em esgotos.

P. freudenrei'chii, espécie de bactéria encontrada no leite cru, no queijo suíço e em outros laticínios; é a espécie típica do gênero P.

P. jensen'ii, espécie de bactéria encontrada em laticínios, na silagem e, algumas vezes, em infecções.

P. propion'icus. SIN *Arachnia propionica.*

pro·pi·on·ic ac·id (pro-pe-on'ik). Ácido propiônico; ácido metilacético; ácido etilfórmico; encontrado no suor; elevado em casos de hiperglicemia cetótica e em casos de deficiência de biotina. SIN propanoic acid.

pro·pi·on·ic ac·i·de·mia (pro-pe-on'ik-as-i-de'me-a). Acidemia propiônica. SIN ketotic *hyperglycinemia.*

pro·pi·o·nyl (pro'pe-o-nil). Propionil; CH$_3$CH$_2$CO–; o radical acil do ácido propiônico. SIN propanoyl.

pro·pi·o·nyl-CoA (pro'pe-o-nil-ko-a). Propionil-CoA; o derivado tioéster da coenzima A do ácido propiônico; um intermediário na degradação da L-valina, L-isoleucina, L-treonina, L-metionina e dos ácidos graxos de cadeia ímpar; acumula-se em indivíduos com deficiência de propionil-CoA carboxilase.

p.-CoA carboxylase, propionil-CoA carboxilase; enzima que catalisa a reação da propionil-CoA com CO$_2$ e ATP para produzir ADP, ortofosfato e D-metilmalonil-CoA; uma enzima biotina-dependente; a deficiência hereditária dessa enzima causará acidemia propiônica e retardo do desenvolvimento.

pro·pi·o·nyl·gly·cine (pro'pe-o-nil-gli'sen). Propionilglicina; um metabólito menor que se acumula em pessoas com acidemia propiônica.

pro·pit·o·caine hy·dro·chlo·ride (pro-pit'o-kan). Cloridrato de propitocaína. SIN prilocaine hydrochloride.

pro·pla·sia (pro-pla'ze-a). Proplasia; o estado da célula ou do tecido em que a atividade está aumentada acima do nível considerado euplasia, isto é, caracterizado por estimulação, reparo ou regeneração. [pro- + G. *plasso*, formar]

pro·plas·ma·cyte (pro-plaz'ma-sit). Proplasmócito; célula observada no processo de diferenciação de um plasmoblasto em um plasmócito maduro.

pro·plex·us (pro-plek'sus). O plexo corióideo no ventrículo lateral do cérebro.

pro·po·fol (pro'po-fol). Propofol; emulsão de óleo em água de 1,6-diisopropilfenol, um hipnótico com ação de início rápido e curta duração; usado por via intravenosa para indução e manutenção de anestesia geral. SIN 2,6-diisopropyl phenol.

pro·pos·i·tus, pl. **pro·po·si·ti** (pro'poz'i-tus, -ti). 1. Probando, geralmente referindo-se ao primeiro caso índice determinado. Cf. consultant. 2. Uma premissa; um argumento. [L. de *propono*, pp. -*positus*, planejar, propor]

pro·pox·y·phene hy·dro·chlo·ride (pro-pok'si-fen). Cloridrato de propoxifeno; analgésico narcótico fraco, efetivo por via oral, não-antipirético, estruturalmente relacionado à metadona e usado para alívio da dor leve a moderada; é menos efetivo que a codeína. SIN dextropropoxyphene hydrochloride.

pro·pox·y·phene nap·syl·ate (pro-pok'si-fen). Napsilato de propoxifeno; analgésico narcótico fraco. SIN dextropropoxyphene napsylate.

pro·pran·o·lol hy·dro·chlo·ride (pro-pran'o-lol). Cloridrato de propranolol; bloqueador de receptores β-adrenérgicos; usado no tratamento da angina de peito, hipertensão arterial, arritmias cardíacas e outros distúrbios.

pro·pri·e·tary name (pro-pri'e-tar-e). Nome comercial; marca registrada; nome patenteado; o nome comercial ou marca registrada protegido, registrado no *Departamento de Marcas e Patentes dos Estados Unidos* (*U.S. Patent Office*), sob o qual um fabricante comercializa seu produto. É escrito com uma inicial maiúscula e freqüentemente discriminado por um R supra-escrito em um círculo (®). Cf. generic name, nonproprietary name. [L. *proprietas*, propriedade]

pro·pri·o·cep·tion (pro-pre-o-sep'shun). Propriocepção; sentido ou percepção, geralmente em nível subconsciente, dos movimentos e da posição do corpo e principalmente de seus membros, independentemente da visão; esse sentido é obtido basicamente por impulsos provenientes das terminações nervosas sensoriais, em músculos e tendões (fusos musculares) e na cápsula fibrosa das articulações, combinados a impulsos do aparelho vestibular.

pro·pri·o·cep·tive (pro'pre-o-sep'tiv). Proprioceptivo; capaz de receber estímulos originados nos músculos, tendões e outros tecidos internos. [L. *proprius*, próprio, + *capio*, tomar]

pro·pri·o·cep·tor (pro'pre-o-sep'ter). Proprioceptor; um dos vários órgãos sensoriais (como o fuso muscular e o órgão neurotendíneo de Golgi) em músculos, tendões e cápsulas articulares que percebem a posição ou o estado de contração.

pro·pri·o·spi·nal (pro'pre-o-spi'nal). Propriospinal; relativo especial ou totalmente à medula espinal; especificamente, designa as células nervosas e suas fibras que ligam os diferentes segmentos da medula espinal entre si (p. ex., espino-espinal).

pro·pro·teins (pro'pro-tenz). Proproteínas; precursores inativos das proteínas; p. ex., proinsulina.

prop·tom·e·ter (prop-tom'e-ter). Proptômetro. SIN exophthalmometer. [pro- + G. *ptosis*, queda, + *metron*, medida]

prop·to·sis (prop-to'sis). Proptose. SIN exophthalmos. [G. *proptosis*, queda para diante]

prop·tot·ic (pro-tot'ik). Proptótico; referente à proptose.

pro·pul·sion (pro-pul'shun). Propulsão; a tendência a cair para frente; responsável pela festinação na paralisia agitante. [G. *pro-pello*, pp. -*pulsus*, impelir]

pro·pyl (Pr) (pro'pil). Propil; o radical alquil do propano, CH$_3$CH$_2$CH$_2$–.

p. alcohol, álcool propílico; solvente para resinas e ésteres de celulose. SIN propanol.

p. gallate, galato de propil; antioxidante para emulsões.

p. hydroxybenzoate, hidroxibenzoato de propil. SIN propylparaben.

pro·pyl·car·bi·nol (pro-pil-kar'bi-nol). Propilcarbinol; álcool butílico primário. SIN butyl alcohol.

pro·py·lene (pro'pi-len). Propileno; metiletileno; um hidrocarboneto olefínico gasoso. SIN propene.

p. glycol, propileno glicol; solvente usado em vários fármacos hidrossolúveis para administração parenteral; um ingrediente de pomada hidrófila; um solvente orgânico viscoso freqüentemente usado em preparações farmacêuticas para dissolver substâncias farmacológicas com solubilidade aquosa limitada; usado em parte no preparo de soluções injetáveis de diazepam, fenitoína, pentobarbital e outros fármacos.

pro·pyl·hex·e·drine (pro-pil-hek'se-dren). Propilexedrina; simpaticomimético e vasoconstritor local; freqüentemente usado por inalação.

pro·pyl·i·o·done (pro-pil-i'o-don). Propiliodona; meio radiopaco usado antigamente para broncografia.

pro·pyl·par·a·ben (pro-pil-par'a-ben). Propilparabeno; agente antifúngico e conservante farmacêutico. SIN propyl hydroxybenzoate.

pro·pyl·thi·o·ur·a·cil (PTU) (pro'pil-thi-o-u'ra-sil). Propiltiouracil; agente antitireóideo que inibe a síntese de hormônios tireóideos; usado no tratamento do hipertireoidismo; um bociogênico.

pro·py·ro·ma·zine (pro-pi-ro'ma-zen). Propiromazina; antiespasmódico intestinal com propriedades anticolinérgicas.

pro rat. aet. Abreviatura do L. *pro ratione aetatis*, de acordo com a idade (do paciente).

pro re na·ta (p.r.n.) (pro re na'ta). Quando surgir a ocasião; quando necessário (SOS). [L.]

pro·ren·nin (pro-ren'in). Pró-renina. SIN prochymosin.

pror·sad (pror'sad). Direcionado para frente. [L. *prorsum*, para frente, + *ad*, para]

pro·ru·bri·cyte (pro-roo'bri-sit). Pró-rubricito; normoblasto basófilo. VER erythroblast. [pro- + rubricyte]

pernicious anemia type p., p. do tipo anemia perniciosa; megaloblasto basófilo. VER erythroblast, megaloblast.

pros (pros). 1. (π) Referente ao átomo de nitrogênio no anel imidazol na histidina que está mais próximo do carbono β. Cf. *tele*. 2. *pros-*; Prefixo para junto de ou na frente. [G. próximo]

pro·scil·lar·i·din (pro-si-lar'i-din). Proscilaridina; preparado de cebola-albarrã, a cebola marinha *Urginea maritima*; agente cardiotônico, usado no tratamento da insuficiência cardíaca congestiva.

pro·sco·lex (pro-sko'leks). Proescólex; termo raramente usado para a forma embrionária de uma tênia. [pro- + G. *skolex*, verme]

pro·se·cre·tin (pro-se-kre'tin). Pró-secretina; secretina inativa.

pro·sect (pro-sekt'). Dissecar um cadáver ou qualquer parte, o que pode servir para demonstração de anatomia durante uma aula. [L. *pro-seco*, pp. -*sectus*, cortar]

pro·sec·tor (pro'sek'ter). Dissector; aquele que realiza a dissecção ou prepara o material para uma demonstração de anatomia em uma aula.

pro·sec·to·ri·um (pro'sek-to're-um). Sala de dissecção; local em que são feitos os preparos anatômicos para demonstração ou para preservação em um museu. [L.]

pros·en·ceph·a·lon (pros-en-sef′ă-lon) [TA]. Prosencéfalo; a vesícula cerebral primitiva anterior e a mais rostral das três vesículas cerebrais primárias do tubo neural embrionário; subdivide-se para formar o diencéfalo e o telencéfalo. SIN forebrain vesicle*, forebrain*, proencephalon. [G. *prosō*, para diante, + *enkephalos*, encéfalo]

Proskauer, Bernhard, bacteriologista alemão, 1851–1915. VER Voges-P. *reaction*.

pros·o·dem·ic (pros-ō-dem′ik). Prosodêmico; designa uma doença transmitida diretamente de uma pessoa para outra. [G. *prosō*, para frente, + *dēmos*, povo]

pros·o·dy (proz′ō-dē). Prosódia; a variação no ritmo, intensidade e freqüência da fala que ajuda a transmitir o significado.

prosop-. VER prosopo-.

pros·o·pag·no·sia (pros′ō-pag-nō′sē-ă). Prosopagnosia; dificuldade em reconhecer faces familiares. [prosop- + G. *a-* priv. + *gnōsis*, reconhecimento]

pros·o·pa·gus (pro-sop′ă-gŭs). Prosópago. SIN prosopopagus.

pros·o·pec·ta·sia (pros′ō-pek-tā′zē-ă). Prosopectasia; aumento da face, como na acromegalia. [prosop- + G. *ektasis*, extensão]

pros·o·pla·sia (pros-ō-plā′zē-ă). Prosoplasia; transformação progressiva, como a transformação das células dos ductos salivares em células secretoras. VER cytomorphosis. [G. *prosō*, para frente, + *plasis*, moldagem]

prosopo-, prosop-. A face. VER TAMBÉM facio-. [G. *prosōpon*]

pros·o·po·a·nos·chi·sis (pros′ō-pō-ă-nos′ki-sis). Prosopoanosquise. SIN facial cleft. [prosopo- + G. *anō*, para cima, + *schisis*, fissura]

pros·o·pop·a·gus (pros-ō-pop′ă-gŭs). Prosópago; gêmeos conjugados diferentes, nos quais o parasita, na forma de uma massa tumoral, está unido à órbita ou bochecha do autósito. VER conjoined *twins*, em *twin*. SIN prosopagus. [prosopo- + G. *pagos*, algo unido]

pros·o·pos·chi·sis (pros-ō-pos′ki-sis). Prosoposquise; fenda facial congênita da boca até o ângulo interno do olho. SIN oblique facial cleft. [prosopo- + G. *schisis*, fissura]

pros·o·po·thor·a·cop·a·gus (pros′ō-pō-thor-ă-kop′ă-gŭs). Prosopotoracópago; gêmeos conjugados unidos pela face e pelo tórax; um tipo de cefalotoracópago. VER conjoined *twins*, em *twin*. [prosopo- + G. *thōrax*, tórax, + *pagos*, algo unido]

pros·ta·cy·clin (pros-tă-sī′klin). Prostaciclina; potente inibidor natural da agregação plaquetária e vasodilatador. SIN epoprostenol, epoprostenol sodium.

pros·ta·glan·din (PG) (pros-tă-glan′din). Prostaglandina; qualquer membro de uma classe de substâncias fisiologicamente ativas, presentes em muitos tecidos, com efeitos como vasodilatação, vasoconstrição, estimulação da musculatura lisa intestinal ou brônquica, estimulação uterina e antagonismo a hormônios que influenciam o metabolismo lipídico. As prostaglandinas são ácidos prostanóicos com cadeias laterais de graus variáveis de insaturação e oxidação. Freqüentemente abreviadas PGA, PGB, PGC, PGD, etc. com subscritos numéricos de acordo com a estrutura. [de líquidos genitais com glândulas acessórias onde foram descobertas]

p. E_1, p. E_1. SIN alprostadil.

p. E_2, p. E_2. SIN dinoprostone.

p. endoperoxide synthase, p. endoperóxido sintase; complexo proteico que catalisa duas etapas na biossíntese da prostaglandina; a atividade da ciclooxigenase (que é inibida pelo ácido acetilsalicílico e pela indometacina) converte o araquidonato e o $2O_2$ em prostaglandina G_2; a atividade hidroperoxidase usa a glutationa para converter prostaglandina G_2 em p. H_2. SIN cyclooxygenase.

p. $F_{2\alpha}$, p. $F_{2\alpha}$. SIN dinoprost.

p. $F_{2\alpha}$ **trometamine,** p. $F_{2\alpha}$ trometamina. SIN dinoprost tromethamine.

pros·ta·no·ic ac·id (pros′tă-nō-ik). Ácido prostanóico; o ácido com 20 carbonos que é o esqueleto das prostaglandinas, com várias substituições hidroxila e ceto nas posições 9, 11 e 15, e ligações duplas nas cadeias alifáticas longas.

pros·ta·noids (pros′tă-nōids). Prostanóides; derivados do ácido prostanóico; p. ex., prostaglandinas, tromboxanos, etc.

prostat-. VER prostato-.

pros·ta·ta (pros′tah-tă) [TA]. Próstata. SIN prostate. [L. mod. do G. *prostatēs*, que está adiante]

pros·ta·tal·gia (pros-tă-tal′jē-ă). Prostatalgia; termo raramente usado para designar a dor na área da próstata. [prostat- + G. *algos*, dor]

pros·tate (pros′tāt) [TA]. Próstata; um corpo em forma de amêndoa, que circunda o início da uretra no homem; consiste em dois lobos laterais unidos, anteriormente, pelo istmo e, posteriormente, por um lobo médio situado acima dos ductos ejaculatórios e entre estes. É formada por 30–50 glândulas tubuloalveolares compostas, entre as quais há estroma abundante, que consiste em fibras colágenas e elásticas e muitos feixes de músculo liso. A secreção glandular é um líquido leitoso eliminado por ductos excretores para a uretra prostática no momento da emissão do sêmen. SIN prostata [TA], glandula prostatica, prostate gland.

female p., termo aplicado algumas vezes às glândulas periuretrais na parte superior da uretra feminina.

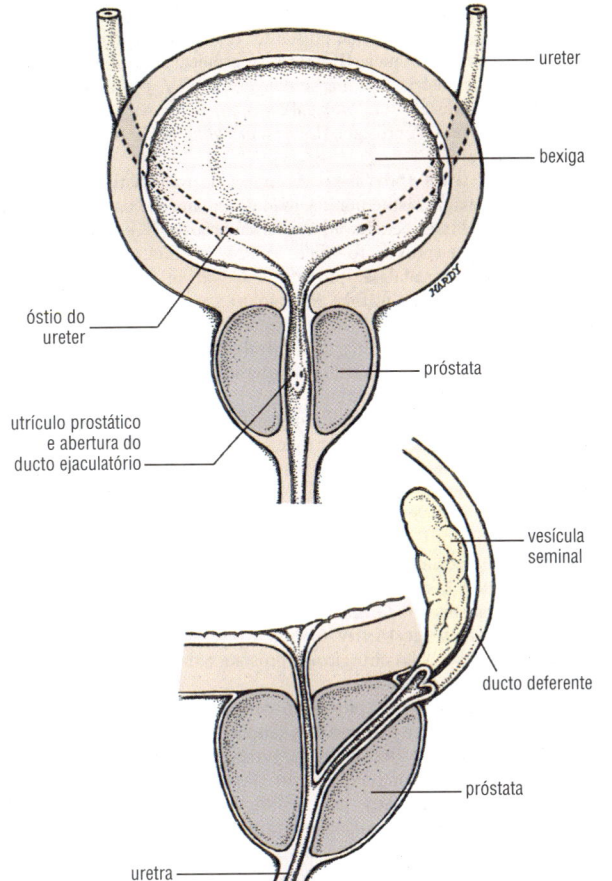

próstata e estruturas adjacentes

pros·ta·tec·to·my (pros-tă-tek′tō-mē). Prostatectomia; remoção de parte da próstata ou de toda ela. [prostat- + G. *ektomē*, excisão]

pros·tat·ic (pros-tat′ik). Prostático; relativo à próstata.

pros·tat·i·co·ves·i·cal (pros-tat′i-kō-ves′i-kăl). Prostaticovesical; relativo à próstata e à bexiga.

pros·ta·tism (pros′tă-tizm). Prostatismo; uma síndrome clínica, observada principalmente em homens idosos, geralmente causada por aumento da próstata e que se manifesta por sinais e sintomas irritativos (nictúria, polaciúria, diminuição do volume eliminado, urgência sensorial e incontinência de urgência) e obstrutivos (hesitação, diminuição do jato, gotejamento terminal, micção dupla e retenção urinária).

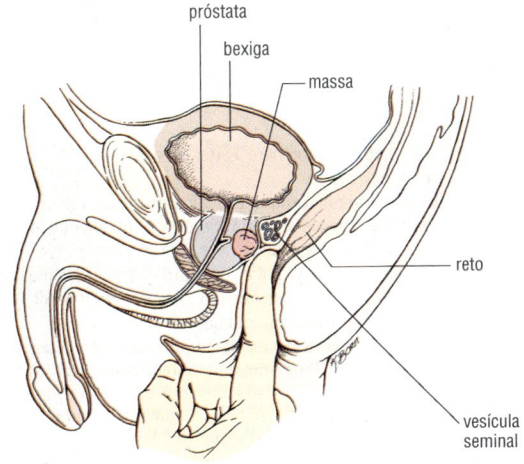

palpação da próstata

pros·ta·ti·tis (pros-tă-tī'tis). Prostatite; inflamação da próstata. O consenso NIH especifica 4 categorias de prostatite: I, prostatite bacteriana aguda; II, prostatite bacteriana crônica; III, prostatite crônica; síndrome de dor pélvica crônica: A, inflamatória, e B, não-inflamatória; e IV, prostatite inflamatória assintomática. [prostat- + G. -itis, inflamação]

prostato-, prostat-. A próstata. [L. med. *prostata* do G. *prostatēs*, que está adiante, protege]

pros·ta·to·cys·ti·tis (pros'tă-tō-sis-tī'tis). Prostatocistite; inflamação da próstata e da bexiga; cistite por extensão de inflamação da uretra prostática. [prostato- + G. *kystis*, bexiga, + -*itis*, inflamação]

pros·ta·to·dyn·ia (pros'tă-tō-din'ē-ă). Prostatodinia; termo raramente usado para designar prostatalgia. [prostato- + G. *odynē*, dor]

pros·tat·o·lith (pros-tat'ō-lith). Prostatólito. SIN prostatic calculus. [prostato- + G. *lithos*, cálculo]

pros·ta·to·li·thot·o·my (pros'tă-tō-li-thot'ō-mē, pros-tat'ō-). Prostatolitotomia; incisão da próstata para remoção de um cálculo. [prostato- + G. *lithos*, cálculo, + *tomē*, incisão]

pros·ta·to·meg·a·ly (pros'tă-tō-meg'ă-lē). Prostatomegalia; aumento da próstata. [prostato- + G. *megas*, grande]

pros·tat·o·my (pros-tat'ō-mē). Prostatotomia. SIN prostatotomy.

pros·ta·tor·rhea (pros'tă-tō-rē'ă). Prostatorréia; eliminação anormal de líquido prostático. [prostato- + G. *rhoia*, fluxo]

pros·ta·to·sem·i·nal·ve·sic·u·lec·to·my (pros'tă-tō-sem'i-năl-ve-sik-ū-lek'tō-mē). Prostatovesiculectomia. SIN prostatovesiculectomy.

pros·ta·tot·o·my (pros'tă-tot'ō-mē). Prostatotomia; incisão da próstata. SIN prostatomy. [prostato- + G. *tomē*, incisão]

pros·ta·to·ve·sic·u·lec·to·my (pros'tă-tō-ve-sik'ū-lek'tō-mē). Prostatovesiculectomia; remoção cirúrgica da próstata e das vesículas seminais. SIN prostatoseminalvesiculectomy.

pros·ta·to·ve·sic·u·li·tis (pros'tă-tō-ve-sik'ū-lī'tis). Prostatovesiculite; inflamação da próstata e das vesículas seminais.

pros·ter·na·tion (pros-ter-nā'shŭn). Prosternação. SIN camptocormia.

pros·the·on (pros'thē-on). Próstio. SIN prosthion.

pros·the·sis, pl. **pros·the·ses** (pros'thē-sis, -sēz; pros-thē'sis). Prótese; substituto fabricado para uma parte danificada ou ausente do corpo. [G. um acréscimo]
  auditory p., p. auditiva; termo genérico para designar dispositivos implantáveis a fim de restaurar a percepção sonora da pessoa surda, sendo o mais comum o implante coclear; está sendo desenvolvido um implante no tronco encefálico para estimular os neurônios do núcleo coclear.
  cardiac valve p., p. valvar cardíaca. VER valve (2).
  cochlear p., p. coclear. SIN cochlear implant.
  definitive p., p. definitiva; p. dental para ser usada durante um período de tempo prescrito.
  dental p., p. dental; substituição artificial de um ou mais dentes e/ou estruturas associadas. VER TAMBÉM denture.
  heart valve p., p. valvar cardíaca; substituição de uma valva cardíaca, retirada devido a doença, por uma valva artificial mecânica ou biológica.
  hybrid p., p. híbrida. SIN overlay denture.
  mandibular guide p., p. com uma extensão projetada para direcionar uma mandíbula ressecada para uma relação funcional com a maxila.
  ocular p., p. ocular; olho artificial ou implante ocular.
  penile p., p. peniana; dispositivo colocado no interior do pênis para correção de disfunção erétil.
  provisional p., p. provisória; p. dental provisória usada por períodos de tempo variáveis.
  surgical p., p. cirúrgica; dispositivo preparado como auxiliar ou como parte de um procedimento cirúrgico, como uma valva cardíaca, placa craniana ou prótese articular.
  testicular p., p. testicular. SIN testicular implant.
  tilting disk valve p., p. valvar de disco basculante; uma valva cardíaca artificial de baixo perfil, empregando um disco preso a um anel, que bascula para se abrir durante a sístole.

pros·thet·ic (pros-thet'ik). Protético. **1.** Relativo a uma prótese ou parte artificial. **2.** VER prosthetic *group*.

pros·thet·ics (pros-thet'iks). Terapia protética; a arte e a ciência de confeccionar e ajustar partes artificiais do corpo humano. VER anaplastology.
  dental p., terapia protética dental. SIN prosthodontics.
  maxillofacial p., terapia protética maxilofacial; ramo da odontologia que fornece próteses ou aparelhos para tratar ou restaurar tecidos do sistema estomatognático e estruturas faciais associadas afetados por doença, traumatismo, cirurgia ou defeito congênito, a fim de proporcionar os melhores resultados funcionais e estéticos possíveis.

pros·the·tist (pros'the-tist). Protético; aquele habilitado para confeccionar e adaptar próteses.

pros·the·to·phac·os (pros'thē-tō-fak'os). Lente intra-ocular protética. SIN lenticulus. [G. *prosthesis*, uma adição, + *phakos*, lente]

pros·thi·on (pros'thē-on). Próstio; o ponto mais anterior sobre o processo alveolar da maxila na linha média. SIN alveolar point, prostheon. [G. neutro de *prosthios*, primeiro]

pros·tho·don·tia (pros-thō-don'shē-ă). Prostodontia. SIN prosthodontics. [L.]

pros·tho·don·tics (pros-thō-don'tiks). Prostodontia; a ciência e a arte de fornecer substitutos adequados para as porções coronais dos dentes, ou para um ou mais dentes perdidos ou ausentes e suas partes associadas, a fim de poder restaurar a função comprometida, o conforto e a saúde do paciente. SIN dental prosthetics, prosthetic dentistry, prosthodontia. [L. *prosthodontia*, do G. *prosthesis* + *odous* (*odont*-), dente]

pros·tho·don·tist (pros-thō-don'tist). Prostodontista; um dentista versado na prática de prostodontia.

Pros·tho·gon·i·mus ma·cror·chis (pros'thō-gon'i-mŭs mak-rōr'kis). Trematódeo digenético (família Prosthogonimidae) localizado no oviduto e na bolsa de Fabrício de aves domésticas da América do Norte, comum sobretudo em estados que fazem fronteira com os Grandes Lagos. [G. *prosthe*, na frente de, + *gonos*, semente, prole; macro- + *orchis*, testículo]

pros·tho·ker·a·to·plas·ty (pros'thō-ker'ă-tō-plas-tē). Prostoceratoplastia; a técnica cirúrgica envolvida na utilização de uma ceratoprótese.

pros·tra·tion (pros-trā'shŭn). Prostração; perda acentuada da força, como na exaustão. [L. *pros-sterno*, pp. *-stratus*, espalhar antes, derrocada]
  heat p., p. pelo calor. VER heat *exhaustion*.

prot-. VER proteo-, proto-.

prot·ac·tin·i·um (Pa) (prō-tak-tin'ē-ŭm). Protactínio; elemento radioativo, de n.º atômico 91, peso atômico 231,03588, formado no decaimento do urânio e do tório; seu isótopo de vida mais longa, Pa^{231}, tem uma meia-vida de 32.500 anos. SIN proactinium, protoactinium. [G. *prōtos*, primeiro]

pro·tal·bu·mose (prō-tal'bū-mōs). Protalbumose; produtos intermediários da digestão das proteínas, derivados da hemialbose; hidrossolúvel e não-coagulável pelo calor, mas precipitada por sulfato de amônio, sulfato cúprico e cloreto de sódio. SIN protoalbumose.

pro·tam·i·nase (prō-tam'i-nās). Protaminase. SIN carboxypeptidase B.

prot·a·mine (prō'tă-mēn, -min). Protamina; qualquer membro de uma classe de proteínas, extremamente básica porque é rica em L-arginina, e sua constituição é mais simples que a das albuminas e globulinas, etc., encontrada em espermatozóides dos peixes associada aos ácidos nucleicos; as protaminas têm uma função semelhante à da histona e são encontradas no esperma de todos os mamíferos; neutraliza a ação anticoagulante da heparina; usada no preparo de vários tipos de insulina de ação prolongada.
  p. sulfate, sulfato de protamina; mistura purificada de princípios proteicos simples do esperma ou dos testículos de espécies adequadas de peixes; é um antagonista da heparina, sendo usado no controle de alguns estados hemorrágicos associados a concentrações aumentadas de substâncias semelhantes à heparina na circulação e no tratamento de *overdose* de heparina.

pro·ta·nom·a·ly (prō'tă-nom'ă-lē). Protanomalia; deficiência da percepção de cores na qual há diminuição do pigmento sensível ao vermelho nos cones. [G. *prōtos*, primeiro, + *anōmalia*, anomalia]

pro·ta·no·pia (prō'tă-nō'pē-ă). Protanopia, protanopsia; forma de dicromatismo caracterizada por ausência dos pigmentos sensíveis ao vermelho nos cones, diminuição da luminosidade para longos comprimentos de onda da luz e confusão no reconhecimento do vermelho e do verde. [G. *prōtos*, primeiro, + *a*- priv. + *ōps* (*ōp*-), olho]

pro·te·an (prō'tē-an). Multiforme; mutável; variável; aquele cuja forma pode ser mudada; que tem a capacidade de mudar a forma do corpo, como a ameba. [G. *Prōteus*, um deus que tinha o poder de mudar de forma]

pro·te·ase (prō'tē-ās). Protease; termo descritivo para enzimas proteolíticas, tanto endopeptidases quanto exopeptidases; enzimas que hidrolisam (rompem) as cadeias polipeptídicas.
  Lon p. Protease de Lon; enzima que degrada uma proteína bacteriana e interrompe a divisão celular até que seja concluído o reparo cromossomial.
  tricorn p., p. tricorne; p. encontrada em organismos que não possuem compartimentos limitados por membrana, que forma o cerne de um sistema proteolítico modular usado para gerar atividades multicatalíticas de modo controlado.

pro·tec·tion (prō-tek'shŭn). Proteção. SIN protective *block*. [ver protective]

protector. Protetor; cobertura ou escudo. [L.L. *protectus*, de pp. *protegere*, proteger, cobrir]
  hearing p.'s, protetores auditivos; dispositivos oclusivos para o canal auditivo externo feitos de material flexível, ou protetores de ouvido cheios de líquido (geralmente glicerina) usados para proteção contra a surdez causada por ruído.

Pro·tee·ae (prō'tē-ē). Tribo pertencente à família de bactérias Enterobacteriaceae, que inclui os três gêneros: *Proteus, Morganella* e *Providencia*.

pro·tein (p) (prō'tēn, prō'tē-in). Proteína; macromoléculas que consistem em longas seqüências de α-aminoácidos [H$_2$N–CHR–COOH] na ligação peptídica (amida) (eliminação de H$_2$O entre o α-NH$_2$ e α-COOH de resíduos sucessivos). A p. representa três quartos do peso seco da maior parte da matéria celular e está envolvida em estruturas, hormônios, enzimas, contração muscular, resposta imunológica e funções vitais essenciais. Os aminoácidos envolvidos geralmente são os 20 α-aminoácidos (glicina, L-alanina, etc.) reconhecidos pelo

protein(p)

código genético. Ligações cruzadas que produzem formas globulares de p. freqüentemente são realizadas através dos grupamentos –SH de dois resíduos L-cisteinil, bem como por forças não-covalentes (ligações de hidrogênio, atrações lipofílicas, etc.). [G. *prōtos*, primeiro, + -in]

p. 4.1, p. 4.1; uma proteína periférica que se liga firmemente à espectrina na membrana da hemácia; também se liga a determinadas glicoforinas e ajuda a determinar o formato e a flexibilidade da hemácia.

p. A, p. A; componente de algumas cepas de *Staphylococcus aureus*.

acute phase p., p. da fase aguda; proteínas plasmáticas associadas à inflamação, incluindo proteína C-reativa (PCR), proteína de ligação da manose, componente amilóide P sérico, α_1-antitripsina, fibrinogênio, ceruloplasmina e componentes do complemento C9 e fator B, cujas concentrações aumentam em resposta às interleucinas 1, 6 e 11.

acyl carrier p. (ACP), p. transportadora de acilas; uma das proteínas do complexo no citoplasma que contém todas as enzimas necessárias para converter acetil-CoA (e, em determinados casos, butiril-CoA ou propionil-CoA) e malonil-CoA em ácido palmítico. Esse complexo está firmemente ligado nos tecidos dos mamíferos e nas leveduras, mas o da *Escherichia coli* é facilmente dissociado. A PCA assim isolada é uma p. termoestável com um peso molecular de aproximadamente 10.000. Contém um –SH livre que se liga aos intermediários acil na síntese de ácidos graxos como tioésteres. Esse grupo –SH é parte de uma 4'-fosfopanteína, acrescentada à apoproteína pela PCA fosfodiesterase, que assim desempenha o mesmo papel que na coenzima A. A PCA participa de cada etapa do processo de síntese de ácidos graxos.

amyloid p., p. amilóide. VER amyloid.

androgen binding p. (ABP), p. de ligação de andrógenios; uma p. secretada pelas células de Sertoli testiculares juntamente com inibina e substância inibidora de Müller. Provavelmente mantém uma alta concentração de androgênio nos túbulos seminíferos.

antitermination p., p. antiterminação; p. que permite que a RNA polimerase transcreva através de determinados sítios de terminação.

antitumor p., p. antitumoral; p. que inibe o crescimento tumoral.

antiviral p. (AVP), p. antiviral; fator humano ou animal, induzido pelo interferon em células infectadas por vírus, que media a inibição da replicação viral pelo interferon.

autologous p., p. autóloga; qualquer p. encontrada normalmente nos líquidos ou tecidos do corpo.

basic p.'s, proteínas básicas; proteínas ricas em aminoácidos básicos; p. ex., histonas.

Bence Jones p.'s, proteínas de Bence Jones; proteínas com termossolubilidade incomum, encontradas na urina de pacientes com mieloma múltiplo, que consistem em cadeias leves de imunoglobulina monoclonal. VER Bence Jones *reaction*. VER TAMBÉM immunoglobulin. [H. Bence Jones, médico inglês, 1813–1873]

bone Gla p. (BGP), p. óssea Gla; osteocalcina. SIN osteocalcin.

p. C, p. C; uma glicoproteína vitamina K-dependente que inibe a coagulação por clivagem enzimática das formas ativas dos fatores V e VIII, e assim interfere com a regulação da formação de coágulo intravascular; a deficiência de proteína C causa comprometimento da regulação da coagulação sanguínea. A deficiência autossômica dominante [MIM*176860], ao contrário da deficiência de antitrombina III e da deficiência de plasminogênio, está associada ao aumento do risco de trombose grave ou prematura.

cAMP receptor p. (CRP), p. receptora de AMPc. SIN catabolite (gene) activator p.

capping p.'s, proteínas de capeamento; proteínas que se ligam a uma extremidade dos filamentos de actina, impedindo tanto a adição quanto a perda de monômeros de actina.

catabolite (gene) activator p. (CAP), p. ativadora de genes do catabolismo; p. que pode ser ativada pelo AMPc e, então, afeta a ação da RNA polimerase por ligação com ela ou próximo dela no DNA a ser transcrito. SIN cAMP receptor p., catabolite gene activator.

cholesterol ester transport p.'s, proteínas transportadoras dos ésteres de colesterol; p. que transporta ésteres de colesterol da HDL para VLDL e LDL; a deficiência dessa proteína está associada a nível elevado de HDL-colesterol.

circumsporozoite p., p. circumsporozoítica; uma das duas proteínas (a outra é a p. adesiva relacionada à trombospondina) envolvidas no reconhecimento de esporozoítas das células hospedeiras na malária.

***cis*-acting p.,** p. *cis*-ativa; p. que atua sobre a molécula de DNA da qual foi expressa.

compound p., p. composta, p. conjugada. SIN conjugated p.

conjugated p., p. conjugada; p. ligada a alguma outra molécula ou moléculas (que não são aminoácidos naturais) de forma diferente de um sal; p. ex., flavoproteínas; cromoproteínas, hemoglobinas. VER TAMBÉM prosthetic *group*. Cf. simple p. SIN compound p.

copper p., p. cúprica; p. contendo um ou mais íons cobre; p. ex., citocromo *c* oxidase, fenol oxidase.

corticosteroid-binding p., p. ligadora dos corticosteróides. Transcortina. SIN transcortin.

C-reactive p. (CRP), p. C-reativa (PCR); β-globulina encontrada no soro de várias pessoas com determinadas doenças inflamatórias, degenerativas e neoplásicas; embora a proteína não seja um anticorpo específico, precipita *in vitro* o polissacarídeo C presente em todos os tipos de pneumococos.

denatured p., p. desnaturada; p. cujas características ou propriedades foram alteradas de alguma forma, como pelo calor, por ação enzimática ou de substâncias químicas e, por isso, perdeu sua atividade biológica.

derived p., p. derivada; um derivado de p. produzido por alteração química, p. ex., hidrólise.

docking p., p. de fixação; no processo de tradução de proteínas que serão exportadas pela célula, a tradução é interrompida até que a cadeia polipeptídica em crescimento, que é ligada por uma partícula específica (partícula de reconhecimento de sinal), entre em contato com essa p. integral do retículo endoplasmático.

encephalithogenic p., p. encefalitogênica; p. importante no sistema nervoso central. SIN myelin p. A1.

eosinophil cationic p. (ECP), p. catiônica eosinofílica; p. cujo nível no soro do sangue coagulado reflete a taxa de ativação dos eosinófilos circulantes.

extrinsic p.'s, proteínas extrínsecas. SIN peripheral p.'s.

fatty acid-binding p., p. ligadora de ácidos graxos. SIN Z p.

fibrous p., p. fibrosa; qualquer p. insolúvel, incluindo os colágenos, elastinas e queratinas, envolvida em tecidos estruturais ou fibrosos.

foreign p., p. heteróloga; p. que difere de todas as proteínas normalmente encontradas no organismo em questão. SIN heterologous p.

G p.'s, proteínas G; proteínas intracelulares associadas à membrana, ativadas por vários receptores (p. ex., β-adrenérgicos); essas proteínas atuam como mensageiros secundários ou transdutores da resposta, iniciada pelo receptor, a elementos intracelulares, como as enzimas, para começar um efeito. Essas proteínas têm alta afinidade por nucleotídeos guanina e, portanto, são denominadas proteínas G. SIN G-p., GTP binding p.'s.

G-p., p. G. SIN G p.'s.

glial fibrillary acidic p., p. ácida fibrilar da glia; uma p. do citoesqueleto, com 51 kd, encontrada em astrócitos fibrosos; colorações para essa proteína freqüentemente são usadas para ajudar no diagnóstico diferencial de lesões neurológicas.

globular p., p. globular; qualquer p. hidrossolúvel, geralmente com acréscimo de ácido, álcali, sal ou etanol, e grosseiramente assim classificada (albuminas, globulinas, histonas e protaminas), ao contrário da proteína fibrosa.

GTP binding p.'s, proteínas G. SIN G p.'s.

heat shock p.'s (hsp), proteínas de choque de calor; proteínas específicas cuja síntese aumenta imediatamente após súbita elevação da temperatura; sua função é ajudar a diminuir os efeitos prejudiciais da alta temperatura.

heterologous p., p. heteróloga. SIN foreign p.

homologous p.'s, proteínas homólogas; proteínas que possuem estruturas primária, secundária e terciária muito semelhantes.

immune p., anticorpo. SIN antibody.

integral p.'s, proteínas integrais, proteínas intrínsecas; proteínas que não podem ser facilmente separadas de uma membrana biológica. SIN intrinsic p.'s.

intrinsic p.'s, proteínas intrínsecas. SIN integral p.'s.

iron-sulfur p.'s, proteínas ferro-enxofre; proteínas que contêm um ou mais átomos de ferro ligados às pontes de enxofre e/ou enxofre de resíduos cisteinil; p. ex., determinadas proteínas na via de transporte de elétrons.

p. kinase C, proteinoquinase C, proteinocinase C; qualquer dentre várias cinases citoplasmáticas ativadas por cálcio, envolvidas em vários processos, incluindo ligação hormonal, ativação plaquetária e promoção de tumor.

p. kinases, proteinoquinases, proteinocinases; classe de enzimas que fosforila outras proteínas; muitas dessas cinases respondem a outros efetores (p. ex., AMPc, GMPc, insulina, fator de crescimento epidérmico, cálcio e calmodulina, cálcio e fosfolipídios).

latent membrane p. (LMP), p. latente da membrana; produto genético do vírus Epstein-Barr.

low molecular weight p.'s (LMP), proteínas de baixo peso molecular; produtos genéticos que são componentes dos proteossomas.

M p., p. M; (1) SIN Streptococcus M *antigen*. VER TAMBÉM β-hemolytic *streptococci*, em *streptococcus, Streptococcus pneumoniae*; (2) SIN monoclonal *immunoglobulin*.

macrophage inflammatory p. (MIP), (mak'rō-fāj in'flam-mă-to-rē), proteína inflamatória de macrófagos; membro da família quimiocina que é quimiotática para determinados subgrupos de linfócitos, como as células T citotóxicas.

mannose-binding p., p. fixadora de manose; p. envolvida na imunidade inata que pode ligar-se a microrganismos manosilados e ativar a via do complemento.

matrix Gla p. (MGP), p. matricial Gla; p. de ligação do cálcio.

microtubule-associated p.'s (MAPs), proteínas associadas aos microtúbulos; proteínas que exibem uma associação específica com α- e/ou β-tubulina; p. ex., tau, MAP1, MAP2; várias delas foram encontradas nas placas observadas na doença de Alzheimer.

monoclonal p., p. monoclonal, P.M. SIN monoclonal *immunoglobulin*.

monocyte chemoattractant p., p. quimioatraente de monócitos; p. quimiotática de monócitos; citocina envolvida na migração dos monócitos.

monocyte chemoattractant p.-1 (MCP-1), p.-1 quimioatraente de monócito; p.-1 quimiotática de monócito; secretada por células endoteliais da parede de um vaso sanguíneo; induz extravasamento de monócitos.

muscle p.'s, proteínas musculares; proteínas presentes no músculo.

myelin p. A1, p. da mielina A1. SIN encephalithogenic p.

native p., p. nativa; o conceito de uma p. em seu estado natural, na célula, inalterada pelo calor, por substâncias químicas, ação enzimática ou pelas exigências da extração.

neutrophil-activating p., p. ativadora de neutrófilos; termo antigo para designar a interleucina-8.

non-heme iron p., p. com ferro não-heme; qualquer p. que contenha ferro, mas não qualquer ferro heme; p. ex., NADH desidrogenase.

nonspecific p., p. inespecífica; substância proteica que induz uma resposta não-mediada por reação antígeno-anticorpo específica.

odorant binding p., p. de ligação odorante; proteínas encontradas no muco nasal que se ligam a moléculas lipofílicas odoríferas e transferem-nas para os receptores olfatórios. Proteínas semelhantes mediariam o paladar.

p. p53, p. p53; p. multifuncional que modula a transcrição genética e controla o reparo do DNA, a apoptose e o ciclo celular.

parathyroid hormonelike p. (PLP), p. semelhante ao paratormônio. SIN parathyroid hormone-related p.

parathyroid hormone-related p., p. relacionada ao paratormônio; uma p. com 140 aminoácidos, secretada por algumas células cancerosas; causa hipercalcemia. SIN parathyroid hormonelike p.

pathologic p.'s, proteínas patológicas. VER paraprotein.

peripheral p.'s, proteínas periféricas; proteínas que podem ser facilmente removidas de uma membrana biológica (p. ex., mediante alteração do pH ou da força iônica). SIN extrinsic p.

phenylthiocarbamoyl p., p. feniltiocarbamoíla; formada pela reação do fenilisotiocianato com um grupamento α-amino terminal de um peptídeo ou proteína. VER TAMBÉM phenylisothiocyanate, phenylthiohydantoin. SIN PhNCS p., PTC p.

PhNCS p., p. PhNCS. SIN phenylthiocarbamoyl p.

p. phosphatases, proteinofosfatases, fosfatases de proteínas; classe de enzimas que catalisam a desfosforilação de proteínas fosforiladas específicas.

placenta p., lactogênio placentário humano. SIN human placental lactogen.

plasma p.'s, proteínas plasmáticas; proteínas dissolvidas (>100) no plasma sanguíneo, principalmente albuminas e globulinas (normalmente 6–8 g/100 mL); retêm líquido nos vasos sanguíneos por osmose e incluem anticorpos e proteínas da coagulação sanguínea. SIN serum p.'s.

prion p. (PrP), príon. SIN prion.

protective p., anticorpo. SIN antibody.

PTC p., p. feniltiocarbamoíla. SIN phenylthiocarbamoyl p.

purified placental p., lactogênio placentário purificado. SIN human placental lactogen.

receptor p., p. receptora; p. intracelular (ou fração proteica) com elevada afinidade específica pela ligação de um estímulo conhecido à atividade celular, como um hormônio esteróide ou adenosina cíclica 3′,5′-fosfato.

retinol-binding p., p. de ligação do retinol; p. plasmática que se liga ao retinol e o transporta.

S p., p. S; o principal fragmento produzido a partir da ribonuclease pancreática pela ação limitada da sutilisina, que cliva a ribonuclease entre os resíduos 20 e 21; o menor fragmento (resíduos 1-20) é o peptídeo S.

p. S, p. S; p. antitrombótica, dependente de vitamina K, que funciona como co-fator para a proteína C ativada.

serum p.'s, proteínas séricas. SIN plasma p.'s.

simple p., p. simples; p. que produz apenas α-aminoácidos ou seus derivados por hidrólise; p. ex., albuminas, globulinas, glutelinas, prolaminas, albuminóides, histonas, protaminas. Cf. conjugated p.

stimulatory p. 1 (SP1), p. estimuladora; um fator de transcrição da RNA polimerase II em vertebrados; liga-se ao DNA em regiões ricas em resíduos G e C; um fator de ligação promotor geral necessário para a ativação de muitos genes.

structure p.'s, proteínas estruturais; proteínas cujo papel é dar estrutura e sustentação ao tecido e à célula; p. ex., os colágenos.

surfactant-specific p.'s, proteínas surfactante-específicas; os componentes proteicos do surfactante pulmonar, incluindo as proteínas surfactantes A, B, C.

Tamm-Horsfall p., p. de Tamm-Horsfall. VER Tamm-Horsfall mucoprotein.

thrombospondin-related adhesive p., p. adesiva relacionada à trombospondina; uma das duas proteínas (a outra é a p. circunsporozoíta) envolvida no reconhecimento, pelos esporozoítas, de células hospedeiras na malária.

thyroxine-binding p. (TBP), p. de ligação da tiroxina; **(1)** SIN thyroxine-binding globulin; **(2)** SIN thyroxine-binding prealbumin.

unwinding p.'s, DNA helicases; enzimas que desenrolam o DNA, permitindo a ocorrência de eventos recombinantes.

vitamin D-binding p. (DBP), p. de ligação da vitamina D; proteína plasmática que se liga à vitamina D.

whey p., p. do soro; a proteína solúvel contida no soro de leite coagulado por renina; p. ex., lactoglobulina, α-lactalbumina, lactoferrina.

Z-p., p. Z; uma proteína de ligação do ácido graxo que participa do movimento intracelular de ácidos graxos. SIN fatty acid-binding p.

pro·tein·a·ceous (prō′tē - nā′shŭs, prō′tē - i - nā′shŭs). Proteináceo; semelhante a uma proteína; que possui, em algum grau, as propriedades físico-químicas características das proteínas.

pro·tein·ase. Proteinase. SIN endopeptidase.

pro·tein hy·drol·y·sate. Hidrolisado de proteínas; solução estéril de aminoácidos e peptídeos de cadeia curta preparados a partir de uma proteína adequada, por hidrólise ácida ou enzimática; usado por via intravenosa, para manter o balanço nitrogenado positivo em doenças graves, e após cirurgia do trato alimentar; ou usado por via oral, nas dietas de lactentes alérgicos ao leite, ou como suplemento quando não pode haver grande ingestão de proteínas em alimentos comuns.

pro·tein·o·gen·ic (prō′ten - ō - jen′ik). Proteinogênico. SIN proteogenic.

pro·tein·oids (prō′ten - oydz; prō′tē - in - oyds). Proteinóides; heteropoli(amino-ácidos) sintetizados artificialmente.

pro·tein·o·sis (pro - tē - nō′sis, prō′tē - i - nō′sis). Proteinose; estado caracterizado por perturbação da formação e distribuição de proteínas, em particular como se manifesta por deposição de proteínas anormais nos tecidos. [protein + G. -osis, condição]

lipoid p. [MIM*247100], p. lipóide; distúrbio do metabolismo lipídico no qual há depósitos de um complexo lipoproteico sobre a língua e nas áreas sublinguais e da fauce, levando à rouquidão, e lesões palpebrais papilomatosas ceratóticas translúcidas; exibe herança autossômica recessiva, freqüentemente com calcificações intracranianas específicas. SIN hyalinosis cutis et mucosae, lipoidosis cutis et mucosae, Urbach-Wiethe disease.

pulmonary alveolar p., p. alveolar pulmonar; doença pulmonar progressiva crônica de adultos, caracterizada por acúmulo alveolar de material proteináceo granular que é PAS-positivo e rico em lipídios, com pouco exsudato celular inflamatório; a causa é desconhecida.

pro·tein·u·ria (prō - tē - noo′rē - ă, prō′tē - i - noo′rē - ă). Proteinúria. **1.** Presença de proteína urinária em quantidades maiores que 0,3 g em uma amostra de urina de 24 horas, ou em concentrações maiores que 1 g/L (1+ a 2+ por métodos turbidométricos padrões) em uma amostra aleatória de urina em duas ou mais ocasiões com intervalo de 6 horas; as amostras devem ser limpas, tomadas do jato médio ou obtidas por cateterização. **2.** SIN albuminuria. [protein + G. ouron, urina]

Bence Jones p., p. de Bence Jones; presença de proteínas de Bence Jones na urina, geralmente indicativa de um processo neoplásico como mieloma múltiplo, amiloidose ou macroglobulinemia de Waldenström.

gestational p., p. gestacional; a presença de proteinúria durante a gravidez, sob a influência desta, na ausência de hipertensão, edema, infecção renal ou doença renovascular intrínseca conhecida.

isolated p., p. isolada; proteinúria em um paciente assintomático, que possui função renal e sedimento urinário normais, e não exibe manifestação de doença sistêmica ao exame inicial.

nonisolated p., p. não-isolada; proteinúria associada a outras anormalidades.

orthostatic p., postural p., p. ortostática, p. postural. SIN orthostatic albuminuria.

pro·ten·si·ty (prō - ten′si - tē). O tempo atribuído a um processo mental; o atributo de um processo mental caracterizado por sua temporalidade ou movimento para diante no tempo. [L. protendo (-tensum), estender]

△ **proteo-, prot-.** Proteo-; proteína.

pro·te·o·clas·tic (prō′tē - ō - klas′tik). Proteoclástico. SIN proteolytic. [proteo- + G. klastos, quebrado]

pro·te·o·gen·ic (prō′tē - ō - jen - ik). Proteogênico; capaz de produzir proteínas. SIN proteinogenic.

pro·te·o·gly·can I. Proteoglicano I. SIN biglycan.

pro·te·o·gly·cans (prō′tē - ō - glī′kanz). Proteoglicanos; glicosaminoglicanos (mucopolissacarídeos) ligados a cadeias proteicas em complexos covalentes; encontrados na matriz extracelular de tecido conjuntivo.

pro·te·o·hor·mone (prō′tē - ō - hōr′mōn). Termo obsoleto para designar um hormônio que possui uma estrutura proteica.

pro·te·o·lip·ids (prō′tē - ō - lip′idz). Proteolipídios; classe de proteínas lipossolúveis encontradas no tecido cerebral; são insolúveis em água, mas solúveis em misturas de clorofórmio–metanol–água.

pro·te·ol·y·sis (prō - tē - ol′i - sis). Proteólise; a decomposição das proteínas; basicamente por hidrólise das ligações peptídicas, tanto enzimaticamente quanto não-enzimaticamente. [proteo- + G. lysis, dissolução]

pro·te·o·lyt·ic (prō′tē - ō - lit′ik). Proteolítico; relativo à proteólise ou que a realiza. SIN proteoclastic.

pro·te·o·met·a·bol·ic (prō′tē - ō - met′ă - bol′ik). Proteometabólico; relativo ao metabolismo das proteínas.

pro·te·o·me·tab·o·lism (prō′tē - ō - mē - tab′ō - lizm). Proteometabolismo. SIN protein metabolism.

proteínas plasmáticas

	função fisiológica	concentração no plasma ou soro (mg/L)	atividade eletroforética	peso molecular (dáltons)
proteínas transportadoras				
albumina	pressão oncótica, transporte de muitas substâncias	35.000–55.000	5,92	66.300
pré-albumina	ligação da tiroxina	100–400	7,6	55.000
transcortina	ligação da cortisona	70	α_1	55.700
haptoglobina (tipos 1-1, 2-1, 2-2)	ligação da hemoglobina, proteína da fase aguda	410–2.460	α_2 4,5	100.000–400.000
hemopexina	liga-se ao heme	500–1.150	β_1 3,1	57.000
proteína de ligação do retinol	liga-se à vitamina A	30–60	α_2	21.000
transcobalaminas I–III	transporte de vitamina B_{12}		α_1–β_1	
α_2-macroglobulina	transporte de hormônio, inibição enzimática, proteína da fase aguda	1.500–4.200	α_2 4,2	725.000
transferrina	transporte de ferro	2.000–4.000	β_1 3,1	76.500
α_1-glicoproteína ácida	proteína da fase aguda	550–1.400	α_1 5,7	41.000
proteína C-reativa	proteína da fase aguda, estimulação da fagocitose	<1		135.000–140.000
imunoglobulinas (Ig)				
IgM	anticorpos iniciais	600–2.800	β/γ 2,1	950.000
IgG	anticorpos tardios	8.000–18.000	γ 1,2	150.000
IgA	anticorpos secretores	900–4.500	β/γ 2,1	160.000 e múltiplos
IgD	anticorpos reguladores	<150	β/γ <2,1	175.000
IgE	reaginas, anticorpos alérgicos	0,3	β/γ 2,3	190.000
sistema complemento				
C1q	(ver em "complemento")	190	γ_2	400.000
C1r		100	β	190.000
C1s		120	α_2	85.000
C2		30	β_2	117.000
C3		1.300	β_1	180.000
C4		430	β_1	206.000
C5		75	β_1	180.000
C6		60	β_2	128.000
C7		10	β_2	121.000
C8		10	γ_1	153.000
C9		10	α_2	79.000
ativadores das vias alternativas				
properdina	ativação do complemento	10–20	β–$\gamma 2$	224.000
proativador de C3 (C3-PA)	através de polissacarídeos ligados à superfície	225	$\beta 2$	93.000
C3-PA convertase		traços		22.000
enzima				
colinesterase	hidrólise de ésteres da colina	5–15	α_2 3,1	348.000
ceruloplasmina	oxidase, ligação ao Cu	150–600	α_2 4,6	132.000
plasminogênio	fibrinólise (proenzima)	100–300	β_1 3,7	91.000
lisozima	protease	5–15	α_1	~15.000
lipase lipoproteica	transporte de gordura	varia	?	?
adenosina desaminase	metabolismo dos nucleotídeos	traços	α/β	?
inibidores de enzimas				
inibidor da C1-esterase	inativação	150–350	α_2	104.000
α_1-antitripsina	inibição da tripsina	2.000–4.000	α_1 5,42	45.000–54.000
inibidor da inter-α-tripsina	inibição da tripsina	200–700	α_1/α_2	~160.000
antiquimotripsina	inibição da quimotripsina	300–600	α_1	68.000
antitrombina III	inibição da trombina	170–300	α_2	65.000
fatores da coagulação				
fator I, fibrinogênio	formação de coagulantes, fase final	2.000–4.500	$\beta/\gamma = \phi$ 2,1	340.000
fator II, protrombina	proenzima	50–100	α	69.000
fatores III–XIII	ver em coagulação (diagrama); ver também fator...			

continua

proteínas plasmáticas (continuação)				
	função fisiológica	concentração no plasma ou soro (mg/L)	atividade eletroforética	peso molecular (dáltons)
lipoproteínas				
α_1-lipoproteína, HDL_2	transporte de lipídios	400–1.200	α_1	
α_1-lipoproteína, HDL_3	transporte de lipídios	220–2.700	α_1	
α_2-lipoproteína, pré-β, lipoproteína de densidade muito baixa (VLDL)	transporte de lipídios	150–2.300	α_2	
β-lipoproteína, lipoproteína de baixa densidade (LDL)	transporte de lipídios	250–8.000	β	

Pro·te·o·myx·id·ia (prō'tē-ō-mik-sid'ē-ă). Nome antigo de Eumycetozoea. [*Proteus* + G. *myxa*, muco]

pro·te·o·pec·tic, pro·te·o·pex·ic (prō'tē-ō-pek'tik, -pek'sik). Proteopéctico; relativo à proteopexia.

pro·te·o·pep·sis (prō'tē-ō-pep'sis). Proteopepsia; a digestão de proteínas. [proteo- + G. *pepsis*, digestão]

pro·te·o·pex·is (prō'tē-ō-pek'sis). Proteopexia; a fixação de proteína nos tecidos. [proteo- + G. *pēxis*, fixação]

pro·te·ose (prō'tē-ōs). Proteose; mistura não descrita de produtos intermediários da proteólise entre a proteína e a peptona.

primary p., p. primária; o primeiro resultado da hidrólise da metaproteína; foram reconhecidos dois estágios: protoproteose e heteroproteose.

secondary p., p. secundária; proteose derivada da proteose primária por hidrólise adicional.

proteosome (prō'tē-ō-sōm). Proteossoma; grupo de genes que codificam componentes do complexo proteolítico do citosol celular, um conjunto de proteínas que parece estar envolvido no processamento celular e no transporte de peptídeos na formação de moléculas classe I do complexo principal de histocompatibilidade. [proteo- + G. *sōma*, corpo]

Pro'teus (prō'tē-ŭs). **1.** Gênero anterior da Sarcodina, agora denominada *Amoeba*. **2.** Gênero de bactérias móveis, peritríquias, não-formadoras de esporos, aeróbicas ou facultativamente anaeróbicas (família Enterobacteriaceae) que contêm bacilos Gram-negativos; em certas condições são encontradas formas cocóides, grandes formas de involução irregular, filamentos e esferoplastos. O metabolismo é fermentativo, produzindo ácido ou ácido e gás visível a partir da glicose; a lactose não é fermentada, e eles rapidamente decompõem a uréia e desaminam a fenilalanina. O *Proteus* é encontrado basicamente na matéria fecal e em materiais em putrefação. A espécie típica é o *P. vulgaris*. [G. *Proteus*, um deus marinho, que tem o poder de mudar de forma]

P. incon'stans, espécie de bactéria encontrada em infecções das vias urinárias e em casos esporádicos de diarréia em seres humanos; algumas cepas causam gastroenterite.

P. mirab'ilis, espécie de bactéria encontrada na carne pútrida, infusões e abscessos; uma causa de infecções urinárias associadas à formação de cálculos renais e vesicais.

P. morgan'ii, nome antigo da *Morganella morganii*, espécie de bactéria encontrada no canal intestinal e em infecções hospitalares.

P. rettge'ri. SIN *Providencia rettgeri*.

P. vulgar'is, a espécie típica do gênero de bactérias *Proteus*, encontrada em materiais em putrefação e abscessos; é patogênica para peixes, cães, cobaias e camundongos; algumas cepas, as cepas X de Weil e Felix, são aglutinadas pelo soro tífico e, portanto, são muito importantes no diagnóstico de tifo; a cepa X-19 é fortemente aglutinada. VER TAMBÉM Weil-Felix *reaction*.

pro·thi·pen·dyl (prō-thī'pen-dil). Protipendil; um antipsicótico.

pro·throm·base (prō-throm'bās). Protrombase. VER *factor* X.

pro·throm·bin (prō-throm'bin). Protrombina; glicoproteína, com peso molecular de aproximadamente 72.500, formada e armazenada nas células do parênquima hepático e presente no sangue em uma concentração de cerca de 20 mg/100 mL. Na presença de tromboplastina e íon cálcio, a protrombina é convertida em trombina que, por sua vez, converte o fibrinogênio em fibrina, sendo a coagulação do sangue o resultado desse processo; a deficiência de protrombina compromete a coagulação sanguínea. SIN serozyme, trombinogen, thrombogen.

pro·throm·bin·ase (prō-throm'bi-nās). Protrombinase. SIN *factor X*.

pro·throm·bi·no·gen (prō-throm'bi-nō-jen). Protrombinogênio. SIN *factor* VII.

pro·throm·bi·no·pe·nia (prō-throm'bi-nō-pē'nē-ă). Protrombinopenia. SIN hypoprothrombinemia.

pro·throm·bo·ki·nase (prō'throm-bō-kī'nās). Protrombocinase. SIN *factor* V, *factor* VIII.

pro·ti·re·lin (prō-tī'rē-lin). Protirelina; forma sintética de tiroliberina.

pro·tist (prō'tist). Protista; membro do reino Protista.

Pro·tis·ta (prō-tis'ta). Reino de organismos unicelulares eucariotos, semelhantes a vegetais e também a animais, seja na forma de organismos solitários, como, p. ex., protozoários, ou de colônias celulares que não possuem tecidos verdadeiros. [G. neutro pl. de *prōtistos*, o primeiro de todos]

pro·ti·um (prō'tē-ŭm). Prótio. SIN hydrogen-1.

⚠ **proto-, prot-.** Proto-; o primeiro em uma série; o de posição mais alta em uma escala. [G. *prōtos*, primeiro]

pro·to·ac·tin·i·um (prō'tō-ak-tin'ē-um). Proto-actínio. SIN protactinium.

pro·to·al·bu·mose (prō-tō-al'bū-mōs). Protoalbumose. SIN protalbumose.

pro·to·al·ka·loid (prō-tō-al'kă-loyd). Protoalcalóide; uma amina biogênica que serve como precursor de um alcalóide.

pro·to·bi·ol·o·gy (prō'tō-bī-ol'ō-jē). Protobiologia. SIN bacteriophagology.

pro·to·cat·e·chu·ic ac·id (prō'tō-kat'ē-choo'ik, -koo'ik). Ácido protocatecóico; produto da oxidação da adrenalina.

pro·to·col (prō'tō-kol). Protocolo; plano detalhado e preciso para o estudo de um problema biomédico ou para um esquema de tratamento.

Bruce p., p. de Bruce; método de prova de esforço graduada, de intensidade crescente, para determinar a intensidade da doença coronariana.

Bruce p., p. de Bruce; protocolo padronizado de exercício monitorado por eletrocardiograma, que utiliza velocidades e elevações crescentes da esteira; um teste para isquemia geralmente causada por doença coronariana. VER TAMBÉM stress *test*.

pro·to·cone (prō'tō-kōn). Protocone; cúspide mesiolingual de um dente molar superior em um mamífero. [proto- + G. *kōnos*, cone]

pro·to·co·nid (prō-tō-kon'ik). Protoconídeo; a cúspide mesiolingual de um dente molar inferior em um mamífero.

pro·to·cop·ro·por·phyr·ia (prō'tō-kop'rō-pōr-fir'ē-ă). Protocoproporfiria; aumento da excreção fecal de proto- e coproporfirinas.

p. heredita'ria, p. hereditária. SIN variegate *porphyria*.

Pro·toc·tis·ta (prō-tok-tis'tă). Reino de eucariotos, incluindo as algas e os protozoários que são os prováveis ancestrais dos reinos dos fungos, vegetais e animais; não possuem o padrão de desenvolvimento originário de uma blástula, típico dos animais, nem o padrão de desenvolvimento do embrião, típico dos vegetais, nem o desenvolvimento de esporos, como nos fungos. Estão incluídos no reino Protoctista as algas nucleadas, os fungos flagelados da água, os fungos gelatinosos e os fungos filamentosos do limo, bem como os protozoários; estão incluídos organismos unicelulares, coloniais e multicelulares, mas o desenvolvimento complexo de tecidos e órgãos de plantas e animais está ausente. O termo Protoctista substitui o termo Protista, que designa microrganismos de uma só célula ou acelulares, enquanto os conjuntos basais pré-vegetais (Protophyta) e pré-animais (Protozoa) incorporados ao Protoctista incluem muitas formas multicelulares, pois a multicelularidade parece ter evoluído independentemente várias vezes dentro desses grupos primitivos. [G. *prōtos*, o primeiro, + *ktizō*, estabelecer]

pro·to·derm (prō'tō-derm). Protoderma; as células indiferenciadas de embriões muito jovens, das quais se desenvolvem as camadas germinativas primárias. [proto- + G. *derma*, pele]

pro·to·di·a·stol·ic (prō'tō-dī-ă-stol'ik). Protodiastólico; no início da diástole, relativo ao começo da diástole cardíaca.

pro·to·du·o·de·num (prō'tō-doo-ō-dē'nŭm, -doo-od'ē-nŭm). Protoduodeno; a primeira parte do duodeno, que se estende do piloro gastroduodenal até a papila maior do duodeno e desenvolve-se a partir da parte caudal do intestino anterior do embrião; não possui pregas circulares e é a sede das glândulas duodenais.

pro·to·e·ryth·ro·cyte (prō'tō-ē-rith'rō-sīt). Protoeritrócito; um eritroblasto primitivo.

pro·to·fil·a·ment (prō-tō-fil'ă-ment). Protofilamento; elemento básico de um microtúbulo flagelar contrátil, com cerca de 5 nm de espessura. [proto- + L. *filum*, filamento]

pro·to·gen, pro·to·gen A (prō′tō-jen). Ácido lipóico. SIN lipoic acid.
pro·to·gon·o·plasm (prō-tō-gon′ō-plazm). Protogonoplasma; massa diferenciada de citoplasma em um protozoário, que forma a substância dos corpos reprodutivos que se desenvolvem posteriormente. [proto- + G. *gonos*, semente, + *plasma*, algo formado]
pro·to·ky·lol hy·dro·chlo·ride (prō-tō-kī′lōl). Cloridrato de protoquilol; derivado do isoproterenol com atividade estimulante seletiva dos β-receptores da substância original; é eficaz por via oral e mais estável no corpo que o isoproterenol; usado como broncodilatador no tratamento da asma brônquica e do estado asmático.
pro·to·leu·ko·cyte (prō-tō-loo′kō-sīt). Protoleucócito; um leucócito primitivo; um leucócito da medula óssea.
pro·tol·y·sate (prō-tol′i-sāt). Protolisado; termo raramente usado para designar um hidrolisado de proteínas.
pro·tom·er (prō′tō-mer). Protômero; subunidade estrutural de uma estrutura maior. Os próprios protômeros podem ser formados por subunidades. Por exemplo, a tubulina, um dímeroαβ, é o protômero dos microtúbulos. [G. *protos*, primeiro, + -mer 1]
pro·tom·e·rite (prō-tom′e-rīt, prō′tō-mer′īt). Protomerito; o segundo segmento (que não possui um núcleo) de uma gregarina septada, entre o epimerito e o deutomerito; torna-se a extremidade anterior do gamonte depois que ele sai de sua célula hospedeira, deixando o epimerito incrustado (geralmente na parede intestinal de um invertebrado infectado). SIN primerite. [proto- + G. *meros*, parte]
pro·to·me·tro·cyte (prō-tō-me′trō-sīt). Protometrócito; a célula ancestral do protoleucócito e protoeritrócito, ou das células da série leucocítica e eritrocítica. [proto- + G. *meter*, mãe, + *kytos*, célula]
pro·ton (p) (prō′ton). Próton; a unidade de carga positiva da massa nuclear; os prótons formam parte (ou, no hidrogênio-1, o todo) do núcleo do átomo, em torno do qual giram os elétrons negativos. [G. neutro de *protos*, primeiro]
pro·to·neu·ron (prō-tō-noor′on). Protoneurônio; neurônio primitivo hipotético que não possui polarização. [proto- + G. *neuron*, nervo]
pro·to·nymph (prō′tō-nimf). Proninfa; em ácaros, o segundo instar.
pro·to·on·co·gene (prō-tō-on′kō-jēn). Protoncogene; gene conservado por muito tempo na escala evolutiva, presente no genoma humano normal, que parece participar da fisiologia celular normal e freqüentemente está envolvido na regulação do crescimento ou proliferação celular normal; em virtude de mutações somáticas, esses genes podem tornar-se oncogênicos; os produtos dos protoncogenes podem desempenhar papéis importantes na diferenciação celular normal.
pro·to·path·ic (prō-tō-path′ik). Protopático; designa um conjunto ou sistema, supostamente primitivo, de fibras nervosas sensitivas periféricas que conduzem baixo grau de sensibilidade álgica e térmica, mal localizada. Cf. epicritic. [proto- + G. *pathos*, que sofre]
pro·to·pec·tin (prō-tō-pek′tin). Protopectina. VER pectin.
pro·to·pi·an·o·ma (prō′tō-pē-an-ō′mă). Protopianoma. SIN mother *yaw*.
pro·to·plasm (prō′tō-plazm). Protoplasma. 1. Matéria viva, de cuja substância são formadas as células animais e vegetais. VER TAMBÉM cytoplasm, nucleoplasm. 2. O material celular total, incluindo organelas celulares. Cf. cytoplasm, cytosol, hyaloplasm. SIN plasmogen. [proto- + G. *plasma*, algo formado]
   totipotential p., p. totipotencial; matéria viva com a menor diferenciação reconhecível de estrutura, mas com o maior potencial, podendo formar todos os órgãos celulares.
pro·to·plas·mat·ic, pro·to·plas·mic (prō′tō-plaz-mat′ik, -plaz′mik). Protoplasmático, protoplásmico; relativo ao protoplasma.
pro·to·plas·mol·y·sis (prō′tō-plaz-mol′i-sis). Protoplasmólise. SIN plasmolysis.
pro·to·plast (prō′tō-plast). Protoplasto. 1. Termo arcaico que significa o primeiro indivíduo de um tipo ou raça. 2. Uma célula bacteriana da qual a parede celular rígida foi completamente removida; a bactéria perde sua forma característica. [proto- + G. *plastos*, formado]
pro·to·por·phyr·ia (prō′tō-pōr-fir′ē-ă). Protoporfiria; aumento da excreção fecal de protoporfirina.
   erythropoietic p. [MIM*177000], p. eritropoética; distúrbio benigno do metabolismo da porfirina causado por uma deficiência de ferroquelatase associada a aumento da excreção fecal de protoporfirina, urina vermelho-púrpura e aumento da protoporfirina IX nas hemácias, plasma e fezes; caracterizada por urticária solar aguda ou eczema solar mais crônico, desenvolve-se rapidamente quando há exposição à luz solar; herança autossômica dominante.
pro·to·por·phy·rin·o·gen type III (prō-tō-pōr′fi-rin′ō-jen). Protoporfirinogênio tipo III; o precursor imediato da protoporfirina III na biossíntese do heme; elevado em casos de porfiria variegada.
   p. t. III oxidase, p. tipo III oxidase; enzima mitocondrial que usa O_2 para converter o protoporfirinogênio tipo III em protoporfirina tipo III na biossíntese do heme; uma deficiência dessa enzima está associada à porfiria variegada.

pro·to·por·phy·rin type III (prō-tō-pōr′fi-rin). Protoporfirina tipo III; a principal protoporfirina encontrada na natureza (1 dentre 15 isômeros possíveis), caracterizada pela presença de quatro grupos metil, dois grupos vinil e duas cadeias laterais de ácido propiônico; um derivado da porfirina que, com o ferro, forma o heme da hemoglobina e os grupos prostéticos da mioglobina, catalase, citocromos, etc.
pro·to·pro·te·ose (prō-tō-prō′tē-ōs). Protoproteose. VER primary *proteose*.
pro·to·salt (prō′tō-sawlt). Protossal. SIN acid salt.
pro·to·spore (prō′tō-spōr). Protoesporo; o produto inicial da clivagem progressiva, no qual é produzido um esporo multinucleado. [proto- + G. *sporos*, semente]
pro·to·sto·ma (prō′tō-stō′mă). Protostoma. SIN blastopore.
pro·tos·tome (prō′tō-stōm). Protostoma. SIN blastopore. [proto- + G. *stoma*, boca]
pro·to·sul·fate (prō-tō-sŭl′fāt). Protossulfato; composto de ácido sulfúrico com um protóxido do metal.
pro·to·tax·ic (prō-tō-tak′sik). Prototáxico; em psiquiatria interpessoal, um termo que se refere à primeira forma de experiência característica do lactente, que é indiferenciada, global e desorganizada. [proto- + G. *taxis*, ordem, arranjo]
Pro·to·the·ca (prō-tō-thē′kă). Gênero de uma alga aclorófila; duas espécies, *P. zopfii* e *P. wickerhamii*, causam prototecose.
pro·to·the·co·sis (prō′tō-thē-kō′sis). Prototecose; infecção cutânea verrucosa rara, bursite do olécrano, ou doença disseminada causada por *Prototheca zopfii* e *Prototheca wickerhamii*.
pro·to·troph (prō′tō-trof, -trōf). Prototrofo; cepa de bactéria que possui as mesmas necessidades nutricionais que a cepa do tipo selvagem da qual provém. VER TAMBÉM wild-type *strain*. [proto- + G. *trophe*, nutrição]
pro·to·tro·phic (prō-tō-trof′ik). Prototrófico. 1. Relativo a um prototrofo. 2. Designa a capacidade de realizar anabolismo ou de obter nutrição de uma única fonte, como do ferro, enxofre ou bactérias nitrificantes ou vegetais que realizam fotossíntese.
pro·to·tro·phism (prō-tō-trof-izm). Prototrofismo; a propriedade de ser prototrófico.
pro·to·type (prō′tō-tīp). Protótipo; a forma primitiva; a primeira forma à qual se adaptam indivíduos subseqüentes da classe ou espécie. [proto- + G. *typos*, tipo]
pro·to·ver·a·trine A and B (prō-tō-ver′ă-trēn). Protoveratrina A e B; uma mistura de dois alcalóides isolados da *Veratrum album*; eles exercem seu principal efeito sobre o sistema cardiovascular através dos receptores do seio carótico e das terminações sensitivas vagais no coração; causam vasodilatação e acredita-se que produzam uma redistribuição para todos os leitos vasculares, induzindo assim uma queda da pressão arterial; usada em determinadas formas de hipertensão; os maleatos possuem as mesmas ações.
pro·to·ver·te·bra (prō′tō-ver′tĕ-bră). Protovértebra. 1. Na literatura antiga, um somito. 2. Mais recentemente aplicado à concentração esclerotômica que se torna o centro de uma vértebra. SIN provertebra.
pro·to·ver·te·bral (prō-tō-ver′tĕ-brăl). Protovertebral; relativo a uma protovértebra.
prot·ox·ide (prō-tok′sīd). Protóxido. SIN suboxide.
Pro·to·zoa (prō-tō-zō′ă). Antigamente considerados um filo, agora considerados como um sub-reino do reino animal, incluindo todas as formas denominadas acelulares ou unicelulares. Consistem em uma única unidade celular funcional ou agregação de células indiferenciadas, frouxamente unidas e que não formam tecidos, distintos da Animalia ou Metazoa, que incluem todos os outros animais. Antigamente, os Protozoa eram divididos em quatro classes: Sarcodina, Mastigophora, Sporozoa e Ciliata; as novas classificações empregam uma taxonomia mais elevada (filo, subfilo e superclasses) e várias grandes subdivisões. [proto- + G. *zōon*, animal]
pro·to·zo·al (prō-tō-zō′ăl). Protozoário. SIN protozoan (2).
pro·to·zo·an (prō-tō-zō′an). Protozoário. 1. Membro do filo Protozoa. SIN protozoon. 2. Relativo aos protozoários. SIN protozoal.
pro·to·zo·i·a·sis (prō′tō-zō-ī′ă-sis). Protozoíase; infecção por protozoários.
pro·to·zo·i·cide (prō-tō-zō′i-sīd). Protozoicida; agente usado para matar protozoários. [protozoa + L. *caedo*, matar]
pro·to·zo·ol·o·gist (prō′tō-zō-ol′ō-jist). Protozoólogo; biólogo especializado em protozoologia.
pro·to·zo·ol·o·gy (prō′tō-zō-ol′ō-jē). Protozoologia; a ciência que estuda todos os aspectos da biologia e do interesse humano em protozoários. [protozoa + G. *logos*, estudo]
pro·to·zo·on, pl. **pro·to·zoa** (prō-tō-zō′on, -zō′ă). Protozoário. SIN protozoan (1).
pro·to·zo·o·phage (prō-tō-zō′ō-fāj). Protozoófago; fagócito que ingere protozoários. [protozoa + G. *phago*, comer]
pro·trac·tion (prō-trak′shŭn). Protração; em odontologia, a extensão dos dentes e outras estruturas maxilares ou mandibulares para uma posição anterior ao normal. [ver protractor]

mandibular p., p. mandibular; tipo de anomalia facial na qual o queixo está situado anterior ao plano orbital.
maxillary p., p. maxilar; tipo de anomalia facial na qual o subnásio situa-se anterior ao plano orbital.
pro·trac·tor (prō-trak′ter, -tōr). Protrator; músculo que puxa uma parte para frente, com ação antagonista à de um retroator; p. ex., o músculo serrátil anterior é um protrator da escápula; o músculo pterigóide lateral é um protrator da mandíbula. [L. *pro-traho*, pp. *-tractus*, fazer sair]
pro·trip·ty·line hy·dro·chlo·ride (prō-trip′ti-lēn). Cloridrato de protriptilina; um antidepressivo.
pro·trude (prō-trood′). Protrair; empurrar para diante ou projetar.
pro·tru·sio ac·e·tab·u·li (prō-troo′sē-ō as-ē-tab′ū-lī). Protrusão do acetábulo. SIN Otto *disease*.
pro·tru·sion (prō-troo′zhun). Protrusão. **1.** O estado de ser empurrado para diante ou projetado. **2.** Em odontologia, uma posição da mandíbula para diante da relação cêntrica. [L. *protrusio*]
bimaxillary p., p. bimaxilar; a projeção para diante excessiva da maxila e da mandíbula em relação à base do crânio. SIN double p.
bimaxillary dentoalveolar p., p. dentoalveolar bimaxilar; o posicionamento de toda a dentição para diante em relação ao perfil facial.
double p., p. dupla. SIN bimaxillary p.
pro·tryp·sin (prō-trip′sin). Tripsinogênio. SIN trypsinogen.
pro·tu·ber·ance (prō-too′ber-ans). [TA]. Protuberância; uma tumefação ou proliferação em forma de botão. Uma parte saliente, tumefata ou protrusa. VER TAMBÉM protuberance. SIN protuberantia [TA]. [L. mod. *protuberantia*]
Bichat p., p. de Bichat. SIN buccal *fat-pad*.
external occipital p. [TA], p. occipital externa; proeminência em torno do centro da superfície externa da porção escamosa do osso occipital, dando fixação ao ligamento nucal. SIN protuberantia occipitalis externa [TA].
internal occipital p. [TA], p. occipital interna; projeção que parte aproximadamente do centro da eminência cruciforme na superfície interna do osso occipital. SIN protuberantia occipitalis interna [TA].
mental p. [TA], p. mentual; a proeminência do queixo na parte anterior da mandíbula. SIN protuberantia mentalis [TA], mental process.
pro·tu·be·ran·tia (prō-too-ber-an′shē-ā). [TA]. Protuberância. SIN protuberance. VER TAMBÉM protuberance, prominence, eminence. [L. mod. de *protubero*, inchar, de *tuber*, um edema]
p. laryn'gea, p. laríngea. SIN laryngeal *prominence*.
p. menta'lis [TA], p. mentual. SIN mental *protuberance*.
p. occipita'lis exter'na [TA], p. occipital externa. SIN external occipital *protuberance*.
p. occipita'lis inter'na [TA], p. occipital interna. SIN internal occipital *protuberance*.
pro·ur·o·kin·ase (prō-ūr-ō-kī′nās). Pró-uroquinase; o precursor de um ativador do plasminogênio, uroquinase.
Proust, Louis J., químico francês, 1755–1826. VER P. *law*.
Proust, T., médico francês do século XIX. VER P. *space*.
pro·ver·te·bra (prō-ver-tē-brā). Provértebra. SIN protovertebra.
Pro·vi·den·cia (prov′i-den′sē-ā). Gênero de bactérias móveis, peritríquias, não-formadoras de esporos, aeróbicas ou facultativamente anaeróbicas (família Enterobacteriaceae) contendo bacilos Gram-negativos. Esses microrganismos não hidrolisam a uréia nem produzem sulfeto de hidrogênio; produzem indol e crescem em meio de citrato de Simmons. Não descarboxilam a lisina, a arginina nem a ornitina. São encontrados em amostras de fontes extra-intestinais, particularmente infecções urinárias; também foram isolados em pequenos surtos e casos esporádicos de doença diarreica. A espécie típica é a *P. alcalifaciens*.
P. alcalifa'ciens, espécie de bactéria encontrada em fontes extra-intestinais, particularmente em infecções urinárias; também foi isolada de pequenos surtos e casos esporádicos de doença diarreica; é a espécie típica do gênero *P.*
P. rettger'i, espécie de bactéria encontrada no cólera de galinhas e na gastroenterite humana. SIN *Proteus rettgeri*.
P. stuar'tii, espécie de bactéria isolada de infecções urinárias e de pequenos surtos e casos esporádicos de doença diarreica.
pro·vi·rus (prō-vī′rus). Provírus; o precursor de um vírus animal, geralmente um retrovírus; teoricamente análogo ao prófago nas bactérias, o provírus é integrado ao núcleo das células infectadas, podendo ser ativado em resposta a certos estímulos.
pro·vi·ta·min (prō-vī′tā-min). Provitamina; substância que pode ser convertida em uma vitamina; p. ex., β-caroteno.
p. A, p. A; nome trivial dos carotenóides que exibem qualitativamente a atividade biológica do β-caroteno; isto é, precursores da vitamina A (α-, β- e γ-caroteno e criptoxantina); encontrados nos óleos de fígado de peixe, espinafre, cenoura, gema do ovo, laticínios e outras folhas verdes ou em vegetais e frutas amarelos.
p. D_2, p. D_2; qualquer substância que possa dar origem ao ergocalciferol (vitamina D_2); p. ex., ergosterol.
p. D_3, p. D_3. SIN 7-dehydrocholesterol.

Prowazek, Stanislas J.M. von, protozoólogo alemão, 1876–1915. VER *Prowazekia*; P. *bodies*, em *body*; P.-Greeff *bodies*, em *body*; Halberstaedter-P. *bodies*, em *body*.
Pro·wa·ze·kia (prō-vă-zē′kē-ā). Gênero de protozoários flagelados coprozóicos, que antigamente faziam parte do gênero *Bodo*; os microrganismos podem ser parasitas, mas, pelo que se sabe, não são patogênicos. [S. *Prowazek*]
Prower. Sobrenome de um paciente no qual foi descoberto pela primeira vez o fator de Stuart-Prower (Stuart-Prower *factor*).
prox-. VER proximo-.
prox·em·ics (prok-sem′iks). Proxêmica; a disciplina científica que estuda os vários aspectos da aglomeração urbana. [L. *proximus*, mais próximo, vizinho]
proxi-. VER proximo-.
prox·i·mad (prok′si-mad). Proximal; em direção a uma parte proximal, ou em direção ao centro; não distal. [L. *proximus*, mais próximo, vizinho, + *ad*, para]
prox·i·mal (prok′si-māl). Proximal. **1.** Mais próximo do tronco ou do ponto de origem, diz-se de uma parte de um membro, de uma artéria ou de um nervo, etc., assim situado. Em direção ao plano médio após a curvatura do arco dental, em contraste com o distal (2). SIN proximalis. **2.** Em anatomia dental, designa a superfície de um dente em relação a seu vizinho, seja mesial ou distal, isto é, mais próximo ou mais distante do plano mediano ântero-posterior. SIN mesial [TA]. [L. mod. *proximalis*, do L. *proximus*, mais próximo, vizinho]
prox·i·ma·lis (prok-si-mā′lis). Proximal. SIN proximal (1). [L. mod.]
prox·i·mate (prok′si-māt). Próximo; imediato; vizinho; proximal.
proximo-, prox-, proxi-. Proximo-, prox-, proxi-; proximal. [L. *proximus*, mais perto, vizinho (a)]
prox·i·mo·a·tax·ia (prok′si-mō-ă-tak′sē-ā). Proximoataxia; ataxia ou ausência de coordenação muscular nas porções proximais dos membros, isto é, braços e antebraços, coxas e pernas. Cf. acroataxia. [proximo- + ataxia]
prox·i·mo·buc·cal (prok′si-mō-buk′al). Proximobucal; relativo às superfícies proximal e bucal de um dente; designando o ângulo formado por sua junção.
prox·i·mo·la·bi·al (prok′si-mō-lā′bē-āl). Proximolabial; relativo às superfícies proximal e labial de um dente; designando o ângulo formado por sua junção.
prox·i·mo·lin·gual (prok′si-mō-ling′gwāl). Proximolingual; relativo às superfícies proximal e lingual de um dente; designando o ângulo formado por sua junção.
prox·y·met·a·caine hy·dro·chlo·ride (prok-si-met′ā-kān). Cloridrato de proximetacaína. SIN proparacaine hydrochloride.
pro·zone (prō′zōn). Prozona; no caso de aglutinação e precipitação, o fenômeno no qual não ocorre reação visível em misturas de antígeno e anticorpo específicos devido ao excesso de anticorpos. SIN prezone.
pro·zy·go·sis (prō-zī-gō′sis). Prozigose. SIN syncephaly. [G. *pro*, antes, + *zygōsis*, união]
PrP Abreviatura de prion *protein*.
PRPP Abreviatura de 5-phospho-α-D-ribosyl-1-pyrophosphate.
PRPP syn·the·tase. PRPP sintetase; enzima que catalisa a reação da α-D-ribose 5-fosfato e do ATP para produzir PRPP e AMP; uma enzima reguladora na biossíntese de purina e pirimidina; o aumento da atividade dessa enzima resulta em aumento da biossíntese de purina, levando à gota.
prune (proon). Ameixa seca; o fruto maduro seco da *Prunus domestica* (família Rosaceae), uma árvore cultivada em regiões quentes, temperadas; um alimento com propriedades laxantes.
Pru·nus (proo′nŭs). Gênero de árvores (família Rosaceae) incluindo a cerejeira, a ameixeira, o pessegueiro e o damasqueiro. [L. ameixeira]
P. seroti'na, a cereja negra silvestre; uma fonte botânica de cereja silvestre. VER *P. virginiana*.
***P. virginia'na,* (1)** casca da cereja negra silvestre, a casca da *P. serotina*, usada como tônico e em misturas contra tosse como sedativo brônquico; **(2)** a cereja silvestre dos Estados Unidos; o principal substituto e adulterante da *P. serotina*.
pru·ri·go (proo-rī′gō). Prurigo; prurigem; doença crônica da pele, caracterizada por erupção papular persistente, com prurido intenso. [L. prurido, de *prurio*, coçar]
actinic p., p. actínico. SIN p. aestivalis.
p. aestiva'lis, p. estival; prurigo que recidiva a cada verão, tornando-se mais intenso à medida que continua o calor. SIN actinic p., summer p.
Besnier p., p. de Besnier; designação européia de prurigo, possivelmente atópico.
p. gestatio'nis, p. gestacional; doença cutânea papular pruriginosa que ocorre em mulheres grávidas, sem afetar adversamente a gravidez do feto.
Hebra p., p. de Hebra; forma grave de dermatite crônica, com infecção secundária, na qual há pápulas e nódulos intensamente pruriginosos, que recidivam constantemente; está freqüentemente associada à atopia.
p. mi′tis, p. leve; forma leve de dermatite crônica caracterizada por pápulas e nódulos intensamente pruriginosos e recorrentes, provavelmente atópicos.
p. nodula'ris, p. nodular; erupção de nódulos endurecidos, em forma de cúpula (nódulos de Picker) na pele, causados pelo ato de coçar e acompanhados

por prurido intenso; ocasionalmente é devido a infecção micobacteriana, mas a causa geralmente é desconhecida.
p. sim'plex, p. simples; forma leve de prurigo com grande tendência a recidivar.
summer p., p. do verão. SIN p. aestivalis.
pru·rit·ic (proo - rit′ik). Pruriginoso; relativo a prurido.
pru·ri·tus (proo - ri′tŭs). Prurido. **1.** SIN itching. **2.** SIN itch (1). [L. prurido, de *prurio,* coçar]
p. aestiva'lis, p. estival; prurido que ocorre no período de calor; pode estar associado a brotoeja. SIN summer itch.
p. a'ni, p. anal; prurido de intensidade variável no ânus; pode ser paroxístico ou constante, associado a dermatite seborreica ou monilíase, com aumento e irritação das veias hemorroidárias, ou pode ocorrer independentemente de quaisquer lesões cutâneas associado a doença sistêmica.
aquagenic p., p. aquagênico; prurido intenso produzido por contato breve com água a qualquer temperatura, sem alterações cutâneas visíveis.
bath p., p. do banho; prurido causado pela retirada inadequada do sabão ou pelo ressecamento excessivo da pele devido ao número exagerado de banhos. SIN bath itch.
essential p., p. essencial; prurido que ocorre independentemente de lesões cutâneas.
p. gravidarum, p. da gravidez; prurido intenso, sem exantema associado, que ocorre durante a gravidez, secundário à colestase intra-hepática e à retenção de sais biliares.
p. hiema'lis, p. invernal. SIN winter itch.
p. seni'lis, senile p., p. senil; prurido associado ao ressecamento da pele nas pessoas idosas.
symptomatic p., p. sintomático; prurido que ocorre como um sintoma de alguma doença sistêmica.
p. vul'vae, p. vulvar; prurido da genitália feminina externa, causado por vários fatores, p. ex., dermatite seborreica, reação a alérgenos de contato, atrofia senil da vulva e, ocasionalmente, doença sistêmica.
Prussak, Alexander, otologista russo, 1839–1897. VER P. *fibers*, em *fiber, pouch, space.*
Prus·sian blue [I.C. 77510]. Azul da Prússia. SIN Berlin blue.
prus·si·ate (prŭsh′e - āt, prŭs′e - āt). Prussiato. **1.** Um cianeto; um sal do ácido hidrociânico. **2.** Um ferricianeto ou ferrocianeto.
prus·sic ac·id (prŭs′ik). Ácido prússico. SIN hydrocyanic acid.
PSA Abreviatura de prostate-specific *antigen*.
psal·ter·i·al (sawl - tĕr′e - ăl). Salterial; relativo ao saltério.
psal·ter·i·um, pl. **psal·ter·ia** (sawl - tĕr′e - ŭm, sawl - tĕr′e - ă). Saltério. SIN commissura fornicis. [G. *psaltērion,* harpa]
△ **psammo-.** Areia. [G. *psammos*]
psam·mo·car·ci·no·ma (sam′o - kar - si - no′mă). Psamocarcinoma; termo obsoleto para designar um carcinoma que contém focos calcificados semelhantes aos corpúsculos de psamoma.
psam·mo·ma (sa - mo′mă). Psamoma; designação obsoleta de meningioma psamomatoso (psammomatous *meningioma*) ou meningioma. [psammo- + G. *-oma,* tumor]
Virchow p., p. de Virchow. SIN psammomatous meningioma.
psam·mo·ma·tous (sa - mo′mă - tŭs). Psamomatoso; que possui ou é caracterizado pela presença de corpos de psamoma; geralmente refere-se a certos tipos de meningioma ou à hiperplasia meníngea com corpos de psamoma.
psam·mous (sam′ŭs). Arenoso. [G. *psammos,* areia]
Psaume, J., médico francês do século XX. VER Papillon-Léage e P. *syndrome.*
PSE Abreviatura de Pidgin Sign English.
psel·lism (sel′izm). Pselismo; gagueira. SIN stammering. [G. *psellismos,* gagueira]
△ **pseud-.** VER pseudo-.
pseud·ac·ro·meg·a·ly (soo - dak - ro - meg′ă - le). Pseudacromegalia; aumento das extremidades e da face não causado por acromegalia.
pseud·a·graph·ia (soo - dă - graf′e - ă). Pseudagrafia; agrafia parcial na qual um indivíduo não consegue escrever um original, mas consegue copiar corretamente. SIN pseudoagraphia. [pseud- + G. *a-* priv. + *graphō,* escrever]
pseud·al·bu·min·u·ria (soo′dal - bū - mi - noo′rē - ă). Pseudo-albuminúria; albuminúria que não está associada a doença renal. SIN pseudoalbuminuria.
Pseud·al·les·che·ria boy·dii (sood′al - es - kē′rē′ă boy′dē - ī). Espécie de fungo que causa micetoma eumicótico e pseudalesqueríase; sua forma de conídio (assexuada) é o *Scedosporium apiospermum*; antigamente denominado *Allescheria boydii.*
pseud·al·les·che·ri·a·sis (sood′al - es - kē′ri - ă - sis). Pseudalesqueríase; variedade de doenças clínicas resultantes de infecção por *Pseudallescheria boydii*; p. ex., colonização brônquica e pneumonite invasiva, bem como ceratite micótica, endoftalmite, endocardite, meningite, sinusite, abscessos cerebrais, infecções cutâneas e subcutâneas, e infecções sistêmicas disseminadas.
Pseu·dam·phis·to·mum (soo - dam - fis′to - mŭm). Gênero de trematódeos digenéticos da família Opisthorchiidae; *P. truncatum* é uma espécie que infecta os ductos biliares do cão e do gato (raramente dos seres humanos) na Europa e na Índia. [psued- + G. *amphi,* que tem dois lados, + *stoma,* boca]

pseud·an·gi·na (soo′dan - ji′nă, soo - dan′ji - nă). Pseudo-angina. SIN angina pectoris vasomotoria.
pseud·an·ky·lo·sis (soo - dang′ki - lo′sis). Pseudo-anquilose. SIN fibrous ankylosis.
pseud·ar·thro·sis (soo - dar - thro′sis). Pseudartrose; articulação nova, falsa, que se origina no local de uma fratura não-consolidada. SIN false joint, pseudoarthrosis. [pseud- + G. *arthrōsis,* articulação]
pseu·del·minth (soo - del′minth). Pseudo-helminto; qualquer coisa que tenha o aspecto de um verme intestinal. [pseud- + G. *helmins,* verme]
pseud·es·the·sia (soo - des - thē′ze - ă). Pseudo-estesia. **1.** SIN paraphia. **2.** Sensação subjetiva que não se origina de um estímulo externo. SIN pseudoesthesia (2). **3.** SIN phantom limb *pain.* [pseud- + G. *aisthēsis,* sensação]
△ **pseudo- (psi), pseud-.** Pseud-, pseudo-; falso (freqüentemente usado a respeito de uma semelhança ilusória). [G. *pseudēs*]
pseu·do·ac·an·tho·sis ni·gri·cans (soo′do - ak - an - thō′sis nī′gri - kanz). Pseudo-acantose nigricante; acantose nigricante secundária à maceração da pele por suor excessivo, ou que ocorre em adultos obesos e de pele escura, ou associada a distúrbios endócrinos; não está associada ao câncer de vísceras.
pseu·do·a·ceph·a·lus (soo′dō - ă - sef′ă - lŭs). Pseudo-acéfalo; gêmeo parasita placentário aparentemente sem cabeça que, contudo, possui estruturas cefálicas rudimentares demonstráveis por dissecção. [pseudo- + G. *a-* priv. + *kephalē,* cabeça]
pseu·do·a·chon·dro·pla·sia (soo′dō - ă - kon - dro - plā′se - ă). Pseudo-acondroplasia; displasia óssea caracterizada por nanismo de membros curtos, com deformidades da perna associadas a *genu varum* ou *genu valgum* e frouxidão ligamentar, permitindo telescopagem das articulações; cabeça e face de aspectos normais. Herança autossômica dominante [MIM*177150 e MIM*177170] causada por mutação no gene da proteína da matriz oligomérica da cartilagem (COMP) em 19p. SIN pseudoachondroplastic spondyloepiphysial dysplasia.
pseu·do·ac·tin·o·my·co·sis (soo′dō - ak′ti - no - mi - kō′sis). Pseudo-actinomicose. SIN para-actinomycosis.
pseu·do·ag·glu·ti·na·tion (soo′dō - ă - gloo - ti - nā′shŭn). Pseudo-aglutinação. **1.** Aglomeração de partículas em soluções que não envolvem combinação antígeno-anticorpo. SIN false agglutination. **2.** SIN rouleaux *formation.*
pseu·do·a·gram·ma·tism (soo′dō - ă - gram′ă - tizm). Pseudo-agramatismo. SIN paraphrasia. [pseudo- + G. *a-* priv. + *gramma,* escrita, + *-ismos,* condição]
pseu·do·a·graph·ia (soo′dō - ă - graf′e - ă). Pseudo-agrafia. SIN pseudagraphia.
pseu·do·ai·nhum (soo′dō - in′ŭm). Pseudo-ainhum; amputação não-espontânea de um dedo, causada por vários distúrbios, como hanseníase neural, siringomielia e ceratodermia palmoplantar.
pseu·do·al·bu·mi·nu·ria (soo′dō - al - bū′mi - noo′rē - ă). Pseudo-albuminúria. SIN pseudalbuminuria.
pseu·do·al·ka·loids (soo′dō - al - kă - loydz). Pseudo-alcalóides; grupo de compostos estruturalmente semelhantes aos alcalóides.
pseu·do·al·lel·ic (soo′dō - ă - le′lik). Pseudo-alélico; relativo ao pseudo-alelismo.
pseu·do·al·lel·ism (soo - dō - ă - lē′lizm). Pseudo-alelismo; relação entre dois ou mais *loci* difíceis de distinguir de um único *locus* por análise genética clássica. Por exemplo, os estados dos componentes D, D e E do *locus* sanguíneo do Rh [MIM*111700] ainda não foram resolvidos.
pseu·do·-al·o·pe·cia ar·e·a·ta (soo′dō - al - ō - pē′she - ă ar - ē - ă′ta). Pseudo-alopecia areata; alopecia na qual surgem alterações inflamatórias leves nos orifícios dos folículos pilosos afetados.
pseu·do·an·a·phy·lac·tic (soo′dō - an - ă - fi - lak′tik). Pseudo-anafilático. SIN anaphylactoid.
pseu·do·an·a·phy·lax·is (soo′dō - an - ă - fi - lak′sis). Pseudo-anafilaxia; condição semelhante à anafilaxia, mas não causada por reação antígeno-anticorpo específica. SIN anaphylactoid crisis (2).
pseu·do·a·ne·mia (soo′dō - ă - nē′me - ă). Pseudo-anemia; palidez da pele e das mucosas sem as alterações sanguíneas da anemia. SIN false anemia.
pseu·do·an·eu·rysm (soo - dō - an′ū - rizm). Pseudo-aneurisma. **1.** Hematoma pulsátil, encapsulado, que se comunica com a luz do vaso roto. **2.** Pseudo-aneurisma ventricular, uma ruptura cardíaca contida e loculada pelo pericárdio, que forma sua parede externa. **3.** Um pseudo-aneurisma cujas paredes consistem na adventícia e no tecido fibroso periarterial e hematoma. SIN communicating hematoma, false aneurysm, pulsatile hematoma.
pseu·do·an·gi·na (soo′dō - an′ji - nă, - an - jī′nă). Pseudo-angina. SIN angina pectoris vasomotoria.
pseu·do·an·o·don·tia (soo′dō - an - ō - don′she - ă). Pseudo-anodontia; ausência clínica dos dentes devido a uma falha da erupção. [pseudo- + G. *an-* priv. + *odous,* dente]
pseu·do·ap·pen·di·ci·tis (soo′dō - ă - pen - di - sī′tis). Pseudo-apendicite; complexo de sintomas que simula apendicite sem inflamação do apêndice.
pseu·do·a·prax·ia (soo′dō - ă - prak′se - ă). Pseudo-apraxia; condição de exagerada inaptidão na qual a pessoa faz uso errado de objetos.
pseu·do·ar·thro·sis (soo′dō - ar - thrō′sis). Pseudo-artrose. SIN pseudarthrosis.

pseu·do·au·then·tic·i·ty (soo'dō-aw-then-ti'si-tē). Pseudo-autenticidade; expressão falsa ou copiada de pensamentos e sentimentos. [pseudo- + G. *authentikos*, original]

pseu·do·ba·cil·lus (soo'dō-bă-sil'ŭs). Pseudobacilo; qualquer objeto microscópico, como um poiquilócito, semelhante a um bacilo.

pseu·do·bac·te·ri·um (soo'dō-bak-tēr'ē-ŭm). Pseudobactéria; qualquer objeto microscópico semelhante a um pequeno organismo bacilar ou outra forma bacteriana.

pseu·do·bul·bar (soo-dō-bŭl'bar). Pseudobulbar; designa uma paralisia supranuclear dos nervos bulbares.

pseu·do·car·ti·lage (soo-dō-kar'ti-lij). Pseudocartilagem. SIN chondroid tissue (1).

pseu·do·car·ti·lag·i·nous (soo'dō-kar-ti-laj'i-nŭs). Pseudocartilaginoso; composto de uma substância com textura semelhante à da cartilagem.

pseu·do·cast (soo'dō-kast). Pseudocilindro. SIN false cast.

pseu·do·cele (soo'dō-sēl). Pseudocele. SIN cavity of septum pellucidum. [pseudo- + G. *koilia*, cavidade]

pseu·do·ce·lom (soo-dō-sē'lom). Pseudoceloma; celoma parcial ou falso, típico de Nematoda (nematódeos) e filos relacionados, no qual a cavidade corporal é revestida por mesoderma ao longo de apenas uma superfície (hypoderme, sob a parede corporal cuticular). Cf. celom, acelom. [pseudo- + G. *koilōma*, cavidade]

pseu·do·ceph·a·lo·cele (soo-dō-sef'a-lō-sēl). Pseudocefalocele; herniação adquirida dos tecidos intracranianos causada por traumatismo ou doença. [pseudo- + G. *kephalē*, cabeça, + *kēlē*, tumor]

pseu·do·chan·cre (soo-dō-shang'ker). Pseudocancro; úlcera endurecida inespecífica, geralmente localizada no pênis, semelhante a um cancro.

pseu·do·cho·lin·es·ter·ase (soo'dō-kol-in-es'ter-ās). Pseudocolinesterase. SIN butyrocholinesterase.
   atypical p. [MIM*177400, MIM*177500, MIM*177600], p. atípica; variante genética da colinesterase que não catalisa a hidrólise da succinilcolina. VER TAMBÉM dibucaine number, fluoride number.
   typical p., p. típica; colinesterase formada no fígado e presente no plasma; catalisa a hidrólise da succinilcolina, primeiro em succinilmonocolina e colina e, depois, em colina e ácido succínico.

pseu·do·cho·rea (soo-dō-kōr'ē'a). Pseudocoréia; afecção espasmódica ou tique extenso semelhante à coréia.

pseu·do·chro·mes·the·sia (soo'dō-krō-mes-thē'zē-ă). Pseudocromestesia; anomalia na qual cada vogal na palavra impressa é vista como colorida. VER TAMBÉM photism, color *hearing*. [pseudo- + G. *chrōma*, cor, + *aisthēsis*, sensação]

pseu·do·chro·mi·dro·sis, pseu·do·chrom·hi·dro·sis (soo'dō-krō-mi-drō'sis, -hi-drō'sis). Pseudocromidrose; a presença de pigmento cutâneo associado à sudorese, mas devido à ação local de bactérias formadoras de pigmentos, e não à excreção de suor colorido. [pseudo- + G. *chrōma*, cor, + *hidrōs*, suor]

pseu·do·chy·lous (soo-dō-kī'lŭs). Pseudoquiloso; semelhante ao quilo.

pseu·do·cir·rho·sis (soo'dō-si-rō'sis). Pseudocirrose. SIN cardiac cirrhosis.

pseu·do·clo·nus (soo-dō-klō'nŭs). Pseudoclônus; resposta clônica não mantida, apesar da força contínua para produzi-la.

pseu·do·co·arc·ta·tion (soo'dō-kō-ark-tā'shŭn). Pseudocoarctação; distorção, freqüentemente com pequeno estreitamento, do arco da aorta ao nível da inserção do ligamento arterial. SIN buckled aorta, kinked aorta.

pseu·do·col·loid (soo-dō-kol'oyd). Pseudocolóide; uma substância mucóide ou semelhante a colóide encontrada em cistos ovarianos e em outras partes.

pseu·do·col·lu·sion (soo'dō-co-loo'zhŭn). Pseudocolusão; em psicanálise, uma sensação aparente de proximidade decorrente de uma transferência. [pseudo- + Fr. *collusion*, do L. *colludo*, jogar junto]

pseu·do·co·ma (soo-dō-kō'mă). Pseudocoma. SIN locked-in syndrome.

pseu·do·cow·pox (soo-dō-kow'poks). Nódulo dos ordenhadores. SIN milkers' nodules, em nodule.

pseu·do·cox·al·gia (soo'dō-kok-sal'jē-ă). Pseudocoxalgia. SIN Legg-Calvé-Perthes *disease*. [pseudo- + L. *coxa*, quadril, + G. *algos*, dor]

pseu·do·cri·sis (soo-dō-krī'sis). Pseudocrise; queda temporária da temperatura em uma doença que, geralmente, termina por crise; não é uma crise verdadeira.

pseu·do·croup (soo-dō-kroop'). Pseudocrupe. SIN laryngismus stridulus.

pseu·do·cryp·tor·chism (soo-dō-krip'tor-kizm). Pseudocriptorquismo. SIN retractile *testis*. [pseudo- + G. *kryptos*, oculto, + *orchis*, testículo]

pseu·do·cu·mene (soo-dō-koo'mēn). Pseudocumeno; líquido incolor obtido do alcatrão; usado na esterilização do categuete. SIN pseudocumol.

pseu·do·cu·mol (soo-dō-koo'mol). Pseudocumol. SIN pseudocumene.

pseu·do·cy·e·sis (soo'dō-si-ē'sis). Pseudociese. SIN false *pregnancy*. [pseudo- + G. *kyēsis*, gravidez]

pseu·do·cyl·in·droid (soo-dō-sil'in-droyd). Pseudocilindróide; fragmento de muco ou de outra substância na urina, semelhante a um cilindro renal.

pseu·do·cyst (soo-dō-sist). Pseudocisto. **1.** Acúmulo de líquido em um lóculo cístico, mas sem revestimento epitelial ou outro revestimento membranoso. SIN

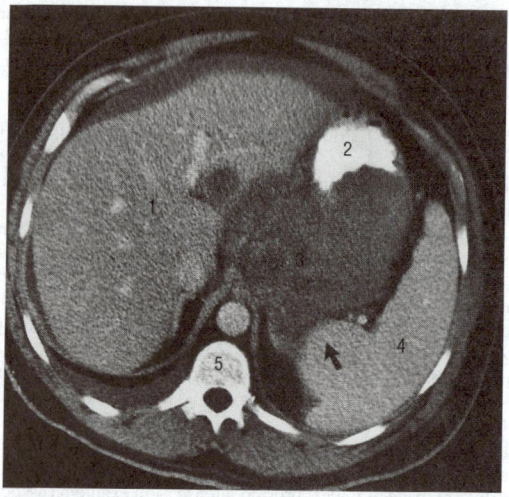

pseudocisto pancreático: TC mostra pseudocisto comprimindo a parede gástrica posterior (seta); (1) fígado, (2) ar no estômago, (3) estômago, (4) pâncreas, (5) vértebra

adventitious cyst, false cyst. **2.** Cisto cuja parede é formada por uma célula hospedeira e não por um parasita. **3.** Massa de 50 ou mais bradizoítas *Toxoplasma*, encontrados em uma célula hospedeira, freqüentemente no encéfalo; antigamente era denominado pseudocisto, mas agora é considerado um cisto verdadeiro encerrado em sua própria membrana dentro da célula hospedeira, que pode romper-se para liberar partículas formadoras de novos cistos, e, aparentemente, é infeccioso para outro hospedeiro vertebrado. VER TAMBÉM bradyzoite. [pseudo- + G. *kystis*, bexiga]

pseu·do·de·cid·u·o·sis (soo'dō-de-sid-ū-ō'sis). Pseudodeciduose; resposta decidual do endométrio na ausência de gravidez. [pseudo- + L. *deciduus*, que cai]

pseu·do·de·men·tia (soo'dō-dē-men'shē-ă). Pseudodemência; condição semelhante à demência, mas geralmente causada por um transtorno depressivo, e não por disfunção cerebral.

pseu·do·dex·tro·car·dia (soo'dō-deks'trō-kar'dē-ă). Pseudodextrocardia; deslocamento do coração para a direita, seja congênito ou causado por traumatismo, com todas as câmaras e vasos em suas posições corretas.

pseu·do·di·a·be·tes (soo'dō-dī-ă-bē'tēz). Pseudodiabetes; condição na qual se observa um teste falso-positivo para açúcar na urina.

pseu·do·di·a·stol·ic (soo'dō-dī-as-tol'ik). Pseudodiastólico; aparentemente associado à diástole cardíaca.

pseu·do·dig·i·tox·in (soo'dō-dij-i-tok'sin). Pseudodigitoxina. SIN gitoxin.

pseu·do·diph·the·ria (soo'dō-dif-thēr'ē-ă). Pseudodifteria. SIN diphtheroid (1).

pseu·do·dip·sia (soo-dō-dip'sē-ă). Pseudodipsia. SIN false *thirst*. [pseudo- + G. *dipsa*, sede]

pseu·do·di·ver·tic·u·lum (soo'dō-dī-ver-tik'ū-loom). Pseudodivertículo; uma evaginação da luz para uma área de necrose central dentro de um grande tumor de músculo liso, ao longo de qualquer parte da parede intestinal.

pseu·do·dom·i·nance (soo-dō-dom'i-nans). Pseudodominância. SIN quasidominance.

pseu·do·dys·en·tery (soo-dō-dis'en-tār-ē). Pseudodisenteria; ocorrência de sintomas indiferenciáveis daqueles da disenteria bacilar, que têm outras causas além da presença dos microrganismos específicos da disenteria bacilar.

pseu·do·e·phed·rine hy·dro·chlo·ride (soo'dō-e-fed'rin). Cloridrato de pseudo-efedrina; o isômero natural da efedrina; uma amina simpaticomimética com ações e empregos semelhantes aos da efedrina.

pseu·do·er·y·sip·e·las (soo'dō-er-i-sip'ē-lăs). Pseudo-erisipela. SIN erysipeloid.

pseu·do·es·the·sia (soo-dō-es-thē'zē-ă). Pseudestesia. **1.** SIN paraphia. **2.** SIN pseudesthesia (2). **3.** SIN phantom limb *pain*.

pseu·do·ex·fo·li·a·tion (soo'dō-eks-fō-lē-ā'shŭn). Pseudo-esfoliação; uma condição que simula a esfoliação em alguns aspectos, mas na qual a camada superficial não está realmente separada.
   p. of lens capsule, p. da cápsula da lente; deposição em todas as partes do olho, incluindo a cápsula da lente, de um material derivado das membranas basais. Se esse material obstrui a rede trabecular, impedindo o efluxo de humor aquoso do olho, pode haver glaucoma. VER exfoliation *syndrome*, pseudoexfoliative *glaucoma*.

pseu·do·fluc·tu·a·tion (soo'dō-flŭk-choo-ā'shŭn). Pseudoflutuação; sensação ondulatória, semelhante à flutuação, obtida por percussão do tecido muscular.

pseu·do·fol·lic·u·li·tis (soo′dō - fo - lik - ū - lī′tis). Pseudofoliculite; pápulas foliculares eritematosas ou, menos comumente, pústulas resultantes da raspagem de pêlos muito crespos; conseqüentemente, as extremidades dos pêlos em crescimento voltam a penetrar na pele adjacente ao folículo, produzindo pêlos que crescem para dentro; a pseudofoliculite na área da barba é muito comum em negros.

pseu·do·frac·ture (soo - dō - frak′choor). Pseudofratura; condição na qual uma radiografia mostra neosteogênese com espessamento do periósteo no local de uma lesão do osso.

pseu·do·fruc·tose (soo - dō - fruk′tōs). Pseudofrutose. SIN psicose.

pseu·do·gan·gli·on (soo - dō - gang′glē - on). Pseudogânglio; espessamento localizado de um tronco nervoso que possui o aspecto de um gânglio.

pseu·do·gene (soo′dō - jēn). Pseudogene. 1. Uma seqüência de nucleotídeos que não é transcrita e, portanto, não tem efeito fenotípico. 2. Um segmento de DNA inativo que se originou por mutação de um gene ativo dos pais.

pseu·do·geu·ses·the·sia (soo′dō - gū - ses - thē′zē - ă). Pseudogeusestesia. SIN color taste. [pseudo- + G. geusis, sabor, + aisthēsis, sensação]

pseu·do·geu·sia (soo - dō - gū′sē - ă). Pseudogeusia; sensação subjetiva de paladar não produzida por um estímulo externo. [pseudo- + G. geusis, paladar]

pseu·do·glan·ders (soo - dō - glan′derz). Pseudomormo. SIN melioidosis.

pseu·do·gli·o·ma (soo′dō - glī - ō′mă). Pseudoglioma; qualquer opacidade intra-ocular que pode ser confundida com um retinoblastoma.

pseu·do·glob·u·lin (soo′dō - glob′oo - lin). Pseudoglobulina; a fração da globulina sérica mais solúvel em uma solução de sulfato de amônio que a fração euglobulina.

pseu·do·glo·mer·u·lus (soo′dō - glō - mer′ū - lŭs). Pseudoglomérulo; uma estrutura dentro de uma neoplasia microscopicamente semelhante a um glomérulo renal, mas que não representa diferenciação glomerular renal.

pseu·do·glu·co·sa·zone (soo′dō - gloo - kō′să - zōn). Pseudoglucosazona; substância, algumas vezes presente na urina normal, que produz uma reação no teste da fenilidrazina.

pseu·do·gout (soo′dō - gowt) [MIM*118600]. Pseudogota; sinovite episódica aguda, causada por depósitos de cristais de pirofosfato de cálcio, em vez de cristais de urato como na gota verdadeira; associada à condrocalcinose articular; a genética é obscura. SIN calcium gout.

pseu·do·gy·ne·co·mas·tia (soo′dō - gī - nĕ - kō - mas′tē - ă, - jin - ĕ - kō-). Pseudoginecomastia; aumento da mama masculina por excesso de tecido adiposo sem qualquer aumento do tecido mamário. [pseudo- + G. gynē, mulher, + mastos, mama]

pseu·do·he·ma·tu·ria (soo′dō - hem - ă - too′rē - ă). Pseudo-hematúria; pigmentação vermelha da urina causada por determinados alimentos ou fármacos e, portanto, que não é realmente hematúria. SIN false hematuria.

pseu·do·he·mop·ty·sis (soo′dō - hē - mop′ti - sis). Pseudo-hemoptise; emissão de sangue que não provém dos pulmões nem dos brônquios. [pseudo- + G. haima, sangue, + ptysis, expectoração]

pseu·do·her·maph·ro·dite (soo′dō - her - maf′rō - dīt). Pseudo-hermafrodita; indivíduo que exibe pseudo-hermafroditismo.

pseu·do·her·maph·ro·dit·ism (soo′dō - her - maf′rō - dī - tizm). Pseudo-hermafroditismo; condição em que não há ambigüidade do sexo gonadal (isto é, o indivíduo possui testículos ou ovários), mas a genitália externa é ambígua. Cf. steroid 5α-reductase. SIN false hermaphroditism.

female p. [MIM*264270], p. feminino; pseudo-hermafroditismo com anomalias ósseas e genitais, mas com gônadas femininas e um cariótipo XX. SIN androgynism, androgyny (1).

male p. [MIM*261550, MIM*264300, MIM*312100], p. masculino; pseudo-hermafroditismo no qual as gônadas são masculinas e o cariótipo é XY, mas exibe anomalias genitais.

pseu·do·her·nia (soo′dō - her′nē - ă). Pseudo-hérnia; inflamação dos tecidos escrotais ou de uma glândula inguinal, simulando uma hérnia estrangulada.

pseu·do·het·er·o·to·pia (su′dō - het - er - ō - tō′pē - ă). Pseudo-heterotopia; aparente deslocamento de alguns tecidos observado após a morte; na verdade, é um artefato, e não uma heterotopia verdadeira.

pseu·do·hy·dro·ceph·a·ly (soo′dō - hī - drō - sef′ă - lē). Pseudo-hidrocefalia; condição caracterizada por aumento da cabeça sem aumento concomitante do sistema ventricular.

pseu·do·hy·dro·ne·phro·sis (soo′dō - hī - drō - ne - frō′sis). Pseudo-hidronefrose; presença de um cisto próximo do rim, simulando hidronefrose.

pseu·do·hy·per·kal·e·mia (soo′dō - hī′per - kal - ē′ē - ă). Pseudo-hipercalemia; falsa elevação da concentração sérica de potássio, que ocorre quando o potássio é liberado in vitro de células em uma amostra de sangue colhida para determinação de potássio. Pode ser conseqüência de uma doença (isto é, distúrbios mieloproliferativos com acentuada leucocitose ou trombocitose) ou decorrente de técnica inadequada de coleta, com hemólise in vitro. [pseudo + G. hyper, acima, + L. kalium, potássio, G. haima, sangue]

pseu·do·hy·per·par·a·thy·roid·ism (soo′dō - hī′per - par - ă - thī′roy - dizm). Pseudo-hiperparatireoidismo; hipercalcemia em um paciente com neoplasia maligna na ausência de metástases ósseas ou hiperparatireoidismo primário; acredita-se que seja causado pela formação de hormônio semelhante ao paratireóideo por tecido tumoral não-paratireóideo.

pseu·do·hy·per·tel·or·ism (soo′dō - hī - per - tel′ōr - izm). Pseudo-hipertelorismo; aparência de excessiva distância entre os olhos (telorismo ocular) causada pelo deslocamento lateral dos cantos internos. VER Waardenburg syndrome.

pseu·do·hy·per·tro·phic (soo′dō - hī - per - trof′ik). Pseudo-hipertrófico; relativo a, ou caracterizado por, pseudo-hipertrofia.

pseu·do·hy·per·tro·phy (soo′dō - hī - per′trō - fē). Pseudo-hipertrofia; aumento do tamanho de um órgão ou parte, causado, não pelo aumento do tamanho ou do número de elementos funcionais específicos, mas de algum outro tecido, adiposo ou fibroso. SIN false hypertrophy.

pseu·do·hy·pha (soo - dō - hī′fă). Pseudo-hifa; cadeia de células fúngicas que se rompem facilmente, intermediária entre uma cadeia de células germinativas e uma hifa verdadeira, caracterizada por constrições, e não por septos nas junções. [pseudo- + G. hyphē, uma membrana (hifa)]

pseu·do·hy·po·na·tre·mia (soo′dō - hī - pō - nă - trē′mē - ă). Pseudo-hiponatremia; baixa concentração sérica de sódio decorrente do deslocamento de volume por grande hiperlipidemia ou hiperproteinemia; também usada para descrever a baixa concentração sérica de sódio que pode ocorrer na presença de altos níveis sanguíneos de glicose.

pseu·do·hy·po·par·a·thy·roid·ism (soo′dō - hī′pō - par - ă - thī′royd - izm) [MIM*103580]. Pseudo-hipoparatireoidismo; distúrbio semelhante ao hipoparatireoidismo, com altos níveis séricos de fosfato e baixos níveis séricos de cálcio, porém com níveis séricos normais ou elevados de hormônio paratireóideo; o defeito é devido à ausência de responsividade do órgão-alvo ao hormônio paratireóideo. Há dois tipos: o tipo I exibe ausência de resposta tubular renal ao paratormônio exógeno, com aumento do AMPc urinário, o tipo Is exibe defeitos ósseos tipo I (SIN Albright hereditary osteodystrophy) e o tipo II está associado a defeito em um locus após a produção de AMPc. Herança dominante ligada ao X causada por mutação no gene que codifica o polipeptídeo 1 com atividade α-estimulante da proteína de ligação do nucleotídeo guanina (GNAS1), que regula a adenil ciclase no cromossoma 20q. Cf. thyrotropin resistance.

p. type Ia, p. tipo Ia; pseudo-hipoparatireoidismo supostamente causado por um defeito na proteína G associada à adenilato ciclase (provavelmente autossômico dominante).

p. type Ib, p. tipo Ib; pseudo-hipoparatireoidismo causado por um defeito no complexo da adenilato ciclase.

pseu·do·ic·ter·us (soo - dō - ik′ter - ŭs). Pseudo-icterícia; coloração amarelada da pele que não é causada por pigmentos biliares, como na doença de Addison. SIN pseudojaundice.

pseu·do·il·e·us (soo - dō - il′ē - ŭs). Pseudo-íleo; obstipação absoluta, semelhante ao íleo paralítico, causada por paralisia da parede intestinal.

pseu·do·in·farc·tion (soo - dō - in - fark′shŭn). Pseudo-infarto; qualquer condição que simule um infarto do miocárdio, p. ex., a pericardite aguda, o aneurisma dissecante da aorta, etc.

pseu·do·in·flu·en·za (soo′dō - in - floo - en′ză). Pseudo-*influenza*; afecção catarral epidêmica semelhante à *influenza*, porém menos grave.

pseu·do·in·tra·lig·a·men·tous (soo′dō - in′tră - lig - ă - men′tŭs). Pseudo-intraligamentar; que produz a falsa impressão de estar situado dentro do ligamento largo; p. ex., um tumor pseudo-intraligamentar.

pseu·do·i·so·chro·mat·ic (soo′dō - ī - sō - krō - mat′ik). Pseudo-isocromático; aparentemente da mesma cor; indica certos mapas que contêm pontos co-

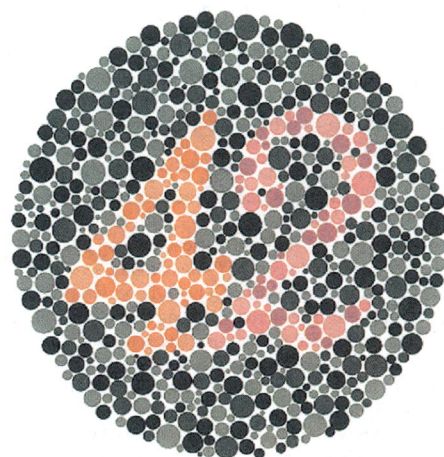

lâmina pseudo-isocromática

loridos misturados com figuras impressas em cores confusas; usado para testar a deficiência visual das cores.

pseu·do·iso·en·zymes (soo'dō-ī-sō-en'zīmz). Pseudo-isoenzimas; múltiplas formas de enzimas que catalisam a mesma reação e possuem a mesma seqüência de aminoácidos; as diferenças são devidas aos efeitos de alguma modificação pós-tradução.

pseu·do·jaun·dice (soo-dō-jawn'dis). Pseudo-icterícia. SIN pseudoicterus.

pseu·do·ker·a·tin (soo-dō-kar'a-tin). Pseudoqueratina; proteína extraída da epiderme e do tecido nervoso (fibrilas gliais), provavelmente envolvida na queratinização.

pseu·do·li·po·ma (soo'dō-li-pō'mă). Pseudolipoma; qualquer tumefação lisa, de consistência mole, circunscrita, geralmente móvel, macroscopicamente semelhante a um lipoma.

pseu·do·li·thi·a·sis (soo'dō-li-thī'a-sis). Pseudolitíase; distúrbio semelhante a uma das síndromes associadas a um cálculo em uma víscera oca ou em outra parte. [pseudo- + G. *lithos*, cálculo]

pseu·do·lo·gia (soo-dō-lō'jē-ă). Pseudologia; mentira patológica no discurso ou na escrita. [pseudo- + G. *logos*, palavra]

  p. phantas'tica, p. fantástica; relato elaborado, muitas vezes fantástico, das proezas de um paciente, que são completamente falsas, mas nas quais o paciente parece acreditar.

pseu·do·lym·pho·cyte (soo-dō-lim'fō-sīt). Pseudoinfócito; pequeno leucócito neutrófilo com um núcleo redondo único, característico da rara anomalia de Pelger-Huët homozigota.

pseu·do·lym·pho·ma (soo'dō-lim-fō'mă). Pseudolinfoma; infiltração benigna de células linfóides ou histiócitos que, microscopicamente, assemelha-se a um linfoma maligno.

  cutaneous p., p. cutâneo. SIN benign *lymphocytoma* cutis.

pseu·do·ly·so·gen·ic (soo'dō-li-sō-jen'ik). Pseudolisogênico; relativo à pseudolisogenia.

pseu·do·ly·sog·e·ny (soo'dō-lī-soj'ē-nē). Pseudolisogenia; a condição em que um bacteriófago é mantido (transportado) em cultura de uma cepa bacteriana, mediante infecção de variantes suscetíveis da cepa, em contraposição à verdadeira lisogenia, na qual o genoma do bacteriófago multiplica-se como parte integrante do genoma bacteriano.

pseu·do·ma·lig·nan·cy (soo'dō-mă-lig'nan-sē). Pseudomalignidade; tumor benigno que parece, clínica ou histologicamente, ser uma neoplasia maligna. VER TAMBÉM pseudotumor.

pseu·do·mam·ma (soo-dō-mam'ă). Pseudomama; designação obsoleta de uma estrutura glandular semelhante à glândula mamária, que ocorre em cistos dermóides.

pseu·do·ma·nia (soo-dō-mā'nē-ă). Pseudomania. **1.** Transtorno mental fictício. **2.** Transtorno mental no qual o paciente alega falsamente ter cometido um crime. **3.** De modo geral, o impulso mórbido de falsificar ou mentir, como na pseudologia.

pseu·do·mas·tur·ba·tion (soo'dō-mas-ter-bā'shŭn). Pseudomasturbação; comportamento que simula estimulação genital.

pseu·do·meg·a·col·on (soo'dō-meg'ah-kō'lon). Pseudomegacolo; aumento da parte distal do colo com função muscular lenta, sem as anormalidades neurológicas do megacolo congênito (Hirschsprung *disease*).

pseu·do·mel·a·no·sis (soo'dō-mel-ă-nō'sis). Pseudomelanose; coloração esverdeado-escura ou enegrecida *postmortem* da superfície das vísceras abdominais, resultante da ação do hidrogênio sulfurado sobre o ferro da hemoglobina desintegrada. [pseudo- + G. *melas*, preto]

pseu·do·mem·brane (soo-dō-mem'brān). Pseudomembrana. SIN false *membrane.*

pseu·do·men·in·gi·tis (soo'dō-men-in-jī'tis). Pseudomeningite. SIN meningism.

pseu·do·men·stru·a·tion (soo'dō-men-stroo-ā'shŭn). Pseudomenstruação; hemorragia uterina sem as alterações endometriais pré-menstruais típicas.

pseu·do·met·a·pla·sia (soo'dō-met-ă-plā'zē-ă). Pseudometaplasia. SIN histologic *accommodation.*

pseu·dom·ne·sia (soo-dom-nē'zē-ă). Pseudomnésia; impressão subjetiva de memória de acontecimentos que não ocorreram. [pseudo- + G. *mnēsis*, memória]

pseu·do·mo·nad (soo-dō-mō'nad). Pseudomônada; termo usado em referência a qualquer membro do gênero *Pseudomonas.*

ⓘ *Pseu·do·mo·nas* (soo-dō-mō'nas). Gênero de bactérias móveis, flageladas polares, não-formadoras de esporos, estritamente aeróbicas (família Pseudomonadaceae), contendo bacilos Gram-negativos retos ou curvos, mas não-helicoidais, encontrados isoladamente. O metabolismo é respiratório, nunca fermentativo. São encontradas comumente no solo, na água doce e em ambientes marinhos. Algumas espécies são patogênicas para vegetais. Outros estão envolvidas em infecções humanas. A espécie típica é o *P. aeruginosa.* [pseudo- + G. *monas*, unidade, mônada]

  P. acido'vorans, espécie de bactéria encontrada na água, no solo e, algumas vezes, em amostras clínicas.

  P. aerugino'sa, espécie de bactéria encontrada no solo, na água e, comumente, em amostras clínicas (infecções de feridas, queimaduras infectadas, infecções urinárias); o agente causador do pus azul; ocasionalmente patogênica para vegetais; em geral causa infecções em seres humanos, nos quais há um defeito nos mecanismos de defesa do hospedeiro. É a espécie típica do gênero *Pseudomonas.* SIN blue pus bacillus.

  P. cepa'cia. SIN *Burkholderia cepacia.*

  P. diminu'ta, espécie de bactéria encontrada basicamente em amostras clínicas, raramente na água.

  P. fluores'cens, espécie de bactéria encontrada no solo e na água; amiúde é encontrada em amostras clínicas e comumente está associada à deterioração de alimentos (ovos, carnes curadas, peixe e leite).

  P. mallei. SIN *Burkholderia mallei.*

  P. maltophil'ia, espécie agora denominada *Xanthomonas maltophilia.* VER *Stenotrophomonas maltophilia.*

  P. piscici'da, espécie de bactéria patogênica para peixes.

  P. pseudoalcalig'enes, espécie de bactéria encontrada na emissão de um seio.

  P. pseudomal'lei. SIN *Burkholderia pseudomallei.* SIN Whitmore bacillus.

  P. putrefa'ciens, designação antiga de *Alteromonas putrefaciens.*

  P. stut'zeri, espécie de bactéria encontrada no solo e na água, freqüentemente em amostras clínicas.

  P. vesicula'ris, espécie de bactéria encontrada em sanguessugas medicinais (*Hirudo medicinalis*) e na água de ribeirões.

pseudomonilethrix (soo'dō-mō-nil'ē-thriks). Pseudomoniletrix; tricodistrofia nodal semelhante ao moniletrix, porém com fraturas nas nodosidades; herança autossômica dominante com início tardio.

pseu·do·mon·o·mo·lec·u·lar (soo-dō-mon-ō-mol-ek'koo-lar). Pseudomonomolecular. SIN pseudounimolecular.

pseu·do·morph (soo'dō-mōrf). Pseudomorfo; mineral encontrado cristalizado em uma forma que não é própria dele, mas de algum outro mineral. [pseudo- + G. *morphē*, forma]

pseu·do·my·ce·li·um (soo'dō-mī-se'lē-ŭm). Pseudomicélio; massa de pseudo-hifas semelhante a um micélio.

pseu·do·my·o·pia (soo'dō-mī-ō'pē-ă). Pseudomiopia; condição que simula a miopia e é causada por espasmo do músculo ciliar.

pseu·do·myx·o·ma (soo'dō-mik-sō'mă). Pseudomixoma; massa gelatinosa semelhante a um mixoma, mas composta de muco.

  p. peritone'i, p. peritoneal; o acúmulo de grandes quantidades de material mucinoso na cavidade peritoneal, em virtude de neoplasias císticas malignas do ovário ou apêndice; freqüentemente persistirá devido ao crescimento de células secretoras de muco dispersas sobre superfícies serosas. SIN gelatinous ascites.

pseu·do·nar·cot·ic (soo'dō-nar-kot'ik). Pseudonarcótico; que induz o sono por um efeito sedativo, mas não diretamente narcótico.

pseu·do·ne·o·plasm (soo-dō-nē'ō-plazm). Pseudoneoplasia. SIN pseudotumor.

pseu·do·neu·ro·ma (soo'dō-noo-rō'mă). Pseudoneuroma. SIN traumatic *neuroma.*

pseu·do·nit (soo'dō-nit). Pseudolêndea. SIN hair *cast.*

pseu·do-os·te·o·ma·la·cia (soo'dō-os'tē-ō-mă-lā'shē-ă). Pseudo-osteomalacia; amolecimento raquítico do osso.

pseu·do-os·te·o·ma·la·cic (soo'dō-os'tē-ō-mă-lā'sik). Pseudo-osteomaláico; caracterizado por pseudo-osteomalacia.

pseu·do·pap·il·le·de·ma (soo'dō-pap-il-e-dē'mă). Pseudopapiledema; elevação anômala do disco óptico; observado na hiperopia grave e drusas do nervo óptico.

pseu·do·pa·ral·y·sis (soo'dō-pă-ral'i-sis). Pseudoparalisia; paralisia aparente causada por inibição voluntária do movimento em virtude de dor, ausência de coordenação ou outra causa, mas sem paralisia real. SIN pseudoparesis (1).

  arthritic general p., p. geral artrítica; doença observada em indivíduos artríticos, que apresentam sintomas semelhantes aos da paresia geral, cujas lesões consistem em alterações difusas de caráter degenerativo e não-inflamatório causadas por ateroma intracraniano.

  congenital atonic p., p. atônica congênita. SIN *amyotonia* congenita.

pseu·do·par·a·ple·gia (soo'dō-par-ă-plē'jē-ă). Pseudoparaplegia; paralisia aparente nos membros inferiores, na qual os reflexos tendíneos e cutâneos e as reações elétricas são normais; a condição é observada algumas vezes no raquitismo.

  Basedow p., p. de Basedow; fraqueza dos músculos da coxa na tireotoxicose; pode ocorrer subitamente e causar a queda do paciente.

pseu·do·par·a·site (soo-dō-par'ă-sīt). Pseudoparasita; falso parasita; pode ser um comensal ou um parasita temporário (sendo este último um microrganismo ingerido acidentalmente e que sobrevive por curto período no intestino).

pseu·do·pa·ren·chy·ma (soo'dō-pă-reng'ki-mă). Pseudoparênquima; em fungos, uma massa de hifas modificadas semelhante a um tecido.

pseu·do·pa·re·sis (soo'dō-pa-rē'sis, -par'ē-sis). Pseudoparesia. **1.** SIN pseudoparalysis. **2.** Condição caracterizada por alterações pupilares, tremores e distúrbios da fala sugestivos de neurossífilis parética inicial, na qual, entretanto, os resultados dos testes sorológicos são negativos.

pseu·do·pe·lade (soo'dō - pē - lahd'). Pseudopelada; tipo cicatricial de alopecia; geralmente ocorre em placas irregulares dispersas; de causa incerta. SIN p. of Brocq. [pseudo- + Fr. *pelade*, doença que causa queda esporádica do cabelo] **p. of Brocq**, p. de Brocq. SIN pseudopelade.

pseu·do·per·i·car·di·tis (soo'dō - per - i - kar - dī'tis). Pseudopericardite; artefato de ausculta semelhante a um atrito, mas devido ao movimento do tecido no espaço intercostal quando o diafragma do estetoscópio é colocado sobre o ápice.

pseu·do·per·ox·i·dase (soo'dō - per - oks - i - dās). Pseudoperoxidase; referente à atividade da peroxidase termoestável, não-enzimática, associada às proteínas do heme.

pseu·do·phac·os (soo'dō - fak'os). Pseudofacos; lentículos. SIN lenticulus. [pseudo- + *phakos*, lente]

pseu·do·pha·kia (soo - dō - fak'ē - ă). Pseudofaquia; pseudofacia; um olho no qual a lente natural é substituída por uma lente intra-ocular. [pseudo- + *phakos*, lentículo (lente)]

pseu·do·pha·ko·do·ne·sis (soo - dō - fā'kō - dō - nē'sis). Pseudofacodonese; mobilidade excessiva de um implante de lente intra-ocular.

pseu·do·pho·tes·the·sia (soo'dō - fō - tes - thē'zē - ă). Pseudofotestesia. SIN photism. [pseudo- + G. *phōs*, luz, + *aisthēsis*, sensação]

pseu·do·phyl·lid (soo - dō - fi'lid). Pseudofilídeo; nome comum de membros da ordem Pseudophyllidea.

Pseu·do·phyl·lid·ea (soo'dō - fi - lid'ē - ă). Ordem de tênias com ciclo vital aquático, que atravessam os estágios coracídio, procercóide e plerocercóide antes de se transformarem em adultos em peixes, mamíferos marinhos ou mamíferos que se alimentam de peixes; inclui a larva tênia dos peixes que infesta os seres humanos, *Diphyllobothrium latum*. [pseudo- + G. *phyllon*, folha]

pseu·do·plate·let (soo - dō - plāt'let). Pseudoplaqueta; qualquer dos fragmentos de neutrófilos que podem ser confundidos com plaquetas, principalmente em esfregaços do sangue periférico de pacientes leucêmicos.

pseu·do·pock·et (soo - dō - pok'et). Pseudobolsa; uma bolsa, adjacente a um dente, resultante de hiperplasia e edema gengival, porém sem migração apical da fixação epitelial.

pseu·do·pod (soo'dō - pod). Pseudópode. SIN pseudopodium.

pseu·do·po·di·um, pl. **pseu·do·po·dia** (soo - dō - pō'dē - ŭm, - pō' - dē - ă). Pseudópode; prolongamento protoplasmático temporário, emitido por um protozoário ameniano ou na fase amebóide, para locomoção ou para preensão de alimento. SIN pseudopod. [pseudo- + G. *pous*, pé]

pseu·do·pol·y·dys·tro·phy (soo'dō - pol - ē - dis'trō - fē). Pseudopolidistrofia. SIN mucolipidosis III.

pseu·do·pol·yp (soo - dō - pol'ip). Pseudopólipo; massa projetada de tecido de granulação, podendo surgir em grande número na colite ulcerativa; pode ser coberta por epitélio regenerativo. SIN inflammatory polyp.

pseu·do·por·phyr·ia (soo'dō - fō - fir'ē - ă). Pseudoporfiria; condição clinicamente idêntica à porfiria, mas sem anormalidade da excreção de porfirina, conseqüente à ingestão de droga ou hemodiálise.

pseu·do·preg·nan·cy (soo - dō - preg'nan - sē). Pseudogravidez. 1. SIN false pregnancy. 2. Condição em que há sintomas semelhantes aos da gravidez, mas que não é gravidez; ocorre após cópula estéril em espécies de mamíferos nas quais a cópula induz a ovulação, e também em cães, nos quais o ciclo estral inclui uma fase lútea acentuada.

pseu·do·prog·na·thism (soo - dō - prog'nă - thizm). Pseudoprognatismo; uma projeção adquirida da mandíbula causada por desarmonias oclusais que forçam a mandíbula para a frente; os côndilos mandibulares estão à frente de sua posição funcional prevista.

pseu·do·pte·ryg·i·um (soo'dō - tē - rij'ē - ŭm). Pseudopterígio; adesão da conjuntiva à córnea, que ocorre após a lesão.

pseu·dop·to·sis (soo - dō - tō'sis, soo - dop'tō - sis). Pseudoptose; condição semelhante à incapacidade de elevar a pálpebra, devida à blefarofimose, blefarocalasia ou alguma outra afecção. SIN false blepharoptosis. [pseudo- + G. *ptōsis*, queda]

pseu·do·pu·ber·ty (soo - dō - pū'ber - tē). Pseudopuberdade; condição caracterizada pelo desenvolvimento precoce de um número variável de alterações somáticas e funcionais típicas da puberdade; comumente causada pelas secreções hormonais de um tumor ovariano (especialmente ovariano ou testicular), surgindo tipicamente antes da idade cronológica da puberdade. Não representa a seqüência puberal normal iniciada por gonadotrofinas hipotalâmico-hipofisárias.
  precocious p., p. precoce; o desenvolvimento de puberdade em crianças muito pequenas; comumente caracterizada por secreção de hormônios gonadais, sem estimulação da gametogênese.

pseu·do·re·ac·tion (soo'dō - rē - ak'shŭn). Pseudo-reação; uma reação falsa; aquela que não tem causas específicas em determinado teste.

pseu·do·rep·li·ca (soo - dō - rep'li - kă). Pseudo-réplica; amostra para exame microscópico eletrônico obtida pela deposição de partículas de uma suspensão contendo vírus sobre uma superfície de agarose, cobrindo a superfície com uma solução contendo plástico, e, após a evaporação do solvente, removendo a película juntamente com partículas emaranhadas, fazendo-as flutuar sobre a superfície de uma solução de acetato de uranil.

pseu·do·ret·i·ni·tis pig·men·to·sa (soo'dō - ret - i - nī'tis pig - men - tō'să). Pseudo-retinite pigmentosa; mosqueamento pigmentar disseminado da retina que pode suceder o traumatismo ocular grave, principalmente por uma lesão penetrante.

pseu·do·rheu·ma·tism (soo - dō - roo'mă - tizm). Pseudo-reumatismo. 1. Sintomas articulares ou musculares sem achados objetivos e sem causas subjacentes aparentes. 2. Sintomas articulares fictícios (obsoleto).

pseu·do·rick·ets (soo - dō - rik'ets). Pseudo-raquitismo. SIN renal rickets.

pseu·do·ro·sette (soo'dō - rō - zet'). Pseudo-roseta; arranjo radial perivascular de células neoplásicas ao redor de um pequeno vaso sanguíneo. VER rosette (2).

pseu·do·ru·bel·la (soo'dō - roo - bel'ă). Pseudo-rubéola, exantema súbito. SIN exanthema subitum.

pseu·do·sar·co·ma (soo - dō - sar - kō'mă). Pseudo-sarcoma; tumor maligno polipóide volumoso do esôfago, composto de células fusiformes com um foco de carcinoma de células escamosas; as células fusiformes podem ser fibroblastos malignos epiteliais ou metaplásicos.

pseu·do·scar·la·ti·na (soo'dō - skar - lă - tē'nă). Pseudo-escarlatina; eritema com febre, devido a outras causas, além do *Streptococcus pyogenes*.

pseu·do·scle·ro·sis (soo'dō - sklēr - ō'sis). Pseudo-esclerose; endurecimento inflamatório ou infiltração adiposa ou de outro tipo, simulando espessamento fibroso. [pseudo- + G. *sklērōsis*, endurecimento]

pseu·do·sei·zure (soo'dō - sē'zher). Pseudoconvulsão; uma convulsão psicogênica.

pseu·do·small·pox (soo - dō - smawl'poks). Pseudovaríola; alastrim. SIN alastrim.

pseu·dos·mia (soo - doz'mē - ă). Pseudosmia; sensação subjetiva de um odor que não existe. [pseudo- + G. *osmē*, odor]

Pseu·do·ster·ta·gia bul·lo·sa (soo'dō - ster - ta'jē - ă bŭl - ō'să). Um dos vermes do estômago médio, localizado no abomaso de ovinos, caprinos e antilocabras; é encontrado principalmente no oeste dos Estados Unidos.

pseu·dos·to·ma (soo - dos'tō - mă). Pseudostoma; abertura aparente em uma célula, membrana ou outro tecido, devida a um defeito na coloração ou a outra causa. [pseudo- + G. *stoma*, boca]

pseu·do·stra·bis·mus (soo'dō - stra - biz'mŭs). Pseudo-estrabismo; o surgimento de estrabismo causado por epicanto, anormalidade da distância interorbital ou reflexo luminoso corneano não-correspondente ao centro da pupila. [pseudo- + G. *strabismos*, estrabismo]

pseu·do·ta·bes (soo - dō - tā'bēz). Pseudotabes; síndrome que exibe as características da neurossífilis tabética, mas não é causada por sífilis. SIN Leyden ataxia.
  pupillotonic p., p. pupilotônica. SIN Adie syndrome.

pseu·do·trun·cus ar·te·ri·o·sus (soo - dō - trŭng'kŭs ar - tēr - ē - ō'sŭs). Pseudotronco arterial; malformação cardiovascular congênita com atresia da valva pulmonar e ausência da artéria pulmonar principal; os pulmões são irrigados com sangue, seja através de um canal permeável ou através de artérias brônquicas originadas na aorta; uma característica da forma mais grave de tetralogia de Fallot.

pseu·do·tu·ber·cle (soo - dō - too'ber - kl). Pseudotubérculo; nódulo histologicamente semelhante a um granuloma tuberculoso, mas devido à infecção por algum outro microrganismo que não o *Mycobacterium tuberculosis*.

pseu·do·tu·ber·cu·lo·sis (soo'dō - too - ber'kū'lō'sis). Pseudotuberculose; doença de uma grande variedade de espécies de animais causada pela bactéria *Yersinia pseudotuberculosis*. Epizootias de p. são comuns em aves e roedores, freqüentemente com elevados índices de casos fatais. Em seres humanos, são reconhecidas sete condições clínicas: infecções focalizadas primárias (pseudo-apendicite, linfadenite mesentérica aguda ou ileíte terminal aguda), infecções generalizadas primárias (septicemia ou febre escarlatiniforme) e fenômenos imunológicos secundários (eritema nodoso ou artralgia). SIN pseudotubercular yersiniosis.

pseu·do·tu·mor (soo'dō - too - mer). Pseudotumor; aumento de caráter não-neoplásico, clinicamente tão semelhante a uma neoplasia verdadeira que, freqüentemente, chega a ser confundido com uma. SIN pseudoneoplasm.
  p. cer'ebri, p. cerebral; distúrbio, comumente associado a obesidade em mulheres jovens, que consiste em edema cerebral com ventrículos pequenos e estreitos, mas com aumento da pressão intracraniana e, freqüentemente, papiledema.
  inflammatory p., p. inflamatório; massa semelhante a um tumor, observada nos pulmões ou em outros locais, composta de tecido fibroso ou de granulação infiltrado por células inflamatórias.

pseu·do·uni·mo·lec·u·lar (soo'dō - oo - nē - mō - lek - oo - lar). Pseudo-unimolecular; referente a uma reação cuja velocidade parece depender da concentração apenas de um substrato; geralmente é causada por um nível de saturação, constante, das outras substâncias. SIN pseudomonomolecular.

pseu·do·u·ri·dine (Ψ, Q) (soo - dō - ū′ri - dēn, - din). Pseudo-uridina; 5-β-D-ribosiluracil; um isômero natural da uridina encontrado em ácidos ribonucleicos de transferência; peculiar porque o ribosil está fixado ao carbono (C-5), e não ao nitrogênio; excretado na urina.

pseu·do·vac·u·ole (soo - dō - vak′ū - ōl). Pseudovacúolo; vacúolo aparente em uma célula, seja um artefato ou um parasita intracelular.

pseu·do·va·ri·o·la (soo′dō - vā - rī′ō - la). Pseudovaríola. SIN alastrim. [pseudo- + L. *variola*, varíola]

pseu·do·ven·tri·cle (soo - dō - ven′tri - kl). Cavidade do septo pelúcido. SIN cavity of septum pellucidum.

pseu·do·vi·ta·min (soo - dō - vī′tă - min). Pseudovitamina; substância com estrutura química muito semelhante à de determinada vitamina, mas que não tem a ação fisiológica habitual.

p. B$_{12}$, p. B$_{12}$; cianeto fosfato de cobamida, 3′-éster com 7-α-D-ribofuranosiladenina, sal interno; vitamina B$_{12}$ com adenina substituindo o dimetilbenzimidazol; uma das várias substâncias produzidas durante a fermentação anaeróbica por determinados microrganismos no conteúdo do rúmen bovino; quimicamente, é muito semelhante à vitamina B$_{12}$ (cianocobalamina), mas, em seres humanos, não exerce a ação fisiológica da vitamina.

pseu·do·vom·it·ing (soo - dō - vom′i - ting). Pseudovômito; regurgitação de material do esôfago ou estômago sem esforço expulsivo.

pseu·do·xan·tho·ma elas·ti·cum (soo′dō - zan - thō′mă e - las′ti - kŭm). [MIM*177850, MIM*177860, MIM*264800]. Pseudoxantoma elástico; distúrbio hereditário do tecido conjuntivo, caracterizado por placas amareladas, pouco elevadas, no pescoço, axilas, abdome e coxas, que surgem na segunda ou terceira década de vida, associadas a estrias angióides da retina, bem como a degeneração do tecido elástico e calcificação nas artérias semelhantes; já foram descritos tipos autossômicos dominantes e autossômicos recessivos, com complicações sistêmicas muito mais leves nestes últimos.

psi (sī). Psi; a 23.ª letra do alfabeto grego (ψ). **2.** (ψ) Símbolo de pseudouridine (pseudo-uridina); pseudo-; wave function (função de onda); o ângulo diédrico de rotação ao redor da ligação C$_1$–C$_\alpha$ associado a uma ligação peptídica. **3.** Libras por polegada quadrada.

psi·cose (sī′kōs). Pseudofrutose; uma ceto-hexose; a D-psicose é epimérica em relação à D-frutose. SIN pseudofructose, ribo-2-hexulose.

psi·lo·cin (sī′lō - sin). Psilocina; agente alucinógeno relacionado à psilocibina.

Psil·o·cy·be (sī - lō - sī′bē). Gênero de cogumelos (família Agaricaceae) que contém muitas espécies com propriedades psicotrópicas ou alucinógenas, incluindo *P. mexicana*, cujos carpóforos são uma fonte do alucinógeno psilocibina.

psi·lo·cy·bin (sī - lō - sī′bin, - sib′in). Psilocibina; o derivado N′, N′-dimetil da 4-hidroxitriptamina; obtida dos carpóforos de *Psilocybe mexicana*, de outras espécies de *Psilocybe* e de *Stropharia*. A psilocibina é um congênere da 5-hidroxitriptamina, com efeitos surpreendentes no sistema nervoso central, sendo facilmente hidrolisada em 4-hidroxibufotenina; usada como alucinógeno (e por indígenas mexicanos para induzir transes). SIN indocybin.

psi·lo·sis (sī - lō′sis). Psilose; queda de cabelo. [G. *psilōsis*, um desnudamento, de *psilos*, despido]

psil·o·thin (sil′ō - thin). Psilotina; emplastro depilatório aplicado quente a uma superfície pilosa e puxado quando frio, arrancando os pêlos. [ver psilosis]

psi·lot·ic (sī - lot′ik). Psilótico. **1.** Relativo à psilose. **2.** SIN epilatory (1).

P-sin·is·tro·car·di·a·le (sin - is - trō - kar - dē - ā′lē). P-sinistrocardíaca; onda P eletrocardiográfica característica de sobrecarga do átrio esquerdo; amiúde é erroneamente denominada P mitral, pois a síndrome pode resultar da sobrecarga do átrio esquerdo de qualquer etiologia.

psit·ta·cine (sit′ă - sēn). Psitacina; referente a aves da família do papagaio (papagaios, periquitos e araras).

psit·ta·co·sis (sit - ă - kō′sis). Psitacose; doença infecciosa em aves psitacinas e seres humanos, causada pela bactéria *Chlamydia psittaci*. A maioria das infecções aviárias é inaparente ou latente, embora haja doença aguda; as infecções humanas podem resultar em doença leve, com uma síndrome gripal, ou em doença grave, principalmente em pessoas idosas, com manifestações de broncopneumonia. SIN Parrot disease (3), parrot fever. [G. *psittakos*, papagaio, + -osis, condição]

pso·as (sō′as). Psoas. VER psoas major (*muscle*), psoas minor (*muscle*). [G. *psoa*, os músculos da região lombar]

pso·mo·pha·gia, pso·moph·a·gy (sō - mō - fā′jē - ă, sō - mof′ă - jē). Psomofagia; a prática de engolir o alimento sem mastigação completa. [G. *psōmos*, bocado, pedaço, + *phagō*, comer]

psor·a·len (sōr′ă - len). Psoraleno; fármaco fototóxico para administração tópica ou oral no tratamento de vitiligo e psoríase. Também é encontrado no perfume do óleo de bergamota e em frutas e vegetais como a lima, que podem causar fotossensibilização. VER TAMBÉM PUVA.

psor·en·ter·i·tis (sōr′en - ter - ī′tis). Psorenterite; edema inflamatório dos folículos linfáticos solitários do intestino. [G. *psōra*, prurido (escabiose), + *enteron*, intestino, + -*itis*, inflamação]

Psor·er·ga·tes (psō - rer′gă - tēz). Gênero de ácaros da sarna (família Cheyletidae) parasitas de bovinos, ovinos e caprinos. *P. bos* é o ácaro da sarna de bovinos, descrito no Novo México; *P. ovis* é o pequeno ácaro da sarna de ovinos nos Estados Unidos, Austrália, Nova Zelândia e África do Sul. [G. *psōra*, prurido]

pso·ri·a·si·form (sō - rī′ă - si - fōrm). Psoriasiforme; semelhante à psoríase.

pso·ri·a·sis (sō - rī′ă - sis). Psoríase; condição hereditária multifatorial comum, caracterizada pela erupção de maculopápulas circunscritas, distintas e confluentes, avermelhadas, de escamas prateadas; as lesões ocorrem predominantemente nos cotovelos, joelhos, couro cabeludo e tronco, exibindo microscopicamente paraceratose característica e alongamento das cristas interpapilares, com encurtamento do tempo de trânsito epidérmico dos ceratinócitos devido à diminuição do monofosfato de guanosina cíclico. [G. *psōriasis*, de *psōra*, o prurido]

p. annula'ris, p. annula'ta, p. anular. SIN p. circinata.

p. arthrop'ica, p. atropática; p. associada a artrite grave, semelhante à artrite reumatóide, embora não haja fator reumatóide sérico.

p. circina'ta, p. circinada; p. em que há cicatrização no centro da lesão enquanto o processo continua na periferia, produzindo uma lesão anular. SIN p. annularis, p. annulata.

p. diffu'sa, diffused p., p. difusa; forma de p. com substancial coalescência das lesões.

exfoliative p., p. esfoliativa; dermatite esfoliativa que se desenvolve a partir da p. crônica, algumas vezes resultando do tratamento excessivo da p.

flexural p., p. flexural; p. que acomete as pregas intertriginosas, p. ex., pele axilar e inguinal, que pode assemelhar-se à dermatite seborreica.

generalized pustular p. of Zambusch, p. pustular generalizada de Zambusch. SIN pustular p. (1).

p. geograph'ica, p. geográfica; p. circinada na qual as lesões sugerem o contorno da costa em um mapa.

p. gutta'ta, p. em gotas; p. que surge abruptamente em placas redondas pequenas; observada em pessoas jovens após infecções estreptocócicas.

p. gyra'ta, p. figurada; p. circinada na qual há coalescência dos anéis, dando origem a figuras de vários contornos.

p. nummula'ris, p. numular; p. na qual as lesões são distintas e discóides.

palmar p., p. palmar; p. hiperceratótica, segmentar, que afeta pontos de contato da superfície volar dos dedos e das palmas das mãos, isoladamente ou associada a p. leve em outras partes; acredita-se que seja uma resposta isomórfica, podendo afetar a região palmar de uma pessoa que pratica esporte ou que tem determinada ocupação.

p. puncta'ta, p. pontilhada; p. em que as lesões individuais são pápulas vermelhas e pontilhadas, com uma única escama branca.

pustular p., p. pustular; **(1)** extensa exacerbação da p., com formação de pústulas na pele normal e psoriática, febre e granulocitose; algumas vezes é precipitada por esteróides orais. SIN generalized pustular p. of Zambusch. **(2)** erupção pustular local nas regiões palmares e plantares, mais comum em um paciente com p.; é difícil distingui-la da acrodermatite contínua.

pso·ri·at·ic (sō - rē - at′ik). Psoriático; relativo à psoríase.

Pso·rop·tes (sō - rop′tēz). Gênero de ácaros da sarna (família Cheyletidae), incluindo a espécie *P. cuniculi* (o ácaro da sarna de coelhos), *P. equi* (o ácaro da sarna de cavalos) e *P. ovis* (o ácaro da sarna comum de ovinos e bovinos). [G. *psōra*, prurido]

PSP Abreviatura de phenolsulfonphthalein (fenolsulfonftaleína).

psych-. VER psycho-.

psy·chal·ga·lia (sī - kal - gā′lē - ă). Psicalgia. SIN psychalgia (1).

psy·chal·gia (sī - kal′jē - ă). Psicalgia. **1.** Sofrimento associado a um esforço mental, observado principalmente na melancolia. SIN phrenalgia (1), psychalgalia. **2.** Dor psicogênica. SIN psychogenic pain. [psych- + G. *algos*, dor]

psy·cha·lia (sī - kā′lē - ă). Termo raramente usado para designar uma condição emocional caracterizada por alucinações auditivas e visuais.

psy·cha·nop·sia (sī′ka - nop′sē - ă). Psicanopsia. SIN mind blindness. [psych- + G. *an-* priv., + *opsis*, visão]

psy·cha·tax·ia (sī - kă - tak′sē - ă). Psicataxia; confusão mental; incapacidade de fixar a atenção ou de fazer qualquer esforço mental contínuo. [psych- + G. *ataxia*, confusão]

psy·che (sī′kē). Psique; termo para designar os aspectos subjetivos da mente, do espírito, da alma; o psicológico ou espiritual, distinto da natureza corporal das pessoas. [G. mente, alma]

psyche-. VER psycho-.

psy·che·del·ic (sī - kē - del′ik). Psicodélico. **1.** Relativo a uma categoria de fármacos algo imprecisa, que atua principalmente no sistema nervoso central e cujos efeitos são ditos de expansão ou elevação da consciência, p. ex., LSD, haxixe, mescalina. **2.** Substância alucinógena, estímulos de espetáculo visual, música ou outros estímulos sensoriais que tenham essa ação. SIN hallucinogenic. [psyche- + G. *dēloō*, manifestar]

psy·chi·at·ric (sī - kē - at′rik). Psiquiátrico; relativo à psiquiatria.

psy·chi·at·rics (sī - kē - at′riks). Psiquiatria. SIN psychiatry.

psy·chi·a·trist (sī - kī′ă - trist). Psiquiatra; médico especializado em psiquiatria.

psy·chi·a·try (sī-kī′ā-trē). **1.** Psiquiatria; a especialidade médica relacionada ao diagnóstico e tratamento de transtornos mentais. **2.** O diagnóstico e tratamento de transtornos mentais. Para alguns tipos de psiquiatria não relacionados adiante, ver também subentradas em therapy, psychotherapy, psychoanalysis. SIN psychiatrics. [psych- + G. *iatreia*, tratamento médico]
analytic p., p. analítica. SIN psychoanalytic p.
biologic p., p. biológica; ramo da p. que enfatiza abordagens moleculares, genéticas e farmacológicas no diagnóstico e tratamento dos transtornos mentais.
child p., p. infantil; ramo da p. que lida com os transtornos emocionais e mentais das crianças.
community p., p. comunitária; p. que se concentra na detecção, prevenção, tratamento precoce e reabilitação de indivíduos com distúrbios emocionais e desvio social quando se desenvolvem na comunidade, de preferência aos casos individuais, no consultório ou em unidades psiquiátricas centralizadas maiores; são enfatizados particularmente os fatores sociais, interpessoais e ambientais que contribuem para a doença mental.
contractual p., p. contratual; designação antiga da intervenção psiquiátrica assumida voluntariamente pelo paciente, que é impelido por dificuldades pessoais ou sofrimento e que retém o controle da interação com o psiquiatra.
cross-cultural p., p. transcultural; campo da p. com interesse no estudo de fenômenos psicológicos e psiquiátricos, expressos de diferentes formas nas culturas de diferentes países.
descriptive p., p. descritiva; aspecto da prática da p. que lida com o diagnóstico de transtornos mentais.
dynamic p., p. dinâmica. SIN psychoanalytic p.
existential p., p. existencial. SIN existential *psychotherapy.*
forensic p., legal p., p. forense, p. judicial; a aplicação da p. em tribunais, p. ex., em determinações de internação, capacidade, competência para ser julgado, responsabilidade por crime.
industrial p., p. industrial; aplicação dos princípios da p. aos problemas observados no comércio e na indústria.
orthomolecular p., p. ortomolecular; proposta da p. que se concentra no uso de grandes doses de vitaminas e nutrientes para tratamento de doenças mentais como os transtornos esquizofrênicos.
psychoanalytic p., p. psicanalítica; teoria e prática da p. que enfatizam os princípios da psicanálise. SIN analytic p., dynamic p.
social p., p. social; proposta da teoria e prática psiquiátricas, enfatizando os aspectos culturais e sociológicos do transtorno mental e do tratamento; a aplicação da p. a problemas sociais. VER TAMBÉM community p.
psy·chic (sī′kik). Psíquico. **1.** Relativo aos fenômenos de consciência, mente ou alma. SIN psychical. **2.** Pessoa supostamente dotada do poder de comunicação com os espíritos; um médium espiritualista. [G. *psychikos*]
psy·chi·cal (sī′ki-kāl). Psíquico. SIN psychic (1).
psy·chism (sī′kizm). Psiquismo; a teoria filosófica do princípio vital que permeia toda a natureza.
psycho-, psych-, psyche-. A mente; mental; psicológico. [G. *psychē*, alma, mente]
psy·cho·a·cous·tics (sī′kō-ā-koos′tiks). Psicoacústica. **1.** Disciplina que combina psicologia experimental e física, que estuda os aspectos físicos do som relacionados à audição, e também a fisiologia e a psicologia dos processos de recepção do som. **2.** A ciência qua aborda os fatores psicológicos que influenciam a consciência de um indivíduo em relação ao som. [psycho- + G. *akoustikos*, relativo à audição]
psy·cho·ac·tive (sī-kō-ak′tiv). Psicoativo; que possui a capacidade de alterar o humor, a ansiedade, o comportamento, os processos cognitivos ou a tensão mental; geralmente aplicado a agentes farmacológicos.
psy·cho·al·ler·gy (sī-kō-al′er-jē). Psicoalergia; termo raramente usado para designar a sensibilização a símbolos emocionalmente carregados.
psy·cho·a·nal·y·sis (sī′kō-ā-nal′i-sis). Psicanálise. **1.** Método de psicoterapia, criado por Freud, destinado a trazer dados pré-conscientes e inconscientes para a consciência, basicamente através da análise de transferência e resistência. SIN psychoanalytic therapy. VER TAMBÉM freudian p. **2.** Método de investigação da mente humana e do funcionamento psicológico, interpretações de resistências, bem como das reações emocionais do paciente ao analista, associado ao uso da associação livre e da análise de sonhos na situação psicanalítica. **3.** Um conjunto integrado de observações e teorias sobre desenvolvimento da personalidade, motivação e comportamento. **4.** Uma escola institucionalizada de psicoterapia, como a psicanálise junguiana ou freudiana. [psycho- + analysis]
active p., p. ativa; designação antiga da p. em que o analista intervém de forma direta e ativa na vida do paciente, p. ex., fazendo proibições, determinando tarefas.
adlerian p., p. de Adler. SIN individual *psychology.*
freudian p., p. freudiana; a teoria e a prática da p. e da psicoterapia da forma desenvolvida por Freud, baseado em: 1) sua teoria da personalidade, que afirma que a vida psíquica consiste em forças instintivas e socialmente adquiridas, ou o id, ego e o superego, cada um deles precisando constantemente acomodar-se aos outros; 2) sua descoberta de que a técnica de associação livre de contar ao analista todos os pensamentos sem qualquer censura é a tática terapêutica que revela as áreas de conflito na personalidade de um paciente; e 3) que o veículo para obter esse *insight* e, a seguir, nessa base, reajustar a personalidade do indivíduo é o aprendizado do paciente ao desenvolver um vínculo emocional tempestuoso com o analista (relação de transferência) e, depois, rompê-lo com sucesso.
jungian p., p. junguiana; a teoria da psicopatologia e a prática da psicoterapia, de acordo com os princípios de Jung, centrados em um sistema de psicologia e psicoterapia que enfatiza a natureza simbólica do ser humano, diferindo da psicanálise freudiana especialmente por dar menos valor aos impulsos instintivos (sexuais). SIN analytical psychology.
psy·cho·an·a·lyst (sī-kō-an′ā-list). Psicanalista; psicoterapeuta, geralmente um psiquiatra ou psicólogo clínico, treinado em psicanálise e que emprega seus métodos no tratamento de transtornos emocionais.
psy·cho·an·a·lyt·ic (sī′kō-an-ā-lit′ik). Psicanalítico; relativo à psicanálise.
psy·cho·au·di·to·ry (sī-kō-aw′di-tōr-ē). Psicoauditivo; relativo à percepção mental e interpretação dos sons. VER psychoacoustics. [psycho- + L. *auditorius*, relativo à audição]
psy·cho·bi·ol·o·gy (sī′kō-bī-ol′ō-jē). Psicobiologia. **1.** O estudo das inter-relações da biologia e psicologia na função cognitiva, incluindo o intelecto, a memória e os processos neurocognitivos relacionados. **2.** Termo de Adolf Meyer para psiquiatria.
psy·cho·ca·thar·sis (sī′kō-kā-thar′sis). Psicocatarse. SIN catharsis (2).
psy·cho·chrome (sī-kō-krōm). Psicocromo; certa cor concebida mentalmente em resposta a uma impressão sensorial. VER TAMBÉM psychochromesthesia. [psycho- + G. *chrōma*, cor]
psy·cho·chro·mes·the·sia (sī′kō-krō-mes-thē′zē-ā). Psicocromestesia; forma de sinestesia em que um determinado estímulo de um dos órgãos especiais do sentido produz a imagem mental de uma cor. VER TAMBÉM photism, color *taste*, pseudogeusesthesia. [psycho- + G. *chrōma*, cor, + *aisthēsis*, sensação]
psy·cho·di·ag·no·sis (sī′kō-dī-ag-nō′sis). Psicodiagnóstico. **1.** Qualquer método usado para descobrir os fatores subjacentes a um comportamento, particularmente um comportamento desajustado ou anormal. **2.** Uma subespecialidade da psicologia clínica que enfatiza o uso de testes e técnicas psicológicas para avaliar a psicopatologia.
Psy·chod·i·dae (sī-kod′i-dē). Família de pequenas moscas ou mosquitos, caracterizada por corpo piloso, semelhante ao de mariposas e pela presença de 7–11 longas nervuras paralelas nas asas, não possuindo nervuras cruzadas; inclui os mosquitos *Phlebotomus* e *Lytzomyia*, vetores de todas as formas conhecidas de leishmaniose. [G. *Psychē*, uma ninfa grega, algumas vezes representada por uma borboleta]
psy·cho·dom·e·try (sī-kō-dom′e-trē). Psicodometria; a medida da velocidade da ação mental. [psycho- + G. *hodos*, caminho, + *metron*, medida]
psy·cho·dra·ma (sī′kō-drah-mā). Psicodrama; método de psicoterapia no qual pacientes encenam seus problemas pessoais, desempenhando espontaneamente, sem ensaio, papéis específicos diagnósticos em representações dramáticas diante de outros pacientes.
psy·cho·dy·nam·ics (sī′kō-dī-nam′iks). Psicodinâmica; o estudo sistematizado e a teoria das forças psicológicas que formam a base do comportamento humano, enfatizando a interação entre motivação inconsciente e consciente e a importância funcional da emoção. VER role-playing. [psycho- + G. *dynamis*, força]
psy·cho·en·do·cri·nol·o·gy (sī′kō-en′dō-krī-nol′ō-jē). Psicoendocrinologia; estudo das relações entre a função endócrina e os estados mentais.
psy·cho·ex·plor·a·tion (sī′kō-eks-plōr-ā′shun). Psicoexploração; estudo das atitudes e da vida emocional de uma pessoa.
psy·cho·gal·van·ic (sī′kō-gal-van′ik). Psicogalvânico; relativo a alterações nas propriedades elétricas da pele; p. ex., alteração da resistência cutânea induzida por estímulo psicológico.
psy·cho·gal·va·nom·e·ter (sī′kō-gal-vā-nom′ē-ter). Psicogalvanômetro; galvanômetro que registra alterações da resistência cutânea relacionadas ao estresse emocional.
psy·cho·gen·der (sī-kō-jen′der). Identificação psicossexual; as atitudes adotadas por uma pessoa em relação à sua identificação como do sexo masculino ou feminino. VER TAMBÉM gender *role*.
psy·cho·gen·e·sis (sī-kō-jen′ē-sis). Psicogênese; a origem e o desenvolvimento dos processos psíquicos, incluindo processos mentais, comportamentais, emocionais, de personalidade e processos psicológicos correlatos. SIN psychogeny. [psycho- + G. *genesis*, origem]
psy·cho·gen·ic, psy·cho·ge·net·ic (sī-kō-jen′ik, -jē-net′ik). Psicogênico, psicogenético. **1.** De origem ou causa mental. **2.** Relativo ao desenvolvimento emocional e psicológico relacionado ou à psicogênese.
psy·chog·e·ny (sī-koj′ē-nē). Psicogenia. SIN psychogenesis.
psy·cho·geu·sic (sī-kō-goo′sik). Psicogêusico; relativo à percepção mental e à interpretação do sabor. [psycho- + G. *geusis*, sabor]

psy·cho·gog·ic (sī-kō-goj′ik). Psicogógico; que atua como estimulante das emoções. [psycho- + G. *agōgos*, condução]

psy·cho·graph·ic (sī-kō-graf′ik). Psicográfico; relativo à psicografia.

psy·chog·ra·phy (sī-kog′ra-fē). Psicografia; a caracterização literária de um indivíduo, real ou fictícia, que emprega categorias e teorias psicanalíticas e psicológicas; uma biografia psicológica ou descrição de caráter. [psycho- + G. *graphē*, escrita]

psy·cho·his·to·ry (sī-kō-his′tōr-ē). Psico-história; o uso combinado da psicologia (principalmente psicanálise) e da história na escrita, principalmente da biografia, como no trabalho de Erik Erikson. VER TAMBÉM psychography.

psy·cho·ki·ne·sis, psy·cho·ki·ne·sia (sī′kō-ki-nē′sis, -nē′zē-a). **1.** Psicocinese, psicocinesia; a influência da mente sobre a matéria, como o uso da "força" mental para mover ou deformar um objeto. **2.** Comportamento impulsivo. [psycho- + G. *kinēsis*, movimento]

psy·cho·lin·guis·tics (sī′kō-ling-gwi′stiks). Psicolingüística; estudo de um grupo de fatores psicológicos associados à fala, incluindo voz, atitudes, emoções e regras gramaticais, que afetam a comunicação e a compreensão da linguagem. [psycho- + L. *lingua*, língua]

psy·cho·log·ic, psy·cho·log·i·cal (sī-kō-loj′ik, -loj′i-kal). Psicológico. **1.** Relativo à psicologia. **2.** Relativo à mente e seus processos. VER psychology.

psy·chol·o·gist (sī-kol′ō-jist). Psicólogo; especialista em psicologia licenciado para a prática profissional de psicologia (p. ex., psicologia clínica), ou qualificado para ensinar psicologia como disciplina escolar (psicologia acadêmica), ou cuja especialidade científica é um subcampo da psicologia (psicologia de pesquisa).

psy·chol·o·gy (sī-kol′ō-jē). Psicologia; a profissão (p. ex., psicologia clínica), disciplina (psicologia acadêmica) e ciência (psicologia de pesquisa) relacionadas ao comportamento de seres humanos e animais, e processos mentais e fisiológicos relacionados. [psycho- + G. *logos*, estudo]

adlerian p., p. de Adler. SIN individual p.

analytical p., p. analítica. SIN jungian *psychoanalysis.*

animal p., p. animal; ramo da p. que estuda o comportamento e as respostas fisiológicas de organismos animais como forma de compreender o comportamento humano; alguns sinônimos incluem p. comparativa, p. experimental e p. fisiológica.

atomistic p., p. atomística; qualquer sistema psicológico baseado na doutrina que afirma serem os processos mentais construídos através da combinação de elementos simples; p. ex., psicanálise, behaviorismo.

behavioral p., behaviorismo. SIN behaviorism.

behavioristic p., p. behaviorista; ramo da p. que usa condutas do behaviorismo, tais como dessensibilização e imersão, ao contrário do aconselhamento e de outras condutas psicodinâmicas para o tratamento de transtornos psicológicos. VER TAMBÉM behavior *therapy*.

child p., p. infantil; ramo da p. cujas teorias e aplicações concentram-se no desenvolvimento cognitivo e intelectual da criança ao contrário do adulto; as subespecialidades incluem p. do desenvolvimento, p. clínica infantil, p. pediátrica e neuropsicologia pediátrica.

clinical p., p. clínica; ramo da p. especializado na descoberta de novos conhecimentos e na aplicação da arte e da ciência de psicologia a pessoas com distúrbios emocionais ou comportamentais; as subespecialidades incluem psicologia clínica infantil e psicologia pediátrica.

cognitive p., p. cognitiva; ramo da p. que tenta integrar em um todo o conhecimento díspar dos subcampos da percepção, aprendizado, memória, inteligência e raciocínio.

community p., p. comunitária; a aplicação da p. a programas comunitários, p. ex., nas escolas, em sistemas penitenciários e de saúde social, e em centros de saúde mental comunitários.

comparative p., p. comparativa; ramo da p. que estuda e compara o comportamento de organismos em diferentes níveis de desenvolvimento filogênico para descobrir as tendências do desenvolvimento.

constitutional p., p. constitucional; a p. do indivíduo relacionada ao biotipo.

counseling p., p. de aconselhamento; p. que enfatiza a facilitação do desenvolvimento e crescimento normais do indivíduo ao defrontar-se com problemas importantes da vida diária, em contraposição à psicologia clínica.

criminal p., p. criminal; o estudo da mente e seu funcionamento em relação ao crime. VER forensic p.

depth p., p. profunda; a p. do inconsciente, principalmente em contraste com a antiga p. acadêmica (século XIX) que lida apenas com o raciocínio consciente; algumas vezes é usada como sinônimo de psicanálise.

developmental p., p. do desenvolvimento; o estudo das alterações psicológicas, fisiológicas e comportamentais em um organismo que ocorrem desde o nascimento até a velhice.

dynamic p., p. dinâmica; abordagem psicológica que estuda as causas do comportamento.

educational p., p. educacional; a aplicação da p. à educação, principalmente a problemas do ensino e do aprendizado.

environmental p., p. ambiental; o estudo e a aplicação por cientistas comportamentais e arquitetos da forma como alterações do espaço físico e estímulos físicos relacionados afetam o comportamento das pessoas. VER TAMBÉM personal *space*.

existential p., p. existencial; teoria da p. baseada nas filosofias da fenomenologia e do existencialismo, afirmando que o estudo apropriado da p. é a experiência humana da seqüência, relação espacial e organização de sua existência no mundo.

experimental p., p. experimental; **(1)** uma subdisciplina da ciência da p. que estuda o condicionamento, o aprendizado, a percepção, a motivação, a emoção, a linguagem e o raciocínio; **(2)** termo que também é usado em relação a áreas de tema-assunto em que são enfatizados métodos experimentais, em contraste com os métodos correlacionais ou sócio-experimentais.

forensic p., p. forense; a aplicação da p. a questões legais em um tribunal.

genetic p., p. genética; ciência que estuda a evolução do comportamento e a relação entre si dos diferentes tipos de atividade mental.

gestalt p., gestaltismo. VER gestaltism.

health p., p. da saúde; o conjunto das contribuições educacionais, científicas e profissionais específicas da disciplina de p. para a promoção e manutenção da saúde, prevenção e tratamento de doenças, identificação de correlatos etiológicos e diagnósticos de saúde, doença e disfunção relacionada, e para a análise e aperfeiçoamento do sistema de saúde.

holistic p., p. holística; qualquer sistema psicológico que afirma que a mente humana ou qualquer processo mental pode ser estudado como uma unidade; p. ex., gestaltismo, psicologia existencial.

humanistic p., p. humanista; qualquer abordagem existencial em p. que enfatiza a peculiaridade, a subjetividade e a capacidade de crescimento psicológico dos seres humanos.

individual p., p. individual; teoria do comportamento humano que enfatiza a natureza social do homem, sua luta pela superioridade e seu esforço para superar, por compensação, sentimentos de inferioridade. SIN adlerian psychoanalysis, adlerian p.

industrial p., p. industrial; a aplicação dos princípios da p. a problemas do comércio e da indústria.

medical p., p. médica; o ramo da p. relacionado à aplicação de princípios psicológicos à prática médica; a aplicação da p. clínica ou da p. de saúde clínica, geralmente em um ambiente hospitalar.

objective p., p. objetiva; p. estudada pela observação do comportamento e das funções mentais em outras pessoas.

subjective p., p. subjetiva; o estudo da própria mente e de suas várias formas de ação como base para deduções psicológicas.

psy·cho·met·rics (sī-kō-met′riks). Psicometria. SIN psychometry.

psy·chom·e·try (sī-kom′e-trē). Psicometria; a disciplina relativa aos testes psicológicos e mentais, e a qualquer análise quantitativa das características ou atitudes psicológicas de uma pessoa ou dos processos mentais. SIN psychometrics. [psycho- + G. *metron*, medida]

psy·cho·mo·tor (sī-kō-mō′ter). Psicomotor. **1.** Relativo aos processos psicológicos associados a movimentos musculares e à produção de movimentos voluntários. **2.** Relativo à combinação de eventos psíquicos e motores, incluindo distúrbios. [psycho- + L. *motor*, motor]

psy·cho·neu·ro·im·mun·o·logy (sī′kō-noo-rō-im′ū-nol′ō-jē). Psiconeuroimunologia; uma área de estudo que focaliza estados emocionais e outros estados psicológicos que afetam o sistema imune, tornando o indivíduo menos ou mais suscetível à doença ou ao curso de uma doença. [psycho- + neuro- + immunology]

psy·cho·neu·ro·sis (sī′kō-noo-rō′sis). Psiconeurose. **1.** Transtorno mental ou comportamental leve ou moderado. **2.** Antigamente, uma classificação de neurose que incluía histeria, psicastenia, neurastenia e distúrbios de ansiedade e fóbicos. [psycho- + G. *neuron*, nervo, + *-osis*, condição]

p. mai′dica, pelagra. SIN pellagra.

psy·cho·neu·rot·ic (sī′kō-noo-rot′ik). Psiconeurótico; relativo à psiconeurose ou que sofre desse transtorno.

psy·cho·nom·ic (sī-kō-nom′ik). Psiconômico; relativo à psiconomia.

psy·chon·o·my (sī-kon′ō-mē). Psiconomia; termo raramente usado referente ao ramo da psicologia que estuda as leis do comportamento. [psycho- + G. *nomos*, lei]

psy·cho·no·sol·o·gy (sī′kō-nō-sol′ō-jē). Psiconosologia; a classificação de doenças mentais e distúrbios do comportamento. SIN psychiatric nosology. [psycho- + G. *nosos*, doença, + *logos*, estudo]

psy·cho·nox·ious (sī-kō-nok′shus). Psiconocivo; termo raramente usado para designar: **1.** O que tem efeito desfavorável sobre a vida emocional e reações mediadas por níveis superiores do sistema nervoso central; pode ser endógeno ou exógeno. **2.** Designa pessoas ou situações que provocam medo, dor, ansiedade ou raiva em um indivíduo. [psycho- + L. *noxius*, nocivo]

psy·cho-on·col·o·gy (sī-kō-ong-kol′ō-jē). Psico-oncologia; os aspectos psicológicos do tratamento do paciente com câncer; combina elementos de psiquiatria, psicologia e medicina com interesse especial nas necessidades psicossociais do paciente e de sua família.

psy·cho·path (sī′kō-path). Psicopata; designação antiga de um indivíduo com personalidade anti-social. VER TAMBÉM antisocial *personality*, sociopath. [psycho- + G. *pathos*, doença]

psy·cho·path·ic (sī-kō-path′ik). Psicopático; relativo a, ou característico de, psicopatia.

psy·cho·pa·thol·o·gist (sī′kō-pă-thol′ō-jist). Psicopatologista; aquele que se especializa em psicopatologia.

psy·cho·pa·thol·o·gy (sī′kō-pă-thol′ō-jē). Psicopatologia. **1.** A ciência que estuda a patologia da mente e do comportamento. **2.** A ciência dos transtornos mentais e comportamentais, incluindo a psiquiatria e a psicologia anormal. [psycho- + G. *pathos*, doença, + *logos*, estudo]

psy·chop·a·thy (sī-kop′ă-thē). Psicopatia; termo antigo e inexato referente a um padrão de comportamento anti-social ou manipulador apresentado por um psicopata. VER TAMBÉM personality *disorder*. [psycho- + G. *pathos*, doença]

psy·cho·phar·ma·ceu·ti·cals (sī′kō-far-mă-soo′ti-kălz). Psicofármacos; medicamentos utilizados no tratamento de distúrbios emocionais.

psy·cho·phar·ma·col·o·gy (sī′kō-far′mă-kol′ō-jē). Psicofarmacologia. **1.** O uso de fármacos no tratamento de transtornos mentais e psicológicos. **2.** A ciência que estuda as relações fármaco-comportamentais. SIN neuropsychopharmacology. [psycho- + G. *pharmakon*, fármaco, + *logos*, estudo]

Com o avanço explosivo dos conhecimentos sobre o cérebro, a partir de 1970, surgiu a maior compreensão do papel que os neurotransmissores desempenham na emoção, no humor e nos estados psicológicos e da forma como erros na síntese ou metabolismo desses agentes podem causar doenças neurológicas e mentais, ou contribuir para essas doenças. Utilizando moléculas marcadas com nucleotídeos como sondas, neuroquímicos identificaram as principais vias neurais e as funções de muitos neurotransmissores, sendo atualmente conhecidos mais de 60 deles. Fundamentados nesses conhecimentos, os neuropsicofarmacologistas tiveram sucesso em criar novos fármacos psicoativos potentes. Até hoje, os que obtiveram maior sucesso foram aqueles destinados ao tratamento de psicoses, transtornos obsessivo-compulsivos, estados de ansiedade e depressão clínica.

psy·cho·phys·i·cal (sī-kō-fiz′i-kăl). Psicofísico. **1.** Relativo à percepção mental de estímulos físicos. VER psychophysics. **2.** Psicossomático. SIN psychosomatic.

psy·cho·phys·ics (sī-kō-fiz′iks). Psicofísica; a ciência da relação entre as características físicas de um estímulo e as características quantitativas, medidas da percepção mental desse estímulo (p. ex., a relação entre alterações no nível de decibéis e as alterações correspondentes na percepção humana do som).

psy·cho·phys·i·o·log·ic (sī′kō-fiz-ē-ō-loj′ik). Psicofisiológico. **1.** Relativo à psicofisiologia. **2.** Designa uma doença denominada psicossomática. **3.** Designa um distúrbio somático com significativa etiologia emocional ou psicológica.

psy·cho·phys·i·ol·o·gy (sī′kō-fiz-ē-ol′ō-jē). Psicofisiologia; a ciência que estuda a relação entre processos psicológicos e fisiológicos; p. ex., elementos de atividade do sistema nervoso autônomo ativados pela emoção.

psy·cho·pro·phy·lax·is (sī′kō-prō-fi-lak′sis). Psicoprofilaxia; psicoterapia voltada para a prevenção de distúrbios emocionais e para a manutenção da saúde mental. [psycho- + prophylaxis]

psy·cho·re·lax·a·tion (sī′kō-rē-lak-sā′shŭn). Psicorrelaxamento; método de tratamento da ansiedade e tensão pela prática de relaxamento corporal geral, como na dessensibilização sistemática.

psy·chor·mic (sī-kōr′mik). Psicoestimulante. SIN psychostimulant. [psycho- + G. *hormaō*, colocar em movimento]

psy·cho·sen·so·ry, psy·cho·sen·so·ri·al (sī′kō-sen′sōr-ē, -sen-sōr′ē-ăl). Psicossensorial. **1.** Designa a percepção mental e a interpretação de estímulos sensoriais. **2.** Designa uma alucinação que, com esforço, a mente é capaz de distinguir da realidade.

psy·cho·sex·u·al (sī-kō-sek′shoo-ăl). Psicossexual; relativo às relações entre os componentes emocional, fisiológico, mental e comportamental do sexo ou do desenvolvimento sexual.

psicofarmacologia	
agentes antipsicóticos	
agentes de baixa potência tradicionais (típicos) clorpromazina, mesoridazina, tioridazina	exercem seu efeito terapêutico, supostamente, por bloqueio dos receptores D_2 (dopamina), mas também têm impacto sobre vários outros receptores, causando efeitos colaterais anticolinérgicos, sedação e hipotensão ortostática
agentes de alta potência flufenazina, haloperidol, loxapina, *molindona, perfenazina, pimozida, tiotixeno, trifluoperazina	exercem seu efeito terapêutico, supostamente, por bloqueio dos receptores D_2 (dopamina); são mais propensos a causar efeitos colaterais neurológicos que os agentes de baixa potência (p. ex., sintomas extrapiramidais, distonia aguda, acinestesia, discinesia tardia)
agentes atípicos clozapina, risperidona, olanzapina, quetiapina	exercem seu efeito terapêutico, supostamente, por seu bloqueio em geral maior dos receptores $5-HT_2$ (serotonina) em relação aos receptores D_2 (dopamina); são menos propensos a causar efeitos colaterais neurológicos que os agentes típicos
agentes antidepressivos	
agentes heterocíclicos amitriptilina, amoxapina, clomipramina, desipramina, doxepina, imipramina, maprotilina, nortriptilina, protriptilina, trimipramina	exercem seu efeito terapêutico, supostamente, por bloqueio da recaptação de serotonina e/ou epinefrina, nos neurônios pré-sinápticos, aumentando a disponibilidade desses neurotransmissores; evidências recentes sugerem que efeitos significativos sobre neurônios pós-sinápticos também podem ser responsáveis pelo efeito terapêutico
inibidores seletivos de recaptação de serotonina citalopram, fluoxetina, fluvoxamina, paroxetina, sertralina	exercem seu efeito terapêutico, supostamente, por bloqueio seletivo (em relação aos outros neurotransmissores) da recaptação de serotonina
inibidores da monoamina oxidase isocarboxazida, fenelzina, tranilcipromina	exercem seu efeito terapêutico, supostamente, por limitação irreversível da atividade da monoamina oxidase, levando a um aumento da disponibilidade de noradrenalina e serotonina na sinapse
agentes novos atualmente bupropiona, mirtazepina, nefazodona, trazodona, venlafaxina	exercem seu efeito terapêutico por várias ações, supostamente aumentando a disponibilidade de serotonina, noradrenalina e/ou dopamina na sinapse
agentes antimaníacos lítio, carbamazepina, gabapentina, **lamotrigina, **ácido valpróico	exercem seu efeito terapêutico de estabilização do humor por meio de ações que ainda não são completamente compreendidas
agentes ansiolíticos	
benzodiazepínicos alprazolam, clorazepato, clordiazepóxido, clonazepam, diazepam, lorazepam, oxazepam	exercem seu efeito terapêutico por atividade agonista no sítio do receptor do ácido γ-aminobutírico, e, em dosagem suficientemente alta, haverá sedação excessiva ou sono; todos podem causar formação de hábito. Outros benzodiazepínicos, devido às suas propriedades farmacológicas, são basicamente úteis como hipnóticos

*também tem a capacidade de bloquear $5-HT_2$ (receptores de serotonina)
** anticonvulsivantes disponíveis há relativamente pouco tempo, com eficácia na estabilização do humor, que não é uma de suas indicações cientificamente comprovadas

psy·cho·sine (sī′kō-sēn). Psicosina; galactosilesfingosina, um constituinte dos cerebrosídeos, formado a partir da UDPgalactose e esfingosina pela UDPgalactose-esfingosina β-D-galactosiltransferase.

psy·cho·sis, pl. **psy·cho·ses** (sī-kō′sis, -sēz). Psicose. **1.** Transtorno mental e do comportamento que causa distorção ou desorganização grosseira da capacidade mental, da resposta afetiva e da capacidade de reconhecer a realidade, comunicar-se e relacionar-se com os outros, a ponto de interferir com a capacidade da pessoa de enfrentar as demandas comuns do dia-a-dia. As psicoses são divididas em duas classificações principais de acordo com suas origens: 1) aquelas associadas a síndromes cerebrais orgânicas (p. ex., síndrome de Korsakoff); 2) aquelas menos claramente orgânicas e que possuem alguns componentes funcionais (p. ex., as esquizofrenias, os distúrbios bipolares). **2.** Termo genérico que designa qualquer uma das assim chamadas insanidades, sendo as formas mais comuns as esquizofrenias. **3.** Um transtorno emocional e comportamental grave. SIN psychotic disorder. [G. animação]

affective p., p. afetiva; p. com predomínio das características afetivas. SIN manic p.

alcoholic psychoses, psicoses alcoólicas; transtornos mentais resultantes do alcoolismo e que envolvem lesão cerebral orgânica, como no *delirium tremens* e na síndrome de Korsakoff.

bipolar p., p. bipolar; transtorno mental caracterizado por um ou mais episódios de mania (depressão maníaca), geralmente acompanhado por um ou mais episódios de depressão (episódio depressivo maior). VER endogenous *depression*, manic-depressive.

Cheyne-Stokes p., p. de Cheyne-Stokes; estado mental caracterizado por ansiedade e agitação, que acompanha a respiração de Cheyne-Stokes.

depressive p., p. depressiva; importante transtorno do humor no qual fatores biológicos parecem desempenhar um papel proeminente. VER depression.

drug p., p. medicamentosa; p. que se segue ou é precipitada pela ingestão de um fármaco (droga), p. ex., LSD.

febrile p., p. febril. SIN infection-exhaustion p.

functional p., p. funcional; termo obsoleto que era usado para designar esquizofrenia e outros transtornos mentais graves antes de a ciência moderna descobrir um componente biológico para alguns aspectos de cada um dos distúrbios.

hysterical p., p. histérica; **(1)** distúrbio psicótico com sintomas predominantemente histéricos; **(2)** distúrbio mental semelhante à histeria de conversão, mas de intensidade psicótica; **(3)** uma p. reativa breve, freqüentemente relacionada à cultura.

ICU p., p. da UTI; episódio(s) psicótico(s), classicamente observado(s) em pacientes com doença coronariana, sem história prévia de p., que ocorre nas 24 horas seguintes à internação em UTI; está relacionada à privação do sono, à estimulação excessiva na UTI e ao tempo gasto em sistemas de suporte da vida, devendo ser distinguida da exacerbação de uma p. preexistente ou de uma p. orgânica, como o delírio.

infection-exhaustion p., p. febril; termo obsoleto para designar uma p. que ocorre após infecção aguda, choque ou intoxicação crônica; começa como delírio seguido por confusão mental grave, com alucinações e delírios não-sistematizados e, algumas vezes, torpor. SIN febrile p.

Korsakoff p., p. de Korsakoff. SIN Korsakoff *syndrome*.

manic p., p. maníaca. SIN affective p. VER bipolar *disorder*, manic-depressive *disorder*, endogenous *depression*.

manic-depressive p., p. maníaco-depressiva. SIN bipolar *disorder*.

posthypnotic p., p. pós-hipnótica; p. que sucede a hipnose ou é por esta precipitada.

postinfectious p., p. pós-infecciosa; distúrbio psicótico com demência após doença febril aguda, como pneumonia ou febre tifóide.

postpartum p., p. pós-parto; distúrbio mental agudo com depressão materna após o parto. SIN puerperal p.

posttraumatic p., p. pós-traumática; p. após traumatismo, principalmente da cabeça. Cf. traumatic p.

pseudo p., pseudopsicose; condição semelhante à psicose; pode ser um distúrbio fictício ou simulação.

puerperal p., p. puerperal. SIN postpartum p.

schizo-affective p., p. esquizoafetiva; distúrbio psicótico no qual há uma mistura de sintomas esquizofrênicos e maníaco-depressivos.

senile p., p. senil; distúrbio mental que ocorre na velhice e relacionado a processos cerebrais degenerativos.

situational p., p. situacional; distúrbio emocional transitório mas grave, provocado em uma pessoa predisposta por uma situação aparentemente insuportável.

toxic p., p. tóxica; p. causada por alguma substância tóxica, seja endógena ou exógena.

traumatic p., p. traumática; p. resultante de lesão física ou choque emocional. Cf. posttraumatic p.

Windigo p., Wittigo p., p. de Windigo, p. de Wittigo; neurose de ansiedade grave, com referência especial aos alimentos, que se manifesta por melancolia, violência e canibalismo obsessivo, observada em índios canadenses.

psy·cho·social (sī-kō-sō′shăl). Psicossocial; que envolve aspectos psicológicos e sociais; p. ex., aspectos de idade, escolaridade, conjugal e outros aspectos relacionados da história de uma pessoa.

psy·cho·so·mat·ic (sī′kō-sō-mat′ik). Psicossomático; relativo à influência da mente ou de funções superiores do encéfalo (p. ex., emoções, medos, desejos) sobre as funções do corpo, principalmente em relação a distúrbios corporais ou doenças. VER psychophysiologic. SIN psychophysical (2). [psycho- + G. *sōma*, corpo]

psy·cho·so·mi·met·ic (sī-kō′sō-mi-met′ik). Psicotomimético. SIN psychotomimetic.

psy·cho·stim·u·lant (sī-kō-stim-ū-lant). Psicoestimulante; agente com propriedades antidepressivas ou de melhora do humor. SIN psychormic.

psy·cho·sur·gery (sī-kō-ser′jer-ē). Psicocirurgia; o tratamento de distúrbios mentais por operação do cérebro, p. ex., lobotomia.

psy·cho·syn·the·sis (sī-kō-sin′thĕ-sis). Psicossíntese; designação de um estilo antigo de tratamento, oposto à psicanálise, que enfatiza a restauração de inibições úteis e do id ao seu lugar legítimo em relação ao ego. [psycho- + synthesis]

psy·cho·tech·nics (sī-kō-tek′niks). Psicotécnica; termo antigo que designa a aplicação prática de métodos psicológicos no estudo da economia, sociologia e outros temas. [psycho- + G. *technē*, arte, habilidade]

psy·cho·ther·a·peu·tic (sī-kō-thār-ă-pū′tik). Psicoterapêutico; relativo à psicoterapia.

psy·cho·ther·a·peu·tics (sī′kō-thār-ă-pū′tiks). Psicoterapêutica. SIN psychotherapy.

psy·cho·ther·a·pist (sī-kō-thār′ă-pist). Psicoterapeuta; uma pessoa, em geral um psiquiatra ou psicólogo clínico, profissionalmente treinada e praticante da psicoterapia. Atualmente, nos EUA, o termo também é aplicado a assistentes sociais, enfermeiros e outros profissionais autorizados pelo estado cuja atuação inclui a psicoterapia.

psy·cho·ther·a·py (sī-kō-thār′ă-pē). Psicoterapia; tratamento de distúrbios emocionais, do comportamento, da personalidade e psiquiátricos com base na comunicação verbal ou não-verbal e em intervenções no paciente, ao contrário dos tratamentos que utilizam medidas químicas e físicas. Ver entradas em psychoanalysis; psychiatry; psychology; therapy. SIN psychotherapeutics. [psycho- + G. *therapeia*, tratamento]

anaclitic p., p. anaclítica; método psicoterapêutico caracterizado por incentivo e utilização da tendência do paciente a depender e confiar no terapeuta como figura de autoridade.

autonomous p., p. autônoma; tipo de p. psicanalítica que enfatiza especialmente o valor da autodeterminação do paciente tanto na situação terapêutica quanto na vida real.

brief p., p. breve; qualquer forma de p. ou aconselhamento destinada a produzir alteração emocional ou comportamental terapêutica em um período mínimo de tempo (geralmente não mais de 20 sessões). A terapia breve geralmente é ativa e diretiva; é mais claramente indicada quando há sintomas ou problemas claramente definidos, e quando os objetivos são limitados e específicos.

contractual p., p. contratual; p. baseada em um sólido acordo ou "contrato" entre o terapeuta e o paciente quanto ao papel de cada um na situação terapêutica.

directive p., p. diretiva; p. que utiliza a autoridade do terapeuta para direcionar o curso do tratamento do paciente, em contraposição à p. não-diretiva.

dyadic p., p. diádica; sessão psicoterapêutica que envolve apenas duas pessoas, o terapeuta e o paciente. Cf. group p. SIN individual therapy.

dynamic p., p. dinâmica. SIN psychoanalytic p.

existential p., p. existencial; tipo de terapia, baseado na filosofia existencialista, que enfatiza a confrontação, basicamente a interação espontânea e as experiências do sentimento em vez do pensamento racional, com menor atenção às resistências do paciente; o terapeuta se envolve no mesmo nível e no mesmo grau que o paciente. SIN existential therapy.

group p., p. de grupo; tipo de tratamento psicológico em que há participação conjunta de vários pacientes, na presença de um ou mais psicoterapeutas que facilitam tanto o relacionamento cognitivo emocional como racional, para alcançar as modificações almejadas no comportamento desajustado do paciente em seus relacionamentos interpessoais diários. Ver também entradas em group.

heteronomous p., p. heterônoma; termo que abrange todas as formas de p. que promovem a dependência do paciente em relação aos outros, principalmente a dependência ao psicoterapeuta, em oposição à p. autônoma.

hypnotic p., p. hipnótica; p. baseada na hipnose.

intensive p., p. intensiva; p. que envolve a exploração completa da história de vida do paciente, conflitos e psicodinâmica relacionada; freqüentemente contrasta com a p. de apoio.

marathon group p., maratona psicoterapêutica; tipo de p. de grupo caracterizada por longas sessões, com duração de horas ou dias, com interrupções mínimas para alimentação e repouso.

nondirective p., p. não-diretiva; p. na qual o terapeuta segue a direção do paciente durante a entrevista, em vez de introduzir suas próprias teorias e guiar o curso da entrevista. VER TAMBÉM client-centered *therapy*.

psychoanalytic p., p. psicanalítica; p. que utiliza princípios freudianos. VER TAMBÉM psychoanalysis. SIN dynamic p.

reconstructive p., p. reconstrutiva; forma de tratamento, como psicanálise, que busca não apenas aliviar os sintomas, mas também produzir alterações na estrutura de caráter desajustado e acelerar novos potenciais de adaptação; esse objetivo é alcançado trazendo-se à consciência a percepção e o discernimento de conflitos, medos, inibições e suas manifestações.

suggestive p., p. sugestiva; termo antigo para designar a p. que utiliza a influência e a autoridade do terapeuta. VER TAMBÉM directive p.

supportive p., p. de apoio; p. que visa reforçar as defesas psicológicas do paciente e promover reafirmação, como na intervenção em uma crise, em vez de devassar provocativamente os conflitos do paciente.

transactional p., p. transacional; p. com ênfase central nas interações (transações) diárias reais entre o paciente e as outras pessoas que participam da sua vida.

psy·chot·ic (sī-kot′ik). Psicótico; relativo à psicose ou afetado por esse transtorno.

psy·chot·o·gen (sī-kot′ō-gen). Psicotógeno; substância que produz manifestações psicóticas. [psychotic + G. *-gen*, que produz]

psy·chot·o·gen·ic (sī-kot-ō-jen′ik). Psicotogênico; capaz de induzir psicose; refere-se particularmente a drogas da série LSD e substâncias semelhantes.

psy·chot·o·mi·met·ic (sī-kot′ō-mi-met′ik). Psicotomimético. **1.** Fármaco ou substância que produz alterações psicológicas e comportamentais semelhantes às da psicose; p. ex., LSD. **2.** Designa um fármaco ou substância desse tipo. SIN psychosomimetic. [psychosis + G. *mimetikos*, mimético]

psy·cho·tro·pic (sī-kō-trop′ik). Psicotrópico; capaz de afetar a mente, as emoções e o comportamento; designa fármacos usados no tratamento de doenças mentais. [psycho- + G. *tropē*, volta]

psychro-. Psicro-; frio. VER TAMBÉM cryo-, crymo-. [G. *psychros*]

psy·chro·al·gia (sī-krō-al′jē-ă). Psicroalgia; sensação dolorosa de frio. [psychro- + G. *algos*, dor]

psy·chro·es·the·sia (sī′krō-es-thē′zē-ă). Psicroestesia. **1.** A forma de sensação que percebe o frio. **2.** Sensação de frio embora o corpo esteja quente; um calafrio. [psychro- + G. *aisthēsis*, sensação]

psy·chrom·e·ter (sī-krom′ĕ-ter). Psicrômetro; dispositivo para medir a umidade da atmosfera pela diferença de temperatura entre dois termômetros, um dos quais tem o bulbo úmido e o outro o tem seco. A evaporação do bulbo úmido reduz a leitura do termômetro; quanto maior a diferença nas leituras, mais seco é o ar; a ausência de diferença indica 100% de umidade relativa. SIN wet and dry bulb thermometer. [psychro- + G. *metron*, medida]

sling p., p. portátil; termômetros de bulbos úmido e seco montados sobre uma alça manual, para usar quando é necessário um psicrômetro portátil pequeno.

psy·chrom·e·try (sī-krom′ĕ-trē). Psicrometria; o cálculo da umidade relativa e das pressões do vapor d'água a partir das temperaturas de bulbo úmido e seco e da pressão barométrica; enquanto a umidade relativa é o valor comumente empregado, a pressão do vapor é a medida do significado fisiológico. SIN hygrometry. [psychro- + G. *metron*, medida]

psy·chro·phile, psy·chro·phil (sī′krō-fīl). Psicrófilo; microrganismo que cresce melhor em baixa temperatura (0 a 32°C), com crescimento ótimo a 15–20°C. [psychro- + G. *phileō*, amar]

psy·chro·phil·ic (sī-krō-fil′ik). Psicrofílico; relativo a um psicrófilo. [psychro- + G. *phileō*, amar]

psy·chro·pho·bia (sī-krō-fō′bē-ă) Psicrofobia. **1.** Extrema sensibilidade ao frio. **2.** Medo mórbido do frio. [psychro- + G. *phobos*, medo]

psy·chro·phore (sī′krō-fōr). Psicróforo; cateter duplo através do qual se faz circular água fria para aplicar frio à uretra ou a outro canal ou cavidade. [psychro- + G. *phoros*, que conduz]

psyl·li·um hy·dro·phil·ic mu·cil·loid (sil′ē-ŭm). Psílio hidrófilo mucilóide. VER *plantago seed*.

psyl·li·um seed (sil′ē-ŭm). Semente de psílio; a semente madura, seca e limpa da *Plantago indica* ou da *P. ovata*. Um catártico leve que atua absorvendo água e fornecendo volume mucilaginoso indigerível para os intestinos. Não deve ser usada na obstrução intestinal. SIN plantago seed, plantain seed.

PT Abreviatura de physical *therapy* (fisioterapia), physical therapist (fisioterapeuta) e prothrombin *time* (tempo de protrombina).

Pt Símbolo de platinum (platina).

PTA Abreviatura de plasma thromboplastin *antecedent* (antecedente de tromboplastina plasmática); phosphotungstic acid (ácido fosfotúngstico); percutaneous transluminal *angioplasty* (angioplastia transluminal percutânea).

PTAH Abreviatura de phosphotungstic acid *hematoxylin* (hematoxilina-ácido fosfotúngstico).

ptar·mic (tar′mik). Ptármico; esternutatório. SIN sternutatory. [G. *ptarmikos*, que leva a espirrar, de *ptarmos*, espirro]

ptar·mus (tar′mŭs). Espirro. [G. *ptarmos*, espirro]

PTC Abreviatura de plasma thromboplastin *component* (componente da tromboplastina plasmática); phenylthiocarbamoyl (feniltiocarbamoil).

PTCA Abreviatura de percutaneous transluminal coronary *angioplasty* (angioplastia coronariana transluminal percutânea).

Ptd Abreviatura de phosphatidyl (fosfatidil).
PtdCho Abreviatura de phosphatidylcholine (fosfatidilcolina).
PtdEth Abreviatura de phosphatidylethanolamine (fosfatidiletanolamina).
PtdIns Abreviatura de phosphatidylinositol (fosfatidilinositol).
PtdIns(4,5)P₂. Símbolo de *phosphatidylinositol* 4,5-bisphosphate (4,5-bifosfato de fosfatidilinositol).
PtdSer Abreviatura de phosphatidylserine (fosfatidilserina).
PTE Abreviatura de pulmonary thromboembolism (tromboembolismo pulmonar) ou pulmonary thromboendarterectomy (tromboendarterectomia pulmonar).
PTEA Abreviatura de pulmonary thromboendarterectomy (tromboendarterectomia pulmonar).

pter-, ptero-. Pter-, ptero-; forma combinante que significa asa; pena. [G. *pteron*, asa, pena]

pter·i·dine (ter′i-dēn, -din). Pteridina; azinopurina; benzotetrazina; pirazino[2,3-d]pirimidina; um composto heterocíclico de dois anéis, encontrado como componente do ácido pteróico e dos ácidos pteroilglutâmico (ácidos fólicos, pteropterina, etc.); derivados simples da pteridina (p. ex., xantopterina, leucopterina) são encontrados como pigmentos nas asas de borboletas, daí o nome.

pter·in (ter′in). Pterina; termo livremente usado para designar qualquer um dos compostos que contêm pteridina; especificamente, 2-amino-4-hidroxipteridina. Algumas pteridinas (p. ex., xantopterina, leucopterina) ainda preservam a raiz pterina.

p. deaminase, p. desaminase; aminoidrolase que catalisa a desaminação hidrolítica da 2-amino-4-hidroxipteridina para formar 2,4-diidroxipteridina e amônia.

pter·i·on (tē′rē-on) [TA]. Ptério; ponto craniométrico na região da fontanela esfenoidal, na junção da asa maior do esfenóide, da parte escamosa do osso temporal e dos ossos frontal e parietal; corta o trajeto da divisão anterior da artéria meníngea média. [G. *pteron*, asa]

pte·ro·ic ac·id (tē-rō′ik). Ácido pteróico; constituinte do ácido fólico que contém ácido *p*-aminobenzóico e pteridina ligada por um grupamento –CH₂– entre o grupamento amino do primeiro e C-6 do último.

pter·op·ter·in (ter-op′ter-in). Pteropterina; um conjugado do ácido fólico, princípio quimicamente semelhante ao ácido fólico, exceto por conter três moléculas de ácido glutâmico, em vez de uma, na ligação γ. SIN fermentation *Lactobacillus casei* factor, pteroyltriglutamic acid.

pter·o·yl·mon·o·glu·tam·ic ac·id (ter′ō-il-mon-ō′gloo-tam′ik). Ácido pteroilmonoglutâmico. SIN folic acid (2).

pter·o·yl·tri·glu·tam·ic ac·id (ter′ō-il-trī′gloo-tam′ik). Ácido pteroiltriglutâmico. SIN pteropterin.

pte·ryg·i·um (tē-rij′ē-ŭm). Pterígio. **1.** Placa triangular de tecido subconjuntival bulbar hipertrofiado que se estende do canto medial até a borda da córnea ou além, com o ápice apontando para a pupila. SIN web eye. **2.** Crescimento anterior da cutícula sobre a placa ungueal, mais comum no líquen plano. SIN p. unguis. **3.** Uma membrana cutânea anormal. [G. *pterygion*, qualquer coisa semelhante a uma asa, uma doença do olho, dim. de *pteryx*, asa]

p. col′li, p. do pescoço; membrana ou faixa firme de pele do pescoço, congênita, geralmente bilateral, que se estende do acrômio até o mastóide, observada nas síndromes de Turner e de Noonan.

p. un′guis, p. ungueal. SIN pterygium (2).

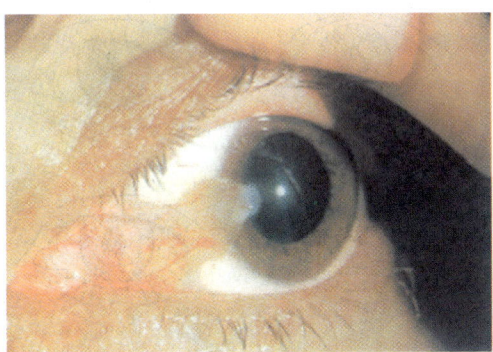

pterígio: vasos e tecido da conjuntiva cresceram sobre a margem da córnea

pterygo-. Pterigo-; em forma de asa, geralmente relativo ao processo pterigóide. [G. *pteryx, pterygos*, asa]

pter·y·goid (ter′i-goyd). Pterigóide; em forma de asa; semelhante a uma asa; termo aplicado a várias partes anatômicas relacionadas com o osso esfenóide. [G. *pteryx (pteryg-)*, asa, + *eidos*, semelhança]

pter·y·go·man·dib·u·lar (ter'i-gō-man-dib'ū-lăr). Pterigomandibular; relativo ao processo pterigóide e à mandíbula.

pte·ry·go·max·il·la·re (ter'i-gō-mak-si-lār'ē). Pterigomaxilar; o ponto onde o processo pterigóide do osso esfenóide e o processo pterigóide da maxila começam a formar a fissura pterigomaxilar; o ponto mais baixo da abertura é usado em cefalometria.

pter·y·go·max·il·lary (ter'i-gō-mak'si-lār-ē). Pterigomaxilar; relativo ao processo pterigóide e a maxila.

pter·y·go·pal·a·tine (ter'i-gō-pal'ă-tīn). Pterigopalatino; relativo ao processo pterigóide e ao osso palatino.

PTF Abreviatura de plasma thromboplastin *factor* (fator tromboplastina plasmática).

PTH Abreviatura de parathyroid *hormone* (paratormônio); phenylthiohydantoin (feniltioidantoína).

PTHC Abreviatura de percutaneous transhepatic *cholangiography* (colangiografia trans-hepática percutânea).

pthi·ri·a·sis (thī-rī'a-sis). Ftiríase. SIN *pediculosis pubis*. [G. *phtheiriasis*, de *phtheir*, piolho]

  p. pu'bis, f. púbica; presença de piolhos no púbis e em outras áreas pilosas do tronco, assim como nos cílios de lactentes e crianças pequenas.

Pthir·us (thī'rŭs). Gênero de piolhos (família Pediculidae) que antigamente eram agrupados no gênero *Pediculus*. A principal espécie é *P. pubis* (antigamente *Pediculus pubis*), o piolho pubiano, um parasita que infesta a região pubiana e as partes pilosas próximas. Amiúde é incorretamente escrito *Phthirus* ou *Phthirius*. [irreg. do G. *phtheir*, piolho]

PTHrP Abreviatura de parathyroid hormone-related *peptide* (peptídeo paratormônio-relacionado).

PTK Acrônimo para phototherapeutic *keratectomy* (ceratectomia fototoerapêutica).

PTMA Abreviatura de phenyltrimethylammonium (feniltrimetilamônio).

pto·maine (tō'mān). Ptomaína; termo indefinido aplicado a substâncias venenosas, p. ex., aminas tóxicas, formadas na decomposição da proteína pela descarboxilação de aminoácidos por ação bacteriana. SIN ptomatine. [G. *ptōma*, cadáver]

pto·mai·ne·mia (tō-mā-nē'mē-ă). Ptomainemia; condição resultante da presença de uma ptomaína no sangue circulante. [ptomaine + G. *haima*, sangue]

pto·ma·tine (tō'mă-tēn). Ptomatina. SIN ptomaine.

pto·mat·ro·pine (tō-mat'rō-pēn). Ptomatropina; ptomaína caracterizada por propriedades venenosas semelhantes às da atropina; formada pela ação de bactérias na descarboxilação de aminoácidos.

ptosed (tōzd). Ptótico. SIN ptotic.

pto·sis, pl. **pto·ses** (tō'sis, tō'sez). **1.** Ptose; queda ou prolapso de um órgão. **2.** Blefaroptose. SIN blepharoptosis. [G. *ptōsis*, queda]

  p. adipo'sa, Blefarocalasia. SIN blepharochalasis.

  aponeurogenic p., Blefaroptose aponeurogênica; queda da pálpebra causada por deiscência do tendão do músculo levantador.

  p. sympathet'ica, p. simpática. SIN Horner *syndrome*.

-ptosis. -Ptose; queda ou prolapso de um órgão. [G. *ptōsis*, queda]

pto.tic (tot'ik). Ptótico; relativo a, ou caracterizado por, ptose. SIN ptosed.

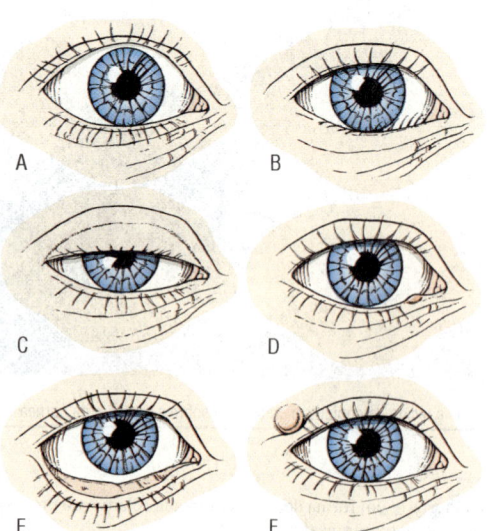

alterações estruturais e distúrbios do olho: (A) exoftalmia, (B) entrópio, (C) ptose, (D) hordéolo, (E) ectrópio, (F) calázio

6-PTS Abreviatura de 6-pyruvoyltetrahydropterin synthase (6-piruvoiltetraidropterina sintase).

PTT Abreviatura de partial thromboplastin *time* (tempo de tromboplastina parcial).

PTU Abreviatura de propylthiouracil (propiltiouracil).

ptyal-, ptyalo-. Ptial-, ptialo-; as glândulas salivares, saliva. VER TAMBÉM sialo-. [G. *ptyalon*]

pty·al·a·gogue (tī-al'ă-gog). Ptialagogo. SIN sialagogue.

pty·a·lec·ta·sis (tī'ă-lek'ta-sis). Ptialectasia. SIN sialectasis. [ptyal- + G. *ektasis*, alongamento]

pty·a·lin (tī'ă-lin). Ptialina. SIN α-amylase.

pty·a·lism (tī'al-izm). Ptialismo. SIN sialorrhea. [G. *ptyalismos*, saliva]

pty·a·lo·cele (tī'ă-lō-sēl). Ptialocele. SIN ranula (2).

pty·a·log·ra·phy (tī-ă-log'ra-fē). Ptialografia. SIN sialography.

pty·a·lo·lith (tī'ă-lō-lith). Ptialólito; sialólito. SIN sialolith.

pty·a·lo·li·thi·a·sis (tī'ă-lō-li-thī'ă-sis). Ptialolitíase. SIN sialolithiasis.

pty·a·lo·li·thot·o·my (tī'ă-lō-li-thot'ō-mē). Ptialolitotomia. SIN sialolithotomy.

pty·cho·tis oil (tī-kō'tis). Óleo de ajowan. SIN ajowan oil.

pty·oc·ri·nous (tī-ok'ri-nŭs). Ptiócrino; secreção por liberação do conteúdo da célula, como nas células mucosas. [G. *ptyō*, cuspir, + *krinō*, separar]

Pu Símbolo de plutonium (plutônio).

pu·bar·che (pū-bar'kē). Pubarca; início da puberdade, particularmente o que se manifesta pelo surgimento de pêlos pubianos. [puberdade + G. *archē*, início]

pu·ber·al, pu·ber·tal (pū'ber-ăl, -ber-tăl). Puberal; relativo à puberdade.

pu·ber·ty (pū'ber-tē). Puberdade; seqüência de eventos pelos quais uma criança torna-se um adulto jovem, caracterizada pelo início da gametogênese, secreção de hormônios gonadais, desenvolvimento de características sexuais secundárias e das funções reprodutivas; o dimorfismo sexual é acentuado. Em meninas, os primeiros sinais de puberdade podem ser evidentes aos 8 anos de idade, estando o processo quase completo aos 16 anos; em meninos, a puberdade comumente começa aos 10–12 anos e está quase completa aos 18 anos. Fatores étnicos e geográficos podem influenciar a época em que ocorrem vários eventos típicos da puberdade. [L. *pubertas*, de *puber*, crescido]

  delayed p., p. tardia; ausência de quaisquer sinais de p. aos 14 anos em ambos os sexos.

  precocious p., p. precoce; condição na qual as alterações puberais começam em uma idade inesperadamente precoce. Esta pode envolver o início das alterações normais do eixo hipotalâmico-hipofisário antes dos 8 anos de idade. A forma idiopática é a mais comum.

  true precocious p., p. precoce verdadeira. SIN hyperovarianism.

seqüência temporal de eventos na puberdade		
idade em anos	**meninas**	**meninos**
9–10	alargamento da pelve, arredondamento dos quadris, adrenarca	
11	telarca, pubarca	adrenarca
12	gonadarca, pico de crescimento	
13	menarca, pêlos axilares	gonadarca, aumento dos testículos
14		pico de crescimento, ginecomastia da puberdade
15	menstruação regular, com ovulação	modificação da voz, pêlos axilares, crescimento da barba
16–17	cessação do crescimento dos ossos longos	pêlos pubianos masculinos, mais pêlos corporais
18–19		cessação do crescimento dos ossos longos

pu·bes (pū'bis) [TA]. **1** [NA]. Pêlo púbico. SIN pubic *hair*. **2.** Púbis. SIN mons pubis. [L. *pubes*, o pêlo sobre a região genital; os órgãos genitais]

pu·bes·cence (pū-bes'ens). Pubescência. **1.** A aproximação da idade da puberdade ou da maturidade sexual. [L. *pubesco*, atingir a puberdade] **2.** Presença de pêlos curtos, finos ou macios. [L. *pubes*, pêlos pubianos]

pu·bes·cent (pū-bes'ent). Pubescente; relativo à pubescência.

pu·bic (pū′bik). Púbico; pubiano; relativo ao púbis.
pu·bi·ot·o·my (pū - bē - ot′ō - mē). Pubiotomia; secção do osso púbis alguns centímetros lateral à sínfise, a fim de aumentar suficientemente a capacidade de uma pelve contraída para permitir a passagem de uma criança viva. [L. *pubis*, osso púbis, + G. *tomē*, incisão]
pubis. Púbis; a porção ântero-inferior do osso do quadril, distinta ao nascimento mas que, depois, se funde ao ílio e ao ísquio; é formado por um corpo que se articula com seu companheiro na sínfise púbica, e por dois ramos; o ramo superior entra na formação do acetábulo, e o ramo inferior funde-se ao ramo do ísquio para formar o ramo isquiopúbico. SIN os pubis.
Pub·lic Health Ser·vice (PHS). Serviço de Saúde Pública. VER *United States Public Health Service*.
pubo-. Pubo-; pubiano, púbis. [L. *pubes*]
pu·bo·cap·su·lar (pū′bō - kap′soo - lăr). Pubocapsular; relativo ao púbis e à cápsula da articulação do quadril.
pu·bo·coc·cy·ge·al (pū - bō - kok - sij′ē - ăl). Pubococcígeo; relativo ao púbis e ao cóccix.
pu·bo·fem·o·ral (pū′bō - fem′ō - răl). Pubofemoral; relativo ao osso púbis e ao fêmur.
pu·bo·pros·tat·ic (pū′bō - pros - tat′ik). Puboprostático; relativo ao osso púbis e à próstata.
pu·bo·rec·tal (pū′bō - rek′tăl). Puborretal; relativo ao osso púbis e ao reto.
pu·bo·ves·i·cal (pū′bō - ves′i - kăl). Pubovesical; relativo ao osso púbis e à bexiga.
Puchtler-Sweat stains. Colorações de Puchtler-Sweat. VER Puchtler-Sweat *stain* for basement membranes, Puchtler-Sweat *stain* for hemoglobin and hemosiderin.
pu·den·da (pū - den′dă). Pudendos; plural de pudendum. [L.]
pu·den·dal (pū - den′dăl). Pudendo; relativo à genitália externa. SIN pudic.
pu·den·dum, pl. **pu·den·da** (pū - den′dŭm, - dă) [TA]. Pudendo; a genitália externa, principalmente a genitália feminina (vulva). Usado também no plural. [L. neutro de *pudendus*, particip. adj. de *pudeo*, sentir-se envergonhado]
  p. femini′num, vulva. SIN vulva.
  p. mulieb′re, termo obsoleto para vulva.
Pudenz, Robert H., neurocirurgião norte-americano, *1911. VER Heyer-P. *valve*.
pu·dic (pū′dik). Pudendo. SIN pudendal. [L. *pudicus*, recatado]
Pud·lak, P., médico tcheco do século XX. VER Hermansky-Pudlak *syndrome*.
pu·er·pe·ra, pl. **pu·er·per·ae** (pū - er′per - ă, - per - ē). Puérpera; mulher que pariu recentemente. [L., de *puer*, criança, + *pario*, parir]
pu·er·per·al (pū - er′per - ăl). Puerperal; relativo ao puerpério, ou período após o parto. SIN puerperant (1).
pu·er·per·ant (pū - er′per - ant). 1. Puerperal. SIN puerperal. 2. Puérpera.
pu·er·pe·ri·um, pl. **pu·er·pe·ria** (pū - er - pēr′ē - ŭm, - ē - ă). Puerpério; período que vai do fim do trabalho de parto até a involução completa do útero, geralmente definido como 42 dias. [L. parto, de *puer*, criança, + *pario*, parir]
Puestow, Charles B., cirurgião norte-americano, 1902–1973. VER P. *procedure*.
puff (pŭf). Um som curto, soprado, à ausculta, geralmente um sopro sistólico auscultado sobre o coração. VER TAMBÉM *chromosome* puffs.
  veiled p., sopro pulmonar fraco, que simula a agitação abafada de uma roupa no vento.
puff·ball (pŭf′bal). SIN Lycoperdon.
Pu·lex (pū′leks). Gênero de pulgas (família Pulicidae, ordem Siphonaptera). [L. pulga]
  P. che′opis, nome antigo da *Xenopsylla cheopis*.
  P. fascia′tus, nome antigo da *Nosopsyllus fasciatus*.
  P. ir′ritans, a pulga humana, uma pulga comum que infesta seres humanos, muitos animais domésticos (principalmente porcos), mamíferos e aves selvagens; um vetor medíocre da peste.
  P. pen′etrans, nome incorreto da *Tunga penetrans*.
  P. serra′ticeps, nome antigo de *Ctenocephalides canis*.
pu·lic·i·cide, pu·li·cide (pū - lis′i - sīd, pū′li - sīd). Pulicida; agente químico destrutivo de pulgas. [L. *pulex* (*pulic-*), pulga, + *caedo*, matar]
pul·ley (pŭl′ē). Tróclea. VER trochlea.
  anular p., parte anular da bainha fibrosa dos dedos da mão e do pé. SIN anular *part* of fibrous digital sheath of digits of hand and foot.
  cruciform p., parte cruciforme da bainha fibrosa dos dedos. SIN cruciform *part* of fibrous digital sheath.
  p. of humerus, tróclea do úmero. SIN *trochlea* of humerus.
  muscular p., tróclea muscular. SIN muscular *trochlea*.
  peroneal p., tróclea fibular. SIN fibular *trochlea* of calcaneus.
  p. of talus, tróclea do tálus. SIN *trochlea* of the talus.
pul·lu·la·nase (pŭl′yū - lă - nās). Pululanase. SIN α-dextrin endo-1,6-α-glucosidase.
pul·lu·late (pŭl′ū - lāt). Pulular; sofrer pululação.
pul·lu·la·tion (pŭl - ū - lā′shŭn). Pululação; o ato de germinação ou de brotamento, como observado em leveduras. [L. *pullulo*, pp. *-atus*, germinar]

pul·mo, gen. **pul·mo·nis**, pl. **pul·mo·nes** (pŭl′mō, pŭl - mō′nis, - mō′nēz) [TA]. Pulmão. SIN lung. [L.]
  p. dex′ter, p. direito.
  p. sinis′ter, p. esquerdo.
pulmo-, pulmon-, pulmono-. Pulmo-, pulmon-, pulmono-; os pulmões. VER TAMBÉM pneum-, pneumo-. [L. *pulmo*, pulmão]
pul·mo·a·or·tic (pŭl′mō - ā - or′tik). Aórtico-pulmonar; relativo à artéria pulmonar e à aorta.
pul·mo·lith (pŭl′mō - lith). Pulmólito. SIN pneumolith. [L. *pulmo*, pulmão, + G. *lithos*, cálculo]
pul·mo·nary (pŭl′mō - nār - ē). Pulmonar; relativo aos pulmões, à artéria pulmonar ou à abertura que vai do ventrículo direito à artéria pulmonar. SIN pneumonic (1), pulmonic (1). [L. *pulmonarius*, de *pulmo*, pulmão]
pul·mo·nec·to·my (pŭl - mō - nek′tō - mē). Pneumectomia. SIN pneumonectomy. [L. *pulmo* (*pulmon-*), pulmão, + G. *ektomē*, excisão]
pul·mon·ic (pŭl - mon′ik). 1. Pulmonar. SIN pulmonary. 2. Designação obsoleta de um remédio para doenças dos pulmões.
pul·mo·ni·tis (pŭl - mō - nī′tis). Pneumonite. SIN pneumonitis.
pulp (pŭlp) [TA]. Polpa. 1. Um sólido macio, úmido, coeso. SIN pulpa [TA]. 2. SIN dental p. 3. SIN chyme. [L. *pulpa*, carne]
  coronal p., p. coronal. SIN crown p.
  crown p. [TA], p. coronal; a parte da polpa do dente contida na câmara pulpar ou cavidade da coroa do dente. SIN pulpa coronalis [TA], coronal p.
  dead p., p. morta. SIN necrotic p.
  dental p. [TA], p. do dente; os tecidos moles na cavidade pulpar, consistindo em tecido conjuntivo que contém vasos sanguíneos, nervos e linfáticos e, na periferia, uma camada de odontoblastos capazes de reparar a dentina internamente. SIN pulp (2) [TA], pulpa dentis [TA], dentinal p., tooth p.
  dentinal p., p. dentinária. SIN dental p.
  digital p., p. digital. SIN p. of finger.
  digital p. of hand, p. digital da mão. SIN p. of finger.
  enamel p., p. do esmalte; camada de células estreladas no órgão do esmalte.
  exposed p., p. exposta; p. que foi exposta ou deixada descoberta por um processo patológico, traumatismo ou instrumento dentário.
  p. of finger, p. do dedo; a massa carnosa na face palmar da extremidade do dedo. SIN digital p. of hand, digital p., pulpa digiti manus.
  mummified p., p. mumificada; designação errada para uma p. tratada com um derivado do formaldeído.
  necrotic p., p. necrótica; necrose da p. dental que, clinicamente, não responde à estimulação térmica; o dente pode ser assintomático ou sensível à percussão e palpação. SIN dead p., nonvital p.
  nonvital p., p. necrótica. SIN necrotic p.
  putrescent p., p. putrescente; p. decomposta, freqüentemente infectada.
  radicular p., p. radicular. SIN root p.
  red p., p. vermelha; p. esplênica observada macroscopicamente como uma substância castanho-avermelhada, devido à abundância de hemácias, que consiste em seios esplênicos e tecido interposto entre elas (cordões esplênicos).
  red p. of spleen [TA], p. vermelha esplênica; tecido vermelho-azulado que constitui cerca de 75% do parênquima esplênico; contém um grande número de seios venosos separados por um retículo fibrocelular rico em fibroblastos e macrófagos; ao corte, tem um aspecto canelado. SIN pulpa rubra splenica [TA].
  root p. [TA], p. radicular; a parte da polpa do dente contida na porção apical ou radicular do dente. SIN pulpa radicularis [TA], radicular p.
  splenic p., p. esplênica; a substância celular macia do baço. SIN pulpa splenica [TA], pulpa lienis.
  p. of toe [TA], p. do dedo do pé; a massa carnosa da face plantar da parte distal do dedo do pé.
  tooth p., p. do dente. SIN dental p.
  vertebral p., p. núcleo pulposo. SIN nucleus pulposus.
  vital p., p. vital; p. composta de tecido viável, normal ou doente, que responde a estímulos elétricos e ao calor e ao frio.
  white p., p. branca; aquela parte do baço que consiste em nódulos e outras concentrações linfáticas.
  white p. of spleen [TA], p. branca do baço; agregações de linfócitos β visíveis macroscopicamente quando o baço fresco é seccionado; apresentam-se como pontos brancos translúcidos, de 1 mm ou menos, que contrastam com a matriz adjacente, de polpa vermelha. SIN pulpa alba splenica [TA].
pul·pa (pŭl′pă) [TA]. Pulpa. SIN pulp (1). [L. pulpa]
  p. alba splenica [TA], p. branca esplênica. SIN white *pulp* of spleen.
  p. corona′lis [TA], p. coronal. SIN crown *pulp*.
  p. den′tis [TA], p. do dente. SIN dental *pulp*.
  p. digiti manus, p. do dedo. SIN *pulp* of finger.
  p. lie′nis, p. esplênica. SIN splenic *pulp*.
  p. radicula′ris [TA], p. radicular. SIN root *pulp*.
  p. rubra splenica [TA], p. vermelha esplênica. SIN red *pulp* of spleen.
  p. splen′ica [TA], p. esplênica. SIN splenic *pulp*. VER TAMBÉM red *pulp*, white *pulp*.
pul·pal (pŭl′păl). Pulpar; relativo à pulpa.

pul·pal·gia (pŭl - pal′jē - ă). Pulpalgia; dor que se origina na polpa do dente. [L. *pulpa*, polpa, + G. *algos*, dor]

pulp·ec·to·my (pŭl - pek′tō - mē). Pulpectomia; remoção de toda a estrutura da polpa de um dente, incluindo o tecido pulpar nas raízes. [L. *pulpa*, polpa, + G. *ektomē*, excisão]

pul·pi·fac·tion (pŭl - pi - fak′shŭn). Polpação; redução a uma condição de polpa. [L. *pulpa*, polpa, + *facio*, pp. *factus*, fazer]

pulp·i·form (pŭl′pi - form). Pulpiforme; semelhante à polpa; polposo.

pulp·i·fy (pŭl′pi - fī). Reduzir a um estado de polpa.

pulp·i·tis (pŭl - pī′tis). Pulpite; inflamação da polpa de um dente. SIN odontitis. [L. *pulpa*, polpa, + G. *-itis*, inflamação]

  hyperplastic p., p. hiperplásica; tecido de granulação hiperplásico que cresce da câmara pulpar exposta de um dente muito cariado. SIN dental polyp, pulp polyp, tooth polyp.

  hypertrophic p., p. hipertrófica; nome errado da pulpite hiperplásica.

  irreversible p., p. irreversível; inflamação da polpa do dente em que a polpa é incapaz de se recuperar; clinicamente, pode ser assintomática ou caracterizada por dor que persiste após estimulação térmica; microscopicamente, caracterizada por inflamação aguda ou crônica acentuada, algumas vezes com necrose parcial da polpa.

  reversible p., p. reversível; inflamação mínima em que a polpa é capaz de se recuperar; caracterizada clinicamente por dor que desaparece rapidamente após a interrupção do estímulo térmico; caracterizada microscopicamente por vasodilatação, hiperemia e edema com diapedese mínima de leucócitos.

  suppurative p., p. supurativa; designação obsoleta de uma pulpite irreversível purulenta.

pulp·less. 1. Sem polpa. **2.** Designa um dente no qual a polpa morreu ou do qual foi retirada. **3.** Designa um dente que não responde a uma prova pulpar elétrica ou térmica.

pulp·o·don·tia (pŭl - pō - don′shē - ă). Pulpodontia; a ciência do tratamento do canal radicular. VER TAMBÉM endodontics. [L. *pulpa*, polpa, + G. *odous*, dente]

pul·po·sus (pŭl - pō′sŭs). Pulposo. SIN pulpy. [L.]

pulp·ot·o·my (pŭl - pot′ō - mē). Pulpotomia; remoção de uma parte da estrutura pulpar de um dente, geralmente a porção coronal. SIN pulp amputation. [L. *pulpa*, polpa, + G. *tomē*, incisão]

pulpy (pŭl′pē). Pulposo; na condição de um sólido macio, úmido. SIN pulposus.

pul·sate (pŭl′sāt). Pulsar; pulsar ou bater ritmicamente; diz-se do coração ou de uma artéria. [L. *pulso*, pp. *-atus*, bater]

pul·sa·tile (pŭl′să - til). Pulsátil; que pulsa ou bate.

pul·sa·tion (pŭl - sā′shŭn). Pulsação; um batimento pulsátil ou rítmico, como o de um pulso ou do coração. [L. *pulsatio*, um batimento]

  balloon counter p., contrapulsação com balão; forma de assistência circulatória na qual um balão é inflado na aorta, durante a diástole, para aumentar a pressão diastólica e esvaziado, durante a sístole, para reduzir a pós-carga ventricular esquerda. Cf. intraaortic balloon *pump*.

  suprasternal p., p. supra-esternal; qualquer pulsação na incisura supra-esternal na face anterior do pescoço.

pul·sa·tor (pŭl - sā′ter, -tōr). Pulsador; máquina ou aparelho que opera de forma pulsátil, vibratória ou rítmica.

pulse (pŭls). Pulso; dilatação rítmica de uma artéria, produzida pelo maior volume de sangue lançado no vaso pela contração do coração. Algumas vezes, também pode ser observado um pulso em uma veia ou órgão vascular, como o fígado. SIN pulsus. [L. *pulsus*]

  abdominal p., p. abdominal; o p. aórtico compressível, mole, que ocorre em determinados distúrbios abdominais. SIN pulsus abdominalis.

  alternating p., p. alternante; alternação mecânica; p. regular, mas com batimentos mais fortes e mais fracos alternados, freqüentemente detectável apenas com o esfigmomanômetro ou outra medida de pressão, geralmente indicando doença miocárdica grave. SIN pulsus alternans.

  anacrotic p., anadicrotic p., p. anacrótico, p. anadicrótico; onda de p. que exibe uma ou mais incisuras ou entalhes em seu ramo ascendente, algumas vezes detectáveis por palpação. SIN pulsus anadicrotus.

  bigeminal p., p. bigeminal; p. em que os batimentos ocorrem em pares. SIN bigemina, coupled p., pulsus bigeminus.

  bisferious p. (bis - fer′ē - ŭs), p. bisférico; p. arterial com picos que podem ser palpáveis. SIN pulsus bisferiens.

  bulbar p., p. bulbar; p. jugular que, supostamente, indica insuficiência tricúspide.

  cannonball p., p. em martelo d'água. SIN water-hammer p.

  capillary p., p. capilar; palidez e ruborização alternadas e rítmicas de uma área capilar, p. ex. sob as unhas ou nos lábios, observado a uma compressão suave; um sinal de dilatação arteriolar, bem observado na insuficiência aórtica. VER TAMBÉM Quincke p.

  carotid p., p. carotídeo; o p. das artérias carótidas no pescoço.

  catacrotic p., p. catacrótico; p. no qual há uma incisura ascendente interrompendo o ramo descendente do esfigmograma. SIN pulsus catacrotus.

  catadicrotic p., p. catadicrótico; pulso catacrótico no qual há duas incisuras ascendentes. SIN pulsus catacrotus.

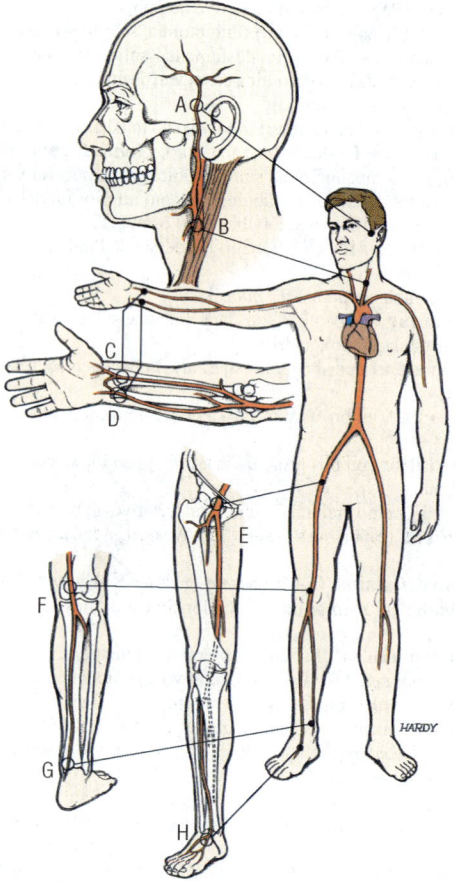

pulsos arteriais periféricos: (A) temporal, (B) carotídeo, (C) radial, (D) ulnar, (E) femoral, (F) poplíteo, (G) tibial posterior, (H) pedioso dorsal

  collapsing p., p. colapsante, p. em martelo d'água. SIN water-hammer p.

  cordy p., p. tenso. SIN tense p.

  Corrigan p., p. de Corrigan. SIN Corrigan *sign*.

  coupled p., p. acoplado. SIN bigeminal p.

  dicrotic p., p. dicrótico; p. caracterizado por um batimento duplo, sendo o segundo, devido a uma onda dicrótica palpável, mais fraco que o primeiro. SIN pulsus duplex.

  entoptic p., p. entóptico; fase intermitente sincrônica com o pulso.

  filiform p., p. filiforme; p. filamentar.

  gaseous p., p. gasoso; p. suave, cheio, mas fraco.

  guttural p., p. gutural; pulsação percebida na garganta.

  hard p., p. duro; p. que golpeia fortemente contra a ponta do dedo e é comprimido com dificuldade, sugerindo hipertensão. SIN pulsus durus.

  intermittent p., p. intermitente; irregularidade cardíaca devida a extra-sístoles fracas demais para abrir as válvulas semilunares; freqüentemente devida à longa pausa existente após o batimento prematuro, pausas excessivamente longas, iguais a dois ciclos regulares, ocorrem regularmente entre os batimentos. SIN pulsus intercidens.

  irregular p., p. irregular; variação na freqüência de impulsos em uma artéria devida à arritmia cardíaca.

  jugular p., p. jugular; o p. venoso observado nas veias jugulares do pescoço, geralmente as veias jugulares profundas.

  labile p., p. lábil; repetidas alterações na freqüência cardíaca.

  long p., p. longo; p. no qual o impacto é percebido por mais tempo que o habitual. SIN sustained p.

  monocrotic p., p. monocrótico; pulso sem qualquer dicrotismo perceptível. SIN pulsus monocrotus.

  mousetail p., p. murino. SIN *pulsus myurus.*

  movable p., p. móvel; o movimento lateral de uma artéria tortuosa que pulsa fortemente.

  nail p., p. ungueal; p. capilar observado através da unha.

  paradoxic p., p. paradoxal; exagero da variação normal no volume do p. arterial sistêmico com a respiração, tornando-se mais fraco com a inspiração e mais forte com a expiração; característico do tamponamento cardíaco, raro na pericardite constritiva; assim denominado porque essas alterações são independentes das alterações na freqüência cardíaca medidas dire-

tamente ou por eletrocardiograma. SIN pulsus paradoxus, pulsus respiratione intermittens.
piston p., p. em pistão. SIN water-hammer p.
plateau p., p. em platô; p. lento, mantido.
quadrigeminal p., p. quadrigêmeo; p. em que os batimentos são agrupados em quatro, com uma pausa após cada quarto batimento. SIN pulsus quadrigeminus.
Quincke p., p. de Quincke; o p. capilar observado nas unhas das mãos e dos pés na insuficiência aórtica; é observado sinal de fluxo e refluxo. SIN Quincke sign.
radial p., p. radial; o p. observado na artéria radial, em geral no punho.
radiofrequency p., p. de radiofreqüência; em ressonância magnética nuclear, um sinal eletromagnético curto usado para mudar a direção do campo magnético. VER sequence p.
respiratory p., p. respiratório; aumento e diminuição de qualquer pulsação produzida pela respiração.
reversed paradoxical p., p. paradoxal invertido; p. cuja amplitude aumenta com a inspiração e diminui com a expiração, como se observa em alguns casos de insuficiência tricúspide e de dissociação AV com arritmia sinusal. SIN Riegel p.
Riegel p., p. de Riegel. SIN reversed paradoxical p.
sequence p., p. seqüencial; em ressonância magnética, a série de sinais de radiofreqüência usados para desviar o campo magnético e, assim, modificar a orientação dos prótons.
soft p., p. suave; p. facilmente extinto por compressão com o dedo.
sustained p., p. longo. SIN long p.
tense p., p. tenso; p. duro, cheio, mas sem excursões muito amplas, semelhante à vibração de um cordão espesso. SIN cordy p.
thready p., p. filiforme; p. pequeno, fino, que parece um pequeno cordão ou fio sob o dedo. SIN pulsus filiformis.
trigeminal p., p. trigeminal; p. no qual os batimentos ocorrem em trios, com uma pausa após cada terceiro batimento. SIN pulsus trigeminus.
triphammer p., p. em martinete. SIN water-hammer p.
undulating p., p. ondulante; p. sem tônus no qual há uma sucessão de ondas sem caráter ou força. SIN pulsus fluens.
unequal p., p. desigual; forças diferentes de p. na mesma artéria entre os lados direito e esquerdo da circulação.
vagus p., p. vagal; p. lento devido à ação inibidora do nervo vago sobre o coração.
venous p., p. venoso; pulsação que ocorre nas veias, principalmente a veia jugular interna. SIN pulsus venosus.
vermicular p., p. vermicular; p. pequeno e rápido, que produz uma sensação vermiforme no dedo.
water-hammer p., p. em martelo d'água; p. com impulso forçado, mas colapso imediato, característico da incompetência aórtica. VER TAMBÉM Corrigan sign. SIN cannonball p., collapsing p., piston p., pulsus celerrimus, triphammer p.
wiry p., p. em arame; p. pequeno, fino, incompressível.
pul·sel·lum (pŭl-sel′ŭm). Pulselo; flagelo posterior que forma o órgão de locomoção em determinados protozoários. [L. mod. dim. do L. *pulsus*, batida]
pul·sim·e·ter, pul·som·e·ter (pŭl-sim′ĕ-ter, -som′ĕ-ter). Pulsímetro; esfigmômetro; instrumento para medir a força e a velocidade do pulso. [L. *pulsus*, pulso, + *metron*, medida]
pul·sion (pŭl′shŭn). Pulsão; impulso para fora ou tumefação. [L. *pulsio*]
pul·sus (pŭl′sŭs). Pulso. VER pulse. [L. golpe, pulso]
  p. abdomina'lis, p. abdominal. SIN abdominal pulse.
  p. alter'nans, p. alternante. SIN alternating pulse.
  p. anadic'rotus, p. anacrótico. SIN anacrotic pulse.
  p. bigem'inus, p. bigêmino. SIN bigeminal pulse.
  p. bisfer'iens, p. bisférico. SIN bisferious pulse.
  p. cap'risans, p. em saltos, irregular tanto na força quanto no ritmo.
  p. catac'rotus, p. catacrótico. SIN catacrotic pulse.
  p. catadic'rotus, p. catadicrótico. SIN catadicrotic pulse.
  p. cel'er, p. célere; batimento de p. que sobe e desce rapidamente.
  p. celer'rimus, p. em martelo d'água. SIN water-hammer pulse.
  p. cor'dis, p. cardíaco; o batimento apical do coração.
  p. deb'ilis, p. débil; um pulso fraco.
  p. dif'ferens, p. diferente; p. incongruente; condição em que os pulsos nas duas artérias radiais ou em outras artérias correspondentes diferem em força. SIN p. incongruens.
  p. du'plex, p. duplo. SIN dicrotic pulse.
  p. du'rus, p. duro. SIN hard pulse.
  p. filifor'mis, p. filiforme. SIN thready pulse.
  p. flu'ens, p. ondulante. SIN undulating pulse.
  p. for'micans, p. formigante; p. muito pequeno, quase imperceptível, sendo a impressão que produz no dedo comparada ao formigamento.
  p. for'tis, p. forte; p. cheio e forte.
  p. fre'quens, p. freqüente; p. rápido.
  p. heterochron'icus, p. heterocrônico; p. arrítmico.

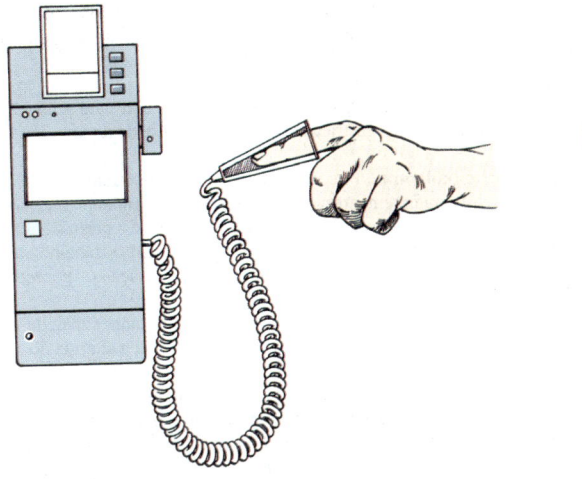

monitor de oxímetro de pulso

  p. inaequa'lis, p. desigual; p. irregular em ritmo e força.
  p. incon'gruens, p. incongruente. SIN p. differens.
  p. infre'quens, p. infreqüente; p. lento.
  p. inter'cidens, p. intermitente. SIN intermittent pulse.
  p. intercur'rens, p. intercorrente; forte onda de p. dicrótica ocasional que dá a impressão de uma contração ventricular intercorrente.
  p. irregula'ris perpet'uus, p. irregular perpétuo; p. permanentemente irregular, amiúde causado por, ou característico de, fibrilação atrial; também pode ser produzido por uma grande variedade de outros ritmos caóticos.
  p. mag'nus, p. amplo; p. grande e cheio.
  p. mol'lis, p. mole; p. mole, facilmente compressível.
  p. monoc'rotus, p. monocrótico. SIN monocrotic pulse.
  p. myu'rus, pulso caracterizado por uma onda cujo ápice é atingido subitamente e que, depois, diminui muito gradualmente. SIN mousetail pulse.
  p. paradoxus (pŭl′sŭs par′a-doks-ŭs). p. paradoxal. SIN paradoxic pulse.
  p. par'vus, p. pequeno; p. de pequena amplitude, como na estenose aórtica.
  p. par'vus et tar'dus (pŭl′sŭs par′vŭs a tar′dŭs), p. pequeno e tardo; considerado típico da estenose aórtica grave.
  p. quadrigem'inus, p. quadrigêmeo. SIN quadrigeminal pulse.
  p. respiratio'ne intermit'tens, p. paradoxal. SIN paradoxic pulse.
  p. tar'dus, p. tardo; p. com ascensão patologicamente gradual, típico da estenose aórtica grave. VER TAMBÉM p. plateau pulse.
  p. trem'ulus, p. trêmulo; pulso fraco e trêmulo.
  p. trigem'inus, p. trigeminal. SIN trigeminal pulse.
  p. vac'uus, p. vazio; p. muito fraco, que mal distende a parede arterial.
  p. veno'sus, p. venoso. SIN venous pulse.
pul·ta·ceous (pŭl-ta′shŭs). Pultáceo; macerado; semelhante a papa. [G. *poltos*, papa]
pul·ver·i·za·tion (pŭl′ver-i-za′shŭn). Pulverização; redução a pó.
pul·ver·ize (pŭl′ver-iz). Pulverizar; reduzir a pó. [L. *pulverizo*, de *pulvis*, *pulveris*, pó]
pul·ver·u·lent (pŭl-ver′u-lent). Pulverulento; em um estado de pó; pulveroso.
pul·vi·nar (pŭl-vi′nar). Pulvinar; a extremidade posterior expandida do tálamo que forma uma proeminência, semelhante a um coxim, sobre os corpos geniculados. Essa estrutura, denominada núcleos pulvinares [TA] (pulvinar nuclei [TA]), é um grupo celular composto, que consiste nos núcleos anterior, inferior, lateral e medial. [L. sofá feito de almofadas, de *pulvinus*, almofada]
pul·vi·nate (pŭl′vi-nat). Pulvinado; elevado ou convexo, que designa uma forma de elevação da superfície de uma cultura bacteriana. [L. *pulvinus*, almofada]
pum·ice (pŭm′is). Pedra-pomes; cinzas vulcânicas moídas em partículas de vários tamanhos; usada em odontologia para polir restaurações ou dentes; um abrasivo. [L. *pumex* (*pumic*-), uma pedra-pomes]
pump (pŭmp). Bomba. **1.** Aparelho para forçar a saída ou entrada de gás ou líquido em qualquer parte. **2.** Qualquer mecanismo para utilizar energia metabólica a fim de realizar transporte ativo de uma substância.
  breast p., b. mamária; dispositivo de sucção para retirar leite da mama.
  calcium p., b. de cálcio; proteína da membrana que consegue transportar íons cálcio através da membrana utilizando energia do ATP.
  calf p., b. da panturrilha; atividade muscular da panturrilha que promove fluxo venoso para o coração.
  Carrel-Lindbergh p., b. de Carrel-Lindbergh; dispositivo de perfusão destinado ao uso em culturas de órgãos completos.

constant infusion p., b. de infusão contínua; dispositivo elétrico para administração, a partir de um reservatório, de um volume constante, freqüentemente muito pequeno, de solução durante um longo período.

dental p., ejetor de saliva. SIN saliva *ejector*.

hydrogen p., b. de hidrogênio; mecanismo molecular para secreção de ácido pelas células parietais gástricas com base na atividade de uma H^+-K^+-ATPase.

intraaortic balloon p., b. com balão intra-aórtico; balão inflável, acionado externa e intermitentemente, colocado na aorta descendente, que, ao ser ativado durante a diástole, aumenta a pressão sanguínea e a perfusão do órgão por sua força pulsátil; depois, ao ser esvaziado, diminui o trabalho cardíaco em cada sístole — o denominado princípio da contrapulsação — por reduzir a pós-carga cardíaca.

ion p., b. iônica; complexo de proteínas da membrana, capaz de transportar íons contra um gradiente de concentração utilizando a energia do ATP.

jet ejector p., b. de ejetor a jato; b. de sucção na qual o líquido sob alta pressão é forçado através de um bico para dentro de um tubo abruptamente maior, onde um jato de alta velocidade, a baixa pressão, de acordo com a lei de Bernoulli, arrasta gás ou líquido da abertura de um tubo lateral, imediatamente após a extremidade do bico para criar sucção; p. ex., a bomba pela qual se emprega o vapor para evacuar uma autoclave, um aspirador de água.

proton p., b. de prótons; mecanismo molecular para o transporte final de prótons através de uma membrana; geralmente envolve a atividade de uma ATPase.

saliva p., ejetor de saliva. SIN saliva *ejector*.

sodium p., b. de sódio; mecanismo biológico que emprega energia metabólica do ATP para obter transporte ativo de sódio através de uma membrana; as bombas de sódio expelem sódio da maioria das células do corpo, algumas vezes associado ao transporte de outras substâncias, e também servem para deslocar sódio através de membranas multicelulares, como as paredes do túbulo renal.

sodium-potassium p., b. de sódio–potássio; transportador ligado à membrana, encontrado em quase todas as células de mamíferos, que transporta íons potássio do líquido extracelular para o citoplasma e, simultaneamente, íons sódio do citoplasma para o líquido extracelular. A bomba transporta ambos os íons contra grandes gradientes de potencial eletroquímico e mantém a concentração de potássio do citoplasma muito acima e a concentração de sódio muito abaixo de seus níveis extracelulares. A b. é uma enzima que transporta dois íons potássio em troca de três íons sódio em uma reação induzida por hidrólise de uma molécula de ATP para formar ADP mais um íon fosfato inorgânico.

stomach p., b. gástrica; aparelho para remover o conteúdo gástrico por meio de sucção.

pump·ox·y·gen·a·tor (pŭmp-ok′si-je-nā′ter). Oxigenador de bomba; aparelho mecânico que pode substituir o coração (bomba) e os pulmões (oxigenador) durante cirurgia cardíaca a céu aberto.

pu·na (poo′nä). Doença das alturas. SIN altitude *sickness*. [Esp., de Quechua *puna*, um planalto alto e seco nos Andes]

punch (pŭnch). Saca-bocado; instrumento para fazer um orifício ou entalhe em algum material sólido ou para retirar um corpo estranho desse material. [L. *pungo*, pp. *punctus*, espetar, puncionar]

punch card. Cartão perfurado; um cartão em que são armazenados dados por meio de orifícios em posições específicas, de forma que os dados possam ser classificados, processados e analisados.

punch·drunk (pŭnch′drŭnk). Aturdido. VER punchdrunk *syndrome*.

punc·ta (pŭngk′tä). Pontos; plural de punctum. [L.]

punc·tate (pŭngk′tāt). Pontilhado; caracterizado por pontos diferenciados da superfície adjacente pela cor, elevação ou textura. [L. *punctum*, ponto]

punc·ti·form (pŭngk′ti-fōrm). Puntiforme; muito pequeno, mas não microscópico, com diâmetro menor que 1 mm. [L. *punctum*, ponto, + *forma*, formato]

punc·tum, gen. **punc·ti,** pl. **punc·ta** (pŭngk′tŭm,-tī,-tä) [TA]. Ponto. **1.** A extremidade de um prolongamento pontiagudo. **2.** Uma mancha minúscula redonda, diferente, na cor ou em outro aspecto, dos tecidos adjacentes. **3.** Ponto no eixo óptico de um sistema óptico. SIN point (1). VER TAMBÉM point, tip, end, center. [L. ponto, pp. neutro de *pungo*, espetar, usado como substantivo]

p. ce'cum, p. cego; o p. cego no campo visual correspondente à localização do disco óptico.

p. coxa'le, p. coxal; o p. mais alto da crista do ílio.

p. doloro'sum, p. doloroso. VER Valleix *points*, em *point*.

p. fixa [TA], p. fixo. SIN fixed *end*.

kissing puncta, condição na qual o p. superior está aposto ao p. inferior quando os olhos estão abertos.

lacrimal p. [TA], p. lacrimal; a pequena abertura circular do canalículo lacrimal, na margem de cada pálpebra próximo da comissura medial. SIN p. lacrimale [TA], lacrimal opening.

p. lacrima'le [TA], p. lacrimal. SIN lacrimal p.

p. lu'teum, mácula lútea da retina. SIN *macula* of retina.

p. mobile [TA], p. móvel. SIN mobile *end*.

p. ossificatio'nis, centro de ossificação. SIN ossification *center*.

p. ossificatio'nis prima'rium, centro primário de ossificação. SIN primary ossification *center*.

p. ossificatio'nis secunda'rium, centro secundário de ossificação. SIN secondary ossification *center*.

p. prox'imum (P.p.), p. próximo. SIN near *point*.

p. remo'tum (P.r.), p. remoto. SIN far *point*.

p. vasculo'sum, um dos pequenos pontos observados ao corte do cérebro, devido a pequenas gotas de sangue nas extremidades seccionadas das artérias.

punc.ture (pŭnk′choor). **1.** Puncionar; fazer um orifício com um pequeno objeto pontiagudo, como uma agulha. **2.** Punção; perfuração ou pequeno orifício feito com um instrumento pontiagudo. [L. *punctura*, de *pungo*, pp. *punctus*, puncionar]

Bernard p., punção de Bernard. SIN diabetic p.

cisternal p., punção da cisterna; introdução de uma agulha oca através da membrana atlantooccipital posterior até a cisterna cerebelobulbar (cerebellomedullary *cistern*).

diabetic p., punção diabética; punção em um ponto no assoalho do quarto ventrículo do encéfalo que causa glicosúria. SIN Bernard p.

lumbar p., p. lombar; punção do espaço subaracnóide da região lombar para retirar líquido cerebrospinal para diagnóstico ou tratamento. SIN Quincke p., rachicentesis, rachiocentesis, spinal p., spinal tap.

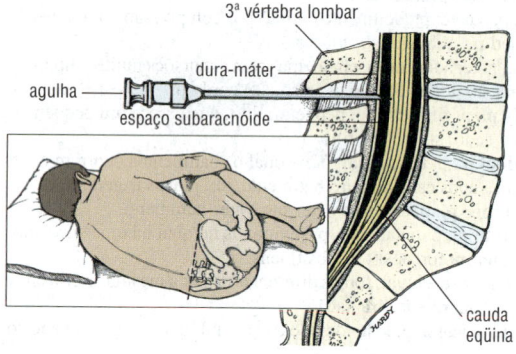

punção lombar: técnica

Quincke p., punção de Quincke. SIN lumbar p.

spinal p., punção lombar. SIN lumbar p.

sternal p., punção esternal; remoção de medula óssea do manúbrio por agulha.

tracheoesophageal p., punção traqueoesofágica; procedimento cirúrgico para restaurar a função vocal em pacientes submetidos a laringectomia, pela criação de uma fístula traqueoesofágica através da qual o paciente laringectomizado força a passagem de ar da traquéia para o esôfago a fim de produzir som, que é articulado em fala.

pun·gent (pŭn′jent). Pungente; agudo; diz-se do sabor ou odor de uma substância. [L. *pungo*, p. pres. *-ens* (*-ent-*), penetrar]

PUO Abreviatura de pyrexia of unknown (or uncertain) origen (pirexia de origem indeterminada [ou incerta]), termo aplicado a doença febril antes do estabelecimento do diagnóstico; também denominada FUO (fever of unknown origin) [febre de origem desconhecida]

pu·pa, pl. **pu·pae** (pū′pä, -pē). Pupa; o estágio de metamorfose de insetos após a larva e anterior ao imago. VER TAMBÉM complete *metamorphosis*. [L. *pupa*, boneca]

pu·pil (p) (pū′pĭl) [TA]. Pupila; o orifício circular no centro da íris, através do qual os raios luminosos entram no olho. SIN pupilla [TA]. [L. *pupilla*]

Adie p., p. de Adie. SIN Adie *syndrome*.

amaurotic p., p. amaurótica; p. em um olho que está cego devido a doença ocular ou do nervo óptico; essa pupila não se contrai exposta à luz, exceto quando o outro olho normal é estimulado pela luz.

Argyll Robertson p., p. de Argyll Robertson; forma de iridoplegia reflexa caracterizada por miose, formato irregular e perda dos reflexos pupilares direto e consensual à luz, com constrição pupilar normal em resposta a um esforço de convergência (dissociação luz-perto); freqüentemente presente na neurossífilis tabética. SIN Robertson p.

artificial p., p. artificial; abertura feita por excisão de uma parte da íris a fim de melhorar a visão em casos de opacidade central da córnea ou lente.

Bumke p., p. de Bumke; dilatação da p. em resposta à ansiedade ou a outros estímulos psíquicos.

catatonic p., p. catatônica; dilatação pupilar transitória associada a ausência de reação pupilar à luz e convergência.

cat's-eye p., p. de gato; p. distorcida, alongada; geralmente causada por anomalia do segmento anterior.
fixed p., p. fixa; p. estacionária que não responde a estímulos.
Gunn p., p. de Gunn. SIN Marcus Gunn p.
Holmes-Adie p., p. de Holmes-Adie. SIN Adie *syndrome*.
Horner p., p. de Horner; p. contraída em virtude de comprometimento da inervação simpática do músculo dilatador da pupila. VER TAMBÉM Horner *syndrome*.
Hutchinson p., p. de Hutchinson; dilatação da p. no lado da lesão como parte de paralisia do terceiro nervo; freqüentemente causada por herniação do úncus do lobo temporal através da incisura do tentório.
keyhole p., p. com um coloboma.
Marcus Gunn p., p. de Marcus Gunn; defeito pupilar aferente relativo (relative afferent *pupillary* defect). SIN Gunn p.
paradoxical p., p. paradoxal. VER paradoxical pupillary *reflex*.
pinhole p., p. puntiforme; pupila extremamente contraída.
Robertson p., p. de Robertson. SIN Argyll Robertson p.
seclusion of p. (se-kloo'zhŭn), seclusão pupilar; a condição resultante de sinéquias anulares posteriores, na qual a íris é limitada em toda a margem pupilar, mas a p. não é ocluída. SIN exclusion of pupil.
tadpole-shaped p., p. em forma de girino; distorção e dilatação breves e intermitentes da p., que fazem com que uma parte da íris forme um pico, de forma que a pupila assemelha-se a um girino; uma condição benigna, temporária, associada à enxaqueca, que pode deixar o paciente com síndrome de Horner.
tonic p., p. tônica; termo geral para designar uma p. com contrações tardias, lentas, de longa duração em resposta à luz e a um esforço de convergência, freqüentemente com dissociação luz-perto; causada por desnervação e reinervação anômala do esfíncter da íris; observada em várias neuropatias autônomas e na síndrome de Adie (Adie *syndrome*).
pu·pil·la, pl. **pu·pil·lae** (pū-pil'ă, pū-pil'ē) [TA]. Pupila. SIN pupil. [L. dim. de *pupa*, uma menina ou boneca]
pu·pil·lary (pū'pi-lār-ē). Relativo à pupila.
 p. light-near dissociation, dissociação pupilar luz-perto; uma resposta mais intensa da p. à convergência que à luz; causada por fracos impulsos pupilomotores, pupila de Argyll-Robertson (Argyll-Robertson *pupil*), síndrome mesencefálica dorsal ou à orientação errada das fibras do músculo ciliar para o esfíncter da íris. SIN light-near dissociation.
 relative afferent p. defect, defeito pupilar aferente relativo; uma assimetria dos impulsos pupilomotores entre os dois olhos; testado alternando-se a luz de um olho para o outro e comparando-se as reações à luz direta.
pupillo-. Pupilo-; as pupilas. [L. *pupilla*, pupila]
pu·pil·log·ra·phy (pū'pi-log'ră-fē). Pupilografia; o registro das reações pupilares. [pupillo- + G. *graphō*, escrever]
pu·pil·lom·e·ter (pū'pi-lom'ĕ-ter). Pupilômetro; instrumento para medir e registrar o diâmetro da pupila. [pupillo- + G. *metron*, medida]
pu·pil·lom·e·try (pū'pi-lom'ĕ-trē). Pupilometria; medida da pupila.
pu·pil·lo·mo·tor (pū'pi-lō-mō'ter). Pupilomotor; relativo às fibras nervosas autônomas que suprem o músculo liso da íris. SIN iridomotor. [pupillo- + L. *motor*, motor]
pu·pil·lo·sta·tom·e·ter (pū'pi-lō-stă-tom'ĕ-ter). Pupiloestatômetro; aparelho para medir a distância entre os centros das pupilas. [pupillo- + G. *statos*, colocado, + *metron*, medida]
pu·pip·a·rous (pū-pip'ă-rŭs). Pupíparo; que transporta pupas; designa os insetos dos quais nascem larvas em estágio final, que já passaram seu desenvolvimento no corpo da fêmea, como ocorre nas moscas das famílias Hippoboscidae e Glossinidae (moscas tsé-tsé). [pupa + L. *pario*, parir]
PUPPP Acrônimo de *pruritic urticarial papules and plaques of pregnancy* (pápulas e placas urticariais pruriginosas da gravidez), erupção muito pruriginosa, ocasionalmente vesicular, que surge no terceiro trimestre da gravidez, sem efeito sobre o feto; há involução espontânea em 10 dias após o termo, e a recorrência é rara em gestações subseqüentes. A microscopia por imunofluorescência da lesão negativa ajuda a excluir herpes gestacional.
Pur Abreviatura de purine (purina).
pure (pūr). Puro; inalterado; livre de mistura ou contaminação por qualquer substância estranha. [L. *purus*]
pur·ga·tion (per-gā'shŭn). Purgação; evacuação do intestino com a ajuda de um purgante ou catártico. SIN catharsis (1). [L. *purgatio*]
pur·ga·tive (per'gă-tiv). Purgativo; agente usado para purgação do intestino. VER TAMBÉM cathartic (2). [L. *purgativus*, purgativo]
 saline p., p. salino; sal de Epsom, sal de Rochelle ou qualquer sal que tenha propriedades purgativas.
purge (perj). **1.** Purgar; causar evacuação copiosa do intestino. **2.** Purgativo; um medicamento catártico. [L. *purgo*, limpar, de *purus*, puro, + *ago*, fazer]
purg·ing cas·sia (perj'ing kash'yă). Cássia purgativa. SIN cassia fistula.
pu·ri·form (pū'ri-fōrm). Puriforme; semelhante ao pus. [L. *pus* (*pur*-), pus, + *forma*, forma]
pu·rine (Pur) (pūr'ēn, -rin). Purina; a substância original da adenina, guanina e outras "bases" purinas que ocorrem naturalmente; não se conhece sua existência como tal em mamíferos.
 p.-nucleoside phosphorylase, p.-nucleosídeo fosforilase; ribosiltransferase que catalisa reversivelmente a fosforólise de um nucleosídeo purina com ortofosfato para produzir uma purina e α-D-ribose 1-fosfato; a deficiência hereditária dessa enzima causa imunodeficiência celular.
 p. ribonucleoside, p. ribonucleosídeo. SIN nebularine.
pu·ri·ne·mia (pū-ri-nē'mē-ă). Purinemia; a presença de bases purina ou xantina no sangue circulante. [purine + G. *haima*, sangue]
pu·ri·ty (pūr'i-tē). Pureza; o estado de ser puro, livre de contaminantes ou poluentes. [L. *puritas*, de *purus*, limpo, imaculado]
 radiochemical p., p. radioquímica; a proporção da atividade total de um radionuclídeo específico em uma forma química ou biológica específica.
 radioisotopic p., p. radioisotópica; termo livre comumente usado para designar a pureza radionuclídica.
 radionuclidic p., p. radionuclídica; a proporção da radioatividade total que existe como um radionuclídeo específico.
 radiopharmaceutical p., p. radiofarmacêutica; a esterilidade e apirogenicidade de um marcador radioativo para uso humano.
Purkinje, Johannes E. von (Jan E. Purkyne), anatomista e fisiologista da Boêmia, 1787–1869. VER P. *conduction, images,* em *image, shift*; subendocardial conducting *system* of heart; P. *cells,* em *cell, corpuscles,* em *corpuscle, fibers,* em *fiber, figures,* em *figure, cell layer, network, phenomenon;* P.-Sanson *images,* em *image*.
Purmann, Matthaeus G., cirurgião alemão, 1649–1721. VER P. *method*.
pu·ro·mu·cous (pū-rō-mū'kŭs). Mucopurulento. SIN mucopurulent. [L. *pus* (*pur*-), pus, + *mucus,* muco]
pu·ro·my·cin (pū-rō-mī'sin). Puromicina; antibiótico produzido pelo crescimento de *Streptomyces alboniger*; usado antigamente no tratamento da amebíase e da tripanossomíase.
pur·ple (per'pl). Púrpura; cor formada por uma mistura de azul e vermelho. Quanto a corantes púrpura individuais, ver nome específico. [L. *purpura*]
 visual p., p. visual, rodopsina. SIN rhodopsin.
pur·pu·ra (pūr'pu-ră). Púrpura; condição caracterizada por hemorragia cutânea. O aspecto das lesões varia com o tipo de púrpura, duração das lesões e intensidade do início. Primeiro, a cor é vermelha, escurece gradualmente até o púrpura, esmaece para um amarelo-acastanhado e, geralmente, desaparece em 2 ou 3 semanas; a cor da pigmentação permanente residual depende principalmente do tipo de pigmento não absorvido do sangue extravasado; também pode haver extravasamentos para as mucosas e órgãos internos. SIN peliosis. [L. do G. *porphyra*, púrpura]
 allergic p., p. alérgica; p. não-trombocitopênica causada por sensibilização a alimentos, fármacos e picadas de insetos. SIN anaphylactoid p. (1).
 anaphylactoid p., p. anafilactóide; **(1)** SIN allergic p.; **(2)** SIN Henoch-Schönlein p.
 p. angioneurot'ica, p. angioneurótica; erupção caracterizada por edema angioneurótico, petéquias e hiperestesia da pele e da mucosa gástrica.
 p. annula'ris telangiecto'des, p. anular telangiectóide; lesões anulares assintomáticas, principalmente nos membros inferiores de meninos adolescentes, nas quais a porção periférica é composta de p. ou petéquias com coloração forte por depósitos de hemossiderina e telangiectasias diminutas.
 factitious p., p. fictícia; equimoses auto-induzidas, freqüentemente dolorosas.
 fibrinolytic p., p. fibrinolítica; p. na qual a hemorragia está associada a rápida fibrinólise do coágulo.
 p. ful'minans, p. fulminante; forma grave e rapidamente fatal de p. hemorrágica, que ocorre principalmente em crianças, com hipotensão, febre e coagulação intravascular disseminada, em geral após uma doença infecciosa.
 Henoch p., p. de Henoch. SIN Henoch-Schönlein p.
 Henoch-Schönlein p., p. de Henoch-Schönlein; erupção de lesões purpúricas palpáveis, não-trombocitopênicas, causadas por vasculite leucocitoclástica dérmica com deposição de IgA nas paredes dos vasos, associada a dor e edema articular, cólica e eliminação de fezes com sangue, ocorrendo caracteristicamente em crianças pequenas. A glomerulonefrite pode ocorrer durante um episódio inicial ou mais tarde. SIN anaphylactoid p. (2), Henoch p., Henoch-Schönlein syndrome, p. rheumatica, Schönlein p., Schönlein-Henoch syndrome.
 hyperglobulinemic p., p. hiperglobulinêmica. SIN Waldenström *macroglobulinemia*.
 idiopathic thrombocytopenic p. (ITP), p. trombocitopênica idiopática; doença sistêmica caracterizada por extensas equimoses e hemorragias das mucosas e número muito baixo de plaquetas; resultante da destruição plaquetária por macrófagos devido a um fator antiplaquetário; em geral, os casos infantis são breves e raramente apresentam-se com hemorragias intracranianas, mas os casos em adultos freqüentemente são recorrentes e possuem uma maior incidência de hemorragia grave, principalmente intracraniana. SIN immune thrombocytopenic p., thrombopenic p.
 immune thrombocytopenic p., p. trombocitopênica imune. SIN idiopathic thrombocytopenic p.
 nonthrombocytopenic p., p. não-trombocitopênica. SIN p. simplex.
 psychogenic p., p. psicogênica; condição psicossomática semelhante à síndrome de auto-sensibilização eritrocitária.

p. pu'licans, p. pulico'sa, p. pulicosa; petéquias causadas pelas picadas de insetos e parasitas animais.
p. rheumat'ica, p. reumática. SIN Henoch-Schönlein p.
Schönlein p., p. de Schönlein. SIN Henoch-Schönlein p.
p. seni'lis, p. senil; a ocorrência de petéquias e equimoses na pele atrófica das pernas em pessoas idosas e debilitadas.
p. sim'plex, p. simples; a erupção de petéquias ou equimoses maiores, geralmente não acompanhada por manifestações constitucionais e não associada a doença sistêmica. SIN nonthrombocytopenic p.
p. symptomat'ica, p. sintomática; erupção petequial na escarlatina e em outros exantemas.
thrombocytopenic p., p. trombocitopênica. VER idiopathic thrombocytopenic p.
thrombopenic p., p. trombopênica. SIN idiopathic thrombocytopenic p.
thrombotic thrombocytopenic p., p. trombocitopênica trombótica; doença rapidamente fatal ou ocasionalmente prolongada, com várias manifestações além da púrpura, incluindo sinais de envolvimento do sistema nervoso central, causada pela formação de trombos de fibrina ou plaquetas nas arteríolas e capilares em muitos órgãos.
p. urti'cans, p. urticante; p. simples acompanhada por uma erupção urticariana.
Waldenström p., p. de Waldenström. SIN Waldenström *macroglobulinemia.*
pur·pu·rea gly·co·sides A, pur·pu·rea gly·co·sides B (per'pū - rē'ă glī'kō - sidz). Glicosídeos purpúricos A e B; os glicosídeos precursores cardioativos da *Digitalis purpurea;* são estruturalmente idênticos aos desacetillanatosídeos A e B, respectivamente. VER TAMBÉM lanatosides A, B and C.
pur·pu·ric (pŭr - poo'rik). Purpúrico; relativo a ou afetado por púrpura.
pur·pu·rin (per'pū - rin). Purpurina. **1.** SIN uroerythrin. **2.** Um corante violeta relacionado à alizarina pela adição de um grupamento 4-OH à alizarina; encontrado na raiz da ruiva e de outros membros da *Rubiaceae;* usada para detectar sais de cálcio, boro e como corante histológico. SIN alizarin purpurin.
pur·pu·ri·nu·ria (per'pū - ri - noo'rē - ă). Purpurinúria. SIN porphyrinuria.
purr (per). Ronronar; um sopro vibratório baixo.
Purtscher, Otmar, oftalmologista alemão, 1852–1927. VER P. *disease.*
pu·ru·lence, pu·ru·len·cy (pūr'ŭ - lens, - len - sē; pūr'ŭ - lens). Purulência; a condição de conter ou formar pus. [L. *purulenta,* supuração, de *pus (pur-),* pus]
pu·ru·lent (pūr'ŭ - lent, pūr'ŭ -). Purulento; que contém, consiste em ou forma pus.
pu·ru·loid (pū'rŭ - loyd). Purulóide; semelhante a pus.
pus (pŭs). Pus; produto líquido da inflamação, consistindo em um líquido contendo leucócitos e os resíduos de células mortas e elementos teciduais liquefeitos pelas enzimas proteolíticas e histolíticas (p. ex., leucoprotease) produzidas por leucócitos polimorfonucleares. [L.]
blue p., p. azul; p. tingido com piocianina, um produto da *Pseudomonas aeruginosa.*
cheesy p., p. caseoso; p. muito espesso, quase sólido, resultante da absorção da parte líquida do pus.
curdy p., p. coagulado; p. que contém flocos de material caseoso.
green p., p. verde; p. azul quando, como acontece algumas vezes, tem mais de um matiz verde.
ichorous p., p. icoroso; p. fino, contendo restos de tecido esfacelado, algumas vezes com odor fétido.
laudable p., p. louvável; termo obsoleto usado quando era considerado improvável que a supuração causasse piemia (intoxicação sanguínea), mas provável que permanecesse localizada.
sanious p., p. sanioso; p. icoroso tinto de sangue.
pus·tu·lant (pŭs'choo - lant). Pustulante. **1.** Que causa uma erupção pustular. **2.** Um agente que produz pústulas.
pus·tu·lar (pŭs'choo - lăr). Pustular; relativo a, ou caracterizado por, pústulas.
pus·tu·la·tion (pŭs'choo - lā'shŭn). Pustulação; a formação ou a presença de pústulas.
pus·tule (pŭs'chool). Pústula; elevação superficial, circunscrita da pele, com até 1,0 cm de diâmetro, contendo material purulento. [L. *pustula*]
malignant p., antraz cutâneo. SIN cutaneous *anthrax.*
spongiform p. of Kogoj, p. espongiforme de Kogoj; p. epidérmica formada por infiltração de neutrófilos na epiderme necrótica, na qual as paredes celulares persistem como uma rede espongiforme; observada na psoríase pustular.
pus·tu·lo·crus·ta·ceous (pŭs'choo - lō - krŭs - tā'shŭs). Pustulocrustáceo, pustulocrustoso; caracterizado por pústulas crostosas com pus seco.
pus·tu·lo·sis (pŭs - choo - lō'sis). Pustulose. **1.** Uma erupção de pústulas. **2.** Termo ocasionalmente usado para designar acropustulose. [L. *pustula,* pústula, + G. *-osis,* condição]
p. palmar'is et plantar'is, p. palmar e plantar; erupção pustular estéril nos dedos das mãos e dos pés, variavelmente atribuída à disidrose, psoríase pustular e infecção bacteriana não identificada. SIN acrodermatitis continua, acrodermatitis perstans, dermatitis repens.
p. vaccinifor'mis acu'ta, p. vaciniforme aguda. SIN *eczema* herpeticum.

pu·ta·men (pū - tā'men) [TA]. Putame; a porção mais externa, maior e de cor cinza mais escura das três em que é dividido o núcleo lentiforme por lâminas de fibras brancas; é unido ao núcleo caudado por faixas interpostas de substância cinzenta que penetram na cápsula interna. Sua estrutura histológica é semelhante à do núcleo caudado, junto com o qual compõe o estriado. VER TAMBÉM striate *body,* lenticular *nucleus.* [L. aquilo que se desprende na poda, de *puto,* podar]
Putnam, James J., neurologista norte-americano, 1846–1918. VER P.-Dana *syndrome.*
pu·tre·fac·tion (pū - tri - fak'shŭn). Putrefação; decomposição ou apodrecimento, a decomposição da matéria orgânica, geralmente por ação bacteriana, resultando na formação de outras substâncias de constituição menos complexa, com a evolução de amônia ou seus derivados e sulfeto de hidrogênio; geralmente caracterizada pela presença de produtos tóxicos ou fétidos. SIN decay (2), decomposition. [L. *putre-facio,* pp. *-factus,* apodrecer]
pu·tre·fac·tive (pū - tri - fak'tiv). Putrefativo; relativo à putrefação ou que a causa.
pu·tre·fy (pū'tri - fī). Putrefazer; tornar podre ou deteriorar-se.
pu·tres·cence (pū - tres'ens). Putrescência; o estado de putrefação.
pu·tres·cent (pū - tres'ent). Putrescente; indicativo ou no processo de putrefação. [L. *putresco,* apodrecer, de *puter,* podre]
pu·tres·cine (pū - tres'ēn). Putrescina; 1,4-diaminobutano; uma poliamina venenosa formada a partir do aminoácido arginina durante a putrefação; encontrada na urina e nas fezes; em algumas células, a putrescina é um precursor do γ-aminobutirato.
pu·trid (pū'trid). Pútrido. **1.** Em estado de putrefação. **2.** Designa putrefação. [L. *putridus*]
Putti, Vittorio, cirurgião italiano, 1880–1940. VER P.-Platt *operation, procedure.*
PUVA Acrônimo para administração oral de *p*soralen e subseqüente exposição à luz *u*ltravioleta de comprimento de onda longo (*uv-a*); usado no tratamento da psoríase.
PVC Abreviatura de polyvinyl chloride (cloreto de polivinil).
PVP Abreviatura de polyvinylpyrrolidone (polivinilpirrolidona).
PVS Abreviatura de persistent vegetative *state* (estado vegetativo persistente).
PWM Abreviatura de pokeweed *mitogen* (mitógeno de erva-dos-cancros).
py·ar·thro·sis (pī - ar - thrō'sis). Piartrose. SIN suppurative *arthritis.* [G. *pyon,* pus, + *arthrōsis,* articulação]
pycno-. VER pykno-.
pyel-. VER pyelo-.
py·e·lec·ta·sis, py·e·lec·ta·sia (pī - ē - lek'tă - sis, pī - ē - lek - tā'zē - ă). Pielectasia; dilatação da pelve renal. [pyel- + G. *ektasis,* extensão]
py·e·lit·ic (pī - ē - lit'ik). Pielítico; relativo à pielite.
py·e·li·tis (pī - ē - lī'tis). Pielite; inflamação da pelve renal. [pyel- + G. *-itis,* inflamação]
pyelo-, pyel-. Pielo; pelve, em geral a pelve renal. [G. *pyelos,* cuba, tina, tanque]
py·e·lo·cal·i·ce·al (pī'ē - lō - kal'i - sē'ăl). Pielocalicial; relativo à pelve renal e aos cálices. SIN pyelocalyceal
py·e·lo·cal·i·ec·ta·sis (pī'ē - lō - kal'ē - ek'tă - sis). Pielocaliectasia. SIN caliectasis.
py·e·lo·cal·y·ce·al (pī - ē - lō - kal'i - sē - ăl). Pielocalicial. SIN pyelocaliceal.
py·e·lo·cys·ti·tis (pī - ē - lō - sis - tī'tis). Pielocistite; inflamação da pelve renal e da bexiga. [pyelo- + G. *kystis,* bexiga, + *-itis,* inflamação]
py·e·lo·flu·o·ros·co·py (pī'ē - lō - flōr - os'kŏ - pē). Pielofluoroscopia; exame fluoroscópico das pelves renais e dos ureteres após a administração de contraste. [pyelo- + L. *fluo,* fluir, + G. *skopeō,* ver]
py·el·o·gram (pī'el - ō - gram). Pielograma; radiografia ou série de radiografias (seriografia) da pelve renal e do ureter, após a injeção de contraste.
py·e·log·ra·phy (pī'ē - log'ră - fē). Pielografia; estudo radiológico do rim, dos ureteres e geralmente da bexiga, realizado com ajuda de um contraste injetado por via intravenosa, ou diretamente através de um cateter ureteral ou de nefrostomia, ou por via percutânea. SIN pelviureterography, pyeloureterography, ureteropyelography. [pyelo- + G. *graphō,* escrever]
antegrade p., p. anterógrada; urografia anterógrada na qual o contraste é injetado nos cálices ou na pelve renal.
intravenous p. (IVP), p. intravenosa; nome antigo da urografia intravenosa (intravenous *urography*).
retrograde p., p. retrógrada; p. na qual o contraste é injetado nos ureteres a partir de um endoscópio na bexiga.
py·e·lo·lith·ot·o·my (pī'ē - lō - li - thot'ō - mē). Pielolitotomia; remoção cirúrgica de um cálculo renal através de uma incisão na pelve renal. SIN pelvilithotomy, pelviolithotomy. [pyelo- + G. *lithos,* cálculo, + *tomē,* incisão]
py·e·lo·lym·phat·ic (pī'ē - lō - lim - fat'ik). Pielolinfático; relativo aos vasos linfáticos da pelve renal.
py·e·lo·ne·phri·tis (pī'ē - lō - ne - frī'tis). Pielonefrite; inflamação do parênquima, cálices e pelve renal, sobretudo a causada por infecção bacteriana local. [pyelo- + G. *nephros,* rim, + *-itis,* inflamação]

pyelonephritis | 1323 | pyknoepilepsy, pyknolepsy

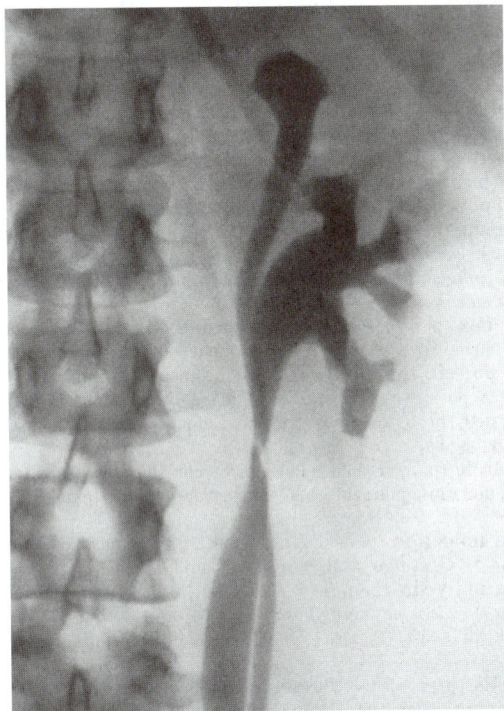

pielografia (urografia anterógrada): pielografia pós-parto de paciente com pielonefrite gravídica exibindo reduplicação da pelve renal e do ureter esquerdos

acute p., p. aguda; inflamação aguda do parênquima e da pelve renais, caracterizada por pequenos abscessos corticais e estrias amareladas na medula decorrentes da existência de pus nos túbulos coletores e no tecido intersticial.
ascending p., p. ascendente; p. causada por infecção bacteriana das vias urinárias inferiores, particularmente por refluxo de urina infectada.
chronic p., p. crônica; inflamação crônica do parênquima e da pelve renais, resultante de infecção bacteriana, caracterizada por deformidades dos cálices e por grandes cicatrizes renais planas sobrejacentes, com distribuição segmentar.
xanthogranulomatous p., p. xantogranulomatosa; condição inflamatória crônica que acomete difusamente todo o rim, e geralmente resultando em grande aumento e ausência de função do rim, que, macroscopicamente, pode assemelhar-se a uma neoplasia ou tuberculose; histologicamente, é caracterizada por uma reação inflamatória com numerosos histiócitos espumosos, cheios de lipídios, misturados a linfócitos e plasmócitos, formando múltiplos granulomas.
py·e·lo·ne·phro·sis (pī′e-lō-ne-frō′sis). Pielonefrose; designação obsoleta dada a qualquer doença da pelve renal. [pyelo- + G. *nephros*, rim, + *-osis*, condição]
py·e·lo·plas·ty (pī′e-lō-plas-tē). Pieloplastia; reconstrução cirúrgica da pelve renal e do ureter para corrigir obstrução na junção ureteropélvica. SIN pelvioplasty. [pyelo- + G. *plastos*, formado]
  capsular flap p., p. com retalho capsular; procedimento reconstrutivo para correção de obstrução ureteropélvica, segundo o qual um retalho de cápsula renal é girado para baixo, a partir do hilo renal, a fim de aumentar a pelve intra-renal e a parte superior do ureter obstruída; usada para corrigir situações que envolvem a perda do tecido pélvico renal e, assim, que impedem o uso da pelve renal para a reconstrução.
  Culp p., p. de Culp; uma técnica de reconstrução para correção de obstrução ureteropélvica, segundo a qual um retalho espiral de pelve renal é trazido para baixo e interposto em uma incisão vertical no ureter. VER TAMBÉM Scardino vertical flap p.
  disjoined p., dismembered p., p. desarticulada, p. desmembrada; procedimento reconstrutivo para correção de obstrução ureteropélvica, pelo qual o segmento obstruído é ressecado e a parte superior do ureter é reanastomosada na pelve renal inferior, em geral utilizando uma técnica de anastomose elíptica modificada.
  Foley Y-plasty p., p. pelo método de Y de Foley; procedimento de reconstrução para correção de obstrução ureteropélvica, pelo qual um retalho em V da pelve renal é levado para baixo até uma incisão vertical na porção superior do ureter, assim alargando a junção ureteropélvica.
  Scardino vertical flap p., p. com retalho vertical de Scardino; técnica de reconstrução para correção de obstrução ureteropélvica, pela qual um retalho vertical de pelve renal é levado para baixo e interposto em uma incisão vertical no ureter. Cf. Culp p.

py·e·lo·pli·ca·tion (pī′e-lō-pli-kā′shŭn). Pieloplicatura; procedimento obsoleto de preguear a parede da pelve renal quando indevidamente dilatada por hidronefrose. [pyelo- + L. *plico*, preguear]
py·e·los·co·py (pī-e-los′ko-pē). Pieloscopia; observação endoscópica ou fluoroscópica da pelve e dos cálices renais. [pyelo- + G. *skopeō*, ver]
py·e·los·to·my (pī-e-los′tō-mē). Pielostomia; formação de uma abertura na pelve renal para estabelecer drenagem urinária. [pyelo- + G. *stoma*, boca]
py·e·lot·o·my (pī-e-lot′ō-mē). Pielotomia; incisão da pelve renal. [pyelo- + G. *tomē*, incisão]
  extended p., p. estendida; extensão de uma p. padrão até o infundíbulo do pólo inferior, através do plano avascular entre as artérias renais segmentares basilar e posterior. SIN Gil-Vernet operation.
py·e·lo·u·re·ter·ec·ta·sis (pī′e-lō-ū-rē′ter-ek′tă-sis). Pieloureterectasia. SIN hydronephrosis. [pyelo- + ureter + G. *ektasis*, estiramento]
py·e·lo·u·re·ter·og·ra·phy (pī′e-lō-ū-rē′ter-og′ră-fē). Pieloureterografia. SIN pyelography.
py·e·lo·ve·nous (pī′e-lō-vē′nŭs). Pielovenoso; designa o fenômeno de drenagem da pelve renal para as veias renais por aumento da pressão intrapélvica. [pyelo- + venous]
py·em·e·sis (pī-em′e-sis). Piêmese; o vômito de pus. [G. *pyon*, pus, + *emesis*, vômito]
py·e·mia (pī-ē′mē-ă). Piemia; septicemia por microrganismos piogênicos causadores de múltiplos abscessos. SIN pyogenic fever. [G. *pyon*, pus, + *haima*, sangue]
  cryptogenic p., p. criptogênica; p. cuja origem não é evidente.
  portal p., p. porta; pileflebite supurativa.
py·e·mic (pī-ē′mik). Piêmico; relativo a, ou que sofre de, piemia.
Py·e·mo·tes tri·ti·ci (pī-e-mō′tēz tri-ti′kī,-sē). O ácaro da sarna da palha ou dos cereais, parasita comum de insetos que vivem em cereais armazenados e causa freqüente de sarna da palha ou dos cereais decorrente de suas picadas; não deve ser confundido com *P. t. ventricosus*, freqüentemente denominado ácaro da sarna da palha, que está associado ao besouro que vive nos móveis *Anobium punctatum* e é inofensivo para os seres humanos. SIN *Pediculoides ventricosus*.
py·en·ceph·a·lus (pī-en-sef′ă-lŭs). Piencéfalo. SIN pyocephalus. [G. *pyon*, pus, + *enkephalos*, encéfalo]
py·e·sis (pī-ē′sis). Piese. SIN suppuration. [G. *pyon*, pus, + *-esis*, condição ou processo]
⚠ **pyg-**. VER pygo-.
py·gal (pī′gal). Relativo às nádegas. [G. *pygē*, nádegas]
py·gal·gia (pī-gal′jē-ă). Pigalgia; termo raramente usado que significa dor nas nádegas. [pyg- + G. *algos*, dor]
pyg·ma·li·on·ism (pig-māl′yon-izm). Pigmalionismo; termo raramente usado para designar o estado de estar apaixonado por um objeto de sua própria criação. [Pigmaleão, personagem da mit. grega]
pyg·my (pig′mē). [MIM*265850]. Pigmeu; anão fisiológico com níveis séricos normais de hormônio do crescimento e somatomedina e refratariedade ao hormônio exógeno; principalmente aquele de uma raça de pessoas semelhantes, como os pigmeus da África Central. SIN pigmy. [G. *pygmaios*, nanismo, de *pygmē*, punho, também uma medida de comprimento do cotovelo até as articulações metacarpofalângicas]
⚠ **pygo-, pyg-**. Pigo-, pig-; as nádegas. [G. *pygē*]
py·go·a·mor·phus (pī′gō-ă-mōr′fŭs). Pigoamorfo; gêmeos conjugados em que o parasita, fixado às nádegas do autósito, é reduzido a uma massa amorfa ou embrioma. VER conjoined *twins*, em *twin*. [pygo- + G. *a-* priv. + *morphē*, forma]
py·go·did·y·mus (pī-gō-did′i-mŭs). Pigodídimo; gêmeos conjugados com uma única região cefalotorácica, mas com as nádegas e partes inferiores duplicadas. VER conjoined *twins*, em *twin*. VER TAMBÉM *duplicitas* posterior. [pygo- + G. *didymos*, gêmeo]
py·gom·e·lus (pī-gom′ē-lŭs). Pigômelo; gêmeos conjugados desiguais nos quais o parasita é representado por uma massa carnosa, ou por um membro mais desenvolvido, fixado à região sacral ou coccígea do autósito. VER conjoined *twins*, em *twin*. [pygo- + G. *melos*, parte]
py·gop·a·gus (pī-gop′ă-gŭs). Pigópago; gêmeos conjugados nos quais os dois indivíduos são unidos pelas nádegas, na maioria das vezes dorso com dorso. VER conjoined *twins*, em *twin*. [pygo- + G. *pagos*, algo fixo]
⚠ **pyk-**. VER pykno-.
pyk·nic (pik′nik). Pícnico; designa um tipo corporal constitucional caracterizado por contornos externos bem arredondados e cavidades corporais amplas; praticamente sinônimo de endomórfico. [G. *pyknos*, espesso]
⚠ **pykno-, pyk-**. Picno-, pic-; espesso, denso, compacto. [G. *pyknos*]
pyk·no·dys·os·to·sis (pik′nō-dis-os-tō′sis). Picnodisostose; condição caracterizada por baixa estatura, fechamento tardio das fontanelas e hipoplasia das falanges terminais. Herança autossômica recessiva. SIN osteopetrosis acroosteolytica. [pykno- + G. *dys-*, difícil, + *osteon*, osso, + *-osis*, condição]
pyk·no·ep·i·lep·sy, pyk·no·lep·sy (pik′nō-ep-i-lep-sē, pik′nō-lep-sē). Picnoepilepsia, picnolepsia; termos obsoletos para ausência. [pykno- + G. *lepsis*, convulsão]

pyk·no·lep·sy. Picnolepsia. SIN childhood absence epilepsy.

pyk·no·mor·phous (pik'nō-mōr'fŭs). Picnomorfo; designa uma célula ou tecido que se cora profundamente porque o material corável apresenta disposição compacta. [pykno- + G. *morphē*, forma]

pyk·no·phra·sia (pik'nō-frā'zē-ă). Picnofrasia; engrossamento da voz. [pykno- + G. *phrasis*, fala]

pyk·no·sis (pik-nō'sis). Picnose; espessamento ou condensação; especificamente, condensação e redução do tamanho da célula ou de seu núcleo, geralmente associada a hipercromatose; a picnose nuclear é um estágio da necrose. [pykno- + G. *-osis*, condição]

pyk·not·ic (pik-not'ik). Picnótico; relativo a, ou caracterizado por, picnose.

py·la (pī'lă). Abertura do aqueduto do mesencéfalo; orifício de comunicação entre o terceiro ventrículo e o aqueduto do mesencéfalo (de Sylvius). [G. *pylē*, portão]

py·lar (pī'lăr). Relativo à abertura do aqueduto do mesencéfalo.

py·le·phle·bi·tis (pī'lē-fle-bī'tis). Pileflebite; inflamação da veia porta ou de qualquer um de seus ramos. [G. *pylē*, portão, + *phleps*, veia, + *-itis*, inflamação]

py·le·throm·bo·phle·bi·tis (pī-lē-throm'bō-phle-bī'tis). Piletromboflebite; inflamação da veia porta com formação de um trombo. [G. *pylē*, portão, + *thrombos*, coágulo, + *phleps*, veia, + *-itis*, inflamação]

py·le·throm·bo·sis (pī'lē-throm-bō'sis). Piletrombose; trombose da veia porta ou de seus ramos. [G. *pylē*, portão, + *thrombos*, coágulo, + *-osis*, condição]

py·lic (pī'lik). Relativo à veia porta.

py·lon (pī'lon). Prótese simples, geralmente sem articulações, para substituir um membro inferior amputado. [G. entrada]

△ **pylor-.** VER pyloro-.

py·lo·ral·gia (pī-lō-ral'jē-ă). Piloralgia; termo raramente usado para designar a dor na região pilórica do estômago. [pylor- + G. *algos*, dor]

py·lo·rec·to·my (pī'lōr-ek'tō-mē). Pilorectomia; excisão do piloro. [pylor- + G. *ektomē*, excisão]

py·lo·ri (pī-lōr'ī). Piloros; plural de pylorus. [L.]

py·lor·ic (pī-lōr'ik). Pilórico; relativo ao piloro.

py·lo·ri·ste·no·sis (pī-lōr'ī-ste-nō'sis). Piloriestenose; estenose ou estreitamento do orifício do piloro. SIN pylorostenosis. [pylor- + G. *stenōsis*, estreitamento]

py·lo·ri·tis (pī-lō-rī'tis). Pilorite; inflamação da extremidade pilórica do estômago. [pylor- + G. *-itis*, inflamação]

△ **pyloro-, pylor-.** Piloro-, pilor-; o piloro. [G. *pyloros*, guarda do portal]

py·lo·ro·du·o·de·ni·tis (pī-lōr'ō-doo'od-ē-nī'tis). Piloroduodenite; inflamação que envolve o piloro e o duodeno. [pyloro- + duodenitis]

py·lo·ro·gas·trec·to·my (pī-lōr'ō-gas-trek'tō-mē). Pilorogastrectomia; ressecção do piloro e de uma parte distal do estômago.

py·lo·ro·my·ot·o·my (pī-lōr'ō-mī-ot'ō-mē). Piloromiotomia; incisão longitudinal através da parede anterior do canal pilórico até o nível da submucosa, a fim de tratar a estenose pilórica hipertrófica. SIN Fredet-Ramstedt operation, Ramstedt operation. [pyloro- + G. *mys*, músculo, + *tomē*, incisão]

py·lo·ro·plas·ty (pī-lōr'ō-plas-tē). Piloroplastia; alargamento do canal pilórico e de qualquer estenose duodenal adjacente por meio de uma incisão longitudinal fechada transversalmente. [pyloro- + G. *plastos*, formado]

Finney p., p. de Finney; incisão longa, de toda a espessura, desde o duodeno, através do piloro e seguindo em sentido proximal até o antro gástrico, com um fechamento em forma de C para proporcionar uma abertura maior entre o estômago e o duodeno.

Heineke-Mikulicz p., p. de Heineke-Mikulicz; p. em que é feita uma incisão longitudinal curta (5 a 8 cm) através do piloro, fechada transversalmente. [pyloro- + G. *plastos*, formado]

Jaboulay p., p. de Jaboulay; uma gastroduodenostomia látero-lateral, útil quando o piloro e o duodeno proximal se apresentam extensamente fibrosados ou endurecidos por úlcera péptica.

py·lor·op·to·sis, py·lor·op·to·sia (pī-lōr-op-tō'sis, -tō'sē-ă). Piloroptose; deslocamento para baixo da extremidade pilórica do estômago. [pyloro- + G. *ptōsis*, ptosis, queda]

py·lo·ro·spasm (pī-lōr'ō-spazm). Pilorospasmo; contração espasmódica do piloro.

py·lo·ro·ste·no·sis (pī-lōr'ō-stē-nō'sis). Pilorostenose. SIN pyloristenosis.

py·lo·ros·to·my (pī-lō-ros'tō-mē). Pilorostomia; estabelecimento de uma fístula da superfície abdominal até o estômago, próximo ao piloro. [pyloro- + G. *stoma*, boca]

py·lo·rot·o·my (pī-lō-rot'ō-mē). Pilorotomia; incisão do piloro. [pyloro- + G. *tomē*, incisão]

py·lo·rus, pl. **py·lo·ri** (pī-lōr'ŭs, pī-lōr'ī), [TA]. Piloro. **1.** Dispositivo muscular ou miovascular para abrir (músculo dilatador) e fechar (músculo esfíncter) um orifício ou a luz de um órgão. **2.** O tecido muscular que circunda e controla a saída aboral do estômago. [L. do G. *pylōros*, porteiro, piloro, de *pylē*, portão, + *ouros*, guardião]

Pym, Sir William, médico inglês, 1772–1861. VER P. *fever*.

△ **pyo-.** Pio-; supuração, acúmulo de pus. [G. *pyon*, pus]

py·o·cele (pī'ō-sēl). Piocele; acúmulo de pus no escroto. [pyo- + G. *kēlē*, tumor, hérnia]

py·o·ce·lia (pī'ō-sē'lē-ă). Pioperitônio. SIN pyoperitoneum. [pyo- + G. *koilia*, cavidade]

py·o·ceph·a·lus (pī'ō-sef'ă-lŭs). Piocéfalo; derrame purulento no crânio. SIN pyencephalus. [pyo- + G. *kephalē*, cabeça]

circumscribed p., p. circunscrito; abscesso cerebral.

external p., p. externo; supuração meníngea.

internal p., p. interno; supuração intraventricular.

py·o·che·zia (pī-ō-kē'zē-ă). Pioquezia; eliminação de pus pelo intestino. [pyo- + G. *chezō*, defecar]

py·o·cin (pī'ō-sin). Piocina; bacteriocina produzida por cepas de *Pseudomonas pyocyaneus*.

py·o·coc·cus (pī'ō-kok'ŭs). Piococo; um dos cocos que causam supuração, principalmente *Streptococcus pyogenes*. [pyo- + G. *kokkos*, coco]

py·o·col·po·cele (pī-ō-kol'pō-sēl). Piocolpocele; tumor ou cisto vaginal que contém pus. [pyo- + G. *kolpos*, vagina, + *kēlē*, tumor, hérnia]

py·o·col·pos (pī-ō-kol'pos). Piocolpo; acúmulo de pus na vagina. [pyo- + G. *kolpos*, vagina]

py·o·cy·an·ic (pī'ō-sī-an'ik). Piociânico; relativo ao pus azul ou ao microrganismo que causa pus azul, *Pseudomonas aeruginosa*. [pyo- + G. *kyanos*, azul]

py·o·cy·a·no·gen·ic (pī'ō-sī'ă-nō-jen'ik). Piocianogênico; que causa pus azul. [pyo- + G. *kyanos*, azul, + *-gen*, que produz]

py·o·cy·a·nol·y·sin (pī'ō-sī-ă-nol'i-sin). Piocianolisina; hemolisina formada por *Pseudomonas aeruginosa*.

py·o·cyst (pī'ō-sist). Piocisto; cisto de conteúdo purulento. [pyo- + G. *kystis*, bexiga]

py·o·cys·tis (pī-ō-sis'tis). Piocisto; desenvolvimento e retenção crônica de volume excessivo de material purulento em uma bexiga que pode ter se tornado afuncional por derivação supravesical prévia. [pyo- + G. *kystis*, bexiga]

py·o·cyte (pī'ō-sīt). Piócito. SIN pus corpuscle. [pyo- + G. *kytos*, célula]

py·o·der·ma (pī-ō-der'mă). Piodermite; qualquer infecção piogênica da pele; pode ser primária, como o impetigo, ou secundária a uma condição pré-existente. [pyo- + G. *derma*, pele]

p. gangreno'sum, pioderma gangrenoso; fagedenismo geométrico; erupção não-infecciosa, crônica, de úlceras que exibem cicatrização central, com infiltração dérmica difusa por neutrófilos; freqüentemente está associado a colite ulcerativa.

secondary p., piodermite secundária; piodermite na qual uma lesão existente (p. ex., eczema, herpes, dermatite seborreica) sofre infecção secundária.

p. veg'etans, piodermite vegetante. SIN dermatitis vegetans.

py·o·gen (pī-ō-jen). Piógeno; agente que causa formação de pus. [pyo- + G. *-gen*, que produz]

py·o·gen·e·sis (pī'ō-jen'ē-sis). Piogênese. SIN suppuration. [pyo- + G. *genesis*, produção]

py·o·gen·ic, py·o·ge·net·ic (pī-ō-jen'ik, -jē-net'ik). Piogênico; que forma pus; relativo à formação de pus. SIN pyogenous.

py·og·e·nous (pī-oj'ē-nŭs). Piogênico. SIN pyogenic.

py·o·he·mia (pī-ō-hē'mē-ă). Pioemia; termo raramente usado para piemia.

py·o·he·mo·tho·rax (pī'ō-hē-mō-thōr'aks). Pioemotórax; presença de pus e sangue na cavidade pleural. [pyo- + G. *haima*, sangue, + tórax]

py·oid (pī'oyd). Pióide; semelhante a pus. [G. *pyōdēs*, de *pyon*, pus, + *eidos*, semelhança]

py·o·me·tra (pī-ō-mē'tră). Piometra; acúmulo de pus na cavidade uterina. [pyo- + G. *metra*, útero]

py·o·me·tri·tis (pī'ō-mē-trī'tis). Piometrite; inflamação da musculatura uterina associada à presença de pus na cavidade uterina. [pyo- + G. *metra*, útero, + *-itis*, inflamação]

py·o·my·o·si·tis (pī'ō-mī-ō-sī'tis). Piomiosite; abscessos, carbúnculos ou seios infectados situados profundamente nos músculos. [pyo- + G. *mys*, músculo, + *-itis*, inflamação]

tropical p., p. tropical; doença observada em Samoa e na África tropical, caracterizada por dor nos membros, febre remitente ou intermitente e abscessos nos músculos de várias partes do corpo (pode resultar em morte por sepse); os microrganismos causadores são *Staphylococcus aureus* e *Streptococcus pyogenes*, mas geralmente a doença está associada a infecções parasitárias. SIN bungpagga, lambo lambo, myositis purulenta tropica, tropical myositis.

py·o·ne·phri·tis (pī'ō-ne-frī'tis). Pionefrite; inflamação supurativa do rim. [pyo- + G. *nephros*, rim, + *-itis*, inflamação]

py·o·neph·ro·li·thi·a·sis (pī'ō-nef'rō-li-thī'ă-sis). Pionefrolitíase; presença de pus e cálculos no rim. [pyo- + G. *nephros*, rim, + *lithos*, cálculo, + *-iasis*, condição]

py·o·ne·phro·sis (pī'ō-ne-frō'sis). Pionefrose; distensão da pelve e dos cálices renais por pus, geralmente associada à obstrução. SIN nephropyosis. [pyo- + G. *nephros*, rim, + *-osis*, condição]

pyo-ova·ri·um (pī'ō-ō-var'ē-ŭm). Pio-ovário; presença de pus no ovário; um abscesso ovariano.

py·o·per·i·car·di·tis (pī′ō-per-i-kar-dī′tis). Piopericardite; inflamação supurativa do pericárdio.
py·o·per·i·car·di·um (pī′ō-per-i-kar′dē-ŭm). Piopericárdio. SIN purulent pericarditis.
py·o·per·i·to·ne·um (pī′ō-per-i-tō-nē′ŭm). Pioperitônio; acúmulo de pus na cavidade peritoneal. SIN pyocelia. [G. *pyon*, pus]
py·o·per·i·to·ni·tis (pī′ō-per-i-tō-nī′tis). Pioperitonite; inflamação supurativa do peritônio. [pyo- + peritonitis]
py·o·phy·so·me·tra (pī′ō-fī-sō-mē′tră). Piofisométrio; presença de pus e gás na cavidade uterina. [pyo- + G. *physa*, ar, + *metra*, útero]
py·o·pneu·mo·cho·le·cys·ti·tis (pī′ō-noo′mō-kō′lē-sis-tī′tis). Piopneumocolecistite; combinação de pus e gás em uma inflamação da vesícula biliar causada por microrganismos produtores de gás ou pela entrada de ar proveniente do duodeno através da árvore biliar. [pyo- + G. *pneuma*, ar, + colecistite]
py·o·pneu·mo·hep·a·ti·tis (pī′ō-noo′mō-hep-ă-tī′tis). Piopneumoepatite; combinação de pus e ar no fígado, geralmente associada a um abscesso. [pyo- + G. *pneuma*, ar, + hepatite]
py·o·pneu·mo·per·i·car·di·um (pī′ō-noo′mō-per-i-kar′dē-ŭm). Piopneumopericárdio; presença de pus e gás no saco pericárdico. [pyo- + G. *pneuma*, ar, + pericárdio]
py·o·pneu·mo·per·i·to·ne·um (pī′ō-noo′mō-per-i-tō-nē′ŭm). Piopneumoperitônio; presença de pus e gás na cavidade peritoneal. [pyo- + G. *pneuma*, ar, + peritônio]
py·o·pneu·mo·per·i·to·ni·tis (pī′ō-noo′mō-per-i-tō-nī′tis). Piopneumoperitonite; peritonite por microrganismos formadores de gás ou por introdução de gás proveniente de uma ruptura intestinal. [pyo- + G. *pneuma*, ar, + peritonite]
py·o·pneu·mo·tho·rax (pī′ō-noo-mō-thōr′aks). Piopneumotórax; a presença de gás juntamente com um derrame purulento na cavidade pleural. [pyo- + G. *pneuma*, ar, + tórax]
  subdiaphragmatic p., subphrenic p., p. subdifragmático, p. subfrênico; abscesso subfrênico associado à perfuração de uma víscera oca, com gás no tórax e abdome.
py·o·poi·e·sis (pī′ō-poy-ē′sis). Piopoese. SIN suppuration. [pyo- + G. *poiēsis*, produção]
py·o·poi·et·ic (pī′ō-poy-et′ik). Piopoético; que produz pus.
py·o·py·e·lec·ta·sis (pī′ō-pī-ē-lek′tă-sis). Piopielectasia; dilatação da pelve renal com inflamação produtora de pus. [pyo- + G. *pyelos*, pelve, + *ektasis*, estiramento]
py·or·rhea (pī-ō-rē′ă). Piorréia; corrimento purulento. [pyo- + G. *rhoia*, fluxo]
py·o·sal·pin·gi·tis (pī′o-sal-pin-jī′tis). Piossalpingite; inflamação supurativa da tuba uterina (de Falópio). [pyo- + salpingitis]
py·o·sal·pin·go-ooph·o·ri·tis (pī-ō-sal′ping-gō-ō-of′ō-rī′tis). Piossalpingo-ooforite]; inflamação supurativa da tuba uterina (de Falópio) e do ovário. SIN pyosalpingo-oothecitis. [pyo- + G. *salpinx*, trompa (tuba), + ooforite]
py·o·sal·pin·go-oo·the·ci·tis (pī-ō-sal′ping-gō-ō′ō-thē-sī′tis). SIN pyosalpingo-oophoritis. [pyo- + G. *salpinx*, trompa (tuba), + L. mod. *ootheca*, ovário, + G. *-itis*, inflamação]
py·o·sal·pinx (pī-ō-sal′pingks). Piossalpinge; distensão de uma tuba uterina (de Falópio) com pus. SIN pus tube. [pyo- + G. *salpinx*, trompa (tuba)]
py·o·se·mia (pī-ō-sē′mē-ă). Piosemia; presença de pus no líquido seminal, freqüentemente associada a prostatite crônica ou a outros distúrbios inflamatórios do trato genital masculino. SIN pyospermia. [pyo- + L. *semen*, semente (masculina)]
py·o·sep·ti·ce·mia (pī′ō-sep-ti-sē′mē-ă). Piossepticemia; infecção do sangue por várias formas de bactérias, denominadas microrganismos piogênicos e, também, não-piogênicos. [pyo- + G. *sēptikos*, putrefato, + *haima*, sangue]
py·o·sis (pī-ō′sis). Piose. SIN suppuration. [G.]
py·o·sper·mia (pī-ō-sper′mē-ă). Piospermia. SIN pyosemia. [pyo- + G. *sperma*, semente, + *-ia*, condição]
py·o·stat·ic (pī-ō-stat′ik). Piostático. **1.** Que interrompe a formação de pus. **2.** Um agente que interrompe a formação de pus. [pyo- + G. *statikos*, que causa parada]
py·o·sto·ma·ti·tis (pī′ō-stō-mă-tī′tis). Piostomatite; erupção inflamatória supurativa da boca. [pyo- + G. *stoma*, boca, + *-itis*, inflamação]
  p. veg'etans, p. vegetante; lesões pustulares confluentes da boca, com erupções proliferativas e verrucosas da mucosa bucal; associada a colite ulcerativa e a outras doenças consuptivas.
py·o·tho·rax (pī-ō-thōr′aks). Piotórax; empiema em uma cavidade pleural.
py·o·u·ra·chus (pī-ō-ū′ră-kŭs). Pioúraco; acúmulo purulento no úraco.
py·o·u·re·ter (pī-ō-ū-rē′ter). Pioureter; distensão de um ureter com pus.
Pyr Abreviatura de pyrimidine (pirimidina); pyroglutamic acid (ácido piroglutâmico).
pyr-. Pir-; fogo, calor. VER TAMBÉM pyreto-, pyro- (1). [G. *pyr*]
pyr·a·cin (pir′ă-sin). Piracina; piridoxolactona, a lactona do ácido 4-piridóxico.

pyr·a·mid (pir′ă-mid) [TA]. Pirâmide. **1.** Termo aplicado a várias estruturas anatômicas que possuem um formato aproximado de uma pirâmide. SIN pyramis [TA]. **2.** Termo que designa a porção petrosa do osso temporal. [G. *pyramis* (*pyramid-*), uma pirâmide]
  anterior p., p. da medula oblonga. SIN p. of medulla oblongata.
  cerebellar p., p. do cerebelo. SIN p. of vermis.
  Ferrein p., p. de Ferrein. SIN medullary ray.
  Lallouette p., p. de Lallouette. SIN pyramidal *lobe* of thyroid gland.
  p. of light, reflexo luminoso. SIN light *reflex* (3).
  Malacarne p., p. de Malacarne; lóbulo na superfície inferior do cerebelo, a porção posterior do verme.
  malpighian p., p. de Malpigh. SIN renal p.'s.
  p. of medulla oblongata, p. da medula oblonga; a proeminência branca, alongada na superfície ventral da medula oblonga de cada lado, ao longo da fissura mediana anterior, correspondente à posição das fibras que formam os tratos corticospinais. SIN pyramis medullae oblongatae [TA], anterior column of medulla oblongata, anterior p.
  medullary p., p. renal. SIN renal p.'s.
  olfactory p., p. olfatória; uma pequena área de substância cinzenta situada entre as raízes dos tratos olfatórios; é contínua caudalmente com a substância perfurada anterior.
  petrous p., parte petrosa do osso temporal. SIN petrous *part* of temporal bone.
  population p., p. populacional; representação gráfica da composição etária e sexual de uma população, construída calculando-se a distribuição percentual da população em cada classe etária e sexual.
  posterior p. of the medulla, fascículo grácil. SIN gracile *fasciculus*.
  renal p.'s [TA], pirâmides renais; massas piramidais observadas ao corte longitudinal do rim; coletivamente, formam as medulas renais e contêm parte dos túbulos secretores e os túbulos coletores. SIN malpighian p., medullary p., pyramides renales, pyramis renalis.

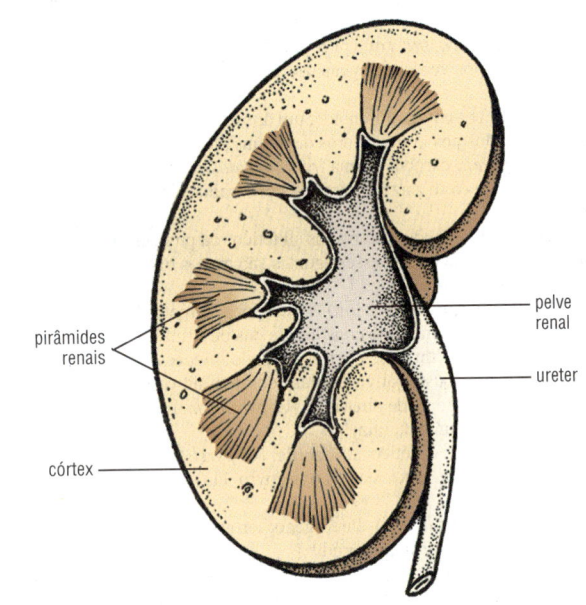

pirâmide renal

  p. of thyroid, lobo piramidal da glândula tireóide. SIN pyramidal *lobe* of thyroid gland.
  p. of tympanum, eminência piramidal. SIN *eminentia* pyramidalis.
  p. of vermis [TA], p. do verme; uma subdivisão do verme inferior do cerebelo entre o túber e a úvula; lóbulo do verme VIII. SIN cerebellar p., pyramis [TA] of cerebellum.
  p. of vestibule [TA], p. do vestíbulo; a extremidade triangular superior da crista do vestíbulo. SIN pyramis vestibuli [TA].
py·ram·i·dal (pi-ram′i-dal). Osso piramidal. **1.** Que tem o formato de uma pirâmide. **2.** Relativo a qualquer estrutura anatômica denominada pirâmide.
py·ra·mi·da·le (pi-ram′i-dā′lē). Osso piramidal. SIN triquetrum. [L. mod.]
py·ra·mi·da·lis. Músculo piramidal. VER pyramidalis (*muscle*).
py·ram·i·dot·o·my (pi-ram′i-dot′ō-mē). Piramidotomia; secção de tratos piramidais, na medula espinal, para alívio de movimentos involuntários. [G. *pyramis*, pirâmide, + *tomē*, incisão]
  medullary p., p. bulbar; tractotomia piramidal bulbar.
  spinal p., p. espinal; tractotomia piramidal espinal.

pyr·a·min, pyr·a·mine (pir′ă-min). Piramina. SIN toxopyrimidine.
pyr·a·mis, pl. **py·ra·mi·des** (pir′ă-mis, pi-ram′i-dēz) [TA]. Pirâmide. SIN pyramid (1). [L. mod. do G. pyramid]
  p. medul′lae oblonga′tae [TA], p. da medula oblonga. SIN pyramid of medulla oblongata.
  p. rena′lis, pl. **pyram′ides rena′les**, p. renal. SIN renal pyramids, em pyramid.
  p. [TA] of cerebellum, p. do cerebelo. SIN pyramid of vermis.
  p. tym′pani, eminência timpânica. SIN eminentia pyramidalis.
  p. vestib′uli [TA], p. do vestíbulo. SIN pyramid of vestibule.
py·ran (pī′ran). Pirano; composto cíclico que pode ser considerado a substância formal que dá origem aos açúcares com uma ponte de oxigênio dos átomos de carbono 1–5 (as piranoses).
pyr·a·none (pir′ă-nōn, pī′-). Piranona. SIN pyrone.
pyr·a·nose (pir′ă-nōs, pī′-). Piranose; forma cíclica de um açúcar na qual a ponte de oxigênio forma um pirano.
py·ran·tel pam·o·ate (pi-ran′tel). Pamoato de pirantel; um anti-helmíntico, particularmente útil nas infecções intestinais simples ou mistas por nematódeos, como *Ascaris*, ancilóstomo, oxiúro e espécies do gênero *Trichostrongylus*.
pyr·a·thi·a·zine hy·dro·chlo·ride (pir-ă-thī′ă-zēn). Cloridrato de piratiazina; um anti-histamínico.
pyr·a·zin·a·mide (pir-ă-zin′ă-mīd). Pirazinamida; medicamento de primeira linha contra a tuberculose, ativo sobretudo contra o *Mycobacterium tuberculosis* em macrófagos. Como todos os medicamentos contra a tuberculose, tem de ser associada a outros medicamentos para ser efetiva na doença ativa. Sua principal toxicidade é hepática.
pyr·az·o·lone (pir-ă-zō′lōn). Pirazolona; classe de antiinflamatórios não-esteróides usados no tratamento de afecções artríticas; p. ex., fenilbutazona.
py·rec·tic (pī-rek′tik). Pirético. SIN febrile.
py·re·ne·mia (pī-rē-nē′mē-ă). Pirenemia; condição caracterizada pela presença de hemácias nucleadas no sangue. [G. *pyrēn*, o caroço de uma fruta, + *haima*, sangue]
Py·re·no·chae·ta ro·me·roi (pī′rē-nō-kē′tă rō′mē-roy). Uma das várias espécies de fungos verdadeiros capazes de causar micetoma em seres humanos.
py·re·noid (pī′rē-noyd). Pirenóide; um dos diminutos corpos brilhantes por vezes observados nos cromatóforos de alguns protozoários, como a *Euglena viridis*. [G. *pyrēn*, caroço de uma fruta, + *eidos*, semelhança]
py·re·thrins (pī-reth′rinz). Piretrinas; constituintes inseticidas das flores do píretro.
py·re·throids. Piretróides; derivados sintéticos da piretrina, usados como inseticidas; como uma classe, esses agentes são menos tóxicos para mamíferos que outros inseticidas eficazes.
py·re·thro·lone (pī-reth′rō-lōn). Piretrolona; 2-metil-4-oxo-3-(2,4-pentanedienil)-2-ciclopentenol, um constituinte das piretrinas.
py·re·thrum (pī-rē′thrŭm). Píretro; a raiz do *Anacyclus pyrethrum* (família Compositae), um arbusto nativo do Marrocos; tem sido usado como sialogogo; suas flores são uma fonte de piretrinas. [G. *pyrethron*, matricária, de *pyr*, fogo, devido ao sabor picante da raiz]
py·ret·ic (pī-ret′ik). Pirético. SIN febrile. [G. *pyretikos*]
♻ **pyreto-**. Pireto-; febre. VER TAMBÉM pyr-, pyro- (1). [G. *pyretos*, febre, de *pyr*, fogo]
py·ret·o·gen (pī-ret′ō-jen). Pirétogeno; termo raramente usado para pirogênio. [pyreto- + G. *-gen*, que produz]
py·re·to·gen·e·sis (pī-rē-tō-jen′ĕ-sis, pī′rē-tō-). Piretogênese; termo raramente usado para designar a origem e o modo de produção da febre. [pyreto- + G. *genesis*, origem]
py·re·to·ge·net·ic, py·re·to·gen·ic (pī′rē-tō-jĕ-net′ik, -jen′ik). Piretogenético. SIN pyrogenic.
py·re·tog·e·nous (pī-rē-toj′ĕ-nŭs). Piretogênico. SIN pyrogenic.
py·re·to·ther·a·py (pī′rē-tō-thār′ă-pē). Piretoterapia. **1.** Sinônimo obsoleto de piroterapia. **2.** Tratamento da febre. SIN artificial fever, induced fever. [pyreto- + G. *therapeia*, tratamento]
py·rex·ia (pī-rek′sē-ă). Pirexia, febre. SIN fever. [G. *pyrexis*, estado febril]
py·rex·i·al (pī-rek′sē-ăl). Piréxico; relativo à febre.
py·rex·i·o·pho·bia (pī-rek′sē-ō-fō′bē-ă). Pirexiofobia; medo mórbido de febre. [G. *pyrexis*, estado febril, + *phobos*, medo]
pyr·i·ben·zyl meth·yl sul·fate (pir-i-ben′zil). Metilsulfato de piribenzil. SIN bevonium methyl sulfate.
pyr·i·dine (pir′i-dēn, -din). Piridina; C_5H_5N; líquido volátil incolor de odor empirreumático e sabor picante, resultante da destilação a seco de matéria orgânica contendo nitrogênio; usada como solvente industrial, em química analítica, e para desnaturação do álcool.
pyridinium. Piridínio; produto da decomposição do colágeno ósseo excretado na urina e determinado para medir a atividade osteoclástica; está aumentado em afecções como doença de Paget, hiperparatireoidismo primário e osteoporose.

pyridinoline. Piridinolina; hidroxipiridínio; produto da decomposição do colágeno ósseo, determinado como o piridínio (q.v.) para medir a atividade osteoclástica.
pyr·i·dof·yl·line (pir-i-dof′i-lin). Piridofilina; composto de sulfato de hidrogênio 7-(2-hidroxietil)teofilina com piridoxol; um vasodilatador coronariano.
pyr·i·do·stig·mine bro·mide (pir′i-dō-stig′mēn). Brometo de piridostigmina; inibidor da colinesterase útil no tratamento da miastenia grave e para reverter o bloqueio neuromuscular produzido pelo curare e agentes semelhantes ao fim de um procedimento cirúrgico.
pyr·i·dox·al (pir-i-dok′săl). Piridoxal; o 4-aldeído da piridoxina, que tem uma ação fisiológica semelhante. VER TAMBÉM pyridoxine.
  p. kinase, p. cinase, p. quinase; enzima que catalisa a fosforilação pelo ATP do piridoxal em piridoxal 5-fosfato e ADP, assim convertendo o nutriente na coenzima ativa.
  p. 5-phosphate (PLP), p. 5-fosfato; coenzima essencial para muitas reações teciduais, notavelmente transaminações e descarboxilações de aminoácidos.
pyr·i·dox·a·mine (pir-i-dok′să-mēn). Piridoxamina; a amina da piridoxina ($-CH_2NH_2$ substituindo $-CH_2OH$ na posição 4), que tem uma ação fisiológica semelhante. VER pyridoxine.
  p. 5-phosphate, p. 5-fosfato; amina do piridoxal 5-fosfato ($-CH_2NH_2$ substituindo $-CHO$ na posição 4), é o intermediário formado em muitas reações catalisadas por enzimas que utilizam piridoxal 5-fosfato.
pyr·i·dox·a·mine-phos·phate ox·i·dase. Piridoxamina-fosfato oxidase; uma oxidorredutase que catalisa a desaminação oxidativa da piridoxamina 5-fosfato (com O_2 e H_2O) para formar piridoxal 5-fosfato, H_2O_2 e NH_3.
4-pyr·i·dox·ic ac·id (pir-i-dok′sik). Ácido 4-piridóxico; o principal produto do metabolismo do piridoxal ($-COOH$ substitui $-CHO$ na posição 4), que aparece na urina.
pyr·i·dox·ine (pir-i-dok′sēn, -sin). Piridoxina; a vitamina B_6 original, cuja denominação atualmente inclui piridoxal e piridoxamina, associada à utilização de ácidos graxos insaturados. Em ratos, sua deficiência provoca dermatite nutricional e acrodinia; em seres humanos, a deficiência pode resultar em aumento da irritabilidade, convulsões e neurite periférica. O cloridrato é usado em preparações farmacêuticas; encontrada em vegetais.
pyr·i·dox·ine 4-de·hy·dro·gen·ase. Piridoxina 4-desidrogenase; uma oxidorredutase que catalisa a oxidação da piridoxina com $NADP^+$ em piridoxal e NADPH.
pyr·i·form (pir′i-fōrm). Piriforme. SIN piriform. [L. *pyrum* (prop. *pirum*), pêra, + *forma*, formato]
pyr·il·a·mine ma·le·ate (pī-ril′ă-mēn, pir′i-lă-). Maleato de pirilamina; um anti-histamínico. SIN mepyramine maleate.
pyr·i·meth·a·mine (pir-i-meth′ă-mēn). Pirimetamina; potente antagonista do ácido fólico usado como agente antimalárico efetivo contra *Plasmodium falciparum*; um supressor útil, ativo contra as formas assexuadas eritrocitária e tecidual; também é usada no tratamento da toxoplasmose.
py·rim·i·dine (Pyr) (pī-rim′i-dēn). Pirimidina; 1,3-diazina; uma substância heterocíclica, a substância original formal de várias "bases" presentes em ácidos nucleicos (uracil, timina, citosina), bem como dos barbitúricos.
  p. 5′-nucleotidase, p. 5′-nucleotidase; enzima que catalisa a hidrólise de um 5′-monofosfato de pirimidina-nucleosídeo para produzir ortofosfato e o nucleosídeo pirimidina; a deficiência dessa enzima resulta em acúmulo de nucleotídeos pirimidina, levando à anemia hemolítica.
  p. transferase, p. transferase. SIN thiamin pyridinylase.
pyrin. Pirina; proteína anormal de neutrófilos codificada pelo gene MEFV na febre familiar do Mediterrâneo. SIN marenostrin.
pyr·i·thi·a·min (pir′i-thī′ă-min). Piritiamina; antimetabólito tiamina, que difere da tiamina porque o anel tiazol da molécula de tiamina é substituído por um anel piridina. SIN neopyrithiamin.
♻ **pyro-**. Piro-. **1.** Forma combinante que significa fogo, calor ou febre. VER TAMBÉM pyr-, pyreto-. **2.** Em química, forma combinante que significa derivados formados por remoção da água (geralmente por calor) para formar anidridos. VER TAMBÉM anhydro-. [G. *pyr*, fogo]
py·ro·bo·ric ac·id (pī-rō-bōr′ik). Ácido pirobórico. SIN tetraboric acid.
py·ro·cal·cif·er·ol (pī′ro-kal-sif′er-ol). Pirocalciferol; produto da decomposição térmica do calciferol.
py·ro·cat·e·chase (pī-rō-kat′ĕ-kās). Pirocatecase. SIN catechol 1,2-dioxygenase.
py·ro·cat·e·chin (pī-rō-kat′ĕ-kin). Pirocatequina. SIN pyrocatechol.
py·ro·cat·e·chol (pī-rō-kat′ĕ-kol). Pirocatecol; 1,2-benzenediol; um constituinte das catecolaminas, epinefrina e norepinefrina, e dopa; usado externamente como anti-séptico. SIN catechol (1), pyrocatechin.
py·ro·gal·lic ac·id (pī-rō-gal′ik). Ácido pirogálico. SIN pyrogallol.
py·ro·gal·lol (pī-rō-gal′ol). Pirogalol; usado externamente no tratamento da psoríase, dermatofitose e outras afecções cutâneas. SIN pyrogallic acid.
py·ro·gal·lol·phthal·e·in (pī′rō-gal-ō-thal′ē-in, -thal′ē-in). Pirogalolftaleína. SIN gallein.

py·ro·gen (pī′rō-jen). Pirogênio; agente causador de febre; os pirogênios são produzidos por bactérias, mofos, vírus e leveduras. [pyro- + G. *-gen*, que produz]

endogenous p. (EP), p. endógeno; proteínas que induzem febre. Já foram identificados vários (cerca de 11), incluindo citocinas formadas por componentes do sistema imune, principalmente macrófagos (p. ex., interleucinas 1 e 6, interferons e fatores de necrose tumoral). SIN leukocytic p.'s.

exogenous p.'s, pirogênios exógenos; fármacos ou substâncias produzidas por microrganismos que causam febre. Entre estas últimas estão os lipopolissacarídeos e o ácido lipoteicóico.

leukocytic p.'s, pirogênios leucocitários. SIN endogenous p.

py·ro·gen·ic (pī-rō-jen′ik). Pirogênico; que causa febre. VER TAMBÉM febrifacient. SIN pyretogenetic, pyretogenic, pyretogenous.

py·ro·glob·u·lins (pī-rō-glob′ū-linz). Piroglobulinas; proteínas séricas (imunoglobulinas), geralmente associadas ao mieloma múltiplo ou macroglobulinemia, que se precipitam irreversivelmente quando aquecidas a 56°C.

py·ro·glu·tam·ic ac·id (Pyr) (pī′rō-gloo-ta′mik). Ácido piroglutâmico. SIN 5-oxoproline.

py·ro·lig·ne·ous (pī-rō-lig′nē-ŭs). Pirolenhoso; relativo à destilação seca da madeira ou por ela produzido. [pyro- + L. *lignum*, madeira]

py·rol·y·sis (pī-rol′i-sis). Pirólise; decomposição de uma substância pelo calor. [pyro- + G. *lysis*, dissolução]

py·ro·ma·nia (pī-rō-mā′nē-ă). Piromania; impulso mórbido de incendiar. SIN incendiarism. [pyro- + G. *mania*, mania]

py·ro·ma·ni·ac (pī-rō-mā′nē-ak). Piromaníaco; aquele afetado por piromania; incendiário.

py·ro·men (pī′rō-men). Piromena. SIN piromen.

py·rom·e·ter (pī-rom′ĕ-ter). Pirômetro; instrumento para medir graus muito altos de calor, além da capacidade de um termômetro de mercúrio ou gás. [pyro- + G. *metron*, medida]

resistance p., p. de resistência. SIN resistance thermometer.

py·rone (pī′ron). Pirona; um ceto derivado do pirano. SIN pyranone.

py·ro·nin (pī′rō-nin). Pironina; corante xanteno básico vermelho fluorescente, o cloreto de tetrametildiaminoxanteno, **p. Y** ou **p. G** (I.C. 45005), ou de tetraetildiaminoxanteno, **p. B** (I.C. 45010). Esses corantes, principalmente a p. Y, são usados em combinação com o verde de metila para coloração diferencial de RNA (vermelho) e DNA (verde); a diferença na coloração provavelmente se deve ao maior grau de polimerização de DNA; a p. Y também é usada como corante traçador do RNA na eletroforese.

py·ro·ni·no·phil·ia (pī′rō-nin-ō-fil′ē-ă). Pironinofilia; afinidade pelos corantes pironina básicos; indicador útil da síntese proteica intensa que acompanha a síntese do RNA, como no citoplasma de um plasmócito ativo. [pyronin + G. *philos*, que tem afinidade com]

py·ro·pho·bia (pī-rō-fō′bē-ă). Pirofobia; medo mórbido de fogo. [pyro- + G. *phobos*, medo]

py·ro·phos·pha·tase (pī-rō-fos′fā-tās). Pirofosfatase; qualquer enzima que cliva uma ligação pirofosfato entre dois grupos fosfóricos, deixando um em cada fragmento; p. ex., pirofosfatase inorgânica, NAD^+ pirofosfatase (cliva NAD, etc., em mononucleotídeos), ATP pirofosfatase (cliva o pirofosfato inorgânico do ATP, deixando AMP. VER TAMBÉM *flavin* adenine dinucleotide. SIN diphosphatase.

inorganic p., p. inorgânica; fosfoidrolase que catalisa a hidrólise do pirofosfato inorgânico em dois ortofosfatos. SIN inorganic diphosphatase.

py·ro·phos·phate (PP, PP_i) (pī-rō-fos′fāt). Pirofosfato; um sal do ácido pirofosfórico; acumula-se em casos de hipofosfatasia; algumas vezes denominado pirofosfato inorgânico (PP_i). SIN diphosphate.

^{99m}Tc p., p. Tc^{99m}; marcador radionuclídeo usado para estudos por imagem do miocárdio isquêmico em medicina nuclear. VER technetium-99m.

py·ro·phos·pho·ki·nas·es (pī′rō-fos-fō-kī′nās-ez). Pirofosfocinases; enzimas (EC 2.7.6.x) que transferem um grupamento pirofosfórico (p. ex., fosfo-α-D-ribosil-pirofosfato sintetase). SIN pyrophosphotransferases.

py·ro·phos·phor·ic ac·id (pī′rō-fos-for′ik). Ácido pirofosfórico; um anidrido do ácido fosfórico obtido por aquecimento deste a 213°C; forma pirofosfatos com bases, e seus ésteres são importantes no metabolismo energético e na biossíntese.

py·ro·phos·pho·ryl·as·es (pī′rō-fos-for′il-ās-ez). Pirofosforilases; nome trivial aplicado às nucleotidiltransferases que catalisam a transferência do AMP do ATP para outro resíduo com a liberação de pirofosfato inorgânico, ou a fixação de um nucleosídeo pirofosfato em um polinucleotídeo com liberação de ortofosfato inorgânico.

py·ro·phos·pho·trans·fer·as·es (pī′rō-fos-fō-trans′fer-ās-ez). Pirofosfotransferases. SIN pyrophosphokinases.

py·ro·poi·ki·lo·cy·to·sis (pī′rō-pōy-kil-ō-si-tō′sis). Piropoiquilocitose; distúrbio recessivo raro que se manifesta por hemólise grave, poiquilocitose acentuada e sensibilidade característica das hemácias à fragmentação induzida pelo calor *in vitro*; aparentemente causada por um defeito na auto-associação da espectrina. SIN hereditary pyropoikilocytosis.

hereditary pyropoikilocytosis, p. hereditária. SIN pyropoikilocytosis.

py·ro·scope (pī′rō-skōp). Piroscópio; instrumento para medir a temperatura comparando-se a luz de um objeto aquecido com um padrão luminoso. [pyro- + G. *skopeō*, ver]

py·ro·sis (pī-rō′sis). Pirose; dor ou sensação de queimação subesternal, geralmente associada à regurgitação de suco gástrico ácido-péptico para o esôfago. SIN heartburn. [G. queimação]

py·ro·ther·a·py (pī′rō-thār′ă-pē). Piroterapia; tratamento de doença por indução de febre artificial no paciente. SIN therapeutic fever.

py·rot·ic (pī-rot′ik). **1.** Pirótico; relativo à pirose. **2.** Cáustico. SIN caustic.

py·ro·tox·in (pī′rō-tok′sin). Pirotoxina; termo obsoleto para designar uma substância tóxica produzida nos tecidos durante o progresso de uma febre.

pyr·ox·y·lin (pī-rok′si-lin). Piroxilina; consiste principalmente em tetranitrato de celulose, obtido pela ação dos ácidos nítrico e sulfúrico sobre o algodão; usado no preparo do colódio. SIN colloxylin, dinitrocellulose, nitrocellulose, soluble gun cotton, xyloidin. [pyro- + G. *xylon*, madeira]

pyr·ro·bu·ta·mine phos·phate (pir-ō-bū′tă-mēn). Fosfato de pirrobutamina; um anti-histamínico.

pyr·ro·lase (pir′ō-lās). Pirrolase. SIN *tryptophan* 2,3-dioxygenase.

pyr·rol blue (pir′ol) [I.C. 42700]. Azul de pirrol; corante triarilmetano ácido empregado como corante vital e como um corante da elastina. SIN Isamine blue.

pyr·role (pir′ōl). Pirrol; divinilenimina; um composto heterocíclico encontrado em muitas substâncias biologicamente importantes. SIN azole, imidole.

pyr·rol·i·dine (pi-rol′i-dēn). Pirrolidina. **1.** Tetraidropirrol; pirrol ao qual foram acrescentados quatro átomos de H; a base estrutural da prolina e da hidroxiprolina. **2.** Uma classe de alcalóides que contém uma porção pirrolidina (1) ou um derivado da pirrolidina.

pyr·rol·i·dine-2-car·box·yl·ate. Pirrolidina-2-carboxilato. SIN proline.

pyr·rol·i·done-5-car·box·yl·ate (pi-rol′i-dōn). Pirrolidona-5-carboxilato. SIN 5-oxoproline.

5-pyr·ro·li·done-2-car·box·yl·ic ac·id. Ácido 5-pirrolidona-2-carboxílico. SIN 5-oxoproline.

pyr·ro·line (pir′ō-lēn). Pirrolina; grupo de isômeros do pirrol aos quais foram adicionados dois átomos de H; a 1-pirrolina tem uma ligação dupla entre o nitrogênio e um carbono adjacente.

1-pyr·ro·line-5-car·box·y·late de·hy·dro·gen·ase. 1-pirrolina-5-carboxilato desidrogenase; enzima que catalisa a reação reversível da 1-pirrolina-5-carboxilato e NAD^+ para formar L-glutamato e NADH; essa enzima participa do metabolismo da prolina e da ornitina; a 1-pirrolina-5-carboxilato está em equilíbrio com o glutamato γ-semialdeído; a deficiência dessa enzima está associada à hiperprolinemia tipo II.

pyr·ro·line-2-car·box·yl·ate re·duc·tase. Pirrolina-2-carboxilato redutase; uma oxidorredutase que reduz a 1-pirrolina-2-carboxilato em L-prolina com NAD(P)H. SIN proline dehydrogenase, proline oxidase.

pyr·ro·line-5-car·box·y·late re·duc·tase. Pirrolina-5-carboxilato redutase; uma oxidorredutase que reduz reversivelmente a 1-pirrolina-5-carboxilato em L-prolina com NAD(P)H; a deficiência dessa enzima está associada à hiperprolinemia tipo I. SIN proline dehydrogenase, proline oxidase.

py·ru·val·dox·ine (pī′roo-val-dok′sen). Piruvaldoxina. SIN isonitrosoacetone.

py·ru·vate (pī′roo-vāt). Piruvato; um sal ou éster do ácido pirúvico.

active p., p. ativo; intermediário formado na descarboxilação oxidativa do piruvato. Cf. p. dehydrogenase (lipoamide). SIN α-lactyl-thiamin pyrophosphate.

p. carboxylase, p. carboxilase; ligase que catalisa a reação do ATP, piruvato e HCO_3^{2-}, para formar ADP, ortofosfato e oxaloacetato; a biotina e o acetil-CoA estão envolvidos; a ausência dessa enzima resulta em perda de neurônios no córtex cerebral, levando a retardo mental.

p. decarboxylase, p. descarboxilase; α-carboxilase; α-cetoácido carboxilase; uma carboxilase do lêvedo, dependente de pirofosfato de tiamina, que catalisa a descarboxilação de um 2-oxoácido (p. ex., piruvato) em um aldeído (p. ex., acetaldeído) sem oxidorredução e sem lipoamida, ao contrário da piruvato desidrogenase (lipoamida).

p. dehydrogenase, p. desidrogenase; conjunto estruturalmente distinto de enzimas que contêm piruvato desidrogenase (lipoamida), diidrolipoil transacetilase e diidrolipoil desidrogenase.

p. dehydrogenase (cytochrome), p. desidrogenase (citocromo), uma oxidorredutase que catalisa a reação entre o ferricitocromo b_1 e o piruvato para produzir acetato e CO_2, e ferrocitocromo b_1.

p. dehydrogenase (lipoamide), p. desidrogenase (lipoamida); oxidorredutase que catalisa a conversão de piruvato e lipoamida (oxidada) em CO_2 e S^6-acetildiidrolipoamida em duas reações sucessivas: a primeira entre o piruvato e o pirofosfato de tiamina para produzir CO_2 e pirofosfato de α-hidroxietiltiamina (pirofosfato ativo); a segunda entre este último e a lipoamida para recuperar o pirofosfato de tiamina e produzir S^6-acetildrolipoamida. Cf. α-ketodecarboxylase.

p. kinase (PK), p. cinase; fosfo*enol*piruvato cinase; uma fosfotransferase que catalisa a transferência de fosfato do fosfo*enol*piruvato para o ADP, formando ATP e piruvato; outros nucleosídeos fosfatos podem participar da reação; uma etapa fundamental na glicólise; a deficiência de piruvato cinase levará a anemia hemolítica.

p. oxidase, p. oxidase; uma oxidorredutase que catalisa a reação de piruvato, fosfato e O_2 para produzir acetil fosfato, CO_2 e H_2O_2.

py·ru·vic ac·id (pī - roo′vik). Ácido pirúvico; ácido 2-oxopropanóico; ácido α-cetopropiônico; ácido acetilfórmico; ácido piroacêmico; o α-cetoácido mais simples; um composto intermediário no metabolismo dos carboidratos; na deficiência de tiamina, sua oxidação é retardada e ele se acumula nos tecidos, principalmente nas estruturas nervosas. A forma enol, ácido *enol* pirúvico, quando fosforilada, tem um papel metabólico importante. VER phospho*enol*pyruvic acid.

py·ru·vic al·de·hyde. Aldeído pirúvico. SIN methylglyoxal.

py·ru·vic-mal·ic car·box·yl·ase. Carboxilase pirúvico-málica. SIN *malate dehydrogenase.*

6-py·ru·vo·yl·tet·ra·hy·drop·ter·in syn·thase (6-PTS). 6-piruvoiltetraidropterina sintase; enzima que catalisa uma etapa na síntese de tetraidrobiopterina; a deficiência dessa enzima resultará em uma forma de hiperfenilalaninemia.

pyr·vin·i·um pam·o·ate (pir - vin′i - ŭm). Pamoato de pirvínio; fármaco altamente eficaz usado na erradicação de oxiúros humanos. SIN viprynium embonate.

Pyth·i·um in·si·di·o·sum (pith′ē - ŭm in - sid′ē - um). Espécie de fungos encontrados na água ou no solo úmido, e uma causa de hifomicose ou pitiose.

py·tho·gen·e·sis (pī - thō - jen′ē - sis). Pitogênese. **1.** Origem a partir de matéria putrefata. **2.** A produção de putrefação. [G. *pythō*, deteriorar, + *genesis*, origem]

py·tho·gen·ic, py·thog·e·nous (pī - thō - jen′ik, pī - thoj′ĕ - nŭs). Pitogênico; que se origina da sujeira ou putrefação.

py·u·ria (pī - ū′rē - ă). Piúria; presença de pus na urina quando eliminada. [G. *pyon*, pus, + *ouron*, urina]

Q

Q Símbolo de coulomb; quantidade; quaternário; glutamina; glutaminil; pseudo-uridina; coenzima Q; carga elétrica; o segundo produto formado em uma reação catalisada por enzima.

Q̇ Símbolo de fluxo sanguíneo. VER flow (3). [quantidade + um ponto no alto que designa o derivado de tempo]

Q_{O_2}, Q_{O_2}. Símbolos de consumo de oxigênio; *oxygen consumption* (1).

Q_{10} Símbolo para o aumento da velocidade de um processo produzido pela elevação da temperatura em 10°C; a velocidade de contração de um coração excisado aproximadamente dobra para cada 10°C (isto é, $Q_{10} = 2$).

Q_{CO_2} Símbolo para os microlitros nas CPTP (condições padrões de temperatura e pressão, tempo seco) de CO_2 produzidos por miligrama de tecido por hora.

-Q_6. Símbolo de ubiquinona-6.

-Q_{10}. Símbolo de ubiquinona-10.

q 1. Em citogenética, símbolo de braço longo de um cromossoma (em contraste com p para o braço curto). 2. Abreviatura de [L.] *quodque*, a cada. 3. *q.* Símbolo de calor.

QALY Acrônimo para anos de vida ajustados para a qualidade, um ajuste que considera a prevalência de limitação da atividade.

Q-band·ing. Bandeamento Q. VER Q-banding *stain*.

q.d. Abreviatura da expressão latina *quaque die*, todos os dias.

QF Abreviatura de fator de qualidade (quality *factor*), o mesmo que efetividade biológica relativa na proteção à radiação.

QH_2 Símbolo de ubiquinol.

q.h. Abreviatura da expressão latina *quaque hora*, a cada hora.

q.i.d. Abreviatura da expressão latina *quater in die*, quatro vezes ao dia.

q.l. Abreviatura da expressão latina *quantum libet*, na quantidade desejada.

QNB Abreviatura de quinuclidinil benzilato.

Q.R. Abreviatura da expressão latina *quantum rectum*, o quanto for correto.

q.s. Abreviatura do L. *quantum sufficiat* ou *satis*, a quantidade suficiente.

Q-TWiST Intervalo de tempo sem sintomas ou toxicidade; uma medida da qualidade de vida. [acrônimo, *quality time without symptoms or toxicity*]

quack (kwak). Charlatão. SIN charlatan. [Abreviatura de quacksalver, holandês *quack*, gabar-se + *salf*, creme]

quack·ery (kwak′er - ē). Charlatanismo. SIN charlatanism.

qua·dran·gu·lar (kwah - drang′ū - lăr). Quadrangular; que possui quatro ângulos. [L. *quadrangularis*, de quadrângulo]

quad·rant (kwah′drant). Quadrante; um quarto de um círculo. Em anatomia, áreas aproximadamente circulares são divididas em quadrantes para fins descritivos. O abdome é dividido em quadrantes superior e inferior direitos e superior e inferior esquerdos por uma linha horizontal e uma vertical que se cruzam no umbigo. Os quadrantes do fundo ocular (nasais superior e inferior, temporais superior e inferior) são demarcados por uma linha horizontal e uma vertical que se cruzam no disco óptico. A membrana timpânica é dividida em quadrantes ântero-superior, ântero-inferior, póstero-superior e póstero-inferior por uma linha traçada através do diâmetro do tímpano no eixo do cabo do martelo e outra cruzando a primeira em ângulos retos no umbigo da membrana do tímpano. [L. *quadrans*, um quarto]

quad·rant·an·o·pia (kwah′drant - an - op′ē - ă). Quadrantanopsia; perda da visão em um quarto do campo visual de um ou ambos os olhos; se bilateral, pode ser homônima ou heterônima, binasal ou bitemporal, ou cruzada, p. ex., envolvendo o quadrante superior de um olho e o quadrante inferior do outro. SIN quadrantic hemianopia.

quad·rate (kwah′drāt). Quadrado; que possui quatro lados iguais. [L. *quadratus*, quadrado]

qua·dra·tus.
quadratus lumborum fascia, fáscia do quadrado lombar, lâmina anterior da aponeurose toracolombar; *termo oficial alternativo para anterior *layer* of thoracolumbar fascia.

quadri-. Quatro. [L. *quattuor*]

quad·ri·ba·sic (kwah - dri - bā′sik). Quadribásico; designa um ácido que possui 4 átomos de hidrogênio que podem ser substituídos por átomos ou radicais de caráter básico.

quad·ri·ceps (kwah′dri-seps). Quadríceps. SIN four-headed *muscle*. [L. de quadri- + *caput*, cabeça]

quad·ri·ceps·plas·ty (kwah - dri - seps′plas - tē). Quadricepsplastia; um procedimento cirúrgico corretivo dos músculo e tendão quadríceps femorais para liberar aderências e melhorar a mobilidade. [quadriceps + G. *plastos*, formado]

quad·ri·cus·pid (kwah - dri - kŭs′pid). Quadricúspide. SIN tetracuspid.

quad·ri·dig·i·tate (kwah - dri - dij′i - tāt). Quadridigitado. SIN tetradactyl. [quadri- + L. *digitus*, dedo]

quad·ri·gem·i·nal (kwah′dri - jem′i - năl). Quadrigêmeo; quádruplo. [quadri- + L. *geminus*, gêmeo]

quad·ri·ge·mi·num (kwah′dri - jem′i - nŭm). Quadrigêmeo; um dos corpos quadrigêmeos.

quad·ri·ge·mi·nus (kwah - dri - jem′i - nŭs). Quadrigêmeo. SIN quadruplet. [L.]

quad·ri·ge·mi·ny (kwah′dri - jem′i - nē). Quadrigeminismo. SIN quadrigeminal *rhythm*.

quad·ri·pa·re·sis (kwah′dri - pă - rē′sis). Quadriparesia. SIN tetraparesis.

quad·ri·ple·gia (kwah′dri - plē′jē - ă). Quadriplegia, tetraplegia; paralisia dos quatro membros. SIN tetraplegia. [quadri- + G. *plēgē*, acidente vascular cerebral]

quad·ri·ple·gic (kwah′dri - plē′jik). Quadriplégico, tetraplégico; relativo a ou afetado por quadriplegia. SIN tetraplegic.

quad·ri·po·lar (kwah′dri - pō′lăr). Quadripolar; que possui quatro pólos.

quad·ri·sect (kwah′dri - sekt). Quadrisseccionar; dividir em quatro partes. SIN quartisect. [quadri- + L. *seco*, pp. *sectus*, cortar]

quad·ri·sec·tion (kwah′dri - sek′shŭn). Quadrissecção; divisão em quatro partes.

quad·ri·tu·ber·cu·lar (kwah′dri - too - ber′kū - lăr). Quadritubercular; possui quatro tubérculos ou cúspides, como um dente molar. [quadri- + L. *tuberculum*, tubérculo]

quad·ri·va·lent (kwah - dri - vā′lent). Quadrivalente, tetravalente; que possui o poder de combinação (valência) de quatro. SIN tetravalent.

quad·ru·ped (kwah′droo - ped). Quadrúpede; um animal de quatro patas. [L. *quattuor*, quatro, + *pes (ped-)*, pé]

quad·rup·let (kwah′drŭp - let, kwa - droo′plet). Quádruplo; quadrigêmeo; uma de quatro crianças nascidas de uma vez. SIN quadrigeminus. [L. *quadruplus*, quatro vezes]

qual·i·ty as·sur·ance. Controle de qualidade; programas de avaliação regular das atividades médicas e de enfermagem para avaliar a qualidade da assistência médica.

Quant, C.A.J., médico holandês do início do século XX. VER Quant *sign*.

quan·ta (kwahn′tă). Plural de *quantum*. [L.]

quan·ti·le (kwon′til). Quantil; divisão de uma distribuição em subgrupos iguais e ordenados; decis são décimos, quartis são quartos, quintis são quintos, tercis são terços, centis são centésimos. [L. *quantum*, quanto, + *-ilis*, sufixo adj.]

quan·tum, pl. **quan·ta** (kwahn′tŭm, - tă). Quantum, pl. quanta. 1. Uma unidade de energia radiante (ε) que varia de acordo com a freqüência (ν) da radiação. 2. Uma certa quantidade definida. [L. quanto]
q. mottle, mosqueado quântico. VER quantum *mottle*. Ver entradas em *mottle*.
q. rectum, o quanto for correto. VER Q.R. [L. tanto quanto seja correto]
q. satis, tanto quanto seja suficiente. VER q.s. [L. tanto quanto seja suficiente]
q. sink, tanto quanto faça diminuir; em estudo radiológico, o estágio em que as informações estatísticas alcançam seu nível mais baixo devido a um baixo fluxo de fótons.
q. sufficiat, tanto quanto seja suficiente. VER q.s. [L. tanto quanto seja suficiente]
q. vis (q.v.), tanto quanto desejar. VER q.v. [L. tanto quanto desejar]

quar·an·tine (kwar′an - tēn). Quarentena. 1. Um período (originalmente 40 dias) de detenção ou isolamento de navios e seus passageiros provenientes de uma área onde exista uma moléstia infecciosa. 2. Deter ou isolar esses navios e seus passageiros até que tenha passado o período de incubação de uma doença infecciosa. 3. Um lugar onde esses navios e seus passageiros são detidos ou isolados. 4. O isolamento de uma pessoa com uma doença contagiosa conhecida ou possível. [It. *quarantina* do L. *quadraginta*, quarenta]

quark (qwark). Quark; uma partícula fundamental que se acredita ser o constituinte primário de todos os mésons e bárions; os quarks possuem uma carga elétrica que é uma fração da carga elétrica de 1 elétron e interagem através de forças eletromagnéticas e nucleares. Acredita-se que existam variantes com os nomes incomuns de *up, down, strange, charmed, bottom* e *top*. [uma palavra de sentido indeterminado usada por James Joyce em seu romance *Finnegans Wake*]

quart (kwōrt). Quarto. 1. Medida de volume; a quarta parte de um galão; o equivalente a 0,9468 litro. Um quarto imperial contém cerca de 20% mais que o quarto comum, ou 1,1359 litro. 2. Uma medida para secos, correspondente a um pouco mais que a medida para líquidos. [L. *quartus*, quarto]

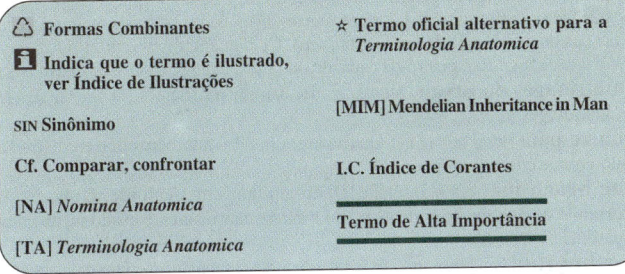

⌬ Formas Combinantes	☆ Termo oficial alternativo para a *Terminologia Anatomica*
🅘 Indica que o termo é ilustrado, ver Índice de Ilustrações	
SIN Sinônimo	[MIM] Mendelian Inheritance in Man
Cf. Comparar, confrontar	I.C. Índice de Corantes
[NA] *Nomina Anatomica*	Termo de Alta Importância
[TA] *Terminologia Anatomica*	

quark — quince

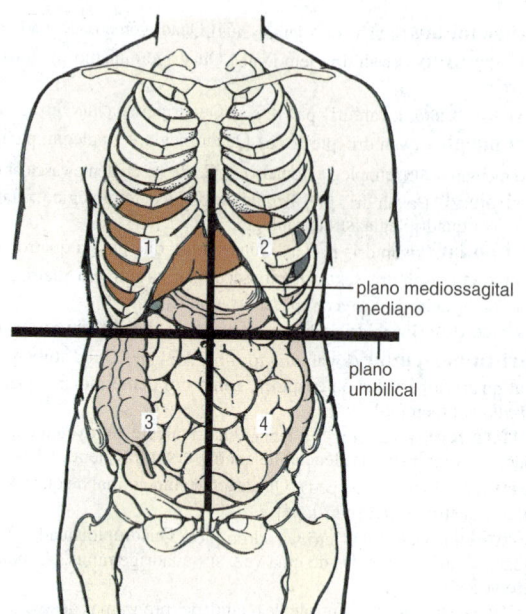

quadrantes: (1) superior direito, (2) superior esquerdo, (3) inferior direito, (4) inferior esquerdo

quar·tan (kwōr′tan). Quartã; que recorre a cada quatro dias, incluindo o primeiro dia de um episódio no cálculo, isto é, após um intervalo livre de dois dias. [L. *quartanus*, relativo a um quarto (objeto)]
 double q., q. dupla; indica a malária com dois grupos independentes de plasmódios, de forma que os paroxismos ocorrem em dois dias sucessivos seguidos por um dia sem febre.
 triple q., q. tripla; indica malária por três grupos independentes de plasmódios, de forma que os paroxismos ocorrem diariamente, assemelhando-se a uma febre terçã dupla ou cotidiana.

quar·ti·sect (kwōr′ti - sekt). Quadrisseccionar. SIN quadrisect. [L. *quartus*, quarto, + *seco*, pp. *sectus*, cortar]

quartz (kwōrtz). Quartzo; uma forma cristalina de dióxido de silício usada em aparelhos químicos e em instrumentos ópticos e elétricos.

qua·si·dom·i·nance (kwā - si - dom′i - nans). Falsa dominância; simulação de herança dominante de um traço recessivo, p. ex., o casamento de um heterozigoto com um homozigoto afetado resultando na manifestação do traço recessivo geração após geração. SIN false dominance, pseudodominance.

qua·si·dom·i·nant (kwā - si - dom′i - nănt). Pseudodominante; designa um traço em um heredograma endogâmico que exibe falsa dominância.

quas·sa·tion (kwah - sā′shŭn). Quassação; redução de matérias-primas de medicamentos, como cascas e troncos, a pedaços pequenos para facilitar a extração e outro tratamento. [L. *quassatio*, fr. *quasso*, pp. *-atus*, agitar violentamente, fr. *quatio*, agitar]

quas·sia (kwah′shē - ā). Quássia; pau-amargo; o cerne da *Picrasma excelsa* (*Picraena excelsa*), também conhecida como q. da Jamaica, ou da *Quassia amara* (família Simarubaceae), conhecida como q. do Suriname; um tônico amargo; a infusão já foi administrada por enema no tratamento de verminoses. [*Quassi*, um residente do Suriname que a usava como tônico]

quater in die (kua′ter - in - dē - ā). Quatro vezes ao dia. VER q.i.d. [L. quatro vezes ao dia]

qua·ter·na·ry (Q) (kwah′ter - năr - ē, kwah - ter′nĕ - rē). Quaternário. **1.** Indica uma substância química que contém quatro elementos; p. ex., $NaHSO_4$. Cf. quaternary *structure*. **2.** Quarto em uma série. **3.** Relativo a compostos orgânicos nos quais algum átomo central está fixado a quatro grupamentos funcionais; aplicado ao nitrogênio geralmente trivalente em seu estado "quaternário", R_4N^+, "nitrogênio quaternário." **4.** Refere-se a um nível de estrutura de macromoléculas nas quais há mais de um biopolímero. Cf. quaternary *structure*. [L. *quaternarius*, de *quaterni*, quatro de cada, de *quattuor*, quatro, + *-arius*, sufixo adj.]

Quatrefages de Breau, Jean L.A. de, naturalista francês, 1810–1892. VER Quatrefages *angle*.

qua·ze·pam (kwā′zĕ - pam). Quazepam; um derivado benzodiazepínico usado como sedativo e hipnótico.

que·brach·ine (kē - brah′chēn). Quebraquina; um alcalóide, $C_{21}H_{26}N_2O_3$, oriundo do quebracho e idêntico à ioimbina; anteriormente usado na dispnéia cardíaca.

que·bra·cho (kē - brah′chō). Quebracho; a casca seca de um gênero de árvores, *Aspidosperma quebrachoblanco* (família Apocynaceae); tem sido usado como estimulante respiratório no enfisema, na dispnéia e na bronquite crônica; os dois principais alcalóides são aspidospermina e quebraquina. [Port. *quebrahacho*, de *quebrar*, quebrar, + *hacha*, machado, referindo-se à dureza da madeira]

Queckenstedt, Hans, neurofisiologista alemão, 1876–1918. VER Q.-Stookey *test*.

quench·ing (kwench′ing). Extinção. **1.** O processo de extinguir, remover ou diminuir uma propriedade física como calor ou luz; p. ex., o resfriamento de um metal quente rapidamente mergulhando-o em água ou óleo. **2.** No contador de cintilação líquida beta, o desvio do espectro de energia de uma energia verdadeira para uma menor; é causada por vários materiais que interferem na solução de contagem, incluindo agentes químicos e corantes estranhos. **3.** O processo de interromper uma reação química ou enzimática. [I. M. *quenchen*, do I. ant. *ācwencan*]
 fluorescence q., e. fluorescente; uma técnica usada em investigações que lidam com a ligação de antígeno (haptenos) por anticorpos purificados, aplicável quando o antígeno ligado (hapteno) absorve (extingue) a luz emitida durante a fluorescência de proteína (anticorpo) excitada por luz ultravioleta.

Quénu, Eduard A.V.A., cirurgião e anatomista francês, 1852–1933. VER Q. hemorrhoidal *plexus*; Q.-Muret *sign*.

quer·ce·tin (kwer′sē - tin). Quercetina; um aglicônio de quercitrina, rutina e outros glicosídeos; ocorre geralmente como o 3-ramnosídeo; usado no tratamento de fragilidade capilar anormal. SIN meletin, sophoretin.

quer·cus (kwer′kŭs). Querco; a casca de *Quercus alba*, carvalho-branco ou carvalho-pedra; usado antigamente como adstringente. [L. carvalho]

quer·u·lent (kwer′ŭ - lent). Queixoso; querelante; designa aquele que é sempre desconfiado, sempre se opõe a qualquer sugestão, queixa-se de ser maltratado e de ser menosprezado ou incompreendido, que se irrita facilmente, e insatisfeito; característica de personalidades paranóides. [L. *querulus*, queixoso, de *queror*, queixar]

Quervain, Fritz de. VER Quervain.

ques·tion·naire (kwes - chŭn - ār′). Questionário; uma lista de perguntas feitas oralmente ou por escrito para obter informações pessoais ou dados estatisticamente úteis.
 Holmes-Rahe q., q. de Holmes-Rahe; um estudo para medir em unidades de modificação de vida o estresse de vários eventos da vida como uma doença aguda, falência, morte de uma pessoa querida, etc.

Quetelet, Lambert Alphonse Jacques, 1796–1857. Astrônomo e matemático belga.

Queyrat, Auguste, dermatologista francês, *1872. VER erythroplasia of Q.

Quick, Armand J., médico norte-americano, 1894–1978. VER Q. *method, test*.

quick (kwik). Ativo; ágil. **1.** Grávida cujo feto tem movimentos detectáveis. **2.** Uma parte sensível, dolorosa ao toque. [A.S. *cwic*, vivo]

quick·en·ing (kwik′ĕn - ing). Sinais de vida percebidos pela mãe em virtude dos movimentos fetais, geralmente observados a partir da 16.ª à 20.ª semana de gravidez. [A.S. *cwic*, vivo]

quick·lime (kwik′līm). Cal virgem, cal viva. VER lime (2).

quick·sil·ver (kwik′sil′ver). Mercúrio. SIN mercury.

qui·es·cent (kwi-es′ent). Quiescente; em repouso ou inativo.

quin-2. (2-[(2-bis-[carboximetil]aono-5-metoxifenil)-metil-6-metoxi-8-bis[carboximetil]aminoquinolina); uma substância fluorescente que se liga firmemente ao Ca^{++}. Os comprimentos de onda da luz que causam fluorescência quando o Ca^{++} está ligado são mais longos que os comprimentos de onda que causam fluorescência quando o Ca^{++} não está ligado. Quando excitados em dois comprimentos de onda diferentes, a razão das intensidades de fluorescência nos dois comprimentos de onda fornece a razão entre as concentrações de Ca^{++} ligado e livre. A concentração de quin-2 livre pode ser medida com precisão, e, assim, a concentração de Ca^{++} livre pode ser calculada com precisão. Quin-2 pode ser injetado em células para medir alterações instantâneas da concentração intracelular de Ca^{++}. VER TAMBÉM aequorin, fura-2.

quin-, quino-. Raiz de quinolina e quinona, usada, portanto, em muitos nomes de substâncias que contêm essas estruturas (p. ex., quinina, quinol).

qui·na (kē′nā, kwē′nā). Quina; casca da cinchona. SIN cinchona. [Esp., de Peruv. *quina* ou *kina*, cinchona]

quin·a·crine hy·dro·chlo·ride (kwin′ā - krēn, - krin). Cloridrato de quinacrina; um derivado da acridina, usado como antimalárico que destrói os trofozoítas de *Plasmodium vivax* e *P. falciparum*, mas não afeta os gametócitos, esporozoítas ou o estágio exoeritrocítico de parasitas; também usado como anti-helmíntico. Como o dicloridrato, é usado como corante em citogenética para demonstrar cromatina Y por microscopia fluorescente. O c. q. intercala-se com o DNA e também desacopla a oxidação e a fotofosforilação. SIN atabrine hydrochloride, mepacrine hydrochloride.

quin·al·dic ac·id (kwin - al′dik). Ácido quináldico; ácido quinolina-2-carboxílico; um produto do catabolismo do L-triptofano, via ácido cinurênico, encontrado na urina humana. SIN quinaldinic acid.

quin·al·dine red (kwin′al - dēn). Vermelho de quinaldina; um iodeto estirenoquinolínico; usado como indicador do pH (torna-se vermelho em pH 3,2) em uma solução de etanol a 1%.

quin·al·din·ic ac·id (kwin-al-din′ik). Ácido quinaldínico. SIN quinaldic acid.

qui·na·qui·na (kē′nā - kē′nā, kwin′ā - kwin′ā). Quinaquina. SIN cinchona. [uma duplicação do Esp. *quina*, cinchona]

qui·nate (kwī′nāt, kwin′āt). Quinato; sal ou éster do ácido quínico.

Quincke

q. dehydrogenase, q. desidrogenase; uma oxidorredutase que catalisa a reação de quinato e NAD$^+$ para formar 3-desidroquinato e NADH.

quin·a·zo·lines (kwin-a-zōl'ēns). Quinazolinas; uma classe de alcalóides derivados biossinteticamente do ácido antranílico.

quince (kwints). Marmelo; o fruto comestível da *Cydonia oblongata* (família Rosaceae); as sementes possuem propriedades demulcentes.

Quincke, Heinrich I., médico alemão, 1842–1922. VER Q. *pulse, puncture, sign.*

quin·es·tra·di·ol, quin·es·tra·dol (kwin'es-trā-dī'ol, kwin-es'trā-dol). Quinestradiol; um estrogênio.

quin·es·trol (kwin-es'trōl). Quinestrol; o éter 3-ciclopentil do etinil estradiol; usado como o componente estrogênico em contraceptivos orais; a substância é armazenada na gordura e pode ser usada semanalmente; um estrogênio.

quin·eth·a·zone (kwin-eth'ā-zōn). Quinetazona; um diurético e anti-hipertensivo.

quin·ges·ta·nol ac·e·tate (kwin-jes'tā-nol). Acetato de quingestanol; um agente progestacional.

quin·hy·drone (kwin-hī'drōn). Quinidrona; uma mistura de quantidades eqüimoleculares de quinona e hidroquinona; usado em determinações do pH (isto é, via uma q. eletrodo).

quin·ic ac·id (kwin'ik). Ácido quínico; ácido L-quínico; o (-) isômero é um ácido encontrado na casca da cinchona e em outras partes dos vegetais; o ácido 5-desidroquínico é um intermediário na biossíntese de L-fenilalanina, L-tirosina e L-triptofano a partir de precursores carboidrato; o a. q. forma uma γ-lactona ao aquecimento. SIN kinic acid.

quin·i·dine (kwin'i-dēn, -din). Quinidina; β-quinina; um dos alcalóides da cinchona, um estereoisômero da quinina (o epímero C-9); usado como antimalárico; também usado no tratamento da fibrilação e do *flutter* atriais, e da taquicardia ventricular paroxística. SIN conquinine.
  q. polygalacturonate, poligalacturonato de q.; um sal de quinidina que pode substituir o sulfato de quinidina; agente antiarrítmico. VER q. sulfate; VER TAMBÉM quinidine.
  q. sulfate, sulfato de q.; o sal de q. que é comumente administrado como antiarrítmico cardíaco; deprime a condução, a contração, a automaticidade e contração miocárdicas; também compromete, por um efeito direto, a condução através do nodo atrioventricular. Possui ação vagolítica que pode aumentar a freqüência cardíaca. VER TAMBÉM quinidine.

qui·nine (kwī'nīn, -nēn, kwin'-īn, -ēn). Quinina; o mais importante dos alcalóides derivados da cinchona, um antimalárico efetivo contra as formas assexuada e eritrocítica do parasita, mas que não tem efeito sobre as formas exoeritrocíticas (teciduais). Não promove cura radical da malária causada por *Plasmodium vivax*, *P. malariae* ou *P. ovale*, mas é usada no tratamento da malária cerebral e de outros ataques graves de malária terçã maligna, bem como na malária provocada por cepas de *P. falciparum* resistentes à cloroquina; também é usada como antipirético, analgésico, agente esclerosante, estomáquico e ocitócico (ocasionalmente), e no tratamento de fibrilação atrial, miotonia congênita e outras miopatias.
  q. bisulfate, bissulfato de q.; o sulfato ácido de q., bastante hidrossolúvel.
  q. carbacrylic resin, resina carbacrílica de q. VER resin.
  q. ethylcarbonate, etilcarbonato de q.; uma forma quase insípida de q. que é mal absorvida pelo trato intestinal.
  q. sulfate, sulfato de q.; o sal de q. mais prescrito.
  q. and urea hydrochloride, cloridrato de q. e uréia; agente esclerosante para tratamento de hemorróidas internas, hidrocele e veias varicosas, contendo não menos que 58% e não mais que 65% de q. anidra.
  q. urethan, q. uretana; uma mistura de uretana e cloridrato de q.; um agente esclerosante para o tratamento de veias varicosas.

qui·nin·ism (kwī'ni-nizm, kwin'i-). Quininismo. SIN cinchonism.

Quinlan test. Teste de Quinlan. Ver em test.

△ **quino-.** VER quin-.

quin·o·cide hy·dro·chlo·ride (kwin'ō-sīd). Cloridrato de quinocida; um antimalárico comparável à primaquina em efetividade e alcance.

quin·ol (kwin'ol). Quinol. VER hydroquinone.

quin·o·line (kwin'ō-lēn,-lin). Quinolina. **1.** Benzo[*b*]piridina; 1-benzazina; uma base nitrogenada volátil obtida pela destilação do alcatrão da hulha, ossos, alcalóides, etc.; uma estrutura básica de muitos corantes e fármacos; também usada como antimalárico. SIN chinoleine, leucoline. **2.** Pertencente a uma classe de alcalóides baseada na estrutura da q. (a).

quin·o·lin·ic ac·id (kwin-ō-lin'ik). Ácido quinolínico; um catabólito do L-triptofano e um precursor do NAD$^+$.

quin·o·lin·ol (kwin-ol'in-ol). Quinolinol. SIN 8-hydroxyquinoline.

quin·o·li·zi·dines (kwin-ol-i-za-dēns). Quinolizidinas; uma classe de alcalóides baseada na estrutura da quinolizidina (norlupinano).

qui·nol·o·gy (kwin-ol'ō-jē). Quinologia; a botânica, a química, a farmacologia e a terapêutica da cinchona e seus alcalóides. [Esp. *quina*, cinchona, + G. *logos*, estudo]

quin·o·lones (kwin'ō-lōnz). Quinolonas; uma classe de agentes antibacterianos sintéticos de amplo espectro que exibem ação bactericida (p. ex., ciprofloxacin). SIN fluoroquinolone.

qui·none (kwin'ōn, kwī'nōn). Quinona. **1.** Nome genérico de compostos aromáticos que possuem dois oxigênios no lugar de dois hidrogênios, geralmente na posição *para*; o produto de oxidação de uma hidroquinona. **2.** SIN 1,4-benzoquinone (1).
  q. reductase, q. redutase. SIN NADPH dehydrogenase (quinone).

qui·no·vose (kwin'ō-vōs). Quinovose. SIN D-epirhamnose.

quin·que·dig·i·tate (kwin'kwē-dij'i-tāt). Qüinqüedigitado. SIN pentadactyl. [L. *quinque*, cinco, + *digitus*, dedo]

quin·que·tu·ber·cu·lar (kwin'kwē-too-ber'kū-lăr). Qüinqüetubercular; que possui cinco tubérculos ou cúspides, como determinados dentes molares. [L. *quinque*, cinco, + *tuberculum*, tubérculo, dim. de *tuber*, uma tumefação]

quin·que·va·lent (kwin-kwē-vā'lent). Qüinqüevalente. SIN pentavalent. [L. *quinque*, cinco, + *valentia*, poder]

quin·qui·na (kwin-kwi'nă). Quinquina. SIN cinchona.

quin·sy (kwin'zē). Esquinência; termo obsoleto para designar abscesso peritonsilar (peritonsillar *abscess*). [I.M. *quinsie* (*quinesie*), uma corrupção do L. *cynanche*, dor de garganta]
  lingual q., e. lingual; inflamação flegmonosa da tonsila lingual e das estruturas adjacentes.

quin·tan (kwin'tan). Quintã; que recorre a cada quinto dia, incluindo o primeiro dia de um episódio no cálculo, isto é, após um intervalo livre de três dias. [L. *quintus*, quinto]

quin·tu·plet (kwin-tŭp'let). Quíntuplo; uma das cinco crianças nascidas do mesmo parto. [L. *quintuplex*, cinco vezes]

qui·nuc·li·din·yl ben·zi·late (QNB) (kwin-oo'-kli-di-nil ben'-zil-āt). Benzilato de quinuclidinil; um agente anticolinérgico muito potente que exibe potência 50 a 100 vezes maior que a da atropina na ligação e no bloqueio dos receptores colinérgicos muscarínicos. Originalmente desenvolvido como um potencial agente incapacitante militar, é amplamente usado hoje como agente radioativo (geralmente -H3-QNB tritiado) para identificar e marcar receptores muscarínicos em estudos farmacológicos.

quis·qua·late (kwiz'kwa-lāt). Quisqualato; um agonista em receptores glutamato do tipo do ácido amino-3-hidroxi-5-metil-isoxazol-4-propiônico (AMPA). O ânion formado quando o ácido quisquálico é dissolvido em água. VER quisqualic acid.

quis·qual·ic ac·id (kwiz'kwa-lik). Ácido quisquálico; aminoácido excitatório (AAE) obtido das sementes de *Quisqualis chinensis*. Usado para identificar um subgrupo específico de receptor do AAE não-*N*-metil D-aspartato (NMDA); tem propriedades anti-helmínticas.

quod·que (q.). A cada. [L.]

quo·tid·i·an (kwō-tid'ē-ăn). Quotidiano; diário; que ocorre todo dia. [L. *quotidianus*, diariamente, de *quot*, tanto quanto, + *dias*, dia]

quo·tient (kwō'shent). Quociente; o número de vezes que uma quantidade está contida em outra; a razão entre dois números. VER TAMBÉM index (2), ratio. [L. *quoties*, com que freqüência]
  achievement q., q. de aproveitamento; uma razão, percentagem ou q. relacionado que designa o grau de aprendizado de uma criança em relação às crianças de sua idade ou escolaridade.
  Ayala q., q. de Ayala. SIN Ayala *index.*
  cognitive laterality q. (CLQ), q. de lateralidade cognitivo; teste que avalia a diferença do desempenho cognitivo dos lados esquerdo e direito do cérebro.
  extremal q., q. de valores extremos; a razão entre a freqüência na jurisdição com a máxima taxa de intervenções como procedimentos cirúrgicos e a freqüência na jurisdição (competência) com a mínima taxa.
  intelligence q. (IQ), q. de inteligência (QI); o índice de inteligência medido pelo psicólogo como parte de uma determinação da inteligência em duas partes, sendo a outra parte um indicador do comportamento adaptativo e incluindo critérios como notas escolares ou desempenho profissional. O QI é um escore, ou índice quantitativo semelhante, usado para indicar a situação de uma pessoa em relação aos seus pares da mesma idade em um teste de capacidade geral, comumente expresso como uma razão entre o resultado obtido por uma pessoa em um determinado teste e o resultado que a pessoa média de idade comparável atingiu no mesmo teste, sendo a razão calculada pelo psicólogo ou determinada por um quadro de padrões para a idade, como as várias escalas de inteligência de Wechsler.
  Meyerhof oxidation q., q. de oxidação de Meyerhof; um índice do efeito do oxigênio sobre a glicólise e a fermentação (isto é, sobre o efeito Pasteur); igual à taxa de fermentação anaeróbica menos a taxa de respiração aeróbica dividida pela taxa de captação de oxigênio.
  P/O q., q. F/O. SIN P/O *ratio.*
  protein q., q. proteico; o número obtido pela divisão da quantidade de globulina do plasma sanguíneo pela quantidade de albumina.
  respiratory q. (R.Q.), q. respiratório; a razão em equilíbrio dinâmico entre o dióxido de carbono produzido por metabolismo tecidual e o oxigênio consumido no mesmo metabolismo; para o corpo inteiro, normalmente cerca de 0,82 em condições basais; no estado de equilíbrio dinâmico, o q. respiratório é igual ao índice de troca respiratória. SIN respiratory coefficient.
  spinal q., q. espinhal. SIN Ayala *index.*

quot. op. sit. Abreviatura de quoties opus sit, com a freqüência necessária.

q.v. Abreviatura de [L.] *quantum>* vis, tanto quanto desejado.

R

ρ 1. Rô, a décima sétima letra do alfabeto grego. **2.** Símbolo de population correlation coefficient (coeficiente de correlação populacional); density (densidade).

R Abreviatura ou símbolo de electrical resistance (resistência elétrica); radical (radical, geralmente um grupamento alquil ou aril, p. ex., ROH corresponde a um álcool, e RNH_2, a uma amina); Réaumur; respiration (respiração); respiratory exchange *ratio* (razão de troca respiratória); roentgen; do restante de uma fórmula química; da unidade calculada que representa a resistência vascular no sistema cardiovascular; da arginine (arginina); arginyl (arginil); purine nucleoside (nucleosídeo purina).

℞ Símbolo de *recipe* (receita) em uma prescrição médica. VER prescription (2).

R_f, R_F Símbolo que indica o movimento de uma substância na cromatografia em papel em *r*elação (R) à *f*rente do solvente (i.e., o fator de retardamento); corresponde à distância da migração de uma substância dividida pela distância da migração da linha de frente do solvente.

R. Abreviatura ou símbolo (em itálico) de molar gas *constant* (constante molar do gás); uma das duas denominações estereoquímicas do sistema de Cahn, Ingold e Prelog; o terceiro produto formado em uma reação catalisada por uma enzima.

r Abreviatura de roentgen; radius (raio).

***r.* 1.** Símbolo de correlation *coefficient*. **2.** Abreviatura de racemic (racêmico), utilizada ocasionalmente na designação dos compostos em lugar dos símbolos mais comuns DL ou (±), p. ex., "*r*-alanina" (o prefixo *rac-* é o mais freqüente).

Ra Símbolo de radium (rádio).

rab·bet·ing (rab′et-ing). Fazer encaixes, entalhes, ranhuras; termo obsoleto dado à técnica que consiste em fazer cortes semelhantes a degraus gradativamente congruentes nas superfícies ósseas em aposição a fim de obter estabilização após impacção. [Fr. *raboter*, nivelar, aplainar]

rab·id. Raivoso; relativo à raiva ou que sofre dela. [L. *rabidus*, delirante, louco, furioso]

ra·bies (rā′bēz). Raiva; doença infecciosa altamente fatal que pode afetar todas as espécies de animais de sangue quente, incluindo os seres humanos; é transmitida pela mordida de animais infectados, como cães, gatos, gambás, lobos, raposas, guaxinins e morcegos, e causada por uma espécie neurotrópica de Lyssavirus, um membro da família Rhabdoviridae, no sistema nervoso central e nas glândulas salivares. Os sinais e sintomas são característicos de um distúrbio profundo do sistema nervoso, p. ex., excitação, agressividade e loucura, seguidos por paralisia e morte. Os corpúsculos de inclusão citoplasmática (corpúsculos de Negri), característicos da doença e encontrados em muitos neurônios, possibilitam a obtenção de um diagnóstico laboratorial rápido. SIN hydrophobia. [L. raiva, fúria, de *rabio*, delirar, enlouquecer]
dumb r., r. paralítica. SIN paralytic r.
furious r., r. furiosa; a forma ou a fase da r. na qual o animal se apresenta muito hiperativo; é caracterizada por períodos de agitação durante os quais o animal se debate, corre, tenta morder ou morde.
paralytic r., r. paralítica; uma forma ou fase da r. caracterizada por paralisia. SIN dumb r.
ra·bi·form (rā′bi-fōrm). Que se assemelha à raiva.

rac-. Rac-; prefixo que significa racêmico (*racemic*).

ra·ce·fem·ine (rā-se-fem′en). Racefemina; utilizada como relaxante uterino para o alívio da dor pós-parto.

rac·e·mase (rā′se-mās). Racemase; enzima capaz de catalisar a racemização, i.e., as inversões de grupamentos assimétricos; quando existe mais de um centro de assimetria, utiliza-se a "epimerase" (p. ex., hidroxiprolina, ribulose fosfato).

rac·e·mate (rā′se-māt). Racemato; um composto racêmico, ou o sal ou o éster de tal composto. VER TAMBÉM racemic.

ra·ceme (rā-sēm′). Um composto químico opticamente inativo. VER TAMBÉM racemic.

⚠ Formas Combinantes	★ Termo oficial alternativo para a *Terminologia Anatomica*
🔲 Indica que o termo é ilustrado, ver Índice de Ilustrações	
SIN Sinônimo	[MIM] Mendelian Inheritance in Man
Cf. Comparar, confrontar	I.C. Índice de Corantes
[NA] *Nomina Anatomica*	
[TA] *Terminologia Anatomica*	Termo de Alta Importância

---

guia para a profilaxia pós-exposição à raiva

tipo de animal	estado do animal	tratamento da pessoa exposta[1]
doméstico cães e gatos	sadio e disponível durante 10 dias para observação	nenhum, a menos que o animal desenvolva manifestações da raiva[2]
	raivoso ou com suspeita de estar com raiva	imunoglobulina anti-rábica humana[3] e vacina anti-rábica de células diplóides humanas ou vacina anti-rábica absorvida[4] imediatamente
	desconhecido (o animal escapou)	consultar as pessoas responsáveis pela saúde pública; se o tratamento for indicado, dar imunoglobulina anti-rábica humana[3] e vacina anti-rábica de células diplóides humanas ou vacina anti-rábica absorvida
selvagem gambás, guaxinins, morcegos, raposas, coiotes e outros carnívoros	considerar o animal raivoso, a menos que se saiba que a área geográfica está livre de raiva ou até que o animal apresente testes laboratoriais[5] negativos para a raiva	imunoglobulina anti-rábica humana[3] e vacina anti-rábica de células diplóides humanas ou vacina anti-rábica absorvida[4] imediatamente
outros aves domésticas, roedores e lagomorfos (coelhos e lebres)	avaliar individualmente; as pessoas responsáveis pela saúde pública local e estadual devem ser consultadas quanto à necessidade de realizar a profilaxia da raiva; as mordidas de esquilos, hamsters, porquinhos-da-índia, gerbos, tâmias, ratos, camundongos e outros roedores, coelhos e lebres quase nunca exigem profilaxia anti-rábica	

as recomendações precedentes compõem apenas um guia; ao aplicá-las, leve em consideração a espécie do animal envolvido, as circunstâncias da mordida ou de outro tipo de exposição, o *status* da vacinação do animal e a existência de raiva na região; ***observação:*** os responsáveis pela saúde pública local ou estadual devem ser consultados, caso surjam dúvidas quanto a necessidade de profilaxia da raiva.

[1]Todas as mordidas e todos os ferimentos devem ser *completamente limpos com água e sabão imediatamente*; se o tratamento contra a raiva for indicado, tanto a imunoglobulina anti-rábica humana como a vacina anti-rábica de células diplóides humanas ou a vacina anti-rábica absorvida devem ser administradas o mais cedo possível, *sem levar em consideração* o tempo decorrido desde a exposição
[2]Durante o habitual período de espera de 10 dias, começar o tratamento com imunoglobulina anti-rábica humana e vacina ao primeiro sinal de raiva em um cão ou gato que mordeu alguém; o animal sintomático deve ser sacrificado imediatamente e submetido a testes
[3]Se a imunoglobulina anti-rábica humana não estiver disponível, utilize o soro anti-rábico eqüino; não utilize uma dose maior do que a recomendada
[4]As reações locais às vacinas são comuns e não contra-indicam a continuidade do tratamento; interrompa a administração da vacina, caso os resultados do teste de anticorpo fluorescente do animal sejam negativos
[5]O animal deve ser sacrificado e submetido a testes o mais cedo possível; o período de espera para a observação do animal não é recomendado

ra·ce·mic (r) (rā-sē′mik, -sem′ik). Racêmico; indica uma mistura opticamente inativa formada por compostos opticamente ativos; é composta por um número igual de substâncias dextrorrotatórias e levorrotatórias, que são separáveis. Os compostos internamente compensados (i.e., que possuem um plano de simetria interno) e que, portanto, não podem ser separados nas formas D e L (ou + e −), são denominados "*meso*".

rac·e·mi·za·tion (rā′sē-mi-zā′shŭn, ras-mi-). Racemização; a conversão parcial de um enantiomorfo em outro (como a de um L-aminoácido no D-aminoácido correspondente), de modo que a rotação óptica específica na mistura resultante é diminuída ou mesmo reduzida a zero.

rac·e·mose (ras′ē-mōs). Racemoso; ramificação com terminações nodulares; que se assemelha a um cacho de uvas. [L. *racemosus*, cheio de cachos]

rac·e·phed·rine hy·dro·chlo·ride (rās-ē-fed′rin). Cloridrato de racefedrina; droga simpaticomimética com efeitos periféricos similares aos da epinefrina e com as mesmas ações e os mesmos usos da efedrina.

rachi-, rachio-. Raqui-, raquio-; a coluna vertebral. [G. *rhachis*, espinha dorsal, coluna vertebral]

ra·chi·al (rā′kē-ăl). Raquial. SIN spinal.

ra·chi·cen·te·sis (rā-kē-sen-tē′sis). Raquicentese, punção lombar. SIN lumbar *puncture*. [rachi- + G. *kentēsis*, punção]

ra·chid·i·al (ră-kid′ē-ăl). Raquidiano, espinal. SIN spinal.

ra·chid·i·an (ră-kid′ē-an). Raquidiano, espinal. SIN spinal.

ra·chil·y·sis (ră-kil′i-sis). Raquilise; a correção forçada de uma curvatura lateral da coluna vertebral pela aplicação de pressão lateral contra a convexidade da curva. [rachi- + G. *lysis*, afrouxamento]

rachio-. Raquio-. VER rachi-.

ra·chi·o·cen·te·sis (rā-kē-ō-sen-tē′sis). Raquiocentese, punção lombar. SIN lumbar *puncture*. [rachio- + G. *kentēsis*, punção]

ra·chi·och·y·sis (rā-kē-ok′i-sis). Raquioquise; derrame subaracnóideo de líquido no canal da coluna vertebral. [rachio- + G. *chysis*, derramar]

ra·chi·op·a·gus (rā-kē-op′ă-gŭs). Raquiópago; gêmeos que se apresentam unidos pelos dorsos, com fusão de suas colunas vertebrais. VER conjoined *twins*, em *twin*. SIN rachipagus. [rachio- + G. *pagos*, algo fixo]

ra·chi·o·ple·gia (rā′kē-ō-plē′jē-ă). Raquioplegia. SIN spinal *paralysis*. [rachio- + G. *plēgē*, ataque]

ra·chi·o·tome (rā′kē-ō-tōm). Raquiótomo; instrumento especialmente desenvolvido para dividir as lâminas das vértebras. SIN rachitome. [rachio- + G. *tomē*, incisão]

ra·chi·ot·o·my (rā-kē-ot′ō-mē). Raquiotomia, laminotomia. SIN laminotomy. [rachio- + G. *tomē*, incisão]

ra·chip·a·gus (ră-kip′ă-gŭs). Raquípago. SIN rachiopagus.

ra·chis, pl. **rach·i·des, ra·chis·es** (rā′kis, rā′ki-dēz, rak-). Raque, coluna vertebral. SIN vertebral *column*. [G. coluna vertebral]

ra·chis·chi·sis (ră-kis′ki-sis). Raquisquise; **1.** Falha embriológica na fusão dos arcos vertebrais e do tubo neural com conseqüente exposição do tecido neural na superfície; espinha bífida cística com mielocele ou mielosquise. **2.** Disrafismo espinal. [G. *rhachis*, coluna vertebral, + *schisis*, divisão]

r. partia′lis, r. parcial. SIN merorachischisis.
r. tota′lis, r. total. SIN holorachischisis.

ra·chit·ic (ră-kit′ic). Raquítico; relativo ao raquitismo ou que sofre dessa doença. SIN rickety.

ra·chi·tis (ră-kī′tis). Raquitismo. SIN rickets. [G. *rhachitis*]
r. feta′lis, r. fetal; r. congênito. SIN r. intrauterina, r. uterina.
r. feta′lis annula′ris, r. fetal anular; aumento congênito das epífises dos ossos longos.
r. feta′lis micromel′ica, r. fetal micromélico; condição congênita na qual o desenvolvimento dos ossos longos é deficiente.
r. intrauteri′na, r. uteri′na, r. intra-uterino, r. uterino. SIN r. fetalis.
r. tar′da, osteomalacia. SIN osteomalacia.

ra·chi·tism (rak′i-tizm). Raquitismo; estado raquítico ou uma tendência ao raquitismo.

rach·i·to·gen·ic (ră-kit-ō-jen′ik). Raquitogênico; que produz ou causa raquitismo. [rachitis + G. *genesis*, produção]

ra·chi·tome (rak′i-tōm). Raquítomo. SIN rachiotome.

rad Rad. **1.** A unidade da dose absorvida de uma radiação ionizante; equivale a 100 ergs por grama de tecido; 100 rad = 1 Gy. **2.** O símbolo de radian (radiano).

ra·dar·ky·mog·ra·phy (rā′dar-kī-mog′ră-fē). Procedimento obsoleto que utiliza uma imagem feita em vídeo do movimento cardíaco obtida por meio de intensificação de imagens e de circuito fechado de televisão durante a fluoroscopia; permitia que o movimento cardíaco fosse avaliado por um registro gráfico linear reproduzível.

ra·dec·to·my (ră-dek′tō-mē). Radectomia. SIN root *amputation*. [L. *radix*, raiz, + G. *ektomē*, excisão]

Radford, Edward P., Jr., fisiologista norte-americano, *1922. VER R. *nomogram*.

ra·di·a·bil·i·ty (rā′dē-ă-bil′i-tē). Radiabilidade; a propriedade de ser radiável.

ra·di·a·ble (rā′dē-ă-bl). Radiável; que pode ser penetrado ou examinado por raios, especialmente pelos raios X.

ra·di·ad (rā′dē-ad). Em direção à face radial.

ra·di·al (rā′dē-ăl). Radial. **1.** Relativo ao rádio (osso do antebraço), a quaisquer estruturas nomeadas a partir dele ou à face radial (ou lateral) do membro superior, quando comparada com a face ulnar (ou medial). SIN radialis [TA]. **2.** Relativo a qualquer raio. **3.** Irradiante; que diverge em todas as direções a partir de um determinado centro. [L. *radialis*, de *radius*, raio, osso lateral do antebraço]

ra·di·a·lis (rā-dē-ā′lis) [TA]. Radial. SIN radial (1). [L. mod.]

ra·di·an (rad) (rā′dē-an). Radiano; unidade suplementar do SI de ângulos planos. [L. *radius*, raio]

ra·di·ant (rā′dē-ant). Radiante. **1.** Que emite raios. **2.** Um ponto a partir do qual a luz se irradia até o olho.

ra·di·ate (rā′dē-āt). Radiar(-se), irradiar(-se); **1.** Propagar-se em todas as direções a partir de um centro. **2.** Emitir radiação. [L. *radio*, pp. *-atus*, brilhar]

ra·di·a·tio, pl. **ra·di·a·ti·o·nes** (rā-dē-ā′shē-ō, -shē-ō′nēz). Radiação; em neuroanatomia, um termo aplicado a qualquer um dos sistemas de fibras talamocorticais que, juntos, compõem a coroa radiada da substância branca do hemisfério cerebral (p. ex., radiação óptica, radiação acústica etc.). SIN radiation (3). [L.]
r. acus′tica [TA], r. acústica. SIN acoustic *radiation*.
r. cor′poris callo′si [TA], r. do corpo caloso. SIN *radiation* of corpus callosum.
r. inferior thalami [TA], r. inferior do tálamo. SIN inferior thalamic *peduncle*.
r. op′tica [TA], r. óptica. SIN optic *radiation*.
r. pyramida′lis, r. piramidal. SIN pyramidal *radiation*.
r. thalami anterior [TA], r. anterior do tálamo. SIN anterior thalamic *radiation*.
r. thalami centralis [TA], r. central do tálamo. SIN central thalamic *radiation*.
r. thalamica posterior [TA], r. posterior do tálamo. SIN posterior thalamic *radiation*.

ra·di·a·tion (rā′dē-ā′shŭn). Radiação. **1.** O ato ou a condição de divergir em todas as direções a partir de um centro. **2.** A emissão de luz, de ondas curtas de rádio, de raios ultravioleta ou de raios X ou de quaisquer outros raios para tratamento ou diagnóstico ou outro propósito. Cf. irradiation (2). **3.** SIN radiatio. **4.** Um raio. **5.** A energia radiante ou um feixe radiante. [L. *radiatio*, de *radius*, raio, feixe]
acoustic r. [TA], r. acústica; as fibras que seguem do corpo geniculado medial até os giros temporais transversos do córtex cerebral, passando pela parte sublentiforme da cápsula interna. SIN radiatio acustica [TA].
afterloading r., r. de pós-carga; técnica de aplicação de r. que consiste na colocação prévia de cateteres locais com posterior introdução da fonte de r.
alpha r., r. alfa; a emissão de um núcleo de energia cinética alta proveniente do núcleo de um átomo que sofreu decaimento radioativo ou fissão.
annihilation r., r. de aniquilação; a r. produzida quando um pósitron proveniente de decaimento beta positivo chega ao repouso. Esse pósitron encontra um elétron e, então, ambos aniquilam-se mutuamente e convertem suas massas restantes em dois raios gama de 0,51 MeV que são emitidos em sentidos exatamente opostos. VER *pair* production.
anterior thalamic r. [TA], r. anterior do tálamo; a r. formada pelas fibras que interligam, através do ramo anterior da cápsula interna, os núcleos talâmicos anterior e medial ao córtex cerebral do lobo frontal (excluindo o giro pré-central que delimita o sulco central). SIN radiatio thalami anterior [TA].

background r., r. de fundo; a radiação proveniente das fontes ambientais, que incluem a crosta terrestre, a atmosfera, os raios cósmicos e os radionuclídeos ingeridos.

> As fontes naturais são responsáveis pela maior parte da radiação recebida pela maioria das pessoas a cada ano (dose anual média de 3,00 mSv), enquanto as fontes médicas e ocupacionais fornecem apenas uma fração (em média menos de 0,60 mSv). Atualmente, acredita-se que o radônio, um gás produzido pelo decaimento do rádio dentro de rochas cristalinas, constitui a principal fonte de radiação de fundo em muitas regiões dos Estados Unidos. O acúmulo de radônio em casas malventiladas pode ser perigoso para a saúde a longo prazo. Os efeitos deletérios da r. de fundo, considerada responsável por 1 a 6% das mutações genéticas espontâneas, aumentam com a dose.

beta r., r. beta; a energia radiante proveniente de uma fonte de raios beta.
central thalamic r. [TA], r. central do tálamo; a r. formada pelas fibras que interligam, através do ramo posterior da cápsula interna, os núcleos ventral lateral, ventral póstero-lateral e ventral póstero-medial, lateral dorsal e lateral posterior com o giro pré-central e o lobo parietal do córtex cerebral. SIN radiatio thalami centralis [TA].
Cerenkov r., r. de Cerenkov; a luz emitida por um meio transparente quando

uma partícula de alta energia atravessa-o a uma velocidade maior do que a da luz naquele meio.

characteristic r., r. característica; r. monocromática produzida quando um elétron é ejetado de um átomo e um outro elétron toma o seu lugar, pulando de uma outra camada; a energia do fóton emitido corresponde à diferença entre as energias de cada camada. VER photoelectric *effect*. SIN characteristic emission.

r. of corpus callosum [TA], r. do corpo caloso; a difusão das fibras do corpo caloso no centro semi-oval de cada hemisfério cerebral. SIN radiatio corporis callosi [TA].

corpuscular r., r. corpuscular; r. que consiste em fluxos de partículas subatômicas, tais como prótons, elétrons, nêutrons etc.

electromagnetic r., r. eletromagnética; r. que se origina em um campo eletromagnético variável; p. ex., as ondas de rádio longas e curtas; a luz, visível e invisível; raios X e raios gama.

gamma r., r. gama; a r. eletromagnética ionizante resultante de processos nucleares, tais como o decaimento radioativo ou a fissão.

geniculocalcarine r., r. geniculocalcarina. SIN optic r.

Gratiolet r., r. de Gratiolet. SIN optic r.

hemibody r., r. do hemicorpo; tratamento paliativo do câncer que consiste na r. de metade do corpo. [hemi- + corpo]

heterogeneous r., r. heterogênea; r. composta por diferentes freqüências, energias diversas ou por várias partículas. VER TAMBÉM polychromatic r.

homogeneous r., r. homogênea; r. composta por uma faixa estreita de freqüências, pela mesma energia ou por um único tipo de partícula.

hyperfractionated r., r. hiperfracionada; frações menores de uma determinada dose de r. que são administradas diariamente e mais de uma vez em um mesmo dia.

hypofractionated r., r. hipofracionada; frações maiores de uma determinada dose que são administradas a intervalos maiores do que um dia.

inferior thalamic r. [TA], r. inferior do tálamo. SIN inferior thalamic *peduncle*.

ionizing r., r. ionizante; r. corpuscular (p. ex., nêutrons, elétrons) ou eletromagnética (p. ex., gama) com energia suficiente para ionizar o material irradiado.

K-r., r. K; geralmente uma forma muito penetrante de radiação X que é excitada por raios catódicos (elétrons com alta velocidade) que colidem com um ânodo metálico, tal como o tungstênio; a energia da r. é uma função da energia de ligação dos elétrons da camada K do ânodo metálico.

L-r., r. L; radiação X com fraco poder de penetração que é excitada por raios catódicos (elétrons com alta velocidade) que colidem com um ânodo metálico; a energia da radiação é uma função da energia de ligação dos elétrons da camada L do ânodo metálico.

monochromatic r., r. monocromática; os raios de luz ou a radiação ionizante com uma faixa muito estreita de comprimento de onda (de preferência, de um único comprimento de onda). Cf. photopeak, characteristic r.

neutron r., r. de nêutrons; emissão de nêutrons provenientes do núcleo de um átomo por decaimento ou fissão.

occipitothalamic r., r. occipitotalâmica. SIN optic r.

optic r. [TA], r. óptica; o sistema de fibras compacto e semelhante a um leque que corre do corpo geniculado lateral do tálamo até o córtex visual (córtex estriado ou calcarino, área 17 de Brodmann); as fibras seguem as partes retrolentiforme e sublentiforme da cápsula interna para a coroa radiada, mas curvam-se de volta ao longo da parede lateral dos cornos temporal e occipital do ventrículo lateral até o córtex estriado na superfície medial e no pólo do lobo occipital. SIN radiatio optica [TA], geniculocalcarine r., geniculocalcarine tract, Gratiolet fibers, Gratiolet r., occipitothalamic r., Wernicke r.

polychromatic r., r. policromática; radiação que contém raios gama (ver *rays*, em *ray*) de muitas energias diferentes; em radiologia diagnóstica, tipicamente a *bremsstrahlung* (= radiação de frenagem).

posterior thalamic r. [TA], r. posterior do tálamo; r. formada pelas fibras que interligam, através da parte retrolentiforme do ramo posterior da cápsula interna, o complexo pulvinar e o núcleo geniculado lateral com os lobos parietal posterior e occipital do córtex cerebral. SIN radiatio thalamica posterior [TA].

primary r., r. primária; um feixe incidente de raios X.

pyramidal r., r. piramidal; as fibras corticoespinais que seguem do córtex para a pirâmide. SIN radiatio pyramidalis.

scattered r., r. dispersa; r. secundária emitida a partir da interação dos raios X com a matéria; em geral sua energia é menor e possui uma distribuição direcional que depende da energia da radiação incidente. SIN secondary r.

secondary r., r. secundária. SIN scattered r.

Wernicke r., r. de Wernicke. SIN optic r.

rad·i·cal (rad′i-kăl). Radical. **1.** Em química, um grupo de elementos ou átomos que em geral passa intato de um composto para outro, mas que em geral é incapaz de existência prolongada em uma forma livre (p. ex., metila, CH_3); em fórmulas químicas, um r. é freqüentemente distinguido por apresentar-se isolado por parênteses ou colchetes. **2.** Completo ou amplo; relativo ou dirigido à extirpação da raiz ou da causa de um processo mórbido; p. ex., uma operação radical. **3.** Indica o tratamento realizado por meio de medidas extremas, drásticas ou inovadoras, em oposição ao tratamento conservador. **4.** Radical livre. SIN free r. [L. *radix* (*radic-*), raiz]

acid r., r. ácido; r. formado a partir de um ácido pela perda de um ou mais íons de hidrogênio; p. ex., SO_4^-, NO_3^-.

color r., r. colorido. SIN chromophore.

free r., r. livre; um r. em sua forma não-combinada (em geral, transitória); um átomo ou grupamento de átomos com um elétron não-pareado e sem carga elétrica; p. ex., a hidroxila (·Ö:H) e a metila

$$\begin{pmatrix} H \\ H:\overset{\cdot}{C}: \\ H \end{pmatrix}$$

Os radicais livres podem participar como intermediários hiperativos e de vida curta em várias reações nos tecidos vivos, notavelmente na fotossíntese. O r. livre do óxido nítrico, NO, é importante na vasodilatação. SIN radical (4).

Os radicais livres ocorrem naturalmente no corpo como resultado de processos metabólicos e podem também ser introduzidos nele (pelo fumo, pela inalação de poluentes ambientais ou pela exposição à radiação ultravioleta). Interagem prontamente com as moléculas vizinhas e podem causar dano celular, inclusive alterações genéticas. Já se aventou que os radicais livres estão envolvidos na formação da placa da aterosclerose, no câncer e nos distúrbios degenerativos, como a doença de Alzheimer e o parkinsonismo. Acredita-se que enzimas naturais, como a superóxido dismutase e a peroxidase, neutralizam os radicais livres, e há evidências de que muitos nutrientes, incluindo as vitaminas C e E e o β-caroteno, também exercem um efeito antioxidante. VER TAMBÉM antioxidant.

oxygen-derived free r.'s, radicais livres derivados do oxigênio; um átomo ou grupo de átomos que possui um elétron não-pareado em um átomo de oxigênio, caracteristicamente derivado do oxigênio molecular. Por exemplo, a redução de um elétron do O_2 produz o radical superóxido, $\overline{O_2}\cdot$; outros exemplos incluem o radical hidroperoxila (HOO·), o radical hidroxila (HO·) e o óxido nítrico (NO·). Esses radicais aparentemente desempenham algum papel na lesão provocada por reperfusão.

ra·di·ces (rā-dī′sēz). Raízes; plural de radix.

rad·i·cle (rad′i-kl). Radícula; uma pequena raiz ou uma estrutura semelhante, como a r. de uma veia (*r. of a vein*), uma diminuta veia que se une a outras para formar uma veia, ou a r. de um nervo (*r. of a nerve*), uma fibra nervosa que se une a outras para formar um nervo. [L. *radicula*, dim. de *radix*, raiz]

rad·i·cot·o·my (rad-i-kot′ō-me). Radicotomia. SIN rhizotomy. [L. *radix* (*radic-*), raiz, + G. *tomē*, incisão]

radicul-. VER radiculo-.

ra·dic·u·la (rā-dik′u-lā). Radícula; uma raiz nervosa espinal. [L. dim. de *radix*, raiz]

ra·dic·u·lal·gia (ra-dik′u-lal′jē-ă). Radiculalgia; neuralgia resultante da irritação da raiz sensitiva de um nervo espinal. [radicul- + G. *algos*, dor]

ra·dic·u·lar (ra-dik′u-lăr). Radicular. **1.** Relativo a uma radícula. **2.** Pertinente à raiz de um dente.

ra·dic·u·lec·to·my (ra-dik′u-lek′tō-me). Radiculectomia. SIN rhizotomy. [radicul- + G. *ektomē*, excisão]

ra·dic·u·li·tis (ra-dik-u-lī′tis). Radiculite. SIN radiculopathy. [radicul- + G. *-itis*, inflamação]

acute brachial r., r. braquial aguda, amiotrofia neurálgica. SIN neuralgic *amyotrophy*.

radiculo-, radicul-. Radiculo-, radicul-; radícula; radicular. [L. *radicula*, radícula, dim. de *radix*, raiz]

ra·dic·u·lo·gang·li·o·ni·tis (ra-dik′u-lō-gang′glē-ō-nī′tis). Radiculoganglionite; comprometimento de raízes e gânglios.

ra·dic·u·lo·me·nin·go·my·e·li·tis (ra-dik′u-lō-mĕ-ning′gō-mī-ĕ-lī′tis). Radiculomeningomielite. SIN rhizomeningomyelitis.

ra·dic·u·lo·my·e·lop·a·thy (ra-dik′u-lō-mī′ĕ-lop′a-the). Radiculomielopatia. SIN myeloradiculopathy.

ra·dic·u·lo·neu·rop·a·thy (ra-dik′u-lō-noo-rop′a-the). Radiculoneuropatia; doença das raízes nervosas e dos nervos espinais.

ra·dic·u·lop·a·thy (ra-dik′u-lop′a-the). Radiculopatia; distúrbio das raízes nervosas espinais. SIN radiculitis. [radiculo- + G. *pathos*, sofrimento]

diabetic thoracic r., r. torácica diabética; um tipo de neuropatia diabética que afeta principalmente pacientes mais velhos com diabetes melito; caracteriza-se clinicamente por dor torácica e abdominal, principalmente anterior, podendo ocorrer irradiação da dor ao redor do tronco a partir da linha média; geralmente unilateral; pode estender-se sobre vários segmentos; é provavelmente resultante de lesão isquêmica de duas ou mais raízes contíguas; um tipo de polirradiculopatia diabética.

ra·di·ec·to·my (rā-dē-ek′tō-mē). Radiectomia. SIN root amputation. [L. *radix*, raiz, + G. *ektomē*, excisão]

ra·dif·er·ous (rā-dif′er-ŭs). Radífero; que contém rádio.

ra·dii (rā′dē-ī). Raios; plural de radius. [L.]

radio-. Radio-. **1.** Radiação, principalmente (em medicina) de raios gama ou raios X. **2.** Radioativo. SIN radioactive. **3.** Raio. SIN radius. [L. *radius*, raio]

ra·di·o·ac·tive (rā′dē-ō-ak′tiv). Radioativo; que possui radioatividade. SIN radio- (2).-

ra·di·o·ac·tive cow. Coloquialismo para "gerador de radionuclídeos" (ver radionuclide *generator*). VER TAMBÉM cow.

ra·di·o·ac·tiv·i·ty (rā′dē-ō-ak-tiv′i-tē). Radioatividade; a propriedade de alguns núcleos atômicos de emitir espontaneamente raios gama ou partículas subatômicas (raios α e β) por meio do processo da desintegração nuclear; é medida por desintegrações por segundo (dps). Uma dps é igual a 1 becquerel, e $3,7 \times 10^{10}$ dps correspondem a 1 curie.

   artificial r., r. artificial; r. de isótopos criada por meio do bombardeamento de isótopos que ocorrem naturalmente por partículas subatômicas ou por altos níveis de raios X ou gama. SIN induced r.

   induced r., r. induzida. SIN artificial r.

ra·di·o·au·to·gram (rā′dē-ō-aw′tō-gram). Radioautograma; termo antigo para auto-radiografia.

ra·di·o·au·tog·ra·phy (rā′dē-ō-aw-tog′ră-fē). Radioautografia. SIN autoradiography.

ra·di·o·bi·cip·i·tal (rā′dē-ō-bī-sip′i-tăl). Radiobicipital; relativo ao rádio e ao músculo bíceps.

ra·di·o·bi·ol·o·gy (rā′dē-ō-bī-ol′ō-jē). Radiobiologia; o estudo dos efeitos biológicos da radiação ionizante sobre o tecido vivo. Cf. radiopathology.

ra·di·o·cal·ci·um (rā′dē-ō-kal′sē-ŭm). Radiocálcio; radioisótopo do cálcio, mais especificamente o cálcio-45.

ra·di·o·car·bon (rā′dē-ō-kar′bon). Radiocarbono; isótopo radioativo do carbono; p. ex., o C^{14}.

ra·di·o·car·di·o·gram (rā′dē-ō-kar′dē-ō-gram). Radiocardiograma; um registro gráfico da concentração de um radioisótopo injetado dentro das câmaras cardíacas.

ra·di·o·car·di·og·ra·phy (rā′dē-ō-kar-dē-og′ră-fē). Radiocardiografia; técnica que consiste no registro ou na interpretação de radiocardiogramas.

ra·di·o·car·pal (rā′dē-ō-kar′păl). Radiocarpal; **1.** Relativo ao rádio e aos ossos do carpo. **2.** Na face radial (ou lateral) do carpo.

ra·di·o·ceph·al·pel·vim·e·try (rā′dē-ō-sef-ăl-pel-vim′e-trē). Radiocefalopelvimetria. SIN pelvimetry. [radio- + cephal- + pelvimetry]

ra·di·o·chem·is·try (rā′dē-ō-kem′is-trē). Radioquímica. **1.** A ciência que utiliza radionuclídeos com o objetivo de sintetizar compostos marcados para pesquisa bioquímica ou biológica ou radiofármacos para estudos diagnósticos clínicos. **2.** O estudo dos métodos para marcação de compostos com radionuclídeos. **3.** A ciência que se ocupa dos efeitos da radiação ionizante ou nuclear sobre reações químicas ou materiais.

ra·di·o·chlo·rine (rā′dē-ō-klōr′ēn). Radiocloro; um isótopo radioativo do cloro, p. ex., o Cl^{36}.

ra·di·o·chol·an·gi·og·ra·phy (rā′dē-ō-kō-lan-jē-og′ră-fē). Radiocolangiografia; colangiografia por administração intravenosa de um radiofármaco excretado. [radio- + colangiografia]

ra·di·o·cho·le·cys·tog·ra·phy (rā′dē-ō-kō-lē-sis-tog′ră-fē). Radiocolecistografia; a visualização da vesícula biliar pelo emprego de contrastes cintilográficos que utilizam um radiofármaco, tal como o derivado do ácido iminodiacético marcado com tecnécio-99m. [radio- + colecistografia]

ra·di·o·cin·e·an·gi·o·car·di·og·ra·phy (rā′dē-ō-sin′ē-an′jē-ō-kar-dē-og′ră-fē). Radiocineangiocardiografia; filme cintilográfico que mostra a passagem de um radiofármaco através do coração e dos grandes vasos. [radio- + cineangiocardiografia]

ra·di·o·cin·e·an·gi·og·ra·phy (rā′dē-ō-sin′ē-an′jē-og′ră-fē). Radiocineangiografia; filmes cintilográficos que mostram a passagem de um radiofármaco através de vasos sangüíneos.

ra·di·o·cin·e·ma·tog·ra·phy (rā′dē-ō-si-nē-mă-tog′ră-fē). Radiocinematografia; a obtenção de um filme dos movimentos dos órgãos ou de outras estruturas, conforme revelado pelo exame fluoroscópico (raios X). [radio- + G. *kinēma*, movimento, + *graphō*, escrever]

ra·di·o·co·balt (rā′dē-ō-kō′balt). Radiocobalto; um isótopo radioativo do cobalto; p. ex., Co^{60}.

ra·di·o·cur·a·ble (rā′dē-ō-kūr′ă-bl). Radiocurável; curável por meio de radioterapia.

ra·di·o·dense (rā′dē-ō-dens). Radiodenso, radiopaco. SIN radiopaque.

ra·di·o·den·si·ty (rā′dē-ō-den′si-tē). Radiodensidade. SIN radiopacity.

ra·di·o·der·ma·ti·tis (rā′dē-ō-der-mă-tī′tis). Radiodermatite; dermatite resultante da exposição aos raios X ou aos raios gama que causa a ionização da água dos tecidos e alterações agudas que se assemelham à lesão pelo calor.

ra·di·o·di·ag·no·sis (rā′dē-ō-dī-ag-nō′sis). Radiodiagnóstico; o diagnóstico obtido pelo emprego dos raios X; ou, mais amplamente, da imagem diagnóstica, que compreende a radiologia, o ultra-som e a ressonância magnética.

ra·di·o·dig·i·tal (rā′dē-ō-dij′i-tăl). Radiodigital; relativo aos dedos da face radial (ou lateral) da mão.

ra·di·o·e·lec·tro·phys·i·ol·o·gram (rā′dē-ō-e-lek′trō-fiz-ē-ol′ō-gram). Radioeletrofisiolograma; o registro obtido por meio do radioeletrofisiológrafo.

ra·di·o·e·lec·tro·phys·i·ol·o·graph (rā′dē-ō-ē-lek′trō-fiz-ē-ol′ō-graf). Radioeletrofisiológrafo; aparelho utilizado no passado que era transportado por um indivíduo e por meio do qual as alterações no potencial elétrico do cérebro ou do coração podiam ser captadas e radiotransmitidas a um eletroencefalógrafo ou a um eletrocardiógrafo. VER telemeter.

ra·di·o·e·lec·tro·phys·i·o·log·ra·phy (rā′dē-ō-ē-lek′trō-fiz′ē-ō-log′ră-fē). Radioeletrofisiologia; técnica utilizada no passado que consistia no registro das alterações no potencial elétrico do cérebro ou do coração por meio do radioeletrofisiológrafo. VER telemetry.

ra·di·o·el·e·ment (rā′dē-ō-el′ē-ment). Radioelemento; qualquer elemento que possui radioatividade.

ra·di·o·ep·i·the·li·tis (rā′dē-ō-ep′i-thē-lī′tis). Radioepitelite; alterações destrutivas no epitélio produzidas por radiação ionizante.

ra·di·o·fre·quen·cy (rā′dē-o-frē′kwen-sē). Radiofreqüência. **1.** A energia radiante de uma determinada faixa de freqüência; p. ex., o rádio e a televisão empregam energia radiante que possui uma freqüência entre 10^5 e 10^{11} Hz, enquanto os raios X utilizados em diagnósticos possuem uma freqüência na faixa de 3×10^{18} Hz. **2.** Nas imagens por ressonância magnética, a energia aplicada para modificar ou criar um gradiente no campo magnético.

ra·di·o·gal·li·um (rā′dē-ō-gal′ē-ŭm). Radiogálio, gálio radioativo; gálio que é radioativo. VER gallium-67, gallium-68.

ra·di·o·gen·e·sis (rā′dē-ō-jen′ē-sis). Radiogênese; a formação ou a produção de radioatividade que resultam da transformação radioativa ou da desintegração de substâncias radioativas. [radio- + G. *genesis*, produção]

ra·di·o·gen·ic (rā′dē-ō-jen′ik). Radiogênico. **1.** Que produz raios de qualquer tipo, especialmente raios eletromagnéticos. **2.** Causado por raios X ou gama.

ra·di·o·gen·ics (rā′dē-ō-jen′iks). A ciência da radiação.

ra·di·o·gold col·loid (rā′dē-ō-gōld kol′oyd). Ouro coloidal radioativo; isótopo radioativo do ouro que emite partículas beta negativas e radiação gama e que possui uma meia-vida de 2,7 dias; antigamente era utilizado para irradiar cavidades serosas fechadas no tratamento paliativo da ascite e do derrame pleural resultante de metástases e em cintilografias hepáticas. SIN ^{198}Au colloid, colloidal radioactive gold.

ra·di·o·gram (rā′dē-ō-gram). Radiograma; termo obsoleto para radiografia. [radio- + G. *gramma*, algo escrito]

ra·di·o·graph (rā′dē-ō-graf). Radiografia; uma imagem negativa impressa em um filme fotográfico e obtida por meio da exposição aos raios X ou aos raios gama que passam através da matéria ou do tecido. SIN roentgenogram, roentgenograph, x-ray (3). [radio- + G. *graphō*, escrever]

   bitewing r., r. interproximal; filme dental intra-oral adaptado para mostrar a porção coronal e o terço cervical das raízes dos dentes em quase oclusão; útil principalmente na detecção de cáries interproximais e na determinação da altura do septo alveolar.

   cephalometric r., r. cefalométrica; incidência radiográfica que exibe a maxila, a mandíbula e o crânio e permite a obtenção de medidas. SIN cephalogram.

   decubitus r., r. em decúbito; r. de um paciente em decúbito lateral, incidência frontal com um feixe de raios X horizontal. SIN lateral decubitus r.

   lateral decubitus r., r. em decúbito lateral. SIN decubitus r.

   lateral oblique r., r. lateral oblíqua; incidência radiográfica da mandíbula que mostra um dos lados desse osso, da sínfise até o côndilo, por meio do deslocamento do outro lado para cima.

   lateral ramus r., r. do ramo lateral; incidência radiográfica do ramo da mandíbula e do côndilo.

   lateral skull r., r. lateral do crânio; a verdadeira incidência radiográfica lateral dos ossos da face e da calvária, mostrando as estruturas ósseas e as passagens que contêm ar.

   maxillary sinus r., r. dos seios maxilares; incidência radiográfica frontal dos seios maxilares, das órbitas, das estruturas nasais e dos zigomas; permite a comparação direta dos lados da face. SIN Waters view r.

   occlusal r., r. oclusal; filme intra-oral posicionado no plano de oclusão e utilizado na visualização de partes inteiras da mandíbula; útil principalmente na exploração de calcificações das glândulas salivares sublinguais.

   panoramic r., r. panorâmica; incidência radiográfica da maxila e da mandíbula que se estende da fossa glenóide esquerda até a direita.

   periapical r., r. periapical; r. que mostra os ápices dos dentes e as estruturas circunjacentes em uma determinada área intra-oral.

   scout r., r. exploradora, r. panorâmica. SIN scout *film*.

   submental vertex r., incidência submentovértice. SIN submentovertex r.

   submentovertex r., incidência submentovértice; incidência radiográfica que mostra a base do crânio, as posições dos côndilos da mandíbula e os arcos zigomáticos. SIN base view, submental vertex r.

   Towne projection r., incidência radiográfica de Towne. VER Towne *projection*.

transcranial r., r. transcraniana; a incidência radiográfica da articulação temporomandibular.
Trendelenburg r., r. de Trendelenburg; r. de um paciente com a cabeça inclinada para trás e em geral em decúbito dorsal; utilizada na detecção de pequenos derrames pleurais.
Waters view r., incidência radiográfica de Waters. SIN maxillary sinus r.
ra·di·og·raph·er (rā-dē-og′ră-fĕr). Técnico em radiografia; técnico treinado para posicionar os pacientes e tirar radiografias ou realizar outros procedimentos radiodiagnósticos.
ra·di·og·ra·phy (rā′dē-og′ră-fē). Radiografia; o exame de qualquer parte do corpo para fins diagnósticos realizado por meio de raios X, com o registro dos achados geralmente impressos sobre um filme fotográfico. SIN roentgenography.

advanced multiple-beam equalization r. (AMBER), r. de equalização de feixes múltiplos avançada; uma variante da r. de equalização de varredura que utiliza vários feixes de raios X.
air-gap r., r. de tórax obtida com um espaço mínimo de 25,4 cm (= 10 polegadas) entre o paciente e o filme. Em vez de utilizar uma grade, esse método emprega a geometria e a absorção dos raios X pelo ar para remover a radiação dispersa.
bedside r., r. portátil. SIN portable r.
computed r. (CR), r. computadorizada; a conversão dos raios X emitidos em luz por meio da utilização de um dispositivo para imagem, tal como uma placa de fósforo fotoestimulável, e a recuperação e o processamento da imagem realizados por um computador digital; a imagem deve, então, ser impressa em um filme ou exibida em uma tela de computador.
digital r. (DR), r. digital; a conversão direta dos raios X emitidos em uma imagem digital por meio da utilização de vários detectores, tal como o selênio ou o silício amorfos, com processamento e exibição computadorizados da imagem. VER DSA.
electron r., obtenção de imagens radiográficas na qual os raios X incidentes no receptor são convertidos em uma imagem latente e depois recuperados por um processo de impressão especial; as vantagens incluem maior liberdade de exposição e maior sensibilidade que as combinações tradicionais de filme-écran. VER xeroradiography, phosphor *plate*.
filmless r., r. sem filme; a aquisição e a distribuição eletrônicas de imagens radiográficas, eliminando assim o manuseio e a armazenagem de filmes. VER TAMBÉM PACS.
magnification r., r. ampliada; r. obtida pelo uso de um tubo de raios X microfocal e pelo aumento da distância entre o paciente e o filme, com o objetivo de fornecer uma ampliação geométrica do paciente sem que ocorra perda significativa de definição e resolução.
mucosal relief r., técnica radiográfica que mostra detalhes delicados da mucosa gastrointestinal após esta ter sido revestida com uma suspensão de bário e o órgão distendido com ar ou gás liberado por um produto (pó) previamente ingerido.
portable r., r. portátil; a obtenção de uma radiografia de um paciente confinado à cama, levando-se um aparelho de raios X móvel até o quarto. SIN bedside r.
scanning equalization r., r. de equalização de varredura; um método aperfeiçoado eletronicamente de obter radiografias no qual um feixe estreito de raios X é passado sobre o paciente enquanto sua atenuação é mensurada, fornecendo, assim, retroalimentação à intensidade do feixe modulado, a fim de igualar a exposição regional do filme de raios X.
sectional r., tomografia. SIN tomography.
serial r., r. seriada; a realização de várias exposições aos raios X de uma única região durante um certo período de tempo, como ocorre na angiografia.
spot-film r., uma radiografia de uma determinada região, em geral em um estudo por meio da fluoroscopia.
ra·di·o·hu·mer·al (rā′dē-ō-hū′mer-ăl). Radioumeral; relativo ao rádio e ao úmero; indica a articulação entre eles.
ra·di·o·im·mu·ni·ty (rā′dē-ō-i-mū′ni-tē). Radioimunidade; sensibilidade diminuída à radiação.
ra·di·o·im·mu·no·as·say (RIA) (rā′dē-ō-im′ŭ-nō-as′sā). Radioimunoensaio; procedimento imunológico (imunoquímico) que se baseia na competição entre o antígeno marcado com radioisótopo ou outra substância e o antígeno não-marcado para anti-soros e que resulta na quantificação do antígeno não-marcado; qualquer método para a detecção ou a quantificação de antígenos ou anticorpos pelo emprego de reagentes radiomarcados. Diminutas quantidades de enzimas, hormônios ou outras substâncias podem ser analisadas.
ra·di·o·im·mu·no·dif·fu·sion (rā′dē-ō-im′ŭ-nō-di-fū′zhŭn). Radiomunodifusão; método que se destina ao estudo de reações antígeno-anticorpo por meio da difusão em gel e que utiliza um antígeno ou anticorpo marcado com radioisótopo.
ra·di·o·im·mu·no·elec·tro·pho·re·sis (rā′dē-ō-im′ŭ-nō-ē-lek′trō-fō-rē′sis). Radiomunoeletroforese; a imunoeletroforese na qual o antígeno ou o anticorpo é marcado com um radioisótopo; p. ex., a detecção dos anticorpos que se ligam à insulina por meio do tratamento do soro a ser testado com insulina marcada com iodo, exposição da mistura (antígeno) à eletroforese,

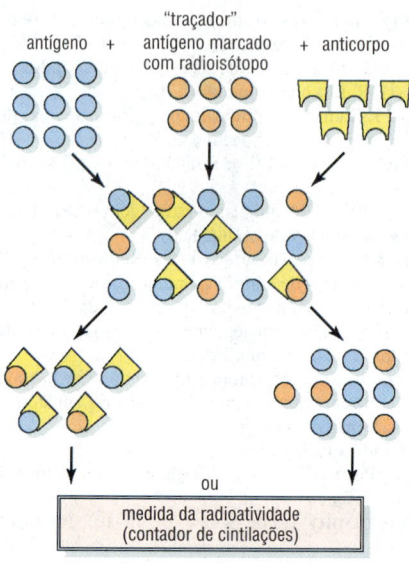

radioimunoensaio

precipitação das imunoglobulinas separadas com anti-soro imunoglobulina-específico e, então, com filme radiossensível (auto-radiografia), a detecção da insulina ligada nos precipitados.
ra·di·o·im·mu·no·pre·cip·i·ta·tion (RIP) (rā′dē-ō-im′ŭ-nō-prē-sip-i-tā′shŭn). Radioimunoprecipitação; imunoprecipitação que utiliza anticorpo ou um antígeno marcado com radioisótopo.
ra·di·o·i·o·din·at·ed (rā′dē-ō-ī′ō-din-ā-ted). Radioiodado; tratado ou combinado com iodo radioativo.
ra·di·o·i·o·dine (rā′dē-ō-ī′ō-dīn). Radioiodo, iodo radioativo; isótopo radioativo do iodo; p. ex., o I^{123}.
ra·di·o·i·ron (rā′dē-ō-ī′ern). Radioferro; isótopo radioativo do ferro; p. ex., o Fe^{59}.
ra·di·o·i·so·tope (rā′dē-ō-ī′sō-tōp). Radioisótopo; isótopo que passa para uma forma mais estável pela emissão de radiação.
ra·di·o·la·beled (rā′dē-ō-lā′bld). Radiomarcado. VER tag (1).
ra·di·o·lead (rā′dē-ō-led′). Radiochumbo, chumbo radioativo; isótopo radioativo do chumbo, geralmente o Pb^{210}. VER lead.
ra·di·o·le·sion (rā′dē-ō-lē′zhŭn). Radiolesão; lesão produzida por radiação ionizante.
ra·di·o·li·gand (rā′dē-ō-lig′and). Radioligante; molécula ligada a um radionuclídeo; é utilizada em geral em procedimentos de radioimunoensaio. [radio- + L. *ligandus*, aquilo que está para ser ligado, de *ligo*, ligar]
ra·di·o·log·ic, ra·di·o·log·i·cal (rā-dē-ō-log′ik,-loj′i-kăl). Radiológico; relativo à radiologia.
ra·di·ol·o·gist (rā-dē-ol′ō-jist). Radiologista; um médico treinado no uso dos raios X, de radionuclídeos e da física e da biologia da radiação para fins diagnósticos e/ou terapêuticos; um radiologista que faz diagnósticos também estaria apto a realizar diagnósticos a partir de exames ultra-sonográficos e de imagens obtidas por ressonância magnética e em física aplicada.
ra·di·ol·o·gy (rā-dē-ol′ō-jē). Radiologia. **1.** A ciência que se ocupa da radiação de alta energia e de suas fontes, assim como dos efeitos químicos, físicos e biológicos de tal radiação; o termo refere-se em geral ao diagnóstico e tratamento de doenças. **2.** Uma disciplina científica da imagenologia médica que utiliza a radiação ionizante, os radionuclídeos, a ressonância magnética nuclear e o ultra-som. SIN diagnostic r. [radio- + G. *logos*, estudo]

cardiovascular r., r. cardiovascular; a subespecialidade clínica da r. que se ocupa do diagnóstico e do tratamento de doenças do sistema vascular.
chest r., r. torácica; a subespecialidade clínica que se ocupa da radiologia diagnóstica das doenças do tórax, principalmente do coração e dos pulmões.
diagnostic r., r. diagnóstica. SIN radiology (2).
interventional r., r. intervencionista; a subespecialidade clínica que utiliza a fluoroscopia, a TC e o ultra-som para guiar os procedimentos percutâneos, tais como a realização de biopsias, a drenagem de líquidos, a inserção de cateteres ou a dilatação de ductos ou vasos estreitados ou a colocação de próteses no interior dos mesmos.
pediatric r., r. pediátrica; a subespecialidade clínica que se ocupa das manifestações radiológicas das doenças das crianças.
therapeutic r., r. terapêutica. SIN radiation oncology.
ra·di·o·lu·cen·cy (rā-dē-ō-loo′sen-sē). Radiotransparência; região de uma radiografia que apresenta exposição aumentada, ou por causa de maior trans-

radiolucency — radix

radiância da parte correspondente do paciente, ou por falta de homogeneidade na fonte da radiação, tal como posicionamento descentralizado.

ra·di·o·lu·cent (rā-dē-ō-loo'sent). Radiotransparente; algo que permite a penetração relativa dos raios X ou de outras formas de radiação. Cf. radiopaque. [radio- + L. *lucens*, brilhante]

ra·di·o·lus (rā-dē'ō-lŭs). Radíolo; estilete para sondar fendas ou uma sonda. [L. dim. de *radius*, raio]

ra·di·om·e·ter (rā-dē-om'e-ter). Radiômetro; dispositivo utilizado na determinação do poder de penetração dos raios X. SIN roentgenometer. [radio- + G. *metron*, medida]

ra·di·o·mi·crom·e·ter (rā'dē-ō-mī-krom'e-ter). Radiomicrômetro; pilha termoelétrica sensível projetada para medir diminutas alterações da energia radiante.

ra·di·o·mi·met·ic (rā'dē-ō-mi-met'ik). Radiomimético; que imita os efeitos biológicos da radiação, como no caso de produtos químicos, tais como as mostardas nitrogenadas. [radio- + G. *mimētikos*, imitador]

ra·di·o·mus·cu·lar (rā'dē-ō-mŭs'kū-lăr). Radiomuscular; relativo ao rádio e aos músculos circunjacentes; indica determinados nervos e ramos musculares da artéria radial.

ra·di·o·ne·cro·sis (rā'dē-ō-ne-krō'sis). Radionecrose; necrose resultante da radiação; p. ex., após exposição excessiva aos raios X ou gama. VER radiation *burn*.

ra·di·o·neu·ri·tis (rā'dē-ō-noo-rī'tis). Radioneurite; neurite causada pela exposição prolongada ou repetida aos raios X ou ao rádio.

ra·di·o·ni·tro·gen (rā'dē-ō-nī'trō-jen). Radionitrogênio; isótopo radioativo do nitrogênio; p. ex., o N^{13}.

ra·di·o·nu·clide (rā'dē-ō-noo'klīd). Radionuclídeo; isótopo de origem natural ou artificial que apresenta radioatividade.

ra·di·o·pac·i·ty (rā'dē-ō-pas'i-tē). Radiopacidade; a imagem radiográfica de um objeto radiopaco. SIN radiodensity.

ra·di·o·pal·mar (rā'dē-ō-pal'măr). Radiopalmar; relativo à face radial (ou lateral) da palma.

ra·di·o·paque (rā-dē-ō-pāk'). Radiopaco; que exibe opacidade relativa ou impenetrabilidade aos raios X ou a qualquer outra forma de radiação. Cf. radiolucent. SIN radiodense. [radio- + Fr. opaque do L. *opacus*, sombreado]

ra·di·o·pa·thol·o·gy (rā'dē-ō-path-ol'ō-jē). Radiopatologia; ramo da radiologia ou da patologia que se ocupa dos efeitos da radiação nas células e nos tecidos. Cf. radiobiology.

ra·di·o·pel·vim·e·try (rā'dē-ō-pel-vim'e-trē). Radiopelvimetria; a medição radiográfica da pelve. VER pelvimetry.

ra·di·o·phar·ma·ceu·ti·cal (rā'dē-ō-far-mă-soo'ti-kal). Radiofármaco; preparação química ou farmacêutica radioativa, marcada com um radionuclídeo que apresenta uma concentração terapêutica ou própria para um traçador e utilizada como agente diagnóstico ou terapêutico.

ra·di·o·pho·bia (rā'dē-ō-fō'bē-ă). Radiofobia; medo mórbido da radiação, como a proveniente dos raios X ou da energia nuclear. [radio- + G. *phobos*, medo]

ra·di·o·phos·pho·rus (rā'dē-ō-fos'fōr-ŭs). Radiofósforo; um isótopo radioativo do fósforo; p. ex., o P^{32}.

ra·di·o·pill (rā'dē-ō-pil). Radiopílula. SIN radiotelemetering *capsule*.

ra·di·o·po·tas·si·um (rā'dē-ō-pō-tas'ē-ŭm). Radiopotássio; um isótopo radioativo do potássio; p. ex., o K^{40}.

radioprotectant (rā'dē-ō-prō-tek'tant). Radioprotetor; substância que impede ou diminui os efeitos da radiação.

ra·di·o·re·cep·tor (rā'dē-ō-rē-sep'ter). Radiorreceptor; **1.** Um receptor que normalmente responde à energia radiante, tal como a luz ou o calor. **2.** Um receptor utilizado como agente de ligação de analito não-marcado ou radiomarcado em um tipo de ensaio de ligação competitiva denominado ensaio de radiorreceptor.

ra·di·o·re·sis·tant (rā'dē-ō-rē-zis'tant). Radiorresistente; termo que se refere às células ou aos tecidos que são menos afetados do que a média das células dos mamíferos, quando expostos à radiação; quando o termo é aplicado às neoplasias, indica que determinada estrutura apresenta menos suscetibilidade aos danos provenientes da radiação terapêutica do que os tecidos hospedeiros circunjacentes.

ra·di·os·co·py (rā'dē-os'kŏ-pē). Radioscopia; termo obsoleto para fluoroscopia. [radio- + G. *skopeō*, visualizar]

ra·di·o·sen·si·tive (rā'dē-ō-sen'si-tiv). Radiossensível; facilmente afetado pela radiação. Cf. radioresistant.

ra·di·o·sen·si·tiv·i·ty (rā'dē-ō-sen-si-tiv'i-tē). Radiossensibilidade; a condição de ser facilmente afetado pela energia radiante.

ra·di·o·sen·si·ti·za·tion (rā'dē-ō-sen-sī-tī-zā'shun). Radiossensibilização; o uso da quimioterapia ou de outros agentes que aumentam a sensibilidade dos tecidos aos efeitos da radioterapia, em geral pela inibição do reparo celular ou pelo aumento da porcentagem de células nas fases mitóticas do ciclo de crescimento.

ra·di·o·sen·si·tiz·er (rā'dē-ō-sen-si-tī'zer). Radiossensibilizador; substância química que aumenta a radiossensibilidade dos tecidos; o restabelecimento da tensão de oxigênio tecidual normal a uma região anóxica é também um método efetivo de radiossensibilização.

ra·di·o·so·di·um (rā'dē-ō-sō'dē-ŭm). Radiossódio; um isótopo radioativo do sódio; p. ex., o Na^{24}.

ra·di·o·ster·e·os·co·py (rā'dē-ō-ster-ē-os'kŏ-pē). Radioestereoscopia; a visualização simultânea de duas radiografias obtidas em projeções levemente distintas, em geral com um dispositivo que reflete a imagem de cada uma em um olho diferente, permitindo, assim, a visão tridimensional de um objeto em relação aos outros. VER stereoradiography, stereoscope. [radio- + G. *stereos*, sólido, + *skopeō*, visualizar]

ra·di·o·stron·ti·um (rā'dē-ō-stron'tē-ŭm). Radioestrôncio, estrôncio radioativo; isótopo radioativo do estrôncio; p. ex., o Sr^{90}.

ra·di·o·sul·fur (rā'dē-ō-sul'fŭr). Radioenxofre; isótopo radioativo do enxofre; p. ex., o S^{35}.

ra·di·o·sur·gery (rā'dē-ō-sŭr-je-rē). Radiocirurgia; radioterapia em um campo bem-delimitado, considerada de maneira otimista equivalente à ressecção da área irradiada.

ra·di·o·te·lem·e·try (rā'dē-ō-tē-lem'e-trē). Radiotelemetria. VER telemetry, biotelemetry.

ra·di·o·ther·a·peu·tic (rā'dē-ō-thăr-ă-pū'tik). Radioterapêutico; relativo à radioterapia ou à radioterapêutica.

ra·di·o·ther·a·peu·tics (rā'dē-ō-thăr-ă-pū'tiks). Radioterapêutica; o estudo e a utilização de agentes radioterapêuticos.

ra·di·o·ther·a·pist (rā'dē-ō-thăr'ă-pist). Radioterapeuta; aquele que pratica a radioterapia ou é versado em radioterapêutica. SIN radiation oncologist.

ra·di·o·ther·a·py (rā'dē-ō-thăr'ă-pē). Radioterapia. SIN radiation *oncology*.
 mantle r., r. em manto; r. realizada com a proteção das estruturas ou dos órgãos radiossensíveis não-envolvidos.

ra·di·o·ther·my (rā'dē-ō-ther'mē). Radiotermia; diatermia produzida pelo calor proveniente de fontes radiantes. [radio- + G. *thermē*, calor]

ra·di·o·thy·roid·ec·to·my (rā'dē-ō-thī'roy-dek'tō-mē). Radiotireoidectomia; a destruição do tecido tireóideo pela administração de iodo radioativo.

ra·di·o·thy·rox·in (rā'dē-ō-thī-rok'sin). Radiotiroxina. SIN radioactive *thyroxine*.

ra·di·o·tox·e·mia (rā'dē-ō-tok-sē'mē-ă). Radiotoxemia; doença causada pela radiação, mais especificamente pelos produtos da desintegração provocada pela ação dos raios X ou de outras formas de radioatividade e pela depleção de determinadas células e sistemas enzimáticos do organismo. [radio- + G. *toxikon*, veneno, + *haima*, sangue]

ra·di·o·trac·er (rā'dē-ō-trā'ser). Radiotraçador; radionuclídeo ou produto químico radiomarcado; traçador radioativo.

ra·di·o·trans·par·ent (rā'dē-ō-trans-par'ent). Radiotransparente; que permite a transmissão relativamente livre de energia radiante. Cf. radiolucent.

ra·di·o·trop·ic (rā'dē-ō-trop'ik). Radiotrópico; afetado pela radiação. [radio- + G. *tropē*, volta]

ra·di·o·ul·nar (rā'dē-ō-ŭl'năr). Radioulnar; relativo ao rádio e à ulna.

ra·di·sec·to·my (rā-dē-sek'tō-mē). Radisectomia. SIN root *amputation*. [L. *radix*, raiz, + G. *ektomē*, excisão]

ra·di·um (Ra) (rā'dē-ŭm). Rádio; elemento metálico com n.º atômico 88, extraído em quantidades muito pequenas da uraninita; o Ra^{226}, o isótopo que apresenta vida mais longa, é produzido como um intermediário da série do urânio pela emissão de uma partícula α do tório-230 (iônio); o Ra^{226} emite partículas α e raios gama com uma meia-vida de 1.599 anos, transformando-se em Rn^{222}; quimicamente, o Ra é um metal alcalino-terroso com propriedades semelhantes às do bário. Sua ação terapêutica é similar à dos raios X porque a emissão α é filtrada. [L. *radius*, raio]

ra·di·us, gen. e pl. **ra·di·i** (rā'dē-ŭs, rā'dē-ī) [TA]. **1.** [NA]. Rádio; o mais curto dos dois ossos do antebraço e que ocupa a posição lateral. **2.** Raio; uma linha reta que vai do centro até a periferia de um círculo. SIN radio- (3). [L. o raio de uma roda, bastão, raio]
 r. fix'us, raio fixo; uma linha traçada desde o hórmio até o ínio.
 radii of lens [TA], raios da lente; nove a doze linhas suaves situadas nas superfícies anterior e posterior da lente que se irradiam dos pólos para o equador; marcam as linhas ao longo das quais as extremidades das fibras da lente se tocam. SIN radii lentis [TA], lens stars (1), lens sutures.
 ra'dii len'tis [TA], raios da lente. SIN radii of lens.

ra·dix, gen. **ra·di·cis**, pl. **ra·di·ces** (rā'diks, rā-di'sis, rā'di-sēz ou rā-dī'sēz) [TA]. Raiz. **1.** SIN root (1). **2.** SIN root of tooth. **3.** O tamanho hipotético de um grupo de pessoas nascidas durante um determinado período de tempo em um quadro de estatística, habitualmente 1.000 ou 100.000. [L.]
 r. accessoria [TA], r. acessória do dente. SIN accessory *root* of tooth.
 r. ante'rior nervi spinalis [TA], r. anterior do nervo espinal. SIN anterior *root* of spinal nerve.
 r. ar'cus ver'tebrae, pedículo do arco vertebral. SIN *pedicle* of arch of vertebra.
 r. bre'vis gan'glii cilia'ris, r. parassimpática do gânglio ciliar. SIN parasympathetic *root* of ciliary ganglion.
 r. buccalis [TA], r. bucal do dente. SIN buccal *root* of tooth.
 r. clin'ica dentis [TA], r. clínica do dente. SIN clinical *root* of tooth.

r. crania'lis nervi accessorii [TA], r. craniana do nervo acessório. SIN cranial root of accessory nerve.
r. den'tis [TA], r. do dente. SIN root of tooth.
r. dorsa'lis nervi spinalis, r. dorsal do nervo espinal. SIN posterior root of spinal nerve.
r. facia'lis, nervo do canal pterigóideo. SIN nerve of pterygoid canal.
r. infe'rior an'sae cervica'lis [TA], r. inferior da alça cervical. SIN inferior root of ansa cervicalis.
r. infe'rior ner'vi vestibulocochlea'ris, r. inferior do nervo vestibulococlear. SIN cochlear root of VIII nerve.
r. latera'lis ner'vi media'ni [TA], r. lateral do nervo mediano. SIN lateral root of median nerve.
r. latera'lis trac'tus op'tici [TA], r. lateral do trato óptico. SIN lateral root of optic tract.
r. lin'guae [TA], r. da língua. SIN root of tongue.
r. lon'ga gan'glii cilia'ris, r. sensitiva do gânglio ciliar. SIN sensory root of ciliary ganglion.
r. media'lis ner'vi media'ni [TA], r. medial do nervo mediano. SIN medial root of median nerve.
r. media'lis trac'tus op'tici [TA], r. medial do trato óptico. SIN medial root of optic tract.
r. mesenter'ii [TA], r. do mesentério. SIN root of mesentery.
r. moto'ria nervi spinalis, r. motora do nervo espinal; *termo oficial alternativo para anterior root of spinal nerve.
r. moto'ria ner'vi trigem'ini [TA], r. motora do nervo trigêmeo. SIN motor root of trigeminal nerve.
r. na'si [TA], r. do nariz. SIN root of nose.
r. nasocilia'ris ganglii ciliaris, r. sensitiva do gânglio ciliar; *termo oficial alternativo para sensory root of ciliary ganglion.
r. ner'vi facia'lis, r. do nervo facial. SIN root of facial nerve.
r. nervi oculomotorii ad ganglion ciliare, r. parassimpática do gânglio ciliar; *termo oficial alternativo para parasympathetic root of ciliary ganglion.
ra'dices ner'vi trigem'ini, raízes do nervo trigêmeo. SIN roots of trigeminal nerve, em root.
r. oculomoto'ria gan'glii cilia'ris, r. parassimpática do gânglio ciliar; *termo oficial alternativo para parasympathetic root of ciliary ganglion.
r. parasympathica ganglii submandibularis, corda do tímpano. SIN chorda tympani.
radices parasympathicae gangliorum pelvicorum, nervos esplâncnicos pélvicos; *termo oficial alternativo para pelvic splanchnic nerves, em nerve.
r. parasympath'ica gan'glii cilia'ris [TA], r. parassimpática do gânglio ciliar. SIN parasympathetic root of ciliary ganglion.
r. parasympathica ganglii otici, nervo petroso menor; *termo oficial alternativo para lesser petrosal nerve.
r. pe'nis [TA], r. do pênis. SIN root of penis.
r. pi'li, r. do pêlo. SIN hair root.
r. poste'rior nervi spinalis [TA], r. posterior do nervo espinal. SIN posterior root of spinal nerve.
r. pulmo'nis [TA], r. do pulmão. SIN root of lung.
r. senso'ria gan'glii cili'aris [TA], r. sensitiva do gânglio ciliar. SIN sensory root of ciliary ganglion.
r. senso'ria gan'glii pterygopalatini [TA], r. sensitiva do gânglio pterigopalatino. SIN sensory root of pterygopalatine ganglion.
r. sensoria ganglii sublingualis [TA], r. sensitiva do gânglio sublingual. SIN sensory root of sublingual ganglion.
r. sensoria ganglii submandibularis [TA], r. sensitiva do gânglio submandibular. SIN sensory root of submandibular ganglion.
r. senso'ria nervi spinalis, r. posterior do nervo espinal; *termo oficial alternativo para posterior root of spinal nerve.
r. senso'ria ner'vi trigem'ini [TA], r. sensitiva do nervo trigêmeo. SIN sensory root of trigeminal nerve.
r. spina'lis nervi accessorii [TA], r. espinal do nervo acessório. SIN spinal root of accessory nerve.
r. supe'rior an'sae cervica'lis [TA], r. superior da alça cervical. SIN superior root of ansa cervicalis.
r. supe'rior ner'vi vestibulocochlea'ris, r. superior do nervo vestibulococlear. SIN vestibular root.
r. sympath'ica gan'glii cilia'ris [TA], r. simpática do gânglio ciliar. SIN sympathetic root of ciliary ganglion.
r. sympathica ganglii otici [TA], r. simpática do gânglio ótico. SIN sympathetic root of otic ganglion.
r. sympathica ganglii pterygopalatini, nervo petroso profundo; *termo oficial alternativo para deep petrosal nerve.
r. sympathica ganglii sublingualis [TA], r. simpática do gânglio sublingual. SIN sympathetic root of sublingual ganglion.
r. sympathica ganglii submandibularis [TA], r. simpática do gânglio submandibular. SIN sympathetic root of submandibular ganglion.
r. un'guis, r. da unha. SIN root of nail.

r. ventra'lis nervi spinalis, r. ventral do nervo espinal. SIN anterior root of spinal nerve.
r. vestibula'ris, r. vestibular. SIN vestibular root.

ra·don (Rn) (rā'don). Radônio; elemento radioativo gasoso, n.º atômico 86, resultante da desintegração do rádio; dos isótopos que apresentam número de massa entre 198 e 228, somente o Rn^{222} possui utilidade médica como um emissor alfa com uma meia-vida de 3,8235 dias; é empregado no tratamento de certas doenças malignas. Casas malventiladas de algumas partes dos EUA acumulam uma quantidade perigosa de gás radônio que ocorre naturalmente. [proveniente do rádio]

Raeder, Georg Johann, oftalmologista norueguês, 1889–1956. VER R. paratrigeminal *syndrome*.

raf·fi·nose (raf'i - nōs). Rafinose; trissacarídeo dextrorrotatório presente na semente do algodão e no melaço de beterraba, composto por D-galactose, D-glucose e D-frutose e formado pela transferência da D-galactose proveniente da UDP-D-galactose para a sucrose; muitas sementes são ricas em r. SIN gossypose, melitose, melitriose.

rage (rāj). Raiva, furor; raiva violenta; descarga total da parte simpática do sistema nervoso autônomo. [Fr., do L. *rabies*, raiva violenta, de *rabo*, delírio, fúria]
sham r., pseudo-raiva; estado quase-emocional caracterizado por manifestações de medo e raiva diante de provocação insignificante; é induzida em animais pela remoção do córtex cerebral (descorticação).

Rahe, Richard H., psiquiatra norte-americano, *1936. VER Holmes-R. *questionnaire*.

Rahn, Hermann, fisiologista respiratório norte-americano, 1912–1990. VER R.-Otis *sample*.

Rail·li·e·ti·na (rī - li - ē - tē'nă). Gênero de tênias (família Davaineidae, ordem Cyclophyllidea); três espécies desse gênero — *R. madagascariensis* ou *R. demerariensis, R. asiatica* e *R. formsana* — já foram encontradas em seres humanos. Contudo, a identificação de muitos desses vermes encontrados em seres humanos tem sido questionada.

rail·li·e·ti·ni·a·sis (rī'li - ē - ti - nī'ă - sis). Railietiníase; infecção por tênias do gênero *Raillietina* que acomete roedores e macacos e ocasionalmente seres humanos.

Rainey, George, anatomista inglês, 1801–1884. VER R. *corpuscles,* em *corpuscle*.

rale (rahl). Estertor; termo ambíguo para um ruído respiratório adventício auscultado sobre os campos pulmonares; é utilizado por alguns para indicar ronco e por outros, crepitação. SIN crackle. [Fr. chocalho]
amphoric r., e. anfórico; som auscultado por meio do estetoscópio e associado ao movimento de líquido em uma cavidade pulmonar que se comunica com um brônquio.
atelectatic r., e. atelectásico; som crepitante suave e transitório que desaparece após respiração profunda ou tosse.
bubbling r., e. bolhoso; som úmido auscultado por meio do estetoscópio e resultante da entrada de ar em partes do tecido pulmonar que contém exsudato e, em conseqüência, da formação de bolhas; está às vezes associado à fase de resolução das pneumonias ou a pequenas cavidades pulmonares.
cavernous r., e. cavernoso; som bolhoso e ressonante provocado pela entrada de ar em uma cavidade parcialmente preenchida com líquido. SIN cavernous rhonchus.
clicking r., e. crepitante; som curto geralmente associado à abertura de pequenos brônquios na respiração profunda, é às vezes auscultado na fase inicial da tuberculose pulmonar.
consonating r., e. consonante; som ressonante produzido em um brônquio e ouvido através de tecido pulmonar condensado.
crackling r. (krak'ling), e. crepitante; sons muito finos produzidos pela presença de líquido em vias aéreas muito pequenas na pneumonia e na insuficiência cardíaca congestiva (congestive heart *failure*).
crepitant r., e. crepitante; som crepitante ou bolhoso fino produzido pela mistura do ar com secreções muito finas em brônquios menores. SIN vesicular r.
dry r., estertor seco; som respiratório áspero ou musical produzido por constrição em um brônquio ou secreção viscosa que estreita o lúmen.
gurgling r., gorgolejo; som grosso auscultado sobre as cavidades grandes ou sobre a traquéia quase completamente preenchida por secreções.
guttural r., e. gutural; som ouvido sobre o pulmão e resultante de obstrução das vias aéreas superiores.
metallic r., e. metálico; ruído com qualidade metálica causado por ressonância em uma grande cavidade.
moist r., estertor úmido; estertor bolhoso provocado pela mistura do ar com um líquido (exsudato) nos brônquios ou em uma cavidade.
mucous r., e. mucoso; estertor bolhoso auscultado sobre os brônquios que contêm muco.
palpable r., e. palpável; vibração que pode ser sentida e que acompanha um e. de tom baixo, rude, musical ou sonoro.
pleural r., atrito pleural. SIN pleural *rub*.
sibilant r., sibilo; som semelhante a um assobio provocado pelo movimento do ar através de uma secreção viscosa que estreita o lúmen de um brônquio. SIN whistling r.

Skoda r., e. de Skoda; e. em um brônquio ouvido através de uma área de tecido consolidado na pneumonia.
sonorous r., e. sonoro; som semelhante a um ronco ou arrulho freqüentemente produzido pela vibração de uma massa saliente de secreção viscosa localizada em um brônquio grande.
subcrepitant r., estertor subcrepitante; estertor crepitante de som muito agudo.
vesicular r., e. crepitante. SIN crepitant r.
whistling r., sibilo. SIN sibilant r.

ral·ox·i·fene (ral-ox'ĭ-fēn). Raloxifeno; modulador seletivo dos receptores de estrógenos (SERM) que apresenta efeitos agonistas do estrógeno sobre os ossos e o metabolismo dos lipídios e efeitos antagonistas do estrógeno sobre as mamas e o útero; é utilizado na profilaxia da osteoporose pós-menopausa.

O r. é um derivado do benzotiofeno que se liga aos receptores de estrógenos. Além de conferir proteção contra a osteoporose após a menopausa, o r. melhora a densidade mineral dos ossos e reduz o risco de fraturas na osteoporose já estabelecida. A diminuição do risco de fraturas é maior do que seria esperado tendo em vista o aumento da densidade óssea. Ao contrário do tamoxifeno, que também reduz o risco de osteoporose, o r. não aumenta o risco de câncer de endométrio. Embora aumente a densidade mineral dos ossos em um grau menor do que os estrógenos, o r. reduz o risco de câncer de mama em vez de aumentá-lo, como talvez faça o estrógeno. Dessa forma, o r. seria a melhor opção para as mulheres que temem o câncer de mama ou que apresentam alto risco de desenvolvê-lo. Como a terapia de reposição hormonal (estrógenos associados a progesterona), o r. diminui os níveis de LDL–colesterol, fibrinogênio e lipoproteína (a) e eleva os de HDL–colesterol, sem aumentar os triglicerídeos. O r. não alivia os fogachos; na verdade, causa-os em 25% das pacientes. Como a terapia de reposição hormonal, o r. está contra-indicado na gravidez e para as mulheres que apresentam história pregressa de tromboembolismo. Ainda não se sabe se o r. protege as pacientes contra as doenças cardiovasculares e a doença de Alzheimer, como fazem os estrógenos.

ra·mal (rā'măl). Relativo a um ramo.
Raman, Sir Chandrasekhara V., físico indiano, laureado com um prêmio Nobel, 1888–1970. VER R. *effect, spectrum.*
Rambourg stains. Colorações de Rambourg. VER Rambourg chromic acid-phosphotungstic acid *stain*, Rambourg periodic acid-chromic methenamine-silver *stain.*
ra·mi (rā'mī). Ramos; plural de ramus. [L.]
ram·i·cot·o·my (ram-i-kot'ō-mē). Ramicotomia. SIN ramisection. [L. *ramus,* ramo, + G. *tomē,* incisão]
ram·i·fi·ca·tion (ram'i-fi-kā'shŭn). Ramificação; o processo de divisão em um padrão semelhante a ramos.
ram·i·fy (ram'i-fī). Ramificar; dividir algo segundo um padrão semelhante a ramos. [L. *ramus,* ramo, + *facio,* fazer]
ram·i·sec·tion (ram-i-sek'shŭn). Ramissecção; a secção dos ramos comunicantes do sistema nervoso simpático. SIN ramicotomy. [L. *ramus,* ramo, + L. *sectio,* secção]
ram·i·tis (ram-ī'tis). Ramite; a inflamação de um ramo. [L. *ramus,* ramo, + G. *-itis,* inflamação]
Ramón y Cajal, VER Cajal.
ra·mose, ra·mous (rā'mōs, rā'mŭs). Ramoso, ramificado. SIN branching. [L. *ramosus,* de *ramus,* um ramo]
ramp. Rampa; em registros elétricos, voltagem ou corrente que aumenta uniformemente. Se recalibrado para zero a intervalos regulares, forma um padrão serrilhado utilizado para fornecer a variação de tempo de um feixe de osciloscópio de raios catódicos; se a volta ao zero se deve a um fenômeno periódico (p. ex., os batimentos cardíacos), a altura das rampas registradas representa o tempo entre os fenômenos.
Ramsay Hunt. VER Hunt.
Ramsden, Jesse, oculista inglês, 1735–1800. VER R. *ocular.*
Ramstedt, Conrad, cirurgião alemão, 1867–1962. VER R. *operation;* Fredet-R. *operation.*
ram·u·lus, pl. **ram·u·li** (ram'ū-lŭs, -lī). Râmulo; pequeno ramo ou graveto; uma das divisões terminais de um ramo. [L. dim. de *ramus,* um ramo]

RAMUS

ra·mus, pl. **ra·mi** (rā'mŭs, rā'mī) [TA]. Ramo; **1.** SIN branch. **2.** Uma das divisões primárias de um nervo ou vaso sangüíneo. Os ramos arteriais e nervosos são também emitidos pelo nervo ou pela artéria principal. VER artery,

nerve. **3.** Parte de um osso com formato irregular (menos delgado que um "processo") que forma um ângulo com o corpo principal (p. ex., o ramo da mandíbula). **4.** Uma das divisões primárias de um sulco cerebral. [L.]
r. accessorius arteriae meningeae mediae [TA], r. acessório da artéria meníngea média. SIN accessory *branch* of middle meningeal artery.
r. acetabula'ris [TA], r. acetabular. SIN acetabular *branch.*
r. acromia'lis arte'riae suprascapula'ris [TA], r. acromial da artéria supraescapular. SIN acromial *branch* of suprascapular artery.
r. acromia'lis arte'riae thoracoacromia'lis [TA], r. acromial da artéria tóraco-acromial. SIN acromial *branch* of thoracoacromial artery.
ra'mi ad pon'tem, artérias da ponte. SIN pontine *arteries,* em *artery.*
ra'mi alveola'res superio'res anterio'res ner'vi infraorbita'lis, nervos alveolares superiores. SIN anterior superior alveolar *nerves,* em *nerve.*
ra'mi alveola'res superio'res posterio'res ner'vi maxilla'ris [TA], ramos alveolares superiores posteriores do nervo maxilar. SIN posterior superior alveolar *branches* of maxillary nerve, em *branch.*
r. alveola'ris supe'rior me'dius ner'vi infraorbita'lis [TA], r. alveolar superior médio do nervo infra-orbital. SIN middle superior alveolar *branch* of infraorbital nerve.
r. anastomot'icus [TA], r. anastomótico. SIN anastomotic *branch.* VER TAMBÉM communicating *branch.*
r. anastomot'icus arte'riae menin'geae me'diae cum arteriae lacrima'li [TA], r. anastomótico da artéria meníngea média com a artéria lacrimal. SIN anastomotic *branch* of middle meningeal artery with lacrimal artery.
r. ante'rior [TA], r. anterior. SIN anterior *branch.*
r. anterior arteriae renalis [TA], r. anterior da artéria renal. VER segmental *arteries* of kidney, em *artery.*
anterior rami of cervical nerves [TA], ramos anteriores dos nervos cervicais. VER anterior r. of spinal nerve. SIN rami anteriores nervorum cervicalium [TA], ventral rami of cervical nerves*, rami ventrales nervorum cervicalium, ventral primary rami of cervical spinal nerves.
r. ante'rior descen'dens, r. descendente da artéria segmentar anterior dos pulmões direito e esquerdo. SIN descending *branch* of anterior segmental artery of left and right lungs.
rami anteriores nervorum cervicalium [TA], ramos anteriores dos nervos cervicais. SIN anterior rami of cervical nerves.
rami anteriores nervorum lumbalium [TA], ramos anteriores dos nervos lombares. SIN anterior rami of lumbar nerves.
rami anteriores nervorum sacralium [TA], ramos anteriores dos nervos sacrais. SIN anterior rami of sacral nerves.
rami anteriores nervorum thoracis [TA], ramos anteriores dos nervos torácicos. SIN anterior rami of thoracic nerves.
r. ante'rior latera'lis, antigo nome do ramo anterior ascendente da artéria pulmonar esquerda (ascending anterior *branch* of the left pulmonary artery).
anterior r. of lateral sulcus of cerebrum [TA], r. anterior do sulco lateral do cérebro. SIN r. anterior sulci lateralis cerebri [TA].
anterior rami of lumbar nerves [TA], ramos anteriores dos nervos lombares. VER anterior r. of spinal nerve. SIN rami anteriores nervorum lumbalium [TA], ventral rami of lumbar nerves*, rami ventrales nervorum lumbalium, ventral primary rami of lumbar spinal nerves.
r. anterior nervi spinalis [TA], r. anterior do nervo espinal. SIN anterior r. of spinal nerve.
anterior rami of sacral nerves [TA], ramos anteriores dos nervos sacrais. VER anterior r. of spinal nerve. SIN rami anteriores nervorum sacralium [TA], ventral rami of sacral nerves*, rami ventrales nervorum sacralium, ventral primary rami of sacral spinal nerves.
anterior r. of spinal nerve [TA], r. anterior do nervo espinal; o maior ramo terminal principal (junto com o ramo posterior) de todos os 31 pares de nervos espinais mistos formado no forame intervertebral e com orientação ântero-lateral. A maioria dos ramos anteriores, principalmente aqueles envolvidos na inervação dos membros, participa da formação dos principais plexos nervosos (cervical, braquial e lombossacral), perdendo, assim, sua identidade. A maioria dos ramos da região torácica, contudo, permanece separada dos ramos adjacentes e transforma-se nos nervos intercostais e subcostais. Os ramos anteriores fornecem a inervação para a parede ântero-lateral do corpo e para o tronco. A Terminologia Anatômica arrola para cada grupo de nervos espinais: 1) r. anteriores do plexo cervical (nervorum cervicalium [TA]), 2) r. anteriores dos nervos torácicos (nervorum thoracicorum [TA]), 3) r. anteriores dos nervos lombares (nervorum lumbalium [TA]), 4) r. anteriores dos nervos sacrais (nervorum sacralium [TA]) e 5) r. anteriores do nervo coccígeo (nervi coccygei [TA]). SIN r. anterior nervi spinalis [TA], r. ventralis nervi spinalis*, ventral r. of spinal nerve*, anterior primary division, ventral primary r. of spinal nerve.
r. anterior sulci lateralis cerebri [TA], r. anterior do sulco lateral do cérebro. SIN anterior r. of lateral sulcus of cerebrum.
anterior rami of thoracic nerves [TA], ramos anteriores dos nervos torácicos. VER anterior r. of spinal nerve. SIN rami anteriores nervorum thoracis [TA], rami ventrales nervorum thoracis*, ventral rami of thoracic nerves*, ventral primary rami of thoracic spinal nerves.

r. apica'lis lo'bi inferio'ris arte'riae pulmona'lis dex'trae, artéria segmentar apical da artéria lobar superior da artéria pulmonar direita; *termo oficial alternativo para apical segmental *artery* of superior lobar artery of right lung.
r. apicalis venae pulmonalis dextrae superioris, veia apical; *termo oficial alternativo para apical *vein*.
r. apicoposte'rior ve'nae pulmona'lis sinis'trae supe'rioris, veia apicoposterior; *termo oficial alternativo para apicoposterior *vein*.
ra'mi articula'res [TA], ramos articulares. SIN articular *branches*, em *branch*.
rami articulares arte'riae descenden'tis genicular'is, ramos articulares da artéria descendente do joelho. VER articular *branches*, em *branch*.
r. ascen'dens [TA], r. ascendente. SIN ascending *branch*.
r. ascendens arteriae superficialis cervicalis [TA], r. ascendente da artéria cervical superficial. SIN ascending *branch* of superficial cervical artery.
r. ascendens sulci lateralis cerebri [TA], r. ascendente do sulco lateral do cérebro. SIN ascending r. of lateral sulcus of cerebrum.
ascending r. of lateral sulcus of cerebrum [TA], r. ascendente do sulco lateral do cérebro. SIN r. ascendens sulci lateralis cerebri [TA].
ra'mi atria'les [TA], ramos atriais. SIN atrial *branches*, em *branch*.
r. atrialis anastomoticus ramus circumflexus arteriae coronariae sinistrae [TA], r. anastomótico atrial do ramo circunflexo da artéria coronária esquerda. SIN atrial anastomotic *branch* of circumflex branch of left coronary artery.
r. atrialis intermedius arteriae coronariae dextrae [TA], r. atrial intermédio da artéria coronária direita. SIN intermediate atrial *branch* of right coronary artery.
ra'mi auricula'res anterio'res arte'riae tempora'lis superficia'lis [TA], ramos auriculares anteriores da artéria temporal superficial. SIN anterior auricular *branches* of superficial temporal artery, em *branch*.
r. auricularis arteriae auricularis posterioris [TA], r. auricular da artéria auricular posterior. SIN auricular *branch* of posterior auricular artery.
r. auricula'ris arte'riae occipita'lis [TA], r. auricular da artéria occipital. SIN auricular *branch* of occipital artery.
r. auricula'ris nervi va'gi, r. auricular do nervo vago. SIN auricular *branch* of vagus nerve.
r. basa'lis ante'rior, artéria segmentar basilar anterior. SIN anterior basal segmental *artery*.
r. basalis anterior venae basalis superioris, veia basilar anterior; *termo oficial alternativo para anterior basal *vein*.
r. basa'lis latera'lis, artéria segmentar basilar lateral. SIN lateral basal segmental *artery*.
r. basa'lis media'lis, artéria segmentar basilar medial. SIN medial basal segmental *artery*.
r. basa'lis poste'rior, artéria segmentar basilar posterior. SIN posterior basal segmental *artery* of left/right lung.
r. basalis tento'rii arte'riae caro'tidis inter'nae [TA], r. basilar do tentório da artéria carótida interna. SIN tentorial basal *branch* of internal carotid artery.
ra'mi bronchia'les, ramos bronquiais da parte torácica da aorta. SIN bronchial *branches* of thoracic aorta, em *branch*.
ra'mi bronchia'les segmento'rum, brônquios intra-segmentares. SIN intrasegmental *bronchi*, em *bronchus*.
ra'mi bucca'les ner'vi facia'lis [TA], ramos bucais do nervo facial. SIN buccal *branches* of facial nerve, em *branch*.
ra'mi calca'nei [TA], ramos calcâneos. SIN calcaneal *branches*, em *branch*.
ra'mi calca'nei latera'les ner'vi sura'lis [TA], ramos calcâneos laterais do nervo sural. SIN lateral calcaneal *branches* of sural nerve, em *branch*.
ra'mi calca'nei media'les ner'vi tibia'lis [TA], ramos calcâneos mediais do nervo tibial. SIN medial calcaneal *branches* of tibial nerve, em *branch*.
r. calcari'nus arte'riae occipita'lis media'lis [TA], r. calcarino da artéria occipital medial. SIN calcarine *branch* of medial occipital artery.
ra'mi cap'sulae inter'nae, ramos para a cápsula interna; os ramos da artéria corióidea anterior que vão para a cápsula interna. SIN branches to internal capsule, genu [TA], branches to internal capsule, posterior limb [TA], rami cruris posterioris capsulae internae [TA], rami genus capsulae internae [TA], rami partis retrolentiformis capsulae internae [TA], branches to internal capsule, retrolentiform limb.
rami capsulares arteriorum intrarenalium [TA], ramos capsulares das artérias intra-renais. SIN capsular *branches* of intrarenal arteries, em *branch*.
ra'mi capsula'res arte'riae rena'lis [TA], ramos capsulares da artéria renal. SIN capsular *branches* of renal artery, em *branch*.
ra'mi cardi'aci cervica'les inferio'res ner'vi va'gi [TA], ramos cardíacos cervicais inferiores do nervo vago. SIN inferior cervical cardiac *branches* of vagus nerve, em *branch*.
ra'mi cardi'aci cervica'les superio'res ner'vi va'gi [TA], ramos cardíacos cervicais superiores do nervo vago. SIN superior cervical cardiac *branches* of vagus nerve, em *branch*.
rami cardiaci thoracici gangliorum thoracicorum [TA], ramos cardíacos torácicos dos glânglios torácicos. SIN thoracic cardiac *branches* of thoracic ganglia, em *branch*.

ra'mi cardi'aci thora'cici ner'vi va'gi [TA], ramos cardíacos torácicos do nervo vago. SIN thoracic cardiac *branches* of vagus nerve, em *branch*.
r. cardi'acus, artéria segmentar basilar medial da artéria pulmonar; termo obsoleto para medial basal *branch* of pulmonary artery.
ra'mi caroticotympan'ici, artérias caroticotimpânicas. SIN caroticotympanic *arteries* (of internal carotid artery), em *artery*.
r. carpa'lis dorsa'lis arte'riae radia'lis [TA], r. carpal dorsal da artéria radial. SIN dorsal carpal *branch* of radial artery.
r. carpa'lis dorsa'lis arte'riae ulna'ris [TA], r. carpal dorsal da artéria ulnar. SIN dorsal carpal *branch* of ulnar artery.
r. carpa'lis palma'ris arte'riae radia'lis [TA], r. carpal palmar da artéria radial. SIN palmar carpal *branch* of radial artery.
r. carpa'lis palma'ris arte'riae ulna'ris [TA], r. carpal palmar da artéria ulnar. SIN palmar carpal *branch* of ulnar artery.
r. car'peus dorsa'lis arte'riae radia'lis, r. carpal dorsal da artéria radial. SIN dorsal carpal *branch* of radial artery.
r. car'peus dorsa'lis arte'riae ulna'ris, r. carpal dorsal da artéria ulnar. SIN dorsal carpal *branch* of ulnar artery.
r. car'peus palma'ris arte'riae radia'lis, r. carpal palmar da artéria radial. SIN palmar carpal *branch* of radial artery.
r. car'peus palma'ris arte'riae ulna'ris, r. carpal palmar da artéria ulnar. SIN palmar carpal *branch* of ulnar artery.
ra'mi cau'dae nu'clei cauda'ti [TA], ramos para a cauda do núcleo caudado; os ramos que vão para a cauda do núcleo caudado. (1) Os ramos provenientes da artéria corióidea anterior ou da artéria comunicante posterior, ou de ambas e que irrigam a cauda do núcleo caudado; (2) um ramo da artéria cerebral média que vai para a cauda do núcleo caudado.
ra'mi celi'aci ner'vi va'gi, ramos celíacos do nervo vago. SIN celiac *branches* of posterior vagal trunk, em *branch*.
rami celiaci trunci vagi posterioris [TA], ramos celíacos do tronco vagal posterior. SIN celiac *branches* of posterior vagal trunk, em *branch*.
ra'mi centra'les anteromedia'les [TA], ramos centrais ântero-mediais. SIN anteromedial central *branches*, em *branch*.
cephalic arterial rami, ramos arteriais cefálicos; os ramos parietais dos troncos simpáticos que conduzem fibras simpáticas pós-sinápticas do gânglio cervical superior até as artérias carótidas para distribuição dentro da cabeça.
r. cervicalis ner'vi facia'lis, r. cervical do nervo facial; *termo oficial alternativo para cervical *branch* of facial nerve.
r. chiasmat'icus [TA], r. quiasmático; um ramo da artéria cerebral anterior que vai para o quiasma óptico.
ra'mi choroi'dei, ramos corióideos. SIN choroid *branches*, em *branch*.
rami choroidei posteriores arteriae cerebri posteriores laterales et mediales [TA], ramos corióideos posteriores laterais e mediais da artéria cerebral posterior. SIN lateral and medial posterior choroidal *branches* of posterior cerebral artery, em *branch*.
r. choroi'dei posterio'res latera'les [TA], ramos corióideos posteriores laterais; os ramos corióideos posteriores laterais da artéria cerebral posterior. VER choroid *branches*, em *branch*.
r. choroi'dei posterio'res media'les [TA], ramos corióideos posteriores mediais; os ramos corióideos posteriores mediais da artéria cerebral posterior. VER choroid *branches*, em *branch*.
r. choroi'dei ventric'uli latera'lis [TA], ramos corióideos do ventrículo lateral; os ramos corióideos da artéria corióidea anterior que vão para o ventrículo lateral. VER choroid *branches*, em *branch*.
r. choroi'dei ventric'uli ter'tii, ramos corióideos para o terceiro ventrículo; os ramos da artéria corióidea anterior que vão para o terceiro ventrículo. VER choroid *branches*, em *branch*.
r. choroi'deus ventric'uli quar'ti [TA], r. corióideo do quarto ventrículo; o ramo corióideo da artéria cerebelar inferior que vai para o quarto ventrículo. VER choroid *branches*, em *branch*.
r. cingula'ris [TA], r. do cíngulo; ramo da artéria calosomarginal que irriga o giro do cíngulo.
r. cingularis arteriae callosomarginalis [TA], r. do cíngulo da artéria calosomarginal. SIN cingular *branch* of callosomarginal artery.
r. circumflex'us arte'riae corona'riae sinis'trae [TA], r. circunflexo da artéria coronária esquerda. SIN circumflex *branch* of left coronary artery.
r. circumflex'us fibula'ris arte'riae tibia'lis posterio'ris [TA], r. circunflexo fibular da artéria tibial posterior. SIN circumflex fibular *branch* (of posterior tibial artery).
r. circumflexus peronealis arteriae tibialis posterioris, r. circunflexo peroneal da artéria tibial posterior; *termo oficial alternativo para circumflex fibular *branch* (of posterior tibial artery).
r. clavicula'ris arte'riae thoracoacromia'lis [TA], r. clavicular da artéria tóraco-acromial. SIN clavicular *branch* of thoracoacromial artery.
rami cli'vales [TA], ramos do clivo; um ramo da parte cerebral da artéria carótida interna que irriga o clivo.
rami clivales partis cerebralis arteriae carotidis internae [TA], ramos do clivo da parte cerebral da artéria carótida interna. SIN clivus *branches* of cerebral part of internal carotid artery, em *branch*.

r. cochlea'ris arte'riae labyrin'thi, r. coclear da artéria do labirinto. SIN cochlear branch of vestibulocochlear artery.
r. cochlearis arteriae vestibulocochlearis [TA], r. coclear da artéria vestibulococlear. SIN cochlear branch of vestibulocochlear artery.
r. colicus arteriae ileocolicae [TA], r. cólico da artéria ileocólica. SIN colic branch of ileocolic artery.
r. collatera'lis arte'riarum intercosta'lium posterio'rum III-XI [TA], r. colateral das artérias intercostais posteriores III-XI. SIN collateral branches of posterior intercostal arteries 3-11, em branch.
r. collateralis nervorum intercostalium [TA], r. colateral dos nervos intercostais. SIN collateral branch of intercostal nerves.
r. col'li ner'vi facia'lis [TA], r. cervical do nervo facial. SIN cervical branch of facial nerve.
r. commu'nicans, pl. **ra'mi communican'tes** [TA], r. comunicante. SIN communicating branch.
r. commu'nicans arte'riae fibula'ris [TA], r. comunicante da artéria fibular. SIN communicating branch of fibular artery.
r. commu'nicans arte'riae perone'ae, r. comunicante da artéria fibular; *termo oficial alternativo para communicating branch of fibular artery.
r. commu'nicans cum chor'da tym'pani [TA], r. comunicante com a corda do tímpano. **(1)** SIN communicating branch of chorda tympani with lingual nerve; **(2)** SIN communicating branch of otic ganglion with chorda tympani.
r. commu'nicans cum ner'vo glossopharyn'geo, r. comunicante com o nervo glossofaríngeo; **(1)** SIN communicating branch of facial nerve with glossopharyngeal nerve; **(2)** SIN communicating branch of tympanic plexus with auricular branch of vagus nerve.
r. commu'nicans fibula'ris ner'vi fibula'ris commu'nis [TA], r. fibular comunicante do nervo fibular comum. SIN sural communicating branch of common fibular nerve.
r. communicans ganglii otici cum chorda tympani, r. comunicante do gânglio ótico com a corda do tímpano. SIN communicating branch of otic ganglion with chorda tympani.
r. commu'nicans gang'lii o'tici cum ner'vo auriculotempora'li, r. comunicante do gânglio ótico com o nervo auriculotemporal. SIN communicating branch of otic ganglion to auriculotemporal nerve.
r. commu'nicans gang'lii o'tici cum ner'vo pterygoi'deo media'li, r. comunicante do gânglio ótico com o nervo pterigóideo medial. SIN communicating branch of otic ganglion with medial pterygoid nerve.
r. commu'nicans gang'lii o'tici cum ra'mo menin'geo nervi mandibula'ris, r. comunicante do gânglio ótico com o ramo meníngeo do nervo mandibular. SIN communicating branch of otic ganglion with meningeal branch of mandibular nerve.
ra'mi communican'tes ner'vi auriculotempora'lis cum ner'vo facia'li [TA], ramos comunicantes do nervo auriculotemporal com o nervo facial. SIN communicating branches of auriculotemporal nerve with facial nerve, em branch.
r. communicans nervi facialis cum nervo glossopharyngeo [TA], r. comunicante do nervo facial com o nervo glossofaríngeo. SIN communicating branch of facial nerve with glossopharyngeal nerve.
r. commu'nicans ner'vi facia'lis cum plex'u tympan'ico, r. comunicante do nervo facial com o plexo timpânico. SIN communicating branch of intermediate nerve with tympanic plexus.
r. communicans nervi fibularis communis cum nervo cutaneo surae mediali, r. comunicante do nervo fibular comum com o nervo cutâneo sural medial; *termo oficial alternativo para sural communicating branch of common fibular nerve.
r. commu'nicans ner'vi glossopharyn'gei cum ra'mo auricula'ri ner'vi vagi, r. comunicante do nervo glossofaríngeo com o ramo auricular do nervo vago. SIN communicating branch of tympanic plexus with auricular branch of vagus nerve.
r. communicans nervi intermedii cum plexu tympanico [TA], r. comunicante do nervo intermédio com o plexo timpânico. SIN communicating branch of intermediate nerve with tympanic plexus.
r. communicans nervi interossei antebrachii anterioris cum nervi ulnari [TA], r. comunicante do nervo interósseo anterior do antebraço com o nervo ulnar. SIN communicating branch of anterior interosseous nerve with ulnar nerve.
r. commu'nicans ner'vi lacrima'lis cum ner'vo zygomat'ico [TA], r. comunicante do nervo lacrimal com o nervo zigomático. SIN communicating branch of lacrimal nerve with zygomatic nerve.
r. communicans nervi laryngei interni cum nervo laryngeo recurrenti [TA], r. comunicante do nervo laríngeo interno com o nervo laríngeo recorrente. SIN communicating branch of internal laryngeal nerve with recurrent laryngeal nerve.
r. commu'nicans ner'vi laryn'gei recurren'tis cum ra'mo laryn'geo inter'no, r. comunicante do nervo laríngeo recorrente com o ramo laríngeo interno. SIN communicating branch of internal laryngeal nerve with recurrent laryngeal nerve.
r. commu'nicans ner'vi laryn'gei superio'ris cum ner'vo laryn'geo recurrenti, r. comunicante do nervo laríngeo superior com o nervo laríngeo recorrente. SIN communicating branch of internal laryngeal nerve with recurrent laryngeal nerve.
r. communicans nervi lingualis cum chorda tympani, r. comunicante do nervo lingual com a corda do tímpano. SIN communicating branch of chorda tympani with lingual nerve.
ra'mi communican'tes ner'vi lingua'lis cum ner'vo hypoglos'so [TA], ramos comunicantes do nervo lingual com o nervo hipoglosso. SIN communicating branches of lingual nerve with hypoglossal nerve, em branch.
r. commu'nicans ner'vi media'ni cum ner'vo ulna'ri, r. comunicante do nervo mediano com o nervo ulnar. SIN communicating branch of median nerve with ulnar nerve.
r. commu'nicans ner'vi nasocilia'ris cum gan'glio cilia'ri, raiz sensitiva do gânglio ciliar; *termo oficial alternativo para sensory root of ciliary ganglion.
r. communicans nervi peronei communis cum nervo cutaneo surae mediali, r. comunicante do nervo fibular comum com o nervo cutâneo sural medial; *termo oficial alternativo para sural communicating branch of common fibular nerve.
r. communicans nervi radialis cum nervi ulnari [TA], r. comunicante do nervo radial com o nervo ulnar. SIN communicating branch of radial nerve with ulnar nerve.
ra'mi communican'tes nervo'rum spina'lium, ramos comunicantes dos nervos espinais. SIN white rami communicantes.
r. commu'nicans perone'us ner'vi pero'nei commu'nis, r. comunicante do nervo fibular comum; *termo oficial alternativo para sural communicating branch of common fibular nerve.
r. communicans plexus tympanici cum ramo auriculari nervi vagi [TA], r. comunicante do plexo timpânico com o ramo auricular do nervo vago. SIN communicating branch of tympanic plexus with auricular branch of vagus nerve.
r. commu'nicans ulna'ris ner'vi radia'lis, r. comunicante do nervo radial com o nervo ulnar. SIN communicating branch of superficial radial nerve with ulnar nerve.
rami communicantes albi [TA], ramos comunicantes brancos. SIN white rami communicantes.
rami communicantes ganglii sublingualis cum nervo linguali, raiz sensitiva do gânglio sublingual; *termo oficial alternativo para sensory root of sublingual ganglion.
rami communicantes grisei [TA], ramos comunicantes cinzentos. SIN gray rami communicantes.
rami communicantes of sympathetic part of autonomic division of nervous system, ramos comunicantes da parte simpática da divisão autônoma do sistema nervoso; são os ramos comunicantes dos nervos espinais e do tronco simpático; correspondem a pequenos feixes de fibras nervosas que unem os nervos espinais aos gânglios simpáticos. As fibras que seguem do gânglio até o nervo espinal não são mielinizadas e são denominadas ramos comunicantes cinzentos; as fibras que seguem no sentido oposto são mielinizadas e chamadas de ramos comunicantes brancos.
communicating rami of sympathetic trunk, ramos comunicantes do tronco simpático. SIN gray rami communicantes.
ra'mi cor'poris amygdaloi'dei [TA], ramos do corpo amigdalóide; os ramos da artéria corióidea anterior que vão para o corpo amigdalóide.
r. cor'poris callo'si dorsa'lis [TA], r. dorsal do corpo caloso; os ramos da artéria occipital medial que vão para o dorso do corpo caloso.
ra'mi cor'poris genicula'ti latera'lis [TA], ramos do corpo geniculado lateral; os ramos da artéria corióidea anterior que vão para o corpo geniculado lateral.
r. costa'lis latera'lis arte'riae thora'cicae inter'nae [TA], r. costal lateral da artéria torácica interna. SIN lateral costal branch of internal thoracic artery.
r. cricothyroi'deus (arteriae thyroideae superioris), r. cricotireóideo (da artéria tireóidea superior). SIN cricothyroid branch of superior thyroid artery.
rami cruris posterioris capsulae internae [TA], ramos do ramo posterior da cápsula interna. SIN rami capsulae internae.
ra'mi cuta'nei anterio'res ner'vi femora'lis [TA], ramos cutâneos anteriores do nervo femoral. SIN anterior cutaneous branches of femoral nerve, em branch.
rami cuta'nei anteriores pectora'lis et abdominalis nervorum intercostalium, ramos cutâneos anterior do tórax e anterior do abdome dos nervos intercostais. SIN thoracoabdominal nerves, em nerve.
ra'mi cuta'nei cru'ris media'les ner'vi saphe'ni [TA], ramos cutâneos crurais mediais do nervo safeno. SIN medial cutaneous nerve of leg.
r. cutaneus anterior abdominalis nervi intercostalis [TA], r. cutâneo anterior do abdome dos nervos intercostais. SIN anterior abdominal cutaneous branch of intercostal nerve.
r. cutaneus anterior pectoralis nervi intercostalis [TA], r. cutâneo anterior do tórax dos nervos intercostais. SIN anterior pectoral cutaneous branch of intercostal nerves.
r. cuta'neus ante'rior ner'vi iliohypogas'trici [TA], r. cutâneo anterior do nervo ilio-hipogástrico. SIN anterior cutaneous branch of iliohypogastric nerve.

r. cuta'neus ante'rior (pectora'lis et abdomina'lis) nervo'rum thoracico'rum, ramo cutâneo anterior do tórax e ramo cutâneo anterior do abdome dos nervos torácicos. SIN thoracoabdominal nerves, em nerve.
r. cuta'neus latera'lis [TA], r. cutâneo lateral. SIN lateral cutaneous branch.
r. cutaneus lateralis abdominalis/pectoralis nervorum intercostalium, ramos cutâneos peitoral lateral e abdominal lateral dos nervos intercostais. SIN lateral abdominal/pectoral cutaneous branches of intercostal nerves, em branch.
r. cuta'neus latera'lis ner'vi iliohypogas'trici, r. cutâneo lateral do nervo ilio-hipogástrico. VER lateral cutaneous branch.
r. cuta'neus latera'lis ramor'um posterior'um arte'riae intercostal'ium, r. cutâneo lateral do ramo posterior das artérias intercostais; o ramo cutâneo lateral do ramo dorsal das artérias intercostais posteriores. VER lateral cutaneous branch.
r. cutaneus medialis rami dorsalis arteriarum intercostalium posteriorum III-XI, r. cutâneo medial do ramo dorsal das artérias intercostais posteriores III-XI. SIN medial cutaneous branch of dorsal branch of posterior intercostal arteries. VER medial cutaneous branch of dorsal branch of posterior intercostal arteries.
r. cuta'neus media'lis ramor'um dorsa'lium nervo'rum thoracico'rum, r. cutâneo medial do ramo dorsal dos nervos torácicos. VER medial cutaneous branch of dorsal branch of posterior intercostal arteries.
r. cutaneus nervi mixti [TA], r. cutâneo do nervo misto. SIN cutaneous branch of mixed nerve.
r. cuta'neus ra'mi anterio'ris ner'vi obturato'rii [TA], r. cutâneo do ramo anterior do nervo obturatório. SIN cutaneous branch of anterior branch of obturator nerve.
r. deltoi'deus [TA], r. deltóideo. SIN deltoid branch.
r. deltoideus arteriae profundae brachii [TA], r. deltóideo da artéria braquial profunda. SIN profunda brachii artery.
r. deltoideus arteriae thoracoacromialis [TA], r. deltóideo da artéria tóraco-acromial. SIN thoracoacromial artery.
dental rami, ramos dentais. SIN dental branches, em branch.
ra'mi denta'les [TA], ramos dentais. SIN dental branches, em branch.
rami denta'les arte'riae alveola'ris inferio'ris, ramos dentais da artéria alveolar inferior. VER dental branches, em branch.
rami denta'les arte'riae alveola'ris superio'ris posterio'ris, ramos dentais da artéria alveolar superior posterior. VER dental branches, em branch.
ra'mi denta'les inferio'res [TA], ramos dentais inferiores. SIN inferior dental branches of inferior dental plexus, em branch. VER dental branches, em branch.
ra'mi denta'les inferio'res plex'us denta'lis inferio'ris [TA], ramos dentais inferiores do plexo dental inferior. SIN inferior dental branches of inferior dental plexus, em branch.
ra'mi denta'les superio'res [TA], ramos dentais superiores. SIN superior dental branches of superior dental plexus, em branch.
rami denta'les superio'res plex'us denta'lis superio'ris [TA], ramos dentais superiores do plexo dental superior. SIN superior dental branches of superior dental plexus, em branch.
r. descen'dens [TA], r. descendente. SIN descending branch.
r. descen'dens arteri'ae circumflex'ae femo'ris latera'lis [TA], r. descendente da artéria circunflexa femoral lateral. SIN descending branch of lateral circumflex femoral artery.
r. descendens arteriae circumflexae femoris medialis [TA], r. descendente da artéria circunflexa femoral medial. SIN descending branch of medial circumflex femoral artery.
r. descen'dens arte'riae occipita'lis [TA], r. descendente da artéria occipital. SIN descending branch of occipital artery.
r. descendens arteriae segmentalis anterioris pulmonis dextri et sinistri [TA], r. descendente da artéria segmentar anterior dos pulmões direito e esquerdo. SIN descending branch of anterior segmental artery of left and right lungs.
r. descendens arteriae segmentalis posterioris pulmonis dextri et sinistri [TA], r. descendente da artéria segmentar posterior dos pulmões direito e esquerdo. SIN descending branch of posterior segmental artery of left and right lungs.
r. descendens rami superficialis arteriae transversae cervicis [TA], r. descendente do ramo superficial da artéria cervical transversa. SIN descending branch of superficial cervical artery.
r. dex'ter [TA], r. direito. SIN right branch.
r. dex'ter arte'riae hepat'icae propri'ae [TA], r. direito da artéria hepática própria. SIN right branch of hepatic artery proper.
r. dex'ter ve'nae por'tae hepa'tis [TA], r. direito da veia porta do fígado. SIN right branch of portal vein.
r. digas'tricus ner'vi facia'lis [TA], r. digástrico do nervo facial. SIN digastric branch of facial nerve.
rami dorsales arteriarum intercostalium posteriorum primae et secundae [TA], ramos dorsais das artérias primeira e segunda intercostal posterior. SIN dorsal branches of first and second posterior intercostal artery, em branch.
rami dorsa'les arte'riae intercosta'lis supre'mae, ramos dorsais da artéria intercostal suprema. SIN dorsal branches of first and second posterior intercostal artery, em branch.
rami dorsa'les arte'riae subcosta'lis, r. dorsal da artéria subcostal. SIN dorsal branch of the subcostal artery.
r. dorsales arteriae subcostalis [TA], r. dorsal da artéria subcostal. SIN dorsal branch of the subcostal artery.
ra'mi dorsa'les lin'guae arte'riae lingua'lis [TA], ramos dorsais da artéria lingual da língua. SIN dorsal lingual branches of lingual artery, em branch.
rami dorsa'les ner'vi ulna'ris [TA], r. dorsal do nervo ulnar. SIN dorsal branch of the ulnar nerve.
r. dorsa'lis, r. dorsal. SIN posterior r. of spinal nerve.
r. dorsa'lis arte'riae lumba'lis [TA], r. dorsal da artéria lombar. SIN dorsal branch of the lumbar artery.
r. dorsa'lis arteria'rum intercostal'ium posterior'um III-XI [TA], r. dorsal das artérias intercostais posteriores III-XI. SIN dorsal branch of the posterior intercostal arteries 3-11.
r. dorsa'lis ner'vi spina'lis, r. posterior do nervo espinal; *termo oficial alternativo para posterior r. of spinal nerve.
r. dorsa'lis vena'rum intercostal'ium posterior'um IV-XI [TA], r. dorsal das veias intercostais posteriores IV-XI. SIN dorsal branch of the posterior intercostal veins 4-11.
dorsal primary r. of spinal nerve, r. posterior do nervo espinal; *termo oficial alternativo para posterior r. of spinal nerve.
rami duodenales arteriae pancreaticoduodenalis superioris anterioris [TA], ramos duodenais da artéria pancreaticoduodenal superior anterior. SIN duodenal branches of anterior superior pancreaticoduodenal artery, em branch.
ra'mi epiplo'icae, ramos epiplóicos. SIN omental branches, em branch.
ra'mi esophagea'les, ramos esofágicos; *termo oficial alternativo para esophageal branches, em branch.
ra'mi esophagea'les aor'tae thora'cicae, ramos esofágicos da aorta torácica; *termo oficial alternativo para esophageal branches of the thoracic aorta, em branch.
ra'mi esophagea'les arte'riae gas'tricae sinis'trae [TA], ramos esofágicos da artéria gástrica esquerda. SIN esophageal branches of the left gastric artery, em branch.
ra'mi esophagea'les arte'riae thyroi'deae inferio'ris [TA], ramos esofágicos da artéria tireóidea inferior. SIN esophageal branches of the inferior thyroid artery, em branch.
rami esophageales gangliorum thoracicorum [TA], ramos esofágicos dos gânglios torácicos. SIN esophageal branches of thoracic ganglia, em branch.
rami esophageales partis thoracicae aortae [TA], ramos esofágicos da parte torácica da aorta. SIN esophageal branches of the thoracic aorta, em branch.
ra'mi esopha'gei [TA], ramos esofágicos. SIN esophageal branches, em branch.
ra'mi esopha'gei ner'vi laryn'gei recurren'tis [TA], ramos esofágicos do nervo laríngeo recorrente. SIN esophageal branches of the recurrent laryngeal nerve, em branch.
ra'mi esopha'gei ner'vi va'gi, ramos esofágicos do nervo vago. SIN esophageal branches of the vagus nerve, em branch.
r. exter'nus ner'vi laryn'gei superio'ris [TA], r. externo do nervo laríngeo superior. SIN external branch of superior laryngeal nerve.
r. externus trunci nervi accessorii [TA], r. externo do tronco do nervo acessório. SIN external branch of trunk of accessory nerve.
ra'mi faucia'les ner'vi lingua'lis, ramos para o istmo das fauces do nervo lingual. SIN branches of lingual nerve to isthmus of fauces, em branch.
r. femora'lis ner'vi genitofemora'lis [TA], r. femoral do nervo genitofemoral. SIN femoral branch of genitofemoral nerve.
r. fronta'lis anteromedia'lis [TA], r. frontal ântero-medial; o ramo frontal ântero-medial da artéria calosomarginal.
r. frontalis anteromedialis arteriae callosomarginalis [TA], r. frontal ântero-medial da artéria calosomarginal. SIN anteromedial frontal branch of callosomarginal artery.
r. frontalis arteriae meningeae mediae [TA], r. frontal da artéria meníngea média. SIN frontal branch of middle meningeal artery.
r. fronta'lis arte'riae tempora'lis superficia'lis [TA], r. frontal da artéria temporal superficial. SIN frontal branch of superficial temporal artery.
r. fronta'lis intermediomedia'lis [TA], r. frontal intermédio-medial; o ramo frontal intermédio-medial da artéria calosomarginal.
r. frontalis intermediomedialis arteriae callosomarginalis [TA], r. frontal intermédio-medial da artéria calosomarginal. SIN intermediomedial frontal branch of callosomarginal artery.
r. fronta'lis posteromedia'lis [TA], r. frontal póstero-medial; o ramo frontal póstero-medial da artéria calosomarginal.
r. frontalis posteromedialis arteriae callosomarginalis [TA], r. frontal póstero-medial da artéria calosomarginal. SIN posteromedial frontal branch of callosomarginal artery.
rami gang'lii submandibula'ris, ramos do gânglio submandibular. SIN glandular branches of submandibular ganglion, em branch.
ra'mi communican'tes gang'lii submandibula'ris cum ner'vo lingua'li, raiz sensitiva do gânglio submandibular; *termo oficial alternativo para sensory root of submandibular ganglion.

r. gang'lii trigemina'lis, ramos ganglionares trigeminais. SIN branches of internal carotid artery to trigeminal ganglion, em branch.
ra'mi gangliona'res, raiz sensitiva do gânglio pterigopalatino. SIN sensory root of pterygopalatine ganglion.
r. ganglionares trigeminales arteriae carotidis internae [TA], ramos ganglionares trigeminais da artéria carótida interna. SIN branches of internal carotid artery to trigeminal ganglion, em branch.
rami ganglio'nici ner'vi maxilla'ris, raiz sensitiva do gânglio pterigopalatino; *termo oficial alternativo para sensory root of pterygopalatine ganglion.
ra'mi gas'trici anterio'res ner'vi va'gi, ramos gástricos anteriores do tronco vagal anterior. SIN anterior gastric branches of anterior vagal trunk, em branch.
rami gastrici anteriores trunci vagalis anterioris [TA], ramos gástricos anteriores do tronco vagal anterior. SIN anterior gastric branches of anterior vagal trunk, em branch.
ra'mi gas'trici posterio'res ner'vi va'gi, ramos gástricos posteriores do tronco vagal posterior. SIN gastric branches of posterior vagal trunk, em branch.
rami gastrici posteriores trunci vagalis posterioris [TA], ramos gástricos posteriores do tronco vagal posterior. SIN posterior gastric branches of posterior vagal trunk, em branch.
r. genita'lis ner'vi genitofemora'lis [TA], r. genital do nervo genitofemoral. SIN genital branch of genitofemoral nerve.
rami genus capsulae internae [TA], ramos do joelho da cápsula interna. SIN rami capsulae internae.
ra'mi gingiva'les inferio'res plex'us denta'lis inferio'ris [TA], ramos gengivais inferiores do plexo dental inferior. SIN inferior gingival branches of inferior dental plexus, em branch.
ra'mi gingiva'les superio'res plex'us denta'lis superio'ris [TA], ramos gengivais superiores do plexo dental superior. SIN superior gingival branches of superior dental plexus, em branch.
ra'mi glandula'res [TA], ramos glandulares. SIN glandular branches, em branch.
r. glandula'res ante'rior/latera'lis/poste'rior arte'riae thyroide'ae superio'ris, ramos glandulares anterior, lateral e posterior da artéria tireóidea superior. SIN anterior/lateral/posterior glandular branches of superior thyroid artery, em branch.
rami glandula'res arte'riae facia'lis [TA], ramos glandulares da artéria facial. SIN glandular branches of facial artery, em branch.
rami glandula'res arte'riae thyroi'deae inferio'ris [TA], ramos glandulares da artéria tireóidea inferior. SIN glandular branches of inferior thyroid artery, em branch.
rami glandular'es gang'lii submandibular'is, ramos glandulares do gânglio submandibular. SIN glandular branches of submandibular ganglion, em branch.
r. glandularis anterior arteriae thyroideae superioris [TA], r. glandular anterior da artéria tireóidea superior. SIN anterior glandular branch of superior thyroid artery.
r. glandularis posterior arteriae thyroideae superioris [TA], r. glandular posterior da artéria tireóidea superior. SIN posterior glandular branch of superior thyroid artery.
ra'mi glo'bi pal'lidi [TA], ramos do globo pálido; os ramos da artéria coriódea anterior que vão para o globo pálido.
gray rami communicantes [TA], ramos comunicantes cinzentos; os nervos curtos que surgem da face lateral do tronco simpático e conduzem fibras nervosas simpáticas pós-sinápticas não-mielinizadas do tronco simpático até as porções iniciais de todos os 31 pares de ramos primários ventrais dos nervos espinais para a sua distribuição por todas as partes do nervo espinal (incluindo o ramo primário dorsal). Os ramos cinzentos correspondem aos ramos parietais dos troncos simpáticos, uma vez que todas as fibras pós-sinápticas distribuídas para a parede do corpo (incluindo os membros) devem passar através deles. SIN rami communicantes grisei [TA], communicating branches of sympathetic trunk, communicating rami of sympathetic trunk.
ra'mi hepat'ici ner'vi va'gi, ramos hepáticos do tronco vagal anterior. SIN hepatic branches of anterior vagal trunk, em branch.
rami hepatici trunci vagi anterior [TA], ramos hepáticos do tronco vagal anterior. SIN hepatic branches of anterior vagal trunk, em branch.
r. hypothalam'icus [TA], r. hipotalâmico; um ramo da artéria cerebral anterior para o hipotálamo.
r. ili'acus arte'riae iliolumba'lis [TA], r. ilíaco da artéria iliolombar. SIN iliacus branch of iliolumbar artery.
r. infe'rior [TA], r. inferior. SIN inferior branch.
r. infe'rior arte'riae glu'teae superio'ris [TA], r. inferior da artéria glútea superior. SIN inferior branch of superior gluteal artery.
inferior dental rami, ramos dentais inferiores. SIN inferior dental branches of inferior dental plexus, em branch.
ra'mi inferio'res ner'vi transver'si cervicalis [col'li], ramos inferiores do nervo cervical transverso. SIN inferior branches of transverse cervical nerve, em branch.

rami inferiores nervi transversi colli, ramos inferiores do nervo cervical transverso; *termo oficial alternativo para inferior branches of transverse cervical nerve, em branch.
r. infe'rior ner'vi oculomoto'rii [TA], r. inferior do nervo oculomotor. SIN inferior branch of oculomotor nerve.
r. inferior ossis pubis [TA], r. inferior do púbis. SIN inferior pubic r.
inferior pubic r. [TA], r. inferior do púbis; a extensão inferior do corpo do púbis que se une ao ramo do ísquio para formar o ramo isquiopúbico. SIN r. inferior ossis pubis [TA].
r. infrahyoi'deus arte'riae thyroi'deae superio'ris [TA], r. infra-hióideo da artéria tireóidea superior. SIN infrahyoid branch of superior thyroid artery.
r. infrapatella'ris ner'vi saphe'ni [TA], r. infrapatelar do nervo safeno. SIN infrapatellar branch of saphenous nerve.
ra'mi inguina'les arte'riarum puden'darum exter'narum profundarum [TA], ramos inguinais da artéria pudenda externa profunda. SIN inguinal branches of deep external pudendal arteries, em branch.
ra'mi intercosta'les anterio'res, ramos intercostais anteriores. SIN anterior intercostal branches of internal thoracic artery, em branch.
rami intercostal'es anterior'es arter'iae thora'cicae inter'nae [TA], ramos intercostais anteriores da artéria torácica interna. SIN anterior intercostal branches of internal thoracic artery, em branch.
ra'mi interglionia'res trunci sympathici [TA], ramos interganglionares do tronco simpático. SIN interganglionic branches of sympathetic trunk, em branch.
r. intermedius arteriae hepaticae propriae [TA], r. intermédio da artéria hepática própria. SIN intermediate branch of hepatic artery proper.
internal r. of accessory nerve, r. interno do nervo acessório. SIN internal branch of trunk of accessory nerve. VER TAMBÉM accessory nerve [CN XI].
r. inter'nus trunci ner'vi accesso'rii [TA], r. interno do tronco do nervo acessório. SIN internal branch of trunk of accessory nerve; VER TAMBÉM accessory nerve [CN XI].
r. inter'nus ner'vi laryn'gei superio'ris [TA], r. interno do nervo laríngeo superior. SIN internal branch of superior laryngeal nerve.
ra'mi interventricula'res septa'les, ramos interventriculares septais. SIN interventricular septal branches of left/right coronary artery, em branch.
rami interventriculares septales arteriae coronariae sinistrae/dextrae, ramos interventriculares septais das artérias coronárias esquerda/direita. SIN interventricular septal branches of left/right coronary artery, em branch.
r. interventricula'ris ante'rior arte'riae corona'riae sinis'trae [TA], r. interventricular anterior da artéria coronária esquerda. SIN anterior interventricular branch of left coronary artery.
r. interventricula'ris poste'rior arte'riae corona'riae dex'trae [TA], r. interventricular posterior da artéria coronária direita. SIN posterior interventricular branch of right coronary artery.
ischial r., r. do ísquio. SIN r. of ischium.
ischiopubic r., r. isquiopúbico; a união do r. inferior do púbis e do r. do ísquio, que juntos formam o limite ínfero-medial do forame obturado.
r. of ischium, r. do ísquio; ramo do ísquio antigamente denominado ramo inferior do ísquio; a parte do osso que passa diante do túber do ísquio para se unir ao r. inferior do púbis, formando, assim, o r. isquiopúbico. SIN r. ossis ischii [TA], ischial r.
ra'mi isth'mi fau'cium ner'vi lingua'lis [TA], ramos do nervo lingual para o istmo da fauces. SIN branches of lingual nerve to isthmus of fauces, em branch.
ra'mi labia'les anterio'res arte'riae puden'dae exter'nae profundae [TA], ramos labiais anteriores da artéria pudenda externa profunda. SIN anterior labial branches of deep external pudendal artery, em branch.
ra'mi labia'les inferio'res ner'vi menta'lis, ramos labiais inferiores do nervo mental. SIN labial branches of mental nerve, em branch.
rami labiales nervi mentalis [TA], ramos labiais do nervo mental. SIN labial branches of mental nerve, em branch.
rami labiales posteriores arteriae perinealis [TA], ramos labiais posteriores da artéria pudenda interna. SIN posterior labial branches of internal perineal artery.
ra'mi labia'les poste'rior'es arte'riae puden'dae inter'nae, ramos labiais posteriores da artéria pudenda interna. SIN posterior labial branches of internal perineal artery.
ra'mi labia'les superio'res ner'vi infraorbita'lis [TA], ramos labiais superiores do nervo infra-orbital. SIN superior labial branches of infraorbital nerve, em branch.
r. labialis inferior arteriae facialis, r. labial inferior da artéria facial. SIN inferior labial branch of facial artery.
r. labialis superior arteriae facialis, r. labial superior da artéria facial. SIN superior labial branch of facial artery.
ra'mi laryngopharyn'gei gang'lii cervica'lis superio'ris [TA], ramos laringofaríngeos do gânglio cervical superior. SIN laryngopharyngeal branches of superior cervical ganglion, em branch.
ra'mi latera'les [TA], ramos laterais. SIN lateral branches, em branch.
rami laterales arteriae pontis [TA], ramos laterais das artérias da ponte. SIN lateral branches of pontine arteries, em branch.

rami latera'les arteria'rum centra'lium anterolatera'lium, ramos laterais das artérias centrais ântero-laterais.
rami laterales arteriarum tuberis cinerei [TA], ramos laterais das artérias do túber cinéreo. SIN lateral branches of artery of tuber cinereum, em branch.
rami latera'les ra'mi sinis'tri ve'nae por'tae hep'atis, ramos laterais do ramo esquerdo da veia porta do fígado. VER lateral branches, em branch.
rami laterales ramorum dorsalium nervorum spinalis, ramos laterais dos ramos primários dorsais dos nervos espinais. VER lateral branches, em branch.
r. latera'lis duc'tus hepa'tici sinis'tri, r. lateral do ducto hepático esquerdo. VER lateral branches, em branch.
r. lateralis interventricularis anterioris arteriae coronariae sinistrae, r. lateral do ramo interventricular anterior da artéria coronária esquerda. VER lateral branches, em branch.
r. lateralis nasi arteriae facialis [TA], r. nasal lateral da artéria facial. SIN lateral nasal branch of facial artery.
r. latera'lis ner'vi supraorbita'lis, r. lateral do nervo supra-orbital. VER lateral branches, em branch.
r. latera'lis ramor'um dorsa'lium nervo'rum thoracico'rum, r. lateral dos ramos dorsais dos nervos torácicos; o ramo cutâneo lateral do ramo dorsal dos nervos torácicos.
r. latera'lis rami lobar'is me'dii arteriae pulmona'lis dextrae, r. lateral do ramo lobar médio da artéria pulmonar direita. VER lateral branches, em branch.
rami liena'les arte'riae liena'lis, ramos esplênicos da artéria esplênica; *termo oficial alternativo para splenic branches of splenic artery, em branch.
rami lingua'les ner'vi glossopharyn'gei, ramos linguais do nervo glossofaríngeo. VER lingual branches, em branch.
rami lingua'les ner'vi hypoglos'si, ramos linguais do nervo hipoglosso. VER lingual branches, em branch.
rami lingua'les ner'vi lingua'lis, ramos linguais do nervo lingual. VER lingual branches, em branch.
ra'mi lingua'les, ramos linguais. SIN lingual branches, em branch.
r. lingual'is ner'vi facia'lis, r. lingual do nervo facial. SIN lingual branch of facial nerve.
r. lingula'ris infe'rior, r. lingular inferior. SIN inferior lingular artery.
r. lingula'ris supe'rior, r. lingular superior. SIN superior lingular artery.
r. lingularis venae pulmonis sinistrae superioris, r. lingular da veia pulmonar esquerda superior; *termo oficial alternativo para lingular vein.
ra'mi lobi cauda'ti rami sinistri venae portae hepatis [TA], ramos do lobo caudado do ramo esquerdo da veia porta do fígado. SIN caudate branches of left branch of portal vein, em branch.
r. lobi medii arteriae pulmonalis dextrae, r. lobar médio da artéria pulmonar direita. VER middle lobe vein.
r. lo'bi me'dii ve'nae pulmona'lis dex'trae superio'ris, r. do lobo médio da veia pulmonar direita superior. SIN middle lobe vein; VER middle lobe vein.
r. lumba'lis arte'riae iliolumba'lis [TA], r. lombar da artéria iliolombar. SIN lumbar branch of iliolumbar artery.
ra'mi malleola'res latera'les arteriae fibularis (peronei) [TA], ramos maleolares laterais da artéria fibular. SIN lateral malleolar branch (of fibular peroneal artery).
ra'mi malleola'res media'les arteriae tibialis posterioris [TA], ramos maleolares mediais da artéria tibial posterior. SIN medial malleolar branches (of posterior tibial artery), em branch.
ra'mi mamma'rii, ramos mamários. VER lateral mammary branches, em branch, medial mammary branches, em branch.
ra'mi mamma'rii latera'les, ramos mamários laterais. SIN lateral mammary branches, em branch.
rami mamma'rii latera'les arte'riae thora'cicae latera'lis [TA], ramos mamários laterais da artéria torácica lateral. SIN lateral mammary branches of lateral thoracic artery, em branch.
rami mamma'rii latera'les ramo'rum cutaneo'rum latera'lium nervo'rum intercosta'lium, ramos mamários laterais do ramo cutâneo lateral dos nervos intercostais. SIN lateral mammary branches of lateral cutaneous branches of thoracic spinal nerves, em branch.
rami mamma'rii latera'les ramo'rum cuta'neorum latera'lis nervo'rum thoracico'rum, ramos mamários laterais do ramo cutâneo lateral dos nervos torácicos. SIN lateral mammary branches of lateral cutaneous branches of thoracic spinal nerves, em branch.
ra'mi mamma'rii media'les, ramos mamários mediais. SIN medial mammary branches, em branch.
rami mammari'i media'les ramo'rum cutaneo'rum anterio'rum nervo'rum intercostal'ium, ramos mamários mediais do ramo cutâneo anterior dos nervos intercostais; os ramos mamários mediais do ramo cutâneo anterior dos ramos primários ventrais dos nervos espinais torácicos. VER medial mammary branches, em branch.
rami mamma'rii media'les ra'mi cuta'nei anterio'ris ramor'um ventral'ium nervo'rum thoraci'corum, ramos mamários mediais do ramo cutâneo anterior dos ramos ventrais dos nervos torácicos; os ramos mamários mediais do ramo cutâneo anterior dos ramos primários ventrais dos nervos espinais torácicos. VER medial mammary branches, em branch.
rami mamma'rii media'les ramo'rum perforan'tium arte'riae thora'cicae inter'nae, ramos mamários mediais dos ramos perfurantes da artéria torácica interna. VER medial mammary branches, em branch.
r. of mandible [TA], r. da mandíbula; a extremidade perpendicular voltada para cima e encontrada em ambos os lados da mandíbula; o músculo masseter insere-se em sua face lateral. SIN r. mandibulae [TA].
r. mandib'ulae [TA], r. da mandíbula. SIN r. of mandible.
r. marginalis [TA], r. marginal. SIN marginal sulcus.
r. marginalis dexter (arteriae coronariae dextrae) [TA], r. marginal direito (da artéria coronária direita). SIN right marginal branch (of right coronary artery).
r. margina'lis mandib'ulae ner'vi facia'lis [TA], r. marginal da mandíbula do nervo facial. SIN marginal mandibular branch of facial nerve.
r. marginalis sinister arteriae coronariae sinistrae [TA], r. marginal esquerdo da artéria coronária esquerda. SIN left marginal artery.
r. marginalis sulci cinguli [TA], r. marginal do sulco do cíngulo. SIN marginal branch of cingulate sulcus.
r. marginalis sulci parietooccipitalis [TA], r. marginal do sulco parietooccipital. SIN marginal branch of parietooccipital sulcus.
r. margina'lis tento'rii arte'riae caro'tidis inter'nae, r. marginal do tentório da artéria carótida interna. SIN tentorial marginal branch of cavernous part of internal carotid artery.
r. marginalis tentorii partis cavernosae arteriae carotidis internae [TA], r. marginal do tentório da parte cavernosa da artéria carótida interna. SIN tentorial marginal branch of cavernous part of internal carotid artery.
ra'mi mastoi'dei arte'riae auricula'ris posterio'ris, ramos mastóideos da artéria auricular posterior. SIN mastoid branches of posterior tympanic artery, em branch.
rami mastoidei arteriae tympanicae posterioris [TA], ramos mastóideos da artéria timpânica posterior. SIN mastoid branches of posterior tympanic artery, em branch.
r. mastoi'deus arte'riae occipita'lis [TA], r. mastóideo da artéria occipital. SIN mastoid branch of occipital artery.
r. mea'tus acus'tici inter'ni, r. do meato acústico interno. SIN labyrinthine artery.
ra'mi media'les [TA], ramos mediais. SIN medial branches, em branch.
rami mediales arteriae pontis [TA], ramos mediais das artérias da ponte. SIN medial branches of pontine arteries, em branch.
rami media'les arteria'rum centra'lium anterolatera'lium, ramos mediais das artérias centrais ântero-laterais. VER medial branches, em branch.
rami mediales arteriarum tuberis cinerei [TA], ramos mediais das artérias do túber cinéreo. SIN medial branches of artery of tuber cinereum, em branch.
r. media'lis duc'tus hepa'tici sinis'tri, r. medial do ducto hepático esquerdo. VER medial branches, em branch.
r. media'lis ner'vi supraorbita'lis, r. medial do nervo supra-orbital. VER medial branches, em branch.
r. media'lis ra'mi loba'ris me'dii arteriae pulmona'lis dextrae, r. medial do ramo lobar médio da artéria pulmonar direita. VER medial branches, em branch.
rami media'les ra'mi sinis'tri ve'nae por'tae hepa'tis, ramos mediais do ramo esquerdo da veia porta do fígado. VER medial branches, em branch.
r. media'lis ramor'um dorsa'lium nervo'rum spinalis. r. medial dos ramos dorsais dos nervos espinais. SIN medial branch of posterior rami of spinal nerves. VER medial branches, em branch.
ra'mi mediastina'les [TA], ramos mediastinais. SIN mediastinal branches, em branch.
rami mediastina'les aor'tae thora'cicae [TA], ramos mediastinais da aorta torácica. SIN mediastinal branches of thoracic aorta, em branch.
rami mediastina'les arte'riae thora'cicae inter'nae [TA], ramos mediastinais da artéria torácica interna. SIN mediastinal branches of internal thoracic artery, em branch.
ra'mi medulla'res latera'les, ramos medulares laterais; os ramos da artéria cerebelar inferior posterior para a parte lateral da medula oblonga.
rami medullares laterales (partis intracranialis) arteriae vertebralis [TA], ramos medulares laterais da (parte intracraniana da) artéria vertebral. SIN lateral medullary branches of (intracranial part of) vertebral artery, em branch.
ra'mi medulla'res media'les, ramos medulares mediais; os ramos da artéria cerebelar inferior posterior para a parte medial da medula oblonga.
rami medullares mediales arteriae vertebralis [TA], ramos medulares mediais da artéria vertebral. SIN medial medullary branches of vertebral artery, em branch.
rami membra'nae tym'pani ner'vi auriculotempora'lis [TA], ramos do nervo auriculotemporal para a membrana timpânica. SIN branches of auriculotemporal nerve to tympanic membrane, em branch.
rami menin'gei [TA], ramos meníngeos. SIN meningeal branches, em branch.
r. meningeus accessorius, r. meníngeo acessório. SIN pterygomeningeal artery.

r. menin'geus accesso'rius arte'riae menin'geae me'diae, r. meníngeo acessório da artéria meníngea média. SIN accessory branch of middle meningeal artery.
r. meningeus anterior arteriae ethmoidalis anterioris [TA], r. meníngeo anterior da artéria etmoidal anterior. SIN anterior meningeal branch (of anterior ethmoidal artery).
r. menin'geus ante'rior arte'riae vertebra'lis, r. meníngeo anterior da artéria vertebral; o ramo meníngeo da artéria vertebral.
r. menin'geus arte'riae carot'idis inter'nae, r. meníngeo da artéria carótida interna. SIN meningeal branch of cavernous part of internal carotid artery.
r. menin'geus arte'riae occipita'lis [TA], r. meníngeo da artéria occipital. SIN meningeal branch of occipital artery.
r. menin'geus me'dius ner'vi maxilla'ris, r. meníngeo médio do nervo maxilar. SIN meningeal branch of maxillary nerve.
r. menin'geus ner'vi mandibula'ris [TA], r. meníngeo do nervo mandibular. SIN meningeal branch of mandibular nerve.
r. meningeus nervi maxillaris [TA], r. meníngeo do nervo maxilar. SIN meningeal branch of maxillary nerve.
r. menin'geus ner'vi va'gi [TA], r. meníngeo do nervo vago. SIN meningeal branch of vagus nerve.
r. menin'geus nervo'rum spina'lium [TA], r. meníngeo dos nervos espinais. SIN meningeal branch of spinal nerves.
r. meningeus partis cavernosae arteriae carotidis internae [TA], r. meníngeo da parte cavernosa da artéria carótida interna. SIN meningeal branch of cavernous part of internal carotid artery.
r. meningeus partis cerebralis arteriae carotidis internae [TA], r. meníngeo da parte cerebral da artéria carótida interna. SIN meningeal branch of cerebral part of internal carotid artery.
r. meningeus (partis intracranialis) arteriae vertebralis [TA], r. meníngeo da (parte intracraniana da) artéria vertebral. SIN meningeal branch of (intracranial part of) vertebral artery.
r. menin'geus poste'rior, r. meníngeo posterior; o ramo meníngeo posterior da artéria vertebral.
r. meningeus recurrens nervi ophthalmici [TA], r. meníngeo recorrente do nervo oftálmico. SIN tentorial nerve.
ra'mi menta'les ner'vi menta'lis [TA], ramos mentuais do nervo mentual. SIN mental branches of mental nerve, em branch.
r. mentalis arteriae alveolaris inferioris [TA], r. mentual da artéria alveolar inferior. SIN mental branch (of inferior alveolar artery).
ra'mi muscula'res [TA], ramos musculares. SIN muscular branches, em branch.
rami musculares arteriae vertebralis [TA], ramos musculares da artéria vertebral. VER muscular branches, em branch.
rami musculares nervi accessorii [TA], ramos musculares do nervo acessório. VER muscular branches, em branch.
rami musculares nervi axillaris [TA], ramos musculares do nervo axilar. VER muscular branches, em branch.
rami musculares nervi fibularis profundi [TA], ramos musculares do nervo fibular profundo. VER muscular branches, em branch.
rami musculares nervi fibularis superficialis [TA], ramos musculares do nervo fibular superficial. VER muscular branches, em branch.
rami musculares nervi interossei antebrachii anterior [TA], ramos musculares do nervo interósseo anterior do antebraço. VER muscular branches, em branch.
rami musculares nervi mediani [TA], ramos musculares do nervo mediano. VER muscular branches, em branch.
rami musculares nervi musculocutanei [TA], ramos musculares do nervo musculocutâneo. VER muscular branches, em branch.
rami musculares nervi radialis [TA], ramos musculares do nervo radial. VER muscular branches, em branch.
rami musculares nervi tibialis [TA], ramos musculares do nervo tibial. VER muscular branches, em branch.
rami musculares nervi ulnaris [TA], ramos musculares do nervo ulnar. VER muscular branches, em branch.
rami musculares nervorum intercostalium [TA], ramos musculares dos nervos intercostais. VER muscular branches, em branch.
rami musculares nervorum perinealium [TA], ramos musculares dos nervos perineais. VER muscular branches, em branch.
rami musculares nervorum spinalium [TA], ramos musculares dos nervos espinais. VER muscular branches, em branch.
rami musculares partis supraclavicularis plexus brachialis [TA], ramos musculares da parte supraclavicular do plexo braquial. VER muscular branches, em branch.
rami musculares rami anterioris nervi obturatorii [TA], ramos musculares do ramo anterior do nervo obturatório. VER muscular branches, em branch.
rami musculares rami posterioris nervi obturatorii [TA], ramos musculares do ramo posterior do nervo obturatório. VER muscular branches, em branch.
r. mus'culi stylopharyn'gei ner'vi glossopharyn'gei [TA], r. do nervo glossofaríngeo para o músculo estilofaríngeo. SIN stylopharyngeal branch of glossopharyngeal nerve.
r. mylohyoi'deus arte'riae alveola'ris inferio'ris [TA], r. milo-hióideo da artéria alveolar inferior. SIN mylohyoid branch (of inferior alveolar artery).
rami nasales anteriores laterales arteriae ethmoidalis anterioris [TA], ramos nasais anteriores laterais da artéria etmoidal anterior. SIN anterior lateral nasal branches of anterior ethmoidal artery, em branch.
rami nasa'les exter'ni ner'vi ethmoida'lis anterio'ris, ramos nasais externos do nervo etmoidal anterior; o ramo nasal externo do nervo nasociliar. VER external nasal branches of infraorbital nerve, em branch.
rami nasa'les exter'ni ner'vi infraorbita'lis, ramos nasais externos do nervo infra-orbital. SIN external nasal branches of infraorbital nerve, em branch. VER external nasal branches of infraorbital nerve, em branch.
ra'mi nasa'les inter'ni [TA], ramos nasais internos. SIN internal nasal branches, em branch.
rami nasa'les inter'ni ner'vi ethmoida'lis anterio'ris, ramos nasais internos do nervo etmoidal anterior; o ramo nasal interno do nervo nasociliar. VER internal nasal branches, em branch.
rami nasa'les inter'ni ner'vi infraorbita'lis, ramos nasais internos do nervo infra-orbital; o ramo nasal interno do nervo infra-orbital. VER internal nasal branches, em branch.
ra'mi nasa'les latera'les ner'vi ethmoida'lis anterio'ris [TA], ramos nasais laterais do nervo etmoidal anterior. SIN lateral nasal branches of anterior ethmoidal nerve, em branch.
ra'mi nasa'les media'les ner'vi ethmoida'lis anterio'ris [TA], ramos nasais mediais do nervo etmoidal anterior. SIN medial nasal branches of anterior ethmoidal nerve, em branch.
ra'mi nasa'les posterio'res inferio'res ner'vi palati'ni majo'ris [TA], ramos nasais póstero-inferiores do nervo palatino maior; SIN posterior inferior nasal nerves, em nerve.
ra'mi nasa'les posterio'res superio'res latera'les gang'lii pterygopalati'ni, ramos nasais posteriores súpero-laterais do gânglio pterigopalatino; SIN posterior superior lateral nasal branches of maxillary nerve, em branch.
rami nasales posteriores superiores laterales nervi maxillaris, ramos nasais posteriores súpero-laterais do nervo maxilar; SIN posterior superior lateral nasal branches of maxillary nerve, em branch.
ra'mi nasa'les posterio'res superio'res media'les gang'lii pterygopalati'ni, ramos nasais posteriores súpero-mediais do gânglio pterigopalatino; SIN posterior superior medial nasal branches of maxillary nerve, em branch.
rami nasales posteriores superiores mediales nervi maxillaris [TA], ramos nasais posteriores súpero-mediais do nervo maxilar; SIN posterior superior medial nasal branches of maxillary nerve, em branch.
r. ner'vi oculomoto'rii arte'riae communican'tis posterio'ris, r. da artéria comunicante posterior para o nervo oculomotor; o ramo para o nervo oculomotor.
r. no'di atriventricula'ris [TA], r. do nó atrioventricular; SIN atrioventricular nodal branch.
r. no'di sinuatria'lis arte'riae corona'riae dex'trae [TA], r. do nó sinoatrial da artéria coronária direita; SIN sinuatrial (S-A) nodal branch of right coronary artery.
ra'mi nucleo'rum hypothalamico'rum [TA], ramos para os núcleos hipotalâmicos; os ramos da artéria corióidea anterior para os núcleos do hipotálamo.
r. obturato'rius arte'riae epigas'tricae inferio'ris, r. obturatório da artéria epigástrica inferior. SIN accessory obturator artery.
r. obturatorius rami pubici arteriae epigastricae inferioris [TA], r. obturatório do ramo púbico da artéria epigástrica inferior. SIN obturator branch of pubic branch of inferior epigastric artery.
rami occipita'les arte'riae auricula'ris posterio'ris, ramos occipitais da artéria auricular posterior. VER occipital branch.
rami occipita'les arte'riae occip'itis, ramos occipitais da artéria occipital; VER occipital branch.
rami occipita'les ner'vi auricula'ris posterio'ris, r. occipital do nervo auricular posterior; VER occipital branch.
r. occipita'lis [TA], r. occipital. SIN occipital branch.
r. occipitotempora'lis [TA], r. occipitotemporal; um ramo da artéria occipital medial para as regiões temporais e occipitais do córtex cerebral.
ra'mi omenta'les [TA], ramos omentais. SIN omental branches, em branch.
rami orbitales nervi maxillaris [TA], ramos orbitais do nervo maxilar. SIN orbital branches of maxillary nerve, em branch.
r. orbita'lis arte'riae menin'geae me'diae [TA], r. orbital da artéria meníngea média. SIN orbital branch of middle meningeal artery.
r. orbita'lis gang'lii pterygopalati'ni, ramos orbitais do gânglio pterigopalatino. SIN orbital branches of maxillary nerve, em branch.
r. os'sis is'chii [TA], r. do ísquio. SIN r. of ischium.
rami ova'rici arte'riae uteri'nae [TA], ramos ováricos da artéria uterina. SIN ovarian branches of uterine artery, em branch.

r. palmaris nervi interossei antebrachii anterioris [TA], r. palmar do nervo interósseo anterior do antebraço. SIN palmar branch of anterior interosseous nerve.

r. palma'ris ner'vi media'ni, r. palmar do nervo mediano. SIN palmar branch of anterior interosseous nerve.

r. palma'ris ner'vi ulna'ris [TA], r. palmar do nervo ulnar. SIN palmar branch of ulnar nerve.

r. palma'ris profun'dus arte'riae ulna'ris [TA], r. palmar profundo da artéria ulnar. SIN deep palmar branch of ulnar artery.

r. palma'ris superficia'lis arte'riae radia'lis [TA], r. palmar superficial da artéria radial. SIN superficial palmar branch of radial artery.

ra'mi palpebra'les ner'vi infratrochlea'ris [TA], ramos palpebrais do nervo infratroclear. SIN palpebral branches of infratrochlear nerve, em branch.

ra'mi pancrea'tici [TA], ramos pancreáticos. SIN pancreatic branches, em branch.

rami pancrea'tici arte'riae pancreaticoduodena'lis superio'ris, ramos pancreáticos da artéria pancreaticoduodenal superior. VER pancreatic branches, em branch.

rami pancrea'tici arte'riae sple'nicae, ramos pancreáticos da artéria esplênica. VER pancreatic branches, em branch.

r. paracentrales [TA], ramos paracentrais. SIN paracentral branches (of pericallosal artery), em branch.

rami paracentrales arteriae callosomarginalis [TA], ramos paracentrais da artéria calosomarginal. SIN paracentral branches of callosomarginal artery, em branch.

ra'mi parieta'les [TA], ramos parietais. SIN parietal branch.

r. parietal'is arte'riae menin'geae me'diae [TA], r. parietal da artéria meníngea média. SIN parietal branch of middle meningeal artery.

r. parietal'is arte'riae occipita'lis media'lis [TA], r. parietal da artéria occipital medial. SIN parietal branch of medial occipital artery.

r. parietal'is arte'riae tempora'lis superficia'lis [TA], r. parietal da artéria temporal superficial. SIN parietal branch of superficial temporal artery.

r. pari'eto-occipita'lis [TA], r. parietooccipital; o ramo parietooccipital da artéria occipital medial.

r. parieto-occipitalis arteriae occipitalis medialis [TA], r. parietooccipital da artéria occipital medial. SIN parieto-occipital branch (of posterior cerebral artery).

ra'mi parotid'ei [TA], ramos parotídeos. SIN parotid branches, em branch.

r. parotid'ei arte'riae tempora'lis superficia'lis, r. parotídeo da artéria temporal superficial. VER parotid branches, em branch.

rami parotid'ei ner'vi auriculotempora'lis, ramos parotídeos do nervo auriculotemporal. VER parotid branches, em branch.

rami parotid'ei ve'nae facia'lis, ramos parotídeos da veia facial; VER parotid branches, em branch.

rami partis retrolentiformis capsulae internae [TA], ramos da parte retrolentiforme da cápsula interna. SIN rami capsulae internae.

ra'mi pectora'les arteri'ae thoracoacromia'lis [TA], ramos peitorais da artéria tóraco-acromial. SIN pectoral branch of thoracoacromial artery, em branch.

ra'mi peduncula'res [TA], ramos pedunculares; os ramos da artéria cerebral posterior para os pedúnculos cerebrais.

r. per'forans [TA], r. perfurante. SIN perforating branches, em branch.

r. per'forans arte'riae fibula'ris [TA], r. perfurante da artéria fibular. SIN perforating branch of fibular artery.

r. perforans arteriae interossei anterioris [TA], r. perfurante da artéria interóssea anterior. SIN perforating branch of anterior interosseous artery.

rami perforantes arcus palmaris profundi [TA], ramos perfurantes do arco palmar profundo. SIN perforating branches of deep palmar arch.

rami perforan'tes arte'riae thorac'icae inter'nae [TA], ramos perfurantes da artéria torácica interna. SIN perforating branches of internal thoracic artery, em branch.

rami perforan'tes arteria'rum metacarpa'lium palma'rium, ramos perfurantes das artérias metacarpais palmares; VER perforating branches of deep palmar arch.

rami perforan'tes arteria'rum metatarsea'rum planta'rium [TA], ramos perfurantes das artérias metatarsais plantares. SIN perforating branches (of plantar metatarsal arteries), em branch.

ra'mi pericardi'aci aor'tae thora'cicae [TA], ramos pericárdicos da aorta torácica. SIN pericardial branch of thoracic aorta, em branch.

r. pericardi'acus ner'vi phren'ici [TA], r. pericárdico do nervo frênico. SIN pericardial branch of phrenic nerve.

ra'mi perinea'les ner'vi cuta'nei fem'oris posterio'ris [TA], ramos perineais do nervo cutâneo femoral posterior. SIN perineal branches of posterior cutaneous nerve of thigh, em branch.

peroneal anastomotic r., r. peroneal anastomótico. SIN sural communicating branch of common fibular nerve.

r. petro'sus arte'riae menin'geae med'iae [TA], r. petroso da artéria meníngea média. SIN petrosal branch of middle meningeal artery.

ra'mi pharyngea'les, ramos faríngeos; *termo oficial alternativo para pharyngeal branches, em branch.

rami pharyngea'les arte'riae pharyn'geae ascenden'tis [TA], ramos faríngeos da artéria faríngea ascendente. SIN pharyngeal branch of the ascending pharyngeal artery.

rami pharyngea'les arte'riae thyroi'deae inferio'ris [TA], ramos faríngeos da artéria tireóidea inferior. SIN pharyngeal branch of inferior thyroid artery.

rami pharyngei [TA], ramos faríngeos. SIN pharyngeal branches, em branch.

rami pharyn'gei ner'vi glossopharyn'gei [TA], ramos faríngeos do nervo glossofaríngeo. SIN pharyngeal branch of glossopharyngeal nerve.

rami pharyngei nervi laryngei recurrentis [TA], ramos faríngeos do nervo laríngeo recorrente. SIN pharyngeal branches of recurrent laryngeal nerve, em branch.

rami pharyn'gei ner'vi va'gi [TA], r. faríngeo do nervo vago. SIN pharyngeal branch of vagus nerve.

r. pharyn'geus arte'riae cana'lis pterygoi'dei [TA], r. faríngeo da artéria do canal pterigóideo. SIN pharyngeal branch of the artery of pterygoid canal.

r. pharyn'geus arte'riae palati'nae descen'dentis [TA], r. faríngeo da artéria palatina descendente. SIN pharyngeal branch of descending palatine artery.

r. pharyn'geus gan'glii pterygopalati'ni, r. faríngeo do gânglio pterigopalatino. SIN pharyngeal nerve.

ra'mi phrenicoabdomina'les ner'vi phre'nici, ramos frenicoabdominais do nervo frênico. SIN phrenicoabdominal branches of phrenic nerve, em branch.

r. planta'ris profun'dus arte'riae dorsa'lis pe'dis, r. plantar profundo da artéria dorsal do pé. SIN deep plantar artery.

r. poste'rior arte'riae obtura'toriae [TA], r. posterior da artéria obturatória. SIN posterior branch of obturator artery.

r. poste'rior arte'riae pancreaticoduodena'lis inferio'ris [TA], r. posterior da artéria pancreaticoduodenal inferior. SIN posterior branch of inferior pancreaticoduodenal artery.

r. poste'rior arte'riae recurren'tis ulna'ris [TA], r. posterior da artéria recorrente ulnar. SIN posterior branch of ulnar recurrent artery.

r. poste'rior arte'riae rena'lis [TA], r. posterior da artéria renal. SIN posterior branch of renal artery; ver segmental arteries of kidney, em artery.

r. poste'rior arte'riae thyroi'deae superio'ris, r. posterior da artéria tireóidea superior. SIN posterior glandular branch of superior thyroid artery.

r. poste'rior descen'dens, r. descendente posterior. SIN descending branch of posterior segmental artery of left and right lungs.

r. poste'rior duc'tus hepa'tici dex'tri [TA], r. posterior do ducto hepático direito. SIN posterior branch of right hepatic duct.

rami posterio'res [TA], ramos posteriores. SIN posterior branches, em branch.

r. poste'rior nervi spina'lis [TA], r. posterior do nervo espinal. SIN posterior r. of spinal nerve.

posterior r. of lateral cerebral sulcus [TA], r. posterior do sulco lateral do cérebro; a continuação longa do sulco lateral do cérebro que se dirige para trás e se estende entre o lobo temporal, inferiormente, e o lobo parietal, superiormente; a parte terminal do r. é circundada pelo giro supramarginal. SIN posterior branch of lateral cerebral sulcus, r. posterior sulci lateralis cerebri.

posterior r. of lateral sulcus of cerebrum [TA], r. posterior do sulco lateral do cérebro. SIN r. posterior sulcus lateralis cerebri [TA].

r. poste'rior ner'vi auricula'ris mag'ni [TA], r. posterior do nervo auricular magno. SIN posterior branch of great auricular nerve.

r. posterior nervi cutanei antebrachii medialis [TA], r. posterior do nervo cutâneo medial do antebraço. SIN posterior branch of medial cutaneous nerve of forearm.

r. poste'rior ner'vi obtura'torii [TA], r. posterior do nervo obturatório. SIN posterior branch of obturator nerve.

r. poste'rior ra'mi dex'tri ve'nae por'tae hepa'tis [TA], r. posterior do ramo direito da veia porta do fígado. SIN posterior branch of right branch of portal vein.

posterior r. of spinal nerve [TA], r. posterior do nervo espinal; o ramo terminal menor de todos os 31 pares de nervos espinais mistos (o ramo anterior é o maior), que se forma no forame intervertebral e se volta abruptamente para trás, dividindo-se em ramos medial e lateral, que inervam os músculos profundos (verdadeiros) do dorso. O ramo medial (rami medialis [TA]) do r. primário dorsal também inerva os ramos articulares que vão para as articulações zigapofiseais e para o periósteo do arco vertebral. No pescoço e na parte superior do dorso, o ramo medial continua-se através dos músculos superficiais e profundos do dorso para inervar a pele suprajacente; na parte inferior do dorso, essa função é desempenhada pelo ramo lateral. A Terminologia Anatômica lista os ramos posteriores (rami dorsales) de cada grupo de nervos espinais: 1) cervical (nervorum cervicalium [TA]), 2) torácico (nervorum thoracicorum [TA]), 3) lombar (nervorum lumbalium [TA]), 4) sacral (nervorum sacralium [TA]) e 5) coccígeo (nervi coccygei [TA]). SIN r. posterior nervi spinalis [TA], dorsal primary r. of spinal nerve*, r. dorsalis nervi spinalis*, dorsal branch (1), posterior primary division, r. dorsalis.

r. poste'rior sul'ci latera'lis cere'bri, r. posterior do sulco lateral do cérebro. SIN posterior r. of lateral cerebral sulcus.

r. posterior sulcus lateralis cerebri [TA], r. posterior do sulco lateral do cérebro. SIN posterior r. of lateral sulcus of cerebrum.

r. posterior venae pulmonalis dextrae superioris [TA], r. posterior da veia pulmonar direita superior. SIN posterior branch of right superior pulmonary vein.

rami precuneales arteriae cerebri anterioris [TA], ramos pré-cuneais da artéria cerebral anterior. SIN precuneal branches (of anterior cerebral artery), em branch.

r. prelaminaris rami spinalis rami dorsalis arteriae intercostalis posterioris [TA], r. pré-laminar dos ramos espinais do ramo dorsal das artérias intercostais posteriores. SIN prelaminar branch of spinal branch of dorsal branch of posterior intercostal artery.

rami profundi arteriae transversae cervicis [TA], r. profundo da artéria cervical transversa. SIN dorsal scapular artery.

r. profundus [TA], r. profundo. SIN deep branch.

r. profundus arteriae circumflexae femoris medialis [TA], r. profundo da artéria circunflexa femoral medial. SIN deep branch of the medial circumflex femoral artery.

r. profundus arteriae gluteae superioris [TA], r. profundo da artéria glútea superior. SIN deep branch of the superior gluteal artery.

r. profundus arteriae plantaris medialis [TA], r. profundo da artéria plantar medial. SIN deep branch of the medial plantar artery.

r. profundus arteriae scapularis descendentis, r. profundo da artéria escapular descendente. SIN dorsal scapular artery.

r. profundus arteriae transversae colli [TA], r. profundo da artéria cervical transversa. SIN dorsal scapular artery.

r. profundus nervi plantaris lateralis [TA], r. profundo do nervo plantar lateral. SIN deep branch of the lateral plantar nerve.

r. profundus nervi radialis [TA], r. profundo do nervo radial. SIN deep branch of radial nerve.

r. profundus nervi ulnaris [TA], r. profundo do nervo ulnar. SIN deep branch of the ulnar nerve.

rami prostatici arteriae rectalis mediae [TA], ramos prostáticos da artéria retal média. SIN prostatic branches of middle rectal artery, em branch.

rami prostatici arteriae vesicalis inferioris [TA], ramos prostáticos da artéria vesical inferior. SIN prostatic branches of inferior vesical artery, em branch.

rami pterygoidei arteriae maxillaris, ramos pterigóideos da artéria maxilar. SIN pterygoid branch of posterior deep temporal artery.

r. pterygoideus arteriae temporalis profundae posterioris [TA], r. pterigóideo da artéria temporal profunda posterior. SIN pterygoid branch of posterior deep temporal artery.

pubic rami, ramos púbicos. VER pubic hair.

r. pubicus arteriae epigastricae inferioris [TA], r. púbico da artéria epigástrica inferior. SIN pubic branch of inferior epigastric artery.

r. pubicus arteriae obturatoriae [TA], r. púbico da artéria obturatória. SIN pubic branch of obturator artery.

r. pubicus venae epigastricae inferioris [TA], r. púbico da veia epigástrica inferior. SIN pubic branch of inferior epigastric vein.

rami pulmonales plexi nervosi pulmonalis [TA], ramos pulmonares do plexo nervoso pulmonar. SIN pulmonary branches of pulmonary nerve plexus, em branch.

rami pulmonales systematis autonomici, ramos pulmonares do sistema nervoso autônomo. SIN pulmonary branch of autonomic nervous system, em branch.

rami pulmonales thoracici gangliorum thoracicorum [TA], ramos pulmonares torácicos dos gânglios torácicos. SIN thoracic pulmonary branches of thoracic ganglia, em branch.

r. pyloricus trunci vagalis anterioris [TA], r. pilórico do tronco vagal anterior. SIN pyloric branch of anterior vagal trunk.

rami radiculares, ramos radiculares. SIN spinal arteries, em artery.

r. atrialis intermedius arteriae coronariae sinistrae [TA], r. atrial intermédio da artéria coronária esquerda. SIN intermediate atrial branch of left coronary artery.

rami renales nervi vagi [TA], ramos renais do nervo vago. SIN renal branch of vagus nerve, em branch.

r. renalis nervi splanchnici minoris [TA], r. renal do nervo esplâncnico menor. SIN renal branch of lesser splanchnic nerve.

rami sacrales laterales arteriae sacralis medianae [TA], ramos sacrais laterais da artéria sacral mediana. SIN lateral sacral branches of median sacral artery, em branch.

r. saphenus arteriae descendentis genicularis [TA], r. safeno da artéria descendente do joelho. SIN saphenous branch of descending genicular artery.

rami scrotales anteriores arteriae pudendae externae profundae [TA], ramos escrotais anteriores da artéria pudenda externa profunda. SIN anterior scrotal branch of deep external pudendal artery.

rami scrotales posteriores arteriae perinealis [TA], ramos escrotais posteriores da artéria perineal. SIN posterior scrotal branches of perineal artery, em branch.

rami scrotales posteriores arteriae pudendae internae, ramos escrotais posteriores da artéria pudenda interna. SIN posterior scrotal branches of perineal artery, em branch.

rami septales, ramos septais; ramos interventriculares septais.

rami septales anteriores arteriae ethmoidalis anterioris [TA], ramos septais anteriores da artéria etmoidal anterior. SIN anterior septal branches of anterior ethmoidal artery, em branch.

r. septi nasi arteriae labialis superioris [TA], r. do septo nasal da artéria labial superior. SIN nasal septal branch of superior labial branch of facial artery.

r. septi posterioris nasalis [TA], r. do septo posterior do nariz. SIN posterior septal branch of nose.

r. sinister [TA], r. esquerdo. SIN left branch.

r. sinister arteriae hepaticae propriae [TA], r. esquerdo da artéria hepática própria. SIN left branch of hepatic artery proper.

r. sinister venae portae hepatis, r. esquerdo da veia porta do fígado.

r. sinus carotici [TA], r. para o seio carótico. SIN carotid branch of glossopharyngeal nerve (CN IX).

r. sinus carotici nervi glossopharyngei CN IX [TA], r. para o seio carótico do nervo glossofaríngeo (IX NC). SIN carotid branch of glossopharyngeal nerve (CN IX).

r. sinus cavernosi, r. do seio cavernoso; um ramo da parte cavernosa da artéria carótida interna que irriga as paredes do seio cavernoso.

r. sinus cavernosi arteriae carotidis internae, r. do seio cavernoso da artéria carótida interna. SIN cavernous branch of cavernous part of internal carotid artery.

r. sinus cavernosi arteriae carotidis internae, r. do seio cavernoso da artéria carótida interna. SIN cavernous branch of cavernous part of internal carotid artery.

r. sinus cavernosi partis cavernosae arteriae carotidis internae [TA], r. do seio cavernoso da parte cavernosa da artéria carótida interna. SIN cavernous branch of cavernous part of internal carotid artery.

rami spinales [TA], ramos espinais; **(1)** SIN spinal branches, em branch; **(2)** as veias tributárias das veias intervertebrais que drenam o sangue das meninges e da medula espinal.

rami splenici arteriae splenicae [TA], ramos esplênicos da artéria esplênica. SIN splenic branches of splenic artery, em branch.

r. stapedius arteriae stylomastoideae, r. do estapédio da artéria estilomastóidea. SIN stapedial branch of posterior tympanic artery.

r. stapedius arteriae tympanicae posterioris [TA], r. do estapédio da artéria timpânica posterior. SIN stapedial branch of posterior tympanic artery.

rami sternales arteriae thoracicae internae [TA], ramos esternais da artéria torácica interna. SIN sternal branches of internal thoracic artery, em branch.

rami sternocleidomastoidei arteriae occipitalis, ramos esternocleidomastóideos da artéria occipital. SIN sternocleidomastoid branches of occipital artery, em branch.

r. sternocleidomastoideus arteriae thyroideae superioris [TA], r. esternocleidomastóideo da artéria tireóidea superior. SIN sternocleidomastoid branch of superior thyroid artery.

r. stylohyoideus nervi facialis [TA], r. estilo-hióideo do nervo facial. SIN stylohyoid branch of facial nerve.

rami subendocardiales fasciculi atrioventricularis [TA], ramos subendocárdicos dos fascículos atrioventriculares. SIN subendocardial branches of atrioventricular bundles, em branch.

rami subscapulares arteriae axillaris [TA], ramos subescapulares da artéria axilar. SIN subscapular branches of axillary artery, em branch.

rami substantiae nigrae [TA], ramos da substância negra; os ramos da artéria corióidea anterior para a substância negra.

r. superficialis [TA], r. superficial. SIN superficial branch.

r. superficialis arteriae circumflexae femoris medialis [TA], r. superficial da artéria circunflexa femoral medial. SIN superficial branch of medial circumflex femoral artery.

r. superficialis arteriae gluteae superioris [TA], r. superficial da artéria glútea superior. SIN superficial branch of the superior gluteal artery.

r. superficialis arteriae plantaris medialis [TA], r. superficial da artéria plantar medial. SIN superficial branch of the medial plantar artery.

r. superficialis arteriae transversae cervicis [TA], r. superficial da artéria cervical transversa. SIN superficial cervical artery.

r. superficialis arteriae transversae colli [TA], r. superficial da artéria cervical transversa. SIN superficial branch of the transverse cervical artery.

r. superficialis nervi plantaris lateralis [TA], r. superficial do nervo plantar lateral. SIN superficial branch of the lateral plantar nerve.

r. superficialis nervi radialis [TA], r. superficial do nervo radial. SIN superficial branch of the radial nerve.

r. superficialis nervi ulnaris [TA], r. superficial do nervo ulnar. SIN superficial branch of the ulnar nerve.

r. superior [TA], r. superior. SIN superior branch.

r. superior arteriae gluteae superioris [TA], r. superior da artéria glútea superior. SIN superior branch of the superior gluteal artery.

superior dental rami, ramos dentais superiores. SIN superior dental branches of superior dental plexus, em branch.
r. supe'rior ner'vi oculomoto'rii [TA], r. superior do nervo oculomotor. SIN superior branch of the oculomotor nerve.
r. supe'rior ner'vi transversa'lis cervica'lis (col'li) [TA], r. superior do nervo cervical transverso. SIN superior branch of the transverse cervical nerve.
r. supe'rior os'sis pu'bis [TA], r. superior do púbis. SIN superior pubic r.
superior pubic r. [TA], r. superior do púbis; uma barra de osso com secção triangular que se estende póstero-superiormente a partir do corpo do púbis para formar o limite superior do forame obturado; após o desenvolvimento, o ramo corresponde a aproximadamente um quinto da face articular do acetábulo. SIN r. superior ossis pubis [TA], superior branch of the pubic bone.
r. supe'rior ve'nae pulmona'lis dex'trae/sinis'trae inferio'ris, r. superior da veia pulmonar direita/esquerda inferior. SIN superior branch of the right and left inferior pulmonary veins.
r. suprahyoi'deus arte'riae lingua'lis [TA], r. supra-hióideo da artéria lingual. SIN suprahyoid branch of lingual artery.
r. sympath'icus (sympathe'ticus) ad gang'lion submandibula're, r. simpático do gânglio submandibular. SIN sympathetic root of submandibular ganglion.
ra'mi tempora'les anterio'res [TA], ramos temporais anteriores; os ramos temporais anteriores da artéria occipital lateral que irrigam o córtex da parte anterior do lobo temporal do cérebro.
ra'mi tempora'les interme'dii [TA], ramos temporais intermédios; os ramos temporais médios (intermédios) da artéria occipital lateral que irrigam o córtex das partes média e medial do lobo temporal do cérebro.
rami temporales intermedii arteriae occipitalis lateralis [TA], ramos temporais intermédios da artéria occipital lateral. SIN intermediate temporal branches of lateral occipital artery, em branch.
rami temporales medii arteriae occipitalis lateralis, ramos temporais médios da artéria occipital lateral; *termo oficial alternativo para intermediate temporal branches of lateral occipital artery, em branch.
ra'mi tempora'les ner'vi facia'lis [TA], ramos temporais do nervo facial. SIN temporal branch of facial nerve, em branch.
ra'mi tempora'les posterio'res [TA], ramos temporais posteriores; os ramos temporais posteriores da artéria occipital lateral que irrigam o córtex da parte posterior do lobo temporal do cérebro.
ra'mi tempora'les superficia'les ner'vi auriculotempora'lis [TA], ramos temporais superficiais do nervo auriculotemporal. SIN superficial temporal branch of auriculotemporal nerve, em branch.
r. temporalis anterior [TA], r. temporal anterior. SIN anterior temporal branch.
r. temporalis medius partis insularis arteriae cerebrae mediae [TA], r. temporal médio da parte insular da artéria cerebral média. SIN middle temporal branch of insular part of middle cerebral artery.
r. temporalis posterior arteriae cerebri mediae [TA], r. temporal posterior da artéria cerebral média. SIN posterior temporal branch of middle cerebral artery.
r. tentor'ii, r. do tentório; *termo oficial alternativo para tentorial nerve.
rami terminales arteriae cerebri medii [TA], ramos terminais da artéria cerebral média. SIN terminal branches of middle cerebral artery, em branch.
ra'mi thalam'ici, ramos talâmicos; os ramos da artéria cerebral posterior para o tálamo, tais como as artérias perfurante do tálamo e talamogeniculada.
r. thalam'icus, r. talâmico; um ramo da artéria cerebral média para o tálamo.
ra'mi thy'mici, ramos mediastinais da artéria torácica interna. SIN mediastinal branches of internal thoracic artery, em branch.
rami thymici arteriae thoracicae internae [TA], ramos tímicos da artéria torácica interna. SIN thymic branches of internal thoracic artery, em branch.
r. thyrohyoi'deus an'sae cervica'lis [TA], r. tíreo-hióideo da alça cervical. SIN thyrohyoid branch of ansa cervicalis.
r. tonsil'lae cerebel'lae [TA], r. da tonsila do cerebelo; um ramo proveniente da artéria cerebelar inferior posterior que irriga a tonsila do cerebelo.
ra'mi tonsilla'res ner'vi glossopharyn'gei, ramos tonsilares do nervo glossofaríngeo. SIN tonsillar branches of glossopharyngeal nerve, em branch.
rami tonsillares nervi palatini minores [TA], ramos tonsilares dos nervos palatinos menores. SIN tonsillar branches of lesser palatine nerves, em branch.
r. tonsilla'ris arte'riae facia'lis [TA], r. tonsilar da artéria facial. SIN tonsillar branch of the facial artery.
ra'mi trachea'les [TA], ramos traqueais. SIN tracheal branches, em branch.
rami trachea'les arte'riae thyroi'deae inferio'ris, ramos traqueais da artéria tireóidea inferior. VER tracheal branches, em branch.
rami trachea'les ner'vi laryn'gei recurren'tis, ramos traqueais do nervo laríngeo recorrente. VER tracheal branches, em branch.
ra'mi trac'tus op'tici [TA], ramos do trato óptico; os ramos da artéria corióidea anterior para o trato óptico.
r. transversus arteriae circumflexae femoris lateralis [TA], r. transverso da artéria circunflexa femoral lateral. SIN transverse branch of lateral femoral circumflex artery.
r. transver'sus arte'riae circumflex'ae fem'oris media'lis, r. transverso da artéria circunflexa femoral medial.

r. tuba'rius [TA], r. tubário. SIN tubal branch.
r. tubarius arteriae ovaricae [TA], r. tubário da artéria ovárica. SIN tubal branch of ovarian artery.
r. tubari'us arte'riae uteri'nae [TA], r. tubário da artéria uterina. SIN tubal branch of the uterine artery.
r. tuba'rius plex'us tympan'ici [TA], r. tubário do plexo timpânico. SIN tubal branch of the tympanic plexus.
ra'mi tu'beris cine'rei [TA], ramos do túber cinéreo; os ramos da artéria corióidea anterior para o túber cinéreo.
r. ulna'ris ner'vi cuta'nei antebra'chii media'lis, r. ulnar do nervo cutâneo medial do antebraço. SIN posterior branch of medial cutaneous nerve of forearm.
ra'mi ureter'ici [TA], ramos uretéricos. SIN ureteric branches, em branch.
rami urete'rici arte'riae ovar'icae [TA], ramos uretéricos da artéria ovárica. SIN ureteric branches of the ovarian artery, em branch.
rami urete'rici arte'riae rena'lis, ramos uretéricos da artéria renal. SIN ureteric branches of the renal artery, em branch.
rami ureterici arteriae suprarenalis inferioris [TA], ramos uretéricos da artéria supra-renal inferior. SIN ureteric branches of the inferior suprarenal artery, em branch.
rami urete'rici arte'riae testicula'ris [TA], ramos uretéricos da artéria testicular. SIN ureteric branches of the testicular artery, em branch.
rami urete'rici par'tis paten'tis arte'riae umbilica'lis [TA], ramos uretéricos da parte patente da artéria umbilical. SIN ureteric branches of the patent part of umbilical artery, em branch.
ventral rami of cervical nerves, ramos anteriores dos nervos cervicais; *termo oficial alternativo para anterior rami of cervical nerves.
rami ventrales nervorum thoracis, ramos anteriores dos nervos torácicos; *termo oficial alternativo para anterior rami of thoracic nerves.
ra'mi ventra'les nervo'rum cervica'lium, ramos anteriores dos nervos cervicais. SIN anterior rami of cervical nerves. VER anterior r. of spinal nerve.
ra'mi ventra'les nervo'rum lumba'lium, ramos anteriores dos nervos lombares. SIN anterior rami of lumbar nerves. VER anterior r. of spinal nerve.
ra'mi ventra'les nervo'rum sacra'lium, ramos ventrais dos nervos sacrais. SIN anterior rami of sacral nerves. VER anterior r. of spinal nerve.
r. ventralis, r. ventral. SIN ventral branch.
r. ventra'lis ner'vi spina'lis, r. ventral do nervo espinal; *termo oficial alternativo para anterior r. of spinal nerve.
ventral rami of lumbar nerves, ramos ventrais dos nervos lombares; *termo oficial alternativo para anterior rami of lumbar nerves.
ventral primary rami of cervical spinal nerves, ramos primários ventrais dos nervos espinais cervicais. SIN anterior rami of cervical nerves.
ventral primary rami of lumbar spinal nerves, ramos primários ventrais dos nervos espinais lombares. SIN anterior rami of lumbar nerves.
ventral primary rami of sacral spinal nerves, ramos primários ventrais dos nervos espinais sacrais. SIN anterior rami of sacral nerves. VER anterior r. of spinal nerve.
ventral primary r. of spinal nerve, r. primário ventral do nervo espinal. SIN anterior r. of spinal nerve.
ventral primary rami of thoracic spinal nerves, ramos primários ventrais dos nervos espinais torácicos. SIN anterior rami of thoracic nerves.
ventral rami of sacral nerves, ramos ventrais dos nervos sacrais; *termo oficial alternativo para anterior rami of sacral nerves.
ventral r. of spinal nerve, r. ventral de nervo espinal; *termo oficial alternativo para anterior r. of spinal nerve.
ventral rami of thoracic nerves, ramos ventrais dos nervos torácicos; *termo oficial alternativo para anterior rami of thoracic nerves.
r. vermis superior [TA], r. superior do verme. SIN superior vermian branch (of superior cerebellar artery).
ra'mi vestibula'res arte'riae labyrin'thi, ramos vestibulares da artéria do labirinto.
r. vestibularis posterior arteriae vestibulocochlearis [TA], r. vestibular posterior da artéria vestibulococlear. SIN posterior vestibular branch of vestibulocochlear artery.
white rami communicantes [TA], ramos comunicantes brancos; nervos curtos que surgem na parte inicial dos ramos primários ventrais dos nervos espinais torácicos e lombares superiores e através dos quais todas as fibras nervosas simpáticas pré-sinápticas devem passar a fim de alcançar os troncos simpáticos; as fibras aferentes (sensitivas) viscerais levadas até os troncos simpáticos pelos nervos esplâncnicos também passam pelos ramos comunicantes brancos. A maioria das fibras conduzidas pelos ramos comunicantes brancos é mielinizada. SIN rami communicantes albi [TA], communicating branches of spinal nerves, rami communicantes nervorum spinalium.
ra'mi zygomat'ici ner'vi facia'lis, ramos zigomáticos do nervo facial. SIN zygomatic branches of facial nerve, em branch.
r. zygomaticofacia'lis ner'vi zygoma'tici [TA], r. zigomaticofacial do nervo zigomático. SIN zygomaticofacial branch of zygomatic nerve.
r. zygomaticotempora'lis ner'vi zygoma'tici [TA], r. zigomaticotemporal do nervo zigomático. SIN zygomaticotemporal branch of zygomatic nerve.

ra·my·cin (ră-mī′sin). Ramicina. SIN fusidic acid.
ran·cid (ran′sid). Rançoso; que apresenta odor e sabor desagradáveis, caracterizando em geral a gordura submetida à oxidação ou à decomposição bacteriana com conseqüente produção de substâncias odoríferas mais voláteis. [L. *rancidus*, fétido, malcheiroso]
ran·cid·i·fy (ran-sid′i-fī). Rancidificar; criar ranço ou tornar-se rançoso.
ran·cid·i·ty (ran-sid′i-tē). Rancidez; o estado de estar rançoso.
Rand, Gertrude, psicóloga visual norte-americana, 1886–1970. VER Hardy-R.-Ritter *test*.
Rand, M.J., farmacologista do século 20. VER Burn and R. *theory*.
Randall, Alexander, urologista norte-americano, *1883. VER R. stone *forceps*.
ran·dom (ran′dom). Aleatório; regido pelo acaso; um processo no qual o resultado (desfecho) é indeterminado e pode assumir qualquer valor de um conjunto de valores (o domínio) com probabilidades previamente especificadas. Enquanto o processo aleatório é amplamente empregado na teoria da probabilidade, a justificativa empírica para o termo é mais complicada. A exigência mínima é de que a repetição do processo esteja baseada em uma distribuição estável ou, se não for metricamente mensurável, em um conjunto estável de freqüências (caso a característica seja apenas classificável). VER random *mechanism*. [I.m. *randon*, rapidez, desvio, do Fr. ant. *randir*, correr, do Al.]
ran·dom·i·za·tion. Randomização; a distribuição aleatória de indivíduos em grupos, p. ex., para métodos de controle e experimentais.
Raney Nic·kel. O nome patenteado de um catalisador de níquel apresentado na forma de um pó fino e preparado a partir da liga de Raney por meio da dissolução do alumínio com um álcali; é utilizado na hidrogenação de substâncias orgânicas. SIN Raney catalyst.
range (rānj). Variação; uma medida estatística da dispersão ou da extensão de valores que é determinada pelos valores situados em cada extremo (o menor e o maior), ou pela diferença entre eles; p. ex., em um grupo de crianças com as idades de 6, 8, 9, 10, 13 e 16 anos, a variação é de 6 a 16 ou, de forma alternativa, 10 (16 menos 6). [Fr. ant. *rang*, linha, do Al.]
therapeutic r., v. terapêutica; refere-se tanto à variação da dose quanto à concentração plasmática ou sérica nas quais geralmente se espera alcançar os efeitos terapêuticos desejados. Alguns pacientes necessitarão de doses (ou concentrações) acima ou abaixo da v. terapêutica; alguns pacientes experimentarão efeitos tóxicos com doses situadas dentro dessa v.
ra·nine (rā′nīn). Ranino; **1.** Relativo à rã. **2.** Relativo à superfície inferior da língua. [L. *rana*, uma rã]
ra·ni·ti·dine (ră-nī′ti-dēn). Ranitidina; um antagonista H_2 da histamina utilizado no tratamento de úlceras gástricas e duodenais e do refluxo gastroesofágico; reduz a secreção de ácido clorídrico.
rank. 1. A posição ordinal de uma observação dentro de um conjunto de observações do qual faz parte. **2.** Ordenar um conjunto de observações de acordo com sua posição.
Ranke, Johannes, antropólogo e médico alemão, 1836–1916. VER R. *angle*.
Ranke, Karl E. von, químico alemão, 1870–1926. VER R. *formula*.
Rankin, Fred Wharton, cirurgião norte-americano, 1886–1954. VER R. *clamp*.
Rankine, William J. McQ., físico escocês, 1820–1870. VER R. *scale*.
Ransohoff, Joseph, cirurgião norte-americano, 1853–1921. VER R. *sign*.
RANTES. Um membro da superfamília interleucina-8 das citocinas. Essa citocina é uma proteína de 8 kD, um quimiotático seletivo para linfócitos T de memória e monócitos. [*R*egulated on *a*ctivation, *n*ormal *T* *e*xpressed and *s*ecreted]
ran·u·la (ran′ū-lă). Rânula; **1.** Hipoglote. **2.** Termo obsoleto dado a qualquer tumor cístico situado na superfície inferior da língua ou no assoalho da boca, principalmente um tumor localizado no assoalho da boca e resultante da obstrução do ducto das glândulas sublinguais. SIN ptyalocele, ranine tumor, sialocele, sublingual cyst. [L. *girino*, dim. de *rana*, rã]
ran·u·lar (ran′ū-lăr). Ranular; relativo a uma rânula.
Ranvier, Louis A., patologista francês, 1835–1922. VER R. *crosses*, em *cross*, *disks*, em *disk*; *node* of R.; R. *plexus*, *segment*.
RAO Abreviatura de right anterior oblique (oblíqua anterior direita), uma incidência radiográfica.
Raoult, François, M., físico francês, 1830–1899. VER R. *law*.
RAPD Abreviatura de rapid analysis of polymorphic DNA (análise rápida de DNA polimórfico).
rape (rāp). **1.** Estupro; forçar relação sexual mediante coação, violência intimidação ou sem consentimento legal (quando a vítima é menor de idade). **2.** Estuprar; a realização de tal ato. [L. *rapio*, agarrar, arrastar para longe]
rape·seed oil (rāp′sēd). Óleo de colza; o óleo extraído das sementes de *Brassica campestris* (família Cruciferae); utilizado na fabricação de sabões, margarina e lubrificantes. [L. *rapa*, nabo]
ra·pha·nia (ră-fā′nē-ă). Rafania; doença espasmódica que se supõe ser causada por envenenamento pelas sementes de *Rhaphanus rhaphanistrum*, o rabanete silvestre. SIN rhaphania.
ra·phe (rā′fē) [TA]. Rafe; a linha de união de duas estruturas contíguas e com simetria bilateral. SIN rhaphe. [G. *rhaphē*, sutura, costura]
amnionic r., r. amniótica; a linha de fusão das pregas amnióticas sobre o embrião de répteis, aves e determinados mamíferos.

r. anococcyg′ea, r. anococcígea. SIN anococcygeal *ligament*.
anogenital r., r. anogenital; no embrião masculino, a linha de fechamento das pregas e saliências genitais que se estendem do ânus até a glande do pênis; no adulto, diferencia-se em três regiões: r. do períneo, r. do escroto e r. do pênis.
r. cor′poris callo′si, r. do corpo caloso; um sulco suave ântero-posterior localizado na linha mediana da superfície superior do corpo caloso.
iliococcygeal r. [TA], r. do músculo iliococcígeo; a parte do corpo anococcígeo formada pela união da metade direita do músculo iliococcígeo à sua metade esquerda na altura da linha média e posteriormente ao canal anal. SIN r. musculi iliococcygeus [TA].
lateral palpebral r., r. lateral da pálpebra; uma faixa fibrosa estreita localizada na parte lateral do músculo orbicular do olho e formada pelo entrelaçamento dos fibras que passam através das pálpebras superior e inferior. SIN palpebral r., r. palpebralis lateralis.
r. lin′guae, r. da língua. SIN median *sulcus* of tongue.
median longitudinal r. of tongue, r. longitudinal mediana da língua. SIN median *sulcus* of tongue.
r. of medulla oblongata, r. da medula oblonga. SIN r. medullae oblongatae.
r. medul′lae oblonga′tae [TA], r. da medula oblonga; a zona mediana da medula oblonga semelhante a uma costura e caracterizada pelo entrecruzamento de feixes de fibras entre os quais estão situados corpos de neurônios. SIN r. of medulla oblongata.
r. musculi iliococcygeus [TA], r. do músculo iliococcígeo. SIN iliococcygeal r.
r. pala′ti [TA], r. do palato. SIN palatine r.
palatine r. [TA], r. do palato; uma pequena elevação um tanto estreita localizada no centro do palato duro e que, a partir da papila incisiva, dirige-se para trás sobre toda a extensão da mucosa do palato duro. SIN r. palati [TA], palatine ridge.
palpebral r., r. da pálpebra. SIN lateral palpebral r.
r. palpebra′lis latera′lis, r. lateral da pálpebra. SIN lateral palpebral r.
penile r., r. do pênis. SIN r. of penis.
r. pe′nis [TA], r. do pênis. SIN r. of penis.
r. of penis [TA], r. do pênis; a continuação da r. do escroto sobre a superfície inferior do pênis. SIN r. penis [TA], penile r.
perineal r. [TA], r. do períneo; a linha central ântero-posterior do períneo, mais acentuada no homem e contínua com a r. do escroto. SIN r. perinei [TA].
r. perine′i [TA], r. do períneo. SIN perineal r.
pharyngeal r. [TA], r. da faringe; a linha central da faringe que se estende para trás e na qual as fibras musculares se encontram e entrelaçam parcialmente. SIN r. pharyngis [TA].
r. pharyn′gis [TA], r. da faringe. SIN pharyngeal r.
r. of pons, r. da ponte. SIN r. pontis.
r. pon′tis [TA], r. da ponte; a continuação da r. da medula oblonga que se dirige para o interior da pars dorsalis (ou tegumento) da ponte. SIN r. of pons.
pterygomandibular r. [TA], r. pterigomandibular; um espessamento tendinoso da fáscia bucofaríngea que dá origem ao músculo bucinador, anteriormente, e ao músculo constritor superior da faringe, posteriormente, isolando-os de outras estruturas. SIN r. pterygomandibularis [TA], pterygomandibular ligament.
r. pterygomandibula′ris [TA], r. pterigomandibular; SIN pterygomandibular r.
r. ret′inae, r. da retina; a linha horizontal que separa a parte superior da inferior da retina temporal e sobre a qual as fibras nervosas da retina não passam.
scrotal r., r. do escroto. SIN r. of scrotum.
r. scro′ti [TA], r. do escroto. SIN r. of scrotum.
r. of scrotum [TA], r. do escroto; uma linha central, semelhante a um cordão, que corre sobre o escroto desde o ânus até a raiz do pênis; assinala a posição do septo do escroto. SIN r. scroti [TA], scrotal r., Vesling line.
Stilling r., r. de Stilling; as interdigitações transversas de feixes de fibras encontradas ao longo da fissura mediana anterior da medula oblonga na decussação dos tratos piramidais.
Rapoport, Abraham, urologista canadense, *1926. VER R. *test*.
Rapoport, Samuel Mitja, bioquímico russo, 1912–1977. VER R.-Luebering *shunt*.
Rappaport, Henry, patologista norte-americano, *1913. VER Rappaport *classification*.
rap·port (rap-ōr′). Relação; **1.** Uma sensação de relacionamento, principalmente quando caracterizada por afinidade emocional. **2.** Um sentimento consciente de harmonia, confiança, empatia e compreensão mútua entre duas ou mais pessoas (p. ex., o médico e o paciente) que estimula o processo terapêutico. [Fr.]
rap·ture of the deep (rap′choor). Êxtase das profundezas. SIN nitrogen *narcosis* (2).
rar·e·fac·tion (rār-ĕ-fak′shŭn). Rarefação; **1.** O processo de tornar-se leve ou menos denso; a condição de ser leve; o oposto de condensação. **2.** Em fisiologia vascular, o processo que resulta na redução da densidade dos capilares em um tecido. [L. *rarus*, ralo, escasso, + *facio*, fazer]
rar·e·fy (rār′ĕ-fī). Rarefazer; tornar leve ou menos denso.
RAS Abreviatura de reticular activating *system*.
ra·sce·ta (ră-sē′tă). Rasceta; o pregueamento transverso localizado na face anterior do pulso. [L. mod. *raseta*, do Ár. *rāhah*, a palma da mão]

rash. Erupção; termo leigo para uma erupção cutânea. [Fr. ant. *rasche*, erupção da pele, do L. *rado*, pp. *rasus*, arranhar, raspar]
 antitoxin r., e. por antitoxina; uma manifestação cutânea da doença do soro.
 black currant r., e. em groselha preta; a erupção cutânea de lentigos observada no xeroderma pigmentoso.
 butterfly r., e. em asa de borboleta. SIN butterfly (2).
 caterpillar r., e. por contato com lagartas. SIN caterpillar *dermatitis*.
 crystal r., e. cristalina. SIN *miliaria* crystallina.
 diaper r., e. por fraldas. SIN diaper *dermatitis*.
 heat r., e. pelo calor, brotoeja. SIN *miliaria* rubra.
 hydatid r., e. hidática; uma erupção tóxica que surge ocasionalmente após a ruptura de um cisto hidático.
 Murray Valley r., e. do Vale Murray. SIN epidemic *polyarthritis*.
 serum r., e. por soro; uma manifestação cutânea da doença do soro.
 summer r., e. do verão. SIN *miliaria* rubra.
 wildfire r., miliária rubra. SIN *miliaria* rubra.
ra·sion (rā′zhŭn). A subdivisão de uma droga em estado bruto por meio de uma lima, a fim de prepará-la para extração. [L. *rasio*, uma raspagem, de *rado*, pp. *rasus*, raspar, aparar]
Rasmussen, Grant L., neuroanatomista americano, *1904. VER *bundle* of Rasmussen, Rasmussen *encephalitis*, Rasmussen *syndrome*.
Rasmussen, Fritz W., médico dinamarquês, 1834–1881. VER R. *aneurysm*.
ras·pa·to·ry (ras′pă-tōr-ē). Rugina; raspador; um instrumento cirúrgico utilizado para alisar as extremidades de um osso partido. [L. *raspatorium*]
RAST Acrônimo de radioallergosorbent *test* (teste radioalergossorvente).

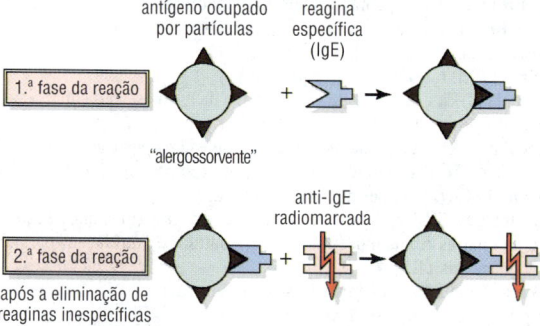

teste radioalergossorvente (RAST)

Rastelli, Gian C. VER R. *operation*.
rat. Rato; um roedor do gênero *Rattus* (família Muridae), que participa da disseminação de algumas doenças, entre elas a peste bubônica.
 albino r.'s, ratos albinos; ratos com pelagem branca e olhos cor-de-rosa; são muito empregados nos experimentos feitos em laboratórios.
 Wistar r.'s, ratos Wistar; uma linhagem consangüínea de ratos, homozigotos na maioria dos *loci*, produzidos pelo cruzamento consangüíneo estritamente entre irmãos por muitas gerações, a fim de se desenvolver animais para pesquisa que apresentem a mesma composição genética geral. [*Wistar* Institute]
rate (rat). Taxa, razão, relação, velocidade, proporção, freqüência, índice; **1.** Um registro da medida de um evento ou processo em função de sua relação com algum padrão fixo; a medida é expressa como a razão entre duas quantidades (p. ex., velocidade, distância por unidade de tempo). **2.** Uma medida da freqüência de um evento em uma população definida; apresenta três componentes: o numerador (número de eventos), o denominador (a população que corre risco de sofrer o evento) e o período de tempo no qual os eventos ocorrem. [L. *ratum*, cálculo, cômputo (ver ratio)]
 abortion r., taxa de abortamento; **(1)** o número de abortamentos induzidos por 1.000 gravidezes que resultaram em um bebê vivo, um natimorto ou que tiveram um término induzido. **(2)** o número de gravidezes interrompidas × 1.000 ÷ idade da população feminina entre 15 e 44 anos.
 age-specific r., taxa específica para a idade; uma taxa para um grupo etário específico, no qual o numerador e o denominador se referem ao mesmo grupo etário.
 attack r., taxa de ataque; uma taxa de incidência cumulativa utilizada para grupos específicos que foram observados durante períodos limitados de tempo e sob circunstâncias especiais, tal como uma epidemia.
 average flow r., taxa de fluxo médio; uma taxa de fluxo determinada pela divisão do volume total de urina eliminado pelo tempo de esvaziamento.
 basal metabolic r. (BMR), taxa de metabolismo basal; SIN basal *metabolism*.
 baseline fetal heart r., freqüência cardíaca fetal basal; a freqüência cardíaca média de um determinado feto durante a fase diastólica das contrações uterinas.
 birth r., taxa de natalidade; uma taxa baseada no número de nascidos vivos em uma população durante um determinado período, em geral um ano; o numerador corresponde ao número de nascidos vivos, e o denominador, à população do meio do período.
 case fatality r., taxa de fatalidade de casos; a proporção de indivíduos que contraem uma doença e morrem dessa doença.
 concordance r., taxa de concordância; a proporção de uma amostra aleatória de pares que são concordantes para uma característica de interesse. Uma alta taxa de concordância pode ser produzida de várias maneiras, muitas das quais podem resultar de uma tendenciosidade (*bias*) irrelevante; contudo, em geral é considerada uma evidência de conexão causal (p. ex., no caso de gêmeos idênticos, um componente genético ou em cônjuges de um acasalamento não-aleatório).
 critical r., freqüência crítica; a freqüência cardíaca na qual ocorre uma aberração ou um bloqueio incompleto; uma conseqüência do encurtamento no comprimento do ciclo de tal modo que o período refratário quase não é registrado.
 death r., taxa de mortalidade; uma estimativa da proporção da população que morre durante um período específico, em geral de um ano; o numerador corresponde ao número de pessoas que morreram, e o denominador, ao número de pessoas da população, em geral uma estimativa do número do meio do período. SIN crude death rate, lethality r., mortality r., mortality (2).
 erythrocyte sedimentation r. (ESR), velocidade de hemossedimentação; a velocidade de sedimentação das células vermelhas do sangue; velocidades elevadas estão freqüentemente associadas a anemia ou a estados inflamatórios.
 fatality r., taxa de fatalidade; a taxa de mortalidade observada em um conjunto definido de pessoas afetadas por um evento simultâneo, tal como uma catástrofe.
 fetal death r., taxa de mortalidade fetal; o número de mortes fetais dividido pela soma de nascidos vivos e de mortes fetais que ocorrem na mesma população durante o mesmo período de tempo. SIN stillbirth r.
 fetal heart r., ritmo cardíaco fetal; no feto, o número de batimentos cardíacos por minuto, normalmente entre 120 e 160.
 five-year survival r., taxa de sobrevida após cinco anos; a proporção de pacientes ainda vivos cinco anos após o diagnóstico ou o término de um tratamento. Em geral, o termo é aplicado à estatística de sobrevida de pacientes com câncer, uma vez que a probabilidade de ocorrência de recidivas é muito menor após cinco anos.
 general fertility r., taxa de fecundidade total; uma medida apurada da fertilidade em uma população; o numerador corresponde ao número de nascidos vivos em um ano, e o denominador, ao número de mulheres em idade fértil, em geral entre 15 e 44 anos (mas que já se admite estender-se até os 49 anos).
 glomerular filtration r. (GFR), taxa de filtração glomerular; o volume de água que é retirado do plasma por meio de filtração através das paredes dos capilares glomerulares localizados no interior das cápsulas de Bowman por unidade de tempo; é considerada equivalente à depuração da inulina.
 gross reproduction r., taxa bruta de reprodução; o número médio de meninas que uma mulher teria caso ela sobrevivesse até o final de sua vida fértil e se, completado esse período, ela estivesse sujeita a um determinado conjunto de taxas de fecundidade específica para a idade e a uma determinada razão de sexos ao nascimento; essa taxa fornece uma medida da substituição da fecundidade de uma população na ausência de mortalidade.
 growth r., taxa de crescimento; o aumento do crescimento absoluto ou relativo, expresso em unidades de tempo.
 growth r. of population, taxa de crescimento da população; uma medida da alteração da população na ausência de migração, englobando a adição de recém-nascidos e a subtração de mortes; o resultado é conhecido como taxa de crescimento natural da população; corresponde à diferença entre a taxa bruta de natalidade e a taxa bruta de mortalidade.
 hazard r., taxa de risco; uma medida teórica do risco de ocorrência de um evento, p. ex., de morte ou de nova doença em um ponto no tempo.
 heart r., freqüência cardíaca; a freqüência dos batimentos cardíacos, expressa pelo número de batimentos por minuto.
 inception r., taxa de incepção; a taxa em que novos ataques de doença ou de casos de uma condição ocorrem em uma população.
 incidence r., taxa de incidência; a taxa em que casos novos surgem em uma população. O numerador corresponde ao número de casos novos que ocorreram em um período definido; o denominador corresponde à população exposta ao evento durante esse período.
 infant mortality r., taxa de mortalidade infantil; uma medida da taxa de mortes de bebês nascidos vivos antes do primeiro aniversário; o numerador corresponde ao número de bebês nascidos vivos, com menos de um ano de idade, de uma região definida e durante o período de um ano que morreram antes de completar um ano de vida; o denominador corresponde ao número total de nascidos vivos; é freqüentemente citada como um indicador útil do nível de saúde de uma comunidade.
 initial r., velocidade inicial. SIN initial *velocity*.
 lethality r., taxa de letalidade. SIN death r.
 maternal death r., taxa de mortalidade materna; o número de mortes maternas que ocorrem como resultado direto do processo reprodutivo por 100.000

nascidos vivos. VER rate; VER TAMBÉM maternal *death*. SIN maternal mortality ratio.

mitotic r., índice mitótico; a proporção de células de um tecido que estão sofrendo mitose, expressa como um índice de mitose ou, *grosso modo*, como o número de células em mitose em cada campo microscópico em grande aumento de cortes de tecidos.

morbidity r., taxa de morbidade; a proporção de pacientes com uma doença específica durante um determinado ano por uma dada unidade de população.

mortality r., taxa de mortalidade. SIN death r.

mucociliary clearance r., taxa de depuração mucociliar; a velocidade do movimento da camada de muco sobre o epitélio respiratório, expressa em geral em mm/hora.

mutation r., taxa de mutação; a probabilidade (ou proporção) de genes dos descendentes com um componente específico do genoma que não está presente em ambos os pais biológicos; é expressa em geral pelo número de mutantes por geração presentes em um gene ou *locus*.

neonatal mortality r., taxa de mortalidade neonatal; o número de mortes ocorridas nos primeiros 28 dias de vida dividido pelo número de nascidos vivos em uma mesma população durante o mesmo período de tempo.

peak flow r., taxa de fluxo de pico; a taxa de fluxo urinário máximo durante o esvaziamento, conforme medido por um urofluxômetro.

perinatal mortality r., taxa de mortalidade perinatal; o número de natimortos com 24 semanas completas ou mais somado ao número de mortes que ocorreram nos primeiros 28 dias de vida dividido pelo número de natimortos com 24 semanas ou mais de gestação somado a todos os bebês nascidos vivos na mesma população, sem levar em conta o período de gestação.

pulse r., freqüência do pulso; a freqüência do pulso, conforme é observada em uma artéria; é expressa em batimentos por minuto.

recurrence r., taxa de recorrência; em aconselhamento genético, o risco que um futuro descendente apresenta de ser afetado por uma dada característica, quando possui um conjunto específico de parentes dos quais pelo menos um já é afetado.

repetition r., taxa de repetição; o número de pulsos por minuto que definem uma produção de energia, p. ex., os pulsos de ultra-som na ecocardiografia em vez dos pulsos dos vasos sangüíneos.

respiratory r., freqüência respiratória; a freqüência da respiração, expressa pelo número de respirações por minuto.

sedimentation r., velocidade de sedimentação; a velocidade na qual se forma um sedimento em uma solução. VER TAMBÉM erythrocyte sedimentation r.

shear r., taxa de cisalhamento; a alteração na velocidade dos planos paralelos em um fluido em movimento separados por uma unidade de distância; suas unidades são expressas em segundos^{-1}.

slew r., taxa de inflexão; em um marca-passo eletrônico, a freqüência máxima de alteração da voltagem de saída do amplificador; uma variável importante que afeta a função cardíaca quando essa é controlada por um marca-passo eletrônico. Os sensores do marca-passo freqüentemente respondem à taxa de inflexão em vez de responderem à amplitude absoluta do pulso da voltagem.

steady-state r., velocidade de equilíbrio. SIN steady-state *velocity*.

steroid metabolic clearance r. (MCR), taxa de depuração metabólica de esteróides; uma medida da taxa de metabolismo de um determinado esteróide dentro do corpo; é em geral expressa em litros de fluido corpóreo que contêm a quantidade de esteróide metabolizada por dia.

steroid production r., taxa de produção de esteróides; a quantidade total de um determinado esteróide formada no corpo; é em geral expressa em miligramas por dia; representa a soma da secreção glandular do esteróide com a formação extraglandular do mesmo a partir de diversos precursores de esteróides.

steroid secretory r., taxa de secreção de esteróides; a taxa de secreção glandular de um determinado esteróide; é em geral expressa em miligramas por dia; não inclui nenhuma quantidade de esteróide formado fora da glândula.

stillbirth r., taxa de natimortalidade; SIN fetal death r.

voiding flow r., taxa de fluxo de esvaziamento; o fluxo urinário como uma função do tempo durante a micção, conforme registrado graficamente por um fluxômetro.

Rathke, Martin H., anatomista, fisiologista e patologista alemão, 1793–1860. VER R. *bundles*, em *bundle*, cleft *cyst*, *diverticulum*, *pocket*, *pouch*, pouch *tumor*.

rating of perceived exertion. Escala de percepção do esforço; uma classificação numérica e subjetiva (escala de 6 a 19) da intensidade do esforço físico, baseada em como um indivíduo se sente em relação ao nível de estresse fisiológico. Uma classificação de 13 ou 14 (esforço sentido como "ligeiramente cansativo") corresponde a uma freqüência cardíaca durante o exercício de cerca de 70% da máxima.

ra·tio (rā′shē-ō). Razão, proporção, relação, índice, quociente; uma expressão da relação entre duas quantidades (p. ex., de uma proporção ou taxa). VER TAMBÉM index (2), quotient. [L. *ratio* (*ration-*) cálculo, razão, de *reor*, pp. *ratus*, calcular, computar]

absolute terminal innervation r., razão da inervação terminal absoluta; o número de placas motoras terminais dividido pelo número de axônios terminais relacionados com elas.

escala de percepção do esforço (EPE)	
6	
7	muito, muito fácil
8	
9	muito fácil
10	
11	relativamente fácil
12	
13	ligeiramente cansativo
14	
15	cansativo
16	
17	muito cansativo
18	
19	muito, muito cansativo

accommodative convergence-accommodation r. (AC/A), relação convergência acomodativa/acomodação (CA/A); a quantidade de convergência (medida em dioptrias prismáticas de convergência) dividida pela quantidade de acomodação (medida em dioptrias) necessária para direcionar ambos os olhos para um objeto.

A/G r., r. A/G; abreviatura de albumin-globulin r.

albumin-globulin r. (A/G r.), relação albumina/globulina; a razão entre a albumina e a globulina no soro ou na urina nas doenças renais; a razão normal no soro é de aproximadamente 1,55.

ALT:AST r., relação ALT/AST; a proporção entre a alanina aminotransferase sérica e a aspartato aminotransferase sérica; níveis séricos elevados de ambas as enzimas caracterizam a doença hepática; quando ambos os níveis estão anormalmente elevados e a proporção entre ALT e AST é maior do que 1,0, é provável a existência de necrose hepática grave ou de doença hepática alcoólica; a proporção menor do que 1,0 indica possível doença hepática aguda não-alcoólica.

amylase-creatinine clearance r., relação depuração da amilase/depuração da creatinina; um teste para o diagnóstico da pancreatite aguda; é determinada pela quantificação da amilase e da creatinina no soro e na urina; em indivíduos aparentemente saudáveis, a depuração (*clearance*) renal da amilase é 5% menor que a da creatinina; diz-se que na pancreatite aguda o valor é maior que 5%.

body-weight r., índice de massa corpórea; o peso do corpo (em gramas) dividido pela estatura (em centímetros).

cardiothoracic r., índice cardiotorácico; a proporção entre o diâmetro horizontal do coração e o diâmetro interno da caixa torácica no seu ponto mais amplo, conforme é determinado em uma radiografia de tórax.

case fatality r., razão de fatalidade de casos; a taxa de mortalidade de uma doença, expressa em geral em números de mortos por 100 casos.

r. of decayed and filled surfaces (RDFS), índice de superfícies cariadas e obturadas; um índice de superfícies permanentes cariadas e obturadas por pessoa, por conjunto de 122 superfícies dentais.

r. of decayed and filled teeth (RDFT), índice de dentes cariados e obturados; um índice de dentes permanentes cariados e obturados por pessoa, por conjunto de 28 dentes.

extraction r. (E), taxa de extração; a fração de uma substância que é removida do fluxo sangüíneo pelos rins; é calculada a partir da fórmula $(A - V)/A$, em que A e V são, respectivamente, as concentrações plasmáticas da substância no sangue arterial e no venoso renal.

fertility r., razão de fertilidade; uma medida da fertilidade de uma população que se baseia na população feminina em idade fértil, ou seja, com idades variando entre 15 e 49 anos.

flux r., razão de fluxo; a razão entre dois fluxos unidirecionais através de uma membrana ou camada limítrofes específicas.

functional terminal innervation r., razão da inervação terminal funcional; o número de fibras musculares dividido pelo número de axônios que as inervam.

grid r., razão da grade; em uma grade antidifusora de raios X, a razão entre a altura e a largura dos intervalos entre as tiras de chumbo; quanto maior é a razão da grade, maior é a quantidade de radiação dispersa removida, mas também maior é o cuidado necessário no posicionamento do tubo de raios X, a fim de evitar o desvio do feixe de radiação primária.

gyromagnetic r., razão giromagnética; em ressonância magnética nuclear, a razão entre o momento do dipolo magnético do núcleo e o momento angular do spin nuclear; a razão giromagnética corresponde a um valor único para cada tipo de núcleo. SIN magnetogyric r.

hand r., razão da mão; a razão entre o comprimento da mão (medido sobre o dorso a partir do processo estilóide da ulna até a extremidade do terceiro dedo) e sua largura através das articulações dos dedos.

international normalized r. (INR), relação normalizada internacional; a relação do tempo da protrombina que teria sido obtida caso um reagente-padrão tivesse sido utilizado na determinação do tempo da protrombina; a relação do tempo da protrombina é expressa pelo tempo da protrombina do paciente dividido pela média do intervalo de referência do tempo da protrombina; a relação do tempo da protrombina é obtida por um reagente preparado no laboratório através do uso de um parâmetro denominado índice de sensibilidade internacional. VER TAMBÉM international sensitivity *index*.

IRI/G r., relação IIR/G; a razão entre a insulina imunorreativa e a glicose sérica e plasmática; nos estados hipoglicêmicos, um valor menor que 0,3 é comum, com exceção da hipoglicemia causada por insulinoma, na qual o valor é freqüentemente maior que 0,3.

K:A r., abreviatura de ketogenic-antiketogenic r.

ketogenic-antiketogenic r. (K:A r.), relação cetogênicos/anticetogênicos (r. C/A); a proporção entre as substâncias que formam as cetonas no corpo e aquelas que formam a D-glicose.

lecithin/sphingomyelin r. (L/S r.), relação lecitina/esfingomielina (r. L/E); uma proporção utilizada na determinação da maturidade pulmonar fetal, obtida por meio da análise do líquido amniótico; quando os pulmões estão maduros, a proporção entre a lecitina e a esfingomielina é de 2 para 1.

L/S r., abreviatura de lecithin/sphingomyelin r.

magnetogyric r. (mag′ne-tō-gy-rik), razão magnetogírica; SIN gyromagnetic r.

mass-action r., razão massa/ação; a razão entre o produto de todas as concentrações dos produtos dividido pelo produto de todas as concentrações dos reagentes de uma reação específica; quando a reação estiver completa (i. e., $t = \infty$), então essa razão é igual à constante de equilíbrio.

maternal mortality r., razão de mortalidade materna; SIN maternal death *rate*.

M:E r., relação M/E; a proporção entre os precursores mielóides e eritróides na medula óssea; normalmente, o valor varia de 2:1 a 4:1; uma proporção elevada é encontrada em infecções, na leucemia mielóide crônica e na hipoplasia eritróide; uma proporção diminuída pode significar uma diminuição na leucopoese ou na hiperplasia normoblástica, dependendo da celularidade global da medula óssea.

mendelian r., proporção mendeliana; a proporção de descendentes com genótipos ou fenótipos específicos esperados de acordo com as leis de Mendel entre a descendência de casais com genótipo ou fenótipos específicos.

molecular weight r. (M_r), relação do peso molecular. SIN molecular *weight*.

nuclear-cytoplasmic r., relação núcleo-citoplasmática; a relação entre o volume do núcleo e o volume do citoplasma, bastante constante para um tipo específico de célula e em geral aumentada nas neoplasias malignas.

nucleolar-nuclear r., relação nucléolo/núcleo; a relação entre o volume do nucléolo e o volume do núcleo, em geral aumentada nas neoplasias malignas.

P/O r., relação fosfato/oxigênio; uma medida da fosforilação oxidativa; a proporção entre os radicais fosfato esterificados (que formam a adenosina 5′-trifosfato a partir da adenosina 5′-difosfato) e os átomos de oxigênio consumidos pelas mitocôndrias; normalmente, a proporção é igual a 3 (começando do NADH). SIN P/O quotient.

respiratory exchange r., razão de troca respiratória; a proporção entre a produção de dióxido de carbono e a simultânea captação de oxigênio em um determinado lugar, ambas expressas em moles ou volumes nas CNTP por unidade de tempo; no estado de equilíbrio, a razão de troca respiratória é igual ao quociente respiratório dos processos metabólicos.

segregation r., proporção de segregação; em genética, a proporção de descendentes com um genótipo ou fenótipo específico provenientes de casais reais (não-hipotéticos) com genótipos específicos. O teste de uma hipótese mendeliana é feito pela comparação da proporção de segregação com a proporção mendeliana.

sex r., proporção de sexos; **(1)** a proporção entre os descendentes machos e fêmeas em alguma fase específica do ciclo de vida, notavelmente na concepção (primária), no nascimento (secundária) ou em qualquer fase entre o nascimento e a morte (terciária); **(2)** a proporção entre o número de homens e mulheres afetados por uma doença ou característica em particular.

signal-to-noise r., relação sinal-ruído; a intensidade relativa de um sinal em relação à variação casual na intensidade do sinal ou no ruído; é utilizada para avaliar muitas técnicas de imagens e sistemas eletrônicos.

standardized mortality r., razão de mortalidade padronizada; a proporção entre o número de casos observados em uma população e o número esperado caso a população tivesse a mesma distribuição, como ocorre em uma população-padrão ou de referência.

systolic/diastolic r., relação sístole/diástole; um cálculo realizado a partir das determinações do ultra-som com Doppler das velocidades do fluxo sangüíneo que reflete a resistência intrínseca em um vaso sangüíneo arterial.

therapeutic r., índice terapêutico; a relação entre a dose máxima tolerada de uma droga e a dose curativa ou efetiva mínima; a DL_{50} dividida pela DE_{50}.

variance r. (F), razão de variação; a distribuição da proporção de duas estimativas independentes da mesma variação a partir de uma distribuição gaussiana, baseada em amostras de tamanhos $(n + 1)$ e $(m + 1)$, respectivamente. As estimativas são, em geral, baseadas em uma determinada amostra analisada de um certo modo, a fim de torná-las independentes; p. ex., a análise da variação e a razão de variação podem ser utilizadas para testar uma hipótese sem validade de que as diferenças observadas entre as médias das amostras não são maiores do que poderiam ser, caso resultassem do acaso.

ventilation/perfusion r. (Va/Q), relação ventilação/perfusão; a relação entre a ventilação alveolar e o simultâneo fluxo sangüíneo nos capilares alveolares em qualquer parte dos pulmões; como tanto a ventilação quanto a perfusão são expressas em unidades de volume de tecido e em unidades de tempo (que se cancelam mutuamente em uma razão), as unidades finais correspondem a litros de gás por litro de sangue.

waist-hip r., relação cintura/quadril; a relação entre a circunferência abdominal na altura do umbigo e a circunferência máxima do quadril e das nádegas.

zeta sedimentation r. (ZSR), velocidade de sedimentação zeta; a relação entre o zetácrito e o hematócrito, que normalmente varia de 0,41 a 0,54 (41 a 54%); é um indicador sensível da velocidade de hemossedimentação (VHS) e, diferentemente da última, não é afetada pela anemia, que tende a elevar a VHS.

ra·tion·al (rash′ŭn-ăl). Racional. **1.** Relativo ao raciocínio ou aos processos de pensamento mais elevados; baseia-se no conhecimento objetivo ou científico, em contraste com o empírico (1). **2.** Que é influenciado pela razão em vez de pela emoção. **3.** Que possui as faculdades do raciocínio; que não está delirante ou comatoso. [L. *rationalis*, de *ratio*, razão]

ra·tion·al·i·za·tion (ra-shŭn-ăl-i-zā′shŭn). Racionalização; mecanismo de defesa psicanalítico postulado por meio do qual o comportamento, os motivos ou os sentimentos irracionais parecem lógicos, razoáveis. [L. *ratio*, razão]

Ratner. VER Kurzrok-Ratner *test*.

rats·bane (rats′bān). Arsênico. SIN arsenic.

rat·tle·snake (rat′l-snăk). Cascavel; um membro dos gêneros *Crotalus* e *Sistrurus*, compostos por crotalídeos caracterizados por um guizo cuticular na extremidade da cauda.

Rat·tus (rat′ŭs). Um gênero de roedores — os ratos — da família Muridae. *R. rattus*, o rato-preto, é a espécie comumente responsável pela transmissão da peste aos humanos por meio da pulga *Xenopsylla cheopis*; é menor e mais escuro que o rato marrom, rato-dos-esgotos ou norueguês (*Rattus norvegicus*) e possui orelhas e cauda mais longas. VER rat.

Rau (Ravius, Raw), Johann J., anatomista holandês, 1668–1719. VER R. *process*; *processus ravii*.

Rauber, August A., anatomista alemão, 1841–1917. VER R. *layer*.

Rauscher, Frank J., oncologista norte-americano do século 20. VER R. *virus*.

Rau·wol·fia (row-wool′fē-ă, raw-, rah-). Um gênero de arbustos e árvores tropicais (família Apocynaceae). A raiz em pó de *R. serpentina* contém alcalóides que produzem ações sedativa, anti-hipertensiva e bradicárdica; cerca de 50% da atividade total devem-se à reserpina. [L. *Rauwolf*, botânico alemão, século 16]

RAV Abreviatura de Rous-associated *virus* (vírus Rous-associado).

Ravius, VER Rau.

ray (rā). Raio. **1.** Um feixe de luz, calor ou outra forma de radiação. Os raios provenientes do rádio e de outras substâncias radioativas são produzidos pela desintegração espontânea do átomo; são partículas com cargas elétricas ou ondas eletromagnéticas com comprimento de onda extremamente curto. **2.** Uma parte ou um ramo que se estende radialmente a partir de uma estrutura. [L. *radius*]

actinic r., r. actínico; um r. de luz em direção a e além da extremidade violeta do espectro que impressiona uma chapa fotográfica e produz outros efeitos químicos. SIN chemical r.

alpha r., partícula alfa. SIN alpha *particle*.

anode r.'s, raios anódicos; os raios que se originam em um tubo de descarga de gás e se movem na direção oposta àquela dos raios catódicos; são compostos por íons com cargas positivas. SIN positive r.'s.

Becquerel r.'s, raios de Becquerel; termo obsoleto da radiação emitida pelo urânio e por outras substâncias radioativas; tais raios incluem os raios α, β e γ.

beta r., r. beta; SIN beta *particle*.

cathode r.'s, raios catódicos; um fluxo de elétrons emitido por um eletrodo negativo (catodo) em um tubo de Crookes; o bombardeamento do ânodo ou da parede de vidro do tubo pelos raios catódicos dá origem aos raios X.

chemical r., r. actínico. SIN actinic r.

cosmic r.'s, raios cósmicos; partículas com alta velocidade e grande quantidade de energia que bombardeiam a Terra a partir do espaço; a "radiação primária" consiste em prótons e núcleos de átomos mais complexos que, ao colidirem com a atmosfera, dão origem a nêutrons, mésons e a outra "radiação secundária" com menor quantidade de energia.

direct r.'s, raios primários. SIN primary r.'s (2).

gamma r.'s, raios gama; a radiação eletromagnética emitida por substâncias radioativas; consistem em raios X de alta energia que se originam no núcleo em vez da camada orbital e não são desviados por um magneto.

glass r.'s, raios de vidro; os raios formados a partir da colisão dos raios catódicos com a parede de um tubo de raios X; um caso especial de raios indiretos e de raios X moles. Obsoleto.

grenz r. (grents), raios X muito moles, que se assemelham aos raios ultravioleta tanto no comprimento de onda (i.e., relativamente longos) quanto na ação biológica sobre os tecidos; são produzidos por um tubo de vácuo especialmente construído com um catodo quente que opera a partir de um transformador que produz não mais do que 8 kw. [Al. *Grenze*, limite, fronteira]
H r.'s, raios H, um feixe de núcleos de hidrogênio, i.e., de prótons.
hard r.'s, raios duros; raios de comprimento de onda curto e grande penetrabilidade.
incident r., r. incidente; o r. que incide na superfície antes da reflexão.
indirect r.'s, raios indiretos; os raios X gerados em uma superfície diferente do seu alvo, o ânodo.
infrared r., r. infravermelho. VER infrared.
intermediate r.'s, raios intermediários; aqueles situados entre os raios ultravioleta e os raios X. SIN W r.'s.
marginal r.'s, raios marginais; em óptica geométrica, aqueles raios que se originam da periferia.
medullary r., r. medular; o centro do lóbulo renal, que apresenta a forma de uma pequena pirâmide composta de partes tubulares retas; essas partes podem ser tanto ramos ascendentes quanto descendentes da alça do néfron ou dos túbulos coletores. SIN Ferrein pyramid, pars radiata lobuli corticalis renis, processus ferreini.
Niewenglowski r.'s, raios de Niewenglowski; a radiação emitida por um corpo fosforescente após exposição à luz solar.
parallel r.'s, raios paralelos; os raios que são paralelos ao eixo de um sistema óptico.
paraxial r.'s, raios paraxiais; em óptica geométrica, aqueles raios que estão focalizados no ponto principal.
positive r.'s, raios positivos. SIN anode r.'s.
primary r.'s, raios primários; **(1)** os raios cósmicos na forma em que se apresentam quando colidem com a atmosfera; **(2)** os raios X gerados no ponto focal do tubo. SIN direct r.'s.
reflected r., r. refletido; r. de luz ou outra forma de energia radiante que é refletido em uma superfície impermeável e não-absorvente; o r. que colide com a superfície antes da reflexão é o r. incidente.
roentgen r., r. de Roentgen. SIN x-ray (1).
secondary r.'s, raios secundários; os raios X gerados quando os raios primários colidem com a matéria; a radiação dispersa.
soft r.'s, raios moles; os raios X com comprimento de onda relativamente longo e pouca penetrabilidade.
supersonic r.'s, raios supersônicos; os raios com comprimento de onda maior do que aquele que pode ser percebido pela orelha humana (> 20.000 Hz).
ultrasonic r.'s, raios ultra-sônicos. VER ultrasonic.
ultraviolet r.'s, raios ultravioleta. VER ultraviolet.
W r.'s, raios W. SIN intermediate r.'s.
x-r., r. X. VER x-ray.
Rayer, Pierre F., médico francês, 1793–1867. VER R. *disease.*
rayl (rāl). Rayl; a unidade de impedância acústica; 1 rayl = 1 kg $\times$ m^{-2} $\times$ s^{-1}. [Barão *Rayleigh* (John W. Strutt), físico inglês]
Rayleigh, Lorde John William Strutt, físico britânico, laureado com um Nobel, 1842–1919. VER R. *equation, test.*
Raynaud, Maurice, médico francês, 1834–1881. VER R. *syndrome, disease, phenomenon, sign.*
Rb Símbolo do rubidium (rubídio).
R-band·ing. VER R-banding *stain.*
rbc, RBC Abreviatura de red blood *cell* (eritrócito, hemácia); red blood count (hemograma).
RBE Abreviatura utilizada em proteção à radiação para relative biologic effectiveness (efetividade biológica relativa). Cf. quality factor, QF.
RBF Abreviatura de renal blood flow (fluxo sangüíneo renal). VER effective renal blood *flow.*
R.C.P. Abreviatura de Royal College of Physicians (da Inglaterra).
R.C.P.(E), R.C.P.(Edin) 1. Abreviatura de Royal College of Physicians (Edimburgo). **2.** Símbolo de reactivity (reatividade)
R.C.P.(I) Abreviatura de Royal College of Physicians (Irlanda).
R.C.P.S.C. Abreviatura de Royal College of Physicians and Surgeons of Canada.
R.C.S. Abreviatura de Royal College of Surgeons (Inglaterra).
R.C.S.(E), R.C.S.(Edin) Abreviatura de Royal College of Surgeons (Edimburgo).
R.C.S.(I) Abreviatura de Royal College of Surgeons (Irlanda).
RCT Abreviatura de randomized controlled *trial* (estudo randomizado com controle).
R.D. Abreviatura de registered dietician (nutricionista).
RDA Abreviatura de recommended daily *allowance* (cota diária recomendada).
RDFS Abreviatura de *ratio* of decayed and filled surfaces (relação entre superfícies cariadas e obturadas).
RDFT Abreviatura de *ratio* of decayed and filled teeth (relação entre dentes com cáries e dentes com obturação).

R.D.H. Abreviatura de Registered Dental Hygienist.
RDPA Abreviatura de right descending pulmonary *artery* (artéria pulmonar descendente direita).
R.E. Abreviatura de right eye (olho direito).
Re Símbolo de rhenium (rênio).
re-. Re-; prefixo que indica "novamente" ou "para trás". [L.]
re·act (rē - akt′) Reagir; tomar parte em ou sofrer uma reação química. [L. mod. *reactus*]
re·ac·tance (*X*) (rē - ak′tans). Reatância; o enfraquecimento de uma corrente elétrica alternada pela passagem através de uma bobina ou de um condensador. SIN inductive resistance.
re·ac·tant (rē - ak′tant). Reagente; uma substância que toma parte em uma reação química.
acute phase r.'s, reagentes de fase aguda; um grupo de proteínas que são produzidas e/ou liberadas em concentrações elevadas durante a reação da fase aguda e que incluem o fibrinogênio, a proteína C reativa, as proteínas B, C3 e C4 do complemento, a α_2 glicoproteína ácida, a amilóide A do soro, os inibidores das proteinases etc.

REACTION

re·ac·tion (rē - ak′shŭn). Reação. **1.** A resposta de um músculo ou outro tecido vivo ou organismo a um estímulo. **2.** A mudança de cor observada no tornassol e em outros pigmentos orgânicos pelo contato com substâncias, tais como ácidos ou álcalis; a propriedade que tais substâncias apresentam de produzir essa mudança. **3.** Em química, a ação intermolecular que ocorre entre duas ou mais substâncias e por meio da qual tais substâncias desaparecem e novas substâncias são formadas em seu lugar (r. química). **4.** Em imunologia, a ação *in vivo* ou *in vitro* de um anticorpo sobre um antígeno específico, com ou sem a participação do complemento ou de outros componentes do sistema imunológico. [L. *re*-, novamente, para trás, + *actio*, ação]
accelerated r., r. acelerada; uma resposta que ocorre em um tempo mais curto do que o esperado; as manifestações cutâneas que ocorrem durante o período entre o segundo e o décimo dia após a vacinação contra a varíola; por ser intermediária entre uma r. primária e uma r. imediata, é considerada uma evidência de algum grau de resistência. SIN vaccinoid r.
acid r., r. ácida; **(1)** qualquer teste que indica a ocorrência de uma r. ácida, tal como a mudança do papel de tornassol azul para vermelho; **(2)** um excesso de íons de hidrogênio em relação aos íons de hidróxido em uma solução aquosa indicado por um valor de pH < 7 (a 22°C). Cf. dissociation *constant* of water.
acute phase r., r. da fase aguda; refere-se às alterações que ocorrem na síntese de determinadas proteínas séricas durante uma resposta inflamatória; essa resposta fornece ao hospedeiro uma proteção rápida contra microrganismos por meio de mecanismos de defesa não-específicos. SIN acute phase response.
acute situational r., r. situacional aguda. SIN stress r.
acute stress r., r. aguda ao estresse. SIN anxiety r.
adverse r., r. adversa; qualquer conseqüência indesejável de um procedimento ou esquema preventivo, diagnóstico ou terapêutico.
alarm r., r. de alarme; fenômenos diversos manifestados pelo corpo, p. ex., estímulo da atividade endócrina, que representam uma resposta adaptativa à lesão ou ao estresse; a primeira fase da síndrome geral da adaptação.
aldehyde r., r. do aldeído; a r. dos derivados do indol com aldeídos aromáticos; p. ex., o triptofano e o *p*-dimetilaminobenzaldeído em H_2SO_4 dão uma cor violeta-avermelhada útil na análise do conteúdo de triptofano nas proteínas. SIN Ehrlich r.
alkaline r., r. alcalina; **(1)** qualquer teste que indica a ocorrência de uma r. alcalina, tal como a mudança do papel de tornassol vermelho para azul; **(2)** excesso de íons de hidróxido em relação aos íons de hidrogênio em uma solução aquosa como indicado por um valor de pH >7 (a 22°C). Cf. dissociation *constant* of water. SIN basic r.
allergic r., r. alérgica; r. local ou generalizada que ocorre após o contato com um alérgeno específico ao qual o organismo tenha sido previamente exposto e pelo qual tenha sido sensibilizado; a interação imunológica entre um antígeno endógeno ou exógeno e um anticorpo ou linfócitos sensibilizados dá origem a inflamação ou a reação tecidual. As reações alérgicas são classificadas em quatro tipos principais: tipo I, anafilática e dependente de IgE; tipo II, citotóxica; tipo III, mediada por complexo imune; tipo IV, mediada por células (tardia). SIN hypersensitivity r.
amphoteric r., r. anfótera; r. dupla observada em certos líquidos que apresentam uma combinação de propriedades ácidas e alcalinas.
anamnestic r., r. anamnésica; a produção aumentada de um anticorpo como conseqüência da exposição prévia do indivíduo ao mesmo antígeno.
anaphylactic r. (an′a - fī - lak′tik), r. anafilática. SIN anaphylaxis.
anaplerotic r., r. anaplerótica. VER anaplerotic.

antigen-antibody r. (AAR), r. antígeno-anticorpo; o fenômeno reversível que consiste na combinação *in vivo* ou *in vitro* de um anticorpo com um antígeno do tipo que estimula a formação do anticopo, resultando, dessa forma, na aglutinação, na precipitação, na fixação de complemento, em maior suscetibilidade à ingestão e à destruição por fagócitos ou na neutralização de exotoxinas. VER TAMBÉM skin *test*.

anxiety r., r. de ansiedade; r. ou experiência psicológica que envolve a apreensão do perigo acompanhada do sentimento de temor e de sinais e sintomas físicos, tais como aumento na freqüência respiratória, taquicardia, na ausência de um estímulo amedrontador claramente identificável; quando essa r. se torna crônica, é denominada transtorno de ansiedade generalizada. VER generalized anxiety *disorder*. VER TAMBÉM panic *attack*. SIN acute stress r.

Arias-Stella r., r. de Arias-Stella. SIN Arias-Stella *phenomenon*.

arousal r., r. de despertar; a alteração no padrão das ondas cerebrais que ocorre quando o indivíduo é subitamente acordado e fica alerta.

Arthus r., r. de Arthus. **(1)** SIN Arthus *phenomenon*; **(2)** r. de tipo Arthus; r. que ocorre em seres humanos e em outras espécies resultante do mesmo mecanismo imunológico (alérgico) básico que evoca, no coelho, o típico fenômeno de Arthus. VER TAMBÉM immune complex *disease*.

Ascoli r., r. de Ascoli; uma técnica para confirmar o diagnóstico de antraz (carbúnculo) por meio de uma r. de precipitina que indica a presença do antígeno termoestável *Bacillus anthracis* no tecido extraído.

associative r., r. associativa; uma r. secundária ou colateral.

basic r., r. básica. SIN alkaline r.

Bence Jones r., r. de Bence Jones; o modo clássico de identificação da proteína de Bence Jones, que se precipita quando a urina (de pacientes com esse tipo de proteinúria) é gradualmente aquecida até 45 a 70°C e torna a dissolver enquanto a urina é aquecida até uma temperatura próxima da fervura; à medida que a amostra esfria, a proteína de Bence Jones precipita-se na faixa de temperatura indicada e volta a dissolver quando a temperatura da amostra cai abaixo de 30 a 35°C.

Berthelot r., r. de Berthelot; a r. da amônia com o fenol e o hipoclorito, originando indofenol; o princípio é utilizado na análise da concentração de amônia nos líquidos corporais.

bi bi r., r. bi bi; uma r. catalisada por uma única enzima e na qual dois substratos e dois produtos estão envolvidos; o mecanismo de pingue-pongue pode estar envolvido em tal r. Cf. mechanism.

Bittorf r., r. de Bittorf; nos casos de cólica renal, a dor que irradia para o rim ao se apertar o testículo ou pressionar o ovário.

biuret r., r. do biureto; a formação de biureto que dá uma cor violeta como conseqüência da r. de um polipeptídeo com mais de três resíduos de aminoácidos com o $CuSO_4$ em uma solução fortemente alcalina; os dipeptídeos e aminoácidos (exceto a histidina, a serina e a treonina) não reagem assim; é utilizada na detecção e quantificação de polipeptídeos, ou proteínas, em líquidos biológicos.

Bloch r., r. de Bloch. SIN dopa r.

Bordet and Gengou r., r. de Bordet e Gengou. VER complement *fixation*.

Brunn r., r. de Brunn; o aumento da absorção de água através da pele de uma rã após receber uma injeção de pituitrina e ser imersa em água; uma das reações fisiológicas utilizadas no estudo e na classificação dos polipeptídeos da pituitária posterior e de seus análogos.

Burchard-Liebermann r., r. de Burchard-Liebermann; a cor azul-esverdeada produzida pela adição de algumas gotas de ácido sulfúrico concentrado a uma solução composta de anidrido acético e colesterol (e outros esteróis) dissolvidos em clorofórmio. VER Liebermann-Burchard *test*.

Cannizzaro r., r. de Cannizzaro; a formação de um ácido e de um álcool pela oxidação simultânea de uma molécula de aldeído e pela redução de outra; a dismutação: $2RCHO \rightarrow RCOOH + RCH_2OH$; quando os aldeídos não são idênticos, tem-se uma reação de Cannizzaro cruzada.

capsular precipitation r., r. de intumescimento capsular. SIN quellung r. (2).

Carr-Price r., r. de Carr-Price; a r. entre o tricloreto de antimônio e a vitamina A que produz uma cor azul brilhante; essa r. forma a base de várias técnicas quantitativas para a determinação da vitamina A.

catalatic r., r. catalática; a decomposição do H_2O_2 em O_2 e H_2O, como ocorre na ação da catalase; análoga à r. da peroxidase.

catastrophic r., r. catastrófica; o comportamento desorganizado que corresponde à resposta a um grave abalo ou a uma situação ameaçadora com os quais a pessoa não consegue lidar.

cell-mediated r., r. mediada por células; a r. imunológica do tipo tardio, que envolve principalmente os linfócitos T, importante na defesa do hospedeiro contra infecções, nas doenças auto-imunes e na rejeição de transplantes. VER TAMBÉM skin *test*.

chain r., r. em cadeia; uma r. contínua na qual um produto de uma etapa da própria r. desencadeia a próxima etapa da r. Cf. autocatalysis.

Chantemesse r., r. de Chantemesse; r. conjuntival, especialmente quando diz respeito à febre tifóide.

cholera-red r., r. vermelha do cólera; um teste para detectar o vibrião do cólera no qual a adição de 3 ou 4 gotas de ácido sulfúrico (concentrado e quimicamente puro) a uma cultura de peptona ou de caldo de carne de 18 horas do microrganismo produz uma cor que varia de cor-de-rosa a vermelha.

chromaffin r., r. cromafim; a produção de uma coloração que varia de marrom-amarelada a marrom em células normais e anormais que contêm epinefrina e norepinefrina, quando cortes de tecido fresco são colocados em uma mistura de cromato-dicromato de um dia para o outro; é útil na detecção do feocromocitoma (medula da supra-renal) e de outros tumores que produzem catecolaminas.

circular r., r. circular; na teoria sensório-motora, a tendência de um organismo a repetir experiências novas.

cocarde r., cockade r., r. da cocarda. VER Römer *test*.

colloidal gold r., r. do ouro coloidal; um teste (agora obsoleto) baseado na precipitação das proteínas do líquido cerebrospinal, quando esse líquido é misturado ao ouro coloidal. Foram observadas alterações nas reações feitas em pacientes com sífilis, esclerose múltipla (ver multiple *sclerosis*), poliomielite e encefalite.

complement-fixation r., r. de fixação do complemento. VER complement *fixation*.

consensual r., r. consensual; a contração da pupila de um dos olhos quando a pupila do outro olho é iluminada. SIN consensual light reflex, indirect pupillary r.

constitutional r., r. constitucional; r. generalizada em contraste com uma r. local ou focal; na alergia, a resposta imediata ou tardia após a introdução de um alérgeno e que ocorre em locais distantes daquele da injeção.

conversion r., r. de conversão. SIN conversion *hysteria*.

cross-r., r. cruzada; uma r. específica que ocorre entre um anti-soro e um complexo antigênico diferente do complexo antigênico que desencadeou os diversos anticorpos específicos do anti-soro. É resultante da presença de pelo menos um determinante antigênico entre os determinantes de outro complexo.

cutaneous graft versus host r., r. enxerto cutâneo *versus* hospedeiro; r. eritematosa maculopapular aguda com formação de bolhas nos casos mais graves; as alterações crônicas podem se assemelhar ao líquen plano ou à esclerodermia.

cytotoxic r., r. citotóxica; r. imunológica (alérgica) na qual anticorpos IgG ou IgM não-citotrópicos se combinam com um antígeno específico localizado na superfície das células; o complexo resultante inicia a ativação do complemento que causa a lise das células ou outra lesão, ou que, na ausência do complemento, pode levar à fagocitose ou aumentar o envolvimento dos linfócitos T, levando à citotoxicidade celular.

Dale r., r. de Dale. VER Schultz-Dale r.

dark r., r. escura; na fotossíntese, a fixação de CO_2 no carboidrato, que não depende do lugar e do momento de absorção de luz.

decidual r., r. decidual; as alterações celulares e vasculares que ocorrem no endométrio no momento da implantação.

delayed r., r. retardada, r. tardia; resposta local ou generalizada que se inicia 24 a 48 horas após a exposição a um antígeno e que envolve as células T. VER cell-mediated r. SIN contact hypersensitivity (2), delayed hypersensitivity (2), late r., tuberculin-type hypersensitivity.

depot r., r. de depósito; coloração avermelhada da pele no local onde ocorreu a penetração da agulha utilizada no teste subcutâneo da tuberculina.

depressive r., r. depressiva. SIN depression (4).

dermotuberculin r., r. dermotuberculínica. SIN Pirquet *test*.

diazo r., r. diazo; a r. entre o ácido sulfanílico diazotado e a bilirrubina que produz azobilirrubina, a qual forma a base para se avaliar a quantidade de bilirrubina presente nos líquidos biológicos. VER van den Bergh *test*. SIN Ehrlich diazo r.

digitonin r., r. da digitonina; a r. dos esteróides de ocorrência natural contendo grupamentos 3β-hidroxila e a digitonina, um glicosídeo esteróide, que resulta na formação de um precipitado insolúvel; é útil na determinação de colesterol e ergosterol.

Dische r., r. de Dische; a análise do DNA por meio da cor azul formada com a difenilamina em ácido (reagente de Dische).

dissociative r., r. dissociativa; r. caracterizada por comportamento dissociativo, tal como amnésia, fugas, sonambulismo e estados oníricos.

dopa r., r. à dopa; coloração escura observada em cortes de tecido fresco aos quais uma solução de dopa foi aplicada e presumivelmente resultante da presença de dopa oxidase no protoplasma de certas células. SIN Bloch r.

dystonic r., r. distônica; estado de tensão ou tônus muscular anormais, similar à distonia, produzido como efeito colateral de certos medicamentos antipsicóticos; uma forma grave, na qual os olhos viram para cima, é denominada crise oculogírica.

early r., r. inicial. SIN immediate r.

echo r., ecolalia. SIN echolalia.

Ehrlich r., r. de Ehrlich. SIN aldehyde r.

Ehrlich benzaldehyde r., r. do benzaldeído de Ehrlich; teste para a detecção de urobilinogênio na urina que consiste na dissolução de 2 g de dimetil-*p*-aminobenzaldeído em 100 mL de ácido clorídrico a 5% e na posterior adição desse reagente à urina; a obtenção de uma cor vermelha a baixas temperaturas indica a presença de uma quantidade excessiva de urobilinogênio.

Ehrlich diazo r., r. diazo de Ehrlich. SIN diazo r.
eosinopenic r., r. eosinopênica; a redução do número de eosinófilos circulantes pelo ACTH ou pelos corticóides da supra-renal.
error-prone polymerase chain r., r. da cadeia da polimerase propensa a erro; a utilização da reação da cadeia da polimerase em condições que favorecem a incorporação errônea de bases, p. ex., quando se busca uma porção de DNA amplificado em mutantes aleatórios.
eye-closure pupil r., r. pupilar ao fechamento dos olhos; a constrição de ambas as pupilas observada quando se faz um esforço para fechar as pálpebras que estão mantidas separadas por meio da força; uma variante da resposta pupilar à observação de um objeto próximo. SIN Galassi pupillary phenomenon, Gifford reflex, lid-closure r., orbicularis phenomenon, orbicularis pupillary reflex, Piltz sign, Westphal pupillary reflex, Westphal-Piltz phenomenon.
false-negative r., r. falso-negativa; uma resposta errônea ou equivocadamente negativa.
false-positive r., r. falso-positiva; uma resposta errônea ou equivocadamente positiva.
Fenton r., r. de Fenton; (1) o uso de H_2O_2 e de sais ferrosos (reagente de Fenton) na oxidação de α-hidroxiácidos a α-cetoácidos ou na conversão de 1,2-glicóis a α-hidroxialdeídos; (2) a formação de OH·, OH^- e Fe^{3+} a partir da r. não-enzimática de Fe^{2+} com H_2O_2; uma r. importante no estresse oxidativo das células sangüíneas e de diversos tecidos.
Fernandez r., r. de Fernandez; r. de hipersensibilidade tardia à lepromina, similar à r. à tuberculina, que ocorre no local da injeção intradérmica do antígeno de Dharmendra no teste da lepromina.
ferric chloride r. of epinephrine, r. da epinefrina ao cloreto férrico; uma cor verde-esmeralda intensa observada em uma solução neutra ou levemente ácida de epinefrina, quando se adiciona cloreto férrico a essa solução; uma r. típica dos catecóis.
Feulgen r., r. de Feulgen. VER Feulgen *stain*.
fight or flight r., r. de luta ou fuga; a teoria de Walter Cannon que afirma que o organismo — o sistema nervoso autônomo e os efetores ligados a ele —, frente a situações de perigo que exigem tanto luta quanto fuga, é provido de um mecanismo que o coloca em prontidão para lidar com emergências, sem dispersão de energia. Também conhecida como teoria da emergência (ver emergency *theory*).
first-order r., r. de primeira ordem; uma r. cuja velocidade é proporcional à concentração da única substância que sofre alteração; o decaimento radioativo é um processo de primeira ordem definido pela equação $dN/dt = kN$, em que N corresponde ao número de átomos sujeitos ao decaimento (reação), t corresponde ao tempo e k corresponde à constante do decaimento de primeira ordem (reação), i.e., a fração de todos os átomos que sofrem decaimento por unidade de tempo. VER TAMBÉM decay *constant*, order.
fixation r., r. de fixação. VER complement *fixation*.
flocculation r., r. de floculação; uma forma de r. de precipitina na qual a precipitação ocorre dentro de uma faixa estreita da proporção antígeno-anticorpo, relacionada principalmente a peculiaridades do anticorpo (precipitina).
focal r., r. focal; r. que ocorre no ponto de entrada de um organismo infectante ou de uma injeção, como observado no fenômeno de Arthus. SIN local r.
Folin r., r. de Folin; a r. que ocorre entre aminoácidos em solução alcalina e 1,2-naftoquinona-4-sulfonato (reagente de Folin) e que produz uma cor vermelha; é útil nos ensaios quantitativos. SIN Folin reagent.
Forssman r., r. de Forssman. SIN Forssman antigen-antibody r.
Forssman antigen-antibody r., r. antígeno-anticorpo de Forssman; a combinação do anticorpo de Forssman com o antígeno heterogenético do tipo Forssman, como ocorre na aglutinação dos eritrócitos de carneiros (os quais contêm o antígeno de Forssman) pelo soro proveniente de uma pessoa com mononucleose infecciosa que contém o anticorpo de Forssman. SIN Forssman r.
fragment r., r. do fragmento; r. utilizada na análise da atividade da peptidil transferase.
Frei-Hoffmann r., r. de Frei-Hoffmann. SIN Frei *test*.
fright r., r. de pavor; após secção e degeneração do nervo facial de um animal, os músculos faciais desnervados contraem-se, quando o animal é amedrontado ou fica enfurecido; é causada pela liberação de acetilcolina na circulação.
fuchsinophil r., r. fucsinofílica; a propriedade apresentada por certos elementos, quando corados com a fucsina ácida, de reter o corante ao serem tratados com álcool do ácido pícrico.
furfurol r., r. do furfurol; a produção de uma cor vermelha ao se adicionar furfurol a uma solução de anilina.
galvanic skin r., r. galvânica da pele. SIN galvanic skin *response*.
gel diffusion r.'s, reações de difusão em gel. SIN gel diffusion precipitin *tests*, em *test*.
Gell and Coombs r.'s, reações de Gell e Coombs. VER allergic r.
gemistocytic r., r. gemistocítica; r. à lesão resultante da proliferação de astrócitos reativos, protoplásticos ou gemistocíticos.
general adaptation r., r. geral de adaptação. VER general adaptation *syndrome*.
Gerhardt r., r. de Gerhardt. SIN Gerhardt *test* for acetoacetic acid.
graft versus host r. (GVHR), r. enxerto *versus* hospedeiro; as alterações histológicas e clínicas da doença do enxerto *versus* hospedeiro que ocorrem em um órgão específico.
group r., r. ao grupo; r. com uma aglutinina ou com outro anticorpo que é comum (embora geralmente em concentrações variáveis) a um grupo inteiro de bactérias correlatas, p. ex., o grupo coli.
Gruber r., r. de Gruber. SIN Widal r.
Gruber-Widal r., r. de Gruber-Widal. SIN Widal r.
Günning r., r. de Günning; a formação de iodofórmio a partir da acetona por meio do iodo e da amônia em álcool.
Haber-Weiss r., r. de Haber-Weiss; a reação do superóxido ($O_2\cdot^-$) com o peróxido de hidrogênio para produzir oxigênio molecular (O_2), radical hidróxido (OH·) e OH^-; é freqüentemente catalisada pelo ferro; uma fonte de estresse oxidativo nas células sangüíneas e em diversos tecidos.
harlequin r., r. de arlequim; o clareamento súbito da metade inferior do corpo de um bebê em decúbito lateral, permanecendo a metade restante do corpo com coloração normal.
heel-tap r., r. à percussão do calcanhar. VER heel *tap*.
hemoclastic r., r. hemoclástica; a hemólise conforme é observada no lavado de sangue.
Henle r., r. de Henle; a coloração castanho-escura observada nas células da medula da supra-renal, quando tratadas com sais de cromo; as células do córtex permanecem não-coradas.
Herxheimer r., r. de Herxheimer; r. inflamatória observada nos tecidos afetados pela sífilis (pele, mucosas, sistema nervoso ou vísceras) e induzida em certos casos pelo tratamento específico com Salvarsan, mercúrio ou antibióticos; acredita-se que seja resultante da rápida liberação do antígeno treponêmico no organismo do paciente associada a reação alérgica. SIN Jarisch-Herxheimer r.
Hill r., r. de Hill; aquela parte da r. fotossintética que envolve a fotólise da água e a liberação de oxigênio e não inclui a fixação do dióxido de carbono. Engloba a adição de oxidantes (quinonas ou ferricianeto) aos cloroplastos; sob iluminação, O_2 é produzido e o oxidante adicionado é reduzido.
homograft r., r. do homoenxerto; a rejeição de um enxerto alogênico pelo hospedeiro.
hunting r., r. da caça; r. incomum dos vasos sangüíneos dos dedos expostos ao frio; ocorre alternância de vasoconstrição e vasodilatação em seqüências repetidas e irregulares, em uma aparente tentativa de equilibrar a temperatura da pele.
hypersensitivity r., r. de hipersensibilidade. SIN allergic r.
id r., ide; uma manifestação alérgica da candidíase, das dermatofitoses e de outras micoses caracterizada por prurido e lesões vesiculares que surgem em resposta às infecções superficiais que estão distantes da própria ide. VER TAMBÉM dermatophytid, -id (1).
r. of identity, r. de identidade. VER gel diffusion precipitin *tests* in two dimensions, em *test*.
immediate r., r. imediata; a resposta local ou generalizada que se inicia alguns minutos a cerca de uma hora após a exposição a um antígeno ao qual a pessoa foi sensibilizada. VER TAMBÉM skin *test*, wheal-and-erythema r. SIN early r.
immediate hypersensitivity r., r. de hipersensibilidade imediata; resposta imune mediada por anticorpos, em geral por IgE, que ocorre alguns minutos após um segundo contato com um mesmo antígeno, resultando na liberação de histamina e subseqüente tumefação e vasodilatação.
immune r., r. imune; r. antígeno-anticorpo que indica um certo grau de resistência, em geral em referência à reação de 36 a 48 horas que ocorre na vacinação contra a varíola; como o grau de resistência indicado pela r. não corresponde à imunidade verdadeira e pode desaparecer de modo relativamente rápido, há uma tendência a referir-se à r. imune como uma r. alérgica.
incompatible blood transfusion r., r. de transfusão de sangue incompatível; síndrome que resulta da hemólise intravascular do sangue transfundido desencadeada pelos anticorpos do soro do receptor, que reagem com um antígeno presente nas hemácias do doador; caracteriza-se por calafrios, febre, dor nas costas ou cãibras musculares, hemoglobinemia, hemoglobinúria e oligúria, que podem levar a insuficiência renal aguda, coagulação intravascular disseminada e morte.
indirect pupillary r., r. consensual. SIN consensual r.
intracutaneous r., intradermal r., r. intracutânea, r. intradérmica; r. após a injeção de um antígeno na pele de uma pessoa sensível, tal como ocorre no caso do teste da tuberculina.
iodate r. of epinephrine, r. da epinefrina ao iodato; r. que depende da oxidação da epinefrina pelo iodo liberado do iodato, o qual é decomposto pelo hormônio; resulta em cor-de-rosa fraca.
iodine r. of epinephrine, r. da epinefrina ao iodo; r. que resulta da oxidação do hormônio; a adição de iodo provoca o surgimento de uma cor-de-rosa fraca.
irreversible r., r. irreversível; r. ou resposta dos tecidos frente a um agente patogênico, caracterizada por alteração patológica permanente.
Jaffe r., r. de Jaffe; um complexo laranja-avermelhado brilhante resultante do tratamento da creatinina com uma solução alcalina de picrato; é a base da maioria dos testes de creatinina de rotina.

Jarisch-Herxheimer r., r. de Jarisch-Herxheimer. SIN Herxheimer r.
Jolly r., r. de Jolly; a perda rápida da resposta à estimulação farádica de um músculo com preservação da resposta galvânica e da força da contração voluntária; uma técnica obsoleta para detectar a miastenia grave. SIN myasthenic r.
Kiliani-Fischer r., r. de Kiliani-Fischer. VER Kiliani-Fischer *synthesis*.
late r., r. tardia. SIN delayed r.
lengthening r., r. de alongamento; no animal descerebrado, o relaxamento um tanto súbito com alongamento dos músculos extensores que ocorre quando um membro é fletido de forma passiva; está associada à espasticidade do tipo canivete.
lepromin r., r. leprominica; r. de hipersensibilidade tardia que ocorre no local de uma injeção intradérmica de uma leproprina, tal como o antígeno de Dharmendra ou o antígeno de Mitsuda, em um teste leprominico; as reações, p. ex., a r. de Fernandez ou a r. de Mitsuda, são variáveis, ocorrendo em 48 horas ou no intervalo de 3 a 5 semanas, mas apresentam-se negativas na hanseníase lepromatosa, na hanseníase dimorfa (*borderline*) e na hanseníase dimorfo-tuberculóide ou dimorfo-lepromatosa.
leukemoid r., r. leucemóide. VER leukemoid reaction.
lid-closure r., r. de fechamento das pálpebras. SIN eye-closure pupil r.
Liebermann-Burchard r., r. de Liebermann-Burchard. VER Burchard-Liebermann r.
ligase chain r., r. da cadeia da ligase; uma técnica para amplificar o DNA, na qual a DNA ligase é utilizada para unir duas amostras de oligonucleotídios complementares que se ligaram a uma seqüência-alvo *in vitro*. O produto da ligação é usado como modelo para a ligação de oligonucleotídios complementares que, por meio de processamento enzimático repetido, permitem o acúmulo logarítmico dos produtos que podem ser empregados na determinação de alvos de interesse.
local r., r. localizada. SIN focal r.
local anesthetic r., r. anestésica local; r. tóxica resultante da absorção de um anestésico local durante uma anestesia regional, que varia de sonolência a convulsões e colapso cardiovascular.
Loewenthal r., r. de Loewenthal; a r. de aglutinação observada na febre recorrente.
Lohmann r., r. de Lohmann; a r. catalisada pela creatinoquinase.
magnet r., r. magnética; uma r. observada em um animal desprovido de cerebelo; quando o animal é colocado em decúbito dorsal com a cabeça fortemente fletida, todas as articulações dos quatro membros tornam-se fletidas. Por causa da estimulação dos receptores das camadas profundas da pele, uma leve pressão feita com o dedo sobre o coxim de um dos dedos do pé desencadeia uma contração reflexa dos músculos extensores dos membros; o membro é, dessa forma, gentilmente pressionado contra o dedo do examinador e, quando o dedo é retirado de modo suave, o examinador tem a sensação de que o dedo está levantando o membro ou o está atraindo como se fosse um ímã.
Marchi r., r. de Marchi; a falha em tingir de preto a bainha de mielina de um nervo, quando essa é submetida à ação do ácido ósmico.
Mazzotti r., r. de Mazzotti. SIN Mazzotti test.
Millon r., r. de Millon; a r. dos compostos fenólicos (p. ex., a tirosina de uma proteína) com $Hg(NO_3)_2$ em HNO_3 (e um traço de HNO_2); o produto apresenta cor vermelha.
miostagmin r., r. da miostagmina; um teste fisioquímico de imunidade projetado por Ascoli que consiste na determinação da tensão superficial de um soro imune ao qual o antígeno específico foi adicionado, antes e após incubação a 37°C durante 2 horas; em uma r. positiva, a tensão superficial está diminuída, conforme indicado por um estalagmômetro.
Mitsuda r., r. de Mitsuda; r. de hipersensibilidade tardia à leproprina que surge na forma de nódulos eritêmato-papulosos no local de uma injeção intradérmica de antígeno de Mitsuda em um teste leprominico.
mixed agglutination r., r. de aglutinação mista; uma aglutinação de base imunológica na qual os agregados contêm células de dois tipos diferentes, mas com determinantes antigênicos comuns a ambos; quando são utilizadas na identificação de isoantígenos, as células do teste são expostas a isoanticorpos apropriados, lavadas e, então, misturadas com eritrócitos indicadores que se combinam aos sítios livres do isoanticorpo ligado às células do teste.
mixed lymphocyte culture r., r. de cultura mista de linfócitos. VER mixed lymphocyte culture *test*.
monomolecular r., r. monomolecular; uma r. que envolve uma única molécula (p. ex., a decomposição, o rearranjo intramolecular, a oxidação ou a redução intramolecular), mesmo quando um agente catalítico — tal como um ácido ou um álcali — estiver presente em excesso na forma molecular, ou quando a reação não for dependente da velocidade; tais reações são em geral reações de primeira ordem. Cf. molecularity. SIN unimolecular r.
myasthenic r., r. miastênica. SIN Jolly r.
Nadi r., r. de Nadi. SIN peroxidase r.
near r., r. próxima; a constrição da pupila associada ao esforço para ver de perto, i.e., com a acomodação e a convergência.

nested polymerase chain r., r. em cadeia da polimerase aninhada; a utilização da r. em cadeia da polimerase de tal modo que um pedaço específico do DNA é amplificado e, em seguida, uma parte contida dentro desse primeiro pedaço é amplificada; a r. é utilizada na presença de quantidades extremamente pequenas de DNA, de problemas de infra-estrutura ou de contaminação do DNA.
Neufeld r., r. de Neufeld. SIN Neufeld capsular *swelling*.
neurotonic r., r. neurotônica; a contração muscular que se mantém após a cessação do estímulo.
neutral r., r. neutra; pH de 7,00; concentrações dos íons H^+ e OH^- iguais a 10^{-7} mol/L a 22°C. Cf. dissociation *constant* of water.
ninhydrin r., r. da ninidrina; um teste para proteínas, peptonas, peptídeos e aminoácidos que possuem grupamentos carboxila e α-amina livres baseado na r. com hidrato de tricetoidrindeno; uma r. de cor azul é utilizada para quantificar os aminoácidos livres (p. ex., após a hidrólise e a separação dos aminoácidos de uma proteína). SIN triketohydrindene r.
nitritoid r., r. nitritóide; uma r. grave semelhante àquela que se segue à administração de nitritos e às vezes observada na administração intravenosa da arsfenamina ou de outras drogas; consiste em rubor da face, edema da língua e dos lábios, vômitos, sudorese profusa, queda da pressão sangüínea e, às vezes, morte.
r. of nonidentity, r. de não-identidade. VER gel diffusion precipitin *tests* in two dimensions, em *test*.
nuclear r., r. nuclear; a interação entre dois núcleos atômicos, ou de um núcleo atômico com uma partícula subatômica, ou de partículas subatômicas dentro de um núcleo atômico, que resulta em uma alteração na natureza dos núcleos envolvidos ou no conteúdo energético dos núcleos ou de ambos, em geral manifestada pela transmutação (acompanhada pela emissão de raios alfa, beta e/ou gama) ou pela fissão ou fusão dos núcleos.
oxidase r., r. da oxidase; (1) a formação de azul de indol quando um esfregaço de sangue contendo leucócitos mielóides é tratado com uma mistura de α-naftol e sulfato de *p*-dimetilanilina; os leucócitos mielóides contêm uma oxidase que catalisa essa r., e os leucócitos linfóides não; (2) em bacteriologia, uma r. que depende da presença de certas oxidases em algumas bactérias que catalisam o transporte de elétrons entre os doadores de elétrons nas bactérias e um corante oxirredutor, tal como a tetrametil-*p*-fenilenodiamina; o corante é reduzido a uma cor azul ou preta.
oxidation-reduction r., r. de oxirredução. VER oxidation-reduction.
pain r., r. à dor; a dilatação da pupila ou qualquer outro ato involuntário que ocorre em resposta a um estímulo que provoca dor aguda em qualquer parte do corpo.
Pandy r., r. de Pandy; um teste para determinar a presença de proteínas (principalmente globulinas) no líquido espinal, pela adição de uma gota de líquido espinal a 1 mL de solução (p. ex., cristais de ácido carbólico em água destilada, cresol ou ácido pirogálico); o produto da r. varia de uma fraca turvação à formação de um precipitado "leitoso" e denso, de acordo com a quantidade de proteínas. SIN Pandy test.
r. of partial identity, r. de identidade parcial; ver gel diffusion precipitin *tests* in two dimensions, em *test*.
passive cutaneous anaphylactic r., r. anafilática cutânea passiva; VER passive cutaneous *anaphylaxis*.
Paul r., r. de Paul; consiste na fricção de pus em uma escarificação feita no olho de um coelho; se o pus for proveniente de uma pústula da varíola ou da vacina contra a varíola, uma condição denominada epiteliose desenvolve-se dentro de 36 a 48 horas; diz-se que a saliva de um paciente com varíola provoca a mesma r. SIN Paul test.
performic acid r., r. do ácido perfórmico; a destruição oxidativa da dupla ligação do etileno (–HC=CH–) que é convertido a um aldeído duplo do reativo de Schiff; é utilizada para indicar a presença de lipídios insaturados, tais como os fosfolipídios e os cerebrosídios, bem como de substâncias ricas em cistina, tais como ceratina, em cortes de tecidos.
periosteal r., r. periostal; osso subperiostal detectável pela radiografia e formado como uma r. aos tecidos moles ou a uma doença óssea.
peroxidase r., r. da peroxidase; a formação de azul de indofenol pela ação de uma enzima oxidante presente em células e tecidos específicos, quando esses são tratados com uma solução de α-naftol e dimetilparafenilenodiamina; por meio dessa técnica, as células da série mielocítica, que tornam a r. positiva, podem ser distinguidas daquelas da série linfocítica, que tornam a r. negativa. SIN Nadi r.
phosphoroclastic r., r. fosfoclástica; a clivagem das ligações C–C que envolve a transferência de fosfato, mas não diretamente a um dos produtos, como ocorre na fosforólise; p. ex., a decomposição de piruvato em acetato + CO_2, na qual o ortofosfato é adicionado a ADP para formar ATP.
Pirquet r., r. de Pirquet. SIN Pirquet test.
plasmal r., r. plasmática; uma técnica histoquímica que utiliza o cloreto de mercúrio para revelar o grupamento aldeído dos acetalfosfatídios e permitir a coloração de Schiff.
pleural r., r. pleural; o espessamento de uma faixa da pleura observado em radiografias de tórax, que indica pleurite, derrame pleural ou fibrose pleural.

polymerase chain r. (PCR) (po-lim′er-ās), r. em cadeia da polimerase; uma técnica enzimática para a cópia repetida de duas fitas de ADN de uma seqüência de genes específica. É amplamente utilizada para amplificar diminutas quantidades de material biológico de modo a fornecer amostras adequadas para estudo laboratorial.

A duplicação do DNA nas células vivas é facilitada pelas polimerases. As duas cadeias de DNA de dupla hélice primeiramente desvencilham-se uma da outra, e, então, a DNA polimerase gera uma cópia de cada fita por meio da adição de nucleotídios livres, a fim de formar uma seqüência de pares de bases complementar à seqüência da fita. A técnica laboratorial conhecida como reação em cadeia da polimerase — que levou o bioquímico americano Kary Mullis a ganhar um Prêmio Nobel de Química em 1993 — explora a capacidade da DNA polimerase de produzir novo DNA. A Taq polimerase, cujo nome provém de sua fonte, o *Thermus aquaticus*, uma bactéria termofílica, é adicionada a uma mistura de nucleotídios livres e primers. (Os primers são unidades especialmente preparadas que contêm tanto RNA quanto DNA com uma terminação livre onde a polimerase reagirá.) A curta seqüência de DNA a ser amplificada é ladeada por dois primers. Uma vez iniciada a reação, a polimerase gera numerosas cópias da seqüência-alvo. As fases da seqüência da reação são iniciadas simplesmente pela execução de um conjunto de alterações estratégicas na temperatura do sistema. Milhões de cópias da seqüência-alvo podem ser geradas pela repetição cíclica — até 30 vezes — dessas alterações de temperatura, e cada fita de DNA produzida em um ciclo dá origem a muitas mais no ciclo seguinte. A técnica é empregada na amplificação de amostras para o diagnóstico tanto de doenças infecciosas quanto genéticas, na realização da impressão digital do DNA e em pesquisas genéticas.

Porter-Silber r., r. de Porter-Silber; a base do teste que quantifica os 17-hidroxicorticosteróides; os esteróides C-21 do córtex da supra-renal, que contêm um grupo diidroxiacetona nos carbonos 19, 20 e 21, reagem com a fenilhidrazina.
Prausnitz-Küstner r., r. de Prausnitz-Küstner; um teste para detectar a presença de hipersensibilidade imediata em seres humanos; o soro do teste, proveniente de uma pessoa atópica, é injetado intradermicamente em uma pessoa normal; após 24 a 48 horas, a pessoa normal é exposta ao antígeno suspeito de desencadear a r. de hipersensibilidade imediata em uma pessoa atópica, em geral na forma de uma pápula eritematosa. SIN P-K test.
precipitin r., r. de precipitina. VER precipitin, precipitin *test*.
primary r., r. primária. SIN vaccinia.
prozone r., r. prozone. VER prozone.
psychogalvanic r., psychogalvanic skin r., r. psicogalvânica, r. psicogalvânica da pele. SIN galvanic skin *response*.
quellung r., r. de quellung; **(1)** SIN Neufeld capsular *swelling*; **(2)** quando pneumococos, tinta-da-índia e anti-soros específicos são misturados, os anticorpos presentes nos soros ligam-se aos antígenos dos polissacarídeos da cápsula dos pneumococos, e a cápsula torna-se mais opaca e tumefeita. Esse teste identifica os pneumococos, bem como os tipos específicos de cápsulas. SIN capsular precipitation r. [Al. *Quellung*, tumefação]
reversed Prausnitz-Küstner r., r. de Prausnitz-Küstner reversa; o surgimento de urticária no local da injeção intradérmica de um soro que contém anticorpos reagínicos em uma pessoa que já apresenta o alérgeno correspondente.
reverse transcriptase polymerase chain r. (RT-PCR), r. em cadeia da polimerase via transcriptase reversa; um processo para a amplificação de RNAm específico no qual a transcriptase reversa adicionada à reação *in vitro* utiliza o RNAm como modelo para produzir um DNAc (DNA complementar), que é, então, amplificado pela reação em cadeia da polimerase.
reversible r., r. reversível; uma r. química que ocorre em ambas as direções, i.e., da esquerda para a direita ou no sentido oposto; a ionização é uma r. desse tipo, assim como as reações que envolvem racemases, isomerases, mutases, transferases etc.
Sakaguchi r., r. de Sakaguchi; guanidinas em solução alcalina desenvolvem uma intensa cor vermelha quando são tratadas com α-naftol e hipoclorito de sódio; um teste qualitativo para detectar a arginina livre ou a que se encontra na estrutura de uma proteína.
Schardinger r., r. de Schardinger; a redução do azul de metileno a branco de metileno pelo formaldeído é rapidamente catalisada pelo leite fresco, mas não pelo leite fervido; o agente catalisador presente no leite fresco é a xantina oxidase (enzima de Schardinger); um exemplo de oxidação na ausência de O_2 com um aceptor orgânico de hidrogênio (o corante).
Schultz r., r. de Schultz. VER Schultz *stain*.
Schultz-Charlton r., r. de Schultz-Charlton; o clareamento característico de uma erupção escarlatiniforme no local da injeção intracutânea de anti-soro da escarlatina. SIN Schultz-Charlton phenomenon.

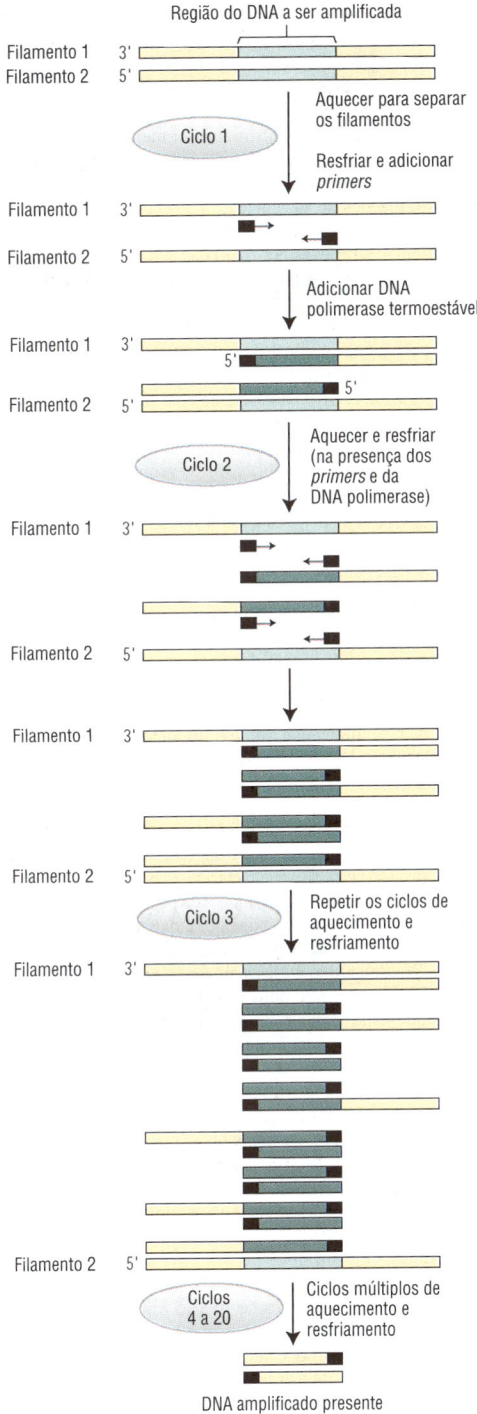

reação da cadeia da polimerase (PCR)

Schultz-Dale r., r. de Schultz-Dale; a contração de uma alça intestinal excisada (Schultz), ou de uma faixa excisada de um útero que nunca se tornou gravídico (Dale) de um animal sensibilizado (cobaia) que ocorre quando esses tecidos são expostos a um antígeno específico.
serum r., r. do soro. SIN serum *sickness*.
shortening r., r. de encurtamento; o encurtamento adaptativo dos músculos extensores dos membros de um animal descerebrado observado quando um membro é estendido após ter sido fletido. Cf. lengthening r.
Shwartzman r., r. de Shwartzman. SIN Shwartzman *phenomenon*.
skin r., r. cutânea. SIN skin *test*.
specific r., r. específica; os fenômenos produzidos por um agente idêntico ou imunologicamente relacionado ao agente que já causou alteração na capacidade de reação do tecido.

startle r., r. de sobressalto. SIN startle *reflex*.
Straus r., r. de Straus; um teste diagnóstico para o mormo. Os porquinhos-da-índia (cobaias) machos são inoculados intraperitonealmente com o material suspeito; quando o organismo causador do mormo está presente, estabelece-se em geral em poucos dias uma inflamação necrosante no saco escrotal, e o organismo específico pode ser confirmado por meio de exame bacteriológico.
stress r., r. de estresse; uma r. emocional aguda relacionada a uma ameaça ou um desafio extremos do ambiente. SIN acute situational r.
supporting r.'s, reações de sustentação; reações descritas por Magnus, que distinguiu dois tipos: **reações de sustentação positivas**, que consistem naquelas contrações musculares reflexas por meio das quais o corpo é sustentado contra a gravidade, observadas de forma exagerada no animal descerebrado; **r. de sustentação negativa**, que consiste na inibição dos músculos extensores e na liberação das articulações que, dessa forma, permitem que o membro seja fletido e movido para uma nova posição. SIN supporting reflexes.
symptomatic r., r. sintomática; uma resposta alérgica semelhante à reação original, mas que ocorre após o uso de uma dose de teste ou terapêutica de um alérgeno ou atopênio.
thermoprecipitin r., r. de termoprecipitina; a formação de um precipitado pela aplicação de calor, como ocorre nos casos de proteinúria.
transcription-based chain r., r. em cadeia baseada na transcrição; uma técnica para realizar a amplificação de DNA ou RNA na qual a transcriptase reversa é empregada na produção de uma molécula de DNA de fita simples para cada DNA ou RNA-alvo; essa molécula é utilizada como um modelo para amplificações posteriores.
***Treponema pallidum* immobilization r.**, r. de imobilização do *Treponema pallidum*. SIN *Treponema pallidum* immobilization *test*.
triketohydrindene r., r. do tricetoidrindeno. SIN ninhydrin r.
type III hypersensitivity r., r. de hipersensibilidade do tipo III; SIN immune complex *disease*.
unimolecular r., r. unimolecular. SIN monomolecular r.
vaccinoid r., r. vacinóide. SIN accelerated r.
Voges-Proskauer r., r. de Voges-Proskauer; r. química utilizada nos testes para a produção de acetilmetilcarbinol por diversas bactérias; consiste na adição de hidróxido de potássio a uma cultura de 24 horas em um meio adequado e completamente misturado; a cultura tratada é exposta ao ar e observada a intervalos de 2, 12 e 24 horas; uma r. positiva caracteriza-se pelo desenvolvimento de uma cor rósea semelhante à da eosina e resultante da produção de acetilmetilcarbinol, que, na presença de um álcali e de oxigênio, é oxidado a diacetil.
Wassermann r. (W. r.), r. de Wassermann. SIN Wassermann *test*.
Weidel r., r. de Weidel; r. que indica a presença de xantina; uma solução composta pela substância suspeita, água clorada e um pouco de ácido nítrico é evaporada em um banho-maria e, em seguida, exposta ao vapor de amônia; o surgimento da cor vermelha ou púrpura indica a presença de xantina.
Weil-Felix r., r. de Weil-Felix. SIN Weil-Felix *test*.
Weinberg r., r. de Weinberg; um teste que consiste na fixação do complemento na presença de doença hidática.
Wernicke r., r. de Wernicke; na hemianopsia, r. resultante de lesão no trato óptico e que consiste na perda da constrição da pupila quando um feixe de luz é dirigido para o lado cego da retina; a constrição da pupila é mantida quando a luz estimula o lado normal. Esse sinal não pode ser observado com um feixe de luz brilhante por causa da difusão intra-ocular sobre a metade normal da retina. SIN Wernicke sign.
wheal-and-erythema r., r. pápula e eritema; a r. imediata e característica observada em um teste cutâneo; cerca de 10 a 15 minutos após a injeção de um antígeno (alérgeno), surge uma pápula irregular, clara e elevada, circundada por uma área eritematosa (rubor). SIN wheal-and-flare r.
wheal-and-flare r., r. pápula e eritema. SIN wheal-and-erythema r.
white r., r. branca; a resposta observada ao se passar levemente um instrumento sem corte sobre a pele de um indivíduo; é atribuída à ação dos capilares.
whitegraft r., r. do enxerto branco; r. imune a um enxerto de tecido incompatível que leva a uma falha na vascularização do enxerto e ao aparecimento de rejeição.
Widal r., r. de Widal; r. de aglutinação observada no teste para o diagnóstico da febre tifóide. SIN Gruber r., Gruber-Widal r.
xanthoprotein r., r. da xantoproteína; teste qualitativo para proteínas; um produto amarelo é formado pelo contato de proteínas reagentes com o ácido nítrico concentrado quente.
Yorke autolytic r., r. autolítica de Yorke; um teste para a hemoglobinúria paroxística; soro é colocado no gelo e mantido a 0°C durante 5 a 7 minutos e, em seguida, em uma incubadora a 37°C juntamente com eritrócitos, durante 1 hora, momento em que, se a r. for positiva, ocorrerá hemólise; se o soro for mantido a 1°C durante uma hora e, em seguida, colocado em uma incubadora com eritrócitos, ocorrerá pouca hemólise.
zero-order r., r. de ordem zero; r. que prossegue a uma velocidade em particular, independentemente da concentração do(s) reagente(s).
Zimmermann r., r. de Zimmermann; r. química que ocorre entre uma solução alcalina de *meta*-dinitrobenzeno e um grupo metileno ativo (carbono 16) dos 17-cetosteróides; é a base do teste para quantificar os 17-cetosteróides; de um modo mais geral, uma r. que ocorre entre as cetonas do metileno e os compostos aromáticos de polinitro em soluções alcalinas. SIN Zimmermann test.

re·ac·ti·vate (rē - ak′ti - vāt). Reativar. **1.** Tornar ativo novamente. **2.** Em particular, diz-se de um soro imune inativado ao qual se adiciona soro normal (complemento).
re·ac·ti·va·tion (rē′ak - ti - vā′shŭn). Reativação. **1.** A restauração da atividade lítica de um soro inativo por meio da adição de complemento. **2.** A restauração da atividade de uma enzima inativada.
re·ac·tiv·i·ty (rē - ak - tiv′i - tē). Reatividade. **1.** A propriedade de reagir, quimicamente ou de qualquer outra forma. **2.** O processo de reagir.
read·ing (rēd′ing). Leitura. **1.** A percepção e o entendimento do significado de símbolos visuais (p. ex., letras ou palavras) por meio da varredura pelos olhos de um texto escrito ou impresso. **2.** Qualquer dos vários modos alternativos de interpretar símbolos, tais como o braile ou a observação cuidadosa dos movimentos faciais do interlocutor.
lip r., leitura labial. SIN speech r.
speech r., leitura labial; utilizada pelas pessoas com deficiência auditiva; consiste na observação dos movimentos da mandíbula e dos lábios, das expressões faciais e de outros gestos feitos pelo interlocutor. SIN lip r.
read·ing frame. Fase de leitura; o agrupamento de três nucleotídeos que forma um códon. VER frame-shift *mutation*.
blocked r. f., f. de l. bloqueada; uma seqüência de DNA que não pode ser traduzida em uma proteína viável; é geralmente resultante da interrupção por um ou mais códons de terminação. SIN closed r. f.
closed r. f., f. de l. fechada. SIN blocked r. f.
open r. f., f. de l. aberta; um gene que se presume ser o responsável pela codificação de uma proteína, mas cujo produto (de gene) ainda não foi identificado; é também conhecida como fase de leitura não-identificada; SIN unidentified r. f.
unidentified r. f. (URF), f. de l. não-identificada. SIN open r. f.
read·through (rēd′throo). Em biologia molecular, a transcrição de uma seqüência de ácido nucléico além de sua seqüência de terminação normal.
re·a·gent (rē - ā′jent). Reativo, reagente; qualquer substância que é adicionada a uma solução formada por outra substância para participar de uma reação química. [L. mod. *reagens*]
amino acid r., r. para aminoácidos; um r. utilizado na identificação e quantificação de aminoácidos.
Benedict-Hopkins-Cole r., r. de Benedict-Hopkins-Cole; glioxalato de magnésio feito a partir de uma mistura de ácido oxálico e magnésio e utilizado em testes para detectar a presença do triptofano em proteínas.
biuret r., r. do biureto; uma solução alcalina de sulfato de cobre.
Cleland r., r. de Cleland. SIN dithiothreitol.
diazo r., r. diazo, diazorreação; solução ácida de ácido sulfanílico e outra de nitrito de sódio, ambas utilizadas no processo da diazotação. SIN Ehrlich diazo r.
Dische r., r. de Dische. VER Dische *reaction*.
Dische-Schwarz r., r. de Dische-Schwarz; um r. utilizado na detecção colorimétrica do RNA.
Drabkin r., r. de Drabkin; uma solução utilizada no método da cianometemoglobina para a quantificação da hemoglobina. Consiste em bicarbonato de sódio, cianeto de potássio e ferricianeto de potássio.
Dragendorff r., r. de Dragendorff; um r. utilizado na detecção de alcalóides.
Edlefsen r., r. de Edlefsen; uma solução alcalina de permanganato utilizada na detecção de açúcar na urina.
Edman r., r. de Edman. SIN phenylisothiocyanate.
Ehrlich diazo r., r. diazo de Ehrlich. SIN diazo r.
Erdmann r., r. de Erdmann; uma mistura de ácidos sulfúrico e nítrico utilizada em testes para detectar alcalóides.
Esbach r., r. de Esbach; ácido pícrico, ácido cítrico e água (na proporção de 1:2:97) utilizados na detecção de albumina na urina.
Exton r., r. de Exton; composto por 50 g de ácido sulfossalicílico e 200 g de $Na_2SO_4 \cdot 10H_2O$ em um litro de água e utilizado em um teste para detectar albumina.
Fehling r., r. de Fehling. SIN Fehling *solution*.
Folin r., r. de Folin. SIN Folin *reaction*.
Fouchet r., r. de Fouchet; uma solução a 25% de ácido tricloroacético que contém 0,9% de cloreto férrico; ao se adicionar uma gota do r. à linha de superfície de um papel filtro impregnado com cloreto de bário e previamente imerso em urina durante 10 s, observa-se o surgimento de uma cor verde, caso a urina contenha bilirrubina. VER TAMBÉM Fouchet *stain*.
Froehde r., r. de Froehde; molibdato de sódio em ácido sulfúrico forte; em contato com alcalóides, esse reagente produz reações de diversas cores.
Frohn r., r. de Frohn; o aquecimento de subnitrato de bismuto (1,5) e água (20,0) até a fervura e, em seguida, a adição de ácido clorídrico (10,0) e iodeto de potássio (7,0); é utilizado nos testes para a detecção de alcalóides e açúcar.

Girard r., r. de Girard; a utilização da hidrazina do cloreto de betaína na extração de esteróides cetônicos por meio da formação de hidrazonas hidrossolúveis com eles.

Günzberg r., r. de Günzberg; a utilização de floroglucina e vanilina como um r. no teste de Günzberg.

Hahn oxine r., r. de oxina de Hahn; uma solução alcoólica de 8-hidroxiquinolina utilizada na determinação do zinco, do alumínio, do magnésio e de outros minerais.

Hammarsten r., r. de Hammarsten; a mistura de 1 parte de uma solução a 25% de ácido nítrico e de 19 partes de uma solução a 25% de ácido clorídrico; a adição de algumas gotas de uma amostra à mistura formada por 1 parte desse r. e por 4 partes de álcool fornece uma cor verde, que indica a presença de bile na amostra.

Ilosvay r., r. de Ilosvay; é composto por 0,5 de ácido sulfanílico dissolvido em 150 de ácido acético diluído, misturados a 1 de naftilamina e dissolvidos em 20 de água fervente; o sedimento azul que se forma é dissolvido em 150 de ácido acético diluído; a adição de algumas gotas desse r. a água, saliva ou a outros líquidos a serem testados produzirá uma cor vermelha, caso esses líquidos contenham nitritos.

Kasten fluorescent Schiff r.'s, reativos de Schiff fluorescente de Kasten; análogos fluorescentes do r. de Schiff que são corantes básicos fluorescentes desprovidos dos grupos laterais ácidos e que contêm um ou mais grupos amina primários; são utilizados na detecção citoquímica do DNA na coloração de Feulgen fluorescente de Kasten e na coloração PAS fluorescente de Kasten e de proteínas na coloração de Schiff-ninidrina; tais análogos incluem a acriflavina, a auramina O e a flavofosfina N.

Lloyd r., r. de Lloyd; silicato de alumínio precipitado que é utilizado na determinação de alcalóides.

Mandelin r., r. de Mandelin; uma solução de vanadato de amônio em ácido sulfúrico que é utilizada nos testes colorimétricos para alcalóides.

Marme r., r. de Marme; solução de iodeto de potássio e iodeto de cádmio utilizada em testes para alcalóides.

Marquis r., r. de Marquis; solução de formaldeído em ácido sulfúrico utilizada nos testes colorimétricos para alcalóides.

Mecke r., r. de Mecke; solução de ácido selenioso em ácido sulfúrico utilizada nos testes colorimétricos para alcalóides.

Meyer r., r. de Meyer; solução de fenolftaleína e hidróxido de sódio em água (destilada); na presença de traços de sangue, a solução torna-se púrpura ou vermelho-azulada.

Millon r., r. de Millon; nitrato de mercúrio e ácido nítrico como são utilizados na reação de Millon.

Nessler r., r. de Nessler; solução de hidróxido de potássio, iodeto de mercúrio e iodeto de potássio; em contato com a amônia, produz uma cor amarela (e um precipitado marrom com quantidades maiores de amônia) que pode ser utilizada em análises quantitativas.

Rosenthaler-Turk r., r. de Rosenthaler-Turk; solução de arseniato de potássio em ácido sulfúrico utilizada na obtenção de testes colorimétricos de diversos alcalóides do ópio.

Sanger r., r. de Sanger. SIN fluoro-2,4-dinitrobenzene.

Schaer r., r. de Schaer; solução alcoólica ou aquosa de hidrato de cloral utilizada como um meio de extração em investigações de alcalóides.

Scheibler r., r. de Scheibler; uma solução de tungstato de sódio em ácido fosfórico utilizada nos testes para alcalóides.

Schiff r., r. de Schiff; solução aquosa de fucsina básica ou de pararrosanilina que é descorada pelo dióxido de enxofre e comumente preparada pela adição de ácido clorídrico a uma solução do corante contendo um sal de metabissulfito ou bissulfito; é utilizada para aldeídos e, em histoquímica, na detecção de polissacarídeos, DNA e proteínas. VER Feulgen *stain*, periodic acid-Schiff *stain*, ninhydrin-Schiff *stain* for proteins.

Scott-Wilson r., r. de Scott-Wilson; solução alcalina de cianeto de mercúrio e nitrato de prata utilizada na detecção da acetona.

sulfhydryl r., r. da sulfidrila; substância que reage com os grupos tióis, sobretudo aqueles presentes nas proteínas.

Sulkowitch r., r. de Sulkowitch; r. utilizado na detecção de cálcio na urina; consiste em 2,5 g de ácido oxálico, 2,5 g de oxalato de amônio, 5 mL de ácido acético glacial e água destilada suficiente para completar 150 mL; ocorre a formação de um precipitado leitoso de oxalato de cálcio quando o r. é adicionado à urina que contém cálcio.

Uffelmann r., r. de Uffelmann; solução preparada pela adição de uma solução a 2% de fenol em água ao cloreto férrico aquoso até a solução tornar-se violeta; a solução passa a amarelo-limão na presença do ácido lático, adquire uma cor opalina em contato com o ácido butírico e é descorada pelo ácido clorídrico.

Wurster r., r. de Wurster; papel filtro impregnado com tetrametil-*p*-fenilenodiamina que se torna azul na presença de ozônio ou de peróxido de hidrogênio.

re·a·gin (rē-ā′jin). Reagina. **1.** O termo dado por Wolff-Eisner para um anticorpo. **2.** Termo antigo para o anticorpo de "Wassermann"; não confundir com o anticorpo de Prausnitz-Küstner. **3.** Os anticorpos que medeiam as reações de hipersensibilidade imediata (IgE nos seres humanos). **4.** SIN homocytotropic *antibody.*

atopic r., r. atópica. SIN Prausnitz-Küstner *antibody.*

re·a·gin·ic (rē-ā-jin′ik). Reagínico; relativo a uma reagina.

REAL Abreviatura de Revised European-American Classification of Lymphoid Neoplasms. VER REAL *classification*.

re·al·i·ty (rē-al′i-tē). Realidade; aquilo que existe objetivamente e de fato e pode ser consensualmente confirmado. [L. *res,* coisa, fato]

re·al·i·ty aware·ness. Consciência da realidade; a capacidade de distinguir objetos externos como sendo diferentes de si próprio.

ream·er (rē′mer). Alargador; um instrumento rotativo para acabamento ou perfuração utilizado para dar forma a ou aumentar um orifício em um osso ou dente. [A.S. *ryman,* alargar]

engine r., alargador com motor; um instrumento dotado de lâminas espiraladas e movido por um motor, utilizado para alargar os canais radiculares dos dentes.

intramedullary r., alargador intramedular; uma lima utilizada para dar forma ao canal intramedular de um osso longo antes da inserção de um dispositivo ou de uma prótese.

re·ar·range·ment (rē-a-rānj′ment). Rearranjo; reestruturação; p. ex., em uma molécula.

Amadori rearrangement, rearranjo de Amadori; uma reestruturação que ocorre em reações de ligações cruzadas e é observada nas glicosilações do colágeno e das proteínas; p. ex., a conversão dos *N*-glicosídeos de aldoses em *N*-glicosídeos das cetoses correspondentes.

reassignment.

sex r., adequação genital; um processo por meio do qual o sexo de um indivíduo é modificado pela combinação de procedimentos psiquiátricos, psicológicos, farmacológicos e cirúrgicos, em geral como parte do tratamento do transexualismo. SIN sex reversal.

re·at·tach·ment (rē-a-tach′ment). Reinserção; nova inserção do tecido epitelial ou conectivo à superfície de um dente que foi cirurgicamente removido e não exposto ao ambiente da cavidade oral.

Réaumur, René A.F. de, físico francês, 1683–1757. VER R. *scale*.

re·base (rē′bās). Reembasar; em odontologia, o ajustamento de uma dentadura por meio da substituição do material da base da dentadura, sem alterar a relação oclusal dos dentes. VER TAMBÉM reline.

re·breath·ing (rē-brēdh′ing). Reinalação; a inalação de parte ou de todos os gases previamente expirados.

Rebuck skin win·dow tech·nique. Técnica da janela cutânea de Rebuck; ver em technique.

RecA. Uma proteína da *Escherichia coli* que reconhece de maneira específica o DNA monofilamentar e fixa-o a uma seqüência complementar em uma dupla hélice que é homóloga. Isso resulta no deslocamento da fita complementar original da dupla hélice.

re·cal·ci·fi·ca·tion (rē-kal′si-fi-kā′shŭn). Recalcificação; a restauração aos tecidos dos sais de cálcio que foram perdidos.

re·call (rē′kawl). Lembrança, recordação; o processo de relembrar pensamentos, palavras e ações de um evento passado em uma tentativa de retomar os acontecimentos reais.

Récamier, Joseph C.A., ginecologista francês, 1774–1852. VER R. *operation*.

re·ca·nal·i·za·tion (rē-kan′ăl-i-zā′-shŭn). Recanalização. **1.** A restauração do lúmen de um vaso sangüíneo que ocorre após a oclusão trombótica por meio da organização do trombo, com a formação de novos canais. **2.** A restauração espontânea da continuidade do lúmen de qualquer ducto ou tubo ocluídos, como ocorre na r. pós-vasectomia.

re·ca·pit·u·la·tion (rē′kă-pit′u-lā′shŭn). Recapitulação. VER recapitulation *theory*.

re·ceiv·er (rē-sē′ver). Receptor; em química, um recipiente que é fixado a um condensador e recebe o produto da destilação. [L. *receptor,* de *recipio,* receber]

re·cep·tac·u·lum, pl. **re·cep·tac·u·la** (rē′sep-tak′ū-lŭm, -lă). Receptáculo; cisterna. SIN reservoir. [L. de *re-cipio,* pp. *-ceptus,* receber, de *capio,* pegar]

r. chy′li, cisterna do quilo. SIN *cisterna* chyli.

r. gan′glii petro′si, fóssula petrosa. SIN petrosal *fossula*.

r. pecquet′i, r. de Pecquet. SIN *cisterna* chyli.

re·cep·tive (rē-sep′tiv). Receptivo; sensível ou responsivo a estímulos.

r. field, campo receptivo; aquela parte da retina cujos fotorreceptores (cones e bastonetes) estão ligados a uma única fibra nervosa óptica. A resposta de um neurônio à estimulação de seu campo receptivo depende do tipo de neurônio e da parte do campo que é iluminada; um neurônio "liga" é estimulado pela luz que incide no centro de seu campo receptivo e inibido pela luz que incide na periferia; um neurônio "desliga" reage de modo exatamente oposto; isto é, ele é inibido pela luz que incide no centro do campo receptivo. Em ambos os casos, a resposta depende de uma ação do tipo liga-desliga (*on-off*) complexa da retina. Quando um campo receptivo inteiro é iluminado igualmente, há predomínio da resposta dos receptores do centro do campo.

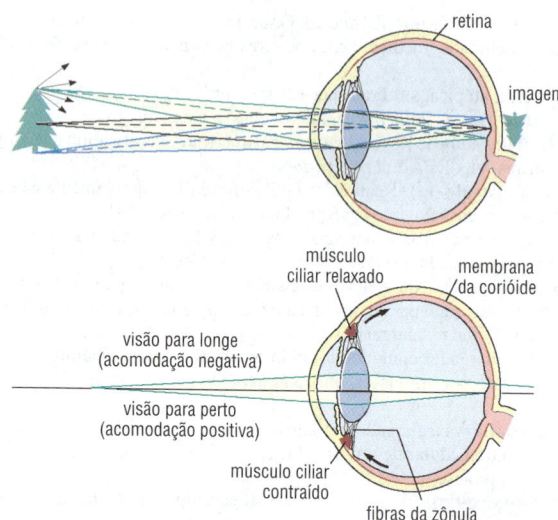

formação da imagem na retina: cada parte do objeto corresponde a parte da imagem na retina; a imagem é uma miniatura invertida do objeto.

re·cep·tor (rē-sep′tŏr, tōr). Receptor. **1.** Uma molécula protéica estrutural localizada na superfície da célula ou dentro de seu citoplasma que se liga a um fator específico, tal como uma droga, um hormônio, um antígeno ou um neurotransmissor. **2.** Termo dado por C. Sherrington para qualquer uma das diversas terminações nervosas sensitivas da pele, dos tecidos profundos, das vísceras e dos órgãos dos sentidos especiais. [L. receptor, de *recipio*, receber]
adrenergic r.'s, receptores adrenérgicos; os componentes reativos dos tecidos efetores; a maioria deles é inervada por fibras pós-ganglionares adrenérgicas do sistema nervoso simpático. Tais receptores podem ser ativados pela norepinefrina e/ou epinefrina e por diversas drogas adrenérgicas; a ativação dos receptores causa uma alteração na função do tecido efetor, como a contração dos músculos das arteríolas ou o relaxamento dos músculos dos brônquios; os receptores adrenérgicos são divididos em receptores α e receptores β, segundo suas respostas aos diversos agentes ativadores e bloqueadores adrenérgicos. SIN adrenoceptor, adrenoreceptors.
α-adrenergic r.'s, receptores α-adrenérgicos; os receptores adrenérgicos localizados nos tecidos efetores que são capazes de ativação e bloqueio seletivos por drogas; são conceitualmente derivados da capacidade de determinados agentes, tal como a fenoxibenzamina, de bloquear apenas alguns receptores adrenérgicos, e de outros agentes, tal como a metoxamina, de ativar apenas os próprios receptores adrenérgicos. Tais receptores são denominados α-receptores. Sua ativação produz respostas fisiológicas, tais como a resistência vascular periférica aumentada, a midríase e a contração dos músculos pilomotores.
β-adrenergic r.'s, receptores β-adrenérgicos; os receptores adrenérgicos localizados nos tecidos efetores que são capazes de ativação e bloqueio seletivos por drogas; são conceitualmente derivados da capacidade de determinados agentes, tal como o propranolol, de bloquear apenas alguns receptores adrenérgicos e de outros agentes, tal como o isoproterenol, de ativar apenas os próprios receptores adrenérgicos. Tais receptores são denominados β-receptores. Sua ativação causa respostas fisiológicas, tais como o aumento da freqüência cardíaca e da força de contração ($β_1$) e o relaxamento da musculatura lisa dos brônquios e dos vasos ($β_2$) contidos no músculo esquelético.
AMPA r., r. de AMPA; um tipo de r. de glutamato que participa da neurotransmissão excitatória e também se liga ao ácido α-amino-3-hidróxi-5-metil-4-isoxazole propiônico e atua como um canal de cátions. SIN quisqualate r.
angiotensin r., r. da angiotensina; os receptores que se ligam à proteína G da superfície das células e que mediam os efeitos da angiotensina II. Conhecem-se dois tipos: AT_1 e AT_2; o primeiro media a poderosa contração dos músculos lisos dos vasos, responsáveis pela resposta hipertensiva produzida pela angiotensina II; o último ainda não é suficientemente compreendido para que se atribua a ele alguma função fisiológica.
ANP r.'s, receptores do PNA; os receptores de superfície de células para o peptídeo natriurético atrial que apresentam um único elemento que atravessa a membrana; esses possuem domínios de cinase e guanilato ciclase integrais.
ANP clearance r.'s, receptores da depuração do PNA; proteínas da superfície celular que se ligam ao peptídeo natriurético atrial e aos fragmentos do PNA, sem iniciar uma ação biológica.
asialoglycoprotein r., r. da asialoglicoproteína; um r. de superfície encontrado nos hepatócitos que se liga às glicoproteínas que apresentam uma galactose em posição terminal; dessa forma, esse r. remove tais proteínas provenientes da circulação, que são, por sua vez, digeridas pelos lisossomas dos hepatócitos.
B cell r.'s, receptores das células B; um complexo que compreende uma molécula de imunoglobulina ligada à membrana associada a duas cadeias (α e β) transdutoras de sinais.
cholinergic r.'s, receptores colinérgicos; os sítios químicos localizados nas células efetoras ou nas sinapses por meio dos quais a acetilcolina exerce sua ação.
epidermal growth factor r. (EGFR), r. do fator de crescimento da epiderme; o r. freqüentemente apresenta-se mais ativo nos tumores epiteliais.
estrogen r., r. de estrógeno; um r. para os estrógenos; sua presença conduz a um prognóstico melhor para os cânceres de mama.
Fas r., r. Fas. VER Fas.
Fc r., r. de Fc; os receptores, presentes em várias células, para o fragmento Fc das imunoglobulinas. Esses receptores reconhecem as imunoglobulinas das classes IgG e IgE.
kainate r., r. do cainato; um tipo de r. de glutamato que participa da neurotransmissão excitatória e também se liga ao cainato e age como um canal de cátions; uma injeção de cainato provoca a morte de neurônios, mas preserva as células gliais e os axônios.
laminin r., r. da laminina; um r. encontrado em muitos tipos de células que se liga à laminina e desempenha um papel importante na união das células e no desenvolvimento da neurite.
L-AP$_4$ r., r. de L-AP$_4$; um tipo de receptor de glutamato que também se liga a um agonista sintético específico e age como um canal de cátions.
low-density lipoprotein r.'s, receptores de lipoproteína de baixa densidade; receptores localizados na superfície das células, principalmente das células do fígado, que se ligam às proteínas de baixa densidade e promovem sua depuração do plasma.
mannose-6-phosphate r.'s (MPR), receptores da manose-6-fosfato; receptores localizados no aparelho de Golgi aos quais se ligam as proteínas recém-sintetizadas que posteriormente penetrarão nos lisossomas.
metabotropic r., r. metabotrópico; um tipo de r. que está associado à produção intracelular de 1,2-diacilglicerol e 1,4,5-trifosfato de inositol. [metabolism + G. *tropē*, volta, inclinação, + -ic]
muscarinic r.'s, receptores muscarínicos; proteínas ligadas à membrana cujo domínio extracelular contém um sítio de reconhecimento para a acetilcolina (ACL); a combinação da acetilcolina com o r. inicia uma alteração fisiológica (lentificação da freqüência cardíaca, aumento da atividade secretória das glândulas e estimulação das contrações da musculatura lisa); as alterações são observadas após um tratamento com a muscarina do alcalóide de cogumelo. Os receptores muscarínicos diferem dos receptores nicotínicos.
nicotinic r.'s, receptores nicotínicos; uma classe de receptores colinérgicos localizados nas células dos músculos esqueléticos que estão associados aos canais de íons presentes na membrana das células.
nicotinic cholinergic r., r. colinérgico nicotínico; uma classe de receptores que respondem à acetilcolina e que também são ativados pela nicotina; os receptores ganglionares (que incluem a medula da supra-renal) e neuromusculares. Existem duas classes: nicotínico-neuronal e nicotínico-muscular.
NMDA r., r. de NMDA; um tipo de r. de glutamato que participa da neurotransmissão excitatória e que também se liga ao *N*-metil-D-aspartato; pode estar particularmente envolvido na lesão celular observada em indivíduos com a doença de Huntington.
opiate r.'s, receptores opióides; regiões do cérebro que apresentam a capaci-

receptores β-adrenérgicos

principais efeitos dos diversos subtipos de receptores β sobre os órgãos

	órgão	função do receptor
tipo β$_1$	coração	aumento da freqüência cardíaca, da contratilidade, da velocidade de condução
	rim	aumento da liberação de renina
	tecido adiposo	aumento da lipólise
Tipo β$_2$	brônquios	dilatação dos brônquios contraídos
	vasos sangüíneos	produção de vasodilatação nos vasos sangüíneos dos músculos esqueléticos
	útero	relaxamento do músculo liso do útero
	pâncreas (células β)	aumento da liberação de insulina
	fígado, músculos esqueléticos	aumento da glicogenólise
	tecido adiposo	aumento da lipólise

dade de se ligar à morfina; alguns receptores estão em áreas relacionadas à dor (ao longo do aqueduto de Sylvius e no centro mediano), mas outros, localizados no estriado, não estão.

orphan r., r. órfão; r. de núcleo ao qual nenhum ligante foi associado ainda.
progesterone r., r. da progesterona; r. intracelular para a progesterona; estão freqüentemente mais ativos no câncer de mama.
quisqualate r., r. do quisqualato. SIN AMPA r.
retinoic acid r., r. do ácido retinóico; r. de núcleo para o ácido retinóico.
retinoid X r., r. do retinóide X; r. para os ácidos retinóicos; apresenta menos afinidade pelo ácido retinóico do que os receptores do ácido retinóico; a função ainda não é bem conhecida.
ryanodine r., r. da rianodina; r. associado ao canal de condutância do cálcio encontrado no retículo sarcoplasmático ou endoplasmático das células, que, ao se ligar à rianodina, faz com que o canal permaneça em um estado subcondutivo, permitindo, assim, a liberação contínua e lenta de íons de cálcio do retículo sarcoplasmático para o interior do citoplasma. Os canais habitualmente são sensíveis aos íons de cálcio e não são sensíveis ao trifosfato de inositol.
scavenger r., r. de varredura; um r. localizado nos macrófagos que se liga preferencialmente à LDL oxidada, fazendo com que os macrófagos englobem a LDL.
sensory r.'s, receptores sensoriais; as terminações periféricas dos neurônios aferentes.
stretch r.'s, receptores de estiramento; os receptores que são sensíveis ao estiramento, em particular aqueles receptores encontrados nos órgãos tendinosos de Golgi e nos fusos musculares, mas também aqueles receptores situados nas vísceras, tais como o estômago, o intestino delgado e a bexiga urinária; esses receptores possuem a função de detectar um estiramento, característica que os distingue dos barorreceptores, que, na verdade, são ativados pelo estiramento da parede dos vasos sangüíneos, mas cuja função é desencadear o mecanismo reflexo central que reduz a pressão sangüínea arterial.
T cell antigen r.'s, receptores dos antígenos das células T; os receptores presentes nas células T que interagem de modo simultâneo tanto com o antígeno processado quanto com os antígenos de histocompatibilidade principal; esses são heterodímeros que consistem em uma cadeia α e outra β, ou em uma cadeia γ e outra δ.

re·cep·to·somes (rē-sep'tō-sōms). Receptossomas; vesículas que "evitam" os lisossomas e liberam seu conteúdo em outros locais dentro da célula.
re·cess (rē'ses) [TA]. Recesso; um pequeno orifício ou recorte. SIN recessus [TA]. [L. *recessus*]
anterior r., r. anterior; um aprofundamento circunscrito da fossa interpeduncular na direção dos corpos mamilares. SIN recessus anterior [TA].
anterior r. of tympanic membrane [TA], r. anterior da membrana timpânica; espaço semelhante a uma fenda localizado na parede do tímpano, entre a prega malear anterior e a membrana timpânica. SIN recessus anterior membranae tympanicae [TA], Tröltsch pockets, Tröltsch r.'s.
azygoesophageal r., r. azigoesofágico; a região situada abaixo do arco da veia ázigos na qual o pulmão direito invade o mediastino, entre o coração e a coluna vertebral, limitada à esquerda pelo esôfago.
cecal r., r. cecal. SIN retrocecal r.
cerebellopontine r., r. cerebelopontino. VER cerebellopontine *angle*.
cochlear r. [TA], r. coclear; pequena depressão localizada na parede interna do vestíbulo do labirinto, na parte da pirâmide do vestíbulo, entre os dois ramos nos quais a crista do vestíbulo se divide posteriormente; é perfurada pelos foramens que dão passagem às fibras que o ramo coclear do nervo vestibulococlear envia para a extremidade posterior do ducto coclear. SIN recessus cochlearis [TA], Reichert cochlear r.
costodiaphragmatic r. [TA], r. costodiafragmático; a extensão da cavidade pleural semelhante a uma fenda e localizada entre o diafragma e a caixa torácica; os derrames pleurais acumulam-se nessa região quando o indivíduo permanece em posição ortostática e, uma vez que o pulmão penetra-a apenas parcialmente, é o local de escolha para a realização da toracocentese. SIN recessus costodiaphragmaticus [TA], phrenicocostal sinus.
costomediastinal r. [TA], r. costomediastinal; o recesso da cavidade pleural situado entre as cartilagens costais e o mediastino. SIN recessus costomediastinalis [TA], costomediastinal sinus.
duodenojejunal r., r. duodenojejunal. SIN superior duodenal *fossa*.
elliptical r. of bony labyrinth [TA], r. elíptico do labirinto ósseo; uma depressão oval localizada no teto e na parede interior do vestíbulo do labirinto que aloja o utrículo. SIN recessus ellipticus labyrinthi ossei [TA], recessus utricularis labyrinthi ossei*, utricular r. of bony labyrinth*, fovea elliptica, fovea hemielliptica.
epitympanic r. [TA], r. epitimpânico; a parte superior da cavidade timpânica situada acima da membrana timpânica; contém a cabeça do martelo e o corpo da bigorna. SIN recessus epitympanicus [TA], attic, epitympanic space, epitympanum, Hyrtl epitympanic r., tympanic attic.
hepatoenteric r., r. hepatoentérico; r. peritoneal localizado na extremidade caudal do r. pneumoentérico embrionário; separa o fígado do estômago, ambos em desenvolvimento.
hepatorenal r. of subhepatic space [TA], r. hepatorrenal do espaço sub-hepático; o recesso profundo do espaço sub-hepático situado no lado direito da cavidade peritoneal e que se estende para cima entre o fígado (frente) e o rim e a supra-renal (atrás); é a parte da cavidade peritoneal que depende da gravidade, quando o indivíduo está na posição supina; os líquidos que drenam da bolsa omental escoam pelo recesso. SIN recessus hepatorenalis, recessus subhepatici [TA], hepatorenal pouch, Morison pouch.
Hyrtl epitympanic r., r. epitimpânico de Hyrtl. SIN epitympanic r.
inferior duodenal r., r. duodenal inferior. SIN inferior duodenal *fossa*.
inferior ileocecal r. [TA], r. ileocecal inferior; uma fossa profunda às vezes encontrada entre a prega ileocecal, o mesoapêndice e o ceco. SIN recessus ileocecalis inferior [TA].
inferior omental r., r. omental inferior. SIN inferior r. of omental bursa.
inferior r. of omental bursa [TA], r. inferior da bolsa omental; um recesso da bolsa omental que se estende entre as camadas anterior e posterior do omento maior. SIN recessus inferior omentalis [TA], inferior omental r.
infundibular r. [TA], r. infundibular; divertículo com forma de funil que se estende da parte anterior do terceiro ventrículo para baixo e para dentro do infundíbulo da hipófise. SIN aditus ad infundibulum [TA], recessus infundibuli [TA].
intersigmoid r. [TA], r. intersigmóideo; um recesso peritoneal triangular situado posterior e inferiormente ao colo sigmóide e criado pela fixação do mesocolo sigmóide que ascende através do psoas esquerdo e, em seguida, vira de modo abrupto, descendo para o interior da pelve; o ureter esquerdo desce pela parede posterior desse recesso. SIN recessus intersigmoideus [TA].
Jacquemet r., r. de Jacquemet; escavação de peritônio situada entre a vesícula biliar e o fígado.
lateral r. of fourth ventricle [TA], r. lateral do quarto ventrículo; o r. estreito do ventrículo que se estende lateralmente sobre o pedúnculo cerebelar inferior e os núcleos cocleares suprajacentes e que desce ao longo da superfície lateral dessas estruturas; em sua extremidade, abre-se através do forame de Luschka para o interior da cisterna interpeduncular do espaço subaracnóideo. Através desse r., parte do plexo corióideo do quarto ventrículo projeta-se para o interior do espaço subaracnóideo. SIN recessus lateralis ventriculi quarti [TA].
mesentericoparietal r., r. mesentericoparietal. SIN parajejunal *fossa*.
optic r., r. óptico. VER supraoptic r.
pancreaticoenteric r., r. pancreaticoentérico; um r. da cavidade peritoneal embrionária que se transforma na bolsa omental no adulto.
paracolic r.'s, recessos paracólicos. SIN paracolic *gutters*, em *gutter*.
paraduodenal r. [TA], r. paraduodenal; recesso ocasional encontrado no peritônio, à esquerda da parte terminal do duodeno e posteriormente a uma prega que contém a veia mesentérica inferior. SIN recessus paraduodenalis [TA], fossa venosa, paraduodenal fossa.
parotid r., r. parotídeo. SIN parotid *space*.
pharyngeal r. [TA], r. faríngeo; depressão semelhante a uma fenda localizada na parede membranácea (não-muscular) da faringe que se estende posteriormente à abertura da tuba auditiva. SIN recessus pharyngeus [TA], recessus infundibuliformis, Rosenmüller fossa, Rosenmüller r.
phrenicomediastinal r. [TA], r. frenicomediastinal; o recesso da cavidade pleural situado entre o diafragma e o mediastino. SIN recessus phrenicomediastinalis [TA].
pineal r. [TA], r. pineal; um divertículo da parte posterior do terceiro ventrículo que se estende para trás, entre a comissura posterior e a comissura habenular; às vezes estende-se para dentro do pedículo da pineal. SIN recessus pinealis [TA].
piriform r., fossa piriforme; *termo oficial alternativo para piriform *fossa*.
pleural r.'s [TA], recessos pleurais; quatro recessos da cavidade pleural, um atrás do esterno e das cartilagens costais (r. costomediastinal), um entre o diafragma e a parede do tórax (r. costodiafragmático), um entre o diafragma e o mediastino (r. frenicomediastinal) e um entre os corpos vertebrais e o mediastino (r. vertebromediastinal). SIN recessus pleurales [TA], pleural sinuses.
pneumatoenteric r., pneumoenteric r., r. pneumoentérico; um r. do celoma embrionário situado entre o broto do pulmão direito e o intestino; está normalmente bastante obliterado antes do nascimento; posteriormente, apenas o r. superior do vestíbulo do saco peritoneal menor permanece como um vestígio.
pontocerebellar r., r. pontocerebelar. SIN cerebellopontine *angle*.
posterior r., r. posterior; aprofundamento da fossa interpeduncular que se dirige à ponte. SIN recessus posterior [TA].
posterior r. of tympanic membrane [TA], r. posterior da membrana timpânica; pequena bolsa situada na parede do tímpano, entre a prega malear posterior e a membrana timpânica. SIN recessus posterior membranae tympanicae [TA], Tröltsch pockets, Tröltsch r.'s.
Reichert cochlear r., r. coclear de Reichert. SIN cochlear r.
retrocecal r. [TA], r. retrocecal; uma das várias bolsas pequenas às vezes encontradas ao longo da margem direita do colo ascendente, próximo ao ceco. SIN recessus retrocecalis [TA], cecal r.
retroduodenal r. [TA], r. retroduodenal; recesso peritoneal ocasionalmente encontrado atrás da terceira parte do duodeno, entre o próprio duodeno e a aorta. SIN recessus retroduodenalis [TA], infraduodenal fossa, retroduodenal fossa.

Rosenmüller r., r. de Rosenmüller. SIN pharyngeal r.
sacciform r. of distal radioulnar joint [TA], r. saciforme da articulação radioulnar distal; uma extensão da cavidade da articulação radioulnar distal, entre os dois ossos. SIN recessus sacciformis articulationis radioulnaris distalis [TA].
sacciform r. of elbow joint [TA], r. saciforme da articulação do cotovelo; uma extensão da cápsula da articulação do cotovelo, no colo do rádio. SIN recessus sacciformis articulationis [TA].
saccular r. of bony labyrinth, r. sacular do labirinto ósseo; *termo oficial alternativo para spherical r. of bony labyrinth.
sphenoethmoidal r. [TA], r. esfenoetmoidal; uma pequena bolsa da cavidade nasal semelhante a uma fenda situada acima da concha nasal superior e para onde drenam os seios esfenoidais. SIN recessus sphenoethmoidalis [TA].
spherical r. of bony labyrinth [TA], r. esférico do labirinto ósseo; depressão arredondada localizada na parede interna do vestíbulo do labirinto, que aloja o sáculo. SIN recessus saccularis labyrinthi ossei*, saccular r. of bony labyrinth*, fovea hemispherica, fovea spherica, recessus sphericus labyrinthi ossei.
splenic r. [TA], r. esplênico; a extensão da bolsa omental que se dirige para o hilo do baço. SIN recessus splenicus [TA], recessus lienalis*.
subhepatic r., r. sub-hepático. SIN subhepatic space.
subphrenic r.'s, recessos subfrênicos. SIN subphrenic space.
subpopliteal r. [TA], r. subpoplíteo; a extensão da cavidade da articulação do joelho entre o tendão do poplíteo e o côndilo lateral do fêmur. SIN recessus subpopliteus [TA], bursa of popliteus.
superior azygoesophageal r., r. azigoesofagiano superior; a região situada acima do arco da veia ázigos na qual o pulmão direito está em contato com o esôfago.
superior duodenal r., fossa duodenal superior; *termo oficial alternativo para superior duodenal fossa.
superior ileocecal r. [TA], r. ileocecal superior; uma escavação rasa ocasionalmente presente entre o íleo terminal, o ceco e a artéria ileocólica, caso essa última esteja presente. SIN recessus ileocecalis superior [TA].
superior r. of lesser peritoneal sac, r. superior do saco peritoneal menor; VER pneumatoenteric r.
superior omental r., r. omental superior. SIN superior r. of omental bursa.
superior r. of omental bursa [TA], r. superior da bolsa omental; a parte do vestíbulo da bolsa omental que se estende para cima, entre a veia cava inferior e o esôfago. SIN recessus superior bursae omentalis [TA], superior omental r.
superior r. of tympanic membrane [TA], r. superior da membrana timpânica; um espaço situado na mucosa sobre a superfície interna da membrana timpânica, entre a parte flácida da membrana e o colo do martelo. SIN recessus superior membranae tympanicae [TA], Prussak pouch, Prussak space.
supraoptic r., r. supra-óptico; um divertículo que se estende para a frente a partir da parte anterior do terceiro ventrículo, acima do quiasma óptico. SIN recessus supraopticus [TA].
suprapineal r. r. suprapineal; divertículo variável da parte posterior do terceiro ventrículo do cérebro que corre para trás, a uma certa distância acima e além do r. pineal. SIN recessus suprapinealis [TA].
supratonsillar r., r. supratonsilar. SIN supratonsillar fossa.
triangular r., r. triangular; evaginação ocasional da parede anterior do terceiro ventrículo do cérebro, situada entre a comissura anterior e os pilares divergentes do fórnice. SIN recessus triangularis.
Tröltsch r.'s, recessos de Tröltsch. SIN anterior r. of tympanic membrane, posterior r. of tympanic membrane.
tubotympanic r., r. tubotimpânico; a parte dorsal da primeira bolsa faríngea endodérmica embrionária; transforma-se na cavidade da orelha média.
r.'s of tympanic cavity [TA], recessos da cavidade timpânica; os espaços da parede timpânica situados ao redor da membrana timpânica. SIN recessus membranae tympanicae [TA].
utricular r. of bony labyrinth, r. utricular do labirinto ósseo; *termo oficial alternativo para elliptical r. of bony labyrinth.
utricular r. of membranous labyrinth [TA], r. utricular do labirinto membranoso; a parte do utrículo que forma uma escavação em fundo cego que se estende para dentro do recesso elíptico (utricular) do labirinto ósseo. SIN recessus utricularis labyrinthi membranacei [TA].
vertebromediastinal r. [TA], r. vertebromediastinal; o recesso pleural formado pela reflexão da parte mediastinal da pleura parietal sobre os corpos vertebrais. SIN recessus vertebromediastinalis [TA].

re·ces·sion (rē-sesh′ŭn). Recessão, retrocesso; um afastamento ou recuo. VER TAMBÉM retraction. [L. *recessio* (ver recessus)]
angle r., recessão do ângulo; laceração na raiz da íris, entre os músculos ciliares longitudinais e circulares; freqüentemente resulta em glaucoma.
clitoral r., recessão do clitóris; procedimento cirúrgico utilizado na redução da proeminência visual do clitóris freqüentemente observada nas mulheres com hiperplasia congênita da supra-renal; é um procedimento que difere da amputação (clitorectomia) e da redução do clitóris. VER TAMBÉM clitoroplasty.
gingival r., r. gengival; a migração apical da gengiva ao longo da superfície do dente, com exposição da superfície do dente. SIN gingival atrophy, gingival resorption.
tendon r., retrocesso do tendão; o deslocamento cirúrgico do tendão de um músculo ocular para uma posição posterior à sua inserção anatômica. SIN curb tenotomy.

re·ces·si·tiv·i·ty (rē′ses-i-tiv′i-tē). Recessividade; o estado de ser recessivo (2).
re·ces·sive (rē-ses′iv). Recessivo. **1.** Que se retira; que recua. **2.** Em genética, indica uma característica resultante de um ou mais alelos específicos, situados em um único *locus*, que não se manifesta, a não ser que existam alelos mutantes em ambos os cromossomas homólogos de um par.
re·ces·sus, pl. **re·ces·sus** (rē-ses′sŭs). [TA]. Recesso. SIN recess. [L. retração, recuo]
r. ante′rior [TA], r. anterior. SIN anterior recess.
r. anterior membra′nae tympa′nicae [TA], r. anterior da membrana timpânica. SIN anterior recess of tympanic membrane.
r. cochlea′ris [TA], r. coclear. SIN cochlear recess.
r. costodiaphragmat′icus [TA], r. costodiafragmático. SIN costodiaphragmatic recess.
r. costomediastina′lis [TA], r. costomediastinal. SIN costomediastinal recess.
r. duodena′lis infe′rior [TA], r. duodenal inferior. SIN inferior duodenal fossa.
r. duodena′lis supe′rior [TA], r. duodenal superior. SIN superior duodenal fossa.
r. ellip′ticus labyrinthi ossei [TA], r. elíptico do labirinto ósseo. SIN elliptical recess of bony labyrinth.
r. epitympan′icus [TA], r. epitimpânico. SIN epitympanic recess.
r. hepatorena′lis recessus subhepatici [TA], r. hepatorrenal do recesso subhepático. SIN hepatorenal recess of subhepatic space.
r. ileoceca′lis infe′rior [TA], r. ileocecal inferior. SIN inferior ileocecal recess.
r. ileoceca′lis supe′rior [TA], r. ileocecal superior. SIN superior ileocecal recess.
r. infe′rior omenta′lis [TA], r. omental inferior. SIN inferior recess of omental bursa.
r. infundib′uli [TA], r. infundibular. SIN infundibular recess.
r. infundibulifor′mis, r. infundibuliforme. SIN pharyngeal recess.
r. intersigmoi′deus [TA], r. intersigmóideo. SIN intersigmoid recess.
r. latera′lis ventric′uli quar′ti [TA], r. lateral do quarto ventrículo. SIN lateral recess of fourth ventricle.
r. liena′lis, r. lienal; *termo oficial alternativo para splenic recess.
r. membranae tympanicae [TA], r. da membrana timpânica. SIN recesses of tympanic cavity, em recess.
r. paraduodena′lis [TA], r. paraduodenal. SIN paraduodenal recess.
r. parotid′eus, r. parotídeo. SIN parotid space.
r. pharyn′geus [TA], r. faríngeo. SIN pharyngeal recess.
r. phrenicomediastina′lis [TA], r. frenicomediastinal. SIN phrenicomediastinal recess.
r. pinea′lis [TA], r. pineal. SIN pineal recess.
r. pirifor′mis [TA], r. piriforme. SIN piriform fossa.
r. pleura′les [TA], r. pleural. SIN pleural recesses, em recess.
r. poste′rior [TA], r. posterior. SIN posterior recess.
r. posterior membra′nae tym′panicae [TA], r. posterior da membrana timpânica. SIN posterior recess of tympanic membrane.
r. retroceca′lis [TA], r. retrocecal. SIN retrocecal recess.
r. retroduodena′lis [TA], r. retroduodenal. SIN retroduodenal recess.
r. sacciformis articulationis [TA], r. saciforme da articulação. SIN sacciform recess of elbow joint.
r. saccifor′mis articulationis radioulnaris distalis [TA], r. saciforme da articulação radioulnar distal. SIN sacciform recess of distal radioulnar joint.
r. saccularis labyrinthi ossei, r. sacular do labirinto ósseo; *termo oficial alternativo para spherical recess of bony labyrinth.
r. sphenoethmoida′lis [TA], r. esfenoetmoidal. SIN sphenoethmoidal recess.
r. spher′icus labyrinthi ossei, r. esférico do labirinto ósseo. SIN spherical recess of bony labyrinth.
r. splenicus [TA], r. esplênico. SIN splenic recess.
r. subhepat′icus [TA], r. sub-hepático. SIN subhepatic space.
r. subphren′icus [TA], r. subfrênico. SIN subphrenic space.
r. subpoplit′eus [TA], r. subpoplíteo. SIN subpopliteal recess.
r. supe′rior bursae omenta′lis [TA], r. superior da bolsa omental. SIN superior recess of omental bursa.
r. superior membra′nae tympa′nicae [TA], r. superior da membrana timpânica. SIN superior recess of tympanic membrane.
r. supraop′ticus [TA], r. supra-óptico. SIN supraoptic recess.
r. suprapinea′lis [TA], r. suprapineal. SIN suprapineal recess.
r. triangula′ris, r. triangular. SIN triangular recess.
r. utricularis labyrinthi membranacei [TA], r. utricular do labirinto membranáceo. SIN utricular recess of membranous labyrinth.
r. utricularis labyrinthi ossei, r. utricular do labirinto ósseo; *termo oficial alternativo para elliptical recess of bony labyrinth.
r. vertebromediastinalis [TA], r. vertebromediastinal. SIN vertebromediastinal recess.

re·cid·i·va·tion (rē-sid-i-vā′shŭn). Recidiva; a recaída em uma doença, um sintoma ou um padrão de comportamento, como uma atividade ilegal pela qual o indivíduo foi previamente detido. [L. *recidivus*, que retrocede, recorrente, de *re- cido*, retroceder, voltar atrás]

re·cid·i·vism (rē-sid′i-vizm). Recidividade; a tendência de um indivíduo à recidiva. [L. *recidivus*, recorrente]

re·cid·i·vist (rē-sid′i-vist). Recidivista; pessoa que tende a apresentar recidivas.

rec·i·pe (℞) (res′i-pē). Receita médica, prescrição médica. **1.** O sobrescrito de uma receita médica, em geral indicado pelo símbolo ℞. **2.** Uma prescrição ou fórmula. [L. imperativo *recipio*, receber]

re·cip·i·ent (rē-sip′ē-ent). Receptor; alguém que recebe, como ocorre na transfusão sangüínea ou nos transplantes de órgãos ou tecidos. [L. *recipiens*, de *recipio*, receber]

re·cip·i·o·mo·tor (rē-sip′ē-ō-mō′ter). Relativo à recepção de estímulos motores. [L. *recipio*, receber, + *motor*, que move]

re·cip·ro·ca·tion (rē-sip-rō-kā′shŭn). Reciprocação; em protodôntica, o modo pelo qual uma parte de um aparelho é elaborada de uma determinada forma, a fim de se opor ao efeito criado pela outra parte. [L. *reciprocare*, pp. *reciprocatus*, mover para a frente e para trás]

re·cir·cu·la·tion (rē-ser-kū-lā′shŭn). Recirculação; o movimento circular da camada de muco de um seio paranasal que resulta da presença de um óstio acessório ou da falha em retirar o óstio natural em uma cirurgia em seios paranasais.

Recklinghausen, Friedrich D. von, histologista e patologista alemão, 1833–1910. VER R. *disease* of bone; von R. *disease*.

rec·li·na·tion (rek-li-nā′shŭn). O deslocamento de uma lente com catarata sobre o vítreo e para o seu interior, a fim de afastá-la da linha de visão; distingue-se da técnica denominada *couching*, na qual a lente é simplesmente deprimida para o interior do vítreo. [L. *reclino*, pp. *-atus*, inclinar-se para trás]

rec·ol·lec·tion (rē-ko-lek′shŭn). Em fisiologia renal, uma técnica na qual um líquido conhecido é infundido na luz do túbulo renal em um local e coletado por uma micropipeta em um local mais adiante para análise. [re- + L. *collectus*, pp. de *colligo*, coletar]

re·com·bi·nant (rē-kom′bi-nant). Recombinante. **1.** Uma célula ou um organismo que recebeu genes de linhagens parentais diferentes. **2.** Relativo a, ou que indica tais organismos. **3.** Nas análises de cruzamentos, uma alteração da fase de pareamento em dois *loci* durante a meiose. Se dois genes sintênicos e não-alelos são herdados dos mesmos pais, eles têm de estar pareados. Uma prole que herda apenas um deles é r. e indica um número ímpar de *cross-overs* entre os *loci*; uma prole que não herda nenhum ou ambos é denominada não-recombinante e pode indicar um mesmo número de *cross-overs* ou nenhum.

re·com·bi·na·tion (rē-kom-bi-nā′shŭn). Recombinação. **1.** O processo de reunião de partes que haviam se separado. **2.** A reversão da fase de pareamento da meiose, conforme avaliado pelo fenótipo resultante. VER TAMBÉM recombinant. **3.** A formação de novas combinações de genes.

  genetic r., r. genética. **(1)** A presença nos descendentes de combinações de genótipos e, talvez, de fenótipos que não estão presentes nos pais e que resultam de *crossing-over*; **(2)** em genética microbiana, a inclusão de uma parte de um cromossoma ou de um elemento extracromossômico de uma cepa de micróbios no cromossoma de outro micróbio; o intercâmbio de partes de cromossomas ou genes entre diferentes cepas de micróbios.

  homologous r., r. homóloga; a troca de partes correspondentes de DNA entre dois cromossomas irmãos.

  site-specific r., r. sítio-específica; a integração de DNA estranho a um sítio específico no genoma do hospedeiro.

re·con (rē′kon). Récon; termo obsoleto para a menor unidade (que corresponde a um único nucleotídeo do DNA) de recombinação ou *crossing-over* entre dois cromossomas homólogos.

re·con·sti·tu·tion (rē′kon-sti-too′shŭn). Reconstituição. **1.** A reconstituição ou o retorno ao estado original de uma substância, ou a combinação das partes com o objetivo de obter o todo. **2.** No caso de um organismo inferior, a restauração de uma parte do corpo por meio da regeneração.

re·con·struc·tion (rē-con-strŭk′shŭn). Reconstrução; a síntese computadorizada de uma ou mais imagens bidimensionais a partir de um conjunto de incidências radiográficas na tomografia computadorizada, ou a partir de um grande número de medidas obtidas pelas imagens por ressonância magnética; várias técnicas são utilizadas; a mais antiga é a retroprojeção, e a mais comum é a transformada bidimensional de Fourier.

  ossicular r., r. da cadeia ossicular; termo geral que indica as diversas técnicas cirúrgicas para restaurar a continuidade da cadeia ossicular da membrana timpânica até a janela oval para permitir a transmissão do som por pressão e, dessa forma, uma melhor audição.

rec·ord (rek′erd). **1.** Prontuário; em medicina, um relato escrito em ordem cronológica que inclui a(s) queixa(s) inicial(is) do paciente e a anamnese, os achados físicos, os resultados de testes e os procedimentos diagnósticos, quaisquer procedimentos e/ou drogas terapêuticos e os subseqüentes acontecimentos durante a evolução da doença. **2.** Em odontologia, um registro das relações da maxila e mandíbula desejadas em material plástico ou dispositivo, de modo a permitir que essas relações sejam transferidas para um articulador. [I.M. *recorden*, do Fr. ant. *recorder*, do L. *recordor*, recordar, de *re-*, de volta, novamente, + *cor*, coração]

  anesthesia r., r. da anestesia; relato escrito ou eletrônico das drogas administradas, dos procedimentos realizados e das respostas fisiológicas durante o curso de uma anestesia cirúrgica ou obstétrica.

  face-bow r., r. com o arco facial; registro que utiliza um arco facial da posição do eixo de rotação e/ou dos côndilos; o r. com o arco facial é empregado na orientação do molde maxilomandibular em relação ao eixo de abertura e fechamento do articulador.

  functional chew-in r., registro intrabucal funcional; r. dos movimentos mastigatórios naturais da mandíbula feito em uma borda oclusal por estiletes inscritores ou dentários.

  hospital r., prontuário hospitalar; o registro feito durante um período de hospitalização, que em geral inclui pareceres médicos, observações feitas por médicos e enfermeiros, tratamento instituído e resultados de todos os testes e/ou procedimentos realizados.

  interocclusal r., registro interoclusal; registro da correlação posicional entre os dentes ou entre a maxila e a mandíbula, realizado por meio da colocação de um material plástico que endurece (tal como gesso ou cera) entre as superfícies oclusais das bordas ou dos dentes; após endurecer, esse material passa a ser o r.; pode ser registrado nas posições cêntrica e excêntrica, como **r. interoclusal cêntrico** (centric interocclusal r.), um r. da relação maxilomandibular cêntrica; **r. interoclusal excêntrico** (eccentric interocclusal r.), um r. da posição maxilomandibular em uma relação diferente da cêntrica; **r. interoclusal lateral** (lateral interocclusal r.), um r. de uma posição maxilomandibular excêntrica lateral; e **r. interoclusal protrusivo** (protrusive interocclusal r.), um r. de uma posição maxilomandibular excêntrica protruída. SIN checkbite.

  maxillomandibular r., r. maxilomandibular; **(1)** r. da relação entre a mandíbula e as maxilas; **(2)** o ato de registrar a relação entre a mandíbula e as maxilas. SIN biscuit bite, maxillomandibular registration.

  medical r., prontuário. VER record (1).

  occluding centric relation r., registro da relação cêntrica em oclusão; um registro da relação cêntrica feito na dimensão vertical oclusal estabelecida.

  preextraction r., registro pré-operatório. SIN preoperative r.

  preoperative r., registro pré-operatório; em odontologia, qualquer registro feito para fins de estudo ou planejamento terapêutico. VER TAMBÉM diagnostic *cast*. SIN preextraction r.

  problem-oriented r. (POR), prontuário orientado para o problema; um sistema de manutenção de registros no qual é feita uma lista dos problemas do paciente, e toda a anamnese, os achados físicos, os dados laboratoriais etc. pertinentes a cada problema são colocados sob a designação dada ao problema; é útil especialmente para os registros ambulatoriais de pacientes que apresentam vários problemas e são acompanhados por longos períodos.

  profile r., registro do perfil; registro do perfil facial de um paciente.

  protrusive r., registro protrusivo; registro da posição da mandíbula, quando esta é projetada para a frente em relação às maxilas.

  terminal jaw relation r., registro da relação mandibular terminal; registro das relações da mandíbula com a maxila feito na relação de oclusão vertical e em posição cêntrica.

  three-dimensional r., registro tridimensional; registro maxilomandibular feito na relação de oclusão.

re·cord·ing (rē-kōrd′ing). Registro; a preservação dos resultados de um estudo.

  clinical r., r. clínico. SIN charting.

  depth r., r. em profundidade; o estudo da atividade elétrica cerebral subcortical após a colocação de eletrodos nessas áreas.

re·cov·er·y (rē-kŏv′er-ē). Recuperação. **1.** Um retorno ou o ato de recobrar algo. **2.** A saída da anestesia geral. **3.** Em ressonância magnética nuclear, refere-se à relaxação. [I.m., do Fr. ant. *recoverer*, do L. *recupero*, recuperar, recobrar, de *re-*, novamente, + *capio*, tomar]

  creep r., r. da fluência; a parte — dependente do tempo — do processo de diminuição da tensão aplicada a um material ou objeto que se segue à retirada do estresse que o deformou.

  inversion r., r. de inversão; em ressonância magnética, uma seqüência de pulsos na qual uma série de inversões do campo magnético de 180° é seguida por uma seqüência de ecos de spin para a detecção do sinal; digno de nota: durante a r., o vetor de magnetização longitudinal passa pelo zero.

  short TI inversion r. (STIR), r. de inversão com tempo de inversão curto; uma seqüência de recuperação de inversão que utiliza um tempo de inversão curto, cerca de 100 ms, entre pulsos de 180°; por meio da seleção adequada do tempo de inversão, o sinal proveniente da água ou da gordura pode ser suprimido.

  spontaneous r., r. espontânea; o retorno da resposta condicionada, após sua aparente extinção, na presença do estímulo condicionado, sem que o estímulo incondicionado esteja também presente. Ver classical *conditioning*.

  ultrasonic egg r., r. do óvulo com ultra-som; a obtenção de um óvulo para a fertilização *in vitro* por meio da aspiração dos folículos ovarianos com uma agulha guiada por ultra-som; pode ser realizada transvesicalmente ou através do fundo-de-saco (*cul-de-sac*).

re·cov·ery room. Sala de recuperação; uma dependência hospitalar com equipamento e pessoal especializados em fornecer assistência pós-operatória imediata aos pacientes, enquanto eles se recuperam de uma anestesia e/ou cirurgia.

re·cru·des·cence (rē-kroo-des′ens). Recrudescência; a retomada de um processo mórbido ou de seus sintomas após um período de remissão. [L. *re-crudesco*, reavivar, surgir outra vez, de *crudus*, cru, rude]

re·cru·des·cent (rē-kroo-des′ent). Recrudescente; que se torna ativo novamente, relativo a uma recrudescência.

re·cruit·ment (rē-kroot′ment). Recrutamento. **1.** Em testes de audição, o aumento maior que o normal da altura do som em resposta a um incremento na intensidade do estímulo acústico em uma orelha que apresenta uma perda de audição sensitiva quando comparada com uma orelha normal. **2.** Em neurofisiologia, a ativação de neurônios adicionais (recrutamento espacial) ou um aumento em sua velocidade de ativação (recrutamento temporal). SIN recruiting response. VER TAMBÉM irradiation. **3.** A adição de canais paralelos de fluxo em qualquer sistema. [Fr. *recrutement*, do L. *re-cresco*, pp. *-cretus*, crescer novamente]

△ **rect-.** VER recto-.
rec·tal (rek′tal). Retal; relativo ao reto.
rec·tal·gia (rek-tal′jē-ă). Retalgia. SIN proctalgia.
rec·tec·to·my (rek-tek′tō-mē). Retectomia. SIN proctectomy.
rec·ti·fi·er (rek′ti-fī-ĕr). Retificador; um dispositivo eletrônico para converter a voltagem alternada em contínua, parte do circuito de uma máquina de raios X. [L. mediev. *rectifico*, tornar reto, de *rectus*, reto, + *facio*, fazer]
rec·ti·fy (rek′ti-fī). Retificar. **1.** Corrigir. **2.** Purificar ou refinar por destilação; em geral, implica destilações repetidas. [L. *rectus*, direito, reto]
rec·ti·tis (rek-tī′tis). Retite. SIN proctitis.
△ **recto-, rect-.** Reto-; o reto. VER TAMBÉM procto-. [L. *rectum*, de *rectus*, reto]
rec·to·ab·dom·i·nal (rek′tō-ab-dom′i-năl). Retoabdominal; relativo ao reto e ao abdome; relativo a um método bimanual de exame no qual uma mão é colocada sobre a parede abdominal e um dedo da outra mão é introduzido no reto.
rec·to·cele (rek′tō-sēl). Retocele. SIN proctocele. [recto- + G. *kēlē*, tumor, hérnia]
rec·toc·ly·sis (rek-tok′li-sis). Retóclise. SIN proctoclysis.
rec·to·coc·cyg·e·al (rek-tō-kok-sij′ē-ăl). Retococcígeo; relativo ao reto e ao cóccix.
rec·to·coc·cy·pexy (rek-tō-kok′si-pek-sē). Retococcipexia. SIN proctococcypexy.
rec·to·co·li·tis (rek′tō-kō-lī′tis). Retocolite. SIN coloproctitis.
rec·to·per·i·ne·al (rek′tō-per-i-nē′ăl). Retoperineal; relativo ao reto e ao períneo.
rec·to·per·i·ne·or·rha·phy (rek′tō-per-i-nē-ōr′ă-fē). Retoperineorrafia. SIN proctoperineoplasty. [recto- + perineo- + G. *rhaphē*, uma costura]
rec·to·pexy (rek′tō-pek-sē). Retopexia. SIN proctopexy.
rec·to·pho·bia (rek-tō-fō′bē-ă). Retofobia. SIN proctophobia. [recto- + G. *phobos*, medo]
rec·to·plas·ty (rek′tō-plas-tē). Retoplastia. SIN proctoplasty.
rec·tor·rha·phy (rek-tōr′ă-fē). Retorrafia. SIN proctorrhaphy.
rec·to·scope (rek′tō-skōp). Retoscópio. SIN proctoscope.
rec·tos·co·py (rek-tos′kō-pē). Retoscopia. SIN proctoscopy.
rec·to·sig·moid (rek′tō-sig′moyd). Retossigmóide; o reto e o colo sigmóide considerados como uma unidade; o termo é também aplicado à junção do colo sigmóide com o reto.
rec·to·ste·no·sis (rek′tō-stē-nō′sis). Retoestenose. SIN proctostenosis.
rec·tos·to·my (rek-tos′tō-mē). Retostomia. SIN proctostomy.
rec·to·tome (rek′tō-tōm). Retótomo. SIN proctotome.
rec·tot·o·my (rek-tot′ō-mē). Retotomia. SIN proctotomy.
rec·to·u·re·thral (rek-tō-ū-rē′thrăl). Retouretral; relativo ao reto e à uretra.
rec·to·u·ter·ine (rek-tō-ū′ter-in). Retouterino; relativo ao reto e ao útero.
rec·to·vag·i·nal (rek-tō-vaj′i-năl). Retovaginal; relativo ao reto e à vagina.
rec·to·ves·i·cal (rek-tō-ves′i-kăl). Retovesical; relativo ao reto e à bexiga.
rec·to·ves·tib·u·lar (rek′tō-ves-tib′ū-lăr). Retovestibular; relativo ao reto e ao vestíbulo da vagina.
rec·tum, pl. **rec·tums**, **rec·ta** (rek′tŭm, rek′tă). Reto; a parte terminal do tubo digestivo, que se estende da junção retossigmóide até o canal anal. (Flexura perineal.) [L. *rectus*, reto, pp. de *rego*, tornar reto]
re·cum·bent (rē-kŭm′bent). Recumbente; que se inclina; que se reclina; que se deita. [L. *recumbo*, recostar-se, reclinar-se, de *re-*, para trás, + *cubo*, deitar-se]
re·cu·per·ate (rē-koo′per-āt). Recuperar; sofrer recuperação. [L. *recupero* (ou *recip-*), pp. *-atus*, pegar novamente, recuperar]
re·cu·per·a·tion (rē-koo-per-ā′shŭn). Recuperação; o restabelecimento ou a restauração do estado normal de saúde e da função. [L. *recuperatio* (ver recuperate)]
re·cur·rence (rē-kŭr′ens). Recorrência. **1.** O retorno dos sintomas, que ocorre como um fenômeno na história natural da doença, conforme é observado na febre recorrente. **2.** SIN relapse. **3.** O surgimento de uma característica genética em um parente genético de um probando. [L. *re-curro*, correr para trás, reaparecer]

re·cur·rent (rē-kŭr′ent). Recorrente. **1.** Em anatomia, que volta sobre si mesmo. **2.** Que indica os sintomas ou as lesões que reaparecem após uma interrupção ou remissão.

re·cur·va·tion (rē-ker-vā′shŭn). Recurvação; uma curvatura ou flexura para trás. [L. *re-curvus*, curvar para trás]

red. Vermelho; uma das cores primárias, que ocupa a extremidade inferior do espectro, na posição oposta à da cor violeta. Para consultar os corantes vermelhos individualmente, ver o nome específico. [A.S. *reád*]

Red Cross. Cruz Vermelha; a cruz vermelha de Genebra sobre um fundo branco, um símbolo internacional para identificar os médicos e outras pessoas que cuidam de doentes e feridos e as dependências destinadas à sua assistência em tempos de guerra; é também o emblema da Cruz Vermelha americana.

re·dia, pl. **re·di·ae** (rē′dē-ă, -dē-ē). Rédia; um dos estágios do desenvolvimento de um trematódeo digenético; é encontrado no interior de um molusco e sucede o estágio de esporocisto primário, o qual se forma após a penetração de um miracídio nos tecidos do caramujo. Originam-se de células situadas dentro do esporocisto, do qual são liberadas, e desenvolvem-se nos tecidos do caramujo (hospedeiro) como organismos musculares, alongados e semelhantes a bolsas, apresentando uma boca e um intestino. As rédias podem produzir uma ou várias gerações no caramujo, mas, no fim, dão origem ao estágio final do desenvolvimento, a cercária. VER TAMBÉM sporocyst (1), miracidium. [F. *Redi*, médico italiano, 1626–1697]

re·dif·fer·en·ti·a·tion (rē-dif′er-en′shē-ā′shŭn). Rediferenciação; o retorno a uma condição completamente especializada para a realização de uma função particular, após um período de atividade não-específica.

re·din·te·gra·tion (rē′din-tē-grā′shŭn). Reintegração. **1.** A restauração de partes lesadas ou perdidas. **2.** A restauração da saúde. **3.** A lembrança de uma experiência inteira baseada somente em algum item ou em alguma parte das circunstâncias ou do estímulo original da experiência. [L. *red-integro*, pp. *-atus*, tornar inteiro novamente, renovar, de *integer*, intacto, inteiro]

Redlich, Emil, neurologista austríaco, 1866–1930. VER Obersteiner-R. *line, zone*.

re·dox (red′oks). Redox; a contração de oxidação-redução. Ver oxidation-reduction *potential*.

re·dresse·ment for·cé (rĕ-dres-mon′ fōr-sā′). Termo obsoleto para o endireitamento, por meio da força, de uma parte deformada, como do joelho valgo [Fr.]

re·dress·ment (rē-dres′ment). **1.** Termo obsoleto para a correção de uma deformidade; o ato de endireitar uma parte. **2.** Um curativo novo em uma ferida.

re·duce (rē-doos′). Reduzir. **1.** Colocar de volta para uma posição de escolha; realizar uma redução (1). **2.** Em química, iniciar uma redução (2). [L. *re-duco*, conduzir de volta, restaurar, reduzir]

re·duc·i·ble (rē-doos′i-bl). Redutível; capaz de ser reduzido.

re·duc·tant (rē-dŭk′tant). Redutor; a substância que é oxidada no decorrer de uma redução.

re·duc·tase (rē-dŭk′tās). Redutase; uma enzima que catalisa uma redução; uma vez que todas as enzimas catalisam reações em ambas as direções, qualquer r. pode, sob condições adequadas, comportar-se como uma oxidase e vice-versa, daí o termo oxirredutase. Para consultar as redutases individualmente, ver os nomes específicos. SIN reducing enzyme.

re·duc·tic ac·id (rē-dŭk′tik). Ácido redútico; um produto redutor potente (antioxidante) formado em soluções de açúcar alcalinas e quentes.

re·duc·tion (rē-dŭk′shŭn). Redução. **1.** A restauração de uma parte à sua relação anatômica normal executada por meio de procedimentos manipulatórios ou cirúrgicos. SIN repositioning (2). **2.** Em química, a reação que envolve o ganho de um ou mais elétrons por uma substância, tal como ocorre quando o ferro passa do estado férrico (3+) para o ferroso (2+), ou quando o hidrogênio é adicionado à dupla ligação de um composto orgânico, ou quando um aldeído é convertido em um álcool. [L. *reductio*, de *re-duco*, pp. *ductus*, conduzir de volta]

r. of chromosomes, r. de cromossomas; o processo observado durante a meiose por meio do qual um membro de cada par de cromossomas homólogos é distribuído para um espermatozóide ou óvulo; o conjunto diplóide de cromossomas (46 nos humanos) é, dessa maneira, reduzido a um conjunto haplóide em cada gameta; a união do espermatozóide com o óvulo em uma única célula — o zigoto — restaura, assim, o número diplóide ou somático de cromossomas.

closed r. of fractures, r. fechada de fraturas; uma r. por meio da manipulação do osso, sem realizar incisão na pele.

r. en masse, r. em massa; a r. de um saco herniário e de seu conteúdo, de tal forma que a obstrução intestinal ainda permanece presente.

open r. of fractures, r. aberta de fraturas; a r. por meio da manipulação do osso, após exposição cirúrgica do local da fratura.

selective r., r. seletiva; uma técnica que consiste na retirada do interior do útero de um ou mais fetos, mantendo um ou mais fetos intactos; é realizada em geral em gravidezes que apresentam anomalias fetais ou em gestações múltiplas. SIN selective termination.

tuberosity r., r. da tuberosidade; a excisão cirúrgica de tecido fibroso ou ósseo excessivos situados na área da tuberosidade maxilar antes da construção de próteses.

re·dun·dan·cy (rē-dun′dăns-ē). Redundância; a ocorrência de seqüências repetidas de DNA bastante idênticas e dispostas linearmente.

terminal r., r. terminal; a condição observada em um cromossoma viral na qual uma informação genética idêntica está presente em cada extremidade do cromossoma.

re·du·pli·ca·tion (rē′doo′pli-kā′shŭn). Reduplicação. **1.** O ato de redobrar. **2.** Uma duplicação, como ocorre com os sons do coração em certos estados mórbidos, ou a presença de duas partes em lugar da parte única habitual. **3.** Uma prega ou duplicatura. [L. *reduplicatio*, de *re-*, novamente, + *duplico*, dobrar, de *duplex*, duplo]

re·du·vid, re·du·vi·id (rē-doo′vĭd -vid). Reduviídeo; um membro da família Reduviidae.

Red·u·vi·i·dae (rē-doo-vī′i-dē). Uma família (ordem Hemiptera) de insetos predadores, os insetos assassinos, que atacam animais e seres humanos. Essa família inclui a subfamília Triatominae, os insetos sugadores ou com tromba em cone, cujo gênero-tipo *Triatoma* engloba as espécies que são vetoras do *Trypanosoma cruzi*.

Reed, Dorothy M., patologista norte-americana, 1874–1964. VER R. *cell*; R.-Sternberg *cell*; Sternberg-R. *cell*.

Reed, Walter, 1851–1902. Cirurgião do Exército norte-americano, que elucidou a epidemiologia da febre amarela. VER Reed-Frost *model*.

reef·ing (rēf′ing). A redução cirúrgica do tamanho de um tecido por meio de pregueamento e fixação com suturas, como em uma plicatura.

stomach r., reefing do estômago; SIN gastroplication.

re·en·act·ment (rē-en-akt′ment). Reinterpretação; em psicodrama, a representação de uma experiência do passado.

re·en·try (rē-en′trē). Reentrada; o retorno do mesmo impulso para uma zona do músculo cardíaco que acabou de ser ativada, porém com atraso, de modo que não está mais refratária, como observado na maioria dos batimentos ectópicos e das taquicardias e nos ritmos recíprocos.

Rees, H. Maynard, médico norte-americano do século 20. VER R.-Ecker *fluid*.

Reese, Algernon B., oftalmologista norte-americano, 1896–1981. VER Cogan-R. *syndrome*.

re·fect (rē-fekt′). Induzir à refeição.

re·fec·tion (rē-fek′shŭn). Refeição; a restauração ao estado normal. [L. *refectio*, de *reficere*, restaurar, de *re-* + *facio*, fazer]

Refetoff, S., endocrinologista norte-americano do século 20. VER R. *syndrome*.

re·fine (rē-fīn′). Refinar; livrar de impurezas.

re·flect (rē-flekt′). Refletir. **1.** Dobrar para trás. **2.** Lançar de volta, p. ex., a energia radiante a partir de uma superfície. **3.** Meditar; pensar sobre um assunto. **4.** Enviar de volta um impulso motor em resposta a um estímulo sensitivo. [L. *re- flecto*, pp. *-flexus*, curvar para trás]

re·flec·tance. Refletância; uma medida da energia acústica refletida como uma função da imitância, como na impedância da orelha média.

re·flec·tion (rē-flek′shŭn). Reflexão. **1.** O ato de refletir. **2.** Aquilo que é refletido. **3.** Em psicoterapia, uma técnica na qual as frases de um paciente são repetidas ou reformuladas, a fim de que o paciente continue a explorar e explicar seu conteúdo emocionalmente significativo. [L. *reflexio*, curvatura para trás]

re·flec·tor (rē-flek′ter). Refletor; qualquer superfície que reflete a luz, o calor ou o som.

REFLEX

re·flex (rē′fleks). Reflexo. **1.** Reação involuntária que ocorre em resposta a um estímulo aplicado na periferia e transmitido aos centros nervosos localizados no cérebro ou na medula espinal. A maioria dos reflexos profundos listados como subentradas é reflexo de estiramento ou reflexo miotático, desencadeados pela percussão de um tendão ou osso, que causa o estiramento, mesmo que suave, do músculo, que, então, se contrai como consequência do estímulo aplicado a seus proprioceptores. VER TAMBÉM phenomenon. **2.** Uma reflexão. [L. *reflexus*, pp. de *reflecto*, curvar-se para trás]

abdominal r.'s, reflexos abdominais; a contração dos músculos da parede abdominal à estimulação da pele (reflexos abdominais superficiais) ou à percussão das estruturas ósseas vizinhas (reflexos abdominais profundos). SIN supraumbilical r. (2).

abdominocardiac r., r. abdominocardíaco; a estimulação mecânica (em geral, a distensão) das vísceras abdominais que causa alterações (em geral, uma lentificação) na freqüência cardíaca ou na ocorrência de extra-sístoles.

Abrams heart r., r. cardíaco de Abrams; a contração do miocárdio que ocorre quando a pele da região precordial é irritada.

accommodation r., r. de acomodação; aumento da convexidade da lente resultante da contração do músculo ciliar e do relaxamento do ligamento suspensor, a fim de manter a imagem da retina distinta.

Achilles r., Achilles tendon r., r.-de-aquiles, r. do tendão-de-aquiles; a contração dos músculos da panturrilha que ocorre quando o tendão do calcâneo é percutido de maneira abrupta. SIN ankle jerk, ankle r., tendo Achillis r., triceps surae r.

acoustic r., r. acústico; a contração do músculo estapédio em resposta a um som intenso, aumentando a impedância da orelha média e, dessa forma, protegendo a orelha interna do som. SIN cochleostapedial r., stapedial r.

acousticopalpebral r., r. acusticopalpebral; SIN cochleopalpebral r.

acquired r., r. adquirido; SIN conditioned r.

acromial r., r. acromial; a contração do músculo bíceps causada pela percussão do acrômio ou do processo coracóide.

adductor r., r. dos adutores; a contração dos adutores da coxa causada pela percussão do tendão do músculo adutor magno enquanto a coxa é abduzida.

allied r.'s, reflexos sinérgicos; os reflexos que, agindo em direção a um propósito comum, podem atravessar juntos a via final comum.

anal r., r. anal; a contração do esfíncter interno que prende o dedo introduzido no reto.

ankle r., r. do tornozelo; SIN Achilles r.

antagonistic r.'s, reflexos antagonistas; os reflexos que não agem em direção a um propósito comum e não podem atravessar juntos a via final comum.

aortic r., r. aórtico; SIN cardiac depressor r.

aponeurotic r., r. aponeurótico; a flexão da planta e dos dedos do pé desencadeada pela percussão da sola do pé, próximo à sua margem externa; apresenta o mesmo significado do r. de flexão dos dedos do pé de Rossolimo. SIN Guillain-Barré r., sole tap r., Weingrow r.

Aschner r., r. de Aschner; SIN oculocardiac r.

Aschner-Dagnini r., r. de Aschner-Dagnini; SIN oculocardiac r.

attitudinal r.'s, reflexos posturais; SIN statotonic r.'s.

auditory r., r. auditivo; qualquer r. que surge em resposta a um som, p. ex., o r. cocleopalpebral.

auditory oculogyric r., r. oculógiro auditivo; a rotação dos olhos em direção à fonte de um som súbito.

auricular r., r. auricular; um movimento das orelhas observado em animais em resposta a um som; parte do r. investigativo.

auriculopalpebral r., r. auriculopalpebral; SIN Kisch r.

auriculopressor r., r. auriculopressor; a vasoconstrição periférica e a elevação da pressão sangüínea em resposta a uma queda da pressão nas grandes veias. SIN Pavlov r.

auropalpebral r., r. auropalpebral; SIN cochleopalpebral r.

axon r., r. axônico; uma resposta desencadeada pela estimulação de um nervo periférico; é atribuída aos impulsos que viajam proximalmente ao longo de axônios motores a partir do local do estímulo, encontram um ponto de ramificação e, então, viajam distalmente por outro ramo, a fim de ativar arteríolas locais (provocando vasodilatação) ou músculos locais (provocando contrações). A latência da resposta diminui com uma estimulação mais proximal; o r. axônico é eliminado pela degeneração dos axônios ou por estímulos fortes, mas não por bloqueios proximais do nervo por anestésicos.

Babinski r., r. de Babinski; SIN Babinski *sign* (1).

back of foot r., dorsum of foot r., r. do dorso do pé. SIN Mendel instep r.

Bainbridge r., r. de Bainbridge; um aumento da freqüência cardíaca causado por uma elevação da pressão sangüínea no interior do átrio direito, resultante de um fluxo e/ou pressão aumentados dentro das grandes veias, junto à entrada do átrio.

Barkman r., r. de Barkman; a contração do músculo reto ipsolateral em resposta a um estímulo aplicado à pele abaixo de um mamilo.

basal joint r., r. da articulação basal; a oposição e adução do polegar com flexão da articulação metacarpofalângica e extensão da articulação interfalângica, quando é realizada a flexão passiva e firme do terceiro, quarto e quinto dedos; o r. está normalmente presente, mas mostra-se ausente nas lesões piramidais. SIN finger-thumb r., Mayer r.

Bechterew-Mendel r., r. de Bechterew-Mendel; a flexão plantar dos dedos do pé causada pela percussão do dorso do pé; está presente na lesão piramidal. SIN dorsum pedis r., Mendel-Bechterew r.

behavior r., r. comportamental; SIN conditioned r.

Benedek r., r. de Benedek; a flexão plantar do pé causada pela percussão da margem anterior da parte inferior da fíbula, enquanto o pé é dorsifletido suavemente.

Bezold-Jarisch r., r. de Bezold-Jarisch; um r. que apresenta vias aferente e eferente no vago, origina-se em quimiorreceptores não-identificados situados no coração e desencadeia bradicardia sinusal, hipotensão e provável vasodilatação periférica.

locais dos corpos dos neurônios dos ramos aferente e eferente dos reflexos representativos

reflexo	célula de origem/ramo aferente	célula de origem/ramo eferente	resposta funcional
abdominal	gânglios da raiz dorsal situados em T_8-T_{11}	neurônios motores do corno ventral situados em T_6-T_{11}	contração dos músculos abdominais com desvio do umbigo na direção do estímulo
de-aquiles (percussão do tornozelo)	gânglios da raiz dorsal situados nos níveis L_5-S_1 da medula espinal	neurônios motores do corno ventral situados nos níveis L_5-S_1 da medula espinal	contração dos músculos gastrocnêmio e sóleo com flexão plantar do pé
de Babinski (sinal de Babinski)	gânglios da raiz dorsal situados nos níveis L_5-S_1 da medula espinal (em geral, apenas no último)	neurônios motores do corno ventral situados nos níveis L_4-S_1 da medula espinal	dorsiflexão do hálux e abertura em forma de leque dos outros dedos do pé após a percussão firme da base do pé; considerado indicativo de doença do SNC após os 14–15 meses de idade, sugerindo lesão do sistema corticoespinal
do seio carótico	gânglio inferior do nervo glossofaríngeo	células pré-ganglionares do núcleo vagal motor dorsal, células pós-ganglionares dos gânglios do coração que agem sobre o músculo atrial	regulação da pressão (arterial) sangüínea
corneal (do piscamento)	gânglio trigeminal	núcleo motor facial	contração dos músculos das pálpebras e fechamento da fissura palpebral em resposta ao toque da córnea
de extensão cruzado	gânglios da raiz dorsal situados em C_7-T_1 (para a mão) e L_5-S_1 (para o pé)	células do corno ventral contralateral situadas em C_5-T_1 (para o braço) e L_2-S_1 (para a perna)	extensão da extremidade no lado oposto a um estímulo nocivo para ajudar a estabilizar o corpo, funciona de comum acordo com o reflexo de retirada
flexor (de retirada)	gânglios da raiz dorsal situados em C_7-T_1 (para a mão) e L_5-S_1 (para o pé)	células do corno ventral ipsolateral situadas em C_5-T_1 (para o braço) e L_2-S_1 (para a perna)	retirada súbita da extremidade de um estímulo nocivo
da ânsia	gânglio inferior do nervo glossofaríngeo e/ou vago	células bilaterais dos núcleos ambíguos	constrição dos músculos faríngeos e elevação do palato mole e da úvula
de Hoffmann (sinal de Hoffmann)	gânglios da raiz dorsal situados nos níveis C_7-C_8 da medula espinal	neurônios motores do corno ventral situados nos níveis C_7-T_1 da medula espinal	o tremor rápido da falange distal do terceiro dedo da mão produz a flexão do polegar e do dedo indicador ou do polegar e de todos os outros dedos
mandibular (de percussão da mandíbula)	núcleo mesencefálico do nervo trigeminal	núcleo motor trigeminal	contração bilateral dos músculos temporal e masseter em resposta a uma leve percussão para baixo do queixo
patelar (de percussão do joelho)	gânglios da raiz dorsal situados nos níveis L_2-L_4 da medula espinal	neurônios motores do corno ventral situados nos níveis L_2-L_4 da medula espinal	contração do músculo quadríceps com extensão da perna
pupilar (à luz)	células ganglionares da retina	células pré-ganglionares do núcleo de Edinger-Westphal, células pós-ganglionares do gânglio ciliar	contração dos músculos do esfíncter da pupila e diminuição do tamanho da pupila em resposta a um feixe de luz que incide sobre o olho; *reação direta* é a contração da pupila ipsolateral ao estímulo, *reação consensual* é a contração da pupila oposta
dos pontos cardeais	gânglio trigeminal	núcleo motor facial	enrugamento dos lábios e rotação da boca em direção à fonte do estímulo; desencadeado ao se friccionar o canto da boca ou a bochecha e observado durante os primeiros meses de vida
salivar	gânglio geniculado (VII NC) e gânglio inferior dos nervos glossofaríngeo e (possivelmente) vago	células pré-ganglionares no núcleo salivatório superior (VII NC) e no núcleo salivatório inferior (IX NC), células pós-ganglionares nos gânglios encontrados dentro (ou sobre as) das glândulas sublinguais e submandibulares e a glândula parótida	vasodilatação e aumento das secreções das glândulas salivares em resposta ao alimento na cavidade oral e conseqüente estimulação dos receptores do paladar

locais dos corpos dos neurônios dos ramos aferente e eferente dos reflexos representativos (continuação)

reflexo	célula de origem/ramo aferente	célula de origem/ramo eferente	resposta funcional
da protrusão labial	gânglio trigeminal	núcleo motor facial	o enrugamento ou pregueamento dos músculos ao redor da boca em resposta a percussão do lábio superior, em geral considerado indicativo de lesão do sistema corticospinal
da deglutição	gânglios inferiores dos nervos glossofaríngeo e vago	núcleo ambíguo para os músculos faríngeos, células pré-ganglionares no núcleo vagal motor dorsal e células pós-ganglionares nos gânglios mioentéricos no esôfago	a contração dos músculos faríngeos e as contrações semelhantes a ondas dos músculos do esôfago movem juntas o alimento através da faringe e para o esôfago
do vômito (faríngeo)	gânglios inferiores dos nervos glossofaríngeo e vago	núcleo ambíguo para a constrição dos músculos faríngeos e o fechamento da epiglote; o núcleo vagal motor dorsal envia fibras pré-ganglionares para as células pós-ganglionares no esôfago e estômago; a coluna de células intermediolateral dos níveis torácicos superiores envia fibras pré-ganglionares para as células pós-ganglionares no esôfago, estômago e esfíncter pilórico, neurônios motores do corno ventral inervam os músculos esqueléticos da parede abdominal	vômito; movimento retrógrado do conteúdo do estômago para o esôfago e para a cavidade oral; o fechamento da epiglote impede o movimento do vômito para os pulmões; a contração dos músculos abdominais auxilia no esvaziamento do estômago; o reflexo do vômito é essencialmente um reflexo da ânsia que se dissemina pelo neuroeixo e influencia um número maior de centros somáticos e viscerais

▪ reflexo relacionado com o tronco cerebral e os nervos cranianos   ▪ reflexo relacionado com a medula espinal   ▪ reflexo com componentes do tronco cerebral e da medula

biceps r., r. bicipital; a contração do músculo bíceps que ocorre quando seu tendão é percutido.
biceps femoris r., r. do bíceps femoral; a contração do bíceps femoral à percussão de sua parte inferior, imediatamente acima de sua inserção na cabeça da fíbula, enquanto o membro é parcialmente flexionado no quadril e no joelho.
Bing r., r. de Bing; quando o pé é dorsifletido passivamente, ocorre a flexão plantar, caso qualquer ponto sobre o tornozelo, entre os dois maléolos, seja percutido.
bladder r., r. da bexiga. SIN micturition r.
blink r., r. do piscamento. VER blink *response.*
body righting r.'s, reflexos posturais; os efeitos reflexos sobre os músculos do pescoço responsáveis pela posição espacial correta da cabeça causados pela estimulação de pressorreceptores situados na parede do corpo, pelo contato com o solo.
brachioradial r., r. do braquiorradial; a percussão próxima à extremidade inferior do rádio, quando o braço está supino a 45°, causa a contração do músculo braquiorradial (supinador longo). SIN radioperiosteal r., styloradial r., supination r., supinator jerk, supinator r., supinator longus r.
Brain r., r. de Brain. SIN quadripedal extensor r.
bregmocardiac r., r. bregmocardíaco; nos bebês, uma pressão sobre a fontanela anterior causa uma lentificação do coração.
Brissaud r., r. de Brissaud; ao se fazer cócegas na sola do pé, ocorre a contração do músculo tensor da fáscia lata, mesmo quando não se observa um movimento responsivo dos dedos do pé.
bulbocavernosus r., r. bulbocavernoso; uma contração abrupta dos músculos bulbocavernoso e isquiocavernoso, quando a glande do pênis é subitamente comprimida ou percutida.
bulbomimic r., r. bulbomímico; em caso de coma resultante de apoplexia grave, uma pressão exercida sobre os globos oculares causa a contração dos músculos faciais da expressão no lado oposto ao da lesão; se o coma é conseqüente de diabetes, uremia ou outra causa tóxica, o r. estará presente em ambos os lados. SIN facial r., Mondonesi r.
Capps r., r. de Capps; epônimo obsoleto para colapso vasomotor no momento da crise na pneumonia.
cardiac depressor r., r. depressor cardíaco; uma queda da pressão sangüínea resultante de vasodilatação periférica e de inibição cardíaca causadas por estímulos nas terminações de um nervo depressor cardíaco situado no arco da aorta e na base do coração. SIN aortic r., depressor r.
carotid sinus r., r. do seio carótico; um r. normal relacionado com a síndrome do seio carótico (carotid sinus *syndrome*), que resulta da hipersensibilidade ou da hiperativação do seio carótico.
celiac plexus r., r. do plexo celíaco; hipotensão arterial que coincide com as manipulações cirúrgicas no abdome superior durante a anestesia geral.
cephalopalpebral r., r. cefalopalpebral; a contração do músculo orbicular desencadeada pela percussão do vértex do crânio.
Chaddock r., r. de Chaddock. SIN Chaddock *sign.*
chain r., r. em cadeia; um conjunto de reflexos cada um servindo como estímulo para o seguinte.
chin r., r. mandibular. SIN jaw r.
Chodzko r., r. de Chodzko; as contrações de vários músculos da cintura escapular e do braço que ocorrem quando o manúbrio do esterno é percutido.
ciliospinal r., r. cilioespinal. SIN pupillary-skin r.
clasping r., a forte flexão dos membros anteriores de anfíbios e de outros animais durante a estação de acasalamento, quando o tórax ou o abdome são estimulados; depende do hormônio sexual masculino.
cochleo-orbicular r., r. cocleoorbicular. SIN cochleopalpebral r.
cochleopalpebral r., r. cocleopalpebral; uma forma de r. do piscamento na qual há uma contração, às vezes muito suave, do músculo orbicular das pálpebras a um som intenso. VER TAMBÉM startle r. SIN acousticopalpebral r., auropalpebral r., cochleo-orbicular r.
cochleopupillary r., r. cocleopupilar; midríase em resposta a um ruído alto, súbito e inesperado; uma resposta normal.
cochleostapedial r., r. cocleoestapedial. SIN acoustic r.
conditioned r. (CR), r. condicionado; um r. que é desenvolvido gradualmente por treinamento e associação através da repetição freqüente de um estímulo definido. VER conditioning. SIN acquired r., behavior r., trained r.
conjunctival r., r. conjuntival; o fechamento dos olhos em resposta à irritação da conjuntiva.
consensual light r., r. consensual à luz. SIN consensual *reaction.*
contralateral r., r. contralateral. SIN Brudzinski *sign* (1).
corneal r., r. corneal, r. corneano; **(1)** a contração das pálpebras que ocorre quando a córnea é tocada suavemente com um pincel de pêlo de camelo. SIN lid r. **(2)** a reflexão da luz na superfície da córnea.
costal arch r., r. do arco costal; a contração do músculo reto do abdome causada pela percussão da margem costal do lado de dentro da linha mamária.
costopectoral r., r. costopeitoral. SIN pectoral r.
cough r., r. da tosse; o r. que media a tosse em resposta à irritação da laringe ou da árvore traqueobrônquica. SIN laryngeal r.

craniocardiac r., r. craniocardíaco; a estimulação das terminações nervosas de certos nervos cranianos (p. ex., o olfatório, o ramo oftálmico do trigêmeo), seguida do r. depressor cardíaco, transmitido pelo ramo cardíaco do vago e manifestado por bradicardia e hipotensão.

cremasteric r., r. cremastérico; uma elevação do escroto e do testículo situado do mesmo lado, quando se estimula a pele que cobre o triângulo de Scarpa ou a face interna da coxa.

crossed r., r. cruzado; um movimento reflexo observado em um lado do corpo em resposta a um estímulo aplicado no lado oposto. SIN crossed jerk.

crossed adductor r., r. adutor cruzado; a contração dos adutores da coxa e a rotação interna do membro desencadeadas pela percussão da sola do pé. SIN crossed adductor jerk.

crossed extension r., r. de extensão cruzado; quando a pata de um animal é estimulada de modo doloroso, ou quando a extremidade central seccionada de um nervo aferente, como o fibular, é estimulada, ocorre a extensão do membro posterior contralateral; às vezes é observado em humanos à percussão da pele.

crossed knee r., r. patelar cruzado; quando o r. patelar é desencadeado, ocorre a contração do quadríceps contralateral. SIN crossed knee jerk.

crossed r. of pelvis, r. cruzado da pelve; a contração dos adutores contralaterais da coxa ao se percutir a espinha ilíaca ântero-superior. SIN crossed spino-adductor r.

crossed spino-adductor r., r. espinoadutor cruzado. SIN crossed r. of pelvis.

cuboidodigital r., r. cuboidodigital; a flexão dos dedos do pé mediante a percussão do osso cubóide; é quase idêntico ao r. de Guillain-Barré e basicamente semelhante ao r. de Rossolimo. SIN metatarsal r.

cutaneous r., r. cutâneo; o enrugamento da pele causado por um estímulo cutâneo, resultante da contração dos músculos eretores dos pêlos.

cutaneous pupil r., cutaneous-pupillary r., r. cutaneopupilar; SIN pupillary-skin r.

darwinian r., r. darwiniano; a tendência dos bebês de agarrar um objeto e mantê-lo suspenso. Cf. grasping r.

deep r., r. profundo; uma contração muscular involuntária que se segue à percussão de um tendão ou osso. SIN jerk (2).

deep abdominal r.'s, reflexos abdominais profundos; a contração dos músculos abdominais desencadeada por um estímulo, tal como a percussão de uma estrutura profunda; p. ex., a margem costal. VER TAMBÉM Galant r., upper abdominal periosteal r.

deep tendon r. (DTR), r. tendinoso profundo. SIN myotatic r.

defense r., r. de defesa. **(1)** SIN flexor r.; **(2)** as reações automáticas observadas em um animal, como a elevação dos pêlos ou das penas, a dilatação das pupilas ou a exposição das garras, quando é amedrontado.

deglutition r., r. da deglutição. SIN swallowing r.

Dejerine r., r. de Dejerine. SIN Dejerine hand *phenomenon*.

delayed r., r. tardio; um r. no qual decorre algum tempo entre o estímulo e a resposta. VER TAMBÉM trace conditioned r.

depressor r., r. depressor. SIN cardiac depressor r.

diffused r., r. difuso; um dos vários reflexos que ocorrem associados ao r. principal.

digital r., r. digital. SIN Hoffmann *sign* (2).

diving r., r. do mergulho; um r. por meio do qual a imersão da face ou do corpo em água, principalmente em água fria, tende a causar bradicardia e vasoconstrição periférica; a pressão aórtica média é pouco afetada, porque a redução do débito cardíaco tende a equilibrar a resistência periférica aumentada que reduz o fluxo sanguíneo periférico. Embora sejam relativamente pequenas na maioria dos humanos, as alterações podem ser profundas em algumas espécies de animais que mergulham, como os patos e as focas.

dorsal r., r. dorsal; a contração dos músculos das costas desencadeada pela estimulação cutânea do músculo eretor da espinha.

dorsum pedis r., r. do dorso do pé. SIN Bechterew-Mendel r.

elbow r., r. do cotovelo. SIN triceps r.

enterogastric r., r. enterogástrico; a contração peristáltica do intestino delgado induzida pela entrada de alimento no estômago. VER TAMBÉM gastrocolic r.

epigastric r., r. epigástrico; a contração da parte superior do músculo reto do abdome que ocorre após a estimulação da pele do epigástrio. SIN supraumbilical r. (1).

erector-spinal r., r. eretor espinal; a contração de parte do músculo eretor da espinha que se segue à estimulação da pele que cobre sua margem externa.

esophagosalivary r., r. esofagossalivar; a salivação desencadeada pela irritação da extremidade inferior do esôfago, como ocorre no carcinoma. SIN Roger r.

external oblique r., r. do oblíquo externo; a contração dos músculos oblíquo externo e reto do abdome após a percussão das partes anterior e externa da parede torácica inferior.

eye r., r. ocular. SIN light r. (2).

eyeball compression r., r. da compressão do globo ocular. SIN eyeball-heart r.

eyeball-heart r., r. globo ocular-coração; a diminuição da freqüência cardíaca como conseqüência dos efeitos vagais resultantes da compressão de um globo ocular. SIN eyeball compression r.

eye-closure r., r. do fechamento dos olhos. SIN wink r.

facial r., r. facial. SIN bulbomimic r.

faucial r., r. faucial. SIN gag r.

femoral r., r. femoral; a estimulação da pele da parte superior da face anterior da coxa provoca a extensão do joelho e a flexão do pé.

femoroabdominal r., r. femoroabdominal; a contração dos músculos abdominais após a percussão da face interna da coxa; está associado ao r. cremastérico. SIN hypogastric r.

Ferguson r., r. de Ferguson; o aumento da atividade uterina como conseqüência da estimulação mecânica da cérvix e do segmento inferior do útero.

finger-thumb r., r. dedo-polegar. SIN basal joint r.

flexor r., r. flexor; a flexão do tornozelo, joelho e quadril após a estimulação dolorosa do pé; ocorre associado ao r. de extensão cruzado. SIN defense r. (1), nociceptive r., withdrawal r.

forced grasping r., r. da preensão forçada. SIN grasping r.

front-tap r., a contração do músculo gastrocnêmio após percussão da canela. SIN periosteal r. (1).

fundus r., r. do fundo do olho. SIN light r. (2).

gag r., r. da ânsia; o contato de um corpo estranho com a membrana mucosa das fauces causa náusea ou desencadeia uma tentativa de vomitar sem êxito. SIN faucial r.

Galant r., r. de Galant; um r. abdominal profundo no qual ocorre a contração dos músculos abdominais após percussão da espinha ilíaca ântero-superior. SIN lower abdominal periosteal r.

galvanic skin r., r. galvânico da pele. SIN galvanic skin *response*.

gastrocolic r., r. gastrocólico; um movimento em massa do conteúdo do colo, freqüentemente precedido por um movimento semelhante no intestino delgado, que às vezes ocorre imediatamente após a entrada de alimento no estômago.

gastroileac r., r. gastroileal; a abertura da válvula ileocólica induzida pela entrada de alimento no estômago.

Geigel r., r. de Geigel; nas mulheres, a contração das fibras musculares situadas na borda superior do ligamento de Poupart à percussão suave da face interna da coxa; análogo ao r. cremastérico nos homens.

Gifford r., r. de Gifford. SIN eye-closure pupil *reaction*.

gluteal r., r. glúteo; a contração dos músculos glúteos que se segue à irritação da pele das nádegas.

Gordon r., r. de Gordon; a flexão dorsal do hálux produzida pela pressão firme e lateral dos músculos da panturrilha. SIN paradoxical flexor r.

grasp r., r. da preensão. SIN grasping r.

grasping r., r. da preensão; a flexão involuntária dos dedos da mão à estimulação tátil ou do tendão da palma da mão, que produz um movimento de preensão involuntário; está em geral associado a lesões do lobo frontal. Cf. darwinian r. SIN forced grasping r., grasp r.

great-toe r., r. do hálux. SIN Babinski *sign* (1).

Guillain-Barré r., r. de Guillain-Barré. SIN aponeurotic r.

gustatory-sudorific r., r. gustativo-sudorífero; a sudorese, principalmente da face, desencadeada pela mastigação de alimentos. VER TAMBÉM auriculotemporal nerve *syndrome*.

H r., r. H; um r. monossináptico obtido de maneira uniforme apenas em adultos normais, pela estimulação do nervo tibial, em geral na fossa poplítea, enquanto é feito um registro do grupo muscular gastrocnêmio-sóleo; é semelhante ao r.-de-aquiles, a não ser pelos fusos neuromusculares que são desviados; é amplamente utilizado nos laboratórios de EMG para diagnosticar radiculopatias em S1 e polineuropatias.

hepatojugular r., r. hepatojugular. VER hepatojugular *reflux*.

Hering-Breuer r., r. de Hering-Breuer; os efeitos dos impulsos aferentes provenientes dos ramos pulmonares do vago sobre o controle da respiração; p. ex., a inflação dos pulmões interrompe a inspiração, que é seguida pela expiração, ao passo que a deflação dos pulmões dá início à inspiração.

Hoffmann r., r. de Hoffmann. SIN Hoffmann *sign* (2).

hypochondrial r., r. hipocôndrico; uma inspiração rápida induzida por forte pressão exercida abaixo da margem costal.

hypogastric r., r. hipogástrico. SIN femoroabdominal r.

inborn r., r. inato. SIN innate r.

innate r., r. inato; um r. instintivo ou não-aprendido, tal como a sucção, que está presente ao nascimento. SIN inborn r.

interscapular r., r. interescapular. SIN scapular r.

intrinsic r., r. intrínseco; uma contração muscular reflexa desencadeada pela aplicação de um estímulo, em geral um estiramento, no próprio músculo, em oposição a uma contração muscular provocada por um estímulo extrínseco, p. ex., na pele, como ocorre nos reflexos cutâneos abdominais.

inverted r., r. invertido. SIN paradoxical r.

inverted radial r., r. radial invertido; a flexão dos dedos sem a flexão do antebraço que se segue à percussão da extremidade inferior do rádio; considerado indicativo de lesão no quinto segmento cervical da medula espinal.

investigatory r., r. investigativo. SIN orienting r.

ipsilateral r., r. ipsilateral; um r. no qual a resposta ocorre no lado do corpo que é estimulado.

Jacobson r., r. de Jacobson; a flexão dos dedos desencadeada pela percussão dos tendões dos músculos flexores situados na articulação do pulso ou da extremidade inferior do rádio.

jaw r., r. mandibular; a contração espasmódica dos músculos temporais que se segue à percussão de cima para baixo da mandíbula que pende relaxadamente. SIN chin jerk, chin r., jaw jerk, mandibular r., masseter r.

jaw-working r., r. do piscamento da mandíbula. SIN jaw-winking *syndrome*.

Joffroy r., r. de Joffroy; a contração dos músculos glúteos que se segue a uma pressão firme sobre as nádegas observada nos casos de paralisia espástica. SIN hip phenomenon.

Kisch r., r. de Kisch; o fechamento do olho em resposta à estimulação da pele do fundo do meato auditivo externo. SIN auriculopalpebral r.

knee r., r. do joelho. SIN patellar r.

knee-jerk r., r. da percussão do joelho. SIN patellar r.

labyrinthine r.'s, reflexos labirínticos; os reflexos iniciados por meio da estimulação dos receptores localizados no utrículo ou nos canais semicirculares. VER TAMBÉM statotonic r.'s, statokinetic r., righting r.'s.

labyrinthine righting r.'s, reflexos de endireitamento do labirinto; a estimulação dos receptores do labirinto provoca alterações no tônus dos músculos do pescoço que posicionam a cabeça.

lacrimal r., r. lacrimal; quando a conjuntiva é irritada, ocorre a secreção de lágrimas.

lacrimogustatory r., r. lacrimogustativo; a secreção de lágrimas desencadeada pela mastigação de alimentos. VER TAMBÉM crocodile tears *syndrome*.

laryngeal r., r. laríngeo. SIN cough r.

laryngospastic r., r. laringoespástico. SIN laryngospasm.

latent r., r. latente; um r. que deve ser considerado normal, mas que em geral aparece apenas em alguma circunstância patológica que diminui seu limiar.

laughter r., r. do riso; riso incontrolado desencadeado por cócegas.

let-down r., r. da descida do leite. SIN milk-ejection r.

lid r., r. palpebral. SIN corneal r. (1).

Liddell-Sherrington r., r. de Liddell-Sherrington. SIN myotatic r.

light r., r. à luz. (1) SIN pupillary r.; (2) um brilho vermelho refletido do fundo do olho quando um feixe de luz é dirigido para a retina, como ocorre na retinoscopia. SIN eye r., fundus r. (3) uma área triangular situada na parte ânteroinferior da membrana timpânica, que se estende do umbo até a periferia e onde pode ser observada a reflexão da luz. SIN cone of light, Politzer luminous cone, pyramid of light, red r., Wilde triangle.

lip r., r. labial; a projeção dos lábios de bebês desencadeada pela percussão próximo ao ângulo da boca.

Lovén r., r. de Lovén; uma reação que consiste na dilatação local de vasos acompanhada de uma vasoconstrição geral; p. ex., quando a extremidade central de um nervo aferente a um órgão é adequadamente estimulada e suas fibras eferentes vasomotoras são mantidas intatas, ocorre uma elevação geral da pressão sangüínea juntamente com uma dilatação dos vasos do órgão.

lower abdominal periosteal r., r. periostal do abdome inferior. SIN Galant r.

magnet r., r. magnético. VER magnet *reaction*.

mandibular r., r. mandibular. SIN jaw r.

mass r., r. em massa; nos casos de lesão macroscópica da medula espinal, enquanto a fase de atividade reflexa sucede a flacidez primária do choque, surge uma condição na qual um estímulo forte aplicado a qualquer parte de um dos membros paralisados é seguido da contração do quadril, joelho e tornozelo situados no mesmo lado e, freqüentemente, em ambos os lados, quando o estímulo é aplicado na linha média do corpo, bem como da contração da parede abdominal e mesmo do esvaziamento da bexiga e da sudorese na área que corresponde ao nível da lesão.

masseter r., r. massetérico. SIN jaw r.

Mayer r., r. de Mayer. SIN basal joint r.

McCarthy r.'s, reflexos de McCarthy. (1) SIN spinoadductor r. (2) SIN supraorbital r.

mediopubic r., r. mediopúbico; a contração dos adutores da coxa à percussão do púbis (osso) próximo à sínfise.

Mendel-Bechterew r., r. de Mendel-Bechterew. SIN Bechterew-Mendel r.

Mendel instep r., r. do dorso do pé de Mendel; quando o pé é firmemente apoiado sobre seu lado interno e se percute de forma abrupta os tendões dorsais, ocorre extensão do segundo ao quinto dedos. SIN back of foot r., dorsum of foot r.

metacarpohypothenar r., r. metacarpo-hipotenar; a flexão do dedo mínimo à percussão do dorso da mão; é observado nas lesões do trato piramidal; é semelhante ao r. de Starling.

metacarpothenar r., r. metacarpotenar. SIN thumb r.

metatarsal r., r. metatarsal. SIN cuboidodigital r.

micturition r., r. da micção; a contração das paredes da bexiga e o relaxamento do trígono e do esfíncter uretral em resposta a uma elevação da pressão no interior da bexiga; o r. pode ser voluntariamente inibido, e a inibição prontamente abolida para controlar a micção. SIN bladder r., urinary r., vesical r.

milk-ejection r., r. da ejeção do leite; a liberação do leite da mama que se segue à estimulação tátil do mamilo; postula-se a existência de uma via aferente que vai do mamilo até o hipotálamo; o ramo eferente é representado pela liberação neuro-hipofisária de ocitocina na circulação sistêmica; a contração dos elementos mioepiteliais no interior da mama, causada pela ocitocina, move o leite para o interior dos ductos coletores e em direção ao mamilo. SIN let-down r., milk let-down r.

milk let-down r., r. da descida do leite. SIN milk-ejection r.

Mondonesi r., r. de Mondonesi. SIN bulbomimic r.

Moro r., r. de Moro. SIN startle r.

muscular r., r. muscular. SIN myotatic r.

myenteric r., r. mioentérico; a contração que ocorre acima e o relaxamento abaixo de um ponto estimulado no intestino. SIN law of intestine.

myotatic r., r. miotático; a contração tônica dos músculos em resposta a uma força de estiramento; é resultante da estimulação dos proprioceptores musculares. SIN deep tendon r., Liddell-Sherrington r., muscular r., stretch r.

nasal r., r. nasal; o espirro causado pela irritação da membrana mucosa nasal.

nasomental r., r. nasomentual; a contração do músculo mentual que se segue à percussão da face lateral do nariz.

near r., r. de proximidade; a constrição pupilar observada quando se realiza um esforço para ver de perto, acompanhada de convergência ou acomodação oculares; trata-se de uma reação associada, e não de um r. verdadeiro.

neck r.'s, reflexos cervicais; as modificações na posição da cabeça causam alterações no tônus dos músculos do pescoço — por meio da estimulação dos proprioceptores situados no labirinto — que trazem a cabeça para a sua posição correta no espaço; a estimulação dos proprioceptores situados nos músculos do pescoço provoca, por sua vez, movimentos reflexos nos membros que trazem o animal para uma posição normal em relação à cabeça.

nociceptive r., r. nociceptivo. SIN flexor r.

nocifensor r., r. nocifensor; a dilatação vascular observada em uma área que circunda uma lesão ou em sua vizinhança.

nose-bridge-lid r., r. ponte do nariz-pálpebra. SIN orbicularis oculi r.

nose-eye r., r. nariz-olho. SIN orbicularis oculi r.

oculocardiac r., r. oculocardíaco; uma diminuição na freqüência do pulso associada à tração dos músculos extra-oculares ou à compressão do globo ocular; é especialmente sensível nas crianças; pode produzir parada cardíaca assistólica. SIN Aschner phenomenon, Aschner r., Aschner-Dagnini r.

oculocephalic r., r. oculocefálico. SIN oculocephalogyric r.

oculocephalogyric r., r. oculocefalógiro; a virada dos olhos e da cabeça na direção da fonte de um estímulo auditivo, visual ou de outra natureza. SIN oculocephalic r.

oculovagal r., r. oculovagal. VER oculocardiac r.

olecranon r., r. do olécrano; a flexão do antebraço causada pela percussão do olécrano. SIN paradoxical triceps r.

Oppenheim r., r. de Oppenheim; a extensão dos dedos do pé induzida pela estimulação da face interna da perna ou pela flexão súbita da coxa sobre o abdome e da perna sobre a coxa; um sinal de irritação cerebral.

optical righting r.'s, reflexos de endireitamento ópticos; os estímulos visuais que capacitam um animal a manter a cabeça em uma posição correta no espaço, por desencadearem movimentos nos músculos do pescoço e dos membros.

orbicularis oculi r., r. orbicular do olho; a contração dos músculos orbiculares dos olhos à percussão da margem da órbita, ou da ponte ou da extremidade do nariz. SIN nose-bridge-lid r., nose-eye r.

orbicularis pupillary r., r. orbicular da pupila. SIN eye-closure pupil *reaction*.

orienting r., r. de orientação; um aspecto da percepção na qual a resposta inicial de um organismo a uma alteração ou a um estímulo novo é tal que o organismo se torna mais sensível à estimulação; p. ex., a dilatação da pupila do olho em resposta à luz fraca. SIN investigatory r., orienting response.

palatal r., palatine r., r. palatal, r. palatino; o r. da deglutição induzido pela estimulação do palato.

palmar r., r. palmar; a flexão dos dedos da mão que se segue às cócegas feitas na palma da mão.

palm-chin r., r. palma-queixo. SIN palmomental r.

palmomental r., r. palmomentual; a contração unilateral (às vezes bilateral) dos músculos mentual e orbicular da boca causada por um estímulo rápido feito sobre a palma da mão ipsolateral. SIN palm-chin r.

parachute r., r. do pára-quedas. SIN startle r.

paradoxical r., r. paradoxal; qualquer r. cuja resposta habitual é inversa ou não está de acordo com a característica-padrão do r. em questão. SIN inverted r.

paradoxical extensor r., r. extensor paradoxal. SIN Babinski *sign* (1).

paradoxical flexor r., r. flexor paradoxal. SIN Gordon r.

paradoxical patellar r., r. patelar paradoxal. (1) a percussão do tendão patelar causa a contração do adutor; (2) a extensão passiva súbita da perna causa uma contração dos músculos extensores da perna.

paradoxical pupillary r., r. pupilar paradoxal; a constrição das pupilas no escuro, ou seja, o inverso do que é esperado. SIN Flynn phenomenon, paradoxical pupillary phenomenon.

paradoxical triceps r., r. tricipital paradoxal. SIN olecranon r.

patellar r., r. patelar; a contração súbita dos músculos anteriores da coxa causada pela percussão do tendão da patela, enquanto a perna pende frouxamente

reflexos tendinosos profundos importantes

tipo	r. do tendão do bíceps	r. tricipital	r. patelar	r.-de-aquiles
estímulo	percussão do dedo que descansa sobre o tendão do bíceps	percussão do tendão do tríceps diretamente acima do olécrano	percussão do tendão da patela	tendão-de-aquiles
efeito	flexão da articulação do cotovelo	extensão da articulação do cotovelo	extensão da articulação do joelho	flexão da planta do pé
segmento espinal	C5–C6	C6–C8	L2–L4	S1–S2

em um ângulo reto com a coxa. SIN knee jerk, knee r., knee-jerk r., patellar tendon r., quadriceps r.

patellar tendon r., r. do tendão patelar. SIN patellar r.

patelloadductor r., r. pateloadutor; a adução cruzada da perna à percussão do tendão do quadríceps.

Pavlov r., r. de Pavlov. SIN auriculopressor r.

pectoral r., r. peitoral; a contração do músculo peitoral maior desencadeada pela percussão da sétima costela, entre as linhas axilares anterior e média, enquanto o braço é abduzido; pode também ocorrer a contração do deltóide e do bíceps. SIN costopectoral r.

Perez r., r. de Perez; quando se percorre de cima para baixo com um dedo a espinha de um bebê apoiado em decúbito ventral, ocorre normalmente a extensão do corpo inteiro do bebê.

pericardial r., r. pericárdico; um r. vagal observado durante as cirurgias que envolvem a manipulação do pericárdio; é caracterizado por sinais de estimulação vagal (bradicardia e hipotensão arterial).

periosteal r., r. periostal. **(1)** SIN front-tap r.; **(2)** a contração muscular no braço que se segue a uma percussão do rádio ou da ulna.

pharyngeal r., r. faríngeo. **(1)** SIN swallowing r. **(2)** SIN vomiting r.

phasic r., r. fásico; uma resposta complexa coordenada, tal como o r. da coçadura no animal espinal.

Phillipson r., r. de Phillipson; a contração dos músculos extensores do joelho observada quando os músculos extensores do joelho oposto são inibidos.

photic-sneeze r., r. fótico de espirro. SIN photoptarmosis.

pilomotor r., r. pilomotor; a contração do músculo liso da pele, levando ao aparecimento da "pele-de-galinha", causada pela aplicação suave de um estímulo tátil ou por resfriamento local.

plantar r., r. plantar; a resposta à estimulação tátil da parte acolchoada do pé, em geral a flexão plantar dos dedos do pé; a resposta patológica corresponde ao sinal de Babinski. VER Babinski *sign* (1). SIN sole r.

plantar muscle r., r. muscular plantar. SIN Rossolimo r.

pneocardiac r., r. pneumocardíaco; uma modificação da pressão sangüínea ou do ritmo cardíaco causada pela inalação de um vapor irritante.

pneopneic r., r. pneumopnéico; uma modificação do ritmo respiratório causada pela inalação de um vapor irritante.

postural r., r. postural; as respostas que controlam a posição do tronco e das extremidades. VER TAMBÉM righting r.'s. SIN static r. (1).

pressoreceptor r., r. pressorreceptor; um r. normal relacionado com a síndrome do seio carótico. Ver carotid sinus *syndrome*.

pronator r., r. pronador. SIN ulnar r.

proprioceptive r.'s, reflexos proprioceptivos; qualquer r. desencadeado pela estimulação dos proprioceptores. VER TAMBÉM proprioceptor.

proprioceptive-oculocephalic r., r. oculocefálico proprioceptivo. SIN vestibuloocular r.

protective laryngeal r., r. laríngeo protetor; o fechamento da glote, a fim de impedir a entrada de substâncias estranhas no interior do trato respiratório.

psychocardiac r., r. psicocardíaco; uma alteração na velocidade da circulação e na consciência subjetiva do coração (freqüentemente do batimento cardíaco) que resulta de uma impressão ou experiência emocional, ou de um estado onírico subconsciente de tal impressão ou experiência.

psychogalvanic r., psychogalvanic skin r., r. psicogalvânico, r. psicogalvânico da pele. SIN galvanic skin *response*.

pulmonocoronary r., r. pulmocoronário; a constrição reflexa das artérias coronárias como conseqüência de estímulos vagais que se originam nos pulmões, como observado na embolia pulmonar.

pupillary r., r. pupilar; uma alteração no diâmetro da pupila como resposta reflexa a qualquer tipo de estímulo; p. ex., a constrição causada pela luz. SIN light r. (1).

pupillary-skin r., r. cutaneopupilar; a dilatação da pupila que se segue à estimulação da pele do pescoço. SIN ciliospinal r., cutaneous pupil r., cutaneous-pupillary r., skin-pupillary r.

quadriceps r., r. do quadríceps. SIN patellar r.

quadripedal extensor r., r. extensor do quadrúpede; a extensão do braço observada quando um paciente hemiplégico é virado de barriga para baixo, como se estivesse sobre quatro patas. SIN Brain r.

radial r., r. radial; após a percussão da extremidade inferior do rádio, ocorre a flexão do antebraço e, às vezes, após forte percussão, a flexão dos dedos da mão. VER TAMBÉM inverted radial r.

radiobicipital r., r. radiobicipital; a contração do músculo bíceps que às vezes ocorre na produção do r. braquiorradial.

radioperiosteal r., r. radioperiostal. SIN brachioradial r.

rectal r., r. retal; a entrada de matéria fecal proveniente do colo sigmóide no reto produz um impulso para defecar.

rectocardiac r., r. retocardíaco; um r. parassimpático que produz bradicardia e hipotensão à estimulação do nervo pélvico, cujo ramo aferente corresponde à parte sacral da divisão parassimpática do sistema nervoso autônomo, e o ramo eferente, ao ramo cardíaco do vago; diz-se que acompanha os exames proctológicos.

rectolaryngeal r., r. retolaríngeo; espasmo laríngeo provocado pela estimulação do esfíncter anal.

red r., r. vermelho. SIN light r. (3).

Remak r., r. de Remak; a flexão plantar dos três primeiros dedos do pé e, às vezes, de todo o pé acompanhada da extensão do joelho desencadeadas pela percussão da face ântero-superior da coxa; ocorre quando as vias de condução da medula espinal são interrompidas.

renal r., r. renal; anúria causada por lesão em uma parte distante do corpo ou por doença ou por lesão em um rim ou ureter.

righting r.'s, reflexos de endireitamento; os reflexos que por meio de diversos receptores — no labirinto, nos olhos, nos músculos ou na pele — tendem a trazer o corpo de um animal para a sua posição normal no espaço e que resistem a qualquer força que tenta colocá-lo em uma posição falsa, p. ex., sobre suas costas. VER TAMBÉM body righting r.'s, labyrinthine righting r.'s, neck r.'s, optical righting r.'s. SIN static r. (2).

Roger r., r. de Roger. SIN esophagosalivary r.

rooting r., r. fundamental; em bebês, o ato de friccionar ou roçar ao redor da boca provoca um enrugamento dos lábios.

Rossolimo r., r. de Rossolimo; a percussão leve da extremidade dos dedos do pé a partir da superfície plantar provoca a flexão dos dedos; um r. de estiramento dos flexores dos dedos do pé observado nas lesões dos tratos piramidais. VER TAMBÉM Starling r. SIN plantar muscle r., Rossolimo sign.

scapular r., r. escapular; a contração dos músculos superiores das costas pela estimulação da área entre as escápulas. SIN interscapular r.

scapulohumeral r., r. escapuloumeral; a contração dos músculos da cintura escapular e do braço provocada pela percussão da parte inferior da margem unilateral da escápula; os músculos que respondem variam de acordo com seu grau de estiramento no momento. SIN scapuloperiosteal r.

scapuloperiosteal r., r. escapuloperiostal. SIN scapulohumeral r.

Schäffer r., r. de Schäffer; nos casos de lesão do trato corticoespinal, o hálux é dorsifletido quando a pele sobre o tendão-de-aquiles é beliscada.

semimembranosus r., semitendinosus r., r. do semimembranáceo, r. do semitendíneo; a contração desses músculos observada ao se percutir a região da tuberosidade da tíbia.

shot-silk r., retina sedosa. SIN shot-silk *retina*.

sinus r., r. do seio carótico. VER carotid sinus *syndrome*.

skin r.'s, reflexos cutâneos. SIN skin-muscle r.'s.

skin-muscle r.'s, reflexos musculocutâneos; os reflexos cutâneos ou superficiais, p. ex., reflexos superficiais do abdome. SIN skin r.'s.

skin-pupillary r., r. cutaneopupilar. SIN pupillary-skin r.

snapping r., r. digital. SIN Hoffmann *sign* (2).

snout r., r. da protrusão labial; a projeção ou o enrugamento dos lábios provocado pela percussão leve dos lábios fechados em sua linha média; é considerado um sinal de disfunção do lobo frontal.

sole r., r. da sola do pé. SIN plantar r.

sole tap r., r. da percussão da sola do pé. SIN aponeurotic r.

spinal r., r. espinal; um arco reflexo que envolve a medula espinal. VER reflex *arc*.

spinoadductor r., r. espinoadutor; a contração dos músculos adutores da coxa à percussão da coluna vertebral. SIN McCarthy r.'s (1).

stapedial r., r. estapediano. SIN acoustic r.

Starling r., r. de Starling; a percussão das superfícies volares dos dedos da mão provoca a flexão dos dedos; é análogo ao r. de Rossolimo, que envolve os dedos do pé.

startle r., r. de moro; a resposta de um lactente (contração dos músculos do pescoço e dos membros) quando é largado por uma curta distância ou se assusta por um ruído ou movimento súbito. SIN Moro r., parachute r., startle reaction. VER TAMBÉM cochleopalpebral r.

static r., r. estático. (**1**) SIN postural r. (**2**) SIN righting r.'s.

statokinetic r., r. estatocinético; um r. que, por meio da estimulação dos receptores situados nos músculos do pescoço e nos canais semicirculares, desencadeia movimentos nos membros e nos olhos apropriados para um determinado movimento da cabeça no espaço.

statotonic r.'s, reflexos estatotônicos; os reflexos nos quais os receptores utriculares, situados no aparelho vestibular, captam as alterações da posição da cabeça no espaço em função da aceleração linear e do campo gravitacional da Terra, enquanto os receptores dos músculos do pescoço captam as alterações da posição da cabeça em relação ao tronco; os impulsos provenientes desses receptores controlam de maneira reflexa o tônus dos músculos dos membros, a fim de manter ou recuperar a postura desejada. SIN attitudinal r.'s.

sternobrachial r., r. esternobraquial; a contração dos adutores do braço observada quando se percute o esterno.

stretch r., r. do estiramento. SIN myotatic r.

Strümpell r., r. de Strümpell; a percussão do abdome ou da coxa provoca a flexão da perna e a adução do pé.

styloradial r., r. estilorradial. SIN brachioradial r.

suckling r., r. da amamentação; a liberação reflexa de prolactina pelo lobo anterior da hipófise desencadeada pela estimulação dos nervos localizados no mamilo durante a amamentação de um animal recém-nascido.

superficial r., r. superficial; qualquer r., p. ex., o r. abdominal ou o cremastérico, que é desencadeado pela estimulação da pele.

supination r., r. de supinação. SIN brachioradial r.

supinator r., supinator longus r., r. do supinador, r. do supinador longo. SIN brachioradial r.

supporting r.'s, reflexos de suporte. SIN supporting *reactions*, em *reaction*.

supraorbital r., r. supra-orbital; a contração do músculo orbicular do olho desencadeada pela estimulação mecânica ou elétrica do nervo supra-orbital. SIN McCarthy r.'s (2), trigeminofacial r.

suprapatellar r., r. suprapatelar; a patela eleva-se quando se percute o tendão do quadríceps situado acima da patela.

supraumbilical r., r. supra-umbilical. (**1**) SIN epigastric r.; (**2**) SIN abdominal r.

swallowing r., r. da deglutição; o ato de deglutir (segundo estágio) desencadeado pela estimulação do palato, das fauces ou da parede posterior da faringe. SIN deglutition r., pharyngeal r. (1).

synchronous r., r. sincrônico; as ações reflexas subsidiárias que ocorrem associadas ao r. indutor ou principal.

tarsophalangeal r., r. tarsofalângico; a extensão de todos os dedos do pé, exceto do primeiro, quando a parte externa do tarso é percutida; em certas doenças cerebrais dá-se o inverso, ou seja, ocorre a flexão dos dedos.

tendo Achillis r., r. do tendão-de-aquiles. SIN Achilles r.

tendon r., r. tendinoso; um r. miotático ou profundo no qual os receptores de estiramento muscular são estimulados pela percussão do tendão de um músculo.

tensor tympani r., r. do tensor do tímpano; em resposta a um som intenso, ocorre a contração do músculo tensor do tímpano, que aumenta a impedância da orelha média e protege, dessa forma, a orelha interna da exposição.

thumb r., r. do polegar; a flexão do polegar observada quando se percute o dorso da mão. SIN metacarpothenar r.

tonic r., r. tônico; a ocorrência de um intervalo considerável de tempo após a produção de um r. e antes do relaxamento, p. ex., a perna permanece elevada durante algum tempo após a percussão do joelho. SIN Gordon symptom.

trace conditioned r., um r. condicionado estabelecido pela aplicação de um estímulo por um curto período de tempo antes do reforço; no r. condicionado de um animal assim preparado, a resposta ocorre no mesmo intervalo de tempo após a aplicação do estímulo, como observado no período de treinamento.

trained r., r. treinado. SIN conditioned r.

triceps r., r. tricipital; a contração súbita do músculo tríceps provocada pela forte percussão de seu tendão, quando o antebraço pende relaxadamente em ângulo reto com relação ao braço. SIN elbow jerk, elbow r.

triceps surae r., r. do tríceps sural. SIN Achilles r.

trigeminofacial r., r. trigeminofacial. SIN supraorbital r.

trochanter r., r. trocantérico; a contração dos músculos adutores da coxa desencadeada por uma percussão sobre o trocanter.

Trömner r., r. de Trömner; o r. de Rossolimo modificado no qual a percussão da face volar da ponta do dedo indicador ou médio, quando os dedos da mão do paciente estão parcialmente fletidos, provoca a flexão dos quatro dedos e do polegar; é observado nas lesões do trato piramidal acompanhadas de espasticidade moderada.

ulnar r., r. ulnar; a pronação e a adução da mão provocadas pela percussão do processo estilóide da ulna. SIN pronator r.

unconditioned r., r. incondicionado; um r. instintivo que não depende de aprendizado ou de experiência prévia.

upper abdominal periosteal r., r. periosteal do abdome superior; a percussão da margem inferior das cartilagens costais na linha mamilar provoca a contração dos músculos abdominais ipsolaterais (inconstante).

urinary r., r. urinário. SIN micturition r.

utricular r.'s, reflexos utriculares. VER statotonic r.'s.

vagovagal r., r. vagovagal; bradicardia e hipotensão arterial, freqüentemente acompanhadas de arritmias supraventriculares; é atribuído à estimulação, principalmente mecânica, das vias aferentes vagais situadas no abdome, no tórax e nas vias aéreas, cujo arco eferente é formado por fibras cardioinibitórias vagais.

vasopressor r., r. vasopressor; vasoconstrição provocada pela estimulação de determinadas fibras aferentes, como as do nervo vago.

venorespiratory r., r. venorespiratório; a estimulação da respiração e o aumento da ventilação pulmonar observados em resposta a um aumento da pressão no interior do átrio direito.

vesical r., r. vesical. SIN micturition r.

vestibuloocular r., r. vestibuloocular; termo genérico dado ao controle reflexo do sistema vestibular sobre a motilidade extra-ocular que, nos testes clínicos, se manifesta como nistagmo. SIN proprioceptive-oculocephalic r.

vestibulospinal r., r. vestibuloespinal; a influência da estimulação vestibular sobre a postura corporal.

visceral traction r., r. da tração visceral; espasmo laríngeo desencadeado pela tração do estômago, da vesícula biliar ou do mesentério do apêndice durante uma cirurgia.

viscerogenic r., r. viscerogênico; qualquer um de vários reflexos, tais como a cefaléia, a tosse, a perturbação do pulso etc., desencadeados por distúrbios em quaisquer vísceras.

visceromotor r., r. visceromotor; a contração dos músculos do tórax ou do abdome observada em resposta a um estímulo proveniente de uma víscera situada em uma dessas regiões.

viscerosensory r., r. viscerossensitivo; uma área de dor ou de sensibilidade à pressão localizada na parede externa do corpo, resultante de doença em uma de suas vísceras. VER TAMBÉM Head *lines*, em *line*.

viscerotrophic r., r. viscerotrófico; uma modificação degenerativa observada nos tecidos moles do esqueleto que resulta de uma condição inflamatória crônica em qualquer uma das vísceras torácicas ou abdominais.

visual orbicularis r., r. orbicular visual; a contração do músculo orbicular do olho provocada por um súbito estímulo visual. VER TAMBÉM wink r.

vomiting r., r. do vômito; o vômito (a contração dos músculos abdominais acompanhada do relaxamento do esfíncter do estômago, do cárdia e dos músculos da garganta) desencadeado por uma variedade de estímulos, principalmente por aqueles aplicados na região das fauces. SIN pharyngeal r. (2).

Weingrow r., r. de Weingrow. SIN aponeurotic r.

Westphal pupillary r., r. pupilar de Westphal. SIN eye-closure pupil *reaction*.

white pupillary r., r. pupilar branco. SIN leukocoria.

wink r., r. do piscamento; termo geral para o r. de fechamento das pálpebras desencadeado por qualquer estímulo. SIN eye-closure r.

withdrawal r., r. de retirada. SIN flexor r.

wrist clonus r., r. clônico do punho; a extensão súbita do pulso provoca um movimento clônico prolongado.

re·flex·o·gen·ic (rē - flek - sō - jen′ik). Reflexogênico; que causa um reflexo. SIN reflexogenous.

re·flex·og·e·nous (rē - flek - soj′ē - nŭs). Reflexógeno. SIN reflexogenic.

re·flex·o·graph (rē-flek'sō-graf). Reflexógrafo; um instrumento utilizado para registrar graficamente um reflexo. [reflex + G. *graphō*, escrever]

re·flex·ol·o·gy (rē-flek-sol'ō-jē). Reflexologia; o estudo dos reflexos. [reflex + G. *logos*, estudo]

re·flex·om·e·ter (rē-flek-som'e-ter). Reflexômetro; um instrumento utilizado para medir a força necessária para desencadear um reflexo. [reflex + G. *metron*, medida]

re·flex·o·phil, re·flex·o·phile (rē-flek'sō-fil, -fīl). Reflexófilo; que possui reflexos exagerados. [reflex + G. *phileō*, amar]

re·flex·o·ther·a·py (rē-flek'sō-thār'ă-pē). Reflexoterapia. SIN reflex *therapy*.

re·flux (rē'flŭks). Refluxo. **1.** Um fluxo retrógrado. VER TAMBÉM regurgitation. **2.** Em química, a fervura sem perda de vapor, em virtude da presença de um condensador, que transforma o vapor em líquido novamente. [L. *re-*, para trás, + *fluxus*, um fluxo]
   abdominojugular r., r. abdominojugular. SIN hepatojugular r.
   esophageal r., gastroesophageal r., r. esofágico, r. gastroesofágico; a regurgitação do conteúdo do estômago para o interior do esôfago e possivelmente da faringe, onde pode ser aspirado entre as cordas vocais e descer para a traquéia; surgem, como conseqüência, os sintomas de dor em queimação e gosto ácido; as complicações pulmonares da aspiração dependem da quantidade, do conteúdo e da acidez do material aspirado.
   hepatojugular r., r. hepatojugular; uma elevação da pressão venosa, visível nas veias jugulares, mensurável nas veias do braço e produzida na insuficiência cardíaca congestiva iminente ou ativa e na pericardite constritiva pela compressão firme do abdome com a mão espalmada. É freqüentemente denominado reflexo hepatojugular, quando a compressão é realizada exclusivamente sobre o fígado. SIN abdominojugular r.
   intrarenal r., r. intra-renal; um r. urinário que segue da pelve renal e dos cálices para o interior dos ductos coletores. É observado como uma vermelhidão da pirâmide renal na cistouretrografia miccional. SIN pyelotubular r.
   pyelotubular r., r. pielotubular. SIN intrarenal r.
   ureterorenal r., r. ureterorrenal; um fluxo retrógrado de urina do ureter para o interior da pelve renal.
   vesicoureteral r., r. vesicoureteral; um fluxo retrógrado de urina da bexiga para o interior do ureter.

re·for·mat (rē-for'mat). Reformatar; em tomografia computadorizada, a recombinação dos dados de uma série de imagens escaneadas transversais contíguas, a fim de produzir imagens em um plano diferente, tais como o sagital ou o coronal.

re·fract (rē-frakt'). Refratar. **1.** Modificar a direção de um raio de luz. **2.** Detectar um erro de refração e corrigi-lo por meio de lentes. [L. *refringo*, pp. *-fractus*, quebrar]

re·frac·ta·ble (ri-frak'ta-bil). Refratável; sujeito à refração. SIN refrangible.

re·frac·tion (rē-frak'shŭn). Refração. **1.** O desvio de um raio de luz observado quando esse raio passa de um meio para um outro com densidade óptica diferente; ao passar de um meio mais denso para outro mais rarefeito, o raio é desviado para longe de uma linha que é perpendicular à superfície do meio refratante; ao passar de um meio mais rarefeito para outro mais denso, o raio inclina-se na direção dessa linha perpendicular. **2.** O ato de determinar a natureza e o grau dos erros de refração do olho e a correção dos mesmos por meio de lentes. SIN refringence. [L. *refractio* (ver refract)]
   double r., dupla r.; a propriedade de possuir mais de um índice refrativo de acordo com a direção da luz transmitida. SIN birefringence.
   dynamic r., r. dinâmica; a r. do olho durante a acomodação.
   static r., r. estática; a r. sem acomodação.

re·frac·tion·ist (rē-frak'shŭn-ist). Refracionista; uma pessoa treinada para medir a refração do olho e para determinar as lentes corretivas adequadas.

re·frac·tion·om·e·ter (rē-frak-shŭn-om'e-ter). Refracionômetro. SIN refractometer.

re·frac·tive (rē-frak'tiv). Refrativo. **1.** Relativo à refração. **2.** Que possui o poder de refratar. SIN refringent.

re·frac·tiv·i·ty (rē-frak-tiv'i-tē). Refratividade; o poder refrativo. SIN refringency.

re·frac·tom·e·ter (rē-frak-tom'e-ter). Refratômetro; um instrumento utilizado para medir o grau de refração das substâncias transparentes, principalmente dos meios oculares. VER refractive *index*. SIN objective optometer, refractionometer. [refraction + G. *metron*, medida]

re·frac·tom·e·try (rē-frak-tom'e-trē). Refratometria. **1.** A medida do índice refrativo. **2.** O uso de um refratômetro para determinar o erro de refração do olho.

re·frac·to·ry (rē-frak'tor-ē). Refratário. **1.** Resistente ao tratamento, como o de uma doença. SIN intractable (1), obstinate (2). **2.** SIN obstinate (1). [L. *refractarius*, de *refringo*, pp. *-fractus*, quebrar em pedaços]

re·frac·ture (rē-frak'choor). Refratura; a quebra de um osso no local de uma fratura prévia já consolidada ou próximo a ela. [re- + fracture]

re·fran·gi·ble (rē-fran'ji-bl). Refrangível. SIN refractable. [L. *refringo*, quebrar em pedaços]

re·fresh (rē-fresh'). **1.** Renovar; recuperar. **2.** Reavivar; VER revivification (2). [Fr. ant. *re-frescher*]

re·frig·er·ant (rē-frij'er-ănt). Refrigerante. **1.** Que refrigera; que reduz levemente a febre. **2.** Um agente que dá uma sensação de frescor ou alivia o estado febril. [L. *re-frigero*, pp. *-atus*, part. pres. *-ans*, esfriar, de *frigus* (*frigor-*), frio]

re·frig·er·a·tion (rē-frij-er-ā'shŭn). Refrigeração; o ato de resfriar ou de reduzir a febre. [L. *refrigeratio* (ver refrigerant)]

re·frin·gence (rē-frin'jens). SIN refraction.

re·frin·gen·cy (rē-frin'jen-sē). Refringência. SIN refractivity.

re·frin·gent (rē-frin'jent). Refringente. SIN refractive.

Refsum, Sigvald, neurologista norueguês, *1907. VER R. *disease, syndrome*.

re·fu·sion (rē-foo'zhŭn). Reperfusão; o retorno da circulação do sangue que foi temporariamente interrompida pela ligadura de um membro. [L. *re-fundo*, pp. *-fusus*, fluir novamente]

re·gain·er (rē-gān'er). Mantenedor de espaço; um dispositivo utilizado na tentativa de recuperar algum espaço nos arcos dentários.

Regaud, Claude, radiologista francês, 1870–1940. VER R. *fixative*; residual *body* of R.

re·gen·er·ate (rē-jen'er-āt). Regenerar; renovar; reproduzir. [L. *re-genero*, pp. *-atus*, reproduzir, de *genus* (*gener-*), nascimento, raça]

re·gen·er·a·tion (rē'jen-er-ā'shŭn). Regeneração. **1.** A reprodução ou a reconstituição de uma parte perdida ou lesada. SIN neogenesis. **2.** Uma forma de reprodução assexuada; p. ex., quando um verme é dividido em duas ou mais partes, cada segmento se regenera, formando um novo indivíduo. [L. *regeneratio* (ver regenerate)]
   aberrant r., r. aberrante; um novo crescimento de fibras nervosas que ocorre em uma direção incorreta; observado, por exemplo, após a lesão do nervo oculomotor. SIN misdirection phenomenon.
   guided tissue r., r. tecidual guiada; uma r. tecidual dirigida pela presença física e/ou pelas atividades químicas de um biomaterial; freqüentemente envolve a colocação de barreiras para excluir um ou mais tipos de células durante a cicatrização ou a r. tecidual.

reg·i·men (rej'i-men). Regime; um programa que utiliza drogas e regula os aspectos do estilo de vida de alguém com um propósito higiênico ou terapêutico; um programa de tratamento; é às vezes denominado erroneamente em inglês *regime*. [L. direção, regra]

REGIO

re·gio, gen. **re·gi·o·nis,** pl. **re·gi·o·nes** (rē'jē-ō, -ō'nis, -ō'nēz) [TA]. Região; SIN region. [L.]
   regio'nes abdo'minis [TA], regiões abdominais. SIN abdominal *regions*, em *region*.
   r. abdominis latera'lis, r. lateral do abdome; *termo oficial alternativo para flank.
   r. ana'lis [TA], r. anal. SIN anal *triangle*.
   r. antebrachia'lis ante'rior, r. antebraquial anterior; *termo oficial alternativo para anterior *region* of forearm.
   r. antebrachia'lis poste'rior, r. antebraquial posterior; *termo oficial alternativo para posterior *region* of forearm.
   r. antebrachii anterior [TA], r. antebraquial anterior. SIN anterior *region* of forearm.
   r. antebrachii posterior [TA], r. antebraquial posterior. SIN posterior *region* of arm.
   r. axilla'ris [TA], r. axilar. SIN axillary *region*.
   r. brachia'lis ante'rior, r. braquial anterior; *termo oficial alternativo para anterior *region* of arm.
   r. brachia'lis poste'rior, r. braquial posterior; *termo oficial alternativo para posterior *region* of arm.
   r. brachii anterior [TA], r. braquial anterior. SIN anterior *region* of arm.
   r. bucca'lis [TA], r. da bochecha. SIN buccal *region*.
   r. calca'nea [TA], r. calcânea. SIN heel *region*.
   regio'nes cap'itis [TA], regiões da cabeça. SIN *regions* of head, em *region*.
   r. carpa'lis ante'rior [TA], r. carpal anterior. SIN anterior *region* of wrist.
   r. carpa'lis poste'rior [TA], r. carpal posterior. SIN posterior *region* of wrist.
   regio'nes cervica'les [TA], regiões cervicais. SIN *regions* of neck, em *region*.
   r. cervica'lis ante'rior [TA], r. cervical anterior. SIN anterior cervical *region*.
   r. cervica'lis latera'lis [TA], r. cervical lateral. SIN lateral cervical *region*.
   r. cervica'lis poste'rior [TA], r. cervical posterior. SIN posterior cervical *region*.
   r. colli posterior, r. cervical posterior; *termo oficial alternativo para posterior cervical *region*.
   regio'nes cor'poris, regiões do corpo. SIN *regions* of body, em *region*.
   r. crura'lis poste'rior [TA], r. crural posterior. SIN posterior *region* of leg.

r. cruris ante′rior [TA], r. crural anterior. SIN anterior region of leg.
r. cubita′lis ante′rior [TA], r. cubital anterior. SIN anterior region of elbow.
r. cubita′lis poste′rior, r. cubital posterior; *termo oficial alternativo para posterior region of elbow.
r. deltoi′dea [TA], r. deltoidea. SIN deltoid region.
regio′nes dorsa′les [TA], regiões dorsais. SIN regions of back, em region.
regiones dorsi, regiões dorsais; *termo oficial alternativo para regions of back, em region.
r. epigas′trica, epigástrio; *termo oficial alternativo para epigastric region.
r. facialis [TA], r. facial. SIN face region.
r. femora′lis poste′rior, r. femoral posterior. SIN posterior region of thigh.
r. femoris [TA], r. femoral. SIN femoral region.
r. femoris ante′rior [TA], r. femoral anterior. SIN anterior region of thigh.
r. femoris posterior [TA], r. femoral posterior. SIN posterior region of thigh.
r. fronta′lis cap′itis [TA], r. frontal da cabeça. SIN frontal region of head.
r. ge′nus ante′rior [TA], r. genicular anterior. SIN anterior region of knee.
r. ge′nus poste′rior [TA], r. genicular posterior. SIN posterior region of knee.
r. glutea′lis [TA], r. glútea. SIN gluteal region.
r. hypochondri′aca, hipocôndrio; *termo oficial alternativo para hypochondriac region.
r. infraclavicula′ris, r. infraclavicular. SIN infraclavicular fossa.
r. inframamma′ria [TA], r. inframamária. SIN inframammary region.
r. infraorbita′lis [TA], r. infra-orbital. SIN infraorbital region.
r. infrascapula′ris [TA], r. infra-escapular. SIN infrascapular region.
r. inguina′lis, r. inguinal; *termo oficial alternativo para groin (1).
r. latera′lis abdominis, r. lateral do abdome; *termo oficial alternativo para flank.
r. lumba′lis, r. lombar. SIN lumbar region.
r. mamma′ria [TA], r. mamária. SIN mammary region.
regio′nes mem′bri inferio′ris [TA], regiões do membro inferior. SIN regions of lower limb, em region.
regio′nes mem′bri superio′ris [TA], regiões do membro superior. SIN regions of upper limb, em region.
r. menta′lis [TA], r. mentual. SIN mental region.
r. nasa′lis [TA], r. nasal. SIN nasal region.
r. nucha′lis, r. cervical. SIN posterior cervical region.
r. occipita′lis cap′itis [TA], r. occipital da cabeça. SIN occipital region of head.
r. olfacto′ria tu′nicae muco′sae na′si, r. olfatória da túnica mucosa do nariz. SIN olfactory region of nasal mucosa.
r. ora′lis [TA], r. oral. SIN oral region.
r. orbita′lis [TA], r. orbital. SIN orbital region.
r. parieta′lis cap′itis [TA], r. parietal da cabeça. SIN parietal region.
r. pectora′lis [TA], r. peitoral. SIN pectoral region.
r. perinea′lis [TA], r. perineal. SIN perineal region.
r. plantaris, planta; *termo oficial alternativo para sole of foot.
r. presterna′lis [TA], r. pré-esternal. SIN presternal region.
r. pu′bica, r. púbica; *termo oficial alternativo para pubic region.
r. respirato′ria tu′nicae muco′sae na′si, r. respiratória da túnica mucosa do nariz. SIN respiratory region of mucosa of nasal cavity.
r. sacra′lis [TA], r. sacral. SIN sacral region.
r. scapula′ris [TA], r. escapular. SIN scapular region.
r. sternocleidomastoi′dea [TA], r. esternocleidomastóidea. SIN sternocleidomastoid region.
r. sura′lis [TA], r. sural. SIN sural region.
r. talocrura′lis, r. talocrural. SIN ankle region.
r. tarsalis [TA], r. tarsal. SIN ankle region.
r. tempora′lis cap′itis [TA], r. temporal da cabeça. SIN temporal region of head.
regiones thoracicae anteriores et laterales [TA], regiões torácicas anteriores e laterais. SIN anterior and lateral thoracic regions, em region.
r. umbilica′lis [TA], r. umbilical. SIN umbilical region.
r. urogenita′lis [TA], r. urogenital. SIN urogenital triangle.
r. vertebra′lis [TA], r. vertebral. SIN vertebral region.
r. zygomat′ica [TA], r. zigomática. SIN zygomatic region.

re·gion (rē′jŭn) [TA]. Região. **1.** Uma parte da superfície do corpo freqüentemente limitada de maneira arbitrária. VER TAMBÉM space, zone. **2.** Uma parte do corpo que possui um suprimento vascular ou nervoso especial, ou uma parte de um órgão que possui uma função especial. VER TAMBÉM area, space, spatium, zone. SIN regio [TA]. [L. regio]
abdominal r.'s [TA], regiões abdominais; as subdivisões topográficas do abdome; baseiam-se na subdivisão do abdome pelos planos mediocalvicular, interespinal e transpilórico; incluem o hipocôndrio direito e esquerdo, o flanco ou a região lateral direita e esquerda, a virilha ou região inguinal direita e esquerda e as regiões ímpares umbilical, púbica e o epigástrio. SIN regiones abdominis [TA], abdominal zones.
anal r., r. anal. SIN anal triangle.
ankle r., r. do tornozelo; [TA] a região do membro inferior situada entre a perna (crus) e o pé (pes). SIN regio tarsalis [TA], regio talocruralis.
anterior antebrachial r., r. antebraquial anterior. SIN anterior r. of forearm.
anterior r. of arm [TA], r. anterior do braço; a área situada entre a região deltóidea, superiormente, e a região anterior do cotovelo, inferiormente. SIN regio brachii anterior [TA], regio brachialis anterior*, anterior surface of arm, facies anterior brachii, facies brachialis anterior.
anterior brachial r., r. braquial anterior; a região anterior do braço.
anterior carpal r., r. carpal anterior. SIN anterior r. of wrist.
anterior cervical r. [TA], r. cervical anterior; a área do pescoço limitada pela mandíbula, pela margem anterior do músculo esternocleidomastóideo e pela linha média anterior do pescoço; é subdividida em trígonos carótico, muscular, submandibular e submentual. SIN regio cervicalis anterior [TA], anterior triangle of neck*, trigonum cervicale anterius*, trigonum colli anterius*, anterior r. of neck.
anterior crural r., r. crural anterior. SIN anterior r. of leg.
anterior cubital r., r. cubital anterior. SIN anterior r. of elbow.
anterior r. of elbow [TA], r. anterior do cotovelo; a área situada na frente do cotovelo, que inclui a fossa cubital. SIN regio cubitalis anterior [TA], anterior cubital r., anterior surface of elbow, facies cubitalis anterior.
anterior r. of forearm [TA], r. anterior do antebraço; a área situada entre as margens radial e ulnar do antebraço, anteriormente. SIN regio antebrachii anterior [TA], regio antebrachialis anterior*, anterior antebrachial r., anterior surface of forearm, facies antebrachialis anterior, facies anterior antebrachii.
anterior hypothalamic r., r. hipotalâmica anterior; *termo oficial alternativo para anterior hypothalamic area.
anterior knee r., r. genicular anterior. SIN anterior r. of knee.
anterior r. of knee [TA], r. anterior do joelho; a região anterior do joelho. SIN regio genus anterior [TA], anterior knee r.
anterior and lateral thoracic r.'s [TA], regiões torácicas anteriores e laterais; as divisões topográficas do tórax: pré-esternal, peitoral e axilar. SIN regiones thoracicae anteriores et laterales [TA], r.'s of chest.
anterior r. of leg [TA], r. anterior da perna; a superfície anterior do membro inferior situada entre o joelho e o tornozelo. SIN regio cruris anterior [TA], anterior crural r., anterior surface of leg, facies anterior cruris, facies cruralis anterior.
anterior r. of neck, r. anterior do pescoço. SIN anterior cervical r.
anterior r. of thigh [TA], r. anterior da coxa; a frente da coxa, que inclui o trígono femoral. SIN regio femoris anterior [TA], anterior surface of thigh, facies femoralis anterior.
anterior r. of wrist [TA], r. anterior do pulso; a parte anterior do pulso. SIN regio carpalis anterior [TA], anterior carpal r.
axillary r. [TA], r. axilar; a região da axila, que inclui a fossa axilar. SIN regio axillaris [TA].
r.'s of back [TA], regiões do dorso; as regiões topográficas do dorso do tronco, que inclui a r. vertebral, a r. sacral, a r. escapular, a r. infra-escapular e a r. lombar. SIN regiones dorsales [TA], regiones dorsi*.
r.'s of body, regiões do corpo; as divisões topográficas do corpo. SIN regiones corporis.
buccal r. [TA], r. da bochecha; a região da bochecha, que corresponde aproximadamente ao contorno do músculo bucinador subjacente. SIN regio buccalis [TA].
calcaneal r., r. calcânea. SIN heel r.
r.'s of chest, regiões do tórax. SIN anterior and lateral thoracic r.'s.
chromosomal r., r. cromossômica; aquela parte de um cromossoma definida pelos detalhes anatômicos, destacadamente o bandeamento, ou pelas suas ligações (grupo de ligação).
complementarity determining r.'s, regiões determinantes de complementaridade; aquela parte da r. variável de um anticorpo ou de um receptor da célula T que se liga ao antígeno ou à molécula de histocompatibilidade principal/do antígeno.
constant r., r. constante. VER immunoglobulin.
deltoid r. [TA], r. deltoidea; a face lateral do ombro demarcada pelo contorno do músculo deltóide. SIN regio deltoidea [TA].
dorsal hypothalamic r., r. hipotalâmica dorsal; *termo oficial alternativo para dorsal hypothalamic area.
epigastric r. [TA], epigástrio; a região do abdome localizada entre as margens costais e o plano subcostal. [A TA lista esse termo como sinônimo de fossa epigástrica (ver epigastric fossa).] SIN epigastrium [TA], regio epigastrica*.
r.'s of face, regiões da face. SIN face r.
face r. [TA], r. facial; as subdivisões topográficas da face, que incluem as regiões nasal, oral, mentual, orbital, infra-orbital, da bochecha, parotídea e zigomática. SIN regio facialis [TA], r.'s of face.
femoral r. [TA], r. femoral; a região da coxa situada entre o quadril e o joelho. SIN regio femoris [TA].
framework r., r. de moldura; em imunologia, a seqüência conservada de aminoácidos situada em ambos os lados das regiões hipervariáveis dos domínios variáveis de uma cadeia da imunoglobulina.
frontal r. of head [TA], r. frontal da cabeça; a região da superfície da cabeça que corresponde ao contorno do osso frontal. SIN regio frontalis capitis [TA].

gluteal r. [TA], r. glútea; a região das nádegas. SIN regio glutealis [TA].

r.'s of head [TA], regiões da cabeça; a divisão topográfica do crânio em relação aos ossos da abóbada craniana; incluem as regiões frontal, parietal, occipital, temporal, auricular, mastóidea e facial. SIN regiones capitis [TA].

heel r., r. calcânea; a região do calcanhar. SIN regio calcanea [TA], calcaneal r.

hinge r., r. da dobradiça; (1) aquela parte da estrutura do RNAt que é deformada, dobrando-se em um modelo em "folha de trevo" (bidimensional) para formar um modelo em "L" (forma cristalizada, como observado à microscopia eletrônica); (2) em uma imunoglobulina, uma seqüência curta de aminoácidos situada entre duas seqüências mais longas e que permite que as últimas se inclinem sobre a primeira.

hypervariable r.'s (hī-per′var-ī-a-ble), regiões hipervariáveis; as regiões da molécula de imunoglobulina que contêm a maioria dos resíduos envolvidos no sítio de ligação do anticorpo.

hypochondriac r., hipocôndrio; a região situada em cada lado do abdome coberta pelas cartilagens costais; é lateral ao epigástrio. SIN hypochondrium [TA], regio hypochondriaca*.

I r., r. I; aquela área do complexo H-2 do camundongo que contém os genes da Classe II do complexo de histocompatibilidade principal.

iliac r., r. ilíaca. SIN groin (1).

r.'s of inferior limb, regiões do membro inferior. SIN r.'s of lower limb.

inframammary r. [TA], r. inframamária; a região do tórax (parte da região peitoral) situada inferiormente à glândula mamária. SIN regio inframammaria [TA].

infraorbital r. [TA], r. infra-orbital; a região facial bilateral, situada abaixo da órbita e lateralmente ao nariz. SIN regio infraorbitalis [TA].

infrascapular r., [TA], r. infra-escapular; a região do dorso situada lateralmente à região vertebral e abaixo da escápula. SIN regio infrascapularis [TA].

inguinal r., r. inguinal; *termo oficial alternativo para groin (1).

r. of interest, r. de interesse; em tomografia computadorizada ou em outro sistema de aquisição de imagens por computador, aquela parte da imagem que é selecionada de modo interativo e cujos valores de pixels individuais ou médios podem ser apresentados numericamente.

intermediate r. [TA], r. intermediária. SIN intermediate column.

intermediate hypothalamic r., r. hipotalâmica intermédia; *termo oficial alternativo para intermediate hypothalamic area.

K r., r. K; os carbonos 9 e 10 do sistema do anel de fenantreno; considerada por alguns o sítio reativo dos diversos carcinógenos de hidrocarbonetos.

lateral abdominal r., r. lateral do abdome; *termo oficial alternativo para flank.

lateral r. of abdominal r., r. lateral do abdome; *termo oficial alternativo para flank.

lateral cervical r. [TA], r. cervical lateral; a região do pescoço limitada pelos músculos esternocleidomastóideo e trapézio e pela margem superior da clavícula, que inclui o trígono omoclavicular. SIN regio cervicalis lateralis [TA], posterior triangle of neck*, trigonum cervicale posterius*, trigonum colli laterale*, lateral r. of neck.

lateral hypothalamic r., r. hipotalâmica lateral; estende-se por toda a maior parte da extensão rostrocaudal do hipotálamo lateral até a coluna do fórnice; engloba os núcleos tuberais laterais, os núcleos túbero-mamilares e populações de células disseminadas.

lateral r. of neck, r. lateral do pescoço. SIN lateral cervical r.

r.'s of lower limb [TA], regiões do membro inferior; as divisões topográficas do membro inferior: r. glútea, do quadril, femoral, do joelho, do membro inferior e do pé. SIN regiones membri inferioris [TA], r.'s of inferior limb.

lumbar r. [TA], r. lombar; a região do dorso situada lateralmente à região vertebral e entre a caixa torácica e a pelve. SIN regio lumbalis [TA].

mammary r. [TA], r. mamária; a região do tórax (região peitoral) que inclui as mamas. SIN regio mammaria [TA].

mental r. [TA], r. mentual; a região do queixo. SIN regio mentalis [TA].

nasal r. [TA], r. nasal; a região do nariz. SIN regio nasalis [TA].

r.'s of neck [TA], regiões do pescoço; as subdivisões topográficas do pescoço. SIN regiones cervicales [TA].

nuchal region, região nucal; SIN posterior cervical r.

nucleolus organizer r., r. organizadora do nucléolo; um arranjo do DNA que codifica a produção de RNA ribossômico (RNAr).

occipital r. of head [TA], r. occipital da cabeça; a região da superfície da cabeça que corresponde ao contorno do osso occipital. SIN regio occipitalis capitis [TA].

r. of olfactory mucosa, r. da mucosa olfatória. SIN olfactory r. of nasal mucosa.

olfactory r. of mucosa of nose [TA], r. olfatória da mucosa do nariz; o epitélio que contém neurônios, cujos axônios formam os filamentos do nervo olfatório; a lâmina própria contém numerosas glândulas olfatórias (Bowman) que se abrem na superfície. SIN olfactory membrane.

olfactory r. of nasal mucosa [TA], r. olfatória da mucosa nasal; uma área receptora olfatória especializada que engloba o terço superior do septo nasal e a parede lateral situada acima da concha superior; é revestida pela mucosa olfatória. SIN pars olfactoria tunicae mucosae [TA], olfactory r. of tunica mucosa of nose, regio olfactoria tunicae mucosae nasi, r. of olfactory mucosa, Schultze membrane.

olfactory r. of nose [TA], r. olfatória do nariz; aquela parte da mucosa nasal que possui células receptoras olfatórias e glândulas de Bowman. SIN olfactory membrane.

olfactory r. of tunica mucosa of nose, r. olfatória da túnica mucosa do nariz. SIN olfactory r. of nasal mucosa.

oral r. [TA], r. oral; a região da face que engloba os lábios e a boca. SIN regio oralis [TA].

orbital r. [TA], r. orbital; a região situada ao redor da órbita. SIN regio orbitalis [TA].

parietal r. [TA], r. parietal; a região da superfície da cabeça que corresponde ao contorno do osso parietal subjacente. SIN regio parietalis capitis [TA].

pectoral r. [TA], r. peitoral; a região do tórax demarcada pelo contorno do músculo peitoral maior; engloba as regiões peitoral lateral, mamilar e inframamária. VER TAMBÉM anterior and lateral thoracic r.'s. SIN regio pectoralis [TA].

perineal r. [TA], r. perineal; a r. da extremidade inferior do tronco situada anteriormente à região sacral e posteriormente à região púbica entre as coxas; é dividida no triângulo anal posteriormente e o triângulo urogenital anteriormente. SIN regio perinealis [TA].

plantar r., r. plantar; *termo oficial alternativo para sole of foot.

popliteal r., r. poplítea. SIN popliteal fossa.

posterior antebrachial r., r. antebraquial posterior. SIN posterior r. of forearm.

posterior r. of arm [TA], r. posterior do braço; o dorso do braço. SIN regio antebrachii posterior [TA], regio brachialis posterior*, facies brachialis posterior, posterior brachial r., posterior surface of arm.

posterior brachial r., r. braquial posterior. SIN posterior r. of arm.

posterior carpal r., r. carpal posterior. SIN posterior r. of wrist.

posterior cervical r. [TA], r. cervical posterior; o dorso do pescoço, que engloba a região suboccipital. SIN regio cervicalis posterior [TA], regio colli posterior*, nuchal region, posterior neck r., posterior r. of neck, regio nuchalis.

posterior crural r., r. crural posterior. SIN posterior r. of leg.

posterior cubital r., r. cubital posterior. SIN posterior r. of elbow.

posterior r. of elbow [TA], r. posterior do cotovelo; o dorso do cotovelo. SIN regio cubitalis posterior*, facies cubitalis posterior, posterior cubital r., posterior surface of elbow.

posterior r. of forearm [TA], r. posterior do antebraço; a área situada na face posterior do antebraço, entre as margens radial e ulnar. SIN regio antebrachialis posterior*, facies antebrachialis posterior, posterior antebrachial r., posterior surface of forearm.

posterior hypothalamic r., r. hipotalâmica posterior; as partes caudais do hipotálamo localizadas internamente na área do corpo mamilar; engloba os núcleos mamilares medial, intermédio e lateral e os núcleos hipotalâmicos posteriores. VER TAMBÉM posterior hypothalamic area.

posterior knee r., r. posterior do joelho. SIN posterior r. of knee.

posterior r. of knee [TA], r. posterior do joelho; a região posterior do joelho, que engloba a fossa poplítea. SIN regio genus posterior [TA], posterior knee r.

posterior r. of leg [TA], r. posterior da perna; o dorso da perna. SIN regio cruralis posterior [TA], facies cruralis posterior, facies posterior cruris, posterior crural r., posterior surface of leg.

posterior r. of neck, r. posterior do pescoço. SIN posterior cervical r.

posterior neck r., r. posterior do pescoço. SIN posterior cervical r.

posterior r. of thigh [TA], r. posterior da coxa; o dorso da coxa. SIN regio femoris posterior [TA], facies femoralis posterior, posterior surface of thigh, regio femoralis posterior.

posterior r. of wrist [TA], r. posterior do punho; a parte posterior do pulso. SIN regio carpalis posterior [TA], posterior carpal r.

preoptic r., r. pré-óptica; a parte mais anterior do hipotálamo que circunda a parte anterior ou pré-óptica do terceiro ventrículo e engloba a lâmina terminal; contém os núcleos pré-ópticos medial e lateral que são contínuos, caudalmente, com os núcleos hipotalâmicos anterior e lateral, respectivamente; a r. pré-óptica é contínua, rostralmente, com o septo pré-comissural e, lateralmente, com a substância inominada. SIN area preoptica [TA], preoptic area [TA].

presternal r. [TA], r. pré-esternal; a parte do tórax situada sobre o esterno. SIN regio presternalis [TA].

presumptive r., r. provável; em embriologia experimental, uma área da blástula da qual se espera o desenvolvimento de um tecido ou órgão específicos.

pretectal r., r. pré-tetal. SIN pretectal area.

pubic r. [TA], r. púbica; a região central inferior do abdome, situada abaixo da região umbilical e acima do monte do púbis. SIN hypogastrium [TA], regio pubica*.

r. of respiratory mucosa, r. da mucosa respiratória. SIN respiratory r. of mucosa of nasal cavity.

respiratory r. of mucosa of nasal cavity [TA], r. respiratória da mucosa da cavidade nasal; a área que começa no vestíbulo do nariz e é revestida pela mucosa respiratória; com a exceção da mucosa olfatória, engloba toda a cavidade nasal. SIN pars respiratoria tunicae mucosae [TA], regio respiratoria tunicae mucosae nasi, r. of respiratory mucosa, respiratory r. of tunica mucosa of nose.

respiratory r. of tunica mucosa of nose, r. respiratória da túnica mucosa do nariz. SIN respiratory r. of mucosa of nasal cavity.

sacral r. [TA], r. sacral; a área do dorso que se situa sobre o sacro. SIN regio sacralis [TA].

scaffold-associated r.'s (SAR), regiões associadas ao *scaffold*; os sítios do DNA que se ligam à topoisomerase II e a outras proteínas *scaffold*; são encontradas nos introns.

scapular r. [TA], r. escapular; a área do dorso que corresponde ao contorno da escápula. SIN regio scapularis [TA].

sternocleidomastoid r. [TA], r. esternocleidomastóidea; a região que se situa sobre o músculo esternocleidomastóideo e engloba a fossa supraclavicular menor. SIN regio sternocleidomastoidea [TA].

suboccipital r., r. suboccipital; a parte superior do dorso do pescoço, localizada inferiormente à região occipital da cabeça e acima do nível da segunda vértebra cervical; situa-se sobre (ou engloba, profundamente) o triângulo suboccipital.

r.'s of superior limb, regiões do membro superior. SIN r.'s of upper limb.

sural r. [TA], r. sural; a saliência muscular do dorso da perna situada abaixo do joelho e formada principalmente pelos ventres dos músculos gastrocnêmio e sóleo. SIN regio suralis [TA].

temporal r. of head [TA], r. temporal da cabeça; a região da superfície da cabeça que corresponde aproximadamente ao contorno do osso temporal. SIN regio temporalis capitis [TA].

umbilical r. [TA], r. umbilical; a região central do abdome, situada ao redor do umbigo. SIN regio umbilicalis [TA].

r.'s of upper limb [TA], regiões do membro superior; as divisões topográficas do membro superior: r. deltóidea, do membro superior, braquial, cubital, antebraquial, carpal e da mão. SIN regiones membri superioris [TA], r.'s of superior limb.

urogenital r., r. urogenital. SIN urogenital *triangle*.

variable r., r. variável. VER immunoglobulin.

vertebral r. [TA], r. vertebral; a região central do dorso, que corresponde à coluna vertebral subjacente. SIN regio vertebralis [TA].

Wernicke r., r. de Wernicke. SIN Wernicke *center*.

zygomatic r. [TA], r. zigomática; a região da face delineada pelo osso zigomático; a proeminência localizada acima da bochecha. SIN regio zygomatica [TA].

re·gion·al (rē′jŭn-ăl). Regional; relativo a uma região.

re·gi·o·nes (rē′jē-ō′nēz). Plural de regio. [L.]

reg·is·ter (rej′is-ter). Registro; um arquivo dos dados concernentes a todos os casos de uma condição específica, tal como o câncer, que ocorrem em uma população definida; registro (*register*) é o documento real, e registro (*registry*) é o sistema de registro de dados (*registration*) contínuo. [L. mediev. *registrum*, do L.L. *regero*, pp. *regestum*, registrar]

reg·is·tra·tion (rej-is-trā′shŭn). Registro; um registro (*record*), ou seja, o ato de gravar ou imprimir dados em um material.

maxillomandibular r., r. maxilomandibular. SIN maxillomandibular *record*.

tissue r., r. dos tecidos; em odontologia, (**1**) o r. acurado da forma dos tecidos sob qualquer condição por meio de um material apropriado; (**2**) uma impressão.

reg·is·try (rej′is-trē). **1.** Uma organização que lista os profissionais em determinados campos. **2.** Uma agência destinada à coleção de material patológico e informação relacionada à organização desses materiais para fins de estudo. **3.** Uma agência destinada à coleção de dados sobre indivíduos que tiveram uma determinada doença, a fim de permitir o acompanhamento e a avaliação da resposta ao tratamento.

reg·nan·cy (reg′nan-sē). A menor unidade de experiência; a unidade composta pelos processos fisiológicos totais que ocorrem em um único momento, os quais constituem as configurações dominantes no cérebro. Um único processo que constitui parte da *regnancy* é referido como um *regnant process*. [L. *regnant-*, *regnans*, part. pres. de *regno*, governar, dominar, reinar]

re·gres·sion (rē-gresh′ŭn). Regressão; **1.** Um abrandamento dos sintomas. **2.** Uma recaída; um retorno dos sintomas. **3.** Qualquer movimento ou ação retrógrados. **4.** O retorno a um modo de comportamento mais primitivo como resultado de uma incapacidade de funcionar em um nível mais adulto de maneira adequada. **5.** A tendência dos descendentes de pais excepcionais a possuir características mais próximas àquelas da população geral. **6.** Um mecanismo de defesa inconsciente por meio do qual ocorre um retorno a padrões de adaptação mais antigos. **7.** A distribuição de uma variável aleatória a partir dos valores específicos de outras variáveis relacionadas com ela, p. ex., uma fórmula para a distribuição do peso como uma função da altura e da circunferência do tórax. O método foi formulado por Galton em seu estudo sobre genética quantitativa. [L. *regredior*, pp. *-gressus*, voltar]

phonemic r., r. fonêmica; decréscimo na inteligibilidade da fala associado ao envelhecimento.

re·gres·sive (rē-gres′iv). Regressivo; relativo a ou caracterizado por regressão.

reg·u·la·tion (reg′ū-lā′shŭn). Regulação. **1.** O controle da velocidade ou da maneira por meio das quais um processo progride ou um produto é formado. **2.** Em embriologia experimental, a capacidade apresentada por um embrião na fase de pré-gástrula de continuar um desenvolvimento quase normal após a manipulação ou a destruição de uma ou mais partes. [L. *regula*, uma regra]

enzyme r., r. enzimática; o controle da velocidade de uma reação catalisada por uma enzima por alguns efetores (p. ex., inibidores ou ativadores) ou pela alteração de alguma condição (p. ex., o pH ou a força iônica).

gene r., r. gênica; o controle da síntese protéica por meio de sua ativação ou inibição.

reg·u·la·tor (reg-ū-lā′tŏr). Regulador; substância ou processo que controla uma outra substância ou um outro processo.

growth r.'s, reguladores do crescimento; as substâncias que podem alterar o crescimento de um organismo vivo.

humoral r., r. humoral; substância cuja ação resulta do contato com estruturas-alvo que são alcançadas através do sangue ou dos líquidos corporais.

reg·u·lon (reg′ū-lon). Régulon; um conjunto de genes estruturais que apresentam a mesma regulação gênica e cujos produtos dos genes estão envolvidos no mesmo caminho da reação.

re·gur·gi·tant (rē-ger′ji-tant). Regurgitante; que regurgita; que flui de volta.

re·gur·gi·tate (rē-ger′ji-tāt). Regurgitar. **1.** Fluir de volta. **2.** Expelir o conteúdo do estômago em pequenas quantidades, menores que no vômito. [L. *re-*, volta, + *gurgito*, pp. *-atus*, inundar, de *gurges* (*gurgit-*), um sorvedouro]

re·gur·gi·ta·tion (rē-ger′ji-tā′shŭn). Regurgitação. **1.** Um fluxo retrógrado, como o do sangue através de uma válvula cardíaca incompetente. **2.** O retorno de gás ou de pequenas quantidades de alimento do estômago. [L. *regurgitatio* (ver regurgitate)]

aortic r., r. aórtica; o refluxo do sangue através de uma válvula aórtica incompetente para o interior do ventrículo esquerdo durante a diástole ventricular. SIN Corrigan disease.

ischemic mitral r., r. mitral isquêmica; uma r. da válvula mitral causada por doença cardíaca isquêmica.

mitral r., r. mitral; o refluxo de sangue através de uma válvula mitral incompetente.

pulmonic r., r. pulmonar; uma incompetência da válvula pulmonar que permite um fluxo retrógrado.

valvular r., r. valvular; o vazamento de uma ou mais válvulas cardíacas, ou seja, o fechamento inadequado de uma ou mais válvulas, permitindo, em conseqüência, a regurgitação do sangue. SIN valvular incompetence, valvular insufficiency.

re·ha·bil·i·ta·tion (rē′hă-bil-i-tā′shŭn). Reabilitação; a restauração da capacidade de funcionar de um modo normal ou próximo ao normal que ocorre após uma doença ou lesão. [L. *rehabilitare*, pp. *-tatus*, adequar, de *re-* + *habilitas*, habilidade]

mouth r., r. bucal; a restauração da forma e da função do aparelho mastigatório a uma condição mais próxima possível da normal.

re·hears·al (rē-her′săl). Repetição; um processo associado ao aumento da memória de curto e longo prazos no qual um indivíduo repete para si mesmo uma ou mais vezes uma informação recém-adquirida, tal como um nome ou uma lista de palavras, a fim de não a esquecer.

Rehfuss, Martin E., médico norte-americano, 1887–1964. VER R. *method*, stomach *tube*.

re·hy·dra·tion (rē-hī-drā′shŭn). Reidratação; o retorno da água para um sistema após sua perda.

Reichel, Friedrich P., ginecologista e cirurgião alemão, 1858–1934. VER R. -Pólya stomach *procedure*.

Reichert, Karl B., anatomista alemão, 1811–1883. VER R. *cartilage*, cochlear *recess*; R.-Meissl *number*.

Reid, Robert W., anatomista escocês, 1851–1939. VER R. base *line*.

Reifenstein, Edward C. Jr., endocrinologista norte-americano, 1908–1975. VER R. *syndrome*.

Reil, Johann C., histologista, neurologista e médico alemão, 1759–1813. VER R. *ansa*, *band*, *ribbon*, *triangle*; limiting *sulcus* of R.; circular *sulcus* of R.; *island* of R.

re·im·plan·ta·tion (rē′im-plan-tā′shŭn). Reimplantação. SIN replantation.

extravesical r., r. extravesical. SIN detrusorrhaphy.

ureteral r., r. ureteral. SIN ureteroneocystostomy.

re·in·fec·tion (rē-in-fek′shŭn). Reinfecção; uma segunda infecção causada pelo mesmo microrganismo após a recuperação de uma infecção primária ou durante sua evolução.

re·in·force·ment (rē-in-fōrs′ment). Reforço. **1.** Um aumento da força ou da resistência; que denota especificamente o aumento da intensidade do reflexo patelar quando, simultaneamente ao reflexo, o paciente fecha o punho com força, tenta estender os dedos fletidos de uma das mãos ou contrai algum outro conjunto de músculos. VER TAMBÉM Jendrassik *maneuver*. **2.** Em odontologia, um aumento ou uma inclusão estruturais utilizados para fornecer força adicional a uma função; p. ex., barras na base de uma dentadura de plástico. **3.** Em condicionamento, a totalidade do processo no qual o estímulo condicionado é seguido pela apresentação de um estímulo incondicionado, que ele pró-

reinforcement

prio desencadeia a resposta a ser condicionada. VER TAMBÉM reinforcer, *schedules* of reinforcement, em *schedule*, classical *conditioning*, operant *conditioning*.
  primary r., r. primário; a satisfação de necessidades ou impulsos fisiológicos, tais como aqueles supridos pela alimentação ou pelo sono.
  secondary r., r. secundário; o r. por meio de algo que, se por um lado não satisfaz a necessidade diretamente, está associado à satisfação direta da necessidade, tal como o efeito sobre o comportamento causado por um comercial de televisão de um alimento ou de cerveja.
re·in·forc·er (rē-in-fōrs′er). Reforço; em condicionamento, um estímulo, objeto ou acontecimento que proporciona prazer ou satisfação (**r. positivo**), ou dor ou insatisfação (**r. negativo**), obtido pela realização de um operante desejado ou predeterminado. VER TAMBÉM reinforcement (3). SIN reward.
Reinke, Friedrich B., anatomista alemão, 1862–1919. VER R. *crystalloids*, em *crystalloid*.
re·in·ner·va·tion (rē-in-ner-vā′shŭn). Reinervação; a restauração do controle nervoso de um músculo paralisado ou de outro órgão efetor por meio de um novo crescimento de fibras nervosas de maneira espontânea ou após uma anastomose.
re·in·oc·u·la·tion (rē′i-nok-ū-lā′shŭn). Reinoculação; reinfecção que ocorre por meio de inoculação.
Reinsch, Adolf, médico alemão, 1862–1916. VER R. *test*.
re·in·te·gra·tion (rē′in-tē-grā′shŭn). Reintegração; nas profissões que se ocupam da saúde mental, o retorno a um funcionamento bem-ajustado após transtornos decorrentes de doença mental.
re·in·ver·sion (re-in-ver′shŭn). Reinversão; a correção espontânea ou cirúrgica de uma inversão, como a do útero.
Reis, Heinrich Maria Wilhelm, oftalmologista alemão, *1872. VER também Reis-Bücklers corneal *dystrophy*.
Reisseisen, Franz D., anatomista alemão, 1773–1828. VER R. *muscles*, em *muscle*.
Reissner, Ernst, anatomista alemão, 1824–1878. VER R. *fiber, membrane*.
Reitan, Ralph M., psicólogo norte-americano, *1922. VER Halstead-R. *battery*.
Reiter, Hans, bacteriologista alemão, 1881–1969. VER R. *test, disease, syndrome*; Fiessinger-Leroy-R. *syndrome*.
re·jec·tion (rē-jek′shŭn). Rejeição; **1.** A resposta imunológica à incompatibilidade que ocorre em um órgão transplantado. **2.** Uma recusa em aceitar, reconhecer ou conceder; uma negativa. **3.** A eliminação de pequenos ecos ultrasônicos do monitor. [L. *rejectio*, lançar de volta]
  accelerated r., r. acelerada; r. de um transplante que se manifesta em menos de 3 dias.
  acute r., r. aguda. SIN acute cellular r.
  acute cellular r., r. celular aguda; r. a um enxerto que geralmente se inicia nos primeiros 10 dias após um enxerto ter sido transplantado em um hospedeiro geneticamente diferente. As lesões no local do enxerto consistem caracteristicamente em um infiltrado com um grande número de linfócitos e macrófagos que causam dano tecidual. VER primary r. SIN acute r.
  allograft r. (al′lō-graft), r. de aloenxerto; a r. do tecido de um indivíduo que foi transplantado em outro da mesma espécie e que é geneticamente diferente. A r. é provocada por linfócitos T que respondem ao complexo de histocompatibilidade principal estranho do enxerto.
  chronic r., r. crônica; uma r. de um transplante que ocorre gradualmente, às vezes após vários meses.
  chronic allograft r., r. crônica de aloenxerto; as lesões mediadas pelo sistema imunológico e observadas em um aloenxerto que ocorrem em geral meses ou anos após o transplante.
  first-set r., r. de primeira fase; o transplante de um aloenxerto para um organismo que não foi previamente sensibilizado pelo tecido do enxerto. A necrose do enxerto inicia-se em geral dentro de 10 dias a partir do transplante.
  hyperacute r., r. hiperaguda; **(1)** uma r. que em geral se desenvolve imediatamente após a implantação de um enxerto vascular; pode ser causada por anticorpos citotóxicos pré-formados contra o enxerto; **(2)** uma forma de dano mediado por anticorpos e geralmente irreversível encontrado em um órgão transplantado, em particular o rim, e que se manifesta predominantemente por lesões trombóticas difusas, em geral confinadas ao próprio órgão e que raramente se disseminam.
  parental r., r. parental; **(1)** o ato de recusar o afeto de um filho ou de negar atenção ao filho; **(2)** o ato praticado por um filho de recusar o afeto de seus pais.
  primary r., r. primária; uma r. que ocorre mais de 7 dias após o transplante, sendo principalmente decorrente de uma resposta imune celular.
  second set r., r. de segunda fase; a r. acelerada de um transplante que ocorre quando um indivíduo foi previamente sensibilizado pelo enxerto.
re·ju·ve·nes·cence (rē-joo-vē-nes′ens). Rejuvenescimento; renovação da juventude; o retorno de uma célula ou de um tecido a um estado apresentado em um estágio anterior da existência. [L. *re-*, novamente, + *juvenesco*, tornar-se jovem, de *juvenis*, um jovem]
re·lapse (rē′laps). Recaída, recidiva, recorrência, reincidência; o retorno das manifestações de uma doença após um intervalo de melhora. SIN recurrence (2). [L. *re-labor*, pp. *-lapsus*, escorregar novamente]
re·laps·ing (rē-lap′sing). Recidivante; recorrente, reincidente; diz-se de uma doença ou de suas manifestações que retornam na forma de um novo ataque após um intervalo de melhora.
re·la·tion (rē-lā′shŭn). Relação. **1.** Uma associação ou conexão entre pessoas ou objetos. VER TAMBÉM relationship. **2.** Em odontologia, o modo de contato dos dentes ou o relacionamento posicional das estruturas orais. [L. *relatio*, trazer de volta]
  acquired centric r., r. cêntrica adquirida. VER centric jaw r.
  acquired eccentric r., r. excêntrica adquirida; r. excêntrica que é assumida pelo hábito, a fim de obter a oclusão dos dentes.
  buccolingual r., r. bucolingual; a posição de um espaço ou dente em r. à língua e à bochecha.
  centric jaw r., centric r., r. maxilomandibular cêntrica, r. cêntrica; **(1)** a r. fisiológica mais recuada da mandíbula em relação à maxila na e a partir da qual o indivíduo pode executar movimentos laterais; condição que pode se manifestar com diferentes graus de separação maxilomandibular e que ocorre ao redor do eixo de rotação terminal; **(2)** a r. mais posterior entre a mandíbula e as maxilas na r. vertical estabelecida. VER TAMBÉM eccentric r. SIN median retruded r., median r.
  dynamic r.'s, relações dinâmicas; os movimentos relativos que ocorrem entre dois objetos, p. ex., a correlação entre a mandíbula e a maxila.
  eccentric r., r. excêntrica; qualquer r. entre a mandíbula e a maxila diferente da r. cêntrica. SIN eccentric position.
  intermaxillary r., r. intermaxilar. SIN maxillomandibular r.
  maxillomandibular r., r. maxilomandibular; qualquer uma das muitas relações existentes entre a mandíbula e as maxilas, como a r. maxilomandibular cêntrica e a r. excêntrica. SIN intermaxillary r.
  median retruded r., median r., r. mediana. SIN centric jaw r.
  occluding r., r. de oclusão; r. maxilomandibular na qual os dentes em oposição estão em oclusão.
  protrusive r., r. protrusiva; a r. existente entre a mandíbula e a maxila quando a mandíbula é projetada para a frente.
  protrusive jaw r., r. maxilomandibular protrusiva; a r. maxilomandibular que resulta da protrusão da mandíbula.
  rest r., r. de repouso; a r. postural entre a mandíbula e a maxila existente quando o paciente descansa confortavelmente na posição ortostática e os côndilos estão em uma posição não-forçada e neutra no interior da fossa glenóide. SIN rest jaw r., unstrained jaw r.
  rest jaw r., r. maxilomandibular de repouso. SIN rest r.
  ridge r., r. inter-rebordos; a r. posicional entre o rebordo mandibular e o rebordo maxilar.
  static r., r. estática; a correlação entre duas partes que não estão em movimento.
  unstrained jaw r., r. maxilomandibular não-forçada. SIN rest r.
re·la·tion·ship (rē-lā′shŭn-ship). Relacionamento, relação; o estado de estar relacionado, associado ou ligado a algo.
  dose-response r., relação dose-resposta; a r. na qual uma alteração na quantidade, intensidade ou duração da exposição está associada a uma mudança no risco de ocorrer um resultado especificado.
  dual r.'s, relacionamentos duais; os relacionamentos nos quais um profissional da área da saúde desempenha concomitantemente duas ou mais categorias de papéis junto a um paciente; tais relacionamentos duais podem ser benignos (como ocorre quando ambos são membros do mesmo grupo social) ou exploratórios (um relacionamento sexual).
  Haldane r., relação de Haldane; relação matemática entre a constante de equilíbrio de uma reação catalisada por uma enzima e todos os parâmetros cinéticos da enzima envolvida, como a V_{max} e a K_m.
  hypnotic r., relação hipnótica; a relação existente entre o hipnotizador e o hipnotizado.
  object r., relação de objeto; nas ciências do comportamento, a ligação emocional existente entre um indivíduo e uma outra pessoa (ou entre dois grupos), em oposição ao interesse do indivíduo (ou do grupo) por si próprio.
  sadomasochistic r., relação sadomasoquista; uma r. caracterizada pelo prazer complementar de infligir e sofrer crueldade.
re·lax (rē-laks′). **1.** Relaxar; aliviar, afrouxar. **2.** Provocar o movimento dos intestinos. [L. *re-laxo*, afrouxar]
re·lax·ant (rē-lak′sănt). **1.** Relaxante; que relaxa; que provoca relaxamento; que reduz a tensão, principalmente a tensão muscular. **2.** Um agente que reduz a tensão muscular ou produz a paralisia dos músculos esqueléticos; geralmente referido como um relaxante muscular.
  depolarizing r., r. despolarizante; um agente, p. ex., a succinilcolina, que induz à despolarização da placa terminal motora e, assim, paralisa a musculatura esquelética por meio de um bloqueio da fase I.
  muscle r., r. muscular; droga com a capacidade de reduzir o tônus muscular; pode ser tanto um r. muscular que atua perifericamente, tal como o curare, e age de modo a produzir um bloqueio na junção neuromuscular (sendo, dessa forma, útil em cirurgias), como um r. muscular que atua centralmente, exer-

relaxant

cendo seus efeitos no interior do cérebro e da medula espinal, de modo a diminuir o tônus muscular (sendo, dessa maneira, útil nos espasmos musculares ou na espasticidade).
  neuromuscular r., r. neuromuscular; um agente, p. ex., o curare ou a succinilcolina, que produz o relaxamento do músculo estriado por meio da interrupção da transmissão dos impulsos nervosos na junção neuromuscular.
  nondepolarizing r., r. não-despolarizante; um agente, p. ex., a tubocurarina, que paralisa o músculo esquelético sem despolarizar a placa terminal motora, como no bloqueio da fase II.
  smooth muscle r., r. da musculatura lisa; um agente, tal como um antiespasmódico, broncodilatador ou vasodilatador, que reduz a tensão ou o tônus do músculo liso (involuntário).
re·lax·a·tion (rē-lak-sā′shŭn). Relaxamento, relaxação; **1.** O afrouxamento, o alongamento ou a diminuição da tensão de um músculo. **2.** Em ressonância magnética nuclear, corresponde ao decaimento da magnetização dos prótons que ocorre após uma mudança na direção do campo magnético circunjacente; as diferentes velocidades de relaxação de núcleos e tecidos são utilizadas para fornecer o contraste na formação da imagem. [L. *relaxatio* (ver relax)]
  cardioesophageal r., r. do cárdia; o r. do esfíncter esofágico inferior, que pode permitir o refluxo do conteúdo gástrico ácido para a parte inferior do esôfago, produzindo esofagite.
  isometric r., r. isométrico; a diminuição da tensão de um músculo que ocorre enquanto o comprimento permanece constante por causa da fixação das extremidades.
  isovolumetric r., r. isovolumétrico. SIN isovolumic r.
  isovolumic r., r. isovolumétrico; aquela parte do ciclo cardíaco situada entre o momento do fechamento da valva da aorta e a abertura da mitral, durante a qual o músculo do ventrículo diminui sua tensão sem se alongar, de modo que o volume ventricular permanece inalterado; o coração nunca permanece precisamente isovolumétrico, exceto durante diástoles longas acompanhadas de um período mesodiastólico de diástase. SIN isovolumetric r.
  longitudinal r., r. longitudinal; em ressonância magnética nuclear, o retorno dos dipolos magnéticos dos núcleos de hidrogênio (vetor de magnetização) ao equilíbrio, ou seja, paralelos ao campo magnético, após terem sido girados em 90°; seu tempo varia para diferentes tecidos, sendo de até 15 s para a água. VER T1. SIN spin-lattice r., spin-spin r.
  spin-lattice r., r. longitudinal. SIN longitudinal r.
  spin-spin r., r. longitudinal. SIN longitudinal r.
  transverse r., r. transversal; em ressonância magnética nuclear, o decaimento do vetor de magnetização nuclear em ângulos retos em relação ao campo magnético após o pulso de 90° ser desligado; o sinal é denominado decaimento de indução livre. VER T2. Cf. longitudinal r.
re·lax·in (rē-lak′sin). Relaxina; hormônio polipeptídeo secretado pelo corpo lúteo de mamíferos durante a gravidez. Facilita o processo de nascimento ao provocar amolecimento e alongamento da sínfise púbica e do colo uterino; inibe também a contração do útero e pode desempenhar algum papel no tempo de parto. SIN cervilaxin, ovarian hormone, releasin. [relax + -in]
re·learn·ing (rē-lern′ing). Reaprendizado; o processo de recuperar uma habilidade ou capacidade que foi parcial ou inteiramente perdida; quando a parte recuperada envolvida no r. é comparada ao aprendizado original, obtém-se um índice do grau de retenção.
re·leas·in. Relaxina. SIN relaxin.
re·li·a·bil·i·ty (rē-lī-ă-bil′i-tē). Confiabilidade; o grau de estabilidade exibido quando uma medição é repetida sob condições idênticas. VER correlation *coefficient*, reliability *coefficient*. [I.m. *relien*, do Fr. ant. *relier*, do L. *religo*, ligar]
  equivalent form r., c. de forma equivalente; em psicologia, a consistência da medição que está baseada na correlação entre as pontuações obtidas em duas formas semelhantes de um mesmo teste que foram realizadas pelo mesmo indivíduo. VER TAMBÉM reliability *coefficient*.
  interjudge r., c. interjuízes; em psicologia, a consistência da medição obtida quando juízes ou examinadores diferentes administram de modo independente o mesmo teste para o mesmo indivíduo. SIN interrater r.
  interrater r., c. interjuízes. SIN interjudge r.
  test-retest r., c. teste-reteste; em psicologia, a consistência da medição que está baseada na correlação entre as pontuações obtidas em um teste e as obtidas em um reteste para um mesmo indivíduo. VER TAMBÉM coefficient, reliability.
re·lief (rē-lēf′). Alívio. **1.** A remoção da dor ou do sofrimento, tanto físicos como mentais. **2.** Em odontologia, a redução ou a eliminação da compressão de uma área específica sob uma base de dentadura. VER TAMBÉM relief *area*, relief *chamber*. [ver relieve]
re·lieve (rē-lēv′). Aliviar; livrar-se parcial ou completamente da dor ou do desconforto, tanto físico como mental. [atr. do Fr. ant. do L. *re-levo*, levantar, aliviar]
re·line (rē′līn′). Reembasar, forrar; em odontologia, a repavimentação da superfície tecidual de uma dentadura com um novo material de base, a fim de ajustá-la de modo mais preciso. VER TAMBÉM rebase.

reno-, reni-.

REM 1. Acrônimo de rapid eye *movements* (movimentos rápidos dos olhos), em *movement*. **2.** Acrônimo de reticular erythematous *mucinosis* (mucinose eritematosa reticular). VER REM *syndrome*.
rem Abreviatura de *roentgen*-equivalent-man (radiação equivalente no homem).
Remak, Ernst J., neurologista alemão, 1848–1911. VER R. *reflex*, *sign*.
Remak, Robert, anatomista e histologista teuto-polonês, 1815–1865. VER R. nuclear *division*, *fibers*, em *fiber*, *ganglia*, em *ganglion*, *plexus*.
re·me·di·a·ble (rē-mē′dē-ă-bl). Remediável; curável. [L. *remediabilis*, de *remedio*, curar]
re·me·di·al (rē-mē′dē-ăl). Remediador; curativo ou que age como um remédio.
rem·e·dy (rem′e-dē). Remédio, medicamento; agente que cura uma doença ou alivia seus sintomas. [L. *remedium*, de *re*-, novamente, + *medeor*, cura]
re·min·er·al·i·za·tion (rē′min′er-ăl-i-zā′shŭn). Remineralização; **1.** O retorno ao organismo ou a uma área local dos constituintes minerais necessários perdidos por causa de uma doença ou por deficiências dietéticas; o termo é normalmente utilizado em referência ao conteúdo de sais de cálcio no osso. **2.** Em odontologia, um processo aprimorado pela presença de fluoreto por meio do qual o esmalte, a dentina e o cemento parcialmente descalcificados se tornam recalcificados pela reposição mineral.
rem·i·nis·cence (rem-i-nis′sens). Reminiscência; em psicologia do aprendizado, uma melhora na lembrança, em relação ao que foi mostrado na última tentativa, do material aprendido de forma incompleta após um intervalo sem prática. [L. *reminiscentiae*, de *reminiscor*, lembrar-se]
re·mis·sion (rē-mish′ŭn) Remissão; **1.** A redução ou diminuição na intensidade dos sintomas de uma doença. **2.** O período durante o qual ocorre tal redução. [L. *remissio*, de *re-mitto*, pp. *-missus*, enviar de volta, afrouxamento, relaxamento]
  spontaneous r., r. espontânea; o desaparecimento dos sintomas sem um tratamento formal.
re·mit (rē-mit′). Remitir; tornar-se menos grave durante um período sem cessar por completo. [ver remission]
re·mit·tence (rē-mit′ens). Remitência; melhora temporária sem a cessação real dos sintomas.
re·mit·tent (rē-mit′ent). Remitente; caracterizado por períodos temporários de redução dos sintomas de uma doença.
rem·nant (rem′nant). Resto, remanescente; alguma coisa que permanece, um resíduo ou vestígio. [Fr. ant. de *remaindre*, permanecer, do L. *remaneo*]
re·mod·el·ing (rē-mod′el-ing). Remodelagem. **1.** Um processo cíclico por meio do qual o osso se mantém em um equilíbrio dinâmico através da reabsorção e formação seqüenciais de uma pequena quantidade de osso em um mesmo local; diferentemente do processo de modelagem, o tamanho e a forma do osso remodelado permanecem inalterados. **2.** Qualquer processo de remodelação ou reorganização.
  heart chamber r., r. da câmara cardíaca; uma mudança arquitetural em qualquer uma das câmaras cardíacas (geralmente em um ou em ambos os ventrículos) que resulta de um estímulo normal (neonatal) ou patológico.
ren, gen. **re·nis,** pl. **re·nes** (ren, rē′nis, rē′nēz). Rim. SIN kidney. [L.]
re·nal (rē′năl). Renal. SIN nephric.
re·nat·ur·a·tion (rē-na-tū-ra′shŭn). Renaturação; a conversão de uma macromolécula inativa e desnaturada de volta à sua configuração bioativa e natural.
ren·cu·lus (ren′koo-lŭs). **1.** SIN cortical lobules of kidney, em *lobule*. **2.** SIN reniculus (2).
Rendu, Henri J.L.M., médico francês, 1844–1902. VER R.-Osler-Weber *syndrome*.
△ **reni-.** Reni-. VER reno-.
ren·i·cap·sule (ren′i-kap′sool). A cápsula do rim. [reni- + L. *capsula*, cápsula]
ren·i·car·di·ac (ren′i-kar′dē-ak). Renocardíaco. SIN cardiorenal. [reni- + G. *kardia*, coração]
re·nic·u·lus, pl. **re·nic·u·li** (rē-nik′u-lŭs, -lī). Renículo. **1.** SIN cortical lobules of kidney, em *lobule*. **2.** Um lobo do rim humano fetal e do rim de alguns animais inferiores nos quais septos fibrosos subdividem o órgão. SIN renculus (2), renunculus (2), [L. dim. de *ren*, rim]
ren·i·form (ren′i-form). Reniforme. SIN nephroid.
re·nin (rē′nin). Renina; um termo originalmente utilizado para indicar uma substância com ação pressora obtida dos rins de coelhos, e atualmente uma enzima que converte o angiotensinogênio em angiotensina I. SIN angiotensinogenase.
ren·i·por·tal (ren′i-pōr′tăl). Reniportal. **1.** Relativo ao hilo do rim. **2.** Relativo à circulação capilar venosa ou portal do rim. [reni- + L. *porta*, portão]
ren·nase (ren′ās). Renase. SIN chymosin.
ren·net (ren′et). Coalho. SIN chymosin.
ren·nin (ren′in). Renina. SIN chymosin.
ren·nin·o·gen, ren·no·gen (rē-nin′ō-jen, ren′ō-jen). Reninogênio. SIN prochymosin. [rennin + -gen, produtor]
△ **reno-, reni-.** Reno-, reni-; o rim. VER TAMBÉM nephro-. [L. *ren*]

re·no·cu·ta·ne·ous (rē'nō - kū - tā'nē - ŭs). Renocutâneo; relativo aos rins e à pele. [reno- + L. *cutis*, pele]

re·no·gas·tric (rē'nō - gas'trik). Renogástrico; relativo aos rins e ao estômago. [reno- + G. *gastēr*, estômago]

re·no·gen·ic (rē - nō - jen'ik). Renogênico; que se origina no rim ou a partir dele.

re·no·gram (rē'nō - gram). Renograma; a avaliação da função renal por meio de detectores de radiação externa após a administração de um radiofármaco que é filtrado e excretado pelo rim. [reno- + G. *gramma*, algo escrito]

re·nog·ra·phy (rē - nog'ra - fē). Renografia; radiografia do rim.

re·no·in·tes·ti·nal (rē'nō - in - tes'ti - nal). Renointestinal; relativo aos rins e ao intestino.

re·no·meg·a·ly (rē'nō - meg'ă - lē). Renomegalia; aumento do rim.

re·nop·a·thy (rē - nop'ă - thē). Renopatia; um termo raramente utilizado para nefropatia.

re·no·pri·val (rē - nō - prī'val). Renoprivo; relativo à, caracterizado pela ou que resulta da perda total da função renal ou da remoção de todo o tecido renal funcionante. [reno- + L. *privus*, desprovido de]

re·no·pul·mo·nary (rē'nō - pŭl'mo - nār - ē). Renopulmonar; relativo aos rins e aos pulmões.

re·no·tro·phic (rē - nō - trof'ik). Renotrófico; relativo a qualquer agente que influencia o crescimento ou a nutrição do rim, ou à ação de tal agente. SIN nephrotrophic, nephrotropic, renotropic. [reno- + G. *trophē*, nutrição]

re·no·tro·phin (rē - nō - trō'fin). Renotrofina; agente que afeta o crescimento ou a nutrição do rim. SIN renotropin.

re·no·tro·pic (rē - nō - trop'ik). Renotrópico. SIN renotrophic. [reno- + G. *tropē*, uma volta]

re·no·tro·pin (rē - nō - trō'pin). Renotropina. SIN renotrophin.

re·no·vas·cu·lar (rē - nō - vas'kū - ler). Renovascular; relativo aos vasos sangüíneos do rim, indicando principalmente uma doença desses vasos.

Renpenning, H., médico canadense do século 20. VER R. *syndrome*.

ren. sem. Abreviatura de [L.] *renovetur semel*, que será renovado (somente) uma vez.

Renshaw, B., neurofisiologista norte-americano do século 20. VER R. *cells*, em *cell*.

re·nun·cu·lus (rē - nŭng'kū - lŭs). Renúnculo. **1.** SIN cortical *lobules* of kidney, em *lobule*. **2.** SIN reniculus (2). [L. dim. de *ren*]

Re·o·vir·i·dae (rē - ō - vir'i - dē). Família de vírus com RNA bifilamentar, alguns dos quais — os Reovirus — foram anteriormente incluídos entre os vírus ECHO e outros — os Orbivirus — entre os arbovírus. Os virions apresentam um diâmetro de 60-80 nm, geralmente não têm envelope e são resistentes ao éter; os genomas contêm RNA segmentado bifilamentar (PM 10-16 × 10⁶); os capsídeos apresentam simetria icosaédrica e duas camadas de capsômeros. A família compreende nove gêneros: Orthoreovirus, Orbivirus, Rotavirus, Coltivirus, Aquareovirus, o grupo dos vírus da poliedrose citoplasmática (Cypovirus) e três grupos de reovírus de vegetais (Phytoreovirus, Fijivirus e Oryzavirus). [*R*espiratory *E*nteric *O*rphan + viridae]

Re·o·vi·rus (rē'ō - vī'rŭs). Gênero de vírus atualmente denominados Orthoreovirus (família Reoviridae) que apresentam um diâmetro de 80 nm, duas camadas distintas de capsômeros e hospedeiros vertebrados; têm sido encontrados em crianças com infecções no trato respiratório superior, febre moderada e, às vezes, diarréia, e em crianças sem infecção aparente, em chimpanzés com coriza, em macacos e camundongos e nas fezes do gado. Existem três tipos humanos antigenicamente diferentes com um antígeno fixador de complemento comum e pelo menos 12 ortorreovírus aviários.

re·pair (rē - pār'). Reparação, reparo; a restauração de tecidos danificados ou afetados por uma doença naturalmente pelos processos de cicatrização, ou artificialmente por meio de procedimentos cirúrgicos. [I.m., do Fr. ant., do L. *reparo*, de *re-*, de volta, novamente, + *paro*, preparar, colocar em boa condição]

chemical r., r. química; a conversão de um radical livre em uma molécula estável.

error-prone r., r. SOS. SIN SOS r.

excision r., r. por excisão; a utilização de um filamento de DNA complementar como um molde para substituir um segmento de DNA danificado.

mismatch r., r. de pareamento incorreto; a substituição dos pares de bases que foram combinadas de forma errônea por meio da remoção da base incorreta e introdução da base correta pela ação da DNA polimerase.

recombinatorial r., r. por recombinação; a incorporação do DNA correspondente de um segmento de DNA a partir de uma molécula de DNA idêntica com o objetivo de substituir um segmento de DNA danificado.

SOS r., r. SOS; um sistema que repara as bases gravemente danificadas do DNA pela retirada e substituição das bases, mesmo quando não houver um modelo para guiar a seleção das bases. Esse processo é o último recurso para o reparo e é freqüentemente a causa de mutações. SIN error-prone r.

re·pand (rē - pand'). Indica uma colônia de bactérias que apresenta bordas marcadas por uma série de segmentos levemente côncavos com projeções angulares nos seus pontos de união. [L. *repandus*, inclinado ou virado para trás, de *re-*, para trás, + *pandus*, curvado]

re·pel·lent (rē - pel'ent). Repelente; **1.** Capaz de afugentar ou repelir; repulsivo. **2.** Um agente que afugenta ou impede o molestamento ou a irritação por pragas de insetos. **3.** Um adstringente ou outro agente que reduz o inchaço. [L. *re-pello*, pp. *-pulsus*, rechaçar]

rep·e·ti·tion-com·pul·sion (rep - e - tish'ŭn - kŏm - pŭl'shŭn). Compulsão à repetição; em psicanálise, a tendência a repetir experiências ou ações passadas em um esforço inconsciente para alcançar um domínio tardio sobre elas; uma necessidade mórbida de repetir um comportamento particular, tal como a lavagem das mãos ou o ato repetido de verificar se uma porta está trancada.

re·place·ment (rē - plās'ment). Recolocação, reposição; substituição. **1.** Restauração. **2.** Substituição.

cephalic r., reposição cefálica; nos casos de distócia do ombro, que impede o parto vaginal, a cabeça fetal é fletida e reinserida na vagina, a fim de restabelecer o fluxo sangüíneo do cordão umbilical, e o parto é realizado por meio de cesariana. SIN Zavanelli maneuver.

re·plant (rē'plant). **1.** Reimplantar; realizar uma reimplantação. **2.** Reimplante; uma parte do corpo ou um órgão assim recolocado ou que está para ser recolocado.

re·plan·ta·tion (rē - plan - tā'shŭn). Reimplantação, reimplante; a reposição de um órgão ou de uma parte do corpo em seu local original e o restabelecimento de sua circulação. SIN reimplantation. [L. *re-*, novamente, + *planto*, pp. *-atus*, plantar, de *planta*, um broto, rebento]

intentional r., r. intencional; a extração eletiva de um dente, a obturação do(s) canal(is) radicular(es) e a recolocação do dente no interior do alvéolo.

re·ple·tion (rē - plē'shŭn). Hipervolemia. SIN hypervolemia. [L. *repletio*, de *re-pleo*, pp. *-pletus*, encher]

rep·li·ca (rep'li - kă). Réplica, cópia; uma amostra para ser examinada sob microscopia eletrônica obtida por meio da cobertura de um arranjo cristalino ou de outro material viral com carbono; o molde (a r.) obtido após o material viral ter sido dissolvido fornece detalhes da estrutura e disposição. [It., do L.L. *re-plico*, dobrar novamente]

rep·li·case (rep'li - kās). Replicase. **1.** Termo descritivo da RNA polimerase dirigida pelo RNA associada à replicação dos vírus de RNA. **2.** Uma enzima que duplica os ácidos nucléicos.

rep·li·cate (rep'li - kāt). Replicar. **1.** Um de vários processos ou observações idênticos. **2.** Repetir; produzir uma cópia exata.

rep·li·ca·tion (rep - li - kā'shŭn). Replicação. **1.** A execução de um experimento ou estudo mais de uma vez, a fim de confirmar os achados originais, aumentar a precisão e obter uma estimativa mais próxima do erro de amostragem. **2.** A auto-reprodução ou a duplicação, como ocorre na mitose ou na biologia celular. VER autoreproduction. **3.** A síntese de DNA dirigida pelo DNA. [L. *replicatio*, uma réplica, de *replico*, pp. *-atus*, dobrar novamente]

bidirectional r., r. bidirecional; uma situação na qual a replicação do DNA avança com duas forquilhas de replicação que se movem em sentidos opostos ao redor de uma estrutura circular ou de uma alça em forma de D.

conservative r., r. conservadora; uma forma hipotética de duplicação na qual um DNA bifilamentar produz dois DNA-filhos de fita dupla, um dos quais é composto pelas duas fitas originais, enquanto o outro DNA-filho é composto por duas cadeias recém-sintetizadas.

semiconservative r., r. semiconservativa; a duplicação na qual um DNA bifilamentar produz dois DNA-filhos de fita dupla, cada um contendo uma das cadeias originais e uma fita recém-sintetizada.

unidirectional r., r. unidirecional; a duplicação na qual ocorre o movimento de uma única forquilha de replicação.

rep·li·ca·tor (rep'li - kā - ter). Replicador; o local específico de um genoma bacteriano (cromossoma) no qual a replicação se inicia.

rep·li·con (rep'li - kon). Réplicon. **1.** Um segmento de um cromossoma (ou do DNA de um cromossoma ou entidade similar) que pode se replicar, acompanhado de seus próprios códons de iniciação e de terminação, independentemente do cromossoma no qual ele está situado. **2.** A unidade de replicação; são encontradas várias unidades por DNA nos sistemas eucarióticos. [*replication* + *-on*]

re·po·lar·i·za·tion (rē'pō - lăr - i - zā'shŭn). Repolarização; o processo por meio do qual a membrana, célula ou fibra, após a despolarização, é polarizada novamente, com cargas elétricas positivas sobre a superfície externa e cargas elétricas negativas sobre a interna.

re·po·si·ti·o. Reposição. SIN reposition.

re·po·si·tion. Reposição; o movimento de retorno da palma e dos dedos da mão da posição contrária; o oposto de oposição. SIN repositio.

re·po·si·tion·ing (rē'pō - zish'ŭn - ing). Reposicionamento. **1.** Colocar em uma outra posição, como ocorre durante uma cirurgia. **2.** SIN reduction (1).

gingival r., r. gengival; o reposicionamento cirúrgico da gengiva inserida para eliminar a patose ou para estabelecer uma forma e função mais aceitáveis.

jaw r., r. mandibular; a alteração de qualquer posição relativa entre a mandíbula e as maxilas, pela modificação da oclusão dos dentes naturais ou artificiais, ou por procedimentos cirúrgicos.

muscle r., r. muscular; o reposicionamento cirúrgico de uma inserção muscular para uma posição mais funcional.

re·pos·i·tor (rē-poz′i-ter, -tōr). Repositor; um instrumento utilizado para reposicionar um órgão deslocado.
representation. Representação.
  internal r., representação interna; termo empregado em programação neurolingüística para indicar o modo como as pessoas utilizam as imagens mentais (visual, auditiva ou cinestésica) para codificar uma experiência, um composto que compreende suas realidades interna e externa.
re·pressed (rē-prest′). Reprimido; que foi submetido a repressão.
re·pres·sion (rē-presh′un). Repressão. **1.** Em psicoterapia, o mecanismo de defesa ou o processo ativo que consiste em manter afastados, expulsar e banir da consciência as idéias ou os impulsos que são inaceitáveis para o ego ou superego. **2.** A expressão diminuída de algum produto do gene. [L. *re-primo*, pp. *-pressus*, pressionar novamente, reprimir]
  catabolite r., r. por catabolito; a expressão diminuída de um operon por causa dos níveis elevados de um catabolito de uma via bioquímica.
  end product r., r. pelo produto final; a r. por catabolito na qual o catabolito é um produto final de uma via específica.
  enzyme r., r. enzimática; inibição da síntese enzimática por alguns metabolitos.
  primal r., r. primal; r. de material que nunca atingiu o pensamento consciente.
re·pres·sor (rē-pres′er). Repressor; o produto de um gene regulador ou repressor.
  active r., r. ativo; um r. que se combina diretamente com um gene operador, a fim de reprimir o operador e seus genes estruturais, reprimindo assim a síntese protéica; um r. ativo pode ser reprimido por um indutor, o que permite a síntese protéica; um mecanismo homeostático para a regulação de sistemas enzimáticos indutíveis.
  inactive r., r. inativo; um r. que, para se combinar com um gene operador, precisa combinar-se primeiramente com um co-repressor (geralmente um produto de uma via protéica); após a ativação, o r. bloqueia a produção de proteínas controlada pelo gene operador; um mecanismo homeostático para a regulação de sistemas enzimáticos repressíveis.
re·pro·duc·i·bil·i·ty (rē-prō-dus′i-bil′i-tē). Reprodutibilidade. **1.** A habilidade para produzir vida novamente ou apresentar algo novamente. **2.** A capacidade de duplicar medições durante longos períodos de tempo por diferentes laboratórios.
re·pro·duc·tion (rē-prō-dŭk′shun). Reprodução. **1.** O processo total por meio do qual os organismos produzem descendentes. SIN generation (1), procreation. **2.** A lembrança e a apresentação na mente dos elementos de uma impressão passada. [L. *re-*, novamente, + *pro-duco*, pp. *-ductus*, conduzir para adiante, produzir]
  asexual r., r. assexuada; r. diferente daquela na qual ocorre a união de células sexuais masculinas e femininas. SIN agamogenesis, agamogony.
  cytogenic r., r. citogênica; r. que ocorre por meio de células germinativas unicelulares; engloba tanto a r. sexuada quanto a r. assexuada por esporos.
  sexual r., r. sexuada; r. que ocorre pela união de gametas masculinos e femininos para formar um zigoto. SIN gamogenesis, syngenesis.
  somatic r., r. somática; a r. assexuada que ocorre por fissão ou brotamento de células somáticas.
  vegetative r., r. vegetativa. VER asexual r.
re·pro·duc·tive (rē′prō-dŭk′tiv). Reprodutivo; relativo a reprodução.
rep·ti·lase (rep′til-as). Reptilase; uma enzima encontrada no veneno de *Bothrops atrox* que coagula o fibrinogênio por meio da cisão de seu fibrinopeptídeo. [reptile + -ase]
Rep·til·ia (rep-til′ē-ă). Uma classe de vertebrados que compreende os jacarés, os crocodilos, os lagartos, os cágados, as tartarugas e as cobras. [L. *reptilis*, neut. *-e*, que rasteja; neut. como subst., réptil]
re·pul·lu·la·tion (rē-pul-ū-lā′shun). Repululação; germinação renovada; o retorno de um processo ou crescimento mórbido. [L. *re-*, novamente, + *pullulo*, pp. *-atus*, germinar]
re·pul·sion (rē-pul′shun). Repulsão. **1.** O ato de repelir ou afastar, em oposição à atração. **2.** Uma forte antipatia; aversão; repugnância. **3.** A fase de pareamento de genes nos *loci* ligados que estão contidos em cromossomas opostos. VER coupling *phase*. [L. *re-pello*, pp. *-pulsus*, rechaçar]
re·quire·ment (rē-kwīr′ment). Necessidade, requisito, exigência. **1.** Algo necessário. **2.** Uma condição.
  minimum protein r., necessidade mínima de proteína; a quantidade, dependente da idade, de proteína exigida diariamente na dieta.
  quantum r., necessidade quântica; o número de quanta de luz absorvida necessário para a transformação de uma molécula; o inverso de rendimento quântico.
RES Abreviatura de reticuloendothelial *system* (sistema reticuloendotelial).
res·a·zu·rin (rē-saz′ū-rin). Resazurina; um composto azul utilizado como indicador de redox no teste da redutase do leite e também como indicador de pH (cor de laranja a 3,8 e violeta a 6,5).
res·cin·na·mine (rē-sin′ă-mēn, -min). Rescinamina; o éster do ácido 3,4,5-trimetoxicinâmico do reserpato de metila; um alcalóide (éster) purificado da fração alseroxilona de espécies de *Rauwolfia*; é química e farmacologicamente relacionado à reserpina, apresentando usos similares.
research (rē-surch, rē′surch). Pesquisa. **1.** (subst.) A busca organizada por novo conhecimento e melhor entendimento, p. ex., do mundo natural, dos determinantes da saúde e da doença. São reconhecidos vários tipos de pesquisa: observacional (empírica), analítica, experimental, teórica e aplicada. **2.** (v) Conduzir tal investigação científica. [Fr. ant. *re-cerche*, de *cerchier*, procurar, do L. *circare*, circular, de *circus*, círculo]
re·sect (rē-sekt′). Ressecar. **1.** Cortar fora ou remover, especialmente cortar fora as extremidades articulares de um ou de ambos os ossos que formam uma articulação. **2.** Excisar um segmento de uma parte. [L. *re-seco*, pp. *sectus*, cortar fora]
re·sect·a·ble (rē-sek′tă-bl). Ressecável; que se presta à ressecção.
re·sec·tion (rē-sek′shun). Ressecção. **1.** Um procedimento realizado para o propósito específico de remover algo, como na remoção das extremidades articulares de um ou ambos os ossos que formam uma articulação. **2.** Remover uma parte. **3.** SIN excision (1).
  abdominoperineal r. (APR), r. abdominoperineal; um tratamento cirúrgico do câncer que consiste na r. do colo sigmóide inferior, do reto, do ânus e da pele circunjacente e na formação de uma colostomia sigmóide; realizado como um procedimento transabdominal e perineal seqüencial ou sincrônico.
  gum r., r. gengival. SIN gingivectomy.
  loop r., r. por alça. SIN loop *excision*.
  muscle r., r. muscular; o encurtamento do tendão de um músculo ocular no estrabismo.
  root r., r. radicular. SIN apicoectomy.
  scleral r., r. escleral; o encurtamento da camada externa do olho que ocorre no descolamento da retina.
  transurethral r., r. transuretral; a remoção via endoscópio de lesões na próstata ou na bexiga, geralmente para aliviar uma obstrução prostática ou tratar tumores malignos da bexiga.
  wedge r., r. em cunha; a remoção de uma parte em forma de cunha do ovário; é utilizada no tratamento dos distúrbios virilizantes de origem ovariana, tal como a síndrome dos ovários policísticos.
re·sec·to·scope (rē-sek′tō-skōp). Ressectoscópio; um instrumento endoscópico especial utilizado na remoção eletrocirúrgica transuretral de lesões que envolvem a bexiga, a próstata ou a uretra.
re·ser·pine (rē-ser′pēn, -pin). Reserpina; alcalóide (éster) isolado da raiz de certas espécies de *Rauwolfia*; diminui as concentrações de 5-hidroxitriptamina e das catecolaminas no sistema nervoso central e nos tecidos periféricos; utilizado em conjunto com outros agentes hipotensivos no tratamento da hipertensão essencial e útil como tranqüilizante em estados psicóticos.
re·serve (rē-zerv′). Reserva; algo disponível, mas guardado para ser utilizado posteriormente, tal como a força ou os carboidratos. [L. *re-servo*, reter, reservar]
  alkali r., r. alcalina; a soma total dos íons básicos (principalmente de bicarbonatos) do sangue e de outros líquidos do organismo que, agindo como tampões, mantém o pH normal do sangue.
  breathing r., r. respiratória; a diferença entre a ventilação pulmonar (i.e., o volume de ar respirado sob condições de repouso comuns) e a capacidade respiratória máxima.
  cardiac r., r. cardíaca; o trabalho que o coração é capaz de realizar — além daquele exigido pelas circunstâncias normais da vida diária — que depende do estado do miocárdio e do grau no qual, dentro dos limites fisiológicos, as fibras do músculo cardíaco podem ser esticadas pelo volume de sangue que chega ao coração durante a diástole.
res·er·voir (rez′ev-wor). Reservatório. SIN receptaculum. [Fr.]
  r. of infection, r. da infecção; o material vivo ou não-vivo no qual um agente infeccioso se multiplica e/ou se desenvolve e do qual tal agente é dependente para sobreviver na natureza.
  Ommaya r., r. de Ommaya; recipiente plástico colocado no espaço subgaleal que se comunica com o ventrículo lateral ou com um cisto tumoral por meio de tubos; é utilizado para instilar medicação no interior do ventrículo ou do cisto tumoral ou para remover líquidos de dentro dessas estruturas.
  Pecquet r., r. de Pecquet. SIN cisterna chyli.
  r. of spermatozoa, r. de espermatozóides; o local onde os espermatozóides são armazenados; a parte distal da cauda do epidídimo e o início do ducto deferente.
  vitelline r., r. vitelínico. SIN vitellarium.
re·set no·dus si·nu·a·tri·a·lis (rē′set nō′dŭs sī′noo-ă-trē-ā′lis). Reajuste do nó sinoatrial; o reajuste do nó sinoatrial produzido pela despolarização (geralmente atrial) quando a soma da duração do ciclo prematuro e do ciclo de retorno é menor que o dobro do comprimento do ciclo espontâneo. Cf. nonreset nodus sinuatrialis. SIN sinus node reset.
res·i·dent (rez′i-dent). Residente; um médico vinculado a um hospital para treinamento clínico; antigamente, alguém que residia de fato no hospital. SIN resident physician. [L. *resideo*, residir]
re·sid·ua (rē-zid′ū-ă). Resíduos; plural de residuum.
re·sid·u·al (rē-zid′ū-ăl). Residual; relativo a ou da natureza de um resíduo.
res·i·due (rez′i-doo). Resíduo; aquilo que permanece após a remoção de uma ou mais substâncias. SIN residuum. [L. *residuum*]

day r., r. do dia; termo psicanalítico para um sonho relacionado a uma experiência do dia anterior.

re·sid·u·um, pl. **re·sid·ua** (rē-zid′ū-ŭm, -ū-ă). Resíduo. SIN residue. [L. neutro de *residuus*, deixado para trás, remanescente, de *re- sideo*, sentar novamente, permanecer para trás]

re·sil·ience (rē-zil′yens). Resiliência. **1.** A energia (por unidade de volume) liberada após suprimir a carga. **2.** Flexibilidade ou elasticidade. [L. *resilio*, tornar a saltar, ricochetear]

res·in (rez′in, roz′in). Resina. **1.** Uma substância frágil e amorfa que consiste na secreção endurecida de várias plantas, provavelmente derivada de um óleo volátil e similar a um estearopteno. **2.** SIN rosin. **3.** Um precipitado formado pela adição de água a certas tinturas. **4.** Um termo amplo utilizado para indicar substâncias orgânicas insolúveis em água; esses monômeros são denominados de acordo com sua composição química, estrutura física e os meios para sua ativação ou polimerização, p. ex., r. acrílica, r. autopolimerizante. [L. *resina*]

acrylic r., r. acrílica; um termo genérico aplicado a um material resinoso de diversos ésteres do ácido acrílico; utilizado como material de base de dentaduras, para outras restaurações dentárias e para moldeiras.

activated r., r. ativada. SIN autopolymer r.

anion-exchange r., r. trocadora de ânions. VER anion exchange, anion exchanger.

autopolymer r., autopolymerizing r., r. autopolimerizante; qualquer r. que pode ser polimerizada por catálise química em vez de pela aplicação de calor ou luz; utilizada em odontologia em restaurações dentárias, reparo de dentaduras e moldeiras de impressão. SIN activated r., cold cure r., cold-curing r., quick cure r., self-curing r.

carbacrylamine r.'s, resinas de carbacrilamina; uma mistura de resinas trocadoras de cátions, r. carbacrílica e r. carbacrílica de potássio (87,5%) e de r. trocadora de ânions e r. poliamina-metileno (12,5%) utilizada para aumentar a excreção fecal de sódio no edema associado à retenção excessiva de sódio pelos rins, p. ex., na insuficiência cardíaca congestiva, na cirrose hepática e na nefrose.

cation-exchange r., r. trocadora de cátions. VER cation exchange, cation exchanger.

chemically cured r., r. quimicamente polimerizada; uma r. que contém um iniciador, em geral o peróxido de benzoíla, e um ativador, geralmente uma amina terciária, em pastas separadas. Quando misturadas, a amina reage com o peróxido de benzoíla para formar radicais livres e ocorrer a polimerização.

cholestyramine r., r. de colestiramina; r. trocadora de ânions fortemente básica na forma de cloreto, que consiste em um copolímero do estireno e do divinilbenzeno com grupos funcionais do amônio quaternário; reduz o colesterol sangüíneo por meio da ligação dos ácidos biliares no intestino, promovendo assim sua excreção nas fezes em vez da reabsorção a partir do intestino; utilizada no tratamento da hipercolesterolemia, da cirrose biliar xantomatosa e de outras formas de xantomatose; liga-se também a numerosas drogas no intestino, reduzindo sua biodisponibilidade.

cold cure r., cold-curing r., r. de polimerização a frio. SIN autopolymer r.

composite r., r. composta; r. sintética geralmente de base acrílica à qual foi adicionado um filtro de vidro ou de sílica natural. Utilizada principalmente em procedimentos de restauração dentária. [L. *compositus*, colocar junto, de *compono*, colocar junto]

copolymer r., r. copolimérica; r. sintética produzida pela polimerização conjunta de dois ou mais monômeros ou polímeros diferentes.

cross-linked r., r. de ligação cruzada. SIN cross-linked polymer.

direct filling r., r. de obturação direta; r. autopolimerizante especialmente projetada como um material para restauração dentária.

dual-cure r., r. de polimerização dual; r. que utiliza tanto a iniciação luminosa quanto a química para ativar a polimerização.

epoxy r., r. epóxi; qualquer r. termopolimerizante que se baseia na reatividade do epóxi; utilizada como adesivo, revestimento protetor e meio de inclusão em microscopia eletrônica.

gum r., goma-resina; o exsudato seco proveniente de várias plantas, que consiste em uma mistura de uma goma e r., sendo a primeira solúvel em água, mas não em álcool, e a segunda solúvel em álcool, mas não em água.

heat-curing r., r. de polimerização a quente; a r. que necessita de calor para iniciar a polimerização.

Indian podophyllum r., r. do podofilo indiano; r. obtida do *Podophyllum emodi*; um catártico e colagogo.

ion-exchange r., r. trocadora de íons. VER ion exchange, ion exchanger.

ipomea r., r. da ipoméia; r. obtida da raiz seca de *Ipomoea orizabensis*; um catártico. VER TAMBÉM scammony.

jalap r., r. da jalapa; r. extraída da raiz tuberosa seca de *Exogonium purga*; um purgativo.

light-activated r., r. ativada pela luz. SIN light-cured r.

light-cured r., r. polimerizada pela luz, r. fotopolimerizada; uma r. que utiliza a luz visível ou ultravioleta para excitar um fotoiniciador, que interage com uma amina para formar radicais livres e iniciar a polimerização; empregada principalmente em odontologia restauradora. SIN light-activated r.

melamine r., r. de melamina; material plástico misturado com gesso comum utilizado em modelos. Esse modelo é mais leve e mais resistente do que aquele feito apenas com gesso comum. SIN melamine formaldehyde.

methacrylate r., r. de metacrilato; material plástico translúcido empregado na fabricação de diversos aparelhos médicos, instrumentos cirúrgicos e componentes de suporte utilizados na substituição total de uma articulação; possui as propriedades ópticas do quartzo fundido e molda-se prontamente quando aquecido; usado no passado na inclusão de tecidos para microscopia eletrônica e, atualmente, suplantado pelas resinas epóxi.

podophyllum r., r. do podofilo; r. extraída de raízes e rizomas secos do *Podophyllum peltatum*, uma erva perene comum em ambientes úmidos e sombreados das regiões situadas ao leste do Canadá e dos Estados Unidos. A droga é utilizada pelos indígenas norte-americanos como vermífugo e emético. Os principais constituintes da r. pertencem ao grupo das ligninas, que são compostos com 118 carbonos relacionados biossinteticamente aos flavonóides e derivados por dimerização de duas unidades C_6-C_3. As resinas mais importantes presentes na r. do podofilo são a podofilotoxina (cerca de 20%), a β-peltatina (cerca de 10%) e a α-peltatina (cerca de 5%). Todas as três ocorrem tanto na forma livre quanto como glicosídeos. A r. é utilizada como purgativo, mas tem sido substituída por agentes mais suaves. É citotóxica e utilizada na forma de um líquido para pincelagem no tratamento de verrugas venéreas frágeis e de outros tipos de verrugas. SIN May apple root, podophyllin, wild mandrake.

polyamine-methylene r., r. de poliamina-metileno; r. sintética que se liga aos ácidos utilizada como antiácido gástrico.

polyester r., r. de poliéster; r. cujos polímeros são insolúveis na maioria dos solventes orgânicos e polimerizados pela luz, pelo calor e pelo oxigênio; utilizada como meio de inclusão de tecidos para microscopia eletrônica.

quick cure r., r. de polimerização rápida. SIN autopolymer r.

quinine carbacrylic r., r. carbacrílica de quinina. SIN azuresin.

self-curing r., r. autopolimerizante. SIN autopolymer r.

res·in ac·ids. Ácidos resínicos; uma classe de compostos orgânicos derivados de várias resinas naturais vegetais; os diterpenos contêm um anel de fenantreno; p. ex., o ácido abiético, o ácido pimárico e as gomas de ésteres. SIN resinic acids.

res·in·ates (rez′in-āts). Resinatos; os sais ou ésteres de ácidos resínicos.

res·ines (rez′ens). Resinas; os ésteres de ácidos resínicos.

res·in·ic ac·ids. Ácidos resínicos. SIN resin acids.

res·in·oid (rez′i-noyd). Resinóide. **1.** Uma substância que contém uma resina ou que se assemelha a uma. **2.** Um extrato obtido pela evaporação de uma tintura. **3.** Que se assemelha a uma resina.

res·in·ols (rez′in-ols). Resinóis; os álcoois resínicos.

res·in·ous (rez′i-nŭs). Resinoso; relativo a ou que deriva de uma resina.

re·sis·tance (rē-zis′tans). Resistência. **1.** A força exercida em oposição a uma força ativa. **2.** A oposição à passagem de uma corrente elétrica em um condutor, por meio do qual há uma perda de energia e uma produção de calor; de modo específico, a diferença de potencial em volts ao longo do condutor por ampère de fluxo de corrente; unidade: ohm. Cf. impedance (1). **3.** A oposição ao fluxo de um líquido através de uma ou mais passagens (p. ex., o fluxo sangüíneo, os gases respiratórios na árvore traqueobrônquica), análogo a (2); as unidades são em geral aquelas da diferença de pressão por unidade de fluxo. Cf. impedance (2). **4.** Em psicanálise, a defesa inconsciente de um indivíduo contra o surgimento na consciência de pensamentos reprimidos. **5.** A capacidade das hemácias de resistir à hemólise e de preservar sua forma quando submetidas a graus variados de pressão osmótica no plasma sangüíneo. **6.** A capacidade natural ou adquirida de um organismo de manter sua imunidade ou resistir aos efeitos de um agente antagônico, p. ex., um microrganismo patogênico, uma toxina, uma droga. [L. *re-sisto*, colocar de pé novamente, resistir a]

airway r., r. das vias aéreas; em fisiologia, a r. ao fluxo dos gases que ocorre durante a ventilação, decorrente de obstrução ou de fluxo turbulento nas vias aéreas superiores e inferiores; deve ser diferenciada, durante a inalação, da r. à insuflação resultante de diminuição na complacência pulmonar e torácica.

bacteriophage r., r. aos bacteriófagos; a r. de uma bactéria mutante a uma infecção por um bacteriófago ao qual a cepa parental da bactéria (tipo selvagem) é susceptível.

dicumarol r. r. ao dicumarol; [MIM*122700], um distúrbio autossômico dominante caracterizado pela r. ao dicumarol, sobre a e acima da variabilidade geral de tolerância à droga; causado por mutação no gene da cumarina 7-hidroxilase (CYP2A6) situado no cromossoma 19p.

drug r., r. à droga, r. medicamentosa; a capacidade dos microrganismos causadores de doenças de resistir a drogas que antes eram tóxicas para eles; obtida por mutação espontânea ou seleção natural após exposição à droga em questão. Os microrganismos patogênicos resistem aos antibióticos por meio de vários mecanismos que incluem a produção de enzimas (p. ex., as β-lactamases), que inativam quimicamente as moléculas dos antibióticos. Nas infecções mistas do trato respiratório, uma β-lactamase (penicilinase) produzida por um microrganismo (p. ex., *Haemophilus influenzae*) pode inativar a penicilina e, dessa forma, bloquear sua eficácia contra os outros organismos causadores da infecção (mista) que não apresentam resistência (p. ex., os estreptococos β-hemolíticos do grupo A). Em geral, um microrganismo que adquiriu resistência a um determinado antibiótico é também resistente a outros da mesma classe química. Algumas bactérias transmitem aos seus descendentes sua r. a um ou vários antibióticos não via cromossomas, e sim via plasmídios, os quais estão situados do lado de fora do núcleo bacteriano, mas que realizam certas funções genéticas. As bactérias de uma espécie podem desenvolver r. a determinados antibióticos ao adquirir plasmídios de bactérias de outras espécies.

A resistência medicamentosa é um problema mundial crescente. Muitas cepas de bactérias, fungos e parasitas desenvolveram resistência, incluindo pneumococos, gonococos, salmonelas, *Mycobacterium tuberculosis*, *Tinea tonsurans* e *Plasmodium falciparum*. Em algumas partes dos Estados Unidos, 40% dos isolados de pneumococos e 90% dos estafilococos são resistentes a penicilina. A prevalência tanto de enterococos resistentes à vancomicina como de *Staphylococcus aureus* resistente à meticilina aumentou 20 vezes desde 1989. Os fatores que favorecem o desenvolvimento da resistência aos antibióticos incluem a prescrição inadequada de antibióticos (p. ex., para tratar de infecções virais), o uso indiscriminado de agentes de espectro estendido recém-desenvolvidos, o tratamento empírico e de amplo espectro de infecções em determinadas populações (p. ex., crianças, idosos e indivíduos que trabalham em instalações de longa permanência), a prescrição de doses subletais e a falha dos pacientes em completar o tratamento com antibióticos. Os centros para controle e prevenção de doenças dos Estados Unidos (*Centers for Disease Control and Prevention*) estimam que os médicos norte-americanos preenchem anualmente 50 milhões de prescrições de antibióticos desnecessárias, incluindo 17 milhões para o tratamento do resfriado comum. Os especialistas em doenças infecciosas e as autoridades responsáveis pela saúde pública têm pedido moderação aos médicos na prescrição de antibióticos, particularmente para as crianças e para infecções do trato respiratório superior não-complicadas e bronquite aguda (quase sempre viral) e também para sinusite aguda e otite média (para as quais não foram estabelecidos critérios diagnósticos confiáveis para infecção bacteriana). Eles têm também realçado a importância da educação pública, uma vez que as expectativas inadequadas dos pacientes ou de seus pais têm sido um fator propulsor para o uso abusivo de antibióticos pelos médicos. A administração de antibióticos ao gado, principalmente para a profilaxia de doenças e a promoção do crescimento, também contribui para o surgimento de cepas de bactérias resistentes.

expiratory r., r. expiratória; a r. ao fluxo de gás para fora dos pulmões ou a r. total ao fluxo de gás durante a fase expiratória do ciclo respiratório.
impact r., r. de impacto; a capacidade de uma lente para uso ocular de resistir ao impacto de uma bola de aço de 3/8 de polegada (= 9,525 mm) que cai de uma altura de 50 pés (= 15,24 m) sem estilhaçar ou quebrar; os critérios para a determinação da r. ao impacto são especificados por regulamentações norte-americanas.
inductive r., r. indutiva. SIN reactance.

insulin r., r. à insulina; a efetividade diminuída da insulina em reduzir os níveis plasmáticos de glicose, definidos arbitrariamente como a necessidade diária de pelo menos 200 unidades de insulina para impedir a hiperglicemia e a cetose; em geral é resultante da ligação de anticorpos à insulina ou aos sítios receptores de insulina; está associada a obesidade, cetoacidose e infecção.

Uma falha na resposta normal das células musculares e de outras células à insulina endógena ou exógena freqüentemente complica a deficiência de insulina endógena que é característica do diabetes melito de tipo 2. É um fenômeno periférico e pode ocorrer mesmo quando a qualidade e a quantidade de insulina produzida pelo pâncreas são normais. É aparentemente resultante de uma diminuição no número de receptores de insulina situados nas células, de uma disfunção do sistema de transporte bioquímico da glicose ou de ambas. A resistência à insulina está com freqüência associada a níveis elevados de anticorpos circulantes contra os receptores de insulina. O fenômeno da resistência à insulina explica por que algumas pessoas com diabetes de tipo 2 exibem hiperinsulinemia em jejum, muitas vezes associada a níveis plasmáticos elevados de glicose. A resistência à insulina correlaciona-se de perto com a obesidade no diabetes. Ocorre com menor freqüência nos diabéticos magros, cujo principal problema é comumente a falência primária na produção de insulina. A resistência à insulina é muitas vezes observada em pessoas com ou sem diabetes franco que possuem outros distúrbios endócrinos ou sistêmicos, incluindo dislipidemias, hipertensão, hiperuricemia e infecção crônica. Algumas mulheres com ovários policísticos, hirsutismo e anovulação também apresentam resistência à insulina e hiperinsulinemia. A troglitazona, o mais recente agente utilizado no tratamento do diabetes melito de tipo 2, melhora a sensibilidade à insulina.

multidrug r., r. a múltiplas drogas; a insensibilidade de diversos tumores a uma variedade de drogas anticancerosas quimicamente correlatas; é mediada por um processo que inativa ou remove a droga das células tumorais-alvo.
mutual r., r. mútua. SIN antagonism.
peripheral r., r. periférica. SIN total peripheral r.
synaptic r., r. sináptica; a facilidade ou dificuldade com a qual um impulso nervoso pode atravessar uma sinapse.
systemic vascular r., r. vascular sistêmica; um índice da complacência ou da constrição arteriolar por todo o corpo; é proporcional à pressão sangüínea dividida pelo débito cardíaco.
thyrotropin r., r. à tireotropina; um distúrbio autossômico recessivo no qual os tireócitos não respondem à tireotropina. Cf. pseudohypoparathyroidism.
total peripheral r. (TPR), r. periférica total; a r. total ao fluxo de sangue no circuito sistêmico; o quociente produzido pela divisão da pressão arterial média pelo volume-minuto cardíaco. SIN peripheral r.
re·sis·tiv·i·ty (rē′zis-tiv′i-tē). Resistividade; a medida da resistência de um material à passagem de corrente elétrica; o oposto de condutividade. [L. *resito*, resistir]
re·sis·tor (rē-zis′ter, -tōr). Resistor; um elemento inserido em um circuito elétrico para fornecer resistência ao fluxo da corrente.
res·o·lu·tion (rez-ō-loo′shŭn). Resolução. **1.** A interrupção de um processo inflamatório sem supuração; a absorção ou a ruptura e remoção dos produtos de uma inflamação ou de uma neoformação. VER line *pairs*, em *pair*. **2.** A capacidade óptica para distinguir detalhes, tal como a separação de objetos vizinhos colocados muito próximos um do outro. SIN resolving power (3). [L. *resolutio*, afrouxar, de *re-solvo*, pp. *-solutus*, desatar, relaxar]
re·sol·vase (rē-sol′vāz). Resolvase; um gene codificado por um transposon que pode catalisar a segunda etapa da transposição, bem como participar da regulação de sua própria expressão. [resolve + -ase]
re·solve (rē-zolv′). Resolver; retornar ou provocar o retorno ao estado normal, especialmente sem supuração; diz-se de um fleimão ou de outra forma de inflamação. [L. *resolvo*, soltar]
re·sol·vent (rē-zol′vent). Resolvente. **1.** Que promove a resolução. **2.** Um agente que interrompe um processo inflamatório ou causa a absorção de uma neoplasia.
res·o·nance (rez′ō-nans). Ressonância. **1.** A vibração do ar natural ou forçada no interior das cavidades situadas acima, abaixo, em frente ou atrás de uma fonte sonora; na fala, a modificação da qualidade (p. ex., harmônicos) de um tom pela passagem do ar através das câmaras do nariz, da faringe e da cabeça, sem aumento da intensidade do som. **2.** O som obtido ao se percurtir uma parte que pode vibrar livremente. **3.** A intensificação e o caráter surdo do som da voz obtido ao se realizar a ausculta sobre uma cavidade. **4.** Em química, a maneira pela qual os elétrons ou as cargas elétricas estão distribuídos entre os átomos nos compostos que são planos e simétricos, especialmente naqueles com ligações duplas conjugadas (alternadas); a existência de r. no último caso reduz o conteúdo de energia e aumenta a estabilidade de um composto. **5.** A freqüência natural ou inerente de qualquer sistema oscilante. **6.** SIN resonant frequency. [L. *resonantia*, eco, de *re-sono*, ressoar, ecoar]
amphoric r., r. anfórica; um som de percussão, como aquele produzido ao se golpear uma garrafa grande e vazia, obtido pela percussão da área situada sobre uma cavidade pulmonar. SIN cavernous r.
bandbox r., r. timpânica. SIN vesiculotympanitic r.
bellmetal r., r. metálica; nos casos em que há uma grande cavidade pulmonar ou um pneumotórax, um som metálico nítido que se obtém pela percussão de uma moeda colocada sobre o tórax por outra moeda, ou pela aplicação de um piparote na parede torácica com a unha; o som é ouvido ao se auscultar a parede torácica do mesmo lado na posição ântero-posterior. SIN anvil sound, bell sound, coin test.
cavernous r., r. cavernosa. SIN amphoric r.
cracked-pot r., r. de panela rachada; um som peculiar, semelhante àquele ouvido ao se percutir uma panela rachada, desencadeado pela percussão da área sobre uma cavidade pulmonar que se comunica com um brônquio, quando a boca do paciente está aberta. SIN cracked-pot sound.
electron paramagnetic r. (EPR), r. paramagnética eletrônica. SIN electron spin r.
electron spin r. (ESR), r. de *spin* eletrônico; uma técnica espectrométrica baseada na medição dos *spins* dos elétrons e dos momentos magnéticos e utilizada na detecção e na avaliação dos radicais livres nas reações e nos sistemas biológicos. SIN electron paramagnetic r.
hydatid r., r. hidática; r. vibrátil peculiar ouvida durante a percussão auscultatória da área sobre um cisto hidático.
nuclear magnetic r. (NMR), r. magnética nuclear; o fenômeno no qual determinados núcleos atômicos que possuem um momento magnético precessam ao redor do eixo de um forte campo magnético externo, com uma freqüência de precessão (freqüência de Larmor) específica para cada núcleo e para a força do campo magnético; os núcleos em rotação induzem seus próprios campos magnéticos oscilantes e, portanto, emitem radiação eletromagnética que pode produzir um sinal detectável na freqüência de Larmor. A r. magnética

nuclear é utilizada como um método para a identificação de ligações covalentes e é usada clinicamente nas imagens por ressonância magnética (ver magnetic resonance *imaging*).

skodaic r., r. de Skoda; um som peculiar, de tonalidade elevada e menos musical do que aquele obtido sobre uma cavidade, desencadeado pela percussão logo acima do nível de um derrame pleural. SIN Skoda sign, Skoda tympany.

tympanitic r., r. timpânica. SIN tympany.

vesicular r., r. vesicular; o som obtido pela percussão da área sobre os pulmões normais.

vesiculotympanitic r., r. vesiculotimpânica; um som peculiar parcialmente timpânico, parcialmente vesicular, obtido pela percussão nos casos de enfisema pulmonar. SIN bandbox r., wooden r.

vocal r. (VR), r. vocal; os sons vocais, conforme são ouvidos na ausculta do tórax.

wooden r., r. de madeira. SIN vesiculotympanitic r.

res·o·na·tor (rez'ō-nā-ter). Ressoador; um dispositivo que possibilita o emprego da indutância para criar uma corrente elétrica de potencial muito alto e volume baixo.

re·sorb (rē-sōrb'). Reabsorver; absorver o que foi excretado, como exsudato ou pus. [L. *re-sorbeo*, sugar novamente]

res·or·cin (rē-zor'sin). Resorcina. SIN resorcinol.

res·or·cin·ol (rē-zōr'si-nol). Resorcinol; um anti-séptico externo para psoríase, eczema, seborréia e tinha; o pirocatecol e a hidroquinona são isômeros do r. SIN resorcin.

  r. monoacetate, monoacetato de r.; utilizado externamente no tratamento da acne, da sicose e da seborréia.

  r. phthalic anhydride, anidrido ftálico de r. SIN fluorescein.

res·or·cin·ol·phtha·lein (rē-zōr'si-nol-thal'ē-in). Resorcinolftaleína. SIN fluorescein.

  r. sodium, r. sódica. SIN *fluorescein* sodium.

re·sorp·tion (rē-sōrp'shŭn). Reabsorção; **1.** O ato de reabsorver. **2.** Uma perda de substância por lise, ou por meios fisiológicos ou patológicos.

  bone r., r. óssea; a remoção de tecido ósseo.

  gingival r., r. gengival. SIN gingival *recession*.

  horizontal r., r. horizontal. SIN horizontal *atrophy*.

  internal r., r. interna; perda da estrutura dentária que se origina dentro da cavidade pulpar.

  ridge r., r. do rebordo; perda de volume e tamanho da parte alveolar da mandíbula ou da maxila.

  root r., r. radicular; a dissolução da raiz de um dente; tanto externa, com perda ou embotamento da parte apical, como interna, com perda de dentina da parte interna (pulpar) da área radicular.

res·pi·ra·ble (re-spīr'a-bl, res'pĭ-ră-bl). Respirável; capaz de ser respirado.

res·pi·ra·tion (res-pi-rā'shŭn). Respiração. **1.** Um processo fundamental vital, característico tanto de animais como de vegetais, no qual o oxigênio é utilizado para oxidar moléculas de combustível orgânico, fornecendo uma fonte de energia, bem como dióxido de carbono e água. Nas plantas verdes, a fotossíntese não é considerada r. **2.** SIN ventilation (2). [L. *respiratio*, de *respiro*, pp. *-atus*, exalar, respirar]

  abdominal r., r. abdominal; a respiração efetuada principalmente pela ação do diafragma.

  aerobic r., r. aeróbica; uma forma de r. na qual há consumo de oxigênio molecular e produção de dióxido de carbono e água.

  amphoric r., r. anfórica; um som semelhante àquele feito ao se soprar o gargalo de uma garrafa, ouvido durante a ausculta em alguns casos nos quais há uma grande cavidade pulmonar ou, ocasionalmente, um pneumotórax.

  anaerobic r., r. anaeróbica; forma de r. na qual não há consumo de oxigênio molecular; p. ex., a r. por nitrato e a r. por sulfato.

  artificial r., ventilação artificial. SIN artificial *ventilation*.

  assisted r., ventilação assistida. SIN assisted *ventilation*.

  Biot r., r. de Biot; um padrão respiratório completamente irregular, que apresenta freqüência e profundidade respiratórias continuamente variáveis; resulta de lesões nos centros respiratórios localizados no tronco encefálico, que se estendem da medula dorsomedial, caudalmente, até o óbex. SIN ataxic breathing, Biot breathing, respiratory ataxia.

  bronchial r., r. brônquica; um som de sopro tubular provocado pela passagem do ar através de um brônquio em uma área de tecido pulmonar consolidado.

  bronchovesicular r., r. broncovesicular; r. brônquica e vesicular combinadas.

  cavernous r., r. cavernosa; um som reverberante e oco ouvido na ausculta da área situada sobre uma cavidade no interior do pulmão.

  Cheyne-Stokes r., r. de Cheyne-Stokes; um padrão respiratório que apresenta aumento gradual na profundidade e, às vezes, na freqüência até um máximo, seguido por uma diminuição que leva a apnéia; os ciclos têm em geral uma duração de 30 segundos a 2 minutos, com 5-30 segundos de apnéia; observado nas lesões profundas e bilaterais do hemisfério cerebral, na encefalopatia metabólica e, caracteristicamente, no coma resultante de acometimento dos centros respiratórios nervosos.

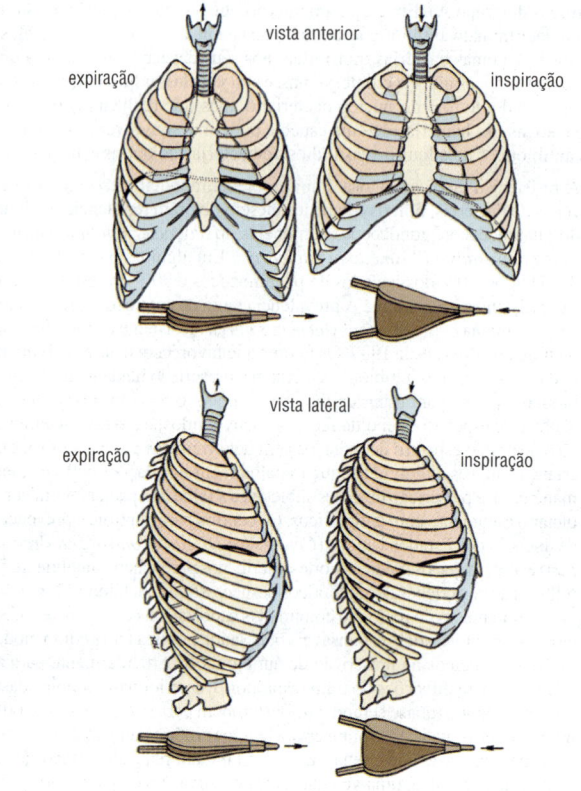

respiração

  cogwheel r., r. em roda dentada; um som inspiratório interrompido por um ou dois intervalos silenciosos. SIN interrupted r., jerky r.

  controlled r., ventilação controlada. SIN controlled *ventilation*.

  costal r., r. costal. SIN thoracic r.

  diffusion r., r. por difusão; a manutenção da oxigenação durante a apnéia por meio de insuflação intratraqueal de oxigênio em taxas de fluxo altas. SIN apneic oxygenation.

  electrophrenic r., r. eletrofrênica; a estimulação elétrica rítmica do nervo frênico por meio de um eletrodo aplicado à pele nos pontos motores desse nervo; é utilizada na paralisia do centro respiratório que resulta da poliomielite bulbar aguda.

  external r., r. externa; a troca dos gases respiratórios que ocorre nos pulmões, em oposição à r. interna ou tecidual.

  forced r., r. forçada; a hiperventilação voluntária.

  internal r., r. interna. SIN tissue r.

  interrupted r., r. interrompida. SIN cogwheel r.

  jerky r., r. entrecortada. SIN cogwheel r.

  Kussmaul r., r. de Kussmaul; r. rápida e profunda, característica da acidose diabética ou de outra origem. SIN Kussmaul-Kien r.

  Kussmaul-Kien r., r. de Kussmaul-Kien. SIN Kussmaul r.

  labored r., r. trabalhosa; respiração difícil, em geral profunda, observada em pacientes com doença cardíaca ou pulmonar que afeta o controle de sistema nervoso da ventilação.

  mouth-to-mouth r., r. boca a boca; um método de ventilação artificial que envolve a sobreposição da boca do paciente (e do nariz, em crianças pequenas) com a boca do socorrista, a fim de insuflar os pulmões do paciente por sopramento, seguida por uma fase expiratória não-assistida desencadeada pela retração elástica do tórax e dos pulmões do paciente; é repetido 12-16 vezes por minuto; quando o nariz do paciente não é coberto pela boca do operador, as narinas devem ser pinçadas com os dedos.

  nitrate r., r. por nitrato; o processo respiratório utilizado por alguns organismos anaeróbicos no qual o nitrato — em vez do oxigênio molecular — é empregado na oxidação de moléculas orgânicas para a obtenção de energia.

  paradoxical r., r. paradoxal; a deflação do pulmão durante a inspiração e a insuflação do pulmão durante a fase de expiração; observada no pulmão situado no mesmo lado de um pneumotórax aberto.

  puerile r., r. infantil; exagero dos sons respiratórios normais, ouvido em crianças e em adultos após esforços físicos.

  stertorous r., r. estertorosa; a respiração ruidosa geralmente ouvida em um paciente comatoso. SIN stertorous breathing.

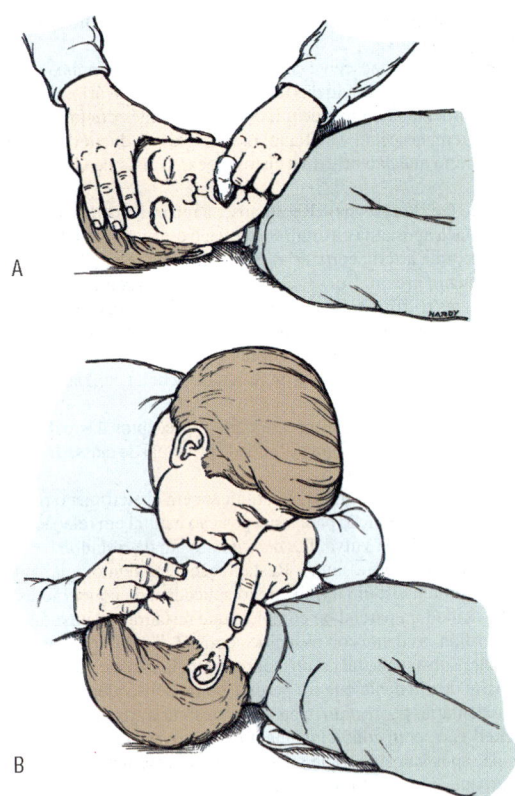

respiração boca a boca: (A) tenta-se remover qualquer corpo estranho da cavidade oral com o dedo indicador envolto em um pedaço de pano ou lenço; (B) inclinar a cabeça da vítima para trás e pinçar o nariz; expirar duas vezes lentamente na cavidade oral da vítima, com os lábios apertados contra os da vítima; expirar até o tórax da vítima elevar-se suavemente

sulfate r., r. por sulfato; o processo respiratório utilizado por alguns organismos anaeróbicos, no qual o sulfato — em vez do oxigênio molecular — é empregado na oxidação de moléculas orgânicas para a obtenção de energia.
thoracic r., r. torácica; a r. realizada principalmente pela ação dos músculos intercostais e por outros músculos que juntos elevam as costelas, provocando a expansão do tórax. SIN costal r.
tissue r., r. tecidual; a troca de gases entre o sangue e os tecidos. SIN internal r.
tubular r., r. tubular; r. brônquica de tom alto.
vesicular r., r. vesicular; o murmúrio respiratório auscultado nos pulmões normais. SIN respiratory murmur, vesicular murmur.
vesiculocavernous r., r. vesiculocavernosa; a r. cavernosa resultante da presença de uma cavidade, misturada ao murmúrio vesicular do tecido pulmonar normal circunjacente.
res·pi·ra·tor (res′pĭ-rā-ter, -tōr). **1.** Respirador; um aparelho para administrar respiração artificial nos casos de falência respiratória. **2.** Um aparelho que se ajusta sobre a boca e o nariz e é utilizado com o propósito de eliminar a poeira, a fumaça ou outros irritantes, ou para modificar o ar antes que ele penetre nas vias aéreas. SIN inhaler (1). SIN ventilator.
cuirass r., r. em couraça; um de vários tipos de respiradores que produzem uma pressão negativa intermitente ao redor da caixa torácica; hoje em dia, raramente utilizado.
Drinker r., r. de Drinker; um r. mecânico no qual o corpo (exceto a cabeça) é encaixado dentro de um tanque de metal, que é selado no pescoço com uma junta hermética; a respiração artificial é induzida, tornando-se negativa a pressão do ar contido no interior do tanque. SIN iron lung, tank r.
pressure-controlled r., r. de pressão controlada; um r. que fornece uma pressão predeterminada aos gases durante a inalação, sendo o volume do gás movido variável, dependente da resistência.
tank r., r. de tanque. SIN Drinker r.
volume-controlled r., r. de volume controlado; um r. que fornece um volume de gases predeterminado durante a inalação, sendo a pressão necessária para mover aquele volume remanescente variável, dependente da resistência.
res·pi·ra·to·ry (res′pĭ-rā-tōr-ē, rĕ-spīr′ă-tōr-ē). Respiratório; relativo à respiração.
re·spire (rĕ-spīr′). **1.** Respirar. **2.** Consumir oxigênio e produzir dióxido de carbono por meio do metabolismo. [L. *respiro*, respirar]
res·pi·rom·e·ter (res-pĭ-rom′ĕ-ter). **1.** Respirômetro; um instrumento para a medição da extensão dos movimentos respiratórios. **2.** Um instrumento para a medição do consumo de oxigênio ou da produção de dióxido de carbono, em geral de um tecido isolado. [L. *respiro*, respirar, + G. *metron*, medida]
Dräger r., r. de Dräger; um medidor inferencial utilizado para determinar o volume corrente e minuto a partir de várias revoluções de uma ventoinha que se movimenta por meio do fluxo de um gás, enquanto esse gás passa através de dois rotores engrenados com forma de losango e de pouco peso.
Wright r., r. de Wright; um medidor inferencial utilizado para determinar o volume corrente e minuto a partir de várias revoluções de uma ventoinha que se movimenta por meio do fluxo de um gás, enquanto esse gás passa através de 10 fendas tangenciais em um anel de estator cilíndrico para girar um rotor com duas pás planas; também denominado espirômetro de Wright.
re·sponse (rē-spons′). Resposta. **1.** A reação de um músculo, um nervo, uma glândula ou outro tecido excitável a um estímulo. **2.** Qualquer ato ou comportamento, ou seus constituintes, que um organismo vivo é capaz de realizar. Os reflexos são em geral excluídos, porque são habitualmente desencadeados por um estímulo que pode ser especificado (natural ou incondicionado), em vez de desencadeados em circunstâncias nas quais o estímulo não pode ser especificado. [L. *responsus*, uma resposta]
acute phase r., r. da fase aguda. SIN acute phase *reaction.*
anamnestic r. (an′am-nes-tik), r. anamnéstica, r. anamnésica. SIN secondary immune r.; VER immune r.
auditory brainstem r. (ABR), r. auditiva do tronco encefálico; medição eletrofisiológica da função auditiva que utiliza as respostas médias obtidas por computador produzidas pelo nervo auditivo e pelas vias auditivas centrais, principalmente do tronco encefálico, a estímulos acústicos repetitivos. Essa resposta é também empregada na localização de uma lesão e na determinação do tipo de dano auditivo (sensitivo *versus* nervoso). SIN brainstem evoked r.
automatic auditory brainstem r., r. auditiva automática do tronco encefálico; uma técnica de r. auditiva do tronco encefálico na qual uma modificação do estímulo é programada com base nas respostas elétricas registradas. O dispositivo determina automaticamente se os limiares predeterminados foram alcançados. É útil na avaliação da audição do recém-nascido.
biphasic r., r. bifásica; **(1)** duas respostas separadas e distintas que são separadas no tempo; **(2)** a reação imediata a um estímulo antigênico seguida por uma recorrência dos sintomas após um intervalo de quiescência.
blink r., r. de piscamento; r. desencadeada durante os estudos da condução nervosa, que consistem em potenciais de ação musculares evocados dos músculos orbiculares dos olhos após uma breve estimulação mecânica ou elétrica da área cutânea inervada pelo ramo oftálmico do nervo trigêmeo. Caracteristicamente, há uma r. inicial (aproximadamente 10 ms após o estímulo), ipsolateral ao local estimulado (rotulada de R1), e respostas tardias bilaterais (aproximadamente 30 ms após o estímulo; rotuladas de R2); as respostas tardias são responsáveis pelo estremecimento visível dos músculos orbiculares dos olhos.
booster r., r. de reforço. SIN secondary immune r. VER immune r.
brainstem evoked r. (BSER), r. evocada do tronco encefálico. SIN auditory brainstem r.
conditioned r., r. condicionada; uma r. que já consta do repertório de um indivíduo, mas que, por meio de pareamentos repetidos com seu estímulo natural, foi adquirida ou novamente condicionada a um estímulo previamente neutro ou condicionado. VER conditioning. Cf. unconditioned r.
Cushing r., r. de Cushing. SIN Cushing *phenomenon.*
depletion r., r. de depleção; r. metabólica subnormal ao trauma observada em uma pessoa cujos processos fisiológicos já estão deprimidos por uma doença.
early-phase r., r. da fase inicial; o início rápido dos sintomas que ocorre após um estímulo antigênico.
evoked r., r. evocada; alteração na atividade elétrica de uma região do sistema nervoso através da qual um estímulo sensitivo aferente está passando; pode ser somatossensitiva, auditiva do tronco encefálico ou visual. VER TAMBÉM evoked *potential.*
flight or fight r., r. de luta ou fuga. VER emergency *theory.*
galvanic skin r. (GSR), r. galvânica da pele; uma medição das alterações do excitamento emocional indicadas por eletrodos fixados em qualquer parte da pele e pelo registro das alterações momento a momento da transpiração e da atividade do sistema nervoso autônomo relacionada. SIN galvanic skin reaction, galvanic skin reflex, psychogalvanic reaction, psychogalvanic skin reaction, psychogalvanic reflex, psychogalvanic skin reflex, psychogalvanic r., psychogalvanic skin r.
Henry-Gauer r., r. de Henry-Gauer; a inibição da secreção do hormônio antidiurético como conseqüência de uma elevação da pressão atrial que estimula os receptores de estiramento atriais.
immune r., r. imune; **(1)** qualquer r. do sistema imune a um antígeno, incluindo a produção de anticorpos e/ou a imunidade mediada por células; **(2)** a r. do sistema imune a um antígeno (imunógeno) que leva à condição de sensibilidade induzida; a r. imune à exposição antigênica inicial (r. imune primária) é detectável, via de regra, somente após um intervalo de vários dias a 2 semanas; a r. imune a um estímulo subseqüente (r. imune secundária) pelo mesmo antígeno é mais rápida do que no caso da r. imune primária.

isomorphic r., r. isomórfica; r. ao trauma no local da lesão em áreas do paciente não-acometidas previamente por doenças cutâneas, tais como a psoríase e o líquen plano, caracterizada tipicamente por lesões lineares nos locais da escoriação ou de uma cicatriz. SIN Köbner phenomenon.
late auditory-evoked r., r. evocada auditiva tardia; a r. do córtex auditivo à estimulação acústica.
late-phase r., r. da fase tardia; a recorrência dos sintomas após um intervalo significativo subseqüente a um estímulo antigênico; precedido por uma r. da fase inicial.
level-dependent frequency r., r. da freqüência dependente do nível; uma das várias estratégias utilizadas em aparelhos auditivos para alterar o equilíbrio da amplificação entre os sons de alta e baixa freqüência.
middle latency r., r. de latência média; r. à estimulação acústica registrada do córtex auditivo do cérebro.
myotonic r., r. miotônica; a falha em obter relaxamento muscular causada pela descarga repetitiva dos potenciais de ação das fibras musculares.
oculomotor r., r. oculomotora; um potencial miogênico disseminado evocado por estímulos visuais.
orienting r., r. de orientação. SIN orienting reflex.
postural sway r., r. de balanço postural; o balanço do corpo induzido por estimulação vestibular.
primary immune r., r. imune primária. VER immune r.
psychogalvanic r. (PGR), psychogalvanic skin r., r. psicogalvânica, r. psicogalvânica da pele. SIN galvanic skin r.
recruiting r., r. de recrutamento. SIN recruitment (2).
relaxation r., r. de relaxamento; reação hipotalâmica integrada que resulta na diminuição da atividade do sistema nervoso simpático que, fisiológica e psicologicamente, é quase uma imagem em espelho das respostas do organismo à teoria da emergência de Cannon (r. de fuga ou luta); pode ser auto-induzida por meio do uso de técnicas associadas à meditação transcendental, à ioga e à biorretroalimentação (biofeedback). VER TAMBÉM emergency theory.
secondary immune r., r. imune secundária. SIN anamnestic r., booster r. VER immune r.
sonomotor r., r. sonomotora; um potencial miogênico disseminado evocado por estimulação do tipo estalido.
stringent r., r. estrita; uma resposta celular à falta de aminoácidos que reduz a quantidade de ribossomas e para a qual os aminoácidos podem ser empregados sob condições nutricionais.
target r., r.-alvo. SIN operant.
triple r., r. tripla; a r. trifásica observada ao se golpear a pele com firmeza. A fase 1 caracteriza-se por um eritema bem demarcado que se segue a um embranquecimento momentâneo da pele e que resulta da liberação de histamina pelos mastócitos. A fase 2 caracteriza-se por rubor vermelho intenso que se estende além das margens da linha de pressão, apresentando, contudo, a mesma configuração, e que resulta da dilatação arteriolar; também denominado rubor axônico por ser mediado pelo reflexo axônico. A fase 3 caracteriza-se pelo aparecimento de uma pápula linear com a configuração do golpe original.
unconditioned r., r. incondicionada; uma r., tal como a salivação, que corresponde a uma parte do repertório humano e animal. Cf. conditioned r.
rest. Descanso, repouso; apoio; resto, remanescente, vestígio, resquício. **1.** Quietude; repouso. [A.S. *raest*] **2.** Repousar; parar de trabalhar. [A.S. *raestan*] **3.** Um grupo de células ou uma parte do tecido fetal que se deslocou e se encontra encravado em um tecido de outra natureza. [L. *restare*, permanecer] **4.** Em odontologia, a extensão de uma prótese que fornece apoio vertical a uma restauração.
adrenal r., remanescente da supra-renal. SIN accessory adrenal.
bed r., repouso no leito; a manutenção da posição inclinada, na cama, a fim de minimizar a atividade e de auxiliar na recuperação de uma doença; extensamente utilizada no passado no tratamento da tuberculose, do infarto do miocárdio e de outras doenças.
cingulum r., apoio no cíngulo; uma parte rígida de uma dentadura parcial removível sustentada por uma área de apoio preparada sobre o cíngulo de um dente anterior ou de uma coroa.
incisal r., apoio incisal; a parte de uma dentadura parcial removível sustentada por uma borda incisal.
lingual r., apoio lingual; uma extensão metálica colocada sobre a superfície lingual de um dente, a fim de fornecer apoio ou retenção indireta para uma dentadura parcial removível.
Malassez epithelial r.'s, restos epiteliais de Malassez; os remanescentes epiteliais da bainha radicular de Hertwig do ligamento periodontal.
Marchand r., remanescente de Marchand. SIN Marchand adrenals, em adrenal.
mesonephric r., remanescente mesonéfrico. SIN wolffian r.
occlusal r., apoio oclusal; uma extensão rígida de uma dentadura parcial removível colocada sobre a superfície oclusal de um dente posterior para sustentação da prótese.
precision r., apoio de precisão; um apoio que consiste em partes intimamente interligadas.
r.'s of Serres, vestígios de Serres; os remanescentes do epitélio da lâmina dental envolvidos por gengiva.
Walthard cell r., remanescente celular de Walthard; um ninho de células epiteliais que ocorre no peritônio das tubas uterinas ou do ovário; quando neoplásico, possivelmente compreende um dos componentes do tumor de Brenner.
wolffian r., remanescente wolffiano; os vestígios do ducto de Wolff do trato genital feminino que dão origem a cistos; p. ex., o cisto de Gartner. SIN mesonephric r.
re·ste·no·sis (rē-sten-ō-sis). Reestenose; a recorrência da estenose em uma válvula cardíaca após uma cirurgia corretiva; o estreitamento de uma estrutura (em geral, de uma artéria coronária) que se segue à remoção ou à redução de um estreitamento prévio. [re-, + G. *stenōsis*, um estreitamento]
res·ti·form (res′ti-fōrm). Restiforme; semelhante a uma corda; com a forma de uma corda; que se refere ao corpo restiforme, a parte maior (lateral) do pedúnculo cerebelar inferior; contém fibras que vão da medula espinal (espinocerebelar) e do bulbo (cuneo-, olivo-, reticulocerebelar etc.) até o cerebelo. [L. *restis*, corda, + *forma*, forma]
rest·i·tope (res′ti-tōp). Restítopo; a parte do receptor das células T que se associa à molécula de histocompatibilidade principal de classe II. [*restric*-tion + -tope]
res·ti·tu·tion (res-ti-too′shǔn). Restituição; em obstetrícia, o retorno da cabeça fetal que sofreu rotação para a sua posição natural em relação aos ombros após sua emergência da vulva. [L. *restitutio*, o ato de restaurar]
res·to·ra·tion (res-tō-rā′shǔn). Restauração; em odontologia: **1.** Uma r. ou um aparelho protéticos; um termo amplo aplicado a qualquer incrustação, coroa, ponte, dentadura parcial ou completa que restaura ou substitui a estrutura dentária perdida, os dentes ou os tecidos orais. **2.** Um tampão ou uma obturação; qualquer substância, tal como o ouro, o amálgama etc., utilizada para restaurar a parte de um dente que foi perdida como conseqüência da remoção de uma cárie dentária. [L. *restauro*, pp. *-atus*, restaurar, reparar]
acid-etched r., r. com condicionamento ácido; a r. da estrutura de um dente com resina, após sua superfície ter sido tratada com uma solução ácida, um tratamento que aumenta a retenção da r.
combination r., r. por combinação; a r. de um dente com dois ou mais materiais aplicados em camadas.
compound r., r. composta; a r. de mais de uma superfície de um dente.
direct acrylic r., r. direta acrílica; uma r. direta com resina acrílica autopolimerizante.
direct composite resin r., r. direta com resina composta. SIN direct resin r.
direct resin r., r. direta com resina; uma r. direta feita por meio da inserção de uma mistura plástica de resinas autopolimerizantes ou fotopolimerizantes no interior de uma cavidade preparada em um dente. SIN direct composite resin r.
overhanging r., r. saliente; uma r. com excesso de material na junção entre a margem da r. e o dente.
permanent r., r. permanente; uma r. definitiva, em oposição a uma r. temporária ou provisória.
provisional r., r. provisória. SIN temporary r.
root canal r., r. do canal radicular; um cone de guta-percha, prata ou plástico que é introduzido em um canal radicular, ou isolado ou associado a um cemento, uma pasta ou um solvente, com o propósito de obturar o espaço do canal.
silicate r., r. de silicato; a restauração da estrutura dentária perdida feita com cimento de silicato.
temporary r., r. temporária; uma r. para ser utilizada por um período limitado de tempo, em oposição a uma r. permanente. SIN provisional r.
re·stor·a·tive (re-stōr′a-tiv). **1.** Restaurativo; que renova a saúde ou a força. **2.** Um agente que promove a renovação da saúde ou da força. [L. *restauro*, restaurar]
re·straint (rē-strānt′). Contenção; em um hospital psiquiátrico, uma intervenção para impedir que um paciente excitado ou violento cause dano a si mesmo ou a outros; pode envolver o uso de uma camisa-de-força. [Fr. ant. *restrainte*]
re·stric·tion (rē-strik′shǔn). Restrição, limitação. **1.** O processo pelo qual um DNA estranho que foi introduzido em uma célula procariótica se torna ineficaz. **2.** Uma limitação.
asymmetric fetal growth r., limitação assimétrica do crescimento fetal; a cabeça fetal com um tamanho normal como conseqüência de desvio preferencial de sangue para o cérebro, acompanhada de circunferência abdominal reduzida por diminuição do tecido adiposo e do tamanho do fígado; condição provavelmente causada por insuficiência placentária.
fetal growth r., limitação do crescimento fetal; peso fetal ≤ 5.º percentil para a idade gestacional. SIN intrauterine growth retardation.
lactase r., limitação da lactase; uma característica herdada na qual há uma redução na atividade da lactase e, por isso, um defeito no metabolismo intestinal da lactose. Cf. lactase *persistence*.
MHC r., limitação do complexo de histocompatibilidade principal; as células T auxiliares somente reconhecem o antígeno que é apresentado aos antígenos de histocompatibilidade principal da classe II, enquanto as células T citotóxicas em geral somente reconhecem o antígeno processado em associação com os antígenos de histocompatibilidade principal da classe I.

symmetric fetal growth r., limitação simétrica do crescimento fetal; a redução proporcional da cabeça fetal e do tamanho do corpo, freqüentemente constitucional ou causada por uma agressão intra-uterina anterior, tal como uma infecção.

re·sus·ci·tate (rē-sŭs′i-tāt). Ressuscitar, reanimar; realizar a ressuscitação ou reanimação. [L. *resuscito*, levantar novamente, reviver]

re·sus·ci·ta·tion (rē-sŭs′i-tā′shŭn). Ressuscitação, reanimação; a revitalização a partir da morte potencial ou aparente. [L. *resuscitatio*]

cardiopulmonary r. (CPR), reanimação cardiopulmonar; a restauração do débito cardíaco e da ventilação pulmonar subseqüente à parada cardíaca e à apnéia, utilizando a respiração artificial e a compressão manual com o tórax fechado ou a massagem cardíaca com o tórax aberto.

mouth-to-mouth r., a respiração boca a boca empregada como parte da reanimação cardiopulmonar de emergência.

re·tain·er (rē-tān′er). Retentor, trava; qualquer tipo de dispositivo usado para a fixação ou estabilização de uma prótese; aparelho usado para evitar o deslocamento dos dentes após tratamento ortodôntico.

continuous bar r., barra de retenção contínua; barra metálica, que geralmente repousa sobre as superfícies linguais dos dentes, para ajudar na estabilização dos mesmos e atuar como r. indireto. SIN continuous clasp.

direct r., r. direto; dispositivo aplicado ao dente-pivô para manter um aparelho removível no lugar.

extracoronal r., r. extracoronário; um r. cujas qualidades retentivas dependem do contato com a circunferência externa da coroa de um dente.

Hawley r., r. de Hawley; um fio removível e um aparelho palatal de acrílico utilizados para reter ou estabilizar os dentes em suas novas posições após o movimento ortodôntico dos dentes; com modificações, pode ser utilizado para mover os dentes como um aparelho ortodôntico ativo. SIN Hawley appliance.

indirect r., r. indireto; a parte de uma dentadura parcial removível que auxilia os retentores diretos na prevenção do deslocamento oclusivo das bases em extensão distal ao atuar como uma alavanca sobre o lado oposto da linha do fulcro.

intracoronal r., r. intracoronário; um r. cujas qualidades retentivas dependem dos componentes colocados no interior da parte coronária de um dente.

matrix r., porta-matriz; um dispositivo mecânico projetado para manter a matriz ao redor de um dente durante os procedimentos restaurativos, em geral pela união das extremidades da banda da matriz e extração da banda bem esticada.

space r., r. de espaço. SIN space *maintainer*.

re·tard·ate (rē-tahr′dāt). Retardado; um termo moderadamente pejorativo, cujo uso tem diminuído, para uma pessoa que apresenta retardamento mental. [L. *retardo*, atrasar, retardar]

re·tar·da·tion (rē-tahr-dā′shŭn). Retardamento, retardo; a lentidão ou limitação do desenvolvimento.

intrauterine growth r., retardo do crescimento intra-uterino. SIN fetal growth *restriction*.

mental r., r. mental; o funcionamento intelectual geral abaixo da média que se origina durante o período de desenvolvimento e está associado a uma falha no comportamento adaptativo. A American Association on Mental Deficiency lista oito classificações médicas e cinco psicológicas; as cinco últimas substituem as três classificações mais antigas: débil mental, imbecil e idiota. A classificação do retardamento mental requer a atribuição de um índice para o desempenho relativo a um amigo da pessoa em dois critérios inter-relacionados: a medição da inteligência (QI) e o comportamento socioadaptativo global (uma avaliação crítica do nível de desempenho relativo de um indivíduo na escola, no trabalho, em casa e na comunidade). Em geral, um QI de 70 ou mais baixo indica um retardamento mental (leve = 50/55-70; moderado = 35/40-50/55; grave = 20/25-35/40; profundo = abaixo de 20/25); um QI de 70-85 indica um funcionamento intelectual limítrofe (*borderline*). SIN amentia (1), mental deficiency, oligophrenia.

psychomotor r., r. psicomotor; atividade psíquica ou motora lenta, ou ambas.

viscoelastic r., r. viscoelástico; uma técnica para a medição do peso molecular das moléculas de DNA grandes; o DNA é esticado por meio de forças de cisalhamento hidrodinâmico, e, quando as moléculas relaxam, o tempo de relaxamento é medido.

re·tard·er (rē-tar′der). Retardador; um agente utilizado para lentificar o endurecimento químico do gesso, de resinas ou de materiais de impressão empregados em odontologia.

retch. Ânsia de vômito; ter ânsia de vômito; fazer um esforço involuntário para vomitar. [A.S. *hraecan*, fazer um esforço para expectorar]

retch·ing. Ânsia de vômito; os movimentos esofágicos e gástricos para vomitar, sem a expulsão do vômito. SIN dry vomiting, vomiturition.

re·te, pl. **re·tia** (rē′tē; rē′shē-ă, -tē-ă). Rede. **1.** SIN network (1). **2.** Uma estrutura composta por uma rede ou malha fibrosa. [L. uma rede]

r. acromia'le arteriae thoracoacromialis [TA], anastomose acromial da artéria tóraco-acromial. SIN acromial *anastomosis* of the thoracoacromial artery.

r. arterio'sum [TA], plexo arterial. SIN arterial *plexus*.

r. articula're cu'biti [TA], r. articular do cotovelo. SIN cubital *anastomosis*.

r. articula're ge'nus [TA], r. articular do joelho. SIN genicular *anastomosis*.

r. calca'neum [TA], r. do calcâneo. SIN calcaneal *anastomosis*.

r. cana'lis hypoglos'si, plexo venoso do canal do nervo hipoglosso. SIN venous *plexus* of canal of hypoglossal nerve.

r. car'pale dorsa'le [TA], r. carpal dorsal. SIN dorsal carpal arterial *arch*.

r. car'pi poste'rius, r. carpal posterior. SIN dorsal carpal arterial *arch*.

r. cuta'neum co'rii, r. cutânea do cório; a rede de vasos paralela à superfície entre o cório e a tela subcutânea.

r. foram'inis ova'lis, plexo venoso do forame oval. SIN venous *plexus* of foramen ovale.

Haller r., r. de Haller. SIN r. *testis*.

r. halleri, r. de Haller. SIN r. *testis*.

r. malleola're latera'le [TA], r. maleolar lateral. SIN lateral malleolar *network*.

r. malleola're media'le [TA], r. maleolar medial. SIN medial malleolar *netwok*.

malpighian r., estrato de Malpighi. SIN malpighian *stratum*.

r. mirab'ile [TA], r. admirável; rede vascular que interrompe a continuidade de uma artéria ou veia, tal como ocorre nos glomérulos do rim (arterial) ou no fígado (venosa).

r. ova'rii, r. do ovário; uma rede temporária de células encontrada no ovário em desenvolvimento; homóloga à rede do testículo (ver r. *testis*).

r. patella're [TA], r. patelar. SIN patellar *anastomosis*.

r. subpapilla're, r. subpapilar; a rede de vasos situada entre os estratos papilar e reticular do cório.

r. tes'tis [TA], r. do testículo; a rede de canais situada na parte terminal dos túbulos retos do mediastino do testículo. SIN Haller r., r. halleri.

r. vasculosum articula're [TA], plexo vascular articular. SIN articular vascular *plexus*.

r. veno'sum dorsa'le ma'nus [TA], r. venosa dorsal da mão. SIN dorsal venous *network* of hand.

r. veno'sum dorsa'le pe'dis [TA], r. venosa dorsal do pé. SIN dorsal venous *network* of foot.

r. veno'sum planta're [TA], r. venosa plantar. SIN plantar venous *network*.

re·ten·tion (rē-ten′shŭn). Retenção. **1.** A permanência no organismo daquilo que normalmente lhe pertence, principalmente a retenção de alimentos e líquidos no interior do estômago. **2.** A permanência no organismo daquilo que normalmente deve ser eliminado, como a urina e as fezes. **3.** A retenção daquilo que foi aprendido, de maneira que possa ser utilizado mais tarde, como na lembrança, no reconhecimento ou, se a retenção for parcial, no reaprendizado. VER TAMBÉM memory. **4.** Resistência ao desalojamento. **5.** Em odontologia, um período passivo subseqüente ao tratamento, quando um paciente está usando um ou mais aparelhos para manter ou estabilizar os dentes em suas novas posições. [L. *retentio*, retenção]

denture r., r. de uma dentadura; os meios pelos quais as dentaduras são mantidas em posição no interior da boca.

direct r., r. direta; em uma dentadura parcial removível, a r. obtida pelo uso de encaixes ou grampos que se opõem à remoção dos dentes de suporte.

indirect r., em uma dentadura parcial removível, a r. obtida por meio do uso de retentores indiretos.

partial denture r., r. de prótese parcial; a fixação de uma dentadura parcial removível por meio do uso de grampos, retentores indiretos ou encaixes de precisão.

re·tia (rē′shē-ă, -tē-ă). Redes; plural de rete. [L.]

re·ti·al (rē′shē-ăl). Reticular, reticulado; relativo a uma rede.

reticul-. VER reticulo-.

re·tic·u·la (re-tik′ū-lă). Retículos; plural de reticulum. [L.]

re·tic·u·lar, re·tic·u·lated (re-tik′ū-lăr, -lāt-ed). Reticular, reticulado; relativo a um retículo.

re·tic·u·la·tion (re-tik-ū-lā′shŭn). Reticulação; a presença ou formação de um retículo ou de uma rede, tal como aquela observada nas hemácias durante a regeneração ativa do sangue. Termo também utilizado para descrever um padrão radiográfico do tórax. VER reticulonodular *pattern*.

re·tic·u·lin (re-tik′ū-lin). Reticulina; nome dado à substância química contida nas fibras reticulares, as quais, no passado, foram consideradas distintas do colágeno por causa de sua estrutura e de suas propriedades tintoriais características, mas que, atualmente, são classificadas como colágeno de tipo III (com seus proteoglicanos e glicoproteínas estruturais associadas).

reticulo-, reticul-. Retículo-, reticul-; retículo; reticular. [L. *reticulum*, uma pequena rede, dim. de *rete*, uma rede]

re·tic·u·lo·cyte (re-tik′ū-lō-sīt). Reticulócito; uma hemácia jovem que contém uma rede citoplasmática basofílica, precipitada pelo azul de cresil brilhante, que representa polirribossomas residuais; essas células tornam-se mais numerosas durante o processo de regeneração ativa do sangue. VER TAMBÉM erythroblast. SIN reticulated corpuscle, skein cell. [reticulo- + G. *kytos*, célula]

re·tic·u·lo·cy·to·pe·nia (re-tik′ū-lō-sī-tō-pē′nē-ă). Reticulocitopenia; a escassez de reticulócitos no sangue. SIN reticulopenia. [reticulocyte + G. *penia*, pobreza]

re·tic·u·lo·cy·to·sis (re-tik′ū-lō-sī-tō′sis). Reticulocitose; um aumento no número de reticulócitos circulantes acima do normal, que é de menos de 1%

do número total de hemácias; ocorre durante a regeneração ativa do sangue (estimulação da medula óssea vermelha) e em certas anemias, principalmente na anemia hemolítica congênita. [reticulocyte + G. *osis*, condição]

re·tic·u·lo·en·do·the·li·al (re-tik′u-lo-en-do-the′le-al). Reticuloendotelial; que indica ou se refere ao reticuloendotélio. Ver reticuloendothelial *system*.

re·tic·u·lo·en·do·the·li·o·ma (re-tik′u-lo-en′do-the-le-o′ma). Reticuloendotelioma; termo obsoleto para reticulose localizada, ou para uma neoplasia derivada do tecido reticuloendotelial. [reticuloendothelium + G. *-oma*, tumor]

re·tic·u·lo·en·do·the·li·um (re-tik′u-lo-en-do-the′le-um). Reticuloendotélio; as células que compõem o sistema reticuloendotelial. [reticulo- + endothelium]

re·tic·u·lo·his·ti·o·cy·to·ma (re-tik′u-lo-his′te-o-si-to′ma). Retículohistiocitoma; um nódulo cutâneo solitário composto por histiócitos grandes multinucleados que contêm glicolipídios; às vezes ocorrem lesões múltiplas associadas a artrite. [reticulo- + histiocytoma]

re·tic·u·lo·his·ti·o·cy·to·sis (re-tik′u-lo-his′te-o-si-to′sis). Retículohistiocitose. VER reticulosis.
  multicentric r., r. multicêntrica; doença rara na qual pápulas cutâneas compostas por histiócitos contendo glicolipídios estão associadas à poliartrite, que freqüentemente leva a um encurtamento dos dedos.

re·tic·u·loid (re-tik′u-loyd). **1.** Reticulóide; semelhante a uma reticulose. **2.** Uma condição que se assemelha à reticulose.
  actinic r., r. actínico; eritema pruriginoso crônico que se inicia nas áreas expostas ao sol em homens idosos, acompanhado de espessamento e sulcagem acentuados da pele exposta, simulando um linfoma; há infiltração de linfócitos T CD8-positivos atípicos.

re·tic·u·lo·pe·nia (re-tik′u-lo-pe′ne-a). Reticulopenia. SIN reticulocytopenia.

re·tic·u·lo·sis (re-tik-u-lo′sis). Reticulose; aumento de histiócitos, monócitos ou de outros elementos reticuloendoteliais. [reticulo- + G. *-osis*, condição]
  benign inoculation r., r. benigna por inoculação. SIN catscratch *disease*.
  leukemic r., r. leucêmica; termo obsoleto da leucemia monocítica (monocytic leukemia).
  malignant midline r., r. maligna da linha média; termo obsoleto da r. polimórfica (polymorphic r.).
  midline malignant reticulosis r., r. maligna da linha média. SIN lethal midline *granuloma*.
  pagetoid r., r. pagetóide; placa verrucosa em geral solitária observada nos membros e caracterizada histologicamente por um infiltrado predominantemente epidérmico de células mononucleares que se assemelham àquelas encontradas na micose fungóide; o prognóstico é bom. SIN Woringer-Kolopp disease.
  polymorphic r., r. polimórfica; lesão linfoproliferativa necrosante com predileção pelo trato respiratório superior; denominada, no passado, granuloma letal da linha média ou reticulose maligna da linha média; o tratamento consiste em radiação.

re·tic·u·lo·spi·nal (re-tik-u-lo-spi′nal). Reticuloespinal; pertinente ao trato reticuloespinal (ver reticulospinal *tract*).

re·tic·u·lot·o·my (re-tik-u-lot′o-me). Reticulotomia; a produção de lesões na formação reticular. [reticulo- + G. *tome*, incisão]

re·tic·u·lum, pl. **re·tic·u·la** (re-tik′u-lum, -la) [TA]. **1.** Retículo; uma fina rede formada por células, por determinadas estruturas situadas no interior das células ou por fibras do tecido conectivo localizadas entre as células. **2.** Neuróglia. SIN neuroglia. **3.** O segundo compartimento do estômago de um ruminante, uma câmara comparativamente pequena que se comunica com o rúmen; às vezes denominada fase de mel, por causa da estrutura característica de suas paredes. [L. dim. de *rete*, uma rede]
  agranular endoplasmic r., r. endoplasmático agranular; o r. endoplasmático que é desprovido de grânulos ribossômicos; está envolvido na síntese de lipídios e de ácidos graxos complexos, na desintoxicação de drogas, na síntese de carboidratos e no seqüestro de Ca^{++}. SIN smooth-surfaced endoplasmic r.
  Ebner r., r. de Ebner; rede de células nucleadas encontrada nos túbulos seminíferos.
  endoplasmic r. (ER), r. endoplasmático; a rede de túbulos ou sacos achatados (cisternas) citoplasmáticos com ribossomas (r. endoplasmático rugoso) ou sem ribossomas (r. endoplasmático liso) sobre a superfície de suas membranas nos eucariotos. SIN endomembrane system.
  Golgi internal r., r. interno de Golgi. SIN Golgi *apparatus*.
  granular endoplasmic r., r. endoplasmático granular; o r. endoplasmático no qual os grânulos ribossômicos estão aplicados sobre a superfície citoplasmática das cisternas; está envolvido na síntese e na secreção de proteínas — via vesículas ligadas às membranas — para o espaço extracelular. SIN chromidial substance, ergastoplasm, rough-surfaced endoplasmic r.
  Kölliker r., r. de Kölliker. SIN neuroglia.
  rough-surfaced endoplasmic r., r. endoplasmático rugoso. SIN granular endoplasmic r.
  sarcoplasmic r., r. sarcoplasmático; o r. endoplasmático do músculo esquelé-

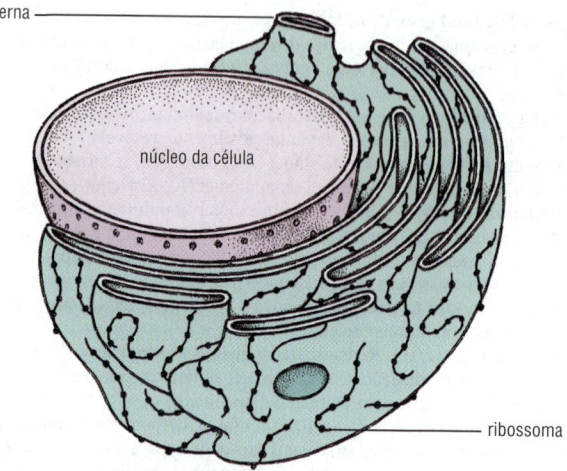

retículo endoplasmático granular (ou rugoso)

tico e cardíaco; o complexo de vesículas, túbulos e cisternas que formam uma estrutura contínua ao redor das miofibrilas estriadas, ocorrendo uma repetição da estrutura no interior de cada sarcômero.
  smooth-surfaced endoplasmic r., r. endoplasmático liso. SIN agranular endoplasmic r.
  stellate r., r. estrelado; malha de células epiteliais disposta no interior de um compartimento preenchido por líquido no centro do órgão do esmalte, entre o epitélio externo e o interno do esmalte.
  trabecular r., r. trabecular. SIN trabecular *tissue* of sclera.
  r. trabecula′re sclerae [TA], r. trabecular da esclera. SIN trabecular *tissue* of sclera.
  trans-Golgi r., face *trans* do r. de Golgi; a parte do aparelho de Golgi que carrega as proteínas recém-processadas e as entrega para as vesículas secretoras, que, em seguida, se fundem a outras biomembranas (p. ex., a membrana plasmática).

ret·i·form (ret′i-form). Retiforme, reticulado; que se assemelha a uma rede ou malha. [L. *rete*, uma rede]

retin-. VER retino-.

ret·i·na (ret′i-na) [TA]. Retina; macroscopicamente, a r. é composta por três partes: a óptica, a ciliar e a irídica. A parte óptica — a porção fisiológica que recebe os raios de luz visuais — é também dividida em duas partes, a pigmentada (epitélio pigmentado) e a nervosa, que estão dispostas nas seguintes camadas: 1) estrato pigmentoso; 2) estrato dos segmentos interno e externo (de bastonetes e cones); 3) estrato limitante externo (na realidade, uma fileira de complexos juncionais); 4) estrato nuclear externo; 5) estrato plexiforme externo; 6) estrato nuclear interno; 7) estrato plexiforme interno; 8) estrato ganglionar; 9) estrato das neurofibras; e 10) estrato limitante interno. As camadas 2-10 compõem o estrato nervoso. No pólo posterior do eixo visual está a mácula e, no centro desta, a fóvea, a área de visão apurada. Aqui, os estratos 6-9 e os vasos sangüíneos estão ausentes, e somente os cones alongados estão presentes. Cerca de 3 mm medialmente à fóvea está o disco óptico, para onde os axônios das células ganglionares convergem para formar o nervo óptico. As partes ciliar e irídica da retina correspondem aos prolongamentos anteriores do estrato pigmentoso e a uma camada de células epiteliais ou colunares de sustentação sobre o corpo ciliar e a superfície posterior da íris, respectivamente. SIN optomeninx. [L. mediev. prov. do L. *rete*, uma rede]
  detached r., descolamento da retina. SIN retinal *detachment*.
  flecked r., r. manchada; r. que exibe *fundus flavimaculatus*, drusas hereditárias ou *fundus albipunctatus*.
  fleck r. of Kandori [MIM*228990], r. manchada de Kandori; um distúrbio autossômico recessivo do epitélio pigmentado da retina caracterizado por manchas retinianas e cegueira noturna, que ocorre entre os japoneses.
  leopard r., r. de leopardo. SIN tessellated *fundus*.
  shot-silk r., r. em seda molhada; o surgimento de numerosos reflexos cintilantes, semelhantes a ondas, como o brilho da seda, às vezes observados na r. de uma pessoa jovem. SIN shot-silk phenomenon, shot-silk reflex.
  tigroid r., r. tigróide. SIN tessellated *fundus*.

ret·i·nac·u·lum, gen. **ret·i·nac·u·li,** pl. **ret·i·nac·u·la** (ret-i-nak′u-lum, -li, -la) [TA]. Retináculo; um freio, ou uma faixa ou ligamento de retenção. [L. uma faixa, um cabresto, de *retineo*, refrear]
  antebrachial flexor r., r. flexor do antebraço; o espessamento da fáscia distal do antebraço próximo à articulação radiocarpal (pulso). É contínuo com o r. extensor nas bordas do antebraço. Essa estrutura difere do ligamento transverso do carpo (ver transverse carpal *ligament*), comumente denominado "retiná-

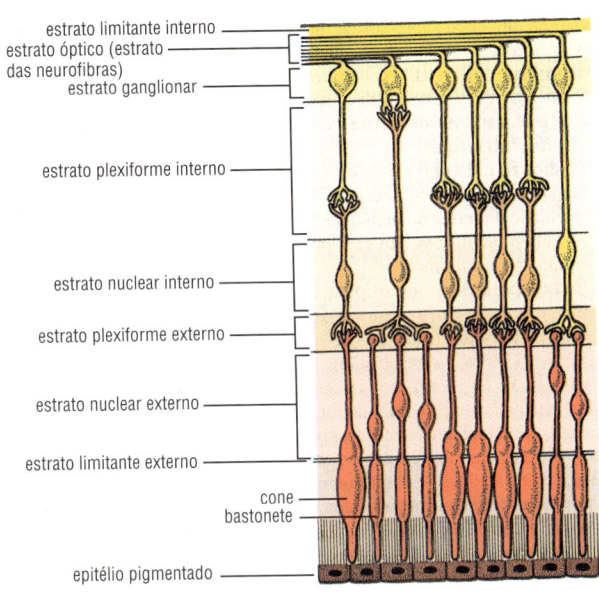

camadas da retina

culo flexor", o qual forma o teto do túnel do carpo. SIN flexor r. of forearm, palmar carpal ligament.
r. of articular capsule of hip, r. da cápsula articular do quadril; uma das várias pregas longitudinais da cápsula articular da articulação do quadril refletida sobre o colo do fêmur; os ramos retinaculares da artéria circunflexa femoral medial passam pela parte mais profunda dessa prega para alcançar a cabeça do fêmur. SIN r. capsulae articularis coxae, Weitbrecht fibers.
r. cap'sulae articula'ris cox'ae, r. da cápsula articular do quadril. SIN r. of articular capsule of hip.
caudal r., r. caudal. SIN r. caudale.
r. cauda'le [TA], r. caudal; as faixas fibrosas, remanescentes da notocorda, que se estendem da pele até o cóccix, formando a fovéola coccígea. SIN caudal ligament, caudal r., ligamentum caudale.
r. cu'tis [TA], ligamento da pele. SIN skin ligaments, em ligament.
r. cutis mammae, ligamentos suspensores das mamas; *termo oficial alternativo para suspensory ligaments of breast, em ligament.
extensor r. [TA], r. extensor; uma faixa fibrosa resistente que se origina de um espessamento da fáscia profunda do antebraço e se estende obliquamente através do dorso do pulso; fixa-se profundamente em cristas situadas na face dorsal do rádio e dos ossos piramidal e pisiforme e liga-se inferiormente aos tendões extensores dos dedos e do polegar. SIN r. musculorum extensorum [TA], dorsal carpal ligament, ligamentum carpi dorsale.
retinacula of extensor muscles, retináculos dos músculos extensores. VER inferior retinaculum of extensor muscles, superior extensor r.
flexor r. [TA], r. flexor; faixa fibrosa resistente que cruza anteriormente o carpo e se liga inferiormente aos tendões flexores dos dedos, ao tendão do músculo flexor radial do carpo e ao nervo mediano, formando, assim, o túnel do carpo. SIN r. musculorum flexorum [TA], deep part of flexor retinaculum, ligamentum carpi transversum, ligamentum carpi volare, transverse carpal ligament, volar carpal ligament.
flexor r. of forearm, r. flexor do antebraço. SIN antebrachial flexor r.
flexor r. of lower limb [TA], r. flexor do membro inferior; faixa larga que passa do maléolo medial até a margem medial e superior do calcâneo e até a superfície plantar, na altura do osso navicular; mantém na posição correta os tendões dos músculos tibial posterior, flexor longo dos dedos e flexor longo do hálux. SIN r. musculorum flexorum membri inferioris [TA], laciniate ligament, ligamentum laciniatum, r. of flexor muscles.
r. of flexor muscles, r. dos músculos flexores; SIN flexor r. of lower limb.
inferior extensor r. [TA], r. extensor inferior; um ligamento em forma de Y que refreia os tendões extensores do pé distalmente à articulação do tornozelo. SIN r. musculorum extensorum inferius [TA], cruciate ligament of leg, inferior r. of extensor muscles, ligamentum cruciatum cruris.
inferior r. of extensor muscles, r. inferior dos músculos extensores. SIN inferior extensor r.
inferior fibular r. [TA], r. fibular inferior; a faixa espessa e larga da fáscia profunda que cobre os tendões dos músculos fibulares longo e curto, à medida que eles passam ao longo da margem lateral do pé, ancorando os tendões e as bolsas em suas posições; corresponde a uma continuação lateral da base do Y, a forma do retináculo extensor inferior, o qual se fixa à tróclea fibular do calcâneo (que se interpõe entre os dois tendões), e, então, continua para se fixar à face ínfero-lateral do calcâneo. SIN r. musculorum fibularium inferius [TA], inferior peroneal r.*, r. musculorum peroneorum inferius*.
inferior peroneal r., r. fibular inferior; *termo oficial alternativo para inferior fibular r.
lateral patellar r. [TA], r. lateral da patela; a parte da aponeurose do músculo vasto lateral que passa lateralmente à patela para se fixar à tuberosidade da tíbia. SIN r. patellae laterale [TA].
medial patellar r. r. medial da patela; a parte da aponeurose do músculo vasto medial que passa medialmente à patela para se fixar ao côndilo medial da tíbia, formando a face ântero-medial da cápsula fibrosa da articulação do joelho. SIN r. patellae mediale [TA].
Morgagni r., r. de Morgagni. SIN frenulum of ileal orifice.
r. musculorum extenso'rum [TA], r. dos músculos extensores. SIN extensor r.
r. musculo'rum extenso'rum infe'rius [TA], r. inferior dos músculos extensores. SIN inferior extensor r.
r. musculo'rum extenso'rum supe'rius [TA], r. superior dos músculos extensores. SIN superior extensor r.
r. musculo'rum fibula'rium, r. dos músculos fibulares. SIN peroneal r.
r. musculorum fibularium inferius [TA], r. inferior dos músculos fibulares. SIN inferior fibular r.
r. musculorum fibularium superius [TA], r. superior dos músculos fibulares; SIN superior fibular r.
r. musculorum flexo'rum [TA], r. dos músculos flexores. SIN flexor r.
r. musculo'rum flexo'rum membri inferioris [TA], r. dos músculos flexores do membro inferior. SIN flexor r. of lower limb.
r. musculo'rum peroneo'rum, r. dos músculos fibulares. SIN peroneal r.
retinacula of nail, retináculos da unha; as fixações fibrosas que se estendem do leito ungueal até a falange subjacente. SIN retinacula unguis.
r. patel'lae latera'le [TA], r. lateral da patela. SIN lateral patellar r.
r. patel'lae media'le [TA], r. medial da patela. SIN medial patellar r.
patellar r., r. da patela; as extensões das aponeuroses dos músculos vastos medial e lateral que passam por ambos os lados da patela, fixando-se às margens da patela e ao ligamento patelar, anteriormente, aos ligamentos colaterais, posteriormente, e aos côndilos da tíbia, distalmente; formam a parte ântero-medial e (juntamente com a expansão fibrosa do trato iliotibial) a parte ântero-lateral da cápsula fibrosa do joelho. VER lateral patellar r., medial patellar r.
peroneal r., r. fibular; as faixas superior e inferior que mantêm os tendões dos músculos peroneais longo e curto em suas posições, à medida que cruzam a face lateral do tornozelo. SIN retinacula of peroneal muscles, r. musculorum fibularium, r. musculorum peroneorum.
r. musculorum peroneorum inferius, r. inferior dos músculos peroneais; *termo oficial alternativo para inferior fibular r.
r. musculorum peroneorum superius, r. superior dos músculos peroneais; *termo oficial alternativo para superior fibular r.
retinacula of peroneal muscles, retináculos dos músculos peroneais. SIN peroneal r.
r. of skin, ligamentos da pele. SIN skin ligaments, em ligament.
superior extensor r. [TA], r. extensor superior; o ligamento que se une inferiormente aos tendões extensores próximo à articulação do tornozelo; é contínuo com (um espessamento de) a fáscia profunda da perna. SIN r. musculorum extensorum superius [TA], ligamentum transversum cruris, superior r. of extensor muscles, transverse crural ligament, transverse ligament of leg.
superior r. of extensor muscles, r. superior dos músculos extensores. SIN superior extensor r.
superior fibular r. [TA], r. fibular superior. SIN r. musculorum fibularium superius [TA], r. musculorum peroneorum superius*, superior peroneal r.*.
superior peroneal r., r. fibular superior; *termo oficial alternativo para superior fibular r.
suspensory r. of breast, r. suspensor da mama; *termo oficial alternativo para suspensory ligaments of breast, em ligament.
r. ten'dinum, r. tendíneo; estrutura ligamentosa que contém os tendões, tais como os retináculos dos flexores e extensores, ou as partes anulares das bainhas fibrosas dos dedos.
retinac'ula un'guis, retináculos da unha. SIN retinacula of nail.
ret·i·nal (ret'i-nal). Retiniano, retínico; retinal. **1.** Relativo à retina. **2.** Retinaldeído; mais comumente referindo-se à forma all-trans.
r. dehydrogenase, retinal desidrogenase; oxirredutase que catalisa a interconversão de retinaldeído e NAD^+ a ácido retinóico e NADH, que, desse modo, afeta o crescimento e a diferenciação. SIN retinaldehyde dehydrogenase.
r. isomerase, retinal isomerase; uma isomerase que catalisa a interconversão cis-trans de all-trans-retinal a 11-cis-retinal(deído); uma parte do ciclo da visão. SIN retinaldehyde isomerase.
r. reductase, retinal redutase; a álcool desidrogenase $NAD(P)^+$.
11-cis-ret·i·nal. 11-cis-retinal; o isômero do retinaldeído que é capaz de se combinar com a opsina para produzir rodopsina; é formado a partir do 11-trans-retinal por meio da retinal isomerase. SIN neoretinal b.

trans-ret·i·nal. Trans-retinal. SIN all-trans-retinal.
ret·i·nal·de·hyde (ret-i-nal'dĕ-hīd). Retinaldeído; o retinol oxidado a um aldeído terminal; o retinal; um caroteno liberado (como all-trans-retinal) no branqueamento da rodopsina pela luz e na dissociação da opsina no ciclo da visão. SIN retinene-1, retinene, vitamin A aldehyde.
 r. dehydrogenase, r. desidrogenase. SIN *retinal* dehydrogenase.
 r. isomerase, r. isomerase. SIN *retinal* isomerase.
 r. reductase, r. redutase; a álcool desidrogenase $(NAD(P)^+)$.
ret·i·nec·to·my (ret'in-ek'tō-mē). Retinectomia; uma excisão cirúrgica de uma parte da retina.
ret·i·nene (ret'i-nēn). Retineno. SIN retinaldehyde.
ret·i·nene-1. Retineno-1. SIN retinaldehyde.
ret·i·nene-2. Retineno-2. SIN dehydroretinaldehyde.
ret·i·ni·tis (ret-i-nī'tis). Retinite; a inflamação da retina. [retina + G. -itis, inflamação]
 albuminuric r., r. albuminúrica. VER hypertensive *retinopathy*.
 circinate r., r. circinada. VER circinate *retinopathy*.
 diabetic r., r. diabética. VER diabetic *retinopathy*.
 exudative r., r. exudati'va, r. exsudativa; anormalidade crônica caracterizada pela deposição de colesterol e de ésteres do colesterol nas camadas externas da retina e no espaço sub-retiniano. É freqüentemente precedida por uveíte nos adultos e por anormalidades vasculares retinianas nas crianças. SIN Coats disease.
 leukemic r., r. leucêmica. VER leukemic *retinopathy*.
 metastatic r., r. metastática; a r. purulenta ou séptica que resulta da parada de êmbolos sépticos no interior dos vasos da retina. SIN purulent r., septic r.
 r. pigmento'sa, r. pigmentar; degeneração progressiva da retina caracterizada por nictalopia bilateral, redução dos campos visuais, anormalidades eletorretinográficas e infiltração pigmentar das camadas internas da retina; pode ser esporádica ou exibir herança autossômica dominante [MIM*180100], autossômica recessiva ou ligada ao cromossoma X [MIM*268000, *312600, *312610]. SIN pigmentary retinopathy.
 r. prolif'erans, r. proliferativa. SIN proliferative *retinopathy*.
 punctate r., r. puntiforme. VER *retinopathy* punctata albescens.
 purulent r., r. purulenta. SIN metastatic r.
 r. sclopeta'ria, r. esclopetária; lesão contundente grave da retina, como aquela causada por um projétil de arma de fogo ou de ar comprimido. [de *sclopetum*, uma arma de fogo medieval]
 secondary r., r. secundária; a r. que ocorre após uma inflamação uveal.
 septic r., r. séptica. SIN metastatic r.
 serous r., r. serosa; edema da retina; inflamação das camadas internas da retina. SIN simple r.
 simple r., r. simples. SIN serous r.
 r. syphilit'ica, syphilitic r., r. sifilítica; r. freqüentemente associada à corioidite sifilítica, especialmente na sífilis congênita.
retino-, retin-. Retino-; a retina. [L. mediev. *retina*]
ret·i·no·blas·to·ma (ret'i-nō-blas-tō'mă) [MIM*180200, MIM*180201, MIM*180202]. Retinoblastoma; neoplasia ocular maligna da infância que se inicia geralmente antes do terceiro ano de vida e que é composta por células arredondadas e pequenas da retina primitiva com núcleos que se coram intensamente e por células alongadas que formam rosetas; há um risco aumentado de desenvolvimento de osteossarcoma em um período posterior da vida. Nos casos familiais, a doença é em geral bilateral, com lesões múltiplas no interior do olho, mas, nos casos esporádicos, raramente isso ocorre. Trata-se de uma herança autossômica dominante causada por uma mutação no gene do retinoblastoma, um gene supressor de tumor situado no cromossoma 13q. [retino- + G. *blastos*, germe, + *-oma*, tumor]

ret·i·no·cho·roid (ret'i-nō-kō'royd). Retinocorióide. SIN chorioretinal.
ret·i·no·cho·roid·i·tis (ret'i-nō-kō-roy'dī'tis). Retinocorioidite; inflamação da retina que se estende até a corióide. SIN chorioretinitis. [retino- choroid + G. *-itis*, inflamação]
 bird shot r., r. do tipo chumbo de caça; vasculite retiniana difusa e bilateral acompanhada de despigmentação de múltiplas áreas da corióide e do epitélio pigmentado da retina na região posterior do equador ocular e freqüentemente associada a papilite ou atrofia óptica; ocasionalmente, ocorre vitiligo. SIN vitiliginous choroiditis.
 r. juxtapapilla'ris, r. justapapilar; r. próxima ao disco óptico. SIN Jensen disease.
ret·i·no·di·al·y·sis (ret'i-nō-dī-al'i-sis). Retinodiálise. SIN *dialysis* retinae. [retino- + G. *dialysis*, separação]
ret·i·no·ic ac·id (ret-i-nō'ik). Ácido retinóico; um ácido da vitamina A_1; o retinal no qual o –CHO terminal foi oxidado a um –COOH; é utilizado topicamente no tratamento da acne; é importante no crescimento e na diferenciação celulares. SIN vitamin A_1 acid.
 13-cis-r. a., ácido 13-*cis*-retinóico; o retinóide mais utilizado nos Estados Unidos para tratar a acne; age reduzindo a secreção de sebo. O uso durante a gravidez é contra-indicado por causa de sua teratogenicidade.
ret·i·noid (ret'i-noyd). **1.** Retinóide; que se assemelha a uma resina; resinoso. [G. *retine*, resina, + *eidos*, semelhança] **2.** Que é semelhante à retina. [L. mediev. *retina*] **3.** Quando no plural, o termo é utilizado para descrever as formas naturais e os análogos sintéticos do retinol.
ret·i·noids (ret'i-noydz). Retinóides; classe de drogas ceratolíticas derivadas do ácido retinóico e utilizadas no tratamento da acne e da psoríase graves.
ret·i·nol (ret'i-nol). Retinol; um hemicaroteno que apresenta a forma β (ou β-ionona) do grupo terminal cíclico e um CH_2OH na posição C-15 (numerado como nos carotenóides) ou na posição 9' (numerado como uma cadeia lateral nonila em um anel do ciclo-hexeno); um intermediário do ciclo da visão que também desempenha um papel no crescimento e na diferenciação celulares. VER TAMBÉM dehydroretinol. SIN vitamin A_1 alcohol, vitamin A_1.
 r. dehydrogenase, r. desidrogenase; oxirredutase que catalisa a interconversão de retinal e NADH em retinol e NAD^+.
11-cis-ret·i·nol. 11-*cis*-retinol; o retinol que apresenta a configuração *cis* na posição 11 (numeração dos carotenóides), ou na posição 5' (numeração do retinol) da cadeia lateral; um intermediário do ciclo da visão. SIN neoretinene B.
ret·i·no·pap·il·li·tis (ret'i-nō-pap-i-lī'tis). Retinopapilite; inflamação da retina que se estende até o disco óptico.
 r. of premature infants, r. dos prematuros. SIN *retinopathy* of prematurity.
ret·i·nop·a·thy (ret-i-nop'ă-the). Retinopatia; doença degenerativa não-inflamatória da retina. [retino- + G. *pathos*, sofrimento]
 arteriosclerotic r., r. arteriosclerótica; r. caracterizada por atenuação das arteríolas retinianas com aumento da tortuosidade, aparência de fio de cobre ou de prata, embainhamento perivascular, irregularidade do lúmen, pequenas hemorragias disseminadas e pequenos depósitos com margens nítidas e sem edema circunjacente.
 central angiospastic r., r. angioespástica central. SIN central serous *choroidopathy*.
 central serous r., r. serosa central. SIN central serous *choroidopathy*.
 circinate r., r. circinada; uma degeneração retiniana caracterizada por um cinturão de exsudatos brancos bem-definidos ao redor de uma mácula edematosa; é em geral bilateral e afeta preferencialmente os idosos.
 compression r., r. por compressão. **(1)** VER Berlin *edema*. VER traumatic r.
 diabetic r., r. diabética; as alterações retinianas que ocorrem no diabetes mellitus, caracterizadas por microaneurismas, exsudatos e hemorragias e, às vezes, neovascularização. SIN fundus diabeticus.

> A doença ocular diabética é responsável por aproximadamente 25% de todos os casos recém-relatados de cegueira nos Estados Unidos. A principal forma é a retinopatia não-proliferativa, que resulta diretamente de alterações degenerativas nos capilares retinianos. As características desse distúrbio, conforme observado no exame fundoscópico, compreendem microaneurismas, exsudatos moles (ou algodonosos) — que correspondem, na realidade, a áreas de microinfarto —, exsudatos duros — que correspondem a depósitos de lipídios e proteínas provenientes de extravasamento capilar — e hemorragias em chama de vela. Alguns pacientes, principalmente aqueles com diabetes de tipo 1, desenvolvem uma retinopatia proliferativa caracterizada por neovascularização (proliferação de novas alças capilares sobre a superfície da retina). O tipo de retinopatia pode prejudicar a visão de forma direta por meio da destruição do tecido retiniano, ou pela predisposição ao edema de retina, ao descolamento da retina e à hemorragia vítrea. Estudos clínicos controlados têm mostrado que a manutenção dos níveis de glicose sangüínea o mais próximo possível do normal em pessoas com diabetes mellitus retarda de

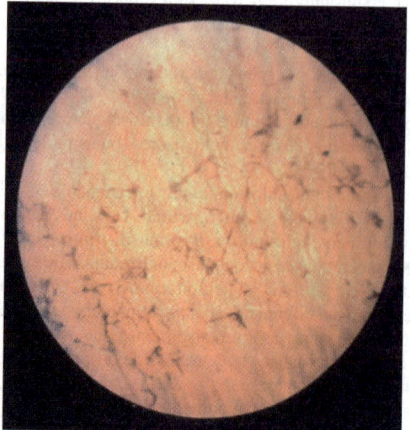

retinite pigmentar (estágio avançado)

maneira substancial o início e a taxa de progressão da retinopatia. A fotocoagulação por laser é eficaz na interrupção da neovascularização na retinopatia diabética proliferativa.

dysproteinemic r., r. por disproteinemia; congestão venosa retiniana resultante de aumento na viscosidade do sangue presente na disproteinemia.
electric r., r. elétrica. SIN photoretinopathy.
external exudative r., r. exsudativa externa. VER exudative *retinitis*.
hypertensive r., r. hipertensiva; condição retiniana que ocorre na hipertensão vascular acelerada, caracterizada por constrição arteriolar, hemorragias em forma de chama de vela, manchas algodonosas, edema em forma de estrela na região da mácula e papiledema.
Leber idiopathic stellate r., r. estrelada idiopática de Leber. VER neuroretinitis.
leukemic r., r. leucêmica; o aspecto da retina em todos os tipos de leucemia, caracterizado por ingurgitamento e tortuosidade das veias, hemorragias disseminadas e edema da retina e do disco.
lipemic r., r. lipêmica; o aspecto leitoso dos vasos da retina (lipemia retiniana) combinado com exsudatos gordurosos com margens delimitadas, observado em pacientes com acidose diabética e hiperlipemia.
macular r., r. macular, maculopatia. SIN maculopathy.
pigmentary r., r. pigmentar. SIN retinitis pigmentosa.
r. of prematurity, r. da prematuridade; a substituição anormal da retina sensitiva por tecido fibroso e vasos sangüíneos, que ocorre principalmente em bebês prematuros com menos de 1.500 g de peso ao nascimento que são colocados em um ambiente rico em oxigênio. SIN retinopapillitis of premature infants, retrolental fibroplasia, Terry syndrome.
proliferative r., r. proliferativa; neovascularização da retina que se estende para o interior do humor vítreo. SIN retinitis proliferans.
r. puncta'ta al'bescens [MIM*136880], doença na qual ambos os fundos dos olhos mostram numerosos pontos ou manchas brancos nas retinas, levando à cegueira noturna; uma herança autossômica dominante, causada pela mutação no gene da "degeneração retiniana lenta" que codifica a periferina no cromossoma 6p. Há também uma forma recessiva [MIM*210370].
Purtscher r., r. de Purtscher; angiopatia retiniana traumática transitória resultante de uma elevação súbita da pressão venosa, como ocorre na compressão do corpo em uma lesão por cinto de segurança; os fundos dos olhos mostram grandes manchas brancas associadas a veias retinianas ao redor do disco ou da mácula, hemorragias e edema de retina; acredita-se que seja resultante de embolia gordurosa proveniente da medula óssea. SIN Purtscher disease, transient r., traumatic r.
renal r., r. renal; r. hipertensiva associada à glomerulonefrite ou à nefroesclerose crônicas.
rubella r., r. por rubéola; as alterações pigmentares periféricas da retina observadas na rubéola congênita, que não afetam a função visual.
sickle cell r., r. falciforme; condição caracterizada por dilatação e tortuosidade das veias da retina e por microaneurismas e hemorragias retinianas; os estágios avançados podem mostrar neovascularização, hemorragia vítrea ou descolamento da retina.
solar r., r. solar. SIN photoretinopathy.
toxemic r. of pregnancy, r. toxêmica da gravidez; angioespasmo súbito das arteríolas da retina, seguido, algum tempo depois, por sinais vasculares retinianos de r. hipertensiva avançada; as alterações vasculares desaparecem rapidamente após o término da gravidez.
toxic r., r. tóxica; as alterações da retina resultantes da administração prolongada de diversas drogas.
transient r., r. transitória. SIN Purtscher r.
traumatic r., r. traumática. SIN Purtscher r.
venous-stasis r., r. por estase venosa; uma retinopatia uniocular associada à oclusão da veia central da retina; uma oclusão não-isquêmica da veia central da retina.
whiplash r., r. por lesão em chicotada; dano retiniano causado por uma lesão por aceleração/desaceleração súbita.
ret·i·no·pexy (ret′i-nō-pek′sē). Retinopexia; um procedimento para manter uma retina descolada em seu lugar; p. ex., a produção de adesões coriorretinianas por congelamento ("criopexia retiniana"). [retino- + G. *pēxis*, fixação]
fluid r., r. por fluido; um procedimento para manter uma retina descolada em seu lugar com o uso de um fluido mais pesado do que o humor vítreo.
gas r., r. por gás; um reparo de descolamento retiniano no qual a retina é mantida em seu lugar por um gás expansível. SIN pneumatic r.
pneumatic r., r. pneumática. SIN gas r.
ret·i·no·pi·e·sis (ret′i-nō-pī-ē′sis). Retinopiese; o reposicionamento de uma retina descolada que consiste em pressioná-la para o seu devido lugar pelo uso de um gás ou líquido. VER retinopexy. [retino- + G. *piesis*, pressão]
ret·i·nos·chi·sis (ret-i-nos′ki-sis). Retinosquise; a cisão degenerativa da retina, com a formação de cistos entre as duas camadas. [retino- + G. *schisis*, divisão]

juvenile r. [MIM*268100], r. juvenil; a r. que ocorre antes dos 10 anos de idade e dentro da camada de fibras nervosas, com freqüente envolvimento macular; inicialmente, a parede interna apresenta-se como uma membrana semelhante a um véu transparente, mas depois torna-se mais densa, podendo deixar a retina branca; uma herança autossômica recessiva. Há uma forma dessa condição que ocorre na meia-idade e é ligada ao cromossoma X [MIM*312700] e uma forma autossômica dominante rara [MIM*180270].
senile r., r. senil; a r. que ocorre mais freqüentemente nos idosos e afeta o estrato plexiforme externo; inicia-se na periferia ínfero-temporal extrema e não apresenta uma progressão significativa; a visão em geral é boa.
ret·i·no·scope (ret′i-nō-skōp). Retinoscópio; dispositivo óptico utilizado para iluminar a retina de um paciente durante a retinoscopia. [retino- + G. *skopeō*, visualizar]
luminous r., r. luminoso; dispositivo óptico portátil que emite um feixe de luz circular ou linear.
reflecting r., r. refletor; espelho plano ou côncavo com uma perfuração central que permite ao observador ver os raios emergindo do olho do paciente.

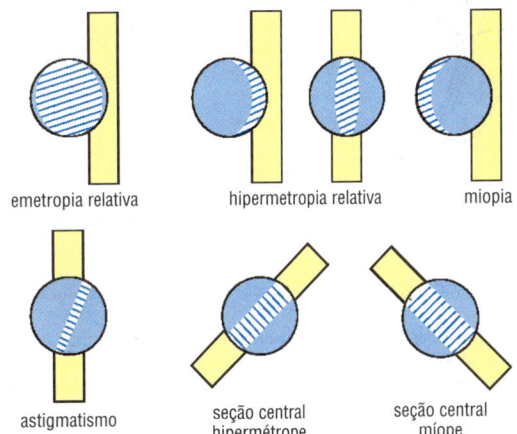

retinoscopia: os aspectos característicos da luz na pupila (as *barras* representam as faixas de luz do retinoscópio)

ret·i·nos·co·py (ret′i-nos′kŏ-pē). Retinoscopia; um método para a determinação dos erros de refração, mediante a iluminação da retina e observação dos raios de luz que emergem do olho. SIN scotoscopy, shadow test, skiascopy. [retino- + G. *skopeō*, visualizar]
cylinder r., r. com cilindro; a determinação dos erros esféricos, astigmáticos e refrativos utilizando lentes cilíndricas.
fogging r., r. com borramento do olho contralateral; um método para reduzir a visão por meio de lentes convexas, até que a acomodação seja interrompida; uma técnica não-ciclopégica e estática.
ret·i·not·o·my (ret′in-ot′ō-mē). Retinotomia; incisão cirúrgica através da retina.
ret·i·nyl phos·phate (ret′i-nil fos′fāt). Fosfato de retinila; o fosfodiéster do all-*trans*-retinol; é essencial para a biossíntese de certas glicoproteínas necessárias para a regulação do crescimento e para a secreção de muco.
ret·o·per·i·the·li·um (rē′to-per-i-thē′lē-ŭm). Reticuloperitélio; as células reticulares relacionadas com a rede de fibras reticulares, como observado no estroma do tecido linfático. [L. *rete*, rede, + G. *peri*, ao redor, + L. mod. *thelium*, do G. *thēlē*, mamilo]
re·tort (rē-tōrt′). 1. Retorta; um recipiente semelhante a um balão com um gargalo longo que se projeta, utilizado, no passado, em destilação. 2. Uma pequena fornalha. [L. mediev. *retorta*, fem. pp. de *retorqueo*, pp. *-tortus*, retorcer ou curvar novamente]
Re·tor·tam·o·nas (rē-tōr-tam′ō-nas). Gênero de protozoários flagelados cuja espécie *R. intestinalis* é, às vezes, encontrada no intestino humano, embora não apresente patogenicidade e seja raramente relatada. [L. *re-torqueo*, retorcer novamente, + G. *monas*, único, uma unidade]
re·tract (rē-trakt′). Retrair; encolher, recuar ou puxar à parte. [L. *re-traho*, pp. *-tractus*, um recuo]
re·trac·tile (rē-trak′til). Retrátil; capaz de ser retraído.
re·trac·tion (rē-trak′shŭn). Retração. 1. Encolhimento, recuo, ou o ato de puxar à parte. 2. O movimento posterior dos dentes, em geral com o auxílio de um aparelho ortodôntico. [L. *retractio*, um recuo]
gingival r., r. gengival; **(1)** o movimento lateral da margem gengival para longe da superfície do dente; pode ser indicativo de inflamação subjacente ou de

formação de uma bolsa; (2) o deslocamento da gengiva marginal para longe do dente por meios mecânicos, químicos ou cirúrgicos.

mandibular r., r. mandibular; um tipo de anomalia facial na qual o gnátion está situado posteriormente ao plano orbital.

re·trac·tor (re-trak'ter, -tōr). Retrator. **1.** Um instrumento utilizado para puxar para um lado as margens de uma ferida ou para reter as estruturas adjacentes ao campo cirúrgico. **2.** Um músculo que puxa uma parte para trás, p. ex., a parte média do músculo trapézio é um r. da escápula; as fibras horizontais do músculo temporal auxiliam na retração da mandíbula.

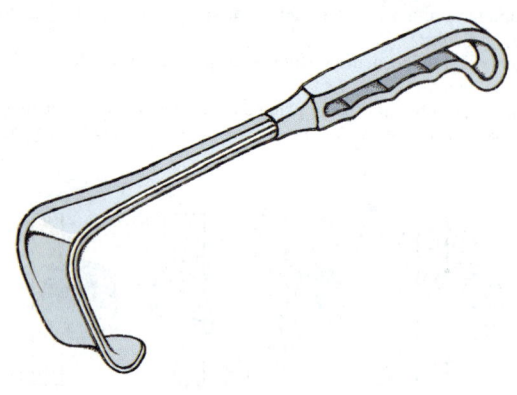

retrator abdominal

Desmarres r., r. de Desmarres; instrumento utilizado para afastar uma pálpebra.

re·trad (re'trad). Para trás, posterior; em direção à parte de trás; direcionado posteriormente. [L. *retro*, para trás, + *ad*, a, para]

re·tra·hens au·rem, re·tra·hens au·ric·u·lam (rēt'ra-henz aw'rem, aw-rik'u-lam). O músculo auricular posterior. VER auricularis posterior (*muscle*). [L. o recuo da orelha ou da aurícula]

re·treat from re·al·i·ty. Fuga da realidade; a substituição de relações com o mundo real por satisfações imaginárias e da fantasia.

re·trench·ment (re-trench'-ment). A retirada de tecido supérfluo. [Fr. *re-*, novamente, + *trancher*, cortar]

re·triev·al (re-tre'val). Recuperação; o terceiro estágio do processo de memorização, após a codificação e o armazenamento, que envolve os processos mentais associados ao ato de trazer a informação armazenada de volta para a consciência. VER TAMBÉM memory.

retro-. Retro-. Para trás ou atrás. [L. para trás]

ret·ro·au·ric·u·lar (re'trō-aw-rik'u-lar). Retroauricular; atrás da aurícula.

ret·ro·buc·cal (re'trō-bŭk'al). Retrobucal; relativo à parte posterior da bochecha ou atrás dela.

ret·ro·bul·bar (re'trō-bŭl'bar). Retrobulbar; atrás do globo ocular. SIN retroocular.

ret·ro·cal·ca·ne·o·bur·si·tis (re'trō-kal-kā'nē-ō-ber-sī'tis). Retrocalcaneobursite. SIN achillobursitis. [retro- + L. *calcaneum*, calcanhar, + bursitis]

ret·ro·ce·cal (re'trō-sē'kal). Retrocecal; posterior ao ceco.

ret·ro·cer·vi·cal (re'trō-ser'vi-kal). Retrocervical; posterior ao colo do útero.

ret·ro·ces·sion (re-trō-sesh'un). Retrocessão. **1.** Um retorno; uma recaída. **2.** A cessação dos sintomas externos de uma doença seguida por sinais de envolvimento de algum órgão ou de alguma parte internos. **3.** Indica uma posição do útero ou de outro órgão mais posterior do que a normal. [L. *retro-cedo*, pp. *-cessus*, retornar, retirar-se]

ret·ro·clu·sion (re-trō-kloo'zhun). Retrooclusão; uma forma de acupressão para impedir um sangramento; a agulha é passada através dos tecidos situados acima da extremidade seccionada da artéria, é girada e, em seguida, é passada de volta embaixo do vaso para surgir próximo ao ponto de entrada. [retro- + L. *claudo* (*cludo*), fechar]

ret·ro·col·ic (re'trō-kol'ik). Retrocólico; posterior ao colo. [retro- + G. *kolon*, colo]

ret·ro·col·lic (re'trō-kol'ik). Retrocervical; relativo ao dorso do pescoço; o movimento da cabeça para trás. [retro- + L. *collum*, pescoço]

ret·ro·con·duc·tion (re-trō-kon-dŭk'shun). Retrocondução. SIN retrograde VA conduction.

ret·ro·cur·sive (re'trō-ker'siv). Retrocursivo; que corre para trás. [retro- + L. *cursus*, uma corrida]

ret·ro·de·vi·a·tion (re'trō-dē-vē-ā'shun). Retrodesvio; uma curvatura ou inclinação para trás.

ret·ro·dis·place·ment (re'trō-dis-plās'ment). Retrodeslocamento; qualquer deslocamento para trás, tal como a retroversão ou a retroflexão do útero.

ret·ro·e·soph·a·ge·al (re'trō-ē-sof'a-jē'al). Retroesofágico; posterior ao esôfago.

ret·ro·fil·ling (re-trō-fil'ing). Retroobturação; a colocação de um material selante no interior do forame apical de uma raiz dentária a partir da extremidade apical.

ret·ro·flect·ed (re'trō-flek-ted). Retrofletido. SIN retroflexed.

ret·ro·flec·tion (re-trō-flek'shun). Retroflexão. SIN retroflexion.

ret·ro·flexed (re'trō-flekst). Retrofletido; curvado para trás ou posteriormente. SIN retroflected. [retro- + L. *flecto*, pp. *flexus*, curvar]

ret·ro·flex·ion (re-trō-flek'shun). Retroflexão; inclinação para trás, como a do útero quando o corpo do útero está fletido para trás, formando um ângulo com o colo. SIN retroflection.

r. of iris, r. da íris; a posição anormal da íris no corpo ciliar após uma concussão grave.

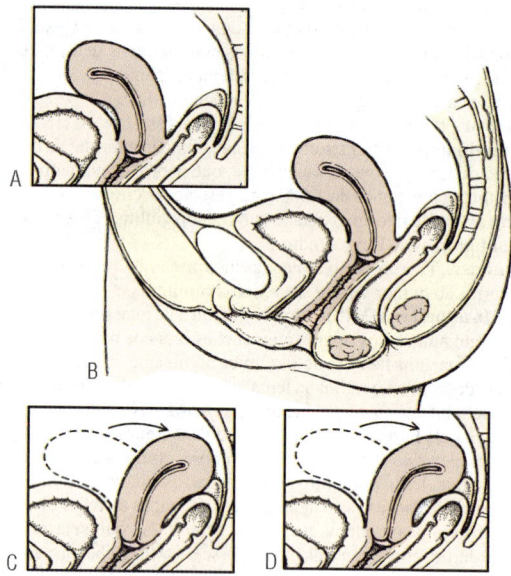

posição do útero: (A) anteflexão, (B) anteversão (normal), (C) retroversão, (D) retroflexão

ret·ro·gnath·ic (re-trō-nath'ik). Retrognático; indica um estado no qual a mandíbula está situada posteriormente à sua posição normal em relação à maxila.

ret·ro·gnath·ism (re-trō-nath'izm). Retrognatismo; desarmonia facial na qual a maxila ou a mandíbula ou o conjunto maxilomandibular está em uma posição posterior à normal em suas relações craniofaciais; o termo é em geral utilizado em referência à mandíbula. [retro- + G. *gnathos*, mandíbula]

ret·ro·grade (ret'rō-grād). Retrógrado. **1.** Que se move para trás. **2.** Em degeneração; revertendo a ordem normal de crescimento e desenvolvimento. [L. *retrogradus*, de retro- + *gradior*, ir]

ret·rog·ra·phy (re-trog'ra-fē). Retrografia. SIN mirror-writing. [retro- + G. *grapho*, escrever]

ret·ro·gres·sion (re-trō-gresh'un). Retrogressão, retrocesso. SIN cataplasia. [L. *retrogressus*, de *retrogradior*, ir para trás]

ret·ro·in·hi·bi·tion (re'trō-in-hi-bish'un). Retroinibição. SIN feedback inhibition.

ret·ro·i·rid·i·an (re'trō-i-rid'ē-an). Retroiridiano; posterior à íris.

ret·ro·jec·tion (re-trō-jek'shun). Retrojeção; a lavagem de uma cavidade pelo fluxo retrógrado de um líquido injetado. [L. *retro*, para trás, + *jacio*, atirar]

ret·ro·jec·tor (re'trō-jek-ter, -tōr). Retrojetor; uma forma de seringa que possui uma conexão tubular longa para o bocal e é utilizada em retrojeção.

ret·ro·len·tal (re'trō-len'tal). Retrolenticular; posterior à lente do olho. SIN retrolenticular (1).

ret·ro·len·tic·u·lar (re'trō-len-tik'u-lar). Retrolenticular. **1.** SIN retrolental. **2.** Atrás do núcleo lentiforme do cérebro.

ret·ro·lin·gual (re'trō-ling'gwal). Retrolingual; relativo à parte posterior da língua; posterior à língua. [retro- + L. *lingua*, língua]

ret·ro·mam·ma·ry (re'trō-mam'a-rē). Retromamário; posterior à mama.

ret·ro·man·dib·u·lar (re'trō-man-dib'u-lar). Retromandibular; posterior à mandíbula. [retro- + L. *mandibula*, mandíbula]

ret·ro·mas·toid (re'trō-mas'toyd). Retromastóideo; posterior ao processo mastóide; relativo às células mastóideas posteriores.

ret·ro·mo·lar (re-tro-mo'lar). Retromolar; distal (ou posterior) ao último dente molar irrompido (ou presente).

ret·ro·mor·pho·sis (re-tro-mor'fo-sis, -mor-fo'sis). Retromorfose. SIN cataplasia. [retro- + G. *morphosis*, processo de formação]

ret·ro·na·sal (re'tro-na'zal). Retronasal; nasal posterior; relativo às narinas posteriores.

ret·ro·oc·u·lar (re'tro-ok'u-lar). Retroocular. SIN retrobulbar.

ret·ro·per·i·to·ne·al (re'tro-per'i-to-ne'al). Retroperitoneal; externo ou posterior ao peritônio.

ret·ro·per·i·to·ne·um (re'tro-per'i-to-ne'um). Retroperitônio. SIN retroperitoneal *space*. [retro- + peritoneum]

ret·ro·per·i·to·ni·tis (ret'ro-per-i-to-ni'tis). Retroperitonite; a inflamação do tecido celular situado atrás do peritônio.

 idiopathic fibrous r., r. fibrosa idiopática. SIN retroperitoneal *fibrosis*.

ret·ro·pha·ryn·ge·al (re'tro-fa-rin'je-al). Retrofaríngeo; posterior à faringe.

ret·ro·phar·ynx (re'tro-far'ingks). Retrofaringe; a parte posterior da faringe.

ret·ro·pla·cen·tal (re'tro-pla-sen'tal). Retroplacentário; atrás da placenta.

ret·ro·pla·sia (ret-ro-pla'ze-a). Retroplasia; o estado de uma célula ou de um tecido no qual a atividade se apresenta diminuída, abaixo daquela considerada normal; associada a alterações retrogressivas (p. ex., lesão, degeneração, morte, necrose). [retro- + G. *plasis*, um molde]

ret·ro·posed (re'tro-pozd). Retroposto; denotando retroposição. [retro- + L. *pono*, pp. *positus*, pôr]

ret·ro·po·si·tion (re'tro-po-zish'un). Retroposição; o deslocamento para trás simples de uma estrutura ou de um órgão, como o útero, sem inclinação, curvatura, retroversão ou retroflexão. [retro- + L. *positio*, posição]

ret·ro·pos·on (re-tro-pos'on). Retroposon; transposição de seqüências que ocorre em um DNA que não se origina no DNA, mas em um RNAm que é transcrito de volta no DNA genômico por transcrição reversa. [retro- + L. *pono*, pp. *positum*, pôr, + -on]

ret·ro·pu·bic (re-tro-pu'bik). Retropúbico; posterior ao púbis.

ret·ro·pul·sion (re-tro-pul'shun). Retropulsão. **1.** O andar ou a corrida para trás involuntária que ocorre em pacientes com síndrome de Parkinson. **2.** O ato de empurrar uma parte qualquer para trás. [retro- + L. *pulsio*, empurrão, de *pello*, pp. *pulsus*, bater, impelir]

ret·ro·spec·tion (re-tro-spek'shun). Retrospecção; o ato ou processo de examinar e rever o passado. [retro- + L. *specto*, pp. *spectatus*, olhar para]

ret·ro·spec·tive (re-tro-spek'tiv). Retrospectivo; relativo à retrospecção.

ret·ro·spon·dy·lo·lis·the·sis (re'tro-spon'di-lo-lis-the'sis). Retrospondilolistese; deslizamento para trás do corpo de uma vértebra, tirando-a de seu alinhamento com as vértebras adjacentes. [retro- + G. *spondylos*, vértebra, + *olisthesis*, deslizamento]

ret·ro·ster·nal (re'tro-ster'nal). Retroesternal; posterior ao esterno.

ret·ro·ste·roid (re-tro-ster'oyd, -ster'oyd). Retroesteróide; termo às vezes utilizado para designar um esteróide no qual as orientações dos elementos situados nos carbonos 9 e 10 são opostas àquelas do composto de referência ou do composto que lhe dá origem.

ret·ro·tar·sal (re'tro-tar'sal). Retrotarsal; posterior ao tarso ou à margem da pálpebra.

ret·ro·u·ter·ine (re'tro-u'ter-in). Retrouterino; posterior ao útero.

ret·ro·ver·si·o·flex·ion (re-tro-ver'se-o-flek'shun, -ver'zho-). Retroversoflexão; a retroversão e a retroflexão combinadas do útero.

ret·ro·ver·sion (re-tro-ver'zhun). Retroversão. **1.** Giro para trás, como o do útero. **2.** A condição na qual os dentes estão situados em uma posição mais posterior do que a normal. [retro- + L. *verto*, pp. *versus*, girar]

ret·ro·vert·ed (re'tro-ver-ted). Retrovertido; indica retroversão.

Ret·ro·vir·i·dae (re-tro-vir'i-de). Família de vírus RNA com envelope e um diâmetro de 80–100 nm; os vírus contêm duas moléculas idênticas de RNA monofilamentar de sentido positivo, com peso molecular de $3-6 \times 10^6$; o RNA genômico serve como molde para a síntese de um DNA complementar, o qual seria integrado ao DNA hospedeiro. Existem atualmente 7 gêneros: os retrovírus de tipo B de mamíferos, os retrovírus de tipo C de mamíferos, os retrovírus de tipo C de aves, os retrovírus de tipo D, os retrovírus HTLV e BLV, os Lentivírus e os Espumovírus.

ret·ro·vi·rus (re'tro-vi'rus). Retrovírus; qualquer vírus da família Retroviridae.

Os retrovírus são poderosos agentes causadores de doenças, mas também têm sido uma valiosa ferramenta de pesquisa em biologia molecular. Em 1979, o biólogo norte-americano Richard Mulligan utilizou um retrovírus geneticamente modificado para desencadear a produção de hemoglobina *in vitro* por células de rins de macacos. Sua técnica de utilização de retrovírus para importar genes estranhos para o interior das células tem sido amplamente empregada. Os pesquisadores da área médica têm também explorado o transporte por retrovírus como um meio de terapia genética. Contudo, evidências sugerindo que os retrovírus podem desempenhar algum papel na carcinogênese têm levantado dúvidas quanto à segurança de seu uso em terapia genética. Ver oncogene.

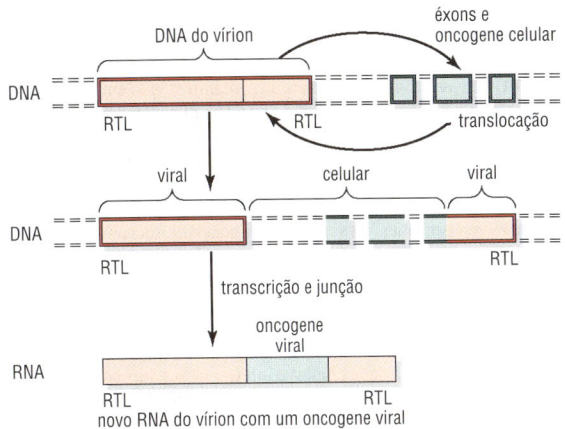

retrovírus: a incorporação de um oncogene celular a um retrovírus, onde se torna um oncogene viral (RTL, repetições terminais longas)

re·tru·sion (re-troo'zhun). Retrusão. **1.** A retração da mandíbula a partir de qualquer ponto. **2.** O movimento para trás da mandíbula. [L. *retrudo*, pp. -*trusus*, empurrar para trás]

Rett, Andreas, pediatra austríaco do século 20. VER R. *syndrome*.

return. Retorno.

 total anomalous pulmonary venous r. (TAPVR), r. venoso pulmonar anômalo total. VER anomalous pulmonary venous *connections*, total ou partial, em *connection*.

 venous r., r. venoso; o sangue que retorna para o coração pelas grandes veias e pelo seio coronário.

Retzius, Anders A., anatomista e antropólogo sueco, 1796–1860. VER R. *cavity*; *cavum* retzii; R. *fibers*, em *fiber*, *gyrus*, *ligament*, *space*; retroperitoneal *veins*, em *vein*.

Retzius, Magnus G., anatomista e antropólogo sueco, 1842–1919. VER R. *striae*, em *stria*; *lines* of R., em *line*; *foramen* of R.; calcification *lines* of R., em *line*; *foramen* of Key-R.; *sheath* of Key and R.

re·u·ni·ent (re-u'ne-ent). Que conecta; indica o *ductus reuniens* (ducto de união). [L. *re*-, novamente, + *unio*, pp. *unitus*, unir]

Reuss, August von, oftalmologista austríaco, 1841–1924. VER R. *formula*, *test*.

re·vac·ci·na·tion (re'vak-si-na'shun). Revacinação; a vacinação de um indivíduo que já foi vacinado com sucesso.

re·vas·cu·lar·i·za·tion (re-vas'ku-lar-i-za'shun). Revascularização; o restabelecimento do suprimento sangüíneo para uma área.

re·ver·ber·a·tion (re'ver-be-ra'shun). Reverberação; ecos ou reflexões múltiplos; em ultra-sonografia, um artefato provocado pelo atraso de um eco que foi refletido para trás e para a frente novamente antes de retornar ao transdutor.

Reverdin, Jacques L., cirurgião suíço, 1842–1929. VER R. *graft*.

re·ver·sal (re-ver'sal). Reversão, inversão. **1.** Virada ou mudança para a direção oposta, como a de um processo, uma doença, um sintoma ou um estado. **2.** A mudança de uma linha escura ou uma linha clara do espectro para o seu oposto. **3.** Indica a dificuldade de algumas pessoas em distinguir a letra *p* minúscula escrita ou impressa da letra *q* ou da *g*, a letra *b* da *d* ou a letra *s* da *z*. **4.** Em psicanálise, a mudança de um instinto ou afeto para o seu oposto, como do amor em ódio. [L. *reverto*, pp. -*versus*, virar para trás ou ao redor]

 adrenaline r., inversão por adrenalina. SIN epinephrine r.

 epinephrine r., inversão por epinefrina; a queda da pressão sangüínea produzida pela epinefrina quando essa é administrada após o bloqueio dos receptores α-adrenérgicos por uma droga apropriada, tal como a fenoxibenzamina; a vasodilatação reflete a capacidade da epinefrina de ativar os receptores β-adrenérgicos que, nos músculos lisos dos vasos, têm ação inibitória; na ausência de bloqueio dos receptores α, a ativação dos receptores β pela epinefrina é mascarada por sua ação predominante (vasoconstritora) sobre os receptores α vasculares. SIN adrenaline r.

 narcotic r., r. por narcóticos; o uso de antagonistas de narcóticos, como a naloxona, para interromper a ação dos narcóticos.

 pressure r., r. da pressão; a cessação da anestesia por meio da pressão hiperbárica; de grande importância na compreensão do modo de ação dos anestésicos.

sex r., r. sexual. SIN sex reassignment.

re·vers·i·ble (rē-ver'si-bl). Reversível; capaz de reversão; diz-se das doenças ou das reações químicas.

re·ver·sion (rē-ver'zhŭn). Reversão. **1.** A manifestação em um indivíduo de certas características, peculiares a um ancestral distante, que foram suprimidas durante uma ou mais gerações intermediárias. **2.** O retorno ao fenótipo original, ou pela restituição do genótipo original (r. verdadeira), ou por uma mutação em um local diferente daquele da primeira mutação, a qual cancela o efeito da primeira mutação (mutação supressiva). [L. *reversio* (ver reversal)]

re·ver·tant (rē-ver'tant). Revertente; em genética microbiana, um mutante que voltou ao seu genótipo antigo (reversão verdadeira) ou ao fenótipo original por meio de uma mutação supressiva. [L. *revertans*, pros. p. de *reverto*, voltar atrás]

review. Revisão.

drug utilization r., r. da utilização das drogas; um programa contínuo, estruturado e autorizado que coleta, analisa e interpreta os padrões de utilização das drogas para melhorar a qualidade do uso das drogas e as conseqüências nos pacientes.

Revilliod, Léon, médico suíço, 1835–1919. VER R. *sign*.

rev·i·ves·cence (re-vi-ves'ens). Revivescência, revivescimento, revivificação. SIN revivification (1). [L. *re-vivesco*, voltar a viver, de *vivo*, viver]

re·viv·i·fi·ca·tion (rē-viv'i-fi-kā'shŭn). Revivificação. **1.** A renovação da vida e da força. SIN revivescence. **2.** O reavivamento das bordas de uma ferida por meio de debridamento ou escarificação, a fim de estimular a cicatrização. SIN vivification. [L. *re-*, novamente, + *vivo*, viver, + *facio*, fazer]

re·vul·sion (rē-vŭl'shŭn). Revulsão; o desvio de sangue de uma parte para outra, como ocorre na contra-irritação. SIN derivation (1). [L. *revulsio*, o ato de afastar, de *revello*, pp. -*vulsus*, arrancar ou puxar para longe]

re·ward (rē-ward'). Recompensa, reforço. SIN reinforcer.

re·warm·ing (rē-warm'ing). Reaquecimento; aplicação de calor para corrigir a hipotermia.

Rexed, Bror A., médico, cientista e funcionário público sueco, *1914. VER *lamina* of Rexed.

Reye, Ralph Douglas Kenneth, patologista australiano do século 20. VER R. *syndrome*.

Reymond. VER Du Bois-Reymond.

Reynolds, Osborne, físico inglês, 1842–1912. VER Reynolds *number*.

RF Abreviatura de releasing *factors* (fatores liberadores); rheumatoid *factors* (fatores reumatóides), em *factor*; replicative *form* (forma replicativa); reticular *formation* (formação reticular).

RFA Abreviatura de right frontoanterior position (posição frontoanterior direita).

RFLP Abreviatura de restriction fragment length *polymorphism* (polimorfismo do comprimento do fragmento de restrição).

RFP Abreviatura de right frontoposterior position (posição frontoposterior direita).

RFT Abreviatura de right frontotransverse position (posição frontotransversa direita).

RH Abreviatura de releasing *hormone* (hormônio liberador).

Rh 1. Símbolo de rhodium (ródio). **2.** Ver Grupo Sangüíneo Rh, no apêndice de Grupos Sangüíneos.

Rha Abreviatura de L-rhamnose (L-ramnose).

rha·bar·ber·one (ra-bar'ber-ōn). Rabarberona. SIN aloe-emodin.

△ **rhabd-.** VER rhabdo-.

rhabditiform. Rabditiforme. VER rhabditiform *larva*.

Rhab·di·tis-like. Semelhante aos membros do gênero *Rhabtidis*. VER rhabditiform *larva*.

△ **rhabdo-, rhabd-.** Rabdo-; bastão; em forma de bastão (rabdóide). [G. *rhabdos*]

rhab·do·cyte (rab'dō-sīt). Rabdócito; termo raramente utilizado para descrever metamielócito ou o leucócito em bastão. [rhabdo- + G. *kytos*, célula]

rhab·doid (rab'doyd). Rabdóide; em forma de bastonete. [rhabdo- + G. *eidos*, semelhança]

rhab·do·my·o·blast (rab-dō-mī'ō-blast). Rabdomioblasto; células grandes, arredondadas, fusiformes ou em forma de alça, com citoplasma fibrilar intensamente eosinofílico que pode exibir estriações cruzadas; encontrado em alguns rabdomiossarcomas. [rhabdo- + G. *mys*, músculo, + *blastos*, germe]

rhab·do·my·ol·y·sis (rab'dō-mi-ol'i-sis). Rabdomiólise; doença aguda, fulminante e potencialmente fatal da musculatura esquelética que acarreta a destruição do músculo, conforme evidenciado por mioglobinemia e mioglobinúria. [rhabdo- + G. *mys*, músculo, + *lysis*, afrouxamento]

acute recurrent r., r. recorrente aguda [MIM*268200]; ataques paroxísticos repetidos de dor e fraqueza musculares seguidos por eliminação de urina castanho-avermelhada escura; é freqüentemente precipitada por uma doença intercorrente e diagnosticada pelo achado de mioglobina na urina; é atribuída à atividade anormal da fosforilase na musculatura esquelética, mas pode haver mais de um tipo biológico; provavelmente a herança é autossômica recessiva. Em alguns casos, pelo menos, existe deficiência de carnitina palmitoil transferase. SIN familial paroxysmal r.

exertional r., r. por esforços físicos; r. produzida em indivíduos suscetíveis por exercício muscular.

familial paroxysmal r., r. paroxística familial. SIN acute recurrent r.

idiopathic paroxysmal r., r. paroxística idiopática, mioglobinúria. SIN myoglobinuria.

rhab·do·my·o·ma (rab'dō-mī-ō'ma). Rabdomioma; neoplasia benigna derivada da musculatura estriada, que acomete o coração de crianças, provavelmente como um processo hamartomatoso. [rhabdo- + G. *mys*, músculo, + *-oma*, tumor]

rhab·do·my·o·sar·co·ma (rab'dō-mī-ō-sar-kō'ma). Rabdomiossarcoma; neoplasia maligna derivada da musculatura esquelética (estriada), que acomete crianças e, menos comumente, adultos; é classificado como alveolar embrionário (composto de agregados frouxos de pequenas células arredondadas), ou pleomórfico (contendo rabdomioblastos). SIN rhabdosarcoma. [rhabdo- + G. *mys*, músculo, + *sarkōma*, sarcoma]

embryonal r., r. embrionário; neoplasia maligna que acomete crianças, consiste em tecido frouxo composto por células fusiformes com raras estriações cruzadas e que surge em muitas partes do organismo, além dos músculos esqueléticos.

rhab·do·pho·bia (rab-dō-fō'bē-a). Rabdofobia; medo mórbido de um bastão (ou chicote) como instrumento de punição. [rhabdo- + G. *phobos*, medo]

rhab·do·sar·co·ma (rab'dō-sar-kō'ma). Rabdossarcoma. SIN rhabdomyosarcoma.

rhab·do·sphinc·ter (rab'dō-sfingk'ter). Rabdoesfíncter; esfíncter constituído de musculatura estriada. SIN striated muscular sphincter. [rhabdo- + G. *sphinktēr*, esfíncter]

Rhab·do·vir·i·dae (rab'dō-vir'i-dē). Família de vírus de vertebrados, insetos e plantas, em forma de bastonete ou projétil, que engloba o vírus da raiva e o vírus da estomatite vesicular (do gado). Os virions (com 100–430 nm por 45–100 nm), formados por brotamento a partir das membranas de superfície das células, são envolvidos por um envelope e são sensíveis ao éter, e apresentam espículas de 5–10 nm de comprimento em sua superfície; os nucleocapsídeos contêm RNA monofilamentar de sentido negativo (PM ~4,4 × 10^6) e exibem simetria helicoidal. Existem cinco gêneros: Vesiculovirus, Lyssavirus, Ephemerovirus, Nucleorhabdovirus e Cytorhabdovirus.

rhab·do·vi·rus (rab'dō-vī'rŭs). Rabdovírus; qualquer vírus da família Rhabdoviridae.

△ **rhachi-.** Raqui-; para as palavras que começam assim, ver rachi-.

Rhad·in·o·vi·rus (rad-ēn'ō-vī-rus). Gênero de herpesvírus, da subfamília Gammaherpesvirinae, associado ao sarcoma de Kaposi.

rhag·a·des (rag'a-dez). Rágades; rachaduras, fendas ou fissuras que acometem as junções mucocutâneas; são observadas nas doenças por deficiência de vitaminas e na sífilis congênita. [G. *rhagas*, pl. *rhagades*, rachaduras]

rha·gad·i·form (ra-gad'i-fōrm). Ragadiforme; que se assemelha às rágades ou que é caracterizado por elas. [G. *rhagas* (*rhagad-*), rachadura, + L. *forma*, forma]

△ **-rhagia.** VER -rrhagia.

L-rham·nose (Rha) (ram'nōs). L-ramnose; metilpentose presente em vários glicosídeos vegetais e encontrada na forma livre no sumagre venenoso, nos lipopolissacarídeos das Enterobacteriaceae e na rutinose (dissacarídeo). SIN isodulcit.

rham·no·side (ram'nō-sīd). Ramnosídeo; um glicosídeo da ramnose.

rham·no·xan·thin (ram-nō-zan'thin). Ramnoxantina, frangulina. SIN frangulin.

Rhamnus (ram'nŭs). Gênero de arbustos e árvores (família Rhamnaceae). A casca e os frutos de *R. cathartica* são catárticos; *R. frangula* é a fonte da frângula; *R. purshiana* é a fonte da cáscara sagrada. SIN buckthorn. [G. *rhamnos*]

rha·pha·nia (ra-fā'nē-a). Rafania. SIN raphania.

rha·phe (rā'fē). Rafe. SIN raphe.

△ **-rhaphy.** VER -rrhaphy.

rhe (rē). rhe; a unidade absoluta de fluidez, a recíproca da unidade de viscosidade. [G. *rheos*, fluxo]

△ **-rhea.** VER -rrhea.

rheg·ma (reg'ma). Regma; rasgão ou fissura. [G. quebra]

rheg·ma·tog·e·nous (reg-ma-toj'e-nŭs). Regmatógeno; que surge da explosão ou fragmentação de um órgão. VER rhegmatogenous retinal *detachment*. [G. *rhēgma*, quebra, + *-gen*, produção]

rhe·ic (rē'ik). Relativo ao gênero *Rheum* (ruibarbo).

Rheinberg mi·cro·scope. Microscópio de Rheinberg. Ver em microscope.

rhe·ni·um (Re) (rē'nē-ŭm). Rênio; elemento metálico do grupo da platina; peso atômico 186,207, n.º atômico 75. [L. mod., do L. *Rhenus*, o rio Reno]

△ **rheo-.** Reo-; fluxo sangüíneo; corrente elétrica. [G. *rheos*, fluxo, corrente]

rhe·o·base (rē'ō-bās). Reóbase; a força mínima de um estímulo elétrico de duração indefinida capaz de causar a excitação de um tecido, p. ex., um músculo ou um nervo. VER TAMBÉM chronaxie. SIN galvanic threshold. [rheo- + G. *basis*, base]

rhe·o·ba·sic (rē-ō-bā'sik). Reobásico; relativo à reóbase ou que possui as características de uma reóbase.

rhe·o·car·di·og·ra·phy (rē'ō - kar - dē - og'ră - phē). Reocardiografia; a pletismografia de impedância aplicada ao coração. [rheo- + cardiography]

rhe·o·chrys·i·din (rē - ō - kris'i - din). Reocrisidina; o éter 3-metila da emodina.

rhe·o·en·ceph·a·lo·gram (rē'ō - en - sef'ă - lō - gram). Reoencefalograma; registro gráfico de alterações na condutividade do tecido da cabeça causadas por fatores vasculares.

rhe·o·en·ceph·a·log·ra·phy (rē'ō - en - sef - ă - log'ră - fē). Reoencefalografia; a técnica de medição do fluxo sangüíneo do cérebro; é comumente utilizada para indicar a r. de impedância que emprega as alterações na impedância e na resistência elétricas como medida de fluxo. [rheo- + encephalography]

rhe·o·gram (rē'ō - gram). Reograma; gráfico da tensão de cisalhamento *versus* a taxa de cisalhamento para um fluido. [rheo- + G. *gramma*, algo escrito]

rhe·ol·o·gist (rē - ol'ō - jist). Reologista; especialista em reologia.

rhe·ol·o·gy (rē - ol'ō - jē). Reologia; o estudo da deformação e do fluxo dos materiais. [rheo- + G. *logos*, estudo]

rhe·om·e·ter (rē - om'e - ter). Reômetro; **1.** Instrumento para medir as propriedades reológicas dos materiais, p. ex., do sangue. **2.** Galvanômetro. [rheo- + G. *metron*, medição]

rhe·om·e·try (rē - om'é - trē). Reometria; medida da corrente elétrica ou do fluxo sangüíneo.

rhe·o·pexy (rē'ō - pek - sē). Reopexia; propriedade de certos materiais na qual uma taxa de cisalhamento elevada favorece um aumento da viscosidade. [rheo- + G. *pēxis*, fixação]

rhe·o·stat (rē'ō - stat). Reostato; resistência variável utilizada para regular a corrente em um circuito elétrico. [rheo- + G. *statos*, estático]

rhe·os·to·sis (rē - os - tō'sis). Reostose; osteíte com hipertrofia e condensação que tende a ocorrer em linhas ou colunas longitudinais, como os pingos de cera em uma vela, e que acomete vários ossos longos. SIN flowing hyperostosis, streak hyperostosis. [rheo- + G. *osteon*, osso, + *-osis*, condição]

rhe·o·tax·is (rē - ō - tak'sis). Reotaxia; uma forma de barotaxia positiva, na qual um microrganismo em um líquido é impelido a se mover contra o fluxo de corrente de seu meio. [rheo- + G. *taxis*, arranjo ordenado]

rhe·ot·ro·pism (rē - ot'rō - pizm). Reotropismo; movimento contrário ao movimento de uma corrente, que engloba uma parte de um organismo em vez do organismo como um todo, como na reotaxia. [rheo- + G. *tropos*, volta]

rhes·to·cy·the·mia (res'tō - sī - thē'mē - ă). Restocitemia; termo obsoleto para a presença de hemácias fragmentadas na circulação periférica. [G. *rhaiō*, destruir, + *kytos*, um orifício (uma célula), + *haima*, sangue]

rhe·sus (rē'sus). Nome genérico para *Macaca mulatta*. [L. mod., do L. *Rhesus*, G. *Rhesos*, um rei mítico da Trácia.]

rheum (room). Reuma; secreção aquosa ou mucosa. [G. *rheuma*, fluxo]

rheu·ma·tal·gia (roo - mă - tal'jē - ă). Reumatalgia; termo obsoleto para a dor reumática. [G. *rheuma*, fluxo, + *algos*, dor]

rheu·mat·ic (roo - mat'ik). Reumático; relativo ao reumatismo ou que é caracterizado por ele. SIN rheumatismal. [G. *rheumatikos*, sujeito ao fluxo, de *rheuma*, fluxo]

rheu·ma·tid (roo'mă - tid). Reumátide; nódulos reumáticos ou outras erupções que podem acompanhar o reumatismo. [G. *rheum*, fluxo, + *-id* (1)]

rheu·ma·tism (roo'mă - tizm). Reumatismo. **1.** Termo obsoleto para a febre reumática (rheumatic *fever*). **2.** Termo indefinido aplicado a diversas condições acompanhadas de dor ou de outros sintomas de origem articular ou relacionados a outros elementos do sistema musculoesquelético. [G. *rheumatismos*, reuma, fluxo]

   articular r., r. articular, artrite. SIN arthritis.
   cerebral r., r. cerebral; os sintomas do sistema nervoso central que resultam de uma doença reumática. Antigamente, ocorria primariamente como uma manifestação da febre reumática (rheumatic *fever*); atualmente, é encontrado com menos freqüência como uma parte de outras doenças, tais como lúpus eritematoso sistêmico (systemic *lupus erythematosus*). VER TAMBÉM Sydenham *chorea*.
   chronic r., r. crônico; distúrbio inespecífico das articulações, com progressão lenta, que provoca espessamento doloroso e contração das estruturas fibrosas, interferindo com o movimento e causando deformidade.
   gonorrheal r., r. gonorréico; artrite que em geral começa como uma poliartrite, mas que com freqüência se localiza em uma articulação na forma de pioartrose causada por infecção sistêmica por gonococos.
   r. of the heart, r. do coração; valvopatia cardíaca reumática, mais freqüentemente das valvas atrioventriculares esquerda (mitral) e da aorta.
   inflammatory r., r. inflamatório; artrite reumatóide ou outra causa de inflamação articular.
   Macleod r., r. de Macleod; artrite reumatóide acompanhada de derrame seroso abundante nas articulações acometidas.
   muscular r., r. muscular, fibrosite. SIN fibrositis (2).
   nodose r., r. nodoso. **(1)** SIN rheumatoid *arthritis*; **(2)** r. articular agudo ou subagudo, caracterizado pela formação de nódulos sobre os tendões, os ligamentos e o periósteo na vizinhança das articulações acometidas.
   subacute r., r. subagudo; forma branda, mas em geral prolongada, de febre reumática aguda, freqüentemente resistente ao tratamento.
   tuberculous r., r. tuberculoso; condição inflamatória das articulações ou dos tecidos fibrosos durante o curso da tuberculose.

rheu·ma·tis·mal (roo - mă - tiz'măl). Reumatismal. SIN rheumatic.

rheu·ma·toid (roo'mă - toyd). Reumatóide; que se assemelha à artrite reumatóide em uma ou mais características. [G. *rheuma*, fluxo, + *eidos*, semelhança]

rheu·ma·tol·o·gist (roo - mă - tol'o - jist). Reumatologista; especialista em reumatologia.

rheu·ma·tol·o·gy (roo - mă - tol'o - jē). Reumatologia; a especialidade médica que se ocupa do estudo, do diagnóstico e do tratamento das condições reumáticas. [G. *rheuma*, fluxo, + *logos*, estudo]

rhi·go·sis (rī - go'sis), a capacidade de sentir frio. [G. *rhigōsis*, calafrio]

rhi·got·ic (rī - go'tik). Relativo a *rhigosis*.

rhIL-11. Interleucina humana recombinante 11. SIN recombinant human *interleukin 11*.

rhin-, rhino-. Rino-; o nariz. [G. *rhis*]

rhi·nal (rī'năl). Nasal, rinal. SIN nasal.

rhi·nal·gia (rī - nal'jē - ă). Rinalgia; dor no nariz. SIN rhinodynia. [rhin- + G. *algos*, dor]

rhin·e·de·ma (rī'ne - dē'mă). Rinedema; tumefação da mucosa nasal. [rhin- + G. *oidēma*, inchaço]

rhin·en·ce·phal·ic (rī'nen - se - fal'ik). Rinencefálico; relativo ao rinencéfalo.

rhin·en·ceph·a·lon (rī'nen - sef'ă - lon). Rinencéfalo; um termo coletivo em grande medida arcaico que se refere às partes do hemisfério cerebral diretamente relacionadas com o sentido do olfato: o bulbo olfatório, o pedúnculo olfatório (juntos ainda arrolados como primeiro nervo craniano ou nervo olfatório, apesar do fato de eles formarem uma parte do sistema nervoso central), o tubérculo olfatório e o córtex olfatório ou piriforme, incluindo o núcleo cortical da amígdala. O termo originalmente abrangia também o hipocampo, toda a amígdala e os giros do cíngulo e para-hipocampal; contudo, não se acredita mais que essas estruturas estejam relacionadas de forma específica com o sentido do olfato. VER TAMBÉM limbic *system*. SIN smellbrain. [rhin- + G. *enkephalos*, cérebro]

rhin·en·chy·sis (rī - nen'kī - sis). Rinenquise; ducha nasal; a lavagem das cavidades nasais. [rhin- + G. *enchysis*, entrar de enxurrada]

rhin·i·on (rin'ē - on). Rínio; um ponto craniométrico: a extremidade inferior da sutura interna. [G. *rhinion*, narina, dim. de *rhis* (rhin-), nariz]

rhi·nism (rī'nizm). Rinolalia, rinofonia. SIN rhinolalia.

rhi·ni·tis (rī - nī'tis). Rinite; inflamação da mucosa nasal. SIN nasal catarrh. [rhin- + G. *-itis*, inflamação]

   acute r., r. aguda; inflamação catarral aguda da mucosa do nariz, caracterizada por espirros, lacrimejamento e abundante secreção de muco aquoso; está em geral associada à infecção por um dos vírus do resfriado comum. SIN coryza, head cold.
   allergic r., r. alérgica; r. associada à febre do feno.
   atrophic r., r. atrófica; r. crônica com adelgaçamento da mucosa; está freqüentemente associada a crostas e secreção fétida. SIN ozena.
   r. caseo'sa, caseous r., r. caseosa; forma de r. crônica na qual as cavidades nasais são quase completamente preenchidas por um material caseoso e fétido.
   chronic r., r. crônica; inflamação lenta e prolongada da mucosa do nariz; nos estágios avançados, a mucosa e suas glândulas podem se apresentar espessas (r. hipertrófica) ou adelgaçadas (r. atrófica).
   gangrenous r., r. gangrenosa. VER *cancrum nasi*.
   hypertrophic r., r. hipertrófica; r. crônica com espessamento permanente da mucosa.
   r. medicamento'sa, r. medicamentosa; inflamação da mucosa do nariz secundária a medicação tópica excessiva ou inadequada.
   scrofulous r., r. escrofulosa; a infecção tuberculosa da mucosa do nariz.
   r. sic'ca, r. seca; forma de r. crônica com pouca ou nenhuma secreção.
   vasomotor r., r. vasomotora; congestão da mucosa nasal e rinorréia sem infecção ou alergia.

rhino-. Rino-. VER rhin-.

rhi·no·an·e·mom·e·ter (rī'nō - an - ē - mom'e - ter). Rinoanemômetro. SIN rhinomanometer. [rhino- + G. *anemos*, vento, + *metron*, medição]

rhi·no·cele (rī'nō - sēl). Rinocele; uma cavidade (ventrículo) do rinencéfalo, a parte olfatória primitiva do telencéfalo. [rhino- + G. *koilia*, cavidade]

rhi·no·ceph·a·ly, rhi·no·ce·pha·lia (rī'nō - sef'ă - lē, - se - fā'lē - ă). Rinencefalia; uma forma de ciclopia na qual o nariz é representado por uma protuberância carnosa semelhante a uma probóscide que surge acima de órbitas semelhantes a fendas, enquanto os lobos rinencefálicos do telencéfalo se apresentam mal desenvolvidos, com certa tendência a tornarem-se fundidos. [rhino- + G. *kephalē*, cabeça]

Rhi·no·clad·i·el·la (rī'nō - klad - ē - el'ă). Gênero de fungos dematiáceos (de cor escura), caracterizados por acroteca, e que provocam cromoblastomicose. VER TAMBÉM *Phialophora*.

rhi·no·clei·sis (rī - nō - klī'sis). Rinoestenose. SIN rhinostenosis. [rhino- + G. *kleisis*, fechamento]

rhi·no·dym·ia (rī-nō-dim′ē-ă). Rinodimia; a duplicação do nariz em uma face sem outras anormalidades. [rhino- + G. *-dymos*, prega]

rhi·no·dyn·ia (rī-nō-din′ē-ă). Rinodinia, rinalgia. SIN rhinalgia. [rhino- + G. *odyne*, dor]

rhi·no·es·tro·sis (rī′nō-es-trō′sis). Rinoestrose; infecção de cavalos e burros — raramente acomete os seres humanos — pelas larvas de *Rhinoestrus purpureus*; a infecção humana é em geral benigna e de curta duração, limitada ao primeiro estágio da larva e que resulta em oftalmomíase branda.

Rhi·no·es·trus pur·pu·re·us (rī-nō-es′trŭs pŭr-poo′rē-ŭs). Uma espécie de mosca da família Oestridae — a mosca-varejeira do nariz — que causa rinoestrose.

rhi·nog·e·nous (rī-noj′ĕ-nŭs). Rinógeno; que se origina no nariz. [rhino- + G. *-gen*, produtor]

rhi·no·ky·pho·sis (rī′nō-kī-fō′sis). Rinocifose; deformidade do nariz em forma de giba. [rhino- + G. *kiphosis*, gibosidade]

rhi·no·la·lia (rī′nō-lā′lē-ă). Rinolalia; fala nasalada. SIN rhinism, rhinophonia. [rhino- + G. *lalia*, fala]
   r. aper′ta, r. aberta; a fala anormal atribuível a fechamento velofaríngeo inadequado.
   r. clau′sa, r. fechada; a fala anormal atribuída a obstrução nasal.

rhi·no·lite (rī′nō-līt). Rinolito. SIN rhinolith.

rhi·no·lith (rī′nō-lith). Rinolito; concreção calcárea na cavidade nasal, encontrada com freqüência ao redor de um corpo estranho. SIN nasal calculus, rhinolite. [rhino- + G. *lithos*, pedra]

rhi·no·li·thi·a·sis (rī′nō-li-thī′ă-sis). Rinolitíase; a presença de um cálculo nasal. [rhinolith + G. *-iasis*, condição]

rhi·no·log·ic (rī-nō-loj′ik) Rinológico; relativo a rinologia.

rhi·nol·o·gist (rī-nol′ō-jist). Rinologista; um especialista em doenças do nariz.

rhi·nol·o·gy (rī-nol′ō-jē). Rinologia; o ramo da ciência médica que se ocupa do nariz, dos seios paranasais e das doenças que acometem essas estruturas. [rhino- + G. *logos*, estudo]

rhi·no·ma·nom·e·ter (rī′nō-mă-nom′ĕ-ter). Rinomanômetro; manômetro utilizado para determinar a presença e a magnitude da obstrução nasal e as relações entre a pressão e o fluxo do ar nasal. SIN rhinoanemometer. [rhino- + manometer]

rhi·no·ma·nom·e·try (rī′nō-mă-nom′ĕ-trē). Rinomanometria. **1.** O uso de um rinomanômetro. **2.** O estudo e a medição do fluxo e das pressões do ar nasal.

rhi·no·ne·cro·sis (rī′nō-ne-krō′sis). Rinonecrose; necrose dos ossos do nariz. [rhino- + necrosis]

rhi·nop·a·thy (rī-nop′ă-thē). Rinopatia; doença do nariz. [rhino- + G. *pathos*, sofrimento]

rhi·no·pha·ryn·ge·al (rī′nō-fă-rin′jē-ăl). Rinofaríngeo. **1.** Nasofaríngeo. SIN nasopharyngeal. **2.** Relativo à rinofaringe.

rhi·no·pha·ryn·go·lith (rī′nō-fă-ring′gō-lith). Rinofaringolito; concreção localizada na nasofaringe. [rhinopharynx + G. *lithos*, pedra]

rhi·no·phar·ynx (rī′nō-far′ingks). Rinofaringe, nasofaringe. SIN nasopharynx. [rhino- + pharynx]

rhi·no·pho·nia (rī′nō-fō′nē-ă). Rinofonia, rinolalia. SIN rhinolalia. [rhino- + G. *phone*, voz]

rhi·no·phy·ma (rī′nō-fī′mă). Rinofima; hipertrofia do nariz acompanhada de dilatação folicular que resulta de hiperplasia das glândulas sebáceas com fibrose e vascularidade aumentada; uma forma de acne rosácea. SIN brandy nose, copper nose, hammer nose, hypertrophic rosacea, potato nose, rum nose, rum-blossom, toper's nose. [rhino- + G. *phyma*, tumor, crescimento]

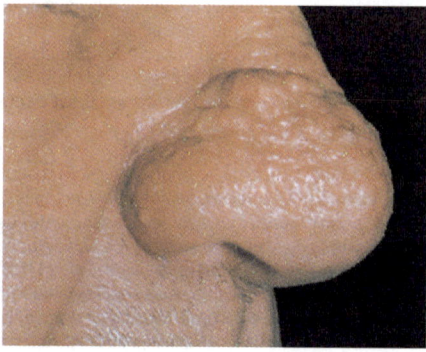

rinofima

rhi·no·plas·ty (rī′nō-plas-tē). Rinoplastia. **1.** A reparação de um defeito do nariz. **2.** A cirurgia plástica para mudar a forma ou o tamanho do nariz. [rhino- + G. *plastos*, formado de]

rhi·no·pneu·mo·ni·tis (rī′nō-noo-mō-nī′tis). Rinopneumonite; inflamação das mucosas do nariz e dos pulmões. [rhino- + G. *pneumon*, pulmão, + *-itis*, inflamação]

rhi·nor·rhea (rī-nō-rē′ă). Rinorréia; secreção oriunda do nariz. [rhino- + G. *rhoia*, fluxo]
   cerebrospinal fluid r., r. liquórica, r. cefalorraquidiana; secreção nasal de líquido cerebrospinal.
   gustatory r., r. gustativa; secreção aquosa nasal associada ao ato de comer.

rhi·no·sal·pin·gi·tis (rī′nō-sal-pin-jī′tis). Rinossalpingite; a inflamação da mucosa do nariz e da tuba auditiva. [rhino- + G. *salpinx*, tuba, + *-itis*, inflamação]

rhi·no·scle·ro·ma (rī′nō-sklĕ-rō′mă). Rinoscleroma; processo granulomatoso crônico que afeta o nariz, o lábio superior, a boca e as vias aéreas superiores; inicia-se em geral com o crescimento de nódulos lisos e duros na porção anterior das narinas que se disseminam para trás, ou seja, para a faringe, a laringe, a traquéia e até mesmo para os brônquios; pode envolver o meato auditivo externo; acredita-se que seja resultante da ação de uma bactéria específica, *Klebsiella rhinoscleromatis*. [rhino- + G. *skleroma*, induração]

rhi·no·scope (rī′nō-skōp). Rinoscópio; pequeno espelho preso a um cabo, semelhante a um bastão, em um ângulo adequado, utilizado na rinoscopia posterior e na nasofaringoscopia.

rhi·no·scop·ic (rī′nō-skop′ik). Rinoscópico; relativo ao rinoscópio ou à rinoscopia.

rhi·nos·co·py (rī-nos′kŏ-pē). Rinoscopia; a inspeção da cavidade nasal. [rhino- + G. *skopeo*, visualizar]
   anterior r., r. anterior; a inspeção da parte anterior da cavidade nasal com ou sem o auxílio de um espéculo nasal.
   median r., r. média; a inspeção do teto da cavidade nasal e das aberturas das células etmoidais posteriores e do seio esfenoidal por meio de um espéculo nasal de lâmina longa ou de um nasofaringoscópio.
   posterior r., r. posterior; a inspeção da nasofaringe e da parte posterior da cavidade nasal por meio de um rinoscópio ou com um nasofaringoscópio. VER TAMBÉM nasopharyngoscopy.

rhi·no·si·nus·i·tis (rī-nō-sī-noo-sī′tis). Rinossinusite; a inflamação da mucosa do nariz e dos seios paranasais.

rhi·no·spo·rid·i·o·sis (rī′nō-spō-rid-ē-ō′sis). Rinosporidiose; a invasão da cavidade nasal e, ocasionalmente, da conjuntiva e de outras estruturas superficiais pelo *Rhinosporidium seeberi*, que resulta em uma doença granulomatosa crônica que produz pólipos ou outras formas de hiperplasia nas mucosas; é encontrada principalmente na Índia e no Sri Lanka.

Rhi·no·spo·rid·i·um see·beri (rī′nōspō-rid′ē-ŭm sē-bē′rī). Um microrganismo semelhante a um fungo, com distribuição universal e posição taxonômica incerta, encontrado em determinados pólipos vasculares nasais que se assemelham a framboesas (rinosporidiose). [rhino- + G. *sporidion*, dim. de *sporos*, sementes]

rhi·no·ste·no·sis (rī′nō-ste-nō′sis). Rinostenose; obstrução nasal. SIN rhinocleisis. [rhino- + G. *stenosis*, um estreitamento]

rhi·not·o·my (rī-not′ō-mē). Rinotomia. **1.** Qualquer cirurgia com incisão do nariz. **2.** Um procedimento cirúrgico no qual é feita uma incisão ao longo de um dos lados do nariz, de modo que ele possa ser afastado, a fim de fornecer uma visão completa das vias nasais para cirurgias radicais dos seios. [rhino- + G. *tome*, incisão, corte]

rhi·no·tra·che·i·tis (rī′nō-trā-kē-ī′tis). Rinotraqueíte; a inflamação das cavidades nasais e da traquéia. [rhino- + trachea + *-itis*, inflamação]

Rhi·no·vi·rus (rī′nō-vī′rŭs). Gênero de vírus ácido-lábeis (família Picornaviridae) com distribuição universal; apresentam genoma composto de RNA monofilamentar e sentido positivo e estão associados ao resfriado comum em seres humanos. Existem mais de 110 tipos antigênicos, antigamente classificados como cepas M (cultiváveis em células de seres humanos e de rins de macacos rhesus) e cepas H (que crescem apenas em culturas de células humanas).

rhi·no·vi·rus. Rinovírus; qualquer vírus do gênero Rhinovirus.
   bovine r.'s, rinovírus bovinos; vírus que causam doenças respiratórias disseminadas subclínicas e, ocasionalmente, doenças clínicas brandas em bezerros nos Estados Unidos e na Europa.
   equine r.'s, rinovírus eqüinos; vírus que causam doença do trato respiratório superior inaparente ou que varia de branda a relativamente grave, nos Estados Unidos e na Europa; a doença é mais prevalente nos estábulos destinados à procriação e está associada a taxa de morbidade alta, mas a taxa de mortalidade insignificante; todos os vírus isolados de eqüinos são sorologicamente relacionados com o vírus isolado original.

Rhi·pi·ceph·a·lus (rī-pi-sef′ă-lŭs). Gênero de carrapatos com escudo sem ornamentação (família Ixodidae) que consiste em cerca de 50 espécies, todas do Velho Mundo, exceto *R. sanguineus*. Olhos e festões estão presentes em ambos os sexos; os palpos curtos e as placas ventrais são encontrados apenas nos machos. O gênero engloba importantes vetores de doenças em seres humanos e animais domésticos. [G. *rhipis*, leque, + *kephale*, cabeça]

R. sanguin′eus, o carrapato marrom do cão; é provavelmente a espécie mais comum e mais cosmopolita encontrada em cachorros nos EUA; pode atacar outros animais, porém raramente pica os seres humanos; é um vetor da febre maculosa das Montanhas Rochosas, no México, e um vetor da riquétsia causadora da febre botonosa.

rhizo-. Rizo-; forma combinante que indica raiz. [G. *rhiza*]

rhi·zoid (rī′zoyd). Rizóide. **1.** Semelhante a uma raiz. **2.** Que se ramifica de maneira irregular, como uma raiz; indica uma forma de crescimento bacteriano. **3.** Em relação aos fungos, as hifas semelhantes a raízes que surgem nos nós das hifas de espécies de *Rhizopus*. [rhizo- + G. *eidos*, semelhança]

rhi·zome (rī′zōm). Rizoma; o caule subterrâneo e rastejante de plantas, tais como a íris, o cálamo e a sangüinária. [G. *rhizōma*, massa de raízes, de *rhiza*, raiz, + *-oma*, massa]

rhi·zo·me·li·a (rī - zō - mē′lē - ă). Rizomelia. **1.** O comprimento desproporcional do segmento mais proximal dos membros (braços e coxas). **2.** Um distúrbio que afeta as articulações do ombro e da coxa. [rhizo- + G. *melos*, membro]

rhi·zo·melic (rī - zō - mel′ik). Rizomélico; das articulações do quadril ou do ombro, ou relativo a elas.

rhi·zo·me·nin·go·my·e·li·tis (rī′zō - mē - ning′gō - mī - ĕ - lī′tis). Rizomeningomielite; a inflamação das raízes nervosas, das meninges e da medula espinal. SIN radiculomeningomyelitis. [rhizo- + G. *meninx*, membrana, + *myelon*, medula, + *-itis*, inflamação]

Rhizomucor (rī - zō - moo - kōr). Gênero de fungos da família Mucoraceae; uma causa de mucormicose.

rhi·zo·plast (rī′zō - plast). Rizoplasto; uma delgada conexão existente entre o flagelo ou blefaroplasto e o núcleo de um protozoário. [rhizo- + G. *plastos*, formado de]

Rhi·zop·o·da (rī - zō - pō′dă). Superclasse do subfilo Sarcodina que engloba as amebas dos seres humanos, que possuem pseudópodes de diversas formas, mas sem filamentos axiais. SIN Rhizopodasida, Rhizopodea. [rhizo- + G. *pous* (*pod-*), pé]

Rhi·zo·po·das·i·da (rī′zō - pō - das′i - dă). SIN Rhizopoda.

Rhi·zo·po·dea (rī - zō - pō′dē - ă). SIN Rhizopoda. [rhizo- + G. *pous* (*pod-*), pé]

rhi·zop·ter·in (rī - zop′ter - in). Rizopterina; um fator do ácido fólico para determinadas bactérias. SIN SLR factor, *Streptococcus lactis* R factor.

Rhi·zo·pus (rī - zō′pŭs). Gênero de fungos (classe dos Zigomicetos, família Mucoraceae); algumas espécies causam mucormicose em seres humanos.

rhi·zot·o·my (rī - zot′ō - mē). Rizotomia; a secção de raízes nervosas espinais para aliviar dor ou paralisia espástica. SIN radicotomy, radiculectomy. [G. *rhiza*, raiz, + *tomē*, secção]

  anterior r., r. anterior; a secção de uma raiz espinal anterior.
  facet r., r. de faceta; a lise da inervação de uma faceta por radiofreqüência percutânea.
  posterior r., r. posterior; a secção de uma raiz espinal posterior. SIN Dana operation.
  trigeminal r., r. trigeminal; a divisão ou secção de uma raiz sensitiva do quinto nervo craniano, executada por meio de abordagem subtemporal (cirurgia de Frazier-Spiller), suboccipital (cirurgia de Dandy) ou transtentorial. SIN retrogasserian neurectomy, retrogasserian neurotomy.

rho (ρ) (rō). **1.** A décima sétima letra do alfabeto grego. **2.** Símbolo de densidade. **3.** VER rho *factor*.

rhod-. VER rhodo-.

rho·da·mine B (rō′dă - mēn, -min) [I.C. 45170]. Rodamina B; um corante de xanteno básico vermelho fluorescente — o cloreto de tetraetilrodamina —, utilizado em histologia como corante de contraste para o azul de metileno e o verde de metila e como fluorocromo vital.

rho·da·nate (rō′dă - nāt). Rodanato, tiocianato. SIN thiocyanate.

rho·da·nese (rō′dă - nēz). Rodanese. SIN *thiosulfate* sulfurtransferase.

rho·dan·ic ac·id (rō - dan′ik). Ácido rodânico, ácido tiociânico. SIN thiocyanic acid.

rho·da·nile blue (rō′dă - nīl). Azul de rodanila; mistura de tinturas — considerada por alguns um sal da rodamina B e do azul do Nilo — utilizada para corar um epitélio ceratinizado (em vermelho) e fibroblastos (em azul), bem como espermatozóides e elementos acidófilos, basófilos e determinados elementos neutrófilos normais e patológicos de células e tecidos; é utilizada como um substituto para a hematoxilina e a eosina.

rho·de·ose (rō′dē - ōs). Rodeose, fucose. SIN fucose.

rho·din (rō′din). Rodina; derivado da diidroporfirina (com os dois hidrogênios adicionais nas posições 17 e 18) do tipo encontrado na clorofila *b* e com um grupamento formila na posição 7 em vez de um grupamento metila.

rho·di·um (Rh) (rō′dē - ŭm). Ródio; elemento metálico de n.º atômico 45 e peso atômico 102,90550. [L. mod. do G. *rhodon*, uma rosa]

Rhod·ni·us (rod′nē - us). Gênero do inseto reduviídeo que é o principal vetor do *Trypanosoma cruzi* na Venezuela, na Colômbia, na Guiana Francesa, na Guiana e no Suriname.
  R. prolixus, inseto reduviídeo, causa importante de tripanossomíase na América do Sul.

rhodo-, rhod-. Rodo-; cor rósea ou vermelha. [G. *rhodon*, rosa]

Rho·do·coc·cus (rō - dō - kok′us). Gênero de bactérias Gram-positivas, aeróbicas, com forma de bastão e parcialmente álcool-ácido-resistentes, encontradas no solo e nas fezes dos herbívoros. Algumas espécies são patogênicas para animais e seres humanos. A espécie-tipo é *Rhodococcus rhodochrous*.
  R. equi, uma espécie de bactéria que causa broncopneumonia e formação de abscessos nos pulmões de potros. Pode causar broncopneumonia em seres humanos imunodeficientes, principalmente naqueles com AIDS/SIDA. SIN *Corynebacterium equi*.

rho·do·gen·e·sis (rō′dō - jen′ĕ - sis). Rodogênese; a produção de rodopsina pela combinação de 11-*cis*-retinal e opsina no escuro. [rhodopsin + G. *genesis*, produção]

rho·do·phy·lac·tic (rō′dō - fī - lak′tik). Rodofilático; relativo à rodofilaxia.

rho·do·phy·lax·is (rō - dō - fī - lak′sis). Rodofilaxia; a ação das células pigmentadas da corióide de manter ou facilitar a reprodução da rodopsina. [rhodopsin + G. *phylaxis*, proteção]

rho·dop·sin (rō - dop′sin). Rodopsina; proteína vermelho-arroxeada, termolábil, com PM de aproximadamente 40.000, encontrada nos segmentos externos dos bastonetes da retina; torna-se branca pela ação da luz, que a converte em opsina e all-*trans*-retinal; é restaurada no escuro pela rodogênese e é a proteína dominante na membrana plasmática das células dos bastonetes. SIN visual purple.
  r. kinase, r. cinase, rodopsinaquinase; uma enzima que regula a função da r. por meio da fosforilação da r. ativada em diversos locais; a r. fotoativada fosforilada liga-se à arrestina.

meta-rho·dop·sin I, *meta-***rho·dop·sin II,** *meta-***rho·dop·sin III.** *meta*-rodopsina I, *meta*-rodopsina II, *meta*-rodopsina III; os precursores da opsina e do all-*trans*-retinal, formados a partir da lumirrodopsina no ciclo da visão.

Rho·do·tor·u·la (rō - dō - tōr′ū - lă). Gênero de leveduras, em geral cor-de-rosa a vermelhas e de patogenicidade questionável, que são, em geral, introduzidas iatrogenicamente em implantes protéticos e em pacientes imunocomprometidos por meio de cateteres intravenosos.

rhomb·en·ceph·a·lon (rom - ben - sef′ă - lon) [TA]. Rombencéfalo; a parte do cérebro em desenvolvimento que corresponde à mais caudal das três vesículas primárias do tubo neural embrionário; em uma etapa posterior, divide-se em metencéfalo e mielencéfalo; o r. engloba a ponte, o cerebelo e a medula oblonga. SIN hindbrain [TA], hindbrain vesicle*. [rhombo- + G. *enkephalos*, encéfalo]

rhom·bic (rom′bik). Rômbico. **1.** SIN rhomboid. **2.** Relativo ao rombencéfalo.

rhombo-. Rombo-; rômbico, rombóide. [G. *rhombos*]

rhom·bo·at·loi·de·us. Romboatlóide. VER *musculus* rhomboatloideus.

rhom·bo·cele (rom′bō - sēl). Rombocele. SIN rhomboidal sinus. [rhombo- + G. *koilia*, um orifício]

rhom·boid, rhom·boi·dal (rom′boyd, rom - boy′dăl). Rombóide, romboidal; que se assemelha a um losango (rombo); i.e., um paralelogramo oblíquo, mas que possui lados desiguais; em anatomia, indica principalmente um ligamento e dois músculos. SIN rhombic (1). [rhombo- + G. *eidos*, semelhança]

rhom·boi·de·us (rom - bō - id′ē - ŭs). Rombóide. VER rhomboid minor (*muscle*).

rhom·bo·mere. Rombômero; os segmentos do tubo neural em desenvolvimento no rombencéfalo; nove rombômeros surgem no humano em desenvolvimento. [rhombencephalon + G. *meros*, parte]

rhon·chal, rhon·chi·al (rong′kăl, rong′kē - ăl). Relativo a, ou característico de, um ronco.

rhon·chus, pl. **rhon·chi** (rong′kŭs, -kī). Ronco; um ruído adventício com um tom musical que ocorre durante a inspiração ou a expiração, ouvido na ausculta do tórax e causado pela passagem do ar através dos brônquios estreitados por inflamação, por espasmo da musculatura lisa ou pela presença de muco no lúmen; quando o ruído possui tom grave, é denominado **r. sonoro** (*sonorous r.*); quando possui tom agudo, semelhante a um assobio ou rangido, **r. sibilante** (*sibilant r.*). [L. do G. *rhenchos*, ronco]
  cavernous r., r. cavernoso. SIN cavernous rale.

rho·phe·o·cy·to·sis (rō - fē - ō - sī - tō′sis). Rofeocitose; o surgimento de vacúolos na superfície de uma célula, sem a formação prévia de projeções citoplasmáticas, por meio dos quais a célula parece aspirar o material circunjacente. VER TAMBÉM pinocytosis. [G. *rhopheō*, engolir, ou aspirar, + *kytos*, célula, + *-osis*, condição]

rhop·try, pl. **rhop·tries** (rōp′trē, - trēs). Roptria; as organelas tubulares ou saculares, elétron-densas e em forma de clava, que se estendem para trás a partir da extremidade anterior de esporozoítos e de outros estágios de certos esporozoários do subfilo Apicomplexa. SIN paired organelles, toxoneme. [G. *rhopalon*, clava]

rho·ta·cism (rō′tă - sizm). Rotacismo; a pronúncia incorreta do som do "r". [G. *rhō*, a letra r]

rhu·barb (roo′barb). Ruibarbo; qualquer planta do gênero *Rheum* (família Polygonaceae), principalmente *R. rhaponticum*, o ruibarbo de jardim, e o *R. officinale* ou *R. palmatum*; as duas últimas espécies, ou seus híbridos, desprovidas dos tecidos peridérmicos, secas e transformadas em pó, são utilizadas por seus efeitos adstringentes, tônicos e laxativos.

Rhus (roos, rŭs). Gênero de plantas trepadeiras e arbustos (família Anacardiaceae) que contêm diversas espécies utilizadas por sua folhagem ornamental; antigamente, eram empregadas no curtimento de peles. Certas espécies venenosas são classificadas como *Toxicodendron*. [L., do G. *rhous*, sumagre]

rhy·po·pho·bia (rī-pō-fō′bē-ă) Riparofobia. SIN mysophobia. [G. *rhypos*, imundície, + *phobos*, medo]

rhythm (rith′ŭm). Ritmo. **1.** O tempo ou o movimento mensurados; a alternância regular de dois ou mais estados diferentes ou opostos. **2.** SIN rhythm method. **3.** A ocorrência regular ou irregular de um evento elétrico no eletrocardiograma ou no eletroencefalograma. VER TAMBÉM wave. **4.** O batimento seqüencial do coração gerado por uma única batida ou seqüência de batidas. [G. *rhythmos*]

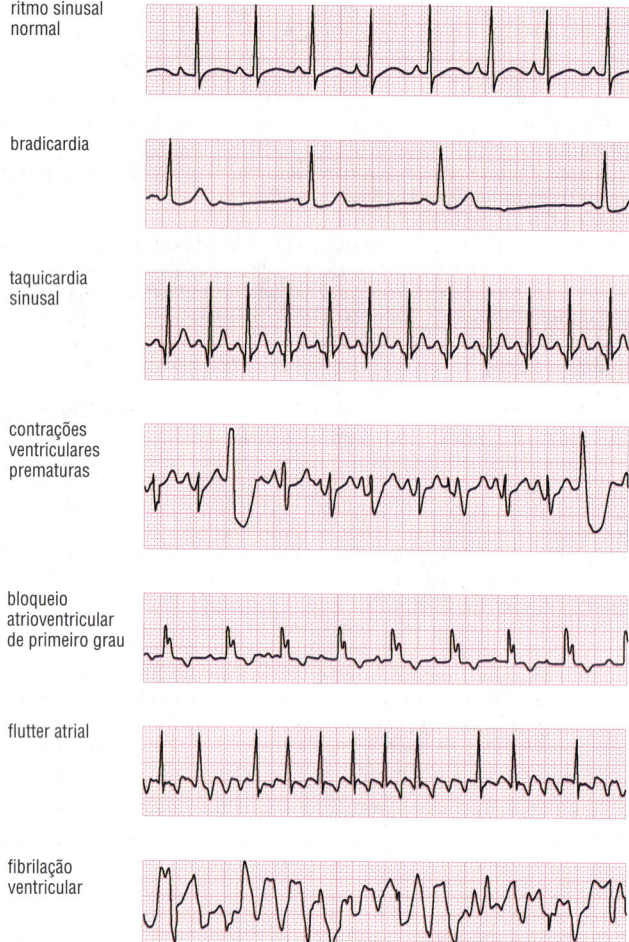

ritmo: traçados de eletrocardiogramas mostrando tipos comuns de arritmia

agonal r., r. agônico; r. idioventricular caracterizado por complexos ventriculares incomumente amplos e bizarros e observado com freqüência em pacientes moribundos.
alpha r., r. alfa; (1) padrão de ondas observado no eletroencefalograma na faixa de freqüência de 8-13 Hz; (2) o r. de 8-13 Hz dominante e posterior encontrado em uma pessoa relaxada, acordada e com os olhos fechados, que é atenuado com a abertura dos olhos. SIN alpha wave, Berger r.
atrioventricular junctional r., r. juncional atrioventricular; o r. cardíaco observado quando o coração é controlado pela junção AV (incluindo o nó); o impulso surge na junção AV, sobe até os átrios e, também, desce para os ventrículos, sendo que cada um desses impulsos apresenta uma velocidade que varia de acordo com o local do marca-passo; o impulso dirige-se apenas para os ventrículos na presença da forma comum de dissociação atrioventricular e do ritmo idiojuncional. SIN AV junctional r., nodal bradycardia, nodal r.
AV junctional r., r. juncional AV. SIN atrioventricular junctional r.
basic electrical r. (BER), r. elétrico básico; onda lenta de despolarização da musculatura lisa que segue do fundo até o piloro e coordena a peristalse e o esvaziamento gástricos.
Berger r., r. de Berger. SIN alpha r.

beta r., r. beta; padrão de onda observado no eletroencefalograma na faixa de freqüência de 18-30 Hz. SIN beta wave.
bigeminal r., r. bigeminado; o r. cardíaco observado quando cada batimento do ritmo dominante (sinusal ou outro) é seguido por um batimento prematuro, resultando em batimentos cardíacos aos pares (bigeminismo). SIN coupled r.
cantering r., r. de galope. SIN gallop.
chaotic r., r. caótico; r. cardíaco completamente irregular com freqüências variáveis. VER TAMBÉM arrhythmia.
circadian r., r. circadiano. VER circadian.
circus r., r. circular. SIN circus movement.
coronary nodal r., r. do nó coronário; termo aplicado, no passado, por alguns especialistas ao padrão eletrocardiográfico de ondas P positivas e normais nas derivações I e II com um intervalo P-R curto.
coronary sinus r., r. do seio coronário; r. atrial ectópico que supostamente se origina em um marca-passo no óstio do seio coronário; é reconhecido no eletrocardiograma por ondas P invertidas nas derivações II, III e aVF com um intervalo P-R normal ou prolongado; ritmo atrial ectópico ("inferior").
coupled r., r. bigeminado. SIN bigeminal r.
delta r., r. delta; padrão de onda encontrado no eletroencefalograma na faixa de freqüência de 1,5-4,0 Hz.
diurnal r., r. diurno. VER diurnal.
ectopic r., r. ectópico; qualquer r. cardíaco que surge em um centro diferente do marca-passo normal.
escape r., r. de escape; três ou mais impulsos consecutivos que ocorrem em uma freqüência que não excede o limite superior do marca-passo natural; a faixa de formação dos impulsos no nó sinoatrial situa-se entre 40 e 180 impulsos por minuto, a da junção atrioventricular é normalmente de 40-60 impulsos por minuto, e a freqüência normal do miocárdio ventricular (ritmo idioventricular) é de 20-40 impulsos por minuto.
gallop r., r. de galope. SIN gallop.
idiojunctional r., r. idiojuncional. SIN idionodal r.
idionodal r., r. idionodal; r. independente, no qual os ventrículos estão sob o controle do nó AV (junção AV). SIN idiojunctional r.
idioventricular r., r. idioventricular; r. ventricular lento e independente que está sob o controle de um centro ventricular (que é, por definição, ectópico). SIN ventricular r.
junctional r., r. juncional; os ritmos que se originam em qualquer lugar dentro da junção AV. Antigamente, eram denominados "ritmos nodais AV" ou simplesmente "ritmos nodais".
nodal r., r. nodal. SIN atrioventricular junctional r.
pendulum r., r. pendular. SIN embryocardia.
quadrigeminal r., r. quadrigeminado; arritmia cardíaca na qual os batimentos cardíacos formam grupos de quatro e cada grupo é geralmente composto por um batimento sinusal seguido de três extra-sístoles; porém qualquer grupo de quatro batimentos que se repete e apresenta uma composição qualquer é considerado quadrigeminado. SIN quadrigeminy.
quadruple r., r. quádruplo; cadência quádrupla dos sons do coração, resultante da fácil audibilidade tanto da terceira como da quarta bulhas cardíacas; é indicativo de doença miocárdica grave. SIN trainwheel r.
reciprocal r., r. recíproco; arritmia cardíaca na qual o impulso que surge na junção AV desce até os ventrículos por uma via intrajuncional, ativando-os e, simultaneamente, sobe em direção aos átrios por vias paralelas; antes de alcançar os átrios, contudo, o impulso é refletido para baixo e ativa novamente os ventrículos, produzindo um eco ou batimento recíproco; é reconhecido no eletrocardiograma por uma onda P invertida na derivação aVF e freqüentemente na derivação II, "espremida", de forma aberrante, entre dois complexos ventriculares, os quais podem ser normais ou compostos por um complexo normal e outro conduzido.
reciprocating r., r. alternante; arritmia cardíaca iniciada por um batimento na junção AV seguido, por sua vez, por um batimento recíproco; o impulso descendente do batimento recíproco é também refletido para trás até os átrios antes de alcançar os ventrículos, e, antes de alcançar os átrios, é refletido para baixo novamente até os ventrículos, de forma que ocorrem tanto ativação atrial retrógrada como ativação ventricular direta.
reversed reciprocal r., r. recíproco invertido; arritmia cardíaca na qual um impulso sinusal normal, antes de alcançar os ventrículos, é refletido para trás até os átrios; dessa forma, no eletrocardiograma, um complexo ventricular permanece "espremido" entre uma onda P sinusal normal e uma onda P retrógrada; se a disritmia continuar, os ciclos subseqüentes serão similares àqueles do ritmo alternante.
sinus r., r. sinusal; o r. cardíaco normal que progride a partir do nó sinoatrial; nos adultos saudáveis, sua freqüência é de 60-90 batimentos/minuto.
systolic gallop r., r. de galope sistólico; termo obsoleto para os sons adicionais, geralmente cliques, ouvidos durante a sístole.
theta r., r. teta; padrão de onda observado no eletroencefalograma na faixa de freqüência de 4-7 Hz. SIN theta wave.
tic-tac r., r. em tique-taque. SIN embryocardia.
trainwheel r., r. quádruplo. SIN quadruple r.

trigeminal r., r. trigeminado; arritmia cardíaca na qual os batimentos estão agrupados em trios, geralmente compostos de um batimento sinusal seguido por duas extra-sístoles. SIN trigeminy.

triple r., r. triplo; cadência tripla dos sons do coração que ocorre em qualquer freqüência cardíaca e resulta da fácil audibilidade da terceira bulha (B_3) (em geral) ou quarta bulha (B_4) cardíacas ou, em freqüências mais rápidas, um somatório decorrente da coincidência da terceira e quarta bulhas cardíacas ("$B_7 = B_3 + B_4$").

ultradian r., r. ultradiano. VER ultradian.

ventricular r., r. ventricular. SIN idioventricular r.

rhytide (rī′tīd). Rítide; uma ruga cutânea. [G. *rhytis*, *-idos*, ruga]

rhyt·i·dec·tomy (rit-i-dek′tō-mē). Ritidectomia; a eliminação de rugas ou a remodelação da face pela excisão da pele em excesso e pelo tensionamento do restante; é também conhecida como *face-lift*. SIN face-lift, rhytidoplasty. [G. *rhytis* (*rhytid-*), uma ruga]

rhyt·i·do·plas·ty (rit′i-dō-plas-tē). Ritidoplastia. SIN rhytidectomy. [G. *rhytis*, uma ruga, + *plastos*, formado de]

rhyt·i·do·sis (rit-i-dō′sis). Ritidose. **1.** O enrugamento da face desproporcional à idade. **2.** A flacidez e o enrugamento da córnea, indicação de morte iminente. SIN rutidosis. [G. um enrugamento, de *rhytis*, uma ruga, + *-osis*, condição]

r. retinae, r. da retina; o enrugamento da retina.

RIA Abreviatura de radioimmunoassay (radioimunoensaio).

Rib Símbolo de ribose.

rib-. VER ribo-.

rib [I-XII]. Costela [I-XII]; um dos 24 ossos curvos e alongados que formam a parte principal da parede óssea do tórax. SIN costa (1). [A.S. *ribb*]

bicipital r., c. bicipital; a fusão da primeira c. torácica com a vértebra cervical.

bifid r., c. bífida; costela cujo corpo se bifurca.

cervical r. [TA], c. cervical; costela supranumerária que se articula com uma vértebra cervical, em geral a sétima, mas que não alcança o esterno anteriormente. VER TAMBÉM cervical rib *syndrome*. SIN costa cervicalis [TA].

false r.'s, costelas falsas; as cinco costelas inferiores situadas em ambos os lados que não se articulam diretamente com o esterno. SIN costae spuriae [VII-XII] [TA], vertebrochondral r.'s.

first r. [I] [TA], primeira costela [I]; costela atípica que possui uma única face articular sobre sua cabeça para a articulação com a vértebra T1 e o corpo mais amplo, mais curto e mais acentuadamente curvo; também apresenta dois sulcos transversos sobre sua face superior para os vasos subclávios, separados pelo tubérculo e pela crista do músculo escaleno. SIN costa prima [I] [TA].

floating r.'s [XI-XII], costelas flutuantes [XI-XII], as duas costelas inferiores situadas em ambos os lados que não estão fixas anteriormente. SIN costae fluctuantes [XI-XII], costae fluitantes, vertebral r.'s.

lumbar r. [TA], c. lombar; c. ocasional que se articula com o processo transverso da primeira vértebra lombar.

r. notching, corrosão da costela; defeito observado na margem inferior de uma ou mais costelas superiores, causado por vasos colaterais intercostais aumentados; com freqüência um sinal de coarctação da aorta.

slipping r., c. deslizante; subluxação de uma cartilagem costal, com separação costocondral.

true r.'s [I-VII], costelas verdadeiras; as sete costelas superiores situadas em ambos os lados cujas cartilagens se articulam diretamente com o esterno. SIN costae verae [I-VII] [TA], vertebrosternal r.'s.

vertebral r.'s, costelas flutuantes. SIN floating r.'s [XI-XII].

vertebrochondral r.'s, costelas falsas. SIN false r.'s.

vertebrosternal r.'s, costelas verdadeiras. SIN true r.'s [I-VII].

ri·ba·vi·rin (rī′ba-vī-rin). Ribavirina; agente antiviral nucleosídico sintético que, por seu efeito inibitório sobre a síntese da guanosina 5′-fosfato, inibe tanto a síntese do DNA quanto do RNA; é utilizado no tratamento da pneumonia viral causada pelo vírus sincicial respiratório.

α-ri·ba·zole (rī′ba-zōl). α-Ribazole; o nucleosídeo benzimidazólico encontrado na vitamina B_{12}.

rib·bon (rib′on). Fita; estrutura em forma de fita. [I.m. *riban*]

Reil r., f. de Reil. SIN medial *lemniscus*.

Ribes, François, médico francês, 1765-1845. VER R. *ganglion*.

ri·bi·tol (rī′bi-tol). Ribitol; produto da redução da ribose (–CHO na posição 1 da ribose reduzido a –CH_2OH). SIN adonitol.

ri·bi·tyl (rī′bi-til). Ribitila; o radical do ribitol; um constituinte da riboflavina.

ribo-. Ribo-. **1.** Ribose. **2.** Quando utilizado como um prefixo em itálico do nome sistemático de um monossacarídeo, *ribo-* indica que a configuração de um conjunto de três grupamentos CHOH (ou assimétricos) consecutivos, mas não necessariamente contíguos, pertence à ribose; p. ex., o nome comum D-ribose corresponde a D-*ribo*-pentose na nomenclatura sistemática. [Al. *Ribose*]

ri·bo·fla·vin, ri·bo·fla·vine (rī′bō-flā-vin). Riboflavina; um fator do complexo da vitamina B que se mantém estável quando aquecido e cujos nucleotídeos da isoaloxazina são coenzimas das flavodesidrogenases. A necessidade diária humana é de 1,7 mg para o homem adulto e de 1,3 mg para a mulher adulta, com uma necessidade diária maior durante a gravidez e a lactação; as fontes dietéticas de riboflavina incluem vegetais verdes, fígado, rins, germe de trigo, leite, ovo, queijo e peixe. SIN flavin (1), flavine, lactoflavin (2), vitamin B_2 (1).

r. kinase, r. cinase; enzima do citosol que catalisa a formação do mononucleotídeo de flavina (fosfato de r.) a partir da r., utilizando ATP como agente fosforilativo. SIN flavokinase.

methylol r., r. de metilol; mistura de derivados do metilol da r. formada pela ação do formaldeído sobre a r. em uma solução fracamente alcalina; apresenta a mesma ação da r., mas é preferida para administração parenteral.

ri·bo·fla·vin 5′-phos·phate. 5′-fosfato de riboflavina. SIN *flavin* mononucleotide.

ri·bo·fu·ra·nose (rī-bō-foor′a-nōs). Ribofuranose; a forma cíclica 1,4 furano da ribose.

9-β-D-ri·bo·fu·ran·o·syl·ad·e·nine (rī′bō-foor-an′o-sil-ad′-ē-nēn). 9-β-D-ribofuranosiladenina. SIN adenosine.

1-β-D-ri·bo·fu·ran·o·syl·cy·to·sine (rī′bō-foor-an′o-sil-sī′tō-sēn). 1-β-D-ribofuranosilcitosina. SIN cytidine.

9-β-D-ri·bo·fu·ran·o·syl·gua·nine (rī′bō-foor-an′o-sil-gwah′nēn). 9-β-D-ribofuranosilguanina. SIN guanosine.

9-β-D-ri·bo·fu·ran·o·syl·pu·rine (rī′bō-foo-ran′o-sil-poo′rēn). 9-β-D-ribofuranosilpurina. SIN nebularine.

ri·bo·fu·ran·o·syl·thy·mine (rī′bō-foor-an′o-sil-thī′mēn). Ribofuranosiltimina. SIN ribothymidine.

1-β-D-ri·bo·fu·ran·o·syl·u·ra·cil (rī′bō-foor-an′o-sil-ūr′a-sil). 1-β-D-ribofuranosiluracila. SIN uridine.

ri·bo-2-hex·u·lose. Ribo-2-hexulose. SIN psicose.

ri·bo·nu·cle·ase (RNase) (rī-bō-noo′klē-ās). Ribonuclease; transferase ou fosfodiesterase que catalisa a hidrólise do ácido ribonucléico. VER TAMBÉM ribonuclease (pancreatic), ribonuclease (*Bacillus subtilis*). SIN ribonucleinase.

RNase A, ribonuclease A; ribonuclease (pancreática).

alkaline RNase, ribonuclease alcalina; ribonuclease (pancreática).

RNase α, ribonuclease α; uma enzima que catalisa a clivagem endonucleolítica do RNA O-metilado, produzindo 5′-fosfomonoésteres.

r. D (RNase D), ribonuclease D; enzima (endonuclease) que retira os 3′-nucleotídeos adicionais presentes no RNAt imaturo.

Escherichia coli **RNase I,** ribonuclease I da *Escherichia coli*. SIN RNase T_2.

RNase I, ribonuclease I; ribonuclease (pancreática).

RNase II, ribonuclease II; uma enzima que promove a clivagem exonucleolítica do RNA na direção 3′ a 5′, produzindo 5′-fosfomononucleotídeos. VER TAMBÉM microbial RNase II.

RNase III, ribonuclease III; enzima que catalisa a clivagem endonucleolítica do RNA bifilamentar, produzindo 5′-fosfomonoésteres.

microbial RNase II, ribonuclease II microbiana. SIN RNase T_2.

RNase N_1, ribonuclease N_1. SIN RNase T_1.

RNase N_2, ribonuclease N_2. SIN RNase T_2.

RNase P, ribonuclease P; enzima que catalisa a clivagem endonucleolítica dos precursores do RNAt para produzir 5′-fosfomonoésteres.

pancreatic RNase, ribonuclease pancreática. VER ribonuclease (pancreatic).

plant RNase, ribonuclease vegetal. SIN RNase T_2.

RNase T_1, ribonuclease T_1; nuclease que cliva endonucleoliticamente os ácidos ribonucléicos na ligação 3′-5′ de um resíduo de 3′-fosfato de guanosina, produzindo oligonucleotídeos que terminam nesse nucleotídeo; uma transferase (endonuclease) na primeira etapa (ciclização) e uma fosfodiesterase na segunda etapa (hidrólise). SIN guanyloribonuclease, RNase N_1.

RNase T_2, enzima que faz a clivagem endonucleolítica de RNA em 3′ nucleotídios, com nucleotídios 2′, 3′- cíclicos como intermediários. SIN *Escherichia coli* RNase I, microbial RNase II, plant RNase, RNase N_2.

RNase U_2, RNase U_2; enzima que promove a clivagem endonucleolítica do RNA, formando 3′-fosfomononucleotídeos e 3′-fosfooligonucleotídeos que terminam em resíduos adenilato ou guanilato com intermediários 2′,3′-fosfato cíclico.

RNase U_4, RNase U_4. SIN yeast RNase.

yeast RNase, RNase de levedura; enzima que catalisa a clivagem exonucleolítica do RNA, produzindo 3′-fosfomononucleotídeos. SIN RNase U_4.

ri·bo·nu·cle·ase (*Ba·cil·lus sub·ti·lis*). Ribonuclease (*Bacillus subtilis*). **1.** Ribonuclease (*Azotobacter agilis*); ribonuclease (*Proteus mirabilis*); enzima que catalisa a clivagem endonucleolítica do RNA para produzir 2′,3′-nucleotídeos cíclicos. **2.** Ribonuclease T_1.

ri·bo·nu·cle·ase (pan·cre·at·ic). Ribonuclease (pancreática); enzima isolada do pâncreas de ruminantes que transfere o 3′-fosfato de um resíduo ribonucleotídeo de pirimidina de um polinucleotídeo da posição 5′ do nucleotídeo adjacente para a posição 2′ do próprio nucleotídeo pirimidina (transferase com ação de endonuclease); desse modo, a ribonuclease quebra a cadeia e forma um 2′,3′-fosfato cíclico de pirimidina e, em seguida (ou independentemente), hidrolisa esse fosfodiéster para liberar um resíduo 3′-fosfato do nucleosídeo de pirimidina (ação de fosfodiesterase); utilizada em citoquímica para degradar seletivamente e remover o RNA como uma forma de controle para a coloração do RNA.

ri·bo·nu·cle·ic ac·id (RNA) (rī′bō-noo-klē′ik). Ácido ribonucléico (RNA); macromolécula que consiste em resíduos ribonucleosídeos ligados por fosfato situado entre a extremidade 3′-hidroxila de um nucleosídeo e a extremidade 5′-hidroxila do nucleosídeo seguinte. O RNA é encontrado em todas as células, tanto nos núcleos como no citoplasma, na forma particulada ou não-particulada, e também em muitos vírus; é a denominação geralmente atribuída aos polinucleotídeos produzidos *in vitro*. As várias frações do RNA são identificadas pelo local onde se encontram, pela forma ou pela função que desempenham.
   acceptor RNA, RNA de transferência (RNAt). SIN transfer RNA.
   antisense RNA, RNA de sentido negativo; o produto da transcrição da fita de DNA com sentido negativo; tal produto pode desempenhar algum papel na inibição da tradução. VER TAMBÉM antisense DNA.
   chromosomal RNA, RNA cromossômico; o RNA que está associado ao cromossoma (e não ao RNAm, ao RNAt ou ao RNAr) e que pode desempenhar algum papel na transcrição.
   heterogeneous nuclear RNA (hnRNA), RNA nuclear heterogêneo; uma forma maldefinida de RNA, de alto peso molecular, que nunca deixa o núcleo e é considerado o precursor do RNA mensageiro.
   informational RNA, RNA mensageiro (RNAm). SIN messenger RNA.
   initiation tRNA, RNAt iniciador; o RNAt de procariontes que contém um resíduo formil-metionil que inicia a tradução. SIN formyl-methionyl-tRNA, starter tRNA.
   messenger RNA (mRNA), RNA mensageiro (RNAm); o RNA que reflete a seqüência exata dos nucleosídeos do DNA geneticamente ativo e carrega a "mensagem" desse DNA — codificada em sua seqüência — para as áreas do citoplasma onde as proteínas são produzidas por meio de seqüências de aminoácidos especificadas pelo RNAm e, portanto, primariamente pelo DNA; os RNA virais são considerados os RNA mensageiros naturais. SIN informational RNA, template RNA.
   messengerlike RNA (mlRNA), RNA semelhante ao RNA mensageiro. VER heterogeneous nuclear RNA.
   nuclear RNA (nRNA), RNA nuclear (RNAn); o RNAn encontrado nos núcleos, ou associado ao DNA ou a estruturas nucleares (nucléolos).
   RNA polymerase, RNA polimerase. VER nucleotidyltransferases.
   ribosomal RNA, RNA ribossômico; o RNA dos ribossomas e polirribossomas.
   small nuclear RNA (snRNA), RNA nuclear pequeno; um RNA pequeno (i.e., com cerca de 90-300 nucleotídeos de comprimento) encontrado no núcleo; acredita-se que desempenhe algum papel no processamento do RNA e na arquitetura celular.
   soluble RNA (sRNA), RNA de transferência (RNAt). SIN transfer RNA. [solúvel em sal molar]
   starter tRNA, RNAt iniciador. SIN initiation tRNA.
   suppressor tRNA, RNAt supressor; o RNAt que está associado a uma mutação supressora.
   template RNA, RNA mensageiro (RNAm). SIN messenger RNA.
   transfer RNA (tRNA), RNA transportador, RNA de transferência; as moléculas do RNA de cadeia curta presentes no interior das células e que apresentam pelo menos 20 variedades; cada variedade consegue combinar-se com um aminoácido específico (ver aminoacyl-tRNA). Transportam resíduos aminoacil e unem-se (por meio de seus anticódons) a locais específicos (os códons) situados ao longo da molécula do RNA mensageiro, levando à formação de moléculas de proteínas com um arranjo de aminoácidos específico, que, na realidade, é ditado por um segmento de DNA localizado nos cromossomas. Cada RNAt possui cerca de 80 nucleotídeos (PM ~ 25.000); a maioria das 20 variedades ocorre em múltiplas formas "isoaceptoras", separáveis pela cromatografia. São encontradas outras subvariedades, p. ex., em cepas distintas de um microrganismo, em organelas subcelulares e em condições metabólicas diferentes. Os RNA transportadores cognatos correspondem aos RNA transportadores que são reconhecidos por aminoacil-RNAt sintetases específicas. SIN acceptor RNA, soluble RNA.

ri·bo·nu·cle·i·nase (rī-bō-noo′klē-i-nās). Ribonucleinase. SIN ribonuclease.

ri·bo·nu·cle·o·pro·tein (RNP) (rī′bō-noo′klē-ō-prō′tēn). Ribonucleoproteína; a combinação do ácido ribonucléico com uma proteína.

ri·bo·nu·cle·o·side (rī-bō-noo′klē-ō-sīd). Ribonucleosídeo; um nucleosídeo cujo componente glicídico é a ribose; os ribonucleosídeos normalmente encontrados no RNA são a adenosina, a citidina, a guanosina e a uridina.

ri·bo·nu·cle·o·tide (rī-bō-noo′klē-ō-tīd). Ribonucleotídeo; um nucleotídeo (fosfato de nucleosídeo) cujo componente glicídico é a ribose; os principais ribonucleotídeos do RNA são o ácido adenílico, o ácido citidílico, o ácido guanílico e o ácido uridílico.
   r. reductase, r. redutase; um complexo protéico que converte os difosfatos de ribonucleotídeo, tais como o ADP e o CDP, a difosfatos de 2′-desoxirribonucleotídeo, tais como os dADP e dCDP. Esse complexo exige tiorredoxina, tiorredoxina redutase e NADPH. É crucial para a síntese do DNA.

ri·bo·pho·rins (rī′-bō-for′inz). Riboforinas; as proteínas receptoras de ribossomas que interagem especificamente com a subunidade ribossômica grande e auxiliam na translocação das proteínas recém-sintetizadas através do retículo endoplasmático. [*ribonucleic acid* + G. *phoros*, transportador, + -in]

ri·bo·pyr·a·nose (rī-bō-pir′ā-nōs). Ribopiranose; a forma 1,5-cíclica da ribose.

ri·bose (Rib) (rī′bōs). Ribose; a pentose que, como o isômero D, está presente no ácido ribonucléico; os epímeros da D-r. são D-arabinose, D-xilose e L-lixose.

ri·bose-5-phos·phate. Ribose-5-fosfato; a ribose fosforilada no carbono 5; um intermediário da via da pentose-fosfato.
   r.-5-p. isomerase, r.-5-f. isomerase; enzima que catalisa a interconversão da D-ribose-5-fosfato em D-ribulose-5-fosfato; de importância no metabolismo da ribose e na via da pentose-fosfato. SIN phosphopentose isomerase, phosphoriboisomerase.

ri·bo·side (rī′bō-sīd). Ribosídeo; o produto formado pela substituição do H da OH do carbono 1 da ribose por um resíduo alcoólico (que pode ser um outro açúcar); difere dos compostos da ribosila e não está presente nos ácidos ribonucléicos, nos quais o radical é uma ribosila (onde falta inteiramente a 1-OH). Ver estrutura do metil β-D-ribofuranosídeo.

ri·bo·some (rī′bō-sōm). Ribossoma; um grânulo de ribonucleoproteína, com um diâmetro de 120-150 Å, que corresponde ao local da síntese protéica — a partir dos aminoacil dos RNA transportadores — conduzida por RNA mensageiros. SIN Palade granule.

ri·bo·su·ria (rī-bō-soo′rē-ă). Ribosúria; excreção urinária aumentada de D-ribose; comumente uma manifestação de distrofia muscular. [ribose + G. *ouron*, urina]

ri·bo·syl (rī′bō-sil). Ribosila; o radical formado pela perda do grupamento OH do hemiacetal de cada uma das duas formas cíclicas da ribose (produzindo os compostos da ribofuranosila e ribopiranosila), pela combinação com um H de um grupo –NH– ou de um grupo –CH–; os nucleosídeos naturais são compostos da ribosila, e não ribosídeos, uma vez que a ligação entre a ribose e a aglicona é C–N ou C–C, e não –C–O–X–.

ri·bo·syl·a·tion (rī-bō-sil-ā-shŭn). Ribosilação; a ligação covalente de um ou mais grupos ribosila a uma molécula (geralmente uma macromolécula).
   ADP r., r. do ADP; a ligação covalente de um radical ADP-ribosila a uma macromolécula; p. ex., a ação da toxina diftérica.

1-ri·bo·syl·or·o·tate (rī′bō-sil-ōr′ō-tāt). 1-ribosilorotato. SIN orotidine.

ri·bo·syl·pur·ine (rī′bō-sil-pūr′ēn). Ribosilpurina. SIN nebularine.

ri·bo·syl·thy·mi·dine. Ribosiltimidina. SIN ribothymidine.

ri·bo·thy·mi·dine (T, Thd) (rī-bō-thī′mi-dēn). Ribotimidina; a 5-metiluridina; o análogo da ribosila encontrado na timidina (desoxirribosiltimidina); nucleosídeo encontrado em pequena quantidade nos ácidos ribonucléicos. SIN ribofuranosylthymine, ribosylthymidine.

ri·bo·thy·mi·dyl·ic ac·id (rTMP, TMP) (rī′bō-thī-mi-dil′ik). Ácido ribotimidílico; a 5′-fosfato ribotimidina; o análogo da ribose do ácido timidílico; um componente raro dos RNA transportadores.

ri·bo·tide (rī′bō-tīd). Ribotídeo; corruptela de ribosídeo, por analogia ao par nucleosídeo-nucleotídeo, que significa ribosila ribonucleotídeo.

ri·bo·vi·rus (rī′bō-vī′rŭs). Ribovírus, vírus RNA. SIN RNA *virus*.

ri·bo·zyme (rī′bō-zīm). Ribozima; biocatalisador não-protéico; algumas ribozimas clivam os precursores do RNAt para produzir RNA transportadores funcionais; outros agem sobre o RNAr; é fundamental nos processos que unem os introns. SIN organic catalyst (1), RNA enzyme. [*ribonucleic acid* + -zyme]

ri·bu·lose (rī′bū-lōs). Ribulose; o isômero 2-ceto da ribose. Na forma r.-5-fosfato, esse isômero participa do desvio (*shunt*) da pentose-monofosfato; na forma r.-1,5-difosfato, combina-se com o CO_2 no início do processo fotossintético nos vegetais verdes ("fixação do dióxido de carbono"); a D-r. é o epímero da D-xilulose.

ri·bu·lose-1,5-bis·phos·phate car·box·yl·ase. Ribulose-1,5-difosfato carboxilase; carboxi-liase que forma dímeros; enzima que catalisa a adição do dióxido de carbono à D-ribulose-1,5-difosfato e a hidrólise do produto da adição em duas moléculas de ácido 3-fosfoglicérico, uma reação-chave na fixação do CO_2 na fotossíntese. SIN carboxydismutase.

ri·bu·lose-phos·phate 3-ep·i·mer·ase. Ribulose-fosfato-3-epimerase; enzima que catalisa a interconversão reversível da D-xilulose-5-fosfato e de seu epímero, a D-ribulose-5-fosfato; etapa da fase não-oxidativa da via da pentose-fosfato. SIN phosphoribulose epimerase.

Ricco, Annibale, astrofísico italiano, 1844–1919. VER R. *law*.

rice (rīs). Arroz; o grão da Oryza *sativa* (família Gramineae), a planta que produz o arroz; um alimento; é também utilizado, na forma de pó fino, como talco. [G. *oryza*]

Rich, Arnold R., patologista norte-americano, 1893–1968. VER Hamman-R. *syndrome*.

Richards, Barry Wyndham, médico inglês do século 20. VER Richards-Rundle *syndrome*.

Richardson, John Clifford, neurologista canadense, *1909. VER Steele-R.-Olszewski *disease*, *syndrome*.

Richter, August G., cirurgião alemão, 1742–1812. VER R. *hernia*; R.-Monro *line*; Monro-R. *line*.

Richter, Maurice N., patologista norte-americano, *1897. VER R. *syndrome*.

ri·cin (rī'sin, ris'in). Ricina; hemaglutinina e lectina altamente tóxica encontrada nas sementes (mamonas) da planta do óleo de rícino (carrapateira), *Ricinus communis*; se ingerida, age como um violento irritante e pode ser fatal; uma N-glicosidase que atua sobre a subunidade 60 S do RNAr.

ric·i·nism (ris'i-nizm). Ricinismo; envenenamento pela ingestão dos princípios tóxicos das sementes (mamonas) ou das folhas da planta do óleo de rícino (carrapateira), o *Ricinus communis*.

ri·cin·o·le·ate (ris-i-nō'lē-āt). Ricinoleato; sal do ácido ricinoléico.

ri·cin·o·le·ic ac·id (ris-i-nō-lē'ik, rī-si-). Ácido ricinoléico; hidroxiácido insaturado presente no óleo de castor.

Ric·i·nus (ris'i-nŭs). Gênero de plantas (família Euphorbiaceae) com uma espécie, *R. communis*, a carrapateira, fonte do óleo de rícino; acredita-se que suas folhas ajam como um galactagogo. SIN castor bean. [L.]

rick·ets (rik'ets). Raquitismo; doença resultante da deficiência de vitamina D, caracterizada por superprodução e calcificação deficiente de tecido osteóide, associada a deformidades esqueléticas, distúrbios do crescimento, hipocalcemia e, às vezes, tetania; é geralmente acompanhada de irritabilidade, apatia e fraqueza muscular generalizada; as fraturas são freqüentes. SIN infantile osteomalacia, juvenile osteomalacia, rachitis. [I. *wrick*, deformar]
  acute r., r. agudo. SIN hemorrhagic r.
  adult r., r. do adulto, osteomalácia. SIN osteomalacia.
  celiac r., r. celíaco; as deformidades ósseas e o atraso do crescimento associados à absorção defeituosa de gordura e de cálcio que ocorre na doença celíaca.
  familial hypophosphatemic r., r. hipofosfatêmico familial. SIN vitamin D-resistant r.
  hemorrhagic r., r. hemorrágico; as alterações ósseas observadas no escorbuto infantil, que consistem em hemorragia subperiosteal e formação deficiente do tecido ósseo; o termo é freqüentemente utilizado para indicar a ocorrência simultânea de r. e escorbuto. SIN acute r.
  hereditary hypophosphatemic r., r. hipofosfatêmico hereditário; acompanhado de hipercalciúria, distúrbio hereditário no qual há um defeito na reabsorção tubular renal.
  late r., r. osteomalácia. SIN osteomalacia.
  refractory r., r. refratário; r. que não responde ao tratamento com as doses usuais de vitamina D e dieta com teores adequados de cálcio e fósforo; é freqüentemente resultante de um distúrbio tubular renal hereditário, p. ex., a síndrome de Fanconi.
  renal r., r. renal; forma de r. observada em crianças que está associada a e é aparentemente causada por uma doença renal acompanhada de hiperfosfatemia. SIN pseudorickets, renal fibrocystic osteosis, renal infantilism, renal osteitis fibrosa.
  scurvy r., escorbuto infantil. SIN infantile *scurvy*.
  vitamin D-resistant r., r. resistente à vitamina D; um grupo de distúrbios metabólicos caracterizados por uma deficiência tubular renal no transporte do fosfato e por anormalidades ósseas que resultam em r. hipofosfatêmico ou osteomalácia; hipocalcemia e tetania não são características dessa doença. Existem uma forma autossômica dominante [MIM*193100] e uma forma dominante ligada ao X [MIM*307800], sendo esta última causada pela mutação no gene regulador do fosfato com homologias às endopeptidases (PHEX) do cromossoma Xp. As duas formas não respondem às doses terapêuticas-padrão de vitamina D, mas podem responder a doses muito grandes de fosfato e/ou vitamina D. Há também uma forma autossômica recessiva [MIM*277440] causada pela mutação no gene receptor da vitamina D, localizado no cromossoma 12q. SIN familial hypophosphatemic r.

Ricketts, Howard T., patologista norte-americano, 1871–1910. VER *Rickettsia*.

Rick·ett·si·a (ri-ket'sē-ă). Gênero de bactérias (ordem Rickettsiales) constituído por microrganismos Gram-negativos, pequenos (não-filtráveis), freqüentemente pleomórficos e em forma de bastonetes ou cocóides que geralmente são encontrados no citoplasma das células de piolhos, pulgas, carrapatos e ácaros e que não crescem nos meios de cultura sem células; as espécies patogênicas infectam seres humanos e outros animais, causando tifo epidêmico, tifo endêmico ou murino, febre maculosa das Montanhas Rochosas, doença de tsutsugamushi, riquetsiose variceliforme e outras doenças; a espécie-tipo é *R. prowazekii*. [Howard T. *Ricketts*]
  R. africae, espécie de R. estudada principalmente no Zimbábue que parece ser transportada pelo carrapato *Amblyomma hebraeum*; causa uma febre maculosa.
  R. ak'ari, espécie de bactéria que causa a riquetsiose variceliforme humana; é transmitida pelo ácaro do camundongo doméstico, o *Liponyssoides sanguineus*; produz uma doença febril branda que dura de 7-10 dias com uma distribuição urbana no nordeste dos EUA e em roedores comensais ou selvagens dos campos da antiga URSS e da África.
  R. austral'is, espécie de bactéria que causa uma febre maculosa, o tifo do norte de Queensland transmitido por carrapato, clínica e sorologicamente similar à doença causada pelo agente da riquetsiose variceliforme; *Ixodes holocyclus* e *I. tasmani* são os prováveis vetores. Há suspeita de que os pequenos marsupiais sejam os reservatórios desse agente, que é encontrado na maior parte do litoral de Queensland, principalmente no cerrado secundário e na savana.
  R. burnet'ii, nome antigo da *Coxiella burnetii*.
  R. canis, nome antigo da *Ehrlichia canis*.
  R. conorii, espécie de bactéria que causa a febre botonosa no sul da Europa, na África e no Oriente Médio; é transmitida por diversos carrapatos, p. ex., *Rhipicephalus sanguineus*, o carrapato do cão.
  R. honei, espécie de bactéria que causa a febre maculosa da Ilha Flinders, na Austrália.
  R. japonica, espécie de bactéria que causa a febre maculosa japonesa.
  R. mooseri, espécie similar a *R. prowazekii*, mas que possui uma aparência menos variável; o tifo endêmico resultante é mais brando e apresenta um início um pouco mais lento.
  R. prowazek'ii, espécie de bactéria que causa o tifo epidêmico e recrudescente e é transmitida pelos piolhos do corpo; é a espécie-tipo do gênero *R*.
  R. psi'ttaci, nome antigo da *Chlamydia psittaci*.
  R. ricketts'ii, espécie de bactéria que causa a febre maculosa das Montanhas Rochosas, a febre da África do Sul transmitida pela picada de carrapato, o tifo exantemático de São Paulo, do Brasil, a febre de Tobia, da Colômbia, e as febres maculosas de Minas Gerais e do México; é transmitida pelos carrapatos ixodídeos infectados, principalmente pelo *Dermacentor andersoni* e pelo *D. variabilis*.
  R. sennet'su, SIN *Ehrlichia sennetsu*.
  R. sibir'ica, espécie de bactéria que causa o tifo siberiano ou do norte da Ásia transmitido por diversos carrapatos ixodídeos, que também servem como reservatórios, possivelmente auxiliados por roedores e lebres; a doença assemelha-se à febre maculosa das Montanhas Rochosas.
  R. slovaca, espécie de bactéria que causa uma riquetsiose recém-identificada que está associada a eritema local e possivelmente a meningoencefalite; é transmitida pelo carrapato *Dermacentor marginatus*.
  R. tsutsugamu'shi, nome antigo da *Orientia tsutsugamushi*.
  R. ty'phi, espécie de bactéria que causa o tifo endêmico ou murino, transmitido pela pulga do rato.

rick·ett·si·al (ri-ket'sē-ăl). Riquetsial; relativo às riquétsias ou causado por elas.

rick·ett·si·al·pox (ri-ket'sē-ăl-poks'). Riquetsiose variceliforme; a infecção causada pela *Rickettsia akari*, que é disseminada por ácaros a partir do reservatório (camundongo doméstico); um processo benigno e autolimitado que foi identificado pela primeira vez em 1946, na área de Kew Gardens, na cidade de Nova York; a partir dessa data, alguns surtos limitados foram observados em outros locais. SIN Kew Gardens fever, mite-born typhus, vesicular rickettsiosis.

rick·ett·si·o·sis (ri-ket-sē-ō'sis). Riquetsiose; a infecção por riquétsias.
  vesicular r., r. variceliforme. SIN rickettsialpox.

rick·ett·si·o·stat·ic (ri-ket'sē-ō-stat'ik). Riquetsiostático; agente que iniba o crescimento das riquétsias. [*Rickettsia* + G. *statikos*, que causa paralisação]

rick·e·ty (rik'ĕ-tē). Raquítico. SIN rachitic.

Rickles, Norman H., patologista oral norte-americano, *1920. VER R. *test*.

RID Abreviatura de radial *immunodiffusion* (imunodifusão radial).

Riddoch, George, médico britânico, 1888–1947. VER Riddoch *phenomenon*. VER TAMBÉM Riddoch *phenomenon*.

Rideal, Samuel, químico e bacteriologista inglês, 1863–1929. VER R.-Walker *coefficient*, *method*.

ridge (rij). Crista. **1.** Uma elevação linear (geralmente áspera). VER TAMBÉM crest. **2.** Em odontologia, qualquer elevação linear localizada na superfície de um dente. **3.** O remanescente do processo alveolar e de seu revestimento de tecido mole após a remoção dos dentes. [A. S. *hyrcg*, dorso, espinha]
  alveolar r., processo alveolar da maxila. SIN alveolar *process* of maxilla.
  apical ectodermal r., c. ectodérmica apical; a camada de células ectodérmicas superficiais situada no ápice do broto embrionário dos membros; acredita-se que exerça uma influência indutiva na condensação do mesênquima subjacente e que seja necessária para o crescimento contínuo do membro.
  basal r., (1) Processo alveolar da maxila. SIN alveolar *process* of maxilla; **(2)** cíngulo do dente. SIN *cingulum* of tooth.
  bicipital r.'s, cristas dos tubérculos. SIN *crest* of greater tubercle, *crest* of lesser tubercle.
  buccocervical r., c. vestibulocervical; convexidade situada dentro do terço cervical da superfície vestibular (bucal) dos molares.
  buccogingival r., c. vestibulogengival; c. nítida situada na superfície vestibular (bucal) de um dente molar decíduo, a aproximadamente 1,5 mm da junção da coroa com a raiz.
  bulbar r., c. bulbar; um dos dois espessamentos subendocárdicos espirais encontrados no bulbo cardíaco embrionário; quando se fundem, dividem o bulbo em aorta e artéria pulmonar.
  bulboventricular r., c. bulboventricular; elevação situada na superfície interna do coração embrionário entre a 4.ª e a 5.ª semana; indica a divisão entre os ventrículos em desenvolvimento e o bulbo cardíaco.
  dental r., c. dentária; a borda proeminente de uma cúspide ou margem de um dente.

dermal r.'s [TA], cristas dérmicas; as cristas superficiais da epiderme das palmas e solas, onde se abrem os poros sudoríferos. SIN cristae cutis [TA], epidermal r.'s, papillary r.'s, skin r.'s.
epidermal r.'s, cristas epidérmicas. SIN dermal r.'s.
epipericardial r., c. epipericárdica; elevação que separa a região faríngea em desenvolvimento do pericárdio embrionário.
external oblique r., linha oblíqua da mandíbula. SIN oblique line of mandible.
ganglion r., c. neural. SIN neural crest.
genital r., c. gonadal. SIN gonadal r.
gluteal r., tuberosidade glútea. SIN gluteal tuberosity.
gonadal r., c. gonadal; elevação do mesotélio espessado e do mesênquima subjacente localizados na margem ventromedial dos mesonefros embrionários; as células germinativas primordiais incrustam-se nela, estabelecendo-a como o primórdio dos testículos ou dos ovários. SIN genital r.
interpapillary r.'s, cristas interpapilares. SIN rete r.
key r., ponto zigomaxilar. SIN zygomaxillare.
lateral epicondylar r., c. supra-epicondilar lateral. SIN lateral supraepicondylar r.
lateral supracondylar r., c. supra-epicondilar lateral; *termo oficial alternativo de lateral supraepicondylar r.
lateral supraepicondylar r. [TA], c. supra-epicondilar lateral; a parte afilada distal da margem lateral do úmero. SIN crista supraepicondylaris lateralis [TA], crista supracondylaris lateralis*, lateral supracondylar r. *, lateral epicondylar crest, lateral epicondylar r., lateral supracondylar crest.
linguocervical r., c. linguocervical. SIN linguogingival r.
linguogingival r., c. linguogengival; c. encontrada na superfície lingual dos dentes incisivos e caninos, próximo ao colo. SIN linguocervical r.
Mall r.'s, cristas de Mall; o epônimo raramente utilizado de pulmonary r.'s.
mammary r., c. mamária; espessamento da ectoderme encontrado no embrião, que se assemelha a uma faixa e se estende em ambos os lados de um ponto abaixo da axila até a região inguinal; nos embriões humanos, as glândulas mamárias surgem dos primórdios situados na parte torácica da c., enquanto o restante da c. desaparece; em alguns mamíferos inferiores que dão à luz uma ninhada, várias glândulas de leite desenvolvem-se ao longo dessas linhas. SIN mammary fold, milk line, milk r.
marginal r., c. marginal do dente. SIN marginal crest of tooth.
medial epicondylar r., c. supra-epicondilar medial. SIN medial supraepicondylar r.
medial supracondylar r., c. supra-epicondilar medial; *termo oficial alternativo de medial supraepicondylar r.
medial supraepicondylar r. [TA], c. supra-epicondilar medial; a parte afilada distal da margem medial do úmero. SIN crista supraepicondylaris medialis [TA], crista supracondylaris medialis*, medial supracondylar r. *, medial epicondylar crest, medial epicondylar r., medial supracondylar crest.
mesonephric r., c. mesonéfrica; c. que, nos embriões humanos mais novos, constitui a c. urogenital inteira; contudo, em uma fase posterior do desenvolvimento, uma c. genital mais medial, a gônada potencial, é demarcada a partir dela. VER TAMBÉM urogenital r. SIN mesonephric fold.
milk r., c. láctea. SIN mammary r.
mylohyoid r., linha milo-hióidea. SIN mylohyoid line.
nasal r., c. do nariz. SIN agger nasi.
oblique r., c. oblíqua; c. situada na superfície mastigatória de um dente molar superior, estendendo-se da cúspide mesiolingual até a distovestibular.
oblique r. of trapezium, tubérculo do trapézio. SIN tuberculum of trapezium bone.
palatine r., rafe do palato. SIN palatine raphe.
papillary r.'s, cristas papilares. SIN dermal r.'s.
Passavant r., c. de Passavant; proeminência situada na parede posterior da nasofaringe, formada pela contração do músculo constritor superior da faringe durante a deglutição. SIN Passavant bar, Passavant cushion, Passavant pad.
pectoral r., c. do tubérculo maior. SIN crest of greater tubercle.
pharyngeal r., fascículo posterior do músculo palatofaríngeo. SIN posterior fascicle of palatopharyngeus muscle.
primitive r., c. primitiva; uma das cristas dispostas aos pares e situadas em ambos os lados do sulco primitivo.
pronator r., c. do pronador; c. oblíqua situada na superfície anterior da ulna, na qual se insere o músculo pronador quadrado.
pterygoid r. of sphenoid bone, c. infratemporal da asa maior do osso esfenóide. SIN infratemporal crest of greater wing of sphenoid.
pulmonary r.'s, cristas pulmonares; um par de cristas que cobrem as veias cardinais comuns e se projetam da parede lateral do corpo para o interior do celoma embrionário; são assim denominadas porque fornecem uma indicação precoce de onde as pregas pleuropericárdicas desenvolver-se-ão.
residual r., c. residual; a parte do processo alveolar da maxila que permanece na boca edêntula após a reabsorção da região que contém os alvéolos.
rete r., c. epidérmica; o espessamento da epiderme que se dirige para baixo entre as papilas dérmicas; o termo inglês "*peg*" (cavilha, estaca, pino) é considerado incorreto, uma vez que as papilas dérmicas são cilíndricas, mas o espessamento epidérmico situado entre as papilas não é. SIN interpapillary r.'s, rete pegs.
skin r.'s, cristas cutâneas. SIN dermal r.'s.
sphenoidal r.'s, cristas esfenoidais; as margens afiladas posteriores das asas menores do osso esfenóide que terminam medialmente no processo clinóide anterior; as cristas esfenoidais separam a fossa anterior do crânio da parte lateral da fossa média do crânio.
superciliary r., arco superciliar. SIN superciliary arch.
supplemental r., c. suplementar; c. encontrada na superfície de um dente e que habitualmente não existe.
supraorbital r., margem supra-orbital. SIN supraorbital margin.
taste r., c. gustativa; uma das cristas que circundam as papilas circunvaladas da língua.
temporal r., linha temporal. SIN inferior temporal line of parietal bone, superior temporal line of parietal bone.
transverse r. [TA], c. transversa. SIN crista transversalis.
transverse palatine r., c. palatina transversa. SIN transverse palatine fold.
transverse r.'s of sacrum [TA], linhas transversas do sacro; uma das quatro cristas que cruzam a superfície pélvica do sacro; essas cristas marcam as posições dos discos intervertebrais situados entre os corpos das cinco vértebras sacrais do osso imaturo. SIN lineae transversae ossis sacri [TA].
trapezoid r., linha trapezóidea. SIN trapezoid line.
triangular r. [TA], c. triangular. SIN crista triangularis.
urogenital r., c. urogenital; uma das cristas longitudinais dispostas aos pares que se desenvolvem na parede dorsal do corpo do embrião, em ambos os lados do mesentério dorsal; inicialmente, a c. é formada pelos mesonefros em crescimento e, posteriormente, pelos mesonefros e pela gônada. SIN genital fold, wolffian r.
wolffian r., c. urogenital. SIN urogenital r.
Ridley, Humphrey, anatomista inglês, 1653–1708. VER R. *circle, sinus; circulus venosus ridleyi.*
Riedel, Bernhard M.C.L., cirurgião alemão, 1846–1916. VER R. *disease, lobe, struma, thyroiditis.*
Rieder, Hermann, patologista alemão, 1858–1932. VER R. *cells,* em *cell, cell leukemia, lymphocyte.*
Riegel, Franz, médico alemão, 1843–1904. VER R. *pulse.*
Rieger, Herwigh, oftalmologista alemão. VER R. *anomaly, syndrome.*
Riehl, Gustav, dermatologista austríaco, 1855–1943. VER R. *melanosis.*
RIF Abreviatura de resistance-inducing *factor* (fator indutor de resistência).
ri·fam·pi·cin (rif′am-pi-sin). Rifampicina, rifampina. SIN rifampin.
rif·am·pin (rif′am-pin). Rifampina, droga antituberculosa de primeira linha; agente bactericida empregado no tratamento da tuberculose e de outras infecções, que, como todas as drogas antituberculosas, não deve ser utilizado isoladamente no tratamento da tuberculose ativa; poderoso indutor das enzimas microssomiais hepáticas. SIN rifampicin.
rif·a·my·cin, rif·o·my·cin (rif-a-mī′sin, rif-ō-). Rifamicina; antibiótico complexo, isolado de *Nocardia mediterranei*, que é ativo contra *Mycobacterium tuberculosis* e *Staphylococcus aureus*; é mal absorvido no trato gastrointestinal e freqüentemente causa irritação e dor intensa nos locais da injeção.
Riga, Antonio, médico italiano, 1832–1919. VER R.-Fede *disease.*
right-eyed (rīt-īd). Destrocular. SIN dextrocular.
right-foot·ed (rīt′fut-ed). Destropedal. SIN dextropedal.
right-hand·ed (rīt′hand-ed). Destrímano, destrômano, destro; indica o uso habitual ou mais hábil da mão direita para escrever e para a maioria das operações manuais. SIN dextral, dextromanual.
ri·gid·i·ty (ri-jid′i-tē). Rigidez. **1.** Dureza ou inflexibilidade. SIN rigor (1). **2.** Em psiquiatria e em psicologia clínica, um aspecto da personalidade caracterizado pela resistência de um indivíduo à mudança. **3.** Em neurologia, um tipo de aumento do tônus muscular; caracterizado por resistência aumentada ao estiramento passivo, independente da velocidade e simétrica ao redor das articulações; aumenta com a ativação dos músculos correspondentes do membro contralateral. Os dois tipos básicos são a r. em roda dentada e a r. em cano de chumbo. VER TAMBÉM nuchal r. [L. *rigidus*, rígido, inflexível]
cadaveric r., r. cadavérica, *rigor mortis.* SIN rigor mortis.
catatonic r., r. catatônica; r. associada aos estados psicóticos catatônicos nos quais todos os músculos exibem flexibilidade cérea (*flexibilitas cerea*).
cerebellar r., r. cerebelar; aumento do tônus dos músculos extensores, relacionado à lesão do verme do cerebelo.
clasp-knife r., espasticidade em canivete. SIN clasp-knife spasticity.
cogwheel r., r. em roda dentada; um tipo de r. observada no parkinsonismo na qual os músculos respondem com espasmos semelhantes ao movimento de uma roda dentada ao uso de uma força constante para flexionar um membro.
decerebrate r., r. da descerebração; mudança postural que ocorre em alguns pacientes comatosos, que consiste em episódios de opistótomo, extensão rígida dos membros, rotação interna das extremidades superiores e acentuada flexão da planta dos pés; é produzida por vários distúrbios cerebrais estruturais e metabólicos. SIN decerebrate state.
decorticate r., r. da decorticação; alteração postural uni ou bilateral, que con-

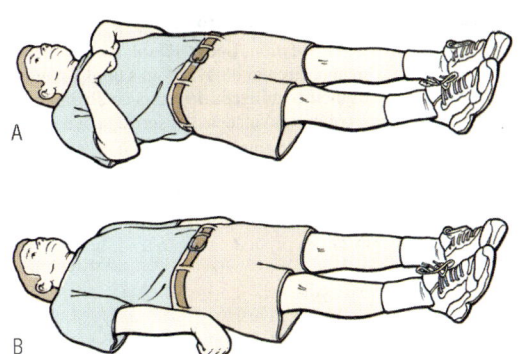

rigidez: (A) de decorticação; (B) de descerebração

siste na flexão e adução dos membros superiores e na extensão rígida dos inferiores; é resultante de lesões estruturais do tálamo, da cápsula interna ou da substância branca do cérebro. SIN decorticate state.
  lead-pipe r., r. em cano de chumbo; um tipo plástico de r. observada em certas formas de parkinsonismo.
  nuchal r., r. da nuca; a dificuldade em flexionar o pescoço resultante de um espasmo dos músculos extensores do pescoço (não é uma r. de fato); é geralmente atribuída a irritação das meninges.
  ocular r., r. ocular; a resistência oferecida pelo globo ocular a uma alteração no volume intra-ocular; manifesta-se como modificação na pressão intra-ocular.
  postmortem r., *rigor-mortis*, r. pós-morte. SIN *rigor mortis.*
  scleral r., r. escleral; uma resistência do olho às alterações em sua forma acompanhada de modificações na pressão intra-ocular.
rig·or (rig′er). **1.** Rigidez. SIN rigidity (1). **2.** Calafrio. SIN chill (2). [L. rigidez]
  acid r., coagulação das proteínas musculares induzida por ácidos.
  calcium r., a parada do coração no estado completamente contraído como resultado de intoxicação por cálcio.
  heat r., coagulação da proteína muscular induzida pelo calor.
  r. mor′tis, *rigor mortis*, r. pós-morte; a rigidez do corpo observada 1-7 horas após a morte e proveniente do enrijecimento dos tecidos musculares como consequência da coagulação do miosinogênio e do paramiosinogênio; desaparece após 1-6 dias ou quando começa a decomposição. SIN cadaveric rigidity, postmortem rigidity.
  myocardial r. mortis, contratura isquêmica do ventrículo esquerdo. SIN ischemic *contracture* of the left ventricle.
Riley, Conrad M., pediatra norte-americano, *1913. VER R.-Day *syndrome*.
Riley, Harris D., Jr., médico norte-americano do século 20. VER Smith-R. *syndrome.*
riluzole (ril′oo-zōl). Riluzol; droga utilizada no tratamento da esclerose lateral amiotrófica; seu mecanismo de ação não é conhecido.
rim. Margem, borda, rebordo, aba; uma margem ou borda, geralmente com forma circular.
  bite r., rolete oclusal, plano oclusal. SIN occlusion r.
  occlusal r., rolete oclusal, plano oclusal. SIN occlusion r.
  occlusion r., rolete oclusal, plano oclusal; as superfícies oclusais construídas nas bases das dentaduras temporárias ou permanentes com o objetivo de fazer os registros da relação maxilomandibular e organizar os dentes. SIN bite r., occlusal r., record r.
  orbital r., margem orbital. SIN orbital *margin.*
  record r., rolete de registro, plano de registro. SIN occlusion r.
ri·ma, gen. e pl. **ri·mae** (rī′mă, rī′mē) [TA]. Rima; fenda ou fissura, ou uma abertura alongada e estreita situada entre duas partes simétricas. [L. uma fenda]
  r. glot′tidis [TA], r. da glote; o intervalo observado entre as cordas vocais verdadeiras. SIN r. vocalis✱, glottis vera, true glottis.
  r. o′ris [TA], r. da boca. SIN oral *fissure.*
  r. palpebra′rum [TA], r. das pálpebras. SIN palpebral *fissure.*
  r. puden′di [TA], r. do pudendo. SIN pudendal *cleft.*
  r. respirato′ria, r. do vestíbulo. SIN r. vestibuli.
  r. vestib′uli [TA], r. do vestíbulo; o intervalo observado entre as cordas vocais falsas ou as pregas vestibulares. SIN false glottis, glottis spuria, r. respiratoria.
  r. voca′lis, r. da glote; ✱termo oficial alternativo de r. glottidis.
  r. vul′vae, r. do pudendo. SIN pudendal *cleft.*
ri·man·ta·dine (ri-man′tă-dēn). Rimantadina; agente antiviral que apresenta uma atividade semelhante à da amantadina, mas aparentemente com menos reações adversas do sistema nervoso central.

Rimini test. Teste de Rimini. VER em test.
ri·mose (rī′mōs). Rimoso; fissurado; marcado por fendas em todas as direções, como as pequenas fissuras observadas na porcelana. [L. *rimosus*, de *rima*, uma fissura]
rim·u·la (rim′u-lă). Rímula; uma diminuta fenda ou fissura. [L. dim. de *rima*]
Rindfleisch, Georg E., médico alemão, 1836–1908. VER R. *folds*, em fold.
ring (rĭng). [TA]. Anel. **1.** Uma faixa circular que circunda uma ampla abertura central; uma estrutura em forma de anel ou circular que circunda uma abertura ou superfície plana. SIN anulus [TA]. **2.** A cadeia fechada (i. e., sem fim) de átomos em um composto cíclico; termo habitualmente utilizado para "cíclico" ou "ciclo". **3.** Um crescimento marginal observado na superfície de um caldo de cultura para bactérias, que adere às paredes do tubo de teste, formando um círculo. SIN annulus. [A.S. *hring*]
  abdominal r., a. inguinal profundo. SIN deep inguinal r.
  amnion r., a. amniótico; o a. formado pela fixação do âmnio ao cordão umbilical no ponto em que este último emerge do umbigo.
  annuloplasty r., a. de anuloplastia; a sutura de um anel protético a um anel dilatado que reduz este último ao seu tamanho sistólico normal.
  anterior limiting r., lâmina limitante anterior. SIN anterior limiting *lamina.*
  Balbani r., a. de Balbani; uma "protuberância" extremamente grande observada em uma banda de um cromossoma politênico.
  benzene r., a. do benzeno; o arranjo dos átomos de carbono e hidrogênio em uma cadeia fechada na molécula do benzeno. VER TAMBÉM cyclic *compound.*
  Bickel r., a. de Bickel. SIN pharyngeal lymphatic r.
  Cannon r., ponto de Cannon. SIN Cannon *point.*
  cardiac lymphatic r., a. linfático do cárdia. SIN *lymph nodes* around cardia of stomach, em *lymph node.*
  casting r., a. de fundição. SIN refractory *flask.*
  choroidal r., a. da coróide; um crescente ou anel levemente pigmentado adjacente ao disco óptico.
  ciliary r., a. ciliar. SIN orbiculus ciliaris.
  common tendinous r. of extraocular muscles [TA], a. tendíneo comum dos músculos extra-oculares; anel fibroso que circunda o canal óptico e a parte medial da fissura orbital superior; dá origem aos quatro músculos retos do olho e está parcialmente fundido à bainha do nervo óptico. SIN anulus of Zinn, anulus tendineus communis, Zinn ligament, Zinn r., Zinn tendon.
  conjunctival r. [TA], a. da conjuntiva; um anel estreito situado na junção da periferia da córnea com a conjuntiva. SIN anulus conjunctivae [TA].
  constriction r., a. de constrição; **(1)** a rigidez espástica verdadeira da cavidade uterina que ocorre quando uma zona do músculo sofre contração tetânica local e forma uma firme constrição ao redor de alguma parte do feto. **(2)** SIN amnionic *band.*
  crural r., a. femoral. SIN femoral r.
  deep inguinal r., a. inguinal profundo; a abertura situada na fáscia transversal através da qual o ducto deferente e os vasos gonadais (ou o ligamento redondo na mulher) penetram no canal inguinal. Localizado a meio caminho entre a espinha ilíaca ântero-superior e o tubérculo púbico, é limitado medialmente pela prega umbilical lateral (vasos epigástricos inferiores) e inferiormente pelo trato iliopúbico. As hérnias inguinais indiretas saem da cavidade abdominal através do a. inguinal profundo. SIN anulus inguinalis profundus [TA], abdominal r., anulus abdominalis, internal inguinal r.
  external inguinal r., a. inguinal superficial. SIN superficial inguinal r.
  femoral r. [TA], a. femoral; a abertura superior do canal femoral, limitada anteriormente pelo ligamento inguinal, posteriormente pelo músculo pectíneo, medialmente pelo ligamento lacunar e lateralmente pela veia femoral. Trata-se de uma passagem por onde muitos vasos linfáticos provenientes do membro inferior passam para o abdome. Acomoda o aumento da veia femoral observado na manobra de Valsalva. É freqüentemente ocupada por um linfonodo (l. de Cloquet) e é o local de aparecimento das hérnias femorais. SIN anulus femoralis [TA], crural r.
  fibrocartilaginous r. of tympanic membrane [TA], a. fibrocartilagíneo da membrana timpânica; a parte espessada da circunferência da membrana timpânica que se fixa ao sulco timpânico. SIN anulus fibrocartilagineus membranae tympani [TA], Gerlach annular tendon.
  fibrous r., a. fibroso. **(1)** (right and left) fibrous r.'s of heart. **(2)** SIN *anulus fibrosus of intervertebral disk.*
  fibrous r. intervertebral disk, a. fibroso do disco intervertebral. SIN *anulus fibrosus of intervertebral disk.*
  Fleischer r., a. de Fleischer; anel incompleto com freqüência presente na base do cone do ceratocone; pode ser amarelo ou esverdeado em virtude da deposição de hemossiderina.
  Fleischer-Strümpell r., a. de Fleischer-Strümpell. SIN Kayser-Fleischer r.
  Flieringa r., a. de Flieringa; a. de aço inoxidável que é suturado na esclera para evitar o colapso do globo nas cirurgias intra-oculares difíceis.
  gestational r., a. gestacional; o a. branco identificado pela ecossonografia por pulsos que sinaliza um estágio inicial da gravidez.
  glaucomatous r., halo glaucomatoso. SIN glaucomatous *halo* (1).
  Graefenberg r., a. de Graefenberg; termo obsoleto para um a. de prata ou de

fio de seda natural projetado para ser inserido na cavidade uterina e utilizado como um meio de contracepção.

greater r. of iris, a. maior da íris. SIN outer *border* of iris.

internal inguinal r., a. inguinal interno. SIN deep inguinal r.

r. of iris, margem da íris. SIN *border* of iris.

Kayser-Fleischer r., a. de Kayser-Fleischer; a. pigmentado amarelo-esverdeado que circunda a córnea, junto à parte interna da margem corneoescleral, observado na degeneração hepatolenticular e resultante da deposição de cobre na membrana de Descemet (ver Descemet *membrane*). SIN Fleischer-Strümpell r.

lesser r. of iris, a. menor da íris. SIN inner *border* of iris.

Liesegang r.'s, anéis de Liesegang; os anéis coloridos de precipitado de cromato de prata formados quando uma gota de nitrato de prata concentrado é adicionada à superfície de um gel (tal como a gelatina, o ágar ou o gel de sílica) que contém dicromato de potássio.

Lower r., a. de Lower. SIN (right and left) fibrous r.'s of heart.

lymphatic r. of cardiac part of stomach, a. linfático da cárdia do estômago. SIN *lymph nodes* around cardia of stomach, em *lymph node*.

neonatal r., a. neonatal. SIN neonatal *line*.

pathologic retraction r., a. de retração patológica; constrição localizada na junção do segmento uterino inferior adelgaçado com o segmento uterino superior retraído e espessado e que resulta da obstrução do trabalho de parto; é um dos sinais clássicos de ameaça de ruptura uterina.

pharyngeal lymphatic r. [TA], a. linfático da faringe; a. fragmentado de tecido linfático, formado pelas tonsilas lingual, palatina, faríngea e tubária. SIN anulus lymphoideus pharyngis [TA], Bickel r., tonsillar r., Waldeyer throat r.

physiologic retraction r., a. de retração fisiológica; uma crista situada na superfície interna do útero, na linha que separa o segmento uterino superior do inferior, e observada no curso do trabalho de parto normal.

polar r., a. polar; um anel espesso e elétron-denso situado na extremidade anterior de certos estágios dos membros do filo Apicomplexa; uma parte do complexo apical característico desses esporozoários.

(right and left) fibrous r.'s of heart [TA], anéis fibrosos (direito e esquerdo) do coração; os dois anéis fibrosos que cercam os orifícios atrioventriculares do coração, proporcionando um local para a fixação dos folhetos das válvulas atrioventriculares e mantendo os orifícios pérvios. Como parte do esqueleto fibroso do coração, os anéis fibrosos também fornecem um local para a origem e inserção do miocárdio. SIN anulus fibrosus (1) [TA], anulus fibrosus dexter/sinister cordis, coronary tendon, fibrous r. (1), Lower r.

Schatzki r., a. de Schatzki; a. de contração ou diafragma incompleto de mucosa situado no terço inferior do esôfago, que é ocasionalmente sintomático.

Schwalbe r., a. de Schwalbe. SIN anterior limiting *lamina*.

scleral r., a. da esclera; o aspecto da esclera junto ao disco óptico observado quando o epitélio pigmentado da retina não se estende até o nervo óptico.

signet r., a. de sinete; o estágio inicial do desenvolvimento dos trofozoítas do parasita da malária na hemácia; quando são utilizados corantes de Romanowsky, o citoplasma do parasita cora-se de azul ao redor de sua margem circular, o núcleo cora-se de vermelho e o vacúolo central fica claro, o que confere ao parasita um aspecto semelhante a um anel.

r. of Soemmerring, a. de Soemmerring; uma massa de fibras lenticulares encerrada entre a parte anterior e a posterior da cápsula lenticular e que deixa a área da pupila relativamente livre.

subcutaneous r., a. inguinal superficial. SIN superficial inguinal r.

superficial inguinal r. [TA], a. inguinal superficial; abertura semelhante a uma fenda situada na aponeurose do músculo oblíquo externo da parede abdominal através da qual o cordão espermático (o ligamento redondo na mulher) e as hérnias inguinais emergem do canal inguinal. VER TAMBÉM *aponeurosis* of external oblique muscle. SIN anulus inguinalis superficialis, external inguinal r., subcutaneous r.

tonsillar r., a. linfático da faringe. SIN pharyngeal lymphatic r.

tracheal r., cartilagem traqueal. SIN tracheal *cartilages*, em *cartilage*.

tympanic r. [TA], a. timpânico; no feto, um anel ósseo mais ou menos completo situado na extremidade medial do meato acústico externo cartilaginoso, no qual se fixa a membrana timpânica. SIN anulus tympanicus, tympanic bone.

umbilical r. [TA], a. umbilical; abertura na linha alba através da qual passam os vasos umbilicais no feto; em embriões mais jovens, fica relativamente perto do púbis, mas gradualmente ascende até o centro do abdome; no adulto, o anel apresenta-se fechado, e seu local é indicado pelo umbigo. SIN anulus umbilicalis, canalis umbilicalis.

vascular r., a. vascular; as artérias anômalas (arcos aórticos) que congenitamente circundam a traquéia e o esôfago e, por vezes, produzem sintomas compressivos.

Vieussens r., a. de Vieussens. SIN *limbus fossae ovalis*.

Vossius lenticular r., a. lenticular de Vossius; opacidade em forma de anel encontrada na cápsula anterior da lente após uma contusão do olho, causada por pigmento e sangue.

Waldeyer throat r., a. faríngeo de Waldeyer. SIN pharyngeal lymphatic r.

Zinn r., a. de Zinn. SIN common tendinous r. of extraocular muscles.

Ringer, Sydney, fisiologista inglês, 1835–1910. VER R. *injection*, *solution*; lactated R. *injection*; Krebs-R. *solution*; Locke-R. *solution*; Ringer *lactate*.

ring-knife (ring-nīf). Um anel circular ou oval com a borda interna cortante, semelhante à plaina de carpinteiro, utilizada na remoção de tumores localizados na cavidade nasal e em outras cavidades. SIN spoke-shave.

ring·worm (ring'werm). Tinha. SIN tinea.

r. of beard, t. da barba. SIN *tinea* barbae.

black-dot r., t. dos pontos pretos; a tinha da cabeça (*tinea capitis*) mais freqüentemente causada por *Trichophyton tonsurans* ou *T. violaceum*.

r. of body, t. do corpo. SIN *tinea* corporis.

crusted r., t. crostosa. SIN *tinea* favus.

r. of foot, t. do pé. SIN *tinea* pedis.

honeycomb r., t. favosa, favo. SIN *favus*.

r. of nails, t. das unhas, onicomicose. SIN *onychomycosis*.

Oriental r., t. oriental. SIN *tinea* imbricata.

r. of scalp, t. do couro cabeludo. SIN *tinea* capitis.

scaly r., t. escamosa. SIN *tinea* imbricata.

Tokelau r., t. de Tokelau. SIN *tinea* imbricata. [Ilhas *Tokelau*, no Oceano Pacífico Sul]

Rinne, Friedrich Heinrich A., otologista alemão, 1819–1868. VER R. *test*.

Riolan, Jean, anatomista e botânico francês, 1577–1657. VER R. *anastomosis*, *arc*, *arcades*, em *arcade*, *bones*, em *bone*, *bouquet*, *muscle*.

RIP. Abreviatura de radioimmunoprecipitation (radioimunoprecipitação).

ri·par·i·an (ri-par'ē-an, rī-). Ripário; relativo a uma margem; marginal.

Ripault, Louis H.A., médico francês, 1807–1856. VER R. *sign*.

rip·en·ing (rī'pen-ing). Envelhecimento; indica a oxidação progressiva das soluções dos corantes, como ocorre no envelhecimento das soluções de hematoxilina a hemateína ou do azul de metileno a corantes de azures.

Ripstein, Charles B., cirurgião norte-americano do século 20. VER Ripstein *operation*.

RISA Abreviatura de radioiodinated serum *albumin* (albumina sérica radioiodada).

risk. Risco; a probabilidade de um evento ocorrer.

attributable r., r. atribuível; a freqüência de uma doença ou outra conseqüência observada em indivíduos expostos que pode ser atribuída à exposição.

competing r., r. competitivo; um evento que remove um indivíduo que ameaça o resultado que está sob investigação.

empiric r., r. empírico; o r. que está baseado apenas na evidência empírica, sem qualquer apelo a uma teoria ou suposição formais.

radiation r.'s, riscos da radiação; os riscos para a saúde atribuídos à exposição à radiação. As fontes de exposição são tanto naturais como artificiais (p. ex., médica ou ocupacional). VER background *radiation*.

> A exposição excessiva à radiação ionizante está associada a risco aumentado de doenças malignas, sobretudo da pele e dos órgãos formadores de sangue; ao risco aumentado de variações anormais nas células reprodutivas, com a possibilidade de anormalidades nos descendentes; e ao risco aumentado de anormalidades fetais resultantes da exposição materna no início da gravidez. Para a maioria das pessoas, as fontes naturais são responsáveis pela maior parte da radiação recebida, enquanto as fontes artificiais adicionam somente uma pequena porcentagem à dose anual média. A percepção pública dos perigos da radiação está freqüentemente em desacordo com as posições científicas sobre o assunto. Os resultados duvidosos das pesquisas (como nas tentativas de estimar o risco adicional de câncer atribuído às mamografias) têm contribuído para criar um receio no público. Alguns estudos levaram à conclusão de que, independentemente de o medo do público com relação às usinas nucleares ser justificado ou não, o estresse adicional causado por tal medo constitui uma ameaça para a saúde.

recurrence r., r. de recorrência; o r. de uma doença ocorrer em outro lugar de uma árvore genealógica, dado que pelo menos um de seus membros (o probando) exibe a doença.

relative r., r. relativo; a razão entre o r. de doença junto àqueles expostos a um fator de r. e o r. junto àqueles não expostos.

Risley, Samuel D., oftalmologista norte-americano, 1845–1920. VER R. rotary *prism*.

ri·so·ri·us (ri-sōr'ē-ŭs). Risório. VER risorius (*muscle*). [L. *risor*, uma risada, de *rideo*, pp. *risus*, rir]

RIST Abreviatura de radioimmunosorbent *test* (teste radioimunossorvente).

ris·to·ce·tin (ris-tō-sē'tin). Ristocetina; antibiótico produzido pela fermentação do *Amycolatopsis orientalis*, subesp. *lurida*, que compreende duas substâncias: a r. A e a r. B; é útil contra as infecções estafilocócicas e enterocócicas refratárias a outros antibióticos.

ri·sus (rī'sŭs). Riso, sorriso, uma gargalhada. [risada]

r. caninus (rī'sŭs kā-nī'nŭs), riso sardônico; o simulacro de um riso forçado produzido por espasmo facial e observado principalmente no tétano, mas também em alguns tipos de envenenamento. SIN canine spasm, r. sardonicus, sardonic grin, trismus sardonicus. [L. *risus*, riso, + *caninus*, semelhante a um cão]

r. sardonicus (sar-don′i-kŭs), r. sardônico. SIN r. caninus. [L. *risus*, riso, + *sardonicus*, do G. *sardanios*, desdenhoso, infl. por *sardonios*, sardo, ref. aos efeitos da *Strychnos nux-vomica*, erva venenosa da Sardenha]

Ritgen, Ferdinand A.M.F. von, obstetra alemão, 1787–1867. VER R. *maneuver*.

ri·to·drine (ri′to-drēn). Ritodrina; agente simpaticomimético com ações estimulantes β₂-adrenérgicas, utilizado como relaxante uterino.

Ritter, Johann W., físico alemão, 1776–1810. VER R. opening *tetanus*; R.-Rollet *phenomenon*.

rit·u·al (rich′oo-ăl). Ritual; em psiquiatria e psicologia, qualquer atividade psicomotora (p. ex., a lavagem mórbida das mãos) realizada por uma pessoa com o objetivo de aliviar a ansiedade ou evitar o seu desenvolvimento; é tipicamente observado no distúrbio obsessivo-compulsivo. [L. *ritualis*, de *ritus*, rito]

rituximab (rit-ŭks′im-ab). Anticorpo monoclonal utilizado no tratamento do linfoma não-Hodgkin.

ri·val·ry (ri′văl-rē). Rivalidade; competição entre dois ou mais indivíduos ou entidades pelo mesmo objeto ou meta. [L. *rivalis*, competidor, rival]

binocular r., r. binocular; alteração na percepção de partes do campo visual que ocorre quando os dois olhos são simultânea e rapidamente expostos a alvos que contêm cores ou bordas diferentes.

r. of retina, r. retiniana; a excitação simultânea de áreas retinianas correspondentes de cada olho por estímulos que diferem quanto ao tamanho, à cor, à forma ou à luminosidade, o que torna impossível a fusão.

sibling r., r. fraterna; a competição ciumenta entre crianças, principalmente por atenção, afeto e estima de seus pais; por extensão, um fator tanto da competitividade normal quanto da anormal por toda a vida.

Riv·ea co·rym·bo·sa (riv′ē-ă ko-rim-bo′să). Uma trepadeira mexicana; planta da família Convolvulaceae cujas sementes foram utilizadas em cerimônias pelos índios astecas, no México, e que contêm amida do ácido lisérgico, ácido isolisérgico, monoetilamida do ácido lisérgico, canoclavina e outros alcalóides do indol; várias centenas de sementes precisam ser ingeridas para que ocorram efeitos alucinatórios e eufóricos. SIN morning glory (2).

Riverius. VER Rivière.

Rivero-Carvallo, José Manuel, cardiologista mexicano, *1905. VER Carvallo *sign*; Rivero-Carvallo *effect*.

Rivers, William H., médico inglês, 1864–1922. VER R. *cocktail*.

Rivière (Riverius), Lazare (Lazarus), médico francês, 1589–1655. VER R. *salt*.

Rivinus (forma latina de Bachmann). August Q., anatomista alemão, 1652–1723. VER Rivinus *canals*, em *canal*, Rivinus *ducts*, em *duct*, Rivinus *gland*, Rivinus *incisure*, Rivinus *membrane*, Rivinus *notch*.

ri·vus la·cri·ma·lis (ri′vŭs lak-ri-mā′lis) [TA]. Rego lacrimal. SIN lacrimal pathway. [L. *rivus*, riacho, corrente, + L. mediev. *lacrimalis*, do L. *lacrima*, uma lágrima]

riz·i·form (riz′i-fōrm). Riziforme, oriziforme; que se assemelha aos grãos de arroz. [De *riz*, arroz]

RLL Abreviatura de right lower lobe (lobo inferior direito do pulmão).

RLQ Abreviatura de right lower quadrant (quadrante inferior direito do abdome).

RMA Abreviatura de right mentoanterior position (posição mentoanterior direita).

RML Abreviatura de right middle lobe (lobo médio direito do pulmão).

RMP Abreviatura de right mentoposterior position (posição mentoposterior direita).

RMT Abreviatura de right mentotransverse position (posição mentotransversa direita).

RMV Abreviatura de respiratory minute *volume* (volume minuto respiratório).

R.N. Abreviatura de registered *nurse*.

Rn Símbolo de radon (radônio).

RNA Abreviatura de ribonucleic acid (ácido ribonucléico). Para consultar os termos formados com essa abreviatura, ver as subentradas em ribonucleic acid.

RNase Abreviatura de ribonuclease. Para consultar os termos formados com essa abreviatura, ver as subentradas em ribonuclease.

RNase D Abreviatura de *ribonuclease* D (ribonuclease D).

RNA splic·ing. Entrelaçamento do RNA. SIN splicing (2).

RNP Abreviatura de ribonucleoprotein (ribonucleoproteína).

ROA Abreviatura de right occipitoanterior position (posição occipitoanterior direita).

Roach, F. Ewing, protodontista norte-americano, 1868–1960. VER R. *clasp*.

Roaf, R. VER R. *syndrome*.

Robert, Heinrich, L.F., ginecologista alemão, 1814–1878. VER R. *pelvis*.

Roberts, J.B., médico norte-americano do século 20. VER R. *syndrome*.

Robertshaw, Frank L., anestesiologista inglês do século 20. VER R. *tube*.

Robertson, VER Argyll R.

Robin, Pierre, pediatra francês, 1867–1950. VER Pierre R. *syndrome*.

Robin, Charles P., médico francês, 1821–1885. VER Virchow-R. *space*.

Robinow, Meinhard, médico norte-americano, *1909. VER Robinow *dwarfism*, Robinow *syndrome*.

Robinson, Brian F., cardiologista britânico do século 20. VER R. *index*.

Robison, Robert, químico inglês, 1884–1941. VER R. *ester*, ester *dehydrogenase*; R.-Embden *ester*.

Robles, Rudolfo (Valverde), dermatologista guatemalteco, 1878–1939.

ro·bot·ic (ro-bot′ik). Robótico; relativo a ou característico de um robô, ou seja, um dispositivo mecânico automático projetado para duplicar uma função humana sem que haja operação direta do homem. [Tcheco *robot*, robô, de *robota*, trabalho penoso, + *-ic*]

Robson. VER Mayo-Robson.

ro·bust·ness (ro-bust′nes). Robustez; em estatística, o grau no qual a probabilidade de se tirar uma conclusão errada a partir do resultado de um teste não é seriamente afetada pelas divergências moderadas de suposições implícitas no modelo no qual o teste está baseado. [L. *robustus*, robusto, forte, de *robur*, carvalho, duro, forte]

ROC Acrônimo de receiver operating *characteristic* (característica operacional do receptor), uma expressão analítica da acurácia diagnóstica. VER ROC *curve*.

roc·cel·lin (rok′sel-in) [I.C. 15620]. Rocelina. SIN archil.

Ro·cha·li·maea (ro-chă-li′mā-ă). Antigo nome da *Bartonella*. [H. da *Rocha-Lima*, microbiologista brasileiro]

Rochalimaea henselae, VER *Bartonella henselae*.

Rochalimaea quintana, VER *Bartonella quintana*.

rod (rod). Bastonete; bastão; haste; prisma. **1.** Uma estrutura ou um dispositivo cilíndrico e delgado. **2.** A parte fotossensível e dirigida para fora de um bastonete que contém rodopsina e se situa no estrato granular externo da retina; milhões de bastonetes, juntamente com os cones, formam a camada fotorreceptora de cones e bastonetes. SIN rod cell of retina. [A.S. *rōd*]

analyzing r., haste analisadora; um dispositivo utilizado com um paralelômetro (delineador) para determinar as posições relativas de superfícies paralelas e reentrâncias, quando se projetam dentaduras parciais removíveis.

Auer r.'s, corpúsculos de Auer. SIN Auer *bodies*, em *body*.

basal r., bastão basal. SIN costa (2).

Corti r.'s, bastonetes de Corti. SIN pillar *cells*, em *cell*.

enamel r.'s, prismas do esmalte. SIN *prismata adamantina*, em *prisma*.

germinal r., esporozoíto. SIN sporozoite.

Maddox r., cilindro de Maddox; um cilindro de vidro, ou um conjunto de cilindros de vidro, que converte a imagem de uma fonte de luz em uma linha de luz perpendicular ao eixo do cilindro. A posição dessa faixa em relação à imagem da fonte de luz observada pelo outro olho indica a presença e a quantidade de heteroforia.

surgical r., haste cirúrgica; um implante cilíndrico, em geral composto de metal, utilizado para alinhar e fixar internamente as fraturas dos ossos longos. VER TAMBÉM nail, pin.

Ro·den·tia (ro-den′shē-ă). Os roedores; a maior ordem de mamíferos placentários (classe Eutheria); todos os membros possuem um par de incisivos superiores, semelhantes a cinzéis, para roer e molares e pré-molares com coroas planas para triturar; engloba os camundongos, ratos, porquinhos-da-índia (as cobaias), esquilos, castores e muitos outros. [L. mod., do L. *rodo*, part. pres. *rodens*, roer]

ro·den·ti·cide (ro-den′ti-sīd). Rodenticida; agente letal para os roedores. [rodent + L. *caedo*, matar]

Roentgen, Wilhelm K., físico alemão laureado com um Nobel, 1845–1923. Em 1901, recebeu o Prêmio Nobel em Física por ter descoberto os raios X, fato que ocorreu em novembro de 1895. VER roentgen; roentgen *ray*.

roent·gen (R, r) (rent′gen, rent′chen). A unidade internacional de dose de exposição aos raios X ou gama; a quantidade de radiação que produz em 1 cc ou 0,001293 g de ar, nas CNTP, $2,08 \times 10^9$ íons de ambos os sinais, cada um totalizando 1 unidade eletrostática de carga; no sistema MKS, corresponde a $2,58 \times 10^{-4}$ coulombs por kg de ar. [W.K. Roentgen]

r.-equivalent-man (rem), dose equivalente no homem (rem); uma unidade de dose que é equivalente à radiação ionizante de qualquer tipo que produz, em seres humanos, o mesmo efeito biológico de 1 rad de raios X ou gama; o número de rems é igual à dose absorvida, medida em rads, multiplicado pelo fator de qualidade da radiação em questão. 100 rem = 1 Sv.

r.-equivalent-physical, dose equivalente nos tecidos vivos; uma unidade de medida obsoleta; a quantidade de radiação ionizante de qualquer tipo que, ao ser absorvida pelo tecido vivo, produz um ganho de energia por grama de tecido que é equivalente àquela produzida por 1 rad de raios X ou gama. VER rad.

roent·gen·ky·mo·gram (rent′gen-ki′mo-gram). Roentgencimograma; registro dos movimentos do coração obtido por meio do roentgencimógrafo.

roent·gen·ky·mo·graph (rent′gen-ki′mo-graf). Roentgencimógrafo; aparelho utilizado para registrar os movimentos do coração e dos grandes vasos ou do diafragma sobre um único filme. Consiste em uma folha de chumbo denominada grade na qual são feitas fendas horizontais ou verticais, geralmente com menos de 1 mm de largura, separadas por 1 a 2 cm. Durante uma exposição aos raios X, que dura o correspondente a vários ciclos cardíacos ou respiratórios, a grade ou o filme é movido verticalmente, a fim de registrar o movimento cardíaco, ou horizontalmente, para registrar o movimento do diafragma.

roent·gen·ky·mog·ra·phy (rent′gen - kī - mog′rȧ - fē). Roentgencimografia; técnica obsoleta que consiste no registro dos movimentos do coração por meio do roentgencimógrafo.

roent·gen·o·gram (rent′gen - ō - gram). Roentgenograma. SIN radiograph.

roent·gen·o·graph (rent′gen - ō - graf). Roentgenógrafo. SIN radiograph.

roent·gen·og·ra·phy (rent′ge - nog′rȧ - fē). Radiografia. SIN radiography.

roent·gen·ol·o·gist (rent′gen - ol′ō - jist). Radiologista; pessoa habilitada na aplicação diagnóstica ou terapêutica dos raios de Roentgen.

roent·gen·ol·o·gy (rent′gen - ol′ō - jē). O estudo dos raios de Roentgen em todas as suas aplicações. Radiologia (radiology) é o termo preferido no contexto da imagenologia médica.

roent·gen·om·e·ter (rent′ge - nom′ē - ter). Roentgenômetro. SIN radiometer.

roent·gen·om·e·try (rent - ge - nom′ē - trē). Roentgenometria; a medição de uma dose diagnóstica ou terapêutica administrada e do poder de penetração dos raios X. SIN x-ray dosimetry.

roent·gen·o·scope (rent′gen - ō - scōp). Roentgenoscópio; termo obsoleto para fluoroscópio.

roent·gen·os·co·py (rent - gen - os′kō - pē). Roentgenoscopia; termo obsoleto para fluoroscopia.

roent·gen·o·ther·a·py (rent′gen - ō - thar′ȧ - pē). Roentgenoterapia; termo obsoleto para radioterapia.

roeth·eln. VER röteln.

Roger, Georges Henri, fisiologista francês, 1860–1946. VER R. *reflex*.

Roger, Henri L., médico francês, 1809–1891. VER R. *disease*, *murmur*; *bruit* de R.; *maladie* de R.

Rogers, Oscar H., médico norte-americano, 1857–1941. VER R. *sphygmomanometer*.

Rohr, Karl, embriologista e ginecologista suíço, *1863. VER R. *stria*.

Röhrer in·dex. Índice de Röhrer. VER em index.

Rokitansky, Karl Freiherr von, patologista austríaco, 1804–1878. VER R. *disease*, *hernia*; R.-Aschoff *sinuses*, em *sinus*; Mayer-R.-Küster-Hauser *syndrome*.

ro·lan·dic (rō - lan′dik). Rolândico; relativo a ou descrito por Luigi Rolando.

Rolando, Luigi, anatomista italiano, 1773–1831. VER R. *angle*, *area*, *cells*, em *cell*, *column*; rolandic *epilepsy*; R. gelatinous *substance*, *tubercle*; *fissure* of R.

role (rōl). Papel; o padrão de comportamento que um indivíduo exibe em relação às pessoas importantes de sua vida; possui suas raízes na infância e é influenciado por pessoas significativas com as quais tal indivíduo tem ou teve um relacionamento primário. [Fr.]

complementary r., p. complementar; um p. no qual o padrão de comportamento se ajusta às expectativas e exigências das outras pessoas.

gender r., p. do gênero sexual; a apresentação pública da identidade sexual; mais especificamente, tudo aquilo que um indivíduo diz e faz que sinaliza aos outros ou a si mesmo que ele é um homem ou uma mulher (ou um ser andrógino). VER sex r., gender *identity*.

noncomplementary r., p. não-complementar; p. que não se ajusta às expectativas e exigências das outras pessoas.

sex r., p. sexual; de um modo específico, o padrão de comportamento e de pensamento relacionados aos órgãos sexuais e à procriação; de uma maneira mais geral, o comportamento e o pensamento que são estereotipicamente classificados como pertencentes a um sexo ou ao outro. VER gender r.

sick r., p. de doente; em sociologia médica, o p. ou padrão de comportamento, aceito culturalmente ou pela família, que é permitido que um indivíduo exiba durante uma doença ou uma condição de invalidez, e que inclui a ausência sancionada da escola ou do trabalho e um relacionamento submisso e dependente em relação à família, à equipe de assistência médica e a outras pessoas importantes para ele.

role-play·ing. Dramatização; um método psicoterapêutico utilizado no psicodrama para entender e tratar conflitos emocionais por meio da encenação ou reencenação de acontecimentos interpessoais estressantes. VER psychodrama.

ro·li·tet·ra·cy·cline (rō′li - tet - rȧ - sī′klēn). Rolitetraciclina; um derivado da tetraciclina que é mais solúvel e menos irritante; apresenta usos e eficácia similares aos da tetraciclina e pode ser administrado por via intravenosa ou intramuscular, o que o torna mais útil quando a administração oral de uma tetraciclina é impossível ou impraticável.

roll (rōl). Rolo, cilindro. **1.** Uma massa ou estrutura com a forma de um rolo. **2.** O processo por meio do qual um elemento redondo é movido por um gradiente de pressão, como, p. ex., um leucócito movendo-se ao longo da parede de um vaso sangüíneo.

iliac r., rolo ilíaco; massa em forma de salsicha, freqüentemente dolorosa e não-flutuante, com convexidade para a direita e palpável na fossa ilíaca esquerda, que resulta do enrijecimento das paredes da flexura sigmóide.

scleral r., esporão da esclera. SIN scleral *spur*.

Roller, Christian F.W., neurologista e psiquiatra alemão, 1802–1878. VER R. *nucleus*.

roll·er (rō′ler). Atadura. VER roller *bandage*.

Rolleston, Sir Humphry D., médico britânico, 1862–1944. VER R. *rule*.

Rollet, Alexander, fisiologista austríaco, 1834–1903. VER R. *stroma*; Ritter-R. *phenomenon*.

Romaña, Cecilio, médico argentino que viveu no Brasil, *1899. VER R. *sign*.

Romano, C., médico italiano do século 20. VER Romano-Ward *syndrome*.

Romanowsky, Dimitri L., médico russo, 1861–1921. VER R. blood *stain*.

Romberg, Moritz H., médico alemão, 1795–1873. VER R. *test*, *disease*; facial *hemiatrophy* of R.; R. *syndrome*, *sign*.

rom·berg·ism (rom′berg - izm). Sinal de Romberg. SIN Romberg *sign*.

Römer, Paul H., bacteriologista alemão, 1876–1916. VER R. *test*.

ron·geur (rawn - zhēr′). Pinça saca-bocado; pinça cortante robusta utilizada para retirar um pedaço de osso de um osso. [Fr. *ronger*, roer]

Rønne, Henning K.T., oftalmologista dinamarquês, 1878–1947. VER R. nasal *step*.

roof (roof) Teto; uma cobertura ou estrutura semelhante a um teto; p. ex., um tentório (tectorium), teto (tectum), tegme (tegmen), tegmento (tegmentum), tegumento (integument). [A.S. *hrōf*]

r. of fourth ventricle [TA], t. do quarto ventrículo. SIN *tegmen* ventriculi quarti.

r. of mouth, palato. SIN palate.

r. of orbit [TA], parede superior da órbita; é formado pela face orbital do osso frontal e pela asa menor do osso esfenóide; o canal óptico abre-se em seu limite posterior; uma reentrância — a fossa da glândula lacrimal — está localizada na parte ântero-lateral do teto. SIN paries superior orbitae [TA], superior wall of orbit.

r. of skull, calvária. SIN calvaria.

r. of tympanic cavity, parede tegmental da cavidade timpânica. SIN tegmental wall of tympanic cavity.

r. of tympanum, tegme timpânico. SIN *tegmen* tympani.

roof·plate (roof′plāt). Lâmina do teto. VER roof *plate*.

room·ing-in (room′ing - in). Alojamento conjunto; a colocação do recém-nascido junto à mãe, em vez de no berçário, durante a permanência hospitalar após o parto.

root (rōōt) [TA]. Raiz. **1.** A parte primária ou inicial de qualquer estrutura, como a de um nervo em sua origem no tronco encefálico ou na medula espinal. SIN radix (1) [TA]. **2.** SIN r. of tooth. **3.** A parte descendente e subterrânea de uma planta, que realiza a absorção de água e substâncias nutritivas, fornece apoio e armazena nutrientes. Para consultar as raízes de importância farmacológica que não estão listadas a seguir, ver os nomes específicos. [A.S. rot]

accessory r. of tooth [TA], r. acessória do dente; raiz dentária adicional anômala. SIN radix accessoria [TA].

anatomical r., r. anatômica; a parte de um dente que se estende da linha cervical até sua extremidade apical.

anterior r. of spinal nerve [TA], r. anterior do nervo espinal; a raiz motora de um nervo espinal. SIN radix anterior nervi spinalis [TA], motor r. of spinal nerve*, radix motoria nervi spinalis*, ventral r. of spinal nerve*, radix ventralis nervi spinalis.

buccal r. of tooth [TA], r. bucal do dente; a raiz de um dente multirradicular que está voltada para a face bucal da crista alveolar. SIN radix buccalis [TA].

clinical r. of tooth [TA], r. clínica do dente; a parte de um dente que está embutida nas estruturas de revestimento; a parte de um dente que não é visível na cavidade oral. SIN radix clinica dentis [TA].

cochlear r. of VIII nerve, r. coclear do VIII nervo; um dos componentes do nervo vestibulococlear; é formado pelos processos centrais dos neurônios bipolares que compõem o gânglio espiral (da cóclea) situado no canal espiral do modíolo, da cóclea óssea; a r. coclear penetra na cavidade craniana em fascículos, passando através do trato espiral foraminoso situado no fundo do meato acústico interno; penetra no tronco encefálico através do sulco bulbopontino, aderindo intimamente à face caudoventral da r. vestibular, e distribui suas fibras para os núcleos cocleares ventral e dorsal situados no assoalho do recesso lateral do quarto ventrículo. SIN radix inferior nervi vestibulocochlearis.

cranial r. of accessory nerve [TA], r. craniana do nervo acessório; as raízes do nervo acessório que emergem do bulbo; as fibras nervosas da r. craniana juntam-se à parte intracraniana do nervo vago e são distribuídas para o plexo faríngeo, fornecendo a inervação motora do palato mole (exceto do músculo tensor do véu palatino) e da faringe. VER TAMBÉM accessory *nerve* [CN XI]. SIN radix cranialis nervi accessorii [TA], pars vagalis nervi accessorii*, vagal part of accessory nerve*, accessory portion of spinal accessory nerve.

Culver r., r. de Culver. SIN leptandra.

dorsal r. of spinal nerve, r. posterior do nervo espinal; *termo oficial alternativo de posterior r. of spinal nerve.

facial r., nervo do canal pterigóideo. SIN nerve of pterygoid canal.

r. of facial nerve, r. do nervo facial; as fibras que correm do núcleo motor facial para cima até o colículo facial, onde se curvam ao redor do núcleo abducente e, em seguida, passam perifericamente entre o núcleo olivar superior e o núcleo sensitivo do trigêmeo, para emergir como nervo facial no sulco bulbopontino. SIN radix nervi facialis.

r. of foot, tarso. SIN tarsus (1).

hair r., r. do pêlo; a parte de um pêlo que está incrustada no folículo piloso; a extremidade carnosa inferior do folículo piloso envolve as papilas dérmicas na parte bulbosa profunda do folículo. SIN radix pili.

inferior r. of ansa cervicalis [TA], r. inferior da alça cervical; as fibras do segundo e terceiro nervos cervicais que passam adiante e para baixo ao longo da veia jugular interna; contribuem para formar a alça cervical e inervam os músculos infra-hióideos. SIN radix inferior ansae cervicalis [TA], inferior limb of ansa cervicalis*, descendens cervicalis.

lateral r. of median nerve [TA], r. lateral do nervo mediano; a parte do nervo mediano que surge do cordão lateral do plexo braquial. SIN radix lateralis nervi mediani [TA].

lateral r. of optic tract [TA], r. lateral do trato óptico; a divisão maior da extremidade posterior do trato óptico que termina no corpo geniculado lateral. SIN radix lateralis tractus optici [TA].

long r. of ciliary ganglion, r. sensitiva do gânglio ciliar. SIN sensory r. of ciliary ganglion.

r. of lung [TA], r. do pulmão; todas as estruturas que penetram no pulmão ou que saem dele através do hilo, formando um pedículo revestido pela pleura; engloba os brônquios, a artéria e as veias pulmonares, as artérias e veias, linfáticos e nervos brônquicos. SIN radix pulmonis [TA].

May apple r., podofilo (resina). SIN podophyllum resin.

medial r. of median nerve [TA], r. medial do nervo mediano; a parte do nervo mediano que se origina no cordão medial do plexo braquial. SIN radix medialis nervi mediani [TA].

medial r. of optic tract [TA], r. medial do trato óptico; a divisão menor da extremidade posterior do trato óptico que desaparece sob o corpo geniculado medial. SIN radix medialis tractus optici [TA].

r. of mesentery [TA], r. do mesentério; a origem do mesentério do intestino delgado (jejuno e íleo) proveniente do peritônio parietal posterior; com cerca de 23 cm de comprimento, estende-se da flexura duodenojejunal (à esquerda da linha média no nível da vértebra L2) até a junção ileocecal (fossa ilíaca). SIN radix mesenterii [TA].

motor r. of ciliary ganglion, r. parassimpática do gânglio ciliar. SIN parasympathetic r. of ciliary ganglion.

motor r. of spinal nerve, r. anterior do nervo espinal; *termo oficial alternativo de anterior r. of spinal nerve.

motor r. of trigeminal nerve [TA], r. motora do nervo trigêmeo; a raiz menor do nervo trigêmeo, composta de fibras que se originam no núcleo motor do nervo trigêmeo e emergem da ponte, medialmente à raiz sensitiva (a raiz maior), para se juntar ao nervo mandibular; transporta fibras motoras e proprioceptivas até os músculos derivados do primeiro arco branquial (mandibular), incluindo os quatro músculos da mastigação e o músculo milo-hióideo, a barriga anterior do músculo digástrico e os músculos tensores do tímpano e do véu palatino. SIN radix motoria nervi trigemini [TA], masticator nerve, portio minor nervi trigemini.

r. of nail, r. da unha; a extremidade proximal da unha, oculta sob uma prega de pele. SIN radix unguis.

nasociliary r. of ciliary ganglion, r. sensitiva do gânglio ciliar; *termo oficial alternativo de sensory r. of ciliary ganglion.

nerve r., r. nervosa; um dos dois feixes de fibras nervosas (raízes anterior e posterior) que emergem da medula espinal e se juntam para formar um único nervo espinal segmentar (misto); alguns dos nervos cranianos são formados de modo semelhante pela união de duas raízes, em particular o nervo trigêmeo (ou quinto nervo craniano).

r. of nose [TA], r. do nariz; a parte superior menos protrusa do nariz externo, situada entre as duas órbitas. SIN radix nasi [TA].

oculomotor r. of ciliary ganglion, r. parassimpática do gânglio ciliar; *termo oficial alternativo de parasympathetic r. of ciliary ganglion.

olfactory r.'s, estrias olfatórias. SIN olfactory striae, em stria.

r.'s of olfactory tract, lateral and medial, raízes medial e lateral do trato olfatório; as duas faixas de fibras que formam a continuação caudal do trato olfatório e que, após divergirem, circundam o tubérculo olfatório.

parasympathetic r. of ciliary ganglion [TA], r. parassimpática do gânglio ciliar; um ramo do nervo oculomotor que envia fibras nervosas parassimpáticas pré-ganglionares para o gânglio ciliar. SIN radix parasympathica ganglii ciliaris [TA], oculomotor r. of ciliary ganglion*, radix nervi oculomotorii ad ganglion ciliare*, radix oculomotoria ganglii ciliaris*, branch of oculomotor nerve to ciliary ganglion, motor r. of ciliary ganglion, radix brevis ganglii ciliaris, short r. of ciliary ganglion.

parasympathetic r. of otic ganglion, nervo petroso menor; *termo oficial alternativo de lesser petrosal nerve.

parasympathetic r. of pelvic ganglia, nervos esplâncnicos pélvicos; *termo oficial alternativo de pelvic splanchnic nerves, em nerve.

parasympathetic r. of pterygopalatine ganglion, nervo petroso maior; *termo oficial alternativo de greater petrosal nerve.

parasympathetic r. of submandibular ganglion, corda do tímpano. SIN chorda tympani.

r. of penis [TA], r. do pênis; a parte fixa e proximal do pênis, que engloba os dois ramos e o bulbo. SIN radix penis [TA].

posterior r. of spinal nerve [TA], r. posterior do nervo espinal; a raiz sensitiva de um nervo espinal; possui o gânglio da r. dorsal, que contém os corpos dos neurônios cujas fibras são conduzidas pela extremidade distal da raiz. SIN radix posterior nervi spinalis [TA], dorsal r. of spinal nerve*, radix sensoria nervi spinalis*, sensory r. of spinal nerve*, radix dorsalis nervi spinalis.

sensory r. of ciliary ganglion [TA], r. sensitiva do gânglio ciliar; as fibras sensitivas que passam do globo ocular através do gânglio ciliar até seus corpos celulares, situados no gânglio trigeminal, via nervo nasociliar. SIN radix sensoria ganglii ciliaris [TA], nasociliary r. of ciliary ganglion*, radix nasociliaris ganglii ciliaris*, ramus communicans nervi nasociliaris cum ganglio ciliari*, communicating branch of nasociliary nerve with ciliary ganglion, long r. of ciliary ganglion, radix longa ganglii ciliaris.

sensory r. of pterygopalatine ganglion [TA], r. sensitiva do gânglio pterigopalatino; os ramos ganglionares, ou seja, os dois ramos sensitivos curtos do nervo maxilar situado na fossa pterigopalatina, cujas fibras passam pelo gânglio pterigopalatino sem fazer sinapse. SIN radix sensoria ganglii pterygopalatini [TA], ganglionic branches of maxillary nerve to pterygopalatine ganglion*, rami ganglionici nervi maxillaris*, ganglionic branches of maxillary nerve, nervi pterygopalatini, nervi sphenopalatini, pterygopalatine nerves, rami ganglionares.

sensory r. of spinal nerve, r. posterior do nervo espinal; *termo oficial alternativo de posterior r. of spinal nerve.

sensory r. of sublingual ganglion [TA], r. sensitiva do gânglio sublingual; o ramo ou os ramos do nervo lingual que conduzem fibras sensitivas para o gânglio sublingual, as quais passam através desse gânglio sem fazer sinapse e se distribuem pelo assoalho da boca. SIN radix sensoria ganglii sublingualis [TA], ganglionic branches of lingual nerve to sublingual ganglion*, ganglionic branches of lingual nerve to submandibular ganglion*, rami communicantes ganglii sublingualis cum nervo linguali*.

sensory r. of submandibular ganglion [TA], r. sensitiva do gânglio submandibular; as raízes motoras do gânglio submandibular; as raízes comunicantes entre o gânglio submandibular e o nervo lingual. SIN radix sensoria ganglii submandibularis [TA], rami communicantes ganglii submandibularis cum nervo linguali*, ganglionic branches of lingual nerve.

sensory r. of trigeminal nerve [TA], r. sensitiva do nervo trigêmeo; a raiz sensitiva (grande) do nervo trigêmeo (ou quinto nervo craniano), que se estende do gânglio semilunar até a ponte através do pedúnculo cerebelar médio ou braço da ponte e está situada em uma posição imediatamente lateral à r. motora (pequena). SIN radix sensoria nervi trigemini [TA], portio major nervi trigemini.

short r. of ciliary ganglion, r. parassimpática do gânglio ciliar. SIN parasympathetic r. of ciliary ganglion.

spinal r. of accessory nerve [TA], r. espinal do nervo acessório; origina-se nos cinco ou seis segmentos cervicais espinais superiores, emerge da superfície lateral da medula espinal e ascende através do forame magno para se juntar à raiz craniana. SIN radix spinalis nervi accessorii [TA], pars spinalis nervi accessorii*, spinal part of accessory nerve*.

superior r. of ansa cervicalis [TA], r. superior da alça cervical; as fibras que surgem do primeiro e segundo nervos cervicais, acompanham o nervo hipoglosso e, em seguida, ramificam-se para encontrar a raiz inferior na alça cervical; inervam os músculos infra-hióideos. SIN radix superior ansae cervicalis [TA], superior limb of ansa cervicalis*, descendens hypoglossi, descending branch of hypoglossal nerve.

sympathetic r. of ciliary ganglion [TA], r. simpática do gânglio ciliar; as fibras pós-ganglionares cujos corpos celulares se situam no gânglio cervical superior, que se ramificam no plexo carótico, passam pelo gânglio ciliar sem fazer sinapse e alcançam o globo ocular. SIN radix sympathica ganglii ciliaris [TA].

sympathetic r. of otic ganglion [TA], r. simpática do gânglio ótico; o ramo que surge do plexo periarterial da artéria meníngea média, conduzindo as fibras pós-sinápticas simpáticas do gânglio cervical superior simpático, as quais passam pelo gânglio sem fazer sinapse e se distribuem para os vasos sangüíneos situados dentro da glândula parótida. SIN radix sympathica ganglii otici [TA].

sympathetic r. of pterygopalatine ganglion, nervo petroso profundo; *termo oficial alternativo de deep petrosal nerve.

sympathetic r. of sublingual ganglion [TA], r. simpática do gânglio sublingual; o ramo que surge do plexo periarterial da artéria facial, conduzindo as fibras pós-sinápticas simpáticas do gânglio cervical superior simpático, as quais passam pelo gânglio sem fazer sinapse e se distribuem pelos vasos sangüíneos da glândula sublingual. SIN radix sympathica ganglii sublingualis [TA].

sympathetic r. of submandibular ganglion [TA], r. simpática do gânglio submandibular; ramo que se dirige para o gânglio submandibular e é composto de fibras pós-sinápticas simpáticas do plexo carótico interno conduzidas principalmente por um plexo periarterial da artéria facial. SIN radix sympathica ganglii submandibularis [TA], ramus sympathicus (sympatheticus) ad ganglion submandibulare, sympathetic branch to submandibular ganglion.

tegmental r. of tympanic cavity, parede tegmental da cavidade timpânica; *termo oficial alternativo de tegmental wall of tympanic cavity.

r. of tongue [TA], r. da língua; a parte fixa e posterior da língua. SIN radix linguae [TA], base of tongue.

r. of tooth [TA], r. do dente; a parte de um dente situada abaixo do colo, coberta por cemento em vez de esmalte e fixada ao osso alveolar pelo ligamento periodontal. SIN radix dentis [TA], radix (2) [TA], root (2) [TA].

r.'s of trigeminal nerve, raízes do nervo trigêmeo; termo coletivo utilizado para as raízes sensitiva e motora do nervo trigêmeo. SIN radices nervi trigemini.

tuberous r., r. tuberosa; uma r. que é tumefeita por causa do armazenamento de nutrientes; as raízes primárias tuberosas são encontradas no acônito, na beterraba e na cenoura; as raízes secundárias tuberosas, nas plantas da família Umbelliferae; e as raízes adventícias tuberosas, na jalapa e na batata doce.

ventral r. of spinal nerve, r. anterior do nervo espinal; *termo oficial alternativo de anterior r. of spinal nerve.

vestibular r., r. vestibular; a r. vestibular do VIII nervo, um termo coletivo utilizado para as fibras sensitivas do oitavo nervo craniano (n. vestibulococlear) que se originam no labirinto vestibular, apresentam seus corpos celulares no gânglio vestibular e atuam na esfera do balanço e equilíbrio; centralmente, essas fibras terminam principalmente nos núcleos vestibulares do tronco encefálico e no cerebelo. SIN radix superior nervi vestibulocochlearis, radix vestibularis, vestibular r. of vestibulocochlear nerve.

vestibular r. of vestibulocochlear nerve, r. vestibular do nervo vestibulococlear. SIN vestibular r.

root·lets (root'lets). Radículas; em neuroanatomia, as radículas nervosas (filamentos radiculares). VER filum. VER TAMBÉM radicular *fila*, em *filum*.

root plan·ing (plān'ing). Aplainamento radicular; em odontologia, a abrasão das superfícies radiculares ásperas, a fim de se obter uma superfície lisa.

ROP Abreviatura de right occipitoposterior position (posição occipitoposterior direita).

ro·pal·o·cy·to·sis (rō-pal'ō-sī-tō'sis). Ropalocitose; a formação de numerosos processos nas células eritróides que, em cortes ultrafinos, apresentam-se em forma de clava, associam-se a vesículas citoplasmáticas e são encontrados em algumas doenças do sangue. [G. *ropalon*, clava, + *kytos*, célula, + *-osis*, condição]

Ropes test. Teste de Ropes. VER em test.

Rorschach, Hermann, psiquiatra suíço, 1884–1922. VER R. *test*.

Ro·sa (rō'za). Gênero de plantas que engloba as rosas (família Rosaceae); o óleo de rosas é obtido de diversas variedades: *R. alba* ou rosa-branca; *R. centifolia* ou rosa-de-cem-folhas (fonte do óleo de rosas oficial); *R. damascena* ou rosa-damascena; e *R. gallica* ou rosa-rubra. [L. rosa]

ro·sa·cea (rō-zā'shē-a). Rosácea; dilatação folicular e vascular crônica que acomete o nariz e as partes contíguas das bochechas; pode variar de um eritema moderado, porém persistente, a uma hiperplasia extensa das glândulas sebáceas; é observada principalmente em homens na forma de rinofima e pápulas e pústulas profundas; é acompanhada por telangiectasia nos locais eritematosos afetados. SIN acne rosacea. [L. *rosaceus*, róseo]

granulomatous r., r. granulomatosa; as lesões papulares encontradas na r. e caracterizadas microscopicamente por granulomas perifoliculares com necrose central e células gigantes disseminadas. O lupus miliaris disseminado da face é provavelmente uma forma de r. granulomatosa. SIN rosacea-like tuberculid, tuberculoid r.

hypertrophic r., rinofima. SIN rhinophyma.

tuberculoid r., r. tuberculóide. SIN granulomatous r.

Rosai, Juan, patologista norte-americano, nascido em 1941. VER Rosai-Dorfman *disease*.

ros·an·i·lin (rō-zan'i-lin) [I.C. 42510]. Rosanilina; composto tri(aminofenil)metil; como a pararrosanilina, a rosanilina é um dos componentes da fucsina básica; é também utilizada como um agente antifúngico.

ro·sap·ros·tol (rō'sa-prost-ol). Rosaprostol; análogo das prostaglandinas com propriedades protetoras para a mucosa gástrica; é similar ao misoprostol e também utilizado como uma droga antiúlcera.

ro·sa·ry (rō'zer-ē). Rosário; arranjo ou estrutura semelhante a uma fileira de pequenas contas.

rachitic r., r. raquítico; uma fileira de nódulos situados na junção das costelas com suas cartilagens e observados com freqüência em crianças raquíticas. SIN beading of the ribs.

Roscoe, Sir Henry E., químico britânico, 1833–1915. VER Bunsen-R. *law*.

Rose, Edmund, médico alemão, 1836–1914. VER R. *position*.

Rose, Harry M., microbiologista norte-americano, *1906. VER R.-Waaler *test*.

rose (rōz). Rosa. 1. Qualquer arbusto do gênero *Rosa*. 2. As pétalas da *Rosa gallica*, coletadas antes de a flor desabrochar; utilizadas em razão de seu odor agradável. [L. *rosa*]

r. hips, o fruto ou as bagas dos arbustos da rosa silvestre e, em particular, da *Rosa canina*, da *R. gallica*, da *R. condita* e da *R. rugosa* (família Rosaceae). Uma fonte rica de vitamina C (ácido ascórbico). SIN hipberries.

r. oil, óleo de rosas; um óleo volátil proveniente da *Rosa centifolia*; é utilizado em perfumaria e ungüentos. SIN attar of rose.

rose ben·gal (rōz' ben'gal) [I.C. 45440]. Rosa bengala; o sal de sódio da tetraiodotetraclorfluoresceína, utilizado como corante para bactérias, como corante no diagnóstico da ceratite seca (*keratitis sicca*) e nos testes para avaliar as funções hepáticas.

Rose-Bradford kid·ney. Rim de Rose-Bradford. VER em kidney.

rose·mary oil (rōz'mār-ē). Óleo de alecrim; o óleo volátil destilado com o vapor proveniente das extremidades recém-floridas de *Rosmarinus officinalis* (família Labiatae); é utilizado como um tempero e em perfumaria.

Rosenbach, Ottomar, médico alemão, 1851–1907. VER R. *law*, *sign*, *test*; R.-Gmelin *test*.

Rosenmüller, Johann C., anatomista alemão, 1771–1820. VER R. *fossa*, *gland*, *node*, *recess*, *valve*; *organ* of R.

Rosenthal, Curt, psiquiatra alemão do século 20. VER Melkersson-R. *syndrome*.

Rosenthal, Friedrich C., anatomista alemão, 1780–1829. VER R. *canal*, *vein*; basal *vein* of R.

Rosenthaler-Turk re·a·gent. Reagente de Rosenthaler-Turk. Ver em reagent.

Rosenthal fi·ber. Fibra de Rosenthal. Ver em fiber.

ro·se·o·la (rō-zē'ō'la). Roséola; erupção simétrica de pequenas manchas intimamente agregadas de cor rosa-avermelhada. Acredita-se que seja causada pelo herpesvírus humano do tipo 6. VER TAMBÉM exanthema subitum. SIN macular erythema. [L. mod. dim. de L. *roseus*, róseo]

epidemic r., rubéola. SIN rubella.

idiopathic r., r. idiopática; a r. que não ocorre como um sintoma de uma doença conhecida.

r. infan'tilis, r. infan'tum, exantema súbito. SIN exanthema subitum.

syphilitic r., r. sifilítica; é geralmente a primeira erupção da sífilis, que ocorre 6 a 12 semanas após a lesão inicial.

Roser, Wilhelm, cirurgião alemão, 1817–1888. VER R.-Nélaton *line*.

ro·sette (rō-zet'). Roseta. 1. O parasita da malária quartã, *Plasmodium malariae*, em sua fase segmentada ou madura. 2. Um agrupamento de células característico das neoplasias de origem neuroblástica, neuroectodérmica ou ependimária; vários núcleos formam um anel a partir do qual neurofibrilas — que podem ser demonstradas por meio de impregnação pela prata — estendem-se para se entrelaçar no centro (roseta de Homer-Wright). 3. O espiralamento em forma de rosa do útero de certas tênias pseudofilídeas, tais como o *Diphyllobothrium latum*. 4. Células de um determinado tipo circundando uma célula de outro tipo. [Fr. uma pequena rosa]

E r. (ro-zet'), r. E; a aderência dos eritrócitos às células. Os eritrócitos de carneiros aderem espontaneamente às células T humanas, formando rosetas.

EAC r., r. EAC; indica a existência de receptores de complemento. Os eritrócitos (E) revestidos com anticorpos (A) e complemento (C) são incubados com células-teste; se as células-teste possuírem receptores de complemento, o complexo EAC aderirá a essas células, formando rosetas.

Homer-Wright r.'s, rosetas de Homer-Wright; as pseudo-rosetas formadas pelo arranjo das células tumorais ao redor de um emaranhado de fibras nervosas imaturas; uma evidência de diferenciação neuroblástica em um meduloblastoma ou tumor neuroectodérmico primitivo.

Wintersteiner r.'s, rosetas de Wintersteiner; as rosetas encontradas apenas em tumores retinianos embrionários e formadas por um grupo de células colunares com uma membrana basal periférica dispostas de maneira radiada ao redor de uma cavidade central, com os raios correspondendo aos fotorreceptores.

ros·in (roz'in). Colofônia; a resina sólida obtida após a destilação a vapor do bálsamo bruto extraído do *Pinus palustris* e de outras espécies de *Pinus* (família Pinaceae); é utilizada em emplastros para torná-los adesivos e também em ungüentos para torná-los localmente estimulantes. SIN colophony, resin (2).

p-**ro·so·lic ac·id** (rō-sol'ik). Ácido p-rosólico. SIN aurin.

Ross, Donald N., cirurgião cardíaco britânico, *1922; introduziu a substituição da valva aórtica por meio da utilização de um auto-enxerto de valva pulmonar. VER R. *procedure*.

Ross, Sir George W., médico canadense, 1841–1931. VER R.-Jones *test*.

Ross, Sir Ronald, médico inglês laureado com um Nobel, 1857–1932. VER R. *cycle*.

Rossolimo, Grigoriy I., neurologista russo, 1860–1928. VER R. *reflex*, *sign*.

ros·tel·lum (ros-tel'ŭm). Rostelo; a parte anterior, fixa e invertível do escólex de uma tênia, freqüentemente provida de uma fileira (ou de várias fileiras) de ganchos. [L. dim. de *rostrum*, um bico]

armed r., r. armado; um r. com uma ou mais fileiras de ganchos.

unarmed r., r. desarmado; um r., desprovido de ganchos.

ros·trad (ros'trad). 1. Que está direcionado para o rostro. 2. Situado muito perto de um rostro ou da extremidade da tromba de um organismo em relação a um ponto de referência específico; o oposto de caudad (2). [L. *rostrum*, bico, + *-ad*, para a frente]

ros·tral (ros'tral) [TA]. Rostral. 1. Relativo a qualquer rostro ou estrutura anatômica que se assemelha a um bico. 2. Na extremidade da cabeça. SIN rostralis [TA]. [L. *rostralis*, de *rostrum*, bico]

ros·tra·lis (ros'trā'lis) [TA]. Rostral. SIN rostral. [L. de *rostrum*, bico]

ros·trate (ros'trāt). Rostrado; que possui um bico ou um gancho. [L. *rostratus*]

ros·tri·form (ros'tri-fōrm). Rostriforme; em forma de bico. [L. *rostrum*, bico]

ros·trum, pl. **ros·tra, ros·trums** (ros'trŭm, -tra) [TA]. Rostro; qualquer estrutura em forma de bico. [L. um bico]

r. cor'poris callo'si [TA], r. do corpo caloso. SIN r. of corpus callosum.

r. of corpus callosum [TA], r. do corpo caloso; a ponta do corpo caloso, a parte recurvada do corpo caloso que segue para trás a partir do joelho até a comissura anterior. SIN r. corporis callosi [TA].

sphenoidal r. [TA], r. esfenoidal; a parte saliente e anterior do corpo do osso esfenóide que se articula com o vômer. SIN r. sphenoidale [TA], r. of the sphenoid bone.

r. sphenoida'le [TA], r. esfenoidal. SIN sphenoidal r.

r. of the sphenoid bone, r. esfenoidal. SIN sphenoidal r.

ROT Abreviatura de right occipitotransverse position (posição occipitotransversa direita).

rot. Apodrecer, decompor, estragar; cariar; deteriorar ou putrefazer. [A.S. *rotian*]

ro·ta·mase (rō′ta-māz). Rotamase; enzima capaz de alterar a conformação rotacional de uma molécula.

ro·ta·mer (rō′ta-mer). Rotâmero; isômero que difere de outra(s) conformação(ões) apenas no posicionamento rotacional de suas partes, tais como as formas cis- e trans-.

ro·tam·e·ter (rō-tam′e-ter). Rotâmetro; um dispositivo utilizado para medir o fluxo de gás ou líquido; o fluido que flui para cima através de um tubo levemente estreitado eleva uma bola ou outro peso que obstrui parcialmente o fluxo, até que o corte transversal mais largo permita que o fluxo passe ao redor da obstrução flutuante. [L. *rota*, roda, + G. *metron*, medida]

ro·ta·tion (rō-tā′shŭn). Rotação; rodízio. **1.** O giro ou movimento de um corpo ao redor de seu eixo. **2.** Uma recorrência em ordem regular de certos eventos, tais como os sintomas de uma doença periódica. **3.** Em educação médica, um período de tempo em um serviço ou especialidade específicos. [L. *rotatio*, de *roto*, pp. *rotatus*, revolver, rodar]

intestinal r., rotação intestinal; a r. da alça intestinal primitiva ao redor de um eixo formado pela artéria mesentérica superior. VER malrotation.

molecular r., rotação molecular; um centésimo do produto entre a r. específica de um composto opticamente ativo e seu peso molecular.

off-vertical r., a r. em volta de um eixo excêntrico ao corpo.

optic r., rotação óptica; a mudança no plano de polarização quando a luz polarizada de um dado comprimento de onda passa através de substâncias opticamente ativas; medida em função da rotação específica por polarimetria, trata-se de uma importante ferramenta no estudo da estrutura química, principalmente dos carboidratos.

specific optic r. ([α]), rotação óptica específica; o arco através do qual o plano da luz polarizada é rodado por 1 g de uma substância por mililitro de água, quando o comprimento do caminho luminoso através da solução é de 1 decímetro e a luz normalmente utilizada corresponde à linha D do sódio.

ro·ta·tor (rō-tā′ter, -tōr). Rotador. SIN rotator *muscle*. VER rotatores (*muscles*), em *muscle*. [L. Ver rotation]

medial r., r. medial; um músculo que gira medialmente uma estrutura. VER TAMBÉM invertor. SIN intortor.

ro·ta·vi·rus (rō′ta-vī′rŭs). Rotavírus; um grupo de vírus de RNA (família Reoviridae) que se assemelham a uma roda e formam um gênero — o Rotavirus — que engloba os vírus da gastroenterite humana (uma causa importante de diarréia infantil em todo o mundo). Separados em grupos de A até F, os rotavírus podem infectar diversos vertebrados. São vírus exigentes, e sua cultura *in vitro* é difícil. SIN duovirus, gastroenteritis virus type B, infantile gastroenteritis virus, reovirus-like agent. [L. *rota*, roda, + virus]

Rotch, Thomas M., médico norte-americano, 1849–1914. VER R. *sign*.

röt·eln, roeth·eln (ruht′eln). Rubéola. SIN rubella. [Al. pequenas manchas vermelhas, de *rot*, vermelho, + *-el*, sufixo diminutivo.]

ro·te·none (rō′te-nōn). Rotenona; o principal componente inseticida da raiz do timbó, *Derris elliptica*, da *D. malaccensis* e outras espécies de *D.*, e da *Lonchocarpus nicou* (família Leguminosae); é utilizado externamente no tratamento da escabiose e da infestação por bichos-de-pé e, em medicina veterinária, no tratamento da sarna folicular e da infestação por piolhos, pulgas e carrapatos; um inibidor da cadeia respiratória.

Roth. VER Benedict-Roth *apparatus*.

Roth, Moritz, patologista e médico suíço, 1839–1914. VER R. *spots*, em *spot*; *vas* aberrans of R.

Roth, Vladimir K., neurologista russo, 1848–1916. VER Bernhardt-R. *syndrome*.

Rothera, Arthur C.H., bioquímico inglês, 1880–1915. VER Rothera nitroprusside *test*.

Roth·ia (roth′ē-ā). Um gênero de bactérias que variam de aeróbicas a anaeróbicas facultativas, imóveis, não-formadoras de esporos e não-álcool-ácido-resistentes (família Actinomycetaceae); contêm células Gram-positivas, cocóides, difteróides e filamentosas; o metabolismo é fermentativo, e a fermentação da glicose produz principalmente ácido lático, mas não ácido propiônico. Esses microrganismos são habitantes normais da cavidade oral humana e são patógenos oportunistas. A espécie-tipo é *R. dentocariosa*. [G. D. *Roth*]

R. dentocariosa, uma causa rara de endocardite infecciosa em humanos.

Rothmund, August von, médico alemão, 1830–1906. VER R. *syndrome*; R.-Thomson *syndrome*.

Rotor, Arturo B., médico internista filipino do século 20. VER R. *syndrome*.

ro·to·sco·li·o·sis (rō′tō-skō-lē-ō′sis). Rotoescoliose; desvios rotacional e lateral combinados da coluna vertebral. [L. *roto*, girar, + G. *skoliōsis*, deformidade]

ro·to·tome (rō′tō-tōm). Instrumento cortante rotatório utilizado em cirurgia artroscópica.

ro·tox·a·mine (rō-tok′sā-mēn). Rotoxamina; o isômero ativo da carbinoxamina; anti-histamínico.

Rouget, Antoine D., fisiologista francês do século 19. VER R. *bulb*.

Rouget, Charles M.B., fisiologista francês, 1824–1904. VER R. *muscle*; R.-Neumann *sheath*.

rough (rŭf). Rugoso; que não é liso; indica a superfície irregular e grosseiramente granular de um certo tipo de colônia de bactérias.

rough·age (rŭf′ij). Substâncias não-digeríveis que auxiliam a digestão; qualquer elemento da dieta, p. ex., o farelo de cereais, que serve como volume estimulante da peristalse intestinal.

Roughton, Francis J.W., cientista britânico, 1899–1972. VER R.-Scholander *apparatus*, *syringe*.

Rougnon de Magny, Nicholas F., médico francês, 1727–1799. VER Rougnon-Heberden *disease*.

rou·leau, pl. **rou·leaux** (roo-lō′). Empilhamento; agregado de eritrócitos dispostos como uma pilha de moedas. A formação de "rouleau" geralmente indica uma elevação das imunoglobulinas plasmáticas. [De carretel, cilindro, de *rouler*, rolar, do L.L. *rotulo*, de *rota*, roda]

round·worm (rownd′werm). Nematelminto; um nematódeo — membro do filo Nematoda —, geralmente limitado às formas parasíticas.

Rous, F. Peyton, patologista norte-americano laureado com o prêmio Nobel, 1879–1970. VER R. *sarcoma*, sarcoma *virus*, *tumor*; R.-associated *virus*.

Roussy, Gustave, patologista francês, 1874–1948. VER R.-Lévy *disease*, *syndrome*; Dejerine-R. *syndrome*.

Rouviere, Henri, anatomista e embriologista francês, *1875. Ver *node* of R.

Roux, César, cirurgião suíço, 1857–1934. VER R.-en-Y *anastomosis*, *operation*.

Roux, Philibert J., cirurgião francês, 1780–1854. VER R. *method*.

Roux, Pierre P.E., bacteriologista francês, 1853–1933. VER Ro *spatula*; R. *stain*.

Rovsing, Niels T., cirurgião dinamarquês, 1862–1927. VER R. *sign*.

RPF Abreviatura de renal plasma flow (fluxo plasmático renal). VER effective renal plasma *flow*.

R.Ph. Abreviatura de Registered Pharmacist.

rpm Abreviatura de revolutions per minute (revoluções ou rotações por minuto).

RPO 1. Abreviatura de right posterior oblique (oblíqua posterior direita), uma incidência radiográfica. **2.** Abreviatura de radiation protection officer.

R.Q. Abreviatura de respiratory *quotient* (quociente respiratório).

-rrhagia. -rragia; secreção excessiva ou incomum; hemorragia. [G. *rhēgnymi*, romper para fora]

-rrhaphy. -rrafia; uma sutura cirúrgica. [G. *rhaphē*, sutura]

-rrhea. -rréia; secreção; um fluxo. [G. *rhoia*, um fluxo]

-rrhoea. VER -rrhea.

rRNA Abreviatura de ribosomal ribonucleic acid (ácido ribonucléico ribossomial).

RSA Abreviatura de right sacroanterior position (posição sacroanterior direita).

RSD Abreviatura de reflex sympathetic *dystrophy* (distrofia simpática reflexa).

RSP Abreviatura de right sacroposterior position (posição sacroposterior direita).

RST Abreviatura de right sacrotransverse position (posição sacrotransversa direita).

RSV Abreviatura de Rous sarcoma *virus* (vírus do sarcoma de Rous); respiratory syncytial *virus* (vírus sincicial respiratório).

RT, rt Abreviatura de room *temperature* (temperatura ambiente).

RT₃ Símbolo de reverse triiodothyronine (triiodotironina).

rTMP Abreviatura de ribothymidylic acid (ácido ribotimidílico).

RT-PCR Abreviatura de reverse transcriptase polymerase chain *reaction* (reação da cadeia da polimerase da transcriptase reversa).

RU-486 Mifepristona. SIN mifepristone.

Ru Símbolo de ruthenium (rutênio).

rub (rŭb). Atrito; a fricção observada ao se mover um corpo que está em contato com outro corpo.

friction r., atrito. SIN friction *sound*.

pericardial r., pericardial friction r., a. pericárdico. SIN pericardial friction *sound*.

pleural r., a. pleural; o ruído de atrito provocado pela inflamação da pleura. SIN pleural friction r., pleural rale.

pleural friction r., atrito pleural. SIN pleural r.

pleuritic r., a. pleurítico; um ruído de fricção produzido pelo contato das superfícies ásperas das pleuras parietal e visceral.

Rubarth, Sven, veterinário sueco, *1905. VER R. disease *virus*.

rub·ber (rŭb'er). Borracha; o suco leitoso, espesso e beneficiado de *Hevea brasiliensis* e de outras espécies de *Hevea* (família Euphorbiaceae), conhecido no comércio como borracha tipo Pará pura; é utilizado na fabricação de diversos emplastros, tecidos, bandagens etc.

rub·ber po·lice·man. VER policeman.

ru·be·an·ic ac·id (roo'bē-an-ik). Ácido rubeânico; a ditiooxamida, que forma complexos completos de cor verde escura a preta com o cobre em solução etanólica alcalina; é utilizada em histoquímica na demonstração de depósitos patológicos de cobre, como observado na doença de Wilson; também reage com o cobalto e o níquel.

ru·be·do (roo-bē'dō). Vermelhidão temporária da pele. [L. vermelhidão, de *ruber*, vermelho]

ru·be·fa·cient (roo-bē-fā'shent). 1. Rubefaciente; que causa a rubefação da pele. 2. Contra-irritante que produz eritema quando aplicado à superfície da pele. [L. *rubi-facio*, de *ruber*, vermelho, + *facio*, fazer]

ru·be·fac·tion (roo-bē-fak'shŭn). Rubefação; o eritema da pele causado pela aplicação local de um contra-irritante. [ver rubefacient]

ru·bel·la (roo-bel'ă). Rubéola, doença exantematosa aguda, porém branda, causada pelo vírus da rubéola (um rubivírus da família Togaviridae) e caracterizada por aumento dos nódulos linfáticos e geralmente pouca febre ou reação constitucional; a alta incidência de defeitos congênitos em crianças resulta de infecção materna durante o primeiro trimestre da vida fetal (síndrome da rubéola congênita). SIN epidemic roseola, German measles, röteln, roetheln, third disease, three-day measles. [L. *rubellus*, fem. *-a*, avermelhado, dim. de *ruber*, vermelho]

ru·bel·lin (roo-bel'in). Rubelina; glicosídeo cardíaco com ação semelhante à dos digitálicos e obtido da *Urginia rubella* (família Liliaceae).

ru·be·o·la (roo-bē'ō-lă, -bē-ō'lă). Sarampo; o mesmo que *measles* (sarampo); o termo *rubeola* (sarampo) não deve ser confundido com *rubella* (rubéola). [L. mod. dim. de *ruber*, vermelho, avermelhado]

ru·be·o·sis (roo-bē-ō'sis). Rubeose; coloração avermelhada, como a da pele. [L. *ruber*, vermelho, + G. *-osis*, condição]

r. i'ridis diabet'ica, r. da íris observada no diabetes; a neovascularização da superfície anterior da íris que ocorre no diabetes mellitus.

ru·bes·cent (roo-bes'ent). Rubescente; que enrubesce. [L. *rubesco*, part. pres. *rubescens*, tornar vermelho]

ru·bid·i·um (Rb) (roo-bid'ē-ŭm). Rubídio; um elemento alcalino com n.° atômico 37 e peso atômico 85,4678; seus sais foram utilizados em medicina para os mesmos propósitos que os sais de sódio e potássio correspondentes. [L. *rubidus*, avermelhado, vermelho escuro, de *rubeo*, ser vermelho]

ru·bid·o·my·cin (dau·no·ru·bi·cin) (roo-bid'ō-mī-sin). Rubidomicina (daunorrubicina); antibiótico utilizado como antineoplásico, particularmente nas leucemias agudas; apresenta atividade antitumoral e cardiotoxicidade cumulativa semelhantes às da doxorrubicina.

Rubin, Isidor C., ginecologista norte-americano, 1883–1958. VER R. *test*.

ru·bin S, ru·bine (roo'bin, bēn) [I.C. 42685]. Rubina S, rubina. SIN acid fuchsin.

Rubinstein, Jack H., pediatra e psiquiatra infantil norte-americano, *1925. VER R.-Taybi *syndrome*.

Ru·bi·vi·rus (roo'bi-vī'rŭs). Gênero de vírus (família Togaviridae) que engloba os vírus da rubéola. [*rubella* + virus]

Rubner, Max, bioquímico e higienista alemão, 1854–1932. VER R. *laws* of growth, em *law, test*.

ru·bor (roo'bōr). Rubor; vermelhidão, um dos quatro sinais da inflamação (rubor, calor, tumor e dor) enunciados por Celsus. [L.]

ru·bra·tox·in (roo-bră-tok'sin). Rubratoxina; micotoxina produzida pelo *Penicillium rubrum* e pelo *P. purpurogenum*, que se forma rapidamente nos grãos de cereais; é responsável por surtos de toxicose nos EUA.

ru·bre·dox·ins (roo-brē-dok'sinz). Rubredoxinas; as ferredoxinas sem enxofre ácido-lábil e com ferro em um arranjo mercaptídico típico.

ru·bri·blast (roo'bri-blast). Rubriblasto. SIN pronormoblast. [L. *ruber*, vermelho, + G. *blastos*, germe]

pernicious anemia type r., r. da anemia perniciosa. SIN promegaloblast. VER erythroblast.

rub·ric. Rubrica; o título da seção ou do capítulo, utilizado com referência a grupos de doenças, como no CID. [I.m. *rubrike*, título ou cabeçalho em vermelho, do L. *ruber*, vermelho]

ru·bri·cyte (roo'bri-sīt). Rubricito; o normoblasto policromático. VER erythroblast. [L. *ruber*, vermelho, + *kytos*, célula]

ru·bro·spi·nal (roo'brō-spī'năl). Rubrospinal; relativo às fibras nervosas que passam do núcleo rubro até a medula espinal: o trato rubrospinal (ver rubrospinal *tract* [TA]).

Ru·bu·la·vi·rus (roo-boo'lă-vī-rus). Gênero da família Paramyxoviridae; causa caxumba. SIN mumpvirus.

ruc·tus (rŭk'tŭs). Arroto, eructação. SIN eructation. [L. de *ructo*, pp. *-atus*, arrotar]

Rud, Einar, médico dinamarquês, *1892. VER R. *syndrome*.

ru·di·ment (roo'di-ment). Rudimento. 1. Um órgão ou uma estrutura que apresenta desenvolvimento incompleto. 2. O primeiro indício de uma estrutura no curso da ontogenia. SIN rudimentum. [L. *rudimentum*, primeiro elemento, rudimento, de *rudis*, que não tem forma]

ru·di·men·ta·ry (roo-di-men'tăr-ē). Rudimentar; relativo a um rudimento. SIN abortive (2).

ru·di·men·tum, pl. **ru·di·men·ta** (roo'di-men'tŭm, -tă). Rudimento. SIN rudiment, rudiment. [L.]

r. hippocam'pi, r. do hipocampo. VER *indusium griseum*.

ruff (rŭf). Rufo; um colar ou prega.

pupillary r., a borda preguedada e castanho-escura da pupila normal, que corresponde ao epitélio pigmentado posterior da íris, que se volta para si mesma na margem da pupila.

Ruffini, Angelo, histologista italiano, 1864–1929. VER R. *corpuscles*, em *corpuscle*; flower-spray *organ* of R.

ru·fous (roo'fŭs). Ruivo; que possui uma compleição avermelhada e cabelo vermelho. SIN erythristic. [L. *rufus*, avermelhado]

ru·ga, pl. **ru·gae** (roo'gă, roo'gē) [TA]. Ruga; prega, crista ou dobra; uma ruga. [L. uma ruga]

rugae of gallbladder, pregas da mucosa da vesícula biliar; ✶termo oficial alternativo de mucosal *folds* of gallbladder, em *fold*.

gastric rugae, pregas gástricas; ✶termo oficial alternativo de gastric *folds*, em *fold*.

r. gas'trica, prega gástrica. SIN gastric *folds*, em *fold*.

r. palati'na, prega palatina transversa. SIN transverse palatine *fold*.

rugae of stomach, pregas gástricas. SIN gastric *folds*, em *fold*.

rugae of vagina, rugas vaginais. SIN vaginal rugae.

vaginal rugae [TA], rugas vaginais; várias cristas transversas localizadas na membrana mucosa da vagina. SIN rugae vaginales [TA], rugae of vagina.

ru'gae vagina'les [TA], rugas vaginais. SIN vaginal rugae.

rugae vesicae biliaris, pregas da mucosa da vesícula biliar; ✶termo oficial alternativo de mucosal *folds* of gallbladder, em *fold*.

ru·gine (roo-zhēn'). 1. SIN periosteal *elevator*. 2. Um raspador. [Fr.]

ru·gi·tus (roo'ji-tŭs). Borborigmo; um ruído de ronco nos intestinos. VER TAMBÉM borborygmus. [L. um rugido, de *rugio*, rugir]

ru·gose (roo'gōs). Rugoso; marcado por rugas; preguedado. SIN rugous. [L. *rugosus*]

ru·gos·i·ty (roo-gos'i-tē). Rugosidade. 1. O estado de apresentar pregas ou dobras. 2. Uma ruga.

ru·gous (roo'gŭs). Rugoso. SIN rugose.

Ruhemann pur·ple. Púrpura de Ruhemann; um corante violeta-azulado formado pela reação da ninidrina com aminoácidos.

RUL Abreviatura de right upper lobe (lobo superior direito do pulmão).

rule (rool). Regra, critério; um padrão ou guia que orienta um procedimento, um arranjo, uma ação etc. VER TAMBÉM law, principle, theorem. [Fr. ant. *reule*, do L. *regula*, um guia, padrão]

Abegg r., r. de Abegg; a tendência da soma da valência positiva máxima e negativa máxima de um elemento específico de tornar-se igual a 8; p. ex., o C pode ter uma valência de +4 e −4, o O de +6 e −2. Afirma-se, às vezes, de modo incorreto, que todos os átomos possuem o mesmo número de valências, como uma conseqüência da tendência das camadas eletrônicas de valência de atingir o valor 8.

American Law Institute r., critério do American Law Institute (uma instituição legal norte-americana); um critério de responsabilidade criminal (1962): "uma pessoa não é responsável pela sua conduta criminosa se, no momento de tal conduta e como resultado de doença ou deficiência mentais, ela carece da capacidade substancial de avaliar a ilegalidade da conduta ou de adaptar sua conduta às exigências da lei".

r. of bigeminy, r. do bigeminismo; a r. que afirma que um batimento ventricular prematuro ocorre após o batimento que finaliza um ciclo longo. O prolongamento súbito do ciclo ventricular, por alteração da refratariedade no sistema de condução, torna uma região periférica de bloqueio bidirecional transitoriamente unidirecional e, dessa forma, abre caminhos potenciais para a ocorrência da reentrância.

Chargaff r., r. de Chargaff; no DNA, o número de unidades de adenina é igual ao número de unidades de timina; do mesmo modo, o número de unidades de guanina é igual ao número de unidades de citosina.

Clark weight r., r. do peso de Clark; uma r. obsoleta para o cálculo da dose aproximada para crianças; o valor é obtido por meio da divisão do peso da criança, em libras, por 150 e por meio da multiplicação do resultado pela dose para adultos.

Cowling r., r. de Cowling; uma r. obsoleta para calcular a dose para crianças: aquela fração da dose para adultos obtida pela divisão da idade da criança no aniversário mais próximo por 24.

Durham r., r. de Durham; um critério norte-americano de responsabilidade criminal (1954) por meio do qual uma pessoa acusada não é considerada criminalmente responsável se seu ato ilegal foi produto de doença ou deficiência mentais.

Gibb phase r., r. das fases de Gibb. SIN phase r.

Goriaew r., r. de Goriaew; termo raramente utilizado para uma regra aplicada a um campo de contagem sangüínea, segundo a qual o campo deve ser separado em vários quadrados e alguns deles devem ser novamente divididos em 16 quadrados menores.

Haase r., r. de Haase; o comprimento do feto, em centímetros, dividido por 5, corresponde à duração da gravidez em meses, i.e., à idade do feto.

Hückel r., r. de Hückel; o número de elétrons despolarizados em um anel aromático é igual a $4n + 2$, em que n corresponde a 0 ou a qualquer número inteiro positivo; a L-tirosina, a L-fenilalanina, o L-triptofano e a L-histidina (quando o anel imidazólico está desprovido de prótons) obedecem a essa regra.

Ingelfinger r., r. de Ingelfinger; um princípio desenvolvido por Franz Ingelfinger para ser empregado nos escritórios editoriais do *New England Journal of Medicine*; tal princípio afirma que os originais submetidos a publicação devem ser revistos mediante a concordância de que a mesma informação não poderá ser publicada em outro meio durante o período de revisão; foi adotado por muitos periódicos médicos revistos por terceiros.

isoprene r., r. do isopreno; a frase antiquada e clássica que afirma que os terpenos de ocorrência natural são produzidos pela condensação de unidades de isopreno por uma ligação 1-4 ("cabeça a cauda") ou por uma ligação 4-4 ("cauda a cauda").

Jackson r., r. de Jackson; após um ataque epiléptico, as funções simples e quase-automáticas são menos afetadas e mais rapidamente restauradas do que as funções mais complexas.

Le Bel-van't Hoff r., r. de Le Bel-van't Hoff; o número de estereoisômeros de um composto orgânico corresponde a 2^n, em que n representa o número de átomos de carbono assimétricos (a menos que exista um plano interno de simetria); um corolário de suas conclusões anunciadas de modo simultâneo, em 1874, que afirmam que a orientação mais provável das ligações de um átomo de carbono ligado a quatro grupos ou átomos está voltada para os ápices de um tetraedro e que tal fato respondia por todos os fenômenos então conhecidos de assimetria molecular (que envolviam um átomo de carbono ligado a quatro diferentes átomos ou grupos). VER TAMBÉM stereoisomerism.

Liebermeister r., r. de Liebermeister; na taquicardia febril do adulto, cerca de oito batimentos cardíacos correspondem a uma elevação de 1°C na temperatura.

Meyer-Overton r., r. de Meyer-Overton; pelo fato de os agentes inalatórios agirem via células do SNC ricas em lipídios, a potência anestésica aumenta de acordo com a liposolubilidade.

M'Naghten r., r. de M'Naghten; o critério inglês clássico de responsabilidade criminal (1843): "ao se estabelecer uma defesa no terreno da insanidade, deve ser claramente provado que, na época em que o ato foi cometido, a parte acusada estava agindo sob uma certa deficiência de raciocínio, resultante de doença mental, como não entender a natureza e a qualidade do ato que estava praticando, ou, se as entendia, que não entendia que estava fazendo o que era errado".

Nägele r., r. de Nägele; a determinação da data estimada para o parto pela adição de 7 dias ao primeiro dia do último período menstrual normal, a subtração de 3 meses e a adição de 1 ano.

New Hampshire r., r. de New Hampshire; o critério pioneiro norte-americano de responsabilidade criminal (1871): "se o ato [criminoso] resultou de insanidade, uma intenção criminosa não o produziu".

r. of nines, r. dos nove; o método utilizado no cálculo da área da superfície corporal envolvida em queimaduras, por meio do qual valores de 9% ou 18% da área da superfície são atribuídos a regiões específicas conforme se segue: cabeça e pescoço, 9%; tórax anterior, 18%; tórax posterior, 18%; braços, 9% cada; pernas, 18% cada; e períneo, 1%.

Ogino-Knaus r., r. de Ogino-Knaus; a época do período menstrual em que é mais provável que a concepção ocorra se encontra a cerca de meio caminho entre dois períodos menstruais; é menos provável que a fertilização do óvulo ocorra pouco antes ou pouco depois da menstruação; a base para o método do ritmo de contracepção.

r. of outlet, uma r. obstétrica para determinar se o canal pélvico permite a passagem de um feto; a soma do diâmetro sagital posterior com o diâmetro transverso da passagem deve ser igual a, pelo menos, 15 cm para que um bebê de cabeça normal passe.

phase r., r. das fases; uma expressão da relação existente entre sistemas em equilíbrio: $P + V = C + 2$, em que P corresponde ao número de fases, V corresponde à variância ou aos graus de liberdade e C, ao número de componentes; logo, a variância corresponde a $V = C + 2 − P$. Para a H_2O em seu ponto triplo, $V = 1 + 2 − 3 = 0$, i.e., tanto a temperatura como a pressão são fixas. SIN Gibb phase r.

Prentice r., r. de Prentice; cada centímetro de descentralização de uma lente resulta em 1 dioptria prismática de desvio de luz para cada dioptria de potência da lente.

Rolleston r., r. de Rolleston; a pressão arterial sistólica do adulto corresponde a 100 mais a metade da idade, ao passo que a pressão fisiológica máxima corresponde a 100 mais a idade; de interesse histórico.

Schütz r., r. de Schütz; a velocidade de uma reação enzimática é proporcional

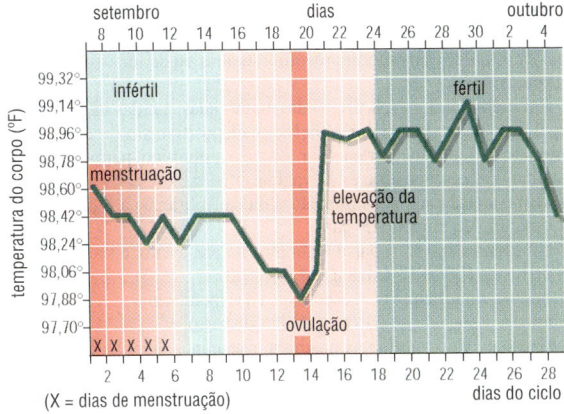

regra de Ogino-Knaus

à raiz quadrada da concentração enzimática; aplicada especificamente à pepsina dentro de uma faixa limitada. SIN Schütz law.

stopping r.'s, em ensaios controlados randomizados e em outros experimentos sistemáticos feitos em seres humanos, as regras apresentadas *a priori* que especificam as condições sob as quais o experimento será finalizado, p. ex., a demonstração inequívoca de que uma regra em um ensaio controlado randomizado é claramente superior a outra, ou que determinada regra é claramente prejudicial.

Trusler r. for pulmonary artery banding, r. de Trusler para a ligadura da artéria pulmonar; um método que fornece um guia quanto à tensão adequada da ligaduras; a medida da ligadura para uma anomalia cardíaca congênita complexa com desvio bidirecional menor do que aquela para as anomalias simples.

Young r., r. de Young; r. obsoleta para determinar a dose para crianças: adiciona-se 12 à idade da criança e divide-se a soma pela idade; a dose para adultos dividida pela quantidade assim obtida fornece a dose apropriada.

rul·er (roo′ler). Régua; uma tira calibrada utilizada para medir superfícies planas.

isometric r., r. isométrica; escala calibrada utilizada para eliminar a distorção na medição de superfícies planas.

rum (rŭm). Rum; bebida alcoólica destilada proveniente do suco fermentado do açúcar da cana.

rum·blos·som (rŭm - blos′ŭm). Rinofima. SIN rhinophyma.

ru·mi·nant (roo′mi - nănt). Ruminante; animal que mastiga novamente o material regurgitado do rúmen; p. ex., carneiro, vaca, veado ou antílope.

ru·mi·na·tion (roo - mi - nā′shŭn). Ruminação; **1.** O processo fisiológico observado em animais ruminantes no qual um alimento ingerido apressadamente é regurgitado do rúmen, remastigado completamente, reduzido a partículas menores, misturado à saliva e engolido novamente. **2.** Um distúrbio da infância caracterizado pela regurgitação repetida do alimento, com perda de peso ou desenvolvimento precário, que surge após um período de funcionamento normal. **3.** A reconsideração periódica do mesmo assunto. [L. *ruminatio*, de *rumino*, mastigar o material regurgitado do rúmen, refletir, de *rumen*, garganta]

ru·mi·na·tive (roo′min - ā - tiv). Ruminativo; caracterizado por uma preocupação com certos pensamentos e idéias.

Ru·mi·no·coc·cus (room′ē - nō - kok′us). Gênero de cocobacilos Gram-positivos e anaeróbicos isolados do trato respiratório de humanos e do trato intestinal de seres humanos e animais. A espécie-tipo é o *Ruminococcus productus*, antigamente denominado *Peptostreptococcus productus*.

Rumpel, Theodor, médico alemão, 1862–1923. VER R.-Leede *sign, test, phenomenon*.

run (rŭn). Um grupo de medições sucessivas em um processo analítico ou durante um período de tempo dentro do qual se espera que a acurácia e a precisão do sistema de medidas sejam estáveis. [I.m. *runnen*, do A.S. *rinnan*, de O.N. *rinna*]

Rundle, A.T., médico britânico. VER Richards-Rundle *syndrome*.

Runeberg, Johan W., médico finlandês, 1843–1918. VER r. *formula*.

run·off (rŭn′awf). A parte demorada do exame angiográfico de um leito vascular, para mostrar a permeabilidade de artérias pequenas.

runt (rŭnt). Um animal raquítico observado mais freqüentemente em espécies que dão à luz grandes ninhadas. [A.S.]

ru·pia (roo′pē - ă). Rupia. **1.** As úlceras da sífilis secundária e tardia, cobertas com crostas amareladas ou castanhas que foram comparadas, quanto à aparência, a conchas de ostras. **2.** Termo utilizado ocasionalmente para designar uma lesão psoriática e escamosa, com infecção secundária. [G. *rhypos*, imundície]

ru·pi·oid (roo′pē - oyd). Rupióide; que se assemelha à rupia. [G. *rhypos*, imundície (rupia), + *eidos*, semelhança]

rup·ture (rŭp'choor). **1.** Hérnia. SIN hernia. **2.** Ruptura, rotura; uma solução de continuidade ou uma laceração; o rompimento de um órgão ou de partes moles. [L. *ruptura*, uma ruptura (de um membro ou de uma veia), de *rumpo*, pp. *ruptus*, romper]
artificial membrane r., r. artificial das membranas; a r. das membranas induzida pelo uso de um rompedor de bolsa ou dispositivo similar.
membrane r., r. das membranas; a r. do saco amniótico, permitindo que o líquido amniótico escape através da vagina.
premature membrane r., r. prematura das membranas; a r. das membranas antes do início do trabalho de parto.
preterm membrane r., r. das membranas no pré-termo; a r. das membranas antes do termo (< de 37 semanas de gestação).
spontaneous membrane r., r. espontânea das membranas; a r. espontânea das membranas, associada ou não ao trabalho de parto.
RUQ Abreviatura de right upper quadrant (quadrante superior direito do abdome).
Rushton, Martin A., patologista britânico, 1903–1970. VER R. *bodies*.
Russell, Albert L., dentista norte-americano, 1905–1985. VER R. Periodontal Index.
Russell, Alexander, pediatra britânico do século 20. VER R. *syndrome*; Silver-R. *dwarfism, syndrome*.
Russell, Gerald F.M., médico inglês do século 20. VER R. *sign*.
Russell, Hamilton, cirurgião australiano do século 20. VER R. *traction*.
Russell, James S. Risien, médico britânico, 1863–1939. VER hooked *bundle* of R.; uncinate *bundle* of R.
Russell, Patrick, médico irlandês que viveu na Índia, 1727–1805. VER R.'s viper *venom, viper*.
Russell, William, médico escocês, 1852–1940. VER R. *bodies*, em *body*.
Russell, William James, químico inglês, 1830–1909. VER R. *effect*.
Russell Per·i·o·don·tal In·dex. Índice Periodontal de Russell; um índice que avalia o grau de doença periodontal presente na boca por meio da medição tanto da perda óssea ao redor dos dentes como da inflamação gengival; é utilizado freqüentemente na investigação epidemiológica da doença periodontal.

Rust, Johann N., cirurgião alemão, 1775–1840. VER r. *phenomenon*.
rusts (rŭsts). Ferrugem; uma espécie de *Puccinia* (fungo) e de outros micróbios que constituem patógenos importantes de plantas, principalmente de grãos de cereais; são alérgenos de relevância para seres humanos quando inalados em grande quantidade, como ocorre durante as colheitas.
ru·the·ni·um (Ru) (roo-thē'nē-ŭm). Rutênio; um elemento metálico do grupo da platina; n.º atômico 44 e peso atômico 101,07; o Ru^{106}, com uma meia-vida de 1.020 anos, foi utilizado no tratamento de certos problemas oculares. [L. mediev. *Ruthenia*, Rússia, onde o Ru foi obtido pela primeira vez]
ru·the·ni·um red. Vermelho de rutênio; o oxicloreto de vermelho de rutênio amoniatado, utilizado em histologia e em microscopia eletrônica como um corante para certos polissacarídeos complexos.
ruth·er·ford (rŭth'er-ferd). Termo obsoleto para uma unidade de radioatividade, que representa a quantidade de material radioativo na qual ocorre um milhão de desintegrações por segundo; 37 rd = 1 mCi. VER Becquerel. [Ernest *Rutherford*, físico britânico laureado com um prêmio Nobel, 1871–1937]
ru·ti·do·sis (roo-ti-dō'sis). Rutidose. SIN rhytidosis.
ru·tin (roo'tin). Rutina; um flavonóide obtido do trigo-mourisco (trigo-mouro ou trigo-sarraceno), que causa diminuição da fragilidade capilar. SIN rutoside.
ru·tin·ose (roo'ti-nōs). Rutinose; dissacarídeo da D-glicose e da L-ramnose e um componente da rutina.
ru·to·side (roo'tō-sīd). Rutinosídeo. SIN rutin.
Ruysch, Frederik, anatomista holandês, 1638–1731. VER R. *membrane, muscle, tube, veins*, em *vein*.
RV Abreviatura de residual *volume* (volume residual).
Ryan, Norbert J., patologista australiano do século 20. VER R. *stain*.
ry·an·o·dine (rī-an'ō-dēn). Rianodina; alcalóide obtido da *Ryania speciosa* (família Flacourtiaceae); possui um efeito disruptivo sobre o armazenamento de cálcio na musculatura esquelética e cardíaca, onde produz contrações prolongadas; utilizado como inseticida.
rye smut (rī'smŭt'). Esporão do centeio. SIN ergot.
Ryle, John A., médico inglês, 1889–1950. VER R. *tube*.

cromasia laranja; utilizado em histologia como corante nuclear, em microbiologia como contracorante no método de Gram e para demonstrar o caráter enterocromafin.

saf·ra·no·phil, saf·ra·no·phile (saf′rã - no - fil, - fīl). Safranófilo; que se cora facilmente com safranina; designa certas células e tecidos.

saf·role (saf′rōl). Safrol; éter metileno do alil pirocatecol; contido no óleo de sassafrás, no óleo de cânfora e em vários outros óleos voláteis; obtido principalmente do óleo de cânfora por destilação fracionada; utilizado como tônico e carminativo. A administração prolongada causa degeneração gordurosa.

sage (sāj). Sálvia. SIN salvia. [L. *salvia,* a planta sálvia, de *salvus,* seguro]

sa·git·ta (saj′i - tă). Otólitos. SIN otoliths.

sag·it·tal (saj′i - tăl). Sagital; semelhante a uma seta; na linha de uma seta atirada de um arco, isto é, em direção ântero-posterior; refere-se a um plano ou sentido sagital. SIN sagittalis [TA]. [L. *sagitta,* seta]

sa·git·ta·lis (saj - i - tā′lis). Sagital. SIN sagittal. [L.]

Saint, Charles F.M., cirurgião africano, *1886. VER S. *triad.*

Saint Anthony fire (sānt anth - ō - nē). **1.** SIN Ergotismo ergotism. **2.** Qualquer uma de várias inflamações ou condições gangrenosas da pele (p. ex., erisipela). [Santo Antônio, monge egípcio, cerca de 250–350 a.C.]

Sakaguchi re·ac·tion. Reação de Sakaguchi. Ver em reaction.

Saksenaea vasiformis. Espécie de fungo que causa mucormicose; essa espécie é notável pela proporção de casos com infecção subcutânea em lugar da doença pulmonar ou dos seios paranasais, que constituem manifestações mais típicas da mucormicose.

Sakurai. Oftalmologista japonês. VER Sakurai-Lisch *nodule.*

sal, pl. **sales** (sal, sal′ēz). Sal. SIN salt. [L.]

  s. alem′broth, produto obtido pela cristalização de uma solução de partes iguais de cloreto de amônio e cloreto mercúrico. SIN salt of wisdom. [termo de origem desconhecida utilizado pelos alquimistas.]

  s. ammo′niac, cloreto de amônio. SIN ammonium chloride.

  s. diuret′icum, acetato de potássio. SIN potassium acetate.

  s. soda, carbonato sódico. SIN sodium carbonate.

  s. vol′atile, s. volátil. SIN aromatic ammonia *spirit.*

Salah, M., cirurgião egípcio do século XX. VER S. sternal puncture *needle.*

sal·bu·ta·mol (sal - bū′tă - mol). Salbutamol. SIN albuterol.

Saldino, Ronald M., radiologista americano.

sal·i·cin (sal′i-sin). Salicina; glicosídeo do *o*-hidroxibenzilálcool, obtido da casca de várias espécies de *Salix* (salgueiro) e *Populus* (choupo); a salicina é hidrolisada a glicose e saligenina (álcool salicílico); antigamente utilizada na artrite reumatóide.

sal·i·cyl (sal′i-sil). Salicil; o radical acil do ácido salicílico.

  s. aldehyde, aldeído salicílico; obtido de *Spirea ulmaria* (rainha-dos-prados) e produzido sinteticamente; utilizado como diurético e anti-séptico, bem como em perfumaria. SIN salicylic aldehyde.

sal·i·cyl·am·ide (sal - i - sil′ă - mīd). Salicilamida; a amida do ácido salicílico, *o*-hidroxibenzamida; analgésico, antipirético e antiartrítico, de ação semelhante ao ácido acetilsalicílico.

sal·i·cyl·an·i·lide (sal′i - sil - an′i - līd). Salicilanilida; agente antifúngico particularmente útil na tinha da cabeça causada por *Microsporum audouinii.*

sal·lic·y·late (să - lis′i - lāt). **1.** Salicilato; sal ou éster do ácido salicílico. **2.** Tratar alimentos com ácido salicílico como conservante. SIN salicylize.

sa·licy·lat·ed (să - lis′i - lāt - ed). Salicilado; tratado pela adição de ácido salicílico como conservante.

sal·i·cyl·az·o·sul·fa·pyr·i·dine (sal′i - sil - az′ō - sool - fă - pir′i - dēn). Salicilazossulfapiridina. SIN sulfasalazine.

sal·i·cyl·ic ac·id (sal - i - sil′ik). Ácido salicílico; componente do ácido acetilsalicílico, derivado da salicina e produzido sinteticamente; utilizado externamente como agente ceratolítico, anti-séptico e fungicida.

sal·i·cyl·ic al·de·hyde (sal - i - sil′ik). Aldeído salicílico. SIN salicyl aldehyde.

sal·i·cyl·ism (sal′i-sil-izm). Salicilismo; intoxicação pelo ácido salicílico ou por qualquer um de seus compostos.

sal·i·cyl·ize (sal′i - sil - īz). Tratar alimentos com ácido salicílico como conservante. SIN salicylate (2).

sal·i·cyl·sal·i·cyl·ic ac·id (sal′i-sil-sal-i-sil′ik). Ácido salicilsalicílico. SIN salsalate.

sal·i·cyl·sul·fon·ic ac·id (sal′i - sil - sūl - fon′ik). Ácido salicilsulfônico. SIN sulfosalicylic acid.

sal·i·cyl·u·ric ac·id (sal′i - sil′ūr′ik). Ácido salicilúrico; o produto de conjugação da glicina com o ácido salicílico; excretado na urina após a administração de ácido salicílico ou de alguns de seus compostos.

sa·lient (sā′lē - ent, sāl′yent). **1.** Saliência. SIN projection. **2.** Em radiologia, termo obsoleto para incidência. [L. *salio,* saltar]

sal·i·fi·a·ble (sal - i - fī′ă - bl). Salificável; capaz de ser transformado em sal; refere-se a uma base que se combina com ácidos para formar sais.

sal·i·fy (sal′i - fī). Salificar; converter em sal.

sal·i·gen·in, sal·i·gen·ol (sal - i - jen′in, sal′i - jen - ol). Saligenina, saligenol; obtido pela hidrólise da salicinina; anestésico local.

sa·lim·e·ter (să - lim′ē - ter). Salímetro; hidrômetro para determinar a densidade ou a concentração de uma solução salina.

sa·line (sā′lēn, - līn). **1.** Salino; relativo a, da natureza de ou contendo sal; salgado. **2.** Solução salina, geralmente de cloreto de sódio. [L. *salinus,* salgado, de *sal,* sal]

  physiologic s., soro fisiológico; solução aquosa isotônica de sais, contendo cloreto de sódio a 0,9%.

sa·li·nom·e·ter (sal - i - nom′ē - ter). Salinômetro; hidrômetro calibrado de modo a fornecer uma leitura direta da percentagem de determinado sal presente em solução.

sa·li·va (să - lī - vă). Saliva; líquido claro, insípido, inodoro, discretamente ácido (pH a 6,8) e viscoso, secretado pelas glândulas salivares parótida, sublingual e submaxilar e pelas glândulas mucosas da cavidade oral; sua função consiste em manter a mucosa da boca úmida, em lubrificar o alimento durante a mastigação e, até certo ponto, em converter o amido em maltose, sendo esta última ação efetuada por uma enzima diastática, a ptialina. SIN spittle. [L. proveniente do G. *sialon*]

  chorda s., s. da corda; secreção da glândula submaxilar obtida por estimulação do nervo corda do tímpano.

  ganglionic s., s. ganglionar; saliva submaxilar obtida por irritação direta da glândula.

  resting s., s. de repouso; saliva encontrada na boca nos intervalos da ingestão e mastigação do alimento.

  sympathetic s., s. simpática; saliva submaxilar obtida por estimulação das fibras simpáticas que inervam a glândula.

sal·i·vant (sal′i-vant). **1.** Salivante, salivar; que produz um fluxo de saliva. **2.** Salivador; agente que aumenta o fluxo de saliva. SIN salivator.

sal·i·vary (sal′i - văr - ē). Salivar; relativo à saliva. SIN sialic, sialine. [L. *salivarius*]

sal·i·vate (sal′i - vāt). Salivar; causar fluxo excessivo de saliva.

sal·i·va·tion (sal′i - vā′shŭn). Salivação. SIN sialorrhea.

sal·i·va·tor (sal′i - vā - ter). Salivador. SIN salivant (2).

sa·li·vo·li·thi·a·sis (sa - li′vō - li - thī′ă - sis). Salivolitíase. SIN sialolithiasis.

Salk, Jonas, imunologista norte-americano, 1914–1995. VER S. *vaccine.*

Sal·mo·nel·la (sal′mō - nel′ă). Gênero de bactérias aeróbicas ou anaeróbicas facultativas (família Enterobacteriaceae) que contém bastonetes Gram-negativos, móveis ou imóveis; as células móveis são peritríquias. Esses microrganismos não liquefazem a gelatina nem produzem indol e variam quanto à sua produção de sulfeto de hidrogênio; utilizam o citrato como única fonte de carbono; seu metabolismo é fermentativo, produzindo ácido e geralmente gás a partir da glicose, porém não atacam a lactose; a maioria é aerogênica, porém *S. typhi* nunca produz gás; são patogênicos para os seres humanos e outros animais. A espécie tipo é *S. choleraesuis.* [Daniel E. *Salmon,* patologista norte-americano, 1850–1914]

  S. enterica subsp. *enterit′idis;* espécie amplamente distribuída, que ocorre em seres humanos e animais domésticos e selvagens, especialmente em roedores; provoca gastroenterite humana.

  S. enterica subsp. *paratyphi A;* espécie bacteriana importante como agente etiológico da febre entérica nos países em desenvolvimento.

  S. enterica subsp. *parathyphi B,* (antigamente conhecida como *S. schottmülleri*); consiste em dois tipos distintos de cepas: as que produzem febre entérica, encontradas primariamente nos seres humanos, e aquelas que provocam gastroenterite nos seres humanos, também encontradas em espécies animais. Essa espécie inclui 56 cepas que podem ser distinguidas através de fagotipagem e/ou biotipagem, características de valor epidemiológico.

  S. enterica subsp. *typhi,* SIN *S. typhi.*

  S. enterica subsp. *typhimu′rium;* espécie que causa intoxicação alimentar no ser humano; trata-se de um patógeno natural de todos os animais de sangue quente, sendo também encontrado em cobras e tartarugas; no mundo inteiro, é a causa mais freqüente de gastroenterite por *S. enterica.*

  S. enterica subsp. *choleraesuis,* espécie encontrada em porcos, nos quais é um importante invasor secundário na cólera suína viral, porém não ocorre como patógeno natural em outros animais; em certas ocasiões, provoca gastroenterite aguda e febre entérica nos seres humanos; trata-se da espécie tipo do gênero *S.*

  S. ty′phi, espécie responsável pela febre tifóide nos seres humanos; transmitida através da ingestão de água ou alimentos contaminados. SIN Eberth bacillus, *S. enterica* subsp. *typhi,* typhoid bacillus.

  S. typho′sa, nome antigo de *S. typhi.*

sal·mo·nel·lo·sis (sal′mō - nel - ō′sis). Salmonelose; infecção por bactérias do gênero *Salmonella;* os pacientes com anemia falciforme e comprometimento do sistema imune são particularmente suscetíveis a essa infecção. [*Salmonella* + G. *-osis,* condição]

sal·ol (sal′ol). fenil salicilato. SIN phenyl salicylate.

△ **salping-.** Salping. VER salpingo-.

sal·pin·gec·to·my (sal - pin - jek′tō - mē). Salpingectomia; remoção da tuba uterina. SIN tubectomy. [salping- + G. *ektomē,* excisão]

abdominal s., s. abdominal; remoção de uma ou de ambas as tubas uterinas através de incisão abdominal.

sal·pin·ges (sal-pin′jēz). Salpinges; plural de salpinx.

sal·pin·gi·an (sal-pin′jē-ăn). Salpingiano, salpíngico; relativo à tuba uterina ou à tuba auditiva.

sal·pin·gi·o·ma (sal-pin-jē-ō′mă). Salpingioma; qualquer tumor que surge nos tecidos de uma tuba uterina. [salping- + G. *-oma*, tumor]

sal·pin·git·ic (sal-pin-jit′ik). Salpingítico; relativo à salpingite.

sal·pin·gi·tis (sal-pin-jī′tis). Salpingite; inflamação da tuba uterina ou auditiva. [salping- + G. *-itis*, inflamação]

  chronic interstitial s., s. intersticial crônica; salpingite em que a fibrose ou infiltração de células mononucleares acomete todas as camadas da tuba uterina ou auditiva.

  foreign body s., s. por corpo estranho; salpingite em que ocorre formação de células gigantes no tecido, em conseqüência da introdução de material estranho na tuba uterina.

  gonorrheal s., s. gonorreica; inflamação da tuba uterina após infecção gonorreica aguda.

  s. isth'mica nodo'sa, s. ístmica nodosa; condição da tuba uterina caracterizada por espessamento nodular da túnica muscular da porção ístmica da tuba, envolvendo duplicações císticas ou semelhantes a glândulas da luz. SIN adenosalpingitis.

  pyogenic s., s. piogênica; forma de salpingite aguda que ocorre habitualmente na infecção puerperal.

⚠ **salpingo-, salping-.** Salpingo-, salping-. Tuba (geralmente uterina ou auditiva). VER TAMBÉM tubo-. [G. *salpinx*, trompa (tubo)]

sal·pin·go·cele (sal-ping′gō-sēl). Salpingocele; hérnia de uma tuba uterina. [salpingo- + G. *kēlē*, hérnia]

sal·pin·go·cy·e·sis (sal-ping′gō-sī-ē′sis). Salpingociese. SIN tubal pregnancy. [salpingo- + G. *kyēsis*, gravidez]

sal·pin·gog·ra·phy (sal-ping-gog′ră-fē). Salpingografia; radiografia das tubas uterinas após a injeção de contraste radiopaco. [salpingo- + G. *graphō*, escrever]

sal·pin·gol·y·sis (sal-ping-gol′i-sis). Salpingólise; liberação de aderências da tuba uterina. [salpingo- + G. *lysis*, afrouxamento]

sal·pin·go·ne·os·to·my (sal-ping′ō-nē-os′tō-mē). Salpingoneostomia; reabertura cirúrgica de uma tuba uterina em baqueta, devido a aderências das fímbrias. [salpingo- + neostomy]

⚠ **salpingo-oophor-, salpingo-oophoro-.** Salpingo-oofor-. A tuba uterina e o ovário. [salpingo- + L. mod. *oophoron*, ovário, do G. *ōophoros*, portador de ovos]

sal·pin·go-o·o·pho·rec·to·my (sal-ping′gō-ō-of-ō-rek′tō-mē). Salpingo-ooforectomia; remoção do ovário e de sua trompa de Falópio. SIN salpingo-ovariectomy, tubo-ovariectomy.

sal·pin·go-o·o·pho·ri·tis (sal-ping′gō-ō-of-ō-rī′tis). Salpingo-ooforite; inflamação da tuba uterina e do ovário. SIN tubo-ovaritis.

sal·pin·go-o·oph·o·ro·cele (sal-ping′gō-ō-of′ō-rō-sēl). Salpingo-ooforocele; hérnia do ovário e da tuba uterina.

sal·pin·go-o·var·i·ec·to·my (sal-ping′gō-ō-var-ē-ek′tō-mē). Salpingo-ovariectomia. SIN salpingo-oophorectomy.

sal·pin·go·per·i·to·ni·tis (sal-ping′gō-per-i-tō-nī′tis). Salpingoperitonite; inflamação da tuba uterina, da perissalpinge e do peritônio. [salpingo- + peritonitis]

sal·pin·go·pexy (sal-ping′gō-pek-sē). Salpingopexia; fixação cirúrgica de um oviduto. [salpingo- + G. *pēxis*, fixação]

sal·pin·go·pha·ryn·ge·al (sal-ping′gō-fă-rin′jē-ăl). Salpingofaríngeo; relativo à tuba auditiva e à faringe.

sal·pin·go·pha·ryn·ge·us. Salpingofaríngeo. VER salpingopharyngeus *(muscle)*.

sal·pin·go·plas·ty (sal-ping′gō-plas-tē). Salpingoplastia; cirurgia plástica das tubas uterinas. SIN tuboplasty (tuboplastia). [salpingo- + G. *plastos*, formado]

sal·pin·gor·rha·gia (sal-ping-gō-rā′jē-ă). Salpingorragia; hemorragia de uma tuba uterina. [salpingo- + G. *rhēgnymi*, irromper]

sal·pin·gor·rha·phy (sal-ping-gōr′ă-fē). Salpingorrafia; sutura da tuba uterina. [salpingo- + G. *rhaphē*, sutura]

sal·pin·gos·co·py (sal-ping-gos′kō-pē). Salpingoscopia; visualização da porção intraluminal das tubas uterinas, geralmente por radiografia ou através de um endoscópio. [salpingo- + G. *skopeō*, ver]

sal·pin·gos·to·my (sal-ping-gos′tō-mē). Salpingostomia; estabelecimento de uma abertura artificial numa trompa de Falópio primariamente como tratamento cirúrgico para a gravidez ectópica. [salpingo- + G. *stoma*, boca]

sal·pin·got·o·my (sal-ping-got′ō-mē). Salpingotomia; incisão de uma tuba uterina. [salpingo- + G. *tomē*, incisão]

  abdominal s., s. abdominal; incisão de uma tuba uterina através de uma abertura na parede abdominal.

sal·pinx, pl. **sal·pin·ges** (sal′pingks, sal-pin′jēz). Salpinge; *termo oficial alternativo para uterine *tube*. [G. trompa (tuba)]

  s. uteri'na, s. uterina. SIN uterine *tube*.

sal·sa·late (sal′să-lāt). Salsalato; combinação de duas moléculas de ácido salicílico em ligação a éster; o composto é hidrolisado durante e após absorção a ácido salicílico que, a exemplo de outros salicilatos, exerce efeitos analgésicos e antiinflamatórios. SIN salicylsalicylic acid.

salt. Sal. **1.** Composto formado pela interação de um ácido e uma base, sendo os átomos de hidrogênio ionizáveis do ácido substituídos pelo íon positivo da base. **2.** Cloreto de sódio, o protótipo do sal. **3.** Catártico salino, principalmente sulfato de magnésio, sulfato de sódio ou sal de Rochelle; freqüentemente referido no plural, sais (salts). SIN sal. [L. *sal*]

  acid s., s. ácido; sal em que nem todo o hidrogênio ionizável do ácido é substituído pelo elemento eletropositivo; p. ex., $NaHSO_4$, KH_2PO_4. SIN protosalt.

  artificial Carlsbad s., s. de Carlsbad artificial; mistura de sulfato de potássio, cloreto de sódio, bicarbonato de sódio e sulfato de sódio seco; laxativo.

  artificial Kissingen s., s. de Kissingen artificial; mistura de cloreto de potássio, cloreto de sódio, sulfato de magnésio anidro e bicarbonato de sódio; antiácido e laxativo.

  artificial Vichy s., s. de Vichy artificial; mistura de bicarbonato de sódio, sulfato de magnésio anidro, carbonato de potássio e cloreto de sódio, antiácido.

  basic s., s. básico; sal em que há um ou mais íons hidroxila não substituídos pelo elemento eletronegativo de um ácido; p. ex., $Fe-(OH)_2Cl$.

  bile s.'s, sais biliares; as formas de sais dos ácidos biliares; p. ex., taurocolato, glicocolato.

  bone s., s. ósseo. VER bone-salt.

  common s., s. comum. SIN sodium chloride.

  diazonium s.'s, sais diazônio; sais de uma base teórica, $R-\overset{+}{N}\equiv N$ ou $R-N=NOH$, útil em histoquímica para demonstrar fenóis teciduais e aril aminas ou com naftóis e naftilaminas liberados enzimaticamente para formar o grupamento azo cromóforo $-N=N-$; os sais diazônio contêm apenas um grupamento $R-\overset{+}{N}\equiv N$, os sais tetrazônio contêm dois e os sais hexazônio contêm três; os exemplos incluem a base GBC granada rápida e o naftol AS.

  double s., s. duplo; sal em que dois íons positivos diferentes estão ligados ao mesmo íon negativo, ou vice-versa; p. ex., $NaKSO_4$.

  effervescent s.'s, sais efervescentes; preparações obtidas pela adição de bicarbonato de sódio e ácidos tartárico e cítrico ao sal ativo; quando colocados em água, os ácidos rompem o bicarbonato de sódio, liberando o gás do ácido carbônico.

  Epsom s.'s, sais de Epson. SIN magnesium sulfate.

  Glauber s., s. de Glauber. SIN sodium sulfate.

  hexazonium s.'s, sais hexazônio; sais diazônio que contêm três grupos azo.

  Reinecke s., s. de Reinecke; sal de amônio preparado pela fusão do tiocianato de amônio com dicromato de amônio; cristais vermelho-escuros; utilizado na detecção e análise das aminas primárias e secundárias, incluindo aminoácidos; também utilizado como reagente para mercúrio.

  Rivière s., s. de Rivière. SIN potassium citrate.

  Rochelle s., s. de Rochelle. SIN potassium sodium tartrate.

  Seignette s., s. de Seignette. SIN potassium sodium tartrate.

  smelling s.'s, sais aromáticos. SIN aromatic ammonia *spirit*.

  s. substitute, s. substituto; aditivo alimentar com baixo conteúdo de sódio que tem sabor semelhante ao sal, como cloreto de potássio; útil como alternativa do sal nos alimentos.

  table s., s. de mesa. SIN sodium chloride.

  tetrazonium s.'s, sais tetrazônio; sais diazônio que contêm dois grupos azo.

  s. of wisdom, s. da sabedoria. SIN sal alembroth.

sal·ta·tion (sal-tā′shŭn). Saltada; ato de dançar ou saltar, como ocorre numa doença (p. ex., coréia) ou função fisiológica (p. ex., condução saltatória). [L. *saltatio*, de *salto*, pp. *-atus*, dançar, de *salio*, saltar]

sal·ta·to·ry (sal′tă-tōr-ē). Saltatório; relativo a, ou caracterizado por, saltada.

Salter, Sir Samuel J.A., dentista inglês, 1825–1897. VER S. incremental *lines*, em *line*.

Salter, Robert B., ortopedista canadense do século XX. VER S.-Harris *classification* of epiphysial plate injuries.

salt·ing in (salt′ing). Aumento da solubilidade (conforme observado para algumas proteínas) por soluções de sais diluídas (em comparação com água pura).

salt·ing out. Precipitação de uma proteína de sua solução por saturação ou por saturação parcial com sais neutros, como cloreto de sódio, sulfato de magnésio ou sulfato de amônio.

salt·pe·ter (salt′pē-ter). Salitre. SIN potassium nitrate.

  Chilean s., s. do Chile. SIN sodium nitrate.

sa·lu·bri·ous (să-loo′brē-ŭs). Salubre; saudável, referindo-se habitualmente ao clima. [L. *salubris*, saudável, de *salus*, saúde]

sal·u·re·sis (sal-ū-rē′sis). Salurese; excreção de sódio na urina. [L. *sal*, sal + G. *ourēsis*, urese (micção)]

sal·u·ret·ic (sal-ū-ret′ik). Salurético; que facilita a excreção renal de sódio.

Salus, Robert, oftalmologista boêmio, *1877. VER Koerber-Salus-Elschnig *syndrome*.

sa·lu·ta·ri·um (sal-ū-tār′ē-ŭm). Sanatório. SIN sanitarium. [L. *salutaris*, saudável, de *salus (salut-)*, saúde]

sal·u·tary (sal′ū-tār-ē). Salutar; saudável; sadio. [L. *salutaris*]

Sal·var·san (sal′var-san). Nome comercial histórico da arsfenamina. [L. *salvare*, preservar + *sanitas*, saúde]

salve (sav). Pomada. SIN ointment. [A.S. *sealf*]

sal·via (sal′vē-ā). Sálvia; as folhas secas de *Salvia officinalis* (família de Labiatae), a sálvia dos jardins ou dos prados; inibe a atividade secretora, especialmente das glândulas sudoríparas; foi também utilizada na bronquite e na inflamação da garganta. SIN sage. [L.]

Salzmann, Maximilian, oftalmologista alemão, 1862–1954. VER S. nodular corneal *degeneration*.

SAM Abreviatura de *S*-adenosyl-L-methionine (*S*-adenosil-L-metionina).

sam·an·da·rine (sa-măn′da-rēn). Samandarina; alcalóide tóxico das salamandras; provoca hemólise.

sa·mar·i·um (Sm) (sā-mār′ē-ŭm). Samário; elemento metálico do grupo dos lantanídeos, de número atômico 62, peso atômico 150,36. [as faixas indicando a sua presença foram encontradas pela primeira vez no espectro da *samarskite*, um mineral assim designado em homenagem ao Col. von Samarski, oficial de minas russo do século XIX]

sam·bu·cus (sam-bū′kŭs). Sambuco; flores secas de *Sambucus canadensis* ou *S. nigra* (família Caprifoliaceae), o sabugueiro comum ou sabugueiro negro; discretamente laxativo. SIN elder, elder flowers. [L. sabugueiro]

sAMP Abreviatura de adenylosuccinic acid (ácido adenilossuccínico).

sam·ple (sam′pel). Amostra. **1.** Amostra de uma entidade global, pequena o suficiente para não ameaçar nem danificar o todo; alíquota. **2.** Subgrupo selecionado de uma população; uma amostra pode ser randômica ou não-randômica (aleatória), representativa ou não-representativa. [I.m. *ensample*, do L. *exemplum*, exemplo]

cluster s., a. de conjunto; cada unidade de amostragem é um grupo de indivíduos.

end-tidal s., a. corrente final; amostra do último gás expirado numa expiração normal, de preferência constituída apenas de gás alveolar.

Haldane-Priestley s., a. de Haldane-Priestley; aproximação do gás alveolar obtida do final de uma expiração máxima súbita num tubo de Haldane.

probability s., a. de probabilidade; cada indivíduo na amostra tem uma probabilidade conhecida e geralmente igual de ser selecionado.

proficiency s.'s, amostras de proficiência; amostras enviadas a um laboratório como amostras desconhecidas para a avaliação externa do desempenho do laboratório; prática freqüente como parte de programas de teste de proficiência para garantir que o laboratório está fornecendo resultados corretos. VER TAMBÉM proficiency *testing*.

Rahn-Otis s., a. de Rahn-Otis; aproximação do gás alveolar continuamente fornecido por um dispositivo simples que admite apenas a última parte de cada expiração.

random s., a. randômica; seleção ao acaso de indivíduos ou itens numa população para pesquisa; a seleção é feita de tal maneira que todos os membros presumivelmente têm a mesma chance de serem escolhidos.

stratified s., a. estratificada; subgrupo de uma população total, definido por algum critério objetivo, como idade ou ocupação.

sam·pling. Amostragem; processo de dedução do comportamento de um grupo ao estudar uma fração do conjunto. [MF essample, de L. exemplum, extração]

biological s., a. biológica; amostragem que pode ser extraída sem prejuízo do organismo integral (p. ex., para estudo hematológico ou bioquímico); devido à complexidade das amostras biológicas, admite-se, em geral, que a fonte da amostra seja completamente misturada e, portanto, representativa; essa pressuposição freqüentemente não é verdadeira, como, por exemplo, em estudos genéticos de pacientes mosaicos.

chemical s., a. química; amostra obtida por qualquer método conveniente e, em seguida, purificado de seus elementos irrelevantes antes da análise; a pressuposição de mistura completa não é necessária.

continuous interleaved s., a. interfoliada contínua; estratégia no processo de fala para implantes cocleares, em que são apresentados breves pulsos a cada eletrodo numa seqüência não-superposta.

haphazard s., a. acidental; reunião de dados de maneira não prescrita e não definida, que não permite nenhuma dedução científica lógica, a não ser o estabelecimento da existência de tipos. (O simples fato de encontrar um unicórnio num conjunto desse tipo estabeleceria que os unicórnios podem existir, porém nenhuma dedução poderia ser feita acerca de sua prevalência.) Cf. random *sample*.

random s., a. randômica; seleção de elementos de uma população, de modo que cada resultado possível seja independente de outros resultados possíveis, de modo que existe uma igual probabilidade de cada membro da população ser escolhido.

snowball s., a. em bola de neve; método através do qual os nomes de indivíduos para entrevista prospectiva para um estudo estatístico são obtidos de indivíduos que já foram entrevistados para o estudo.

Sanarelli, Giuseppe, bacteriologista italiano, 1865–1940. VER S. *phenomenon*; S.-Shwartzman *phenomenon*.

san·a·tive (san′a-tiv). Sanativo; que tem tendência a curar. [L. *sano*, curar, cicatrizar]

san·a·to·ri·um (san′ā-tōr′ē-ŭm). Sanatório; instituição para o tratamento de distúrbios crônicos e local para recuperação sob supervisão médica. Cf. sanitarium. [L. mod. neutro de *sanatorius*, curativo, de *sano*, curar, cicatrizar]

san·a·to·ry (san′a-tōr-ē). Sanativo; que confere saúde, que leva à saúde. [L. mod. *sanatorius*]

Sanchez Salorio, Manuel, oftalmologista espanhol, *1930. VER Sanchez Salorio *syndrome*.

sand. Areia; as finas partículas granulares de quartzo e outras rochas cristalinas ou material arenoso semelhante à areia. [A.S.]

brain s., a. cerebral. SIN corpora arenacea, em *corpus*.

hydatid s., a. hidática; os escóleces, cistos filhos, ganchos e corpúsculos calcários das tênias *Echinococcus* no líquido dentro de um cisto hidático primário ou filho.

intestinal s., a. intestinal; cálculos minúsculos ou material arenoso que ocorre nas fezes; é composta de sabões, pigmento biliar, colesterol, sais de magnésio, ácido succínico, etc.

urinary s., a. urinária; múltiplas partículas calculosas pequenas eliminadas na urina de pacientes com nefrolitíase; em geral, cada partícula é pequena demais para causar sintomas significativos ou para ser identificada como verdadeiro cálculo.

san·dal·wood oil (san′dăl-wood). Óleo de sândalo. SIN santal oil.

sand·fly (sand′flī). Mosquito-pólvora; pequeno díptero picador do gênero *Phlebotomus* ou *Lutzomyia;* vetor da leishmaniose.

Sandhoff K., bioquímico alemão contemporâneo. VER S. *disease*.

Sandison, J. Calvin, cirurgião norte-americano, *1899. VER S.-Clark *chamber*.

Sandström, I., anatomista sueco, 1852–1889. VER S. *bodies*, em *body*.

sand·worm (sand′werm). Qualquer um dos vários ancilóstomos do cão e do gato cujas larvas causam larva migrans cutânea.

sane (sān). São; que indica sanidade. [L. *sanus*]

Sanfilippo, Sylvester J., pediatra norte-americano do século XX. VER S. *syndrome*.

Sanger, Frederick, bioquímico inglês e duas vezes ganhador do Prêmio Nobel, *1918. VER S. *reagent, method*.

♻ **sangui-, sanguin-, sanguino-.** Sangui-, sanguin-, sanguíneo-. Sangue, sanguíneo. [G. *sanguis*]

san·gui·fa·cient (sang-gwi-fā′shent). Sanguifaciente. SIN hemopoietic [sangui- + L. *facio*, fazer]

san·guif·er·ous (sang-gwif′er-ŭs). Sanguífero; que contém ou transporta sangue. SIN circulatory (2). [sangui- + L. *fero*, carregar, transportar]

san·gui·fi·ca·tion (sang′gwi-fi-kā′shun). Sanguificação. SIN hemopoiesis. [sangui- + L. *facio*, fazer]

san·guin·a·rine (sang-gwi-nā′rēn). Sanguinarina; alcalóide obtido da planta *Sanguinaria canadensis*, utilizado no tratamento e remoção da placa dentária.

san·guine (sang′gwin). Sanguíneo. **1.** SIN plethoric. **2.** Antigamente, referia-se a um temperamento caracterizado por compleição clara, pulso cheio, boa digestão, aspecto otimista e temperamento ativo, porém não duradouro. SIN sanguineous (3). [L. *sanguineus*]

san·guin·e·ous (sang-gwin′ē-ŭs). Sanguíneo. **1.** Relativo ao sangue; sanguinolento. **2.** Pletórico. SIN plethoric. **3.** Sanguíneo. SIN sanguine (2). [L. *sanguineus*]

san·guin·o·lent (sang-gwin′ō-lent). Sanguinolento; misturado de sangue. [L. *sanguinolentus*]

san·gui·no·pu·ru·lent (sang′gwi-nō-poo′roo-lent). Sanguinopurulento; refere-se ao exsudato ou à matéria contendo sangue e pus. [sanguino- + L. *purulentus*, supurativo, de *pus*, pus]

San·gui·su·ga (sang-gwi-soo′gā). Nome antigo de *Hirudo*. [L. sanguessuga, de *sanguis*, sangue + *sugo*, pp. s*uctus;* sugar]

san·guiv·or·ous (sang-gwiv′er-ŭs). Sanguívoro; que suga sangue, aplicado a determinados morcegos, sanguessugas, insetos, etc. [sangui- + L. *voro*, devorar]

sa·ni·es (sā′nē-ēz). Sânie; corrimento purulento ralo e sanguinolento. [L.]

sa·ni·o·pu·ru·lent (sā′nē-ō-poo′roo-lent). Saniopurulento; caracterizado por pus sanguinolento. [L. *sanies*, matéria sanguinolenta rala + *purulentus*, supurativo, de *pus*, pus]

sa·ni·o·se·rous (sā′nē-ō-sēr′ŭs). Sanioseroso; caracterizado por soro tinto de sangue.

sa·ni·ous (sā′nē-ŭs). Sanioso; relativo a sânie; icoroso e tinto de sangue.

san·i·tar·i·an (san-i-tār′ē-an). Sanitarista; pessoa especializada em sanitarismo e saúde pública. [L. *sanitas*, saúde, de *sanus*, são]

san·i·tar·i·um (san-i-tār′ē-ŭm). Clínica; estância de saúde. Cf. sanatorium. SIN salutarium. [L. *sanitas*, saúde]

san·i·tary (san′i-tār-ē). Salutar; saudável; que conduz à saúde; referindo-se, em geral, a um ambiente limpo. [L. *sanitas*, saúde]

san·i·ta·tion (san-i-tā'shŭn). Saneamento; uso de medidas destinadas a promover a saúde e evitar a doença; desenvolvimento e estabelecimento de condições ambientais favoráveis à saúde. [L. *sanitas*, saúde]

san·i·ti·za·tion (san'i-ti-zā'shŭn). Sanitização; processo de tornar algo sanitário.

san·i·ty (san'i-tē). Sanidade; estado saudável da mente, das emoções e do comportamento; grau normal de saúde mental. [L. *sanitas*, saúde]

San Jose, Hermenia, patologista chileno do século XX. VER Maldonado-San Jose *stain*.

Sansom, Arthur E., médico inglês, 1839–1907. VER S. *sign*.

Sanson, Louis J., médico francês, 1790–1841. VER S. *images*, em *image*; Purkinje-S. *images*, em *image*.

san·tal oil (san'tăl). Óleo de sândalo; óleo volátil destilado da madeira do *Santalum album* (família Santalaceae), uma árvore da Índia; antigamente utilizado na bronquite subaguda e na gonorréia. SIN sandalwood oil.

san·to·nin (san'tō-nin). Santonina; anidrido interno ou lactona do ácido santonínico, obtido da santônica, os capítulos florais não abertos de *Artemisia cina* e de outras espécies de *Artemisia* (família Compositae); tem sido utilizada para a eliminação de nematódeos (*Ascaris lumbricoides*), bem como no tratamento da incontinência urinária. [G. *santonikon*, absinto]

Santorini, Giandomenico (Giovanni Domenico), anatomista italiano, 1681–1737. VER S. *canal, cartilage,* major *caruncle,* minor *caruncle, concha, duct, fissures,* em *fissure, incisures,* em *incisure, labyrinth, muscle, tubercle, vein; incisura* santorini.

sap. Seiva; suco ou líquido tecidual de um organismo vivo.
   cell s., s. celular; conteúdo dos vacúolos.
   nuclear s., s. nuclear. SIN karyolymph.

sa·phe·na (să-fē'nă). Safena. VER vein. [L. mod. atribuído por alguns como derivado do Ar. *safin*, ficar de pé; por outros, do G. *saphēnēs*, manifesto, claramente visível]

saph·e·nec·to·my (saf-ĕ-nek'tō-mē). Safenectomia; excisão de uma veia safena. [saphena + G. *ektomē*, excisão]

sa·phe·nous (să-fē'nŭs). Safeno; relativo ou associado a uma veia safena; indica algumas estruturas na perna. [ver saphena]

⚠ **sapo-, sapon-.** Sapo-, sapon-. Sabão. [L. *sapo*]

sap·o·gen·in (să-poj'ĕ-nin). Sapogenina; a aglicona de uma saponina; membro de uma família de esteróides do tipo espirostano (um 16,22:22,26-diepoxicolestano).

sap·o·na·ceous (sap-ō-nā'shŭs). Saponáceo; relativo ou semelhante a sabão.

sap·o·na·tus (sap-ō-nā'tŭs). Misturado com sabão. [L.]

sa·pon·i·fi·ca·tion (să-pon'i-fi-kā'shŭn). Saponificação; conversão em sabão, referindo-se à ação hidrolítica de um álcali sobre a gordura, especialmente sobre triacilgliceróis; em histoquímica, a saponificação é utilizada para desmetilar ou reverter o bloqueio de ácido carboxílico, permitindo, assim, a ocorrência de basofilia. [sapo- (*sapon-*) +L. *facio*, fazer]

sa·pon·i·fy (să-pon'i-fī). Saponificar; efetuar ou sofrer saponificação.

sap·o·nins (sap'ō-ninz). Saponinas; glicosídeos de origem vegetal, caracterizados pelas propriedades de formar espuma na água e provocar lise celular (como na hemólise, quando são injetadas saponinas na corrente sanguínea); surfactantes poderosos; muitas exibem atividade antibiótica.

Sappey, Marie P.C., anatomista francesa, 1810–1896. VER S. *fibers,* em *fiber, plexus, veins,* em *vein*.

sap·phism (saf'izm). Safismo. SIN lesbianism. [*Sapphō*, poetisa grega homossexual, rainha da ilha de Lesbos]

⚠ **sapr-.** Sapr-. VER sapro-.

sa·pre·mia (să-prē'mē-ă). Sapremia; termo obsoleto para septicemia. [sapr- + G. *haima*, sangue]

⚠ **sapro-, sapr-.** Sapro-, sapr-. Apodrecido, pútrido, decomposto. [G. *sapros*]

sap·robe (sap'rōb). Sapróbio; organismo que depende de matéria orgânica morta; esse termo é preferível a saprófita, visto que as bactérias e os fungos não são mais considerados vegetais. [sapro- + G. *bios*, vida]

sa·pro·bic (sap-rō'bik). Sapróbico; relativo a um sapróbio.

sap·ro·don·tia (sap-rō-don'shē-ă). Saprodontia. SIN dental *caries*. [sapro- + G. *odous*, dente]

sap·ro·gen (sap'rō-jen). Saprógeno; organismo que depende de matéria orgânica morta e que causa sua decomposição. [sapro- + G. *-gen,* que produz]

sap·ro·gen·ic, sa·prog·e·nous (sap-rō-jen'ik, să-proj'ĕ-nŭs). Saprogênico, saprógeno; que causa ou resulta de decomposição.

sa·proph·i·lous (să-prof'i-lŭs). Saprófilo; que cresce em matéria orgânica em decomposição. [sapro- + G. *philos*, amigo]

sap·ro·phyte (sap'rō-fīt). Saprófita; organismo que cresce em matéria orgânica morta, vegetal ou animal. VER saprobe. SIN necroparasite. [sapro- + G. *phyton*, planta]
   facultative s., s. facultativo; organismo, geralmente parasita, que ocasionalmente vive e cresce como saprófita.

sap·ro·phyt·ic (sap-rō-fit'ik). Saprofítico; relativo a saprófita.

sap·ro·zo·ic (sap-rō-zō'ik). Saprozóico; que vive em matéria orgânica em decomposição; refere-se especialmente a determinados protozoários. [sapro- + G. *zōikos*, relativo a animais]

sap·ro·zo·o·no·sis (sap'rō-zō-ō-nō'sis). Saprozoonose; zoonose cujo agente exige tanto um hospedeiro vertebrado quanto um reservatório não-animal (alimento, solo, planta) ou local de desenvolvimento para completar seu ciclo de vida; podem ser utilizados termos combinados, como saprometazoonoses, para infecções por trematódeos, quando as metacercárias se encistam em plantas, ou saprociclozoonoses para infestações por carrapatos, cujos agentes completam parte de seu ciclo de vida no solo. [sapro- + G. *zōon,* animal + *nosos,* doença]

SAR Abreviatura de scaffold-associated *regions* (regiões associadas a estrutura), em *region*.

Sar Abreviatura de sarcosine (sarcosina).

sar·al·a·sin ac·e·tate (sar-al'ă-sin). Acetato de saralasina; antagonista da angiotensina II utilizado no tratamento da hipertensão essencial.

α-sar·cin (sar'sin). α-sarcina; toxina fúngica que atua sobre a subunidade grande do rRNA e inativa o ribossoma.

Sar·ci·na (sar'si-nă). Gênero de bactérias imóveis e estritamente anaeróbicas (família Peptococcaceae) contendo cocos Gram-positivos, com 1,8–3,0 μm de diâmetro, que se dividem em três planos perpendiculares, produzindo grupos regulares de oito ou mais células; o metabolismo desses microrganismos quimiorganotróficos é fermentativo; existem espécies saprofíticas e parasitas facultativas; a espécie típica é S. *ventriculi*. [L. *sarcina*, porção, feixe, de *sarcio,* remendar]
   S. ventric'uli, espécie encontrada no solo, na lama, no conteúdo de estômago humano doente, conteúdo gástrico de coelho e cobaia e na superfície de sementes de cereais; trata-se da espécie típica do gênero S.

sar·cine (sar'sēn). Sarcina; termo obsoleto para hipoxantina.

⚠ **sarco-.** Sarco-. Forma combinante que indica substância muscular ou semelhança com carne. [G. *sarx (sark-),* carne]

sar·co·blast (sar'kō-blast). Sarcoblasto. SIN myoblast. [sarco- + G. *blastos,* germe]

Sar·co·cys·tis (sar-kō-sis'tis). Gênero de protozoário parasita, relacionado aos gêneros de esporozoários *Eimeria, Isospora* e *Toxoplasma,* incluído numa família distinta, Sarcocystidae, porém com os gêneros já citados na mesma subordem, Eimeriina, na subclasse Coccidia, classe Sporozoea e filo Apicomplexa. Os estágios teciduais do *Sarcocystis* são habitualmente observados como cistos cilíndricos ou fusiformes muitas vezes extremamente grandes (1 cm ou mais), de paredes espessas (tubos de Miescher), no músculo estriado de répteis, aves ou mamíferos. Os cistos são lisos, no camundongo, doméstico ou com espinhas radiais (citofâneros) em carneiros ou coelhos; o conteúdo pode ser compartimentalizado por septos. Os esporos de formas variáveis (corpúsculos de Rainey) provavelmente são células arredondadas periféricas (esporoblastos, citômeros), que se dividem para formar "esporos" maduros (bradizoítos), corpúsculos móveis quando liberados do cisto; foram descritos estágios sexuados em culturas de tecido. Esses parasitas são abundantes, mas raramente têm importância patogênica. Os seres humanos que ingerem carne contendo os sarcocistos maduros atuam como hospedeiros definitivos; foi relatada a ocorrência de febre, diarréia intensa, dor abdominal e perda de peso num pequeno número de hospedeiros imunocomprometidos. Quando seres humanos ingerem acidentalmente oocistos de fontes fecais de outros animais, os sarcocistos que se desenvolvem no músculo humano não parecem causar nenhuma resposta inflamatória. [sarco- + G. *kystis,* bexiga]
   S. bovih'ominis, SIN S. *hominis.*
   S. fusifor'mis, espécie encontrada no músculo estriado e cardíaco de bovinos e búfalos aquáticos.
   S. hom'inis, espécie atualmente reconhecida como causadora de uma infecção com dois hospedeiros, com o boi servindo como hospedeiro intermediário, fonte de cistos teciduais infecciosos para os seres humanos, que servem como hospedeiro final. Ocorrem gamogonia e esporogonia nas células da mucosa do intestino delgado humano; os bois tornam-se infectados a partir de fezes humanas contaminadas com esporocistos de S. *hominis.* SIN S. *bovih'ominis.*
   S. lindeman'ni, espécie descrita em raras ocasiões nos músculos estriado e cardíaco dos seres humanos, provavelmente como infecção causada por várias espécies, possivelmente de cães domésticos ou de outros hospedeiros finais, a partir dos quais os oocistos ou esporocistos infectantes são transmitidos para os seres humanos através da água ou de exposição direta; nesses casos, os seres humanos servem como hospedeiro intermediário, em vez de hospedeiro final.
   S. miescheria'na, espécie comum de distribuição mundial, encontrada no músculo estriado e cardíaco de porcos; trata-se da espécie típica do gênero S.
   S. suihom'inis, forma de S. em que os seres humanos servem como hospedeiro final, enquanto o porco atua como hospedeiro intermediário, a fonte de tecido infectado para os seres humanos. O ciclo de vida e a doença moderada

provocada seguem o padrão do *S. hominis,* embora a doença pareça ser algo mais patogênica. A infecção humana é disseminada, e sua ocorrência foi relatada na Europa, no Mediterrâneo, na África Ocidental, na Indonésia e na América do Sul.

S. tenel'la, espécie extremamente comum de distribuição mundial, encontrada no músculo estriado e cardíaco de ovinos e caprinos.

sar·co·cys·to·sis (sar'kō-sis-tō'sis). Sarcossistose; infecção por protozoários parasitas do gênero *Sarcocystis.*

sar·code (sar'kōd). Sarcode; termo de interesse histórico (1835), aplicado ao protoplasma de protozoários antes da criação do termo protoplasma. [sarco- + G. *eidos,* semelhança]

Sar·co·di·na (sar'kō-di'nă, -dē'nă). As amebas; subfilo de protozoários no filo Sarcomastigophora, em que os microrganismos possuem pseudópodes ou um fluxo protoplasmático locomotivo para o seu movimento. Inclui formas que possuem flagelos durante o desenvolvimento e formas com uma carapaça ou esqueleto interno ou externo e outras que carecem dessa estrutura; ocorre reprodução assexuada por fissão, enquanto a reprodução sexuada, quando presente, ocorre por gametas flagelados ou amebóides; a maioria das espécies é de vida livre. [L. mod. do G. *sarx,* carne]

sar·cog·lia (sar-kog'lē-ă). Sarcóglia; acúmulo de células do neurolema na placa terminal motora. [sarco- + G. *glia,* cola]

sar·coid (sar'koyd). Sarcóide. SIN sarcoidosis. [sarco- + G. *eidos,* semelhança]

Boeck s., s. de Boeck. SIN sarcoidosis.

Spiegler-Fendt s., s. de Spiegler-Fendt. SIN benign *lymphocytoma cutis.*

sar·coid·o·sis (sar-koy-dō'sis). Sarcoidose; doença granulomatosa sistêmica, de causa desconhecida, que acomete principalmente os pulmões, com consequente fibrose intersticial, mas que também afeta os linfonodos, a pele, o fígado, o baço, os olhos, as falanges e as glândulas parótidas; os granulomas são compostos de células epitelióides e células gigantes multinucleadas com pouca ou nenhuma necrose. SIN Besnier-Boeck-Schaumann disease, Besnier-Boeck-Schaumann syndrome, Boeck disease, Boeck sarcoid, sarcoid, Schaumann syndrome. [sarcoid + G. *-osis,* condição]

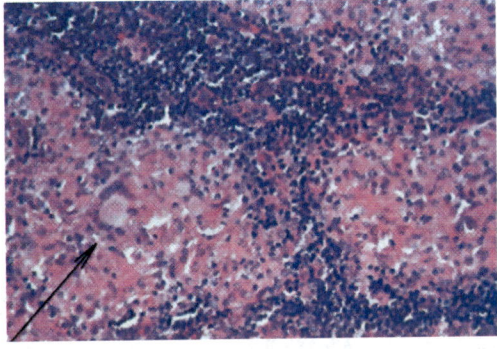

sarcoidose: corte microscópico de linfonodo mostrando grupos de células epitelióides e uma célula gigante solitária (seta)

hypercalcemic s., s. hipercalcêmica; sarcoidose com hipercalcemia de causa desconhecida, não necessariamente associada a comprometimento ósseo detectável pela sarcoidose.

sar·co·lem·ma (sar'kō-lem'ă). Sarcolema; membrana plasmática de uma fibra muscular; antigamente, para alguns, esse termo também se aplicava ao tecido conjuntivo delicado do endomísio. SIN myolemma. [sarco- + G. *lemma,* casca).

sar·co·lem·mal, sar·co·lem·mic, sar·co·lem·mous (sar'kō-lem'al, -lem'ik, -lem'ŭs). Sarcolêmico; relativo ao sarcolema.

sar·col·o·gy (sar-kol'ō-jē). Sarcologia. **1.** SIN myology. **2.** A anatomia das partes moles, distinta da osteologia. [sarco- + G. *logos,* estudo]

sar·co·ly·sine (sar-kō-li'sēn). Sarcolisina. SIN merphalan.

sar·co·ma (sar-kō'mă). Sarcoma; neoplasia do tecido conjuntivo, em geral extremamente maligna, formada pela proliferação de células mesodérmicas. [G. *sarkōma,* excrescência carnosa, de *sarx,* carne + *-oma,* tumor]

alveolar soft part s., s. alveolar de partes moles; tumor maligno formado por estroma reticular de tecido conjuntivo envolvendo agregados de grandes células redondas ou poligonais; ocorre em tecidos subcutâneos e fibromusculares.

ameloblastic s., s. ameloblástico. SIN ameloblastic *fibrosarcoma.*

angiolithic s., s. angiolítico; termo obsoleto para psammomatores *meningioma* (meningioma psammatoso).

avian s., s. aviário. SIN Rous s.

botryoid s., s. botrióide; forma polipóide de rabdomiossarcoma embrionário que ocorre em crianças, mais freqüentemente nas vias urogenitais, caracterizado pela formação de agregados de tecido neoplásico macroscopicamente aparentes e semelhantes a cachos de uva, que consistem em rabdomioblastos e células fusiformes e estreladas num estroma mixomatoso; as neoplasias desse tipo crescem com relativa rapidez e são extremamente malignas.

endometrial stromal s., s. do estroma endometrial; termo algumas vezes utilizado para referir-se a um sarcoma relativamente raro, que se acredita seja uma forma de endometriose, em que as lesões formam múltiplos focos no miométrio e em espaços vasculares em outros locais e que consistem em elementos histológicos e citológicos que se assemelham àqueles do estroma do endométrio.

Ewing s., s. de Ewing. SIN Ewing *tumor.*

fascicular s., s. fascicular. SIN spindle cell s.

giant cell s., s. de células gigantes; tumor maligno de células gigantes do osso.

giant cell monstrocellular s. of Zülch, s. monstrocelular de células gigantes de Zülch. SIN giant cell *glioblastoma multifome.*

granulocytic s., s. granulocítico; tumor maligno de células mielóides imaturas, freqüentemente subperiósteo, associado à leucemia granulocítica ou que a precede. VER TAMBÉM chloroma. SIN myeloid s.

immunoblastic s., s. imunoblástico; termo obsoleto para immunoblastic *lymphoma.*

Jensen s., s. de Jensen; tumor de camundongo transmissível por inoculação.

juxtacortical osteogenic s., s. osteogênico justacortical; forma de sarcoma osteogênico de malignidade relativamente baixa, que, provavelmente, se origina do periósteo e, no início, acomete o osso cortical e tecido conjuntivo adjacente; ocorre em adultos de meia-idade, bem como em adultos jovens, afetando mais comumente a parte inferior da diáfise do fêmur. SIN periosteal s.

Kaposi s., s. de Kaposi; neoplasia maligna multifocal de tecido vasoformador primitivo, que ocorre na pele e, algumas vezes, em linfonodos ou vísceras; consiste em células fusiformes e pequenos espaços vasculares irregulares freqüentemente infiltrados por macrófagos pigmentados por hemossiderina e eritrócitos extravasados; clinicamente, manifesta-se por lesões cutâneas, que consistem em máculas, placas ou nódulos cuja cor varia de púrpura-avermelhado a azul-escuro; observado mais comumente em homens acima de 60 anos de idade e em pacientes com AIDS/SIDA como doença oportunista associada à infecção pelo herpes vírus humano 8. SIN multiple idiopathic hemorrhagic s.

leukocytic s., s. leucocítico. SIN leukemia.

lymphatic s., s. linfático; termo obsoleto para lymphosarcoma.

medullary s., s. medular; sarcoma de consistência mole e extremamente vascular.

multiple idiopathic hemorrhagic s., s. hemorrágico idiopático múltiplo. SIN Kaposi s.

myelogenic s., s. mielogênico; sarcoma que se origina na medula óssea.

myeloid s., s. mielóide. SIN granulocytic s.

osteogenic s., s. osteogênico; o mais comum e maligno dos sarcomas ósseos, originário de células formadoras de osso e afetando principalmente as extremidades dos ossos longos; sua maior incidência é observada entre os 10 e 25 anos de idade. SIN osteosarcoma.

periosteal s., s. osteogênico justacortical. SIN juxtacortical osteogenic s.

reticulum cell s., s. de células reticulares; termo obsoleto para histiocytic *lymphoma* (linfoma histiocítico).

round cell s., s. de células redondas; termo obsoleto para uma neoplasia maligna indiferenciada, supostamente de origem mesenquimatosa, composta sobretudo de células redondas densamente agrupadas.

Rous s., s. de Rous; fibrossarcoma, originalmente observado numa galinha Plymouth Rock; atualmente considerado como expressão de infecção por certos vírus do complexo leucose–sarcoma aviário na família Retroviridae. SIN avian s., Rous tumor.

spindle cell s., s. de células fusiformes; neoplasia maligna de origem mesenquimatosa, composta de células alongadas e fusiformes. SIN fascicular s.

synovial s., s. sinovial; tumor maligno raro, de origem sinovial, que acomete mais comumente a articulação do joelho; composto de células fusiformes que, geralmente, envolvem fendas ou espaços pseudoglandulares que podem ser revestidos por células epiteliformes dispostas radialmente.

telangiectatic osteogenic s., s. osteogênico telangiectásico; variante cística lítica do sarcoma osteogênico, composta de espaços aneurismáticos cheios de sangue, revestidos por células do sarcoma que produzem osteóide.

Sar·co·mas·ti·goph·o·ra (sar'kō-mas-ti-gof'ō-ră). Filo do sub-reino Protozoa, caracterizado por flagelos, pseudópodes ou ambos os tipos de organelas locomotoras; inclui tanto os flagelados (subfilo Mastigophora) quanto as amebas (subfilo Sarcodina) num único grande grupo. [sarco- + G. *mastix (mastig-),* chicote + *phoros,* carregar]

sar·co·ma·toid (sar-kō'mă-toyd). Sarcomatóide; semelhante a um sarcoma. [sarcoma + G. *eidos,* semelhança]

sar·co·ma·to·sis (sar'kō-mă-tō'sis). Sarcomatose; ocorrência de várias proliferações sarcomatosas em diferentes partes do corpo. [sarcoma + G. *-osis*, condição]

sar·com·a·tous (sar-kō'mă-tŭs). Sarcomatoso; relativo a ou da natureza do sarcoma.

sar·co·mere (sar'kō-mēr). Sarcômero; o segmento de uma miofibrila entre duas linhas Z adjacentes, representando a unidade funcional do músculo estriado. [sarco- + G. *meros*, parte]

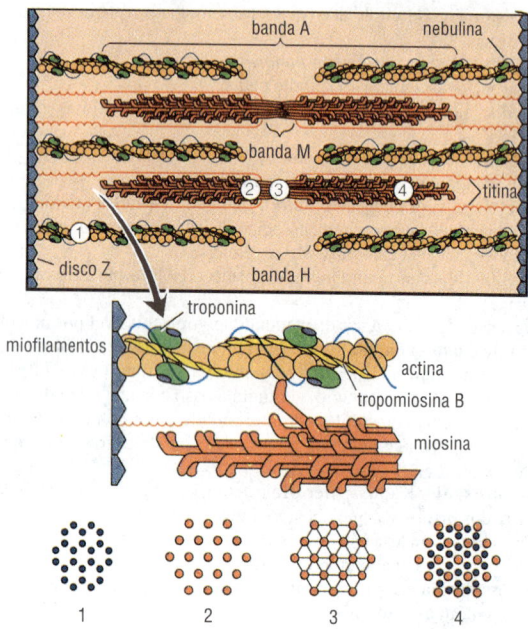

sarcômero: estrutura molecular; cada filamento espesso é circundado por uma série hexagonal de filamentos delgados

sar·co·neme (sar'kō-nēm). Sarconema. SIN microneme. [sarco- + G. *nēma*, filamento]

sar·co·plasm (sar'kō-plazm). Sarcoplasma; o citoplasma não-fibrilar de uma fibra muscular. [sarco- + G. *plasma*, algo formado]

sar·co·plas·mic (sar-kō-plaz'mik). Sarcoplásmico, sarcoplasmático; relativo ao sarcoplasma.

sar·co·plast (sar'kō-plast). Sarcoplasto. SIN satellite cell of skeletal muscle. [sarco- + G. *plastos*, formado]

sar·co·poi·et·ic (sar'kō-poy-et'ik). Sarcopoético; formador de músculo. [sarco- + G. *poiēsis*, fazer]

Sar·cop·syl·la pen·e·trans (sar-kō-sil'ă pen'ĕ-tranz). SIN *Tunga penetrans.*

Sar·cop·syl·li·dae (sar-kop-sil'li-dē). Nome antigo de Tungidae. [sarco- + G. *psylla*, pulga]

Sar·cop·tes sca·bi·ei (sar-kop'tēz skā'bē-ī). Antigamente *Acarus scabiei*, o ácaro do prurido, cujas variedades encontram-se distribuídas por todo o mundo, afetando seres humanos, cavalos, bois, porcos, carneiros, cães, gatos e muitos animais selvagens; as infecções graves e fatais não são raras em animais não tratados. Embora sejam considerados como pertencentes a uma única espécie, não se transmitem facilmente de um hospedeiro para outro de uma espécie animal diferente; entretanto, ocorrem infecções transitórias desse tipo, especialmente de vários animais para o homem, sendo a transmissão por contato direto. O ácaro escava a pele e deposita seus ovos no sulco; ocorrem prurido intenso e exantema próximo à escavação em cerca de um mês. VER scabies, mange. [sarco- + G. *koptō*, cortar; L. *scabies*, descamação]

sar·cop·tic (sar-kop'tik). Sarcóptico; relativo a, ou causado por, ácaros do gênero *Sarcoptes* ou por outros membros da família Sarcoptidae.

sar·cop·tid (sar-kop'tid). Sarcoptídeo; nome comum para designar membros da Sarcoptidae, uma família de ácaros que inclui os gêneros *Sarcoptes*, *Knemidokoptes* e *Notoedres.*

sar·co·sine (Sar) (sar'kō-sēn). Sarcosina; *N*-metilglicina; um intermediário no metabolismo da colina; pode doar um grupamento metil para o tetraidrofolato, produzindo N^5,N^{10}-metilenotetraidrofolato; a desmetilação pela sarcosina desidrogenase produz formaldeído, glicina e um aceptor reduzido; presença de níveis elevados em certos distúrbios hereditários.

s. dehydrogenase, s. desidrogenase; enzima que cliva a sarcosina utilizando algum aceptor para produzir glicina, formaldeído e uma molécula aceptora reduzida; a deficiência dessa enzima resulta em sarcosinemia.

sar·co·si·ne·mia (sar'kō-si-nē'mē-ă). [MIM* 268900]. Sarcosinemia; distúrbio do metabolismo dos aminoácidos, devido à deficiência de sarcosina desidrogenase, causando elevação dos níveis plasmáticos de sarcosina e sua excreção na urina; alguns lactentes afetados apresentam deficiência do desenvolvimento, são irritáveis, podem apresentar tremores musculares e exibem retardo do desenvolvimento motor e mental; herança autossômica recessiva. SIN hypersarcosinemia.

sar·co·sis (sar-kō'sis). Sarcose. **1.** Aumento anormal de carne. **2.** Crescimento múltiplo de tumores carnosos. **3.** Sarcoma difuso que acomete todo um órgão. [G. *sarkōsis*, crescimento de carne, de *sarx*, carne]

sar·co·some (sar'kō-sōm). Sarcossoma. **1.** Antigamente, qualquer grânulo numa fibra muscular. **2.** Atualmente, termo algumas vezes utilizado como sinônimo de miomitocôndria. [sarco- + G. *soma*, corpo]

sar·cos·to·sis (sar-kos-tō'sis). Sarcostose; ossificação do tecido muscular. [sarco- + G. *osteon*, osso + *-osis*, condição]

sar·cot·ic (sar-kot'ik). Sarcótico. **1.** Relativo à sarcose. **2.** Que causa aumento carnoso.

sar·co·trip·sy (sar'kō-trip-sē). Sarcotripsia; termo raramente empregado para referir-se ao uso de pinças compressoras para interromper a hemorragia. [sarco- + G. *tripsis*, atrito]

sar·co·tu·bules (sar-kō-too'boolz). Sarcotúbulos; o sistema contínuo de túbulos membranosos no músculo estriado, que corresponde ao retículo endoplasmático liso de outras células.

sar·cous (sar'kŭs). Sarcoso; relativo ao tecido muscular; carnoso. [G. *sarx*, carne]

sar·don·ic grin (sar-don'ik). Riso sardônico. SIN risus caninus.

sargramostim (sar-gra-mos'tim). Sargramostima; fator de estimulação de colônias de granulócitos-macrófagos (FEC-GM) humano recombinante; utilizada para proteger o indivíduo contra a infecção na leucemia mielógena aguda e em transplantes de medula óssea.

sa·rin (zah-rēn'). Sarina; veneno nervoso semelhante ao diisopropril fluorofosfato e tetraetil pirofosfato; inibidor muito potente e irreversível da colinesterase, e gás nervoso mais tóxico do que o tabun ou soman. [Ger.]

sar·mas·sa·tion (sar-mă-sā'shŭn). Compressão, massagem ou carícia erótica dos tecidos e órgãos femininos. [G. *sarx*, carne, + *massō*, amassar]

sar·sa·pa·ril·la (sar'să-per-il'ă, sas-per-il'ă). Salsaparrilha; a raiz seca de *Smilax aristolochiaefolia* (salsaparrilha mexicana), *S. regelii* (salsaparrilha hondurenha), *S. febrifuga* (salsaparrilha equatoriana) ou de espécies indeterminadas de *Smilax* (família Liliaceae), um arbusto espinhoso amplamente distribuído em todas as regiões tropicais e semitropicais; tem sido utilizada no tratamento da psoríase, gota, reumatismo e sífilis, sendo a usada popularmente como "purificador do sangue". [Esp. *zarza*, arbusto espinhoso]

SART Abreviatura de sinoatrial recovery *time* (tempo de recuperação sinoatrial).

sar·to·ri·us (sar-tōr'ē-ŭs). Sartório. VER sartorius (*muscle*). [L. *sartor*, alfaiate, sendo o músculo utilizado ao cruzar as pernas na posição do alfaiate, de *sarcio* pp. *sartus*, remendar]

Sartwell, Philip, epidemiologista norte-americano, *1908. VER S. incubation *model.*

sas·sa·fras (sas'ă-fras). Sassafrás; a casca seca da raiz de *Sassafras albidum* (família Lauraceae), uma árvore do leste dos Estados Unidos; agente aromatizante, diurético e diaforético; óleo de sassafrás, um óleo volátil obtido por destilação da casca de *S. albidum* e *S. variifolium*, utilizado como agente carminativo, anti-séptico tópico, pediculicida e aromatizante.

sat. Abreviatura de saturated ou saturation (saturado ou saturação), como em O_2 sat (sat. O_2).

sat·el·lite (sat'ĕ-līt). Satélite. **1.** Pequena estrutura que acompanha outra mais importante ou maior; p. ex., uma veia que acompanha uma artéria, ou uma lesão pequena ou secundária adjacente a uma maior. **2.** Membro posterior de um par de gametócitos gregarinos na sizígia, vários dos quais podem ser encontrados em algumas espécies. VER TAMBÉM primite. [L. *satelles* (*sattelit-*), acompanhante]

chromosome s., cromossoma satélite; pequeno segmento cromossômico separado do corpo principal do cromossoma por uma constrição secundária; nos seres humanos, está habitualmente associado ao braço curto de um cromossoma acrocêntrico.

perineuronal s., s. perineuronal; célula da oligodendróglia que circunda o neurônio.

sat·el·lit·o·sis (sat'ĕ-li-tō'sis). Satelitose. **1.** Condição caracterizada pelo acúmulo de células da neuróglia ao redor dos neurônios do sistema nervoso central. **2.** Presença de lesões satélites ou estruturas menores, como, por exemplo, melanoma metastático na pele adjacente ao tumor primário ou linfócitos em contato com um ceratinócito lesado na reação aguda de enxerto cutâneo *versus* hospedeiro. [L. *satelles* (*satellit-*), acompanhante +G. *-ōsis*, condição]

sa·ti·a·tion (sā-shē-ā'shŭn). Saciedade; o estado produzido pela satisfação de uma necessidade específica, como fome ou sede. [L. *satio*, pp. *-atus*, preencher, satisfazer]

sat. sol., sat. soln. Abreviatura de saturated *solution* (solução saturada).
Sattler, Hubert, oftalmologista austríaco, 1844–1928. VER S. elastic *layer, veil.*
sat·u·rate (satch′ŭ - rāt). Saturar. **1.** Impregnar inteiramente. **2.** Neutralizar; preencher todas as afinidades químicas de uma substância (como ao converter todas as ligações duplas em ligações simples). **3.** Dissolver uma substância até uma concentração além da qual a adição de mais substância resulta em duas fases. [L. *saturo,* pp. *-atus,* preencher, de *satur,* saciado]
sat·u·ra·tion (satch - ŭ - rā′shŭn). Saturação. **1.** Impregnação de uma substância por outra na maior extensão possível. **2.** Neutralização, como a de um ácido por um álcali. **3.** A concentração de uma substância dissolvida que não pode ser excedida. **4.** Em óptica, ver saturated *color.* **5.** Preenchimento de todos os locais disponíveis de uma molécula de enzima por seu substrato ou de uma molécula de hemoglobina por oxigênio (símbolo S_{O_2}) ou monóxido de carbono (símbolo S_{CO}). [L. *saturatio,* de *saturo,* preencher, de *satis,* suficiente]
   secondary s., s. secundária; técnica de anestesia com óxido nitroso que consiste na suspensão abrupta do oxigênio na mistura inalada para produzir um plano profundo de anestesia, após o que o oxigênio é administrado para corrigir a hipoxia.
sat·ur·nine (sat′er - nīn). Saturnino. **1.** Relativo a um chumbo. **2.** Devido a ou sintomático da intoxicação por chumbo. [L. mediev. *saturninus,* saturninos, de *saturnus,* chumbo, do L. *saturnus,* o deus e planeta Saturno]
sat·urn·ism (sat′er-nizm). Saturnismo. SIN lead *poisoning.* [L. mediev. *saturnus,* termo utilizado pelos alquimistas para o chumbo]
sat·y·ri·a·sis (sat - i - rī′ā - sis). Satiríase; satiromania, satirismo; excitação e comportamento sexuais excessivos no homem, o equivalente da ninfomania na mulher. SIN satyriasis. [G. *satyros,* sátiro]
sat·y·rism (sat′i-rizm). Satirismo. SIN satyriasis.
sau·cer·i·za·tion (saw′ser - i - zā′shŭn). Craterização; escavação de tecido para formar uma depressão superficial, efetuada no tratamento de feridas para facilitar a drenagem de áreas infectadas. SIN craterization.
Saundby, Robert, médico inglês, 1849–1918. VER S. *test.*
sau·ri·a·sis (saw - rī′ā - sis). Ictiose. SIN ichthyosis. [G. *sauros,* lagarto + *-iasis,* condição]
Savage, Henry, anatomista e ginecologista inglês, 1810–1900. VER S. perineal *body.*
saw. Serra; instrumento de metal utilizado em operação que possui uma borda de projeções pontiagudas e semelhantes a dentes, para secção de osso, cartilagem ou gesso; as bordas podem ser fixadas a uma faixa rígida, fio ou corrente flexível ou a um oscilador motorizado. [A.S. *saga*]
   Gigli s., s. de Gigli; serra de arame manual para uso em craniotomia.
   Stryker s., s. de Stryker; serra de oscilação rápida, utilizada para cortar osso ou aparelhos de gesso; corta material duro, mas os tecidos moles cedem e, portanto, não são lesados.
sax·i·tox·in (sak-si-tok′sin). Saxitoxina; neurotoxina potente encontrada em moluscos, como o mexilhão ou marisco, produzida pelo dinoflagelado *Gonyaulax catenella,* que é ingerido pelo molusco; responsável por casos de envenenamento em conseqüência da ingestão de mexilhão da Califórnia (*Mytilus californianus*), vieiras e marisco do Alasca (*Saxidomus giganteus*).
Sayre, George P., oftalmologista norte-americano, *1911. VER Kearns-S. *syndrome.*
Sb Símbolo do antimony (antimônio).
SBE Abreviatura de subacute bacterial *endocarditis* (endocardite bacteriana subaguda).
SBS Abreviatura de shaken baby *syndrome* (síndrome do bebê sacudido).
Sc Símbolo do scandium (escândio).
s.c. Abreviatura de subcutaneous (subcutâneo); subcutaneously (por via subcutânea).
scab (skab). Casca ou crosta de ferida; crosta formada pela coagulação do sangue, pus, soro ou uma combinação desses elementos na superfície de uma úlcera, erosão ou outro tipo de ferida. [A.S. *scaeb*]
scab·i·ci·dal (skā - bi - sī′dăl). Escabicida; que destrói os ácaros causadores da sarna.
scab·i·cide (skā′bi - sīd). Escabicida; agente letal para os ácaros causadores da sarna.
sca·bies (skā′bēz). Escabiose, sarna. **1.** Erupção causada pelo ácaro *Sarcoptes scabiei* var. *hominis;* a fêmea escava a pele, produzindo uma erupção vesicular com intenso prurido entre os dedos das mãos, na genitália masculina ou feminina, nas nádegas e em outras partes do tronco e dos membros. **2.** Em animais, o termo escabiose ou sarna é habitualmente aplicado à acaríase cutânea em ovinos, que pode ser causada por *Sarcoptes, Psoroptes* ou *Chorioptes.* [L. *scabo,* coçar]
   crusted s., e. crostosa, e. norueguesa. SIN Norwegian's.
   Norwegian s., e. norueguesa; forma grave de escabiose com presença de inúmeros ácaros no estrato córneo espessado; tem sido associada a deficiência imune celular, incluindo AIDS/SIDA. SIN crusted s., Norway itch.
sca·brit·i·es (skā - brish′i - ēz). Escabrícia; estado rugoso da pele. [L. de *scaber,* escamoso]
   s. un′guium, escabrícia ungueal; espessamento e deformação das unhas.
sca·la, pl. **sca·lae** (skā′lă, -lē). Escala, rampa; uma das cavidades da cóclea, tornando-se espiralada ao redor do modíolo. [L. *escada*]
   Löwenberg s., escala de Löwenberg. SIN cochlear *duct.*
   s. me′dia, ducto coclear. SIN cochlear *duct.*
   s. tym′pani [TA], rampa do tímpano; a divisão do canal espiral da cóclea situada no lado basal da lâmina espiral.
   s. vestib′uli [TA], rampa do vestíbulo; a divisão do canal espiral da cóclea situada no lado apical da lâmina espiral e membrana vestibular. SIN vestibular canal.
scald (skawld). **1.** Escaldar; queimar por contato com vapor ou líquido quente. **2.** Escaldadura, escaldo; lesão resultante desse contato. [L. *excaldo,* lavar com água quente]
scald·ing (skawl′ding). Ardência; dor em queimação durante a micção.
scale (skāl). **1.** Escala; teste padronizado para medir características psicológicas, da personalidade ou do comportamento. VER TAMBÉM score, test. **2.** Escama. SIN squama. **3.** crosta; pequena placa fina de epitélio córneo, semelhante às escamas de peixe, retirada da pele. **4.** Descamar. **5.** Raspar; remover tártaro dos dentes. **6.** Escala; dispositivo através do qual se mede alguma propriedade. [L. *scala,* escada]
   absolute s., escala absoluta; termo obsoleto para Kelvin s. (e. de Kelvin).
   activities of daily living s., escala de atividades da vida diária; escala para avaliar a atividade física e suas limitações, baseada em respostas a perguntas simples relativas à locomoção, cuidados pessoais, capacidade de se arrumar, etc; amplamente utilizada em geriatria, reumatologia, etc.
   adaptive behavior s.'s, escalas de comportamento adaptativo; dispositivo de avaliação comportamental para quantificar os níveis de habilidades de indivíduos com retardo mental e retardo do desenvolvimento em sua interação com o ambiente; consiste em três fatores relacionados de desenvolvimento: (1) auto-suficiência pessoal, como, por exemplo, comer, vestir-se; (2) auto-suficiência comunitária, como, por exemplo, fazer compras, comunicar-se; (3) responsabilidade pessoal e social, como, por exemplo, uso de tempo de lazer, desempenho no trabalho. VER intelligence.
   Ångström s., escala de Ångström; tabela de comprimentos de onda de grande número de raios luminosos correspondendo a um igual número de linhas de Fraunhofer no espectro.
   Baumé s., escala de Baumé; escala hidrométrica para determinar a densidade de líquidos mais pesados e mais leves do que a água, respectivamente: para líquidos mais leves do que a água, dividir 140 por 130 mais o grau de Baumé; para os líquidos mais pesados do que a água, dividir 145 por 145 menos o grau de Baumé.
   Bayley s.'s of Infant Development, escalas de Bayley de desenvolvimento de lactentes; teste psicológico utilizado para medir o progresso do desenvolvimento de lactentes durante os primeiros dois anos e meio de vida; consiste em três escalas: registro mental, motor e comportamental.
   Binet s., escala de Binet; medida da inteligência tanto para crianças quanto para adultos.
   Binet-Simon s., escala de Binet-Simon; precursora dos testes de inteligência individual, sobretudo a escala de inteligência de Stanford-Binet; algumas vezes denominada escala de Binet.
   Brazelton Neonatal Behavioral Assessment s.'s, escalas de avaliação do comportamento neonatal de Brazelton; escala utilizada por obstetras, pediatras e psicólogos pediatras para avaliar o desenvolvimento sensorial, motor, emocional e físico do recém-nascido, geralmente aplicada ao nascimento ou no primeiro mês de vida.
   Cattell Infant Intelligence S., escala de inteligência do lactente de Cattell; escala padronizada para avaliação do desenvolvimento cognitivo de lactentes entre 3 e 30 meses de idade.
   Celsius s., escala de Celsius; escala de temperatura baseada no ponto triplo da água (definido como 273,16 K), ao qual se atribui o valor de 0,01°C; substituiu a escala centígrada, visto que o ponto triplo da água pode ser medido com mais acurácia do que o ponto de congelamento, embora, para fins práticos, as duas escalas sejam equivalentes.
   centigrade s., escala centígrada; escala de termômetro na qual existem 100 graus entre o ponto de congelamento da água (ao qual se atribui o valor de 0,0°C) e o ponto de ebulição da água a nível do mar; tecnicamente suplantada pela escala de Celsius. Cf. Celsius s.
   Charrière s., escala de Charrière. SIN French s.
   Columbia Mental Maturity S., escala de maturidade mental de Colúmbia; teste de inteligência, administrado individualmente, que fornece uma estimativa da capacidade intelectual de crianças; estipula idades mentais que variam de 3–12 anos e não exige resposta verbal, com resposta motora mínima. [Columbia University, NY]
   coma s., escala de coma, escala clínica para avaliar o comprometimento da consciência; a avaliação pode incluir a responsividade motora, o desempenho verbal e a abertura dos olhos, como na escala de coma de Glasgow (Escócia), ou os mesmos três itens e disfunção dos nervos cranianos, como na escala de coma de Maryland (Estados Unidos).

scale · scalpel

escala de coma de Glasgow		
desempenho monitorado	**reação**	**escore**
abertura dos olhos	espontânea	4
	abertos em resposta à voz	3
	abertos em resposta à dor	2
	nenhuma reação	1
desempenho verbal	coerente	5
	confuso, desorientado	4
	palavras desconexas	3
	sons incompreensíveis	2
	nenhuma reação verbal	1
resposta motora	obedece a instruções	6
	evita a dor	5
	movimento motor grande	4
	sinergismo flexor	3
	sinergismo extensor	2
	nenhuma reação	1

digital gray s., latitude. SIN latitude.
expanded disability status s. (EDSS), escala expandida do estado de incapacidade; sistema de avaliação comumente utilizado para estimar o grau de comprometimento neurológico na esclerose múltipla com base nos achados neurológicos, e não nos sintomas; ao todo, existem 10 graus, em etapas e meias etapas (p. ex., 4, 4,5, 5), em que o "1" indica neurologicamente normal, e o "10", morte. SIN Kurtzke multiple sclerosis disability s.
Fahrenheit s., e. Fahrenheit; escala de termômetro na qual o ponto de congelamento da água é de 32° F, e o ponto de ebulição, de 212°F; 0°F indica a menor temperatura Fahrenheit que se poderia obter pela mistura de gelo e sal em 1.724; °C = 5/9(°F − 32).
French s. (F), escala francesa; escala para graduar os tamanhos de sondas, tubos e cateteres, com base num diâmetro de 1/3 mm igual a 1 F na escala (p. ex., 3 F = 1 mm); a graduação da escala é feita utilizando uma placa de metal com orifícios cujo diâmetro varia de 1/3 mm a 1 cm. SIN Charrière s.
Gaffky s., e. de Gaffky. SIN Gaffky *table*.
gray s., latitude. SIN latitude. VER gray-scale *ultrasonography*.
Guttman s., escala de Guttman; escala de medida que avalia as categorias de resposta a uma pergunta, em que cada unidade representa uma expressão cada vez mais forte de um atributo, como dor ou incapacidade.
Hamilton anxiety rating s., escala de graduação da ansiedade de Hamilton; lista de sintomas específicos utilizada como medida da intensidade da ansiedade.
Hamilton depression rating s., escala de graduação da depressão de Hamilton, lista de sintomas específicos utilizada como medida da intensidade da depressão.
hardness s., escala de dureza; escala qualitativa em que os minerais são classificados por ordem de sua dureza crescente, com base no fato de que o mais duro de dois materiais riscará o mais mole e não será riscado por ele. A escala relaciona 15 substâncias: 1, talco; 2, gesso; 3, calcita; 4, fluorita; 5, apatita; 6, ortoclase, periclase; 7, sílica pura vítrea; 8, quartzo, estelite; 9, topázio; 10, granada; 11, carboreto de tântulo, zircônio fundido; 12, alumínio fundido; 13, carboreto de silício; 14, carboreto de bório; 15, diamante. SIN Mohs s.
homigrade s., escala homígrada; escala de termômetro especial em que 100° indicam a temperatura normal do homem (98,6°F, 37°C), 0° indica o ponto de congelamento e 270°, o ponto de ebulição da água.
interval s., escala de intervalo; à semelhança de uma escala de temperatura em unidades centígrados ou Fahrenheit, trata-se de uma escala em que os intervalos são iguais, mas cujo ponto zero é arbitrário; p. ex., os valores do quociente de inteligência são valores ao longo de uma escala de intervalo.
Karnofsky s., escala de Karnofsky; escala de desempenho para avaliar as atividades habituais de uma pessoa; utilizada para avaliar o progresso do paciente após procedimento terapêutico.
Kelvin s., escala de Kelvin; escala de temperatura na qual se atribui ao ponto triplo da água o valor de 273,16 K; °C = K − 273,15.
Kurtzke multiple sclerosis disability s., escala de incapacidade de Kurtzke para esclerose múltipla. SIN expanded disability status s.
Leiter International Performance S., escala de desempenho internacional de Leiter; teste não-verbal (de desempenho) para medir a inteligência, que contém normas para cada idade entre 2 e 18 anos; originalmente desenvolvida como método de avaliação das capacidades intelectuais comparativas de crianças caucasianas, chinesas e japonesas; todavia, hoje em dia é algumas vezes utilizada para avaliar pessoas com aprendizado lento e pessoas cegas, surdas ou com déficit verbal.

Likert s., escala de Likert; escala ordinal de respostas a uma questão ou declaração, disposta em seqüência hierárquica do fortemente negativo para o fortemente positivo. Utilizada principalmente na ciência comportamental e em psiquiatria.
masculinity-femininity s., escala de masculinidade–feminilidade; qualquer escala, num teste psicológico, que avalia a masculinidade ou feminilidade relativa de um indivíduo; as escalas variam e podem concentrar-se, p. ex., na identificação básica com um dos sexos ou na preferência por determinado papel sexual.
Mohs s., escala de Mohs. SIN hardness s.
ordinal s., escala ordinal; escala baseada na classificação de pessoas ou coisas em categorias qualitativas, como estados socioeconômico.
pH s., escala de pH. SIN Sörensen s.
Rahe-Holmes social readjustment rating s., escala de graduação de reajuste social de Rahe-Holmes; escala amplamente utilizada na ciência social e do comportamento que atribui valores a acontecimentos significativos da vida, como casamento, nascimento de filhos, perdas, perda do emprego; esses eventos correlacionam-se a estados emocionais.
Rankin s., escala de Rankine; escala de termômetro em que cada grau Rankine (°Rank) é igual ao Fahrenheit, porém aplicado à escala de temperatura absoluta, com seu ponto zero no zero absoluto; °Rank = °F + 459,67.
ratio s., escala-razão; escala que envolve unidades físicas e demonstra suas relações.
Réaumur s., escala de Réaumur; escala de termômetro em que grau Réaumur (°R) corresponde a 1/80 da diferença de temperatura entre o ponto de congelamento e o ponto de ebulição da água pura a 1 atm, estando o 0°R no ponto de congelamento, enquanto 80°R corresponde ao ponto de ebulição da água.
Shipley-Hartford s., escala de Shipley-Hartford; teste de aptidão intelectual e conceitual. [*Hartford* Retreat, CT, onde Shipley trabalhava]
Sörensen s., escala de Sörensen; logaritmo negativo da concentração de íons hidrogênio, utilizada como escala para expressar a acidez e alcalinidade. VER TAMBÉM pH. SIN pH s.
Stanford-Binet intelligence s., escala de inteligência de Stanford-Binet; teste padronizado para a medida da inteligência, que consiste numa série de perguntas, graduadas de acordo com a inteligência de crianças normais em diferentes idades, cujas respostas indicam a idade mental da pessoa testada; basicamente utilizada em crianças; todavia, contém também normas para adultos, padronizadas contra faixas etárias de adultos, e não contra as de crianças, como ocorria antigamente. SIN Binet test.
Wechsler-Bellevue s., escala de Wechsler-Bellevue; medida de inteligência geral substituída pela escala de inteligência do adulto de Wechsler e sua revisão subseqüente. VER TAMBÉM Wechsler intelligence s.'s.
Wechsler intelligence s.'s, escalas de inteligência de Wechsler; escalas padronizadas, continuamente revistas e atualizadas, para a medida da inteligência geral em crianças pré-escolares (escala de inteligência pré-escolar e primária), em crianças (escala de inteligência de Wechsler para crianças) e em adultos (escala de inteligência de Wechsler para adultos, a sucessora da escala de Wechsler-Bellevue).
Zubrod s., escala de Zubrod; escala de 5 pontos, semelhante à escala de Karnofsky de 10 pontos; ambas medem o estado de desempenho da natureza ambulatorial de um paciente, desde uma atividade normal até a total dependência de outros para efetuar os cuidados pessoais. VER TAMBÉM Karnofsky s.

sca·lene (skā′lēn). Escaleno. **1.** Que possui lados de comprimentos desiguais, referindo-se a um triângulo assim formado. **2.** Um dos vários músculos assim denominados. VER scalenus anterior (*muscle*), *musculus* scalenus anticus, scalenus medius (*muscle*), scalenus minimus (*muscle*), scalenus posterior (*muscle*), *musculus* scalenus posticus. SIN scalenus. [G. *skalēnos*, desigual]
sca·le·nec·to·my (skā′lē - nek′tō - mē). Escalenectomia; ressecção dos músculos escalenos. [scalene + G. *ektomē*, excisão]
sca·le·not·o·my (skā′lē - not′ō - mē). Escalenotomia; divisão ou secção do músculo escaleno anterior. [scalene + G. *tomē*, incisão]
sca·le·nus (skā - lē′nŭs). Escaleno. SIN scalene. [L.]
scal·er (skā′ler). **1.** Raspador; instrumento para remover tártaro dos dentes. **2.** contador; dispositivo para a contagem de impulsos elétricos, como no ensaio de materiais radioativos.
hoe s., raspador em forma de enxada com lâmina muito curta.
ultrasonic s., raspador ultra-sônico; dispositivo ultra-sônico que utiliza a vibração de alta freqüência para remover depósitos aderentes dos dentes.
scal·ing (skā′ling). Raspagem; em odontologia, remoção de concreções das coroas e raízes dos dentes com o uso de instrumentos especiais.
scal·lop·ing (skal′ō - ping). Recorte; série de entalhes ou erosões na margem normalmente lisa de uma estrutura.
scalp (skalp). Escalpo; a pele e o tecido subcutâneo, normalmente com cabelos, que recobrem o neurocrânio. [I. m. do Escand. *skalpr*, bainha]
scal·pel (skal′pl). Escalpelo; bisturi utilizado em dissecação cirúrgica. [L. *scalpellum*; dim. de *scalprum*, faca]
plasma s., e. plasmático; escalpelo que utiliza para corte um jato gasoso fino em alta temperatura, em vez de uma lâmina.

scal·pri·form (skal′pri-fōrm). Escalpriforme; em forma de cinzel. [L. *scalprum*, cinzel + *forma*, forma]

scal·prum (skal′prŭm). Escalpro. **1.** Escapelo grande e forte. **2.** Raspador. [L. chisel, canivete, de *scalpo*, pp. *scalptus*, entalhar]

scaly (skā′lē). Escamoso. SIN squamous.

scam·mo·ny (skam′ō-nē). Escamônia; a planta *Convolvulus scammonia* (família Convolvulaceae), cuja raiz seca contém uma resina catártica. VER TAMBÉM ipomea. [G. *skammōnia*]

scan (skan). **1.** Examinar com um dispositivo sensor ativo ou passivo. **2.** Imagem, registro ou dados obtidos ao exame, geralmente identificada pela tecnologia ou dispositivo empregados; p. ex., TC, cintilografia, ultra-sonografia, etc. **3.** Forma abreviada de cintilografia, geralmente identificada pelo órgão ou estrutura examinados; p. ex., cintilografia cerebral, cintilografia óssea, etc.

  CT s., TC. VER tomography.
  duplex Doppler s., Doppler dúplex; método de visualização e avaliação seletiva dos padrões de fluxo das artérias e veias periféricas utilizando a ultra-sonografia e Doppler com pulsos.
  EMI s., historicamente, termo comumente utilizado para referir-se à tomografia computadorizada da cabeça, a técnica planejada por Hounsfield, que trabalhava como cientista na EMI, uma firma eletrônica inglesa.
  Meckel s., cintigrafia de Meckel; uso do pertecnetato de tecnécio^{99m} numa cintilografia do intestino delgado para detectar a mucosa gástrica ectópica no divertículo de Meckel; o íon pertecnetato é secretado por células epiteliais na mucosa gástrica.
  multiple-gated acquisition s. (MUGA), c. de aquisição com regulação múltipla; estudo de medicina nuclear do reservatório de sangue cardíaco através de aquisição de imagens com regulagem múltipla; utilizada para a avaliação da fração de ejeção (ejection *fraction*) e movimento da parede. VER TAMBÉM radionuclide ejection *fraction*.
  renal cortical s., cintigrafia cortical renal; técnica de imagem que consiste na injeção de um radiofármaco para localização do córtex renal (p. ex., Tc^{99m}-DMSA, Tc^{99m}-glicoepatanato) para visualização do córtex renal na detecção de fibrose ou pielonefrite.
  sector s., em ultra-sonografia, sistema em que o transdutor ou feixe de ultra-som transmitido efetua uma rotação através de um ângulo, resultando numa imagem em forma de fatia de torta.
  ventilation-perfusion s., cintigrafia de ventilação–perfusão; prova de função pulmonar, especialmente útil para embolia pulmonar, que utiliza um radionuclídeo inalado para ventilação e um radionuclídeo intravenoso para perfusão; suas distribuições respectivas no pulmão são registradas na cintilografia.

scan·di·um (Sc) (skan′dē-ŭm). Escândio; elemento metálico de número atômico 21, peso atômico 44,955910. [L. *Scandia*, Escandinávia, onde foi descoberto]

scan·ner (skan′er). Escaneador, *scanner*; dispositivo ou instrumento para varredura.

scan·ning (skan′ing). Varredura; exame atravessando com um dispositivo sensor ativo ou passivo, freqüentemente identificado pela tecnologia ou dispositivo empregado.
  transvaginal s., ultra-sonografia transvaginal; ultra-sonografia da pelve feminina com o transdutor colocado no interior da vagina.

scan·o·gram (skan′ō-gram). Escanometria; técnica radiográfica para fornecer as verdadeiras dimensões ao mover um feixe ortogonal estreito de raios X ao longo do comprimento da estrutura que está sendo medida, como, por exemplo, os membros inferiores. [scan- + G. *gramma*, algo escrito]

Scanzoni, Friedrich W., obstetra alemão, 1821–1891. VER S. maneuver.

sca·pha (skaf′ă, skā′fă). Escafa. **1.** [TA]. Depressão longitudinal entre a hélice e a antélice da orelha. SIN fossa of helix. **2.** Termo obsoleto para referir-se à scaphoid *fossa* (fossa escafóide). [L. do G. *skaphē*, esquife]

scapho-. Escafo-. Escafa, escafóide. [G. *skaphē*, esquife, barco]

scaph·o·ce·phal·ic (skaf-ō-se-fal′ik). Escafocefálico; que indica escafocefalia ou que se refere a esta. SIN escaphocephalous, tectocephalic.

scaph·o·ceph·a·lism (skaf-ō-sef′ă-lizm). Escafocefalismo. SIN scaphocephaly.

scaph·o·ceph·a·lous (skaf-ō-sef′ă-lŭs). Escafocéfalo. SIN scaphocephalic.

scaph·o·ceph·a·ly (skaf-ō-sef′ă-lē). Escafocefalia; forma de craniocinostose que resulta em cabeça longa e estreita, com ausência das eminências parietais e proeminência das protrusões frontal e occipital; pode haver uma crista indicando o local de uma sutura sagital de fechamento pré-natal; algumas vezes acompanhada de retardo mental. SIN cymbocephaly, sagittal synostosis, scaphocephalism, tectocephaly. [scapho- + G. *kephalē*, cabeça]

scaph·o·hy·dro·ceph·a·lus, scaph·o·hy·dro·ceph·a·ly (skaf′ō-hī′drō-sef′ă-lŭs, -lē). Escafoidrocefalia; ocorrência de hidrocefalia num indivíduo com escafocefalia.

scaph·oid (skaf′oyd) [TA]. Escafóide; navicular; côncavo. VER scaphoid (*bone*). [scapho- + G. *eidos*, semelhança]

scap·u·la, gen. e pl. **scap·u·lae** (skap′ū-lă, -lē) [TA]. Escápula; grande osso triangular achatado situado sobre as costelas, posteriormente de cada lado, que se articula lateralmente com a clavícula na articulação acromioclavicular e com o úmero na articulação do ombro. Forma uma articulação funcional com a parede torácica, a articulação escapulotorácica. SIN blade bone, shoulder blade. [L. *scapulae*, escápulas]
  s. ala′ta, e. alada. SIN winged s.
  s. eleva′ta, e. elevada. SIN Sprengel *deformity*.
  winged s., e. alada; condição em que a borda medial da escápula projeta-se, afastando-se do tórax; a protrusão é posterior e lateral quando a escápula sofre rotação medial; mais comumente causada por paralisia do músculo serrátil anterior. SIN s. alata.

scap·u·lal·gia (skap′ū-lal′jē-ă). Escapulalgia; termo raramente utilizado para referir-se à dor nas escápulas. SIN scapulodynia. [scapula + G. *algos*, dor]

scap·u·lar (skap′ū-lăr). Escapular; relativo à escápula.

scap·u·lary (skap′ū-lăr-ē). Escapulário; forma de atadura ou suspensório para manter um cinto ou uma atadura no corpo no local.

scap·u·lec·to·my (skap′ū-lek′tō-mē). Escapulectomia; excisão da escápula. [scapula + G. *ektomē*, excisão]

scapulo-. Escápulo-; escápula, escapular. [L. *scapulae*, escápulas]

scap·u·lo·cla·vic·u·lar (skap′ū-lō-klă-vik′ū-lăr). **1.** Acromioclavicular. SIN acromioclavicular. **2.** Coracoclavicular. SIN coracoclavicular.

scap·u·lo·dyn·ia (skap′ū-lō-din′ē-ă). Escapulodinia. SIN scapulalgia. [scapulo- + G. *odynē*, dor]

scap·u·lo·hu·mer·al (skap′ū-lō-hū′mer-ăl). Escapuloumeral; relativo à escápula e ao úmero. VER TAMBÉM glenohumeral.

scap·u·lo·pexy (skap′ū-lō-pek-sē). Escapulopexia; fixação cirúrgica da escápula à parede torácica ou ao processo espinhoso das vértebras. [scapulo- + G. *pēxis*, fixação]

sca·pus, pl. **sca·pi** (skā′pŭs, -pī). Escapo; haste ou pedúnculo. [L. haste, pedículo]
  s. pe′nis, corpo do pênis. SIN body of penis.
  s. pi′li, haste pilosa. SIN hair *shaft*.

scar (skar). Cicatriz; tecido fibroso que substitui tecidos normais destruídos por lesão ou doença. [G. *eschara*, crosta]
  cigarette-paper s.'s, cicatrizes "em papel de cigarro", cicatrizes papiráceas; cicatrizes atróficas na pele em locais de laceração mínima nos joelhos, pernas e cotovelos de indivíduos com síndrome de Ehlers-Danlos. SIN papyraceous s.'s.
  hypertrophic s., c. hipertrófica; cicatriz elevada que se assemelha a um quelóide, mas que não se propaga para os tecidos circundantes; raramente é dolorosa e sofre regressão espontânea; os feixes de colágeno dispõem-se paralelamente à superfície da pele.
  papyraceous s.'s, cicatrizes papiráceas. SIN cigarette-paper s.'s.
  radial s., c. radial. SIN radial sclerosing *lesion*.

Scardino, Peter T., urologista norte-americano, *1915. VER S. vertical flap *pyeloplasty*.

Scarff, John E., neurocirurgião norte-americano, 1898–1978. VER Stookey-S. *operation*.

scar·i·fi·ca·tion (skar-i-fi-kā′shŭn). Escarificação; ato de efetuar várias incisões superficiais na pele. [L. *scarifico*, raspar, do G. *skariphos*, estilete para esboço]

scar·i·fy (skar′i-fī). Escarificar; produzir escarificação.

scar·la·ti·na (skar′lă-tē′nă). Escarlatina; doença exantematosa, causada pela infecção por estreptococos que produzem uma toxina eritrogênica; caracterizada por febre e outros distúrbios constitucionais e por erupção generalizada de pontos ou pequenas máculas densamente agregadas, de cor vermelho-brilhante, seguidas de descamação em grandes lâminas, tiras ou escamas; a mucosa da boca e das fauces geralmente está também afetada. SIN scarlet fever. [através do It. do L. mediev. *scarlatum*, escarlate, roupa escarlate]
  anginose s., s. angino′sa, e. anginosa; forma de e. em que a afecção da garganta é inusitadamente grave. SIN Fothergill *disease* (2).
  s. hemorrhag′ica, e. hemorrágica; forma de e. em que o sangue extravasa para a pele e mucosas, dando à erupção uma tonalidade fosca; ocorre também sangramento freqüente do nariz e do intestino.
  s. la′tens, latent s., e. latente; forma de e. em que não há erupção cutânea; entretanto, ocorrem outras complicações da infecção estreptocócica, como nefrite aguda.
  s. malig′na, e. maligna; e. grave em que o paciente é rapidamente dominado pela intensidade da intoxicação sistêmica.
  s. rheumat′ica, dengue. SIN dengue.
  s. sim′plex, e. simples; forma leve da doença.

scar·la·ti·nal (skar-lă-tē′năl). Escarlatinoso; relativo à escarlatina.

scar·la·ti·nel·la (skar-lă-ti-nel′ă). Escarlatinela. SIN Filatov-Dukes *disease*. [dim. de *scarlatina*]

scar·la·ti·ni·form (skar-lă-tē′ni-fōrm, -tin′i-fōrm). Escarlatiniforme; semelhante à escarlatina, referindo-se a uma erupção cutânea. SIN scarlatinoid (1).

scar·la·ti·noid (skar-lă-tē′noyd, skar-lat′i-noyd). Escarlatinóide. **1.** SIN scarlatiniform. **2.** SIN Filatov-Dukes *disease*. [scarlatina + G. *eidos*, semelhança]

scar·let (skar′let). Escarlate; que apresenta cor vermelho-brilhante tendendo para o laranja. [L. mediev. *scarlatum*, roupa escarlate]

scar·let red [C.I. 26905]. Vermelho-escarlate; corante azo; pó vermelho-acastanhado escuro, solúvel em óleos, gorduras e clorofórmio, porém insolúvel em água; utilizado em medicina como vulnerário, em histologia para coloração da gordura em cortes teciduais e proteínas básicas em pH elevado, e na imunoeletroforese. SIN Biebrich scarlet red, medicinal scarlet red, scharlach red, Sudan IV.

scar·let red sul·fo·nate. Sulfonato de vermelho-escarlate; corante azo que tem sido utilizado para estimular a cicatrização de úlceras e feridas superficiais crônicas.

Scarpa, Antonio, anatomista, ortopedista e oftalmologista italiano, 1747–1832. VER *canals* of S., em *canal*; membranous *layer* of subcutaneous tissue of abdomen; S. *fluid, foramina,* em *foramen; fossa* scarpae major; S. *ganglion, habenula, hiatus, liquor, membrane, method, sheath, staphyloma, triangle.*

Scatchard, George, químico e bioquímico norte-americano, 1892–1973. VER S. *plot.*

sca·te·mia (skă-tē′mē-ă). Escatemia; auto-intoxicação intestinal. [scato- + G. *haima,* sangue]

△ **scato-.** Escato-. Fezes. VER TAMBÉM copro-, sterco-. [G. *skōr (skat-),* excremento]

scat·o·log·ic (skat-ō-loj′ik). Escatológico; relativo à escatologia.

sca·tol·o·gy (skă-tol′o-jē). Escatologia. **1.** Estudo científico e análise das fezes para fins fisiológicos e diagnósticos. SIN coprology. **2.** O estudo relativo aos aspectos psiquiátricos do excremento ou da função excremental (anal). [scato- + G. *logos,* estudo]

sca·to·ma (ska-tō′mă). Escatoma. SIN fecaloma. [scato- + G. *-oma,* tumor]

sca·toph·a·gy (skă-tof′ă-jē). Escatofagia. SIN coprophagia. [scato- + G. *phagō,* comer]

sca·tos·co·py (skă-tos′kō-pē). Escatoscopia; exame das fezes para fins de diagnóstico. [scato- + G. *skopeō,* ver]

scat·ter (skat′er). Dispersão. **1.** Mudança na direção de um fóton ou de uma partícula subatômica em conseqüência de colisão ou interação. **2.** A radiação secundária decorrente da interação da radiação primária com a matéria.
  Compton s., d. de Compton; mecanismo de dispersão denominado efeito de Compton.

scat·ter·gram (skat-er-gram). Gráfico da distribuição de duas variáveis em relação uma com a outra. [scatter + G. *gramma,* algo escrito]

scat·u·la (skat′ū-lă). Escátula; caixa quadrada para pílulas. [L. mediev. figura retangular cuja largura corresponde a um décimo de seu comprimento]

Scedosporium (se-dō-spōr′ē-um). Fungo imperfeito da classe Hyphomycetes; anamorfo de *Pseudallescheria.*
  S. apiosper′mum (sked-os-pōr′ē-ŭm). O estado imperfeito do fungo *Pseudallescheria boydii,* uma das 16 espécies de fungos verdadeiros que podem causar micetoma nos seres humanos ou infecção grave em pacientes imunossuprimidos.
  S. infla′tum, VER *S. prolificans.*
  S. proli′ficans, fungo filamentoso; causa rara de infecção fúngica profunda. Antigamente denominado *S. inflatum.*

sce·lal·gia (se-lal′jē-ă). Escelalgia; dor na perna. [G. *skelos,* perna + *algos,* dor]

scene. Cena.
  primal s., c. primal; em psicanálise, a observação verdadeira ou fantasiada de relação sexual por uma criança, particularmente entre os pais.

scent (sent). Fragrância. SIN odor. [I.m., do Fr. A., do L. *sentio,* sentir]

Schacher, Polycarp G., médico alemão, 1674–1737. VER S. *ganglion.*

Schaer re·a·gent. Reagente de Schaer. Ver em reagent.

Schäfer, Sir Edward A. Sharpey-, fisiologista e histologista inglês, 1850–1935. VER S. *method.*

Schäffer, Max, neurologista alemão, 1852–1923. VER S. *reflex.*

Schaffer test. Teste de Schaffer. Ver em test.

Schamberg, Jay F., dermatologista norte-americano, 1870–1934. VER Schamberg *fever.*

Schapiro, Heinrich, médico russo, 1852–1901. VER S. *sign.*

Schardinger, Franz, cientista austríaco, 1853–1920. VER S. *dextrins,* em *dextrin, enzyme, reaction.*

schar·lach red (shar′lak). Vermelho-escarlate. SIN scarlet red.

Schatzki, Richard, radiologista norte-americano, 1901–1992. VER Schatzki *ring.*

Schaudinn, Fritz R., bacteriologista alemão, 1871–1906. VER S. *fixative.*

Schaumann, Jörgen N., médico sueco, 1879–1953. VER S. *bodies,* em *body, lymphogranuloma, syndrome;* Besnier-Boeck-S. *disease, syndrome.*

Schaumberg, H.H., neuropatologista norte-americano, *1912.

Schauta, Friedrich, ginecologista austríaco, 1849–1919. VER S. vaginal *operation.*

Schede, Max, cirurgião alemão, 1844–1902. VER S. *method.*

sched·ule (sked′jool). Esquema, programa. Plano de procedimentos para um objetivo proposto, especialmente a seqüência e o tempo atribuídos a cada item ou operação necessários para sua conclusão. [L. *scheda,* de *scida,* uma tira de papiro, folha de papel]
  s.'s of reinforcement, programas de reforço; na psicologia de condicionamento, procedimentos ou seqüências estabelecidos para reforçar o comportamento operante; p. ex., numa situação em que é necessário pressionar uma alavanca, cada deslocamento da alavanca fornecerá uma porção de alimento ou reforço comparável (**continuous reinforcement s.,** programa de reforço contínuo), ou o reforço aparecerá a cada 5 segundos, independentemente do número de deslocamentos efetuados anteriormente (**fixed-interval reinforcement s.,** programa de reforço a intervalos fixos), a cada décimo deslocamento (**fixed-ratio reinforcement s.,** programa de reforço com relação fixa) ou numa média de cada 5 segundos (**variable-interval reinforcement s.,** programa de reforço a intervalos variáveis), ou o reforço virá de forma não-contínua, em que menos de 100% dos deslocamentos levarão ao reforço (**intermittent reinforcement s.,** programa de reforço intermitente).

Scheele, Karl W., químico sueco, 1742–1786. VER S. *green.*

Scheibe, A. médico norte-americano, *1875. VER Scheibe *hearing impairment.*

Scheibler re·a·gent. Reagente de Scheibler. Ver em reagent.

Scheie, Harold G., oftalmologista norte-americano, *1909. VER S. *syndrome.*

Scheiner, Christoph, físico alemão, 1575–1650. VER S. *experiment.*

Schellong, Fritz, médico alemão, 1891–1953. VER S. *test;* S.-Strisower *phenomenon.*

sche·ma, pl. **sche·ma·ta** (skē′mă, skē-mah′tă). Esquema. **1.** Plano, esboço ou disposição. SIN scheme. **2.** Em teoria sensorimotora, a unidade organizada de experiência cognitiva. [G. *schēma,* forma]
  body s., imagem corporal. SIN body *image.*

sche·mat·ic (skē-mat′ik). Esquemático; feito de acordo com um tipo definido de fórmula; que representa de modo geral, mas não com exatidão absoluta; refere-se a um desenho ou modelo anatômico. [G. *schēmatikos,* em exibição externa, de *schēma,* forma]

sche·mat·o·graph (skē-mat′ō-graf). Esquematógrafo; instrumento para fazer um traçado do contorno do corpo em tamanho reduzido. [G. *schēma,* forma + *graphō,* escrever]

scheme (skēm). Esquema, Sistema. SIN schema (1).
  occlusal s., sistema oclusivo. SIN occlusal *system.*

sche·mo·chromes (skē-mō-krōmz). Esquemocromos. SIN structural *color.*

Schenck, Benjamin R., cirurgião norte-americano, 1873–1920. VER S. *disease.*

Scheuermann, Holger W., cirurgião dinamarquês, 1877–1960. VER S. *disease.*

Schick, Bela, pediatra austríaca nos Estados Unidos, 1877–1967. VER S. *method, test, test toxin.*

Schiff, Hugo, químico alemão em Florença, 1834–1915. VER S. *base, reagent;* Kasten fluorescent S. *reagents,* em *reagent; periodic acid-*S. *stain;* ninhydrin-S. *stain for proteins.*

Schiff, Moritz, fisiologista alemão, 1823–1896. VER S.-Sherrington *phenomenon.*

Schilder, Paul Ferdinand, neurologista austríaco, 1886–1940.

Schiller, Walter, patologista austríaco nos Estados Unidos, 1887–1960. VER S. *test.*

Schilling, Victor, hematologista alemão, 1883–1960. VER S. *blood count,* band *cell, index, test,* type of monocytic *leukemia.*

schin·dy·le·sis (skin-dī-lē′sis) [TA]. Esquindilese; forma de articulação fibrosa em que a borda cortante de um osso penetra numa fenda na borda do outro osso, como na articulação do vômer com o rostro do esfenóide (sutura esfenovomeral). SIN schindyletic joint, wedge-and-groove joint, wedge-and-groove suture. [G. *schindylēsis,* lasca]

Schiötz, Hjalmar, médico norueguês, 1850–1927. VER S. *tonometer.*

Schirmer, Otto W.A., oftalmologista alemão, 1864–1917. VER S. *test.*

△ **schisto-.** Esquisto-. Fenda, separação. VER TAMBÉM schizo-. [G. *schistos,* fenda, divisão]

schis·to·ce·lia (skis-tō-sē′lē-ă). Esquistocelia; fissura congênita da parede abdominal. [schisto- + G. *koilia,* cavidade]

schis·to·cor·mia (skis-tō-kōr′mē-ă). Esquistocormia; fenda congênita do tronco, geralmente com desenvolvimento imperfeito dos membros inferiores do feto. SIN schistosomia. [schisto- + G. *kormos,* tronco de uma árvore]

schis·to·cys·tis (skis-tō-sis′tis). Esquistocisto; fissura da bexiga. [schisto- + G. *kystis,* bexiga]

schis·to·cyte (skis′tō-sīt). Esquistócito; variedade de poiquilócito cuja forma anormal se deve à fragmentação que ocorre à medida que a célula flui através de pequenos vasos lesados. SIN schizocyte. [schisto- + G. *kytos,* célula]

schis·to·cy·to·sis (skis′tō-sī-tō′sis). Esquistocitose; ocorrência de numerosos esquistócitos no sangue. SIN schizocytosis.

schis·to·glos·sia (skis-tō-glos′ē-ă). Esquistoglossia; fissura ou fenda congênita da língua. [schisto- + G. *glōssa,* língua]

schis·to·me·lia (skis′tō-mel′ē-ă). Esquistomelia; fenda congênita de um membro.

schis·tor·rha·chis (skis-tōr′ă-kis). Esquistorraque. SIN *spina* bifida. [schisto- + G. *rhachis,* coluna vertebral]

Schis·to·so·ma (skis-tō-sō′mă). Gênero de trematódeos digenéticos, incluindo os importantes trematódeos sanguíneos do homem e de animais domésticos, que causam a esquistossomose; caracterizados pela sua forma alongada, sexos separados com acentuado dimorfismo sexual, localização incomum nos vasos sanguíneos menores do hospedeiro e utilização de caramujos de água como hospedeiros intermediários. [schisto- + G. *sōma,* corpo]

S. haemato'bium, o trematódeo sanguíneo vesical, uma espécie com ovos com espinhos terminais que ocorre como parasita no sistema porta e nas veias mesentéricas da bexiga (causando a esquistossomose hematóbica humana) e no reto; comum no delta do Nilo, porém encontrado também ao longo de canais, valas de irrigação ou riachos em toda a África e em partes do Oriente Médio; o hospedeiro intermediário é *Bulinus truncatus* no Egito; em outras partes, outros caramujos da subfamília Bulininae (*Bulinus, Physopsis, Pyrgophysa*) estão envolvidos.

S. intercala'tum, espécie de trematódeo sanguíneo relacionada ao *S. haematobium*, de distribuição local no Zaire e em outras regiões da África Central, responsável por disenteria leve e dores abdominais, com aumento de tamanho do baço e do fígado; o hospedeiro intermediário é um caramujo planorbídeo, *Bulinus (Physopsis) africanus.*

S. japon'icum, o trematódeo sanguíneo oriental ou japonês, uma espécie cujos ovos apresentam pequenos espinhos laterais, geralmente apenas com uma pequena protuberância; causa a esquistossomose oriental, com patologia extensa devido à encapsulação dos ovos, sobretudo no fígado; trata-se da mais patogênica das três espécies comuns de esquistossoma que acometem os seres humanos, possivelmente devido à maior produção de ovos por fêmea; é também a mais refratária ao tratamento e a de controle mais difícil, visto que os hospedeiros intermediários são caramujos anfíbios (espécies de *Oncomelania*, da família Hydrobiidae) que podem deixar a água para evitar os moluscocidas, e também pelo fato de muitos outros animais, como porcos, bois, gado e cães, servirem como hospedeiros reservatórios.

S. malayen'sis, membro do complexo *S. japonicum*, descrito no roedor *Rattus muelleri*, na Malásia peninsular. O caramujo aquático *Robertsiella kaporensis* e duas outras espécies desse gênero são naturalmente infectadas. *S. malayensis* é considerado mais relacionado ao *S. mekongi*. Foram relatadas infecções humanas, baseadas em evidências sorológicas, em nativos da Malásia peninsular central.

S. manso'ni, espécie comum de trematódeo, caracterizada por grandes ovos com acentuado espinho lateral; a espécie é transmitida por caramujos planorbídeos do gênero *Biomphalaria*; provoca esquistossomose mansônica em seres humanos na África, em regiões do Oriente Médio, América do Sul e certas ilhas do Caribe.

S. mat'theei, espécie encontrada nas veias porta e mesentérica de ruminantes, primatas (incluindo seres humanos), zebras e roedores na África.

S. mekon'gi, espécie descrita no delta do Mekong, no sul do Laos e norte do Camboja. As taxas de infecção são maiores na faixa etária de 7–15 anos; os cães parecem ser o principal hospedeiro reservatório; o hospedeiro intermediário é o caramujo operculídeo *Tricula aperta*. A patogenia assemelha-se à do *S. japonicum*, porém é geralmente menos grave.

schis·to·some (skis′tō-sōm). Esquistossoma; nome comum para os membros do gênero *Schistosoma*.

schis·to·so·mia (skis-tō-sō′mē-ă). Esquistossomia. SIN schistocormia. [schisto- + G. *sōma*, corpo]

schis·to·so·mi·a·sis (skis′tō-sō-mī′ă-sis). Esquistossomose, esquistossomíase; infecção por uma espécie de *Schistosoma*; as manifestações dessa doença, freqüentemente crônica e debilitante, variam de acordo com a espécie infectante, mas dependem, em grande parte, da reação tecidual (granulação e fibrose) aos ovos depositados em vênulas e nos espaços porta hepáticos, resultando em hipertensão porta e varizes esofágicas, bem como em lesão hepática com conseqüente cirrose. VER tropical *diseases*, em *disease*. VER TAMBÉM schistosomal *dermatitis*, Symmers clay pipestem *fibrosis*. SIN bilharziasis, bilharziosis, hemic distomiasis, snail fever.

Asiatic s., e. asiática. SIN s. japonica.
bladder s., e. vesical. SIN s. haematobium.
cutaneous s. japonica, e. cutânea oriental. SIN s. japonica.
ectopic s., e. ectópica; forma clínica de esquistossomose que ocorre fora do local normal de parasitismo (veia mesentérica ou espaços porta hepáticos); pode resultar do transporte hematogênico acidental de ovos de esquistossoma ou, raramente, de vermes adultos para diversos locais incomuns, como a pele, o cérebro ou a medula espinal.
s. haemato'bium, infecção causada por *Schistosoma haematobium*, cujos ovos invadem as vias urinárias, causando cistite e hematúria e, possivelmente, probabilidade aumentada de câncer vesical. SIN bladder s., Egyptian hematuria, endemic hematuria, urinary s.
s. intercalatum, infecção causada por *Schistosoma intercalatum*; ocorre apenas na África Ocidental; poucos sintomas relatados e nenhum caso reconhecido de fibrose hepática.
intestinal s., e. intestinal. SIN s. mansoni.
s. japon'ica, Japanese s., e. oriental; infecção causada por *Schistosoma japonicum*, caracterizada por disenteria, aumento doloroso do fígado e do baço, hidropisia, urticária e anemia progressiva. SIN Asiatic s., cutaneous s. japonica, kabure itch, kabure, Katayama syndrome, Kinkiang fever, Oriental s., rice itch, urticarial fever, Yangtze Valley fever.
Manson s., e. mansônica. SIN s. mansoni.
s. manso'ni, e. mansônica; infecção causada por *Schistosoma mansoni*, cujos ovos invadem a parede do intestino grosso e o fígado, causando irritação, inflamação e, por fim, fibrose. SIN intestinal s., Manson disease, Manson s.
s. mekon'gi, infecção causada por *Schistosoma mekongi*, que acomete principalmente crianças no delta do Mekong, onde foi descoberta; a doença assemelha-se à e. japonesa.
Oriental s., e. oriental. SIN s. japonica.
pulmonary s., manifestações pulmonares da infecção por *Schistosoma*, geralmente por *Schistosoma mansoni*, a qual ocorre quando os esquistossomas, que se desenvolvem na pele a partir das cercárias que penetraram com água infestada, migram através da corrente sanguínea para os pulmões, em direção ao trato gastrointestinal e à veia porta; em geral, os sintomas limitam-se a tosse.
urinary s., e. urinária. SIN s. haematobium.

schis·to·som·u·lum, pl. **schis·to·som·u·la** (skis-tō-sō′mū-lŭm, -lă). Esquistossômulo; estágio no ciclo de vida de um trematódeo sanguíneo do gênero *Schistosoma* imediatamente após a sua penetração na pele sob a forma de cercária; caracterizado pela perda da cauda e mudanças fisiológicas, permitindo a sua sobrevivência na corrente sanguínea de um mamífero.

schis·to·ster·nia (skis-tō-ster′nē-ă). Esquistosternia. SIN schistothorax. [schisto- + G. *sternon*, esterno]

schis·to·tho·rax (skis-tō-thō′raks). Esquistotórax; fenda congênita da parede torácica. SIN schistosternia. [schisto- + G. *thōrax*, tórax]

schiz-. Esquiz-. VER schizo-.

schiz·am·ni·on (skiz-am′nē-on). Esquizâmnio; âmnio que se desenvolve, como no embrião humano, pela formação de uma cavidade sobre a massa celular interna ou no interior desta. [schiz- + amnion]

schiz·ax·on (skiz-ak′son). Esquizaxônio; axônio dividido em dois ramos. [schiz- + G. *axōn*, eixo]

schiz·en·ceph·a·ly (skiz-en-sef′ă-lē). Esquizencefalia; divisões ou fendas anormais da substância cerebral. [schiz- + G. *enkephalos*, cérebro]

schizo-, schiz-. Esquizo-, esquiz-. Fenda, divisão; esquizofrenia. VER TAMBÉM schisto-. [G. *schizō*, dividir ou clivar]

schiz·o·af·fec·tive (skiz′ō-ă-fek′tiv). Esquizoafetivo; que possui uma mistura de sintomas sugestivos de esquizofrenia e transtorno afetivo (do humor).

schiz·o·cyte (skiz′ō-sīt). Esquizócito. SIN schistocyte. [schizo- + G. *kytos*, célula]

schiz·o·cy·to·sis (skiz′ō-sī-tō′sis). Esquizocitose. SIN schistocytosis.

schiz·o·gen·e·sis (skiz-ō-jen′ĕ-sis). Esquizogênese; reprodução por fissão. SIN fissiparity, scissiparity. [schizo- + G. *genesis*, origem]

schi·zog·o·ny (ski-zog′ō-nē). Esquizogonia; fissão múltipla em que o núcleo divide-se em primeiro lugar e, a seguir, a célula divide-se em tantas partes quantos são os núcleos; denominada merogonia se as células-filhas forem merozoítas; esporogonia, se as células-filhas forem esporozoítas; ou gametogonia, se as células-filhas forem gametas. SIN agamocytogeny. [schizo- + G. *gonē*, geração]

schiz·o·gy·ria (skiz-ō-jī′rē-ă, -jir′ē-ă). Esquizogiria; deformidade das convoluções cerebrais, caracterizada por interrupções ocasionais de sua continuidade. [schizo- + G. *gyros*, círculo (convolução)]

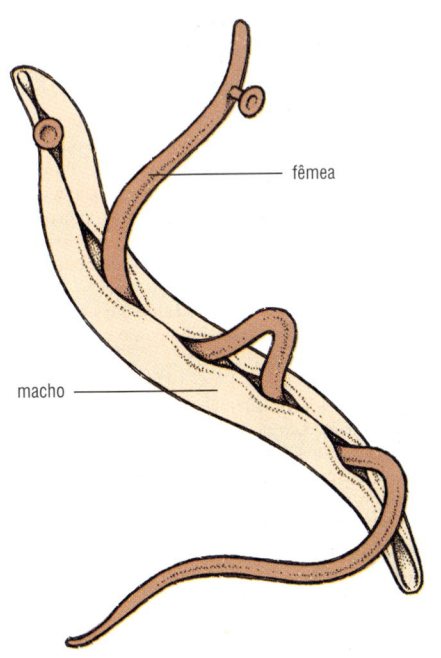

Schistosoma mansoni: copulação

schiz·oid (skiz′oyd). Esquizóide; socialmente isolado, retirado, que possui poucos (ou nenhum) amigos ou relações sociais; semelhante aos aspectos da personalidade característicos da esquizofrenia, porém numa forma mais leve. VER TAMBÉM schizoid *personality*. [schizo(phrenia), + G. *eidos*, semelhança]

schiz·oid·ism (skiz′oy-dizm). Esquizoidismo; estado esquizóide; a manifestação de tendências esquizóides.

schiz·o·my·cete (skiz′ō-mī-sēt). Esquizomiceto; membro da classe Schizomycetes; uma bactéria.

schiz·o·my·cet·ic (skiz-ō-mī-sē′tik). Esquizomicético; relativo a, ou causado por, fungos (bactérias) que se dividem por cissiparidade.

schiz·ont (skiz′ont). Esquizonte; trofozoíta de esporozoário (forma vegetativa), que se reproduz por esquizogonia, produzindo um número variado de trofozoítas ou merozoítas. VER TAMBÉM meront, segmenter. SIN agamont, segmenting body. [schizo- + G. *ōn* (*ont-*), ser]

schi·zon·ti·cide (ski-zon′ti-sīd). Esquizonticida; agente que destrói esquizontes. [schizont + L. *caedo*, matar]

schiz·o·nych·ia (skiz-ō-nik′ē-ă). Esquizoniquia; fissura das unhas. [schizo- + G. *onyx*, unha]

schiz·o·pha·sia (skiz-ō-fā′zē-ă). Esquizofasia; termo raramente empregado para referir-se à fala desordenada (salada de palavras) do indivíduo esquizofrênico. [schizo- + G. *phasis*, fala]

schiz·o·phre·nia (skiz-ō-frē′nē-ă, skit′sō-). Esquizofrenia; termo criado por Bleuler, sinônimo que substitui a expressão demência precoce (*dementia praecox*); tipo comum de psicose, que se caracteriza por anormalidades na percepção, no conteúdo do pensamento e nos processos mentais (alucinações e delírios) e por substancial retraimento de interesse do indivíduo em relação a outras pessoas e ao mundo externo, com enfoque excessivo na própria vida mental; hoje em dia, a esquizofrenia é considerada como um grupo ou espectro de distúrbios, e não como uma entidade única, algumas vezes sendo feita distinção entre esquizofrenia processual e esquizofrenia reativa. A personalidade "dividida" da esquizofrenia, em que as funções ou componentes psíquicos individuais dividem-se e tornam-se autônomos, é identificada popularmente, porém de forma incorreta, como personalidade múltipla, em que 2 ou mais personalidades relativamente completas dominam sucessivamente a vida psíquica de um indivíduo. [schizo- + G. *phrēn*, mente]

A esquizofrenia é a psicose mais prevalente que acomete cerca de 2 milhões de norte-americanos. O custo anual da doença para a economia norte-americana é estimado em U$65 bilhões, dos quais U$46 bilhões estão relacionados à perda de produtividade dos pacientes e de seus cuidadores. O risco de incidência durante a vida é de cerca de 1%. O início é tipicamente gradual, sem nenhuma causa precipitante óbvia. Os sintomas iniciais consistem em redução do tempo de atenção, déficit de memória e menor capacidade de tomar decisões. Os pacientes ficam doentes, em sua maioria, antes dos 40 anos de idade. Os sintomas psicóticos persistem por vários meses ou anos, e existe um risco permanente de recidiva. As disfunções cognitivas são tipicamente acompanhadas de redução do nível de energia, afeto embotado ou deprimido, anedonia e abulia. Praticamente todos os pacientes exibem empobrecimento do conteúdo dos pensamentos, isolamento social e comprometimento da função ocupacional, e, até mesmo com psicoterapia intensiva e tratamento farmacológico, cerca de 25% necessitam de cuidados sob custódia ou em clínicas. Embora alguns indivíduos com esquizofrenia se tornem assassinos ou cometam assassinatos em massa, a grande maioria não representa nenhuma ameaça para a sociedade, e cerca de 10% cometem suicídio. Os estudos neurofisiológicos realizados mostraram anormalidades generalizadas do lobo límbico e córtex pré-frontal, tamanho pequeno anormal do tálamo e alterações na intensidade de sinais na substância branca adjacente. As técnicas de imagens do cérebro revelam inconsistentemente anormalidades estruturais ou fisiológicas no córtex pré-frontal, córtex do cíngulo, córtex temporal e formação hipocampal. A melhora ou a exacerbação da esquizofrenia produzidas por certos agentes farmacológicos parecem indicar que o distúrbio representa uma disfunção de sistemas neuronais que utilizam a dopamina, a serotonina, o glutamato e o ácido γ-aminobutírico (GABA) como transmissores ou moduladores. Estudos genéticos sugerem que a suscetibilidade à esquizofrenia é herdada como um complexo de variações que afetam diversos genes. De acordo com a hipótese de neurodesenvolvimento, já existe uma lesão cerebral ou esta é adquirida no início da vida, porém não se manifesta integralmente até o final da adolescência ou início da vida adulta, quando desencadeia anormalidades na proliferação neuronal, crescimento axonal, migração celular, sobrevida das células, regressão sináptica ou mielinização. A psicoterapia e a terapia comportamental são inconsistentemente efetivas no tratamento da esquizofrenia. Os agentes neurolépticos reduzem os episódios de psicose aguda, limitam a necessidade de cuidados em clínicas e diminuem o risco de recidiva, porém o seu uso prolongado está associado a efeitos colaterais graves, particularmente discinesia tardia. Os agentes mais recentes, como clozapina, olanzipina, quetiapina e risperidona, são mais efetivos na melhora da função cognitiva e é menos provável que induzam efeitos colaterais extrapiramidais. Os indivíduos com esquizofrenia freqüentemente interrompem seus medicamentos, e estima-se que, em determinado momento, apenas metade desses indivíduos está recebendo tratamento ou supervisão médica.

acute s., e. aguda; distúrbio em que os sintomas de esquizofrenia surgem abruptamente; podem regredir ou tornar-se crônicos com o decorrer do tempo. SIN acute schizophrenic episode.

ambulatory s., e. ambulatorial; forma mais leve de esquizofrenia, em que o paciente consegue manter-se na sociedade e não precisa ser hospitalizado.

catatonic s., e. catatônica; esquizofrenia caracterizada por distúrbio pronunciado, podendo incluir torpor, negativismo, rigidez, excitação ou alterações da postura; algumas vezes, ocorre rápida alternância entre os extremos de excitação e torpor. As características associadas incluem comportamento estereotípico, maneirismos e flexibilidade acentuada; o mutismo é particularmente comum.

childhood s., e. infantil. SIN infantile *autism*.

disorganized s., e. desorganizada; forma grave de esquizofrenia, caracterizada pela predominância de incoerência, afeto embotado, inapropriado ou tolo e ausência de delírios sistematizados. SIN hebephrenic s.

hebephrenic s., e. hebefrênica. SIN disorganized s.

latent s., e. latente; suscetibilidade preexistente a desenvolver esquizofrenia franca sob forte estresse emocional.

paranoid s., e. paranóide; esquizofrenia caracterizada predominantemente por delírios de perseguição e megalomania.

process s., e. processual; termo obsoleto para as formas de distúrbios esquizofrênicos graves, em que as condições biológicas progressivas e crônicas no cérebro são consideradas a causa primária e cujo prognóstico é sombrio, com início insidioso numa idade jovem, em contraste com a esquizofrenia reativa.

pseudoneurotic s., e. pseudoneurótica; esquizofrenia em que o processo psicótico subjacente é mascarado por queixas habitualmente consideradas neuróticas.

reactive s., e. reativa; formas de distúrbios esquizofrênicos graves que são distinguidas da esquizofrenia processual pelo seu início mais agudo, maior relação com o estresse ambiental e melhor prognóstico.

residual s., e. residual; afeto embotado ou inapropriado, isolamento social, comportamento excêntrico ou associações frouxas, porém sem sintomas psicóticos proeminentes, como os vestígios dos sintomas psicóticos anteriores da esquizofrenia.

simple s., e. simples; esquizofrenia caracterizada por retraimento, apatia, indiferença e empobrecimento dos relacionamentos humanos, sem manifestações psicóticas francas.

schiz·o·phren·ic (skiz-ō-fren′ik, -frē′nik, skit-sō-). Esquizofrênico; relativo a, caracterizado por ou que sofre de uma das esquizofrenias.

schiz·o·to·nia (skiz-ō-tō′nē-ă). Esquizotonia; divisão da distribuição do tônus nos músculos. [schizo- + G. *tonos*, tensão, tônus]

schiz·o·trich·ia (skiz-ō-trik′ē-ă). Esquizotriquia; fios de cabelo com pontas quebradas. SIN scissura pilorum. [schizo- + G. *thrix*, cabelo]

Schiz·o·tryp·a·num cru·zi (skiz-ō-trī′pan-ŭm kroo′zī). Designação genérica distinta utilizada para o *Trypanosoma cruzi*, freqüentemente empregada por trabalhadores na área endêmica da tripanossomíase da América do Sul; também utilizada como designação subgenérica, isto é, *Trypanosoma (Schizotrypanum) cruzi*. [schizo- + G. *trypanon*, perfurador, escavador]

schiz·o·zo·ite (skiz-ō-zō′īt). Esquizozoíta; merozoíta anterior à esquizogonia, como na fase exoeritrocitária do desenvolvimento do *Plasmodium*, após invasão do hepatócito por esporozoítas e antes da divisão múltipla. [schizo- + G. *zōon*, animal]

schlamm·fie·ber (shlăm′fē-ber). Nome dado a um surto de leptospirose perto de Breslau, na Alemanha, possivelmente devido à infecção por *Leptospira grippotyphosa*.

Schlatter, Carl B., cirurgião suíço, 1864–1934. VER Osgood-S. *disease*.

Schlemm, Friedrich, anatomista alemão, 1795–1858. VER S. *canal*.

Schlesinger, Hermann, médico austríaco. 1868–1934. VER S. *sign;* Pool-S. *sign.*

schlieren (schlēr′en). VER schlieren *optics*.

Schmid, Rudi, internista e bioquímico suíço-norte-americano, *1922. VER McArdle-S.-Pearson *disease*.

Schmid, W. VER S.-Fraccaro *syndrome*.

Schmidel, Kasimir C., anatomista alemão, 1718–1792. VER S. *anastomoses*, em *anastomosis*.

Schmidt, Gerhard, bioquímico norte-americano, *1900. VER S.-Thannhauser *method*.

Schmidt, Henry D., anatomista e patologista norte-americano, 1823–1888. VER S.-Lanterman *clefts*, em *cleft, incisures*, em *incisure*.

Schmidt, Johann F.M., laringologista alemão, 1838–1907. VER S. *syndrome*.

Schmidt, Martin Benno, médico alemão, 1863–1949. VER S. *syndrome.*
Schmorl, Christian G., patologista alemão, 1861–1932. VER S. *nodule,* ferric-ferricyanide reduction *stain,* picrothionin *stain, jaundice.*
Schneider, C.V., anatomista alemão, 1614–1680. VER schneiderian *membrane.*
Schneider, Franz C., químico alemão, 1813–1897. VER S. *carmine.*
Schneider, Kurt, psiquiatra alemão, 1887–1967.
Schnei·der·sitz (shni′der-zitz). Posição sentada típica com as pernas cruzadas na frente, exibida por pacientes gravemente afetados com fenilcetonúria e semelhante à posição comumente atribuída a alfaiates. [Ger.]
Schnitzler, L., médico europeu do século XX. VER S. *syndrome.*
Scholander, Per F., fisiologista norueguês, 1905–1980. VER S. *apparatus;* Roughton-S. *apparatus, syringe.*
Scholz, Willibald, neurologista alemão, 1889–1971. VER S. *disease.*
Schönbein, Christian F., químico alemão, 1799–1868. VER S. *test.*
Schönlein, Johann L., médico alemão, 1793–1864. VER S. *purpura;* Henoch-S. *purpura.*
school (skool). Escola; conjunto de crenças, ensinamentos, métodos, etc. [I. ant. *scōl*]
  biometrical s., e. biométrica; grupo de geniticistas ingleses, seguidores de Galton e Karl Pearson, cuja abordagem da genética era mais quantitativa do que enumerativa.
  dogmatic s., e. dogmática; antiga escola grega ou tradição na medicina, cujos membros foram os sucessores ou seguidores de Hipócrates; basearam seus conceitos de doença na teoria humoral e sua prática na experiência e raciocínio lógico; eram comparativamente livres de excentricidades, teorias especulativas e dogmas, cujo termo dogmático falsamente sugere.
  dynamic s., e. dinâmica; grupo de teorias fundado por G.E. Stahl, que ensinava a crença de que toda ação vital resulta de uma força interna independente de qualquer coisa externa ao corpo.
  hippocratic s., e. hipocrática; os seguidores dos ensinamentos de Hipócrates. VER TAMBÉM dogmatic s.
  iatromathematical s., e. iatromatemática; grupo de acadêmicos, dos quais Descartes foi um dos primeiros proponentes, que afirmava que todos os processos fisiológicos resultavam de leis físicas. SIN mechanistic s.
  mechanistic s., e. mecanística. SIN iatromathematical s.
Schott, Theodor, 1850–1921, médico alemão em Bad Nauheim. VER S. *treatment.*
schra·dan (schrā′dan). Potente organofosforado inibidor irreversível da colinesterase, utilizado como inseticida. Foi preparado para uso potencial como gás nervoso. A intoxicação produz uma crise colinérgica que pode ser fatal. SIN octamethyl pyrophosphoramide. [Gerhard *Schrader,* químico alemão, + -an).
Schreger, Christian H.T., anatomista e químico alemão, 1768–1833. VER S. *lines,* em *line;* Hunter-S. *bands,* em *band, lines,* em *line.*
Schridde, Hermann R.A., patologista alemão, *1876. VER S. cancer *hairs,* em *hair.*
Schroeder, Karl L.E., ginecologista alemão, 1838–1887. VER S. *operation.*
Schuchardt, Karl A., cirurgião alemão, 1856–1902. VER S. *operation.*
Schüffner, Wilhelm, patologista alemão em Sumatra, 1867–1949. VER S. *granules,* em *granule, dots,* em *dot.*
Schüller, Artur, neurologista austríaco, *1874. VER S. *disease, phenomenon, syndrome;* Hand-S.-Christian *disease.*
Schüller, Karl H.L.A., Max, cirurgião alemão, 1843–1907. VER S. *ducts,* em *duct.*
Schultes, Johann. VER Scultetus.
Schultz, Arthur R.H., médico alemão, *1890. VER S. *reaction, stain.*
Schultz, Werner, internista alemão, 1878–1947. VER S.-Charlton *phenomenon, reaction;* S.-Dale *reaction.*
Schultze, Bernhard S., obstetra alemão, 1827–1919. VER S. *fold, mechanism, phantom, placenta.*
Schultze, Max J.S., histologista e zoólogo alemão, 1825–1874. VER S. *cells,* em *cell, membrane, sign;* comma *bundle* of S.; comma *tract* of S.
Schütz, Erich, bioquímico alemão, *1902. VER S. *law, rule.*
Schütz, Hugo, anatomista alemão do século XX. VER S. *bundle.*
Schwabach, Dagobert, otologista alemão, 1846–1920. VER S. *test.*
Schwalbe, Gustav A., anatomista alemão, 1844–1916. VER S. *corpuscle, nucleus, ring, spaces,* em *space.*
Schwann, Theodor, histologista e fisiologista alemão, 1810–1882. VER S. *cells,* em *cell, cell unit, white substance; sheath* of S.
schwan·no·ma (shwah-nō′mă). Schwanoma; neoplasia encapsulada benigna, cujo componente fundamental é estruturalmente idêntico a um sincício de células de Schwann; as células neoplásicas proliferam no endoneuro, e o perineuro forma cápsula. A neoplasia pode originar-se de um nervo periférico ou simpático, bem como de vários nervos cranianos, sobretudo o oitavo nervo; quando o nervo é pequeno, é geralmente encontrado (quando o é) na cápsula da neoplasia; se o nervo for grande, o neurolemoma pode desenvolver-se na bainha do nervo, cujas fibras podem disseminar-se então sobre a superfície da cápsula à medida que a neoplasia aumenta. Microscopicamente, o neurilemoma é composto de combinações de dois padrões, os tipos A e B de Antoni, e qualquer um dos dois pode ser predominante em vários exemplos de neurilemomas. VER TAMBÉM neurofibroma. SIN neurilemoma, neuroschwannoma. [Theodor *Schwann* + -oma]
  acoustic s., s. do acústico. SIN vestibular s.
  vestibular s., s. vestibular; tumor benigno, porém potencialmente fatal, que surge a partir de células de Schwann, geralmente da divisão vestibular do oitavo nervo craniano; no estágio inicial, provoca perda auditiva, tinido e distúrbios vestibulares e, nos estágios tardios, sinais cerebelares, do tronco cerebral e de outros nervos cranianos, bem como aumento da pressão intracraniana. SIN acoustic neurinoma, acoustic neuroma, acoustic s., acoustic tumor, cerebellopontine angle tumor, eighth nerve tumor.
schwan·no·sis (shwah-nō′sis). Schwanose; proliferação não-neoplásica de células de Schwann nos espaços perivasculares da medula espinal; observada sobretudo em pacientes idosos, especialmente naqueles com diabetes melito.
Schwartz, Henry G., neurocirurgião norte-americano, *1909. VER S. *tractotomy.*
Schwartz, Oscar, pediatra norte-americano, *1919. VER S. *syndrome.*
Schweigger-Seidel, Franz, fisiologista alemão, 1834–1871. VER *sheath* of Schweigger-Seidel.
Schweninger, Ernst, dermatologista alemão, 1850–1924. VER S.-Buzzi *anetoderma;* S. *method.*
sci·age (sē-ahzh′). Movimento de vai-e-vem da mão, semelhante ao de uma serra, durante a massagem. [Fr. *scie,* serra]
sci·at·ic (sī-at′ik). Ciático. 1. Relativo a ou situado próximo ao ísquio ou quadril. Isquiático ou ciático. SIN ischiadic, ischial, ischiatic. 2. Relativo à ciática. SIN ischiadicus. [L. mediev. *sciaticus,* corruptela do G. *ischiadikos,* de *ischion,* a articulação do quadril]
sci·at·i·ca (sī-at′i-kă). Ciática; dor na região lombar e no quadril que se irradia ao longo da face posterior da coxa até a perna, inicialmente atribuída à disfunção do nervo ciático (daí o termo); todavia, hoje em dia sabe-se que a dor é habitualmente causada por hérnia de disco lombar que compromete uma raiz nervosa, mais comumente a raiz L5 ou S1. SIN sciatic neuralgia, sciatic neuritis. [ver sciatic]
SCID Abreviatura de severe combined *immunodeficiency* (imunodeficiência combinada grave).
SCID mice Abreviatura de severe combined immunodeficient mice (camundongos com imunodeficiência combinada grave).
sci·ence (sī′ens). Ciência. 1. Ramo de conhecimento que fornece explicações teóricas dos fenômenos naturais com base em experimentos e observações. 2. Uma área desse conhecimento restrita para explicar uma classe limitada de fenômenos. [L. *scientia,* conhecimento, de *scio,* conhecer]
scientometrics (sī-en-tō-met′riks). Cientimetria; medida da produção científica e impacto dos achados científicos, como, por exemplo, sobre a política pública. [L. *scientia,* ciência, conhecimento, de *scio,* conhecer + G. *metron,* medida + -ics]
scil·la (sil′ă). Cila. SIN squill. [G.]
scil·la·ren (sil′lă-ren). Cilareno; mistura de glicosídeos presentes na cila, que exercem ações semelhantes aos digitálicos.
  s. A, c. A.; glicosídeo esteróide cristalino (*Scilla maritima*), presente na cila, que pode ser hidrolisado a glicose e proscilaridina A; esta última pode ser hidrolisada a ramnose e no esteróide aglicona cilaridina A; possui as mesmas ações e usos dos glicosídeos digitálicos. SIN transvaalin.
  s. B, c. B; fração glicosídica amorfa obtida da cila, consistindo em pelo menos sete glicosídeos cardioativos: glicocilareno A, cilifeosídeo, glicocilifeosídeo, cilicriptosídeo, ciliglaucosídeo, cilicianosídeo e cilazorosídeo.
scil·lar·i·cide (sil′ar-i-sīd). Cilaricida; princípio tóxico da cila utilizado como rodenticida.
scil·lir·o·side (sil′ir-ō-sīd). Cilirosídeo; glicosídeo da cila vermelha, a variedade vermelha de *Urginea maritima* (família Liliaceae). Utilizado como rodenticida.
scin·ti·cis·tern·og·ra·phy (sin′ti-sis-tern-og′ră-fē). Cinticisternografia; cisternografia efetuada com um radiofármaco e registrada com um dispositivo de imagens de radionuclídeo.
scin·ti·gram (sin′ti-gram). Cintilograma. SIN scintiscan. [L. *scintilla,* centelha + G. *gramma,* algo escrito]
scin·ti·graph·ic (sin′ti-graf′ik). Cintilográfico; relativo a, ou obtido por, cintilografia.
scin·tig·ra·phy (sin-tig′ră-fē). Cintilografia, cintigrafia; procedimento diagnóstico que consiste na administração de um radionuclídeo com afinidade pelo órgão ou tecido de interesse, seguida do registro da distribuição da radioatividade com uma câmara de cintilação externa estacionária ou de varredura. VER gamma *camera.*
scin·til·la·scope (sin-til′ă-skōp). Cintilascópio; termo obsoleto para *counter* (contador). [L. *scintilla,* centelha + G. *skopeō,* observar]
scin·ti·la·tion (sin-ti-lā′shun). Cintilação. 1. Emissão de faísca ou centelha; sensação subjetiva, como lampejos ou centelhas de luz. 2. Em medida de radiação, a luz produzida por um evento ionizante num fósforo, como num cristal ou cintilador líquido. VER TAMBÉM scintillation *counter.* [L. *scintilla,* centelha]

scin·til·la·tor (sin′ti-lā-ter, -tōr). Cintilador; substância que emite luz visível quando atingida por uma partícula subatômica ou por raios X ou gama. VER TAMBÉM scintillation counter.
  liquid s., c. líquido; líquido com as propriedades de um cintilador, em que a substância cuja radioatividade se pretende medir pode ser dissolvida e colocada em contador.
scin·til·lom·e·ter (sin-ti-lom′e-ter). Cintilômetro. SIN scintillation counter. [L. scintilla, centelha + G. metron, medida]
scin·ti·mam·mog·ra·phy (sin′te-mam-og′ra-fē). Cintilomamografia; técnicas de imagem das mamas que utilizam radionuclídeo para detecção de câncer.
scin·ti·pho·to·graph (sin-ti-fō′tō-graf). Cintilofotografia; imagem obtida por cintilofotografia; termo obsoleto. VER TAMBÉM scintiscan.
scin·ti·pho·tog·ra·phy (sin′ti-fō-tog′ra-fē). Cintilofotografia; processo de obtenção de um registro fotográfico da distribuição de um radiofármaco administrado internamente com o uso de uma câmara gama; termo obsoleto. SIN scintography.

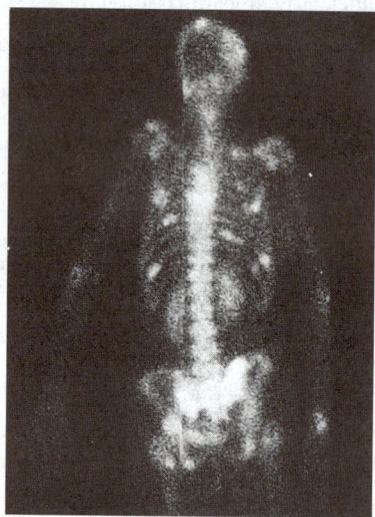

cintilofotografia: metástases disseminadas numa paciente com câncer de mama

scin·ti·scan (sin′ti-skan). Cintilograma; o registro obtido por cintilografia ou cintigrafia. VER TAMBÉM scan. SIN photoscan, scintigram.
scin·ti·scan·ner (sin′ti-skan′er). Cintilógrafo; aparelho utilizado para efetuar uma cintilografia.
scint·og·ra·phy (sin-tog′ra-fē). Cintilografia, cintigrafia. SIN scintiphotography.
sci·on (sī′on). Em embriologia experimental, parte ou tecido embrionário enxertado em outro embrião da mesma espécie ou de outra espécie. VER TAMBÉM chimera. [Fr. ant. sion, broto, rebento, do L. seco, cortar]
scir·rhos·i·ty (skir-os′i-tē, sir-). Cirrosidade; estado cirroso ou dureza de um tumor.
scir·rhous (skir′us, sir′). Cirroso; duro; relativo a um cirro.
scir·rhus (skir′us, sir′). Cirro; termo obsoleto para referir-se a qualquer área fibrosa endurecida, principalmente um carcinoma endurecido. [G. skirrhos, duro, tumor duro]
scis·sion (sizh′un). Cissão, cisão. **1.** Separação, divisão ou clivagem, como na fissão. **2.** SIN cleavage (2). [L. scissio, de scindo, pp. scissus, clivar]
scis·si·par·i·ty (sis-i-par′i-tē). Cissiparidade. SIN schizogenesis. [L. scissio, clivagem, + pario, parir, produzir]
scis·sors (siz′erz). Tesoura; instrumento com duas lâminas que se movem em torno de um eixo, cortando uma contra a outra. SIN shears. [L. scindo, pp. scissus, cortar]
  de Wecker s., t. de Wecker; pequena tesoura com pontas agudas para corte intra-ocular da íris e cápsula da lente.
  Smellie s., t. de Smellie; termo obsoleto para referir-se a uma tesoura com ponta em lança, com bordas externas cortantes, utilizada para craniotomia fetal.
scis·sors-shad·ow. Imagem deformada observada no astigmatismo misto por retinoscopia.
scis·su·ra, pl. **scis·su·rae** (si-soo′ră, -rē). Cissura. **1.** Fenda ou fissura. **2.** Divisão. SIN scissure. [L.]
  s. pilo′rum, esquizotriquia. SIN schizotrichia.
scis·sure (sish′oor). Cissura. SIN scissura.
scler-. Escler-. VER sclero-.
scle·ra, pl. **scle·ras, scler·ae** (skler′ă, -ăz, -ē) [TA]. Esclera, esclerótica; porção da camada fibrosa que forma o envoltório externo do globo ocular, à exceção do sexto anterior, que consiste na córnea. SIN sclerotic coat, sclerotica, tunica albuginea oculi, tunica sclerotica. [L. mod. do G. skleros, duro]
  blue s., e. azul; aspecto do tecido uveal através de uma esclerótica fina, observada em diversas condições, incluindo miopia, buftalmia, estafiloma escleral (scleral staphyloma), síndrome de Ehlers-Danlos (Ehlers-Danlos syndrome), síndrome de Marfan (Marfan syndrome), osteogênese imperfeita (osteogenesis imperfecta), doença de Paget (Paget disease) e síndrome de Pierre Robin (Pierre Robin syndrome).
scler·ad·e·ni·tis (skler′ad-ĕ-nī′tis). Escleradenite; endurecimento inflamatório de uma glândula. [scler- + G. aden, glândula + -itis, inflamação]
scle·ral (skler′al). Escleral; relativo à esclera ou esclerótica. SIN sclerotic (2).
scle·ra·tog·e·nous (skler-ă-toj′e-nŭs). Escleratógeno. SIN sclerogenous.
scle·rec·ta·sia (skler-ek-tā′ze-ă). Esclerectasia; saliência localizada da esclera ou esclerótica. SIN scleral ectasia. [scler- + G. ektasis, extensão]
  partial s., e. parcial; protrusão parcial de uma porção da esclera, tipicamente observada na miopia acentuada. VER staphyloma.
  total s., e. total; estiramento uniforme de toda a esclera, tipicamente observado na buftalmia.
scle·rec·to·my (sklē-rek′tō-mē). Esclerectomia. **1.** Excisão de uma porção da esclera ou esclerótica. **2.** Remoção das aderências fibrosas formadas na otite média crônica. [scler- + G. ektome, excisão]
scle·re·de·ma (skler-e-dē′mă). Escleredema; edema duro não-depressível que ocorre na pele da face dorsal da parte superior do corpo e membros, conferindo um aspecto sério e sem demarcação nítida; observado em diabéticos e no escleredema do adulto. [scler- + G. oidema, tumefação (edema)]
  s. adulto′rum, e. do adulto; endurecimento disseminado benigno da pele do tecido subcutâneo, possivelmente de origem estreptocócica, que pode ocorrer após uma doença febril, com aparecimento de espessamento e endurecimento não-depressível da pele por depósitos de colágeno e de mucina, inicialmente na cabeça e no pescoço, estendendo-se depois pelo tronco; termo incorreto, visto que a doença não se restringe a adultos. SIN Buschke disease.
scle·re·ma (skle-rē′mă). Esclerema; endurecimento da gordura subcutânea. [scler- + edema]
  s. neonato′rum, e. do recém-nascido; esclerema que surge ao nascimento ou nos primeiros meses de vida, geralmente em prematuros e lactentes hipotérmicos, na forma de placas endurecidas bem demarcadas e branco-amareladas, que habitualmente acometem as bochechas, nádegas, ombros e panturrilhas; a gordura subcutânea exibe uma alta proporção de ácidos graxos saturados; ao exame microscópico, há espessamento do tecido fibroso interlobular e formação de cristais de triglicerídeos e células gigantes de corpo estranho; o prognóstico é sombrio para as lesões disseminadas, enquanto as lesões localizadas podem regredir lentamente no decorrer de um período de muitos meses.
scle·ren·ceph·a·ly, scle·ren·ce·pha·lia (skler-en-sef′ă-lē, -en-sĕ-fā′lē-ă). Esclerencefalia; esclerose e retração da substância cerebral. [scler- + G. enkephalos, cérebro]
scle·ri·tis (sklē-rī′tis). Esclerite; inflamação da esclera ou esclerótica.
  anterior s., e. anterior; inflamação da esclera adjacente à córnea.
  anular s., e. anular; inflamação freqüentemente prolongada da porção anterior da esclera, formando um anel ao redor do limbo córneo-escleral.
  brawny s., e. gelatinosa; tumefação de aspecto gelatinoso que circunda a córnea, com tendência a acometer a sua periferia. SIN gelatinous s.
  deep s., e. profunda; inflamação intensa da esclera, com comprometimento da úvea subjacente.
  gelatinous s., e. gelatinosa. SIN brawny s.
  malignant s., e. maligna; inflamação progressiva da esclera anterior e coróide adjacente, com uveíte associada.
  necrotizing s., e. necrosante; degeneração fibrinóide e necrose da esclera.
  nodular s., e. nodular; áreas firmes e imóveis, isoladas ou múltiplas de esclerite localizada.
  posterior s., e. posterior; inflamação freqüentemente monocular da esclera adjacente ao nervo óptico, com extensão freqüente na retina e coróide.
sclero-, scler-. Esclero-, escler-. Dureza (endurecimento), esclerose, relação com a esclera. [G. skleros, duro]
scle·ro·at·ro·phy (sklēr-ō-at′rō-fē). Escleroatrofia. SIN sclerotylosis.
scle·ro·blas·te·ma (sklēr-ō-blas-tē′mă). Escleroblastema; tecido embrionário que entra na formação do osso. [sclero- + G. blastema, broto]
scle·ro·cho·roi·dal (sklēr-ō-kō-roy′dăl). Esclerocoriódie; relativo à esclera e à coróide.
scle·ro·cho·roid·i·tis (sklēr′ō-kō-roy-dī′tis). Esclerocorioidite; inflamação da esclera e da coróide.
  s. ante′rior, e. anterior; inflamação secundária da esclera por extensão de um processo da úvea.
  s. poste′rior, e. posterior. SIN posterior staphyloma.
scle·ro·con·junc·ti·val (sklēr′ō-kon-jŭngk-tī′val). Escleroconjuntival; relativo à esclera e conjuntiva.
scle·ro·cor·nea (sklēr-ō-kōr′nē-ă). Esclerocórnea. **1.** A córnea e a esclera consideradas como formando juntas a camada externa dura do olho, a túnica

fibrosa do olho. **2.** Anomalia congênita em que toda a córnea ou parte dela torna-se opaca e assemelha-se à esclera; com freqüência, existem outras anormalidades oculares.

scle·ro·dac·ty·ly, scle·ro·dac·tyl·ia (sklēr-ō-dak′ti-lē, -dak-til′ē-ā). Esclerodactilia. SIN acrosclerosis. [sclero- + G. *daktylos*, dedo da mão ou do pé]

scle·ro·der·ma (sklēr-ō-der′mă). Esclerodermia; espessamento e endurecimento da pele em consequência da formação de novo colágeno, com atrofia dos folículos pilosos; manifestação da esclerose sistêmica progressiva ou localizada (morféia). VER systemic *sclerosis*, morphea. SIN systemic s., systemic sclerosis (2). [sclero- + G. *derma*, pele]

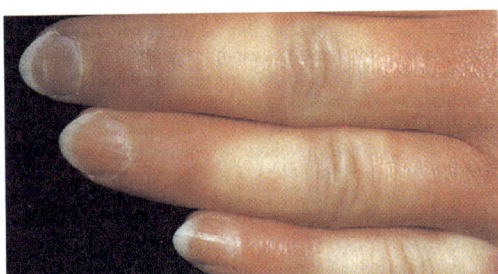

esclerodermia: estágio inicial

linear s., e. linear; esclerodermia localizada com lesões da pele semelhantes a faixas, com endurecimento, atrofia, hiper ou hipopigmentação, podendo ser desfigurante, com extensão para os tecidos subjacentes e contraturas articulares. O acometimento da fronte e do couro cabeludo tem sido denominado "coup de sabre" (q.v.). SIN morphea linearis.
localized s., e. localizada. SIN morphea.
progressive familial s., [MIM*181750], e. progressiva familiar; síndrome caracterizada por calcinose cutânea, fenômeno de Raynaud, esclerodactilia e telangiectasia; geralmente devida a esclerodermia; forma autossômica dominante de esclerose sistêmica progressiva.
systemic s., e. sistêmica. SIN scleroderma.

scle·ro·der·ma·tous (sklēr-ō-der′mă-tŭs). Esclerodermatoso; caracterizado por ou semelhante à esclerodermia.

scle·rog·e·nous, scle·ro·gen·ic (skle-roj′e-nŭs, sklēr-ō-jen′ik). Esclérogeno, esclerogênico; que produz tecido duro ou esclerótico; que causa esclerose. SIN scleratogenous. [sclero- + G. *-gen*, produtor]

scle·roid (sklēr′oyd). Esclerôide; endurecido ou esclerótico, de textura incomumente firme, semelhante a couro ou com textura semelhante a uma cicatriz. SIN sclerosal, sclerous. [sclero- + G. *eidos*, semelhança]

scle·ro·i·ri·tis (sklēr′ō-ī-rī′tis). Escleroirite; inflamação da esclera e da íris.

scle·ro·ker·a·ti·tis (sklēr′ō-ker-ă-tī′tis). Escleroceratite; inflamação da esclera e da córnea. [sclero- + G. *keras*, corno]

scle·ro·ker·a·to·i·ri·tis (sklēr-ō-ker′ă-tō-ī-rī′tis). Escleroceratoirite; inflamação da esclera, da córnea e da íris.

scle·ro·ma (skle-rō′mă). Escleroma; foco endurecido circunscrito de tecido de granulação na pele ou na mucosa. [G. *sklērōma*, endurecimento]
respiratory s., e. respiratório; rinoscleroma em que a lesão acomete a mucosa da maior parte do trato respiratório superior ou de todo ele.

scle·ro·ma·la·cia (sklēr′ō-mă-lā′shē-ă). Escleromalacia; adelgaçamento degenerativo da esclera, que ocorre em indivíduos com artrite reumatóide e outros distúrbios do colágeno. [sclero- +G. *malakia*, amolecimento]

scle·ro·mere (sklēr′ō-mēr). Esclerômero. **1.** Qualquer metâmero do esqueleto, como um segmento vertebral. **2.** Metade caudal de um esclerótomo. [sclero- + G. *meros*, parte]

scle·rom·e·ter (sklē-rom′e-ter). Esclerômetro; dispositivo para determinar a densidade ou a dureza de qualquer substância. [sclero- + G. *metron*, medida]

scle·ro·myx·e·de·ma (sklēr′ō-mik-se-dē′mă). Escleromixedema; líquen mixedematoso generalizado, com espessamento difuso da pele subjacente às pápulas.

scle·ro·nych·ia (sklēr-ō-nik′ē-ă). Escleroniquia; endurecimento e espessamento das unhas. [sclero- + G. *onyx*, unha + *-ia*, condição]

scle·ro·o·o·pho·ri·tis (sklēr′ō-ō-of′ō-rī′tis). Esclero-ooforite; endurecimento inflamatório do ovário. [sclero- + L. mod. *oophoron*, ovário + G. *-itis*, inflamação]

scle·roph·thal·mia (sklēr-of-thal′mē-ă). Escleroftalmia; anormalidade em que a maior parte da córnea normalmente transparente assemelha-se à esclera opaca. [sclero- + G. *ophthalmos*, olho]

scle·ro·plas·ty (sklēr′ō-plas-tē). Escleroplastia; cirurgia plástica da esclera ou esclerótica. [sclero- + G. *plastos*, formado]

scle·ro·pro·tein (sklēr-ō-prō′tēn). Escleroproteína. SIN albuminoid (3). VER TAMBÉM fibrous *protein*.

scle·ro·sal (sklē-rō′săl). Escleroso. SIN scleroid.

scle·ro·sant (sklēr-ō-sant). Esclerosante; substância irritante injetável utilizada no tratamento de varizes para a produção de trombos em seu interior.

scle·rose (sklē-rōz′). Esclerosar; endurecer; sofrer esclerose.

scle·ro·sis, pl. **scle·ro·ses** (sklē-rō′sis, -sēz). Esclerose. **1.** Induração. SIN induration (2). **2.** Em neuropatia, o endurecimento de estruturas nervosas ou outras estruturas por hiperplasia do tecido conjuntivo glial ou fibroso intersticial. [G. *sklērōsis*, dureza]
Alzheimer s., e. Alzheimer; degeneração hialina dos vasos sanguíneos de calibre médio e menores do cérebro.
amyotrophic lateral s. (ALS), e. lateral amiotrófica; doença degenerativa fatal que acomete os neurônios corticobulbares, corticospinais e motores espinais, manifestando-se na forma de fraqueza e debilitação progressivas dos músculos inervados pelos neurônios afetados; é comum a ocorrência de fasciculações e cãibras. O distúrbio é de natureza esporádica em 90–95% dos casos (embora alguns casos sejam herdados como caráter autossômico dominante [MIM*105400]), afeta adultos (tipicamente, idosos) e costuma ser fatal dentro de 2 a 5 anos após o seu início. Trata-se do subgrupo mais comum de doença dos neurônios motores e o único a se manifestar por uma combinação de anormalidades superiores e inferiores. As variantes incluem: 1) paralisia bulbar progressiva, em que ocorre comprometimento motor do tronco cerebral inferior isolado ou predominante; 2) esclerose lateral primária, em que são observadas apenas anormalidades dos neurônios motores superiores; e 3) atrofia progressiva dos músculos espinais, em que se observa apenas uma disfunção dos neurônios motores inferiores. SIN Aran-Duchenne disease, Charcot disease, Duchenne-Aran disease, Lou Gehrig disease, progressive muscular atrophy, progressive spinal amyotrophy.
arterial s., arteriosclerose. SIN arteriosclerosis.
arteriocapillary s., e. arteriocapilar; arteriosclerose, especialmente dos vasos mais finos.
arteriolar s., arteriolosclerose. SIN arteriolosclerosis.
bone s., eburnação. SIN eburnation.
Canavan s., doença de Canavan. SIN Canavan *disease.*
central areolar choroidal s., e. corioidal areolar central. SIN areolar *choroidopathy.*
combined s., e. combinada. SIN subacute combined *degeneration* of the spinal cord.
diffuse infantile familial s., e. infantil familiar difusa. SIN globoid cell *leukodystrophy.*
disseminated s., e. disseminada. SIN multiple s.
endocardial s., e. endocárdica. SIN endocardial *fibrosis.*
glomerular s., e. glomerular. SIN glomerulosclerosis.
hippocampal s., e. hipocampal; perda de neurônios corticais e astrocitose reativa nas regiões do hipocampo de alguns indivíduos com epilepsia.
idiopathic hypercalcemic s. of infants, e. hipercalcêmica idiopática dos lactentes. VER idiopathic *hypercalcemia* of infants.
insular s., e. insular. SIN multiple s.
laminar cortical s., e. cortical laminar; degeneração de fibras nervosas na coroa radiada em um padrão laminar.
lateral spinal s., e. espinal lateral. SIN primary lateral s.
lobar s., e. lobar. SIN Pick *atrophy.*
mantle s., e. em manto; lesão cerebral comum nos estados paralíticos do início da vida, caracterizada por atrofia cortical nodular.
menstrual s., e. menstrual. SIN physiologic s.
Mönckeberg s., e. de Mönckeberg. SIN Mönckeberg *arteriosclerosis.*
multiple s. (MS). e. múltipla (EM); distúrbio desmielinizante comum do sistema nervoso central, caracterizado por placas de esclerose no cérebro e na medula espinal; ocorre primariamente em adultos jovens e exibe manifestações clínicas multiformes, dependendo da localização e do tamanho da placa; os sintomas típicos incluem perda da visão, diplopia, nistagmo, disartria, fraqueza, parestesias, anormalidades vesicais e alterações do humor; tipicamente, as placas estão "separadas no tempo e no espaço" e, clinicamente, os sintomas sofrem exacerbações e remissões. SIN disseminated s., insular s.
nodular s., e. nodular. SIN atherosclerosis.
nuclear s., e. nuclear; aumento da refratividade da porção central do cristalino do olho. VER nuclear *cataract.*
ovulational s., e. ovular. SIN physiologic s.
physiologic s., e. fisiológica; esclerose lentamente progressiva das paredes das artérias ovarianas que começa após a puberdade. SIN menstrual s., ovulational s.
posterior s., e. posterior. SIN tabetic *neurosyphilis.*
posterior spinal s., e. espinal posterior. SIN tabetic *neurosyphilis.*
primary lateral s., e. lateral primária; considerada por muitos como um subgrupo da doença dos neurônios motores; trata-se de um distúrbio degenerativo lentamente progressivo dos neurônios motores do córtex cerebral, resultando em fraqueza disseminada com origem nos neurônios motores superiores; ocorrem espasticidade, hiper-reflexia e sinais de Babinski, mas não potenciais de fasciculação, nem qualquer evidência eletrodiagnóstica de lesão dos neurônios motores inferiores. SIN lateral spinal s.

systemic s., e. sistêmica; **(1)** doença sistêmica caracterizada pela formação de tecido fibroso colagenoso hialinizado e espessado, com espessamento da pele e adesão aos tecidos subjacentes (especialmente das mãos e da face), disfagia em decorrência da perda do peristaltismo e fibrose submucosa do esôfago, dispnéia devido a fibrose pulmonar, fibrose do miocárdio e alterações vasculares renais que se assemelham àquelas da hipertensão maligna; os achados comuns incluem fenômeno de Raynaud, atrofia dos tecidos moles e osteoporose das falanges distais (acrosclerose), algumas vezes com gangrena nas pontas dos dedos. O termo esclerose sistêmica progressiva é comumente utilizado e mostra-se apropriado para descrever casos com comprometimento cutâneo inicialmente disseminado, incluindo o tronco. Todavia, quando o acometimento da pele se limita às partes distais dos membros e à face, há freqüentemente atraso prolongado no aparecimento das manifestações viscerais. VER TAMBÉM CREST *syndrome;* **(2)** SIN scleroderma.

tuberous s. [MIM*191100], e. tuberosa; facomatose caracterizada pela formação de hamartomas multissistêmicos que produzem convulsões, retardo mental e angiofibromas da face; as lesões cerebrais e retinianas consistem em nódulos gliais; outras lesões cutâneas incluem máculas hipopigmentadas, placas chagrem e fibromas periungueais; herança autossômica dominante com expressão variável, causada por mutação no gene da esclerose tuberosa (TSC1) no cromossoma 9q ou do TSC2 no cromossoma 16p. SIN Bourneville disease, epiloia.

unicellular s., e. unicelular; proliferação de tecido fibroso entre células individuais de uma parte, isolando-as umas das outras.

valvular s., e. valvar; fibrose, freqüentemente com calcificação valvar, considerada uma alteração do processo de envelhecimento, e não causada por doença valvar primária.

vascular s., e. vascular. SIN arteriosclerosis.

s. of white matter, e. da substância branca. SIN leukodystrophy.

scle·ro·ste·no·sis (sklēr-ō-ste-nō'sis). Esclerostenose; endurecimento e contração dos tecidos. [sclero- + G. *stenōsis,* estreitamento]

Scle·ros·to·ma (sklē-ros'tō-mă). Denominação genérica antiga dos nematódeos do gênero estrôngilo e tricostrôngilos de cavalos; hoje em dia, foi substituído por outros gêneros, porém ainda é utilizado como termo coletivo para referir-se a esse grupo. As espécies incluem *S. duodenale (Ancylostoma duodenale)* e *S. syngamus (Syngamus trachea)* [sclero- + G. *stoma,* boca]

scle·ros·to·my (sklĕ-ros'tō-mē). Esclerostomia; perfuração cirúrgica da esclera, como a efetuada para alívio de glaucoma. [sclero- + G. *stoma,* boca]

scle·ro·ther·a·py (sklēr-ō-thăr'ă-pē). Escleroterapia; terapia envolvendo a injeção de uma solução esclerosante nos vasos ou tecidos. SIN sclerosing therapy.

scle·ro·thrix (sklēr'ō-thriks). Esclerotriquia; endurecimento e fragilidade do cabelo. SIN sclerotrichia. [sclero- + G. *thrix,* cabelo]

scle·rot·ic (sklĕ-rot'ik). **1.** Esclerótico; relativo a, ou caracterizado por, esclerose. **2.** Escleral. SIN scleral.

scle·rot·i·ca (sklĕ-rot'i-kă). Esclera; esclerótica. SIN sclera. [L. mod. *scleroticus,* duro]

scle·ro·ti·um, pl. **scle·ro·tia** (sklĕ-rō'shē-ŭm, -shē-ă). Esclerócio. **1.** Nos fungos, corpo em repouso de tamanho variável, composto de uma massa endurecida de hifas com ou sem tecido hospedeiro, geralmente com revestimento externo escuro, a partir do qual pode haver desenvolvimento de corpos frutíferos, estromas, conidióforos ou micélios. **2.** Condição de repouso endurecida do plasmódio de Myxomycetes.

scle·ro·tome (sklēr'ō-tōm). Esclerótomo. **1.** Instrumento utilizado na esclerotomia. **2.** Grupo de células mesenquimatosas que surgem da parte ventromedial de um somito e migram para a notocorda. As células do esclerótomo de somitos adjacentes fundem-se em massas localizadas entre os somitos, constituindo os primórdios dos centros das vértebras. [sclero- + G. *tomē,* corte]

scle·rot·o·my (sklĕ-rot'ō-mē). Esclerotomia; incisão através da esclera. [sclero- + G. *tomē,* incisão]

anterior s., e. anterior; incisão na câmara anterior do olho.

posterior s., e. posterior; incisão feita através da esclera no humor vítreo.

scle·ro·trich·ia (sklēr-ō-trik'ē-ă). Esclerotriquia. SIN sclerothrix.

scle·ro·ty·lo·sis (sklēr'ō-tī-lō'sis) [MIM*181600]. Esclerotilose; fibrose atrófica da pele, hipoplasia das unhas e ceratodermia palmoplantar; associada a cânceres da pele e gastrointestinais; herança autossômica dominante. SIN scleroatrophy. [sclero- + G. *tylosis,* o processo de tornar-se caloso]

scle·rous (sklēr'ŭs). Escleroso. SIN scleroid. [G. *sklēros,* duro]

SCM Abreviatura de sternocleidomastoid (*muscle*) (músculo esternocleidomastóideo).

scol·e·ces (skō'le-sez). Escóleces; plural de scolex.

scol·e·ci·a·sis (skō-lē-sī'ă-sis). Escoleciáse; infecção do intestino por larvas de lepidópteros (mariposas e borboletas). [G. *skōlēx,* verme, + *-iasis,* condição]

sco·le·ci·form (skō-lē'si-form). Escoleciforme, escolecóide. SIN scolecoid.

sco·le·coid (skō'le-koyd). Escolecóide. **1.** Semelhante ao escólex de uma tênia. **2.** Semelhante a um verme. VER TAMBÉM lumbricoid (1), vermiform. SIN scoleciform. [G. *skōlēkoeidēs,* de *skōlēx,* verme + *eidos,* aparência]

sco·le·col·o·gy (skō-lē-kol'ō-jē). Escolecologia. SIN helminthology. [G. *skōlēx,* verme + *logos,* estudo]

sco·lex, pl. **scol·e·ces, scol·i·ces** (skō'leks, skō'le-sēz, skō'li-sēz). Escólex, escólece; a cabeça ou extremidade anterior de uma tênia fixada por ventosas e freqüentemente por ganchos rostelares à parede do intestino; forma-se no interior do cisto hidático de *Echinococcus,* no interior de um cisticerco na *Taenia,* cisticercóide no *Hymenolepis* e através de pleurocercóide, como no *Diphyllobothrium latum.* A forma do escólex varia enormemente, sendo a forma mais comum arredondada ou claviforme, com quatro ventosas musculares circulares e um rostelo armado ou desarmado, ou um escólex achatado espatulado, com um par de ventosas semelhantes a fendas (bótrios) sem rostelo, como no *Diphyllobothrium* e espécies afins. Outros helmintos possuem formas complexas, semelhantes a folhas, caliciformes ou fimbriadas, ou probóscides retráteis com múltiplos espinhos. Essas formas variadas caracterizam as ordens dos cestóides, que são particularmente bem desenvolvidas como parasitas de tubarões e arraias. [G. *skōlēx,* verme]

sco·li·o·ky·pho·sis (skō'lē-ō-kī-fō'sis). Escoliocifose, cifoescoliose. SIN kyphoscoliosis. [G. *scolios,* curvado + *kyphōsis,* cifose]

sco·li·om·e·ter (skō-lē-om'e-ter). Escoliômetro; instrumento para medir curvas, especialmente aquelas na curvatura lateral da coluna vertebral. [G. *skolios,* curvo + *metron,* medida]

sco·li·o·sis (skō-lē-ō'sis). [TA]. Escoliose; curvatuva lateral e rotacional anormal da coluna vertebral. Dependendo da etiologia, pode haver uma curva ou curvas compensatórias primárias ou secundárias; a escoliose pode ser "fixa", em conseqüência de deformidade muscular e/ou óssea, ou "móvel", resultante de contração muscular desigual. [G. *skoliōsis,* curvatura]

coxitic s., e. coxítica; escoliose na coluna lombar em decorrência da inclinação da pelve na vigência de doença do quadril.

empyemic s., e. empiêmica; esclerose devido à retração de um lado do tórax após empiema.

habit s., e. postural; esclerose supostamente devida à postura em pé ou sentada habitual numa posição imprópria.

myopathic s., e. miopática; curvatura lateral devido à fraqueza dos músculos espinhais, como na poliomielite.

ocular s., ophthalmic s., e. ocular, e. oftálmica; esclerose supostamente decorrente da inclinação da cabeça, causada por disfunção oftalmológica.

osteopathic s., e. osteopática; curvatura lateral da coluna em virtude de doença vertebral.

paralytic s., e. paralítica; curvatura lateral da coluna, devido à paralisia dos músculos espinais.

rachitic s., e. raquítica; esclerose que ocorre em conseqüência de raquitismo.

sciatic s., e. ciática; esclerose causada por espasmo assimétrico dos músculos espinais, geralmente associada à ciática, manifestando-se como inclinação para um lado.

static s., e. estática; curvatura lateral da coluna vertebral, devido a desigualdade no comprimento das pernas.

sco·li·ot·ic (skō'lē-ot'ik). Escoliótico; relativo a ou que sofre de escoliose.

sco·li·o·tone (skō'lē-ō-tōn). Escoliótono; aparelho para estiramento da coluna vertebral e redução da curva na escoliose. [G. *skolios,* curvo + *tonos,* tensão]

Scol·o·pen·dra (skō-lō-pen'dră). Gênero de lacraia, caracterizado por 21–23 pares de pernas. As espécies comuns nos Estados Unidos são *S. heros* (a lacraia doméstica ocidental) e *S. morsitans.* [L. mod. do G. *skōlopendra,* multípede]

s-cone. Cone S; cone sensível a um comprimento de onda curto (cone azul).

scoop (skoop). Cureta; instrumento estreito, semelhante a uma colher, para extrair o conteúdo de cavidades ou cistos. [A.S. *skopa*]

△ **scope.** -Scópio. Indica um instrumento para visualização, mas que foi estendido para incluir outros métodos de exame (p. ex., estetoscópio). [G. *skopeō,* ver]

sco·pine (skō'pen). Escopina; escopalamina menos a cadeia lateral de ácido trópico, isto é, 6,7-epoxitropina ou 6,7-epoxi-3-hidroxitropano.

sco·pol·a·mine (skō-pol'ă-mēn, -min). Escopolamina; alcalóide encontrado nas folhas e sementes de *Hyoscyamus niger, Duboisia myopoides, Scopolia japonica, Scopolia carniolica, Atropa belladonna* e outras plantas solanáceas; o 6,7-epóxido de atropina, isto é, tropato de 6,7-epoxitropina. Exerce ações anticolinérgicas semelhantes à atropina; acredita-se que exerça efeitos mais acentuados sobre o sistema nervoso central; útil na prevenção da cinetose. SIN hyoscine.

s. hydrobromide, bromidrato de e.; ação anticolinérgica semelhante à da atropina. SIN hyoscine hydrobromide.

s. methylbromide, metilbrometo de e.; derivado de amônio quaternário da escopalamina; utilizado quando se deseja obter efeitos espasmolíticos ou antisecretores.

sco·po·lia (skō-pō'lē-ă). Escopólia; rizoma e raízes secos de *Scopolia carniolica* (família Solanaceae), uma erva da Áustria e países vizinhos da Europa; assemelha-se à beladona na sua ação farmacológica. [G.A. *Scopoli,* naturalista italiano, 1723–1788]

S. japon'ica, beladona japonesa cujas folhas, raízes e sementes contêm escopolamina.

sco·po·line (skō′pō-lēn). Escopolina; produto de decomposição da escopalamina e isômero da escopina, visto que os grupos epóxi e hidroxila encontram-se em diferentes locais.

sco·pom·e·ter (skō-pom′e-ter). Escopômetro; aparelho para determinar a densidade de um precipitado pelo grau de transparência de um líquido que o contém. VER TAMBÉM nephelometer. [G. *skopeō*, ver + *metron*, medida]

sco·po·phil·ia (skō-pō-fil′ē-ā). Escopofilia. SIN voyeurism. [G. *skopeō*, ver + *philos*, amigo]

sco·po·pho·bia (skō-pō-fō′bē-ā). Escopofobia; medo mórbido de ser visto. [G. *skopeō*, ver + *phobos*, medo]

Scop·u·lar·i·op·sis (skō′pū-lar-ē-op′sis). Gênero de fungos filamentosos raramente patogênicos para os seres humanos; diversas espécies foram implicadas na onicomicose, granuloma ulcerativo e outras condições "mitóticas". Semelhante ao *Penicillium*, é comum na natureza e constitui geralmente um contaminante em culturas laboratoriais de tecidos humanos. [L. mod. *scopula*, pequena vassoura + G. *opsis*, aspecto]

-scopy. -Scopia. Ação ou atividade envolvendo o uso de um instrumento para visualização. [G. *skopeō*, ver]

scor·bu·tic (skōr-bū′tik). Escorbútico; relativo a, que sofre de ou que se assemelha ao escorbuto.

scor·bu·ti·gen·ic (skōr-bū-ti-jen′ik). Escorbutigênico; que produz escorbuto.

scor·bu·tus (skōr-bū′tus). Escorbuto. SIN scurvy. [L. mediev. forma do Teutônico *schorbuyck*, escorbuto]

scor·di·ne·ma (skōr′di-nē′ma). Escordinema; sensação de peso da cabeça acompanhada de bocejo e espreguiçamento, que ocorre como pródromo de uma doença infecciosa. [G. *skordinēma*, bocejo]

score (skōr). Escore, índice; avaliação, em geral expressa numericamente, do estado, realização ou condição em determinado conjunto de circunstâncias. [I.m. *scor*, incisura, talha]

APACHE s., e. APACHE; *acute physiology and chronic health evaluation* (avaliação da fisiologia aguda e da saúde crônica). Método mais utilizado para avaliação da gravidade da doença em pacientes com quadro agudo na unidade de tratamento intensivo.

Apgar s., índice de Apgar; avaliação do estado físico do recém-nascido ao atribuir valores numéricos (0–2) a cada um destes cinco critérios: 1) freqüência cardíaca, 2) esforço respiratório, 3) tônus muscular, 4) resposta a estímulos e 5) cor da pele; um escore de 8–10 indica a melhor condição possível.

escore de Apgar				
depois de 60 segundos	escore	0	1	2
freqüência cardíaca	....	ausente	abaixo de 100	acima de 100
esforço respiratório	....	ausente	lento, irregular	bom (choro forte)
tônus muscular	....	flácido	bom nos membros	movimento ativo
reação ao cateter na narina	....	nenhuma resposta	careta	tosse ou espirro
cor da pele	....	pálida	tronco róseo, membros azuis	rósea
escore	....	(total de pontos: 8–10 normal)		

Bishop s., e. de Bishop; sistema para determinar a induzibilidade do colo uterino na gestante, com base na dilatação, apagamento, posição parada e consistência e posição cervical.

discrimination s., e. de discriminação; percentagem de palavras que um indivíduo consegue repetir corretamente a partir de uma lista de palavras foneticamente equilibradas apresentadas 25–40 dB acima do limiar de recepção da fala.

Dubowitz s., e. de Dubowitz; método de avaliação clínica da idade gestacional no recém-nascido que inclui critérios neurológicos para determinar sua maturidade e outros critérios físicos para determinar sua idade gestacional; útil desde o nascimento até 5 dias de vida.

Gleason s., e. de Gleason. VER Gleason tumor *grade*.

Jarman s., e. de Jarman; índice de privação social e médica, utilizada principalmente por médicos da família, especialmente no Reino Unido.

Logistic Organ Dysfunction S., E. de Disfunção Orgânica Logístico; método de avaliação utilizado em tratamento intensivo, que enumera o nível de disfunção de cada sistema orgânico, bem como entre sistemas orgânicos; inclui a avaliação do grau de disfunção dos sistemas cardiovascular, hepático, hematológico, pulmonar, renal e nervoso.

raw s., e. bruto; o escore, medida ou valor real obtido antes da aplicação de qualquer estatística. Cf. standard s.

recovery s., e. de recuperação; número que expressa a condição de um lactente em vários intervalos estipulados maiores que 1 minuto após o nascimento, baseando-se nas mesmas características avaliadas pelo escore de Apgar nos 60 segundos após o nascimento.

standard s., e. padrão; escore estatisticamente derivado ou com referências, que representa o desvio de um escore bruto a partir de sua média em unidades de desvio padrão.

symptom s., e. sintomático; sistema de pontuação da *American Urological Association* para avaliação da obstrução prostática.

scor·pi·on (skōr′pē-on). Escorpião; membro da ordem Scorpionida; inclui o escorpião do diabo, *Vejovis*, e o escorpião peludo, *Hadrurus*. [G. *skorpios*]

Scor·pi·on·i·da (skōr-pē-on′i-dā). Os escorpiões; ordem de artrópodes aracnídeos predadores e venenosos, caracterizados por um abdome ósseo nitidamente segmentado, que termina num aguilhão bastante recurvado, equipado com uma glândula de veneno; sua picada é muito dolorosa, porém raramente fatal. Os gêneros na América do Norte incluem *Centruroides*, *Hadrurus* e *Vejovis*. [L. mod.]

scoto-. Escoto-. Escuridão. [G. *skotos*]

scot·o·chro·mo·gens (skō′tō-krō′mō-jenz). Escotocromógenos. SIN Runyon group II *mycobacteria*. [scoto- + G. *chrōma*, cor, + -*gen*, que produz]

scot·o·graph (skō′tō-graf). Escotógrafo; aparelho para ajudar uma pessoa a escrever em linhas retas no escuro ou para ajudar o cego a escrever, utilizado pelo historiador W.H. Prescott. SIN noctograph. [scoto- + G. *graphō*, escrever]

sco·to·ma, pl. **sco·to·ma·ta** (skō-tō′ma, skō-tō′ma-ta). Escotoma. **1.** Área isolada de tamanho e forma variáveis dentro do campo visual, na qual a visão está ausente ou diminuída. **2.** Ponto cego na consciência psicológica. [G. *skotōma*, vertigem, de *skotos*, escuridão]

absolute s., e. absoluto; e. em que não há percepção de luz.

anular s., e. anular; e. circular que circunda o centro do campo visual. VER ring s.

arcuate s., e. arqueado; e. que se estende a partir do ponto cego e curva-se no campo nasal, seguindo as linhas das fibras do nervo retiniano.

Bjerrum s., e. de Bjerrum; e. em forma de cometa, que ocorre no glaucoma, fixado na extremidade temporal ao ponto cego ou dele separado por uma lacuna estreita; o defeito alarga-se à medida que se estende para cima e curva-se nasalmente ao redor do ponto de fixação, estendendo-se, em seguida, para baixo e terminando exatamente no meridiano horizontal nasal. SIN Bjerrum sign, sickle s.

cecocentral s., e. cecocentral; e. que envolve a área do disco óptico (mancha cega) e as fibras papilomaculares; existem três formas: 1) o defeito cecocentral, que se estende desde o ponto cego em direção à área de fixação ou para o seu interior; 2) angioscotoma; 3) e. de feixe de fibras nervosas glaucomatoso, devido ao comprometimento de feixes de fibras nervosas na borda do disco óptico. VER TAMBÉM Bjerrum s., Ronne nasal *step*.

central s., e. central; escotoma que envolve o ponto de fixação.

color s., e. colorido; área de diminuição da visão colorida no campo visual.

flittering s., e. cintilante. SIN scintillating s.

glaucomatous nerve-fiber bundle s., e. do feixe de fibras nervosas glaucomatoso. VER cecocentral s.

hemianopic s., e. hemianópico; escotoma que envolve metade do campo central.

mental s., e. mental; ausência de discernimento ou incapacidade de compreender itens relativos a um assunto cujo conteúdo é extremamente emocional para o indivíduo. SIN blind spot (2).

negative s., e. negativo; e. que não é normalmente percebido, sendo apenas detectado ao exame do campo visual.

paracentral s., e. paracentral; e. adjacente ao ponto de fixação.

pericentral s., e. pericentral; e. que circunda o ponto de fixação de modo mais ou menos simétrico.

peripheral s., e. periférico; e. fora dos 30 graus centrais do campo visual.

physiologic s., e. fisiológico; e. negativo no campo visual, correspondendo ao disco óptico. SIN blind spot (1).

positive s., e. positivo; e. que é percebido como mancha negra no campo visual.

quadrantic s., e. quadrântico; e. que envolve um quarto do campo visual central.

relative s., e. relativo; e. em que há depressão visual, mas não há perda completa da percepção da luz.

ring s., e. anular; área anular de cegueira no campo visual que circunda o ponto de fixação na degeneração pigmentar da retina e no glaucoma.

scintillating s., e. cintilante; área localizada de cegueira circundada por luzes trêmulas de cores brilhantes (teicopsia); em geral, trata-se de um sintoma prodrômico de enxaqueca. VER TAMBÉM fortification *spectrum*. SIN flittering s.

Seidel s., e. de Seidel; forma de e. de Bjerrum. VER TAMBÉM Seidel *sign*.

sickle s., e. falciforme. SIN Bjerrum s.

zonular s., e. zonular; e. curvo que não corresponde ao trajeto das fibras nervosas retinianas.

sco·to·ma·ta (skō-tō′mă-tă). Escotomas; plural de scotoma.
sco·tom·a·tous (skō-tō′mă-tŭs). Escotomatoso; relativo a escotoma.
sco·tom·e·ter (skō-tom′ĕ-ter). Escotômetro; instrumento para determinar o tamanho, a forma e a intensidade de um escotoma.
sco·tom·e·try (skō-tom′ĕ-trē). Escotometria; plotagem e medida de um escotoma. [scoto- + G. *metron,* medida]
scot·o·phil·ia (skō-tō-fil′ē-ă). Escotofilia. SIN nyctophilia. [scoto- + G. *philos,* amigo]
scot·o·pho·bia (skō-tō-fō′bē-ă). Escotofobia. SIN nyctophobia. [scoto- + G. *phobos,* medo]
sco·to·pia (skō-tō′pē-ă). Escotopia. SIN scotopic *vision.* [scoto- + G. *opsis,* visão]
sco·top·ic (skō-tō′pik, -top′ik). Escotópico; refere-se à baixa iluminação na qual o olho se adapta ao escuro. VER scotopic *vision.*
sco·top·sin (skō-top′sin). Escotopsina; parte proteica do pigmento nos bastonetes da retina.
sco·tos·co·py (skō-tos′kō-pē). Escotoscopia. SIN retinoscopy. [scoto- + G. *skopeō,* ver]
Scott, Charles I., Jr., pediatra norte-americano, *1934. VER Aarskog-S. *syndrome.*
Scott, Henry William Jr., cirurgião norte-americano, *1916. VER S. *operation.*
Scott-Wilson, H., cientista inglês. VER Scott-Wilson *reagent.*
scot·ty dog (scot′tē dawg). Refere-se ao aspecto irregular das facetas articulares na incidência oblíqua de radiografias da coluna lombar semelhante a um terrier escocês; o colo do cão é a parte interarticular, local do defeito mais comum na espondilólise.
scrape. Raspado. SIN scraping.
scrap·ie (skrap′ē, skrā′pē). *Scrapie;* encefalopatia espongiforme trasmissível do sistema nervoso central de ovinos e caprinos, causada por um príon e caracterizada por um período de incubação muito longo, seguido de prurido, anormalidades da marcha e, invariavelmente, morte; assemelha-se à doença de Creutzfeldt-Jakob e ao kuru nos seres humanos. [de scraping, ato de os animais afetados esfregarem-se contra objetos para aliviar o prurido]
scrap·ing (skrāp′ing). Raspado; amostra raspada de uma lesão ou local específico para exame citológico. VER TAMBÉM smear. SIN scrape.
screen (skrēn). **1.** Tela; lâmina de qualquer substância utilizada para proteger um objeto de qualquer influência, como calor, luz, raios X, etc. **2.** Tela sobre a qual uma imagem é projetada. **3.** Antigamente, efetuar um exame fluoroscópico. **4.** Em psicanálise encobrimento, como uma imagem ou memória encobrindo outra. VER TAMBÉM screen *memory.* **5.** Triagem; examinar, avaliar; processar um grupo para selecionar ou separar certos indivíduos. **6.** Fina camada de cristais que converte os raios X em fótons luminosos para expor o filme; utilizada no chassi para produzir imagens radiográficas no filme. [Fr. *écran*]
Bjerrum s., tela de Bjerrum. SIN tangent s.
s.-film contact, contato tela–filme; a proximidade e uniformidade entre o filme de raios X em um chassi e a tela (screen, 6). A resolução da imagem depende dessa propriedade.
fluorescent s., tela fluorescente; tela recoberta de cristais fluorescentes, como o tungstato de cálcio utilizado no fluoroscópio.
Hess s., tela de Hess; tela utilizada na medida do desvio ocular.
intensifying s., t. intensificadora; tela (screen, 6) utilizada em radiografia.
multiple marker s., triagem com múltiplos marcadores; uso de dois ou mais marcadores no soro materno para determinar o risco relativo de um feto anormal. VER TAMBÉM triple s.
rare-earth s., tela de terra rara; tela intensificadora (6) feita de uma terra rara, óxido de fósforo, mais eficiente do que o tungstato de cálcio, especialmente nas quilovoltagens maiores utilizadas na moderna radiografia.
tangent s., tela tangente; superfície plana e habitualmente preta, utilizada para medir os 30 graus centrais do campo visual. SIN Bjerrum s.
triple s., triagem tripla; determinação da α-fetoproteína, da gonadotropina coriônica e do estrogênio não conjugado no soro materno para indicação de risco aumentado de anormalidade fetal, especialmente trissomia do 21.
vestibular s., tela vestibular; tela feita de resina acrílica que recobre as superfícies labial ou bucal de uma ou de ambas as arcadas dentárias; utilizada no tratamento de hábitos orais e para estimular o movimento dos dentes ao usar a força dos músculos periorais.
screen·ing (skrēn′ing). **1.** Examinar (screen 5). **2.** Triagem, rastreamento; exame de um grupo de indivíduos habitualmente assintomáticos para detectar aqueles que têm alta probabilidade de apresentar determinada doença, tipicamente através de um exame diagnóstico de baixo custo. **3.** Na saúde mental, refere-se à avaliação inicial do paciente, que inclui história clínica e psiquiátrica, avaliação do estado mental e formulação diagnóstica para determinar a adequabilidade do paciente a determinada modalidade de tratamento.
carrier s., triagem de portadores; exame indiscriminado de membros de uma população para detectar heterozigotos para distúrbios graves e fornecer um aconselhamento sobre os riscos de casamento com outros portadores, bem como diagnóstico pré-natal quando ambos os cônjuges são portadores; com freqüência, sacrifica a especificidade em favor da sensibilidade e aplica-se com maior eficácia a populações reconhecidas de alto risco.
cytologic s., t. citológica; triagem para detecção de doença em seu estágio inicial, geralmente câncer, através do exame microscópico de uma amostra celular, com inspeção de cada célula e estrutura presente, utilizando, em geral, um aumento de 100 vezes com platina mecânica, de modo que todas as áreas possam ser examinadas; os achados são avaliados, e as anormalidades significativas são assinaladas (p. ex., marcando a lamínula com pontos) para avaliação posterior por um citopatologista. Essa triagem é habitualmente efetuada por um citotecnólogo, mas, algumas vezes, é feita por uma máquina automática de pré-triagem.
familial s., t. familiar; triagem efetuada em parentes próximos de probandos com doenças que podem permanecer latentes, como nos traços dominantes dependentes da idade, ou que podem envolver um risco para a progênie, como traços ligados ao X.
mass s., t. em massa; exame de uma grande população para detectar a manifestação de uma doença, a fim de iniciar o tratamento ou evitar a sua disseminação, como parte de uma campanha de saúde pública.
multiphasic s., t. multifásica; uso rotineiro de múltiplos testes, habitualmente bioquímicos, com a finalidade de detectar uma doença num estágio passível de prevenção ou cura.
neonatal s., t. neonatal; teste de recém-nascidos para detecção de doença passível de prevenção ou cura, ou para diagnóstico de doença genética.
prenatal s., t. pré-natal; triagem para detecção de doença fetal, geralmente através de ultra-sonografia ou exame do líquido amniótico obtido por amniocentese. Outras técnicas de triagem incluem testes efetuados no soro materno e biopsia placentária.
screw (skroo). Parafuso; cilindro com sulco helicoidal para prender dois objetos ou para ajustar a posição de um objeto fixado sobre uma extremidade do parafuso.
afterloading s., dispositivo para estabelecer o comprimento de um músculo em contração ao encontrar uma pós-carga.
screw-worm (skroo′werm). Larva do díptero *Cochliomyia hominivorax* e outras formas semelhantes, que causam miíase humana em animal.
primary s.-w., larva obrigatória que consegue penetrar nos tecidos normais e alimentar-se como invasor primário. As importantes moscas da miíase humana que servem como larvas primárias são *Cochliomyia hominivorax, Chrysomyia bezziana* e *Wohlfahrtia magnifica.*
secondary s.-w., larva acidental ou facultativa que penetra numa ferida ou condição supurada e alimenta-se de tecidos infectados (não dos tecidos intactos). Muitos dípteros estão incluídos, como *Calliphora vicina, Phaenicia sericata, Phormia regina, Cochliomyia macellaria, Chrysomyia* e outras moscas varejeiras.
scribe (skrīb). **1.** Riscar; escrever, traçar ou marcar fazendo uma linha com um marcador ou instrumento pontiagudo, como na confecção de um molde dentário para prótese removível. **2.** Formar, através de instrumentação, áreas negativas em um molde para produzir uma moldura positiva na estrutura de uma dentadura parcial removível ou a área de fechamento palatino posterior para uma dentadura completa. [L. *scribo,* pp. *scripto,* escrever]
Scribner, Belding H., nefrologista norte-americano, *1921. VER S. *shunt.*
scro·bic·u·late (skrō-bik′ū-lāt). Escrobiculado; que apresenta pequenas cavidades; caracterizado por minúsculas depressões. [L. *scrobiculus,* dim. de *scrobis,* fosso, vala]
scro·bic·u·lus cor·dis (skrō-bik′ū-lŭs kōr′dis). Fossa epigástrica. SIN epigastric *fossa.* [L. depressão ou fossa do coração]
scrof·u·la (skrof′ū-lă). Escrófula; termo histórico para designar a linfadenite tuberculosa cervical. [L. *scrofulae* (pl. apenas), tumefação glandular, escrófula de *scrofa,* porca reprodutora]
scrof·u·lo·der·ma (skrof′ū-lō-der′mă). Escrofulodermia; tuberculose resultante da extensão de infecção por micobactérias atípicas subjacentes na pele, mais comumente de linfonodos cervicais em crianças com infecção tonsilar pelo bacilo da tuberculose bovino. [scrofula + G. *derma,* pele]
scrof·u·lous (skrof′ū-lŭs). Escrofuloso; relativo a ou que sofre de escrófula.
scro·tal (skrō′tăl). Escrotal; relativo ao escroto. SIN oscheal.
scro·tec·to·my (skrō-tek′tō-mē). Escrotectomia; remoção total ou parcial do escroto. [scrotum, + G. *ektomē,* excisão]
scro·ti·form (skrō′ti-form). Escrotiforme; que possui a forma de um escroto.
scro·ti·tis (skrō-tī′tis). Escrotite; inflamação do escroto.
scro·to·plas·ty (skrō′tō-plas-tē). Escrotoplastia; reconstrução cirúrgica do escroto. SIN oscheoplasty. [scrotum + G. *plastos,* formado]
scro·tum, pl. **scro·ta, scro·tums** (skrō′tŭm, -tă, -tŭmz). [TA]. Escroto; saco musculocutâneo que contém os testículos; é formado de pele, contendo uma rede de fibras musculares não-estriadas (túnica dartos), que também forma o septo escrotal internamente. SIN marsupium (1). [L.]
lymph s. elefantíase escrotal. SIN *elephantiasis* scroti.
watering-can s., escroto em regador; fístulas urinárias no escroto e períneo, em decorrência de doença da uretra perineal. VER TAMBÉM watering-can *perineum.*
scru·ple (skroo′pl). Escrúpulo; peso farmacêutico de 20 grãos ou um terço de uma dracma. [L. *scrupulus,* pequena pedra pontiaguda; um peso, a vigé-

sima quarta parte de uma onça, um escrúpulo, dim. de *scrupus,* pedra pontiaguda]
SCUBA Acrônimo de *s*elf-*c*ontained *u*nderwater *b*reathing *a*pparatus (aparelho subaquático autônomo de respiração).
Scultetus (Scul·tet), originalmente Schultes, Johann, cirurgião alemão, 1595–1645. VER S. *bandage, position.*
scum (skŭm). Escuma; película de material insolúvel que sobe até a superfície de um líquido, como na epistase. [l.m.]
scurf (skerf). Caspa. SIN dandruff. [A.S.]
scur·vy (sker′vē). Escorbuto; doença caracterizada por inanição, debilidade, anemia e edema das partes pendentes; condição esponjosa, algumas vezes com ulceração das gengivas e perda dos dentes, hemorragia na pele proveniente das mucosas e de órgãos internos e cicatrização deficiente de feridas; decorrente de dieta com deficiência de vitamina C. SIN scorbutus, sea s. [do A.S. *scurf*]
  Alpine s., pelagra. SIN pellagra.
  hemorrhagic s., e. hemorrágico; escorbuto com hemorragias substanciais nas gengivas, na pele e em outros tecidos, que ocorrem tipicamente no estágio grave da doença.
  infantile s., e. infantil; osteopatia hemorrágica do lactente; condição caquética em lactentes, resultante de desnutrição e caracterizada por palidez, hálito fétido, língua saburrosa, diarréia e hemorragias subperiósteas; trata-se, provavelmente, de uma combinação de escorbuto e raquitismo, decorrente de deficiência combinada das vitaminas C e D. SIN Barlow disease, Cheadle disease, osteopathia hemorrhagica infantum, scurvy rickets.
  land s., e. terrestre; antigamente, e. que ocorria em pessoas que não tinham ido para o mar.
  sea s., escorbuto. SIN scurvy.
scu·tate (skoo′tāt). Escutiforme. SIN scutiform.
scute (skoot). Placa; lâmina ou placa fina. SIN scutum (1). [L. *scutum,* escudo]
  tympanic s., lâmina timpânica; a delgada placa óssea que separa o recesso epitimpânico das células mastóideas.
scu·ti·form (skoo′ti-form). Escutiforme; que apresenta forma de escudo. SIN scutate. [L. *scutum,* escudo, + *forma,* forma]
Scu·tig·e·ra (skoo-tij′er-ă). Gênero de centopéia comumente encontrado no leste dos Estados Unidos; a centopéia doméstica oriental é um membro da espécie *S. cleopatra.* [L. *scutum,* escudo oblongo]
scu·tu·lum, pl. **scu·tu·la** (skoo′tū-lŭm, -lă; skoo′choo-loom). Escútulo; crosta discóide amarela, lesão característica do favo, que consiste numa massa de hifas, pus e escamas. [L. dim. de *scutum,* escudo]
scu·tum, pl. **scu·ta** (skoo′tŭm, -tă). Placa, escudo. **1.** SIN scute. **2.** Nos carrapatos ixodídeos (duros), placa que recobre, em grande parte ou totalmente, o dorso do macho e forma um escudo anterior atrás do capítulo da fêmea ou de carrapatos imaturos. [L. shield]
scyb·a·la (sib′ă-lă). Cíbalos; plural de scybalum.
scyb·a·lous (sib′ă-lŭs). Cibaloso; relativo a cíbalos.
scyb·a·lum, pl. **scyb·a·la** (sib′ă-lŭm, -lă). Cíbalo; coprólito; massa dura e arredondada de fezes espessadas. [G. *skybalon,* excremento]
scy·phi·form (sī′fi-form). Cifióideo. SIN scyphoid. [G. *skyphos,* taça, cálice + L. *forma,* forma]
scy·phoid (sī′foyd). Cifióideo; em forma de taça. SIN scyphiform. [G. *skyphos,* taça + *eidos,* semelhança]
SD Abreviatura de streptodornase (estreptodornase); standard *deviation* (desvio padrão).
SDA Abreviatura de specific dynamic *action* (ação dinâmica específica).
SDS Abreviatura de *sodium* dodecyl sulfate (sulfato sódico de dodecila).
Se Símbolo de (selênio).
seal (sēl). Selo. **1.** Fechamento hermético. **2.** Efetuar fechamento hermético.
  border s., s. periférico; contato da borda da dentadura com os tecidos subjacentes ou adjacentes para evitar a passagem de ar ou de outras substâncias. SIN peripheral s.
  palatal s., s. palatino. SIN posterior palatal s.
  peripheral s., s. periférico. SIN border s.
  posterior palatal s., s. palatino posterior; o s. na borda posterior de uma dentadura. VER TAMBÉM posterior palatal seal *area.* SIN palatal s., post dam, postdam, postpalatal s.
  postpalatal s., s. pós-palatino. SIN posterior palatal s.
  velopharyngeal s., s. velofaríngeo; fechamento entre as cavidades oral e nasofaríngea.
seal·ant (sē′lănt). Selante; material empregado para efetuar um fechamento hermético.
  dental s., s. dentário. SIN fissure s.
  fissure s., s. de fissura; material dentário habitualmente feito pela interação entre o bisfenol e glicidil metacrilato; esses selantes são utilizados para selar depressões e fissuras não-fundidas e não-cariadas nas superfícies dos dentes. SIN dental s.
sea nettle (sē net′il). Urtiga-do-mar, água-viva. SIN *Chrysaora quinquecirrha.*
search·er (ser′cher). Explorador; forma de sonda utilizada para determinar se há cálculo na bexiga.

Seashore, Carl E., psicólogo norte-americano, 1866–1949. VER S. *test.*
sea·sick·ness (sē′sik-nes). Enjôo do mar; forma de náusea causada pelo movimento de uma plataforma flutuante, como navio, barco ou jangada. SIN mal de mer, naupathia, vomitus marinus.
sea·son (sē′zon). Estação; fase particular de algum fenômeno cíclico lento, principalmente o ciclo anual das estações.
seat (sēt). Assento; superfície contra a qual um objeto pode repousar para apoiar-se.
  basal s., a. basal. SIN denture foundation *area.*
  rest s., a. de repouso. SIN rest *area.*
seat·worm (sēt′werm). Oxiúro. SIN pinworm.
sea wasp. SIN *Chiropsalmus quadrumanus.*
♻ **seb-.** Seb-. VER sebo-.
se·ba·ceous (sē-bā′shŭs). Sebáceo; relativo a sebo; oleoso, gorduroso. SIN sebaceus. [L. *sebaceus*]
se·ba·ceus (sē-bā′shŭs). Sebáceo. SIN sebaceous. [L.]
seb·i·a·gog·ic (seb′ē-ă-goj′ik). Sebiagogo. SIN sebiferous. [sebi- + G. *agōgos,* que conduz]
se·bif·er·ous (sē-bif′er-ŭs). Sebífero; que produz material sebáceo. SIN sebiagogic, sebiparous. [sebi- + L. *fero,* transportar]
Sebileau, Pierre, anatomista francês, 1860–1953. VER S. *hollow, muscle.*
se·bip·a·rous (sē-bip′ă-rŭs). Sebíparo. SIN sebiferous. [sebi- + L. *pario,* produzir]
♻ **sebo-, seb-, sebi-.** Sebo-, seb-, sebi-; sebo, sebáceo. [L. *sebum,* sebo]
seb·or·rhea (seb-ō-rē′ă). Seborréia; hiperatividade das glândulas sebáceas, resultando em quantidade excessiva de sebo. [sebo- + G. *rhoia,* fluxo]
  s. cap′itis, s. da cabeça; s. do couro cabeludo.
  eczematoid s., s. eczematóide; eczema seborreico em que as lesões perderam a definição e tornaram-se confluentes, habitualmente em decorrência de traumatismo e/ou do uso excessivo de sabão e medicação.
  s. facie′i, s. of face, s. da face; s. que afeta especialmente o nariz e a fronte.
  s. furfura′cea, s. furfurácea. SIN s. sicca (1).
  s. oleo′sa, s. oleosa; condição gordurosa da pele, devido à secreção excessiva das glândulas sebáceas.
  s. sic′ca, s. seca; **(1)** acúmulo de escamas secas sobre a pele, principalmente no couro cabeludo. SIN s. furfuracea. **(2)** Caspa. SIN dandruff.
  s. squamo′sa neonato′rum, s. escamosa do recém-nascido; dermatite seborreica em lactentes.
seb·or·rhe·ic (seb-ō-rē′ik). Seborreico; relativo à seborréia.
se·bum (sē′bŭm). Sebo; a secreção das glândulas sebáceas. [L. sebo]
sec Abreviatura de second (segundo).
Se·cer·nen·tas·i·da (se-ser-nen-tas′i-dă). Classe de nematódeos que possuem canais laterais que se abrem para o sistema excretor e fasmídeos; inclui a maioria dos parasitas nematódeos familiares dos seres humanos e animais domésticos, destacando-se os nematódeos do solo, estrongilídeos e filárias. VER TAMBÉM Adenophorasida. SIN Phasmidia, Secernentia. [L. *secerno,* separar, ocultar]
Se·cer·nen·tia (se-ser-nen′shē-ă). SIN Secernentasida.
Seckel, Helmut P.G., médico alemão, *1900. VER S. *dwarfism syndrome.*
sec·o·bar·bi·tal (sē-kō-bar′bi-tahl). Secobarbital; sedativo e hipnótico de ação curta que está se tornando obsoleto; substituído, em grande parte, pelos benzodiazepínicos.
sec·on·dar·ies (sek′on-dār-ēz). **1.** Metástases. SIN metastasis. **2.** As lesões da sífilis secundária.
se·cos·te·roid (sek′ō-stēr′oyd). Secosteróide; composto derivado de um esteróide em que houve clivagem de um anel. [L. *seco,* cortar + steroid]
se·cre·ta (se-krē′tă). Secreções. [L. neuter pl. de *secretus,* pp. de *se-cerno,* separar]
se·cre·ta·gogue (se-krē′tă-gog). Secretagogo; agente que promove a secreção; p. ex., acetilcolina, gastrina, secretina. SIN secretogogue. [secreta + G. *agōgos,* que impele]
se·cre·tase (sē-krē′tās). Secretases; termo utilizado para descrever uma proteinase que atua sobre uma proteína precursora amilóide para produzir peptídeos que não contêm toda a proteína amilóide β (importante componente das placas encontradas na doença de Alzheimer), que são solúveis e que não precipitam para produzir amilóide.
se·crete (se-krēt′). Secretar; elaborar ou produzir alguma substância fisiologicamente ativa (p. ex., enzima, hormônio, metabólito) por uma célula e liberá-la no sangue, numa cavidade corporal, ou suco, por difusão direta, por exocitose celular ou através de um ducto. [L. *se-cerno,* pp. *-cretus,* separar]
se·cre·tin (se-krē′tin). Secretina; hormônio formado pelas células epiteliais do duodeno sob o estímulo do conteúdo ácido do estômago, que estimula a secreção de suco pancreático; utilizada como auxiliar no diagnóstico de doença do pâncreas exócrino e como adjuvante na obtenção de células pancreáticas descamadas para exame citológico. SIN oxykrinin. [secrete + -in]
  s. family, família de secretinas; classe de hormônios que são semelhantes, do ponto de vista estrutural e funcional, à secretina; p. ex., glucagon, polipeptídeo inibitório gástrico, polipeptídeo intestinal vasoativo e glicentina.

se·cre·tion (se-krē'shun). Secreção. **1.** Produção por uma célula ou grupo de células (uma glândula) de uma substância fisiologicamente ativa e sua saída da célula ou do órgão em que foi formada. **2.** O produto sólido, líquido ou gasoso de atividade celular ou glandular, que é armazenado ou utilizado pelo organismo no qual é produzido. Cf. excretion. [L. *se-cerno*, pp. *-cretus*, separar]
    cytocrine s., s. citócrina; a transferência de material secretor de uma célula para outra, como a transferência de grânulos de melanina dos melanócitos para as células epidérmicas.
    external s., s. externa; substância formada por uma célula e transportada fora da parede celular como meio de livrá-la da substância ou como mensageiro para afetar a função de outras células.
    neurohumoral s., s. neuro-humoral; transmissão de um impulso nervoso através de uma sinapse ou para um órgão terminal através da secreção de uma diminuta quantidade de transmissor químico, como a acetilcolina.
se·cre·to·gogue (se-krē'tō-gog). Secretagogo. SIN secretagogue.
se·cre·to·mo·tor, se·cre·to·mo·tory (se-krē'tō-mō'ter, -mō'ter-ē). Secretomotor; que estimula a secreção. [secrete + *motor*, motor]
se·cre·tor (se-krē'ter, tōr). Secretor; indivíduo cujos líquidos corporais (saliva, sêmen, secreções vaginais) contêm uma forma hidrossolúvel dos antígenos do grupo sanguíneo ABO. Os secretores constituem 80% da população. Em medicina forense, o exame dos líquidos tem melhorado a capacidade dos funcionários da justiça em obter informações para a identificação de criminosos e estreitar o campo de suspeitos.
se·cre·to·ry (se-krēt'e-rē, se'krē-tōr-ē). Secretor, secretório; relativo à secreção ou secreções.
sec·tile (sek'til, tīl). Séctil. **1.** Capaz de ser cortado ou seccionado. **2.** Que tem o aspecto de ter sido seccionado. [L. *sectilis*, de *seco*, cortar]
sec·tio, pl. **sec·ti·o·nes** (sek'shē-ō, sek-shē-ō'nēz) [TA]. Secção; em anatomia, subdivisão ou segmento. [L.]
sec·tion (sek'shun). Secção. **1.** Ato de cortar. **2.** Corte ou divisão. **3.** Segmento ou parte de qualquer órgão ou estrutura delimitada do restante. **4.** Superfície de corte. **5.** Fatia fina de tecido, células, microrganismos ou qualquer material para exame ao microscópio. SIN microscopic s. [L. *sectio*, corte, de *seco*, cortar]
    abdominal s., celiotomia. SIN celiotomy.
    attached cranial s., craniotomia ligada. SIN attachéd *craniotomy*.
    axial s., s. axial. SIN transverse s.
    cesarean s., cesariana; incisão através da parede abdominal e do útero (histerotomia abdominal) para extração do feto.
    classical cesarean s., cesariana clássica; cesariana em que o útero é penetrado através de uma incisão vertical no seu fundo.
    coronal s., corte coronal; corte transversal obtido ao efetuar um corte, real ou através de técnicas de imagem, do corpo, de qualquer parte do corpo ou de qualquer estrutura anatômica no plano coronal ou frontal, isto é, num plano vertical perpendicular ao plano mediano ou sagital. Como a s. real no plano coronal resulta numa parte anterior e numa posterior, o corte coronal anatômico seria uma vista bidimensional da superfície de corte da face posterior da parte anterior ou da face anterior da parte posterior. SIN frontal s.
    cross s., corte transversal; **(1)** vista, diagrama ou imagem planar ou bidimensional da estrutura interna do corpo, de parte do corpo ou de qualquer estrutura anatômica obtida ao efetuar um corte, verdadeiro ou através de técnicas de imagem (radiográfica, de ressonância magnética ou microscópica), do corpo ou de qualquer estrutura ao longo de determinado plano. Tradicionalmente, o "corte transversal" referia-se a vistas obtidas ao efetuar um corte em ângulos retos ao eixo longitudinal da estrutura (axial ou transaxial); todavia, o termo, como é atualmente utilizado, refere-se ao corte da estrutura em qualquer plano determinado; **(2)** fatia ou secção de determinada espessura obtida através de cortes paralelos seriados através de uma estrutura ou mediante o uso de uma técnica de imagem.
    detached cranial s., craniotomia livre. SIN detached *craniotomy*.
    diagonal s., corte oblíquo. SIN oblique s.
    frontal s., corte frontal. SIN coronal s.
    frozen s., corte por congelamento; fatia fina de tecido obtida de uma amostra congelada, freqüentemente utilizada para diagnóstico microscópico rápido.
    Latzko cesarean s., s. cesariana de Latzko; secção cesariana em que o útero é penetrado por dissecção romba paravesical sem penetração da cavidade peritoneal.
    longitudinal s., corte longitudinal; corte transversal obtido ao efetuar um corte, real ou através de técnicas de imagem, em qualquer plano paralelo ao longo do eixo maior ou vertical do corpo, de qualquer parte do corpo ou de qualquer estrutura anatômica. Os cortes longitudinais incluem os cortes mediano, sagital e coronal, mas não se limitam a eles.
    lower uterine segment cesarean s., cesariana do segmento uterino inferior; cesariana em que o útero é penetrado em seu segmento inferior por uma abordagem transperitoneal.
    median s., corte mediano; corte transversal obtido ao efetuar um corte, verdadeiro ou através de técnicas de imagem, no plano medial do corpo ou de qualquer parte do corpo ocupando ou atravessando o plano mediano ao ao cortar qualquer estrutura anatômica geralmente simétrica, como um dedo da mão ou célula, em sua linha média. Como a verdadeira secção do plano mediano resulta numa metade direita e numa metade esquerda, um corte mediano anatômico seria uma vista bidimensional da superfície de corte na face medial das duas metades. SIN midsagittal s.
    microscopic s., corte microscópico. SIN section (5).
    midsagittal s., corte mediano, corte mediossagital. SIN median s.
    oblique s., corte oblíquo; corte transversal diagonal obtido ao efetuar um corte, real ou através de técnicas de imagem, do corpo, de qualquer parte do corpo ou de qualquer estrutura anatômica em qualquer plano não-paralelo ao eixo longitudinal ou sem intersecção em ângulo reto, isto é, que não é longitudinal (vertical) nem transversal (horizontal). SIN diagonal s.
    parasagittal s., s. parassagital. SIN sagittal s.
    perineal s., s. perineal; qualquer secção através do períneo, seja litotomia lateral ou mediana (operações de importância histórica) ou uretrotomia externa.
    pituitary stalk s., s. do pedículo hipofisário; transecção da conexão neurovascular entre o hipotálamo e a hipófise.
    Saemisch s., s. de Saemisch; procedimento de transfixação da córnea sob uma úlcera, removendo-a, em seguida, através da base.
    sagittal s., corte sagital; corte transversal obtido ao efetuar um corte, verdadeiro ou através de técnicas de imagem, do corpo, de qualquer parte do corpo ou de qualquer estrutura anatômica no plano sagital, isto é, num plano vertical paralelo ao plano mediano. Como a secção verdadeira no plano sagital resulta numa parte direita e numa parte esquerda, um corte sagital anatômico pode consistir numa vista bidimensional da superfície de corte na face medial de ambas as partes. SIN parasagittal s.
    serial s., s. seriada; uma entre diversas secções microscópicas consecutivas.
    thin s., ultrathin s., corte fino, corte ultrafino; secção de tecido para exame ao microscópio eletrônico; a amostra é fixada, tipicamente em glutaraldeído e/ou tetróxido de ósmio, imersa numa resina plástica e seccionada com espessura de menos de 0,1 μm com bisturi de vidro ou diamante num ultramicrótomo.
    transverse s., corte transversal; corte transversal obtido ao efetuar um corte, verdadeiro ou através de técnicas de imagem, do corpo, de qualquer parte do corpo ou de qualquer parte da estrutura do corpo num plano horizontal, isto é, num plano que cruza o eixo longitudinal em ângulo reto. Como a secção verdadeira no plano transversal resulta numa parte inferior e numa parte superior, um corte transversal anatômico seria uma vista bidimensional da superfície de corte na face inferior da parte superior ou na face superior da parte inferior. Por convenção, nas técnicas de imagem, os cortes transversais mostram a face inferior da parte superior, a não ser que indicado especificamente. SIN axial s.
sec·tor·an·o·pia (sek'tor-an-ō'pē-ā). Setoranopia; perda da visão num setor do campo visual. [sector + G. *an-* priv. + *opsis*, visão]
sec·to·ri·al (sek-tōr'ē-āl). Setorial. **1.** Relativo a um setor. **2.** Que corta ou está adaptado para cortar; designa os dentes molares ou pré-molares cortantes ou dilacerantes dos carnívoros. [L. *sector*, cortador]
se·cun·di·grav·i·da (sek'un-di-grav'i-dā). Secundípara. VER gravida.
se·cun·di·na, pl. **se·cun·di·nae** (sek-un-dī'nā, -nē). Secundinas. SIN afterbirth. [L. *secundinae*, o pós-parto, de *secundus*, segundo]
se·cun·dines (sek'un-dēnz). Secundinas. SIN afterbirth. [L. *secundinae*, o pós-parto]
se·cun·dip·a·ra (sek'un-dip'ā-rā). Secundípara. VER para.
se·date (se-dāt'). Sedar; submeter à influência de um sedativo. [L. *sedatus*; ver sedation]
se·da·tion (se-dā'shun). Sedação. **1.** Ato de acalmar, especialmente pela administração de um sedativo. **2.** O estado de ser calmo. [L. *sedatio*, acalmar, aquietar]
sed·a·tive (sed'ā-tiv). Sedativo. **1.** Calmante; tranqüilizante. **2.** Fármaco que reduz a excitação nervosa; designado de acordo com o órgão ou o sistema sobre o qual a ação específica é exercida; p. ex., cardíaco, cerebral, nervoso, respiratório, espinal. [L. *sedativus*; ver sedation]
SEDC Abreviatura de spondyloepiphyseal *dysplasia* congenita (displasia espondiloepifisária congênita).
se·dig·i·tate (se-dij'i-tāt). Sexdigital. SIN sexdigitate. [L. *sex*, seis + *digitus*, dedo]
sed·i·ment (sed'i-ment). **1.** Sedimento; material insolúvel que tende a precipitar no fundo de um líquido, como na hipostase. SIN sedimentum. **2.** Sedimentar; causar ou efetuar a formação de um sedimento ou depósito, como no caso de centrifugação ou ultracentrifugação. SIN sedimentate. [L. *sedimentum*, depósito, de *sedeo*, sentar, depositar]
sed·i·men·tate (sed'i-men'tāt). Sedimentar. SIN sediment (2).
sed·i·men·ta·tion (sed'i-men-tā'shun). Sedimentação; formação de um sedimento.
sed·i·men·ta·tor (sed'i-men-tā'ter, tōr). Sedimentador; centrífuga.
sed·i·men·tom·e·ter (sed'ī-men-tom'e-ter). Sedimentômetro; aparelho fotográfico para o registro automático da velocidade de hemossedimentação [sediment + G. *metron*, medida]
sed·i·men·tum (sed-i-men'tŭm). Sedimento. SIN sediment (1). [L.]
    s. laterit'ium, s. laterício. SIN brickdust *deposit*.

se·do·hep·tu·lose (sē-dō-hep′tū-lōs). Sedoeptulose; uma 2-cetoeptulose formada metabolicamente na via de pentose monofosfato como 7-fosfato por condensação de D-xilulose 5-fosfato e D-ribose 5-fosfato, liberando D-gliceraldeído 3-fosfato; o açúcar não fosforilado é encontrado em *Sedum* (erva-pinheira). SIN D-*altro*-2-heptulose.

sedoxantrone trihydrochloride (se-doks′an-trōn trī-hī-drō-klōr-īd). Tricloridrato de sedoxantrona; inibidor da topoisomerase II na quimioterapia antineoplásica.

seed (sēd). **1.** Semente; elemento reprodutivo de uma planta com flores; o óvulo maduro. SIN semen (2). **2.** Semear; em bacteriologia, inocular um meio de cultura com microrganismos. [A.S. *soed*]

Seeligmüller, Otto L.G.A., neurologista alemão, 1837–1912. VER S. *sign.*

Seessel, Albert, embriologista norte-americano, 1850–1910. VER S. *pocket, pouch.*

seg·ment (seg′ment) [TA]. **1.** Segmento; secção; parte de um órgão ou outra estrutura delimitada de forma natural, artificial ou por invaginação do restante. SIN segmentum [TA]. VER TAMBÉM metamere. **2.** Segmento; território de um órgão que possui função, suprimento ou drenagem independente. **3.** Segmentar; dividir ou dividir novamente em pequenas partes iguais. [L. *segmentum*, de *seco*, cortar]

A1 s. of anterior cerebral artery, parte pré-comunicante da artéria cerebral anterior; *termo oficial alternativo para precommunicating *part* of anterior cerebral artery.

A2 s. of anterior cerebral artery, parte pós-comunicante da artéria cerebral anterior; *termo oficial alternativo para postcommunicating *part* of anterior cerebral artery.

abnormal ST s., período isoelétrico. SIN isoelectric *period.*

anterior s. [TA], s. anterior; parte ou secção delimitada de um órgão ou outra estrutura situado na frente das outras partes ou secções semelhantes, ou ventralmente. VER anterior (bronchopulmonary) s. [S III], anterior basal (bronchopulmonary) s. [S VIII], anterior inferior renal s., anterior superior renal s., anterior ocular s. SIN segmentum anterius [TA].

anterior basal (bronchopulmonary) s. [S VIII], s. basilar anterior do pulmão [S VIII]; dos quatro segmentos broncopulmonares dos lobos inferiores do pulmão direito ou do pulmão esquerdo que entram em contato com o diafragma, o segmento basal anterior situa-se em frente, isto é, mais próximo das cartilagens costais; suprido pelo brônquio segmentar basilar anterior a [B VIII] e pela artéria (pulmonar) segmentar basilar anterior. SIN segmentum (bronchopulmonale) basale anterius [S VIII].

anterior (bronchopulmonary) s. [S III] [TA], s. anterior do pulmão [S III]; dos três segmentos broncopulmonares que compreendem o lobo superior dos pulmões direito e esquerdo, o segmento anterior situa-se mais próximo das cartilagens costais, suprido pelo brônquio segmentar anterior [B III] e pela artéria (pulmonar) segmentar anterior. SIN segmentum (bronchopulmonale) anterius S III [TA].

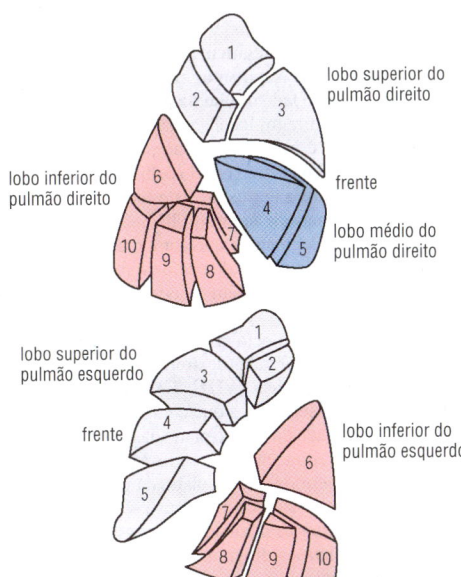

segmentos broncopulmonares: vistas laterais; (1) segmento (s.) apical, (2) s. posterior (no pulmão esquerdo, 1 + 2 = s. apicoposterior, antigamente "apicobasal"), (3) s. anterior, (4) s. lateral do pulmão direito (para o pulmão esquerdo, s. lingular superior), (5) s. medial do pulmão direito (para o pulmão esquerdo, s. lingular inferior), (6) s. apical (ou superior), (7) s. basal medial (ou s. cardíaco do pulmão direito; inconstante no pulmão esquerdo), (8) s. basal anterior, (9) s. basal lateral, (10) s. basal posterior

anterior inferior renal s., s. ântero-inferior do rim; parte do rim exclusivamente suprida pela artéria (renal) do segmento ântero-inferior do rim. SIN segmentum renale anterius inferius.

anterior ocular s., s. anterior do bulbo do olho; parte do bulbo do olho constituída pela córnea, íris e lente e câmaras associadas (anterior e posterior), preenchidas com humor aquoso. SIN segmentum oculare anterius [TA].

anterior superior renal s. [TA], s. ântero-superior do rim; parte do rim suprida exclusivamente pela artéria (renal) do segmento ântero-superior do rim. SIN segmentum renale anterius superius.

apical (bronchopulmonary) s. [S I], s. apical do pulmão [S I]; dos três segmentos broncopulmonares que compreendem o lobo superior do pulmão direito, é aquele que se estende para o nível mais alto (para a pleura parietal cervical), suprido pelo brônquio segmentar apical [B I] e pela artéria (pulmonar) segmentar apical. SIN segmentum bronchopulmonale apicale S I.

apicoposterior (bronchopulmonary) s. [SI + SII], s. apicoposterior do pulmão [SI + SII]; dos quatro segmentos broncopulmonares que tipicamente compreendem o lobo superior do pulmão esquerdo, é o mais superior e posterior, suprido pelo brônquio segmentar apicoposterior esquerdo [B I + II]; correspondem aproximadamente, quanto à sua posição, aos segmentos broncopulmonares separados apical e posterior do lobo superior do pulmão direito. SIN segmentum (bronchopulmonale) apicoposterius [SI + II].

arterial s.'s of kidney, segmentos renais. SIN renal s.'s.

s. bronchopulmonale basale posterius S X [TA], s. basilar posterior do pulmão S X. SIN posterior basal bronchopulmonary s. S X.

bronchopulmonary s. [TA], s. broncopulmonar; a menor subdivisão dos lobos dos pulmões passível de ressecção cirúrgica, suprida exclusivamente por um brônquio terciário (segmentar) e pelo ramo terciário correspondente da artéria pulmonar (artéria pulmonar segmentar); tipicamente, o pulmão direito possui dez segmentos broncopulmonares, e o esquerdo, oito ou nove, devido à fusão dos segmentos apical e posterior do lobo superior e dos segmentos basilares anterior e medial do lobo inferior. SIN segmentum bronchopulmonale.

cardiac s., s. medial do pulmão [S VII]. SIN medial basal bronchopulmonary s. S VII.

cervical s.'s of spinal cord [C1–C8], parte cervical da medula espinal [C1–C8]; *termo oficial alternativo para cervical *part* of spinal cord.

coccygeal s. of spinal cord [Co], parte coccígea da medula espinal; segmento mais inferior da medula espinal que dá a origem ao par coccígeo de nervos espinais e constitui a parte coccígea da medula espinal. SIN segmentum medullae spinalis coccygeum [Co] [TA].

hepatic s.'s [TA], segmentos hepáticos; partes cirurgicamente ressecáveis do fígado supridas por ramos independentes da veia porta e artéria hepática e drenadas por ramos lobulares independentes dos ductos biliares hepáticos; por conseguinte, a denominação e a numeração dos oito segmentos hepáticos na TA baseiam-se na distribuição portobilioarterial: segmentos posterior [I], lateral [II], ântero-lateral esquerdo [III] e medial [IV] da (parte) esquerda do fígado e segmentos ântero-medial [V], ântero-lateral direito [VI], póstero-lateral [VII] e póstero-medial [VIII] da (parte) direita do fígado; os segmentos hepáticos são separados pelos planos verticais das três veias hepáticas principais (direita, intermediária e esquerda); os segmentos da (parte) direita do fígado também são separados pelo plano horizontal da divisão direita da árvore portobilioarterial. VER anterior s., lateral s., medial s., posterior s. SIN segmenta hepatis [TA], s.'s of liver.

s. I, s. I; *termo oficial alternativo para posterior hepatic s. I.

inferior s. [TA], s. inferior; parte ou secção delimitada de um órgão ou outra estrutura situada no nível mais baixo (mais próximo aos pés) em comparação com as outras partes ou secções semelhantes. SIN segmentum inferius [TA].

inferior lingular (bronchopulmonary) s. [S V], s. lingular inferior (broncopulmonar) [S V]; dos quatro segmentos broncopulmonares que, tipicamente, compreendem o lobo superior do pulmão esquerdo, trata-se do mais inferior, suprido pelo brônquio lingular inferior [B V] e pela artéria (pulmonar) segmentar lingular inferior; corresponde aproximadamente, quanto à sua posição, ao segmento medial [S V] do lobo médio do pulmão direito; a língula é uma característica dessa parte do pulmão esquerdo. SIN segmentum lingulare bronchopulmonale inferius S V [TA].

inferior renal s., s. inferior do rim; parte do rim exclusivamente suprida pela artéria (renal) segmentar inferior. SIN segmentum renale inferius [TA].

interannular s., s. interanular. SIN internodal s.

intermaxillary s., s. intermaxilar; a massa primordial de tecido formada pela fusão das proeminências nasais mediais do embrião; contribui para a porção intermaxilar do maxilar, porção pró-labial do lábio superior e palato primário.

internodal s., s. internodal; a porção de uma fibra nervosa mielinizada entre dois nodos sucessivos. SIN interannular s., internode, Ranvier s., segmentum internodale.

Lanterman s.'s, segmentos de Lanterman; as divisões da fibra nervosa entre as incisuras de Schmidt-Lanterman.

lateral s. [TA], s. lateral; parte ou secção delimitada de um órgão ou outra estrutura situada o mais afastado à esquerda ou à direita em relação às outras partes ou secções semelhantes. VER lateral bronchopulmonary s. S IV, lateral

basal (bronchopulmonary) s. [S IX], (left anterior) lateral hepatic s. [III], (left posterior) lateral hepatic s. III, right anterior lateral hepatic s. [VI] (right) posterior lateral hepatic s. [VII]. SIN segmentum laterale [TA].
lateral basal (bronchopulmonar) s. [S IX], s. (broncopulmonar) basal lateral [S IX]; dos quatro segmentos broncopulmonares do lobo inferior dos pulmões direito e esquerdo que entram em contato com o diafragma, o segmento basal lateral é o mais distante à direita no pulmão direito e mais distante à esquerda no pulmão esquerdo, suprido pelo brônquio segmentar pigmentar basal lateral [B IX] e pela artéria (pulmonar) segmentar basal lateral. SIN segmentum (bronchopulmonale) basale laterale [S IX].
lateral bronchopulmonary s. S IV [TA], s. broncopulmonar lateral [S IV]; dos dois segmentos broncopulmonares que compreendem o lobo médio do pulmão direito, o s. lateral é aquele situado do lado direito, suprido pelo brônquio segmentar lateral [B IV] e pela artéria (pulmonar) segmentar lateral. SIN segmentum bronchopulmonale laterale S IV [TA].
(left anterior) lateral hepatic s. [III] [TA], s. lateral hepático (anterior esquerdo) do fígado [III]; um dos três segmentos hepáticos que constituem a (parte) esquerda do fígado, situado à esquerda da porção inferior do ligamento falciforme, tipicamente superposto ao estômago anteriormente, suprido pelo ramo lateral inferior da parte umbilical do ramo esquerdo da veia porta hepática. SIN lateral inferior hepatic area [TA], segmentum hepatis anterius laterale sinistrum [III] [TA], segmentum III*.
(left) medial hepatic s. [IV] [TA], s. medial (esquerdo) do fígado; dos três segmentos hepáticos que constituem a (parte) esquerda do fígado, o segmento medial situa-se à direita do ligamento falciforme; localiza-se entre esse ligamento e o plano vertical da veia hepática direita, demarcada na superfície diafragmática do fígado por uma linha extrapolada da fossa da vesícula biliar até a veia cava inferior; o lobo quadrado da superfície visceral do fígado também faz parte do segmento hepático medial; o segmento medial é suprido pelos ramos mediais da parte umbilical do ramo esquerdo da veia porta. SIN segmentum hepatis mediale (sinistrum) [IV] [TA], segmentum IV*.
(left posterior) lateral hepatic s. III [TA], s. lateral (posterior esquerdo) do fígado [S III]; um dos três segmentos hepáticos que constituem a (parte) esquerda do fígado, situado à esquerda da porção superior do ligamento falciforme e da fissura para o ligamento venoso; tipicamente, localiza-se superiormente ao estômago e é irrigado pelo ramo lateral superior da parte umbilical do ramo esquerdo da veia porta hepática. SIN lateral superior hepatic area [TA], segmentum hepatis posterius laterale sinistrum [III] [TA], segmentum II*.
s.'s of liver, segmentos do fígado. SIN hepatic s.'s.
lower uterine s., s. uterino inferior; a porção inferior ou istmo do útero, cuja extremidade inferior une-se ao canal cervical e, durante a gravidez, expande-se para transformar-se na parte inferior da cavidade uterina. Não representa a porção do útero que sofre contração ativa.
lumbar s.'s L1–L5 of spinal cord, segmentos lombares L1–L5 da medula espinal. SIN lumbar part of spinal cord.
lumbar s.'s of spinal cord L1–L5, segmentos da medula espinal lombar L1–L5; os cinco segmentos da medula espinal que dão origem aos cinco pares de nervos espinais lombares [L1–L5] e constituem a parte lombar da medula espinal que, no adulto, situa-se entre a porção do canal vertebral formado pelas vértebras T11–L1. SIN segmenta medullae spinalis lumbaria L1–L5.
medial s. [TA], s. medial; parte ou secção delimitada de um órgão ou outra estrutura que se localiza mais próximo à linha mediana em relação às outras partes ou secções semelhantes. VER medial bronchopulmonary s. S V, medial basal bronchopulmonary s. S VII, (left) medial hepatic s. [IV], (right) posterior medial hepatic s. [VIII], (right) anterior medial hepatic segment [V]. SIN segmentum mediale [TA].
medial basal bronchopulmonary s. S VII [TA], s. broncopulmonar basal medial [VII]; dos quatro segmentos broncopulmonares dos lobos inferiores dos pulmões direito e esquerdo que entram em contato com o diafragma, o segmento basal medial possui uma localização diretamente inferior ao hilo do pulmão em contato com a parte média da face lateral do mediastino, suprido pelo brônquio segmentar basal medial [B VII] e pela artéria (pulmonar) segmentar basal medial. SIN segmentum bronchopulmonale basale mediale S VII [TA], cardiac s., segmentum cardiacum.
medial bronchopulmonary s. S V [TA], s. broncopulmonar medial [S V]; dos dois segmentos broncopulmonares que compreendem o lobo médio do pulmão direito, o s. medial localiza-se à esquerda, suprido pelo brônquio segmentar medial [B V] e pela artéria (pulmonar) segmentar medial. SIN segmentum bronchopulmonale mediale S V [TA].
mesoblastic s., s. mesoblástico. SIN somite.
M2 s. of middle cerebral artery, ramos terminais da artéria cerebral média; *termo oficial alternativo para terminal branches of middle cerebral artery, em branch.
neural s., s. neural. SIN neuromere.
posterior s. [TA], s. posterior; parte ou secção delimitada de um órgão ou outra estrutura situada posterior ou dorsalmente às outras partes ou secções semelhantes. VER posterior bronchopulmonary s. S II, posterior basal bronchopulmonary s. S X, posterior hepatic s. I, (right) posterior lateral hepatic s. [VII], (right) posterior medial hepatic s [VIII], posterior renal s. SIN segmentum posterius [TA].
posterior basal bronchopulmonary s. S X [TA], s. broncopulmonar basal posterior [S X]; dos quatro segmentos broncopulmonares dos lobos inferiores dos pulmões direito e esquerdo que entram em contato com o diafragma, o segmento basal posterior localiza-se mais próximo da coluna vertebral, suprido pelo brônquio segmentar basal posterior [B X] e pela artéria (pulmonar) segmentar basal posterior. SIN s. bronchopulmonale basale posterius S X [TA].
posterior bronchopulmonary s. S II [TA], s. broncopulmonar posterior; dos três segmentos broncopulmonares que compreendem o lobo superior do pulmão direito, o s. posterior localiza-se mais próximo da coluna vertebral, suprido pelo brônquio segmentar posterior [B II] e pela artéria (pulmonar) segmentar posterior. SIN segmentum bronchopulmonale posterius S II [TA].
posterior hepatic s. I [TA], s. posterior do fígado; a parte relativamente pequena do fígado suprida pelos ramos caudados dos ramos esquerdo (ou esquerdo e direito) da veia porta, demarcada pela superfície visceral do fígado como lobo caudado. SIN segmentum hepatis posterius I [TA], caudate lobe*, lobus caudatus*, posterior liver*, posterior part of liver*, s. I*, segmentum I*, Spigelius lobe.
posterior renal s. [TA], s. posterior do rim; parte do rim exclusivamente suprida pela artéria (renal) segmentar posterior. SIN segmentum renale posterius [TA].
P1 s. of posterior cerebral artery, da artéria cerebral posterior. SIN precommunicating part of posterior cerebral artery.
P2 s. of posterior cerebral artery, da artéria cerebral posterior; *termo oficial alternativo para postcommunicating part of posterior cerebral artery.
P3 s. of posterior cerebral artery [TA], s. P3 da artéria cerebral posterior. SIN lateral occipital artery.
P4 s. of posterior cerebral artery, s. P4 da artéria cerebral posterior; *termo oficial alternativo para medial occipital artery.
PR s., s. PR; parte da curva eletrocardiográfica entre o final da onda P e o início do complexo QRS.
precommunical s. of anterior cerebral artery, parte pré-comunicante da artéria cerebral anterior. SIN precommunicating part of anterior cerebral artery.
precommunical s. of posterior cerebral artery, parte pré-comunicante da artéria cerebral posterior. SIN precommunicating part of posterior cerebral artery.
Ranvier s., s. de Ranvier. SIN internodal s.
renal s.'s [TA], s. renais; regiões do rim supridas por artérias terminais que se ramificam a partir das artérias renais; são denominados: s. ântero-inferior, s. ântero-superior, s. inferior, s. posterior e s. superior. SIN segmenta renalia [TA], arterial s.'s of kidney.
right anterior lateral hepatic s. [VI] [TA], s. hepático lateral anterior direito [VI]; dos quatro segmentos que compreendem a (parte) direita do fígado (isto é, aqueles situados do lado direito do plano da veia hepática média), o segmento lateral anterior direito também se localiza à direita do plano da veia hepática direita e inferiormente ao plano da porção transversa do ramo direito da veia porta hepática; é suprido pelo ramo anterior lateral da veia porta. SIN segmentum hepatis anterius laterale dextrum [VI] [TA].
(right) anterior medial hepatic segment [V] [TA], segmento hepático medial anterior (direito); dos quatro segmentos que compreendem a (parte) direita do fígado (isto é, situados do lado direito do plano da veia hepática média), o segmento medial anterior (direito) localiza-se entre este último plano e o plano da veia hepática direita e inferiormente ao plano da porção transversa do ramo direito da veia porta hepática; é suprido pelo ramo anterior medial da veia porta. SIN segmentum hepatis anterius mediale (dextrum) [V] [TA].
(right) posterior lateral hepatic s. [VII] [TA], s. hepático lateral posterior (direito) [VII]; dos quatro segmentos que compreendem a (parte) direita do fígado (isto é, situados no lado direito do plano da veia hepática média), o segmento lateral posterior (direito) também se localiza à direita do plano da veia hepática direita e superiormente ao plano da porção transversa do ramo direito da veia porta hepática; é suprido pelo ramo posterior lateral da veia porta. SIN segmentum hepatis posterius laterale (dextrum) [VII] [TA].
(right) posterior medial hepatic s. [VIII] [TA], s. hepático medial posterior (direito) [VIII]; dos quatro segmentos que compreendem a (parte) direita do fígado (isto é, situados do lado direito do plano da veia hepática média), o segmento medial posterior direito localiza-se entre este último plano e o plano da veia hepática direita e superiormente ao plano da porção transversa do ramo direito da veia porta hepática; é suprido pelo ramo posterior medial da veia porta. SIN segmentum hepatis posterius mediale (dextrum) [VIII] [TA].
RST s., s. RST; parte do eletrocardiograma entre o complexo QRS e a onda T. Praticamente nunca é distinto no coração normal, em que forma a parte inicial da onda T sem ponto final aceito. SIN ST s.
s.'s of spinal cord [C1-Co] [TA], segmentos da medula espinhal [C1–Co]; uma das 31 porções da medula espinal, dando origem, cada uma delas, às raízes anterior e posterior que se combinam para formar um par de nervos espinais. Esses segmentos são: os segmentos da medula espinal cervical [C1–C8]; os segmentos da medula espinal torácica [T1–T12]; os segmentos da medula espinal lombar [L1–L5]; os segmentos da medula espinal sacral [S1–S5] e o seg-

mento da medula espinal coccígea [Co]. SIN segmenta medullae spinalis C1–Co [TA].
s.'s of spleen, segmentos do baço; territórios esplênicos que recebem suprimento arterial independente ou que são drenados por raízes independentes da veia esplênica. SIN segmenta lienis.
ST s., s. ST. SIN RST s.
subapical s., s. subapical; segmento inconstante do lobo inferior dos pulmões direito e esquerdo. SIN segmentum subapicale, segmentum subsuperius, subsuperior s.
subsuperior s., s. subsuperior. SIN subapical s.
superior s., s. superior; o segmento superior do rim.
superior lingular bronchopulmonary s. S IV [TA], s. broncopulmonar lingular superior [S IV]; dos quatro segmentos broncopulmonares que tipicamente compreendem o lobo superior do pulmão esquerdo, o segmento de localização central e posterior, suprido pelo brônquio lingular superior [B IV] e pela artéria (pulmonar) segmentar lingular superior; corresponde aproximadamente, quanto à sua posição, ao segmento lateral [S IV] do lobo médio do pulmão direito. SIN segmentum bronchopulmonale lingulare superius [S IV] [TA].
superior renal s. [TA], s. superior do rim; porção do rim suprida apenas pela artéria (renal) segmentar superior. SIN segmentum renale superius [TA].
sympathetic s., s. simpático; uma divisão dos troncos simpáticos baseada nas origens dos ramos comunicantes cinzentos.
upper uterine s., s. uterino superior; a principal porção do corpo do útero grávido, cuja contração proporciona a principal força de expulsão no trabalho de parto.
venous s.'s of the kidney, segmentos venosos do rim; segmentos anatômicos do rim drenados por tributárias da veia renal; não é uma distribuição segmentar verdadeira, visto que existe uma comunicação cruzada entre as várias tributárias no rim.
seg·men·ta (seg-men'ta). Segmentos; plural de segmentum.
seg·men·tal (seg-men'tal). Segmentar; relativo a um segmento.
seg·men·ta·tion (seg'men-tā'shŭn). 1. Segmentação; o ato de dividir em segmentos; o estado de estar dividido em segmentos. 2. Divisão mitótica. SIN cleavage (1).
seg·men·tec·to·my (seg-men-tek'tō-mē). Segmentectomia; excisão de um segmento anatômico de qualquer órgão ou glândula.
seg·men·ter (seg'men-ter). Segmentador; esquizonte; termo habitualmente aplicado ao parasita da malária que se desenvolve num eritrócito após ter sofrido divisão nuclear e citoplasmática, logo antes da ruptura celular e liberação dos merozoítas.
Seg·men·ti·na (seg-men-tī'nă). Gênero de caramujos pulmonados de água doce (família Planorbidae, subfamília Segmentininae); inclui a espécie *S. hemisphaerula*, um importante hospedeiro intermediário de *Fasciolopsis buski*. [L. *segmentum*, de *seco*, cortar]
seg·men·tum, pl. **seg·men·ta** (seg-men'tŭm, -tă). [TA] Segmento. SIN segment (1). [L. segment]
 s. A1 arteriae cerebri anterioris, parte pré-comunicante da artéria cerebral anterior; *termo oficial alternativo para precommunicating part of anterior cerebral artery.
 s. A2 arteriae cerebri anterioris, parte pós-comunicante da artéria cerebral anterior; *termo oficial alternativo para postcommunicating part of anterior cerebral artery.
 s. ante'rius [TA], s. anterior. SIN anterior segment.
 s. apica'le, s. apical; segmento apical do lobo inferior dos pulmões direito e esquerdo.
 s. bronchopulmona'le [TA], s. broncopulmonar. SIN bronchopulmonary segment.
 s. (bronchopulmonale) anterius S III [TA], s. (broncopulmonar) anterior S III. SIN anterior (bronchopulmonary) segment [S III].
 s. bronchopulmonale apicale S I, s. broncopulmonar apical S I. SIN apical (bronchopulmonary) segment [S I].
 s. (bronchopulmonale) basa'le latera'le [S IX], s. (broncopulmonar) basal lateral [S IX]. SIN lateral basal (bronchopulmonary) segment [S IX].
 s. bronchopulmonale basale mediale S VII [TA], s. broncopulmonar basal medial [S VII]. SIN medial basal bronchopulmonary segment S VII.
 s. bronchopulmonale laterale S IV [TA], s. broncopulmonar lateral S IV. SIN lateral bronchopulmonary segment S IV.
 s. bronchopulmonale lingulare superius [S IV] [TA], s. broncopulmonar lingular superior [S IV]. SIN superior lingular bronchopulmonary segment S IV.
 s. bronchopulmonale mediale S V [TA], s. broncopulmonar medial S V. SIN medial bronchopulmonary segment S V.
 s. bronchopulmonale posterius S II [TA], s. broncopulmonar posterior S II. SIN posterior bronchopulmonary segment S II.
 s. (bronchopulmonale) apicoposte'rius [SI + II], s. (broncopulmonar) apicoposterior (SI + II]. SIN apicoposterior (bronchopulmonary) segment [SI + SII].
 s. cardi'acum, s. cardíaco. SIN medial basal bronchopulmonary segment S VII.
 segmenta cervicalia C1–C5, parte cervical da medula espinal. SIN cervical part of spinal cord.

segmen'ta cervica'lia medul'lae spina'lis [TA], parte cervical da medula espinal. SIN cervical part of spinal cord.
segmen'ta coccyg'ea medul'lae spina'lis [TA], parte coccígea da medula espinal. SIN coccygeal part of spinal cord.
segmen'ta hep'atis [TA], segmentos hepáticos. SIN hepatic segments, em segment.
 s. hepatis anterius laterale dextrum [VI] [TA], s. hepático anterior lateral direito [VI]. SIN right anterior lateral hepatic segment [VI].
 s. hepatis anterius laterale sinistrum [III] [TA], s. hepático anterior lateral esquerdo [III]. SIN (left anterior) lateral hepatic segment [III].
 s. hepatis anterius mediale (dextrum) [V] [TA], s. hepático anterior medial (direito) [V]. SIN (right) anterior medial hepatic segment [V].
 s. hepatis mediale (sinistrum) [IV] [TA], s. hepático medial (esquerdo) [IV]. SIN (left) medial hepatic segment [IV].
 s. hepatis posterius I [TA], s. hepático posterior I. SIN posterior hepatic segment I.
 s. hepatis posterius laterale sinistrum [II] [TA], s. hepático posterior lateral esquerdo [II]. SIN (left posterior) lateral hepatic segment II.
 s. hepatis posterius laterale (dextrum) [VII] [TA], s. hepático posterior lateral (direito) [VII]. SIN (right) posterior lateral hepatic segment [VII].
 s. hepatis posterius mediale (dextrum) [VIII] [TA], s. hepático posterior medial (direito) [VIII]. SIN (right) posterior medial hepatic segment [VIII].
 s. I, s. I; *termo oficial alternativo para posterior hepatic segment I.
 s. II, s. II; *termo oficial alternativo para (left posterior) lateral hepatic segment II.
 s. III, s. III; *termo oficial alternativo para (left anterior) lateral hepatic segment [III].
 s. inferius [TA], s. inferior. SIN inferior segment.
 s. internoda'le, s. internodal. SIN internodal segment.
 s. IV, s. IV; *termo oficial alternativo para (left) medial hepatic segment [IV].
 s. latera'le [TA], s. lateral. SIN lateral segment.
segmen'ta lien'is, segmentos lienais. SIN segments of spleen, em segment.
 s. lingulare bronchopulmonale inferius S V [TA], s. broncopulmonar lingular inferior S V. SIN inferior lingular (bronchopulmonary) segment [S V].
segmenta lumbalia L1–L5, segmentos lombares L1–L5. SIN lumbar part of spinal cord.
segmenta lumbalia medullae spinalis, parte lombar da medula espinal. SIN lumbar part of spinal cord.
 s. media'le [TA], s. medial. SIN medial segment.
segmenta medullae spinalis C1–Co [TA], segmentos da medula espinal C1–Co. SIN segments of spinal cord [C1–Co], em segment.
segmenta medullae spinalis cervicalia C1–C8 [TA], segmentos da medula espinal cervical C1–C8. SIN cervical part of spinal cord.
 s. medullae spinalis coccygeum [Co] [TA], s. da medula espinal coccígea. SIN coccygeal segment of spinal cord [Co].
segmenta medullae spinalis lumbaria L1–L5, segmentos da medula espinal lombar L1–L5. SIN lumbar segments of spinal cord L1–L5, em segment.
 s. oculare anterius [TA], s. ocular anterior. SIN anterior ocular segment.
 s. P4 arteriae cerebri posterioris, s. P4 da artéria cerebral posterior; *termo oficial alternativo para medial occipital artery.
 s. P3 arteriae cerebri posterioris [TA], s. P3 da artéria cerebral posterior. SIN lateral occipital artery.
 s. P1 arteriae cerebri posterioris, s. P1 da artéria cerebral posterior; *termo oficial alternativo para medial occipital artery.
 s. poste'rius [TA], s. posterior. SIN posterior segment.
 s. renale ante'rius infe'rius, s. renal ântero-inferior. SIN anterior inferior renal segment.
 s. renale ante'rius supe'rius, s. renal ântero-superior. SIN anterior superior renal segment.
 s. renale inferius [TA], s. renal inferior. SIN inferior renal segment.
segmen'ta rena'lia [TA], segmentos renais. SIN renal segments, em segment.
 s. renale posterius [TA], s. renal posterior. SIN posterior renal segment.
 s. renale superius [TA], s. renal superior. SIN superior renal segment.
segmen'ta sacra'lia medul'lae spina'lis [TA], parte sacral da medula espinal. SIN sacral part of spinal cord.
 s. (bronchopulmonale) basale anterius [S VIII], s. (broncopulmonar) basal anterior [S VIII]. SIN anterior basal (bronchopulmonary) segment [S VIII].
 s. subapica'le, s. subapical. SIN subapical segment.
 s. subsupe'rius, s. subsuperior. SIN subapical segment.
segmen'ta thora'cica medul'lae spina'lis [TA], parte torácica da medula espinal. SIN thoracic part of spinal cord.
seg·re·ga·tion (seg-rē-gā'shŭn). Segregação. 1. Remoção de determinadas partes de uma massa, p. ex., as pessoas com doenças infecciosas. 2. Separação de caracteres contrastantes na prole de heterozigotos. 3. Separação do estado emparelhado dos genes, que ocorre na divisão de redução da meiose; apenas um membro de cada par de genes somáticos é normalmente incluído em cada espermatozóide ou óvulo; p. ex., um indivíduo heterozigoto para um par de genes, *Aa*, formará metade dos gametas contendo o gene *A* e metade contendo

gene a. **4.** Restrição progressiva das potências no zigoto para o embrião seguinte. [L. *segrego,* pp. *-atus,* separar do grupo, separar]

seg·re·ga·tor (seg′re - gā - ter, tor). Segregador. SIN separator (2).

Seidel, Erich, oftalmologista alemão, 1882–1946. VER S. *scotoma, sign.*

Seignette, Pierre, farmacêutico francês, 1660–1719. VER S. *salt.*

Seiler, Carl, laringologista e anatomista suíço nos Estados Unidos, 1849–1905. VER S. *cartilage.*

Seip, Martin, médico escandinavo do século XX. VER Lawrence-S. *syndrome;* S. *syndrome.*

seis·mo·car·di·o·gram (sīz′mō - kar′dē - ō - gram). Sismocardiograma; registro das vibrações cardíacas na medida em que afetam o corpo inteiro, através de várias técnicas. [G. *seismos,* agitação + cardiogram]

seis·mo·ther·a·py (sīz - mō - thār′a - pē). Sismoterapia. SIN vibratory *massage.* [G. *seismos,* agitação, vibração]

sei·zure (sē′zher). **1.** Ataque; início súbito de uma doença ou de determinados sintomas. **2.** Crise epiléptica. SIN convulsion (2). [Fr. ant. *seisir,* agarrar, do germânico]

absence s., crise de ausência; crise caracterizada por distúrbio da percepção de interação com, ou da memória de, eventos externos ou internos ao indivíduo; pode apresentar os seguintes elementos: confusão mental, diminuição da percepção do ambiente, incapacidade de responder a estímulos internos ou externos e amnésia. (O termo ausência foi utilizado pela primeira vez por Louis-Florentin Calmeil (1798–1895) para introduzir o conceito de ausência epiléptica, referindo-se à perda de consciência ou confusão de curta duração observada em pacientes epilépticos.)

akinetic s., crise acinética. SIN atonic s.

anosognosic s.'s, ataque anosognósico. SIN anosognosic *epilepsy.*

astatic s., ataque astático; ataque que causa perda da postura ereta.

atonic s., crise atônica; crise caracterizada por perda súbita e breve (1–2 s.) do tônus muscular, afetando os músculos posturais; em geral, o termo aplica-se a eventos bilateralmente sincrônicos. SIN akinetic s.

atypical absence s., crise de ausência atípica; crise de ausência associada a um padrão EEG ponta-onda irregular ou lento em menos de 2,5 Hz ou a atividade rápida paroxística num EEG basal anormalmente lento.

audiogenic s., crise audiogênica; crise reflexa precipitada por ruídos altos, rara em seres humanos. As crises audiogênicas em roedores constituem um modelo animal de epilepsia.

automotor s., crise automotora; crise caracterizada por automatismo afetando predominantemente a porção distal dos membros.

autonomic s., crise autônoma; crise caracterizada por disfunção objetivamente documentada do sistema nervoso autônomo, afetando geralmente as funções cardiovascular, gastrointestinal ou sudomotora.

clonic s., convulsão clônica; convulsão caracterizada por contrações rítmicas repetitivas de todo o corpo ou parte dele.

complex motor s., ataque motor complexo; ataque caracterizado pela contração assincrônica e seqüencial dos músculos de cada membro, produzindo um movimento que pode assemelhar-se a uma atividade voluntária.

complex partial s., ataque parcial complexo; ataque com comprometimento da consciência, que ocorre num paciente com epilepsia focal.

convulsive s., crise convulsiva; crise com atividade motora clônica ou tônico-clônica.

dileptic s., crise diléptica; crise caracterizada por comprometimento da consciência de eventos, de sua interação com esses eventos ou da memória deles.

early s., crise precoce; crise que ocorre na semana seguinte a um traumatismo cranioencefálico.

electrographic s., crise eletrográfica. SIN subclinical s.

epileptic s., crise epiléptica; manifestações clínicas e/ou laboratoriais de um ataque epiléptico.

febrile s., convulsão febril. SIN febrile *convulsion.*

focal motor s., crise focal motora; crise parcial simples com atividade motora localizada.

gelastic s., crise gelástica; crise caracterizada por episódios de risada ou gargalhada involuntária, geralmente sem caráter afetivo apropriado; mais freqüentemente relacionada a lesões hipotalâmicas, como hamartomas.

generalized s., crise generalizada; caracterizada por manifestações clínicas generalizadas.

generalized tonic-clonic s., crise tônico-clônica generalizada; crise generalizada caracterizada pelo súbito início de contração tônica dos músculos freqüentemente associada a grito ou gemido e levando muitas vezes a queda ao chão. A fase tônica da crise é gradualmente substituída por movimentos convulsivos clônicos de ocorrência bilateral e sincrônica antes de diminuir e, por fim, cessar, seguida de um período variável de inconsciência e recuperação gradual. SIN cryptogenic epilepsy, generalized tonic-clonic epilepsy, grand mal s., grand mal, idiopathic epilepsy (2), major epilepsy.

grand mal s., crise de grande mal. SIN generalized tonic-clonic s.

hypermotor s., crise hipermotora; crise caracterizada por automatismos afetando predominantemente os músculos proximais dos membros e produzindo acentuada luxação.

hypomotor s., crise hipomotora; crise caracterizada por interrupção completa ou parcial da atividade motora num paciente cujo nível de consciência não pode ser determinado de modo acurado (p. ex., recém-nascidos, lactentes, pacientes com retardo mental).

jacksonian s., crise jacksoniana; crise motora que acomete inicialmente parte do corpo e, a seguir, estende-se progressivamente para outras partes do corpo do mesmo lado; pode tornar-se generalizada; com freqüência, origina-se no neocórtex rolândico contralateral ou próximo a ele. SIN jacksonian epilepsy.

late s., crise tardia; crise que ocorre por mais de uma semana após traumatismo craniocerebral ou agressão do SNC.

major motor s., crise motora maior; crise de grande mal ou outra crise convulsiva.

minor motor s., crise motora menor; termo antigo para referir-se à crise não-convulsiva observada em pacientes com epilepsia generalizada secundária.

myoclonic s., crise mioclônica; crise caracterizada por contrações súbitas e de curta duração (200-ms) de fibras musculares, músculos ou grupos de músculos de topografia variável (partes axial, proximal ou distal dos membros).

negative myoclonic s., crise mioclônica negativa; crise caracterizada por cessação abrupta e de curta duração da atividade muscular, algumas vezes precedida de contração mioclônica; termo habitualmente aplicado a músculos distais unilaterais.

nonconvulsive s., crise não-convulsiva; crise sem atividade clônica ou tônica ou outra atividade motora convulsiva. VER TAMBÉM complex partial s., absence s.

nonepileptic s., crise não-epiléptica; qualquer comportamento semelhante a uma crise, mas não-epiléptica, isto é, não associada a uma atividade cerebral anormal no EEG. VER TAMBÉM psychogenic s.

partial s., crise parcial; crise caracterizada por início ictal cerebral localizado. Os sintomas que aparecem dependem da área cortical do início ictal ou da disseminação da crise.

petit mal s., crise de pequeno mal; termo obsoleto para referir-se a uma crise cerebral não manifestada por movimentos tônico-clônicos (isto é, grande mal); antigamente, acreditava-se que fossem as manifestações clínicas apenas de uma ponta de 3s no padrão de ondas, conforme observado no eletroencefalograma; entretanto, sabe-se hoje em dia que está associada a diversos padrões EEG diferentes.

psychic s., crise psíquica; crise parcial simples caracterizada por um ataque de fenômenos psíquicos, como estado de devaneio, *déjà vu,* sensação autônoma ou emoção; geralmente, mas não exclusivamente, associada à epilepsia do lobo temporal.

psychogenic s., crise psicogênica; acesso clínico que se assemelha a uma crise epiléptica, porém não causada por epilepsia. O EEG apresenta-se normal durante um ataque e o comportamento está freqüentemente relacionado a distúrbio psiquiátrico, como transtorno de conversão.

psychomotor s., crise psicomotora; crise caracterizada por manifestação psíquica e crise complexa motora. VER psychic s.

secondarily generalized tonic-clonic s., crise tônico-clônica secundariamente generalizada; crise tônico-clônica generalizada que começa com uma crise parcial e evolui para uma crise tônico-clônica generalizada.

simple partial s., crise parcial simples; crise parcial que não está associada a comprometimento da consciência; observada em pacientes com epilepsia focal.

subclinical s., crise subclínica; crise detectada por EEG, sem nenhuma correlação clínica, isto é, uma crise EEG apenas. SIN electrographic s.

tonic s., crise tônica; ataque caracterizado por um aumento duradouro do tônus muscular, início e *offset* abruptos ou graduais, de poucos segundos a um minuto de duração, geralmente de 10–20 s; as crises tônicas que afetam os músculos proximais bilateralmente muitas vezes levam à adoção de uma postura.

tonic-clonic s., crise tônico-clônica; crise caracterizada por uma seqüência que consiste numa fase tônico-clônica; quando generalizada, constitui o que conhecemos como crise de "grande mal".

versive s., crise versiva; crise caracterizada por desvio ocular conjugado forçado e cefálico e/ou troncular duradouro.

se·la·pho·bia (sē - lā - fō′bē - ā). Selafobia. Termo raramente utilizado para referir-se ao medo mórbido de um clarão de luz. [G. *selas,* luz + *phobos,* medo]

Sel·din·ger, Sven Ivar, radiologista sueco, *1921. VER Seldinger *technique.*

se·lec·tin (sel-ek′tin). Selectina; molécula de superfície celular envolvida na adesão imune e trânsito de células. [L. *se-ligo,* pp. *se-lectum,* selecionar, escolher + -in]

E selectin, E-selectina; receptor de superfície celular produzido pelo endotélio.

L selectin, L-selectina; receptor de superfície celular produzido por leucócitos.

P selectin, P-selectina; receptor de superfície celular presente no endotélio, que está envolvido na migração dos neutrófilos até o tecido inflamado.

se·lec·tion (sē - lek′shun). Seleção; o efeito combinado das causas e das conseqüências de fatores genéticos determinantes do número médio da prole de uma espécie que atinge a maturidade sexual; os fenótipos que são letais no início da vida (p. ex., doença de Tay-Sachs), que causam esterilidade (p. ex., síndrome de Turner) ou que produzem uma progênie estéril são contra-selecionados. Quando a seleção é utilizada em heredogramas individuais, outros fatores, notavelmente a variância do número da prole e do número que sobrevive até a maturidade, constituem considerações importantes; em grandes populações, esses fatores equilibram-se e apenas a média é importante. [L. *se-ligo,* separar, selecionar, de *se,* separado + *lego,* selecionar]

artificial s., s. artificial; interferência do homem na seleção natural através do cruzamento proposital de animais ou plantas de genótipo ou fenótipo específico para produzir uma cepa com características desejadas; p. ex., o cruzamento do gado leiteiro para aumentar a produção de leite.

medical s., s. médica; preservação, através de assistência e tratamento médico, de indivíduos com genótipos patológicos que, de outro modo, não se reproduziriam, o que tende a aumentar a freqüência de genes patológicos na população; inversamente, redução da freqüência de genes patológicos ao impedir a reprodução de indivíduos de genótipo específico por esterilização cirúrgica ou outros métodos.

natural s., s. natural; "sobrevivência do mais apto", o princípio de que, na natureza, os indivíduos com maior capacidade de adaptar-se ao meio sobreviverão e se reproduzirão, enquanto aqueles menos capazes morrerão sem progênie, com conseqüente aumento na freqüência dos genes presentes nos sobreviventes. Esse princípio é mais heurístico do que rigoroso, visto que não pode ser testado, sendo o resultado tautológico com a definição empírica de aptidão.

sexual s., s. sexual; forma de seleção natural em que, de acordo com a teoria de Darwin, o macho ou a fêmea são atraídos por determinadas características, forma, cor, comportamento, etc., presentes no sexo oposto; em conseqüência, são produzidas modificações de natureza especial na espécie.

se·le·gi·line (sē-lej'e-lēn). Selegilina; inibidor da enzima monoaminaoxidase; como inibe apenas a isozima tipo B, o consumo de alimentos ou bebidas contendo tiramina tem menos tendência a induzir crises de hipertensão em indivíduos tratados com selegilina do que em indivíduos cujo tratamento consiste em inibidores não-seletivos da monoamina-oxidase. O fármaco é utilizado no tratamento da doença de Parkinson. SIN deprenyl.

se·le·ne un·gui·um (sē-lē'nē ung'gwi-ŭm). Lúnula. SIN lunule of nail. [G. *selēnē,* lua; gen. pl. do L. *unguis,* unha]

se·le·ni·um (Se) (sē-lē'nē-ŭm). Selênio; elemento metálico quimicamente semelhante ao enxofre, de número atômico 34, peso atômico de 78,96; oligoelemento essencial, tóxico em grandes quantidades; necessário para a glutationa-peroxidase e algumas outras enzimas; o Se^{75} (com meia-vida de 119,78 dias) é utilizado na cintilografia do pâncreas e das glândulas paratireóides. [G. *selēnē,* lua]

s. sulfide, sulfeto de selênio; mistura de monossulfeto de selênio cristalino e soluções sólidas de selênio e enxofre numa forma amorfa, contendo 52–55,5% de Se; utilizado no tratamento da seborréia do couro cabeludo ou caspa; aplicado ao couro cabeludo na forma de suspensão.

se·le·no·cys·teine (sē-lē-nō-sis'tēn). Selenocisteína; cisteína contendo selênio em lugar de um átomo de enxofre.

se·len·o·dont (sē-lē'nō-dont). Selenodonte; refere-se a um animal ou ser humano que possui dentes, como os molares humanos, com cristas longitudinais em forma de crescente. [G. *selēnē,* lua, + *odous (odont-),* dente]

se·le·no·me·thi·o·nine (sē-lē'nō-me-thī'ō-nēn). Selenometionina; metionina contendo selênio em lugar de enxofre.

Se·le·no·mo·nas (sē-lē'nō-mō'nas). Gênero de bactérias de afiliação taxonômica incerta, contendo bacilos curvos a crescênticos ou helicoidais, Gramnegativos e estritamente anaeróbios, que são móveis e exibem movimento de rolamento ativo. Existem vários flagelos num tufo, freqüentemente próximo ao centro do lado côncavo. A espécie típica, *S. sputigena,* é encontrada na cavidade bucal humana. [G. *selēnē,* lua + *monas,* único (unidade)]

self. Próprio. **1.** Somatório das atitudes, sentimentos, memórias, traços e predisposições comportamentais que formam a personalidade. **2.** O indivíduo representado em sua própria consciência e no seu ambiente. **3.** Em imunologia, refere-se aos componentes celulares autólogos de um indivíduo, em contraste com constituintes não-próprios ou estranhos; o mecanismo básico subjacente ao reconhecimento entre próprio e não-próprio permanece desconhecido, mas serve para proteger o hospedeiro de um ataque imunológico de seus próprios constituintes antigênicos, em oposição à destruição ou eliminação de antígenos estranhos pelo sistema imune.

subliminal s., mente subconsciente; a soma dos processos mentais que ocorrem sem o conhecimento consciente do indivíduo. SIN subconscious mind.

self-ac·cu·sa·tion. Auto-acusação; sintoma psiquiátrico comum, encontrado mais tipicamente na depressão agitada.

self-a·nal·y·sis. Auto-análise. SIN autoanalysis.

self-a·ware·ness. Autoconhecimento; percepção dos sentimentos e da experiência emocional atual; importante objetivo de toda a psicoterapia.

self-cen·tered·ness. Autocentrismo. SIN autosynnoia.

self-com·mit·ment. Auto-internação; hospitalização voluntária em clínica para doentes mentais.

self-con·trol. Autocontrole. **1.** Auto-regulação do comportamento de acordo com as crenças, objetivos, atitudes e expectativas sociais do indivíduo. **2.** Uso de estratégias de adaptação ativas por um indivíduo para lidar com situações problemáticas, em contraste com estratégias de condicionamento passivas, que fazem as coisas para o indivíduo e não exigem nenhuma ação por parte da pessoa.

self-dif·fer·en·ti·a·tion. Autodiferenciação; diferenciação resultante da ação de causas intrínsecas.

self-dis·cov·e·ry. Autodescoberta; em psicanálise, a libertação do ego reprimido numa pessoa criada para ser submissa àqueles que a cercam.

self-ef·fi·ca·cy. Auto-eficácia; estimativa ou discernimento pessoal da própria capacidade do indivíduo em atingir uma meta específica, como, por exemplo, deixar de fumar ou perder peso, ou uma meta mais geral, como, por exemplo, continuar mantendo um peso prescrito.

self-fer·til·i·za·tion. Autofertilização; fecundação dos óvulos pelo pólen da mesma flor, ou dos ovos pelos espermatozóides do mesmo animal nas formas hermafroditas; refere-se a um tipo extremo de cruzamento observado em certas formas vegetais e animais que produzem gametas tanto masculinos quanto femininos.

self-in·fec·tion. Auto-infecção. SIN autoinfection.

self-knowl·edge. Autoconhecimento. SIN autognosis.

self-lim·it·ed. Autolimitado; refere-se a uma doença que tende a cessar após um período de tempo definido; p. ex., pneumonia.

self-love. Amor próprio. SIN narcissism.

self-poi·son·ing. Auto-envenenamento. SIN autointoxication.

self-reg·u·la·tion. Auto-regulação; estratégia em três estágios para ensinar os pacientes a interromper comportamentos que põem em risco a saúde, como o tabagismo e o excesso de alimentação: 1. automonitorização (auto-observação), o primeiro estágio na auto-regulação envolve o acompanhamento e registro deliberados do comportamento do indivíduo; 2. auto-avaliação, o segundo estágio, em que o indivíduo avalia o que aprendeu na automonitorização, como, por exemplo, a freqüência com que fuma e o local onde fuma, e passa a utilizar esses dados de observação para estabelecer metas ou critérios de saúde; e 3. auto-reforço, o terceiro estágio, em que o indivíduo se gratifica por cada sucesso comportamental em direção à meta estabelecida, aumentando, assim, a probabilidade de atingi-la.

self-stim·u·la·tion. Auto-estimulação; técnica de estimulação elétrica dos nervos periféricos, da medula espinal ou do cérebro pelo paciente para aliviar a dor.

self-tolerance. Autotolerância. SIN horror autotoxicus.

Selivanoff, Feodor, químico russo, *1859. VER S. *test.*

sel·la (sel'ă). Sela. SIN saddle (1). [L. sela]

empty s., sela vazia; sela turca, freqüentemente aumentada, que não contém hipótese discernível; pode ser primariamente decorrente de diafragma da sela incompetente, com compressão da hipófise pela pia-aracnóide herniada, ou secundariamente devido a cirurgia ou radioterapia.

s. tur'cica [TA], s. turca; proeminência óssea semelhante a uma sela na superfície superior do osso esfenóide, constituindo a parte média da fossa craniana média em forma de borboleta; inclui o tubérculo da sela, anteriormente, e o dorso da sela, posteriormente; com seu revestimento de dura-máter, constitui a fossa hipofisária que acomoda a hipófise ou glândula pituitária. SIN pars sellaris, Turkish saddle.

sel·lar (sel'ăr). Selar; relativo à sela turca.

Sellick, Brian A., anestesista inglês do século XX. VER S. *maneuver.*

Selye, Hans, endocrinologista austríaco radicado no Canadá, 1907–1982. VER adaptation *syndrome* of S.

SEM Abreviatura de standard error of the *mean* (erro padrão da média).

se·man·tics (se-man'tiks). Semântica; ramo da semiótica: **1.** O estudo da importância e do desenvolvimento do significado das palavras. **2.** O estudo das relações entre sinais e aquilo a que se referem; as relações entre os sinais de um sistema; e a reação comportamental humana aos sinais, incluindo atitudes inconscientes, influências de instituições sociais e suposições epistesmológicas e lingüísticas. [G. *sēmainō,* mostrar]

Sémélaigne, Georges, pediatra francês do século XX. VER Debré-S. *syndrome;* Kocher-Debré-S. *syndrome.*

sem·el·in·ci·dent (sem-el-in'si-dent). Termo obsoleto para referir-se a algo que ocorre apenas uma vez; diz-se de uma doença infecciosa que confere imunidade permanente. [L. *semel,* uma vez + *incido,* acontecer, de *cado,* cair]

se·men, pl. **sem·i·na, se·mens** (sē'men, sē-mi'nă, sē'menz). **1.** [NA]. Sêmen. O ejaculado do pênis; líquido espesso e viscoso, branco amarelado, que contém espermatozóides; mistura produzida por secreções dos testículos, vesículas seminais, próstata e glândulas bulbouretrais. SIN seminal fluid. **2.** Semente. SIN seed (1). [L. *semen (semin-),* semente (de plantas, do homem, de animais)]

se·me·nu·ria (sē-mě-noo'rē-ă). Espermatúria; excreção de urina contendo sêmen. SIN seminuria, spermaturia.

♻ **semi-.** Semiponto, metade; parcialmente. Cf. hemi-. [L. *semis,* metade]

sem·i·al·de·hyde (sem-ē-al'dē-hīd). Semi-aldeído; o monoaldeído de um ácido dicarboxílico, assim denominado porque metade dos grupamentos COOH do ácido original é reduzida a aldeído, enquanto a outra metade permanece inalterada; p. ex., γ- semi-aldeído do ácido glutâmico, OHC–

$CH_2CH_2CH(NH_3)^+ –COO^-$. Muitos semi-aldeídos são intermediários na biossíntese e na degradação metabólica de aminoácidos (p. ex., L-prolina, L-lisina, L-glutamato).

sem·i·ca·nal (sem′ē-kă-nal′). Semicanal; metade de um canal; sulco profundo na borda de um osso que, unindo-se com um sulco ou parte semelhante de um osso adjacente, forma um canal completo. SIN semicanalis.
  s. of auditory tube, s. da tuba auditiva. SIN canal for pharyngotympanic (auditory) tube.
  s. for tensor tympani muscle, s. para o músculo tensor do tímpano. SIN canal for tensor tympani muscle.

sem·i·ca·na·lis, pl. **sem·i·ca·na·les** (sem′ē-kă-nal′is, -ēz). Semicanal. SIN semicanal. [L.]
  s. mus′culi tensor′is tym′pani [TA], s. para o músculo tensor do tímpano. SIN canal for tensor tympani muscle.
  s. tu′bae auditi′vae [TA], s. da tuba auditiva. SIN canal for pharyngotympanic (auditory) tube.
  s. t′ubae audito′riae, s. da tuba auditiva. SIN canal for pharyngotympanic (auditory) tube.

sem·i·car·ti·lag·i·nous (sem′ē-kar-ti-laj′i-nŭs). Semicartilaginoso; composto parcialmente de cartilagem.

sem·i·cir·cu·lar (sem′ē-sir′kū-lăr). Semicircular; que forma meio círculo ou um círculo incompleto. SIN semiorbicular.

sem·i·co·ma (sem′ē-kō′ma). Semicoma. VER semicomatose.

sem·i·com·a·tose (sem′ē-kō′ma-tōs). Semicomatoso; termo impreciso para um estado de sonolência e inação, em que pode ser necessário mais do que um estímulo normal para induzir uma resposta, podendo esta ser tardia ou incompleta. SIN semiconscious.

sem·i·con·duc·tor (sem′ē-kon-dŭk′ter). Semicondutor; metalóide, numa forma ou em outra, que conduz a eletricidade mais facilmente do que um verdadeiro não-metal, porém menos facilmente do que um metal; p. ex., silício, germânio.

sem·i·con·scious (sem′ē-kon′shŭs). Semiconsciente. SIN semicomatose.

sem·i·con·serv·a·tive. Semiconservador; processo de replicação do DNA em que os dois filamentos permanecem intactos, são separados e copiados, dirigindo-se, cada um deles, para cada célula-filha.

sem·i·cris·ta (sem′ē-kris′tă). Semicrista. Crista pequena ou imperfeita. [semi- + L. *crista,* crista, tufo]
  s. incisi′va, s. incisiva. SIN nasal crest.

sem·i·de·cus·sa·tion (sem′ē-dē-kŭs-sā′shŭn). Semidecussação; decussação incompleta, como a que ocorre no quiasma óptico humano.

sem·i·flex·ion (sem-ē-flek′shŭn). Semiflexão; posição de uma articulação ou segmento de um membro a meio caminho entre a extensão e a flexão.

sem·i·lu·nar (sem-ē-loo′năr). Semilunar. SIN lunar (2). [semi- + L. *luna,* lua]

sem·i·lu·na·re (sem-ē-loo-nā′rē). Semilunar. VER lunate *(bone).*

sem·i·lux·a·tion (sem-ē-lŭk-sā′shŭn). Subluxação. SIN subluxation.

sem·i·mem·bra·no·sus (sem′ē-mem-bră-nō′sŭs). Semimembranáceo. VER semimembranosus *(muscle).*

sem·i·mem·bra·nous (sem′ē-mem′bră-nŭs). Semimembranáceo; que consiste parcialmente em membrana; refere-se ao músculo semimembranáceo.

sem·i·nal (sem′i-năl). Seminal. **1.** Relativo ao sêmen. **2.** Original ou que influencia futuros desenvolvimentos.

sem·i·na·tion (sem-i-nā′shŭn). Inseminação. SIN insemination.

sem·i·nif·er·ous (sem′i-nif′er-ŭs). Seminífero; que transporta ou conduz o sêmen; designa os túbulos do testículo. [L. *semen,* semente (sêmen) + *fero,* transportar]

sem·i·no·ma (sem-i-nō′mă). Inseminoma; neoplasia maligna radiossensível que habitualmente se origina de células germinativas nos testículos de adultos jovens, metastatizando para os linfonodos paraaórticos; equivalente ao disgerminoma do ovário. [L. *semen,* semente (sêmen) + G. *-oma,* tumor]
  spermacytic s., i. espermacítico; tipo de i. testicular de crescimento relativamente lento e localmente invasivo, que não metastatiza e não tem equivalente ovariano.

se·mi·no·ma·tous (sem-i-nō′mă-tŭs). Inseminomatoso; relativo a um inseminoma.

sem·i·nor·mal (N/2). (sem-ē-nōr′mal). Seminormal; refere-se a uma solução com metade da concentração de uma solução normal (0,5 N).

sem·i·nu·ria (sē-mi-noo′rē-ă). Espermatúria. SIN semenuria.

sem·i·o·path·ic, se·mei·o·path·ic (sē′mē-ō-paht′ik). Semiopático; refere-se ao uso desordenado de símbolos. [G. *sēmeion,* sinal + *pathos,* doença]

sem·i·or·bic·u·lar (sē-mē-ōr-bik′ū-lăr). Semi-orbicular. SIN semicircular.

se·mi·o·sis, se·mei·o·sis (sē-mē-ō′sis). Semiose; processo mental ou simbólico em que algo (p. ex., palavra, símbolo, indicação não-verbal) funciona como sinal para o organismo. [G. *sēmeiōsis,* de *sēmeion,* sinal]

se·mi·ot·ic, se·mei·ot·ic (sē-mē-ot′ik, sem-ē-). Semiótico. **1.** Relativo à semiótica. **2.** Relativo aos sinais, lingüísticos ou corporais. [G. *sēmeiōtikos,* de *sēmeion,* sinal]

se·mi·ot·ics, se·mei·ot·ics (sē-mē-ot′iks, sem-e-). Semiótica. **1.** A teoria filosófica geral dos sinais e símbolos na comunicação, que possui três ramos: sintática, semântica e pragmática. **2.** Termo obsoleto para referir-se à sintomatologia. [ver semiotic]

se·mi·pen·nate (sem′ē-pen′at) [TA]. Semipenado. **1.** Que apresenta um arranjo em pena em um dos lados; que se assemelha à metade de uma pena. **2.** Refere-se a certos músculos cujas fibras seguem um trajeto em ângulo agudo com um lado de um tendão. SIN unipennate*, demipenniform.

sem·i·pen·ni·form (sem′ē-pen′i-fōrm). Semipeniforme; peniforme de um lado. VER semipennate *muscle.*

sem·i·per·me·a·ble (sem-ē-per′mē-ă-bl). Semipermeável; livremente permeável à água (ou outro solvente), porém relativamente impermeável a solutos. Dependendo do contexto, o termo tem sido utilizado para referir-se à impermeabilidade a todos os solutos, exceto moléculas muito pequenas sem carga elétrica (p. ex., membrana celular) ou, simplesmente, à impermeabilidade a moléculas muito grandes, como as proteínas (p. ex., membrana capilar).

sem·i·pro·na·tion (sem′ē-prō-nā′shŭn). Semipronação; atitude ou adoção de decúbito ventral parcial, como na posição de Sims.

sem·i·prone (sem-ē-prōn′). Semiprono; que se refere à semipronação.

sem·i·qui·none (sem-ē-kwin′on). Semiquinona; radical livre que resulta da remoção de um átomo de hidrogênio com seu elétron durante o processo de desidrogenação de uma hidroquinona a quinona ou composto semelhante (p. ex., flavina mononucleotídeo).

sem·i·spi·nal (sem-ē-spī′nal). Semi-espinal; designa os músculos inseridos, em parte, nos processos espinhosos das vértebras.

Sem·i·sul·co·spi·na (sem-ē-sŭl-kō-spī′nă). Gênero de caramujos operculados (família Pleuroceriidae, subclasse Prosobranchiata). Uma forma oriental, *S. libertina,* serve de primeiro hospedeiro intermediário de diversos trematódeos, incluindo *Paragonimus westermani.* [semi- + L. *sulcus,* sulco + *spina,* espinho]

sem·i·sul·cus (sem′ē-sŭl′kŭs). Semi-sulco; sulco discreto na borda de um osso ou outra estrutura que, ao se unir com um sulco semelhante na estrutura adjacente correspondente, forma um sulco completo.

sem·i·su·pi·na·tion (sem′ē-soo-pi-nā′shŭn). Semi-supinação; atitude ou adoção de decúbito dorsal parcial.

sem·i·su·pine (sem-ē-soo-pīn′). Semi-supino; que se refere à semi-supinação.

sem·i·syn·thet·ic (sem′ē-sin-thet′ik). Semi-sintético; descreve o processo de síntese de determinada substância química utilizando uma substância química natural como material de partida, evitando, assim, parte de uma síntese total; p. ex., a conversão do colesterol (obtido de uma fonte natural) em corticosteróide.

sem·i·sys·tem·at·ic name (sem′ē-sis-tē-mat′ik). Nome semi-sistemático; nome de uma substância química que, pelo menos em parte, é sistemático e, pelo menos em parte, não o é (ou seja, é trivial). Por exemplo, o calciferol inclui o sufixo -ol, que indica um radical –OH, enquanto calcifer-, que não tem nenhum significado sistemático, é utilizado apenas nessa palavra. O termo cortisona contém o sufixo -ona, que indica um grupamento cetona, enquanto o restante do termo deriva do córtex (supra-renal). O ácido hipúrico (trivial) pode ser definido como *N*-benzoilglicina (nome semitrivial); o termo benzoil é sistemático para o radical $C_6H_5–CO–$, enquanto glicina é o nome trivial para o ácido α-aminoacético (ou ácido 2-aminoetanóico, para ser totalmente sistemático), enquanto o *N* refere-se ao benzoil fixado no nitrogênio da glicina; com base nisso, a estrutura $C_6H_5–CO–NH–CH_2–COOH$ é exclusivamente definida. Muitos nomes genéricos ou não-comerciais de drogas, incluindo USAN, hormônios, etc., são semitriviais nesse sentido químico, embora freqüentemente sejam considerados nomes triviais; com freqüência, não se faz uma distinção entre trivial e semitrivial. SIN semitrivial name.

sem·i·ten·di·no·sus (sem′ē-ten-di-nō′sŭs). Semitendinoso. SIN semitendinous. [L.]

sem·i·ten·di·nous (sem′ē-ten′di-nŭs). Semitendinoso; composto em parte de tendão; refere-se ao músculo semitendinoso. SIN semitendinosus. [L. *semitendinosus*]

sem·i·ter·tian (sem-ē-ter′shē-ăn, -ter′shŭn). Semiterçã; parcialmente terçã, particularmente cotidiana; refere-se à malária, na qual ocorrem dois paroxismos em um dia e outro no dia seguinte.

sem·i·triv·i·al name (sem-ē-triv′ē-ăl). Nome semitrivial. SIN semisystematic name.

sem·i·va·lent (sem-ē-vā′lent). Semivalente; refere-se à capacidade de formar uma ligação com um elétron.

Semon, Richard W., biologista alemão, 1859–1918. VER S.-Hering *theory.*

Semple, Sir David, médico inglês, 1856–1937. VER S. *vacine.*

se·mus·tine (se-mus′ten). Semustina. SIN methyl-CCNU.

Senear, Francis E., dermatologista norte-americano, 1889–1958. VER S.-Usher *disease, syndrome.*

Se·ne·cio (sē-nē′sē-ō, -shē-ō). **1.** Grande gênero de plantas (família Compositae) das quais muitas espécies contêm alcalóides que provocam necrose hepática. **2.** Erva daninha comum do leste dos Estados Unidos, antigamente utilizada no tratamento da amenorréia e de outras irregularidades menstruais. [L. uma planta, tasneira, de *senecio,* homem idoso]

se·ne·ci·o·ic ac·id (sĕ-nē′si-ō-ik). Ácido senecióico; precursor polímero e precursor dos compostos isoprenóide e terpeno; o componente ácido do binapacril no qual é esterificado com 4,6-dinitro-2-(1-metilpropil)fenol; o derivado coenzima A é um intermediário na degradação da L-leucina; utilizado como fungicida e acaricida.

se·ne·ci·o·sis (sĕ-nē-sē-ō′sis). Seneciose; degeneração e necrose hepáticas causadas pela ingestão de plantas do gênero *Senecio*, como tasneira; foram observadas propriedades tóxicas semelhantes após a ingestão de alguns tipos de *Crotalaria* e *Heliotropium*.

sen·e·ga (sen′ĕ-gă). Sênega; a raiz seca de *Polygala senega* (família Polygalaceae), uma erva do leste e do centro da América do Norte; expectorante. SIN Seneca snakeroot. [*Seneca*, uma tribo indígena]

se·nes·cence (se-nes′ens). Senescência; o estado de ficar velho. [L. *senesco*, envelhecer, de *senex*, idoso]
 dental s., s. dentária; condição dos dentes e estruturas associadas em que há deterioração devido a processos de envelhecimento normais ou prematuros.

se·nes·cent (sĕ-nes′ent). Senescente; que envelhece.

Sengstaken, Robert W., neurocirurgião norte-americano, *1923. VER S.-Blakemore *tube*.

se·nile (sē′nīl, sen′īl). Senil; relativo a ou característico de idade avançada. [L. *senilis*]

se·nil·i·ty (se-nil′i-tē). Senilidade; velhice; termo geral para referir-se a uma variedade de distúrbios orgânicos, tanto físicos quanto mentais, que ocorrem na idade avançada. [ver senile]

se·ni·um (sē′nē-ŭm). Termo raramente utilizado para referir-se à velhice; indica especialmente a debilidade da idade avançada. [L. fraqueza da idade, de *seneo*, ficar velho, frágil]

sen·na (sen′ă). Sene; as folhas pequenas ou leguminosas de *Cassia acutifolia* (s. Alexandrina) e de *C. angustifolia* (s. de Tinnevelly ou índia); laxativo. [Ar. *senā*]

sen·no·side A, sen·no·side B (sen′ō-sīd). Senosídeo A, senosídeo B; dois glicosídeos da antraquinona que constituem os princípios laxativos da sene.

sen·sate (sen′sāt). Capaz de perceber o toque e outras sensações; termo utilizado para referir-se a pacientes que sofreram lesões parciais de nervos ou da medula espinal.

sen·sa·tion (sen-sā′shŭn). Sensação; sentimento; a tradução, para a consciência, dos efeitos de um estímulo que está excitando qualquer um dos órgãos do sentido. [L. *sensatio*, percepção, sensação, de *sentio*, perceber, sentir]
 delayed s., s. tardia; sensação que só é percebida depois de transcorrido um intervalo de tempo apreciável após a aplicação do estímulo.
 general s., s. geral; sensibilidade referida no corpo como um todo, e não em qualquer parte específica.
 girdle s., s. de constrição em cinto. SIN zonesthesia.
 primary s., s. primária; sensação que resulta diretamente de um estímulo.
 referred s., s. referida; s. percebida em um local em resposta a um estímulo aplicado em outro local.

sense (sens). Sentido, sensibilidade; a faculdade de perceber qualquer estímulo. [L. *sentio*, pp. *sensus*, sentir, perceber]
 chemical s.'s, sentidos químicos; os sentidos do olfato e paladar.
 color s., sensibilidade à cor; capacidade de perceber variações de tonalidade, luminosidade e saturação de luz.
 s. of equilibrium, sentido do equilíbrio; sentido que torna possível uma postura fisiológica normal. SIN static s.
 geometric s., sentido geométrico; uma de duas direções ao longo de uma curva em que algo se move, como, por exemplo, sentido horário ou sentido anti-horário.
 joint s., sensibilidade articular. SIN articular *sensibility*.
 kinesthetic s., sentido cinestésico; a sensação percebida no músculo ao se contrair; consciência do movimento ou da atividade nos músculos ou articulações; sentido de posição ou movimento mediado, em grande parte, pelas colunas posteriores e lemnisco medial. VER TAMBÉM bathyesthesia. SIN deep sensibility, muscular s., myesthesia, myoesthesis, myoesthesia.
 light s., sensibilidade à luz; capacidade de perceber variações no grau de luz ou brilho.
 muscular s., sentido muscular. SIN kinesthetic s.
 obstacle s., sensibilidade a obstáculos; capacidade freqüentemente encontrada no cego de evitar objetos sem alerta visual.
 position s., sentido de posição. SIN posture s.
 posture s., sentido de postura; capacidade de reconhecer a posição na qual um membro é passivamente colocado, com os olhos fechados. SIN position s.
 pressure s., sensibilidade à pressão; faculdade de discriminar vários graus de pressão sobre a superfície. SIN baresthesia, weight s.
 seventh s., sétimo sentido. SIN visceral s.
 space s., sentido espacial; a faculdade de perceber as posições relativas de objetos no mundo externo.
 special s., sentido especial; um dos cinco sentidos relacionados, respectivamente, aos órgãos da visão, audição, olfato, paladar e tato.
 static s., sentido estático. SIN s. of equilibrium.
 tactile s., sentido tátil. SIN touch (1).
 temperature s., sentido de temperatura. SIN thermoesthesia.
 thermal s., thermic s., sentido térmico. SIN thermoesthesia.
 time s., sentido temporal; faculdade pela qual se percebe a passagem do tempo.
 visceral s., sentido visceral; percepção da existência dos órgãos internos. SIN seventh s., splanchnesthesia, splanchnesthetic sensibility.
 weight s., sentido de peso. SIN pressure s.

sen·si·bil·i·ty (sen-si-bil′i-tē). Sensibilidade; a consciência da sensação; capacidade de perceber estímulos sensíveis. [L. *sensibilitas*]
 articular s., s. articular; percepção de sensações nas superfícies articulares. SIN arthresthesia, joint sense.
 bone s., s. óssea. SIN pallesthesia.
 cortical s., s. cortical; a integração de estímulos sensoriais pelo córtex cerebral.
 deep s., s. profunda. SIN bathyesthesia, kinesthetic *sense*.
 dissociation s., s. de dissociação; a perda do sentido da dor e sentido térmico, com preservação da sensibilidade tátil, ou vice-versa.
 electromuscular s., s. eletromuscular; sensibilidade do tecido muscular à estimulação pela eletricidade.
 epicritic s., s. epicrítica. VER epicritic.
 pallesthetic s., s. palestésica. SIN pallesthesia.
 proprioceptive s., s. proprioceptiva. VER proprioceptive.
 protopathic s., s. protopática. VER protopathic.
 splanchnesthetic s., s. esplancnestésica. SIN visceral *sense*.

sensação			
modalidade de sensação	objeto de percepção	natureza dos estímulos	tipo de receptores
sentido da visão	claridade, escuridão, cores	radiação eletromagnética 4.000–7.000 Å	fotorreceptores
sentido de temperatura	frio, calor	radiação eletromagnética 7.000–9.000 Å, transporte do calor por convecção	termorreceptores
sentido do tato	pressão, toque		
sentido da audição	som, freqüências		
sentido estatocinético	posição absoluta do corpo, velocidade do corpo, posição relativa do corpo e movimento de partes do corpo e das articulações, sensação de força	modificação dos mecanorreceptores por objetos sólidos ou transmissão de mudanças na pressão do ar	mecanorreceptores
sentido do olfato	odores	substâncias químicas	
sentido do paladar	azedo, salgado, doce, amargo	íons	quimiorreceptores
sentido da dor	dor	lesão tecidual mecânica	nociceptores

vibratory s., s. vibratória, percepção vibratória. SIN pallesthesia.

sen·si·ble (sen'si-bl). Sensível. **1.** Perceptível aos sentidos. **2.** Capaz de sentir. **3.** SIN sensitive. **4.** Que possui razão ou julgamento; inteligente. [L. *sensibilis*, de *sentio*, sentir, perceber]

sen·sif·er·ous (sen-sif'er-ŭs). Sensífero; que conduz uma sensação. [L. *sensus*, sentido + *fero*, transportar]

sen·sig·e·nous (sen-sij'e-nŭs). Senságeno; que origina sensação. [L. *sensus*, sentido + G. *-gen*, produzir]

sen·sim·e·ter (sen-sim'e-ter). Sensímetro; instrumento que mede graus de sensação cutânea. [L. *sensus*, sentido + G. *metron*, medida]

sensing. Percepção.

  quorum s., *sensiquorum;* fenômeno observado em bactérias, que limita a ocorrência de determinados comportamentos apenas acima de uma densidade populacional específica.

sen·si·tive (sen'si-tiv). Sensitivo, sensível. **1.** Capaz de perceber sensações. **2.** Que responde a determinado estímulo. **3.** Que percebe agudamente situações interpessoais. **4.** Aquele que é facilmente hipnotizável. **5.** Facilmente submetido a uma alteração química, porém com pouca alteração nas condições ambientais, como um reagente sensível. **6.** Em imunologia, refere-se: 1) a um *antígeno* sensibilizado (*sensitized antigen*); 2) a um indivíduo (ou animal) que se tornou suscetível a reações imunológicas em consequência de exposição prévia ao antígeno envolvido. SIN sensible (3).

sen·si·tiv·i·ty (sen-si-tiv'i-tē). Sensibilidade. **1.** A capacidade de perceber através de um ou mais sentidos. **2.** Estado de ser sensível. SIN esthesia (2). **3.** Em patologia clínica e triagem médica, a proporção de indivíduos afetados que apresentam um teste positivo para a doença que o teste pretende revelar, isto é, os resultados positivos verdadeiros divididos pelos resultados verdadeiro-positivos e falso-negativos totais, geralmente expressos em percentagem. Cf. specificity (2). [L. *sentio*, pp. *sensus*, sentir]

  acquired s., s. adquirida. SIN allergy (1).

  analytical s., s. analítica; **(1)** limite de detecção mínima; **(2)** grau de resposta a uma mudança na concentração do analisado que está sendo medido num ensaio.

  antibiotic s., s. a antibióticos; suscetibilidade microbiana a antibióticos. VER TAMBÉM antibiotic sensitivity *test*, minimal inhibitory *concentration*.

  clinical s., s. clínica; positividade de um teste na presença de doença; capacidade de um teste de identificar corretamente uma doença. VER TAMBÉM diagnostic s.

  contrast s., s. de contraste; s. a contrastes; em óptica, a capacidade de perceber a diferença no brilho de áreas adjacentes; em radiologia, reação alérgica a contraste radiográfico iodado.

  diagnostic s., s. diagnóstica; a probabilidade (P) de que, considerando a presença de doença (D), um resultado de teste anormal (T) indique a presença de doença; isto é, P(T/D). VER TAMBÉM clinical s.

  idiosyncratic s., s. idiossincrásica; atopia, reação alérgica tipo I.

  induced s., s. induzida. SIN allergy (1).

  multiple chemical s., s. a múltiplas substâncias químicas; conjunto de sintomas de apresentação variável, atribuídos à exposição recorrente a substâncias químicas ambientais conhecidas, em doses geralmente inferiores aos níveis estabelecidos como nocivos; as queixas incluem múltiplos sistemas orgânicos. SIN environmental illness.

  pacemaker s., s. do marcapasso; a atividade cardíaca mínima necessária para deflagrar, de forma consistente, um gerador de pulso.

  photoallergic s., s. fotoalérgica. VER photosensitization.

  phototoxic s., s. fototóxica. VER photosensitization.

  primaquine s., s. à primaquina; sensibilidade congênita não-imunológica à primaquina, que provoca hemólise após exposição a essa droga, devido à deficiência de glicose 6-fosfato-desidrogenase nos eritrócitos.

  relative s., s. relativa; a sensibilidade de uma prova de triagem clínica, conforme determinado através de comparação com o mesmo tipo de teste; p. ex., sensibilidade de um novo teste sorológico em relação à sensibilidade de um teste sorológico estabelecido.

  salt s., s. ao sal; tendência de determinadas suspensões bacterianas a sofrer aglutinação espontânea em solução salina fisiológica.

  spectral s., s. espectral; a recíproca da quantidade de radiação monocromática que produz uma resposta fixa.

sen·si·ti·za·tion (sen'si-ti-zā'shŭn). Sensibilização; imunização, sobretudo em relação a antígenos (imunógenos) não associados a infecção; indução de sensibilidade adquirida ou de alergia.

  autoerythrocyte s., s. auto-eritrocitária. VER autoerythrocyte sensitization *syndrome*.

  covert s., s. oculta; condicionamento ou treinamento aversivo para livrar-se de um comportamento não desejado, em que se ensina o paciente a imaginar consequências desagradáveis e aversivas relacionadas enquanto enfoca o hábito indesejado.

  photodynamic s., s. fotodinâmica; a ação pela qual certas substâncias, notavelmente os corantes fluorescentes (acridina, eosina, azul de metileno, rosa de bengala, absorvem a luz visível e emitem energia em comprimentos de onda que são prejudiciais aos micróbios ou outros organismos na suspensão contendo corante, ou provocam destruição seletiva das células cancerosas sensibilizadas pela administração de porfirina intravenosa expostas à luz laser vermelha. SIN photosensitization (2).

sen·si·tize (sen'si-tīz). Sensibilizar; tornar-se sensível; induzir uma sensibilidade adquirida, imunizar. VER TAMBÉM sensitized *antigen*.

sen·si·tiz·er (sen'si-tīz-er). **1.** Sensibilizador; substância que provoca alergia ou dermatite após alteração (sensibilização) da pele por exposição prévia à substância em questão. **2.** SIN antibody.

sens·i·tom·e·try (sen-si-tom'e-trē). Sensitometria; em radiologia, procedimento de medir a resposta do filme à radiação. [sensibilidade + G. *metron*, medida]

sen·so·mo·bile (sen-sō-mō'bel). Sensomóvel; capaz de efetuar um movimento em resposta a um estímulo.

sen·so·mo·bil·i·ty (sen-sō-mō-bil'i-tē). Sensomobilidade; estado de ser sensomóvel.

sen·so·mo·tor (sen-sō-mō'ter). Sensomotor. SIN sensorimotor.

sen·sor (sen'sŏr). Sensor; dispositivo projetado para responder a estímulos físicos, como temperatura, luz, magnetismo ou movimento, bem como para transmitir os impulsos resultantes para interpretação, registro, movimento ou controle operacional. VER sense.

⚠ **sensori-.** Sensori-. Sensório, sensorial. [L. *sensorius*]

sen·so·ri·al (sen-sōr'ē-ăl). Sensorial; relativo ao sensório.

sen·so·ri·glan·du·lar (sen'sŏr-i-glan'dū-lăr). Sensoriglandular; relativo à secreção glandular excitada por estimulação dos nervos sensoriais.

sen·so·ri·mo·tor (sen'sŏr-i-mō'ter). Sensorimotor; tanto sensorial quanto motor; refere-se a um nervo misto com fibras aferentes e eferentes. SIN sensomotor.

sen·so·ri·mus·cu·lar (sen'sŏr-i-mŭs'kū-lăr). Sensorimuscular; refere-se à contração muscular que ocorre em resposta a um estímulo sensorial.

sen·so·ri·um, pl. **sen·so·ria, sen·so·ri·ums** (sen-sōr'ē-ŭm, -ă, -ŭmz). Sensório. **1.** Órgão dos sentidos. **2.** A "sede da sensação" hipotética. SIN perceptorium. **3.** Em biologia e psicologia humanas, a consciência; algumas vezes utilizado como termo genérico para as funções intelectuais e cognitivas. [L. ant.]

sen·so·ri·vas·cu·lar (sen'sŏr-i-vas'kū-lăr). Sensorivascular. SIN sensorivasomotor.

sen·so·ri·vas·o·mo·tor (sen'sŏr-i-vas-ō-mō'ter). Sensorivasomotor; refere-se à contração ou dilatação dos vasos sanguíneos, que ocorrem como reflexo sensorial. SIN sensorivascular.

sen·so·ry (sen'sŏ-rē). Sensorial; relativo à sensação. [L. *sensorius*, de *sensus*, sentido]

sen·su·al (sen'shoo-ăl). Sensual. **1.** Relativo ao corpo e aos sentidos, distinto do intelecto ou do espírito. **2.** Refere-se ao prazer corporal ou sensorial, não necessariamente sexual. [L. *sensualis*, dotado de sentimento]

sen·su·al·ism (sen'shoo-ăl-izm). Sensualismo. **1.** Dominação pelas emoções. **2.** Indulgência nos prazeres sensoriais. [L. *sensualis*, dotado de sentimento, de *sentio*, sentir]

sen·su·al·i·ty (sen-shū-al'i-tē). Sensualidade; o estado ou qualidade de ser sensual.

sen'su la'to. De sentido amplo. [L.]

sen'su stri'cto. Em sentido estrito. [L.]

sen·tient (sen'shent, sen'shē-ent). Senciente; capaz de, ou caracterizado por, sensação. [L. *sentiens*, p. pres. de *sentio*, sentir, perceber]

sen·ti·ment (sen'ti-ment). Sentimento. **1.** Sentimento ou emoção em relação a uma idéia. **2.** Disposição ou organização complexa de uma pessoa em relação a determinado objeto (uma pessoa, uma coisa ou uma idéia abstrata) que torna o objeto aquilo que representa para a pessoa. [L. *sentio*, sentir]

sen·ti·sec·tion (sen-ti-sek'shŭn). Sentissecção; vivissecção de um animal não anestesiado. [L. *sentio*, sentir + *sectio*, corte]

sep·a·ra·tion (sep'ă-rā'shŭn). Separação. **1.** Ato de manter afastado ou dividido, ou estado de ser mantido afastado. **2.** Em odontologia, o processo de ganhar pequenos espaços entre os dentes na preparação para tratamento.

  jaw s., s. da mandíbula; espaço entre a mandíbula e o maxilar em qualquer grau de abertura.

  s. of retina, descolamento da retina. SIN retinal *detachment*.

  sternochondral s., s. esternocondral; separação da cartilagem costal do esterno, especialmente da segunda até a sétima vértebras, que são articulações verdadeiras revestidas por membranas sinoviais.

  s. of teeth, s. dos dentes; **(1)** perda do contato proximal dos dentes; **(2)** em ortodontia, a criação de espaços interproximais para adaptação de um aparelho.

sep·a·ra·tor (sep'er-ā-ter). Separador. **1.** Aquilo que divide ou mantém afastadas duas ou mais substâncias ou que impede a sua mistura. **2.** Em odontologia, instrumento para forçar o afastamento de dois dentes, de modo a ter acesso às paredes proximais adjacentes. SIN segregator. [L. *se-paro*, pp. *-atus*, separar, de *se*, afastado + *paro*, preparar]

Se·pha·dex (sef'a-deks). Nome comercial de certas polidextranas utilizadas na cromatografia de coluna.

sep·sis, pl. **sep·ses** (sep'sis, -sēz). Sepse, sépsis; presença de diversos microrganismos patogênicos ou suas toxinas no sangue ou nos tecidos; a septicemia é um tipo comum de sepse. [G. *sēpsis*, putrefação]

intestinal s., s. intestinal; s. associada a auto-intoxicação de origem intestinal.
s. len'ta, s. lenta; infecção de desenvolvimento lento e mais ou menos localizada.
puerperal s., s. puerperal. SIN puerperal *fever.*

sept-. Sept-. VER septi-, septico-, septo-.

sep·ta (sep'tă). Septos; plural de septum. [L.]
intra-alveolar septa, septos intra-alveolares. SIN interradicular *septa* of maxilla and mandible, under *septum.*

sep·tal (sep'tăl). Septal; relativo a um septo.

sep·tan (sep'tăn). Septã; refere-se a uma febre malárica cujos paroxismos sofrem recidiva a cada sétimo dia, considerando o dia de ocorrência como o primeiro dia, isto é, com intervalo assintomático de cinco dias. [L. *septem,* sete]

Sep·ta·ta (sep-tā'tă). Membro recém-descrito de protozoário do filo Microspora, encontrado no intestino de um indivíduo imunocomprometido. A espécie descrita é *S. intestinalis.* Esse microrganismo foi reclassificado como *Encephalitozoon intestinalis.* VER TAMBÉM *Encephalitozoon intestinalis.*

sep·tate (sep'tāt). Septado; que possui um septo; dividido em compartimentos. [L. *saeptum,* septo]

sep·tec·to·my (sep-tek'tō-mē). Septectomia; remoção cirúrgica total ou parcial de um septo, especificamente o septo nasal. [L. *saeptum,* septo + G. *ektomē,* excisão]

sep·te·mia (sep-tē'mē-ă). Termo raramente utilizado para septicemia.

septi-, sept-. Septi-, sept-. Sete. [L. *septem*]

sep·tic (sep'tik). Séptico; relativo a, ou causado por, sepse.

sep·ti·ce·mia (sep-ti-sē'mē-ă). Septicemia; doença sistêmica causada pela disseminação de microrganismos e suas toxinas através do sangue circulante; antigamente denominada "envenenamento do sangue". VER TAMBÉM pyemia. SIN septic fever, septic intoxication. [G. *sēpsis,* putrefação + *haima,* sangue]
acute fulminating meningococcal s., s. meningocócica fulminante aguda. SIN Waterhouse-Friderichsen *syndrome.*
anthrax s., antracemia. SIN anthracemia.
cryptogenic s., s. criptogênica; forma de septicemia em que não se consegue encontrar nenhum foco primário de infecção.
metastasizing s., s. metastatizante; sepse com entrada de microrganismos na corrente sanguínea, resultando na formação de abscesso distante do local de origem da infecção.
morphine injector's s., s. do dependente de morfina; infecção da corrente sanguínea de um indivíduo que se auto-injeta narcóticos, geralmente por via intravenosa, devido à contaminação bacteriana do equipamento utilizado. Observada mais freqüentemente com a heroína e narcóticos do que com a morfina.
plague s., s. da peste; infecção pelo microrganismo da peste, *Yersinia pestis,* com infecção da corrente sanguínea.
puerperal s., s. puerperal; infecção grave da corrente sanguínea em conseqüência de parto ou procedimento obstétrico.
typhoid s., s. tifóide; febre tifóide durante a fase em que o microrganismo pode ser cultivado do sangue. SIN typhosepsis.

sep·ti·ce·mic (sep-ti-sē'mik). Septicêmico; relativo a, que sofre de ou que resulta de septicemia.

septico-, septic-. Septico-, septic-. Sepse, séptico. [G. *sēptikos,* em putrefação, de *sēpsis,* putrefação]

sep·ti·co·py·e·mia (sep'ti-kō-pī-ē'mē-ă). Septicopiemia; piemia e septicemia concomitantes.

sep·ti·co·py·e·mic (sep'ti-kō-pī-ē'mik). Septicopiêmico; relativo à septicopiemia.

sep·ti·va·lent (sep-ti-vā'lent, sep-tiv'ă-lent). Septivalente, que possui um poder de combinação (valência) de sete.

septo-, sept-. Septo. [L. *saeptum*]

sep·to·der·mo·plas·ty (sep-tō-der'mō-plas-tē). Septodermoplastia; operação para enxertar epitélio escamoso e derme para substituir a mucosa do septo nasal, sobretudo em pacientes com telangiectasia hemorrágica hereditária [sépto- + dermo- + G. *plastos,* formado]

sep·to·mar·gi·nal (sep'tō-mar'ji-năl). Septomarginal; relativo à margem de um septo ou ao septo e a uma margem.

sep·to·na·sal (sep'tō-nā'săl). Septonasal; relativo ao septo nasal.

sep·to·plas·ty (sep'tō-plas-tē). Septoplastia; operação para corrigir defeitos ou deformidades do septo nasal, freqüentemente através de alteração ou remoção parcial de estruturas esqueléticas. [septo- + G. *plastos,* formado]

sep·to·rhi·no·plas·ty (sep-tō-rī'nō-plas-tē). Septorrinoplastia; operação combinada para reparo de defeitos ou deformidades do septo nasal e do nariz externo. [septo- + G. *rhis,* nariz + *plastos,* formado]

sep·tos·to·my (sep-tos'tō-mē). Septostomia; criação cirúrgica de um defeito septal. [septo- + G. *stoma,* boca]
atrial s., s. atrial; estabelecimento de uma comunicação entre os dois átrios do coração. SIN atrioseptostomy.
balloon s., s. em balão; s. efetuada por cateterismo cardíaco com uso de um balão inflado colocado através do septo interatrial pelo forame oval; utilizada em casos de transposição dos grandes vasos ou atresia tricúspide.

sep·tu·lum, pl. **sep·tu·la** (sep'tū-lŭm, -lă). Séptulo; pequeno septo. [L. mod. dim. de *septum*]
s. tes'tis, s. do testículo. SIN septula of testis.

septula of testis, séptulos do testículo; uma das trabéculas do testículo; septos imperfeitos e cordões fibrosos que se irradiam do mediastino do testículo em direção à superfície da glândula. SIN s. testis, trabecula testis.

SEPTO

sep·tum, gen. **sep·ti,** pl. **sep·ta** (sep'tŭm, -tī, -tă). Septo. **1.** [TA]. Parede delgada que divide duas cavidades ou massas de tecido mais mole. VER septal *area,* transparent s. **2.** Nos fungos, uma parede; geralmente uma parede transversal numa hifa. [L. *saeptum,* divisão]
s. accesso'rium, s. acessório; crista adicional que forma a borda inferior do limbo da fossa oval.
alveolar s., s. alveolar. SIN interalveolar s.
anteromedial intermuscular s. [TA], s. intermuscular anterior medial da coxa; triângulo fascial denso que se estende da borda medial inferior do músculo adutor magno até o músculo vasto medial. Juntamente com o músculo sartório, esse septo denso forma o teto da metade inferior do canal adutor e, como os vasos femorais penetram profundamente nele, é muitas vezes confundido com o hiato dos adutores. SIN s. intermusculare vastoadductorium [TA], subsartorial fascia, vastoadductor fascia.
aortopulmonary s., s. aortopulmonar; septo espiral que, durante o desenvolvimento, separa o tronco arterial em tronco pulmonar ventral e aorta dorsal. VER TAMBÉM bulbar *ridge.*
atrioventricular s. [TA], s. atrioventricular; pequena parte do septo membranoso do coração, logo acima da válvula septal da valva atrioventricular direita, que separa o átrio direito do ventrículo esquerdo. SIN s. atrioventriculare [TA].
s. atrioventricula're [TA], s. atrioventricular. SIN atrioventricular s.
Bigelow s., s. de Bigelow. SIN calcar *femorale.*
bony nasal s. [TA], s. nasal ósseo da cavidade nasal óssea; os ossos que sustentam a parte óssea do septo nasal; são eles: a lâmina perpendicular do etmóide, o vômer, o rostro esfenoidal, a crista nasal, a espinhal frontal e a crista mediana formada pela aposição dos ossos maxilar e palatino. SIN s. nasi osseum [TA].
bulbar s., termo obsoleto para spiral s.
s. bul'bi ure'thrae, s. do pênis; septo fibroso no bulbo do pênis, que o divide em dois hemisférios.
s. cana'lis musculotuba'rii, s. do canal musculotubário. SIN s. of pharyngotympanic (auditory) tube.
cartilaginous s., cartilagem do septo nasal. SIN septal nasal *cartilage.*
s. cervica'le interme'dium [TA], s. cervical intermédio. SIN intermediate cervical s.
s. clitor'idis, s. dos corpos cavernosos do clitóris. SIN s. of corpora cavernosa of clitoris.
Cloquet s., s. de Cloquet. SIN femoral s.
comblike s., s. pectiniforme. SIN pectiniform s.
s. of corpora cavernosa of clitoris [TA], s. dos corpos cavernosos do clitóris; septo fibroso incompleto entre os corpos cavernosos do clitóris. SIN s. corporum cavernosorum clitoridis [TA], s. clitoridis.
s. cor'porum cavernoso'rum clitor'idis [TA], s. do corpo cavernoso do clitóris. SIN s. of corpora cavernosa of clitoris.
crural s., s. femoral. SIN femoral s.
distal spiral s., s. espiral distal. VER spiral s.
endovenous s., s. endoveno'sum, s. endovenoso; remanescente da separação primitiva entre veias que se fundiram para formar um tronco definitivo, como o tronco que leva às veias ilíaca comum esquerda e renal esquerda.
femoral s. [TA], s. femoral; massa de tecido conjuntivo que ocupa o canal femoral, fechando efetivamente o canal, mas permitindo a passagem de vasos linfáticos que drenam o membro inferior. SIN s. femorale [TA], Cloquet s., crural s.
s. femora'le [TA], s. femoral. SIN femoral s.
s. of frontal sinuses [TA], s. dos seios frontais; divisão óssea entre os seios frontais direito e esquerdo; freqüentemente defletido para um lado da linha média. SIN sinuum frontalium [TA].
gingival s., papila gengival. SIN gingival *papilla.*
s. glan'dis [TA], s. da glande. SIN s. of glans penis.
s. of glans penis [TA], s. da glande; divisão fibrosa que se estende da superfície inferior da túnica albugínea, através da glânde do pênis, até a uretra. SIN s. glandis [TA].
hanging s., s. pendente; deformidade causada por largura anormal da porção septal das cartilagens alares.
interalveolar s. [TA], s. interalveolar; **(1)** tecido interposto entre dois alvéolos pulmonares adjacentes; consiste numa rede capilar densa recoberta, nas duas

superfícies, por células epiteliais alveolares muito delgadas; (2) uma das divisões ósseas entre os alvéolos dentários da mandíbula e maxilar (septos interalveolares da mandíbula e do maxilar). SIN s. interalveolare [TA], alveolar s., septal bone.

s. interalveola're, pl. **sep'ta interalveola'ria** [TA], s. interalveolar. SIN interalveolar s.

interatrial s. [TA], s. interatrial; a parede entre os átrios do coração. VER TAMBÉM s. primum, s. secundum. SIN s. interatriale [TA].

s. interatria'le [TA], s. interatrial. SIN interatrial s.

interdental s., s. interdentário; a porção óssea que separa dois dentes adjacentes numa arcada dentária.

interlobular s., s. interlobular; o tecido conjuntivo entre os lóbulos pulmonares secundários que, habitualmente, contém uma veia e vasos linfáticos; observado radiograficamente quando espessado como linha B de Kerley ou linha septal.

intermediate cervical s. [TA], s. cervical intermédio; septo delgado composto de fibras gliais e tecido conjuntivo leptomeníngeo na medula cervical, marcando a borda entre os fascículos grácil e cuneiforme do funículo posterior. SIN s. cervicale intermedium [TA].

s. interme'dium, s. intermédio; termo antigo para referir-se ao septo do canal atrioventricular do coração embrionário formado pela fusão dos coxins dorsal e ventral do canal atrioventricular.

intermuscular s. [TA], s. intermuscular; termo aplicado aos folhetos aponeuróticos que separam vários músculos dos membros; são eles: os septos intermusculares anterior e posterior da perna (septa intermuscularis cruris anterius et posterius), os septos intermusculares lateral e medial da coxa (septa intermuscularis femoris laterale et mediale), os septos intermusculares lateral e medial do braço (septa intermuscularis brachii laterale et mediale). SIN s. intermusculare [TA].

s. intermuscula're [TA], s. intermuscular. SIN intermuscular s.

s. intermuscula're va'stoadducto'rium [TA], s. anterior medial da coxa. SIN anteromedial intermuscular s.

interpulmonary s., s. interpulmonar. SIN mediastinum (2).

sep'ta interradicula'ria mandi'bulae et ma'xillae [TA], septos inter-radiculares da maxila e da mandíbula. SIN interradicular septa of maxilla and mandible.

interradicular septa of maxilla and mandible [TA], septos inter-radiculares da maxila e mandíbula; as divisões ósseas que se projetam para os alvéolos entre as raízes dos dentes molares. SIN septa interradicularia mandi'bulae et ma'xillae [TA], intra-alveolar septa.

interventricular s. [TA], s. interventricular; a parede entre os ventrículos do coração. SIN s. interventricullare [TA], ventricular s.

s. interventricula're [TA], s. interventricular. SIN interventricular s.

s. lin'guae [TA], s. da língua. SIN lingual s.

lingual s. [TA], s. da língua; divisão fibrosa vertical mediana da língua que se funde posteriormente na aponeurose da língua. SIN s. linguae [TA], s. of tongue.

s. lu'cidum, s. pelúcido. SIN s. pellucidum.

s. mediastina'le, s. mediastinal. SIN mediastinum (2).

s. membrana'ceum ventriculo'rum, parte membranácea do septo interventricular. SIN membranous *part* of interventricular septum.

membranous s., (1) parte membranácea do septo nasal. SIN membranous *part* of nasal septum; (2) parte membranácea do septo interventricular. SIN membranous *part* of interventricular septum.

s. mo'bile na'si, s. móvel do nariz. SIN mobile *part* of nasal septum.

s. muscula're ventriculo'rum, parte muscular do septo interventricular. SIN muscular *part* of interventricular septum (of heart).

s. of musculotubal canal, s. do canal musculotubário. SIN s. of pharyngotympanic (auditory) tube.

nasal s. [TA], s. nasal; a parede que divide a cavidade nasal em metades; é composta de um esqueleto de sustentação central recoberto, de cada lado, por uma mucosa. SIN s. nasi [TA].

s. na'si [TA], s, nasal. SIN nasal s.

s. na'si oss'eum [TA], s. ósseo nasal da cavidade nasal óssea. SIN bony nasal s.

orbital s. [TA], s. orbital; membrana fibrosa fixada à margem da órbita, que se estende nas pálpebras, contendo a gordura orbital e constituindo, em grande parte, a fáscia posterior do músculo orbicular do olho. SIN s. orbitale [TA].

s. orbita'le [TA], s. orbital. SIN orbital s.

pectiniform s., s. pectinifor'me, s. pectiniforme; a porção anterior do septo do pênis que é interrompida por diversas perfurações semelhantes a fendas. SIN comblike s.

s. pellu'cidum [TA], s. pelúcido; delgada placa de tecido cerebral que contém células nervosas e numerosas fibras nervosas, sendo distendida como uma lâmina vertical plana entre a coluna e o corpo do fórnix, abaixo, e o corpo caloso, acima e anteriormente; em geral, funde-se no plano mediano com seu análogo no lado oposto, formando uma delgada divisão mediana entre os cornos frontais esquerdo e direito dos ventrículos laterais; em menos de 10% dos seres humanos, existe um espaço cego, em forma de fenda e preenchido por líquido entre os dois septos pelúcidos, a cavidade do septo pelúcido. O septo pelúcido é contínuo ventralmente, através do intervalo entre o corpo caloso e a comissura anterior, com o septo pré-comissural e giro subcaloso. VER TAMBÉM cavity of septum pellucidum, septal *area.* SIN s. lucidum, transparent s.

s. pe'nis [TA], s. do pênis; porção da túnica albugínea que separa incompletamente os dois corpos cavernosos do pênis.

s. of pharyngotympanic (auditory) tube [TA], s. do canal musculotubário; placa horizontal muito fina de osso formando dois semicanais, o superior, de menor tamanho, para o músculo tensor do tímpano, e o inferior, de maior tamanho, para a tuba auditiva; sua terminação no ouvido médio é o processo cocleariforme. SIN s. canalis musculotubarii, s. of musculotubal canal, s. tubae.

placental septa, septos placentários; divisões incompletas entre os cotilédones placentários; são recobertos por trofoblasto e contêm um cerne de tecido materno.

precommissural s., s. pré-comissural. VER septal *area.*

s. pri'mum, s. *primum*; septo em crescente, no coração embrionário, que se desenvolve sobre a parede dorsocefálica do átrio originalmente ímpar e começa sua divisão em câmaras direita e esquerda; as pontas do septo avançam e fundem-se com os coxins do canal atrioventricular.

proximal spiral s., s. espiral proximal. VER spiral s.

rectovaginal s. [TA], s. retovaginal; a camada de fáscia entre a vagina e a parte inferior do reto. SIN s. rectovaginale [TA].

s. rectovagina'le [TA], s. retovaginal. SIN rectovaginal s.

rectovesical s. [TA], s. retovesical; camada de fáscia que se estende superiormente a partir do tendão central do períneo até o peritônio, entre a próstata e o reto. SIN s. rectovesicale [TA], Denonvilliers aponeurosis, rectovesical fascia, Tyrrell fascia.

s. rectovesica'le [TA], s. retovesical. SIN rectovesical s.

scrotal s. [TA], s. do escroto; parede incompleta de tecido conjuntivo e músculo não-estriado (túnica dartos) que divide o escroto em dois sacos, cada um contendo um testículo. SIN s. scroti [TA].

s. scro'ti [TA], s. escrotal. SIN scrotal s.

s. secun'dum, s. *secundum*; a segunda das duas principais estruturas septais envolvidas na divisão do átrio, que se desenvolve depois do s. *primum* e localiza-se à sua direita; assim como o s. *primum*, possui forma em crescente, porém suas pontas estão orientadas para o seio venoso, e é mais densamente muscular; permanece como uma divisão incompleta até depois do nascimento, constituindo a sua área não-fechada o forame oval.

sinus s., s. sinusal; pequena prega que forma a extremidade medial da válvula da veia cava inferior; desenvolve-se a partir da parede dorsal do seio venoso embrionário.

s. sin'uum fronta'lium [TA], s. dos seios frontais. SIN s. of frontal sinuses.

s. sin'uum sphenoida'lium [TA], s. dos seios esfenoidais. SIN s. of sphenoidal sinuses.

s. of sphenoidal sinuses [TA], s. dos seios esfenoidais; a divisão óssea entre os dois seios esfenoidais, freqüentemente defletida para um lado da linha média. SIN s. sinuum sphenoidalium [TA].

spiral s., s. espiral; septo que divide o bulbo cardíaco embrionário em tratos de saída pulmonar e aórtico no coração em desenvolvimento; o septo espiral distal deriva dos coxins endocárdicos direito e esquerdo e, assim, separa os orifícios pulmonar e aórtico; o septo espiral proximal é a porção do septo que se incorpora à parede membranácea do septo interventricular.

spiral bulbar s., s. bulbar espiral. VER spiral s.

s. spu'rium, s. espúrio; septo no átrio direito do coração embrionário, formado pela válvula venosa direita e sua continuação na parede dorsocefálica do átrio; em embriões humanos, atinge seu desenvolvimento completo durante o terceiro mês e, a seguir, regride, não participando da divisão atrial (daí sua designação como falso); porções reduzidas persistem na forma da valva da veia cava inferior e valva do seio coronário.

s. of testis, mediastino do testículo. SIN *mediastinum* of testis.

s. of tongue, s. da língua. SIN lingual s.

transparent s., s. pelúcido. SIN s. pellucidum.

transverse s., (1) crista ampular. SIN ampullary *crest;* (2) seio transverso; a massa mesodérmica que separa as cavidades pericárdica e peritoneal; é recoberta por mesotélio, exceto onde está intimamente associada ao fígado, que originalmente se desenvolve no seu interior; o septo é definitivamente incorporado ao diafragma como o centro tendíneo do diafragma.

s. tu'bae, s. do canal musculotubário. SIN s. of pharyngotympanic (auditory) tube.

urogenital s., s. urogenital; a crista de localização coronal, formada pela porção caudal das cristas urogenitais que se unem na linha média do embrião; situa-se entre o intestino posterior, dorsalmente, e a bexiga, ventralmente.

urorectal s., s. urorretal; em embriões, uma divisão da cloaca numa porção dorsal retal e numa porção ventral, denominada seio urogenital; ao alcançar a membrana cloacal aproximadamente no momento de sua desintegração, o septo urorretal divide a saída cloacal num orifício anal e num orifício urogenital. SIN urorectal fold.

ventricular s., s. interventricular. SIN interventricular s.

se·que·la, pl. **se·que·lae** (sē-kwel′ă, sē-kwel′ē). Seqüela; condição que ocorre em consequência de uma doença. [L. *sequela,* seqüela, de *sequor,* seguir]

se·quence (sē′kwens). Seqüência; a sucessão de uma coisa ou evento após outro. [L. *sequor,* seguir]
 Alu s.'s, seqüências Alu; no genoma humano, uma seqüência repetida e relativamente conservada de cerca de 300 bp (pares de bases), que freqüentemente contém um local de clivagem para a enzima de restrição AluI próximo ao centro; cerca de 1 milhão de cópias no genoma humano.
 chi s., s. qui; seqüência octomérica de bases no DNA, que participa na recombinação genética mediada por RecBc.
 coding s., s. de codificação; a porção do DNA que codifica transcrição do RNA mensageiro. VER exon.
 insertion s., s. de inserção; seqüências distintas do DNA de nucleotídeos que são repetidos em vários locais em cromossomas bacterianos, certos plasmídeos e bacteriófagos e que pode mover-se de um local para outro do cromossoma, para outro plasmídeo na mesma bactéria ou para um bacteriófago.
 intervening s., s. interposta. SIN intron.
 s. ladder, escala de seqüência; série de bandas, que se tornam visíveis por marcação, quando o DNA fragmentado por endonucleases é submetido a eletroforese em gel; corresponde à seqüência de nucleotídeos.
 leader s., seqüências-líder; seqüências, no final de ácidos nucleicos (DNA e RNA) ou de proteínas, que têm de ser clivadas para permitir o desempenho de uma função específica da molécula madura.
 long terminal repeat s.'s (LTR), seqüências de repetição terminal longa (LTR); regiões do genoma do RNA associadas a regulação, integração e expressão de retrovírus.
 monotonic s., s. monotônica; seqüência em que cada valor de um conjunto é maior do que o valor precedente.
 palindromic s., s. palindrômica. VER palindrome.
 pulse s., s. de pulsos; na ressonância magnética, uma série de alterações no campo magnético induzido, que incluem os gradientes de codificação de fase e freqüência e funções de leitura.
 regulatory s., s. reguladora; qualquer seqüência de DNA responsável pela regulação da expressão gênica, como promotores e operadores.
 Shine-Dalgarno s., s. de Shine-Dalgarno; região não-traduzida e rica em purinas de mRNA no códon de iniciação nos procariotas; auxilia no alinhamento do mRNA sobre o ribossoma.
 termination s., s. de terminação. SIN termination *codon.*
 twin reversed arterial perfusion s. (TRAP), s. de perfusão arterial invertida gemelar; anomalia circulatória em gêmeos monozigóticos, caracterizada por anastomoses arterioarteriais e venovenosas placentárias e anomalias umbilicais, sendo um dos fetos perfundido com sangue desoxigenado; o feto receptor desenvolve-se como acefálico acardíaco, e o gêmeo doador corre risco de insuficiência cardíaca.

se·quenc·ing (sē′kwens-ing). Seqüenciamento; determinação da seqüência de subunidades numa macromolécula.
 dideoxy sequencing, seqüenciamento didesoxi; método de seqüenciamento do DNA que utiliza 2′,3′-didesoxirribonucleosídeo trifosfatos.
 Maxim-Gilbert sequencing, seqüenciamento de Maxim-Gilbert; método de seqüenciamento do DNA que utiliza dimetil sulfato e hidrazinólise.

se·quen·tial (sē-kwen′shăl). Seqüencial; que ocorre em seqüência.
se·ques·tra (sē-kwes′tră). Seqüestros; plural de sequestrum.
se·ques·tral (sē-kwes′trăl). Relativo a um seqüestro.
se·ques·tra·tion (sē-kwes-trā′shŭn). Seqüestração, seqüestro. **1.** Formação de um seqüestro. **2.** Perda de sangue ou de seu conteúdo líquido em espaços corporais, de modo que é retirado do volume circulante, resultando em comprometimento hemodinâmico, hipovolemia, hipotensão e redução do retorno venoso ao coração. [L. *sequestratio,* de *sequestro,* pp. *-atus,* colocar de lado]
 bronchopulmonary s., s. broncopulmonar; anomalia congênita em que uma massa de tecido pulmonar torna-se isolada do resto do pulmão durante o desenvolvimento; os brônquios na massa estão habitualmente dilatados ou císticos e não estão conectados à árvore brônquica; é suprida por um ramo da aorta.

se·ques·trec·to·my (sē-kwes-trek′tō-mē). Seqüestrectomia; remoção cirúrgica de um seqüestro. SIN sequestrotomy. [sequestrum + G. *ektomē,* excisão]
se·ques·trot·o·my (sē-kwes-trot′ō-mē). Seqüestrectomia. SIN sequestrectomy. [sequestrum + G. *tomē,* incisão]
se·ques·trum, pl. **se·ques·tra** (sē-kwes′trŭm, -tră). Seqüestro; pedaço de tecido necrótico, geralmente osso, que foi separado do tecido saudável circundante. [L. mod. uso do L. mediev. *sequestrum,* algo colocado de lado, do L. *sequestro,* colocar de lado, separar]
 primary s., s. primário; s. totalmente destacado.

se·quoi·o·sis (sē-kwoy-ō′sis). Sequoiose; alveolite alérgica extrínseca causada pela inalação de serragem de secóia, contendo esporos de *Graphium, Pullularia, Aureobasidium* e outros fungos. [*Sequoia* (nome do gênero) para *Sequoah* (George Guess), sábio Cherokee, + G. *-osis,* condição]

SER Abreviatura de somatosensory evoked response (resposta evocada somatossensorial). VER TAMBÉM evoked *response.*

Ser Símbolo de serine (serina) e seu radical.
se·ra (ser′ă). Soros; plural de serum.
ser·al·bu·min (ser-al-bū′min). Soroalbumina, albumina sérica. SIN serum albumin.
ser·en·dip·i·ty (ser-en-dip′i-tē). Descoberta acidental. Em ciência, encontrar uma coisa ao procurar outra, como a descoberta da penicilina por Fleming. [Termo criado por Horace Walpole e relacionado com a obra *The Three Princes of Serendip,* da grafia alternativa de *Serendib,* nome antigo de Sri Lanka]
Sergent, Emile, médico francês, 1867–1943. VER S. white *line;* Bernard-S. *syndrome.*
se·ries, pl. **se·ries** (ser′ēz). Série. **1.** Sucessão de objetos semelhantes e consecutivos, no espaço ou no tempo. **2.** Em química, refere-se a um grupo de substâncias, elementos ou compostos, que possuem propriedades semelhantes ou que diferem entre si quanto à sua composição por uma relação constante. [L. de *sero,* unir]
 aromatic s., s. aromática; todos os compostos derivados do benzeno ou compostos cíclicos semelhantes que obedecem à regra de Hückel, diferenciados dos compostos que são acíclicos ou que contêm anéis sem a estrutura de dupla ligação conjugada característica do benzeno.
 erythrocytic s., s. eritrocítica; as células, nos vários estágios de desenvolvimento na medula óssea vermelha, que levam à formação do eritrócito, como, por exemplo, eritroblastos, normoblastos, eritrócitos.
 fatty s., s. gordurosa; os alcanos; todos os compostos acíclicos no grupo do metano, etano, propano, etc., distintos da série aromática.
 granulocytic s., s. granulocítica; as células, nos vários estágios de desenvolvimento na medula óssea, que levam à formação do granulócito maduro da circulação, como, por exemplo, mieloblastos, diferentes estágios do mielócito, granulócitos.
 Hofmeister s., s. de Hofmeister; a série de cátions Mg^{2+}, Ca^{2+}, Sr^{2+}, Ba^{2+}, Li^+, Na^+, K^+, Rb^+, Cs^+ e de ânions citrato^{3-}, tartarato^{2-}, SO_4^{2-}, acetato$^-$, NO_3^-, ClO_3^-, I^-, CNS^- (entre outros), estando cada série disposta em ordem de capacidade decrescente para: 1) precipitar a substância dispersa de sóis liofílicos; 2) precipitar substâncias orgânicas (p. ex., anilina, acetato de etila) de soluções aquosas; ou 3) inibir a tumefação de géis. Esses efeitos, entre outros relacionados, são atribuíveis à extração e ligação da água por esses íons (isto é, hidratação), que também diminui na ordem citada, de modo que (na série de cátions monovalentes), o Li^+, com o menor raio de cristal, tem o maior raio hidratado, e vice-versa para o Cs^+. SIN lyotropic s.
 homologous s., s. homóloga; uma série de compostos orgânicos cujos membros sucessivos diferem entre si pelo radical CH_2 (como na série gordurosa).
 lymphocytic s., lymphoid s., s. linfocítica, s. linfóide; as células em vários estados de desenvolvimento no tecido linfóide dos linfócitos maduros, como, por exemplo, linfoblastos, linfócitos jovens, linfócitos maduros.
 lyotropic s., s. liotrópica. SIN Hofmeister s.
 myeloid s., s. mielóide; a série granulocítica e eritrocítica.
 small bowel s., seriografia do intestino delgado; exame radiográfico do intestino delgado após a administração oral de contraste, geralmente sulfato de bário. Cf. small bowel *enema.*
 thrombocytic s., s. trombocítica; as células de estágios sucessivos no desenvolvimento trombocítico (plaquetário) na medula óssea, como, por exemplo, tromblastos, trombócitos.
 upper GI s., seriografia GI alta, seriografia esôfago–estômago–duodeno (SEED); estudo radiográfico contrastado do esôfago, estômago e duodeno.

ser·ine (S, Ser) (ser′ēn). Serina; ácido 2-amino-3-hidroxipropanóico; o L-isômero é um dos aminoácidos presentes nas proteínas.
 s. deaminase, s. desaminase. SIN *threonine* dehydratase.
 s. dehydrase, s. desidrase. SIN L-S. dehydratase.
 L- dehydratase, L-s. desidratase; L-hidroxiaminoácido desidratase; uma hidrolase de desaminação que converte a L-serina em piruvato e NH_3; parte do catabolismo dos aminoácidos. VER TAMBÉM *threonine* dehydratase. SIN s. dehydrase.
 s. sulfhydrase, s. sulfidrase. SIN cystathionine β-synthase.

se·ri·o·graph (ser′ē-ō-graf). Seriógrafo; aparelho para realizar uma série de radiografias; utilizado, por exemplo, na angiografia cerebral; termo obsoleto para referir-se a um rápido trocador de filme. [series + G. *graphō,* escrever]
se·ri·og·ra·phy (ser-ē-og′ra-fē). Seriografia; realização de uma série de radiografias através do seriógrafo.
se·ri·os·co·py (ser-ē-os′kō-pē). Serioscopia; antigamente, uma série de radiografias de uma região efetuadas em diferentes direções e posteriormente combinadas. [series + G. *skopeō,* ver]
ser·i·scis·sion (ser-i-sish′ŭn). Termo raramente utilizado para referir-se à secção do pedículo de um tumor ou outro tecido por uma ligadura de seda. [L. *sericum,* seda + *scissio,* clivagem]

SERM Abreviatura de selective estrogen receptor *modulator* (modulador seletivo do receptor de estrogênio).

sero-. Soro, seroso. [L. *serum,* soro do leite]
se·ro·co·li·tis (ser′ō-kō-li′tis). Serocolite. SIN pericolitis. [L. mod. *serosa,* membrana serosa + colitis]

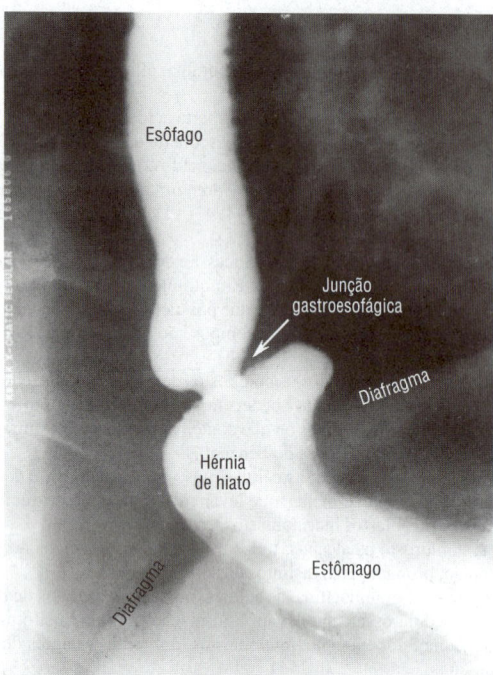

seriografia gastrointestinal superior: radiografia mostrando hérnia de hiato

se·ro·con·ver·sion (sēr′ō - kon - ver′zhŭn). Soroconversão; desenvolvimento de anticorpos específicos detectáveis no soro em conseqüência de infecção ou imunização.

se·ro·cys·tic (sēr - ō - sis′tik). Serocístico; relativo a um ou mais cistos serosos.

se·ro·di·ag·no·sis (sēr′ō - dī - ag - nō′sis). Sorodiagnóstico; diagnóstico estabelecido através de reações sorológicas, utilizando soro sanguíneo ou outros líquidos serosos do corpo.

se·ro·en·ter·i·tis (sēr′ō - en - ter - ī′tis). Soroenterite. SIN perienteritis. [L. mod. *serosa*, serosa + enteritis]

se·ro·ep·i·de·mi·ol·o·gy (sēr′ō - ep - i - dē - mē - ol′ō - jē). Soroepidemiologia; estudo epidemiológico baseado na detecção de infecção por teste sorológico.

se·ro·fast (sēr′ō - fast). Serorresistente. SIN serum-fast.

se·ro·fi·brin·ous (sēr - ō - fī′bri - nŭs). Serofibrinoso; relativo a um exsudato composto de soro e fibrina.

se·ro·fi·brous (sēr - ō - fī′brŭs). Serofibroso; relativo a uma serosa e tecido fibroso.

serogroup (ser′ō - groop, sēr). Sorogrupo. **1.** Grupo de bactérias contendo um antígeno comum, utilizado na classificação de certos gêneros. **2.** Grupo de espécies virais que estão estreitamente relacionadas do ponto de vista antigênico.

se·ro·log·ic (sēr - ō - loj′ik). Sorológico, serológico; relativo à sorologia.

se·rol·o·gy (sē - rol′ō - jē). Sorologia, serologia; ramo da ciência relacionado com o soro, especialmente soros imunes ou líticos específicos, e com a medida de antígenos ou anticorpos no soro. [sero- + G. *logos*, estudo]

se·ro·ma (sē - rō′mă). Seroma; massa ou tumefação causada pelo acúmulo localizado de soro no interior de um tecido ou órgão. [sero- + G. *-oma*, tumor]

se·ro·mem·bra·nous (sēr′ō - mem′bră - nŭs). Seromembranoso; relativo a uma serosa.

se·ro·mu·coid (sēr - ō - mū′koyd). Seromucóide; termo geral para referir-se a uma mucoproteína (glicoproteína) do soro.
  acid s., s. ácido. SIN orosomucoid.

se·ro·mu·cous (sēr - ō - mū′kŭs). Seromucoso; relativo a uma mistura de material aquoso e mucinoso, como a de certas glândulas.

ser·o·my·ot·o·my (se′rō - mī - ot′ō - mē). Seromiotomia; incisão na parede de uma víscera oca que envolve a serosa e a muscular, mas não a mucosa. [serosa (1) + G. *mys*, músculo + *tomē*, corte]

se·ro·neg·a·tive (sēr - ō - neg′ă - tiv). Soronegativo; que carece de um anticorpo de tipo específico no soro; utilizado para indicar ausência de infecção prévia por um agente específico (p. ex., vírus da rubéola), desaparecimento de anticorpos após tratamento de uma doença (p. ex., sífilis) ou ausência de anticorpos habitualmente encontrados em determinada síndrome (p. ex., artrite reumatóide sem fator reumatóide).

se·ro·pos·i·tive (sēr - ō - poz′i - tiv). Soropositivo; que contém anticorpo de um tipo específico no soro; utilizado para indicar a presença de evidências imunológicas de infecção específica (p. ex., doença de Lyme, sífilis) ou presença de anticorpo útil para o diagnóstico (p. ex., artrite reumatóide com fator reumatóide).

se·ro·pu·ru·lent (sēr′ō - poo′roo - lent). Soropurulento; composto de ou que contém soro e pus; refere-se a uma secreção de pus aquoso (soropus).

se·ro·pus (sēr′ō - pŭs). Soropus; soropurulento, isto é, pus diluído, em grande parte, com soro.

se·ro·re·ver·sion (sir - ō - rē - vur′zhŭn). Reversão sorológica; perda de reatividade sorológica; pode ser espontânea ou em resposta ao tratamento.

se·ro·sa (se - rō′să). [TA]. **1.** Túnica serosa; o revestimento ou camada serosa mais externa de uma estrutura visceral encontrada nas cavidades corporais do abdome ou do tórax; consiste numa camada superficial do mesotélio reforçada por tecido conjuntivo fibroelástico irregular. **2.** Serosa; a parte mais externa das membranas extra-embrionárias que encerra o embrião e todas as suas outras membranas; consiste em somatopleura, isto é, ectoderma reforçado por mesoderma somático; a serosa de embriões de mamíferos é freqüentemente denominada trofoderma. SIN membrana serosa (2). VER TAMBÉM chorion. SIN tunica serosa [TA], serous coat*, membrana serosa (1), serous membrane, serous tunic. [fem. do L. mod. *serosus*, seroso]
  s. of colon, s. do intestino grosso. SIN s. of large intestine.
  s. of esophagus [TA], túnica serosa do esôfago; camada serosa da parte abdominal do esôfago. SIN tunica serosa esophagi [TA].
  s. of gallbladder [TA], túnica serosa da vesícula biliar; camada serosa da vesícula biliar; o peritônio visceral que recobre as porções da vesícula biliar que não está em contato direto com o fígado. SIN tunica serosa vesicae biliaris [TA], tunica serosa vesicae felleae*.
  s. of large intestine [TA], s. do intestino grosso; camada serosa do colo; o peritônio visceral do intestino grosso. SIN tunica serosa intestini crassi [TA], s. of colon, tunica serosa coli.
  s. of liver [TA], túnica serosa do fígado; camada serosa do fígado; revestimento peritoneal do fígado, encerrando quase todo o órgão, exceto uma área triangular em sua superfície posterior (a "área nua do fígado") e uma área menor onde o fígado e a vesícula biliar estão em contato direto. SIN tunica serosa hepatis [TA].
  s. of parietal pleura [TA], s. da pleura parietal; superfície interna brilhante da pleura parietal. SIN tunica serosa pleurae perietalis [TA].
  s. of peritoneum, túnica serosa do peritônio; epitélio escamoso simples que forma a superfície brilhante das camadas parietal e visceral do peritônio. SIN tunica serosa peritonei [TA], serous coat of peritoneum*, serous layer of peritoneum.
  s. of serous pericardium [TA], túnica serosa do pericárdio seroso; camada única de células achatadas que reveste o saco pericárdico e o coração; essa camada, juntamente com a tela subserosa, constitui o pericárdio seroso. SIN tunica serosa pericardii serosi [TA].
  s. of small intestine [TA], túnica serosa do intestino delgado; camada serosa do intestino delgado; o revestimento peritoneal da superfície externa do intestino delgado. SIN tunica serosa intestini tenuis [TA].
  s. of the spleen [TA], túnica serosa do baço; peritônio visceral que recobre o baço. SIN tunica serosa splenis [TA].
  s. of stomach [TA], túnica serosa do estômago; camada serosa do estômago; peritônio visceral que recobre a superfície externa do estômago. SIN tunica serosa gastricae [TA], tunica serosa ventriculi.
  s. of (urinary) bladder [TA], túnica serosa da bexiga; camada serosa da bexiga; o peritônio visceral que recobre o teto e as paredes laterais da bexiga. SIN tunica serosa vesicae (urinariae) [TA].
  s. of uterine tube [TA], túnica serosa da tuba uterina; camada serosa da tuba uterina; o peritônio visceral que forma a superfície externa das tubas uterinas. SIN tunica serosa tubae uterinae [TA].
  s. of uterus [TA], túnica serosa do útero; camada serosa do útero; o peritônio visceral que recobre o fundo e o corpo posterior do útero. SIN tunica serosa uteri [TA].
  s. of visceral pleura [TA], túnica serosa da pleura visceral; camada única de células achatadas que reveste e, assim, forma a superfície externa brilhante dos pulmões. SIN tunica serosa pleurae visceralis [TA].

se·ro·sa·mu·cin (se - rō - să - mū′sin). Serosamucina; material mucóide encontrado em líquidos serosos, como, por exemplo, no líquido ascítico ou sinovial.

se·ro·san·guin·e·ous (sēr′ō - sang - gwin′ē - ŭs). Serossanguíneo, sorossanguíneo; relativo a um exsudato ou secreção constituída por soro e sangue ou contendo esses elementos.

se·ro·se·rous (sēr - ō - sēr′ŭs). Serosseroso. **1.** Relativo a duas superfícies serosas. **2.** Refere-se a uma sutura, como a do intestino, em que as bordas da ferida estão dobradas para dentro, de modo a colocar as duas superfícies serosas em aposição.

se·ro·si·tis (sēr - ō - sī′tis). Serosite; inflamação de uma serosa.
  multiple s., s. múltipla, polisserosite. SIN polyserositis.

se·ros·i·ty (se - ros′i - tē). Serosidade. **1.** Líquido seroso ou soro. **2.** Condição de ser seroso. **3.** A qualidade serosa de um líquido.

se·ro·syn·o·vi·al (sēr′ō - si - nō′vē - ăl). Serossinovial; relativo ao soro e, também, à sinóvia.

se·ro·syn·o·vi·tis (sēr'ō-sin-ō-vī'tis). Serossinovite; sinovite acompanhada de derrame seroso copioso.

se·ro·tax·is (sēr-ō-tak'sis). Serotaxia; edema da pele induzido pela aplicação de um forte irritante cutâneo. [sero- + G. *taxis*, disposição]

se·ro·ther·a·py (sēr-ō-thār'ă-pē). Seroterapia, soroterapia; tratamento de uma doença infecciosa pela injeção de uma antitoxina ou soro contendo anticorpo específico. SIN serum therapy.

se·ro·ti·na (sēr'ō-tī'nă). Serotino. VER decidua. [L. fem. de *serotinus*, tardio]

se·ro·to·ner·gic (sēr-ō-tō-ner'jik, sēr-). Serotoninérgico; relativo à ação da serotonina ou seu precursor, o L-triptofano. [serotonin + G. *ergon*, tabalho]

se·ro·to·nin (sēr-ō-tō'nin). Serotonina; vasoconstritor liberado pelas plaquetas sanguíneas, que inibe a secreção gástrica e estimula o músculo liso; presente em concentrações relativamente altas em algumas áreas do sistema nervoso central (hipotálamo, núcleos da base); ocorre em muitos tecidos e células periféricas, bem como em tumores carcinóides. SIN 5-hydroxytryptamine, enteramine, thrombocytin, thrombotonin. [sero- + G. *tonos*, tônus, tensão + -in]

se·ro·type (sēr'ō-tīp). Sorotipo, sorovariante. SIN serovar.
 heterologous s., s. heterólogo; anticorpo que foi induzido por um antígeno e que reage com outro antígeno.
 homologous s., s. homólogo; anticorpo induzido por determinado antígeno e que reage com o antígeno em questão.

se·rous (sēr'ŭs). Seroso, soroso; relativo a, contendo ou produzindo soro ou uma substância apresentando consistência fluida e aquosa.

se·ro·vac·ci·na·tion (sēr'ō-vak-si-nā'shŭn). Sorovacinação; processo para produzir imunidade mista através da injeção de um soro, de modo a garantir imunidade passiva, e através de vacinação com uma cultura modificada ou morta para adquirir posteriormente imunidade ativa.

se·ro·var (sēr'ō-var). Sorovariante; subdivisão de uma espécie ou subespécie distinguível de outras cepas abrangidas por elas com base na antigenicidade. SIN serotype. [sero- + *variant*]

se·ro·zyme (sēr'ō-zīm). Serozima, protrombina. SIN prothrombin.

ser·pen·tar·ia (ser-pen-tā'rē-ă, -tar'ē-ă). Serpentária; o rizoma e as raízes dessecados de *Aristolochia serpentaria*, a serpentária-da-Virgínia, ou de *A. reticulata*, a serpentária-do-Texas (família Aristolochiaceae), estomáquico. SIN snakeroot. [L. snakeweed]

ser·pig·i·nous (ser-pij'i-nŭs). Serpiginoso; rastejante; designa uma úlcera ou outra lesão cutânea que se estende com uma borda arciforme; a margem possui uma borda ondulante ou semelhante a uma serpente. [L. mediev. *serpigo-(-gin-)*, tinha, do L. *serpo*, rastejar]

ser·pi·go (ser-pī'gō). 1. Tinha. SIN tinea. 2. Herpes. SIN herpes. 3. Qualquer erupção serpiginosa. [L. mediev. *serpigo (-gin-)*, tinha, do L. *serpo*, rastejar]

ser·pins. Inibidores da serina protease. SIN serine protease *inhibitors*, em *inhibitor*. [serine *protease inhibitors*]

ser·rate, ser·rat·ed (ser'āt, -ā'ted). Serreado; dentado, sérreo, serrátil. [L. *serratus*, de *serra*, uma serra]

Ser·ra·tia (se-rā'shē-ă). Gênero de bactérias aeróbicas a facultativamente anaeróbicas, móveis e peritríquias (família Enterobacteriaceae) que contém pequenos bastonetes Gram-negativos. Algumas cepas são encapsuladas. Muitas cepas produzem um pigmento rosado, vermelho ou magenta; seu metabolismo é fermentativo, e esses microrganismos são saprófitas em materiais vegetais e animais em decomposição. A espécie típica é *S. marcescens*. [Serafino *Serrati*, físico italiano do século XVIII]
 S. marces'cens, espécie encontrada na água, no solo, no leite, em alimentos e no bicho-da-seda e outros insetos; trata-se de uma causa significativa de infecção hospitalar, especialmente em pacientes com comprometimento da imunidade; é espécie típica do gênero *S*.

ser·ra·tion (se-rā'shŭn). Serração. **1.** Estado de ser serreado ou chanfrado. **2.** Qualquer um dos processos numa formação serreada ou dentada. [L. *serra*, serra]

serre·fine (ser-e-fēn'). Pequena pinça utilizada para aproximar as bordas de uma ferida ou para fechar temporariamente uma artéria durante uma cirurgia. [Fr.]

ser·re·no·eud (ser-e-no-ood'). Instrumento para apertar uma ligadura. [Fr. *serrer*, pressionar + *noeud*, nó]

Serres, Antoine E.R.A., anatomista francês, 1786–1868. VER S. *angle, glands,* em *gland; rests* of S., em *rest.*

ser·ru·late, ser·ru·lat·ed (ser'ū-lāt, -lā'ted). Serrilhado, picotado; finamente serreado. [L. *serrula*, uma pequena serra, dim. de *serra*]

Sertoli, Enrico, histologista italiano, 1842–1910. VER *Sertoli* cell *tumor;* S. *cells,* em *cell, columns,* em *column;* S.-cell-only *syndrome;* Sertoli-Leydig cell *tumor;* Sertoli-stromal cell *tumor.*

ser·tra·line (ser'tră-lēn). Sertralina; antidepressivo que bloqueia seletivamente a recaptação de serotonina; semelhante à fluoxetina.

se·rum, pl. **se·rums, se·ra** (sēr'ŭm, -ŭmz, -ă). Soro. **1.** Líquido aquoso claro, principalmente aquele que umedece a superfície das serosas ou exsudato na inflamação de qualquer uma dessas membranas. **2.** A porção líquida do sangue obtida após remoção do coágulo de fibrina e das células sanguíneas, distinguida do plasma no sangue circulante. Termo algumas vezes utilizado como sinônimo de anti-soro ou antitoxina. [L. soro do leite]
 anticomplementary s., s. anticomplementar; soro que destrói ou inativa o complemento.
 antiepithelial s., s. antiepitelial, anti-soro (citotoxina) para as células epiteliais.
 antilymphocyte s. (ALS), s. antilinfocítico; anti-soro contra linfócitos, utilizado para suprimir a rejeição de enxertos ou transplantes de órgãos; quando utilizado no homem, administra-se habitualmente a fração globulínica do soro heterólogo (preparado no cavalo ou em outros animais) em associação a outros agentes imunossupressores (drogas ou substâncias químicas), por um período limitado de tempo. SIN antilymphocyte globulin.
 antirabies s., s. anti-rábico; solução estéril contendo anticorpos obtidos do soro sanguíneo ou do plasma de um animal sadio ou ser humano que foi imunizado contra a raiva através de vacina; administrado imediatamente após mordeduras graves ou múltiplas de animais domésticos com suspeita de raiva e após mordeduras de animais selvagens, seguido de um esquema de vacina anti-rábica.
 antireticular cytotoxic s., s. citotóxico anti-reticular; anti-soro específico para células do sistema reticuloendotelial.
 antitoxic s., s. antitóxico; uma antitoxina.
 bacteriolytic s., s. bacteriolítico; anti-soro (bacteriolisina) que sensibiliza uma bactéria à ação lítica do complemento.
 blood s., s. sanguíneo. VER serum (2).
 convalescent s., s. convalescente; soro de pacientes recentemente recuperados de uma doença; útil para diagnóstico ao demonstrar um aumento de quatro vezes dos títulos de anticorpos específicos ou na prevenção ou modificação por imunização passiva da mesma doença em indivíduos suscetíveis expostos.
 Coombs s., s. de Coombs. SIN antihuman *globulin.*
 dried human s., s. humano seco; soro preparado por desidratação do soro humano líquido através de congelamento–secamento ou por qualquer outro método que evitará a desnaturação das proteínas e produzirá um produto facilmente solúvel em um volume de água igual ao volume de soro humano líquido a partir do qual foi preparado.
 foreign s., s. estranho; soro derivado de um animal e injetado em animal de outra espécie ou em seres humanos.
 human s., s. humano. VER dried human s., normal human s.
 human measles immune s., s. imune do sarampo humano; soro obtido do sangue de um indivíduo sadio que sobreviveu a um episódio de sarampo. SIN measles convalescent s.
 human pertussis immune s., s. imune da coqueluche humana; o soro estéril preparado do sangue misturado de adultos sadios que receberam repetidos esquemas de vacina contra coqueluche da fase I; administrado por via intravenosa ou intramuscular para a profilaxia ou tratamento da coqueluche.
 human scarlet fever immune s., s. imune da escarlatina humana; soro convalescente da escarlatina, obtido de indivíduos sadios que sobreviveram à escarlatina.
 hyperimmune s., s. hiperimune; anti-soro com elevado título de anticorpos produzido através de injeções repetidas de antígenos.
 immune s., s. imune. SIN antiserum.
 inactivated s., s. inativado; soro que foi aquecido a 56°C durante 30 min para destruir a atividade lítica do complemento.
 s. lactis, s. do leite. SIN whey.
 liquid human s., s. humano líquido; mistura de líquidos separados do sangue colhido de seres humanos e coagulado na ausência de qualquer anticoagulante; no máximo, são misturadas 10 doações diferentes; as contribuições de doadores dos grupos A, O e B ou AB são representadas numa proporção aproximada de 9:9:2.
 measles convalescent s., s. convalescente do sarampo. SIN human measles immune s.
 muscle s., s. muscular; o líquido que permanece após a coagulação de plasma muscular e a separação da miosina.
 nonimmune s., s. não-imune; soro de um indivíduo que não é imune; soro sem anticorpos contra determinado antígeno.
 normal s., s. normal; soro não-imune, referindo-se em geral a um soro obtido antes de imunização.
 normal horse s., s. eqüino normal; o soro estéril e filtrado de um cavalo sadio não-vacinado.
 normal human s., s. humano normal; soro estéril obtido pela mistura de volumes aproximadamente iguais da porção líquida do sangue total coagulado de oito ou mais indivíduos sem qualquer doença transmissível por transfusão.
 polyvalent s., s. polivalente; anti-soro obtido por inoculação de um animal com vários antígenos, ou espécies ou cepas diferentes de bactérias.
 pooled s., pooled blood s., s. misturado; o soro misturado obtido de vários indivíduos.
 salted s., salgado. SIN salted *plasma.*
 specific s., s. específico; anti-soro monovalente, isto é, aquele obtido por inoculação de um animal com um antígeno ou com uma espécie ou cepa de bactéria.
 thyrotoxic s., s. tireotóxico; anti-soro obtido por injeção das nucleoproteínas da glândula tireóide em animais.

truth s., s. da verdade; designação coloquial de uma droga, como o amobarbital sódico ou o tiopental sódico, injetada por via intravenosa com escopolamina com o propósito de obter informações do indivíduo sob a sua influência; designação incorreta, visto que as revelações feitas pelo indivíduo podem ou não ser verdadeiras, de modo que a sua situação e uso para fins legais são questionáveis.

se·rum·al (sēr'ŭm-ăl). Soral; relativo ao soro ou derivado dele.

se·rum-fast (sēr'ŭm-fast). Soro-resistente. 1. Relativo a um soro no qual há pouca ou nenhuma alteração nos títulos de anticorpos, mesmo em condições de tratamento ou de estimulação imunológica. 2. Resistente ao efeito destrutivo do soro. SIN serofast.

se·rum glu·tam·ic-ox·a·lo·ace·tic trans·am·i·nase (SGOT). Transaminase glutâmico-oxaloacética sérica (TGO). SIN *aspartate* aminotransferase.

se·rum glu·tam·ic-py·ru·vic trans·am·i·nase (SGPT). Transaminase glutâmico-pirúvica sérica (TGP). SIN *alanine* aminotransferase.

ser·va·tion (ser-vā'shŭn). Uso ou função de um órgão.

Servetus (Servet, Servide), Miguel, anatomista e teólogo espanhol, 1511–1553. VER S. *circulation*.

ser·vo·mech·a·nism (ser'vō-mek'ă-nizm). Servomecanismo, servossistema. 1. Sistema de controle que utiliza o mecanismo de retroalimentação negativa para operar outro sistema. 2. Processo que se comporta como um dispositivo auto-regulador; p. ex., a reação da pupila à luz. [L. *servus,* servo + G. *mēchanē,* invento]

ser·yl (ser'il). Seril; radical da serina.

ses·a·me (sĕs'ă-mē). Sésamo; o gergelim, uma erva, *Sesamum indicum* (família Pedaliaceae), cujas sementes são utilizadas como alimento, constituindo a fonte do óleo de sésamo. [G. *sēsamē,* sésamo, uma planta leguminosa oriental]
s. oil, óleo de Sésamo; o óleo fixo refinado obtido da semente de uma ou mais variedades cultivadas de *Sesamum indicum;* solvente para injeções intramusculares. SIN benne oil, gingili oil, teel oil.

ses·a·moid (sĕs'ă-moyd). Sesamóide. 1. Semelhante, quanto ao tamanho ou à forma, a um grão de sésamo. 2. Refere-se a um osso sesamóide. [G. *sēsamoeidēs,* semelhante ao sésamo]

♻ **sesqui-.** Sesqui-. Prefixo que significa 3/2; antigamente utilizado em química para indicar uma relação de 3:2 entre as duas partes de um composto (p. ex., sesquissulfeto, sesquibásico); todavia, hoje em dia, é apenas utilizado para sesquiidratos e sesquiterpenos. [L.]

ses·qui·hy·drates (ses-kwi-hī'drāts). Sesquiidratos; compostos que cristalizam com (nominalmente) uma molécula e meia de água.

ses·qui·ter·penes (ses-kwi-ter'pēnz). Sesquiterpenos; compostos formados a partir de três unidades de isopreno; podem ser acíclicos, mono, di ou tricíclicos; sintetizados a partir do farnesilpirofosfato (p. ex., tricotecina, nicina).

ses·sile (sĕs'il). Séssil; que possui uma ampla base de fixação; não-pedunculado. [L. *sessilis,* de crescimento lento, de *sedeo,* pp. *sessus,* sentar]

ses·ter·ter·penes (sĕs'ter-ter-pēnz). Sesterterpenos; compostos formados a partir de cinco unidades isopreno; com freqüência, possuem uma estrutura tricíclica; formados a partir de geranilfarnesilpirofosfato (p. ex., cocliobolina B). [L. *sestertius,* dois e meio, de *semis,* metade + *tertius,* terceiro + terpene]

set. 1. Prontidão para perceber ou responder de alguma maneira; atitude que facilita ou predetermina um resultado; p. ex., o preconceito ou o fanatismo como disposição para responder de modo negativo, independentemente dos méritos do estímulo. **2.** Reduzir uma fratura; isto é, trazer os ossos de volta a uma posição ou alinhamento normal. **3.** Conjunto; grupo definido de eventos, objetos, dados, distinguível de outros grupos. [I.m. *sette,* do Fr. ant., do L. med. *secta,* curso, de *sequor,* seguir]
haploid s., conjunto haplóide; conteúdo genético de um gameta normal em que cada *locus* autossômico é representado por um único alelo e por um único conjunto completo de genes ligados ao cromossoma X ou um conjunto completo de genes ligados ao cromossoma Y; a célula somática adulta normal contém dois conjuntos haplóides.
learning s., disposição ao aprendizado, prontidão ou predisposição a aprender, desenvolvida a partir de experiências prévias de aprendizado, como, por exemplo, quando um organismo aprende a resolver cada problema sucessivo (de dificuldade igual ou crescente) com menos tentativas.
postural s., disposição postural; prontidão motora global a responder, como um corredor instruído a ficar preparado na linha de partida.

se·ta, pl. **set·ae** (sē'tă, -tē). Cerda; estrutura delgada e rígida, setiforme. SIN chaeta. [L. *saeta,* ou *seta,* pêlo duro ou cerda]

se·ta·ceous (sē-tā'shŭs). **1.** Setáceo, cerdoso; que possui cerdas. **2.** Cerdáceo, setiforme; semelhante a uma cerda. [L. *seta,* cerda]

Se·tar·ia (sē-tā'rē-ă, -tar'ē-ă). Gênero de nematódeos da família Stephanofilariidae (superfamília Filarioidea). Os adultos são longos e delgados, tipicamente encontrados na cavidade peritoneal e produzem microfilárias embanhadas no sangue, que são transmitidas para outros hospedeiros após desenvolvimento cíclico em hospedeiros mosquitos apropriados. São parasitas de gado bovino ou eqüinos (selvagens ou domésticos) e, em geral, não são patogênicos, embora, em certas ocasiões, os vermes jovens possam ser encontrados na câmara anterior do olho. [L. *seta,* cerda]

S. cer'vi, espécie que ocorre na cavidade abdominal do gado bovino, búfalo, bisão, iaque e vários cervídeos, porém raramente em ovinos.
S. equi'na, espécie que é parasita comum de cavalos e outros eqüídeos em todas as partes do mundo; são filamentos delgados e esbranquiçados, com vários centímetros de comprimento, habitualmente encontrados livres na cavidade peritoneal, mas, em certas ocasiões, observados na cavidade pleural, nos pulmões, no escroto, no olho e no intestino.

set·back (set'bak). Operação cirúrgica para tratamento de fenda palatina bilateral, em que o pré-maxilar é movido posteriormente; com freqüência, o procedimento é acompanhado de enxerto ósseo.

se·tif·er·ous (sē-tif'er-ŭs). Setífero. Cerdoso ou que possui cerdas. SIN setigerous (setígero). [L. *seta,* cerda + *fero,* transportar]

se·tig·er·ous (sē-tij'er-ŭs). Setígero. SIN *setiferous*. [L. *seta,* cerda + *gero,* produzir]

se·ton (sē'ton). Sedenho; mecha de fios, faixa de gaze, pedaço de fio ou outro material estranho passado através dos tecidos subcutâneos ou de um cisto para formar um seio ou uma fístula. [L. *seta,* cerda]

set·ting. Endurecimento, como do amálgama.

set·up. 1. Disposição de dentes numa base de dentadura provisória. **2.** Procedimento em análise de casos dentários que envolve a retirada e o reposicionamento de dentes nas posições desejadas sobre um molde de gesso.

se·vere com·bined im·mu·no·de·fi·cient mice (SCID mice). Camundongos com imunodeficiência combinada grave (camundongos IDCG); camundongos sem linfócitos T e B utilizados para transplante e estudo de tecidos linfóides humanos, resultando numa quimera de IDCG humana e de camundongo. VER TAMBÉM severe combined *immunodeficiency*.

Severinghaus, John W., fisiologista e anestesiologista norte-americano, *1922. VER S. *electrode*.

se·vo·flu·rane (sev-ō-floor'ān). Sevoflurano; éter halogenado para anestesia por inalação.

se·vum (sē'vŭm). Sebo. [L.]

sex (seks). Sexo. **1.** O caráter ou qualidade biológica que distingue o macho da fêmea, expresso pela análise das características gonadais, morfológicas (tanto internas quanto externas) cromossômicas e hormonais do indivíduo. Cf. gender. **2.** Os processos fisiológicos e psicológicos de um indivíduo que determinam o comportamento relacionado à procriação ou ao prazer erótico. [L. *sexus*]
s. assignment, especificação sexual: processo pelo qual o sexo de um recém-nascido intersexual (hermafrodita) é inicialmente especificado.
safe s., s. seguro; práticas sexuais que limitam o risco de transmissão ou aquisição de doença infecciosa através da troca de sêmen, sangue e outros líquidos orgânicos, como, por exemplo, uso de preservativo, masturbação mútua ou abstinência de relação anal.

sex·dig·i·tate (seks-dij'i-tāt). Sexdigital; que tem seis dedos em uma ou em ambas as mãos ou pés. SIN sedigitate. [L. *sex,* seis + *digitus,* dedo]

sex-in·flu·enced. Influenciado pelo sexo; refere-se a uma classe de distúrbios genéticos em que o mesmo genótipo apresenta diferentes manifestações nos dois sexos; a variação pode ser racional (p. ex., o câncer de mama ocorre menos freqüentemente em homens) ou ter apenas suporte empírico (p. ex., o padrão de calvície comporta-se como um traço dominante no homem e como um traço recessivo na mulher). VER TAMBÉM sex-influenced *inheritance*.

sex·i·va·lent (sek-sī-vā'lent, sek-siv'ă-lent). Hexavalente; que possui valência de seis. [L. *sex,* seis + *valencia,* força]

sex-lim·it·ed. Limitado a um sexo apenas; que ocorre apenas em um sexo. VER sex-limited *inheritance*.

sex-linked. Ligado ao sexo. VER sex *linkage*.

sex·ol·o·gy (sek-sol'ō-jē). Sexologia; o estudo científico de todos os aspectos do sexo, incluindo diferenciação e dimorfismo e, em particular, comportamento sexual. [L. *sexus,* sexo + G. *logos,* estudo]

sex·tan (seks'tan). Sextã; refere-se a uma febre malárica cujos paroxismos recidivam a cada sexto dia, considerando o dia do episódio como primeiro, isto é, com um intervalo assintomático de quatro dias. [L. *sextus,* sexto]

sex·u·al (sek'shoo-ăl). Sexual; relativo a sexo, incluindo estimulação, responsividade e funcionamento dos órgãos sexuais. [L. *sexualis,* de *sexus,* sexo]

sex·u·al·i·ty (sek-shoo-al'i-tē). Sexualidade. **1.** A soma dos comportamentos e tendências sexuais de uma pessoa, e a força dessas tendências. **2.** Grau de atratividade sexual do indivíduo. **3.** Qualidade de possuir funções ou implicações sexuais.
infantile s., s. infantil; na teoria da personalidade psicanalítica, o conceito relacionado ao desenvolvimento psicosexual em lactentes e crianças; inclui as fases oral, anal e fálica superpostas durante os primeiros cinco anos de vida.

sex·u·al·i·za·tion (sek'shoo-ăl-i-zā'shŭn). Sexualização. **1.** O estado caracterizado pela presença de energia ou impulso sexual. **2.** O ato de adquirir energia ou impulso sexual. **3.** O ato de atribuir um significado ou qualidade sexual a indivíduos ou comportamentos.

sex·u·al pref·er·ence. Preferência sexual. **1.** O sexo procurado em parceiros sexuais. **2.** Modo particular de comportamento que leva a uma satisfação sexual.

Sézary, Albert, dermatologista francês, 1880–1956. VER S. *cell, erythroderma, syndrome*.

SFO Abreviatura de subfornical *organ* (órgão subfornicial).
S.G.O. Abreviatura de Surgeon General's Office.
SGOT Abreviatura de serum glutamic-oxaloacetic transaminase (transaminase glutâmico-oxaloacética sérica).
SGPT Abreviatura de serum glutamic-pyruvic transaminase (transaminase glutâmico-pirúvica sérica).
SH 1. Abreviatura de serum *hepatitis* (hepatite sérica). **2.** Abreviatura de sulfhydryl (sulfidrila).
shad·ow (shăd'ō). **1.** Sombra; área de superfície definida pela intercepção de luz ou raios X por um corpo. VER TAMBÉM density (3). **2.** Em psicologia junguiana, o arquétipo que consiste nos instintos animais coletivos. **3.** Acromócito. SIN achromocyte.
   acoustic s., sombra acústica; aspecto ultra-sonográfico de amplitude de eco reduzida de regiões situadas além de um objeto atenuante. Cf. acoustic *enhancement*.
   Gumprecht s.'s, sombras de Gumprecht. SIN smudge cells, em cell.
   hilar s., imagem hilar; hilo do pulmão em radiografia; imagem radiográfica composta das artérias e veias pulmonares centrais, com paredes brônquicas e linfonodos associados no pulmão direito ou esquerdo.
   Ponfick s., s. de Ponfick. SIN achromocyte.
   radiographic parallel line s., imagem radiográfica de linhas paralelas. SIN tram lines, em line.
shad·ow-cast·ing. Evaporação a vácuo e deposição de uma película de carbono ou determinados metais, como paládio, platina ou cromo, sobre um objeto microscópico contornado, a fim de permitir que o objeto seja observado em relevo ao microscópio eletrônico ou, algumas vezes, ao microscópio óptico.
Shaffer, A., bioquímico norte-americano, 1881–1960. VER S.-Hartmann *method*.
shaft [TA]. Diáfise. SIN diaphysis. [A.S. *sceaft*]
   s. of clavicle [TA], d. da clavícula; corpo alongado e semelhante a um bastão da clavícula. SIN corpus claviculae [TA], body of clavicle*.
   s. of femur [TA], d. do fêmur; a diáfise cilíndrica do osso da coxa. SIN corpus ossis femoris [TA], body of femur*, body of thigh bone, corpus femoris.
   s. of fibula [TA], d. da fíbula; corpo da fíbula; porção alongada da fíbula que compreende a maior parte de seu comprimento. SIN corpus fibulae [TA], body of fibula*.
   hair s., haste do pêlo; porção de um pêlo que não cresce, que se projeta da pele, isto é, do folículo. SIN scapus pili.
   s. of humerus [TA], d. do úmero; a porção alongada do úmero entre o colo cirúrgico, proximalmente, e o aparecimento das cristas supracondilares, distalmente. SIN corpus humeri [TA], body of humerus*.
   s. of metacarpal [TA], d. metacarpal; a porção alongada do osso metacarpal. SIN corpus metacarpale [TA], body of metacarpal*.
   s. of metatarsal [TA], d. metatarsal; a porção alongada do osso metatarsal. SIN corpus metatarsale [TA], body of metatarsal*.
   s. of phalanx [TA], d. da falange; a diáfise de cada falange da mão ou do pé. SIN corpus phalangis [TA], body of phalanx*.
   s. of radius [TA], d. do rádio; o corpo triangular do rádio localizado entre as extremidades expandidas proximal e distal do osso. SIN corpus radii [TA], body of radius*.
   s. of tibia [TA], d. da tíbia; o corpo triangular da tíbia entre as extremidades expandidas proximal e distal. SIN corpus tibiae [TA], body of tibia*.
   s. of ulna [TA], d. da ulna; a diáfise da ulna entre a extremidade proximal e a cabeça. SIN corpus ulnae [TA], body of ulna*.
shakes. Tremedeira, calafrio; termo vernacular para referir-se a um paroxismo associado a uma febre intermitente.
   smelter's shakes, febre do fundidor de minério. SIN smelter's *fever*.
shank. 1. Tíbia; canela; perna. **2.** Haste; a porção de um instrumento que liga a porção cortante ou funcional a um cabo; nos instrumentos rotatórios, como brocas e furadeiras, a extremidade que se encaixa no mandril. [A. S. *sceanca*]
shap·ing (shāp'ing). No condicionamento operante, quando a resposta do operante não está no repertório do organismo, procedimento em que o experimentador divide a resposta nas partes que aparecem com mais freqüência, começa a reforçá-las e, a seguir, suspende lenta e sucessivamente o reforço até que seja emitido mais e mais do operante.
shark liv·er oil. Óleo de fígado de tubarão; óleo extraído do fígado de tubarões, principalmente da espécie *Hypoprion brevirostris;* trata-se de uma rica fonte de vitaminas A e D.
Sharpey, William, fisiologista e histologista escocês, 1802–1880. VER S. *fibers,* em *fiber*.
Sharpey-Schäfer. VER Schäfer.
Shaver, Cecil Gordon, médico canadense, *1901. VER S. *disease*.
SHBG Abreviatura de sex hormone-binding *globulin* (globulina de ligação dos hormônios sexuais).
shear (shēr). Cisalhamento; deformação de um corpo por duas forças paralelas de direção oposta. A deformação consiste no deslizamento de planos imaginários (dentro do corpo) um sobre o outro, paralelos aos planos das forças. [A.S.]
shears (shērz). Tesoura. SIN scissors.
   Liston s., t. de Liston; tesoura forte para cortar o gesso das ataduras gessadas.

sheath (shēth). **1.** Qualquer estrutura de envoltório, como o revestimento membranáceo de um músculo, nervo ou vaso sanguíneo. Qualquer estrutura semelhante a uma bainha. SIN vagina (1). **2.** O prepúcio de animais machos, principalmente do cavalo. **3.** Instrumento tubular especialmente projetado através do qual podem ser introduzidos obturadores ou instrumentos de corte especiais, para retirada de coágulos sanguíneos, fragmentos de tecido, cálculos, etc. **4.** Tubo utilizado como aparelho ortodôntico, geralmente nos molares. [A.S. *scaeth*]
   anterior tarsal tendinous s.'s [TA], bainhas dos tendões anteriores do tarso; bainhas sinoviais tendíneas que permitem o movimento de tendões através da fase anterior dos ossos do tarso, profundamente até os retináculos dos músculos extensores; estão incluídas as bainhas dos tendões (vagina tendini musculi...) do: (1) (músculo) tibial anterior [TA] (...tibialis anterioris [TA]), (2) (músculo) extensor longo do hálux [TA] (...extensoris hallucis longi [TA]) e (3) (músculo) extensor longo dos dedos [TA] (...extensoris digitorum longi [TA]). SIN vaginae tendinum tarsales anteriores [TA].
   axillary s., b. axilar; bainha neurovascular fibrosa, formada como extensão da camada pré-vertebral da fáscia cervical profunda através do canal cervicoaxilar, que envolve a primeira parte da artéria axilar, veia axilar e plexo braquial.
   carotid s. [TA], b. carótica; o revestimento fibroso denso da artéria carótida, da veia jugular interna e do nervo vago de cada lado do pescoço, profundamente até o músculo esternocleidomastóideo; as camadas da fáscia cervical fundem-se com ela. SIN vagina carotica [TA].
   carpal tendinous s.'s [TA], bainhas dos tendões do carpo; bainhas tendíneas que ocorrem em relação ao punho, permitindo o deslizamento livre dos tendões através dos ossos e formações ósseas do punho quando mantidos no local pelos retináculos dos músculos flexores e extensores. SIN vaginae tendinum carpalium [TA].
   caudal s., b. caudal; grupo de microtúbulos dispostos cilindricamente ao redor do pólo caudal do núcleo num espermatozóide em desenvolvimento.
   common flexor s. (of hand) [TA], b. comum dos tendões dos músculos flexores (da mão); a bainha tendínea palmar sinovial do carpo que circunda os oito tendões dos flexores superficiais e profundos dos dedos da mão quando atravessam o canal do carpo; em geral, é contínua com a bainha sinovial do quinto dedo. SIN vagina communis tendinum musculorum flexorum (manus) [TA], ulnar bursa.
   common peroneal tendon s., b. comum dos tendões dos músculos fibulares; a bainha que circunda os tendões dos músculos fibulares longo e curto em sua passagem ao longo do tornozelo. SIN vagina communis tendinum musculorum fibularium communis [TA], vagina tendinum musculorum fibularium communis, vagina tendinum musculorum peroneorum communis.
   crural s., b. crural. SIN femoral s.
   dentinal s., b. dentinária; camada de tecido relativamente resistente à ação de ácidos, que forma as paredes do túbulos dentinários. SIN Neumann s.
   dorsal carpal tendinous s.'s [TA], bainha dos tendões dorsais do carpo; bainhas sinoviais tendíneas que permitem o movimento de tendões através da face posterior do punho, profundamente até o retináculo dos extensores; são seis bainhas dos tendões (vaginae tendinum... [TA]): (1) dos (músculos) abdutor longo e extensor curto do polegar [TA] (...musculorum abductoris longi et extensoris pollicis brevis [TA]); (2) dos (músculos) extensores radiais do punho [TA] (...musculi extensorum carpi radialium [TA]); (3) do (músculo) extensor longo do polegar [TA] (...musculi extensoris pollicis longi [TA]); (4) dos (músculos) extensores dos dedos e extensor do indicador [TA] (...musculorum extensoris digitorum et extensoris indicis [TA]); (5) do (músculo) extensor curto do dedo mínimo (...musculi extensoris digiti minimi [TA] e (6) do (músculo) extensor ulnar do punho [TA] (...musculi extensoris carpi ulnaris [TA]). SIN vaginae tendinum carpalium dorsalium [TA].
   dural s., b. dural; extensão da dura-máter que reveste as raízes dos nervos espinais ou, mais particularmente, a vagina externa dos nervos ópticos.
   dural s. of optic nerve, bainha externa do nervo óptico. SIN outer s. of optic nerve.
   enamel rod s., b. do bastonete de esmalte; cobertura orgânica do bastonete de esmalte individual.
   external s. of optic nerve, b. externa do nervo óptico. SIN outer s. of optic nerve.
   external root s., b. radicular externa. VER root s.
   s. of eyeball, b. do bulbo do olho. SIN fascial s. of eyeball.
   fascial s.'s of extraocular muscles, fáscias musculares dos músculos extrínsecos do bulbo do olho. SIN muscular *fascia* of extraocular muscle.
   fascial s. of eyeball [TA], b. do bulbo do olho; condensação de tecido conjuntivo na face externa da esclerótica da qual está separada por um espaço episcleral estreito semelhante a uma fenda; a bainha está fixada à esclerótica, próximo à junção esclerocorneana, e une-se com a fáscia dos músculos extra-oculares. SIN vagina bulbi [TA], capsula bulbi, eye capsule, fascia bulbi, s. of eyeball, Tenon capsule, vagina oculi.
   femoral s., b. femoral; a fáscia que envolve os vasos femorais, formada pela fáscia transversal, anteriormente, e pela fáscia ilíaca, posteriormente; dois septos dividem a bainha em três compartimentos: o lateral, que contém a artéria femoral e o ramo femoral do nervo genitofemoral, o médio, que contém a veia femoral; e o medial, que é o canal femoral. SIN crural s., infundibuliform s.

sheath

fenestrated s., b. fenestrada; bainha com uma janela cortada na ponta ou convexidade lateral, através da qual podem ser introduzidos instrumentos de corte especiais.

fibrous s.'s, bainhas fibrosas. VER fibrous tendon s., fibrous s.'s of digits of hand, fibrous digital s.'s of toes.

fibrous digital s.'s of foot, bainhas fibrosas dos dedos do pé. SIN fibrous digital s.'s of toes.

fibrous digital s.'s of hand, bainhas fibrosas dos dedos da mão. SIN fibrous s.'s of digits of hand.

fibrous digital s.'s of toes [TA], bainhas fibrosas dos dedos do pé; a camada fibrosa tubular que envolve a bainha sinovial e os tendões dos flexores longo e curto dos dedos e flexor longo do hálux nos dedos; são compostas de partes anular e cruciforme. SIN vaginae fibrosae digitorum pedis [TA], fibrous digital s.'s of foot.

fibrous s.'s of digits of hand [TA], bainhas fibrosas dos dedos da mão; as camadas fibrosas tubulares que envolvem as bainhas sinoviais e os tendões flexores superficial e profundo, assim como o tendão do flexor longo do polegar em sua passagem ao longo de seus respectivos dedos; são compostas de partes anular e cruciforme. SIN vaginae fibrosae digitorum manus [TA], fibrous digital s.'s of hand.

fibrous tendon s. [TA], b. fibrosa dos tendões; bainha fibrosa de um tendão. SIN stratum fibrosum vaginae tendinis*, vagina fibrosa tendinis.

fibular tarsal tendinous s.'s [TA], bainhas dos tendões fibulares do tarso; bainhas sinoviais dos tendões flexores que permitem o movimento dos tendões posteriormente ao maléolo lateral e através dos ossos do tarso, passando profundamente até os retináculos dos músculos fibulares; incluem: (1) a bainha comum dos tendões dos músculos fibulares [TA] (vagina communis tendineum musculorum fibularum (peroneum) [TA]); e (2) a bainha do tendão plantar do (músculo) fibular longo [TA] (vagina plantaris tendinis musculi fibularis (peronei) longi [TA]). SIN vaginae tendinum tarsales fibulares [TA].

Henle s., b. de Henle. SIN endoneurium.

Hertwig s., b. de Hertwig; as camadas epiteliais externa e interna unidas do órgão do esmalte; estende-se além da região da coroa anatômica e inicia a formação de dentina na raiz de um dente em desenvolvimento; sofre atrofia à medida que a raiz é formada, e as células que persistem são denominadas remanescentes epiteliais de Malassez.

Huxley s., b. de Huxley. SIN Huxley layer.

infundibuliform s., b. infundibuliforme. SIN femoral s.

inner s. of optic nerve [TA], b. interna do nervo óptico; a bainha mais interna ao redor do nervo óptico, contínua com as leptomeninges (pia-aracnóide) e incluindo um espaço intervaginal repleto de líquido cefalorraquidiano, contínuo com o espaço subaracnóide. SIN vagina interna nervi optici [TA], internal s. of optic nerve.

internal s. of optic nerve, b. interna do nervo óptico. SIN inner s. of optic nerve.

internal root s., bainha radicular interna. VER root s.

intertubercular tendon s. [TA], b. tendínea intertubercular; a extensão da membrana sinovial da articulação do ombro para baixo, no sulco intertubercular, circundando o tendão da cabeça longa do músculo bíceps. SIN vagina tendinis intertubercularis [TA].

s. of Key and Retzius, b. de Key e Retzius. SIN endoneurium.

Mauthner s., b. de Mauthner. SIN axolemma.

medullary s., b. de mielina. SIN myelin s.

microfilarial s., b. microfilarial; a membrana que circunda os embriões de certas microfilárias transportadas pelo sangue, como *Wuchereria*, *Brugia* e *Loa* dos seres humanos; acredita-se que seja derivada da membrana vitelina.

mitochondrial s., b. mitocondrial; as mitocôndrias dispostas em espiral na porção média de um espermatozóide; fornece a energia necessária para o movimento da cauda.

mucous s. of tendon, b. sinovial do tendão. SIN synovial tendon s.

myelin s., b. de mielina; o envoltório lipoproteináceo nos vertebrados que circunda a maioria dos axônios com mais de 0,5 μm de diâmetro; consiste numa dupla camada plasmática firmemente enrolada em torno do axônio, num número variável de voltas, sendo suprida por células da oligodendróglia (no cérebro e na medula espinal) ou células de Schwann (nos nervos periféricos); quando desenrolada, a membrana dupla aparece como uma expansão celular semelhante a uma lâmina, que carece de citoplasma, à exceção de alguns filamentos citoplasmáticos estreitos que correspondem a interrupções aparentes da estrutura regular de mielina, as incisuras de Schmidt-Lanterman; a bainha de mielina de cada axônio é composta de uma seqüência longitudinal bastante regular de segmentos, correspondendo cada um ao comprimento da bainha suprida por uma única célula da oligodendróglia ou de Schwann; no curto intervalo entre cada dois segmentos vizinhos, os nodos de Ranvier, o axônio é desmielinizado, embora envolto por complexas expansões plasmáticas digitiformes das células vizinhas da oligodendróglia ou de Schwann. SIN medullary s.

Neumann s., b. de Neumann. SIN dentinal s.

neurovascular s., b. neurovascular; tecido fibroso que circunda e junta artérias com suas veias acompanhantes (*venae comitantes*) e nervos; com freqüência, trata-se meramente do tecido adventício das estruturas neurovasculares, mas pode estar muito desenvolvida na forma de camada fascial distinta (p. ex., no caso das bainhas carótida ou axilar).

notochordal s., b. da notocorda; o revestimento fibroso externo da notocorda.

outer s. of optic nerve [TA], bainha externa do nervo óptico; a bainha externa ao redor do nervo óptico, contínua com a dura-máter. SIN vagina externa nervi optici [TA], dural s. of optic nerve, external s. of optic nerve.

palmar carpal tendinous s.'s [TA], bainhas dos tendões palmares do carpo; três bainhas sinoviais tendíneas que permitem o movimento dos tendões através da face anterior do punho, profundamente até o retináculo dos músculos flexores; são elas: (1) a b.°do tendão do (músculo) flexor longo do polegar [TA] (vagina tendinis musculi flexoris pollicis longi [TA]); (2) b. do tendão do (músculo) flexor radial do carpo [TA] (vagina tendinis musculi flexoris carpi radialis [TA]); e (3) b. comum dos tendões dos músculos flexores [TA] (vagina communis tendineum musculorum flexorum [TA]). SIN vaginae tendinum carpales palmares [TA].

parotid s., fáscia parotídea. SIN parotid *fascia*.

periarterial lymphatic s. (PALS), b. linfática periarterial; o acúmulo de linfócitos envolvendo as artérias centrais do baço e compreendendo a polpa branca.

plantar tendon s. of fibularis longus muscle, b. do tendão plantar do músculo fibular longo; a bainha sinovial que envolve o tendão do músculo fibular longo em seu trajeto através da planta do pé. SIN vagina tendinis musculi fibularis longi plantaris [TA], plantar tendon s. of peroneus longus muscle*, vagina tendinis musculi peronei longi plantaris*.

plantar tendon s. of peroneus longus muscle, b. do tendão plantar do músculo fibular longo; *termo oficial alternativo para plantar tendon s. of fibularis longus muscle.

prostatic s., b. prostática; envoltório fibroso frouxo e parcialmente vascular da próstata e sua cápsula fibrosa densa (verdadeira); continua-se inferiormente com a fáscia superior do diafragma urogenital e, posteriormente, torna-se parte do septo retovesical; contém o plexo venoso prostático.

rectus s. [TA], b. do músculo reto do abdome; formada pelas aponeuroses dos três músculos ântero-laterais da parede abdominal que se dividem para envolver o músculo reto, sofrendo fusão medial para formar a linha alba; consiste numa lâmina anterior e numa lâmina posterior, estando a última ausente abaixo da linha arqueada. VER TAMBÉM *aponeurosis* of external oblique muscle, *aponeurosis* of internal oblique muscle. SIN vagina musculi recti abdominis [TA].

resectoscope s., b. do ressectoscópio; bainha operatória através da qual pode-se efetuar a eletrorressecção transuretral de tumores vesicais ou da próstata.

root s. b. radicular; uma das camadas epidérmicas do folículo piloso: a bainha radicular externa é contínua com o estrato basal e estrato espinhoso da epiderme; a bainha radicular interna compreende a cutícula das raízes internas, camada de Huxley e camada de Henle.

Rouget-Neumann s., b. de Rouget-Neumann; a substância fundamental amorfa existente entre um osteócito e a parede lacunar ou canalicular.

Scarpa s., b. de Scarpa. SIN cremasteric *fascia*.

s. of Schwann, b. de Schwann. SIN neurilemma.

s. of Schweigger-Seidel, b. de Schweigger-Seidel. SIN ellipsoid.

s. of styloid process [TA], b. do processo estilóide; uma crista de osso (borda da porção timpânica do osso temporal) que se estende da frente e lado medial do processo mastóide até a espinha do esfenóide; divide-se para embainhar a base do processo estilóide. SIN vagina processus styloidei [TA], vaginal process.

synovial s. [TA], b. sinovial. VER synovial tendon s., *vagina* synovialis trochleae, synovial s.'s of digits of hand, synovial s.'s of toes. SIN vagina synovialis [TA].

synovial s.'s of digits of foot, bainhas sinoviais dos dedos do pé. SIN synovial s.'s of toes.

synovial s.'s of digits of hand [TA], bainhas sinoviais dos dedos da mão; bainhas sinoviais que envolvem os tendões flexores dos dedos da mão e revestem o interior das bainhas fibrosas. SIN vaginae synoviales digitorum manus [TA].

synovial tendon s. [TA], b. sinovial dos tendões; bainha de membrana sinovial que envolve alguns tendões; contém um pequeno volume de líquido sinovial. SIN vagina synovialis tendinis [TA], mucous s. of tendon, theca tendinis, vagina mucosa tendinis, vaginal synovial membrane.

synovial s.'s of toes [TA], bainhas sinoviais dos dedos do pé; de estrutura semelhante às bainhas correspondentes da mão. SIN vaginae tendinum digitorum pedis [TA], synovial s.'s of digits of foot.

tail s., b. caudal; o envoltório fibroso na cauda de um espermatozóide.

tendinous s. of abductor pollicis longus and extensor pollicis brevis muscles [TA], b. dos tendões dos músculos abdutor longo e extensor curto do polegar; a bainha sinovial dos tendões dorsais do carpo que reveste o compartimento do retináculo dos músculos extensores contendo os tendões dos músculos abdutor longo do polegar e extensor curto do polegar. SIN vagina tendinum musculorum abductoris long et extensoris brevis pollicis [TA].

tendinous s. of extensor carpi radialis muscles [TA], b. dos tendões dos músculos extensores radiais do carpo; a bainha sinovial dos tendões dorsais do carpo que reveste o compartimento do retináculo dos músculos extensores contendo os tendões dos músculos extensores radiais do carpo (longo e curto). SIN vagina tendinum musculorum extensorum carpi radialium [TA].

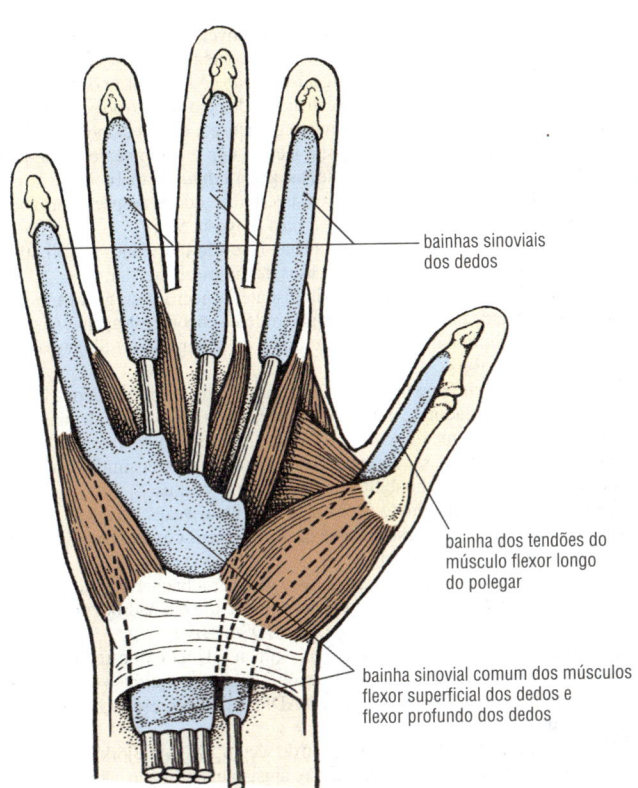

bainhas dos tendões dos flexores: a mão

tendinous s. of extensor carpi ulnaris muscle [TA], b. do tendão do músculo extensor ulnar do carpo; a bainha sinovial tendínea do carpo dorsal que circunda o tendão do músculo extensor ulnar do carpo em seu trajeto profundo até o retináculo dos extensores. SIN vagina tendinis musculi extensoris carpi ulnaris [TA], peritenon.
tendinous s. of extensor digiti minimi muscle [TA], b. do tendão do músculo extensor do dedo mínimo; a bainha sinovial do tendão dorsal do carpo que circunda o tendão do músculo extensor do dedo mínimo em seu trajeto profundo até o retináculo dos músculos extensores. SIN vagina tendinis musculi extensoris digiti minimi [TA].
tendinous s. of extensor digitorum and extensor indicis muscles [TA], b. dos tendões dos músculos extensores dos dedos e extensor do indicador; a b. sinovial do tendão dorsal do carpo que circunda os quatro tendões do músculo extensor dos dedos e o tendão do músculo extensor do indicador profundamente, até o retináculo dos músculos extensores. SIN vagina tendinum musculorum extensoris digitorum et extensoris indicis [TA].
tendinous s. of extensor digitorum longus muscle of foot [TA], b. dos tendões do músculo extensor longo dos dedos do pé; a bainha sinovial dos tendões anteriores do tarso que circunda os tendões do músculo extensor longo dos dedos e músculo fibular terceiro em seu trajeto através do tornozelo. SIN vagina tendinum musculi extensoris digitorum pedis longi [TA].
tendinous s. of extensor hallucis longus muscle [TA], b. do tendão do músculo extensor longo do hálux; a bainha sinovial dos tendões anteriores do tarso que circunda o tendão do músculo extensor longo do hálux em seu trajeto através do tornozelo. SIN vagina tendinis musculi extensoris hallucis longi [TA].
tendinous s. of extensor pollicis longus muscle [TA], b. do tendão do músculo extensor longo do polegar; a bainha sinovial dos tendões dorsais do carpo que circunda o tendão do músculo extensor longo do polegar em seu trajeto profundo até o retináculo dos extensores. SIN vagina tendinis musculi extensoris pollicis longi [TA].
tendinous s. of flexor carpi radialis muscle [TA], b. do tendão do músculo flexor radial do carpo; a bainha sinovial dos tendões palmares do carpo que envolve o tendão do músculo flexor radial do carpo quando atravessa o punho. SIN vagina tendinis musculi flexoris carpi radialis [TA].
tendinous s. of flexor digitorum longus muscle (of foot) [TA], b. dos tendões do músculo flexor longo dos dedos (do pé); a bainha sinovial dos tendões tibiais do tarso que envolve os tendões do músculo flexor longo dos dedos quando passam pelo pé, profundamente, até o retináculo dos músculos flexores. SIN vagina tendinum musculi flexoris digitorum pedis longi [TA].
tendinous s. of flexor hallucis longus muscle [TA], b. do tendão do músculo flexor longo do hálux; a bainha sinovial dos tendões tibiais do tarso que envolve o tendão do músculo flexor longo do hálux em seu trajeto para o pé, profundamente, até o retináculo dos músculos flexores. SIN vagina tendinis musculi flexoris hallucis longi [TA].
tendinous s. of flexor pollicis longus muscle [TA], b. do tendão do músculo flexor longo do polegar; a bainha sinovial dos tendões palmares do carpo que envolve o tendão do músculo flexor longo do polegar em seu trajeto através do canal do carpo; continua-se com a bainha digital do polegar, sendo as duas geralmente consideradas como uma bainha. SIN vagina tendinis musculi flexoris pollicis longi [TA], radial bursa.
tendinous s. of superior oblique muscle [TA], b. do tendão do músculo oblíquo superior; a bainha sinovial que envolve o tendão do músculo oblíquo superior quando passa através da tróclea. SIN vagina tendinis musculi obliqui superioris [TA], synovial trochlear bursa, trochlear synovial bursa, vagina synovialis trochleae.
tendinous s. of tibialis anterior muscle [TA], b. do tendão do músculo tibial anterior; a bainha sinovial do tarso anterior, profunda em relação ao retináculo dos músculos extensores, que circunda o tendão do músculo tibial anterior quando este cruza o tornozelo. SIN vagina tendinis musculi tibialis anterioris [TA].
tendinous s. of tibialis posterior muscle [TA], b. do tendão do músculo tibial posterior; a bainha sinovial dos tendões tibiais do tarso que circunda o tendão do músculo tibial posterior quando este passa pelo pé, profundamente, até o retináculo dos músculos flexores. SIN vagina tendinis musculi tibialis posterioris [TA].
s. of thyroid gland, b. da glândula tireóide; revestimento da glândula tireóide externamente à sua cápsula, formado por uma divisão da camada pré-traqueal da fáscia cervical profunda na borda posterior da glândula; a lâmina anterior recobre a glândula em sua face ântero-lateral, fixando-se ao arco da cartilagem cricóide superiormente ao istmo da glândula (fazendo com que se mova com a traquéia durante a elevação/depressão da laringe); a lâmina posterior passa posteriormente ao esôfago para unir-se à fáscia bucofaríngea; inferiormente, a bainha estende-se ao longo das veias tireóideas inferiores para abrir-se no mediastino superior (em conseqüência, a expansão da tireóide, como a decorrente de bócio, pode seguir essa direção).
tibial tarsal tendinous s.'s [TA], bainhas dos tendões tibiais do tarso; bainhas sinoviais tendíneas que permitem o movimento dos tendões através do lado medial dos ossos do tarso, profundamente até o retináculo dos flexores; incluem: a bainha dos tendões (vagina tendinis/tendinum musculi…) (1) do (músculo) flexor longo dos dedos [TA] (…flexoris digitorum longi [TA]); (2) do (músculo) tibial posterior [TA] (…tibialis posterioris [TA]); e (3) do (músculo) flexor longo do hálux [TA] (…flexoris hallucis longi [TA]). SIN vaginae tendinum tarsales tibialis [TA].
vascular s.'s, bainhas vasculares; envoltórios fibrosos que envolvem as artérias com suas veias acompanhantes e, algumas vezes, também os nervos. SIN s.'s of vessels, vaginae vasorum.
s.'s of vessels, bainhas dos vasos. SIN vascular s.'s.
Waldeyer s., b. de Waldeyer; espaço tubular entre a parede vesical e a porção intramural do ureter quando este segue o seu trajeto obliquamente através dessa estrutura; na verdade, trata-se de um espaço, e não de uma verdadeira bainha. SIN Waldeyer space.
Sheehan, Harold L., patologista inglês, *1900. VER S. *syndrome.*
Sheldon, J.H., pediatra inglês, 1920–1964. VER Freeman-S. *syndrome.*
shelf. Prateleira; em anatomia, refere-se a uma estrutura semelhante a uma prateleira.
Blumer s., p. de Blummer. SIN rectal s.
dental s., p. dentária. SIN dental *ledge.*
palatal s., p. palatal; crescimento do maxilar embrionário em direção medial; quando fundida com seu número oposto, forma o palato secundário.
rectal s., p. retal; prateleira palpável ao exame retal, devido a células tumorais metastáticas provenientes de um câncer abdominal, crescendo na bolsa retovesical ou retouterina. SIN Blumer s.
vocal s., corda vocal. SIN vocal *fold.*
shell. Camada, concha, cobertura externa.
cytotrophoblastic s., c. citotrofoblástica; camada externa de células trofoblásticas derivadas do feto na superfície materna da placenta.
diffusion s., c. de difusão; um pequeno vaso constituído de uma membrana semipermeável através da qual a peptona, mas não a albumina sérica, consegue passar; utilizada na realização do teste de Abderhalden.
K s., camada atômica K; órbita ou camada eletrônica mais interna; pode compreender dois elétrons.
L s., camada atômica L; o próximo nível energético mais baixo de elétrons no átomo, depois do nível K. (q.v.).
M s., camada atômica M; o nível energético mais baixo em que transições de elétrons dão origem aos raios X.
O s., camada atômica O; a camada mais externa de elétrons, assim denominada porque o deslocamento de elétrons produz uma emissão no espectro visível ou óptico.

shel·lac (shĕ-lak′). Goma-laca; excreção resinosa de um inseto, *Laccifer (Tachardia) lacca* (família Coccidae). Os insetos sugam a seiva de várias árvores resiníferas asiáticas (principalmente indianas) e excretam e depositam "laca pegajosa". A goma-laca torna-se mais macia em temperatura baixa. Tem muitas aplicações não-medicinais e também é utilizada para revestir electuários e comprimidos, bem como em materiais dentários, como, por exemplo, composto de impressão e placas de base de dentadura. SIN lacca.

Shemin, David, bioquímico norte-americano, *1911. VER S. *cycle.*
Shenton, Edward W.H., radiologista inglês, 1872–1955. VER S. *line.*
Shepherd, Francis J., cirurgião canadense, 1851–1929. VER S. *fracture.*
Sherman, Henry C., bioquímico norte-americano, 1875–1955. VER S. *unit;* S. Bourquin *unit* of vitamin B_2; S.-Munsell *unit.*
Sherrington, Sir Charles S., fisiologista inglês e Prêmio Nobel, 1857–1952. VER S. *phenomenon, law;* Schiff-S. *phenomenon;* Liddell-S. *reflex.*

shield (shēld). Escudo; tela protetora; placa de chumbo para proteger o operador e o paciente dos raios X. [A.S. *scild*]
  embryonic s., disco embrionário; área espessada do blastoderma embrionário a partir da qual se desenvolve o embrião.
  nipple s., e. mamilar; cobertura colocada sobre o mamilo para protegê-lo durante a amamentação.
  oral s.'s, escudos orais; aparelhos removíveis utilizados no tratamento ortodôntico, geralmente colocados entre a mucosa labial e bucal e os dentes.

shift. Mudança, desvio, deslocamento. SIN change. VER TAMBÉM deviation.
  antigenic s., deslocamento antigênico; mutação, isto é, súbita alteração na estrutura molecular do RNA/DNA em microrganismos, especialmente vírus, que produz novas cepas; os hospedeiros anteriormente expostos a outras cepas têm pouca ou nenhuma imunidade adquirida às novas cepas; acredita-se que o deslocamento antigênico seja a explicação para o aparecimento de novas cepas do vírus influenza, que ocorrem por recombinação ou rearranjo genético de duas cepas virais diferentes em determinado hospedeiro, estando associado a epidemias de larga escala.
  axis s., desvio de eixo. SIN axis deviation.
  chemical s., desvio químico; dependência da freqüência de ressonância de um núcleo sobre a ligação química do átomo ou molécula em que está contido. VER chemical shift *artifact.*
  chloride s., desvio de cloreto; quando o CO_2 proveniente dos tecidos penetra no sangue, passa para o interior do eritrócito e é convertido em bicarbonato (HCO_3^-) pela carbonato desidratase; o íon HCO_3^- vai para o plasma, enquanto o Cl^- migra para o eritrócito. Ocorrem alterações inversas nos pulmões quando o CO_2 é eliminado do sangue. SIN Hamburger phenomenon.
  Doppler s., desvio Doppler; a magnitude da mudança de freqüência em hertz quando o som e o observador estão em movimento relativo afastando-se ou aproximando-se um do outro. VER TAMBÉM Doppler *effect.*
  s. to the left, desvio para a esquerda; (1) aumento acentuado na percentagem de células imaturas presentes no sangue circulante, com base na premissa hematológica de que a medula óssea com suas células mielóides imaturas encontra-se à esquerda, enquanto o sangue circulante com seus neutrófilos maduros está à direita. SIN deviation to the left. (2) VER maturation *index.*
  luteoplacental s., desvio luteoplacentário; mudança no local de produção de estrogênio e progesterona essencial para a gravidez humana do corpo lúteo para a placenta; a ovariectomia sempre interrompe a gravidez na maioria dos mamíferos, visto que suas placentas nunca produzem estrogênio e progesterona em quantidades suficientes; todavia, depois da sexta semana de gravidez, a placenta humana pode produzir esses hormônios numa quantidade suficiente para evitar o aborto, apesar da ovariectomia.
  permanent threshold s., desvio do limiar permanente; perda irreversível da audição que resulta da exposição a impulsos intensos ou som contínuo, em oposição ao desvio do limiar temporário reversível, que também resulta dessa exposição.
  phase s., mudança de fase; em ressonância magnética nuclear, a mudança de fase causada pelo movimento dos *spins,* que pode ser utilizada para mostrar o fluxo de líquido.
  Purkinje s., desvio de Purkinje. SIN Purkinje phenomenon.
  s. to the right, desvio para a direita; (1) na contagem diferencial dos leucócitos do sangue periférico, a ausência de formas jovens e imaturas. SIN deviation to the right. (2) VER maturation *index.*
  temporary threshold s., desvio do limiar temporário; perda reversível da audição que resulta da exposição a impulsos intensos ou som contínuo, em oposição ao desvio do limiar permanente irreversível, que pode resultar dessa exposição.
  threshold s., desvio do limiar; o grau de perda ou comprometimento da audição em termos de um desvio de decibel em relação a um audiograma prévio do indivíduo. Após exposição a som intenso, pode haver um desvio do limiar temporário com recuperação em poucas horas ou dias ou desvio do limiar permanente (noise-induced *hearing loss* [perda auditiva induzida por ruído]).

Shiga, Kiyoshi, bacteriologista japonês, 1870–1957. VER *Shigella;* S. *bacillus;* S.-Kruse *bacillus.*

Shi·gel·la (shē-gel′la). Gênero de bactérias imóveis, aeróbicas ou anaeróbicas facultativas (família Enterobacteriaceae), que contém bastonetes não-encapsulados Gram-negativos. Esses microrganismos não podem utilizar o citrato como única fonte de carbono; seu crescimento é inibido pelo cianeto de potássio, e seu metabolismo é fermentativo; fermentam a glicose e outros carboidratos, com produção de ácido, mas não de gás; a lactose não é comumente fermentada, embora algumas vezes seja lentamente atacada; o *habitat* normal consiste no trato intestinal de seres humanos e macacos superiores; todas as espécies provocam disenteria. A espécie típica é *S. dysenteriae.* [Kiyoshi *Shiga*]
  S. *boy'dii,* espécie encontrada apenas nas fezes de indivíduos sintomáticos; ocorre numa pequena proporção de casos de disenteria bacilar.
  S. *dysenter'iae,* espécie que provoca disenteria necrosante grave em seres humanos induzida por uma toxina shiga virulenta encontrada apenas nas fezes de indivíduos sintomáticos; a espécie típica do gênero S. SIN Shiga bacillus, Shiga-Kruse bacillus.
  S. *flexne'ri,* espécie encontrada nas fezes de indivíduos sintomáticos e de convalescentes ou portadores; trata-se de uma causa comum de epidemias de disenteria, especialmente na Ásia e no Oriente Médio. Atualmente reconhecida pela sua capacidade de ser algumas vezes sexualmente transmitida através de relação anal. SIN Flexner bacillus, paradysentery bacillus.
  S. *son'nei,* espécie que provoca disenteria, algumas vezes mais leve do que a causada por outras espécies. Trata-se da espécie mais comum de S. causadora de doença nos Estados Unidos.

shig·el·lo·sis (shig-ĕ-lō′sis). Shigelose; disenteria bacilar causada por bactérias do gênero *Shigella,* que freqüentemente ocorre em padrões epidêmicos; infecção oportunista em indivíduos com AIDS/SIDA.

shi·kim·ate de·hy·dro·gen·ase (shi-kim′āt). Uma óxido-redutase que é responsável pela reação reversível do ácido 3-desidrochiquímico com NADPH ácido, produzindo ácido chiquímico e $NADP^+$ na biossíntese da L-fenilalanina e L-tirosina.

Shiley, D.B., engenheiro norte-americano do século XX. VER Björk-Shiley *valve.*

shim (shim). Na ressonância magnética, o ajustamento fino do campo magnético para melhorar a uniformidade.

shin. Borda anterior da tíbia. SIN anterior border of tibia. [A.S. *scina*]
  saber s., t. em sabre; tíbia convexa anteriormente com borda bem definida na sífilis congênita.
  toasted s.'s, dermatite pelo calor. SIN erythema ab igne.

Shine, J., biologista molecular australiano contemporâneo.

shin·gles (shing′glz). Herpes zoster. SIN herpes zoster. [L. *cingulum,* cintura]

shin·splints. Dor espontânea e à palpação associada a endurecimento e aumento de volume dos músculos pré-tibiais, após esforço atlético excessivo por indivíduo não-treinado; pode ser uma forma leve da síndrome do compartimento tibial anterior.

ship. Estrutura semelhante ao casco de um navio.
  Fabricius s., os contornos dos ossos esfenóide, occipital e frontal, em virtude de sua suposta semelhança com o casco de um navio.

Shipley, Walter C., psiquiatra norte-americano, *1903. VER S.-Hartford *scale.*
Shirodkar, N. V., obstetra e ginecologista indiano, 1900–1971. VER S. *operation.*

shiv·er. 1. Ter calafrios ou tremer, especialmente de frio. **2.** Tremor; discreto calafrio.

shiv·er·ing. Tremor de frio ou de medo.

shock (shok). Choque. **1.** Condição em que as células do organismo recebem volumes inadequados de oxigênio secundariamente a alterações da perfusão; mais comumente secundária à perda de sangue ou sepse. **2.** Distúrbio físico ou bioquímico súbito que resulta em fluxo sanguíneo e oxigenação inadequados para os órgãos vitais de um animal. **3.** Estado de profunda depressão mental e física em conseqüência de grave lesão física ou distúrbio emocional. **4.** Estado caracterizado por fluxo sanguíneo inadequado em todo o corpo a ponto de ocorrer lesão das células teciduais; se o choque for prolongado, o próprio sistema cardiovascular é afetado e começa a deteriorar, resultando num ciclo vicioso que leva à morte. VER diastolic s., systolic s. [Fr. *choc,* do germânico]
  anaphylactic s., c. anafilático; forma grave e freqüentemente fatal de choque, caracterizada pela contração dos músculos lisos e dilatação capilar desencadeadas por anticorpos citotrópicos (da classe IgE); tipicamente, trata-se de um fenômeno associado a anticorpos (reação alérgica tipo I). VER TAMBÉM anaphylaxis, serum *sickness.*
  anaphylactoid s., c. anafilactóide; reação semelhante ao choque anafilático, mas que não exige o período de incubação característico da sensibilidade induzida (anafilaxia); não está relacionado a reações antígeno-anticorpo. SIN anaphylactoid crisis (1), pseudoanaphylactic s.
  anesthetic s., c. anestésico; choque produzido pela administração de agente(s) anestésico(s), habitualmente em *overdose* relativa.
  break s., c. por interrupção; choque produzido pela interrupção de uma corrente constante passando através do corpo.
  cardiac s., c. cardiogênico. SIN cardiogenic s.
  cardiogenic s., c. cardiogênico; choque que resulta do declínio do débito cardíaco secundário a cardiopatia grave, geralmente infarto do miocárdio. SIN cardiac s.

chronic s., c. crônico; o estado de insuficiência circulatória periférica que se desenvolve em pacientes idosos portadores de doença debilitante, como, por exemplo, carcinoma; um volume sanguíneo subnormal torna o paciente suscetível ao choque hemorrágico em decorrência de uma perda de sangue até mesmo moderada, como a que pode ocorrer durante uma cirurgia.
counter s., desfibrilação cardíaca. VER countershock.
cultural s., c. cultural; forma de estresse associada ao início da assimilação, pelo indivíduo, de uma nova cultura muito diferente daquela em que foi criado.
declamping s., fenômeno de desgrampeamento. SIN declamping *phenomenon*.
deferred s., delayed s., c. tardio; estado de choque que surge muito tempo após sofrer a lesão.
diastolic s., c. diastólico; o impacto anormalmente palpável, verificado por uma das mãos sobre a parede torácica, de uma terceira bulha cardíaca muito intensa.
electric s., c. elétrico; impressão súbita e violenta causada pela passagem de uma corrente de eletricidade através de qualquer parte do corpo.
endotoxin s., c. endotóxico; choque induzido pela liberação de endotoxinas de bactérias Gram-negativas, especialmente *Escherichia coli*.
hemorrhagic s. c. hemorrágico; choque hipovolêmico resultante de hemorragia aguda, caracterizado por hipotensão, taquicardia, pele pálida, fria e úmida e oligúria.
histamine s., c. histamínico; o estado de choque produzido em animais pela injeção de histamina; caracteriza-se por espasmo bronquiolar na cobaia e por constrição das veias hepáticas no cão.
hypovolemic s., c. hipovolêmico; choque causado por redução do volume sanguíneo, como na hemorragia ou na desidratação.
insulin s., c. insulínico; hipoglicemia grave produzida pela administração de insulina; manifesta-se por sudorese, tremor, ansiedade, vertigem e diplopia, seguidos de delírio, convulsões e colapso. SIN wet s.
irreversible s., c. irreversível; choque que evoluiu por causa de lesão celular além do estágio em que existe a possibilidade de recuperação.
nitroid s., c. nitróide; síndrome semelhante àquela produzida pela administração de uma grande dose de nitrito, algumas vezes causada por uma injeção intravenosa excessivamente rápida de arsfenamina ou alguma outra droga. VER nitritoid *reaction*.
oligemic s., c. oligêmico; choque associado a queda pronunciada do volume sanguíneo, algumas vezes em decorrência do aumento de permeabilidade dos vasos sanguíneos.
osmotic s., c. osmótico; alteração súbita da pressão osmótica à qual é submetida uma célula, geralmente para provocar a sua lise.
primary s., c. primário; choque de natureza principalmente nervosa, por dor, ansiedade, etc., que ocorre quase imediatamente após uma lesão grave.
protein s., c. proteico; reação sistêmica após a administração parenteral de uma proteína.
pseudoanaphylactic s., c. anafilactóide. SIN anaphylactoid s.
reversible s., c. reversível; choque que responderá ao tratamento e cuja recuperação é possível.
septic s., c. séptico; **(1)** choque associado a infecção que liberou quantidades suficientemente grandes de toxinas ou substâncias vasoativas, incluindo citocinas, para estar associado a hipotensão; **(2)** choque associado a septicemia causada por bactérias Gram-negativas.
serum s., c. sérico; choque anafilático ou anafilactóide causado por injeção de soro antitóxico ou outro soro estranho.
shell s., fadiga de batalha. SIN battle *fatigue*.
spinal s., c. medular; depressão ou abolição transitória da atividade reflexa abaixo do nível de transecção ou lesão aguda da medula espinal.
systolic s., c. sistólico; o impacto anormalmente palpável, verificado por uma das mãos sobre a parede torácica, de uma primeira bulha acentuada.
toxic s., c. tóxico. VER toxic shock *syndrome*.
vasogenic s., c. vasogênico; choque resultante da atividade deprimida dos centros vasomotores superiores no tronco cerebral e bulbo, produzindo vasodilatação sem perda de líquido, de modo que o recipiente é desproporcionalmente grande. No choque oligêmico, o volume sanguíneo está reduzido; em ambos, o retorno do sangue venoso é inadequado.
wet s., c. insulínico. SIN insulin s.

Shone, John D., cardiologista inglês do século XX. VER S. *anomaly, complex, syndrome*.
shook jong (shuk-yong′). Koro. SIN koro.
Shope, Richard E., patologista norte-americano, 1902–1966. VER S. *fibroma*, fibroma *virus, papilloma*, papilloma *virus*.
short-chain ac·yl-CoA de·hy·dro·gen·ase. Desidrogenase da acil-CoA de cadeia curta. VER acyl-CoA dehydrogenase (NADPH).
short·sight·ed·ness (shōrt′sit-ed-nes). Miopia. SIN myopia.
shot-feel (shot′fēl). Sensação peculiar, como de descarga nervosa ou choque elétrico, passando rapidamente do topo da cabeça até os pés, algumas vezes descrita como uma sensação de ser atingido por um raio, que ocorre na acromegalia.
shoul·der (shōl′der). **1.** Ombro; a porção lateral da região escapular, onde a escápula se une à clavícula e ao úmero, sendo recoberta pela massa arredondada do músculo deltóide. **2.** Em odontologia, a plataforma formada pela junção das paredes gengival e axial em preparações restauradoras extracoronárias. [A.S. *sculder*]
frozen s., o. congelado. SIN adhesive *capsulitis*.
shoul·der blade (shōl′der blād). Escápula. SIN scapula.
show (shō). **1.** Aparecimento, manifestação. **2.** Primeiro aparecimento de sangue no início da menstruação. **3.** Sinal de trabalho de parto iminente, caracterizado pela emissão vaginal de pequeno volume de muco tinto de sangue, representando extrusão do tampão mucoso que preencheu o canal cervical durante a gravidez. [A.S. *scéawe*]
Shprintzen, R.J. VER Shprintzen *syndrome*.
Shrapnell, Henry J., anatomista inglês, 1761–1841. VER S. *membrane*.
shud·der (shŭd′er). Estremecimento; tremor convulsivo e involuntário. [I.m. *shodderen*]
carotid s., e. carotídeo; vibrações na crista do traçado do pulso carotídeo, observadas na estenose aórtica.
Shulman, Lawrence E., reumatologista norte-americano, *1919. VER S. *syndrome*.
Shumway, Norman, cirurgião norte-americano, *1923, desenvolveu um método para tratar a rejeição de tecido relacionada a transplantes cardíacos.
shunt (shŭnt). **1.** Derivar ou desviar. **2.** Derivação ou desvio de líquido para outro sistema contendo líquido para fistulação ou dispositivo protético. A nomenclatura inclui comumente a origem e o destino da derivação; p. ex., derivação atriovenosa, esplenorrenal, ventriculocisternal. VER TAMBÉM bypass. [I.m. *shunten*, retrair-se]
arteriovenous s. (A-V s.), d. arteriovenosa; a passagem de sangue diretamente das artérias para as veias, sem passar pela rede capilar.
Blalock s., d. de Blalock; derivação da artéria subclávia para a artéria pulmonar para aumentar a circulação pulmonar na cardiopatia cianótica, com redução do fluxo pulmonar.
Blalock-Taussig s., d. de Blalock-Taussig; anastomose paliativa da artéria subclávia com a artéria pulmonar.
cavopulmonary s., d. cavopulmonar. SIN cavopulmonary *anastomosis*.
Denver s., d. de Denver; tubo colocado por via subcutânea que conecta a cavidade abdominal de um paciente portador de ascite com a veia cava superior de baixa pressão. Essa derivação não apenas possui uma válvula unidirecional, como também uma câmara manualmente compressível para facilitar o fluxo.
dialysis s., d. de diálise; derivação arteriovenosa que conecta as cânulas arterial e venosa no braço ou na perna.
Dickens s., d. de Dickens. SIN pentose phosphate *pathway*.
distal splenorenal s., d. esplenorrenal distal; anastomose da veia esplênica com a veia renal esquerda, geralmente término-lateral, para controle da hipertensão porta. SIN renal-splenic venous s., Warren s.
Glenn s., d. de Glenn. SIN cavopulmonary *anastomosis*.
H s., d. em H; derivação látero-lateral entre vasos adjacentes, que utiliza um condutor conector; essa derivação é mais comumente colocada entre a veia mesentérica superior e a veia cava superior em pacientes com hipertensão porta. SIN H. graft.
hexose monophosphate s., d. de hexose monofosfato. SIN pentose phosphate *pathway*.
jejunoileal s., d. jejunoileal. SIN jejunoileal *bypass*.
left-to-right s., d. da esquerda para a direita; derivação de sangue do lado esquerdo do coração para o lado direito (como através de um defeito septal) ou da circulação sistêmica para a pulmonar (como através de um canal arterial persistente).
LeVeen s., d. de LeVeen; tubo colocado por via subcutânea, com válvula unidirecional, utilizado para transportar o líquido ascítico do abdome através da veia jugular para a veia cava superior.
mesocaval s., d. mesocava; **(1)** anastomose do lado da veia mesentérica superior com a extremidade proximal da veia cava inferior dividida para controle da hipertensão porta; **(2)** anastomose em H da veia cava inferior com a veia mesentérica superior, utilizando um conduto sintético ou veia autóloga.
pentose monophosphate s., d. de pentose monofosfato. SIN pentose phosphate *pathway*.
peritoneovenous s., d. peritoneovenosa; derivação, geralmente por um cateter, entre a cavidade peritoneal e o sistema venoso central torácico.
pleuroperitoneal s., d. pleuroperitoneal; cateter cirurgicamente implantado para transporte de líquido de um espaço pleural na cavidade peritoneal (peritoneal *cavity*) onde é absorvida; utilizada principalmente para o tratamento de derrames pleurais malignos.
pleurovenous s., d. pleurovenosa; cateter cirurgicamente implantado para transporte de líquido de um espaço pleural para o sistema venoso; raramente utilizada, principalmente para tratamento de derrames pleurais malignos.
portacaval s., d. portocava; **(1)** anastomose cirúrgica entre as veias porta e sistêmicas; **(2)** anastomose cirúrgica entre a veia porta e a veia cava.
portasystemic s., d. portossistêmica; derivação entre quaisquer partes dos sistemas venosos porta e sistêmico, incluindo derivações portocava, mesocava, esplenorrenal, ou derivações de ocorrência espontânea.

proximal splenorenal s., d. esplenorrenal proximal; anastomose da extremidade proximal da veia esplênica seccionada com o lado da veia renal esquerda para controle da hipertensão porta; considerada como derivação venosa visceral central ou completa.
Rapoport-Luebering s., d. de Rapoport-Luebering; parte da via glicolítica característica dos eritrócitos humanos, em que ocorre formação do 2,3-difosfoglicerato (2,3,-P_2Gri) como intermediário entre 1,3-P_2Gri e 3-fosfoglicerato; 2,3-P_2Gri é um importante regulador da afinidade da hemoglobina pelo oxigênio.
renal-splenic venous s., d. venosa esplenorrenal. SIN distal splenorenal s.
reversed s., d. invertida; derivação da direita para a esquerda que, previamente, era uma derivação da esquerda para a direita; raramente o oposto.
right-to-left s., d. da direita para a esquerda; passagem de sangue do lado direito do coração para o lado esquerdo (como através de um defeito septal) ou da artéria pulmonar para a aorta (como através de um canal arterial persistente); essa derivação só ocorre quando a pressão do lado direito excede a do lado esquerdo, como na estenose pulmonar avançada, ou quando a pressão da artéria pulmonar excede a pressão aórtica, como numa forma da síndrome de Eisenmenger ou na atresia tricúspide.
Scribner s., d. de Scribner; conexão de uma artéria, habitualmente a radial, com a veia cefálica através de um cateter extracorpóreo curto.
Torkildsen s., d. de Torkildsen; derivação ventriculocisternal. VER shunt (2).
tracheoesophageal s., derivação traqueoesofágica. VER tracheoesophageal puncture.
transjugular intrahepatic portosystemic s. (TIPS), d. portossistêmica intra-hepática transjugular; procedimento radiológico de intervenção para alívio da hipertensão porta.
Warburg-Dickens-Horecker s., d. de Warburg-Dickens-Horecker. SIN pentose phosphate *pathway.*
Warburg-Lipmann-Dickens-Horecker s., d. Warburg-Lipmann-Dickens-Horecker. SIN pentose phosphate *pathway.*
Warren s., d. de Warren. SIN distal splenorenal s.
Waterston s., d. de Waterston; criação de uma abertura estreita (cerca de 3 mm) entre a aorta ascendente e a artéria pulmonar direita subjacente para aumentar a circulação pulmonar na cardiopatia cianótica com redução do fluxo pulmonar.
shut·tle (shut'il). Transporte bidirecional; movimento regular de vai-e-vem; termo utilizado em relação a certos processos de transporte através de uma biomembrana.
glycerophosphate s., transporte bidirecional de glicerofosfato; mecanismo de transferência de equivalentes redutores do citosol para as mitocôndrias; o NADH é utilizado para síntese de glicerol 3-fosfato no citosol; a seguir, esse composto é transportado para as mitocôndrias, onde é convertido em diidroxi-acetona fosfato (DHAP), utilizando FAD; a seguir, DHAP retorna ao citosol para completar o ciclo; ocorre no tecido cerebral, no tecido adiposo marrom e no músculo branco.
malate-aspartate s., transporte bidirecional de malato-aspartato; mecanismo de transferência de equivalentes redutores do citosol para as mitocôndrias utilizando duas isozimas de malato desidrogenase e aspartato transaminase.
Shwachman, Harry, pediatra norte-americano, 1910–1986. VER Shwachman *syndrome,* Shwachman-Diamond *syndrome.*
Shwartzman, Gregory, bacteriologista russo nos Estados Unidos, 1896–1965. VER S. *phenomenon, reaction;* generalized S. *phenomenon;* Sanarelli-S. *phenomenon.*
Shy, George Milton, neurologista norte-americano, 1919–1967. VER S.-Drager *syndrome.*
Shy Abreviatura de 6-mercaptopurine (6-mercaptopurina).
SI Abreviatura de International System of Units (Système International d'Unités, Sistema Internacional de Unidades).
Si Símbolo de silicon (silício).
sI Abreviatura de 6-mercaptopurine ribonucleoside (ou 6-thioinosine) (ribonucleosídeo de 6-mercaptopurina ou 6-tioinosina).
Sia Abreviatura de sialic acids (ácidos siálicos).
SIADH Abreviatura de *syndrome* of inappropriate secretion of antidiuretic hormone (síndrome de secreção inapropriada de hormônio antidiurético).
⚠ **sial-.** Sial-. VER sialo-.
si·al·a·den (sī-al'ă-den). Glândula salivar. [sial- + G. *adēn,* glândula]
si·al·ad·e·ni·tis (sī'al-ad-ĕ-nī'tis). Sialadenite; inflamação de uma glândula salivar. SIN sialoadenitis. [sial- + G. *adēn,* glândula + *-itis,* inflamação]
si·al·ad·e·no·tro·pic (sī'al-ad'ĕ-nō-trop'ik). Sialadenotrópico; que influencia as glândulas salivares. [sial- + G. *adēn,* glândula + *tropē,* uma volta]
si·al·a·gogue (sī-al'ă-gog). Sialagogo. **1.** Que promove o fluxo de saliva. **2.** Agente que possui essa ação (p. ex., agentes anticolinesterásicos). SIN ptyalagogue, sialogogue. [sial- + G. *agōgos,* impelir]
si·al·ec·ta·sis (sī'ă-lek'tă-sis). Sialectasia; dilatação de um ducto salivar. SIN ptyalectasis. [sial- + G. *ektasis,* estiramento]
si·al·em·e·sis, si·al·e·me·sia (sī'al-em'ē-sis, -ē-mē'zē-ă). Sialêmese; vômito de saliva ou vômito causado por secreção excessiva de saliva ou acompanhando-a. [sial- + G. *emesis,* vômito]

si·al·ic (sī-al'ik). Siálico, salivar. SIN salivary.
si·al·ic ac·ids (Sia) (sī-al'ik). Ácidos siálicos; ésteres e outros derivados *N*- e *O*-acil do ácido neuramínico; os radicais dos ácidos siálicos são sialoil, se o OH do COOH for removido, e sialosil, se o OH provém do carbono anomérico (C-2) da estrutura cíclica; p. ex., ácido *N*-acetil-neuramínico.
si·al·i·dase (sī-al'i-dās). Sialidase; enzima que cliva resíduos acetilneuramínicos terminais de oligossacarídeos, glicoproteínas ou glicolipídios; presente no antígeno de superfície de mixovírus; utilizada em histoquímica para a remoção seletiva de sialomucinas, como das glândulas mucosas brônquicas e do intestino delgado; a deficiência dessa enzima resulta em sialidose. SIN neuraminidase.
si·al·i·do·sis (sī-al-i-dō'sis). Sialidose. SIN cherry-red spot myoclonus syndrome.
si·a·line (sī'ă-lēn). Sialina. SIN salivary.
si·a·lism, si·a·lis·mus (sī'ă-lizm, sī'ă-liz'mŭs). Sialismo. SIN sialorrhea. [G. *sialismos*]
⚠ **sialo-, sial-.** Sialo-, sial-. Saliva, glândulas salivares. VER TAMBÉM ptyal-. Cf. ptyal-. [G. *sialon*]
si·a·lo·ad·e·nec·to·my (sī'ă-lō-ad-ĕ-nek'tō-mē). Sialoadenectomia; excisão de uma glândula salivar. [sialo- + G. *adēn,* glândula + *ektomē,* excisão]
si·a·lo·ad·e·ni·tis (sī'ă-lō-ad-ĕ-nī'tis). Sialoadenite. SIN sialadenitis.
si·a·lo·ad·e·not·o·my (sī'ă-lō-ad-ĕ-not'ō-mē). Sialoadenotomia; incisão de uma glândula salivar. [sialo- + G. *adēn,* glândula + *tomē,* incisão]
si·a·lo·aer·oph·a·gy (sī'ă-lō-ār'of-ă-jē). Sialoaerofagia; hábito de deglutição freqüente pelo qual saliva e ar são levados ao estômago. SIN aerosialophagy. [sialo- + G. *aēr,* ar + *phagō,* comer]
si·a·lo·an·gi·ec·ta·sis (sī'ă-lō-an-jē-ek'tă-sis). Sialoangiectasia; dilatação dos ductos salivares. [sialo- + G. *angeion,* vaso + *ektasis,* estiramento]
si·a·lo·an·gi·i·tis (sī'ă-lō-an-jē-ī'tis). Sialoangiite; inflamação de um ducto salivar. [sialo- + G. *angeion,* vaso + *-itis,* inflamação]
si·a·lo·cele (sī'ă-lō-sēl). Sialocele. SIN ranula (2). [sialo- + G. *kēlē,* tumor]
si·a·lo·do·chi·tis (sī'ă-lō-dō-kī'tis). Sialodoquite; inflamação do ducto de uma glândula salivar. [sialo- + G. *dochē,* receptáculo + *-itis,* inflamação]
si·a·lo·do·cho·plas·ty (sī'ă-lō-dō'kō-plas'tē). Sialodocoplastia; reparo de um ducto salivar. [sialo- + G. *dochē,* receptáculo + *plassō,* modelar]
si·a·log·e·nous (sī'ă-loj'ē-nŭs). Sialógeno; que produz saliva. VER TAMBÉM sialagogue. [sialo- + G. *-gen,* que produz]
si·a·lo·glyc·o·sphin·go·lip·id. Sialoglicoesfingolipídio. SIN ganglioside.
si·a·lo·gogue (sī-al'ă-gog). Sialogogo. SIN sialagogue.
si·a·lo·gram (sī-al'ō-gram). Sialograma; imagem obtida por sialografia. [sialo- + G. *gramma,* escrever]
si·a·log·ra·phy (sī-ă-log'ră-fē). Sialografia; radiografia das glândulas e ductos salivares após a introdução de contraste nos ductos. SIN ptyalography. [sialo- + G. *graphō,* escrever]
si·a·lo·lith (sī'ă-lō-lith). Sialólito; cálculo salivar. SIN ptyalolith. [sialo- + G. *lithos,* pedra]
si·a·lo·li·thi·a·sis (sī'ă-lō-li-thī'ă-sis). Sialolitíase; formação ou presença de cálculo salivar. SIN ptyalolithiasis, salivolithiasis. [sialolith + G. *-iasis,* condição]
si·a·lo·li·thot·o·my (sī'ă-lō-li-thot'ō-mē). Sialolitotomia; incisão de um ducto ou glândula salivar para remoção de cálculo. SIN ptyalolithotomy. [sialolith + G. *tomē,* incisão]
si·al·o·met·a·pla·sia (sī'ă-lō-met-ă-plā'zē-ă). Sialometaplasia; metaplasia de células escamosas nos ductos salivares. [sialo- + metaplasia]
necrotizing s., s. necrotizante; metaplasia de células escamosas dos ductos e lóbulos das glândulas salivares, com necrose dos lóbulos das glândulas salivares; observada mais freqüentemente no palato duro.
si·a·lom·e·try (sī-ă-lom'ē-trē). Sialometria; medida da secreção salivar, geralmente para comparação de uma glândula desnervada ou doente com seu equivalente saudável. [sialo- + G. *metron,* medida]
si·a·lor·rhea (sī'ă-lō-rē'ă). Sialorréia; fluxo excessivo de saliva. SIN hygrostomia, ptyalism, salivation, sialism, sialismus, sialosis. [sialo- + G. *rhoia,* fluxo]
si·a·los·che·sis (sī'ă-los'kĕ-sis). Sialosquese; supressão da secreção de saliva. [sialo- + G. *schesis,* retenção]
si·a·lo·se·mi·ol·o·gy, si·a·lo·se·mei·ol·o·gy (sī-ă-lō-sē-mē-ol'ō-jē). Sialossemiologia; estudo e análise da saliva como exame complementar ao diagnóstico. [sialo- + G. *sēmeion,* sinal + *logos,* estudo]
si·a·lo·sis (sī'ă-lō'sis). Sialose. SIN sialorrhea.
si·a·lo·ste·no·sis (sī'ă-lō-ste-nō'sis). Sialoestenose; estreitamento de um ducto salivar. [sialo- + G. *stenōsis,* estreitamento]
sib. Irmãos, germano; membro de uma família. SIN sibling.
sib·i·lant (sib'i-lănt). Sibilante, que tem o caráter de silvo; refere-se a uma forma de ronco. [L. *sibilans (-ant-),* p. pres. de *sibilo,* sibilar]
sib·i·lus (sib'i-lŭs). Sibilo; estertor sibilante. [L. sibilo]
sib·ling. Irmãos, germano. SIN sib. [A.S. *sib,* relação + *-ling,* diminutivo]
sib·ship. Irmãos, germano. **1.** Estado recíproco entre indivíduos que possuem os mesmos pais. **2.** Irmãos; toda a prole de um casal. [A.S. *sib,* relação]

Sibson, Francis, anatomista inglês, 1814–1876. VER S. *aponeurosis, fascia, groove, muscle,* aortic *vestibule.*

Sicard, Jean A., médico francês, 1872–1929. VER Collet-S. *syndrome.*

sic·cant (sik′ant). Secante, sicativo. **1.** Que seca; que remove a umidade de substâncias adjacentes. **2.** Substância que possui essas propriedades. SIN siccative. [L. *siccans* (*-ant-*), p. pres. de *sicco,* pp. *-atus,* secar]

sic·ca·tive (sik′ă-tiv). Sicativo, secante. SIN siccant.

sic·cha·sia (sĭ-kā′zē-ă). **1.** Náusea. SIN nausea. **2.** Aversão a alimentos. [G. *sikchasia,* aversão, de *sikchos,* enjoado]

sic·co·la·bile (sik-ō-lā′bil, -bĭl). Sicolábil; sujeito a alteração ou destruição por ressecamento. [L. *siccus,* seco + *labilis,* perecível]

sic·co·sta·bile, sic·co·sta·ble (sik-ō-stā′bil; -bl). Sicoestável; não sujeito a alteração ou destruição por ressecamento. [L. *siccus,* seco + *stabilis,* estável]

sick (sik). **1.** Doente, enfermo; que sofre de doença. **2.** Nauseado, enjoado. SIN nauseated. [A.S. *seóc*]

sick·le·mia (sik-lē′mē-ă). Falcemia; presença de eritrócitos falciformes ou em forma de crescente no sangue periférico; observada na anemia falciforme e no traço falciforme.

sick·ling (sik′ling). Afoiçamento; produção de eritrócitos falciformes na circulação, como na anemia falciforme.

sick·ness (sik′nes). Doença, enfermidade, moléstia, mal. SIN disease (1).
  acute African sleeping s., d. do sono africana aguda. SIN Rhodesian *trypanosomiasis.*
  aerial s., náusea aérea. SIN altitude s.
  African sleeping s., d. do sono africana. VER Gambian *trypanosomiasis,* Rhodesian *trypanosomiasis.*
  air s., náusea aérea; forma de cinetose causada ao voar em avião.
  altitude s., náusea das alturas; síndrome causada por baixa pressão de oxigênio inspirado (como em grandes altitudes) e caracterizada por náuseas, cefaléia, dispnéia, mal-estar e insônia; nos casos graves, podem ocorrer edema pulmonar e síndrome de angústia respiratória do adulto. SIN Acosta disease, mountain s., puna, soroche. SIN aerial s., altitude disease.
  balloon s., náusea de balão; forma de cinetose que ocorre em indivíduos em decorrência da subida num balão.
  black s., leishmaniose visceral. SIN visceral *leishmaniasis.*
  caisson s., mal-do-caixão, mal-dos-mergulhadores; doença causada por rápida descompressão; assim denominado pela sua ocorrência em trabalhadores construindo túneis ou suportes para pontes, trabalhando em unidades fechadas sob alta pressão atmosférica para impedir a entrada de água circundante, denominadas "caissons". VER decompression s.
  car s., náusea do automóvel; forma de cinetose causada ao viajar em trem, automóvel ou ônibus.
  cave s., doença das cavernas; histoplasmose adquirida pela inalação do microganismo *Histoplasma capsulatum* em cavernas (enquanto praticam espeleologia) ou poços de minas contendo poleiros para aves ou morcego, condições favoráveis para o crescimento dos microrganismos.
  chronic African sleeping s., d. do sono africana crônica. SIN Gambian *trypanosomiasis.*
  chronic mountain s., mal-das-montanhas crônico; perda da tolerância a altitudes elevadas após exposição prolongada (p. ex., por residência), caracterizada por policitemia extrema, hipoxemia exagerada e redução da capacidade física e mental; aliviada com a descida. SIN altitude erythremia, chronic soroche, Monge disease.
  decompression s., d. da descompressão; um complexo de sintomas causado pelo escapamento de bolhas de nitrogênio da solução nos líquidos corporais, originalmente absorvidas em alta pressão atmosférica, em decorrência da redução abrupta da pressão atmosférica (rápida ascensão para grandes altitudes ou rápido retorno de um ambiente de ar comprimido); caracteriza-se por cefaléia, dor nos braços, pernas, articulações e epigástrio, prurido cutâneo, vertigem, dispnéia, tosse, sufocação, vômitos, fraqueza e, algumas vezes, paralisia e colapso circulatório periférico grave; podem ocorrer infartos ósseos devido a bolhas nos vasos nutrientes, resultando em seqüelas em longo prazo. VER TAMBÉM caisson s. SIN caisson disease, decompression disease, diver's palsy.
  East African sleeping s., d. do sono africana oriental. SIN Rhodesian *trypanosomiasis.*
  falling s., epilepsia. SIN epilepsy.
  green s., clorose. SIN chlorosis.
  green tobacco s., d. do tabaco verde; doença dos trabalhadores que colhem tabaco, caracterizada por cefaléia, tonteira e vômitos.
  Indian s., proctite gangrenosa epidêmica. SIN epidemic gangrenous *proctitis.*
  Jamaican vomiting s., d. do vômito jamaicana. SIN ackee *poisoning.*
  milk s., d. do leite; doença humana causada pela ingestão de leite contaminado de vacas que sofrem de paralisia agitante; as manifestações clínicas consistem em vômitos intensos, respiração difícil, delírio, convulsões, coma e morte; a recuperação da doença não-letal é lenta. SIN lactimorbus.
  morning s., êmese gravídica; as náuseas e os vômitos do início da gravidez. SIN morning vomiting, nausea gravidarum.
  motion s., cinetose; a síndrome da palidez, náuseas, fraqueza e mal-estar, que pode evoluir para vômitos e incapacitação, causada pela estimulação dos canais semicirculantes durante viagens ou movimentos como os de barco, avião, trem, automóvel, balanço ou brinquedo que gira. SIN kinesia.
  mountain s., d. das montanhas. SIN altitude s.
  radiation s., d. por radiação; condição sistêmica causada por irradiação corporal total significativa, observada após explosões ou acidentes nucleares, raramente após radioterapia. As manifestações dependem da dose, incluindo desde anorexia, náuseas, vômitos e leucopenia leve até trombocitopenia, com hemorragia, leucopenia pronunciada com infecção, anemia, lesão do sistema nervoso central e morte. SIN radiation poisoning.
  sea s., enjôo do mar; cinetose que ocorre em indivíduos que viajam de barco.
  serum s., d. do soro; doença por imunocomplexos que surge alguns dias (em geral, 1–2 semanas) após a injeção de soro ou proteína sérica estranhos, com reações locais e sistêmicas, como urticária, febre, linfadenopatia geral, edema, artrite e, em certas ocasiões, albuminúria ou nefrite grave; originalmente descrita em pacientes que recebiam soroterapia. O termo é algumas vezes empregado para descrever reações alérgicas a drogas clinicamente semelhantes. SIN serum disease, serum reaction.
  sleeping s., d. do sono. VER Gambian *trypanosomiasis,* Rhodesian *trypanosomiasis.*
  space s., d. espacial; tonteira em conseqüência de alterações no ouvido interno devido à ausência de gravidade. SIN physiologic vertigo.
  West African sleeping s., d. do sono africana ocidental. SIN Gambian *trypanosomiasis.*

side (sīd). Lado; uma das duas margens ou superfícies laterais de um corpo, a meio caminho entre a frente e as costas. [A.S. *sīde*]
  balancing s., l. de equilíbrio; em odontologia, o lado não-funcionante a partir do qual a mandíbula se move durante a mordida.
  working s., l. operacional; em odontologia, o segmento lateral de uma dentição em direção ao qual a mandíbula se move durante a função oclusiva.

side ef·fect. Efeito colateral; resultado de uma droga ou outra terapia além do efeito terapêutico desejado; em geral, mas não necessariamente, indica um efeito indesejado. Embora, tecnicamente, o efeito terapêutico além do limite desejado (p. ex., hemorragia causada por anticoagulante) seja um efeito colateral, o termo refere-se, com mais freqüência, aos resultados farmacológicos do tratamento não-relacionados ao objetivo habitual (p. ex., desenvolvimento de sinais de síndrome de Cushing com a esteroidoterapia).

sid·er·a·tion (sid-er-ā′shŭn). Sideração; qualquer crise súbita, como de apoplexia. [L. *sideror,* pp. *sideratus,* ser fulminado ou paralisado por uma constelação, de *sidus* (*sider-*), constelação, firmamento]

sidero-. Sidero-. Ferro. [G. *sidēros*]

sid·er·o·blast (sid′er-ō-blast). Sideroblasto; eritroblasto contendo grânulos de ferritina corados pela reação com azul-da-Prússia. [sidero- + G. *blastos,* germe]

sid·er·o·cyte (sid′er-ō-sīt). Siderócito; eritrócito que contém grânulos de ferro livre, detectados pela reação com azul-da-Prússia no sangue de fetos normais, onde representam 0,10–4,5% dos eritrócitos. [sidero- + G. *kytos,* célula]

sid·er·o·fi·bro·sis (sid′er-ō-fī-brō′sis). Siderofibrose; fibrose associada a pequenos focos nos quais ocorre deposição de ferro.

sid·er·og·en·ous (sid-er-oj′ē-nŭs). Siderógeno; formador de ferro. [sidero- + G. *-gen,* que produz]

sid·er·o·pe·nia (sid′er-ō-pē′nē-ă). Sideropenia; nível anormalmente baixo de ferro sérico. [sidero- + G. *penia,* pobreza]

sid·er·o·pe·nic (sid′er-ō-pē′nik). Sideropênico; caracterizado por sideropenia.

sid·er·o·phage (sid′er-ō-fāj). Siderófago. SIN siderophore. [sidero- + G. *phagō,* comer]

sid·er·o·phil, sid·er·o·phile (sid′er-ō-fil, -fīl). Siderófilo. **1.** Que absorve o ferro. SIN siderophilous. **2.** Célula ou tecido que contém ferro. [sidero- + G. *philos,* amigo]

sid·er·oph·i·lins (sid-er-ō-fil′in, -of′ĭ-lin). Siderofilinas; proteínas não-hêmicas de ligação do ferro; existem três classes principais de siderofilinas: a transferrina (1) (no sangue de vertebrados), a lactoferrina (no leite e outras secreções de mamíferos) e a conalbumina ou ovotransferrina (sangue e clara do ovo de aves).

sid·er·oph·i·lous (sid-er-of′ĭ-lŭs). Siderófilo. SIN siderophil (1).

sid·er·o·phore (sid′er-ō-for). Sideróforo; grande fagócito mononuclear extravasado que contém grânulos de hemossiderina, encontrado no escarro ou nos pulmões de indivíduos com congestão pulmonar de longa data em decorrência de insuficiência ventricular esquerda. VER TAMBÉM heart failure *cell.* SIN siderophage. [sidero- + G. *phoros,* portador]

sid·er·o·sil·i·co·sis (sid′er-ō-sil′ĭ-kō′sis). Siderossilicose; silicose devida à inalação de poeira contendo ferro e sílica. SIN silicosiderosis. [sidero- + silicosis]

sid·er·o·sis (sid-er-ō′sis). Siderose. **1.** Forma de pneumoconiose devida à presença de poeira de ferro. **2.** Pigmentação de qualquer parte em conseqüên-

siderosis

cia da deposição de pigmento contendo ferro; em geral, denominada hemossiderose. **3.** Excesso de ferro no sangue circulante. **4.** Degeneração da retina, da lente e da úvea em conseqüência da deposição intra-ocular de ferro. [sidero- + G. -*osis,* condição]

pulmonary s., s. pulmonar. SIN *pneumoconiosis siderotica.*

sid·er·ot·ic (sid-er-ot′ik). Siderótico; relativo à siderose; pigmentado por ferro ou contendo excesso de ferro.

SIDS Abreviatura de sudden infant death *syndrome* (síndrome de morte súbita do lactente).

Siegert, Ferdinand, pediatra alemão, 1865–1946. VER S. *sign.*

Siegle, Emil, otologista alemão, 1833–1900. VER S. *otoscope.*

sie·mens (S) (sē′menz). Siemens; a unidade de condutância elétrica do SI; a condutância de um corpo com uma resistência elétrica de 1 ohm, permitindo o fluxo de 1 ampère de corrente por volt aplicado; igual a 1 mho. SIN mho. [Sir William *Siemens,* engenheiro inglês nascido na Alemanha, 1823–1883]

Siemerling, Ernst, médico alemão, 1857–1931.

sieve (siv). Peneira; dispositivo reticulado ou perfurado para separar partículas finas de partículas mais grosseiras. [I. ant. *sive*]

molecular s., peneira molecular; material semelhante a gel com poros cujas dimensões excluem moléculas acima de determinados tamanhos; utilizada no fracionamento ou na purificação de macromoléculas.

sie·vert (Sv) (sē′vert). Sievert; a unidade de dose efetiva de radiação ionizante do SI, igual à dose absorvida em gray, pesada tanto para a qualidade de radiação em questão quanto para resposta do tecido à radiação. A unidade é o joule por quilograma e 1 Sv = 100 rem. VER effective *dose,* equivalent *dose.*

SIF Abreviatura de somatotropin release-inhibiting *factor* (fator inibidor da liberação de somatotropina).

Sig. Abreviatura do L. *signa,* rotular, escrever, ou *signetur,* aviar.

Siggaard-Andersen, Ole, bioquímico clínico dinamarquês, *1932. VER Siggaard-Andersen *nomogram.*

sigh (sī). **1.** Suspiro; inspiração e expiração audíveis sob a influência de alguma emoção. **2.** Suspirar. [A.S. *sīcan*]

sight (sīt). Visão; a capacidade ou faculdade de ver. VER TAMBÉM vision. [A.S. *gesihth*]

day s., v. diurna, nictalopia. SIN nyctalopia.
far s., hiperopia. SIN hyperopia.
long s., hiperopia. SIN hyperopia.
near s., miopia. SIN myopia.
night s., v. noturna. SIN hemeralopia.
second s., segunda visão; melhora da miopia no idoso em conseqüência do aumento da refratividade do núcleo da lente. SIN senile lenticular myopia.
short s., miopia. SIN myopia.

sig·ma (sig′mă). Sigma; a décima oitava letra do alfabeto grego, σ.

sig·ma·tism (sig′mă-tizm). Sigmatismo. SIN lisping. [G. *sigma,* a letra S]

sig·moid (sig′moyd). Sigmóide; semelhante ao contorno da letra S ou a uma das formas do sigma grego. [G. *sigma,* a letra S + *eidos,* semelhança]

♻ **sigmoid-.** Sigmoid-. VER sigmoido-.

sig·moi·dec·to·my (sig-moy-dek′tō-mē). Sigmoidectomia; excisão do colo sigmóide. [sigmoid- + G. *ektomē,* excisão]

sig·moid·ic·i·ty (sig′moyd-i-sa-tē). Sigmoidicidade; que descreve uma curva em forma de S; p. ex., a forma das curvas de cinética enzimática para enzimas que exibem cooperatividade homotrópica positiva.

sig·moid·i·tis (sig-moy-dī′tis). Sigmoidite; inflamação do colo sigmóide. [sigmoid- + G. *-itis,* inflamação]

♻ **sigmoido-, sigmoid-.** Sigmoido-, sigmoid-. Sigmóide, referindo-se habitualmente ao colo sigmóide. [G. *sigma,* a letra σ + *eidos,* semelhança]

sig·moi·do·pexy (sig-moy′dō-pek-sē). Sigmoidopexia; fixação cirúrgica do colo sigmóide a uma estrutura firme para corrigir o prolapso retal. [sigmoido- + G. *pēxis,* fixação]

sig·moi·do·proc·tos·to·my (sig-moy′dō-prok-tos′tō-mē). Sigmoidoproctostomia; anastomose entre o colo sigmóide e o reto. SIN sigmoidorectostomy. [sigmoido- + G. *prōktos,* ânus + *stoma,* boca]

sig·moi·do·rec·tos·to·my (sig-moy′dō-rek-tos′tō-mē). Sigmoidorretostomia. SIN sigmoidoproctostomy.

sig·moi·do·scope (sig-moy′dō-skōp). Sigmoidoscópio; endoscópio para visualizar a luz do colo sigmóide. SIN sigmoscope. [sigmoido- + G. *skopeō,* ver]

sig·moi·dos·co·py (sig′moy-dos′ko-pē). Sigmoidoscopia; inspeção, através de um endoscópio, do interior do colo sigmóide.

sig·moi·dos·to·my (sig′moy-dos′tō-mē). Sigmoidostomia; estabelecimento de um ânus artificial através de abertura no colo sigmóide. [sigmoido- + G. *stoma,* boca]

sig·moi·dot·o·my (sig′moy-dot′ō-mē). Sigmoidotomia; abertura cirúrgica do sigmóide. [sigmoido- + G. *tomē,* incisão]

sig·mo·scope (sig′mō-skōp). Sigmoscópio. SIN sigmoidoscope.

SIGN

sign (sīn). Sinal. **1.** Qualquer anormalidade indicando doença, passível de ser descoberta ao exame do paciente; indicação objetiva de doença, em contraste com um sintoma, que constitui uma indicação subjetiva de doença. **2.** Abreviatura ou símbolo. **3.** Em psicologia, qualquer objeto ou artefato (estímulo) que representa algo específico ou que transmite uma idéia específica para a pessoa que o percebe. [L. *signum,* marca]

Aaron s., s. de Aaron; na apendicite aguda, dor referida ou sensação de desconforto no epigástrio ou na região precordial com pressão firme e contínua sobre o ponto de McBurney.

Abadie s. of tabes dorsalis, s. de Abadie da tabes dorsal; falta de sensibilidade à compressão do tendão de Aquiles (tendão do calcâneo).

Abrahams s., s. de Abrahams; sinal obsoleto. **(1)** Estertores e outros ruídos adventícios, alterações dos sons respiratórios e aumento de sons sussurrados que podem ser ouvidos à ausculta sobre a extremidade acromial da clavícula algum tempo antes de se tornarem audíveis no ápice; ouvido primariamente na tuberculose pulmonar que afeta a porção apical do pulmão; **(2)** som maciço sem ressonância, isto é, aquele entre a macicez normal no ápice direito e a ausência absoluta de ressonância, ouvido à percussão naquela região, indicando evolução da tuberculose incipiente para avançada.

accessory s., s. acessório; achado freqüentemente, mas nem sempre, numa doença. SIN assident s.

antecedent s., s. prodrômico. SIN prodromic s.

assident s., s. acessório. SIN accessory s.

Auenbrugger s., s. de Auenbrugger; proeminência epigástrica observada em casos de derrame pericárdico volumoso.

Aufrecht s., s. de Aufrecht; sons respiratórios diminuídos ou ruidosos na traquéia, logo acima da incisura jugular, em casos de estenose.

Auspitz s., s. de Auspitz; achado típico da psoríase, em que a remoção de uma escama de pele provoca sangramento puntiforme.

Babinski s., s. de Babinski; **(1)** extensão do hálux e abdução dos outros dedos do pé em lugar do reflexo de flexão normal à estimulação plantar, considerado como indicador de comprometimento do trato piramidal (Babinski "positivo"). SIN Babinski phenomenon, Babinski reflex, great-toe reflex, parodoxical extensor reflex, toe phenomenon. **(2)** Na hemiplegia, fraqueza do platisma do lado acometido, conforme evidenciado em ações como soprar ou abrir a boca; **(3)** quando o paciente está em decúbito dorsal, com os braços cruzados na frente do tórax, e tenta sentar, a coxa do lado de uma paralisia orgânica (*organic paralysis*) é flexionada e o calcanhar elevado, enquanto o membro do lado sadio permanece plano; **(4)** na hemiplegia, o antebraço do lado afetado passa para uma posição de pronação quando colocado numa posição de supinação.

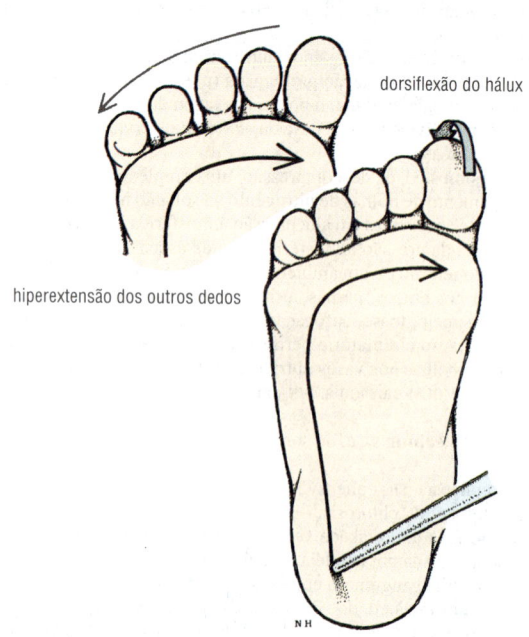

sinal de Babinski: com estimulação da planta do pé, a extensão do hálux com abertura dos outros dedos em leque constitui uma resposta normal até seis meses de idade, porém anormal posteriormente; a obtenção de uma resposta positiva é considerada indicadora de comprometimento do trato piramidal

Baccelli s., s. de Baccelli; sinal obsoleto: boa condução do sussurro em derrames pleurais não-purulentos. SIN aphonic pectoriloquy.

Ballance s., s. de Ballance; som maciço à percussão em ambos os flancos, constante do lado esquerdo, porém modificando-se com a mudança de posição do lado direito, considerado como indicação de ruptura do baço; a maciez se deve ao sangue líquido do lado direito, porém coagulado do lado esquerdo.

Bamberger s., s. de Bamberger; (1) pulso jugular na insuficiência tricúspide; (2) aloquiria. SIN allochiria; (3) macicez à percussão no ângulo da escápula, que desaparece quando o paciente se inclina para a frente, indicando pericardite com derrame. SIN Bamberger-Pins-Ewart.

Bamberger-Pins-Ewart s., s. de Bamberger-Pins-Ewart. SIN Bamberger s.

banana s., s. da banana; a curvatura anormal do cerebelo observada na ultra-sonografia num feto com malformação de Arnold-Chiari (Arnold-Chiari *malformation*).

Bárány s., s. de Bárány; nos casos de doença do ouvido, em que o vestíbulo está sadio, a injeção de água abaixo da temperatura corporal, no meato acústico externo, provoca nistagmo rotatório para o lado oposto; quando o líquido injetado está acima da temperatura corporal, os olhos giram para o lado injetado; se o labirinto estiver comprometido ou não-funcional, pode haver redução ou ausência do nistagmo.

Barré s., s. de Barré; um indivíduo hemiplégico colocado em decúbito ventral com os membros flexionados nos joelhos não consegue manter a posição de flexão do lado da lesão: estende a perna.

Bassler s., s. de Bassler; na apendicite crônica, o pinçamento do apêndice entre o polegar e o músculo ilíaco provoca dor aguda.

Bastedo s., s. de Bastedo; sinal obsoleto; na apendicite crônica, dor espontânea e à palpação na fossa ilíaca direita com insuflação de ar no colo.

Battle s., s. de Battle; equimose pós-auricular em casos de fratura da base do crânio.

B6 bronchus s., s. brônquico B6; na radiologia de pulmão, aparecimento de um broncograma aéreo do brônquio segmentar superior do lobo inferior, devido a atelectasia segmentar ou consolidação.

beak s., s. do bico; no esofagograma de contraste, o aspecto do esôfago distal na acalasia; também utilizado para descrever a porção proximal do canal pilórico em seriografias GI altas na estenose pilórica congênita.

Bechterew s., s. de Bechterew; paralisia de movimentos faciais automáticos, com preservação da capacidade de movimento voluntário.

Beevor s., s. de Beevor; na paralisia das porções inferiores do músculo reto do abdome, o umbigo desloca-se para cima.

Bergman s., s. de Bergman; achado radiográfico em que 1) o ureter está dilatado distalmente a uma obstrução ureteral e 2) um cateter, introduzido de modo retrógrado, enrola-se no ureter dilatado. SIN catheter coiling s.

Biederman s., s. de Biederman; enantema pardacento da porção inferior dos pilares anteriores das fauces em certos casos de sífilis.

Bielschowsky s., s. de Bielschowsky; na paralisia de um músculo oblíquo superior, a inclinação da cabeça para o lado do olho acometido provoca a rotação desse olho para cima.

Biot s., s. de Biot; padrão respiratório anormal caracterizado por períodos de apnéia e períodos em que o indivíduo tem várias incursões respiratórias de volume semelhante; observado quando a pressão intracraniana está aumentada.

Biot breathing s., s. respiratório de Biot; períodos irregulares de apnéia que alternam com quatro ou cinco incursões respiratórias profundas; observado quando a pressão intracraniana está aumentada.

Bird s., s. de Bird; uma zona de macicez à percussão, com ausência de sinais respiratórios no cisto hidático do pulmão.

Bjerrum s., s. de Bjerrum. SIN Bjerrum *scotoma*.

blue dot s., sinal da mácula azul; mácula azul ou preta visível sob a pele na face cranial do testículo ou epidídimo. Trata-se de um apêndice testicular torcido, que habitualmente é muito hipersensível.

Blumberg s., s. de Blumberg; dor que surge à descompressão súbita de uma área suspeita do abdome, indicando peritonite.

Bonhoeffer s., s. de Bonhoeffer; perda do tônus muscular normal na coréia.

Bozzolo s., s. de Bozzolo; vasos pulsantes na mucosa nasal, observados ocasionalmente no aneurisma torácico.

Branham s., s. de Branham; bradicardia que ocorre após compressão ou excisão de uma fístula arteriovenosa.

Braxton Hicks s., s. de Braxton Hicks; contrações uterinas irregulares que ocorrem depois do terceiro mês de gravidez.

Broadbent s., s. de Broadbent; retração da parede torácica, sincrônica com a sístole cardíaca, visível em qualquer parte, porém particularmente na linha axilar posterior esquerda; sinal de aderência pericárdica.

Brockenbrough s., s. de Brockenbrough; redução absoluta da pressão diferencial do batimento imediatamente após um batimento prematuro; sinal de estenose subaórtica hipertrófica idiopática.

Brudzinski s., s. de Brudzinski; (1) na meningite, com a flexão passiva de uma perna do paciente, observa-se um movimento semelhante na perna oposta. SIN contralateral reflex, contralateral s. (2) Na meningite, flexão involuntária dos joelhos e quadris após flexão do pescoço do paciente em decúbito dorsal. SIN neck s.

burning drops s., s. das gotas queimantes; em certos casos de úlcera gástrica perfurada, sensação de gotas de líquido quente caindo na cavidade abdominal ou de líquido intensamente quente sendo derramado na cavidade.

calcium s., s. do cálcio; na radiografia de tórax, deslocamento da linha da íntima calcificada da aorta para longe de sua parede externa, um achado numa pequena percentagem de casos de dissecção de sangue na média da aorta; prefere-se a expressão "calcificação deslocada da íntima" ao termo sinal do cálcio. VER aortic *dissection*.

Calkins s., s. de Calkins; mudança da forma discóide do útero para ovóide, indicando separação placentária da parede uterina.

Cantelli s., s. de Cantelli. VER doll's eye s.

Carman s., s. de Carman; em radiologia gástrica, o aspecto de uma úlcera maligna preenchida por contraste, que não se estende além da linha da parede gástrica, como o faz uma úlcera benigna; apresenta também uma borda espessa e pendente de tecido tumoral.

Carnett s., s. de Carnett; desaparecimento da dor abdominal à palpação quando os músculos abdominais anteriores são contraídos, indicando dor de origem intra-abdominal; sua persistência sugere uma origem na parede abdominal, que também é indicada quando a hipersensibilidade é produzida por delicado pinçamento de uma dobra de pele e gordura entre o polegar e o indicador.

Carvallo s., s. de Carvallo; aumento da intensidade do sopro pansistólico da regurgitação tricúspide durante a inspiração ou no final, que distingue o comprometimento tricúspide do mitral.

catheter coiling s., s. do cateter enrolado. SIN Bergman s.

Chaddock s., s. de Chaddock; quando a área cutânea do maléolo externo é irritada, ocorre extensão do hálux em casos de doença orgânica das vias reflexas corticospinais. SIN Chaddock-reflex.

Chadwick s., s. de Chadwick; coloração azulada do colo uterino e da vagina, um sinal de gravidez.

chandelier s., s. do candelabro; termo coloquial para referir-se à dor intensa produzida durante o exame pélvico de pacientes com doença inflamatória pélvica, em que a paciente responde ao estender-se para cima, em direção ao teto, para alívio.

Chaussier s., s. de Chaussier; dor intensa no epigástrio, um pródromo de eclampsia; pode ser de origem central ou causada por distensão da cápsula do fígado por hemorragia.

Chvostek s., s. de Chvostek; irritabilidade facial na tetania, sendo o espasmo unilateral do músculo orbicular do olho ou da boca excitado por leve percussão sobre o nervo facial, logo à frente do meato acústico externo. SIN Weiss s.

Claybrook s., s. de Claybrook; na ruptura de víscera abdominal, a transmissão de sons respiratórios e cardíacos através da parede abdominal.

clenched fist s., s. do punho cerrado; na angina de peito, a pressão do punho cerrado contra o tórax para indicar a qualidade constritiva e de compressão da dor.

Collier s., s. Collier; retração unilateral ou bilateral das pálpebras devido a lesão do mesencéfalo; ocorre em qualquer idade. VER setting sun s., Epstein s. SIN Collier tucked lid s.

Collier tucked lid s., s. de Collier. SIN Collier s.

colon cutoff s., s. de corte do colo; sinal radiográfico de doença (geralmente) inflamatória, impedindo a distensão da porção distal do colo transverso.

Comby s., s. de Comby; sinal precoce de sarampo, que consiste em placas finas e esbranquiçadas sobre as gengivas e mucosa oral, formadas de células epiteliais descamativas.

comet s., s. do cometa. SIN comet tail s.

comet tail s., s. da cauda de cometa; em radiologia de tórax, o aspecto curvado das artérias e veias pulmonares em associação a atelectasia redonda, fibrose associada a pleurisia organizada. SIN comet s.

commemorative s., s. comemorativo; fenômeno indicando a existência prévia de alguma outra doença além daquela presente no momento.

contralateral s., s. contralateral. SIN Brudzinski s. (1).

conventional s.'s, sinais convencionais; sinais que adquirem sua função através de costume social (lingüístico); p. ex., palavras, símbolos matemáticos. VER TAMBÉM symbol (4).

Corrigan s., s. de Corrigan; pulso cheio e forte, seguido de colapso súbito facilmente palpável, que ocorre na regurgitação aórtica. SIN Corrigan pulse.

Courvoisier s., lei de Courvoisier. SIN Courvoisier *law*.

crescent s., s. do crescente; (1) em radiografia de pulmão, um crescente de gás próximo ao ápice de uma lesão expansiva, indicando cavitação com um espaço acima dos resíduos; observado no aspergiloma, hidatidoma; (2) na tomografia computadorizada (computed *tomography*), uma alta camada atenuante de sangue recente num aneurisma; indica a ruptura de aneurisma da aorta abdominal; (3) na ultra-sonografia diagnóstica (diagnostic *ultrasound*), uma camada sonotransparente em crescente numa massa tumoral, tipicamente necrose em tumores de estroma do intestino delgado; (4) na ultra-sonografia diagnóstica, crescente hiperecóico, representando a borda penetrante de uma intussuscepção; também conhecido como "crescente numa rosca"; (5) em osteorradiologia, crescente transparente subcortical na cabeça do fêmur, indicando osteonecrose. SIN meniscus s.

Cruveilhier-Baumgarten s., s. de Cruveilhier-Baumgarten; sopro sobre o umbigo freqüente quando há "cabeça de medusa", resultante de hipertensão porta, habitualmente na cirrose hepática; a recanalização da veia umbilical com fluxo sanguíneo invertido do fígado para a parede abdominal cria o sopro.

Cullen s., s. de Cullen; escurecimento da pele periumbilical devido à presença de sangue, um sinal de hemorragia intraperitoneal, especialmente na ruptura de gravidez ectópica.

Dalrymple s., s. de Dalrymple; retração da pálpebra superior na doença de Graves, causando alargamento anormal da fissura palpebral.

Dance s., s. de Dance; discreta retração na adjacência da fossa ilíaca direita em alguns casos de intussuscepção.

Danforth s., s. de Danforth; dor no ombro à inspiração, devido à irritação do diafragma por hemoperitônio na ruptura de gravidez ectópica.

Darier s., s. de Darier; urticação ao tocar lesões cutâneas da urticária pigmentosa (mastocitose).

Dejerine s., s. de Dejerine; agravamento dos sintomas de irritação radicular com a tosse, espirro ou esforço para defecar.

Delbet s., s. de Delbet; em caso de aneurisma de uma artéria principal, circulação colateral eficiente se a nutrição da parte inferior estiver bem preservada, a despeito do desaparecimento do pulso.

de Musset s., s. de Musset. SIN Musset s.

D'Éspine s., s. de D'Éspine; sinal obsoleto (1) broncofonia sobre os processos espinhosos ouvida, em nível mais baixo do que no indivíduo sadio, na tuberculose pulmonar, (2) sussurro ecoado após uma palavra falada, ouvido com o estetoscópio colocado sobre a sétima vértebra cervical, ou primeira ou segunda vértebra dorsal, em casos de tuberculose das glândulas mediastínicas.

dimple s., da depressão; no dermatofibroma, depressão produzida quando a lesão é comprimida.

doll's eye s., s. do olho de boneca; movimento reflexo dos olhos na direção oposta àquela da cabeça; p. ex., os olhos dirigem-se para baixo quando a cabeça é elevada, e vice-versa (sinal de Cantelli); indicação da integridade funcional das vias tegmentares do tronco cerebral e nervos cranianos envolvidos no movimento ocular.

Dorendorf s., s. de Dorendorf; plenitude de um sulco supraclavicular no aneurisma do arco aórtico.

double-bubble s., s. da bolha dupla; em radiologia pediátrica, aspecto do estômago dilatado repleto de ar e bulbo duodenal, associado a atresia ou membrana duodenal, menos freqüentemente a vôlvulo do intestino médio.

double ring s., s. do anel duplo; dois anéis concêntricos em torno do nervo óptico, característicos da hipoplasia do nervo óptico.

double track s., s. do duplo rastro; em radiologia pediátrica, um sinal menos comum de estenose pilórica congênita, quando o bário é retido entre as pregas mucosas no piloro hipertrofiado.

drawer s., s. da gaveta; no exame do joelho, o deslizamento anterior ou posterior da tíbia com aplicação de estresse, indicando frouxidão ou laceração dos ligamentos cruzados anteriores (deslizamento anterior) ou posteriores (deslizamento posterior) do joelho. SIN drawer test.

drooping lily s., s. do lírio caído; em urografia, sinal de um sistema coletor renal duplo com obstrução do sistema superior causando depressão dos cálices opacificados do sistema inferior, de modo que parecem estar caindo.

Drummond s., s. de Drummond; em determinados casos de aneurisma aórtico, um sopro sincrônico com a sístole cardíaca, proveniente das narinas, quando a boca está fechada.

Duchenne s., s. de Duchenne; afundamento do epigástrio durante a inspiração na paralisia do diafragma.

Dupuytren s., s. de Dupuytren; (1) na luxação congênita, ocorre movimento livre para cima e para baixo da cabeça do fêmur com tração intermitente; (2) sensação de crepitação à pressão sobre o osso em certos casos de sarcoma.

Duroziez s., s. de Duroziez. SIN Duroziez murmur.

Ebstein s., s. de Ebstein; no derrame pericárdico, macicez à percussão do ângulo cárdio-hepático.

s. of edema of lower eyelid, s. de edema da pálpebra inferior; edema da pálpebra inferior observado na insuficiência cardíaca congestiva, no mixedema ou na nefrose.

Epstein s., s. de Epstein; retração palpebral num lactente, conferindo-lhe uma expressão aterrorizada e "olhar selvagem". VER setting sun s., Collier s.

Ewart s., s. de Ewart; em derrames pericárdicos grandes, área de macicez com respiração brônquica e broncofonia abaixo do ângulo da escápula esquerda. SIN Pins s.

Ewing s., s. de Ewing; hipersensibilidade à palpação no ângulo interno superior da órbita, no ponto de fixação da inserção do músculo oblíquo superior, indicando fechamento da saída do seio frontal.

Faget s., s. de Faget; pulso lento com temperatura elevada, freqüentemente observado na febre amarela.

fan s., s. do leque; afastamento dos dedos dos pés no sinal de Babinski completo.

Fischer s., s. de Fischer; sinal obsoleto: na tuberculose das glândulas mediastínicas ou peribrônquicas, após curvar ao máximo a cabeça do paciente para trás, a ausculta sobre o manúbrio do esterno revela, algumas vezes, um sopro alto contínuo produzido pela pressão das glândulas aumentadas sobre os grandes vasos do mediastino. SIN Fischer symptom.

fissure s., s. da fissura; na cintilografia de perfusão dos pulmões, captação diminuída de radionuclídeo na periferia de cada lobo, tornando as fissuras visíveis; produzido por uma variedade de doenças e artefatos.

flag s., s. da bandeira; faixas de coloração dos cabelos (avermelhados, louros ou cinza, dependendo da cor original), em decorrência de flutuações nutricionais características do *kwashiorkor*, bem como em doenças com depleção protéica, como a colite ulcerativa.

Forchheimer s., s. de Forchheimer; presença, no sarampo, de erupção maculopapular avermelhada no palato mole.

Fothergill s., s. de Fothergill; no hematoma da bainha do músculo reto, o hematoma produz uma massa que não cruza a linha mediana e permanece palpável quando o músculo reto está tenso.

Friedreich s., s. de Friedreich; no pericárdio aderente, colapso súbito das veias previamente distendidas do pescoço em cada diástole do coração.

Froment s., s. de Froment; flexão da falange distal do polegar quando uma folha de papel é mantida entre o polegar e o indicador na paralisia do nervo ulnar.

Gaenslen s., s. de Gaenslen; dor à hiperextensão do quadril com a pelve fixada por flexão do quadril oposto; provoca estresse por torção nas articulações sacroilíaca e lombossacra.

Gauss s., s. de Gauss; mobilidade acentuada do útero nas primeiras semanas de gravidez.

Glasgow s., s. de Glasgow; sopro sistólico ouvido sobre a artéria braquial no aneurisma da aorta.

gloved-finger s., sinal do dedo-luva; em radiologia de tórax, o aspecto da impactação mucóide dos brônquios ramificados.

Goggia s., s. de Goggia; a fibrilação do músculo bíceps, quando pinçado e percutido, restringe-se a uma área limitada em casos de doença debilitante, enquanto é geral no indivíduo sadio.

Goldstein toe s., s. do hálux de Goldstein; aumento do espaço entre o hálux e seu vizinho, observado na síndrome de Down, algumas vezes no cretinismo e como variante normal.

Goodell s., s. de Goodell; amolecimento do colo do útero e da vagina, indicando geralmente gravidez.

Gordon s., s. de Gordon. SIN finger *phenomenon*.

Gorlin s., s. de Gorlin; facilidade incomum em tocar a ponta do nariz com a língua, observada na síndrome de Ehlers-Danlos.

Gower s., s. de Gower; uso dos músculos dos membros para assumir uma posição sentada, em que o paciente utiliza as mãos para "elevar" as pernas; observada em condições de fraqueza da cintura pélvica e dos músculos proximais da perna.

Graefe s., s. de Graefe; na doença de Graves, retardo da pálpebra superior ao acompanhar a rotação do globo ocular para baixo. SIN von Graefe s.

Grasset s., s. de Grasset; contração normal do músculo esternocleidomastóideo do lado paralisado em casos de hemiplegia.

Grey Turner s., s. de Grey Turner; áreas locais de pigmentação em torno do umbigo e na região da virilha, na pancreatite hemorrágica aguda e em outras causas de hemorragia retroperitoneal.

Griesinger s., s. de Griesinger; eritema e edema na parte posterior do processo mastóide, devido à trombose séptica da veia emissária mastóidea, indicando tromboflebite do seio sigmóide.

Grocco s., s. de Grocco; (1) dilatação aguda do coração após esforço muscular, descrita na doença de Graves, ocorre também em várias formas de miocardiopatia; (2) extensão da macicez hepática vários centímetros para a esquerda da linha média espinal em casos de aumento do fígado.

groove s., s. do sulco; linfonodos grandes, duros, fixos e extremamente hipersensíveis à palpação na virilha, acima e abaixo do ligamento inguinal, com um sulco ao longo do ligamento; característico do linfogranuloma venéreo.

Gunn s., s. de Gunn; (1) compressão da veia subjacente em cruzamentos arteriovenosos observada na oftalmoscópio na esclerose arteriolar; (2) com estimulação alternada com luz, a pupila de um olho com defeito de transmissão do nervo óptico sofre pouca constrição, ou até mesmo dilata-se quando estimulada (defeito pupilar aferente relativo). SIN Marcus Gunn s.

Gunn crossing s., s. de cruzamento de Gunn; cruzamento arteriovenoso retiniano com compressão venosa na doença hipertensiva.

Guyon s., s. de Guyon; (1) rechaço do rim em casos de nefroptose, especialmente quando existe também um tumor renal; (2) o nervo hipoglosso localiza-se diretamente sobre a artéria carótida externa, de modo que esse vaso pode ser distinguido da carótida interna quando há necessidade de ligadura.

halo s., s. do halo; elevação da camada de gordura subcutânea sobre o crânio de um feto morto ou moribundo; considerado sinal radiológico mais comum de morte fetal.

halo s. of hydrops, s. do halo da hidropisia; sinal radiológico desacreditado de hidropisia fetal causado por edema do couro cabeludo, de modo que o crânio é circundado por uma coroa definida.
Hamman s., s. de Hamman; ruído de crepitação áspero, sincrônico com o batimento cardíaco, ouvido sobre o precórdio e, algumas vezes, a certa distância do tórax no enfisema mediastinal (mediastinal *emphysema*).
Hawkins impingement s., sinal de compressão de Hawkins; dor produzida pela rotação medial forçada do úmero em 90° de abdução.
Hegar s., s. de Hegar; amolecimento e compressibilidade do segmento inferior do útero no início da gravidez (em torno da sétima semana) que, ao exame bimanual, é percebido pelo dedo na vagina como se o colo e o corpo do útero estivessem separados ou apenas conectados por uma fina faixa de tecido.
Heim-Kreysig s., s. de Heim-Kreysig; no pericárdio aderente, uma retração dos espaços intercostais, sincrônica com a sístole cardíaca. SIN Kreysig s.
Hennebert s., s. de Hennebert; nistagmo produzido por pressão aplicada a um canal auditivo externo obliterado; pode ser observado na fístula labiríntica ou com membrana timpânica íntegra no comprometimento sifilítico da cápsula ótica.
Higoumenakia s., s. de Higoumenakia; tumefação esternoclavicular na sífilis congênita tardia.
Hill s., s. de Hill; na insuficiência aórtica, pressão arterial sistólica maior nas pernas do que nos braços; a pressão sistólica arterial normal na perna é 10–20 mm Hg maior que no braço, ao passo que, na insuficiência aórtica, a diferença pode ser de 60–100 mm Hg. SIN Hill phenomenon.
Hoagland s., s. de Hoagland; edema das pálpebras na mononucleose infecciosa.
Hoffmann s., s. de Hoffmann; **(1)** na tetania latente, a estimulação mecânica leve do nervo trigêmeo provoca dor intensa; **(2)** flexão da falange terminal do polegar e da segunda e terceira falanges de um ou mais dedos da mão quando a superfície volar da falange terminal dos dedos é percutida. SIN digital reflex, Hoffmann reflex, snapping reflex.
Homans s., s. de Homans; dor na panturrilha quando o tornozelo é submetido a dorsiflexão lenta e suave (com o joelho flexionado), indicando trombose incipiente ou estabelecida nas veias da perna.
Hoover s.'s, sinais de Hoover; **(1)** quando se pede a um indivíduo em decúbito dorsal que eleve uma das pernas, ele involuntariamente cria uma contrapressão com o calcanhar da outra perna; se essa perna estiver paralisada, qualquer força muscular nela preservada será exercida dessa maneira; ou, se o paciente tentar levantar uma perna paralisada, a contrapressão será feita com o outro calcanhar, independentemente da ocorrência ou não de qualquer movimento no membro paralisado; não observado na histeria ou no fingimento; **(2)** modificação do movimento das bordas costais durante a respiração, causada por achatamento do diafragma; sugere a possibilidade de empiema ou de outra condição intratorácica causando uma alteração no contorno do diafragma.
iconic s.'s, sinais icônicos; sinais que adquirem sua função através da semelhança com seu significado; p. ex., uma fotografia como sinal da pessoa representada.
impingement s., s. de compressão; dor em pacientes com tendinite ou laceração do manguito rotator no espaço subacromial, produzida por manobras provocativas ao exame físico.
indexical s.'s, sinais indicadores; sinais que adquirem sua função através de uma conexão causal com seu significado; p. ex., fumaça como sinal de fogo.
inferior triangle s., s. do triângulo inferior; na radiologia de tórax, deslocamento lateral da pleura mediastínica próximo ao diafragma, associado a colapso do lobo superior, geralmente do lado direito. Cf. superior triangle s.
Jackson s., s. de Jackson; durante a respiração silenciosa, o movimento do lado paralisado do tórax pode ser maior que o do lado oposto, ao passo que, na respiração forçada, o lado paralisado movimenta-se menos do que o outro.
Joffroy s., s. de Joffroy; distúrbio da faculdade aritmética (o indivíduo é incapaz de fazer cálculos simples de adição ou multiplicação) nos estágios iniciais de doença cerebral orgânica.
Kehr s., s. de Kehr; dor violenta no ombro esquerdo em caso de ruptura do braço.
Kerandel s., s. de Kerandel; sensação tardia de dor indicando tripanossomíase africana.
Kernig s., s. de Kernig; quando o indivíduo está em decúbito dorsal com a coxa em flexão formando um ângulo reto com o eixo do tronco, a extensão completa da perna sobre a coxa é impossível; presente em várias formas de meningite.
Kestenbaum s., s. de Kestenbaum; redução do número de arteríolas que atravessam as margens do disco óptico como sinal de neurite óptica.
knuckle s., s. da falange; na radiografia de tórax, afilamento abrupto de uma grande artéria pulmonar causado por embolia pulmonar.
Kocher s., s. de Kocher; na doença de Graves, com o olhar para cima, o globo não acompanha o movimento da pálpebra superior.
Kreysig s., s. de Kreysig. SIN Heim-Kreysig s.
Kussmaul s., s. de Kussmaul; na pericardite constritiva, aumento paradoxal da distensão e pressão venosas ou ausência de colapso durante a inspiração; sinal observado ocasionalmente na pericardite com derrame constritiva, quando o líquido pericárdico, causando tamponamento, situa-se acima de uma epicardite constritiva.
Lancisi s., s. de Lancisi; grande onda venosa jugular sistólica causada por regurgitação tricúspide, substituindo a depressão sistólica negativa normal (colapso "x").
Landolfi s., s. de Landolfi; na insuficiência aórtica, contração sistólica e dilatação diastólica da pupila.
Lasègue s., s. de Lasègue; quando o indivíduo está em decúbito dorsal com flexão do quadril e extensão do joelho, a dorsiflexão do tornozelo ao causar dor ou espasmo muscular na face posterior da coxa, indica irritação da raiz lombar ou do nervo ciático.
Legendre s., s. de Legendre; na hemiplegia facial de origem central, quando o examinador levanta as pálpebras dos olhos ativamente fechados, a resistência é menor do lado acometido.
lemon s., s. do limão; na ultra-sonografia, achado de recorte do osso frontal associado à malformação de Arnold-Chiari (Arnold-Chiari *malformation*).
Leri s., s. de Leri; a flexão voluntária do cotovelo é impossível em caso de hemiplegia, quando o punho do mesmo lado é passivamente fletido.
Leser-Trélat s., s. de Leser-Trélat; o súbito aparecimento e rápido aumento no número e tamanho de ceratoses seborreicas com prurido; associado a neoplasia maligna interna.
Lhermitte s., s. de Lhermitte, choques súbitos semelhantes a choques elétricos que descem pela coluna ao flexionar a cabeça.
local s., s. local; a característica de uma sensação que permite distingui-la de outra sensação através da localização de sua posição no espaço.
Lorenz s., s. de Lorenz; sinal obsoleto: rigidez da coluna torácica na tuberculose pulmonar inicial.
Lovibond profile s., s. do perfil de Lovibond. SIN Lovibond *angle.*
Macewen s., s. de Macewen; a percussão do crânio produz um som de pote rachado em casos de hidrocefalia. SIN Macewen symptom.
Magendie-Hertwig s., s. de Magendie-Hertwig; desvio oblíquo dos olhos nas lesões cerebelares agudas. SIN Magendie-Hertwig syndrome.

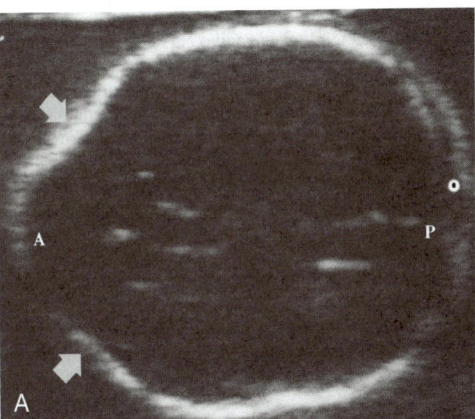

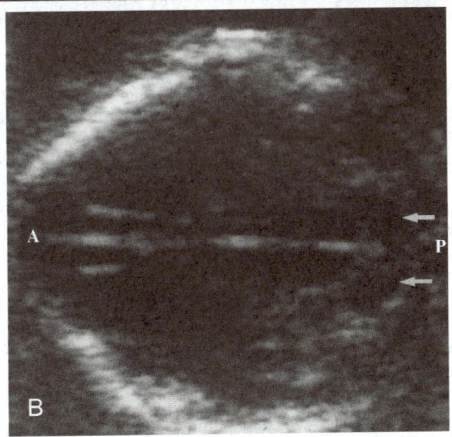

sinais do limão e da banana: (A) sinal do limão; a concavidade dos ossos frontais (setas) confere ao crânio fetal a forma de um "limão" em incidências no plano axial; esse aspecto sugere a possibilidade de espinha bífida; (B) sinal da banana; a compressão dos hemisférios cerebelares associada à herniação do tronco cerebral para baixo e à malformação de Chiari II resulta numa "banana" hipoecóica (setas) na face posterior do crânio fetal no plano axial (A indica anterior; P indica posterior)

Magnan s., s. de Magnan; parestesia na psicose de viciados em cocaína, que imaginam possuir um corpo estranho, no formato de um pó ou areia fina sob a pele, que está constantemente modificando sua posição.

Magnus s., s. de Magnus; sinal obsoleto: após a morte, a constrição de um membro ou de um de seus segmentos não é seguida de congestão venosa da parte distal.

Mannkopf s., s. de Mannkopf; aceleração do pulso quando um ponto doloroso é pressionado.

Marañón s., s. de Marañón; na doença de Graves, reação vasomotora que ocorre após estimulação da pele sobre a garganta.

Marcus Gunn s., s. de Marcus Gunn. SIN Gunn s.

McBurney s., s. de McBurney; hipersensibilidade a dois terços de distância entre o umbigo e a espinha ilíaca ântero-superior; observado na apendicite.

meniscus s., s. do menisco. SIN crescent s.

Metenier s., s. de Metenier; eversão fácil da pálpebra superior na síndrome de Ehlers-Danlos.

Mirchamp s., s. de Mirchamp; sintoma premonitório de caxumba; se uma substância de sabor forte for colocada sobre a língua, ocorre secreção reflexa dolorosa de saliva na glândula que é o local da infecção incipiente.

Möbius s., s. de Möbius; comprometimento da convergência ocular na doença de Graves.

Mosler s., s. de Mosler; hipersensibilidade sobre o esterno num paciente com anemia mieloblástica aguda.

Muehrcke s., s. de Muehrcke. SIN Muehrcke bands, em band.

Müller s., s. de Müller; na insuficiência aórtica, movimentos pulsáteis rítmicos da úvula, sincrônicos com a ação cardíaca; acompanhados de edema e eritema do véu palatino e das tonsilas.

Munson s., s. de Munson; no ceratocone, o arqueamento adicional da pálpebra inferior causado pela córnea deformada quando o olho roda para baixo.

Murphy s., s. de Murphy; dor à palpação na área subcostal direita durante a inspiração, freqüentemente associada a colecistite aguda.

Musset s., s. de Musset; na incompetência da valva aórtica, a inclinação rítmica da cabeça, sincrônica com o batimento cardíaco. SIN de Musset s.

neck s., s. do pescoço. SIN Brudzinski s. (2).

Neer impingement s., s. de compressão de Neer; dor produzida pela elevação passiva máxima do ombro superior.

Néri s., s. de Néri; na hemiplegia, o joelho curva-se espontaneamente quando a perna é estendida passivamente.

Nikolsky s., s. de Nikolsky; vulnerabilidade peculiar da pele no pênfigo vulgar; a epiderme aparentemente normal pode ser separada na camada basal e removida quando pressionada com movimento de deslizamento.

objective s., s. objetivo; sinal que é evidente ao examinador.

s. of the orbicularis, s. do orbicular; na hemiplegia, a incapacidade de fechar voluntariamente o olho do lado paralisado, exceto em conjunção com o fechamento do outro olho. SIN Revilliod s.

Osler s., s. de Osler. SIN Osler node.

painful arc s., s. do arco doloroso; dor produzida durante a abdução ativa do membro inferior entre 60° e 120°.

Pastia s., s. de Pastia; linhas transversais róseas ou vermelhas no ângulo do cotovelo no estágio pré-eruptivo da escarlatina; persistem durante a estágio eruptivo e permanecem como linhas pigmentadas após a descamação. SIN Thomson s.

patellar apprehension s., s. de apreensão patelar; achado físico em que o deslocamento lateral forçado da patela provoca ansiedade e resistência em pacientes com história de instabilidade patelar lateral.

Payr s., s. de Payr; dor à compressão da planta do pé; sinal de tromboflebite.

Perez s., s. de Perez; estertores audíveis sobre a parte superior do tórax quando os braços são elevados e abaixados alternadamente; comum em casos de mediastinite fibrosa e, também, de aneurisma do arco aórtico.

Pfuhl s., s. de Pfuhl; a pressão exercida pelo pus no interior de um abscesso subfrênico aumenta durante a inspiração e diminui durante a expiração, o contrário do que ocorre no caso de uma coleção purulenta acima do diafragma; quando o diafragma está paralisado, essa distinção é perdida.

physical s., s. físico; sinal observado à, ou produzido por, inspeção, palpação, percussão ou ausculta.

Piltz s., s. de Piltz. SIN eye-closure pupil reaction.

Pins s., s. de Pins. SIN Ewart s.

Pitres s., s. de Pitres. (1) SIN haphalgesia; (2) redução da sensação nos testículos e no escroto no tabes dorsal.

placental s., s. placentário; sangramento endometrial discreto que ocorre em certos animais e, algumas vezes, em mulheres no momento da implantação do ovo fertilizado. Nas mulheres, em que o sangue aparece externamente, pode ser confundido com um período menstrual escasso.

Pool-Schlesinger s., s. de Pool-Schlesinger. SIN Pool phenomenon (1).

Potain s., s. de Potain; na dilatação da aorta, macicez à percussão que se estende do manúbrio do esterno em direção ao segundo espaço intercostal e terceira cartilagem costal à direita, estendendo-se o limite superior a partir da base do esterno no segmento de um círculo à direita.

prodromic s., s. prodrômico; sinal que aparece durante o pródromo de uma doença. SIN antecedent s.

pseudo-Graefe s., s. pseudo-Graefe; fenômeno de retração palpebral semelhante ao sinal de Graefe, porém devido à regeneração aberrante de fibras do nervo oculomotor no músculo elevador da pálpebra superior.

puddle s., s. do piparote; sinal de líquido abdominal livre: o paciente fica na posição de quatro apoios; um flanco é percutido por repetidos piparotes leves de intensidade constante, enquanto se coloca um estetoscópio tipo Bowles sobre a porção mais baixa do abdome, deslocando-o gradualmente em direção ao flanco oposto à percussão; um súbito aumento na intensidade do som captado pelo estetoscópio indica o nível do líquido.

pyramid s., s. da pirâmide; quaisquer sintomas ou sinais indicativos de lesão dos tratos piramidais, como o sinal de Babinski ou sinal de Gordon, paralisia espinal espástica, clônus do pé, etc.

Quant s., s. de Quant; depressão em forma de T no osso occipital que ocorre em muitos casos de raquitismo, especialmente em lactentes deitados constantemente na cama (compressão do occipúcio).

Quénu-Muret s., s. de Quénu-Muret; no aneurisma, a circulação colateral bem mantida indicada pelo fluxo de sangue quando a artéria principal do membro é comprimida e se efetua uma punção na periferia.

Quincke s., s. de Quincke. SIN Quincke pulse.

Ransohoff s., s. de Ransohoff; pigmentação amarela na região umbilical na ruptura do colédoco.

Raynaud s., s. de Raynaud. SIN acrocyanosis.

red, white, and blue s., s. vermelho, branco e azul; a ocorrência simultânea de eritema, isquemia e necrose numa ferida, como no loxoscelismo.

Remak s., s. de Remak; dissociação da sensibilidade tátil e sensação de dor na tabes dorsal e na polineurite.

reversed-three s., s. do três invertido; no esofagograma de um paciente com coarctação da aorta, a forma do esôfago preenchido por contraste produzida pelo arco aórtico (convexidade superior) e dilatação pós-estenótica (convexidade inferior); a cúspide do três para trás encontra-se no nível da própria coarctação.

Revilliod s., s. de Revilliod. SIN s. of the orbicularis.

Ripault s., s. de Ripault; sinal de morte, que consiste em alteração permanente da forma da pupila produzida por pressão unilateral do bulbo do olho.

Romaña s., s de Romaña; edema acentuado de uma ou de ambas as pálpebras, geralmente edema palpebral unilateral, considerado uma resposta de sensibilização à picada do triatomíneo infectado por *Trypanosoma cruzi*, e como forte indício de doença de Chagas aguda.

Romberg s., s. de Romberg; com os pés aproximados, o indivíduo fica com os olhos abertos e, a seguir, fechados; se o fechamento dos olhos aumentar o desequilíbrio, indica uma perda do controle proprioceptivo, e o sinal é positivo. SIN Romberg test, rombergism, station test.

Rosenbach s., s. de Rosenbach, s. de Rosenbach; perda do reflexo abdominal em casos de inflamação aguda das vísceras.

Rossolimo s., reflexo de Rossolimo. SIN Rossolimo reflex.

Rotch s., s. de Rotch; no derrame pericárdico, macicez à percussão no quinto espaço intercostal à direita.

Rovsing s., s. de Rovsing; dor no ponto de McBurney induzida em casos de apendicite por pressão exercida sobre o colo descendente.

Rumpel-Leede s., s. de Rumpel-Leede. SIN capillary fragility test.

Russell s., s. de Russell; abrasões e cicatrizes no dorso das mãos de indivíduos com bulimia, geralmente devido a tentativas manuais de auto-indução do vômito.

Sansom s., s. de Sansom; na estenose mitral, duplicação aparente da segunda bulha cardíaca.

scarf s., s. do cachecol; sinal utilizado na escala de Dubowitz (q.v.) para avaliação da idade de desenvolvimento e tônus muscular em recém-nascidos. O braço do recém-nascido é puxado lateralmente, cruzando o tórax; no neonato hipotônico, o cotovelo cruza a linha média, enquanto, no recém-nascido a termo com tônus normal, o cotovelo não atinge a linha média.

Schapiro s., sinal de Schapiro; na falência do miocárdio, não ocorre redução do pulso quando o paciente se deita.

Schlesinger s., s. Schlesinger. SIN Pool phenomenon (1).

Schultze s., s. de Schultze; na tetania latente, a percussão da língua causa a sua depressão com dorso côncavo. SIN tongue phenomenon.

scimitar s., s. da cimitarra; estrutura curvilínea observada radiograficamente no pulmão e associada a anormalidade da drenagem venosa pulmonar, sugerindo a forma de um sabre; também utilizado para referir-se à forma recortada do sacro no disrafismo espinal com meningocele anterior.

Seeligmüller s., s. de Seeligmüller; contração da pupila no lado afetado na neuralgia facial.

Seidel s., s. de Seidel; escotoma falciforme que aparece como extensão superior ou inferior do ponto cego.

sentinel loop s., s. da alça sentinela; em radiologia gastrointestinal, dilatação de um segmento do intestino delgado ou grosso, indicando íleo paralítico localizado decorrente de inflamação adjacente.

setting sun s., sinal do pôr-do-sol; retração da pálpebra superior sem olhar para cima, de modo que a íris parece "pôr-se" abaixo da pálpebra inferior; sinal sugestivo de lesão neurológica no recém-nascido, geralmente desaparecendo sem deixar seqüelas. VER Collier s., Epstein s.

S s. of Golden, s. do S de Golden; em radiologia pulmonar, a combinação de um lobo atelectático e de uma massa obstrutiva central, produzindo uma concavidade e uma convexidade, semelhante à letra S.

Shibley s., s. de Shibley; à auscultação do tórax, o som "i" é ouvido como "ah" sobre uma área de consolidação pulmonar ou imediatamente acima de um derrame pleural.

shoulder apprehension s., s. de apreensão do ombro; achado físico em que a colocação do úmero na posição de abdução de 90° e rotação lateral máxima produz ansiedade e resistência em pacientes com história de instabilidade glenoumeral anterior. SIN anterior apprehension test (1).

Siegert s., s. de Siegert; encurtamento e curvatura para dentro da falange terminal dos quintos dedos das mãos na síndrome de Down.

silhouette s. of Felson, s. da silhueta de Felson; em radiologia pulmonar, a obliteração de uma interface ar–tecidos moles normal, como a silhueta cardíaca, quando o líquido ocupa a parte adjacente do pulmão.

Skoda s., s. de Skoda. SIN skodaic *resonance.*

Snellen s., s. de Snellen; ruído ouvido à auscultação sobre o olho num paciente com doença de Graves (Graves *disease*), devido à circulação hiperdinâmica.

spinal s., s. espinal; na pleurisia, os músculos espinais encontram-se num estado de contração tônica do lado afetado.

spine s., s. da coluna; resistência à flexão da coluna em casos de meningite.

Steinberg thumb s., s. do polegar de Steinberg; na síndrome de Marfan, quando o polegar é cruzado sobre a palma da mesma mão, ele se projeta além da superfície ulnar da mão.

Stellwag s., s. de Stellwag; pestanejar infreqüente e incompleto na doença de Graves.

Sternberg s., s. de Sternberg; hipersensibilidade ou desconforto unilateral à palpação dos músculos do cíngulo superior num paciente com pleurisia no mesmo lado.

Stewart-Holmes s., s. de Stewart-Holmes; na doença cerebelar, a incapacidade de verificar um movimento quando a resistência passiva é subitamente liberada. SIN rebound phenomenon (1).

Stierlin s., s. de Stierlin; esvaziamento repetido do ceco, observado radiograficamente, com permanência do bário na parte terminal do íleo e no colo transverso; devido à irritação do ceco, algumas vezes causada por cecite tuberculosa (tiflite).

Straus s., s. de Straus; na paralisia facial, a lesão é periférica se uma injeção de pilocarpina é seguida de sudorese do lado afetado mais tarde do que do outro lado.

string s., s. do barbante; em radiologia gastrointestinal pediátrica, o estreitamento do canal pilórico observado na estenose pilórica congênita; também utilizado para descrever um segmento estreitado na ileíte regional em seriografia do intestino delgado.

subjective s., s. subjetivo; sinal que só é percebido pelo paciente.

Sumner s., s. de Sumner; aumento discreto do tônus dos músculos abdominais, constituindo uma indicação precoce de inflamação do apêndice, cálculo no rim ou no ureter ou torção do pedículo de um cisto ovariano; é detectado por palpação extremamente delicada da fossa ilíaca direita ou esquerda.

superior triangle s., s. do triângulo superior; em radiologia do tórax, alargamento do mediastino superior, geralmente à direita, associado a colapso do lobo inferior, tracionando a pleura mediastínica. Cf. inferior triangle s.

ten Horn s., s. de ten Horn; dor causada por tração delicada do cordão espermático direito, indicando apendicite.

Thomson s., s. de Thomson. SIN Pastia s.

Tinel s., s. de Tinel; sensação de formigamento ou de "alfinetes e agulhas", no local da lesão ou mais distalmente, ao longo do trajeto de um nervo, quando este é percutido; indica uma lesão parcial ou regeneração inicial do nervo. SIN distal tingling on percussion.

Toma s., s. de Toma; distingue a ascite inflamatória da não-inflamatória: em condições inflamatórias do peritônio, o mesentério se contrai, levando o intestino para o lado direito; por conseguinte, quando o paciente se encontra em decúbito dorsal, ocorre timpanismo do lado direito e macicez do lado esquerdo.

Topolanski s., s. de Topolanski; congestão da região pericorneana do olho na doença de Graves.

Tournay s., s. de Tournay. SIN Tournay *phenomenon.*

Traube s., s. de Traube; som ou sopro duplo ouvido à auscultação sobre as artérias (sobretudo as artérias femorais) na regurgitação aórtica significativa.

Trendelenburg s., s. de Trendelenburg; achado ao exame físico associado a várias anormalidades do quadril (p. ex., luxação congênita, fraqueza do abdutor do quadril, artrite reumática, osteoartrite) em que a pelve desce do lado oposto ao lado afetado durante a fase de apoio simples no lado afetado; durante a marcha, ocorre compensação ao inclinar o tronco para o lado afetado durante a fase de apoio sobre o membro afetado. SIN Trendelenburg gait.

Tresilian s., s. de Tresilian; proeminência avermelhada no orifício do ducto de Stenson, observada na caxumba.

trough s., s. do sulco; defeito glenóide ântero-medial resultante de luxação posterior do ombro.

Trousseau s., s. de Trousseau; na tetania latente, a ocorrência de espasmo carpopedal acompanhado de parestesia produzida quando o braço é comprimido, como, por exemplo, por um torniquete ou por um manguito do esfingmomanômetro.

Trunecek s., s. de Trunecek; impulso palpável da artéria subclávia próximo ao ponto de origem do músculo esternomastóideo em casos de esclerose aórtica.

Uthoff s., s. de Uthoff. VER Uthoff *sympton.*

Vierra s., s. de Vierra; tonalidade amarelada e canalização da unha no fogo selvagem.

Vipond s., s. de Vipond; adenopatia generalizada que ocorre durante o período de incubação de vários dos exantemas da infância, proporcionando um sinal diagnóstico precoce em caso de exposição conhecida.

vital s.'s, sinais vitais; determinação da temperatura, freqüência respiratória e pressão arterial.

von Graefe s., s. de von Graefe. SIN Graefe s.

Weber s., s. de Weber. SIN Weber *syndrome.*

Weiss s., s. de Weiss. SIN Chvostek s.

Wernicke s., s. de Wernicke. SIN Wernicke *reaction.*

Westermark s., s. de Westermark; em radiografia do tórax, diminuição da trama pulmonar devido a oligemia causada por embolia pulmonar.

Wilder s., s. de Wilder; discreta contração do bulbo do olho ao mudar o movimento de abdução para adução, ou o inverso, observada na doença de Graves.

Winterbottom s., s. de Winterbottom; aumento de volume dos linfonodos cervicais posteriores, característico dos estágios iniciais da tripanossomíase africana; útil para levantamentos ou controle de migrações de áreas endêmicas de indivíduos com infecções pré-clínicas.

wrist s., s. do punho; na síndrome de Marfan, quando o punho é agarrado pela mão oposta, o polegar e o quinto dedo superpõem-se consideravelmente.

sig·nal (sig'nal). **1.** Algo que produz uma ação. **2.** Seqüência de modelo de DNA que altera a transcrição da RNA polimerase. **3.** O produto final observado quando ocorre deleção de uma seqüência específica de DNA ou RNA por algum método.

arrest s., seqüência de parada; seqüência de DNA que determina a parada de transcrição da RNA polimerase.

contralateral routing of s.'s, trajeto contralateral de sinais; aparelho auditivo para perda auditiva mais acentuada numa orelha do que na outra, em que o som é captado pelo microfone no ouvido com audição mais comprometida e transferido para o ouvido de melhor audição.

pause s., s. de pausa; seqüência de DNA que produz pausa na transcrição da RNA polimerase.

termination s., codon de terminação. SIN termination *codon.*

sig·na·ture (sig'nă-choor, -toor). A parte de uma prescrição que contém as orientações para o paciente. [L. mediev. *signatura*, do L. *signum*, sinal, marca]

Signed English. Sistema de comunicação que constitui uma representação semântica do inglês em que os sinais da *American Sign Language* são utilizados na organização das palavras em inglês, com uso de sinais adicionais para inflexão; utilizado principalmente na educação de crianças com menos de 6 anos de idade.

sig·nif·i·cant (sig-nif'i-kant). Significante, significativo; em estatística, refere-se à confiabilidade de um achado ou, inversamente, à probabilidade de o achado ser o resultado do acaso (geralmente menos de 5%). [L. *significo*, tornar conhecido, significar, de *signum*, sinal + *facio*, fazer]

sig·u·a·tera (sēg-wă-tā'ă). Ciguatera. VER ciguatera.

SIH Abreviatura de somatotropin release-inhibiting *hormone* (hormônio inibidor da liberação de somatotropina).

Silber, Robert H., bioquímico norte-americano, *1915. VER Porter-S. *chromogens*, em *chromogen, reaction,* chromogens *test.*

sil·den·a·fil (sil-den'ă-fil). Sildenafil; inibidor seletivo da fosfodiesterase tipo 5 (PDE5) GMPc-específica; relaxa o músculo no pênis, resultando em maior fluxo sanguíneo e ereção; utilizado no tratamento da impotência masculina; potencializa os efeitos hipotensores dos nitratos.

si·lent (sī'lent). Silencioso; que não produz sinais ou sintomas detectáveis, referindo-se a certas doenças ou processos mórbidos.

sil·i·ca (sil'ĭ-kă). Sílica; o principal constituinte da areia e, portanto, do vidro. SIN silicic anhydride, silicon dioxide. [L. mod. do L. *silex (silic-),* silex]

s. gel, gel de sílica; forma precipitada do ácido silícico, utilizado para adsorção de vários gases.

sil·i·cate (sil'ĭ-kāt). Silicato. **1.** Sal do ácido silícico. **2.** Termo algumas vezes aplicado a restaurações dentárias de porcelana sintética.

sil·i·ca·to·sis (sil'ĭ-kă-tō'sis). Silicatose. SIN silicosis.

si·li·ceous (si-lish'ŭs). Silício; que contém sílica. SIN silicious.

si·lic·ic (si-lis′ik). Silícico; relativo à sílica ou ao silício.

si·lic·ic ac·id. Ácido silícico; obtido na água como colóide através do tratamento de silicatos; o ácido silícico precipitado é o gel de sílica.

si·lic·ic an·hy·dride. Anidrido silícico. SIN silica.

si·li·cious (si-lish′ŭs). Silicoso. SIN siliceous.

sil·i·co·an·thra·co·sis (sil′ĭ-ko-an′thră-ko-sis). Silicoantracose; pneumoconiose consistindo numa combinação de silicose e antracose, observada em mineiros de antracito.

sil·i·co·flu·o·ride (sil′ĭ-ko-flōr′id). Silicofluoreto; composto de silício de flúor com outro elemento.

sil·i·con (Si) (sil′ĭ-kon). Silício; elemento não-metálico muito abundante, de número atômico 14 e peso atômico 28,0855, que ocorre na natureza na forma de sílica e silicatos; em sua forma pura, é utilizado como semicondutor e em baterias solares; também encontrado em certas estruturas de polissacarídeos nos tecidos de mamíferos. [L. *silex,* sílex]

amorphous s., s. amorfo; material fotossensível utilizado em radiografia digital (digital *radiography*) (q.v.) e fluoroscopia (q.v.).

sil·i·con di·ox·ide. Dióxido de silício. SIN silica.

colloidal s. d., dióxido de silício coloidal; sílica gasosa submicroscópica preparada pela hidrólise em fase de vapor de um composto de silício; utilizado como diluente de comprimidos e como agente de suspensão e espessante.

sil·i·cone (sil′ĭ-kon). Silicone; polímero de óxidos de silício orgânicos, que podem estar na forma de líquido, gel ou sólido, dependendo da extensão de polimerização; outrora amplamente utilizado em implantes cirúrgicos, em tubos intracorpóreos para conduzir líquidos, como material de impressão dentária, como substância lubrificante ou seladora, como revestimento do interior de recipientes de vidro para colheita de sangue e em vários procedimentos oftalmológicos.

s.-related disease problems, problemas de doença relacionados ao silicone; doença que, supostamente, resulta da liberação de silicone no corpo.

sil·i·co·pro·te·i·no·sis (sil′ĭ-ko-pro′tē-i-no′sis). Silicoproteinose; distúrbio pulmonar agudo, que se assemelha, do ponto de vista radiológico e histológico, à proteinose alveolar pulmonar, resultante de exposição relativamente curta a altas concentrações de poeira de sílica; os sintomas pulmonares têm início rápido, e a condição é invariavelmente fatal.

sil·i·co·sid·er·o·sis (sil′ĭ-ko-sid′er-o′sis). Silicossiderose. SIN siderosilicosis.

sil·i·co·sis (sil-i-ko′sis). Silicose; forma de pneumoconiose resultante de exposição ocupacional e inalação de poeira de sílica durante um período de vários anos; caracteriza-se por fibrose lentamente progressiva dos pulmões, podendo resultar em comprometimento da função pulmonar; a silicose predispõe à tuberculose pulmonar. SIN pneumosilicosis, silicatosis, stone-mason's disease. [L. *silex,* sílex + *-osis,* condição]

sil·i·co·tu·ber·cu·lo·sis (sil′ĭ-ko-too-ber-ku-lo′sis). Silicotuberculose; silicose associada a lesões pulmonares tuberculosas.

si·li·qua oli·vae (sil′ĭ-kwa o-li′ve). Sílica da oliva; as fibras arqueadas que parecem circundar a oliva inferior do bulbo. [L. a casca da oliva]

silk. Seda; as fibras ou filamentos obtidos do casulo do bicho-da-seda.

floss s., fio dental. SIN dental *floss.*

surgical s., fio de seda cirúrgico; fio preparado a partir dos filamentos de goma viscosa dos casulos que são tecidos pelo bicho-da-seda da amoreira *Bombyx mori;* podem ser obtidos em vários tamanhos e utilizados como material de sutura.

virgin s., fio de seda virgem; material de sutura oftálmico extremamente fino, que consiste em dois a sete filamentos naturais unidos por sericina, um adesivo natural.

Silver, Henry K., pediatra norte-americano, *1918. VER S.-Russell *dwarfism, syndrome.*

sil·ver (Ag). Prata; L. *argentum*; elemento metálico de número atômico 47 e peso atômico de 107,8682. Muitos sais possuem aplicações clínicas. SIN argentum. [A.S. *seolfor*]

s. chloride, cloreto de p.; utilizado na preparação de compostos anti-sépticos de prata.

colloidal s. iodide, iodeto de p. coloidal; anti-séptico utilizado no tratamento da inflamação das mucosas.

s. fluoride, fluoreto de p.; $AgF_2 \cdot H_2O$; anti-séptico.

fused s. nitrate, nitrato de p. fundido. SIN toughened s. nitrate.

s. iodate, iodato de p.; reagente para determinação do cloreto.

s. lactate, lactato de p.; antigamente utilizado como adstringente e anti-séptico.

mild s. protein, proteína de p. leve; complexo preparado pela reação do óxido de prata com gelatina ou albumina sérica. Os cristais brilhantes pretos liberam prata e eram outrora amplamente utilizados como antiinfecciosos tópicos nas mucosas. Contém 19–25% de prata, dos quais apenas uma pequena fração é ionizável. Pode produzir pigmentação preta ou castanha, devido à deposição de prata reduzida nos tecidos. SIN argyrol, silvol.

s. nitrate, nitrato de p.; anti-séptico e adstringente; utilizado externamente, em solução, na prevenção da oftalmia neonatal (hoje em dia, utiliza-se freqüentemente penicilina); também utilizado na coloração especial do sistema nervoso, espiroquetas, fibras reticulares, aparelho de Golgi, região organizadora nucleolar e cálcio.

s. oxide, óxido de p.; tem sido utilizado na epilepsia e na coréia; é explosivo quando misturado com substâncias facilmente combustíveis.

s. picrate, picrato de p.; sal ionizável de prata; tem sido utilizado no tratamento da tricomoníase e monilíase da vagina.

strong s. protein, proteína de p. forte; composto de prata e proteína contendo não menos de 7,5 e não mais de 8,5% de prata; utilizado externamente como anti-séptico, desprovido de propriedades adstringentes e quase desprovido de propriedades irritantes.

s. sulfadiazine, sulfadiazina de p.; o derivado de prata da sulfadiazina, utilizado externamente como agente antibacteriano tópico na prevenção e no tratamento de infecções em queimaduras.

toughened s. nitrate, nitrato de p. endurecido; nitrato de prata misturado com cloreto de prata, que se deixa secar. Geralmente aplicado às extremidades de pequenos aplicadores de madeira ou na forma de lápis. Esses aplicadores são utilizados após umedecimento como químico cáustico para remoção de verrugas. SIN fused s. nitrate, lunar caustic.

sil·ver im·preg·na·tion. Impregnação pela prata; complexos de prata empregados para demonstrar a reticulina em tecidos normais e doentes, bem como a neuróglia, neurofibrilas, células argentafins e aparelho de Golgi.

Silverman, Leslie, engenheiro norte-americano, 1914–1966. VER S.-Lilly *pneumotachograph.*

Silverman, William A., pediatra norte-americano do século XX. VER Caffey-S. *syndrome.*

Silverskiöld, Nils G., ortopedista sueco. 1888–1957. VER S. *syndrome.*

sil·vol (sil′vol). Silvol. SIN mild *silver* protein.

si·meth·i·cone (si-meth′i-kon). Simeticona; mistura de dimetil polisiloxinos e gel de sílica; antiflatulento.

si·mi·lia si·mi·li·bus cur·an·tur (si-mil′e-ă si-mil′i-bŭs ker-an′ter). O conceito homeopático que expressa a lei dos semelhantes (literalmente, "os semelhantes são curados pelos semelhantes"); a doutrina segundo a qual qualquer substância capaz de provocar sintomas mórbidos no indivíduo sadio eliminará sintomas semelhantes que ocorrem com expressão de uma doença. Outra leitura do conceito, empregada por Hahnemann, o fundador da homeopatia, é *similia similibus curentur,* "deixemos os semelhantes serem curados pelos semelhantes". [L. os semelhantes são curados por semelhantes]

si·mil·i·mum, si·mil·li·mum (si-mil′i-mŭm). Em homeopatia, o remédio indicado em determinado caso porque a mesma substância, quando administrada a uma pessoa sadia, produzirá o complexo de sintomas mais próximo daquele da doença em questão. [L. *simillimus,* mais semelhante, superl. de *similis* semelhante]

Simmonds, Morris, médico alemão, 1855–1925. VER S. *disease.*

Simmons, James S., bacteriologista norte-americano, 1890–1954. VER S. citrate *medium.*

Simon, Gustav, cirurgião alemão, 1824–1876. VER S. *position.*

Simon, Richard, oncologista norte-americano do século XX. VER Norton-S. *hypothesis.*

Simon, Théodore, médico francês, 1873–1961. VER Binet-S. *scale.*

Simonart, Pierre J.C., obstetra belga, 1816–1846. VER S. *bands,* em *band, ligaments,* em *ligament.*

Simons, Arthur, médico alemão, *1877. VER S. *disease.*

Simonsiella (si′mon-se-el′ah). Gênero de bactérias deslizantes não-fotossintéticas, Gram-negativas, quimioorganotrópicas que ocorrem na forma de filamentos multicelulares com o eixo longitudinal de células individuais perpendicular ao eixo longitudinal do filamento. As células são achatadas e curvadas, produzindo uma simetria convexo-côncava em forma de crescente. Isoladas da cavidade oral de mamíferos. A espécie típica é *Simonsiella muelleri.*

sim·ple (sim′pl). **1.** Simples; não complexo ou composto. **2.** Em anatomia, composto de um número mínimo de partes. **3.** Erva medicinal. [L. *simplex*]

Sim·plex·vi·rus (sim′pleks-vi′rus). Virus herpes simples. SIN herpes simplex.

Sim·pli·fied Oral Hy·giene In·dex (OHI-S). Índice Simplificado de Higiene Oral; índice que mede o estado atual de higiene oral com base na quantidade de resíduos e tártaro que ocorrem em seis superfícies dentárias representativas na boca; freqüentemente utilizado em pesquisas de campo de doença periodontal.

Simpson, Sir James Y., obstetra escocês, 1811–1870. VER S. uterine *sound, forceps.*

Simpson, William, engenheiro civil inglês, †1917.

Sims, James Marion, ginecologista norte-americano, 1813–1883. VER S. *position,* uterine *sound.*

sim·u·la·tion (sim-u-la′shŭn). Simulação. **1.** Imitação; diz-se de uma doença ou sintoma semelhante a outro ou da simulação da doença, como na doença fictícia ou simulação. **2.** Em radioterapia, uso de um sistema radiográfico geometricamente semelhante ou computador para planejar a localização das portas de terapia. [L. *simulatio,* de *simulo,* pp. *-atus,* imitar, de *similis,* semelhante]

computer s., s. computadorizada. SIN computer *model.*

sim·u·la·tor (sim′ū-lā-ter, tōr). Simulador; aparelho projetado para produzir efeitos que simulam aqueles de condições ambientais específicas; utilizado em experimentação e treinamento.

Sim·u·lium (si-mū′lē-ŭm). Gênero de mosquitos de cor escura, pernas curtas e asas largas, cujas fêmeas se alimentam do sangue de vertebrados; da família de dípteros Simuliidae (simulíídeos). As larvas aquáticas exigem rios de fluxo rápido ou águas muito oxigenadas para o seu desenvolvimento, um fator epidemiológico decisivo no papel desses insetos como vetores de doenças. Nas Américas Central e do Sul, no México e através da África Central, várias espécies transmitem *Onchocerca volvulus*, o agente da oncocercíase humana. SIN *Eusimulium*. [L. *simulo*, simular]

S. damno'sum, espécie que é um importante vetor da oncocercíase na África Central.

S. neav'ei, espécie que é um importante vetor da oncocercíase no leste da África, onde suas larvas e pupas se fixam às conchas de caranguejos do gênero *Potamonantes*.

S. ochra'ceum, espécie que é um vetor da oncocercíase humana na África Central.

S. ruggle'si, espécie que é um vetor do *Leucocytozoon simondi* no Canadá e norte dos Estados Unidos.

simultagnosia (sī-mŭl-tag-nō′sē-ā). Simultagnosia. SIN simultanagnosia.

si·mul·tan·ag·no·sia (sī-mŭl-tan-ag-nō′sē-ā). Simultanagnosia; incapacidade de reconhecer múltiplos elementos numa apresentação visual, isto é, a capacidade de apreciar um objeto ou alguns elementos de uma cena, mas não a cena como um todo. SIN simultagnosia. [simultaneous + agnosia]

SIMV Abreviatura de synchronized intermittent mandatory *ventilation* (ventilação mandatória intermitente sincronizada).

sim·va·sta·tin (sim′vă-sta-tin). Sinvastatina; potente inibidor da HMG-CoA-redutase (a enzima que limita a velocidade na biossíntese do colesterol). Utilizada no tratamento da hiperlipidemia; semelhante à lovastatina.

sin·ca·lide (sin′kă-līd). Sincalídeo; o octapeptídeo C-terminal da colecistocinina; provoca contração do músculo liso da vesícula biliar e do intestino delgado, relaxamento da junção coledocoduodenal e estimula as secreções pancreática e gástrica; também utilizado como auxiliar diagnóstico para obter bile para análise.

sin·cip·i·tal (sin-sip′i-tăl). Sincipital; relativo ao sincipúcio.

sin·ci·put, pl. **sin·cip·i·ta, sin·ci·puts** (sin′si-put, sin-sip′i-tă). Sincipúcio; parte ântero-superior do crânio; *termo oficial alternativo para forehead. [L. metade da cabeça]

SINES Abreviatura de short interspersed *elements* (elementos intercalados curtos), em *element*.

sin·ew (sin′oo). Tendão. SIN tendon. [A.S. *sinu*]

Singer, Mark I., laringologista norte-americano, *1945. VER Blom-S. *valve*.

sin·gle·ton (sing′gel-tun). **1.** Feto que se desenvolve sozinho. **2.** SIN sport. [desconhecido]

sin·gul·ta·tion (sing′gŭl-tā′shŭn). Soluço. VER hiccup. [L. *singulto*, pp. *-atus*, soluçar]

sin·gul·tous (sing-gŭl′tŭs). Singultoso; relativo a soluços.

sin·gul·tus (sing-gŭl′tŭs). Singulto. SIN hiccup. [L.]

sin·i·grase, sin·i·gri·nase (sin′i-grās, -gri-nās). Sinigrase, sinigrinase. SIN thioglucosidase.

sin·is·ter (si-nis′ter) [TA]. Sinistro; à esquerda. [L.]

sin·is·trad (sin′is-trad, si-nis′trad). Sinistro; para a esquerda. [L. *sinister*, esquerdo + *ad*, para]

sin·is·tral (sin′is-trăl, sī-nis′trăl). Sinistro. **1.** Relativo ao lado esquerdo. SIN sinistrous. **2.** Refere-se a uma pessoa canhota.

sin·is·tral·i·ty (sin-is-trăl′i-tē). Sinistralidade; a condição de ser canhoto.

sinistro-. Sinistro-. À esquerda. [L. *sinister*]

sin·is·tro·car·dia (sin′is-trō-kar′dē-ă). Sinistrocardia; deslocamento do coração além de sua posição normal no lado esquerdo. [sinistro- + G. *kardia*, coração]

sin·is·tro·ce·re·bral (sini′s-trō-ser′ē-brăl). Sinistrocerebral; relativo ao hemisfério cerebral esquerdo. [sinistro- + L. *cerebrum*, cérebro]

sin·is·troc·u·lar (sin-is-trok′ū-lăr). Sinistrocular; termo raramente empregado para designar aquele que prefere o olho esquerdo no trabalho monocular, como, por exemplo, no uso de um microscópio. Cf. dominant *eye*. [sinistro- + L. *oculus*, olho]

sin·is·tro·gy·ra·tion (sin′is-trō-jī-rā′shŭn). Sinistrógiro, levógiro. SIN sinistrotorsion. [sinistro- + L. *gyratio*, uma volta (giro)]

sin·is·tro·man·u·al (sin′is-trō-man′ū-ăl). Sinistrômano. SIN left-handed. [sinistro- + L. *manus*, mão]

sin·is·trop·e·dal (sin-is-trop′ē-dăl). Sinistropedal; designa aquele que usa de preferência a perna esquerda. SIN left-footed. [sinistro- + L. *pes (ped-)*, pé]

sin·is·tro·ro·ta·tion (sin′is-trō-rō-tā′shŭn). Sinistrorrotação. SIN sinistrotorsion.

sin·is·trorse (sin′is-trors). Sinistrorso; que gira para a esquerda. [L. *sinistrorsus*, do lado esquerdo, de *sinister*, esquerda + *verto*, pp. *versus*, virar]

sin·is·tro·tor·sion (sin′is-trō-tōr′shŭn). Sinistrotorção, levorrotação; giro ou torção para a esquerda. SIN levocycleduction, levorotation (2), levotorsion (1), sinistrogyration, sinistrorotation. [sinistro- + L. *torsio*, giro (torção)]

sin·is·trous (sin′is-trŭs, si-nis′trŭs). Sinistro. SIN sinistral (1).

si·no·a·tri·al (sī′nō-ā′trē-ăl). Sinoatrial. SIN sinuatrial.

si·nog·ra·phy (sī-nog′ră-fē). Sinografia; uso radiológico de contraste para opacificação de uma fístula. [sinus + G. *graphō*, escrever]

si·no·pul·mo·nary (sī′nō-pŭl′mō-nār-ē). Sinopulmonar; relativo aos seios paranasais e às vias aéreas pulmonares.

si·no·vag·i·nal (sī-nō-vaj′i-năl). Sinovaginal; relativo à parte da vagina derivada do seio urogenital.

sin·ter (sin′ter). Concrecionar; aquecer uma substância pulverizada sem liquefazê-la por completo, causando sua fusão numa massa sólida, porém porosa. [Al. transformar em escória]

si·nu·a·tri·al (S-A) (sin′ū-ā′trē-ăl, sī′noo-). Sinoatrial; relativo ao seio venoso e ao átrio direito do coração. SIN sinoatrial.

SINUS

si·nus, pl. **si·nus, si·nus·es** (sī′nŭs, -ēz). Seio. **1.** [TA]. Um canal para passagem de sangue ou de linfa, sem os revestimentos de um vaso comum; p. ex., passagens de sangue no útero grávido ou aquelas nas meninges cerebrais. **2.** [TA]. Cavidade ou espaço oco no osso ou em outro tecido. **3.** [TA]. Dilatação de um vaso sanguíneo. **4.** Fístula ou trato que leva a uma cavidade supurativa. [L. *sinus*, cavidade, canal, concavidade]

s. a'lae par'vae, s. esfenoparietal. SIN sphenoparietal s.

anal sinuses [TA], seios anais; **(1)** os sulcos entre as colunas anais; SIN Morgagni s. (1). **(2)** bolsas ou criptas na zona colunar do canal anal entre a linha anocutânea e a linha anorretal; os seios conferem à mucosa um aspecto recortado. SIN s. anales [TA], anal crypts, Morgagni crypts, rectal sinuses.

s. ana'les [TA], seios anais. SIN anal sinuses.

anterior sinuses, células etmoidais anteriores. SIN anterior ethmoidal *cells*, em *cell*.

s. aor'tae [TA], s. da aorta. SIN aortic s.

aortic s. [TA], s. da aorta; o espaço entre a face superior de cada válvula da valva aórtica e a porção dilatada da parede da aorta ascendente, imediatamente acima de cada válvula. SIN s. aortae [TA], Petit s., Valsalva s.

Arlt s., s. de Arlt; depressão inconstante na porção inferior da superfície interna do saco lacrimal.

barber pilonidal s., s. pilonidal dos barbeiros; seio pilonidal que ocorre em barbeiros, geralmente na membrana interdigital, devido ao encravamento de pêlos exógenos em virtude do afrouxamento e retesamento alternados dos tecidos da mão pela manipulação das tesouras.

basilar s., plexo basilar dos seios da dura-máter. SIN basilar venous *plexus*.

Breschet s., s. de Breschet. SIN sphenoparietal s.

s. carot'icus [TA], s. carótico. SIN carotid s.

carotid s. [TA], s. carótico; discreta dilatação da artéria carótida comum em sua bifurcação nas carótidas externa e interna; contém barorreceptores que, quando estimulados, causam redução da freqüência cardíaca, vasodilatação e queda da pressão arterial; inervado primariamente pelo nervo glossofaríngeo. SIN s. caroticus [TA], carotid bulb.

s. caverno'sus [TA], s. cavernoso. SIN cavernous s.

cavernous s. [TA], s. cavernoso; seio venoso da dura-máter, par de cada lado da sela turca, estando os dois conectados por anastomoses, o seio intercavernoso anterior da dura-máter (sinus intercavernosus anterior [TA]) e o seio intercavernoso posterior da dura-máter [TA] (sinus intercavernosus posterior [TA]), em frente e atrás da hipófise, respectivamente, tornando assim o seio circular; o seio cavernoso é peculiar entre os seios venosos da dura-máter por ser trabeculado; no interior do seio passam a artéria carótida interna e o nervo abducente. SIN s. cavernosus [TA].

cerebral sinuses, seios venosos da dura-máter . SIN dural venous sinuses.

cervical s., s. cervical; em embriões pequenos de mamíferos, refere-se a uma depressão na região da nuca, caudalmente ao arco hióide, com o terceiro e o quarto arcos branquiais e sulcos ectodérmicos em seu assoalho; normalmente, é obliterado depois do segundo mês; todavia, em certas ocasiões, há persistência de fístulas cervicais como vestígios. SIN precervical s.

circular s., (1) formação venosa da dura-máter que circunda a hipófise, composta pelos seios cavernosos direito e esquerdo e pelos seios intercavernosos. SIN circulus venosus ridleyi, Ridley circle; **(2)** um seio venoso na periferia da placenta; **(3)** seio venoso da esclera. SIN scleral venous s.

s. circula'ris, s. venoso da esclera. SIN scleral venous s.

coccygeal s., s. coccígeo; fístula que se abre na região do cóccix. VER TAMBÉM pilonidal s.

s. corona'rius [TA], s. coronário. SIN coronary s.

coronary s. [TA], s. coronário; tronco curto que recebe a maioria das veias cardíacas; começando na junção da veia cardíaca magna com a veia oblíqua do átrio esquerdo, segue seu trajeto na parte posterior do sulco coronário e deságua no átrio direito, entre a veia cava inferior e o orifício atrioventricular. SIN s. coronarius [TA].
costomediastinal s., s. recesso costomediastinal. SIN costomediastinal *recess*.
cranial sinuses, seios venosos da dura-máter. SIN dural venous sinuses.
dermal s., s. dérmico; seio revestido com epiderme e anexos cutâneos, que se estende da pele até alguma estrutura mais profunda, mais freqüentemente a medula espinal.
s. du'rae ma'tris [TA], seios venosos da dura-máter. SIN dural venous sinuses.
dural venous sinuses [TA], seios venosos da dura-máter; canais venosos revestidos de endotélio na dura-máter. SIN s. durae matris [TA], cerebral sinuses, cranial sinuses, sinuses of dura mater, venous sinuses.
sinuses of dura mater, seios venosos da dura-máter. SIN dural venous sinuses.
Englisch s., s. de Englisch. SIN inferior petrosal s.
s. epididym'idis [TA], s. do epidídimo. SIN s. of epididymis.
s. of epididymis [TA], s. do epidídimo; um espaço estreito entre o corpo do epidídimo e o testículo. SIN s. epididymidis [TA].
ethmoidal sinuses, células etmoidais. SIN ethmoid *cells*, em *cell*.
s. ethmoida'les, células etmoidais. SIN ethmoid *cells*, em *cell*.
s. ethmoidales anterio'res, células etmoidais anteriores. SIN anterior ethmoidal *cells*, em *cell*.
s. ethmoidales me'diae, células etmoidais médias. SIN middle ethmoidal *cells*, em *cell*.
s. ethmoidales posterio'res, células etmoidais posteriores. SIN posterior ethmoidal *cells*, em *cell*.
frontal s. [TA], s. frontal; seio paranasal oco formado de cada lado na parte inferior da escama do osso frontal; comunica-se pelo infundíbulo etmoidal com o meato médio da cavidade nasal do mesmo lado. SIN s. frontalis [TA].
s. fronta'lis [TA], s. frontal. SIN frontal s.
Guérin s., s. de Guérin; fundo-de-saco ou divertículo atrás da valva da fossa navicular.
Huguier s., s. de Huguier. SIN *fossa* of oval window.
inferior longitudinal s., s. sagital inferior da dura-máter. SIN inferior sagittal s.
inferior petrosal s. [TA], s. petroso inferior da dura-máter; par de seios venosos durais seguindo seu trajeto no sulco sobre a fissura petroccipital que conecta o seio cavernoso com o bulbo superior da veia jugular interna. SIN s. petrosus inferior [TA], Englisch s.
inferior sagittal s. [TA], s. sagital inferior da dura-máter; seio venoso dural ímpar na margem inferior da foice do cérebro, que segue seu trajeto paralelamente ao seio sagital superior e une-se com a veia magna do cérebro para formar o seio reto da dura-máter. SIN s. sagittalis inferior [TA], inferior longitudinal s.
s. intercaverno'si anterior et posterior [TA], seios intercavernosos anterior e posterior. SIN intercavernous sinuses.
intercavernous sinuses, seios intercavernosos; as anastomoses anterior e posterior entre os seios cavernosos, que passam anterior e posteriormente à hipófise e formam, com os seios cavernosos, o seio circular. VER TAMBÉM cavernous s. SIN s. intercavernosi anterior et posterior [TA], Ridley s.
jugular s., s. jugula'ris, bulbo jugular; uma das três dilatações das veias jugulares; o bulbo jugular externo situa-se entre os dois grupos de válvulas; os bulbos jugulares internos estão na origem (bulbo superior) e próximo ao término (bulbo inferior).
s. lactif'eri [TA], s. lactífero. SIN lactiferous s.
lactiferous s. [TA], s. lactífero; dilatação fusiforme circunscrita do ducto lactífero imediatamente antes de entrar no mamilo. Em mães que amamentam, essa dilatação armazena uma gotícula de leite que é espremida pela compressão quando o lactente começa a sugar; acredita-se que isso estimule a sucção contínua até haver o reflexo de ejeção do leite. SIN s. lactiferi [TA], ampulla lactifera, ampulla of lactiferous duct, ampulla of milk duct, lactiferous ampulla.
laryngeal s., ventrículo da laringe. SIN laryngeal *ventricle*.
s. laryn'geus, ventrículo da laringe. SIN laryngeal *ventricle*.
lateral s., s.transverso. SIN transverse s.
s. lie'nis, s. esplênicos. SIN splenic s.
longitudinal s., s. sagital. VER inferior sagittal s., superior sagittal s.
longitudinal vertebral venous s., plexo venoso vertebral longitudinal; grandes veias plexiformes que formam porções do plexo venoso vertebral interno anterior, situadas sobre as superfícies posteriores dos corpos vertebrais, de cada lado do ligamento longitudinal posterior. SIN s. vertebrales longitudinales.
Luschka s., s. de Luschka; seio venoso na sutura petroescamosa.
lymph s., s. linfático. SIN lymphatic s.
lymphatic s., s. linfático; os canais, num linfonodo, atravessados por um retículo de células e fibras e delimitados por células litorais; existem seios subcapsulares, trabeculares e medulares. SIN lymph s.
Maier s., s. de Maier; depressão infundibuliforme na superfície interna do saco lacrimal, que recebe os canalículos lacrimais.
marginal sinuses of placenta, seios marginais da placenta; lagos venosos descontínuos na margem da placenta.
mastoid sinuses, células mastóideas. SIN mastoid *cells*, em *cell*.
s. maxilla'ris [TA], s. maxilar. SIN maxillary s.
maxillary s. [TA], s. maxilar; o maior dos seios paranasais; ocupa o corpo da maxila, comunicando-se com o meato médio do nariz. SIN s. maxillaris [TA], antrum of Highmore, genyantrum, maxillary antrum.
Meyer s., s. de Meyer; pequena concavidade no assoalho do canal auditivo externo, próximo à membrana timpânica.
middle ethmoidal sinuses, células etmoidais médias. SIN middle ehtmoidal *cells*, em *cell*.
Morgagni s., s. de Morgagni; **(1)** SIN anal sinuses (1); **(2)** SIN prostatic *utricle*; **(3)** SIN laryngeal *ventricle*.
s. of nail, s. ungueal. SIN s. unguis.
oblique pericardial s. [TA], s. oblíquo do pericárdio; o recesso na cavidade pericárdica posterior à base do coração, delimitado, lateralmente, pelas reflexões pericárdicas nas veias pulmonares e veia cava inferior e, posteriormente, pelo pericárdio sobrejacente à face anterior do esôfago. SIN s. obliquus pericardii [TA], oblique s. of pericardium.
oblique s. of pericardium, s. oblíquo do pericárdio. SIN oblique pericardial s.
s. obli'quus pericar'dii [TA], s. oblíquo do pericárdio. SIN oblique pericardial s.
occipital s. [TA], s. occipital; seio venoso dural ímpar que começa na confluência dos seios e segue para baixo, na base da foice do cerebelo até o forame magno. SIN s. occipitalis [TA].
s. occipita'lis [TA], s. occipital. SIN occipital s.
Palfyn s., s. de Palfyn; espaço dentro da crista etmoidal descrito como comunicando-se com os seios etmoidal e frontal.
paranasal sinuses [TA], seios paranasais; cavidades pares cheias de ar nos ossos da face, revestidas por mucosa contínua com a da cavidade nasal; esses seios são o frontal, o esfenoidal, o maxilar e o etmoidal. SIN s. paranasales [TA].

os seios venosos da dura-máter

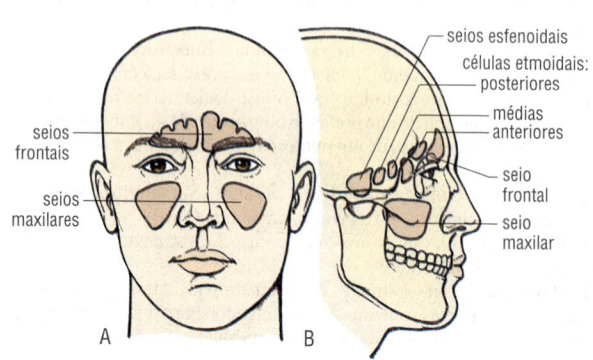

seios paranasais: vistas (A) anterior e (B) lateral da cabeça

s. paranasa'les [TA], seios paranasais. SIN paranasal sinuses.
parasinoidal sinuses, lacunas laterais do seio sagital superior da dura-máter. SIN lateral *lacunae* of superior sagital sinus, em *lacuna.*
Petit s., s. de Petit. SIN aortic s.
petrosal s., s. petroso. VER inferior petrosal s., superior petrosal s.
s. petro'sus infe'rior [TA], s. petroso inferior. SIN inferior petrosal s.
s. petro'sus supe'rior [TA], s. petroso superior. SIN superior petrosal s.
phrenicocostal s., recesso costodiafragmático. SIN costodiaphragmatic *recess.*
pilonidal s., s. pilonidal; fístula ou depressão, na região sacral, que se comunica com o exterior, contendo pêlos que podem atuar como corpo estranho, produzindo inflamação crônica. SIN pilonidal fistula.
piriform s., recesso da parte laríngea da faringe; piriforme. SIN piriform *fossa.*
pleural sinuses, recessos pleurais. SIN pleural *recesses,* em *recess.*
s. pocula'ris, utrículo prostático. SIN prostatic *utricle.*
s. poste'rior cavi tympani [TA], s. posterior da cavidade timpânica. SIN posterior s. of tympanic cavity.
posterior s. of tympanic cavity [TA], s. posterior da cavidade timpânica; sulco profundo, acima da eminência piramidal, que se estende até a fossa da bigorna na parede posterior da cavidade timpânica. SIN s. posterior cavi tympani [TA].
preauricular s., s. pré-auricular; fístula ou depressão, na pele periauricular, como resultado do defeito de desenvolvimento do primeiro e do segundo arcos branquiais. SIN preauricular pit.
precervical s., s. pré-cervical. SIN cervical s.
prostatic s. [TA], s. prostático; o sulco existente de cada lado da crista uretral na parte prostática da uretra, em que se abrem os ductos prostáticos. SIN prostaticus [TA].
s. prostat'icus [TA], s. prostático. SIN prostatic s.
pulmonary sinuses, seios do tronco pulmonar. SIN s. of pulmonary trunk.
s. of pulmonary trunk [TA], s. do tronco pulmonar; o espaço na origem do tronco pulmonar entre a parede dilatada do vaso e cada válvula da valva pulmonar. SIN s. trunci pulmonalis [TA], pulmonary sinuses.
rectal sinuses, seios anais. SIN anal sinuses.
s. rec'tus [TA], s. reto da dura-máter. SIN straight s.
renal s. [TA], s. renal; a cavidade do rim que contém os cálices e a pelve do ureter e os vasos segmentares mergulhados numa matriz gordurosa. Os seios renais fazem com que os rins tenham um aspecto oco ou em forma de C nos cortes transversais ou nas técnicas de imagem. SIN s. renalis [TA].
s. rena'lis [TA], s. renal. SIN renal s.
s. reu'niens, termo obsoleto para seio venoso.
rhomboidal s., s. rhomboidalis, ventrículo terminal da medula espinal; dilatação do canal central da medula espinal na região lombar. SIN rhombocele.
Ridley s., s. de Ridley. SIN intercavernous sinuses.
Rokitansky-Aschoff sinuses, seios de Rokitansky-Aschoff; pequenas dilatações saculares da mucosa da vesícula biliar que se estendem através da camada muscular; podem ser congênitos.
s. sagitta'lis infe'rior [TA], s. sagital inferior. SIN inferior sagittal s.
s. sagitta'lis supe'rior [TA], s. sagital superior. SIN superior sagittal s.
scleral venous s. [TA], s. venoso da esclera; a estrutura vascular que circunda a câmara anterior do olho e através da qual o humor aquoso retorna à circulação sanguínea. SIN s. venosus sclerae [TA], circular s. (3), Fontana canal, Lauth canal, Schlemm canal, s. circularis, venous s. of sclera.
sigmoid s. [TA], s. sigmóideo da dura-máter; seio venoso da dura-máter, em forma de S, situado profundamente ao processo mastóide do osso temporal e imediatamente posterior à parte petrosa do osso temporal; continua-se com o seio transverso e deságua na veia jugular interna quando passa através do forame jugular. SIN s. sigmoideus [TA].
s. sigmoi'deus [TA], s. sigmóideo. SIN sigmoid s.
sphenoidal s. [TA], s. esfenoidal; um seio de um par de seios paranasais, no corpo do osso esfenóide, que se comunica com a cavidade nasal posterior superior ou recesso esfenoetmoidal. SIN s. sphenoidalis [TA].
s. sphenoida'lis [TA], s. esfenoidal. SIN sphenoidal s.
sphenoparietal s. [TA], s. esfenoparietal da dura-máter; seio venoso da dura-máter, pareado, que começa no osso parietal, segue seu trajeto ao longo das cristas esfenoidais e deságua no seio cavernoso. SIN s. sphenoparietalis [TA], Breschet s., s. alae parvae.
s. sphenoparieta'lis [TA], s. esfenoparietal. SIN sphenoparietal s.
splenic s., s. esplênico; canal venoso alongado, de 12–40 μm de largura, revestido por células em bastão. SIN s. lienis.
straight s. [TA], s. reto da dura-máter; seio venoso da dura-máter, ímpar, na parte posterior da foice do cérebro, onde está fixado à fenda do cerebelo; formado anteriormente pela união da veia magna do cérebro com o sagital inferior, seguindo um trajeto horizontal e posterior até a confluência dos seios. SIN s. rectus [TA], tentorial s.
superior longitudinal s., s. sagital superior. SIN superior sagittal s.
superior petrosal s. [TA], s. petroso superior; seio venoso dural par no sulco ao longo da crista da parte petrosa do osso temporal, conectando o seio cavernoso com a terminação do seio transverso ou início do seio sigmóide. SIN s. petrosus superior [TA].

superior sagittal s. [TA], s. sagital superior da dura-máter; seio venoso da dura-máter, ímpar no sulco sagital, que começa no forame cego e termina na confluência dos seios, onde se une com o seio reto; recebe as veias cerebrais superiores e possui extensões laterais, as lacunas laterais venosas. SIN s. sagittalis superior [TA], superior longitudinal s.
tarsal s. [TA], s. do tarso; cavidade ou canal formado pelo sulco do talo e sulco interósseo do calcâneo ocupado pelo ligamento talocalcâneo interósseo. SIN s. tarsi [TA], tarsal canal.
s. tar'si [TA], s. do tarso. SIN tarsal s.
tentorial s., s. reto da dura-máter. SIN straight s.
terminal s., s. termina'lis, s. terminal; a veia que limita a área vascular no blastoderma.
s. tonsilla'ris, fossa tonsilar. SIN tonsillar *fossa.*
Tourtual s., s. de Tourtual. SIN supratonsillar *fossa.*
transverse s. [TA], s. transverso da dura-máter; s. venoso da dura-máter, pareado, que drena na confluência dos seios, seguindo seu trajeto ao longo da fixação occipital da tenda do cerebelo, terminando no seio sigmóideo. SIN s. transversus [TA], lateral s.
transverse pericardial s. [TA], s. transverso do pericárdio; passagem no saco pericárdico entre as origens dos grandes vasos, isto é, posteriormente às porções intrapericárdicas do tronco pulmonar e aorta ascendente e anteriormente à veia cava superior e superiormente aos átrios; formado em conseqüência da flexura do tubo cardíaco, aproximando parcialmente os grandes vasos venosos e arteriais. SIN s. transversus pericardii [TA], Theile canal, transverse s. of pericardium.
transverse s. of pericardium, s. transverso do pericárdio. SIN transverse pericardial s.
s. transver'sus [TA], s. transverso da dura-máter. SIN transverse s.
s. transver'sus pericar'dii [TA], s. transverso do pericárdio. SIN transverse pericardial s.
s. trun'ci pulmona'lis [TA], s. do tronco pulmonar. SIN s. of pulmonary trunk.
s. tym'pani [TA], s. do tímpano. SIN tympanic s.
tympanic s. [TA], s. do tímpano; depressão na cavidade timpânica, posterior ao promontório do tímpano. SIN s. tympani [TA].
s. un'guis, s. ungueal; a fenda profunda que abriga a raiz da unha. SIN s. of nail.
urogenital s., (1) s. urogenital; a parte ventral da cloaca após a sua separação do reto pelo crescimento do septo urorretal; a partir daí, desenvolvem-se a parte inferior da bexiga em ambos os sexos, a porção prostática da uretra masculina e a uretra e o vestíbulo no sexo feminino; (2) cloaca persistente. SIN persistent *cloaca.*
s. urogenita'lis, s. urogenital. SIN persistent *cloaca.*
uterine s., s. uterino; pequeno canal vascular irregular no endométrio que se forma durante a gravidez. SIN uterine sinusoid.
uteroplacental sinuses, seios uteroplacentários; espaços vasculares irregulares na zona de fixação coriônica à decídua basal.
Valsalva s., s. de Valsalva. SIN aortic s.
s. of the vena cava [TA], s. das veias cavas; a porção da cavidade do átrio direito do coração que recebe o sangue da veia cava; é separado do resto do átrio pela crista terminal. SIN s. venarum cavarum [TA].
s. vena'rum cava'rum [TA], s. das veias cavas. SIN s. of the vena cava.
s. veno'sus [TA], s. venoso; cavidade na extremidade caudal do tubo cardíaco embrionário em que se unem as veias dos arcos circulatórios intra e extra-embrionário; durante o desenvolvimento, forma a porção do átrio direito conhecida, na anatomia do adulto, como seio da veia cava. SIN saccus reuniens.
s. veno'sus scle'rae [TA], s. venoso da esclera. SIN scleral venous s.
venous sinuses, seios venosos da dura-máter. SIN dural venous sinuses.
venous s. of sclera, s. venoso da esclera. SIN scleral venous s.
s. vertebra'les longitudina'les, s. vertebrais longitudinais. SIN longitudinal vertebral venous, s.

si·nus·i·tis (sī-nŭ-sī'tis). Sinusite; inflamação da mucosa de qualquer seio, especialmente um dos seios paranasais. [sinus + G. *-itis,* inflamação]
si·nus·oid (sī'nŭ-soyd). Sinusóide. **1.** Semelhante a um seio. **2.** Capilar sinusoidal; vaso sanguíneo terminal de paredes finas, cujo calibre é irregular e maior do que o de um capilar comum; suas células endoteliais possuem grandes lacunas, e a lâmina basal é descontínua ou ausente. SIN sinusoidal capillary. [sinus + G. *eidos,* semelhança]
   uterine s., s. uterino. SIN uterine *sinus.*
si·nus·oi·dal (sī-nŭ-soy'dăl). Sinusoidal; relativo a um sinusóide.
si·nus·ot·o·my (sin-ŭ-sot'o-mē). Sinusotomia; incisão num seio. [sinus + G. *tome,* incisão]
si op. sit Abreviatura do L. *si opus sit,* se necessário.
si·phon (sī'fon). Sifão; tubo curvo com dois ramos de comprimentos diferentes, utilizado para remover líquido de uma cavidade ou vaso por pressão atmosférica. [G. *siphōn,* tubo]
si·phon·age (sī'fon-ij). Sifonagem; esvaziamento do estômago ou de outra cavidade por meio de um sifão.

Si·pho·na ir·ri·tans (si̅-fo̅′nă ir′i-tanz). A mosca dos chifres, uma mosca muscóide hematófaga que causa grande irritação e perturbação ao gado e transmite *Stephanofilaria stilesi*. [G. *siphōn*, tubo]

Si·pho·nap·tera (si̅-fo̅-nap′te-ră). As pulgas, uma ordem de insetos ectoparasitas sem asas, altamente adaptados para a sobrevida no pêlo dos mamíferos; são insetos lateralmente achatados, espinhosos e equipados com patas metatorácicas bem desenvolvidas para saltar. [G. *siphōn*, tubo + G. *a-* priv. + *pteron*, asa]

Sipho·vir·i·dae (sif′o̅-vi̅′ră-dă). Família de vírus bacterianos com longas caudas não-contráteis e cabeças isométricas ou alongadas, contendo DNA de filamento duplo (PM 25-79 × 10⁶); inclui o grupo do fago temperado λ e, provavelmente, outros gêneros. [L. *sipho*, pequeno tubo, cachimbo, de G. *siphōn*, + vírus]

Sipple, John H., médico norte-americano, *1930. VER S. *syndrome*.
Sippy, Bertram W., médico norte-americano, 1866–1924. VER S. *diet*.
si·ren·i·form (si̅-ren′i-fōrm). Sireniforme; refere-se a uma malformação com aspecto de sirenomelia.
si·re·no·me·lia (si̅′rĕ-no̅-me̅′lē-ă). Sirenomelia; fusão das pernas com união completa ou parcial dos pés. VER TAMBÉM Sympus. SIN mermaid malformation, symmelia. [L. *siren*, G. *seirēn*, sereia]
si·ri·a·sis (si-ri̅′ă-sis). Siríase. SIN sunstroke. [G. *seriasis*, de *seiriao*, estar quente]
Siris, Evelyn, radiologista norte-americana, *1914. VER Coffin-S *syndrome*.
sir·up (sir′ŭp). Xarope. SIN syrup.
sis·mos·ther·a·py (sis-mo̅-thar′ă-pē). Sismoterapia. SIN vibratory *massage*. [G. *seismos*, agitação, de *seio̅*, fut. *seiso̅*, agitar]
sis·o·mi·cin sul·fate (sis-o̅-mi̅′sin). Sulfato de sisomicina; antibiótico produzido por *Micromonospora inyoensis*, com espectro de atividade e aplicação semelhantes aos da gentamicina.
sis·ter. Irmã; na Grã-Bretanha e países da Comunidade: **1.** Título de uma enfermeira-chefe num hospital público ou numa enfermaria ou sala de cirurgia de um hospital. **2.** Qualquer enfermeira registrada na prática particular.
Sistrunk, Walter Ellis, cirurgião norte-americano, 1880–1933. VER S. *operation*.
site (sit). Local, sítio, localização ou *locus*. SIN situs. [L. *situs*].
  acceptor s., s. aceptor; o local de ligação ribossomal para o aminoacil-tRNA durante a síntese de proteínas.
  acceptor splicing s., local aceptor de junção. SIN right splicing *junction*.
  active s., local ativo; porção de uma molécula de enzima em que ocorre a reação verdadeira; acredita-se que consiste em um ou mais resíduos ou átomos num arranjo especial, permitindo a interação com o substrato para efetuar a reação deste último.
  allosteric s., local alostérico; considerado o local numa enzima, diferente do local ativo, onde um composto, que pode ser o produto final da via de biossíntese envolvendo a enzima, pode ligar-se e influenciar a atividade enzimática ao modificar a configuração da enzima; a influência do CTP (citidina 5′-trifosfato) sobre a atividade da aspartato carbamoiltransferase exemplifica o conceito de um local alostérico numa proteína alostérica.
  antibody-combining s., local de combinação do anticorpo. SIN paratope.
  antigen-binding s., local de ligação do antígeno. SIN paratope.
  cleavage s., local de clivagem. SIN restriction s.
  fragile s. [MIM*136540, MIM*136670], local frágil; lacuna que não se cora num ponto específico de um cromossoma, envolvendo geralmente ambas as cromátides, sempre no mesmo ponto em cromossomas de diferentes células de um indivíduo ou família; resulta na produção *in vitro* de fragmentos acêntricos, cromossomas com deleção ou outras anomalias cromossômicas; herdado como marcador cromossômico dominante.
  immunologically privileged s.'s, locais imunologicamente privilegiados; locais onde os enxertos não são facilmente rejeitados e onde os tumores escapam da vigilância imune, provavelmente porque essas áreas particulares têm pouca drenagem linfática e não são facilmente acessíveis às células efetoras do sistema imune.
  ligand-binding s., local de ligação do ligante; o local, na superfície de uma proteína, que se liga a um ligante; equivalente ao local ativo se o ligante for o substrato de uma enzima.
  privileged s., local privilegiado; área anatômica que carece de drenagem linfática, como o cérebro, a córnea e a bolsa bucal do *hamster*, em que tumores homólogos podem crescer, visto que o hospedeiro não se torna sensibilizado.
  receptor s., local receptor; ponto de fixação dos vírus, hormônios e outros ativadores às membranas celulares.
  replication s., local de replicação; o local *in vivo* de replicação do DNA.
  restriction s., local de restrição; local, no ácido nucleico, em que as bases limitantes são de um tipo que as torna vulneráveis à ação de clivagem de uma endonuclease. SIN cleavage s.
  sequence-tagged s.'s (STSs), locais de seqüência marcados; segmentos curtos de seqüências de DNA que podem ser detectados pelo uso da reação em cadeia da polimerase.

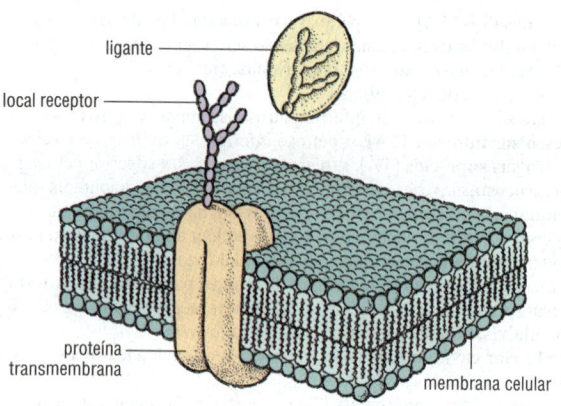

local receptor celular

  switching s., local de mudança; o ponto de ruptura, numa seqüência de DNA, em que um segmento gênico une-se a outro segmento gênico, como na produção das imunoglobulinas.
sito-. Sito-. Alimento, cereal. [G. *sitos, sition*]
si·to·stane (si̅′to̅-stān). Sitostano. SIN stigmastane.
β-si·tos·ter·ol (si̅-to̅-ster′ol). β-Sitosterol; um sitosterol e anticolesterêmico. SIN cinchol.
sitosterolemia (si̅-to̅-ster-o̅-lē-mē-ă). Sitosterolemia. SIN phytosterolemia.
si·to·tax·is (si̅-to̅-tak′sis). Sitotaxia. SIN sitotropism. [sito- + G. *taxis*, arranjo ordenado]
si·to·tox·in (si̅-to̅-tok′sin). Sitotoxina; qualquer toxina alimentar, especialmente a que se desenvolve em cereais. [sito- + G. *toxikon*, veneno]
si·to·tox·ism (si̅-to̅-tok′sizm). Sitotoxismo. **1.** Envenenamento por cereais estragados ou com fungos. **2.** Intoxicação alimentar em geral. [sito- + G. *toxikon*, veneno]
si·tot·ro·pism (si̅-tot′ro̅-pizm). Sitotropismo; movimento das células vivas aproximando-se ou afastando-se do alimento. SIN sitotaxis. [sito- + G. *tropē*, uma volta]
sit·u·a·tion (sich-u̅-ā′shŭn). Situação; conjunto de fatores biológicos, psicológicos e sócio-biológicos que afetam o padrão de comportamento de um indivíduo.
  psychoanalytic s., s. psicanalítica; a relação, tipicamente restrita ao consultório do terapeuta, entre paciente e terapeuta.
si·tus (si̅′tŭs). Sítio, *situs*. SIN site. [L.]
  s. inver′sus, s. *situs inversus*; inversão de posição ou localização. SIN s. transversus.
  s. inversus viscerum, *situs inversus viscerum*, inversão visceral; transposição de vísceras, como, por exemplo, desenvolvimento do fígado do lado esquerdo ou do coração do lado direito. SIN visceral inversion.
  s. perver′sus, posição incorreta de qualquer víscera.
  s. sol′itus, disposição normal das vísceras.
  s. transver′sus, *situs inversus*. SIN s. inversus.
Siwe, Sture A., pediatra sueco, 1897–1966. VER Letterer-S. *disease*.
siz·er (si̅′zer). Calibrador, medidor; cilindro de diâmetro variável, com extremidades arredondadas, utilizado para medir o diâmetro interno do intestino na preparação para grampeamento.
Sjögren, Henrik C., oftalmologista sueco, 1899–1986. VER S. *disease, syndrome*; Gougerot-S. *disease*.
Sjögren, Torsten, médico sueco, 1859–1939. VER S.-Larsson *syndrome*; Torsten S. *syndrome*; Marinesco-Sjögren *syndrome*.
Sjöqvist, O., neurocirurgião sueco, 1901–1954. VER S. *tractotomy*.
SK Abreviatura de streptokinase (estreptoquinase).
skato-. Escato-. Forma obsoleta de scato-.
skat·ole (skat′ōl). Escatol; 3-metil-1*H*-indol, formado no intestino pela decomposição bacteriana do L-triptofano e encontrado na matéria fecal, à qual confere seu odor característico.
skat·ox·yl (skă-tok′sil). Escatoxil; 3-hidroximetilindol formado no intestino pela oxidação do escatol; uma parte sofre conjugação no corpo com os ácidos sulfúrico ou glicurônico, sendo excretada na urina na forma conjugada.
skein (skān). Espirema; os filamentos espiralados de cromatina observados na prófase da mitose. [Gael. *sgeinnidh*, fio do cânhamo]
  choroid s., glomo corióideo. SIN choroid *enlargement*.
skel·e·tal (skel′ĕ-tăl). Esquelético; relativo ao esqueleto.
skel·e·tol·o·gy (skel-ĕ-tol′o̅-jē). Esqueletologia; ramo da anatomia e da mecânica que trata do esqueleto.

skel·e·ton (skelʹē-tŏn). Esqueleto. **1.** A estrutura óssea do corpo nos vertebrados (endoesqueleto) ou o envoltório externo rígido dos insetos (exoesqueleto ou dermoesqueleto). **2.** Todas as partes secas que permanecem após a destruição e remoção de todas as partes moles; inclui os ligamentos e as cartilagens, bem como os ossos. **3.** Todos os ossos do corpo em conjunto. **4.** Estrutura não-óssea, rígida ou semi-rígida, que funciona como arcabouço de suporte de determinada estrutura. [G. *skeletos*, seco, n. *skeleton*, múmia, esqueleto]
 appendicular s. [TA], e. apendicular; os ossos dos membros, incluindo os cíngulos dos membros superiores e inferiores. SIN s. appendiculare [TA].
 s. appendicula're [TA], e. apendicular. SIN appendicular s.
 articulated s., e. articulado; esqueleto montado, estando as várias partes conectadas de modo a demonstrar as relações normais e permitir o movimento entre seus componentes, como ocorre no corpo vivo.
 axial s. [TA], e. axial; os ossos articulados da cabeça e da coluna vertebral, isto é, cabeça e tronco, em oposição ao esqueleto apendicular, constituído pelos ossos articulados dos membros superiores e inferiores. SIN s. axiale [TA].
 s. axia'le [TA], e. axial. SIN axial s.
 cardiac s., e. fibroso cardíaco. SIN fibrous s. of heart.
 cardiac fibrous s., e. fibroso cardíaco. SIN fibrous s. of heart.
 s. of eyelid, tarso. SIN tarsus (2).
 facial s., viscerocrânio; *termo oficial alternativo para viscerocranium.
 fibrous s. of heart, e. fibroso do coração; arcabouço complexo de colágeno denso formando quatro anéis fibrosos (*annuli fibrosi*) que circundam os óstios das valvas, um trígono fibroso direito e esquerdo, formado pela conexão dos anéis, e as porções membranáceas dos septos interatrial e interventricular; encontrado em associação à base dos ventrículos, isto é, ao nível do sulco coronário; suas funções incluem: 1) reforço dos óstios valvares enquanto atua como inserção para os folhetos e as válvulas das valvas; 2) proporciona a origem e a inserção para o miocárdio; e 3) serve como um tipo de "isolante" elétrico, separando os impulsos eletricamente conduzidos dos átrios e ventrículos e proporcionando uma passagem para o feixe atrioventricular de tecido de condução através do trígono fibroso direito e septo interventricular membranáceo. SIN cardiac fibrous s., cardiac s., s. of heart.
 s. of free inferior limb, e. do membro inferior livre; os ossos do membro inferior, exceto os ossos do quadril, isto é, todos os ossos dos membros inferiores, incluindo o fêmur e distalmente a ele.
 s. of free superior limb, e. do membro superior livre; os ossos do membro superior, exceto a escápula e a clavícula, isto é, todos os ossos dos membros superiores, incluindo úmero e distalmente a ele.
 gill arch s., e. dos arcos branquiais; cartilagens associadas à porção visceral do condrocrânio de mamíferos embrionários, representando os esqueletos dos arcos branquiais, conforme observado em peixes do tipo do tubarão; são os primórdios da cartilagem de Meckel, das cartilagens estilóide, hióide, cricóidea, tireóidea e aritenóidea e dos ossículos da audição. VER TAMBÉM branchial *arches*, em *arch*.
 s. of heart, e. fibroso do coração. SIN fibrous s. of heart.
 jaw s., e. da viscerocrânio. SIN viscerocranium.
 thoracic s. [TA], e. torácico; os ossos e a cartilagem que formam o gradil torácico. SIN s. thoracis [TA], s. thoracicus.
 s. thoracicus, e. do tórax. SIN thoracic s.
 s. thoracis [TA], e. do tórax. SIN thoracic s.
 visceral s., e. visceral. SIN visceroskeleton (2).
Skene, Alexander J.C., ginecologista norte-americano, 1837–1900. VER S. *glands*, em *gland*, *tubules*, em *tubule*; *ducts* of S. *glands*, em *duct*.
ske·nei·tis, ske·ni·tis (skē-nīʹtis). Esqueneíte, esquenite; inflamação das glândulas de Skene.
skene·o·scope (skēnʹō-skōp). Esqueneoscópio; tipo de endoscópio para inspeção das glândulas de Skene.
skew (skū). Desvio; assimetria; em estatística, afastamento da simetria de uma distribuição de freqüência.
skia-. Esquia-, cio-. Sombra; substituído por radio-. [G. *skia*]
ski·as·co·py (skī-asʹkō-pē). Retinoscopia. SIN retinoscopy.
Skillern, Penn Gaskell Jr., cirurgião norte-americano, *1882. VER S. *fracture*.
skin [TA]. Pele; a membrana protetora que cobre o corpo, consistindo em epiderme e cório (derme). SIN cutis [TA]. [A.S. *scinn*]
 alligator s., ictiose. SIN ichthyosis.
 bronzed s., p. bronzeada; a pele escura na doença de Addison.
 deciduous s., ceratólise. SIN keratolysis (2).
 elastic s., p. elástica. VER Ehlers-Danlos *syndrome*.
 farmer's s., pele do fazendeiro; pele seca e enrugada com ceratoses pré-malignas secas; observada mais comumente em pessoas de pele clara e olhos azuis expostas ao sol por períodos prolongados e durante muitos anos devido à sua ocupação ou à prática de esportes. SIN golfer's s., sailor's s.
 fish s., ictiose. SIN ichthyosis.

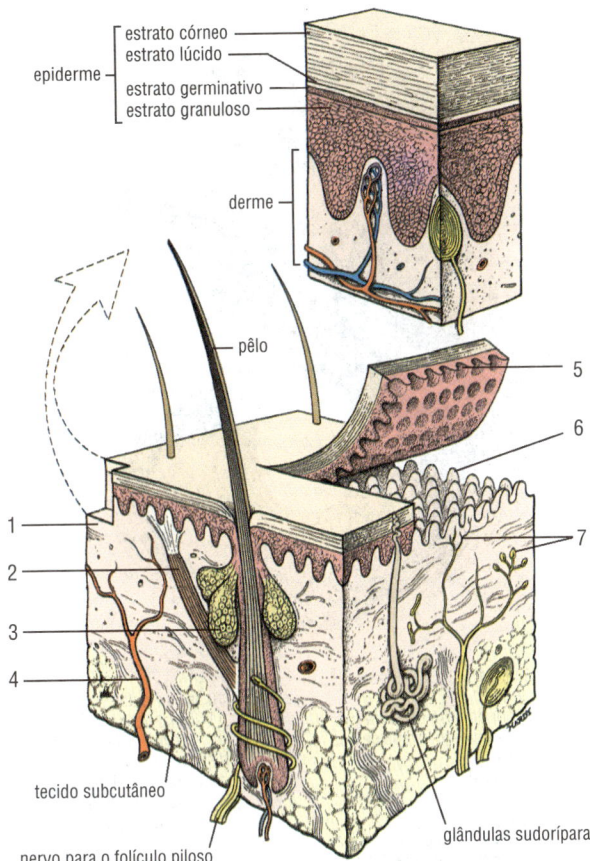

componentes e camadas da pele: (1) derme, (2) músculo eretor dos pêlos, (3) glândula sebácea, (4) vaso sanguíneo, (5) epiderme levantada para mostrar as papilas da derme, (6) papilas, (7) terminações nervosas

 glabrous s., p. glabra; pele normalmente desprovida de pêlos.
 glossy s., atrofodermatose neurítica; atrofia brilhante da pele, habitualmente das mãos, após lesão nervosa; tipo de atrofia neurotrófica. SIN atrophoderma neuriticum.
 golfer's s., pele do jogador de golfe. SIN farmer's s.
 hidden nail s., eponíquia, eponíquio. SIN eponychium (2).
 loose s., dermatocalasia. SIN dermatochalasis.
 parchment s., p. apergaminhada; aparência de pergaminho da pele causada pela perda do tecido conjuntivo e elástico subjacente ou pela perda relativamente rápida e persistente de água da camada córnea.
 piebald s., p. malhada. SIN piebaldism.
 pig s., p. de porco; pele mole em que os folículos estão muito dilatados; observada no mixedema pré-tibial.
 porcupine s., p. hiperceratose epidermolítica. SIN epidermolytic hyperkeratosis.
 sailor's s., p. de marinheiro. SIN farmer's s.
 shagreen s., p. de chagrém; placa nevóide elevada e oval, da cor da pele ou, em certas ocasiões, pigmentada, lisa ou enrugada, que aparece no tronco ou na região lombar nos primeiros anos de vida; algumas vezes observada com outros sinais de esclerose tuberosa. SIN shagreen patch.
 s. of teeth, cutícula do esmalte. SIN enamel *cuticle*.
 thick s., p. espessa; pele das palmas das mãos e plantas dos pés, assim denominada em virtude de sua epiderme relativamente espessa.
 thin s., p. fina; pele de áreas do corpo, à exceção das palmas das mãos e plantas dos pés, assim denominada em virtude de sua epiderme relativamente fina.
 toad s., frinoderma. SIN phrynoderma.
 yellow s., (1) Xantocromia. SIN xanthochromia; (2) Xantoderma. SIN xanthoderma (2).
Skinner, Burrhus F., psicólogo norte-americano, 1904–1990. VER skinnerian *conditioning*; S. *box*.
skin writ·ing. Dermatografismo. SIN dermatographism.
Sklowsky, E.L., médico alemão do século XX. VER S. *symptom*.
Skoda, Joseph, clínico da Boêmia, atuando em Viena, 1805–1881. VER skodaic *resonance*; S. *rale*, *sign*, *tympany*.
sko·da·ic (skō-dāʹik). Skodaico; relativo a Skoda.
skull (skŭl). Crânio. SIN cranium. [Ing. ant. *skulle*, tigela]

skull ... smallpox

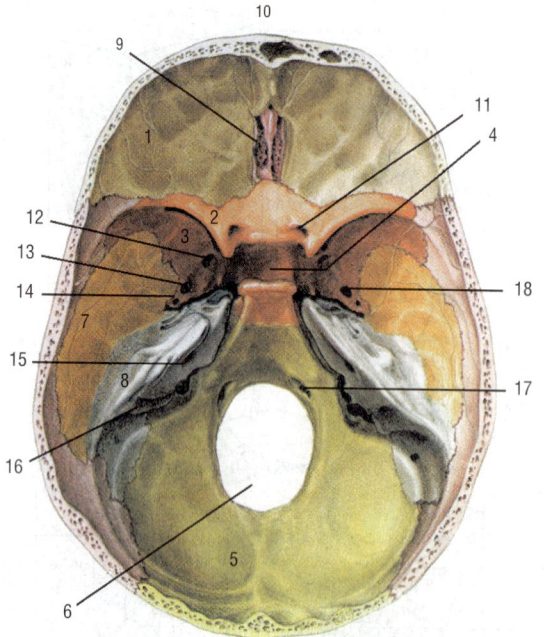

crânio: visão interna da base
1. osso frontal
2. asa menor do osso esfenóide
3. asa maior do osso esfenóide
4. sela turca
5. osso occipital
6. forame magno
7. osso temporal
8. porção petrosa do osso temporal
9. placa cribriforme do osso etmóide
10. seio frontal
11. canal óptico
12. forame rotundo
13. forame oval
14. forame espinhoso
15. meato acústico interno
16. forame jugular
17. canal hipoglosso
18. canal carótido

cloverleaf s., c. em trevo. VER cloverleaf skull *syndrome.*
maplike s., c. geográfico; vários defeitos no crânio, especialmente no osso temporal, na fossa anterior e nas órbitas, formando contornos irregulares semelhantes às fronteiras dos países num atlas.
natiform s., c. natiforme; nódulos ósseos palpáveis na superfície do crânio em lactentes com sífilis congênita (congenital *syphilis*).
steeple s., tower s., oxicefalia. SIN *oxycephaly.*
skull·cap (skŭl′kap). Calota craniana, calvária. SIN *calvaria.*
sky blue (skī′ bloo′). Azul-céu; mistura de pigmentos de estanato de cobalto e sulfato de cálcio; utilizado biologicamente como massa de injeção.
SL Abreviatura de spinal *lenght* (comprimento espinal).
sl Símbolo de slyke.
slab-off. Processo pelo qual o prisma é produzido no campo de leitura de uma lente de óculos através de polimento bicêntrico.
SLE Abreviatura de systemic *lupus* erythematosus (lúpus eritematoso sistêmico).
sleep (slēp). Sono; estado fisiológico de inconsciência relativa e inatividade dos músculos voluntários, cuja necessidade reaparece periodicamente. Os estágios do sono foram variadamente definidos em termos de profundidade (leve, profundo), características do EEG (ondas delta, sincronização), características fisiológicas (REM, NREM) e nível anatômico pressuposto (pontino, mesencefálico, rombencefálico, rolândico, etc.). [A.S. *slaep*]
  electric s., s. elétrico; condição de convulsões e inconsciência induzida pela passagem de uma corrente elétrica através do cérebro.
  electrotherapeutic s., s. eletroterapêutico. VER electrotherapeutic sleep *therapy.*
  hypnotic s., hipnose. SIN *hypnosis.*
  light s., s. leve. SIN *dysnystaxis.*
  paroxysmal s., narcolepsia. SIN *narcolepsy.*
  rapid eye movement s., REM s., s. de movimento rápido dos olhos, s. REM, s. paradoxal; estado de sono profundo em que ocorrem movimentos oculares rápidos, padrão EEG de vigília e sonhos; várias funções centrais e autônomas são distintas durante esse estado.
  s. terror, terror noturno. SIN *night terrors.*
  winter s., s. hibernação. SIN *hibernation.*
sleep·i·ness (slēp′i-nes). Sonolência. SIN *somnolence (1).*
sleep·less·ness (slēp′les-nes). Insônia. SIN *insomnia.*
sleep·talk·ing. Soniloquismo. **1.** Soniloqüência. SIN *somniloquence (1).* **2.** SIN *somniloquy.*
sleep·walk·er. Sonâmbulo. SIN *somnambulist.*
sleep·walk·ing. Sonambulismo. SIN *somnambulism (1).*

slide (slīd). Lâmina; lâmina de vidro retangular sobre a qual se coloca um objeto a ser examinado ao microscópio.
sling. Tipóia; bandagem de apoio ou dispositivo suspensório; especialmente uma alça pendurada no pescoço, que sustenta o antebraço flexionado.
slit. Fenda; abertura ou incisão longa e estreita.
  Cheatle s., f. de Cheatle; incisão longitudinal na borda antimesentérica do intestino delgado que, quando fechada transversalmente, cria uma luz maior do que seria possível por simples anastomose término-terminal; atualmente modificada para incluir incisões longitudinais nas extremidades seccionadas do intestino delgado transeccionado ou outras estruturas tubulares, permitindo a realização de uma anastomose elíptica de grande calibre.
  filtration s.'s, poros de filtração. SIN *slit pores,* em *pore.*
  pudendal s., f. interglútea. SIN *pudendal cleft.*
  vulvar s., f. interglútea. SIN *pudendal cleft.*
slit·lamp. Lâmpada de fenda; em oftalmologia, um instrumento que consiste num microscópio associado a uma fonte luminosa retangular, que pode ser estreitada numa fenda. SIN biomicroscope, Gullstrand s.
  Gullstrand s., lâmpada de fenda de Gullstrand. SIN *slitlamp.*
slope (slōp). Inclinação.
  lower ridge s., i. da crista inferior; a inclinação da crista residual mandibular no segundo e terceiro molares, conforme observado pelo lado bucal.
slough (slŭf). **1.** Crosta; tecido necrosado separado da estrutura viva. **2.** Esfolar; separar do tecido vivo, referindo-se a uma parte morta ou necrosada. [I.m. *slughe*]
Sluder, Greenfield, laringologista norte-americano, 1865–1928.
Sluder neu·ral·gia. Neuralgia de Sluder. ver em neuralgia.
sludge (slŭdj). Lama; sedimento lodoso. VER TAMBÉM sludged *blood.*
  activated s., l. ativada. VER activated sludge *method.*
sluice (sloos). Comporta, eclusa. SIN *waterfall.*
sluice·way (sloos′wā). Boca de eclusa, conduto de evacuação. SIN *spillway.*
slur·ry (sler′ē). Massa semifluida; suspensão semilíquida fina de um sólido em um líquido.
slyke (sl) (slīk). Unidade de valor de tamponamento, a inclinação da curva de titulação ácido-básica de uma solução; os milimoles de ácido ou de base forte que devem ser adicionados por unidade de mudança no pH. [D.D. Van *Slyke*, médico e químico norte-americano, 1883–1971].
Sm Símbolo de samarium (samário).
SMA Abreviatura de sequential multichannel *autoanalyzer,* spinal muscular *atrophy* (auto-analisador seqüencial multicanal; atrofia da musculatura espinal).

small·pox (smawl′poks). Varíola; doença contagiosa eruptiva aguda, causada por um poxvírus (Orthopoxvirus, membro da família Poxviridae) e caracterizada, no início, por calafrios, febre alta, dor nas costas e cefaléia; em 2–5 dias, os sintomas constitucionais desaparecem, e surge uma erupção cutânea na forma de pápulas, que se transformam em vesículas umbilicadas e, a seguir, em pústulas, que secam e formam crostas, as quais, ao caírem, deixam uma marca permanente na pele; o período de incubação médio é de 8–14 dias. Em decorrência de programas de vacinação cada vez mais agressivos, conduzidos no decorrer de um período de cerca de 200 anos, a varíola está atualmente erradicada. SIN variola major, variola. [E. *small pocks,* ou pústulas]

> A varíola foi um flagelo universalmente temido por mais de 3 milênios, com taxas de mortalidade que, algumas vezes, ultrapassavam 20%. A varíola, que, em muitos aspectos, era uma doença singular, não tinha nenhum reservatório não-humano e nenhum estado de portador humano. Inicialmente submetida a algum controle através do processo de variolação na Índia e na China, no século X, foi gradativamente suprimida no mundo industrializado após a marcante descoberta feita por Edward Jenner, em 1776, de que a infecção pelo vírus inócuo da varíola bovina (vacínia) torna os seres humanos imunes ao vírus da varíola. A Organização Mundial de Saúde iniciou, em 1966, um programa de erradicação global, e o último caso de ocorrência natural da doença foi relatado na Somália, em 1977. Hoje em dia, a doença possui principalmente interesse histórico.

  confluent s., v. confluente; forma grave em que as lesões aproximam-se umas das outras, formando grandes áreas supurativas.
  discrete s., v. distinta; forma habitual em que as lesões são separadas e distintas umas das outras.
  fulminating s., v. fulminante. SIN *hemorrhagic s.*
  hemorrhagic s., v. hemorrágica; forma grave e freqüentemente fatal de varíola, acompanhada de extravasamento de sangue para a pele, no estágio inicial, ou nas pústulas num estágio posterior, freqüentemente acompanhada de epistaxe e hemorragia por outros orifícios do corpo. SIN fulminating s., variola hemorrhagica.
  malignant s., v. maligna. SIN *variola maligna.*

modified s., varicelloid s., v. modificada, v. varicelóide. SIN varioloid (2).
West Indian s., v. da Índia Ocidental, alastrim. SIN alastrim.

smear (smēr). Esfregaço; amostra delgada para exame; em geral, o material é espalhado uniformemente sobre uma lâmina de vidro, sendo fixado e, a seguir, corado antes do exame.
alimentary tract s., e. do trato alimentar; conjunto de amostras citológicas contendo material da boca (e. oral), esôfago e estômago (e. gástrico), duodeno (e. paraduodenal) e colo (e. colônico), obtido por técnicas de lavagem especializadas; utilizado principalmente para o diagnóstico de câncer dessas áreas.
bronchoscopic s., e. broncoscópico, e. das vias respiratórias baixas. SIN lower respiratory tract s.
buccal s., e. bucal; esfregaço citológico contendo material obtido por raspagem da mucosa bucal lateral acima da linha denteada, efetuando-se o esfregaço e fixando-o imediatamente; utilizado principalmente para a determinação do sexo somático, conforme indicado pela presença do cromocentro sexual (corpúsculo de Barr).
cervical s., e. cervical; denominação genérica para diferentes tipos de esfregaços do colo uterino, como, por exemplo, ectocervical, endocervical, pancervical; utilizado principalmente para triagem cervical.
colonic s., e. colônico. VER alimentary tract s.
cul-de-sac s., e. do fundo-de-saco; amostra citológica de material obtida por aspiração da bolsa de Douglas (escavação retouterina) do fórnice vaginal posterior, preparada através da realização de esfregaço, centrifugação ou filtração; utilizado principalmente no diagnóstico de câncer de ovário.
cytologic s., e. citológico; tipo de amostra citológica efetuada por esfregaço de uma amostra (obtida de diversos locais por uma variedade de métodos), com fixação e coloração, geralmente em álcool etílico a 95% e coloração de Papanicolaou. SIN cytosmear.
duodenal s., e. duodenal. VER alimentary tract s.
ectocervical s., e. ectocervical; esfregaço citológico de material obtido da ectocérvix, habitualmente por raspagem; utilizado principalmente para o diagnóstico de cânceres tardios envolvendo a ectocérvix.
endocervical s., e. endocervical; esfregaço citológico de material obtido do canal endocervical por *swab*, aspiração ou raspagem; utilizado principalmente para a detecção de câncer cervical em seu estágio inicial.
endometrial s., e. endometrial; conjunto de esfregaços citológicos contendo material obtido diretamente do endométrio por aspiração, lavagem ou escovado da cavidade uterina.
esophageal s., e. esofágico. VER alimentary tract s.
fast s., e. rápido; esfregaço citológico contendo material da região vaginal e raspados pancervicais, misturados e preparados numa lâmina de microscópio, com realização do esfregaço e fixação imediata; utilizado principalmente para triagem de rotina dos ovários, do endométrio, do colo uterino, da vagina e dos estados hormonais.
gastric s., e. gástrico. VER alimentary tract s.
lateral vaginal wall s., e. da parede lateral da vagina; e. citológico contendo material obtido através de raspagem da parede lateral da vagina, próximo à junção de seu terço superior e médio; utilizado para avaliação cito-hormonal.
lower respiratory tract s., e. das vias respiratórias inferiores; conjunto de amostras citológicas contendo material das vias respiratórias inferiores e consistindo principalmente em escarro (espontâneo, induzido) e material obtido na broncoscopia (aspirado, lavado, escovado); utilizado para estudo citológico do câncer e de outras doenças do pulmão. SIN bronchoscopic s., sputum s.
oral s., e. oral. VER alimentary tract s.
pancervical s., e. pancervical; esfregaço citológico de material obtido do canal endocervical, do orifício externo e da ectocérvix através de raspagem dessas áreas com uma espátula cervical apropriada; utilizado principalmente para a detecção precoce do câncer cervical.
Pap s., e. de Papanicolaou; esfregaço de células vaginais ou cervicais obtidas para estudo citológico. SIN Papanicolaou s.
Papanicolaou s., e. de Papanicolaou. SIN Pap s.
sputum s., e. de escarro. SIN lower respiratory tract s.
urinary s., e. urinário; conjunto de amostras citológicas contendo urina processada obtida da bexiga, dos ureteres ou da pelve renal; utilizado para o estudo citológico do câncer e de outras doenças das vias urinárias.
vaginal s., e. vaginal; esfregaço de fragmentos da luz vaginal de tênias de mamíferos, utilizado para determinar o estágio de seu ciclo reprodutivo. É mais útil em mamíferos subprimatas cujos ciclos estrais são curtos; as células epiteliais nucleadas e os leucócitos prevalecem no esfregaço durante o diestro e o proestro, enquanto predominam as células cornificadas durante o estro.
VCE s., e. VCE; esfregaço citológico de material obtido da vagina, da ectocérvix e da endocérvix, com esfregaços realizados separadamente (nessa ordem) numa lâmina e fixados imediatamente; utilizado principalmente para detecção de câncer do colo uterino e identificação dos locais de doenças nessas áreas, bem como para avaliação hormonal.

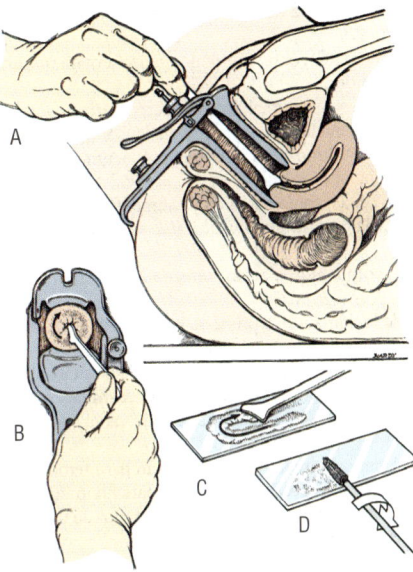

esfregaço de Papanicolaou (ou de Pap): (A) espéculo no lugar e espátula de Ayre em posição no orifício cervical; (B) a ponta da espátula é aplicada no orifício cervical, e efetua-se uma rotação de 360°; (C) o material celular aderido à espátula é então espalhado uniformemente sobre a lâmina de vidro, que é imediatamente colocada em solução de fixador; (D) faz-se girar a escova citológica no orifício cervical, que é, em seguida, girada sobre a lâmina de vidro

smeg·ma (smeg′mă). Esmegma; acúmulo pastoso e fétido de células epidérmicas descamadas e sebo nas áreas úmidas da genitália. [G. unguent]
s. clitor′idis, e. do clitóris; a secreção das glândulas apócrinas do clitóris, em combinação com células epiteliais em descamação.
s. prepu′tii, e. do prepúcio; secreção esbranquiçada que se acumula sob o prepúcio do pênis ou do clitóris; composto principalmente de células epiteliais descamadas.
smeg·ma·lith (smeg′mă-lith). Esmegmólito; concreção calcária no esmegma. [smegma + G. *lithos*, pedra]
smell. 1. Cheirar; perceber um odor por meio do aparelho olfativo. 2. Olfação. SIN olfaction (1). 3. Odor, cheiro. SIN odor.
smell-brain (smel′brān). Rinencéfalo. SIN rhinencephalon.
Smellie, William, obstetra inglês, 1698–1763. VER S. *scissors*.
Smith, David W., pediatra norte-americano, 1926–1981. VER S.-Lemli-Opitz *syndrome*.
Smith, Henry, cirurgião militar inglês, nascido na Irlanda e radicado na Índia, 1862–1948. VER S. *operation*; S.-Indian *operation*.
Smith, M.J.V., urologista norte-americano do século XX.
Smith, Robert W., cirurgião irlandês, 1807–1873. VER S. *fracture*.
Smith, Theobald, patologista norte-americano, 1859–1934. VER Theobald S. *phenomenon*.
Smith, William R., médico norte-americano do século XX. VER S.-Riley *syndrome*.
Smith-Petersen, Marius N., cirurgião norte-americano, 1886–1953. VER Smith-Petersen *nail*.
smog. *Smog*; poluição do ar caracterizada por uma atmosfera de névoa, freqüentemente muito irritante, resultante de uma mistura de nevoeiro com fumaça e outros poluentes do ar. [smoke + fog]
smut (smŭt). Alforra; alfonsia, ferrugem; doença fúngica de grãos de cereais, causada por espécies do gênero *Ustilago* e caracterizada por massas castanho-escuras ou pretas de esporos nas plantas; p. ex., alforra do milho (*U. maydis*); alforra frouxa do trigo (*U. nuda*).
Sn Símbolo de tin (estanho).
^{113}**Sn** Símbolo de tin-113 (estanho-113).
sn-. Prefixo que significa numerado estereoespecificamente; sistema de numeração dos átomos de carbono do glicerol em lipídios, de modo que os números permanecem constantes, independentemente de substituições químicas, ao contrário da numeração sistemática.
snail (snāl). Caramujo; nome comum dos membros da classe Gastropoda (filo Mollusca). Os caramujos pulmonados de água doce (não-operculados, de respiração aérea) (subclasse Pulmonata, ordem Basommatophora) incluem a maioria dos hospedeiros intermediários de parasitas trematódeos dos seres humanos e de aves e mamíferos domésticos, principalmente nas famílias Lymnaeidae e Planorbidae. A subclasse Prosobranchiata, os caramujos operculados, inclui a ordem Neogastropoda, que compreende os caramujos cônicos venenosos (gênero *Conus*), e a ordem Mesogatropoda, cuja família Hydrobii-

snail

dae compreende a maioria dos caramujos hospedeiros de importância clínica [I.m. *snaile*]

snake (snāk). Serpente, cobra; réptil alongado, sem membros e com escamas da subordem Ophidia.

snake·root (snāk′root). Serpentária. SIN serpentaria.
   Canada s., s.-do-Canadá. SIN *Asarum canadense*.
   European s., s.-da-Europa. SIN *Asarum europaeum*.
   Seneca s., Sênega. SIN senega.
   Texas s., s.-do-Texas; fonte botânica da serpentária.
   Virginia s., s.-da-Virgínia; *Aristolochia serpentaria;* fonte botânica da serpentária.

snap. Estalido; som agudo e curto; refere-se especialmente aos ruídos cardíacos.
   closing s., e. de fechamento; a primeira bulha cardíaca acentuada da estenose mitral, relacionada ao fechamento da valva anormal.
   opening s., e. de abertura; estalido agudo e alto no início da diástole, habitualmente audível com maior nitidez entre o ápice cardíaco e a borda esternal esquerda inferior, relacionado com a abertura da valva anormal em casos de estenose mitral.

snare (snār). Alça, laço metálico; instrumento para remoção de pólipos e outras projeções de uma superfície, especialmente no interior de uma cavidade; consiste numa alça metálica que é passada ao redor da base do tumor e gradualmente apertada. [A.S. *snear*, cordão]
   cold s., alça fria; alça não-aquecida.
   galvanocaustic s., hot s., alça galvanocáustica, alça quente; alça cujo metal é aquecido a uma temperatura elevada por uma corrente elétrica.

SNE Abreviatura de *subacute necrotizing encephalomyelopathy* (encefalomielopatia necrosante subaguda).

Sneddon, Ian B., dermatologista inglês do século XX. VER S. *syndrome;* S.-Wilkinson *disease*.

sneeze (snēz). **1.** Espirrar; expelir ar do nariz e da boca por uma contração espasmódica involuntária dos músculos da expiração. **2.** Espirro; ato de espirrar; reflexo desencadeado por irritação da mucosa do nariz ou, algumas vezes, por uma luz forte incidindo no olho. [A.S. *fneōsan*]

Snell, Simeon, oftalmologista inglês, 1851–1909. VER S. *law*.

Snellen, Hermann, oftalmologista holandês, 1834–1908. VER S. *sign, test types*.

snore (snōr). **1.** Ronco; ruído inspiratório rude e estrondoso produzido pela vibração do palato pendular, algumas vezes das cordas vocais, durante o sono ou o coma. VER TAMBÉM stertor, rhonchus. **2.** Roncar; respirar ruidosamente ou com um ronco. [A.S. *snora*]

snow (snō). Neve. VER *carbon dioxide snow*.

snRNA Abreviatura de *small nuclear RNA* (RNA nuclear pequeno).

snuff (snŭf). **1.** Inalação, fungada; inalar forçadamente através do nariz. **2.** Rapé; tabaco finamente pulverizado utilizado por inalação através do nariz ou aplicado às gengivas. **3.** Qualquer pó medicinal aplicado por insuflação à mucosa nasal. [echoic]

snuff·box (snŭf′boks). Tabaqueira. VER *anatomic snuffbox*.

snuf·fles (snŭf′lz). Respiração nasal obstruída, especialmente no recém-nascido, algumas vezes devido à sífilis congênita.

Snyder, Marshall L., microbiologista norte-americano, 1907–1969. VER S. *test*.

SOAP Acrônimo de *subjective, objective, assessment,* and *plan* (avaliação e planejamento subjetivos, objetivos); utilizado em registros orientados para o problema, a fim de organizar dados de acompanhamento, avaliação e planejamento.

soap (sōp). Sabão; sais de sódio ou de potássio de ácidos graxos de cadeia longa (p. ex., estearato de sódio); utilizado como emulsificador para fins de limpeza e como excipiente na fabricação de pílulas e supositórios. [A.S. *sape,* L. *sapo,* G. *sapōn*]
   animal s., s. animal; sabão feito com hidróxido de sódio e uma gordura animal purificada, que consiste principalmente em estearina; utilizado em farmácia no preparo de certos linimentos. SIN curd s., domestic s., tallow s.
   Castile s., s. de Castile. SIN hard s.
   curd s., domestic s., s. animal. SIN animal s.
   green s., s. verde. SIN medicinal soft s.
   hard s., s. duro, s. de pedra; sabão fabricado com óleo de oliva ou algum outro óleo ou gordura apropriado e hidróxido de sódio; utilizado como detergente, bem como na forma de supositório ou enema de espuma de sabão para constipação; utilizado também como excipiente em pílulas. SIN Castile s.
   insoluble s., s. insolúvel; sabão feito com um ácido graxo e uma base terrosa ou metálica (sais de ferro ou cálcio de ácidos graxos).
   marine s., s. marinho; sabão feito de óleo de palma ou de coco para uso com água do mar, na qual é solúvel. SIN salt water s.
   medicinal soft s., s. mole medicinal; sabão feito com óleos vegetais, hidróxido de potássio, ácido oleico, glicerina e água purificada; utilizado como agente de limpeza e como estimulante em doenças cutâneas crônicas. SIN green s., soft s.
   salt water s., s. de água salgada. SIN marine s.
   soft s., s. mole medicinal. SIN medicinal soft s.
   soluble s., s. solúvel; qualquer sabão feito com hidróxido de potássio, sódio ou amônio; sabão animal comum, sabão de Castile, sabão verde, etc.
   superfatted s., s. supergorduroso; sabão que contém um excesso (3–5%) de gordura acima daquela necessária para neutralizar por completo todo o álcali; utilizado na fabricação do sabão medicinal, bem como no tratamento de doenças cutâneas.
   tallow s., s. animal. SIN animal s.

soap·stone (sōp′stōn). Pedra-sabão, esteatita. SIN talc.

Soave, F., cirurgião pediátrico italiano do século XX. VER S. *operation*.

so·cal·o·in (sō-kal′ō-in). Socaloína; uma aloína obtida do aloés da Ilha de Socotra.

so·cia (sō′shē-ă). Porção ectópica, supranumerária ou acessória de um órgão.
   socia parotidis (sō′shē-ă pa-rot′i-dis). Glândula parótida acessória. SIN accessory parotid *gland*. [L. companheiro da parótida]

so·cial·i·za·tion (sō′shăl-i-zā′shŭn). Socialização. **1.** Processo de aprendizado de atitudes e habilidades interpessoais e interativas que estão de acordo com os valores de determinada sociedade. **2.** Em terapia de grupo, maneira de aprender a participar efetivamente no grupo. [L. *socius,* parceiro, companheiro]

socio-. Sócio-. Social, sociedade. [L. *socius,* companheiro]

so·ci·o·ac·u·sis (sō-sē-ō-ak-ū′sis). Socioacusia; perda da audição produzida por exposição a ruído não-ocupacional, como pequenas armas disparadas na caça e na prática ao alvo. [socio- + G. *akousis,* audição]

so·ci·o·cen·tric (sō′sē-ō-sen′trik). Sociocêntrico; sociável; reativo ao meio social ou cultural. [socio- + L. *centrum,* centro]

so·ci·o·cen·trism (sō′sē-ō-sen′trizm). Sociocentrismo; consideração do próprio social como padrão através do qual os outros são avaliados.

so·ci·o·cosm (sō′sē-ō-kozm). Sociocosmo; a totalidade que inclui a sociedade humana, o pensamento humano e a relação dos seres humanos com a natureza. [socio- + G. *kosmos,* universo]

so·ci·o·gen·e·sis (sō′sē-ō-jen′ĕ-sis). Sociogênese; a origem do comportamento social a partir de experiências interpessoais passadas. [socio- + G. *genesis,* origem]

so·ci·o·gram (sō′sē-ō-gram). Sociograma; representação diagramática das valências e graus de atração e aceitação de cada indivíduo de acordo com as interações interpessoais entre membros de um grupo; diagrama em que as interações do grupo são analisadas com base em atrações mútuas ou antipatias entre os membros do grupo. [socio- + G. *gramma,* algo escrito]

so·ci·o·med·i·cal (sō′sē-ō-med′i-kăl). Sócio-médico; pertinente à relação entre a prática da medicina e a sociedade.

so·ci·om·e·try (sō-sē-om′ĕ-trē). Sociometria; o estudo das relações interpessoais num grupo. [socio- + G. *metron,* medida]

so·ci·o·path (sō′sē-ō-path). Sociopata; designação de uma pessoa com distúrbio de personalidade anti-social. VER TAMBÉM antisocial *personality,* psychopath.

so·ci·op·a·thy (sō-sē-op′ă-thē). Sociopatia; termo para referir-se ao padrão comportamental exibido por pessoas com distúrbio de personalidade anti-social. VER TAMBÉM personality *disorder*. [socio- + G. *pathos,* sofrimento]

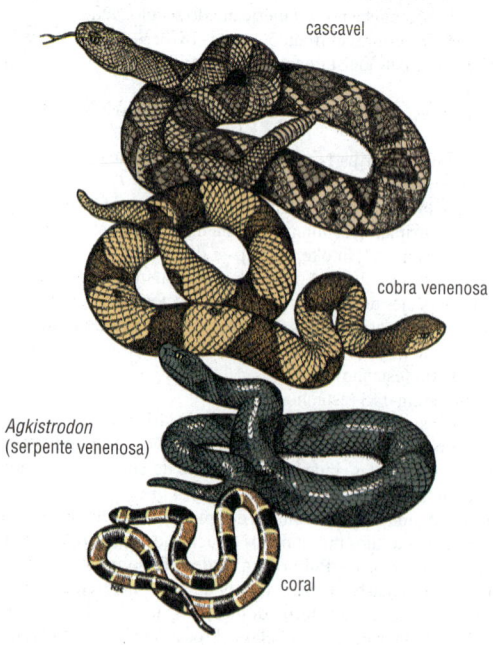

serpentes venenosas

sock·et (sok'et). Alvéolo, cavidade, gonfose. SIN gomphosis. **1.** A parte oca de uma articulação; a escavação em um osso de uma articulação que recebe a extremidade articular do outro osso. **2.** Qualquer concavidade na qual se encaixa outra parte, como a órbita. [atr. Fr. ant. do L. *soccus,* sapato, meia]
dry s., cavidade, alvéolo. SIN alveoalgia.
eye s., órbita; em geral a órbita, embora a verdadeira "concavidade" para o bulbo do olho, na qual seria inserida uma prótese ocular, seja formada pela bainha fascial do bulbo do olho. SIN orbit.
tooth s. [TA], alvéolo dentário; cavidade no processo alveolar do maxilar ou da mandíbula, no interior da qual cada dente se encaixa e está fixado por meio do ligamento periodontal. SIN alveolus dentalis [TA], alveolus (4) [NA].
SOD Abreviatura de *superoxide* dismutase (superóxido dismutase).
so·da (sō'dă). Soda. SIN *sodium* carbonate. [It., possivelmente do L. medev. barrilheira]
baking s., bicarbonato de sódio. SIN *sodium* bicarbonate.
caustic s., s. cáustica; hidróxido de sódio. SIN *sodium* hydroxide.
s. lime, cal de soda; mistura de hidróxidos de cálcio e de sódio utilizada para absorver dióxido de carbono em situações nas quais ocorre nova respiração; p. ex., em determinações basais ou em certos tipos de circuitos anestésicos.
washing s., carbonato de sódio. SIN *sodium* carbonate.
so·dic (sō'dik). Sódico; relativo a ou que contém soda ou sódio.
sodio-. Sódio-. Composto que contém sódio; como o citrato de sódio, o tartarato de sódio, um citrato ou tartarato de algum elemento que contém sódio.

SODIUM

so·di·um (Na) (sō'dē-ŭm). Sódio; elemento metálico, de número atômico 11, peso atômico 22,989768; metal alcalino que se oxida prontamente no ar ou na água; seus sais são encontrados em sistemas biológicos naturais, sendo muito utilizados na medicina e na indústria. O íon sódio é o íon extracelular mais abundante do corpo. Para os sais de sódio orgânicos não relacionados a seguir, VER sob o nome da porção ácida orgânica. SIN natrium. [L. mod. de *soda*]
s. acetate, acetato de s.; alcalinizante sistêmico e urinário, expectorante e diurético.
s. acid carbonate, carbonato ácido de s. SIN s. bicarbonate.
s. acid citrate, citrato ácido de s. SIN s. citrate.
s. acid phosphate, fosfato ácido de s. SIN s. biphosphate.
s. alginate, alginato de s. SIN algin.
s. *p*-aminohippurate, *p*-amino-hipurato de s.; utilizado por via intravenosa em provas de função renal, para determinar o fluxo plasmático renal e a excreção tubular.
s. *p*-aminophenylarsonate, *p*-aminofenilarsonato de s.; composto que foi um dos primeiros arsenicais pentavalentes modernos. SIN s. arsanilate.
s. aminosalicylate, aminosalicilato de s.; utilizado para os mesmos propósitos do que o ácido aminosalicílico.
s. antimonylgluconate, antimonilgliconato de s. SIN stibogluconate *sodium* (2).
s. antimonyl tartrate, antimonil tartarato de s. SIN antimony sodium tartrate.
s. arsanilate, arsanilato de s. SIN s. *p*-aminophenylarsonate.
s. ascorbate, ascorbato de s.; mesmas ações e usos do ácido ascórbico; é preferido para administração intramuscular.
s. aurothiomalate, aurotiomalato de s. SIN gold sodium thiomalate.
s. aurothiosulfate, aurotiossulfato de s. SIN gold sodium thiosulfate.
s. benzoate, benzoato de s.; utilizado no reumatismo agudo e crônico, como prova de função hepática e como conservante.
s. bicarbonate, bicarbonato de s.; NaHCO$_3$; utilizado como antiácido gástrico e sistêmico, para alcalinizar a urina e para lavagens de cavidades corporais. SIN baking soda, s. acid carbonate, s. hydrogen carbonate.
s. biphosphate, bifosfato de s.; utilizado para aumentar a acidez urinária. SIN primary s. phosphate, s. acid phosphate, s. dihydrogen phosphate.
s. bisulfite, bissulfito de s.; NaHSO$_3$; sulfito sódico ácido, utilizado na fermentação gástrica e intestinal, externamente no tratamento de doenças parasitárias e como antioxidante em determinadas injeções (metabissulfito de sódio). SIN s. hydrogen sulfite, s. pyrosulfite.
s. borate, borato de s.; utilizado em loções, gargarejos, colutórios e como detergente. SIN borax, s. pyroborate, s. tetraborate.
s. bromide, brometo de s.; NaBr hipnótico e sedativo obsoleto; em certas ocasiões, utilizado na epilepsia e em outros distúrbios funcionais do sistema nervoso.
s. cacodylate, cacodilato de s.; utilizado na anemia, na leucemia e na malária. SIN s. dimethylarsenate.
s. carbonate, carbonato de s.; utilizado no tratamento de doenças cutâneas descamativas; raramente tem outras aplicações na medicina devido à sua ação irritante. SIN sal soda, soda, washing soda.

s. carboxymethyl cellulose, carboximetil celulose de s.; o sal sódico de um éter policarboximetil da celulose; utilizado como laxativo devido à sua não-digestibilidade e ligação à água no trato gastrointestinal.
s. chloride, cloreto de s.; NaCl o principal componente do sangue de outros líquidos corporais, bem como da urina; utilizado para tornar soluções salinas isotônicas e fisiológicas, no tratamento da depleção de sal e, topicamente, para lesões inflamatórias. SIN common salt, table salt.
s. citrate, citrato de s.; utilizado como diurético, antilítico, alcalinizante sistêmico e urinário, expectorante e anticoagulante (in vitro). SIN s. acid citrate.
s. citrate, acid, citrato ácido de s.; possui as mesmas ações e usos do citrato de sódio; além disso, pode ser utilizado em soluções de glicose sem produzir caramelização da última durante a auto clavagem.
s. cromoglycate, cromoglicato de s. SIN cromolyn sodium.
s. dehydrocholate, desidrocolato de s.; colagogo; também utilizado para determinar o tempo de circulação.
s. diatrizoate, diatrizoato de s.; composto de iodo orgânico hidrossolúvel, utilizado antigamente na urografia intravenosa e na angiografia.
dibasic s. phosphate, fosfato de s. dibásico. SIN s. phosphate.
s. dihydrogen phosphate, fosfato diidrogenado de s. SIN s. biphosphate.
s. dimethylarsenate, dimetilarsenato de s. SIN s. cacodylate.
s. dodecyl sulfate (SDS), sulfato sódico de dodecila. SIN s. lauryl sulfate.
effervescent s. phosphate, fosfato de s. efervescente; fosfato de sódio 200 dessecado, bicarbonato de sódio 477, ácido tartárico 252 e ácido cítrico 162, misturados e passados através de uma peneira para produzir um sal granulado.
exsiccated s. sulfite, sulfito de s. dessecado; sulfito de sódio anidro, utilizado como preservativo em preparações farmacêuticas.
s. fluoride, fluoreto de s.; utilizado como profilático dentário contra cáries na água potável, bem como topicamente na forma de solução a 2% aplicada aos dentes.
s. fluosilicate, fluossilicato de s. SIN s. hexafluorosilicate.
s. folate, folato de s.; o sal sódico do ácido fólico; suas ações e usos são iguais aos do ácido fólico, porém é preferido para administração parenteral. SIN s. pteroylglutamate.
s. fusidate, fusidato de s. SIN fusidate sodium.
s. glycerophosphate, gliceroforfato de s.; tem sido utilizado como tônico.
s. hexafluorosilicate, hexafluorosilicato de s.; Na$_2$SiF$_6$ utilizado (em soluções diluídas) como anti-séptico e desodorante, bem como para fluoração da água potável. SIN s. fluosilicate, s. silicofluoride.
s. hydrogen carbonate, carbonato hidrogenado de s. SIN s. bicarbonate.
s. hydrogen sulfite, sulfito hidrogenado de s. SIN s. bisulfite.
s. hydroxide, hidróxido de s.; NaOH utilizado externamente como cáustico. SIN caustic soda.
s. hypochlorite, hipoclorito de s.; oxidante forte; explosivo quando na forma anidra. Decompõe-se ao absorver dióxido de carbono do ar; libera cloro e oxigênio; utilizado em solução aquosa como alvejante e desinfetante. Trata-se do componente ativo de muitos alvejantes domésticos, como, por exemplo, Clorox.
s. hypophosphite, hipofosfito de s.; antigamente utilizado como tônico dos nervos.
s. hyposulfite, hipossulfito de s. SIN s. thiosulfate.
s. ichthyolsulfonate, ictiossulfonato de s.; alterativo e anti-séptico.
s. indigotin disulfonate, dissulfonato sódico de indigotina. SIN indigo carmine.
s. iodide, iodeto de s.; NaI; utilizado como fonte de iodo.
s. lactate, lactato de s.; alcalinizante sistêmico e urinário.
s. lauryl sulfate, sulfato sódico de lauril; agente tensoativo do tipo aniônico, utilizado em pastas dentifríceas. SIN s. dodecyl sulfate.
s. levothyroxine, levotiroxina sódica; sal sódico do isômero natural da tiroxina, um hormônio tireóideo. É duas vezes mais eficaz do que a forma racêmica. Utilizada no tratamento do hipotireoidismo em seres humanos e animais, bem como para tratar a fertilidade diminuída em touros e para estimular a lactação em animais.
s. liothyronine, liotironina sódica; L-triiodotironina, o isômero fisiologicamente ativo da triiodotironina, duas vezes mais ativo do que a forma racêmica; utilizada no tratamento das síndromes de deficiência da tireóide. Trata-se de um metabólito da tiroxina.
s. metabisulfite, metabissulfito de s.; utilizado como antioxidante em soluções injetáveis.
s. methicillin, meticilina sódica. SIN methicilin sodium.
s. methylarsonate, metilarsonato de s.; antigamente utilizado na tuberculose, na coréia e em outras afecções nas quais se usavam cacodilatos.
s. nitrate, nitrato de s.; NaNO$_3$; antigamente utilizado no tratamento da disenteria e como diurético. SIN Chilean saltpeter, cubic niter.
s. nitrite, nitrito de s.; NaNO$_2$ utilizado para reduzir a pressão arterial sistêmica, aliviar espasmos vasomotores locais, especialmente na angina de peito e na doença de Raynaud, para relaxar os espasmos brônquicos e intestinais e como antídoto para o envenenamento por cianeto.
s. nitroferricyanide, nitroferricianeto de s. SIN s. nitroprusside.
s. nitroprusside, nitroprussiato de s.; potente vasodilatador arterial e venoso de ação rápida, utilizado em emergências hipertensivas e administrado por via

intravenosa. Atua de modo semelhante aos nitratos e nitritos vasodilatadores através da doação de óxido nítrico que produz vasodilatação; também utilizado como reagente para detecção de compostos orgânicos na urina. SIN s. nitroferricyanide.

s. orthophosphate, ortofosfato de s. SIN s. phosphate.

s. perborate, perborato de s.; utilizado na preparação extemporânea de peróxido de hidrogênio; uma solução a 2% equivale, na sua ação germicida, a 0,4% de peróxido de hidrogênio.

s. peroxide, peróxido de s.; Na_2O_2; utilizado externamente como pasta ou sabão no tratamento de comedões e da acne.

s. pertechnetate, pertecnetato de s.; $NaTC^{99m}O_4$; radiofármaco utilizado na cintilografia do cérebro, da tireóide e das glândulas salivares.

s. phosphate, fosfato de s.; laxativo. SIN dibasic s. phosphate, s. orthophosphate.

s. phosphate ^{32}P, fosfato de sódio P^{32}; fósforo radioativo aniônico na forma de uma solução de fosfato ácido de sódio e fosfato básico de sódio; emissor beta com meia-vida de 14,3 dias; após a sua administração, as maiores concentrações são encontradas nos tecidos de rápida proliferação; utilizado no tratamento da policitemia vera, leucemia mielógena crônica e metástases ósseas. VER TAMBÉM chromic phosphate ^{32}P colloidal *suspension*.

s. polyanhydromannuronic acid sulfate, sulfato sódico do ácido polianidromanurônico; anticoagulante preparado a partir do ácido algínico, com ação semelhante à da heparina.

s. polystyrene sulfonate, sulfonato sódico de polistireno; resina de troca catiônica utilizada na hiperpotassemia.

s. potassium tartrate, tartarato de potássio e s. SIN *potassium* sodium tartrate.

pravastatin s., pravastatina sódica; agente anti-hiperlipoproteinêmico. Inibidor da HMG-Co redutase, que se assemelha à lovastatina e sinvastatina; inibe a formação de colesterol.

primary s. phosphate, fosfato de s. primário. SIN s. biphosphate.

s. propionate, propionato de s.; o sal sódico do ácido propiônico; utilizado nas infecções fúngicas da pele, habitualmente em combinação com propionato de cálcio; utilizado como conservante.

s. psylliate, psiliato de s.; o sal sódico dos ácidos graxos líquidos do óleo psílio, preparado por dissolução do ácido graxo em solução diluída de hidróxido de sódio; utilizado como morruato de sódio como agente esclerosante no tratamento das vias varicosas.

s. pteroylglutamate, pteroilglutamato de s. SIN s. folate.

s. pyroborate, piroborato de s. SIN s. borate.

s. pyrosulfite, pirossulfito de s. SIN s. bisulfite.

s. rhodanate, rodanato de s. SIN s. thiocyanate.

s. ricinoleate, s. ricinate, ricinoleato de s., ricinato de s.; o sal sódico do ácido ricinoleico; agente esclerosante de ação semelhante à do morruato de sódio.

s. salicylate, salicilato de s.; analgésico, antipirético e anti-reumático.

s. silicofluoride, silicofluoreto de s. SIN s. hexafluorosilicate.

s. stearate, estearato de s.; o sal sódico do ácido esteárico, utilizado como adjuvante farmacêutico em pomadas, cremes e supositórios.

s. sulfate, sulfato de s.; componente de muitas das águas laxativas naturais, também utilizado como catártico hidragogo, primariamente em animais de grande porte. SIN Glauber salt.

s. sulfite, sulfito de s.; tem sido utilizado para o alívio da fermentação intestinal e externamente na estomatite aftosa.

s. sulfocyanate, sulfocianato de s. SIN s. thiocyanate.

s. sulforicinate, s. sulforicinoleate, sulforicinato de s., sulforicinoleato de s.; produzido pela combinação do óleo de rícino, ácido sulfúrico e hidróxido e cloreto de sódio; utilizado como solvente para iodo, iodofórmio, resorcinol, pirogalol e várias outras substâncias para uso externo.

s. tartrate, tartarato de s.; laxante.

s. taurocholate, taurocolato de s.; o sal sódico do ácido taurocólico, extraído da bile de carnívoros; colagogo.

s. tetraborate, tetraborato de s. SIN s. borate.

s. tetradecyl sulfate, tetradecil sulfato de s.; agente tensoativo aniônico utilizado pelas suas propriedades umidificantes para aumentar a ação superficial de determinadas soluções anti-sépticas; também utilizado como agente esclerosante semelhante ao morruato de sódio no tratamento das veias varicosas.

s. thiocyanate, tiocianato de s.; antigamente utilizado no tratamento da hipertensão essencial. SIN s. rhodanate, s. sulfocyanate.

s. thiosulfate, tiossulfato de s.; antídoto no envenenamento por cianeto juntamente com o nitrito de sódio; utilizado como agente profilático contra infecções causadas por tinha em piscinas e banheiros, bem como para medir o volume de líquido extracelular do corpo. SIN s. hyposulfite.

s. tungstoborate, tungstoborato de s.; utilizado em microscopia eletrônica como corante negativo.

so·di·um-24 (^{24}Na). Sódio-24; o isótopo do sódio com peso atômico de 24 e meia-vida de 14,96 h; emite raios beta e gama, sendo mais fácil de preparar do que o Na^{22} emissor de pósitrons de meia-vida mais longa (meia-vida de 2,605 anos). É utilizado para medir o líquido extracelular por diluição de indicador.

so·di·um group. Grupo do sódio; os metais alcalinos: césio, lítio, potássio, rubídio e sódio.

so·do·ku (sō-dō'koo). Sodoku. SIN rat-bite *fever*. [Jap. veneno de rato]

sod·om·ist, sod·om·ite (sod'ō-mist, -mīt). Sodomita; aquele que pratica sodomia. [G. *sodomitēs*, habitante da cidade bíblica de Sodoma, que foi destruída pelo fogo por causa da luxúria de seu povo]

sod·o·my (sod'ōm-ē). Sodomia; termo que designa várias práticas sexuais variadamente condenadas pela lei, especialmente bestialidade, contato orogenital e coito anal. SIN buggery. [ver sodomist]

Soemmerring, Samuel Thomas von, anatomista alemão, 1755–1830. VER S. *ganglion, ligament, muscle, spot; ring* of S.

Soffer, Louis J., internista norte-americano, *1904. VER Sohval-S. *syndrome*.

soft·ware. *Software*; o programa ou as instruções de um computador.

Sohval, Arthur R., internista norte-americano, *1904. VER S.-Soffer *syndrome*.

soil (soyl). Sujeira, excremento.

night s., fezes humanas utilizadas como fertilizante.

so·ja (sō'yah). Soja. SIN soybean.

so·ko·sho ((sō-kō'shō). Sokosho. SIN rat-bite *fever*. [Jap. *so*, rato + *ko*, mordida + *sho*, doença]

sol. Sol. **1.** Dispersão coloidal de um sólido num líquido. Cf. gel. **2.** Abreviatura de solution (solução).

So·la·na·ce·ae (sō-lă-nā'sē-ē). Família de plantas que inclui o gênero *Solanum* (erva-moura) e cerca de 84 outros gêneros que compreendem 1.800 espécies, incluindo beladona, tomate e batata.

so·la·na·ceous (sō-lă-nā'shŭs, sol'ă-). Solanáceo; relativo a plantas da família Solanaceae ou a drogas delas derivadas.

sol·a·no·chro·mene (sol'ă-nō-krō'mēn). Solanocromeno. SIN plastochromenol-8.

so·lap·sone (sō-lap'sōn). Solapsona. SIN solasulfone.

sol·a·sul·fone (sol-ă-sŭlf'ōn). Solassulfona; agente leprostático. SIN solapsone.

sol·a·tion (sol-ā'shŭn). Solação; em química coloidal, a transformação de um gel em sol, como ocorre na liquefação da gelatina.

sol·der (sod'er). Solda. **1.** Liga de metal fundível empregada para unir bordas ou superfícies de duas peças de metal de maior ponto de fusão; as soldas duras, que em geral contêm ouro ou prata como principal componente, costumam ser utilizadas em odontologia para unir ligas de metal nobre. **2.** Unir duas peças de metal com essa liga. [L. *solido*, tornar sólido, através do Fr., várias formas]

sol·der·ing (sod'er-ing). Soldagem; técnica de laser para fazer aderir um tecido a outro.

sole (sōl) [TA]. Planta, sola. A superfície plantar ou parte inferior do pé. SIN planta [TA], pelma. [A.S.]

s. of foot [TA], planta do pé; face inferior ou base do pé, cuja maior parte está em contato com o chão na posição ortostática; recoberta com pele glabra habitualmente não-pigmentada, particularmente espessada e com cristas epidérmicas nas áreas de sustentação do peso. SIN planta pedis [TA], plantar region*, regio plantaris*, plantar surface of foot.

So·le·nog·ly·pha (sō-lē-nog'li-fă). Importante categoria de serpentes, que inclui as famílias da víbora e da cascavel. [L., do G. *solēn*, tubo, cano + *glyphō*, entalhar]

so·le·noid (sol'ē-noyd). Solenóide; espiral de fio eletricamente energizado para produzir um campo magnético, que induz uma corrente em qualquer condutor colocado dentro da espiral ou próximo a ela.

So·le·no·po·tes cap·il·la·tus (sō-lē-nop'ō-tēz kap-i-lā'tŭs). Piolho sugador de bovinos, conhecido como o pequeno piolho azul do gado bovino nos Estados Unidos e como piolho transmissor da tuberculose na Austrália. [G. *solen*, tubo + *potos*, bebida)

so·le·nop·sin A (sō-lē-nop'sin). Solenopsina A; um dos vários — provavelmente cinco — alcalóides presentes no veneno da formiga-de-fogo, *Solenopsis saevissima;* o veneno possui propriedades necrotóxicas, hemolíticas, inseticidas e antibióticas.

Solenopsis (sōl-ē-nop'sis). Gênero de formigas conhecidas como formigas-de-fogo (lava-pés), cujas picadas dolorosas causam queimação e reações locais e, em certas ocasiões, sistêmicas.

S. invicta, a formiga-de-fogo vermelha importada, uma espécie proveniente da América do Sul que se propagou bastante no sudeste dos Estados Unidos, onde passou a constituir uma importante praga tanto para os seres humanos quanto para os animais; pica seres humanos, produzindo tumefação e prurido locais, com formação de uma pústula no local da picada, podendo, em raros casos, causar choque anafilático com morte por parada respiratória ou cardíaca. VER TAMBÉM *S. richteri*. SIN red imported fire ant.

S. richteri, a formiga-de-fogo negra importada, uma espécie proveniente da América do Sul, porém que está menos amplamente estabelecida nos Estados Unidos do que a *S. invicta*. VER TAMBÉM *S. invicta*. SIN black imported fire ant.

so·le·us (sō-lē'ŭs). Sóleo. VER soleus (*muscle*). [L. mod. do L. *solea*, sandália, planta do pé (de animais), de *solum*, base, assoalho, chão]

sol·id. Sólido. **1.** Firme; compacto; não-fluido; sem interstícios ou cavidades; não-esponjoso. **2.** Corpo que preserva sua forma quando não confinado; que não é fluido, nem líquido nem gasoso. [L. *solidus*]

sol·id·ism (sol'i-dizm). Solidismo; a teoria proposta por Asclepiades e seus seguidores segundo a qual a doença era causada por um desequilíbrio entre partículas sólidas (átomos) do corpo e os espaços (poros) entre elas, uma doutrina que se opunha ao conceito humoral de Hipócrates. SIN methodism.

sol·id·ist (sol'i-dist). Solidista; seguidor da doutrina do solidismo.

sol·id·is·tic (sol-i-dis'tik). Solidístico; relativo ao solidismo.

sol·i·dus (sol'i-dūs). Sólido; a linha, num diagrama de organização, que indica a temperatura abaixo da qual todo o metal é sólido.

sol·i·ped (sol'i-ped). Solípede; animal de casco sólido, como o cavalo. [L. *solidus*, sólido + *pes*, pé]

sol·ip·sism (sō'lip-sizm, sol'ip-). Solipsismo; conceito filosófico segundo o qual tudo que existe é o produto do desejo e das idéias do indivíduo que percebe. [L. *solus*, só + *ipse*, próprio]

soln. Abreviatura de solution (solução).

sol·u·bil·i·ty (sol-ū-bil'i-tē). Solubilidade; a propriedade de ser solúvel.

sol·u·ble (sol'ū-bl). Solúvel; capaz de ser dissolvido. [L. *solubilis*, de *solvo*, dissolver]

so·lum (sō'lŭm). Fundo; a parte inferior. [L.]

sol·ute (sol'ūt, sō'loot). Soluto; a substância dissolvida numa solução. [L. *solutus*, dissolvido, pp. de *solvo*, dissolver]

so·lu·tio (sō-loo'shē-ō). Solução. SIN solution. [L.]

so·lu·tion (sol., soln.) (sō-loo'shun). Solução. **1.** A incorporação de um sólido, líquido ou gás em um líquido ou sólido não-cristalino, resultando numa fase única homogênea. VER dispersion, suspension. **2.** Em geral, uma solução aquosa de uma substância não-volátil. **3.** Na linguagem da Farmacopéia, uma solução aquosa de uma substância não-volátil é denominada solução ou líquor; uma solução aquosa de uma substância volátil é uma água (aqua); uma solução alcoólica de uma substância não-volátil é uma tintura (tinctura); uma solução alcoólica de uma substância volátil é um espírito (spiritus); uma solução em vinagre é um vinagre (acetum); uma solução em glicerina é um glicerol (glyceritum); uma solução em vinho é um vinho (vinum); uma solução de açúcar em água é um xarope (syrupus); uma solução de uma substância mucilaginosa é uma mucilagem (mucilago); uma solução de um alcalóide ou óxido metálico em ácido oleico é um oleato (oleatum). **4.** O término de uma doença por uma crise. **5.** Ruptura, corte ou laceração dos tecidos sólidos. VER s. of contiguity, s. of continuity. SIN solutio. [L. *solutio*].

acetic s., s. acética; um vinagre.

amaranth s., s. de amaranto; uma solução a 1% de amaranto (ácido naftol sulfônico trissódico), um corante vermelho-vivo sintético, estável em ácido e intensificado em solução de hidróxido de sódio; utilizado como corante vermelho ou rosado em produtos farmacêuticos líquidos.

aqueous s., s. aquosa; solução contendo água como solvente; os exemplos incluem água de cal, água de rosas, solução salina e grande número de soluções para administração intravenosa.

Benedict s., s. de Benedict; solução aquosa de citrato de sódio, carbonato de sódio e sulfato de cobre cuja cor azul normal modifica-se para laranja, vermelho ou amarelo na presença de açúcar redutor, como a glicose. VER TAMBÉM Benedict *test* for glucose.

Burow s., s. de Burow; preparação de subacetato de alumínio e ácido acético glacial, utilizada pela sua ação anti-séptica e adstringente sobre a pele.

chemical s., s. química. VER solution (1).

colloidal s., s. coloidal; um dispersóide, emulsóide ou suspensóide. SIN colloidal dispersion.

s. of contiguity, s. de contigüidade; ruptura da contigüidade; luxação ou deslocamento de duas partes normalmente contíguas.

s. of continuity, s. de continuidade; divisão de ossos ou partes moles normalmente contínuas produzida, p. ex., por fratura, laceração ou incisão. SIN dieresis.

Dakin s., s. de Dakin; irrigante bactericida para feridas. SIN Dakin fluid.

disclosing s., s. reveladora; solução que cora seletivamente todos os resíduos moles, películas e placa bacteriana sobre os dentes; utilizada como auxiliar na identificação da placa bacteriana após enxágüe com água.

Earle s., s. de Earle; meio de cultura tecidual contendo $CaCl_2$, $MgSO_4$, KCl, $NaHCO_3$, NaCl, $NaH_2PO_4 \cdot H_2O$ e glicose.

ethereal s., s. etérea; solução de qualquer substância em éter.

Fehling s., s. de Fehling; solução de tartarato de cobre alcalina antigamente utilizada para detecção de açúcares redutores. SIN Fehling reagent.

ferric and ammonium acetate s., s. de acetato férrico e de amônio; líquido claro, aromático e castanho-avermelhado que tem sido utilizado na anemia ferropriva em animais e seres humanos; fonte de ferro. SIN Basham mixture.

Fonio s., s. de Fonio; diluente com sulfato de magnésio, empregado para esfregaços corados de plaquetas sanguíneas.

Gallego differentiating s., s. diferenciadora de Gallego; solução diluída de formaldeído e ácido acético usada numa coloração de Gram modificada para diferenciar e aumentar a ligação da fucsina básica aos microrganismos Gram-negativos.

Gey s., s. de Gey; solução salina habitualmente utilizada em combinação com substâncias orgânicas de ocorrência natural (p. ex., soro sanguíneo, extratos teciduais) e/ou soluções nutritivas quimicamente definidas e mais complexas para cultura de células animais.

Hanks s., s. de Hanks; solução salina habitualmente utilizada em combinação com substâncias orgânicas de ocorrência natural (p. ex., soro sanguíneo, extratos teciduais) e/ou soluções nutritivas quimicamente definidas e mais complexas para cultura de células animais; duas variações contêm $CaCl_2$, $MgSO_4 \cdot 7H_2O$, KCl, KH_2PO_4, $NaHCO_3$, NaCl, $Na_2HPO_4 \cdot 2H_2O$ e D-glicose.

Hartman s., s. de Hartman; solução empregada para dessensibilizar a dentina em cirurgias dentárias; contém timol, álcool etílico e éter sulfúrico.

Hartmann s., s. de Hartmann. SIN lactated Ringer s.

Hayem s., s. de Hayem; diluente sanguíneo utilizado antes da contagem de eritrócitos.

Krebs-Ringer s., s. de Krebs-Ringer; uma modificação da solução de Ringer, preparada misturando-se NaCl, KCl, $CaCl_2$, $MgSO_4$ e tampão fosfato, pH 7,4.

lactated Ringer s., s. de Ringer lactato; solução contendo NaCl, lactato de sódio, $CaCl_2$ (diidrato) e KCl em água destilada; utilizada para os mesmos propósitos da solução de Ringer. SIN Hartmann s.

Lange s., s. de Lange; solução de ouro coloidal utilizada para demonstrar anormalidades das proteínas no líquido espinal. VER Lange *test*.

Locke s.'s, soluções de Locke; soluções contendo, em quantidades variáveis, NaCl, $CaCl_2$, KCl, $NaHCO_3$ e D-glicose; usadas para irrigar o coração de mamíferos e outros tecidos em experimentos laboratoriais; também utilizadas em combinação com substâncias orgânicas de ocorrência natural (p. ex., soro sanguíneo, extratos teciduais) e/ou soluções nutritivas quimicamente definidas e mais complexas para cultura de células animais.

Locke-Ringer s., s. de Locke-Ringer; solução contendo NaCl, $CaCl_2$, KCl, $MgCl_2$, $NaHCO_3$, D-glicose e água; usada em laboratório para experimentos fisiológicos e farmacológicos.

Lugol iodine s., s. iodada de Lugol; solução de iodo-iodeto de potássio empregada como agente oxidante, para remoção de artefatos de fixação mercuriais e, também, em histoquímica e para corar amebas.

molecular dispersed s., dispersóide. SIN dispersoid.

Monsel s., s. de Monsel; solução de subsulfato férrico utilizada para coagular o sangramento superficial, como aquele que ocorre após biopsia cutânea.

normal s., s. normal. VER normal (3).

ophthalmic s.'s, soluções oftálmicas; soluções estéreis, livres de partículas estranhas e apropriadamente misturadas e dispensadas para instilação no olho.

Ringer s., s. de Ringer; **(1)** solução semelhante ao soro sanguíneo em seus componentes salinos; contém 8,6 g de NaCl, 0,3 g de KCl e 0,33 g de $CaCl_2$ em cada 1.000 mL de água destilada; utilizada na forma de infusão intravenosa para reposição hidroeletrolítica; **(2)** solução salina habitualmente utilizada em combinação com substâncias orgânicas de ocorrência natural (p. ex., soro sanguíneo, extratos teciduais) e/ou soluções nutritivas quimicamente definidas e mais complexas para cultura de células animais. SIN Ringer lactate. VER Ringer *injection*.

saline s., (1) solução salina; uma solução de qualquer sal. SIN salt s. **(2)** especificamente, uma solução isotônica de cloreto de sódio; 0,85–0,9 por 100 mL de água.

salt s., s. salina. SIN saline s. (1).

saturated s. (sat. sol., sat. soln.), s. saturada; solução que contém a quantidade máxima de uma substância capaz de se dissolver; solução de uma substância em equilíbrio com um excesso de substância não-dissolvida.

standard s., standardized s., s. padrão, s. padronizada; solução de concentração conhecida, usada como padrão de comparação ou análise.

supersaturated s., s. supersaturada; solução contendo maior quantidade do sólido do que o do líquido que normalmente seria dissolvida no líquido; produzida por aquecimento do solvente quando se adiciona a substância, sendo esta última retida sem precipitação com o resfriamento; a adição de um cristal ou sólido de qualquer tipo geralmente resulta em precipitação do excesso do soluto, deixando uma solução saturada.

test s., s. de teste; solução de algum reagente, em concentração definida, utilizada em análise química ou testes.

Tyrode s., s. de Tyrode; solução de Locke modificado; contém 8 g de NaCl, 0,2 g de KCl, 0,2 g de $CaCl_2$, 0,1 g de $MgCl_2$, 0,05 g de NaH_2PO_4, 1 g de $NaHCO_3$, 1 g de D-glicose e água até 1.000 mL; utilizada para irrigação da cavidade peritoneal, bem como em estudos laboratoriais.

volumetric s. (VS), s. volumétrica; solução produzida pela mistura de volumes medidos dos componentes.

Weigert iodine s., s. de iodo de Weigert; mistura de iodo e iodeto de potássio usada como reagente para alterar violeta cristal e metil, de modo que sejam retidos por determinadas bactérias e fungos.

sol·vate (sol'vāt). Solvato; solução não-aquosa ou dispersóide na qual existe uma combinação não-covalente ou facilmente reversível entre solvente e soluto, ou meio de dispersão e fase dispersa; quando a água é o solvente ou meio de dispersão, denomina-se hidrato.

sol·va·tion (sol-vā'shŭn). Solvatação; combinação não-covalente ou facilmente reversível de um solvente com um soluto ou de um meio de dispersão com a fase dispersa; se o solvente for água, a solvatação é denominada hidratação. A solvatação afeta o tamanho dos íons em solução; assim, o Na^+ é muito maior na H_2O do que em NaCl sólido.

sol·vent. Solvente; líquido que mantém outra substância em solução, isto é, que a dissolve. [L. *solvens*, p. pres. de *solvo*, dissolver]
   amphiprotic s., s. anfiprótico; s. capaz de atuar como ácido ou como base; p. ex., H_2O. VER solvolysis.
   fat s.'s, solventes lipídicos; líquidos orgânicos notáveis pela sua capacidade de dissolver lipídios; em geral, mas nem sempre, imiscíveis em água; p. ex., éter dietílico, tetracloreto de carbono. SIN nonpolar s.'s.
   nonpolar s.'s, solventes não-polares. SIN fat s.'s.
   polar s.'s, solventes polares; solventes que exercem forças polares sobre os solutos, devido ao elevado momento dipolo, ampla separação de cargas elétricas ou associação forte; p. ex., água, álcoois, ácidos.
   universal s., s. universal; substância buscada pelos alquimistas e que alguns afirmaram ter encontrado, supostamente capaz de dissolver todas as substâncias; termo algumas vezes aplicado, em sentido fisiológico, à água.

sol·vol·y·sis (sol-vol'i-sis). Solvólise; a reação de um sal dissolvido com o solvente para formar um ácido e uma base; o inverso (parcial) da neutralização. Se o solvente for água, um solvente anfiprótico, a solvólise é denominada hidrólise.

so·ma (sō'mă). Soma. **1.** A parte axial do corpo, isto é, cabeça, pescoço, tronco e cauda, excluindo os membros. **2.** Tudo de um organismo, à exceção das células germinativas. VER TAMBÉM body. **3.** O corpo de uma célula nervosa do qual se projetam axônios, dendritos etc. [G. *sōma*, corpo]

so·man (sō'man). Inibidor extremamente potente da colinesterase. VER TAMBÉM sarin, tabun.

so·mas·the·nia (sō-mas-thē'nē-ă). Somastenia. SIN somatasthenia.

△ **somat-.** VER somato-.

so·ma·tag·no·sia (sō'mă-tag-nō'sē-ă). Somatagnosia. SIN somatotopagnosis. [somat- + G. *a-* priv. + *gnōsis*, reconhecimento]

so·ma·tal·gia (sō-mă-tal'jē-ă). Somatalgia. **1.** Dor no corpo. **2.** Dor com causas orgânicas, em oposição à dor psicogênica. [somat- + G. *algos*, dor]

so·ma·tas·the·nia (sō'mă-tas-thē'nē-ă). Somatastenia; condição de fraqueza física crônica e fatigabilidade. SIN somasthenia. [somat- + G. *astheneia*, fraqueza]

so·ma·tes·the·sia (sō'mă-tes-thē'zē-ă). Somatestesia; sensação corporal, a percepção consciente do corpo. SIN somesthesia. [somat- + G. *aisthēsis*, sensação]

so·mat·es·the·tic (sō'mat-es-thet'ik). Somatestético; relativo à somatestesia.

so·mat·ic (sō-mat'ik). Somático. **1.** Relativo ao soma ou tronco, à parede da cavidade corporal ou ao corpo em geral. SIN parietal (2). **2.** Relativo a ou envolvendo o esqueleto ou musculatura esquelética (voluntária) e inervação desta última, em oposição as vísceras ou musculatura visceral (involuntária) e sua inervação (autônoma). SIN parietal (3). **3.** Relativo às funções vegetativas, em oposição às funções geradoras. [G. *sōmatikos*, corporal]

so·mat·i·co·splanch·nic (sō-mat-i-kō-splangk'nik). Somaticoesplâncnico; relativo ao corpo e às vísceras. SIN somaticovisceral. [G. *sōmatikos*, relativo ao corpo + *splanchnikos*, relativo às vísceras]

so·mat·i·co·vis·cer·al (sō-mat-i-kō-vis'er-ăl). Somaticovisceral. SIN somaticosplanchnic.

so·ma·tist (sō'mă-tist). Somatista; termo mais antigo para referir-se àquele que considera as neuroses e psicoses como manifestações de doença orgânica.

so·ma·ti·za·tion (sō'mat-i-zā'shŭn). Somatização; o processo pelo qual as necessidades psicológicas se expressam em sintomas físicos; p. ex., a expressão ou conversão em sintomas físicos de ansiedade, ou o desejo de ganho material associado a uma ação legal após lesão ou necessidade psicológica relacionada. VER TAMBÉM somatization *disorder*.

△ **somato-, somat-, somatico-.** O corpo, corporal. [G. *sōma*, corpo]

so·ma·to·chrome (sō-mat'ō-krōm). Somatocromo; designa o grupo de neurônios ou células nervosas em que existe uma abundância de citoplasma, circundando o núcleo por completo. [somato- + G. *chrōma*, cor]

so·ma·t·o·crin·in (sō'mă-tō-crin'in). Somatocrinina; hormônio liberador do hormônio do crescimento hipotalâmico, GHRH. [somato- + G. *krinō*, secretar + *-in*]

so·ma·to·gen·ic (sō'mă-tō-jen'ik). Somatogênico. **1.** Que se origina no soma ou corpo sob a influência de forças externas. **2.** Que tem origem nas células corporais. [somato- + G. *genesis*, origem]

so·ma·to·lib·er·in (sō'mă-tō-lib'er-in). Somatoliberina; um decapeptídeo liberado pelo hipotálamo, que induz a liberação do hormônio de crescimento humano (somatotropina). SIN growth hormone-releasing factor, growth hormone-releasing hormone, somatotropin-releasing factor, somatotropin-releasing hormone. [somatotropin + L. *libero*, liberar + *-in*]

so·ma·tol·o·gy (sō-mă-tol'o-jē). Somatologia; a ciência que estuda o corpo; inclui tanto a anatomia quanto a fisiologia. [somato- + G. *logos*, estudo]

so·ma·to·mam·mo·tro·pin (sō'mă-tō-mam'ō-trō-pin). Somatomamotropina; hormônio peptídico estreitamente relacionado à somatotropina em suas propriedades biológicas, produzido pela placenta normal e por determinadas neoplasias. [somato- + L. *mamma*, mama + G. *tropē*, uma volta, + *-in*]
   human chorionic s. (HCS), s. coriônica humana. SIN human placental *lactogen*.

so·ma·to·me·din (sō'mă-tō-mē'din). Somatomedina; a somatomedina A é um peptídeo (PM de cerca de 4.000) sintetizado no fígado e, provavelmente, no rim, capaz de estimular determinados processos anabólicos no osso e na cartilagem, como a síntese de DNA, RNA e proteína (incluindo a condromucoproteína) e a sulfatação de mucopolissacarídeos; sabe-se que a secreção e/ou a atividade biológica da somatomedina dependem da somatotropina. VER TAMBÉM insulinlike growth *factor*. [*somato*, tropina + *mediator* + *-in*]

so·ma·to·me·dins. Somatomedinas. SIN insulinlike growth *factor*.

so·ma·tom·e·try (sō-mă-tom'e-trē). Somatometria; classificação dos indivíduos de acordo com a forma do corpo e relação dos tipos com características fisiológicas e psicológicas. [somato- + G. *metron*, medida]

so·ma·top·a·gus (sō-mă-top'ă-gŭs). Somatópago; gêmeos unidos em suas regiões corporais. VER conjoined *twins*, em twin. [somato- + G. *pagos*, algo fixado]

so·ma·to·path·ic (sō'mă-tō-path'ik). Somatopático; relativo a doença corporal ou orgânica, em oposição ao distúrbio mental (psicológico). [somato- + G. *pathos*, sofrimento]

so·ma·top·a·thy (sō-mă-top'ă-thē). Somatopatia; termo obsoleto para referir-se a qualquer doença do corpo. [somato- + G. *pathos*, sofrimento]

somatopause. Somatopausa; diminuição nas atividades do eixo hormônio do crescimento–fator de crescimento insulino-símile associada ao envelhecimento.

so·ma·to·phre·nia (sō'mă-tō-frē'nē-ă). Somatofrenia; termo mais antigo para referir-se a uma tendência a imaginar ou exagerar doenças corporais. [somato- + G. *phrēn*, mente]

so·ma·to·plasm (sō-mat'ō-plazm). Somatoplasma; conjunto de todas as formas de protoplasma especializadas que entram na composição do corpo, à exceção do plasma germinativo. [somato- + G. *plasma*, algo formado]

so·ma·to·pleure (sō'mă-tō-ploor). Somatopleura; camada embrionária formada pela associação da camada parietal do mesoderma lateral com o ectoderma. [somato- + G. *pleura*, lado]

so·ma·to·pros·thet·ics (sō'ma-tō-pros-thet'iks). Somatoprotética; a arte e a ciência de substituir partes externas do corpo ausentes ou deformadas por próteses. [somato- + G. *prosthesis*, uma adição]

so·ma·to·psy·chic (sō'mă-tō-sī'kik). Somatopsíquico; relativo à relação corpo-mente; o estudo dos efeitos do corpo sobre a mente, em oposição à psicossomática, que é o estudo dos efeitos da mente sobre o corpo. [somato- + G. *psychē*, alma]

so·ma·to·psy·cho·sis (sō'mă-tō-sī-kō'sis). Somatopsicose; distúrbio emocional associado a uma doença orgânica. [somato- + G. *psychōsis*, animação]

so·ma·tos·co·py (sō-mă-tos'kō-pē). Somatoscopia; exame do corpo. [somato- + G. *skopeō*, ver]

so·ma·to·sen·so·ry (sō'mă-tō-sen'sō-rē). Somatossensorial; sensação relativa às partes superficiais e profundas do corpo em contraste com os sentidos especializados, como a visão.

so·ma·to·sex·u·al (sō'mă-tō-sek'shoo-ăl). Somatossexual; designa os aspectos somáticos da sexualidade, em oposição a seus aspectos psicossociais.

so·ma·to·stat·in (sō'mă-tō-stat'in). Somatostatina; tetradecapeptídeo capaz de inibir a liberação da somatotropina pelo lobo anterior da hipófise; a somatostatina possui meia-vida curta; inibe também a liberação de insulina e de gastrina. SIN growth hormone-inhibiting hormone, somatotropin release-inhibiting factor, somatotropin release-inhibiting hormone. [somatotropin + G. *stasis*, permanecer quieto + *-in*]

so·ma·to·stat·i·no·ma (sō'mă-tō-stat-i-nō'mă). Somatostatinoma; tumor das ilhotas pancreáticas secretor de somatostatina.

so·ma·to·ther·a·py (sō'mă-tō-thār'ă-pē). Somatoterapia. **1.** Terapia direcionada para distúrbios físicos. **2.** Em psiquiatria, inúmeras intervenções terapêuticas que empregam métodos químicos ou físicos, em oposição a métodos psicológicos.

so·ma·to·top·ag·no·sis (sō'mă-tō-top'ag-nō'sis). Somatotopagnose; a incapacidade de identificar qualquer parte do corpo, seja do próprio corpo ou de outro. Cf. autotopagnosia. SIN somatagnosia. [somato- + top- + G. *a-* priv. + G. *gnōsis*, conhecimento]

so·ma·to·top·ic (sō-mă-tō-top'ik). Somatotópico; relativo à somatotopia.

so·ma·tot·o·py (sō-mă-tot'ō-pē). Somatotopia; a associação topográfica de relações de posição de receptores no corpo através das respectivas fibras nervosas à sua distribuição terminal em áreas funcionais específicas do córtex cerebral; a continuação dessas relações de posição em todos os estágios de ascensão dessas fibras nervosas através do sistema nervoso central permite ao cérebro e à medula espinal funcionar numa base de unidades designadas espacialmente. [somato- + G. *topos*, lugar]

so·ma·to·tropes (sō-mă'tō-trōps). Somatotropos; subclasse de células acidofílicas da hipófise, local de síntese do hormônio do crescimento.

so·ma·to·troph (sō′mat′ō - trof). Somatotrofo; célula da adeno-hipófise que produz somatotropina.

so·ma·to·tro·phic (sō′mă - tō - trof′ik). Somatotrófico. SIN somatotropic. [somato- + G. *trophē*, nutrição]

so·ma·to·tro·pic (sō′mă - tō - trop′ik). Somatotrópico; que exerce efeito estimulante sobre o crescimento do corpo. SIN somatotrophic. [somato- + G. *tropē*, uma volta]

so·ma·to·tro·pin (sō′mă - tō - trō′pin). Somatotropina; hormônio proteico do lobo anterior da hipófise produzido pelas células acidófilas, que promove o crescimento do corpo, a mobilização de gorduras e a inibição da utilização da glicose; diabetogênico quando presente em excesso; a deficiência de somatotropina está associada a diversos tipos de nanismo (o tipo III é um distúrbio ligado ao X). SIN growth hormone, pituitary growth hormone, somatotropic hormone. [para *somatotrophin*, de somato- + G. *trophē*, nutrição; corrompido de -tropin e reanalisada como proveniente do G. *tropē*, uma volta]

so·ma·to·type (sō′mă - tō - tīp). Somatotipo. **1.** O tipo constitucional ou corporal de um indivíduo. **2.** O tipo constitucional ou corporal particular associado a um tipo de personalidade específico.

so·ma·to·ty·pol·o·gy (sō′mă - tō - tī - pol′ō - jē). Somatotipologia; o estudo dos somatotipos. [somato- + G. *typos*, forma + *logos*, estudo]

so·ma·trem (sō′mă - trem). Somatrem; hormônio do crescimento *N*-L-metionil (humano); hormônio polipeptídico purificado, produzido por técnicas de DNA recombinante, que contém a seqüência idêntica de 191 aminoácidos que constitui a somatropina natural, mais um aminoácido adicional, a metionina; utilizado no tratamento em longo prazo de crianças com deficiência de somatotropina.

somatropin (so - ma - trō′pin). Somatropina; fármaco idêntico ao hormônio do crescimento (GH) humano; utilizado no tratamento de distúrbios do crescimento decorrentes de secreção insuficiente do hormônio do crescimento em crianças ou em adultos, ou em associação à disgenesia gonadal (síndrome de Turner) e de distúrbios do crescimento em crianças pré-puberais com insuficiência renal crônica.

som·es·the·sia (sō - mes - thē′zē - ă). Somestesia. SIN somatesthesia.

so·mite (sō′mīt). Somito; uma das massas celulares pares, de disposição metamérica, formadas no mesoderma paraxial embrionário inicial; começando na terceira ou no início da quarta semana na região do metencéfalo, desenvolvem-se em direção caudal, tipicamente, até que sejam formados 42 pares. SIN mesoblastic segment. [G. *sōma*, corpo + -*ite*]

occipital s., s. occipital; um dos quatro somitos mais rostrais; tornam-se incorporados à região occipital do crânio embrionário.

som·nam·bu·lance (som - nam′bū - lans). Sonambulismo. SIN somnambulism (1).

som·nam·bu·lism (som - nam′bū - lizm). Sonambulismo. **1.** Distúrbio do sono que envolve complexos atos motores; ocorre primariamente durante o primeiro terço da noite, mas não durante o sono com movimentos rápidos dos olhos (sono REM). SIN oneirodynia activa, sleepwalking, somnambulance. **2.** Forma de histeria em que o indivíduo esquece o comportamento intencional. [L. *somnus*, sono + *ambulo*, andar]

som·nam·bu·list (som - nam′bū - list). Sonâmbulo; que está sujeito ao sonambulismo (1). SIN sleepwalker.

som·ni·fa·cient (som - ni - fā′shent). Sonifaciente. SIN soporific (1). [L. *somnus*, sono + *facio*, fazer]

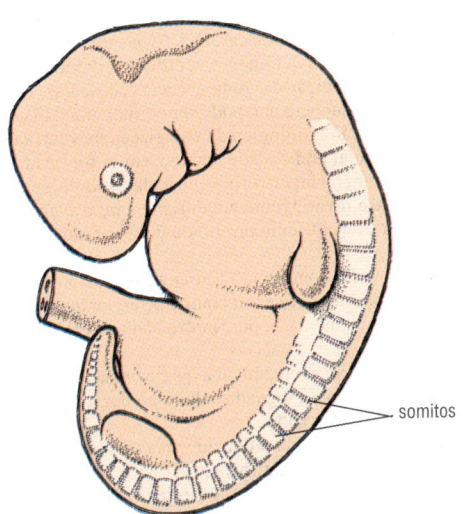

somitos: num embrião humano de 29 dias

som·nif·er·ous (som - nif′er - ŭs). Sonífero. SIN soporific (1). [L. *somnus*, sono + *fero*, trazer]

som·nif·ic (som - nif′ik). Sonífico. SIN soporific (1).

som·nil·o·quence, som·nil·o·quism (som - nil′ō - kwens, - kwizm). Soniloqüência. **1.** Falar ou murmurar durante o sono. SIN sleeptalking (1). **2.** SIN somniloquy. [L. *somnus*, sono + *loquor*, falar]

som·nil·o·quist (som - nil′ō - kwist). Soniloquista; que habitualmente fala dormindo.

som·nil·o·quy (som - nil′ō - kwē). Soniloquia; que fala sob a influência de sugestão hipnótica. SIN sleeptalking (2), somniloquence (2), somniloquism. [L. *somnus*, sono + *loquor*, falar]

som·no·lence, som·no·len·cy (som′nō - lens, - len - sē). Sonolência. **1.** Tendência a dormir. SIN sleepiness. **2.** Estado de torpor. SIN somnolentia (1). [L. *somnolentia*]

som·no·lent (som′nō - lent). Sonolento. **1.** Que tem tendência a dormir. **2.** Numa condição de sono incompleto; meio adormecido, semicomatoso. [L. *somnus*, dormir]

som·no·len·tia (som - nō - len′shē - ă). Sonolência. **1.** SIN somnolence. **2.** SIN sleep *drunkenness*. [L.]

som·no·les·cent (som - nō - les′ent). Sonolento; inclinado a dormir.

som·no·lism (som′nō - lizm). Hipnotismo. SIN hypnotism (1).

Somogyi, Michael, bioquímico norte-americano, 1883–1971. VER S. *effect, method, unit*.

Sondermann, R., oftalmologista alemão do século XX. VER S. *canal*.

sone (sōn). Sone; unidade de intensidade; um tom puro de 1.000 Hz a 40 dB acima do limiar normal de audibilidade possui uma intensidade de 1 s. [L. *sonus*, som]

son·ic (son′ik). Sônico; relativo a, ou determinado por, som; p. ex., vibração sônica. [L. *sonus*, som]

son·i·cate (son′i - kāt). Expor uma suspensão de células ou micróbios ao efeito de ruptura da energia de ondas sonoras de alta freqüência.

son·i·ca·tion (son - i - kā′shŭn). O processo de ruptura de materiais biológicos pelo uso da energia das ondas sonoras.

son·i·fi·ca·tion (son′i - fi - kā′shŭn). A produção de som ou de ondas sonoras.

son·i·fi·er (son′i - fī - er). Instrumento que produz ondas sonoras, especialmente aquelas das freqüências utilizadas em procedimentos de produção de som.

son·i·fy (son′i - fī). Produzir som.

Sonne, Carl, bacteriologista dinamarquês, 1882–1948.

son·o·chem·is·try (son - ō - kem′is - trē). Sonoquímica; ramo da química relacionado com as alterações químicas causadas por ou envolvendo o som, particularmente o ultra-som.

son·o·gram (son′ō - gram). Sonograma, ultra-sonograma. SIN ultrasonogram. [L. *sonus*, som + G. *gramma*, desenho]

son·o·graph (son′ō - graf). Sonógrafo. SIN ultrasonograph. [L. *sonus*, som + G. *graphō*, escrever]

so·nog·ra·pher (sō - nog′ră - fer). Sonógrafo. SIN ultrasonographer.

so·nog·ra·phy (sō - nog′ră - fī). Sonografia. SIN ultrasonography. [L. *sonus*, som + G. *graphō*, escrever]

son·o·lu·cent (son - o - lu′sent). Sonotransparente; em ultra-sonografia, que contém poucos ecos ou nenhum eco; termo incorreto para transônico ou anecóico. VER anechoic. [L. *sonus*, som + L. *luceo*, brilhar]

son·o·mi·crom·e·ter (son′ō - mī - krom′e - ter). Sonomicrômetro; um calibrador de dimensão ultra-sônico cirurgicamente implantado para medir o espessamento e o movimento da parede do coração.

son·o·mo·tor (son - ō - mō′ter). Sonomotor; relacionado aos movimentos causados pelo som. VER sonomotor *response*.

so·phis·ti·cate (sō - fis′ti - kāt). Sofismar; adulterar. [L. mod. *sophisticare*, pp. *sophisticatus*, alterar enganosamente, do G. *sophistikos*, enganoso]

soph·o·re·tin (sof - ō - rē′tin). Soforetina. SIN quercetin.

so·por (sō′pōr). Sopor; sono profundo não-natural, sono mórbido. [L.]

so·po·rif·er·ous (sō - pōr - if′er - ŭs, sop′ōr-). Soporífero. SIN soporific. [L. *soporifer*, de *sopor*, sono profundo + *fero*, trazer]

so·po·rif·ic (sō - pōr - if′ik, sop′ōr-). **1.** Soporífico, soporífero; que provoca sono. SIN somnifacient, somniferous, somnific, soporiferous. **2.** Hipnótico. SIN hipnotic (2). [L. *sopor*, sono profundo, + *facio*, induzir]

sop·o·rose, so·po·rous (sō′pō - rōs, - rŭs). Soporoso; relativo a ou que causa sono profundo não-natural. [L. *sopor*, sono profundo]

sor·be·fa·cient (sōr - bē - fā′shent). **1.** Que causa absorção. **2.** Agente que causa ou que facilita a absorção. [L. *sorbeo*, sugar, + *facio*, fazer]

sor·bic ac·id (sōr′bik). Ácido ascórbico; obtido das bagas da sorveira-brava, *Sorbus aucuparia* (família Rosaceae) ou preparado sinteticamente; inibe o crescimento das leveduras e do mofo, sendo quase atóxico para o ser humano; utilizado como conservante.

sor·bin (sōr′bin). Sorbina. SIN L-sorbose.

sor·bin·ose (sōr - bin - ōs). Sorbinose. SIN L-sorbose.

sor·bi·tan (sōr′bi - tan). Sorbitan; sorbitol ou sorbose e compostos relacionados em combinação éster com ácidos graxos e com cadeias laterais oligo (óxido de etileno) curtas e uma terminação oleato para formar detergentes, como o polissorbato 80.

sor·bite (sōr′bīt). Sorbitol. SIN sorbitol.
sor·bi·tol (sōr′bi - tol). Sorbitol; produto da redução da glicose e sorbose encontradas nas bagas da sorveira-brava, *Sorbus aucuparia* (família Rosaceae), e em muitas frutas e algas. Possui vários usos industriais e farmacêuticos; em medicina, é utilizado como laxativo e adoçante, sendo quase totalmente metabolizado (a CO_2 e H_2O); acumula-se no diabetes melito tipo I; a presença de níveis elevados pode causar lesão osmótica. SIN sorbite.
D-sor·bi·tol-6-phos·phate de·hy·dro·gen·ase. D-sorbitol-6-fosfato desidrogenase; óxido redutase que catalisa a interconversão do D-sorbitol 6-fosfato e NAD^+ em D-frutose 6-fosfato e NADH. Etapa-chave no metabolismo da frutose no cristalino. SIN ketose reductase.
sor·bi·tose (sōr′bi - tōs). Sorbitose. SIN L-sorbose.
L-sor·bose (sōr′bōs). L-sorbose; 2-cetoexose redutora muito doce, porém não-fermentável, obtida das bagas da sorveira-brava, *Sorbus aucuparia* (família Rosaceae), e do sorbitol por fermentação com *Acetobacter suboxydans;* a L-sorbose é epimérica com a D-frutose, sendo usada na fabricação da vitamina C. SIN sorbin, sorbinose, sorbitose.
sor·des (sōr′dēz). Saburra, sarro; coleção crostosa castanho-escura ou enegrecida nos lábios, nos dentes e nas gengivas de uma pessoa com desidratação associada a uma doença debilitante crônica. [L. filth, de *sordeo,* estar sujo]
sore (sōr). 1. Ferida, úlcera ou qualquer lesão cutânea aberta. 2. Doloroso; sensível. [A.S. *sār*]
  bed s., úlcera de decúbito. VER bedsore.
  canker s., estomatite aftosa. SIN aphtha (2).
  cold s., coloquialismo para referir-se ao herpes simples (*herpes* simplex).
  Delhi s., úlcera de Delhi. SIN Oriental s.
  desert s., úlcera do deserto; qualquer uma das várias úlceras cutâneas inespecíficas crônicas, mais comumente nas pernas, joelhos, mãos e antebraços, e provavelmente uma variante do ectima, que ocorrem em regiões tropicais e em desertos. SIN veldt s.
  hard s., cancro. SIN chancre.
  Lahore s., úlcera de Lahore. SIN Oriental s.
  Natal s., úlcera de Natal; lesão da leishmaniose cutânea.
  Oriental s., úlcera oriental. VER cutaneous *leishmaniasis.* SIN Delhi s., Lahore s.
  pressure s., úlcera de decúbito. SIN decubitus *ulcer.*
  soft s., cancróide. SIN chancroid.
  tropical s., úlcera tropical. SIN tropical *ulcer* (1). VER cutaneous *leishmaniasis.*
  veldt s., úlcera da savana; úlcera do deserto. SIN desert s.
  venereal s., cancróide. SIN chancroid.
sore·mouth (sōr′mowth). Orf. SIN orf.
Sörensen, Sören P.L., químico dinamarquês, 1868–1939. VER S. *scale.*
Soret, C., radiologista francês, †1931. VER S. *band, phenomenon.*
so·ro·che (sō - rō′chē). Mal das montanhas. SIN altitude *sickness.* [Esp. (orig. minério, antigamente atribuído às emanações tóxicas de minérios em montanhas)]
  chronic s., mal das montanhas crônico. SIN chronic mountain *sickness.*
sorp·tion (sōrp′shun). Adsorção ou absorção.
Sorsby, Arnold, oftalmologista inglês, 1900–1980. VER S. macular *degeneration, syndrome.*
s.o.s. Abreviatura do L. *si opus sit,* se necessário.
so·ta·lol hy·dro·chlo·ride (sō′tă - lol). Cloridrato de sotalol; agente bloqueador dos receptores β, com usos semelhantes aos do propranolol; possui também propriedades de bloqueio dos canais de potássio.
Sotos, J.F., pediatra norte-americano, *1927. VER S. *syndrome.*
Sottas, Jules, neurologista francês, 1866–1943. VER Dejerine-S *disease.*
souf·fle (soo′fl). Sopro, som suave que se ouve ao escutar o coração. [Fr. *souffler,* soprar]
  cardiac s., s. cardíaco; sopro cardíaco suave.
  fetal s., s. fetal; murmúrio soprado, sincrônico com o batimento cardíaco fetal, algumas vezes apenas sistólico, outras vezes contínuo, ouvido à ausculta sobre o útero grávido. SIN funic s., funicular s., umbilical s.
  funic s., funicular s., s. fetal. SIN fetal s.
  mammary s., s. mamário; sopro ouvido no final da gravidez e durante a lactação na borda medial da mama, algumas vezes apenas sistólico, outras vezes contínuo.
  placental s., s. uterino. SIN uterine s.
  umbilical s., s. fetal. SIN fetal s.
  uterine s., s. uterino; sopro sincrônico com a sístole da mãe, ouvido à ausculta do útero grávido. SIN placental s.
Soulier, Jean Pierre, hematologista francês, 1915–1985. VER Bernard-S. *disease, syndrome.*
sound (sownd). 1. Som; as vibrações produzidas por um corpo que emite som, transmitidas pelo ar ou por outro meio e percebidas pelo ouvido interno. 2. Sonda; instrumento de metal cilíndrico alongado, geralmente curvo, utilizado para explorar a bexiga ou outras cavidades do corpo, para dilatar estreitamentos da uretra, do esôfago ou de outro canal, para medir o calibre da luz de uma cavidade corporal ou para detectar a presença de um corpo estranho numa cavidade corporal. 3. Sondar; explorar ou medir o calibre de uma cavidade com uma sonda. 4. Sadio, íntegro; não-doente ou não-lesado.
  adventitious breath s.'s, sons respiratórios adventícios; sons ouvidos à ausculta de pulmões anormais. VER TAMBÉM rale, rhonchus, crackle, crepitation, wheeze, rub, crunch.
  after-s., audição tardia. VER aftersound.
  amphoric voice s., voz anfórica. VER amphoric *voice.*
  anvil s., som de bigorna. SIN bellmetal *resonance.*
  atrial s., quarta bulha cardíaca ($β_4$). SIN fourth heart s.
  auscultatory s., s. auscultatório; estertor, sopro, ruído, frêmito ou outro som ouvido à ausculta do tórax ou do abdome.
  bell s., som de sino. SIN bellmetal *resonance.*
  bowel s.'s, ruídos intestinais; ruídos abdominais relativamente de alta intensidade produzidos pela propulsão do conteúdo intestinal através do trato alimentar inferior.
  breath s.'s, sons respiratórios; sopro, ruído, frêmito, roncos ou estertores detectados à ausculta sobre os pulmões ou qualquer parte do trato respiratório. SIN respiratory s.'s.
  bronchial breath s.'s, sons respiratórios brônquicos; sons respiratórios altos, agudos e de tom abafado ouvidos à ausculta, principalmente sobre o esterno; quando ouvidos em outra parte do tórax, podem indicar consolidação pulmonar ou outra condição patológica.
  bronchovesicular breath s.'s, sons respiratórios broncovesiculares; sons intermediários entre os sons respiratórios brônquicos e vesiculares; podem ser anormais, porém são normais quando ouvidos entre o primeiro e o segundo espaços intercostais, anterior e posteriormente entre as escápulas.
  Campbell s., sonda de Campbell; sonda miniatura com bico curto de ponta redonda, especialmente curvado para a uretra profunda do homem jovem.
  cannon s., ruído de canhão. SIN bruit de canon.
  cardiac s., bulha cardíaca. SIN heart s.'s.
  cavernous voice s., som de voz cavernosa. VER cavernous *voice.*
  coconut s., som de coco; som semelhante àquele produzido quando se percute um coco rachado; produzido pela percussão do crânio de um paciente com osteíte deformante.
  complex s., s. complexo; som composto de diversos sons de freqüências diferentes.
  cracked-pot s., som de pote rachado. SIN cracked-pot *resonance.*
  Davis interlocking s., sonda interligada de Davis; sonda constituída de dois instrumentos com extremidades macho e fêmea curvas, utilizada para introduzir um cateter na bexiga no tratamento da ruptura da uretra; a sonda macho é introduzida na uretra distal através do meato, enquanto a sonda fêmea é passada através do colo vesical até a uretra proximal por meio de uma cistotomia a céu aberto; as extremidades dos dois instrumentos são encaixadas, com a sonda fêmea guiando a sonda macho para cima até a bexiga; a seguir, um cateter é suturado à extremidade da sonda macho e retirado através da uretra para restabelecer a continuidade de sua luz.
  double-shock s., som de duplo choque. SIN bruit de rappel.
  eddy s.'s, sons em contracorrente; sons que assinalam o sopro contínuo da persistência do canal arterial, conferindo-lhe uma qualidade tipicamente "desigual".
  ejection s.'s, ruídos de ejeção; sons semelhantes a um estalido durante a ejeção de uma aorta ou artéria pulmonar hipertensa ou associados a estenose (particularmente congênita) da valva aórtica ou pulmonar.
  first heart s. (S_1), primeira bulha cardíaca ($β_1$); ocorre na sístole ventricular, sendo produzida principalmente pelo fechamento das valvas atrioventriculares.
  fourth heart s. (S_4), quarta bulha cardíaca ($β_4$); som produzido no final da diástole em associação ao enchimento ventricular, devido à sístole atrial e relacionado com a diminuição da complacência ventricular. Trata-se de uma oscilação de baixa freqüência que pode ser normal numa idade mais avançada, devido ao declínio fisiológico da complacência ventricular; todavia, é quase sempre anormal numa idade mais jovem se for de alta intensidade ou palpável. É comum na hipertrofia ventricular, sobretudo com hipertensão, ocorrendo quase invariavelmente durante o infarto agudo do miocárdio. $β_4$ pode surgir do ventrículo direito ou do esquerdo, ou de ambos. SIN atrial s.
  friction s., ruído de atrito; som ouvido à ausculta, produzido pelo atrito de duas superfícies serosas opostas que se tornaram ásperas por um exsudato inflamatório ou, em caso de cronicidade, por fibrose não-aderente. SIN friction murmur, friction rub.
  gallop s., ruído de galope; a terceira ou a quarta bulha cardíaca anormal que, quando somada à primeira e à segunda bulhas, produz a cadência tripla do ritmo de galope. VER TAMBÉM gallop.
  heart s.'s, bulha cardíaca; ruído produzido pela contração muscular e fechamento das valvas cardíacas durante o ciclo cardíaco. VER first heart s., second heart s., third heart s., fourth heart s. SIN cardiac s., heart tones.
  hippocratic succussion s., som de sucussão hipocrática; som de pancada produzido ao sacudir um paciente com hidro ou piopneumotórax, estando a orelha do médico aplicada ao tórax.

Jewett s., sonda de Jewett; sonda reta e curta para dilatação da uretra anterior.

Korotkoff s.'s, ruídos de Korotkoff; sons ouvidos sobre uma artéria quando a pressão exercida sobre ela é reduzida abaixo da pressão arterial sistólica, como na determinação da pressão arterial pelo método de ausculta.

Le Fort s., sonda de Le Fort; sonda curva para uma vela filiforme, utilizada para dilatação de estenoses uretrais no homem quando um pequeno calibre ou a presença de falsas passagens impede a passagem segura de uma sonda ou cateter padrão.

McCrea s., sonda de McCrea; sonda discretamente curva empregada para dilatar a uretra em lactentes ou crianças.

Mercier s., sonda de Mercier; cateter cujo bico é curto e inclinado quase em ângulo reto.

muscle s., som muscular; ruído ouvido à ausculta sobre o ventre de um músculo em contração.

percussion s., som de percussão; qualquer som produzido por percussão de uma das cavidades do corpo.

pericardial friction s., ruído de atrito pericárdico; som áspero, de lixa ou, raramente, rangido, contínuo, ouvido sobre o coração em alguns casos de pericardite, devido ao atrito das superfícies pericárdicas inflamadas quando o coração se contrai e relaxa; durante o ritmo sinusal normal, é habitualmente trifásico. Durante qualquer ritmo, pode ser bifásico ou unifásico. SIN pericardial rub, pericardial friction rub.

pistol-shot s., ruído de tiro de pistola; som criado pela ligeira compressão de uma artéria durante a regurgitação aórtica; algumas vezes audível sem compressão.

pistol-shot femoral s., ruído femoral de tiro de pistola; ruído sistólico semelhante a um tiro ouvido sobre a artéria femoral nos estados de alto débito, especialmente na insuficiência aórtica; provavelmente devido ao súbito estiramento da parede elástica da artéria; os ruídos de tiro de pistola também podem ser ouvidos sobre outras artérias de calibre relativamente grande (p. ex., braquial, radial).

posttussis suction s., ruído de aspiração pós-tosse; ruído produzido após queda de uma gota de muco ou pus de volta à cavidade pulmonar após ter sido esvaziada pela tosse.

respiratory s.'s, sons respiratórios. SIN breath s.'s.

sail s., som de vela; som comparado ao estalido de uma vela; a primeira bulha cardíaca anormal em alguns pacientes com anomalia de Ebstein.

Santini booming s., som ressoante de Santini; ruído sonoro ouvido à percussão auscultatória de um cisto hidático.

second s., segunda bulha. SIN second heart s.

second heart s. (S_2), segunda bulha cardíaca (β_2); a segunda bulha ouvida à ausculta do coração; indica o início da diástole e é devida ao fechamento das valvas semilunares. SIN second s.

Simpson uterine s., sonda uterina de Simpson; bastão de metal flexível e delgado utilizado para medir o calibre ou dilatar o canal cervical, ou para manter o útero em várias posições durante a cirurgia ginecológica.

Sims uterine s., sonda uterina de Sims; sonda flexível e delgada com uma pequena projeção a cerca de 7 cm de sua extremidade; utilizada para estimar o tamanho e o calibre da cavidade uterina.

splitting of heart s.'s, desdobramento das bulhas cardíacas; a produção dos principais componentes da primeira e da segunda bulhas cardíacas (raramente da terceira e da quarta), devido à contribuição das valvas do lado esquerdo e do lado direito; assim, a primeira bulha cardíaca deve ter um componente mitral e um componente tricúspide, e a segunda bulha cardíaca, um componente aórtico (A_2) e pulmonar (P_2). Estes últimos são mais bem percebidos durante a respiração, em que a inspiração retarda P_2 e produz um componente aórtico mais precoce.

succussion s., ruído de sucussão; ruído produzido pela presença de líquido com ar sobrejacente quando agitado, como ocorre na dilatação gástrica ou na presença de líquido e ar numa cavidade pleural (hidropneumotórax).

tambour s., som de tambor. SIN *bruit* de tambour.

third s., terceira bulha. SIN third heart s.

third heart s. (S_3), terceira bulha cardíaca (β_3); ocorre no início da diástole e corresponde ao término da primeira fase de enchimento ventricular rápido; normal em crianças e indivíduos jovens, porém anormal em outras pessoas. SIN third s.

tic-tac s.'s, ruídos de tique-taque. SIN embryocardia.

to-and-fro s., ruído de vaivém; duplicação de um sopro anormal geralmente na sístole e na diástole e antigamente aplicado a atritos pericárdicos.

tracheal breath s.'s, sons respiratórios traqueais; sons respiratórios altos, ásperos e abafados, habitualmente ouvidos apenas sobre o pescoço.

van Buren s., sonda de van Buren; sonda padrão disponível em vários calibres, com uma ponta discretamente curva, projetada para acompanhar o contorno da uretra bulbosa no homem; utilizada para medida do calibre ou dilatação da uretra.

vesicular breath s.'s, murmúrio vesicular, o ruído suave da respiração normal auscultado na maior parte dos campos pulmonares; a fase inspiratória é geralmente mais prolongada do que a expiratória.

waterwheel s., ruído de roda d'água; ruído produzido pelo movimento cardíaco induzindo pancadas na presença de líquido e de ar no interior do saco pericárdico.

water-whistle s., som borbulhante ouvido à ausculta sobre uma fístula brônquica ou pulmonar.

Winternitz s., sonda de Winternitz; cateter de corrente dupla em que a água circula em qualquer temperatura desejada.

xiphisternal crunching s., ruído de esmagamento xifoesternal. VER Hamman *sign*.

Southern, M.E., biólogo inglês do século XX. VER Southern blot *analysis*.

Southey, Reginald, médico inglês, 1835–1899. VER S. *tubes,* em *tube*.

soy·a (soy′a). Soja. SIN soybean. [Hind. *soya,* funcho]

soy·bean (soy′ben). Soja; vagem da trepadeira *Glycine soja* ou *G. hispida* (família Leguminosae); vagem rica em proteína e que contém pouco amido; constitui a fonte do óleo de soja; a farinha de soja é utilizada no preparo de um pão para diabéticos, em leites artificiais para lactentes que não toleram o leite de vaca e para adultos alérgicos ao leite de vaca. SIN soja, soya. [Hind. *soya,* funcho]

s. oil, óleo de soja; obtido da soja por expressão ou extração em solvente; contém triglicerídeos dos ácidos linoleico, oleico, linolênico e ácidos graxos saturados; utilizado como alimento e na fabricação de margarinas e outros produtos alimentares.

SP Abreviatura de sacroposterior *position* (posição sacroposterior).

SP1 Abreviatura de stimulatory *protein* 1 (proteína estimuladora 1).

sp. Abreviatura de espécie; a forma no plural é spp. [L. *spiritus, spirit.,* espírito]

spa (spah). Spa; balneário, estação de águas, especialmente aquela em que há uma ou mais fontes de águas minerais que possuem propriedades terapêuticas. [*Spa,* estação de águas minerais localizada na Bélgica]

SPACE

space (spās) [TA]. Espaço. Qualquer parte demarcada do corpo, seja uma área de superfície, um segmento de tecidos ou uma cavidade. VER TAMBÉM area, region, zone. SIN spatium [TA]. [L. *spatium,* sala, espaço]

alveolar dead s., e. morto alveolar; a diferença entre o espaço morto fisiológico e o espaço morto anatômico, representa a parte do espaço morto fisiológico resultante da ventilação de alvéolos relativamente hipoperfundidos ou não-perfundidos; difere especificamente por estar colocado de modo a encher e esvaziar paralelamente com alvéolos funcionais, e não por estar interposto nos tubos de condução entre alvéolos funcionais e o meio externo.

anatomic dead s., e. morto anatômico; o volume das vias aéreas de condução do meio externo (no nariz e na boca) até o nível em que o gás inspirado troca oxigênio e dióxido de carbono com o sangue capilar pulmonar; a princípio, acreditava-se que se estendia até o início do epitélio alveolar nos bronquíolos respiratórios; entretanto, evidências mais recentes indicam que a troca gasosa efetiva estende-se por alguma distância até as vias aéreas de condução de paredes mais espessas, devido à rápida mistura longitudinal. Cf. alveolar dead s., physiologic dead s. SIN anatomic airway.

antecubital s., fossa cubital. SIN cubital *fossa*.

anterior clear s., espaço retroesternal. SIN retrosternal s.

apical s., e. apical; espaço entre a parede alveolar e o ápice da raiz de um dente, onde geralmente se origina um abscesso alveolar.

axillary s., axilar. SIN axilla.

Berger s., e. de Berger; espaço entre a fossa hialóidea do vítreo e a lente.

Bogros s., e. de Bogros. SIN retroinguinal s.

Böttcher s., e. de Böttcher. SIN endolymphatic *sac*.

Bowman s., e. de Bowman. SIN capsular s.

Burns s., e. de Burns. SIN suprasternal s.

capsular s., e. capsular; espaço semelhante a uma fenda entre as camadas visceral e parietal da cápsula do corpúsculo renal; abre-se no túbulo proximal do nefron, no colo do túbulo. SIN Bowman s., filtration s.

cartilage s., e. cartilaginoso; lacuna na matriz de cartilagem. SIN cartilage *lacuna*.

cavernous s. [TA], caverna; cavidade anatômica com muitas câmaras interconectadas. SIN cavern, caverna.

cavernous s.'s of corpora cavernosa [TA], cavernas dos corpos cavernosos; espaços vasculares do corpo cavernoso que, juntamente com as trabéculas fibrosas intervenientes, formam o tecido erétil do pênis ou do clitóris. SIN cavernae corporum cavernosorum [TA], caverns of corpora cavernosa, cavities of corpora cavernosa.

cavernous s.'s of corporus spongiosum [TA], cavernas do corpo esponjoso; espaços vasculares que formam o tecido erétil do corpo esponjoso do pênis, no sexo masculino, e do bulbo do vestíbulo, no sexo feminino. SIN cavernae corporis spongiosi [TA], caverns of corpus spongiosum, cavities of corpus spongiosum.

central palmar s., e. palmar central; o mais medial dos espaços palmares centrais delimitado, medialmente, pelo compartimento hipotenar; relacionado distalmente com as bainhas tendíneas sinoviais do terceiro e quarto dedos e, proximalmente, com a bainha flexora comum. SIN medial midpalmar s., middle palmar s.

Chassaignac s., e. de Chassaignac; espaço potencial entre o músculo peitoral maior e a glândula mamária.

Cloquet s., e. de Cloquet; espaço entre a zônula ciliar e o corpo vítreo.

Colles s., e. de Colles. SIN superficial perineal s.

corneal s., e. corneano; um dos espaços estrelados entre as lamelas da córnea, contendo, cada um, uma célula ou corpúsculo corneano. SIN lacuna (4).

Cotunnius s., e. de Cotunnius. SIN endolymphatic sac.

(cranial) extradural s. [TA], e. extradural (craniano); espaços entre os ossos cranianos e a camada periósteo externa da dura; torna-se um verdadeiro espaço apenas patologicamente, como em caso de hemorragia extra ou epidural formando um hematoma.

dead s., e. morto; **(1)** cavidade, virtual ou real, que permanece após o fechamento de uma ferida que não é obliterada por técnica cirúrgica; **(2)** VER anatomic dead s., physiologic dead s.

deep perineal s., e. profundo do períneo; região imediatamente superior à membrana do períneo, ocupada pela parte membranácea da uretra; a glândula bulbouretral (no homem), os músculos transverso profundo do períneo e esfíncter da uretra e o nervo dorsal e a artéria do pênis ou do clitóris. SIN deep perineal pouch, spatium perinei profundum.

denture s., e. da dentadura; **(1)** a porção da cavidade oral que é ou pode ser ocupada por dentadura(s) maxilar e/ou mandibular; **(2)** espaço entre as cristas residuais disponível para dentaduras. VER TAMBÉM interarch disease.

disk s., e. discal; em radiografias da coluna, a região radiotransparente entre dois corpos vertebrais.

Disse s., e. de Disse. SIN perisinusoidal s.

s. of Donders, e. de Donders; espaço entre o dorso da língua e o palato duro quando a mandíbula se encontra em posição de repouso após o ciclo expiratório da respiração.

endolymphatic s. [TA], e. endolinfático; espaço preenchido de endolinfa contido pelo labirinto membranáceo. SIN spatium endolympha'ticum [TA].

epidural s., e. extradural; espaço entre as paredes do canal vertebral e a dura-máter da medula espinal. SIN extradural s. [TA], spatium extradurale [TA], spatium extradura'le*, cavum epidurale, epidural cavity.

episcleral s. [TA], e. episcleral; espaço entre a bainha fascial do bulbo do olho e a esclera. SIN spatium episclerale [TA], interfascial s., spatium interfasciale, spatium intervaginale bulbi oculi, Tenon s.

epitympanic s., recesso epitimpânico da cavidade timpânica. SIN epitympanic recess.

extradural s. [TA], e. extradural. SIN epidural s.

extraperitoneal s. [TA], e. extraperitoneal; espaço areolar frouxo (potencial apenas em muitos locais) ou plano imediatamente externo ao peritônio; na cirurgia, esse plano permite a dissecção na parede corporal, porém externamente ao peritônio. VER TAMBÉM retroperitoneal s. SIN spatium extraperitonea'le [TA].

filtration s., e. de filtração. SIN capsular s.

Fontana s., espaços de Fontana. SIN s.'s of iridocorneal angle.

freeway s., e. interoclusal; espaço entre as superfícies oclusivas dos dentes maxilares e mandibulares quando a mandíbula se encontra em posição de repouso fisiológica. SIN interocclusal clearance, interocclusal distance (2), interocclusal gap, interocclusal rest s. (2).

gingival s., e. gengival. SIN gingival sulcus.

haversian s.'s, espaços de Havers; espaços no osso formados pelo aumento dos canais de Havers.

Henke s., espaço de Henke. SIN retropharyngeal s.

His perivascular s., e. perivascular de His. SIN Virchow-Robin s.

infraglottic s., cavidade infraglótica. SIN infraglottic cavity.

interalveolar s., e. interalveolar. SIN interarch distance.

intercostal s. [TA], e. episcleral; intervalo entre as costelas ocupado por músculos intercostais, veias, artérias e nervos. SIN spatium intercostale [TA].

interfascial s., e.episcleral SIN episcleral s.

interglobular s., e. interglobular; um dentre vários espaços irregulares ramificados próximos à periferia da dentina da coroa de um dente, através dos quais passam as ramificações dos túbulos; são causados pela falha de calcificação da dentina. SIN interglobular s. of Owen, spatium interglobulare.

interglobular s. of Owen, e. interglobular de Owen. SIN interglobular s.

intermembrane s., e. intermembrana; espaço entre as duas membranas numa célula ou organela delimitadas por uma dupla membrana biológica; p. ex., o espaço entre as membranas interna e externa das mitocôndrias; algumas vezes designado como matriz externa.

interocclusal rest s., **(1)** distância interoclusal (1). SIN interocclusal distance (1); **(2)** e. interoclusal. SIN freeway s.

interosseous metacarpal s.'s [TA], espaços interósseos do metacarpo; espaços entre os ossos metacarpais na mão. SIN spatia interossea metacarpi [TA].

interosseus metatarsal s.'s [TA], espaços interósseos do metatarso; espaços entre os ossos metatarsais no pé. SIN spatia interossea metatarsi [TA].

interpleural s., e. interpleural. SIN mediastinum (2).

interproximal s., e. interproximal; espaço entre dentes adjacentes numa arcada dentária; é dividido no vão oclusal para a área de contato e no espaço septal gengival para a área de contato.

interradicular s., e. inter-radicular; espaço entre as raízes de dentes com múltiplas raízes.

interseptovalvular s., e. interseptovalvular; o intervalo no coração embrionário em desenvolvimento entre o septo primum e a válvula esquerda do seio venoso.

intersheath s.'s of optic nerve, espaço intervaginal subaracnóideo do nervo óptico. SIN intervaginal subarachnoid s. of optic nerve.

intervaginal subarachnoid s. of optic nerve [TA], e. intervaginal subaracnóideo do nervo óptico; espaço dentro da bainha interna do nervo óptico; entre as camadas aracnóide-máter e pia-máter, preenchido por líquido cefalorraquidiano e contínuo com o espaço subaracnóideo. SIN spatium intervaginale subarachnoidale nervi optici [TA], intersheath s.'s of optic nerve, Schwalbe s.'s.

intervillous s.'s, espaços intervilosos; espaços que contêm sangue materno, localizados entre as vilosidades placentárias; são revestidos de sincício trofoblasto.

intraretinal s., e. intra-retiniano; a fenda virtual entre as camadas pigmentada e neural da retina; representa a cavidade da vesícula óptica embrionária; ocorre descolamento retiniano devido à abertura desse espaço.

s.'s of iridocorneal angle [TA], espaços do ângulo iridocorneal; espaços de forma irregular e revestidos de endotélio no interior do retículo trabecular, através dos quais o humor aquoso filtra para alcançar o seio venoso da esclerótica. SIN spatia anguli iridocornealis [TA], ciliary canals, Fontana s.'s.

Kiernan s., e. de Kiernan; espaço interlobular no fígado.

Kretschmann s., e. de Kretschmann; discreta depressão no recesso epitimpânico abaixo do recesso superior da membrana timpânica.

Kuhnt s.'s, espaços de Kuhnt; divertículos ou recessos superficiais, entre o corpo ciliar e a zônula ciliar, que se abrem na câmara posterior do olho.

lateral central palmar s., e. palmar central lateral; o mais lateral (radial) dos espaços palmares centrais, delimitado lateralmente pelo compartimento tenar; relacionado, distalmente, com a bainha sinovial do tendão do dedo indicador e, proximalmente, com a bainha flexora comum. SIN lateral midpalmar s., thenar s.

lateral midpalmar s., e. palmar médio lateral. SIN lateral central palmar s.

lateral pharyngeal s. [TA], e. laterofaríngeo; parte do espaço perifaríngeo localizada nos lados da faringe. SIN spatium lateropharyngeum [TA], spatium pharyngeum laterale [TA].

leeway s., e. marginal; a diferença entre as larguras mesiodistais combinadas das cúspides decíduas e molares e seus sucessores.

leptomeningeal s., e. leptomeníngeo, e. subaracnóideo. SIN subarachnoid s. SIN spatium leptomeningeum [TA].

lymph s., e. linfático; espaço, no tecido ou num vaso, preenchido por linfa.

Magendie s.'s, espaços de Magendie; espaços entre a pia-máter e a aracnóide-máter ao nível das fissuras cerebrais.

Malacarne s., e. de Malacarne. SIN posterior perforated substance.

masticator s., e. mastigador; espaço subtendido pela camada superficial da fáscia cervical profunda, que se divide em faixas lateral e medial na borda inferior da mandíbula para envolver o músculo masseter, parte do músculo temporal e os músculos pterigóideo lateral e medial antes de se fixar ao arco zigomático e à base do crânio.

Meckel s., e. de Meckel. SIN trigeminal cave.

medial midpalmar s., e. palmar médio medial. SIN central palmar s.

mediastinal s., e. mediastínico. SIN mediastinum (2).

medullary s., e. medular; a cavidade central e os intervalos celulares entre as trabéculas ósseas, preenchidos por medula óssea.

middle palmar s., e. palmar médio. SIN central palmar s.

midpalmar s., e. palmar médio; um dos dois espaços palmares centrais (medial ou lateral).

Mohrenheim s., e. de Mohrenheim. SIN infraclavicular fossa.

muscular s. of retroinguinal compartment [TA], lacuna dos músculos; o compartimento lateral abaixo do ligamento inguinal (Poupart) para a passagem do músculo iliopsoas e nervo femoral; é separado da lacuna dos vasos pelo arco iliopectíneo. SIN lacuna musculorum retroinguinalis, lacuna musculorum, muscular lacuna.

Nuel s., e. de Nuel; intervalo no órgão espiral (de Corti) entre as células pilares externas, de um lado, e as células falângicas e ciliadas, do outro.

paraglottic s., e. paraglótico; o espaço, de cada lado da glote, delimitado lateralmente pelo pericôndrio da cartilagem tireóidea e membrana cricotireóidea e, posteriormente, pela mucosa do seio piriforme; ântero-superiormente, estende-se no espaço pré-epiglótico. Trata-se de uma importante via de disseminação transglótica e extralaríngea do carcinoma de laringe.

parapharyngeal s. [TA], e. laterofaríngeo. SIN pharyngomaxillary s. SIN spatium parapharyngeum.

Parona s., e. de Parona; espaço entre o músculo pronador quadrado profundo e os tendões flexores sobrejacentes do antebraço, que é contínuo com o espaço palmar central médio através do túnel do carpo.

parotid s., e. parotídeo; sulco profundo no lado da face, flanqueando a face posterior do ramo da mandíbula, com seus músculos inseridos, ocupado pela glândula parótida; é revestido por lâminas fasciais (a bainha da parótida) derivadas da camada da fáscia cervical profunda; as estruturas que delimitam o espaço constituem, em seu conjunto, o leito parotídeo. Os cirurgiões que operam essa área tiram proveito do fato de que as dimensões ântero-posteriores do espaço parotídeo aumentam com a protrusão da mandíbula. SIN bed of parotid gland, parotid recess, recessus parotideus.

perforated s., substância. perfurada. VER anterior perforated *substance*, posterior perforated *substance*.

perichoroid s., e. pericorióideo. SIN perichoroidal s.

perichoroidal s. [TA], e. pericorióideo; o intervalo entre a corióide e a esclera preenchido pelas redes frouxas da lâmina fosca da esclera e lâmina supracorióide. SIN spatium perichoroideum [TA], perichoroid s.

perilymphatic s. [TA], e. perilinfático; espaço entre as porções óssea e membranácea do labirinto. SIN spatium perilymphaticum [TA], cisterna perilymphatica.

perineal s.'s, espaços do períneo. VER deep perineal s., superficial perineal s.

perinuclear s., e. perinuclear. SIN cisterna caryothecae.

peripharyngeal s. [TA], e. perifaríngeo; espaço preenchido por tecido areolar frouxo ao redor da faringe; é dividido em duas partes, o espaço parafaríngeo (laterofaríngeo) e o espaço retrofaríngeo. SIN spatium peripharyngeum [TA].

periportal s. of Mall, s. periporta de Mall; espaço tecidual entre a lâmina limitante e o canal porta no fígado.

perisinusoidal s., e. perissinusoidal; espaço extravascular virtual entre os sinusóides hepáticos e as células do parênquima hepático. SIN Disse s.

perivitelline s., e. perivitelino; espaço entre a membrana vitelina e a zona pelúcida, que aparece no óvulo imediatamente após a fertilização.

personal s., e. pessoal; termo empregado na ciência do comportamento para designar a área física que circunda imediatamente um indivíduo próximo a um ou mais indivíduos, sejam eles conhecidos ou desconhecidos, servindo como zona de tamponamento corporal nessas transações interpessoais.

pharyngeal s., recesso faríngeo; a área ocupada pela faringe (naso-, oro- e laringofaringe). Não deve ser confundido com o espaço retrofaríngeo.

pharyngomaxillary s., e. laterofaríngeo; espaço limitado pela parede lateral da faringe, pelas vértebras cervicais e pelo músculo pterigóide medial. SIN parapharyngeal s. [TA].

physiologic dead s. (V_D), e. morto fisiológico; a soma dos espaço morto anatômico e alveolar; o espaços morto calculado quando a pressão de dióxido de carbono no sangue arterial sistêmico é utilizada em lugar da pressão do gás alveolar na equação de Bohr; trata-se de um volume virtual ou aparente que leva em consideração o comprometimento da troca gasosa em virtude de distribuições desiguais na ventilação e perfusão pulmonares.

plantar s., e. plantar; uma das quatro áreas entre as camadas fasciais no pé, onde pode haver acúmulo de pus quando o pé está infectado.

pleural s., cavidade pleural. SIN pleural *cavity*.

pneumatic s., e. pneumático; qualquer um dos seios paranasais.

Poiseuille s., e. de Poiseuille. SIN still *layer*.

popliteal s., fossa poplítea. SIN popliteal *fossa*.

postpharyngeal s., e. retrofaríngeo. SIN retropharyngeal s.

preepiglottic s., e. pré-epiglótico; o espaço anterior à epiglote, delimitado, anteriormente, pela membrana tireo-hióidea e pelas partes superiores da lâmina da cartilagem tireóidea, superiormente, pelo ligamento hioepiglótico e, inferiormente, pelo ligamento tireoepiglótico; lateralmente, estende-se nos espaços paraglóticos. O carcinoma da porção infra-hióidea da epiglote estende-se freqüentemente para o espaço pré-epiglótico.

Proust s., e. de Proust. SIN rectovesical *pouch*.

Prussak s., e. de Prussak. SIN superior *recess* of tympanic membrane.

pterygomandibular s., e. pterigomandibular; a área entre o ramo mandibular e o processo pterigóide do osso esfenóide.

quadrangular s., e. quadrangular; formação musculotendínea que proporciona a passagem para o nervo axilar, artéria circunflexa umeral posterior e veias que seguem seu trajeto da axila para a parte posterior superior do braço; no local de entrada das estruturas neurovasculares na formação, anteriormente, é delimitada superiormente pela articulação do ombro, medialmente pela borda lateral do músculo subescapular, lateralmente pelo colo cirúrgico do úmero e, inferiormente, pelo tendão do músculo latíssimo do dorso; no local de saída dos vasos na formação, posteriormente, é delimitada superiormente pelo músculo redondo menor, medialmente pela cabeça longa do tríceps, lateralmente pela cabeça lateral do tríceps e, inferiormente, pelo músculo redondo maior ou seu tendão; quando emergem, as estruturas neurovasculares seguem, em sua maioria, na superfície profunda do músculo deltóide que suprem. SIN quadrilateral s.

quadrilateral s., e. quadrilateral. SIN quadrangular s.

Reinke s., e. de Reinke; espaço virtual entre a lâmina própria e a lâmina elástica externa da corda vocal. O edema nesse espaço provoca rouquidão na inflamação crônica.

respiratory dead s., e. morto respiratório; a parte das vias respiratórias ou de uma respiração em que não ocorre troca de oxigênio e de dióxido de carbono com o sangue capilar pulmonar; termo inespecífico que não permite distinguir entre espaço morto anatômico e espaço morto fisiológico.

retroadductor s., e. retroadutor; espaço virtual entre os músculos adutor do polegar e primeiro interósseo dorsal.

retroinguinal s. [TA], e. retroinguinal; espaço triangular entre o peritônio e a fáscia transversal, em cujo ângulo inferior está o ligamento inguinal; contém a porção inferior da artéria ilíaca externa. SIN spatium retroinguinale [TA], Bogros s.

retromylohyoid s., e. retromilo-hióideo; sulco na extremidade posterior da linha milo-hióidea.

retroperitoneal s. [TA], e. retroperitoneal; espaço entre o peritônio parietal e os músculos e ossos da parede abdominal posterior. SIN spatium retroperitoneale [TA], retroperitoneum.

retropharyngeal s. [TA], e. retrofaríngeo; parte do espaço perifaríngeo localizada posteriormente à faringe. SIN spatium retropharyngeum [TA], Henke s., postpharyngeal s.

retropubic s. [TA], e. retropúbico; a área de tecido conjuntivo frouxo entre a bexiga com sua fáscia relacionada e o púbis e a parede abdominal anterior. SIN spatium retropubicum [TA], cavum retzii, Retzius cavity, Retzius s.

retrosternal s., e. retroesternal; na incidência lateral (perfil) de radiografias de tórax é a região posterior ao esterno e anterior à aorta ascendente. SIN anterior clear s.

retrozonular s. [TA], e. retrozonular; espaço potencial da câmara do bulbo do olho imediatamente posterior à zônula e anterior ao corpo vítreo. SIN spatium retrozonulare [TA].

Retzius s, e. de Retzius. SIN retropubic s.

Schwalbe s.'s, espaços de Schwalbe. SIN intervaginal subarachnoid s. of optic nerve.

(spinal) epidural space [TA], espaço extradural (espinal); espaço preenchido por gordura imediatamente externo à dura-máter envolvendo a medula espinal; contém o plexo venoso vertebral (epidural) interno e constitui o local-alvo para anestesia epidural. SIN spatium peridurale*.

subarachnoid s. [TA], e. subaracnóideo; espaço entre a aracnóide-máter e a pia-máter, atravessado por delicadas trabéculas fibrosas e preenchido por líquido cefalorraquidiano. Como a pia-máter adere imediatamente à superfície do cérebro e da medula espinal, o espaço é acentuadamente alargado nos locais onde a superfície cerebral exibe uma depressão profunda (p. ex., entre o cerebelo e o bulbo); esses alargamentos são denominados cisternas; os grandes vasos sanguíneos que suprem o cérebro e a medula espinal situam-se no espaço subaracnóideo. SIN spatium subarachnoideum [TA], cavum subarachnoideum, leptomeningeal s., subarachnoid cavity.

subchorial s., lago subcorial; parte da placenta adjacente abaixo da placa coriônica; une-se com canais irregulares, formando os lagos marginais. SIN subchorial lake.

subdural s. [TA], e. subdural; originalmente considerado como um estreito intervalo preenchido por líquido entre a dura-máter e a aracnóide-máter; hoje em dia, sabe-se que se trata de um e. artificial criado pela separação da aracnóide-máter da dura-máter em conseqüência de traumatismo ou de algum processo patológico atual; no estado de saúde, a aracnóide está pouco aderida à dura-máter (mantida nessa posição pela pressão do líquido cefalorraquidiano), e não há espaço subdural de ocorrência natural. SIN spatium subdurale [TA], cavum subdurale, subdural cavity, subdural cleavage, subdural cleft.

subgingival s., e. subgengival. SIN gingival *sulcus*.

subhepatic s. [TA], recesso sub-hepático do peritônio; parte da cavidade peritoneal entre a superfície visceral do fígado e o colo transverso. SIN recessus subhepaticus [TA], subhepatic recess.

subphrenic s. [TA], recesso subfrênico do peritônio; os recessos na cavidade peritoneal entre a parte anterior do fígado e o diafragma, separados em direito e esquerdo pelo ligamento falciforme. SIN recessus subphrenicus [TA], subphrenic recesses, suprahepatic s.'s.

superficial perineal s. [TA], e. superficial do períneo; o compartimento superficial do períneo; o espaço delimitado, superiormente, pela membrana perineal (antigamente a fáscia inferior do diafragma urogenital, hoje em dia obsoleta) e, inferiormente, pela fáscia perineal superficial (de Colles); contém a estrutura da raiz do pênis ou do clitóris e musculatura associada, mais o músculo transverso superficial do períneo e, apenas na mulher, as glândulas vestibulares maiores. SIN spatium perinei superficiale [TA], Colles s., superficial perineal pouch.

suprahepatic s.'s, recesso sub-hepático do peritônio. SIN subphrenic s.

suprasternal s. [TA], e. supra-esternal; intervalo estreito entre as camadas profunda e superficial da fáscia cervical acima do manúbrio do esterno, através do qual passam as veias jugulares anteriores. SIN spatium supraspinale [TA], Burns s.

Tarin s., e. de Tarin. SIN interpeduncular *cistern*.
Tenon s., e. de Tenon. SIN episcleral s.
thenar s., e. tenar. SIN lateral central palmar s.
Traube semilunar s., e. semilunar de Traube; espaço crescêntico de cerca de 12 cm de largura, delimitado, medialmente, pela borda esquerda do esterno, acima por uma linha oblíqua, que se estende da sexta cartilagem costal até a borda inferior da oitava ou nona costela, na linha axilar média, e, abaixo, pela reborda costal; a percussão aqui é normalmente timpânica, devido ao estômago subjacente, porém é modificada por enfisema pulmonar, derrame pleural ou aumento do baço.
Trautmann triangular s., e. triangular de Trautmann; área do osso temporal delimitada pelo seio sigmóideo da dura-máter, seio petroso superior da dura-máter e por uma tangente ao canal semicircular posterior.
vascular s. of retroinguinal compartment [TA], lacuna dos vasos; o compartimento medial abaixo do ligamento inguinal, para a passagem dos vasos femorais; é separado do espaço muscular pelo arco iliopectíneo. SIN lacuna vasorum retroinguinalis [TA], lacuna vasorum, vascular lacuna.
vertebral epidural s., e. extradural. VER spinal *dura mater*.
Virchow-Robin s., e. de Virchow-Robin; extensão do espaço subaracnóideo semelhante a um túnel, circundando os vasos sanguíneos que seguem do espaço subaracnóide para o cérebro ou medula espinal; o revestimento do canal é composto de pia-máter e pés gliais de astrócitos; provavelmente não ocorre continuação do espaço ao redor dos capilares e das células nervosas. SIN His perivascular s.
Waldeyer s., e. de Waldeyer. SIN Waldeyer *sheath*.
Westberg s., e. de Westberg; espaço que circunda a origem da aorta, revestida por pericárdio.
zonular s.'s [TA], espaços zonulares; espaços entre as fibras da zona ciliar no equador da lente. SIN spatia zonularia [TA], Petit canals.

spacing (spā'sing). Espaçamento; formação de espaços, especialmente a intervalos.
third spacing, terceiro espaço; perda de líquido extracelular do compartimento vascular para outros compartimentos corporais.
spa·gyr·ic (spā - jir'ik). Espagírico; relativo ao sistema de Paracelso ou de alquimia de medicina, que defendia o tratamento das doenças por vários tipos de substâncias químicas. [G. *spao*, dilacerar + *ageiro*, reunir]
spag·y·rist (spaj'ī - rist). Espagirista; médico do século XVI, seguidor dos ensinamentos de Paracelso, que acreditava na importância essencial do conhecimento químico ou alquímico para a compreensão e tratamento das doenças.
spall (spawl). **1.** Fragmento. **2.** Quebrar em fragmentos.
Spallanzani, Lazaro, padre e cientista italiano, 1729–1799. VER S. *law*.
spall·a·tion (spaw - lā'shŭn). Fragmentação. **1.** SIN fragmentation. **2.** Reação nuclear em que os núcleos, ao serem bombardeados por partículas de alta energia, liberam diversos prótons e partículas alfa. [I.m. *spalle*, fragmento]
span. Amplitude; espaço de tempo; a distância ou comprimento entre dois pontos; a extensão total ou alcance de algo.
attention s., tempo de atenção; o tempo durante o qual uma pessoa consegue concentrar-se num assunto.
memory s., o número máximo de itens lembrados após uma única apresentação (auditiva ou visual).
spar·ga·no·ma (spar - gă - nō'mă). Esparganoma; massa localizada resultante da esparganose.
spar·ga·no·sis (spar - gă - nō'sis). Esparganose; infecção pelo plerocercóide ou espargano de uma tênia pseudofilídea, habitualmente numa ferida da derme em decorrência da aplicação de carne infectada como cataplasma; pode ocorrer também infecção devido à ingestão de carne crua de rã, cobra, mamífero ou ave, que servem de hospedeiro intermediário ou de transporte do espargano, mas não de peixe com larvas de *Diphyllobothrium*, visto que a esparganose é uma infecção por tênias pseudofilídeas não-humanas, geralmente espécies de *Spirometra*. A esparganose também pode desenvolver-se em conseqüência da ingestão de água contendo *Cyclops* infectados por procercóides.
ocular s., e. ocular; infestação das órbitas pelo espargano de *Spirometra mansoni*; caracterizada por eritema e edema das pálpebras, lacrimejamento e blefaroptose; adquirida pela aplicação de carne crua de rã infectada sobre o olho como cataplasma.
spar·ga·num (spar'gă - nŭm). Espargano; originalmente descrito como gênero, porém atualmente restrito ao estágio plerocercóide de determinadas tênias. [G. *sparganon*, bandagem, de *spargo*, enfaixar]
spar·te·ine (spar'tē - ēn, - tē - in). Esparteína; alcalóide obtido do escopário, *Cytisus scoparius* e *Lupinus luteus*; o sulfato de escarpeína já foi utilizado como droga oxitócica. SIN lupinidine.
spasm (spazm). Espasmo; contração involuntária súbita de um ou mais músculos; inclui cãibras, contraturas. SIN muscle s., spasmus. [G. *spasmos*]
s. of accommodation, e. de acomodação; contração excessiva do músculo ciliar.

affect s.'s, espasmos de afeto; termo raramente empregado para ataques espasmódicos de riso, choro e gritos, acompanhados de taquipnéia acentuada.
anorectal s., e. anorretal. SIN proctalgia fugax.
Bell s., e. de Bell. SIN facial *tic*.
cadaveric s., e. cadavérico; *rigor mortis* que ocorre irregularmente nos diferentes músculos, causando movimentos dos membros.
canine s., e. canino. SIN risus caninus.
carpopedal s., e. carpopedal; espasmo das mãos e dos pés observado na hiperventilação, deficiência de cálcio e tetania: flexão das mãos nos punhos e dos dedos nas articulações metacarpofalângicas e extensão dos dedos nas articulações falângicas; os pés estão em dorsiflexão nos tornozelos, e os dedos dos pés apresentam flexão plantar.
diffuse esophageal s., e. esofágico; difuso; contração anormal da parede muscular do esôfago, causando dor e disfagia, freqüentemente em resposta à regurgitação do conteúdo de ácido gástrico.
epidemic transient diaphragmatic s., e. diafragmático transitório epidêmico. SIN epidemic *pleurodynia*.
epileptic s., e. epiléptico; caracterizado por súbita flexão-extensão ou extensão-flexão mista, predominantemente proximal (incluindo os músculos do tronco), que costuma ser mais prolongado do que um movimento mioclônico, mas não tão duradouro quanto uma convulsão tônica. Ocorre freqüentemente em salvas, e os episódios individuais variam na sua duração, desde componentes mioclônicos até tônicos.
esophageal s., e. esofágico; distúrbio da motilidade do esôfago, caracterizado por dor ou eructações pronunciadas após a deglutição de alimento. As contrações musculares do esôfago são excessivas tanto em força quanto duração. A dor torácica pode ser confundida com sintomas de origem cardíaca ou outra origem.
facial s., e. facial. SIN facial *tic*.
habit s., e. habitual. SIN tic.
hemifacial s., e. hemifacial; distúrbio nervoso facial, de início na vida adulta avançada, caracterizado por episódios de contrações mioclônicas irregulares, algumas vezes dolorosas, de vários músculos faciais; desencadeado por movimentos voluntários ou reflexos da face, o espasmo começa tipicamente no músculo orbicular do olho e, a seguir, dissemina-se; em certas ocasiões, seqüela da paralisia de Bell, porém, mais freqüentemente, o resultado de compressão proximal do nervo facial por um vaso sanguíneo aberrante ou por uma neoplasia.
infantile s., e. do lactente; espasmos musculares breves (1–3 segundos) em lactentes com síndrome de West, que freqüentemente aparecem como espasmos de anuência ou salamaleque. SIN salaam convulsions.
intention s., e. intencional; contração espasmódica dos músculos que ocorre quando se procura efetuar um movimento voluntário.
masticatory s., e. mastigatório; contração muscular convulsiva involuntária que afeta os músculos da mastigação.
mobile s., e. móvel; e. tônico que ocorre na hemiplegia espástica do lactente na tentativa de um movimento.
muscle s., e. muscular. SIN spasm.
nictitating s., e. nictante; pestanejar espasmódico involuntário. SIN spasmus nictitans, winking s.
nodding s., e. de anuência; **(1)** em lactentes, queda da cabeça sobre o tórax, devido à perda do tônus nos músculos do pescoço, como na epilepsia de anuência, ou ao espasmo tônico dos músculos anteriores do pescoço, como na síndrome de West; **(2)** em adultos, cabeceio da cabeça devido a espasmos clônicos dos músculos esternocleidomastóideos. SIN salaam attack, salaam s., spasmus nutans (1).
salaam s., e. de salamaleque. SIN nodding s.
saltatory s., e. saltatório; afecção espasmódica dos músculos dos membros inferiores. SIN Bamberger disease (1), Gowers disease (1).
winking s., e. nictante. SIN nictitating s.
spasmo-. Espasmo. [G. *spasmos*]
spas·mod·ic (spaz - mod'ik). Espasmódico; relativo a, ou caracterizado por, espasmo. [G. *spasmodes*, convulsivo, de *spasmos*, + *eidos*, forma]
spas·mo·gen (spaz'mō - jen). Espasmógeno; substância que causa contração do músculo liso; por exemplo, histamina.
spas·mo·gen·ic (spaz - mō - jen'ik). Espasmogênico; que causa espasmos. [spasmo- + G. *-gen*, que produz]
spas·mol·y·sis (spaz - mol'i - sis). Espasmólise; interrupção de um espasmo ou convulsão. [spasmo- + G. *lysis*, dissolução]
spas·mo·lyt·ic (spaz'mō - lit'ik). Espasmolítico. **1.** Relativo à espasmólise. **2.** Refere-se a um agente químico que alivia os espasmos da musculatura lisa.
spas·mo·phil·ic (spaz - mō - fil'ik). Espasmofílico; relativo à espasmofilia.
spas·mus (spaz'mŭs). Espasmo. SIN spasm. [L. do G. *spasmos*, espasmo]
s. coordina'tus, e. coordenado; movimentos compulsivos, como tiques imitativos ou mímicos, festinação, etc.
s. glot'tidis, e. da glote. SIN laryngismus stridulus.
s. nic'titans, e. nictante ou nictitante. SIN nictitating *spasm*.

s. nu·tans, e. **(1)** Espasmo de anuência. SIN nodding *spasm;* **(2)** nistagmo fino algumas vezes rotatório, outras vezes monocular, associado a movimentos de anuência da cabeça.

spas·tic (spas'tik). Espástico. **1.** SIN hypertonic (1). **2.** Relativo a espasmo ou a espasticidade. [L. *spasticus*, de G. *spastikos*, fechando]

spas·tic·i·ty (spas-tis'i-tē). Espasticidade; um tipo de aumento do tônus muscular em repouso; caracterizada por aumento da resistência ao estiramento passivo, velocidade dependente e assimétrica em torno das articulações (isto é, maior nos músculos flexores no cotovelo e músculos extensores no joelho). Outras manifestações incluem reflexos tendinosos profundos exagerados e clono. VER TAMBÉM clasp-knife s.

clasp-knife s., e. em canivete; resistência inicial aumentada ao estiramento dos músculos extensores de uma articulação, que cedem subitamente, permitindo que a articulação seja então facilmente flexionada; a rigidez se deve a um exagero do reflexo de estiramento. VER TAMBÉM lengthening *reaction.* SIN clasp-knife effect, clasp-knife rigidity.

spa·tia (spā'shē-ā). Espaços; plural de spatium. [L.]

spa·tial (spā'shăl). Espacial; relativo ao espaço ou a um espaço.

spa·ti·um, pl. **spa·tia** (spā'shē-ŭm, -shē-ā). [TA]. Espaço. SIN space. [L.]

spa'tia an'guli iridocor'nea'lis [TA], espaços do ângulo iridocorneal. SIN *spaces* of iridocorneal angle, em *space.*

s. endolympha'ticum [TA], e. endolinfático. SIN endolymphatic *space.*

s. episclera'le [TA], e. episcleral. SIN episcleral *space.*

s. extradura'le, e. extradural; *termo oficial alternativo para epidural *space.*

s. extradurale [TA], e. extradural. SIN epidural *space.*

s. extraperitonea'le [TA], e. extraperitoneal. SIN extraperitoneal *space.*

s. intercosta'le [TA], e. intercostal. SIN intercostal *space.*

s. interfascia'le, e. episcleral. SIN episcleral *space.*

s. interglobula're, pl. **spa'tia interglobula'ria,** e. interglobular. SIN interglobular *space.*

spa'tia interos'sea metacar'pi [TA], espaços interósseos do metacarpo. SIN interosseous metacarpal *spaces,* em *space.*

spa'tia interos'sea metatar'si [TA], espaços interósseos do metatarso. SIN interosseous metatarsal *spaces,* em *space.*

s. intervagina'le bulb'i oc'uli, e. episcleral. SIN episcleral *space.*

s. intervagina'le subarachnoidale ner'vi op'tici [TA], e. intervaginal subaracnóideo do nervo óptico. SIN intervaginal subarachnoid *space* of optic nerve.

s. lateropharyn'geum [TA], e. laterofaríngeo. SIN lateral pharyngeal *space.* VER TAMBÉM retropharyngeal *space.*

s. leptomeningeum [TA], e. leptomeníngeo. SIN leptomeningeal *space.*

s. parapharyngeum, e. laterofaríngeo. SIN parapharyngeal *space.*

s. perichoroideum [TA], e. pericoróide. SIN perichoroidal *space.*

s. peridurale, e. extradural; *termo oficial alternativo para (spinal) epidural *space.*

s. perilymphat'icum [TA], e. perilinfático. SIN perilymphatic *space.*

s. perine'i profun'dum, e. profundo do períneo. SIN deep perineal *space.*

s. perine'i superficia'le [TA], e. superficial do períneo. SIN superficial perineal *space.*

s. peripharyn'geum [TA], e. perifaríngeo. SIN peripharyngeal *space.*

s. pharyngeum laterale [TA], e. laterofaríngeo. SIN lateral pharyngeal *space.*

s. retroinguina'le [TA], e. retroinguinal. SIN retroinguinal *space.*

s. retroperitonea'le [TA], e. retroperitoneal. SIN retroperitoneal *space.*

s. retropharyn'geum [TA], e. retrofaríngeo. SIN retropharyngeal *space;* VER TAMBÉM lateral pharyngeal *space.*

s. retropu'bicum [TA], e. retropúbico. SIN retropubic *space.*

s. retrozonulare [TA], e. retrozonular. SIN retrozonular *space.*

s. subarachnoideum [TA], e. subaracnóideo. SIN subarachnoid *space.*

s. subdura'le [TA], e. subdural. SIN subdural *space.*

s. supraspinale [TA], e. supra-esternal. SIN suprasternal *space.*

spa'tia zonula'ria [TA], espaços zonulares. SIN zonular *spaces,* em *space.*

spat·u·la (spach'ŭ-lă). Espátula; lâmina plana, como a lâmina de uma faca, porém sem borda cortante, utilizada em farmácia para espalhar emplastros e pomadas e como auxiliar na mistura de ingredientes num almofariz e pilão. [L. dim. de *spatha*, instrumento de madeira largo e plano, do G. *spathē*]

iris s., e. para íris; instrumento cirúrgico plano utilizado para reposicionamento de íris que sofreu prolapso através de uma ferida.

Ro s., e. de Ro; espátula muito pequena de aço niquelado para transferir fragmentos de material infectado, como membrana diftérica, para tubos de cultura.

spat·u·late (spach'ŭ-lāt). **1.** Espatulado; que tem a forma de uma espátula. **2.** Espatular; manipular ou misturar com uma espátula. **3.** Incisar a extremidade seccionada de uma estrutura tubular longitudinalmente e abri-la para permitir a criação de uma anastomose elíptica de maior circunferência do que seria possível com anastomoses convencionais transversais ou oblíquas (em bisel) término-terminais. SIN spatulated.

spat·u·lat·ed (spach'ŭ-lāt-ed). Espatulado. SIN spatulate.

spat·u·la·tion (spach'ŭ-lā'shŭn). Espatulação; manipulação de material com uma espátula.

Spatz, Hugo, neurologista e psiquiatra alemão, 1888–1969. VER Hallervorden-S. *disease, syndrome.*

spay (spā). Castrar; remover os ovários de um animal. [Gael. *spoth,* castrar ou G. *spadōn,* eunuco]

SPCA Abreviatura de serum prothrombin conversion *accelerator* (acelerador da conversão de protrombina sérica).

spear·mint (spēr-mint). Hortelã; as folhas e as sumidades de *Mentha viridis* ou *M. cardiaca* (família Labiatae); agente carminativo e aromatizante.

s. oil, óleo de hortelã; o óleo volátil destilado com vapor das partes frescas da planta em floração de *Mentha viridis* ou *M. cardiaca,* um agente aromatizante.

spe·cial·ist (spesh'ă-list). Especialista; aquele que adquiriu experiência profissional em determinada especialidade ou área.

spe·cial·i·za·tion (spesh'ă-li-zā'shŭn). Especialização. **1.** Atenção profissional limitada a determinada especialidade ou área para estudo, pesquisa e/ou tratamento. **2.** SIN differentiation (1).

spe·cial·ize (spesh'ă-līz). Especializar; empenhar-se numa especialização (1).

spe·cial·ty (spesh'al-tē). Especialidade; a área ou ramo particular da ciência médica ao qual alguém dedica atenção profissional. [L. *specialitas,* de *specialis,* especial]

spe·ci·a·tion (spē-shē-ā'shŭn). Especiação; o processo evolutivo pelo qual diversas espécies de animais ou plantas são formadas a partir de uma espécie ancestral comum.

spe·cies, pl. **spe·cies** (spē'shēz). Espécie. **1.** Divisão biológica entre o gênero e uma variedade ou o indivíduo; um grupo de organismos que geralmente possuem estreita semelhança entre si nas características mais essenciais de sua organização e que se reproduzem efetivamente, dando origem a uma prole fértil. **2.** Classe de preparações farmacêuticas que consistem numa mistura de plantas secas, não-pulverizadas, porém em divisão fina o suficiente para o uso conveniente no preparo de decocções ou infusões extemporâneas, como um chá. [L. aparência, forma, tipo, de *specio*, olhar para]

type s., espécie típica; o nome da espécie isolada ou de uma das espécies de um gênero ou subgênero quando o nome do gênero ou subgênero foi originalmente publicado de forma válida.

spe·cies-spe·cif·ic. Espécie-específico; característico de determinada espécie; soro produzido pela injeção de imunógenos num animal e que só atua sobre as células, proteínas, etc., de um membro da mesma espécie na qual foi obtido o antígeno original.

spe·cif·ic (spē-sif'ik). Específico. **1.** Relativo a uma espécie. VER TAMBÉM specific *epithet.* **2.** Relativo a uma doença infecciosa individual, causada por um microrganismo especial. **3.** Remédio que possui ação terapêutica definida em relação a uma doença ou sintoma específico, como a quinina em relação à malária. [L. *specificus,* de *species* + *facio,* fazer]

spec·i·fic·i·ty (spes-i-fis'i-tē). Especificidade. **1.** A condição ou estado de ser específico, de possuir uma relação fixa com uma causa única ou um resultado definido; manifesta-se na relação de uma doença com seu microrganismo patogênico, de uma reação com determinada união química ou de um anticorpo com seu antígeno ou o inverso. **2.** Em patologia clínica e triagem médica, a proporção de indivíduos com resultados negativos de testes para a doença que o teste pretende revelar, isto é, resultados verdadeiro-negativos como proporção do total de resultados verdadeiro-negativos e falso-positivos. Cf. sensitivity (2).

analytical s., e. analítica; liberdade de interferência por qualquer elemento ou composto, a não ser o analisado.

diagnostic s., e. diagnóstica; a probabilidade (P) de que, dada a ausência de doença (D), um resultado normal do teste (T) exclua a doença; isto é, P(T/D).

relative s., e. relativa; a especificidade de um teste de triagem médica determinada por comparação com o mesmo tipo de teste (p. ex., especificidade de um novo teste sorológico em relação à especificidade de um teste sorológico estabelecido).

substrate s., e. de substrato; capacidade de uma enzima de reconhecer seu substrato e ligar-se a ele, tipicamente medida pelas relações $V_{máx}/K_m$ ou k_{cat}/K_m.

spe·cil·lum, pl. **spe·cil·la** (spe-sil'ŭm, -lă). Especilho; pequena sonda. [L. uma sonda, de *specio*, olhar para]

spec·i·men (spes'i-men). Amostra; espécime, pequena parte ou exemplar de qualquer substância ou material obtido para exame. [L. de *specio,* olhar para]

cytologic s., a. citológica; amostra que pode ser obtida por uma variedade de métodos a partir de muitas áreas do corpo, incluindo o trato genital feminino, as vias respiratórias, as vias urinárias, o trato alimentar e as cavidades corporais; utilizada para exame citológico e diagnóstico (p. ex., esfregaços citológicos, preparações filtradas, botões centrifugados).

SPECT Abreviatura de single photon emission computed *tomography* (tomografia computadorizada com emissão fotônica única).

spec·ta·cles (spek'tĭ-klz). Óculos; lentes colocadas numa armação que as segura na frente dos olhos, usadas para corrigir erros de refração ou para proteger os olhos. As partes dos óculos são: as *lentes;* a *ponte* entre as lentes, que repousa sobre o nariz; os *aros,* que circundam as lentes; as *hastes,* que passam pelo lado da cabeça até as orelhas; as *curvas,* as extremidades curvas nas têmporas; os *ombros,* barras curtas fixadas aos aros ou às lentes e unidas com os lados. SIN eyeglasses, glasses (1). [L. *specto,* pp. -*atus,* observar]

bifocal s., o. bifocais; o. com lentes bifocais. VER lens.
clerical s., o. para leitura. SIN half-glass s.
divers' s., o. de mergulho; lentes fortemente convexas para visão nítida sob a água.
divided s., o. dividido. SIN Franklin s.
Franklin s., o. de Franklin; forma primitiva de óculos bifocais, em que a metade inferior da lente é para a visão de perto, enquanto a metade superior é para a visão a distância. SIN divided s.
half-glass s., o. de meia-lente; óculos utilizados para leitura, nos quais a porção superior das lentes é removida. SIN clerical s., pantoscopic s., pulpit s.
hemianopic s., o. hemianópico; óculos com prisma ou espelho para permitir que o indivíduo com hemianopsia homônima veja objetos no meio campo cego.
lid crutch s., o. de masselon; óculos com pequenas ramificações de metal de bordas lisas, que se encaixam acima da pálpebra superior e a mantém elevada acima da pupila em casos de blefaroptose paralítica. SIN Masselon s.
Masselon s., o. de Masselon. SIN lid crutch s.
orthoscopic s., o. ortoscópicos; lentes convexas com prismas com base interna para trabalho de perto.
pantoscopic s., o. pantoscópicos. SIN half-glass s.
photochromic s., o. fotocromáticos; óculos com lentes que escurecem na exposição à luz ultravioleta.
protective s., o. protetores ou de segurança; óculos que protegem contra raios ultravioleta ou infravermelhos ou contra lesões mecânicas. SIN safety s.
pulpit s., o. de púlpito. SIN half-glass s.
safety s., o. de segurança. SIN protective s.
stenopeic s., stenopaic s., o. estenopeicos, o. estenopaicos; (1) discos opacos com fendas estreitas no centro para permitir apenas a entrada de uma quantidade mínima de luz; utilizados como proteção contra cegueira da neve; (2) óculos que possuem discos opacos com múltiplas perfurações, utilizados para auxiliar na visão na catarata incipiente e em opacidades distintas da córnea; em certas ocasiões, utilizados como substitutos de lentes corretivas ou de óculos escuros.
telescopic s., o. telescópicos; óculos de aumento obtidos pelo uso de uma lente objetiva convexa e uma ocular côncava separadas pela diferença de seus comprimentos focais.
spec·ti·no·my·cin hy·dro·chlo·ride (spek'ti-nō-mī'sin). Cloridrato de espectinomicina; agente antibacteriano antibiótico.
spec·tra (spek'tra). Espectros; plural de spectrum. [L.]
spec·tral (spek'tral). Espectral; relativo a um espectro.
spec·trin (spek'trin). Espectrina; proteína contrátil filamentosa que, juntamente com a actina e outras proteínas do citoesqueleto, forma uma rede que confere à membrana do eritrócito a sua forma e flexibilidade; a existência de um defeito ou uma deficiência de espectrina está associada à esferocitose hereditária e eliptocitose hereditária; principal componente do esqueleto da membrana dos eritrócitos. Constituída de duas subunidades, uma unidade alfa com PM de 240.000 [MIM*182860] e uma unidade beta com PM de 225.000 [MIM*182870].
spectro-. Espectro-. Um espectro. [L. *spectrum*, uma imagem]
spec·tro·chem·is·try (spek'trō-kem'is-trē). Espectroquímica; o estudo de substâncias e sua identificação por meio de espectroscopia, isto é, pela luz emitida ou absorvida.
spec·tro·col·or·im·e·ter (spek'trō-kŏl-er-im'ē-ter). Espectrocolorímetro; colorímetro que utiliza uma fonte de luz de uma porção selecionada do espectro, isto é, de comprimento de onda selecionado.
spec·tro·flu·o·rom·e·ter (spek-trō-flōr-om'ē-ter). Espectrofluorômetro; instrumento para medir a intensidade e a qualidade da fluorescência.
spec·tro·gram (spek'trō-gram). Espectrograma; representação gráfica de um espectro. [spectro- + G. *gramma*, algo escrito]
spec·tro·graph (spek'trō-graf). Espectrógrafo; instrumento utilizado em espectografia.
mass s., e. de massa; instrumento que submete íons com cargas elétricas e acelerados (atômicos ou moleculares) a um campo magnético que confere uma via curva que difere para cada relação massa-carga elétrica, separando, assim, espécies individuais; utilizado na detecção e na análise de relações isotópicas e nas determinações da estrutura molecular.
spec·trog·ra·phy (spek-trog'ră-fē). Espectrografia; o procedimento de fotografar ou traçar um espectro. [spectro- + G. *grapho*, escrever]
spec·trom·e·ter (spek-trom'ē-ter). Espectrômetro; instrumento para determinar o comprimento de onda ou a energia da luz ou de outra emissão eletromagnética. [spectro- + G. *metron*, medida]
spec·trom·e·try (spek-trom'ē-trē). Espectrometria; procedimento de observar e medir os comprimentos de onda da luz ou de outras emissões eletromagnéticas.
clinical s., e. clínica. SIN biospectrometry.
spec·tro·pho·bia (spek-trō-fō'bē-ă). Espectrofobia; medo mórbido de espelhos ou da imagem refletida no espelho. [spectro- + G. *phobos*, medo]
spec·tro·pho·to·flu·o·rim·e·try (spek'trō-fō'tō-flōr-im'ē-trē). Espectrofotofluorimetria; medida da intensidade da qualidade da fluorescência por meio de um espectofotômetro.
spec·tro·pho·tom·e·ter (spek'trō-fō-tom'ē-ter). Espectrofotômetro; instrumento para medir a intensidade da luz de um comprimento de onda definido, transmitida por uma substância ou solução, fornecendo uma medida quantitativa do material na solução que absorve a luz; colorímetro com uma escolha de comprimento de onda e medida fotométrica. [spectro- + photometer]
spec·tro·pho·tom·e·try (spek'trō-fō-tom'ē-trē). Espectrofotometria; análise por meio de um espectrofotômetro.
atomic absorption s., e. de absorção atômica; determinação da concentração pela capacidade dos átomos de absorver energia radiante de comprimentos de onda específicos.
flame emission s., e. de emissão de chama; determinação da concentração de um elemento pela medida da luz emitida quando esse elemento é excitado por energia na forma de calor.
spec·tro·po·lar·im·e·ter (spek'trō-pō-lar-im'ē-ter). Espectropolarímetro; instrumento para medir a rotação do plano da luz polarizada de comprimento de onda específico com a sua passagem através de uma solução ou sólido translúcido. [spectro- + polarimeter]
spec·tro·scope (spek'trō-skōp). Espectroscópio; instrumento para resolução da luz de qualquer corpo luminoso dentro de seu espectro, bem como para a análise do espectro assim formado. Consiste num prisma que produz refração da luz ou numa grade para difração da luz, um arranjo para tornar os raios paralelos e um telescópio que aumenta o espectro. [spectro- + G. *skopeō*, ver]
direct vision s., e. de visão direta; e. que consiste num tubo único contendo uma série de prismas; uma extremidade do tubo é colocada em maior contato possível com a substância a ser examinada, enquanto o observador olha pela extremidade oposta; pode ser utilizado para fazer um exame espectroscópico do sangue *in vivo*, como no lobo da orelha ou na membrana interdigital do polegar.
spec·tro·scop·ic (spek-trō-skop'ik). Espectroscópico; relativo a, ou realizado por meio de, um espectroscópio.
spec·tros·co·py (spek-tros'kō-pē). Espectroscopia; observação e estudo dos espectros de luz absorvida ou emitida por meio de um espectroscópio.
clinical s., e. clínica. SIN biospectroscopy.
infrared s., e. de infravermelho; o estudo da absorção específica na região infravermelha do espectro eletromagnético; utilizada no estudo das ligações químicas no interior das moléculas.
magnetic resonance s., e. de ressonância magnética; detecção e medida dos espectros de ressonância de espécies moleculares num tecido ou numa amostra.
spectrum, pl. **spec·tra, spec·trums** (spek'trŭm, -ă, -ŭmz). Espectro. 1. Faixa de cores apresentada quando a luz branca é decomposta em suas cores constituintes pela sua passagem através de um prisma ou através de uma grade de difração: vermelho, laranja, amarelo, verde, azul, índigo e violeta, dispostas de acordo com a sua freqüência crescente de vibração ou comprimento de onda decrescente. 2. Em termos figurativos, a gama de microrganismos patogênicos contra a qual um antibiótico ou outro agente antibacteriano é ativo. 3. A plotagem da intensidade *vs.* comprimento de onda da luz emitida ou absorvida por uma substância, geralmente característica da substância e utilizada em análise qualitativa e quantitativa. 4. A faixa de comprimentos de onda apresentada quando um feixe de energia radiante é submetido a dispersão e enfocado. [L. uma imagem, de *specio*, olhar para]
absorption s., e. de absorção; o espectro observado após a passagem da luz através de uma solução ou substância translúcida e sua absorção parcial por essa solução ou substância; muitos grupamentos moleculares exibem padrões característicos de absorção da luz, que podem ser utilizados para detecção e ensaio quantitativo.
antimicrobial s., e. antimicrobiano. VER *spectrum* (2).
broad s., e. amplo; termo que indica uma ampla faixa de atividade de um antibiótico contra uma grande variedade de microrganismos.
chromatic s., e. cromático; o *continuum* de cores formado pela luz branca ao atravessar um prisma ou uma grade de difração. SIN color s.
color s., e. colorido, e. cromático. SIN chromatic s.
continuous s., e. contínuo; espectro em que não há nenhuma banda ou linha de absorção.
excitation s., e. de excitação; fluorescência produzida sobre uma faixa de comprimentos de onda da luz excitante.
fluorescence s., e. de fluorescência; fluorescência produzida numa faixa de comprimentos de onda quando o comprimento de onda de excitação é máximo.
fortification s., e. de fortificação; a disposição de faixas em ziguezague de luz, semelhantes às paredes de torres medievais fortificadas, que marca a margem do escotoma cintilante da enxaqueca. SIN fortification figures, telehopsias.
frequency s., e. de freqüência; a faixa de freqüências num sinal, utilizada para descrever o poder de resolução de um sistema de imagem em radiologia.
infrared s., e. infravermelho; parte do espectro invisível de comprimentos de onda um pouco maiores que os da luz visível. SIN thermal s.

invisible s., e. invisível; a radiação localizada de cada lado da luz visível, isto é, a luz infravermelha e a ultravioleta.
Raman s., e. de Raman; a disposição característica da luz produzida pelo efeito de Raman.
thermal s., e. térmico, e. infravermelho. SIN infrared s.
ultraviolet s., e. ultravioleta; o espectro eletromagnético nos comprimentos de onda mais curtos do que a extremidade violeta do espectro visível.
visible s., e. visível; a parte da radiação eletromagnética que é visível ao olho humano; estende-se do vermelho extremo, 7.606 Å (760,6 nm), ao violeta extremo, 3.934 Å (393,4 nm).
vocal s., e. vocal; a freqüência e faixas de intensidade da voz.
wide s., e. largo. VER *spectrum* (3).

spec·u·lum, pl. **spec·u·la** (spek′ū-lŭm, -lă). Espéculo; instrumento para expor a abertura de qualquer canal ou cavidade para facilitar a inspeção de seu interior. [L. um espelho, de *specio,* olhar para]

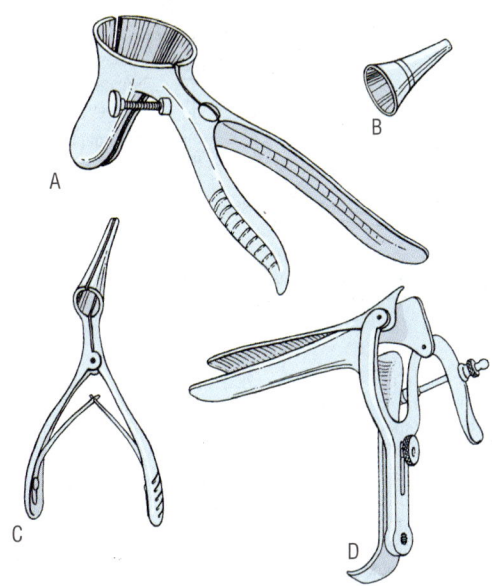

espéculo: (A) retal, (B) auricular, (C) nasal, (D) vaginal em bico de pato

bivalve s., e. bivalve; espéculo como duas lâminas ajustáveis.
Cooke s., e. de Cooke; espéculo de três lâminas para exame e cirurgias retais.
duckbill s., e. em bico de pato; espéculo bivalve, cujas lâminas são largas e achatadas, lembrando um bico de pato; utilizado na inspeção da vagina e do colo uterino.
eye s., e. ocular, blefarostato; instrumento para manter as pálpebras abertas durante a inspeção ou operação do olho. SIN blepharostat.
Kelly rectal s., e. retal de Kelly; espéculo tubular com obturador para exame retal.
Pedersen s., e. de Pedersen; espéculo plano e estreito utilizado em vaginas com intróito estreito.
stop-s., e. de interrupção; espéculo dilatador, semelhante a um espéculo palpebral, que possui um dispositivo para impedir a sua abertura excessiva.
Spee, Ferdinand Graf von, embriologista alemão, 1855–1937. VER *curve* of S.
SPEECH1. Gene que, ao sofrer mutação, é responsável por dispraxia motora.
speech. Fala; o uso da voz para comunicar idéias. [A.S. *spaec*]
 alaryngeal s., f. alaríngea; forma de fala que ocorre após laringectomia ao utilizar uma fonte vibratória externa ou o segmento faringoesofágico como fonte vibratória interna. VER TAMBÉM esophageal s. A fala traqueoesofágica pode ser produzida após laringectomia mediante desvio cirúrgico do ar exalado para faringe por uma fístula traqueoesofágica construída permanente.
 cerebellar s., f. cerebelar; forma explosiva de expressão vocal, com lentidão das palavras.
 clipped s., f. titubeante. SIN scamping s.
 cued s., f. sugerida; sistema de comunicação com uma pessoa portadora de acentuado comprometimento auditivo, em que se utiliza a comunicação gestual com as mãos para sugerir sons, a fim de suplementar a linguagem falada.
 echo s., ecolalia. SIN echolalia.
 esophageal s., f. esofágica; técnica para falar após laringectomia total; consiste na deglutição de ar no esôfago e sua regurgitação, produzindo uma vibração na hipofaringe.
 explosive s., f. explosiva; fala alta e súbita relacionada a uma lesão do sistema nervoso. SIN logospasm (2).
 helium s., f. do hélio; fala peculiar alta, freqüentemente ininteligível, produzida quando o indivíduo respira uma mistura de até 80% de hélio e 20% de oxigênio.
 mirror s., f. espelhada; inversão da ordem das sílabas numa palavra, análoga à escrita espelhada.
 scamping s., f. titubeante; forma de lalismo em que as consoantes ou sílabas de pronúncia difícil são omitidas. SIN clipped s.
 scanning s., f. escandida; fala medida e freqüentemente lenta, com interrupções.
 slurring s., f. indistinta; articulação incorreta dos sons das letras mais difíceis.
 spastic s., f. espástica; fala difícil relacionada ao aumento do tônus muscular.
 staccato s., f. em *staccato*; expressão vocal abrupta, em que cada sílaba é enunciada separadamente; observada especialmente na esclerose múltipla. SIN syllabic s.
 subvocal s., f. subvocal; movimentos pequenos dos músculos da fala relacionados ao pensamento, porém sem produzir nenhum som.
 syllabic s., f. silábica. SIN staccato s.
 tracheoesophageal s., f. traqueoesofágica; forma de fala alaríngea obtida por uma técnica cirúrgica que cria uma derivação entre a traquéia e o esôfago, permitindo que o ar pulmonar produza vibrações na mucosa esofágica superior e faríngea como substituto das vibrações das cordas vocais quando a laringe é cirurgicamente removida.
speed (spēd). Velocidade; a magnitude da velocidade sem considerar a sua direção. Cf. velocity.
spe·len·ceph·a·ly (spē-len-sef′ă-lē). Espelencefalia. SIN porencephaly. [*spēlaion,* caverna + *enkephalos,* cérebro]
Spens, Thomas, médico escocês, 1769–1842. VER S. *syndrome.*
sperm. Espermatozóide. SIN spermatozoon. [G. *sperma,* semente]
sperma-, spermato-, spermo-. Esperma-, espermato-, espermo-. Sêmen, espermatozóides. [G. *sperma,* semente]
sper·ma·ce·ti (sper-mă-set′ē). Espermacete; substância gordurosa e cérea peculiar, principalmente cetina (palmitato de cetila), obtida da cabeça do cachalote, *Physeter macrocephalus;* utilizada para conferir firmeza às bases das pomadas. SIN cetaceum. [sperma- + G. *ketos,* baleia]
sperm·ag·glu·ti·na·tion (sperm′ă-gloo-ti-nā′shŭn). Espermaglutinação; aglutinação dos espermatozóides.
sperm-as·ter (sperm′-as-ter). Espermaster; citocentro com raios estrelados no citoplasma de um óvulo inseminado; produzido pelo espermatozóide que penetra, transformando-se no fuso mitótico da primeira divisão. [sperm + G. *aster,* uma estrela]
sper·mat·ic (sper-mat′ik). Espermático; relativo ao esperma ou ao sêmen.
sper·ma·tid (sper′mă-tid). Espermátide; célula num estágio avançado de desenvolvimento do espermatozóide; trata-se de uma célula haplóide derivada do espermatócito secundário, que se transforma em espermatozóide através da espermiogênese. SIN nematoblast. [spermat- + *-id* (2)]
sper·ma·tin (sper′mă-tin). Espermatina; nome proposto para um albuminóide no líquido seminal.
spermato-. Espermato-. VER sperma-.
sper·ma·to·blast (sper′mă-tō-blast). Espermatoblasto, espermatogônio. SIN spermatogonium. [spermato- + G. *blastos,* germe]
sper·ma·to·cele (sper′mă-tō-sēl). Espermatocele; cisto do epidídimo contendo espermatozóides. SIN spermatocyst. [spermato- + G. *kēlē,* tumor]
sper·ma·to·ci·dal (sper′mă-tō-sī′dăl). Espermaticida, espermicida; que destrói os espermatozóides. SIN spermicidal.
sper·ma·to·cide (sper′mă-tō-sid). Espermaticida; agente destrutivo para os espermatozóides. SIN spermicide. [spermato- + L. *caedo,* matar]
sper·ma·to·cyst. Espermatocisto. SIN spermatocele.
sper·ma·to·cy·tal (sper′mă-tō-sī′tal). Espermatocitário; relativo aos espermatócitos.
sper·ma·to·cyte (sper′mă-tō-sīt). Espermatócito; célula-mãe de uma espermátide, derivada de uma espermatogônia por divisão mitótica. [spermato- + G. *kytos,* célula]
 primary s., e. primário; espermatócito derivado de uma espermatogônia através de uma fase de crescimento, que sofre a primeira divisão da meiose.
 secondary s., e. secundário; espermatócito derivado de um espermatócito primário através da primeira divisão meiótica; cada espermatócito secundário produz duas espermátides através da segunda divisão meiótica.
sper·ma·to·cy·to·gen·e·sis (sper′mă-tō-sī′tō-jen′ĕ-sis). Espermatocitogênese. SIN spermatogenesis.
sper·ma·to·gen·e·sis (sper′mă-tō-jen′ĕ-sis). Espermatogênese; todo o processo através do qual as células-tronco ou primordiais (espermatogônias) dividem-se e diferenciam-se em espermatozóides. VER TAMBÉM spermiogenesis. SIN spermatocytogenesis, spermatogeny. [spermato- + G. *genesis,* origem]

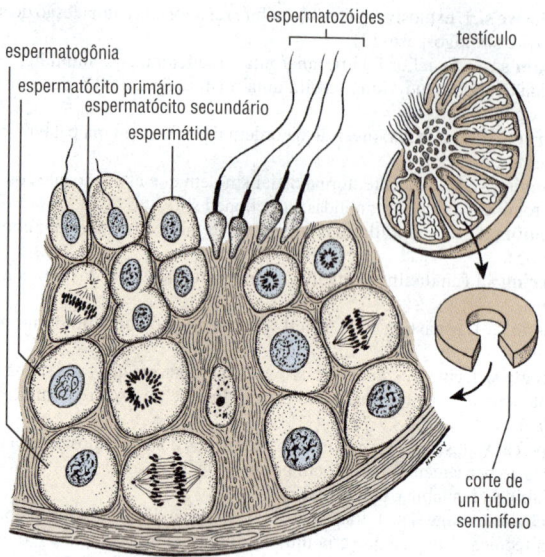

espermatogênese: vários estágios observados ao corte de um túbulo seminífero

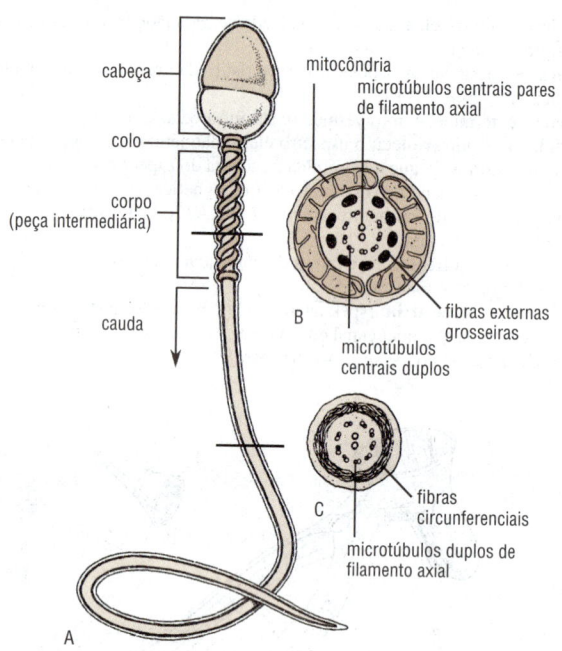

espermatozóide humano: corte longitudinal (A); cortes transversais do corpo (B) e da cauda (C)

sper·ma·to·ge·net·ic (sper′mă-tō-jĕ-net′ik). Espermatogenético. SIN spermatogenic.

sper·ma·to·gen·ic (sper′mă-tō-jen′ik). Espermatogênico; relativo à espermatogênese; produtor de espermatozóides. SIN spermatogenetic, spermatogenous, spermatopoietic (1).

sper·ma·tog·e·nous (sper-mă-toj′ĕ-nŭs). Espermatógeno. SIN spermatogenic.

sper·ma·tog·e·ny (sper-mă-toj′ĕ-nē). Espermatogenia. SIN spermatogenesis.

sper·ma·to·gone (sper′mă-tō-gōn). Espermatogônia. SIN spermatogonium.

sper·ma·to·go·ni·um (sper′mă-tō-gō′nē-ŭm). Espermatogônia; a célula espermática primitiva derivada da célula germinativa por divisão mitótica; aumentando várias vezes de tamanho, transforma-se num espermatócito primário. VER TAMBÉM spermatid. SIN spermatoblast, spermatogone. [spermato- + G. *gonē*, geração]

sper·ma·toid (sper′mă-tōid). Espermatóide. 1. Semelhante a um espermatozóide, a uma cauda de espermatozóide ou sêmen. 2. Forma masculina ou flagelada do microparasita da malária. [spermato + G. *eidos*, forma]

sper·ma·tol·o·gy (sper-mă-tol′ō-jē). Espermatologia; ramo da histologia, fisiologia e embriologia relacionado ao estudo dos espermatozóides e/ou secreção seminal. [spermato- + G. *logos*, estudo]

sper·ma·tol·y·sin (sper-mă-tol′i-sin). Espermatolisina; lisina específica (anticorpo) formada em resposta à injeção repetida de espermatozóides.

sper·ma·tol·y·sis (sper-mă-tol′i-sis). Espermatólise; destruição dos espermatozóides, com dissolução. SIN spermolysis. [spermato- + G. *lysis*, dissolução]

sper·ma·to·lyt·ic (sper′mă-tō-lit′ik). Espermatolítico; relativo à espermatólise.

sper·ma·to·pho·bia (sper′mă-tō-fō′bē-ă). Espermatofobia; medo mórbido de espermatorréia ou perda de sêmen. [spermato- + G. *phobos*, medo]

sper·ma·to·phore (sper′mă-tō-fōr). Espermatóforo; cápsula que contém espermatozóides; encontrado em vários invertebrados. [spermato- + G. *phoros*, que transporta]

sper·ma·to·poi·et·ic (sper′mă-tō-poy-et′ik). Espermatopoético. 1. SIN spermatogenic. 2. Que secreta sêmen. [spermato- + G. *poieō*, fazer]

sper·ma·tor·rhea (sper′mă-tō-rē′ă). Espermatorréia; secreção involuntária de sêmen, sem orgasmo. [spermato- + G. *rhoia*, fluxo]

sper·ma·tox·in (sper′mă-tok′sin). Espermatoxina; anticorpo citotóxico específico contra espermatozóides. SIN spermotoxin.

sper·ma·to·zoa (sper′mă-tō-zō′ă). Espermatozóides; plural de spermatozoon.

sper·ma·to·zo·al, sper·ma·to·zo·an (sper′ma-tō-zō′ăl, -zō′ăn). Espermatozóico; relativo a espermatozóides.

sper·ma·to·zo·on, pl. **sper·ma·to·zoa** (sper′mă-tō-zō′on, -zō′ă). Espermatozóide; gameta masculino ou célula sexual que contém a informação genética a ser transmitida pelo macho, apresenta autocinesia e tem a capacidade de efetuar a zigose com um ovo. O espermatozóide humano é composto de uma cabeça e uma cauda, sendo a cauda dividida em colo, peça intermediária, peça principal e peça terminal; a cabeça, com 4–6 μm de comprimento, é um corpo achatado e amplamente oval, que contém o núcleo; a cauda tem cerca de 55 μm de comprimento. SIN sperm cell, sperm. [G. *sperma*, semente + *zōon*, animal]

sper·ma·tu·ria (sper-mă-too′rē-ă). Espermatúria. SIN semenuria.

sper·mia (sper′mē-ă). Espérmios; plural de spermium.

sper·mi·ci·dal (sper-mi-sī′dăl). Espermicida. SIN spermatocidal.

sper·mi·cide (sper′mi-sīd). Espermicida. SIN spermatocide.

sper·mi·dine (sper′mi-dēn). Espermidina; poliamina encontrada com a espermina numa ampla variedade de organismos e tecidos; encontrada no esperma humano; importante no crescimento das células e tecidos.

sper·mi·duct (sper′mi-dŭkt). 1. Ducto deferente. SIN *ductus* deferens. 2. Ducto ejaculatório. SIN ejaculatory *duct*.

sperm·ine (sper′mēn). Espermina; poliamina encontrada em algumas bactérias; associada aos ácidos nucleicos em alguns vírus; encontrada no esperma humano; importante no crescimento de células e tecidos. SIN gerontine, musculamine, neuridine.

sper·mi·o·gen·e·sis (sper′mē-ō-jen′ĕ-sis). Espermiogênese; fase da espermatogênese durante a qual as espermátides imaturas transformam-se em espermatozóides. [sperm- + G. *genesis*, origem]

sperm·ism (sper′mizm). Espermismo; a crença dos pré-formacionistas de que a célula sexual masculina (espermatozóide) contém um corpo pré-formado em miniatura denominado homúnculo.

sperm·ist. Espermista; pré-formacionista que acreditava no conceito do espermismo. Cf. ovist.

sper·mi·um, pl. **sper·mia** (sper′mē-ŭm, -ă). Espérmio; termo proposto por H.W.G. Waldeyer para a célula germinativa masculina madura ou espermatozóide.

spermo-. Espermo-. VER sperma-.

sper·mo·lith (sper′mō-lith). Espermólito; concreção no canal deferente. [spermo- + G. *lithos*, pedra]

sper·mol·y·sis (sper-mol′i-sis). Espermólise. SIN spermatolysis.

Sper·moph·il·us (sper-mof′il-us). Gênero de esquilo terrícola. *S. beecheyi, S. grammurus, S. pygmaeus, S. townsendi* e várias outras espécies atuam como importantes reservatórios de *Yersinia pestis*.

sper·mo·tox·in (sper-mō-tok′sin). Espermatoxina. SIN spermatoxin.

SPF. Abreviatura de sun protection *factor* (fator de proteção solar).

sp. gr. Abreviatura de specific *gravity* (densidade).

sph. Abreviatura de spherical ou spherical *lens* (lente esférica).

sphac·e·late (sfas′ĕ-lāt). Esfacelar; tornar gangrenoso ou necrótico. [G. *sphakelos*, gangrena]

sphac·e·la·tion (sfas-ĕ-lā′shŭn). Esfacelamento. 1. O processo de tornar-se gangrenoso ou necrótico. 2. Gangrena ou necrose. [G. *sphakelos*, gangrena]

sphac·el·ism (sfas′ĕ-lizm). Esfacelismo; condição manifestada por um esfácelo.

sphac·e·lous (sfas′ĕ-lŭs). Esfacelado; descamativo, gangrenoso ou necrótico.

sphac·e·lus (sfas′ĕ-lŭs). Esfácelo; massa de material descamado, gangrenoso ou necrótico. [G. *sphakelos*, gangrena]

Sphaer·ol·tilus (sfēr-ol′til-us). Gênero de bactéria estreitamente relacionado a *Leptothrix*, encontrado na água doce; *S. natans* cresce numa esteira de película biológica espessa em água contendo sulfito, especialmente drenada de fábrica de papel.

sphen·eth·moid (sfē-neth′moyd). Esfenoetmóide. SIN sphenoethmoid.

sphe·ni·on (sfē′nē-on). Esfênio; a extremidade do ângulo esfenoidal do osso parietal; ponto craniométrico. [L. mod. do G. *sphēn*, cunha + dim. -*ion*]

spheno-. Esfeno-. Cunha, cuneiforme; o osso esfenóide. [G. *sphēn*, cunha]

sphe·no·bas·i·lar (sfē′nō-bas′i-lăr). Esfenobasilar; relativo ao osso esfenóide e à parte basilar do osso occipital. SIN sphenoccipital, sphenooccipital.

sphe·noc·cip·i·tal (sfē-nok-sip′i-tăl). Esfenobasilar. SIN sphenobasilar.

sphe·no·ceph·a·ly (sfē′nō-sef′ă-lē). Esfenocefalia; condição caracterizada por deformação do crânio, conferindo-lhe um aspecto cuneiforme. [spheno- + G. *kephalē*, cabeça]

sphe·no·eth·moid (sfē-nō-eth′moyd). Esfenoetmóide; relativo aos ossos esfenóide e etmóide. SIN sphenethmoid.

sphen·o·eth·moi·dec·to·my (sfē′nō-eth-moy-dek′tō-mē). Esfenoetmoidectomia; cirurgia para remover o tecido enfermo dos seios esfenoidal e etmoidal.

sphe·no·fron·tal (sfē′nō-fron′tăl). Esfenofrontal; relativo aos ossos esfenóide e frontal.

sphe·noid (sfē′noyd). **1.** Esfenoidal, esfenóide. SIN sphenoidal. **2.** Esfenóide. SIN sphenoid (*bone*). [G. *sphēnoeidēs*, de *sphēn*, cunha + *eidos*, semelhança]

sphe·noi·dal (sfē-noy′dăl). **1.** Esfenoidal; relativo ao osso esfenóide. **2.** Esfenóide; cuneiforme. SIN sphenoid (1) [TA].

sphe·noi·da·le (sfē-noy-dā′lē). O ponto de maior convexidade entre o contorno anterior da sela turca e o plano esfenoidal.

sphe·noid·i·tis (sfē-noy-dī′tis). Esfenoidite. **1.** Inflamação do seio esfenóide. **2.** Necrose do osso esfenóide. [sphenoid + G. -*itis*, inflamação]

sphe·noi·dos·to·my (sfe-noy-dos′tō-mē). Esfenoidostomia; abertura cirúrgica feita na parede anterior do seio esfenoidal. [sphenoid + G. *stoma*, boca]

sphe·noi·dot·o·my (sfē′noy-dot′ō-mē). Esfenoidotomia; qualquer operação no osso ou no seio esfenóide. [sphenoid + G. *tomē*, incisão]

sphe·no·ma·lar (sfē′nō-mā′lăr). Esfenozigomático. SIN sphenozygomatic.

sphe·no·max·il·lary (sfē′nō-mak′si-lār-ē). Esfenomaxilar; relativo ao osso esfenóide e ao maxilar.

sphe·no·oc·cip·i·tal (sfē′nō-ok-sip′i-tăl). Esfenobasilar. SIN sphenobasilar.

sphe·no·pal·a·tine (sfē-nō-pal′ă-tīn). Esfenopalatino; relativo aos ossos esfenóide e palatino.

sphe·no·pa·ri·e·tal (sfē′nō-pă-rī′ă-tăl). Esfenoparietal; relativo aos ossos esfenóide e parietal.

sphe·no·pe·tro·sal (sfē′nō-pe-trō′săl). Esfenopetroso; relativo ao osso esfenóide e à porção petrosa do osso temporal.

sphe·nor·bit·al (sfē-nōr′bi-tăl). Esfenorbital; designa as porções do osso esfenóide que contribuem para as órbitas.

sphe·no·sal·pin·go·staph·y·li·nus (sfē′nō-sal-ping′gō-staf-i-lī′nŭs). Esfenossalpingostafilino. VER tensor veli palati (*muscle*). [L.]

sphe·no·squa·mo·sal (sfē′nō-skwā-mō′săl). Escamoesfenóide. SIN squamosphenoid.

sphe·no·tem·po·ral (sfē′nō-tem′pŏ-răl). Esfenotemporal; relativo aos ossos esfenóide e temporal.

sphe·not·ic (sfē-nō′tik). Esfenótico; relativo ao osso esfenóide e à caixa óssea da orelha. [spheno- + G. *ous*, orelha]

sphe·no·tur·bi·nal (sfē′nō-ter′bi-năl). Esfenoturbinal; designa a concha esfenoidal.

sphe·no·vo·mer·ine (sfē′nō-vō′mer-ēn, -īn). Esfenovomerino; relativo ao osso esfenóide e ao vômer.

sphe·no·zy·go·mat·ic (sfē′nō-zī-gō-mat′ik). Esfenozigomático; relativo aos ossos esfenóide e zigomático. SIN sphenomalar.

sphere (sfēr). Esfera; uma bola ou corpo globular. [G. *sphaira*]

attraction s., e. de atração. SIN astrosphere.

Morgagni s.'s, esferas de Morgagni. SIN Morgagni *globules*, em *globule*.

spher·i·cal (sph.) (sfēr′i-kăl). Esférico; relativo ou de forma semelhante a uma esfera.

sphero-. Esfero-. Esférico, uma esfera. [G. *sphaira*, globo]

sphe·ro·cyl·in·der (sfēr′ō-sil′in-der). Lente esferocilíndrica. SIN spherocylindrical *lens*.

sphe·ro·cyte (sfēr′ō-sīt). Esferócito; pequeno eritrócito esférico. [sphero- + G. *kytos*, célula]

sphe·ro·cy·to·sis (sfēr′ō-sī-tō′sis). Esferocitose; presença de eritrócitos esféricos no sangue. SIN microspherocytosis. [spherocyte + G. -*osis*, condição]

hereditary s. [MIM*182900], e. hereditária; defeito congênito da espectrina [MIM*182860], o principal componente da membrana do eritrócito, que se torna anormalmente permeável ao sódio, resultando em eritrócitos espessados e quase esféricos, frágeis e suscetíveis a hemólise espontânea, com redução da sobrevida na circulação; resulta em anemia crônica com reticulocitose, episódios de icterícia leve devido a hemólise e crises agudas com cálculos biliares, febre e dor abdominal; as manifestações são extremamente variáveis; herança autossômica dominante, causada pela mutação no gene da ancirina (ANK1)

em 8p. Todavia, como no caso da eliptocitose, existe uma forma autossômica recessiva [MIM*270970], causada pela mutação do gene da alfa-espectrina 1 (SPTA1) no cromossoma 1q. SIN chronic acholuric jaundice, chronic familial icterus, chronic familial jaundice, congenital hemolytic icterus, congenital hemolytic jaundice, spherocytic anemia.

sphe·roid, sphe·roi·dal (sfēr′oyd, sfir-; sfē-royd′ăl). Esferóide; que tem forma semelhante a uma esfera. [L. *spheroideus*]

sphe·rom·e·ter (sfēr-om′ĕ-ter). Esferômetro; instrumento para determinar a curvatura de uma esfera ou de uma lente esférica. VER Geneva lens *measure*. [sphero- + G. *metron*, medida]

sphe·ro·pha·ki·a (sfēr-ō-fā′kē-ă). Esferofaquia; aberração bilateral congênita em que as lentes dos olhos são pequenas, esféricas e sujeitas subluxação; pode ocorrer como anomalia independente ou estar associada à síndrome de Weill-Marchesani. [sphero- + G. *phakos*, lente]

sphe·ro·plast (sfēr′ō-plast). Esferoplasto; célula bacteriana cuja parede celular rígida foi incompletamente removida. A bactéria perde a sua forma característica e torna-se redonda. [sphero- + G. *plastos*, formado]

sphe·ro·prism (sfēr′ō-prizm). Esferoprisma; lente esférica descentralizada para produzir um efeito prismático, ou lente esférica e prisma combinados.

sphe·ro·sper·mia (sfēr′ō-sper′mē-ă). Esferospermia; espermatozóides esferóides sem cauda alongada, em contraste com o espermatozóide de cauda filiforme dos seres humanos e outros mamíferos (nematospermia). [sphero- + G. *sperma*, semente]

spher·ule (sfer′ool). Esférula. **1.** Pequena estrutura esférica. **2.** Estrutura semelhante a um esporângio, preenchida com endosporos na maturidade, produzida no interior do tecido e *in vitro* por *Coccidioides immitis*. [L. ant. *sphaerula*, dim. do L. *sphaera*, esfera, bola]

sphinc·ter (sfingk′ter) [TA]. Esfíncter; músculo que circunda um ducto, um tubo ou um orifício de modo que a sua contração diminui a luz ou orifício. SIN musculus sphincter [TA], sphincter muscle [TA]. [G. *sphinktēr*, uma faixa ou um cordão]

s. of ampulla, músculo s. da ampola hepatopancreática; *termo oficial alternativo para s. of hepatopancreatic ampulla.

anatomic s., e. anatômico; acúmulo de fibras circulares musculares ou fibras oblíquas especialmente dispostas, cuja função é reduzir, parcial ou totalmente, a luz de um tubo, orifício de um órgão ou a cavidade de uma víscera; o componente de fechamento do piloro.

s. angula'ris, angular s., músculo esfíncter do piloro; espessamento da camada muscular circular, formando um suposto esfíncter intermediário ao nível da incisura angular do estômago. Embora o espessamento do músculo circular possa indicar o início do antro pilórico, não se observa uma verdadeira atividade esfincteriana funcional distinta das outras contrações peristálticas do estômago, embora algumas delas possam, de fato, fechar temporariamente o antro do restante da luz do estômago. SIN antral s., midgastric transverse s., s. antri, s. intermedius, s. of antrum, s. of gastric antrum.

s. a'ni, anal s., e. do ânus. VER external anal s., internal anal s.

s. a'ni, ter'tius, terceiro e. anal; o terceiro esfíncter do anorreto, um esfíncter fisiológico na junção sigmoidorretal.

antral s., músculo esfíncter do piloro. SIN s. angularis.

s. an'tri, músculo esfíncter do piloro. SIN s. angularis.

s. of antrum, músculo esfíncter do piloro. SIN s. angularis.

anular s., e. anular; espessamento curto de fibras musculares circulantes, semelhante a um anel; esfíncter anular em oposição a um esfíncter segmentar.

artificial s., e. artificial; esfíncter produzido por procedimentos cirúrgicos para reduzir a velocidade do fluxo no sistema digestivo ou para manter a continência do intestino.

basal s., e. basal; espessamento da camada muscular circular na base da papila ileal no íleo terminal. SIN sphincteroid tract of ileum.

bicanalicular s., e. bicanalicular; esfíncter que circunda dois canais, como as porções terminais do ducto colédoco e do ducto pancreático principal.

s. of biliaropancreatic ampulla, músculo e. da ampola hepatopancreática; *termo oficial alternativo para s. of hepatopancreatic ampulla.

Boyden s., e. de Boyden. SIN s. of (common) bile duct.

canalicular s., e. canalicular; esfíncter localizado em algum ponto ao longo do trajeto de um órgão, um tubo ou um ducto, em oposição ao esfíncter ostial.

choledochal s., músculo e. do ducto colédoco. SIN s. of (common) bile duct.

colic s., e. cólico; um dos esfíncteres fisiológicos do colo.

s. of (common) bile duct [TA], músculo e. do ducto colédoco; esfíncter de músculo liso do colédoco, imediatamente proximal à ampola hepatopancreática e organizado em esfíncter superior e inferior; é esse esfíncter que controla o fluxo de bile no duodeno. SIN musculus sphincter ductus choledochi [TA], musculus sphincter ductus biliaris*, Boyden s., choledochal s., sphincter muscle of common bile duct.

s. constric'tor car'diae, e. esofágico inferior. SIN inferior esophageal s.

duodenal s., e. duodenal; um dos esfíncteres fisiológicos descritos no duodeno.

duodenojejunal s., e. duodenojejunal; o esfíncter supostamente presente na flexura duodenojejunal.

external anal s. [TA], músculo e. externo do ânus; um anel fusiforme de fibras musculares estriadas que circunda o ânus, fixado posteriormente ao cóccix e anteriormente ao tendão central do períneo; é subdividido, freqüentemente de modo indistinto, numa parte subcutânea, numa parte superficial e numa parte profunda para fins descritivos. SIN musculus sphincter ani externus [TA], external sphincter muscle of anus.

external urethral s. [TA], músculo esfíncter externo da uretra; músculo que constringe a parte membranácea da uretra para reter a urina na bexiga; inervação, pudendo. SIN s. urethrae externus [TA], Guthrie muscle, musculus constrictor urethrae, musculus sphincter urethrae externus, sphincter muscle of urethra, Wilson muscle (1).

external urethral s. of female [TA], músculo e. externo da uretra feminina; composto de músculo estriado (voluntário) e, mais apropriadamente, de um esfíncter urogenital; uma parte forma um verdadeiro esfíncter anular em torno da uretra, outra parte se estende superiormente até o colo da bexiga, outra passa anteriormente à uretra, que se fixa aos ramos isquiáticos (músculo compressor da uretra), e outra parte, semelhante a uma faixa, circunda tanto a uretra como a vagina (esfíncter uretrovaginal). SIN musculus sphincter urethrae externus femininae [TA].

external urethral s. of male [TA], músculo e. externo da uretra masculina; composto de músculo estriado (voluntário), inclui uma porção tubuliforme que circunda a parte membranácea da uretra, bem como uma grande porção, em forma de canaleta, que ascende à face anterior da uretra prostática até o colo da bexiga, e uma parte que passa anteriormente à uretra membranosa e fixa-se aos ramos isquiáticos em ambos os lados (músculo compressor da uretra). SIN musculus sphincter urethrae externus masculinae [TA].

extrinsic s., e. extrínseco; esfíncter produzido por fibras musculares circulares extrínsecas ao órgão.

first duodenal s., primeiro e. duodenal; o esfíncter supostamente localizado ao nível da extremidade aboral do bulbo duodenal.

functional s., e. funcional. SIN physiologic s.

s. of gastric antrum, músculo e. da ampola hepatopancreática. SIN s. angularis.

Glisson s., e. de Glisson. SIN s. of hepatopancreatic ampulla.

s. of hepatic flexure of colon, e. da flexura hepática do colo; esfíncter fisiológico ao nível da flexura cólica direita.

hepatopancreatic s., músculo e. da ampola hepatopancreática. SIN s. of hepatopancreatic ampulla.

s. of hepatopancreatic ampulla [TA], músculo e. da ampola hepatopancreática; o esfíncter de músculo liso da ampola hepatopancreática na papila duodenal. SIN musculus sphincter ampullae hepatopancreaticae [TA], musculus sphincter ampullae biliaropancreaticae*, musculus sphincter ampullae*, s. of ampulla*, s. of biliaropancreatic ampulla*, Glisson s., hepatopancreatic s., Oddi s.

hypertensive upper esophageal s., acalasia cricofaríngea. SIN cricopharyngeal achalasia.

Hyrtl s., e. de Hyrtl; faixa, geralmente incompleta, de fibras musculares circulares no reto, cerca de 10 cm acima do ânus (ampola do reto superior).

ileal s., e. ileal; espessamento da musculatura circular na margem livre da papila ileal. SIN ileocecocolic s., marginal s., operculum ilei, Varolius s.

ileocecocolic s., e. ileocecocólico. SIN ileal s.

iliopelvic s., e. iliopélvico. SIN midsigmoid s.

inferior esophageal s., e. esofágico inferior; esfíncter fisiológico ao nível da junção esofagogástrica; trata-se, de fato, de um esfíncter extrínseco formado pela musculatura circundante do hiato esofágico do pilar direito do diafragma; produz constrição normal na junção esofagogástrica, que pode ser observada com deglutição de bário. SIN s. constrictor cardiae.

s. intermedius, músculo e. do piloro. SIN s. angularis.

internal anal s. [TA], músculo e. interno do ânus; anel de músculo liso formado por aumento das fibras circulares do reto, situado na extremidade superior do canal anal, internamente ao músculo esfíncter externo voluntário do ânus. O músculo esfíncter interno do ânus sofre contração máxima quando a ampola retal está "em repouso"—vazia e relaxada para acomodar uma massa fecal. É inibido com o enchimento da ampola, aumento da distensão e peristaltismo. SIN musculus sphincter ani internus [TA], internal sphincter muscle of anus.

internal urethral s. [TA], músculo e. interno da uretra; o colar completo de células musculares lisas do colo da bexiga, que se estende distalmente para circundar a porção pré-prostática da uretra masculina. Não existe nenhuma estrutura comparável no colo da bexiga feminina; o esfíncter uretral interno existiria para impedir o refluxo de sêmen para a bexiga. SIN musculus sphincter urethrae internus*, preprostatic s.*, supracollicular s.*, anulus urethralis, muscular s. supracollicularis, musculus sphincter vesicae, preprostate urethral s., proximal urethral s., sphincter muscle of urinary bladder, s. vesicae.

intrinsic s., e. intrínseco; espessamento das fibras musculares da túnica muscular de um órgão.

lower esophageal s. (LES), e. esofágico inferior (EEI); musculatura da junção gastroesofágica que é tonicamente ativa, exceto durante a deglutição.

macroscopic s., e. macroscópico; esfíncter visível a olho nu.

marginal s., e. marginal. SIN ileal s.

mediocolic s., e. mediocólico; esfíncter fisiológico localizado a meio caminho no colo ascendente.

microscopic s., e. microscópico; e. visível apenas ao microscópio.

midgastric transverse s., músculo e. do piloro. SIN s. angularis.

midsigmoid s., e. mesossigmóide; e. fisiológico a meio caminho no colo sigmóide. SIN iliopelvic s.

muscular s. supracollicularis, músculo e. interno da uretra. SIN internal urethral s.

myovascular s., e. miovascular; e. que possui um componente muscular e vascular (habitualmente venoso). VER myovenous s.

myovenous s., e. miovenoso; e. que possui um componente muscular e venoso, como, por exemplo, na junção faringoesofágica e no canal anal.

Nélaton s., e. de Nélaton. VER transverse *folds* of rectum, em *fold*. SIN Nélaton fibers.

O'Beirne s., e. de O'Beirne. SIN rectosigmoid s.

s. oc'uli, músculo orbicular do olho. SIN orbicularis oculi (*muscle*).

Oddi s., e. de Oddi. SIN s. of hepatopancreatic ampulla.

s. o'ris, músculo orbicular da boca. SIN orbicularis oris (*muscle*).

ostial s., e. osteal; espessamento de fibras musculares circulares ao nível de um orifício.

palatopharyngeal s., fascículo posterior do músculo palatofaríngeo; *termo oficial alternativo para posterior *fascicle* of palatopharyngeus muscle.

pancreatic s., músculo e. do ducto pancreático. SIN s. of pancreatic duct.

s. of pancreatic duct [TA], músculo e. do ducto pancreático; esfíncter de músculo liso do ducto pancreático principal imediatamente proximal à ampola hepatopancreática. SIN musculus sphincter ductus pancreatici, pancreatic s., sphincter muscle of pancreatic duct.

pathologic s., e. patológico; espessamento da musculatura circular causado por doença.

pelvirectal s., e. pelvirretal. SIN rectosigmoid s.

s. of the pharyngeal isthmus, fascículo posterior do músculo palatofaríngeo. SIN posterior *fascicle* of palatopharyngeus muscle.

physiologic s., e. fisiológico; corte de uma estrutura tubular que atua como se tivesse uma faixa de músculo circular para contraí-la, embora não se possa encontrar esse tipo de estrutura especializada ao exame morfológico. SIN functional s., radiologic s.

postpyloric s., e. pós-pilórico; a porção duodenal do e. ou mecanismo de fechamento do piloro gastroduodenal.

prepapillary s., e. pré-papilar; esfíncter do duodeno descrito na localização oral à papila duodenal principal.

preprostate urethral s., músculo esfíncter interno da uretra. SIN internal urethral s.

preprostatic s., músculo esfíncter interno da uretra; *termo oficial alternativo para internal urethral s.

prepyloric s., e. pré-pilórico; faixa de fibras musculares circulares na parede do estômago, próximo ao piloro gastroduodenal.

proximal urethral s., músculo e. interno da uretra. SIN internal urethral s.

s. pupil'lae [TA], músculo e. da pupila; anel de fibras musculares lisas que circunda a borda pupilar da íris. SIN musculus sphincter pupillae [TA], sphincter muscle of pupil.

pyloric s. [TA], músculo e. do piloro; espessamento da camada circular da musculatura gástrica que circunda a junção gastroduodenal. SIN musculus sphincter pylori [TA], sphincter muscle of pylorus.

radiologic s., e. radiológico. SIN physiologic s.

rectosigmoid s., e. retossigmóide; faixa circular de fibras musculares na junção retossigmóide. SIN O'Beirne s., O'Beirne valve, pelvirectal s.

segmental s., e. segmentar; esfíncter de um segmento de um órgão, um tubo ou um canal, mais longo do que um esfíncter anular.

smooth muscular s., e. de músculo liso. SIN lissosphincter.

striated muscular s., e. de músculo estriado. SIN rhabdosphincter.

superior esophageal s., músculo constritor inferior da faringe. SIN inferior constrictor (*muscle*) of pharynx. VER inferior constrictor (*muscle*) of pharynx.

supracollicular s., músculo e. interno da uretra; *termo oficial alternativo para internal urethral s.

s. of third portion of duodenum, e. da terceira porção do duodeno; e. fisiológico supostamente localizado na porção horizontal (inferior) do duodeno.

unicanalicular s., e. unicanalicular; e. limitado a um canal ou tubo visceral.

s. ure'thrae externus [TA], músculo e. externo da uretra. SIN external urethral s.

urethrovaginal s. [TA], músculo e. uretrovaginal; parte voluntária, semelhante a uma faixa, do e. externo da uretra feminina, que circunda tanto a uretra quanto a vagina superiormente à membrana perineal. SIN musculus sphincter urethrovaginalis [TA].

s. vagi'nae, músculo bulboespanjoso. SIN bulbospongiosus (*muscle*).

Varolius s., e. de Varolius. SIN ileal s.

velopharyngeal s., fascículo posterior do músculo palatofaríngeo. SIN posterior *fascicle* of palatopharyngeus muscle.

s. vesi'cae, músculo e. interno da uretra. SIN internal urethral s.

s. vesi'cae biliaris, e. da vesícula biliar; o esfíncter da vesícula biliar, na transição entre o colo da vesícula biliar e o ducto cístico.

sphinc·ter·al (sfingk′ter-ăl). Esfincteriano; relativo a um esfíncter. SIN sphincterial, sphincteric.

sphinc·ter·al·gia (sfingk-ter-al′jē-ă). Esfincteralgia; dor nos músculos do esfíncter anal. [sphincter + G. *algos*, dor]

sphinc·ter·ec·to·my (sfingk-ter-ek′tō-mē). Esfincterectomia. 1. Excisão de uma porção da borda pupilar da íris. 2. Remoção de qualquer músculo esfincteriano. [sphincter + G. *ektomē*, excisão]

sphinc·te·ri·al, sphinc·ter·ic (sfingk-tēr′ē-ăl, -ter-ik). Esfincteriano. SIN sphincteral.

sphinc·ter·is·mus (sfingk-ter-iz′mŭs). Esfincterismo; contração espasmódica dos músculos esfíncteres do ânus.

sphinc·ter·i·tis (sfingk′ter-ī′tis). Esfincterite; inflamação de qualquer esfíncter.

sphinc·ter·oid (sfingk′ter-oyd). Esfincteróide; indica semelhança com um esfíncter. [sphincter + G. *eidos*, semelhança]

sphinc·ter·ol·y·sis (sfingk-ter-ol′i-sis). Esfincterólise; cirurgia para liberar a íris da córnea nos casos de sinéquia anterior envolvendo apenas a borda pupilar. [sphincter, + G. *lysis*, afrouxamento]

sphinc·ter·o·plas·ty (sfingk′ter-ō-plas-tē). Esfincteroplastia; cirurgia em qualquer músculo esfincteriano. [sphincter + G. *plastos*, formado]

sphinc·ter·o·scope (sfingk′ter-ō-skōp). Esfincteroscópio; espéculo para facilitar a inspeção do músculo esfíncter interno do ânus. [sphincter + G. *skopeō*, ver]

sphinc·ter·os·co·py (sfingk′ter-os′kō-pē). Esfincteroscopia; exame visual de um esfíncter.

sphinc·ter·o·tome (sfingk′ter-ō-tōm). Esfincterótomo; instrumento para incisão de um esfíncter.

sphinc·ter·ot·o·my (sfingk-tē-rot′ō-mē). Esfincterotomia; incisão ou divisão de um músculo esfíncter. [sphincter + G. *tomē*, incisão]
  external s., e. externa; incisão transuretral do esfíncter uretral externo.
  transduodenal s., e. transduodenal; divisão do esfíncter de Oddi; cirurgia para abrir a extremidade inferior do ducto comum para remover cálculos impactados ou aliviar o espasmo ou a estenose dos ductos pancreático e biliar terminal.

sphin·ga·nine (sfing′gă-nēn). Esfinganina; diidroespingosina; constituinte dos esfingolipídios.

(4E)-sphin·gen·ine (sfing′gen-ēn). (4E)-esfingenina. SIN sphingosine.

sphing·ol (sfing′gol). Esfingol. SIN sphingosine.

sphin·go·lip·id (sfing′gō-lip-id). Esfingolipídio; qualquer lipídio contendo uma base de cadeia longa semelhante à da esfingosina (p. ex., ceramidas, cerebrosídeos, gangliosídeos, esfingomielinas); constituinte do tecido nervoso.

sphin·go·lip·i·do·sis (sfing′gō-lip-i-dō′sis). Esfingolipidose; designação coletiva de várias doenças caracterizadas pelo metabolismo anormal dos esfingolipídios, p. ex., gangliosidose, doença de Gaucher, doença de Niemann-Pick. SIN sphingolipodystrophy.
  cerebral s., e. cerebral; grupo de doenças hereditárias caracterizadas por retardo de desenvolvimento, hipertonicidade, paralisia espástica progressiva, perda da visão e cegueira, geralmente com degeneração macular e atrofia óptica, convulsões e deterioração mental; associada a armazenamento anormal de esfingomielina e lipídios correlatos no cérebro. São reconhecidos quatro tipos clínica e enzimaticamente distintos: 1) **tipo do lactente** (doença de Tay-Sachs, gangliosidose G_{M2}), decorrente de deficiência de hexosaminidase A; 2) **tipo juvenil precoce** (doença de Jansky-Bielschowsky ou Bielschowsky); 3) **tipo juvenil tardio** (doença de Spielmeyer-Vogt; doença de Spielmeyer-Sjögren; doença de Batten-Mayou, lipofuscinose ceróide; e 4) **tipo adulto** (doença de Kufs). SIN cerebral lipidosis.

sphin·go·lip·o·dys·tro·phy (sfing′gō-lip-ō-dis′trō-fē). Esfingolipodistrofia. SIN sphingolipidosis.

sphin·go·my·e·li·nase (sfing′gō-mī′e-li-nās). Esfingomielinase. SIN sphingomyelin phosphodiesterase.

sphin·go·my·e·lin phos·pho·di·es·ter·ase (sfing′gō-mī′e-lin). Esfingomielina fosfodiesterase; enzima que catalisa a hidrólise da esfingomielina a *N*-acilesfingosina (uma ceramida) e fosfocolina; a deficiência dessa enzima está associada à doença de Niemann-Pick. SIN sphingomyelinase.

sphin·go·my·e·lins (sfing′gō-mī′e-linz). Esfingomielinas; grupo de fosfolipídios encontrados no cérebro, na medula espinal, no rim e na gema do ovo, contendo 1-fosfocolina (colina *O*-fosfato) combinada com uma ceramida (um ácido graxo de cadeia longa ligado ao nitrogênio de uma base de cadeia longa, como a esfingosina). SIN ceramide 1-phosphorylcholine, phosphosphingosides.

sphin·go·sine (sfing′gō-sēn). Esfingosina; (4E)-esfengenina, esfingol; a principal base de cadeia longa encontrada nos esfingolipídios. SIN (4E)-sphingenine, sphingol.

sphygm-. Espigme-. VER sphygmo-.

sphygm·ic (sfig′mik). Esfígmico; relativo ao pulso.

sphygmo-, sphygm-. Esfigmo-, esfigm-. Pulso. [G. *sphygmos*]

sphyg·mo·car·di·o·graph (sfig′mō-kar′dē-ō-graf). Esfigmocardiógrafo; polígrafo que registra tanto os batimentos cardíacos quanto o pulso radial. SIN sphygmocardioscope. [sphygmo- + G. *kardia*, coração + *graphō*, escrever]

sphyg·mo·car·di·o·scope (sfig′mō-kar′dē-ō-skōp). Esfigmocardioscópio. SIN sphygmocardiograph. [sphygmo- + G. *skopeō*, ver]

sphyg·mo·chron·o·graph (sfig′mō-kron′ō-graf). Esfigmocronógrafo; esfigmógrafo modificado, que representa graficamente as relações de tempo entre o batimento cardíaco e o pulso; registra o caráter e a velocidade do pulso. [sphygmo- + G. *chronos*, tempo + *graphō*, escrever]

sphyg·mo·gram (sfig′mō-gram). Esfigmograma; curva gráfica feita por um esfigmógrafo. SIN pulse curve. [sphygmo- + G. *gramma*, algo escrito]

sphyg·mo·graph (sfig′mō-graf). Esfigmógrafo; instrumento que consiste numa alavanca, cuja extremidade curta repousa sobre a artéria radial do punho, enquanto a extremidade longa é provida de um estilete que registra as excursões do pulso numa fita móvel de papel enfumaçado. [sphygmo- + G. *graphō*, escrever]

sphyg·mo·graph·ic (sfig-mō-graf′ik). Esfigmográfico; relativo a, ou feito por, um esfigmógrafo; refere-se ao traçado esfigmográfico ou esfigmograma.

sphyg·mog·ra·phy (sfig-mog′ră-fē). Esfigmografia; uso do esfigmógrafo no registro do caráter do pulso.

sphyg·moid (sfig′moyd). Esfigmóide; semelhante ao pulso. [sphygmo- + G. *eidos*, semelhança]

sphyg·mo·ma·nom·e·ter (sfig′mō-mă-nom′e-ter). Esfigmomanômetro; instrumento para medir a pressão arterial, consistindo num manguito insuflável, num bulbo de insuflação e num calibrador que mostra a pressão arterial. SIN sphygmometer. [sphygmo- + G. *manos*, fino, escasso + *metron*, medida]
  Mosso s., e. de Mosso; aparelho para medir a pressão arterial nas artérias digitais.
  Riva-Rocci s., e. de Riva-Rocci; aparelho original de pressão arterial utilizado pela primeira vez para medida não-invasiva da pressão arterial.
  Rogers s., e. de Rogers; esfigmomanômetro com barômetro aneróide.

sphyg·mo·ma·nom·e·try (sfig′mō-mă-nom′e-trē). Esfigmomanometria; determinação da pressão arterial através de um esfigmomanômetro.

sphyg·mom·e·ter (sfig-mom′e-ter). Esfigmômetro. SIN sphygmomanometer.

sphyg·mo·met·ro·scope (sfig-mō-met′rō-skōp). Esfigmometroscópio; instrumento para ausculta do pulso, utilizado especialmente no método auscultatório de leitura da pressão arterial, sobretudo a pressão diastólica. [sphygmo- + G. *metron*, medida + *skopeō*, ver]

sphyg·mo·os·cil·lom·e·ter (sfig′mō-os′i-lom′e-ter). Esfigmooscilômetro; aparelho semelhante a um esfigmomanômetro aneróide utilizado na medida da pressão arterial sistólica e diastólica. [sphygmo- + L. *oscillo*, oscilar + G. *metron*, medida]

sphyg·mo·pal·pa·tion (sfig′mō-pal-pa′shŭn). Esfigmopalpação; palpação do pulso. [sphygmo- + L. *palpatio*, palpação]

sphyg·mo·phone (sfig′mō-fōn). Esfigmofone; instrumento por meio do qual é produzido um som a cada batimento do pulso. [sphygmo- + G. *phōnē*, som]

sphyg·mo·scope (sfig′mō-skōp). Esfigmoscópio; instrumento pelo qual os batimentos do pulso tornam-se visíveis ao produzir a elevação de um líquido num tubo de vidro, por meio de um espelho que projeta um feixe de luz, ou simplesmente pelo movimento de uma alavanca, como no esfigmógrafo. [sphygmo- + G. *skopeō*, ver]
  Bishop s., e. de Bishop; instrumento para medir a pressão arterial, com referência especial à pressão diastólica; o tubo é preenchido com uma solução de

esfingolipidoses

classificadas de acordo com a substância de armazenamento e defeito enzimático correspondente (nem todas as variantes estão incluídas)

doença	substância armazenada	enzima deficiente
doença de Niemann-Pick (esfingomielinose, tipo A)	esfingomielina	esfingomielinase
doença de Gaucher	glicocerebrosídeo	β-glucosidase
leucodistrofia de células globóides	galactocerebrosídeo	cerebrosídeo β-galactosidase
leucodistrofia metacromática	sulfatídeo	cerebrosídeo sulfatase, arilsulfatase A
doença de Fabry	ceramida triexosídeo	α-galactosidase
gangliosidoses	gangliosídeos	β-galactosidase hexosaminidase *N*-acetilgalactosaminil transferase

borotungstato de cádmio, e a escala é o inverso daquela de um manômetro de mercúrio, sendo a pressão produzida diretamente pelo peso do líquido, e não por ar comprimido.

sphyg·mos·co·py (sfig-mos'kŏ-pē). Esfigmoscopia; exame do pulso. [sphygmo- + G. *skopeō*, ver]

sphyg·mo·sys·to·le (sfig-mō-sis'tō-lē). Esfigmossístole; termo obsoleto para referir-se ao segmento da onda de pulso que corresponde à sístole cardíaca. [sphygmo- + G. *systolē*, uma contração]

sphyg·mo·ton·o·graph (sfig-mō-tō'nō-graf). Esfigmotonógrafo; instrumento para registrar graficamente tanto o pulso quanto a pressão arterial. [sphygmo- + G. *tonos*, tensão + *graphō*, escrever]

sphyg·mo·to·nom·e·ter (sfig-mō-tō-nom'ĕ-ter). Esfigmotonômetro; instrumento, semelhante ao esfigmotonógrafo, para determinar o grau da pressão arterial. [sphygmo- + G. *tonos*, tensão + *metron*, medida]

sphyg·mo·vis·co·sim·e·try (sfig-mō-vis-kō-sim'ĕ-trē). Esfigmoviscosimetria; medida da pressão e da viscosidade do sangue.

spi·ca, pl. **spi·cae** (spī'kă, spī'kē). Atadura. VER bandage. [L. ponta, espiga]

spic·u·la (spik'ū-lă). Espículas; plural de spiculum. [L.]

spic·u·lar (spik'ū-lăr). Espicular; relativo a ou que possui espículas.

spic·ule (spik'ūl). Espícula. **1.** Pequeno corpo em forma de agulha. **2.** Estrutura reprodutiva acessória em nematódeos machos; útil na identificação da espécie. [L. *spiculum,* dim de *spica* ou *spicum,* ponta]

spic·u·lum, pl. **spic·u·la** (spik'ū-lŭm, -lă). Espícula; pequena espiga. [L.]

spi·der (spī'der). Aranha. **1.** Artrópode da ordem Araneida (subclasse Arachnida), que se caracteriza por quatro pares de patas, um cefalotórax, um abdome globoso e liso e um complexo de fiandeiras para tecer teias. Entre as aranhas venenosas encontradas no Novo Mundo estão a viúva-negra, *Latrodectus mactans;* a viúva de pernas vermelhas, *Latrodectus bishopi;* a tarântula peruana, *Glyptocranium gasteracanthoides;* a aranha castanha chilena, *Loxosceles laeta;* a aranha castanha peruana, *Loxosceles rufiper;* a aranha reclusa castanha da América do Norte, *Loxosceles reclusus.* **2.** Proliferação obstrutiva na teta de uma vaca. [I. ant. *spinnan,* girar]

   arterial s., a. arterial. SIN spider angioma.
   vascular s., a. vascular. SIN spider angioma.

spi·der-burst (spī'der-berst). Teia de aranha; linhas capilares vermelho-escuras que se irradiam na pele da perna, geralmente sem quaisquer veias varicosas visíveis ou palpáveis, decorrentes de dilatação venosa profunda. [*spider*web + sun*burst*]

Spiegelberg, Otto, ginecologista alemão, 1830–1881. VER S. *criteria,* em *criterion.*

Spieghel, Adrian van der. VER Spigelius.

Spiegler, Eduard, dermatologista austríaco, 1860–1908. VER cutaneous *pseudolymphomas;* S.-Fendt *sarcoid.*

Spielmeyer, Walter, neurologista de Munique, 1879–1935. VER S. acute *swelling;* S.-Stock *disease;* S.-Vogt *disease.*

spi·ge·li·an (spī-jē'lē-an). Espigeliano; relativo a, ou descrito por, Spigelius.

Spigelius, Adrian (van der Spieghel), anatomista flamengo radicado em Pádua, 1578-1625. VER spigelian *hernia;* S. *line, lobe.*

spike. 1. Ponta; breve evento elétrico de 3–25 ms que, no eletroencefalograma, produz a aparência de uma linha vertical ascendente e descendente. **2.** Pico; na eletroforese, uma deflexão ascendente acentuadamente oblíqua no traçado densitométrico.

   ponto-geniculo-occipital s., pico, ponto geniculooccipital; picos EEG durante o sono REM que surgem na ponte e passam para o corpo geniculado lateral e córtex occipital.

spill. Derramamento; fluxo excessivo; transbordamento de líquido ou substância finamente dividida.

   cellular s., d. celular; disseminação de células através da linfa ou do sangue, resultando, assim, em metástases ou implantação de tecido estranho em qualquer parte ou órgão.

Spiller, William G., neurologista norte-americano, 1863–1940. VER Frazier-S. *operation.*

spill·way. Rego; sulco ou canal através do qual o alimento pode passar a partir das superfícies oclusivas dos dentes durante o processo da mastigação.

spi·lus (spī'lŭs). Nevo achatado. SIN nevus spilus. [L. mod. do G. *spilos,* mancha]

spin-. Espin-. VER spino-.

spi·na, gen. e pl. **spi·nae** (spī'nă, -nē) [TA]. Espinha. SIN spine (1). [L. um espinho, a coluna vertebral, espinha]

   s. angula'ris, e. do osso esfenóide. SIN spine of sphenoid bone.
   s. bif'ida, e. bífida; defeito embriológico de fusão de um ou mais arcos vertebrais; os subtipos de espinha bífida baseiam-se no grau e no padrão de malformação associada com comprometimento do neuroectoderma. SIN hydrocele spinalis, schistorrhachis.
   s. bif'ida aper'ta, e. bífida aberta. SIN s. bifida cystica.
   s. bif'ida cys'tica, e. bífida cística; espinha bífida associada a um cisto meníngeo (meningocele) ou um cisto contendo tanto as meninges como a

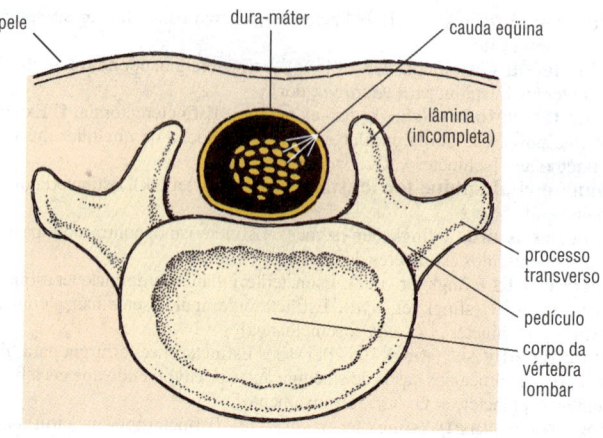

espinha bífida oculta

medula espinal (meningomielocele) ou apenas a medula espinal (mielocele). SIN s. bifida aperta, s. bifida manifesta.
   s. bif'ida manifes'ta, e. bífida manifesta. SIN s. bifida cystica.
   s. bif'ida occul'ta, e. bífida oculta; espinha bífida na qual existe um defeito espinal, porém sem protrusão da medula espinal ou de suas membranas, embora haja freqüentemente alguma anormalidade no seu desenvolvimento.
   s. dorsa'lis, coluna vertebral. SIN vertebral *column.*
   s. fronta'lis, e. nasal do osso frontal. SIN nasalis ossis frontalis.
   spinae geniorum inferior et superior, espinhas genianas inferior e superior. SIN mental *spine.*
   s. hel'icis [TA], e. da hélice. SIN *spine* of helix.
   s. ili'aca ante'rior infe'rior [TA], e. ilíaca ântero-inferior. SIN anterior inferior iliac *spine.*
   s. ili'aca ante'rior supe'rior [TA], e. ilíaca ântero-superior. SIN anterior superior iliac *spine.*
   s. ili'aca poste'rior infe'rior [TA], e. ilíaca póstero-inferior. SIN posterior inferior iliac *spine.*
   s. ili'aca poste'rior supe'rior [TA], e. ilíaca póstero-superior. SIN posterior superior iliac *spine.*
   s. ischiad'ica [TA], e. isquiática. SIN ischial *spine.*
   s. mea'tus, e. do meato. SIN suprameatal *spine.*
   s. menta'lis (inferior et superior) [TA], e. geniana (inferior e superior). SIN mental *spine.*
   s. nasa'lis ante'rior corporis maxillae [TA], e. nasal anterior da maxilar. SIN anterior nasal *spine* of maxilla.
   s. nasa'lis os'sis fronta'lis [TA], e. nasal do osso frontal. SIN nasal *spine* of frontal bone.
   s. nasa'lis poste'rior laminae horizontalis ossis palatini [TA], e. nasal posterior da lâmina horizontal do osso palatino. SIN posterior nasal *spine* of horizontal plate of palatine bone.
   s. os'sis sphenoida'lis [TA], e. do osso esfenóide. SIN *spine* of sphenoid bone.
   spi'nae palati'nae [TA], espinhas palatinas. SIN palatine *spines,* em *spine.*
   s. peronea'lis, tróclea fibular do calcâneo. SIN fibular *trochlea* of calcaneus.
   s. pu'bis, tubérculo púbico. SIN pubic *tubercle.*
   s. scap'ulae [TA], e. da escápula. SIN *spine* of scapula.
   s. suprameatalis, e. suprameática; *termo oficial alternativo para suprameatal *spine.*
   s. supramea'tica, e. suprameática. SIN suprameatal *spine.*
   s. trochlea'ris [TA], e. troclear. SIN trochlear *spine.*
   s. tympan'ica ma'jor [TA], e. timpânica maior. SIN greater tympanic *spine.*
   s. tympan'ica mi'nor [TA], e. timpânica menor. SIN lesser tympanic *spine.*

spi·nal (spī'năl). Espinal, espinhal. **1.** Relativo a qualquer espinha ou processo espinhoso. **2.** Relativo à coluna vertebral. SIN rachial, rachidial, rachidian, spinalis. [L. *spinalis*]

spi·na·lis (spī-nā'lis). Espinal. SIN spinal. [L.]

spi·nate (spī'nāt). Espinhoso; que possui espinhos.

spin·dle (spin'dl). Fuso; em anatomia e patologia, qualquer célula ou estrutura fusiforme. [A.S.]

   aortic s., f. aórtico; dilatação fusiforme da aorta imediatamente além do istmo. SIN His s.
   central s., f. central; grupo central de microtúbulos (fibras contínuas) que seguem seu trajeto de modo ininterrupto, entre os ásteres, em contraste com os microtúbulos fixados aos cromossomas individuais (fibras do fuso).
   cleavage s., f. de clivagem; fuso formado durante a clivagem de um zigoto ou seus blastômeros.

His s., f. de His. SIN aortic s.
Krukenberg s., f. de Krukenberg; área fusiforme vertical de pigmentação de melanina na superfície posterior da córnea central.
Kühne s., f. de Kühne. SIN neuromuscular s.
mitotic s., f. mitótico; a figura fusiforme característica de uma célula em divisão; consiste em microtúbulos (fibras do fuso), algumas das quais se fixam a cada cromossoma em seu centrômero e estão envolvidas no movimento cromossômico; outros microtúbulos (fibras contínuas) passam de um pólo a outro. SIN nuclear s.
muscle s., f. muscular. SIN neuromuscular s.
neuromuscular s., f. neuromuscular; órgão terminal fusiforme no músculo esquelético em que terminam as fibras nervosas aferentes e algumas eferentes; contém 3–10 fibras musculares estriadas (fibras intrafusais), que são muito menores do que as fibras musculares comuns, delas separadas por uma cápsula que encerra o órgão e inervadas pelo delgado axônio de um motoneurônio gama (fibra motora gama); as terminações sensoriais que ocorrem nas fibras intrafusais são anuloespirais ou em ramalhete; esse órgão terminal sensorial é particularmente sensível ao estiramento passivo do músculo em que está encerrado. SIN Kühne s., muscle s.
neurotendinous s., f. neurotendíneo. SIN Golgi tendon *organ.*
nuclear s., f. nuclear. SIN mitotic s.
sleep s., f. do sono; o registro eletroencefalográfico de salvas de ondas com freqüência de 14 por segundo, observados no exame EEG.
spine (spin) [TA]. **1.** Espinha; processo curto e pontiagudo de osso, semelhante a um espinho; um processo espinhoso. SIN spina [TA]. **2.** coluna vertebral. SIN vertebral *column.* [L. *spina*]
alar s., e. do osso esfenóide. SIN s. of sphenoid bone.
angular s., e. do osso esfenóide. SIN s. of sphenoid bone.
anterior inferior iliac s. [TA], e. ilíaca ântero-inferior; espinha na borda anterior do ílio entre a espinha ilíaca ântero-superior e o acetábulo; local de origem da cabeça direta do músculo reto femoral. SIN spina iliaca anterior inferior [TA].
anterior nasal s. (ANS), e. nasal anterior da maxila. SIN anterior nasal s. of maxilla.
anterior nasal s. of maxilla [TA], e. nasal anterior da maxila; projeção pontiaguda na extremidade anterior da sutura intermaxilar; a ponte, conforme observado numa radiografia cefalométrica lateral, é utilizada como marco cefalométrico. SIN spina nasalis anterior corporis maxillae [TA], anterior nasal s.
anterior superior iliac s. [TA], e. ilíaca ântero-superior; a extremidade anterior da crista ilíaca, que proporciona a inserção do ligamento inguinal e do músculo sartório. SIN spina iliaca anterior superior [TA].
bamboo s., e. em bambu; em radiologia, o aspecto da espinha torácica ou lombar na espondilite anquilosante.
cleft s., e. bífida. VER *spina* bifida.
dendritic s.'s, espinhas dendríticas; excrescências de comprimento variável de dendritos de células nervosas, variando, na sua forma, desde pequenos nódulos a processos espinhosos ou filamentosos, geralmente mais numerosos em arborizações dendríticas distais do que na parte proximal dos troncos dendríticos; constituem um local preferencial de contato axodendrítico sináptico; escassas ou ausentes em alguns tipos de células nervosas (neurônios motores, as grandes células do globo pálido, as células estreladas do córtex cerebral), extremamente numerosas em outras, como as células piramidais do córtex cerebral e as células de Purkinje do córtex cerebelar. SIN dendritic thorns, gemmule (2).
dorsal s., coluna vertebral. SIN vertebral *column.*
greater tympanic s. [TA], e. timpânica maior; a borda anterior da incisura timpânica (de Rivinus). SIN spina tympanica major [TA].
s. of helix [TA], e. da hélice; espinha dirigida anteriormente na extremidade da raiz da hélice da orelha. SIN spina helicis [TA], apophysis helicis.
hemal s., e. hemática; o ponto médio no lado inferior do arco hemático de uma vértebra nos vertebrados inferiores; considerada, por alguns, como representada pelo esterno nos seres humanos.
Henle s., e. de Henle. SIN suprameatal s.
iliac s., e. ilíaca. VER anterior inferior iliac s., anterior superior iliac s., posterior inferior iliac s., posterior superior iliac s.
ischiadic s., e. isquiática. SIN ischial s.
ischial s. [TA], e. isquiática; processo pontiagudo da borda posterior do ísquio em nível com a borda inferior do acetábulo; fornece a inserção para o músculo coccígeo e ligamento sacroespinhoso; o nervo pudendo passa dorsalmente à espinha isquiática, que é palpável pela vagina ou reto, sendo portanto utilizada como alvo para a ponta da agulha na administração de bloqueio do nervo pudendo. SIN spina ischiadica [TA], ischiadic s., sciatic s.
lesser tympanic s. [TA], e. timpânica menor; a borda posterior da incisura timpânica (de Rivinus). SIN spina tympanica minor [TA].
meatal s., e. suprameática. SIN suprameatal s.
mental s. [TA], e. geniana; projeção discreta, algumas vezes duas (superior e inferior), na linha média da superfície posterior do corpo da mandíbula, fornecendo inserção ao músculo genio-hióideo (abaixo) e genioglosso (acima). SIN spina mentalis (inferior et superior) [TA], genial tubercle, spinae geniorum inferior et superior.
nasal s. of frontal bone [TA], e. nasal do osso frontal; projeção do centro da parte nasal do osso frontal, localizada entre os ossos nasais e a lâmina perpendicular do etmóide e articulando-se com eles. SIN spina nasalis ossis frontalis [TA].
neural s., e. neural; o ponto médio do arco neural da vértebra típica, representada pelo processo espinhoso.
palatine s.'s [TA], espinhas palatinas; as cristas longitudinais ao longo dos sulcos palatinos na superfície inferior do processo palatino do maxilar. SIN spinae palatinae [TA].
poker s., e. da espondilite; coluna vertebral rígida resultante de imobilidade articular generalizada ou de espasmo muscular maciço, como a que pode ser provocada por osteomielite de uma vértebra ou espondilite reumatóide.
posterior inferior iliac s. [TA], e. ilíaca póstero-inferior; espinha na extremidade inferior da borda posterior do ílio, entre a espinha ilíaca póstero-superior e a incisura isquiática maior; forma a borda superior desta última. SIN spina iliaca posterior inferior [TA].
posterior nasal s. of horizontal plate of palatine bone [TA], e. nasal posterior da lâmina horizontal do osso palatino; a extremidade posterior pontiaguda da crista nasal do palato duro. SIN spina nasalis posterior laminae horizontalis ossis palatini [TA], posterior palatine s.
posterior palatine s., e. nasal posterior da lâmina horizontal do osso palatino. SIN posterior nasal s. of horizontal plate of palatine bone.
posterior superior iliac s. [TA], e. ilíaca póstero-superior; a extremidade posterior da crista ilíaca, o ponto mais alto de fixação dos ligamentos sacrotuberal e sacroilíaco posterior; existe uma depressão facilmente visível na pele que recobre a espinha ilíaca póstero-superior, clinicamente útil como indicação do nível da vértebra S2, o nível do limite inferior do espaço subaracnóideo. SIN spina iliaca posterior superior [TA].
pubic s., tubérculo. púbico SIN pubic *tubercle.*
s. of scapula [TA], e. da escápula; a crista triangular proeminente na face dorsal da escápula, fornecendo a fixação para os músculos trapézio e deltóide e separando as fossas supra-espinal e infra-espinal; o acrômio é uma extensão lateral da espinha. SIN spina scapulae [TA].
sciatic s., e. isquiática. SIN ischial s.
sphenoidal s., e. do osso esfenóide. SIN s. of sphenoid bone.
s. of sphenoid bone [TA], e. do osso esfenóide; projeção posterior e inferior da asa maior do osso esfenóide de cada lado, localizada póstero-lateralmente ao forame espinhoso, assim denominado devido à sua proximidade com a espinha do esfenóide; fornece a fixação para o ligamento esfenomandibular. SIN processus spinosus [TA], spina ossis sphenoidalis [TA], alar s., angular s., sphenoidal s., spina angularis, spinous process of sphenoid.
Spix s., e. de Spix. SIN *lingula* of mandible.
suprameatal s. [TA], e. suprameática; pequena proeminência óssea anterior à depressão suprameastóide na margem póstero-superior do meato acústico ex-

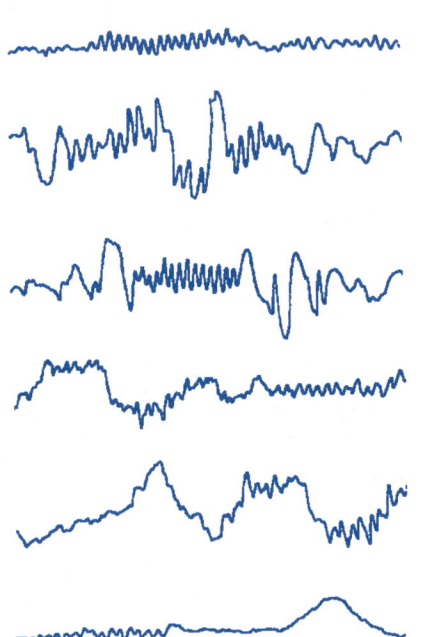

fuso do sono: EEG mostrando os traçados fusiformes do ritmo alfa (9–14 Hz) no primeiro e terceiro traçados

terno ósseo. SIN spina suprameatalis*, Henle s., meatal s., spina meatus, spina suprameatica.

thoracic s., a região torácica da coluna vertebral; as vértebras torácicas [T1–T12] como um todo; parte da coluna vertebral que entra na formação do tórax.

trochlear s. [TA], e. troclear; espícula óssea que se origina na borda da fóvea troclear, fornecendo fixação à tróclea do músculo oblíquo superior do bulbo do olho. SIN spina trochlearis [TA].

Spinelli, Pier G., ginecologista italiano, 1862–1929. VER S. *operation.*

spinn·bar·keit (spin′bahr - kīt). O caráter filamentoso e elástico do muco cervical durante o período ovulatório; em contraste com outras fases do ciclo menstrual, as secreções cervicais no meio do ciclo são claras, abundantes e de baixa viscosidade. [Al. *Spinnbarkeit*, viscosidade, capacidade de formar um filamento]

△ **spino-, spin-.** Espino-, espin-. **1.** A coluna vertebral. **2.** Espinhoso. [L. *spina*]

spi·no·bul·bar (spī′nō - bul′bar). Espinobulbar. SIN bulbospinal.

spi·no·cer·e·bel·lum (spī′nō - sār - ĕ - bel′ŭm) [TA]. Espinocerebelo. SIN paleocerebellum.

spi·no·col·lic·u·lar (spī′nō - col - ik′ū - lar). Espinocolicular. SIN spinotectal.

spi·no·cos·ta·lis (spī′nō - kos - tā′lis). Espinocostal; os músculos serráteis posteriores superior e inferior considerados como um. [L.]

spi·no·gle·noid (spī′nō - glē′noyd). Espinoglenóide; relativo à coluna e à cavidade glenóide da escápula.

spi·no·mus·cu·lar (spī′nō - mŭs′kū - lar). Espinomuscular; relativo à medula espinal e aos músculos supridos pelos nervos espinais.

spi·no·neu·ral (spī - nō - noo′ral). Espinoneural; relativo à medula espinal e aos nervos que dela partem.

spi·nose (spī′nōs). Espinhoso. SIN spinous.

spi·no·tec·tal (spī - nō - tek′tal). Espinotectal; que ascende da medula espinal até o teto. SIN spinocollicular.

spi·no·trans·ver·sar·i·us (spī′nō - trans - ver - sār′ē - ŭs). Espinotransverso; os músculos esplênio e oblíquos da cabeça considerados como um.

spi·nous (spī′nŭs). Espinhoso; relativo ou com forma semelhante a espinho, ou que possui um espinho ou espinhos. SIN spinose.

spin·thar·i·con (spin - thār′i - kon). Espintariscópio; câmara de cintilação utilizada para registrar a distribuição de emissões de baixa energia por radiofármacos administrados internamente, sobretudo para cintilografias da tireóide utilizando iodo-125. [G. *spinthēr*, centelha]

spin·thar·i·scope (spin - thār′i - skōp). Espintariscópio. SIN scintillation counter. [G *spinthēr*, centelha + *skopeō*, ver]

spip·e·rone (spip′ē - rōn). Espiperona; antipsicótico.

△ **spir-.** Espir-. VER spiro-.

spi·ra·cle (spī′ra - kl, spir-). Espiráculo; abertura para respiração em artrópodes (estigma) e em tubarões e peixes relacionados. [L. *spiraculum*, de *spiro*, respirar]

spi·rad·e·no·ma (spī - rad - ĕ - nō′ma). Espiradenoma; tumor benigno das glândulas sudoríparas. [G. *speira*, espiral + adenoma]

eccrine s., e. écrino; tumor cutâneo benigno, tipicamente doloroso, composto de dois tipos celulares derivados da parte secretora das glândulas sudoríparas écrinas.

spi·ral (spī′ral). Espiral. **1.** Enrolado; enrolado em torno de um centro, como uma mola de relógio; enrolado e ascendente como uma mola. **2.** Uma estrutura em forma de espiral. [L. mediev. *spiralis*, do G. *speira*, espiral]

Curschmann s.'s, espirais de Curschmann; massas espiraladas de muco que aparecem no escarro na asma brônquica.

s. of Tillaux, e. de Tillaux; linha imaginária que conecta as inserções dos músculos retos do bulbo do olho.

spir·a·my·cin (spir - ă - mī′sin). Espiramicina; substância antibiótica (quase idêntica à leucomicina) produzida por *Streptomyces ambofaciens*; agente antimicrobiano.

spi·rem, spi·reme (spī′rem, spī′rēm). Espirema; termo outrora aplicado ao primeiro estágio da mitose ou meiose (prófase), quando os filamentos cromossômicos estendidos têm o aspecto de uma bola frouxa de lã, com a suposição incorreta de que os filamentos eram contínuos e, posteriormente, rompiam-se para formar cromossomas individuais. [G. *speirēma*, uma espiral]

spi·ril·la (spī - ril′a). Espirilos; plural de spirillum.

Spi·ril·la·ce·ae (spī - ri - lā′sē - ē). Família de bactérias aeróbicas a facultativamente anaeróbicas, habitualmente móveis (ordem Pseudomonadales), que consistem em células Gram-negativas em forma de bastonete, curvas ou espiraladas. As células móveis contêm um único flagelo polar ou um tufo de flagelos polares. Esses microrganismos são primariamente formas aquáticas, apesar de alguns serem parasitas ou patogênicos dos seres humanos e de outros animais superiores. O gênero típico é *Spirillum*. VER *Spirillum.*

spi·ril·lar (spī - ril′ar). Espirilar; em forma de S; refere-se a uma célula bacteriana com forma de S.

spi·ril·li·ci·dal (spī - ril - i - sī′dal). Espirilicida; que destrói espirilos ou espiroquetas. [spirilla + L. *caedo*, matar]

spi·ril·lo·sis (spī′ri - lō′sis). Espirilose; qualquer doença causada pela presença de espirilos no sangue ou nos tecidos.

Spi·ril·lum (spī - ril′ŭm). Gênero de bactérias Gram-negativas grandes (1,4–1,7 μm de diâmetro), rígidas e helicoidais (família Spirillaceae), que se movimentam por meio de fascículos de flagelos bipolares. Esses microrganismos de água doce são obrigatoriamente microaerófilos e quimiorganotróficos, possuindo um metabolismo estritamente respiratório; não oxidam nem fermentam carboidratos. A espécie-tipo é *S. volutans*. [L. mod. dim. do L. *spira*, espiral, do G. *speira*]

S. mi'nus, espécie de classificação taxonômica incerta que provoca uma forma de febre por mordida de rato (sodoku). Essa espécie nunca foi cultivada.

S. volu'tans, espécie encontrada na água doce; trata-se da espécie típica de *S.*

spi·ril·lum, pl. **spi·ril·la** (spī - ril′ŭm, - ă). Espirilo; membro do gênero *Spirillum.*

Obermeier s., e. de Obermeier. SIN *Borrelia recurrentis.*

Vincent s., e. de Vincent; espirilo ou espiroqueta encontrado em associação ao bacilo de Vincent. *Fusobacterium nucleatum* é freqüentemente o único bacilo isolado.

spir·it (spir′it). **1.** Bebida alcoólica mais forte do que o vinho, obtida por destilação. **2.** Qualquer líquido destilado. **3.** Solução alcoólica ou hidroalcoólica de substâncias voláteis; alguns são utilizados como agentes aromatizantes, enquanto outros têm valor medicinal. SIN spiritus. [L. *spiritus*, respiração, alma, de *spiro*, respirar]

ardent s.'s, aguardentes; *brandy*, uísque e outras formas de bebidas alcoólicas destiladas.

aromatic ammonia s., sais aromáticos; solução hidroalcoólica contendo cerca de 2% de amônia e 4% de carbonato de amônio e os seguintes aromatizantes: óleo de limão, óleo de lavanda e óleo de noz-moscada. Utilizado principalmente por inalação para produzir estimulação reflexa em indivíduos que desmaiaram ou que correm risco de síncope. SIN sal volatile, smelling salts.

industrial methylated s., methylated s., álcool desnaturado. SIN denatured alcohol.

neutral s.'s, destilados de matérias-primas apropriadas; consistem em etanol a 95% (v/v), isto é, com pelo menos 190° quando destilados. Utilizados para misturar com uísque puro e para fazer gim, licores e vodca. VER TAMBÉM alcohol.

proof s., bebida alcoólica; álcool diluído, de densidade 0,920, contendo 49,5% por peso (57,27% por volume) de C_2H_5OH a 15,56°C. Originalmente, na Grã-Bretanha, era o álcool mais fraco capaz de permitir a ignição da pólvora umedecida com ele. A bebida alcoólica britânica possui uma densidade de 0,9198 e contém 49,2% de C_2H_5OH por peso ou 57,1% por volume, na temperatura de 10,56°C.

pyroligneous s., pyroxylic s., álcool metílico, metanol. SIN methyl *alcohol.*

rectified s., etanol, álcool e etílico. SIN alcohol (2).

vital s.'s, princípios vitais; nos ensinamentos de Galeno, uma essência ou princípio vital supostamente gerado a partir do ar ou pneuma no ventrículo esquerdo do coração; transportado no sangue até o cérebro e convertido em espíritos animais que então fluíam ao longo dos nervos de todas as partes do corpo.

wine s., álcool etílico, etanol. SIN alcohol (2).

wood s., álcool metílico. SIN methyl *alcohol.*

spir·i·tu·ous (spir′i - choo - ŭs). Alcoólico; que contém álcool em grande quantidade, referindo-se a bebidas alcoólicas.

spir·i·tus, gen. e pl. **spir·i·tus** (spir′i - tŭs). SIN spirit. [L.]

△ **spiro-, spir-.** Espiro-, espir-. **1.** Espiral, espiralado. [G. *speira*] **2.** Respiração. [L. *spiro*, respirar]

Spi·ro·cer·ca lu·pi (spi - rō - ser′kă loo′pī). O verme esofágico de cães e outros carnívoros, um nematódeo espirúroide vermelho que ocorre em nódulos na parede do esôfago, do estômago e da aorta de cães, raposas e lobos; os hospedeiros intermediários são vários besouros coprofágicos. Os sintomas clínicos só aparecem nas infecções muito maciças, que estão associadas a carcinomas esofágicos em cães e a osteoartropatia pulmonar hipertrófica. [L. do G. *speira*, espiral + G. *kerkos*, cauda; L. *lupus*, lobo]

ℹ **Spi·ro·chae·ta** (spī′rō - kē′ta). Gênero de bactérias móveis (ordem Spirochaetales) contendo provavelmente bastonetes Gram-negativos, flexíveis, ondulantes e espiralados, que podem ou não apresentar extremidades afiladas e flageliformes. O protoplasto enrola-se em espiral num filamento axial. Não há membrana periplástica óbvia nem estriações transversais. Esses microrganismos locomovem-se através de um movimento serpiginoso sobre as superfícies de objetos de sustentação. Não são parasitas, mas são encontrados na forma de vida livre na lama em água doce ou salgada; são comumente encontrados no esgoto e em águas sujas. Atualmente, o gênero contém cinco espécies. A espécie típica é *S. plicatilis*. [L. mod. do G. *speira*, espiral + *chaitē*, pêlo]

S. obermei'eri, SIN *Borrelia recurrentis.*

S. plicat'ilis, uma espécie muito grande (algumas vezes com comprimento de até 200 μm) de bactéria; não é parasita pelo que se sabe; trata-se da espécie típica do gênero *S.*

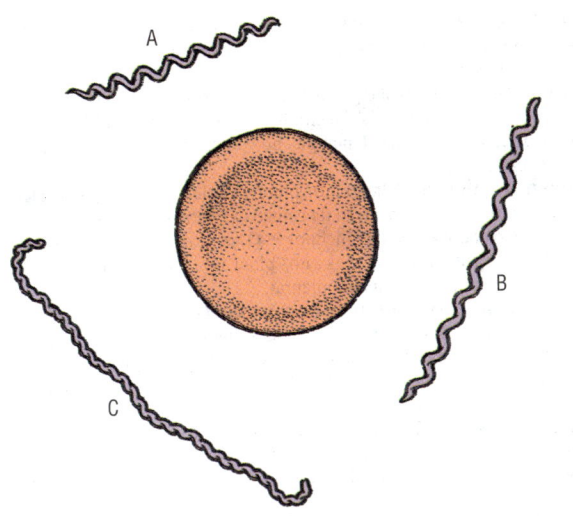

espiroquetas: (mostrados com um eritrócito para comparação do tamanho) (A) *Treponema*; (B) *Borrelia*; (C) *Leptospira*.

Spi·ro·chae·ta·ce·ae (spī-rō-kē-tā′sē-ē). Família de bactérias (ordem Spirochaetales) que consistem em células espiraladas grosseiras de 30–50 μm de comprimento, dotadas de estruturas protoplasmáticas definidas. Esses microrganismos são encontrados em água estagnada, doce ou salgada e nas vias intestinais de moluscos bivalves. O gênero típico é *Spirochaeta*. VER *Spirochaeta*.

Spi·ro·chae·ta·les (spī-rō-kē-tā′lēz). Ordem de bactérias que contêm células delgadas e flexíveis, de 6–500 μm de comprimento, na forma de espirais com pelo menos uma volta completa. Algumas espécies podem possuir um filamento axial, uma crista lateral ou estriações transversais. Todos esses microrganismos são móveis, girando ao redor do eixo longitudinal, de modo que o microrganismos é impelido para frente ou para trás. Existem formas de vida livre, saprófitas e parasitas. A família típica é Spirochaetaceae.

spi·ro·chet·al (spī-rō-kē′tăl). Espiroquético; relativo às espiroquetas, especialmente à infecção causada por esses microrganismos.

spi·ro·chete (spī′rō-kēt). Espiroqueta; termo vernacular utilizado para referir-se a qualquer microrganismo semelhante a *Leptospira*, *Spirochaeta* ou *Treponema*.

spi·ro·chet·e·mia (spī′rō-kē-tē′mē-ă). Espiroquetemia; presença de espiroquetas no sangue. [spirochete + G. *haima*, sangue]

spi·ro·che·ti·cide (spī-rō-kē′tĭ-sīd). Espiroqueticida; agente que destrói espiroquetas. [spirochete + L. *caedo*, matar]

spi·ro·che·tol·y·sis (spī′rō-kē-tol′ĭ-sis). Espiroquetólise; destruição de espiroquetas através de fármacos ou de anticorpos específicos. [spirochete + G. *lysis*, afrouxamento]

spi·ro·che·to·sis (spī′rō-kē-tō′sis). Espiroquetose; qualquer doença causada por espiroqueta.

   bronchopulmonary s., e. broncopulmonar. SIN *hemorrhagic bronchitis.*

spi·ro·che·tot·ic (spī′rō-kē-tot′ik). Espiroquetótico; relativo a, ou caracterizado por, espiroquetose.

spi·ro·gram (spī′rō-gram). Espirograma; traçado feito pelo espirógrafo.

spi·ro·graph (spī′rō-graf). Espirógrafo; dispositivo para representar graficamente a profundidade e a velocidade dos movimentos respiratórios. [L. *spiro*, respirar + G. *graphō*, escrever]

spi·ro·in·dex (spī′rō-in-deks). Índice respiratório; capacidade vital dividida pela altura do indivíduo.

spi·rom·e·ter (spī-rom′ĕ-ter). Espirômetro; na prática clínica e em pesquisa, qualquer dispositivo utilizado para medir fluxos e volumes, inspirados e expirados pelos pulmões, avaliando, assim, a função pulmonar. Considerado o dispositivo de medida mais básico da função pulmonar. [L. *spiro*, respirar + G. *metron*, medida]

   chain-compensated s., e. compensado por cadeia; espirômetro de Tissot em que a compensação para a mudança na flutuabilidade da campânula é feita automaticamente por uma cadeia suspensa de massa correta por unidade de comprimento.

   Krogh s., e. de Krogh; espirômetro com fecho hidráulico em que a campânula consiste numa grande caixa retangular rasa fazendo uma ligeira rotação em torno de um eixo horizontal que se estende ao longo de uma borda, com um braço estendendo-se além desse eixo até um peso de equilíbrio; comparável a um espirômetro em cunha.

   Tissot s., e. de Tissot; espirômetro muito grande com fecho hidráulico projetado para acumular gás expirado durante um longo período de tempo; o equilíbrio da campânula (quase sem atrito) é compensado pela mudança da campânula na flutuabilidade quando emerge da água, mantendo o gás contido precisamente na pressão atmosférica ambiente.

   wedge s., e. em cunha; espirômetro sem água constituído de duas grandes placas retangulares com bordas conectadas por borracha sanfonada, de modo que as grandes mudanças de volume são acomodadas por pequenas alterações no ângulo agudo do interior cuneiforme, percebidas por um transdutor elétrico; projetado para rápida resposta ao reduzir a aceleração das partes móveis.

Spi·ro·me·tra (spī-rō-mē′tră). Gênero de tênias pseudofilídeas. [G. *speira*, espiral + *mētra*, útero]

   S. manso′ni, espécie de tênias pseudofilídeas de gatos selvagens e ferozes, cuja forma larvar (espargano) pode sobreviver nos tecidos humanos; era comumente encontrada em seres humanos no Oriente, mas também é descrita em outras áreas amplamente dispersas; a infecção dos seres humanos pelo espargano ocorre por migração ativa da larva de rãs infectadas recentemente partidas utilizadas como cataplasma para feridas, inflamações oculares (como na esparganose ocular), contusões ou ulcerações; é também provável que os seres humanos possam ser infectados por larvas do espargano ao ingerir qualquer vertebrado que albergue esses plerocercóides. SIN *Diphyllobothrium linguloides*, *Diphyllobothrium mansoni*.

   S. mansonoi′des, espécie de tênias pseudofilídeas da América do Norte, cuja larva (espargano) seria uma causa de esparganose em seres humanos na Flórida e nos estados do Golfo do México. SIN *Diphyllobothrium mansonoides*.

spi·rom·e·try (spī-rom′ĕ-trē). Espirometria; realização de medidas pulmonares com espirômetro.

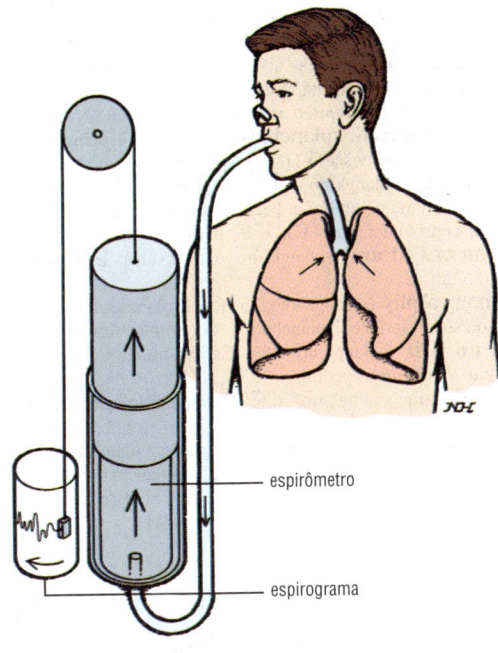

espirometria: princípio de espirometria de circuito fechado

   forced s., e. forçada; inspiração e, mais particularmente, expiração em que o volume é representado graficamente contra o tempo, fornecendo uma medida da função pulmonar. O volume de ar expelido em um segundo (VEF) é freqüentemente considerado a medida isolada mais importante em fisiologia respiratória clínica.

spi·ro·no·lac·tone (spī′rō-nō-lak′tōn). Espironolactona; diurético que bloqueia as ações tubulares renais da aldosterona. Aumenta a excreção urinária de sódio e de cloreto, diminui a excreção de potássio e amônio e reduz a acidez titulável da urina; utilizado mais efetivamente para potencializar a ação natriurética e reduzir a excreção de potássio produzida por outros diuréticos.

spi·ro·scope (spī′rō-skōp). Espiroscópio; dispositivo para medir a capacidade aérea dos pulmões. [L. *spiro*, respirar + G. *skopeō*, ver]

spi·ro·stan (spī′rō-stan). Espirostano; um 16,22:22,26-diepoxicolestano.

spi·ru·roid (spī′roo-royd). Espiruróide; nome comum de um membro da superfamília Spiruroidea.

Spi·ru·roi·dea (spī-roo-roy′dē-ă). Superfamília de parasitas nematódeos transmitidos por artrópodes do trato digestivo, sistema respiratório ou cavidades orbitárias, nasais ou orais de vertebrados. Trata-se de parasitas comuns, freqüentemente patogênicos, de mamíferos e aves domésticos, produzindo ulcerações em consequência da penetração da extremidade anterior desses vermes espinhosos através do revestimento do tubo digestivo; inclui as famílias Acuariidae, Gnathostomatidae, Rictulariidae, Seuratidae, Physalopteridae, Spiruridae e Thelaziidae. [G. *speiroeidēs*, espiral]

spis·si·tude (spis′i-tood). Espessidão; estado de estar espessado; condição de um líquido espessado quase até o estado sólido por evaporação ou espessamento. [L. *spissitudo*, de *spissus*, espesso]

spit·ting. Cuspir, escarrar, expectorar. SIN expectoration (2).

spit·tle (spit′l). Saliva. SIN saliva. [A.S. *spātl*]

Spitz, Sophie, patologista norte-americana do século XX. VER S. *nevus*.

Spitzer, Alexander, anatomista austríaco, 1868–1943. VER S. *theory*.

Spitzka, Edward C., neurologista norte-americano, 1852–1914. VER S. *nucleus*, marginal *tract*, marginal *zone*; *column* of S.-Lissauer.

Spix, Johann B., anatomista alemão, 1781–1826. VER S. *spine*.

SPL Abreviatura de sound pressure *level* (nível de pressão sonora).

splanchn-. Esplanc-. VER splanchno-.

splanch·nap·o·phys·i·al, splanch·nap·o·phys·e·al (splangk′na-pō-fiz′ē-ăl). Esplancnapofisário; relativo a uma esplancnapófise.

splanch·na·poph·y·sis (splangk′na-pof′i-sis). Esplancnapófise; uma apófise da vértebra típica, do lado oposto à apófise neural, ou qualquer processo ósseo, fornecendo fixação para uma víscera ou parte do trato digestivo. [splanchn- + G. *apophysis*, protuberância]

splanch·nec·to·pia (splangk-nek-tō′pē-ă). Esplancnectopia; deslocamento de qualquer víscera. [splanchn- + G. *ektopos*, fora de lugar]

splanch·nes·the·sia (splangk-nes-thē′zē-ă). Esplancnestesia. SIN visceral sense. [splanch- + G. *aisthēsis*, sensação]

splanch·nic (splangk′nik). Esplâncnico. SIN visceral.

splanch·ni·cec·to·my (splangk-ni-sek-tō-mē). Esplancnicectomia; ressecção dos nervos esplâncnicos e, em geral, do gânglio celíaco também. [splanchni- + G. *ektomē*, excisão]

splanch·ni·cot·o·my (splangk-ni-kot′ō-mē). Esplancnicotomia; secção de um nervo ou nervos esplâncnicos, um procedimento cirúrgico outrora utilizado no tratamento da hipertensão arterial. [splanchni- + G. *tomē*, incisão]

splanchno-, splanchn-, splanchni-. Esplancno-, esplanc-, esplancni-. As vísceras. VER TAMBÉM viscero-. [G. *splanchnon*, víscera]

splanch·no·cele (splangk′nō-sēl). Esplancnocele. **1.** A cavidade corporal primitiva ou celoma no embrião. [G. *koilos*, cavidade] **2.** Hérnia de qualquer uma das vísceras abdominais. [G. *kēlē*, hérnia]

splanch·no·cra·ni·um (splangk-nō-krā′nē-ŭm). Esplancnocrânio. SIN viscerocranium.

splanch·nog·ra·phy (splangk-nog′ra-fē). Esplancnografia; tratado sobre as vísceras ou sua descrição. [splanchno- + G. *graphō*, escrever]

splanch·no·lith (splangk′nō-lith). Esplancnólito; cálculo intestinal. [splanchno- + G. *lithos*, pedra]

splanch·no·lo·gia (splangk′nō-lō′jē-ă). Esplancnologia. SIN splanchnology, splanchnology.

splanch·nol·o·gy (splangk-nol′ō-jē). Esplancnologia; ramo da ciência médica que trata das vísceras. SIN splanchnologia. [splanchno- + G. *logos*, estudo]

splanch·no·meg·a·ly (splangk-nō-meg′a-lē). Esplancnomegalia. SIN visceromegaly. [esplanchno- + G. *megas*, grande]

splanch·no·mic·ria (splangk-nō-mik′rē-ă). Esplancnomicria; condição em que os órgãos esplâncnicos são menores do que o normal. [splanchno- + G. *mikros*, pequeno]

splanch·nop·a·thy (splangk-nop′a-thē). Esplancnopatia; qualquer doença das vísceras abdominais. [splanchno- + G. *pathos*, doença]

splanch·no·pleu·ral (splangk-nō-ploor′ik). Esplancnopleural. SIN splanchnopleuric.

splanch·no·pleure (splangk′nō-ploor). Esplancnopleura; a camada embrionária formada por associação da camada visceral do mesoderma da placa lateral com o endoderma. [splanchno- + G. *pleura*, lado]

splanch·no·pleu·ric (splangk-nō-ploor′ik). Esplancnopleural; relativo à esplancnopleura. SIN splanchnopleural.

splanch·nop·to·sis, splanch·nop·to·sia (splangk′no-tō′sis, -tō′sē-ă). Esplancnoptose. SIN visceroptosis. [splanchno- + G. *ptōsis*, queda]

splanch·no·scle·ro·sis (splangk′nō-skle-rō′sis). Esplancnosclerose; endurecimento, através de proliferação do tecido conjuntivo, de qualquer víscera. [splanchno- + G. *sklērōsis*, endurecimento]

splanch·no·skel·e·tal (splangk-nō-skel′ē-tăl). Esplancnoesquelético. SIN visceroskeletal.

splanch·no·skel·e·ton (splangk-nō-skel′ē-tŏn). Esplancnoesqueleto. SIN visceroskeleton (2).

splanch·no·so·mat·ic (splangk′nō-sō-mat′ik). Esplancnossomático. SIN viscerosomatic. [splanchno- + G. *sōma*, corpo]

splanch·not·o·my (splangk-not′ō-mē). Esplancnotomia; dissecção das vísceras por incisão. [splanchno- + G. *tomē*, incisão]

splanch·no·tribe (splangk′nō-trīb). Esplancnótribo; instrumento semelhante a um grande angiótribo utilizado para oclusão temporária do intestino, antes da ressecção. [splanchno- + G. *tribō*, esfregar, contundir]

splay (splā). **1.** Abrir a extremidade de uma estrutura tubular por meio de uma incisão longitudinal para aumentar o seu diâmetro potencial. VER TAMBÉM spatulate. **2.** O arredondamento do ângulo no gráfico que relaciona a taxa de secreção ou reabsorção tubular renal de uma substância com a sua concentração plasmática arterial, devido primariamente ao fato de que alguns néfrons atingem seu máximo tubular antes de outros.

spleen (splēn) [TA]. Baço; grande órgão linfático vascular, localizado na parte superior da cavidade abdominal, do lado esquerdo, entre o estômago e o diafragma, composto de polpas branca e vermelha; a polpa branca consiste em nódulos linfáticos e tecido linfático difuso; a polpa vermelha consiste em sinusóides venosos entre os quais se encontram cordões esplênicos; o estroma da polpa vermelha e da polpa branca consiste em fibras reticulares e células. Um arcabouço de trabéculas fibroelásticas que se estendem a partir da cápsula subdivide o órgão em lóbulos mal definidos. Trata-se de um órgão hematopoético no início da vida e, posteriormente, de um órgão de armazenamento para eritrócitos e plaquetas; devido ao grande número de macrófagos, atua também como filtro sanguíneo, identificando e destruindo eritrócitos anormais. SIN splen [TA], lien*. [G. *splēn*]

accessory s. [TA], b. acessório; uma das pequenas massas globulares de tecido esplênico algumas vezes encontradas na região do baço, em uma das pregas peritoneais ou em outra parte. SIN splen accessorius [TA], lien accessorius*,

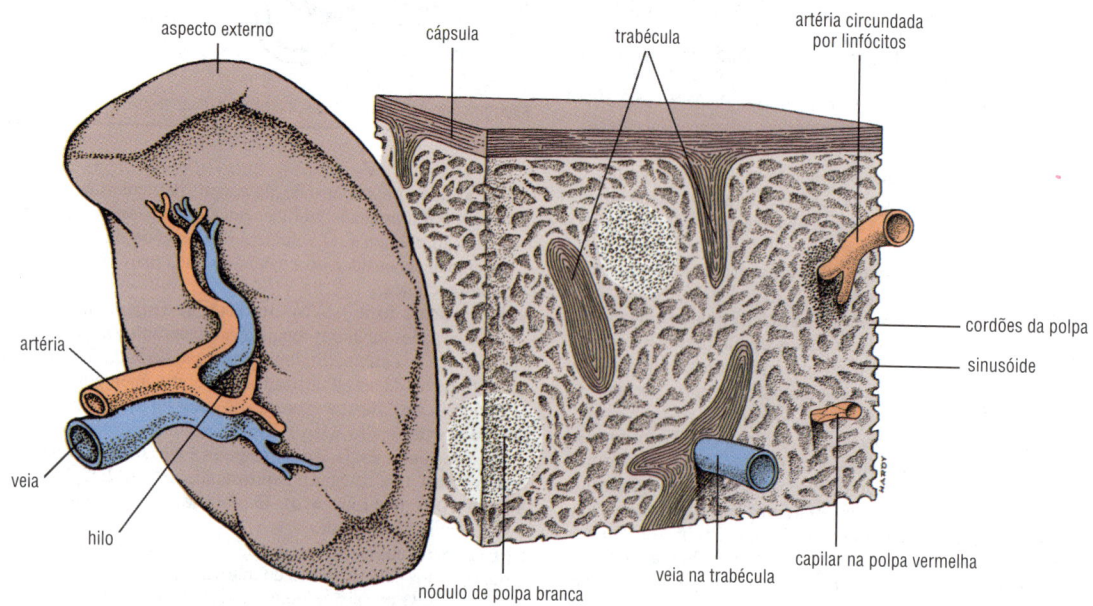

corte do baço: disposição geral do tecido esplênico

lien succenturiatus, lienculus, lienunculus, spleneolus, spleniculus, splenule, splenulus, splenunculus.
diffuse waxy s., b. céreo difuso; condição de degeneração amilóide do baço, que afeta principalmente os espaços teciduais extra-sinusoidais da polpa.
floating s., b. flutuante; baço palpável em virtude de sua mobilidade excessiva devido a um pedículo relaxado ou alongado, e não devido a aumento. SIN lien mobilis, movable s.
lardaceous s., b. lardáceo, b. céreo. SIN waxy s.
movable s., b. móvel. SIN floating s.
sago s., amiloidose no baço, que afeta principalmente os corpos de Malpigui.
sugar-coated s., hialoserosite que acomete o baço.
waxy s., b. céreo; amiloidose do baço. SIN lardaceous s.
splen [TA]. Baço. SIN spleen. [G. *splen,* baço]
s. accessorius [TA], b. acessório. SIN accessory spleen.
splen-. Esplen-. VER spleno-.
sple·nal·gia (splē-nal'jē-ă). Esplanalgia; termo raramente empregado para referir-se a uma condição dolorosa do baço. SIN splenodynia. [splen- + G. *algos,* dor]
Splendore, Alfonso, médico italiano do século XX. VER S.-Hoeppli *phenomenon;* Lutz-S.-Almeida *disease.*
sple·nec·to·my (splē-nek'tō-mē). Esplenectomia; remoção do baço. [splen- + G. *ektomē,* excisão]
sple·nec·to·pia, sple·nec·to·py (splen'ek-tō'pē-ă, splē-nek'tō-pē). Esplenectopia. 1. Deslocamento do baço, como no baço flutuante. 2. A presença de restos de tecido esplênico, geralmente na região do baço. [splen- + G. *ektopos,* fora do lugar]
sple·nel·co·sis (splen-el-kō'sis). Esplenelcose; abscesso do baço. [splen- + G. *helkōsis,* ulceração]
sple·ne·o·lus (splē-nē'ō-lŭs). Esplenéolo. SIN accessory spleen. [L. mod. dim. do G. *splēn*]
sple·net·ic (splē-net'ik). 1. Esplênico. SIN splenic. 2. Mal-humorado.
sple·ni·al (splē'nē-ăl). Esplenial. 1. Relativo ao esplênio. 2. Relativo ao músculo esplênio. [G. *splēnion,* bandagem]
splen·ic (splen'ik). Esplênico; relativo ao baço. SIN lienal, splenetic (1).
sple·ni·cu·lus (splen-ik'ū-lŭs). Esplenículo. SIN accessory spleen. [L. mod.]
splen·i·form (splen'i-form, splē'ni-). Espleniforme. SIN sphenoid.
splen·i·ser·rate (splen'i-ser'āt). Espleniosserrátil; relativo aos músculos esplênio e serrátil.
sple·ni·tis (splē-nī'tis). Esplenite; inflamação do baço. [splen- + G. *-itis,* inflamação]
sple·ni·um, pl. **sple·nia** (splē'nē-ŭm, -ă). 1. Compressa ou bandagem. 2. [TA]. Esplênio; estrutura semelhante a uma parte enfaixada. [L. mod. do G. *splēnion,* bandagem]
s. cor'poris callo'si [TA], e. do corpo caloso. SIN s. of corpus callosum.
s. of corpus callosum [TA], e. do corpo caloso; a extremidade posterior espessada do corpo caloso. SIN s. corporis callosi [TA], tuber corporis callosi.
sple·ni·us (splē'nē-ŭs). Esplênio. VER splenius *muscle* of head, splenius *muscle* of neck. [L. mod. do G. *splēnion,* bandagem]
spleno-, splen-. Espleno-, esplen-. O baço. [G. *splēn*]
sple·no·cele (splē'nō-sēl). Esplenocele; hérnia esplênica. [spleno- + G. *kēlē,* tumor, hérnia]
sple·no·clei·sis (splē-nō-klī'sis). Esplenoclise; indução da formação de novo tecido fibroso na superfície do baço por atrito ou envolvimento com gaze. [spleno- + G. *kleisis,* fechamento]
sple·no·col·ic (splē'nō-kol'ik). Esplenocólico; relativo ao baço e ao colo; designa um ligamento ou dobra de peritônio que passa entre as duas vísceras.
sple·no·dyn·ia (splē'nō-din'ē-ă). Esplenodinia. SIN splenalgia. [spleno- + G. *odynē,* dor]
sple·no·he·pa·to·meg·a·ly, sple·no·he·pa·to·me·ga·lia (splē'nō-hep'ă-tō-meg'ă-lē, -mē-gā'lē-ă). Espleno-hepatomegalia, hepatoesplenomegalia; aumento do baço e do fígado. [spleno- + G. *hēpar,* fígado + *megas,* grande]
sple·noid (splē'noyd). Esplenóide; semelhante ao baço. SIN spleniform. [spleno- + G. *eidos,* semelhança]
sple·no·lym·phat·ic (splē'nō-lim-fat'ik). Esplenolinfático; relativo ao baço e aos linfonodos.
sple·no·ma (splē-nō'mă). Esplenoma; termo geral inespecífico para referir-se a um baço aumentado. [spleno- + G. *-oma,* tumor]
sple·no·ma·la·cia (splē'nō-mă-lā'shē-ă). Esplenomalacia; amolecimento do baço. [spleno- + G. *malakia,* amolecimento]
sple·no·med·ul·lary (splē-nō-med'ŭ-lār-ē). Esplenomedular. SIN splenomyelogenous. [spleno- + L. *medulla,* medula]
sple·no·meg·a·ly, sple·no·me·ga·lia (splē-nō-meg'ă-lē, -mē-gā'lē-ă). Esplenomegalia; aumento do baço. SIN megalosplenia. [spleno- + G. *megas* (*megal-*), grande]
congestive s., e. congestiva; aumento do baço em virtude de congestão passiva; termo algumas vezes utilizado como sinônimo de síndrome de Banti.

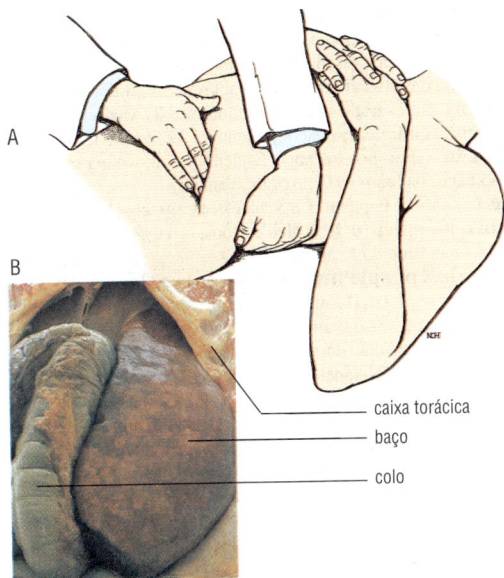

esplenomegalia: (A) técnica de palpação utilizada no diagnóstico; (B) esplenomegalia devido a leucemia granulocítica, observada à necropsia (peso do baço: 4.200 g)

Egyptian s., e. egípcia; termo algumas vezes empregado como sinônimo de esquistossomose mansônica, embora a hepatomegalia e a fibrose sejam mais consistentemente encontradas do que o aumento do baço.
hemolytic s., e. hemolítica; esplenomegalia associada a icterícia hemolítica.
hyperreactive malarious s., e. malárica hiper-reativa; síndrome caracterizada por esplenomegalia persistente, níveis séricos excepcionalmente elevados de IgM e anticorpos antimaláricos e linfocitose sinusoidal hepática; acredita-se que seja um distúrbio no controle pelos linfócitos T da resposta humoral à malária recorrente. SIN tropical splenomegaly syndrome.
Niemann s., e. de Niemann; aumento do baço observado na doença de Niemann-Pick.
tropical s., leishmaniose visceral. SIN visceral leishmaniasis.
sple·no·my·e·log·e·nous (splē'nō-mī-ĕ loj'ĕ-nŭs). Esplenomielógeno; que se origina no baço e na medula óssea, referindo-se a uma forma de leucemia. SIN lienomedullary, lienomyelogenous, splenomedullary. [spleno- + G. *myelos,* medula + *-gen,* produtor]
sple·no·my·e·lo·ma·la·cia (splē'nō-mī'ĕ-lō-mă-lā'shē-ă). Esplenomielomalacia; amolecimento patológico do baço e da medula óssea. [spleno- + G. *myelos,* medula + *malakia,* amolecimento]
sple·no·neph·ric (splē'nō-nef'rik). Esplenonéfrico. SIN splenorenal. [spleno- + G. *nephros,* rim]
sple·no·pan·cre·at·ic (splē'nō-pan-krē-at'ik). Esplenopancreático; relativo ao baço e ao pâncreas. SIN lienopancreatic.
sple·nop·a·thy (splē-nop'ă-thē). Esplenopatia; qualquer doença do baço. [spleno- + G. *pathos,* sofrimento]
sple·no·pex·y, sple·no·pex·ia (splē'nō-pek-sē, splē-nō-pek'sē-ă). Esplenopexia; sutura no local um baço ectópico ou flutuante. SIN splenorrhaphy (2). [spleno- + G. *pēxis,* fixação]
sple·no·phren·ic (splē'nō-fren'ik). Esplenofrênico; relativo ao baço e ao diafragma; designa um ligamento ou dobra de peritônio que se estende entre as duas estruturas. [spleno- + G. *phrēn,* diafragma]
sple·no·por·to·gram (splē-nō-pōr'tō-gram). Esplenoportograma; registro radiográfico das veias esplênicas e porta e suas colaterais após injeção direta de meio de contraste hidrossolúvel no baço.
sple·no·por·tog·ra·phy (splē'nō-pōr-tog'ră-fē). Esplenoportografia; introdução de material radiopaco no baço para obter uma visualização radiográfica das veias esplênicas e principais veias porta da circulação porta. SIN splenic portal venography. [spleno- + portography]
sple·nop·to·sis, sple·nop·to·sia (splē-nop-tō'sis, -tō'sē-ă). Esplenoptose; deslocamento do baço para baixo, como no baço flutuante. [spleno- + G. *ptōsis,* queda]
sple·no·re·nal (splē'nō-rē'năl). Esplenorrenal; relativo ao baço e ao rim; designa um ligamento ou dobra de peritônio que se estende entre as duas estruturas. SIN lienorenal, splenonephric.
sple·nor·rha·gia (splē'nō-rā'jē-ă). Esplenorragia; hemorragia a partir de baço roto. [spleno- + G. *rhēgnymi,* irromper]
sple·nor·rha·phy (splē-nōr'ă-fē). Esplenorrafia. 1. Sutura do baço roto. 2. Esplenopexia. SIN splenopexy. [spleno- + G. *rhaphē,* sutura]

sple·no·sis (splē-nō'sis). Esplenose; implantação e crescimento subseqüente de tecido esplênico no abdome, em conseqüência de ruptura do baço.
thoracic s., e. torácica; presença de tecido esplênico no tórax em decorrência de traumatismo envolvendo o tórax e o abdome, seguido de esplenectomia.

sple·not·o·my (splē-not'ō-mē). Esplenotomia. **1.** Anatomia ou dissecção do baço. **2.** Incisão cirúrgica do baço. [spleno- + G. *tomē*, incisão]

sple·no·tox·in (splē-nō-tok'sin). Esplenotoxina; toxina específica para as células do baço. [spleno- + G. *toxikon*, veneno]

splen·ule (splen'ūl). Esplênulo. SIN *accessory spleen*. [L. mod. *splenulus*]

splen·u·lus, pl. **splen·u·li** (splen'ū-loos, -lī). Esplênulo. SIN *accessory spleen*. [L. mod. dim. do L. *splen*, baço]

sple·nun·cu·lus, pl. **sple·nun·cu·li** (splē-nŭng'kū-lŭs, -lī). Esplenúnculo. SIN *accessory spleen*. [L. mod. dim. do L. *splen*, baço]

splice·o·some (splī'sē-ō-sŏm). Estrutura especializada que participa na remoção de introns e reunião dos exons remanescentes do mRNA; além da transcrição primária do mRNA, pelo menos quatro RNA nucleares pequenos (snRNA) e algumas proteínas estão envolvidos. [splice + -some]

splic·ing (splīs'ing). *Splicing;* junção. **1.** Fixação de uma molécula de DNA a outra. SIN gene splicing. **2.** Remoção de introns de precursores do mRNA e a reunião ou fixação de exons. SIN RNA splicing.
alternative s., junção alternativa; diferentes maneiras de montagem de exons para produzir diferentes mRNA maduros.

splint. 1. Aparelho, tala; aparelho para impedir o movimento de uma articulação ou para fixação de partes deslocadas ou móveis. **2.** A fíbula. [Hol. médio *splinte*]
acid etch cemented s., a. cimentado com ácido cáustico; a. de metal pesado que é cimentado às superfícies labiais dos dentes com qualquer uma das técnicas de cimento de ácido cáustico; utilizado para estabilização de dentes deslocados por traumatismo com doença periodontal.
active s., a. ativo, a. dinâmico. SIN *dynamic s.*
air s., a. insuflável; a. de plástico insuflado por ar, utilizado para imobilizar parte de um membro ou todo ele. SIN inflatable s.
airplane s., a. em "aeroplano"; a. complicado que mantém o braço em abdução aproximadamente ao nível do ombro, com o antebraço em flexão parcial, geralmente com suporte axilar.

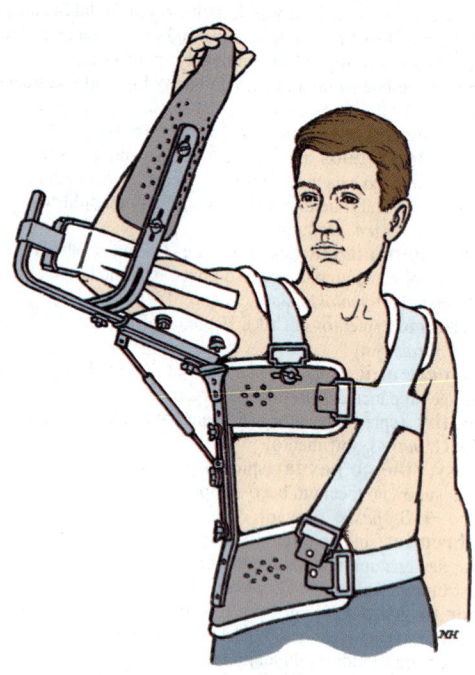

aparelho em "aeroplano"

anchor s., a. de ancoragem; a. utilizado em fratura da mandíbula, com fios metálicos ao redor dos dentes e um bastão para mantê-lo no lugar.
Anderson s., a. de Anderson; a. de tração esquelética com pinos inseridos nas extremidades proximal e distal de uma fratura; a redução é obtida por um bastão externo fixado aos pinos; também descrito como de fixação externa.
backboard s., a. de respaldo; prancha com aberturas para fixação do corpo com alças; os mais curtos são utilizados para lesões do pescoço, e os mais longos, para lesões das costas.
Balkan s., a. de Balkan. SIN *Balkan frame.*
cap s., jaquetas; a. de plástico ou metálico com fendas para cobrir as coroas dos dentes e geralmente cimentado a elas.
coaptation s., a. de coaptação; a. curto projetado para evitar o cavalgamento das extremidades de um osso fraturado, habitualmente suplementado por um aparelho mais longo para fixar todo o membro. Utilizado mais comumente para reparo de fraturas de diáfise do úmero.
Cramer wire s., a. de Cramer. SIN *ladder s.*
Denis Browne s., a. de Denis Browne; a. de alumínio leve aplicado à face lateral da perna e do pé; utilizado para deformidades de torsão da perna, do tornozelo ou do pé em crianças.
dynamic s., a. dinâmico; a. que utiliza molas ou faixas elásticas que auxiliam os movimentos iniciados pelo paciente ao controlar o plano e o arco de movimento. SIN active s., functional s. (1).
Essig s., a. de Essig; fio de ácido inoxidável passado labial e lingualmente ao redor de um segmento da arcada dentária e mantido em posição por fios de ligadura individuais ao redor das áreas de contato dos dentes; utilizado para estabilizar dentes fraturados ou reposicionados, bem como o osso alveolar acometido.
Frejka pillow s., suporte com almofada de Frejka, suporte com almofada utilizado para abdução e flexão dos fêmures no tratamento da displasia ou da luxação congênita do quadril em lactentes.
functional s., a. funcional; **(1)** SIN *dynamic s.* **(2)** união de dois ou mais dentes numa unidade rígida por meio de restaurações fixas que recobrem todos os dentes de sustentação ou parte deles.
Gunning s., a. de Gunning; prótese fabricada a partir de modelos de arcadas maxilares e mandibulares edentadas para auxiliar na redução e fixação de uma fratura.
inflatable s., a. inflável. SIN *air s.*
interdental s., a. interdentário; a. para mandíbula fraturada que consiste em duas faixas metálicas ou de resina acrílica fixadas por fios metálicos aos dentes do maxilar e da mandíbula, respectivamente, e unidas para manter as mandíbulas imóveis.
Kingsley s., a. de Kingsley; a. maxilar dotado de asas, utilizado para aplicar uma tração, para reduzir fraturas maxilares, bem como para imobilizá-las ao fixar as asas a um aparelho colocado na cabeça com elásticos. SIN reverse Kingsley s.
labial s., a. labial; a. de plástico, metal ou de uma combinação de ambos, projetado para adaptar-se à face externa da arcada dentária e utilizado no tratamento de lesões da mandíbula e da face.
ladder s., a. em escada; a. flexível que consiste em dois fios metálicos paralelos resistentes, com fios transversais mais finos. SIN Cramer wire s.
lingual s., a. lingual; semelhante ao a. labial, porém ajusta-se à face interna da arcada dentária.
plaster s., a. gessado; a. constituído por ataduras impregnadas com gesso.
reverse Kingsley s., a. inverso de Kingsley. SIN *Kingsley s.*
Stader s., a. de Stader; a. utilizado primariamente em medicina veterinária; com pinos metálicos através dos segmentos proximal e distal de uma fratura de osso longo, a fixação dos pinhos é mantida pelo a., que é externo ao membro.
surgical s., a. cirúrgico; termo geral para referir-se a um dispositivo utilizado para manter os tecidos numa nova posição após a cirurgia.
Taylor s., a. de Taylor. SIN *Taylor back brace.*
Thomas s., a. de Thomas; a. longo para perna, que se estende desde um anel no quadril até abaixo do pé, permitindo a tração de uma perna fraturada, para emergências e transporte.
Tobruk s., a. de Tobruk; a. de Thomas aplicado e imobilizado com ataduras gessadas; utilizado pela primeira vez durante a II Guerra Mundial para imobilizar o membro durante condições perigosas, como transporte de barcos pequenos para barcos grandes. [porto de *Tobruk,* na Líbia]
wire s., a. metálico; a. utilizado para estabilizar dentes afrouxados por acidente ou por uma condição periodontal no maxilar ou na mandíbula; dispositivo para reduzir e estabilizar fraturas do maxilar ou da mandíbula através de sua aplicação a ambos, conectando-os por fios metálicos ou faixas de borracha intermaxilares.

splint·ing. Imobilização. **1.** Aplicação de um aparelho ou tratamento utilizando uma tala. **2.** Em odontologia, a união de dois ou mais dentes numa unidade rígida por meio de restaurações ou aparelhos fixos ou removíveis. **3.** Enrijecimento de parte do corpo para evitar a dor causada pelo movimento dessa parte, como numa fratura ou outra lesão. **4.** Em psiquiatria, o exercício feito pela família, por amigos e colaboradores das várias estratégias, destinado a minimizar o comprometimento e aumentar a função de uma pessoa com função cortical superior diminuída.

splints. Exostoses que ocorrem ao longo do trajeto dos pequenos ossos do metacarpo e metatarso do cavalo. VER splint.

split·ting. Desdobramento, clivagem; em química, a clivagem de uma ligação covalente, fragmentando a molécula envolvida.

spm Abreviatura de um gene que leva à *su*pressão e *m*utação de alelos instáveis.

spo·dog·e·nous (spō-doj'e-nŭs). Espodógeno; causado por escórias. [G. *spodos*, cinzas + *-gen,* produzindo]

spod·o·gram (spŏ′dō-gram). Espodograma; padrão de resíduo de cinzas formado por microincineração de uma amostra de tecido diminuta, geralmente um corte fino. [G. *spodos*, cinzas + *gramma*, desenho]

spo·dog·ra·phy (spō-dog′-ră-fē). Espodografia. SIN microincineration. [G. *spodos*, cinzas + *graphō*, escrever]

spo·doph·o·rous (spō-dof′ō-rŭs). Espodóforo; que remove ou retira as escórias do corpo. [G. *spodos*, cinzas + *phoros*, que transporta]

spoke-shave (spōk′-shāv). Rasoura. SIN ring-knife.

spon·da·ic (spon-dā′ik). Espondaico; relativo ao espondeu.

spon·dee (spon′dē). Espondeu; palavra dissílaba com acentuação geralmente equivalente em cada uma das duas sílabas; utilizada no teste da audição da fala. [Fr.]

spondyl-. Espondil-. VER spondylo-.

spon·dy·lal·gia (spon-di-lal′jē-ă). Espondilalgia; dor na coluna vertebral. [spondyl- + G. *algos*, dor]

spon·dy·lar·thri·tis (spon-dil-ar-thrī′tis). Espondilartrite; inflamação das articulações intervertebrais. [spondyl- + G. *arthron*, articulação + -*itis*, inflamação]

spon·dy·lit·ic (spon-di-lit′ik). Espondilítico; relativo à espondilite.

spon·dy·li·tis (spon-di-lī′tis). Espondilite; inflamação de uma ou mais vértebras. [spondyl- + G. -*itis*, inflamação]

  ankylosing s., e. ancilosante, e. anquilosante; artrite da coluna vertebral, semelhante à artrite reumatóide, que pode evoluir para ancilose óssea, com formação de rebordos nas margens vertebrais; a doença é mais comum nos homens, freqüentemente com ausência do fator reumatóide e presença do antígeno HLA. Existe uma notável associação com o tipo tecidual B27, e a acentuada agregação familiar sugere um importante fator genético, talvez herdado como caráter autossômico dominante [MIM*106300]; todavia, o mecanismo permanece obscuro. SIN Marie-Strümpell disease, rheumatoid s., Strümpell-Marie disease.

  s. defor′mans, e. deformante; artrite e osteíte deformante acometendo a coluna vertebral; caracterizada por depósitos nodulares nas bordas dos discos intervertebrais, com ossificação dos ligmanetos e ancilose óssea das articulações intervertebrais, resultando em cifose arredondada com rigidez. SIN Bechterew disease, poker back, Strümpell disease (1).

  rheumatoid s., e. reumatóide. SIN ankylosing s.

  tuberculous s., e. tuberculosa; infecção tuberculosa da coluna vertebral associada a uma angulação aguda da coluna no local da doença. SIN Pott disease.

spondylo-, spondyl-. Espôndilo-, espondil-. As vértebras. [G. *spondylos*, vértebra]

spon·dy·lo·lis·the·sis (spon′di-lō-lis-thē′sis). Espondilolistese; movimento para a frente do corpo de uma das vértebras lombares inferiores sobre a vértebra abaixo dela ou sobre o sacro. SIN spondyloptosis. [spondylo- + G. *olisthēsis*, deslizamento e queda]

spon·dy·lo·lis·thet·ic (spon′di-lō-lis-thet′ik). Espondilolistético; relativo à espondilolistese ou caracterizado por ela.

spon·dy·lol·y·sis (spon-di-lol′i-sis). Espondilólise; degeneração ou desenvolvimento deficiente de parte da vértebra; em geral, acomete a parte interarticular, podendo resultar em espondilolistese. [spondylo- + G. *lysis*, afrouxamento]

spon·dy·lo·ma·la·cia (spon-di-lō-mă-lā′shē-ă). Espondilomalacia; amolecimento das vértebras com colapso de múltiplos corpos vertebrais. [spondylo- + G. *malakia*, amolecimento]

spon·dy·lop·a·thy (spon-di-lop′ă-thē). Espondilopatia; qualquer doença das vértebras ou da coluna vertebral. [spondylo- + G. *pathos*, sofrimento]

spon·dy·lop·to·sis (spon′di-lō-tō′sis). Espondiloptose, espondilolistese. SIN spondylolisthesis. [spondylo- + G. *ptōsis*, queda]

spon·dy·lo·py·o·sis (spon′di-lō-pī-ō′sis). Espondilopiose; inflamação supurativa de um ou mais corpos vertebrais. [spondylo- + G. *pyōsis*, supuração]

spon·dy·los·chi·sis (spon-di-los′ki-sis). Espondilosquise; falha embriológica da fusão do arco vertebral. VER spina bifida. [spondylo- + G. *schisis*, fissura]

spon·dy·lo·sis (spon-di-lō′sis). Espondilose; ancilose das vértebras; termo freqüentemente aplicado de modo inespecífico a qualquer lesão da coluna vertebral de natureza degenerativa. [G. *spondylos*, vértebra]

  cervical s., e. cervical; e. que afeta as vértebras cervicais, os discos intervertebrais e o tecido mole circundante.

  hyperostotic s., e. hiperostótica. SIN diffuse idiopathic skeletal *hyperostosis*.

spon·dy·lo·syn·de·sis (spon′di-lō-sin-dē′sis). Espondilossíndese. SIN spinal *fusion*. [spondylo- + G. *syndesis*, união]

spon·dy·lo·tho·rac·ic (spon′di-lō-thō-ras′ik). Esponditorácico; relativo às vértebras e ao tórax.

spon·dy·lous (spon′di-lŭs). Espondiloso; relativo a uma vértebra.

sponge (spŭnj). Esponja. **1.** Material absorvente, como gaze ou algodão preparado, utilizado para absorver líquidos. **2.** Membro do filo Porifera, cujo endoesqueleto celular é uma fonte de esponjas comerciais. SIN spongia. [G. *spongia*]

  absorbable gelatin s., e. de gelatina absorvível; e. com base gelatinosa hidrossolúvel, absorvível e estéril, utilizada para controlar o sangramento capilar em cirurgias; é colocada *in situ* e absorvida em 4 a 6 semanas.

  Bernays s., e. de Bernays; disco comprimido de algodão asséptico que aumenta de volume quando umedecido; utilizado no enchimento de cavidades.

  compressed s., e. comprimida; esponja impregnada com mucilagem fina de acácia, envolvida com cordão até o formato desejado e, em seguida, seca; utilizada para dilatar seios, o óstio uterino, etc., porque absorve a umidade após sua inserção. SIN sponge tent.

  contraceptive s., e. contraceptiva; esponja hidrofílica elástica de espuma de poliuretano, impregnada com espermicida; a contracepção é obtida pela ação do espermicida; não é mais fabricada nos Estados Unidos.

spon·gia (spŭn′jē-ă). Esponja. SIN sponge. [G.]

spon·gi·form (spŭn′ji-form). Espongiforme. SIN spongy.

spongio-. Espôngio-. Esponja, semelhante a esponja, esponjoso. [G. *spongia*]

spon·gi·o·blast (spŭn′jē-ō-blast). Espongioblasto; célula do epêndima filiforme, neuroepitelial, que se estende por toda a espessura da parede do cérebro ou da medula espinal, isto é, da membrana limitante interna até a externa; os espongioblastos transformam-se em células da neuróglia e ependimárias. VER TAMBÉM glioblast. [spongio- + G. *blastos*, germe]

spon·gi·o·blas·to·ma (spŭn′jē-ō-blas-tō′mă). Espongioblastoma. **1.** Glioma que consiste em células (alongadas, fusiformes e, algumas vezes, pleomórficas, com um ou dois prolongamentos fibrilares) que se assemelham a espongioblastos embrionários, ocorrendo normalmente em torno do canal neural do embrião humano; seu crescimento é relativamente lento, originando-se, em geral, no tronco cerebral, no quiasma óptico ou no infundíbulo; infiltra estruturas adjacentes ou provoca compressão do terceiro e do quarto ventrículos. Antigamente, os espongioblastos eram subclassificados em e. polar e e. unipolar. **2.** Termo obsoleto para glioblastoma multiforme. [spongioblast + G. -*oma*, tumor]

spon·gi·o·cyte (spŭn′jē-ō-sīt). Espongiócito. **1.** Célula da neuróglia. **2.** Célula na zona fasciculada da supra-renal, contendo numerosas gotículas de material lipídico que, após coloração com hematoxilina e eosina, exibem acentuada vacuolização. [spongio- + G. *kytos*, célula]

spon·gi·oid (spŭn′jē-oyd). Espongióide. SIN spongy. [spongio- + G. *eidos*, semelhança]

spon·gi·ose (spŭn′jē-ōs). Esponjoso.; semelhante a ou característico de uma esponja. [L. *spongiosus*]

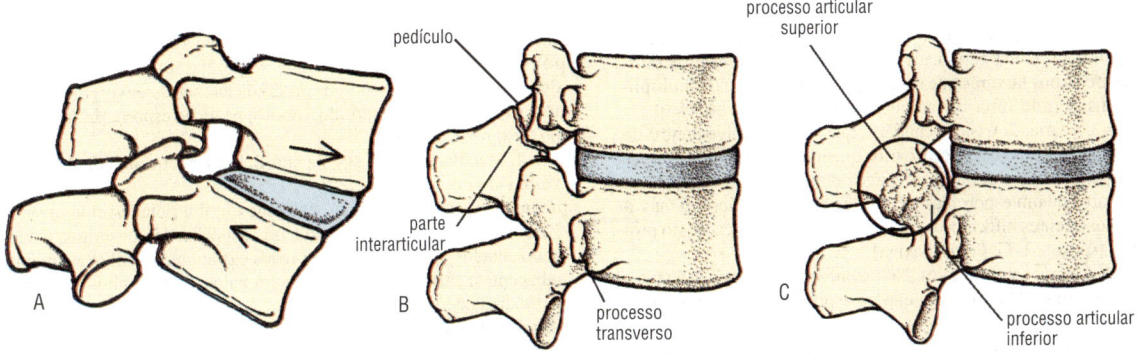

espondilolistese: (A) mostrando o deslizamento anterior das vértebras lombares; **espondilólise:** (B) mostrando a fratura da parte interarticular; **espondilose:** (C) mostrando a fixação dos processos articulares

spon·gi·o·sis (spŭn-jē-ō′sis). Espongiose; edema intercelular inflamatório da epiderme.

spon·gi·o·si·tis (spŭn-jē-ō-sī′tis). Espongiosite; inflamação do corpo esponjoso ou do corpo cavernoso da uretra.

spongy (spŭn′jē). Esponjoso; que possui textura ou aspecto esponjoso. SIN spongiform, spongioid.

spon·ta·ne·ous (spon-tā′nē-ŭs). Espontâneo; sem causa aparente; diz-se de processos mórbidos ou remissões. [L. *spontaneus*, voluntário, caprichoso]

spoon (spoon). Colher; instrumento com um cabo e uma pequena extremidade em forma de tigela ou taça. [A.S. *spōn*, lasca]
  cataract s., c. de catarata; pequeno instrumento côncavo para remover uma lente afetada por catarata.
  Daviel s., c. de Davie; pequeno instrumento ovóide para remoção dos remanescentes de uma catarata após discissão.
  sharp s., c. cortante; instrumento com uma pequena extremidade em forma de taça dotado de bordas cortantes, utilizado para raspar lesões cutâneas.
  Volkmann s., c. de Volkmann; colher com borda cortante para raspar o osso cariado ou outro tecido doente.

△ **spor-.** Espor-. VER sporo-.

spo·rad·ic (spō-rad′ik). Esporádico. **1.** Que indica um padrão temporal de ocorrência de doença numa população de animais ou na população humana, em que a doença surge apenas raramente, sem regularidade. VER endemic, epidemic, enzootic, epizootic. **2.** No contexto genético, indica um singleto. Esse termo abrange diversos fenômenos muito diferentes e distintos, incluindo uma nova mutação; não-paternidade oculta; a probabilidade de um caráter recessivo em dois genitores portadores com uma pequena família; variabilidade extrema na expressão de um gene; fenocópia ambiental; genocópia multilocal, etc. Não é possível prever nenhuma propriedade útil em todos os mebros dessa classe, sendo o termo inútil especulativamente. **3.** Que ocorre de modo irregular, ao acaso. [G. *sporadikos*, esporádico]

spo·ra·din (spŏr′a-din). Esporadina; estágio de gametócito de um parasita gregarino após ter perdido seu epimerito ou mucro.

spo·ran·gi·o·phore (spō-ran′jē-ō-fōr). Esporangióporo; nos fungos, hifa especializada que possui um esporângio em sua extremidade. [sporangium + G. *phoros*, portador]

spo·ran·gi·um (spō-ran′jē-ŭm). Esporângio; estrutura (célula) saculiforme no interior de um fungo, em que se formam esporos assexuados por clivagem progressiva. [L. do G. *sporos*, semente + *angeion*, vaso]

spore (spōr). Esporo. **1.** O corpo reprodutor assexuado ou sexuado dos fungos ou protozoários esporozoários. **2.** Célula de um vegetal de organização inferior às plantas espermatofíticas que possuem sementes. **3.** Forma resistente de certas espécies de bactérias. **4.** O corpo reprodutivo muito modificado de certos protozoários, como nos filos Microspora e Myxozoa. [G. *sporos*, semente]
  black s., e. negro; parasita da malária ou outro parasita do sangue em degeneração no corpo do mosquito.

spo·ri·ci·dal (spōr-i-sī′dal). Esporicida; letal para esporos. [spori- + L. *caedo*, matar]

spo·ri·cide (spōr′i-sīd). Esporicida; agente que mata esporos.

spo·rid·i·um, pl. **spo·rid·ia** (spō-rid′ē-ŭm, -ă). Esporídio; esporo protozoário; microrganismo protozoário embrionário. [L. mod. dim. do G. *sporos*, semente]

△ **sporo-, spori-, spor-.** Esporo-, spori-, spor-. Semente, esporo. [G. *sporos*]

spo·ro·ag·glu·ti·na·tion (spōr′ō-a-gloo-ti-nā′shŭn). Esporoaglutinação; método diagnóstico em relação às micoses, baseado no fato de que o sangue de pacientes com doenças causadas por fungos contém aglutininas específicas que causam a agregação dos esporos desses organismos.

spo·ro·blast (spōr′ō-blast). Esporoblasto; estágio inicial no desenvolvimento de um esporocisto, antes da diferenciação dos esporozoítas. VER TAMBÉM oocyst, sporocyst (2), pansporoblast. SIN zigotomere. [sporo- + G. *blastos*, germe]

spo·ro·cyst (spōr′ō-sist). Esporocisto. **1.** Forma larvar do trematódeo digenético que se desenvolve no corpo de um molusco, seu hospedeiro intermediário, geralmente um caramujo; o esporocisto forma uma estrutura saculiforme simples com células germinativas que brotam internamente e transformam-se em outros tipos larvares que continuam esse processo de multiplicação larvar (considerado uma forma de poliembrionia). VER TAMBÉM miracidium, redia, cercaria. **2.** Cisto secundário que se desenvolve dentro do oocisto de Coccidia, um grupo de esporozoários que inclui muitos dos agentes patológicos mais importantes de animais e aves domésticos; o esporocisto desenvolve-se a partir de um esporoblasto e produz no seu interior um ou vários esporozoítas, os agentes infecciosos para infecção e multiplicação no próximo hospedeiro. [sporo- + G. *kystis*, bexiga]

Spo·ro·cys·tin·ea (spōr′ō-sis-tin′ē-ă). Nos esquemas de classificação mais antigos, uma subordem de Coccidia em que os esporoblastos desenvolvem esporocistos. [sporo- + G. *kystis*, bexiga]

spo·ro·do·chi·um (spō-rō-dō′kē-ŭm). Esporodóquio; nos fungos, estroma em forma de coxim, recoberto por conidióforos.

spo·ro·gen·e·sis (spōr-ō-jen′ĕ-sis). Esporogênese. SIN sporogony. [sporo- + G. *genesis*, produção]

spo·rog·e·nous (spō-roj′ĕ-nŭs). Esporógeno; relativo a ou envolvido na esporogonia.

spo·rog·e·ny (spō-roj′ĕ-nē). Esporogenia. SIN sporogony.

spo·rog·o·ny (spō-rog′ō-nē). Esporogonia; a formação de esporozoítas em protozoários esporozoários, um processo de divisão assexuada dentro do esporoblasto, que se transforma no esporocisto dentro de um oocisto; segue-se a fusão dos gametas (gametogonia) e a formação do zigoto (esporonte). SIN sporogenesis, sporogeny. [sporo- + G. *goneia*, geração]

spo·ront (spōr′ont). Esporonte; o estágio de zigoto no interior da parede do oocisto no ciclo de vida dos coccídeos; origina esporoblastos, que formam esporocistos, no interior dos quais são produzidos os esporozoítas infectantes. [sporo- + G. *ōn* (*ont*-), ser]

spo·ro·phore (spōr′ō-fōr). Esporóforo; quaisquer hifas especializadas em fungos que dão origem a esporos. [sporo- + G. *phoros*, portador]

spo·ro·plasm (spōr′ō-plazm). Esporoplasma; o protoplasma de um esporo. [sporo- + G. *plasma*, algo formado]

spo·ro·the·ca (spōr′ō-thē′kă). Esporoteca; o envoltório que encerra os minúsculos esporos em forma de agulha de certos esporozoários. [sporo- + G. *thēkē*, caixa]

Spo·ro·thrix (spōr′ō-thriks). Gênero de fungos imperfeitos dimórficos, incluindo a espécie *S. schenckii*, um microrganismo de distribuição mundial e agente etiológico da esporotricose nos seres humanos e animais, que cresce no solo ou na vegetação, especialmente em arbustos espinhosos, adquirida pelo homem quando espinhos infectados são introduzidos em tecidos subcutâneos; a 37°C, cresce como levedura e parasita os tecidos nessa forma. [L. mod. do G. *sporos*, semente + *thrix*, pêlo]

spo·ro·tri·cho·sis (spōr′ō-tri-kō′sis). Esporotricose; micose cutânea que se dissemina através dos linfáticos; causada por inoculação do *Sporothrix schenckii*, tipicamente raro em cortes histológicos, porém de rápido crescimento em culturas. A esporotricose extracutânea origina-se provavelmente nos pulmões, mas dissemina-se, causando doença osteoarticular ou outra doença visceral. A doença pulmonar cavitária crônica constitui outra manifestação. SIN Schenck disease.

Spo·ro·tri·chum (spō-rot′ri-kŭm). Gênero de fungos imperfeitos (Hyphomycetes), que são habitualmente contaminantes comuns. [L. mod. do G. *sporos*, semente + *thrix*, pêlo]

spo·ro·zo·an (spōr-ō-zō′an). Esporozoário. **1.** Microrganismo da classe Sporozoea. SIN sporozoon. **2.** Relativo aos Sporozoea.

Spo·ro·zo·as·i·da (spōr′ō-zō-as′i-dă). SIN Sporozoea.

Spor·o·zo·ea (spōr-ō-zō′ē-ă). Grande classe de protozoários (filo Apicomplexa, sub-reino Protozoa), consistindo em parasitas obrigatórios com esporos simples, que não possuem filamentos polares; não há cílios nem flagelos (exceto nos microgametas, encontrados em alguns grupos), e a locomoção é feita por ondulação, deslizamento ou flexão do corpo; a sexualidade, quando presente, é por singamia, formando oocistos com esporozoítas infectantes por esporogonia. A classe inclui os gregarinos e os coccídeos, abrangendo estes últimos muitos agentes causadores de doença humana e animal, como os plasmódios da malária. SIN Sporozoasida, Telosporea. [L. mod. do G. *sporos*, semente + *zōon*, animal]

spo·ro·zo·ite (spōr-ō-zō′īt). Espozoíto; um dos minúsculos corpos alongados produzidos pela divisão repetida do oocisto durante a esporogonia. No caso do parasita da malária, trata-se da forma que se concentra nas glândulas salivares e é introduzido no sangue pela picada de um mosquito; penetra nos hepatócitos (ciclo exoeritrocitário), cuja prole, os merozoítos, infecta os eritrócitos, iniciando a malária clínica. SIN germinal rod, zoite, zygotoblast. [sporo- + G. *zōon*, animal]

spo·ro·zo·on (spōr-ō-zō′on). Esporozoário. SIN sporozoan (1).

sport (spōrt). Organismo que varia, no todo ou em parte, sem razão aparente, dos demais de seu tipo; essa variação pode ser transmitida aos descendentes, ou estes últimos podem voltar ao tipo original. SIN singleton (2). [I. m. *disporte*, do Fr. ant. *desport*, diversão]

spor·u·lar (spōr′ū-lăr). Esporular; relativo a um esporo ou espórulo.

spor·u·la·tion (spōr′oo-lā′shŭn). Esporulação; processo pelo qual as leveduras sofrem miose, sendo os produtos da meiose envolvidos em invólucros.

spor·ule (spōr′ool). Espórulo; esporo; pequeno esporo. [L. mod. *sporula*; dim do G. *sporos*, semente]

spot. 1. Mácula, mancha. SIN macula. **2.** Perder pequeno volume de sangue através da vagina.
  acoustic s., mácula acústica. VER *macula* of utricle, *macula* of saccule.
  Bitot s., manchas de Bitot; pequenos depósitos circunscritos, foscos, branco-acinzentados, espumosos, gordurosos e triangulares sobre a conjuntiva bulbar adjacente à córnea, na área da fissura palpebral de ambos os olhos; ocorre na deficiência de vitamina A.
  blind s., (1) SIN physiologic *scotoma;* **(2)** SIN mental *scotoma;* **(3)** SIN optic *disk.*
  blood s.'s, folículos de Graaf hemorrágicos observados em ovários de fêmeas de camundongos, causados pela injeção de urina de gestantes; resultado positivo no teste de Aschheim-Zondek atualmente obsoleto para gravidez.

blue s., (1) mancha azulada. SIN *macula cerulea*; (2) mancha mongólica. SIN *mongolian s.*
Brushfield s.'s, manchas de Brushfield; condensações de cor clara na superfície da íris; observadas na síndrome de Down.
café-au-lait s.'s, manchas café-com-leite; lesões cutâneas pigmentadas, de castanho-claras a castanho-escuras, produzidas por excesso de melanossomas nas células de Malpighi, e não por excesso de melanócitos; as manchas café-com-leite constituem uma das principais manifestações cutâneas da neurofibromatose (doença de von Recklinghausen); na neurofibromatose tipo 1 (periférica), podem-se observar quase sempre 6 ou mais dessas manchas, em que pelo menos algumas têm um diâmetro de mais de 1,5 cm. Essas manchas são freqüentemente acompanhadas de manchas semelhantes a sardas nas axilas.
cherry-red s., mancha vermelho-cereja; aspecto oftalmoscópico da coróide normal sob a fóvea central, aparecendo como uma mancha vermelha circundada por edema retiniano branco no fechamento da artéria central ou como infiltração lipídica na esfingolipidose. SIN Tay cherry-red s.
corneal s., mancha corneana. SIN *macula corneae*.
cotton-wool s.'s, manchas algodonosas. SIN *cotton-wool patches, em patch*.
De Morgan s.'s, manchas de De Morgan. SIN *senile hemangioma*.
Elschnig s.'s, manchas de Elschnig; manchas amarelas ou vermelho-brilhantes isoladas na coróide, com flocos de pigmento negro em suas bordas, observadas ao exame oftalmoscópico na retinopatia hipertensiva avançada.
flame s.'s, manchas em chama; áreas hemorrágicas que ocorrem na camada de fibras nervosas da retina.
focal s., mancha focal; local de bombardeio de elétrons e emissão de raios X do anodo de um tubo de raios X. VER TAMBÉM focal spot size.
Fordyce s.'s, manchas de Fordyce; condição caracterizada por numerosos corpos ou grânulos pequenos, branco-amarelados, na superfície interna e borda vermelha dos lábios; histologicamente, as lesões são glândulas sebáceas ectópicas. SIN Fordyce disease, Fordyce granules.
Fuchs black s., mancha negra de Fuchs; área de proliferação pigmentar na região macular na miopia degenerativa.
hot s., mancha quente; região em um gene na qual existe uma taxa de mutação ou recombinação supostamente elevada.
hypnogenic s., mancha hipnogênica; ponto sensível à pressão no corpo de determinadas pessoas suscetíveis que, quando pressionado, causa a indução do sono.
Koplik s.'s, manchas de Koplik; pequenas manchas vermelhas na mucosa oral, em cujo centro pode-se observar um minúsculo ponto branco-azulado sob luz intensa; essas manchas ocorrem no início do sarampo, antes da erupção cutânea, e são consideradas um sinal patognomônico da doença.
liver s., lentigo senil. SIN *senile lentigo*.
Mariotte blind s., mancha cega de Mariotte. SIN *optic disk*.
milk s.'s, manchas de leite; (1) placas brancas de tecido fibroso hialinizado situadas no epicárdio sobre o ventrículo direito do coração, onde não está recoberto pelo pulmão. SIN soldier's patches. (2) áreas macroscópicas brancas no omento, devido ao acúmulo de macrófagos e linfócitos. SIN tache laiteuse (1).
mongolian s., mancha mongólica; qualquer uma das diversas manchas arredondadas ou ovais de cor azul-escura ou amora, na região sacral, devido à presença ectópica de melanócitos espalhados na derme. Essas lesões congênitas são freqüentes em filhos de negros, índios norte-americanos e asiáticos, entre 2 e 12 anos de idade, quando então começam a desaparecer gradualmente; não desaparecem à pressão e, algumas vezes, são confundidas com equimoses causadas por maus-tratos. SIN blue s. (2).
mulberry s.'s, manchas em amora; a erupção cutânea abdominal na febre tifóide.
rose s.'s, manchas róseas; exantema característico da febre tifóide; 10–20 pequenas pápulas rosadas, na parte inferior do tronco, que permanecem por alguns dias e deixam uma área de hiperpigmentação.
Roth s.'s, manchas de Roth; mancha redonda e branca na retina, circundada por hemorragia na endocardite bacteriana, bem como em outras condições hemorrágicas da retina.
saccular s., mácula do sáculo. SIN *macula of saccule*.
Soemmerring s., mancha de Soemmerring. SIN *macula of retina*.
spongy s., SIN *vascular zone*.
Tardieu s.'s, equimoses de Tardieu. SIN *Tardieu ecchymoses, em ecchymosis*.
Tay cherry-red s., mancha vermelho-cereja de Tay. SIN *cherry-red s.*
temperature s., mancha térmica; uma de várias manchas de disposição definida na pele sensível ao calor e ao frio, mas não à pressão comum ou a estímulos dolorosos.
tendinous s., mancha tendínea. SIN *macula albida*.
Trousseau s., mancha de Trousseau. SIN *meningitic streak*.
utricular s., mácula do utrículo. SIN *macula of utricle*.
white s., mancha branca. SIN *macula albida*.
yellow s., mácula lútea. SIN *macula of retina*.
spp. Abreviatura do plural de species (espécies).
sprain (sprān). **1.** Entorse; lesão de um ligamento em decorrência da aplicação de forças anormais ou excessivas a uma articulação, porém sem luxação ou fratura. **2.** Causar entorse de uma articulação.

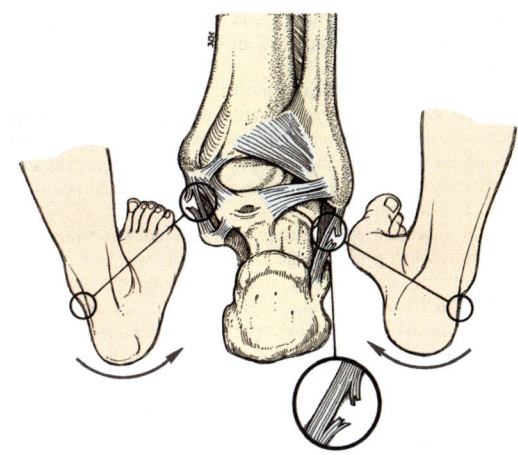

entorse: acometendo os ligamentos do tornozelo

spray (sprā). *Spray*, borrifo, aerossol; jato de líquido em finas gotas, maiores que as do vapor; produzido ao forçar a passagem do líquido por uma minúscula abertura num vaporizador, misturando com ar.
spread·er (spred'er). **1.** Espalhador, espátula; instrumento utilizado para distribuir uma substância sobre uma superfície ou área. **2.** Afastador, dispositivo para afastar ou dividir estruturas.
gutta-percha s., e. guta-percha; instrumento utilizado em odontologia para condensar a guta-percha lateralmente num canal radicular.
rib s., afastador de costelas; retrator para alargar o espaço entre as costelas em cirurgias intratorácicas.
root canal s., afastador do canal radicular; instrumento afilado utilizado para condensar lateralmente materiais de enchimento da raiz.
Sprengel, Otto G.K., cirurgião alemão, 1852–1915. VER S. *deformity*.
sprout (sprowt). Broto; estrutura semelhante ao broto de uma planta.
syncytial s., b. sincicial. SIN *syncytial knot*.
sprue (sproo). **1.** Espru; má absorção intestinal primária com esteatorréia. SIN cachexia aphthosa. **2.** Jito; em odontologia, um cano de cera ou metal empregado para formar a(s) abertura(s) para que o metal fundido flua para o molde; refere-se também ao metal que posteriormente preenche o(s) orifício(s) do jito. [D. *spruw*]
celiac s., e. celíaco. SIN *celiac disease*.
nontropical s., e. não-tropical; espru que ocorre em indivíduos distantes dos trópicos; geralmente denominado doença celíaca; devido a enteropatia induzida por glúten.
tropical s., e. tropical; espru que ocorre nos trópicos, freqüentemente associado a infecção entérica e deficiência nutricional; com freqüência, complicado pela deficiência de folato com anemia macrocítica. SIN tropical diarrhea.
sprue-form·er (sproo-fōr'mer). A base à qual o jito (sprue) (2) é fixado enquanto o molde de cera recebe um revestimento refratário num frasco de modelagem; algumas vezes denominado formador de cadinho.
spud (spŭd). Faca triangular utilizada para remover corpos estranhos da córnea.
Spu·ma·vir·i·nae (spoo'mă-vir'i-nē). Antigamente, uma subfamília de vírus (família Retroviridae) que inclui os vírus (agentes) espumosos de primatas e outros mamíferos; atualmente incluídos no gênero Spumavirus. Em comum com outros retrovírus, possuem DNA polimerases RNA-dependentes (transcriptase reversa). [L. *spuma*, espuma]
Spu·ma·vi·rus (spoo'mă-vī-rŭs). Gênero de vírus que compreende um grupo pouco caracterizado de retrovírus que causam vacuolização (espuma) das células cultivadas; em geral, produzem infecções persistentes, porém silenciosas, em seus hospedeiros naturais; não foi identificada nenhuma doença causada por esses agentes.
spur (sper) [TA], esporão. SIN *calcar*. [A.S. *spora*]
calcarine s. [TA], *Calcar avis*; a menor das duas elevações na parede medial do corno posterior do ventrículo lateral do cérebro produzidas pela profundidade do sulco calcarino. SIN calcar avis [TA], Haller unguis, hippocampus minor, minor hippocampus, Morand s., unguis avis.
Fuchs s., e. de Fuchs; proliferação epitelial do músculo dilatador da pupila aproximadamente a meia distância na largura do esfíncter; parte da inserção do músculo dilatador no esfíncter da íris.
Grunert s., e. de Grunert; crescimento epitelial do músculo dilatador da pupila na junção da íris com o corpo ciliar; parte da origem do músculo dilatador da íris.
heel s., e. do calcâneo; espessamento ósseo da superfície flexora do calcâneo associado a dor intensa na posição ortostática.

Michel s., e. de Michel; crescimento epitelial do músculo dilatador da pupila na borda periférica do esfíncter; parte da inserção do músculo dilatador no esfíncter da íris.

Morand s., e. de Morand. SIN calcarine s.

scleral s. [TA], e. da esclera; crista circular da esclera na face interna da junção corneoescleral; em corte transversal, aparece como um processo semelhante a um gancho profundamente ao seio venoso escleral; relativamente rígido, fornece a fixação (origem) para as fibras meridionais do corpo ciliar. SIN calcar sclerae [TA], scleral roll.

vascular s., e. vascular; septo parcial entre vasos (artérias e veias) ao nível da fusão ou ramificação em ângulo agudo. VER TAMBÉM calcar (1).

spu·ri·ous (spoo'rē-ŭs). Espúrio; falso; não-genuíno. [L. *spurius*]

spu·tum, pl. **spu·ta** (spū'tŭm-ta). Esputo; escarro. **1.** Material expectorado, especialmente muco ou material mucopurulento expectorado em doenças das vias aéreas. VER TAMBÉM expectoration (1). **2.** Massa individual desse material. [L. *sputum,* de *spuo,* pp. *sputus,* cuspir]

s. aerogeno'sum, expectoração verde observada algumas vezes na icterícia, devido à coloração do escarro por pigmentos biliares. SIN green s.

globular s., e. globular. SIN nummular s.

green s., e. verde. SIN s. aerogenosum.

nummular s., e. numular; massa espessa e coerente expectorada em forma globular, que não corre no fundo do recipiente, mas que forma uma massa discóide numular. SIN globular s.

prune-juice s., e. em suco de ameixa; expectoração fina avermelhada, característica de necrose do tecido pulmonar, geralmente por infecção; devido à hemorragia causada pela destruição do parênquima pulmonar; algumas vezes observado em tumores pulmonares. SIN prune-juice expectoration.

rusty s., e. ferruginoso; expectoração tinta de sangue, castanho-avermelhada, característica da pneumonia pneumocócica lobar.

SQ Abreviatura de subcutaneous (subcutâneo).

squalamine lactate (skwal'a-mēn lak'tāt). Lactato de esqualamina; agente antiangiogênico não-citotóxico utilizado no tratamento de tumores sólidos.

squa·lene (skwā'lēn). Esqualeno; hidrocarboneto hexaisoprenóide (triterpenóide) encontrado no óleo de tubarão e em algumas plantas; intermediário na biossíntese do colesterol e de outros esteróis e triterpenos.

s. epoxidase, e. epoxidase; enzima que catalisa a conversão do esqualeno em esqualeno-2,3-óxido no retículo endoplasmático; etapa necessária para a ocorrência de ciclização, levando à síntese do primeiro esterol, o lanosterol, na esteroidogênese; utiliza NADPH.

s. synthase, e. sintase; enzima que catalisa a formação do esqualeno a partir de duas moléculas de farnesilpirofosfato utilizando NADPH e produção concomitante de duas moléculas de pirofosfato.

squa·ma, pl. **squa·mae** (skwā'mă, skwā'mē). Escama. **1.** Placa delgada de osso. **2.** Escama epidérmica. SIN squame. SIN scale (2). [L. uma escama]

frontal s., escama occipital. SIN squamous part of frontal bone.

s. fronta'lis [TA], e. frontal. SIN squamous part of frontal bone.

s. occipita'lis, occipital s. [TA], e. occipital. SIN squamous part of occipital bone.

temporal s., parte escamosa do temporal. SIN squamous part of temporal bone.

s. tempora'lis, parte escamosa do temporal. SIN squamous part of temporal bone.

squa·ma·ti·za·tion (skwā'mă-ti-zā'shŭn). Escamatização; transformação de outros tipos de células em células escamosas.

squame (skwām). Escama. SIN squama (2).

♳ **squamo-.** Escamo-; escama, escamoso. [L. *squama,* uma escama]

squa·mo·cel·lu·lar (skwā-mō-sel'ū-lăr). Escamocelular; relativo a ou que possui epitélio escamoso.

squa·mo·co·lum·nar (skwā-mō-kol'ŭm-năr). Escamocolunar; refere-se à junção entre uma superfície epitelial escamosa estratificada e uma superfície revestida por epitélio colunar; p. ex., o cárdia do estômago ou ânus.

squa·mo·fron·tal (skwā'mō-frŏn'tăl). Escamofrontal; relativo à parte escamosa do osso frontal.

squa·mo·mas·toid (skwā'mō-mas'toyd). Escamomastóide; relativo às partes escamosa e petrosa do osso temporal.

squa·mo·oc·cip·i·tal (skwā'mō-ok-sip'i-tăl). Escamoccipital; relativo à parte escamosa do osso occipital, desenvolvendo-se, em parte, na membrana e, em parte, na cartilagem.

squa·mo·pa·ri·e·tal (skwā'mō-pă-rī'ē-tăl). Escamoparietal; relativo ao osso parietal e à parte escamosa do osso temporal.

squa·mo·pe·tro·sal (skwā'mō-pē-trō'săl). Escamopetroso. SIN petrosquamosal.

squa·mo·sa, pl. **squa·mo·sae** (skwā-mō'să, -sē). As partes escamosas dos ossos frontal, occipital ou temporal, sobretudo a última. [L. *squamosus,* escamoso, de *squama,* escama]

squa·mo·sal (skwā-mō'săl). Escamoso; relativo principalmente à parte escamosa do osso temporal.

squa·mo·sphe·noid (skwā'mō-sfē'noyd). Escamoesfenóide; relativo ao osso esfenóide e à parte escamosa do osso temporal. SIN sphenosquamosal.

squa·mo·tem·po·ral (skwā'mō-tem'pŏ-răl). Escamotemporal; relativo à parte escamosa do osso temporal.

squa·mo·tym·pan·ic (skwā'mō-tim-man'ik). Escamotimpânico. SIN tympanosquamosal.

squa·mous (skwā'mŭs). Escamoso; relativo a, ou coberto por, escamas. SIN scaly. [L. *squamosus*]

squa·mo·zy·go·mat·ic (skwā'mō-zī-gō-mat'ik). Escamozigomático; relativo à parte escamosa do osso temporal e ao processo zigomático do osso temporal.

squill (skwil). Cila; as escamas internas carnosas cortadas e secas do bulbo da variedade branca de *Urginea maritima* (Cila do Mediterrâneo) ou de *U. indica* (Cila indiana) (família Liliaceae); a porção central do bulbo é excluída durante o seu processamento; a cila contém glicosídeos cardíacos (cilareno-A e cilareno-B) e cilaricida, um rodenticida. SIN scilla. [L. *squilla* ou *scilla*]

squint (skwint). **1.** Estrabismo. SIN strabismus. **2.** Sofrer de estrabismo.

convergent s., e. convergente. SIN esotropia.

divergent s., e. divergente. SIN exotropia.

external s., e. externo. SIN exotropia.

internal s., e. interno. SIN esotropia.

^{87m}**Sr** Abreviatura do estrôncio-87m.

Sr Símbolo de strontium (estrôncio).

sr. Abreviatura de steradian (esteradiano).

^{85}**Sr** Abreviatura de strontium-85 (estrôncio-85).

^{89}**Sr** Símbolo de strontium-89 (estrôncio-89).

^{90}**Sr** Símbolo de strontium-90 (estrôncio-90).

SRF Abreviatura de somatotropin-releasing *factor* (fator liberador da somatotropina).

SRF-A Abreviatura de slow-reacting *factor* of anaphylaxis (fator de reação lenta da anafilaxia).

SRH Abreviatura de somatotropin-releasing *hormone* (hormônio liberador de somatotropina).

SRIF Abreviatura de somatotropin release-inhibiting *factor* (fator inibidor da liberação da somatotropina).

sRNA Abreviatura de soluble RNA (RNA solúvel). Ver entradas em ribonucleic acid.

S ro·ma·num (rō-mā'nŭm). Termo arcaico para colo sigmóide.

SRP Abreviatura de signal recognition *particle* (partícula reconhecedora de sinal).

SRS Abreviatura de slow-reacting *substance* (substância de reação lenta).

SRS-A Abreviatura de slow-reacting *substance* of anaphylaxis (substância de reação lenta da anafilaxia).

ss Abreviatura de single-stranded (monofilamentar), steady *state* (equilíbrio dinâmico).

SSPE Abreviatura de subacute sclerosing *panencephalitis* (panencefalite esclerosante subaguda).

SSPL Abreviatura de saturation sound pressure *level* (nível de saturação da pressão sonora).

SSS Abreviatura de soluble specific *substance* (substância específica solúvel).

stab. Perfurar com um instrumento pontiagudo, como uma faca ou adaga. [Gael. *stob*]

sta·bi·late (stā'bi-lāt). Amostra de microrganismos preservados vivos numa única ocasião, isto é, por congelamento.

sta·bile (stā'bĭl, -bil). Estável, fixo; referindo-se a: 1) determinados constituintes do soro que não são afetados por graus comuns de calor; 2) um eletrodo mantido constantemente sobre uma parte durante a passagem de uma corrente elétrica. Cf. labile. [L. *stabilis*]

stab·i·lim·e·ter (stā-bi-lim'ē-ter). Estabilímetro; instrumento para medir o balanço do corpo quando em posição ortostática, com os pés juntos e, em geral, com os olhos fechados. [L. *stabilitas,* firmeza + G. *metron,* medida]

sta·bil·i·ty (stă-bil'i-tē). Estabilidade; a condição de ser estável ou resistente a mudanças.

denture s., e. da prótese dentária; a qualidade de uma prótese dentária de ser firme, estável, constante e resistente a mudanças de posição quando são aplicadas forças funcionais. SIN stabilization (2).

detrusor s., e. do detrusor; propriedade do detrusor de acomodar um volume vesical crescente sem aumento significativo da pressão do detrusor e sem a sua contração involuntária.

dimensional s., e. dimensional; a propriedade de um material de preservar seu tamanho e sua forma.

endemic s., e. endêmica; situação em que todos os fatores que influenciam a ocorrência de doença são relativamente estáveis, resultando em pouca flutuação na incidência da doença com o decorrer do tempo; as alterações em um ou mais desses fatores (p. ex., redução na proporção de

indivíduos com imunidade à exposição a determinado agente infeccioso) podem levar a uma situação instável na qual ocorrem grandes surtos de doença. SIN enzootic s.
  enzootic s., e. enzoótica. SIN endemic s.
  suspension s., e. de suspensão; velocidade de sedimentação muito lenta.
sta·bi·li·za·tion (stā′bi-li-zā′shŭn). **1.** Estabilização; a obtenção de um estado estável. **2.** Estabilidade. SIN denture *stability.*
sta·bi·liz·er (stā′bi-lī-zer). Estabilizador. **1.** Aquilo que torna algo mais estável. **2.** Agente que retarda o efeito de um acelerador, preservando, assim, um equilíbrio químico. **3.** Uma parte que possui a qualidade de rigidez ou de criar rigidez quando adicionada a outra parte.
  endodontic s., e. endodôntico; pino implantado que atravessa o ápice de um dente a partir do canal radicular e que se estende bem até o osso subjacente para proporcionar a imobilização dos dentes com comprometimento periodontal.
sta·ble (stā′bl). Estável; firme; não-variável; resistente a alterações. VER TAMBÉM stabile.
stach·ybot·ry·o·tox·i·co·sis (stak-ē-bot′rē-ō-tok-si-kō′sis). Estaquibotriotoxicose; tipo de micotoxicose observada em cavalos e gado bovino após a ingestão de feno e forragem contaminados pelo fungo *Stachybotrys atra*; pode ocorrer também em seres humanos expostos ao feno por inalação ou pela absorção da toxina através da pele, manifestando-se por erupção cutânea, faringite e leucopenia leve.
stach·y·drine (stak′i-drēn). Estaquidrina; betaína da L-prolina encontrada na alfafa, no crisântemo e em plantas cítricas.
stach·y·ose (stak′ē-ōs). Estaquiose; rafinosegalactopiranosídeo, um tetrassacarídeo que, ao sofrer hidrólise, produz D-glicose, D-frutose e 2 moles de D-galactose; presente em certos tubérculos e em outros tecidos vegetais.
stac·tom·e·ter (stak-tom′ē-ter). Estalagmômetro. SIN stalagmometer. [G. *staktos*, gotejamento, de *stazō*, deixar cair em gotas + *metron*, medida]
Stader, Otto, cirurgião veterinário norte-americano, *1894. VER S. *splint.*
Staderini, Rutilio, neuroanatomista italiano do século XIX. VER S. *nucleus.*
sta·di·om·e·ter (stā-dē-om′ē-ter). Estadiômetro; instrumento para medir a altura de pé ou sentado. [L. *stadium*, do G. *stadion*, comprimento fixo + G. *metron*, medida]
sta·di·um, pl. **sta·dia** (stā′dē-ŭm, -dē-ă). Estádio; termo obsoleto para referir-se a um estágio na evolução de uma doença, especialmente de uma doença febril aguda. [L. de G. *stadion,* um comprimento padrão fixo]
staff. 1. Equipe; grupo específico de pessoas que trabalham. **2.** Chefe de um serviço. SIN director (1). [A.S. *staef*]
  attending s., e. de assistência; médicos e cirurgiões que são membros de uma e. hospitalar e que atendem regularmente seus pacientes no hospital; além disso, podem supervisionar e ensinar os plantonistas, pós-graduandos e estudantes de medicina.
  consulting s., e. consultora; especialistas afiliados a um hospital que dão pareceres à equipe de assistência.
  house s., e. de residentes; médicos e cirurgiões em treinamento na sua especialidade num hospital que cuidam dos pacientes sob a direção e supervisão da equipe de assistência.
staff of Aes·cu·la·pi·us. Bastão de Esculápio; bastão circundado por uma serpente; símbolo da medicina e emblema da *American Medical Association, Royal Army Medical Corps* (Inglaterra) e *Royal Canadian Medical Corps.* VER TAMBÉM caduceus. [L. *Aesculapius,* G. *Asklēpios,* Deus da medicina]
Stafne, Edward C., patologista oral norte-americano, 1894–1981. VER S. bone *cyst.*
stage (stāj). **1.** Estágio; período na evolução de uma doença; descrição do comprometimento de um processo mórbido ou das condições de um paciente com uma doença específica, como a distribuição e o grau de disseminação de uma doença neoplásica maligna; refere-se também ao ato de determinar o estágio de uma doença, especialmente câncer. VER TAMBÉM period. **2.** Platina; parte de um microscópio sobre a qual se coloca uma lâmina com o objeto a ser examinado. **3.** Estágio; determinada etapa, fase ou posição num processo de desenvolvimento. Para os estágios psicossexuais, Ver subentradas em phase. [I. m. através do Fr. ant. *estage,* do L. *sto,* pp. *status,* ficar de pé]
  algid s., e. o estágio de colapso na cólera.
  Arneth s.'s, estágios de Arneth; classificação diferencial dos neutrófilos polimorfonucleares de acordo com o número de lobos em seus núcleos, isto é, células com 1, 2, 3, 4 ou 5 (ou mais) lobos, designados, respectivamente, como classe I, II, e assim por diante. VER TAMBÉM Arneth *formula.*
  bell s., e. em sino; terceiro estágio no desenvolvimento dos dentes, em que as células formam o epitélio do esmalte interno, o estrato intermédio, o retículo estrelado e o epitélio do esmalte externo; o órgão do esmalte assume a forma de um sino.
  bud s., primeiro estágio no desenvolvimento dos dentes; desenvolvimento dos primórdios dos órgãos do esmalte, os botões dos dentes.
  cap s., o segundo estágio no desenvolvimento dos dentes, em que ocorre desenvolvimento do epitélio do esmalte interno e externo.
  cold s., o estágio de calafrio num paroxismo de malária.
  defervescent s., e. defervescente. VER defervescence.
  end s., e. final; a fase tardia e totalmente desenvolvida de uma doença; p. ex., na doença renal terminal, presença de um rim contraído e fibrosado que pode resultar de várias de doenças crônicas, cujos efeitos sobre o rim se tornaram indistinguíveis.
  eruptive s., e. eruptivo; o estágio de uma doença exantematosa, em que ocorre exantema.
  exoerythrocytic s., e. exoeritrocitário; estágio de desenvolvimento do parasita da malária (*Plasmodium*) nas células do parênquima hepático do hospedeiro vertebrado antes da invasão dos eritrócitos. A geração inicial produz criptozoítos, e a geração seguinte, metacriptozoítos; aparentemente, não ocorre reinfecção dos hepatócitos a partir das células sanguíneas. O desenvolvimento tardio do esporozoíto (hipnozoíto) do *Plasmodium vivax* e do *P. ovale* parece ser responsável pela recidiva da malária que pode ocorrer com esses agentes patológicos.
  genital s., e. genital; que se refere à organização psíquica e que é característica do período genital freudiano da organização psicossocial do lactente. VER genitality. VER TAMBÉM anality, orality.
  imperfect s., e. imperfeito; termo de micologia utilizado para descrever a fase do ciclo de vida assexuada de um fungo. VER anamorph.
  incubative s., período de incubação. SIN incubation *period* (1).
  intuitive s., e. intuitivo; em psicologia, um estágio de desenvolvimento, habitualmente observado entre 4 e 7 anos de idade, em que os processos mentais de uma criança são determinados pelos aspectos mais proeminentes dos estímulos aos quais é exposta, e não por alguma forma de pensamento lógico.
  s. of invasion, período de invasão. SIN incubation *period* (1).
  s.'s of labor, fases do trabalho de parto. VER labor.
  latent s., e. latente. SIN incubation *period* (1).
  perfect s., e. perfeito; termo de micologia utilizado para descrever a fase do ciclo de vida sexuada de um fungo, em que ocorre formação dos esporos após fusão nuclear. SIN teleomorph.
  preconceptual s., e. pré-conceitual; em psicologia, o e. de desenvolvimento na vida de um lactente, antes do raciocínio conceitual real, em que predomina a atividade sensorimotora.
  prodromal s., e. prodrômico; estágio/sintomas iniciais de doença antes do aparecimento dos sintomas característicos.
  resting s., e. de repouso; o e. quiescente de uma célula ou de seu núcleo, durante o qual não ocorrem alterações cariocinéticas. SIN vegetative s.
  Tanner s., e. de Tanner; e. da puberdade no gráfico de crescimento de Tanner, baseado no crescimento dos pêlos púbicos, desenvolvimento da genitália no sexo masculino e desenvolvimento das mamas no sexo feminino.
  trypanosome s., e. de tripanossoma. VER trypomatigote.
  tumor s., e. tumoral; a extensão da disseminação de uma neoplasia maligna a partir de seu local de origem. VER TAMBÉM TNM *staging.*
  vegetative s., e. vegetativo. SIN resting s.
stag·ger (stag′er). Cambalear; caminhar de modo instável; balançar.
stag·gers (stag′erz). Forma de doença de descompressão, cujos principais sintomas consistem em vertigem, confusão mental e fraqueza muscular.
stag·ing (stāj′ing). Estadiamento. **1.** A determinação ou classificação das fases ou períodos distintos na evolução de uma doença ou processo patológico. **2.** Determinação da extensão específica de um processo mórbido num paciente.
  Jewett and Strong s., e. de Jewett e Strong; termo obsoleto para o estadiamento do carcinoma vesical: O, não-invasivo; A, com invasão da submucosa; B, com invasão muscular; C, com invasão da gordura perivascular; D, com metástases para os linfonodos.
  TNM s., e. TNM; sistema de avaliação clinicopatológica de tumores com base na extensão do comprometimento tumoral no local primário (T, seguido de um número, para indicar o tamanho e a profundidade da invasão) e no comprometimento dos linfonodos (N) e metástases (M), todos seguidos de um número que começa em 0 para a ausência de metástases evidentes; os números usados dependem do órgão acometido e influenciam o prognóstico e a escolha do tratamento.
stag·na·tion (stag-nā′shŭn). Estagnação; retardo ou cessação do fluxo sanguíneo nos vasos, como na congestão passiva; acentuada redução ou acúmulo em qualquer parte de um líquido normalmente circulante. [L. *stagnum,* lago, poço]
Stahl, Friedrich K., médico alemão, 1811–1873. VER S. *ear.*
Stahl, George E., médico e químico alemão, 1660–1734. Promulgou a teoria do flogístico. VER phlogiston.
Stähli, Jean, oftalmologista suíço, *1890. VER Hudson-S. *line.*

sistema de estadiamento de Ann Arbor	
estágio I	comprometimento em uma única região de linfonodos ou uma única localização extralinfática
estágio II	comprometimento de duas ou mais regiões de linfonodos no mesmo lado do diafragma comprometimento contíguo localizado apenas de um local extralinfático e região de linfonodos (estágio IIE)
estágio III	comprometimento de regiões de linfonodos em ambos os lados do diafragma; pode incluir o baço
estágio IV	comprometimento disseminado de um ou mais órgãos extralinfáticos, com ou sem comprometimento de linfonodos

estadiamento TNM			
T	—	tumor primário	
TX		tumor primário que não pode ser avaliado	
T0		nenhuma base para um tumor primário	
Tis		carcinoma/tumor *in situ*	
T1, T2, T3, T4		tamanhos e/ou graus crescentes de invasão tumoral primária	
N	—	linfonodos regionais	
NX		linfonodos regionais que não podem ser avaliados	
N0		nenhuma metástase para linfonodos regionais	
N1, N2, N3		invasão crescente de linfonodos regionais	
M	—	metástase	
MX		a existência de metástases não pode ser avaliada	
M0		nenhuma metástase	
M1		presença de metástases	
		a categoria M1 pode ser subdividida da seguinte maneira:	
		pulmão PUL	medula óssea MAR
		osso OSS	costelas PLE
		fígado HEP	peritônio PER
		cérebro BRA	pele SKI
		linfonodos LYM	outros órgãos OTH
R	—	tumor residual (pós-operatório)	
R0		nenhum tumor residual	
R1		tumor residual microscópico	
R2		tumor residual macroscópico	
G	—	grau (graduação) de diferenciação histopatológica	
GX		o grau de diferenciação não pode ser determinado	
G1		bem diferenciado	
G2		moderadamente diferenciado	
G3		pouco diferenciado	
G4		indiferenciado	

STAIN

stain (stān). **1.** Descolorar. **2.** Colorir; corar. **3.** Descoloração. **4.** Corante utilizado em técnicas histológicas e bacteriológicas. **5.** Procedimento em que um corante ou uma combinação de corantes e reagentes são utilizados para colorir os constituintes das células e dos tecidos. Quanto aos corantes ou substâncias de coloração individuais, VER os nomes específicos. [l.m. *steinen*]
Abbott s. for spores, corante de Abbott para esporos; os esporos coram-se de azul com azul-de-metileno alcalino; os corpos dos bacilos tornam-se rosados com a contracoloração pela eosina.
aceto-orcein s., corante de aceto-orceína; corante utilizado para cromossomas em material citológico seco ao ar ou esmagado.
acid s., corante ácido; corante em que o ânion é o componente colorido da molécula de corante, como, p. ex., eosinato de sódio (eosina).
Ag-AS s., corante Ag-As. SIN silver-ammoniac silver s.
Albert s., corante de Albert; corante para bacilos da difteria e seus grânulos metacromáticos; contém azul-de-toluidina, verde metil, ácido acético glacial, álcool e água destilada.
Altmann anilin-acid fuchsin s., corante de anilina de Altmann-fucsina ácida; mistura de ácido pícrico, anilina e fucsina ácida que cora as mitocôndrias em carmim contra um fundo amarelo.

auramine O fluorescent s., corante fluorescente de auramina O; técnica rápida e acurada para *Mycobacterium tuberculosis,* que utiliza auramina O-fenol e uma contracoloração pelo azul-de-metileno.
basic s., corante básico; corante em que o cátion é o componente colorido da molécula do corante que se liga a grupos aniônicos dos ácidos nucleicos ($PO_4^=$) ou mucopolissacarídeos ácidos (p. ex., sulfato de condroitina).
basic fuchsin-methylene blue s., corante de fucsina básica-azul-de-metileno; corante para cortes epóxi intactos; os cortes de espessura média de tecidos imersos em plástico possuem núcleos corados de púrpura; o colágeno, a lâmina elástica e o tecido conectivo coram-se de azul; as mitocôndrias, a mielina e as gotículas de lipídio, em vermelho; o citoplasma, as células musculares lisas, o axoplasma e os condroblastos, em rosa.
Bauer chromic acid leucofuchsin s., corante de leucofucsina-ácido crômico de Bauer; corante para glicogênio e fungos que utiliza o ácido crômico como agente oxidante de polissacarídeos, seguido pelo reagente de Schiff; o glicogênio e as paredes celulares dos fungos aparecem em cor vermelha intensa.
Becker s. for spirochetes, corante de Becker para espiroquetas; corante aplicado a esfregaços finos fixados em formaldeído-ácido acético; as preparações são tratadas sucessivamente com tanino, ácido carbólico e carbol fucsina.
Bennhold Congo red s., corante de vermelho-Congo de Bennhold; corante amilóide útil para detecção de amilóide em tecido patológico; confere ao amilóide uma coloração vermelha; além disso, induz birrefringência verde no amilóide sob luz polarizada.
Berg s., corante de Berg; método de coloração para espermatozóides que utiliza uma solução de carbol fucsina seguida de ácido acético diluído e azul-de-metileno; os espermatozóides coram-se de vermelho-brilhante, enquanto a maioria das outras estruturas aparecem coradas de azul a púrpura.
Best carmine s., corante carmim de Best; método para demonstração de glicogênio nos tecidos.
Bielschowsky s., corante do Bielschowsky; método de tratamento dos tecidos com nitrato de prata para demonstrar fibras reticulares, neurofibrilas, axônios e dendritos.
Biondi-Heidenhain s., corante de Biondi-Heidenhain; corante obsoleto para espiroquetas que utiliza fucsina ácida e orange G.
Birch-Hirschfeld s., corante de Birch-Hirschfeld; corante obsoleto para demonstrar o amilóide, utilizando castanho de Bismarck e cristal violeta; o amilóide cora-se habitualmente de vermelho-rubi brilhante, enquanto o citoplasma das células não é corado, e os núcleos aparecem castanhos.
Bodian copper-PROTARGOL s., corante de cobre de Body-PROTARGOL; corante que emprega um complexo de proteinato de prata (PROTARGOL) para demonstrar cilindros do eixo e neurofibrilas.
Borrel blue s., corante azul de Borrel; corante para demonstrar espiroquetas, treponemas e *Borrelia,* utilizando óxido de prata (preparado através de soluções mistas de nitrato de prata e bicarbonato de sódio) e azul-de-metileno.
Bowie s., corante de Bowie; corante para grânulos justaglomerulares, em que os cortes de rim são corados numa mistura de vermelho-escarlate de Biebrich e violeta etílico; os grânulos justaglomerulares e as fibras elásticas coram-se de púrpura intenso; os eritrócitos, de âmbar; e o tecido de fundo, em tons de vermelho.
Brown-Brenn s., corante de Brown-Brenn; método para coloração diferencial de bactérias Gram-positivas e Gram-negativas em cortes histológicos; utiliza uma coloração de Gram modificada de cristal violeta, iodo de Gram e fucsina básica.
Cajal astrocyte s., corante para astrócitos de Cajal; método para demonstrar os astrócitos por impregnação numa solução contendo cloreto de ouro e cloreto de mercúrio.
carbol-thionin s., corante de carbol tionina; corante útil para demonstração de bacilos tifóides em esfregaços e cortes, bem como para a substância de Nissl.
C-banding s., corante de banda C; corante de banda seletivo para cromossomas, utilizado em citogenética humana, que emprega a coloração de Giemsa após desnaturação ou extração do DNA por tratamento com álcali, ácido, sal ou calor; apenas as regiões heterocromáticas próximas aos centrômeros e ricas em DNA satélite coram-se, à exceção do cromossoma Y, cujo braço longo cora-se habitualmente por completo. SIN centromere banding s.
centromere banding s., corante de bandas do centrômero. SIN C-banding s.
chromate s. for lead, corante de cromato para chumbo; método em que tecidos preservados em fixadores contendo cromato, como os fixadores de Regaud ou Orth, precipitam o chumbo na forma de cristais de cromato de chumbo amarelos; os cortes fixados em formol são tratados com cromato de potássio acidificado com ácido acético.
chrome alum hematoxylin-phloxine s., corante de hematoxilina de alume de cromo-floxina; corante utilizado para demonstrar as células das ilhotas pancreáticas; as células alfa coram-se de vermelho, enquanto as células beta tornam-se azuis ou não se coram.
Ciaccio s., corante de Ciaccio; método para demonstrar lipídios intracelulares insolúveis complexos utilizando a fixação em solução de formol-dicromato, com imersão em parafina, coloração com sudão III ou IV e exame em montagem aquosa.

contrast s., corante diferencial; corante utilizado para colorir parte de um tecido ou célula que não foi afetada quando a outra parte foi corada por um corante de cor diferente. SIN differential s.

Cresylecht violet s., corante violeta de Cresylecht; corante utilizado para a identificação de *Pneumocystis carinii*.

Da Fano s., corante de Da Fano; corante de prata que produz um enegrecimento dos elementos de Golgi após fixação dos tecidos numa mistura de nitrato e formol.

Dane s., corante de Dane; corante para a pré-queratina, queratina e mucina, que emprega hemalume, floxina, azul de Alcian e orange G; os núcleos exibem coloração laranja a castanha, os mucopolissacarídeos ácidos aparecem azul-pálidos, as queratinas, laranja a vermelho-alaranjado.

DAPI s., corante DAPI; sonda fluorescente sensível para DNA, 4'6-diamidino-2-fenilindol·2HCl, utilizado em microscopia de fluorescência para a detecção do DNA em mitocôndrias de leveduras, cloroplastos, vírus, micoplasmas e cromossomas; o DNA é visualizado em células vivas com coloração vital e após fixação das células em formaldeído.

diazo s. for argentaffin granules, corante diazo para grânulos argentafins; nas células enterocromafins, são utilizados vários sais diazônio para enegrecê-las.

Dieterle s., corante de Dieterle; corante utilizado para demonstrar espiroquetas e corpúsculos de Leishman-Donovan; emprega nitrato de prata e nitrato de urânio.

differential s., corante diferencial. SIN contrast s.

double s., corante duplo; mistura de dois corantes em que cada um deles cora diferentes porções de um tecido ou de uma célula.

Ehrlich acid hematoxylin s., corante de hematoxilina ácida de Ehrlich; tipo de alume de corante hematoxilina utilizado como método de coloração regressiva para núcleos, seguida de diferenciação para a intensidade de coloração necessária; pode-se deixar a solução amadurecer naturalmente à luz do sol ou ser parcialmente oxidada com iodato de sódio.

Ehrlich aniline crystal violet s., corante de anilina violeta cristal de Ehrlich; corantes para bactérias Gram-positivas.

Ehrlich triacid s., corante triácido de Ehrlich; corante leucocitário diferencial que compreende soluções saturadas de orange G, fucsina ácida e verde de metila.

Ehrlich triple s., corante triplo de Ehrlich; mistura de indulina, eosina Y e aurantia.

Einarson gallocyanin-chrome alum s., corante de galocianina-alume de cromo de Einarson; método para a coloração tanto do RNA quanto do DNA em azul intenso; com controles apropriados, pode-se estimar o conteúdo de ácido nucleico das células e núcleos corados por citofotometria; também útil para substância de Nissl.

Eranko fluorescence s., corante fluorescente de Eranko; exposição de cortes congelados ao formaldeído, que produz uma forte fluorescência amarelo-esverdeada nas células que contêm norepinefrina.

Feulgen s., corante de Feulgen; reação citoquímica seletiva para DNA, em que os cortes ou as células são inicialmente hidrolisados com ácido clorídrico para produzir ácido apurínico, sendo então corados com o reagente de Schiff para produzir núcleos de cor magenta; em geral, a concentração de DNA nos nucléolos e nas mitocôndrias é muito baixa para permitir a sua detecção por esse corante. VER TAMBÉM Kasten fluorescent Feulgen s.

Field rapid s., corante rápido de Field; corante que permite um rápido diagnóstico positivo de malária em áreas endêmicas com o uso de esfregaços espessos; emprega o azul-de-metileno e o azur B em tampão de fosfato, sendo a preparação contracorada por eosina em um tampão fosfato.

Fink-Heimer s., corante de Fink-Heimer; método utilizado para a demonstração histológica de degeneração de fibras nervosas e terminações do sistema nervoso central (preto sobre um fundo amarelo).

Flemming triple s., corante triplo de Flemming; corante constituído de safranina, violeta de metila e orange G.

fluorescence plus Giemsa s., corante fluorescente mais Giemsa; corante utilizado para demonstrar a troca de cromátides-irmãs; as células são cultivadas em 5-bromodesoxiuridina, seguidas de preparação cromossômica, coloração em HOECHST 33258, exposição à luz e coloração pelo método de Giemsa; os cromossomas exibem um aspecto de "arlequim".

fluorescent s., corante fluorescente; corante ou procedimento de coloração que utiliza um corante ou uma substância fluorescente que combinar-se-á seletivamente com determinados componentes histológicos e, a seguir, emitirá fluorescência à irradiação com luz ultravioleta ou azul-violeta.

Fontana s., corante de Fontana; método tradicional para impregnação com prata de treponemas e outras formas de espiroquetas.

Fontana-Masson silver s., corante de prata de Fontana-Masson. SIN Masson-Fontana ammoniac silver s.

Foot reticulin impregnation s., impregnação da reticulina de Foot; corante de prata em que a reticulina cora-se de negro, e o colágeno, de castanho-dourado; os cortes são colocados flutuando sobre a superfície de soluções para evitar a contaminação com resíduos de prata.

Fouchet s., corante de Fouchet; reagente de Fouchet empregado para demonstrar pigmentos biliares; os cortes em parafina são utilizados para pigmentos biliares conjugados, e os cortes por congelamento, para os pigmentos biliares não-conjugados.

Fraser-Lendrum s. for fibrin, corante de Fraser-Lendrum para fibrina; procedimento de coloração múltipla, após fixação de Zenker, em que a fibrina, a ceratina e alguns grânulos citoplasmáticos adquirem coloração vermelha, os eritrócitos coram-se de laranja, e o colágeno, de verde.

Friedländer s. for capsules, corante de Friedländer para cápsulas; corante obsoleto que emprega violeta de genciana.

G-banding s., coloração de bandas G; técnica de coloração de cromossomas utilizada em citogenética humana para identificar cromossomas individuais, que produz bandas características; utiliza a fixação em ácido acético, secagem ao ar, desnaturação leve dos cromossomas com enzimas proteolíticas, sais, calor, detergentes ou uréia e, finalmente, coloração pelo método de Gram; as bandas cromossômicas têm aspecto semelhante àquelas fluorocromadas pela coloração das bandas Q. SIN Giemsa chromosome banding s.

Giemsa s., corante de Giemsa; composto contendo eosina–azul-de-metileno e azul-de-metileno, utilizado para demonstrar corpúsculos de Negri, espécies de *Tunga*, espiroquetas e protozoários, bem como para coloração diferencial de esfregaços sanguíneos; também utilizado para cromossomas, algumas vezes após hidrólise da preparação citológica em ácido clorídrico quente, bem como para revelar as bandas G dos cromossomas; freqüentemente utilizado em solução tampão de glicerol-metanol.

Giemsa chromosome banding s., coloração das bandas de cromossomas pelo método de Giemsa. SIN G-banding s.

Glenner-Lillie s. for pituitary, corante de Glenner-Lillie para hipófise; modificação do corante de azul-de-metileno–eosina de Mann, que modifica as proporções do corante, tamponando a mistura de corante e corando a 60°C; os basófilos coram-se de azul a negro, os acidófilos, de vermelho-escuro, os grânulos cromófobos, de cinza a rosado, e os eritrócitos, de laranja; com a modificação, o método também é útil para células enterocromafins, células caliciformes, células de Paneth e células das ilhotas pancreáticas.

Golgi s., corante de Golgi; qualquer um dos vários métodos de coloração de células nervosas, fibras nervosas e neuróglia, utilizando fixação e endurecimento em combinações de formol-dicromato ósmico para vários tecidos, sendo o processo seguido de impregnação com nitrato de prata.

Gomori aldehyde fuchsin s., corante de fucsina aldeído de Gomori; corante utilizado para demonstrar as células beta do pâncreas, a forma de armazenamento do hormônio tireotrópico em células β da adeno-hipófise, substância neurossecretora hipofisária, mastócitos, grânulos, fibras elásticas, mucinas sulfatadas e células gástricas principais.

Gomori chrome alum hematoxylin-phloxine s., corante de hematoxilina de alume de cromo-floxina de Gomori; técnica utilizada para demonstrar os grânulos citoplasmáticos, após fixação de Bouin ou de formol-Zenker, utilizando hematoxilina oxidada mais floxina; no pâncreas, as células β apresentam-se azuis, e as células α e Δ, vermelhas, enquanto os grânulos de zimogênio são vermelhos ou não se coram; na hipófise, as células α tornam-se rosadas; as células β e os cromófobos, cinza-azulado; e os núcleos, púrpura a azuis.

Gomori-Jones periodic acid-methenamine-silver s., corante de ácido periódico-metenamina-prata de Gomori-Jones; método de coloração que utiliza metenamina-prata, ácido periódico, cloreto de ouro, hematoxilina e eosina para delinear a membrana basal, a reticulina, o colágeno e os núcleos; utilizado em histopatologia renal. VER TAMBÉM Rambourg periodic acid-chromic methenamine-silver s.

Gomori methenamine-silver s.'s (GMS), corantes de metenamina-prata de Gomori; técnicas para 1) *células argentafins:* método que utiliza uma solução de metenamina-prata em combinação com cloreto de ouro, tiossulfato de sódio e safranina O; os grânulos argentafins aparecem castanho-pretos contra um fundo verde; 2) *uratos:* cortes a quente tratados diretamente com uma solução de metenamina-prata quente para produzir enegrecimento dos uratos; 3) *fungos* ver Grocott-Gomori methenamine-silver s.; 4) *melanina,* que reduz o nitrato de prata.

Gomori nonspecific acid phosphatase s., corante para fosfatase ácida inespecífica de Gomori; método em que os cortes por congelamento fixados em formol são incubados num substrato contendo β-glicerofosfato sódico e nitrato de chumbo em pH 5,0; o fosfato de chumbo insolúvel produzido é tratado com sulfeto de amônio para produzir um sulfeto de chumbo negro.

Gomori nonspecific alkaline phosphatase s., corante para fosfatase alcalina inespecífica de Gomori; método de cálcio-sulfeto de cobalto que utiliza cortes por congelamento ou cortes em parafina fixados com formol ou acetona fria, mais β-glicerofosfato sódico como substrato em pH de 9,0–9,5 com Mg^{2+} como ativador; os íons cálcio precipitam o fosfato liberado, o sal de cobalto substitui o fosfato de cálcio e o sulfeto de amônio converte o produto num sulfeto de cobalto negro.

Gomori one-step trichrome s., coloração tricrômica em uma etapa de Gomori; a coloração do tecido conectivo que utiliza hematoxilina e uma mistura de corantes contendo cromotropo 2R e verde-claro ou azul-anilina; as fibras musculares tornam-se vermelhas, o colágeno é verde (ou azul, se for utilizado azul-anilina), enquanto os núcleos são azuis a negros.

Gomori silver impregnation s., coloração por impregnação pela prata de Gomori; método seguro para a reticulina, como auxílio no diagnóstico de neoplasias e cirrose incipiente do fígado; a solução de coloração utiliza nitrato de prata, hidróxido de potássio e amônia, devendo ser cuidadosamente preparada para evitar a precipitação da prata.

Goodpasture s., corante de Goodpasture; corante para bactérias Gram-negativas que utiliza fucsina anilina.

Gordon and Sweet s., corante de Gordon e Sweet; corante para a reticulina que utiliza permanganato de potássio acidificado, ácido oxálico, alume férrico, nitrato de prata, formaldeído, cloreto de ouro e tiossulfato de sódio.

Gram s., coloração de Gram; método para coloração diferencial das bactérias; os esfregaços são fixados por flambagem, corados em solução de cristal violeta, tratados com solução de iodo, enxaguados, descorados e, a seguir, contracorados com safranina O; os microrganismos Gram-positivos coram-se de púrpura-escuro, enquanto os microrganismos Gram-negativos coram-se de rosa; útil na taxonomia e na identificação das bactérias, bem como na indicação de diferenças fundamentais na estrutura da parede celular.

Gram-chromotrope s., coloração cromotrópica de Gram; coloração tricrômica modificada para esporos de microsporídios que combina os reagentes da coloração de Gram no procedimento.

green s., coloração verde; depósito produzido por bactérias cromogênicas encontrado nas partes cervicolabiais dos dentes, geralmente em crianças. VER TAMBÉM acquired *pellicle*.

Gridley s., coloração de Gridley; método de coloração pela prata para o retículo.

Gridley s. for fungi, coloração de Gridley para fungos; método para cortes histológicos fixados, baseado na coloração pela leucofucsina–ácido crômico de Bauer, com adição do corante de fucsina-aldeído de Gomori e amarelo metanil como contracorantes; contra um fundo amarelo, as hifas, os conídios, as cápsulas das leveduras, a elastina e a mucina aparecem em diferentes tonalidades de azul e púrpura.

Grocott-Gomori methenamine-silver s., corante de metenamina-prata de Grocott-Gomori; modificação do corante de metenamina de Gomori para fungos, em que os cortes são pré-tratados com ácido crômico antes da adição da solução de metenamina-prata e, a seguir, contracorados com verde-claro para demonstrar os fungos castanho-enegrecidos contra um fundo verde-pálido.

Hale colloidal iron s., corante de ferro coloidal de Hale; corante utilizado para distinguir os mucopolissacarídeos ácidos, como o ácido hialurônico; pode ser combinado com PAS (ácido periódico de Schiff) para visualizar também proteínas contendo carboidratos e glicoproteínas.

Heidenhain azan s., corante azan de Heidenhain; técnica que utiliza azocarmina B ou G seguida de azul-anilina para corar os núcleos e os eritrócitos de vermelho, o músculo de laranja, as fibrilas da glia de avermelhado, a mucina de azul e o colágeno e retículo de azul-escuro. [*az*ocarmina + *an*ilina azul]

Heidenhain iron hematoxylin s., corante de hematoxilina férrica de Heidenhain; corante de hematoxilina de alume de ferro utilizado para corar estriações musculares e estruturas mitóticas em azul-enegrecido.

hematoxylin and eosin s., coloração pela hematoxilina e eosina; trata-se, provavelmente, do mais útil de todos os métodos de coloração para tecidos; os núcleos coram-se de azul intenso com hematoxilina, enquanto o citoplasma cora-se de rosa após contracoloração com eosina, geralmente em água.

hematoxylin-malachite green-basic fuchsin s., corante de hematoxilina-verde malaquita-fucsina básica; corante para cortes extraídos em resina epóxi; os cortes de espessura média têm seu plástico dissolvido, e o tecido residual é corado seqüencialmente com os vários corantes; os núcleos e os astrócitos tornam-se rosa-púrpura, e a mielina, as gotículas de lipídios, os nucléolos e os oligodendrócitos aparecem verde-azulados brilhantes.

hematoxylin-phloxine B s., coloração pela hematoxilina-floxina B; coloração para cortes de epóxi intactos; os cortes de espessura média dos tecidos imersos em plástico apresentam as seguintes estruturas coradas em azul a negro: cromatina, nucléolo, citoplasma basófilo, mitocôndrias, membranas plasmáticas e nucleares, miofibrilas anisotrópicas, grânulos dos mastócitos e membranas elásticas dos vasos sanguíneos; em rosa a vermelho: fibrilas de colágeno, retículo, mucinas das células caliciformes, matriz da cartilagem hialina, estereocílios, citoplasma e eritrócitos; as gotículas de lipídios e a matriz pericondrocítica aparecem verdes.

Hirsch-Peiffer s., corante de Hirsch-Peiffer; corante utilizado para demonstração citológica de leucodistrofia metacromática; os sulfatídeos em excesso coram-se metacromaticamente (castanho-dourado) com violeta de cresil em ácido acético.

Hiss s., corante de Hiss; corante para a demonstração das cápsulas de microrganismos, utilizando violeta de genciana ou fucsina básica, seguida de lavagem com sulfato de cobre.

Holmes s., coloração de Holmes; método de coloração pelo nitrato de prata para fibras nervosas.

Hortega neuroglia s., coloração de Hortega para a neuróglia; um os vários métodos de coloração pelo carbonato de prata para demonstrar os astrócitos, a olidendróglia e a micróglia.

Hucker-Conn s., corante de Hucker-Conn; mistura de cristal de violeta e oxalato de amônio utilizada na coloração de Gram.

immunofluorescent s., coloração imunofluorescente; coloração que resulta da combinação de anticorpo fluorescente com um antígeno específico para esse anticorpo.

India ink capsule s., coloração pela tinta nanquim para cápsulas; coloração negativa para bactérias transparentes em que as células adquirem uma cor púrpura (cristal de violeta de Gram), enquanto as cápsulas aparecem claras contra um fundo escuro.

intravital s., coloração intravital; corante que é captado pelas células vivas após administração parenteral, como, por exemplo, por via intravenosa ou subcutânea.

iodine s., coloração pelo iodo; coloração para a detecção de amilóide, celulose, quitina, amido, carotenos e glicogênio e para corar amebas em virtude de seu conteúdo de glicogênio; as fezes e outras preparações a fresco são coradas diretamente com solução iodada de Lugol; os esfregaços são tratados com fixador de Schaudinn e, a seguir, corados com iodo alcoólico, seguido de hematoxilina férrica de Heidenhain.

Jenner s., corante de Jenner; eosinato de azul-de-metileno semelhante à coloração de Wright, mas que difere por não utilizar azul-de-metileno policromado; empregado para a coloração de esfregaços sanguíneos.

Kasten fluorescent Feulgen s., corante de Feulgen fluorescente de Kasten; modificação fluorescente do corante de Feulgen que utiliza qualquer um dos vários corantes básicos fluorescentes aos quais se adiciona SO_2; a fluorescência brilhante torna esse método muito sensível e adaptável à quantificação citofluorométrica do DNA.

Kasten fluorescent PAS s., corante PAS fluorescente de Kasten; modificação fluorescente do corante ácido periódico de Schiff (PAS) para polissacarídeos que utiliza um dos reagentes de Schiff fluorescentes de Kasten.

Kinyoun s., coloração de Kinyoun; método para a demonstração de microrganismos álcool-ácido-resistentes que utiliza carbol fucsina, álcool ácido e azul-de-metileno; os microrganismos álcool-ácido-resistentes aparecem corados de vermelho contra um fundo azul.

Kleihauer s., coloração de Kleihauer; combinação de azul-anilina e vermelho-escarlate de Biebrich utilizada para a detecção de células fetais no sangue materno.

Klinger-Ludwig acid-thionin s. for sex chromatin, coloração de tionina ácida de Klinger-Ludwig para cromatina sexual; método que utiliza um tratamento ácido preliminar em esfregaços bucais, antes da coloração com tionina tamponada, para diferenciar o corpúsculo de Barr.

Klüver-Barrera Luxol fast blue s., corante azul resistente de Klüver-Barrera Luxol; em combinação com violeta de cresil, corante útil para a demonstração da mielina e da substância de Nissl.

Kokoskin s., corante de Kokoskin; corante tricrômico modificado para esporos de microsporídios em que se utiliza o calor para diminuir os tempos de coloração.

Kossa s., corante de Kossa. SIN von Kossa s.

Kronecker s., corante de Kronecker; corante de cloreto de sódio a 5% tornado fracamente alcalino com carbonato de sódio, utilizado no exame de tecidos frescos ao microscópio.

lactophenol cotton blue s., corante de azul algodão de lactofenol; solução composta de cristais de fenol, glicerol, ácido láctico e água destilada à qual se adicionam azul de algodão ou cristal violeta; utilizado como corante em micologia.

Laquer s. for alcoholic hyalin, corante de Laquer para hialina alcoólica; combinação do corante fucsina ácida-anilina de Altmann com corante tricrômico de Masson que, num fundo castanho acinzentado, cora a hialina alcoólica de vermelho, o colágeno de verde e os núcleos de castanho.

lead hydroxide s., coloração pelo hidróxido de chumbo; coloração para microscopia eletrônica; após fixação com aldeído, o hidróxido de chumbo alcalino cora preferencialmente o RNA; entretanto, após fixação com OsO_4 reage, em grande parte, com o ósmio nos tecidos, produzindo uma coloração geral; além de ligar-se às citomembranas, cora também os carboidratos (p. ex., glicogênio).

Leishman s., corante de Leishman; corante de eosina policromada e azul-de-metileno, utilizado no exame de esfregaços sanguíneos.

Lendrum phloxine-tartrazine s., corante de floxina-tartrazina de Lendrum; corante para demonstrar corpúsculos de inclusão acidofílicos, que aparecem em vermelho sobre um fundo amarelo; os núcleos coram-se de azul, enquanto os corpúsculos de Negri não se coram.

Lepehne-Pickworth s., coloração de Lepehne-Pickworth; técnica de coloração para hemoglobina e outras substâncias contendo heme em criostato ou cortes por congelamento, que utiliza a presença de peroxidase tecidual para oxidar a benzidina a uma quinidrona azul.

Levaditi s., corante de Levaditi; corante de nitrato de prata para escurecimento dos espiroquetas em cortes histológicos.

Lillie allochrome connective tissue s., coloração alocrômica de Lillie do tecido conjuntivo; procedimento que utiliza PAS, hematoxilina, ácido pícrico e azul-de-metila; utilizada para distinguir entre membrana basal e reticulina, bem como para a demonstração de lesões arterioscleróticas.

Lillie azure-eosin s., corante de azur-eosina de Lillie; coloração em que se utiliza uma solução de eosinato de azur para corar bactérias e riquétsias em tecidos.

Lillie ferrous iron s., corante de ferro ferroso de Lillie; método que utiliza ferrocianeto de potássio em ácido acético para demonstração das melaninas, que adquirem coloração verde intensa; as lipofuscinas e os pigmentos hêmicos não são reativos.

Lillie sulfuric acid Nile blue s., coloração pelo azul do Nilo e ácido sulfúrico de Lillie; técnica para a demonstração de ácidos graxos quando presentes em altas concentrações.

Lison-Dunn s., coloração de Lison-Dunn; técnica que utiliza azul patente leuco V e peróxido de hidrogênio para demonstrar a peroxidase da hemoglobina em cortes e esfregaços.

Loeffler s., corante de Loeffler; corante para flagelos; a amostra é tratada com uma mistura de sulfato ferroso, ácido tânico e fucsina alcoólica e, a seguir, corada com anilina-fucsina hídrica ou violeta de genciana tornada alcalina com solução de hidróxido de sódio.

Loeffler caustic s., corante cáustico de Loeffler; corante para flagelos que utiliza uma solução aquosa de tanino e sulfato ferroso, com adição de um corante fucsina alcoólica.

Luna-Ishak s., coloração de Luna-Ishak; método de coloração que utiliza azul-celeste e fucsina ácida, em que os canalículos biliares coram-se de rosa a vermelho.

Macchiavello s., coloração de Macchiavello; seqüência de fucsina básica, ácido cítrico e azul-de-metileno em esfregaços que produz coloração vermelha das riquétsias e dos corpúsculos de inclusão, enquanto os núcleos coram-se de azul.

MacNeal tetrachrome blood s., corante tetracrômico de MacNeal para sangue; corante para esfregaços sanguíneos composto de uma mistura de azul-de-metileno, azur A, violeta-de-metileno e eosina Y.

malarial pigment s., coloração para pigmento da malária; coloração que utiliza a seqüência de floxina e azul-de-toluidina O; o pigmento da malária e os núcleos aparecem azulados; os eritrócitos e o citoplasma coram-se de vermelho a laranja; encontrado em células fagocíticas do sistema reticuloendotelial.

Maldonado-San Jose s., coloração de Maldonato-San Jose; método de coloração para corar as células das ilhotas pancreáticas, que utiliza uma seqüência de floxina, azur B e hematoxilina; as células alfa tornam-se púrpuras, as células beta coram de azul-violeta, as células delta, de azul-claro, e as células exócrinas, de azul-acinzentado com grânulos de secreção vermelhos.

Mallory s. of actinomyces, coloração de Mallory para actinomicetos; coloração que utiliza hematoxilina de alume, seguida de eosina; imersão em corante de cristal violeta anilina de Ehrlich e solução de iodo de Weigert; os micélios coram-se de azul, e os bastões, de vermelho.

Mallory aniline blue s., corante de azul-anilina de Mallory. SIN Mallory trichrome s.

Mallory collagen s., coloração de Mallory para colágeno; um de vários métodos de coloração que utilizam o ácido fosfomolíbdico ou fosfotúngstico como corante ácido, como azul-anilina ou hematoxilina para coloração do tecido conjuntivo.

Mallory s. for hemofuchsin, coloração de Mallory para hemofucsina; os cortes são corados seqüencialmente em hematoxilina de alume e fucsina básica; o pigmento semelhante à lipofuscina e o ceróide coram-se de vermelho-brilhante, os núcleos de azul, enquanto a melanina e a hemossiderina não se coram, exibindo sua cor castanha natural.

Mallory iodine s., coloração de Mallory pelo iodo; o amilóide apresenta-se castanho-avermelhado após iodo de Gram e, a seguir, violeta e azul após irrigação com ácido sulfúrico diluído.

Mallory phloxine s., coloração de Mallory pela floxina; técnica baseada na retenção da floxina pela hialina após supercoloração e, a seguir, descoloração com carbonato de lítio associada a hematoxilina de alume para obter uma coloração nuclear; a hialina apresenta-se vermelha; a hialina mais antiga, rosada a incolor; o amilóide, rosa-pálido; e os núcleos, azul-enegrecidos.

Mallory phosphotungstic acid hematoxylin s., coloração e Mallory pela hematoxilina-ácido fosfotúngstico. SIN phosphotungstic acid *hematoxylin*.

Mallory trichrome s., coloração tricrômica de Mallory; método particularmente apropriado para o estudo do tecido conjuntivo; os cortes são corados em fucsina ácida, solução de azul-anilina e laranja G e ácido fosfotúngstico; as fibrilas de colágeno coram-se de azul; a fibróglia, a neuróglia e as fibras musculares, de vermelho; e as fibras de elastina, de rosa ou amarelo. SIN Mallory aniline blue s., Mallory triple s.

Mallory triple s., coloração tripla de Mallory. SIN Mallory trichrome s.

Mann methyl blue-eosin s., coloração de Mann pelo azul-de-metila-eosina; coloração útil para a adeno-hipófise e os corpúsculos de inclusão virais; uma mistura dos dois corantes cora os grânulos das células alfa em vermelho, os grânulos das células β em azul-escuro, os cromófobos em cinza-rosa, o colóide em vermelho, os eritrócitos em vermelho-alaranjado e as fibras colágenas em azul; esse método também é útil para as células enterocromafins, caliciformes,

de Paneth e das ilhotas pancreáticas; os corpúsculos de Negri aparecem em vermelho, enquanto os seus núcleos e grânulos centrais são azuis.

Marchi s., coloração de Marchi; método de coloração em que a amostra é endurecida durante 8–10 dias em fixador de Müller modificado, seguida de imersão durante 1–3 semanas no mesmo, com adição de ácido ósmico; a gordura e as fibras nervosas em degeneração coram-se de preto.

Masson argentaffin s., corante argentafin de Masson; corante utilizado para corar os grânulos enterocromafins em castanho-enegrecido.

Masson-Fontana ammoniac silver s., coloração de Masson-Fontana pela prata amoniacal; coloração utilizada para demonstrar a melanina e os grânulos argentafins. SIN Fontana-Masson silver s.

Masson trichrome s., coloração de tricrômica de Masson; composição original para preparações histológicas multicoloridas, incluindo vermelho de xilidina, fucsina ácida, hematoxilina de alume férrica e azul-anilina ou verde resistente FCF; a cromatina cora-se em negro, o citoplasma adquire tons de vermelho, os grânulos dos eosinófilos e mastócitos adquirem uma vermelha intensa, os eritrócitos aparecem negros, as fibras elásticas coram-se de vermelho, e as fibras de colágeno e o muco, de vermelho-escuro (azul-anilina) ou verde (verde resistente FCF); as modificações substituem certos corantes por outros, como o vermelho-escarlate de Biebrich e o verde-claro.

Maximow s. for bone marrow, corante de Maximow para a medula óssea; corante de alume-hematoxilina e azur II-eosina utilizado para distinguir os leucócitos com grânulos, os mastócitos e a cartilagem.

Mayer hemalum s., corante de hemalume de Mayer; corante nuclear progressivo também utilizado como contracorante.

Mayer mucicarmine s., corante mucicarmin de Mayer. VER mucicarmine.

Mayer mucihematein s., corante de muciemateína de Mayer. VER mucihematein.

May-Grünwald s., corante de May-Grünwald; equivalente alemão do corante de Jenner, utilizado para a coloração do sangue e em citologia; freqüentemente associado à coloração de Giemsa; útil para a demonstração de flagelados parasitas.

metachromatic s., corante metacromático; corante, como azul-de-metileno, tionina ou azur A, que tem a capacidade de produzir diferentes cores com várias estruturas histológicas ou citológicas.

methenamine silver s., corante de metenamina-prata; corante utilizado para cistos de *Pneumocystis carinii*.

methyl green-pyronin s., corante de verde de metila-pironina; método de coloração útil para a identificação de plasmócitos intensamente pironinofílicos; uma mistura de corante verde e corante vermelho que tem a propriedade de corar o ácido nucleico (DNA) extremamente polimerizado em verde e os ácidos nucleicos de baixo peso molecular (RNA) em vermelho. VER Unna-Pappenheim s.

modified acid-fast s., coloração álcool-ácido-resistente modificada; coloração para coccídeos (*Cryptosporidium, Cyclospora, Isospora*) em que o descolorante é um ácido muito diluído (ácido sulfúrico a 1–3%); é menos provável que remova corante demais.

modified trichrome s., coloração tricrômica modificada; coloração desenvolvida a partir da modificação de Wheatley da coloração tricrômica de Gomori, que utiliza 10 vezes mais corante cromótropo 2R para esporos de microsporídios, que se coram de rosa a vermelho.

Mowry colloidal iron s., corante de ferro coloidal de Mowry; corante utilizado para a demonstração de mucopolissacarídeos ácidos.

MSB trichrome s., coloração tricrômica MSB; coloração para fibrina que utiliza amarelo de Martius, cristal escarlate brilhante 6R e azul solúvel; a fibrina cora-se seletivamente de vermelho, enquanto o tecido conjuntivo apresenta-se azul.

multiple s., corante múltiplo; mistura de vários corantes em que cada um deles exerce uma ação seletiva independente sobre uma ou mais partes do tecido.

Nair buffered methylene blue s., coloração pelo azul-de-metileno tamponado de Nair; coloração utilizada para revelar os detalhes nucleares de trofozoítos protozoários quando utilizado em pH baixo (3,6–4,8).

Nakanishi s., coloração de Nakanishi; método para coloração vital de bactérias em que a lâmina é tratada com uma solução de azul-de-metileno quente até adquirir uma cor azul-celeste; em seguida, coloca-se uma gota de uma emulsão das bactérias sobre a lamínula que é aplicada à lâmina; as bactérias coram-se de modo diferencial, algumas partes mais intensamente do que outras.

Nauta s., coloração de Nauta; coloração para axônios em degeneração que se coram pela prata e aparecem como fibras fragmentadas e tumefeitas.

negative s., coloração negativa; coloração que forma um fundo opaco ou colorido contra o qual o objeto a ser demonstrado aparece como uma área translúcida ou incolor; em microscopia eletrônica, utiliza-se um material elétron-opaco como o ácido fosfotúngstico ou fosfotungstato de sódio, para fornecer detalhes da estrutura superficial.

Neisser s., coloração de Neisser; coloração para os núcleos polares do bacilo da difteria que utiliza uma mistura de azul-de-metileno e cristal violeta.

neutral s., corante neutro; composto de um corante ácido e um corante básico, como o eosinato de azul-de-metileno, em que o ânion e o cátion contêm, cada um, um grupo cromóforo. SIN salt dye.

Nicolle s. for capsules, coloração de Nicolle para cápsula; coloração numa mistura de uma solução saturada de violeta de genciana em álcool fenólico.

ninhydrin-Schiff s. for proteins, coloração de ninidrina-Schiff para proteínas; as proteínas são reveladas através do uso de ninidrina ou aloxano para produzir aldeídos a partir de aminas alifáticas primárias por desaminação oxidativa; os aldeídos são mostrados pela reação com o reagente de Schiff.

Nissl s., coloração de Nissl; (1) método para coloração de células nervosas com fucsina básica; (2) método para coloração de agregados de retículo endoplasmático rugoso e ribossomas em corpos celulares de neurônios e dendritos com corantes básicos, como cresil violeta (ou cresil verdadeiro), tionina, azul-de-toluidina O ou azul-de-metileno.

Noble s., coloração de Noble; técnica de coloração com fucsina básica e orange G para detecção de corpúsculos de inclusão virais em tecidos fixados.

nuclear s., coloração nuclear; coloração para núcleos celulares, geralmente baseada na ligação de um corante básico ao DNA ou nucleoistona.

Orth s., corante de Orth; corante de carmim de lítio para as células nervosas e seus processos.

Padykula-Herman s. for myosin ATPase, coloração de Padykula-Herman para miosina ATPase; técnica semelhante àquela da coloração para fosfatase alcalina inespecífica de Gomori, porém a incubação é efetuada com ATP como substrato em pH 9,4, na ausência de Mg^{2+}; a atividade enzimática é demonstrada na forma de depósitos enegrecidos na banda A dos sarcômeros do músculo estriado; são necessários cortes histológicos de controle sem substrato, contendo inibidores sulfidrílicos.

Paget-Eccleston s., coloração de Paget-Eccleston; técnica de coloração modificada com aldeído, tionina, PAS e orange G para identificar sete tipos celulares diferentes na hipófise anterior.

panoptic s., coloração panóptica; coloração em que se combina um corante tipo Romanowsky com outro corante; essa combinação melhora a coloração dos grânulos citoplasmáticos e outros corpúsculos.

Papanicolaou s., coloração de Papanicolaou; coloração multicromática utilizada principalmente em amostras citológicas esfoliadas e baseada no uso de hematoxilina aquosa com múltiplos contracorantes em álcool etílico a 95%, conferindo uma grande transparência e delicadeza dos detalhes; importante na triagem do câncer, especialmente de esfregaços ginecológicos.

Pappenheim s., coloração de Pappenheim; corante de verde metila e pironina, utilizado originalmente para corar linfócitos.

paracarmine s., corante paracarmim; líquido corante que consiste numa solução de cloreto de cálcio e ácido carmínico em álcool em 75%.

PAS s., método de PAS. SIN periodic acid-Schiff s.

periodic acid-Schiff s. (PAS), método do ácido periódico de Schiff; procedimento de coloração histológica em que os grupamentos 1,2-glicol são inicialmente oxidados com ácido periódico a aldeídos, que então reagem com o reagente leucofucsina sulfito de Schiff, adquirindo uma cor vermelho-violeta; ocorre coloração intensa com polissacarídeos, como glicogênio, e mucopolissacarídeos de mucinas epiteliais, membranas basais e tecido conjuntivo. SIN PAS s.

Perls Prussian blue s., coloração pelo azul-da-Prússia de Perls; corante para o ferro férrico, como aquele presente nas hemossiderinas, utilizando ferro cianeto de potássio em ácido acético ou ácido clorídrico diluído, seguido de contracorante vermelho, como safranina O ou vermelho neutro; várias hemossiderinas e a maioria dos ferros minerais produzem uma reação azul-esverdeada, enquanto os núcleos coram-se de vermelho.

peroxidase s., coloração para peroxidase; método para demonstração de grânulos de peroxidase em alguns neutrófilos e eosinófilos; a enzima promove a oxidação da benzidina pelo peróxido de hidrogênio; os tecidos tratados com peroxidase de rábano-bastardo também podem ter a enzima detectada à microscopia eletrônica.

phosphotungstic acid s., corante de ácido fosfotúngstico; o primeiro corante geral utilizado para microscopia eletrônica; corante seletivo para componentes extracelulares, como a elastina, o colágeno e os mucopolissacarídeos da membrana basal; a coloração pode ser seguida de acetato de uranil ou chumbo. SIN PTA s.

picrocarmine s., corante de picrocarmim; pó cristalino vermelho derivado de uma solução de carmim, amônia e ácido pícrico, que é evaporada, deixando pó (hidrossolúvel); produz excelente coloração dos grânulos cerato-hialinos.

picro-Mallory trichrome s., coloração picro-tricrômica de Mallory; modificação da coloração tricrômica de Mallory que envolve a adição de ácido pícrico.

picronigrosin s., corante de picronigrosina; solução de nigrosina em ácido pícrico, utilizada para coloração do tecido conjuntivo.

plasma s., plasmatic s., plasmic s., corante plasmático; corante cuja principal afinidade é pelo citoplasma das células.

plastic section s., coloração de corte plástico; (1) para microscopia eletrônica, um corante (p. ex., ácido ósmico, PTA, permanganato de potássio) utilizado em cortes finos de tecidos imersos em plástico, utilizando a fixação diferencial de átomos pesados a várias estruturas celulares e teciduais, de modo que os elétrons possam ser absorvidos e dispersos por essas estruturas, produzindo uma imagem; para obter uma coloração diferencial, o corante deve penetrar nas incrustações plásticas não-umedecíveis; (2) para microscopia óptica, utiliza-se um corante (p. ex., azul-de-toluidina alcalina, metenamina-prata) em tecidos imersos em plástico para obter uma maior resolução e maiores detalhes do que o normalmente possível; os cortes de espessura média (0,5–1,5 μm) são úteis sobretudo para os exames histopatológicos do rim, principalmente em combinação com microscopia de fase.

port-wine s., mancha em vinho-do-Porto. SIN nevus flammeus.

positive s., coloração positiva; ligação direta de um corante com componente tecidual para produzir contraste; em microscopia eletrônica, são utilizados metais pesados, como uranil e sais de chumbo, para ligação a constituintes celulares seletivos, produzindo aumento da densidade no feixe de elétrons, isto é, contraste.

Prussian blue s., coloração pelo azul-da-Prússia; coloração que emprega ferrocianeto de potássio ácido para demonstração do ferro, como em siderócitos.

PTA s., corante PTA. SIN phosphotungstic acid s.

Puchtler-Sweat s. for basement membranes, coloração de Puchtler-Sweat para membranas basais; método de coloração que utiliza resorcina-fucsina e soluções de vermelho resistente nucleares após fixação de Carnoy; as membranas basais tornam-se cinza ou negras, e os núcleos, rosados a vermelhos.

Puchtler-Sweat s. for hemoglobin and hemosiderin, coloração de Puchtler-Sweat para hemoglobina e hemossiderina; método de coloração complexa em que, sobre um fundo amarelo, a hemoglobina cora-se de vermelho, a hemossiderina de azul a verde, e as fibras elásticas de rosa.

Q-banding s., corante para bandas Q; coloração fluorescente para cromossomas que produz padrões específicos de bandas para cada par de cromossomas homólogos; o derivado do corante acridina, cloridrato de quinacrina, ou outros derivados, como o dicloridrato mostarda da quinacrina, produzem uma fluorescência verde-amarelada em pH de 4,5 nos segmentos cromossômicos ricos em heterocromatina constitutiva, com bases de desoxiadenilato-desoxitimidilato (A-T) de DNA; as regiões dos centrômeros dos cromossomas humanos 3, 4 e 13 coram-se especificamente, bem como os satélites de alguns cromossomas acrocêntricos e a extremidade do braço longo do cromossoma Y; os padrões de bandas assemelham-se aos obtidos com a coloração das bandas G; são obtidos resultados semelhantes de coloração fluorescente com os antibióticos adriamicina e daunomicina, bem como com os corantes terciários butil proflavina e DAPI e o corante bisbenzimidazol, HOECHST 33258. SIN quinacrine chromosome banding s.

quinacrine chromosome banding s., corante de quinacrina para bandas cromossômicas. SIN Q-banding s.

Rambourg chromic acid-phosphotungstic acid s., coloração de Rambourg pelo ácido crômico-ácido fosfotúngstico; coloração para glicoproteínas, utilizada com microscópio eletrônico, com a qual cortes histológicos ultrafinos revelam carboidratos complexos nas mesmas localizações mostradas pela coloração de Rambourg com ácido periódico-metenamina crômica-prata.

Rambourg periodic acid-chromic methenamine-silver s., coloração de Rambourg pelo ácido periódico-metenamina crômica-prata; coloração para glicoproteínas, utilizada com microscópio eletrônico, adaptada da coloração de Gomori-Jones pelo ácido periódico-metenamina-prata; produz depósitos de prata em sáculos maduros do aparelho de Golgi, vesículas lisossômicas, revestimento celular e membranas basais.

R-banding s., coloração das bandas R; método de coloração inversa das bandas cromossômicas de Giemsa que produz bandas complementares às bandas G; induzida por tratamento com altas temperaturas, pH baixo ou coloração pelo laranja de acridina; freqüentemente utilizado juntamente com a coloração das bandas G no cariótipo humano para detectar a ocorrência de deleções.

Romanowsky blood s., corante de Romanowsky para sangue; protótipo dos corantes de eosina e azul-de-metileno para esfregaços sanguíneos, utilizando soluções aquosas constituídas de uma mistura de azul-de-metileno (saturado) e eosina. Os corantes tipo Romanowsky dependem de sua ação sobre compostos formados pela interação do azul-de-metileno e eosina; a maioria não tem utilidade se houver água no álcool, visto que os corantes neutros precipitam.

Roux s., coloração de Roux; dupla coloração para bacilos diftéricos, que emprega cristal violeta ou dália e verde de metila.

Ryan s., coloração de Ryan; coloração tricrômica modificada para esporos de microsporídios, em que a concentração do cromotropo 2R corresponde a 10 vezes a concentração usada nas colorações tricrômicas para amostras de fezes, sendo o contracorante azul-anilina.

Schaeffer-Fulton s., coloração de Schaeffer-Fulton, coloração para esporos bacterianos que utiliza o verde de malaquita e a safranina, de modo que os corpos bacterianos tornam-se vermelhos a rosados, enquanto os esporos são verdes.

Schmorl ferric-ferricyanide reduction s., coloração de redução férrica-ferricianeto de Schmorl; coloração para testar substâncias redutoras nos tecidos, incluindo melanina, grânulos argentafins, colóide tireóide, ceratina, ceratoialina e pigmentos de lipofuscina; o ferricianeto é convertido em ferrocianeto, que é convertido em azul-da-Prússia insolúvel na presença de íons férricos.

Schmorl picrothionin s., corante de picrotionina de Schmorl; coloração para o osso compacto que emprega soluções de tionina e ácido pícrico para produzir uma coloração azul a azul-enegrecida dos canalículos e células ósseas; a matriz óssea torna-se amarelada, enquanto a substância fundamental da cartilagem é púrpura.

Schultz s., coloração de Schultz; coloração para colesterol; teste histoquímico relativamente específico, porém insensível, para o colesterol e ésteres do colesterol, em que cortes por congelamento de tecidos fixados com formol são oxidados em alume de ferro, peróxido de hidrogênio ou iodato de sódio, tratados, a seguir, com ácido sulfúrico para produzir uma cor azul-esverdeada a vermelha numa reação positiva; a presença de glicerol inibe a reação.

selective s., corante seletivo; corante que cora parte de um tecido ou de uma célula exclusivamente ou com mais intensidade do que as partes remanescentes.

Semichon acid carmine s., coloração de carmim ácido de Semichon; coloração para trematódeos adultos.

silver s., coloração pela prata; qualquer uma de várias colorações (p. ex., colorações de Bielschowsky, pela prata de Gomori, de impregnação) que utilizam soluções alcalinas de nitrato de prata para corar as fibras do tecido conjuntivo (reticulina, colágeno), depósitos de sais de cálcio, espiroquetas, tecido neurológico e regiões organizadoras nucleolares.

silver-ammoniac silver s., coloração pela prata-prata amoniacal; coloração para o componente proteico ácido de regiões nucleolares ativas ou que foram ativas por transcrição na interfase precedente; utiliza nitrato de prata, prata amoniacal e formol. SIN Ag-AS s.

silver protein s., coloração por proteinato de prata; complexo de proteinato de prata utilizado na coloração de fibras nervosas, terminações nervosas e protozoários flagelados; também utilizada para demonstrar a fagocitose em animais vivos pelas células do sistema reticuloendotelial.

Stirling modification of Gram s., modificação de Stirling da coloração de Gram; coloração estável com anilina-cristal violeta.

supravital s., coloração supravital; procedimento em que o tecido vivo é removido do corpo, e as células são colocadas numa solução corante atóxica, permitindo, assim, o estudo de seus processos vitais.

Taenzer s., corante de Taenzer; solução de orceína utilizada para a coloração do tecido elástico. SIN Unna-Taenzer s.

Takayama s., corante de Takayama; corante que contém piridina, hidrato de sódio e dextrose; utilizado para a identificação de colorações do sangue; uma gota adicionada a uma coloração do sangue suspeita resulta na formação de cristais hemocromógenos.

telomeric R-banding s., coloração da bandas R teloméricas; coloração modificada das bandas R em que os telômeros se tornam fortemente corados, aparecendo ainda bandas R fracas no restante dos cromossomas; utiliza lâminas secas ao ar, com envelhecimento durante vários dias e coloração pelo corante de Giemsa de fosfato tamponado quente.

thioflavine T s., corante tioflavina T; corante utilizado para a detecção do amilóide que induz uma fluorescência amarela específica; os cortes de tecido são inicialmente colocados em alume-hematoxilina para apagar a fluorescência nuclear e, a seguir, corados com tioflavina T.

Tizzoni s., corante de Tizzoni; corante utilizado para testar a presença de ferro no tecido; o tecido é tratado com uma solução de ferrocianeto de potássio e, a seguir, com ácido clorídrico diluído; a observação de uma coloração azul indica a presença de ferro.

Toison s., corante de Toison; diluente sanguíneo e corante de leucócitos que contém violeta de metila, cloreto de sódio, sulfato de sódio e glicerina; também utilizado para a contagem de eritrócitos.

toluidine blue s., coloração pelo azul-de-toluidina; coloração utilizada para trofozoítos de *Pneumocystis carinii*.

trichrome s., coloração tricrômica; combinações de coloração habitualmente contendo três corantes de cores contrastantes, selecionados para corar o tecido conjuntivo, o músculo, o citoplasma e os núcleos em cores brilhantes; em geral, os cortes de tecido são inicialmente corados em hematoxilina férrica antes de serem tratados com os outros corantes.

trypsin G-banding s., coloração das bandas G com tripsina. VER G-banding s.

ultrafast Pap s., coloração de Papanicolaou ultra-resistente; coloração modificada de Papanicolaou apropriada para uso em situações em que é necessário tomar rápidas decisões, com os cortes por congelamento podendo não ser confiáveis ou práticos o suficiente. VER TAMBÉM Papanicolaou s.

Unna s., corante de Unna; (1) corante de azul-de-metileno alcalino para plasmócitos; (2) corante de azul-de-metileno policrômico que cora os mastócitos de vermelho (metacromáticos).

Unna-Pappenheim s., corante de Unna-Pappenheim; corante de contraste que consiste numa solução de verde de metila-pironina; originalmente utilizado para gonococos, porém posteriormente empregado para a detecção do RNA e DNA em cortes histológicos; o RNA cora-se de vermelho, enquanto o DNA apresenta-se verde; utilizado para demonstrar plasmócitos durante a inflamação crônica. VER methyl green-pyronin s.

Unna-Taenzer s., corante de Unna-Taenzer. SIN Taenzer s.

uranyl acetate s., corante de acetato de uranil; corante utilizado em microscopia eletrônica; o acetato de uranil liga-se especificamente a ácidos nucleicos, mas tende seletivamente a ser abolido por fixação em ósmio; as proteínas são bem coradas, enquanto as citomembranas são pouco coradas.

urate crystals s., coloração dos cristais de urato; coloração que utiliza prata-metenamina para a detecção de cristais, que polarizam a luz em contraste com os cristais de cálcio; útil no diagnóstico da gota e de infartos renais resultantes do acúmulo de ácido úrico.

van Ermengen s., coloração de van Ermengen; método para corar flagelos que utiliza ácido acético glacial, ácido ósmico, ácido tânico, nitrato de prata, ácido gálico e acetato de potássio.

van Gieson s., corante de van Gieson; mistura de fucsina ácida em solução saturada de ácido pícrico; utilizado na coloração do colágeno.

Verhoeff elastic tissue s., coloração de Verhoeff para tecido elástico; coloração para cortes histológicos em que se utiliza uma mistura de hematoxilina, cloreto férrico e solução iodada de Lugol; o tecido pode ser contracorado, se desejado, com eosina ou com o corante de van Gieson; as fibras elásticas e os núcleos tornam-se azul-enegrecidos a negro, enquanto o colágeno e outros componentes exibem tons de rosa a vermelho.

vital s., corante vital; corante aplicado a células ou a parte de células enquanto vivas.

von Kossa s., coloração de von Kossa; coloração para o cálcio no tecido mineralizado; utiliza uma solução de nitrato de prata seguida de tiossulfato de sódio; o osso calcificado, mas não o osteóide, cora-se de castanho a negro. SIN Kossa s.

Wachstein-Meissel s. for calcium-magnesium-ATPase, coloração de Wachstein-Meissel para a cálcio-magnésio-ATPase; método semelhante ao da coloração de Gomori para fosfatase ácida inespecífica, porém a incubação é efetuada com ATP como substrato em pH neutro; a atividade enzimática é geralmente demonstrada nas membranas celulares.

Warthin-Starry silver s., coloração pela prata de Warthin-Starry; coloração para espiroquetas em que as preparações são incubadas em solução de nitrato de prata a 1%, seguida de revelador.

Weber s., coloração de Weber; coloração tricrômica modificada para esporos de microsporídios em que a concentração do cromotropo 2R é 10 vezes maior do que a utilizada nas colorações tricrômicas para amostras de fezes, sendo o contracorante o vermelho resistente.

Weigert s. for actinomyces, coloração de Weigert para actinomicetos; método de coloração que utiliza imersão numa solução de orselina vermelho-escura em álcool; a seguir, efetua-se a coloração em solução de cristal violeta. VER TAMBÉM iron *hematoxylin*.

Weigert s. for elastin, coloração de Weigert para a elastina; solução de coloração de fucsina, resorcina e cloreto férrico; as fibras elásticas coram-se em azul-enegrecido.

Weigert s. for fibrin, coloração de Weigert para fibrina; método de coloração que utiliza soluções de anilina-cristal violeta e iodo-iodeto de potássio, descolorando, a seguir, em óleo de anilina e xilol; a fibrina cora-se em azul-escuro.

Weigert-Gram s., coloração de Weigert-Gram; coloração para bactérias em tecidos cujos cortes são corados em alume-hematoxilina e, a seguir, eosina, anilina, violeta de metila e solução de Lugol.

Weigert iron hematoxylin s., coloração da hematoxilina férrica de Weigert; solução para coloração nuclear contendo hematoxilina, cloreto férrico e ácido clorídrico; útil em combinação com a coloração de van Gieson, especialmente para demonstração dos elementos do tecido conjuntivo ou de *Entamoeba histolytica* em cortes.

Weigert s. for myelin, coloração de Weigert para mielina; método de coloração que utiliza cloreto férrico e hematoxilina; a mielina cora-se em azul intenso, enquanto as porções degeneradas adquirem uma cor amarelada suave.

Weigert s. for neuroglia, coloração de Weigert para a neuróglia; processo complicado em que o tratamento final assemelha-se àquele para coloração da fibrina; a neuróglia e os núcleos coram-se de azul.

Wilder s. for reticulum, coloração de Wilder para a reticulina; técnica de impregnação pela prata em que o retículo aparece na forma de fibras negras bem definidas, sem formação de contas, com um fundo relativamente claro.

Williams s., coloração de Williams; coloração para os corpúsculos de Negri que utiliza ácido pícrico, fucsina e azul-de-metileno; os corpúsculos de Negri coram-se em magenta, os grânulos e as células nervosas em azul, e os eritrócitos em cor amarelada.

Wright s., corante de Wright; mistura de eosinatos de azul-de-metileno policromado utilizada na coloração de esfregaços sanguíneos.

Ziehl s., corante de Ziehl; solução de carbol-fucsina de fenol e fucsina básica utilizada para demonstrar bactérias e núcleos celulares.

Ziehl-Neelsen s., coloração de Ziehl-Neelsen; método para corar bactérias álcool-ácido-resistentes (BAAR) utilizando corante de Ziehl, descolorando em álcool-ácido e efetuando uma contracoloração com azul-de-metileno; os microrganismos álcool ácido-resistentes apresentam-se vermelhos, enquanto outros elementos teciduais coram-se de azul-claro; uma modificação dessa coloração é também utilizada para *Actinomycetes* e *Brucella*.

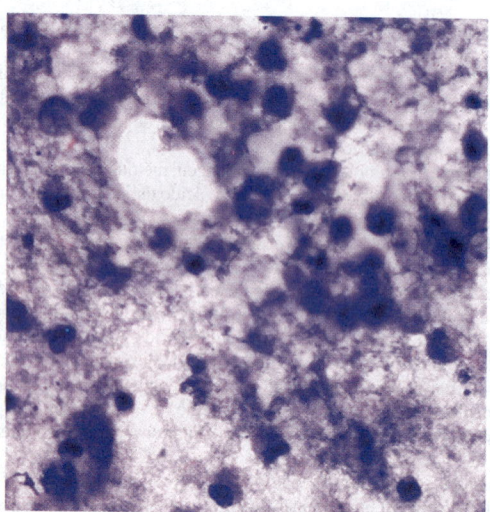

coloração de Ziehl-Neelsen: utilizada aqui para demonstrar a inflamação granulomatosa em aspirado de fígado

stain·ing (stān'ing). Coloração. **1.** O ato de aplicar um corante. VER TAMBÉM stain. **2.** Em odontologia, modificação da cor do dente ou da base da dentadura.
  progressive s., c. progressiva; procedimento em que a coloração é mantida até atingir a intensidade desejada de coloração dos elementos teciduais.
  regressive s., c. regressiva; tipo de coloração em que os tecidos são excessivamente corados, e o excesso de corante é então removido seletivamente até se obter a intensidade desejada.
stains-all (stainz'awl). Corante que colore as fosfoproteínas de azul, as proteínas de vermelho, os ácidos nucleicos de púrpura e as mucoproteínas e mucopolissacarídeos de várias cores em géis de acrilaminda; também utilizado em cortes histológicos.
stair·case (stār'kās). Em escada; uma série de reações sucessivas de intensidade progressivamente crescente ou decrescente, de modo que o gráfico que as representa mostra uma ascensão ou queda contínua. VER treppe.
stal·ag·mom·e·ter (stal-ă-gom'ē-ter). Estalagmômetro; instrumento para determinar exatamente o número de gotas em determinada quantidade de líquido; utilizado como medida da tensão superficial de um líquido (quanto menor a tensão, menores as gotas e, conseqüentemente, mais numerosas em determinado volume do líquido). SIN stactometer. [G. *stalagma*, uma gota + *metron*, medida]
stalk (stawk). Pedículo, pedúnculo; conexão estreita com uma estrutura ou órgão.
  allantoic s., p. alantóico; conexão estreita entre a porção intra-embrionária do alantóide e a vesícula alantóica extra-embrionária.
  body s., p. corporal; o precursor extra-embrionário do pedículo de conexão ou cordão umbilical pelo qual o embrião está fixado ao cório trofoblástico. SIN connecting s.
  connecting s., p. de conexão. SIN body s.
  s. of epiglottis, p. da epiglote; a extremidade inferior ou pedículo da cartilagem da epiglote fixado à incisura superior da cartilagem tireóidea. SIN petiolus epiglottidis.
  infundibular s., p. infundibular. SIN infundibular *stem.*
  optic s., p. óptico; a porção proximal constrita da vesícula óptica no embrião; contribui para o nervo óptico.
  pineal s., p. pineal; a fixação do corpo pineal ao teto do terceiro ventrículo; contém o recesso pineal do terceiro ventrículo.
  pituitary s., p. hipofisário; processo compreendendo a parte tuberal que reveste o pedúnculo infundibular que fixa a hipófise ao tuber cinéreo na base do cérebro.
  yolk s., p. vitelino; conexão estreita entre o intestino intra-embrionário e o saco vitelino; suas paredes são esplancnopleura. SIN umbilical duct, vitelline duct, vitellointestinal duct.
stam·mer (stam'er). Tartamudear, gaguejar. **1.** Hesitar na fala, parar, repetir e errar na pronúncia devido a embaraço, agitação ou falta de familiaridade com o assunto, ou de causa fisiológica ainda não definida. Cf. stutter. **2.** Pronunciar errado ou transpor certas consoantes na fala. [A. S. *stamur*].
stam·mer·ing (stam'er-ing). Tartamudez, gagueira. **1.** Distúrbio da fala caracterizado por hesitação e repetição de palavras ou por erro de pronúncia ou transposição de certas consoantes, especialmente *l*, *r* e *s*. **2.** Outros sons, além da fala, que se assemelham à tartamudez. SIN paralalia literalis, psellism.
  s. of the bladder, hesitação vesical. SIN urinary *stuttering.*
Stam·no·so·ma (stam-nō-sō'mă). Gênero de trematódeos da família Heterophyidae, idêntico ao *Centrocestus*. Duas espécies, *S. armatum* e *S. formosanum,* foram descritas como infectantes ocasionais de seres humanos. [G. *stamnos*, frasco + *sōma*, corpo]
stan·dard (stan'dard). Padrão. **1.** Refere-se a algo que serve como base para comparação; especificação técnica ou relato feito por especialistas. **2.** VER standard *substance*. [I.m. do Fr. ant. *estandard*, local de reunião, do frâncico *standan*, ficar de pé + *hard*, duro, rápido]
stan·dard·i·za·tion (stan'dard-i-zā'shun). Padronização. **1.** Preparo de uma solução de concentração definida que pode ser utilizada para comparação, bem como em testes. **2.** Preparo de qualquer droga ou outra preparação conforme o tipo ou padrão. **3.** Conjunto de técnicas utilizadas para remover o mais rápido possível os efeitos de diferenças na idade ou outras variáveis confusas, quando se comparam duas ou mais populações.
  s. of a test, p. de um teste; em psicologia, seguir procedimentos definidos para administração, pontuação, avaliação e relato dos resultados de um novo teste em fase de desenvolvimento.
stand·still. Parada. Cessação da atividade.
  atrial s., parada atrial; cessação das contrações atriais, caracterizada pela ausência de ondas atriais no eletrocardiograma. SIN auricular s.
  auricular s., parada atrial. SIN atrial s.
  cardiac s., parada cardíaca, assistolia. SIN asystole.
  sinus s., parada sinusal; cessação da atividade do nódulo sinusal, caracterizada pela ausência de ondas P normais no eletrocardiograma.
  ventricular s., parada ventricular; cessação das contrações ventriculares, caracterizada pela ausência de complexos ventriculares no eletrocardiograma.
Stanley, Edward, cirurgião inglês, 1793–1862. VER S. cervical *ligaments,* em *ligament.*
stan·nic (stan'ik). Estânico; relativo ao estanho, especialmente quando em combinação com a sua maior valência. [L. *stannum*, estanho]
stan·nic chlo·ride. Cloreto estânico; $SnCl_4$; líquido que produz vapor (espírito de Libavius), de densidade específica 2,23, ponto de ebulição de 115°C, que forma vários hidratos; o pentaidrato (manteiga de estanho) é utilizado como mordente e para "falsificar" ou "dar peso" à seda.
stan·nic ox·ide. Óxido de estanho; SnO_2; utilizado na indústria; trata-se de uma causa de pneumoconiose. SIN tin oxide.
Stannius, Herman F., biólogo alemão, 1808–1883. VER S. *ligature.*
stan·nous (stan'ŭs). Estanhoso; relativo ao estanho, especialmente quando em combinação na sua valência menor. [L. *stannum*, estanho]
stan·nous flu·o·ride. Fluoreto estanhoso; preparação que contém não menos de 71,2% de estanho estanhoso e não menos de 22,3% nem mais de 25,5% de fluoreto; utilizado como profilático contra cáries em odontologia.
stan·num (stan'ŭm). Estanho. SIN tin. [L.]
stan·o·lone (stan'ō-lōn). Estanolona; andrógenio com as mesmas ações e usos da testosterona; utilizado pelos seus efeitos anabólicos e supressores tumorais, especificamente no carcinoma de mama. SIN dihydrotestosterone.
stan·o·zo·lol (stan-ō'zō-lol, -lōl). Estanozolol; estanozol, 17α-metil-5α-androstan-17β-ol, que possui um anel pirazol (=CH—NH—N=) ligado a C-2 e C-3 (ver esteróides para a estrutura do androstano). Agente anabólico semi-sintético, efetivo por via oral.
sta·pe·dec·to·my (stā-pē-dek'tō-mē). Estapedectomia; operação para remover o estribo no todo ou em parte, com substituição por prótese de metal ou plástico; efetuada para otosclerose com fixação do estribo para tratamento de surdez condutiva. [stapes + G. *ektomē*, excisão]
sta·pe·di·al (stā-pē'dē-ăl). Estapédico; relativo ao estribo.
sta·pe·di·o·te·not·o·my (stā-pē'dē-ō-te-not'ō-mē). Estapediotenotomia; divisão do tendão do músculo estapédio. [stapedius + G. *tenōn*, tendão + *tomē*, incisão]
sta·pe·di·o·ves·tib·u·lar (stā-pē'dē-ō-ves-tib'ū-lăr). Estapediovestibular; relativo ao estribo e ao vestíbulo da orelha.
sta·pe·di·us, pl. **sta·pe·dii** (stā-pē'dē-ŭs, stā-pē'dē-ī). Estapédio. SIN stapedius (*muscle*). [L. mod.]
sta·pe·dot·o·my (stā-pē-dot'ō-mē). Estapedotomia; técnica cirúrgica para melhorar a audição na otosclerose; efetua-se um orifício na base do estribo, através do qual se coloca a extremidade de uma prótese em forma de pistão, sendo a outra extremidade fixada ao ramo longo da bigorna.
sta·pes, pl. **sta·pes, sta·pe·des** (stā'pēz, stā'pē-dēz) [TA]. Estribo. O menor dos três ossículos da audição; sua base encaixa-se na janela vestibular (oval), enquanto sua cabeça articula-se com o processo lenticular do ramo longo da bigorna. SIN stirrup. [L. mod. stirrup]
♳**staphyl-.** Estafil-. VER staphylo.
staph·y·lec·to·my (staf-i-lek'tō-mē). Estafilectomia. SIN uvelectomy. [staphyl- + G. *ektomē*, excisão]
staph·yl·e·de·ma (staf'il-e-dē'mă). Estafiledema; edema da úvula. [staphyl- + G. *oidēma*, tumefação (edema)]
staph·y·line (staf'i-lin, -lēn). Estafilina. SIN botryoid.
sta·phyl·i·on (stă-fil'ē-on). Estafílio; o ponto médio da borda posterior do palato duro; ponto craniométrico. VER TAMBÉM posterior nasal *spine* of horizontal plate of palatine bone. [G. dim. de *staphylē*, um cacho de uva]

staphylo-, staphyl-. Estafilo-, estafil-. Semelhança com uma uva ou cacho de uvas, referindo-se, habitualmente, a estafilococos ou, em termo obsoletos, à úvula palatina. VER TAMBÉM uvulo-. [G. *staphylē*, um cacho de uvas]

staph·y·lo·coc·cal (staf′i-lō-kok′ăl). Estafilocócico; relativo a, ou causado por, qualquer microrganismo do gênero *Staphylococcus*.

staph·y·lo·coc·ce·mia (staf′i-lō-kok-sē′mē-ă). Estafilococcemia; presença de estafilococos no sangue circulante. [staphylo- + G. *haima*, sangue]

staph·y·lo·coc·ci (staf′i-lō-kok′sī). Estafilococos; plural de staphylococcus.

staph·y·lo·coc·cic (staf′i-lō-kok′sik). Estafilocócico; relativo a, ou causado por, qualquer espécie de *Staphylococcus*.

staph·y·lo·coc·col·y·sin (staf′i-lō-kŏ-kol′i-sin). Estafilococolisina. SIN staphyloly sin

staph·y·lo·coc·col·y·sis (staf′i-lō-kŏ-kol′i-sis). Estafilococólise; lise ou destruição de estafilococos. [staphylo- + G. *lysis*, dissolução]

staph·y·lo·coc·co·sis, pl. **staph·y·lo·coc·co·ses** (staf′i-lō-kok-ō′sis, -sēz). Estafilococose; infecção por espécies de *Staphylococcus*.

Sta·phy·lo·coc·cus (staf′i-lō-kok′ŭs). Gênero de bactérias imóveis, não-formadoras de esporos, aeróbicas ou anaeróbicas facultativas (família Micrococcaceae), contendo células Gram-positivas esféricas, de 0,5–1,5 μm, que se dividem em mais de um plano para formar grupos irregulares. Trata-se de microrganismos quimiorganotróficos, de metabolismo respiratório e fermentativo. Em condições anaeróbicas, produzem ácido láctico a partir da glicose; em condições aeróbicas, ocorre produção de ácido acético e pequenas quantidades de CO_2. As cepas coagulase-positivas produzem várias toxinas e, portanto, são potencialmente patogênicas, podendo causar intoxicação alimentar. Em geral, esses microrganismos são sensíveis a antibióticos como os β-lactâmicos e macrolídios, as tetraciclinas, a novobiocina e o cloranfenicol, porém são resistentes à polimixina e aos poliênicos. São sensíveis a antibacterianos, como fenóis e seus derivados, compostos tensoativos, salicilanilidas, carbanilidas e halogênios (cloro e iodo) e seus derivados, como cloraminas e iodóforos. São encontrados na pele, nas glândulas cutâneas, nas mucosas nasais e outras mucosas de animais homeotérmicos, bem como em vários produtos alimentares. A espécie típica é *S. aureus*. [staphylo- + G. *kokkos*, baga]

S. au′reus, espécie comum encontrada especialmente na mucosa nasal e na pele (folículos pilosos); espécie bacteriana que produz exotoxinas, incluindo as que causam a síndrome do choque tóxico, resultando em erupção cutânea e em doença renal, hepática e do sistema nervoso central, bem como uma exotoxina associada à intoxicação alimentar; provoca furunculose, celulite, piemia, pneumonia, osteomielite, endocardite, supuração de feridas e outras infecções; constitui também uma causa de infecção em queimados; os seres humanos constituem o principal reservatório. Trata-se da espécie típica do gênero *S*. SIN *S. pyogenes aureus*.

S. epider′midis, espécie de bactéria, a mais comum do grupo de estafilococos coagulase-negativos.

S. haemoly′ticus, estafilococo coagulase-negativo, residente em hospedeiros humanos e mamíferos.

S. hominis, estafilococo coagulase-negativo, residente em hospedeiros humanos e mamíferos.

S. pyog′enes al′bus, nome antigamente aplicado aos microrganismos que, hoje em dia, são considerados mutantes do *S. aureus* que formam colônias brancas.

S. pyog′enes au′reus. SIN *S. aureus.*

S. saprophyticus, espécie coagulase-negativa que provoca infecções das vias urinárias.

S. simulans, estafilococo coagulase-negativo, residente em hospedeiros humanos e mamíferos.

S. species, **coagulase-negative,** espécies de *S.* coagulase-negativas; grupo de espécies encontradas como flora normal da pele, das vias respiratórias e mucosas dos seres humanos. Apesar de serem comensais normais, as cepas constituem causas proeminentes de infecções hospitalares, sobretudo em pacientes com implantação de dispositivos de acesso intravenoso; algumas cepas formam abscessos e causam diversas infecções, incluindo sinusite, infecções de feridas e osteomielite.

staph·y·lo·coc·cus, pl. **staph·y·lo·coc·ci** (staf′i-lō-kok′ŭs, kok′sī). Estafilococo; termo do vernáculo utilizado para referir-se a qualquer membro do gênero *Staphylococcus*.

staph·y·lo·di·al·y·sis (staf′i-lō-dī-al′i-sis). Estafilodiálise. SIN uvuloptosis. [staphylo- + G. *dialysis*, uma separação]

staph·y·lo·he·mia (staf′i-lō-hē′mē-ă). Estafiloemia; termo obsoleto para estafilococcemia.

staph·y·lo·he·mo·ly·sin (staf′i-lō-hē-mol′i-sin). Estafiloemolisina; mistura de hemolisinas (alfa, beta, gama e delta), incluídas na exotoxina estafilocócica; a hemolisina α exerce acentuado efeito sobre o músculo vascular.

staph·y·lo·ki·nase (staf′i-lō-kī′nās). Estafilocinase; metaloenzima microbiana do *Staphylococcus aureus*, com ação semelhante à da urocinase e estreptocinase, que pode converter o plasminogênio em plasmina, mas que necessita de Ca^{2+}; separada em formas A, B e C.

staph·y·lol·y·sin (staf-i-lol′i-sin). Estafilolisina. **1.** Hemolisina elaborada por um estafilococo. **2.** Anticorpo que causa lise de estafilococos. SIN staphylococcolysin.

staph·y·lo·ma (staf-i-lō′mă). Estafiloma; projeção da córnea ou da esclera contendo tecido uveal. [staphylo- + G. *-ōma*, tumor]

anterior s., e. anterior; projeção próximo ao pólo anterior do globo ocular. SIN corneal s.

anular s., e. anular; e. que se estende ao redor da periferia da córnea.

ciliary s., e. ciliar; e. escleral que ocorre na região do corpo ciliar.

corneal s., e. corneano. SIN anterior s.

equatorial s., e. equatorial; e. que ocorre na área de saída das veias do vórtice. SIN scleral s.

intercalary s., e. intercalar; e. escleral encontrado entre a inserção do corpo ciliar e a raiz da íris.

posterior s., e. posterior; projeção próxima ao pólo posterior do globo ocular devido a alterações degenerativas na miopia grave. SIN Scarpa s., sclerochoroiditis posterior.

Scarpa s., e. de Scarpa. SIN posterior s.

scleral s., e. escleral. SIN equatorial s.

uveal s., e. uveal; termo raramente empregado para referir-se à protrusão da íris através de uma ruptura da esclera.

staph·y·lom·a·tous (staf-i-lō′mă-tŭs). Estafilomatoso; relativo a, ou caracterizado por, um estafiloma.

staph·y·lo·phar·yn·gor·rha·phy (staf′i-lō-far-in-gōr′ă-fē). Estafilofaringorrafia; reparo cirúrgico de defeitos na úvula ou palato mole e na faringe. SIN palatopharyngorrhaphy. [staphylo- + pharynx + G. *rhaphē*, sutura]

staph·y·lo·plas·ty (staf′i-lō-plas-tē). Estafiloplastia. SIN palatoplasty. [staphylo- + G. *plassō*, formar]

staph·y·lop·to·sis (staf′i-lop-tō′sis). Estafiloptose. SIN uvuloptosis. [staphylo- + G. *ptōsis*, queda]

staph·y·lor·rha·phy (staf-i-lōr′ă-fē). Estafilorrafia. SIN palatorrhaphy. [staphylo- + G. *rhaphē*, sutura]

staph·y·lo·tox·in (staf′i-lō-tok′sin). Estafilotoxina; a toxina elaborada por qualquer espécie de *Staphylococcus*. VER TAMBÉM staphylohemolysun. [staphylo- + G. *toxikon*, veneno]

sta·pling (stāp′ling). Grampeamento; uso de um dispositivo de grampeamento que une dois tecidos, como as duas extremidades do intestino, através da aplicação de uma fileira ou círculo de grampos.

gastric s., g. gástrico; divisão do estômago por fileiras de grampos; utilizado no tratamento da obesidade grave.

star (stăr). Estrela; qualquer estrutura em forma de estrela. VER TAMBÉM aster, astrosphere, stella, stellula. [A.S. *steorra*]

daughter s., estrela-filha; uma das figuras que formam o diáster. SIN polar s.

lens s.'s (1) Raio da lente. SIN *radii* of lens, em *radius;* **(2)** Estrelas da lente; cataratas congênitas com opacidades ao longo das linhas de sutura da lente; podem ser anteriores e/ou posteriores.

mother s., estrela-mãe. SIN monaster.

polar s., e. polar. SIN daughter s.

venous s., e. venosa; pequeno nódulo vermelho formado por uma veia dilatada na pele; causada por aumento da pressão venosa.

Verheyen s.'s, estrelas de Verheyen. SIN *venulae* stellatae, em *venula.*

Winslow s.'s, estrelas de Winslow. SIN *stellulae* winslowii, em *stellula.*

starch. Amido; polissacarídeo de alto peso molecular, formado de resíduos de D-glicose em ligação α-1,4, que difere da celulose pela presença de ligações α- e não β-glicosídicas, encontrado na maioria dos tecidos vegetais; convertido em dextrina, quando submetido à ação do calor seco e em dextrina e D-glicose por amilases e glicoamilases presentes na saliva e no suco pancreático; utilizado como pó secante, emoliente e ingrediente em comprimidos medicinais, bem como importante material bruto para a fabricação de álcool, acetona, *n*-butanol, ácido láctico, ácido cítrico, glicerina e ácido glicônico por fermentação; principal carboidrato de armazenamento na maioria das plantas superiores. SIN amylum. [A.S. *stearc,* forte]

animal s., glicogênio. SIN glycogen.

liver s., glicogênio. SIN glycogen.

moss s., liquenina. SIN lichenin.

rice s., a. de arroz; produto do arroz utilizado como suplemento em muitas formulações empregadas para cultura de protozoários intestinais (p. ex., *Entamoeba histolytica*).

soluble s., a. solúvel; dextrina hidrossolúvel, de alto peso molecular, produzida pela hidrólise ácida parcial do amido; útil em iodimetria, visto que produz um ponto final púrpura-escuro facilmente visível na presença de iodo livre.

starch-eat·ing. Amilofagia. SIN amylophagia.

stare (stār). Olhar fixo. **1.** Olhar intencional ou fixamente. **2.** Olhar intencional. [A.S. *starian*]

Stargardt, Karl, oftalmologista alemão, 1875–1927. VER S. *disease.*

Starling, Ernest H., fisiologista inglês, 1866–1927. VER S. *curve, hypothesis, law, reflex;* Frank-S. *curve.*

Starr, Albert, médico norte-americano, *1926. VER Starr-Edwards *valve.*
Starry. VER Warthin-Starry silver *stain.*
start·er (start′er). Iniciador. SIN primer (1).
star·va·tion (star - vā′shŭn). Inanição; privação prolongada e contínua de alimento.
starve. Submeter à fome. **1.** Sofrer carência alimentar. **2.** Privar de alimento, de modo a causar sofrimento ou morte. **3.** Antigamente, morrer de frio. [A.S. *steorfan,* morrer]
Stas, Jean-Servais, químico belga, 1813–1891. VER S.-Otto *method.*
stas·i·mor·phia (stas - i - mōr′fē - ă). Estasimórfia; dismorfogênese devida à interrupção do desenvolvimento. [G. *stasis,* parada + *morphē,* forma]
sta·sis, pl. **sta·ses** (stā′sis, stas′is; -ēz). Estase; estagnação do sangue ou de outros líquidos. [G. parada]
   intestinal s., e. intestinal. SIN enterostasis.
   papillary s., e. papilar; termo obsoleto para papiledema.
   pressure s., e. por compressão. SIN traumatic *asphyxia.*
   venous s., e. venosa; congestão e redução da circulação nas veias, devido a bloqueio por obstrução ou por pressão elevada no sistema venoso, geralmente acometendo mais os pés e as pernas.
stat. Abreviatura do L. *statim,* imediatamente.
△ **stat-.** Stat-. Prefixo aplicado a unidades elétricas no sistema eletrostático CGS para distingui-las das unidades no sistema eletromagnético CGS (prefixo ab-) e daquelas no sistema métrico ou SI (sem prefixo).
△ **-stat.** Estat. Agente que tem por objetivo impedir a mudança, o fluxo ou o movimento de algo. [G. *states,* estacionário]
stat·am·pere (stat - am′pēr). Estatampère; unidade eletrostática de corrente; o fluxo de uma unidade eletrostática de carga (1 statcoulomb) por segundo; igual a $3{,}335641 \times 10^{-10}$ ampère. [G. *statos,* ficar de pé (estacionário) + ampère]
stat·cou·lomb (stat - koo′lom). Statcoulomb; unidade eletrostática de carga, de modo que dois objetos, exibindo cada um essa carga e separados (centro a centro) por 1 cm em vácuo, repelem-se com uma força de 1 dina (ou 10^{-5} newton); igual a $3{,}335641 \times 10^{-10}$ coulomb. [G. *statos,* ficar de pé (estacionário) + coulomb]
state (stāt). Estado; condição, situação ou estado. [L. *status,* condição, estado]
   absent s., e. de ausência. SIN dreamy s.
   activated s., e. ativado. SIN excited s.
   anxiety tension s., e. de ansiedade de tensão; forma mais leve de distúrbio de ansiedade. VER anxiety *disorders,* em *disorder.*
   apallic s., e. apálico; **(1)** degeneração bilateral e difusa do córtex cerebral causada por lesão cranioencefálica, anoxia ou encefalite; **(2)** estado de ausência persistente de responsividade, como o mutismo acinético, causado por lesão cerebral. VER TAMBÉM vegetative. SIN apallic syndrome, apallic.
   carrier s., e. de portador; o estado de ser portador de microrganismos patogênicos, isto é, aquele que está infectado mas não apresenta doença.
   central excitatory s., e. de excitação central; o desenvolvimento de influências excitatórias produzidas por impulsos individuais causa, finalmente, a deflagração do neurônio seguinte.
   convulsive s., epilepsia. SIN epilepsy.
   decerebrate s., rigidez de descerebração. SIN decerebrate *rigidity.*
   decorticate s., rigidez de descorticação. SIN decorticate *rigidity.*
   dreamy s., e. onírico; o estado de semiconsciência associado a um ataque epiléptico. SIN absent s.
   eunuchoid s., e. eunucóide; condição delineada de modo impreciso de um indivíduo do sexo masculino com sinais de secreção inadequada de androgênios durante o crescimento adolescente, independentemente da causa; em geral, refere-se a pernas longas, tronco curto e face imberbe semelhante à de um menino.
   excited s., e. de excitação; a condição de um átomo ou molécula após absorver energia, que pode resultar de exposição à luz, eletricidade, temperatura elevada ou reação química; essa ativação pode ser um prelúdio necessário para uma reação química ou para a emissão de luz. SIN activated s.
   ground s., e. fundamental; o estado inativado e normal de um átomo a partir do qual, mediante ativação, são derivados os estados singleto e tripleto, bem como outros estados de excitação.
   hypnoid s., e. hipnóide; estado de sonolência ou de sono artificialmente induzido por um hipnotizador em indivíduos com níveis de sugestionabilidade maiores do que a média. VER hypnosis.
   hypnotic s., e. hipnótico. SIN hypnosis.
   hypometabolic s., e. hipometabólico; estado raro de redução do metabolismo com sintomas semelhantes ao hipotireoidismo, porém com resultados normais em algumas provas de função da glândula tireóide; termo também utilizado para descrever a atividade metabólica reduzida observada no hipotireoidismo verdadeiro.
   imperfect s., e. imperfeito; nos fungos, refere-se ao estado ou estágio no qual são formados apenas esporos assexuados, como os conídios, a maioria dessas espécies é classificada como Deuteromycetes (Fungi Imperfecti).
   lacunar s., e. lacunar; presença de lacunas no cérebro; um dos principais fatores subjacentes à doença vascular cerebral; alta correlação com a hipertensão e a aterosclerose. As formas sintomáticas incluem síndrome de hemiplegia motora pura e hemissensorial pura; a ocorrência de múltiplos infartos lacunares constitui a causa mais comum de paralisia pseudobulbar.
   local excitatory s., e. de excitação local; aumento da irritabilidade de uma fibra nervosa ou fibra muscular, produzido por um estímulo elétrico subliminar; pode ocorrer somação dos estímulos, resultando em impulso propagado se dois ou mais estímulos subliminais forem aplicados em rápida sucessão.
   multiple ego s.'s, estados múltiplos do ego; vários estados organizacionais psicológicos, refletindo diferentes personas ou experiências de vida.
   perfect s., e. perfeito; nos fungos, parte do ciclo de vida em que são formados esporos após a fusão nuclear.
   persistent vegetative s. (PVS), e. vegetativo persistente; estado vegetativo (q.v.) de duração prolongada (definido, em diferentes fontes, como tendo duração de mais de 1 mês, 1 ano ou 2 anos); geralmente permanente. VER TAMBÉM vegetative.
   post-steady s., e. pós-equilíbrio dinâmico; qualquer período de tempo, particularmente numa reação catalisada por enzima, após o intervalo de estado de equilíbrio dinâmico; p. ex., quando a velocidade de formação de produtos está declinando numa reação catalisada por enzimas.
   pre-steady s., e. pré-equilíbrio dinâmico; as condições e o intervalo de tempo que precedem o estabelecimento do estado de equilíbrio dinâmico.
   refractory s., e. refratário; excitabilidade subnormal imediatamente após uma resposta à excitação prévia; o estado é dividido em fases absoluta e relativa.
   singlet s., e. singleto; estado excitado e transitório de uma molécula (p. ex., de clorofila, após a absorção de luz) que pode liberar energia na forma de calor ou de luz (fluorescência) e, assim, retornar ao estado inicial (fundamental); alternativamente, pode assumir um estado um pouco mais estável, porém ainda excitado (e. tripleto), com um elétron ainda deslocado como antes, porém com *spin* inverso.
   steady s. (ss, s), e. de equilíbrio dinâmico; **(1)** estado obtido no exercício muscular moderado, quando a remoção de ácido láctico por oxidação acompanha sua produção, sendo o suprimento de oxigênio adequado, e os músculos não sofrem débito de oxigênio; **(2)** qualquer condição em que a formação ou a introdução de substâncias acompanha o ritmo de sua destruição ou remoção, de modo que todos os volumes, as concentrações, as pressões e os fluxos permanecem constantes; **(3)** em cinética enzimática, condições nas quais a velocidade de mudança na concentração de qualquer espécie enzimática (p. ex., enzima livre ou complexo binário enzima–substrato) é zero ou bem abaixo da velocidade de formação do produto. [freqüentemente com subscrito s ou ss]
   triplet s., e. tripleto; um segundo estado de excitação de uma molécula (p. ex., clorofila) produzido pela absorção de luz para originar o estado singleto, seguido de perda de alguma energia (fluorescência) para atingir o estado tripleto de maior duração. A molécula pode permanecer por tempo suficientemente longo no estado tripleto para que um segundo *quantum* de luz ativador seja eficaz na produção de um "segundo estado tripleto", que, obviamente, ainda se encontra num nível maior de excitação e, portanto, de reatividade. Alternativamente, pode perder a energia do estado tripleto diretamente e retornar ao estado fundamental.
   twilight s., e. crepuscular; condição de perturbação da consciência, durante a qual as ações podem ser realizadas sem a vontade consciente do indivíduo e sem a memória dessas ações. Cf. somnambulic *epilepsy.*
   vegetative s., e. vegetativo; condição clínica em que ocorre ausência completa de consciência do *self* e do ambiente, acompanhada de ciclos de sono–vigília, porém com preservação parcial ou completa das funções autônomas hipotalâmicas e do tronco cerebral; pode ser transitório ou permanente. Existem múltiplas causas, todas envolvendo o cérebro, incluindo lesões traumáticas e não-traumáticas, distúrbios metabólicos e degenerativos e malformações congênitas.
stat·far·ad (stat - fa′rad). Statfarad; unidade eletrostática de capacitância, igual a $1{,}112650 \times 10^{-12}$ farad.
stat·hen·ry (stat - hen′rē). Stathenry; unidade eletrostática de indutância, igual a $8{,}987552 \times 10^{11}$ henry.
stath·mo·ki·ne·sis (stath′mō - ki - nē′sis). Estatmocinese; condição de interrupção da mitose após tratamento com determinado agente, como colchicina, que altera efetivamente o fuso mitótico, impedindo o rearranjo típico dos cromossomas antes da divisão celular. [G. *stathmos,* lugar para ficar de pé + *kinēsis,* movimento]
sta·tim (stā′tim). Imediatamente. [L.]
stat·ins (stat′ins). Estatinas. SIN releasing *factors.*
sta·tion. O grau de descida da parte de apresentação do feto através da pélvis materna, medido em relação às espinhas isquiáticas da pélvis materna.
sta·tis·ti·cal sig·nif·i·cance. Significância estatística; métodos estatísticos que permitem uma estimativa da probabilidade do grau observado de associação entre variáveis, a partir da qual pode ser expressa a significância estatística, geralmente em termos do valor P.
sta·tis·tics (stă - tis′tiks). Estatística. **1.** Coleção de valores numéricos, dados ou outros fatos que são numericamente agrupados em classes definidas e submetidos a análise, particularmente análise da probabilidade de os achados

empíricos resultantes serem devidos ao acaso. **2.** A ciência e arte de coletar, resumir e analisar dados sujeitos a variação randômica.

descriptive s., e. descritiva; valores numéricos, como média, mediana e modo, que descrevem as principais características de um grupo de pontuações, sem considerar uma população maior.

inferential s., e. dedutiva; estatística a partir da qual é feita uma dedução sobre a natureza de uma população; o objetivo é fornecer uma generalização sobre a população, com base em dados da amostra selecionada da população.

vital s., e. vital; informações reunidas sistematicamente em tabelas sobre nascimentos, casamentos, divórcios, separações e mortes, com base no número de registros oficiais desses acontecimentos; o ramo da estatística que lida com esses dados.

stat·o·a·cou·stic (stat′o-ă-koo′stik). Estatoacústico; relativo ao equilíbrio e à audição. SIN vestibulocochlear (2). [G. *statos*, estacionário + *akousticos*, acústico]

stat·o·co·nia, sing. **stat·o·co·ni·um** (stat′o-ko′ne-ă, -ne-ŭm) [TA]. Estatocônios. SIN otoliths. [L. do G. *statos*, estacionário, *konis*, poeira]

stat·o·ki·net·ic (stat′o-ki-net′ik). Estatocinética; relativo à estatocinética.

stat·o·ki·net·ics (stat′o-ki-net′iks). Estatocinética; o ajuste feito pelo corpo em movimento para manter o equilíbrio estável. [G. *statos*, estacionário + *kinesis*, movimento]

stat·o·liths (stat′o-liths). Estatólitos. SIN otoliths. [G. *statos*, estacionário + *lithos*, pedra]

sta·tom·e·ter (stă-tom′e-ter). Estatômetro. SIN exophthalmometer. [G. *statos*, estacionário + *metron*, medida]

stat·o·sphere (stat′o-sfer). Estatosfera. SIN centrosphere.

stat·ure (statch′er). Estatura; a altura de uma pessoa. [L. *statura*, de *statuo*, pp. *statutus*, fazer ficar de pé]

sta·tus (sta′tŭs, stat′ŭs). Estado; estado ou condição. [L. uma forma de posição]

s. angino′sus, e. anginoso; angina de peito prolongada, refratária ao tratamento.

s. arthrit′icus, e. artrítico; termo obsoleto para referir-se a diátese ou predisposição gotosa.

s. asthamat′icus, e. asmático; condição de asma prolongada e grave.

s. cholera′icus, e. colérico; o estágio frio de choque e depressão na cólera, devido à perda de líquidos e eletrólitos e conseqüente hipovolemia; caracterizado por pulso fraco, pele fria e pegajosa, confusão e depressão.

s. chore′icus, e. coreico; forma muito grave de coréia em que a persistência dos movimentos impede o sono, podendo o paciente morrer de exaustão.

s. cribro′sus, e. crivoso; condição caracterizada por dilatações dos espaços perivasculares no cérebro.

s. crit′icus, e. crítico; forma muito grave e persistente de crise na tabes dorsal.

s. dysmyelinisa′tus, e. desmielinizado. SIN Hallervorden-Spatz *syndrome*.

s. dysra′phicus, e. disráfico; condição em que há falha na fusão das estruturas da linha média, especialmente falha do fechamento do tubo neural. SIN arrhaphia.

s. epilep′ticus, e. de mal epiléptico; crise repetida ou prolongada, com duração de pelo menos 30 min; pode ser convulsivo (tônico-clônico), não-convulsivo (ausência ou parcial complexo), parcial (epilepsia parcial contínua) ou subclínico (estado de mal epiléptico eletrográfico).

s. hemicra′nicus, e. hemicrânico; condição em que as crises de enxaqueca se sucedem com intervalos tão curtos que ela se torna quase contínua.

s. hypnot′icus, e. hipnótico; termo raramente utilizado para hipnose.

s. lacuna′ris, e. lacunar; condição observada na arteriosclerose cerebral em que existem numerosas áreas pequenas de degeneração no cérebro.

s. lymphat′icus, e. linfático. SIN s. thymicolymphaticus.

s. marmora′tus, e. marmóreo; condição congênita decorrente do desenvolvimento anormal do corpo estriado associado a coreoatetose, em que os núcleos estriados possuem aspecto marmóreo causado por alteração da mielinização.

nonreassuring fetal s., e. fetal ameaçador; anormalidade da freqüência cardíaca ou ritmo do feto na monitorização eletrônica, sugerindo isquemia fetal. SIN fetal distress.

performance s., e. de desempenho; medida do bem-estar de um paciente, definido como a atividade normal que ele consegue executar.

s. prae′sens, e. presente; termo obsoleto para referir-se à parte da história de um caso que descreve a condição do paciente por ocasião de sua observação inicial.

s. spongio′sus, e. esponjoso; múltiplos espaços de tamanho microscópico, repletos de líquido na substância branca cerebral; observado em certas doenças hipóxicas, tóxicas e metabólicas.

s. ster′nuens, e. de esternutação; estado de espirros contínuos.

s. thymicolymphat′icus, e. timicolinfático; termo obsoleto para referir-se a uma síndrome de suposto aumento de tamanho do timo e dos linfonodos em lactentes e crianças pequenas, antigamente associada a morte súbita inexplicada; acreditava-se, também erroneamente, que a pressão do timo sobre a traquéia pudesse causar morte durante a anestesia. A proeminência dessas estruturas é hoje considerada normal em crianças pequenas, incluindo aquelas que morrem subitamente sem doenças precedentes passíveis de levar à atrofia do tecido linfóide. VER TAMBÉM sudden infant death *syndrome*. SIN s. lymphaticus, s. thymicus.

s. thy′micus, e. tímico. SIN s. thymicolymphaticus.

s. vertigino′sus, e. vertiginoso; condição em que ocorrem episódios de vertigem em rápida sucessão. SIN chronic vertigo.

stat·volt (stat′volt). Stat-volt; unidade eletrostática de potencial ou força eletromotriz, igual a 299,7925 V. [G. *statos*, ficar de pé (estacionário) + volt]

Staub, Hans, internista suíço, 1890–1967. VER S.-Traugott *effect*, *phenomenon*.

stau·ri·on (staw′re-on). Estáurio; ponto craniométrico na interseção das suturas palatinas mediana e transversal. [G. dim. de *stauros*, cruz]

STD Abreviatura de sexually transmitted *disease* (doença sexualmente transmissível).

steal (stel). Roubo; desvio de sangue por vias alternativas ou inversão do fluxo de um leito vascular para outro, causando freqüentemente sintomas no órgão a partir do qual o fluxo sanguíneo foi desviado. [I.m. *stelen*, do A.S. *stelan*]

coronary s., roubo coronário; desvio causado pela origem anormal da artéria coronária a partir da artéria pulmonar.

iliac s., roubo ilíaco; redução do fluxo numa artéria ilíaca comum quando ocorre liberação de uma oclusão na outra artéria ilíaca comum.

renal-splanchnic s., roubo renal-esplâncnico; desvio de sangue da artéria renal direita, através do ramo supra-renal inferior, para colaterais esplâncnicas distais a uma estenose do eixo celíaco.

subclavian s., roubo subclávio; obstrução da artéria subclávia proximal à origem da artéria vertebral; o fluxo sanguíneo através da artéria vertebral é invertido, de modo que a artéria subclávia "rouba" sangue cerebral, causando sintomas de insuficiência vértebro-basilar (síndrome de roubo subclávio); manifesta-se durante o uso vigoroso de um membro superior.

ste·ap·sin (ste-ap′sin). Esteapsina. SIN triacylglycerol lipase.

♻ **stear-.** Estear-. VER stearo-.

ste·a·ral (ste′ă-ral). Estearal; octadecanal (deído); o aldeído do ácido esteárico. SIN stearaldehyde.

ste·a·ral·de·hyde (ste-ă-ral′de-hid). Estearaldeído. SIN stearal.

ste·a·rate (ste′ă-rat). Estearato; sal do ácido esteárico.

ste·ar·ic ac·id (ste′ă-rik). Ácido esteárico; ácido *n*-octadecanóico; um dos mais abundantes ácidos graxos encontrados em lipídios animais; utilizado em preparações farmacêuticas, pomadas, sabões e supositórios.

ste·a·rin (ste′ă-rin). Estearina; tristearoilglicerol; o "triglicerídeo" do ácido esteárico presente em gorduras animais sólidas e em algumas gorduras vegetais; fonte do ácido esteárico; a estearina comercial também contém algum ácido palmítico. SIN tristearin.

Stearns, A. Warren, médico norte-americano, 1885–1959.

♻ **stearo-, stear-.** Estearo-, estear-. Forma combinante que significa gordura. VER TAMBÉM steato-. [G. *stear*, sebo]

ste·ar·rhea (ste-ă-re′ă). Estearréia. SIN steatorrhea.

ste·a·ryl al·co·hol (ste′ă-ril). Álcool esteárilico; ingrediente de pomada hidrofílica e petrolato hidrofílico; também utilizado no preparo de cremes.

ste·a·ryl-CoA, ste·a·ryl-co·en·zyme A. Estearil-CoA, estearil-coenzima A; o tioéster coenzima A do ácido esteárico; precursor do ácido oléico e, no cérebro, dos ácidos graxos C_{22} e C_{24} presentes nas esfingomielinas; no cérebro, o uso de estearil-CoA aumenta durante a mielinização.

s.-CoA desaturase, estearil-CoA dessaturase; complexo proteico importante na síntese dos ácidos graxos insaturados; introduz uma dupla ligação em Δ^9; os altos níveis de ácidos graxos insaturados na dieta diminuem a atividade dessa enzima no fígado; diversos agentes induzem a enzima (p. ex., insulina, hidrocortisona e triiodotironina)

ste·a·tite (ste′ă-tit). Esteatito; saponito; talco na forma de massa.

ste·a·ti·tis (ste-ă-ti′tis). Esteatite; inflamação do tecido adiposo. [G. *stear* (*steat*-), sebo + *-itis*, inflamação]

♻ **steato-.** Esteato-; forma combinante que significa gordura. VER stearo-. [G. *stear* (*steat*-), sebo]

ste·a·to·cys·to·ma (ste′ă-to-sis-to′mă). Esteatocistoma; cisto com células de glândulas sebáceas em sua parede.

s. mul′tiplex, e. múltiplo; cistos de paredes finas, múltiplos e disseminados na pele, que são revestidos de epitélio escamoso, incluindo lóbulos de células sebáceas.

ste·a·to·gen·e·sis (ste′ă-to-jen′e-sis). Esteatogênese; biossíntese de lipídios. O termo é utilizado especificamente para designar o acúmulo de lipídios nos testículos de vertebrados não-mamíferos ao termo da espermatogênese no período de reprodução. [steato- + G. *genesis*, produção]

ste·a·tol·y·sis (ste-ă-tol′i-sis). Esteatólise; a hidrólise ou emulsão da gordura no processo de digestão. [steato- + G. *lysis*, dissolução]

ste·a·to·lyt·ic (ste-ă-to-lit′ik). Esteatolítico; relativo à esteatólise.

ste·a·to·ne·cro·sis (ste′ă-to-ne-kro′sis). Esteatonecrose. SIN fat *necrosis*. [steato- + G. *nekrosis*, morte]

ste·a·to·py·ga, ste·a·to·py·gia (ste′ă-to-pi′gă, -pij′e-ă). Esteatopigia; acúmulo excessivo de gordura nas nádegas. [steato- + G. *pyge*, nádegas]

ste·a·to·py·gous (ste-ă-top′ă-gŭs). Esteatopígeo; que apresenta excesso de gordura nas nádegas.

ste·a·tor·rhea (stē′ă-tō-rē′ă). Esteatorréia; eliminação de grandes quantidades de gordura nas fezes, devido à falta de sua digestão e absorção; ocorre na doença pancreática e nas síndromes de má absorção. SIN fat indigestion. SIN stearrhea. [steato- + G. *rhoia*, fluxo]
  biliary s., e. biliar; esteatorréia em conseqüência da ausência de bile no intestino; habitualmente acompanhada de icterícia.
  intestinal s., e. intestinal; esteatorréia causada por má absorção resultante de doença intestinal. VER TAMBÉM sprue, celiac *disease*.
  pancreatic s., e. pancreática; esteatorréia devida à ausência de suco pancreático no intestino.

ste·a·to·sis (stē-ă-tō′sis). Esteatose. 1. SIN adiposis. 2. SIN fatty *degeneration*. [steato- + G. *-osis*, condição]
  s. cardiaca, e. cardíaca; presença de gordura em excesso no pericárdio, invadindo o músculo cardíaco.
  s. cor'dis, e. cardíaca; degeneração gordurosa do coração.
  hepatic s., e. hepática. SIN fatty *liver*.

ste·a·to·zo·on (stē′ă-tō-zō′on). Esteatozoário; nome comum do *Demodex folliculorum*. [steato- + G. *zōon*, animal]

Steele, John C., neurologista canadense, 1951–1968. VER S.-Richardson-Olszewski *disease, syndrome*.

Steell, Graham, médico inglês, 1851–1942. VER Graham Steell *murmur*.

Steenbock, Harry, fisiologista e químico norte-americano, 1886–1967. VER S. *unit*.

ste·ge (stē′gē). Pilar interno do órgão de Corti. [G. *stegos*, teto, casa]

steg·no·sis (steg-nō′sis). Estegnose. 1. Interrupção de qualquer uma das secreções ou excreções. 2. Constrição ou estenose. [G. stoppage]

steg·not·ic (steg-not′ik). Estegnótico. 1. Adstringente ou constipante. 2. Agente adstringente ou constipante.

Stein, Irving F., ginecologista norte-americano, *1887. VER S.-Leventhal *syndrome*.

Stein, Stanislav A.F. von, otologista russo, *1855. VER S. *test*.

Steinberg, I. VER S. thumb *sign*.

Steinbrinck, W., médico alemão do século XX. VER Chédiak-S.-Higashi *anomaly, syndrome*.

Steinert, Hans, médico alemão, *1875. VER S. *disease*.

Steinmann, Fritz, cirurgião suíço, 1872–1932. VER S. *pin*.

stein·stras·se (stīn′stra-se). Complicação da litotripsia extracorpórea por ondas de choque para cálculos do trato urinário, em que os fragmentos do cálculo bloqueiam o ureter, formando uma "rua de pedras". [Al. *Stein*, pedra + *Strasse*, rua]

STEL Abreviatura de short-term exposure *limit* (limite de exposição em curto prazo).

stel·la, pl. **stel·lae** (stel′ă, -ē). Estrela; estrela ou figura em forma de estrela. [L. mod.]
  s. len'tis hyaloi'dea, e. hialóidea da lente; o pólo posterior da lente. VER *radii* lentis, em *radius*.
  s. len'tis irid'ica, e. irídica da lente; o pólo anterior da lente. VER *radii* lentis, em *radius*.

stel·late (stel′āt). Estrelado; em forma de estrela. [L. *stella*, estrela]

stel·lec·to·my (stel-ek′tō-mē). Estrelectomia; excisão do gânglio estrelado (cervicotorácico).

stel·lu·la, pl. **stel·lu·lae** (stel′ū-lă, -lē). Pequena estrela ou figura em forma de estrela. [L. dim. de *stella*, estrela]
  stel'lulae vasculo'sae, estrelas vasculares. SIN stellulae winslowii.
  stel'lulae verheyen'ii, estrelas de Verheyen. SIN venulae stellatae, em *venula*.
  stel'lulae winslo'wii, estrelas de Winslow; espirais capilares na lâmina coroideocapilar a partir das quais se originam as veias vorticosas. SIN stellulae vasculosae, Winslow stars.

Stellwag, Carl von C., oftalmologista austríaco, 1823–1904. VER S. *sign*.

stem. Tronco; estrutura de sustentação semelhante ao caule de uma planta.
  brain s., t. encefálico. VER brainstem.
  infundibular s., pedículo infundibular; o componente neural do pedículo hipofisário contendo os tratos nervosos que se estendem do hipotálamo até a parte nervosa. SIN infundibular stalk.

sten. Termo estatístico que utiliza o desvio-padrão para a conversão dos dados em pontuações padronizadas, que definem 10 etapas ao longo de uma distribuição normal, com cinco etapas em cada lado da média.

Stender, Wilhelm P., fabricante de aparelhos científicos de Leipzig no século XIX. VER S. *dish*.

Stenger test. Teste de Stenger. Ver em test.

ste·ni·on (sten′ē-on). Estênio; a extremidade, na fossa temporal, do menor diâmetro transversal do crânio; um ponto craniométrico. [G. *stenos*, estreito + dim, *-ion*]

Steno. VER Stensen.

steno-. Esteno-; estreitamento, constrição; oposto de eury-. [G. *stenos*, estreito]

sten·o·breg·mat·ic (sten′ō-breg-mat′ik). Estenobregmático; designa um crânio estreito anteriormente, na parte onde se encontra o bregma. [steno- + G. *bregma*]

sten·o·car·dia (sten-ō-kar′dē-ă). Estenocardia. SIN angina pectoris. [steno- + G. *kardia*, coração]

sten·o·ce·pha·lia (sten-ō-se-fā′lē-ă). Estenocefalia. SIN stenocephaly.

sten·o·ceph·a·lous, sten·o·ce·phal·ic (sten-ō-sef′ă-lŭs, -se-fal′ik). Estenocéfalo, estenocefálico; relativo a ou que se caracteriza por, estenocefalia.

sten·o·ceph·a·ly (sten-ō-sef′ă-lē). Estenocefalia; estreitamento acentuado da cabeça. SIN stenocephalia. [steno- + G. *kephalē*, cabeça]

sten·o·cho·ria (sten-ō-kō′rē-ă). Estenocoria; contração anormal de qualquer canal ou orifício, especialmente dos ductos lacrimais. [G. *stenochōria*, estreitamento, de steno- + *chōra*, local, sala]

sten·o·com·pres·sor (sten′ō-kom-pres′er, or). Estenocompressor; instrumento para comprimir os ductos das glândulas parótidas (ducto de Stensen) para reter a saliva durante cirurgias dentárias.

sten·o·crot·a·phy, sten·o·cro·ta·phia (sten′ō-krot′ă-fē, -krō-tā′fē-ă). Estenocrotafia; estreitamento do crânio na região temporal; a condição de um crânio estenobregmático. [steno- + G. *krotaphos*, têmpora]

Stenon. VER Stensen. [*Stenonius*, forma latina de Stensen]

sten·o·pe·ic, sten·o·pa·ic (sten-ō-pē′ik, sten-ō-pā′ik). Estenopeico, estenopaico; provido de uma abertura ou fenda estreita, como nos óculos estenopeicos. [steno- + G. *opē*, abertura]

ste·no·sal (ste-nō′săl). Estenótico. SIN stenotic.

ste·nosed (sten′ōzd). Estenosado; estreitado; contraído; com estritura.

ste·no·sis, pl. **ste·no·ses** (ste-nō′sis, -sēz). Estenose; estreitamento de qualquer canal ou orifício. [G. *stenōsis*, estreitamento]
  aortic s., e. aórtica; estreitamento patológico do orifício da valva aórtica.
  bronchial s., e. brônquica; estreitamento da luz de um tubo brônquico. SIN bronchiostenosis.
  buttonhole s., e. em casa de botão; estreitamento extremo, geralmente da valva mitral.
  calcific nodular aortic s., e. aórtica nodular calcificada; tipo mais comum de estenose aórtica, que ocorre habitualmente em homens idosos, em que as válvulas contêm nódulos fibrosos calcificados nas duas superfícies; as causas incluem febre reumática, aterosclerose, degeneração relacionada com a idade e valva aórtica congenitamente bicúspide.
  congenital pyloric s., e. pilórica congênita. SIN hypertrophic pyloric s.
  coronary ostial s., e. do óstio coronário; estreitamento dos orifícios das artérias coronárias em decorrência de aortite sifilítica ou aterosclerose.
  Dittrich s., e. de Dittrich. SIN infundibular s.
  double aortic s., e. aórtica dupla; estenose subaórtica associada à estenose da própria valva, sendo ambas lesões congênitas.
  fish-mouth mitral s., e. mitral em boca de peixe; estenose mitral extrema.
  hypertrophic pyloric s., e. pilórica hipertrófica; hipertrofia muscular do esfíncter pilórico, associada a vômitos em projétil, que surge nas primeiras semanas de vida, mais comumente em meninos. SIN congenital pyloric s.
  idiopathic hypertrophic subaortic s., e. subaórtica hipertrófica idiopática; obstrução do trato de saída do ventrículo esquerdo em virtude de hipertrofia, geralmente congênita, do septo interventricular. SIN muscular subaortic s.
  idiopathic subglottic s., e. subglótica idiopática; estreitamento da luz infraglótica, de causa desconhecida; aparentemente, ocorre apenas em mulheres.
  infundibular s., e. infundibular; estreitamento do trato de saída do ventrículo direito abaixo da valva pulmonar; pode ser decorrente de um diafragma fibroso localizado imediatamente abaixo da valva ou, mais comumente, de um canal fibromuscular estreito e longo. SIN Dittrich s.
  laryngeal s., e. laríngea; estreitamento ou estritura de qualquer uma das áreas da laringe ou de todas elas; pode ser congênita ou adquirida.
  mitral s. (MS), e. mitral; estreitamento patológico do orifício da valva mitral.
  muscular subaortic s., e. subaórtica hipertrófica idiopática. SIN idiopathic hypertrophic subaortic s.
  pulmonary s., e. pulmonar; estreitamento da abertura do ventrículo direito para a artéria pulmonar.
  pyloric s., e. pilórica; estreitamento do piloro gástrico, especialmente por hipertrofia muscular congênita ou fibrose resultante de uma úlcera péptica. VER TAMBÉM hypertrophic pyloric s.
  subaortic s., e. subaórtica; estreitamento congênito do trato de saída do ventrículo esquerdo por um anel de tecido fibroso ou por hipertrofia do septo muscular abaixo da valva aórtica. SIN subvalvar s.
  subvalvar s., e. subaórtica. SIN subaortic s.
  subvalvular aortic s., e. aórtica subvalvar; estreitamento congênito, abaixo das valvas aórticas, decorrente de membrana ou hipertrofia muscular, freqüentemente confundido com estenose aórtica valvular.
  supravalvar s., e. supravalvar; estreitamento da aorta, acima da valva aórtica, por um anel constritivo ou prateleira, ou por coarctação ou hipoplasia da aorta ascendente.
  supravalvular s., e. supravalvular; estenose distal à valva aórtica, geralmente decorrente de membrana congênita. Em geral, os pacientes apresentam um tipo de fácies de elfo e assemelham-se muito mais entre si do que com os membros de sua família.

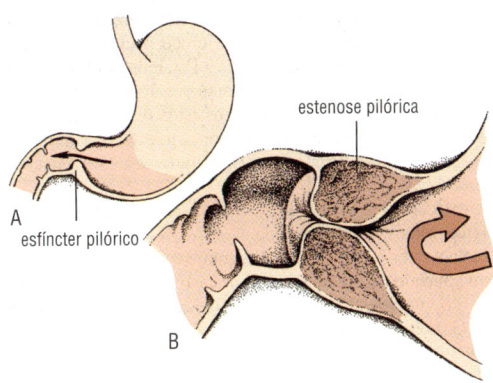

estenose pilórica: (A) passagem normal pelo esfíncter pilórico, (B) interrupção do fluxo devido à estenose do esfíncter

---

tricuspid s., e. tricúspide; estreitamento patológico do orifício da valva tricúspide.
sten·o·ste·no·sis (sten′ō-stĕ-nō′sis). Estenostenose; estreitamento do ducto parotídeo (ducto de Steno ou Stensen).
sten·o·sto·mia (sten-ō-stō′mē-ă). Estenotosmia; estreitamento da cavidade oral. [steno- + G. *stoma,* boca]
sten·o·ther·mal (sten-ō-ther′mal). Estenotérmico; termoestável numa estreita faixa de temperatura; capaz de resistir apenas a pequenas alterações da temperatura. [steno- + G. *therme,* calor]
sten·o·tho·rax (sten′ō-thōr′aks). Estenotórax; tórax estreito e contraído.
ste·not·ic (stĕ-not′ik). Estenótico; estreitado; acometido por estenose. SIN stenosal.
Sten·o·tro·pho·mo·nas (sten′ō-trō-fō-mōn′as). Gênero de bacilos Gram-negativos que, tipicamente, residem no solo e na água e não fazem parte da flora humana normal.
S. maltophilia, patógeno bacteriano ocular oportunista que provoca ceratite, ceratopatia e conjuntivite; bastonete Gram-negativo que não forma esporos, um importante patógeno hospitalar emergente, de importância especial em unidades de tratamento intensivo, em parte devido à sua resistência à maioria das penicilinas e às cefalosporinas e aminoglicosídeos. Antigamente denominado *Xanthomonas maltophilia* e *Pseudomonas maltophilia*.
sten·ox·e·nous (sten-ok′sĕ-nŭs). Estenoxênico; designa um parasita com estreita gama de hospedeiros; p. ex., *Eimeria* (entre os Coccidia), ancilóstomos, piolhos picadores e sugadores. [steno- + G. *xenos,* estrangeiro, forasteiro]
Stensen (Steno, Stenon, Stenonius). Niels (Nicholaus), anatomista dinamarquês, 1638–1686. VER Stensen *duct,* Stensen *foramen,* Stensen *plexus,* Stensen *veins,* em *vein*.
Stent, Charles R., dentista inglês, †1901. VER stent; S. *graft*.
stent. 1. *Stent;* fio, bastão ou cateter, localizado dentro da luz de estruturas tubulares, utilizado para proporcionar sustentação durante ou após a sua anastomose, ou para assegurar a desobstrução de uma luz intacta, porém contraída. **2.** O processo de colocar um *stent*. **3.** Dispositivo utilizado para manter um orifício ou cavidade durante um enxerto de pele. **4.** Imobilizar um enxerto cutâneo após a sua colocação. [Charles R. *Stent*]
expandable s., s. expansível; *stent* colocado na luz de uma estrutura, freqüentemente por via percutânea, que se encurta longitudinalmente e aumenta de diâmetro, aumentando, assim, a dimensão interna da estrutura.
step (stĕp). **1.** Em odontologia, projeção em rabo de andorinha, ou forma semelhante, de uma cavidade preparada em um dente, numa superfície perpendicular à parte principal da cavidade, com o objetivo de impedir o deslocamento da restauração pela força da mastigação. **2.** Mudança de direção semelhante a um degrau em uma linha, uma superfície ou construção de um corpo sólido.
Krönig s.'s, extensão da parte inferior da borda direita da macicez cardíaca absoluta na hipertrofia do coração direito.
Rønne nasal s., degrau nasal de Rønne; defeito do campo visual nasal com uma margem correspondente ao meio horizontal da retina; observado no glaucoma.
ste·pha·ni·al (stĕ-fā′nē-ăl). Estefânico; relativo ao estefânio.
ste·pha·ni·on (stĕ-fā′nē-on). Estefânio; ponto craniométrico em que a sutura coronal cruza a linha temporal inferior. [G. dim. de *stephanos,* coroa]
Steph·a·no·fi·lar·ia (stef′ă-nō-fĭ-lār′ē-ă). Gênero de nematódeos filaróides da família Stephanofilariidae, parasitas subcutâneos de grandes mamíferos, especialmente gado bovino.
S. stilesi, espécie de filária que infecta a pele, parasita do gado bovino e transmitida pela mosca *Haematobia irritans;* trata-se da única espécie conhecida que ocorre nos Estados Unidos; caracteriza-se por uma fileira de espinhos atrás da boca do verme adulto, cuja fêmea tem 6–8 mm e o macho 2–3 mm. Tanto os adultos quanto as larvas são encontrados em lesões cutâneas granulomatosas

no gado bovino, geralmente na face inferior do abdome. [G. *stephanos,* coroa + *filaria*]
Steph·a·nu·rus den·ta·tus (stef′ă-noo′rŭs). O verme renal ou da gordura dos suínos, uma espécie de parasita nematódeo estrongilóide, que também ocorre, ainda que raramente, no fígado do gado bovino. Os vermes adultos nos suínos vivem na gordura perirrenal, na pelve renal ou como formas erráticas em muitas outras localizações. Os ovos são eliminados através da urina, e a infecção é direta, por ingestão de larvas infectantes ou por infecção cutânea ou indireta, através da ingestão de minhocas nas quais as larvas conseguem sobreviver. [G. *stephanos,* coroa + *oura,* cauda]
step·page (step′aj). Marcha de passos altos. SIN steppage *gait.* [Fr.]
ste·ra·di·an (sr) (stĕ-rā′dē-an). Esterorradiano; a unidade de ângulo sólido; o ângulo sólido que abrange uma área, na superfície de uma esfera, equivalente ao quadrado do raio da esfera. [G. *stereos,* sólido + *radion,* raio]
ster·ane (ster′an, stēr′an). Esterano; a molécula original hipotética de qualquer hormônio esteróide; hidrocarboneto saturado que não contém oxigênio. O nome foi originalmente concebido para alcançar formas de nomenclatura sistemática, porém hoje é suplantado pelas variantes fundamentais: gonano, estrano, androstano, norandrostano (etiano), colano, colestano, ergostano e estigmastano. VER TAMBÉM steroids.
sterco-. Esterco-. Fezes. VER TAMBÉM corpo-, scato-. [L. *stercus,* excremento]
ster·co·bi·lin (ster′kō-bī′lin, -bil′in). Estercobilina; produto de degradação da hemoglobina, de cor castanha, presente nas fezes. VER TAMBÉM bilirubinoids.
***l*-ster·co·bi·lin·o·gen** (ster′kō-bī-lin′ō-jen). *L*-estercobilinogênio; produto de redução do *l*-urobilinogênio, precursor da *l*-estercobilina nos estágios finais no metabolismo da bilirrubina; excretado nas fezes, onde é oxidado a estercobilina. VER TAMBÉM bilirubinoids.
ster·co·lith (ster′kō-lith). Estercólito. SIN fecalith. [sterco- + G. *lithos,* pedra]
ster·co·ra·ceous (ster-kō-rā′shŭs). Estercoráceo; relativo a ou que contém fezes. SIN stercoral, stercorous.
ster·co·ral (ster′kō-răl). Estercoral. SIN stercoraceous.
ster·co·rin (ster′kō-rin). Estercorina. SIN coprosterol.
ster·co·ro·ma (ster-kō-rō′mă). Estercoroma. SIN fecaloma. [sterco- + G. *-oma,* tumor]
ster·co·rous (ster′kō-rŭs). Estercoroso. SIN stercoraceous.

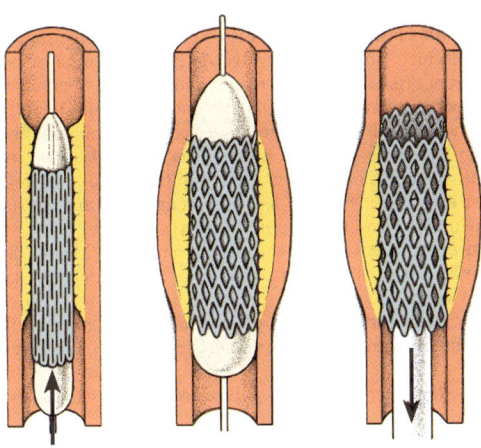

***stent* vascular**

---

ster·cus (ster′kŭs). Fezes. SIN feces. [L. *feces,* excremento]
stere (stēr, star). Estere, estéreo; medida de capacidade; equivalente a um metro cúbico ou um quilolitro; igual a 1,307951 jardas cúbicas. [Fr. do G. *stereos,* sólido]
stereo-. Estéreo-. **1.** Um sólido; uma condição ou estado sólido. **2.** Qualidades espaciais, tridimensionalidade. [G. *stereos,* sólido]
ster·e·o·ag·no·sis (ster′ē-ō-ag-nō′sis). Agnosia tátil. SIN tactile *agnosia*.
ster·e·o·an·es·the·sia (ster′ē-ō-an-es-thē′zē-ă). Agnosia tátil. SIN tactile *agnosia*. [stereo- + G. *an-* priv. + *aisthesis,* sensação]
ster·e·o·ar·throl·y·sis (ster′ē-ō-ar-throl′i-sis). Estereoartrólise; produção de uma nova articulação com mobilidade em casos de ancilose óssea. [stereo- + G. *arthron,* articulação + *lysis,* frouxamento]
ster·e·o·cam·pim·e·ter (ster′ē-ō-kam-pim′ē-ter). Estereocampímetro; aparelho para estudar os campos visuais centrais enquanto o outro olho mantém-se fixo. [stereo- + L. *campus,* campo + G. *metron,* medida]
ster·e·o·chem·i·cal (ster′ē-ō-kem′i-kăl). Estereoquímico; relativo à estereoquímica.
ster·e·o·chem·is·try (ster-ē-ō-kem′is-trē). Estereoquímica; ramo da química que trata das relações tridimensionais espaciais de átomos em molécu-

las, isto é, as posições dos átomos em um composto em relação uns aos outros no espaço.

ster·e·o·cil·i·um, pl. **ster·e·o·cil·ia** (sterʹē-ō-silʹē-ŭm, -ă). Estereocílio; microvilosidade longa imóvel. [stereo- + L. *cilium*, pálpebra]

ster·e·o·cin·e·flu·o·rog·ra·phy (sterʹē-ō-sinʹē-flōr-ogʹră-fē). Estereocinefluorografia; prática obsoleta de registrar em filme as imagens obtidas por fluoroscopia estereoscópica; são obtidas vistas tridimensionais.

ster·e·o·col·po·gram (sterʹē-ō-kolʹpō-gram). Estereocolpograma; fotografia efetuada com o estereocolposcópio.

ster·e·o·col·po·scope (sterʹē-ō-kolʹpō-skōp). Estereocolposcópio; instrumento que proporciona ao observador uma inspeção macroscópica tridimensional ampliada da vagina e do colo do útero. [stereo- + G. *kolpos*, uma cavidade (vagina) + *skopeō*, ver]

ster·e·o·e·lec·tro·en·ceph·a·log·ra·phy (ster-ē-ō-ē-lekʹtrō-en-sef-ă-logʹră-fē). Estereoeletroencefalografia; registro da atividade elétrica em três planos do cérebro, isto é, com eletrodos superficiais e profundos.

ster·e·o·en·ceph·a·lom·e·try (sterʹē-ō-en-sefʹă-lomʹē-trē). Estereoencefalometria; a localização das estruturas cerebrais através do uso de coordenadas tridimensionais.

ster·e·og·no·sis (sterʹē-ogʹnōʹsis). Estereognose, estereognosia; a apreciação da forma de um objeto através do tato. [stereo- + G. *gnōsis*, conhecimento]

ster·e·og·nos·tic (sterʹē-og-nosʹtik). Estereognóstico; relativo à estereognose.

ster·e·o·gram (sterʹē-ō-gram). Estereograma; imagem radiográfica estereoscópica de um par.

ster·e·o·graph (sterʹē-ō-graf). Estereógrafo; aparelho de raios X estereoscópico.

ster·e·og·ra·phy (ster-ē-ogʹră-fē). Estereografia. SIN stereoradiography.

ster·e·o·i·so·mer (sterʹē-ō-īʹsō-mer). Estereoisômero; molécula que contém o mesmo número e tipo de agrupamentos de átomos do que outra, porém em diferente arranjo espacial; os estereoisômeros não são interconversíveis, a não ser que as ligações sejam rompidas e reformadas, razão pela qual exibem diferentes propriedades ópticas, como, por exemplo, entre os D- e L-aminoácidos, 5α e 5β-esteróides. Cf. isomer. [stereo- + G. *isos*, igual + *meros*, parte]

ster·e·o·i·so·mer·ic (sterʹē-ō-ī-sō-merʹik). Estereoisomérico; relativo ao estereoisomerismo.

ster·e·o·i·som·er·ism (sterʹē-ō-ī-somʹer-izm). Estereoisomerismo; assimetria molecular; isomerismo envolvendo diferentes arranjos espaciais dos mesmos grupos (p. ex., androsterona e isoandrosterona, diferindo apenas pelo fato de que um possui uma 3α-OH, e o outro, uma 3β-OH). VER TAMBÉM stereoisomer, Le Bel-van't Hoff *rule*. SIN stereochemical isomerism.

ster·e·ol·o·gy (sterʹē-olʹō-jē). Estereologia; estudo dos aspectos tridimensionais de uma célula ou estrutura microscópica. [stereo- + G. *logos*, estudo]

ster·e·om·e·ter (ster-ē-omʹē-ter). Estereômetro; instrumento utilizado em estereometria. [stereo- + G. *metron*, medida]

ster·e·om·e·try (ster-ē-omʹē-trē). Estereometria. **1.** Medida de um objeto sólido ou da capacidade cúbica de um vaso. **2.** Determinação da densidade específica de um líquido.

ster·e·o·or·thop·ter (ster-ē-ō-ōr-tropʹter). Estereortóptero; tipo de estereoscópio utilizado no treinamento visual. [stereo- + G. *orthos*, reto + *optikos*, óptico]

ster·e·op·a·thy (ster-ē-opʹă-thē). Estereopatia; pensamento estereotipado persistente.

ster·e·o·pho·rom·e·ter (sterʹē-ō-fō-romʹē-ter). Estereoforômetro; forômetro com fixação estereoscópica.

ster·e·o·pho·to·mi·cro·graph (sterʹē-ō-fō-tō-mīʹkrō-graf). Estereofotomicrografia; fotomicrografia estereoscópica que, quando observada com um estereoscópio, aparece tridimensional.

ster·e·op·sis (ster-ē-opʹsis). Estereopsia. SIN stereoscopic vison. [stereo- + G. *opsis*, visão]

ster·e·o·ra·di·og·ra·phy (sterʹē-ō-rā-dē-ogʹră-fē). Estereorradiografia; preparação de um par de radiografias com deslocamento apropriado do tubo de raios X ou filme, de modo que as imagens possam ser vistas estereoscopicamente para proporcionar um aspecto tridimensional. SIN stereography, stereoroentgenography.

ster·e·o·roent·gen·og·ra·phy (sterʹē-ō-rentʹgen-ogʹră-fē). Estereoradiografia. SIN stereoradiography.

ster·e·o·scope (sterʹē-ō-skōp). Estereoscópio; instrumento que produz duas imagens horizontalmente separadas do mesmo objeto, fornecendo uma única imagem com aspecto de profundidade. [stereo- + G. *skopeō*, ver]

ster·e·o·scop·ic (sterʹē-ō-skopʹik). Estereoscópico; relativo a um estereoscópio ou que fornece a aparência de três dimensões.

ster·e·os·co·py (ster-ē-osʹkō-pē). Estereoscopia. **1.** Técnica óptica através da qual duas imagens do mesmo objeto são reunidas em uma, conferindo uma aparência tridimensional à imagem única. **2.** VER radiostereoscopy.

ster·e·o·se·lec·tive (sterʹē-ō-sē-lekʹtiv). Estereosseletivo; quando aplicado a uma reação, designa um processo em que, dentre dois ou mais produtos estereoisoméricos possíveis, apenas um deles predomina; um processo estereosseletivo não é necessariamente estereoespecífico.

ster·e·o·spe·cif·ic (sterʹē-ō-spē-sifʹik). Estereoespecífico; quando aplicado a uma reação, designa um processo em que materiais iniciais estereoisomericamente diferentes dão origem a produtos estereoisomericamente diferentes; por conseguinte, um processo estereoespecífico é necessariamente estereosseletivo, mas nem todos os processos estereosseletivos são estereoespecíficos.

ster·e·o·tac·tic, ster·e·o·tax·ic (sterʹē-ō-takʹtik, -takʹsik). Estereotático, estereotáxico, relativo à estereotaxia.

ster·e·o·tax·is (sterʹē-ō-takʹsis). **1.** Arranjo tridimensional. **2.** Estereotropismo, porém aplicado mais exatamente aos casos em que o organismo como um todo, mais do que apenas uma parte, reage. **3.** Estereotaxia. SIN stereotaxy. [stereo- + G. *taxis*, arranjo ordenado]

ster·e·o·taxy (sterʹē-ō-takʹsē). Estereotaxia; método preciso de identificação de estruturas anatômicas não-visualizadas mediante o uso de coordenadas tridimensionais; mais freqüentemente utilizado para cirurgia de cérebro ou medula espinal. SIN stereotactic surgery, stereotaxic surgery, stereotaxis (3).

ster·e·o·tro·pic (sterʹē-ō-tropʹik). Estereotrópico; relativo a ou que exibe esteotropismo.

ster·e·ot·ro·pism (sterʹē-otʹrō-pizm). Estereotropismo; crescimento ou movimento de uma planta ou animal em direção a um corpo sólido (**estereotropismo positivo**) ou afastando-se dele (**estereotropismo negativo**), habitualmente aplicado aos casos em que uma parte do organismo, mais do que o todo, reage. [stereo- + G. *tropos*, uma volta]

ster·e·o·ty·py (sterʹē-ō-tī-pē). Estereotipia. **1.** Manutenção de uma atitude por longo período de tempo. **2.** Repetição constante de determinados gestos ou movimentos sem significado, como em determinadas formas de esquizofrenia. [stereo- + G. *typos*, impressão, tipo]

oral s., e. oral, verbigeração. SIN verbigeration.

ste·ric (sterʹik, stēr-). Estérico; relativo à estereoquímica.

s. hindrance, bloqueio estérico; interferência ou inibição de uma reação aparentemente possível (geralmente sintética), devido ao tamanho de um ou outro reagente, que impede a sua aproximação até a distância interatômica necessária.

ster·id (sterʹid, stēr). Estereódeo. SIN steroid (2).

ste·rig·ma, pl. **ste·rig·ma·ta** (ste-rigʹma, -mă-tă). Esterigma; estrutura pontiaguda e delgada que surge de um basídio sobre o qual irá desenvolver-se um basiosporo. [G. *sterigma*, suporte]

ster·ile (sterʹil). Estéril; relativo a, ou caracterizado por, esterilidade. [L. *sterilis*, improdutivo]

ste·ril·i·ty (stĕ-rilʹi-tē). Esterilidade. **1.** Em geral, a incapacidade de fertilização ou de reprodução. VER female s., male s. **2.** Condição de ser asséptico ou desprovido de qualquer microrganismo vivo. [L. *sterilitas*]

aspermatogenic s., e. aspermatogênica; e. decorrente de falha na produção de espermatozóides vivos.

dysspermatogenic s., e. dispermatogênica; e. masculina decorrente de alguma anormalidade na produção de espermatozóides.

female s., e. feminina; a incapacidade da mulher de conceber, decorrente de inadequação na estrutura ou função dos órgãos genitais. SIN infecundity.

male s., e. masculina; a incapacidade do homem de fertilizar o óvulo; pode ou não estar associada a impotência.

normospermatogenic s., e. normospermatogênica; e. masculina decorrente de uma causa diferente da incapacidade de produzir espermatozóides normais e vivos, como, por exemplo, bloqueio das vias seminíferas.

ster·il·i·za·tion (sterʹī-li-zāʹshŭn). Esterilização. **1.** O ato ou processo pelo qual o indivíduo torna-se incapaz de fertilização ou reprodução, p. ex. através de vasectomia, salpingectomia parcial ou castração. **2.** A destruição de todos os microrganismos no interior ou ao redor de um objeto, através de vapor (fluido ou pressurizado), agentes químicos (álcool, fenol, metais pesados, gás óxido de etileno), bombardeio com elétrons em alta velocidade, calor ou radiação ultravioleta.

discontinuous s., e. descontínua. SIN fractional s.

fractional s., e. fracionada; exposição a uma temperatura de 100°C (fluxo de vapor) por um período definido, habitualmente uma hora, durante vários dias; a cada aquecimento, as bactérias desenvolvidas são destruídas; os esporos, que não são afetados, germinam durante os períodos de intervalo e são subseqüentemente destruídos. SIN discontinuous s., intermittent s., tyndallization.

intermittent s., e. intermitente. SIN fractional s.

ster·il·ize (sterʹī-līz). Esterilizar; produzir esterilidade.

ster·il·iz·er (sterʹi-lī-zer). Esterilizador; aparelho para tornar os objetos estéreis.

glass bead s., e. com contas de vidro; esterilizador para equipamento endodôntico; o calor é transmitido aos instrumentos, pontos absorventes ou algodão por meio de contas de vidro.

hot salt s., e. com sal aquecido; esterilizador para equipamento endodôntico, em que o sal de mesa é aquecido num recipiente a 218–246°C. O calor seco é transmitido aos instrumentos para tratamento canal, pontos absorventes ou algodão para rápida esterilização (5–10 segundos).

Stern, Heinrich, médico norte-americano, 1868–1918. VER S. *posture*.

stern-. Estern-. VER sterno-.

ster·na (ster'nă). Esternos; plural de sternum.

ster·nad (ster'nad). Em direção ao esterno.

ster·nal (ster'năl). Esternal; relativo ao esterno.

ster·nal·gia (ster-nal'jē-ă). Esternalgia; dor no esterno ou na região esternal. SIN sternodynia. [stern- + G. *algos*, dor]

ster·na·lis (ster-nā'lis) Esternal. VER sternalis (*muscle*).

Sternberg, George M., bacteriologista norte-americano, 1838–1915. VER S. *cell*; S.-Reed *cell*; Reed-S. *cell*.

ster·ne·bra, pl. **ster·ne·brae** (ster'nē-bră, -brē). Estérnebra; um dos quatro segmentos do esterno primordial do embrião, cuja fusão leva à formação do corpo do esterno adulto. [L. mod. de stern(um) + (vert)ebra]

ster·nen. Relativo ao esterno, independentemente de quaisquer outras estruturas. [stern- + G. *en*, em]

sterno-, stern-. Esterno-, estern-; esterno, esternal. [G. *sternon*, tórax]

ster·no·chon·dro·sca·pu·la·ris (ster'nō-kon'drō-skap-ū-lā'ris). Esternocondroescapular. VER sternochondroscapular *muscle*. [L. mod.]

ster·no·cla·vic·u·lar (ster'nō-kla-vik'ū-lăr). Esternoclavicular; relativo ao esterno e à clavícula.

ster·no·cla·vi·cu·la·ris (ster'nō-kla-vik'ū-lā'ris). Esternoclavicular. VER sternoclavicular *muscle*.

ster·no·clei·dal (ster'nō-klī'dăl). Esternocleido; relativo ao esterno e à clavícula. [sterno- + G. *kleis*, chave (clavícula)]

ster·no·clei·do·mas·toid (ster'nō-klī'dō-mas'toyd). Esternocleidomastóideo; relativo ao esterno, à clavícula e ao processo mastóide.

ster·no·clei·do·mas·toi·de·us (ster'nō-klī'dō-mas-tō-id'ē-ŭs). Esternocleidomastóideo. VER sternocleidomastoid (*muscle*). [L. mod]

ster·no·cos·tal (ster'nō-kos'tăl). Esternocostal; relativo ao esterno e às costelas. [L. *costa*, costela]

ster·no·dyn·ia (ster-nō-din'ē-ă). Esternodinia. SIN sternalgia. [sterno- + G. *odyne*, dor]

ster·no·fas·ci·a·lis (ster'nō-fash-ē-ā'lis). Esternofascial. VER *musculus* sternofascialis.

ster·no·glos·sal (ster-nō-glos'ăl). Esternoglosso; designa fibras musculares que, ocasionalmente, se estendem a partir do músculo esterno-hióideo para unir-se ao músculo hioglosso.

ster·no·hy·oi·de·us (ster'nō-hī-oyd'ē-ŭs). Esterno-hióideo. VER sternohyoid (*muscle*). [L. mod.]

ster·noid (ster'noyd). Esternóide; semelhante ao esterno. [sterno- + G. *eidos*, semelhança]

ster·no·mas·toid (ster'nō-mas'toyd). Esternomastóide; relativo ao esterno e ao processo mastóide do osso temporal; aplica-se ao músculo esternocleidomastóideo.

ster·no·pa·gia (ster-nō-pā'jē-ă). Esternopagia; condição apresentada por gêmeos unidos pelos esternos ou mais extensamente pelas paredes ventrais do tórax. VER conjoined *twins*, em *twin*. [sterno- + G. *pagos*, algo fixo]

ster·no·per·i·car·di·al (ster'nō-per'i-kar'dē-ăl). Esternopericárdico; relativo ao esterno e ao pericárdio.

ster·nos·chi·sis (ster-nos'ki-sis). Esternosquise; fenda congênita do esterno. [sterno- + G. *schisis*, clivagem]

ster·no·thy·roi·de·us (ster'nō-thī-royd'ē-ŭs) Esternotireóideo. VER sternothyroid (*muscle*). [L. mod.]

ster·not·o·my (ster-not'ō-mē). Esternotomia; incisão no esterno ou através dele. [sterno- + G. *tome*, incisão]

median s., e. mediana; incisão feita através da linha média do esterno, geralmente para ter acesso ao coração, às estruturas mediastinais e aos grandes vasos.

ster·no·tra·che·al (ster'nō-trā'kē-ăl). Esternotraqueal; relativo ao esterno e à traquéia.

ster·no·try·pe·sis (ster'nō-trī-pē'sis). Esternotripese; perfuração do esterno. [sterno- + G. *trypesis*, perfuração]

ster·no·ver·te·bral (ster'nō-ver'tĕ-brăl). Esternovertebral; relativo ao esterno e às vértebras; designa as costelas verdadeiras ou as sete costelas superiores de cada lado, que se articulam com as vértebras e com o esterno. SIN vertebrosternal.

ster·num, gen. **ster·ni,** pl. **ster·na** (ster'nŭm, -nī, -nă) [TA]. Esterno; osso plano e longo que se articula com as cartilagens das sete primeiras vértebras e com a clavícula, formando a parte média da parede anterior do tórax; consiste em três partes: o corpo, o manúbrio e o processo xifóide. SIN breast bone. [L. mod. do G. *sternon*, tórax]

ster·nu·ta·tion (ster'noo-tā'shŭn). Esternutação, espirro; o ato de espirrar. [L. *sternutatio*, de *sternuo* (*sternuto*), pp. *sternutatus*, espirrar]

ster·nu·ta·tor (ster'noo-tā-ter, -tōr). Esternutatório; substância, como um gás, que provoca espirros. SIN sneezing gas.

ster·nu·ta·to·ry (ster-noo'tă-tōr-ē). Esternutatório. **1.** Que causa espirro. **2.** Agente que provoca espirros. SIN ptarmic.

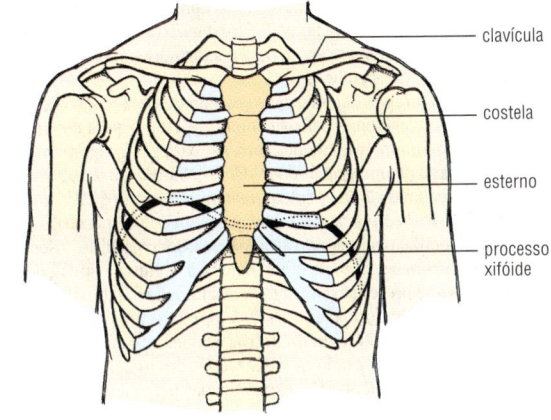

esterno e estruturas circundantes

ste·roid (stēr'oyd, ster'oyd). Esteróide. **1.** Relativo aos esteróides. SIN steroidal. Cf. steroids. **2.** Um dos esteróides. SIN sterid. **3.** Designação genérica dos compostos de estrutura estreitamente relacionada à dos esteróides, como esteróis, ácidos biliares, glicosídeos cardíacos, androgênios, estrogênios, corticosteróides e precursores das vitaminas D.

anabolic s., e. anabólico; composto esteróide com a capacidade de aumentar a massa muscular; compostos com propriedades androgênicas que aumentam a massa muscular e são utilizados no tratamento de emaciação. Algumas vezes utilizados por atletas num esforço de aumentar o tamanho, a força e a resistência dos músculos. Os exemplos incluem metiltestosterona, nandrolona, metandrostenolona e estanozolol.

s. hydroxylases, e. hidroxilases. SIN s. monooxigenases.

s. 21-monooxygenase, e. 21-monoxigenase; enzima que catalisa a reação de um esteróide, O_2 e algum composto reduzido para produzir água, o composto oxidado e um 21-hidroxiesteróide; a deficiência dessa enzima resulta em diminuição da síntese de cortisol, das quais existem três tipos (forma perdedora de sal, virilizante simples e não-clássica).

s. monooxygenases, e. monoxigenases; enzimas que catalisam a adição de grupamentos hidroxila aos anéis esteróides utilizando O_2; diferenciadas, p. ex., em esteróide 11β-monoxigenase, esteróide 17α-monoxigenase e esteróide 21-monoxigenase, de acordo com a posição do grupamento hidroxila introduzido de modo catalítico. SIN s. hydroxylases.

s. 5α-reductase, e. 5α-redutase; enzima que utiliza NADPH para reduzir certos esteróides (p. ex., a conversão da testosterona em diidrotestosterona); a deficiência dessa enzima está associada a uma forma de pseudo-hermafroditismo masculino, em que indivíduos genéticos masculinos possuem órgãos genitais masculinos, bem como genitália externa feminina.

s. sulfatase deficiency, deficiência de e. sulfatase. SIN X-linked *ichthyosis*.

ste·roi·dal (stēr'oy-dăl, ster'oy'). Esteróide. SIN steroid (1).

ste·roi·do·gen·e·sis (stēr'oy-dō-jen'ĕ-sis, ster'). Esteroidogênese; a formação de esteróides; refere-se comumente à síntese biológica de hormônios esteróides, mas não à produção desses compostos em laboratório químico. [steroid- + G. *genesis*, produção]

ste·roids (stēr'oydz, ster-). Esteróides; grande família de substâncias químicas, que compreende numerosos hormônios, constituintes corporais e drogas, contendo, cada um deles, o esqueleto ciclopenta[*a*]fenantreno tetracíclico. O estereoisomerismo entre esteróides não é apenas comum, mas de suma importância biológica. As convenções em termos de nomenclatura são as de que o núcleo é apresentado como se estivesse projetado no plano do papel, com os grupamentos situados acima desse plano denotados por ligações espessadas e denominadas β, e aqueles localizados abaixo desse plano denotados por ligações interrompidas e denominados α; a letra ξ indica orientação espacial desconhecida ou inespecífica. As principais classes de esteróides, com os nomes para as formas de hidrocarbonetos saturadas não-substituídas, que estão claramente relacionadas a funções ou origens fisiológicas são: 1) gonanos (em que os grupamentos metila em C-18 e C-19 foram substituídos por H), 2) estranos (em que os grupamentos metila C-19 foram substituídos por H), 3) androstanos (equivalente à Fórmula II), 4) norandrostanos (em que os grupamentos metila, tipicamente em C-18, foram substituídos por H) 5) colanos (com $-CH(CH_3)(CH_2)_2CH_3$ ligado ao C-17), 6) colestanos (com $-CH-(CH_3)_2(CH_2)_3CH(CH_3)_2$ em C-17, 7) ergostanos (com $-CH-(CH_3)_2(CH_2)_2$ $(CH_3)CH(CH_3)_2$ em C-17) e 8) estigmastanos (com $-CH(CH_3)(CH_2)_2CH-(CH_2CHCH_3)CH(CH_3)_2$ em C-17). Além disso, cada uma das classes pode estar numa série 5α ou 5β.

Os derivados esteróides conhecidos como cardanolídeos são androstanos com uma lactona de cinco membros ligada ao C-17. Os venenos de sapo, conhecidos como bufanolídeos, são androstanos com uma lactona de seis membros ligada ao C-17. Os espirostanos e furostanos (as estruturas básicas de muitas "geninas", incluindo as sapogeninas) são androstanos que apresentam certos componentes éteres cíclicos.

Os derivados naturais e sintéticos são designados pela adição de prefixos e sufixos químicos convencionais para substituos, p. ex., -ol para um grupamento hidroxila, -on(a) para um grupamento ceto, -al para um grupamento aldeído. "Nor" indica a perda de um grupamento –CH$_2$–; "homo", a adição de um grupamento –CH$_2$–; cada um é precedido pela letra indicando qual o anel contraído ou expandido, respectivamente, ou, no caso em que há perda do –CH$_2$– de um grupamento metila, o número do átomo de carbono perdido. "Seco" indica fissão de um anel com a adição de átomos de hidrogênio nas posições indicadas por numerais que precedem o termo. A insaturação é indicada, como habitualmente, pelo uso de termos apropriados, p. ex., -en(o), -in(o), -adien(o), substituindo as partes -ano ou -an do hidrocarboneto ou dos nomes da classe original, com numerais indicando as localizações das ligações insaturadas. As localizações das ligações duplas são especificadas pelo menor dos dois números (consecutivos) dos átomos de carbono envolvidos. Quando se forma uma ligação dupla entre dois átomos de carbono não-consecutivos, o segundo é indicado entre parênteses depois do primeiro; p. ex., o estriol e os estradióis possuem três ligações duplas entre C-1 e C-2, entre C-3 e C-4 e entre C-5 e C-10, respectivamente.

Os alcalóides esteróides podem ser designados a partir do esteróide original, conforme já indicado aqui, ou a partir dos nomes familiares triviais, terminando geralmente em -anina, se o esteróide for saturado, ou em -enina, -adienina, etc., se não for saturado (p. ex., conanina, tomatanina).

ste·rol (ster'ol). Esterol; esteróide com um grupamento OH (álcool); os nomes sistemáticos contêm o prefixo hidroxi- ou o sufixo -ol, p. ex., colesterol, ergosterol.

ster·tor (ster'tor). Estertor; inspiração ruidosa que ocorre no coma ou no sono profundo, algumas vezes devido à obstrução da laringe ou das vias aéreas superiores. [L. *sterto*, roncar]

hen-cluck s., e. em cacarejo; ruído respiratório semelhante ao cacarejar de uma galinha, algumas vezes ouvido em casos de abscesso retrofaríngeo.

ster·to·rous (ster'tor-us). Estertoroso; relativo a, ou caracterizado por, estertor ou ronco.

⚠ **steth-.** Estet-. VER stetho-.

ste·thal·gia (ste-thal'je-a). Estetalgia; dor no tórax. [steth- + G. *algos*, dor]

steth·ar·te·ri·tis (steth'ar-ter-i'tis). Estetarterite; inflamação da aorta ou de outras artérias no tórax. [steth- + L. *arteria*, artéria + G. *-itis*, inflamação]

⚠ **stetho-, steth-.** Esteto-, estet-; formas combinantes que designam o tórax. [G. *stethos*]

steth·o·graph (steth'o-graf). Estetógrafo; aparelho para registrar os movimentos respiratórios do tórax. [stetho- + G. *grapho*, escrever]

steth·o·my·i·tis (steth'o-mi-i'tis). Estetomiite; inflamação dos músculos da parede torácica. SIN stethomyositis. [stetho- + G. *mys*, músculo + *-itis*, inflamação]

steth·o·my·o·si·tis (steth'o-mi-o-si'tis). Estetomiosite. SIN stethomyitis.

steth·o·pa·ral·y·sis (steth'o-pa-ral'i-sis). Estetoparalisia; paralisia dos músculos respiratórios.

steth·o·scope (steth'o-skop). Estetoscópio; instrumento originalmente projetado por Laennec para ajudar na ausculta dos ruídos respiratórios e cardíacos no tórax, porém atualmente modificado de diversas maneiras e utilizado na ausculta de qualquer ruído vascular ou outros ruídos em qualquer parte do corpo. [stetho- + G. *skopeo*, ver]

binaural s., e. biauricular; estetoscópio em que as duas peças destinadas a ouvir conectam-se com uma única campânula.

Bowles type s., e. do tipo Bowles; estetoscópio em que a peça torácica é uma cúpula de metal rasa, de cerca de 4,5 cm de diâmetro, cuja boca é recoberta por uma borracha rígida ou diafragma de celulóide.

differential s., e. diferencial; estetoscópio que possui duas peças para o tórax, de modo que dois sons em diferentes partes do tórax podem ser ouvidos e comparados simultaneamente.

steth·o·scop·ic (steth-o-skop'ik). Estetoscópico. **1.** Relativo a ou efetuado por meio de um estetoscópio. **2.** Relativo a um exame do tórax.

ste·thos·co·py (ste-thos'ko-pe). Estetoscopia. **1.** Exame de tórax por meio de ausculta, mediata ou imediata, e percussão. **2.** Ausculta mediata com o estetoscópio.

Stevens, Albert M., pediatra norte-americano, 1884–1945. VER S.-Johnson *syndrome*.

Stewart, Fred Waldorf, médico norte-americano, 1894–1991. VER S.-Treves *syndrome*.

Stewart, George N., cientista canadense-norte-americano, 1860–1930. VER S. *test*; Stewart-Hamilton *method*.

Stewart, R.M., neurologista inglês do século XX. VER S.-Morel *syndrome*.

Stewart, Thomas Grainger, neurologista inglês do século XX, 1877–1957. VER S.-Holmes *sign*.

STH Abreviatura de somatotropic *hormone* (hormônio somatotrópico).

sthe·nia (sthe'ne-a). Estenia; condição de atividade e força aparente, como na febre estênica aguda. [G. *sthenos*, força + *-ia*, condição]

sthen·ic (sthen'ik). Estênico; ativo; caracterizado por estenia; diz-se de uma febre com pulso alternante forte, temperatura alta e delírio ativo.

⚠ **stheno-.** Esteno-; força, resistência, poder. [G. *sthenos*]

sthe·nom·e·ter (sthe-nom'e-ter). Estenômetro; instrumento para medir a força muscular. [stheno- + G. *metron*, medida]

sthe·nom·e·try (sthe-nom'e-tre). Estenometria; a medida da força muscular. [stheno- + G. *metrin*, medir]

stib·a·mine glu·co·side (stib'a-men). Glicosídeo de estibamina; glicosídeo nitrogenado de *p*-aminobenzenostibonato sódico; composto de antimônio pentavalente; era usado na leishmaniose (calazar) e em algumas outras doenças tropicais, porém não é mais comercializado.

stib·e·nyl (stib'e-nil). Estibenil; o primeiro antimonial pentavalente utilizado no tratamento da leishmaniose (calazar).

stib·i·al·ism (stib'e-a-lizm). Estibialismo; intoxicação crônica por antimônio. [L. *stibium*, antimônio]

stib·i·a·ted (stib'e-a-ted). Estibiado; impregnado por ou contendo antimônio.

stib·i·a·tion (stib-e-a'shun). Estibiação; impregnação por antimônio.

stib·i·um (stib'e-um). Antimônio. SIN antimony. [L. do G. *stibi*]

stib·o·cap·tate (stib-o-kap'tat). Estibocaptato. SIN *antimony* dimercaptosuccinate.

stib·o·glu·co·nate s. s. (stib-o-gloo'ko-nat). **1.** Estibogliconato sódico pentavalente utilizado no tratamento de todos os tipos de leishmaniose; é freqüente a ocorrência de efeitos tóxicos. SIN antimony sodium gluconate. **2.** Gliconato sódico de antimônio trivalente, utilizado no tratamento da esquistossomose; é freqüente a ocorrência de efeitos tóxicos. SIN sodium antimonylgluconate.

sti·bo·ni·um (sti-bo'ne-um). Estibônio; o radical hipotético SbH$_4^+$, análogo ao amônio.

stib·o·phen (stib'o-fen). Estibofeno; composto de antimônio trivalente orgânico; utilizado no tratamento da esquistossomose, filaríase, leishmaniose e linfogranuloma inguinal.

stich·o·chrome (stik'o-krom). Esticromo; designa uma célula nervosa em que a substância cromófila, ou material corável, está disposta em fileiras ou linhas aproximadamente paralelas. [G. *stichos*, uma fileira + *chroma*, cor]

Stickler, Gunnar B., médico norte-americano, *1925. VER S. *syndrome*.

Stieda, Alfred, cirurgião alemão, 1869–1945. VER Pellegrini-S. *disease*.

Stieda, Ludwig, anatomista alemão, 1837–1918. VER S. *process*.

Stierlin, Eduard, cirurgião alemão, 1878–1919. VER S. *sign*.

stig·ma, pl. **stig·mas, stig·ma·ta** (stig'ma, -ma-ta). Estigma. **1.** Evidência visível de uma doença. **2.** SIN follicular s. **3.** Qualquer mancha ou defeito na pele. **4.** Mancha hemorrágica na pele, considerada uma manifestação de histeria de conversão. **5.** O ocelo alaranjado de certos protozoários portadores de clorofila, como *Euglena viridis*, que serve como filtro de luz, absorvendo determinados comprimentos de onda. **6.** Marca de vergonha ou descrédito. [G. uma marca, de *stizo*, picar]

follicular s., e. folicular; ponto onde o folículo de Graaf está prestes a sofrer ruptura na superfície do ovário. SIN macula pellucida, stigma (2).

malpighian stigmas, estigmas de Malpighi; os pontos de entrada das veias menores nas veias maiores do baço.

s. ventric'uli, uma dentre várias equimoses miliares da mucosa gástrica.

stig·mas·tane (stig-mas'tan). Estigmastano; a substância original do citosterol. SIN sitostane.

stig·ma·ta (stig'ma-ta). Estigmas; plural alternativo de stigma.

stig·mat·ic (stig-mat'ik). Estigmático; relativo a, ou caracterizado por, um estigma.

stig·ma·tism (stig'ma-tizm). Estigmatismo; a condição de ter um estigma. SIN stigmatization

stig·ma·ti·za·tion (stig'ma-ti-za'shun). Estigmatização. **1.** SIN stigmatism. **2.** Produção de estigmas, especialmente de natureza estérica. **3.** Depreciação de uma pessoa ao atribuir-lhe uma característica negativa ou outro estigma.

stil·bam·i·dine (stil-bam'i-den). Estilbamidina; composto utilizado no tratamento da leishmaniose (calazar), em infecções causadas por *Blastomyces dermatitidis*, e na actinomicose; também utilizado no mieloma múltiplo para alívio da dor óssea.

stil·baz·i·um io·dide (stil-baz'e-um). Iodeto de estilbázio; anti-helmíntico.

stil·bene (stil'ben). Estilbeno. **1.** $C_6H_5CH=CHC_6H_5$; α,β-difeniletileno; hidrocarboneto insaturado, o núcleo do estilbestrol e de outros compostos estrogênicos sintéticos. **2.** Classe de compostos baseada no estilbeno (1).

stil·bes·trol (stil-bes'trol). Estilbestrol. SIN diethylstilbestrol.

Stiles, Walter S., físico inglês, 1901–1985. VER S.-Crawford *effect*.

sti·let, sti·lette (sti'let, sti-let'). Estilete. VER stylet.

Still, Sir George F., médico inglês, 1868–1941. VER S. *disease, murmur*; S.-Chauffard *syndrome*.

still·birth (stil'berth). Nascimento de um feto que morreu antes do parto.

still·born (stil'born). Natimorto; nascido morto; designa um feto morto ao nascimento.

Stilling, Benedict, anatomista alemão, 1810–1879. VER S. *canal, column, nucleus, raphe,* gelatinous *substance*.

sti·lus (stī′lŭs). Estilo. VER stylus.

stim·u·lant (stim′ū-lănt). Estimulante. **1.** Estimulante; que excita à ação. **2.** Agente que desperta atividade orgânica, fortalece a ação do coração, aumenta a vitalidade e promove uma sensação de bem-estar; classificado de acordo com as partes sobre as quais atua principalmente: cardíaco, respiratório, gástrico, hepático, cerebral, espinal, vascular, genital. SIN excitor, stimulator. VER TAMBÉM stimulus. SIN excitant. [L. *stimulans,* p. pres. de *stimulo,* pp. *-atus,* incitar, estimular, de *stimulus,* um estímulo]

  diffusible s., e. difusível; estimulante que produz efeito rápido, porém temporário.

  general s., e. geral; estimulante que afeta todo o corpo.

  local s., e. local; estimulante cuja ação é restrita à parte à qual é aplicado.

stim·u·la·tion (stim-ū-lā′shŭn). Estimulação. **1.** Incitação do corpo ou de qualquer de suas partes ou órgãos a um aumento de atividade funcional. **2.** A condição de ser estimulado. **3.** Em neurofisiologia, a aplicação de um estímulo a uma estrutura responsiva, como nervo ou músculo, a despeito de a intensidade do estímulo ser suficiente para produzir excitação. [ver stimulant]

  dorsal column s., e. da coluna dorsal; estimulação elétrica, seja percutânea ou por aplicação direta de eletrodos, das colunas dorsais da medula espinal.

  fetal scalp s., e. do couro cabeludo fetal; teste intraparto do bem-estar fetal; a aceleração da freqüência cardíaca do feto em resposta à estimulação digital ou com fórceps do couro cabeludo está associada a um pH sanguíneo normal do couro cabeludo.

  Ganzfeld s., e. de Ganzfeld; iluminação de toda a retina no eletrorretinograma. [Al. *Ganzfeld,* campo inteiro]

  percutaneous s., e. percutânea; estimulação elétrica dos nervos periféricos ou da medula espinal através da aplicação de eletrodos à pele.

  photic s., e. fótica; uso de uma luz bruxuleante em várias freqüências para influenciar o padrão do eletroencefalograma occipital e também para ativar anormalidades latentes.

  vagal nerve s., e. do nervo vago; tratamento adjuvante para pacientes com epilepsia refratária, sobretudo crises complexas parciais ou secundariamente generalizadas; a estimulação é aplicada ao nervo vago esquerdo no pescoço, geralmente em salvas de 30 s a cada 5 1/2 minutos por um estimulador implantado na parede torácica anterior.

stim·u·la·tor (stim′ū-lā-ter, -tōr). Estimulador. SIN stimulant (2).

  long-acting thyroid s. (LATS), e. tireóideo de ação prolongada; substância encontrada no sangue de alguns pacientes com hipertireoidismo, que exerce um efeito estimulador prolongado sobre a glândula tireóide; associado no plasma à fração IgG (γ-globulina 7 S); parece ser um anticorpo ou, talvez, um imunocomplexo.

stim·u·lus, pl. **stim·u·li** (stim′ū-lŭs, -lī). Estímulo. **1.** Um estimulante. **2.** Aquilo que pode produzir ou despertar uma ação (resposta) num músculo, nervo, glândula ou outro tecido excitável, ou causar um aumento da ação em qualquer função ou processo metabólico. [L. aguilhão]

  adequate s., e. adequado, e. ao qual um receptor específico responde efetivamente e que origina uma sensação característica; p. ex., as ondas luminosas e sonoras que estimulam, respectivamente, os receptores visuais e auditivos.

  aversive s., e. aversivo; e. nocivo, como choque elétrico, utilizado no treinamento (aversive *training*) ou condicionamento aversivo. VER TAMBÉM aversive *training*.

  conditioned s., e. condicionado; **(1)** e. aplicado a um dos órgãos do sentido (p. ex., receptores da visão, audição, tato) que constituem parte essencial e integrante do mecanismo neural subjacente a um reflexo condicionado. VER classical *conditioning,* higher order *conditioning*; **(2)** e. neutro, quando associado ao e. não-condicionado em apresentação simultânea a um organismo, capaz de desencadear determinada resposta.

  discriminant s., e. discriminante; e. que pode ser diferenciado de todos os outros estímulos no ambiente, visto que foi e continua sendo um indicador de um reforçador potencial.

  heterologous s., e. heterólogo; e. que atua sobre qualquer parte do aparelho sensorial ou trato nervoso.

  heterotopic s., e. heterotópico; qualquer atividade elétrica de um local anormal.

  homologous s., e. homólogo; e. que atua apenas sobre as terminações nervosas num órgão especial dos sentidos.

  inadequate s., e. inadequado, e. subliminar. SIN subthreshold s.

  liminal s., e. liminar. SIN threshold s.

  maximal s., e. máximo; e. forte o suficiente para provocar uma resposta máxima.

  square wave stimuli, estímulos de onda quadrada; estimulação elétrica em que a intensidade da corrente alcança subitamente determinado nível, sendo mantida nesse nível até ocorrer uma súbita interrupção; esse tipo de e. é particularmente útil na obtenção de uma curva de intensidade–duração.

  subliminal s., e. subliminar. SIN subthreshold s.

  subthreshold s., e. subliminar; e. muito fraco para desencadear uma resposta. SIN inadequate s., subliminal s.

  supramaximal s., e. supramáximo; e. cuja intensidade está significativamente acima daquela necessária para ativar todas as fibras nervosas ou musculares em contato com o eletrodo; utilizado quando se deseja obter uma resposta de todas as fibras.

  threshold s., e. limiar; e. de intensidade limiar, isto é, aquele de intensidade apenas suficiente para excitar. VER TAMBÉM adequate s. SIN liminal s.

  train-of-four s., e. em série de quatro; método para medir a magnitude e o tipo de bloqueio neuromuscular, com base na relação entre a amplitude da quarta resposta mecânica induzida e da primeira, quando são aplicadas quatro correntes elétricas de 2-Hz supramáximas durante 2 s a um nervo motor periférico.

  unconditioned s., e. incondicionado; e. que produz uma resposta incondicionada; p. ex., o alimento é um estímulo incondicionado para a salivação que, por sua vez, representa uma resposta incondicionada num animal com fome. VER classical *conditioning*.

stim·u·lus word. Palavra de estímulo; a palavra utilizada em testes de associação para provocar uma resposta.

sting. 1. Dor aguda momentânea, mais comumente produzida pela punção da pele por numerosas espécies de artrópodes, incluindo hexápodes, miriápodes e aracnídeos; pode ser também produzida por água-viva, ouriço-do-mar, esponjas, moluscos e várias espécies de peixes venenosos, como a arraia-lixa, o peixe-saco e o bagre. **2.** O aparelho venenoso de um animal capaz de picar ou ferroar, que consiste numa espícula quitinosa ou num espinho ósseo e uma glândula ou saco de veneno. **3.** Introduzir (ou processo de introduzir) um veneno através de picada. [I. ant. *stingan*]

sting·ers (sting′erz). Episódios de dor em caráter de queimação no membro superior. SIN burners.

stink weed. Estramônio. SIN *Datura stramonium.*

stip·pling (stip′ling). Pontilhado. **1.** Salpicamento de uma célula sanguínea ou outra estrutura com pontos finos quando exposta à ação de um corante básico, devido à presença de grânulos basofílicos livres no protoplasma da célula. SIN punctate basophilia. **2.** Aspecto de casca de laranja da gengiva fixada. **3.** Rugosidade das superfícies de uma base de dentadura para estimular o pontilhado gengival natural.

  geographic s. of nails, p. geográfico das unhas; pontilhado longitudinal de disposição regular, encontrado comumente na psoríase e, em certas ocasiões, na alopecia em áreas. VER TAMBÉM nail *pits,* em *pit*.

  Ziemann s., p. de Ziemann. SIN Ziemann *dots,* em *dot*.

STIR Acrônimo de short TI inversion *recovery* (inversão-recuperação com tau curto).

Stirling, William, histologista e fisiologista inglês, 1851–1932. VER S. modification of Gram *stain*.

stir·rup (ster′ŭp, stir′ŭp). Estribo. SIN stapes. [A.S. *stirāp*]

stitch. 1. Dor aguda semelhante a uma picada, de duração momentânea. **2.** Ponto de sutura. **3.** Suturar. SIN suture (2). [A.S. *stice,* picada]

  lock s., sutura contínua. SIN locking *suture*.

STM Abreviatura de short-term *memory* (memória de curto prazo).

Stock, Wolfgang, oftalmologista alemão, 1874–1956. VER Spielmeyer-S *disease*.

stock (stok). Todas as populações de organismos derivadas de um organismo isolado, sem qualquer implicação de homogeneidade ou caracterização [A.S. *stoc*]

Stocker, Frederick William, oftalmologista norte-americano, 1893–1974. VER S. *line*.

Stoffel, Adolf, cirurgião ortopédico alemão, 1880–1937. VER S. *operation*.

stoi·chi·ol·o·gy (stoy-kē-ol′-ō-jē). Estequiologia; a ciência que trata dos elementos ou princípios em qualquer ramo de conhecimento, especialmente em química, citologia ou histologia. [G. *stoicheion,* elemento (lit. um dentre uma série), de *stoichos,* uma fileira + *logos,* estudo]

stoi·chi·o·met·ric (stoy′kē-ō-met′rik). Estequiométrico; relativo à estequiometria.

stoi·chi·om·e·try (stoy-kē-om′e-trē). Estequiometria; determinação das quantidades relativas das substâncias envolvidas em qualquer reação química; p. ex., com as leis das proporções definidas em química, como nas proporções molares numa reação. [G. *stoicheion,* elemento + *metron,* medida]

stokes (stōk). Stokes; unidade de viscosidade cinemática, referindo-se àquela de um líquido com viscosidade de 1 poise e densidade de 1 g/ml; igual a 10^{-4} m²/s. [Sir George Gabriel *Stokes*]

Stokes, Sir George Gabriel, físico e matemático inglês, 1819–1903. VER stoke; S. *law* (2), *law* (3).

Stokes, William, médico irlandês, 1804–1878. VER S. *law* (1); Cheyne-S. *psychosis, respiration;* S.-Adams *disease;* Adam-S. *disease;* Morgagni-Adams-S. *syndrome*.

Stokes, Sir William, cirurgião irlandês, 1839–1900. VER S. *amputation;* Gritti-S. *amputation*.

sto·lon (stō′lon). Estolho; hifa aérea em broto ou conectiva que forma um grupo de rizóides quando entra em contato com o substrato e, a seguir, emite outros brotos para produzir o micélio aéreo e os esporangiósforos típicos de *Rhizopus.* [L. *stolo,* ramo, rebento, broto]

stom-. Estom-. VER stomato-.

sto·ma, pl. **sto·mas, sto·ma·ta** (stō′mă, stō′maz, stō′mă-tă). Estoma. **1.** Abertura minúscula ou poro. **2.** Abertura artificial entre duas cavidades ou canais ou entre estes e a superfície do corpo. [G. uma boca]
  Fuchs stomas, estomas de Fuchs; pequena depressão na superfície da íris próximo à margem da pupila.
  loop s., e. em alça; estoma especializado do intestino ou do ureter pelo qual passa uma alça da víscera oca através de uma abertura na parede abdominal, com criação de uma abertura no ápice da víscera para permitir a saída de seu conteúdo.

stom·ach (stŭm′ŭk). [TA]. Estômago; grande saco irregularmente piriforme entre o esôfago e o intestino delgado, localizado logo abaixo do diafragma, quando distendido, tem 25–28 cm de comprimento e 10–10,5 cm em seu maior diâmetro, com capacidade de cerca de 1 L. Sua parede é formada de quatro camadas ou túnicas: mucosa, submucosa, muscular e peritoneal; a camada muscular é composta de três camadas, com fibras correndo longitudinalmente na camada externa, circularmente na camada média e obliquamente na camada interna. SIN gaster (1) [TA], ventriculus (1) [TA]. [G. *stomachos*, L. *stomachus*]

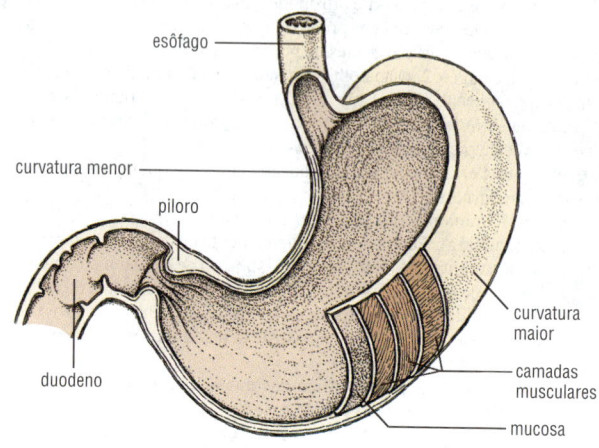

estômago

  bilocular s., e. bilocular. SIN hourglass s.
  s. bubble, bolha do estômago; o gás no fundo do estômago observada numa radiografia em posição ortostática.
  cascade s., e. em cascata; descrição radiográfica: quando o contraste é deglutido com o paciente na posição ortostática, o fundo gástrico atua como reservatório até o contraste extravasar para o antro; uma variante normal no estômago horizontal.
  drain-trap s., SIN water-trap s.
  hourglass s., e. em ampulheta; condição em que existe uma constrição central da parede do estômago, dividindo-o em duas cavidades: a cárdica e a pilórica. SIN bilocular s., ectasia ventriculi paradoxa.
  leather-bottle s., e. em odre; acentuado espessamento e rigidez da parede gástrica, com redução da capacidade da luz, embora freqüentemente sem obstrução; quase sempre decorrente de carcinoma cirroso, como na linite plástica. SIN sclerotic s.
  miniature s., e. em miniatura. SIN Pavlov *pouch*.
  Pavlov s., e. de Pavlov. SIN Pavlov *pouch*.
  powdered s., e. pulverizada; a parede sem gordura, seca e pulverizada do estômago do porco, *Sus scrofa*; contém fatores termolábeis, incluindo vitamina B_{12} nativa e fator intrínseco; era utilizado no tratamento da anemia perniciosa.
  sclerotic s., e. esclerótico. SIN leather-bottle s.
  thoracic s., e. torácico; condição em que parte do estômago ou todo ele está contido no tórax, devido a uma hérnia de hiato paraesofágica.
  trifid s., e. trífido; condição em que o estômago é dividido por duas constrições em três bolsas.
  wallet s., e. em carteira; forma de estômago dilatado, caracterizada por distensão geral semelhante a uma bolsa, em que o antro e o fundo são indistinguíveis.
  water-trap s., estômago ptótico e dilatado, que possui uma saída pilórica relativamente alta (embora normalmente localizada), que é sustentada pelo ligamento gastroepático. SIN drain-trap s.

stom·ach·al (stŭm′ă-kăl). Estomacal; relativo ao estômago. SIN stomachic (1).
stom·a·chal·gia (stŭm-ă-kal′jē-ă). Estomacalgia; termo obsoleto para gastralgia (stomach *ache*). [stomach + G. *algos*, dor]
sto·mach·ic (stō′mak′ĭk). Estomáquico. **1.** SIN stomachal. **2.** Agente que melhora o apetite e a digestão.
stom·a·cho·dyn·ia (stŭm′ă-kō-din′ē-ă). Estomacodinia; termo obsoleto para gastralgia (stomach *ache*). [stomach + G. *odynē*, dor]

sto·mal (stō′măl). Estomal; relativo a um estoma.
stomat-. Estomat-. VER stomato-.
sto·ma·ta (stō′mă-tă). Estomas; plural alternativo de stoma.
sto·ma·tal (stō′mă-tal). Estomatal; relativo a um estoma.
sto·ma·tal·gia (stō-mă-tal′jē-ă). Estomatalgia; dor na boca. SIN stomatodynia. [stomat- + G. *algos*, dor]
sto·mat·ic (stō-mat′ĭk). Estomático; relativo à boca; oral.
sto·ma·ti·tis (stō-mă-tī′tis). Estomatite; inflamação da mucosa da boca. [stomat- + G. *-itis*, inflamação]
  angular s., e. angular. SIN angular *cheilitis*.
  aphthous s., e. aftosa. SIN aphtha (2).
  epidemic s., e. epidêmica; infecção oral contagiosa, geralmente causada por vírus Coxsackie do grupo A. VER TAMBÉM herpangina.
  fusospirochetal s., e. fusoespiroquética; infecção da boca por espiroquetas, geralmente em associação a outros microrganismos anaeróbicos. VER TAMBÉM Vincent *angina*.
  gangrenous s., e. gangrenosa; estomatite caracterizada por necrose do tecido oral. VER noma.
  gonococcal s., e. gonocócica; lesões orais inflamatórias e ulcerativas resultantes de infecção por *Neisseria gonorrhoeae*; geralmente primária em decorrência de contato orogenital; todavia, em certas ocasiões, resulta de gonococcemia.
  lead s., e. por chumbo; manifestação oral da intoxicação por chumbo; consiste numa linha negro-azulada que acompanha os contornos da gengiva marginal, onde ocorreu precipitação do sulfeto de chumbo devido ao ambiente inflamado.
  s. medicamento′sa, e. medicamentosa; alterações inflamatórias da mucosa oral associadas a uma alergia sistêmica a drogas; as lesões podem consistir em eritema, vesículas, bolhas, ulcerações ou edema angioneurótico.
  mercurial s., e. mercurial; alterações da mucosa oral em decorrência de intoxicação crônica por mercúrio; podem consistir em eritema e edema da mucosa, ulceração e deposição de sulfeto de mercúrio nos tecidos inflamados, resultando em pigmentação oral semelhante àquela da estomatite por chumbo.
  nicotine s., e. por nicotina; lesões estimuladas pelo calor, geralmente no palato, que começam com eritema e progridem para múltiplas pápulas brancas com ponto vermelho no centro. O ponto vermelho representa um orifício dilatado e inflamado do ducto salivar.
  primary herpetic s., e. herpética primária; primeira infecção dos tecidos orais pelo vírus do herpes simples; caracterizada por inflamação gengival, vesículas e úlceras. SIN primary herpetic gingivostomatitis.
  recurrent aphthous s., e. aftosa recorrente. SIN aphtha (2).
  recurrent herpetic s., e. herpética recorrente; reativação da infecção pelo vírus do herpes simples, caracterizada por vesículas e ulceração limitadas ao palato duro e à gengiva fixa.
  recurrent ulcerative s., e. ulcerativa recorrente. SIN aphtha (2).
  ulcerative s., e. ulcerativa. SIN aphtha (2).
  vesicular s., e. vesicular; doença vesicular de cavalos, bois, suínos e, em certas ocasiões, dos seres humanos, causada por um vesiculovírus (vírus da estomatite vesicular) da família Rhabdoviridae; nos cavalos e no gado, a doença geralmente provoca na boca vesículas que, nos bois, não podem ser clinicamente diferenciadas daquelas da doença do pé-e-boca.

stomato-, stom-, stomat-. Estomato-, estom-, estomat-; boca. [G. *stoma*]
sto·ma·to·cyte (stō′mă-tō-sīt). Estomatócito; eritrócito que exibe uma palidez em forma de fenda ou de boca em lugar da palidez central no esfregaço seco ao ar; p. ex., células nulas Rh. [stomato- + G. *kytos*, célula]
sto·ma·to·cy·to·sis (stō′mă-tō-sī-tō′sis). Estomatocitose; deformação hereditária dos eritrócitos, que estão tumefeitos e com forma de taça, causando anemia hemolítica congênita. VER TAMBÉM Rh null *syndrome*.

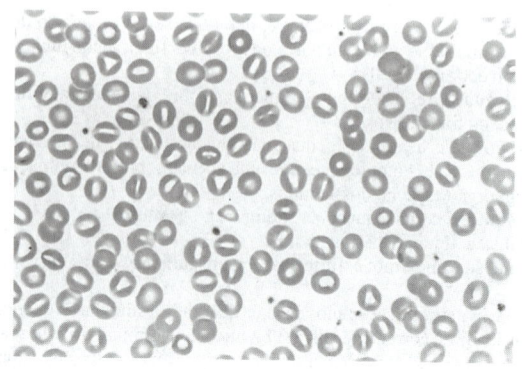

estomatocitose: o sangue periférico de um paciente com estomatocitose hereditária revela eritrócitos com áreas de palidez semelhantes a uma fenda ou boca [estoma = boca] (aumento original 250×)

sto·ma·to·de·um (stō′mă-tō-dē′ŭm). Estomodeu. SIN stomodeum (1).

sto·ma·to·dyn·ia (stō′mă-tō-din′ē-ă). Estomatodinia. SIN stomatalgia. [stomato- + G. *odynē*, dor]

sto·ma·to·dys·o·dia (stō′mă-tō-di-sō′dē-ă). Estomatodisodia. SIN halitosis. [stomato- + G. *dysōdia*, odor ruim]

sto·ma·to·gnath·ic (stō′mă-tog-nath′ik). Estomatognático; relativo à boca e mandíbula. [stomato- + G. *gnathos*, mandíbula]

sto·ma·to·log·ic (stō′mă-tō-loj′ik). Estomatológico; relativo à estomatologia.

sto·ma·tol·o·gist (stō-mă-tol′ō-jist). Estomatologista; especialista em doenças da cavidade oral.

sto·ma·tol·o·gy (stō-mă-tol′ō-jē). Estomatologia; o estudo das estruturas, funções e doenças da boca. [stomato- + G. *logos*, estudo]

sto·ma·to·ma·la·cia (stō′mă-tō-mă-lā′shē-ă). Estomatomalacia; amolecimento patológico de qualquer uma das estruturas da boca. [stomato- + G. *malakia*, amolecimento]

sto·ma·to·my·co·sis (stō′mă-tō-mī-kō′sis). Estomatomicose; doença da boca causada por fungo. [stomato- + G. *mykēs*, fungo + *-osis*, condição]

sto·ma·to·ne·cro·sis (stō′mă-tō-nĕ-krō′sis). Estomatonecrose. SIN noma. [stomato- + G. *nekrōsis*, morte]

sto·ma·top·a·thy (stō′mă-top′ă-thē). Estomatopatia; qualquer doença da cavidade oral. SIN stomatosis. [stomato- + G. *pathos*, sofrimento]

sto·ma·to·plas·ty (stō′mă-tō-plas-tē). Estomatoplastia; termo antigo para cirurgia corretiva da boca. [stomato- + G. *plastos*, formado]

sto·ma·tor·rha·gia (stō-mă-tō-rā′jē-ă). Estomatorragia; sangramento das gengivas ou de outra parte da cavidade oral. [stomato- + G. *rhēgnymi*, impelir]

sto·ma·to·scope (stō′mă-tō-skōp). Estomatoscópio; aparelho para iluminar o interior da boca, a fim de facilitar o seu exame. [stomato- + G. *skopeō*, ver]

sto·ma·to·sis (stō-mă-tō′sis). Estomatose. SIN stomatopathy. [stomato- + G. *-osis*, condição]

sto·mi·on (stō′mē-on). Estômio; o ponto mediano da fenda oral quando os lábios estão fechados.

sto·mo·ceph·a·lus (stō′mō-sef′ă-lŭs). Estomocéfalo; indivíduo malformado com mandíbula não desenvolvida e boca semelhante a um bico; tende a estar associado a um tipo etmocefálico de ciclopia. [G. *stoma*, boca + *kephalē*, cabeça]

sto·mo·de·al (stō′mō-dē′ăl). Estomodeal; relativo a um estomodeu.

sto·mo·de·um (stō-mō-dē′ŭm). Estomodeu. **1.** Depressão ectodérmica na linha média, ventralmente ao cérebro embrionário e circundada pelo arco mandibular; quando a membrana bucofaríngea desaparece, torna-se contínua com o intestino anterior e forma a boca. SIN stomatodeum. **2.** A porção anterior do canal alimentar dos insetos, que consiste em boca, cavidade bucal, faringe, esôfago, papo (freqüentemente um divertículo) e pró-ventrículo. [L. mod. do G. *stoma*, boca + *hodaios*, a caminho, de *hodos*, um caminho]

Sto·mox·ys cal·ci·trans (stō-mok′sis kal′si-tranz). Mosca-de-estábulo, uma espécie de mosca que pica, cujo tamanho e aparência geral assemelham-se aos da mosca-doméstica comum, constitui uma praga para os seres humanos e animais domésticos em todo o mundo, estando envolvida na transmissão mecânica de doenças. [L. mod. do G. *stoma*, boca + *oxys*, agudo; L. pres. p. de *calcitro*, chutar, de *calx*, calcanhar]

-stomy. -Stomia. Abertura artificial ou cirúrgica. VER stomato-. [G. *stoma*, boca]

stone (stōn). **1.** Cálculo, pedra. SIN calculus. **2.** Unidade inglesa de peso do corpo humano, igual a 14 libras. [A.S. *stān*]

   artificial s., derivado do gesso especialmente calcinado semelhante ao gesso de Paris, porém mais forte, visto que os grãos não são porosos.

   bladder s.'s, cálculos vesicais; cálculos do trato urinário na bexiga. Em toda a história do homem, constituiu a forma predominante de doença calculosa das vias urinárias, mencionada no juramento de Hipócrates, dando origem ao procedimento cirúrgico antigo comum, a litotomia. Em grande parte do mundo, a doença por cálculos vesicais tornou-se rara, enquanto os cálculos renais e ureterais (que têm origens diferentes) passaram a ser mais comuns. Hoje em dia, os cálculos vesicais são observados tipicamente em pacientes com bexiga neurogênica, reconstrução do trato urinário ou obstrução infravesical. SIN bladder calculus.

   philosopher's s., p. filosofal; pedra procurada pelos alquimistas da Idade Média, que, supostamente, tinha a capacidade de transmutar metais em ouro, produzir pedras preciosas e curar todas as enfermidades e, assim, conferir longevidade; acreditava-se também ser um solvente universal.

   pulp s., p. da polpa. SIN endolith.

   tear s., cálculo lacrimal. SIN dacryolith.

   vein s., cálculo venoso. SIN phlebolith.

Stookey, Byron P., neurocirurgião norte-americano, 1887–1966. VER S.-Scarff *operation*; Queckenstedt-S. *test*.

stool (stool). **1.** Evacuação do intestino. **2.** Fezes; a matéria eliminada numa evacuação. SIN evacuation (2). SIN motion (3), movement (3). [A.S. *stōl*, assento]

   butter s.'s, fezes gordurosas; fezes que ocorrem especialmente na esteatorréia.

   currant jelly s., fezes em geléia de groselha; fezes que contêm sangue e produtos de inflamação, conferindo-lhes o aspecto de geléia de groselha; consideradas um sinal de intussuscepção.

   fatty s., fezes gordurosas; fezes que contêm quantidades excessivas de gordura.

   rice-water s., fezes em água de arroz; líquido aquoso contendo flóculos esbranquiçados, eliminado do intestino na cólera e, em certas ocasiões, em outros casos de diarréia serosa.

   spinach s.'s, fezes em espinafre; fezes verde-escuras semelhantes a um mingau, lembrando espinafre picado.

   Trélat s.'s, fezes de Trélat; fezes viscosas com estrias de sangue, que ocorre na proctite.

stops. Curvaturas ou fios soldados a um arco para limitar a passagem através de um suporte ou tubo.

stor·age (stōr′ij). Armazenamento; o segundo estágio no processo da memória, após codificação, anterior à recuperação, envolvendo processos mentais associados à retenção de estímulos que foram registrados e modificados por codificação. VER memory.

sto·rax (stōr′aks). Estoraque; bálsamo líquido obtido da madeira e da casca interna de *Liquidamber orientalis*, uma árvore da Ásia Menor, ou de *L. styraciflua* (família Hamamelidaceae); era utilizado no tratamento da inflamação crônica das mucosas e externamente na escabiose. SIN styrax. [G. *styrax*, resina de odor adocicado]

STORCH Revisão do acrônimo TORCH (q.v.) para incluir a sífilis (syphilis) como causa de infecções congênitas.

sto·ri·form (stōr′i-fōrm). Estoriforme; que possui um padrão em roda de carroça, como as células fusiformes com núcleos alongados irradiando-se de um centro. [L. *storea*, esteira entrelaçada + *-formis*, forma]

storm (stōrm). Tempestade; exacerbação dos sintomas ou crise durante a evolução de uma doença.

   thyroid s., t. tireóidea. SIN thyrotoxic *crisis*.

Stout wir·ing. Ver em wiring.

STPD Abreviatura indicando que um volume de gás foi expresso como se estivesse em temperatura padrão (0°C), pressão padrão (760 mm Hg absoluto) e seco; nessas condições, um mol de gás ocupa 22,4 L.

stra·bis·mal (stra-biz′mal). Estrábico; relativo ou acometido de estrabismo. SIN strabismic.

stra·bis·mic (stra-biz′mik). Estrábico. SIN strabismal.

stra·bis·mol·o·gist (stra-biz-mol′ah-jist). Estrabismologista; médico especializado em oftalmologia pediátrica, com ênfase no tratamento do estrabismo e ambliopia.

stra·bis·mus (stra-biz′mŭs). Estrabismo; ausência manifesta de paralelismo dos eixos visuais dos olhos. SIN crossed eyes, heterotropia, heterotropy, squint (1). [L. mod. do G. *strabismos*, estrabismo]

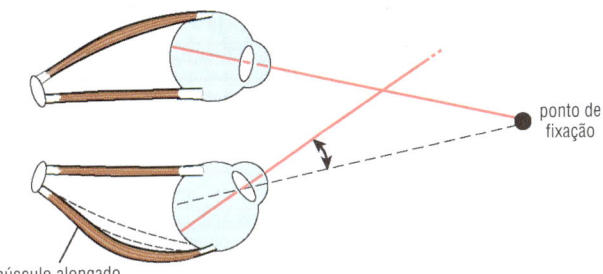

estrabismo convergente (esotropia): neste caso, o olho direito desvia-se para dentro, devido ao músculo reto lateral alongado

   A-s., estrabismo A; **(1)** estrabismo em que a esotropia é mais acentuada ao olhar para cima do que para baixo; **(2)** estrabismo em que a exotropia é mais acentuada ao olhar para baixo do que para cima. SIN A-pattern s.

   accommodative s., e. acomodativo; estrabismo em que a intensidade do desvio varia com a acomodação.

   alternate day s., e. em dias alternados. SIN cyclic *esotropia*.

   alternating s., e. alternante; uma forma de estrabismo em que ocorre fixação de um dos olhos.

   A-pattern s., e. de padrão A. SIN A-s.

   comitant s., e. concomitante; condição em que o grau de estrabismo é igual em todas as direções do olhar. SIN concomitant s.

   concomitant s., e. concomitante. SIN comitant s.

   convergent s., e. convergente. SIN esotropia.

   cyclic s., e. cíclico; estrabismo que aparece e desaparece de forma rítmica, mais freqüentemente a intervalos de 48 horas.

   divergent s., e. divergente. SIN exotropia.

   incomitant s., e. paralítico. SIN paralytic s.

   kinetic s., e. cinético; e. decorrente de espasmo de um músculo extrínseco do bulbo do olho.

   manifest s., e. manifesto; desvio evidente de um olho ou do outro; pode ser alternante ou monocular.

mechanical s., e. mecânico; e. decorrente de restrição da ação do músculo ocular dentro da órbita.
paralytic s., e. paralítico; estrabismo decorrente de fraqueza de um músculo ou músculos oculares. SIN incomitant s.
vertical s., e. vertical; uma forma de e. em que o eixo visual de um olho desvia-se para cima (e. *sursum vergens*) ou para baixo (s. *deorsum vergens*).
X-s., estrabismo X; e. em que a exotropia é mais acentuada ao olhar para cima ou para baixo do que ao olhar reto para a frente.

strain (strān). **1.** Cepa, estirpe; uma população de organismos homogêneos dotados de um conjunto de características definidas; em bacteriologia, refere-se ao grupo de descendentes que mantêm as características do ancestral; os membros de uma cepa que, subseqüentemente, diferem do organismo isolado original são considerados como pertencentes a uma subcepa da cepa original ou a uma nova cepa. **2.** Célula hospedeira específica designada ou selecionada para otimizar a produção de produtos recombinantes. [A.S. *strēon*, progênie]. **3.** Fazer um esforço além do limite da própria resistência. **4.** Lesar por uso excessivo ou impróprio (referindo-se, em geral, a uma laceração muscular). **5.** Ato de esforçar-se. **6.** Lesão resultante de esforço ou uso excessivo. [L. *stringere, estirar*] **7.** A mudança de forma sofrida por um corpo quando submetido a uma força externa. **8.** Filtrar; coar.
auxotrophic s.'s, cepas auxotrópicas; cepas derivadas da cepa prototófica, mas que exigem fatores de crescimento adicionais.
carrier s., cepa portadora; cepa bacteriana que é contaminada por um bacteriófago de baixa infectividade. SIN pseudolysogenic s.
cell s., cepa celular; em cultura de tecido, células derivadas de uma cultura primária ou de uma única célula (clone), exibindo uma característica específica, como cromossoma marcador, antígeno ou resistência a um vírus.
congenic s., cepa congênica; cepa endogâmica de animais produzida por cruzamento contínuo de um gene de uma linhagem com o de outra linhagem endogâmica (isogênica).
HFR s., Hfr s., cepa HFR; cepa ou clone em que um plasmídio conjugado (como F'), integrado no genoma bacteriano, é útil na transferência (juntamente com o DNA do plasmídio) do DNA bacteriano integrado numa forma seqüencial para um receptor apropriado. [*h*igh *f*requency of *r*ecombination, alta freqüência de recombinação]
hypothetical mean s. (HMS), cepa média hipotética; cepa hipotética que possui as características de um organismo médio calculado.
isogenic s., cepa isogênica; cepa de animais endogâmicos durante muitas gerações e homozigotos de alta probabilidade para determinados genes especificados.
lysogenic s., cepa lisogênica; cepa de bactéria infectada por um bacteriófago temperado. VER lysogeny.
neotype s., cepa neotípica; cepa aceita por consenso internacional para substituir uma cepa típica que não existe mais ou para servir como cepa típica se esta não foi designada e se não existir nenhuma cepa que possa ser designada como tipo. SIN neotype culture.
prototrophic s.'s, cepas prototróficas; cepas que possuem as mesmas exigências nutricionais que a cepa típica selvagem.
pseudolysogenic s., cepa pseudolisogênica. SIN carrier s.
recombinant s., cepa recombinante. VER recombinant (1).
stock s., cepa-tronco; cepa bacteriana ou de outro micróbio que foi mantida em condições laboratoriais como representante de seu tipo.
type s., cepa típica; a nomenclatura de uma espécie ou subespécie.
wild-type s., cepa típica selvagem; cepa encontrada na natureza ou cepa padrão. VER TAMBÉM auxotrophic s.'s, prototrophic s's.

strait (strāt). Estreito; passagem estreita. **Inferior s.,** abertura inferior da pelve; *apertura pelvis inferior*; **superior s.,** abertura superior da pelve; *apertura pelvis superior*. [I. m. *streit* através do Fr. ant. do L. *strictus*, unido, apertado]

strait·jack·et (strāt′jak-et). Camisa de força; dispositivo semelhante a uma roupa com mangas compridas que pode ser utilizado para imobilizar uma pessoa violentamente perturbada. SIN camisole.

stra·mo·ni·um (stra-mō′nē-ŭm). Estramônio; as folhas e sumidades floridas ou com frutos secos da *Datura stramonium* ou *D. tatula* (família Solanaceae), uma erva abundante em países temperados e subtropicais; contém um alcalóide, a datirina; idêntico à hiosciamina. Trata-se de um antiespasmódico, que era utilizado no tratamento da asma e do parquinsonismo; quando utilizado em excesso ou tomado de modo inadvertido, pode causar uma psicose tóxica semelhante à da atropina. [L. mod.]

strand. Filamento; em microbiologia, uma estrutura filamentosa, filamentar ou filiforme.
anticoding s., f. anticodificador; o filamento do DNA duplo que é utilizado como modelo para a síntese do mRNA. SIN antisense s.
antiparallel s., f. antiparalelo; filamento macromolecular orientado na direção oposta a um filamento vizinho.
antisense s., f. anti-sentido. SIN anticoding s.
coding s., f. codificador; filamento de DNA duplo que possui a mesma seqüência do mRNA (porém, o mRNA contém ribonucleotídeos em lugar de desoxirribonucleotídeos). SIN sense s.
complementary s., f. complementar. VER replicative *form*.
minus s., f. negativo. VER replicative *form*.
plus s., f. positivo. VER replicative *form*.
sense s., f. de sentido. VER coding s.
viral s., f. viral. VER replicative *form*.

Strandberg, James Victor, dermatologista sueco, *1883. VER Grönblad-S. *syndrome*.

stran·gal·es·the·sia (strang′gal-es-thē′zē-ă). Estrangalaestesia. SIN zonesthesia. [G. *strangalē*, corda + *aisthēsis*, sensação]

stran·gle (strang′gl). Estrangular; sufocar; obstruir; comprimir a traquéia para impedir a passagem suficiente de ar. [G. *strangaloō*, estrangular, de *strangalē*, corda]

stran·gu·lat·ed (strang′gū-lā-ted). Estrangulado; constrito de modo a impedir a passagem suficiente de ar, como através da traquéia, ou interromper o retorno venoso e/ou o fluxo arterial de modo a comprometer a viabilidade, como no caso de uma hérnia. [L. *strangulo*, pp. -*atus*, estrangular, do G. *strangaloō*, (estrangular)]

stran·gu·la·tion (strang′gū-lā′shŭn). Estrangulamento; o ato de estrangular ou a condição de ser estrangulado, em qualquer sentido: compressão, constrição, herniação.

stran·gu·ry (strang′gū-rē). Estrangúria; dificuldade na micção, com esforço para urinar; a urina pode ser eliminada intermitentemente, com dor e tenesmo. [G. *stranx* (strang-), algo extraído, uma gota + *ouron*, urina]

strap. 1. Tira de emplastro adesivo. **2.** Aplicar tiras de emplastro adesivas superpostas. [A.S. *stropp*]

Strassburg, Gustav A., fisiologista alemão, *1848. VER S. *test*.

strat·i·fi·ca·tion (strat′i-fi-kā′shŭn). Estratificação; o processo ou resultado de separar uma amostra em subamostras, de acordo com critérios específicos, como grupos etários ou ocupacionais. [L. *stratum*, camada + *facio*, fazer]

strat·i·fied (strat′i-fīd). Estratificado; disposto na forma de camadas ou extratos.

stra·tig·ra·phy (stra-tig′ră-fē). Tomografia. SIN tomography. [L. *stratum*, camada + G. *graphē*, algo escrito]

STRATUM

stra·tum, gen. **stra·ti,** pl. **stra·ta** (strat′ŭm, tă; strā′tŭm; tī). Estrato; uma das camadas de tecido diferenciado, cuja agregação forma qualquer estrutura determinada, como a retina ou a pele. VER TAMBÉM lamina, layer. [L. *sterno*, pp. *stratus*, espalhar, neutro do pp. como substantivo, *stratum*, lençol, camada]
s. aculea′tum, e. aculeado; termo obsoleto para referir-se ao e. espinhoso.
s. basa′le, e. basal; **(1)** a camada mais externa do endométrio que sofre apenas alterações mínimas durante o ciclo menstrual. SIN basal layer. **(2)** SIN s. basale epidermidis.
s. basa′le epider′midis, e. basal da epiderme; a camada mais profunda da epiderme, composta de células-tronco em divisão e células de ancoragem. SIN basal cell layer, columnar layer, germinative layer, palisade layer, s. basale (2), s. cylindricum, s. germinativum.
s. cerebra′le ret′inae, e. cerebral da retina. SIN cerebral layer of retina.
s. cine′reum collic′uli superio′ris, e. cinzentos do colículo superior. SIN gray layers of superior colliculus, em layer.
s. circula′re membra′nae tym′pani, camada circular da membrana timpânica; fibras circulares profundas em relação à camada radiada da membrana, que são mais abundantes próximo à periferia; ausente na parte flácida. SIN circular layer of tympanic membrane.
s. circulare musculi detrusoris vesicae [TA], camada circular do músculo detrusor da bexiga. SIN circular layer of detrusor (muscle) of urinary bladder.
s. circula′re tu′nicae muscula′ris [TA], camada circular da túnica muscular. SIN circular layer of muscular coat.
s. circula′re tu′nicae muscula′ris co′li, camada circular da túnica muscular do colo; camada circular da túnica muscular do colo.
s. circulare tunicae muscularis intestini tenuis [TA], camada helicoidal da túnica muscular do intestino delgado. SIN circular layer of muscle coat of small intestine.
s. circula′re tu′nicae muscula′ris rec′ti, camada circular da túnica muscular do reto.
s. circula′re tu′nicae muscula′ris ventric′uli, camada circular da túnica muscular do estômago.
s. compac′tum, e. compacto; a camada superficial de tecido decidual no útero grávido em que predomina o tecido interglandular. SIN compacta.
s. cor′neum epider′midis, e. córneo da epiderme; a camada externa da epiderme, que consiste em várias camadas de células não-nucleadas queratinizadas planas. SIN corneal layer of epidermis, horny layer of epidermis.

stratum

s. cor'neum un'guis, e. córneo da unha; a camada córnea externa da unha. SIN cornified layer of nail, horny layer of nail.

s. cuta'neum membra'nae tym'pani, e. cutâneo da membrana do tímpano; a camada delgada de pele na superfície externa da membrana do tímpano. SIN cutaneous layer of tympanic membrane.

s. cylin'dricum, e. cilíndrico. SIN s. basale epidermidis.

s. disjunc'tum, e. disjunto; a camada de células parcialmente destacadas na superfície livre do e. córneo, conforme observado em cortes ao microscópio; trata-se, provavelmente, de um artefato de fixação.

s. fibrosum vaginae tendinis, bainha fibrosa do tendão; *termo oficial alternativo para fibrous tendon sheath.

s. fibrosum [TA], cápsula fibrosa. SIN fibrous capsule.

s. fibro'sum capsulae articularis, camada fibrosa da cápsula articular. SIN fibrous layer of joint capsule, fibrous capsule.

s. fibrosum panniculi adiposi telae subcutaneae [TA], e. fibroso do panículo adiposo da tela subcutânea. SIN fibrous layer in or on deep aspect of fatty layer of subcutaneous tissue.

s. functiona'le, e. funcional; o endométrio, exceto o e. basal; antigamente acreditava-se que fosse perdido durante a menstruação; todavia, hoje em dia, acredita-se que sofra apenas ruptura parcial.

s. gangliona're ner'vi op'tici, e. ganglionar do nervo óptico. SIN ganglionic layer of optic nerve.

s. ganglionicum [TA], e. ganglionar. SIN ganglionic layer.

s. germinati'vum, e. germinativo. SIN s. basale epidermidis.

s. germinati'vum un'guis, e. germinativo da unha; a camada mais profunda da unha que é contínua com o e. germinativo da pele circundante e a partir da qual a placa ungueal se forma continuamente. SIN germinative layer of nail.

s. granulare [TA], e. granuloso. SIN granular layer. VER layers of dentate gyrus, em layer.

s. granulo'sum corticis cerebel'li [TA], e. granuloso do cerebelo. SIN granular layer of cerebellum.

s. granulo'sum epider'midis, e. granuloso da epiderme. SIN granular layer of epidermis.

s. granulo'sum follic'uli ova'rici vesiculo'si, e. granuloso do folículo ovariano vesicular; a camada de células pequenas que forma a parede de um folículo ovariano. SIN granular layer of a vesicular ovarian follicle, granulosa, membrana granulosa, s. granulosum ovarii.

s. granulo'sum ova'rii, e. granuloso do ovário. SIN s. granulosum folliculi ovarici vesiculosi.

s. gris'eum collic'uli superio'ris, e. cinzento do colículo superior. SIN gray layers of superior colliculus, em layer.

s. gris'eum interme'dium [TA], e. cinzento intermédio. VER gray layers of superior colliculus, em layer.

s. gris'eum profun'dum [TA], e. cinzento profundo. VER gray layers of superior colliculus, em layer.

s. griseum profundum colliculis superioris [TA], e. cinzento profundo do colículo superior. SIN deep gray layer of superior colliculus.

s. gris'eum superficia'le [TA], e. cinzento superficial. VER gray layers of superior colliculus, em layer.

strata gyri dentati [TA], estratos do giro denteado. SIN layers of dentate gyrus, em layer.

s. helicoidale brevis gradus, camada helicoidal de passo curto; *termo oficial alternativo para circular layer of muscle coat of small intestine.

s. helicoidale longi gradus, camada helicoidal de passo longo; *termo oficial alternativo para longitudinal layer of muscle coat of small intestine.

strata hippocampi [TA], estratos do hipocampo. SIN layers of hippocampus, em layer.

s. interoliva're lemnis'ci, e. interolivar do lemnisco; a região medial da medula oblonga entre os núcleos olivares direito e esquerdo, atravessada longitudinalmente pelo lemnisco medial esquerdo e direito e, transversalmente, pelas fibras olivocerebelares em decussação.

s. lemnis'ci, e. do lemnisco; camada em grande parte fibrosa (e, portanto, esbranquiçada) do colículo superior, que separa a camada cinzenta média do colículo superior da camada cinzenta profunda e contendo, entre outras, fibras dos lemniscos espinal e trigeminal. SIN fillet layer.

s. limitans externum [TA], e. limitante externo. SIN outer limiting layer.

s. limitans internum [TA], e. limitante interno. SIN inner limiting layer.

s. longitudina'le tu'nicae muscula'ris [TA], e. longitudinal da túnica muscular. SIN longitudinal layer of muscular coat.

s. longitudina'le tu'nicae muscula'ris co'li, e. longitudinal da túnica muscular do colo.

s. longitudina'le tu'nicae muscula'ris intesti'ni ten'uis [TA], camada helicoidal de passo longo do intestino delgado. SIN longitudinal layer of muscle coat of small intestine.

s. longitudina'le tu'nicae muscula'ris rec'ti, e. longitudinal da túnica muscular do reto.

s. longitudina'le tu'nicae muscula'ris ventric'uli, e. longitudinal da túnica muscular do estômago.

s. lu'cidum, e. lúcido; camada de corneócitos de coloração clara no nível mais profundo do e. córneo; encontrada primariamente na epiderme espessa da pele palmar e plantar. SIN clear layer of epidermis.

strata magnocellularia [TA], estratos magnocelulares. VER lateral geniculate body.

malpighian s., e. de Malpighi; a camada viva da epiderme que compreende o e. basal, o e. espinhoso e o e. granuloso. SIN malpighian layer, malpighian rete.

s. medullare intermedium [TA], e. medular intermédio. SIN intermediate white layer [TA] of superior colliculus.

s. medullare profundum [TA], e. medular profundo. SIN deep white layer of superior colliculus.

s. molecula're, e. molecular. SIN molecular layer.

s. molecula're corticis cerebel'li, e. molecular do cerebelo. SIN molecular layer of cerebellar cortex.

s. moleculare et substratum lacunosum [TA], e. molecular e substrato lacunar. SIN lacunar-molecular layer. VER layers of hippocampus, em layer.

s. molecula're ret'inae, estratos plexiformes da retina. SIN molecular layer of retina.

s. multiforme [TA], estratos cinzentos do colículo superior. SIN multiform layer. VER layers of dentate gyrus, em layer.

s. musculosum panniculi adiposi telae subcutaneae [TA], e. muscular do panículo adiposo da tela subcutânea. SIN muscle layer in fatty layer of subcutaneous tissue.

s. neuroepithelia'le ret'inae, e. neuroepitelial da retina. SIN neuroepithelial layer of retina.

s. neurofibrarum [TA], camada de fibras nervosas. SIN layer of nerve fibers.

s. neurono'rum pirifor'mium, termo obsoleto para Purkinje cell layer (estrato purkinjense).

s. nucleare externum [TA], e. nuclear externo. SIN outer nuclear layer.

s. nucleare internum [TA], e. nuclear interno. SIN inner nuclear layer.

strata nuclea'ria exter'na et inter'na ret'inae, estratos nucleares externo e interno da retina. SIN nuclear layers of retina, em layer.

s. op'ticum [TA], e. óptico. SIN optic layer.

s. oriens [TA], e. de orientação. SIN oriens layer. VER layers of hippocampus, em layer.

s. papilla're cor'ii, e. papilar do cório; a camada mais superficial do cório, cujas papilas se interdigitam com a epiderme. SIN corpus papillare, papillary layer.

strata parvocellularia [TA], estratos parvocelulares. VER lateral geniculate body.

s. pigmen'ti bul'bi, e. pigmentoso do bulbo. SIN pigmented layer of retina.

s. pigmen'ti cor'poris cilia'ris, e. pigmentoso do corpo ciliar; a continuação da camada pigmentada da retina até a face posterior do corpo ciliar. SIN pigmented layer of ciliary body.

s. pigmen'ti i'ridis, e. pigmentoso da íris; a dupla camada de epitélio pigmentado na superfície posterior da íris. SIN pigmented layer of iris.

s. pigmen'ti ret'inae, e. pigmentoso da retina. SIN pigmented layer of retina.

s. plexiforme externum, e. plexiforme externo. SIN plexiform layers of retina, em layer.

s. plexiforme externum [TA], e. plexiforme externo. SIN outer plexiform layer.

s. plexiforme internum [TA], e. plexiforme interno. SIN plexiform layers of retina, em layer.

s. plexiforme internum [TA], e. plexiforme interno. SIN inner plexiform layer.

s. purkinjense corticis cerebelli [TA], e. purkinjense do cerebelo. SIN Purkinje cell layer.

s. pyramidale [TA], e. piramidal. SIN pyramidal layer. VER layers of hippocampus, em layer.

s. radiatum [TA], e. radiado. SIN radiant layer. VER layers of hippocampus, em layer.

s. radia'tum membra'nae tym'pani, e. radiado da membrana do tímpano, a camada de tecido conjuntivo da membrana do tímpano sob o e. cutâneo, cujas fibras se irradiam do manúbrio do martelo até o anel fibrocartilaginoso periférico da membrana; ausente na parte flácida. SIN radiate layer of tympanic membrane.

s. reticula're co'rii, e. reticular do cório; a camada profunda mais espessa do cório, consistindo em tecido conjuntivo denso de disposição irregular. SIN reticular layer of corium, s. reticulare cutis, tunica propria corii.

s. reticula're cu'tis, e. reticular da cútis. SIN s. reticulare corii.

s. segmentorum externorum et internorum [TA], e. dos segmentos externo e interno. SIN layer of inner and outer segments.

s. spino'sum epider'midis, e. espinhoso da epiderme; a camada de células poliédricas na epiderme; os artefatos de retração e a adesão dessas células em suas junções desmossômicas conferem um aspecto espinhoso. SIN prickle cell layer, spinous layer.

s. spongio'sum, e. esponjoso; a camada média do endométrio formada principalmente por estruturas glandulares dilatadas; é flanqueado pelo extrato compacto, na face luminal e pelo extrato basal, na face miometrial.

s. subcuta'neum, tecido subcutâneo. SIN subcutaneous tissue.

s. synovia'le, membrana sinovial. SIN synovial membrane, synovial membrane.

s. zona'le [TA], e. zonal. SIN zonular layer.

Straus, Isidore, médico francês, 1845–1896. VER S. *reaction*, *sign*.
Strauss, Lotte, patologista norte-americano, *1913. VER Churg-S. *syndrome*.
Sträussler. VER Gerstmann-Sträussler-Scheinker *syndrome*.
streak (strēk). Estria; linha, estria ou tira, especialmente quando indistinta ou evanescente. [A.S. *strica*]
   angioid s., estrias angióides; calcificação da lâmina basilar da corióide visível no fundo ocular peripapilar; associadas ao pseudo à xantoma elástico, à anemia falciforme e à doença de Paget; predispondo à neovascularização da corióide. SIN elastosis dystrophica, Knapp s.'s, Knapp striae.
   germinal s., linha germinativa. SIN primitive s.
   gonadal s., estria gonadal; forma de aplasia em que o ovário é substituído por um tecido não-funcional, como aquele encontrado na síndrome de Turner. SIN streak gonad.
   Knapp s.'s, estrias de Knapp. SIN angioid s.'s.
   meningitic s., linha meningítica; linha de eritema resultante do desenho de um ponto através da pele, notável sobretudo nos casos de meningite. SIN Trousseau spot.
   Moore lightning s.'s, faixas luminosas de Moore; fotopsia que se manifesta por clarões luminosos verticais, observados habitualmente na face temporal do olho afetado, causada pela retração involutiva do humor vítreo.
   primitive s., linha primitiva; crista de epiblasto na linha mediana, na extremidade caudal do disco embrionário, a partir da qual surge o mesoderma intraembrionário e o endoderma definitivo; surge por migração interna e, a seguir, lateral de células; nos embriões humanos, aparece aos 15 dias e proporciona uma evidência visual do eixo cefalocaudal. SIN germinal s.
stream (strēm). Corrente. SIN flumen.
   hair s.'s, fluxos dos cabelos; as linhas curvas ao longo das quais se distribuem os cabelos na cabeça e em várias partes do corpo, especialmente perceptíveis no feto. SIN flumina pilorum.
stream·ing (strēm'ing). Fluxo. VER ameboid *movement*.
streb·lo·dac·ty·ly (streb-lō-dak'ti-lē). Camptodactilia. SIN camptodactyly. [G. *streblos*, torcido + *daktylos*, dedo]
Streeter, George L., embriologista norte-americano, 1873–1948. VER S. *developmental horizon(s)*.
Streeter de·vel·op·men·tal ho·ri·zon(s). Horizonte(s) de desenvolvimento de Streeter; termo tomado emprestado à geologia e arqueologia por Streeter para definir 23 estágios de desenvolvimento nos embriões humanos em fase inicial de desenvolvimento, desde a fertilização até os primeiros 2 meses; cada horizonte estendia-se por 2–3 dias e enfatizava características anatômicas específicas para evitar discrepâncias na determinação e das dimensões corporais. [G.L. Streeter]
Streiff, Enrico Bernard, oftalmologista suíço, *1908. VER Hallermann-S. *syndrome*; Hallermann-S.-François *syndrome*.
strength. 1. Força, potência; a qualidade de ser forte ou potente. 2. Grau de intensidade. 3. Resistência; a propriedade apresentada pelos materiais de resistir à aplicação de uma força sem ceder nem quebrar.
   associative s., poder associativo; em psicologia, o poder de ligação da resposta a um estímulo, medido pela freqüência com que um estímulo provoca determinada resposta. VER conditioning.
   biting s., força de mastigação. SIN force of mastication.
   compressive s., resistência à tração, exceto por o estresse estar na compressão.
   fatigue s., grau de fadiga; o nível de estresse abaixo do qual um componente particular sobreviverá a um número indefinido de ciclos de carga (tipicamente cerca de 50% da potência final do componente).
   ionic s. (I), força iônica; simbolizada por $\Gamma/2$ ou I e estabelecida como sendo igual a $0,5 \Sigma m_i z_i^2$, onde m_i é igual à concentração molar e z_i é igual à carga de cada íon presente na solução; se forem utilizadas concentrações molares (c_i) em lugar da molalidade (e a solução estiver diluída), então $I = 0,5(1/\rho_o) \Sigma c_i z_i^2$, onde ρ_o é a densidade do solvente; diversos eventos bioquimicamente importantes (p. ex., solubilidade das proteínas e taxas de ação enzimática) variam com a força iônica de uma solução.
   tensile s., resistência à tração; o estresse ou a carga de tensão máxima que um material é capaz de suportar; geralmente expressa em libras por polegada quadrada.
   ultimate s., limite de ruptura; estresse máximo alcançado antes da falha de um componente com uma única aplicação da carga.
   yield s., intensidade ou força de deformação; a tensão na qual uma deformação permanente (plástica) em um componente torna-se mensurável (geralmente considerada como 0,2% da tensão permanente).
streph·o·sym·bo·lia (stref'ō-sim-bō'lē-ă). Estrefossimbolia. 1. Em geral, a percepção de objetos invertidos, como num espelho. 2. Especificação, dificuldade em distinguir letras escritas com o impressas que se estendem em direções opostas, mas que são semelhantes nos demais aspectos, como *p* e *d*, ou tipos relacionados de inversão especular. [G. *strephō*, girar + *symbolon*, uma marca ou sinal]
stre·pi·tus (strep'i-tŭs). Estrépito; termo raramente utilizado para referir-se a um ruído, geralmente um ruído percebido à ausculta.
streptavidin (strep-ta-vī'din). Estreptavidina; proteína bacteriana utilizada como sonda em ensaios imunológicos, em virtude de sua forte afinidade e especificidade pela biotina; a estreptavidina é utilizada como ponte para ligar um cromógeno a um substrato biotinilado específico para substâncias de interesse. [*strept*ococcus + *avidin*]
strep·ti·ce·mia (strep-ti-sē'mē-ă). Estrepticemia; termo obsoleto para streptococcemia (estreptococcemia).
strep·ti·dine (strep'ti-dēn). Estreptidina; componente aglicônico da estreptomicina.
strepto-. Estrepto-. Curvo ou torcido (referindo-se habitualmente a organismos assim descritos). [G. *streptos*, torcido, de *strephō*, torcer]
Strep·to·ba·cil·lus (strep-tō-ba-sil'ŭs). Gênero de bactérias aeróbicas a anaeróbicas facultativas, não-formadoras de esporos e imóveis (família Bacteroidaceae), contendo células Gram-negativas pleomórficas, que variam desde bastonetes curtos a filamentos longos entrelaçados, com tendência a sofrer fragmentação em cadeias de elementos bacilares e cocobacilares. Esses microrganismos podem ser patogênicos para ratos, camundongos e outros mamíferos. A espécie típica é *S. moniliformis*. [strepto- + *bacillus*]
   S. monilifor'mis, espécie bacteriana comumente encontrada como residente da nasofaringe de ratos; ocorre como agente etiológico de uma poliartrite séptica epizoótica em camundongos e como tipo de febre da mordedura do rato; trata-se da espécie típica do gênero *S*.
strep·to·bi·o·sa·mine (strep'tō-bī-ō'să-mēn). Estreptobiosamina; dissacarídeo metilamino (estreptose + *N*-metil-L-glicosamina), com a ligação do oxigênio entre o C-2 da estreptose e o C-1 da glicosamina; com a estreptidina, forma a estreptomicina.
strep·to·bi·ose (strep-tō-bī'ōs). Estreptobiose; termo antigo para referir-se à streptose (estreptose).
strep·to·cer·ci·a·sis (strep'tō-ser-kī'ă-sis). Estreptocercíase; infecção de seres humanos e primatas superiores pelo nematódeo *Mansonella streptocerca*.
strep·to·coc·cal (strep'tō-kok'ăl). Estreptocócico; relativo a, ou causado por, qualquer microrganismo do gênero *Streptococcus*.
strep·to·coc·ce·mia (strep'tō-kok-sē'-mē-ă). Estreptococcemia; presença de estreptococos no sangue. SIN streptosepticemia. [*streptococcus* + G. *haima*, sangue]
strep·to·coc·ci (strep'tō-kok'sī). Estreptococos; plural de streptococcus.
strep·to·coc·cic (strep'tō-kok'sik). Estreptocócico; relativo a, ou causado por, qualquer microrganismo do gênero *Streptococcus*.
strep·to·coc·co·sis (strep'tō-kō-kō'sis). Estreptococose; qualquer infecção estreptocócica.
Strep·to·coc·cus (strep-tō-kok'ŭs). Gênero de bactérias aeróbicas a anaeróbicas facultativas, não-formadoras de esporos e imóveis (com poucas exceções) (família Lactobacillaceae), contendo células Gram-positivas esféricas ou ovóides, que ocorrem em pares ou em cadeias curtas ou longas. O ácido láctico dextrorrotatório constitui o principal produto de fermentação dos carboidratos. Esses microrganismos são encontrados regularmente na boca e no intestino de seres humanos e outros animais, em laticínios e outros alimentos e nos sucos vegetais em fermentação. Algumas espécies são patogênicas. A espécie típica é *S. pyogenes*. [strepto- + G. *kokkos*, baga (coco)]
   S. agalac'tiae, espécie encontrada no leite e tecidos do úbere de vacas com mastite; também relatada em associação a várias infecções humanas, especialmente as do trato urogenital.
   S. angino'sus, espécie α-hemolítica encontrada na garganta, nos seios, em abscesso, na vagina, na pele e nas fezes de seres humanos; essa bactéria é uma causa comum de abscessos hepáticos isolados.
   S. bo'vis, espécie encontrada no trato alimentar bovino; esse microrganismo também pode ser encontrado no sangue e em lesões cardíacas em casos de endocardite subaguda.
   S. constella'tus, espécie α-hemolítica encontrada nas amígdalas, na pleurite purulenta, no apêndice, no nariz, na garganta e nas gengivas e, raramente, na pele e na vagina.
   S. dur'ans, espécie encontrada no leite em pó e no intestino de seres humanos e outros animais.
   S. faeca'lis, SIN *Enterococcus faecalis*.
   S. intermedius, uma espécie de um grupo heterogêneo de estreptococos, geralmente encontrada na boca ou nas vias respiratórias superiores; a classificação é geralmente estabelecida pelos padrões de fermentação, pela análise da composição dos carboidratos da parede celular e pelo uso dos padrões de produção de carboidratos. SIN *Peptostreptococcus intermedius*.
   S. lac'tis, espécie encontrada comumente como contaminante no leite e em laticínios; trata-se de uma causa de acidificação e coagulação do leite; algumas cepas produzem nisina, um poderoso antibiótico que inibe o crescimento de muitos outros microrganismos Gram-positivos.
   S. milleri, termo utilizado para referir-se ao grupo do *S. intermedius*, que contém três espécies distintas de estreptococo, incluindo *S. intermedius*, *S. constellatus* e *S. anginosus*. Essas bactérias são encontradas na cavidade oral de seres humanos e têm sido associadas a várias infecções, incluindo bacteriemia, endocardite e infecções torácicas, orais e do SNC.
   S. mi'tis, espécie encontrada na boca, garganta e nasofaringe de seres humanos; habitualmente, não é considerada patogênica, porém esse microrganismo

pode ser isolado de dentes e seios ulcerados, bem como do sangue e de lesões cardíacas em casos de endocardite subaguda.

S. morbillorum, SIN *Peptostreptococcus morbillorum.*

S. mu'tans, espécie associada à produção de cáries dentárias nos seres humanos e em alguns outros animais e à endocardite subaguda.

S. pneumo'niae, espécie de cocos e diplococos Gram-positivos, em forma de lanceta, que freqüentemente ocorrem em cadeias; as células são rapidamente lisadas por sais biliares. As formas virulentas estão encerradas em cápsulas de polissacarídeos tipo-específicas, que constituem a base de uma vacina efetiva. São habitantes normais do trato respiratório e constituem a causa mais comum de pneumonia lobar, sendo os agentes causais mais comuns da meningite e pneumonia no mundo inteiro; além disso, causam sinusite e outras infecções. Trata-se da espécie típica do gênero mais antigo *Diplococcus*. SIN Fraenkel pneumococcus, pneumococcus, pneumonococcus.

S. pyog'enes, espécie encontrada na boca, na garganta e no trato respiratório de seres humanos e em exsudatos inflamatórios, na corrente sanguínea e em lesões celulíticas em doenças humanas; algumas vezes, a espécie é encontrada no úbere de vacas e na poeira de quartos de doentes, enfermarias de hospitais, escolas, teatros e outros locais públicos; causa formação de pus, septicemia fatal e fasciite e miosite necrosante. Existe também um antígeno somático específico (proteína M) para cada um dos cerca de 85 tipos. Trata-se da espécie típica do gênero S.

S. saliva'rius, espécie encontrada na boca, garganta e nasofaringe de seres humanos, associada a doença dentária.

S. san'guis, espécie originalmente encontrada na denominada vegetação em valvas cardíacas de casos de endocardite bacteriana subaguda; em certas ocasiões, é encontrada em fístulas e dentes infectados, bem como na poeira doméstica.

S. vir'idans, nome aplicado não a uma espécie distinta, porém ao grupo de estreptococos α-hemolíticos como um todo; estreptococos viridans foram isolados da boca e do intestino de seres humanos, do intestino de cavalos, do leite e das fezes de vacas e de laticínios. SIN viridans streptococci.

strep·to·coc·cus, pl. **strep·to·coc·ci** (strep'tō - kok'ŭs, - kok'sī). Estreptococo; termo utilizado para referir-se a qualquer membro do gênero *Streptococcus*.

group A streptococci (GAS), estreptococos do grupo A; bactéria comum, que constitui a causa de faringite estreptocócica, escarlatina, impetigo, celulite-erisipela, febre reumática, nefrite glomerular aguda, endocardite e fasciite necrosante por estreptococos do grupo A. O protótipo é *Streptococcus pyogenes*.

group B streptococci, estreptococos do grupo B; causa principal de uma forma de sepse neonatal com taxa de mortalidade de 10–20%, em que grande número dos sobreviventes apresenta lesão cerebral; trata-se também de uma importante causa de meningite.

hemolytic streptococci, estreptococos hemolíticos. SIN β-hemolytic streptococci.

α-hemolytic streptococci, estreptococos α-hemolíticos; estreptococos que formam uma variedade verde de hemoglobina reduzida na área da colônia em meio de ágar-sangue. VER TAMBÉM *Streptococcus viridans*.

β-hemolytic streptococci, estreptococos β-hemolíticos; estreptococos produtores de hemolisinas ativas (O e S) que causam uma zona de hemólise clara em meio de ágar-sangue na área da colônia; os estreptococos β-hemolíticos são divididos em grupos (A a O) com base no carboidrato C da parede celular (ver Lancefield *classification*); o grupo A (nas cepas patogênicas para o homem) compreende mais de 50 tipos (designados por algarismos arábicos) determinados pela proteína M da parede celular, que parece estar estreitamente associada à virulência e que é produzida principalmente por cepas com colônias foscas ou mucóides, em contraste com as cepas não-virulentas, produtoras de colônias brilhantes; outros antígenos proteicos de superfície, como R e T (substância T), e a fração nucleoproteica (substância P) parecem ser menos importantes. As mais de 20 substâncias extracelulares elaboradas por cepas de estreptococos β-hemolíticos incluem a toxina eritrogênica (elaborada apenas por cepas lisogênicas), a desoxirribonuclease (estreptodornase), hemolisinas (estreptolisinas O e S), hialuronidase e estreptocinase. SIN hemolytic streptococci.

viridans streptococci, estreptococos viridans. SIN *Streptococcus viridans.*

strep·to·dor·nase (SD) (strep - tō - dōr'nās). Estreptodornase; uma "dornase" (desoxirribonuclease) obtida de estreptococos; utilizada com a estreptocinase para facilitar a drenagem em condições cirúrgicas sépticas.

strep·to·fu·ra·nose (strep - fōor'ă - nōs). Estreptofuranose. SIN streptose.

strep·to·ki·nase (SK) (strep - tō - kī'nās). Estreptocinase; estreptoquinase; metaloenzima extracelular de estreptococos hemolíticos que cliva o plasminogênio, produzindo plasmina, responsável pela liquefação da fibrina (atividade igual à da estafilocinase e urocinase); por conseguinte, é utilizada na remoção de coágulos. SIN plasminokinase, streptococcal fibrinolysin.

strep·to·ki·nase-strep·to·dor·nase. Estreptocinase-estreptodornase; mistura purificada contendo estreptocinase, estreptodornase e outras enzimas proteolíticas; utilizada por aplicação tópica ou injeção em cavidades corporais para remover o sangue coagulado e acúmulos fibrinosos e purulentos de exsudato; por conseguinte, é utilizada na remoção de coágulos.

strep·to·ly·sin (strep - tol'i - sin). Estreptolisina; hemolisina produzida por estreptococos.

s.O, Estreptolisina O; hemolisina produzida por estreptococos β-hemolíticos e hemoliticamente ativa apenas no estado reduzido; a antiestreptolisina O (ASO) produzida durante a infecção possui importância diagnóstica.

Strep·to·my·ces (strep - tō - mī'sēz). Gênero de bactérias Gram-positivas aeróbicas e imóveis (família Streptomycetaceae), que crescem na forma de um micélio muito ramificado; os conídios são produzidos em cadeias sobre hifas aéreas. Esses microrganismos (várias centenas de espécies no gênero) são formas do solo predominantemente saprofíticas; algumas são parasitas de vegetais ou animais; muitos desses microrganismos produzem antibióticos. A espécie típica é *S. albus*. [strepto- + G. *mykēs*, fungo]

S. al'bus, espécie encontrada na poeira, no solo, em grãos e na palha; algumas cepas produzem actinomicetina; outras produzem tioluitina ou endomicina; trata-se da espécie típica do gênero S.

S. gibso'nii, espécie encontrada em infecções humanas. SIN *Nocardia gibsonii*.

S. somalien'sis, espécie que causa o micetoma branco de Bouffardi.

Strep·to·my·ce·ta·ce·ae (strep'tō - mī - se - ta'sē - ē). Família de bactérias Gram-positivas aeróbicas (ordem Actinomycetales) produtoras de um micélio vegetativo que não se fragmenta em formas bacilares ou cocóides; produzem conídios que são transportados em esporóforos. Esses microrganismos ocorrem basicamente no solo; alguns são termófilos encontrados no estrume em decomposição, outros são parasitas e muitos deles produzem antibióticos. O gênero típico é *Streptomyces*.

strep·to·my·cete (strep'tō - mī'sēt). Estreptomiceto; termo utilizado para referir-se a um membro do gênero *Streptomyces*; algumas vezes é utilizado impropriamente para referir-se a qualquer membro da família Streptomycetaceae.

strep·to·my·cin (strep - tō - mī'sin). Estreptomicina; agente antibiótico obtido de *Streptomyces griseus*, que é ativo contra o bacilo da tuberculose e grande número de bactérias Gram-positivas e Gram-negativas; a estreptomicina também é utilizada na forma de diidroestreptomicina (aldeído da estreptomicina reduzido a CH_2OH). É um glicosídeo que contém estreptidina e estreptobiosamina ligadas por uma ponte de oxigênio entre o C-4 do resíduo inositol e o C-1 do resíduo estreptose; a estreptomicina B possui um resíduo de manose fixado à glicosamina e é um produto natural, com menos atividade do que a estreptomicina A. É utilizada quase exclusivamente no tratamento da tuberculose; a toxicidade inclui lesão do oitavo nervo craniano, resultando em surdez e/ou disfunção vestibular. SIN streptomycin A.

strep·to·my·cin A. Estreptomicina A. SIN streptomycin.

strep·to·my·co·sis (strep'tō - mī - kō'sis). Estreptomicose; termo antigo para referir-se à estreptococcemia. [strepto- + G. *mykēs*, fungo + -*osis*, condição]

strep·to·ni·vi·cin (strep'tō - ni - vī'sin). Estreptonivicina. SIN novobiocin.

strep·tose (strep'tōs). Estreptose; L-pentose incomum que é um componente da estreptobiosamina e, portanto, da estreptomicina. SIN streptofuranose.

strep·to·sep·ti·ce·mia (strep'tō - sep - ti - sē'mē - ă). Estreptossepticemia. SIN streptococcemia.

strep·to·thri·cho·sis (strep'tō - thri - kō'sis). Estreptotricose. SIN dermatophilosis.

strep·to·tri·chi·a·sis (strep'tō - tri - kī'ă - sis). Estreptotriquíase. SIN dermatophilosis.

strep·to·tri·cho·sis (strep'tō - tri - kō'sis). Estreptotricose. SIN dermatophilosis.

strep·to·zo·cin (strep - tō - zō'sin). Estreptozocina; agente antineoplásico utilizado no tratamento do carcinoma metastático de células das ilhotas do pâncreas. SIN streptozotocin.

streptozotocin (strep'tō - zō - toks'in). Estreptozotocina. SIN streptozocin.

stress (stres). Estresse, tensão. **1.** Reações do corpo a forças de natureza deletéria, a infecções e a vários estados anormais que tendem a perturbar seu equilíbrio fisiológico normal (homeostasia). **2.** Em odontologia, as forças exercidas nos dentes, suas estruturas de sustentação e estruturas que restauram ou substituem dentes, em consequência da força de mastigação. **3.** A força ou pressão aplicada ou exercida entre partes de um corpo ou corpos, geralmente expressa em libras por polegada quadrada. **4.** Em reologia, a força num material transmitida por unidade de área a camadas adjacentes. **5.** Em psicologia, um estímulo físico ou psicológico, como calor excessivo, crítica pública ou outro agente ou experiência nociva, que, ao atuar sobre determinados indivíduos, provoca tensão ou desequilíbrio psicológico. [L. *strictus*, apertado, de *stringo*, reunir]

life s., estresse da vida; acontecimentos ou experiências que provocam grave tensão, p. ex., fracasso no emprego, separação conjugal, perda de um ente amado.

shear s., força de cisalhamento; a força que atua no fluxo de cisalhamento expressa por unidade de área; unidades no sistema CGS: dinas/cm².

tensile s., esforço de tensão, esforço de tração; força que atua sobre um corpo por unidade de área transversal, de modo a alongar o corpo.

yield s., tensão de escoamento, tensão de deformação; a tensão crítica que precisa ser aplicada a um material antes que este comece a escoar, como num plástico de Bingham.

stress break·er. Amortecedor de tensão; dispositivo que alivia os dentes de apoio, aos quais está fixada uma dentadura parcial fixa ou removível, de toda ou parte da força gerada pela oclusão.

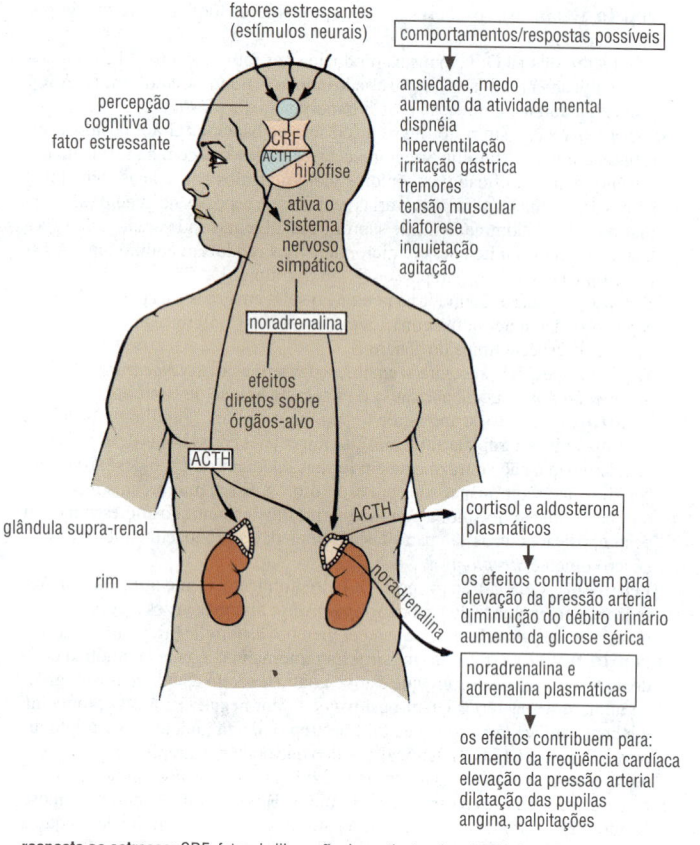

resposta ao estresse: CRF, fator de liberação da corticotropina; ACTH, hormônio adrenocorticotrópico

---

stress ris·er. Criador de tensão, concentrador de tensões locais; defeito mecânico, como um orifício, no osso ou em outros materiais, que concentra estresse na área e aumenta o risco de falência do osso ou do material nesse local.
stress shield·ing. Osteopenia que ocorre no osso em conseqüência da remoção do estresse normal oriundo do osso por um implante.
stretch·er (stre′cher). **1.** Maca, padiola; geralmente consistindo num lençol de lona estendido numa armação com quatro pegadores, utilizada para o transporte de doentes ou feridos. **2.** Maca com quatro rodas e parte superior plana para o transporte de pacientes, geralmente em hospitais. [A.S. *streccan*, estender]
stri·a, gen. e pl. **stri·ae** (strī′a, strī′e). **1.** Estriação, estria; tira, faixa, listra ou linha que se distingue pela cor, textura, depressão ou elevação do tecido em que é encontrada. SIN striation. **2.** SIN striae cutis distensae. [L. canal, sulco]
acoustic striae, estrias medulares do quarto ventrículo. SIN medullary striae of fourth ventricle.
anterior acoustic s. [TA], e. coclear anterior; esses axônios originam-se no núcleo coclear ventral, atravessam a linha média como parte do corpo trapezóide, unem-se ao lemnisco lateral e terminam, em grande parte, no complexo olivar superior. SIN s. cochlearis anterior [TA], ventral acoustic s. [TA].
stri′ae atroph′icae, estrias atróficas. SIN striae cutis distensae.
auditory striae, estrias acústicas do quarto ventrículo. SIN medullary striae of fourth ventricle.
brown striae, estrias de Retzius. SIN Retzius striae.
stri′ae cilia′res, pregas ciliares; sulcos radiais rasos na superfície do orbículo ciliar, que se estendem dos dentes da ora serrata e vão até as depressões entre os processos ciliares.
s. cochlearis anterior [TA], estria coclear anterior. SIN anterior acoustic s.
s. cochlearis intermedia [TA], estria coclear intermédia. SIN intermediate acoustic s.
s. cochlearis posterior [TA], estria coclear posterior. SIN posterior acoustic s.
stri′ae cu′tis disten′sae, atrofodermatose estriada, estrias atróficas; faixas de pele fina e enrugada, inicialmente vermelhas, mas que se tornam púrpuras e brancas, que ocorrem comumente no abdome, nas nádegas e nas coxas na puberdade e/ou durante e após a gravidez; resultam da atrofia da derme e hiperextensão da pele; também associadas a ascite e à síndrome de Cushing. SIN atrophoderma striatum, lineae atrophicae, linear atrophy, stretch marks, stria (2), striae atrophicae, striate atrophy of skin, traction atrophy.
diagonalis s., estria diagonal. VER Broca diagonal band.

s. diagonalis [TA], estria diagonal. SIN Broca diagonal band.
s. externa medullae renalis [TA], estrias externas da medula renal. SIN outer stripes of renal medulla, em stripe.
s. for′nicis, estria medular do tálamo. SIN medullary s. of thalamus.
Gennari s., estria (linha) de Gennari, e. occipital. SIN line of Gennari.
stri′ae gravida′rum, estrias gravídicas; estrias por distensão da pele relacionadas com a gravidez.
intermediate acoustic s. [TA], estria coclear intermédia; esses axônios surgem nos núcleos cocleares; algumas fibras cruzam adjacentes ao corpo trapezóide, outras ascendem do mesmo lado; terminam nos núcleos perioliveres e núcleos do lemnisco lateral; modulariam a atividade do trato olivococlear. SIN s. cochlearis intermedia [TA].
s. of internal granular layer [TA], estria da lâmina granular interna do isocórtex. VER Baillarger lines, em line.
s. of internal pyramidal layer [TA], estria da lâmina piramidal interna do isocórtex. VER Baillarger lines, em line.
s. interna medullae renalis [TA], estria interna da medula renal. SIN inner stripes of renal medulla, em stripe.
Knapp striae, estrias de Knapp. SIN angioid streaks, em streak.
s. laminae granularis internae [TA], estria da lâmina granular interna do isocórtex. SIN Baillarger lines, em line.
s. laminae molecularis [TA], estria da lâmina molecular do isocórtex. SIN band of Kaes-Bechterew.
s. laminae pyramidalis internae [TA], estria da lâmina piramidal interna. SIN Baillarger lines, em line.
stri′ae lanci′si, estrias de Lancisi; a estria longitudinal lateral e a estria longitudinal medial.
Langhans s., estria de Langhans; substância fibrinóide que se acumula na placa coriônica entre as bases das vilosidades placentárias durante a primeira metade da gravidez.
lateral longitudinal s. [TA], estria longitudinal lateral; faixa longitudinal delgada de fibras nervosas acompanhada pela substância cinzenta, próximo a cada borda externa da superfície superior do corpo caloso, sob a cobertura do giro do cíngulo. SIN s. longitudinalis lateralis [TA], s. tecta, tectal s.
s. longitudina′lis latera′lis [TA], estria longitudinal lateral. SIN lateral longitudinal s.
s. longitudina′lis media′lis [TA], estria longitudinal medial. SIN medial longitudinal s.
s. mallea′ris [TA], estria malear. SIN malleolar s.
malleolar s. [TA], estria malear; linha brilhante observada através da membrana timpânica, produzida pela fixação do manúbrio do martelo. SIN s. mallearis [TA], mallear stripe.
medial longitudinal s., estria longitudinal medial; faixa longitudinal delgada de fibras nervosas acompanhada por substância cinzenta, que percorre a superfície do corpo caloso de cada lado da linha mediana. Juntamente com a estria longitudinal lateral, forma parte de uma delgada camada de substância cinzenta na superfície dorsal do corpo caloso, o indúsio cinzento, um componente rudimentar do hipocampo. SIN s. longitudinalis medialis [TA].
stri′ae medulla′res ventric′uli quar′ti [TA], estrias medulares do quarto ventrículo. SIN medullary striae of fourth ventricle.
s. medulla′ris thal′ami [TA], estria medular do tálamo. SIN medullary s. of thalamus.
medullary striae of fourth ventricle [TA], estrias medulares do quarto ventrículo; fascículos delgados de fibras que se estendem transversalmente, abaixo do assoalho ependimário do ventrículo, a partir do sulco mediano, para penetrarem no pedúnculo cerebelar inferior. Originam-se dos núcleos arqueados na superfície ventral da pirâmide medular. SIN striae medullares ventriculi quarti [TA], acoustic striae, auditory striae, Bergmann cords, medullary teniae, taeniae acusticae.
medullary s. of thalamus [TA], estria medular do tálamo; feixe de fibras compacto e estreito que se estende ao longo da linha de fixação do teto do terceiro ventrículo até o tálamo de cada lado, terminando posteriormente no núcleo habenular. É composta de fibras que se originam na área septal, na substância perfurada anterior, no núcleo pré-óptico lateral e no segmento medial do globo pálido. SIN s. medullaris thalami [TA], s. fornicis, s. ventriculi tertii.
s. of molecular layer [TA], estria da lâmina molecular do isocórtex. SIN band of Kaes-Bechterew.
s. na′si transver′sa, sulco nasal transverso; sulco horizontal profundo único ao nível das asas, sem defeitos associados. SIN transverse nasal groove.
Nitabuch s., estria de Nitabuch. SIN Nitabuch membrane.
s. occipitalis [TA], estria occipital. SIN line of Gennari.
stri′ae olfacto′riae [TA], estrias olfatórias. SIN olfactory striae.
olfactory striae [TA], estrias olfatórias; três faixas de fibras distintas (estria medial, estria intermédia, estria lateral) que estendem caudalmente o trato olfatório além de sua fixação ao trígono olfatório. A estria olfatória medial [TA] (s. olfactoria medialis [TA]) curva-se dorsalmente na tênia tectal; a intermédia, quase sempre dificilmente visível, estende-se numa reta para trás e termina no

tubérculo olfatório; a estria olfatória lateral [TA] (s. olfactoria lateralis [TA]), a maior das três, passa ao longo da face lateral do tubérculo olfatório, curvando-se lateralmente até o límen da ínsula e, a seguir, agudamente, em sentido medial, para alcançar o unco do giro para-hipocampal, onde termina na camada plexiforme do córtex olfatório. VER TAMBÉM medial longitudinal s. SIN striae olfactoriae [TA], olfactory roots.
   stri'ae paral'lelae, estrias de Retzius. SIN Retzius striae.
   posterior acoustic s. [TA], estria coclear posterior; esses axônios originam-se do núcleo coclear posterior, cruzam a linha média dorsalmente ao corpo trapezóide e unem-se ao lemnisco lateral; algumas fibras podem terminar no núcleo olivar superior, porém a maioria passa diretamente para o colículo inferior ou faz sinapse nos núcleos do lemnisco lateral *enroute*. SIN s. cochlearis posterior [TA].
   striae ret'inae, estrias da retina; linhas concêntricas na superfície de uma retina normal. SIN Paton lines.
   Retzius striae, estrias de Retzius; linhas concêntricas escuras que cruzam os prismas de esmalte dos dentes, observadas em cortes transversais axiais do esmalte. SIN brown striae, striae parallelae.
   Rohr s., estria de Rohr; camada de fibrinóide nos espaços intervilosos da placenta.
   s. spino'sa, estria espinhosa; sulco fraco ocasionalmente produzido pelo nervo corda do tímpano sobre a espinha do esfenóide. SIN Lucas groove, sulcus spinosus.
   s. tec'ta, estria longitudinal lateral. SIN lateral longitudinal s.
   tectal s., estria longitudinal lateral. SIN lateral longitudinal s.
   terminal s. [TA], estria terminal; feixe de fibras compacto e delgado que conecta os corpos amigdalóides com o hipotálamo e com outras estruturas basilares do telencéfalo. Originando-se na tonsila, o feixe segue inicialmente em sentido caudal no teto do corno temporal do ventrículo lateral; percorre o lado medial do núcleo caudado anteriormente no assoalho da parte central (ou corpo) do ventrículo, até alcançar o forame interventricular, em cuja parede posterior curva-se acentuadamente para penetrar no hipotálamo, com fibras seguindo em direção rostral e caudal até a comissura anterior. O feixe, cujo percurso segue caudalmente na parte medial do hipotálamo, termina nos núcleos hipotalâmicos anterior e ventromedial. SIN s. terminalis [TA], Foville fasciculus, Tarin tenia, tenia semicircularis.
   s. termina'lis [TA], estria terminal. SIN terminal s.
   s. vascularis of cochlear duct [TA], estria vascular do ducto coclear; o epitélio estratificado que reveste a parte superior do ligamento espiral do ducto coclear; é penetrada por capilares, e acredita-se que seja o local de produção da endolinfa. SIN s. vascularis ductus cochlearis [TA], psalterial cord, vascular stripe.
   s. vascula'ris duc'tus cochlea'ris [TA], estria vascular do ducto coclear. SIN s. vascularis of cochlear duct.
   ventral acoustic s. [TA], estria coclear ventral. SIN anterior acoustic s.
   s. ventric'uli ter'tii, estria medular do tálamo. SIN medullary s. of thalamus.
   Wickham striae, estrias de Wickham; linhas finas esbranquiçadas, com disposição reticular, na superfície de pápulas do líquen plano.
   striae of Zahn, estrias de Zahn. SIN lines of Zahn, em line.
stri·a·tal (strī′ă-tăl). Relativo ao corpo estriado.
stri·ate (strī′āt). Estriado, Sulcado; caracterizado ou provido de estrias. [L. *striatus*, estriado]
stri·a·tion (strī-ā′shŭn). 1. Estria. SIN stria (1). 2. Aspecto estriado. 3. Estriação, estriamento; o ato de estriar ou fazer estrias.
   basal s.'s, estriações basais; as estriações infranucleares verticais devidas à membrana plasmática invaginada e mitocôndrias; são observadas nos túbulos renais e em certos ductos salivares intralobulares.
   tabby cat s., estriação tigróide. SIN tigroid s.
   tigroid s., estriação tigróide; marcas lineares esbranquiçadas ou amareladas no músculo cardíaco com degeneração gordurosa. SIN tabby cat s.
stri·a·to·ni·gral (strī-ă-tō-nī′gral). Estriadonigral; refere-se à conexão eferente do estriado com a substância negra (*substantia* nigra).
stri·a·tum (strī-ā′tŭm). [TA], Estriado; nome coletivo para o núcleo caudado e putame que, juntamente com o globo pálido, formam o corpo estriado. SIN neostriatum*. [L. neut. de *striatus*, estriado]
   dorsal s. [TA], estriado dorsal; partes do núcleo caudado e, especialmente, o putame localizados geralmente em posição dorsal a um plano representando a comissura anterior; pode funcionar em atividades motoras com origens cognitivas. SIN s. dorsale [TA].
   s. dorsale [TA], estriado dorsal. SIN dorsal s.
   ventral s. [TA], estriado ventral; partes do estriado localizadas geralmente em posição ventral a um plano representando a comissura anterior; inclui o *nucleus acumbens* e alguns núcleos do tubérculo olfatório; pode funcionar em atividades motoras com origens emocionais ou motivacionais. SIN s. ventrale [TA].
   s. ventrale [TA], estriado ventral. SIN ventral s.
stric·ture (strik′choor). Estreitamento ou estenose circunscrita de uma estrutura oca, consistindo em contratura cicatricial ou na deposição de tecido anormal. [L. *strictura*, de *stringo*, pp. *strictus*, apertar, unir]
   anastomotic s., e. anastomótica; estreitamento, geralmente por fibrose, de uma linha de sutura anastomótica.
   anular s., e. anular; constrição anular que circunda a parede de um canal.
   bridle s., e. em brida; estreitamento de um canal por uma faixa de tecido que se estende através de parte de sua luz.
   contractile s., e. contrátil. SIN recurrent s.
   functional s., e. funcional. SIN spasmodic s.
   organic s., e. orgânica; estenose decorrente de tecido cicatricial ou de outro tecido novo; não-espasmódica. SIN permanent s.
   permanent s., e. permanente. SIN organic s.
   recurrent s., e. recorrente; estenose causada por tecido contrátil que pode ser dilatado, mas logo retorna à sua posição. SIN contractile s.
   spasmodic s., e. espasmódica; e. decorrente de espasmo localizado de fibras musculares na parede do canal. SIN functional s., temporary s.
   temporary s., e. temporária. SIN spasmodic s.
   urethral s., e. uretral; lesão estenosante da uretra, causada geralmente por inflamação ou instrumentação iatrogênica, resultando em redução do calibre da uretra, que pode ser focal ou envolver praticamente toda a extensão da uretra.
stric·tur·o·plas·ty (strik′chur-plas′tē). Procedimento cirúrgico para alargamento de um segmento de intestino estreitado, que envolve incisão e fechamento em direções opostas. [stricture + G. *plastos*, formado]
stric·tur·o·tome (strik′choor-ō-tōm). Instrumento para uso na divisão de uma estenose.
stric·tur·ot·o·my (strik′-choor-ot′ō-mē). Abertura ou divisão cirúrgica de uma estenose. [stricture + G. *tomē*, incisão]
stri·dent (strī′dent). Estridente; estridor; rangido; ruído áspero; designa um ruído ou estertor à ausculta. [L. *stridens*, pres. p. de *strideo*, ranger]
stri·dor (strī′dōr). Estridor; respiração ruidosa, alta, semelhante ao sopro do vento; trata-se de um sinal de obstrução respiratória, especialmente na traquéia ou na laringe. [L. som áspero, rangido]
   congenital s., e. congênito, e. laríngeo; inspiração ruidosa que ocorre ao nascimento ou nos primeiros meses de vida; algumas vezes sem causa aparente, outras vezes decorrente de flacidez anormal da epiglote ou aritenóides. SIN laryngeal s.
   s. den'tium, e. dentário; rangido dos dentes.
   expiratory s., e. expiratório; som canoro decorrente de cordas vocais semi-aproximadas que oferecem resistência à saída de ar ou de obstrução da traquéia ou dos brônquios.
   inspiratory s., e. inspiratório; som durante a fase inspiratória da respiração decorrente de patologia afetando as vias respiratórias superiores, especialmente a epiglote ou laringe.
   laryngeal s., e. laríngeo, e. congênito. SIN congenital s.
   s. serrat'icus, som áspero semelhante ao de uma serra.
strid·u·lous (strī′ū-lŭs). Estriduloso, estridente; que apresenta som agudo e penetrante ou rangido. [L. *stridulus*, de *strideo*, ranger, sibilar]
string. Corda; corda fina ou estrutura semelhante a uma corda.
   auditory s., cordões auditivos; feixes de filamentos paralelos na zona pectinada da lâmina basilar da cóclea; o comprimento dos cordões varia de 64 μm na espiral basal até 480 μm no ápice.
stri·o·la (strī′ō-la). Estriola da membrana dos estatocônios da mácula do ducto utriculossacular; a área central estreita da mácula do utrículo, onde as orientações dos estereocílios e cinocílios mais comprimidos mudam. [L. *stria*, tira + -*ola*, sufixo dim.]
strip. 1. Ordenhar; espremer o conteúdo de um tubo ou canal passível de colapso, como a uretra, correndo-se o dedo ao longo dele. SIN milk (4). 2. Excisão subcutânea de uma veia em seu eixo longitudinal, efetuada com um fleboextrator. 3. Tira, fita; qualquer peça estreita, relativamente longa e de largura uniforme. [A.S. *strypan*, roubar]
   abrasive s., f. abrasiva; pedaço de linho semelhante a uma fita, com partículas abrasivas em um dos lados; utilizada em odontologia para delinear e polir superfícies proximais de restaurações.
   amalgam s., f. de amálgama; fita de linho sem abrasivo utilizada para alisar os contornos proximais de restaurações recém-colocadas.
   celluloid s., f. de celulóide; fita de plástico transparente utilizada como matriz quando se insere um cimento ou resina em preparações de cavidades proximais de dentes anteriores.
   lightning s., f. de abrandamento; fita de metal com abrasivo em um dos lados, utilizada para abrir contatos ásperos ou impróprios de restaurações proximais.
stripe (strīp). Estria. 1. Em anatomia, uma listra, linha, faixa ou estria. 2. Em radiografia, opacidade linear cuja densidade difere das partes adjacentes da imagem; em geral, representa a imagem tangencial de uma estrutura planar, como a pleura ou o peritônio. VER TAMBÉM psoas *margin*. [l.m.]
   s. of Gennari, estria (linha) de Gennari, estria occipital. SIN line of Gennari.

Hensen s., faixa de Hensen; faixa na superfície inferior da membrana tectória do ducto coclear.
inner s.'s of renal medulla [TA], estrias internas da medula renal; a parte mais profunda ou mais central da medula externa do rim, reconhecível em corte sagital através da pirâmide de uma amostra recente; difere estruturalmente da estria externa, visto que é atravessada por porções tanto delgadas quanto espessas (ramos) dos túbulos dos néfrons. SIN stria interna medullae renalis [TA].
malleolar s., estria malear. SIN *malleolar stria.*
Mees s.'s, linhas de Mees. SIN Mees *lines,* em *line.*
occipital s. [TA], estria occipital. SIN *line* of Gennari.
outer s.'s of renal medulla [TA], estrias externas da medula renal; a porção mais superficial ou mais periférica da medula externa do rim, reconhecível em corte sagital através da pirâmide de uma amostra recente; difere estruturalmente da estria interna, uma vez que é atravessada apenas por porções espessas (ramos) dos túbulos dos néfrons. SIN stria externa medullae renalis [TA].
pleural s., linha pleural. SIN pleural *lines,* em *line.*
tracheal wall s., linha da parede traqueal; em radiografia de tórax, a opacidade linear entre o ar na traquéia e no lobo superior direito.
vascular s., estria vascular do ducto coclear. SIN *stria* vascularis of cochlear duct.
strip·per. Extrator.
vein s., fleboextrator; instrumento utilizado para remover uma veia ao amarrá-la em uma das extremidades e ao puxá-la, separando-a de seus ramos e, assim, extirpando-a do corpo.

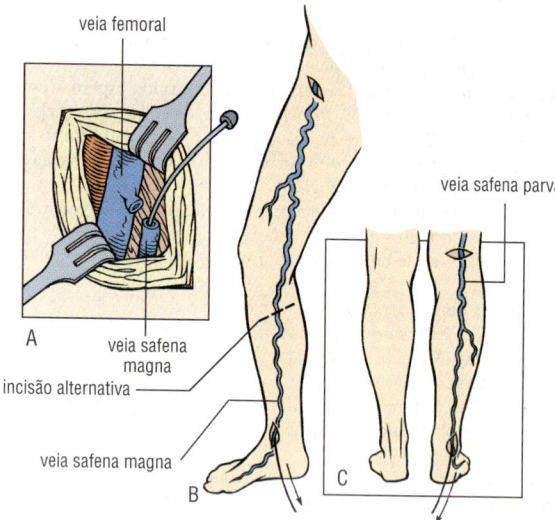

extirpação das veias safenas: (A) tributários da veia safena ligados, com ligadura da veia safena na junção safenofemoral; (B) fleboextrator introduzido no tornozelo superiormente até a virilha, com extirpação da veia de cima para baixo; (C) veia safena parva extirpada de sua junção com a veia poplítea até um ponto posterior ao maléolo lateral

strip·ping. Extirpação; remoção, freqüentemente de um revestimento.
membrane s., e. das membranas; separação das membranas gestacionais do segmento uterino inferior mediante introdução de um dedo através do óstio do útero para desencadear o reflexo de Ferguson ou a liberação de prostaglandinas da decídua e acelerar o trabalho de parto.
Strisower. VER Schellong-Strisower *phenomenon.*
stro·bi·la, pl. **stro·bi·lae** (strō'bi-la, -lē). Estróbilo; cadeia de segmentos, menos o escólex e a porção não-segmentada do colo de uma tênia; nas tênias monozóicas (subclasse Cestodaria e alguns membros da subclasse Cestoda), pode consistir numa única proglote. [G. *stobile,* fio torcido]
stro·bi·lo·cer·cus (strō'bi-lō-ser'kŭs). Estrobilocerco; larva de tênia do tipo cisticerco, porém com colo segmentado conspícuo; pequena bexiga terminal e escólex evertido; a forma larvar da *Taenia taeniaeformis,* denominada *Cysticercus fascilolaris.* [G. *strobile,* fio torcido + *kerkos,* cauda]
stro·bi·loid (strō'bi-loyd). Estrobilóide; semelhante a uma cadeia de segmentos de uma tênia. [G. *strobile,* estróbilo + *eidos,* semelhança]
stro·bo·scope (strō'bō-skōp). Estroboscópio; instrumento eletrônico que produz clarões intermitentes de freqüência controlada; utilizado para influenciar a atividade elétrica do córtex cerebral.
stro·bo·scop·ic (strō-bō-skop'ik). Estroboscópico; relativo à ilusão de movimento, retardado ou acelerado, produzido por imagens visuais observadas intermitentemente, em rápida sucessão. [G. *strobos,* torção ao redor, de *strephō,* torcer + *skopeō,* ver]

stro·bos·co·py (strō-bos'kō-pē). Estroboscopia; endoscopia realizada com luz intermitente, numa freqüência que se aproxima da freqüência de movimento do objeto visualizado, de modo que pareça imóvel; útil na análise da estrutura e movimento das cordas vocais.

stroke (strōk) **1.** Acidente vascular cerebral; qualquer evento clínico agudo relacionado a comprometimento da circulação cerebral, de mais de 24 horas de duração. SIN apoplexy, brain attack. **2.** Descarga prejudicial de um raio, sobretudo quando afeta o ser humano. **3.** Pulsação, batimento. **4.** Afagar; passar a mão ou qualquer instrumento suavemente sobre uma superfície. VER TAMBÉM stroking. **5.** Alisar; movimento de deslizamento sobre uma superfície. [A.S. *strāc*]

Os déficits neurológicos agudos decorrentes de comprometimento circulatório, que sofrem resolução em 24 horas, são denominados ataques isquêmicos transitórios (AIT). A maioria dos AIT dura apenas 15–20 minutos. Em contrapartida, o acidente vascular cerebral (AVC) envolve lesão cerebral irreversível, com o tipo e gravidade dos sintomas dependendo da localização e da extensão do tecido cerebral cuja circulação foi comprometida. A evolução de um AVC varia desde comprometimento mínimo até coma de instalação rápida, seguido prontamente por morte. O AVC é a terceira causa de morte em adultos nos Estados Unidos, depois da cardiopatia isquêmica e do câncer. Nos Estados Unidos, cerca de 700.000 pessoas são anualmente vítimas de AVC, e, em qualquer momento determinado, a população inclui cerca de 3 milhões de sobreviventes de acidente vascular cerebral. A incidência dessa afecção declinou gradualmente nesta última geração. Os fatores de risco associados ao AVC incluem hipertensão, valvopatia cardíaca, fibrilação atrial, hiperlipidemia, diabetes melito, tabagismo (cigarro) e história familiar de AVC. Além disso, estudos recentes mostraram que níveis plasmáticos elevados de homocisteína, baixos níveis circulantes de ácido fólico e piridoxina (vitamina B_6), doença periodontal e bronquite crônica são fatores de risco independentes.

O AVC isquêmico, que é responsável por cerca de 85% de todos os casos de acidente vascular cerebral, é geralmente causado por aterotrombose ou embolia de uma importante artéria cerebral. As causas menos comuns de AVC isquêmico incluem doença vascular não-ateromatosa e distúrbios da coagulação. A isquemia aguda e grave no tecido nervoso ocasiona alterações celulares (influxo de cálcio, ativação da protease), que podem causar rapidamente uma lesão irreversível (infarto). Ao redor da zona de infarto encontra-se uma "área de penumbra" (tecido isquêmico e eletricamente silencioso) que pode ser recuperada através de reperfusão imediata. A taxa de mortalidade do AVC isquêmico é de 15–30% nos primeiros 30 dias. O AVC hemorrágico, que é responsável pelos outros 15%, possui prognóstico mais grave, com uma taxa de mortalidade de 40–80% em 30 dias. A avaliação diagnóstica do paciente com acidente vascular cerebral inclui anamnese, exame físico, hemograma, bioquímica sanguínea, coagulograma, eletrocardiograma e técnicas de imagem. Apesar de a TC do crânio ser o procedimento de escolha para a identificação de hemorragia subaracnóidea, a RMN é um indicador mais sensível de hemorragia parenquimatosa, bem como de isquemia e infarto. Cerca de 20% dos indivíduos inicialmente considerados acometidos por acidente vascular cerebral tiveram, na verdade, algum outro distúrbio, e até 20% dos casos de AVC não são detectados na avaliação inicial por médicos do Pronto-Socorro. O tratamento precoce e agressivo é de suma importância para limitar a lesão do tecido cerebral e obter um desfecho ótimo. No AVC isquêmico, foi constatado que a administração intravenosa do ativador do plasminogênio tecidual (TPA) nas primeiras 3 horas, com o propósito de dissolver um trombo causador de obstrução, melhora a evolução global em 90 dias. Os fatores limitantes do uso de agentes trombolíticos são a necessidade de afastar a possibilidade de AVC hemorrágico (cujo diagnóstico é por vezes difícil com os métodos disponíveis de imagem) e o fato de que a própria terapia pode induzir hemorragia. À exceção do TPA, os agentes trombolíticos intravenosos são menos efetivos, além de apresentarem maior tendência a causar hemorragia. Em estudos limitados, foi constatado que a injeção intra-arterial de pró-urocinase dentro de até 6 horas após o início do AVC influenciou favoravelmente a evolução. Durante a fase aguda do AVC, o suporte respiratório e circulatório e a atenção ao equilíbrio hidroeletrolítico e à alimentação são de importância vital. A hipotermia e a administração intravenosa de heparina e de magnésio também melhoram o desfecho em casos selecionados. As conseqüências em longo prazo dependeriam da agressividade e da persistência da fisioterapia e reabilitação.

As medidas efetivas na profilaxia contra o AVC incluem controle agressivo da hipertensão, da hiperlipidemia e do diabetes melito, interrupção do fumo de cigarros e farmacoprofilaxia em indivíduos de alto risco. A administração de AAS (ácido acetilsalicílico) inibe profilaticamente a agregação plaquetária ao suprimir o tromboxano A_2. Uma metanálise de estudos clínicos controlados e randomizados, envolvendo um total de mais de 50.000 pessoas, indicou que a administração de AAS em dose baixa (80–325 mg/dia) reduz o risco de AVC isquêmico em 39 eventos por 10.000 indivíduos, porém aumenta o risco de acidente vascular cerebral hemorrágico em 12 eventos por 10.000 indivíduos. Outros estudos sugerem que o AAS em doses mais altas (1,3 g/dia em doses fracionadas) protege os homens, mas não as mulheres, do AVC isquêmico, visto que, nas mulheres, o AAS também suprime a prostaciclina, um inibidor natural da agregação plaquetária. A profilaxia com outros agentes antiplaquetários (clopidogrel, ticlopidina) é igualmente efetiva em ambos os sexos e, pelo menos, tão protetora quanto o AAS. Na fibrilação atrial não-valvular, a profilaxia com warfarina reduz em dois terços o risco de acidente vascular cerebral. A maioria dos estudos mostra que, em indivíduos com estenose da artéria carótida de pelo menos 60%, a endarterectomia da carótida diminui o risco de AVC. A *National Stroke Association* recomendou a adoção do termo *infarto cerebral* para o acidente vascular cerebral, em analogia com o termo familiar *infarto do miocárdio*, para enfatizar tanto a localização da lesão quanto a urgência da necessidade de avaliação e tratamento. VER TAMBÉM tissue plasminogen activator.

effective s., batimento efetivo; o rápido movimento dos cílios para frente.
heart s., impacto do ápice do coração contra a parede do tórax.
heat s., intermação, hiperpirexia maligna. VER heatstroke.
recovery s., batimento de recuperação; o movimento de retorno lento dos cílios.
spinal s., início abrupto de disfunção focal da medula espinal decorrente de distúrbio de seu suprimento sanguíneo.
sun s., insolação. VER sunstroke.
strok·ing (strōk'ing). Afago; carícia não-verbal e carinho dispensados a lactentes ou as formas não-verbais e verbais de aceitação, segurança e reforço positivo dispensadas a crianças e adultos, seja por um indivíduo a si próprio ou a outra pessoa, a fim de satisfazer uma necessidade biopsicológica básica de todo o ser humano em desenvolvimento; acredita-se que várias condições psicopatológicas ocorrem quando esse afago está ausente ou deficiente.
stro·ma, pl. **stro·ma·ta** (strō'ma, strō'ma - tā). Estroma. **1.** O arcabouço, geralmente de tecido conjuntivo, de um órgão, glândula ou outra estrutura, distinto do parênquima ou substância específica da parte. **2.** Fase aquosa dos cloroplastos, isto é, a matriz do cloroplasto. **3.** Forma arcaica para referir-se à matriz mitocondrial. [G. *strōma*, leito]
s. glan'dulae thyroi'deae, e. da glândula tireóide. SIN s. of thyroid gland.
s. i'ridis, e. da íris. SIN s. of iris.
s. of iris, e. da íris; o tecido conjuntivo vascular delicado situado entre a superfície anterior da íris e a parte irídica da retina. SIN s. iridis.
lymphatic s., e. linfático; a rede de fibras reticulares e células reticulares associadas do tecido linfático.
nerve s., e. dos nervos; o tecido conjuntivo que sustenta as estruturas das fibras nervosas periféricas, consistindo em endoneuro, perineuro e epineuro.
s. ova'rii, e. do ovário. SIN s. of ovary.
s. of ovary, e. do ovário; o tecido fibroso da medula do ovário. SIN s. ovarii.
Rollet s., e. de Rollet; o estroma incolor dos eritrócitos.
s. of thyroid gland, e. da glândula tireóide; o tecido conjuntivo que sustenta os lóbulos e folículos da glândula tireóide. SIN s. glandulae thyroideae.
s. of vitreous, e. do vítreo; a delicada estrutura do corpo vítreo imersa no humor vítreo ou que o circunda. SIN s. vitreum.
s. vit'reum, e. do vítreo. SIN s. of vitreous.
stro·mal (strō'mal). Estromal; relativo ao estroma de um órgão ou outra estrutura. SIN stromic.
stro·ma·tin (strō'ma - tin). Estromatina; proteína insolúvel no estroma dos eritrócitos.
stro·ma·tol·y·sis (strō - mă - tol'i - sis). Estromatólise; destruição da membrana envoltória de uma célula, como o eritrócito. [stroma + G. *lysis*, dissolução]
strom·ic (strō'mik). Estromal. SIN stromal.
stro·muhr (strōm'oor). Instrumento para medir o volume de sangue que flui através de um vaso sanguíneo por unidade de tempo. [Al. *Strom*, corrente + *Uhr*, relógio]
Ludwig s., um dos primeiros aparelhos para medir o fluxo em vasos sanguíneos.
thermo-s., VER thermostromuhr.
Strong, Edward K., Jr., psicólogo norte-americano, *1884. VER S. vocational interest *test*.
stron·gyle (stron'jil). Estrôngilo; denominação comum dos membros da família Strongylidae. [G. *strongylos*, redondo]
Stron·gyl·i·dae (stron - jil'i - dē). Família de vermes nematódeos parasitas (ordem Strongyloidea), que inclui os gêneros *Strongylus* e *Oesophagostomum*. [ver *Strongyloides*]
Stron·gy·loi·dea (stron - ji - loy'dē - ă). Superfamília de parasitas nematódeos estrôngilos, que inclui os gêneros *Ancylostoma*, *Necator*, *Ostertagia*, *Haemonchus* e *Strongylus*, bem como as tênias de galinhas, os vermes pulmonares de carnívoros e alguns dos mais importantes helmintos patógenos dos seres humanos e de animais domésticos. [ver *Strongyloides*]
Stron·gy·loi·des (stron - ji - loy'dēz). Gênero de pequenos parasitas nematódeos (superfamília Rhabditoidea), comumente encontrado no intestino delgado de mamíferos (particularmente ruminantes), caracterizados por um ciclo biológico incomum que envolve uma ou várias gerações de vermes adultos de vida livre. A infecção humana é causada principalmente por *S. stercoralis*, o pequeno nematódeo do homem, disseminado em todas as regiões tropicais, ou por *S. fuelleborni*, um parasita de primatas não-humanos, na região tropical da África e Ásia e de seres humanos na África tropical. A subespécie *S. fuelleborni kellyi* ocorre na Nova Guiné, onde provoca infecção disseminada. A infecção fatal em lactentes de 2 meses de idade, possivelmente infectados por transmissão transmamária, produz a condição conhecida localmente como doença da barriga inchada ou síndrome da barriga inchada, que causa acentuada distensão do abdome, invariavelmente fatal nesses lactentes. Outras espécies incluem *S. papillosus*, em bovinos, ovinos e caprinos, e *S. ransomi* em suínos. [G. *strongylos*, redondo + *eidos*, semelhança]
stron·gy·loi·di·a·sis (stron'ji - loy - dī'a - sis). Estrongiloidíase; infecção por nematódeos do solo do gênero *Strongyloides*, considerado como fêmea parasita partogenética. As larvas eliminadas no solo desenvolvem-se passando por quatro estágios larvários, formando adultos de vida livre, ou transformam-se do primeiro e segundo estágios de vida livre em larvas estrongiliformes ou filariformes de terceiro estágio infecciosas, que penetram na pele ou na mucosa oral através da ingestão de água. Pode ocorrer infecção através de larvas de uma nova geração desenvolvida no solo (ciclo indireto), através de larvas infectantes que se desenvolveram sem estágio adulto interposto (ciclo direto) ou através de larvas que se desenvolvem diretamente nas fezes dentro do intestino do hospedeiro, penetram na mucosa e passam por migração retrógrada do sangue/escarro pulmonar para o intestino (auto-reinfecção); a maioria das infecções humanas graves e quase todos os casos fatais resultam de auto-reinfecção e infecção disseminada subseqüente, que ocorrem comumente após imunossupressão por esteróides, ACTH ou outros agentes imunossupressores. A auto-reinfecção também pode ocorrer em pacientes com AIDS/SIDA. SIN strongyloidosis.
stron·gy·loi·do·sis (-dō'sis). Estrongiloidíase. SIN strongyloidiasis.
stron·gy·lo·sis (stron - ji - lō'sis). Estrongilose; doença causada pela infecção por uma espécie do nematódeo *Strongylus*; os efeitos podem ser extremos em consequência de lesões, nódulos e aneurismas causados pelo verme.
Stron·gy·lus (stron'ji - loos). Um gênero de grandes nematódeos estrôngilos (subfamília Strongylinae, família Strongylidae) parasita de cavalos e outros eqüídeos, constituindo a causa da estrongilose. [G. *strongylos*, redondo]
S. asi'ni, espécie que ocorre no intestino grosso do jumento e de outros eqüídeos selvagens.
S. edenta'tus, espécie hematófaga encontrada no ceco e no colo de cavalos, jumentos, mulas e zebras.
S. equi'nus, espécie hematófaga cosmopolita encontrada no ceco e (raramente) no colo de cavalos e outros eqüídeos.
S. radia'tus, SIN *Cooperia oncophora*.
S. ventrico'sus, SIN *Cooperia oncophora*.
S. vulga'ris, espécie hematófaga encontrada principalmente no ceco de cavalos e outros eqüídeos; durante a sua migração, as larvas costumam alojar-se na parede da aorta posterior, causando lesão da parede e desenvolvimento de aneurismas verminosos nesse vaso, principalmente nas artérias mesentéricas anteriores.
stron·ti·um (Sr) (stron'shē - ŭm). Estrôncio; elemento metálico, de número atômico 38, peso atômico 87,62; pertence à série dos alcalinos terrosos e assemelha-se ao cálcio nas suas propriedades químicas e biológicas. Vários sais de estrôncio são utilizados terapeuticamente por seus ânions; p. ex., brometo, iodeto e lactato de estrôncio. [*Strontian*, uma cidade na Escócia]
stron·ti·um-85 (^{85}Sr). Estrôncio-85; isótopo radioativo do estrôncio com meia-vida de 64,84 dias; utilizado em cintigrafia óssea.
stron·ti·um-87m (^{87m}Sr). Estrôncio-87; isótopo radioativo do estrôncio com meia-vida de 2,80 h; utilizado em cintigrafia óssea.
stron·ti·um-89 (^{89}Sr). Estrôncio-89; isótopo radioativo do estrôncio; emissor β com meia-vida de 50,52 dias; utilizado como marcador em estudos de absorção do estrôncio pelo corpo, incorporação do estrôncio aos ossos, etc.
stron·ti·um-90 (^{90}Sr). Estrôncio-90; isótopo radioativo do estrôncio; emissor β com meia-vida de 29,1 anos; importante componente (cerca de 5%) dos produtos de fissão do urânio; incorpora-se ao tecido ósseo, onde a renovação é lenta; utilizado na terapia de certos distúrbios oculares (p. ex., pterígio).
stro·phan·thin (strō - fan'thin). Estrofantina; glicosídeo ou mistura de glicosídeos do *Strophanthus kombé*; tônico cardíaco, semelhante à ouabaína (G-s.); extremamente tóxica.
Stro·phan·thus (strō - fan'thŭs). Gênero de trepadeiras do leste da África (família Apocynaceae); as sementes maduras secas de *S. kombé* ou *S. hispidus* contêm o glicosídeo cardíaco estrofantina e eram utilizadas como veneno de flechas; as sementes de *S. gratus* constituem a fonte vegetal da ouabaína. [G. *strophos*, cordão torcido + *anthos*, flor]
stroph·o·ceph·a·ly (strof - ō - sef'ă - lē). Estrofocefalia; condição caracterizada por distorção congênita da cabeça e da face, com tendência a ciclopia e malformação da região oral. [G. *strophē*, torção + *kephalē*, cabeça]

stroph·o·so·mia (strof-ō-sō'mē-ă). Estrofossomia; forma grave de fissura ventral congênita, extremamente rara nos seres humanos. [G. *strophē*, torção + *sōma*, corpo]

struc·tura (strook-too'ra). Estrutura. SIN structure.

structurae oculi accessoriae [TA], estrutura ocular acessória. SIN accessory visual *structures*, em *structure*.

struc·tur·al (strŭk'choor-ăl). Estrutural; relativo à estrutura de determinada parte; que possui uma estrutura. SIN anatomical (2).

struc·tur·al·ism (strŭk'choor-ăl-izm). Estruturalismo; ramo da psicologia interessado na estrutura básica e nos elementos da consciência.

struc·ture (strŭck'choor). Estrutura. **1.** O arranjo dos detalhes de uma parte; o modo de formação de uma parte. **2.** Tecido ou formação constituídos por partes diferentes, porém relacionadas. **3.** Em química, as conexões específicas dos átomos em determinada molécula. SIN structura. [L. *structura*, de *struo*, pp. *structus*, construir]

accessory s.'s [TA], estruturas acessórias; partes acessórias do órgão ou estrutura principal. SIN accessory organs (1), adnexa, annexa.

accessory visual s.'s [TA], estruturas oculares acessórias; as pálpebras, com cílios e sobrancelhas, aparelho lacrimal, saco conjuntival e músculos extrínsecos do globo ocular. SIN structurae oculi accessoriae [TA], accessory organs of the eye, accessory visual apparatus, adnexa oculi, appendages of eye, organa oculi accessoria.

brusch heap s., entrelaçamento aleatório de fibrilas em material de impressão em gel ou hidrocolóide.

chi s., e. chi; união entre duas moléculas duplas de DNA. VER TAMBÉM chi *sequence*.

cointegrate s., e. co-integrada; uma estrutura do DNA produzida pela fusão de dois replicons, possuindo um deles um transposon.

complementary s.'s, estruturas complementares; estruturas em que uma define a outra, p. ex., os dois filamentos de DNA duplo.

crystal s., e. cristalina; a disposição no espaço e as distâncias interatômicas e ângulos dos átomos nos cristais, geralmente determinada por medidas de difração de raios X.

denture-supporting s.'s, estruturas de sustentação da dentadura; os tecidos, dentes e/ou cristas residuais que servem como base para dentaduras removíveis parciais ou completas.

fine s., ultra-estrutura. SIN ultrastructure.

gel s., e. gel; estrutura entrelaçada de fibrilas, conferindo firmeza a hidrocolóides.

Holliday s., junção de Holliday. SIN Holliday *junction*.

primary s., e. primária; uma macromolécula, a seqüência de subunidades que compõem a macromolécula; p. ex., a seqüência de aminoácidos numa proteína.

quaternary s., e. quaternária; o arranjo e a constituição tridimensionais de uma macromolécula multimérica (isto é, substância contendo mais de um biopolímero), p. ex., o tetrâmero $\alpha_2\beta_2$ da hemoglobina A.

secondary s., e. secundária; o arranjo localizado no espaço de regiões de um biopolímero; com freqüência, esses tipos de estruturas são regulares e repetem-se ao longo de uma dimensão; p. ex., a hélice α freqüentemente encontrada em proteínas.

tertiary s., e. terciária; a configuração tridimensional de um biopolímero.

tuboreticular s., e. tuborreticular; túbulos de 20–30 nm de comprimento que se localizam no interior das cisternas do retículo endoplasmático liso; observados em doenças do tecido conjuntivo, como o LES, e em vários cânceres e infecções virais.

stru·ma, pl. **stru·mae** (stroo'mă, -mē). Estruma. **1.** Bócio. SIN goiter. **2.** Antigamente, termo utilizado para indicar qualquer aumento de um tecido. [L. tumor escrofuloso, de *struo*, empilhar, construir]

s. aberra'ta, bócio aberrante. SIN aberrant *goiter*.

s. colloi'des, bócio colóide. SIN colloid *goiter*.

Hashimoto s., tireoidite de Hashimoto. SIN Hashimoto *thyroiditis*.

ligneous s., tireoidite de Riedel. SIN Riedel *thyroiditis*.

s. lymphomato'sa, tireoidite de Hashimoto. SIN Hashimoto *thyroiditis*.

s. malig'na, termo obsoleto para câncer da glândula tireóide.

s. medicamento'sa, bócio produzido pelo uso de algum agente terapêutico.

s. ova'rii, tumor ovariano raro, considerado teratomatoso, em que o tecido tireóideo excedeu os outros elementos; ocasionalmente associado ao hipertireoidismo.

Riedel s., tireoidite de Riedel. SIN Riedel *thyroiditis*.

stru·mi·form (stroo'mi-fōrm). Semelhante a um bócio. [struma + L. *forma*, forma]

stru·mi·tis (stroo-mī'tis). Inflamação, com edema, da glândula tireóide. VER TAMBÉM thyroiditis. [struma + G. *-itis*, inflamação]

stru·mous (stroo'mŭs). Estrumoso; relativo a, ou caracterizado por, estruma.

Strümpell, Ernst Adolf von, médico alemão, 1853–1925. VER S. *disease, phenomenon, reflex*; Fleischer-Strümpell *ring*; S.-Marie *disease*; Marie-S. *disease*.

Strutt, VER Rayleigh.

stru·vite (stroo'vīt). Estruvita; o hexaidrato de fosfato de magnésio e amônio; encontrado em alguns cálculos renais. Cf. bobierrite, newberyite. [H.C.G. von Struve, diplomata russo + *-ite*]

strych·nine (strik'nin, -nēn, -nīn) Estricnina; alcalóide de *Strychnos nux-vomica*; cristais incolores de sabor intensamente amargo, quase insolúveis em água. Estimula todas as partes do sistema nervoso central e era utilizada como estomáquico, como antídoto para venenos depressores e no tratamento da miocardite. A estricnina bloqueia o neurotransmissor inibitório glicina e, por conseguinte, pode causar convulsões. Os sais de estricnina utilizados antigamente eram o cloridrato de estricnina, o fosfato de estricnina e o sulfato de estricnina. Trata-se de uma substância química potente, capaz de provocar envenenamento agudo ou crônico em seres humanos ou animais.

strych·nin·ism (strik'nin-izm). Estricninismo; envenenamento crônico pela estricnina, cujos sintomas decorrem da estimulação do sistema nervoso central; os primeiros sinais consistem em tremores e contrações, progredindo para convulsões graves e parada respiratória.

Strych·nos (strik'nos). Gênero de arbustos ou árvores tropicais (família Loganiaceae); a maioria das espécies da América do Sul contém principalmente alcalóides bloqueadores neuromusculares quaternários, p. ex., curare; as espécies africanas, asiáticas e australianas contêm alcalóides terciários semelhantes à estricnina (p. ex., alcalóides do tipo estricnina, brucina e yoimbina). [G. erva-moura]

Stryker, Garold V., patologista norte-americano, *1896. VER S.-Halbeisen *syndrome*.

Stryker, Homer H., cirurgião ortopédico norte-americano. VER S. *frame, saw*.

STSs Abreviatura de sequence-tagged *sites* (locais marcados por seqüências), em *site*.

Stuart. Sobrenome do paciente no qual foi descoberto pela primeira vez o fator de Stuart (S. *factor*) ou Stuart-Prower (Stuart-Prower *factor*).

Stu·dent. Pseudônimo de William Sealy Gosset, estatístico e químico inglês, 1876–1937. VER Student's *t test*.

study (stŭd'ē). Estudo; pesquisa, exame detalhado e/ou análise de um organismo, objeto ou fenômeno. [L. *studium*, estudo, pesquisa]

analytic s., e. analítico; em epidemiologia, estudo destinado a examinar associações, geralmente relações supostas ou causais hipotéticas; em geral, tem por objetivo identificar ou medir os efeitos dos fatores de risco ou os efeitos de exposições específicas sobre a saúde.

blind s., e. cego, e. com incógnita; estudo em que o investigador não sabe quais os grupos submetidos a determinados procedimentos.

case control s., e. de controle de casos; método epidemiológico que começa pela identificação de indivíduos com a doença ou condição que se pretende estudar (os casos) e que compara a sua história pregressa de exposição a fatores de risco identificados ou suspeitos com a história pregressa de exposições semelhantes entre indivíduos que se assemelham aos casos, mas que não têm a doença ou condição em questão (os controles).

cohort s., e. de coortes; estudo que utiliza métodos epidemiológicos, como um estudo clínico, em que uma coorte com determinado atributo (p. ex., fumantes, receptores de uma droga) é acompanhada prospectivamente e comparada quanto à algum resultado (p. ex., doença, cura) com outra coorte que não possui o atributo. SIN follow-up s. (1).

cross-over s., e. cruzado; estudo em que o indivíduo submetido a um procedimento experimental é transferido para o procedimento de controle (ou vice-versa).

cross-sectional s., e. transversal, e. sincrônico; estudo em que grupos de indivíduos de diferentes tipos são reunidos numa grande amostra e estudados apenas em determinado momento no tempo (p. ex., levantamento em que todos os membros de uma determinada população, independentemente da idade, religião, sexo ou localização geográfica, são reunidos para uma determinada característica ou achado num dia específico). SIN synchronic s.

diachronic s., e. longitudinal. SIN longitudinal s.

double blind s., e. duplo-cego, e. com dupla incógnita; estudo em que nem os pacientes, nem o investigador ou qualquer outro avaliador dos resultados sabem quais os indivíduos submetidos a determinados procedimentos, ajudando, assim, a garantir que nem a tendenciosidade nem as expectativas influenciarão os resultados.

ecologic s., e. ecológico; estudo epidemiológico em que as unidades de análise consistem em populações ou grupos de pessoas, em vez de indivíduos.

flow-volume loop s.'s, estudos de alça de fluxo–volume; métodos diagnósticos em que as curvas de fluxo–volume inspiratório e expiratório são utilizadas para determinar a localização de uma obstrução na árvore traqueobrônquica.

follow-up s., e. de acompanhamento; **(1)** SIN cohort s; **(2)** estudo em que indivíduos expostos a um risco ou aos quais se ministra um esquema profilático ou terapêutico são observados no decorrer de um período ou a determinados intervalos para estabelecer o resultado da exposição ou do esquema ministrado.

Framingham Heart S., o primeiro grande estudo da epidemiologia da doença cardiovascular nos Estados Unidos, iniciado em Framingham, Massachusetts, em 1948, sob os auspícios do *National Heart Institute* (hoje em dia, *National Heart, Lung and Blood Institute*) e que ainda está em andamento. A princípio, os investigadores do estudo Framingham recrutaram mais de 5.000

indivíduos entre 30 e 60 anos de idade para estudar a evolução da cardiopatia e identificar fatores de risco para o ataque cardíaco. Em 1971, os filhos dos participantes originais do estudo começaram a ser recrutados para uma segunda geração de observações.

O estudo de Framingham teve grande impacto na moderna compreensão da doença cardiovascular e na profilaxia e no tratamento não apenas do infarto do miocárdio, mas também do acidente vascular cerebral. Durante a década de 1960, o tabagismo, os níveis elevados de colesterol, a hipertensão, a obesidade e a falta de exercício físico foram todos estatisticamente confirmados como fatores de risco de infarto do miocárdio. Nos anos subseqüentes, o estudo forneceu informações de inestimável valor sobre os triglicerídeos, LDL-colesterol, prolapso da valva mitral, insuficiência cardíaca, fibrilação atrial, acidente vascular cerebral, diabetes, fatores de risco cardiovasculares em minorias étnicas e papel do estrogênio na prevenção do infarto do miocárdio em mulheres após a menopausa. Após 50 anos, o estudo continua fornecendo novos indícios sobre a causa e a prevenção da cardiopatia e de outras doenças cardiovasculares.

longitudinal s., e. longitudinal; estudo da evolução natural de uma vida ou distúrbio em que uma coorte de indivíduos é observada de forma seriada, durante determinado período de tempo, sem a necessidade de fazer suposições sobre a estabilidade do sistema. SIN diachronic s.
multivariate s.'s, estudos multivariados; uso de técnicas estatísticas para a investigação simultânea da influência de diversas variáveis.
synchronic s., e. sincrônico, e. transversal. SIN cross-sectional s.
stump (stŭmp). Coto. 1. A extremidade de um membro que permanece após amputação. 2. O pedículo que permanece após a remoção do tumor a ele fixado. [I.m. *stumpe*]
stun (stŭn). Atordoar; estupeficar; tornar inconsciente por traumatismo cerebral. [A.S. *stunian*, produzir um ruído alto]
stupe (stoop). Compressa; compressa ou tecido embebido em água quente, geralmente impregnado com terebintina ou outro irritante, aplicada à superfície para produzir contra-irritação. [L. estopa]
stu·por (stoo'per). Estupor, torpor; estado de comprometimento da consciência em que o indivíduo mostra acentuada diminuição de reatividade a estímulos ambientais, podendo ser despertado somente através de estimulação contínua. [L. de *stupeo*, estar inconsciente]
benign s., e. benigno; síndrome torporosa cuja recuperação é a regra, em oposição ao e. maligno. SIN depressive s.
catatonic s., e. catatônico; estupor associado à catatonia.
depressive s., e. depressivo. SIN benign s.
malignant s., e. maligno; condição torporosa cuja recuperação é infreqüente, em oposição ao estupor benigno.
stu·por·ous (stoo'per-ŭs). Estuporoso, torporoso; relativo a, ou caracterizado por, estupor. SIN carotic.
Sturge, William A., médico inglês, 1850–1919. VER S.-Weber *syndrome*, *disease*.
Sturm, Johann C., 1635–1703. VER S. *conoid*, *interval*.
Sturmdorf, Arnold, ginecologista norte-americano, 1861–1934. VER S. *operation*.
stut·ter (stŭt'er). Tartamudear, gaguejar; falar sem fluência; enunciar certas palavras com dificuldade e com freqüentes paradas e repetição da consoante inicial de uma palavra ou sílaba. [freqüentativo de *stut.*, do gótico *stautan*, bater]
stut·ter·ing (stŭt'er-ing). Tartamudez, gagueira; distúrbio da fonação ou articulação que, tipicamente, começa na infância, com intensa ansiedade sobre a eficiência da comunicação oral e caracterizado pela falta de fluência: hesitações, repetições e prolongamentos de sons e sílabas, interjeições, palavras cortadas, circunlocuções e palavras produzidas com excessiva tensão. SIN logospasm (1).
urinary s., t. urinária; interrupção involuntária freqüente que ocorre durante o ato da micção. SIN stammering of the bladder.
sty, stye, pl. **sties, styes** (sti, stīz). Terçol, hordéolo externo. SIN *hordeolum externum*.
meibomian s., t. de Meibomius. SIN *hordeolum internum*.
zeisian s., t. de Zeis; inflamação de uma das glândulas de Zeis.
style (stīl). Estilete. SIN stylet.
sty·let, sty·lette (stī'let, stī-let'). Estilete. 1. Bastão metálico flexível inserido na luz de um cateter flexível para enriquecê-lo e dar-lhe forma durante sua passagem. 2. Sonda delgada. SIN style, stylus (3), stilus. [It. *stilletto*, adaga; dim. do L. *stilus* ou *stylus*, estaca, caneta]
endotracheal s., e. endotraqueal; bastão de metal flexível utilizado para manter a curva desejada de um tubo para sua inserção na traquéia.
sty·li·form (stī'li-fōrm). Estiliforme, estilóide. SIN styloid. [L. *stilus* (*stylus*), estaca + *forma*, forma]
♲ **stylo-**. Estilo-; estilóide (especificamente, o processo estilóide do osso temporal). [G. *stylos*, pilar, poste]
sty·lo·au·ri·cu·la·ris (stī'lō-aw-rik-ū-lā'ris). Estiloauricular. VER styloauricular (*muscle*).

sty·lo·glos·sus (stī'lō-glos'ŭs). Estiloglosso; relativo ao processo estilóide e à língua. VER styloglossus (*muscle*).
sty·lo·hy·al (stī-lō-hī'al). Estilo-hióideo; relativo ao processo estilóide do osso temporal e ao osso hióide. SIN stylohyoid (1).
sty·lo·hy·oid (stī-lō-hī'oyd). Estilo-hióideo. 1. SIN stylohyal. 2. Relativo ao músculo estilo-hióideo.
sty·loid (stī'loyd). Estilóide; em forma de coluna; designa um dos vários processos ósseos delgados. VER styloid *process* of third metacarpal bone, styloid *process* of temporal bone, styloid *process* of radius, styloid *process* of ulna. SIN styliform. [stylo- + G. *eidos*, semelhança]
sty·loi·di·tis (stī-loy-dī'tis). Estiloidite; inflamação de um processo estilóide.
sty·lo·la·ryn·ge·us (stī'lō-lar-in-jē'ŭs). Estilolaríngeo. VER *musculus* stylolaryngeus.
sty·lo·man·dib·u·lar (stī'lō-man-dib'ū-lar). Estilomandibular; relativo ao processo estilóide do osso temporal e da mandíbula; designa o ligamento estilomandibular. SIN stylomaxillary.
sty·lo·mas·toid (stī'lō-mas'toyd). Estilomatóide; relativo aos processos estilóide e mastóide do osso temporal; designa especialmente uma pequena artéria e um forame.
sty·lo·max·il·lary (stī'lō-mak'si-lar-ē). Estilomaxilar. SIN stylomandibular.
sty·lo·pha·ryn·ge·us (stī'lō-far-in-jē'ŭs). Estilofaríngeo. VER stylopharyngeus (*muscle*).
sty·lo·po·di·um (stī-lō-pō'dē-ŭm). Estilopódio; o segmento intermediário proximal do esqueleto do membro, úmero e fêmur, no embrião. [stylo- + G. *podion*, pé pequeno]
sty·lo·staph·y·line (stī-lō-staf'i-līn). Estilostafilina; relativo ao processo estilóide do osso temporal e úvula.
sty·los·te·o·phyte (stī-los'tē-ō-fīt). Estilosteófito; crescimento ósseo em forma de estaca. [G. *stylos*, coluna + *osteon*, osso + *phyton*, crescimento]
sty·lus, sti·lus (stī'lŭs, stī'lŭs). 1. Qualquer estrutura em forma de lápis. 2. Preparação medicinal em forma de lápis para aplicação externa; p. ex., vela de medicamento, lápis ou bastão de nitrato de prata ou outra substância cáustica. 3. Estilete. SIN stylet. [L. *stilus* ou *stylus*, estaca ou caneta]
stype (stīp). Um tampão. [G. *stypē*, estopa]
styp·tic (stip'tik). Estíptico. 1. Que possui efeito adstringente ou hemostático. 2. Agente adstringente utilizado topicamente para interromper o sangramento. SIN hemostyptic. [G. *styptikos*, adstringente]
styr·a·mate (stī'ra-māt). Estiramato; relaxante muscular esquelético efetivo por via oral, com ação de duração relativamente longa.
sty·rax (stī'raks). Estoraque. SIN storax.
sty·rene (stī'rēn). Estireno; feniletileno; o monômero a partir do qual são produzidos poliestirenos, plásticos e borracha sintética; juntamente com o divinilbenzeno (para ligação cruzada), constitui a base de muitos trocadores iônicos sintéticos. SIN cinnamene, ethenylbenzene, styrol, vinylbenzene.
sty·rol (stī'rol). Estirol. SIN styrene.
sty·rone (stī'rōn). Estirona; $C_9H_{10}O$; obtida do estoraque por destilação com hidróxido de potássio; utilizada como desodorante em solução de glicerina a 12% e como agente descolorante em histologia. SIN cinnamic alcohol.
♲ **sub-**. Sub-; sob, menos do que o normal ou típico, inferior. Cf. hypo-. [L. *sub*, sob]
sub·ab·dom·i·nal (sŭb-ab-dom'i-nal). Subabdominal; abaixo do abdome.
sub·ab·dom·i·no·per·i·to·ne·al (sŭb-ab-dom'i-nō-per-i-tō-nē'-al). Subabdominoperitoneal; sob o peritônio abdominal, para distingui-lo do peritônio pélvico. SIN subperitoneoabdominal.
sub·ac·e·tate (sŭb-as'e-tāt). Subacetato; mistura ou complexo de uma base e seu acetato.
sub·a·cro·mi·al (sŭb-ā-krō'mē-al). Subacromial; abaixo do acrômio.
sub·a·cute (sŭb-ā-kūt'). Subagudo; entre agudo e crônico; refere-se à evolução de uma doença de duração ou gravidade moderada.
sub·al·i·men·ta·tion (sŭb'al-i-men-tā'shŭn). Subalimentação; condição de nutrição insuficiente. SIN hypoalimentation.
sub·a·nal (sŭb-ā'nal). Subanal; abaixo do ânus.
sub·a·or·tic (sŭb'ā-ōr'tik). Subaórtico; abaixo da aorta.
sub·ap·i·cal (sŭb-ap'i-kal). Subapical; abaixo do ápice de qualquer parte.
sub·ap·o·neu·rot·ic (sŭb-ap-ō-noo-rot'ik). Subaponeurótico; sob uma aponeurose.
sub·a·rach·noid (sŭb-ā-rak'noyd). Subaracnóide; sob a membrana aracnóide.
sub·ar·cu·ate (sŭb-ar'kū-āt). Subarqueado; um pouco arqueado ou curvo.
sub·a·re·o·lar (sŭb-ā-rē'ō-lar). Subareolar; sob uma aréola, especialmente a aréola da mama.
sub·as·trag·a·lar (sŭb-as-trag'a-lar). Subtalar; sob o calcâneo (tálus).
sub·a·tom·ic (sŭb-ā-tom'ik). Subatômico; relativo a partículas que constituem a estrutura intra-atômica; p. ex., prótons, elétrons, nêutrons.
sub·au·ral (sŭb-aw'ral). Subaural; sob a orelha.
sub·au·ric·u·lar (sŭb-aw-rik'ū-lar). Subauricular; sob a orelha; especialmente a concha ou pavilhão da orelha.
sub·ax·i·al (sŭb-ak'sē-al). Subaxial; sob o eixo do corpo ou de qualquer parte.
sub·ax·il·lary (sŭb-ak'si-lar-ē). Subaxilar; sob a fossa axilar. SIN infraaxillary.

sub·bas·al (sŭb-bā′sǎl). Sub-basal; sob qualquer base ou membrana basal. SIN infraaxillary.

sub·brach·y·ce·phal·ic (sŭb-brak-ē-se-fal′ik). Sub-braquicefálico; um pouco braquicefálico, que possui índice cefálico de 80,01–83,33.

sub·cal·ca·rine (sŭb-kal′ka-rīn). Subcalcarino; abaixo da fissura calcarina; designa o giro lingual.

sub·cal·lo·sal (sŭb-ka-lō′sǎl). Abaixo do corpo caloso; designa o giro ou fascículo subcaloso.

sub·cap·su·lar (sŭb-kap′soo-lǎr). Subcapsular; sob qualquer cápsula.

sub·car·bon·ate (sŭb-kar′bon-āt). Subcarbonato; mistura ou complexo de uma base e seu carbonato.

sub·car·di·nal (sŭb-kar′di-nǎl). Subcardinal; situado ventralmente às veias cardinais anterior ou posterior no embrião.

sub·car·ti·lag·i·nous (sŭb′kar-ti-laj′i-nŭs). Subcartilaginoso. 1. Parcialmente cartilaginoso. 2. Sob uma cartilagem.

sub·ce·cal (sŭb-sē′kǎl). Subcecal; sob o ceco; designa uma fossa.

sub·cel·lu·lar (sŭb-sel′ū-lǎr). Subcelular. SIN noncellular (1).

sub·cep·tion (sŭb-sep′shŭn). Subcepção; percepção subliminal, como a reação a um estímulo não totalmente percebido. VER subliminal. [sub- + L. -ceptum, percebido]

sub·chlo·ride (sŭb-klōr′īd). Subcloreto; o cloreto de uma série que contém proporcionalmente a maior quantidade do outro elemento no composto; p. ex., o subcloreto de mercúrio é Hg_2Cl_2, enquanto o cloreto ou percloreto de mercúrio é $HgCl_2$.

sub·chon·dral (sŭb-kon′drǎl). Subcondral; sob ou abaixo das cartilagens das costelas.

sub·cho·ri·on·ic (sŭb′kō-rē-on′ik). Subcoriônico; sob o cório.

sub·cho·roi·dal (sŭb-kō-roy′dǎl). Subcorioidal; sob a túnica corióide do olho.

sub·class (sŭb′klas). Subclasse; na classificação biológica, uma divisão entre classe e ordem.

sub·cla·vi·an (sŭb-klā′vē-an). Subclávio. 1. Sob a clavícula. SIN infraclavicular. 2. Relativo à artéria ou veia subclávia.

sub·cla·vic·u·lar (sŭb-kla-vik′ū-lǎr). Subclavicular; relativo à região sob a clavícula.

sub·cla·vi·us (sŭb-klā′vē-ŭs). Subclávio. VER subclavius (muscle).

sub·clin·i·cal (sŭb-klin′i-kǎl). Subclínico; designa uma doença sem sintomas manifestos; pode representar um estágio inicial na evolução de uma doença.

sub·clon·ing (sŭb′klōn-ing). Subclonagem; processo pelo qual um clone de DNA é clivado em partes menores e reclonado; a análise das regiões superpostas desses fragmentos menores de DNA pode confirmar toda a seqüência do clone de DNA original.

sub·col·lat·er·al (sŭb-kō-lat′er-ǎl). Subcolateral; sob a fissura colateral; designa uma convolução ou giro cerebral.

sub·con·junc·ti·val (sŭb-kon-jŭnk-tī′vǎl). Subconjuntival; sob a conjuntiva.

sub·con·junc·ti·vi·tis (sŭb′kon-jŭnk-ti-vī′tis). Subconjuntivite. SIN episcleritis periodica fugax.

sub·con·scious (sŭb-kon′shŭs). Subconsciente. 1. Não totalmente consciente. 2. Designa uma idéia ou impressão que está presente na mente, mas da qual não há, no momento, conhecimento ou percepção consciente. 3. A parte da mente que está fora da percepção consciente.

sub·con·scious·ness (sŭb-kon′shŭs-nes). Subconsciência. 1. Inconsciência parcial. 2. O estado em que os processos mentais ocorrem sem a percepção consciente do indivíduo.

sub·cor·a·coid (sŭb-kōr′a-koyd). Subcoracóide; sob o processo coracóide.

sub·cor·tex (sŭb-kōr′teks). Subcórtex; qualquer parte do cérebro situada abaixo do córtex cerebral e não organizada como córtex.

sub·cor·ti·cal (sŭb-kōr′ti-kǎl). Subcortical; relativo ao subcórtex; sob o córtex cerebral.

sub·cos·tal (sŭb-kos′tǎl). Subcostal. 1. Sob uma costela ou costelas. SIN infracostal. 2. Designa certas artérias, veias e nervos.

sub·cos·tal·gia (sŭb-kos-tal′jē-ǎ). Subcostalgia; dor na região subcostal. [subcostal + G. algos, dor]

sub·cos·to·ster·nal (sŭb-kos′tō-ster′nǎl). Subcostoesternal; sob ou abaixo das costelas e do esterno.

sub·cra·ni·al (sŭb-krā′nē-ǎl). Subcraniano; sob ou abaixo do crânio.

sub·crep·i·tant (sŭb-krep′i-tǎnt). Subcrepitante; quase, mas não francamente, crepitante; designa um estertor.

sub·crep·i·ta·tion (sŭb′krep-i-tā′shŭn). Subcrepitação. 1. Presença de estertores subcrepitantes. 2. Som de caráter próximo ao da crepitação.

sub·cru·ra·lis (sŭb-kroo-rā′lis). Músculo articular do joelho. SIN articularis genus (muscle).

sub·cru·re·us (sŭb-kroo-rē-ŭs). Músculo articular do joelho. SIN articularis genus (muscle). [sub- + L. crus, perna]

sub·cul·ture (sŭb-kŭl′choor). Subcultura. 1. Cultura efetuada mediante transferência de uma cultura prévia para um meio fresco de microrganismos; método utilizado para prolongar a vida de determinada cepa, em que existe uma tendência à degeneração em culturas mais antigas. 2. Efetuar uma cultura fresca com material obtido de uma anterior.

sub·cu·ra·tive (sŭb-kūr′a-tiv). Subcurativo; designa uma dose menor do que a necessária para obter um efeito curativo.

sub·cu·ta·ne·ous (sc., SQ) (sŭb-koo-tā′nē-ŭs). Subcutâneo; sob a pele. SIN hypodermic (1). [sub- + L. cutis, pele]

sub·cu·tic·u·lar (sŭb-koo-tik′ū-lǎr). Subcuticular; abaixo da cutícula ou epiderme. SIN subepidermal, subepidermic.

sub·cu·tis (sŭb-kū′tis). Tecido subcutâneo. SIN subcutaneous tissue.

sub·de·lir·i·um (sŭb-dē-lir′ē-ŭm). Termo raramente utilizado para descrever um delírio leve ou descontínuo.

sub·del·toid (sŭb-del′toyd). Subdeltóide; sob o músculo deltóide; designa uma bolsa.

sub·den·tal (sŭb-den′tǎl). Subdentário; sob as raízes dos dentes.

sub·di·a·phrag·mat·ic (sŭb′dī-ǎ-frag-mat′ik). Subdiafragmático; sob o diafragma. SIN infradiaphragmatic, subphrenic.

sub·dor·sal (sŭb-dōr′sǎl). Subdorsal; abaixo da região dorsal.

sub·duce, sub·duct (sŭb-doos′, sŭb-dŭkt′). Impelir ou empurrar para baixo. [L. sub-duco, pp. -ductus, levar]

sub·du·ral (sŭb-doo′rǎl). Subdural; sob a dura-máter ou entre ela e a aracnóide-máter. VER spatium, subdurale.

sub·en·do·car·di·al (sŭb-en-dō-kar′dē-ǎl). Subendocárdico. Sob o endocárdio.

sub·en·do·the·li·al (sŭb-en-dō-thē′lē-ǎl). Subendotelial; sob o endotélio.

sub·en·do·the·li·um (sŭb′en-dō-thē′lē-ŭm). Subendotélio; o tecido conjuntivo entre o endotélio e a membrana elástica interna na íntima das artérias.

sub·en·dy·mal (sŭb-en′di-mǎl). Subendimário, subependimário; sob o êndima ou epêndima. SIN subependymal.

sub·ep·en·dy·mal (sŭb-ep-en′di-mal). Subependimário. SIN subendymal.

sub·ep·en·dy·mo·ma (sŭb-ep-en-di-mō′ma). Subependimoma; nódulos ependimários lobulados distintos nas paredes do terceiro ventrículo anterior ou quarto ventrículo posterior, comumente encontrados na necropsia.

sub·ep·i·der·mal, sub·ep·i·der·mic (sŭb′ep-i-der′mǎl, -der′mik). Subepidérmico. SIN subcuticular.

sub·ep·i·the·li·al (sŭb′ep-i-thē′lē-ǎl). Subepitelial; sob o epitélio.

sub·ep·i·the·li·um (sŭb′ep-i-thē′lē-ŭm). Subepitélio; qualquer estrutura sob o epitélio.

sub·e·ric ac·id (soo-ber′ik). Ácido subérico; utilizado em plásticos e na ligação cruzada de biopolímeros; encontrado na urina como produto da ω oxidação de ácidos graxos. SIN octandioic acid. [L. suber, sobreiro + -ic]

su·ber·o·sis (soo-ber-ō′sis). Suberose; alveolite alérgica extrínseca causada pela inalação de esporos de fungos da cortiça contaminada. [L. suber, cortiça + G. -osis, condição]

sub·fam·i·ly (sŭb-fam′i-lē). Subfamília; na classificação biológica, uma divisão entre família e tribo ou entre família e gênero.

sub·fas·cial (sŭb-fash′ē-ǎl). Subfascial; sob uma fáscia.

sub·fer·til·i·ty (sŭb-fer-til′i-tē). Subfertilidade; capacidade de reprodução inferior ao normal.

sub·fis·sure (sŭb-fish′er). Subfissura; uma fissura cerebral sob a superfície, oculta por convoluções superpostas.

sub·fo·li·um (sŭb-fō′lē-ŭm). Subfólio; divisão secundária de uma folha do cerebelo.

sub·gal·late (sŭb-gal′āt). Subgalato; ácido gálico parcialmente neutralizado; galato básico, como o subgalato de bismuto.

sub·gem·mal (sŭb-jem′ǎl). Sob uma gema ou botão (p. ex., botão gustativo).

sub·ge·nus (sŭb-jē′nŭs). Subgênero; na classificação biológica, divisão entre gênero e espécie.

sub·gin·gi·val (sŭb-jin′ji-vǎl). Subgengival; sob a margem gengival.

sub·gle·noid (sŭb-glē′noyd) Subglenóide. SIN infraglenoid.

sub·glos·sal (sŭb-glos′ǎl). Subglosso; sob ou abaixo da língua. SIN sublingual.

sub·glot·tic (sŭb-glot′ik). Subglótico. SIN infraglottic.

sub·gran·u·lar (sŭb-gran′oo-lǎr). Subgranular; um pouco granular.

sub·grun·da·tion (sŭb-grŭn-dā′shŭn). A depressão de um fragmento de osso craniano fraturado abaixo do outro. [sub- + A.S. grund, fundo, fundação]

sub·he·pat·ic (sŭb-he-pat′ik). Sub-hepático; abaixo do fígado. SIN infrahepatic.

sub·hy·a·loid (sŭb-hī′ǎ-loyd). Sub-hialóide; sob, no lado vítreo, a membrana hialóide (vítrea).

sub·hy·oid, sub·hy·oid·e·an (sŭb-hī′oyd, sŭb-hī-oyd′ē-an). Sub-hióide. SIN infrahyoid.

sub·ic·ter·ic (sŭb-ik′ter-ik). Subictérico; níveis séricos ligeiramente elevados de bilirrubina, sem evidências clínicas de icterícia. [sub- + G. ikterikos, amarelado]

su·bic·u·lar (soo-bik′ū-lǎr, sŭ-bik′). Subicular; relativo ao subículo.

su·bic·u·lum, pl. **su·bic·u·la** (soo-bik′ū-lŭm, sŭ-bik′; -lǎ) [TA]. Subículo. 1. Um suporte. 2. [TA]. A zona de transição entre o giro para-hipocampal e o corno de Ammon do hipocampo. [L. dim. de subex, suporte]

s. promonto'rii [TA], s. do promontório; suporte do promontório; crista óssea que se liga à fóssula das janelas cocleares, posteriormente. SIN ponticulus promontorii.

sub·il·i·ac (sūb-il'ē-ak). Subilíaco. **1.** Abaixo do ílio. **2.** Relativo ao subílio.

sub·il·i·um (sūb-il'ē-ŭm). Subílio; parte do ílio que contribui para o acetábulo.

sub·in·fec·tion (sŭb-in-fek'shŭn). Subinfecção; infecção secundária que ocorre num indivíduo exposto a uma epidemia de outra doença infecciosa e à qual resiste com sucesso.

sub·in·flam·ma·to·ry (sŭb-in-flam'ă-tō-rē). Subinflamatório. designa irritação discretamente inflamatória dos tecidos.

sub·in·ti·mal (sŭb-in'ti-măl). Subíntimo; sob a íntima.

sub·in·trant (sŭb-in'trant). Subintrante, intermitente, recorrente. SIN proleptic. [L. *sub-intro*, pres. p. *-ans*, entrar furtivamente]

sub·in·vo·lu·tion (sŭb-in-vō-loo'shŭn). Subinvolução; parada da involução normal do útero após o parto, em que o órgão permanece anormalmente grande.

sub·i·o·dide (sŭb-ī'ō-dīd). Subiodeto; aquele de uma série de compostos do iodo com determinado cátion contendo o iodo em sua menor valência; análogo ao subcloreto.

sub·ja·cent (sŭb-jā'sent). Subjacente; sob ou abaixo de outra parte. [L. *subjaceo*, situado sob]

sub·ject (sŭb'jekt). Indivíduo ou organismo objeto de pesquisa, tratamento, experimentação ou dissecção. [L. *subjectus*, situado sob]

sub·jec·tive (sŭb-jek'tiv). Subjetivo. **1.** Percebido apenas pelo indivíduo e não evidente ao examinador; diz-se de determinados sintomas, como a dor. **2.** Modificado pelas crenças e atitudes pessoais do indivíduo. Cf. objective (2). [L. *subjectivus*, de *subjicio*, lançar sob]

sub·jec·tive as·sess·ment da·ta. Dados de avaliação subjetivos; fatos apresentados pelo cliente que revela sua percepção, compreensão e interpretação do que está ocorrendo.

sub·ju·gal (sŭb-joo'găl). Subjugal; sob o osso zigomático (jugal).

sub·king·dom (sŭb-king'dom). Sub-reino; na classificação biológica, uma divisão entre reino e filo.

sub·la·tion (sŭb-lā'shŭn). Descolamento, elevação e remoção de uma parte. [L. *sublatio*, levantamento]

sub·le·thal (sŭb-lē'thăl). Subletal; não totalmente letal.

sub·leu·ke·mia (sŭb-loo-kē'mē-ă). Subleucemia. SIN subleukemic *leukemia*.

sub·li·mate (sŭb'lim-āt). **1.** Sublimar; realizar uma sublimação. **2.** Sublimado, qualquer substância que foi submetida a sublimação. [L. *sublimo*, pp. *-atus*, elevar no alto, de *sublimis*, alto]

corrosive s., s. corrosivo (HgCl₂). SIN mercuric chloride.

sub·li·ma·tion (sŭb-lim-ā'shŭn). Sublimação. **1.** O processo de converter um sólido em gás sem passar pelo estado líquido; análogo à destilação. **2.** Em psicanálise, um mecanismo de defesa inconsciente em que impulsos e desejos instintivos inaceitáveis são modificados em canais mais aceitáveis ao nível pessoal e social.

sub·lime (sŭb-līm'). **1.** Sublimar. **2.** Sofrer um processo de sublimação.

sub·lim·i·nal (sŭb-lim'i-năl). Subliminal, subliminar; abaixo do limiar da percepção ou excitação; abaixo do limite ou limiar da consciência. [sub- + L. *limen* (*limin*-), limiar]

sub·li·mis (sŭb-lī'mis). **1.** Sublime; no ápice. **2.** Superficial. SIN superficialis. [L.]

sub·lin·gual (sŭb-ling'gwăl). Sublingual. SIN subglossal.

sub·lob·u·lar (sŭb-lob'ū-lăr). Sublobular; sob um lóbulo, como o do fígado.

sub·lum·bar (sŭb-lŭm'băr). Sublombar; abaixo da região lombar.

sub·lu·mi·nal (sŭb-loo'mi-năl). Subluminal; sob ou abaixo da estrutura voltada para a luz de um órgão.

sub·lux·a·tion (sŭb-lŭk-sā'shŭn). Subluxação; luxação incompleta; embora haja alteração de uma relação, o contato entre as superfícies articulares permanece. SIN semiluxation. [sub- + L. *locatio*, luxação]

arytenoid s., subluxação aritenóidea. SIN arytenoid *dislocation*.

sub·lym·phe·mia (sŭb-lim-fē'mē-ă). Termo obsoleto para um estado do sangue caracterizado por acentuado aumento na proporção de linfócitos, embora o número total de leucócitos esteja normal. [sub- + L. *lympha*, linfa + G. *haima*, sangue]

sub·mam·ma·ry (sŭb-mam'ă-rē). Submamário. **1.** Localizado profundamente em relação à glândula mamária. **2.** SIN inframammary.

sub·man·dib·u·lar (sŭb-man-dib'ū-lăr). Submandibular; sob a mandíbula. SIN inframandibular, submaxillary (2).

sub·mar·gin·al (sŭb-mar'ji-năl). Submarginal; próximo à margem de qualquer parte.

sub·max·il·la (sŭb-mak-sil'ă). Mandíbula. SIN mandible.

sub·max·il·lary (sŭb-mak'si-lār-ē). **1.** Mandibular. SIN mandibular. **2.** Submandibular. SIN submandibular.

sub·me·di·al, sub·me·di·an (sŭb-mē'dē-ăl, sŭb-mē'dē-an). Submedial, submediano; quase, mas não exatamente, no meio.

sub·mem·bra·nous (sŭb-mem'bră-nŭs). Submembranoso; parcialmente ou quase membranoso.

sub·men·tal (sŭb-men'tăl). Submental, submentual; sob o queixo.

sub·merged (sŭb-merjd'). Submergido, submerso; em odontologia, descreve um campo de operação coberto por saliva.

sub·met·a·cen·tric (sŭb'met-ă-sen'trik). Submetacêntrico. VER submetacentric *chromosome*.

sub·mi·cron·ic (sŭb-mī-kron'ik). Submicrônico; menor do que 1 mícron.

sub·mi·cro·scop·ic (sŭb'mī-krō-skop'ik). Submicroscópico; demasiado pequeno para ser visível ao microscópio óptico. SIN amicroscopic, ultramicroscopic.

sub·mor·phous (sŭb-mōr'fŭs). Submorfo; nem definidamente amorfo nem definidamente cristalino, referindo-se à estrutura de determinados cálculos.

sub·mu·co·sa (sŭb-moo-kō'să). Submucosa, tela submucosa; uma camada de tecido sob uma mucosa; a camada de tecido conjuntivo sob a túnica mucosa. SIN tela submucosa, tunica submucosa.

sub·mu·cous (sŭb-moo'kŭs). Submucoso; sob uma mucosa.

sub·nar·co·tic (sŭb-nar-kot'ik). Subnarcótico; um pouco narcótico.

sub·na·sal (sŭb-nā'săl). Subnasal; sob o nariz.

sub·na·si·on (sŭb-nā'zē-on). Subnásio; o ponto do ângulo entre o septo do nariz e a superfície do lábio superior.

sub·neu·ral (sŭb-noo'răl). Subneural; abaixo do eixo neural.

sub·ni·trate (sŭb-nī'trāt). Subnitrato; um nitrato básico; um sal do ácido nítrico que possui um ou mais átomos da base ainda capaz de se combinar com o ácido.

sub·nor·mal (sŭb-nōr'măl). Subnormal; abaixo do padrão normal de determinada qualidade.

sub·nor·mal·i·ty (sŭb-nōr-mal'i-tē). Subnormalidade; estado ou condição subnormal.

sub·no·to·chor·dal. Subnotocordal; situado sob a notocorda.

sub·nu·cle·us (sŭb-noo'klē-ŭs). Subnúcleo; núcleo secundário.

sub·oc·cip·i·tal (sŭb-ok-sip'i-tăl). Suboccipital; abaixo do occipúcio ou do osso occipital.

sub·op·ti·mal (sŭb-op'ti-măl). Subótimo; abaixo ou menor do que o ótimo.

sub·or·bit·al (sŭb-ōr'bi-tăl). Suborbitário, suborbital, infra-orbital. SIN infraorbital.

sub·or·der (sŭb-ōr'der). Subordem; na classificação biológica, uma divisão entre ordem e família.

sub·ox·i·da·tion (sŭb'oks-i-dā'shŭn). Suboxidação; oxidação deficiente.

sub·ox·ide (sŭb-ok'sīd). Subóxido; aquele de uma série de óxidos que contém o menos oxigênio. SIN protoxide.

sub·pa·ri·e·tal (sŭb-pa-rī'ē-tăl). Subparietal; sob ou abaixo de qualquer estrutura denominada parietal: osso, lobo, camada de uma membrana serosa, etc.

sub·pa·tel·lar (sŭb-pa-tel'ăr). Subpatelar. **1.** Profundamente à patela. **2.** SIN infrapatellar.

sub·pec·to·ral (sŭb-pek'tō-răl). Subpeitoral; sob o músculo peitoral.

sub·pel·vi·per·i·to·ne·al (sŭb-pel'vi-per-i-tō-nē'ăl). Subpelviperitoneal; sob o peritônio pélvico, distinto do abdominal. SIN subperitoneopelvic.

sub·per·i·car·di·al (sŭb-per-i-kar'dē-ăl). Subpericárdico; sob o pericárdio.

sub·per·i·os·te·al (sŭb-per-ē-os'tē-ăl). Subperiósteo; sob o periósteo.

sub·per·i·to·ne·al (sŭb-per-i-tō-nē'ăl). Subperitoneal; sob o peritônio.

sub·per·i·to·ne·o·ab·dom·i·nal (sŭb-per-i-tō-nē'ō-ab-dom'i-năl). Subperitoneoabdominal. SIN subabdominoperitoneal.

sub·per·i·to·ne·o·pel·vic (sŭb-per-i-tō-nē'ō-pel'vik). Subperitoneopélvico. SIN subpelviperitoneal.

sub·pe·tro·sal (sŭb-pe-trō'săl). Subpetroso. **1.** Designa o petroso inferior. **2.** Designa um seio venoso dural.

sub·pha·ryn·ge·al (sŭb-fă-rin'jē-ăl). Subfaríngeo; abaixo da faringe.

sub·phren·ic (sŭb-fren'ik). Subfrênico. SIN subdiaphragmatic.

sub·phy·lum (sŭb-fī'lŭm). Subfilo; na classificação biológica, uma divisão entre filo e classe.

sub·pi·al (sŭb-pī'ăl). Subpial; sob a pia-máter.

sub·pla·cen·tal (sŭb-pla-sen'tăl). Subplacentário; sob a placenta; designa a decídua basal.

sub·pleu·ral (sŭb-plu'răl). Subpleural; sob a pleura.

sub·plex·al (sŭb-plek'săl). Sob ou abaixo de qualquer plexo.

sub·pre·pu·tial (sŭb-prē-pū'shē-ăl). Subprepucial; sob o prepúcio.

sub·pu·bic (sŭb-pū'bik). Subpúbico; sob o arco púbico; designa um ligamento, o ligamento arqueado do púbis, que conecta os dois ossos púbicos abaixo do arco.

sub·pul·mo·nary (sŭb-pŭl'mō-nār-ē) Subpulmonar; abaixo dos pulmões.

sub·py·ram·i·dal (sŭb-pi-ram'i-dăl). Subpiramidal. **1.** Abaixo de qualquer pirâmide, refere-se especialmente ao seio do tímpano. **2.** De forma piramidal.

sub·ret·i·nal (sŭb-ret'i-năl). Sub-retiniano. **1.** Entre a retina sensorial e o epitélio pigmentar da retina. **2.** Entre o epitélio pigmentar da retina e a coróide.

sub·salt (sŭb-salt). Sal básico; sal em que a base não foi completamente neutralizada pelo ácido.

sub·sar·to·ri·al (sŭb-sar-tō'rē-ăl). Subsartorial; sob o músculo sartório; refere-se a um plexo nervoso e fáscia.

sub·scap·u·lar (sŭb-skap'ŭ-lăr). Subescapular. **1.** Profundamente à escápula. **2.** SIN infrascapular.
sub·scap·u·la·ris (sŭb-skap-ū-lā'ris). Subescapular. VER subscapularis (*muscle*).
sub·scle·ral (sŭb-sklē'răl). Subescleral; sob a esclera do olho, isto é, sobre o lado corioidal dessa camada. SIN subsclerotic (1).
sub·scle·rot·ic (sŭb-skle-rot'ik). Subesclerótico. **1.** SIN subsclera. **2.** Parcial ou pouco esclerótico ou esclerosado.
sub·scrip·tion (sŭb-skrip'shŭn). A parte de uma receita que precede a assinatura, na qual estão as orientações sobre a composição. [L. *subscriptio*, de *subscribo*, pp. *-scriptus*, escrever sob, subscrever]
sub·ser·osa [TA]. Subserosa, tela subserosa; a camada de tecido conjuntivo sob uma serosa, como a do peritônio ou pericárdio. SIN tela subserosa [TA], subserous layer*.
sub·se·rous, sub·se·ro·sal (sŭb-sē'rŭs, sŭb-se-rō'săl). Subseroso; sob uma serosa.
sub·sib·i·lant (sŭb-sib'i-lănt). Termo raramente utilizado que designa um estertor com uma qualidade entre o sopro e o sibilo.
sub·si·dence (sŭb-sī'dens). Afundamento; depressão ou assentamento no osso, como no caso de um componente de prótese de um implante articular total.
sub·spi·na·le (sŭb-spi-nā'lē). Subespinal; em cefalometria, o ponto mais posterior da linha média sobre a pré-maxila, entre a espinha nasal anterior e o próstio. SIN point A.
sub·spi·nous (sŭb-spī'nŭs). Subespinhoso. **1.** SIN infraspinous. **2.** Tendência a espinhosidade.
sub·stage (sŭb'stāj). Subplatina; fixação a um microscópio, abaixo da platina, que sustenta o condensador ou outro acessório.
sub·stance (sŭb'stans). Substância; matéria; material. SIN substantia [TA], matter. [L. *substantia*, essência, material, de *sub-sto*, ficar embaixo, estar presente]
alpha s., s. reticular. SIN reticular s. (1).
anterior perforated s. [TA], s. perfurada anterior; uma região na base do cérebro através da qual numerosos e pequenos ramos das artérias cerebrais anterior e média (artérias lenticuloestriadas) penetram profundamente no hemisfério cerebral; é ladeada medialmente pelo quiasma óptico e pela metade anterior do trato óptico, rostral e lateralmente pelas estrias olfatórias laterais; sua parte ântero-medial corresponde ao tubérculo olfatório. SIN substantia perforata anterior [TA], locus perforatus anticus, olfactory area, substantia perforata rostralis.
autacoid s., s. autacóide. SIN autacoid.
bacteriotropic s., s. bacteriotrópica; opsonina ou outra substância que altera as células bacterianas de tal forma que elas se tornam mais suscetíveis à ação fagocítica.
basophil s., s. basófila. SIN Nissl s.
basophilic s., s. basofílica. SIN Nissl s.
blood group s., antígeno de grupo sanguíneo. SIN blood group antigen.
blood group-specific s.'s A and B, substâncias A e B específicas de grupo sanguíneo; solução de complexos de polissacarídeos e aminoácidos que reduz o título de isoaglutininas anti-A e anti-B no soro de indivíduos do grupo O; utilizadas para tornar o sangue de grupo O razoavelmente seguro para transfusão em indivíduos de grupo A, B ou AB, mas que não afeta qualquer incompatibilidade decorrente de vários outros fatores, como o fator Rh.
cementing s., s. de cementação; depósito de matriz mineralizada amorfa circundando os ósteons do osso compacto.
central gray s., s. cinzenta central; **(1)** em geral: a substância cinzenta constituída predominantemente de pequenas células, adjacente a ou circundando o canal central da medula espinal e o terceiro e quarto ventrículos do tronco cerebral; **(2)** em particular: a espessa manga de substância cinzenta que circunda o aqueduto do mesencéfalo, continuando-se em direção rostral, com o núcleo posterior do hipotálamo; em cortes corados para mielina, destaca-se do teto e do tegmento adjacentes pela escassez de suas fibras mielinizadas. SIN substantia grisea centralis [TA], periaqueductal gray s.
central and lateral intermediate s.'s, s. intermédia central e lateral; a substância cinzenta central da medula espinal que circunda o canal central. SIN anterior gray column, Stilling gelatinous s., substantia gelatinosa centralis.
chromidial s., retículo endoplasmático granular. SIN granular endoplasmic reticulum.
chromophil s., s. cromófila. SIN Nissl s.
compact s., s. compacta. SIN compact bone.
controlled s., s. controlada; substância sujeita ao *Controlled Substances Act* (1970), que regula a prescrição e a dispensação, bem como a fabricação, o armazenamento, a venda ou a distribuição de substâncias classificadas em cinco classes, de acordo com 1) seu potencial ou evidência de abuso, 2) potencial de dependência psíquica ou fisiológica, 3) contribuição para um risco de saúde pública, 4) efeito farmacológico prejudicial ou 5) seu papel como precursor de outras substâncias controladas.
cortical s., s. cortical. SIN cortical bone.
exophthalmos-producing s. (EPS), s. produtora de exoftalmia; fator encontrado em extratos não-purificados de tecido hipofisário que produz exoftalmia em animais de laboratório (especialmente peixes). Sua existência e o seu papel na produção da exoftalmia na doença de Graves (Graves *disease*) são questionados.
filar s., s. reticular. SIN reticular s. (1).
gelatinous s. [TA], s. gelatinosa; a parte apical do corno posterior (corno dorsal; coluna cinzenta posterior) da substância cinzenta da medula espinal, composta, em grande parte, de células nervosas muito pequenas; seu aspecto gelatinoso deve-se a seu conteúdo muito baixo de fibras nervosas mielinizadas; lâmina espinal II (de Rexed). SIN substantia gelatinosa [TA], lamina spinalis II*, spinal lamina II*, Rolando gelatinous s., Rolando s.
glandular s. of prostate, s. glandular da próstata; o tecido glandular da próstata, distinto do estroma e da cápsula. SIN substantia glandularis prostatae.
gray s. [TA], s. cinzenta. SIN gray matter.
ground s., s. fundamental, s. amorfa; o material amorfo no qual ocorrem os elementos estruturais; no tecido conjuntivo, compõem-se de proteoglicanos, constituintes plasmáticos, metabólitos, água e íons presentes entre células e fibras. SIN substantia fundamentalis.
H s., s. H; designação dada por Sir Thomas Lewis a uma substância difusível na pele, cuja ação é indistinguível daquela da histamina, que é liberada em consequência de lesão e provoca resposta tripla. SIN released s.
innominate s. [TA], s. inominada da parte basilar do telencéfalo; região do prosencéfalo situada ventralmente à metade anterior do núcleo lentiforme, estendendo-se no plano frontal da zona pré-óptico-hipotalâmica lateral, lateralmente sobre o trato óptico até a amígdala (corpo amigdalóide); rostralmente, termina em ponta sobre a borda dorsal do tubérculo olfatório e, caudalmente, termina no local onde a cápsula interna alcança a superfície para formar o pedúnculo cerebral ou pé do pedúnculo. Notável entre sua população de células polimórficas é o núcleo basal de grandes células de Meynert. Esses elementos magnocelulares na substância inominada são encontrados no septo medial e na faixa diagonal de Broca, porém ocorrem em maior número ventralmente ao globo pálido. As evidências histoquímicas indicam que os elementos magnocelulares distribuem fibras colinérgicas amplamente no córtex cerebral e que essas células sofrem degeneração seletiva na doença de Alzheimer. SIN substantia innominata [TA].
Kendall s., s. de Kendall. SIN Kendall compounds, em compound.
s. of lens of eye [TA], s. da lente do bulbo do olho; substância que constitui a lente do bulbo do olho, composta de um núcleo e um córtex e recoberta por epitélio. SIN substantia lentis [TA].
medullary s., s. medular; **(1)** o material lipídico presente na bainha de mielina das fibras nervosas. SIN Schwann white s.; **(2)** medula dos ossos e de outros órgãos. SIN substantia medullaris (2).
müllerian inhibiting s. (MIS), s. inibidora de Müller; glicoproteína de 535 aminoácidos secretada pelas células de Sertoli do testículo. Está relacionada à inibina. SIN anti-müllerian hormone, müllerian inhibiting factor.
muscular s. of prostate, s. muscular da próstata; músculo liso no estroma da próstata. SIN musculus prostaticus, substantia muscularis prostatae.
neurosecretory s., s. neurossecretora; a secreção dos corpos das células nervosas localizados no hipotálamo; a substância é transportada pelas fibras do trato hipotálamo-hipofisário até a neuro-hipófise, onde as terminações das fibras nervosas contêm a secreção. Conforme observado à microscopia óptica nas fibras e terminações, a substância aparece como corpúsculos de Herring ou corpúsculos hialinos da hipófise. VER hyaline *bodies* of pituitary, em *body*.
Nissl s., s. de Nissl; material que consiste em retículo endoplasmático granuloso e ribossomas, encontrado em corpos de células nervosas e dendritos. SIN basophil s., basophilic s., chromophil s., Nissl bodies, Nissl granules, substantia basophilia, tigroid bodies, tigroid s.
s. P, s. P; neurotransmissor peptídico composto de 11 resíduos aminoácidos (com o grupamento carboxila amidado), normalmente presente em minúsculas quantidades no sistema nervoso e no intestino dos seres humanos e de vários animais e encontrada no tecido inflamado, que está primariamente envolvido na transmissão da dor e constitui um dos compostos mais potentes que afetam o músculo liso (dilatação dos vasos sanguíneos e contração do intestino), desempenhando, supostamente, um papel na inflamação.
periaqueductal gray s., s. cinzenta central. SIN central gray s.
P s. of Lewis, fator P de Lewis. SIN factor P.
posterior perforated s. [TA], s. perfurada posterior; o fundo da fossa interpeduncular, na base do mesencéfalo, que se estende da borda anterior da ponte para a frente até os corpos mamilares, contendo numerosas aberturas para a passagem de ramos perfurantes das artérias cerebrais posteriores. SIN substantia perforata posterior [TA], locus perfuratus posticus, Malacarne space.
pressor s., base pressora. SIN pressor base.
proper s., s. própria. VER *substantia* propria of cornea, *substantia* propria membrane tympani, *substantia* propria of sclera.
Reichstein s., s. de Reichstein; um dos vários esteróides; p. ex., substância F de Reichstein (cortisona), substância H de Reichstein (corticosterona), substância M de Reichstein (cortisol), substância Q de Reichstein (cortexona) e substância S de Reichstein (cortexolona). SIN Reichstein compound.
released s., s. H. SIN H s.

reticular s., s. reticular; (1) material plasmático filamentoso que apresenta grânulos, demonstrável através de coloração vital nos eritrócitos imaturos. SIN alpha s., filar mass, filar s., substantia reticularis (1), substantia reticulofilamentosa. (2) Formação reticular. SIN reticular formation.
Rolando gelatinous s., Rolando s., s. gelatinosa de Rolando, s. de Rolando. SIN gelatinous s.
Schwann white s., s. branca de Schwann. SIN medullary s. (1).
slow-reacting s. (SRS), slow-reacting s. of anaphylaxis (SRS-A), s. de reação lenta, s. de reação lenta da anafilaxia; lipoproteína de baixo peso molecular composta de leucotrienos, que é liberada no choque anafilático e provoca contração mais lenta e mais prolongada do músculo do que a histamina; é ativa na presença de anti-histamínicos (mas não de epinefrina) e parece não ocorrer na forma pré-formada nos mastócitos, porém como resultado de uma reação antígeno-anticorpo nos grânulos; induz o efeito observado nas reações anafiláticas. Cf. peptidyl leukotrienes. SIN slow-reacting factor of anaphylaxis.
soluble specific s. (SSS), s. específica solúvel, s. capsular específica. SIN specific capsular s.
specific capsular s., s. capsular específica; polissacarídeo tipo-específico solúvel, produzido durante o crescimento ativo de pneumococos virulentos, que compreende grande parte da cápsula. SIN pneumococcal polysaccharide, soluble specific s., specific soluble polysaccharide, specific soluble sugar.
spongy s., s. esponjosa. SIN substantia spongiosa.
standard s., s. padrão; substância autêntica e pura utilizada para fins de identificação.
Stilling gelatinous s., s. gelatinosa de Stilling. SIN central and lateral intermediate s.'s.
threshold s., s. limiar; qualquer material (p. ex., glicose) excretado na urina apenas quando a sua concentração plasmática excede determinado valor, denominado limiar. SIN threshold body.
tigroid s., s. tigróide. SIN Nissl s.
vasodepressor s., s. vasodepressora; substância química não totalmente caracterizada, aparentemente produzida durante a lesão hepática, que tende a diminuir a pressão vascular e a relaxar as paredes arteriais.
white s., s. branca. SIN white matter.
zymoplastic s., s. tromboplastina. SIN thromboplastin.

sub·stan·tia, pl. **sub·stan·ti·ae** (sŭb-stan'shē-ă, -shē-ē) [TA]. Substância. SIN substance. [L.]
s. adamanti'na, esmalte. SIN enamel.
s. al'ba, s. branca. SIN white matter.
basal s. [TA], s. basilar; estruturas basilares associadas ao complexo amigdalóide e suas conexões; inclui o núcleo basilar [TA] (nucleus basalis [TA]), também denominado núcleo de Ganser, parte sublenticular da amígdala [TA] (pars sublenticularis amygdalae [TA]) e núcleo da estria terminal [TA] (nucleus stria terminalis [TA]). SIN s. basalis [TA].
s. basalis [TA], s. basilar. SIN basal s.
s. basophi'lia, s. basófila. SIN Nissl substance.
s. cine'rea, s. cinza. SIN gray matter.
s. compac'ta [TA], s. compacta. SIN compact bone.
s. compac'ta os'sium, s. compacta. SIN compact bone.
s. cortica'lis [TA], s. cortical. SIN cortical bone.
s. ebur'nea, dentina. SIN dentine.
s. ferrugin'ea, locus ceruleus. SIN locus caeruleus.
s. fundamenta'lis, s. fundamental, s. amorfa. SIN ground substance.
s. gelatino'sa, s. gelatinosa. SIN gelatinous substance.
s. gelatino'sa centra'lis, s. intermédia central e lateral. SIN central and lateral intermediate substances, em substance.
s. glandula'ris pros'tatae, s. glandular da próstata. SIN glandular substance of prostate.
s. gris'ea [TA], s. cinzenta. SIN gray matter.
s. gris'ea centra'lis [TA], s. cinzenta central. SIN central gray substance.
s. innomina'ta [TA], s. inominada da parte basilar do telencéfalo. SIN innominate substance.
s. interme'dia centra'lis [TA], s. intermédia central. VER central and lateral intermediate substances, em substance.
s. intermedia lateralis [TA], s. intermédia lateral. SIN lateral intermediate substance. VER central and lateral intermediate substances, em substance.
s. len'tis [TA], s. da lente. SIN substance of lens of eye.
s. medulla'ris, (1) Medula. SIN medulla; **(2)** Medula óssea. SIN medullary substance.
s. muscula'ris prosta'tae, s. muscular da próstata. SIN muscular substance of prostate.
s. ni'gra [TA], s. negra; uma grande massa celular, em forma de crescente em corte transversal, que se estende para frente sobre a superfície dorsal dos pilares do cérebro, da borda rostral da ponte até à região subtalâmica; é composta de um setor dorsal de células pigmentadas (isto é, contendo melanina) próximas, que é a parte compacta da s. negra [TA], uma região ventral maior de células afastadas, a parte reticulada da s. negra, [TA] e regiões menores e menos distintas, a parte lateral da s. negra [TA] e a parte retrorrubral da s. negra [TA]; a parte compacta, em particular, inclui numerosas células que se projetam para a frente até o estriado (núcleo caudado e putame) e contém dopamina, que atua como transmissor em suas terminações sinápticas; outras células aparentemente não-dopaminérgicas da s. negra projetam-se para uma parte rostral do núcleo ventral do tálamo, até as camadas médias do colículo superior e para partes restritas da formação reticular do mesencéfalo; a projeção negroestriada é retribuída por um sistema maciço de fibras estriatonegras com múltiplos neurotransmissores, entre os quais o principal é o ácido γ-aminobutírico (GABA); a s. negra recebe projeções aferentes menores do núcleo subtalâmico, do segmento lateral do globo pálido, do núcleo dorsal da rafe e do núcleo pedúnculo pontino do mesencéfalo. A parte reticulada forma parte do sistema eferente para o corpo estriado. A s. negra está envolvida nos distúrbios metabólicos associados à doença de Parkinson e à doença de Huntington. SIN locus niger, nucleus niger, Soemmering ganglion.
s. os'sea den'tis, cemento. SIN cement (1).
s. perfora'ta ante'rior [TA], s. perfurada anterior. SIN anterior perforated substance.
s. perforata rostralis, s. perfurada anterior. SIN anterior perforated substance.
s. perfora'ta poste'rior [TA], s. perfurada posterior. SIN posterior perforated substance.
s. propria of cornea, s. própria da córnea; tecido conjuntivo transparente modificado entre cujas camadas se encontram espaços abertos ou lacunas quase totalmente preenchidos por células ou corpúsculos corneanos. SIN s. propria corneae.
s. pro'pria cor'neae, s. própria da córnea. SIN s. propria of cornea.
s. pro'pria membra'nae tym'pani, s. própria da membrana timpânica; a camada de fibras colágenas radiais e circulares da membrana timpânica.
s. propria of sclera [TA], s. própria da esclera; o tecido fibroso branco denso, disposto em feixes entrelaçados, que forma a massa principal da esclera, contínua anteriormente com a substância própria da córnea. SIN s. propria sclerae [TA].
s. pro'pria scle'rae [TA], s. própria da esclera. SIN s. propria of sclera.
s. reticula'ris, (1) s. reticular (1). SIN reticular substance (1); **(2)** Formação reticular. SIN reticular formation.
s. reticulofilamento'sa, s. reticular (1). SIN reticular substance (1).
s. spongio'sa [TA], s. esponjosa; osso cujas espículas ou trabéculas formam uma rede tridimensional (osso esponjoso) com os interstícios preenchidos por tecido conjuntivo embrionário ou medula óssea. SIN spongy bone (1) [TA], s. trabecularis*, trabecular bone*, cancellous bone, spongy substance.
s. trabecula'ris, s. esponjosa; *termo oficial alternativo para s. spongiosa.
s. vit'rea, esmalte. SIN enamel.

sub·ster·nal (sŭb-ster'năl). Subesternal. 1. Profundamente ao externo. 2. SIN infrasternal.
sub·ster·no·mas·toid (sŭb-ster'nō-mas'toyd). Subesternomastóideo; sob o músculo esternomastóideo; designa um grupo de linfonodos cervicais profundos.
sub·sti·tute (sŭb'sti-toot). Substituto. 1. Qualquer coisa que tome o lugar de outra. 2. Em psicologia, um sub-rogado.
blood s., s. do sangue; qualquer material (p. ex., plasma humano, albumina sérica ou uma solução dessas substâncias, como dextrana) utilizado para transfusão na hemorragia e no choque.
plasma s., s. do plasma; solução de uma substância (p. ex., dextrana) utilizada para transfusão na hemorragia ou no choque como substituto do plasma. SIN plasma expander.
volume s., s. de volume; infusão de líquidos sem células ou expansores de volume, como a dextrana, para reposição de líquido perdido da circulação, como parte da profilaxia ou tratamento do choque circulatório.
sub·sti·tu·tion (sŭb-sti-too'shŭn). Substituição. 1. Em química, a substituição de um átomo ou grupamento em um composto por outro átomo ou grupamento (p. ex., a substituição do H por Cl no CH_4 produz CH_3Cl. 2. Em psicanálise, mecanismo de defesa inconsciente através do qual um objetivo, objeto ou emoção inaceitável ou inatingível é substituído por outro mais aceitável ou alcançável; o processo é mais agudo e direto e menos sutil do que a sublimação. [L. substitutio, por no lugar de outro]
generic s., s. genérica; a dispensação de uma droga quimicamente equivalente, porém de menor custo no lugar de um produto comercial cujo prazo de patente expirou.
stimulus s., condicionamento clássico. SIN classical conditioning.
symptom s., s. de sintoma; processo psicológico inconsciente pelo qual o impulso reprimido manifesta-se indiretamente através de um sintoma específico, p. ex., ansiedade, compulsão, depressão, alucinação, obsessão. SIN symptom formation.
sub·strate (S) (sŭb'strāt). Substrato. 1. A substância sobre a qual atua uma enzima, modificando-a; o reagente "atacado" numa reação química. 2. A base sobre a qual um microrganismo vive ou cresce; p. ex., o substrato sobre o qual crescem microrganismos e células numa cultura de células. [L. sub-sterno, pp. -stratus, espalhar debaixo]
insulin receptor s.-1 (IRS-1), s. do receptor de insulina 1; proteína citoplasmática que atua como s. direto do receptor de insulina ativado, cinase. A expo-

sição da insulina resulta em sua rápida fosforilação em múltiplos resíduos tirosina. Os locais fosforilados associam-se com alta afinidade a determinadas proteínas celulares. Por conseguinte, o IRS-1 atua como uma molécula adaptadora que liga o receptor cinase a diversas atividades celulares que são reguladas pela insulina. O IRS-1 também é fosforilado após estimulação pelo fator de crescimento insulino-símile 1 e por várias interleucinas.

suicide s., s. suicida; inibidor competitivo que é convertido em inibidor irreversível no sítio ativo da enzima. SIN mechanism-based inhibitor, suicide inhibitor.

sub·stra·tum (sŭb-strā'tŭm). Substrato; qualquer camada ou estrato situado sob outro. [L. ver substrate]

sub·struc·ture (sŭb-strŭk'choor). Subestrutura; tecido ou estrutura situado parcial ou totalmente sob a superfície.

implant denture s., s. de implantação dentária; o arcabouço de metal que é colocado sob os tecidos moles em contato com o osso ou imerso nele com o propósito de sustentar uma superestrutura de implantação dentária.

sub·sul·fate (sŭb-sŭl'fāt). Subsulfato, sulfato básico; sulfato que contém alguma base não-neutralizada e ainda capaz de combinar-se com o ácido.

sub·tar·sal (sŭb-tar'săl). Subtarsal; sob o tarso.

sub·ten·to·ri·al (sŭb-ten-tō'rē-ăl). Subtentorial; sob o tentório do cerebelo.

sub·ter·mi·nal (sŭb-ter'mi-năl). Subterminal; situado próximo à extremidade de um corpo oval ou em forma de bastão.

sub·te·tan·ic (sŭb-te-tan'ik). Subtetânico; designa os espasmos musculares tônicos ou convulsões que não são totalmente mantidos, mas que apresentam remissões breves.

sub·tha·lam·ic (sŭb-thă-lam'ik). Subtalâmico; relacionado à região do subtálamo ou ao núcleo subtalâmico.

sub·thal·a·mus (sŭb-thal'ă-mŭs) [TA]. Subtálamo; a parte do diencéfalo situada entre o tálamo na face dorsal e o pedúnculo cerebral ventralmente, lateral à metade dorsal do hipotálamo do qual não pode ser bem delineada. É composto do núcleo subtalâmico (corpo de Luysi), da zona incerta e dos campos de Forel; lateralmente, expande-se como uma asa até o núcleo reticular do tálamo; caudalmente, continua-se com o tegmento do mesencéfalo. SIN ventral thalamus.

sub·thy·roid·e·us (sŭb-thī-royd'ē-ŭs). Subtireóideo; feixe muscular formado de fibras derivadas dos músculos tireoaritenóideo e vocal.

sub·til·i·sin (sŭb-ti-lī'sin). Subtilisina; proteinase formada pelo *Bacillus subtilis* e por outras espécies, semelhante às proteinases séricas de outros fungos e bactérias; catalisa a hidrólise de algumas ligações peptídicas específicas em determinadas proteínas, convertendo, assim, o quimiotripsinogênio em quimotripsina e a ovalbumina em placalbumina, e cliva a ribonuclease pancreática em peptídio S e proteína S. SIN subtilopeptidase.

sub·ti·lo·pep·ti·dase (sŭb'ti-lō-pep'ti-dās). Subtilopeptidase. SIN subtilisin.

sub·trac·tion (sŭb-trak'shŭn). Subtração; técnica utilizada para melhorar a detectabilidade de estruturas anatômicas opacificadas em imagens radiográficas ou cintilográficas; o negativo de uma imagem obtida antes da introdução do contraste ou de radionuclídeo é fotográfica ou eletronicamente removido de uma imagem posterior; comumente utilizada na angiografia do cérebro. VER TAMBÉM digital subtraction *angiography*, mask.

energy s., s. de energia; radiografia digital que utiliza exposições de maior e menor energia, através de dupla exposição em níveis de 2 kV ou através da interposição de um filtro de cobre que absorve os fótons de menor energia entre duas placas de fósforo, com cálculo computadorizado das imagens de alto Z ou baixo Z (osso e tecidos moles, respectivamente); recorre ao fato de que os raios X de menor energia são absorvidos por substâncias de Z mais alto, como cálcio e cobre, devido ao efeito fotoelétrico (photoelectric *effect*). VER TAMBÉM Z, photoelectric *effect*, phosphor *plate*.

sub·tra·pe·zi·al (sŭb-tra-pē'zē-ăl). Subtrapezial; sob o músculo trapézio; designa um plexo nervoso.

sub·tribe (sŭb-trīb). Subtribo; na classificação biológica, uma divisão entre tribo e gênero.

sub·tro·chan·ter·ic (sŭb-trō-kan-ter'ik). Subtrocantérico; sob qualquer trocanter.

sub·troch·le·ar (sŭb-trok'lē-ar). Subtroclear; sob qualquer tróclea.

sub·tu·ber·al (sŭb-too'ber-ăl). Subtuberal; situado sob qualquer tuberosidade.

sub·tym·pan·ic (sŭb-tim-pan'ik). Subtimpânico; sob a cavidade timpânica.

sub·um·bil·i·cal (sŭb-ŭm-bil'i-kăl). Subumbilical. SIN infraumbilical.

sub·un·gual, sub·un·gui·al (sŭb-ŭng'gwăl, sŭb-ŭng'gwi-ăl). Subungueal; sob a unha do dedo da mão ou do pé. SIN hyponychial (1). [L. *unguis*, unha]

sub·u·nit (sŭb'oo-nit). Subunidade. **1.** Uma unidade que forma uma parte distinta de uma estrutura maior. VER TAMBÉM monomer. **2.** A proteína ou cadeia polipeptídica individual que pode ser separada de uma proteína oligomérica sem a clivagem de ligações covalentes, a não ser fontes de dissulfeto entre resíduos cisteinil. **3.** Biopolímero isolado separado de uma estrutura multimérica maior.

sub·u·re·thral (sŭb-ū-rē'thrăl). Suburetral; sob a uretra masculina ou feminina.

sub·vag·i·nal (sŭb-vaj'i-năl). Subvaginal. **1.** Sob a vagina. **2.** Sobre a face interna de qualquer membrana tubular que serve como bainha.

sub·val·var, sub·val·vu·lar (sŭb-val'văr, sŭb-val'vū-lăr). Subvalvar, subvalvular; sob qualquer valva.

sub·ver·te·bral (sŭb-ver'tē-brăl). Subvertebral; sob a face ventral (ou na face ventral) de uma vértebra ou da coluna vertebral.

sub·vir·ile (sŭb-vir'il). Subviril; deficiente em virilidade.

sub·vir·ion (sŭb-vir'ē-on). Subvírion; partícula viral incompleta. [sub- + virion]

sub·vit·ri·nal (sŭb-vit'ri-năl). Subvítreo; sob o corpo vítreo.

sub·wak·ing (sŭb-wāk'ing). Subvigília; designa o estado mental entre o sono e a vigília.

sub·zon·al (sŭb-zō'năl). Subzonal; sob qualquer zona, como a zona radiada ou a zona pelúcida.

sub·zy·go·mat·ic (sŭb-zī-gō-mat'ik). Subzigomático; sob ou abaixo do osso ou arco zigomático.

suc·ca·gogue (sŭk'ă-gog). Sucagogo. **1.** Que estimula o fluxo de suco. **2.** Agente que possui esse efeito. [L. *succus*, suco + G. *agōgos*, que impele]

suc·ce·da·ne·ous (sŭk-sē-dā'nē-ŭs). Sucedâneo. **1.** Relativo a um sucedâneo. **2.** Relativo aos dentes permanentes ou secundários que substituem os dentes decíduos ou primários. [ver succedaneum]

suc·ce·da·ne·um (sŭk-sē-dā'nē-ŭm). Sucedâneo; substituto; droga ou qualquer agente terapêutico que possui as propriedades de outro e que pode ser utilizado em seu lugar. [L. *succedaneus*, seguindo depois, substituindo, de *succedo*, seguir, tomar o lugar de, de *sub*, sob + *cedo*, ir]

suc·cen·tu·ri·ate (sŭk-sen-tū'rē-āt). Em anatomia, que substitui algum órgão ou atua como acessório. [L. *suc-centurio*, pp. *-atus*, substituir]

suc·ci·nate (sŭk'si-nāt). Succinato; sal do ácido succínico.

active s., s. ativo. SIN succinyl-coenzyme A.

s. dehydrogenase, succinato desidrogenase; flavoenzima que catalisa a remoção de hidrogênio do ácido succínico, convertendo-o em ácido fumárico; p. ex., succinato + FAD ↔ fumarato + FADH$_2$; esse complexo faz parte do ciclo do ácido tricarboxílico. SIN fumarate reductase (NADH), fumaric hydrogenase.

suc·ci·nate sem·i·al·de·hyde (sŭk'sin-āt sem-ē-al-dē-hīd). Succinato semialdeído; um intermediário no catabolismo do γ-aminobutirato.

s. s. dehydrogenase, succinato semialdeído desidrogenase; enzima que catalisa a reação do succinato semialdeído com NAD$^+$ ou NADP$^+$ para formar succinato e NADH (ou NADPH); a deficiência dessa enzima está associada à acidúria 4-hidroxibutírica.

suc·cin·ic ac·id (sŭk-sin'ik). Ácido succínico; intermediário no ciclo do ácido tricarboxílico; vários de seus sais têm sido utilizados de modo variado na medicina.

suc·cin·ic thi·o·ki·nase. Tiocinase (tioquinase) succínica. SIN succinyl-CoA synthetase.

suc·cin·i·mide (sŭk'sin-ă-mīd). Succinimida; classe química de drogas da qual derivam os agentes antiepilépticos etosuximida, metosuximida e fensuximida. A succimida não-substituída tem sido utilizada como antiurolítico.

suc·ci·nyl·ac·e·tone (sŭk'sin-il-ăs'e-tōn). Succinil acetona; metabólito de pouca importância que está elevado em indivíduos com tirosinemia IA.

***N*-suc·cin·yl·ad·en·yl·ic ac·id** (sŭk-sin-il-ăd-ē-nil'ik). Ácido *N*-succiniladenílico. SIN adenylocuccinic acid.

suc·ci·nyl·cho·line (sŭk'si-nil-kō'lēn). Succinilcolina; relaxante neuromuscular de curta ação que, tipicamente, despolariza primeiro a placa motora terminal (bloqueio de fase I), mas que muitas vezes está posteriormente associado a bloqueio neuromuscular não-despolarizante e semelhante ao do curare (bloqueio de fase II); utilizado para produzir relaxamento para intubação traqueal e durante a anestesia cirúrgica. SIN diacetylcholine, suxamethonium.

suc·ci·nyl-CoA (sŭk'sin-il). Succinil-CoA. SIN succinyl-coenzyme A.

s.-CoA synthetase, succinil-CoA sintetase; **(1)** ligase envolvida na reação reversível do succinato e da CoA com ATP para produzir ADP, fosfato inorgânico e succinato-CoA-CoA; **(2)** sintetase semelhante, porém capaz de utilizar o itaconato, bem como o succinato e GTP (ou ITP) no lugar de ATP; faz parte do ciclo do ácido tricarboxílico. SIN succinic thiokinase, succinyl-CoA ligase.

suc·ci·nyl-CoA li·gase. Succinil-CoA ligase. SIN succinyl-CoA synthetase.

suc·ci·nyl-co·en·zyme A (sŭk'si-nil-kō-en'zīm). Succinil-coenzima A; o produto de condensação do ácido succínico com CoA; um dos intermediários do ciclo do ácido tricarboxílico e um precursor na síntese do heme. SIN active succinate, succinyl-CoA.

suc·ci·nyl·di·cho·line (sŭk'si-nil-dī-kō'lēn). Succinildicolina; cloreto de succinilcolina.

***O*-suc·ci·nyl·ho·mo·ser·ine (thi·ol)·ly·ase** (sŭk'si-nil-hō'mō-ser'ēn). *O*-succinil-homosserina (tiol)-liase; enzima que catalisa a reação entre a cistationina e o succinato para formar L-cisteína e *O*-succinil-L-homosserina. SIN cystathionine γ-synthase.

suc·ci·nyl·sul·fa·thi·a·zole (sŭk'si-nil-sŭl'fă-thī'ă-zōl). Succinilsulfatiazol; a mais efetiva das sulfonamidas bacteriostáticas pouco absorvidas utilizadas na esterilização do trato intestinal.

suc·ci·sul·fone im·i·no·di·eth·a·nol (sŭk - si - sŭl'fōn). Succissulfona iminodietanol; agente antimicrobiano.

suc·cor·rhea (sŭk - ō - rē'ă). Sucorréia; aumento anormal na secreção de um líquido digestivo. [L. *succus*, suco + G. *rhoia*, fluxo]

suc·cu·bus (sŭk'ū - bŭs). Súcubo; demônio, em forma de mulher, que se acreditava manter relações sexuais com um homem durante o sono. Cf. incubus. [L. *succubo*, ficar sob]

suc·cuss (sŭ - kŭs'). Sacudir, abalar; produzir sucussão.

suc·cus·sion (sŭk - kŭsh'ŭn). Sucussão; procedimento diagnóstico que consiste em agitar o corpo do paciente de modo a produzir um ruído de pancada na água numa cavidade contendo tanto gás quanto líquido. [L. *sucussio*, de *succutio* (*subc*-), pp. -*cussus*, agitar, sacudir, de *quatio*, agitar, sacudir]

  hippocratic s., s. hipocrática; ruído de pancada na água produzido pela agitação do corpo quando há gás ou ar e líquido no estômago ou no intestino, ou gás e líquido livres no peritônio, tórax e, raramente, pericárdio.

suck (sŭk). Sugar, aspirar. **1.** Puxar um líquido através de um tubo ao extrair o ar na sua frente. **2.** Aspirar um líquido até a boca; especificamente, extrair leite da mama. [A.S. *sūcan*]

suck·le (sŭk'l). **1.** Amamentar; alimentar com leite da mama. **2.** Mamar; obter sustento a partir da mama.

Sucquet, J. P., anatomista francês, 1840–1870. VER S. *anastomoses*, em *anastomosis*, *canals*, em *canal*; S.-Hoyer *anastomoses*, em *anastomosis*, *canals*, em *canal*.

su·cral·fate (soo - kral'fāt). Sucralfato; complexo de octossulfato (sulfato de hidrogênio) de sacarose e alumínio; polissacarídeo com atividade antipéptica, utilizado no tratamento de úlceras duodenais ao proporcionar um revestimento protetor que permite a cicatrização.

su·crase (soo'krās). Sacarase. SIN sucrose α-D-glucohydrolase.

su·crate (soo'krāt). Sacarato; composto da sacarose.

su·crose (soo'krōs). Sacarose; dissacarídeo não-redutor constituído de D-glicose e D-frutose, obtido da cana de açúcar, *Saccharum officinarum* (família Gramineae), de várias espécies de sorgo e da beterraba, *Beta vulgaris*, (família Chenopodiaceae); o adoçante comum, utilizado em farmácia na fabricação de xarope, eletuários, etc. SIN saccharose, saccharum.

  s. octaacetate, octacetato de sacarose; desnaturante do álcool.

su·crose α-D-glu·co·hy·dro·lase. Sacarose α-D-glicoidrolase; enzima que hidrolisa a sacarose e a maltose num complexo com isomaltase; por conseguinte, hidrolisa tanto a sacarose quanto a isomaltose; encontrada na mucosa intestinal; a deficiência dessa enzima resulta na digestão deficiente de sacarose e de α1,4-glicanos lineares. SIN sucrase.

su·cro·se·mia (soo - krō - sē'mē - ă). Sacarosemia; presença de sacarose no sangue. [sucrose + G. *haima*, sangue]

su·cro·su·ria (soo - krō - soo'rē - ă). Sacarosúria; excreção de sacarose na urina. [sucrose + G. *ouron*, urina]

suc·tion (sŭk'shŭn). Sucção; o ato ou processo de sugar. VER TAMBÉM aspiration (1), aspiration (2). [L. *sugo*, pp. *suctus*, sugar]

  posttussive s., s. pós-tosse; ruído de sucção ouvido à ausculta sobre uma cavidade pulmonar no final de uma tosse.

  Wangensteen s., s. de Wangensteen; sifão modificado que mantém uma pressão negativa constante, utilizado com um tubo duodenal para alívio da distensão gástrica e intestinal. SIN Wangensteen tube.

suc·to·ri·al (sŭk - tō'rē - ăl). Relativo à sucção ou ao ato de sugar; adaptado para sugar.

su·da·men, pl. **su·dam·i·na** (soo - dā'men, - dam'i - nă). Sudâmina; minúscula vesícula formada em conseqüência da retenção de líquido num folículo sudoríparo ou na epiderme. [L. mod. do L. *sudo*, suar]

su·dam·i·na (soo - dam'i - nă). **1.** Sudâminas; plural de sudamen. **2.** Miliaria cristalina. SIN miliaria crystallina.

Su·dan III [C.I. 26100]. Sudão III; corante vermelho utilizado para a gordura neutra em técnica histológica; cora também o envoltório lipídico do bacilo da tuberculose. SIN Sudan red III.

Su·dan IV [C.I. 26105]. Sudão IV. SIN scarlet red.

Su·dan black B [C.I. 26150]. Sudão negro B; corante diazo utilizado como corante para gorduras.

Su·dan brown [C.I. 12020]. Sudão castanho; corante castanho, derivado da α-naftilamina e utilizado como corante para gorduras.

su·dan·o·phil·ia (soo - dan - ō - fil'ē - ă). Sudanofilia. **1.** Afinidade por um corante lipossolúvel ou sudão. **2.** Condição em que os leucócitos contêm minúsculas gotículas lipídicas que se coram de vermelho-brilhante quando tratadas com sudão III a 0,2% e azul de cresil a 0,1% em álcool absoluto.

su·dan·o·phil·ic (soo - dan - ō - fil'ik). Sudanofílico; que se cora facilmente com corantes sudão, referindo-se, em geral, aos lipídios nos tecidos.

su·dan·o·pho·bic (soo - dan - ō - fō'bik). Sudanofóbico; designa um tecido que não se cora com um corante sudão ou lipossolúvel.

Su·dan red III. Sudão vermelho III. SIN Sudan III.

Su·dan yel·low. Sudão amarelo; metadioxiazobenzeno; corante amarelo para lipídios.

su·da·tion (soo - dā'shŭn). Sudação. SIN perspiration (1). [L. *sudatio*, de *sudo*, pp. -*atus*, suar]

Sudeck, Paul H. M., cirurgião alemão, 1866–1938. VER S. *atrophy*, critical *point*, *syndrome*.

su·do·mo·tor (soo - dō - mō'ter). Sudomotor; designa os nervos autônomos (simpáticos) que estimulam a atividade das glândulas sudoríparas. [L. *sudor*, suor + *motor*, motor]

su·dor (soo'dōr). Suor. SIN perspiration (3). [L.]

  s. anglicus, SIN English sweating *disease*.

sudor-. Sudor-; suor, transpiração. [L. *sudor*]

su·do·re·sis (soo - dō - rē'sis). Sudorese; suor profuso. [sudor- + G. -*ēsis*, condição]

su·do·rif·er·ous (soo - dō - rif'er - ŭs). Sudorífero; que transporta ou produz suor. [sudor- + L. *fero*, transportar]

su·do·rif·ic (soo - dō - rif'ik). Sudorífico, diaforético; que causa suor. [sudor- + L. *facio*, fazer]

su·do·rom·e·ter (soo - dō - rom'ē - ter). Sudorômetro; instrumento para medir a quantidade de transpiração. [sudor- + G. *metron*, medir]

su·dor·rhea (soo - dō - rē'ă). Hiperidrose. SIN hyperhidrosis. [sudor- + G. *rhoia*, fluxo]

su·et (soo'et). Sebo; a gordura dura ao redor dos rins de bovinos e ovinos; quando derretida, fornece o sebo.

  prepared s., s. preparado; a gordura interna do abdome do ovino, *Ovis aries*, purificada por liquefação e filtração; antigamente, era utilizada em farmácia na produção de pomadas. SIN prepared mutton tallow.

su·fen·ta·nil cit·rate (soo - fen'tă - nil). Citrato de sufentanil; narcótico injetável de curta ação semelhante ao fentanil; utilizado na "anestesia balanceada".

suf·fo·cate (sŭf'ō - kāt). Sufocar. **1.** Impedir a respiração; asfixiar. **2.** Ser incapaz de respirar; sofrer de asfixia. [L. *suffoco* (*subf*-), pp. -*atus*, sufocar, estrangular]

suf·fo·ca·tion (sŭf - ō - kā'shŭn). Sufocação; o ato ou a condição de sufocar ou de asfixiar.

suf·fu·sion (sŭ - fū'zhŭn). **1.** Sufusão; o ato de verter um líquido sobre o corpo. **2.** Ruborização da superfície. **3.** Condição de estar molhado por um líquido. **4.** Extravasar. SIN extravasate (2). [L. *suffusio*, de *suffundo* (*subf*-), despejar]

sug·ar (shu - ger). Açúcar; um dos açúcares, q.v.; as formas farmacêuticas consistem em açúcar compressível e açúcar de confeiteiros. VER TAMBÉM sugars. [G. *sakcharon*; L. *saccharum*]

  amino s.'s, aminoaçúcares; açúcares cujo grupo hidroxila foi substituído por um grupo amino; p. ex., D-glicosamina.

  beechwood s., a. de madeira de faia; D-xilose. VER xylose.

  beet s., a. de beterraba; D-sacarose. VER sucrose.

  blood s., D-glicose. VER D-glicose.

  brain s., D-galactose. VER galactose.

  cane s., a. de cana; D-sacarose. VER sucrose.

  corn s., a. de milho. VER D-glucose.

  deoxy s., desoxiaçúcar; açúcar que contém menos átomos de oxigênio do que de carbono e no qual, consequentemente, um ou mais carbonos na molécula carecem de grupo hidroxila ligado. SIN desoxy s.

  desoxy s., desoxiaçúcar. SIN deoxy s.

  fruit s., D-frutose. VER fructose.

  gelatin s., glicina. SIN glycine.

  grape s., a. de uva. VER D-glucose.

  invert s., a. invertido; mistura de partes iguais de D-glicose e D-frutose, produzida por hidrólise da sacarose (inversão).

  s. of lead, acetato de chumbo. SIN lead acetate.

  malt s., maltose. SIN maltose.

  manna s., manitol. SIN mannitol.

  maple s., a. de bordo; sacarose extraída da seiva do bordo, *Acer saccharinum*. SIN saccharum canadense.

  milk s., a. do leite, lactose. SIN lactose.

  oil s., oleossacarato. SIN oleosaccharum.

  pectin s., D-arabinose. VER arabinose.

  reducing s., a. redutor; a., como a glicose na urina, que tem a propriedade de reduzir vários íons inorgânicos, notavelmente o íon cúprico a íon cuproso.

  specific soluble s., substância capsular específica. SIN specific capsular *substance*.

  starch s., a. de amido. VER D-glucose.

  wood s., a. de madeira; D-xilose. VER xylose.

sug·ar ac·ids. Ácidos de açúcar; ácidos, como os ácidos glicônico, glicurônico e sacárico, produzidos pela oxidação da glicose.

sug·ar al·co·hol. Álcool do açúcar; o poliálcool resultante da redução do grupo carbonila num monossacarídeo a um grupamento hidroxila.

sug·ar al·de·hyde. Aldeído de açúcar; açúcar que contém um acetal interno.

sug·ars (shug'erz). Açúcares; os carboidratos (sacarídeos) que apresentam a composição geral $(CH_2O)_n$ e derivados simples. Embora os açúcares monoméricos simples (glicoses) sejam freqüentemente escritos como polihidroxi aldeídos ou cetonas, como, p. ex., $HOCH_2$—$(CHOH)_4$—CHO para as aldoexoses (p. ex., glicose) ou $HOCH_2—(CHOH)_3—CO—CH_2OH$ para as 2-cetoses (p. ex., frutose), a ciclização pode dar origem a estruturas variadas, conforme descrito adiante. Em geral, os açúcares são identificados pela terminação -ose ou, se estiverem em combinação com um não-açúcar (aglicona), -osídeo ou -osil. Os açúcares, em particular a D-glicose, constituem a principal fonte de energia por oxidação na natureza; eles e seus derivados (p. ex., D-glicosamina, ácido D-glicurônico), na forma polimérica, são importantes constituintes das mucoproteínas, das paredes celulares bacterianas e do material estrutural vegetal (p. ex., celulose). Os açúcares são freqüentemente encontrados em combinação com esteróides (glicosídeos esteróides) e outras agliconas.

Fischer projection formulas of s., fórmulas de projeção dos açúcares de Fischer; representações, por projeção, de açúcar cíclico ou derivados, em que a cadeia de carbono é representada verticalmente. O átomo de carbono assimétrico de menor numeração (C-1 nas aldoses; C-2 nas 2-cetoses, p. ex., frutose) é representado no topo, sendo os restantes átomos de carbono da cadeia representados em seqüência abaixo do átomo de carbono do topo. Para cada átomo de carbono, representado em projeção como situado no plano do papel, as ligações carbono–carbono, que, na verdade, afastam-se do observador, são representadas como linhas verticais. As ligações à esquerda e à direita de cada átomo de carbono, que realmente apontam para o observador, são, em projeção, representadas como linhas horizontais.

As convenções para as fórmulas de Fischer dos açúcares cíclicos são as seguintes: 1) se o átomo de carbono assimétrico de maior numeração tem seu OH (ou sua substituição) situado à direita, como a 2-OH do D-gliceraldeído, o açúcar possui a configuração D; se a OH estiver à esquerda, o açúcar possui a configuração L; 2) no átomo de carbono anomérico (C-1 nas aldoses; C-2 nas 2-cetoses), uma OH ou OH substituída situada à direita, com a OH do átomo de carbono assimétrico de maior numeração também à direita, é definida como α; se estiver à esquerda, com a OH do átomo de carbono de maior numeração à direita, é β; ocorre o inverso se a última OH estiver à esquerda; 3) a orientação de um grupo CH_2OH terminal nas aldoses não tem nenhum significado em termos de configuração, visto que não contém nenhum átomo de carbono assimétrico.

Haworth conformational formulas of cyclic s., fórmulas conformacionais de Haworth dos açúcares cíclicos; para as piranoses, representam as formas (conformações) em que nenhum, um ou dois átomos do anel localizam-se fora do plano do anel. Se houver dois desses átomos *para* entre si, podem situar-se: 1) nos lados opostos do plano (*trans*), produzindo "formas em cadeira", ou 2) no mesmo lado do plano (*cis*), produzindo "formas em barco".

De forma semelhante, existem seis configurações "em barco". Se os dois átomos exoplanares (*trans*) forem *meta* entre si, a conformação é oblíqua; se os dois átomos forem *orto* entre si, a conformação é uma forma de meia-cadeira.

Para as furanoses, as conformações em envoltório apresentam um átomo do anel exoplanar. Se houver três átomos do anel coplanares adjacentes (os dois átomos do anel exoplanares nos lados opostos do plano), as conformações consistem em formas torcidas.

Haworth perspective formulas of cyclic s., fórmulas em perspectiva de Haworth dos açúcares cíclicos; representações em perspectiva das estruturas da furanose ou piranose como pentágonos ou hexágonos, respectivamente, com as ligações sombreadas de modo que possam aparecer como se o plano do anel estivesse num ângulo de 30° em relação ao plano do papel, estando as ligações ao H e OH em ângulos retos com o plano do anel. Essas fórmulas representam a conformação planar, uma situação que, habitualmente, não é observada. Outras fórmulas conformacionais, como, p. ex., as fórmulas conformacionais de Haworth dos açúcares cíclicos, representam os diversos desvios da planaridade.

As convenções básicas nas fórmulas de Haworth dos açúcares cíclicos (glicoses cíclicas) são as seguintes: 1) o átomo de carbono do anel assimétrico de menor numeração é representado à direita; 2) se o átomo de carbono assimétrico de maior numeração for D, o açúcar é D; a fórmula de uma L-glicose pode ser derivada daquela de seu isômero D por inversão da direção para cima ou para baixo de todos os grupos ligados aos átomos de carbonos do anel; 3) se o grupo hidroxila fixado ao carbono anomérico (C-1 nas aldoses, C-2 nas 2-cetoses) estiver abaixo do plano do anel de uma D-glicose, é α; se estiver acima, é β; o inverso é observado se o açúcar for L. VER TAMBÉM Fischer projection formulas of s.

sug·gest·i·bil·i·ty (sŭg - jes'tĭ - bĭl'i - tē). Sugestibilidade; responsividade ou susceptibilidade a um processo psicológico, como comando hipnótico, através do qual uma idéia é introduzida num indivíduo ou adotada por ele sem argumentação, comando ou coerção. SIN sympathism.

sug·gest·i·ble (sŭg - jes'tĭ - bl). Sugestionável; suscetível a sugestão.

sug·ges·tion (sŭg - jes'chŭn). Sugestão; a implantação de uma idéia na mente de outra pessoa por alguma palavra ou ato de alguém, sendo a conduta ou condição física do indivíduo influenciadas, em certo grau, pela idéia implantada. VER TAMBÉM autosuggestion. [L. *sug-gero* (*subg-*), pp. -*gestus*, pôr debaixo, fornecer]

hypnotic s., s. hipnótica; orientação feita a um indivíduo em transe que é efetuada durante ou após o transe. VER TAMBÉM minor *hypnosis*.

posthypnotic s., s. pós-hipnótica; sugestão dada a um indivíduo sob hipnose para a realização de determinadas ações após "despertar" do transe hipnótico.

sug·ges·tive (sŭg - jes'tiv). Sugestivo; relativo à sugestão.

sug·gil·la·tion (sŭg - ji - lā'shŭn, sŭj - i -). Sugilação; termo obsoleto para referir-se a equimose ou livedo. VER TAMBÉM contusion. [L. *sugillo*, pp. *-atus*, ficar preto e azul devido a pancada]

postmortem s., s. *post-mortem*. SIN postmortem *livedo*.

Sugiura, M., cirurgião japonês do século XX. VER S. *procedure*.

SUI Abreviatura de stress urinary *incontinence* (incontinência urinária de esforço).

su·i·cide (soo'i - sīd). **1.** Suicídio; ato de tirar a própria vida. **2.** Suicida; pessoa que comete esse ato. [L. *sui*, próprio + *caedo*, matar]

physician-assisted s., suicídio assistido por médico; término voluntário da própria vida através da administração de uma substância letal, com assistência direta ou indireta de um médico. O suicídio assistido por médico deve ser diferenciado da interrupção das medidas de suporte da vida ou da recusa de mantê-las nos estados terminais ou vegetativos, em que o paciente morre da doença subjacente, e da administração de analgésicos narcóticos no câncer terminal, que pode acelerar indiretamente a morte. VER TAMBÉM end-of-life *care*, advance *directive*.

Polêmicas e controvérsias acerca do suicídio assistido propagaram-se pela comunidade médica e sociedade em geral. A Suprema Corte dos Estados Unidos, numa decisão de 9–0, decretou que o cidadão não tem nenhum direito constitucional ao suicídio assistido por médico, porém não impôs nenhum obstáculo à legalização da prática por legislaturas estaduais. De acordo com a lei do Oregon, qualquer residente mentalmente competente nesse estado, que tenha atingido 18 anos de idade e que sofra de doença terminal prenunciando a morte em 6 meses, pode tomar a decisão informada e voluntária de pôr termo à vida mediante administração de uma superdose letal de medicamento oral prescrito por um médico para esse propósito. O médico é isento de qualquer acusação ou denúncia civil ou criminal. A despeito da legalização do suicídio assistido por médico em pelo menos um estado, e apesar das atividades extremamente divulgadas dos "médicos da morte" em outros estados, a *American Medical Association* e a *American Nurses Association* dos Estados Unidos publicaram relatórios oficiais contra o suicídio assistido em todas as circunstâncias. Entre as objeções proclamadas por oponentes da legalização do suicídio assistido por médico e sua integração na prática médica, destacam-se o desgaste da confiança pública nos profissionais de saúde; a mudança radical na relação tradicional entre médico e paciente; a preocupação de que, se o suicídio assistido por médico se tornar uma opção aceita para o "tratamento" de determinadas doenças, os médicos poderão ver-se obrigados a oferecê-la aos pacientes como alternativa, que poderia ser apoiada por seguros de saúde (inclusive no *managed care*) por ser uma opção de menor custo; e o medo de que, uma vez legalizado, o suicídio assistido por médico seja permitido para condições não-terminais e que outras pessoas além do paciente sejam autorizadas a tomar essa decisão. A polêmica acerca do suicídio assistido por médico chamou a atenção para numerosas deficiências na assistência de pacientes moribundos e para a obrigação preeminente dos profissionais de saúde em proporcionar uma assistência responsável, com atitude de respeito apropriada e eticamente correta.

su·i·cid·ol·o·gy (soo'i - sī - dol'ō - jē). Suicidologia; ramo das ciências do comportamento dedicado ao estudo da natureza, dás causas e da prevenção do suicídio. [suicide + G. *logos*, estudo]

su·int (swint). Suarda; a gordura natural existente na lã de ovinos, da qual se extrai a gordura de lã oficial (lanolina anidra) [Fr. gordura de lã]

suit (soot). Traje; vestuário externo destinado à proteção contra condições ambientais específicas.

anti-G s., t. anti-G; vestuário com partes infláveis que se expandem para aplicar uma pressão externa ao abdome e aos membros inferiores durante manobras em G positiva durante o vôo ou numa centrífuga humana; o traje anti-G é utilizado para evitar o acúmulo de sangue e aumenta a capacidade do usuário de resistir à exposição a forças G maiores.

sul·bac·tam (sŭl - bak'tam). Sulbactam; inibidor da β-lactamase com ação antibacteriana fraca; quando associado a penicilinas (p. ex., ampicilina) com pouca ação inibidora da β-lactamase, o sulbactam aumenta muito sua efetividade contra microrganismos que, habitualmente, não seriam suscetíveis.

sul·ben·tine (sŭl - ben'tēn). Sulbetina. SIN dibenzthione.

sul·cal (sŭl'kal). Relativo a um sulco.

sul·cate (sŭl'kāt). Sulcado; marcado por um sulco ou sulcos.

sul·ci·form (sŭl'si - fōm). Sulciforme; que possui a forma de um sulco.

sul·cu·lus, pl. **sul·cu·li** (sŭl'kŭ - lŭs, -lī). Súlculo; pequeno sulco. [L. mod. dim. do L. *sulcus*, sulco]

SULCUS

sul·cus, gen. e pl. **sul·ci** (sool′kŭs, sŭl′sī). Sulco, incisura. **1.** [TA]. Um dos sulcos na superfície do cérebro que limitam as várias convoluções ou giros; uma fissura. VER TAMBÉM fissure. **2.** [NA]. Qualquer sulco estreito e longo ou depressão leve. VER TAMBÉM groove. **3.** Sulco ou depressão na cavidade oral ou sobre a superfície de um dente. [L. sulco ou vala]

alveolobuccal s., s. alveolobucal. SIN alveolobuccal groove.
alveololabial s., s. alveololabial. SIN alveololabial groove.
alveololingual s., s. alveololingual. SIN alveololingual groove.
s. ampulla'ris [TA], s. ampular. SIN ampullary groove.
ampullary s., s. ampular. SIN ampullary groove.
s. angula'ris, incisura angular. SIN angular incisure.
anterior intermediate s., s. intermédio anterior; sulco ocasionalmente observado no adulto entre a fissura mediana anterior e o sulco lateral anterior da medula espinal, mas geralmente presente apenas no feto. Indica a borda lateral do fascículo corticospinal anterior. SIN anterior intermediate groove, s. intermedius anterior.
anterior interventricular s., [TA], interventricular anterior; sulco na superfície ântero-superior do coração, marcando a localização do septo entre os dois ventrículos. SIN s. interventricularis anterior [TA], anterior interventricular groove, crena cordis (1).
anterior parolfactory s., s. para-olfatório anterior; fissura que marca a borda anterior da área para-olfatória. SIN s. parolfactorius anterior.
anterolateral s., s. ântero-lateral; sulco indistinto sobre a superfície central da medula espinal e da medula oblonga, marcando, em cada lado, a linha de saída das raízes nervosas anteriores. SIN s. anterolateralis [TA], ventrolateral s.*, anterolateral groove.
s. anterolatera'lis [TA], s. ântero-lateral. SIN anterolateral s.
s. anthel'icis transver'sus, s. antélice transverso. SIN transverse anthelicine groove.
aortic s., impressão aórtica. SIN aortic impression of left lung.
a. aor'ticus, impressão aórtica. SIN aortic impression of left lung.
s. arte'riae occipita'lis [TA], s. da artéria occipital. SIN occipital groove.
s. arteriae subclaviae costae primae [TA], s. da artéria subclávia da primeira costela. SIN groove of first rib for subclavian artery.
s. arte'riae tempora'lis me'diae [TA], s. da artéria temporal média. SIN groove for middle termporal artery.
s. arte'riae vertebra'lis [TA], s. da artéria vertebral. SIN groove for vertebral artery.
sul'ci arterio'si [TA], sulcos arteriais. SIN arterial grooves, em groove.
atrioventricular s., s. coronário. SIN coronary s.
s. for auditory tube, s. para tuba auditiva. SIN s. for pharyngotympanic tube.
s. auric'ulae ante'rior, incisura anterior da orelha. SIN anterior notch of auricle.
basilar s. [TA], s. basilar da ponte. SIN basilar pontine s.
s. basila'ris [TA], s. basilar da ponte. SIN basilar pontine s.
basilar pontine s., s. basilar da ponte; sulco mediano, na superfície ventral da ponte, no qual se situa a artéria basilar. SIN basilar s. [TA], s. basilaris [TA].
s. bicipita'lis latera'lis [TA], s. bicipital lateral da região braquial. SIN lateral bicipital groove.
s. bicipita'lis media'lis [TA], s. bicipital medial da região braquial. SIN medial bicipital groove.
s. bicipitalis radialis, s. bicipital lateral da região braquial; *termo oficial alternativo para lateral bicipital groove.
s. bicipitalis ulnaris, s. bicipital medial da região braquial; *termo oficial alternativo para medial bicipital groove.
s. bulbopontis [TA], s. bulbopontino. SIN medullopontine s.
calcaneal s. [TA], s. do calcâneo; o sulco na parte superior do calcâneo que, com um sulco correspondente no tálus, forma o seio do tarso. SIN s. calcanei [TA], interosseous groove of calcaneus, interosseous groove (1).
s. calca'nei [TA], s. do calcâneo. SIN calcaneal s.
calcarine s. [TA], s. calcarino; fissura profunda, na face medial do córtex cerebral, que se estende sobre a linha arqueada do istmo do giro fornicado para trás até o pólo occipital, marcando a borda entre o giro lingual, abaixo, e o cúneo, acima. O córtex na profundidade do sulco corresponde ao meridiano horizontal da metade contralateral do campo visual. SIN s. calcarinus [TA], calcarine fissure, fissura calcarina, posthippocampal fissure.
s. calcari'nus [TA], s. calcarino. SIN calcarine s.
callosal s., s. do corpo caloso. SIN s. of corpus callosum.
callosomarginal s., s. do cíngulo. SIN cingulate s.
s. callosomargina'lis, s. do cíngulo. SIN cingulate s.
s. carot'icus [TA], s. carótico. SIN cavernous groove.
carotid s., s. carótico. SIN cavernous groove.
s. car'pi [TA], s. do carpo. SIN carpal groove.

central s. [TA], s. central; fissura em forma de duplo S que se estende obliquamente para cima e para trás, na superfície lateral de cada hemisfério cerebral, no limite entre os lobos frontal e parietal. SIN s. centralis [TA], fissure of Rolando.
central s. of insula [TA], s. central da ínsula; sulco que atravessa o córtex insular e o divide numa parte anterior, os giros curtos, e numa parte posterior, os giros longos. SIN s. centralis insulae [TA].
s. centra'lis [TA], s. central. SIN central s.
s. centralis insulae [TA], s. central da ínsula. SIN central s. of insula.
cerebellar sulci, fissuras do cerebelo; sulcos entre as folhas do cerebelo.
cerebral sulci [TA], sulcos do cerebelo; os sulcos entre os giros ou convoluções cerebrais. SIN sulci cerebri [TA].
sul'ci cer'ebri [TA], sulcos do cérebro. SIN cerebral sulci.
chiasmatic s., s. pré-quiasmático. SIN prechiasmatic s.
cingulate s. [TA], s. do cíngulo; fissura, na superfície mesial do hemisfério cerebral, que delimita a superfície superior do giro do cíngulo (convolução calosa); a parte anterior é denominada parte subfrontal; a parte posterior, que se curva para cima até a margem súpero-medial do hemisfério e forma uma borda com o lóbulo paracentral posteriormente, é o ramo marginal. SIN s. cinguli [TA], calloso-marginal fissure, callosomarginal s., s. callosomarginalis, s. of cingulum.
s. cin'guli [TA], s. do cíngulo. SIN cingulate s.
s. of cingulum, s. do cíngulo. SIN cingulate s.
circular s. of insula [TA], s. circular da ínsula; fissura semicircular que separa a ínsula dos opérculos acima, abaixo e atrás. SIN s. circularis insulae [TA], circular s. of Reil, limiting s. of Reil.
s. circula'ris in'sulae [TA], s. circular da ínsula. SIN circular s. of insula.
circular s. of Reil, s. circular de Reil. SIN circular s. of insula.
collateral s. [TA], s. colateral; fissura sagital longa e profunda, sobre a superfície inferior do lobo temporal, marcando a borda entre o giro occipitotemporal lateral, lateralmente, e os giros hipocampal e lingual, medialmente; a grande profundidade do sulco colateral resulta em abaulamento do assoalho do corno occipital e temporal do ventrículo lateral, a eminência colateral. SIN occipitotemporal s. [TA], s. collateralis [TA], s. occipitotemporalis [TA], collateral fissure, fissura collateralis.
s. collatera'lis [TA], s. colateral. SIN collateral s.
s. corona'rius [TA], s. coronário. SIN coronary s.
coronary s. [TA], s. coronário; sulco, na superfície externa do coração, que marca a divisão entre os átrios e os ventrículos. SIN s. coronarius [TA], atrioventricular groove, atrioventricular s., auriculoventricular groove, coronary groove.
s. cor'poris callo'si [TA], s. do corpo caloso. SIN s. of corpus callosum.
s. of corpus callosum [TA], s. do corpo caloso; fissura entre o corpo caloso e o giro do cíngulo. SIN s. corporis callosi [TA], callosal s.
s. cos'tae [TA], incisuras costais. SIN costal groove.
s. costae arte'riae subcla'viae, s. da artéria subclávia da primeira costela. SIN. groove of first rib for subclavian artery.
costophrenic s., s. costofrênico; o recesso entre as costelas e a parte mais lateral do diafragma, parcialmente ocupado pela parte mais caudal do pulmão; observado em radiografias como ângulo costofrênico.
s. cru'ris heli'cis [TA], s. do ramo da hélice. SIN groove of crus of helix.
sul'ci cu'tis [TA], sulcos da pele. SIN skin sulci.
dorsal intermediate s., s. intermédio posterior da medula espinal. SIN posterior intermediate s.
dorsal median s., s. mediano posterior da medula oblonga; *termo oficial alternativo para posterior median s. of medulla oblongata.
dorsolateral s., s. póstero-lateral; *termo oficial alternativo para posterolateral s.
s. ethmoida'lis [TA], s. etmoidal. SIN ethmoidal groove.
external spiral s., s. espiral externo do labirinto vestibular. SIN outer spiral s.
fimbriodentate s. [TA], s. fibriodentado; sulco superficial entre as fímbrias e o giro dentado do hipocampo. SIN s. fibriodentatus [TA].
s. fimbriodenta'tus [TA], s. fibriodentado. SIN fimbriodentate s.
s. fronta'lis infe'rior [TA], s. frontal inferior. SIN inferior frontal s.
s. fronta'lis me'dius, s. frontal médio. SIN middle frontal s.
s. fronta'lis supe'rior [TA], s. frontal superior. SIN superior frontal s.
s. frontomargina'lis, s. frontomarginal. VER middle frontal s.
gingival s. [TA], s. gengival; espaço entre a superfície do dente e a gengiva livre. SIN s. gingivalis [TA], gingival crevice, gingival groove, gingival space, subgingival space.
s. gingiva'lis [TA], s. gengival. SIN gingival s.
gingivobuccal s., s. alveolobucal. SIN alveolobuccal groove.
gingivolabial s., s. alveololabial. SIN alveololabial groove.
gingivolingual s., s. gengivolingual. SIN alveololingual groove.
s. glu'teus [TA], s. glúteo. SIN gluteal fold.
s. for greater palatine nerve, s. palatino maior. SIN greater palatine groove.
habenular s. [TA], s. habenular; pequeno sulco localizado entre o trígono habenular e o tálamo dorsal adjacente. SIN s. habenularis.

s. habenularis, s. habenular. SIN habenular s.
s. ham'uli pterygoi'dei [TA], s. do hâmulo pterigóideo. SIN groove for pterygoid hamulus.
hippocampal s. [TA], s. hipocampal; sulco superficial entre o giro dentado e para-hipocampal; os remanescentes de uma fissura que se estendem profundamente no hipocampo, entre o corno de Ammon e o giro dentado, sofrendo obliteração durante o desenvolvimento fetal. SIN s. hippocampalis [TA], dentate fissure, fissura dentata, fissura hippocampi, hippocampal fissure.
s. hippocam'palis [TA], s. hipocampal. SIN hippocampal s.
hypothalamic s. [TA], s. hipotalâmico; sulco na parede lateral do terceiro ventrículo, de cada lado, que se estende do forame interventricular até a abertura do aqueduto do mesencéfalo; limite demarcado por sulco entre o tálamo dorsal e o hipotálamo. SIN s. hypothalamicus [TA], Monro s.
s. hypothalam'icus [TA], s. hipotalâmico. SIN hypothalamic s.
inferior frontal s. [TA], s. frontal inferior; fissura sagital, na superfície convexa lateral de cada lobo frontal do cérebro, que demarca o meio a partir do giro frontal inferior. SIN s. frontalis inferior [TA].
inferior petrosal s., s. do seio petroso inferior. SIN groove for inferior petrosal sinus.
inferior temporal s. [TA], s. temporal inferior; sulco, na face basilar do lobo temporal, que separa o giro occipitotemporal lateral do giro temporal inferior em sua face lateral. SIN s. temporalis inferior [TA], Clevenger fissure.
s. infraorbita'lis [TA], s. infra-orbital. SIN infraorbital groove.
infrapalpebral s., s. infrapalpebral; cavidade ou sulco abaixo da pálpebra inferior. SIN s. infrapalpebralis.
s. infrapalpebra'lis, s. infrapalpebral. SIN infrapalpebral s.
inner spiral s. [TA], s. espiral interno do labirinto vestibular; concavidade, no assoalho do ducto coclear, formada pelo lábio do limbo vestibular suprajacente. SIN s. spiralis internus [TA], internal spiral s.
s. interme'dius ante'rior, s. intermédio anterior. SIN anterior intermediate s.
s. interme'dius poste'rior [TA], s. intermédio posterior. SIN posterior intermediate s.
internal spiral s., s. espiral interno do labirinto vestibular. SIN inner spiral s.
interparietal s., s. intraparietal. SIN intraparietal s.
intertubercular s. [TA], s. intertubercular; sulco que desce pela diáfise do úmero entre os dois tubérculos, alojando o tendão da cabeça longa do bíceps e proporcionando fixação em seu assoalho ao músculo latíssimo do dorso. SIN intertubercular groove [TA], s. intertubercularis [TA], bicipital groove*.
s. intertubercula'ris [TA], s. intertubercular. SIN intertubercular s.
s. interventricula'ris ante'rior [TA], s. interventricular anterior. SIN anterior interventricular s.
s. interventricula'ris cor'dis, s. interventricular do coração. VER anterior interventricular s., posterior interventricular s.
s. interventricula'ris poste'rior [TA], s. interventricular posterior. SIN posterior interventricular s.
intragracile s., s. fissura lunográcil; fissura entre os lóbulos paramediano e semilunar inferior do cerebelo. SIN s. intragracilis.
s. intragra'cilis, fissura lunográcil. SIN intragracile s.
intraparietal s. [TA], s. intraparietal; sulco horizontal que se estende para trás, a partir do sulco pós-central, por certa distância, a seguir dividindo-se perpendicularmente em dois ramos, de modo a formar, com o sulco pós-central, a figura da letra H. Divide o lobo parietal em lóbulos parietais superior e inferior. SIN s. intraparietalis [TA], interparietal s., intraparietal s. of Turner, Turner s.
s. intraparieta'lis [TA], s. intraparietal. SIN intraparietal s.
intraparietal s. of Turner, s. intraparietal de Turner. SIN intraparietal s.
labial s., s. labial; sulco entre o lábio e a gengiva em desenvolvimento. SIN labiodental s., lip s., primary labial groove.
labiodental s., s. labiodental. SIN labial s.
s. lacrima'lis [TA], s. lacrimal. SIN lacrimal groove.
lateral s., s. lateral do mesencéfalo; o mais profundo e mais proeminente dos sulcos corticais, que se estende da substância perfurada anterior, a princípio lateralmente, na incisura profunda entre os lobos frontal e temporal, a seguir caudal e um pouco dorsal, na face lateral do hemisfério cerebral; o giro temporal superior forma o seu banco inferior, a ínsula, o seu assoalho amplamente expandido, e os opérculos frontal e parietal, seu banco superior. O sulco é composto de três partes: um ramo posterior grande [TA] (ramus posterior [TA]), comumente denominado o sulco lateral; um ramo anterior curto [TA] (ramus posterior [TA]), localizado entre a parte orbital e a parte triangular do giro frontal inferior; e um ramo ascendente curto [TA] (ramus ascendens [TA]), localizado entre a parte triangular e a parte opercular. SIN s. lateralis [TA], fissura cerebri lateralis, lateral cerebral fissure, sylvian fissure, fissure of Sylvius.
s. latera'lis [TA], s. lateral do mesencéfalo. SIN lateral s.
lateral occipital s., s. occipital lateral; um dos vários sulcos variáveis, na face lateral do lobo occipital de cada hemisfério cerebral, delimitando as convoluções occipitais laterais. SIN s. occipitalis lateralis.
s. lim'itans [TA], s. limitante do quarto ventrículo. SIN limiting s.
s. lim'itans ventriculi quar'ti [TA], s. limitante do quarto ventrículo. SIN limiting s. of fourth ventricle.

limiting s., s. limitante; sulco longitudinal medial, na superfície interna do tubo neural, que separa as placas alar e basal. SIN s. limitans [TA].
limiting s. of fourth ventricle [TA], s. limitante do quarto ventrículo; sulco lateral que percorre toda a extensão do assoalho da fossa rombóide de cada lado da linha mediana, representando os remanescentes do sulco que demarca a placa alar (dorsal) da placa basal (ventral) do rombencéfalo embrionário; a posição do sulco indica a separação geral dos núcleos motores dos nervos cranianos (de localização medial) dos núcleos sensitivos dos nervos cranianos (de localização lateral). SIN s. limitans ventriculi quarti [TA].
limiting s. of Reil, s. limitante de Reil. SIN circular s. of insula.
lip s., s. labial. SIN labial s.
longitudinal s. of heart, s. longitudinal do coração. VER anterior interventricular s., posterior interventricular s.
lunate s., s. semilunar; pequeno sulco semilunar inconstante, na convexidade cortical, próximo ao pólo occipital, marcando a borda anterior do córtex visual ou estriado (área 17), considerado homólogo ao sulco principal do mesmo nome, que constitui uma característica mais constante do córtex cerebral em macacos e chimpanzés. SIN lunate fissure [TA], s. lunatus [TA], simian fissure.
s. luna'tus [TA], s. semilunar. SIN lunate s.
malleolar s., s. maleolar. SIN malleolar groove.
s. malleola'ris [TA], s. maleolar. SIN malleolar groove.
marginal s. [TA], ramo marginal do sulco do cíngulo; sulco de localização imediatamente caudal ao giro paracentral posterior: a parte ascendente posterior do sulco do cíngulo. SIN ramus marginalis [TA], s. marginalis [TA], marginal branch [TA] of cingulate sulcus.
s. marginalis [TA], ramo marginal do sulco do cíngulo. SIN marginal s.
s. ma'tricis un'guis, s. da matriz ungueal; sulco cutâneo no qual está situada a borda lateral da unha. SIN groove of nail matrix, vallecula unguis.
medial s. of crus cerebri, s. do nervo oculomotor no mesencéfalo. SIN oculomotor s. of mesencephalon.
s. media'lis cru'ris cer'ebri, s. do nervo oculomotor no mesencéfalo. SIN oculomotor s. of mesencephalon.
median s. of fourth ventricle [TA], s. mediano do quarto ventrículo; sulco raso na linha média, no assoalho do ventrículo. SIN s. medianus ventriculi quarti [TA].
median s. of tongue [TA], s. mediano da língua; discreta depressão longitudinal que segue para frente, na superfície dorsal da língua, a partir do forame cego, dividindo o dorso em metades direita e esquerda. SIN s. medianus linguae [TA], median groove of tongue, median longitudinal raphe of tongue, raphe linguae.
s. media'nus lin'guae [TA], s. mediano da língua. SIN median s. of tongue.
s. media'nus poste'rior medul'lae oblonga'tae [TA], s. mediano posterior da medula oblonga. SIN posterior median s. of medulla oblongata.
s. media'nus poste'rior medul'lae spina'lis [TA], s. mediano posterior da medula espinal. SIN posterior median s. of spinal cord.
s. media'nus ventric'uli quar'ti [TA], s. mediano do quarto ventrículo. SIN median s. of fourth ventricle.
medullopontine s. [TA], s. bulbopontino; sulco transverso, na face ventral do tronco cerebral, que demarca a medula oblonga da ponte e contém as raízes emergentes dos sexto, sétimo e oitavo nervos cranianos. SIN s. bulbopontis [TA].
mentolabial s., s. mentolabial; linha indistinta que separa o lábio inferior do queixo. SIN mentolabial furrow, s. mentolabialis.
s. mentolabia'lis, s. mentolabial. SIN mentolabial s.
middle frontal s., s. frontal médio; fissura sagital relativamente superficial do cérebro, que divide a convolução frontal média em partes superior e inferior; esse sulco é encontrado apenas nos seres humanos e em macacos antropóides; em sua extremidade anterior, bifurca-se, e os dois ramos distribuem-se lateralmente, constituindo o sulco frontomarginal. SIN s. frontalis medius.
middle temporal s., s. temporal médio; sulco entre o giro temporal médio e o giro temporal inferior. SIN s. temporalis medius.
s. for middle temporal artery, s. da artéria temporal média. SIN groove for middle temporal artery.
Monro s., s. de Monro. SIN hypothalamic s.
s. mus'culi subcla'vii [TA], s. do músculo subclávio na clavícula. SIN subclavian groove.
s. mylohyoi'deus [TA], s. milo-hióideo. SIN mylohyoid groove.
nasolabial s. [TA], s. nasolabial; sulco entre a asa do nariz e o lábio. SIN s. nasolabialis [TA], nasolabial groove.
s. nasolabia'lis [TA], s. nasolabial. SIN nasolabial s.
s. nervi oculomotorii [TA], s. do nervo oculomotor no mesencéfalo. SIN oculomotor s. of mesencephalon.
s. ner'vi petro'si majo'ris [TA], s. do nervo petroso maior no temporal. SIN groove for greater petrosal nerve.
s. ner'vi petro'si mino'ris [TA], s. do nervo petroso menor. SIN groove of lesser petrosal nerve.
s. ner'vi radia'lis [TA], s. do nervo radial no úmero. SIN radial groove.
s. ner'vi spina'lis [TA], s. do nervo espinal na vértebra. SIN groove for spinal nerve.
s. ner'vi ulna'ris [TA], s. do nervo ulnar no úmero. SIN groove for ulnar nerve.

nymphocaruncular s., s. ninfocaruncular; sulco entre o lábio menor e a borda do remanescente do hímen, no qual está a abertura do ducto da glândula vestibular maior de cada lado. SIN nymphohymenal s., s. nymphocaruncularis.
s. nymphocaruncula'ris, SIN nymphocaruncular s.
s. nymphohymenal, s. ninfocaruncular. SIN nymphocaruncular s.
nymphohymenal s., s. ninfocaruncular. SIN nymphocaruncular s.
s. obturato'rius [TA], s. obturatório. SIN obturator groove.
s. of occipital artery, s. da artéria occipital. SIN occipital groove.
s. occipita'lis latera'lis, s. occipital lateral. SIN lateral occipital s.
s. occipita'lis supe'rior, s. occipital superior. SIN superior occipital s.
s. occipita'lis transver'sus [TA], s. occipital transverso. SIN transverse occipital s.
occipitotemporal s. [TA], s. occipitotemporal. SIN collateral s.
s. occipitotempora'lis [TA], s. occipitotemporal. SIN collateral s.
oculomotor s. of mesencephalon [TA], s. do nervo oculomotor no mesencéfalo; sulco na parede lateral da fossa interpeduncular do mesencéfalo a partir do qual emergem as radículas do nervo oculomotor. SIN s. nervi oculomotorii [TA], medial s. of crus cerebri, s. medialis cruris cerebri, s. of the oculomotor nerve.
s. of the oculomotor nerve, s. do nervo oculomotor no mesencéfalo. SIN oculomotor s. of mesencephalon.
s. olfacto'rius [TA], s. olfatório. SIN olfactory s.
s. olfacto'rius cavi na'si [TA], s. olfatório na cavidade nasal. SIN olfactory groove of nasal cavity.
olfactory s. [TA], s. olfatório; sulco sagital, na superfície inferior ou orbital de cada lobo frontal do cérebro, demarcando o giro reto do giro orbital, recoberto, na superfície orbital, pelo bulbo e trato olfatório. SIN s. olfactorius [TA], olfactory groove.
olfactory s. of nasal cavity, s. olfatório na cavidade nasal. SIN olfactory groove of nasal cavity.
orbital sulci [TA], sulcos orbitais; diversos sulcos variáveis, de disposição irregular, que dividem a superfície inferior ou orbital de cada lobo frontal do cérebro nos giros orbitais. SIN sulci orbitales [TA].
sul'ci orbita'les [TA], sulcos orbitais. SIN orbital sulci.
outer spiral s. [TA], s. espiral externo do labirinto vestibular; concavidade na parede externa do ducto coclear, entre a proeminência espiral e o órgão espiral. SIN s. spiralis externus [TA], external spiral s.
sulci palati'ni [TA], sulcos palatinos. SIN palatine grooves, em groove.
s. palati'nus ma'jor [TA], s. palatino maior. SIN greater palatine groove.
s. palatovagina'lis [TA], s. palatovaginal. SIN palatovaginal groove.
paracentral s. [TA], s. paracentral; sulco na superfície medial do hemisfério, algumas vezes considerado como ramo do sulco do cíngulo, localizado entre as partes anteriores do lóbulo paracentral e partes mediais do giro frontal superior. SIN s. paracentralis [TA].
s. paracentralis [TA], s. paracentral. SIN paracentral s.
sul'ci paraco'lici [TA], sulcos paracólicos. SIN paracolic gutters, em gutter.
paraglenoid s., incisura anterior da orelha. SIN preauricular groove.
s. paraglenoida'lis, incisura anterior da orelha. SIN preauricular groove.
sulci paraolfactorii [TA], sulcos paraolfatórios. SIN parolfactory sulci.
parietooccipital s. [TA], s. parietoccipital; fissura muito profunda e de orientação quase vertical, na superfície medial do córtex cerebral, que marca a borda entre a parte pré-cúnea do lobo parietal e o cúneo do lobo occipital; sua parte inferior curva-se para a frente e funde-se com a extensão anterior da fissura calcarina (sulco calcarino); a grande profundidade dessa fissura combinada produz uma saliência na parede medial do corno occipital do ventrículo lateral, o calcar avis. SIN s. parieto-occipitalis [TA], fissura parietooccipitalis, parietooccipital fissure.
s. parieto-occipita'lis [TA], s. parietoccipital. SIN parietooccipital s.
s. parolfacto'rius ante'rior, s. paraolfatório anterior. SIN anterior parolfactory s.
s. parolfacto'rius poste'rior, s. paraolfatório posterior. SIN posterior parolfactory s.
parolfactory sulci [TA], sulcos paraolfatórios; pequenos sulcos encontrados na área paraolfatória localizada imediatamente rostral à lâmina terminal; com frequência, consistem nos sulcos anterior e posterior. VER TAMBÉM anterior parolfactory s. SIN sulci paraolfactorii [TA].
periconchal s., fossa anti-hélica SIN fossa antihelica.
s. for pharyngotympanic tube [TA], s. da tuba auditiva; sulco na superfície interna da borda superior da asa maior do osso esfenóide para a parte cartilagínea da tuba auditiva. SIN s. tubae auditoriae [TA], groove for auditory tube, pharyngotympanic groove, s. for auditory tube.
s. poplit'eus [TA], s. poplíteo. SIN groove for popliteus.
postcentral s. [TA], s. pós-central; sulco que demarca o pós-central dos lóbulos parietais superior e inferior. SIN s. postcentralis [TA].
s. postcentra'lis [TA], s. pós-central. SIN postcentral s.
s. poste'rior auric'ulae [TA], s. posterior da orelha. SIN posterior auricular groove.
posterior intermediate s. [TA], s. intermédio posterior da medula espinal; sulco longitudinal entre os sulcos mediano posterior e póstero-lateral da medula espinal na região cervical, separando o fascículo grácil do fascículo cuneiforme. SIN s. intermedius posterior [TA], dorsal intermediate s., posterior intermediate groove.
posterior interventricular s. [TA], s. interventricular posterior; sulco na superfície diafragmática do coração, marcando a localização do septo entre os dois ventrículos. SIN s. interventricularis posterior [TA], crena cordis (2), posterior interventricular groove.
posterior median s. of medulla oblongata [TA], s. mediano posterior da medula oblonga; sulco longitudinal que marca a linha mediana posterior da medula oblonga; contínuo abaixo com o sulco mediano posterior da medula espinal. SIN s. medianus posterior medullae oblongatae [TA], dorsal median s.*, posterior median fissure of the medulla oblongata.
posterior median s. of spinal cord [TA], s. mediano posterior da medula espinal; sulco superficial na linha mediana da superfície posterior da medula espinal. SIN s. medianus posterior medullae spinalis [TA], posterior median fissure of spinal cord.
posterior parolfactory s. [TA], s. paraolfatório posterior; sulco superficial na superfície medial do hemisfério, demarcando o giro subcaloso ou o septo pré-comissural da área paraolfatória. SIN s. parolfactorius posterior.
posterolateral s. [TA], s. póstero-lateral; sulco longitudinal, situado de cada lado do sulco mediano posterior da medula espinal, marcando a linha de entrada das raízes nervosas posteriores. SIN s. posterolateralis [TA], dorsolateral s.*, posterolateral groove.
s. posterolatera'lis [TA], s. póstero-lateral. SIN posterolateral s.
preauricular s., s. incisura anterior da orelha. SIN preauricular groove.
precentral s. [TA], s. pré-central; fissura interrompida anterior e, em geral, paralela ao sulco central, marcando a borda anterior do giro pré-central. SIN s. precentralis [TA], s. verticalis.
s. precentra'lis [TA], s. pré-central. SIN precentral s.
prechiasmatic s. [TA], s. pré-quiasmático; sulco na superfície superior do osso esfenóide, de percurso transversal entre os canais ópticos, delimitado, anteriormente, pelo limbo esfenoidal e, posteriormente, pelo tubérculo da sela; forma-se em relação ao quiasma óptico. SIN s. prechiasmaticus [TA], chiasmatic groove, chiasmatic s., optic groove.
s. prechiasma'ticus [TA], s. pré-quiasmático. SIN prechiasmatic s.
s. promonto'rii cavitatis tympanicae [TA], s. do promontório na cavidade timpânica. SIN groove of promontory of labyrinthine wall of tympanic cavity.
s. of promontory of tympanic cavity, s. do promontório na cavidade timpânica. SIN groove of promontory of labyrinthine wall of tympanic cavity.
s. of pterygoid hamulus, s. do hâmulo pterigóideo. SIN groove for pterygoid hamulus.
s. pterygopalati'nus, s. palatino maior. SIN greater palatine groove.
s. pulmona'lis [TA], s. pulmonar. SIN pulmonary groove.
pulmonary s., s. pulmonar. SIN pulmonary groove.
rhinal s. [TA], s. rinal; a continuação rostral superficial do sulco colateral que delimita a parte rostral do giro para-hipocampal do giro fusiforme ou occipitotemporal lateral. Um dos mais antigos sulcos do pálio, marca a borda entre o neocórtex e o alocortical (olfatório). SIN s. rhinalis [TA], rhinal fissure.
s. rhina'lis [TA], s. rinal. SIN rhinal s.
sagittal s., s. do seio sagital superior. SIN groove for superior sagittal sinus.
s. of sclera, s. do seio da esclera. SIN s. sclerae.
s. scle'rae [TA], s. da esclera; sulco discreto, na superfície externa do bulbo do olho, indicando a linha de união da esclera com a córnea (junção corneoescleral ou limbo da córnea). SIN scleral s., s. of sclera.
scleral s., s. da esclera. SIN s. sclerae.
sigmoid s., s. do seio sigmóide. SIN groove for sigmoid sinus.
s. si'nus petro'si inferio'ris [TA], s. do seio petroso inferior. SIN groove for inferior petrosal sinus.
s. si'nus petro'si superio'ris [TA], s. do seio petroso superior. SIN groove for superior petrosal sinus.
s. si'nus sagitta'lis superio'ris, s. do seio sagital superior. SIN groove for superior sagittal sinus.
s. si'nus sigmoi'dei [TA], s. do seio sigmóide. SIN groove for sigmoid sinus.
s. si'nus transver'si [TA], s. do seio transverso. SIN groove for transverse sinus.
skin sulci [TA], sulcos da pele; os numerosos sulcos de profundidade variável na superfície da epiderme. SIN sulci cutis [TA], skin furrows, skin grooves.
s. spino'sus, s. espinhoso. SIN stria spinosa.
s. spira'lis exter'nus [TA], s. espiral externo do labirinto vestibular. SIN outer spiral s.
s. spira'lis inter'nus [TA], s. espiral interno do labirinto vestibular. SIN inner spiral s.
subclavian s., s. da veia subclávia na primeira costela. subclávio. SIN subclavian groove.
s. subclavia'nus, s. da veia subclávia na primeira costela. SIN subclavian groove.
s. subcla'vius, s. da artéria subclávia no pulmão. SIN groove of lung for subclavian artery.
subparietal s. [TA], s. subparietal; sulco que se continua na direção do sulco do cíngulo, a partir do qual a parte marginal dessa fissura curva-se para

cima; forma o limite superior da parte posterior do giro do cíngulo. SIN s. subparietalis [TA].
s. subparieta'lis [TA], s. subparietal. SIN subparietal s.
superior frontal s. [TA], s. frontal superior; fissura sagital, na superfície superior de cada lobo frontal do cérebro, que começa a partir do sulco pré-central; forma o limite lateral da convolução frontal superior. SIN s. frontalis superior [TA].
superior longitudinal s., s. do seio sagital superior. SIN groove for superior sagittal sinus.
superior occipital s., s. occipital superior; um dos vários sulcos pequenos e variáveis que limitam os giros occipitais superiores na face superior do lobo occipital do cérebro. SIN s. occipitalis superior.
superior petrosal s., s. do seio petroso superior. SIN groove for superior petrosal sinus.
superior temporal s. [TA], s. temporal superior; sulco longitudinal que separa os giros temporais superior e médio. SIN s. temporalis superior [TA], superior temporal fissure.
supraacetabular s., s. supra-acetabular. SIN supra-acetabular groove.
s. supraacetabula'ris [TA], s. supra-acetabular. SIN supra-acetabular groove.
talar s., s. do tálus. SIN s. tali.
s. ta'li [TA], s. do tálus; sulco na superfície inferior do tálus que, juntamente com um sulco correspondente no calcâneo, forma o seio do tarso. SIN interosseous groove of talus, interosseus groove (2), talar s.
sul'ci tempora'les transver'si, sulcos temporais transversos. SIN transverse temporal s.
s. tempora'lis infe'rior [TA], s. temporal inferior. SIN inferior temporal s.
s. tempora'lis me'dius, s. temporal médio. SIN middle temporal s.
s. tempora'lis supe'rior [TA], s. temporal superior. SIN superior temporal s.
s. temporalis transversus [TA], s. temporal transverso. SIN transverse temporal s.
s. ten'dinis mus'culi fibula'ris lon'gi [TA], s. do tendão do músculo fibular longo. SIN groove for tendon of fibularis longus.
s. ten'dinis mus'culi flexo'ris hal'lucis lon'gi [TA], s. do tendão do músculo flexor longo do hálux. SIN groove for tendon of flexor hallucis longus.
s. ten'dinis mus'culi perone'i lon'gi, s. do tendão do músculo fibular longo; (1) *termo oficial alternativo para groove for tendon of fibularis longus; (2) sulco distal à tuberosidade do osso cubóide.
terminal s. [TA], s. terminal. SIN s. terminalis.
s. terminalis cordis [TA], s. terminal do coração; sulco, na superfície do átrio direito do coração, marcando a junção do seio venoso primitivo com o átrio. SIN s. terminalis atrii dextri [TA].
s. termina'lis [TA], s. terminal; sulco que demarca a extremidade de uma estrutura (e, em geral, o início de outra). SIN terminal s. [TA].
s. terminalis atrii dextri [TA], s. terminal do coração. SIN s. terminalis cordis.
s. terminalis linguae [TA], s. terminal da língua. SIN terminal s. of tongue.
terminal s. of tongue [TA], s. terminal da língua; sulco em forma de V cujo ápice aponta para trás, na superfície da língua, marcando a separação entre as partes anterior (oral ou horizontal) e posterior (faríngea ou vertical). SIN s. terminalis linguae [TA].
tonsillolingual s., s. tonsilolingual; o espaço entre a tonsila palatina e a língua.
transverse occipital s., s. occipital transverso; ramo vertical posterior do sulco intraparietal. SIN s. occipitalis transversus [TA].
s. for transverse sinus, s. do seio transverso. SIN groove for transverse sinus.
transverse temporal s. [TA], s. temporal transverso; sulco superficial que demarca os giros temporais transversos na superfície opercular do giro temporal superior. Esse sulco em geral consiste em mais de um sulco, dependendo da configuração exata do giro (giros) temporais transversos. SIN s. temporalis transversus [TA], sulci temporales transversi.
s. tu'bae auditoriae [TA], s. da tuba auditiva. SIN s. for pharyngotympanic tube.
Turner s., s. de Turner. SIN intraparietal s.
tympanic s. [TA], s. timpânico; sulco na face interna da parte timpânica do osso temporal, no qual se fixa a membrana do tímpano. SIN s. tympanicus [TA], tympanic groove.
s. tympan'icus [TA], s. timpânico. SIN tympanic s.
s. of umbilical vein, s. da veia umbilical; sulco, no fígado fetal, ocupado pela veia umbilical. SIN s. venae umbilicalis.
s. for vena cava [TA], s. da veia cava no fígado; sulco na superfície posterior do fígado, entre o lobo caudato e o lobo direito, que dá passagem à veia cava inferior. SIN s. venae cavae [TA], fossa venae cavae, groove for inferior venae cava.
s. ve'nae ca'vae [TA], s. da veia cava no fígado. SIN s. for vena cava.
s. ve'nae ca'vae crania'lis, s. da veia cava. SIN groove for superior vena cava.
s. ve'nae subcla'viae [TA], s. da veia subclávia na primeira costela. SIN groove for subclavian vein.
s. ve'nae umbilica'lis [TA], s. da veia umbilical. SIN s. of umbilical vein.
sul'ci veno'si [TA], sulcos venosos. SIN venous grooves, em groove.
s. ventra'lis, fissura mediana anterior da medula espinal. SIN anterior median fissure of spinal cord.

ventrolateral s., s. ântero-lateral da medula espinal; *termo oficial alternativo para anterolateral s.
s. for vertebral artery, s. da artéria vertebral. SIN groove for vertebral artery.
s. vertica'lis, s. pré-central. SIN precentral s.
vomeral s., s. do vômer. SIN vomerine groove.
s. vomera'lis, s. do vômer. SIN vomerine groove, vomerine groove.
s. vo'meris [TA], s. do vômer. SIN vomerine groove.
s. vomerovagina'lis [TA], s. vomerovaginal. SIN vomerovaginal groove.

△ **sulf-, sulfo-**. Sulf-, sulfo-. 1. Prefixo que indica que o composto a cujo nome está ligado contém um átomo de enxofre. Trata-se da grafia preferida pela *American Chemical Society* (em lugar de sulph-, sulpho-) que foi adotada pela USP e NF, mas não pela BP. 2. Prefixo do ácido sulfônico ou sulfonato.
sul·fa (sŭl'fă). Sulfa; designa os fármacos à base de sulfa ou sulfonamidas.
sul·fa·benz·am·ide (sŭl-fă-ben'ză-mīd). Sulfabenzamida; antimicrobiano do grupo das sulfonamidas. SIN N-sulfanylbenzamide.
sul·fa·cet·a·mide (sŭl-fă-set'ă-mīd). Sulfacetamida; agente antibacteriano do grupo das sulfonamidas, primariamente de uso tópico; a s. sódica tem as mesmas aplicações que a sulfacetamida e também é utilizada localmente para infecções oculares e na profilaxia da oftalmia gonorreica em recém-nascidos. SIN N-sulfanylacetamide.
sulf·ac·id (sŭlf - as'id). Sulfácido. SIN thioacid.
sul·fa·cy·tine (sŭl - fă - sī'tēn). Sulfacitina; sulfonamida utilizada como antibiótico oral no tratamento de infecções do trato urinário.
sul·fa·di·a·zine (sŭl - fă - dī'ă - zēn). Sulfadiazina; um de um grupo de derivados diazina da sulfanilamida, o análogo pirimidínico da sulfapiridina e do sulfatiazol; um dos componentes da mistura de sulfonamida tripla. Trata-se de um inibidor da síntese de ácido fólico das bactérias que tem sido bastante efetivo contra infecções pneumocócicas, estafilocócicas e estreptocócicas, contra infecções causadas por *Escherichia coli* e *Klebsiella pneumoniae*, e no tratamento da artrite gonocócica aguda; a sulfadiazina sódica tem os mesmos usos.
sul·fa·di·me·thox·ine (sŭl'fă - dī - mē - thok'sēn). Sulfadimetoxina; sulfonamida de ação longa, que sofre rápida absorção após administração oral e é lentamente excretada pelo rim; acumula-se no tecido e exige doses menores do que as outras sulfonamidas para atingir concentrações teciduais efetivas.
sul·fa·dim·i·dine (sŭl - fă - dim'i - dēn). Sulfadimidina. SIN sulfamethazine.
sul·fa·dox·ine (sŭl - fă - dok'sēn). Sulfadoxina; sulfonamida de ação longa, utilizada com quinina e pirimetamina para reduzir a taxa de recidiva da malária. SIN sulformethoxine.
sul·fa·eth·i·dole (sŭl - fă - eth - i - dōl). Sulfaetidol; sulfonamida utilizada no tratamento de infecções sistêmicas e do trato urinário.
sul·fa·fur·a·zole (sŭl - fă - fūr'ă - zōl). Sulfafurazol. SIN sulfisoxazole.
sul·fa·gua·ni·dine (sŭl - fă - gwahn'i - dēn). Sulfaguanidina; o derivado guanidina da sulfanilamida. É pouco absorvida pelo trato gastrointestinal; útil para infecções bacterianas do trato intestinal inferior e para esterilização pré-operatória do trato intestinal; bociógeno. SIN sulfaguine.
sul·fa·guine (sŭl'fă - guīn). Sulfaguinidina. SIN sulfaguanidine.
sul·fa·lene (sŭl'fă - lēn). Sulfaleno; sulfonamida de ação muito longa que aumenta, como o fazem outras sulfonamidas e sulfonas, a eficácia de agentes antimaláricos, como pirimetamina, cloroguanida ou cicloguanil.
sul·fa·mer·a·zine (sŭl - fă - mer'ă - zēn). Sulfamerazina; um dos componentes das misturas de sulfonamida triplas.
sul·fa·me·ter (sŭlf'ă - mē - ter). Sulfâmetro; sulfonamida excretada lentamente, outrora utilizada no tratamento de infecções agudas e crônicas do trato urinário. SIN sulfamethoxydiazine.
sul·fa·meth·a·zine (sŭl - fă - meth'ă - zēn). Sulfametazina; um dos componentes da mistura de sulfonamida tripla. SIN sulfadimidine.
sul·fa·meth·i·zole (sŭl - fă - meth'i - zōl). Sulfametizol; sulfonamida útil no tratamento de infecções do trato urinário, em virtude de sua alta solubilidade.
sul·fa·meth·ox·a·zole (sŭl'fă - meth - ok'să - zōl). Sulfametoxazol; sulfonamida quimicamente relacionada ao sulfisoxazol, com espectro antibacteriano semelhante, porém com absorção mais lenta pelo trato gastrointestinal e excreção urinária.
sul·fa·me·thox·y·di·a·zine (sŭl'fă - me - thok'si - dī'ă - zēn). Sulfametoxidiazina. SIN sulfameter.
sul·fa·me·thox·y·py·rid·a·zine (sŭl'fă - me - thok'si - pi - rid'ă - zēn). Sulfametoxipiridazina; sulfonamida de ação longa que exige uma única dose diária para manter concentrações teciduais eficazes. A sulfametoxipiridazina acetil é uma preparação apropriada para uso pediátrico, uma vez que é insípida; é também utilizada para aumentar as ações da quinina e de outros agentes supressores na farmacoprofilaxia da malária.
sul·fa·mox·ole (sŭl - fă - mok'sōl). Sulfamoxol; agente antimicrobiano do grupo das sulfonamidas.
p-sul·fa·myl·ac·e·tan·il·ide (sŭl'fă - mil - as - e - tan'il - īd). p-sulfamilacetanilida. SIN N^4-acetylsulfanilamide.
sul·fa·nil·a·mide (sŭl - fă - nil'ă - mīd). Sulfanilamida; a primeira sulfonamida utilizada pelo seu efeito farmacoterápico em infecções causadas por alguns estrep-

tococos β-hemolíticos, meningococos, gonococos, *Clostridium welchii* e em certas infecções do trato urinário, especialmente aquelas causadas por *Escherichia coli* e *Proteus vulgaris*, sendo menos efetiva que a sulfapiridina no tratamento de infecções pneumocócicas, estafilocócicas e por *Klebsiella pneumoniae*. As manifestações tóxicas incluem acidose, cianose, anemia hemolítica e agranulocitose.

N-sul·fan·i·lyl·ac·et·a·mide (sŭl-fan′i-lil-ă-set′ă-mīd). *N*-sulfanililacetamida. SIN sulfacetamide.

N-sul·fan·i·lyl·benz·a·mide (sŭl-fan′i-lil-ben′ză-mīd). *N*-sulfanililbenzamida. SIN sulfabenzamide.

sul·fa·phen·a·zole (sŭl-fa-fen′ă-zōl). Sulfafenazol; sulfonamida de ação longa que sofre rápida absorção após administração oral; é suficiente uma dose para manter concentrações teciduais efetivas durante 24 horas.

sul·fa·pyr·a·zine (sŭl-fă-pir′ă-zēn). Sulfapirazina; agente antibacteriano do grupo das sulfonamidas.

sul·fa·pyr·i·dine (sŭl-fă-pir′i-dēn). Sulfapiridina; agente antibacteriano do grupo das sulfonamidas.

sul·fa·sal·a·zine (sŭl-fă-sal′ă-zēn). Sulfassalazina; sulfonamida (composto ácido-azossulfa) com acentuada afinidade pelos tecidos conjuntivos, especialmente aqueles ricos em elastina, utilizada na colite ulcerativa crônica; sofre decomposição no organismo a ácido aminossalicílico e sulfapiridina. SIN salicylazosulfapyridine.

sul·fa·tase (sŭl′fă-tās). Sulfatase. **1.** Nome trivial de enzimas no grupo EC 3.1.6, as hidrolases de éster sulfúrico, que catalisam a hidrólise de ésteres sulfúricos (sulfatos) nos álcoois correspondentes e sulfato inorgânico; inclui as aril-, esterol-, glicol-, condroitina-, colina-, celulose-, cerobrosídeo- e condrosulfatases. **2.** SIN arylsulfatase.
multiple s. deficiency, deficiência múltipla de s.; distúrbio hereditário (autossômico recessivo) caracterizado por falha na hidrolisação de sulfatídeos e mucopolissacarídeos sulfatados; essa deficiência leva a seu acúmulo nos tecidos neurais e extraneurais, causando desmielinização, sulfatidúria, dismorfismo facial e esquelético, etc.

sul·fate (sŭl′fāt). Sulfato; sal ou éster do ácido sulfúrico.
acid s., s. ácido. SIN bisulfate.
active s., s. ativo. SIN adenosine 3′-phosphate 5′-phosphosulfate.
s. adenylyltransferase, s. adenililtransferase; enzima que catalisa uma etapa na via de síntese de sulfato ativo; a enzima atua na reação do ATP com sulfato, produzindo pirofosfato e adenosina 5′-fosfossulfato (APS). SIN ATP sulfurylase.
codeine s., s. de codeína; sal hidrossolúvel da codeína, freqüentemente utilizado em formas farmacêuticas sólidas. Também utilizado em preparações antitussígenas, nas quais o fármaco suprime o reflexo da tosse.
dermatan s., s. de dermatan; anticoagulante com propriedades semelhantes à heparina, que compartilha com esta uma estrutura de mucopolissacarídeo sulfatado; polímero de repetição de ácido L-idurônico e *N*-acetil-D-galactosamina. Ocorre *O*-sulfação de resíduos de ácido idurônico na posição C-2 e de resíduos de galactosamina nas posições C-4 e C-6 em graus variáveis. SIN chondroitin sulfate B.
iron s., s. de ferro; sal solúvel de ferro, freqüentemente utilizado como suplemento de ferro em comprimidos e preparações líquidas como hematínico. SIN ferrous sulfate.
polysaccharide s. esters, ésteres de sulfato de polissacarídeos; ésteres de sulfato de polissacarídeos freqüentemente encontrados nas paredes celulares.

sul·fa·thi·a·zole (sŭl-fă-thī′ă-zōl). Sulfatiazol; agente antibacteriano do grupo das sulfonamidas.

sul·fa·ti·dates (sŭl′fă-ti-dāts). Sulfatidatos. SIN sulfatides.

sul·fa·tides (sŭl′fă-tīdz). Sulfatidos; ésteres sulfúricos de cerebrosídeos contendo um ou mais grupamentos sulfato na porção açúcar da molécula. SIN sulfatidates.

sul·fa·ti·do·sis (sŭl′fă-ti-dō′sis) [MIM*272200]. Sulfatidose; combinação de leucodistrofia metacromática e mucopolissacaridose causadas pela deficiência de enzimas sulfatases, como arilsulfatases A, B e C e esteróides sulfatases; caracterizada por traços faciais grosseiros, ictiose, hepatoesplenomegalia e anormalidades esqueléticas, com excreção urinária aumentada de sulfatos de dermatan e heparan; herança autossômica recessiva. VER TAMBÉM metachromatic *leukodystrophy*.

sul·fa·tion (sŭl-fā′shŭn). Sulfatização; adição de grupos sulfato na forma de ésteres a moléculas preexistentes.

sulf·he·mo·glo·bin (sŭlf-hē′mō-glō-bin). Sulfemoglobina. SIN sulfmethemoglobin.

sulf·he·mo·glo·bi·ne·mia (sŭlf-hē′mō-glō-bi-nē′mē-ă). Sulfemoglobinemia; condição mórbida decorrente da presença de sulfemoglobina no sangue; caracterizada por cianose persistente, apesar de o hemograma não revelar qualquer anormalidade especial; acredita-se que seja causada pela ação do sulfeto de hidrogênio absorvido do intestino.

sulf·hy·drate (sŭlf-hī′drāt). Sulfidrato; composto (hidrossulfeto) contendo o íon HS⁻. SIN sulfohydrate.

sulf·hy·dryl (SH) (sŭlf-hī′dril). Sulfidrila; o radical –SH contido na glutationa, cisteína, coenzima A, lipoamida (todas no estado reduzido) e nos mercaptanos (R–SH). SIN thiol.

sul·fide (sŭl′fīd). Sulfeto; composto de enxofre em que este possui uma valência de −2; p. ex., Na₂S, HgS; além disso, trata-se de um tioéter (isto é, R–S–R′, como a lantionina). SIN sulfuret.

sul·fi·ki·nase (sŭl′fi-kīn′ās). Sulficinase, sulfiquinase. SIN sulfotransferase.

sul·fin·di·got·ic ac·id (sŭl′fin-dī-got′ik). Ácido sulfindigótico; formado pela ação do ácido sulfúrico sobre o índigo, uma reação que também produz índigo carmim.

sul·fin·py·ra·zone (sŭl-fin-pir′ă-zōn). Sulfimpirazona; analgésico e agente uricosúrico, útil na gota, que promove a excreção de ácido úrico, provavelmente ao interferir na reabsorção tubular de ácido úrico.

β-sul·fi·nyl·py·ru·vic ac·id (sŭl′fi-nil-pī-roo′vik). Ácido β-sulfinilpirúvico; produto intermediário do catabolismo da L-cisteína nos tecidos de mamíferos.

sul·fi·so·mi·dine (sŭl-fi-sō′mi-dēn). Sulfisomidina; isômero estrutural da sulfametazina utilizado no tratamento de infecções sistêmicas e do trato urinário.

sul·fi·sox·a·zole (sŭl-fi-sok′să-zōl). Sulfissoxazol; sulfonamida utilizada principalmente em infecções bacterianas do trato urinário. SIN sulfafurazole.
s. diolamine, s. diolamina; o sal 2,2′-iminodietanol do sulfissoxazol; utilizado por via intravenosa, subcutânea ou intramuscular.

sul·fite (sŭl′fīt). Sulfito; sal do ácido sulfuroso; elevado nos casos de deficiência do co-fator molibdênio.
s. dehydrogenase, s. desidrogenase; óxido redutase que catalisa a reação do sulfeto com 2–ferricitocromo *c* e água, produzindo sulfato e 2–ferrocitocromo *c*.
s. oxidase, s. oxidase; óxido redutase (hemoproteína) hepática, que catalisa a reação do íon sulfeto inorgânico com O₂ e água para produzir íons sulfato e H₂O₂; observa-se menor atividade dessa enzima nos casos de deficiência do co-fator molibdênio.
s. reductase, s. redutase; óxido redutase que catalisa a redução do sulfito a H₂S, utilizando algum aceptor reduzido.

sul·fi·tu·ria (sulf′it-oor-ē-ă). Sulfitúria; níveis elevados de sulfetos na urina.

sulf·met·he·mo·glo·bin (sŭlf-met-hē′mō-glō-bin). Sulfemetemoglobina; o complexo formado por H₂S (ou sulfetos) e íon férrico na metemoglobina. SIN sulfhemoglobin.

sulfo-. Sulfo-. VER sulf-.

sul·fo·ac·id (sŭl′fō-as-id). Sulfoácido. **1.** SIN thioacid. **2.** SIN sulfonic acid.

3-sul·fo·al·a·nine (sŭl-fō-al′ă-nēn). 3-Sulfoalanina. SIN cysteic acid.

sul·fo·bro·mo·phtha·lein so·di·um (sŭl′fō-brō-mō-thal′ē-in). Sulfobromoftaleína sódica; derivado trifenilmetano excretado pelo fígado, utilizada em provas de função hepática, sobretudo pelas células reticuloendoteliais. SIN bromosulphthalein, bromsulphthalein.

sul·fo·cy·a·nate (sŭl-fō-sī′ă-nāt). Sulfocianato. SIN thiocyanate.

sul·fo·cy·an·ic ac·id (sŭl-fō-sī-an′ik) Ácido sulfociânico. SIN thiocyanic acid.

S-sul·fo·cys·teine (sŭl-fō-sis′tē-ēn). *S*-sulfocisteína; derivado sulfatado da cisteína, cujos níveis estão elevados em indivíduos com deficiência do co-fator molibdênio.

3-sul·fo·ga·lac·to·syl·cer·a·mide. 3-Sulfogalactosilceramida; sulfatido que se acumula em indivíduos com leucodistrofia metacromática.

sul·fo·gel (sŭl′fō-jel). Sulfogel; hidrogel com ácido sulfúrico em lugar de água como meio de dispersão.

sul·fo·hy·drate (sŭl-fō-hī′drāt). Sulfoidrato. SIN sulfhydrate.

sul·fo·ki·nase (sŭl′fō-kīn-ās). Sulfocinase; sulfoquinase. SIN sulfotransferase.

sul·fol·y·sis (sul-fol′i-sis). Sulfólise; lise produzida ou acelerada pelo ácido sulfúrico.

sul·fo·mu·cin (sŭl-fō-mū′sin). Sulfomucina; mucina que contém ésteres sulfúricos em seus mucopolissacarídeos ou glicoproteínas.

sul·fo·myx·in so·di·um (sŭl-fō-mik′sin). Sulfomixina sódica; mistura de polimixina B sulfometilada e bissulfeto de sódio; agente antibacteriano.

sul·fon·a·mides (sŭl-fon′ă-mīdz). Sulfonamidas; as sulfas, um grupo de drogas bacteriostáticas que contêm o grupamento sulfanilamida (sulfanilamida, sulfapiridina, sulfatiazol, sulfadiazina e outros derivados da sulfanilamida).

sul·fo·nate (sŭl′fō-nāt). Sulfonato; sal ou éster do ácido sulfônico.

sul·fone (sŭl-fōn). Sulfona; composto com estrutura geral R′–SO₂–R″.

sul·fon·ic ac·id (sŭl-fon′ik). Ácido sulfônico; qualquer um dos compostos em que um átomo de hidrogênio de um grupamento CH é substituído pelo grupamento do ácido sulfônico, –SO₃H; fórmula geral: R–SO₃H. SIN sulfoacid (2).

sul·fo·ni·um salts (sŭl-fō′nē-um). Sais de sulfônio; compostos que contêm enxofre ligado de forma covalente a três componentes; por exemplo, RS⁺(R′)R‴, como *S*-adenosil-L-metionina.

sul·fo·nyl·u·re·as (sŭl′fō-nil-ū-rē′ăz). Sulfoniluréias; derivados da isopropiltiodiazilsulfanilamida, quimicamente relacionada às sulfonamidas, que possuem ação hipoglicêmica. A essa série pertencem as seguintes drogas: acetoexamida, azepinamida, clorpropamida, flufempramida, glimidina, hidroxiexamida, heptolamida, indilamida, tioexamida, tolazamida e tolbutamida.

sul·fo·pro·tein (sŭl-fō-prō′tēn). Sulfoproteína; molécula de proteína que contém grupamentos sulfato.

6-sul·fo·qui·no·vo·syl di·ac·yl·glyc·er·ol (sūl′fō-kwī′nō-vō-sil.-kwin′ō). 6-Sulfoquinovosil diacilglicerol; quinovose contendo SO$_3$H em C-6 e um glicerol duplamente substituído em C-1; o sulfolipídio encontrado em todos os tecidos fotossintéticos.

sul·fo·rho·da·mine B (sūl-fō-rō′dă-mēn) [C.I. 45100]. Sulforrodamina B; derivado do corante xanteno, um fluorocromo utilizado para juntar proteínas por uma condensação sulfamida; empregada em imunofluorescência, isoladamente ou em combinação com isotiocianato de fluoresceína, para a detecção microscópica simultânea de dois antígenos através das cores vermelha e verde contrastantes. SIN lissamine rhodamine B 200.

sul·for·me·thox·ine (sūl′fŏr-me-thok′sēn). Sulformetoxina. SIN sulfadoxine.

sul·fo·sal·i·cyl·ic ac·id (sūl′fō-sal-i-sil′ik). Ácido sulfossalicílico; utilizado como teste para albumina e íon férrico. SIN salicylsulfonic acid.

sul·fo·sol (sūl′fō-sol). Sulfossol; hidrossol com ácido sulfúrico em lugar de água como meio de dispersão.

sul·fo·trans·fer·ase (sūl-fō-trans′fer-ās). Sulfotransferase; designação genérica de enzimas na subclasse EC 2.8.2, que catalisam a transferência de um grupamento sulfato do 3′-fosfoadenilil sulfato (sulfato ativo) para o grupamento hidroxila de um aceptor, produzindo o derivado sulfatado e 3′-fosfoadenosina 5′-fosfato. SIN sulfikinase, sulfokinase.

sulf·ox·ide (sūl-fok′sīd). Sulfóxido; o análogo sulfúrico de uma cetona, R′–SO–R′′.

sulf·ox·one so·di·um (sūl-fok′sōn). Sulfoxona sódica; antileprótico.

sul·fur (S) (sūl′fer). Enxofre; elemento de número atômico 16, peso atômico 32,066, que se combina com oxigênio para formar dióxido de enxofre (SO$_2$) e trióxido de enxofre (SO$_3$); ambos se combinam com água para formar ácidos fortes, bem como com diversos metais e elementos não-metálicos para formar sulfetos, discretamente laxativo; era utilizado no tratamento do reumatismo, da gota e da bronquite e, externamente, no tratamento de doenças cutâneas. SIN brimstone. [L. *sulfur*, enxofre]

  s. dioxide, dióxido de enxofre; SO$_2$; gás incolor não-inflamável, de odor forte e sufocante; poderoso agente redutor utilizado para evitar a deterioração oxidativa de produtos alimentares e medicinais. VER TAMBÉM sulfurous oxide.

  s. iodide, iodeto de enxofre; outrora utilizado no tratamento de determinadas doenças da pele.

  liver of s., potassa sulfurada. SIN sulfurated potash.

  precipitated s., e. precipitado; enxofre sublimado fervido com água de cal, sendo esta removida do precipitado mediante lavagem com ácido clorídrico diluído; utilizado na preparação de pomada de enxofre e no tratamento de vários distúrbios cutâneos. SIN lac sulfuris, milk of sulfur.

  roll s., pedra de enxofre; enxofre sublimado fundido e moldado em moldes cilíndricos; algumas vezes denominado *brimstone*.

  soft s., e. mole; forma alotrópica obtida por gotejamento de enxofre fundido muito quente em água; possui temporariamente consistência viscosa ou cérea.

  sublimed s., e. sublimado; utilizado no preparo de pomada de enxofre e no tratamento de vários distúrbios cutâneos. SIN flowers of sulfur.

  s. trioxide, trióxido de enxofre; SO$_3$; forma ácido sulfúrico, H$_2$SO$_4$, através de sua reação com água. SIN sulfuric oxide.

  vegetable s., e. vegetal. SIN lycopodium.

  washed s., e. lavado; enxofre sublimado macerado em amônia diluída em água para remover o ácido livre; mesmas aplicações terapêuticas que o enxofre sublimado.

  wettable s., e. umedecível; enxofre preparado a partir de solução de polissulfeto de cálcio contendo um colóide protetor, como a caseína; é facilmente disperso e suspenso em água.

sul·fur-35 (^{35}S). Enxofre-35 (S^{35}); isótopo radioativo do enxofre; emissor beta com meia-vida de 87,2 dias; utilizado como marcador no estudo do metabolismo da cisteína, cistina, metionina, etc.; também utilizado para avaliar, com sulfato marcado, os volumes de líquido extracelular.

sul·fu·ret (sūl′fer-et). Sulfeto. SIN sulfide.

sul·fur group. Grupo do enxofre; os elementos enxofre, selênio e telúrio; formam ácidos dibásicos com hidrogênio e seus oxiácidos também são dibásicos.

sul·fur·ic (sūl-fū′rik). Sulfúrico; relacionado ao ácido sulfúrico.

sul·fu·ric ac·id (sūl-fūr′ik). Ácido sulfúrico; H$_2$SO$_4$; líquido incolor, quase inodoro, pesado, oleoso e corrosivo, que contém 96% de ácido absoluto; utilizado ocasionalmente como cáustico. SIN oil of vitriol.

  fuming s. a., a. sulfúrico fumegante. SIN Nordhausen s.a.

  Nordhausen s. a., a. sulfúrico de Nordhausen; ácido sulfúrico contendo gás de ácido sulfuroso em solução. SIN fuming s.a [nome dado em homenagem a *Nordhausen*, uma cidade na Saxônia onde foi preparado pela primeira vez]

sul·fu·ric ether. Éter sulfúrico. SIN diethyl ether.

sul·fu·ric ox·ide. Óxido sulfúrico. SIN *sulfur* trioxide.

sul·fu·rous (sūl′fūr-ūs). Sulfuroso; designa um composto de enxofre em que o enxofre possui valência +4, em contraste com os compostos sulfúricos nos quais apresenta valência +6 ou sulfetos (−2).

sul·fu·rous ac·id. Ácido sulfuroso; solução de dióxido de enxofre com cerca de 6% em água; utilizado principalmente como desinfetante e alvejante; tem sido utilizado externamente pelo seu efeito parasiticida em várias doenças cutâneas.

sul·fu·rous ox·ide. Óxido sulfuroso. SIN *sulfur* dioxide.

sul·fu·ryl (sūl′fūr-il). Sulfuril; o radical bivalente –SO$_2$– .

sul·fy·drate (sūl-fī′drăt). Sulfidrato; composto de SH$^-$.

sul·in·dac (sūl-in′dak). Sulindac; agente antiinflamatório não-esteróide com ações analgésica e antipirética. O sulindac é uma pró-droga que é reduzida a droga ativa.

sul·i·so·ben·zone (soo-lī′sō-ben′zōn). Sulisobenzona; protetor solar.

Sulkowitch, Hirsh W., médico norte-americano, *1906. VER S. *reagent*.

△ **sulph-, sulpho-.** Sulf-, sulfo-. VER sulf-.

sul·pir·ide (sūl′pir-īd). Sulpiridag; agente antidepressivo.

sul·thi·ame (sūl-thī′ām). Sultiame; inibe a anidrase carbônica; anticonvulsivante utilizado no tratamento da epilepsia do lobo temporal e da epilepsia do tipo grande mal com convulsões psicomotoras; pode causar ataxia, parestesias e episódios psicóticos.

Sulzberger, Marion B., dermatologista norte-americano, 1895–1983. VER Bloch-S. *disease*; syndrome; S.-Garbe *disease, syndrome*.

sum·ma·tion (sŭm-ā′shŭn). Somação; somatório; a agregação de vários impulsos ou estímulos neurais semelhantes. [L. mediev. *summatio*, de *summo*, pp. *-atus*, somar, de L. *summa*, soma]

  s. of stimuli, s. de estímulos; efeitos musculares ou neurais cumulativos produzidos pela freqüente repetição de estímulos.

Sumner, F.W., cirurgião inglês do século XX. VER S. *sign*.

sun·burn (sŭn′bern). Queimadura solar; eritema com ou sem formação de vesículas, causado pela exposição a quantidades críticas de luz ultravioleta, geralmente na faixa de 260–320 nm da luz solar (UVB). SIN erythema solare.

sun·down·ing (sŭn′down-ing). Fenômeno crepuscular; início ou exacerbação de delírio à tarde ou à noite, com melhora ou desaparecimento durante o dia; mais freqüentemente observado nos estágios intermediários e avançados de distúrbios de demência, como a doença de Alzheimer.

sun·flow·er seed oil (sŭn′flow-er). Óleo de semente de girassol; óleo das sementes de *Helianthus annuus* (família Compositae); os glicerídeos consistem principalmente nos triglicerídeos mistos, contendo, cada um deles, um ou dois radicais de ácido linoleico; utilizado como alimento e em suplementos dietéticos.

sun·screen (sŭn′skrēn). Protetor solar; produto tópico que protege a pele do eritema induzido pela luz ultravioleta e que resiste à lavagem; seu uso também diminui a formação de ceratoses solares e reduz o melanoma e outros cânceres de pele, bem como o enrugamento, induzidos pelo ultravioleta B.

sun·stroke (sŭn′strōk). Insolação. Forma de intermação resultante da exposição indevida aos raios solares, provavelmente causada pela ação dos raios actínicos em combinação com a temperatura elevada; os sintomas são aqueles da intermação, porém freqüentemente sem febre. SIN heliosis, ictus solis, insolation (2), siriasis, solar fever (2).

△ **super-.** Super-; em excesso, acima, superior ou na parte superior de; possui freqüentemente o mesmo uso que L. supra-. Cf. hyper-. [L. *super*, acima, além]

su·per·ab·duc·tion (soo-per-ab-dŭk′shŭn). Superabdução; abdução de um membro além do limite normal. SIN hyperabduction.

su·per·a·cid·i·ty (soo′per-a-sid′i-tē). Superacidez; excesso de ácido; acidez excessiva.

su·per·a·cro·mi·al (soo-per-ă-krō′mē-ăl). Supra-acromial; acima do acrômio. SIN supra-acromial.

su·per·ac·tiv·i·ty (soo-per-ak-tiv′i-tē). Superatividade, hiperatividade; atividade anormalmente grande. SIN hyperactivity (1).

su·per·a·cute (soo′per-ă-kūt′). Superagudo; extremamente agudo, caracterizado por extrema gravidade dos sintomas e rápida progressão, como na evolução de uma doença.

su·per·al·i·men·ta·tion (soo′per-al′i-men-tā′shŭn). Superalimentação, hiperalimentação. SIN hyperalimentation.

su·per·a·nal (soo-per-ā′nal). Supra-anal. SIN supra-anal.

su·per·an·ti·gen. Superantígeno; antígeno que interage com o receptor de células T num domínio fora do sítio de reconhecimento do antígeno. Essa interação induz a ativação de maior número de células T do que aquele induzido por antígenos apresentados no sítio de reconhecimento de antígeno, resultando na liberação de numerosas citocinas. VER TAMBÉM antigen.

su·per·cil·i·ary (soo-per-sil′ē-ār-ē). Supraciliar; relativo a ou na região do supercílio. SIN supraciliary.

su·per·cil·i·um, pl. **su·per·cil·ia** (soo′per-sil′ē-ŭm, -ă). Supercílio. SIN eye-brow. [L. de *super*, acima + *cilium*, pálpebra]

su·per·coil·ing. Superespiral. SIN superhelicity.

su·per·di·crot·ic (soo-per-dī-krot′ik). Superdicrótico. SIN hyperdicrotic.

su·per·dis·ten·tion (soo′per-dis-ten′shŭn). Superdistensão. SIN hyperdistention.

su·per·duct (sooper-dŭkt). Elevar ou impelir para cima. [L. *super-duco*, pp. *-ductus*, conduzir para cima]

su·per·e·go (soo-per-ē′gō). Superego; em psicanálise, um dos três componentes do aparelho psíquico na estrutura froidiana, sendo os outros dois o ego e o id. Trata-se de um produto do ego que se identificou inconscientemente com pessoas importantes, como os pais, desde o início da vida, e que resulta da incorporação dos valores e desejos dessas pessoas e, subseqüentemente, de normas sociais como parte dos próprios padrões para formar a "consciência".

su·per·e·rup·tion. Movimento de um dente além do plano normal de oclusão, devido à perda de seu antagonista.

su·per·ex·ci·ta·tion (soo-per-ek-si-tā'shŭn). Superexcitação; sobreexcitação. **1.** Ato de excitar ou de estimular indevidamente. **2.** Condição de extrema excitação ou estimulação.

su·per·ex·ten·sion (soo-per-eks-ten'shŭn). Superextensão. SIN hyperextension.

su·per·fat·ted (soo'per-fat'ed). Supergorduroso; com acréscimo de gordura adicional, como no caso do sabão.

su·per·fe·ta·tion (soo'per-fe-tā'shŭn). Superfetação; presença de dois fetos de idades diferentes, não-gêmeos, no útero, devido à implantação de dois óvulos liberados em períodos sucessivos da ovulação; conceito obsoleto. SIN hypercyesis, hipercyesia, multifetation, superimpregnation.

su·per·fi·cial (soo-per-fish'ăl) [TA]. Superficial. **1.** Rápido; não-completo. **2.** Relativo ou situado próximo à superfície. **3.** SIN superficialis. [L. *superficialis*, de *superficies*, superfície]

su·per·fi·ci·a·lis (soo'per-fish-ē-ā'lis) [TA]. Superficial; situado mais próximo da superfície do corpo em relação a um ponto de referência específico. Cf. profundus. SIN superficial (3) [TA], sublimis (2). [L.]
s. vo'lae, ramo palmar superficial da artéria radial. SIN superficial palmar *branch of radial artery.*

su·per·fi·cies (su-per-fish'ĭ-ēz). Exterior, aparência; superfície externa; fácies. [L. superfície superior, de *super*, acima + *facies*, figura, forma]

su·per·flex·ion (soo-per-flek'shŭn). Superflexão. SIN hyperflexion.

su·per·fuse (soo-per-fūs'). Superfundir; lavar a parte superior de um tecido com líquido. Cf. perfuse, perifuse.

su·per·fu·sion (soo-per-fū'zhŭn). Superfusão; ato de superfundir.

su·per·gen·u·al (soo-per-jen'ū-ăl). Acima do joelho.

su·per·hel·ic·i·ty (soo'per-hē-li'si-tē). Superenrolamento; refere-se à estrutura dupla do DNA nativo, na qual ocorre enrolamento adicional da dupla hélice. SIN supercoiling.

su·per·im·preg·na·tion (soo'per-im-preg-nā'shŭn). Superimpregnação. SIN superfetation.

su·per·in·duce (soo'per-in-doos). Superinduzir; induzir ou adicionar a algo já existente.

su·per·in·fec·tion (soo'per-in-fek'shŭn). Superinfecção; infecção nova acrescentada a outra já presente.

su·per·in·vo·lu·tion (soo'per-in-vō-loo'shŭn). Superinvolução; extrema redução no tamanho do útero após o parto, atingindo um tamanho abaixo do normal do órgão não-grávido.

su·pe·ri·or (soo-pēr'ē-ōr). Superior. **1.** Situado acima ou dirigido para cima. **2.** [NA]. Em anatomia humana, situado mais próximo do vértice da cabeça em relação a um ponto de referência específico; oposto de inferior. SIN cranial (2). [L. comparativo de *superus*, acima]

su·per·lac·ta·tion (soo'per-lak-tā'shŭn). Superlactação; continuação da lactação além do período normal. SIN hyperlactation.

su·per·lig·a·men (soo-per-lig'ă-men). Curativo de retenção; bandagem que mantém um curativo cirúrgico no lugar. [L. *ligamen*, bandagem]

su·per·me·di·al (soo-per-mē'dē-ăl). Supermedial; acima do meio de qualquer parte.

su·per·mo·til·i·ty (soo'per-mō-til'i-tē). Supermotilidade. SIN hyperkinesis.

su·per·na·tant (soo-per-nā'tănt). Sobrenadante. VER supernatant *fluid.* [super- + L. *natare*, nadar]

su·per·nu·mer·ar·y (soo-per-noo'mer-ār-ē). Supranumerário; acima do número normal. Não espectal. [super- + L. *numerus*, número]

su·per·nu·tri·tion (soo'per-noo-trish'ŭn). Supernutrição; alimentação excessiva que leva à obesidade. SIN hypernutrition.

su·per·o·lat·er·al (soo-per-ō-lat'er-ăl). Súpero-lateral; ao lado e acima.

su·per·ov·u·la·tion (soo'per-ō-vū-lā'shŭn). Superovulação; ovulação de um número de óvulos maior que o normal; em geral, constitui o resultado da administração de gonadotropinas exógenas.

su·per·ox·ide (soo-per-oks'īd). Superóxido; um radical livre de oxigênio, O_2^-, que é tóxico para as células.
s. dismutase (SOD), s. dismutase; enzima que catalisa a reação de dismutação, $2O_2^- + 2H^+ \rightarrow H_2O_2 + O_2$; existem três isoenzimas da SOD: uma forma extracelular (ECSOD), que contém cobre e zinco; uma forma citoplasmática, que também contém cobre e zinco; e uma forma mitocondrial, que contém manganês; a deficiência de SOD está associada à esclerose lateral amiotrófica.

su·per·par·a·site (soo-per-par'ă-sīt). Superparasita; membro de uma grande população de parasitas que vivem num hospedeiro, geralmente uma larva de himenóptero parasita no seu inseto hospedeiro. VER TAMBÉM parasitoid.

su·per·par·a·sit·ism (soo-per-par'ă-si-tizm). Superparasitismo. **1.** Associação entre Hymenoptera parasita e seus insetos hospedeiros. **2.** Excesso de parasitas da mesma espécie num hospedeiro, sobrecarregando o mecanismo de defesa até atingir um grau que leva a doença ou morte, em contraste com o parasitismo múltiplo.

su·per·pe·tro·sal (soo-per-pe-trō'săl). Superpetroso; acima ou na porção superior da parte petrosa do osso temporal.

su·per·sat·u·rate (soo-per-sach'ū-rāt). Supersaturar; fazer uma solução reter mais sal ou outra substância em solução do que a sua capacidade de dissolvê-lo quando em equilíbrio com esse sal na fase sólida; essas soluções são habitualmente instáveis em relação à precipitação do excesso de sal ou substância e à saturação.

su·per·scrip·tion (soo'per-skrip'shŭn). Sobrescrito; o início de uma prescrição, que consiste na injunção, *recipe,* tomar, geralmente indicada pelo sinal ℞. [L. *super-scribo,* pp. *-scriptus,* escrever sobre]

su·per·son·ic (soo'per-son'ik). Supersônico. **1.** Relativo a, ou caracterizado por, uma velocidade maior que a do som. VER TAMBÉM hypersonic. **2.** Relativo a vibrações sonoras de alta freqüência, acima do nível de audibilidade humana. VER TAMBÉM ultrasonic. [super- + L. *sonus,* som]

su·per·struc·ture (soo-per-strŭk'choor). Superestrutura; estrutura acima da superfície.
implant denture s., s. de implante da dentadura; a dentadura que é retida e estabilizada pela subestrutura de implante da dentadura.

su·per·ten·sion (soo-per-ten'shŭn). Supertensão; tensão extrema; termo utilizado incorretamente como sinônimo de pressão arterial elevada ou hiperpiese.

su·per·volt·age (soo'per-vol'tij). Supervoltagem; em radioterapia, termo descritivo para uma radiação de alta energia acima de 1.000 V.

su·pi·nate (soo'pi-nāt). Supinar. **1.** Assumir ou ser colocado em posição supina (com a face para cima) ou decúbito dorsal. **2.** Efetuar a supinação do antebraço ou do pé. [L. *supino,* pp. *-atus,* curvar-se para trás, colocar-se nas costas, de *supinus,* supino]

su·pi·na·tion (soo'pi-nā'shŭn) [TA]. Supinação; a condição de estar em posição supina; o ato de assumir ou ser colocado em posição supina.
s. of the foot, s. do pé; inversão e abdução do pé, causando elevação da borda medial.
s. of the forearm, s. do antebraço; rotação do antebraço de modo que a palma da mão esteja voltada para a frente, quando o braço está em posição anatômica, ou para cima, quando o braço está em extensão, fazendo um ângulo reto com o corpo.

su·pi·na·tor (soo'pi-nā-ter, -tōr) [TA]. Supinador. SIN supinator *(muscle).* VER supinator *(muscle),* biceps brachii *(muscle).*

su·pine (soo-pīn'). Supino. **1.** Designa o corpo quando deitado com a face para cima (decúbito dorsal). **2.** Supinação do antebraço ou do pé. [L. *supinus*]

sup·port (sŭ-pōrt'). **1.** Acrescentar na tentativa de proporcionar maior força. **2.** VER supporter. **3.** Em odontologia, termo utilizado para indicar uma resistência aos componentes verticais da força de mastigação. [L. *supporto,* conduzir]

sup·port·er (sŭ-pōrt'er). Suporte; aparelho destinado a manter no lugar uma parte pendente ou pendular, um órgão prolapsado ou uma articulação. SIN support (2). [ver support]

sup·pos·i·to·ry (sŭ-poz'i-tōr-ē). Supositório; pequeno corpo sólido de forma apropriada para fácil introdução em um dos orifícios do corpo, exceto a cavidade oral (p. ex., reto, uretra, vagina), composto de uma substância, geralmente medicinal, que é sólida em temperatura comum, mas que derrete à temperatura corporal. As bases de supositório geralmente utilizadas são o óleo de cacau, gelatina glicerinada, óleos vegetais hidrogenados, misturas de polietileno glicóis e vários pesos moleculares e ésteres de ácidos graxos do polietileno glicol. [L. *suppositorium,* de *suppositorius,* colocado sob]
glycerin s., s. de glicerina; forma posológica translúcida cônica destinada a administração retal para alívio da constipação; freqüentemente utilizado em crianças pequenas. Contém glicerina e um agente endurecedor, como estearato de sódio (sabão). A ação é produzida por lubrificação, retenção de água e irritação local.

sup·pres·sion (sŭ-presh'ŭn). Supressão. **1.** Excluir deliberadamente do pensamento consciente. Cf. repression. **2.** Parada da secreção de um líquido, como urina ou bile. Cf. retention (2). **3.** Interrupção do fluxo ou secreção anormal, como na supressão de uma hemorragia. **4.** O efeito de uma segunda mutação que suprime uma alteração fenotípica causada por uma mutação prévia num diferente ponto no cromossoma. VER epistasis. **5.** Inibição da visão em um olho quando imagens diferentes incidem em pontos correspondentes da retina. [L. subprimo (subp-), pp. *-pressus,* pressionar para baixo]
fixation s., s. por fixação; redução no nistagmo induzido ou espontâneo que ocorre com a fixação visual.
immune s., imunossupressão; supressão da resposta imune por algum composto ou agente.
intergenic s., s. intergênica. VER suppressor *mutation* (2).
intragenic s., s. intragênica. VER suppressor *mutation* (2).

sup·pres·sor (sŭ-pres'or). Supressor; composto que suprime os efeitos de mutações ou o que deveria ser uma seqüência normal de eventos.
amber s., s. âmbar; gene mutante que codifica um tRNA cujo anticódon foi alterado, de modo que o tRNA alterado também responde a códons UAG.

sup·pu·rant (sŭp′ŭr - ant). Supurativo. **1.** Que provoca ou induz supuração. **2.** Agente que exerce essa ação. [L. *suppurans*, que causa supuração]

sup·pu·rate (sŭp′yūr - āt). Supurar; formar pus. [L. *sup-puro* (*subp-*), pp. *-atus*, formar *pus* (*pur*), pus]

sup·pu·ra·tion (sŭp′yu - rā′shŭn). Supuração; formação de pus. SIN pyesis, pyogenesis, pyopoiesis, pyosis. [L. *suppuratio* (ver suppurate)]

sup·pu·ra·tive (sŭp′yūr - ā - tiv). Supurativo; que forma pus.

△ **supra-**. Supra-; posição acima da parte indicada pela palavra à qual o prefixo está unido; nesse sentido, o mesmo que super-; oposto de infra-. [L. *supra*, na face superior]

su·pra·a·cro·mi·al (soo - pră - ă - krō′me - ăl). Supra-acromial. SIN supera-cromial.

su·pra·a·nal (soo - pră - ā′năl). Supra-anal; acima do ânus. SIN superanal.

su·pra·au·ric·u·lar (soo - pră - aw - rik′u - lăr). Supra-auricular; acima da orelha.

su·pra·ax·il·lary (soo′prā - ak′si - lār′e). Supra-axilar; acima da axila.

su·pra·buc·cal (soo - prā - bŭk′ăl). Suprabucal; acima da bochecha.

su·pra·bulge (soo′prā - bŭlj). Porção da coroa de um dente que converge em direção à superfície oclusiva do dente.

su·pra·car·di·nal (soo - prā - kar′di - năl). Supracardinal; situado dorsalmente às veias cardinais anterior e posterior no embrião.

su·pra·cer·e·bel·lar (soo - prā - ser - e - bel′ar). Supracerebelar; sobre ou acima da superfície do cerebelo.

su·pra·ce·re·bral (soo - prā - ser′e - brăl, -sĕ - rē′brăl). Supracerebral; sobre ou acima da superfície do cérebro.

su·pra·cho·roid (soo - prā - kō′royd). Supracorióide; sobre a face externa da corióide do olho.

suprachoroidea. Lâmina supracorióide da esclera. SIN suprachoroid *lamina of sclera*.

su·pra·cil·i·ary (soo - prā - sil′ē - ār - e). Supraciliar. SIN superciliary.

su·pra·cla·vic·u·lar (soo - prā - kla - vik′u - lăr). Supraclavicular; acima da clavícula, referindo-se a alguns nervos cutâneos.

su·pra·cla·vic·u·lar·is (soo′prā - kla - vik′u - lār′is). Supraclavicular. VER supraclavicular *muscle*.

su·pra·con·dy·lar (soo - prā - kon′di - lăr). Supracondilar; acima de um côndilo. SIN supracondyloid.

su·pra·con·dy·loid (soo′ - prā - kon′di - loyd). Supracondilóide. SIN supracondylar.

su·pra·cos·tal (soo - prā - kos′tăl). Supracostal; acima das costelas.

su·pra·cot·y·loid (soo - prā - kot′i - loyd). Supracotilóide; acima da cavidade cotilóide ou acetábulo.

su·pra·cris·tal (soo - prā - kris′tăl). Acima de uma crista; termo especificamente utilizado para referir-se a uma linha ou plano através dos ápices das cristas ilíacas.

su·pra·di·a·phrag·mat·ic (soo - prā - dī - ā - frag - mat′ik). Supradiafragmático; acima do diafragma.

su·pra·duc·tion (soo - prā - dŭk′shŭn). Supradução; sursundução; a rotação de um olho para cima. SIN sursumduction.

su·pra·ep·i·con·dy·lar (soo - prā - ep′i - kon′di - lăr). Supra-epicondilar; acima de um epicôndilo.

su·pra·gle·noid (soo - prā - glē′noyd). Supraglenóide; acima da cavidade ou fossa glenóide.

su·pra·glot·tic (soo - prā - glot′ik). Supraglótico; acima da glote.

su·pra·glot·ti·tis (soop′ra - gla - tī′tis). Supraglotite; inflamação infecciosa e edema do tecido laríngeo acima da glote, especialmente da epiglote, que se torna vermelha e esférica, resultando em obstrução das vias aéreas superiores.

su·pra·he·pat·ic (soo - prā - he - pat′ik). Supra-hepático; acima do fígado.

su·pra·hy·oid (soo - prā - hī′oyd). Supra-hióideo; acima do osso hióide, designando, entre outras coisas, um grupo de músculos.

su·pra·in·gui·nal (soo - prā - ing′gwin - ăl). Supra-inguinal; acima da região inguinal ou virilha.

su·pra·in·tes·ti·nal (soo - prā - in - tes′ti - năl). Supra-intestinal; acima do intestino.

su·pra·lim·i·nal (soo - prā - lim′i - năl). Supraliminal; mais do que apenas perceptível; acima do limiar para a percepção consciente. Cf. subliminal. [supra- + L. *limen*, limiar]

su·pra·lum·bar (soo - prā - lŭm′bar). Supralombar; acima da região lombar.

su·pra·mal·le·o·lar (soo - prā - mal - ē - ō - lăr). Supramaleolar; acima de um maléolo.

su·pra·mam·ma·ry (soo - prā - mam′ā - rē). Supramamário; acima da glândula mamária.

su·pra·man·dib·u·lar (soo - prā - man - dib′u - lăr). Supramandibular; acima da mandíbula.

su·pra·mar·gin·al (soo - prā - mar′jin - ăl). Supramarginal; acima de qualquer margem; designa especialmente o giro supramarginal.

su·pra·mas·toid (soo - prā - mas′toyd). Supramastóideo; acima do processo mastóide do osso temporal.

su·pra·max·il·la (soo′prā - mak - sil′ā). Termo obsoleto para maxila.

su·pra·max·il·lary (soo - prā - mak′si - lăr - ē). Supramaxilar; acima da maxila.

su·pra·men·tal (soo - prā - men′tăl). Supramental; supramentoniano, supramentual; acima do queixo.

su·pra·men·ta·le (soo′prā - men - tā′le). Supramental; em cefalometria, o ponto mais posterior na linha média; acima do queixo, sobre a mandíbula, entre o infradentado e o pogônio. SIN point B. [supra- + L. *mentum*, queixo]

su·pra·na·sal (soo - prā - nā′săl). Supranasal; acima do nariz.

su·pra·neu·ral (soo - prā - noo′răl). Supraneural; acima do eixo neural.

su·pra·nu·cle·ar (soo - prā - noo′klē - er). Supranuclear; acima (cranial) do nível dos neurônios motores dos nervos espinais ou cranianos; as vias das fibras nervosas supra-segmentares seguem seu trajeto para alcançar os corpos celulares motores no tronco cerebral; quando utilizado em neurologia clínica, o termo supranuclear indica distúrbios de movimento causados por destruição ou comprometimento funcional de outras estruturas cerebrais além dos neurônios motores, como córtex motor, trato piramidal ou corpo estriado; p. ex., a paralisia supranuclear, distinta da paralisia nuclear (ou flácida ou "neurônio motor inferior") que resulta da destruição ou do comprometimento funcional dos neurônios motores e seus axônios num nervo periférico.

su·pra·oc·clu·sion (soo′prā - ō - kloo′zhŭn). Supra-oclusão; relação oclusiva que se estende além do plano de oclusão.

su·pra·or·bit·al (soo - prā - ōr′bi - tăl). Supra-orbital; acima da órbita, na face ou no crânio; designa numerosas estruturas. VER canal, foramen, notch, nerve.

su·pra·or·bi·to·me·a·tal (soo - prā - or - bit - ō - mē - at′al). Supra-orbitomeatal; acima ou no ápice de ambas as órbitas e meato acústico externo; designa uma linha ou plano.

su·pra·pa·tel·lar (soo - prā - pă - tel′ăr). Suprapatelar; acima da patela, referindo especialmente a uma bolsa.

su·pra·pel·vic (soo - prā - pel′vik). Suprapélvico; acima da pelve.

su·pra·phys·i·o·log·ic, su·pra·phys·i·o·log·i·cal (soo′prā - fiz - ē - ō - loj′ik, - loj′i - kăl). Suprafisiológico; designa qualquer dose (de um agente químico que é ou imita um hormônio, neurotransmissor ou outro agente de ocorrência natural) maior ou mais potente do que a que ocorre naturalmente, ou os efeitos dessa dose. Cf. homeopathic (2), pharmacologic (2), physiologic (4).

su·pra·pu·bic (soo - prā - pū′bik). Suprapúbico; acima do púbio.

su·pra·re·nal (soo′prā - rē′năl). Supra-renal. **1.** Acima do rim. SIN surrenal. **2.** Referente às glândulas supra-renais. [supra- + L. *ren*, rim]

su·pra·scap·u·lar (soo - prā - skap′u - lăr). Supra-escapular; acima da escápula, designando especialmente uma artéria, veia e nervo.

su·pra·scle·ral (soo - prā - sklēr′al). Supra-escleral; sobre a face externa da esclera, designando o espaço supra-escleral ou periscleral entre a esclera e a fáscia do bulbo.

su·pra·sel·lar (soo - prā - sel′ar). Supra-selar; acima da ou sobre a sela turca.

su·pra·spi·nal (soo - prā - spī′năl). Supra-espinal; acima da coluna vertebral ou de qualquer espinha.

su·pra·spi·na·lis (soo - prā - spi - nā′lis). Supra-espinal. VER supraspinalis (*muscle*).

su·pra·spi·na·tus (soo - prā - spi - nā′tŭs). Supra-espinal. VER supraspinatus (*muscle*).

su·pra·spi·nous (soo - prā - spī′nŭs). Supra-espinal; acima de qualquer espinha; especialmente acima de uma ou mais das espinhas vertebrais (p. ex., ligamento supra-espinal) ou da espinha da escápula.

su·pra·sta·pe·di·al (soo - prā - sta - pēd′ē - ăl). Supra-estapedial; acima do estribo.

su·pra·ster·nal (soo - prā - ster′năl). Supra-esternal; acima do esterno.

su·pra·syl·vi·an (soop - ra - sil′vē - an). Supra-silviano; acima da fissura de Sylvius ou sulco lateral.

su·pra·sym·phys·ary (soo - prā - sim - phiz′ā - rē). Supra-sinfisário; acima da sínfise púbica.

su·pra·tem·po·ral (soo - prā - tem′po - răl). Supratemporal; acima da região temporal.

su·pra·ten·to·ri·al (soo′prā - ten - tōr′e - ăl). Supratentorial; designa o conteúdo craniano localizado acima do tentório do cerebelo; termo freqüentemente utilizado para descrever sintomas funcionais.

su·pra·tho·rac·ic (soo - prā - thō - ras′ik). Supratorácico; acima ou na parte superior do tórax.

su·pra·ton·sil·lar (soo - prā - ton′si - lăr). Supratonsilar; acima da tonsila; designa um recesso acima e ligeiramente atrás da tonsila.

su·pra·troch·le·ar (soo - prā - trok′lē - ăr). Supratroclear; acima de uma tróclea, designando um nervo.

su·pra·tur·bi·nal (soo - prā - ter′bi - năl). Concha nasal suprema. SIN supreme nasal *concha*.

su·pra·tym·pan·ic (soo - prā - tim - pan′ik). Supratimpânico; acima da cavidade do tímpano.

su·pra·vag·i·nal (soo - prā - vaj′i - năl). Supravaginal; acima da vagina ou de qualquer bainha.

su·pra·val·var (soo-pră-val'văr). Supravalvar; acima das valvas, pulmonar ou aórtica. SIN supravalvular.
su·pra·val·vu·lar (soo-pră-val'vū-lăr). Supravalvar. SIN supravalvar.
su·pra·ven·tric·u·lar (soo-pră-ven-trik'u-lăr). Supraventricular; acima dos ventrículos; termo especialmente aplicado a ritmos que se originam de centros proximais aos ventrículos, isto é, no átrio, nodo AV ou junção AV, em contraste com os ritmos que se originam nos próprios ventrículos.
su·pra·ver·sion (soo-pră-ver'zhŭn). Supraversão. **1.** Uma volta (versão) para cima. **2.** Em odontologia, a posição de um dente quando está fora da linha de oclusão numa direção oclusiva; supermordida profunda. **3.** Em oftalmologia, rotação conjugada binocular para cima. [supra- + L. *verto*, pp. *versus*, girar]
su·pro·fen (soo-prō'fen). Suprofeno; agente antiinflamatório não-esteróide com propriedades antipiréticas e analgésicas; semelhante ao ibuprofeno.
su·ral (soo'răl). Sural; relativo à panturrilha (sura).
sur·al·i·men·ta·tion (ser-al'i-men-tā'shŭn). Superalimentação. SIN hyperalimentation. [Fr. *sur*, do L. *super*, acima]
sur·a·min so·di·um (soo'ră-min), Suramina sódica; derivado complexo da uréia; utilizada no tratamento da tripanossomíase, oncocercíase e pênfigo.
sur·face (ser'făs) [TA]. Superfície, face; a parte externa de qualquer sólido. SIN face (2) [TA], facies (2) [TA]. [F. do L. *superficius*, ver superficial]
acromial articular s. of clavicle, face articular acromial da clavícula. SIN acromial *facet of clavicle*.
anterior s. [TA], s. anterior; a superfície de uma estrutura ou parte do corpo voltada para a frente. A TA reconhece uma superfície anterior (facies anterior...) das seguintes estruturas: coração (... cordis [TA]); córnea (... corneae [TA]); corpo da maxila (... corporis maxillae [TA]); lente (... lentis [TA]); pálpebras (... palpebrae [TA]); parte petrosa do osso temporal (... pars petrosi ossis temporalis [TA]); rim (... renis [TA]); íris (... iridis [TA]); patela (... patellae [TA]); próstata (... prostatae [TA]); rádio (... radii [TA]); glândula supra-renal (... glandulae suprarenalis [TA]); ulna (... ulnae [TA]); útero (... uteri [TA]). SIN facies anterior [TA].
anterior s. of arm, s. anterior do braço. SIN anterior *region* of arm.
anterior articular s. of dens [TA], s. articular anterior do dente do áxis; a faceta articular curva na face anterior do dente do áxis que se articula com a faceta do dente do áxis do arco anterior do atlas. SIN facies articularis anterior dentis [TA].
anterior s. of cornea [TA], face anterior da córnea; a superfície externa da córnea. SIN facies anterior corneae [TA].
anterior s. of elbow, região anterior do cotovelo. SIN anterior *region* of elbow.
anterior s. of eyelids, face anterior das pálpebras. SIN *facies* anterior palpebrarum.
anterior s. of forearm, região anterior do antebraço. SIN anterior *region* of forearm.
anterior s. of iris [TA], face anterior da íris; face da íris do bulbo do olho visível através da córnea. SIN facies anterior iridis [TA].
anterior s. of kidney [TA], face anterior do rim; face do rim voltada para a cavidade abdominal. SIN facies anterior renis [TA].
anterior s. of leg, região anterior da perna. SIN anterior *region* of leg.
anterior s. of lens [TA], face anterior da lente; a face da lente do bulbo do olho que forma o limite posterior do segmento anterior preenchido com humor aquoso. SIN facies anterior lentis [TA].
anterior s. of lower limb [TA], face anterior do membro inferior; face ventral ou flexora do membro inferior. SIN facies anterior membri inferioris [TA].
anterior s. of maxilla [TA], face anterior da maxila; a superfície da maxila abaixo da órbita e lateralmente à abertura nasal. SIN facies anterior corporis maxillae [TA].
anterior s. of patella [TA], face anterior da patela; face subcutânea da patela. SIN facies anterior patellae [TA].
anterior s. of petrous part of temporal bone [TA], face anterior da parte petrosa do osso temporal; a superfície da parte petrosa do osso temporal que contribui para o assoalho da fossa craniana média. SIN facies anterior partis petrosae ossis temporalis [TA].
anterior s. of prostate [TA], s. anterior da próstata; face da próstata voltada para a sínfise púbica. SIN facies anterior prostatae [TA].
anterior s. of radius [TA], s. anterior do rádio; a face ventral do rádio, cuja maior parte fornece a fixação para o músculo flexor longo do polegar. SIN facies anterior radii [TA].
anterior s. of suprarenal gland [TA], s. anterior da glândula supra-renal; face da glândula supra-renal voltada para a cavidade abdominal. SIN facies anterior glandulae suprarenalis [TA].
anterior talar articular s. of calcaneus [TA], s. articular talar anterior do calcâneo; subjacente à cabeça do talo e contribuindo para a articulação talo-calcâneo-navicular. SIN facies articularis talaris anterior calcanei [TA].
anterior s. of thigh, região anterior da coxa. SIN anterior *region* of thigh.
anterior s. of ulna [TA], face anterior da ulna; superfície anterior da ulna. SIN facies anterior ulnae [TA].
anterior s. of uterus [TA], face anterior do útero; superfície ventral do útero; em sua posição normal (antevertido e antifletido), constitui, na realidade, uma superfície em sua maior parte inferior. SIN facies anterior uteri [TA].
anteroinferior s. of pancreas [TA], face ântero-inferior do corpo do pâncreas, a superfície do corpo do pâncreas voltada para a frente e para baixo. SIN facies anteroinferior corporis pancreatis [TA].
anterolateral s. of arytenoid cartilage [TA], face ântero-lateral da cartilagem aritenóide; das três superfícies não-articulares da cartilagem aritenóide piramidal, a convexa e mais áspera que apresenta as fóveas oblonga e triangular, fornecendo a primeira a inserção para os músculos vocal e cricoartenóide lateral, e a última, para o ligamento vestibular. SIN facies anterolateralis cartilaginis arytenoideae [TA].
anterolateral s. of (shaft of) humerus [TA], face ântero-medial do úmero (diáfise); a superfície do úmero lateral ao sulco intertubercular. SIN facies anterolateralis corporis humeri [TA], facies anterior lateralis corporis humeri.
anteromedial s. of shaft of humerus [TA], face ântero-medial da diáfise do úmero; a superfície do úmero entre as bordas anterior e medial do osso. SIN facies anteromedialis corporis humeri [TA], facies anterior medialis corporis humeri.
anterosuperior s. of body of pancreas [TA], face ântero-superior do corpo do pâncreas; das três superfícies do corpo do pâncreas em forma de prisma, a voltada (em contato) para o estômago, sendo separada dele pelo espaço potencial da bolsa omental. SIN facies anterosuperioris corporis pancreatis [TA].
approximal s. of tooth [TA], face aproximal; superfície de um dente voltada para um dente adjacente no arco dental; a superfície de contato mais próxima da linha mediana anterior do arco dental é a superfície mesial do dente; a mais distante é a superfície distal. SIN interproximal s. of tooth*, contact s. of tooth, facies approximalis dentis, facies contactus dentis.
articular s. [TA], s. articular, face articular; qualquer superfície articular. SIN facies articularis [TA].
articular s. of acromion, face articular da clavícula do acrômio. SIN clavicular articular *facet* of acromion.
articular s. of arytenoid cartilage [TA], face articular da cartilagem aritenóidea; a superfície oval na superfície inferior do processo muscular da cartilagem aritenóidea para a articulação com a cartilagem cricóidea. SIN facies articularis cartilaginis arytenoideae [TA].
articular s. of mandibular fossa of temporal bone [TA], face articular da fossa mandibular do osso temporal; a parte lisa da fossa articular mandibular e eminência do osso temporal que se articula com o disco da articulação temporomandibular. SIN facies articularis fossae mandibularis ossis temporalis [TA].
articular s. on calcaneus for cuboid bone [TA], face articular do cubóide do calcâneo; a superfície em forma de sela na extremidade anterior do calcâneo para articulação do cubóide (osso). SIN facies articularis cuboidea ossis calcanei [TA], cuboidal articular s. of calcaneus.
articular s. of patella [TA], face articular da patela; a superfície posterior da patela, coberta com cartilagem hialina e subdividida por uma crista vertical numa superfície lateral maior e superfície medial menor para articulação com os côndilos correspondentes do fêmur. SIN facies articularis patellae [TA].
arytenoidal articular s. of cricoid [TA], face articular aritenóidea da cartilagem cricóidea; uma das duas facetas ovais na margem súpero-lateral da lâmina cricóidea para a articulação com as cartilagens aritenóideas. SIN facies articularis arytenoidea cricoideae [TA].
auricular s. of ilium [TA], face auricular da face sacropélvica do ílio, a superfície articular irregular, em forma de L, na face medial do ílio; que se articula com o sacro. SIN facies auricularis ossis ilii [TA].
auricular s. of sacrum [TA], s. auricular da parte lateral do sacro; a superfície articular rugosa; na face lateral do sacro, que se articula com o ílio de cada lado. SIN facies auricularis ossis sacri [TA].
axial s.'s, faces axiais; superfícies de um dente paralelas ao seu eixo longitudinal; são as faces vestibular (labial ou bucal), a lingual e a de contato (mesial ou distal).
balancing occlusal s., s. oclusal de equilíbrio. SIN balancing *contact*.
basal s., face basal; a superfície da dentadura cujo detalhe é determinado pela impressão e que repousa sobre o assento basal.
buccal s., face bucal; **(1)** parte da bochecha da face vestibular do dente; **(2)** a mucosa da bochecha; **(3)** em protodontia, a face de uma dentadura adjacente à bochecha.
calcaneal articular s. of talus [TA], face articular calcânea do tálus; uma das três facetas articulares no tálus para união com o calcâneo: face articular calcânea anterior (facies articularis calcanea anterior tali [TA]), face articular calcânea média (facies articularis calcanea media tali [TA]) e face articular calcânea posterior (facies articularis calcanea posterior tali [TA]). SIN facies articularis calcanea tali [TA].
carpal articular s. of radius [TA], face articular carpal do rádio; a superfície distal bicôncava do rádio para articulação com o osso escafóide, lateralmente, e o semilunar, medialmente. SIN facies articularis carpi radii [TA].
cerebral s., face cerebral; a superfície interna de certos ossos cranianos; são eles (a asa maior do) escafóide (facies cerebralis alae majoris ossis sphenoidale [TA]) e (a parte escamosa do) osso temporal (facies cerebralis partis squamosae ossis temporale [TA]). SIN facies cerebralis.
colic s. of spleen, impressão cólica do baço. SIN colic *impression* of spleen.

contact s. of tooth, face aproximal. SIN approximal s. of tooth.
costal s. [TA], face costal; a superfície de certas estruturas voltadas para as costelas; são as superfícies costais dos pulmões (facies costalis pulmonis [TA]) e da escápula (facies costalis scapulae [TA]). SIN facies costalis [TA].
costal s. of lung [TA], face costal do pulmão; a superfície de cada pulmão que está em contato com a pleura costal. SIN facies costalis pulmonis [TA].
costal s. of scapula [TA], face costal da escápula; a face côncava do corpo da escápula voltada para o tórax e que se aloja principalmente no músculo subescapular, dando origem a ele. SIN facies costalis scapulae [TA].
cuboidal articular s. of calcaneus, face articular cubóide do calcâneo. SIN articular s. on calcaneus for cuboid bone.
denture basal s., s. basal da dentadura. SIN denture foundation s.
denture foundation s., s. de alicerce da dentadura; parte da superfície de uma dentadura que tem seu contorno determinado pela impressão e sustenta a maior parte da carga oclusal. SIN denture basal s.
denture impression s., s. de impressão da dentadura; parte da superfície de uma dentadura que tem seu contorno determinado pela impressão; inclui as bordas da dentadura e estende-se até a superfície polida
denture occlusal s., face oclusal da dentadura; parte da superfície de uma dentadura que faz contato ou quase contato com a superfície correspondente de uma dentadura ou dente oposto. SIN facies occlusalis dentis [TA], occlusal s. of tooth (2) [TA], facies masticatoria, grinding s., masticating s., masticatory s.
denture polished s., s. polida da dentadura; parte da dentadura que se estende em direção oclusal a partir da borda da dentadura e que inclui a superfície palatina; trata-se da parte da base da dentadura que costuma ser polida e inclui as superfícies bucal e lingual dos dentes.
diaphragmatic s. [TA], face diafragmática; a superfície de um órgão em contato com o diafragma (facies diaphragmatica...), como a do coração (... cordis [TA]); fígado (... hepatis [TA]); pulmões (... pulmonis [TA]) e baço (... splenica [TA]). SIN facies diaphragmatica [TA].
distal s. of tooth [TA], face distal do dente; a superfície de contato de um dente que se afasta do plano mediano do arco dental; oposta à superfície mesial de um dente. SIN facies distalis dentis [TA].
dorsal s. [TA], face dorsal; a superfície dorsal de uma estrutura, como o sacro, os dedos das mãos ou dos pés. SIN facies dorsalis [TA].
dorsal s. of digit (of hand or foot) [TA], face dorsal do dedo (da mão ou do pé); a superfície dorsal de um dedo da mão ou do pé. SIN facies digitalis dorsalis (manus et pedis) [TA].
dorsal s. of sacrum [TA], face dorsal do sacro; face póstero-superior do sacro marcada por uma crista sacral mediana e duas cristas laterais, entre as quais se localizam quatro forames sacrais dorsais de cada lado. SIN facies dorsalis ossis sacri [TA].
dorsal s. of scapula, s. posterior da escápula. SIN posterior s. of scapula.
external s. [TA], face externa do frontal ou do parietal; a superfície convexa externa do osso frontal ou parietal. SIN facies externa [TA].
external s. of cochlear duct [TA], parede externa do ducto coclear; a face do ducto voltada para o lado externo (ligamento espiral) da cóclea. SIN paries externus ductus cochlearis [TA], external wall of cochlear duct.
external s. of cranial base [TA], base externa do crânio; face externa da base do crânio. SIN basis cranii externa [TA], external base o skull, norma basilaris, norma inferior, norma ventralis.
external s. of frontal bone [TA], face externa da escama externa do osso frontal; a superfície externa convexa do osso frontal. SIN facies externa ossis frontalis [TA].
external s. of parietal bone [TA], face externa do osso parietal; a superfície externa convexa do osso parietal. SIN facies externa ossis parietalis [TA].
facial s. of tooth, face vestibular do dente. SIN vestibular s. of tooth.
fibular articular s. of tibia, face articular fibular da tíbia. SIN fibular articular facet of tibia.
gastric s. of spleen, impressão gástrica do baço. SIN gastric impression on spleen.
glenoid s., fossa mandibular. SIN mandibular fossa.
gluteal s. of ilium [TA], face glútea do ílio; a superfície externa da asa do ílio marcada pelas linhas glúteas anterior, posterior e inferior, que separam as origens dos músculos glúteos. SIN facies glutea ossis ilii [TA].
grinding s., face oclusal do dente. SIN denture occlusal s.
incisal s., margem incisal. SIN incisal margin.
inferior articular s. of atlas [TA], face articular inferior do atlas; uma das duas superfícies côncavas, nas massas laterais do atlas, que se articulam com as superfícies correspondentes do áxis. SIN facies articularis inferior atlantis [TA], fovea articularis inferior atlantis, inferior articular facet of atlas, inferior articular pit of atlas.
inferior articular s. of tibia [TA], face articular inferior da tíbia; a superfície quadrilátera da extremidade distal da tíbia para articulação com o tálus; é côncava na parte ântero-posterior e mais larga anteriormente. SIN facies articularis inferior tibiae [TA].
inferior s. of cerebellar hemisphere, face inferior do hemisfério do cerebelo; repousa na fossa craniana posterior e sobrepõe-se à medula; inclui o semilunar inferior, o lóbulo biventri, tonsila cerebelar e o flóculo. SIN facies inferior hemispherii cerebri [TA].
inferior cerebral s., s. cerebral inferior. SIN base of brain.
inferior s. of petrous part of temporal bone [TA], s. inferior da parte petrosa do osso temporal; a porção da parte petrosa do osso temporal que contribui para a base externa do crânio. SIN facies inferior partis petrosae ossis temporalis [TA].
inferior s. of tongue [TA], face inferior da língua; a superfície da língua voltada para o assoalho da cavidade oral, cuja mucosa é fina, lisa e desprovida de papilas. SIN facies inferior linguae [TA].
inferolateral s. of prostate [TA], face ínfero-lateral da próstata; a superfície da próstata voltada para o corpo do púbis e o diafragma pélvico. SIN facies inferolateralis prostate [TA].
infratemporal s. of (body of) maxilla [TA], face infratemporal da maxila; a superfície póstero-lateral convexa do corpo da maxila que forma a parede anterior da fossa infratemporal. SIN facies infratemporalis corporis maxillae [TA].
infratemporal s. of greater wing of sphenoid [TA], face infratemporal da asa maior do esfenóide; superfície da asa maior do esfenóide, orientada inferiormente, que forma um teto para fossa infratemporal. SIN facies infratemporalis alaris majoris ossis sphenoidalis [TA].
interlobar s.'s of lung [TA], faces interlobares do pulmão; superfície de um lobo do pulmão adjacente (em contato com) à superfície do outro lobo; as duas superfícies são separadas por uma fissura interlobar nas fissuras interlobares do pulmão. SIN facies interlobares pulmonis.
internal s. [TA], face interna; a superfície côncava interna do osso frontal ou parietal. SIN facies interna [TA].
internal s. of cranial base [TA], base interna do crânio; a face interior da base do crânio sobre a qual repousa o cérebro; o assoalho da cavidade craniana. SIN basis cranii interna [TA], internal base of skull.
internal s. of frontal bone [TA], face interna do osso frontal; a superfície do osso frontal que contribui para a parede da cavidade craniana. SIN facies interna ossis frontalis [TA].
internal s. of parietal bone [TA], face interna do osso parietal; a superfície côncava do osso parietal que forma parte da parede da cavidade craniana. SIN facies interna ossis parietalis [TA].
interproximal s. of tooth, face aproximal; *termo oficial alternativo para approximal s. of tooth.
intestinal s. of uterus [TA], face intestinal do útero; a superfície póstero-superior do útero com a qual as alças intestinais entram em contato. SIN facies intestinalis uteri [TA].
lateral s. [TA], face lateral; superfície de uma parte do corpo que se afasta da linha mediana; a TA reconhece uma superfície lateral nas seguintes estruturas: fíbula, ovário, rádio, testículo, tíbia, osso zigomático. SIN facies lateralis [TA].
lateral s. of arm, face lateral do braço; a superfície lateral do braço. SIN facies lateralis brachii.
lateral s. of fibula [TA], face lateral da fíbula; a superfície lateral da fíbula. SIN facies lateralis fibulae [TA].
lateral s. of finger, face lateral do dedo da mão; a superfície lateral de um dedo da mão. SIN facies lateralis digiti manus.
lateral s. of leg, face lateral da perna; a superfície lateral da parte do membro inferior entre o joelho e o tornozelo. SIN facies lateralis cruris.
lateral s. of lower limb, face lateral do membro inferior; a superfície lateral do membro inferior. SIN facies lateralis membri inferioris.
lateral malleolar s. of talus, face maleolar lateral do tálus. SIN lateral malleolar facet of talus.
lateral s. of ovary [TA], face lateral do ovário; a superfície do ovário voltada para a parede pélvica. SIN facies lateralis ovarii [TA].
lateral s. of testis [TA], face lateral do testículo; a superfície de orientação lateral do testículo. SIN facies lateralis testis [TA].
lateral s. of tibia [TA], face lateral da tíbia; a superfície lateralmente orientada da tíbia. SIN facies lateralis tibiae [TA].
lateral s. of toe, face lateral do dedo do pé; a superfície lateral de um dedo do pé. SIN facies lateralis digiti pedis.
lateral s. of zygomatic bone [TA], face lateral do zigomático; a superfície lateral do osso zigomático. SIN facies lateralis ossis zygomatici [TA].
lingual s. of tooth [TA], face lingual do dente; superfície de um dente voltada para a língua; oposta à superfície vestibular do dente. SIN facies lingualis dentis [TA].
lunate s. of acetabulum [TA], face semilunar do acetábulo; a superfície articular curva que circunda a fossa acetabular e articula-se com a cabeça do fêmur. SIN facies lunata acetabuli [TA].
malleolar articular s. of fibula, s. articular do maléolo lateral. SIN articular facet of lateral malleolus.
malleolar articular s. of tibia, s. articular do maléolo medial. SIN articular facet of medial malleolus.
masticating s., fase oclusal do dente. SIN denture occlusal s.
masticatory s., face oclusal do dente. SIN denture occlusal s.
maxillary s. of greater wing of sphenoid bone [TA], face maxilar da asa maior do esfenóide; parte da superfície anterior da asa maior do osso esfenóide que é

perfurada pelo forame redondo e forma o limite posterior da fossa pterigopalatina. SIN facies maxillaris alaris majoris ossis sphenoidalis [TA].
maxillary s. of palatine bone, face maxilar do palatino; a superfície lateral da placa perpendicular do osso palatino. SIN facies maxillaris ossis palatini [TA].
medial s. [TA], face medial; superfície de uma parte do corpo voltada para a linha mediana. A TA reconhece uma superfície medial nas seguintes estruturas: cartilagem aritenóidea, hemisfério cerebral, fíbula, ovário, testículo, tíbia, ulna. SIN facies medialis [TA].
medial s. of arytenoid cartilage [TA], face medial da cartilagem aritenóidea; a superfície da cartilagem aritenóidea voltada para o seu par contralateral. SIN facies medialis cartilaginis arytenoideae [TA].
medial cerebral s., face medial do hemisfério cerebral. SIN medial s. of cerebral hemisphere.
medial s. of cerebral hemisphere [TA], face medial do hemisfério cerebral; volta-se para cima, bem como anterior e posteriormente ao corpo caloso, foice do cérebro; abaixo dela estão o mesencéfalo e a parede medial, coberta pela dura-máter, da fossa craniana média. SIN facies medialis hemispherii cerebri [TA], medial cerebral s.
medial s. of fibula [TA], face medial da fíbula; a superfície da fíbula voltada para linha média. SIN facies medialis fibulae [TA].
medial s. of lung, face mediastinal do pulmão. SIN mediastinal s. of lung.
medial s. of ovary [TA], face medial do ovário; a superfície do ovário voltada para a cavidade pélvica. SIN facies medialis ovarii [TA].
medial s. of testis, face medial do testículo. SIN *facies medialis testis.*
medial s. of tibia, face medial da tíbia. SIN *facies medialis tibiae.*
medial s. of toes [TA], face medial dos dedos dos pés; a superfície medial de um dedo do pé. SIN facies medialis digiti pedis [TA].
medial s. of ulna, face medial da ulna. SIN *facies medialis ulnae.*
mediastinal s. of lung [TA], face mediastinal do pulmão; parte da superfície medial de um pulmão em contato com o mediastino. SIN facies mediastinalis pulmonis [TA], facies medialis pulmonis, medial s. of lung, mediastinal part of lung, pars mediastinalis pulmonis.
mesial s. of tooth [TA], face mesial do dente; superfície de contato de um dente que está dirigida para o plano mediano do arco dental; oposta à superfície distal do dente. SIN facies mesialis dentis [TA].
middle talar articular s. of calcaneus [TA], face articular talar média do calcâneo; subjacente à cabeça do tálus, contribuindo para a articulação talocalcaneonavicular. SIN facies articularis talaris media calcanei [TA].
nasal s. of maxilla [TA], face nasal da maxila; a superfície da maxila que forma parte da parede nasal lateral com um grande defeito (hiato maxilar) posteriormente e o sulco lacrimal em sua porção média. SIN facies nasalis maxillae [TA].
nasal s. of palatine bone [TA], face nasal do palatino; **(1)** a superfície nasal da lâmina perpendicular do osso palatino, que forma parte da parede lateral da cavidade nasal (facies nasalis lamina perpendicularis ossis palatini [TA]); **(2)** a superfície nasal da lâmina horizontal do osso palatino, que forma parte do assoalho da cavidade nasal (facies nasalis lamina horizontalis ossis palatini [TA]). SIN facies nasalis ossis palatini [TA].
navicular articular s. of talus [TA], face articular navicular do tálus; a grande superfície convexa na cabeça do tálus para articulação com o osso navicular. SIN facies articularis navicularis tali [TA].
occlusal s. of tooth [TA], face oclusal do dente; **(1)** a superfície de um dente que oclui ou contacta uma superfície oposta de um dente na mandíbula oposta; **(2)** SIN denture occlusal s.
orbital s. [TA], face orbital; a superfície de um osso que contribui para as paredes da órbita. A TA reconhece uma superfície orbital (facies orbitalis... [TA]) nos seguintes ossos: asa maior do esfenóide (... alaris majoris ossis sphenoidale [TA]); corpo da maxila (... corporis maxillae [TA]; frontal (... ossis frontalis [TA]); zigomático (... ossis zigomatici [TA]). SIN facies orbitalis [TA].
palatine s. of horizontal plate of palatine bone [TA], face palatina da placa horizontal do osso palatino; a superfície inferior da placa horizontal do osso palatino. SIN facies palatina laminae horizontalis ossis palatini [TA].
palmar s.'s of fingers [TA], faces palmares dos dedos das mãos; a superfície palmar dos dedos das mãos; a superfície flexora ou anterior dos dedos das mãos. SIN facies palmares digitorum [TA], facies digitalis palmaris, facies digitalis ventralis, ventral s. of digit.
patellar s. of femur [TA], face patelar do fêmur; o sulco formado anteriormente, entre as partes ântero-superiores dos côndilos femorais, que acomoda a patela. SIN facies patellaris femoris [TA], trochlea femoris.
pelvic s. of sacrum [TA], face pélvica do sacro; superfície do sacro voltada para baixo e para diante, formando o teto e parte da parede posterior da cavidade pélvica. SIN facies pelvica ossis sacri [TA].
Petzval s., s. de Petzval; o plano de imagem curvo sobre o qual qualquer objeto linear estendido é focado por uma lente; é curvado para as bordas de uma lente convexa e afasta-se das bordas de uma lente côncava (concave *lens.*) VER barrel *distortion,* pincushion *distortion.*
plantar s. of foot, face plantar do pé. SIN *sole* of foot.
plantar s. of toe, face plantar dos dedos dos pés. SIN facies digitalis plantaris.

popliteal s. of femur [TA], face poplítea do fêmur; a superfície posterior da extremidade inferior do fêmur entre os lábios divergentes da linha áspera. SIN facies poplitea femoris [TA], planum popliteum, popliteal plane of femur.
posterior s. [TA], face posterior; a superfície de uma parte do corpo voltada para a parte posterior do corpo. A TA reconhece uma superfície posterior das seguintes estruturas: cartilagem aritenóidea, córnea, pálpebra, fíbula, úmero, íris, rim, lente, pâncreas, parte petrosa do osso temporal, próstata, rádio, escápula, glândula supra-renal, tíbia, ulna, útero. SIN facies posterior [TA].
posterior s. of arm, região posterior do braço. SIN posterior *region* of arm.
posterior articular s. of dens, face articular posterior do dente do áxis. SIN posterior articular *facet* of dens.
posterior s. of arytenoid cartilage [TA], face posterior da cartilagem aritenóidea; face côncava da cartilagem aritenóidea que fornece fixação para o músculo aritenóide e dirige-se para a laringofaringe. SIN facies posterior cartilaginis arytenoideae [TA].
posterior s. of cornea [TA], face posterior da córnea; a superfície profunda ou interna da córnea em contato com o humor aquoso. SIN facies posterior corneae [TA].
posterior s. of elbow, região posterior do cotovelo. SIN posterior *region* of elbow.
posterior s. of eyelids [TA], face posterior das pálpebras; a superfície interna das pálpebras, coberta pela conjuntiva. SIN facies posterior palpebrarum [TA].
posterior s. of fibula [TA], face posterior da fíbula; face da fíbula que forma, com a tíbia e a membrana interóssea, o limite anterior do compartimento posterior da perna. SIN facies posterior fibulae [TA].
posterior s. of forearm, região posterior do antebraço. SIN posterior *region* of forearm.
posterior s. of iris [TA], face posterior da íris; a face da íris coberta com retina não-visual, formando o limite anterior da câmara posterior do bulbo do olho. SIN facies posterior iridis [TA].
posterior s. of kidney [TA], face posterior do rim; a face do rim voltada para a parede abdominal posterior. SIN facies posterior renis [TA].
posterior s. of leg, região posterior da perna. SIN posterior *region* of leg.
posterior s. of lens [TA], face posterior da lente; a face da lente que forma o limite anterior da câmara postremal e é adjacente ao corpo vítreo. SIN facies posterior lentis [TA].
posterior s. of lower limb, face posterior do membro inferior; a superfície posterior do membro inferior. SIN facies posterior membri inferioris.
posterior s. of pancreas [TA], face posterior do pâncreas; a face do pâncreas voltada para a parede abdominal posterior. SIN facies posterior pancreatis [TA].
posterior s. of petrous part of temporal bone [TA], face posterior da parte petrosa do temporal; a superfície da parte petrosa do osso temporal que contribui para a fossa craniana posterior. SIN facies posterior partis petrosae ossis temporalis [TA].
posterior s. of prostate [TA], face posterior da próstata; a face da próstata voltada para o reto, separada dele pela fáscia retroprostática. SIN facies posterior prostatae [TA].
posterior s. of radius [TA], face posterior do rádio; a face dorsal do rádio. SIN facies posterior radii [TA].
posterior s. of scapula [TA], face posterior da escápula; a face externa do corpo da escápula, subdividida pela espinha proeminente da escápula em fossa supra-espinal menor e fossa infra-espinal maior. SIN dorsal s. of scapula, facies dorsalis scapulae.
posterior s. of shaft of humerus [TA], face posterior da diáfise do úmero; a porção do úmero que marca a linha áspera e à qual se fixam os septos intermusculares da inserção da coxa. SIN facies posterior corporis humeri [TA].
posterior s. of suprarenal gland [TA], face posterior da glândula supra-renal; a superfície póstero-medial da glândula supra-renal que entra em contato com o pilar do diafragma. SIN facies posterior glandulae suprarenalis [TA].
posterior talar articular s. (of calcaneus) [TA], face articular talar posterior (do calcâneo); articula-se com o tálus (articulação subtalar) posteriormente ao seio do tarso. SIN facies articularis talaris posterior calcanei [TA].
posterior s. of thigh, região posterior da coxa. SIN posterior *region* of thigh.
posterior s. of tibia [TA], face posterior da tíbia; a face da tíbia que, com a superfície posterior da fíbula e a membrana interóssea, forma o limite anterior do compartimento posterior da perna. SIN facies posterior tibiae [TA].
posterior s. of ulna [TA], face posterior da ulna; a face dorsal da ulna. SIN facies posterior ulnae [TA].
renal s. of spleen, impressão renal do baço. SIN renal *impression* of spleen.
renal s. of suprarenal gland [TA], face renal da glândula supra-renal; superfície da glândula supra-renal em contato com o rim. SIN facies renalis glandulae suprarenalis [TA].
right/left pulmonary s.'s of heart, faces pulmonares direita/esquerda do coração; as superfícies laterais do coração dirigidas para os pulmões; à esquerda, encontra-se principalmente a parede ventricular esquerda; à direita, a parede atrial direita e a parte superior da parede ventricular direita. SIN facies pulmonales cordis dextra/sinistra.
sacropelvic s. of ilium [TA], face sacropélvica do ílio; a superfície medial do ílio atrás e abaixo da fossa ilíaca; inclui a tuberosidade ilíaca, a superfície au-

ricular e a superfície pélvica abaixo e em frente da superfície auricular. SIN facies sacropelvina ossis ilii [TA].

sternal articular s. of clavicle, face articular esternal da clavícula. SIN sternal facet of clavicle.

sternocostal s. of heart [TA], face esternocostal do coração; a face anterior do coração, formada principalmente pelo ventrículo direito e, em menor grau, pelo ventrículo esquerdo. SIN facies sternocostalis cordis [TA].

subocclusal s., face subocclusal; parte da superfície oclusal de um dente abaixo do nível da parte oclusal do dente.

superior articular s. of atlas [TA], face articular superior do atlas; uma das duas superfícies articulares côncavas, na face superior das massas laterais do atlas, que se articulam com os côndilos occipitais. SIN facies articularis superior atlantis [TA], fovea articularis superior atlantis, superior articular facet of atlas, superior articular pit of atlas.

superior articular s. of tibia [TA], face articular superior da tíbia; a superfície articular na extremidade proximal da tíbia, que é dividida em partes medial e lateral, para a articulação dos côndilos do fêmur. SIN facies articularis superior tibiae [TA].

superior s. of cerebellar hemisphere, face superior do hemisfério do cerebelo; localiza-se contra a superfície inferior do tentório e inclui a asa dos lóbulos central, o lóbulo quadrangular, o lóbulo simples e o lóbulo semilunar superior. SIN facies superior hemispherii cerebelli.

superior s. of talus, face superior do tálus. SIN superior facet of trochlear of tálus.

superolateral cerebral s., face súpero-lateral do hemisfério cerebral. SIN superolateral s. of cerebrum.

superolateral s. of cerebrum [TA], face súpero-lateral do hemisfério cerebral; a face do hemisfério cerebral que está em contato com os ossos planos do crânio; inclui partes dos lobos frontal, parietal, temporal e occipital. SIN facies superolateralis hemispherii cerebri [TA], superolateral face of cerebral hemisphere [TA], cortical convexity, superolateral cerebral s.

symphysial s. of pubis [TA], face sinfisial do púbis; a superfície medial, oval e alongada do púbis voltada para o seu par contralateral, com o qual se articula por meio do disco interpúbico, formando a sínfise púbica. SIN facies symphysialis [TA].

talar articular s.'s of calcaneus [TA], faces articulares talares do calcâneo; as três facetas do calcâneo que se articulam com o tálus sobrejacente; a face articular talar anterior e a média contribuem para a articulação talocalcaneonavicular e são separadas pelo seio do tarso da face articular talar posterior, que penetra na articulação subtalar. SIN facies articularis talaris calcanei [TA].

temporal s. [TA], face temporal; a superfície de um osso que contribui para a fossa temporal, isto é, a asa maior do esfenóide, a parte escamosa dos ossos temporal, frontal e zigomático. SIN facies temporalis [TA].

tentorial s., face tentorial; as áreas do lobo occipital (face inferior) e do cerebelo (face superior) apostas às superfícies superior e inferior, respectivamente, do tentório do cerebelo.

thyroid articular s. of cricoid (cartilage) [TA], face articular tireóidea da (cartilagem) cricóidea; uma das duas pequenas facetas circulares na superfície lateral da cartilagem cricóidea, próximo à margem inferior da junção do arco e da lâmina para articulação com os cornos inferiores da cartilagem tireóidea. SIN facies articularis thyroidea cricoideae [TA].

tympanic s. of cochlear duct [TA], parede timpânica do ducto coclear; a parede que separa o ducto coclear da rampa do tímpano; consiste na lâmina espiral óssea e na membrana basilar. SIN paries tympanicus ductus cochlearis [TA], membrana spiralis*, spiral membrane*, tympanic wall of cochlear duct.

urethral s. of penis [TA], face uretral do pênis; a superfície do pênis oposta a seu dorso. SIN facies urethralis penis [TA].

ventral s. of digit, face palmar do dedo. SIN palmar s.'s of fingers.

vesical s. of uterus [TA], face vesical do útero; a superfície do útero voltada para a bexiga e dela separada pela bolsa uterovesical do peritônio. SIN facies vesicalis uteri [TA].

vestibular s. of cochlear duct [TA], face vestibular do ducto coclear; a membrana que separa o ducto coclear do canal vestibular; consiste em células epiteliais escamosas com microvilosidades voltadas para o ducto, numa membrana basal e numa fina camada de tecido conjuntivo para a rampa. SIN paries vestibularis ductus cochlearis [TA], membrana vestibularis ductus cochlearis*, vestibular membrane*, Reissner membrane, vestibular wall of cochlear duct.

vestibular s. of tooth [TA], face vestibular do dente; a superfície de um dente voltada para a mucosa bucal ou labial do vestíbulo da boca; oposta à superfície lingual do dente. SIN facies vestibularis dentis [TA], facial s. of tooth, facies facialis dentis.

visceral s. of liver [TA], face visceral do fígado; a superfície póstero-inferior do fígado voltada para órgãos abdominais adjacentes; a porta do fígado e a vesícula biliar estão localizadas nessa superfície. SIN facies visceralis hepatis [TA].

visceral s. of the spleen [TA], face visceral do baço; a superfície do baço em contato com vísceras adjacentes. SIN facies visceralis splenis [TA].

working occlusal s.'s, faces oclusais ativas; as superfícies dos dentes sobre as quais pode ocorrer a mastigação.

sur·face-ac·tive (ser′fās-ak′tiv). Tensoativo; indica a propriedade de determinados agentes de alterar a natureza físico-química de superfícies e interfaces, causando redução da tensão interfacial; em geral, possuem grupos tanto lipofílicos quanto hidrofílicos. VER TAMBÉM surfactant.

sur·fac·tant (ser-fak′tănt). Surfactante. **1.** Agente tensoativo, incluindo substâncias comumente designadas como agentes umidificantes, depressores da tensão superficial, detergentes, agentes dispersantes, emulsificantes, anti-sépticos de amônio quaternário, etc. **2.** Os agentes tensoativos, que formam uma camada monomolecular sobre as superfícies alveolares dos pulmões; as lipoproteínas, incluindo lecitinas e esfingomielinas que estabilizam o volume alveolar ao reduzirem a tensão superficial e ao alterarem a relação entre tensão superficial e área de superfície. [*sur*face *a*ctive *a*ge*nt*]

nonionic s., s. não-iônico; surfactante sem componente apresentando carga.

zwitterionic s., s. zuiteriônico; surfactante dipolar.

sur·geon (ser-jŭn). Cirurgião, médico que trata doenças, lesões e deformidades através de operação ou manipulação. [G. *cheirougos*; L. *chirurgus*]

attending s., c. de atendimento; cirurgião membro da equipe de atendimento de um hospital.

dental s., c. dentista; profissional geral de odontologia; nos Estados Unidos, dentista com grau D.D.S ou D.M.D.

genitourinary s., urologista. SIN urologist.

oral s., c. oral; dentista especializado em cirurgia oral.

sur·geon gen·er·al. O principal oficial médico no exército, na marinha e na aeronáutica dos Estados Unidos ou no Serviço de Saúde Pública. Em alguns serviços militares estrangeiros, qualquer membro do corpo médico que ocupe o posto de general, não necessariamente o principal oficial médico.

sur·gery (ser′jer-ē). Cirurgia. **1.** O ramo da medicina relacionado ao tratamento de doenças, lesões e deformidades através de operação ou manipulação física. **2.** A realização ou os procedimentos de uma operação. [L. *chirurgia*; G. *cheir*, mão + *ergon*, trabalho]

ambulatory s., c. ambulatorial; procedimentos cirúrgicos realizados em pacientes que são internados e recebem alta no mesmo dia.

aseptic s., s. asséptica; a realização de uma c. com mãos e instrumentos esterilizados, utilizando precauções contra a introdução de microrganismos infecciosos do meio externo.

closed s., c. fechada; c. sem incisão da pele, p. ex., redução de uma fratura ou luxação.

cosmetic s., c. cosmética; c. em que o principal objetivo é melhorar a aparência. SIN esthetic s.

craniofacial s., c. craniofacial; procedimento simultâneo no crânio e ossos faciais.

endolymphatic sac s., c. do saco endolinfático; designação genérica para várias operações realizadas no saco endolinfático para tratamento da doença de Ménière.

esthetic s., c. estética. SIN cosmetic s.

functional endoscopic sinus s. (FESS), c. endoscópica funcional dos seios paranasais; grupo de operações efetuadas nos seios paranasais, com iluminação e aumento através de um endoscópio.

keratorefractive s., c. ceratorrefrativa, ceratoplastia de refração. SIN refractive keratoplasty.

laparoscopic s. c. laparoscópica; procedimento cirúrgico realizado com uma técnica cirúrgica minimamente invasiva para exposição, que evita a incisão tradicional; a visualização é obtida com o uso de um instrumento de fibra óptica fixado a uma câmara de vídeo.

laparoscopically assisted s., c. laparoscopicamente assistida; procedimento cirúrgico realizado com o uso de técnicas laparoscópica e aberta combinadas.

left ventricular volume reduction s., c. de redução do volume do ventrículo esquerdo; cirurgia em que o volume de um ventrículo esquerdo dilatado não-aneurismático é reduzido por ressecção miocárdica para melhorar a geometria e a função mecânica do ventrículo e, conseqüentemente, tratar a insuficiência cardíaca congestiva de estágio terminal. SIN Battista operation, partial left ventriculectomy, reduction left ventriculoplasty.

lung volume reduction s., c. de redução do volume pulmonar; procedimento pelo qual o tecido pulmonar não-funcional é removido em pacientes com enfisema, permitindo um maior espaço na cavidade torácica para o tecido relativamente sadio e, assim, melhorando teoricamente a função pulmonar. VER TAMBÉM emphysema.

major s., c. de grande porte. VER major *operation*.

microscopically controlled s., c. microscopicamente controlada. SIN Mohs chemosurgery.

minimally invasive s., c. minimamente invasiva; procedimento cirúrgico realizado de modo a resultar na menor incisão possível ou na ausência total de incisão; inclui procedimentos cirúrgicos laparoscópicos, laparoscopicamente assistidos, toracoscópicos e endoscópicos.

minor s., c. de pequeno porte. VER minor *operation*.
Mohs s., c. de Mohs. SIN Mohs *chemosurgery.*
Mohs micrographic s., c. micrográfica de Mohs. SIN Mohs *chemosurgery.*
open heart s., c. cardíaca a céu aberto; procedimento(s) cirúrgico(s) realizado(s) sobre ou dentro do coração exposto, geralmente com derivação cardiopulmonar.
oral s., c. oral; o ramo da odontologia relacionado ao diagnóstico e tratamento cirúrgico e auxiliar de doenças, lesões e deformidades da região oral e maxilofacial.
orthognathic s., c. ortognática. SIN surgical *orthodontics.*
orthopedic s., c. ortopédica; o ramo da cirurgia que inclui o tratamento de distúrbios agudos e crônicos do sistema musculoesquelético, incluindo lesões, doenças, disfunção e deformidades (originalmente deformidades em crianças) nos membros e na coluna vertebral. VER TAMBÉM orthopaedics.
plastic s., c. plástica; a especialidade ou procedimento cirúrgico relacionado com a restauração, construção, reconstrução ou aperfeiçoamento da forma e da aparência de estruturas do corpo ausentes, defeituosas, lesadas ou malformadas.
reconstructive s., c. reconstrutiva. VER plastic s.
skull base s., c. da base do crânio; designação genérica para referir-se a uma especialidade da cirurgia e a um grupo de operações, técnicas de abordagens de lesões afetando a base do crânio ou seu conteúdo.
stereotactic s., c. estereotática. SIN stereotaxy.
stereotaxic s., c. estereotática. SIN stereotaxy.
thoracoscopic s., c. toracoscópica; cirurgia no tórax utilizando um toracoscópio; antigamente, instrumento de visualização direta utilizado principalmente para procedimentos simples, como terapia do colapso e biopsia pleural; hoje, utiliza técnicas e instrumentos videoendoscópicos minimamente invasivos e é utilizada para procedimentos mais complexos. Cf. video-assisted thoracic s.
transsexual s., c. transexual; procedimentos destinados a alterar as características sexuais externas de um paciente, de forma que se assemelhem ao outro sexo.
ventricular reduction s., c. de redução ventricular. SIN Batista *procedure.*
video-assisted thoracic s. (VATS), c. torácica videoassistida; c. torácica realizada com o uso de câmaras endoscópicas, sistemas ópticos e vídeos, bem como instrumentos e grampeadores cirúrgicos especialmente projetados; a capacidade de efetuar pequenas incisões sem expansão das costelas constitui uma vantagem sobre a toracotomia padrão; tem sido aplicada à maioria dos procedimentos torácicos.

sur·gi·cal (ser'ji-kăl). Cirúrgico, relativo à cirurgia.
sur·re·nal (ser'rē'năl). Supra-renal. SIN suprarenal (1).
sur·ro·gate (ser'ō-gāt). Substituto, suplente, sub-rogado. **1.** Pessoa que atua na vida de outra como substituto de uma terceira pessoa, como um parente que assume o sustento e outras responsabilidades dos pais ausentes. **2.** Pessoa que lembra outra pessoa, de modo que é usada como substituto emocional da segunda. [L. *surrogo*, colocar em outro lugar]
 mother s., s. materno; pessoa que substitui ou toma o lugar da mãe.
sur·round (ser'-ownd'). Ambiente; meio.
 acoustical s., campo acústico. SIN sound *field.*
sur·sum·duc·tion (ser'-sŭm-dŭk'shŭn). Sursundução. SIN supraduction. [L. *sursum*, para cima + *duco*, pp. *-ductus*, puxar]
sur·sum·ver·sion (ser'-sŭm-ver'zhŭn). Sursunversão; ato de rotação dos olhos para cima. [L. *sursum*, para cima + *verto*, pp. *versus*, girar]
sur·veil·lance (ser-vā'lans). Vigilância, supervisão. **1.** A coleta, o cotejo, a análise e a disseminação de dados; tipo de estudo de observação que envolve a monitorização contínua da ocorrência de doença numa população. **2.** Inspeção, que utiliza geralmente métodos caracterizados mais pela sua praticabilidade, uniformidade ou rapidez do que pela sua acurácia completa. [Fr. *surveiller*, observar, do L. *super-* + *vigilo*, vigiar]
 immune s., imunovigilância; teoria segundo a qual o sistema imune reconhece e destrói células tumorais que estão surgindo constantemente durante a vida do indivíduo. SIN immunological s.
 immunological s., vigilância imunológica. SIN immune s.
 post-marketing s., vigilância pós-comercialização; procedimento implementado após licenciamento de uma droga para uso público, destinado a fornecer informações sobre o uso e a ocorrência de efeitos colaterais, efeitos adversos, etc.
sur·vey (ser'vā). Levantamento, inspeção, sondagem. **1.** Investigação em que a informação obtida é sistematicamente coletada, porém sem o uso do método experimental. **2.** Exame abrangente ou grupo de exames para triagem de um ou mais achados. **3.** Série de perguntas formuladas a uma amostra de indivíduos numa população. [Fr. ant. *surveeir*, do L. mediev. *supervideo*, de *super*, sobre + *video*, ver]
 field s., sondagem de campo; coleta planejada de dados entre pessoas não-institucionalizadas na população geral.
 skeletal s., exame esquelético; exame radiográfico de todo o esqueleto ou de partes selecionadas à procura de fraturas ocultas, metástases, etc.

sur·vey·ing (ser-vā'ing). Em odontologia, o procedimento de localizar e delinear o contorno e a posição dos dentes de apoio e estruturas associadas antes de planejar uma dentadura parcial removível.
sur·vey·or (ser-vā'er, or). Em odontologia, o instrumento utilizado na localização.
sur·viv·al (ser-vī'văl). Sobrevida; persistência da vida.
sus·cep·ti·bil·i·ty (su-sep-ti-bil'i-tē). Suscetibilidade. **1.** Tendência do indivíduo a desenvolver efeitos prejudiciais devido a um agente externo, como *Mycobacterium tuberculosis*, grandes altitudes ou temperatura ambiental. **2.** Na ressonância magnética, a perda do sinal de magnetização causada pela rápida dispersão de fase devido à acentuada homogeneidade local do campo magnético, como nas múltiplas interfaces ar–tecido mole nos pulmões.
sus·pen·sion (sŭs-pen'shŭn). Suspensão. **1.** Interrupção temporária de qualquer função. **2.** Pendurar em um suporte, como aquele utilizado no tratamento de curvaturas da coluna vertebral ou durante a aplicação de um aparelho de gesso. **3.** Fixação de um órgão, como o útero, a outro tecido para suporte. **4.** Dispersão de um sólido através de um líquido em partículas finamente divididas de tamanho suficientemente grande para serem detectadas por meios puramente ópticos; se as partículas forem demasiado pequenas para serem observadas ao microscópio, porém ainda grandes o suficiente para causar dispersão da luz (fenômeno de Tyndall), permanecerão dispersas indefinidamente e são ainda denominadas suspensão coloidal. SIN coarse dispersion. **5.** Classe de preparações da farmacopéia de drogas não-dissolvidas finamente divididas (p. ex., pós para suspensão) dispersas em veículos líquidos para uso oral ou parenteral. [L. *suspensio*, de *suspendo*, pp. *-pensus*, pendurar, suspender.
 amorphous insulin zinc s., s. de insulina zíncica amórfica. SIN prompt insulin zinc s.
 chromic phosphate ^{32}P colloidal s., s. coloidal de fosfato crômico P^{32}; radiofármaco coloidal puro β-emissor, não-absorvível, administrado nas cavidades corporais, como os espaços pleural ou peritoneal, para controlar derrames malignos. VER TAMBÉM sodium phosphate ^{32}P.
 Coffey s., s. de Coffey; técnica cirúrgica após excisão parcial do corno uterino, como na salpingectomia, em que os ligamentos largo e redondo são suturados sobre a ferida para restaurar a continuidade do peritônio e suspender o útero do lado operado.
 crystalline insulin zinc s., s. de insulina zíncica cristalina. SIN extended insulin zinc s.
 extended insulin zinc s., s. de insulina zíncica de ação prolongada; suspensão de insulina de ação longa obtida do boi, com tempo aproximado de início de 7 horas e duração de ação de 36 horas. SIN crystalline insulin zinc s.
 insulin zinc s., s. de insulina zíncica; suspensão tamponada estéril com cloreto de zinco contendo habitualmente 100 unidades por ml; a fase sólida da suspensão consiste numa mistura de 7 partes de insulina cristalina e 3 partes de insulina amorfa. SIN lente insulin.
 magnesia and alumina oral s., s. oral de magnésio e alumínio; mistura de hidróxido de magnésio e quantidades variáveis de óxido de alumínio; utilizada como antiácido.
 prompt insulin zinc s., s. de insulina zíncica imediata; suspensão estéril de insulina em água tamponada para injeção, modificada pela adição de cloreto de zinco, de modo que a fase sólida da suspensão é amorfa; em geral, contém 100 unidades por ml; a duração da ação é equivalente à da injeção de insulina. SIN amorphous insulin zinc s., semilente insulin.
sus·pen·soid (sŭs-pen'soyd). Suspensóide; solução coloidal em que as partículas dispersas são sólidas e liófobas ou hidrófobas e, portanto, nitidamente demarcadas do líquido no qual estão suspensas. SIN hydrophobic colloid, lyophobic colloid, suspension colloid. [suspension + G. *eidos*, semelhança]
sus·pen·so·ry (sŭs-pen'sō-rē). Suspensor. **1.** Que suspende; que sustenta; designa um ligamento, um músculo ou uma outra estrutura que mantém um órgão ou outra parte no lugar. **2.** Um suporte aplicado para levantar uma parte pendente, como o escroto ou uma mama pendular.
sus·ten·tac·u·lar (sŭs-ten-tak'ū-lăr). Sustentacular; relativo a um sustentáculo; que sustenta.
sus·ten·tac·u·lum, pl. **sus·ten·tac·u·la** (sŭs'ten-tak'ū-lŭm, -lă). Sustentáculo; estrutura que serve como alicerce ou suporte para outra. [L. um prop, de *sustento*, manter ereto]
 s. lienis, ligamento frenoesplênico. SIN phrenicosplenic *ligament.*
 s. ta'li, s. do tálus; suporte do tálus, uma projeção lateral semelhante a prateleira, a partir da superfície medial do calcâneo, cuja face superior apresenta uma faceta para a articulação com o tálus.
su·sur·rus (su-ser'ŭs). Sussurro. SIN murmur (1). [L.]
 s. au'rium, sussurro no ouvido; murmúrio no ouvido.
Sutter blood group. Grupo sanguíneo de Sutter. Ver apêndice de Grupos Sanguíneos.
Sutton, Richard L., dermatologista norte-americano, 1878–1952. VER S. *nevus.*
Sutton, Richard L., Jr., dermatologista norte-americano, *1908. VER S. *disease, ulcer.*

SUTURA

su·tu·ra, pl. **su·tu·rae** (soo'too'ră, -rē) [TA]. Sutura. SIN suture (1). [L. costura, sutura, de *suo*, pp. *sutus*, costurar]
  s. corona'lis [TA], s. coronal. SIN coronal *suture*.
  sutu'rae cra'nii [TA], suturas do crânio. SIN cranial *sutures*, em *suture*
  s. ethmoidolacrima'lis [TA], s. etmoidolacrimal. SIN ethmoidolacrimal *suture*.
  s. ethmoidomaxilla'ris [TA], s. etmoidomaxilar. SIN ethmoidomaxillary *suture*.
  s. fronta'lis, s. frontal. SIN frontal *suture*.
  s. frontalis persistens, s. frontal persistente; *termo oficial alternativo para metopic *suture*.
  s. frontoethmoida'lis [TA], s. frontoetmoidal. SIN frontoethmoidal *suture*.
  s. frontolacrima'lis [TA], s. frontolacrimal. SIN frontolacrimal *suture*.
  s. frontomaxilla'ris [TA], s. frontomaxilar. SIN frontomaxillary *suture*.
  s. frontonasa'lis [TA], s. frontonasal. SIN frontonasal *suture*.
  s. frontozygomat'ica [TA], s. frontozigomática. SIN frontozygomatic *suture*.
  s. incisi'va [TA], s. incisiva. SIN incisive *suture*.
  s. infraorbita'lis [TA], s. infra-orbital. SIN infraorbital *suture*.
  s. intermaxilla'ris [TA], s. intermaxilar. SIN intermaxillary *suture*.
  s. internasa'lis [TA], s. internasal. SIN internasal *suture*.
  s. interparieta'lis, s. sagital. SIN sagittal *suture*.
  s. lacrimoconcha'lis [TA], s. lacrimoconchal. SIN lacrimoconchal *suture*.
  s. lacrimomaxilla'ris [TA], s. lacrimomaxilar. SIN lacrimomaxillary *suture*.
  s. lambdoi'dea [TA], s. lambdóidea. SIN lambdoid *suture*.
  s. meto'pica [TA], s. metópica. SIN metopic *suture*.
  s. nasofronta'lis, s. frontonasal. SIN frontonasal *suture*.
  s. nasomaxilla'ris [TA], s. nasomaxilar. SIN nasomaxillary *suture*.
  s. no'tha (nō'tă), s. falsa. SIN false *suture*. [G. fem. de *nothos*, espúrio]
  s. occipitomastoi'dea [TA], s. occipitomastóidea. SIN occipitomastoid *suture*.
  s. palati'na media'na [TA], s. palatina mediana. SIN median palatine *suture*.
  s. palati'na transver'sa [TA], s. palatina transversa. SIN transverse palatine *suture*.
  s. palatoethmoida'lis [TA], s. palatoetmoidal. SIN palatoethmoidal *suture*.
  s. palatomaxilla'ris [TA], s. palatomaxilar. SIN palatomaxillary *suture*.
  s. parietomastoi'dea [TA], s. parietomastóidea. SIN parietomastoid *suture*.
  s. pla'na [TA], s. plana. SIN plane *suture*.
  s. sagitta'lis [TA], s. sagital. SIN sagittal *suture*.
  s. serra'ta [TA], s. serrátil. SIN serrate *suture*.
  s. sphenoethmoida'lis [TA], s. esfenoetmoidal. SIN sphenoethmoidal *suture*.
  s. sphenofronta'lis [TA], s. esfenofrontal. SIN sphenofrontal *suture*.
  s. sphenomaxilla'ris [TA], s. esfenomaxilar. SIN sphenomaxillary *suture*.
  s. spheno-orbita'lis, s. esfeno-orbital. SIN spheno-orbital *suture*.
  s. sphenoparieta'lis [TA], s. esfenoparietal. SIN sphenoparietal *suture*.
  s. sphenosquamo'sa [TA], s. esfenoescamosa. SIN sphenosquamous *suture*.
  s. sphenovomeria'na [TA], s. esfenovomeral. SIN sphenovomerine *suture*.
  s. sphenozygoma'tica [TA], s. esfenozigomática. SIN sphenozygomatic *suture*.
  s. squamoparietalis, (1) s. escamosa. SIN squamous *suture*; **(2)** s. escamoparietal. SIN squamoparietal *suture*.
  s. squamosomastoi'dea [TA], s. escamomastóidea. SIN squamomastoid *suture*.
  s. temporozygomat'ica [TA], s. temporozigomática. SIN temporozygomatic *suture*.
  s. zygomaticofronta'lis, s. frontozigomática. SIN frontozygomatic *suture*.
  s. zygomaticomaxilla'ris [TA], s. zigomaticomaxilar. SIN zygomaticomaxillary *suture*.
  s. zygomaticotempora'lis, s. temporozigomática. SIN temporozygomatic *suture*.

su·tur·al (soo'choor-ăl). Sutural; relativo a uma sutura em qualquer sentido.

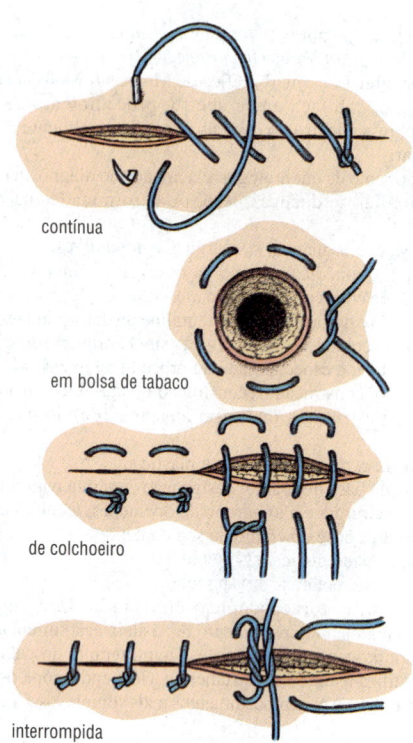

contínua

em bolsa de tabaco

de colchoeiro

interrompida

suturas cirúrgicas

SUTURE

su·ture (soo'choor) [TA]. **1.** Sutura; uma forma de articulação fibrosa em que dois ossos formados em membrana são unidos por uma membrana fibrosa contínua com o periósteo. SIN sutura [TA], suture joint. **2.** Suturar; unir duas superfícies por costura. SIN stitch (3). **3.** Fio de sutura; o material (fio de seda, metal, material sintético, etc.) com o qual duas superfícies são mantidas em aposição. **4.** A costura assim formada, uma sutura cirúrgica. [L. *sutura*, costura]
  absorbable surgical s., fio de sutura absorvível; fio de s. cirúrgico preparado a partir de uma substância que pode ser dissolvida pelos tecidos do corpo e, portanto, não é permanente; disponível em vários diâmetros e resistência a tensões; a velocidade de desaparecimento da resistência depende das características do fio de s.
  Albert s., s. de Albert; s. de Czerny modificada, em que a primeira fileira de pontos atravessa toda a espessura da parede do intestino.
  apposition s., s. de aposição; s. apenas da pele. SIN coaptation s.
  approximation s., s. de aproximação; s. que aproxima os tecidos profundos.
  atraumatic s., s. atraumática; fio de s. preso à extremidade de uma agulha sem orifício.
  blanket s., s. caseada; ponto duplo contínuo utilizado para aproximar a pele de uma ferida.
  bridle s., s. de contenção; s. através do músculo reto superior para rotação do bulbo do olho para baixo em cirurgia oftalmológica.
  Bunnell s., s. de Bunnell; método de tenorrafia que utiliza um fio metálico distendido afixado a botões.
  buried s., s. oculta; qualquer s. colocada totalmente abaixo da superfície da pele.
  button s., s. de botão; s. em que os fios são passados através dos orifícios de um botão e, a seguir, amarrados; utilizada para reduzir o risco de os fios cortarem a carne.
  catgut s., fio categute. VER catgut.
  coaptation s., s. de coaptação. SIN apposition s.
  cobbler's s., suturas de sapateiro. SIN doubly armed s.
  Connell s., s. de Connell; s. contínua utilizada para inverter a parede gástrica ou a intestinal na realização de uma anastomose.
  continuous s., s. contínua, s. em espiral; série ininterrupta de pontos utilizando um único fio de s.; o ponto é preso em cada extremidade por um nó. SIN spiral s., uninterrupted s.
  control release s., s. de liberação de controle; sutura com o fio preso a uma agulha sem orifício, de modo que os dois se separam quando se aplica tensão ao fio.
  coronal s. [TA], s. coronal; a linha de junção do osso frontal com os dois ossos parietais do crânio. SIN sutura coronalis [TA].
  cranial s.'s [TA], suturas cranianas; as suturas entre os ossos do crânio. SIN suturae cranii [TA].
  Cushing s., s. de Cushing; s. de colchoeiro horizontal utilizada para aproximar duas superfícies adjacentes.
  Czerny s., s. de Czerny; a primeira fileira da sutura intestinal de Czerny-Lembert; a agulha penetra na serosa e atravessa a submucosa ou muscular e, a seguir, entra na submucosa ou muscular do lado oposto, emergindo da serosa.
  Czerny-Lembert s., s. de Czerny-Lembert; s. intestinal em duas fileiras, que combina a sutura de Czerny (primeira) e a de Lembert (segunda).
  delayed s., s. tardia; s. de uma ferida depois de um intervalo de dias.
  dentate s., s. serrátil. SIN serrate s.

doubly armed s., s. duplamente armada, s. de sapateiro; sutura com uma agulha fixada em ambas as extremidades. SIN cobbler's s.
Dupuytren s., s. de Dupuytren; sutura de Lembert contínua.
end-on mattress s., sutura de colchoeiro vertical utilizada para aproximação exata da pele.
ethmoidolacrimal s. [TA], s. etmoidolacrimal; a linha de união da lâmina orbital do etmóide com a margem posterior do osso lacrimal. SIN sutura ethmoidolacrimalis [TA].
ethmoidomaxillary s. [TA], s. etmoidomaxilar; linha de aposição da superfície orbital do corpo da maxila com a lâmina orbital do osso etmóide. SIN sutura ethmoidomaxillaris [TA].
Faden s., s. de Faden; sutura efetuada entre um músculo reto do bulbo do olho e a porção posterior da esclera para limitar a ação excessiva do bulbo do olho. [Al. *Faden*, fio]
false s., s. falsa; s. cujas margens opostas são lisas ou apresentam apenas algumas projeções mal definidas. SIN sutura notha.
far-and-near s., s. de longe e de perto; s. interrompida que utiliza pontos alternados próximos e distantes, usada para aproximar bordas fasciais.
figure-of-8 s., s. em forma de 8; s. que utiliza pontos cruzados para aproximar bordas faciais ou as camadas musculofascial e externa de uma ferida abdominal.
frontal s., s. frontal; s. entre as duas metades do osso frontal, habitualmente obliterada em torno do sexto ano de vida; quando persistente, é denominada sutura metópica ou sutura frontal persistente. SIN sutura frontalis.
frontoethmoidal s. [TA], s. frontoetmoidal; linha de união entre a lâmina cribriforme do etmóide e a lâmina orbital e margem posterior do processo nasal do osso frontal. SIN sutura frontoethmoidalis [TA].
frontolacrimal s. [TA], s. frontolacrimal; linha de união entre a margem superior do osso lacrimal e a lâmina orbital do osso frontal. SIN sutura frontolacrimalis [TA].
frontomaxillary s. [TA], s. frontomaxilar; articulação do processo frontal da maxila com o osso frontal. SIN sutura frontomaxillaris [TA].
frontonasal s. [TA], s. frontonasal; linha de união do osso frontal e dos dois ossos nasais. SIN sutura frontonasalis [TA], sutura nasofrontalis.
frontozygomatic s. [TA], s. frontozigomática; linha de união entre o processo zigomático do frontal e o processo frontal do osso zigomático. SIN sutura frontozygomatica [TA], sutura zygomaticofrontalis.
Frost s., s. de Frost; s. intermarginal entre as pálpebras para proteger a córnea.
Gély s., s. de Gély; s. de sapateiro utilizada no fechamento de feridas intestinais.
glover s., s. de luveiro; s. contínua em que cada ponto atravessa a alça do ponto precedente.
Gould s., s. de Gould; s. de colchoeiro intestinal, em que cada alça é invaginada de modo que o tecido na alça fica saliente, tornando-se convexo em vez de côncavo.
Gussenbauer s., s. de Gussenbauer; s. em forma de 8 para o intestino, que se assemelha à sutura de Czerny-Lembert, mas que não inclui a mucosa.
Halsted s., s. de Halsted; s. que atravessa a fáscia subcuticular; utilizada para aproximação exata da pele.
harmonic s., s. plana. SIN plane s.
implanted s., s. implantada; passagem de um pino através de cada lado da ferida paralelamente à linha de incisão, sendo os pinos então unidos com fios de sutura.
incisive s. [TA], s. incisiva; linha de união das duas porções da maxila (pré- e pós-maxila); presente ao nascimento, podendo persistir na idade avançada. SIN sutura incisiva [TA], premaxillary s.
infraorbital s. [TA], s. infra-orbital; s. inconstante que segue o forame infra-orbital até o sulco infra-orbital. SIN sutura infraorbitalis [TA].
intermaxillary s. [TA], s. intermaxilar; a linha de união das duas maxilas. SIN sutura intermaxillaris [TA].
internasal s. [TA], s. internasal; linha de união entre os dois ossos nasais. SIN sutura internasalis [TA].
interparietal s., s. sagital. SIN sagittal s.
interrupted s., s. interrompida; série de pontos isolados, sendo as extremidades de cada um amarradas.
Jobert de Lamballe s., s. de Jobert de Lamballe; s. intestinal interrompida, utilizada para invaginar as margens dos intestinos da enterorrafia circular.
lacrimoconchal s. [TA], s. lacrimoconchal; linha de união do osso lacrimal com a concha nasal inferior. SIN sutura lacrimoconchalis [TA].
lacrimomaxillary s. [TA], s. lacrimomaxilar; linha de união, na parede medial da órbita, entre a margem anterior e inferior do osso lacrimal e a maxila. SIN sutura lacrimomaxillaris [TA].
lambdoid s. [TA], s. lambdóidea; linha de união em forma de λ invertido entre os ossos occipital e parietal. SIN sutura lambdoidea [TA].
Lembert s., s. de Lembert; a segunda fileira da s. intestinal de Czerny-Lembert; s. invertida para cirurgia intestinal, utilizada como sutura contínua ou interrompida, produzindo aposição da serosa e incluindo a camada submucosa colagenosa, porém sem penetrar na luz do intestino.
lens s.'s, raios da lente. SIN *radii* of lens, em *radius*.

locking s., s. de bloqueio; s. contínua em que o fio de sutura passa através da alça feita pelo ponto anterior. SIN lock stitch.
mattress s., s. de colchoeiro; s. utilizando um ponto duplo que forma uma alça ao redor do tecido de ambos os lados de uma ferida, produzindo eversão das bordas quando apertada. SIN quilted s.
median palatine s. [TA], s. palatina mediana; linha de união entre as lâminas horizontais dos ossos palatinos, continuando a sutura intermaxilar posteriormente. SIN sutura palatina mediana [TA].
metopic s. [TA], s. metópica; s. frontal persistente, algumas vezes discernível a curta distância acima da sutura frontonasal. VER TAMBÉM frontal s. SIN sutura metopica [TA], persistent frontal s.*, sutura frontalis persistens*.
nasomaxillary s. [TA], s. nasomaxilar; linha de união da margem lateral do osso nasal com o processo frontal da maxila. SIN sutura nasomaxillaris [TA].
nerve s., neurorrafia. SIN neurorrhaphy.
neurocentral s., sincondrose neurocentral. SIN neurocentral *synchondrosis*.
nonabsorbable surgical s., s. cirúrgica não-absorvível; fio de sutura cirúrgico que relativamente não é afetado pelas atividades biológicas dos tecidos do corpo e, portanto, permanente, a não ser que removido; p. ex., aço inoxidável, seda, algodão, náilon e outros materiais sintéticos.
occipitomastoid s. [TA], s. occipitomastóidea; continuação da s. lambdóidea entre a borda posterior da parte petrosa do osso temporal e o osso occipital. SIN sutura occipitomastoidea [TA].
palatoethmoidal s. [TA], s. palatoetmoidal; linha de junção do processo orbital do osso palatino e da lâmina orbital do etmóide. SIN sutura palatoethmoidalis [TA].
palatomaxillary s. [TA], s. palatomaxilar; linha de união, no assoalho da órbita, entre o processo orbital do osso palatino e a superfície orbital da maxila. SIN sutura palatomaxillaris [TA].
Paré s., s. de Paré; a aproximação das bordas de uma ferida através da passagem de tiras de tecido até a superfície, com sutura destas em lugar da pele.
parietomastoid s. [TA], s. parietomastóidea; a articulação do ângulo póstero-inferior do osso parietal com o processo mastóide do osso temporal. SIN sutura parietomastoidea [TA].
Parker-Kerr s., s. de Parker-Kerr; sutura contínua e invertida utilizada para fechar uma extremidade aberta do intestino.
persistent frontal s., s. frontal persistente; *termo oficial alternativo para metopic s.
petrosquamous s., fissura petroescamosa. VER petrosquamous *fissure*.
plane s. [TA], s. plana; aposição firme simples de duas superfícies lisas de ossos, sem superposição, como a observada na sutura lacrimomaxilar. SIN sutura plana [TA], harmonia, harmonic s.
pledgetted s., s. com compressa; s. sustentada por um pequeno pedaço de tecido, de modo que não se romperá através do tecido.
premaxillary s., s. pré-maxilar. SIN incisive s.
purse-string s., s. em bolsa de tabaco; s. contínua colocada de forma circular para inversão (como para um coto apendicular) ou fechamento (como para uma hérnia).
quilted s., s. de colchoeiro. SIN mattress s.
relaxation s., s. de relaxamento; pontos de sutura dispostos de modo que a sutura possa ser afrouxada se a tensão exercida pela ferida se tornar excessiva.
retention s., s. de retenção; s. de reforço densa colocada profundamente nos músculos e nas fáscias da parede abdominal para aliviar a tensão sobre a linha de s. primária. SIN tension s.
sagittal s. [TA], s. sagital; união na linha média entre os dois ossos parietais. SIN sutura sagittalis [TA], interparietal s., sutura interparietalis.
secondary s., s. secundária; fechamento tardio de uma ferida.
serrate s. [TA], s. serrátil; s. cujas margens opostas apresentam entalhes profundos semelhantes aos dentes de uma serra, como grande parte da sutura sagital. SIN sutura serrata [TA], dentate s.
shotted s., s. perolada; s. em que as extremidades são apertadas mediante passagem através de um grão de chumbo dividido (bala de chumbo parcialmente dividida), que é então comprimido.
sphenoethmoidal s. [TA], s. esfenoetmoidal; linha de união entre a crista do osso esfenóide e as lâminas perpendicular e cribriforme do etmóide. SIN sutura sphenoethmoidalis [TA].
sphenofrontal s. [TA], s. esfenofrontal; linha de união entre a lâmina orbital e o osso frontal e as asas menores do esfenóide de cada lado. SIN sutura sphenofrontalis [TA].
sphenomaxillary s. [TA], s. esfenomaxilar; s. inconstante entre o processo pterigóideo do osso esfenóide e o corpo da maxila. SIN sutura sphenomaxillaris [TA].
sphenooccipital s., sincondrose esfeno-occipital. SIN sphenooccipital *synchondrosis*.
spheno-orbital s., s. esfeno-orbital; articulação entre o processo orbital do osso palatino e a superfície externa do corpo do esfenóide. SIN sutura spheno-orbitalis.
sphenoparietal s. [TA], s. esfenoparietal; linha de união da borda inferior do osso parietal com a borda superior da asa maior do esfenóide. SIN sutura sphenoparietalis [TA].

sphenosquamous s. [TA], s. esfenoescamosa; articulação da asa maior do esfenóide com a parte escamosa do osso temporal. SIN sutura sphenosquamosa [TA].
sphenovomerine s. [TA], s. esfenovomeral; linha de união do processo vaginal do esfenóide com a asa do vômer. SIN sutura sphenovomeriana [TA].
sphenozygomatic s. [TA], s. esfenozigomática; junção do osso zigomático com a asa maior do esfenóide. SIN sutura sphenozygomatica [TA].
spiral s., s. em espiral. SIN continuous s.
squamomastoid s. [TA], s. escamosomastóidea; linha de união das partes escamosa e petrosa do osso temporal durante o desenvolvimento; algumas vezes, persiste na região do processo mastóide. SIN sutura squamosomastoidea [TA].
squamoparietal s., s. escamoparietal; a articulação do osso parietal com a parte escamosa do osso temporal. SIN sutura squamoparietalis (2).
squamous s. [TA], s. escamosa; s. semelhante a uma escama, cujas margens opostas são semelhantes a escamas e superpostas. SIN sutura squamoparietalis (1).
subcuticular s., s. subcuticular. VER Halsted s.
temporozygomatic s., s. temporozigomática; linha de junção do processo zigomático do osso temporal com o processo temporal do osso zigomático. SIN sutura temporozygomatica [TA], sutura zygomaticotemporalis, zygomaticotemporal s.
tendon s., tenorrafia. SIN tenorrhaphy.
tension s., s. de retenção, s. de tensão. SIN retention s.
transfixion s., s. de transfixação; (1) ponto cruzado colocado de modo a controlar o sangramento de uma superfície tecidual ou de um pequeno vaso quando apertado; (2) s. utilizada para fixar a colunela ao septo nasal.
transverse palatine s. [TA], s. palatina transversa; linha de união dos processos palatinos da maxila com as lâminas horizontais dos ossos palatinos. SIN sutura palatina transversa [TA].
tympanomastoid s., fissura timpanomastóidea. SIN tympanomastoid fissure.
uninterrupted s., s. ininterrupta. SIN continuous s.
wedge-and-groove s., esquindilese. SIN schindylesis.
zygomaticomaxillary s. [TA], s. zigomaticomaxilar; articulação do osso zigomático com o processo zigomático da maxila. SIN sutura zygomaticomaxillaris [TA].
zygomaticotemporal s., s. temporozigomática. SIN temporozygomatic s.

su·tur·ec·to·my (soo-choor-ek'tō-mē). Suturectomia; remoção de sutura craniana.
suxamethonium. Suxametônio, succinilcolina. SIN succinylcholine.
Suzanne, Jean G., médico francês, *1859. VER S. gland.
SV Abreviatura de simian virus (vírus de símios) numerados seriadamente; p. ex., SV1.
SV40 Símbolo do simian vacuolating virus No. 40 (vírus vacuolizante de símios n.º 40).
Sv Abreviatura de sievert.
Svedberg, Theodor, químico sueco e Prêmio Nobel, 1884–1971. VER S. equation, ou flotation, unit.
Svedberg of flo·ta·tion. Constante de flutuação. SIN flotation constant.
swab (swob). Swab; chumaço de algodão, gaze ou outro material absorvente fixado à extremidade de um bastão, utilizado para aplicação ou remoção de substância de uma superfície.
swage (swāj). 1. Fundir o fio de sutura a agulhas de sutura. 2. Moldar metal martelando ou adaptando-o a um molde, utilizando freqüentemente um contramolde. [Fr. ant. souage]

swal·low (swawl'ō). Deglutir; passar qualquer coisa através das fauces, faringe e esôfago até o estômago; efetuar o ato da deglutição. [A.S. swelgan]
Gastrografin s., esofagograma ou seriografia esôfago-estômago-duodeno (SEED) utilizando contraste iodado solúvel (no caso, diatrizoato de meglumina). SIN hypaque s.
hypaque s., seriografia esôfago-estômago-duodeno usando o contraste Hypaque (diatrizoato de meglumina). SIN Gastrografin s.
somatic s., d. somática; padrão de deglutição com contrações musculares que parecem estar sob o controle da pessoa em nível subconsciente; distinta da deglutição visceral.
visceral s., d. visceral; o padrão de deglutição imaturo de um lactente ou de uma pessoa com impulso da língua, lembrando as contrações musculares peristálticas semelhantes a ondas observadas no intestino; a deglutição do adulto ou madura é mais volitiva e, portanto, somática.
Swan, Harold James C., cardiologista norte-americano, *1922. VER S.-Ganz catheter.
swarm·ing (swōrm'ing). Propagação progressiva de bactérias móveis sobre a superfície de um meio de cultura sólido. [A.S. swearm]
Sweat, Faye, patologista do século XX. VER Puchtler-S. stains. VER Puchtler-S. stains.
sweat (swet). 1. Suor; perspiração (3), especialmente transpiração sensível. 2. Transpirar. [A.S. swāt]
night s.'s, suor noturno; sudorese profusa à noite, que ocorre na tuberculose pulmonar e em outras afecções debilitantes crônicas com febre baixa.
red s., s. vermelho; vermelhidão do suor, especialmente na axila, devido a um pigmento produzido por Streptomyces roseofulvis. VER TAMBÉM chromidrosis.
sweat·ing (swet'ing). Sudorese. SIN perspiration (1).
sweep (swēp). Varredura; movimento do feixe de um osciloscópio de raios catódicos da esquerda para a direita, representando o eixo de tempo, produzido por uma voltagem denteada (com formato em dentes de serra) gerada artificialmente.
Sweet, Robert Douglas, dermatologista inglês do século XX. VER S. disease.
Sweet. VER Gordon e Sweet stain.
swell·ing (swel'ing). Tumefação, intumescência, saliência, aumento de volume. 1. Aumento, p. ex., protuberância ou tumor. 2. Em embriologia, uma elevação primordial que se desenvolve numa prega, crista ou proeminência.
albuminous s., t. albuminosa. SIN cloudy s.
arytenoid s., saliência aritenóide; elevações primordiais pares, de cada lado da laringe embrionária, no interior das quais se formam as cartilagens aritenóideas.
brain s., t. cerebral; entidade patológica, localizada ou generalizada, caracterizada por aumento de volume do tecido cerebral, devido à expansão dos compartimentos intravascular (congestão) ou extravascular (edema), que podem coexistir ou ocorrer separadamente, sendo clinicamente indistinguíveis; as manifestações clínicas dependem da perturbação da função neuronal em virtude da tumefação local, deslocamento das estruturas intracranianas e efeitos da hipertensão intracraniana ou distúrbio circulatório.
Calabar s., loíase. SIN loiasis.
cloudy s., degeneração granular; tumefação de células devido à lesão das membranas, afetando a transferência iônica; provoca acúmulo de água intracelular. SIN albuminous s., granular degeneration, hydropic degeneration, parenchymatous degeneration.
fugitive s., loíase. SIN loiasis.
genital s.'s, saliências genitais; elevações primordiais bilaterais que flanqueiam o tubérculo genital e o orifício urogenital do embrião; desenvolvem-se nas pregas labioescrotais, que se transformam nos lábios maiores do pudendo na mulher, e unem-se para formar a bolsa escrotal do homem. SIN labioscrotal s.'s.

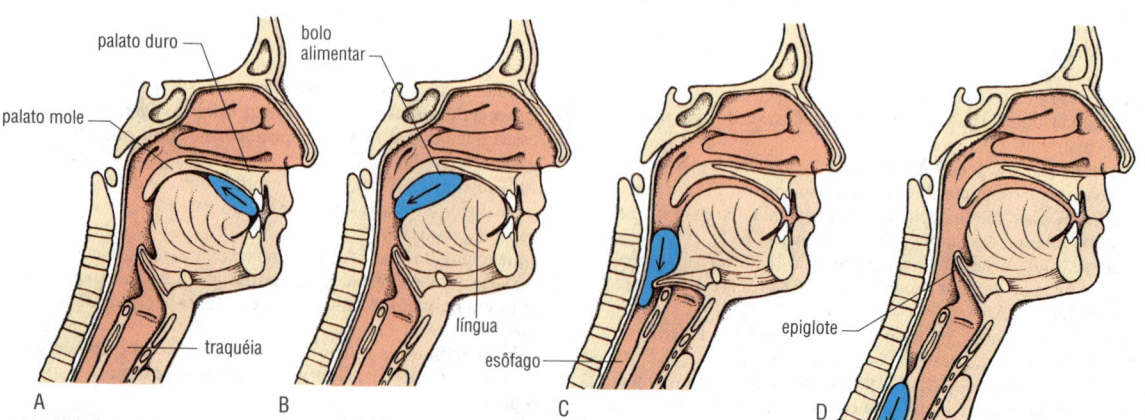

deglutição: (A) o bolo alimentar é empurrado para trás; (B) a nasofaringe se fecha; (C) a epiglote fecha a traquéia; (D) o bolo alimentar é propelido pelo esôfago

hunger s., edema da inanição causado por muitos fatores, primariamente a redução da albumina sérica.

labial s., saliência labial; a tumefação genital embrionária feminina que se alonga para tornar-se o lábio maior do pudendo definitivo. VER TAMBÉM genital s.'s.

labioscrotal s.'s, saliências genitais. SIN genital s.'s.

lateral lingual s.'s, tumefações linguais laterais; no embrião, elevações ovais bilaterais que aparecem no assoalho da boca, ao nível do arco mandibular; as elevações primordiais, compostas de mesênquima recoberto por ectoderma de origem estomodeal, fundem-se para formar a maior parte dos dois terços anteriores da língua.

levator s., toro do levantador. SIN *torus levatorius.*

Neufeld capsular s., intumescimento capsular de Neufeld; aumento da opacidade e da visibilidade da cápsula de microrganismos encapsulados expostos a anticorpos anticapsulares aglutinantes específicos. SIN Neufeld reaction, quellung phenomenon, quellung reaction (1), quellung test.

scrotal s., saliência escrotal; tumefação formada após a fusão das saliências genitais embrionárias esféricas, situada na base do pênis; pouco antes do nascimento, os testículos passam a localizar-se em seu interior.

Spielmeyer acute s., t. aguda de Spielmeyer; forma de degeneração das células nervosas em que o corpo celular e seus prolongamentos aumentam de volume e coram-se pálida e difusamente.

switch·ing (swich'ing). Mudança, desvio. **1.** Fazer um desvio ou mudança. **2.** Movimento de uma região definida do DNA no interior de um genoma.

  class s., mudança de classe; mudança na expressão da região C de uma cadeia pesada de imunoglobulina.

Swyer, Paul R., pediatra norte-americano, *1921. SIN Swyer-James *syndrome*; S.-James-MacLeod *syndrome*.

sy·co·sis (sī-kō'sis). Sicose; foliculite pustular, sobretudo da área coberta com barba. [G. *sykōsis*, de *sykōn*, figo + *-osis*, condição]

Sydenham, Thomas, médico inglês, 1624–1689. VER S. *chorea, disease.*

Sydney crease. Prega de Sydney. Ver em crease.

Sydney line. Linha de Sydney. Ver em line.

syl·la·ble-stum·bling (sil'a̅-bl-stum'bling). Dissilabia; forma de tartamudez em que o indivíduo se detém em certas sílabas que considera difícil de pronunciar. SIN dyssyllabia. [L. *syllabē*, várias letras ou sons considerados em conjuntos]

syl·vat·ic (sil-vat'ik). Silvático; que ocorre em ou que afeta animais selvagens. [L. *silva*, florestas]

Sylvest, Ejnar, médico norueguês, 1880–1931. VER S. *disease.*

syl·vi·an (sil've̅-an). Silviano; relativo a Franciscus ou Jacobus Sylvius ou a qualquer uma das estruturas descritas por um deles.

Sylvius, Jacobus (Jacques), anatomista francês, 1478–1555. VER *caro quadrata sylvii; os sylvii.*

Sylvius, Le Böe, Franciscus (François), médico, anatomista e fisiologista holandês, 1614–1672. VER sylvian *angle*; sylvian *aqueduct*; sylvian *fissure*; sylvian *line*; sylvian *point*; sylvian *valve*; sylvian *ventricle*; *fossa* of S.; *vallecula sylvii.*

♲ **sym-.** Sim-. VER sym-.

sym·bal·lo·phone (sim-bal'ō-fōn). Simbalofone; estetoscópio que possui duas campânulas, projetado para lateralizar o som e produzir um efeito estereofônico. [G. *symballō*, arremessar + *phōnē*, som]

sym·bi·on, sym·bi·ont (sim'bē-on, -ont). Simbionte; organismo associado a outro em simbiose. SIN mutualist, symbiote. [G. *symbion*, neut. de *symbiōs*, que vive junto]

sym·bi·o·sis (sim-bē-ō'sis). Simbiose. **1.** A associação biológica de duas ou mais espécies, com benefício mútuo. Cf. commensalim, mutualistic s., parasitism. **2.** A cooperação mútua ou interdependência de duas pessoas, como mãe e lactente ou marido e mulher; termo algumas vezes utilizado para designar uma interdependência excessiva ou patológica de duas pessoas. [G. *symbiōsis*, estado de viver junto, de sym- + *bios*, vida + *-osis*, condição]

  dyadic s., s. diádica; s. entre uma criança e um dos pais.

  mutualistic s., s. mutualística; simbiose em que todos os parceiros obtêm uma vantagem.

  triadic s., s. triádica; simbiose entre uma criança e ambos os pais.

sym·bi·ote (sim'bē-ōt). Simbiota. SIN symbion.

sym·bi·ot·ic (sim-bē-ot'ik). Simbiótico; relativo a simbiose.

sym·bleph·a·ron (sim-blef'a̅-ron). Simbléfaro; aderência de uma ou de ambas as pálpebras ao bulbo do olho, parcial ou completa, em decorrência de queimaduras ou outro traumatismo; raramente congênita. SIN artretoblepharia. [sym- + G. *blepharon*, pálpebra]

  anterior s., s. anterior; união entre a pálpebra e o bulbo do olho por uma faixa fibrosa, sem envolver o fórnice.

  posterior s., s. posterior; aderência entre o bulbo do olho e a pálpebra, envolvendo o fórnice.

sym·bol (sim'bŏl). Símbolo. **1.** Sinal convencional que serve como abreviação. **2.** Em química, abreviatura do nome de um elemento, radical ou composto, expressando em fórmulas químicas, um átomo ou uma molécula desse elemento (p. ex., H e O na H_2O); em bioquímica, abreviatura de nomes triviais de moléculas utilizada primariamente em combinação com outros símbolos semelhantes para construir conjuntos maiores (p. ex., Gly para glicerina, Ado para adenosina, Glc para glicose). **3.** Em psicanálise, um objeto ou ação interpretado para representar algum desejo reprimido ou inconsciente, freqüentemente sexual. **4.** Sinal filosófico-lingüístico. VER TAMBÉM conventional *signs*, em *sign*. [G. *symbolon*, marca ou sinal, de *sym-ballō*, arremessar conjuntamente]

sym·bo·lia (sim-bō'lē-a̅). Simbolia; a capacidade de reconhecer a forma e a natureza de um objeto pelo tato. [G. *symbolon*, marca ou sinal]

sym·bol·ism (sim'bō-lizm). Simbolismo. **1.** Em psicanálise, o processo envolvido na representação disfarçada na consciência de conteúdo ou eventos inconscientes ou reprimidos. **2.** Estado mental em que tudo o que acontece é considerado pelo indivíduo como simbólico de seus próprios pensamentos. **3.** A descrição da vida e das experiências emocionais em termos abstratos.

sym·bol·i·za·tion (sim'bō-li-zā'shŭn). Simbolização; mecanismo mental inconsciente através do qual um objeto ou idéia é representado por outro.

sym·brach·y·dac·ty·ly (sim-brak'i-dak'ti-lē). Simbraquidactilia; condição em que dedos das mãos anormalmente curtos são unidos ou possuem membranas interdigitais em suas porções proximais. [sym- + G. *brachys*, curto + *daktylos*, dedo]

Syme, James, cirurgião escocês, 1799–1870. VER S. *amputation, operation.*

Symington, Johnson, anatomista escocês, 1851–1924. VER S. anococcygeal *body.*

sym·me·lia (si-mē'lē-a̅). Simelia. SIN sirenomelia. [sym- + G. *melos*, membro]

Symmers, W. St. C., patologista inglês, 1863–1937. VER S. clay pipestem *fibrosis.*

sym·me·try (sim'ĕ-trē). Simetria; igualdade ou correspondência na forma de partes distribuídas ao redor de um centro ou de um eixo, nas extremidades ou pólos ou nas faces opostas de qualquer corpo. [G. *symmetria*, de sym- + *metron*, medida]

  inverse s., s. inversa; correspondência do lado direito ou esquerdo de um indivíduo assimétrico com o lado esquerdo ou direito de outro.

♲ **sympath-, sympatheto-, sympathico-, sympatho-.** Simpat-, simpateto-, simpatico-, simpato-; a parte simpática do sistema nervoso autônomo. [ver sympathetic]

sym·pa·thec·to·my (sim-pă-thek'tō-mē). Simpatectomia; excisão de um segmento de um nervo simpático ou de um ou mais gânglios simpáticos. SIN sympathetectomy, sympathicectomy. [sympath- + G. *ektomē*, excisão]

  chemical s., s. química; destruição dos nervos simpáticos periarteriais, como na operação de Doppler, por um corrosivo, como o fenol.

  periarterial s., s. periarterial; desnervação simpática por descorticação arterial. SIN histoneurectomy, Leriche operation.

  presacral s., s. pré-sacral. SIN presacral *neurectomy.*

sym·pa·the·tec·to·my (sim-pă-thē-tek'tō-mē). Simpatectomia. SIN sympathectomy.

sym·pa·thet·ic (sim-pă-thet'ik). Simpático. **1.** Relativo a ou que exibe simpatia. **2.** Designa a parte simpática do sistema nervoso autônomo. SIN sympathic. [G. *sympathētikos*, de *sympatheō*, simpatizar, de *syn*, com + *pathos*, sofrimento]

sym·pa·thet·o·blast (sim-pă-thet'ō-blast). Simpatetoblasto. SIN sympathoblast.

sym·pa·thic (sim-path'ik). Simpático. SIN sympathetic.

sym·path·i·cec·to·my (sim-path'i-sek'tō-mē). Simpaticectomia. SIN sympathectomy.

♲ **sympathico-.** Simpático-. VER sympath-.

sym·path·i·co·blast (sim-path'i-kō-blast). Simpaticoblasto. SIN sympathoblast.

sym·path·i·co·neu·ri·tis (sim-path'i-kō-noo-rī'tis). Simpaticoneurite; inflamação dos nervos autônomos.

sym·path·i·cop·a·thy (sim-path-i-kop'a̅-thē). Simpaticopatia; doença decorrente de um distúrbio do sistema nervoso autônomo. [sympathico- + G. *pathos*, sofrimento]

sym·path·i·co·to·nia (sim-path'i-kō-tō'nē-a̅). Simpaticotonia; condição em que há aumento do tônus do sistema simpático e acentuada tendência ao espasmo vascular e elevação da pressão arterial; oposto da vagotonia. [sympathico- + G. *tonos*, tônus, tensão]

sym·path·i·co·ton·ic (sim-path'i-kō-ton'ik). Simpaticotônico; relativo a, ou caracterizado por, simpaticotonia.

sym·path·i·co·trip·sy (sim-path'i-kō-trip'sē). Simpaticotripsia; esmagamento cirúrgico do gânglio simpático. [sympathico- + G. *tripsis*, atrito]

sym·pa·thin (sim'pă-thin). Simpatina; a substância que se difunde para a circulação a partir das terminações nervosas simpáticas quando estão ativas. O termo foi introduzido por W.B. Cannon, que acreditava que essa substância diferia do mediador produzido pela terminação nervosa (hoje em dia, sabe-se que isso está incorreto); o próprio mediador (norepinefrina) difunde-se para a circulação. SIN sympathetic hormone.

sym·pa·thism (sim'pă-thizm). Simpatismo. SIN suggestibility. [G. *sympatheia*, simpatia]

sym·pa·thiz·er (sim'pă-thī-zer). Simpatizante. **1.** Olho acometido de oftalmia simpática. **2.** Aquele que exibe simpatia.

sympatho-. Simpato-. VER sympath-.
sym·pa·tho·ad·re·nal (sim'pă-thō-ă-drē'năl). Simpatoadrenal; relativo à parte simpática do sistema nervoso autônomo e à medula da glândula supra-renal, como os neurônios pós-ganglionares.
sym·pa·tho·blast (sim'pă-thō-blast). Simpatoblasto; célula primitiva derivada da glia da crista neural; junto com os feocromoblastos, os simpatoblastos entram na formação da medula supra-renal e dos gânglios simpáticos. SIN sympathetoblast, sympathicoblast. [sympatho- + G. *blastos*, germe]
sym·pa·tho·go·nia (sim'pă-thō-gō'nē-ă). Simpatogonia; as células completamente indiferenciadas do sistema nervoso simpático. [sympatho- + G. *gonē*, semente]
sym·pa·tho·lyt·ic (sim'pă-thō-lit'ik). Simpatolítico; designa antagonismo à atividade nervosa adrenérgica ou inibição da mesma. VER TAMBÉM adrenergic blocking *agent*, antiadrenergic. [sympatho- + G. *lysis*, afrouxamento]
sym·pa·tho·mi·met·ic (sim'pă-thō-mi-met'ik). Simpatomimético; refere-se à imitação da ação do sistema simpático. VER TAMBÉM adrenomimetic. [sympatho- + G. *mimikos*, que imita]
sym·pa·thy (sim'pă-thē). Simpatia. 1. A relação mútua, fisiológica ou patológica, entre dois órgãos, sistemas ou partes do corpo. 2. Contágio mental, como aquele observado na histeria, na massa ou no bocejo induzido pela observação de outra pessoa bocejando. 3. Apreciação sensitiva expressa ou preocupação emocional e ato de compartilhar o estado mental e emocional de outra pessoa. Cf. empathy (1). [G. *sympatheia*, de sym- + *pathos*, sofrimento]
sym·per·i·to·ne·al (sim'per-i-tō-nē'ăl). Simperitoneal; relativo à indução cirúrgica de aderência entre duas partes do peritônio.
sym·pha·lan·gism, sym·pha·lan·gy (sim-fal'an-jizm, sim-fal'an-jē). Sinfalangismo. 1. Sindactilia. SIN syndactyly. 2. Ancilose das articulações dos dedos das mãos e dos pés. [sym- + phalanx]
sym·phys·i·al, sym·phys·e·al (sim-fiz'ē-ăl). Sinfisial; que crescem juntos; relativo a uma sínfise; fundido. SIN symphysic.
sym·phys·ic (sim-fiz'ik). Sinfísico. SIN symphysial.
sym·phys·i·on (sim-fiz'ē-on). Sinfísio; ponto craniométrico, o ponto mais anterior do processo alveolar da mandíbula.
sym·phys·i·o·tome, sym·phys·e·o·tome (sim-fiz'ē-ō-tōm). Sinfisiótomo; instrumento para uso em sinfisiotomia.
sym·phys·i·ot·o·my, sym·phys·e·ot·o·my (sim-fiz-ē-ot'ō-mē). Sinfisiotomia; divisão da articulação púbica de modo a aumentar a capacidade de uma pelve contraída e permitir a passagem de uma criança viva. SIN synchondrotomy. [symphysis + G. *tomē*, incisão]
sym·phy·sis, gen. **sym·phy·ses** (sim'fi-sis, -sēz) [TA]. Sínfise. 1. [NA]. Forma de articulação cartilaginosa em que a união entre dois ossos é efetuada por meio de fibrocartilagem. SIN amphiarthrosis. 2. Uma união, ponto de encontro ou comissura de duas estruturas. 3. Aderência patológica ou crescimento conjunto. SIN secondary cartilaginous joint [TA]. [G. que cresce junto]
intervertebral s. [TA], s. intervertebral; a união entre corpos vertebrais adjacentes compostos do núcleo pulposo, ligamento anular e ligamentos longitudinais anterior e posterior. SIN s. intervertebralis [TA].
s. intervertebra'lis [TA], s. intervertebral. SIN intervertebral s.
s. mandib'ulae [TA], s. mandibular. SIN mandibular s.
mandibular s. [TA], s. mandibular; a união fibrocartilaginosa das duas metades da mandíbula no feto; transforma-se em união óssea durante o primeiro ano de vida. SIN s. mandibulae [TA], mental s., s. mentalis, s. menti.
manubriosternal s. [TA], s. manubriesternal; a união posterior, por fibrocartilagem, do manúbrio com o corpo do esterno; começa como uma sincondrose e torna-se uma sínfise, fundindo-se ocasionalmente para transformar-se em sinostose. SIN s. manubriosternalis [TA], sternomanubrial junction.
s. manubriosterna'lis [TA], s. manubriesternal. SIN manubriosternal s.
mental s., s. mandibular, mentual. SIN mandibular s.
s. menta'lis, s. mandibular, mentual. SIN mandibular s.
s. men'ti, s. mandibular. SIN mandibular s.
pericardial s., s. pericárdica; aderência entre as camadas parietal e visceral do pericárdio.
pubic s. [TA], s. púbica; a articulação fibrocartilaginosa firme entre os dois púbis. SIN s. pubica [TA], s. pubis.
s. pu'bica [TA], s. púbica. SIN pubic s.
s. pu'bis, s. púbica. SIN pubic s.
s. sacrococcyg'ea, articulação sacrococcígea. SIN sacrococcygeal *joint*.
s. xiphosternalis [TA], s. xifosternal. SIN xiphisternal *joint*.
sym·plas·mat·ic (sim-plaz-mat'ik). Simplasmático; relativo à união do protoplasma, como na formação de células gigantes. [G. *sym- plassō*, modelar em conjunto]
sym·plast (sim'plast). Simplasto; célula multinucleada que se formou por fusão de células separadas. [sym- + G. *plastos*, formado]
sym·po·dia (sim-pō'dē-ă). Simpodia; condição caracterizada pela união dos pés. VER TAMBÉM sirenomelia, sympus. [sym- + G. *pous*, pé]
sym·port (sim'pōrt). Simporte; transporte acoplado de duas moléculas ou íons diferentes através de uma membrana, na mesma direção, por um mecanismo transportador comum (simportador). Cf. antiport, uniport. [sym- + L. *porto*, transportar]
sym·port·er (sim-pōrt'er). Simportador; a proteína responsável por mediar o simporte.
symp·tom (simp'tŏm). Sintoma; qualquer fenômeno mórbido ou desvio normal na estrutura, função ou sensação, apresentado pelo paciente e indicador de doença. VER TAMBÉM phenomenon (1), reflex (1), sign (1), syndrome. [G. *symptōma*]
abstinence s.'s, sintomas de abstinência. SIN withdrawal s.'s.
accessory s., s. acessório; sintoma que geralmente, mas nem sempre, acompanha determinada doença, distinto de um sintoma patognomônico. SIN assident s., concomitant s.
accidental s., s. acidental; qualquer fenômeno mórbido que ocorre concomitantemente na evolução de uma doença, mas que não tem nenhuma relação com ela.
assident s., s. acessório. SIN accessory s.
Baumès s., s. de Baumès; dor atrás do esterno na angina de peito.
Bolognini s., s. de Bolognini; sensação de crepitação com aumento gradual da pressão sobre o abdome em casos de sarampo.
cardinal s., s. cardinal; o s. primário de importância diagnóstica.
concomitant s., s. concomitante. SIN accessory s.
constitutional s., s. constitucional; s. que indica o efeito sistêmico de uma doença; p. ex., perda de peso.
deficiency s., s. de deficiência; manifestação de carência, em graus variáveis, de alguma substância (p. ex., hormônio, enzima, vitamina) necessária para a estrutura e/ou função normais de um organismo.
Demarquay s., s. de Demarquay; ausência de elevação da laringe durante a deglutição, considerada como indicação de endurecimento sifilítico da traquéia.
Epstein s., s. de Epstein. VER Epstein *sign*.
equivocal s., s. equívoco; s. que não aponta definitivamente para qualquer doença especial, estando associado a qualquer um de vários estados mórbidos ou cuja presença é incerta ou indefinida.
first rank s.'s (FRS), sintomas de primeiro grau. SIN Schneider first rank s.'s.
Fischer s., sinal de Fischer. SIN Fischer *sign*.
Gordon s., s. de Gordon. SIN tonic *reflex*.
incarceration s., s. de encarceramento. SIN Dietl *crisis*.
induced s., s. induzido; s. desencadeado por droga, exercício ou outros meios, muitas vezes intencionalmente para fins diagnósticos.
local s., s. local; s. de extensão limitada, causado por doença de determinado órgão ou parte.
localizing s., s. de localização; s. que indica claramente o local do processo mórbido.
Macewen s., s. de Macewen. SIN Macewen *sign*.
negative s., s. negativo; um dos sintomas de déficit da esquizofrenia, resultando da diminuição da volição e função de execução, incluindo inércia, anergia, falta de envolvimento com o ambiente, pobreza de pensamento, isolamento social e afeto embotado.
objective s., s. objetivo; s. que é evidente para o observador.
pathognomonic s., s. patognomônico; s. que, quando presente, indica definitivamente a presença de determinada doença.
positive s., s. positivo; um dos sintomas agudos ou floridos da esquizofrenia, incluindo alucinações, delírios, distúrbio do pensamento, associações desconexas, ambivalência ou labilidade afetiva.
Pratt s., s. de Pratt; termo raramente utilizado para referir-se à rigidez nos músculos de um membro lesado, que precede a ocorrência de gangrena.
presenting s., s. principal; a queixa apresentada pelo paciente como principal motivo de procurar assistência médica; em geral, sinônimo de chief *complaint* (queixa principal).
rainbow s., s. do arco-íris. SIN glaucomatous *halo* (2).
reflex s., s. reflexo; distúrbio da sensação ou da função em determinado órgão ou parte mais ou menos distante da condição mórbida que o originou; p. ex., espasmo muscular devido a inflamação articular. SIN sympathetic s.
Schneider first rank s.'s, sintomas de primeiro grau de Schneider; sintomas que, quando presentes, indicam a probabilidade de diagnóstico de esquizofrenia, contanto que seja excluída uma etiologia orgânica ou tóxica: ilusão de controle, disseminação do pensamento, retraimento do pensamento, inserção do pensamento, ouvir os próprios pensamentos em voz alta, alucinações auditivas que comentam sobre o comportamento do próprio indivíduo e alucinações auditivas em que duas vozes conversam. SIN first rank s.'s, schneiderian first rank s.'s.
schneiderian first rank s.'s, sintomas de primeiro grau de Schneider. SIN Schneider first rank s.'s.
Sklowsky s., s. de Sklowsky; a ruptura de uma vesícula de varicela produzida por pressão muito leve com o dedo, sendo necessária uma maior pressão para romper as vesículas da varíola, do herpes ou de outras afecções.
subjective s., s. subjetivo; sintoma apenas aparente para o paciente.
sympathetic s., s. simpático. SIN reflex s.
Trendelenburg s., sinal de Trendelenburg; marcha anserina na paresia dos músculos glúteos, como na distrofia muscular progressiva.

Uhthoff s., s. de Uhthoff; entorpecimento transitório dependente da temperatura, fraqueza ou perda da visão. Ocorre interrupção da condução em qualquer nervo se a temperatura sofrer elevação excessiva. Em um nervo lesado (p. ex., desmielinização), essa temperatura de colapso é reduzida e pode aproximar-se da temperatura corporal normal. Pode surgir, então, uma disfunção neurológica transitória com uma chuveirada quente, prática de exercício físico ou ocorrência de febre. SIN Uhthoff syndrome.

Wartenberg s., s. de Wartenberg; (1) flexão do polegar quando o paciente tenta flexionar os quatro dedos contra a resistência, um "sinal piramidal"; (2) prurido intenso na ponta do nariz e das narinas em casos de tumor cerebral.

withdrawal s.'s, sintomas de abstinência; conjunto de sintomas mórbidos, incluindo excitabilidade e irritabilidade, que ocorrem em um dependente privado da dose habitual do agente de dependência. SIN abstinence s.'s.

symp·to·mat·ic (simp-to-mat′ik). Sintomático, indicativo; relacionado a uma doença ou que constitui o conjunto de seus sintomas.

symp·tom·a·tol·o·gy (simp′to-mă-tol′o-jē). Sintomatologia. **1.** A ciência dos sintomas de doença, sua produção e as indicações que fornecem. **2.** O conjunto de sintomas de uma doença. [symptom + G. *logos*, estudo]

symp·to·mat·o·lyt·ic (simp′to-mat-o-lit′ik). Sintomatolítico; que elimina os sintomas. SIN symptomolytic. [symptom + G. *lytikos*, que dissolve]

symp·to·mo·lyt·ic (sim-to-mo-lit′ik). Sintomatolítico. SIN symptomatolytic.

symp·to·sis (sim-to′sis). Simptose; debilitação localizada ou generalizada do corpo. [G. queda em conjunto, colapso, de *syn*, junto + *ptosis*, queda]

sym·pus (sim′pŭs). Simpodia, indivíduo com fusão das pernas e dos pés na linha mediana. [G. *sympous*, de sym- + *pous*, pé]

 s. a'pus, s. sem pés; sirenômelo sem pés.
 s. di'pus, s. com pés; sirenômelo com ambos os pés mais ou menos distintos.
 s. mo'nopus, s. com um pé; sirenômelo com apenas um pé externamente visível.

Syms, Parker, cirurgião norte-americano, 1860–1933. VER S. *tractor*.

syn-. Sin-; junto, com, unido; aparece como sim- antes de b, p ou m; corresponde ao L. com-. [G. *syn*, com, junto]

syn·a·del·phus (sin-ă-del′fŭs). Sinadelfo; gêmeos unidos com uma única cabeça, tronco parcialmente unido e quatro membros superiores e quatro inferiores. VER conjoined *twins*, em *twin*. [syn- + G. *adelphos*, irmão]

synanamorph (sin-an′ă-morf). Sinanamorfo; a mesma espécie de fungo que cresce numa forma diferente.

syn·a·nas·to·mo·sis (sin′an-as-to-mo′sis). Sinanastomose; anastomose entre vários vasos sanguíneos.

syn·an·dro·gen·ic (sin′an-dro-jen′ik). Sinandrogênico; relativo a qualquer agente ou condição que aumenta os efeitos dos androgênios.

sy·nan·them, syn·an·the·ma (si-nan′them, sin′an-the′mă). Sinantema; exantema que consiste em várias formas diferentes de erupção. [G. *syn- antheo*, florescer junto]

sy·naph·o·cep·tors (si-naf-o-sep′terz). Sinaforreceptores; receptores estimulados por contato direto. [G. *synaphe*, contato + L. *recipio*, receber]

syn·apse, pl. **syn·aps·es** (sin′aps, si-naps′; si-nap′sēz). Sinapse; o contato funcional entre membranas da célula nervosa com outra célula nervosa, com um efetor (músculo, glândula) ou com uma célula receptora sensitiva. A sinapse serve para transmissão de impulsos nervosos, comumente de uma terminação axônica de tamanho variável (1–12 μm), geralmente em forma de protuberância arredondada ou bastão (elemento pós-sináptico) para a placa circunscrita da membrana plasmática da célula receptora (elemento pós-sináptico) na qual ocorre a sinapse. Na maioria dos casos, o impulso é transmitido através de uma substância química transmissora (como acetilcolina, ácido γ-aminobutírico, dopamina, norepinefrina) liberada numa fenda sináptica (de 15–50 nm de largura), que separa a membrana pré-sináptica da pós-sináptica; o transmissor é armazenado, na forma quantal, em vesículas sinápticas: vacúolos redondos ou elipsóides delimitados por membrana (10–50 nm de diâmetro) no elemento pré-sináptico. Em outras sinapses, a transmissão ocorre por propagação direta do potencial bioelétrico da membrana pré-sináptica para a pós-sináptica; nessas sinapses eletrotônicas ("junções intercelulares"), a fenda sináptica não possui mais do que cerca de 2 nm de largura. Na maioria dos casos, a transmissão sináptica ocorre apenas em uma direção ("polaridade dinâmica" da sinapse); todavia, em algumas sinapses, ocorrem vesículas sinápticas em ambas as faces da fenda sináptica, sugerindo a possibilidade de transmissão química recíproca. [syn- + G. *hapto*, prender]

 axoaxonic s., s. axoaxônica; junção sináptica entre uma terminação axônica de um neurônio e o segmento axônico inicial ou uma terminação axônica de outra célula nervosa.
 axodendritic s., s. axodendrítica; o contato sináptico entre uma terminação axônica de uma célula nervosa e um dendrito de outra célula nervosa.
 axosomatic s., s. axossomática; junção sináptica de uma terminação axônica de uma célula nervosa com o corpo celular de outra célula nervosa. SIN pericorpuscular s.
 electrotonic s., s. eletrotônica. SIN gap *junction*. VER TAMBÉM synapse.
 pericorpuscular s., s. pericorpuscular. SIN axosomatic s.

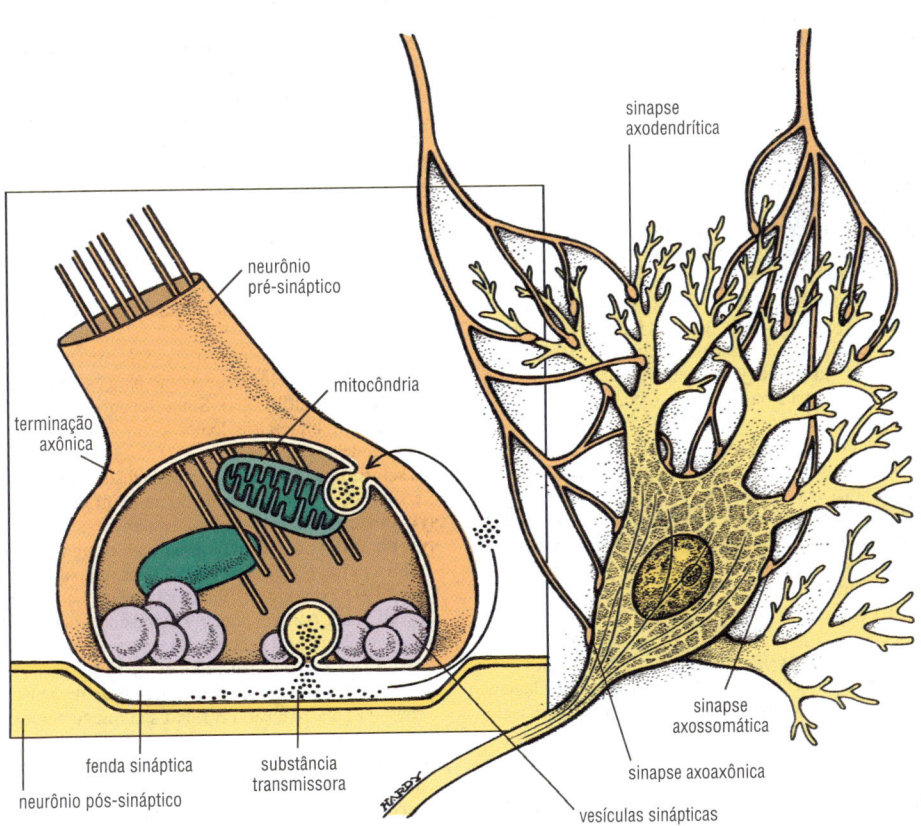

sinapses

syn·ap·sin I (si-nap′sin). Sinapsina I; fosfoproteína fibrosa que liga vesículas sinápticas entre si na terminação axônica; a sinapsina I é um substrato de determinadas cinases; a fosforilação da sinapsina I permite a liberação de neurotransmissores.

syn·ap·sis (si-nap′sis). Sinapse; o pareamento, ponto por ponto, de cromossomas homólogos durante a prófase da meiose. SIN synaptic phase. [G. conexão, junção]

syn·ap·tic (si-nap′tik). Sináptico. **1.** Relativo a uma sinapse. **2.** Relativo a sinapse.

syn·ap·tol·o·gy (sin′ap-tol′o-je). Sinaptologia; estudo da sinapse.

syn·ap·to·phys·in (si-nap′to-fi′sin). Sinaptofisina; proteína de membrana integral encontrada em muitos tipos de neurônios ativos; acredita-se que forma um hexâmero que cria um canal iônico e está envolvido na captação de neurotransmissores; a sinaptofisina é encontrada na membrana apenas após a estimulação dos neurônios.

syn·ap·to·some (si-nap′to-som). Sinaptossoma; saco delimitado por membrana, contendo vesículas sinápticas, que se separa das terminações axônicas quando o tecido cerebral é homogeneizado em condições controladas; essas partículas podem ser separadas de outras partículas subcelulares por centrifugação diferencial e por gradiente de densidade. [synapse + G. *soma*, corpo]

syn·ar·thro·dia (sin′ar-thro′de-a). Sinartrodia, articulação fibrosa. SIN fibrous joint.

syn·ar·thro·di·al (sin-ar-thro′de-al). Sinartrodial; relativo a sinartrose; designa uma articulação sem cavidade articular.

syn·ar·thro·phy·sis (sin-ar-thro-fi′sis). Sinartrófise; o processo de ancilose. [syn- + G. *arthron*, articulação + *physis*, crescimento]

syn·ar·thro·sis, pl. **syn·ar·thro·ses** (sin′ar-thro′sis, -sez) [TA]. Sinartrose; união imóvel ou quase imóvel de componentes rígidos do sistema esquelético, incluindo articulações fibrosas, articulações cartilaginosas e uniões ósseas (sinostoses). VER articulation. [G. de *syn*, junto + *arthrosis*, articulação]

syn·can·thus (sin-kan′thus). Sincanto; aderência do bulbo do olho a estruturas orbitais. [syn- + L. *canthus*, roda]

syn·car·y·on (sin-kar′e-on). Sincário. SIN synkaryon.

syn·ceph·a·lus (sin-sef′a-lus). Sincéfalo, monocéfalo; gêmeos unidos que possuem uma única cabeça com dois corpos. VER conjoined *twins*, em *twin*. Cf. craniopagus, janiceps. SIN monocephalus, monocranius. [syn- + G. *kephale*, cabeça]

s. asymmet′ros, s. assimétrico, janicéfalo assimétrico. SIN janiceps asymmetrus.

syn·ceph·a·ly (sin-sef′a-le). Sincefalia; a condição exibida por um sincéfalo. SIN prozygosis.

syn·chei·lia (sin-ki′le-a). Sinquilia; aderência mais ou menos completa dos lábios; atresia da boca. SIN synchilia. [syn- + G. *cheilos*, lábio]

syn·chei·ria (sin-ki′re-a). Sinquiria; forma de disquiria em que o indivíduo refere um estímulo aplicado a um lado do corpo a ambos os lados. SIN synchiria. [syn- + G. *cheir*, mão]

syn·chi·lia. Sinquilia. SIN syncheilia.

syn·chi·ria. Sinquiria. SIN syncheiria.

syn·chon·dro·se·ot·o·my (sin-kon′dro-se-ot′o-me). Sincondroseotomia; operação de corte através de uma sincondrose; especificamente, secção através dos ligamentos sacroilíacos e fechamento forçado do arco do púbis; utilizada no tratamento da extrofia da bexiga. [synchondrosis + G. *tome*, corte]

syn·chon·dro·sis, pl. **syn·chon·dro·ses** (sin′kon-dro′sis, -sez) [TA]. Sincondrose; articulação cartilaginosa em que os dois ossos são unidos por cartilagem hialina ou fibrocartilagem. SIN synchondrodial joint [TA]. [L. mod. do G. *syn*, junto + *chondros*, cartilagem + -*osis*, condição]

anterior intraoccipital s. [TA], s. intra-occipital anterior; união cartilaginosa no recém-nascido entre as partes lateral e basilar do osso occipital. SIN s. intraoccipitalis anterior [TA], anterior intraoccipital joint.

s. arycornicula′ta, s. aricorniculada. SIN arycorniculate s.

arycorniculate s., s. aricorniculada; a junção da cartilagem corniculada (de Santorini) com a aritenóidea. SIN s. arycorniculata.

cranial synchondroses [TA], sincondroses do crânio; as articulações cartilaginosas do crânio; incluem a s. esfenoetmoidal, a s. esfenoccipital, a s. esfenopetrosa, a s. petroccipital, a s. intra-occipital anterior e s. intra-occipital posterior. SIN synchondroses cranii [TA].

synchondro′ses cra′nii [TA], sincondroses do crânio. SIN cranial synchondroses.

s. epiphy′seos, linha epifisial. SIN epiphysial line.

synchondroses intersternebra′les, sincondroses intersternebrais; cartilagens persistentes que unem os elementos ósseos do esterno, conforme observado em alguns animais domésticos, como o cão. SIN intersternebral joints.

s. intraoccipita′lis ante′rior [TA], s. intra-occipital anterior. SIN anterior intraoccipital s.

s. intraoccipita′lis poste′rior [TA], s. intra-occipital posterior. SIN posterior intraoccipital s.

s. manubrioster′nal·is [TA], sínfise manubrioesternal, sincondrose manubrioesternal. SIN manubriosternal joint.

neurocentral s., s. neurocentral; a união cartilaginosa de cada lado entre o corpo e o arco de uma vértebra na criança de pouca idade. SIN neurocentral joint, neurocentral suture.

petrooccipital s. [TA], s. petrooccipital; fibrocartilagem que preenche a fissura petrooccipital. SIN s. petro-occipitalis [TA], petrooccipital joint.

s. petro-occipita′lis [TA], s. petrooccipital. SIN petrooccipital s.

posterior intraoccipital s. [TA], s. intra-occipital posterior; união cartilaginosa entre as partes escamosa e lateral do osso occipital no recém-nascido. SIN s. intraoccipitalis posterior [TA], Budin obstetrical joint, posterior intraoccipital joint.

sphenoethmoidal s. [TA], s. esfenoetmoidal; união cartilaginosa entre o corpo do esfenóide e a parte posterior do labirinto etmoidal. SIN s. sphenoethmoidalis [TA].

s. sphenoethmoida′lis [TA], s. esfenoetmoidal. SIN sphenoethmoidal s.

sphenooccipital s. [TA], s. esfenoccipital; união cartilaginosa entre o corpo do esfenóide e a parte basilar do occipital; está fundida aos 20 anos de idade e, portanto, tem importância particular na antropologia forense; incorretamente denominada sphenoccipital suture. SIN s. spheno-occipitalis [TA], sphenoccipital joint, sphenoccipital suture.

s. spheno-occipita′lis [TA], s. esfenoccipital. SIN sphenooccipital s.

s. sphenopetro′sa [TA], s. esfenopetrosa. SIN sphenopetrosal s.

sphenopetrosal s., **sphenopetrous s.** [TA], s. esfenopetrosa; fibrocartilagem que preenche a fissura esfenopetrosa. SIN s. sphenopetrosa [TA].

sternal synchondroses [TA], sincondroses esternais; as junções cartilaginosas entre o corpo do esterno e o manúbrio (articulação ou sínfise manubrioesternal) e entre o corpo do esterno e o processo xifóide (articulação ou sínfise xifosternal); em animais domésticos, pode haver várias delas, p. ex., articulações manubrioesternal, interesternebral e xifosternal. SIN synchondroses sternales [TA], sternal joints.

synchondro′ses sterna′les [TA], sincondroses esternais. SIN sternal synchondroses.

s. xiphosterna′lis, s. xifosternal. SIN xiphisternal joint.

syn·chon·dro·to·my (sin-kon-drot′o-me). Sincondrotomia. SIN symphysiotomy.

syn·cho·ri·al (sin-kor′e-al). Sincorial; relativo a córios fundidos, como aqueles encontrados em gestações de múltiplos fetos. [syn- + chorion]

syn·chro·nia (sin-kro′ne-a). Sincronia. **1.** Sincronismo. SIN synchronism. **2.** Origem, desenvolvimento, involução ou funcionamento de tecidos ou órgãos na época habitual desse evento. Cf. heterochronia. [syn- + G. *chronos*, tempo]

syn·chron·ic (sin′kron-ik). Sincrônico; refere-se ao estudo da história natural de uma doença pelo seu estado e distribuição numa população em determinado momento. As deduções quanto à evolução longitudinal a partir desse estudo são apenas justificadas em condições especiais, notavelmente o fato de que a evolução longitudinal da doença é, em si, inalterável e de que os indivíduos na amostra constituem uma amostra representativa dos sobreviventes.

syn·chro·nism (sin′kro-nizm). Sincronismo; ocorrência de dois ou mais eventos ao mesmo tempo; a condição de ser simultâneo. SIN synchronia (1). [syn- + G. *chronos*, tempo]

syn·chro·nous (sin′kro-nus). Sincrônico; que ocorre simultaneamente. SIN homochronous (1). [G. *synchronos*]

syn·chro·ny (sin′kro-ne). Sincronia; o aparecimento simultâneo de dois eventos separados. [syn- + G. *chronos*, tempo]

bilateral s., s. bilateral; atividade eletroencefalográfica registrada simultaneamente em ambos os hemisférios; termo geralmente utilizado para referir-se à atividade ponta-onda.

syn·chro·tron (sin′kro-tron). Síncrotron; máquina para gerar elétrons ou prótons de alta velocidade, como para estudos nucleares.

syn·chy·sis (sin′ki-sis). Sínquise; colapso da estrutura colagenosa do humor vítreo, com liquefação do corpo vítreo. [G. uma mistura conjunta, de syn- + *chysis*, despejar]

s. scintil′lans, s. cintilante; aparência de pontos brilhantes no olho, devido aos cristais de colesterol flutuando num vítreo líquido.

syn·ci·ne·sis (sin-si-ne′sis). Sincinese. SIN synkinesis.

syn·cli·nal (sin′kli-nal). Sinclinal; designa duas estruturas inclinadas uma para a outra. [G. *syn*- *klino*, inclinar juntos]

syn·clit·ic (sin-klit′ik) Sinclítico; relativo a, ou caracterizado por, sinclitismo.

syn·cli·tism (sin′kli-tizm). Sinclitismo; condição de paralelismo entre os planos da cabeça fetal e da pelve, respectivamente. [G. *synklino*, inclinar juntos]

syn·co·pal (sin′ko-pal). Sincopal; relativo a síncope. SIN syncopic.

syn·co·pe (sin′ko-pe). Síncope; perda da consciência e do tônus postural causada pela redução do fluxo sanguíneo cerebral. [G. *synkope*, interrupção, desmaio]

Adams-Stokes s., s. de Adams-Stokes; s. devido a bloqueio AV completo. SIN Morgagni-Adams-Stokes s.

cardiac s., s. cardíaca; desmaio com inconsciência de qualquer causa cardíaca.

carotid sinus s., s. do seio carótico; s. resultante da hiperatividade do seio carótico; as crises podem ser espontâneas ou produzidas por pressão sobre um seio carótico sensível.

deglutition s., s. de deglutição; desmaio ou inconsciência com a deglutição. Essa condição deve-se quase sempre a um efeito vagal excessivo sobre o coração, que já pode apresentar bradicardia ou bloqueio atrioventricular. SIN swallow s.
hysterical s., s. histérica; desmaio devido a um estresse emocional ou para evitá-lo.
laryngeal s., s. laríngea; neurose paroxística que se caracteriza por episódios de tosse, com sensações incomuns, como cócegas na garganta, seguidas de breve período de inconsciência.
local s., s. localizada; parestesia limitada a uma parte, sobretudo dedos das mãos; um dos sintomas, geralmente associado a asfixia local, da doença de Raynaud.
micturition s., s. de micção; s. que ocorre em associação ao ato de esvaziar a bexiga.
Morgagni-Adams-Stokes s., s. de Morgagni-Adams-Stokes. SIN Adams-Stokes s.
postural s., s. postural; s. ao assumir a posição ortostática, causada pela falha dos mecanismos vasoconstritores normais.
swallow s., s. de deglutição. SIN deglutition s.
tussive s., s. da tosse; desmaio em consequência de um acesso de tosse, causado pela elevação persistente da pressão intratorácica, diminuindo o retorno venoso ao coração e, portanto, reduzindo o débito cardíaco; com mais freqüência, ocorre em homens fumantes inveterados que apresentam bronquite crônica. SIN Charcot vertigo, laryngeal vertigo.
vasodepressor s., s. vasodepressora; desmaio ou perda da consciência devido à redução reflexa da pressão arterial. SIN vasovagal s.
vasovagal s., s. vasovagal. SIN vasodepressor s.
syn·cop·ic (sin-kop′ik). Sincópico. SIN syncopal.
syn·cre·tio (sin-krē′shē-ō). Sincreção; desenvolvimento de aderência entre superfícies opostas inflamadas. [L. mod. do G. *synkrētizō*, unir as cidades de Creta, reanalisado como syn- + L. *cresco*, pp. *cretum*, crescer]
syn·cy·a·nin (sin-sī′ă-nin). Sincianina; pigmento azul produzido por *Pseudomonas syncyanea*.
syn·cy·tial (sin-sish′ăl, -sish′ē-ăl, -sit′ē-ăl). Sincicial; relativo a um sincício.
syn·cy·ti·o·tro·pho·blast (sin-sish′ē-ō-trō′fō-blast). Sinciciotrofoblasto; a camada externa sincicial de trofoblasto; local de síntese da gonadotropina coriônica humana. VER TAMBÉM trophoblast. SIN placental plasmodium, plasmodial trophoblast, plasmodiotrophoblast, syncytial trophoblast, syntrophoblast. [syncytium + trophoblast]
syn·cy·ti·um, pl. **syn·cy·tia** (sin-sish′ē-ŭm, -ă, -sit′ē-ŭm). Sincício; massa protoplasmática multinucleada formada pela união secundária de células originalmente separadas. [L. mod. de syn- + G. *kytos*, célula]
syn·dac·tyl, syn·dac·tyle (sin-dak′til, -dak′til). Sindáctilo. SIN syndactylous.
syn·dac·tyl·ia, syn·dac·ty·lism (sin-dak-til′ē-ă, -dak′ti-lizm). Sindactilia. SIN syndactyly.
syn·dac·ty·lous (sin-dak′ti-lŭs). Sindáctilo; que apresenta fusão dos dedos das mãos ou dos pés ou dedos aderentes por meio de membrana. SIN syndactyl, syndactyle.
syn·dac·ty·ly (sin-dak′ti-lē). Sindactilia; qualquer grau de fusão ou aderência por meio de membrana dos dedos das mãos ou dos pés, envolvendo apenas as partes moles ou incluindo estruturas ósseas; em geral, herança autossômica dominante. SIN symphalangism (1), symphalangy, syndactylia, syndactylism. [syn- + G. *daktylos*, dedo da mão ou do pé]
syn·dein (sin-dē′in). Sindeína. SIN ankyrin. [G. *syndeō*, ligar + -in]
△ **syndesm-**. Sindesm-. VER syndesmo-.
syn·des·mec·to·my (sin-dez-mek′tō-mē). Sindesmectomia; secção de uma porção de um ligamento. [syndesm- + G. *ektomē*, excisão]
syn·des·mi·tis (sin-dez-mī′tis). Sindesmite; inflamação de um ligamento. [syndesm- + G. *-itis*, inflamação]
s. metatar′sea, s. metatarsal; inflamação dos ligamentos do metatarso.
△ **syndesmo-, syndesm-**. Sindesmo-; sindesm-; ligamento, ligamentoso. [G. *syndesmos*, fixação, de *syndeō*, ligar]
syn·des·mo·cho·ri·al (sin-dez-mō-kōr′ē-ăl). Sindesmocorial; relativo à placenta em animais ruminantes. [syndesmo- + G. *chorion*, membrana]
syn·des·mo·di·al (sin-des-mō′dē-ăl). Sindesmodial. SIN syndesmotic.
syn·des·mog·ra·phy (sin-dez-mog′ră-fē). Sindesmografia; tratado sobre os ligamentos ou a sua descrição. [syndesmo- + G. *graphō*, escrever]
syn·des·mo·lo·gia (sin-dez′mō-lō′jē-ă). Sindesmologia. SIN arthrology.
syn·des·mol·o·gy (sin-dez-mol′ō-jē). Sindesmologia. SIN arthrology. [syndesmo- + G. *logos*, estudo]
syn·des·mo·phyte (sin-dez′mō-fīt). Sindesmófito; excrescência óssea fixada a um ligamento. [syndesmo- + G. *phyton*, planta]
syn·des·mo·sis, pl. **syn·des·mo·ses** (sin′dez-mō′sis, -sēz) [TA]. Sindesmose; forma de articulação fibrosa em que as superfícies opostas, que são relativamente afastadas, são unidas por ligamentos; p. ex., a união do processo estilóide do osso temporal com o osso hióide através do ligamento estilo-hióideo, e a união fibrosa entre o rádio e a ulna (sindesmose radiolunar) e a tíbia e a fíbula (sindesmose tibiofibular). SIN syndesmodial joint, syndesmotic joint. [syndesmo- + G. *-osis*, condição]

radioulnar s. [TA], s. radioulnar; a união fibrosa do rádio e da ulna, que consiste no cordão oblíquo e na membrana interóssea. SIN s. radioulnaris [TA], middle radioulnar joint.
s. radioulna′ris [TA], s. radioulnar. SIN radioulnar s.
tibiofibular s. [TA], s. tibiofibular; a união fibrosa da tíbia e da fíbula, que consiste na membrana interóssea e nos ligamentos tibiofibulares anterior, interósseo e posterior nas extremidades distais dos ossos. SIN s. tibiofibularis [TA], distal tibiofibular joint, inferior tibiofibular joint, tibiofibular articulation (2).
s. tibiofibula′ris [TA], s. tibiofibular. SIN tibiofibular s.
tympanostapedial s. [TA], s. timpanoestapedial; a conexão da base do estribo com a janela do vestíbulo (oval). SIN s. tympanostapedialis [TA], tympanostapedial junction.
s. tympanostapedia′lis [TA], s. timpanoestapedial. SIN tympanostapedial s., tympanostapedial s.
syn·des·mot·ic (sin-des-mot′ik). Sindesmótico; relativo à sindesmose. SIN syndesmodial.

SYNDROME

syn·drome (sin′drōm). Síndrome; o conjunto de sinais e sintomas associados a qualquer processo mórbido que, juntos, formam o quadro da doença. VER TAMBÉM disease. [G. *syndromē*, corrida junto, reunião tumultuada; (in med.) uma confluência de sintomas, de *syn-*, junto + *dromos*, corrida]
Aagenaes s., s. de Aagenaes; forma idiopática de colestase intra-hepática familiar associada a linfedema dos membros inferiores.
Aarskog-Scott s., s. de Aarskog-Scott. SIN faciodigitogenital dysplasia.
abdominal muscle deficiency s., [MIM*100100, MIM*264140], s. de deficiência muscular abdominal; ausência congênita (parcial ou completa) dos músculos abdominais, em que o contorno dos intestinos é visível através da parede abdominal protuberante; nos homens, são também encontradas anomalias genitourinárias (dilatação do trato urinário e criptorquidismo); genética não-definida. VER TAMBÉM prune belly s. SIN prune belly.
abstinence s., s. de abstinência; conjunto de alterações fisiológicas apresentadas por indivíduos ou animais que se tornaram fisicamente dependentes de uma droga ou substância química devido a seu uso prolongado em doses elevadas e que são abruptamente privados da substância em questão. A s. de abstinência varia de acordo com a dependência a determinada droga. Em geral, os efeitos observados seguem uma direção oposta aos produzidos pela droga; p. ex., a s. de abstinência de depressores do sistema nervoso central, como barbitúricos e benzodiazepínicos, consiste em insônia, inquietação, tremores, alucinações e, em casos extremos, convulsões tônico-clônicas que podem ser fatais. O momento de início e a gravidade de abstinência dependem da velocidade de desaparecimento da droga do corpo.
Achard s. [MIM*100700], s. de Achard; aracnodactilia com pequena mandíbula recuada, crânio largo e frouxidão articular limitada às mãos e aos pés; genética não-definida.
Achard-Thiers s., s. de Achard-Thiers; forma de distúrbio virilizante de origem adrenocortical em mulheres, caracterizada por masculinização e distúrbios menstruais em associação a manifestações de diabetes melito, como glicosúria.
Achenbach s., s. de Achenbach; hematoma da polpa do dedo da mão com edema acompanhante; de causa desconhecida na ausência de distúrbios dos mecanismos da coagulação sanguínea.
acquired immunodeficiency s., s. de imunodeficiência adquirida (AIDS/SIDA). SIN AIDS.
acrofacial s., s. acrofacial. SIN acrofacial dysostosis.
acroparesthesia s., s. de acroparestesia; sensação anormal, como entorpecimento e formigamento nas mãos, geralmente em mulheres de meia-idade; sabe-se, agora, que se trata de um sintoma clássico da síndrome do túnel do carpo.
acute organic brain s., s. cerebral orgânica aguda. SIN organic brain s.
acute radiation s., s. de radiação aguda; síndrome causada pela exposição do corpo a grandes quantidades de radiação (p. ex., em decorrência de determinadas formas de terapia, acidentes e explosões nucleares); classificada em três formas principais, que são, por ordem crescente de gravidade: a hematológica, a gastrointestinal e a do sistema nervoso central-cardiovascular; suas manifestações clínicas são divididas em estágios prodrômico, latente, manifesto e de recuperação.
acute respiratory distress s., s. de angústia respiratória aguda. SIN adult respiratory distress s.
Adams-Stokes s., s. de Adams-Stokes; s. caracterizada por pulso lento ou ausente, vertigem, síncope, convulsões e, algumas vezes, respiração de Cheyne-Stokes; em geral, resulta de bloqueio AV avançado ou de síndrome do nó sinoatrial. SIN Adams-Stokes disease, Morgagni disease, Morgagni-Adams-Stokes s., Spens s., Stokes-Adams disease, Stokes-Adams s.

adaptation s. of Selye, s. de adaptação de Selye; adaptação inespecífica geral do organismo em resposta a estímulos específicos que desencadeiam um ciclo de alterações fisiológicas substanciais no sistema endócrino e em outros sistemas de órgãos, devido a estresse prolongado e intenso. VER general adaptation s.

addisonian s., s. addisoniana. SIN chronic adrenocortical *insufficiency.*

adherence s., s. de aderência; ação de restrição de um músculo ocular, devido a aderências entre o músculo e sua bainha fascial.

Adie s. [MIM*100300], s. de Adie; desnervação pós-ganglionar idiopática dos músculos intra-oculares inervados pelo parassimpático, geralmente complicada por sinais de regeneração aberrante desses nervos; reação fraca à luz com paralisia segmentar do esfíncter da íris, resposta forte e lenta de perto. Os reflexos tendinosos profundos muitas vezes estão assimetricamente reduzidos. VER TAMBÉM tonic *pupil.* SIN Adie pupil, Holmes-Adie pupil, Holmes-Adie s., pupillotonic pseudotabes.

adiposogenital s., s. adiposo genital. SIN adiposogenital *dystrophy.*

adrenal cortical s., s. adrenocortical; termo inexato (e obsoleto) que tem sido aplicado à síndrome de Cushing, doença de Addison ou s. adrenogenital.

adrenal virilizing s., s. virilizante supra-renal. SIN adrenal *virilism.*

adrenogenital s., s. adrenogenital; designação genérica de um grupo de distúrbios causados por hiperplasia adrenocortical ou tumores malignos e caracterizados por masculinização das mulheres, feminização dos homens ou desenvolvimento sexual precoce das crianças; representativa de padrões secretores excessivos ou anormais de esteróides adrenocorticais, especialmente aqueles com efeitos androgênicos ou estrogênicos.

adulto respiratory distress s. (ARDS), s. de angústia respiratória do adulto (SARA); lesão pulmonar aguda com várias causas, caracterizada por edema intersticial e/ou alveolar e hemorragia, além de edema pulmonar perivascular associado à formação de membrana hialina, proliferação de fibras colágenas e tumefação do epitélio com aumento da pinocitose. SIN acute respiratory distress, s. diffuse alveolar damage, wet lung (2), white lung.

afferent loop s., s. da alça aferente; obstrução crônica do duodeno e do jejuno proximalmente à gastrojejunostomia efetuada numa gastrectomia do tipo Billroth II; a alça aferente distendida de jejuno e duodeno provoca dor e plenitude associados à ingestão de alimento; é comum haver perda de peso. SIN gastrojejunal loop obstruction s.

aglossia-adactylia s. [MIM*103300], s. de aglossia-adactilia; ausência ou hipoplasia congênita da língua, associada à ausência dos dedos.

Aircardi s. [MIM*304050], s. de Aircardi; distúrbio dominante ligado ao X com letalidade em homens hemizigotos; caracterizada por agenesia do corpo caloso, anormalidade coriorretiniana com "orifícios", fenda labial associada ou não a fenda palatina, convulsões e alterações características do EEG.

Alagille s. [MIM 118450], s. de Alagille; s. autossômica dominante que se torna aparente na infância e está associada à icterícia devido à escassez de ductos biliares intra-hepáticos; as características incluem face estreita e queixo pontudo, testa larga, nariz longo e reto, olhos profundos, embriotoxo posterior do olho, anormalidades cardiovasculares, defeitos vertebrais e nefropatia.

Albright s., s. de Albright; (1) SIN McCune-Albright s; (2) SIN Albright hereditary *osteodystrophy.*

alcohol amnestic s., s. amnéstica por alcoolismo; s. amnéstica decorrente de alcoolismo; *blackouts* alcoólicos. Cf. Korsakoff s.

Aldrich s., s. de Aldrich. SIN Wiskott-Aldrich s.

Alice in Wonderland s., s. de Alice no País das Maravilhas; a ilusão de sonhos, sensação de levitação e alteração na percepção da passagem do tempo, algumas vezes associadas a enxaqueca, epilepsia e várias doenças do lobo parietal do cérebro.

Allen-Masters s., s. de Allen-Masters; dor pélvica resultante de laceração antiga do ligamento largo do útero sofrida durante o parto.

Allgrove s., s. de Allgrove. SIN triple A s.

Alport s., s. de Alport; distúrbio geneticamente heterogêneo, caracterizado por nefrite associada a hematúria microscópica e progressão lenta da insuficiência renal, perda da audição neurossensorial e anormalidades oculares, como lenticone e maculopatia; existem formas autossômica dominante [MIM*104200, MIM*153640 e MIM*153650], autossômica recessiva [MIM*203780] e recessiva ligada ao X [MIM*301050 e MIM*303630]. A forma ligada ao X é causada por mutação no gene alfa-5 do colágeno tipo IV (COL4A5) no cromossoma Xq; a forma autossômica recessiva é causada por mutação no gene alfa-3 do colágeno tipo IV (COL4A3) ou no gene alfa-4 (COL4A4) no cromossoma 2q.

Alström s. [MIM*203800], s. de Alström; degeneração da retina com nistagmo e perda da visão central, associada a obesidade na infância; em geral, ocorrem perda da audição neurossensorial e diabetes melito depois dos 10 anos de idade; herança autossômica recessiva.

amenorrhea-galactorrhea s., s. de amenorréia-galactorréia; lactação não-fisiológica de causas endocrinológicas ou em decorrência de tumor hipofisário.

amnestic s., s. amnéstica; (1) SIN Korsakoff s; (2) s. cerebral orgânica com distúrbio da memória de curto prazo (mas não imediata), independentemente da etiologia.

amnionic band syndrome, síndrome da banda amniótica. SIN amnionic *band.*

amnionic fluid s., s. do líquido amniótico; fenômenos embólicos pulmonares atribuídos à infusão de líquido amniótico contendo escamas epiteliais nos vasos sanguíneos maternos; o processo é seguido de choque, podendo ocorrer morte súbita. VER amnionic fluid *embolism.*

Amsterdam s., s. de Amsterdam. SIN de Lange s. [*Amsterdam,* países baixos]

androgen insensitivity s., s. de insensibilidade aos androgênios. SIN androgen resistance s.'s.

androgen resistance s.'s, síndromes de resistência aos androgênios; classe de distúrbios associados à deficiência da 5α-esteróide redutase, feminização testicular e distúrbios relacionados. Cf. *steroid* 5α-reductase, Reifenstein s., infertile male s., testicular feminization s. SIN androgen insensitivity s.

Angelman s., s. de Angelman; microdeleção do 15q-13, de origem materna, resultando em retardo mental, ataxia, paroxismos de gargalhada, convulsões, face característica e fala mínima. VER Prader-Willi s.

Angelucci s., s. de Angelucci; extrema excitabilidade, distúrbios vasomotores e palpitação associados a conjuntivite primaveril.

angioosteohypertrophy s., s. de angiosteo-hipertrofia. SIN Klippel-Trenaunay-Weber s.

ankyloglossia superior s., s. de anciloglossia superior; condição congênita em que a língua adere ao palato duro; nenhuma evidência de fatores genéticos.

anorectal s., s. anorretal; ulceração, ardência, prurido ou outra irritação do reto, juntamente com eritema ao redor do ânus, algumas vezes acompanhado de diarréia, ocorrendo como efeito tóxico da administração oral de determinados antibióticos de amplo espectro.

anterior chamber cleavage s. [MIM*261540], s. de clivagem da câmara anterior; distúrbio congênito em decorrência da separação defeituosa de estruturas embrionárias; resulta em opacidades centrais bilaterais da córnea, com fixação anular anterior da borda pupilar da íris e cataratas polares anteriores; associada a nanismo de membros curtos; herança autossômica dominante. VER iridocorneal endothelial s. SIN Peters anomaly.

anterior tibial compartment s., s. do compartimento tibial anterior; isquemia dos músculos do compartimento tibial anterior da perna, presumivelmente causada por compressão transitória do fluxo sanguíneo arterial por músculos edematosos dentro de um compartimento fascial fechado, após atividade física vigorosa.

antibody deficiency s., s. de deficiência de anticorpos; qualquer um de um grupo de distúrbios associados à produção deficiente de anticorpos em decorrência de defeitos no sistema de linfócitos do tipo B ou nos linfócitos tipo T; a principal manifestação consiste em aumento da susceptibilidade a infecção por vários microrganismos. VER agamaglobulinemia, hipogammaglobulinemia, immunodeficiency. SIN antibody deficiency disease.

Anton s., s. de Anton; na cegueira cortical, ausência da consciência de estar cego.

anxiety s., s. de ansiedade; o conjunto de sinais e sintomas do sistema nervoso autônomo que acompanham a apreensão de perigo e pavor. VER anxiety.

aortic arch s., s. do arco aórtico; obliteração ateromatosa e/ou trombótica dos ramos do arco da aorta, levando a uma redução ou ausência dos pulsos no pescoço e nos braços. VER TAMBÉM Takayasu *arteritis,* reversed *coarctation.* SIN Martorell s.

apallic s., SIN apallic *state.*

Apert s. [MIM*101200], s. de Apert; distúrbio caracterizado por craniossinostose e sindactilia de todos os dedos das mãos e, em geral, também dos dedos dos pés; os polegares permanecem livres, o retardo mental é uma manifestação variável. Mutação autossômica dominante, sendo a maioria dos casos esporádica e causada por mutação no gene do receptor 2 do fator de crescimento dos fibroblastos (FGFR2, *fibroblast growth factor receptor 2*) no cromossoma 10q. VER TAMBÉM acrocephalosyndactyly. SIN type I acrocephalosyndactyly.

s. of approximate relevant answers, s. das respostas relevantes aproximadas. SIN Ganser s.

Arnold-Chiari s., s. de Arnold-Chiari. SIN Arnold-Chiari *malformation*

arterial thoracic outlet s., s. do desfiladeiro torácico arterial; distúrbio raro devido à compressão da artéria subclávia (com conseqüente dilatação pós-estenótica) por uma costela cervical totalmente formada ou por uma primeira costela torácica anormal; formam-se trombos no segmento arterial distal dilatado, e pode ocorrer isquemia do membro distal devido a eventos tromboembólicos.

Ascher s. [MIM*109900], s. de Ascher; condição em que um lábio duplo congênito está associado a blefarocalasia e aumento atóxico da glândula tireóide.

Asherman s., s. de Asherman. SIN traumatic *amenorrhea.*

asplenia s., s. de asplenia; s. observada em pacientes que carecem de baço funcional, devido à sua remoção cirúrgica ou doença (p. ex., anemia falciforme); inclui aumento da susceptibilidade a infecções bacterianas, especialmente infecção pneumocócica.

ataxia telangiectasia s., s. de ataxia telangiectasia. SIN *ataxia* telangiectasia.

auriculotemporal nerve s., s. do nervo auriculotemporal; rubor e sudorese localizados da orelha e da bochecha em resposta à alimentação. SIN Frey s., gustatory sweating s.

autoerythrocyte sensitization s., s. de auto-sensibilização eritrocitária; condição que, habitualmente, afeta mulheres, a pessoa acometida apresenta equimoses facilmente (púrpura simples), que tendem a aumentar e a afetar tecidos adjacentes, resultando em dor nas partes acometidas; assim denominada devido à produção de lesão semelhantes por inoculação do sangue ou de vários componentes dos eritrócitos do indivíduo; acredita-se que seja uma forma de auto-sensibilização localizada, embora não haja nenhum anticorpo específico demonstrável. SIN Gardner-Diamond s.

Avellis s., s. de Avellis, paralisia unilateral da laringe e do palato mole, com perda contralateral da sensibilidade álgica e térmica nas porções abaixo. SIN jugular foramen s.

A-V strabismus s., s. do estrabismo A-V; estrabismo em que o ângulo de desvio é mais acentuado no olhar para cima ou para baixo. VER TAMBÉM A-pattern *esotropia*, V-pattern *esotropia*, A-pattern *exotropia*, V-pattern *exotropia*.

Ayerza s., s. de Ayerza; esclerose das artérias pulmonares no *cor pulmonale* crônico; associada a cianose intensa, trata-se de uma condição que se assemelha à policitemia vera, mas que resulta de arteriosclerose pulmonar primária ou hipertensão pulmonar primária; caracterizada por lesões plexiformes das arteríolas. SIN Ayerza disease, cardiopathia nigra, plexogenic pulmonary arteriopathy.

Babinski s., s. de Babinski; a combinação de manifestações cardíacas, arteriais e do sistema nervoso central da sífilis tardia (late *syphilis*).

baby bottle s., s. da mamadeira. SIN nursing bottle *caries*.

Balint s., s. de Balint; entidade caracterizada por ataxia óptica (optic *ataxia*) e simultanagnosia. Essa dificuldade em aplicar o sistema visual a uma tarefa visual deve-se geralmente a lesão das áreas temporooccipitais superiores em ambos os hemisférios.

Bamberger-Marie s., s. de Bamberger-Marie. SIN hypertrophic pulmonary *osteoarthropathy*.

Bannwarth s., s. de Bannwarth; manifestações neurológicas da doença de Lyme, também denominada meningite linfocítica crônica e meningopolineurite transmitida por carrapato.

Banti s., s. de Banti; esplenomegalia congestiva crônica que ocorre primariamente em crianças como seqüela de hipertensão nas veias porta ou esplênicas, geralmente em conseqüência de trombose dessas veias; em geral, ocorrem anemia, esplenomegalia e episódios regulares de sangramento gastrointestinal, com ascite, icterícia, leucopenia e trombocitopenia, que se desenvolvem em várias combinações. SIN Banti disease, splenic anemia.

Bardet-Biedl s. [MIM*209900], s. de Bardet-Biedl; retardo mental, retinopatia pigmentar, polidactilia, obesidade e hipogenitalismo; herança autossômica recessiva. VER TAMBÉM Laurence-Moon s.

bare lymphocyte s., s. do linfócito nu; ausência de antígenos HLA nas células mononucleares periféricas, podendo resultar em imunodeficiência.

Barlow s. [MIM*157700], s. de Barlow; sopro telessistólico apical ou estalido sistólico (denominado "mesotele") ou ambos, devido à protuberância do folheto anterior e/ou posterior (mural) da valva mitral na cavidade atrial esquerda (também conhecida como síndrome da valva frouxa); ao exame eletrocardiográfico, verifica-se freqüentemente a coexistência de alterações ST-T numa distribuição póstero-inferior, semelhantes às da isquemia do miocárdio, por razões desconhecidas; podem coexistir distúrbios do ritmo com essa síndrome, sem relação patogenética demonstrável.

Barrett s., s. de Barrett; ulceração péptica crônica da parte inferior do esôfago, que é revestida de epitélio colunar, lembrando a mucosa do cárdia; adquirida em decorrência de esofagite crônica de longa duração; foi também relatada a ocorrência de estenose esofágica com refluxo e adenocarcinoma. SIN Barrett esophagus, Barrett metaplasia.

Bart s. [MIM*132000], s. de Bart; forma de epidermólise bolhosa com formação de vesículas nos membros e nas áreas intertriginosas, ausência localizada congênita de pele, erosões da boca e unhas distróficas; com freqüência, ocorre melhora espontânea sem cicatrização residual; herança autossômica dominante, causada por mutação no gene do colágeno tipo VII (COL7A1) no cromossoma 3p.

Barth s., s. de Barth; s. ligada ao X caracterizada por crescimento deficiente, neutropenia, miocardiopatia e excreção urinária excessiva de ácido 3-metilglutacônico; alguns pacientes também apresentam fraqueza muscular esquelética.

Bartter s. [MIM*241200], s. de Bartter; distúrbio devido a um defeito na reabsorção ativa de cloreto na alça de Henle; caracterizada por hiperplasia primária das células justaglomerulares, com hiperaldosteronismo secundário, alcalose hipopotassêmica, hipercalciúria, níveis elevados de renina ou de angiotensina, pressão arterial normal ou baixa e retardo do crescimento; ausência de edema. Herança autossômica recessiva, devido a uma mutação no gene do co-transportador de Na-K-2Cl (SLC12A1) no cromossoma 15q ou no gene do canal de K(+) (KCNJ1) no cromossoma 11q.

basal cell nevus s. [MIM*109400], s. do nevo de células basais, s. do nevo basocelular; síndrome com miríades de nevos de células basais, com desenvolvimento de carcinomas de células basais na vida adulta, ceratocistos odontogênicos, depressões eritematosas nas palmas das mãos e plantas dos pés, calcificação da foice do cérebro e, com freqüência, anomalias esqueléticas, particularmente das costelas, que são bífidas ou alargadas anteriormente; herança autossômica dominante, causada por mutação no gene PTCH, o homólogo humano do gene *"patched"* de *Drosophila* no cromossoma 9q. SIN Gorlin s.

Bassen-Kornzweig s., s. de Bassen-Kornzweig. SIN abetalipoproteinemia.

battered child s., s. da criança espancada; manifestação clínica de abuso de crianças: várias lesões do esqueleto, dos tecidos moles ou órgãos de uma criança em decorrência de repetidos maus-tratos ou espancamento, geralmente por um indivíduo responsável pela sua criação.

battered spouse s., s. do cônjuge espancado; lesões físicas, psicológicas e emocionais numa pessoa que sofre abuso de um cônjuge ou parceiro; geralmente associada ao alcoolismo no cônjuge que pratica o abuso.

Bauer s., s. de Bauer; aortite e endocardite aórtica como manifestação pouco reconhecida de artrite reumatóide.

Bazex s., s. de Bazex. SIN paraneoplastic *acrokeratosis*.

Beckwith-Wiedemann s. [MIM*130650], s. de Beckwith-Wiedemann; síndrome de crescimento excessivo caracterizada por exonfalia, macroglossia e gigantismo, freqüentemente com hipoglicemia neonatal; existe uma associação com hemi-hipertrofia e tumor de Wilms. Herança autossômica dominante, com a maioria dos casos sendo esporádica; influenciada por impressão genômica e dissomia uniparental; causada por mutação no gene P57 (KIP2) no cromossoma 11p. SIN EMG s.

Behçet s. [MIM*109650], s. de Behçet; s. caracterizada pela ocorrência simultânea ou sucessiva de episódios recorrentes de ulcerações genitais e orais (aftas) e uveíte ou iridociclite com hipópio, muitas vezes com artrite; uma fase de um distúrbio generalizado, que ocorre mais freqüentemente em homens do que em mulheres, com manifestações variáveis, incluindo dermatite, eritema nodoso, tromboflebite e comprometimento cerebral. SIN Behçet disease, cutaneomucouveal s., iridocyclitis septica, oculobuccogenital s., recurrent hypopyon, triple symptom complex, uveoencephalitic s.

Behr s. [MIM*210000], s. de Behr; caracterizada por atrofia óptica bilateral com defeitos do campo temporal, nistagmo, ataxia, espasticidade e retardo mental; provavelmente, herança autossômica recessiva. SIN Behr disease.

Benedikt s., s. de Benedikt; hemiplegia com espasmo clônico ou tremor e paralisia oculomotora do lado oposto.

Beradinelli s., s. de Beradinelli; crescimento acelerado, lipodistrofia com hipertrofia muscular, hepatomegalia e lipemia.

Berardinelli s., s. de Berardinelli. SIN congenital total *lipodystrophy*.

Bernard-Horner s., s. de Bernard-Horner. SIN Horner s.

Bernard-Sergent s., s. de Bernard-Sergent. SIN acute adrenocortical *insufficiency*.

Bernard-Soulier s., s. de Bernard-Soulier; distúrbio da coagulação caracterizado por trombocitopenia, plaquetas gigantes e tendência hemorrágica.

Bernhardt-Roth s., s. de Bernhardt-Roth. SIN meralgia *paresthetica*.

Bernheim s., s. de Bernheim; congestão sistêmica que se assemelha as conseqüências da insuficiência cardíaca direita (aumento do fígado, distensão das veias do pescoço e edema) sem congestão pulmonar em indivíduos com aumento do ventrículo esquerdo de qualquer causa; observa-se redução no tamanho da cavidade ventricular direita nas técnicas de imagem contrastadas ou na ecocardiografia ou *postmortem*, devido à invasão pelo septo interventricular hipertrofiado ou aneurismático.

Besnier-Boeck-Schaumann s., s. de Besnier-Boeck-Schaumann. SIN sarcoidosis.

Beuren s., s. de Beuren; estenose aórtica supravalvar com múltiplas áreas de estenose periférica da artéria pulmonar, retardo mental e anomalias dentárias.

Biemond s. [MIM*210350], s. de Biemond; coloboma da íris, retardo mental, obesidade, hipogenitalismo e polidactilia pós-axial; provavelmente, trata-se de um distúrbio de herança autossômica recessiva, semelhante às síndromes de Laurence-Moon e Bardet-Biedel s.'s.

billowing mitral valve s., s. de prolapso da valva mitral. SIN mitral valve *prolapse* s.

Björnstad s. [MIM*262000], s. de Björnstad; pêlos tortos (pili torti) associados a perda da audição neurossensorial, estando a intensidade da distorção e fragilidade dos cabelos correlacionada com o grau de comprometimento da audição; herança autossômica dominante.

Blatin s., s. de Blatin. SIN hydatid *thrill*.

blind loop s., s. da alça cega; estagnação do conteúdo intestinal com hiperproliferação de bactérias produtoras de substâncias que interferem na absorção de gordura, vitaminas e outros nutrientes; em geral, ocorre numa parte do intestino delgado que foi excluída do fluxo de quimo.

Bloch-Sulzberger s., s. de Bloch-Sulzberger. SIN incontinentia *pigmenti*.

Bloom s. [MIM*210900], s. de Bloom; eritema telangiectásico congênito, primariamente de distribuição em asa de borboleta, na face e, em certas ocasiões, nas mãos e antebraços, com sensibilidade das lesões cutâneas ao sol e nanismo com proporções corporais normais, exceto por uma face estreita e dolicocefalia; os cromossomas são excessivamente instáveis, e existe uma predisposição a neoplasia maligna; herança autossômica recessiva, causada por mutação no gene da síndrome de Bloom (BLM) no cromossoma 15q.

syndrome

blue diaper s., s. da fralda azul; distúrbio da absorção de triptofano; o triptofano não-absorvido em excesso no intestino é metabolizado a indóis e indicans, que são absorvidos e resultam na excreção urinária de indican, que é oxidado a índigo na fralda. Os pacientes também apresentam hipercalcemia e nefrocalcinose.

blue toe s., s. do dedo do pé azul; lesão tecidual progressiva ou gangrena por microtromboembolia na presença de pulsos pedais palpáveis.

Boerhaave s., s. de Boerhaave; ruptura do esôfago causada por aumento da pressão intraluminal durante o vômito seco ou vômito com glote fechada; resulta em mediastinite e, algumas vezes, sofre ruptura no espaço pleural esquerdo.

Bonnet-Dechaume-Blanc s., s. de Bonnet-Dechaume-Blanc. SIN Wyburn-Mason s.

Bonnier s., s. de Bonnier; causada por lesão do núcleo de Deiters e sua conexão. As manifestações incluem distúrbios oculares (p. ex., paralisia de acomodação, nistagmo, diplopia), bem como surdez, náuseas, sede, anorexia e sintomas relacionados ao comprometimento dos centros vagais.

Böök s. [MIM*112300], s. de Böök; aplasia pré-molar, hiperidrose e encanecimento prematuro; caráter autossômico dominante.

BOR s., s. BOR. SIN branchiootorenal *dysplasia*.

Börjeson-Forssman-Lehmann s. [MIM*301900], s. de Börjeson-Forssman-Lehmann; condição caracterizada por deficiência mental, epilepsia, hipogonadismo, hipometabolismo, obesidade, orelhas grandes e fissuras palpebrais estreitas; herança recessiva ligada ao X.

bowel bypass s., s. de derivação intestinal; febre recorrente, calafrios, mal-estar e pápulas e pústulas cutâneas inflamatórias nos membros e na parte superior do tronco, com infiltração difusa de neutrófilos, algumas vezes com poliartralgia ou poliartrite após cirurgia de derivação intestinal.

Bradbury-Eggleston s., s. de Bradbury-Eggleston. SIN pure autonomic *failure*.

bradytachycardia s. (brā-dē-tă-kē-car'dē'ă), s. de taquibradicardia; freqüências cardíacas rápidas e lentas alternadas, que podem representar qualquer distúrbio do ritmo em qualquer combinação, geralmente relacionada a doença do nó sinoatrial. SIN tachybradycardia s.

branchiootorenal s., s. branquiootorrenal; distúrbio autossômico dominante, caracterizado por anomalias dos derivados dos arcos branquiais, comprometimento auditivo sensorial e anormalidades renais.

Briquet s., s. de Briquet; distúrbio mental crônico, porém flutuante, em geral acometendo mulheres jovens, caracterizado por queixas freqüentes de doença física afetando simultaneamente múltiplos sistemas orgânicos.

Brissaud-Marie s., s. de Brissaud-Marie; espasmo unilateral da língua e dos lábios, de natureza histérica.

Brock s., s. de Brock. SIN middle lobe s.

bronze baby s., s. do bebê bronzeado; pigmentação castanha ou bronzeada da pele que pode ocorrer em crianças com hiperbilirrubinemia submetidas a fototerapia.

Brown s., s. de Brown. SIN tendon sheath s.

Brown-Séquard s., s. de Brown-Séquard; s. com lesões unilaterais da medula espinal, perda da propriocepção e fraqueza de ocorrência ipsilateral à lesão, enquanto podem ocorrer dor e temperatura contralaterais. SIN Brown-Séquard paralysis.

Budd s., s. de Budd. SIN Chiari s.

Budd-Chiari s., s. de Budd-Chiari. SIN Chiari s.

Bürger-Grütz s., s. de Bürger-Grütz. SIN type I familial *hyperlipoproteinemia*.

burner s., s. de queimação; múltiplos episódios de dor em queimação nos membros superiores, algumas vezes acompanhados de fraqueza do cíngulo do membro superior, que ocorrem durante esportes de contato, especialmente futebol, com cada pancada vigorosa na cabeça ou no ombro; atribuída a uma plexopatia braquial da parte superior do tronco.

Burnett s., s. de Burnett. SIN milk-alkali s.

burning foot s., s. do pé em queimação; distúrbio observado em prisioneiros de guerra durante a II Guerra Mundial, hoje considerado decorrente de deficiência de pantotenato.

burning mouth s., s. da boca em queimação; condição clínica em que o paciente se queixa de sensação de queimação na cavidade oral, embora o aspecto da mucosa oral seja normal; a causa ainda não foi determinada.

burning tongue s., s. da língua em queimação; s. de dor na língua sem qualquer lesão aparente, freqüentemente associada a ageusia; mais comum em mulheres idosas.

burning vulva s., s. da vulva em queimação; vulvodinia persistente na qual não foi identificada nenhuma causa física.

Buschke-Ollendorf s., s. de Buschke-Ollendorf. SIN osteodermatopoikilosis.

Caffey s., s. de Caffey. SIN infantile cortical *hyperostosis*.

Caffey-Kempe s., s. de Caffey-Kempe. VER battered child s.

Caffey-Silverman s., s. de Caffey-Silverman. SIN infantile cortical *hyperostosis*.

camptomelic s., s. camptomélica; também associada a face plana, vértebras curtas, escápula hipoplásica e tíbia arqueada. SIN osteochondrodysplasia.

Capgras s., s. de Capgras; crença ilusória de que uma pessoa (ou pessoas) próxima(s) ao paciente esquizofrênico foi (foram) substituída(s) por um ou mais impostores; pode ter uma etiologia orgânica. SIN Capgras phenomenon, illusion of doubles.

Caplan s., s. de Caplan; nódulos intrapulmonares, histologicamente semelhantes aos nódulos reumatóides subcutâneos, associados a artrite reumatóide e pneumoconiose em mineiros de carvão. SIN Caplan nodules.

carbonic anhydrase II deficiency s., s. de deficiência da anidrase carbônica II; deficiência herdada da anidrase carbônica II, resultando em osteopetrose e acidose metabólica. SIN osteopetrosis with renal tubular acidosis.

carcinoid s., s. carcinóide; combinação de sintomas e lesões geralmente produzidos pela liberação de serotonina por tumores carcinóides do trato gastrointestinal que metastatizaram para o fígado; consiste em rubor mosqueado irregular, angiomas planos da pele, estenose tricúspide e pulmonar adquirida, freqüentemente com regurgitação, algumas vezes com algum comprometimento menor das valvas no lado esquerdo do coração, diarréia, espasmo brônquico, aberração mental e excreção de grandes quantidades de ácido 5-hidroxindolacético. SIN malignant carcinoid s., metastatic carcinoid s.

cardiofacial s., s. cardiofacial; **(1)** paresia facial inferior parcial unilateral, transitória ou persistente, que acompanha alguma cardiopatia congênita; **(2)** grupo de síndromes caracterizadas por anormalidades congênitas cardiovasculares, ósseas, dos tecidos moles e da face. Os exemplos incluem a s. de Rubinstein-Taybi, a s. de Noonan e a s. de Williams.

Caroli s., s. de Caroli; malformação congênita dos ductos biliares no fígado, levando à formação de dilatações císticas multifocais.

carotid sinus s., s. do seio carótico; estimulação de um seio carótico hiperativo, causando acentuada queda da pressão arterial, devido a vasodilatação e/ou redução da freqüência cardíaca; pode ocorrer síncope, com ou sem convulsões ou bloqueio AV. SIN Charcot-Weiss-Baker s.

carpal tunnel s., s. do túnel do carpo; a s. de compressão de nervos mais comum, caracterizada por parestesia e dor noturnas na mão e, algumas vezes, perda sensorial e debilitação na distribuição do nervo mediano; afeta mais as mulheres do que os homens e costuma ser bilateral; causada por compressão crônica do nervo mediano no punho, no interior do túnel do carpo.

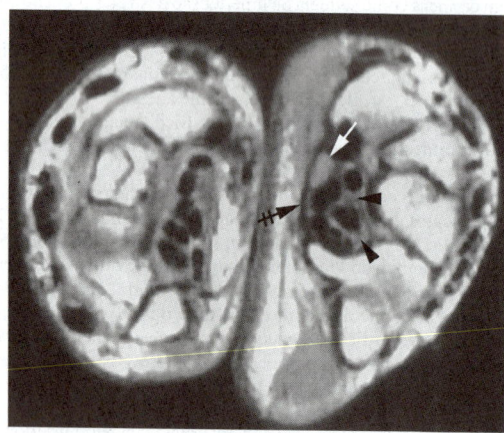

síndrome do túnel do carpo: RMN de ambos os punhos; aumento do nervo mediano direito (seta branca), aumento do volume de líquido entre os tendões flexores no túnel (cabeças de seta pretas) e ligeira curvatura do retináculo dos flexores (seta com cruz)

Carpenter s., s. de Carpenter; a associação de hipotireoidismo primário, insuficiência adrenocortical primária e diabetes melito. [C.C.J. Carpenter]

cataract-oligophrenia s., s. de catarata-oligofrenia. SIN Marinesco-Garland s.

cat's cry s., s. do miado-de-gato. SIN cri-du-chat s.

cat's-eye s. [MIM*115470], s. do olho de gato; distúrbio cromossômico caracterizado por colobomas da íris (semelhantes às pupilas verticais do gato), fissuras palpebrais inclinadas para baixo, atresia anal, proeminências e/ou depressões pré-auriculares, malformações cardíacas e renais e, em certas ocasiões, leve retardo mental; associada à tetrassomia parcial 22. SIN Schmid-Fraccaro s.

cauda equina s., s. da cauda eqüina; comprometimento freqüentemente assimétrico de múltiplas raízes que formam a cauda eqüina (isto é, raízes L2-S3), manifestado por dor, parestesia e fraqueza; com freqüência, a função dos esfíncteres vesical e intestinal não é afetada, devido à preservação sacral (ausência de comprometimento das raízes S2, S3 e S4).

cavernous sinus s., s. do seio cavernoso; síndrome causada por trombose do seio intracraniano cavernoso, caracterizada por edema das pálpebras e conjuntivas e por paralisia do terceiro, quarto e sexto nervos.

Ceelen-Gellerstedt s., s. de Ceelen-Gellerstedt. SIN idiopathic pulmonary *hemosiderosis*.

celiac s., s. celíaca. SIN celiac *disease*.

cellular immunity deficiency s., s. de deficiência da imunidade celular; síndrome caracterizada por aumento da suscetibilidade a infecções, especialmente virais, associada ao funcionamento deficiente do mecanismo responsável pela imunidade adquirida do tipo mediado por células. VER TAMBÉM immunodeficiency.

central cord s., s. medular central; tetraparesia que acomete mais gravemente a parte distal dos membros superiores, com ou sem perda sensorial e disfunção vesical, geralmente devido a isquemia por compressão osteofítica ou traumática da parte central da medula espinal cervical e/ou artéria.

cerebellar s., s. cerebelar; os sinais e sintomas de disfunção cerebelar: dismetria, disartria, assinergia, nistagmo, ataxia, marcha bamboleante e adiadococinesia.

cerebellomedullary malformation s., s. de malformação cerebelobulbar. SIN Arnold-Chiari *malformation.*

cerebellopontine angle s., s. do ângulo cerebelopontino; síndrome causada mais comumente por lesão na região entre o cerebelo e a ponte, que pode afetar múltiplos nervos cranianos; pode caracterizar-se por perda da audição, zumbido, vertigem, ataxia ou fraqueza facial.

cerebrohepatorenal s. [MIM*214100, MIM*211410], s. cerebro-hepatorrenal. SIN Zellweger s.

cervical compression s., s. de compressão cervical. SIN cervical disk s.

cervical disk s., s. do disco cervical; dor, parestesias e, algumas vezes, fraqueza na área de distribuição de uma ou mais raízes cervicais, devido à pressão de um disco intervertebral cervical protruso. SIN cervical compression s.

cervical fusion s., s. de fusão cervical. SIN Klippel-Feil s.

cervical rib s., s. da costela cervical; termo indefinido, igualmente aplicável a duas síndromes diferentes: 1) s. do desfiladeiro torácico arterial, em que a artéria subclávia é comprimida por uma costela cervical totalmente formada, e 2) s. do desfiladeiro torácico neurogênica verdadeira, em que o tronco inferior proximal do plexo braquial é comprometido por uma faixa translúcida que se estende de uma costela cervical rudimentar até a primeira costela.

cervical rib and band s., s. da faixa e costela cervical. SIN true neurogenic thoracic outlet s.

cervical tension s., s. da tensão cervical. SIN posttraumatic neck s.

cervicooculoacoustic s. [MIM*314600], s. cervicooculoacústica; distúrbio caracterizado por pescoço congenitamente curto com fusão das vértebras cervicais (anomalia de Klippel-Feil), paralisia do sexto nervo craniano com retração do bulbo do olho e estreitamento da fissura palpebral em adução (paralisia de Duane) e surdez neurossensorial; acredita-se que a herança seja multifatorial, limitada às mulheres. SIN Wildervanck s.

Cestan-Chenais s., s. de Cestan-Chenais; hemiplegia, hemianestesia e perda da sensibilidade álgica e térmica contralaterais, com hemiacinergia e lateropulsão ipsolaterais, paralisia da laringe e do palato mole, enoftalmia, miose e ptose, devido a lesões do tronco cerebral.

chancriform s., s. cancriforme; lesão ulcerativa no local de infecção primária por microrganismos, com aumento dos linfonodos regionais; ocorre não apenas em infecções cancróides, mas também em várias infecções bacterianas e fúngicas.

Chandler s., s. de Chandler; atrofia da íris com edema da córnea. SIN iridocorneal syndrome.

Charcot s., s. de Charcot. SIN intermittent *claudication.*

Charcot-Weiss-Baker s., s. de Charcot-Weiss-Baker. SIN carotid sinus s.

CHARGE s., s. CHARGE. SIN CHARGE *association.*

Chauffard s., s. de Chauffard; os sintomas da doença de Still em um indivíduo que sofre de forma bovina ou outra forma não-humana de tuberculose. SIN Still-Chauffard s.

Chédiak-Higashi s. [MIM*214500 e MIM*214450], s. de Chédiak-Higashi; distúrbio genético associado a anormalidades da granulação e estrutura nuclear de todos os tipos de leucócitos, com presença de grânulos peroxidase-positivos, inclusões citoplasmáticas e corpúsculos de Dohle; caracteriza-se por hepatoesplenomegalia, linfadenopatia, neutropenia, albinismo parcial, nistagmo, fotofobia e suscetibilidade a infecções e linfomas; em geral, a morte ocorre na infância; acomete bisões, bois, camundongos, orcas e seres humanos; herança autossômica recessiva, causada por mutação do gene de Chediak-Higashi (CHS) no cromossoma 1q. SIN Béguez César disease, Chédiak-Higashi disease, Chédiak-Steinbrinck-Higashi anomaly, Chédiak-Steinbrinck-Higashi s.

Chédiak-Steinbrinck-Higashi s. [MIM*214500, MIM*214450], s. de Chédiak-Steinbrinck-Higashi. SIN Chédiak-Higashi s.

Cheney s., s. de Cheney; acrosteólise com osteoporose e alterações do crânio e da mandíbula.

cherry-red spot myoclonus s., s. de mioclonia com mancha vermelho-cereja; distúrbio de armazenamento neuronal em crianças, caracterizado por mancha vermelho-cereja na mácula, mioclonia progressiva e convulsões de fácil controle; constitui o resultado da deficiência de sialidase. O tipo 1 caracteriza-se por biotipo normal, mácula vermelho-cereja, mioclonia e níveis normais de β-galactosidase; o tipo 2, por estatura baixa, anormalidades ósseas e deficiência de β-galactosidase. SIN sialidosis.

Chiari s., s. de Chiari; trombose da veia hepática, com grande aumento do fígado e desenvolvimento extenso de vasos colaterais, ascite intratável e hipertensão porta grave. SIN Budd s., Budd-Chiari s., Chiari disease, Chiari-Budd s., Rokitansky disease (2).

Chiari-Budd s., s. de Chiari-Budd. SIN Chiari s.

Chiari-Frommel s., s. de Chiari-Frommel; lactação não-fisiológica e amenorréia após a gravidez, mas não causada pela amamentação do lactente; caracterizada por hiperprolactinemia e adenoma hipofisário.

Chiari II s., s. de Chiari II; deslocamento da medula oblonga e das tonsilas cerebelares e verme através do forame magno para o canal espinal superior; freqüentemente associada a outras anomalias cerebrais.

chiasma s., s. do quiasma; s. caracterizada por defeito bitemporal do campo visual e atrofia do nervo óptico, devido a uma lesão no quiasma ou ao seu redor.

Chilaiditi s., s. de Chilaiditi; interposição do colo entre o fígado e o diafragma.

CHILD s., s. CHILD; hemidisplasia congênita com eritroderma ictiosiforme e defeitos dos membros (*c*ongenital *h*emidysplasia with *i*chthyosiform erythroderma and *l*imb *d*efects).

Chinese restaurant s., s. do restaurante chinês; desenvolvimento de dor torácica, sensações de pressão facial e de ardência sobre partes variáveis da superfície do corpo após a ingestão de alimento contendo L-glutamato monossódico (MSG) por pessoas sensíveis a esse aditivo alimentar.

Chotzen s. [MIM*101400], s. de Chotzen. SIN Saethre-Chotzen s.

Christian s., s. de Christian. SIN Hand-Schüller-Christian *disease.*

chromosomal s., s. cromossômica; designação geral para as síndromes decorrentes de aberrações cromossômicas; tipicamente, estão associadas a retardo mental e anomalias congênitas múltiplas.

chromosomal instability s.'s, chromosomal breakage s.'s, síndromes de instabilidade cromossômica, síndromes de ruptura cromossômica; grupo de condições mendelianas associadas a instabilidade e ruptura cromossômica *in vitro*, que freqüentemente manifestam maior tendência a determinados tipos de neoplasias malignas. VER Bloom s., *xeroderma* pigmentosum.

chronic hyperventilation s., s. de hiperventilação crônica; redução do conteúdo de CO_2 do sangue (hipocapnia) em conseqüência de hiperventilação de duração prolongada; pode ocorrer em estados de ansiedade e em algumas doenças orgânicas crônicas, geralmente cardiovasculares; podem ocorrer alcalemia, parestesia e tetania.

Churg-Strauss s., s. de Churg-Strauss; asma, febre, eosinofilia e sinais e sintomas variados de vasculite, afetando primariamente as pequenas artérias, com granulomas vasculares e extravasculares. SIN allergic granulomatosis, allergic granulomatous angiitis.

Cianca s., s. de Cianca; forma grave de esotropia infantil, caracterizada por fixação cruzada e músculo reto medial do bulbo do olho tenso.

Clarke-Hadfield s., s. de Clarke-Hadfield. SIN cystic *fibrosis.*

classic cervical rib s., s. da costela cervical clássica. SIN true neurogenic thoracic outlet s.

Claude s., s. de Claude; síndrome mesencefálica com paralisia oculomotora no lado da lesão e incoordenação do lado oposto.

click s., s. do estalido; s., particularmente das valvas atrioventriculares, em que a sístole provoca uma súbita tensão do entalhe de uma valva ou de toda uma cúspide, produzindo estalido auscultatório.

climacteric s., s. climatérica. SIN menopausal s.

cloverleaf skull s. [MIM*148800], s. do crânio em folha de trevo; displasia óssea intra-uterina e sinostose das suturas coronal e lambdóidea, produzindo uma cabeça de forma trilobar, algumas vezes associada a exoftalmia e várias anomalias craniofaciais e dos ossos longos; a condição é esporádica.

Cobb s., s. de Cobb; malformação capilar cutânea, geralmente numa distribuição de dermátomo no tronco, associada a uma anormalidade vascular da medula espinal e conseqüentes sintomas neurológicos. SIN cutaneomeningospinal angiomatosis.

Cockayne s. [MIM*216400 e MIM*216411], s. de Cockayne; nanismo, aspecto precocemente senil, degeneração pigmentar da retina, atrofia óptica, surdez, sensibilidade à luz solar, microcefalia e retardo mental; herança autossômica recessiva associada a um reparo de excisão defeituoso do DNA. Existem vários grupos de complementação. SIN Cockayne disease.

Coffin-Lowry s. [MIM*303600], s. de Coffin-Lowry; caracterizada por traços faciais grosseiros com nariz bulboso, orelhas grandes e lábios espessos, estatura baixa; dedos das mãos afilados; anomalias esqueléticas e retardo mental. Herança recessiva ligada ao X, causada por mutação do gene da S6 cinase ribossomial (RSK) no cromossoma Xp.

Coffin-Siris s. [MIM*135900], s. de Coffin-Siris; caracterizada por retardo mental, nariz bulboso, ponte do nariz plana, hirsutismo moderado e anomalias digitais com ausência ou hipoplasia das unhas e falange terminal do quinto dedo da mão ou do pé; provavelmente de herança autossômica dominante. SIN fifth digit s.

Cogan s., s. de Cogan. SIN oculovestíbulo-auditory s.

Cogan-Reese s., s. de Cogan-Reese. SIN iridocorneal endothelial s.

cold agglutinin s., s. da crioaglutinina. SIN cold hemagglutinin *disease.*

Collet-Sicard s., s. de Collet-Sicard; lesões unilaterais do nono, décimo, décimo primeiro e décimo segundo nervos cranianos, produzindo a síndrome de Vernet e paralisia da língua do mesmo lado.

combined immunodeficiency s., s. de imunodeficiência combinada; imunodeficiência primária grave que afeta tanto as células T quanto as células B.
compartment s., s. do compartimento; condição em que o aumento da pressão em um espaço anatômico confinado afeta adversamente a circulação e ameaça a função e a viabilidade dos tecidos nesse local.
complete androgen insensitivity s., s. de insensibilidade completa aos androgênios. SIN testicular feminization.
compression s., s. de compressão. SIN crush s.
congenital rubella s., s. de rubéola congênita; infecção fetal pelo vírus da rubéola durante o primeiro trimestre de gravidez, provocando várias anormalidades congênitas, incluindo cardiopatia, surdez e cegueira.
Conn s., s. de Conn. SIN primary aldosteronism.
Conradi-Hünermann s., s. de Conradi-Hünermann; uma das síndromes de condrodisplasia pontilhada (q.v.), autossômica dominante, com distúrbios variáveis de ceratinização cutânea e anormalidades faciais, cardíacas, ópticas e do sistema nervoso central; ocorre também pontilhado epifisário.
Cornelia de Lange s., s. de Cornelia de Lange. SIN de Lange s.
corpus luteum deficiency s., s. de deficiência do corpo lúteo; distúrbios funcionais causados por luteinização ovariana insuficiente; reflete-se por uma resposta endometrial inadequada na fase lútea.
Costen s., s. de Costen; complexo sintomático de perda da audição, otalgia, zumbido, tontura, cefaléia e sensação de queimação na garganta, língua e parte lateral do nariz; originalmente atribuída à disfunção da articulação temporomandibular em decorrência de desarmonia oclusal; todavia, atualmente acredita-se que essa hipótese não esteja bem fundamentada em princípios anatômicos e fisiológicos.
costochondral s., s. costocondral; dor no tórax, com hipersensibilidade à palpação de uma ou mais junções costocondrais.
costoclavicular s., s. costoclavicular; uma das predecessoras da s. do desfiladeiro torácico, em que se acreditava que a artéria e veia subclávias, bem como, em relatórios posteriores, o plexo braquial fossem comprimidos entre a clavícula e a primeira costela normal ao assumir determinadas posturas corporais, p. ex., a posição militar.
Cotard s., s. de Cotard; depressão psicótica envolvendo a ilusão da existência do próprio corpo, juntamente com idéias de negação e impulsos suicidas.
Crandall s. [MIM*262000], s. de Crandall; caracterizada por pêlos tortos, surdez neurossensorial e hipogonadismo; traço familiar em que há deficiência de hormônio luteinizante e hormônio do crescimento. VER TAMBÉM Björnstad s.
CREST s., s. CREST; variante da esclerose sistêmica, caracterizada por calcinose, fenômeno de Raynaud, distúrbios da motilidade esofágica, esclerodactilia e telangiectasia.
cri-du-chat s., cri du chat s., cat-cry s., s. do miado-do-gato; distúrbio devido à deleção do braço curto do cromossoma 5, caracterizado por microcefalia, hipertelorismo, fissuras palpebrais antimongolóides, pregas epicânticas, micrognatia, estrabismo, retardo mental e físico e choro característico agudo, semelhante a um miado. SIN cat's cry s., Lejeune s.
Crigler-Najjar s. [MIM*218800], s. de Crigler-Najjar; defeito raro na capacidade de formar glicuronídeo de bilirrubina, devido à deficiência de bilirrubina-glicuronídeo glicuronosiltransferase; caracteriza-se por icterícia não-hemolítica familiar e, na sua forma grave, por lesão cerebral irreversível na lactância, que se assemelha ao *kernicterus* e pode ser fatal; herança autossômica recessiva, causada por mutação no gene da uridina difosfato glicosiltransferase 1 (UGT1) no cromossoma 1q. Existe uma forma autossômica dominante, denominada s. de Gilbert, também causada por mutação no gene UGT1. SIN Crigler-Najjar disease.
crocodile tears s., s. das lágrimas de crocodilo; fluxo de lágrimas, geralmente unilateral, durante a alimentação ou na sua antecipação; ocorre quando as fibras nervosas originalmente destinadas a uma glândula salivar são lesadas e voltam a crescer de modo aberrante na glândula lacrimal.
Cronkhite-Canada s. [MIM*175500], s. de Cronkhite-Canada; síndrome de ocorrência esporádica de pólipos gastrointestinais com alopecia difusa e distrofia ungueal; provavelmente não-genética.
Crouzon s. [MIM*123500], s. de Crouzon; craniossinostose com alargamento da fronte, hipertelorismo ocular, exoftalmia, nariz em bico e hipoplasia da maxila; herança autossômica dominante causada por mutação no gene do receptor do fator de crescimento dos fibroblastos 2 (FGFR2) no cromossoma 10q. A síndrome de Crouzon com acantose nigricans é causada por mutação no gene do receptor do fator de crescimento dos fibroblastos 3 (FGFR3) no cromossoma 4p. SIN craniofacial dysostosis, Crouzon disease.
Crow-Fukase s., s. de Crow-Fukase. SIN POEMS.
crush s., s. de esmagamento; estado semelhante ao choque que ocorre após a liberação de um membro ou membros ou do tronco e da pelve após um período prolongado de compressão, como aquele exercido por um objeto pesado; caracteriza-se por supressão da função renal, provavelmente em conseqüência da lesão dos túbulos renais pela mioglobina liberada dos músculos lesados. SIN compression s.
Cruveilhier-Baumgarten s., s. de Cruveilhier-Baumgarten; cirrose do fígado com veias umbilicais ou paraumbilicais ou paraumbilicais permeáveis e veias periumbilicais varicosas (cabeça de medusa). SIN Cruveilhier-Baumgarten disease.
cryptophthalmus s., s. de criptoftalmia. SIN Fraser s.
cubital tunnel s., s. do túnel cubital; grupo de sintomas que se desenvolvem em decorrência da compressão do nervo ulnar no interior do túnel cubital no cotovelo; pode incluir parestesia no quarto e quinto dedos da mão e fraqueza dos músculos intrínsecos da mão.
Cushing s., s. de Cushing; distúrbio resultante do aumento da secreção adrenocortical de cortisol (produzindo o quadro clínico da doença de Cushing [Cushing *disease*]) devido a qualquer uma de várias fontes: hiperplasia ou tumor adrenocortical ACTH-dependente, tumor secretor de ACTH ectópico ou administração excessiva de esteróides; caracterizada por obesidade do tronco, face de lua cheia, acne, estrias abdominais, hipertensão, diminuição da tolerância aos carboidratos, catabolismo das proteínas, distúrbios psiquiátricos e osteoporose, amenorréia e hirsutismo nas mulheres; quando associada a um adenoma produtor de ACTH, é denominada doença de Cushing. SIN Cushing basophilism.
Cushing s. medicamentosus, s. de Cushing medicamentosa; número variável dos sinais e sintomas da síndrome de Cushing; produzida pela administração crônica de grandes doses de qualquer esteróide que seja um potente glicocorticóide.
cutaneomucouveal s., s. cutaneomucoueval. SIN Behçet s.
Dandy-Walker s. [MIM*304340], s. de Dandy-Walker; anomalia de desenvolvimento do quarto ventrículo associada a atresia dos forames de Luschka e Magendie, que resulta em hipoplasia cerebelar, hidrocefalia e formação de cistos na fossa posterior.
dead arm s., s. do braço morto; diminuição ou perda sensorial no braço após luxação ou subluxação anterior do ombro.
dead fetus s., s. do feto morto; síndrome caracterizada por retenção intra-uterina prolongada de um feto morto, geralmente com mais de 4 semanas, com desenvolvimento de hipofibrinogenemia e, em certas ocasiões, coagulopatia intravascular disseminada.
dead-in-bed s., s. da morte no leito; achado de diabético jovem insulino-dependente sem doença prévia ou controle anormal da glicose morto no leito pela manhã. Acredita-se que seja devido à hipoglicemia, porém tem sido difícil estabelecer esse fato *postmortem*. Em geral, ocorrem em diabéticos que tomam três doses diárias de insulina, sugerindo a administração inadvertida de dose incorreta, com ausência da percepção de hipoglicemia durante o sono.
Debré-Sémélaigne s., s. de Debré-Sémélaigne. SIN Kocher-Debré-Sémélaigne s.
de Clerambault s., s. de Clerambault; erotomania acompanhada de crença ilusória de que determinada pessoa está apaixonada por você.
Degos s., s. de Degos. SIN malignant atrophic papulosis.
Dejerine-Klumpke s., s. de Dejerine-Klumpke. SIN Klumpke palsy.
Dejerine-Roussy s., s. de Dejerine-Roussy. SIN thalamic s.
de Lange s. [MIM 122470], s. de Lange; s. de anomalias congênitas múltiplas, caracterizada por retardo mental, face característica com microcefalia, sinofre, baixa linha de implantação anterior dos fios de cabelo, depressão da ponte do nariz, narinas antevertidas, filtro longo, boca de carpa, lábio superior fino e orelhas de implantação baixa, retardo do crescimento pré- e pós-natal, hirsutismo e, com freqüência, anomalias dos membros. A genética não está bem estabelecida, embora alguns casos pareçam ser de herança autossômica dominante. SIN Amsterdam s., Cornelia de Lange s.
Del Castillo s., s. de Del Castillo. SIN Sertoli-cell-only s.
de Morsier s., s. de Morsier. SIN septooptic dysplasia.
dengue shock s., s. de choque do dengue; febre de dengue de grau III ou IV.
Denys-Drash s., s. de Denys-Drash; s. consistindo em nefropatia, tumor de Wilms e anormalidades genitais.
depersonalization s., s. de despersonalização. SIN depersonalization.
depressive s., s. depressiva. SIN depression (4).
dermatitis-arthritis-tenosynovitis s., s. de dermatite-artrite-tenossinovite; infecção disseminada por *Neisseria gonorrhoeae*, causando lesões cutâneas (freqüentemente pustulares ou necróticas), juntamente com sinovite das grandes articulações (como joelho, tornozelo, cotovelo) e bainhas tendíneas.
De Sanctis-Cacchione s. [MIM*278800], s. de De Sanctis-Cacchione; xerodermia pigmentosa com deficiência mental, nanismo e hipoplasia gonadal; herança autossômica recessiva associada a um reparo defeituoso do DNA após lesão por irradiação ultravioleta.
s. of deviously relevant answers, s. de respostas divergentemente relevantes. SIN Ganser s.
dialysis disequilibrium s., s. de desequilíbrio da diálise; náuseas, vômitos e hipertensão, algumas vezes com convulsões, que surgem dentro de várias horas após o início da hemodiálise para insuficiência renal; aparentemente causada pela remoção muito rápida da uréia do compartimento de líquido extracelular, com movimento da água para o interior das células e edema cerebral.
dialysis encephalopathy s., s. de encefalopatia da diálise; encefalopatia difusa progressiva e freqüentemente fatal, que ocorre em alguns pacientes submetidos a hemodiálise crônica; deve ser diferenciada da síndrome de desequilíbrio da diálise autolimitada e relativamente aguda. SIN dialysis dementia.

Diamond-Blackfan s., s. de Diamond-Blackfan. SIN congenital hypoplastic anemia.

diencephalic s. of infancy, s. diencefálica do lactente; profunda emaciação após crescimento normal inicial, hiperatividade locomotora e euforia, geralmente com palidez cutânea, hipotensão e hipoglicemia; em geral, causada por neoplasia afetando o hipotálamo anterior.

Di Ferrante s. [MIM*253230], s. de Di Ferrante; associada a deficiência de N-acetilglicosamina 6-sulfatase e à excreção urinária de sulfato de heparan e sulfato de ceratan. SIN type VII mucopolysaccharidosis (2).

DiGeorge s. [MIM*188400], s. de DiGeorge; condição decorrente de defeito de desenvolvimento da terceira e da quarta bolsas faríngeas, resultando em ausência ou desenvolvimento deficiente do timo e das glândulas paratireóides, associada a anormalidades do trato de fluxo do coração, face característica, hipoparatireoidismo, hipocalcemia com tetania e deficiência da imunidade das células T; trata-se de uma s. de deleção gênica contígua envolvendo o cromossoma 22q11; herança autossômica dominante. SIN congenital aplasia of thymus, immunodeficiency with hypoparathyroidism, pharyngeal pouch s., third and fourth pharyngeal pouch s., thymic hypoplasia.

Di Guglielmo s. [MIM*133180], s. de Di Guglielmo. SIN Di Guglielmo *disease*.

disconnection s., s. de desconexão; designação geral para vários distúrbios neurológicos, devido à interrupção das vias de fibras do cérebro.

disk s., s. do disco; conjunto de sinais e sintomas, incluindo dor, parestesias, perda sensorial, fraqueza e reflexos diminuídos, devido a radiculopatia causada por compressão do disco intervertebral.

disputed neurogenic thoracic outlet s., s. contestada do desfiladeiro torácico neurogênico; distúrbio muito controvertido em que o plexo braquial está supostamente reprimido em um ou mais locais ao longo de seu trajeto, particularmente no triângulo interescaleno e entre a primeira costela torácica normal e algumas outras estruturas; freqüentemente atribuída a traumatismo (em particular, a acidentes automobilísticos) e diagnosticada, com mais freqüência, em mulheres jovens e de meia-idade; nenhuma manifestação clínica característica, embora a dor torácica seja característica; não há achados objetivos definidos, e não se dispõe de nenhum estudo diagnóstico auxiliar incontestável.

distal intestinal obstructive s., s. obstrutiva intestinal distal; síndrome observada na fibrose cística secundária à impacção com fezes e muco espessado.

Donohue s., s. de Donohue. SIN leprechaunism.

Doose s., s. de Doose; tipo familiar raro de epilepsia astática mioclônica generalizada primária, caracterizada por complexos ponta-onda de 2–3 ou 4–6 Hz no EEG; em geral, a condição responde à medicação.

Dorfman-Chanarin s. [MIM*275630], s. de Dorfman-Chanarin; ictiose congênita, vacúolos leucocitários e comprometimento variável de outros sistemas orgânicos. SIN neutral lipid storage disease.

dorsal midbrain s., s. mesencefálica dorsal. SIN Parinaud s.

Down s., s. de Down; s. de disgenesia cromossômica consistindo em um conjunto variável de anormalidades causadas por triplicação ou translocação do cromossoma 21. As anormalidades incluem retardo mental, retardo do crescimento, face hipoplásica plana com nariz curto, pregas cutâneas epicânticas proeminentes, orelhas pequenas de baixa implantação com antélice proeminente, fissura e espessamento da língua, frouxidão dos ligamentos articulares, displasia pélvica, mãos e pés largos, dedos atarracados e prega palmar transversa. É comum a ocorrência de opacidades lenticulares e cardiopatia. A incidência de leucemia está aumentada, e a ocorrência de doença de Alzheimer é quase inevitável aos 40 anos de idade. SIN trisomy 21.

Dressler s., s. de Dressler; pericardite recorrente após infarto do miocárdio agudo.

dry eye s., s. do olho seco. SIN keratoconjunctivitis sicca.

Duane s., s. de Duane. SIN retraction s.

Dubin-Johnson s. [MIM*237500], s. de Dubin-Johnson; defeito herdado da função excretora hepática, caracterizado por icterícia com níveis séricos de bilirrubina de até cerca de 6 mg/dL, dos quais mais da metade está na forma conjugada, e pela excreção urinária de proporções anormais de coproporfirina I. Ocorre também retenção de um pigmento escuro nos hepatócitos, que deriva da melanina ou das catecolaminas; entretanto, a histologia hepática está normal sob os demais aspectos. Na colecistografia oral não se consegue visualizar a vesícula biliar, e a excreção de substâncias-teste (p. ex., bromossulfoftaleína) pelo fígado é anormal. O defeito básico parece residir no transporte canalicular. Não há necessidade de terapia; herança autossômica recessiva causada por mutação no gene do transportador de ânions orgânicos multiespecífico canalicular (CMOAT) no cromossoma 10q. SIN chronic idiopathic jaundice.

Dubreuil-Chambardel s., s. de Dubreuil-Chambardel; cáries simultâneas dos dentes incisivos superiores, que ocorrem em ambos os sexos entre 14 e 17 anos de idade; depois de um intervalo de duração variável, os outros dentes também são afetados.

dumping s., s. do esvaziamento rápido; s. que ocorre após a alimentação, mais freqüentemente observada em pacientes com derivações do canal alimentar superior; caracterizada por rubor, sudorese, tontura, fraqueza e colapso vasomotor, em decorrência da passagem rápida de grandes quantidades de alimento no intestino delgado, com efeito osmótico que remove o líquido do plasma e causa hipovolemia. SIN early dumping s., postgastrectomy s.

Duncan s., s. de Duncan. SIN X-linked lymphoproliferative s.

Dyggve-Melchior-Clausen s. [MIM*223800], s. de Dyggve-Melchior-Clausen; displasia esquelética que exibe alguma semelhança clínica com a s. de Morquio, porém sem mucopolissacaridúria; caracterizada por retardo mental, nanismo com tronco curto, saliência progressiva do esterno, restrição da mobilidade articular, marcha anserina e achados radiográficos de cristas ilíacas irregulares e achatamento dos corpos vertebrais; herança autossômica recessiva. Existe uma forma ligada ao X [MIM*304950].

dysarthria-clumsy hand s., s. de disartria-mão desajeitada; distúrbio caracterizado por disartria e inabilidade de uma das mãos, causado por acidente vascular cerebral lacunar na parte basilar da ponte.

dyskinesia s. [MIM*242650], s. de discinesia; a eliminação de muco é lenta, e a bronquiectasia é prevalente e intratável. Há evidências de que o defeito reside na dineína, uma proteína dos cílios. O padrão de herança é aparentemente autossômico recessivo.

dysmnesic s., s. dismnésica. SIN Korsakoff s.

dysplastic nevus s., s. do nevo displásico. VER dysplastic *nevus*.

Eagle-Barrett s., s. de Eagle-Barrett. SIN prune belly s.

early dumping s., s. do esvaziamento precoce. SIN dumping s.

Eaton-Lambert s., s. de Eaton-Lambert. SIN Lambert-Eaton s.

ectopic ACTH, s. do ACTH ectópico; associação da s. de Cushing com neoplasia não-hipofisária, geralmente um carcinoma de pulmão que produz ACTH.

ectrodactyly—ectodermal dysplasia—clefting s., s. de ectrodactilia—displasia ectodérmica—fenda palatina; distúrbio autossômico recessivo resultando em defeitos das mãos e dos pés; a displasia ectodérmica causa pele clara, anodontia e fenda palatina.

Edwards s., s. de Edwards. SIN trisomy 18 s.

egg-white s., s. da clara de ovo; dermatite, queda dos pêlos e perda da coordenação muscular produzidas em ratos por dietas contendo grandes quantidades de clara de ovo crua, cuja avidina combina-se com a biotina, provocando deficiência desta última. SIN egg-white injury.

Ehlers-Danlos s. (EDS), s. de Ehlers-Danlos (SED); grupo de distúrbios do tecido conjuntivo, caracterizados por hiperelasticidade e fragilidade da pele, hipermobilidade das articulações e fragilidade dos vasos sanguíneos cutâneos e, algumas vezes, das grandes artérias, devido a uma deficiência na qualidade ou quantidade de colágeno; os tipos mais comuns são herdados de modo au-

síndrome de Down

freqüência de alguns sinais e sintomas orgânicos

ordem de freqüência relativa	característica	percentagem dos casos com a característica
1	retardo do desenvolvimento	99%
2	face mongolóide	90%
3	fissura palpebral	86,5%
4	braquicefalia	75%
5	clinodactilia V	50–70%
6	epicanto	67%
7	boca aberta	65%
8	prega palmar transversa	59%
9	lacuna entre o primeiro e o segundo dedos dos pés	53%
10	nariz curto e plano	53%
11	língua escrotal	51%
12	manchas de Brushfield	50%
13	deformidade da orelha externa	50%
14	macroglossia	41%
15	defeitos cardíacos congênitos	40–60%
16	hipotonia muscular	31%
17	braquidactilia	29%
18	estrabismo	14–23%

tossômico dominante, causados por mutação em um dos seguintes genes: o gene do colágeno V alfa-1 (COL5A1) no cromossoma 9q, ou o gene do colágeno V alfa-2 (COL5A2) no cromossoma 2q, ou o gene COL3A1 no cromossoma 2q.

Eisenmenger s., s. de Eisenmenger; insuficiência cardíaca com derivação da direita para a esquerda significativa, produzindo cianose devido à maior pressão no lado direito da derivação. Em geral, devido ao complexo de Eisenmenger, um defeito do septo interventricular com hipertrofia e dilatação do ventrículo direito, hipertensão pulmonar grave e freqüente acavalgamento do defeito por uma raiz aórtica de posição incorreta.

Ekbom s., s. de Ekbom. SIN restless legs s.
elfin facies s., s. da face de elfo. SIN Williams s.
Ellis-van Creveld s., s. de Ellis-van Creveld. SIN chondroectodermal *dysplasia*.
E-M s., s. E-M. SIN eosinophilia-myalgia s.
EMG s., s. EMG. SIN Beckwith-Wiedemann s.
encephalotrigeminal vascular s., s. vascular encefalotrigeminal; angiomatose do cérebro, acompanhada de nevos na área trigeminal. VER TAMBÉM Sturge-Weber s.

eosinophilia-myalgia s., s. de eosinofilia-mialgia; provável distúrbio auto-imune precipitado por comprimidos contaminados de L-triptofano e caracterizado por fadiga, febre baixa, mialgias, hipersensibilidade e cãibras musculares, fraqueza, parestesias dos membros e endurecimentos cutâneos; há eosinofilia acentuada nos estudos do sangue periférico e aumento da aldolase sérica; as biopsias de nervo periférico, músculo, pele e fáscia revelam microangiopatia e inflamação no tecido conjuntivo. SIN E-M s.

episodic dyscontrol s., s. de descontrole episódico. SIN intermittent explosive *disorder*.

erythrodysesthesia s., s. de eritrodisestesia; sensação de formigamento nas palmas das mãos e plantas dos pés, evoluindo para dor intensa e hipersensibilidade à palpação, com eritema e edema; causada por terapia de infusão contínua.

euthyroid sick s., s. do doente eutireóideo; anormalidades nos níveis dos hormônios e provas de função relacionados à glândula tireóide, que ocorrem em pacientes com doença sistêmica grave. Na verdade, a função tireóidea está normal nesses pacientes, e não se sabe ao certo se o tratamento dessas anormalidades seria benéfico. SIN sick thrombocytopenia.

Evans s., s. de Evans; anemia hemolítica adquirida e trombocitopenia.
exfoliation s., s. esfoliação. SIN pseudoexfoliation s.
extrapyramidal s., s. extrapiramidal; anormalidades do movimento relacionadas a lesão de vias motoras diferentes do trato piramidal.
Faber s., s. de Faber. SIN achlorhydric *anemia*.

false memory s., s. de memória falsa; memória aparente de um evento imaginado, geralmente traumático e remoto no tempo; em geral, utilizada pejorativamente para implicar que a memória foi gerada pelo terapeuta ao facilitar a sua recuperação; conceito controvertido.

familial aortic ectasia s., s. de ectasia aórtica familiar; ocorrência, como caráter autossômico dominante, de valva aórtica bicúspide, freqüentemente com calcificação prematura, ectasia e dissecção da aorta e, raramente, coarctação da aorta. Assemelha-se superficialmente à síndrome de Marfan. SIN familial aortic ectasia.

familial chylomicronemia s., s. de quilomicronemia familiar; distúrbio herdado que resulta em acúmulo de quilomícrons e triacilgliceróis. VER TAMBÉM chylomicronemia.

Fanconi s. [MIM*227650–227660], s. de Fanconi; **(1)** SIN Fanconi *anemia*; **(2)** grupo de condições com distúrbios característicos da função tubular renal, que podem ser classificados em: 1) cistinose, uma doença autossômica recessiva do início da infância; 2) s. de Fanconi do adulto, uma forma hereditária rara, provavelmente causada por um gene recessivo diferente daquele encontrado na cistinose, caracterizada por disfunção tubular observada na cistinose e por osteomalacia, porém sem depósito de cistina nos tecidos; 3) s. de Fanconi adquirida, que pode estar associada a mieloma múltiplo ou resultar de intoxicação química, traumatismo ou lesão persistente do epitélio tubular proximal de várias causas, levando a múltiplos defeitos da função tubular.

FAPA s., s. FAPA; síndrome de etiologia desconhecida que provoca surtos periódicos de febre, adenite, faringite e úlceras aftosas (*f*ever, *a*denitis, *p*haryngitis e *a*phthous ulcers).

Farber s. [MIM*228000], s. de Farber. SIN disseminated *lipogranulomatosis*.
Favre-Racouchot s., s. de Favre-Racouchot. SIN Favre-Racouchot *disease*.
Felty s., s. de Felty; artrite reumatóide com esplenomegalia e leucopenia.
fetal alcohol s., s. alcoólica fetal; padrão de malformação com deficiência do crescimento, anomalias craniofaciais e déficits funcionais, incluindo retardo mental, observada na prole de mães alcoólatras.

fetal aspiration s., s. de aspiração fetal; s. resultante da aspiração intra-uterina de líquido amniótico e mecônio pelo feto, geralmente causada por hipoxia e levando, com freqüência, a pneumonia por aspiração. SIN meconium aspiration s.

fetal face s., s. da face fetal; s. de fácies semelhante a um feto em desenvolvimento inicial, com antebraços curtos e hipoplasia genital ao nascimento, porém sem qualquer evidência de acondroplasia; leva ao nanismo sem retardo mental.

fetal hydantoin s., s. da hidantoína fetal; s. que resulta da ingestão materna de análogos da hidantoína (p. ex., fenitoína), caracterizada por deficiência do crescimento, deficiência mental, face dismórfica, fenda palatina e/ou lábio leporino, defeitos cardíacos e genitália anormal.

fetal trimethadione s., s. da trimetadiona fetal; s. resultante da ingestão pela mãe de trimetadiona durante as primeiras semanas de gravidez e caracterizada por atraso do desenvolvimento, sobrancelhas em forma de V, epicanto, orelhas de implantação baixa com hélice anteriormente dobrada, anomalia do palato e dentes irregulares.

fetal warfarin s., s. da warfarina fetal; sangramento fetal, hipoplasia nasal, atrofia óptica e morte em decorrência da ingestão de warfarina pela gestante.

fibrinogen-fibrin conversion s., s. de conversão do fibrinogênio em fibrina; s. caracterizada por hipofibrinogenemia com sangue incoagulável; pode ser observada no descolamento prematuro da placenta, retenção prolongada de feto morto numa mãe isossensibilizada ao fator Rh, reações sanguíneas hemolíticas, necrose bilateral do córtex renal e casos de traumatismo.

fibromyalgia s., s. de fibromialgia. SIN fibromyalgia.
Fiessinger-Leroy-Reiter s., s. de Fiessinger-Leroy-Reiter. SIN Reiter s.
fifth digit s., s. do quinto dedo. SIN Coffin-Siris s.
first arch s., s. do primeiro arco; termo genérico que inclui síndromes de malformações afetando derivados do primeiro arco branquial, com ou sem malformações associadas; inclui disostose mandibulofacial, micrognatia com peromelia, disostose otomandibular, disostose acrofacial e outras malformações.

Fisher s., s. de Fisher; s. caracterizada por oftalmoplegia, ataxia e arreflexia; forma de polineurorradiculite.

Fitz-Hugh and Curtis s., s. de Fitz-Hugh e Curtis; peri-hepatite em mulheres com história de salpingite gonocócica ou por clamídias.

flashing pain s. [MIM*190400], s. da dor fugaz; breves episódios súbitos, intermitentes e intensos de dor, sem causa aparente, na distribuição de um dermátomo espinal; assemelha-se, quanto ao caráter, à dor do tique doloroso. Cf. *tic* douloureux.

flecked retina s. [MIM*228980], s. da retina manchada; distúrbio retiniano hereditário com transmissão anormal de fluorescência através do epitélio pigmentar da retina na angiografia.

floppy valve s., s. da valva flácida; deslizamento retrógrado de folhetos da valva mitral ou tricúspide no orifício valvar além do ponto de fechamento durante a sístole do ventrículo esquerdo; uma característica da síndrome de Barlow.

Flynn-Aird s. [MIM*136300], s. de Flynn-Aird; s. familiar caracterizada por consunção muscular, ataxia, demência, atrofia cutânea, cáries dentárias, rigidez articular, retinite pigmentosa e perda progressiva da audição neurossensorial; herança autossômica dominante.

Foix-Alajouanine s., s. de Foix-Alajouanine; tromboflebite das veias espinais, resultando em paralisia flácida dolorosa ascendente subaguda devido a mielite necrótica.

Foix-Cavany-Marie s., s. de Foix-Cavany-Marie; conjunto de diplegia faciofaringoglossomastigatória com dissociação voluntária automática, sem demência associada ou riso ou grito forçados geralmente causados por infartos bilaterais de grandes artérias do córtex opercular.

folded-lung s., atelectasia redonda. SIN rounded *atelectasis*.
Forbes-Albright s., s. de Forbes-Albright; tumor hipofisário em pacientes sem acromegalia, que secreta quantidades excessivas de prolactina (LTH) e produz lactação persistente.

Foster Kennedy s., s. de Foster Kennedy. SIN Kennedy s.
Foville s., s. de Foville; forma de hemiplegia alternante caracterizada por paralisia do abducente de um lado e paralisia dos membros do outro lado.

fragile X s., s. do X frágil; s. recessiva ligada ao X [MIM*309550] que consiste em retardo mental, face característica e macroorquidismo; a análise do DNA revela repetições de trinucleotídeos anormais no cromossoma X, próximo à extremidade do braço longo, em Xq27.3; pode-se demonstrar uma constrição nesse local na cariotipagem após cultura em meio deficiente em folato. SIN FMR1, marker X s., Martin-Bell s.

> A incidência da s. do X frágil (cerca de 1:2.000 nos homens) ocupa o segundo lugar depois da s. de Down entre as causas geneticamente identificáveis de retardo mental. A expressão fenotípica é variável, enquanto o retardo mental é a manifestação mais comum. A face é longa e estreita, com orelhas grandes, sínfise mandibular proeminente e palato com arco alto. É comum a macrocefalia absoluta ou relativa. O macroorquidismo aparece na puberdade ou antes; os estudos histológicos revelam apenas edema dos testículos. As anormalidades do tecido conjuntivo podem manifestar-se por hipermobilidade dos dedos das mãos e de outras articulações, pé plano, dilatação da aorta e prolapso da valva mitral. Além do comprometimento intelectual, os achados neuropsiquiátricos incluem hiperatividade, curto tempo de atenção, contato ocular deficiente, comportamento semelhante ao do altista, fala jocosa, ecolalia e incoordenação motora. O QI pode sofrer deterioração com a idade. Alguns homens com esse defeito genético e cerca de dois terços das mulheres são fenotipicamente normais. A expressão depende de uma mutação que

ocorre em duas ou mais etapas e que é instável tanto na meiose quanto na mitose. A transmissão é complexa e varia de acordo com o sexo do probando e do genitor transmissor. O *locus* cromossômico frágil representa um sítio de amplificação anormal com número variável de repetições CGG. Essas repetições bloqueiam a transcrição do gene FMR1 (retardo mental familiar), que normalmente codifica a proteína FMR1; a expressão clínica deve-se à ausência de síntese da proteína FMR1 e à metilação anormal de seqüências do DNA distalmente ao sítio frágil.

Fraley s., s. de Fraley; dilatação dos cálices renais do pólo superior devido à estenose do infundíbulo superior, geralmente causada por compressão de vasos que suprem os segmentos superior e médio do rim.
Franceschetti s., s. de Franceschetti; disostose mandibulofacial (mandibulofacial *dysostosis*), quando completa ou quase completa.
Franceschetti-Jadassohn s., s. de Franceschetti-Jadassohn. SIN Naegeli s.
Fraser s. [MIM*219000], s. de Fraser; associação de criptoftalmia com múltiplas anomalias, incluindo malformações das orelhas média e externa, fenda palatina, deformidade laríngea, deslocamento do umbigo e dos mamilos, malformações digitais, separação da sínfise púbica, desenvolvimento defeituoso dos rins e masculinização da genitália no sexo feminino; herança autossômica recessiva. SIN cryptophthalmus s.
Freeman-Sheldon s., s. de Freeman-Sheldon. SIN craniocarpotarsal *dystrophy*.
Frey s., s. de Frey. SIN auriculotemporal nerve s.
Friderichsen-Waterhouse s., s. de Friderichsen-Waterhouse. SIN Waterhouse-Friderichsen s.
Fröhlich s., s. de Fröhlich. SIN adiposogenital *dystrophy*.
Froin s., s. de Froin; alteração do líquido cefalorraquidiano, que é amarelado e sofre coagulação espontânea alguns segundos após a sua coleta, devido ao conteúdo acentuadamente aumentado de proteína (albumina e globulina); observada em porções loculadas do espaço subaracnóideo isoladas da circulação do líquido cefalorraquidiano por obstrução inflamatória ou neoplásica.
Fuchs s. [MIM*136800], s. de Fuchs; s. caracterizada por degeneração da córnea, heterocromia da íris, iridociclite, precipitados ceráticos e catarata; provavelmente de herança autossômica dominante. SIN Fuchs heterochromic cyclitis.
functional prepubertal castration s., s. de castração pré-puberal funcional; s. caracterizada pela ausência de testículos no escroto, porém pela presença, em seu lugar, de derivados do ducto mesonéfrico, ginecomastia pronunciada e biotipo eunucóide, com aumento dos níveis plasmáticos e da excreção urinária de gonadotropinas.
G s. [MIM*145410], s. G; s. de fácies característica associada a hipospadia, curvatura ventral do pênis e disfagia. Aparentemente, a mesma s. BBB de Opritz *et al.* Herança autossômica dominante. [primeira letra do sobrenome da pessoa afetada descrita]
Gaisböck s., s. de Gaisböck. SIN polycythemia hipertonica.
Ganser s., s. de Ganser; condição de tipo psicótico, sem os sinais e sintomas de uma psicose tradicional, ocorrendo tipicamente em prisioneiros que simulam insanidade; p. ex., a pessoa, quando solicitada a multiplicar 6 por 4, responde 23, ou dará uma chave o nome de fechadura. VER malingering, factitious *disorder*. SIN nonsense s., s. of approximate relevant answers, s. of deviously relevant answers.
Gardner s. [MIM*175100-0006], s. de Gardner; polipose múltipla que predispõe ao carcinoma do colo; além disso, múltiplos tumores, osteomas do crânio, cistos epidermóides e fibromas; herança autossômica dominante, causada por mutação no gene da polipose adenomatosa do colo (APC) no cromossoma 5q. Esse distúrbio é alélico à *polipose* adenomatosa familiar (FAP).
Gardner-Diamond s., s. de Gardner-Diamond. SIN autoerythrocyte sensitization s.
gastrocardiac s., s. gastrocardíaca; distúrbios da ação cardíaca em virtude da ação deficiente do sistema digestivo, especialmente do estômago.
gastrojejunal loop obstruction s., s. de obstrução da alça gastrojejunal. SIN afferent loop s.
gay bowel s., s. do intestino *gay*; desconforto gastrointestinal apresentado por homens homossexuais; inclui dor abdominal, cólicas, distensão, flatulência, náuseas, vômitos ou diarréia causada por bactérias entéricas, vírus, fungos, zooparasitas ou traumatismo.
Gélineau s., s. de Gélineau. SIN narcolepsy.
gender dysphoria s., s. de disforia sexual; s. em que um indivíduo sofre acentuado estresse pessoal, devido à sensação de que, apesar de possuir a genitália e os caracteres sexuais secundários de um sexo, existe um senso de compatibilidade e maior identidade com o outro sexo; o indivíduo pode ser submetido a cirurgia para reconstruir a anatomia do outro sexo.
general adaptation s., s. de adaptação geral; termo introduzido por Hans Selye para descrever alterações fisiológicas pronunciadas em vários sistemas orgânicos do corpo, especialmente o sistema hipofisário-endócrino, em conseqüência da exposição a estresse físico ou psicológico prolongado, com progressão das alterações corporais através de três estágios que o autor descreveu como reação de alarme, resistência e, finalmente, exaustão.

Gerstmann s., s. de Gerstmann; agnosia digital, agrafia, confusão da lateralidade do corpo e acalculia; causada por lesões entre a área occipital e o giro angular.
Gerstmann-Sträussler-Scheinker s., s. de Gerstmann-Sträussler-Scheinker; forma cerebelar crônica de encefalopatia espongiforme.
Gianotti-Crosti s., s. de Gianotti-Crosti; manifestação cutânea de hepatite B que ocorre em crianças pequenas; exantema consistindo em pápulas pardacentas não-pruriginosas nas pernas, nádegas e extensores dos braços; a s. de Gianotti-Crosti dura 2–8 semanas e está associada a adenopatia, hepatomegalia anictérica e mal-estar. SIN papular acrodermatitis of childhood.
Gilbert s., s. de Gilbert. SIN familial nonhemolytic *jaundice*.
Gilles de la Tourette s. [MIM*137580], s. de Gilles de la Tourette. SIN Tourette s.
Gillespie s., s. de Gillespie; s. de ausência congênita da íris, retardo mental e ataxia cerebelar; etiologia desconhecida.
Gitelman s., s. de Gitelman; distúrbio observado em crianças de mais idade e adultos jovens, caracterizado por hipopotassemia, hipomagnesemia, hipocalciúria e, algumas vezes, tetania.
glucagonoma s., s. do glucagonoma; eritema migratório necrolítico ou dermatite intertriginosa ou periorofacial, estomatite, anemia, perda de peso e hiperglicemia em decorrência de tumores das células das ilhotas pancreáticas secretores de glucagon.
Goldenhar s. [MIM*257700], s de Goldenhar. SIN oculoauriculovertebral *dysplasia*.
Goldmann-Favre s., s. de Goldmann-Favre, degeneração vitreotapetorretiniana progressiva, autossômica recessiva.
gold-myokymia s., s. de miocimia por ouro; o complexo sintomático de miocimia disseminada, dor muscular e distúrbios autônomos (sudorese excessiva, hipotensão ortostática) que pode resultar da terapia com ouro.
Goltz s., s. de Goltz. SIN focal dermal *hypoplasia*.
Goodpasture s. [MIM*233450], s. de Goodpasture; glomerulonefrite do tipo antimembrana basal, associada a ou precedida de hemoptise; em geral, a nefrite progride rapidamente, causando morte por insuficiência renal, e os pulmões, à necropsia, revelam hemossiderose extensa ou hemorragia recente.
Gopalan s., s. de Gopalan; desconforto intenso dos pés associado a temperatura cutânea elevada e sudorese excessiva.
Gorham s., s. de Gorham. SIN disappearing bone *disease*.
Gorlin s., s. de Gorlin. SIN basal cell nevus s.
Gorlin-Chaudhry-Moss s. [MIM*233500], s. de Gorlin-Chaudhry-Moss; disostose craniofacial, persistência do canal arterial, hipertricose, hipoplasia dos lábios maiores do pudendo e anormalidades dentais e oculares. VER TAMBÉM Weill-Marchesani s.
Gougerot-Carteaud s., s. de Gougerot-Carteaud. SIN confluent and reticulate *papillomatosis*.
Gowers s., s. de Gowers; s. que consiste em palpitação, dor torácica, dificuldades respiratórias e distúrbios da motilidade gástrica; outrora atribuída à estimulação vagal; hoje em dia, considerada psicogênica (neurose de ansiedade). SIN vagal attack, vasovagal attack, vasovagal s.
gracilis s., s. grácil; osteonecrose do púbis após traumatismo.
Gradenigo s., s. de Gradenigo; s. que consiste em otorréia, cefaléia, diplopia e dor retroorbital na petrosite, devido a um abscesso epidural no ápice da superfície anterior da pirâmide petrosa, causando compressão do nervo abducente no canal de Dorello e irritação do gânglio trigeminal.
gray s., gray baby s., s. cinzenta, s. do bebê cinzento; aspecto acinzentado de um recém-nascido e durante o período neonatal, que pode ser causado por efeitos tóxicos transplacentários da droga cloranfenicol usada pela mãe no final da gravidez; a síndrome pode ser fatal.
Greig s., s. de Greig. SIN ocular *hypertelorism*.
Greig cephalopolysyndactyly s. [MIM*175700], s. de cefalopolissindactilia de Greig; distúrbio autossômico dominante caracterizado por polissindactilia das mãos e dos pés, macrocefalia, bossa frontal, hipertelorismo e ponte do nariz plana, causado por mutação do gene GLI3 no cromossoma 7p13.
Grönblad-Strandberg s., s. de Grönblad-Strandberg; estrias angióides da retina, juntamente com pseudoxantoma elástico da pele.
Gubler s., s. de Gubler; forma de hemiplegia alternante, caracterizada por hemiplegia contralateral e paralisia facial ipsilateral. SIN Gubler paralysis, Millard-Gubler s.
Guillain-Barré s., s. de Guillain-Barré; distúrbio agudo imunologicamente mediado de nervos periféricos, raízes espinais e nervos cranianos, que comumente se manifesta como fraqueza ascendente rapidamente progressiva, arreflexiva e relativamente simétrica da musculatura dos membros, tronco, respiratória, faríngea e facial, com disfunção sensitiva e autônoma variável; tipicamente, atinge seu ponto mais baixo dentro de 2–3 semanas, seguido, inicialmente, por um período de platô de duração semelhante e, subsequentemente, de recuperação gradual, porém completa, na maioria dos casos. A s. de Guillain-Barré é freqüentemente precedida de infecção respiratória ou gastrointestinal e está associada a uma dissociação albuminocitológica do líquido cefalorraquidiano cerebral. Embora classicamente considerada, do ponto de vista his-

topatológico, uma polirradiculoneuropatia desmielinizante inflamatória aguda (q.v.), recentemente foram reconhecidas formas puras de degeneração axônica. SIN acute idiopathic polyneuritis, acute inflammatory polyneuropathy, infectious polyneuritis, Landry paralysis, Landry s., Landry-Guillain-Barré s., myeloradiculopolyneuronitis, postinfectious polyneuritis.

Gulf War s., s. da Guerra do Golfo; designação aplicada freqüentemente, porém de modo inapropriado, a diversos problemas de saúde apresentados por militares norte-americanos após servir no conflito do Golfo Pérsico de 1991; foram relatadas fadiga, dor musculoesquelética, cefaléia, dispnéia, perda da memória e diarréia, porém uma comissão do NIH concluiu que faltavam evidências de doença específica. SIN Persian Gulf s.

Gunn s., s. de Gunn. SIN jaw-winking s.

gustatory sweating s., s. da sudorese gustativa. SIN auriculotemporal nerve s.

Guyon tunnel s., s. do túnel de Guyon; compressão do nervo ulnar no canal de Guyon quando passa no punho.

Haber s., s. de Haber; rubor permanente e telangiectasia das bochechas, nariz, fronte e queixo, com aberturas foliculares proeminentes, pequenas pápulas com descamação e diminutas áreas deprimidas; em certas ocasiões, acompanhada de lesões descamativas e ceratóticas do tronco.

HAIR-AN s., s. HAIR-AN; hiperandrogenismo, resistência a insulina e acantose nigricans; virilização em meninas puberais associada a níveis acentuadamente elevados de insulina e níveis normais de hormônio luteinizante e hormônio folículo-estimulante. [*h*yperandrogenism, *i*nsulin *r*esistance, *a*canthosis *n*igricans]

Hallermann-Streiff s., s. de Hallermann-Streiff. SIN dyscephalia mandibulo-oculofacialis.

Hallermann-Streiff-François s., s. de Hallermann-Streiff-François. SIN dyscephalia mandibulo-oculofacialis.

Hallervorden s., s. de Hallervorden. SIN Hallervorden-Spatz s.

Hallervorden-Spatz s., s. de Hallervorden-Spatz; distúrbio caracterizado por distonia com outras disfunções extrapiramidais, que aparecem nas duas primeiras décadas de vida; associada a grandes quantidades no ferro pálido e na substância negra. SIN Hallervorden s., Hallervorden-Spatz disease, status dysmyelinisatus.

Hallgren s., s. de Hallgren; ataxia vestibulocerebelar, distrofia pigmentar da retina, surdez congênita e catarata.

Hamman s., s. de Hamman; enfisema mediastinal espontâneo, resultante de ruptura dos alvéolos. SIN Hamman disease.

Hamman-Rich s., s. de Hamman-Rich. SIN idiopathic pulmonary fibrosis.

hand-and-foot s., s. da mão e do pé; tumefação dolorosa recorrente das mãos e dos pés que ocorre em lactentes e crianças pequenas com anemia falciforme. SIN sickle cell dactylitis.

hand-foot s., s. mão-pé; s. descamativa dolorosa associada ao 5-fluorouracil, especialmente quando administrado de modo contínuo e em combinação com citarabina.

Hanhart s., s. de Hanhart. SIN micrognathia with peromelia.

hantavirus pulmonary s., s. pulmonar por hantavírus; doença febril causada por diversas espécies de hantavírus (vírus dos Andes, de Bayou, do Black Creek Canal, de Nova York e Sin Nombre) na América do Norte e América do Sul, caracterizada por trombocitopenia, leucocitose e extravasamento capilar nos pulmões, sendo a morte causada por choque e complicações cardíacas.

happy puppet s. [MIM*234400], s. da boneca feliz; s. caracterizada por retardo mental, ataxia, hipotonia, convulsões epilépticas, espasmos de riso facilmente provocados e prolongados, prognatismo e expressão com boca aberta.

Harada s., s. de Harada; edema bilateral da retina, uveíte, coroidite e descolamento da retina, com surdez temporária ou permanente, encanecimento dos cabelos (poliose) e alopecia; relacionada à s. de Voft-Koyanagi e à oftalmia simpática. SIN Harada disease, uveoencephalitis, uveomeningitis s.

Harris s., s. de Harris; produção excessiva de insulina com hipoglicemia, fome, nervosismo, taquicardia e rubor, que ocorre em determinadas condições, como distúrbios funcionais do pâncreas, hiperplasia das ilhotas de Langerhans ou insulinoma.

Hartnup s., s. de Hartnup. SIN Hartnup disease.

Hayem-Widal s., s. de Hayem-Widal; termo obsoleto para a icterícia hemolítica adquirida (acquired hemolytic icterus). SIN Widal s.

head-bobbing doll s., s. da cabeça pendular da boneca; movimento pendular da cabeça, geralmente devido a cistos no interior ou ao redor do terceiro ventrículo.

Hegglin s., s. de Hegglin; dissociação entre sístole eletromecânica (intervalo QSII) e sístole elétrica (intervalo QT), de modo que a segunda bulha cardíaca (SII) é registrada antes do final da onda T; descrita por Hegglin como insuficiência cardíaca dinâmica durante o coma diabético e outros distúrbios metabólicos.

HELLP s., s. HELLP; tipo de pré-eclâmpsia grave envolvendo hemólise, elevação das provas de função hepática e baixa contagem de plaquetas (*h*emolysis, *e*levated *l*iver function, and *l*ow *p*latelets).

Helweg-Larssen s. [MIM*125050], s. de Helweg-Larssen; distúrbio autossômico dominante caracterizado por displasia ectodérmica anidrótica e perda auditiva, com desenvolvimento desta última na quarta ou quinta década de vida.

hemolytic uremic s., s. hemolítico-urêmica; anemia hemolítica e trombocitopenia que ocorrem na insuficiência renal aguda; em crianças, caracteriza-se por início súbito de sangramento gastrointestinal, hematúria, oligúria e anemia hemolítica microangiopática; em adultos, associada a complicações da gravidez após parto normal ou ao uso de anticoncepcionais orais ou à presença de infecção; freqüentemente causada pela infecção por *Escherichia coli*.

Henoch-Schönlein s., s. de Henoch-Schönlein. SIN Henoch-Schönlein purpura.

hepatorenal s., hepatonephric s., s. hepatorrenal, s. hepatonéfrica; ocorrência de insuficiência renal aguda em pacientes com doença do fígado ou das vias biliares, aparentemente devido à redução do fluxo sanguíneo renal e a condições que lesam ambos os órgãos, como intoxicação por tetracloreto de carbono e leptospirose.

Herlitz s., s. de Herlitz. SIN epidermolysis bullosa lethalis.

Hermansky-Pudlak s., s. de Hermansky-Pudlak; forma de albinismo oculocutâneo (autossômico recessivo) com acúmulo de ceróide nos lisossomas, com doença pulmonar restritiva, colite granulomatosa, insuficiência renal, miocardiopatia e plaquetas com deficiência de armazenamento. VER oculocutaneous *albinism*.

heroin overdose s., s. da superdose (overdose) de heroína. SIN opiate intoxication s.

Herrmann s. [MIM*172500], s. de Herrmann; distúrbio multissistêmico que começa no final da infância ou no início da adolescência, com fotomioclonia e perda da audição, seguidas de diabetes melito, demência progressiva, pielonefrite e glomerulonefrite; a perda da audição neurossensorial progressiva tem início mais tardio; provavelmente de herança autossômica dominante com penetrância incompleta.

Hinman s., s. de Hinman. SIN nonneurogenic neurogenic bladder.

HIV wasting s., s. de debilitação por HIV. SIN wasting s. (2).

holiday s., s. do feriado; regressão, desenvolvimento de ansiedade difusa, sentimentos de desamparo, irritabilidade e depressão; nos Estados Unidos, diz-se que ocorre em determinados pacientes psicanalíticos antes do dia de ação de graças e continua durante o feriado natalino, terminando alguns dias após o primeiro dia de janeiro.

holiday heart s., s. cardíaca do feriado; arritmias cardíacas, algumas vezes aparentes após férias ou um final de semana distante do trabalho, após consumo excessivo de álcool; geralmente transitória.

Holmes-Adie s., s. de Holmes-Adie. SIN Adie s.

Holt-Oram s. [MIM*142900], s. de Holt-Oram; defeito do septo interatrial em associação a polegar ausente ou semelhante aos outros dedos da mão e a outras deformidades do antebraço; herança autossômica dominante, causada pela mutação no gene T-box5 (TBX5) no cromossoma 12q.

Horner s., s. de Horner; ptose, miose e anidrose no lado da paralisia assimpática. A enoftalmia é mais aparente do que real. A pupila afetada sofre visivelmente dilatação lenta no escuro; causada por uma lesão da cadeia simpática cervical ou de suas vias centrais. SIN Bernard-Horner s., ptosis sympathetica.

Houssay s., s. de Houssay; melhora do diabetes melito pela lesão destrutiva na hipófise ou sua remoção cirúrgica.

Houston-Harris s., s. de Houston-Harris. SIN Type IA achondrogenesis.

Hughes-Stovin s., s. de Hughes-Stovin; s. caracterizada por aneurismas das grandes e pequenas artérias pulmonares e por trombose das veias periféricas e seios durais.

Hunt s. [MIM*159700], s. de Hunt; (1) tremor intencional que começa em um membro, aumenta gradualmente de intensidade e, subseqüentemente, afeta outras partes do corpo. SIN progressive cerebellar tremor; (2) paralisia facial, otalgia e herpes zoster em decorrência de infecção viral do sétimo nervo craniano e gânglio geniculado; (3) forma de paralisia agitante juvenil associada a atrofia primária do sistema do pálido. SIN paleostriatal s., pallidal s. SIN Ramsay Hunt s. (1).

Hunter s. [MIM*309900], s. de Hunter; erro do metabolismo dos mucopolissacarídeos, caracterizado pela deficiência de iduronato sulfatase, com excreção urinária de sulfato de dermatan e sulfato de heparan; clinicamente semelhante à síndrome de Hurler, porém diferenciada por alterações esqueléticas menos graves, ausência de turvação da córnea e herança recessiva ligada ao X; causada por mutação no gene da iduronato sulfatase (IDS) no cromossoma Xq. SIN type II mucopolysaccharidosis.

Hurler s. [MIM*252800], s. de Hurler; mucopolissacaridose em que ocorrem deficiência de α-L-iduronidase, acúmulo de material intracelular anormal e excreção urinária de sulfato de dermatan e sulfato de heparan; caracteriza-se por anormalidade acentuada no desenvolvimento da cartilagem óssea e do osso, com nanismo, cifose, membros deformados, limitação da mobilidade articular, mão espatulada, turvação da córnea, hepatoesplenomegalia, retardo mental e fácies semelhante a uma gárgula; herança autossômica recessiva, causada por mutação no gene da α-L-iduronidase (IDUA) no cromossoma 4p. VER TAMBÉM mucolipidosis. SIN Hurler disease, lipochondrodystrophy, Pfaundler-Hurler s., type IH mucopolysaccharidosis.

Hurler-Scheie s., s. de Hurler-Scheie; síndrome fenotípica intermediária entre a síndrome de Hurler e a síndrome de Scheie; deficiência de α-L-iduronidase. SIN type I H/S mucopolysaccharidosis.

Hutchinson-Gilford s., s. de Hutchinson-Gilford. SIN progeria.
Hutchison s., s. de Hutchison; neuroblastoma supra-renal de lactentes com metástase para a órbita; outrora, acreditava-se erroneamente que se originava predominantemente da glândula supra-renal esquerda. VER TAMBÉM Pepper s.
hyaline membrane s., s. da membrana hialina. SIN hyaline membrane *disease of the newborn.*
hydralazine s., s. da hidralazina. SIN drug-induced *lupus.*
17-hydroxylase deficiency s. [MIM*202110], s. da deficiência de 17-hidroxilase; deficiência congênita da esteróide C-17α-hidroxilase córtico-supra-renal e, possivelmente, ovariana; a conseqüente secreção excessiva de corticosterona e de desoxicorticosterona provoca amenorréia, genitália ambígua, hipertensão e alcalose hipopotassêmica; herança autossômica recessiva, causada por mutação em um dos genes do citocromo P450 (CYP17) no cromossoma 10q.
hyperabduction s., s. hiperabdução; (1) diminuição ou perda dos pulsos distais do membro superior com a hiperabdução do membro; (2) uma das predecessoras da s. do desfiladeiro torácico, em que a artéria subclávia ou a axilar, no plexo braquial, poderia estar comprimida no espaço costoclavicular ou sob o tendão do peitoral menor, durante a hiperabdução do membro. SIN subcoracoid-pectoralis minor tendon s., Wright s.
hyperactive child s., s. da criança hiperativa. SIN attention deficit hyperactivity *disorder.*
hypereosinophilic s., s. hipereosinofílica; eosinofilia periférica persistente com infiltração eosinofílica na medula óssea, coração e outros sistemas orgânicos; acompanhada de sudorese noturna, tosse, anorexia e perda ponderal, prurido e várias lesões cutâneas, bem como sintomas de endocardite de Löffler.
hyper-IgM s., s. da hiper-IgM; distúrbio de imunodeficiência ligado ao X, caracterizado por concentrações séricas muito baixas de IgG e IgA, com concentração normal ou acentuadamente elevada de IgM policlonal; os meninos afetados desenvolvem infecções bacterianas recorrentes no primeiro ou segundo ano de vida.
hyperimmunoglobulin E s., s. da hiperimunoglobulina E; distúrbio de imunodeficiência caracterizado por altos níveis plasmáticos de IgE, defeito quimiotático dos leucócitos e infecções estafilocócicas recorrentes da pele, das vias respiratórias superiores e de outros locais. SIN Job s.
hyperkinetic s., s. hipercinética; condição caracterizada por energia patologicamente excessiva, observada algumas vezes em crianças pequenas com lesão cerebral, doença mental e distúrbio de déficit de atenção, bem como em epilépticos; as principais características consistem em hipermotilidade e instabilidade emocional; comumente acompanhada de distratibilidade, desatenção e ausência de timidez e de medo.
hyperkinetic heart s., s. do coração hipercinético; imprecisamente, s. em que o coração parece estar "trabalhando excessivamente", isto é, batendo excessivamente rápido e/ou causando uma percepção subjetiva de atividade cardíaca contínua.
hyperornithinemia-hyperammonemia-hypercitrullinuria s., s. de hiperornitinemia-hiperamonemia-hipercitrulinúria; raro distúrbio hereditário, caracterizado por comprometimento do transporte da ornitina nas mitocôndrias. VER TAMBÉM lysinuric protein *intolerance.*
hypersensitive xiphoid s., s. de hipersensibilidade do xifóide; hipersensibilidade anormal do xifóide à palpação, freqüentemente associada a dores espontâneas no tórax, parte superior do abdome e ombros.
hyperventilation s., s. de hiperventilação. VER chronic hyperventilation s.
hyperviscosity s., s. de hiperviscosidade; resultante do aumento da viscosidade do sangue; o aumento das proteínas séricas pode estar associado a hemorragia das mucosas, retinopatia e sintomas neurológicos; algumas vezes observada na macroglobulinemia de Waldenström e no mieloma múltiplo; um aumento da viscosidade secundário a policitemia pode estar associado à congestão de órgãos e diminuição da perfusão capilar.
hypometabolic s., s. hipometabólica; situação clínica que sugere hipotireoidismo ou mixedema, em que algumas provas de função tireóidea podem ser normais e a glândula não exibe atrofia ou doença evidente; indica falta de sensibilidade dos tecidos periféricos ao hormônio tireóideo.
hypoparathyroidism s., s. de hipoparatireoidismo; síndrome caracterizada por fadiga, fraqueza muscular, parestesia e cãibras dos membros, tetania e estridor laríngeo; deve-se à hipocalcemia decorrente da ausência de paratormônio (PTH); pode ser idiopática, pós-operatória ou causada por lesões orgânicas das paratireóides.
hypophysial s., s. hipofisária. SIN adiposogenital *dystrophy.*
hypophysiosphenoidal s., s. hipofisária-esfenoidal; invasão neoplásica da base do crânio na região do seio esfenoidal, freqüentemente com destruição do dorso da sela.
hypoplastic left heart s. [MIM*241550], s. do coração esquerdo hipoplásico; associação de subdesenvolvimento das câmaras cardíacas esquerdas com atresia ou estenose da valva aórtica e/ou mitral e hipoplasia da aorta ascendente.
iliotibial band s., s. da banda iliotibial; s. de dor no joelho, que pode resultar de inflamação devido à fricção mecânica da banda iliotibial e epicôndilo femoral lateral.
iliotibial band friction s., s. de fricção da banda iliotibial; condição dolorosa que afeta o quadril, a coxa ou o joelho; produzida pela irritação do trato iliotibial quando desliza sobre o trocanter maior, a espinha ilíaca ântero-superior, o tubérculo de Gerdy ou o côndilo femoral lateral; algumas vezes associada a uma sensação de estalo ou rangido.
Imerslünd-Grasbeck s., s. de Imerslünd-Grasbeck; má absorção de cobalamina pelos enterócitos.
immotile cilia s. [MIM*242650], s. dos cílios imóveis; distúrbio hereditário caracterizado por infecções sinopulmonares recorrentes, redução da fertilidade em mulheres e esterilidade em homens, devido à incapacidade das estruturas ciliadas de se movimentarem de maneira efetiva, em virtude da ausência de um ou de ambos os braços de dineína; herança autossômica recessiva. Cf. Kartagener s.
immunodeficiency s., s. de imunodeficiência; deficiência ou distúrbio imunológico, cujo principal sintoma consiste em aumento de suscetibilidade a infecções, dependendo o padrão de suscetibilidade do tipo de deficiência. VER TAMBÉM immunodeficiency.
impingement s., s. do impacto. SIN supraspinatus s.
s. of inappropriate secretion of antidiuretic hormone (SIADH), s. de secreção inapropriada do hormônio antidiurético (SIHAD); secreção contínua de hormônio antidiurético (HAD), apesar da baixa osmolalidade sérica e do volume extracelular expandido.
indifference to pain s., s. de indiferença à dor; insensibilidade congênita à dor, possivelmente devido a uma ausência de terminações nervosas organizadas na pele.
infertile male s., s. do homem infértil; distúrbio hereditário da proteína receptora de androgênios, resultando em atividade androgênica deficiente. VER TAMBÉM Reifenstein s.
inspissated bile s., s. da bile espessada; icterícia persistente em recém-nascidos com anemia hemolítica, com elevações da bilirrubina tanto direta quanto indireta.
internal capsule s., s. da cápsula interna; hemianopsia com hemianestesia contralateral da face.
inversed jaw-winking s., s. do piscar e da mandíbula invertida; quando ocorrem lesões supranucleares do nervo trigêmeo, o toque da córnea pode produzir um movimento brusco da mandíbula para o lado oposto.
iridocorneal endothelial s., s. endotelial iridocorneana; s. de glaucoma, atrofia da íris, diminuição do endotélio da córnea, sinéquias periféricas anteriores e múltiplos nódulos na íris. SIN Cogan-Reese s., iris-nevus s.
iridocorneal syndrome, s. iridocorneana. SIN Chandler s.
iris-nevus s., s. da íris-nevo. SIN iridocorneal endothelial s.
Irvine-Gass s., s. de Irvine-Gass; edema macular, afacia e humor vítreo aderente à incisão para extração de catarata.
Isaac s., s. de Isaac; distúrbio raro que resulta de atividade muscular espontânea anormal de origem neural, manifestado como rigidez muscular contínua e relaxamento tardio após exercício, freqüentemente acompanhado de dor, cãibras, fasciculações, hiperidrose e hipertrofia muscular (no EMG, manifesta-se como miocimia). Em geral, a síndrome de Isaac começa nos membros inferiores, mas pode afetar os músculos abdominais, dos membros superiores, vocais e respiratórios; com mais freqüência, a síndrome é esporádica, embora tenha sido relatada uma herança autossômica dominante. Trata-se, provavelmente, de uma doença auto-imune, com anticorpos dirigidos contra os canais de potássio dos nervos periféricos. SIN Isaac-Merton s.
Isaac-Merton s., s. de Isaac-Merton. SIN Isaac s.
Ivemark s. [MIM*208530], s. de Ivemark. SIN polysplenia.
Jadassohn-Lewandowski s., s. de Jadassohn-Lewandowski. SIN *pachyonychia congenita.*
Jahnke s., s. de Jahnke; s. de Sturge-Weber sem glaucoma.
jaw-winking s. [MIM*154600], s. da mandíbula-piscar; aumento da largura das fissuras palpebrais durante a mastigação, algumas vezes com elevação rítmica do lábio superior, quando a boca está aberta, e ptose, quando a boca está fechada. SIN Gunn phenomenon, Gunn s., jaw-winking phenomenon, jaw-working reflex, Marcus Gunn phenomenon, Marcus Gunn s.
Jeghers-Peutz s., s. de Jeghers-Peutz. SIN Peutz-Jeghers s.
Jervell and Lange-Nielsen s. [MIM*220440 e MIM*176261], s. de Jervell e Lange-Nielsen; prolongamento do intervalo QT registrado no eletrocardiograma de certas crianças congenitamente surdas vítimas de episódios de inconsciência em decorrência de convulsões de Adams-Stokes e fibrilação ventricular; herança autossômica recessiva causada por homozigosidade de uma mutação no gene dos canais de potássio (KVLQT1) no cromossoma 11 ou no gene dos canais de íons potássio mínimo (KCNE1) no cromossoma 21. SIN surdocardiac s.
Jeune s., s. de Jeune. SIN asphyxiating thoracic *dystrophy.*
Job s., s. de Job. SIN hyperimmunoglobulin E s. [*Job*, personagem bíblico]
Johanson-Blizzard s., s. de Johanson-Blizzard; s. clínica manifestada por insuficiência pancreática, defeitos do couro cabeludo, aplasia das asas do nariz, surdez, baixo peso ao nascer, microcefalia, retardo psicomotor, hipotireoidismo, nanismo e ausência de dentes permanentes.

Joubert s. [MIM*213300], s. de Joubert; agenesia do verme do cerebelo, caracterizada clinicamente por ataques de taquipnéia ou apnéia prolongada, movimentos oculares anormais, ataxia e retardo mental.

jugular foramen s., s. do forame jugular. SIN Avellis s.

Kallmann s., s. de Kallmann. SIN hypogonadism with anosmia.

Kanner s., s. de Kanner. SIN infantile autism,

Kartagener s. [MIM*244400], s. de Kartagener; situs inversus completo, associado a bronquiectasia, e sinusite crônica associada a dismotilidade ciliar e comprometimento do transporte de muco ciliar no epitélio respiratório; herança autossômica recessiva com penetrância variável. O mecanismo da reversão da lateralidade permanece obscuro, mas parece ser estritamente uma abolição (indiferença) de lateralidade, mais do que uma verdadeira reversão. VER TAMBÉM immotile cilia s. SIN Kartagener triad, Zivert s.

Kasabach-Merritt s., s. de Kasabach-Merritt; s. em que as plaquetas são aprisionadas; associada a púrpura trombocitopênica.

Kast s., s. de Kast. SIN Maffucci s.

Katayama s., s. de Katayama. SIN schistosomiasis japonica.

Kawasaki s., s. de Kawasaki. SIN Kawasaki disease.

Kearns-Sayre s. [MIM*165100], s. de Kearns-Sayre; forma de oftalmoplegia externa progressiva crônica com defeitos associados da condução cardíaca, estatura baixa e perda da audição; miopatia mitocondrial de ocorrência esporádica que se manifesta na infância.

Kennedy s., s. de Kennedy; atrofia óptica ipsolateral com escotoma central e estase papilar contralateral ou papiledema, causada por meningioma do nervo óptico ipsolateral. SIN Foster Kennedy s.

Kenny-Caffey s., s. de Kenny-Caffey; distúrbio caracterizado por hipocalcemia intermitente (associada a anormalidades da secreção de hormônio paratireóideo) e anormalidades ósseas e oculares; existem formas de herança autossômica dominante e autossômica recessiva.

Kimmelstiel-Wilson s., s. de Kimmelstiel-Wilson; s. nefrótica e hipertensão em diabéticos, associada a glomerulosclerose diabética. SIN Kimmelstiel-Wilson disease.

Kleine-Levin s. [MIM*148840], s. de Kleine-Levin; forma rara de hipersonia periódica, associada a bulimia, que ocorre em homens entre 10 e 25 anos de idade, caracterizada por períodos de apetite voraz alternando com sono prolongado (de até 18 horas), juntamente com distúrbios do comportamento, comprometimento dos processos mentais e alucinações; uma doença aguda ou a ocorrência de fadiga podem preceder um episódio, que pode ocorrer até várias vezes por ano.

Klinefelter s., s. de Klinefelter; anomalia cromossômica com 47 cromossomas e constituição XXY dos cromossomas sexuais; as células bucais e outras células geralmente são positivas para a cromatina sexual; os pacientes são do sexo masculino quanto ao desenvolvimento, mas apresentam disgenesia dos túbulos seminíferos, níveis plasmáticos e urinários elevados de gonadotropinas, ginecomastia variável e aspecto eunucóide; alguns pacientes são mosaicos cromossômicos, com duas ou mais linhagens celulares de diferente constituição cromossômica; o gato casco de tartaruga macho (gato calico) é um modelo animal. SIN XXY s.

Klippel-Feil s. [MIM*148900], s. de Klippel-Feil; defeito congênito que se manifesta na forma de pescoço curto, fusão das vértebras cervicais e anormalidades do tronco cerebral e do cerebelo; herança autossômica dominante, com a maioria dos casos esporádicos. SIN cervical fusion s.

Klippel-Trenaunay-Weber s. [MIM*149000], s. de Klippel-Trenaunay-Weber; anomalia dos membros em que existe uma combinação de angiomatose e desenvolvimento anômalo do osso e do músculo subjacentes, algumas vezes associada a gigantismo localizado; provavelmente de herança autossômica dominante, com a maioria dos casos esporádica. SIN angioosteohypertrophy s., congenital dysplastic angiectasia, hemangiectatic hypertrophy.

Klüver-Bucy s., s. de Klüver-Bucy; s. caracterizada por cegueira psíquica ou hiper-reatividade a estímulos visuais, aumento da atividade oral e sexual e depressão do impulso e das reações emocionais; descrita em macacos após ablação bitemporal do lobo temporal, porém raramente relatada em seres humanos.

Kniest s. [MIM*156550 e MIM*120140], s. de Kniest; condrodisplasia caracterizada por face plana e redonda, aumento e rigidez das articulações, contraturas articulares, escoliose, miopia com deslocamento da retina, perda palatina, surdez e achados radiográficos característicos de alargamento metafisário dos ossos longos, achatamento e fenda coronal das vértebras; herança autossômica dominante, causada por mutação no gene do colágeno tipo II (COL2A1) no cromossoma 12q.

Kobberling-Dunnigan s., s. de Kobberling-Dunnigan. SIN familial partial lipodystrophy.

Kocher-Debré-Sémélaigne s., s. de Kocher-Debré-Sémélaigne; cretinismo atireótico de herança autossômica recessiva, associado a pseudo-hipertrofia muscular. SIN Debré-Sémélaigne s.

Koenig s., s. de Koenig; episódios alternados de constipação e diarréia, com cólica; meteorismo e ruídos hidroaéreos na fossa ilíaca direita, considerados sintomáticos de tuberculose cecal.

Koerber-Salus-Elschnig s., s. de Koerber-Salus-Elschnig. SIN convergence-retraction nystagmus.

Kohlmeier-Degos s., s. de Kohlmeier-Degos; dustúrbio oclusivo vascular que acomete predominantemente as pequenas artérias da pele e do intestino, com sintomas do sistema nervoso central secundários a fibrose arterial e trombose em cerca de um quinto dos pacientes.

Korsakoff s., s. de Korsakoff; s. amnésica alcoólica caracterizada por confusão e grave comprometimento da memória, especialmente para eventos recentes, compensada pelo paciente por meio de confabulação; tipicamente observada em alcoólatras crônicos; a síndrome pode ser precedida de delirium tremens, e, com freqüência, verifica-se a coexistência da s. de Wernicke; a patogenia precisa é incerta, porém os efeitos tóxicos diretos do álcool provavelmente são menos importantes do que as deficiências nutricionais graves freqüentemente associadas ao alcoolismo crônico. SIN amnestic s. (1), dysmnesic s., Korsakoff psychosis.

Kostmann s., s. de Kostmann; agranulocitose infantil grave, um distúrbio hereditário da lactância caracterizado por graves infecções recorrentes e neutropenia.

Kuskokwim s., s. de Kuskokwim; contraturas articulares congênitas que se assemelham à artrogripose; encontrada em Inuits (esquimós) do delta do Rio Kuskokwim no Alasca.

Laband s. [MIM*135500 e 135300]; s. de Laband; fibromatose das gengivas associada a hipoplasia das falanges distais, displasia ungueal, hipermotilidade articular e, algumas vezes, hepatoesplenomegalia; herança autossômica dominante.

Lady Windemere's syndrome, s. de Lady Windemere; doença pulmonar micobacteriana não-tuberculosa numa mulher frágil e idosa, freqüentemente com peito escavado ou escoliose. [nome derivado do principal personagem na peça de Oscar Wilde, Lady Windemere's Fan]

LAMB s. [MIM*160980], s. LAMB; presença concomitante de lentigos, mixoma atrial, mixomas mucocutâneos e nevos azuis (lentigines, atrial myxoma, mucocutaneous myxomas, and blue nevi). VER TAMBÉM NAME s.

Lambert s., s. de Lambert. SIN Lambert-Eaton s.

Lambert-Eaton s. (LES), s. de Lambert-Eaton (SLE); distúrbio generalizado da transmissão neuromuscular, causado por um defeito na liberação de quanta de acetilcolina das terminações nervosas pré-sinápticas; freqüentemente associado ao carcinoma de pequenas células do pulmão, particularmente em homens idosos com longa história de tabagismo. Em contraste com a miastenia grave, a fraqueza tende a afetar apenas os músculos axiais, os músculos das cinturas e, com menos freqüência, os músculos dos membros; é comum a ocorrência de distúrbios autônomos, como, por exemplo, boca seca e impotência; os reflexos tendíneos profundos não podem ser evocados. Em estudos de condução motora, as respostas à estimulação inicial têm amplitude muito baixa, porém exibem acentuada facilitação pós-tetânica depois de alguns segundos de exercício. A s. de Lambert-Eaton é causada pela perda dos canais de cálcio sensíveis à voltagem localizados na terminação nervosa motora pré-sináptica. VER myasthenic s. SIN carcinomatous myopathy, Eaton-Lambert s., Lambert s., myasthenic s.

Landau-Kleffner s., s. de Landau-Kleffner; distúrbio infantil caracterizado por convulsões generalizadas e psicomotoras associadas a afasia adquirida; espículas multifocais e descargas em espículas e ondas no eletroencefalograma. SIN acquired epileptic aphasia.

Landry s., s. de Landry. SIN Guillain-Barré s.

Landry-Guillain-Barré s., s. de Landry-Guillain-Barré. SIN Guillain-Barré s.

Langer-Saldino s., s. de Langer-Saldino. SIN Type II achondrogenesis.

Larsen s., s. de Larsen; s. caracterizada por múltiplas luxações congênitas com anomalias ósseas, incluindo face achatada característica e fenda do palato mole.

Lasègue s., s. de Lasègue; na histeria de conversão, incapacidade de movimentar um membro anestesiado, exceto sob controle da visão.

late dumping s., s. do esvaziamento rápido tardio; s. observada em pacientes submetidos à ablação do mecanismo do esfíncter pilórico; associada a rubor, sudorese, tontura, fraqueza e colapso vasomotor dentro de 2–3 horas após uma refeição e causada por hipoglicemia em decorrência da rápida absorção de uma grande carga de carboidratos, que estimula a liberação de insulina. VER TAMBÉM dumping s.

lateral medullary s., s. medular lateral. SIN posterior inferior cerebellar artery s.

Launois-Bensaude s., s. de Launois-Bensaude. SIN multiple symmetric lipomatosis.

Launois-Cléret s., s. de Launois-Cléret. SIN adiposogenital dystrophy.

Laurence-Moon s. [MIM*245800], s. de Laurence-Moon; distúrbio caracterizado por retardo mental, retinopatia pigmentar, hipogenitalismo e paraplegia espástica; herança autossômica recessiva. Essa síndrome deve ser diferenciada da s. de Bardet-Biedl [MIM*209900]: no passado, as duas foram reunidas sob a designação de s. de Laurence-Moon-Bardet-Biedl.

Lawrence-Seip s., s. de Lawrence-Seip. SIN lipoatrophy.

Lejeune s., s. de Lejeune. SIN cri-du-chat s.

Lenègre s., s. de Lenègre, lesão isolada do sistema de condução cardíaca em consequência de lesão esclerodegenerativa; caracterizada habitualmente como

fibrose idiopática do nó atrioventricular, feixe de His ou ramo, com correspondente bloqueio de condução. SIN Lenègre disease.
Lennox s., s. de Lennox. SIN Lennox-Gastaut s.
Lennox-Gastaut s., s. de Lennox-Gastaut; epilepsia astática mioclônica generalizada em crianças, com retardo mental, em decorrência de várias afecções cerebrais, como hipoxia perinatal, hemorragia cerebral, encefalites, desenvolvimento defeituoso ou distúrbios metabólicos do cérebro; caracterizada por múltiplos tipos de convulsões (tônica generalizada, tônica, mioclônica, tônico-clônica e ausência atípica) e lentificação de base e padrão ponta-onda lento no EEG. SIN Lennox s.
LEOPARD s., s. LEOPARD; s. que consiste em lentigos (múltiplos), anormalidades eletrocardiográficas, hipertelorismo ocular, estenose pulmonar, anormalidades da genitália, retardo do crescimento e surdez (neurossensorial) (*l*entigines, *e*letrocardiographic abnormalities, *o*cular hypertelorism, *p*ulmonary stenosis, *a*bnormalities of genitalia, *r*etardation of growth, and *d*eafness). Herança autossômica dominante. SIN multiple lentigines s.
Leriche s., s. de Leriche; doença oclusiva aortoilíaca (aortoiliac occlusive *disease*), produzindo sinais e sintomas isquêmicos distais.
Leri-Weill s., s. de Leri-Weill. SIN dyschondrosteosis.
Lermoyez s., s. de Lermoyez; perda progressiva da audição e zumbido precedendo um episódio de vertigem, seguido de melhora da audição. Variante da doença de Ménière (Ménière *disease*).
Lesch-Nyhan s. [MIM*308000 several kinds], s. de Lesch-Nyhan; distúrbio do metabolismo da purina, devido à deficiência de hipoxantina-guanina fosforribosil transferase (HPRT); caracterizada por hiperuricemia, cálculos renais de ácido úrico, retardo mental, espasticidade, coreatetose e automutilação dos dedos das mãos e dos lábios por mordidas; herança ligada ao X, causada por mutação no gene HPRT no cromossoma Xq.
Lev s., s. de Lev; bloqueio de ramo num paciente com miocárdio normal e artérias coronárias normais, em decorrência de fibrose ou calcificação, incluindo o sistema de condução; afeta o septo membranoso, o ápice do septo muscular e, com freqüência, os anéis das valvas mitral e aórtica. SIN Lev disease.
Libman-Sacks s., s. de Libman-Sacks. SIN Libman-Sacks *endocarditis*.
Li-Fraumeni cancer s. [MIM*151623 e 191170], s. cancerosa de Li-Fraumeni; câncer de mama familiar em mulheres jovens, com sarcomas de tecidos moles em crianças, tumores cerebrais e outros cânceres em parentes próximos; herança autossômica dominante, causada por mutação no gene P53 no cromossoma 17p.
liver kidney s., s. do fígado-rim; acentuada perda das funções hepática e renal, observada em várias doenças, freqüentemente com evolução fatal. Observada particularmente na insuficiência hepática de estágio avançado, devido a cirrose ou hepatite, bem como em várias infecções virais.
locked-in s., s. de bloqueio; infarto da base da ponte, resultando em quadriplegia, oftalmoplegia horizontal, disfagia e diplegia facial com preservação da consciência; causada por oclusão da artéria basilar. SIN pseudocoma.
loculation s., s. de loculação. SIN Froin s.
Loeffler s. I, s. de Loeffler I; infiltrados pulmonares eosinofílicos, freqüentemente associados a migração parasitária; também associada a reações a alguns antibióticos, ao L-triptofano ou ao *crack*. SIN eosinophilic pneumonia.
Loeffler s. II, s. de Loeffler II; endocardite/miocardite eosinofílica.
Löffler s., s. de Löffler; **(1)** SIN simple pulmonary *eosinophilia*; **(2)** SIN Löffler *endocarditis*.
long QT s.'s, síndromes do QT longo; grupo de doenças congênitas e adquiridas em que o intervalo QT eletrocardiográfico é mais longo do que as medidas estabelecidas para a idade e sexo; os intervalos QT longos são um prenúncio de arritmias e morte súbita. VER TAMBÉM QT *interval*.
Lorain-Lévi s., s. de Lorain-Lévi. SIN pituitary *dwarfism*.
Louis-Bar s., s. de Louis-Bar; SIN ataxia telangiectasia.
Lowe s., s. de Lowe. SIN oculocerebrorenal s.
Lowe-Terrey-MacLachlan s., s. de Lowe-Terrey-MacLachlan. SIN oculocerebrorenal s.
Lown-Ganong-Levine s., s. de Lown-Ganong-Levine; s. eletrocardiográfica de um intervalo PR curto, com duração normal do complexo QRS; não possui a onda delta arrastada da síndrome de Wolff-Parkinson-White, porém assemelha-se a ela na sua associação freqüente (controvertida) à taquicardia paroxística, qualificando-a como síndrome; de outro modo, pode ocorrer um intervalo PR curto em indivíduos sem outros problemas de saúde.
low salt s., low sodium s., s. do sal reduzido, s. do sódio reduzido; s. resultante da restrição de sal e do uso de diuréticos no tratamento da insuficiência cardíaca congestiva e hipertensão, caracterizada por fraqueza, sonolência, cãibras musculares e redução da filtração glomerular, com conseqüente retenção de nitrogênio, insuficiência renal e, algumas vezes, morte; ocorre também na cirrose hepática com ascite e na insuficiência supra-renal. SIN salt depletion s.
lupus-like s., s. semelhante ao lúpus; s. clínica que se assemelha ao lúpus eritematoso sistêmico (systemic *lupus* erithematosus), porém devida a alguma outra causa.

Lutembacher s., s. de Lutembacher; anormalidade cardíaca congênita que consiste num defeito do septo interatrial, estenose mitral e aumento do átrio direito.
Lyell s., s. de Lyell. SIN toxic epidermal *necrolysis*.
lymphoproliferative s., s. linfoproliferativa. SIN Duncan *disease*.
Lynch s., s. de Lynch; câncer colorretal familiar do tipo I, que geralmente ocorre na juventude; câncer colorretal familiar tipo II que ocorre na juventude, juntamente com câncer genital feminino ou cânceres em outros locais proximais ao intestino.
Macleod s., s. de Macleod. SIN unilateral lobar *emphysema*.
Mad Hatter s., s. do Chapeleiro Louco; manifestações gastrointestinais e do sistema nervoso central da intoxicação crônica por mercúrio, incluindo estomatite, diarréia, ataxia, tremor, hiper-reflexia, comprometimento neurossensorial e instabilidade emocional; previamente observada em trabalhadores que confeccionavam chapéus de feltro e que colocavam na boca material contendo mercúrio para torná-los mais flexíveis. [do personagem de *Alice no País das Maravilhas*]
Maffucci s. [MIM*166000], s. de Maffucci; encondromas dos membros em associação a malformação venosa e linfático-venosa; tendência a desenvolver outros tumores benignos ou malignos. SIN dyschondroplasia with hemangiomas, Kast s.
Magendie-Hertwig s., s. de Magendi-Hertwig. SIN Magendic-Hertwig *sign*.
malabsorption s., s. de malabsorção; estado caracterizado por diversas manifestações, como diarréia, fraqueza, edema, cansaço, perda ponderal, apetite deficiente, abdome protuberante, palidez, tendências hemorrágicas, parestesias, cãibras musculares e esteatorréia; causada por qualquer uma de várias condições caracterizadas por absorção não-efetiva de nutrientes, como, por exemplo, espru, enteropatia induzida por glúten, gastroileostomia, tuberculose e determinadas fístulas.
malignant carcinoid s., s. carcinóide maligna. SIN carcinoid s.
malignant mole s. [MIM*155600], s. do nevo maligno; nevos de forma irregular, cor variável e distintamente melanocíticos, de 5-10 mm, que ocorrem em grande número (>100) primariamente no tronco e nos membros, com alto risco de neoplasia maligna; provavelmente herança autossômica dominante. VER TAMBÉM dysplastic *nevus*.
Mallory-Weiss s., s. de Mallory-Weiss; hemorragia gastrointestinal superior em decorrência de laceração da mucosa na junção gastroesofágica, geralmente induzida por ânsia de vômitos ou vômitos. SIN Mallory-Weiss lesion, Mallory-Weiss tear.
mandibulofacial dysostosis s., s. de disostose mandibulofacial. SIN mandibulofacial *dysostosis*.
mandibulo-oculofacial s., s. mandíbulo-oculofacial. SIN dyscephalia mandibulo-oculofacialis.
Marchiafava-Micheli s., s. de Marchiafava-Micheli. SIN paroxysmal nocturnal *hemoglobinuria*.
Marcus Gunn s., s. de Marcus-Gunn. SIN jaw-winking s.
Marfan s. [MIM*154700], s. de Marfan; distúrbio multissistêmico do tecido conjuntivo, caracterizado por alterações esqueléticas (aracnodactilia, membros longos, frouxidão articular, alterações do tórax), defeitos cardiovasculares (aneurisma da aorta, que pode dissecar, prolapso da valva mitral) e ectopia da lente; herança autossômica dominante causada por mutação no gene da fibrilina-1 (FBN1) no cromossoma 15q. SIN Marfan disease.
Marie-Robinson s., s. de Marie-Robinson; insônia e melancolia leve associadas a levulosúria alimentar.
Marine-Lenhart s., s. de Marine-Lenhart; bócio multinodular tóxico.
Marinesco-Garland s. [MIM*248800], s. de Marinesco-Garland; distúrbio neurológico raro, caracterizado por ataxia cerebelar, cataratas congênitas e retardo mental e do crescimento; herança autossômica recessiva. SIN cataractoligophrenia s., Marinesco-Sjögren s., Torsten Sjögren s.
Marinesco-Sjögren s., s. de Marinesco-Sjögren. SIN Marinesco-Garland s.
marker X s., s. do X marcador. SIN fragile X s.
Maroteaux-Lamy s. [MIM*253200], s. de Maroteaux-Lamy; erro do metabolismo dos mucopolissacarídeos, caracterizado por excreção urinária de sulfato de dermatan, retardo do crescimento, cifose lombar, protrusão do esterno, joelho valgo, geralmente hepatoesplenomegalia e ausência de retardo mental; o início é observado depois dos 2 anos de idade; herança autossômica recessiva, causada por mutação no gene da arilsulfatase B (ARSB) no cromossoma 5q. SIN arylsulfatase B deficiency, type VI mucopolysaccharidosis.
Marshall s. [MIM*154780], s. de Marshall; síndrome de hipoplasia da face média, catarata, perda da audição neurossensorial e hipoidrose. Há polêmica quanto ao fato de essa síndrome ser distinta da síndrome de Stickler.
Martin-Bell s., s. de Martin-Bell. SIN fragile X s.
Martorell s., s. de Martorell. SIN aortic arch s.
MASS s., s. MASS; s. muito semelhante à s. de Marfan e s. de Barlow. Entretanto, não ocorre luxação da lente, nem alterações aneurismáticas da aorta, e o prolapso da valva mitral não é de modo algum invariável. No momento, a síndrome não recebeu nenhum número MIM separado e compartilha o da s. de Barlow [MIM*157700] [prolapso da valva mitral, anomalias da aorta, altera-

ções esqueléticas e alterações cutâneas (*m*itral valve prolapse, *a*ortic anomalies, *s*keletal changes and *s*kin changes)]

massive bowel resection s., s. da ressecção maciça do intestino; malabsorção após substancial ressecção do intestino, sobretudo do intestino delgado, caracterizada por diarréia, esteatorréia, hipoproteinemia e desnutrição.

maternal deprivation s., s. de privação materna; falha do desenvolvimento observado em lactentes e crianças pequenas e manifestada como um conjunto de sinais físicos, sintomas e comportamentos, geralmente associada a perda, ausência ou negligência materna; caracterizada pela falta de responsividade ao ambiente e, com freqüência, por depressão.

Mauriac s., s. de Mauriac; nanismo com obesidade e hepatoesplenomegalia em crianças com diabetes melito inadequadamente controlado.

Mayer-Rokitansky-Küster-Hauser s., s. de Mayer-Rokitansky-Küster-Hauser; amenorréia primária devido à agenesia dos ductos de Müller, resultando em ausência da vagina ou presença de uma bolsa vaginal curta e ausência do útero, com cariótipo e ovários normais. SIN müllerian agenesis, Rokitansky-Küster-Hauser s.

May-White s., s. de May-White; epilepsia mioclônica progressiva com lipomas, surdez e ataxia; trata-se, provavelmente, de uma forma familiar de encefalomiopatia mitocondrial.

McArdle s., s. de McArdle. SIN type 5 *glycogenosis*.

McCune-Albright s., s. de McCune-Albright; displasia fibrosa poliostótica com placas castanhas irregulares de pigmentação cutânea e disfunção endócrina, especialmente puberdade precoce em meninas. VER TAMBÉM pseudohypoparathyroidism. SIN Albright disease, Albright s. (1).

Meadows s., s. de Meadows; miocardiopatia que se desenvolve durante a gravidez ou o puerpério.

Meckel s., s. de Meckel. SIN dysencephalia splanchnocystica.

Meckel-Gruber s., s. de Meckel-Gruber. SIN dysencephalia splanchnocystica.

meconium aspiration s., s. de aspiração do mecônio. SIN fetal aspiration s.

meconium blockage s., s. de bloqueio por mecônio; obstrução intestinal baixa em recém-nascidos, devido ao bloqueio do mecônio.

megacystic s., s. megacística; associação de bexiga grande, lisa e de paredes finas, refluxo vesicoureteral e ureteres dilatados.

megacystitis-megaureter s., s. de megacistite-megaureter; achados radiológicos de bexiga de grande capacidade e paredes finas e refluxo vesicoureteral maciço, sem obstrução ou neuropatia subjacente ou micção disfuncional.

megacystitis-microcolon-intestinal hypoperistalsis s., s. de megacistite-microcolo-hipoperistaltismo intestinal; condição rara caracterizada por distensão abdominal, frouxidão da musculatura abdominal, rotação intestinal incompleta e peristaltismo intestinal deficiente. A bexiga é grande e, com freqüência, há refluxo vesicoureteral. Afeta tipicamente recém-nascidas e costuma ser fatal no primeiro ano de vida.

Meigs s., s. de Meigs; fibromioma do ovário associado a hidroperitônio e hidrotórax.

Meischer s., s. de Meischer. SIN *cheilitis* granulomatosa.

Melkersson-Rosenthal s. [MIM*155900], s. de Melkersson-Rosenthal; queilite granulomatosa, fissura da língua e paralisia do nervo facial recorrente.

Melnick-Needles s., s. de Melnick-Needles. SIN osteodysplasty.

Ménétrier s., s. de Ménétrier. SIN Ménétrier *disease*.

Ménière s., s. de Ménière. SIN Ménière *disease*.

Menkes s., s. de Menkes. SIN kinky-hair *disease*.

menopausal s., s. da menopausa; sintomas recidivantes apresentados por algumas mulheres durante o período do climatério; incluem fogachos, calafrios, cefaléia, irritabilidade e depressão. SIN climacteric s.

Meretoja s., s. de Meretoja; forma familiar de amiloidose sistêmica com distrofia da córnea (corneal *dystrophy*), paralisia de nervos cranianos e nervos periféricos, protrusão dos lábios, fácies semelhante a uma máscara e orelhas frouxas.

metastatic carcinoid s., s. carcinóide metastática. SIN carcinoid s.

methionine malabsorption s., s. de má absorção de metionina; distúrbio hereditário caracterizado por incapacidade de absorção intestinal de L-metionina.

Meyenburg-Altherr-Uehlinger s., s. de Meyenburg-Altherr-Uehlinger. SIN relapsing *polychondritis*.

Meyer-Betz s., s. de Meyer-Betz. SIN myoglobinuria.

middle lobe s., s. do lobo médio; atelectasia com pneumonite crônica do lobo médio do pulmão (direito), devido à compressão do brônquio do lobo médio, geralmente por linfonodos aumentados, que podem ser tuberculosos; os principais sinais e sintomas consistem em tosse crônica, sibilos, infecções respiratórias recorrentes, hemoptise, dor torácica, mal-estar, fatigabilidade fácil e perda ponderal; algumas vezes confundida com acúmulo interlobar de líquido na incidência lateral. SIN Brock s.

Mikulicz s., s. de Mikulicz; os sintomas característicos da doença de Mikulicz que ocorrem como complicação de alguma outra doença, como linfoma, leucemia ou febre uveoparotídea.

milk-alkali s., s. leite-álcali; distúrbio crônico caracterizado pela deposição patológica de cálcio em muitos locais, especialmente nos rins, reversível nos estágios iniciais e induzido pela ingestão de grandes quantidades de cálcio e de álcali, antigamente utilizados no tratamento da úlcera péptica; pode evoluir para a insuficiência renal. SIN Burnett s.

Milkman s., s. de Milkman; osteomalacia com múltiplas pseudofraturas, habitualmente bilaterais e simétricas, podendo ocorrer fraturas patológicas verdadeiras.

Millard-Gubler s., s. de Millard-Gubler. SIN Gubler s.

minimal-change nephrotic s., s. nefrótica por lesão mínima; s. nefrótica com alterações glomerulares mínimas à microscopia óptica ou eletrônica, que ocorre mais freqüentemente em crianças, caracterizada por edema, albuminúria e aumento do colesterol no sangue, porém com função renal muito boa sob os demais aspectos; o epitélio tubular é vacuolado por gotículas de colesterol, porém os glomérulos exibem apenas fusão dos pedicelos das células epiteliais glomerulares, provavelmente em decorrência da proteinúria; desconhece-se a causa do aumento da permeabilidade glomerular às proteínas plasmáticas.

Mirizzi s., s. de Mirizzi; obstrução benigna dos ductos hepáticos, devido a espasmo e/ou fibrose do tecido conjuntivo circundante; freqüentemente associada a um cálculo no ducto cístico e colecistite crônica.

mitral valve prolapse s., s. de prolapso da valva mitral; o conjunto clínico de achados, com ou sem sintomas, devido ao prolapso da valva mitral: estalido sistólico que não é de ejeção acentuado na posição ortostática, algumas vezes múltiplo, outras vezes com ocorrência de regurgitação mitral numa fase relativamente tardia na sístole; acompanhada de evidências ecocardiográficas de prolapso da valva mitral, geralmente com espessamento dos folhetos da valva. Os sintomas são inespecíficos e podem incluir dor torácica vaga e dispnéia de esforço. SIN billowing mitral valve s.

Möbius s. [MIM*157900], s. de Möbius; paralisia facial bilateral que ocorre durante o desenvolvimento, habitualmente associada a distúrbios oculomotores ou outros distúrbios neurológicos. SIN congenital facial diplegia.

Mohr s., s. de Mohr; síndrome orofacial digital autossômica recessiva.

Monakow s., s. de Monakow; hemiplegia contralateral, hemianestesia e hemianopsia homônima, devido à oclusão da artéria corióidea anterior.

monofixation s., s. de monofixação; estrabismo de pequeno ângulo (menos de 10 dioptrias do prisma) com fixação central pelo olho preferido, supressão central do olho se desviando e fusão binocular da visão periférica.

Morgagni s. [MIM*144800], s. de Morgagni; hiperostose frontal interna em mulheres idosas, com obesidade e distúrbios neuropsiquiátricos de causa incerta; pelo menos algumas de causa familiar. SIN metabolic craniopathy, Stewart-Morel s.

Morgagni-Adams-Stokes s., s. de Morgagni-Adams-Stokes. SIN Adams-Stokes s.

morning glory s. [MIM*120330], s. da hipoméia; nervo óptico hipoplásico afunilado com um ponto de tecido branco em seu centro; circundado por anel elevado de pigmento coriorretiniano.

Morquio s. [MIM*253000, MIM*253010, MIM*230500], s. de Morquio; erro do metabolismo dos mucopolissacarídeos com excreção de sulfato de ceratan na urina; caracterizada por graves defeitos esqueléticos com estatura baixa, acentuada deformidade da coluna e do tórax, ossos longos com epífises irregulares, porém com diáfises de comprimento normal, articulações aumentadas, ligamentos fláccidos e marcha bamboleante; herança autossômica recessiva; a mucopolissacaridose tipo IVA deve-se à ausência de galactose-1-sulfatase e é causada por mutação no gene da *N*-acetilgalactosamina-6-sulfato sulfatase (GALNS) no cromossoma 16q, enquanto o tipo IVB deve-se à deficiência de β-galactosidase e é causada por mutação no gene da β-galactosidase (GLB1) no cromossoma 3p. SIN Brailsford-Morquio disease, Morquio disease, Morquio-Ullrich disease, type IVA, B mucopolysaccharidosis.

Morton s., s. de Morton; encurtamento congênito do primeiro metatarso, causando metatarsalgia.

Mounier-Kuhn s., s. de Mounier-Kuhn. SIN tracheobronchomegaly.

Muckle-Wells s. [MIM*191900], s. de Muckle-Wells; s. caracterizada por amiloidose, afetando notavelmente os rins, com perda progressiva da audição neurossensorial e períodos de urticária febril associados a dor nas articulações e músculos dos membros; herança autossômica dominante.

mucocutaneous lymph node s., s. do linfonodo mucocutâneo. SIN Kawasaki *disease*.

Muir-Torre s., s. de Muir-Torre. SIN Torre s.

multiple endocrine deficiency s., s. de deficiência endócrina múltipla; deficiência adquirida da função de várias glândulas endócrinas, geralmente de base auto-imune, como na s. de Schmidt (2). SIN multiple glandular deficiency s., polyendocrine deficiency s., polyglandular deficiency s.

multiple endocrine neoplasia s., type 1, s. de neoplasia endócrina múltipla, tipo 1; predisposição autossômica dominante a tumores das glândulas paratireóides, adeno-hipófise, pâncreas endócrino e, menos comumente, outros órgãos. SIN multiple endocrine neoplasia, type 1, Wermer s.

multiple endocrine neoplasia s., type 2A, s. de neoplasia endócrina múltipla, tipo 2A; predisposição autossômica dominante a tumores de células C da tireóide (carcinoma medular), medula supra-renal (feocromocitoma) e hiperplasia nodular das glândulas paratireóides. SIN multiple endocrine neoplasia, type 2A.

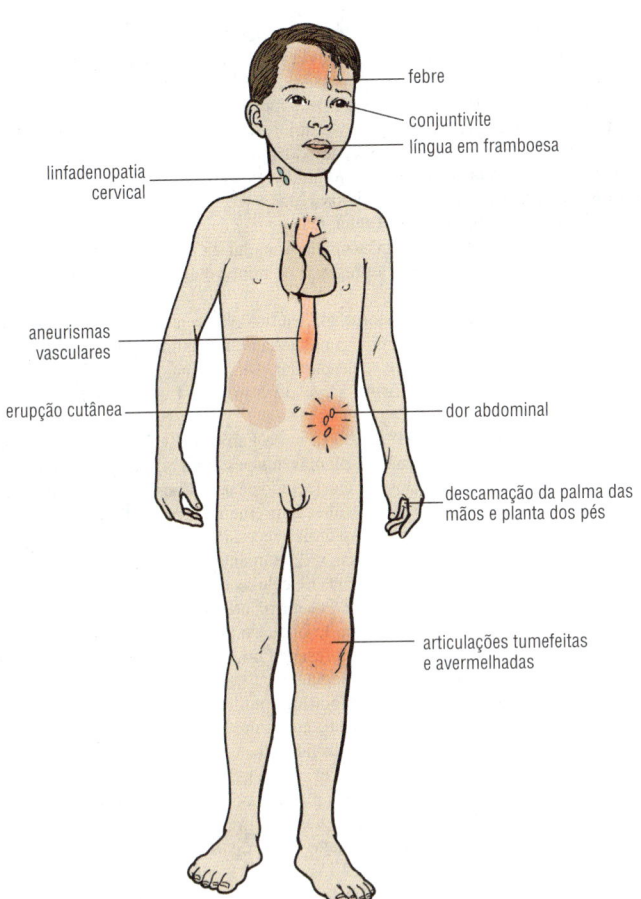

síndrome do linfonodo mucocutâneo (doença de Kawasaki): sinais e sintomas comuns

multiple endocrine neoplasia s., type 2B, s. de neoplasia endócrina múltipla, tipo 2B; predisposição autossômica dominante a tumores de células C da tireóide (carcinoma medular), medula supra-renal (feocromocitoma), nervos periféricos (neurinoma mucoso) e ganglioneuromatose intestinal; associada a um biotipo alto e magro.
multiple glandular deficiency s., s. de deficiência glandular múltipla. SIN multiple endocrine deficiency s.
multiple hamartoma s., s. de hamartomas múltiplos. SIN Cowden disease.
multiple lentigines s., s. de lentigos múltiplos. SIN LEOPARD s.
multiple mucosal neuroma s., s. de múltiplos neuromas da mucosa; neuromas ou neurofibromas submucosos múltiplos da língua, dos lábios e das pálpebras em pessoas jovens; algumas vezes associada a tumores da tireóide ou da medula supra-renal ou a neurofibromatose subcutânea.
Munchausen s., s. de Munchausen; maquinação repetida de simulações clinicamente convincentes de doença com o propósito de receber atenção médica; termo que se refere a pacientes que peregrinam de um hospital a outro fingindo ter uma doença clínica ou cirúrgica aguda e fornecendo informações falsas e irreais acerca de sua história clínica e social sem motivo aparente, a não ser o de receber atenção. VER factitious *disorder*.
Munchausen s. by proxy, s. de Munchausen por procuração; forma de maus-tratos ou abuso de criança por um responsável (geralmente a mãe), com maquinação de sintomas e/ou indução de sinais de doença, levando a investigações e intervenções desnecessárias, algumas vezes com graves conseqüências para a saúde, incluindo morte da criança. SIN factitious illness by proxy.
Münchhausen s., s. de Münchhausen. VER Munchausen s.
myasthenic s. (MS), s. miastênica (SM). SIN Lambert-Eaton s.
myelodysplastic s., s. mielodisplásica. SIN preleukemia.
myeloproliferative s.'s, síndromes mieloproliferativas; grupo de condições resultantes de um distúrbio na velocidade de formação das células na medula óssea, incluindo leucemia granulocítica crônica, eritremia, mielosclerose, panmielose e mielose eritrêmica e eritroleucemia.
myofascial s., s. miofascial; irritação dos músculos e da fáscia do dorso e do pescoço, causando dor aguda e crônica não associada a evidências neurológicas ou ósseas de doença; pressupõe-se que seja primariamente decorrente de alterações pouco compreendidas nos próprios músculos e fáscia.
myofascial pain-dysfunction s., s. de dor-disfunção miofascial; disfunção do aparelho mastigatório relacionada ao espasmo dos músculos da mastigação, precipitado por desarmonia oclusal ou alteração na dimensão vertical da mandíbula e exacerbada por estresse emocional; caracterizada por dor na região pré-auricular, hipersensibilidade dos músculos à palpação, estalido na articulação temporomandibular e limitação do movimento da mandíbula. SIN temporomandibular joint pain-dysfunction s.
Naegeli s. [MIM*161000], s. de Naegeli; pigmentação cutânea reticular, redução da sudorese, hipodontia, hiperceratose das palmas das mãos e plantas dos pés e formação de vesículas; pode ser confundida com a incontinência pigmentar (*incontinentia* pigmenti), porém afeta igualmente ambos os sexos; herança autossômica dominante. SIN Franceschetti-Jadassohn s.
Naffziger s., s. de Naffziger; síndrome scalenus-anticus.
nail-patella s. [MIM*161200], s. da unha-patela; distúrbio esquelético caracterizado por ausência ou hipoplasia da patela, cornos ilíacos, displasia das unhas dos dedos das mãos e dos pés e espessamento da lâmina densa glomerular; as extremidades inferiores do fêmur possuem uma forma muito semelhante à deformidade em frasco de Erlenmeyer; herança autossômica dominante, causada por mutação no gene que codifica a proteína de homeodomínio LIM (LMX1B) no cromossoma 9q.
NAME s., s. NAME; ocorrência concomitante de *n*evos, mixoma *a*trial, neurofibromas *m*ixóides e *e*félides.
Nance-Insley s., s. de Nance-Insley. SIN *chondrodystrophy* with sensorineural deafness.
Nelson s., s. de Nelson; s. de hiperpigmentação, lesão do terceiro nervo e aumento da sela turca; causada por adenomas hipofisários presumivelmente presentes antes da supra-renalectomia para tratamento da s. de Cushing, mas que aumentam e tornam-se posteriormente sintomáticos. SIN postadrenalectomy s.
nephritic s., s. nefrítica; os sinais e sintomas clínicos de glomerulonefrite aguda, particularmente hematúria, hipertensão e insuficiência renal.
nephrotic s., s. nefrótica; estado clínico caracterizado por edema, albuminúria, redução da albumina plasmática, corpúsculos duplamente refratários na urina e, em geral, aumento do colesterol sanguíneo; pode haver gotículas de lipídios nas células dos túbulos renais, porém a lesão básica consiste em aumento da permeabilidade das membranas basais capilares glomerulares, de causa desconhecida ou em decorrência de glomerulonefrite, glomerulosclerose diabética, lúpus eritematoso sistêmico, amiloidose, trombose da veia renal ou hipersensibilidade a vários agentes tóxicos. SIN nephrosis (3).
Netherton s. [MIM*256500], s. de Netherton; eritrodermia ictiosiforme congênita ou ictiose linear circunscrita associada a fios de cabelo em bambu, atopia, urticária, aminoacidúria intermitente e retardo mental; provavelmente um caráter autossômico recessivo que, muitas vezes, regride ou melhora na adolescência.
neural crest s., s. da crista neural; s. que consiste em perda da sensibilidade álgica, disfunção autônoma, anormalidades pupilares, anidrose neurogênica, instabilidade vasomotora, aplasia do esmalte dentário, espessamento das meninges, hiperflexão e certo grau de albinismo, pode refletir anormalidades da crista neural durante o desenvolvimento.
neurocutaneous s., s. neurocutânea; a ocorrência de nevos e, algumas vezes, de várias deformidades esqueléticas, com manifestações de gliose ou abiotrofia do sistema nervoso central.
neuroleptic malignant s., s. maligna neuroléptica; hipertermia com distúrbios extrapiramidais e autônomos, que podem levar à morte, após o uso de agentes neurolépticos.
Nezelof s., s. de Nezelof. SIN cellular *immunodeficiency* with abnormal immunoglobulin synthesis.
Noack s., s. de Noack. SIN Pfeiffer s.
nonsense s., s. do absurdo. SIN Ganser s.
Noonan s. [MIM*163950, MIM*163955], s. de Noonan; s. observada em ambos os sexos, com fenótipo lembrando o da s. de Turner; caracterizada por hipertelorismo, inclinação das fissuras palpebrais para baixo, pescoço alado, estatura baixa e cardiopatia congênita, especialmente estenose pulmonar; cariótipo cromossômico normal; herança autossômica dominante.
Nothnagel s., s. de Nothnagel; tontura, marcha bamboleante e em balanço, com formas irregulares de paralisia oculomotora e, com freqüência, nistagmo; observada em casos de tumor do mesencéfalo.
numb chin s., s. de parestesia mental; parestesia e perda sensorial afetando um lado do queixo e lábio inferior, em decorrência de infiltração neoplásica do nervo mentual ipsolateral; as causas comuns incluem mieloma múltiplo e carcinoma de mama ou de próstata.
nystagmus blockage s., s. de bloqueio do nistagmo; estrabismo com olhos e cabeça numa posição para minimizar o nistagmo associado.
OAV s., s. OAV. SIN oculoauriculovertebral *dysplasia*.
occipital horn s., s. do corno occipital; distúrbio recessivo ligado ao X em que ocorre excreção biliar deficiente de cobre, resultando em deficiência de lisil oxidase, que causa frouxidão cutânea e articular.

ocular-mucous membrane s., s. da membrana ocular-mucosa; síndrome de Stevens-Johnson com lesões oculares associadas (conjuntivite, pan-oftalmite, irite), lesões orais (bolhas, erosões, úlceras superficiais) e lesões genitais (uretrite, balanite circinada, bolhas).

oculobuccogenital s., s. oculobucogenital. SIN Behçet s.

oculocerebrorenal s. [MIM*309000], s. oculocerebrorrenal; s. congênita com hidroftalmia, cataratas, retardo mental, aminoacidúria, redução da produção de amônia pelo rim e raquitismo resistente à vitamina D; herança recessiva ligada ao X, causada por mutação no gene oculocerebrorrenal (OCRL) no cromossoma Xq. SIN Lowe s., Lowe-Terrey-MacLachlan s.

oculocutaneous s., s. oculocutânea. SIN Vogt-Koyanagi s.

oculomandibulofacial s., s. s. oculomandibulofacial. SIN *dyscephalia mandibulo-oculofacialis.*

oculopharyngeal s. [MIM*164300], s. oculofaríngea; distúrbio miopático com blefaroptose lentamente progressiva e disfagia, começando numa fase tardia da vida; herança autossômica dominante causada por mutação no gene que codifica a proteína de ligação de poli(A)-2 (PABP2) no cromossoma 14q.

oculovertebral s., s. oculovertebral. SIN oculovertebral *dysplasia.*

oculovestibulo-auditory s., s. oculovestibulo-auditiva; ceratite intersticial não-sifilítica, caracterizada por início abrupto, com vertigem e zumbido seguidos de comprometimento da audição; cerca de 50% dos pacientes apresentam doença sistêmica associada, mais comumente poliarterite nodosa. SIN Cogan s.

OFD s., s. OFD. SIN orofaciodigital s.

Ogilvie s., s. de Ogilvie; pseudo-obstrução, predominantemente do colo, parecendo resultar de distúrbio da motilidade; sem obstrução física.

Oldfield s., s. de Oldfield; polipose familiar do colo.

Olmsted s., s. de Olmsted; ceratodermia palmar, plantar e periorificial congênita, resultando em contraturas em flexão e amputação espontânea de dedos.

Omenn s. [MIM*603554], s. de Omenn; doença por imunodeficiência rapidamente fatal, caracterizada por eritrodermia, diarréia, infecções repetidas, hepatoesplenomegalia e leucocitose com eosinofilia; herança autossômica recessiva, causada por mutação no gene ativador de recombinação 1 (RAG1) ou no gene RAG2 adjacente no cromossoma 11p.

opiate intoxication s., s. de intoxicação por opiáceos; a tríade de miose com depressão da consciência e da freqüência respiratória; a s. recebe freqüentemente o nome do opiáceo específico responsável, p. ex., síndrome de intoxicação por heroína. SIN heroin overdoses.

Opitz BBB s., s. BBB de Opitz. SIN ocular *hypertelorism.*

Opitz G s., s. G de Opitz. SIN ocular *hypertelorism.*

Oppenheim s., s. de Oppenheim. SIN *amyotonia congenita.*

organic brain s. (OBS), s. cerebral orgânica (SOC); conjunto de sinais e sintomas de comportamento ou psicológicos, incluindo problemas relacionados com a atenção, concentração, memória, confusão, ansiedade e depressão, devido a disfunção transitória ou permanente do cérebro. SIN acute organic brain s.

organic mood s., s. de humor orgânica; síndrome atribuída a um fator orgânico, caracterizada por humor depressivo ou maníaco. VER bipolar *disorder.*

orofaciodigital s., s. orofaciodigital; s. hereditária, letal no sexo masculino, com combinações variáveis de defeitos da cavidade oral, da face das mãos, incluindo língua lobulada ou bífida, fenda ou pseudofenda palatina, tumores da língua, dentes ausentes ou mal posicionados, cartilagem hipoplásica da asa do nariz, depressão da ponte do nariz, braquidactilia, clinodactilia, sindactilia incompleta e, com freqüência, retardo mental; herança autossômica recessiva [MIM 252100 e MIM 258850] ou ligada ao X [MIM 311200]. SIN OFD s., orodigitofacial dysostosis, Papillon-Léage and Psaume s.

osteomyelofibrotic s., s. osteomielofibrótica. SIN *myelofibrosis.*

Ostrum-Furst s., s. de Ostrum-Furst; sinostose congênita do pescoço.

Othello s., s. de Othello; crença ilusória na infidelidade do cônjuge. [*Othello*, personagem de Shakespeare]

otomandibular s., s. otomandibular. SIN otomandibular *dysostosis.*

otopalatodigital s. [MIM*311300], s. oropalatodigital; comprometimento da audição de condução, fenda palatina, raiz do nariz larga e bossa frontal, grande espaçamento entre os dedos dos pés, polegar e hálux largos e, com freqüência, outros sinais de displasia óssea generalizada; herança recessiva ligada ao X.

ovarian vein s., s. da veia ovariana; condição caracterizada por dor abdominal intermitente, causada por compressão ureteral da veia ovariana direita, que ocorre mais freqüentemente do lado direito; acredita-se que seja devida ao cruzamento aberrante da veia ovariana direita sobre o ureter, geralmente ao nível da primeira vértebra sacral; presume-se que a dilatação da veia ovariana, durante a gravidez, e a ptose unilateral do rim sejam fatores contribuintes, resultando em obstrução ureteral intermitente e surtos recorrentes de dor e pielonefrite.

pacemaker s., s. do marca-passo; ocorrência de sintomas relacionados com a perda da sincronia atrioventricular em pacientes com marca-passo ventricular ou de sintomas causados por ritmo inadequado das contrações atriais e ventriculares em pacientes com marca-passo.

pachydermoperiostosis s., s. de paquidermoperiostose. VER pachydermoperiostosis.

Paget-von Schrötter s., s. de Paget-von Schrötter; trombose por estresse ou trombose espontânea da veia subclávia ou axilar; síndrome de desfiladeiro torácico. SIN effort-induced thrombosis.

painful arc s., s. do arco doloroso. SIN supraspinatus s.

painful-bruising s., s. da equimose dolorosa; reação inflamatória intensa a ligeiro extravasamento de sangue, devido a sensibilidade alérgica aos eritrócitos; observada mais comumente em mulheres adultas.

paleostriatal s., s. paleoestriatal. SIN Hunt s. (3).

pallidal s., s. do pálido. SIN Hunt s. (3).

Pancoast s., s. de Pancoast; plexopatia braquial da parte inferior do tronco e síndrome de Horner, devido à presença de tumor maligno na região do sulco pulmonar superior.

pancreatorenal s., s. pancreatorrenal; insuficiência renal aguda que ocorre em pacientes com pancreatite aguda grave; taxa de mortalidade elevada.

papillary muscle s., s. do músculo papilar. SIN papillary muscle *dysfunction.*

Papillon-Léage and Psaume s., s. de Papillon-Léage e Psaume. SIN orofaciodigital s.

Papillon-Lefèvre s. [MIM*245000], s. de Papillon-Lefèvre; hiperceratose congênita das palmas das mãos e plantas dos pés, com destruição progressiva do osso alveolar ao redor dos dentes decíduos e permanentes, que começa aos 2 anos de idade, e também com esfoliação prematura dos dentes e calcificação da foice do cérebro; herança autossômica recessiva.

paraneoplastic s., s. paraneoplásica; s. diretamente resultante de neoplasia maligna, mas não decorrente da presença de células tumorais nas partes afetadas.

Parenti-Fraccaro s., s. de Parenti-Fraccaro. SIN Type IB *achondrogenesis.*

Parinaud s., s. de Parinaud; paralisia do olhar conjugado para cima, com lesão ao nível dos colículos superiores; presença do fenômeno de Bell. SIN dorsal midbrain s., Parinaud ophthalmoplegia.

Parinaud oculoglandular s., s. oculoglandular de Parinaud; granuloma conjuntival unilateral com adenopatia pré-auricular na tularemia, no cancro, na tuberculose e na doença do miado-do-gato.

Parkes Weber s., s. de Parkes Weber; existência concomitante de múltiplas fístulas arteriovenosas congênitas ou malformações arteriovenosas com coloração capilar e anomalias linfaticovenosas num membro aumentado.

Parsonage-Turner s., s. de Parsonage-Turner. SIN neuralgic *amyotrophy.*

Patau s., s. de Patau. SIN trisomy 13 s.

patellofemoral s., s. patelofemoral; dor na parte anterior do joelho, devido a um distúrbio estrutural ou funcional na relação entre a patela e a parte distal do fêmur.

patellofemoral stress s., s. do estresse patelofemoral. SIN runner's *knee.*

Paterson-Brown-Kelly s., s. de Paterson-Brown-Kelly. SIN tendon sheath s.

Paterson-Kelly s., s. de Paterson-Kelly. SIN Plummer-Vinson s.

pathologic startle s.'s, síndromes de estremecimento patológico; grupo de distúrbios caracterizados por reflexo do estremecimento acentuadamente exagerado e outras respostas exageradas induzidas por estímulos. Inclui a hiperexplexia e, provavelmente, latah e a doença saltadora do Maine.

Pellizzi s., s. de Pellizzi. SIN *macrogenitosomia praecox.*

Pendred s. [MIM*274600], s. de Pendred; caracterizada por comprometimento auditivo neurossensorial congênito com bócio (geralmente pequeno), devido à ligação orgânica deficiente do iodo na tireóide; os indivíduos acometidos são habitualmente eutireóideos; herança autossômica recessiva, causada por mutação no gene da síndrome de Pendred (PDS), que codifica a pendrina no cromossoma 7q.

Pepper s., s. de Pepper; epônimo obsoleto para o neuroblastoma da glândula supra-renal com metástases no fígado; antigamente, acreditava-se que ocorria mais freqüentemente quando o tumor primário situava-se na supra-renal direita, enquanto os tumores da supra-renal esquerda tendiam a metastatizar para o crânio (síndrome de Hutchison).

pericolic membrane s., s. da membrana pericólica; complexo sintomático simulando a apendicite crônica, causado por constrição congênita das membranas pericólicas.

Perrault s., s. de Perrault; disgenesia gonadal XX associada a surdez neurossensorial.

Persian Gulf s., s. do Golfo Pérsico. SIN Gulf War s.

persistent müllerian duct s., s. do ducto de Müller persistente; distúrbio familiar com presença de tuba uterina, útero e testículo num indivíduo do sexo masculino. Deficiência da substância inibitória de Müller secundária a um defeito das células de Sertoli. SIN hernia uteri inguinale.

pertussis s., s. da coqueluche. SIN pertussis.

pertussis-like s., s. coqueluche-símile; s. caracterizada por episódios intensos de tosse, semelhantes à coqueluche (whooping *cough*).

petrosphenoidal s., s. petroesfenoidal; infiltração neoplásica do ápice do osso petroso e da parte anterior do forame lacerado.

Peutz s., s. de Peutz. SIN Peutz-Jeghers s.

Peutz-Jeghers s. [MIM*175200], s. de Peutz-Jeghers; polipose múltipla hamartomatosa generalizada do trato intestinal, acometendo consistentemente o jejuno, associada a pontos de melanina nos lábios, na mucosa bucal e nos dedos da mão; herança autossômica dominante, causada por mutação no gene da serina/treonina cinase (STK11) no cromossoma 19p. SIN Jeghers-Peutz s., Peutz s.

Pfaundler-Hurler s., s. de Pfaundler-Hurler. SIN Hurler s.

Pfeiffer s. [MIM*101600], s. de Pfeiffer; distúrbio caracterizado por polegares e háluces largos e curtos, freqüentemente com duplicação dos háluces e sindactilia variável dos dedos; a craniossinostose é uma característica variável. Herança autossômica dominante, causada por mutação no gene do receptor do fator de crescimento dos fibroblastos 1 (FGFR1) no cromossoma 8p ou no gene FGFR2 no cromossoma 10q. SIN Noack s., type V acrocephalosyndactyly.

pharyngeal pouch s., s. da bolsa faríngea. SIN DiGeorge s.

phospholipid s., s. dos fosfolipídios; combinação de anticorpos antifosfolipídios e eventos oclusivos arteriais ou venosos, como trombose.

Picchini s., s. de Picchini; forma de polisserosite afetando as três grandes serosas em contato com o diafragma, algumas vezes também as meninges, a túnica vaginal do testículo, as bainhas sinoviais e bolsas, causada pela presença de um tripanossoma.

Pick s., s. de Pick. SIN Pick *disease*.

pickwickian s., s. de Pickwick; combinação de obesidade acentuada e grotesca, sonolência e debilidade geral, teoricamente resultante de hipoventilação induzida pela obesidade; pode resultar em hipercapnia, hipertensão pulmonar e *cor pulmonale*. [nome do "menino gordo" na história de Dickens, *Pickwick Papers*]

Pierre Robin s. [MIM*261800], s. de Pierre Robin; micrognatia e fenda palatina em forma de U, glossoptose, freqüentemente associada a obstrução das vias aéreas superiores e dificuldades na alimentação; evidências fracas de herança autossômica recessiva. SIN Robin s.

pigment dispersion s., s. de dispersão do pigmento; resistência aumentada ao fluxo de humor aquoso através da pupila da câmara anterior para a câmara posterior, resultando em arqueamento posterior da íris periférica contra as zônulas; um possível mecanismo no glaucoma pigmentar.

Pins s., s. de Pins; macicez, diminuição do frêmito toracovocal e do murmúrio vesicular e discreto sopro cardíaco, auscultado na região póstero-inferior do tórax, no lado esquerdo, em casos de derrame pericárdico; algumas vezes, há também estertores finos nessa região, porém todos os sinais auscultatórios adventícios desaparecem quando o paciente assume a posição genopeitoral.

placental dysfunction s., s. de disfunção placentária; desnutrição e hipoxia fetais em decorrência do comprometimento da transferência de oxigênio e de vários nutrientes da mãe para o feto.

placental transfusion s., s. de transfusão placentária; transfusão de sangue *in utero* de um gêmeo para outro, de modo que o doador torna-se anêmico e com retardo do crescimento, enquanto o receptor torna-se policitêmico e desenvolve hidropisia. VER TAMBÉM twin-twin *transfusion*.

Plummer-Vinson s., s. de Plummer-Vinson; anemia ferropriva, disfagia, estenose esofágica e glossite atrófica. SIN Paterson-Kelly s., sideropenic dysphagia.

POEMS s., s. POEMS; condição caracterizada por *p*olineuropatia, *o*rganomegalia, *e*ndocrinopatia, gamopatia *m*onoclonal e alterações cutâneas (*s*kin).

Poland s., s. de Poland; anomalia que consiste na ausência dos músculos peitoral maior e peitoral menor, hipoplasia mamária ipsolateral e ausência de dois a quatro segmentos de costelas.

polycystic ovary s. [MIM*184700], s. do ovário policístico; condição comumente caracterizada por hirsutismo, obesidade, anormalidades menstruais, infertilidade e aumento dos ovários; acredita-se que reflete a secreção excessiva de androgênio de origem ovariana. SIN sclerocystic disease of the ovary, Stein-Leventhal s.

polyendocrine deficiency s., polyglandular deficiency s., s. de deficiência poliendócrina, s. de deficiência poliglandular. SIN multiple endocrine deficiency s.

polysplenia s., s. de polisplenia. SIN bilateral *left-sidedness*.

popliteal entrapment s., s. de compressão poplítea; s. de esmagamento resultante de compressão da artéria poplítea e comprometimento de seu fluxo sanguíneo por estruturas do espaço poplíteo.

postadrenalectomy s., s. pós-adrenalectomia. SIN Nelson s.

postcardiotomy s., s. pós-cardiotomia. SIN postpericardiotomy s.

postcholecystectomy s., s. pós-colecistectomia; recidiva ou persistência de sinais e sintomas que levaram à remoção da vesícula biliar, porém após colecistectomia.

postcommissurotomy s., s. pós-comissurotomia. SIN postpericardiotomy s.

postconcussion s., s. pós-concussão. SIN posttraumatic s.

posterior inferior cerebellar artery s., s. da artéria cerebelar póstero-inferior; s. habitualmente causada por trombose, caracterizada por disartria, disfagia, marcha bamboleante e vertigem e marcada por hipotonia, incoordenação do movimento voluntário, nistagmo, s. de Horner ipsolateral e perda da sensibilidade álgica e térmica do lado do corpo oposto à lesão. SIN lateral medullary s., Wallenberg s.

posterior leukoencephalopathy s., s. de leucoencefalopatia posterior; s. clínico-radiológica reversível, caracterizada por confusão, cefaléia, convulsões, cegueira cortical e outras anormalidades visuais, vômitos e sinais motores, associada a evidências, na RMN ou na TC, de edema bilateral da substância branca afetando as regiões cerebrais parietooccipitais.

postgastrectomy s., s. pós-gastrectomia. SIN dumping s.

post-lumbar puncture s., s. pós-punção lombar. SIN spinal *headache*.

postmalaria neurologic s., s. neurológica pós-malária; distúrbio autolimitado do sistema nervoso central que se desenvolve pouco depois da recuperação de um episódio grave de malária por *P. falciparum*, caracterizado principalmente por estado agudo de confusão ou psicose, convulsões generalizadas ou ambas, de 1–10 dias de duração e associado a esfregaços sanguíneos negativos para o parasita da malária; s. ligada à terapia prévia com mefloquina.

postmaturity s., s. pós-maturidade; gestação que se estende por 43 semanas ou mais; algumas vezes associada a imaturidade fetal.

postmyocardial infarction s. (PMIS), s. pós-infarto do miocárdio (SPIM); complicação que surge vários dias a várias semanas após infarto do miocárdio; as manifestações clínicas consistem em febre, leucocitose, dor torácica e sinais de pericardite, algumas vezes com pleurite e pneumonite, com forte tendência a recidiva; provavelmente de origem imunopatogênica.

postpartum pituitary necrosis s., s. de necrose hipofisária pós-parto. SIN Sheehan s.

postpericardiotomy s., s. pós-pericardiotomia; pericardite, com ou sem febre e freqüentemente em episódios repetidos, dentro de semanas a meses após cirurgia cardíaca. SIN postcardiotomy s., postcommissurotomy s.

postphlebitic s., s. pós-flebítica; estado caracterizado por edema, dor, dermatite de estase, celulite e veias varicosas e, nos estágios tardios, associado a ulceração da perna, mais freqüentemente como seqüela de trombose venosa profunda do membro inferior.

postrubella s., s. pós-rubéola; grupo de defeitos congênitos resultantes de rubéola materna durante o primeiro trimestre de gravidez, incluindo microftalmia, cataratas, surdez, retardo mental, persistência do canal arterial e estenose da artéria pulmonar.

postthrombotic s., s. pós-trombótica; s. que ocorre após trombose vascular. Termo habitualmente utilizado para indicar dificuldades, como edema persistente, após trombose venosa.

posttraumatic s., s. pós-traumática; distúrbio clínico que, freqüentemente, ocorre após lesão craniana, caracterizado por cefaléia, tontura, neurastenia, hipersensibilidade a estímulos e diminuição da concentração.

posttraumatic neck s., s. pós-traumática do pescoço; complexo clínico de dor, hipersensibilidade à palpação, rigidez da musculatura cervical, instabilidade vasomotora e sintomas mal definidos, como tontura e borramento visual, em conseqüência de traumatismo do pescoço. Também denominada neuralgia ou neurite occipital ou suboccipital; síndrome de tensão cervical, mioespasmo cervical, miosite ou fibrosite. SIN cervical fibrositis, cervical tension s.

posttraumatic stress s., s. de estresse pós-traumático; distúrbio que aparece após um evento física ou psicologicamente traumático fora do âmbito da experiência humana habitual (p. ex., séria ameaça à própria vida ou presenciar a morte de um ente amado), caracterizado por sintomas de nova experiência do evento, embotamento da responsividade ao ambiente, resposta de alarme exagerada, sentimentos de culpa, comprometimento da memória e dificuldades na concentração e no sono.

Potter s., s. de Potter; agenesia renal com hipoplasia pulmonar e angústia respiratória neonatal associada, instabilidade hemodinâmica, acidose, cianose, edema e fáceis característica (de Potter); a morte geralmente ocorre por insuficiência respiratória, que se desenvolve antes da uremia.

Prader-Willi s. [MIM*176270], s. de Prader-Willi; s. congênita caracterizada por estatura baixa, retardo mental, polifagia com acentuada obesidade e infantilismo sexual; a hipotonia muscular acentuada e a responsividade precária a estímulos externos diminuem com a idade; é possível demonstrar uma pequena deleção no cromossoma 15q11-13 de origem paterna em muitos casos; alguns casos são devidos a dissomia materna (isto é, ambos os cromossomas 15 provêm da mãe).

precordial catch s., s. de dificuldade pré-cordial; s. benigna de origem incerta, caracterizada por dor súbita e aguda na região do ápice cardíaco à inspiração, porém habitualmente aliviada ao efetuar uma respiração mais profunda; não há hipersensibilidade à palpação.

preexcitation s., s. de pré-excitação. SIN Wolff-Parkinson-White s.

preinfarction s., s. pré-infarto; desenvolvimento abrupto de angina de peito ou agravamento da angina existente em decorrência de aumento de sua freqüência ou intensidade; algumas vezes, prenúncio de infarto do miocárdio.

premature senility s., s. de senilidade prematura. SIN progeria.

premenstrual s. (PMS), s. pré-menstrual (SPM); em mulheres de idade fértil, conjunto de sinais e sintomas emocionais, comportamentais e físicos que surgem na fase lútea (pré-menstrual) do ciclo menstrual e desaparecem com o início da menstruação; caracterizada por edema e ganho ponderal, devido à retenção de líquido, hipersensibilidade das mamas, irritabilidade, flutuação do humor, ansiedade, depressão, sonolência, fadiga, dificuldade de concentração e alterações no apetite e na libido. SIN late luteal phase dysphoria, late luteal phase dysphoric disorder, menstrual molimina, premenstrual tension s., premenstrual tension.

Cerca de 80% das mulheres entre 25–40 anos de idade que menstruam apresentam alguns sintomas de SPM em pelo menos alguns ciclos menstruais, enquanto cerca de 5% exibem sintomas intensos e incapacitantes. Não foi identificada nenhuma causa biológica específica. Anormalidades relatadas no metabolismo da serotonina levaram à hipótese de que, em mulheres com SPM, as flutuações hormonais normais do ciclo menstrual interagem com uma desregulação do neurotransmissor, desencadeando sintomas de mau humor e ansiedade. Nenhuma terapia farmacológica foi aprovada pela FDA para o tratamento da SPM. Entretanto, os anticoncepcionais e os antidepressivos serotoninérgicos são amplamente utilizados para essa indicação. A redução da cafeína e da ingestão de sal pode diminuir o mal-estar e a depressão associados, e a prática regular de exercício e uma dieta rica em carboidratos complexos podem ajudar a minimizar a gravidade dos episódios. Em um grande estudo, o consumo diário de 1,2 g de cálcio em suplemento mastigável reduziu os sintomas em maior grau do que no grupo placebo. Após a sua inclusão na edição de 1987 do *Diagnostic and Statistical Manual of Mental Disorders (DSM-III)*, a SPM tornou-se objeto de polêmica entre feministas, que questionaram a sua qualificação como verdadeiro distúrbio. A SPM foi utilizada como defesa aceita num julgamento de homicídio no Reino Unido.

premenstrual salivary s., s. salivar pré-menstrual; anormalidades glandulares que ocorrem antes do início da menstruação, incluindo edema dos tecidos mamários e aumento das glândulas salivares.
premenstrual tension s., s. de tensão pré-menstrual. SIN premenstrual s.
premotor s., s. pré-motora; hemiplegia com espasticidade, reflexo de Rossolimo, porém sem sinal de Babinski, juntamente com apreensão forçada e distúrbios vasomotores.
pronator teres s., s. do pronador quadrado; compressão do nervo mediano na parte proximal do antebraço, geralmente onde o nervo passa entre as duas cabeças do músculo pronador quadrado.
Proteus s., s. de Proteus; distúrbio esporádico de possível origem genética, de fenótipo variável; caracterizado por aumento grosseiro das mãos e dos pés, crescimento anormal deformado e gigantismo da cabeça; freqüentemente confundido com neurofibromatose tipo I. SIN elephant man's disease (1).
prune belly s., s. de deficiência dos músculos abdominais; síndrome de deficiência da musculatura abdominal, testículos não descidos, bexiga hipotônica grande e ureteres dilatados e sinuosos. SIN Eagle-Barrett s.
pseudoexfoliation s., s. pseudo-esfoliação; condição freqüentemente levando ao glaucoma, em que depósitos na superfície da lente assemelham-se à esfoliação da cápsula da lente. VER TAMBÉM *pseudoexfoliation* of lens capsule. SIN exfoliation s.
psychogenic nocturnal polydipsia s., PNP s., s. de polidipsia noturna psicogênica, s. de PNP; ingestão excessiva de água emocionalmente induzida à noite.
pterygium s. [MIM*178110, MIM*265000, MIM*312150], s. de pterígio; pescoço alado, fossas antecubitais e fossas poplíteas com deformidades em flexão dos membros e anomalias das vértebras; já foram descritos casos de herança autossômica dominante, autossômica recessiva e recessiva ligada ao X.
pulmonary dysmaturity s., s. de imaturidade pulmonar; distúrbio respiratório que ocorre em prematuros pequenos, incapazes de ventilação pulmonar normal e que, freqüentemente, morrem de hipoxia depois de uma doença de 6–8 semanas; os pulmões contêm bolhas enfisematosas focais disseminadas, e o parênquima possui paredes alveolares espessadas; diagnosticada baseando-se principalmente na história clínica, nos achados da radiografia de tórax e achados à necropsia, que devem incluir a ausência de alterações histopatológicas características de outros distúrbios pulmonares comumente encontrados nessa faixa etária. SIN Wilson-Mikity s.
punchdrunk s., s. de encefalopatia dos boxeadores; condição observada em boxeadores, quase sempre vários anos após abandono dos ringues e presumivelmente causada por lesão cerebral repetida; caracterizada por fraqueza dos membros inferiores, instabilidade da marcha, lentidão dos movimentos musculares, tremores das mãos, disartria e raciocínio lento.
Putnam-Dana s., s. de Putnam-Dana. SIN subacute combined *degeneration* of the spinal cord.
radial aplasia-thrombocytopenia s., s. de aplasia radial-trombocitopenia; síndrome de trombocitopenia e ausência dos rádios.
radial tunnel s., s. do túnel radial; dor na face lateral do cotovelo e antebraço, sem qualquer déficit motor ou sensorial, em decorrência da compressão do nervo radial em qualquer dos vários locais ao longo de seu trajeto, quando passa pelo cotovelo e parte proximal do antebraço.
radicular s., s. radicular; grupo de sintomas decorrentes de qualquer interferência na porção intradural de uma ou mais raízes dos nervos espinais; os principais sinais e sintomas consistem em dor, parestesia, hipoestesia ou hiperestesia, distúrbios motores, tróficos e reflexos.

Raeder paratrigeminal s., s. paratrigeminal de Raeder; síndrome de Horner pós-ganglionar associada a disfunção do nervo trigêmeo causada por comprometimento do plexo simpático carótido, próximo do cavo de Mechel.
Ramsay Hunt s., s. de Ramsay Hunt; (1) SIN Hunt s; (2) SIN *herpes* zoster oticus.
Rasmussen s., s. de Rasmussen. SIN rasmussen *encephalitis.*
Raynaud s., s. de Raynaud; cianose bilateral paroxística idiopática dos dedos, devido à contração arterial e arteriolar; causada pelo frio ou por emoção. VER TAMBÉM Raynaud *phenomenon*. SIN Raynaud disease, symmetric asphyxia.
Refetoff s., s. de Refetoff; condição caracterizada por bócio e níveis séricos elevados de hormônios tireóideos, sem manifestações de tireotoxicose, devido à falta de responsividade do órgão-alvo aos hormônios tireóideos.
Refsum s., s. de Refsum. SIN Refsum *disease.*
Reifenstein s. [MIM*312300 e MIM*313700], s. de Reifenstein; sensibilidade androgênica parcial; forma familiar de pseudo-hermafroditismo masculino, caracterizada por graus variáveis de genitália ambígua ou hipospadias, desenvolvimento pós-puberal de ginecomastia e infertilidade associada à esclerose dos túbulos seminíferos; pode haver criptorquidismo, e a hipofunção das células de Leydig pode levar à impotência em anos posteriores; os estudos cromossômicos revelam um cariótipo 46,XY; herança recessiva ligada ao X, causada por mutação no gene do receptor de androgênio (AR) no cromossoma Xq.
Reiter s., s. de Reiter; associação de uretrite, iridociclite, lesões mucocutâneas e artrite, algumas vezes com diarréia; uma ou mais dessas condições podem sofrer recidiva a intervalos de meses ou anos, enquanto a artrite pode ser persistente. SIN Fiessinger-Leroy-Reiter s., Reiter disease.
REM s., s. REM; dermatite eritematosa reticular da parte superior do tronco, mais comum em mulheres, caracterizada por infiltrado perivascular de linfócitos, pequeno número de plasmócitos e depósitos de mucina na derme superior; sofre agravamento com exposição à luz ultravioleta. SIN reticular erytematous mucinosis.
Rendu-Osler-Weber s., s. Rendu-Osler-Weber. SIN hereditary hemorrhagic *telangiectasia.*
Renpenning s. [MIM*309500], s. de Renpenning; retardo mental ligado ao X com estatura baixa e microcefalia, não associado ao cromossoma X frágil; ocorre mais freqüentemente no sexo feminino, embora algumas mulheres também possam ser afetadas.
residual ovary s., s. do ovário residual; desenvolvimento de massa pélvica, dor pélvica e, em certas ocasiões, dispareunia após histerectomia sem remoção de ambos os ovários.
resistant ovary s. [MIM*176440], s. do ovário resistente; amenorréia associada a hipergonadotropismo e, em geral, folículos ovarianos normais; pode ser de herança autossômica dominante.
respiratory distress s. of the newborn, s. de angústia respiratória do recém-nascido. SIN hyaline membrane *disease* of the newborn.
respiratory distress s. type II, s. de angústia respiratória tipo II. SIN transient *tachypnea* of the newborn.
restless legs s., s. das pernas inquietas; sensação de indescritível desconforto, contrações ou inquietação nas pernas após o indivíduo deitar-se, levando freqüentemente à insônia e podendo ser aliviada temporariamente pelo ato de caminhar; acredita-se que seja causada por circulação inadequada ou como efeito colateral de medicação antipsicótica. VER TAMBÉM akathisia. SIN Ekbom s., restless legs.
retraction s., s. de retração do globo e pseudoptose ao efetuar uma adução; devida à co-inervação dos retos horizontais. Algumas vezes existe uma incapacidade de abduzir o olho afetado (tipo 1) ou aduzir o olho afetado (tipo 2) ou ambas as condições (tipo 3). SIN Duane s.
Rett s. [MIM*312750], s. de Rett; (1) distúrbio de desenvolvimento difuso, caracterizado pelo desenvolvimento de vários déficits específicos após um período pré-natal e perinatal aparentemente normal, incluindo desaceleração do crescimento da cabeça, perda das habilidades manuais com deterioração dos movimentos manuais estereotípicos, comprometimento da linguagem expressiva e receptiva e retardo psicomotor significativo; (2) diagnóstico do DSM estabelecido quando são preenchidos critérios específicos.
Reye s., s. de Reye; encefalopatia adquirida de crianças de pouca idade após uma doença febril aguda, geralmente influenza ou varicela; caracterizada por vômitos recorrentes, agitação e letargia, que podem levar ao coma, com hipertensão intracraniana; elevação da amônia e das transaminases séricas; a morte pode resultar de edema cerebral e conseqüente herniação cerebral.
Rh null s. [MIM*268150], s. do Rh nulo; condição caracterizada por ausência de todos os antígenos Rh, anemia hemolítica compensada e estomatocitose; herança autossômica recessiva, causada por mutação no gene do polipeptídeo associado a Rhesus de 50-kD (RH50A) no cromossoma 6p.
Richards-Rundle s. [MIM*245100], s. de Richards-Rundle; distúrbio neurológico que começa no início da infância, com perda auditiva neurossensorial progressiva e grave, ataxia, nistagmo por debilitação muscular, ausência dos reflexos tendíneos profundos, retardo mental, falha no desenvolvimento das características sexuais secundárias e cetoacidúria; herança autossômica recessiva.

Richter s., s. de Richter; linfoma de alto grau, que se desenvolve durante a evolução da leucemia linfocítica crônica; associada a caquexia, pirexia, disproteinemia e linfomas com células tumorais multinucleadas.

Rieger s. [MIM*180500], s. de Rieger; disgenesia mesenquimatosa iridocorneana, combinada com hipodontia ou anodontia e hipoplasia maxilar; herança autossômica dominante; ocorrem atraso do desenvolvimento sexual e hipotireoidismo.

Riley-Day s., s. de Riley-Day. SIN familial *dysautonomia.*

Roaf s., s. de Roaf; distúrbio craniofacial-esquelético não-hereditário, caracterizado por descolamento da retina congênito ou precoce, cataratas, miopia, encurtamento dos ossos longos e retardo mental; a perda auditiva neurossensorial progressiva tem início mais tardio.

Roberts s. [MIM*268300], s. de Roberts; focomelia ou graus menores de hipomelia, microbraquicefalia, defeito mesofacial, deficiência de crescimento pré-natal e criptorquidismo; associada a anormalidades centroméricas dos cromossomas; herança autossômica recessiva.

Robin s., s. de Robin. SIN Pierre Robin s.

Robinow s. [MIM*180700], s. de Robinow; displasia esquelética caracterizada por protrusão da fronte, hipertelorismo, depressão da ponte do nariz (algumas vezes denominada face fetal), boca larga, encurtamento acromesomélico dos membros, hemivértebras e hipoplasia da genitália; existe também uma forma autossômica recessiva [MIM*268310]. VER TAMBÉM fetal face s. SIN Robinow dwarfism.

Rokitansky-Küster-Hauser s., s. de Rokitansky-Küster-Hauser. SIN Mayer-Rokitansky-Küster-Hauser s.

Romano-Ward s. [MIM*192500], s. de Romano-Ward; prolongamento do intervalo Q-T no eletrocardiograma, em crianças sujeitas a ataques de inconsciência, que resultam de arritmias ventriculares, incluindo fibrilação ventricular; herança autossômica dominante, com uma forma causada por mutação no gene dos canais de potássio (KVLQT1) no cromossoma 11p. Cf. Jervell and Lange-Nielsen s. SIN Ward-Romano s.

Romberg s., s. de Romberg. SIN facial *hemiatrophy.*

Rothmund s. [MIM*268400], s. de Rothmund; atrofia, pigmentação e telangiectasia da pele, habitualmente com catarata juvenil, nariz em sela, defeitos ósseos congênitos, distúrbio do crescimento dos pêlos, hipogonadismo; herança autossômica recessiva. SIN poikiloderma atrophicans and cataract, poikiloderma congenitale, Rothmund-Thomson s.

Rothmund-Thomson s., s. de Rothmund-Thomson. SIN Rothmund s.

Rotor s., s. de Rotor; icterícia que aparece na infância, devido ao comprometimento da excreção biliar; a maior parte da bilirrubina plasmática está conjugada, as provas de função hepática são habitualmente normais, e não há pigmentação hepática.

Roussy-Lévy s., s. de Roussy-Lévy. SIN Roussy-Lévy *disease.*

Rubinstein-Taybi s. [MIM*180849], s. de Rubinstein-Taybi; retardo mental, polegar e hálux largos, fenda antimongolóide dos olhos, nariz fino e adunco, microcefalia, fronte proeminente, orelhas de implantação baixa, palato arqueado alto e anomalia cardíaca; pode existir um defeito cromossômico submicroscópico, mas não há evidências de que essa síndrome seja devida a uma mutação do gene que codifica o coativador transcricional, a proteína de ligação de CREB (CREB), no cromossoma 16p.

Rud s. [MIM*308200], s. de Rud; eritrodermia ictiosiforme associada a acantose nigricans, nanismo, hipogonadismo e epilepsia; principalmente esporádica, embora possa existir um traço recessivo ligado ao X.

runting s., s. de nanismo; quando camundongos recém-nascidos são timectomizados, não ganham peso e o seu tecido linfóide sofre atrofia. SIN wasting s. (1).

Russell s., s. de Russell; retardo do crescimento de lactentes e crianças pequenas devido a lesões supra-selares, comumente astrocitomas do terceiro ventrículo anterior; embora o hormônio do crescimento possa estar elevado, a criança apresenta-se magra e com perda da gordura corporal. VER TAMBÉM pseudoachondroplasia.

Saethre-Chotzen s., s. de Saethre-Chotzen; condição caracterizada por craniossinostose, assimetria do crânio (plagiocefalia), ptose, ramo da hélice proeminente e sindactilia cutânea dos dedos da mão 2–3 e dedos do pé 3–4; herança autossômica recessiva, causada por mutação no gene do fator de transcrição TWIST no cromossoma 7p. SIN Chotzen s., type III acrocephalosyndactyly.

salt depletion s., s. de depleção de sal. SIN low salt s.

salt-losing s., s. perdedora de sal. SIN salt-losing *nephritis.*

Samter s., s. de Samter; tríade de asma, pólipos nasais e intolerância à aspirina.

Sanchez Salorio s., s. de Sanchez Salorio; s. caracterizada por distrofia pigmentar da retina, catarata, hipotricose dos cílios, deficiências mentais e atraso do desenvolvimento somático.

Sandifer s., s. de Sandifer; torcicolo (q.v.) em lactentes, associado a refluxo gastroesofágico; seria um mecanismo para proteger as vias aéreas ou reduzir a dor associada ao refluxo de ácido.

Sanfilippo s., [MIM*252900, MIM*252920, MIM*252930], s. de Sanfilippo; erro do metabolismo dos mucopolissacarídeos, com excreção de grandes quantidades de sulfato de heparan na urina; caracterizada por grave retardo mental com hepatomegalia; o esqueleto pode ser normal ou exibir alterações leves semelhantes àquelas da síndrome de Hurler; já foram identificados vários tipos diferentes (A, B, C e D), de acordo com a deficiência enzimática; herança autossômica recessiva. SIN type III mucopolysacchridosis.

Savage s., s. de Savage; termo obsoleto para referir-se à síndrome do ovário resistente [sobrenome da primeira paciente descrita]

scalded mouth s., s. da boca escaldada; s. em que o paciente se queixa de sensação de queimação da língua, dos lábios, da garganta ou do palato relacionadas à escaldadura causada por líquidos quentes; clinicamente, os tecidos possuem aspecto normal; tem sido associada ao uso de inibidores da enzima conversora de angiotensina (iECA).

scalded skin s., s. da pele escaldada. VER staphylococcal scalded skin s.

scalenus anterior s., s. do escaleno anterior; uma das precursoras da questionada s. de desfiladeiro torácico neurogênica; causa popular de desconforto dos membros superiores no final da década de 1930 e década de 1940, com base no conceito, não-comprovado, de que o tronco inferior do plexo braquial e a artéria subclávia podem ser comprimidos no triângulo intra-escaleno por hipertrofia do músculo escaleno anterior, em que a compressão afeta, por sua vez, os nervos, estabelecendo um círculo vicioso. Esse conceito foi essencialmente abandonado na década de 1950, quando foram reconhecidas causas reais, como radiculopatia cervical e síndrome do túnel do carpo, para os sintomas nos membros inferiores, porém reapareceu na década de 1980, sem atribuição, como etiologia da contestada síndrome do desfiladeiro torácico neurogênica do tipo do plexo superior.

scapulocostal s., s. escapulocostal; dor de desenvolvimento insidioso, na parte superior ou posterior do ombro, que se irradia para o pescoço e occipúcio, desce para o braço ou ao redor do tórax; pode haver dormência ou formigamento dos dedos das mãos; atribuída a uma alteração da relação normal entre a escápula e a parte posterior do tórax.

Schaumann s., s. de Schaumann. SIN sarcoidosis.

Scheie s. [MIM*252800], s. de Scheie; forma alélica à s. de Hurler, porém com fenótipo muito mais leve; caracterizada por deficiência de α-L-iduronidase, turvação da córnea, deformidade das mãos, comprometimento da valva aórtica e inteligência normal; herança autossômica recessiva, causada por mutação no gene da α-L-iduronidase (IUDA) no cromossoma 4p. SIN type IS mucopolysaccharidosis.

Schmid-Fraccaro s., s. de Schmid-Fraccaro. SIN cat's-eye s.

Schmidt s., s. de Schmidt; (1) paralisia unilateral de uma corda vocal, do palato mole, do trapézio e do esternocleidomastóideo. [J.F.M. Schmidt]; (2) a associação de hipotireoidismo primário, insuficiência córtico-supra-renal primária e diabetes melito insulino-dependente [M.B. Schmidt]

Schnitzler s., s. de Schnitzler; urticária crônica generalizada, dor articular ou óssea e gamopatia monoclonal do tipo kappa.

Schönlein-Henoch s., s. de Schönlein-Henoch. SIN Henoch-Schönlein *purpura.*

Schüller s., s. de Schüller. SIN Hand-Schüller-Christian *disease.*

Schwartz s. [MIM*255800], s. de Schwartz; distúrbio congênito caracterizado por miopatia miotônica, distrofia das cartilagens epifisárias resultando em nanismo, contraturas articulares, blefarofimose e fácies característica; herança autossômica recessiva.

Seckel s. [MIM*210600], s. de Seckel; distúrbio autossômico recessivo caracterizado por baixo peso ao nascimento, nanismo, microcefalia, olhos grandes, nariz aduncho, mandíbula recuada e retardo mental moderado. SIN Seckel dwarfism.

Seip s., s. de Seip. SIN congenital total *lipodystrophy.*

Senear-Usher s., s. de Senear-Usher. SIN *pemphigus* erythematosus.

sepsis s., s. de sepse; evidências clínicas de infecção aguda com hipertermia ou hipotermia, taquicardia, taquipnéia e evidências de função ou perfusão orgânica inadequada, manifestada pelo menos por uma das seguintes alterações: alteração do estado mental, hipoxemia, acidose, oligúria ou coagulação intravascular disseminada.

Sertoli-cell-only s. [MIM*305700], s. de células de Sertoli apenas; ausência de epitélio germinativo nos túbulos seminíferos dos testículos, com presença de células de Sertoli apenas; ocorre esterilidade devido à azoospermia, porém sem outra anormalidade sexual; as células de Leydig são normais, e ocorre aumento dos níveis plasmáticos e urinários das gonadotropinas; representa provavelmente uma forma de disgenesia dos túbulos seminíferos. SIN Del Castillo s.

Sézary s., s. de Sézary; dermatite esfoliativa com intenso prurido, resultante de infiltração cutânea por células mononucleares atípicas (linfócitos T com núcleos acentuadamente convolutos ou cerebriformes), também encontradas no sangue periférico, associada a alopecia, edema e alterações ungueais e pigmentares, uma variante da micose fungóide. SIN Sézary erythroderma.

---

shaken baby s. (SBS), s. do bebê sacudido (SBS); s. de lesão neurológica ou outras lesões, de manifestação variável, causada por violenta sacudida de um lactente.

A s. do bebê sacudido constitui uma forma cada vez mais reconhecida de abuso de crianças. O ato de sacudir vigorosamente um lactente, com ou sem violência direta contra a cabeça, pode resultar em lesão da medula espinal ou sangramento intracraniano, com lesão cerebral irreversível, cegueira, surdez, convulsões, incapacidade de aprendizagem, paralisia ou morte. A SBS ocorre mais freqüentemente antes de 1 ano de idade e raramente depois dos 2 anos. Os lactentes com menos de 6 meses são particularmente vulneráveis, devido às suas cabeças desproporcionalmente pesadas, fraqueza dos músculos do pescoço e crânios finos. Nos Estados Unidos, cerca de 1.000 bebês são hospitalizados anualmente com esse diagnóstico; cerca de 25% morrem, e cerca de 25% dos sobreviventes sofrem de lesão cerebral irreversível. É mais provável que os homens causem lesões ao sacudir o lactente. Os meninos têm mais tendência a ser vítimas do que as meninas, e os gêmeos correm maior risco do que os filhos únicos. A maioria dos casos ocorre como resposta impulsiva do cuidador ao choro persistente da criança. No incidente típico, não há testemunhas, a não ser o cuidador e a vítima. Pode haver uma história pregressa de abuso ou sinais de lesão prévia. O agressor pode inventar uma história de lesão acidental para explicar os achados. Os sinais da SBS variam amplamente, desde uma manifestação gripal ou letargia até vômitos, convulsões ou coma inexplicados. Com freqüência, não existe a tríade clássica de hematoma subdural, edema cerebral e hemorragia retiniana ou sub-hialóidea. Podem ser encontradas marcas dos dedos das mãos do cuidador na parede torácica ou nos ombros da criança, mas, com freqüência, não há sinais externos de lesão. Metade dos pacientes com hematoma subdural não apresenta fratura de crânio. A prevenção da s. do bebê sacudido exige educação dos pais e de outros encarregados dos cuidados de crianças pequenas quanto ao grave perigo de sacudir um bebê. Os novos pais devem ser informados de que todos os bebês choram e que o ato de sacudi-los nunca é uma resposta apropriada. É necessário planejar maneiras alternativas de lidar com o estresse causado por um bebê que chora. Os pacientes também devem ter cautela na escolha de *baby sitters*, creches ou agências de cuidados de crianças. Todos os encarregados pelos cuidados da criança devem ser proibidos de tocar uma criança quando estão com raiva. Os profissionais de saúde precisam estar atentos quanto aos sinais sutis da SBS e de outras formas de abuso de criança.

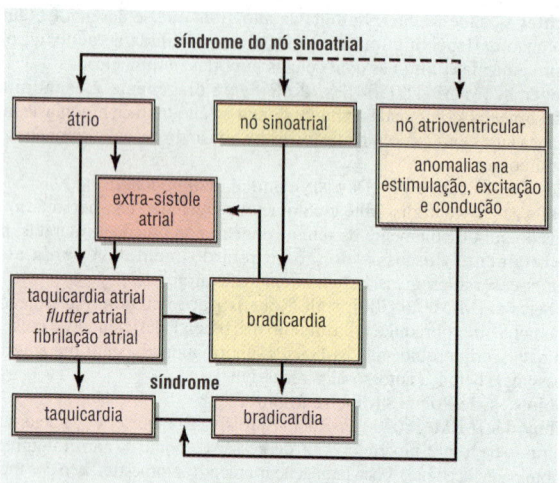

síndrome do nó sinoatrial: diagrama esquemático da patogenia da síndrome do nó sinoatrial, mostrando as anomalias de taquicardia e bradicardia

Sheehan s., s. de Sheehan; hipopituitarismo que se desenvolve após o parto em conseqüência de necrose hipofisária; causado por isquemia em decorrência de um episódio de hipotensão durante o parto. SIN pituitary cachexia, postpartum pituitary necrosis s., Simmonds disease, thyrohypophysial s.
Shone s., s. de Shone; associação de lesões obstrutivas do complexo da valva mitral, incluindo anel supravalvar e valva mitral em pára-quedas, com obstrução do fluxo ventricular esquerdo e coarctação da aorta.
short-bowel s., s. do intestino curto; má absorção e má digestão em decorrência de doença ou ressecção de grandes porções do intestino delgado.
shoulder-girdle s., s. do cíngulo do membro superior. SIN neuralgic *amyotrophy*.
shoulder-hand s., s. ombro-mão. SIN reflex sympathetic *dystrophy*.
Shprintzen s., s. de Shprintzen. SIN velocardiofacial s.
Shulman s., s. de Shulman. SIN eosinophilic *fasciitis*.
Shwachman s. [MIM*260400], s. de Shwachman; distúrbio autossômico recessivo caracterizado por sinusite, bronquiectasia, insuficiência pancreática resultando em malabsorção, neutropenia com defeito da quimiotaxia dos neutrófilos, estatura baixa e alterações esqueléticas com achados radiográficos de alargamento metafisário dos ossos longos. SIN Shwachman-Diamond s.
Shwachman-Diamond s., s. de Shwachman-Diamond. SIN Shwachman s.
Shy-Drager s. [MIM*146500], s. de Shy-Drager; termo atualmente obsoleto para a atrofia sistêmica múltipla, em que predomina uma insuficiência do sistema nervoso autônomo.
sicca s., s. seca. SIN Sjögren s.
sick building s., s. do "edifício doente"; termo antigo para building-related illness.
sick euthyroid s., s. do enfermo eutireóideo. SIN euthyroid sick s.
sick sinus s. [MIM*182190], s. do nó sinoatrial; sintomas que incluem desde tontura até inconsciência, devido à atividade atrial caótica ou ausente, freqüentemente com bradicardia alternada com taquicardia, batimentos ectópicos recidivantes, incluindo batimentos de escape, salvas de arritmias supraventriculares e ventriculares, parada sinusal e bloqueio sinoatrial.
Silver-Russell s. [MIM*270050], s. de Silver-Russell; distúrbio caracterizado por baixo peso ao nascimento, fechamento tardio da fontanela anterior, assimetria bilateral do corpo, clinodactilia dos quintos dedos da mão, fácies triangular e boca de carpa; poucas evidências genéticas úteis. SIN Silver-Russell dwarfism.
Silverskiöld s., s. de Silverskiöld; tipo de osteocondrodistrofia com alterações vertebrais apenas discretas, porém com ossos longos dos membros curvos e encurtados.
Sinding-Larsen-Johansson s., s. de Sinding-Larsen-Johansson; apofisite do pólo distal da patela.

sinus venosus s., s. do seio cavernoso; associação de conexão pulmonar-venosa anormal parcial e pequeno defeito do septo interatrial do tipo venoso.
Sipple s. [MIM*171400], s. de Sipple; feocromocitoma, carcinoma medular da tireóide e adenomas paratireóideos; herança autossômica dominante, causada por mutação no oncogene RET no cromossoma 10q.
Sjögren s., s. de Sjögren; ceratoconjuntivite seca, ressecamento das mucosas, telangiectasias ou manchas purpúricas na face e aumento bilateral das parótidas; observada em mulheres na menopausa e freqüentemente associada a artrite reumatóide, fenômeno de Raynaud e cáries dentárias; ocorrem alterações das glândulas lacrimais e salivares semelhantes às da doença de Mikulicz. SIN Gougerot-Sjögren disease, sicca s., Sjögren disease. [H.S.C. Sjögren]
Sjögren-Larsson s. [MIM*270200], s. de Sjögren-Larsson; ictiose congênita em associação com oligofrenia e paraplegia espástica; herança autossômica recessiva, causada por mutação no gene da aldeído desidrogenase de lipídios (FALDH) no cromossoma 17p.
sleep apnea s., s. de apnéia no sono; distúrbio caracterizado por múltiplos episódios de interrupção parcial ou completa da respiração durante o sono.
sleep phase delay s., s. de retardo da fase do sono; distúrbio em que o ritmo circadiano de sono e vigília exibe uma relação tardia, porém estável, com indícios cronológicos externos de dia e noite.
SLE-like s., s. LES-símile; doença com manifestações sugestivas de lúpus eritematoso sistêmico, sem preencher os critérios diagnósticos dessa doença; designação algumas vezes utilizada para o lúpus fármaco-induzido.
slit ventricle s., s. do ventrículo em fenda; em pacientes dependentes de derivação, estado caracterizado por cefaléias intermitentes ou crônicas, ventrículos pequenos e fluxo lento do mecanismo valvar.
Sly s., s. de Sly; distúrbio autossômico recessivo causado pela deficiência de uma β-glicuronidase; degradação lisossomial deficiente de sulfato de dermatan, sulfato de heparan e sulfato de condroitina; função celular afetada na maioria dos tecidos. SIN type VII mucopolysaccharidosis (1).
Smith-Lemli-Opitz s. [MIM*270400], s. de Smith-Lemli-Opitz; retardo mental, estatura baixa, narinas antevertidas, ptose, anomalias genitais masculinas e sindactilia do segundo e do terceiro dedos dos pés, freqüentemente em bebês nascidos em apresentação pélvica com atividade fetal tardia; herdada por caráter autossômico recessivo.
Smith-Riley s., s. de Smith-Riley; hemangiomas múltiplos, macrocefalia e discos ópticos borrados; os angiomas surgem ao nascimento ou mais tarde, e aumentam e multiplicam-se.
Sneddon s., s. de Sneddon; arteriopatia cerebral de etiologia desconhecida, caracterizada por hiperplasia não-inflamatória da íntima dos vasos de calibre médio, associada a livedo reticular cutâneo difuso.
Sohval-Soffer s. [MIM*307500], s. de Sohval-Soffer; hipogonadismo, ginecomastia, anomalias esqueléticas e retardo mental; herança provavelmente ligada ao X.
Sorsby s., s. de Sorsby; coloboma macular congênito e distrofia apical das extremidades.
Sotos s. [MIM*117550], s. de Sotos; gigantismo cerebral e músculos grandes generalizados na infância, com retardo mental e coordenação deficiente; etiologia desconhecida. A maioria dos casos tem sido esporádica, representando talvez novas mutações dominantes com baixa competência; todavia, existe um grupo de gêmeos idênticos concordantes registrado.

space adaptation s., s. de adaptação espacial; alterações da fisiologia normal que ocorrem durante exposição prolongada à ausência da ação da gravidade, a não ser que sejam tomadas medidas preventivas. Caracterizada por atrofia muscular, perda do mineral dos ossos, alterações cardiovasculares, etc.
Spens s., s. de Spens. SIN Adams-Stokes s.
splenic flexure s., s. da flexura esplênica; dor, gases, distensão, sensação de plenitude no quadrante superior esquerdo do abdome, algumas vezes abaixo das costelas, irradiando-se para cima em alguns casos e, em outros, provocando dor torácica anterior central ou predominantemente à esquerda. Pode ser induzida experimetalmente por introdução e retenção de ar na flexura esplênica.
staphylococcal scalded skin s., s. da pele escaldada estafilocócica; doença que acomete lactentes, em que grandes áreas de pele descamam como numa queimadura de segundo grau, em consequência de infecção estafilocócica das vias respiratórias superiores, apesar de as lesões cutâneas serem estéreis; o nível de separação da pele é subcorneano, ao contrário de uma queimadura ou da necrólise epidérmica tóxica clinicamente semelhante, que ocorre em crianças e adultos e que envolve clivagem subepidérmica. SIN Lyell disease.
Stauffer s., s. de Stauffer; elevação das provas de função hepática na ausência de doença metastática, devido à colestase em pacientes com câncer de células renais.
Steele-Richardson-Olszewski s., s. de Steele-Richardson-Olszewski. SIN progressive supranuclear *palsy.*
Stein-Leventhal s., s. de Stein-Leventhal. SIN polycystic ovary s.
steroid withdrawal s., s. de suspensão de esteróides; condição apresentada por pessoas que, previamente, estavam recebendo grandes doses terapêuticas de hormônios glicocorticóides por longos períodos; há manifestações de insuficiência hipofisário-córtico-supra-renal, particularmente durante situações de estresse, por um período de até um ano ou mais depois, podendo-se observar graus variáveis de distúrbio emocional.
Stevens-Johnson s., s. de Stevens-Johnson; forma bolhosa de eritema multiforme, que pode ser extensa, acometendo as mucosas e grandes áreas do corpo; pode provocar sintomas subjetivos graves e levar a morte. VER TAMBÉM ocular-mucous membrane s. SIN erythema multiforme bullosum, erythema multiforme exudativum, erythema multiforme major.
Stewart-Morel s., s. de Stewart-Morel. SIN Morgagni s.
Stewart-Treves s., s. de Stewart-Treves; angiossarcoma que surge em braços afetados por linfedema pós-mastectomia.
Stickler s., s. de Stickler. SIN hereditary progressive *arthroophthalmopathy.*
stiff heart s., s. do coração rígido; qualquer condição, habitualmente aguda, que provoca restrição do coração em diástole, afetando principalmente os ventrículos; antigamente, uma complicação da cirurgia cardíaca.
stiff man s., s. do homem rígido; distúrbio raro manifestado clinicamente por contração isométrica contínua de muitos músculos somáticos; as contrações costumam ser vigorosas e dolorosas e, com mais frequência, acometem a musculatura do tronco, embora os músculos dos membros possam ser afetados. Trata-se de uma doença auto-imune, com anticorpos circulantes contra a enzima de síntese do GABA e a descarboxilase do ácido glutâmico, entre outros tipos de anticorpos presentes.
Still-Chauffard s., s. de Still-Chauffard. SIN Chauffard s.
Stockholm s., s. de Estocolmo; forma de vínculo entre cativo e seqüestrador, em que o cativo começa a identificar-se com o seqüestrador, podendo até mesmo simpatizar com ele. [*Stockholm*, Suécia, onde foi relatado o primeiro caso]
Stokes-Adams s., s. de Stokes-Adams. SIN Adams-Stokes s.
straight back s., s. das costas retas; desaparecimento da concavidade normal da coluna toracolombar, com dimensão do tórax ântero-posterior estreitada, resultando em compressão do coração entre a coluna e o esterno, com conseqüentes pulsações precordiais proeminentes, sopro de ejeção e imagem radiológica cardíaca alargada (coração em panqueca).
streptococcal toxic shock s., s. do choque tóxico estreptocócico; s. tóxica caracterizada por hipotensão e por vários sinais e sintomas indicando insuficiência de múltiplos órgãos, incluindo disfunção cerebral, insuficiência renal, s. de angústia respiratória aguda, miocardiopatia tóxica e disfunção hepática. A síndrome é geralmente precipitada por infecções locais da pele ou dos tecidos moles por estreptococos; foi relatada uma taxa de mortalidade de 30%.
Stryker-Halbeisen s., s. de Stryker-Halbeisen; erupção macular avermelhada e descamativa na cabeça e na parte superior do tronco, decorrente de deficiência de vitaminas do complexo B; associada a anemia macrocítica.
Sturge-Kalischer-Weber s., s. de Sturge-Kalischer-Weber. SIN Sturge-Weber s.
Sturge-Weber s. [MIM*185300], s. de Sturge-Weber; em sua forma completa, tríade de ocorrência unilateral de 1) malformação capilar congênita (nevo flâmeo) na distribuição do nervo trigêmeo; 2) malformações vasculares leptomeníngeas, com calcificação intracraniana e sinais neurológicos; e 3) malformações vasculares da coróide, freqüentemente com glaucoma secundário. A herança não está bem estabelecida, e a maioria dos casos é esporádica. VER TAMBÉM encephalotrigeminal vascular s. SIN cephalotrigeminal angiomatosis, encephalotrigeminal angiomatosis, Sturge-Kalischer-Weber s., Sturge-Weber disease.

subclavian steal s., s. do roubo subclávio; sinais e sintomas de insuficiência vertebrobasilar em decorrência de roubo subclávio.
subcoracoid-pectoralis minor tendon s., s. de hiperabdução. SIN hyperabduction s.

---

sudden infant death s. (SIDS), s. de morte súbita do lactente (SMSL); morte súbita de um lactente aparentemente sadio, que permanece inexplicada após exclusão de todas as causas conhecidas possíveis na necropsia, investigação do local da morte e revisão da história médica. SIN cot death, crib death.

> A SMSL é a principal causa de morte em lactentes entre 1 semana e 1 ano de idade, com taxa aproximada de 2 por 1.000 nascimentos vivos; 6.000–7.000 bebês morrem de SMSL a cada ano nos Estados Unidos. O pico é observado entre 2 e 4 meses, e a maioria das mortes ocorre durante os meses de inverno (de outubro a abril no hemisfério norte). A definição dos casos exclui especificamente a morte causada por drogas ou venenos, apnéia, infecções respiratórias, sufocação, aspiração de vômito, asfixia, estrangulamento acidental e abuso de crianças. A maioria das vítimas tem aspecto sadio antes da morte, que ocorre rapidamente, em geral durante o sono. A SMSL atinge família de todas as raças e níveis socioeconômicos. É um pouco mais comum no sexo masculino, e o segundo filho é mais suscetível do que o primeiro. Algumas teorias sugerem um defeito congênito ou de desenvolvimento, porém o fenômeno não exibe agregação familiar. No atual estado de nossos conhecimentos, a SMSL não pode ser prevista, evitada ou revertida. Entretanto, estudos estatísticos identificaram certos fatores de risco, entre os quais o fumo de cigarros pela mãe antes e depois do nascimento da criança, cuidados pré-natais inadequados, baixo peso ao nascer, mãe jovem e uso de drogas pesadas pela mãe. Alguns estudos, mas nem todos, sugeriram que o aleitamento materno reduz um pouco o risco. A infecção gástrica por *Helicobacter pylori* foi especulativamente implicada em alguns casos. Até o momento, o fator de risco mais importante identificado foi a criança dormir em decúbito ventral. Dormir de lado é menos perigoso do que em decúbito ventral, porém mais perigoso do que em decúbito dorsal. A razão dessas diferenças não é conhecida, porém a incidência de SMSL declinou acentuadamente desde 1992, quando a *American Academy of Pediatrics* começou a recomendar que os lactentes sadios fossem colocados para dormir em decúbito dorsal. Para lactentes com refluxo gastroesofágico, disfunção da deglutição ou paralisia unilateral de cordas vocais, o decúbito ventral pode ser a posição preferida. Para lactentes sadios, o decúbito dorsal não aumenta o risco de vômitos e de aspiração. A prática clínica atual salienta haver uma redução do risco ao evitar o decúbito ventral para dormir e o tabagismo materno, bem como a necessidade de orientação, aconselhamento e apoio emocional dos pais das vítimas.

Sudeck s., s. de Sudeck. SIN Sudeck *atrophy.*
Sulzberger-Garbe s., s. de Sulzberger-Garbe. SIN exudative discoid and lichenoid *dermatitis.*
sump s., s. do coletor; complicação da coledocoduodenostomia látero-lateral, em que a extremidade inferior do ducto colédoco atua algumas vezes como um divertículo, com conseqüente estase, retenção de partículas alimentares e infecção.
superior cerebellar artery s., s. da artéria cerebelar superior; s. decorrente de trombose da artéria cerebelar superior que supre o trato espinotalâmico e o pedúnculo cerebelar superior; ocorre incoordenação na realização de movimentos que exigem habilidade, com perda da sensibilidade álgica e térmica no lado da face e do corpo oposto ao da lesão.
superior mesenteric artery s., s. da artéria mesentérica superior; vômitos que se acredita sejam secundários à compressão do duodeno pela artéria mesentérica superior; associada a rápida perda ponderal. SIN Wilkie disease.
superior vena cava s., s. da veia cava superior; obstrução parcial ou completa da veia cava superior, habitualmente por câncer, causando edema e ingurgitamento dos vasos da face, do pescoço e dos braços, tosse improdutiva, sintomas cerebrais e dispnéia.
supine hypotensive s., s. da hipotensão supina; na gestante a termo ou próxima do termo, em decúbito dorsal, hipotensão materna; a hipotensão materna deve-se à obstrução da veia cava inferior pelo útero grávido, com conseqüente redução do retorno venoso ao coração; a hipoxia fetal resulta da hipotensão materna e obstrução da aorta materna pelo útero grávido, com conseqüente diminuição da perfusão placentária.
supraspinatus s., s. do supra-espinal; dor à elevação do ombro e hipersensibilidade à compressão profunda do tendão do músculo supra-espinal; deve-se a lesão ou inflamação do tendão, ou inflamação da bolsa subacromial que entra em contato com o processo acromial sobrejacente ou o comprime, estando o braço elevado acima do nível do ombro. SIN impingement s., painful arc s.
supravalvar aortic stenosis s. [MIM*185500], s. de estenose aórtica supravalvar; estenose aórtica supravalvar (habitualmente membranácea) algumas vezes as-

sociada a estenose da valva pulmonar ou arterial periférica, porém com fácies e mentalidade normais; herança autossômica dominante, causada por mutação no gene da elastina (ELN) no cromossoma 7q. Cf. Williams s.

supravalvar aortic stenosis-infantile hypercalcemia s. [MIM*194050], s. de estenose aórtica supravalvar-hipercalcemia infantil. SIN Williams s.

surdocardiac s., s. surdocardíaca. SIN Jervell and Lange-Nielsen s.

sweaty feet s., s. dos pés suados. SIN isovaleric acidemia.

swollen belly s., s. da barriga inchada. SIN swollen belly disease.

Swyer s., s. de Swyer; disgenesia gonadal em mulheres fenotípicas com genótipo XY.

Swyer-James s., s. de Swyer-James; (1) enfisema lobar unilateral. SIN unilateral lobar emphysema; (2) hipertransparência de um pulmão por bronquiolite obliterante, habitualmente causada por infecção por adenovírus na infância, com diminuição do tamanho e da vascularidade do pulmão; diferenciada de outras causas de hipertransparência unilateral pela demonstração da retenção de ar sem obstrução central.

Swyer-James-MacLeod s., s. de Swyer-James-MacLeod. SIN unilateral lobar emphysema.

systemic capillary leak s., s. de extravasamento capilar sistêmico; distúrbio raro, de causa desconhecida, que se manifesta como hipotensão episódica, hemoconcentração e hipoalbuminemia; freqüentemente associada a gamopatia monoclonal.

tachybradycardia s., s. taquibradicardia. SIN bradytachycardia s.

tachycardia-bradycardia s., s. taquicardia-bradicardia; períodos alternados de batimentos cardíacos lentos e rápidos, freqüentemente associada a distúrbios de condução sinoatrial e atrioventricular. VER TAMBÉM sick sinus s.

Takayasu s., s. de Takayasu. SIN Takayasu arteritis.

Tapia s., s. de Tapia; paralisia unilateral da laringe, do palato mole e da língua, com atrofia da última.

tarsal tunnel s., s. do túnel do tarso; s. causada por neuropatia de compressão dos ramos terminais do nervo tibial posterior (nervos plantar medial, plantar lateral e calcaneal) no tornozelo.

Taussig-Bing s., s. de Taussig-Bing; transposição completa da aorta, que se origina do ventrículo direito, com artéria pulmonar esquerda cavalgando o ventrículo esquerdo e com defeito do septo interventricular, hipertrofia do ventrículo direito, aorta de localização anterior e artéria pulmonar de localização posterior. SIN Taussig-Bing disease.

tegmental s., s. tegmentar; s. habitualmente causada por lesão vascular no tegmento; caracterizada por hemiplegia contralateral e paresia ocular ipsilateral.

temporomandibular s., s. temporomandibular; desconforto e dor causados pela perda da dimensão vertical, ausência de oclusão posterior ou outra má oclusão, trismo, tremor muscular, artrite ou traumatismo direto da articulação temporomandibular.

temporomandibular joint pain-dysfunction s., s. de dor-disfunção da articulação temporomandibular. SIN myofascial pain-dysfunction s.

tendon sheath s., s. da bainha tendínea; elevação limitada do olho na adução, que aparece clinicamente como paresia do músculo oblíquo inferior, devido à fáscia que contrai o músculo oblíquo superior do mesmo lado. SIN Brown s., Paterson-Brown-Kelly s.

Terry s., s. de Terry. SIN retinopathy of prematurity.

Terson s., s. de Terson; hemorragias vítreas, retinianas e sub-hialóideas associadas a hemorragia subaracnóidea.

testicular feminization s. [MIM*313700], s. de feminização testicular; tipo de pseudo-hermafroditismo masculino, caracterizado por genitália externa feminina (que pode ser ambígua se a síndrome for incompleta), desenvolvimento incompleto da vagina, freqüentemente com útero e tubas uterinas rudimentares, biotipo feminino na puberdade, porém com pêlos axilares e púbicos escassos ou ausentes e amenorréia, testículos presentes no abdome ou nos canais inguinais ou lábios maiores do pudendo; epidídimo e canal deferente habitualmente presentes; ocorre formação de androgênios e estrogênios, porém os tecidos-alvo são, em grande parte, não-responsivos aos androgênios; os indivíduos apresentam cariótipo masculino normal; herança recessiva ligada ao X, causada por mutação no gene do receptor de androgênio (AR) no cromossoma Xq.

tethered cord s., s. da medula espinal fixada; posicionamento baixo anormal (abaixo da vértebra L_2) da porção distal da medula espinal (cone medular) pelo filo terminal. Pode estar associada a incontinência, comprometimento motor e sensorial progressivo nas pernas, dor e escoliose.

thalamic s., s. talâmica; síndrome produzida por infarto do tálamo póstero-inferior; causa hemiparesia transitória, acentuada perda da sensibilidade superficial e profunda, com preservação da percepção grosseira de dor nos membros hipoálgicos, que freqüentemente apresentam distúrbios vasomotores ou tróficos. SIN Dejerine-Roussy s.

Thiemann s., s. de Thiemann, necrose avascular das epífises das falanges dos dedos das mãos ou dos pés, geralmente familiar, que começa na infância ou na adolescência, resultando em deformidade dos dedos da mão; também denominada artropatia familiar dos dedos das mãos ou dos pés. SIN Thiemann disease.

third and fourth pharyngeal pouch s., s. da terceira e da quarta bolsas faríngeas. SIN DiGeorge s.

thoracic outlet s. (TOS), s. do desfiladeiro torácico; designação coletiva de diversas condições atribuídas ao comprometimento de vasos sanguíneos ou fibras nervosas (plexo braquial) em qualquer ponto entre a base do pescoço e a axila; antigamente classificadas com base na suposta estrutura ou mecanismo afetado, isto é, s. do escaleno anterior, s. de hiperabdução, s. costoclavicular; hoje em dia, são classificadas com base na estrutura reconhecida ou supostamente comprometida e divididas em dois grupos principais: vasculares e neurológicas (o comprometimento simultâneo de estruturas tanto neurais quanto vasculares é raro); as subdivisões vasculares incluem arterial e venosa.

Thorn s., s. de Thorn. SIN salt-losing nephritis.

thrombocytopenia-absent radius s., TAR s. [MIM*274000], s. de trombocitopenia e ausência do rádio, s. TAR; ausência congênita do rádio associada a trombocitopenia, que é sintomática na lactância, mas que melhora posteriormente; em alguns casos, ocorrem cardiopatia congênita e anomalias renais; herança autossômica recessiva.

thrombopathic s., s. trombopática; termo indefinido que descreve qualquer uma de várias doenças hemorrágicas em que a formação do coágulo é deficiente, e não aquelas em que existe um defeito orgânico dos vasos sanguíneos.

thyrohypophysial s., s. tireo-hipofisária. SIN Sheehan s.

Tietz s., s. de Tietz; herança autossômica dominante de albinismo e surdez causados, pelo menos em alguns subgrupos de famílias, por uma mutação do gene do fator de transcrição da microftalmia.

Tietze s., s. de Tietze; inflamação e tumefação não-supurativa dolorosa e hipersensível de uma junção costocondral. SIN peristernal perichondritis.

Tolosa-Hunt s., s. de Tolosa-Hunt; s. do seio cavernoso produzida por granuloma idiopático.

tooth-and-nail s. [MIM*189500], s. do dente e da unha; hipodontia associada a unhas ausentes ou muito pequenas ao nascimento. Comum em menonitas holandeses no Canadá.

TORCH s., s. TORCH; grupo de infecções observadas em neonatos que atravessaram a barreira placentária, exibindo manifestações clínicas semelhantes, embora os sintomas possam variar quanto ao grau e momento de aparecimento: *t*oxoplasmose, *o*utras infecções, *r*ubéola, infecção por *c*itomegalovírus e *h*erpes simples.

Tornwaldt s., s. de Tornwaldt; secreção nasofaríngea, cefaléia occipital e rigidez dos músculos cervicais posteriores, com halitose, devido à infecção crônica da bolsa faríngea.

Torre s., s. de Torre; múltiplos adenomas das glândulas sebáceas associados a múltiplas neoplasias malignas viscerais, freqüentemente carcinoma colorretal. SIN Muir-Torre s.

Torsten Sjögren s., s. de Torsten Sjögren. SIN Marinesco-Garland s.

Tourette s., s. de Tourette; distúrbio com tiques que surge na infância, caracterizado por múltiplos tiques motores e tiques vocais presentes há mais de 1 ano. Pode haver comportamento obsessivo-compulsivo, distúrbio de déficit de atenção e outros distúrbios psiquiátricos associados; raramente ocorrem coprolalia e ecolalia; herança autossômica dominante. SIN Gilles de la Tourette disease, Gilles de la Tourette s., Tourette disease.

toxic shock s. (TSS), s. do choque tóxico (SCT); infecção por estafilococos produtores de toxina; ocorre mais freqüentemente na vagina de mulheres menstruadas que utilizam tampões superabsorventes, mas também prevalente em muitas infecções dos tecidos moles e caracterizada por febre alta, vômitos, diarréia, exantema escarlatiniforme seguido de descamação e declínio da pressão arterial e choque, podendo resultar em morte; ocorre também hiperemia das mucosas conjuntival, orofaríngea e vaginal.

transplant lung s., s. pulmonar de transplante; s. associada a febre e infiltração pulmonar bilateral difusa, principalmente na base ou no hilo do pulmão; pode acompanhar a rejeição de transplante de órgão (rim, fígado, etc.) ou ocorrer após uma redução na dose de um agente imunossupressor.

transurethral resection s., s. de ressecção transuretral; absorção de glicina da solução de irrigação durante a ressecção transuretral, que não pode ser metabolizada pelo fígado, resultando em aumento dos níveis séricos de amônia. SIN TUR s.

Treacher Collins s. [MIM*154500], s. de Treacher Collins; disostose mandibulofacial (mandibulofacial dysostosis) quando limitada à região orbital e malar.

trichorhinophalangeal s., s. tricorrinofalangeal; condição caracterizada por pêlos finos escassos, nariz largo, com filtro longo, falanges médias intumescidas com epífises cônicas e retardo do crescimento. Parecem existir pelo menos três distúrbios semelhantes, dois dominantes [MIM*150230 e MIM 190350] e um recessivo [MIM*275500].

triple A s. [MIM*231550], s. do A triplo; s. recessiva autossômica associada a *a*calasia do cárdia e *a*lacrimia; os problemas associados incluem anormalidades do sistema nervoso, como retardo mental e disfunção autônoma. SIN Allgrove s.

triple X s., s. do X triplo; trissomia do cromossoma X; as observações originais (efetuadas em instituições para doentes mentais) foram seriamente tendenciosas, e as alterações fenotípicas, espúrias. A inteligência pode estar situada na faixa inferior da normalidade, a estatura é habitualmente alta e pode haver problemas da fala e do comportamento. A característica proeminente da s. consiste na presença de corpúsculos de Barr gêmeos numa célula típica.

trisomy 8 s., s. de trissomia do 8; a trissomia do 8 completa está habitualmente associada a letalidade precoce, porém a maioria dos indivíduos afetados são mosaicos, com dismorfismo craniofacial, pescoço curto e largo, tronco cilíndrico e estreito, múltiplas anormalidades articulares e digitais e pregas profundas das palmas das mãos e plantas dos pés.

trisomy 13 s., s. de trissomia do 13; distúrbio cromossômico habitualmente fatal em 2 anos; caracterizado por retardo mental, malformação das orelhas, lábio leporino ou fenda palatina, microftalmia ou coloboma, mandíbula pequena, polidactilia, defeitos cardíacos, convulsões, anomalias renais, hérnia umbilical, má rotação do intestino e anomalias dermatoglíficas. SIN Patau s., trisomy D s.

trisomy 18 s., s. de trissomia do 18; distúrbio cromossômico habitualmente fatal em 2–3 anos; caracterizado por retardo mental, forma anormal do crânio, orelhas de implantação baixa e malformadas, mandíbula pequena, defeitos cardíacos, esterno curto, hérnia diafragmática ou inguinal, divertículo de Meckel, flexão anormal dos dedos das mãos e anomalias dermatoglíficas. SIN Edwards s.

trisomy 20 s., s. de trissomia do 20; distúrbio cromossômico caracterizado por retardo mental profundo, fácies grosseira, macrostomia e macroglossia, pequenas anomalias das orelhas, displasia pigmentar da pele, cifoescoliose dorsal e outros defeitos esqueléticos.

trisomy 21 s., s. de trissomia do 21. SIN Down s.

trisomy C s., s. de trissomia do C; trissomia de qualquer cromossoma do grupo C, dos números 6–12, mais freqüentemente do número 8.

trisomy D s., s. de trissomia do D. SIN trisomy 13 s.

trochanteric s., s. trocantérica; tendinite e bursite ao redor do trocanter maior.

trophic s., s. trófica; ulceração de uma área desnervada, freqüentemente secundária ao mexer com os dedos na superfície anestésica.

tropical splenomegaly s., s. de esplenomegalia tropical. SIN hyperreactive malarious splenomegaly.

Trousseau s., s. de Trousseau; tromboflebite migratória associada a câncer visceral.

true neurogenic thoracic outlet s., s. do desfiladeiro torácico neurogênica verdadeira; plexopatia braquial por perda axônica muito crônica, causada pelo comprometimento das fibras do tronco inferior por uma banda congênita que se estende desde uma costela cervical rudimentar até a primeira costela torácica; distúrbio raro, encontrado principalmente em mulheres (desde a juventude até à meia-idade), que se manifesta como desgaste e fraqueza unilaterais da musculatura da mão, acometendo particularmente a iminência tenar lateral; algumas vezes acompanhada de desconforto intermitente ao longo da parte medial do antebraço e da mão. SIN cervical rib and band s., classic cervical rib s.

tumor lysis s., s. de lise tumoral; hiperfosfatemia, hipocalcemia, hiperpotassemia e hiperuricemia que ocorrem após quimioterapia de indução de neoplasias malignas; atribuída à liberação de produtos intracelulares por lise das células.

TUR s., s. de RTU. SIN transurethral resection s.

Turcot s. [MIM* 276300], s. de Turcot; forma rara e distinta de polipose intestinal múltipla associada a tumores cerebrais; herança autossômica recessiva, causada por mutação em um dos genes de reparo de combinação imprópria: MLH1 no cromossoma 3p, PMS2, no cromossoma 7p ou o gene da polipose adenomatosa do colo (APC) no cromossoma 5q.

Turner s., s. de Turner; s. com 45 cromossomas e apenas um cromossoma X; as células bucais e outras células geralmente são negativas para cromatina sexual; as anomalias incluem nanismo, pescoço alado, deformidade em valgo dos cotovelos, peito de pombo, desenvolvimento sexual infantil e amenorréia; o ovário não possui folículos primordiais e pode ser representado apenas por uma faixa fibrosa; alguns indivíduos são mosaicos cromossômicos, com duas ou mais linhagens celulares de diferente constituição cromossômica; observada em muitas espécies de animais; na ratazana dos prados é o estado normal da fêmea. SIN XO s.

twiddler's s., s. do giro; condição em que um fio de marcapasso cardíaco é removido de sua posição no coração com a rotação do marcapasso subcutâneo pelo paciente ao "fazer um giro".

Uhthoff s., s. de Uhthoff. SIN Uhthoff symptom.

Ullmann s., s. de Ullmann; angiomatose sistêmica devido a múltiplas malformações arteriovenosas.

Ulysses s., s. de Ulysses; os efeitos deletérios de extensas investigações diagnósticas conduzidas em virtude da obtenção de um resultado falso-positivo no decorrer de uma triagem laboratorial de rotina. [L. *Ulysses*, do G. *Odysseus*, figura da mitologia.]

uncombable hair s., s. do cabelo não-penteável; s. genética em que os cabelos, que freqüentemente são louro-prateados, são rebeldes e não permanecem lisos devido às suas hastes de forma irregular. SIN spun glass hair.

Unna-Thost s., s. de Unna-Thost. SIN diffuse *hyperkeratosis* of palms and soles.

unroofed coronary sinus s., s. do seio coronário dissecado; espectro de anomalias cardíacas em que parte ou toda a parede comum entre o seio coronário e o átrio direito está ausente.

urethral s., s. uretral; condição de etiologia não-estabelecida, caracterizada por polaciúria, urgência, disúria na ausência de infecção específica, obstrução ou disfunção. Além disso, podem ocorrer dor suprapúbica, hesitação e dor nas costas. Geralmente observada em mulheres.

Usher s. [MIM*276900, MIM* 276901], s. de Usher; herança autossômica recessiva com heterogeneidade genética; podem ser distinguidas três formas com base nos dados de ligação: o tipo 1 provoca perda da audição neurossensorial, perda da função vestibular e retinite pigmentar; os tipos 2 e 3 caracterizam-se por surdez e retinite pigmentosa.

uveocutaneous s., s. uveocutânea. SIN Vogt-Koyanagi s.

uveoencephalitic s., s. uveoencefálica. SIN Behçet s.

uveomeningitis s., s. de uveomeningite. SIN Harada s.

VACTERL s., s. VACTERL; anormalidades das *v*értebras, do *a*nus, da árvore *c*ardiovascular, da *t*raquéia, do *e*sôfago, do sistema *r*enal e dos brotos dos membros (*l*imb) associadas à administração de esteróides sexuais no início da gravidez.

van Buchem s. [MIM*239100], s. de van Buchem; displasia esquelética osteoesclerosante, caracterizada por aumento da mandíbula, espessamento das diáfises e calvária e aumento dos níveis séricos de fosfatase alcalina; herança autossômica recessiva. SIN generalized cortical hyperostosis.

van der Hoeve s., s. de van der Hoeve; subtipo de osteogênese imperfeita (*osteogenesis* imperfecta), em que a perda de audição condutiva progressiva começa na infância, devido à fixação do estribo.

vanished testis s. s. do testículo desaparecido; ausência de ambos os testículos num indivíduo do sexo masculino com cromossomas normais (XY) e genitália normal sob os demais aspectos ao nascimento e na infância. Os testículos estavam presentes pelo menos no primeiro trimestre de gravidez, porém desapareceram depois.

vanishing lung s., s. do pulmão evanescente; diminuição progressiva da opacidade radiográfica do pulmão causada pelo desenvolvimento acelerado de enfisema ou rápida destruição cística do pulmão por infecção.

Van Lohuizen s., s. de Van Lohuizen. SIN *cutis* marmorata telangiectatica congenita.

vasculocardiac s. of hyperserotonemia, s. vasculocardíaca de hiperserotonemia; termo obsoleto para a síndrome carcinóide.

vasovagal s., s. vasovagal. SIN Gowers s.

velocardiofacial s. [MIM*192430], s. velocardiofacial; s. com fala hipernasal, traços faciais dismórficos (face média longa, nariz cilíndrico, cantos da boca voltados para baixo) e anormalidade cardíacas; mesma anormalidades cromossômica observada na síndrome de DiGeorge (microdeleção no cromossoma 22q11); herança dominante. SIN Shprintzen s.

Verner-Morrison s., s. de Verner-Morrison; diarréia aquosa, hipopotassemia e acloridria associadas à secreção de polipeptídeo intestinal vasoativo por um tumor das ilhotas pancreáticas na ausência de hipersecreção gástrica. SIN WDHA s.

Vernet s., s. de Vernet; s. caracterizada por paralisia dos componentes motores dos nervos cranianos glossofaríngeo vago e acessório, quando localizados na fossa posterior; resulta mais comumente de lesão cefálica.

vertical retraction s., s. de retração vertical. VER retraction s.

vibration s., s. de vibração; formigamento, dormência e empalidecimento dos dedos das mãos em decorrência do uso de instrumentos vibratórios seguros com a mão; pode persistir sem exposição adicional à vibração.

virus-associated hemophagocytic s., s. hemofagocítica associada a vírus; s. muito semelhante à histiocitose maligna, porém potencialmente reversível, que ocorre após infecção por vírus do grupo herpes, como vírus Epstein-Barr.

vitreoretinal choroidopathy s., [MIM* 193220] s. de coroidopatia vitreorretiniana; condição ocular caracterizada por retinopatia pigmentar periférica, anormalidades vasculares da retina, opacidades do vítreo, atrofia da coróide e cataratas pré-senis; herança autossômica dominante.

vitreoretinal traction s., s. da tração vitreorretiniana; tração sobre a membrana limitante interna da retina por fibrilas vítreas aderentes no descolamento do humor vítreo.

Vogt s., s. de Vogt. SIN double *athetosis*. [Cècile e Oscar Vogt]

Vogt-Koyanagi s., s. de Vogt-Koyanagi; uveíte bilateral com irite e glaucoma, encanecimento prematuro dos cabelos, alopecia, vitiligo e disacusia; relacionada à síndrome de Harada e à oftalmopatia simpática. SIN oculocutaneous s., uveocutaneous s.

Vohwinkel s., s. de Vohwinkel. SIN mutilating *keratoderma*.

voice fatigue s., s. de fadiga da voz; fraqueza e perda da voz, habitualmente no final do dia, devido a seu uso por um período excessivamente longo e falando muito alto.

von Hippel-Lindau s. [MIM*193300], s. de von Hippel-Lindau; tipo de facomatose, consistindo em malformações vasculares retinianas, que podem ser múltiplas e bilaterais, associadas a hemangioblastomas primariamente do cerebelo e das paredes do quarto ventrículo, acometendo, em certas ocasiões, a medula espinal; algumas vezes associada a carcinomas de células renais ou cistos ou hamartomas do rim, da supra-renal ou de outros órgãos; herança autossômica dominante, devido à mutação no gene de von Hippel-Lindau (VHL) no cromossoma 3p. SIN cerebroretinal angiomatosis, Lindau disease.

vulnerable child s., s. da criança vulnerável; reação caracterizada por distúrbio do desenvolvimento psicossocial, ocorrendo freqüentemente em crianças cujos pais esperam ou tenham morte prematura.

Waardenburg s. [MIM*193500, MIM*193510], s. de Waardenburg; distúrbio caracterizado por deslocamento lateral dos cantos internos (distopia dos cantos), raiz do nariz larga, heterocromia da íris, surdez coclear, topete branco e sinófris; herança autossômica dominante, com diferenciação entre o tipo I e o tipo II pela presença de distopia dos cantos. O tipo I é causado por mutação no gene PAX3 no cromossoma 2q, enquanto alguns casos do tipo II são produzidos por mutação no gene do fator de transcrição associado à microftalmia (MITF) no cromossoma 3p.

Wagner s., s. de Wagner. SIN hyaloideoretinal degeneration.

WAGR s., s. WAGR; acrônimo para tumor de Wilms, aniridia, malformações genitourinárias e retardo mental.

Waldenström s., s. de Waldenström. SIN Waldenström macroglobulinemia.

Wallenberg s., s. de Wallenberg. SIN posterior inferior cerebellar artery s.

Ward-Romano s., s. Ward-Romano. SIN Romano-Ward s.

wasting s., s. de consunção; (1) SIN runting s.; (2) perda ponderal involuntária e progressiva observada em pacientes com infecção por HIV; pode ser decorrente de vários fatores atuando isoladamente ou em combinação, incluindo ingestão inadequada de alimento, alteração do estado metabólico e/ou má absorção. Não responde ao aumento da ingestão calórica. Definida como uma acentuada perda ponderal involuntária superior a 10% do peso corporal basal, juntamente com diarréia crônica (pelo menos duas evacuações de fezes pastosas por dia durante > 30 dias ou fraqueza crônica e febre documentada (durante > 30, intermitente ou constante), na ausência de qualquer doença ou condição concomitante, que não seja a infecção por HIV passível de explicar esses achados (como câncer, tuberculose, criptosporidiose ou outra enterite específica). SIN HIV wasting s.

Waterhouse-Friderichsen s., s. de Waterhouse-Friderichsen, condição que ocorre principalmente em crianças com menos de 10 anos de idade, caracterizada por vômitos, diarréia, púrpura extensa, cianose, convulsões tônico-clônicas e colapso circulatório, geralmente com meningite e hemorragia nas glândulas supra-renais. SIN acute fulminating meningococcal septicemia, Friderichsen-Waterhouse s.

WDHA s., s. WDHA. SIN Verner-Morrison s. [watery diarrhea, hypokalemia, achlorydria (diarréia aquosa, hipopotassemia, acloridria)]

Weber s., s. de Weber; lesão do tegmento do mesencéfalo, caracterizada por paresia do nervo oculomotor ipsolateral e paralisia contralateral dos membros, da face e da língua. SIN Weber sign.

Weber-Cockayne s. [MIM*131800], s. de Weber-Cockayne; epidermólise bolhosa (*epidermolysis* bolhosa) das mãos e dos pés; herança autossômica dominante, causada por mutação no gene da ceratina 5 (KRT5) no cromossoma 12q ou no gene da ceratina 14 (KRT14) no cromossoma 17q.

Weil-Marchesani s. [MIM*277600], s. de Weil-Marchesani; ectopia da lente (lente anormalmente redonda e pequena), estatura baixa e braquidactilia; herança autossômica recessiva.

Wells s., s. de Wells. SIN eosinophilic cellulitis.

Wermer s., s. de Wermer. SIN multiple endocrine neoplasia s., type 1.

Werner s. [MIM*277700], s. de Werner; envelhecimento prematuro que consiste em alterações cutâneas semelhantes a esclerodermia, cataratas juvenis bilaterais, progeria e hipogonadismo e diabetes melito; herança autossômica recessiva, causada por mutação no gene WRN, que codifica uma proteína helicase no cromossoma 8p.

Wernicke s., s. de Wernicke; condição freqüentemente observada em alcoólatras crônicos, causada, em grande parte, por deficiência de tiamina e caracterizada por distúrbios da motilidade ocular, alterações pupilares, nistagmo e ataxia com tremores; com freqüência, psicose orgânico-tóxica é um achado associado, com coexistência freqüente de síndrome de Korsakoff; patologia celular característica observada em várias áreas do cérebro. SIN superior hemorrhagic polioencephalitis, Wernicke disease, Wernicke encephalopathy.

Wernicke-Korsakoff s., s. de Wernicke-Korsakoff; coexistência das síndromes de Wernicke e de Korsakoff.

West s., s. de West; encefalopatia na lactância, caracterizada por espasmos infantis, parada do desenvolvimento psicomotor e hipsarritmia.

Weyers-Thier s., s. de Weyers-Thier. SIN oculovertebral dysphasia.

whistling face s., s. da face assobiadora. SIN craniocarpotarsal dystrophy.

white-out s., s. do branco total; psicose que ocorre em exploradores do Ártico ou outros indivíduos igualmente expostos a privação de estímulos em um ambiente coberto de neve. VER TAMBÉM sensory deprivation.

Widal s., s. de Widal. SIN Hayem-Widal s.

Wildervanck s., s. de Wildervanck. SIN cervicooculoacoustic s.

Williams s. [MIM*194050], s. de Williams; distúrbio caracterizado por fácies distinta com cristas supra-orbitais superficiais, afunilamento medial das sobrancelhas, padrão estrelado da íris, pequeno nariz com narinas antevertidas, hipoplasia malar com bochechas pendentes, lábios grossos, estenose aórtica supravalvar, hipocalcemia neonatal, retardo mental leve e personalidade loquaz. Herança autossômica dominante; trata-se de uma s. de deleção de genes contíguos, em que um dos genes que sofre mutação é o gene da elastina (ELN) no cromossoma 7q. SIN elfin facies s., supravalvar aortic stenosis-infantile hypercalcemia s., Williams-Beuren s.

Williams-Beuren s., s. de Williams-Beuren. SIN Williams s.

Wilson-Mikity s., s. de Wilson-Mikity. SIN pulmonary dysmaturity s.

Wiskott-Aldrich s. [MIM*301000], s. de Wiskott-Aldrich; distúrbio de imunodeficiência que ocorre em meninos, caracterizado por trombocitopenia, eczema, melena e suscetibilidade a infecções bacterianas recorrentes; ocorre morte por hemorragia grave ou infecção maciça; herança recessiva ligada ao X, causada por mutação no gene da síndrome de Wiskott-Aldrich (WASP) no cromossoma Xp. SIN Aldrich s.

Wissler s., s. de Wissler; febre intermitente alta, erupção macular e maculopapular irregularmente recorrente da face, do tórax e dos membros, leucocitose, artralgia, ocasionalmente eosinofilia e elevação da velocidade de hemossedimentação; acomete crianças e adolescentes, com duração variável.

withdrawal s., s. de abstinência; desenvolvimento de uma síndrome especificamente relacionada a substâncias, que surge após a interrupção ou a redução do uso de uma substância psicoativa da qual o indivíduo previamente fazia uso regular; por exemplo, a síndrome clínica de desorientação, distúrbio perceptual e agitação motora que sucede à interrupção do uso crônico de quantidades excessivas de álcool é denominada síndrome de abstinência de álcool. A síndrome que se desenvolve varia de acordo com a substância psicoativa utilizada. Os sintomas comuns consistem em ansiedade, inquietação, irritabilidade, insônia e redução da atenção. VER TAMBÉM abstinence s.

Wolff-Parkinson-White s. [MIM*194200], s. de Wolff-Parkinson-White; padrão eletrocardiográfico algumas vezes associado a taquicardia paroxística; consiste em intervalo PR curto (em geral, 0,1 segundo ou menos; algumas vezes normal), juntamente com prolongamento do complexo QRS, com componente inicial arrastado (onda delta). SIN preexcitation s.

Wolfram s. (DIDMOD), s. de Wolfram (DIDMOD); s. que consiste em diabetes insípido, diabetes melito, atrofia óptica e surdez (*deafness*); a anormalidade genética localiza-se no cromossoma 4p, herança autossômica recessiva.

Wright s., s. de Wright. SIN hyperabduction s.

Wyburn-Mason s., s. de Wyburn-Mason; malformação arteriovenosa no córtex cerebral, malformação arteriovenosa da retina e nevo facial que geralmente ocorre em indivíduos com retardo mental. SIN Bonnet-Dechaume-Blanc s.

X-linked lymphoproliferative s., s. linfoproliferativa ligada ao X; imunodeficiência e doença linfoproliferativa recessivas ligadas ao X, causadas por mutação no gene da proteína 1A do domínio SH2 (SH2D1A) no cromossoma Xq; a s. caracteriza-se por uma resposta imune celular ou humoral deficiente ao vírus Epstein-Barr; as manifestações consistem em mononucleose infecciosa fulminante, neoplasias malignas de células B e hipogamaglobulinemia. SIN Duncan disease, Duncan s., X-linked lymphoproliferative disease.

XO s., s. XO. SIN Turner s.

XXY s., s. de XXY. SIN Klinefelter s.

XYY s., s. de XYY; anomalia cromossômica com 47 cromossomas, com um cromossoma Y supranumerário; as evidências controvertidas associam a ocorrência de estatura elevada, agressividade e acne a essa condição.

yellow nail s., s. da unha amarela. SIN yellow nail.

Young s., s. de Young; azoospermia obstrutiva e infecções sinopulmonares crônicas.

Zellweger s., s. de Zellweger; distúrbio metabólico de início neonatal, caracterizado por fácies distinta, hipotonia muscular, hepatomegalia com icterícia, cistos renais, pontilhado epifisário das patelas, desmielinização cerebral e defeitos de migração neuronal e retardo psicomotor; observa-se uma perturbação na biogênese peroxissomal; herança autossômica recessiva, causada por mutação em qualquer um dos vários genes de peroxina (PEX) no cromossoma 6, 7, 8 ou 12. SIN cerebrohepatorenal s.

Zieve s., s. de Zieve; icterícia transitória, anemia hemolítica e hiperlipemia associadas a alcoolismo agudo em pacientes com cirrose ou esteatose hepática.

Zivert s., s. de Zivert. SIN Kartagener s.

Zollinger-Ellison s. [MIM*131100], s. de Zollinger-Ellison; úlcera péptica com hipersecreção gástrica e gastrinoma do pâncreas ou do duodeno, algumas vezes associada a adenomatose endócrina múltipla familiar tipo 1.

---

syn·drom·ic (sin-drom′ik, -drō′mik). Sindrômico; relativo a uma síndrome.

syn·ech·ia, pl. **syn·ech·i·ae** (si-nek′ē-ā, -kē-ē; si-nē′kē-ā). Sinéquia; qualquer aderência; especificamente, sinéquia anterior ou posterior. [G. *synecheia*, continuidade, de *syn*, junto + *echo*, ter, reter]

anterior s., s. anterior; aderência da íris à córnea.

anular s., s. anular; aderência de toda a margem pupilar da íris à cápsula da lente.
peripheral anterior s., s. anterior periférica. SIN goniosynechia.
posterior s., s. posterior; aderência da íris à cápsula da lente.
total s., s. total; aderência de toda a superfície da íris à cápsula da lente.

syn·ech·i·ot·o·my (si-nek′e-ot′o-me). Sinequiotomia; divisão das aderências na sinéquia. [synechia + G. *tome*, incisão]

syn·ech·o·tome (si-nek′o-tom). Sinecótomo; pequeno bisturi para uso na sinequiotomia.

syn·ec·ten·ter·ot·o·my (si-nek′ten-ter-ot′o-me). Sinectenterotomia; divisão de aderências intestinais. [G. *synektos*, manter unido (ver synechia) + *enteron*, intestino + *tome*, incisão]

syn·en·ceph·a·lo·cele (sin-en-sef′a-lo-sel). Sinencefalocele; protrusão da substância cerebral através de um defeito no crânio, com aderências impedindo a redução. [syn- + G. *enkephalos*, cérebro + *kele*, hérnia]

syn·er·e·sis (si-ner′e-sis). Sinérese. **1.** A contração de um gel, p. ex., um coágulo sanguíneo, através da qual parte da dispersão do meio é expelida. **2.** Degeneração do humor vítreo com perda da consistência gel, tornando-se parcial ou completamente líquido. [G. *synairesis*, tomar ou impelir juntos]

syn·er·get·ic (sin-er-jet′ik). Sinérgico. SIN synergistic.
syn·er·gia (si-ner′je-a). Sinergia. SIN synergism.
syn·er·gic (si-ner′jik). Sinérgico. SIN synergistic.

syn·er·gism (sin′er-jizm). Sinergismo; ação coordenada ou correlacionada de duas ou mais estruturas, agentes ou processos fisiológicos, de tal modo que a ação combinada é maior do que a soma de cada uma separadamente. Cf. antagonism. SIN synergia, synergistic effect, synergy. [G. *synergia*, de *syn*, junto + *ergon*, trabalho]

syn·er·gist (sin′er-jist). Sinergista; estrutura, agente ou processo fisiológico que auxilia a ação de outro. Cf. antagonist.

syn·er·gis·tic (sin-er-jis′tik). Sinérgico. **1.** Relativo ao sinergismo. **2.** Designa um sinergista. SIN synergetic, synergic.

syn·er·gy (sin′er-je). Sinergia. SIN synergism.

syn·es·the·sia (sin-es-the′ze-a). Sinestesia. **1.** Condição em que um estímulo, além de excitar a sensação habitual e normalmente localizada, dá origem a uma sensação subjetiva de caráter ou localização diferente; p. ex., audição da cor, sabor da cor. **2.** Numa perspectiva neurolingüística, condicionamento estímulo-resposta, como aquele observado numa fobia. [syn- + G. *aisthesis*, sensação]
s. al′gica, s. álgica. SIN synesthesialgia.

syn·es·the·si·al·gia (sin′es-the-ze-al′je-a). Sinestesialgia; sinestesia dolorosa. SIN synesthesia algica.

Syn·gam·i·dae (sin-gam′i-de). Família de nematódeos (ordem Strongyloidea) parasitas do sistema respiratório de aves e mamíferos. [ver *Syngamus*]

Syn·gamus (sin′ga-mus). Gênero de nematódeos estrôngilos hematófagos da família Syngamidae.
S. laryngeus, infestação da laringe por nematódeos do gênero *Syngamus*, causando tosse, hemoptise, sensação de corpo estranho e dispnéia.

syn·ga·my (sin′ga-me) Singamia; conjugação dos gametas na fertilização. [syn- + G. *gamos*, casamento]

syn·ge·ne·ic (sin′je-ne′ik). Singênico; relativo a indivíduos geneticamente idênticos. SIN isogeneic, isogenic, isologous, isoplastic, syngenic. [G. *syngenes*, congênito]

syn·gen·e·sis (sin-jen′e-sis). Singênese. SIN sexual reproduction. [syn- + G. *genesis*, origem]

syn·ge·net·ic (sin-je-net′ik). Singenético; relativo à singênese.

syn·gen·ic (sin-jen′ik). Singênico. SIN syngeneic.

syn·gna·thia (sin-nath′e-a). Singnatia; aderência congênita da maxila e mandíbula por faixas fibrosas. [syn- + G. *gnathos*, mandíbula]

syn·graft (sin′graft). Sinenxerto; tecido ou órgão transplantado entre indivíduos geneticamente idênticos. SIN isogeneic graft, isograft, isologous graft, isoplastic graft, syngeneic graft.

syn·i·dro·sis (sin-i-dro′sis). Sinidrose; condição em que a sudorese excessiva faz parte do quadro clínico. [syn- + G. *hidrosis*, sudorese]

syn·i·ze·sis (sin-i-ze′sis). Sinizese. **1.** Fechamento ou obliteração da pupila. **2.** O acúmulo de cromatina em um lado do núcleo, que ocorre habitualmente no início da sinapse. [G. colapso]

syn·kar·y·on (sin-kar′e-on). Sincário; o núcleo formado pela fusão dos dois pró-núcleos na cariogamia. SIN syncaryon. [syn- + G. *karyon*, cerne (núcleo)]

syn·ki·ne·sis (sin-ki-ne′sis). Sincinesia; movimento involuntário que acompanha um voluntário, como movimento de um olho fechado após o do olho descoberto, ou o movimento observado num músculo paralisado que acompanha o movimento em outra parte. SIN syncinesis. [syn- + G. *kinesis*, movimento]

syn·ki·net·ic (sin-ki-net′ik). Sincinético; relativo a, ou caracterizado por, sincinesia.

syn·ne·ma·tin B (sin-e-ma′tin, si-ne′ma-tin). Sinematina B. SIN cephalosporin N.

syn·o·nych·ia (sin-o-nik′e-a). Sinoníquia; fusão de duas ou mais unhas dos dedos, como na sindactilia. [sin- + G. *onyx (onych-)*, unha]

syn·o·nym (sin-o-nim). Sinônimo; em nomenclatura biológica, termo empregado para designar um de dois ou mais nomes para a mesma espécie ou grupo taxonômico (taxon).
objective s., sinônimos objetivos; diferentes nomes para o mesmo organismo, baseado em um e no mesmo tipo de nomenclatura, como nos casos em que uma espécie é transferida de um gênero para outro (p. ex., a transferência de *Diplococcus pneumoniae* para o gênero *Streptococcus* como *Streptococcus pneumoniae*), em contraste com os sinônimos objetivos.
senior s., s. antigo; o primeiro nome publicado entre dois ou mais nomes disponíveis para o mesmo organismo, geralmente utilizado como nome correto (lei da prioridade).
subjective s.'s, sinônimos subjetivos; nomes diferentes, baseados em diferentes tipos de nomenclatura, para organismos originalmente considerados diferentes, mas que depois passaram a ser considerados idênticos ou quase, como questão de opinião pessoal, em contraste com os sinônimos objetivos.

syn·oph·rys (sin-of′ris). Sinofre; hipertrofia e fusão das sobrancelhas. [syn- + G. *ophrys*, sobrancelha]

syn·oph·thal·mia (sin-of-thal′me-a). Sinoftalmia. SIN cyclopia. [sin- + G. *ophthalmos*, olho]

syn·oph·thal·mus (-mus). Sinoftalmia. SIN cyclopia.

syn·op·to·phore (sin-op′to-for). Sinoptóforo; forma modificada de estereoscópio de Wheatstone utilizada no treinamento ortóptico. [syn- + G. *ops*, olho + *phoros*, que conduz]

syn·or·chi·dism, syn·or·chism (sin-or′ki-dizm, sin-or′kizm). Sinorquidismo; fusão congênita dos testículos no abdome ou no escroto. [syn- + G. *orchis* testículo]

syn·os·che·os (sin-os′ke-os). Sinósqueo; aderência parcial ou completa do pênis ou do escroto, uma malformação no hermafroditismo. [syn- + G. *osche*, escroto]

syn·os·te·ol·o·gy (sin-os′te-ol′o-je). Sinosteologia. SIN arthrology. [syn- + G. *osteon*, osso + *logos*, estudo]

syn·os·te·o·sis (sin-os-te-o′sis). Sinostose. SIN synostosis.

syn·os·to·sis (sin-os-to′sis) [TA]. Sinostose; união óssea entre dois ossos que supostamente não são unidos; refere-se comumente à formação de um feixe ósseo entre o rádio e a ulna após fratura desses dois ossos. SIN bony ankylosis, synosteosis, true ankylosis. [syn- + G. *osteon*, osso + -*osis*, condição]
sagittal s., s. sagital. SIN scaphocephaly.
tribasilar s., s. tribasilar; fusão, no início da vida, dos três ossos na base do crânio, resultando em interferência no desenvolvimento do cérebro.

syn·os·tot·ic (sin-os-tot′ik). Sinostótico; relativo à sinostose.

sy·no·tia (si-no′she-a). Sinotia; fusão ou aproximação anormal dos lobos das orelhas na otocefalia. [syn- + G. *ous*, orelha]

syn·o·vec·to·my (sin-o-vek′to-me). Sinovectomia; excisão de parte da membrana sinovial de uma articulação ou de toda ela. [synovia + G. *ektome*, excisão]
radiopharmaceutical s., s. radiofarmacêutica; tratamento de membranas sinoviais anormais por radiação proveniente da instilação, na articulação, de um radiofármaco, como um radioativo.

syn·o·via (si-no′ve-a) [TA], líquido sinovial. SIN synovial *fluid*. [L. mod., uma palavra criada por Paracelsus, do G. *syn*, junto + *oon* (L. *ovum*), ovo]

syn·o·vi·al (si-no′ve-al). Sinovial. **1.** Relativo a, que contém ou que consiste em sinóvia. **2.** Relativo à membrana sinovial.

syn·o·vip·a·rous (sin′o-vip′a-rus). Sinovíparo; que produz sinóvia. [synovia + L. *pario*, produzir]

syn·o·vi·tis (sin-o-vi′tis). Sinovite; inflamação de uma membrana sinovial, especialmente a de uma articulação; em geral, quando não qualificada, significa o mesmo que artrite. [synovia + G. -*itis*, inflamação]
bursal s., bursite. SIN bursitis.
chronic hemorrhagic villous s., s. vilosa hemorrágica crônica. SIN pigmented villonodular s.
dry s., s. seca; sinovite com pouco derrame seroso ou purulento. SIN s. sicca.
filarial s., s. filarial; inflamação sinovial freqüentemente seguida de anquilose fibrótica, devido à presença de microfilárias na articulação.
pigmented villonodular s., s. vilonodular pigmentada; proliferações difusas da membrana sinovial de uma articulação, geralmente o joelho, composta de vilosidades sinoviais e nódulos fibrosos infiltrados por macrófagos contendo hemossiderina e lipídios e por células gigantes multinucleadas; a condição pode ser inflamatória, apesar da tendência à recidiva após remoção incompleta. SIN chronic hemorrhagic villous s.
purulent s., artrite supurativa. SIN suppurative *arthritis*.
serous s., s. serosa; sinovite com grande derrame de líquido não-purulento.
s. sic′ca, s. seca. SIN dry s.
suppurative s., artrite supurativa. SIN suppurative *arthritis*.
tendinous s., tenossinovite. SIN tenosynovitis.

syn·o·vi·um (si-no′ve-um). Sinóvia. SIN synovial *membrane*.

syn·pol·y·dac·ty·ly (sin′pol-e-dak′ti-le). Simpolidactilia; sindactilia e polidactilia associadas.

syn·tac·tics (sin-tak′tiks). Sintática; ramo da semiótica que trata das relações formais entre sinais, da abstração de seu significado e de seus intérpretes. [syn- + G. *taxis*, ordem]

syn·tal·i·ty (sin-tal′i-tē). Sintalidade; o comportamento coerente e previsível de um grupo social. [provavelmente uma condensação de syn- + mentality]

syn·tec·tic (sin-tek′tik). Sintético; relativo a, ou caracterizado por, síntese.

syn·ten·ic (sin-ten′ik). Sintênico; relativo a sintenismo.

syn·te·ny (sin′ten-ē). Sintenismo; a relação entre dois *loci* genéticos (não genes) representada no mesmo par de cromossomas ou (para cromossomas haplóides) no mesmo cromossoma; trata-se mais de uma relação anatômica do que segregacional. [syn- + G. *tainia*, fita]

syn·tex·is (sin-tek′sis). Sintaxe; emaciação ou debilitação. [G. *syn-texis*, fusão]

syn·thase (sin′thās). Sintase; nome trivial utilizado no Enzyme Commission Report para designar uma reação liase na direção inversa (NTP-independente). Quanto às sintases individuais, ver os nomes específicos. VER TAMBÉM synthetase.

syn·ther·mal (sin-ther′mal). Sintérmico; que possui a mesma temperatura. [syn- + G. *thermē*, calor]

syn·the·sis, pl. **syn·the·ses** (sin′thĕ-sis, -sēz). Síntese. **1.** Construção, reunião, composição. **2.** Em química, a formação de compostos pela união de compostos mais simples ou elementos. **3.** Estágio no ciclo celular (cell *cycle*) em que o DNA é sintetizado como estágio preliminar da divisão celular. [G. de *syn*, junto + *thesis*, arranjo]

 s. of continuity, s. de continuidade; cicatrização das bordas de uma ferida ou fratura.

 enzymatic s., s. enzimática; s por enzimas. VER biosynthesis.

 Kiliani-Fischer s., s. de Kiliani-Fischer; procedimento sintético para a extensão da cadeia de átomos de carbono de aldoses mediante tratamento com cianeto; hidrólise das cianoidrinas seguida de redução da lactona produz a aldose homóloga; com esse método, a D-glicose e a D-manose podem ser sintetizadas a partir de D-arabinose.

 Merrifield s., s. de Merrifield; a síntese de peptídeos e proteínas através de um sistema automático em polímeros transportadores.

 protein s., s. de proteínas; o processo em que aminoácidos individuais, seja de origem exógena ou endógena, são unidos um a outro através de ligação peptídica, numa ordem específica determinada pela seqüência de nucleotídeos no DNA; essa seqüência orientadora é transferida para o aparelho de síntese nos ribossomas pelo mRNA, formado pelo pareamento de bases no molde de DNA.

syn·the·size (sin′thĕ-sīz). Sintetizar; produzir algo por síntese, isto é, sinteticamente.

syn·the·tase (sin′thĕ-tās). Sintetase; enzima que catalisa a síntese de uma substância específica. A sintetase é limitada, no *Enzyme Commission Report*, para uso como nome trivial das ligases (EC classe 6); estas, por sua vez, são as enzimas sintetizadoras que exibem a clivagem de uma ligação pirofosfato no ATP ou composto semelhante. A inversão das reações de liase (EC classe 4), produzindo uma síntese, é indicada (em nomes triviais) por sintetase; essas reações não envolvem a clivagem do pirofosfato. Para as sintetases individuais, ver os nomes específicos.

syn·thet·ic (sin-thet′ik). Sintético; relativo a, ou produzido por, síntese.

syn·tho·rax (sin-thōr′aks). Sintórax. SIN thoracopagus.

syn·ton·ic (sin-ton′ik). Sintônico; que possui tom ou temperamento uniforme; traço de personalidade caracterizado por elevado grau de responsividade emocional ao ambiente. [G. *syntonos*, em harmonia, de *syn*, junto + *tonos*, tom]

syn·tro·phism (sin′trō-fizm). Sintrofismo; estado de dependência mútua, com referência ao suprimento de alimentos, de órgãos ou células de uma planta ou animal. [syn- + G. *trophē*, nutrição]

syn·tro·pho·blast (sin-trō′fō-blast, -trof′ō-). Sintrofoblasto. SIN syncytiotrophoblast.

syn·tro·pic (sin-trop′ik). Sintrópico; relativo à sintropia.

syn·tro·py (sin′trō-pē). Sintropia. **1.** Tendência algumas vezes observada em que duas doenças coalescem em uma. **2.** Estado de associação harmoniosa com outras. **3.** Em anatomia, diversas estruturas semelhantes inclinadas numa direção geral; p. ex., os processos espinhosos de uma série de vértebras, as costelas. [syn- + G. *tropē*, uma volta]

 inverse s., s. inversa; situação em que a presença de uma doença tende a diminuir a possibilidade de outra.

syn·zyme (sin′zīm). Sinzima; macromolécula sintética que possui atividade enzimática. SIN enzyme analog.

Sy·pha·cia (si-fā′shē-ă). Gênero de nematódeos oxiurídeos de roedores; *S. obvelata* é o oxiúro cecal de camundongos, e *S. muris*, de ratos. VER TAMBÉM *Aspiculuris tetraptera*. [do L. *siphon*, tubo]

△ **syphil-.** Sifil-. VER syphilo-.

syph·i·le·mia (sif-i-lē′mē-ă). Sifilemia; estado em que o microrganismo específico, *Treponema pallidum*, encontra-se na corrente sanguínea. [syphilis + G. *haima*, sangue]

syph·i·lid (sif′i-lid). Sifílide; termo histórico para qualquer um dos vários tipos de lesões cutâneas e mucosas da sífilis secundária e terciária. SIN syphiloderm, syphiloderma. [syphilis + -*id* (1)]

syph·i·lim·e·try (sif-i-lim′ĕ-trē). Sifilimetria; teste desenvolvido para determinar a intensidade da infecção sifilítica, p. ex., teste sorológico titulado. [syphilis + G. *metron*, medida]

🅘 **syph·i·lis** (sif′i-lis). Sífilis; doença infecciosa e crônica causada pela bactéria *Treponema pallidum* e transmitida por contato direto, geralmente através de relação sexual. Depois de um período de incubação de 12–30 dias, a primeira manifestação consiste no aparecimento de um cancro, seguido de febre baixa e outros sintomas constitucionais (sífilis *primária*), vindo a seguir erupção cutânea de vários aspectos com placas mucosas e linfadenopatia generalizada (sífilis *secundária*) e, subseqüentemente, formação de gomas, infiltração celular e anormalidades funcionais geralmente decorrentes de lesões cardiovasculares e do sistema nervoso central (sífilis *terciária*). SIN lues venerea, malum venereum. [L. mod. *syphilis* (syphilid-), (?) de um poema, *Syphilis sive Morbus Gallicus*, de Fracastorius, em que *Syphilus* é um pastor e o principal personagem.]

 cardiovascular s., s. cardiovascular; comprometimento do sistema cardiovascular observado na s. tardia, resultando geralmente em aortite, formação de aneurisma e insuficiência da valva aórtica.

 congenital s., s. congênita; s. adquirida pelo feto *in utero* e, portanto, presente ao nascimento. SIN hereditary s., s. hereditaria.

 s. d'emblée, s. imediata; s. que ocorre sem cancro inicial. [Fr. imediatamente]

 early s., s. inicial; s. latente primária, secundária ou inicial, antes do aparecimento de qualquer manifestação terciária.

 early latent s., s. latente inicial; infecção por *Treponema pallidum*, o microrganismo causador da sífilis, após regressão das fases primária e secundária, durante o primeiro ano após a infecção, antes do aparecimento de qualquer manifestação de s. terciária.

 endemic s., s. endêmica. SIN nonvenereal s.

 s. heredita'ria, s. hereditária. SIN congenital s.

 s. heredita'ria tar'da, s. hereditária tardia; s. considerada congênita, mas que só se manifesta vários anos após o nascimento.

 hereditary s., s. hereditária. SIN congenital s.

 late s., s. tardia; comprometimento do sistema cardiovascular ou do sistema nervoso central, ou desenvolvimento de goma em qualquer órgão, devido à infecção por *Treponema pallidum*; em geral, dentro de vários anos a 2–3 décadas após a infecção inicial. SIN tertiary s.

 late benign s., s. benigna tardia; sífilis tardia manifestada por evidências sorológicas de infecção, porém sem qualquer manifestação clínica.

 late latent s., s. latente tardia; geralmente infecciosa apenas em mulheres grávidas, que podem transmitir a infecção para o feto.

 latent s., s. latente; infecção por *Treponema pallidum*, após regressão das manifestações da sífilis primária e secundária (ou que nunca foram observadas), antes do aparecimento de qualquer manifestação de sífilis terciária.

 meningovascular s., s. meningovascular; manifestação rara de sífilis secundária ou terciária, caracterizada por inflamação crônica não-supurativa leve das leptomeninges e por angiíte intracraniana ou espinhal.

 nonvenereal s., s. não-venérea; sífilis causada por microrganismos estreitamente relacionados ao *Treponema pallidum*, transmitida por contato pessoal, mas não necessariamente sensual; habitualmente adquirida na infância, mais comum em áreas de pobreza e aglomeração excessiva; rara nos Estados Unidos; inclui framboesia, pinta e bejel. SIN s. endemic s.

 primary s., s. primária; o primeiro estágio da sífilis. VER syphilis.

 quaternary s., s. quaternária. SIN parasyphilis.

 secondary s., s. secundária; o segundo estágio da sífilis. VER syphilis.

 tertiary s., s. terciária. SIN late s.

syph·i·lit·ic (sif-i-lit′ik). Sifilítico; relativo a, causado por ou que sofre de sífilis. SIN luetic.

△ **syphilo-, syphil-, syphili-.** sifilo-; sifil-, sifili-; sífilis. [ver syphilis]

syph·i·lo·derm, syph·i·lo·der·ma (sif′i-lō-derm, -dĕr′mă). Sifiloderma. SIN syphilid. [syphilo- + G. *derma*, pele]

syph·i·loid (sif′i-loyd). Sifilóide; semelhante à sífilis. [syphilo- + G. *eidos*, semelhança]

syph·i·lol·o·gist (sif-i-lol′ō-jist). Sifilologista; especialista no estudo, no diagnóstico e no tratamento da sífilis.

syph·i·lol·o·gy (sif-i-lol′ō-jē). Sifilologia; ramo da ciência médica relacionado com a origem, prevenção e tratamento da sífilis. [syphilo- + G. *logos*, estudo]

syph·i·lo·ma (sif-i-lō′mă). Sifiloma. SIN gumma. [syphilo- + G. -*oma*, tumor]

 s. of Fournier, s. de Fournier. SIN Fournier *disease*.

syr Abreviatura do L. mod. *syrupus*, xarope.

sy·rig·mus (sī-rig′mŭs). Sirigmo. SIN tinnitus aurium. [L. do G. *syrigmos*, silvo]

△ **syring-.** Siring-. VER syringo-.

syr·ing·ad·e·no·ma (sir′ing-ad-ĕ-nō′mă). Siringoadenoma; tumor benigno das glândulas sudoríparas que exibe diferenciação glandular típica de células secretoras. SIN syringoadenoma. [syring- + G. *adēn*, glândula + -*oma*, tumor]

syr·ing·ad·e·no·sus (sir′ing-ad-ĕ-nō′sŭs). Siringadenoso; relativo a glândulas sudoríparas. [L. de syring- + G. *adēn*, glândula]

sy·ringe (sĭ-rĭnj', sĭr'ĭnj). Seringa; instrumento utilizado para a injeção ou retirada de líquidos, constituído de tambor e êmbolo. [G. *syrinx*, tubo]
  air s., s. de ar. SIN chip s.
  chip s., s. de ar; tubo metálico afilado através do qual o ar é forçado a partir de um bulbo de borracha ou tanque de pressão para remover detritos ou para secar uma cavidade no preparo de dentes para restauração. SIN air s.
  control s., s. de controle; tipo de seringa Luer-Lok com anéis para o polegar e o indicador fixados à extremidade proximal do cilindro e à ponta do êmbolo, permitindo a operação da seringa com apenas uma das mãos. SIN ring s.
  Davidson s., s. de Davidson; tubo de borracha, armado com um bocal apropriado, atravessado por um bulbo compressível, com válvulas dispostas de modo que a pressão força o líquido, em que uma das extremidades do tubo está mergulhada, para a extremidade do bocal.
  dental s., s. dentária; s. com estojo metálico carregado por trás ao qual se adapta uma ampola de vidro hermeticamente fechada contendo a solução anestésica.
  fountain s., s. de fonte; aparelho que consiste num reservatório para retenção de líquido, em cujo fundo está fixado um tubo com bocal apropriado; utilizada para injeções vaginais ou retais, irrigação de feridas, etc., sendo a força do fluxo regulada pela altura do reservatório acima do ponto de descarga.
  hypodermic s., s. hipodérmica; pequena s. com um cilindro (que pode ser calibrado), êmbolo perfeitamente ajustado e ponta; utilizada com uma agulha oca para injeções subcutâneas e para aspiração. SIN hypodermic (3).
  Luer s., s. de Luer; s. de vidro com uma ponta de metal e dispositivo de trava para segurar a agulha; utilizada para fins hipodérmicos e intravenosos. SIN Luer-Lok s.
  Luer-Lok s., s. de Luer-Lok. SIN Luer s.
  Neisser s., s. de Neisser; s. uretral utilizada no tratamento da uretrite gonocócica.
  probe s., s. de sonda; s. com ponta em forma de oliva, utilizada no tratamento de doenças das vias lacrimais.
  ring s., s. anular. SIN control s.
  Roughton-Scholander s., s. de Roughton-Scholander. SIN Roughton-Scholander *apparatus.*
  rubber-bulb s., s. com bulbo de borracha; seringa com bulbo de borracha oco e cânula provida de uma válvula de retenção, utilizada para obter um jato de ar ou de água.
sy·rin·ge·al (sĭ-rĭn'jē-ăl). Siríngico; relativo a uma siringe.
sy·rin·gec·to·my (si-rin-jĕk'tō-mē). Siringectomia. SIN fistulectomy. [syring- + G. *ektomē*, excisão]
sy·rin·gi·tis (si-rin-jī'tis). Siringite; inflamação da trompa de Eustáquio. [syring- + G. *-itis*, inflamação]
♻ **syringo-, syring-.** Siringo-, siring-; siringe, fístula, tubo; siringeal. [G. *syrinx*, cano ou tubo]
sy·rin·go·ad·e·no·ma (sĭ-rĭng'gō-ad-ĕ-nō'mă). Siringoadenoma. SIN syringadenoma.
sy·rin·go·bul·bia (sĭ-rĭng'gō-bŭl'bē-ă). Siringobulbia; cavidade do tronco cerebral repleta de líquido, análoga à siringomielia. [syringo- + L. *bulbus*, bulbo (medula oblonga)]
sy·rin·go·car·ci·no·ma (sĭ-rĭng'gō-kar-si-nō'mă). Siringocarcinoma; termo obsoleto para referir-se a uma neoplasia epitelial maligna que sofreu alteração cística (carcinoma cístico). [syringo- + carcinoma]
sy·rin·go·cele (sĭ-rĭng'gō-sēl). Siringocele. 1. SIN central *canal.* 2. Meningomielocele em que existe uma cavidade na medula espinal ectópica. [syringo- + G. *koilia*, uma cavidade]
sy·rin·go·cys·tad·e·no·ma (sĭ-rĭng'gō-sis-tad-ĕ-nō'mă). Siringocistadenoma; tumor cístico benigno das glândulas sudoríparas. [syringo- + cystadenoma]
  s. papillif'erum, s. papilífero; s. caracterizado por numerosas projeções digitiformes de células epiteliais neoplásicas proliferadas em duas camadas sobre um cerne de estroma de tecido conjuntivo fibroso infiltrado por plasmócitos, ocorrendo isoladamente ou como parte de um nevo sebáceo.
sy·rin·go·cys·to·ma (sĭ-rĭng'gō-sis-tō'mă). Siringocistoma. SIN hidrocystoma. [syringo- + cystoma]
sy·rin·go·en·ceph·a·lo·my·e·lia (sĭ-rĭng'gō-en-sef'ă-lō-mī-ē'lē-ă). Siringoencefalomielia; cavidade tubular envolvendo tanto o cérebro quanto a medula espinal e não relacionada, do ponto de vista etiológico, com insuficiência vascular. [syringo- + G. *enkephalos*, cérebro + *myelos*, medula]
sy·rin·goid (sĭ-rĭng'goyd). Siringóide; semelhante a um tubo ou a uma fístula. [syringo- + G. *eidos*, semelhança]
sy·rin·go·ma (si-rĭng-gō'mă). Siringoma; neoplasia benigna, freqüentemente múltipla e algumas vezes eruptiva, dos ductos das glândulas sudoríparas, composta de cistos redondos muito pequenos. [syringo- + G. *-ōma*, tumor]
  chondroid s., s. condróide; tumor benigno das glândulas sudoríparas, com estroma mucóide exibindo metaplasia cartilaginosa. SIN mixed tumor of skin.
sy·rin·go·me·nin·go·cele (sĭ-rĭng'gō-mĕ-ning'gō-sēl). Siringomeningocele; forma de espinha bífida em que o saco dorsal consiste principalmente em membranas, com muito pouca substância medular, envolvendo uma cavidade que se comunica com uma cavidade siringomiélica. [syringo- + meningocele]

sy·rin·go·my·e·lia (sĭ-rĭng'gō-mī-ē'lē-ă). Siringomielia; presença, na medula espinal, de cavidades longitudinais revestidas por tecido gliógeno denso, que não são causadas por insuficiência vascular. A siringomielia caracteriza-se clinicamente por dor e parestesia, seguida de atrofia muscular das mãos e analgesia com termoanestesia das mãos e dos braços, porém com preservação da sensibilidade tátil; posteriormente, caracteriza-se por paroníquias indolores, paralisia espástica nos membros inferiores e escoliose da coluna lombar. Alguns casos estão associados a astrocitomas de baixo grau ou a malformações vasculares da medula espinal. SIN hydrosyringomyelia, Morvan disease, syringomyelus. [syringo- + G. *myelos*, medula]
sy·rin·go·my·e·lo·cele (sĭ-rĭng'gō-mī'ĕ-lō-sēl). Siringomielocele; forma de espinha bífida que consiste em protrusão das membranas e da medula espinal através de um defeito dorsal na coluna vertebral, em que o líquido da siringe da medula está aumentado e expandindo o tecido medular num saco de paredes finas que, a seguir, se expande através do defeito vertebral. [syringo- + myelocele]
si·rin·go·my·e·lus (sĭ-rĭng'gō-mī'ĕ-lus). Siringomielia. SIN syringomyelia. [syringo- + G. *myelos*, medula]
sy·rin·go·pon·tia (sĭ-rĭng'gō-pon'shē-ă). Siringopontia; formação de cavidade na ponte, da mesma natureza que a siringomielia. [syringo- + L. *pons*, ponte]
sy·rin·go·tome (sĭ-rĭn'gō-tōm). Siringótomo. SIN fistulatome.
sy·rin·got·o·my (si-rin-gŏt'ō-mē). Siringotomia. SIN fistulotomy.
syr·inx, pl. **sy·ring·es** (sĭr'ĭngks, sĭ-rĭn'jēz). Siringe. 1. Sinônimo raramente utilizado de fístula. 2. Cavidade tubular patológica no cérebro ou na medula espinal. [G. tubo, canal]
sy·ro·sing·o·pine (sĭr-ō-sĭng'gō-pēn). Sirosingopina; preparado da reserpina por hidrólise e reesterificação; agente anti-hipertensivo com ações semelhantes às da reserpina.
syr·up (sĕr'ŭp, sĭr'ŭp). Xarope. 1. Melado refinado; solução de sacarina não-cristalizável que permanece após a refinação do açúcar. 2. Qualquer líquido doce; solução de açúcar em água, em qualquer proporção. 3. Preparação líquida de substâncias medicinais ou aromatizantes em solução aquosa concentrada de um açúcar, habitualmente sacarose; outros polióis, como a glicerina ou sorbitol, podem estar presentes para retardar a cristalização da sacarose e, assim, aumentar a solubilidade dos ingredientes adicionados. Quando o xarope contém uma substância medicinal, denomina-se xarope medicamentoso; embora um xarope tenha tendência a resistir à contaminação por fungos ou bactérias (devido a seu conteúdo muito elevado [aproximadamente 85%] de sacarose), pode conter agentes antimicrobianos para evitar o crescimento de bactérias e fungos. SIN sirup, syrupus. [L. mod. *syrupus*, do Ár. *sharāb*]
  ipecac s., x. de ipeca; preparação medicinal líquida adoçada contendo extrato de ipeca em pó, incluindo os alcalóides emitina e cefalina; utilizado como emético em certos casos de envenenamento e (em doses menores) como expectorante.
syr·u·pus (syr) (sĭr'ŭ-pŭs). Xarope. SIN syrup. [L. mod.]
syr·upy (sĕr'ŭ-pē, sĭr'). Xaroposo; relativo a xarope; da consistência do xarope.
sys·sar·co·sic (sis'ar-kō-sik). Sissarcósico. SIN syssarcotic.
sys·sar·co·sis (sis'ar-kō'sis). Sissarcose; articulação muscular; união de ossos por músculo; p. ex., nos seres humanos, as conexões musculares da patela. [G. *syssarkōsis, crescimento* carnoso excessivo, de *syn*, com + *sarx*, carne]
sys·sar·cot·ic (sis'ar-kot'ik). Sissarcódico; relativo a, ou caracterizado por, sissarcose. SIN syssarcosic.

SYSTEM

ℹ **sys·tem** (sis'tĕm). Sistema. 1. [TA]. Conjunto consistente e complexo constituído de partes correlacionadas e semi-independentes. Complexo de estruturas anatômicas funcionalmente relacionadas. 2. O organismo como um todo visto como uma complexa organização de partes. 3. Qualquer complexo de estruturas anatomicamente relacionadas (p. ex., sistema vascular) ou funcionalmente relacionadas (p. ex., sistema digestivo). 4. Esquema de teoria médica. VER TAMBÉM apparatus, classification. 5. S. seguido de uma ou mais letras indica transportadores de aminoácidos específicos; o s. N é um transportador sódio-dependente de aminoácidos específicos, como L-glutamina, L-asparagina e L-histidina; s. y$^+$ é um transportador sódio-independente de aminoácidos catiônicos. SIN systema [TA]. [G. *systēma*, um todo organizado]
  absolute s. of units, s. absoluto de unidades; sistema baseado em unidades absolutas aceitas como fundamentais (comprimento, massa, tempo) e das quais são derivadas outras unidades (força, energia ou trabalho, potência); esses sistemas em uso comum são os sistemas pé-libra-segundo, centímetro-grama-segundo e metro-quilograma-segundo.
  absorbent s., s. absorvente. SIN lymphoid s.
  alimentary s. [TA], s. alimentar; trajeto digestivo desde a boca até o ânus, com todas as suas glândulas e órgãos associados. SIN systema digestorium [TA],

alimentary apparatus, apparatus digestorius, digestive apparatus, digestive s., systema alimentarium.

anterolateral s., s. ântero-lateral; feixe composto de fibras, localizado na parte ventrolateral do funículo lateral, contendo fibras espinotalâmicas, espino-hipotalâmicas, espinorreticulares e espinomesencefálicas (espinotectais, espinhais para a substância cinzenta periaquedutal, etc.); ocupa as áreas combinadas da substância branca espinal historicamente dividida em tratos espinotalâmicos anterior e lateral; localizado na substância branca ventral ao ligamento denticulado, daí a base anatômica da cordotomia ântero-lateral; relacionado com a transmissão da informação nociceptiva e térmica e com o tato não-discriminativo. VER TAMBÉM spinothalamic *tract*. SIN anterolateral tract, tractus anterolaterales.

arch-loop-whorl s. (ALW), s. do arco-alça-verticilo. VER Galton system of classification of *fingerprints*, under *fingerprint*.

association s., s. de associação; grupos ou tratos de fibras nervosas que interconectam diferentes regiões de uma e da mesma grande subdivisão do sistema nervoso central, como as várias áreas do córtex cerebral e os vários segmentos da medula espinal.

autonomic nervous s. (ANS), s. nervoso autônomo (SNA). SIN autonomic division of nervous system.

Bethesda s., s. Bethesda, s. para relatar os achados citológicos cervicais ou diagnóstico. SIN Bethesda classification. [*Bethesda*, Maryland, local do NIH]

George Papanicolaou dividiu os achados citológicos em esfregaços cervicais corados em cinco classes, de I (normal) a V (carcinoma). As classes II–IV representavam graus crescentes de atipia pré-maligna das células escamosas. Posteriormente, o sistema foi modificado por pesquisadores, com a introdução dos termos displasia (leve, moderada, grave) e neoplasia intra-epitelial cervical (*CIN, cervical intraepithelial neoplasia*) (graus 1–3). Os achados dos esfregaços de Pap relatados com base nessa nomenclatura apresentavam pouca reprodutibilidade entre observadores e, até mesmo, entre leituras separadas pelo mesmo observador. Além disso, havia pouca correlação entre categorias diagnósticas e opções de tratamento. Em 1988, o *National Cancer Institute* patrocinou um *workshop* em Bethesda, Maryland, para desenvolver um sistema mais útil. O sistema Bethesda foi utilizado pela primeira vez em 1991 e, hoje em dia, tornou-se o padrão em todo o mundo. Esse sistema substitui as designações numéricas por diagnósticos descritivos de alterações celulares. O quadro anexo compara o sistema de Bethesda com classificações

	sistema nervoso autônomo			
órgão	função do sistema nervoso simpático	nervo(s) simpático(s)	função do sistema nervoso parassimpático	nervo(s) parassimpático(s)
olho	dilatação da pupila, contração do músculo ciliar para acomodação	fibras pós-ganglionares do gânglio cervical superior (nervo carótico interno)	constrição da pupila	fibras pós-ganglionares do gânglio ciliar através dos nervos ciliares curtos
glândula lacrimal	leve ou sem efeito	fibras pós-ganglionares do gânglio cervical superior (nervo carótico externo)	secreção	fibras pós-ganglionares do gânglio pterigopalatino através do nervo zigomaticotemporal
glândulas salivares	secreção espessa viscosa	nervo carótico externo	secreção aquosa abundante	fibras pós-ganglionares do gânglio submandibular e gânglio ótico
coração	aumento da freqüência e da força dos batimentos cardíacos, dilatação dos vasos coronários (indiretamente?), redução do tempo de condução	nervos cardíaco cervical e cardíaco torácico	contração dos vasos coronários (indiretamente?), aumento do tempo de condução	fibras pós-ganglionares dos gânglios terminal/intermural através do nervo vago
pulmões	broncodilatação, inibição da secreção	nervos pulmonares	constrição brônquica, estimulação da secreção	fibras pós-ganglionares dos gânglios terminal/intramural através do nervo vago
trato digestório	inibição peristáltica, vasoconstrição	nervos esplâncnicos maior, menor, imo e ramos dos gânglios celíaco, mesentérico superior e mesentérico inferior	estimulação do peristaltismo e da secreção	fibras pós-ganglionares dos gânglios terminal/intermural através dos nervos valgo e pélvico
fígado e vesícula biliar	Liberação de glicose	ramos do gânglio celíaco	excreção de bile	fibras pós-ganglionares dos gânglios terminal/intramural através do nervo vago
medula supra-renal	secreção de adrenalina	nervo esplâncnico menor	nenhuma conexão	nenhum nervo
rim	vasoconstrição, inibição da formação de urina	ramos do gânglio córtico-renal	nenhum efeito (?)	nenhum nervo
Bexiga	retenção de urina	ramos do gânglio mesentérico inferior (através do plexo hipogástrico)	liberação de urina	fibras pós-ganglionares dos gânglios terminal/intramural através dos nervos pélvicos
genitália	ejaculação	ramos do gânglio mesentérico inferior (através do plexo hipogástrico)	ereção do pênis e do clitóris	fibras pós-ganglionares dos gânglios terminal/intramural através dos nervos pélvicos
glândulas sudoríparas	secreção	fibras pós-ganglionares dos gânglios da cadeia simpática	nenhuma conexão	nenhum nervo
vasos sanguíneos periféricos	constrição do músculo liso	fibras pós-ganglionares dos gânglios da cadeia simpática	nenhuma conexão, à exceção de dilatação na área genital	nenhum nervo
músculo esquelético	constrição dos músculos lisos nos vasos sanguíneos	fibras pós-ganglionares dos gânglios da cadeia simpática	dilatação	nenhum nervo

anteriores. O formato padronizado para relatar os achados de citologia cervical de acordo com o sistema Bethesda compreende três elementos: 1) estado de adequação da amostra (satisfatória, não-satisfatória ou satisfatória, porém limitada, p. ex., pela ausência de células endocervicais); 2) categorização geral (dentro de limites normais, alterações celulares benignas ou anormalidade das células epiteliais); e 3) diagnóstico descritivo, elaborado na categorização geral e incluindo a menção de todas as anormalidades significativas, bem como o estado hormonal da paciente (quando existem células vaginais no esfregaço). As alterações celulares benignas incluem aquelas causadas por infecção (*Candida, Trichomonas*, herpes simples), atrofia, radioterapia ou presença de DIU. As anormalidades das células epiteliais podem envolver células escamosas ou glandulares. As células escamosas anormais de importância indeterminada (ASCUS, *abnormal squamous cells of undetermined significance*) mostram atipia celular, porém nenhuma evidência bem definida de alteração pré-maligna. Cerca de 20% das mulheres com ASCUS acabam desenvolvendo lesões intra-epiteliais escamosas ou carcinoma invasivo. As alterações das células escamosas antigamente denominadas displasia leve ou CIN 1 (incluindo atipia celular característica da infecção por papilomavírus humano) são atualmente designadas como lesão intra-epitelial escamosa de baixo grau. A categoria de lesão intra-epitelial escamosa de alto grau engloba o que antigamente era denominado displasia moderada e grave ou CIN 2 e CIN 3. As anormalidades das células glandulares são categorizadas de modo semelhante.

blood group s.'s, sistemas de grupo sanguíneo. Ver apêndice de Grupos Sanguíneos.
blood-vascular s., s. vascular sanguíneo. SIN cardiovascular s.
bulbosacral s., s. bulbossacral. SIN parasympathetic *part* of autonomic division of peripheral nervous system.
cardiovascular s. [TA], s. cardiovascular; o coração e os vasos sanguíneos considerados como um todo. SIN systema cardiovasculare [TA], blood-vascular s.
caudal neurosecretory s., s. neurossecretor caudal; uro-hipófise.
centimeter-gram-second s. (CGS, cgs), s. centímetro-grama-segundo (CGS, cgs); o s. científico de expressão das unidades físicas fundamentais de comprimento, massa e tempo e as unidades delas derivadas, em centímetros, gramas e segundos; atualmente, está sendo substituído pelo Sistema Internacional de Unidades, baseado no metro, quilograma e segundo.
central nervous s. (CNS) [TA], s. nervoso central (SNC); o cérebro e a medula espinal. SIN pars centralis systematis nervosi [TA], systema nervosum centrale*.
cerebrospinal s., s. cerebroespinal; o sistema nervoso central e sistema nervoso periférico combinados.
charge transfer s., s. de transferência de carga. SIN charge transfer *complex*.
chromaffin s., s. cromafin; as células do corpo que se coram com sais de cromo e ocorrem na parte medular da supra-renal, paragânglios e em relação a determinados nervos simpáticos.
circulatory s., s. circulatório. SIN vascular s.
closed s., s. fechado; s. em que não há troca de material, energia ou informação com o ambiente.
colloid s., s. colóide; combinação das duas fases, interna e externa, de uma solução colóide; os vários sistemas são: gás + líquido (espuma); gás + sólido (magnesita); líquido + gás (*fog*); sólido + gás (fumaça); sólido + líquido (sol); líquido + sólido (gel); líquido + líquido (emulsão); sólido + sólido (vidro colorido).
complement s., s. complemento; um grupo de mais de 20 proteínas séricas, algumas das quais são seriadamente ativadas e participam numa cascata, resultando em lise celular; o s. complemento também atua na quimiotaxia, opsonização e fagocitose.

sistema Bethesda

classe de Papanicolaou	displasia	CIN	categoria Bethesda
I–II	negativa	negativa	dentro de limites normais
III	—	—	ASCUS
III	leve	1	LGSIL
III	moderada	2	HGSIL
IV	grave	3	HGSIL
IV	carcinoma *in situ*	3	HGSIL
V	carcinoma	carcinoma	carcinoma

conducting s. of heart [TA], s. de condução do coração; o s. de fibras musculares modificadas atípicas que compreende o nó sinoatrial, o nó e o fascículo atrioventriculares, os ramos direito e esquerdo e suas ramificações subendocárdicas terminais (rede de Purkinje). SIN complexus stimulans cordis [TA], systema conducens cordis*.
craniosacral nervous s., s. nervoso craniossacral. SIN parasympathetic *part of autonomic division of peripheral nervous system.*
cytochrome s., s. citocromo. SIN respiratory *chain*.

cytochrome P-450 s., s. citocromo P-450; grupo heterogêneo de enzimas que catalisam diversas reações oxidativas no fígado, intestino, rim, pulmão e sistema nervoso central humanos; essas enzimas estão envolvidas no metabolismo de numerosos substratos endógenos e exógenos, incluindo drogas, toxinas, hormônios e produtos vegetais naturais. As enzimas do citocromo P-450 são classificadas com base na sua estrutura química (seqüência de aminoácidos). Cada enzima recebe a designação de CYP seguido de um algarismo indicando a família a que pertence, uma letra para a subfamília e, algumas vezes, um segundo algarismo para a enzima individual.

O constante aumento no número e na variedade de agentes farmacêuticos disponíveis para o tratamento de infecções, afecções degenerativas e malignas, transtornos mentais e outras doenças levou à polifarmácia, com seus riscos associados de interações farmacológicas indesejáveis. As alterações na função do sistema do citocromo P-450 estão sendo cada vez mais reconhecidas como importantes causas dessas interações. Quando uma droga aumenta a formação de uma enzima P-450, outras drogas metabolizadas por esta enzima são eliminadas mais rapidamente, podendo não produzir os efeitos terapêuticos desejados. Por outro lado, uma droga que inibe a atividade enzimática P-450 pode retardar o metabolismo de drogas que atuam como substrato, com conseqüente elevação dos níveis séricos e teciduais e aumento dos efeitos da droga, incluindo efeitos colaterais. Em geral, a inibição envolve uma competição entre drogas pelo mesmo sítio de ligação numa molécula de enzima. A inibição reversível constitui o mecanismo mais comum de interações farmacológicas envolvendo o sistema P-450. Em geral, as drogas competem por uma isoenzima P-450 específica. Exemplos de agentes que causam interações através de inibição reversível incluem: fluoroquinolonas, antibióticos, cimetidina, cetoconazol e inibidores da protease utilizados no tratamento da AIDS/SIDA. A CYP3A, a mais abundante das enzimas do citocromo P-450 humano, é responsável por 30% das enzimas encontradas no fígado. Seus substratos incluem numerosos medicamentos psicoativos, cetoconazol, eritromicina e inibidores da protease. Essa enzima é inibida por alguns antidepressivos, antifúngicos azóis, cimetidina, eritromicina e outras drogas. A formação aumentada da CYP3A é induzida pela carbamazepina, fenobarbital, fenitoína e rifampicina. Diferenças étnicas na expressão de CYP2D6 explicam por que os indivíduos brancos têm mais tendência do que os negros e asiáticos a sofrer intoxicação em decorrência do acúmulo e dos níveis séricos excessivos de drogas metabolizadas por essa enzima, como antidepressivos tricíclicos, ISRS, antipsicóticos e beta-bloqueadores.

digestive s., s. digestório. SIN alimentary s.
ecological s., s. ecológico. SIN ecosystem s.
electron-transport s., s. de transporte de elétrons. SIN respiratory *chain*.
endocrine s., s. endócrino. SIN endocrine *glands*, em *gland*.
endomembrane s., s. endomembrana. SIN endoplasmic *reticulum*.
esthesiodic s., s. estesiódico; sistema de neurônios e tratos na medula espinal e no cérebro que servem à sensação.
exterofective s., s. exterofectivo; nome aplicado por Cannon ao sistema nervoso somático, oposto ao sistema interfectivo ou autônomo.
extrapyramidal motor s., s. motor extrapiramidal; literalmente: todas as estruturas do cérebro que afetam o movimento do corpo (somático), excluindo os neurônios motores, o córtex motor e o trato piramidal (corticobulbar e corticospinal). A despeito de sua conotação literal muito ampla, o termo é utilizado mais freqüentemente para designar em particular o corpo estriado (gânglios da base), suas estruturas associadas (substância negra, núcleo subtalâmico) e suas conexões descendentes com o mesencéfalo.
feedback s., s. de retroalimentação; (1) um complexo de circuitos neuronais em que uma parte da via eferente retorna à eferente para modular sua atividade, atuando, assim, como orientador do sistema; (2) VER feedback.
foot-pound-second s. (FPS, fps), s. pé-libra-segundo; s. de unidades absolutas baseadas no pé, na libra e no segundo.
gamma motor s., s. motor gama. SIN gamma *loop*.
genital s. [TA], s. genital; o complexo s. que consiste nas gônadas masculinas ou femininas, ductos associados e genitália externa dedicados à função de reproduzir a espécie. SIN systema genitalia [TA], reproductive s.

genitourinary s., s. genitourinário. SIN urogenital s.
geographic information s., s. de informações geográficas; s. computadorizado que combina habilidades cartográficas com processamento de dados eletrônicos para produzir rapidamente mapas para uso em estudos epidemiológicos.
glandular s., s. glandular; todas as glândulas do corpo.
haversian s., s. de Havers. SIN osteon.
health information s., s. de informações sanitárias; combinação de dados estatísticos vitais e sanitários de múltiplas fontes, utilizados para obter informações acerca das necessidades e recursos sanitários, uso de serviços sanitários e resultados de seu uso pela pessoa numa região ou jurisdição específica.
hematopoietic s., s. hematopoético; os órgãos formadores de sangue; no embrião em diferentes idades, esses órgãos consistem no saco vitelino, fígado, timo, baço, linfonodos e medula óssea; após o nascimento, são constituídos principalmente pela medula óssea, baço, timo e linfonodos.
hepatic portal s., s. porta hepático; sistema porta venoso, em que a veia porta recebe sangue, através de suas tributárias, dos capilares da maioria das vísceras abdominais e drena nos sinusóides hepáticos.
heterogeneous s., s. heterogêneo; em química, sistema que contém várias partes ou fases distintas e mecanicamente separáveis; p. ex., uma suspensão ou emulsão.
hexaxial reference s., s. de referência hexaxial; a figura obtida quando linhas de derivação das derivações unipolares dos membros do eletrocardiograma são adicionadas ao sistema de referência triaxial.
His-Tawara s., s. de His-Tawara; o complexo sistema de fibras de Purkinje entrelaçadas dentro do miocárdio ventricular. VER TAMBÉM conducting s. of heart.
homogeneous s., s. homogêneo; em química, sistema cujas partes não podem ser mecanicamente separadas, sendo, portanto, uniforme, exibindo, em cada parte, propriedades físicas idênticas; p. ex., uma solução de cloreto em água.
hypophyseoportal s., s. porta hipofisário. SIN portal hypophysial circulation.
hypophysial portal s., s. porta hipofisário. SIN portal hypophysial circulation.
hypophysioportal s., s. porta hipofisário. SIN portal hypophysial circulation.
hypothalamohypophysial portal s., s. porta hipotálamo-hipofisário; **(1)** SIN portal hypophysial circulation; **(2)** SIN renal portal s.
hypoxia warning s., s. de alarme de hipoxia; dispositivo projetado para produzir um sinal auditivo ou visual em um nível predeterminado de pressão parcial de oxigênio; a situação ideal seria que o sistema desse o alarme de hipoxia iminente a tempo para serem tomadas medidas corretivas.
immune s., s. imune; complexo intrincado de componentes celulares, moleculares e genéticos inter-relacionados que proporcionam uma defesa (resposta imune) contra substâncias ou organismos estranhos e células nativas aberrantes.
indicator s., s. indicador; em testes imunológicos *in vitro*, associação de reagentes utilizados para determinar o grau de combinação dos reagentes imunológicos (p. ex., eritrócitos sensibilizados em testes de fixação do complemento; enzima e substrato em ensaios imunoabsorventes ligados a enzimas).

information s., s. de informação; combinação de dados estatísticos vitais e sanitários de múltiplas fontes, utilizados para obter informações e tomar decisões sobre as necessidades e recursos sanitários, custos, uso e resultados da assistência sanitária.
integumentary s., s. tegumentar. SIN integument.
intermediary s., s. intermediário. SIN interstitial *lamella*.
International S. of Units, Sistema Internacional de Unidades. SIN International System of Units.
interofective s., s. interofectivo; termo aplicado por W. Cannon ao sistema nervoso autônomo, em oposição ao sistema nervoso somático ou sistema exterofectivo.
involuntary nervous s., s. nervoso involuntário. SIN autonomic *division* of nervous system.
kallikrein s., s. da calicreína; sistema sérico do sangue, cuja atividade é iniciada pelo fator XII (fator de Hageman), levando à produção do ativador précalicreína e, a seguir, da calicreína que, após ativação pela plasmina, libera a bradicinina do cininogênio.
kinetic s., s. cinético; **(1)** termo proposto por G.W. Crile para designar cadeia de órgãos através dos quais a energia latente é transformada em movimento e calor: inclui o cérebro, a tireóide, as supra-renais, o fígado, o pâncreas e os músculos; **(2)** a parte do sistema neuromuscular em que os movimentos ativos são afetados; diferenciado do sistema estático.
limbic s., s. límbico; termo coletivo para referir-se a um conjunto heterogêneo de estruturas cerebrais na borda (limbo) da parede medial do hemisfério cerebral ou próximo a ela, em particular o hipocampo, a amígdala e o *gyrus fornicatus*; o termo é freqüentemente utilizado para incluir também as interconexões dessas estruturas, bem como suas conexões com a área septal, o hipotálamo e uma zona medial do tegmento mesencefálico. Através destas últimas conexões, o s. límbico exerce uma importante influência sobre os sistemas endócrino e motor autônomo; suas funções também parecem afetar os estados de motivação e o humor. SIN visceral brain.
linnaean s. of nomenclature, s. de nomenclatura de Linné; o s. de nomenclatura em que os nomes das espécies são constituídos de duas partes: um nome genérico e um epíteto específico (nome da espécie, em botânica). SIN binary nomenclature, binomial nomenclature. [Carl von *Linné*]
lymphatic s., s. linfático. SIN lymphoid s.
lymphoid s. [TA], s. linfóide; consiste em vasos linfáticos, linfonodos e tecido linfóide; deságua nas veias ao nível da abertura superior do tórax. SIN systema lymphoideum [TA], absorbent s., lymphatic s., systema lymphaticum.
s. of macrophages, s. de macrófagos. SIN mononuclear phagocyte s.
masticatory s., s. mastigatório; os órgãos e as estruturas que funcionam primariamente na mastigação: a mandíbula, a maxila, os dentes com suas estruturas de sustentação, a articulação temporomandibular, os músculos da mastigação, a língua, os lábios, as bochechas e a mucosa oral. SIN dental apparatus, masticatory apparatus (1).
metameric nervous s., s. nervoso metamérico; parte do s. nervoso que inerva estruturas do corpo desenvolvidas, na ontogenia, a partir dos somitos de disposição segmentar ou, na região da cabeça, dos arcos branquiais. O termo fornece uma referência aos mecanismos neurais intrínsecos da medula espinal e do tronco cerebral (representado pelos núcleos sensitivos, grupos de células neuronais motores e seus interneurônios associados na formação reticular); por definição estrita, deve excluir o s. nervoso autônomo.
meter-kilogram-second s., s. metro-quilograma-segundo; sistema absoluto baseado no metro, no quilograma e no segundo; constitui a base do Sistema Internacional de Unidades.
metric s., s. métrico; sistema de pesos e medidas, universal para uso científico, baseado no metro, que originalmente era considerado um décimo milionésimo de um quadrante do meridiano da terra, sendo atualmente baseado no comprimento atravessado pela luz no vácuo em determinado período de tempo (ver metro). Os prefixos do metro (e outros padrões) refletem frações ou múltiplos do metro e são idênticos ao sistema internacional de unidades (q.v.). A unidade de peso é o grama, que é o peso de um centímetro cúbico de água, equivalente a 15,432358 grãos. A unidade de volume é o litro ou um decímetro cúbico, igual a 1,056688 quartos de líquido U.S.; um centímetro cúbico corresponde a cerca de 16,23073 mínimos U.S.
mononuclear phagocyte s. (MPS), s. fagocítico mononuclear; conjunto amplamente distribuído de macrófagos livres e fixos derivados de células precursoras da medula óssea através de monócitos; sua atividade fagocítica significativa é mediada por imunoglobulinas e pelo sistema de complemento sérico. Tanto no tecido conjuntivo quanto no tecido linfóide, podem ocorrer na forma de macrófagos livres e fixos; nos sinusóides hepáticos, na forma de células de Kupffer; no pulmão, na forma de macrófagos alveolares; e, no sistema nervoso, como micróglia. SIN s. of macrophages.
muscular s., s. muscular; todos os músculos do corpo coletivamente.
nervous s. [TA], s. nervoso; todo o aparelho nervoso, composto de uma parte central, o cérebro e a medula espinal, e de uma parte periférica, os nervos cranianos e espinais, os gânglios autônomos e os plexos. SIN systema nervosum [TA].

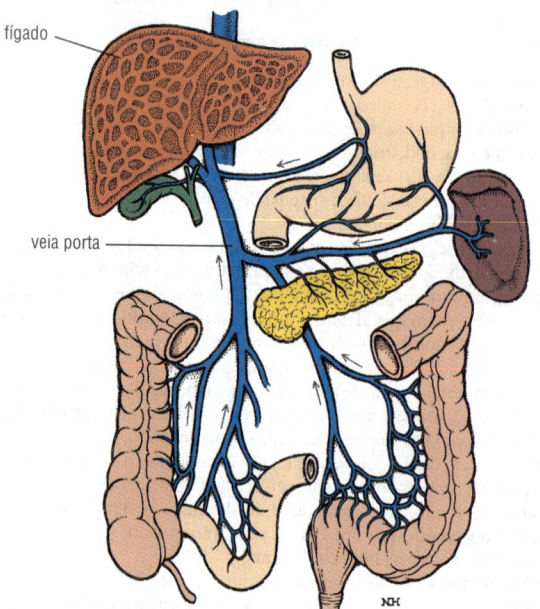

sistema porta hepático

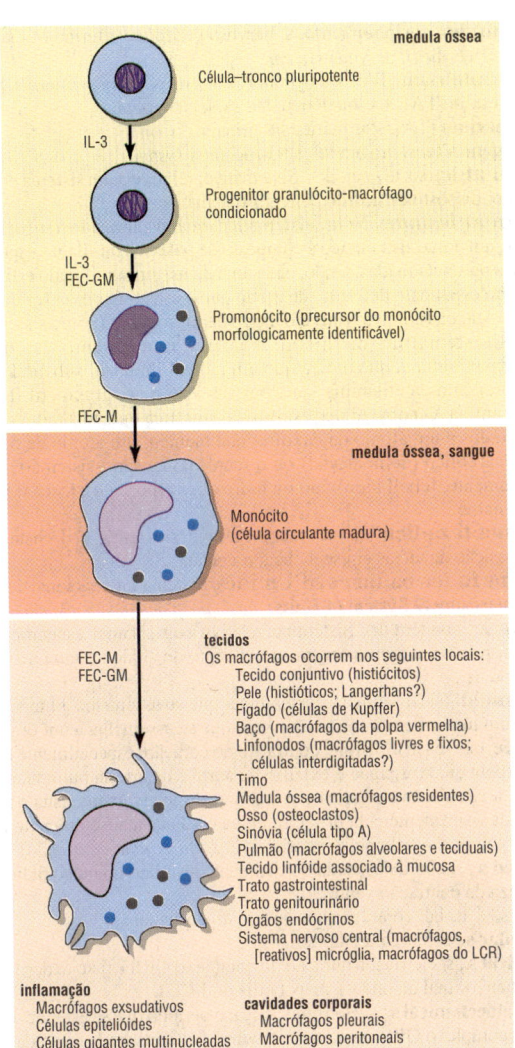

células que pertencem ao **sistema fagocítico mononuclear**: IL = interleucina; FEC–GM = fator de estimulação de colônias de granulócitos-macrófagos

---

neuromuscular s., s. neuromuscular; os músculos do corpo coletivamente e os nervos que os suprem.
nonspecific s., s. inespecífico. SIN reticular activating s.
occlusal s., s. oclusal; forma ou projeto e disposição das unidades oclusais e incisais de uma dentição ou dos dentes numa dentadura. SIN occlusal scheme.
oculomotor s., s. oculomotor; parte do sistema nervoso central relacionada com os movimentos oculares; é composta de vias que conectam várias regiões do cérebro, tronco cerebral e núcleos oculares, utilizando articulações multissinápticas.
open s., s. aberto; sistema em que ocorre troca contínua de material, de energia e informações com o ambiente.
O-R s., s. O-R; abreviatura do sistema de oxidação-redução.
oxidation-reduction s. (O-R s.), s. de oxidação-redução; sistema enzimático existente nos tecidos, através do qual a oxidação e a redução ocorrem simultaneamente através da transferência de hidrogênio ou de um ou mais elétrons de um metabólito para outro. VER TAMBÉM oxidation-reduction. SIN redox s.
parasympathetic nervous s., s. nervoso parassimpático. SIN parasympathetic *part* of autonomic division of peripheral nervous system, autonomic *division* of nervous system.
pedal s., s. podálico; fibras eferentes que conectam o proencéfalo com estruturas mais caudais.
periodic s., s. periódico; a disposição dos elementos químicos numa ordem definida, conforme indicado pelos seus respectivos números atômicos, de tal modo que grupos de elementos com propriedades químicas semelhantes (número de elétrons da camada de valência semelhante) são agrupados juntos. VER Mendeléeff *law*.
peripheral nervous s. [TA], s. nervoso periférico; a parte periférica do sistema nervoso externa ao cérebro e à medula espinal, desde suas raízes até suas terminações periféricas. Inclui os gânglios, tanto sensitivos quanto autônomos, bem como quaisquer plexos através dos quais passam as fibras nervosas. VER TAMBÉM autonomic *division* of nervous system. SIN pars peripherica systematis nervosi [TA], systema nervosum periphericum *, peripheral part of nervous system.
Pinel s., s. de Pinel; abolição da contenção à força no tratamento do paciente mental hospitalar.
portal s., s. porta; s. de vasos em que o sangue, após atravessar um leito capilar, é conduzido através de uma segunda rede capilar, como no sistema porta hepático, no qual o sangue proveniente do intestino passa através dos sinusóides hepáticos.
pressoreceptor s., s. pressorreceptor; as áreas pressorreceptoras que, com suas fibras aferentes e conexões com o sistema autônomo, reagem a uma elevação da pressão arterial e servem para tamponá-la ao inibirem a freqüência cardíaca e o tônus vascular. VER TAMBÉM baroreceptor.
projection s., s. de projeção; o s. de axônios que conduzem estímulos de uma parte do sistema nervoso para outras partes.
properdin s., s. da properdina; s. imunológico que constitui a via alternativa do complemento, constituído de várias proteínas distintas que reagem de modo seriado e ativam C3 (terceiro componente do complemento), aparentemente sem utilizar os componentes C1, C4 e C2; além da properdina, o sistema inclui os Fatores B, D, H e I. O sistema pode ser ativado, na ausência de anticorpo específico, por endotoxinas bacterianas; por uma variedade de polissacarídeos e lipopolissacarídeos, e por um componente do veneno de *naja*.
Purkinje s., s. de Purkinje. SIN subendocardial conducting s. of heart.
redox s., s. redox. SIN oxidation-reduction s.
renal portal s., s. porta renal; s. porta arterial em que as arteríolas glomerulares eferentes recebem sangue dos capilares dos glomérulos renais e o transportam até o plexo capilar peritubular que circunda os túbulos contornados proximais e distais. SIN hypothalamohypophysial portal s. (2).
renin-angiotensin s., s. de renina-angiotensina; regulador seletivo da via de biossíntese da aldosterona; atua através de aumento da produção de aldosterona e retenção de sódio em decorrência da depleção de volume, com conseqüente aumento da produção de renina no rim e conversão, no plasma, da angiontensina I em angiotensina II.
renin-angiotensin-aldosterone s., s. renina-angiotensina-aldosterona; os hormônios renina, angiotensina e aldosterona atuam em conjunto para regular a pressão arterial. A ocorrência de uma queda persistente da pressão arterial determina a liberação de renina pelo rim. Esse processo leva à formação de angiotensina na circulação. A seguir, a angiotensina eleva diretamente a pressão arterial por constrição arteriolar e estimula a glândula supra-renal a produzir aldosterona, que promove a retenção de sódio e de água no rim, com conseqüente aumento do volume sanguíneo e da pressão arterial.
reproductive s., s. reprodutor. SIN genital s.
respiratory s. [TA], s. respiratório; todas as passagens de ar do nariz até os alvéolos pulmonares. SIN systema respiratorium [TA], apparatus respiratorius, respiratory apparatus.
reticular activating s. (RAS), s. de ativação reticular; termo fisiológico designativo da parte da formação reticular do tronco encefálico que desempenha um papel central no estado de alerta orgânico e comportamental do organismo; estende-se como um aparelho neural difusamente organizado através da região central do tronco encefálico até o subtálamo e os núcleos intralaminares do tálamo; através de suas conexões ascendentes, afeta a função do córtex cerebral no sentido de responsividade comportamental; suas conexões descendentes (reticulospinais) transmitem sua influência ativadora sobre a postura corporal e os mecanismos reflexos (p. ex., tônus muscular), em parte através dos neurônios motores gama. VER TAMBÉM reticular *formation*. SIN nonspecific s.
reticuloendothelial s. (RES), s. reticuloendotelial (SRE); conjunto de supostos macrófagos, descritos pela primeira vez por Aschoff, que incluía a maioria dos macrófagos verdadeiros (agora classificados como sistema fagocítico mononuclear) e as células que revestem os sinusóides do baço, dos linfonodos e da medula óssea, bem como as células reticulares fibroblásticas dos tecidos hematopoéticos; todas estas últimas células são apenas fracamente fagocíticas e não constituem macrófagos verdadeiros. O termo persiste na literatura e, com freqüência, é utilizado como sinônimo do sistema fagocítico mononuclear.
second signaling s., s. de sinalização secundária; termo de Pavlov para a fala, em que as palavras são consideradas os "sinais secundários" capazes de produzir respostas condicionadas.
skeletal s. [TA], s. esquelético; os ossos e as cartilagens do corpo. SIN systema skeletale [TA].
somesthetic s., s. somestésico; dados sensoriais provenientes da pele, dos músculos e dos órgãos do corpo, em contraste com aqueles derivados dos cinco sentidos especiais.
static s., s. estático; a parte do sistema neuromuscular que faz o organismo animal ser mantido em postura e equilíbrio, neutralizando as forças da gravidade e da pressão atmosférica; distinto do sistema cinético (2).

stomatognathic s., s. estomatognático; todas as estruturas envolvidas na fala e na recepção, na mastigação e na deglutição do alimento. VER TAMBÉM masticatory s. SIN masticatory apparatus (2).

subendocardial conducting s. of heart, s. de condução subendocárdico do coração; ramificações terminais nos ventrículos do sistema de condução especializado do coração. SIN Purkinje s.

sympathetic nervous s., s. nervoso simpático. SIN sympathetic part of autonomic division of peripheral nervous system.

T s., s. T; os túbulos transversos que são contínuos com o sarcolema nas fibras musculares esqueléticas e cardíacas.

thoracolumbar s., s. toracolombar. VER autonomic division of nervous system, sympathetic part of autonomic division of peripheral nervous system.

thoracolumbar nervous s., s. nervoso toracolombar. SIN sympathetic part of autonomic division of peripheral nervous system.

triaxial reference s., s. de referência triaxial; a figura resultante do rearranjo das linhas de derivação das três derivações padrões dos membros do eletrocardiograma (representado no triângulo de Einthoven), de modo que, em lugar de formar os lados de um triângulo eqüilátero, seccionam uma à outra. SIN Dieuaide diagram.

urinary s. [TA], s. urinário; todos os órgãos envolvidos com a formação, armazenamento e eliminação da urina, incluindo rins, ureteres, bexiga e uretra. SIN systema urinarium [TA], urinary apparatus, uropoietic s.

urogenital s., s. urogenital; inclui todos os órgãos envolvidos na reprodução e na formação e eliminação da urina. SIN apparatus urogenitalis, genitourinary apparatus, genitourinary s., systema urogenitale, urogenital apparatus.

uropoietic s., s. uropoético. SIN urinary s.

vascular s., s. vascular; os sistemas cardiovascular e linfático em conjunto. SIN circulatory s.

vegetative nervous s., s. nervoso vegetativo. SIN autonomic division of nervous system.

vertebral-basilar s., s. vertebrobasilar; o complexo arterial constituído pelas duas artérias vertebrais que se unem para formar a artéria basilar e seus ramos imediatos.

vertebral venous s., s. venoso vertebral; qualquer uma das quatro redes venosas interligadas que circundam a coluna vertebral; o plexo venoso vertebral externo anterior [TA] (plexus vertebralis externus anterior [TA]), o pequeno plexo ao redor dos corpos vertebrais; o plexo venoso vertebral externo posterior [TA] (plexus vertebralis internus anterior [TA]), o plexo extenso ao redor dos processos vertebrais; o plexo venoso vertebral interno anterior [TA] (plexus vertebralis internus posterior [TA]), o plexo que corre ao longo do canal vertebral anteriormente à dura; o plexo venoso vertebral interno posterior, o plexo que corre ao longo do canal vertebral posteriormente à dura; estes dois últimos constituem o plexo venoso epidural. SIN Batson plexus, plexus venosus vertebralis, vertebral venous plexus.

visceral motor s., s. motor visceral. SIN autonomic division of nervous system.

visceral nervous s., s. nervoso visceral. SIN autonomic division of nervous system.

Zaffaroni s., s. de Zaffaroni; s. cromatográfico para separação dos esteróides.

sys·te·ma (sis'tē'mă) [TA]. Sistema. SIN system. VER TAMBÉM system, apparatus. [L. do G. *systēma*]

s. alimenta'rium, s. alimentar. SIN alimentary system.

s. cardiovasculare [TA], s. cardiovascular. SIN cardiovascular system.

s. conducens cordis, s. de condução do coração; *termo oficial alternativo para conducting system of heart.

s. digesto'rium [TA], s. digestório. SIN alimentary system.

s. genitalia [TA], s. genital. SIN genital system.

s. lymphat'icum, s. linfático. SIN lymphoid system.

s. lymphoideum [TA], s. linfóide. SIN lymphoid system.

s. nervo'sum [TA], s. nervoso. SIN nervous system.

s. nervo'sum autonom'icum, s. nervoso autônomo. SIN autonomic division of nervous system.

s. nervo'sum centra'le, s. nervoso central; *termo oficial alternativo para central nervous system.

s. nervo'sum peripher'icum, s. nervoso periférico; *termo oficial alternativo para peripheral nervous system.

s. respirato'rium [TA], s. respiratório. SIN respiratory system.

s. skeleta'le [TA], s. esquelético. SIN skeletal system.

s. urinarium [TA], s. urinário. SIN urinary system.

s. urogenita'le, s. urogenital. SIN urogenital system.

sys·tem·at·ic (sis'tĕ-mat'ik). Sistemático; relativo a um sistema em qualquer sentido; disposto de acordo com um sistema.

sys·tem·at·ic name. Nome sistemático; quando aplicado a substâncias químicas, um nome sistemático é composto de palavras ou sílabas especialmente criadas ou selecionadas, tendo, cada uma delas, um significado estrutural químico precisamente definido, de modo que a estrutura possa ser deduzida do nome. A água (nome trivial) é o óxido de hidrogênio (nome sistemático). O nome sistemático da histamina (um nome semi-sistemático) é imidazoletilamina, que indica que um radical imidazol substitui um átomo de hidrogênio da etilamina, que, por sua vez, é um grupo etil fixado a um grupo amina. O nome dimetil sulfóxido significa que dois radicais metil estão fixados a um átomo de enxofre, que mantém um átomo de oxigênio. O ácido carbólico (nome trivial) ou o fenol (nome semi-sistemático) é, sistematicamente, fenoil hidróxido ou hidroxibenzeno. VER TAMBÉM semisystematic name.

sys·tem·a·ti·za·tion (sis-tĕ-mat'i-zā'shŭn, sis-tem'ă-ti-). Sistematização; a disposição de idéias em seqüência ordenada.

Sys·tème In·ter·na·tion·al d'Un·i·tés. Sistema Internacional de Unidades. VER International System of Units.

sys·tem·ic (sis-tem'ik). Sistêmico; relativo a um sistema; especificamente somático, relativo a todo o organismo, distinto de qualquer uma de suas partes individuais.

sys·te·moid (sis'tĕ-moyd). Sistemóide; que se assemelha a um sistema; designa um tumor de estrutura complexa, que se assemelha a um órgão.

sys·to·le (sis'tō-lē). Sístole; contração do coração, especialmente dos ventrículos, pela qual o sangue é expulso da aorta e da artéria pulmonar para atravessar a circulação sistêmica e pulmonar, respectivamente; sua ocorrência é indicada fisicamente pela primeira bulha cardíaca à ausculta, pelo batimento apical palpável e pelo pulso arterial. [G. *systolē*, uma contra*ção*]

aborted s., s. abortada; perda do batimento sistólico no pulso radial devido à fraqueza da contração ventricular.

atrial s., s. atrial; contração dos átrios. SIN auricular s.

auricular s., s. auricular. SIN atrial s.

electrical s., s. elétrica; a duração do complexo QRST (isto é, desde a onda Q inicial até o final da onda T mais tardia do ECG).

electromechanical s., s. eletromecânica; o período que se estende desde o início do complexo QRS até a primeira vibração (aórtica) da segunda bulha cardíaca. SIN QS_2 interval.

extra-s., extra-sístole. VER extrasystole.

late s., s. tardia. SIN prediastole.

premature s., extra-sístole. SIN extrasystole.

ventricular s., s. ventricular; contração dos ventrículos.

sys·tol·ic (sis-tol'ik). Sistólico; relativo a ou que ocorre durante a sístole cardíaca.

sys·to·lom·e·ter (sis'tō-lom'ĕ-ter). Sistolômetro. **1.** Aparelho para determinar a força da contração cardíaca. **2.** Instrumento para analisar os sons do coração. [systole + G. *metron*, medida]

sys·trem·ma (sis-trem'ă). Sistrema; cãibra muscular na panturrilha da perna, em que os músculos contraídos formam uma bola dura. [G. algo torcido]

sy·zyg·i·al (si-zij'ē-ăl). Sizigial; relativo a uma sizígia.

sy·zyg·i·ol·o·gy (si-zij'ē-ol'ō-jē). Sizigiologia; o estudo das inter-relações ou interdependências, especialmente do todo, composição ao estudo das partes separadas ou funções isoladas. [G. *syzygios*, unido, emparelhado (ver syzygy), + *logos*, estudo]

sy·zyg·i·um (si-zij'ē-ŭm). Sizígia. SIN syzygy.

syz·y·gy (siz'i-jē). Sizígia. **1.** A associação de protozoários gregarinos de extremidade a extremidade ou em pareamento lateral (sem fusão sexual). **2.** Pareamento de cromossomas na meiose. SIN syzygium. [G. *syzygios*, unido, ligado entre si, de *syn*, junto + *zygon*, julgo]

T

τ A décima nona letra do alfabeto grego, tau; símbolo de tempo de relaxamento (relaxation *time*).

θ, Θ. A oitava letra do alfabeto grego, teta; símbolo de ângulo (angle).

T 1. Símbolo de ribotimidina (ribothymidine); tensão (tension, T+, tensão aumentada; T−, tensão diminuída); tera-; tesla, a unidade de força do campo magnético; trítio (tritium); treonina (threonine); torqu (torque); transmitância (transmittance). 2. Como subscrito, refere-se ao volume corrente (tidal *volume*). 3. Abreviatura de vértebra torácica (T1–T12); tocoferol (tocopherol).

α-T, Símbolo do α - tocopherol (α - tocoferol).

β-T Símbolo de β - tocopherol (β-tocoferol).

γ-T. Símbolo de γ - tocopherol (γ-tocoferol).

T1. Na ressonância magnética, o intervalo de tempo para ocorrerem 63% de relaxamento longitudinal; o valor é uma função da força do campo magnético e do ambiente químico do núcleo de hidrogênio; para prótons em lipídio e em água, num magneto 1,5T, cerca de 250 ms e 3000 ms, respectivamente. Uma imagem T1-ponderada (ou ponderada em T1) terá um sinal brilhante para lipídios.

T2. Na ressonância magnética, o intervalo de tempo para ocorrerem 63% de relaxamento transversal; o valor é uma função da força do campo magnético e do ambiente químico do núcleo de hidrogênio; para prótons em lipídio e em gordura, num magneto 1,5T, cerca de 60 ms e 250 ms, respectivamente. Uma imagem T2-ponderada (ou ponderada em T2) terá um sinal brilhante na água.

2,4,5-T Abreviatura de [(2,4,5-trichlorophenoxy)] acetic acid [ácido (2,4,5-triclorofenoxi) acético].

T Símbolo de temperatura absoluta (absolute *temperature*) (kelvin).

T_m Símbolo de *temperature midpoint* (ponto térmico médio) (kelvin); ponto de fusão (melting *point*).

T_3 Símbolo de 3,5,3′-triiodothyronine (3,5,3′-triiodotironina).

T_4 Símbolo de thyroxine (tiroxina).

t Abreviatura de metric ton (tonelada métrica); tempo (time).

t Símbolo de temperature (temperatura Celsius); trítio (tritium).

t_m Símbolo de *temperature midpoint* (ponto térmico médio) (Celsius).

TA Abreviatura de *Terminologia Anatomica*.

Ta Símbolo de tantalum (tântalo).

tab·a·nid (tab′ă-nid). Tabanídeo; nome comum das moscas (mutucas) da família Tabanidae. [L. *tabanus,* moscardo]

Ta·ban·i·dae (tă-ban′i-dē). Família de moscas hematófagas (mutucas) que inclui os gêneros *Tabanus* (mutuca) e *Chrysops,* envolvidas na transmissão de vários parasitas transportados pelo sangue. [L. *tabanus,* moscardo]

Ta·ba·nus (tă-bā′nŭs). *Tabanus.* Os moscardos e as mutucas; gênero de moscas que picam, das quais algumas espécies transmitem a surra, a anemia infecciosa eqüina, o antraz e outras doenças. [L. moscardo]

ta·bar·dil·lo (tah-bar-dē′yō). Tabardilho; termo mexicano para o tifo exantemático. [Esp. do L.L. *tabardilii,* pústulas]

ta·ba·tière an·a·to·mique (tab-ah-tē-ār′ an-ah-to-mēk′). Tabaqueira anatômica. SIN anatomic snuffox. [Fr. tabaqueira]

ta·bel·la, pl. **ta·bel·lae** (tă-bel′lă, -lē). Comprimido ou pastilha medicinal. [L. dim. de *tabula,* comprimido]

ta·bes (tā′bēz). Tabes, tabe; debilitação ou emaciação progressivas. [L. definhamento]

 t. infan′tum, t. do lactente; t. em lactentes com sífilis congênita.

 t. mesenter′ica, t. mesentérica; tuberculose dos linfonodos mesentéricos e retroperitoneais.

ta·bes·cence (ta-bes′ens). Tabescência; o estado de debilitação progressiva.

ta·bes·cent (ta-bes′ent). Tabescente, tábido; característico da tabes. [L. *tabesco,* definhar, de *tabes,* definhamento]

ta·bet·ic (ta-bet′ik). Tabético; relativo a ou que sofre de tabes, especialmente tabes dorsal. SIN tabic, tabid.

ta·bet·i·form (ta-bet′i-fōrm). Tabetiforme; semelhante à tabes, especialmente tabes dorsal. [irreg. formado do L. *tabes,* definhamento + *forma,* forma]

tab·ic (tab′ik). Tábido, tabético, tabescente. SIN tabetic.

tab·id (tab′id), Tábido, tabescente, tabético. SIN tabetic. [L. *tabidus,* definhamento]

tab·la·ture (tab-lā-choor). Tablatura; estado de divisão dos ossos cranianos em duas lâminas separadas pela díploe. [L. *tabula,* tablete]

ta·ble (tā′bl). 1. Uma das duas placas ou lâminas, separadas pela díploe, na qual os ossos cranianos são divididos. 2. Quadro, tabela. Arranjo de dados em colunas paralelas, mostrando os fatos essenciais de uma forma que pode ser facilmente avaliada. 3. Mesa; plataforma sobre a qual podem ser colocados itens. [L. *tabula*]

 Aub-DuBois t., tabela de Aub-DuBois; tabela das taxas metabólicas basais em calorias por metro quadrado de superfície corporal por hora ou dia para diferentes idades.

 contingency t., tabela de contingência; classificação tabular de dados, de tal modo que as subcategorias de uma característica são indicadas em fileiras (horizontais) e as subcategorias de outra característica são indicadas em colunas (verticais).

 examining t., mesa de exame; mesa sobre a qual o paciente se deita durante um exame médico.

 external t. of calvaria [TA], lâmina externa da calvária; a camada compacta externa dos ossos cranianos. SIN lamina externa calvaria [TA], lamina externa cranii, outer t. of skull.

 Gaffky t., tabela de Gaffky; graduação numérica para classificação da tuberculose de acordo com o número de bacilos da tuberculose no escarro, estendendo-se de 1 (um a quatro microrganismos em todo o esfregaço) a 9 (média de 100 por campo). SIN Gaffky scale.

 inner t. of skull, lâmina interna do crânio. SIN internal t. of calvaria.

 internal t. of calvaria [TA], lâmina interna da calvária; a camada compacta interna dos ossos cranianos. SIN lamina interna calvariae [TA], inner t. of skull, lamina interna cranii.

 life t., tábuas da vida; representação dos prováveis anos de sobrevida de uma população definida de indivíduos; como sobrevida é alterada por novos métodos de prevenção ou tratamento, utiliza-se comumente um estudo diacrônico, visto que o principal interesse reside na estrutura composta da população atual. (No resumo da técnica usada para descrever o padrão de mortalidade e de sobrevida em determinada população, os sobreviventes até a idade *x* são designados pelo símbolo 1*x,* e a expectativa de vida na idade *x,* pelo símbolo *x.*)

 occlusal t., tábua oclusal; as superfícies oclusal ou de trituração dos dentes bicúspides e molares.

 operating t., mesa de operação; uma mesa sobre a qual o paciente se deita durante uma cirurgia.

 outer t. of skull, lâmina externa do crânio. SIN external t. of calvaria.

 tilt t., mesa inclinada; mesa cujo tampo consegue girar sobre seu eixo transverso, de modo que um paciente deitado sobre ela pode ser colocado na posição ortostática, quando desejado; usada na investigação experimental e em fisioterapia.

 vitreous t., lâmina interna da calvária; a lâmina interna de um dos ossos cranianos; é mais compacta e mais dura do que a lâmina externa. SIN lamina interna ossium cranii.

ta·ble·spoon (tā′bl-spoon). Colher de sopa; colher grande utilizada como medida da dose de um medicamento, equivalente a cerca de 15 ml ou 4 dracmas líquidas ou 1/2 onça líquida.

tab·let. Tablete, drágea, comprimido; apresentação posológica sólida (pó) contendo substâncias medicinais com ou sem excipientes apropriados; pode variar quanto à forma, ao tamanho e ao peso e pode ser classificado, de acordo com o método de fabricação, como comprimido. SIN tabule. [Fr. *tablette,* L. *tabula*]

 buccal t., comprimido oral; em geral, pequeno comprimido achatado desenvolvido para ser introduzido na cavidade achatado, onde o ingrediente ativo é absorvido diretamente através da mucosa oral; esse comprimido dissolve-se ou sofre erosão lentamente.

 compressed t., comprimido preparado, geralmente em larga escala, sob grande pressão; a maioria desses comprimidos consiste no ingrediente ativo e num excipiente, quelante, desintegrador e lubrificante.

 dispensing t., comprimido farmacêutico; comprimido preparado por moldagem ou por compressão; utilizado pelo farmacêutico para obter determinadas substâncias potentes numa forma conveniente para composição acurada. Antigamente usado na preparação de soluções de substâncias químicas germicidas, como, por exemplo, bicloreto de mercúrio. Não se destina a uso interno.

 enteric coated t., comprimido com revestimento entérico; forma posológica oral em que o pó é revestido por um material destinado a impedir ou minimizar a sua dissolução no estômago, porém permitindo a sua dissolução no intestino delgado. Esse tipo de formulação protege o estômago de uma substância potencialmente irritante (p. ex., ácido acetilsalicílico) ou protege a substância (p. ex., eritromicina) de sua degradação parcial no ambiente ácido do estômago.

 hypodermic t., comprimido para uso injetável; comprimido preparado por compressão ou moldagem que se dissolve completamente em água para formar uma solução injetável.

 prolonged action t., repeat action t., comprimido de ação prolongada. SIN sustained action t.

△ Formas Combinantes	☆ Termo oficial alternativo para a *Terminologia Anatomica*
▯ Indica que o termo é ilustrado, ver Índice de Ilustrações	[MIM] Mendelian Inheritance in Man
SIN Sinônimo	
Cf. Comparar, confrontar	I.C. Índice de Corantes
[NA] *Nomina Anatomica*	
[TA] *Terminologia Anatomica*	Termo de Alta Importância

sublingual t., comprimido sublingual; em geral, pequeno comprimido achatado para ser colocado sob a língua, onde o ingrediente ativo é absorvido diretamente através da mucosa oral; esse comprimido (p. ex., nitroglicerina) dissolve-se rapidamente.
sustained action t., sustained release t., comprimido de ação prolongada, comprimido de liberação prolongada; formulação de uma substância que fornece a dose necessária inicialmente e, a seguir, a mantém ou repete a intervalos desejados. SIN prolonged action t., repeat action t.
t. triturate, triturado de comprimido; pequeno disco habitualmente cilíndrico, moldado ou comprimido, de tamanho variável, contendo um excipiente que, em geral, consiste em glicose ou numa mistura de lactose e sacarose em pó e agente umidificante ou excipiente, como álcool diluído.

ta·boo, ta·bu (tă-boo′). Tabu; restrito, proibido ou interditado; rejeitado por motivos religiosos ou cerimoniais. [Tongan, rejeitado]

tab·u·lar (tab′ū-lăr). Tabular. **1.** Semelhante a uma tábua. **2.** Disposto na forma de quadro ou tabela (2). [L. *tabularis,* de *tabula,* tabela]

tab·ule (tab′ūl). Tablete, drágea, comprimido. SIN tablet. [L. *tabula*]

ta·bun (tă′bŭn). Inibidor da colinesterase extremamente potente; acredita-se que a dose letal para seres humanos seja de apenas 0,01 mg/kg; a dose letal mediana (respiratória) é de cerca de 40 mg/min/m^3 para indivíduos em repouso.

Tac (tak). Polipeptídio de 55 kD que constitui uma das duas cadeias que formam o receptor de IL-2.

tache (tash). Mácula, mancha; coloração circunscrita da pele ou da mucosa, como mácula ou efélide. [Fr. mancha]
t. blanche, mácula branca. SIN macula albida.
t. laiteuse, (1) mácula láctea. SIN milk spots, em spot; **(2)** mácula álbida. SIN macula albida. [Fr. mancha leitosa]

ta·chis·to·scope (tă-kis′tŏ-skōp). Taquistoscópio; instrumento para determinar o menor tempo de exposição necessária de um objeto para que seja percebido. [G. *tachistos,* muito rápido, de *tachys,* rápido + *skopeō,* ver]

tach·o·gram (tak′ō-gram). Tacograma; registro feito por um tacômetro. [G. *tachos,* velocidade + *gramma,* marca]

tach·o·graph (tak′ō-graf). Tacógrafo; tacômetro projetado para fornecer um registro contínuo de velocidade ou freqüência. [G. *tachos,* velocidade + *graphō,* escrever]

ta·chog·ra·phy (tă-kog′ră-fē). Tacografia; registro de velocidade ou freqüência. [G. *tachos,* velocidade + *graphō,* escrever]

ta·chom·e·ter (tă-kom′ĕ-ter). Tacômetro; instrumento para medir a velocidade ou freqüência; por exemplo, revoluções de um eixo, freqüência cardíaca (cardiotacômetro), fluxo sangüíneo arterial (hemotacômetro), fluxo gasoso respiratório (pneumotacômetro). [G. *tachos,* velocidade + *metron,* medida]

△ **tachy-.** Taqui-; rápido. [G. *tachys,* rápido]

tach·y·ar·rhyth·mia (tak′ē-ă-ridh′mē-ă). Taquiarritmia; qualquer distúrbio do ritmo cardíaco, regular ou irregular, resultando, por convenção, numa freqüência de mais de 100 batimentos por minuto (bpm) durante um exame físico. [tachy- + G. *a-* priv. + *rhythmos,* ritmo]

tach·y·aux·e·sis (tak′ē-awk-sē′sis). Taquiauxese; tipo de crescimento em que uma parte cresce mais rapidamente do que o todo. [tachy- + G. *auxō,* aumentar]

tach·y·car·dia (tak′ĭ-kar′dē-ă). Taquicardia; batimento rápido do coração, aplicado, convencionalmente, a freqüências acima de 90 batimentos por minuto (bpm). SIN polycardia, tachyrhythmia, tachysystole. [tachy- + G. *kardia,* coração]
atrial t., t. atrial; t. paroxística que se origina em um foco ectópico no átrio. SIN auricular t.
atrial chaotic t., t. atrial caótica; origem multifocal de t. no átrio; freqüentemente confundida com fibrilação atrial durante o exame físico. SIN multifocal atrial t.
atrioventricular junctional t., t. juncional atrioventricular; t. que se origina na junção AV. SIN junctional t., nodal t.
auricular t., t. atrial. SIN atrial t.
AV junctional t., t. juncional AV. SIN atrioventricular junctional t.
bidirectional ventricular t., t. ventricular bidirecional; t. ventricular em que os complexos QRS no eletrocardiograma são, alternadamente, principalmente positivos e principalmente negativos; muitos desses casos seriam uma t. ventricular com formas alternantes de condução ventricular aberrante.
Coumel t., t. de Coumel; t. recíproca juncional persistente, que habitualmente utiliza uma via póstero-septal de condução lenta para a transmissão retrógrada.
double t., t. dupla; t. simultânea de dois marca-passos ectópicos, p. ex., t. atrial e juncional.
ectopic t., t. ectópica; t. que se origina em outro foco diferente do nó sinoatrial, p. ex., t. atrial, t. juncional AV ou t. ventricular.
t. en salves, t. em salvas; curtos episódios de t. paroxística do tipo Gallavardin. Cf. Gallavardin *phenomenon.* [De *taquicardia em salvas*]
essential t., t. essencial; termo obsoleto para a ação rápida persistente do coração, devido a lesão orgânica não-detectável.
t. exophthal′mica, t. exoftálmica; ação cardíaca rápida que ocorre como uma das manifestações do bócio exoftálmico.
fetal t., t. fetal; freqüência cardíaca fetal ≥160 batimentos por minuto (bpm).
junctional t., t. juncional; t. supraventricular que se origina na junção atrioventricular (antigamente denominada t. nodal).
multifocal atrial t. (MAT), t. atrial multifocal. SIN atrial chaotic t.
nodal t., t. juncional. SIN atrioventricular junctional t.
orthostatic t., t. ortostática; aumento da freqüência cardíaca ao passar para a posição ortostática.
paroxysmal t., t. paroxística; episódios recorrentes de t., geralmente com início abrupto e, com freqüência, também com término abrupto, que se originam de um foco ectópico que pode ser atrial, juncional AV ou ventricular.
reflex t., t. reflexa; aumento da freqüência cardíaca em resposta a algum estímulo transmitido através dos nervos cardíacos.
sinus t., t. sinusal; taquicardia que se origina no nó sinoatrial.
supraventricular t., t. supraventricular; freqüência cardíaca rápida devido a um marca-passo em qualquer ponto acima do nível ventricular, isto é, nó sinoatrial, átrio, junção atrioventricular. Os complexos QRS são sempre estreitos, a não ser que haja alguma aberrância relacionada à freqüência ou algum retardo preexistente da condução intraventricular.
ventricular t., t. ventricular; t. paroxística que se origina em um foco ectópico no ventrículo. VER TAMBÉM torsade de pointes.

tach·y·car·di·ac (tak-i-kar′dē-ak). Taquicardíaco; relativo a ou que sofre de ação cardíaca excessivamente rápida.

tach·y·car·dic (tak-i-kar′dik). Taquicárdico; relativo à freqüência cardíaca rápida.

tach·y·crot·ic (tak′i-krot′ik). Taquicrótico; relativo a, que causa ou que se caracteriza por um pulso rápido. [tachy- + G. *krotos,* que toca]

tach·y·ki·nin (tak-ē-kī′nin). Taquicinina; qualquer membro de um grupo de polipeptídios, amplamente espalhados nos tecidos de vertebrados e invertebrados, que possuem em comum quatro dos cinco aminoácidos terminais: Phe-Xaa-Gli-Leu-Met-NH$_2$; do ponto de vista farmacológico, todos causam hipotensão nos mamíferos, contração da musculatura lisa intestinal e vesical e secreção de saliva. [G. *tachys,* rápido + *kineō,* mover + *-in*]

tach·y·pac·ing (tak′ī-pā′sing). Taquiestimulação; estimulação rápida do coração por um marca-passo eletrônico artificial que opera mais rápido do que a freqüência cardíaca básica.

tach·y·phy·lax·is (tak′i-fi-lak′sis). Taquifilaxia; rápido aparecimento de diminuição progressiva da resposta a determinada dose após administração repetida de uma substância farmacológica ou fisiologicamente ativa. [tachy- + G. *phylaxis,* proteção]

tach·yp·nea (tak-ip-nē′ă). Taquipnéia; respiração rápida. SIN polypnea. [tachy- + G. *pnoē (pnoiē),* respiração]

transient t. of the newborn, t. transitória do recém-nascido; síndrome de t. geralmente leve em recém-nascidos sadios sob os demais aspectos, que geralmente dura apenas cerca de 3 dias. SIN respiratory distress syndrome type II.

tach·y·rhyth·mia (tak-i-ridh′mē-ă). Taquirritmia. SIN tachycardia. [tachy- + G. *rhythmos,* ritmo]

ta·chys·ter·ol (tă-kis′ter-ōl). Taquisterol; esterol (esteróis) formado(s) por irradiação ultravioleta de qualquer 5,7-dieno-3β-esterol, que rompe a ligação 9,10, mas geralmente a partir do ergosterol e/ou do lumisterol para produzir t.$_2$ [ertacalciol, (6*E*,22*E*)-9,10-secoergosta-5(10),6,8,22-tetraen-3β-ol) e a partir do 7-desidrocolesterol para produzir t.$_3$ (tacalciol, (6*E*,3*S*)-9,10-secocolesta-5(10),6,8,trien-3β-ol). Quando reduzido à forma 5,7-dieno (ou 5,7,22-trieno), diidrotaquisterol$_3$ (10,19-diidrocalciol) ou diidrotaquisterol$_2$ (10,19-diidroercalciol), surge a ação anti-raquítica. Essa propriedade tem sido de interesse terapêutico, porém o t. está sendo substituído pelo hormônio vitamina D verdadeiro (calcitriol) e seus derivados.

tach·y·sys·to·le (tak-i-sis′tō-lē). Taquicardia SIN tachycardia. [tachy- + G. *systolē,* que contrai]

tach·y·zo·ite (tak-ĭ-zō′it). Taquizoíta; estágio de rápida multiplicação no desenvolvimento da fase tecidual de determinadas infecções por coccídeos, como no desenvolvimento do *Toxoplasma gondii* em infecções agudas de toxoplasmose. [tachy- + G. *zōon,* animal]

tac·rine (tak′rēn). Tacrina; agente anticolinesterásico com efeitos estimuladores inespecíficos sobre o sistema nervoso central; utilizado nos estágios iniciais da doença de Alzheimer.

tac·tile (tak′til). Tátil; relativo ao toque ou ao sentido do tato. [L. *tactilis,* de *tango,* pp. *tactus,* tocar]

tac·tion (tak′shŭn). **1.** O sentido do tato. **2.** Toque; o ato de tocar. [L. *tactio,* de *tango,* pp. *tactus,* tocar]

tac·tom·e·ter (tak-tom′ĕ-ter). Tactômetro. SIN esthesiometer. [L. *tactus,* toque + G. *metron,* medida]

tac·tor (tak′tăr, -tōr). Órgão terminal tátil. [L. aquele ou aquilo que toca]

tac·tu·al (tak′chool). Relativo a ou causado pelo toque.

TAD Acrônimo de transient acantholytic *dermatosis* (dermatose acantolítica transitória).

Taenia (tē′nē-ā). Gênero de cestóides que antigamente incluía a maioria das tênias, mas que hoje em dia se limita às espécies que infectam carnívoros com cisticercos encontrados nos tecidos de vários herbívoros, roedores e outras presas. VER TAMBÉM tapeworm. [ver taenia]

T. africa'na, tênia encontrada em nativos africanos, cujo cisticerco é desconhecido.

T. arma'ta, SIN *T. solium.*

T. crassic'ollis. SIN *T. taeniaeformis.*

T. demerarien'sis, designação antiga de *Davainea madagascariensis.*

T. denta'ta. SIN *T. solium.*

T. equi'na. SIN *Anoplocephala perfoliata.*

T. hom'inis, forma incomum de *T. saginata.*

T. hydatig'ena, tênia de cães, gatos, lobos, raposas e outros carnívoros; a larva é conhecida como *Cysticercus tenuicollis.*

T. madagascarien'sis, designação antiga de *Davainea madagascariensis.*

T. min'ima, designação antiga de *Hymenolepis nana.*

T. o'vis, tênia de cães e raposas cuja forma larvar é encontrada nos músculos de carneiros; as infecções larvares maciças em carneiros podem ter graves consequências econômicas, devido à condenação das carcaças durante as inspeções da Vigilância Sanitária.

T. philippi'na, forma atípica de *T. saginata.*

T. pisifor'mis, tênia comum de cães, raposas e outros carnívoros; a forma larvar é *Cysticercus pisiformis.*

T. quadriloba'ta. SIN *Anoplocephala perfoliata.*

T. sagina'ta, a tênia do boi, sem acúleos, que infecta seres humanos; adquirida pela ingestão de carne de vaca insuficientemente cozida e infectada por *Cysticercus bovis.*

T. so'lium, a tênia do porco, com acúleos, ou "solitária" de seres humanos, adquirida pela ingestão de carne de porco insuficientemente cozida e infectada por *Cysticercus cellulosae;* a eclosão dos ovos no intestino humano pode resultar no estabelecimento de cisticercos nos tecidos humanos, levando a cisticercose. SIN *T. armata, T. dentata.*

T. taeniaefor'mis, uma das tênias comuns de gatos domésticos; a forma larvar é denominada *Cysticercus fasciolaris.* SIN *Hydatigera taeniaeformis, T. crassicollis.*

tae·nia (tē′nē-ā). **1.** Tênia; estrutura anatômica espiralada, semelhante a uma faixa. VER tenia (1). **2.** Nome comum para uma tênia ("solitária",) especialmente do gênero *Taenia.* SIN tenia (2). [L., do G. *tainia,* faixa, fita e tênia]

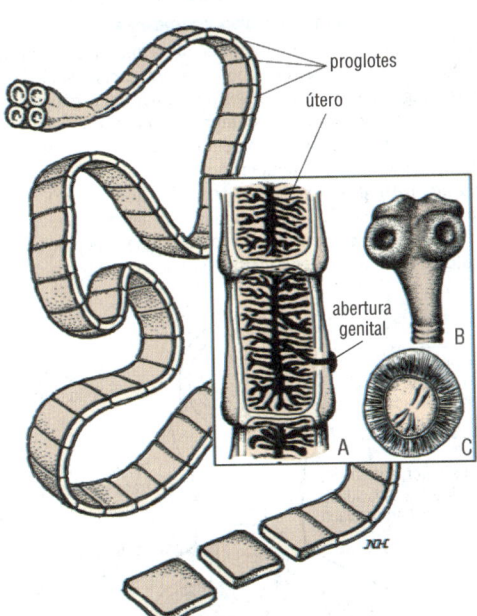

Taenia saginata (tênia do boi): (A) segmento corporal mostrando os órgãos reprodutores (1,7×), (B) escólex (12×), (C) ovo (550×).

Tae·ni·a·rhyn·chus (tē′nē-ā-ring′kŭs). Gênero estabelecido para espécies de *Taenia* que possuem um rostelo rudimentar, mas que carecem dos ganchos rostelares típicos de *Taenia.* O exemplo mais conhecido é *Taeniarhynchus saginatus,* porém a designação antiga, *Taenia saginata,* é mais comumente utilizada. [G. *tainia,* faixa + *rhynchos,* focinho]

tae·ni·a·sis (tē-nē-ī′ā-sis). Teníase; infecção por cestóides do gênero *Taenia.*

tae·ni·id (tē-nē′id). Tenídio; designação comum de um membro da família Taeniidae.

Tae·ni·i·dae (tē-nē′i-dē). Família de cestóides parasitas (ordem Cyclophyllidea), que inclui os gêneros *Taenia, Taeniarhynchus, Multiceps* e *Echinococcus.*

tae·ni·oid (tē′nē-oyd). Tenióide; designa membros do gênero *Taenia.*

Tae·ni·o·rhyn·chus (tē-nē-ō-ring′kŭs). Gênero e subgênero de mosquitos atualmente considerado sinônimo de *Mansonia.* [G. *tainia,* faixa, + *rhynchos,* focinho]

Taenzer, Paul R., dermatologista alemão, 1858–1919. VER T. *stain;* Unna-T. *stain.*

TAF Abreviatura de tumor angiogenic *factor* (fator angiogênico tumoral).

tag. 1. Marcador. VER label, tracer. **2.** Excrescência, apêndice. Pequena proeminência ou pólipo. **3.** Em ressonância magnética, faixa de saturação que pode ser seguida para detectar o movimento tecidual.

anal skin t., pólipo cutâneo anal; pólipo fibroso da pele imediatamente fora do ânus.

epiploic t.'s, apêndices omentais do colo. SIN omental *appendices,* em *appendix.*

sentinel t., apêndice sentinela; projeção de pele edematosa na extremidade inferior de uma fissura anal.

skin t., apêndice cutâneo; **(1)** proliferação polipóide da epiderme e do tecido fibrovascular dérmico; **(2)** em embriologia, projeção recoberta de pele, que pode ou não conter cartilagem; tipicamente localizada numa linha entre o trago e o canto da boca e associada a anomalias da orelha externa. SIN acrochordon, fibroepithelial polyp, fibroma molle, papilloma molle, soft papilloma.

tag·a·tose (tag′ā-tōs). Tagatose; ceto-hexose; a D-tagatose é epimérica com a D-frutose.

tag·li·a·co·ti·an (tal-yah-cō′shē-an). Tagliacotiano; relativo a ou descrito por Tagliacozzi.

Tagliacozzi, Gaspare, cirurgião italiano, 1546-1599.

tail (tāl) [TA]. Cauda. **1.** Qualquer cauda ou estrutura semelhante a uma cauda ou extremidade afilada ou alongada de um órgão ou outra parte. SIN cauda [TA]. **2.** Em anatomia veterinária, um apêndice livre representando a extremidade caudal da coluna vertebral; coberto por pele e pêlos, penas ou escamas. [A.S. *taegl.*]

t. of caudate nucleus [TA], c. do núcleo caudado; extensão posterior alongada do núcleo caudado, que é paralela ao corpo e ao corno inferior do ventrículo lateral. SIN cauda nuclei caudati [TA], cauda striati.

t. of dentate gyrus, c. do giro denteado. SIN uncus *band* of Giacomini.

t. of epididymis [TA], c. do epidídimo; parte inferior do epidídimo que leva ao ducto deferente; parte do reservatório de espermatozóides. SIN cauda epididymidis [TA], cauda epididymis, globus minor.

t. of helix [TA], c. da hélice; processo achatado que termina na cartilagem da hélice da orelha, posterior e inferiormente. SIN cauda helicis [TA].

t. of pancreas [TA], c. do pâncreas; extremidade esquerda do pâncreas dentro do ligamento esplenorrenal. SIN cauda pancreatis [TA].

tail·gut (tāl′gŭt). Intestino terminal. SIN postanal *gut.*

Tait, Robert L., ginecologista inglês, 1845–1899. VER T. *law.*

Ta·ka·di·as·tase (tă′ka-dī′as-tās). Takadiastase. SIN α-amylase.

Takahara, Shigeo, otolaringologista japonês do século 20. VER T. *disease.*

Takayama, Masao, médico japonês, *1872. VER T. *stain.*

Takayasu (Takayashu), Michishige, oftalmologista japonês, *1872. VER Takayasu *arteritis,* Takayasu *disease,* Takayasu *syndrome.*

take (tāk). Pega; enxerto ou vacinação bem-sucedida.

ta·lal·gia (tă-lal′jē-ā). Talalgia; dor no tornozelo. [L. *talus,* tornozelo, G. *algos,* dor]

ta·lar (tā′lar). Talar; relativo ao tálus.

Talbot, William Henry Fox, cientista inglês, 1800–1877. VER Plateau-T. *law.*

talc (tălk). Talco; silicato de magnésio hidratado nativo, contendo, algumas vezes, pequenas proporções de silicato de alumínio, purificado por ebulição do talco pulverizado com ácido clorídrico em água; utilizado em farmácia como auxiliar de filtro, como pó para polvilhar e em preparações cosméticas. SIN French chalk, soapstone, talcum. [Ár. *talq*]

tal·co·sis (tal-kō′sis). Talcose; distúrbio pulmonar relacionado à silicose que ocorre em trabalhadores expostos ao talco misturado com silicatos; caracterizada por distúrbios restritivos ou obstrutivos da respiração ou por ambos em associação. [talc + G. *-osis,* condição]

pulmonary t., t. pulmonar; pneumoconiose em decorrência da inalação de poeira de talco.

tal·cum (tal′kŭm). Talco. SIN talc. [L.]

tal·i·on (tal′ē-on, tal′yŭn). Talião; talionato; o princípio de retribuição no comportamento intrapsíquico. [Galês *tal,* compensação]

t. dread, medo de talião; as ansiedades simbólicas que representam o medo inconsciente de penalidades por um ato.

tal·i·ped·ic (tal-i-ped′ik). Talipédico; que possui pé torto.

tal·i·pes (tal′i-pēz). Tálipe, talipe; qualquer deformidade do pé afetando o tálus. [L. *talus,* tornozelo + *pes,* pé]

t. calcaneoval′gus, t. calcaneovalgo; tálipe calcâneo e tálipe valgo combinado; o pé apresenta-se em dorsiflexão, eversão e abdução.

t. calcaneoa′rus, t. calcaneovaro; t. calcâneo e t. varo combinados; o pé apresenta-se em dorsiflexão, inversão e adução.

t. calca′neus, t. calcâneo; deformidade devido a fraqueza ou ausência dos músculos da panturrilha, em que o eixo do calcâneo se torna orientado verticalmente; observado comumente na poliomielite. SIN calcaneus (2).

t. ca′vus, t. cavo; exagero do arco normal do pé. SIN contracted foot, pes cavus, t. plantaris.

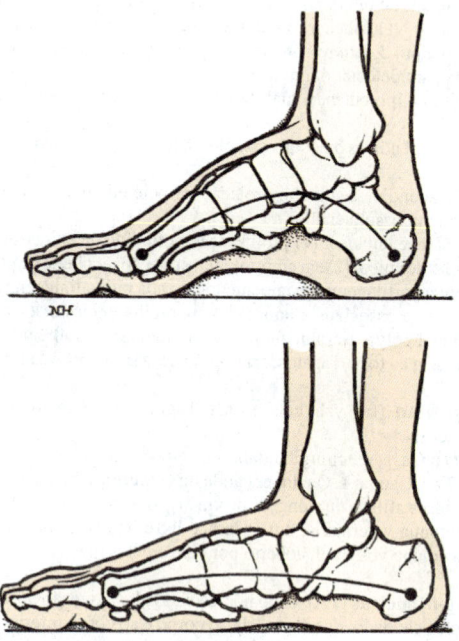

talipe cavo (em cima) e **talipe plano** (embaixo)

t. equinoval′gus, t. eqüinovalgo; t. eqüino e t. valgo combinados; o pé apresenta-se em flexão plantar, evertido e em abdução. SIN equinovalgus, pes equinovalgus.

t. equinova′rus, t. eqüinovaro; t. eqüino e t. varo combinados; o pé apresenta-se em flexão plantar, invertido e em adução. SIN clubfoot, equinovarus, pes equinovarus.

t. equi′nus, t. eqüino; flexão plantar permanente do pé, de modo que apenas o antepé toca o chão; comumente combinado com t. varo.

t. planta′ris, t. plantar, t. cavo. VER t. cavus.

t. pla′nus, pé plano. SIN *pes planus.*

t. transversopla′nus, t. transversoplano. SIN *metatarsus latus.*

t. val′gus, t. valgo; eversão permanente do pé, em que apenas a face interna da planta toca o chão; habitualmente combinado com retificação do arco plantar. SIN pes abductus, pes pronatus, pes valgus.

t. va′rus, t. varo; inversão do pé, com apenas a face externa da planta tocando o chão; em geral, existe algum grau de t. eqüino associado e, com freqüência, t. cavo. SIN pes adductus, pes varus.

tal·low (tal′o). Sebo; a gordura derretida das vísceras de carneiro.

prepared mutton t., s. de carneiro preparado. SIN prepared suet.

talo-. Talo-; o tálus. [L. *talus,* tornozelo, tálus]

ta·lo·cal·ca·ne·al, ta·lo·cal·ca·ne·an (ta-lo-kal-ka′ne-ăl, ta-lo-kal-ka′-ne-an). Talocalcâneo; relativo ao tálus e ao calcâneo.

ta·lo·cru·ral (ta′lo-kroo′ral). Talocrural; relativo ao tálus e aos ossos da perna; designa a articulação do tornozelo.

ta·lo·fib·u·lar (ta′lo-fib′u-lar). Talofibular; relativo ao tálus e à fíbula.

ta·lo·na·vic·u·lar (ta′lo-na-vik′u-lar). Talonavicular; relativo ao tálus e ao osso navicular. SIN astragaloscaphoid, taloscaphoid.

ta·lo·scaph·oid (ta′-lo-skaf′oyd). Talonavicular. SIN talonavicular.

tal·ose (tal′os). Talose; aldo-hexose, isomérica com glicose; a D-t. é epimérica com a D-galactose.

ta·lo·tib·i·al (ta′lo-tib′e-ăl). Talotibial; relativo ao tálus e à tíbia.

ta·lus, gen. **ta·li** (ta′lŭs, -li). [TA]. Tálus; o osso do pé que se articula com a tíbia e a fíbula para formar a articulação do tornozelo. SIN ankle bone, ankle (3). [L. osso do tornozelo, calcanhar]

tam·a·rind (tam′ă-rind). Tamarindo; a polpa da fruta da *Tamarindus indica* (família Leguminosae), uma grande árvore da Índia; levemente laxativo. [L. Mediev. do Ár. *tamr*]

tam·bour (tahm-bur′) Tambor; a parte registradora de um aparelho gráfico, como um esfigmógrafo, que consiste numa membrana esticada através da extremidade aberta de um cilindro e o estilete de registro fixado a ela. [Fr. tambor]

Tamm, Igor, virologista norte-americano, *1922. VER T.-Horsfall *mucoprotein, protein.*

ta·mox·i·fen cit·rate (ta-mok′si-fen). Citrato de tamoxifeno; antagonista estrogênico não-esteróide sintético utilizado na profilaxia e no tratamento do câncer de mama.

Ao competir com o estrogênio de ocorrência natural pelos sítios de ligação nas células teciduais, o tamoxifeno inibe o efeito estimulante do estrogênio sobre o câncer de mama. É mais provável que os tumores que, através de ensaio bioquímico, demonstraram ser ricos em receptores de estrogênio respondam ao tratamento. Desde 1985, o t. vem sendo utilizado em pacientes submetidas a cirurgia ou a irradiação para câncer de mama, a fim de retardar ou evitar a recidiva. Foi constatada a efetividade do fármaco na redução do risco de recidiva do câncer ou de progressão da doença em mulheres com ou sem metástases nos linfonodos axilares. Nas mulheres com doença extensa, a terapia com t. mostrou-se tão efetiva quanto a ooforectomia no retardo da progressão. Em 1992, o Breast Cancer Prevention Trial (BCPT) do National Cancer Institute recrutou mais de 13.000 mulheres nos Estados Unidos e no Canadá para estudar o valor preventivo do t. Todas as mulheres que participaram foram consideradas de alto risco para câncer de mama devido à idade (>60), história familiar forte ou diagnóstico prévio de carcinoma lobular *in situ.* Em março de 1998, a diferença na incidência de câncer de mama entre o grupo tratado com t. e o grupo placebo era tão grande, que os investigadores concluíram que a necessidade ética de informar as participantes sobre os benefícios claros da profilaxia farmacológica ativa superava quaisquer benefícios possíveis de prosseguir o estudo controlado. As mulheres incluídas nas categorias de maior risco exibiram uma redução de 45% na incidência de câncer de mama. Entretanto, esse estudo não demonstrou qualquer efeito sobre a taxa de mortalidade, e, em dois estudos clínicos semelhantes conduzidos na Europa, o t. não demonstrou um efeito protetor estatisticamente significativo. As mulheres que tomam t. correm risco aumentado de carcinoma endometrial, trombose venosa profunda, embolia pulmonar e cataratas. O perigo dessas conseqüências adversas é maior em mulheres com mais de 50 anos de idade. O uso prolongado do fármaco está associado a candidíase vaginal recorrente. O t. está contra-indicado durante a gravidez, devido ao risco de dano fetal.

tam·pon. 1. Tampão; cilindro ou bola de algodão, gaze ou outra substância frouxa; utilizado como tampão ou compressa num canal ou numa cavidade para deter a hemorragia, absorver secreções ou manter um órgão deslocado na sua posição. **2.** Inserir esse tampão ou compressa. [Fr. Ant.]

Corner t., t. de Corner; tampão de omento colocado numa ferida do estômago ou do intestino como tampão temporário.

tam·pon·ade, tam·pon·age (tam-po-nad′, tam′po-nij). **1.** Compressão patológica de um órgão. **2.** Tamponamento. SIN tamponing.

cardiac t., t. cardíaco; compressão do coração em virtude de um aumento crítico do volume de líquido no pericárdio. SIN heart t.

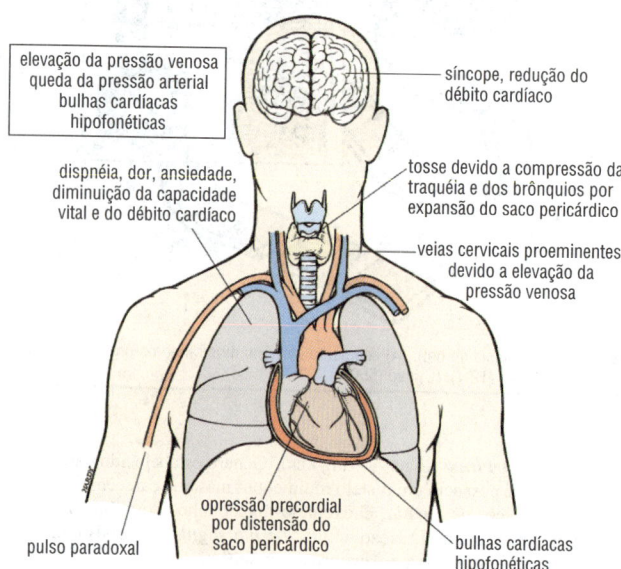

avaliação do **tamponamento cardíaco** secundário a derrame pericárdico

tamponade, tamponage

chronic t., t. crônico; compressão cardíaca por longo período de tempo, devido a um aumento patológico do líquido no saco pericárdico.
heart t., t. cardíaco. SIN cardiac t.
tam·pon·ing, tam·pon·ment (tam′pon-ing, tam-pon′ment). Tamponamento; o ato de inserir um tampão. SIN tamponade (2), tamponage.
ta·nace·tol, tan·a·ce·tone (ta-nās′tol, tan-ā-sē′tōn). Tanacetol, tanacetona. SIN thujone.
tan·dem (tan′dem), Termo utilizado para descrever múltiplas cópias da mesma seqüência num ácido polinucléico situadas uma adjacente à outra.
tan·gen·ti·al·i·ty (tan-jen′shē-al′i-tē). Tangencialidade; distúrbio do processo mental associativo, em que o indivíduo tende a desviar-se facilmente de um tópico em discussão para outros tópicos que surgem no curso de associações; observada no distúrbio bipolar e na esquizofrenia, bem como em determinados tipos de distúrbios cerebrais orgânicos. Cf. circumstantiality. [fora de uma tangente, do L. *tango,* tocar]
tan·gle (tang′l). Emaranhado; novelo; pequeno nó irregular.
neurofibrillary t., novelo neurofibrilar; acúmulos intraneuronais de filamentos helicoidais com padrões contorcidos; encontrado em células do hipocampo e do córtex cerebral em indivíduos com doença de Alzheimer.
tank. Tanque, reservatório; dispositivo para receber e/ou manter líquidos.
Hubbard t., t. de Hubbard; grande tanque, geralmente com água morna, utilizado para exercícios terapêuticos num programa de fisioterapia.
tan·nase (tan′ās). Tanase; tanino acil-hidrolase, uma enzima produzida em culturas de *Penicillium glaucum* e encontrada em determinadas plantas produtoras de tanino; hidrolisa o digalato em galato e também atua sobre ligações éster em outros taninos.
tan·nate (tan′āt) Tanato; sal do ácido tânico.
Tanner growth chart. Tabela de crescimento de Tanner. Ver em chart.
Tanner stage. Estágio Tanner. Ver em stage.
tan·nic (tan′ik). Tânico; relativo a curtume (casca de carvalho) ou ao tanino.
tan·nic ac·id. Ácido tânico; um tanino, $C_{76}H_{52}O_{46}$, encontrado em muitas plantas, sobretudo na casca de carvalhos e outros membros das Fagaceae; utilizado com o estíptico e adstringente, bem como no tratamento da diarréia; também disponível na forma de glicerito de ácido tânico. Algumas vezes utilizado como sinônimo de tanino.
tan·nin (tan′in). Tanino; qualquer um de um grupo de constituintes vegetais não-uniformes e complexos, que podem ser classificados em taninos hidrolisáveis (ésteres de um açúcar, geralmente glicose, e um ou vários ácidos triidroxibenzenocarboxílicos) e taninos condensados (derivados de flavonóis). Os taninos são utilizados no curtume, na coloração, em fotografia e como agentes de clarificação para cerveja e vinho. Termo algumas vezes empregado como sinônimo de ácido tânico. Os taninos formam corantes pretos na presença de ferro.
tan·nyl·ac·e·tate (tan-il-as′e-tāt). Tanil acetato. SIN acetyltannic acid.
tan·ta·lum (Ta) (tan′tă-lŭm). Tântalo; metal pesado do grupo do vanádio, de número atômico 73, peso atômico 180,9479; utilizado em próteses cirúrgicas, em virtude de suas propriedades não-corrosivas. [G. rei mitológico da Lídia, *Tantalus*]
tan·trum (tan′trŭm). Ataque de cólera; ataque de mau humor, especialmente em crianças.
tan·y·cyte (tan′i-sīt). Tanicito; variedade de célula ependimária encontrada principalmente nas paredes do terceiro ventrículo do cérebro; os tanicitos podem exibir prolongamentos ramificados ou não-ramificados, alguns dos quais terminam em capilares ou neurônios.
tan·y·pho·nia (tan-i-fō′nē-ă). Tanifonia; voz fraca e fina resultante de tensão dos músculos vocais. [G. *tanyō,* distender + *phonē,* som]
TAP. Proteína que transporta um peptídio do citoplasma para a luz do retículo endoplasmático.
tap. **1.** Puncionar; retirar líquido de uma cavidade por meio de um trocarte e cânulo, agulha oca ou cateter. **2.** Percutir levemente com o dedo ou um instrumento semelhante a um martelo na percussão ou para produzir um reflexo tendíneo. **3.** Golpe leve. **4.** Febre das Índias Orientais de natureza indeterminada. **5.** Instrumento para fazer roscas em um orifício no osso antes da inserção de um parafuso. [M.E. *tappe,* do A.S. *taeppa*]
heel t., movimento reflexo dos dedos dos pés quando o calcanhar é percutido, presente na esclerose múltipla e em outras doenças do trato piramidal.
mitral t., golpe mitral; **(1)** o equivalente palpável do estalido de abertura da valva mitral; **(2)** a primeira bulha cardíaca hiperfonética palpável da estenose mitral; freqüentemente confundido com batimento apical.
pericardial t., punção pericárdica, pericardiocentese. SIN pericardiocentesis.
pleural t., punção pleural, toracocentese. SIN thoracocentesis.
spinal t., punção lombar. SIN lumbar *puncture*.
tape (tāp). Fita; faixa fina e achatada de fáscia ou tendão ou de material sintético, empregada como ligadura ou sutura. [A.S. *taeppe*]
adhesive t., f. adesiva, esparadrapo; tecido ou película uniformemente recoberto de um lado com uma mistura adesiva sensível à pressão.
ta·pe·to·cho·roi·dal (tă-pē′tō-kō-roy′dăl). Tapetocorioidal; relativo ao tapete e à corióide.

ta·pe·to·ret·i·nal (tă-pē′tō-ret′i-năl). Tapetorretiniano; relativo ao epitélio pigmentar da retina e à retina sensorial.
ta·pe·to·ret·in·op·a·thy (tă-pē′tō-ret-in-op′ă-thē). Tapetorretinopatia; degeneração hereditária da retina sensorial e do epitélio pigmentar; observada na retinopatia pigmentar, corioideremia, atrofia circinada, nictalopia congênita, amaurose congênita e degeneração heredomacular. [tapetum + retinopathy]
ta·pe·tum, pl. **ta·pe·ta** (tă-pē′tŭm, -tă). Tapete. **1.** Em geral, qualquer camada ou revestimento membranoso. **2.** [TA]. Em neuroanatomia, lâmina delgada de fibras na parede lateral dos cornos temporal e occipital do ventrículo lateral, contínua com o corpo caloso. SIN Fielding membrane, membrana versicolor. **3.** Camada densa na corióide do olho de muitas espécies de mamíferos, incluindo o gato e o cão, mas não os seres humanos, que forma uma área distinta ou difusa de células refletivas, pequenos bastonetes e fibras; suas propriedades de reflexão da luz intensa produzem o tom metálico e o brilho desses olhos no escuro. [L. *tapeta,* tapete]
t. alve′oli, periodonto. SIN periodontium.
t. ni′grum, estrato pigmentoso da retina. SIN pigmented *layer* of retina.
t. oc′uli, estrato pigmentoso da retina. SIN pigmented *layer* of retina.
tape·worm (tāp′werm). Tênia; verme parasita intestinal, cujos adultos são encontrados no intestino de vertebrados; o termo é geralmente restrito a membros da classe Cestoidea. As tênias são constituídas de um escólex, diversamente equipado com estruturas espinhosas ou de sucção por meio das quais o verme se fixa à parede intestinal do hospedeiro, e de estróbilos, que possuem várias a numerosas proglotes, sem tubo digestivo em qualquer estágio de seu desenvolvimento. Ao alcançar o intestino de um hospedeiro intermediário apropriado, o ovo eclode e libera o hexacanto, penetra na parede intestinal e transforma-se numa forma larvar específica (p. ex., cisticercóide, cisticerco, hidátide, estrobilocerco), que se transforma num adulto quando o hospedeiro intermediário é ingerido pelo hospedeiro final apropriado. Nos ciclos de vida aquáticos, observa-se um ciclo constituído de três hospedeiros, com coracídio natatório, larva procercóide e pleurocercóide (espárgano) e verme adulto intestinal, como no *Diphyllobothrium latum* e em outros cestóides pseudofiládeos. Outras espécies importantes de tênia incluem *Echinococcus granulosus, Hymenolepis nana* ou *H. nana* var. *fraterna, Taenia saginata, T. solium* e *Thysanosoma actinoides.*
taph·o·phil·ia (taf-ō-fil′ē-ă). Tafofilia; atração mórbida por túmulos. [G. *taphos,* túmulo + *phileō,* amar]
taph·o·pho·bia (taf-ō-fō′bē-ă). Tafofobia; medo mórbido de ser enterrado vivo. [G. *taphos,* túmulo + *phobos,* medo]
Tapia, Antonio G., otolaringologista espanhol, 1875–1950. VER T. *syndrome.*
tap·i·no·ce·phal·ic (tap′i-nō-sē-fal′ik, tă-pī′nō-). Tapinocefálico; que possui cabeça achatada e baixa; relativo à tapinocefalia.
tap·i·no·ceph·a·ly (tă-pi-nō-sef′ă-lē). Tapinocefalia; condição de achatamento da cabeça, em que o crânio possui um índice vertical inferior a 72; semelhante à camecefalia. [G. *tapeinos,* baixo + *kephalē,* cabeça]
tap·i·o·ca (tap′ē-ō′kă). Tapioca; amido da raiz de *Janipha manihot* e de outras espécies de *J.* (família Euphorbiaceae), plantas da América tropical; trata-se de um amido de fácil digestão, desprovido de propriedades irritantes. SIN cassava starch. [Bras. *tipioca*]
ta·pote·ment (tă-pot-mawn′). Tapotagem; movimento de massagem que consiste em golpear com a parte lateral da mão, habitualmente com os dedos parcialmente flexionados. SIN tapping. [Fr. de *tapoter,* dar pancadinhas]
tap·ping (tap′ing). **1.** Tapotagem. SIN tapotement. **2.** Paracentese. SIN paracentesis.
TAPVC Abreviatura de total anomalous pulmonary venous connection (conexão venosa pulmonar anômala total). VER anomalous pulmonary venous *connections,* total or partial, em *connection.*
TAPVR Abreviatura de total anomalous pulmonary venous *return* (retorno venoso pulmonar anômalo total). VER anomalous pulmonary venous *connections,* total or partial, em *connection.*
TAR Acrônimo de *t*hrombocytopenia and *a*bsent *r*adius (trombocitopenia e ausência do rádio). VER thrombocytopenia-absent radius *syndrome.*
tar. Alcatrão; massa espessa, semi-sólido e castanho-enegrecida, composta de hidrocarbonetos complexos, obtida pela destilação destrutiva de materiais carbonáceos. Para os alcatrões individuais, ver os nomes específicos.
rectified t. oil, óleo de alcatrão retificado; óleo volátil destilado do alcatrão de pinheiro; utilizado externamente no tratamento de doenças cutâneas, como eczema e psoríase.
tar·an·tism (tar′an-tizm). Tarantismo; forma de histeria coletiva que surgiu em Taranto, Itália, no final da Idade Média, como mania de dançar para curar a loucura supostamente causada pela picada de uma tarântula.
ta·ran·tu·la (tă-ran′choo-lă) Tarântula; aranha muito grande e peluda, considerada muito venenosa, e que costuma ser muito temida; todavia, a sua picada geralmente não causa maior dano do que a picada de uma abelha, e a criatura é relativamente inofensiva. VER tarantism.
American t., t. americana; *Eurypelma hentzii,* a t. do Arkansas; embora muito temida, sua picada é relativamente incomum e inofensiva para os seres humanos.

black t., t. negra; *Sericopelma communis,* grande t. negra do Panamá e da Zona do Canal, cuja picada é venenosa, apesar de o efeito ser localizado.
European t., t. européia; *Lycosa tarentula,* a grande aranha armadeira européia ou t. verdadeira. Antigamente, acreditava-se que sua picada causava loucura, o que inspirou contorções e danças frenéticas para livrar o corpo do veneno, embora a picada seja, na verdade, inofensiva, como a da maioria das grandes "tarântulas" peludas dos trópicos.
Peruvian t., t. peruana; *Glyptocranium gasteracanthoides,* uma aranha peruana venenosa cuja picada provoca gangrena local, hematúria e sintomas neurotóxicos.

ta·rax·a·cum (tă-rak'să-kŭm). Taraxaco; o rizoma e a raiz secos de *Taraxacum officinale* (família Compositae), o dente-de-leão, uma planta selvagem de ampla distribuição por todas as regiões temperadas do hemisfério norte; considerado tônico e estimulante hepático. [L. Mod. do Ár. *tarakshagūn,* chicória selvagem]

Tardieu, Ambroise A., médico francês, 1818–1879. VER T. *ecchymoses,* em *ecchymosis, petechiae,* em *petechiae, spots,* em *spot.*

tar·dive (tar'div). Tardio; tarde; moroso.
cyanose t., cianose tardia. SIN late cyanosis.

tar·get (tar'get). **1.** Alvo; objeto fixado como meta ou ponto de exame. **2.** No oftalmômetro, a mira. **3.** Órgão-alvo. SIN target *organ.* **4.** Anodo de um tubo de raios X. VER TAMBÉM x-ray. [It. *targhetta,* um pequeno escudo]

tar·get·ing (tar'get-ing). Marcação; processo pelo qual determinadas proteínas contêm sinais específicos, de modo que as proteínas são dirigidas especificamente para determinados locais celulares, p. ex., o lisossoma. Cf. processing.

targretin (tar'gre-tin). Targretina; análogo retinóide sintético novo que se liga a membros da subclasse RXR de receptores; possui baixa toxicidade e induz a apoptose em vários tipos de células tumorais.

Tarin (Tarini, Tarinus), Pierre, anatomista francês, 1725–1761. VER T. *space, tenia, valve; valvula* semilunaris tarini; *velum* tarini.

ta·rir·ic ac·id (tă-rī'rik). Ácido tarírico; ácido de 18 carbonos, notável pela presença de uma ligação tripla.

Tarlov, Isadore Max, cirurgião norte-americano, *1905. VER T. *cyst.*

Tarnier, Étienne Stephane, obstetra francês, 1828–1897. VER T. *forceps.*

tar·ra·gon oil (tar'ă-gon). Óleo de tarragona; óleo volátil destilado a partir das folhas *Artemisia dranculus* (família Compositae); aromatizante. SIN estragon oil.

△ **tars-.** Tars-. VER tarso-.

tar·sal (tar'săl). Tarsal; relativo ao tarso em qualquer sentido.

tar·sa·le, pl. **tar·sa·lia** (tar-să'lē, tar-să'lē-ă) [TA]. Tarsal. SIN tarsal *bones,* em *bone.* [L. Mod. do G. *tarsos,* planta do pé]

tars·al·gia (tar-sal'jē-ă). Tarsalgia. SIN podalgia. [tarsus + G. *algos,* dor]

tar·sa·lis (tar-să'lis). Músculo tarsal. VER inferior tarsal *muscle,* superior tarsal *muscle.*

tars·ec·to·my (tar-sek'tō-mē). Tarsectomia; excisão do tarso do pé ou de um segmento do tarso de uma pálpebra. [tarsus + G. *ektomē,* excisão]

tar·sec·to·pia, tar·sec·to·py (tar-sek-tō'pē-ă, -sek'tō-pē). Tarsectopia; subluxação de um ou mais ossos do tarso. [tarsus + G. *ektopos,* fora do lugar]

tar·sen. Dentro do tarso; relativo ao tarso, independente de outras estruturas. [tarsus + G. *en,* dentro]

tar·si·tis (tar-sī'tis). Tarsite. **1.** Inflamação do tarso do pé. **2.** Inflamação da borda tarsal de uma pálpebra.

△ **tarso-, tars-.** Tarso-, tars. Tarso. [Ver tarsus]

tar·so·cla·sia, tar·soc·la·sis (tar-sō-klā'zē-ă, tar-sok'lă-sis). Tarsoclasia; fratura instrumental do tarso para a correção do tálipe eqüinovaro. [tarso- + G. *klasis,* ruptura]

tar·so·ma·la·cia (tar'sō-mă-lā'shē-ă). Tarsomalacia; amolecimento das cartilagens tarsais das pálpebras. [tarso- + G. *malakia,* amolecimento]

tar·so·meg·a·ly (tar-sō-meg'ă-lē). Tarsomegalia; desenvolvimento congênito anormal e crescimento excessivo de um osso do tarso ou do carpo. SIN dysplasia epiphysialis hemimelia. [tarso- + G. *megas,* grande]

tar·so·met·a·tar·sal (tar-sō-met'ă-tar'săl). Tarsometatarsal; relativo aos ossos do tarso e do metatarso; designa as articulações entre dois grupos de ossos e os ligamentos correspondentes.

tar·so·or·bit·al (tar'sō-ōr'bi-tăl). Tarso-orbital; relativo às pálpebras e à órbita.

tar·so·pha·lan·ge·al (tar-sō-fă-lan'jē-ăl). Tarsofalângico; relativo ao tarso e às falanges.

tar·so·rha·phy (tar-sōr'ă-fē). Tarsorrafia; a sutura das margens palpebrais, parcial ou completa, para reduzir a fissura palpebral ou para proteger a córnea na ceratite ou na paralisia do músculo orbicular do olho. [tarso- + G. *rhaphē,* sutura]

tar·so·tar·sal (tar'sō-tar'săl). Tarsotarsal. SIN intertarsal.

tar·so·tib·i·al (tar'sō-tibē-al). Tarsotibial. SIN tibiotarsal.

tar·sot·o·my (tar-sot'ō-mē). Tarsotomia. **1.** Incisão da cartilagem tarsal de uma pálpebra. **2.** Termo raramente utilizado para qualquer operação no tarso do pé. [tarso- + G. *tomē,* incisão]

tar·sus, gen. e pl. **tar·si** (tar'sŭs, -sī). Tarso. **1.** Como divisão do esqueleto, os sete ossos do tarso do pé. SIN root of foot. VER tarsal *bones,* em *bone.* [G. *tarsos,* superfície plana, planta do pé, borda da pálpebra]. **2.** As placas fibrosas que conferem solidez e forma às bordas das pálpebras; com freqüência, incorretamente denominadas cartilagens tarsais ou ciliares. SIN skeleton of eyelid. VER TAMBÉM inferior t., superior t.
t. infe'rior [TA], t. inferior da pálpebra. SIN inferior t.
inferior t. [TA], t. inferior; a placa fibrosa na pálpebra inferior. SIN t. inferior [TA].
t. supe'rior [TA], t. superior da pálpebra. SIN superior t.
superior t. [TA], t. superior ; a placa fibrosa na pálpebra superior. SIN t. superior [TA].

tar·tar (tar'tăr). Tártaro. **1.** Crosta no interior dos barris de vinho, que consiste essencialmente em bitartarato de potássio. **2.** Depósito branco, castanho ou castanho-amarelado na margem gengival dos dentes ou abaixo dela, principalmente hidroxiapatita numa matriz orgânica. SIN dental calculus (2). [L. Mediev. *tartarum,* etim. desconhecida]
cream of t., bitartarato de potássio. SIN potassium bitartrate.
t. emetic., t. emético. SIN antimony potassium tartrate.
soluble t., tartarato de potássio. SIN potassium tartrate.

tar·tar·ic ac·id (tar-tar'ik). Ácido tartárico; produzido a partir do tártaro bruto; laxativo e refrigerante; utilizado na fabricação de vários pós, comprimidos e grânulos efervescentes.

tar·trate (tar'trāt). Tartarato; sal do ácido tartárico.
acid t., t. ácido; sal do ácido tartárico que contém um grupamento ácido ainda capaz de se combinar com uma base; p. ex., bitartarato.
normal t., t. normal; t. que contém grupamentos ácidos não-combinados.

tar·trat·ed (tar'trāt-ed). Tartarado; combinado com ou que contém tártaro ou ácido tartárico.

tar·tra·zine (tar'tră-zēn). [C.I. 19140]. Tartrazina; corante ácido amarelo utilizado em lugar do orange G numa variante da coloração azul anilina de Mallory para colágeno e corpúsculos de inclusão celulares. SIN hydrazine yellow.

tas·tant (tās'tant). Qualquer substância química que estimula as células sensoriais num botão gustativo.

taste (tāst). **1.** Saborear; perceber através do sistema gustatório. **2.** Sabor, gosto, paladar; sensação produzida por um estímulo apropriado aplicado aos botões gustativos. [It. *tastare;* L. *tango,* tocar]
after-t., paladar tardio. VER aftertaste.
color t., paladar colorido; forma de sinestesia em que o sentido das cores e o paladar estão associados, com a estimulação de qualquer desses sentidos induzindo uma sensação subjetiva no sentido associado. SIN pseudogeusesthesia.
franklinic t., sabor franklínico; sabor metálico ou amargo produzido pela aplicação de eletricidade estática à língua. SIN voltaic t.
voltaic t., sabor voltaico. SIN franklinic t.

TAT Abreviatura de thematic apperception *test* (teste de percepção temática).

tat·too (tă-too'). **1.** Tatuagem; implante ou injeção ornamental deliberada de pigmentos indeléveis na pele ou o efeito tintorial de implantação acidental. **2.** Tatuar; produzir esse efeito. O procedimento, histórica e geograficamente difundido, está associado a riscos de infecção. A remoção é difícil, e o tratamento com laser em pulsos oferece baixo risco de cicatriz. [Taiti, *tatu*]
amalgam t., t. de amálgama; lesão macular negro-azulada ou cinzenta da mucosa oral, causada por implante acidental de amálgama de prata no tecido durante uma restauração ou extração de dente.

tau (τ). **1.** A décima nona letra do alfabeto grego. **2.** Símbolo de tele (distância); relaxation time (tempo de relaxamento). **3.** Proteína que se associa a microtúbulos e outros elementos do citoesqueleto; o t. acelera a polimerização da tubulina e estabiliza os microtúbulos; é também encontrado na placa observada em indivíduos com doença de Alzheimer e em neurônios cerebrais em outros distúrbios neurodegenerativos.

tau·rine (taw'rin, -rēn). **1.** Taurina; ácido aminossulfônico, sintetizado a partir de L-cisteína e utilizado em diversas funções, incluindo na síntese de determinados sais biliares. **2.** Taurino; característico de ou que designa um touro. [L. *taurinus,* de touros, de *taurus,* touro + sufixo *-inus,* pertencente a]

tau·ro·cho·late (taw-rō-kō'lāt). Taurocolato; sal do ácido taurocólico.

tau·ro·cho·lic ac·id (taw-rō-kō'lik). Ácido taurocólico; coliltaurina; *N*-coloiltaurina; composto de ácido cólico e taurina, envolvendo o grupo carboxila do primeiro e o grupo amino da segunda; sal biliar comum em carnívoros. SIN cholaic acid.

tau·ro·don·tism (taw-rō-don'tizm). Taurodontismo; anomalia de desenvolvimento que envolve os dentes molares, nos quais a bifurcação ou trifurcação das raízes está muito próxima do ápice, resultando numa câmara pulpar anormalmente grande e longa, com canais pulpares excessivamente curtos. [L. *taurus,* touro + G. *odous,* dente]

Taussig, Helen B., pediatra norte-americana, 1898–1986. VER T.-Bing *disease, syndrome;* Blalock-T. *operation, shunt.*

tau·to·mer·ic (taw-tō-mer'ik). Tauromérico. **1.** Relativo à mesma parte. **2.** Relativo a ou caracterizado por tautomerismo. [G. *tautos,* o mesmo + *meros,* parte]

tau·tom·er·ism (taw-tom′er-izm). Tautomerismo; fenômeno em que uma substância química existe em duas formas de estruturas diferentes (isômeros) em equilíbrio, diferindo, as duas formas, geralmente na posição de um átomo de hidrogênio; por exemplo, tautomerismo ceto-enol, R–CH_2–C(O)–R′↔R–CH=C(OH)–R′. [G. *tautos*, o mesmo + *meros*, parte]

Tawara, K. Sunao, patologista japonês, 1873–1952. VER T. *node;* His-T. *system; node* of Aschoff and T.

taxa (tak′sā). Táxons; plural de taxon.

taxanes (taks′anz). Taxanos; classe de agentes antitumorais derivados diretamente ou de forma semi-sintética de *Taxus brevifolius*, o teixo do Pacífico; os exemplos incluem o paclitaxel e o docetaxel.

tax·is (tak′sis). Taxia. **1.** Redução de uma hérnia ou de uma luxação de qualquer parte por meio de manipulação. **2.** Classificação sistemática ou arranjo ordenado. **3.** A reação do protoplasma a um estímulo, através do qual animais e vegetais são levados a mover-se ou a agir em determinadas formas definidas em relação a seu ambiente; os vários tipos de taxia são designados por um prefixo que indica o estímulo que os determina; por exemplo, quimiotaxia, eletrotaxia, termotaxia. [G. disposição sistemática]
  negative t., t. negativa; a repulsão do protoplasma em relação a um estímulo.
  positive t., t. positiva; a atração do protoplasma em direção a um estímulo.

tax·on, pl. **taxa** (tak′son, tak′sā). Táxon; nome dado a determinado nível ou agrupamento numa classificação sistemática de coisas ou organismos vivos (taxonomia). [G. *taxis*, ordem, disposição + -on]

tax·o·nom·ic (tak-sō-nom′ik). Taxonômico; relativo a taxonomia.

tax·on·o·my (tak-san′o-mē). Taxonomia; a classificação sistemática de coisas ou organismos vivos. Os reinos dos organismos vivos são divididos em grupos (táxons) para mostrar graus de semelhança ou supostas relações evolutivas, sendo as categorias superiores maiores, mais inclusivas e mais amplamente definidas, enquanto as categorias inferiores são mais restritas, com menor número de espécies mais intimamente relacionadas. As divisões abaixo do reino são, em ordem decrescente: filo, classe, ordem, família, gênero, espécie e subespécie (variedade). As categorias infra- e supra- ou sub- e super- podem ser utilizadas quando necessário; outras categorias, como tribo, seção, nível, grupo etc., também são utilizadas. [G. *taxis*, disposição ordenada, + *nomos*, lei]

taxonomia	
classificação taxonômica de *Leptospira interrogans*	
reino	Procaryotae
filo	Gracillicutes
classe	Scotobacteria
ordem	Spirochaetales
família	Leptospiraceae
gênero	*Leptospira*
espécie	*Leptospira interrogans*
subespécie sorovariante	p. ex., *Leptospira interrogans* icterohemorrhagiae

  chemical t., t. química; abordagem para classificação dos organismos com base na distribuição de produtos naturais.
  numerical t., t. numérica; abordagem para classificação de organismos que lutam pela objetividade, em que são atribuídos pesos iguais às características dos organismos (classificação adansoniana), sendo as relações dos organismos •numericamente determinadas, em geral com auxílio de um computador.

Taxus (taks′us). Gênero de plantas que incluem o teixo do Pacífico (*Taxus brevifolius*); sua casca fornece agentes antitumorais do grupo taxano.

Tay, Warren, médico inglês, 1843–1927. VER T. cherry-red *spot*; T.-Sachs *disease*.

Taybi, Hooshang, pediatra e radiologista norte-americano, *1919. VER Rubinstein-T. *syndrome*.

Taylor, Charles F., cirurgião ortopédico norte-americano, 1827–1899. VER T. back *brace, apparatus, splint*.

Taylor, Robert W., dermatologista norte-americano, 1842–1908. VER T. *disease*.

TB Abreviatura coloquial de tuberculosis (tuberculose).

Tb Símbolo de terbium (térbio).

TBG Abreviatura de thyroxine-binding *globulin* (globulina ligadora de tiroxina).

tBoc Abreviatura de *tert*-butyloxycarbonyl (butiloxicarbonil/terciário).

TBP Abreviatura de thyroxine-binding *protein* (proteína ligadora de tiroxina).

TBPA Abreviatura de thyroxine-binding *prealbumin* (pré-albumina ligadora de tiroxina).

TBV Abreviatura de total blood volume (volume sanguíneo total).

TBW Abreviatura de total body *water* (água corporal total).

Tc Símbolo de technetium (tecnécio).

Tc Abreviatura de T cytotoxic *cells* (células T citotóxicas), em *cell*.

^{99m}Tc Símbolo de technetium-99m (tecnécio-99m).

^{99}Tc Símbolo de technetium-99 (tecnécio-99).

2,3,7,8-TCDD. Abreviatura de 2,3,7,8-tetrachlorodibenzo[b,e]-[1,4]dioxin (2,3,7,8-tetraclorodibenzo[b,e]-[1,4]dioxina). VER dioxin (3).

^{99m}Tc-dimercaptosuccinic acid. Ácido dimercaptossuccínico - Tc^{99m}; radiofármaco que localiza o córtex renal em técnicas de imagem para determinação de fibrose ou pielonefrite.

^{99m}Tc-DMSA Abreviatura de ^{99m}Tc-dimercaptosuccinic acid (ácido dimercaptossuccínico - Tc^{99m}).

TCG Abreviatura de time compensation *gain* (ganho de compensação temporal).

^{99m}Tc-glucoheptanate. Gluco-heptanato-Tc^{99m}; radiofármaco que possui propriedades de localização do córtex renal e de controle da excreção; pode ser utilizado para técnicas de imagem do córtex renal a fim de determinar se existe fibrose ou a função renal por renografia.

TCID$_{50}$, TCD$_{50}$ Abreviatura de tissue culture infectious *dose* (dose infecciosa em cultura de tecido).

TDF Abreviatura de testis-determining *factor* (fator determinante de testículos).

TDP Abreviatura de ribothymidine 5′-diphosphate (5′-difosfato de ribotimidina); o análogo timidínico do dTDP.

TdT Abreviatura de terminal deoxynucleotidyl *transferase* (transferase da desoxinucleotidil terminal).

TE Em seqüências de pulsos eco de spin na ressonância magnética, o tempo para o eco, quando o sinal de magnetização é recebido.

Te Símbolo de tellurium (telúrio).

tea (tē). Chá. **1.** As folhas secas de vários gêneros da família Theaceae, incluindo *Thea* (*T. senensis), Camellia* e *Gordonia*, um arbusto nativo da China, do Sul e Sudeste da Ásia e do Japão. Seu principal constituinte, do qual depende, em grande parte, sua ação estimulante, é o alcalóide cafeína, que está presente na quantidade de 1-4%; existe também a teofilina, um alcalóide quimicamente relacionado. **2.** A infusão feita ao despejar água fervendo sobre as folhas de chá. **3.** Qualquer infusão ou decocção feita de modo extemporâneo. VER TAMBÉM species (2). SIN thea. [Chinês (dial. Amoy) *t'e*, L. Mod. *thea*]
  Hottentot t., c. de Hottentot. SIN buchu.
  Jesuit t., Mexican t., c. de jesuíta, c. mexicano. SIN chenopodium.
  Paraguay t., c. do Paraguai. SIN maté.

Teale, Thomas P., cirurgião inglês, 1801–1868.

tear (tār). Laceração; descontinuidade na substância de uma estrutura. Cf. laceration.
  bucket-handle t., l. em alça de balde; laceração e separação na parte central de uma cartilagem semilunar com as extremidades intactas, que produz uma figura semelhante à alça de um balde.

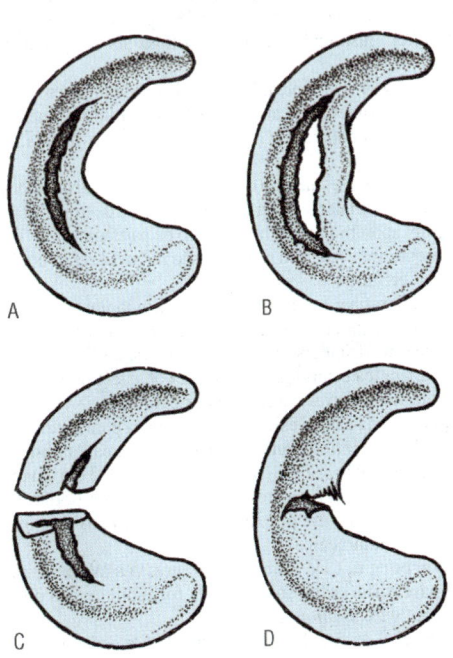

lacerações do menisco: (A) longitudinal, (B) em alça de balde, (C) horizontal, (D) em bico de papagaio

Mallory-Weiss t., t. de Mallory-Weiss. SIN Mallory-Weiss *syndrome.*

tear (tēr). Lágrima; o líquido secretado pelas glândulas lacrimais por meio do qual a conjuntiva e a córnea são mantidas úmidas. [A.S. *teár*]
  artificial t.'s, lágrimas artificiais; misturas de compostos líquidos para substituir as lágrimas produzidas naturalmente.
  crocodile t.'s, lágrimas de crocodilo. VER crocodile tears *syndrome.*

tear·ing (tēr'ing). Epífora. SIN epiphora.

tease (tēz). Separar as partes estruturais de um tecido por meio de uma agulha com o objetivo de prepará-lo para exame microscópico. [A.S. *taesan*]

tea·spoon (tē'spoon). Colher de chá; colher pequena, com capacidade de 1 dracma (cerca de 5 ml de líquido); utilizada como medida na dosagem de medicamentos líquidos.

teat (tēt). **1.** Mamilo. SIN nipple. **2.** Mama. SIN breast. **3.** Papila. SIN papilla. [A.S. *tit*]

teb·u·tate (teb'ū-tāt). Tebutato; contração aprovada pela USAN para o butilacetato terciário, $(CH_3)_3C-CH_2-CO_2^-$.

tech·ne·ti·um (Tc) (tek-nē'shē-um). Tecnécio; elemento radioativo artificial, de número atômico 43, peso atômico 99, produzido em 1937 por bombardeio do molibdênio por dêuterons; trata-se também de um produto da fissão do U^{235}; utilizado como marcador radiográfico em estudos de imagem de órgãos internos. [G. *technetos,* artificial]

tech·ne·ti·um-99 (^{99}Tc). Tecnécio-99; radioisótopo do tecnécio que é o produto da desintegração do tecnécio-99m e que possui emissão beta fraca e meia-vida física de 213.000 anos.

tech·ne·ti·um-99m (^{99m}Tc). Tecnécio-99m (Tc^{99m}); radioisótopo do tecnécio que sofre desintegração por transição isomérica, emitindo um raio gama essencialmente monoenergético de 142 keV, com meia-vida de 6,01 h. Em geral, é obtido a partir de um gerador de radionuclídios de molibdênio-99 e é utilizado no preparo de radiofármacos para cintilografia do cérebro, das parótidas, da tireóide, dos pulmões, de acúmulo de sangue, do fígado, do coração, do baço, dos rins, do aparelho de drenagem lacrimal, dos ossos e da medula óssea.

^{99m}Tc diphosphonate, difosfonato de Tc^{99m}; complexo de radionuclídio utilizado para cintilografias ósseas.

^{99m}Tc-DTPA, Tc^{99m}-DTPA; complexo de quelato de radionuclídios utilizado para obter imagens e avaliação da função dos rins; também conhecido como pentatato de Tc^{99m}. [*d*iethylene *t*riamine *p*enta*a*cetic *a*cid]

^{99m}Tc sestamibi, sestamibi Tc^{99m}; complexo catiônico lipofílico de um isonitrito marcado com Tc^{99m}, utilizado como radionuclídio em diversos órgãos (por exemplo, cérebro, osso, tireóide, mama) para detecção de câncer, ou no coração para a identificação de oclusão da artéria coronária. Substituiu T1-201 nos métodos de imagens cardíacas e nas mamas (experimental).

^{99m}Tc sulfur colloid, colóide de enxofre Tc^{99m}; complexo de radionuclídios particulados captado pelo sistema reticuloendotelial; utilizado para obter imagens do fígado e do baço.

tech·nic (tek-nik'). Técnica. SIN technique.

tech·ni·cal (tek'ni-kal). Técnico. **1.** Relativo a técnica. **2.** Relativo à alguma arte, ciência ou negócio específico. **3.** Associado a uma substância química, indica que a substância contém quantidades apreciáveis de impurezas.

tech·ni·cian (tek-nish'ŭn). Técnico, tecnólogo. SIN technologist. [G. *technē,* uma arte]

tech·nique (tek-nēk'). Técnica; forma de desempenho ou os detalhes de qualquer cirurgia, experimento ou ato mecânico. VER TAMBÉM method, operation, procedure. SIN technic. [Fr., do G. *technikos,* relativo a *technē,* arte, habilidade]
  airbrasive t., t. abrasiva; método de triturar, cortar a estrutura do dente ou tornar a superfície de um dente natural ou a superfície de uma restauração áspera por meio de um aparelho que utiliza um jato de partículas finas de Al_2O_3 impelidas por gás que, após baterem no dente, são removidas por um aspirador. VER TAMBÉM microetching t.
  air·gap t., radiografia de tórax efetuada utilizando um espaço entre o indivíduo e o filme em lugar de uma placa para absorver a radiação dispersa; exige habitualmente uma distância do filme de 300 cm.
  atrial-well t., técnica cirúrgica semifechada obsoleta para reparo de defeitos do septo interatrial e outras anormalidades cardíacas.
  ballpoint pen t., t. da caneta esferográfica; técnica para medir a induração dos testes tuberculínicos intradérmicos; utiliza-se uma caneta esferográfica para traçar duas linhas opostas sobre a pele, começando 1-2 cm a partir do local da reação dérmica nos lados opostos, parando quando a borda de induração é percebida. A distância entre as extremidades proximais das linhas é a extensão registrada da induração.
  Barcroft-Warburg t., t. de Barcroft-Warburg. VER Warburg *apparatus.*
  Begg light wire differential force t., t. da força diferencial do fio elétrico de Begg. VER light wire *appliance.*
  cellulose tape t., t. da fita de celulose; uso de um pedaço de fita de celulose transparente aplicado a uma lâmina para obter amostras perianais para identificação de ovos de oxiúros.
  direct t., t. direta. SIN direct *method* for making inlays.
  Ficoll-Hypaque t., t. de Ficoll-Hypaque; técnica de centrifugação por gradiente de densidade para separar os linfócitos de outros elementos figurados do sangue; a amostra é depositada sobre um gradiente de Ficoll-metrizoato sódico de densidade específica; após centrifugação, os linfócitos são coletados da interface plasma-Ficoll.
  flicker fusion frequency t., perimetria de oscilação. SIN flicker *perimetry.*
  fluorescent antibody t., t. do anticorpo fluorescente; técnica utilizada para testar um antígeno com anticorpo fluorescente, geralmente efetuada por um de dois métodos: *direto,* em que a imunoglobulina (anticorpo) conjugada com um corante fluorescente é adicionada ao tecido e combina-se com um antígeno específico (micróbio ou outro antígeno), sendo o complexo antígeno-anticorpo resultante localizado por microscopia de fluorescência; ou *indireto,* em que a imunoglobulina não-marcada (anticorpo) é adicionada ao tecido e combina-se com um antígeno específico, podendo o complexo antígeno-anticorpo ser subseqüentemente marcado com anticorpo antiimunoglobulina conjugado com fluoresceína, sendo o complexo triplo resultante localizado por microscopia fluorescente.
  flush t., t. de ruborização; técnica para determinar a pressão arterial sistólica em lactentes; o membro elevado tem o sangue "ordenhado" da mão ou do pé em sentido proximal; a seguir, o manguito de pressão arterial é insuflado acima da pressão sistólica provável, e o membro é então abaixado; o manguito de pressão é então gradualmente liberado até haver ruborização do membro pálido.
  Hampton t., t. de Hampton; designação obsoleta para exame fluoroscópico atraumático, sem palpação do trato gastrintestinal superior na úlcera péptica com hemorragia ativa.
  Hartel t., t. de Hartel; método para alcançar o gânglio de Gasser introduzindo-se uma agulha pela boca, inserindo-a aproximadamente no nível do dente molar médio superior e levando-a para dentro até o ponto que alcança o osso na frente e até a face externa do forame oval, com injeção de álcool para alívio da neuralgia do trigêmeo.
  high-kV t., t. de alta kV; radiografia de tórax que utiliza uma quilovoltagem de pelo menos 125 kVp, geralmente 140-150 kVp, para reduzir a dose do paciente e aumentar a latitude.
  Ilizarov t., t. de Ilizarov; método para promover a osteogênese controlada com a finalidade de alongar o osso e corrigir deformidades angulares e de rotação, em que se aplica uma força gradualmente crescente a fragmentos apostos de um osso cirurgicamente dividido por uma estrutura de fixação externa (aparelho de Ilizarov).
  immunoperoxidase t., t. da imunoperoxidase; teste imunológico que utiliza anticorpos quimicamente conjugados com a enzima peroxidase.
  indirect t., t. indireta. SIN indirect *method* for making inlays.
  Jerne t., t. de Jerne; técnica para medir a imunocompetência através da quantificação de células esplênicas formadoras de anticorpos encontradas num camundongo sensibilizado a eritrócitos de carneiro. O número de placas formadas correlaciona-se com o número de células esplênicas formadoras de anticorpos.
  Judkins t., t. de Judkins; método de cateterismo seletivo da artéria coronária que utiliza técnica padrão de Seldinger através de punção percutânea da artéria femoral.
  Knott t., t. de Knott; procedimento de concentração que utiliza sangue e formol diluído; destinado a detectar microfilárias.
  long cone t., t. do cone longo; uso da distância de um cone de 35 cm ou mais na realização de radiografias orais.
  McGoon t., t. de McGoon; reconstrução plástica de uma valva mitral incompetente, quando a incompetência se deve a ruptura da cordoalha até o folheto posterior, por plicatura do folheto redundante.
  Merendino t., t. de Merendino; reconstrução plástica de uma valva mitral incompetente utilizando fios de sutura grossos para estreitar o anel na região da comissura medial.
  microetching t., t. de microcorrosão; método para tornar a superfície de um dente natural ou uma restauração áspera utilizando um jato de partículas finas abrasivas impelidas por gás. Aumenta a fixação de cimentos de resina ou materiais de restauração à superfície. VER TAMBÉM airbrasive t.
  Mohs fresh tissue chemosurgery t., t. de quimiocirurgia de tecido fresco de Mohs; quimiocirurgia em que se efetua a excisão de cânceres superficiais após fixação *in vivo.*
  Ouchterlony t., t. de Ouchterlony; técnica em que ambos os componentes da reação (antígeno e anticorpo) difundem-se um para o outro num gel, numa reação de precipitação.
  PAP t., t. de PAP; método de peroxidase com anticorpo não-marcado, que reage tanto com o anticorpo antiperoxidase de rábano bastardo do coelho quanto com a peroxidase livre do rábano bastardo para formar um complexo solúvel de peroxidase-antiperoxidase ou PAP; método imuno-histoquímico muito sensível aplicável a tecidos imersos em parafina.
  rebreathing t., t. de reinalação; uso de um circuito de respiração ou anestesia, em que o ar expirado é subseqüentemente inalado, com ou sem absorção de CO_2 do ar expirado.

Rebuck skin window t., t. da janela cutânea de Rebuck; teste *in vivo* da resposta inflamatória, em que a pele é escoriada, e aplica-se uma lâmina à área escoriada para permitir a visualização da mobilização dos leucócitos.
sealed jar t., t. do recipiente fechado; técnica para produzir suspensão da animação em pequenos animais experimentais, que consiste em fechar o animal num recipiente que é então refrigerado.
Seldinger t., t. de Seldinger; método de inserção percutânea de um cateter num vaso sangüíneo ou espaço: utiliza-se uma agulha para puncionar a estrutura e introduz-se um fio-guia através da agulha; quando esta é retirada, o cateter é passado sobre o fio; este é então retirado, deixando-se o cateter no lugar.
sterile insect t., t. do inseto estéril; técnica utilizada para controle ou erradicação de pragas ou vetores, utilizando a indução por irradiação de letalidade dominante nos cromossomas dos insetos liberados.
vacuum pack t., t. da compressa a vácuo; fechamento temporário do abdome por meio de uma folha de plástica fenestrada sobre o intestino, porém sob a parede abdominal anterior, seguido da colocação de tampões umedecidos com cateter de sucção no interior da ferida. Todo o defeito é então coberto por uma folha de plástico não-porosa; permite a drenagem da cavidade abdominal por sucção, enquanto mantém a rigidez da parede abdominal anterior.
washed field t., t. do campo lavado; corte de preparações de cavidade nos dentes utilizando um irrigante constante, que é imediatamente removido da boca através de um dispositivo a vácuo.
tech·no·cau·sis (tek-nō-kaw′sis) Tecnocause. SIN actual *cautery*. [G. *technē*, arte + *kausis*, queimadura]
tech·nol·o·gist (tek-nol′ō-jist). Tecnólogo; técnico; indivíduo treinado e que utiliza as técnicas de uma profissão, arte ou ciência. SIN technician.
tech·nol·o·gy (tek-nol′ō-jē). Tecnologia; o conhecimento e o uso de técnicas de uma profissão, arte ou ciência. [G. *technē*, arte + *logos*, estudo]
assisted reproductive t., t. da reprodução assistida; originalmente, um conjunto de técnicas para manipulação de ovos e espermatozóides para superar a infertilidade. Abrange tratamentos farmacológicos para estimular a ovulação; métodos cirúrgicos para remoção dos ovos (p. ex., laparoscopia e aspiração transvaginal guiada por ultra-som) e para reimplante de embriões (p. ex., transferência intratubária do zigoto (ou ZIFT, *zygote intrafallopian transfer*); fertilização *in vitro* e *in vivo* (p. ex., inseminação artificial ou transferência intratubária de gameta (ou GIFT, *gamete intrafallopian transfer*); cirurgia fetal *ex utero* e *in utero*; bem como métodos laboratoriais para congelamento e triagem de espermatozóides e embriões e micromanipulação e clonagem de embriões. VER eugenics.
tec·lo·thi·a·zide (tek-lō-thī′a-zīd). Teclotiazida. SIN tetrachlormethiazide.
tec·tal (tek′tal). Relativo a um teto.
tec·ti·form (tek′ti-fōrm). Em forma de teto.
Tec·ti·vi·ri·dae (tek′tē-vī′rā-dā). Nome de uma família de bacteriófagos de DNA de duplo filamento sem envoltório, icosaédricos, que possuem capsídios duplos. [L. *tectum*, teto, cobertura, + vírus]
tec·to·ce·phal·ic (tek′tō-se-fal′ik). Escafocefálico. SIN scaphocephalic. [L. *tectum*, teto + G. *kephalē*, cabeça]
tec·to·ceph·a·ly (tek′to-sef′a-lē). Escafocefalia. SIN scaphocephaly.
tec·tol·o·gy (tek-tol′ō-jē). Tectonologia; morfologia estrutural. [G. *tektōn*, construtor + -*logia*]
tec·ton·ic (tek-ton′ik). Tectônico; relativo a variações na estrutura do olho, sobretudo da córnea. [G. *tektonikos*, relativo a uma construção]
tec·to·ri·al (tek-tōr′ē-al). Tectorial; relativo a ou característico de uma membrana tectória.
tec·to·ri·um (tek-tōr′ē-um). 1. Estrutura sobrejacente. 2. Membrana tectória do ducto coclear. SIN tectorial *membrane* of cochlear duct. [L. uma superfície sobrejacente (reboco, estuque), de *tego*, pp. *tectus*, cobrir]
tec·to·spi·nal (tek-tō-spī′nal). Tetospinal; designa fibras nervosas que se estendem do teto do mesencéfalo até a medula espinal.
tec·tum, pl. **tec·ta** (tek′tum, tek′ta). Teto; qualquer cobertura ou estrutura semelhante a um teto. [L. teto, estrutura com teto, de *tego*, pp. *tectus*, cobrir]
t. mesenceph′ali [TA], lâmina do t. do mesencéfalo. SIN lamina of mesencephalic tectum.
t. of midbrain, lâmina do t. do mesencéfalo. SIN lamina of mesencephalic tectum.
TEDD Abreviatura de total end-diastolic *diameter* (diâmetro diastólico final total).
teel oil (tēl). Óleo de sésamo ou de gergelim. SIN sesame oil.
teeth (tēth). Dentes; plural de tooth.
acoustic teeth [TA], dentes acústicos do limbo espiral do ducto coclear; formações ou cristas em forma de dente que ocorrem no lábio vestibular do limbo espiral do ducto coclear. SIN dentes acustici [TA], auditory teeth, Corti auditory teeth, Huschke auditory teeth.
teeth·ing (tē′thing). Dentição; erupção dos dentes, especialmente dos dentes decíduos. SIN odontiasis.
tef·lu·rane (tef′loo-rān). Teflurano; anestésico inalatório não-explosivo e não-inflamável de potência moderada.

teg·men, gen. **teg·mi·nis,** pl. **teg·mi·na** (teg′men, -mi-nis, -mi-nă). Tegme; teto; estrutura que recobre ou serve como teto de uma parte. [L. uma cobertura, de *tego*, cobrir]
t. cru′ris, designação antiga de *tegmentum* mesencephali (tegmento do mesencéfalo).
t. mastoi′deum, a lâmina óssea que serve como teto das células mastóideas.
t. tym′pani [TA], tegme timpânico; o teto da orelha média, formado pela superfície anterior adelgaçada da parte petrosa do osso temporal. Sua borda anterior está inserida na fissura petroescamosa, de modo que pode ser observada como cunha de osso subdividindo a fissura em fissura escamotimpânica e fissura petrotimpânica. SIN roof of tympanum.
t. ventric′uli quar′ti [TA], teto do quarto ventrículo; teto do quarto ventrículo, formado em sua parte superior pelo véu medular superior, que se estende entre os dois braços conjuntivos (pedúnculos cerebelares superiores) e, em sua parte inferior, pelo véu medular inferior, composto da membrana coróidea e do plexo coróideo do quarto ventrículo. SIN roof of fourth ventricle [TA].
teg·men·tal (teg-men′tal). Tegmentar; relativo a, característico de ou colocado ou orientado em direção a um tegmento ou tegme.
teg·men·tot·o·my (teg-men-tot′ō-mē). Tegmentotomia; produção de lesões na formação reticular do tegmento do mesencéfalo. [tegmentum + G. *tomē*, incisão]
teg·men·tum, pl. **teg·men·ta** (teg-men′tum, -tă). Tegmento. 1. Estrutura de revestimento. 2. Tegmento do mesencéfalo. SIN mesencephalic t. [L. estrutura de cobertura, de *tego*, cobrir]
t. mesenceph′ali [TA], t. do mesencéfalo. SIN mesencephalic t.
mesencephalic t., t. do mesencéfalo; a principal parte da substância do mesencéfalo, que se estende da substância negra até o nível do aqueduto cerebral. SIN t. mesencephali [TA], t. of midbrain [TA], midbrain t., tegmentum (2).
midbrain t., t. do mesencéfalo. SIN mesencephalic t.
t. of midbrain [TA], t. do mesencéfalo. SIN mesencephalic t.
t. of pons [TA], t. da ponte. SIN dorsal *part* of pons.
t. pontis [TA], t. da ponte. SIN dorsal *part* of pons.
t. rhombenceph′ali, t. do rombencéfalo. SIN rhombencephalic t.
rhombencephalic t., t. do rombencéfalo; a porção da ponte contínua com o teto do mesencéfalo; consiste na formação reticular, tratos e núcleos dos nervos cranianos e forma a parte dorsal da ponte (pars dorsalis pontis). SIN t. of rhombencephalon, t. rhombencephali.
t. of rhombencephalon, t. do rombencéfalo. SIN rhombencephalic t.
teg·u·ment (teg′ū-ment). Tegumento. 1. SIN integument. 2. SIN integument (2). [L. *tegumentum*, forma colateral de *tegmentum*]
teg·u·men·tal, teg·u·men·ta·ry (teg-ū-men′tal, teg-ū-men′tă-rē). Tegumentar, tegumentário; relativo ao tegumento.
Teichmann, Ludwig, histologista alemão, 1823–1895. VER T. *crystals,* em crystal.
tei·cho·ic ac·ids (tī-kō′ik). Ácidos teicóicos; uma de duas classes (sendo a outra constituída pelos ácidos murâmicos ou mucopeptídeos) de polímeros que constituem as paredes celulares de bactérias Gram-positivas, mas que também são encontrados no meio intracelular; polímeros lineares de um poliol (fosfato de ribitol ou fosfato de glicerol) que transportam resíduos D-alanil esterificados por grupamentos OH com ligação glicosídica.
tei·chop·si·a (tī-kop′sē-ă). Teicopsia; sensação visual tremeluzente recortada, semelhante às fortificações de uma torre medieval; o escotoma cintilante da enxaqueca. [G. *teichos*, parede, + *opsis*, visão]
tel-, tele-, telo-. Tel-, tele-, telo-; distância, extremidade, outra extremidade. [G. *tēle*, distante, *telos*, extremidade]
te·la, gen. e pl. **te·lae** (tē′lă, tē′lē). Tela. 1. Qualquer estrutura fina semelhante a uma rede. 2. Um tecido; especialmente aquele de formação delicada. [L. teia]
t. choroi′dea [TA], t. corióidea; parte da pia-máter que recobre o teto ependimário ou, no caso do ventrículo lateral, a parede medial de um ventrículo cerebral. SIN choroid membrane [TA].
t. choroi′dea of fourth ventricle [TA], t. corióidea do quarto ventrículo; o folheto da pia-máter que recobre a parte inferior do teto ependimário do quarto ventrículo. SIN t. choroidea ventriculi quarti [TA], t. choroidea inferior.
t. choroi′dea infe′rior, t. corióidea do quarto ventrículo. SIN t. choroidea of fourth ventricle.
t. choroi′dea supe′rior, t. corióidea do terceiro ventrículo. SIN t. choroidea of third ventricle.
t. choroi′dea of third ventricle, t. corióidea do terceiro ventrículo; prega dupla da pia-máter, encerrando trabéculas subaracnóideas, entre o fórnice acima e o teto epitelial do terceiro ventrículo e o tálamo abaixo; em cada margem lateral, existe uma franja vascular que se projeta na fissura corióidea do ventrículo lateral; em sua superfície inferior, existem várias projeções vasculares pequenas que preenchem as pregas do teto ependimário do terceiro ventrículo. SIN t. choroidea ventriculi tertii [TA], t. choroidea superior, triangular lamella, velum interpositum, velum triangulare.
t. choroi′dea ventric′uli quar′ti [TA], t. corióidea do quarto ventrículo. SIN t. choroidea of fourth ventricle.

t. choroi'dea ventric'uli ter'tii [TA], t. corióidea do terceiro ventrículo. SIN t. choroidea of third ventricle.
t. conjuncti'va, tecido conjuntivo. SIN connective tissue.
t. elas'tica, tecido elástico. SIN elastic tissue.
t. subcuta'nea [TA], tecido subcutâneo. SIN subcutaneous tissue.
t. subcuta'nea penis [TA], t. subcutânea do pênis. SIN subcutaneous tissue of penis.
t. subcuta'nea perinei [TA], t. subcutânea do períneo. SIN subcutaneous tissue of perineum.
t. submuco'sa, t. submucosa. SIN submucosa.
t. submuco'sa pharyn'gis, fáscia faringobasilar. SIN pharyngobasilar fascia.
t. subsero'sa [TA], t. subserosa. SIN subserosa.
t. vasculo'sa, plexo corióideo. SIN choroid plexus.

Te·la·dor·sa·gia dav·ti·ani (tē'lä-dōr-sä'jē-ä dav-shē-än'ī). Uma das espécies de vermes do estômago médio (família Trichostrongylidae) de carneiros, cabras e cervos, que ocorre no abomaso; semelhante a *Ostertagia trifurcata.* [tele- + L. *dorsum,* dorso]

tel·al'gia (tel-al'jē-ä). Telalgia, dor referida. SIN referred pain. [G. *tēle,* distante, + *algos,* dor]

tel·an·gi·ec·ta·sia (tel-an'jē-ek-tā'zē-ä). Telangiectasia; dilatação dos vasos pequenos ou terminais previamente existentes de uma parte. SIN angiotelectasis, angiotelectasia. [G. *telos,* fim + *angeion,* vaso, + *ektasis,* ação de estender]

cephalo-oculocutaneous t., t. cefaloculocutânea; angioma que acomete a pele da face, a órbita, as meninges e o cérebro. VER TAMBÉM Sturge-Weber *syndrome.*

essential t., t. essencial; **(1)** dilatação capilar localizada de origem indeterminada; **(2)** SIN angioma serpiginosum.

hereditary benign t., t. benigna hereditária; distúrbio autossômico dominante em que a face, a parte superior do tronco e os braços desenvolvem telangiectasias.

hereditary hemorrhagic t. [MIM*187300], t. hemorrágica hereditária; doença que surge habitualmente após a puberdade, caracterizada por múltiplas e pequenas telangiectasias e vênulas dilatadas que se desenvolvem lentamente sobre a pele e as mucosas; os locais freqüentes incluem a face, os lábios, a língua, a nasofaringe e a mucosa intestinal, e pode ocorrer sangramento recorrente; herança autossômica dominante, causada por mutação no gene (ENG) que codifica a endoglina no cromossoma 9q. SIN Rendu-Osler-Weber syndrome.

t. lymphat'ica, linfangiectasia. SIN lymphangiectasis.
t. macula'ris erupti'va per'stans, t. macular eruptiva persistente; erupção disseminada de telangiectasias associadas a máculas eritematosas e edematosas.

primary t., t. primária. SIN angioma serpiginosum.
secondary t., t. secundária; telangiectasia relacionada a uma causa conhecida de dilatação vascular prolongada na derme, como luz solar, veias varicosas e doenças do tecido conjuntivo; freqüentemente associada à atrofia da pele.
spider t., t. aracniforme. SIN spider angioma.
t. verruco'sa, angioceratoma. SIN angiokeratoma.

tel·an·gi·ec·ta·sis, pl. **tel·an·gi·ec·ta·ses** (tel-an'jē-ek'tä-sis, -sēz). Telangiectasia; lesão formada por um capilar ou artéria terminal dilatados, mais comumente na pele. VER telangiectasia.

tel·an·gi·ec·tat·ic (tel-an'jē-ek-tat'ik). Telangiectásico; relativo a ou caracterizado por telangiectasia.

tel·an·gi·ec·to·des (tel-an'jē-ek-tō'dēz). Telangiectóides; termo utilizado para qualificar tumores bastante vascularizados. [telangiectasis + G. -*ōdes,* de *eidos,* semelhança]

tel·an·gi·o·ma (tel-an'jē-ō'mä). Telangioma; angioma decorrente de dilatação dos capilares ou das arteríolas terminais.

tel·an·gi·on (tel-an'jē-on). Telângio; uma das arteríolas terminais ou um vaso capilar. SIN trichangion. [G. *telos,* fim, + *angeion,* vaso]

tel·an·gi·o·sis (tel'an-jē-ō'sis). Telangiose; qualquer doença dos capilares e das artérias terminais.

tele (tel'ē). Tele; refere-se ao átomo de nitrogênio do anel imidazólico da histidina, que é o mais distante do carbono β. Cf. *pros.* [G. *longe*]

♻ **tele-.** Tele-. VER tel-.

tel·e·can·thus (tel-ē-kan'thŭs). Telecanto; aumento da distância entre os cantos mediais das pálpebras. SIN canthal hypertelorism. [G. *tēle,* distante, + *kanthos,* canto]

tel·e·car·di·o·gram (tel-ē-kar'dē-ō-gram). Telecardiograma. SIN telelectrocardiogram.

tel·e·car·di·o·phone (tel-ē-kar'dē-ō-fōn). Telecardiofone; estetoscópio especialmente construído por meio do qual as bulhas cardíacas podem ser ouvidas por pessoas a certa distância do paciente. [G. *tēle,* distante, + *kardia* + coração, + *phōnē,* som]

tel·e·co·balt (tel'ē-kō'bawlt). Telecobalto; teleterapia que utiliza cobalto radioativo como fonte.

tel·e·di·ag·no·sis (tel'ē-dī-ag-nō'sis). Telediagnóstico; detecção de uma doença através da avaliação de dados transmitidos a uma estação de recepção, um processo que normalmente envolve instrumentos de monitorização do paciente e uma ligação de transferência a um centro de diagnóstico a determinada distância do paciente.

tel·e·di·a·stol·ic (tel'ē-dī-ä-stol'ik). Telediastólico; relativo a ou que ocorre próximo ao final da diástole ventricular. [G. *telos,* fim, + *diastolē,* dilatação]

telehopsias. Espectro de fortificação. SIN fortification *spectrum.*

tel·e·lec·tro·car·di·o·gram (tel'ē-lek-trō-kar'dē-ō-gram). Teleletrocardiograma; eletrocardiograma (ECG) registrado a uma certa distância do indivíduo que está sendo examinado; p. ex., o ECG obtido através de telemetria ou, como no caso de um galvanômetro no laboratório, conectado por um fio ao paciente em outra sala. SIN telecardiogram. [G. *tēle,* distante, + electrocardiogram]

te·lem·e·ter (tē-lem'ē-ter). Telêmetro; instrumento eletrônico que percebe e mede determinada quantidade e, a seguir, transmite sinais de rádio até uma estação distante para registro e interpretação. [G. *tēle,* distante, + *metron,* medida]

te·lem·e·try (tē-lem'ē-trē). Telemetria; a ciência de medir determinada quantidade, transmitindo os resultados por sinais de rádio até uma estação distante, onde são interpretados, indicados e/ou registrados os resultados. VER TAMBÉM biotelemetry.
cardiac t., t. cardíaca; transmissão de sinais cardíacos (elétricos ou derivados da pressão) a um local receptor, onde são apresentados para monitoração.

tel·en·ce·phal·ic (tel'en-se-fal'ik). Telencefálico; relativo ao telencéfalo.
tel·en·ceph·al·i·za·tion (tel-en-sef'äl-i-zā'shŭn). Telencefalização. SIN corticalization.

tel·en·ceph·a·lon (tel-en-sef'ä-lon). [TA]. Telencéfalo; a divisão anterior do prosencéfalo, que se transforma nos lobos olfatórios, no córtex dos hemisférios cerebrais e nos núcleos telencefálicos subcorticais e gânglios da base (núcleos), sobretudo o estriado e a amígdala. SIN endbrain. [G. *telos,* final, + *enkephalos,* cérebro]

te·le·ol·o·gy (tel-ē-ol'ō-jē). Teleologia; a doutrina filosófica segundo a qual os eventos, especialmente em biologia, são explicados, em parte, por referência a causas ou objetivos finais; a doutrina segundo a qual os objetivos e estados finais têm uma influência causal sobre os eventos atuais e segundo a qual tanto o futuro quanto o passado afetam o presente. [G. *telos,* final, + *logos,* estudo]

tel·e·o·mi·to·sis (tel'ē-ō-mī-tō'sis). Teleomitose; mitose concluída. [G. *teleos,* completo, + *mitosis*]

tel·e·o·morph (tel'ē-ō-morf). Teleomorfo; estrutura reprodutiva de um fungo, resultado de plasmogamia e recombinação nuclear; estado sexual (reprodução sexuada). SIN perfect stage.

tel·e·o·nom·ic (tel'ē-ō-nom'ik). Teleonômico. **1.** Relativo à teleonomia. **2.** Em psicologia, designa os padrões de comportamento que são uma função de um propósito ou motivo inferido; por exemplo, o padrão de comportamento de uma criança pode ser classificado, do ponto de vista teleonômico, por um observador como para chamar a atenção.

tel·e·on·o·my (tel-ē-on'ō-mē). Teleonomia; doutrina segundo a qual a vida se caracteriza pelo envolvimento com um projeto ou propósito; isto é, a existência de uma determinada estrutura ou função num organismo implica que teve valor em termos de sobrevivência na evolução. [G. *telos,* final, + *nomos,* lei]

tel·e·op·sia (tel-ē-op'sē-ä). Teleopsia; erro no julgamento da distância de objetos, devido a lesões na região parietotemporal. [G. *tēle,* distante, + *opsis,* visão]

tel·e·or·gan·ic (tel'ē-ōr-gan'ik). Teleorgânico; que manifesta a vida. [G. *teleos,* completo, + *organikos,* orgânico]

tel·e·path·ine (tel-ē-path'en). Telepatina. SIN harmine.

te·lep·a·thy (tē-lep'ä-thē). Telepatia; transmissão ou recepção de pensamentos por outros meios diferentes dos sentidos normais, como uma forma de percepção extra-sensorial. SIN extrasensory thought transference, mind-reading. [G. *tēle,* distante, + *pathos,* sentimento]

tel·e·ra·di·og·ra·phy (tel-ē-rā-dē-og'rä-fē). Telerradiografia; radiografia com o tubo de raios X posicionado acerca de 2 m do filme, garantindo, assim, um paralelismo dos raios X para minimizar a deformação geométrica; a configuração padrão para a radiografia de tórax. Cf. air-gap *technique.* SIN teleroentgenography. [G. *tēle,* distante, + radiography]

tel·e·ra·di·ol·o·gy (tel-ē-rā-dē-ol'ō-jē). Telerradiologia; a interpretação das imagens diagnósticas digitadas transmitidas por modem em linhas telefônicas. [tele- + radiology]

tel·e·ra·di·um (tel'ē-rā'dē-ŭm). Telerrádio. VER teleradium *therapy.*

tel·e·re·cep·tor (tel'ē-rē-sep'ter, -tōr). Telerreceptor; órgão, como o olho, que pode receber estímulos sensoriais a distância.

tel·er·gy (tel'er-jē). Telergia. SIN automatism. [G. *tēle,* distante, + *ergon,* trabalho]

tel·e·roent·gen·og·ra·phy (tel'ē-rent-gen-og'rä-fē). Telerradiografia. SIN teleradiography.

tel·e·roent·gen·ther·a·py (tel'ē-rent'gen-thār'ä-pē). Telerradiografia. SIN teletherapy.

telescope. Telescópio.
  Hopkins rod-lens t., t. de Hopkins; telescópio endoscópico em que os espaços contendo ar entre a série convencional de lentes são substituídos por bastões de vidro com extremidades polidas, separados por pequenas "lentes-ar". Esse sistema transmite mais luz, proporciona maior aumento, bem como maior profundidade e largura de campo do que os sistemas de lentes convencionais.
tel·e·sis (tel-ē'sis). Telese; objetivo a ser alcançado através de conduta planejada. [G. *telos,* final, + *-osis,* condição]
tel·e·sys·tol·ic (tel'ē-sis-tol'ik). Telessistólico; relativo ao final da sístole ventricular. [G. *telos,* final, + *systolē,* contração]
tel·e·ther·a·py (tel-ē-thār'a-pē). Teleterapia; radioterapia administrada com a fonte a determinada distância do corpo. Cf. interstitial *therapy.* SIN teleroentgentherapy. [G. *tēle,* distante, + *therapeia,* tratamento]
TeLinde, Richard W., ginecologista norte-americano, *1894. VER T. *operation.*
tel·lu·ric (te-loor'ik). Telúrico. **1.** Relativo a ou que se origina na terra. **2.** Relativo ao elemento telúrio, especialmente em seu estado de valência 6+. [L. *tellus* (*tellur*-), a terra]
tel·lu·rism (tel'oo-rizm). Telurismo; a suposta influência das emanações do solo na produção de doença. [L. *tellus* (*tellur*-), a terra]
tel·lu·ri·um (Te) (tel-oo'rē-ŭm). Telúrio; elemento semimetálico raro, de número atômico 52, peso atômico 127,60, pertencente ao grupo do enxofre. [L. *tellus* (*tellur*-), a terra]
telo-. Telo-. VER tel-.
tel·o·den·dron (tel-ō-den'dron). Telodendro; termo anômalo que se refere à arborização terminal de um axônio. SIN end-brush. [G. *telos,* extremidade, + *dendron,* árvore]
tel·o·gen (tel'ō-jen). Telógeno; fase de repouso do ciclo piloso. [G. *telos,* extremidade, + *-gen,* que produz]
te·log·lia (tē-log'lē-ă). Teloglia; acúmulo de células neurolêmicas na junção mioneural. [G. *telos,* extremidade, + *glia,* cola]
tel·og·no·sis (tel-og-nō'sis). Telognose; termo obsoleto que designa o diagnóstico por meio de radiografias ou outros exames diagnósticos transmitidos por telefone ou rádio. VER teleradiology. [G. *tēle,* distante, + *gnōsis,* conhecimento]
tel·o·ki·ne·sia (tel'ō-ki-nē'zē-ă). Telocinesia. SIN telophase. [G. *telos,* final, + *kinēsis,* movimento]
tel·o·lec·i·thal (tel-ō-les'i-thăl). Telolécito; designa um ovo em que grande quantidade de deuteroplasma ou vitelo acumula-se no pólo vegetativo, como nos ovos das aves e dos répteis. [G. *telos,* extremidade, + G. *lekithos,* vitelo]
tel·o·me·rase (tel-ō'mer-ās). Telomerase; transcriptase reversa que compreende um modelo de RNA, que atua como molde (padrão) para a seqüência TTAGGG, e um componente protéico catalítico, que não é encontrado nas células somáticas normais em processo de envelhecimento. A telomerase medeia o reparo ou a preservação de regiões do telômero (seqüências terminais) dos cromossomas.

> O processo de envelhecimento ocorre nas células somáticas normais, e o limite natural do número de vezes que essas células podem sofrer mitose está associado a um encurtamento seqüencial dos telômeros, devido à falta de replicação das seqüências terminais durante a mitose. As células em que esse encurtamento não ocorre (células cancerosas, células germinativas, células-tronco hematopoéticas e outras células) exibem uma expressão transitória da telomerase, que não apenas retarda a erosão dos telômeros como também acrescenta efetivamente bases de DNA aos telômeros. A transfecção experimental de um gene para o componente catalítico da telomerase em células normais em processo de envelhecimento resulta na extensão dos telômeros. A restauração do comprimento dos telômeros parece restabelecer a expressão gênica, a morfologia celular e o tempo de vida de replicação. Em consequência, foi sugerido que esses procedimentos podem permitir uma modificação terapêutica dos mecanismos celulares subjacentes a doenças relacionadas com a idade, como a aterosclerose, a osteoartrite, a degeneração macular e a demência de Alzheimer. Entretanto, o envelhecimento celular é apenas um elemento do processo de envelhecimento clínico, sendo os outros constituídos pela hereditariedade e pelo ambiente. Apesar da expressão da telomerase representar um importante marcador de neoplasia maligna, ele não constitui em si a causa do câncer. A expressão da telomerase e o alongamento dos telômeros aparentemente não alteram o controle dos ciclos celulares normais, o complemento cromossômico ou a morfologia das células.

tel·o·mere (tel'ō-mēr). Telômero; a extremidade distal do braço de um cromossoma. [G. *telos,* extremidade + *meros,* parte]
tel·o·pep·tide (tel-ō-pep'tīd). Telopeptídio; peptídio ligado de forma covalente numa proteína ou sobre ela, projetando-se da mesma e, portanto, estando sujeito ao ataque enzimático à modificação por maturação ou ligação cruzada, e que confere especificidade imunogênica.
tel·o·phase (tel'ō-fāz). Telófase; o estágio final da mitose ou da meiose, que começa quando a migração dos cromossomas para os pólos da célula está concluída; os cromossomas alongam-se progressivamente, enquanto as membranas nucleares das duas células filhas são reconstruídas, e uma membrana celular no equador completa a separação das duas células filhas. SIN telokinesia. [G. *telos,* extremidade, + *phasis,* aparência]
Te·lo·spo·re·a (tel-ō-spō'rē-ă). SIN Sporozoea.
Te·lo·spo·rid·i·a (tel'ō-spō-rid'ē-ă). Antiga ordem de Sporozoea. [G. *telos,* extremidade, + *sporos,* semente]
tel·o·tism (tel'ō-tizm). Telotismo; o desempenho perfeito de uma função, como o da visão ou da audição. [G. *telos,* extremidade]
TEM Abreviatura de triethylenemelamine (trietilenomelamina).
te·maz·e·pam (te-maz'ē-pam). Temazepam; benzodiazepínico sedativo-hipnótico primariamente utilizado para alívio da insônia.
tem·per. 1. Humor; disposição; em geral, qualquer estado mental característico ou específico. SIN temperament (2). **2.** Temperamento; demonstração de irritação ou raiva. VER tantrum. **3.** Temperar; tratar um metal pela aplicação de calor, com no recozimento ou resfriamento.
tem·per·a·ment (tem'per-ă-ment). Temperamento. **1.** A organização psicológica ou biológica peculiar ao indivíduo, incluindo as predisposições de caráter ou de personalidade, que influenciam a forma do pensamento e as ações, bem como a visão geral da vida. **2.** SIN temper (1). [L. *temperamentum,* medida apropriada, moderação, disposição]
tem·per·ance (tem'per-ans). Temperança; moderação em todas as coisas; em particular, abstinência do uso de bebidas alcoólicas. [L. *temperantia,* moderação]
tem·per·ate (tem'per-āt). Temperado; moderado; restrito na indulgência de qualquer apetite ou atividade.
tem·per·a·ture (tem'per-ă-chŭr). Temperatura; a intensidade perceptível de calor de qualquer substância; a manifestação da energia cinética média das moléculas que constituem uma substância, devido à agitação pelo calor. VER TAMBÉM scale. [L. *temperatura,* medida apropriada; temperatura, de *tempero,* em proporção adequada]
  absolute t. (*T*), t. absoluta; t. medida em Kelvins a partir do zero absoluto.
  basal body t., t. corporal basal; a t. em repouso, geralmente medida ao acordar pela manhã, sem qualquer influência que possa elevá-la; pode fornecer uma prova indireta de ovulação.
  critical t., t. crítica; a t. de um gás acima da qual não é mais possível por meio de qualquer pressão, ainda que grande, convertê-lo em líquido.
  denaturation t. of DNA, t. de desnaturação do DNA; t. na qual, na presença de um determinado conjunto de condições, o DNA de duplo filamento é transformado (50%) em DNA de filamento único; em condições padrões, é possível estimar a composição de bases do DNA a partir da temperatura de desnaturação, visto que, quanto maior a temperatura de desnaturação, maior o conteúdo de guanina-mais-citosina (isto é, o conteúdo de GC) do DNA. SIN melting t. of DNA.
  effective t., t. efetiva; índice ou escala de conforto que leva em consideração a t. do ar, seu grau de umidade e movimento.
  equivalent t., t. equivalente; a t de um recinto termicamente uniforme no qual, em condições de ar parado, um corpo negro "bastante grande" perde calor na mesma velocidade do que no ambiente não-uniforme.
  eutectic t., t. eutética; a t. em que uma mistura eutética se torna líquida (funde-se).
  fusion t. (wire method), t. de fusão (método do arame); **(1)** a temperatura registrada na qual um fio metálico de calibre 20 se dobra sob uma carga de 3 onças (~90 g); **(2)** a temperatura registrada na qual a porcelana se torna vitrificada.
  maximum t., t. máxima; em bacteriologia, designa uma t. acima da qual não ocorrerá crescimento.
  mean t., t. média; a t. atmosférica média em qualquer localidade por um período específico de tempo, como um mês ou um ano.
  melting t., t. de fusão. SIN t. midpoint.
  melting t. of DNA, t. de desnaturação (fusão) do DNA. SIN denaturation t. of DNA.
  t. midpoint (T_m, t_m), t. do ponto central; o ponto médio na alteração das propriedades ópticas (absorbância, rotação) de um polímero estruturado (p. ex., DNA) com o aumento progressivo da temperatura. SIN melting t.
  minimum t., t. mínima; em bacteriologia, designa uma t. abaixo da qual não ocorrerá crescimento.
  optimum t., t. ideal; a t. em que qualquer operação, como a cultura de qualquer microrganismo especial, é mais bem efetuada.
  room t. (RT, rt), t. ambiente; a t. comum (65°F a um pouco menos de 80°F, 18,3°C-26,7°C) da atmosfera no laboratório; uma cultura mantida em t. ambiente é aquela mantida no laboratório, e não numa incubadora.
  sensible t., t. sensível; a t. atmosférica percebida pelo indivíduo, supostamente a registrada pelo termômetro de bulbo úmido.
  standard t., t. padrão; t. de 0°C ou 273,15° absolutos (Kelvin).
tem·plete (tem'plāt). Molde, modelo. **1.** Um padrão ou guia que determina a forma de uma substância. **2.** Metaforicamente, a natureza que especifica uma macromolécula, geralmente ácido nucléico ou polinucleotídio em relação à estrutura primária do ácido nucléico ou polinucleotídio ou proteína produzidos a partir dela *in vivo* ou *in vitro.* **3.** Em odontologia, uma lâmina curva ou plana utilizada como auxílio na colocação dos dentes. **4.** Contorno utilizado para marcar dentes, ossos ou tecidos moles, a fim de padronizar sua forma. **5.**

Padrão ou guia que determina a especialidade de globulinas anticorpos. [Fr. *templet*, tempereiro de um tear, do L. *templum*, pequena prancha]
surgical t., m. cirúrgico; **(1)** base de resina fina e transparente, moldada para duplicar a forma da superfície de impressão de uma dentadura imediata, utilizada como guia para moldagem cirúrgica do processo alveolar para encaixar uma dentadura imediata; **(2)** guia para vários procedimentos de osteotomia; **(3)** guia para duplicar o tamanho e a forma para enxerto gengival autógeno (livre).

tem·ple (tem'pl). **1.** [TA]. Têmpora a área da fossa temporal do lado da cabeça, acima do arco zigomático. **2.** A parte de uma armação de óculos que passa sobre a orelha. [L. *tempus* (*tempor*-), tempo, têmpora]

tem·po·la·bile (tem-pō-lā'bil, -bīl). Tempolábil; que sofre mudança ou destruição espontânea durante a passagem do tempo. [L. *tempus*, tempo, + *labilis*, perecível]

tem·po·ra (tem'pō-ră). As têmporas. [L. pl. de *tempus*]

tem·po·ral (tem'pō-răl). Temporal. **1.** Relativo ao tempo; limitado quanto ao tempo; temporário. **2.** Relativo à têmpora. VER temporal *region of head*. [L. *temporalis*, de *tempus* (*tempor*-), tempo, têmpora]

tem·po·ra·lis (tem-pō-rā'lis). Músculo temporal. SIN temporalis (muscle). [L.]

♻ **temporo-.** Temporo-. Temporal (2). [L. *temporalis*, temporal]

tem·po·ro·au·ric·u·lar (tem'pō-rō-aw-rik'ū-lăr). Temporoauricular; relativo à região temporal e à aurícula.

tem·po·ro·hy·oid (tem'pō-rō-hī'oyd). Têmporo-hióideo; relativo aos ossos ou às regiões temporal e hióide.

tem·po·ro·ma·lar (tem'pō-rō-mā'lăr). Temporozigomático. SIN temporozygomatic.

tem·po·ro·man·dib·u·lar (tem'pō-rō-man-dib'ū-lăr). Temporomandibular; relativo ao osso temporal e à mandíbula; designa a articulação da mandíbula. SIN temporomaxillary (2).

tem·po·ro·max·il·lary (tem'pō-rō-mak'si-lār'ē). **1.** Temporomaxilar; relativo às regiões dos ossos temporal e maxilar. **2.** Temporomandibular. SIN temporomandibular.

tem·po·ro·oc·cip·i·tal (tem'pō-rō-ok-sip'i-tăl). Temporoccipital; relativo aos ossos ou regiões temporal e occipital.

tem·po·ro·pa·ri·e·tal (tem'pō-rō-pa-rī'e-tăl). Temporoparietal; relativo aos ossos ou regiões temporal e parietal.

tem·po·ro·pon·tine (tem-pō-rō-pon'tin). Temporopontino; refere-se às fibras de projeção do lobo temporal do córtex cerebral até a parte basilar da ponte.

tem·po·ro·sphe·noid (tem'pō-rō-sfē'noyd). Temporesfenóide; relativo aos ossos temporal e esfenóide.

tem·po·ro·zy·go·mat·ic (tem'pō-rō-zī'gō-mat'ik). Temporozigomático; relativo aos ossos ou regiões temporal e zigomático. SIN temporomalar.

tem·po·sta·bile, tem·po·sta·ble (tem-pō-stā'bil, -stā'bl). Tempoestável; não sujeito a alteração ou destruição espontânea. [L. *tempus*, tempo, + *stabilis*, estável]

temps utile (temp' oo-tēl'). Tempo de utilização. SIN utilization time. [Fr. tempo de serviço ou de utilização]

tem·pus, gen. **tem·po·ris**, pl. **tem·po·ra** (tem'pŭs, -pō-ris, -pō-ră). **1.** A têmpora. **2.** Tempo. SIN time. [L. tempo]

TEN Abreviatura de toxic epidermal *necrolysis* (necrólise epidérmica tóxica).

te·na·cious (tĕ-nā'shŭs). Tenaz; viscoso; que indica tenacidade. [L. *tenax* (*tenac*-), de *teneo*, segurar]

te·nac·i·ty (tĕ-nas'i-tē). Tenacidade; adesividade; o caráter ou a propriedade de segurar firmemente. [L. *tenacitas*, de *teneo*, segurar]
cellular t., t. celular; a propriedade inerente de todas as células de persistir em determinada forma ou direção de atividade.

te·nac·u·lum, pl. **te·nac·u·la** (tĕ-nak'ū-lŭm, -lă). Tenáculo; gancho cirúrgico projetado para segurar ou prender tecido durante a dissecção, geralmente utilizado para segurar o colo do útero. [L. segurador, de *teneo*, segurar]
tenac'ula ten'dinum, estrutura tendínea de restrição, como um retináculo extensor ou flexor; historicamente aplicado a vínculos tendíneos que, entretanto, não são estruturas de restrição.

te·nal·gia (te-nal'jē-ă). Tenalgia; termo obsoleto para a dor referida a um tendão. SIN tenodynia. [G. *tenōn*, tendão, + *algos*, dor]
t. crep'itans, t. crepitante. SIN tenosynovitis crepitans.

ten·as·cin (ten-as'sin). Tenascina; proteína presente no mesênquima, que circunda os epitélios em órgãos em fase de desenvolvimento nos embriões; acredita-se que participa na indução da diferenciação dos epitélios.

ten·der. Hipersensível; sensível ou dolorido em consequência de compressão ou contato, que não são suficientes para causar desconforto em tecidos normais. [L. *tener*, macio, delicado]

ten·der·ness (ten'dĕr-nes). Hipersensibilidade; a condição de ser hipersensível ou doloroso à compressão ou contato.
pencil t., hipersensibilidade bem-localizada, produzida por pressão exercida com a ponta de borracha de um lápis, p. ex., em casos de fratura incompleta ou subperióstea.
rebound t., descompressão dolorosa; hipersensibilidade percebida quando a pressão, particularmente aquela exercida sobre o abdome, é subitamente liberada.

ten·di·ni·tis (ten-di-nī'tis). Tendinite. SIN tendonitis.

ten·di·no·plas·ty (ten'din-ō-plas-tē). Tendinoplastia; cirurgia reparadora ou plástica dos tendões. SIN tenontoplasty, tenoplasty. [L. Mediev. *tendo* (*tendin*-), tendão, + G. *plastos*, formado]

ten·di·no·su·ture (ten'di-nō-soo'choor). Tendinossutura. SIN tenorrhaphy.

ten·di·nous (ten'di-nŭs). Tendíneo, tendinoso; relativo a, composto de ou semelhante a um tendão.

ten·do, gen. **ten·di·nis**, pl. **ten·di·nes** (ten'dō, -di-nis, -di-nēz) [TA]. Tendão. SIN tendon. Para descrição histológica, ver tendon. [L. Mediev., do L. *tendo*, estirar, estender]
t. Achil'lis, tendão-de-aquiles, t. do calcâneo. SIN calcaneal *tendon*.
t. calca'neus [TA], t. do calcâneo. SIN calcaneal *tendon*.
t. calca'neus commu'nis, t. comum do calcâneo. VER hamstring (2).
t. conjuncti'vus, t. conjuntivo; *termo oficial alternativo para inguinal *falx*.
t. cricoesopha'geus [TA], t. cricoesofágico. SIN cricoesophageal *tendon*.
t. oc'uli, ligamento palpebral medial. SIN medial palpebral *ligament*.
t. palpebra'rum, ligamento palpebral medial. SIN medial palpebral *ligament*.

♻ **tendo-.** Tendo-. Tendão. VER TAMBÉM teno-. [L. *tendo*]

ten·dol·y·sis (ten-dol'i-sis). Tenólise. SIN tenolysis. [tendo- + G. *lysis*, dissolução]

ten·do·mu·cin, ten·do·mu·coid (ten-dō-mū'sin, -mū'koyd). Tendomucina, tendomucóide; forma de mucina encontrada em tendões.

ℹ **ten·don** (ten'dŏn) [TA]. Tendão; cordão ou faixa fibrosa não-distensível de comprimento variável que faz parte do músculo, que conecta a parte carnosa (contrátil) do músculo à sua inserção no osso ou a outra estrutura; pode unir-se à parte carnosa do músculo em sua extremidade ou pode seguir ao longo da face lateral ou no centro da parte carnosa por uma maior ou menor distância, recebendo as fibras musculares ao longo de sua borda; na determinação do comprimento de um músculo, o comprimento do tendão é incluído, bem como a parte carnosa; consiste em fascículos de fibras colágenas de disposição muito densa, quase paralelas, fileiras de fibrócitos alongados e quantidade mínima de substância fundamental. SIN tendo [TA], sinew. [L. *tendo*]

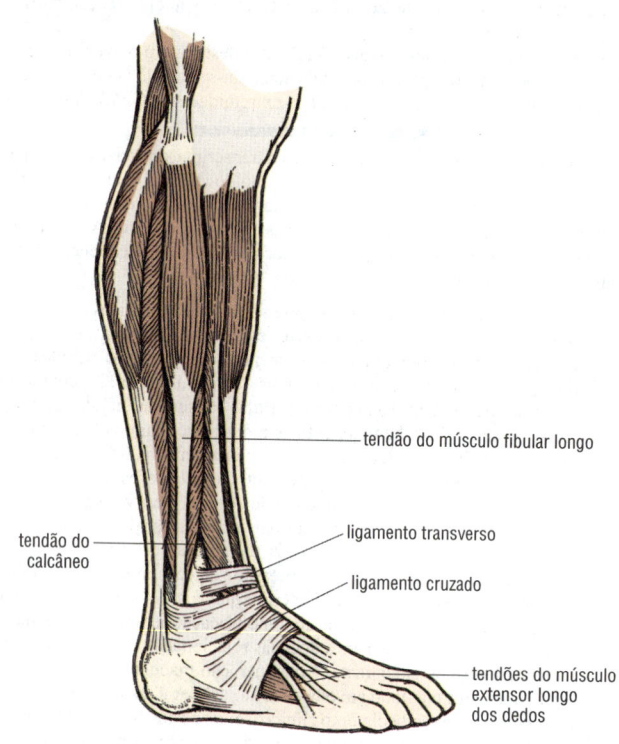

tendões e ligamentos da perna

Achilles t., t.-de-aquiles. SIN calcaneal t.
calcaneal t. [TA], t. do calcâneo; o tendão espesso de inserção do músculo tríceps sural (gastrocnêmio e sóleo) na tuberosidade do calcâneo. SIN tendo calcaneus [TA], Achilles t., chorda magna, heel t., tendo Achillis.
central t. of diaphragm [TA], centro tendíneo do diafragma; lâmina fibrosa trilobada que ocupa o centro do diafragma; superiormente, funde-se com o pericárdio fibroso que fornece a fixação (inserção) para a extremidade móvel das fibras musculares. SIN centrum tendinum diaphragmatis [TA], trefoil t.
central t. of perineum [TA], corpo do períneo; massa fibromuscular entre o canal anal e o diafragma urogenital no plano medial, em que vários músculos

perineais se inserem (músculo bulboesponjoso, esfíncter anal externo, músculo transverso profundo do períneo e músculo transverso superficial do períneo); as episiotomias na linha mediana estendem-se nessa estrutura. SIN centrum tendineum perinei [TA], perineal body, Savage perineal body.
conjoined t., foice inguinal. SIN inguinal *falx.*
conjoint t., foice inguinal; *termo oficial alternativo para inguinal *falx.* VER TAMBÉM *aponeurosis* of internal oblique muscle.
coronary t., anéis fibrosos (direito/esquerdo) do coração. SIN (right and left) fibrous *rings* of heart, em *ring.*
cricoesophageal t. [TA], t. cricoesofágico; fibra longitudinal do esôfago que se fixa à face posterior da cartilagem cricóidea da laringe. SIN tendo cricoesophageus [TA], Gillette suspensory ligament, suspensory ligament of esophagus.
Gerlach annular t., t. anular de Gerlach. SIN fibrocartilaginous *ring* of tympanic membrane.
hamstring t., t. poplíteo. VER hamstring.
heel t., t. do calcâneo. SIN calcaneal t.
Todaro t., t. de Todaro; estrutura tendínea inconstante que se estende do trígono fibroso do coração em direção à valva da veia cava inferior.
trefoil t., t. trifólio. SIN central t. of diaphragm.
Zinn t., t. de Zinn. SIN common tendinous *ring* of extraocular muscles.

ten·don·i·tis (ten-dō-nī′tis). Tendinite; inflamação de um tendão. SIN tendinitis, tenonitis (2), tenontitis.
ten·doph·o·ny (ten-dof′ō-nē). Tenofonia. SIN tenophony.
ten·do·syn·o·vi·tis (ten′dō-si-no-vī′tis). Tenossinovite. SIN tenosynovitis.
ten·dot·o·my (ten-dot′ō-mē). Tenotomia. SIN tenotomy.
ten·do·vag·i·nal (ten-dō-vaj′i-nal). Tenovaginal; relativo a um tendão e sua bainha. [tendo- + L. *vagina,* bainha]
ten·do·vag·i·ni·tis (ten′dō-vaj-i-nī′tis). Tenossinovite. SIN tenosynovitis. [tendo- + L. *vagina,* bainha, + G. *-itis,* inflamação]
radial styloid t., t. estilóide radial. SIN de Quervain *disease.*
te·nec·to·my (tē-nek′tō-mē). Tenectomia; ressecção de parte de um tendão. SIN tenonectomy. [G. *tenōn,* tendão, + *ektome,* excisão]
te·nes·mic (tē-nez′mik). Tenésmico; relativo a ou caracterizado por tenesmo.
te·nes·mus (te-nez′mŭs). Tenesmo; espasmo doloroso do diafragma urogenital com desejo urgente de evacuar o intestino ou a bexiga, esforço involuntário de defecação e eliminação de pouco material fecal ou urina. [G. *teinesmos,* esforço ineficaz para defecar, de *teinō,* estirar]
ten Horn, C., cirurgião holandês. VER t. H. *sign.*
te·nia, pl. **te·ni·ae** (tē′nē-ă, tē′nē-ē). Tênia. **1.** Estria; qualquer estrutura anatômica semelhante a uma fita. **2.** SIN taenia (2). [L. do G. *tainia,* faixa, fita, tênia]
tae′niae, acus′ticae, estrias medulares do quarto ventrículo. SIN medullary *striae* of fourth ventricle, em *stria.*
t. choroi′dea [TA], t. corióidea; a linha ligeiramente espessada ao longo da qual se fixa uma membrana ou plexo corióideo à borda de um ventrículo cerebral. SIN choroid line [TA], t. telae.
te′niae co′li [TA], tênias do colo; as três faixas nas quais se reúnem as fibras musculares longitudinais do intestino grosso, exceto o reto; são elas: a tênia mesocólica (t. mesocolica [TA]), situada no local que corresponde à fixação mesentérica; a tênia livre (t. libera [TA]), oposta à tênia mesocólica; e a tênia omental (t. omentalis [TA]), no local que corresponde ao local de aderência do omento maior ao colo transverso. SIN bands of colon, colic teniae, teniae of Valsalva.
colic teniae, tênias do colo. SIN teniae coli.
t. fim′briae, t. do fórnice. SIN t. fornicis.
t. for′nicis [TA], t. do fórnice; a linha de fixação do plexo corióideo do ventrículo lateral ao fórnice. SIN t. fimbriae, t. of the fornix.
t. of the fornix, t. do fórnice. SIN t. fornicis.
t. of fourth ventricle, estrias medulares do quarto ventrículo. SIN t. ventriculi quarti.
free t. [TA], t. livre. VER teniae coli. SIN t. libera [TA].
t. hippocam′pi, fimbrias do hipocampo. SIN *fimbria* hippocampi.
t. lib′era [TA], t. livre. SIN free t. VER teniae coli.
medullary teniae, estrias medulares do quarto ventrículo. SIN medullary *striae* of fourth ventricle, em *stria.*
mesocolic t., t. mesocólica. VER teniae coli. SIN t. mesocolica [TA].
t. mesocol′ica [TA], t. mesocólica. SIN mesocolic t.
omental t. [TA], t. omental. VER teniae coli. SIN t. omentalis [TA].
t. omenta′lis [TA], t. omental. SIN omental t. VER teniae coli.
t. semicircula′ris, estria terminal. SIN terminal *stria.*
Tarin t., t. de Tarin. SIN terminal *stria.*
t. tec′ta, indúsio cinzento. VER *indusium* griseum.
t. te′lae, t. corióidea. SIN t. choroidea.
t. termina′lis, crista terminal do átrio direito. SIN *crista* terminalis of right atrium.
t. thal′ami [TA], t. do tálamo; a borda ou ângulo agudo entre as superfícies superior e medial do tálamo, em ambos os lados; a ela está fixada a lâmina epitelial que forma o teto do terceiro ventrículo. SIN t. ventriculi tertii, thalamic t.

thalamic t., t. do tálamo. SIN t. thalami.
teniae of Valsalva, tênias de Valsalva. SIN teniae coli.
t. ventric′uli quar′ti, t. do quarto ventrículo; a linha de fixação do teto da corióidea à borda do quarto ventrículo. SIN t. of fourth ventricle.
t. ventric′uli ter′tii, t. do terceiro ventrículo. SIN t. thalami.

te·ni·a·cide (tē′nē-ă-sīd). Tenicida; agente que destrói as tênias. SIN tenicide. [L. *taenia,* tênia + *caedo,* matar]
te·ni·a·fuge (tē′nē-ă-fooj). Tenífugo; agente que causa a expulsão das tênias. SIN tenifuge. [L. *taenia,* tênia, + *fugo,* pôr em fuga]
ten·i·al (ten′ē-al). **1.** Relativo a uma tênia. **2.** Relativo a uma das estruturas denominadas tênias.
te·ni·a·sis (tē-nī′ă-sis). Teníase; presença de tênias no intestino.
somatic t., t. somática; invasão do corpo pelo cisticerco de um verme tenióide.
ten·i·cide (ten′i-sīd). Tenicida. SIN teniacide.
ten·i·form (ten′i-fōrm). Teniforme. SIN tenioid.
te·nif·u·gal (te-nif′ū-găl). Tenífugo; que tem a capacidade de expelir tênias.
ten·i·fuge (ten′i-fūj). Tenífugo. SIN teniafuge.
te·ni·oid (tē′nē-oyd). Tenióide. **1.** Em forma de faixa; em forma de fita. **2.** Semelhante a uma tênia. SIN teniform. [G. *tainia,* fita, + *eidos,* semelhança]
te·ni·o·la (tē-nī′ō-lă). Teníola; tênia delgada ou estrutura semelhante a uma fita. [L. dim. de *taenia,* fita]
t. cor′poris callo′si, t. do corpo caloso. SIN rostral *lamina.*

♻ **teno-, tenon-, tenont-, tenonto-.** Teno-, tenon-, tenont-, tenonto-; tendão. VER TAMBÉM tendo-. [G. *tenōn*]
te·no·de·sis (tē-nodē′-sis, ten′ō-dē′sis). Tenodese; estabilização de uma articulação através de fixação dos tendões que movimentam essa articulação, impedindo, assim, qualquer excursão dos tendões. [teno- + G. *desis,* ligação]
ten·o·dyn·ia (ten-ō-din′ēa). Tenodinia. SIN tenalgia. [teno- + G. *odynē,* dor]
ten·o·fi·bril (ten-ō-fī′bril). Tonofibrila. SIN tonofibril. [teno- + L. Mod. *fibrilla,* pequena fibra]
ten·ol·y·sis (ten-ol′i-sis). Tenólise; liberação de um tendão de suas aderências. SIN tendolysis.
ten·o·my·o·plas·ty (ten-ō-mī′ō-plas-tē). Tenomioplastia. SIN tenontomyoplasty.
ten·o·my·ot·o·my (ten-ō-mī-ot′ō-mē). Tenomiotomia. SIN myotenotomy.
Tenon, Jacques R., patologista e oftalmologista francês, 1724–1816. VER T. *capsule, space.*

♻ **tenon-.** Tenon-. VER teno-.
ten·o·nec·to·my (ten-ō-nek′tō-mē). Tenectomia. SIN tenectomy. [tenon- + G. *ektome,* excisão]
ten·o·ni·tis (ten-ō-nī′tis). **1.** Tenonite; inflamação da cápsula de Tenon ou do tecido conjuntivo no interior do espaço de Tenon. **2.** Tendinite. SIN tendonitis. [tenont- + G. *-itis,* inflamação]
ten·on·ti·tis (ten′on-tī′tis). Tenotite. SIN tendonitis. [tenont- + G. *-itis,* inflamação]

♻ **tenonto-.** Tenonto-. VER teno-.
te·non·tog·ra·phy (ten′on-tog′ră-fē). Tenontografia; tratado sobre os tendões ou sua descrição. [tenonto- + G. *graphe,* descrição]
te·non·tol·o·gy (ten′on-tol′ō-jē). Tenontologia; o ramo da ciência relacionado aos tendões. [tenonto- + G. *logos,* estudo]
te·non·to·my·o·plas·ty (te-non′tō-mī′ō-plas′tē). Tenontomioplastia; termo obsoleto para uma tenontoplastia e mioplastia combinadas, utilizadas na correção radical de uma hérnia. SIN tenomyoplasty. [tenonto- + G. *mys,* músculo + *plastos,* formado]
te·non·to·my·ot·o·my (te-non′tō-mī-ot′ō-mē). Tenontomiotomia. SIN myotenotomy.
te·non·to·plas·tic (te-non′tō-plas-tik). Tenontoplástico; relativo à tenontoplastia.
te·non·to·plas·ty (te-non′tō-plas-tē). Tenontoplastia. SIN tendinoplasty. [tenonto- + G. *plastos,* formado]
te·noph·o·ny (te-nof′ō-nē). Tenofonia; sopro cardíaco supostamente devido a uma condição anormal das cordas tendíneas. SIN tendophony. [teno- + G. *phōnē,* som]
ten·o·phyte (ten′ō-fit). Tenófito; crescimento ósseo ou cartilaginoso no interior de um tendão ou sobre ele. [teno- + G. *phyton,* planta]
ten·o·plas·tic (ten-ō-plas′tik). Tenoplástico; relativo à tenoplastia.
ten·o·plas·ty (ten′ō-plas-tē). Tenoplastia. SIN tendinoplasty.
ten·o·re·cep·tor (ten′ō-rē-sep′ter, -tōr). Tenorreceptor; receptor existente num tendão, ativado por aumento da tensão.
te·nor·rha·phy (te-nōr′ă-fē). Tenorrafia; sutura das extremidades seccionadas de um tendão. SIN tendinosuture, tendon suture, tenosuture. [teno- + G. *raphē,* sutura]
ten·os·to·sis (ten-os-tō′sis). Tenostose; ossificação de um tendão. [teno- + G. *osteon,* osso, + *-osis,* condição]
ten·o·sus·pen·sion (ten′ō-sŭs-pen′shŭn). Tenossuspensão; uso de um tendão como ligamento suspensor, algumas vezes como enxerto livre ou em continuidade.

ten·o·su·ture (ten-ō-soo′choor). Tenossutura. SIN tenorrhaphy.
ten·o·syn·o·vec·to·my (ten′ō-sin-ō-vek′tō-mē). Tenossinovectomia; excisão de uma bainha tendínea. [teno- + synovia + G. *ektomē*, excisão]
ten·o·syn·o·vi·tis (ten′ō-sin-ō-vī′tis). Tenossinovite; inflamação de um tendão e de sua bainha. SIN tendinous synovitis, tendosynovitis, tendovaginitis, tenovaginitis. [teno- + synovia + G. *-itis*, inflamação]
  t. crep'itans, t. crepitante; inflamação de um bainha tendínea, em que o movimento do tendão é acompanhado de um som de estalido. SIN tenalgia crepitans.
  de Quervain t., t. de Quervain; inflamação dos tendões do primeiro compartimento dorsal do punho, incluindo o músculo abdutor longo do polegar e o músculo extensor curto do polegar; diagnosticada através de um teste provocativo específico (teste de Finkelstein).
  localized nodular t., t. nodular localizada. SIN giant cell *tumor* of tendon sheath.
  pigmented villonodular t., t. vilonodular pigmentada. SIN villous t.
  stenosing t., t. estenosante; inflamação de um tendão e sua bainha, resultando em contratura da bainha, com conseqüente obstrução do deslizamento do tendão; pode ser uma causa de dedo em gatilho.
  villous t., t. vilosa; condição que se assemelha à sinovite vilonodular pigmentada, mas que surge mais no tecido mole periarticular do que na sinóvia articular; ocorre mais comumente nas mãos. SIN pigmented villonodular t.
te·not·o·my (te-not′ō-mē). Tenotomia; secção cirúrgica de um tendão para aliviar uma deformidade causada por encurtamento congênito ou adquirido de um músculo, como no pé torto ou no estrabismo. SIN tendotomy. [teno- + G. *tomē*, incisão]
  curb t., recessão de tendão. SIN tendon *recession*.
  graduated t., t. graduada; incisões parciais do tendão de um músculo ocular para a correção do estrabismo.
  subcutaneous t., t. subcutânea; secção de um tendão por meio de um pequeno bisturi pontiagudo introduzido através da pele e do tecido subcutâneo, sem operação aberta.
ten·o·vag·i·ni·tis (ten′ō-vaj-i-nī′tis). Tenovaginite. SIN tenosynovitis. [teno- + L. *vagina*, bainha, + G. *-itis*, inflamação]
tense (tens). Tenso; rígido ou forçado; caracterizado por ansiedade e tensão psicológica. [L. *tensus*, pp. de *tendo*, estirar]
ten·si·om·e·ter (ten-sē-om′ē-ter). Tensiômetro; aparelho para medir a tensão. [L. *tensio*, tensão, + G. *metron*, medida]
ten·sion (ten′-shŭn). Tensão, pressão. **1.** O ato de estirar. **2.** A condição de estar estirado ou tenso, ou uma força de estiramento ou tração. **3.** A pressão parcial de um gás, especialmente a de um gás dissolvido em líquido, como o sangue. **4.** Tensão mental, emocional ou nervosa; relações tensas ou hostilidade dificilmente controladas entre pessoas ou grupos. [L. *tensio*, de *tendo*, pp. *tensus*, estirar]
  arterial t., pressão arterial; a pressão do sangue dentro de uma artéria.
  interfacial surface t., t. de superfície na interface; a t. ou resistência à separação apresentada pela película de líquido entre duas superfícies bem-adaptadas, como a fina película de saliva entre a base da dentadura e os tecidos.
  ocular t. (Tn), pressão ocular; resistência das túnicas do olho à deformação; pode ser estimada digitalmente ou medida por meio de tonômetro.
  premenstrual t., t. pré-menstrual. SIN premenstrual *syndrome*.
  surface t. (γ, σ), t. superficial; a expressão da atração intermolecular na superfície de um líquido, em contato com ar ou outro gás, de um sólido ou outro líquido imiscível, que tende a atrair as moléculas do líquido da superfície para dentro; fórmula dimensional: mt^{-2}.
  tissue t., t. tecidual; condição teórica de equilíbrio entre os tecidos e as células, através da qual a hiperatividade de qualquer parte é restrita pela tração da massa.
ten·sor, pl. **ten·so·res** (ten′sōr, ten-sō′rēz). Tensor; músculo cuja função é tornar uma parte firme e tensa. [L. Mod. do L. *tendo*, pp. *tensus*, estirar]
tent. 1. Tenta; dossel sobre o leito usado em vários tipos de terapia inalatória para controlar a umidade e a concentração de oxigênio no ar inspirado. **2.** Cilindro de algum material, geralmente absorvente, introduzido num canal ou seio para manter a sua perviedade ou para dilatá-lo. **3.** Elevar ou erguer um segmento de pele, fáscia ou tecido em determinado ponto, conferindo-lhe o aspecto de uma tenda. [L. *tendo*, pp. *tensus*, estirar]
  oxygen t., t. de oxigênio; dossel transparente, suspenso sobre o leito e que envolve o paciente, utilizado para proporcionar uma alta concentração de oxigênio.
  sponge t., tampão de esponja. SIN compressed *sponge*.
ten·ta·cle (ten′tă-kl). Tentáculo; prolongamento delgado para percepção, preensão ou locomoção nos invertebrados. [L. Mod. *tentaculum*, antena, de *tento*, sentir]
ten·to·ri·al (ten-tō′rē-ăl). Tentorial; relativo a um tentório.
ten·to·ri·um, pl. **ten·to·ria** (ten-tō′rē-ŭm, -rē-ă) [TA]. Tentório; revestimento membranáceo ou divisória horizontal. [L. *tent*, de *tendo*, estirar]
  t. cerebel'li [TA], t. do cerebelo; prega resistente de dura-máter que serve de teto para a fossa posterior do crânio, com uma abertura mediana anterior, a incisura do tentório, através da qual passa o mesencéfalo; o tentório do cerebelo está fixado ao longo da linha mediana à foice do cérebro e separa o cerebelo da superfície basilar dos lobos occipital e temporal do hemisfério cerebral. SIN cerebellar r. [TA].
  cerebellar t. [TA], t. do cerebelo. SIN t. cerebelli.
  t. of hypophysis, diafragma da sela. SIN *diaphragma sellae*.
TEPA Abreviatura de triethylenephosphoramide (trietilenofosforamida).
teph·ro·ma·la·cia (tef′rō-mă-lā′shē-ă). Tefromalacia; amolecimento da substância cinzenta do cérebro ou da medula espinal. [G. *tephros*, cinza, + *malakia*, amolecimento]
teph·ry·lom·e·ter (tef′-ri-lom′ē-ter). Tefrilômetro; instrumento para medir a espessura do córtex cerebral; consiste num tubo graduado de vidro fino, que é inserido na substância cerebral, de modo que a profundidade da substância cinzenta possa ser lida na escala. [G. *tephros*, cinza, + *hylē*, matéria, + *metron*, medida]
TEPP Abreviatura de tetraethyl pyrophosphate (pirofosfato de tetraetila).
tep·ro·tide (te′prō-tīd). Teprotídio; nonapeptídio no qual a glicina é substituída por triptofano, em que a leucina e a primeira prolina estão ausentes, e a lisina é substituída por glutamina; inibidor da enzima conversora de angiotensina. SIN bradykinin-potentiating peptide.
tera- (T). Tera-. **1.** Prefixo utilizado nos sistemas SI e métrico para significar um trilhão. **2.** Forma combinante que designa um monstro. VER TAMBÉM terato-. [G. *teras*, monstro]
ter·as, pl. **ter·a·ta** (ter′as, ter′ă-tă). Concepto com partes deficientes, redundantes, incorretamente posicionadas ou flagrantemente malformadas. [G.]
ter·at·ic (ter-at′ik). Terático; relativo a um monstro.
ter·a·tism (ter′ă-tizm). Teratismo. SIN teratosis. [G. *teratisma*, de *teras*]
terato-. Terato-; monstro. VER TAMBÉM tera- (2). [G. *teras*, monstro]
ter·a·to·blas·to·ma. Teratoblastoma; tumor que contém tecido embrionário que se diferencia de um teratoma porque não apresenta todas as camadas germinativas.
ter·a·to·car·ci·no·ma (ter′ă-tō-kar-si-nō′mă). Teratocarcinoma. **1.** Teratoma maligno, que ocorre mais comumente no testículo em associação com carcinoma embrionário. **2.** Tumor epitelial maligno que se origina num teratoma.
te·rat·o·gen (ter′ă-tō-jen). Teratógeno; droga ou outro agente que causa desenvolvimento pré-natal anormal. [terato- + G. *-gen*, que produz]
ter·a·to·gen·e·sis (ter′ă-tō-jen′ē-sis). Teratogênese; a origem ou o modo de produção de um feto malformado; os processos de crescimento afetados envolvidos na produção de um recém-nascido malformado. [terato- + G. *genesis*, origem]
ter·a·to·gen·ic, ter·a·to·ge·net·ic (ter′ă-tō-jen′ik, -jē-net′ik). Teratogênico, teratogenético. **1.** Relativo à teratogênese. **2.** Que causa desenvolvimento pré-natal anormal.
ter·a·to·ge·nic·i·ty (ter′ă-tō-jē-nis′i-tē). Teratogenicidade; a propriedade ou capacidade de produzir malformação. [terato- + G. *genesis*, geração]
ter·a·toid (ter′ă-toyd). Teratóide; semelhante a um monstro. [G. *teratōdēs*, de *teras (terat-)*, monstro, + *eidos*, semelhança]
ter·a·to·log·ic (ter′ă-tō-loj′ik). Teratológico; relativo à teratologia.
ter·a·tol·o·gy (ter-ă-tol′ō-jē). Teratologia; o ramo da ciência relacionado com a produção, o desenvolvimento, a anatomia e a classificação de fetos malformados. VER TAMBÉM dysmorphology. [terato- + G. *logos*, estudo]
ter·a·to·ma (ter-ă-tō′mă). Teratoma; neoplasia composta de múltiplos tecidos, incluindo tecidos normalmente não encontrados no órgão do qual se origina. Os teratomas ocorrem mais freqüentemente no ovário, onde são habitualmente benignos e formam cistos dermóides; no testículo, onde costumam ser malignos; e, raramente, em outros locais, especialmente na linha média do corpo. SIN teratoid tumor. [terato- + G. *-oma*, tumor]
  t. or'bitae, t. da órbita. SIN orbitopagus.
  sacrococcygeal t., t. sacrococcígeo; t. encontrado na região do botão caudal. Tumor mais comum no período neonatal.
  triphyllomatous t., t. trifilomatoso; t. composto de tecidos derivados de todas as três camadas germinativas. SIN tridermoma.
ter·a·tom·a·tous (ter′ă-tō′mă-tŭs). Teratomatoso; relativo a ou da natureza de um teratoma.
ter·a·to·pho·bia (ter′ă-tō-fō′bē-ă). Teratofobia; medo mórbido de carregar e dar à luz um feto malformado. [terato- + G. *phobos*, medo]
ter·a·to·sis (ter′ă-tō′sis). Teratose; anomalia que produz um monstro. SIN teratism. [terato- + G. *-osis*, condição]
  atresic t., t. atrésica; t. em que qualquer um dos orifícios normais, como as narinas, a boca, o ânus ou a vagina, é imperfurado.
  ceasmic t., t. ceásmica; t. na qual não há união das metades laterais de uma parte, como na fenda palatina.
  ectogenic t., t. ectogênica; t. em que existe uma deficiência de partes.
  ectopic t., t. ectópica; t. em que os órgãos ou outras partes estão malcolocados.
  hypergenic t., t. hipergênica; t. em que existe redundância de partes.
  symphysic t., t. sinfísica; t. em que há fusão de partes normalmente separadas.
ter·a·to·sper·mia (ter′ă-tō-sper′mē-ă). Teratospermia. SIN teratozoospermia. [terato- + G. *sperma*, semente]

teratozoospermia (ter'ă-tō-zō-ō-sperm'ē-ă). Teratozoospermia; condição caracterizada por espermatozóides malformados no sêmen. SIN teratospermia. [terato- + *zôos*, vivo, + *sperma*, semente, sêmen, + -ia]

te·ra·zo·sin hy·dro·chlo·ride (tĕ-rā'zō-sin). Cloridrato de terazosina; antiandrogênico de ação periférica, utilizado no tratamento da hipertrofia prostática benigna e da hipertensão arterial.

ter·bi·um (Tb) (ter'bē-ŭm). Térbio; elemento metálico da série dos lantanídeos ou terras raras, de número atômico 65, peso atômico 158,92534. [de *Ytterby*, uma aldeia da Suécia]

ter·bu·ta·line sul·fate (ter-bū'tă-lēn). Sulfato de terbutalina; agente simpatomimético com atividade β₂-agonista relativamente seletiva, prescrito principalmente como agente broncodilatador ou tocolítico.

ter·e·bene (ter'ĕ-bēn). Terebeno; líquido incolor, fino e de odor e sabor aromáticos, uma mistura de hidrocarbonetos terpênicos, principalmente dipenteno e terpineno, obtidos do óleo de terebintina; utilizado como expectorante e na cistite e uretrite.

ter·e·bin·thi·nate (ter-ĕ-bin'thĭ-nāt). Terebintinato. **1.** Que contém ou é impregnado de terebintina. **2.** Preparação contendo terebintina. SIN terebinthine. [G. *terebinthos*, terebinto ou árvore da terebintina]

ter·e·bin·thine (ter-ĕ-bin'thin). Terebintina. SIN terebinthinate.

ter·e·bin·thin·ism (ter-ĕ-bin'thin-izm). Terebintinismo. SIN turpentine poisoning.

ter·e·brant, ter·e·brat·ing (ter'ĕ-brant, -brā'-ting). Terebrante; perfurante; utilizado figurativamente, como na expressão dor terebrante. [L. *terebro*, pp. *-atus*, perfurar, de *terebra*, escavador]

ter·e·bra·tion (ter-ĕ-brā'shŭn). Terebração. **1.** O ato de perfurar ou de trepanar. **2.** Dor perfurante. [L. *terebro*, perfurar, de *terebra*, escavador]

te·res, gen. **ter·e·tis,** pl. **ter·e·tes** (ter'ez, -tĕr-; ter'ĕ-tis; ter'ĕ-tēz). Redondo e longo; designa determinados músculos e ligamentos. VER teres minor (*muscle*), teres major (*muscle*), round *ligament* of uterus, round *ligament* of liver, pronator teres (*muscle*). [L. redondo, liso, de *tero*, deslizar]

ter·fen·a·dine (ter-fen'ă-dēn). Terfenadina; anti-histamínico H₁ utilizado no tratamento de várias condições alérgicas; possui menos efeitos sedativos do que outros anti-histamínicos; todavia, em combinação com vários outros fármacos, pode causar arritmias cardíacas graves.

ter·gal (ter'găl). Tergal, dorsal. SIN dorsal (1). [L. *tergum*, dorso]

ter·gum (ter'gŭm). Tergo, o dorso. SIN dorsum. [L.]

term. Termo. **1.** Período definido ou limitado. **2.** Nome ou palavra ou frase descritivas. VER TAMBÉM terminus, term *infant*. [L. *terminus*, limite, término]

ter·mi·nad (ter'mi-nad). Em direção ao término.

ter·mi·nal (ter'mi-năl). Terminal. **1.** Relativo ao término; final. **2.** Relativo à extremidade ou ao final de qualquer corpo; p. ex., a extremidade de um biopolímero. **3.** Terminação, extremidade ou final. [L. *terminus*, limite]
  amino-t., amino-terminal. VER amino-terminal.
  axon t.'s, terminações axônicas; terminações algo dilatadas e, com freqüência, em forma de clava, através das quais os axônios fazem contatos sinápticos com outras células nervosas ou com células efetoras (células musculares ou glandulares). Quando isoladas, por homogeneização do cérebro ou da medula espinal, contêm acetilcolina e enzimas correlatas. As terminações axônicas contêm neurotransmissores de vários tipos, algumas vezes mais de um. Esses neurotransmissores podem ser demonstrados por análise química e por métodos imunocitoquímicos. VER TAMBÉM synapse. SIN axonal terminal boutons, end-feet, neuropodia, pieds terminaux, synaptic boutons, synaptic endings, synaptic t.'s. terminal boutons, bouton terminaux.
  carboxy t., carboxi-terminal. VER C. *terminus*.
  synaptic t.'s, terminações sinápticas. SIN axon t.'s.

ter·mi·nal de·ox·y·nu·cle·o·ti·dyl trans·fer·ase (dē-ok'sē-noo'klē-ō-tĭ-dil-trans'fer-ās). Desoxinucleotidil transferase terminal. SIN DNA nucleotidylexotransferase.

ter·mi·na·tio, pl. **ter·mi·na·ti·o·nes** (ter'mi-nā'shē-ō, -ō'nēz) [TA]. Terminação. SIN termination. VER TAMBÉM ending. [L.]
  terminatio'nes nervo'rum li'berae, terminações nervosas livres. SIN free nerve *endings*, em *ending*.

ter·mi·na·tion (ter'mi-nā'shŭn). Terminação; extremidade ou final; uma terminação ou extremidade, particularmente uma terminação nervosa. VER ending. SIN terminatio [TA]. [L. *terminatio*]
  selective t., t. seletiva. SIN selective *reduction*.

ter·mi·na·ti·o·nes (ter-mi-nā-she-ō'nēz). Terminações; plural de terminatio. [L.]

Terminologia Anatomica (TA). Terminologa Anatômica (TA); sistema de nomenclatura anatômica que consiste em cerca de 7.500 termos, elaborados e aprovados pela International Federation of Associations of Anatomists (IFAA; Federação Internacional de Associações de Anatomistas, FIAA) e promulgada em agosto de 1997, em São Paulo, Brasil.

Desde a sua criação, em 1903, a IFAA tem feito convenções periódicas para a padronização de conceitos e terminologia anatômicos. Em 1989, a Federação nomeou uma Federative Committee on Anatomical Terminology (FCAT; Comissão Federativa da Terminologia Anatômica) de doze membros, consistindo em especialistas de 11 países, para empreender uma revisão em grande escala da última edição (sexta) da *Nomina Anatomica* (NA VI). Com a eleição de membros adicionais, em 1994, a FCAT reuniu representantes de 16 países e 5 continentes. A comissão solicitou sugestões de anatomistas e outros especialistas do mundo inteiro, e, a partir de mais de 10.000 termos para introdução ou manutenção, formulou e publicou uma lista daqueles considerados valiosos. Durante oito anos de deliberações, escolheram os termos mais simples e mais exatos, dando preferência aos termos descritivos de forma ou função aos semanticamente dúbios. Cerca de 10% dos termos previamente aceitos foram rejeitados ou alterados por não serem acurados ou por serem ambíguos ou inapropriados. Foram introduzidos cerca de 1.000 novos termos, incluindo alguns para estruturas não oficialmente designadas em sistemas anteriores de nomenclatura. Muitos desses termos já tinham sido adotados informalmente em vários países. Espera-se que a adoção da nova terminologia seja difundida. Como o inglês é falado em muitos países e serve como língua comum para a comunicação científica e médica, existe uma publicação que fornece os equivalentes dos termos latinos em inglês. Entretanto, apenas os termos latinos possuem valor oficial. O FCAT está atualmente trabalhando em formulações complementares da terminologia relativa à histologia, citologia, embriologia, odontologia e antropologia.

ter·mi·nus, pl. **ter·mi·ni** (ter'mi-nŭs, -nī). Término, terminação; fronteira ou limite. [L.]
  C t., terminação C; a extremidade de um peptídio ou proteína que possui um grupamento carboxila (-COOH) livre.
  ter'mini genera'les, termos gerais; palavras que são de uso geral em anatomia descritiva.
  N t., terminação N. VER amino-terminal.

ter·mo·lec·u·lar (ter-mō-lek'oo-lar). Trimolecular; designa três moléculas; p. ex., uma reação termolecular exige a presença de três moléculas para que ocorra a reação. [L. *ter*, três vezes, + molecular]

ter·mone (ter'mōn). Termônio; tipo de ectormônio, secretado por alguns organismos invertebrados, que estimula a gametogênese. [L. *ter*, três vezes, triplo, + hormone]

ter·na·ry (ter'nār-ē). Ternário; que designa ou que é constituído de três compostos, elementos, moléculas etc. [L. *ternarius*, de três]

Ter·ni·dens (Ter'nē-denz). Gênero de nematódeo encontrado no intestino de várias espécies de símios na África, na Índia e na Indonésia, bem como em seres humanos em partes da África; diferenciado dos ancilóstomos pela cápsula bucal orientada anteriormente, protegida por uma dupla coroa de cerdas resistentes; esse gênero é encontrado na parede do intestino grosso, onde pode produzir nódulos císticos.
  T. deminutus, espécie de nematódeo cujas larvas desenvolvem-se no solo; provavelmente infeccioso para seres humanos; o ciclo de vida é desconhecido.

ter·ox·ide (ter-ok'sīd). Teróxido. SIN trioxide.

ter·pene (ter'pēn). Terpeno; um de uma classe de hidrocarbonetos com fórmula empírica $C_{10}H_{16}$, ocorre em óleos essenciais e resinas. Os terpenos acíclicos podem ser considerados isômeros e polímeros de unidades de isopreno; as formas cíclicas incluem o mentano, o bornano e canfeno. Os terpenos que contêm 15, 20, 30, 40 etc. átomos de carbono são denominados sesquiterpenos, diterpenos, triterpenos, tetrapertenos etc.

***p*-ter·phen·yl** (ter-fen'il). *p*-terfenil; $C_6H_5-C_6H_4-C_6H_5$; útil como cintilador primário na contagem de cintilação líquida.

ter·pin. Terpina; álcool terpeno cíclico, $C_{10}H_{18}(OH)_2$, obtido pela ação do ácido nítrico e ácido sulfúrico diluído sobre óleo de pinheiro.
  t. hydrate, hidrato de terpina; monoidrato de terpina; supostamente um expectorante. SIN terpinol.

ter·pin·e·ol (ter-pin'ē-ol). Terpineol; terpeno alcoólico insaturado obtido por aquecimento do hidrato de terpina com ácido fosfórico diluído; anti-séptico e aroma.

ter·pi·nol (ter'pin-ol). Terpinol. SIN terpin hydrate.

ter·race (ter'as). Sutura por planos; suturar em várias fileiras, no fechamento de uma ferida através de uma considerável espessura de tecido. [atrav. do Fr. Ant. do L. *terra*, terra]

ter·ra ja·pon·i·ca (ter'ră jă-pon'i-kă). Terra japonesa. VER gambir.

Terrey, Mary, médica norte-americana do século 20. VER Lowe-T.-Mac-Lachlan *syndrome*.

Terrien, Louis-Felix, cirurgião francês, 1837–1908. VER T. *valve,* marginal *degeneration*.

ter·ri·to·ri·al·i·ty (ter'i-tor-ē-al'i-tē). Territorialidade. **1.** A tendência de indivíduos ou de grupos de defender um domínio ou esfera particular de interesse ou influência. **2.** A tendência de um animal a definir um espaço limitado como seu próprio hábitat, do qual afugenta animais de sua própria espécie que possam invadi-lo.

Terry, Theodore L., oftalmologista norte-americano, 1899–1946. VER T. *syndrome.*

Terson, Albert, oftalmologista francês, 1867–1935. VER T. *glands,* em *gland.*

ter·tian (ter′shan). Terçã; que sofre recidiva a cada terceiro dia, contando o dia de um episódio como o primeiro; na verdade, ocorre a cada 48 horas ou em dias alternados. [L. *tertianus,* de *tertius,* terceiro]

    double t., t. dupla; designa infecções por dois grupos diferentes de plasmódios que produzem paroxismos diários. VER TAMBÉM quotidian *malaria.*

ter·ti·a·rism, ter·ti·a·ris·mus (ter′shē-a-rizm, -riz′mŭs). Terciarismo; todos os sintomas do estágio terciário da sífilis em conjunto.

TESD Abreviatura de total end-systolic *diameter* (diâmetro sistólico final total).

Tesla, Nikola, engenheiro elétrico sérvio-americano, 1856–1943. VER tesla; T. *current.*

tesla (T) (tes′lă). Tesla; no sistema SI, a unidade de densidade do fluxo magnético expressa em kg s^{-2} A^{-1}; igual a 1 Wb/m². [N. *Tesla*]

tes·sel·lat·ed (tes′ĕ-lāt-ed). Enxadrezado; constituído de pequenos quadrados; quadriculado. [L. *tessella,* pequena pedra quadrada]

Tessier, Paul, médico francês do século 20. VER Tessier *classification.*

TEST

test. 1. Testar; provar; experimentar uma substância; determinar a natureza química de uma substância por meio de reagentes. **2.** Teste, prova, método de exame, p. ex., para determinar a presença ou ausência de uma doença definida ou de alguma substância em qualquer um dos líquidos, tecidos ou excreções do corpo ou para determinar a presença ou o grau de um traço psicológico ou comportamental. **3.** Reagente utilizado na realização de um teste. **4.** VER testa (1). VER TAMBÉM assay, reaction, reagent, scale, stain. [L. *testum,* um vaso de barro]

acetone t., prova da acetona; teste para cetonúria; a urina suspeita é agitada com algumas gotas de nitroprussiato de sódio; a seguir, despeja-se delicadamente água amoniacal concentrada sobre a mistura; na presença de acetona, forma-se um anel magenta na linha de contato; hoje em dia, são utilizados mais comumente comprimidos contendo nitroprussiato de sódio e álcali.

achievement t., teste de desempenho; teste padronizado utilizado para medir o aprendizado adquirido como, por exemplo, a competência numa área específica, como leitura ou aritmética, em contraste com o teste de inteligência, que é um indicador útil de capacidade ou aprendizado potencial.

acidified serum t., teste do soro acidificado; lise dos eritrócitos do paciente em soro fresco acidificado, específico para a hemoglobinúria paroxística noturna. SIN Ham t.

acid perfusion t., teste de perfusão com ácido. SIN Bernstein t.

acid phosphatase t. for semen, teste da fosfatase ácida para sêmen; prova de triagem para o sêmen através da determinação do conteúdo de fosfatase ácida; como o líquido seminal contém altas concentrações de fosfatase ácida, enquanto outros líquidos orgânicos e material estranhos possuem concentrações muito baixas, a obtenção de valores elevados da fosfatase ácida em aspirado ou lavado vaginal ou no líquido de lavagem de colorações torna a identificação do sêmen positiva, mesmo se o homem apresentar aspermia.

acid reflux t., teste do refluxo de ácido; teste para a detecção de refluxo gastroesofágico mediante monitorização do pH esofágico por um eletrodo na porção distal do esôfago, em condições basais ou após a instilação de ácido no estômago.

acoustic stimulation t., teste de estimulação acústica; teste para avaliação do bem-estar fetal através do uso de um aparelho acústico para estimular o feto e produzir aceleração da freqüência cardíaca fetal.

ACTH stimulation t., teste de estimulação com ACTH; prova de função córtico-supra-renal; a administração de ACTH por infusão intravenosa contínua ou por via intramuscular provoca elevação do cortisol plasmático nos indivíduos normais; na insuficiência córtico-supra-renal, o aumento esperado do cortisol plasmático é limitado ou inexistente.

Addis t., contagem de Addis. VER Addis *count.*

adhesion t., teste de adesão; aplicação diagnóstica do fenômeno de adesão imune. SIN erythrocyte adherence t., immune adhesion t., red cell adherence t.

Adler t., teste de Adler. SIN benzidine t.

Adson t., teste de Adson; teste para a síndrome do desfiladeiro torácico; o paciente senta com a cabeça estendida e voltada para o lado da lesão; com a inspiração profunda, ocorre redução ou perda total do pulso radial do lado afetado. Nem todos os pacientes com teste de Adson positivo apresentam a síndrome do desfiladeiro torácico. SIN Adson maneuver.

agglutination t., teste de aglutinação; qualquer um de vários testes que dependem da agregação de células, microrganismos ou partículas quando misturados com anti-soro específico.

Albarran t., teste de Albarran; prova para insuficiência renal, em que a ingestão de grandes quantidades de água provoca aumento proporcional no volume de urina se os rins estiverem normais, mas não se houver lesão do epitélio dos túbulos secretores. SIN polyuria t.

alkali denaturation t., teste de desnaturação em álcali; teste para a hemoglobina F (Hb F), baseado no fato de que as hemoglobinas, à exceção da Hb F, sofrem desnaturação por álcalis em hematina alcalina; o teste é sensível à presença de 2% ou mais de Hb F.

Allen t., teste de Allen; **(1)** para fenol: com a adição de 5 ou 6 gotas de ácido clorídrico e, a seguir, uma de ácido nítrico ao líquido suspeito, surge uma cor vermelha; [A.H. Allen] **(2)** para estricnina: o líquido é extraído com éter, que é então evaporado por meio de pipetagem "gota a gota" num prato ou cadinho de porcelana aquecido; o resíduo é tratado com uma pequena quantidade de dióxido de manganês e ácido sulfúrico diluído; surge uma cor azul-avermelhada ou violeta na presença de estricnina. [A.H. Allen] **(3)** teste para desobstrução radial ou ulnar; a artéria radial ou ulnar é comprimida digitalmente pelo examinador após forçar a saída de sangue da mão cerrando o punho; a ausência de difusão de sangue para a mão quando aberta indica que a artéria não-comprimida está ocluída. [Edgar Van Nuys Allen]

Allen-Doisy t., teste de Allen-Doisy; teste para atividade estrogênica; o material a ser investigado é injetado repetidamente em ratos ou camundongos imaturos ou castrados; o desaparecimento de leucócitos do esfregaço vaginal e o aparecimento de células cornificadas constituem uma reação positiva.

Almén t. for blood, teste de Almén para sangue; teste obsoleto em que são adicionados ácido acético glacial, solução de resina de guáiaco e peróxido de hidrogênio a uma suspensão aquosa da coloração suspeita; na presença de sangue oculto ou pigmento sangüíneo, surge uma cor azul. SIN guaiac t., Schönbein t., van Deen t.

Alpha t.'s, testes alfa; conjunto de testes mentais administrados com lápis e papel utilizados pela primeira vez no exército dos Estados Unidos, em 1917–1918, para determinar a capacidade mental de recrutas alfabetizados; o conjunto inclui oito tipos diferentes de testes: isto é, instruções, problemas aritméticos, julgamento prático, sinônimos e antônimos, orações na ordem inadequada, séries de números a completar, analogias e informações; são planejados especialmente para avaliar simultaneamente grandes grupos de indivíduos e para rápido processamento de máquinas; distintos dos testes Beta do exército, um conjunto complementar de testes para administração a recrutas que não podem ler ou escrever inglês, em que as instruções são fornecidas em sinais e o material do teste é ilustrado. VER Beta t.'s. SIN Army Alpha t.

alternate binaural loudness balance t., ABLB t., teste de equilíbrio de intensidade binaural alternada, teste ABLB; teste para recrutamento em uma orelha; a comparação da intensidade relativa de uma série de intensidades apresentadas alternadamente a cada orelha.

alternate cover t., teste da cobertura alternada; teste para detecção de foria ou estrabismo; a atenção é dirigida para um pequeno objeto de fixação, e um dos olhos é coberto durante vários segundos; a seguir, o outro olho é imediatamente coberto; se o olho se mover quando descoberto, significa a presença de estrabismo ou foria. SIN cover-uncover t.

alternating light t., teste com luz alternada; teste para detectar um defeito aferente relativo em um olho ao observar os movimentos pupilares. Quando o paciente está fixando a distância, a luz é mantida em cada olho por cerca de um segundo e rapidamente deslocada para o outro olho. Pressupondo-se que não há defeito de inervação do esfíncter da íris em um olho (que produziria anisocoria na luz), o olho com resposta mais fraca à luz apresenta um defeito pupilar aferente relativo. Essa assimetria de influxo pupilomotor pode ser estimada mantendo-se filtros de densidade neutra na frente do melhor olho até haver equilíbrio das respostas pupilares dos dois olhos. SIN swinging light t.

Ames t., teste de Ames; prova de triagem para possíveis carcinógenos utilizando cepas de *Salmonella typhimurium,* que são incapazes de sintetizar histidina; se a substância do teste produzir mutações que recuperam a capacidade de sintetizar histidina, a substância é carcinogênica. SIN Ames assay.

Amsler t., teste de Amsler; projeção de um defeito do campo visual em um gráfico de Amsler.

Anderson-Collip t., procedimento obsoleto para avaliação da atividade tireotrópica de um extrato da adeno-hipófise, indicada por aumento do metabolismo basal ou por evidências histológicas de estimulação da glândula tireóide no rato hipofisectomizado no qual foi injetado o extrato do teste.

Anderson and Goldberger t., teste de Anderson e Goldberger; teste obsoleto para tifo, em que o sangue do paciente é injetado na cavidade peritoneal de uma cobaia. Na presença de tifo, observa-se uma curva de temperatura típica.

anoxemia t., teste de anoxemia; teste obsoleto para insuficiência coronariana; o paciente respira uma mistura de oxigênio a 10% e nitrogênio a 90%; se esse procedimento induzir dor anginosa ou anormalidades eletrocardiográficas, o teste é positivo. SIN hypoxemia t.

anterior apprehension t., teste da apreensão anterior; **(1)** SIN shoulder apprehension *sign;* **(2)** teste de estabilidade do ombro; a apreensão com abdução e rotação lateral da articulação sugere instabilidade anterior. SIN crank test.

antibiotic sensitivity t., teste de sensibilidade a antibióticos, antibiograma; teste *in vitro* de culturas bacterianas com antibióticos para determinar a suscetibilidade de bactérias à antibioticoterapia. VER TAMBÉM Bauer-Kirby t.
antiglobulin t., teste da antiglobulina. SIN Coombs t.
antihuman globulin t., teste da antiglobulina humana. VER Coombs t.
antithrombin t., teste da antitrombina; procedimento para avaliar o efeito inibitório de uma amostra de plasma desfibrinado sobre a ação da trombina na conversão do fibrinogênio em fibrina.
Apt t., teste de Apt; teste para identificação do sangue fetal mediante adição de hidróxido de sódio e água a uma amostra.
aptitude t., teste de aptidão; teste de inteligência de orientação ocupacional utilizado para avaliar as capacidades, os talentos e as habilidades de uma pessoa; particularmente valioso no aconselhamento vocacional.
Army Alpha t., teste Alfa do exército. SIN Alpha t.'s.
Army Beta t.'s, testes Beta do exército. SIN Beta t.'s.
Army General Classification T., teste de classificação geral do exército; teste de triagem de seleção de capacidade intelectual global administrado para admissão de recrutas ao exército, utilizado na determinação de qualificações para admissão em uma da ampla variedade de posições nas quais cada indivíduo é colocado ao final do treinamento básico.
Ascoli t., teste de Ascoli; teste de precipitina para antraz que utiliza um extrato tecidual e anti-soro contra antraz.
ascorbate-cyanide t., teste do ascorbato-cianeto; teste para eritrócitos com deficiência de glicose-6-fosfato; o sangue é incubado com cianeto de sódio e ascorbato; o peróxido de hidrogênio gerado é livre para oxidar a hemoglobina a metemoglobina, visto que o cianeto inibe a catalase; forma-se uma cor castanha mais rapidamente nas células com deficiência de glicose-6-fosfato.
association t., teste de associação; teste em que uma palavra (palavra de estímulo) é dita ao indivíduo, que deve responder imediatamente com outra palavra (palavra de reação) sugerida pela primeira; utilizado como auxílio diagnóstico em psiquiatria e psicologia, sendo os indícios fornecidos pelo tempo (tempo de associação) levado entre as palavras de estímulo e de reação, bem como pela natureza das palavras de reação.
Astwood t., teste de Astwood. SIN metrotrophic t.
atropine t., teste da atropina. SIN Dehio t.
augmented histamine t., teste de aumento da histamina. SIN histamine t.
aussage t., teste de declaração; teste para avaliar a capacidade de reproduzir corretamente algo que foi visto por um breve intervalo de tempo. [Alemão *Aussage*, declaração]
autohemolysis t., teste de auto-hemólise; quando se incuba sangue desfibrinado estéril a 37°C, os eritrócitos normais sofrem hemólise lentamente; as células com defeitos da membrana ou defeitos metabólicos o fazem em maior grau.
Bachman t., teste de Bachman; teste cutâneo para triquinose, em que um extrato de larvas de *Trichinella* é suspenso em solução salina e injetado por via intradérmica. A observação de uma reação imediata de pápula e eritema ou de resposta tardia indica infecção.
Bachman-Petit t., teste de Bachman-Petit; modificação do teste de Kober para detecção do estradiol e de hormônios estrogênicos semelhantes na urina.
Bagolini t., teste de Bagolini; teste para correspondência retiniana, em que o indivíduo observa uma figura através de duas lentes estriadas.
Bárány caloric t., teste calórico de Bárány; teste para avaliação da função vestibular, que consiste em irrigar o meato auditivo externo com água quente ou fria; isso normalmente causa estimulação do aparelho vestibular, resultando em nistagmo e desvio na prova do indicador; na presença de doença vestibular, a resposta pode estar reduzida ou ausente. SIN caloric t., nystagmus t.
Barlow t., teste de Barlow. SIN Barlow *maneuver.*
Bauer-Kirby t., teste de Bauer-Kirby; teste padronizado para suscetibilidade microbiológica, que consiste em transferir uma cultura pura padronizada do microrganismo de interesse para uma placa de sensibilidade (placa de Petri com *ágar* Mueller-Hinton) e na observação do crescimento na presença de discos contendo antibióticos.
BEI t., teste do BEI. SIN butanol-extractable iodine t.
belt t., teste do cinturão; teste obsoleto; a pressão firme para cima exercida sobre a parte inferior do abdome remove a sensação de desconforto em casos de enteroptosia.
Bender gestalt t., teste de gestalt de Bender; teste psicológico utilizado por neurologistas e psicólogos clínicos para medir a capacidade do indivíduo de copiar visualmente um conjunto de desenhos geométricos; útil para medir a coordenação visuoespacial e visuomotora para detectar lesão cerebral. SIN Bender Visual Motor Gestalt t.
Bender Visual Motor Gestalt t., teste de Gestalt Visual Motor de Bender. SIN Bender gestalt t.
Benedict t. for glucose, teste de Benedict para glicose; teste de redução do cobre para glicose na urina, que envolve o tiocianato além do sulfato de cobre para uso qualitativo ou quantitativo.
bentiromide t., teste da bentiromida; prova de função exócrina pancreática que não exige intubação duodenal; a bentiromida administrada por via oral é clivada pela quimiotripsina na luz do intestino delgado e libera ácido *p*-aminobenzóico, que é absorvido e excretado na urina; a excreção urinária diminuída de ácido *p*-aminobenzóico sugere insuficiência pancreática.
bentonite flocculation t., teste de floculação da bentonita; teste de floculação obsoleto para artrite reumatóide, que consiste na adição de partículas de bentonita sensibilizadas ao soro inativado; a prova é positiva quando metade das partículas sofre agregação, enquanto a outra metade permanece em suspensão.
benzidine t., teste da benzidina; teste para sangue; o líquido suspeito é tratado com ácido acético glacial e éter; a seguir, esse último é decantado e tratado com peróxido de hidrogênio e uma solução de benzidina em ácido acético; a presença de sangue é indicada por uma cor azulada que se transforma em púrpura. SIN Adler t.
Bernstein t., t. de Bernstein; teste para estabelecer que a dor subesternal é causada por esofagite de refluxo; consiste na instilação de uma solução fraca de ácido clorídrico diretamente na parte inferior do esôfago através de uma sonda; os sintomas desaparecem quando a solução ácida é substituída por solução salina normal. SIN acid perfusion t.
Berson t., t. de Berson; prova de depuração tireóidea do ^{131}I do plasma pela glândula tireóide.
Beta t.'s, testes Beta; conjunto de testes mentais administrados visualmente, utilizados pela primeira vez em 1917–1918 pelo exército dos Estados Unidos para determinar a capacidade mental relativa de recrutas analfabetos ou com deficiência em ler e escrever inglês; as instruções são fornecidas através de sinais, sendo o material do teste de natureza ilustrativa; distintos dos testes Alfa, que foram administrados ao mesmo tempo a recrutas alfabetizados. SIN Army Beta t.'s.
Betke-Kleihauer t., teste de Betke-Kleihauer; teste em lâmina para a presença de eritrócitos fetais entre os eritrócitos da mãe; as hemoglobinas diferentes da Hb F são eluídas dos eritrócitos num esfregaço de sangue seco ao ar por um tampão de pH 3,3.
Bettendorff t., teste de Bettendorff; teste para arsênico; após misturar o líquido suspeito com ácido clorídrico, adiciona-se uma solução de cloreto estanhoso; quando se adiciona um pedaço de folha de estanho, forma-se um precipitado castanho.
Bial t., teste de Bial; teste obsoleto para pentose com orcinol. SIN orcinol t.
bile acid tolerance t., teste de tolerância aos ácidos biliares; prova sensível de disfunção hepática; após a administração oral de ácido biliar marcado ou não-marcado, determina-se a taxa de desaparecimento fracionado ou a retenção em 10 minutos.
bile esculin t., teste da esculina biliar; teste bioquímico utilizado para caracterizar estreptococos do grupo O, baseado na capacidade dos microrganismos de crescer em meio contendo bile e de hidrolisar a esculina.
bile solubility t., teste de solubilidade da bile; procedimento que diferencia o *Streptococcus pneumoniae* de outros estreptococos α-hemolíticos ao demonstrar a sua suscetibilidade à lise na presença de bile.
binaural alternate loudness balance t., teste do equilíbrio de intensidade alternada binaural; teste para recrutamento em uma orelha; a comparação da intensidade relativa de uma série de intensidades apresentadas alternadamente a cada orelha.
Binet t., teste de Binet. SIN Stanford-Binet intelligence *scale.*
bithermal caloric t., teste calórico bitermal; prova de função vestibular em que cada canal auditivo é irrigado alternada ou simultaneamente com água a 7°C acima ou abaixo da temperatura corporal; o nistagmo produzido pode ser monitorizado por direção, amplitude, velocidade do componente lento e duração.

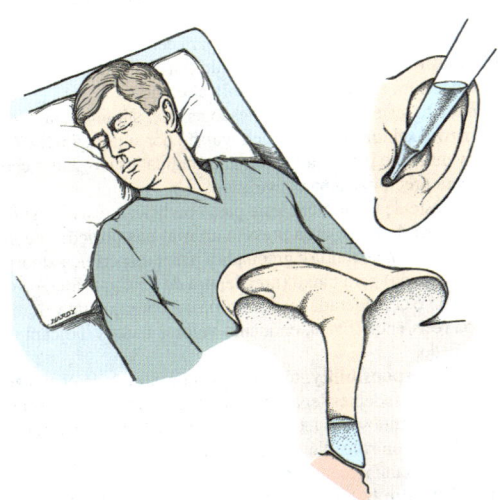

teste calórico de Bárány: para função vestibular

biuret t., teste do biureto; teste para determinação das proteínas séricas, baseado na reação de um reagente de cobre alcalino com substâncias contendo duas ou mais ligações peptídicas, produzindo uma cor azul-violeta.

blind t., teste cego; método de testagem em que um observador independente registra os resultados de qualquer teste, droga, placebo ou procedimento sem conhecer a identidade das amostras ou o resultado esperado.

block design t., teste de desenho em blocos; teste de desempenho que utiliza blocos coloridos que o indivíduo deve utilizar para combinar desenhos retratados; um dos subtestes das escalas de inteligência de Wechsler.

Bonney t., teste de Bonney. SIN Marshall t.

breath t., teste respiratório; qualquer teste diagnóstico em que são medidos materiais endógenos ou exógenos em amostras de respiração como meio de identificar processos patológicos; os exemplos incluem o teste respiratório de hidrogênio para intolerância à lactose ou teste de depuração respiratória da uréia para detectar a colonização gástrica por *Helicobacter pylori*. SIN breath analysis.

breath-holding t., teste de pausa apnéica; índice grosseiro da reserva cardiopulmonar medida pelo tempo em que um indivíduo pode voluntariamente interromper a respiração; a duração normal é de 30 segundos ou mais; a existência de redução da reserva cardíaca ou pulmonar é indicada por uma duração de 20 segundos ou menos.

Brigg t., teste de Brigg; teste que utiliza a redução do molibdato para avaliar a excreção de ácido homogentísico.

bromphenol t., teste do bromofenol; teste colorimétrico para medida da proteína, albumina e globulina na urina através do uso de fitas reagentes.

bromsulphalein t., teste de bromossulfaleína; prova obsoleta de função hepática (capacidade excretora hepática) que consiste na injeção intravenosa de uma quantidade conhecida de corante, geralmente 5 mg/kg de peso corporal; subseqüentemente (em geral, depois de 45 minutos), determina-se a quantidade de corante que permanece no soro; uma concentração de 0,4 mg ou menos de bromossulfaleína por 100 ml de soro ou menos do que 4% do corante injetado é considerada normal; pode ocorrer retenção de bromossulfaleína após redução do fluxo sangüíneo hepático ou obstrução biliar, bem como na lesão das células hepáticas. SIN BSP t.

BSP t., teste de BSP. SIN bromsulphalein t.

butanol-extractable iodine t., teste do iodo extraído em butanol; prova de função tireóidea obsoleta, efetuada em pacientes aos quais foram administradas grandes quantidades de iodo ou produtos iodados. SIN BEI t.

California psychological inventory t., teste de inventário psicológico da Califórnia; inventário de personalidade, utilizado com indivíduos normais, em que são enfatizadas variáveis de interação social.

Calmette t., teste de Calmette; reação conjuntival à tuberculina.

caloric t., teste calórico. SIN Bárány caloric t.

CAMP t., teste CAMP; teste para identificar estreptococos do grupo B com base na formação de uma substância (fator CAMP) que aumenta a área de hemólise formada pela β-hemólise estreptocócica. [*C*hristie, *A*tkins e *M*unch-*P*etersen, criadores do teste]

cancer antigen 125 t. (CA125), teste do antígeno de câncer 125 (CA125); teste para antígeno de superfície celular presente em derivados do epitélio celômico. Os níveis elevados desse antígeno estão associados a neoplasia ovariana e a doença pélvica benigna, como endometriose.

capillary fragility t., teste de fragilidade capilar; teste do torniquete utilizado para determinar a presença de deficiência de vitamina C ou trombocitopenia; um círculo de 2,5 cm de diâmetro, cuja borda superior está 4 cm abaixo da dobra do cotovelo, é traçado na face interna do antebraço; aplica-se uma pressão a meio caminho entre a pressão sistólica e diastólica acima do cotovelo durante 15 minutos, e efetua-se a contagem das petéquias presentes dentro do círculo: 10, normal; 10-20, marginal; mais de 20, anormal. SIN capillary resistance t., Rumpel-Leede sign, Rumpel-Leede t., vitamin C t.

capillary resistance t., teste de resistência capilar. SIN capillary fragility t.

carbohydrate utilization t., teste de utilização dos carboidratos; teste para identificação definitiva de leveduras e microrganismos leveduriformes clinicamente importantes.

carotid sinus t., teste do seio carótico; estimulação de um seio carótico (mas nunca ambos) para produzir efeitos reflexos que podem diminuir a freqüência cardíaca e/ou reduzir a pressão sistólica para diagnóstico ou, no caso de determinadas arritmias, para fins terapêuticos.

Carr-Price t., teste de Carr-Price; teste quantitativo para vitamina A, baseado na reação com tricloreto de antimônio em clorofórmio.

Casoni intradermal t., teste intradérmico de Casoni; teste para doença hidática, que consiste em injeção intracutânea de líquido hidático; a observação de uma reação de pápula e eritema imediata ou tardia constitui um resultado positivo. SIN Casoni skin t.

Casoni skin t., teste cutâneo de Casoni. SIN Casoni intradermal t.

CF t., teste de FC. SIN complement *fixation t.*

Chick-Martin t., teste de Chick-Martin; método para avaliar a eficiência *in vitro* de um agente bactericida; uma cultura padrão de *Salmonella typhi* à qual foi adicionada uma quantidade fixa de fezes esterilizadas ou levedura é testada durante um determinado período (30 minutos) contra várias concentrações de solução de fenol e várias concentrações do desinfetante; o resultado é expresso na forma de relação: o coeficiente de fenol, que é a maior diluição do desinfetante do teste em que as bactérias são destruídas, dividido pela maior diluição do fenol que esteriliza a solução no mesmo período de tempo.

chi-square t., teste do qui-quadrado; método estatístico para avaliar a significância de uma diferença, como no caso em que os dados de duas ou mais amostras, como o número de homens e mulheres em cada um de duas faculdades, são representados por um número distinto. SIN χ^2 t.

cis/trans t., teste *cis/trans*; teste sobre a configuração relativa na expressão de duas mutações.

Clauberg t., teste de Clauberg; teste de atividade progestacional; são administradas oito injeções diárias de estrogênio a coelhas imaturas; a seguir, administram-se cinco injeções diárias da substância do teste; a quantidade necessária para produzir alterações progestacionais definidas no endométrio é considerada a unidade; é equivalente a 0,75 mg de progesterona.

clomiphene t., teste do clomifeno; prova de reserva hipofisária de gonadotropinas que utiliza clomifeno.

clonidine growth hormone stimulation t., teste de estimulação do hormônio do crescimento com clonidina; a administração do agonista dos receptores α-2-adrenérgicos, clonidina, não consegue elevar os níveis de hormônio do crescimento em pacientes com atrofia com múltiplos sistemas; os níveis aumentam nos indivíduos normais.

coccidioidin t., teste da coccidioidina; teste intracutâneo para pesquisa de infecção pelo fungo *Coccidioides immitis;* uma reação de hipersensibilidade tardia indica uma prova positiva e é interpretada como infecção pregressa ou atual pelo fungo.

coin t., teste da moeda. SIN bellmetal *resonance.*

cold bend t., teste da curvatura a frio; teste da capacidade de um fio de ser modelado; efetuado através da contagem do número de vezes em que um fio pode ser curvado até formar um ângulo reto e devolvido ao mesmo ponto antes de sofrer ruptura; importante no estabelecimento de especificações para fios ortodônticos.

cold pressor t., teste de pressão com frio; teste provocativo cardiocirculatório convencionalmente efetuado ao se imergir uma das mãos em água gelada durante dois minutos ou mais (conforme tolerado) para produzir uma elevação aguda da pressão arterial; impondo, a seguir, uma resistência à ejeção de sangue do ventrículo esquerdo para o sistema arterial sistêmico, com conseqüente aumento agudo da pós-carga (pós-carga = aumento do estresse da parede ventricular esquerda). SIN Hines-Brown t.

colloidal gold t., teste do ouro coloidal. VER Lange t.

colorimetric caries susceptibility t., teste colorimétrico de suscetibilidade a cáries. SIN Snyder t.

complement-fixation t., teste de fixação do complemento; teste imunológico para determinar a presença de um antígeno ou anticorpo específico quando se sabe da presença de um deles, com base no fato de que o complemento é "fixado" na presença de antígeno e de seu anticorpo específico. VER TAMBÉM Bordet-Gengou *phenomenon.*

contraction stress t., teste de estresse de contração. SIN oxytocin challenge t.

Coombs t., teste de Coombs; teste para anticorpos, o denominado teste antiglobulina humana que utiliza as provas de Coombs direta ou indireta. SIN antiglobulin t.

Corner-Allen t., t. de Corner-Allen; prova de atividade progestacional; coelhas adultas são acasaladas durante o estro e castradas dentro de 18 horas; a substância do teste é injetada por via subcutânea em 5 dias sucessivos; a quantidade mínima necessária para produzir proliferação progestacional completa do endométrio é considerada a unidade, equivalente a 1,25 mg de progesterona.

cover t., teste da cobertura; teste utilizado para demonstração objetiva de desvio ocular no estrabismo; pode ser efetuado por dois métodos: o teste de cobertura-descobertura e o teste de cobertura alternada.

cover-uncover t., teste de cobertura-descobertura. SIN alternate cover t.

CO_2-withdrawal seizure t., teste de convulsão por supressão de CO_2; utilização de hiperventilação para demonstrar anormalidades nas ondas cerebrais ou até mesmo para precipitar uma convulsão.

Crampton t., teste de Crampton; teste para condição e resistência física; efetua-se um registro do pulso e da pressão arterial nas posições de decúbito e ortostática, e a diferença obtida é graduada a partir da perfeição teórica de 100 (raramente alcançada) para baixo (uma leitura de 75 é considerada excelente, enquanto a de 65 é considerada insatisfatória); a obtenção de valores altos indica uma boa resistência física, enquanto valores baixos indicam um estado não-condicionado.

t.'s of criminal responsibility, testes de responsabilidade criminal; em psiquiatria forense, precedentes legais nos quais são baseadas decisões relativas à insanidade de criminosos. VER TAMBÉM American Law Institute *rule,* Durham *rule,* M'Naghten *rule,* New Hampshire *rule.*

cutaneous t., teste cutâneo. SIN skin t.

cutaneous tuberculin t., teste cutâneo da tuberculina. VER tuberculin t.

cyanide-nitroprusside t., teste de cianeto-nitroprussiato; teste qualitativo para o diagnóstico de cistinúria; a adição de cianeto de sódio fresco formado por nitroprussiato de sódio a uma amostra de urina produz uma cor vermelho-púrpura estável se houver cistina.

cytotropic antibody t., teste do anticorpo citotrópico; teste de roseta para anticorpo citotrópico de macrófagos: camadas únicas de macrófagos são expostas inicialmente a anticorpo citotrópico para macrófagos e, a seguir, ao antígeno (contra o qual o anticorpo é específico) e hemácias de carneiro indicadoras; se o anticorpo for específico para hemácias de carneiro, estas formam uma roseta diretamente ao redor dos macrófagos; caso contrário, se o antígeno for solúvel, este deve ser acoplado às hemácias de carneiro por um agente, como benzidina bis-diazotizada.

DA pregnancy t., teste de gravidez por AD; teste de aglutinação direta (AD) no látex para gravidez. VER immunologic pregnancy t.

Day t., teste de Day; pesquisa de sangue que consiste na adição do líquido suspeito ou do lavado de uma coloração suspeita com tintura de guáiaco e, a seguir, peróxido de hidrogênio; a presença de sangue resulta em cor azul.

D-dimer t., teste do D-dímero; teste para detectar o fragmento de degradação da fibrina de ligação cruzada, o D-dímero. São observadas elevações desse fragmento na fibrinólise primária e secundária; durante a terapia trombolítica ou de desfibrinação com ativador do plasminogênio tecidual; ou em doenças trombóticas, como trombose venosa profunda, embolia pulmonar ou CID; na crise vasoclusiva da anemia falciforme, em neoplasias malignas e na cirurgia.

Dehio t., teste de Dehio; se uma injeção de atropina alivia a bradicardia, a condição deve-se à ação do nervo vago; caso contrário, a condição pode ser devida a uma afecção do próprio coração. SIN atropine t.

dehydrocholate t., teste do desidrocolato; método para determinar a velocidade da circulação sangüínea; injeta-se uma solução de desidrocolato de sódio por via intravenosa, e registra-se o tempo decorrido até a percepção de sabor amargo na boca; a média desse tempo é normalmente de cerca de 13 segundos.

Denver Developmental Screening T., Teste de Triagem de Desenvolvimento de Denver; escala empregada por psicólogos e pediatras para avaliar a maturidade de desenvolvimento, intelectual, motora e social de crianças em qualquer idade, entre o nascimento e a adolescência.

dexamethasone suppression t., teste de supressão com dexametasona; teste para detecção e diagnóstico da síndrome de Cushing; após a administração de 1,0 mg de dexametasona às 23 horas, os indivíduos normais apresentam supressão do cortisol plasmático para baixos níveis, o que não ocorre nos pacientes com síndrome de Cushing. Esquemas de doses maiores permitem diferenciar a síndrome de Cushing causada por tumor daquela causada por hiperplasia.

Dick t., teste de Dick; teste intracutâneo de suscetibilidade à toxina eritrogênica de *Streptococcus pyogenes*, responsável pela erupção cutânea e por outras manifestações da escarlatina. SIN Dick method.

differential renal function t., prova de função renal diferencial. SIN differential ureteral catheterization t.

differential ureteral catheterization t., prova de cateterismo uteral diferencial; estudo realizado para determinar vários parâmetros funcionais de um rim em comparação com o rim contralateral; são inseridos catéteres ureterais (por cistoscopia) no ureter ou na pelve renal bilateralmente; e efetuam-se medidas simultâneas da velocidade do fluxo urinário, da insulina ou do PAH (se infundido), creatinina endógena e vários solutos urinários. SIN differential renal function t., split renal function t.

dinitrophenylhydrazine t., teste da dinitrofenilidrazina; pesquisa da doença da urina em xarope de bordo; a adição de 2,4-dinitrofenilidrazina em HCl à urina produz um precipitado branco cretáceo na presença de cetoácidos.

direct Coombs t., prova de Coombs direta; prova para detecção de eritrócitos sensibilizados na eritroblastose fetal e em casos de anemia hemolítica imune adquirida: os eritrócitos do paciente são lavados com solução salina para remover o soro e anticorpos não-fixados; a seguir, são incubados com antiglobulina humana de Coombs (em geral, soro de coelho ou de cabra previamente imunizado com globulina humana), e, após incubação, o sistema é centrifugado e examinado à procura de aglutinação, o que indica a presença dos denominados anticorpos incompletos ou univalentes na superfície dos eritrócitos.

direct fluorescent antibody t., teste do anticorpo fluorescente direto. VER fluorescent antibody *technique*.

discontinuation t., teste de suspensão; teste para determinar se determinada droga é responsável por uma reação através da observação de uma remissão dos sintomas após interrupção de seu uso.

Doerfler-Stewart t., teste de Doerfler-Stewart; exame da capacidade do paciente de responder a palavras na presença de um ruído mascarador do tipo dente de serra; utilizado especialmente na diferenciação entre surdez funcional e orgânica. SIN D-S t.

double (gel) diffusion precipitin t. in one dimension, teste de dupla difusão (em gel) de precipitina unidimensional. VER gel diffusion precipitin t.'s in one dimension.

double (gel) diffusion precipitin t. in two dimensions, teste de dupla difusão (em gel) de precipitina bidimensional. VER gel diffusion precipitin t.'s in two dimensions.

Dragendorff t., teste de Dragendorff; teste qualitativo obsoleto para bile; um jogo de cores é produzido pela ação de uma gota de ácido nítrico a um papel de filtro branco ou porcelana não-vitrificada, umedecido com líquido contendo pigmentos biliares. O teste é essencialmente idêntico ao teste de Gmelin para bile na urina.

drawer t., sinal da gaveta. SIN drawer *sign*.

D-S t., teste de D-S. SIN Doerfler-Stewart t.

Ducrey t., teste de Ducrey; teste intradérmico que utiliza *Haemophilus ducreyi* inativado para o diagnóstico de cancróide; a obtenção de uma reação tardia positiva indica infecção presente ou pregressa; ocorrem resultados falso-positivos.

Duke bleeding time t., teste do tempo de sangramento de Duke; teste que consiste na realização de uma incisão no lóbulo da orelha e na medida do tempo decorrido até a interrupção do sangramento.

dye disappearance t., teste de desaparecimento do corante. SIN fluorescein instillation t.

dye exclusion t., teste de exclusão de corante; teste para determinar a viabilidade celular, que consiste na mistura de uma solução diluída de determinados corantes (p. ex., azul tripano, eosina Y, nigrosina, azul Alcian) com uma suspensão de células vivas; as células que excluem o corante são consideradas vivas, enquanto as células coradas são consideradas mortas; o teste nem sempre é acurado, visto que indica apenas a integridade estrutural da membrana celular.

Ebbinghaus t., teste de Ebbinghaus; teste psicológico em que o paciente é solicitado a completar certas sentenças das quais foram retiradas diversas palavras.

Ellsworth-Howard t., teste de Ellsworth-Howard; determinação do fósforo sérico e urinário após a administração intravenosa de extrato paratireóideo; utilizado no diagnóstico de pseudo-hipoparatireoidismo.

E-rosette t., teste da roseta E; teste para identificar linfócitos T, que consiste em misturar linfócitos sangüíneos purificados com soro e hemácias de carneiro; formam-se rosetas de eritrócitos em torno dos linfócitos T humanos com incubação.

erythrocyte adherence t., teste de aderência eritrocitária. SIN adhesion t.

erythrocyte fragility t., teste de fragilidade eritrocitária. SIN fragility t.

exercise t., teste do exercício; qualquer teste que utiliza o exercício físico para determinar as respostas e/ou a condição física do paciente.

Farnsworth-Munsell color t., teste da cor de Farnsworth-Munsell; teste para percepção das cores; a tarefa consiste em dispor 84 discos coloridos (em quatro fileiras separadas de 20-22 discos) numa seqüência com separação mínima de tonalidade entre discos adjacentes.

fern t., teste da samambaia; **(1)** teste para atividade estrogênica; os esfregaços de muco cervical formam um padrão em samambaia nos períodos de elevação da secreção de estrogênio, como no momento da ovulação; foram relatadas alterações semelhantes na saliva; **(2)** teste para detectar a ruptura das membranas amnióticas.

ferric chloride t., teste do cloreto férrico; teste qualitativo para a detecção de fenilcetonúria; a adição de cloreto férrico à urina produz uma cor verde-azulada na presença de fenilcetonúria.

Finckh t., teste de Finckh; teste psicológico em que o paciente é solicitado a explicar determinadas expressões proverbiais, como "queimar a vela nas duas pontas", "o pássaro madrugador pega a minhoca" etc.

finger-nose t., teste dedo-nariz; teste de coordenação e propriocepção do membro superior; o indivíduo é solicitado a tocar lentamente a ponta do nariz com o dedo indicador esticado; avalia a função cerebelar.

finger-to-finger t., teste dedo-dedo; teste de coordenação e propriocepção dos membros superiores; o indivíduo é solicitado a aproximar as pontas dos dedos indicadores; avalia a função cerebelar.

Finkelstein t., teste de Finkelstein; teste para detectar a tenossinovite de de Quervain, em que o polegar é flexionado na palma e coberto pelos quatro dedos; a seguir, o punho é desviado para o lado ulnar; o teste positivo produz dor e crepitação ao longo da via do tendão afetado.

Fishberg concentration t., teste de concentração de Fishberg; prova de conservação renal de água; após privação de água durante a noite, efetua-se a coleta de amostras de urina pela manhã e determina-se a densidade.

Fisher exact t., teste exato de Fisher; teste para associação numa tabela 2 × 2, baseado na distribuição exata das freqüências na tabela.

fistula t., teste da fístula; a compressão ou a rarefação do ar no canal auditivo externo excita o nistagmo se houver erosão da cápsula ótica, contanto que o labirinto ainda seja capaz de funcionar.

FIT t., teste FIT. SIN fusion-inferred threshold t.

Fleitmann t., teste de Fleitmann; teste obsoleto para arsênico; o hidrogênio é gerado num tubo de ensaio contendo líquido suspeito; o líquido é aquecido, e um pedaço de papel de filtro umedecido com solução de nitrato de prata é mantido sobre o topo; se houver arsênico, o papel umedecido torna-se negro.

flocculation t., teste de floculação. VER flocculation *reaction*.

fluorescein instillation t., teste de instilação de fluoresceína; teste para desobstrução do sistema lacrimal; a fluoresceína instilada no saco conjuntival pode ser recuperada do meato nasal inferior. SIN dye disappearance t., Jones t.

fluorescein string t., teste do cordão de fluoresceína; teste raramente utilizado, que consiste na deglutição de um cordão por um paciente com sangramento gastrintestinal; administra-se fluoresceína por via intravenosa; se houver fluorescência do cordão após sua remoção, significa que houve contaminação por sangue desde a injeção de fluoresceína; utilizado para determinar o local da lesão hemorrágica.

fluorescent antinuclear antibody t., FANA t., teste do anticorpo antinuclear fluorescente; teste para componentes de anticorpos antinucleares; utilizado particularmente para o diagnóstico de colagenoses.

fluorescent treponemal antibody-absorption t., teste de absorção de anticorpo treponêmico fluorescente; prova sorológica sensível e específica para sífilis que utiliza uma suspensão da cepa Nichols de *Treponema pallidum* como antígeno; a presença ou ausência de anticorpos no soro do paciente é indicada por uma técnica de anticorpo fluorescente indireta. SIN FTA-ABS t.

foam stability t., teste de estabilidade da espuma; teste para maturidade pulmonar fetal, determinada pela capacidade do surfactante pulmonar no líquido amniótico de produzir espuma estável na presença de etanol após agitação mecânica. SIN shake t.

Folin t., teste de Folin; (1) teste quantitativo para ácido úrico com base na cor produzida com ácido fosfotúngstico e uma base; (2) teste quantitativo para uréia; a uréia sofre decomposição por fervura com cloreto de magnésio, e a amônia liberada é medida.

Folin-Looney t., teste de Folin-Looney; teste obsoleto para tirosina, que produz uma cor azul em solução alcalina com um reagente que consiste em tungstato de sódio, ácido fosfomolíbdico e ácido fosfórico.

formol-gel t., teste de formol-gel; teste para detectar o acentuado aumento das proteínas séricas na leishmaniose visceral; acrescenta-se uma gota de formalina de formol de concentração total a 1 mL de soro, sendo a reação positiva indicada pela ocorrência de coagulação rápida e completa.

Fosdick-Hansen-Epple t., teste de Fosdick-Hansen-Epple; teste para determinar a atividade das cáries dentárias, com base numa solução de esmalte humano pulverizado numa mistura de saliva-glicose-esmalte.

Foshay t., teste de Foshay; teste intradérmico para a doença da arranhadura do gato ou para a tularemia, que utiliza material preparado a partir de linfonodos supurativos de indivíduos que tiveram a doença (não disponível comercialmente).

fragility t., teste de fragilidade; teste que mede a resistência dos eritrócitos à hemólise em soluções salinas hipotônicas; os eritrócitos a serem testados são adicionados a concentrações variáveis de solução salina (em geral, variando de cloreto de sódio a 0,85-0,10%, com aumentos de 0,05%), e mede-se a hemólise inicial e completa; os eritrócitos normais sofrem hemólise inicial em concentrações de 0,45-0,39% e hemólise completa em 0,33-0,30%; na esferocitose hereditária, a fragilidade dos eritrócitos está acentuadamente aumentada, ao passo que, na talassemia, anemia falciforme e icterícia obstrutiva, a fragilidade dos eritrócitos geralmente está reduzida. SIN erythrocyte fragility t.

Frei t., teste de Frei; teste diagnóstico intracutâneo para linfogranuloma venéreo: o antígeno de Frei é habitualmente uma preparação estéril de clamídias inativadas de aves domésticas; a observação de uma reação de tipo tardio positiva não é específica para o diagnóstico de linfogranuloma venéreo e raramente é utilizada. SIN Frei-Hoffmann reaction.

FTA-ABS t., teste de FTA-ABS. SIN fluorescent treponemal antibody-absorption t.

fusion-inferred threshold t., teste de limiar deduzido por fusão; emprego do fenômeno de fusão cerebral de sons binaurais para substituir o mascaramento convencional no teste de audição. SIN FIT t.

Gaddum and Schild t., teste de Gaddum e Schild; método sensível para identificação de adrenalina em tecido ou outro material, baseado na fluorescência da adrenalina exposta à luz ultravioleta na presença de álcali e oxigênio; a sensibilidade varia de 1:50 a 1:100 milhões.

galactose tolerance t., teste de tolerância à galactose; prova de função hepática baseada na capacidade do fígado de converter a galactose em glicogênio, medida pela taxa de excreção da galactose após ingestão ou injeção intravenosa de uma quantidade conhecida; normalmente, aparecem menos de 3 g na urina dentro de 5 horas após a ingestão de 40 g.

gel diffusion precipitin t.'s, testes de precipitina com difusão em gel; testes de precipitina em que o precipitado imune se forma em um meio de gel (habitualmente ágar), no qual ocorreu difusão de um ou de ambos os reagentes; em geral, classificados em dois tipos: unidimensional e bidimensional. SIN gel diffusion reactions.

gel diffusion precipitin t.'s in one dimension, testes da precipitina com difusão em gel unidimensional; testes de precipitina em que a solução de antígeno e o anticorpo incorporado em ágar são depositados em tubos, permitindo a difusão efetiva na dimensão vertical; o ágar contendo anticorpo pode ser sobreposto diretamente com solução de antígeno (difusão única (gel) unidimensional).

gel diffusion precipitin t.'s in two dimensions, testes de precipitina com difusão em gel bidimensional; testes de precipitina efetuados em uma camada de ágar, permitindo a difusão radial de um ou de ambos os reagentes em ambas as direções horizontais. A dupla difusão (gel) em duas dimensões (teste, técnica ao método de Ouchterlony) incorpora soluções de antígeno e de anticorpo colocadas em orifícios separados numa lâmina de ágar, permitindo a difusão radial de ambos os reagentes; esse método é amplamente utilizado para determinar relações antigênicas; as faixas de precipitado que se formam onde os reagentes se encontram em concentração ideal são de três padrões, denominados reação de identidade, reação de identidade parcial (reação cruzada) e reação de não-identidade.

Gellé t., teste de Gellé; aplica-se um diapasão vibrando sobre o processo mastóideo; se for ouvido, o ar no meato acústico externo é comprimido por meio de um tubo de borracha inserido no canal e um bulbo manual, fixando, assim, o estribo na janela oval, e o som deixa de ser ouvido, porém é novamente percebido se a pressão do ar for removida; teste de mobilidade dos ossículos.

Gerhardt t. for acetoacetic acid, teste de Gerhardt para ácido acetoacético; na urina fresca, surge uma cor vermelha após a adição de $FeCl_3$. Não há coloração se a urina tiver sido fervida; esse teste possui baixa especificidade e sensibilidade. SIN Gerhardt reaction.

Gerhardt t. for urobilin in the urine, teste de Gerhardt para urobilina na urina; a urobilina é extraída com clorofórmio e, a seguir, é tratada com iodo e hidrato de potássio, com produção de uma cor verde fluorescente.

germ tube t., teste do tubo de germes; teste para a identificação de *Candida albicans;* após incubação de 3 horas em soro, um inóculo de *Candida* desenvolve apêndices semelhantes a tubos.

glucose oxidase paper strip t., teste da fita reagente de glicose oxidase; teste qualitativo para glicose na urina em que a glicose é oxidada a ácido glicônico pela glicose oxidase; teste específico, exceto na presença de ácido ascórbico.

glucose tolerance t., teste de tolerância à glicose; teste para diabetes ou para estados hipoglicêmicos, como os que raramente podem ser observados em pacientes com insulinomas. Após a ingestão de 75 g de glicose com o paciente em jejum, o nível de glicemia aumenta imediatamente e, a seguir, volta ao normal dentro de 2 horas; nos diabéticos, a elevação é maior, e o retorno a valores normais é inusitadamente prolongado; em pacientes hipoglicêmicos, podem-se observar níveis reduzidos de glicose nas medidas de 3, 4 ou 5 horas.

glycerol dehydration t., teste de desidratação com glicerol; melhora transitória da audição em alguns indivíduos com doença de Ménière após administração de uma dose oral de glicerol, resultando em diurese osmótica.

Gmelin t., teste de Gmelin; teste obsoleto para bile na urina ou em outro líquido corporal; adiciona-se cuidadosamente ácido nítrico, com um pouco de ácido nitroso, a alguns mililitros do material a ser testado; se houver bile (bilirrubina), esta é oxidada em graus variáveis, resultando, assim, em zonas semelhantes a discos que são (da interface para fora) amarela, vermelha, violeta, azul e verde; o desenvolvimento das camadas verde e violeta é essencial para a validade do teste. SIN Rosenbach-Gmelin t.

Gofman t., t. de Gofman; teste para várias lipoproteínas séricas que contêm colesterol, como índice da tendência ao desenvolvimento de lesões ateromatosas e de arteriosclerose; o teste baseia-se na flutuação diferencial de moléculas de vários tamanhos quando o soro é tratado numa ultracentrífuga.

Goldscheider t., t. de Goldscheider; determinação da percepção da temperatura ao aplicar à pele um bastão metálico pontiagudo aquecido em graus variáveis.

gold sol t., teste do ouro coloidal. SIN Lange t.

Goodenough draw-a-man t., teste do desenho de um homem de Goodenough; teste rápido para avaliar o nível de inteligência de um indivíduo, baseado no grau de acurácia do desenho e do número de elementos incluídos por uma criança ou por um adulto ao qual são fornecidos um lápis e uma folha de papel branco e ao qual é solicitado fazer o desenho de um homem, segundo a sua habilidade máxima de fazê-lo. Também denominado teste de desenho de uma pessoa de Goodenough e, na sua forma atual, teste do desenho de Goodenough-Harris.

goodness of fit t., teste de boa qualidade de adequação; teste estatístico sobre a hipótese de que dados coletados ou obtidos aleatoriamente de uma população seguem uma determinada distribuição teórica.

Göthlin t., teste de Göthlin; teste de fragilidade capilar para determinar a presença ou a ausência de escorbuto.

Graham-Cole t., teste de Graham-Cole. SIN cholecystography.

group t., teste de grupo; em psicologia, teste destinado a ser aplicado a mais de um indivíduo de cada vez; por exemplo, teste de desempenho escolar, teste de admissão a uma escola de medicina.

guaiac t., prova de guáiaco. SIN Almén t. for blood.

Günzberg t., teste de Günzberg; teste para ácido clorídrico, que utiliza floroglucina com vanilina (reagente de Günzberg), com a qual é produzida uma cor vermelho-viva na presença do ácido.

Guthrie t., teste de Guthrie; ensaio de inibição bacteriana para medida direta da fenilalanina sérica; de uso disseminado para detecção da fenilcetonúria no recém-nascido.

Gutzeit t., teste de Gutzeit; teste obsoleto para arsênico; consiste na adição de um pedaço de zinco e de uma pequena quantidade de ácido sulfúrico ao líquido suspeito, que é então fervido; um pedaço de papel de filtro com uma solu-

Ham t., teste de Ham. SIN acidified serum t.
Hardy-Rand-Ritter t., teste de Hardy-Rand-Ritter; teste para deficiência da visão colorida que utiliza cartões pseudo-isocromáticos.
Harrington-Flocks t., teste de Harrington-Flocks; teste rápido de triagem para defeitos do campo visual; os padrões são observados taquistoscopicamente, sendo visíveis apenas quando iluminados por um *flash* de luz ultravioleta.
Harris t., teste de Harris. SIN Harris and Ray t.
Harris and Ray t., teste de Harris e Ray; teste obsoleto para vitamina C na urina; teste de microtitulação da urina contra um volume conhecido de solução aquosa a 0,05% do corante 2,6-dicloroindofenol em ácido acético a 10% (em geral, utiliza-se 0,05 mL do corante, o que equivale aproximadamente a 0,025 mg de ácido ascórbico). SIN Harris t.
head-dropping t., teste da cabeça caída; teste utilizado no diagnóstico de doença do sistema extrapiramidal ou do estriado (p. ex., parkinsonismo, doença de Wilson); com o paciente em decúbito dorsal, relaxado e com atenção desviada, o examinador eleva subitamente a cabeça do paciente com a mão direita e, a seguir, permite que caia sobre a palma de sua mão esquerda; a cabeça de uma pessoa normal cai subitamente como um peso morto; na doença do estriado, a cabeça cai lenta e suavemente, quase de forma hesitante.
heat coagulation t., teste de coagulação por calor; teste para determinação da proteína na urina; a albumina e a globulina são coaguladas pelo calor em pH ácido, e a intensidade da turvação presente fornece uma estimativa qualitativa do grau de proteinúria.
heat instability t., teste de instabilidade térmica; teste para a presença de hemoglobinas instáveis; os eritrócito frescos lisados em água destilada desenvolvem um precipitado dentro de 1 hora a 50°C na presença de hemoglobina instável.
heel-tap t., teste de percussão do calcanhar. VER heel *tap*.
heel-to-knee-to-toe t., teste calcanhar-joelho-dedo do pé. SIN heel-to-shin t.
heel-to-shin t., teste calcanhar-tíbia; teste de coordenação e propriocepção dos membros inferiores; o indivíduo coloca o calcanhar sobre o joelho oposto e, a seguir, o faz deslizar distalmente ao longo da tíbia até o tornozelo oposto. SIN heel-to-knee-to-toe t.
Heinz body t., teste dos corpúsculos de Heinz; teste para eritrócitos com deficiência de glicose-6-fosfato desidrogenase; adiciona-se um oxidante (acetilfenilidrazina) ao sangue; após incubação a 37°C, as amostras com deficiência de glicose-6-fosfato desidrogenase apresentam mais de 30% de corpúsculos de Heinz.
hemadsorption virus t., teste de hemadsorção viral; método para detecção de vírus hemaglutinantes, baseado na aderência de eritrócitos a células infectadas.
hemagglutination t., teste de hemaglutinação; teste sensível para medir determinados antígenos, anticorpos ou vírus, que utiliza sua capacidade de aglutinar certos eritrócitos.
Hemoccult t., teste de Hemoccult; nome comercial de um teste qualitativo para pesquisa de sangue oculto nas fezes, baseado na detecção da atividade de peroxidase da hemoglobina; pode-se utilizar um *kit* de teste em casa, sendo as amostras (em geral, 3 amostras obtidas em dias seqüenciais) remetidas a um laboratório para avaliação.
Hering t., teste de Hering; teste de visão binocular; o indivíduo olha através de um aparelho que tem em sua extremidade mais distante um fio perto do qual há uma pequena esfera pendente; com a visão binocular, o observador reconhece a localização da esfera em frente ou atrás do fio, o que não é possível com a visão monocular.
Hershberg t., teste de Hershberg; teste para esteróides anabólicos, em que ratos machos castrados são tratados com a substância testada.
Hines-Brown t., teste de Hines-Brown. SIN cold pressor t.
Hinton t., teste de Hinton; teste de precipitina (floculação) outrora amplamente utilizado para sífilis, em que o "antígeno" consistia em glicerol, colesterol e extrato de coração bovino.
Hirschberg t., teste de Hirschberg; teste de alinhamento motor binocular em que se acende uma pequena lanterna do tamanho de uma caneta diante dos olhos e observa-se a posição do reflexo luminoso na córnea, permitindo uma estimativa do desvio, quando presente.
Histalog t., t. Histalog; teste para medida da produção máxima de acidez gástrica ou de sua ausência; assemelha-se ao teste da histamina, porém utiliza Histalog (cloridrato de betazol); um análogo da histamina. SIN maximal Histalog t.
histamine t., t. da histamina; teste para a produção máxima de acidez gástrica ou de sua ausência; após administração preliminar de um anti-histamínico, injeta-se fosfato ácido de histamina por via subcutânea, numa dose de 0,04 mg/kg de peso corporal, seguido de análise do conteúdo gástrico. VER TAMBÉM Histalog t. SIN augmented histamine t.
histoplasmin-latex t., teste de histoplasmina-látex; teste de aglutinação passiva para histoplasmose; são utilizadas partículas de látex, sensibilizadas com antígeno extraído do *Histoplasma capsulatum,* numa reação de floculação com o soro do paciente.

Hollander t., teste de Hollander. SIN insulin hypoglycemia t.
Holmgren wool t., teste da lã de Holmgren; teste para cegueira para cores, em que o indivíduo combina variadamente meadas de lã coloridas.
homovanillic acid t., teste do ácido homovanílico; teste para o ácido homovanílico, baseado na presença de dopamina no tecido nervoso simpático como precursor da norepinefrina; como a norepinefrina possui uma via metabólica que produz ácido homovanílico, certos tumores, como neuroblastomas e ganglioneuromas, podem causar elevações dos níveis urinários de dopamina e de ácido homovanílico. SIN HVA t.
Howard t., teste de Howard; teste obsoleto, que consiste em cateterismo ureteral diferencial através da inserção de cateteres ureterais bilaterais para medir simultaneamente o volume urinário e a concentração de sódio em pacientes com suspeita de hipertensão vascular renal.
Huhner t., t. de Huhner. SIN postcoital t.
HVA t., teste do HVA. SIN homovanillic acid t.
17-hydroxycorticosteroid t., teste dos 17-hidroxicorticosteróides; teste que depende da reação de Porter-Silber, utilizada como medida da função adrenocortical e realizada em amostra de urina. São observados baixos valores na doença de Addison e no hipopituitarismo, enquanto ocorrem valores elevados na síndrome de Cushing e no estresse extremo. SIN 17-OH-corticoids t., Porter-Silber chromogens t.
hyperventilation t., prova de hiperventilação; consiste na produção de alcalose respiratória por hiperventilação para (1) produzir anormalidades clínicas, como, por exemplo, convulsões tetânicas; (2) causar anormalidades EEG; (3) causar anormalidades EMG.
hypoxemia t., teste de hipoxemia. SIN anoxemia t.
immune adhesion t., teste de imunoaderência. SIN adhesion t.
immunologic pregnancy t., teste imunológico para gravidez; denominação genérica dos testes para detecção de aumento da gonadotropina coriônica humana no plasma ou na urina por técnicas imunológicas, incluindo aglutinação de partículas de látex, inibição da hemaglutinação, radioimunoensaio, ensaios de radiorreceptores e imunoensaios enzimáticos.
impingement t., teste do impacto; teste diagnóstico que consiste na injeção de anestésico local num espaço subacromial de um paciente com sinais de impacto; o alívio da dor após a injeção durante manobras provocativas é útil para confirmar o espaço subacromial como origem dos sintomas.
indirect t., teste indireto. VER Prausnitz-Küstner *reaction*.
indirect Coombs t., prova de Coombs indireta; prova realizada rotineiramente na prova cruzada do sangue ou na investigação de reações transfusionais; o soro do paciente é incubado com uma suspensão de hemácias do doador; na presença de anticorpos específicos, estes se fixam ao antígeno nas células do doador; após lavagem com solução salina, adiciona-se antiglobulina humana de Coombs; a ocorrência de aglutinação nesse ponto indica que os anticorpos presentes no soro do teste original realmente fixaram-se aos eritrócitos do doador.
indirect fluorescent antibody t., teste do anticorpo fluorescente indireto. VER fluorescent antibody *technique*.
indirect hemagglutination t., teste de hemaglutinação indireta. SIN passive hemagglutination.
indole t., teste do indol; teste utilizado para identificar membros da família *Enterobacteriaceae* e outros bacilos Gram-negativos, baseado na capacidade dos microrganismos de produzir indol a partir do triptofano.
inkblot t., teste de Rorschach. SIN Rorschach t.
insulin hypoglycemia t., teste de hipoglicemia induzida por insulina; teste raramente utilizado para determinar a totalidade da vagotomia; após cirurgia, administra-se insulina para produzir hipoglicemia; se a vagotomia for completa, a secreção de ácido do estômago após a administração de insulina é significativamente menor que aquela antes da administração de insulina; se não houver nenhuma alteração do nível, é provável que haja vagotomia incompleta. As complicações da hipoglicemia são muito graves, de modo que o teste foi, em grande parte, abandonado. SIN Hollander t.
intelligence t., teste de inteligência; teste que utiliza itens bem-pesquisados e que envolve um método sistemático de administração e contagem dos pontos, utilizado para avaliar a aptidão geral ou o nível de competência potencial do indivíduo, em contraste com um teste de desempenho.
intradermal t., teste intradérmico. SIN skin t.
iodine t., teste do iodo; teste para detectar amido, baseado na sua reação com iodo.
Ishihara t., teste de Ishihara; teste para deficiência da visão para cores, que utiliza uma série de placas pseudo-isocromáticas sobre as quais estão impressos números ou letras em pontos de cores primárias, circundados por pontos de outras cores; as figuras são distinguíveis por indivíduos com visão normal para cores.
isopropanol precipitation t., teste de precipitação em isopropanol; teste que utiliza o princípio de que as ligações internas da hemoglobina são enfraquecidas por solventes não-polares; assim, as hemoglobinas instáveis precipitam mais rapidamente do que outras hemoglobinas em isopropanol.
^{131}I uptake t., teste de captação de I^{131}; prova de função tireóidea que consiste na administração oral de I^{131}-iodeto; depois de 24 horas, a quantidade presente

na glândula tireóide é medida e comparada com valores normais. SIN radioactive iodide uptake t., RAI t.

Ivy bleeding time t., teste do tempo de sangramento de Ivy; prova de tempo de sangramento que consiste na inflação de um esfigmomanômetro até 40 mm Hg ao redor do braço, na realização de uma incisão profunda de 5 mm na superfície flexora do antebraço e na medida do tempo levado para a cessação do sangramento.

Jacquemin t., teste de Jacquemin; teste para fenol; consiste na adição ao líquido suspeito de uma quantidade igual de anilina e, após mistura completa, de uma pequena quantidade de solução de hipoclorito de sódio; o líquido adquire uma coloração azul na presença de fenol.

Jaffe t., teste de Jaffe; **(1)** teste quantitativo para creatinina, baseado em sua reação com picrato alcalino; **(2)** teste qualitativo para a presença de indicanúria; após a adição de uma quantidade igual de HCl à urina, a adição posterior de clorofórmio e de CaCl$_2$ produz gotículas de clorofórmio de cor azul ou púrpura, que precipitam na presença de indican.

Janet t., teste de Janet; teste para anestesia funcional ou orgânica; pede-se ao paciente (com os olhos fechados) para dizer "sim" ou "não" quando sentir (ou não) o toque do dedo do examinador; no caso de anestesia funcional, o paciente pode dizer "não" quando uma área anestesiada for tocada, mas não dirá nada e não terá consciência de que está sendo tocado em caso de anestesia orgânica.

Jolles t., teste de Jolles; teste para bile; obtém-se um precipitado mediante agitação com clorofórmio, uma solução de cloreto de bário e ácido clorídrico; o precipitado é então removido, e a adição de uma ou de duas gotas de ácido sulfúrico produzirá um jogo de cores na presença de pigmentos biliares.

Jones t., teste de Jones. SIN fluorescein instillation t.

Jones I t., teste de Jones I. SIN primary dye t.

Jones II t., teste de Jones II. SIN secondary dye t.

Katayama t., teste de Katayama; prova colorimétrica qualitativa para carboxiemoglobina no sangue.

ketogenic corticoids t., teste dos corticóides cetogênicos. SIN 17-ketogenic steroid assay t.

17-ketogenic steroid assay t., teste de ensaio dos esteróides 17-cetogênicos; prova colorimétrica baseada na reação de Zimmermann, que indica os metabólitos ou esteróides supra-renais e testiculares excretados na forma de 17-cetonas na urina; os valores aumentados são mais notáveis nos tumores adrenocorticais, e os valores diminuídos, na doença de Addison ou no pan-hipopituitarismo. SIN ketogenic corticoids t.

Knoop hardness t., teste de dureza de Knoop. VER Knoop hardness *number*.

Kober t., teste de Kober; teste para estrogênios naturais, baseado na produção de uma cor rosada (absorção máxima: 520 μm) quando um estrogênio é aquecido numa mistura de fenol e ácido sulfúrico.

Kolmer t., teste de Kolmer; método quantitativo padrão antigo para o teste de Wassermann, com numerosas modificações (principalmente no que diz respeito ao antígeno).

Korotkoff t., teste de Korotkoff; teste de circulação colateral; enquanto a artéria acima de um aneurisma é comprimida, determina-se a pressão arterial na circulação distal; se estiver bastante alta, significa uma boa circulação colateral.

Krimsky t., teste de Krimsky; teste de alinhamento motor binocular, em que uma pequena lanterna é acesa diante dos olhos e a posição do reflexo luminoso centralizada com um prisma, indicando assim a quantidade de desvio.

Kurzrok-Ratner t., teste de Kurzrok-Ratner; teste para estrogênios na urina; a urina é extraída com acetato de etila, e, após purificação, o extrato é submetido a bioensaio, como no teste de Allen-Doisy.

Kveim t., teste de Kveim; teste intradérmico para detecção de sarcoidose, que consiste na injeção do antígeno de Kveim (obtido de baços de indivíduos com sarcoidose) e no exame de biopsias cutâneas depois de 3 a 6 semanas; a positividade do teste é indicada pelo aparecimento de nódulos típicos exibindo evidências de tecido sarcóide. SIN Kveim-Siltzbach t., Nickerson-Kveim t.

Kveim-Siltzbach t., teste de Kveim-Siltzbach. SIN Kveim t.

Lachman t., teste de Lachman; manobra para detectar a deficiência do ligamento cruzado anterior; com o joelho flexionado em 20-30º, a tíbia é deslocada anteriormente em relação ao fêmur; um ponto final mole ou um deslocamento de mais de 4 mm indica um teste positivo (anormal).

Lancaster red green t., teste de vermelho e verde de Lancaster; teste para medir desvios oculares em vários campos visuais em pacientes adultos com estrabismo adquirido e diplopia; consiste em colocar um filtro vermelho sobre o olho direito e um filtro verde sobre o olho esquerdo, seguido de alinhamento, pelo paciente, de uma luz vermelha ou verde com a luz da cor oposta projetada pelo examinador.

Landsteiner-Donath t., t. de Landsteiner-Donath. VER Donath-Landsteiner *phenomenon*.

Lange t., teste de Lange; teste obsoleto e inespecífico para proteínas alteradas no líquido cefalorraquidiano. Conforme originalmente utilizado por Lange, em 1912, o teste era considerado específico para neurossífilis; entretanto, isso provou ser incorreto. São efetuadas diluições do líquido cefalorraquidiano em solução salina, às quais se adiciona uma solução de ouro coloidal; se houver proteínas alteradas, observa-se uma mudança de cor ou a formação de precipitado. SIN gold sol t., Zsigmondy t.

latex agglutination t., teste de aglutinação do látex; teste de aglutinação passiva, em que o antígeno é adsorvido a partículas de látex que sofrem agregação na presença de anticorpo específico contra o antígeno adsorvido. SIN latex fixation t.

latex fixation t., teste de fixação do látex. SIN latex agglutination t.

LE cell t., teste da célula LE; a incubação *in vitro* de sangue ou de medula óssea de pacientes com lúpus eritematoso sistêmico ou a ação de seu soro sobre leucócitos normais levam à formação de células LE características. SIN lupus erythematosus cell t.

Legal t., teste de Legal; teste para acetona; a urina torna-se alcalina mediante a adição de algumas gotas de uma solução de hidróxido de potássio, à qual são adicionadas duas ou três gotas de uma solução de nitroprussiato de sódio a 10% recém-preparada; a urina torna-se vermelha e, a seguir, amarela; então, são aplicadas algumas gotas de ácido acético à parede lateral do tubo de ensaio, e, na linha de junção dos dois líquidos, verifica-se a formação de um anel carmim ou púrpura.

leishmanin t., teste da leishmanina; teste de hipersensibilidade tardia para leishmaniose cutânea; o teste é positivo quando a induração granulomatosa ultrapassa 5 mm depois de 2-3 dias no local de inoculação intradérmica de uma suspensão de leishmanias em formol. SIN Montenegro t. [leishmania + sufixo -*in*, componente, derivado]

lepromin t., teste de lepromina; teste que consiste na injeção intradérmica de uma lepromina, como o antígeno de Dharmendra ou de Mitsuda, para classificar o estágio da hanseníase com base na reação da lepromina, como a reação de Fernandez ou a reação de Mitsuda; diferencia a lepra tuberculóide, em que se observa uma reação tardia positiva no local da injeção, da lepra lepromatosa, em que não há reação (isto é, resultado negativo), apesar da infecção maligna ativa por *Mycobacterium leprae*; o teste não é diagnóstico, visto que os indivíduos não-infectados normais podem reagir.

leukocyte adherence assay t., ensaio de aderência leucocitária; teste para detectar a capacidade de aderência dos leucócitos a bactérias, efetuado *in vitro* utilizando fibras de náilon para medir a aderência.

leukocyte bactericidal assay t., ensaio bactericida dos leucócitos; teste de leucócitos para determinar sua capacidade de matar uma cultura de bactérias vivas.

Liebermann-Burchard t., teste de Liebermann-Burchard; prova colorimétrica para esteróides insaturados, notavelmente o colesterol; observa-se o desenvolvimento de uma cor esverdeada quando essas substâncias são adicionadas a anidrido acético e ácido sulfúrico em clorofórmio.

limulus lysate t., teste do lisado de *Limulus;* teste para rápida detecção de meningite por bactérias Gram-negativas; a endotoxina de microrganismos Gram-negativos induz a formação de gel de lisados de *Limulus polyphemus* (límulo).

line t., teste da linha; teste para raquitismo, baseado na observação das linhas de calcificação nas extremidades em crescimento de ossos longos raquíticos em ratos aos quais foram administradas preparações de vitamina D em condições de teste padronizadas; utilizado no ensaio biológico da vitamina D pela USP.

lipase t., teste da lipase; teste diagnóstico baseado na determinação da lipase no sangue e na urina como indicador de doença pancreática.

Lombard voice-reflex t., teste do reflexo vocal de Lombard; a observação de flutuações na intensidade da voz do paciente quando um ruído de mascaramento é aumentado ou diminuído; teste útil na avaliação da perda de audição funcional.

Lücke t., teste de Lücke; teste para ácido hipúrico; adiciona-se ácido nítrico quente à urina, que é evaporado até secar; a presença de ácido hipúrico é indicada por um odor de nitrobenzol após aquecimento adicional.

lupus band t., teste de faixa lúpica; técnica de imunofluorescência direta para demonstrar uma faixa de imunoglobulinas na junção dermoepidérmica da pele de pacientes com lúpus eritematoso.

lupus erythematosus cell t., teste da célula do lúpus eritematoso. SIN LE cell t.

Machado-Guerreiro t., teste de Machado-Guerreiro; teste de fixação do complemento para infecção por *Trypanosoma cruzi*.

Maclagan t., teste de Maclagan. SIN thymol turbidity t.

Maclagan thymol turbidity t., teste de turvação do timol de Maclagan. SIN thymol turbidity t.

macrophage migration inhibition t., teste de inibição da migração de macrófagos. SIN migration inhibitory factor t.

Mantel-Haenszel t., teste de Mantel-Haenszel; teste do qui-quadrado resumido, desenvolvido por Mantel e Haenszel para dados estratificados.

Mantoux t., teste de Mantoux. VER tuberculin t.

Marshall t., teste de Marshall; deslocamento manual do colo vesical durante o esforço ou a tosse para verificar se existe incontinência urinária de estresse. SIN Bonney t., Marshall-Marchetti t.

Marshall-Marchetti t., teste de Marshall-Marchetti. SIN Marshall t.

Master t., teste de Master; prova de exercício utilizada há muito tempo para identificar cardiopatia isquêmica, utilizando dois degraus de 24 cm de altura com uma plataforma no alto; o número de subidas e descidas pelo paciente é arbitrariamente escolhido e relacionado com a idade e o peso corporal. VER TAMBÉM two-step exercise t. SIN Master two-step exercise t.

Master two-step exercise t., teste do exercício de dois degraus de Master. SIN Master t.

maximal Histalog t., teste Histalog máximo. SIN Histalog t.

Mazzotti t., teste de Mazzotti; teste para oncocercíase, que utiliza uma dose de teste oral de dietilcarbamazina (50 ou 100 mg), resultando no aparecimento de exantema agudo em 2-24 horas a partir da morte das microfilárias na pele. SIN Mazzotti reaction.

McMurray t., teste de McMurray; rotação da tíbia sobre o fêmur para determinar a presença de lesão de estruturas do menisco.

McNemar t., teste de McNemar; forma de teste do qui-quadrado para dados pareados combinados.

McPhail t., teste de McPhail; teste obsoleto para progesterona e substâncias semelhantes; consiste no tratamento de coelhos fêmeas imaturas com 150 UI de estrona durante um período de 6 dias; a seguir, o material do teste é administrado em cinco doses subcutâneas diárias; observa-se a proliferação gestacional do endométrio, e os resultados são estimados de acordo com uma escala de 0 a ++++; a quantidade necessária para produzir uma resposta média (++) é considerada uma unidade, equivalente a 0,25 mg de progesterona.

Meinicke t., teste de Meinicke; a primeira aplicação bem-sucedida (1917–1918) da imunoprecipitação ao diagnóstico de sífilis, atualmente obsoleta.

Meltzer-Lyon t., teste de Meltzer-Lyon; teste utilizado no diagnóstico de afecções da vesícula biliar: são administrados 25 mL de solução de sulfato de magnésio a 25% na região do esfíncter de Oddi através de uma sonda duodenal, causando contração da vesícula biliar, relaxamento do esfíncter e expulsão da bile do ducto colédoco e da vesícula biliar; a bile do ducto colédoco é relativamente pálida e a primeira a ser expelida, seguida da bile da vesícula biliar; as amostras aspiradas do tubo são examinadas à procura de piócitos, grânulos de pigmento, células epiteliais, colesterol etc.

metabisulfite t., teste do metabissulfito; teste para hemoglobina falciforme (Hb S); a desoxigenação das células contendo Hb S é intensificada pela adição de metabissulfito de sódio ao sangue, causando afoiçamento visível numa lâmina; algumas outras hemoglobinas anormais (Hb C_{Harlem} e Hb I) também sofrem afoiçamento nesse teste.

methacholine challenge t., teste de estimulação com metacolina; teste que consiste na inalação de concentrações crescentes de metacolina, um potente broncoconstritor, em pacientes com possível hiper-reatividade brônquica; geralmente efetuado quando o diagnóstico de asma ou de doença pulmonar broncoespástica não é clinicamente óbvio.

3-methoxy-4-hydroxymandelic acid t., teste do ácido 3-metoxi-4-hidromandélico. SIN vanillylmandelic acid t.

metrotrophic t., teste metrotrófico; teste obsoleto para análise de substâncias estrogênicas; o hormônio é injetado por via subcutânea a ratos fêmeas imaturas (25-49 g), que são sacrificadas depois de 6 horas, quando o aumento do peso uterino (devido, em grande parte, à absorção de água) é considerado critério de atividade estrogênica. SIN Astwood t.

MHA-TP t., teste de MHA-TP. SIN microhemagglutination-Treponema pallidum t.

microhemagglutination-Treponema pallidum t., teste de micro-hemaglutinação do *Treponema pallidum*; versão de microtitulação do teste de hemaglutinação do *Treponema pallidum*. SIN MHA-TP t.

microprecipitation t., teste de microprecipitação; teste de precipitação em que são utilizadas quantidades reduzidas de reagentes do teste.

migration inhibition t., teste de inibição da migração. SIN migration inhibitory factor t.

migration inhibitory factor t., teste do fator de inibição da migração; teste que mede a presença do fator de inibição da migração, uma linfocina de 25-kD. Em geral, são colocados macrófagos peritoneais num tubo capilar, na presença ou ausência de sobrenadante de células T ativadas em resposta a estímulo imunogênico. Na presença de MIF, a migração de monócitos/macrófagos é reduzida. SIN macrophage migration inhibition t., migration inhibition t.

milk-ring t., teste do anel leitoso; forma especial de teste de aglutinação efetuado no leite armazenado de muitas vacas, geralmente de rebanhos inteiros, para a detecção de rebanhos contendo animais infectados por brucelose bovina.

Millon Clinical Multiaxial Inventory t., Teste do Inventário Multiaxial Clínico de Millon; teste efetuado com lápis e papel, que consiste em 20 escalas clínicas derivadas de 175 afirmações autodescritivas e desenvolvido, em 1977, para uso na avaliação da psicopatologia e dos padrões mais resistentes de personalidade; especialmente projetado para corresponder com alguns dos distúrbios de personalidade incluídos no Diagnostic and Statistical Manual of Mental Disorders, utilizado no diagnóstico por profissionais de saúde mental. SIN Millon clinical multiaxial inventory.

Millon-Nasse t., teste de Millon-Nasse; teste para proteína, cuja tirosina reage com nitrito após tratamento breve com íon mercúrio em ácido para produzir uma cor.

Minnesota Multiphasic Personality Inventory t. (MMPI), Teste do Inventário de Personalidade Multifásico de Minnesota; tipo de teste psicológico na forma de questionário para idades a partir dos 16 anos, com 550 afirmações do tipo verdadeiro-falso, codificadas em 4 escalas de validade e 10 escalas de personalidade, que pode ser administrado tanto a indivíduos quanto a grupos. SIN Minnesota Multiphasic Personality Inventory.

mixed agglutination t., teste de aglutinação mista. VER mixed agglutination *reaction*.

mixed lymphocyte culture t., teste de cultura de linfócitos mistos; teste para histocompatibilidade de antígenos HL-A, em que os linfócitos do doador e do receptor são misturados em cultura; o grau de incompatibilidade é indicado pelo número de células que sofreram transformação e mitose ou pela captação de timidina marcada com isótopo radioativo. SIN MLC t.

MLC t., teste de MLC. SIN mixed lymphocyte culture t.

Molisch t., teste de Molisch; teste colorido para açúcar, que se condensa com α-naftol ou timol na presença de ácido sulfúrico concentrado, que converte o açúcar em derivados furfúricos.

Moloney t., teste de Moloney; teste para detectar um elevado grau de sensibilidade ao toxóide diftérico; a observação de mais de uma reação local mínima a toxóide diluído (1:20), administrado por via intradérmica, indica que o toxóide profilático deve ser inoculado em doses fracionadas a intervalos apropriados.

Montenegro t., teste de Montenegro. SIN leishmanin t.

Mörner t., teste de Mörner; **(1)** para cisteína, que produz uma cor púrpura brilhante com nitroprussiato de sódio; **(2)** para tirosina, que produz uma cor verde à fervura com ácido sulfúrico contendo formaldeído.

Moschcowitz t., teste de Moschcowitz; demonstração de isquemia do membro inferior por oclusão da circulação arterial durante 5 min com um torniquete ou uma bandagem de Esmarch. Após liberação, a cor da pele normalmente volta em poucos segundos; na presença de obstrução arterial (por exemplo, arteriosclerótica), a cor retorna mais lentamente.

Mosenthal t., teste de Mosenthal; teste raramente utilizado para avaliar a capacidade de concentração renal ao medir a gravidade da urina a cada 2 horas durante a ingestão de uma dieta controlada.

motility t., teste de motilidade; teste baseado em observação microscópica ou na propagação do crescimento em ágar semi-sólido, utilizado para determinar a motilidade de um microrganismo.

Motulsky dye reduction t., teste de redução do corante de Motulsky; teste para deficiência de glicose-6-fosfato desidrogenase no sangue, que utiliza uma mistura de azul cresil brilhante, glicose-6-fosfato e NADP.

mucin clot t., teste do coágulo de mucina; teste que reflete a polimerização do hialuronato do líquido sinovial; a adição de algumas gotas de líquido sinovial ao ácido acético forma um coágulo; ocorre formação de coágulo deficiente numa variedade de distúrbios inflamatórios, incluindo artrite séptica, artrite gotosa e artrite reumatóide. SIN Ropes t.

Mulder t., teste de Mulder. VER xanthoprotein *reaction*.

multiple puncture tuberculin t., teste tuberculínico de múltipla punção; tipo de teste com pua. VER tuberculin t.

multiple sleep latency t., teste de múltiplas latências do sono; teste para propensão a dormir, realizado através de polissonografia durante múltiplas e breves oportunidades de sono.

mumps sensitivity t., teste de sensibilidade à caxumba; teste cutâneo para sensibilidade à caxumba, em que o vírus da caxumba inativado é utilizado como antígeno.

Nagel t., teste de Nagel; teste de visão para cores, em que o observador determina as quantidades relativas de vermelho e verde necessárias para formar o amarelo espectral; utiliza-se um instrumento denominado anomaloscópio de Nagel.

NBT t., teste do NBT; abreviatura de nitroblue tetrazolium t.

neutralization t., teste de neutralização. SIN protection t.

niacin t., teste da niacina; teste da capacidade de micobactérias de produzir niacina; utilizado para distinguir *Mycobacterium tuberculosis* de outras cepas.

Nickerson-Kveim t., teste de Nickerson-Kveim. SIN Kveim t.

nitroblue tetrazolium t. (NBT t.), teste do nitroazul tetrazólio; teste para detectar a capacidade fagocítica dos leucócitos polimorfonucleares ao medir a capacidade bactericida leucocitária oxigênio-dependente.

nitroprusside t., teste do nitroprussiato; teste qualitativo para cistinúria; após a adição de cianeto de sódio à urina, a adição posterior de nitroprussiato produz uma cor vermelho-púrpura se o cianeto tiver reduzido qualquer cistina presente a cisteína.

nonstress t., teste de não-estresse; teste para avaliar o bem-estar fetal ao avaliar a resposta da freqüência cardíaca do feto ao movimento fetal; um teste de não-estresse reativo consiste numa aceleração da freqüência cardíaca fetal em resposta ao movimento fetal.

nystagmus t., teste do nistagmo. SIN Bárány caloric t.

Ober t., teste de Ober; teste para avaliar o trato iliotibial tenso, contraído ou inflamado; o paciente fica em decúbito lateral sobre o lado não-afetado, e o quadril afetado é abduzido pelo examinador à medida que o joelho é flexionado a 90°; efetua-se a adução passiva do quadril; o grau de abdução ou a produção de dor ao longo do trato iliotibial podem ajudar a identificar o local de inflamação ou de contratura.

Obermayer t., teste de Obermayer; teste para indican; os sólidos na urina são precipitados por meio de uma solução de acetato de chumbo a 20% e, a seguir, filtrados, adicionando-se ao filtrado ácido clorídrico fumegante contendo uma pequena quantidade de solução de cloreto férrico; na presença de indican, a adição de clorofórmio causa a formação de índigo, indicado pela cor azul.

17-OH-corticoids t., teste dos 17-OH-corticóides. SIN 17-hydroxycorticosteroid t.

oral lactose tolerance t., prova de tolerância à lactose oral; prova para deficiência de lactose; a resposta da glicose plasmática a uma carga oral de lactose é medida como na prova de tolerância à glicose (oral).

orcinol t., teste do orcinol. SIN Bial t.

Ortolani t., teste de Ortolani. SIN Ortolani *maneuver*.

Ouchterlony t., teste de Ouchterlony; teste de difusão dupla (gel) em duas dimensões. VER gel diffusion precipitin t.'s in two dimensions. SIN Ouchterlony method.

oxidase t., teste da oxidase; teste para a presença de citocromo oxidase intracelular, baseado na reação com *p*-fenilenodiamina; auxilia na identificação de espécies de *Neisseria* e Pseudomonadaceae.

oxytocin challenge t., teste provocativo com oxitocina; teste de estresse de contração efetuado com a administração de uma solução diluída de oxitocina por via intravenosa para estimular as contrações. SIN contraction stress t.

Pachon t., teste de Pachon; em caso de aneurisma, a determinação da circulação colateral através da estimativa da pressão arterial.

Palmer acid t. for peptic ulcer, teste do ácido para úlcera péptica de Palmer; na úlcera duodenal, a administração de ácido por sonda duodenal provoca dor intensa.

palmin t., palmitin t., teste da palmina, teste da palmitina; prova de eficiência pancreática, baseada no fato de que a presença de gordura no estômago provoca abertura do piloro e permite a passagem de suco gástrico; em conseqüência, ocorre clivagem da palmina, de modo que o exame do conteúdo gástrico, após uma refeição de teste contendo palmina, irá revelar a presença de ácidos graxos.

pancreozymin-secretin t., teste de pancreozimina-secretina. VER secretin t.

Pandy t., teste de Pandy. SIN Pandy *reaction*.

Pap t., teste de Pap; exame microscópico de células esfoliadas ou raspadas de uma superfície mucosa após coloração pelo método de Papanicolaou; utilizado especialmente para a detecção de câncer do colo do útero. SIN Papanicolaou smear t.

Papanicolaou smear t., teste de esfregaço de Papanicolaou. SIN Pap t.

parallax t., teste de paralax; medida do desvio no estrabismo pelo teste de cobertura alternada, combinado com neutralização do desvio utilizando prismas.

parametric t., teste paramétrico; teste estatístico que depende de uma pressuposição acerca da distribuição dos dados, como, por exemplo, a pressuposição de que os dados estão normalmente distribuídos.

passive cutaneous anaphylaxis t., teste de anafilaxia cutânea passiva; injeta-se um anticorpo (habitualmente IgE) por via intradérmica a um animal, que é subseqüentemente estimulado com uma mistura de antígeno e corante de azul de Evans por via intravenosa dentro de 24-48 horas. O aparecimento de uma área escura indica uma reação positiva devido ao extravasamento do corante no local da reação antígeno-anticorpo.

patch t., teste de contato; teste de sensibilidade cutânea: um pequeno pedaço de papel, esparadrapo ou ventosa, umedecido com líquido do teste diluído não-irritante, é aplicado à pele da região dorsal superior ou face externa do braço, e, depois de 48 horas, a área coberta é comparada com a superfície não-coberta; observa-se uma reação eritematosa com vesículas quando a substância provoca alergia de contato. VER TAMBÉM photo-patch t.

Patrick t., teste de Patrick; teste para determinar a presença ou ausência de doença sacroilíaca; com o paciente em decúbito dorsal, a coxa e o joelho são flexionados e o maléolo externo é colocado sobre a patela da perna oposta; essa manobra normalmente pode ser efetuada sem causar dor, mas, ao exercer pressão sobre o joelho, ocorre imediatamente dor na presença de doença sacroilíaca.

Paul t., teste de Paul. SIN Paul *reaction*.

Paul-Bunnell t., teste de Paul-Bunnell; teste para detecção de anticorpos heterófilos na mononucleose infecciosa. VER Forssman *antigen*.

PBI t., teste PBI. SIN protein-bound iodine t.

pentagastrin t., teste da pentagastrina; alternativa da histamina para estimulação da secreção ácida na análise gástrica.

performance t., teste de desempenho; teste, como cinco dos 11 subtestes da escala de inteligência de adultos de Wechsler, que exige pouca ou nenhuma instrução verbal do examinador e praticamente nenhuma resposta verbal do examinado.

Perls t., teste de Perls; teste para hemossiderina, utilizando o *corante* azul da Prússia de Perls.

personality t., teste de personalidade; qualquer um da categoria de testes psicológicos projetados para testar as características da personalidade, estado emocional, distúrbio mental etc., em contraste com um teste de inteligência.

Perthes t., teste de Perthes; teste para perviedade da veia femoral profunda; com o paciente na posição ortostática, aplica-se um torniquete acima do joelho; após caminhar, se a circulação profunda for competente, as varicosidades superficiais permanecem inalteradas; se houver oclusão da circulação profunda, as pernas tornam-se dolorosas.

phentolamine t., teste da fentolamina; teste para feocromocitoma; a administração intravenosa de fentolamina (5 mg) reduz a hipertensão causada por feocromocitoma, mas não aquela devida a outras causas, como, por exemplo, hipertensão essencial; nessa última forma de hipertensão, o fármaco eleva a pressão arterial.

photo-patch t., teste de fotossensibilização por contato; após a aplicação de um emplastro com o sensibilizador suspeito durante 48 horas em dois locais, se não houver nenhuma reação, uma das áreas é exposta a uma dose fraca de luz solar ou luz ultravioleta para induzir eritema; se for positiva, desenvolve-se uma reação com vesiculação mais grave na área exposta do que no local da pele não-exposta.

photostress t., teste de fotoestresse; medida da acuidade visual antes e depois da exposição dos olhos a luz intensa.

phrenic pressure t., teste da pressão frênica; aplica-se uma pressão ao nervo frênico de cada lado, acima das clavículas, onde o nervo passa sobre o músculo escaleno anterior; se o paciente sentir dor e inclinar a cabeça para o lado doloroso, o problema localiza-se no espaço pleural; se a cabeça não for inclinada para um lado, o problema está localizado na cavidade abdominal.

Pirquet t., teste de Pirquet; teste tuberculínico cutâneo. VER tuberculin t. SIN dermotuberculin reaction, Pirquet reaction.

pivot shift t., teste do deslocamento do pivô; manobra para detectar uma deficiência do ligamento cruzado anterior do joelho; quando o joelho é estendido, uma súbita subluxação do côndilo tibial lateral sobre o fêmur distal é positiva.

P-K t., teste P-K. SIN Prausnitz-Küstner *reaction*.

plasmacrit t., teste de plasmácrito; método de triagem sorológica utilizado como auxiliar no diagnóstico da sífilis; após a coleta de apenas algumas gotas de sangue heparinizado (obtido de punção no dedo) em um tubo capilar especial, este é centrifugado para coletar o plasma, que é então misturado com uma gota de 0,01 ml de antígeno (cardiolipina previamente tratada com cloreto de colina como antiinibidor, a fim de evitar a obtenção de resultados falso-negativos que podem ocorrer com plasma ou soro mal-aquecidos). Após agitação mecânica da mistura antígeno-plasma durante 4 min, observa-se a presença ou não de floculação. A obtenção de um resultado positivo não deve ser considerada diagnóstico conclusivo, enquanto um resultado negativo exclui a probabilidade de sífilis.

platelet aggregation t., teste de agregação plaquetária; teste que avalia a capacidade das plaquetas de aderir umas às outras e, assim, de formar um tampão hemostática para impedir o sangramento; ocorre falha da agregação em diversas condições, por exemplo, trombastenia, doença de Von Willebrand e após a administração de aspirina, fenilbutazona e indometacina; o teste é conduzido mediante quantificação da redução de turvação que ocorre no plasma rico em plaquetas após a adição *in vitro* de um ou mais agentes agregadores plaquetários (por exemplo, ADP, epinefrina ou serotonina).

polyuria t., teste de poliúria. SIN Albarran t.

Porges-Meier t., teste de Porges-Meier; teste de floculação antigo para sífilis; importante por ter introduzido como antígenos frações de tecido insolúveis em acetona e solúveis em álcool e lecitina.

Porter-Silber chromogens t., teste dos cromógenos de Porter-Silber. SIN 17-hydroxycorticosteroid t.

postcoital t., teste pós-coito; teste efetuado em muco cervical aproximadamente na época da ovulação para avaliar sua receptividade aos espermatozóides. SIN Huhner t.

precipitation t., teste de precipitação. SIN precipitin t.

precipitin t., teste de precipitina; teste *in vitro* em que o antígeno encontra-se na forma solúvel e precipita quando combinado com anticorpo específico adicionado na presença de um eletrólito. VER TAMBÉM gel diffusion precipitin t.'s, ring precipitin t. SIN precipitation t.

primary dye t., teste do corante primário; avaliação da drenagem lacrimal após o teste de instilação de fluoresceína ao procurar recobrir o corante de fluoresceína abaixo da concha nasal inferior utilizando um *swab*. SIN Jones I t.

prism cover t., teste da cobertura com prisma; medida do desvio no estrabismo pelo teste da cobertura alternada combinado com neutralização para o desvio utilizando prismas.

prism vergence t., teste de vergência com prismas; medida da amplitude de fusão pela colocação de prismas de potência gradualmente crescente na direção testada até que ocorra diplopia.

progesterone challenge t., teste de estímulo da progesterona; administração de um agente progestacional em caso de amenorréia para detectar a presença de endométrio preparado por estrogênio.

projective t., teste projetivo; teste psicológico livremente estruturado contendo muitos estímulos ambíguos que exigem que o indivíduo revele seus sentimentos, personalidade ou psicopatologia em resposta a eles; por exemplo, teste de Rorschach, teste de apercepção temática.

protection t., teste de proteção; teste para determinar a atividade antimicrobiana de um soro ou para identificar determinado organismo através da inoculação de uma mistura do soro e do vírus ou de outro micróbio que está sendo testado num animal suscetível ou numa cultura de células. SIN neutralization t.

protein-bound iodine t., teste do iodo ligado à proteína; prova de função tireóidea utilizada antigamente, que consiste na determinação do iodo ligado à proteína sérica para obter uma estimativa do hormônio ligado à proteína no sangue periférico. SIN PBI t.

prothrombin t., teste da protrombina; teste quantitativo para a protrombina no sangue, com base no tempo de coagulação do plasma sangüíneo na presença de tromboplastina e cloreto de cálcio; avalia a integridade das vias extrínseca e comum da coagulação. VER TAMBÉM prothrombin time. SIN Quick method, Quick t.

prothrombin and proconvertin t., teste da protrombina e da proconvertina; teste utilizado antigamente por alguns para controlar a terapia anticoagulante com bis-hidroxicumarina e indandiona.

provocative t., teste provocativo; qualquer procedimento em que uma anormalidade fisiopatológica suspeita é deliberadamente induzida através da manipulação de condições que reconhecidamente provocam a anormalidade.

provocative Wassermann t., teste provocativo de Wassermann; teste obsoleto que possui apenas interesse histórico; o uso do teste de Wassermann de um ou dois dias ou de uma ou duas semanas após a administração de arsfenamina ou de neoarsfenamina; o resultado pode ser então positivo quando era negativo antes da administração de arsfenamina.

psychological t.'s, testes psicológicos; testes destinados a medir as realizações, a inteligência, as funções neuropsicológicas, as habilidades, a personalidade ou as características individuais ou ocupacionais ou potencialidades de uma pessoa. VER TAMBÉM scale.

psychomotor t.'s, testes psicomotores; testes psicológicos que, apesar de baseados em outros processos psicológicos (por exemplo, sensorial, perceptivo), exigem uma reação motora, como copiar desenhos, construir com blocos ou manipular controles.

pulp t., teste da polpa. SIN vitality t.

Q tip t., teste da ponta Q; teste para determinar a mobilidade da uretra.

Queckenstedt-Stookey t., teste de Queckenstedt-Stookey; a compressão da veia jugular num indivíduo sadio provoca aumento da pressão do líquido cefalorraquidiano na região lombar dentro de 10-12 segundos e uma queda igualmente rápida para valores normais após retirada da pressão exercida sobre a veia; quando há bloqueio dos canais subaracnóideos, a compressão da veia provoca pouca ou nenhuma elevação da pressão no líquido cefalorraquidiano.

quellung t., teste quellung. SIN Neufeld capsular swelling.

Quick t., teste de Quick. SIN prothrombin t.

quinine carbacrylic resin t., teste da resina carbacrílica de quinina; teste para ausência de acidez gástrica. VER azuresin.

Quinlan t., teste de Quinlan; teste para bile; quando se examina uma fina camada de bile através de um espectroscópio, as linhas de absorção surgem no violeta.

radioactive iodide uptake t., teste de captação de iodeto radioativo. SIN ^{131}I uptake t.

radioallergosorbent t. (RAST), teste radioalergoadsorvente (RAST); radioimunoensaio para detectar anticorpos IgE específicos responsáveis pela hipersensibilidade: o alérgeno é ligado a material insolúvel, e o soro do paciente reage com esse conjugado; se o soro tiver anticorpos contra o alérgeno, ocorrerá formação de um complexo com o alérgeno. Adiciona-se um anticorpo anti-IgE humana marcado para reagir com a IgE ligada. A quantidade de radioatividade é proporcional à IgE sérica.

radioimmunosorbent t. (RIST), teste radioimunoadsorvente (RIST); teste de competição efetuado *in vitro*, destinado a medir a IgE específica contra determinado antígeno. Quantidades conhecidas de IgE marcada com isótopo radioativo competem com a IgE não-marcada do paciente pela sua ligação a uma superfície recoberta com anti-IgE. A redução da IgE marcada devido à presença de IgE no soro do paciente pode ser determinada por comparação com padrões de IgE conhecidos; assim, pode-se determinar a quantidade de IgE sérica total do paciente.

RAI t., teste de RAI. SIN ^{131}I uptake t.

rapid plasma reagin t., teste da reagina plasmática rápida; grupo de provas sorológicas para sífilis, em que o soro ou o plasma não-aquecido reage com um antígeno de teste padronizado contendo partículas de carvão; os testes positivos produzem floculação. Uma modificação desse teste, denominada teste de cartão (círculo) RPR, é amplamente utilizada como teste de triagem. SIN RPR t.

Rapoport t., teste de Rapoport; teste de cateterismo ureteral diferencial utilizado para avaliação de suspeita de hipertensão vascular renal; são obtidas amostras de urina de cada rim por cateterismo ureteral bilateral, e determina-se a relação da fração de rejeição tubular medindo-se as concentrações de sódio e de creatinina na urina de cada rim.

Rayleigh t., teste de Rayleigh. SIN Rayleigh *equation.*

red cell adherence t., teste de aderência eritrocitária. SIN adhesion t.

Reinsch t., teste de Reinsch; teste para arsênico em que uma fita de cobre é colocada no líquido suspeito, que é então acidulado com ácido clorídrico e fervido; se houver arsênico, ocorre um depósito cinza sobre o cobre, que, ao ser aquecido, é sublimado e depositado na forma de uma camada cristalina sobre um pedaço de vidro mantido acima da fita de cobre.

Reiter t., teste de Reiter; teste de fixação do complemento para sífilis, que utiliza como antígeno um material preparado a partir da cepa Reiter do *Treponema pallidum;* o teste foi substituído na medicina laboratorial em grande parte pelo teste de absorção de anticorpo treponêmico fluorescente (FTA-ABS) t.

relocation t., teste de reposicionamento; teste para instabilidade anterior do ombro; com o paciente em decúbito dorsal, o examinador efetua uma abdução e rotação lateral do úmero contra a borda da mesa, como fulcro; os pacientes com perda da estabilidade anterior tornam-se apreensivos com a pressão exercida.

resorcinol t., teste do resorcinol; teste para frutosúria; a urina fresca tratada com resorcinol em ácido produz um precipitado vermelho na presença de frutose; o precipitado deve formar uma solução vermelha em etanol. SIN Selivanoff t.

Reuss t., teste de Reuss; teste para atropina; a adição de agentes oxidantes e de ácido sulfúrico a um líquido contendo atropina produz um odor de flores de laranjeira e rosas.

Rh blocking t., teste de bloqueio do Rh; teste para anticorpos Rh não-aglutinantes; em primeiro lugar, efetua-se um teste de aglutinação do Rh; se o teste para aglutininas Rh for negativo, mistura-se uma gota de soro aglutinante anti-Rh$_0$ de título moderado com o soro do paciente contendo células de teste Rh-positivas; se, após incubação durante 1-2 h a 37°C, não houver aglutinação, considera-se a presença de anticorpos bloqueadores Rh$_0$ no soro do paciente.

Rickles t., teste de Rickles; prova colorimétrica para prever a atividade de cáries dentárias mediante incubação da saliva em sacarose e determinação das alterações do pH.

Rimini t., teste de Rimini; teste obsoleto para formaldeído na urina, no leite e em outros líquidos, com o uso de solução diluída de cloridrato de fenilidrazina, nitroprussiato de sódio e hidróxido de sódio.

ring t., teste do anel. SIN ring precipitin t.

ring precipitin t., teste do anel de precipitina; teste da precipitina, em que a solução de antígeno é cuidadosamente depositada sobre a solução de anticorpos em um tubo; à medida que ocorre difusão, forma-se um disco de precipitado no local onde a relação de anticorpos é ótima. SIN ring t.

Rinne t., teste de Rinne; (1) um diapasão posto em vibração é mantido em contato com o crânio (em geral, com o processo mastóideo) até que o som seja perdido; a seguir, suas hastes são aproximadas do orifício auditivo, quando o indivíduo novamente irá ouvir um som fraco se a audição estiver normal; expresso como a condução de ar maior do que a condução óssea e indicador de mecanismo normal de condução do som através da orelha média; (2) um diapasão posto em vibração é ouvido por mais tempo e com maior intensidade quando em contato com o crânio do que quando mantido próximo ao orifício auditivo, expresso como a condução óssea maior do que a condução de ar, indicando algum distúrbio do mecanismo de condução do som.

Romberg t., teste de Romberg. SIN Romberg *sign.*

Römer t., teste de Römer; teste de interesse histórico; injeta-se tuberculina, pura ou diluída, por via intracutânea numa cobaia; se o animal tiver tuberculose, aparece uma grande pápula com centro hemorrágico necrótico em cerca de 24 horas (reação em roseta ou cocar).

Ropes t., teste de Ropes. SIN mucin clot t.

Rorschach t., teste de Rorschach; teste psicológico projetivo em que o indivíduo revela suas atitudes, emoções e personalidade ao relatar o que vê em cada um de 10 quadros de manchas de tinta. SIN inkblot t.

rose bengal radioactive (^{131}I) t., teste do rosa-bengala radioativo (I^{131}); prova de função hepática utilizada como meio de medir o fluxo sangüíneo hepático e para cintilografia do fígado, a fim de determinar o tamanho e o contorno do fígado, ou a presença de massas expansivas no fígado.

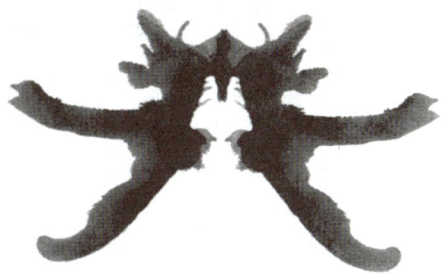

teste de Rorschach: exemplo de imagem utilizada no teste

Rosenbach t., teste de Rosenbach; teste obsoleto para bile na urina; a urina suspeita é filtrada várias vezes através do mesmo papel de filtro, que é então seco e sobre o qual se aplica uma gota de ácido nítrico ligeiramente fumegante; a presença de bile é indicada pelo jogo resultante de cores característico dos pigmentos biliares (mancha amarela circundada por anéis em vermelho, violeta, azul e verde).

Rosenbach-Gmelin t., teste de Rosenbach-Gmelin. SIN Gmelin t.

rosette t., teste das rosetas; teste para células formadoras de rosetas (linfócitos T), que consiste na incubação dessas células e de hemácias de carneiro e leve centrifugação; a seguir, a amostra é examinada ao microscópio à procura de formação de rosetas ou aderência dos eritrócitos aos linfócitos T.

Rose-Waaler t., teste de Rose-Waaler; teste de interesse histórico; quando as hemácias de carneiro são recobertas por uma concentração de anti-soro contra hemácias de carneiro, que é muito baixa para causar aglutinação, a adição de soro de um paciente com artrite reumatóide provoca aglutinação.

Ross-Jones t., teste de Ross-Jones; teste obsoleto para excesso de globulina no líquido cefalorraquidiano; deposita-se cuidadosamente 1 ml de líquido cefalorraquidiano sobre 2 ml de uma solução concentrada de sulfato de amônio; se houver excesso de globulina, surge um delicado anel branco na linha de junção em cerca de 3 min.

Rothera nitroprusside t., teste do nitroprussiato de Rothera; teste para corpos cetônicos; 5 ml de urina fresca são saturados com sulfato de amônio sólido e misturados com 10 gotas de solução de nitroprussiato de sódio a 2% recém-preparada, que é então misturada com 10 gotas de água amoniacal concentrada e mantida em repouso durante 15 min; a presença de ácido acetoacético ou de maiores concentrações de acetona é indicada pelo desenvolvimento de uma cor azul-púrpura.

RPR t., teste da RPR. SIN rapid plasma reagin t.

rubella HI t., teste de IH para rubéola; teste de inibição da hemaglutinação (IH) para rubéola, freqüentemente realizado de modo rotineiro como parte da avaliação pré-natal da gestante; a presença de um título detectável de IH na ausência de doença indica infecção prévia e imunidade à reinfecção; se não for detectado nenhum anticorpo IH, a paciente é considerada potencialmente suscetível, devendo ser acompanhada de acordo. VER TAMBÉM hemagglutination *inhibition*.

Rubin t., teste de Rubin; teste obsoleto de perviedade das tubas uterinas; uma cânula é introduzida no colo do útero, e administra-se dióxido de carbono através da cânula por meio de uma seringa fixada a um manômetro; se as tubas estiverem desobstruídas, o escape de gás na cavidade abdominal é evidenciado por um som borbulhante agudo ouvido à ausculta sobre a parte inferior do abdome, ou pode-se demonstrar a presença de gás livre sob o diafragma em radiografia.

Rubner t., teste de Rubner; teste obsoleto para a lactose ou glicose na urina; adiciona-se acetato de chumbo à urina suspeita, que é então filtrada; adiciona-se amônia até a formação de um precipitado permanente; na presença de lactose, o precipitado adquire uma cor rosada a vermelha quando o líquido é aquecido; na presença de glicose, a cor torna-se amarela a castanha.

Rumpel-Leede t., teste de Rumpel-Leede. SIN capillary fragility t.

Sabin-Feldman dye t., teste do corante de Sabin-Feldman; método para a detecção de anticorpo antitoxoplasma no soro, baseado no fato de que as células de *Toxoplasma gondii* (de exsudato peritoneal em camundongos) coram-se razoavelmente bem com azul-de-metileno alcalino, enquanto os microrganismos em soro contendo anticorpo específico não exibem nenhuma afinidade pelo corante; além disso, as células normais de toxoplasma tornam-se arredondadas, e tanto o núcleo quanto o citoplasma coram-se intensamente quando tratadas com azul-de-metileno; por outro lado, quando o corante é misturado com microrganismos e anticorpos, as células preservam sua forma em crescente e apenas o endossoma nuclear retraído é corado.

Sachs-Georgi t., teste de Sachs-Georgi; o primeiro teste de precipitina para sífilis de caráter diagnóstico prático; a inovação significativa foi a adição de colesterol ao antígeno lipóide (extrato tecidual alcoólico) utilizado no teste de Meinicke mais antigo.

Saundby t., teste de Saundby; teste para sangue nas fezes; consiste na adição de 30 gotas de uma solução de peróxido de hidrogênio a 20 volumes a uma mistura de 10 gotas de uma solução de benzidina saturada e pequena quantidade de fezes em tubo de ensaio; a observação de uma cor azul-escura persistente indica a presença de sangue.

scarification t., teste de escarificação; por exemplo, teste de Pirquet, em que o material é introduzido na pele através de picada ou arranhadura.

Schaffer t., teste de Schaffer; teste para nitritos na urina; a urina é descorada com carvão animal, e, a seguir, são adicionados 4 ml de uma solução de ácido acético a 10% e 3 gotas de uma solução de ferro cianeto de potássio a 5%; na presença de nitritos, surge uma cor amarela intensa.

Schellong t., teste de Schellong; teste para função circulatória; pede-se ao indivíduo ficar em posição ortostática durante 10-20 min; durante esse período, mede-se continuamente a pressão arterial; a ocorrência de queda da pressão sistólica de 20 mm Hg ou mais indica uma função circulatória deficiente.

Schick t., teste de Schick; teste de suscetibilidade à toxina de *Corynebacterium diphtheriae*; injeta-se 0,1 ml da toxina de teste de Schick na pele de um antebraço (local de teste), e a mesma quantidade do mesmo material, porém inativado pelo calor, na pele do outro antebraço (local de controle); os indivíduos com anticorpos neutralizadores da toxina não apresentam nenhuma reação em ambos os locais de injeção (teste negativo) ou podem exibir uma pseudo-reação devido a anticorpos dirigidos contra substâncias (antígenos) presentes nos materiais do teste, diferentes da toxina diftérica; os indivíduos que carecem de anticorpos neutralizadores da toxina podem apresentar uma reação positiva, que consiste no aparecimento de uma área de vermelhidão apenas no local do teste dentro de 24-36 horas, que persiste por 4-5 dias. SIN Schick method.

Schiller t., teste de Schiller; teste para áreas sem glicogênio da parte vaginal do colo do útero, que podem constituir o local de carcinoma de estágio inicial; essas áreas não se coram de marrom-escuro com solução de iodo; a perda de glicogênio devido à erosão e a outras condições benignas também pode produzir um resultado positivo.

Schilling t., teste de Schilling; procedimento para determinar a quantidade de vitamina B_{12} excretada na urina, utilizando cianocobalamina marcada com um radioisótopo do cobalto.

Schirmer t., teste de Schirmer; teste para produção de lágrimas que utiliza um pedaço de papel de filtro; fornece uma medida da função basal e reflexa das glândulas lacrimais.

Schober t., teste de Schober; medida da mobilidade da coluna lombar, em que são traçadas linhas horizontais paralelas acima e 5 cm abaixo da junção lombossacra no indivíduo em posição ortostática; com uma flexão anterior máxima, a distância entre as linhas aumenta em pelo menos 5 cm nos indivíduos normais, porém o aumento é bem menor em pacientes com espondilite ancilosante.

Schönbein t., teste de Schönbein. SIN Almén t. for blood.

Schwabach t., teste de Schwabach; utiliza-se uma série de cinco diapasões de diferentes tons e observa-se o número de segundos em que o paciente pode ouvir cada um deles por condução aérea e óssea.

scratch t., teste de escarificação; forma de teste cutâneo em que o antígeno é aplicado através de uma escarificação na pele.

screening t., teste de triagem; qualquer procedimento de teste projetado para separar pessoas ou objetos de acordo com uma determinada característica ou propriedade, com a intenção de detectar evidências precoces de doença.

Seashore t., teste de Seashore; teste em que o indivíduo deve discriminar entre dois sons, ou em que podem ser medidos o sentido de altura, intensidade, ritmo e outros componentes da habilidade musical inata. VER Halstead-Reitan *battery*.

secondary dye t., teste do corante secundário; localização de obstrução da drenagem lacrimal após instilação de fluoresceína e teste do corante primário por intubação através do ponto lacrimal inferior e canalículo e irrigação com solução salina. VER Jones II t.

secretin t., teste da secretina; prova de função pancreática exócrina, variavelmente realizada e padronizada, em que são determinados o bicarbonato, a amilase e o volume do aspirado duodenal após administração intravenosa de secretina.

Selivanoff t., teste de Selivanoff. SIN resorcinol t.

shadow t., teste de sombra. SIN retinoscopy.

shake t., teste de agitação. SIN foam stability t.

sickle cell t., teste da célula falciforme; numa preparação úmida anaeróbica contendo quantidades iguais de sangue e bissulfito de sódio a 2%, os eritrócitos que contêm hemoglobina S sofrem uma alteração de sua morfologia, assumindo a forma de célula em foice; determina-se o número de células falciformes por 1000 eritrócitos, sendo o resultado expresso em percentagem.

single (gel) diffusion precipitin t. in one dimension, teste de difusão (gel) simples de precipitina unidimensional. VER gel diffusion precipitin t.'s in one dimension.

single (gel) diffusion precipitin t. in two dimensions, teste de difusão (gel) simples de precipitina bidimensional. VER gel diffusion precipitin t.'s in two dimensions.

SISI t., teste de SISI; abreviatura de small increment sensitivity index t.

situational t., teste situacional; em psicologia e psiquiatria, uma situação de teste em que se observa um indivíduo enquanto ele executa uma tarefa ou um exemplo real da profissão ou do papel a ser desempenhado; por exemplo, teste utilizado para a seleção de pessoas para o Office of Strategic Services durante a Segunda Guerra Mundial e para cargos gerenciais hoje em dia.

skin t., teste cutâneo; método para determinar a sensibilidade induzida (alergia) através da aplicação de um antígeno (alérgeno) à pele ou sua inoculação na pele; a sensibilidade induzida (alergia) ao antígeno específico é indicada por uma reação inflamatória de dois tipos gerais: 1) imediata, que aparece dentro de poucos minutos e depende de imunoglobulinas circulantes (anticorpos); 2) tardia, que aparece dentro de 12-48 horas e não depende dessas substâncias solúveis, mas de uma resposta celular e da ocorrência de infiltração. SIN cutaneous t., intradermal t., skin reaction.

skin-puncture t., teste de punção da pele; teste para síndrome de Behçet; após punção da pele com agulha estéril, surge uma pustulação dentro de 24 horas, devido à sensibilidade dérmica nessa doença.

small increment sensitivity index t. (SISI t.), teste do índice de sensibilidade em pequenos incrementos (teste de SISI); o som de um tom 20 dB acima do limiar, seguido de uma série de tons de 200 ms 1 dB acima, cuja percepção indica lesão coclear; a percentagem de pequenos incrementos detectados pelo indivíduo é o índice de sensibilidade em pequenos incrementos. Na perda auditiva sensorial, apresenta-se elevado, e, na audição normal e na perda auditiva neural, apresenta-se baixo.

sniff t., teste de fungação; em fluoroscopia, prova de função diafragmática; o movimento paradoxal de um hemidiafragma quando o paciente funga vigorosamente revela paralisia do nervo frênico ou paresia do hemidiafragma.

Snyder t., teste de Snyder; prova colorimétrica para determinar a atividade de cáries dentárias ou suscetibilidade a elas, com base na taxa de produção de ácido por microrganismos orais acidogênicos (por exemplo, lactobacilos) em meio de glicose, utilizando verde bromocresol como indicador e produzindo uma mudança da cor verde para amarela. SIN colorimetric caries susceptibility t.

solubility t., teste de solubilidade; teste de triagem para hemoglobina falciforme (Hb S), que é reduzida pela ditionita e insolúvel em tampão inorgânico concentrado; a adição de sangue contendo Hb S ao tampão e à ditionita provoca opacidade da solução.

spironolactone t., teste da espironolactona; administração de espironolactona (400 mg por via oral) durante 4 dias consecutivos; a ocorrência de um aumento do potássio sérico durante o teste, seguido de redução, sugere fortemente aldosteronismo primário.

split renal function t., prova de função renal diferencial. SIN differential ureteral catheterization t.

spot t. for infectious mononucleosis, teste em lâmina amplamente utilizado para o diagnóstico de mononucleose infecciosa, baseado no princípio de que os anticorpos heterófilos que ocorrem no soro de pacientes com mononucleose infecciosa são absorvidos por hemácias de boi, mas não por células renais de cobaia; assim, quando hemácias de cavalo (que provocam anticorpos heterófilos) são misturadas com o soro do paciente e ocorre aglutinação na presença de hemácias bovinas, estabelece-se o diagnóstico presuntivo de mononucleose infecciosa.

Spurling t., teste de Spurling; avaliação de compressão de raiz nervosa cervical, em que o examinador estende o pescoço do paciente e faz uma rotação, com inclinação lateral da cabeça para o lado sintomático; a seguir, exerce uma força de compressão axial sobre a cabeça do paciente; o teste é considerado positivo quando a manobra produz a dor radicular típica no braço.

staggered spondaic word t., teste de palavras espondaicas escalonadas; teste de integridade da via auditiva central, em que são apresentadas palavras espondaicas dicoticamente.

standard serologic t.'s for syphilis, STS for syphilis, provas sorológicas padronizadas para sífilis; testes com antígeno não-treponêmico que fornecem evidências presuntivas, mas não conclusivas, de sífilis, incluindo as provas de Wassermann e VDRL.

standing t., teste ortostático; teste para o efeito de uma droga hipotensora, efetuado pelo paciente: após tomar o medicamento, o paciente deve permanecer totalmente imóvel durante 1 minuto a partir do momento em que a ação máxima do fármaco deve manifestar-se; se a dose for adequada, o paciente deve apresentar uma leve reação hipotensiva.

standing plasma t., teste do plasma em repouso; se o plasma for armazenado a 4°C em tubo de ensaio na posição vertical, os quilomicrons flutuarão na superfície, formando uma camada cremosa.

starch-iodine t., teste de amido-iodo; teste para sudorese, em que a pele é pintada com iodo em óleo, seguida de pulverização com pó de amido, que se torna negro-azulado na presença de iodo e de umidade.

station t., teste de posição. SIN Romberg sign.

Stein t., teste de Stein; em casos de doença do labirinto, o paciente é incapaz de permanecer em posição ortostática ou de saltar sobre um pé com os olhos fechados.

Stenger t., teste de Stenger; teste para detectar a simulação de comprometimento auditivo unilateral, em que um tom abaixo do limiar admitido é apresentado à orelha testada, enquanto um tom de menor intensidade é apresentado à outra orelha. Se o indivíduo estiver fingindo uma perda auditiva, o tom menor não pode ser percebido.

Stewart t., teste de Stewart; estimativa da quantidade de circulação colateral, em caso de aneurisma da artéria principal de um membro, através de um calorímetro.

Strassburg t., teste de Strassburg; teste obsoleto para bile na urina; a albumina, quando presente, é precipitada; a seguir, adiciona-se cana-de-açúcar, mergulha-se um papel de filtro no líquido e deixa-se secar; na presença de pigmentos biliares na urina, o ácido sulfúrico faz com que o papel de filtro adquira uma cor violeta avermelhada.

stress t., teste de estresse; qualquer procedimento padronizado para avaliar o efeito do estresse sobre a função cardíaca e a perfusão do miocárdio; o estresse pode ser induzido através de exercício físico ou simulado através da administração de vasodilatador coronário; a freqüência, a pressão arterial e o eletrocardiograma são monitorizados antes, no decorrer e depois da prova; outras observações algumas vezes efetuadas incluem: medida do consumo de oxigênio, ecocardiografia, cardiografia de impedância, avaliação da perfusão miocárdica e mobilidade da parede cardíaca por marcador radionuclídio e cateterismo cardíaco.

Embora não seja tão sensível nem tão específico quanto os procedimentos invasivos, o teste de esforço físico tornou-se uma maneira padronizada de identificar e graduar a coronariopatia em indivíduos com angina de peito típica e atípica, bem como naqueles que se dedicam a certas ocupações críticas (pilotos de aviação, bombeiros). Esse teste demonstrou ser útil para a estratificação do risco em sobreviventes de infarto do miocárdio (IM), bem como no planejamento e na monitorização da reabilitação após IM, cirurgia de derivação coronária ou angioplastia com balão. É também utilizado para avaliar a segurança de programas de exercícios para indivíduos que correm risco de coronariopatia, devido à idade ou a uma história pessoal ou familiar. O teste de dois degraus de Master, que consiste em subir e descer repetidamente um banco com degrau, foi suplantado por métodos mais aprimorados e reprodutíveis. O teste de esforço padrão emprega um esforço físico graduado numa esteira que funciona eletricamente, com inclinações e velocidades variáveis. Os métodos alternativos incluem uma máquina mecânica de subir escadas, uma bicicleta ergométrica estacionária e (para aqueles com certas incapacidades físicas) uma máquina para exercício do braço (manivela manual). São utilizados diversos protocolos e parâmetros finais para medir o resultado do teste de esforço. As cargas de trabalho são medidas em equivalentes metabólicos (MET), em que 1 MET é a quantidade de oxigênio consumida em repouso no leito (3,5 mL/kg/min). No teste de esforço máximo (limitado pela presença de sintomas), o indivíduo continua a prova em níveis crescentes de esforço até a ocorrência de desconforto torácico, hipertensão ou hipotensão significativa, determinadas arritmias, fadiga, problemas da marcha ou dispnéia intensa. O protocolo de Bruce, um protocolo padrão de exercício máximo em esteira, começa numa velocidade de 1,7 mph e grau de inclinação de 10°, para obter uma carga de trabalho de 4,6 MET, com aumentos tanto na velocidade quanto no grau de inclinação a cada 3 min. No teste de esforço submáximo (limitado pelo pulso), o indivíduo continua a prova até atingir uma determinada freqüência cardíaca baseada na idade, na história de saúde e no estado físico do indivíduo (a não ser que seja necessário interromper a prova mais cedo, devido ao aparecimento de sintomas). A duração do teste de esforço é habitualmente de 6-10 min. A ocorrência de elevação ou depressão de segmentos ST em mais de 1 mm durante o exercício é fortemente sugestiva de coronariopatia. Outras alterações sugestivas incluem inversão da onda T, arritmias, queda da pressão arterial sistólica e elevação pronunciada da pressão diastólica. Os protocolos do teste de esforço atingem uma acurácia de 85-90% na identificação de indivíduos sem coronariopatia. Cerca de 5% dos adultos assintomáticos apresentam testes positivos, porém apenas um terço deles apresenta coronariopatia demonstrável na angiografia. São obtidos testes falso-positivos mais freqüentemente nas mulheres. O teste do esforço está contra-indicado na presença de infarto agudo do miocárdio, insuficiência cardíaca congestiva grave, hipertensão grave, doença valvular ou arritmia hemodinamicamente significativa, doença tromboembólica ativa e obesidade extrema. Como alternativa ao teste de esforço, pode-se efetuar uma prova farmacológica mediante infusão intravenosa de dipiridamol ou dobutamina. Além da monitorização ECG contínua, os efeitos cardíacos do estresse ou da prova farmacológica podem ser avaliados através de cintilografia do miocárdio após injeção intravenosa de tálio-201; cineangiografia após a injeção de tecnécio-99m, com ou sem imageamento de coleção de sangue por aquisição de controle múltiplo (MUGA); ou tomografia computadorizada com emissão de fóton único (SPECT).

string t., teste da corda; (1) teste raramente utilizado para localização de hemorragia gastrintestinal; uma corda pesada é repetidamente deglutida e removida, permitindo, a cada vez, que a corda alcance maior distância no intestino, até encontrar a presença de sangue; (2) procedimento semelhante para obter uma amostra da luz intestinal.

Strong vocational interest t., teste de interesse vocacional de Strong; teste que compara as preferências, aversões e interesses específicos de um indivíduo com aqueles característicos de pessoas que trabalham em cada uma de várias vocações.

Student's t t., teste t de Student; teste de significação estatística para avaliar a diferença ou a igualdade de dois ou mais meios populacionais.

Stypven time t., teste do tempo de Stypven; teste que mede o tempo de coagulação do plasma após a adição de *veneno* da víbora de Russell, útil na avaliação de pacientes com deficiências de fator X. [Nome comercial *styp*tic + *ven*om]

sucrose hemolysis t., teste de hemólise da sacarose; a sacarose isotônica promove a ligação do complemento aos eritrócitos; na hemoglobinúria paroxística noturna, uma proporção das células mostra-se sensível à lise mediada pelo complemento, com conseqüente hemólise.

sulcus t., sinal do sulco; teste para instabilidade multidirecional do ombro; o úmero do paciente sentado é tracionado distalmente, e a mobilidade inferior indica um resultado positivo.

sulfosalicylic acid turbidity t., teste de turvação do ácido sulfossalicílico; teste para determinação da proteína na urina; o ácido sulfossalicílico precipita a proteína na urina, com turvação que é aproximadamente proporcional à concentração de proteína numa solução.

sweat t., teste do suor; teste para fibrose cística do pâncreas, em que os eletrólitos são medidos no suor coletado; uma concentração de cloreto de sódio superior a 50 mEq/L (crianças) ou a 60 mEq/L (adultos) é positiva.

sweating t., teste da sudorese; teste para localizar o nível de uma lesão na medula espinal; quando o corpo é aquecido ou se administra um diaforético ao paciente, a secreção de suor está ausente abaixo do nível da lesão.

swinging light t., teste da luz oscilante. SIN alternating light t.

t **t.,** teste *t*; teste que utiliza uma estatística que, sob a hipótese nula, tem a distribuição *t* para testar se dois meios diferem significativamente.

Tactual Performance T., teste de desempenho tactual. SIN Halstead-Reitan battery.

thematic apperception t. (TAT), teste de apercepção temática; teste psicológico projetivo em que se pede ao indivíduo para contar uma história sobre quadros ambíguos padronizados que ilustram situações da vida para revelar suas próprias atitudes e sentimentos.

thermostable opsonin t., teste da opsonina termoestável; teste para atividade opsônica de anticorpo na ausência de efeito do complemento termolábil.

Thompson t., teste de Thompson; **(1)** teste para detectar a ruptura do tendão do calcâneo; com o paciente ajoelhado numa cadeira e os pés pendentes, cada panturrilha é comprimida; se houver ruptura do tendão do calcâneo, não ocorrerá flexão plantar. **(2)** teste obsoleto para gonorréia na urina; a urina é colocada em dois copos; se forem encontrados gonococos e filamentos gonorréicos apenas no primeiro copo, a probabilidade é de que o processo esteja limitado à uretra anterior. SIN two-glass t.

Thormählen t., teste de Thormählen; teste para melanina; o líquido suspeito é tratado com nitroprussiato de sódio, potassa cáustica e ácido acético; na presença de melanina, a solução adquire uma cor azul-intensa.

Thorn t., teste de Thorn; prova suposta de função do córtex supra-renal; a estimulação de um córtex supra-renal com função normal pelo hormônio adrenocorticotrópico é seguida de redução no número de eosinófilos e linfócitos circulantes e aumento na excreção de ácido úrico. O teste carece de especificidade suficiente e raramente é utilizado.

three-glass t., teste dos três copos; a bexiga é esvaziada eliminando a urina numa série de três tubos de ensaio de 90 mL, e examina-se o conteúdo do primeiro e do último; o primeiro tubo contém os lavados da uretra anterior, o segundo, o material da bexiga, e o terceiro, o material da uretra posterior, próstata e vesículas seminais. SIN Valentine t.

thymol turbidity t., t. de turvação do timol; precipitação de proporções anormais de albumina e globulina do soro de pacientes com hepatopatia mediante adição de timol. Apesar de sua popularidade no passado, foi suplantado pela determinação quantitativa de proteínas específicas e determinação direta das enzimas hepáticas. SIN Maclagan t., Maclagan thymol turbidity t.

thyroid-stimulating hormone stimulation t., TSH-stimulating t., teste de estimulação do hormônio tireoestimulante, teste de estimulação do TSH; teste que mede a captação de I^{131} pela glândula tireóide antes e depois da administração de hormônio tireoestimulante; útil para diferenciar o hipertireoidismo primário (aumento das concentrações séricas de TSH) do hipertireoidismo secundário ou terciário (baixas concentrações séricas de TSH).

thyroid suppression t., teste de supressão da tireóide; prova de função tireóidea utilizada para o diagnóstico de casos difíceis de hipertireoidismo, agora substituída, em grande parte, pelo teste de estimulação com o hormônio de liberação da tireotropina; administra-se triiodotironina durante uma semana a 10 dias, e a resposta normal consiste numa redução de sua captação pela glândula tireóide para menos da metade da captação inicial. SIN Werner t.

thyrotropin-releasing hormone stimulation t., TRH-stimulation t., teste de estimulação com hormônio de liberação da tireotropina, teste de estimulação com TRH; teste da resposta hipofisária à injeção de hormônio de liberação da tireotropina, que normalmente estimula a secreção hipofisária de hormônio tireoestimulante (TSH, tireotropina), utilizado primariamente para diferenciar as causas hipofisárias das causas hipotalâmicas de distúrbios da tireóide; o TSH não aumenta em casos de disfunção hipofisária, mas exibe elevação em casos de distúrbios hipotalâmicos.

tilt t., teste de inclinação; qualquer medida da resposta durante a inclinação do corpo, geralmente com a cabeça para cima, mas também para baixo. O teste pode ser monitorado através de cateterismo, ecocardiografia, medidas eletrofisiológicas, eletrocardiografia ou mecanocardiografia.

tine t. VER tuberculin t.

titratable acidity t., teste de acidez titulável; o número de mililitros de NaOH 0,1 N necessários para neutralizar uma amostra de urina de 24 h.

tolbutamide t., teste da tolbutamida; teste para detectar tumores produtores de insulina; após uma dose intravenosa de 1 g de tolbutamida, são determinados os níveis plasmáticos de insulina e de glicose a intervalos de até 3 h; as respostas maiores da insulina e os valores mais baixos da glicose caracterizam pacientes com esses tumores.

tone decay t., teste de declínio do tom; o som de um tom contínuo no limiar durante 1 min; se for necessário aumentar a intensidade em mais de 5 dB para a percepção contínua, indica perda auditiva neural.

total catecholamine t., teste das catecolaminas totais; determinação das catecolaminas em amostras de urina de 24 horas; são observados valores elevados em pacientes com feocromocitoma e neuroblastoma.

tourniquet t., teste do torniquete. VER capillary fragility t.

TPHA t., teste de TPHA. SIN *Treponema pallidum* hemagglutination t.

TPI t., teste de TPI. SIN *Treponema pallidum* immobilization t.

Trendelenburg t., manobra de Trendelenburg; teste das válvulas das veias das pernas; a perna é elevada acima do nível do coração até esvaziamento das veias e, a seguir, rapidamente abaixada; na presença de varicosidade e incompetência das válvulas, as veias sofrem distensão imediata, porém a colocação de um torniquete ao redor da perna impede a distensão das veias abaixo dos perfuradores incompetentes ou válvulas abaixo do torniquete.

***Treponema pallidum* hemagglutination t.,** teste de hemaglutinação do *Treponema pallidum*; teste altamente sensível e específico para o diagnóstico sorológico da sífilis; hemácias taninizadas de carneiro são recobertas com o antígeno de *Treponema pallidum* e, após absorção de anticorpo sérico inespecífico do paciente, uma reação positiva com hemácias taninizadas de carneiro e o soro do paciente indica a presença de anticorpo específico contra *Treponema pallidum* no soro do paciente. SIN TPHA t.

***Treponema pallidum* immobilization t., TPI t.,** teste de imobilização do *Treponema pallidum*, teste de TPI; teste para sífilis em que um anticorpo diferente do anticorpo de Wassermann está presente no soro de um paciente sifilítico; na presença de complemento, causa a imobilização do *Treponema pallidum* ativamente móvel, obtido dos testículos de um coelho infectado por sífilis. SIN TPI t., *Treponema pallidum* immobilization reaction.

triiodothyronine uptake t., teste de captação da triiodotironina; prova de função tireóidea, em que se adiciona triiodotironina (T_3) ao soro do paciente *in vitro* para medir as afinidades relativas das proteínas séricas e de uma substância competitiva adicionada para T_3; as captações maiores de T_3 estão associadas ao hipertireoidismo. SIN T_3 uptake t.

tuberculin t., teste da tuberculina; aplicação do teste cutâneo ao diagnóstico da infecção por *Mycobacterium tuberculosis* em que a tuberculina ou seu derivado protéico "purificado" atua como antígeno (alérgeno); a injeção de doses graduadas de tuberculina ou de derivado protéico purificado na pele, mais freqüentemente através de agulha e seringa (teste de Mantoux) ou por meio de dentes (teste do dente); o material do teste também pode ser aplicado através de um "emplastro" no qual é absorvido, porém esse método (teste do emplastro) é considerado menos confiável; a leitura do teste é feita com base na ocorrência de induração e eritema, sendo a primeira considerada mais diagnóstica de infecção pelo bacilo da tuberculose (*M. tuberculosis*); o teste não distingue entre infecção numa pessoa resistente sem doença e num indivíduo com manifestações clínicas de doença.

T_3 uptake t., teste de captação de T_3. SIN triiodothyronine uptake t.

two-glass t., teste dos dois copos. SIN Thompson t.

two-step exercise t., teste do exercício de dois degraus; teste utilizado principalmente para insuficiência coronária; a depressão significativa do RST no eletrocardiograma é considerada anormal e sugere insuficiência coronária.

two-tail t., teste bicaudal; teste estatístico baseado na pressuposição de que os dados estão distribuídos em ambas as direções a partir de algum valor central.

Tzanck t., teste de Tzanck; exame do líquido de uma lesão bolhosa à procura de células de Tzanck (células epiteliais alteradas, redondas e desprovidas de fixações intercelulares). A periferia dessas células é basofílica, e o núcleo apresenta-se esférico e aumentado, com nucléolos proeminentes; são características de lesões produzidas por varicela, herpes zoster, herpes simples e pênfigo vulgar.

urea clearance t., teste de depuração da uréia; prova de função renal baseada na depuração da uréia.

urease t., teste da urease; **(1)** teste para uréia baseado na conversão da uréia em carbonato de amônio pela enzima urease; **(2)** teste para a produção de urease; utilizado na identificação de *cryptococci* e *Helicobacter pylori*.

urecholine supersensitivity t., teste de supersensibilidade à urecolina; teste urodinâmico que visa a produzir um cistometrograma anormal após a injeção subcutânea de uma droga, a urecolina. A urecolina pode aumentar a resposta de pressão do detrusor durante o enchimento em pacientes com alguns tipos de bexiga neuropática.

urinary concentration t., teste de concentração urinária; prova de função tubular renal em que o paciente é desidratado por um período definido de tempo, com determinação subseqüente da densidade da urina.

vaginal cornification t., teste de cornificação vaginal; teste para atividade estrogênica em que o aparecimento de células epiteliais cornificadas num esfregaço vaginal de um animal de teste fornece uma indicação da ação de um estrogênio.

vaginal mucification t., teste de mucificação vaginal; teste para atividade progestacional; estimulação da produção de muco pelo epitélio vaginal em fêmeas de ratos, cobaias ou camundongos por progestógenos.

Valentine t., teste de Valentine. SIN three-glass t.

Valsalva t., prova de Valsalva; o coração é monitorado por ECG, registro da pressão ou outros métodos, enquanto o paciente realiza a manobra de Valsalva; o coração torna-se menor nas pessoas normais, mas pode dilatar-se no paciente com comprometimento da reserva miocárdica; observa-se uma seqüência complexa característica de eventos cardiocirculatórios, cujo afastamento indica a existência de doença ou disfunção.

van Deen t., teste de van Deen. SIN Almén t. for blood.

van den Bergh t., teste de van den Bergh; teste para pigmentos biliares (bilirrubina) por meio de reação com ácido sulfanílico diazotizado (reação diazo).

van der Velden t., teste de van der Velden; teste para ácido clorídrico livre, cuja presença faz com que uma solução adicionada de azul-de-metileno violeta se torne violeta.

vanillylmandelic acid t., teste do ácido vanililmandélico; teste para tumores secretores de catecolaminas (feocromocitoma e neuroblastoma) efetuado numa amostra de urina de 24 horas; baseia-se no fato de o ácido vanililmandélico ser o principal metabólito urinário da norepinefrina e da epinefrina. SIN 3-methoxy-4-hydroxymandelic acid t., VMA t.

VDRL t, teste VDRL; teste de floculação para sífilis que utiliza o antígeno cardiolipina-lecitina-colesterol desenvolvido pelo Venereal Disease Research Laboratory do United States Public Health Service.

vitality t., teste de vitalidade; grupo de testes térmicos e elétricos utilizados para ajudar a avaliação da saúde da polpa dentária. SIN pulp t.

vitamin C t., teste da vitamina C. SIN capillary fragility t.

VMA t., teste do VMA. SIN vanillylmandelic acid t.

Volhard t., teste de Volhard; prova de função renal; o paciente ingere 1500 mL de água com o estômago vazio. Se o paciente não foi desidratado anteriormente e os rins estão normais, esse líquido deverá ser excretado ao final de 4 horas, com densidade da urina de 1,001 a 1,004.

Vollmer t., teste de Vollmer; teste tuberculínico com emplastro.

Wada t., teste de Wada; injeção de amobarbital unilateral na carótida interna para determinar a lateralidade da fala; a injeção no lado dominante provoca afasia ou mutismo transitório; utilizado antes do tratamento cirúrgico da epilepsia.

Waldenström t., teste de Waldenström; teste para porfobilinogênio ou urobilinogênio na urina que utiliza o reagente aldeído de Ehrlich para produzir uma cor vermelha se uma das duas substâncias estiver presente na urina.

Wang t., teste de Wang; teste quantitativo para indican, que é transformado em índigo-ácido sulfúrico e, a seguir, titulado por uma solução de permanganato de potássio.

washout t., teste de *washout*; meio de estimar a obstrução renal pela velocidade de desaparecimento de material radioativo excretado do rim.

Wassermann t., reação de Wassermann; teste de fixação do complemento utilizado no diagnóstico da sífilis; originalmente, o "antígeno" era um extrato hepático de um feto sifilítico; todavia, posteriormente, foi constatada a presença da substância ativa, denominada cardiolipina, em tecidos normais, incluindo o coração, que foi identificada como difosfatidilglicerol. SIN Wassermann reaction.

water-drinking t., teste da ingestão de água; teste para avaliação do glaucoma de ângulo aberto, que mede a pressão intra-ocular após a ingestão de 0,95 L de água em 5 min.

Watson-Schwartz t., teste de Watson-Schwartz; teste de triagem qualitativo para o diagnóstico de porfiria intermitente aguda pela adição do reagente de Ehrlich e acetato de sódio saturado a uma amostra de urina; a observação de uma cor rosada ou vermelha indica a presença de porfobilinogênio ou urobilinogênio; o primeiro indica a porfiria, mas não o segundo; por conseguinte, os resultados positivos exigem extração diferencial posterior com butanol e clorofórmio para eliminar os resultados falso-positivos devido ao urobilinogênio.

Weber t. for hearing, teste de Weber para audição; a aplicação de um diapasão posto em vibração a um de vários pontos na linha mediana da cabeça ou da face para determinar em que orelha o som é ouvido por condução óssea, sendo essa orelha afetada se o mecanismo de condução do som da orelha média estiver com algum problema, porém normal se houver perda auditiva neurossensorial na outra orelha.

Webster t., teste de Webster; teste para trinitrotolueno na urina.

Weil-Felix t., teste de Weil-Felix; teste para a presença e o tipo de riquetsiose, com base na aglutinação de cepas X de *Proteus vulgaris* com riquétsias suspeitas no soro de um paciente. SIN Weil-Felix reaction.

Werner t., teste de Werner. SIN thyroid suppression t.

Wheeler-Johnson t., teste de Wheeler-Johnson; a citosina ou o uracil, quando tratados com bromo, produzem ácido dialúrico, que produz uma cor verde na presença de excesso de hidróxido de bário.

whiff t., teste de exalação; teste para o odor de peixe detectável quando se aplica KOH a uma amostra de corrimento vaginal em caso de vaginose bacteriana.

Whitaker t., teste de Whitaker; teste de pressão-perfusão nas vias urinárias superiores para determinar um impedimento do fluxo.

Wormley t., teste de Wormley; teste para alcalóides, que consiste em tratar a solução com ácido pícrico e uma solução diluída de iodo-potássio-iodeto, sendo a presença de alcalóides demonstrada por uma reação colorimétrica.

Wurster t., teste de Wurster; teste obsoleto para tirosina; a substância é dissolvida em água fervente e adiciona-se quinona; na presença de tirosina, ocorre uma reação de cor rubi, passando a solução para uma cor marrom depois de algumas horas.

χ^2 t., teste χ^2. SIN chi-square t.

xylose t., teste da xilose; auxílio laboratorial no diagnóstico da pentosúria alimentar ou essencial, condições nas quais ocorre excreção de xilose (pentose); a xilose pode ser identificada pela rápida redução da solução de Benedict, por não-fermentação por leveduras ou por um teste de Bial positivo para pentose.

Yvon t., teste de Yvon; **(1)** para alcalóides; adiciona-se à solução suspeita uma mistura de subnitrato de bismuto, iodeto de potássio e ácido clorídrico em água; uma reação positiva é indicada pelo aparecimento de uma cor vermelha; **(2)** para acetanilida na urina; o líquido suspeito é extraído com clorofórmio e aquecido com nitrato amarelo de mercúrio; na presença de acetanilida, o líquido torna-se verde.

Zimmermann t., teste de Zimmermann. SIN Zimmermann reaction.

Zsigmondy t., teste de Zsigmondy. SIN Lange t.

tes·ta (tes′tā). Testa, concha, carapaça. **1.** Em protozoologia, denominada testa; envoltório de determinadas formas de protozoários amebóides que consiste em vários materiais terrosos unidos a uma base quitinosa (como nos risópodes da subclasse Testacealobosia) ou os esqueletos calcários, silicosos, orgânicos ou de sulfato de estrôncio na subclasse dos risópodes Foraminifera. **2.** Em botânica, o revestimento externo, algumas vezes o único, de uma semente. [L. concha, casca]

Tes·ta·ce·a·lo·bo·sia (tes-tā′shē-ā-lō-bō′zē-ā). Subclasse do subfilo Sarcodina (amebas), cujas células possuem um envoltório quitinoso firme, contendo freqüentemente material terroso, com uma abertura através da qual se projetam os pseudópodes. [L. *testa*, concha, casca]

tes·tal·gia (tes-tal′jē-ā). Testalgia. SIN orchialgia. [testis + G. *algos*, dor]

test·cross (test′kros). Cruzamento de um genótipo desconhecido com um homozigoto recessivo, de modo que o fenótipo da progênie corresponde diretamente aos cromossomas transportados pelos genitores de genótipo desconhecido. SIN backcross (2).

tes·tec·to·my (tes-tek′tō-mē). Testectomia. SIN orchiectomy. [testis + G. *ektomē*, excisão]

tes·tes (tes′tēz). Testículos. Plural de testis. [L.]

tes·ti·cle (tes′tĭ-kl). Testículo. SIN testis. [L. *testiculus*, dim. de *testis*]

tes·tic·u·lar (tes-tik′ū-lăr). Testicular. Relativo aos testículos.

tes·tic·u·lus (tes-tik′ū-lŭs). Testículo. SIN testis. [L.]

test·ing. Teste, análise. VER test.

bench t., teste de um dispositivo contra especificações num ambiente simulado (não-vivo).

contrast sensitivity t., teste de sensibilidade a contrastes; exame do reconhecimento visual da variação na luminosidade de um objeto.

genetic t., análise genética; estudos laboratoriais do sangue ou de outros tecidos humanos com o propósito de identificar distúrbios genéticos. As anormalidades cromossômicas relativamente grandes, como deleção ou transposição, são identificadas através do exame microscópico dos cromossomas de uma célula em mitose (cariotipagem). As aberrações mais sutis podem ser detectadas por sondas de DNA (extensões fabricadas de DNA de filamento simples, que correspondem a partes do gene conhecido). A análise genética em seu sentido mais amplo inclui testes bioquímicos para substâncias anormais ou concentrações anormalmente altas ou baixas de substâncias normais, que atuam como marcadores de deficiência ou anormalidade genética. SIN DNA diagnostics.

A análise genética tornou-se um procedimento padronizado em diversas situações: triagem para doenças genéticas, como hemocromatose, triagem para casais que planejam ter filhos quanto ao estado de portador da fibrose cística e triagem de mutações genéticas que reconhecidamente aumentam o risco de determinados cânceres, como retinoblastoma e câncer de mama de início precoce. Além disso, o perfil genético ("impressão genética") pode estabelecer ou excluir a identidade de origem de duas amostras de material humano ou o parentesco entre duas pessoas, com probabilidade de 99,9%. A disponibilidade de testes para estabelecer o diagnóstico ou antecipar distúrbios sem tratamento, como a coréia de Huntington, bem como para identificar indivíduos com risco aumentado de doença maligna, levantou muitas questões sociais, psicológicas, terapêuticas e legais. As autoridades recomendam que as pessoas que pretendem submeter-se a análise genética recebam antes um aconselhamento acerca das implicações dos resultados positivos ou negativos dos testes. Os leigos freqüentemente interpretam erroneamente o conceito de predisposição ou risco, particularmente no que concerne aos oncogenes. O desenvolvimento de câncer, na maioria dos casos, decorre de mutação genética espontânea no indivíduo, e não de qualquer risco aumentado, e, entre os que herdam o risco, nem todos desenvolvem câncer. A descoberta de que certas populações, como judeus asquenaze, mórmons e amish, apresentam uma incidência muito maior de determinados distúrbios genéticos ameaçou reativar ou reforçar preconceitos étnicos, raciais e religiosos. Os grupos sociais que têm maior tendência a abrigar mutações genéticas facilmente identificadas são, por definição, aqueles cujas composições de genes são mais distintas, em virtude de sua tendência a unir-se por casamento, mais do que a misturar-se com outras populações. Os 1,3% de judeus asquenaze que compartilham uma mutação no gene supressor tumoral BRCA2 podem ser todos descendentes de uma única pessoa (efeito fundador). A possibilidade de identificar a predisposição genética de uma pessoa a doenças graves, crônicas ou incapacitantes enseja a possibilidade de discriminação por empregadores e seguradoras de saúde, vida e invalidez. Os governos estaduais e o governo federal dos Estados Unidos estabeleceram regras que limitam o acesso de empregadores e seguradoras, efetivos e potenciais, ao perfil genético de uma pessoa e que proíbem qualquer estigmatização, discriminação profissional e recusa a fornecer seguros ou assegurar de acordo com os padrões, devido ao perfil genético.

histocompatibility t., prova de histocompatibilidade; sistema de provas para antígenos HLA de suma importância no transplante.

proficiency t., teste de proficiência; programa em que amostras de material para controle da qualidade são periodicamente enviadas a membros de um grupo de laboratórios para análise, sendo os resultados de cada laboratório comparados com os dos outros laboratórios. VER TAMBÉM proficiency *samples,* em *sample.*

reality t., teste de realidade; em psiquiatria e psicologia, a função do ego pela qual o mundo objetivo ou real e a relação subjetivamente percebida do indivíduo com este mundo são avaliadas e apreciadas; a capacidade de distinguir eventos internos dos externos.

susceptibility t., teste de sensibilidade; determinação da capacidade de um antibiótico de matar ou inibir o crescimento das bactérias.

tes·tis, pl. **tes·tes** (tes'tis, -tēz) [TA]. Testículo. Uma das duas glândulas reprodutivas masculinas, localizadas na cavidade do escroto. VER TAMBÉM *appendix* testis. SIN didymus, genital gland (1), male gonad, orchis, testicle, testiculus. [L.]

abdominal t., s. abdominal; testículo não-descido que nunca desceu de sua origem retroperitoneal/abdominal através do anel inguinal interno.

cryptorchid t., t. criptorquídico. SIN undescended t.

ectopic t., t. ectópico; variante de testículo não-descido, em que a posição testicular está fora da via normal de descida. VER TAMBÉM testis *ectopia.*

movable t., t. móvel. SIN retractile t.

peeping t., testículo não-descido que migra para trás e para a frente num anel inguinal interno.

retractile t., t. retrátil; condição em que existe uma tendência do testículo a ascender até a parte superior do escroto ou ao canal inguinal, em contraste com o testículo não-descido. SIN movable t., pseudocryptorchism.

undescended t., t. não-descido; testículo que não desceu do escroto; existem variantes palpáveis e não-palpáveis. SIN cryptorchid t.

tes·ti·tis (tes-tī'tis). Testite. SIN orchitis.

test let·ter. Letra de teste. VER test types.

tes·toid (tes'toyd). Testóide. **1.** SIN androgenic. **2.** SIN androgen. [testis + G. *eidos,* semelhança]

tes·to·lac·tone (tes-tō-lak'tōn). Testolactona. Agente androgênico utilizado como agente antineoplásico no tratamento do carcinoma de mama.

tes·tos·ter·one (tes-tos'tĕ-rōn). Testosterona. O mais potente androgênio de ocorrência natural, formado em maiores quantidades pelas células intersticiais dos testículos e possivelmente secretado também pelo ovário e pelo córtex supra-renal; pode ser produzido em tecidos não-glandulares a partir de precursores, como a androstenediona; utilizada no tratamento do hipogonadismo, do criptorquidismo, de determinados carcinomas e da menorragia.

t. cypionate, cipionato de t.; preparação com as mesmas ações e usos que o propionato de testosterona, porém com duração de ação prolongada.

t. enanthate, enantato de t.; preparação com as mesmas ações e usos que a testosterona, porém de duração de ação prolongada, sendo administrado em óleo.

t. phenylpropionate, fenilpropionato de t.; preparação alternativa para o propionato.

t. propionate, propionato de t.; preparação que possui ação semelhante, porém mais acentuada e prolongada que a da testosterona; utilizado no tratamento dos testículos não-descidos e na menorragia.

tes·to·tox·i·co·sis (tes'tō-toks-ē-kō'sis). Testotoxicose. Doença por mutação da proteína G, resultando em superprodução autônoma de testosterona, com puberdade precoce.

test sym·bols. Símbolos de teste. VER test types.

test types. Optótipos. Letras de vários tamanhos, utilizadas para testar a acuidade visual.

Jaeger t. t., o. de Jaeger; tipos de diferentes tamanhos utilizados para testar a acuidade da visão para perto.

point system t. t., o. de sistema de pontos; um cartão de teste de visão para perto, em que os vários optótipos são múltiplos de um ponto (1/72 polegada), sendo as letras minúsculas metade do tamanho do ponto designado; a leitura de 4 pontos a 40,5 cm é normal e designada N-4.

Snellen t. t., o. de Snellen; símbolos quadrados pretos empregados no teste de acuidade da visão a distância; o tamanho das letras varia de tal modo que cada uma subtende o ângulo visual de 5′ a determinada distância.

tetan-. Tetan-. VER tetano-.

te·tan·ic (te-tan'ik). Tetânico. Relativo a ou caracterizado por contração muscular mantida, como no tétano. [G. *tetanikos*]

te·tan·i·form (te-tan'i-fōrm). Tetaniforme. SIN tetanoid (1).

tet·a·nig·e·nous (tet-ă-nij'ĕ-nŭs). Tetanígeno. Que causa tétano ou espasmos tetaniformes. [tetanus + G. *-gen,* que produz]

tet·a·nism (tet'ă-nizm). Tetanismo. SIN neonatal *tetany.*

tet·a·ni·za·tion (tet'ă-ni-zā'shŭn). Tetanização. **1.** O ato de tetanizar os músculos. **2.** Condição de espasmo tetaniforme.

tet·a·nize (tet'ă-nīz). Tetanizar. Estimular o músculo por uma rápida série de estímulos, de modo que as respostas musculares (contrações) individuais são fundidas numa contração contínua; causa tétano (2) num músculo.

tetano-, tetan-. Tetano-, tetan-. Formas combinantes que significam tétano, tetania. [G. *tetanos,* tensão convulsiva]

tet·a·noid (tet'ă-noyd). Tetanóide. **1.** Semelhante a ou da natureza do tétano. SIN tetaniform. **2.** Semelhante à tetania. [tetano- + G. *eidos,* semelhança]

tet·a·no·ly·sin (tet-ă-nol'i-sin). Tetanolisina. Princípio hemolítico, elaborado por *Clostridium tetani,* que parece não desempenhar nenhum papel na etiologia do tétano.

tet·a·nom·e·ter (tet-ă-nom'ĕ-ter). Tetanômetro. Instrumento para medir a força de espasmos musculares tônicos. [tetano- + G. *metron,* medida]

tet·a·no·mo·tor ((tet'ă-nō-mō'ter). Tetanomotor. Instrumento por meio do qual são produzidos espasmos tônicos através da irritação mecânica de um martelo que golpeia o nervo motor do músculo afetado. [tetano- + L. *motor,* motor]

tet·a·no·spas·min (tet'ă-nō-spaz'min). Tetanospasmina. A neurotoxina do *Clostridium tetani,* que causa os sinais e sintomas característicos do tétano; a principal ação é observada nas células do corno anterior, e os espasmos parecem ser devidos à sua ação em sinapses inibitórias.

tet·a·no·tox·in (tet'ă-nō-tok'sin). Tetanotoxina. SIN tetanus *toxin.* [tetano- + G. *toxikon,* veneno]

tet·a·nus (tet'ă-nŭs). Tétano. **1.** Doença caracterizada por contrações musculares tônicas dolorosas, causada pela toxina neurotrópica (tetanospasmina) do *Clostridium tetani,* que atua sobre o sistema nervoso central. Cf. lockjaw, trismus. **2.** Contração muscular contínua causada por uma série de estímulos nervosos repetidos tão rapidamente que as respostas musculares individuais são fundidas, produzindo uma contração tetânica contínua. VER emprosthotonos, opisthotonos. [L. do G. *tetanos,* tensão convulsiva]

acoustic t., t. acústico; tétano experimental induzido por uma corrente farádica, cuja velocidade é estimada pelo tom das vibrações.

cephalic t., t. cefálico; tipo de tétano local que ocorre após feridas da face e da cabeça; depois de um breve período de incubação (1-2 dias), os músculos faciais e oculares sofrem paresia, mas apresentam espasmos tetânicos repetidos. Os músculos da garganta e da língua também podem ser afetados. SIN cerebral t.

cerebral t., t. cerebral. SIN cephalic t.

complete t., t. completo; tétano em que estímulos para um determinado músculo são repetidos tão rapidamente que não se pode detectar uma redução de tensão entre os estímulos.

drug t., t. medicamentoso; espasmos tônicos causados por estricnina ou outro tetânico. SIN toxic t.

generalized t., t. generalizado; o tipo mais comum de tétano, freqüentemente com trismo como manifestação inicial; os músculos da cabeça, do pescoço, do tronco e dos membros tornam-se persistentemente contraídos, com superposição de contrações tônicas paroxísticas dolorosas (convulsões tetânicas); a elevada taxa de mortalidade (50%) é devida a asfixia ou insuficiência cardíaca.

incomplete t., t. incompleto; tétano (2) em que cada estímulo provoca uma contração iniciada quando o músculo sofreu apenas relaxamento parcial da contração anterior.

local t., t. local; o tipo mais benigno de tétano; os músculos em estreita proximidade de uma ferida infectada desenvolvem contrações involuntárias persistentes, freqüentemente com espasmos superpostos intensos e transitórios desencadeados por diversos estímulos. Os músculos mais distais dos membros superiores são mais freqüentemente afetados; é típica uma recuperação gradual, porém completa.

neonatal t., t. neonatal. SIN t. neonatorum.

t. neonatorum, t. neonatal; tétano que ocorre em recém-nascidos, geralmente devido à infecção da área umbilical por *Clostridium tetani,* freqüentemente como resultado de práticas ritualistas; possui elevada taxa de mortalidade (cerca de 60%). SIN neonatal t.

postpartum t., t. pós-parto. SIN puerperal t.

puerperal t., t. puerperal; tétano que ocorre durante o puerpério em conseqüência de infecção da ferida obstétrica. SIN postpartum t., uterine t.

Ritter opening t., t. da abertura de Ritter; contração tetânica que ocorre em certas ocasiões quando uma corrente intensa, atravessando uma longa extensão de nervo, é subitamente interrompida.

toxic t., t. tóxico. SIN drug t.

traumatic t., t. traumático; tétano que ocorre após infecção de ferida.

uterine t., t. uterino. SIN puerperal t.

tet·a·ny (tet′ă-nē). Tetania. Síndrome neurológica clínica caracterizada por contrações musculares, cãibras e espasmos carpopedais e, quando grave, laringoespasmo e convulsões; esses achados refletem a irritabilidade dos sistemas nervosos central e periférico, habitualmente devido a baixos níveis séricos de cálcio ionizado ou, menos comumente, magnésio. As causas incluem hiperventilação, hipoparatireoidismo, raquitismo e uremia. SIN intermittent cramp. [G. *tetanos,* tétano]

t. of alkalosis, t. da alcalose; tetania em decorrência de perda de ácido do organismo ou de um aumento de álcalis, resultando em diminuição do cálcio ionizado no plasma e nos líquidos orgânicos, por exemplo, tetania da hiperventilação (perda de CO_2), tetania gástrica (perda de HCl por vômitos) ou injeção ou ingestão de quantidades excessivas de bicarbonato de sódio.

gastric t., t. gástrica; tetania associada a um distúrbio gástrico, especialmente com perda de HCl por vômitos.

hyperventilation t., t. da hiperventilação; tetania causada por respiração forçada, devido à uma redução do CO_2 no sangue.

hypoparathyroid t., t. hipoparatireóidea. SIN parathyroid t.

infantile t., t. infantil; tetania de lactentes que ocorre habitualmente em associação ao raquitismo, devido a uma deficiência dietética de vitamina D.

manifest t., t. manifesta; tetania de qualquer causa, em que a hiperexcitabilidade neuromuscular está claramente evidente, ao contrário da tetania latente. SIN symptomatic t.

neonatal t., t. neonatal; tetania hipocalcêmica que ocorre em neonatos ou lactentes de pouca idade, devido ao hipoparatireoidismo funcional transitório no consumo de leite de vaca (elevado conteúdo de fósforo). SIN myotonia neonatorum, tetanism.

parathyroid t., t. paratireóidea; tetania devido à ausência de função paratireóidea, espontânea ou após excisão das glândulas paratireóides. SIN hypoparathyroid t., parathyprival t.

parathyroprival t., t. paratireopriva. SIN parathyroid t.

phosphate t., t. por fosfato; tetania causada pela ingestão de um excesso de fosfatos alcalinos (Na_2HPO_4 ou K_2HPO_4); mais comumente produzida de forma experimental em animais através da injeção de fosfato alcalino, que reduz o cálcio ionizado do sangue.

postoperative t., t. pós-operatória; tetania paratireóidea causada por lesão ou excisão das paratireóides durante procedimentos no pescoço.

symptomatic t., t. sintomática. SIN manifest t.

tetra-. Tetra-. Quatro. [G. *tetra-,* quatro]

tet·ra·a·me·lia (tet′ră-ă-mē′lē-ă). Tetramelia; ausência dos membros superiores e inferiores. [tetra- + G. *a-* priv. + *melos,* membro]

tet·ra·ba·sic (tet-ră-bā′sik). Tetrabásico; designa um ácido com quatro grupos ácidos e, portanto, capaz de neutralizar 4 Eq de base.

tet·ra·ben·a·zine (tet′ră-ben′ă-zen). Tetrabenazina; antigamente utilizada como tranqüilizante; assemelha-se à reserpina em suas ações, porém com duração mais curta dos efeitos.

tet·ra·bo·ric ac·id (tet′ră-bōr′ik). Ácido tetrabórico; ácido perbórico ou pirobórico. SIN pyroboric acid.

tet·ra·bra·chi·us (tet′ră-brā′kē-ŭs). Tetrabráquio; indivíduo com quatro braços. [tetra- + G. *brachion,* braço]

tet·ra·bro·mo·phe·nol·phthal·ein so·di·um (tet′ră-brō′mō-fē′nol-thal′ēn, -ē-in). Tetrabromofenolftaleína sódica; o sal sódico de um corante de bromoteo; antigamente utilizado no desenvolvimento da colecistografia.

tet·ra·caine hy·dro·chlo·ride (tet′ră-kān). Cloridrato de tetracaína; anestésico local altamente potente utilizado para raquianestesia, bloqueio nervoso e anestesia tópica.

tet·ra·chi·rus (tet′ră-kī′rŭs). Tetráquiro; indivíduo com quatro mãos. [tetra- + G. *cheir,* mão]

tet·ra·chlor·eth·y·lene (tet′ră-klōr-eth′i-lēn). Tetracloroetileno; anti-helmíntico contra ancilóstomos e outros nematódeos. SIN carbon dichloride, ethylene tetrachloride, tetrachloroethylene.

tet·ra·chlor·me·thi·a·zide (tet′ră-klōr-me-thī′ă-zīd). Tetraclormetiazida; diurético do tipo tiazídico. SIN teclothiazide.

tet·ra·chlo·ro·eth·ane (tet′ră-klōr-ō-eth′an). Tetracloroetano. Tetracloreto de acetileno; solvente não-inflamável para gorduras, óleos, ceras, resinas etc.; utilizado na fabricação de removedores de tintas e vernizes, filmes fotográficos, lacas e inseticidas. Sua toxicidade é maior que a do clorofórmio e do tetracloreto de carbono, produzindo narcose, lesão hepática, lesão renal e gastroenterite. SIN cellon.

tet·ra·chlo·ro·eth·yl·ene (tet′ră-klōr-ō-eth′i-lēn). Tetracloroetileno. SIN tetrachlorethylene.

tet·ra·chlo·ro·meth·ane (tet′ră-klōr-ō-meth′an). Tetraclorometano. SIN carbon tetrachloride.

tet·ra·coc·cus, pl. **tet·ra·coc·ci** (tet′ră-kok′ŭs, -kok′sī). Tetracoco; termo antigo para descrever uma bactéria esférica que se divide em dois planos e tipicamente forma grupos de quatro células. [tetra- + G. *kokkos,* baga]

tet·ra·co·sac·tide, tet·ra·co·sac·tin (tet′ră-kō-sak′tid, -tin). Tetracosactida, tetracosactina. SIN cosyntropin.

n-tet·ra·co·sa·no·ic ac·id (tet′ră-kō-să-nō′ik). Ácido *n*-tetracosanóico. SIN lignoceric acid.

tet·ra·crot·ic (tet′ră-krot′ik). Tetracrótico; designa uma curva de pulso com quatro ascensões no ciclo. [tetra- + G. *krotos,* golpe]

tet·ra·cus·pid (tet-ră-kŭs′pid). Tetracúspide; que possui quatro cúspides. SIN quadricuspid.

tet·ra·cy·cline (tet-ră-sī′klen, -klin). Tetraciclina; antibiótico de amplo espectro (derivado do naftaceno) que dá origem à oxitetraciclina, preparado a partir da clortetraciclina e também obtido a partir do filtrado de culturas de várias espécies de *Streptomyces;* também disponível como complexo de cloridrato de tetraciclina e fosfato de tetraciclina. A fluorescência da tetraciclina foi utilizada em estudos de tumores em crescimento e deposição de cálcio nos ossos e dentes em desenvolvimento.

tet·rad (tet′rod). Tétrade. **1.** Conjunto de quatro coisas que possuem algo em comum, como uma deformidade combinada com quatro características, como, por exemplo, tetralogia de Fallot. SIN tetralogy. **2.** Em química, elemento quadrivalente. **3.** Em hereditariedade, um cromossoma bivalente que se divide em quatro cromátides durante a meiose. [G. *tetras* (tetrad-), o número quatro]

Fallot t., t. de Fallot. SIN tetralogy of Fallot.

narcoleptic t., t. narcoléptica; síndrome clínica de narcolepsia, cataplexia, paralisia do sono e alucinações hipnagógicas.

tet·ra·dac·tyl (tet-ră-dak′til). Tetradáctilo; que possui apenas quatro dedos em uma das mãos ou dos pés. SIN quadridigitate. [tetra- + G. *daktylos,* dedo da mão ou do pé]

tet·ra·dec·a·no·ic ac·id (tet′ră-dek-ă-nō′ik). Ácido tetradecanóico. SIN myristic acid.

12-*O***-tet·ra·dec·a·no·yl·phor·bol 13-ac·e·tate (TPA, tPA)** (tet′ră-dek′ă-nō-il-fōr′bol). 13-acetato de 12-*O*-tetradecanoilforbol; éster duplo de forbol encontrado no óleo de cróton; co-carcinógeno ou promotor de tumor.

te·trad·ic (te-trad′ik). Tetrádico; relativo a uma tétrade.

tet·ra·eth·yl·am·mo·ni·um chlo·ride (tet-ră-eth′il-ă-mō′nē-ŭm). Cloreto de tetraetilamônio; composto de amônio quaternário que bloqueia parcialmente a transmissão de impulsos através dos gânglios simpáticos e parassimpáticos; utilizado em estudos farmacológicos para bloquear a transmissão ganglionar, porém de utilidade clínica limitada; antigamente utilizado como agente anti-hipertensivo.

tet·ra·eth·yl·lead (tet′ră-eth′i-led). Chumbo tetraetila; composto antidetonante adicionado ao combustível de motores; possui ação tóxica, causando anorexia, náusea, vômitos, diarréia, tremores, fraqueza muscular, insônia, irritabilidade, nervosismo e ansiedade; pode ocorrer morte. SIN lead tetraethyl.

tet·ra·eth·yl·mon·o·thi·o·no·py·ro·phos·phate (ter-ră-eth′il-mon-ō-thī′ō-nō-pī-rō-fos′fat). Tetraetilmonotionopirofosfato; agente anticolinesterásico utilizado no tratamento do glaucoma mediante instilação local no olho.

tet·ra·eth·yl py·ro·phos·phate (TEPP) (tet′ră-eth′il). Tetraetil pirofosfato; composto fosfórico orgânico utilizado como inseticida; potente inibidor irreversível da colinesterase.

tet·ra·eth·yl·thi·u·ram di·sul·fide (ter′ră-eth-il-thī′u-ram). Dissulfeto de tetraetiltiuram. SIN disulfiram.

tet·ra·gas·trin (tet-ră-gas′trin). Tetragastrina. **1.** Tetrapeptídio (Trp-Met-Asp-Phe-NH_2) utilizado para avaliar a secreção de suco digestivo. **2.** Derivado da pterina, um co-fator necessário para diversas enzimas; por exemplo, na conversão da L-fenilalanina em L-tirosina; a incapacidade de sintetizar tetraidrobiopterina está associada a formas de hiperfenilalaninemia maligna.

tet·ra·gly·cine hy·dro·per·i·o·dine (tet-ră-glī′sēn). Hidroperiodeto de tetraglicina. Dissolve-se em água até a proporção de 380 g/L; utilizado para desinfecção de emergência da água potável em quantidades para produzir 8 ppm de iodo ativo.

tet·ra·gon, tet·ra·go·num (tet′ră-gon, tet′ră-gō′nŭm). Tetrágono. Quadrilátero; figura que possui quatro lados. [tetra- + G. *gonia,* ângulo]

t. lumba′le, t. lombar; espaço quadrangular limitado lateralmente pelo músculo oblíquo externo do abdome, medialmente pelo eretor da espinha, acima pelo serrátil posterior inferior e abaixo pelo oblíquo interno do abdome.

tet·ra·go·nus (tet′rã - gō′nŭs). Tetrágono; termo obsoleto para platisma. [*músculo*]

tet·ra·hy·dric (tet - rã - hī′drik). Tetraídrico; designa um composto que contém quatro átomos de hidrogênio ionizáveis (quatro grupos ácidos).

♲ **tetrahydro-.** Tetraidro-. Prefixo que designa a fixação de quatro átomos de hidrogênio; p. ex., tetraidrofolato (H_4 folato).

tet·ra·hy·dro·can·nab·i·nol (THC) (tet′rã - hī′drō - kã - nab′i - nol). Tetraidrocanabinol; o isômero Δ^1-3,4-*trans* e o isômero Δ^6-3-4-*trans* que se acredita sejam os isômeros ativos presentes na *Cannabis*, isolados da maconha. VER TAMBÉM cannabis, dronabinol.

5,6,7,8-tet·ra·hy·dro·fo·late de·hy·dro·gen·ase (tet′rã - hī - drō - fō′lāt). 5,6,7,8-tetraidrofolato desidrogenase. SIN dihydrofolate reductase.

tet·ra·hy·dro·fo·late meth·yl·trans·fer·ase (tet′rã - hī - drō - fōl′āt). Tetraidrofolato metiltransferase. SIN methionine synthase.

tet·ra·hy·dro·fo·lic ac·id (FH_4) (tet′rã - hī - drō - fōl′ik). Ácido tetraidrofólico; a forma coenzimática ativa do ácido fólico; participa no metabolismo de um carbono. SIN coenzyme F.

tet·ra·hy·droz·o·line hy·dro·chlo·ride (tet - rã - hī - droz′ō - lēn). Cloridrato de tetraidrozolina; agente simpatomimético relacionado à efedrina, utilizado como descongestionante tópico nasal e conjuntival; o seu uso excessivo crônico pode converter uma congestão aguda em hiperemia reativa crônica.

Tet·ra·hy·me·na pyr·i·for·mis (tet - rã - hī′mē - nã pir - i - fōr′mis). Ciliado pertencente a um grande grupo caracterizado por três membranas de um lado da cavidade bucal e uma do outro lado; assemelha-se ligeiramente ao paramécio e, como este, é facilmente cultivado e extensamente utilizado para estudos experimentais. [tetra- + G. *hymēn*, membrana]

tet·ra·i·o·do·phe·nol·phthal·ein so·di·um (tet′rã - ī - ō′dō - fē′nol - thal′ēn, -thal′ē - in). Tetraiodofenolftaleína sódica. SIN iodophthalein.

te·tral·o·gy (te - tral′ō - jē). Tetralogia. SIN tetrad (1). [G. *tetralogia*]

Eisenmenger t., t. de Eisenmenger. SIN Eisenmenger *complex*.

t. of Fallot, t. de Fallot; conjunto de defeitos cardíacos congênitos, incluindo defeito do septo interventricular, estenose da valva pulmonar ou estenose infundibular e destroposição da aorta, que passa por cima do septo interventricular e recebe sangue venoso, bem como sangue arterial. A hipertrofia ventricular direita é considerada parte da tetralogia, embora seja reativa aos outros defeitos. SIN Fallot tetrad.

tet·ra·mas·tia (tet′rã - mas′tē - ã). Tetramastia; presença de quatro mamas em um indivíduo. [tetra- + G. *mastos*, mama]

tet·ra·mas·ti·gote (tet - rã - mas′ti - gōt). Tetramastigota; protozoário ou outro microrganismo que possui quatro flagelos. [tetra- + G. *mastix*, chicote]

tet·ra·mas·tous (tet′rã - mas′tŭs). Tetramasto; que possui quatro mamas.

te·tram·e·lus (tē - tram′e - lŭs). Tetrâmelo; gêmeos unidos que possuem quatro braços (tetrabráquio) ou quatro pernas (tetráscelo). VER conjoined *twins*, em *twin*. [tetra- + G. *melos*, membro]

Tet·ra·me·res (tet - ram′e - rēz). Gênero de nematódeos parasitas (família Spiruridae) que infectam o estômago de aves. Quando repleta de ovos, a fêmea apresenta-se muito aumentada e possui aspecto globular, vermelho-sangue. As espécies incluem *T. americana*, encontrado no pró-ventrículo de galinhas (algumas vezes gravemente patogênico em pintos pequenos), perus, galos silvestres e codornas e transmitido por baratas e gafanhotos infectados, e *T. fissispina*, encontrado no pró-ventrículo de patos, gansos, aves aquáticas selvagens e pombos, porém raramente em galináceos. [ver tetrameric]

tet·ra·mer·ic, te·tram·er·ous (tet′rã - mer′ik, tē - tram′e - rŭs). Tetramérico; que possui quatro partes ou partes dispostas em grupos de quatro, ou capaz de existir em quatro formas. [tetra- + G. *meros*, parte]

tet·ra·meth·yl·am·mo·ni·um io·dide (tet - rã - meth′il - ã - mō′nē - ŭm). Iodeto de tetrametilamônio; dissolve-se na água até uma proporção de 0,25 g/L; utilizado para a desinfecção de emergência da água potável.

tet·ra·meth·yl·di·ar·sine (tet′rã - meth′il - dī - ãr′sēn). Tetrametildiarsina. SIN cacodyl.

tet·ra·meth·yl·pu·tres·cine (tet - rã - meth′il - pū - tres′ēn). Tetrametilputrescina; derivado da putrescina, $C_8H_{20}N_2$, semelhante à muscarina na sua ação.

tet·ra·ni·trol (tet - rã - nī′trol). Tetranitrol. SIN erythrityl tetranitrate.

tet·ra·nu·cle·o·tide (tet′rã - noo′klē - ō - tīd). Tetranucleotídio; composto de quatro nuclídios; outrora considerado representante da verdadeira estrutura do ácido nucléico (teoria do tetranucleotídio).

tet·ra·ot·us (tet′rã - ō′tus). Tetraoto. SIN tetrotus.

tet·ra·pa·re·sis (tet′rã - pã - rē′sis). Tetraparesia; fraqueza dos quatro membros. SIN quadriparesis.

tet·ra·pep·tide (tet′rã - pep′tīd). Tetrapeptídio; composto de quatro aminoácidos em ligação peptídica.

tet·ra·pe·ro·me·lia (tet′rã - pē - rō - mē′lē - ã). Tetraperomelia; peromelia que acomete todos os quatro membros. [tetra- + G. *peros*, mutilado, + *melos*, membro]

tet·ra·pho·co·me·lia (tet′rã - fō - kō - mē′lē - ã). Tetrafocomelia; focomelia com acometimento de todos os quatro membros.

tet·ra·ple·gia (tet′rã - plē′jē - ã). Tetraplegia. SIN quadriplegia. [tetra- + G. *plēgē*, golpe]

tet·ra·ple·gic (tet′rã - plē′jik). Tetraplégico. SIN quadriplegic.

tet·ra·ploid (tet′rã - ployd). Tetraplóide. VER polyploidy. [G. *tetraploos*, quatro vezes, + *eidos*, forma]

tet·ra·pus (tet′rã - pŭs). Tetrápode; indivíduo malformado com quatro pés. [G. *tetrapous*, de tetra, + *pous*, pé]

tet·ra·pyr·role (tet′rã - pir′ōl). Tetrapirrol; molécula que contém quatro núcleos de pirrol; p. ex., porfirina.

tet·ra·sac·cha·ride (tet′rã - sak′ã - rīd). Tetrassacarídeo; açúcar contendo quatro moléculas de um monossacarídeo; p. ex., estaquiose.

te·tras·ce·lus (te - tras′e - lŭs). Tetráscelo; indivíduo malformado com quatro pernas. [tetra- + G. *skelos*, perna]

tet·ra·so·mic (tet′rã - sō′mik). Tetrassômico; relativo a um núcleo celular em que um cromossoma é representado quatro vezes, enquanto todos os outros estão presentes em número normal. [tetra- + chromosome]

tet·ras·ter (tet - ras′ter). Tetráster; figura que ocorre excepcional e anormalmente na mitose, em que existem quatro ásteres. [tetra- + G. *astēr*, estrela]

tet·ra·sti·chi·a·sis (tet′rã - sti - kī′ã - sis). Tetrastiquíase; duplicação do crescimento dos cílios (em quatro fileiras). [tetra- + G. *stichos*, fileira]

tet·ra·ter·penes (tet′rã - ter′pēnz). Tetraterpenos; hidrocarbonetos ou seus derivados formados pela condensação de oito unidades de isoprenos (isto é, quatro terpenos), contendo, portanto, 40 átomos de carbono; p. ex., vários carotenóides.

tet·ra·tom·ic (tet′rã - tom′ik). Tetratômico; designa um elemento ou radical quadrivalente. [tetra- + G. *atomos*, átomo]

Tet·ra·trich·o·mo·nas (tet′rã - tri - kom′ō - nas). Gênero de protozoários flagelados parasitas, outrora parte do gênero *Trichomonas*, porém separados, hoje em dia, num gênero distinto pela presença de quatro flagelos anteriores e um flagelo rastejante, um pelta, e um corpúsculo parabasal em forma de disco. VER *Trichomonas*. [tetra- + *Trichomonas*]

T. o'vis, espécie que ocorre no ceco ou no rúmen de ovinos domésticos.

tet·ra·va·lent (tet′rã - vã′lent). Tetravalente. SIN quadrivalent. [tetra- + L. *valentia*, força]

tet·ra·zole (tet′rã - zōl). Tetrazol; o composto CN_4H_2 com a estrutura do tetrazólio.

tet·ra·zo·li·um (tet′rã - zō′lē - ŭm). Tetrazólio; qualquer um de um grupo de sais orgânicos que possuem a estrutura geral que, à redução (com clivagem da ligação 2,3), produz um formazan insolúvel colorido; utilizado como reagente na histoquímica enzimática oxidativa.

nitroblue t. (NBT), nitroazul de tetrazólio; corante amarelo-pálido que é convertido, por redução, em formazans coloridos na demonstração histoquímica de desidrogenases; utilizado em hematologia para a coloração dos neutrófilos, a fim de ajudar a indicar a presença de infecções bacterianas.

tet·ro·do·tox·in (TTX) (tet′rō - dō - tok′sin). Tetrodotoxina; potente neurotoxina encontrada no fígado e nos ovários do baiacu japonês, *Sphoeroides rubripes*, de outras espécies de baiacu e de determinados tritões; produz bloqueios axonais das fibras colinérgicas pré-ganglionares e dos nervos motores somáticos. A tetradotoxina bloqueia os canais de Na^+ regulados por voltagem em tecidos excitáveis.

tet·rose (tet′rōs). Tetrose; monossacarídeo que contém apenas quatro átomos de carbono na cadeia principal; p. ex., eritrose, treose, eritrulose.

te·tro·tus (te - trō′tŭs). Tetroto; indivíduo malformado com quatro orelhas, quatro olhos, duas faces e duas cabeças quase separadas. SIN tetraotus. [tetra- + G. *ous* (*ōt-*) orelha]

te·trox·ide (te - trok′sīd). Tetróxido; óxido que contém quatro átomos de oxigênio; por exemplo, OsO_4.

tet·ter (tet′er). Termo coloquial antiquado, popularmente aplicado à tínea e ao eczema e, em certas ocasiões, a outras erupções. [A.S. *teter*]

Teutleben, F.E.K. von, anatomista alemão, 1842-?. VER T. *ligament*.

tex·ti·form (teks′tī - fōrm). Testiforme; semelhante a uma rede. [L. *textum*, algo tecido]

tex·tur·al (teks′chŭr - ãl). Textural; relativo à textura dos tecidos.

tex·ture (teks′choor). Textura; a composição ou estrutura de um tecido ou órgão. [L. *textura*, de *texo*, pp. *textus*, tecer]

tex·tus (teks′tŭs) Tecido. [L.]

TGC Abreviatura de time-varied gain *control* (controle de ganho que varia com o tempo); time-gain *compensation* (compensação de ganho que varia com o tempo).

TGF Abreviatura de transforming growth *factors* (fator transformador de crescimento), em *factor*.

TGFα Abreviatura de transforming growth *factor* α (fator transformador de crescimento α).

TGFβ Abreviatura de transforming growth *factor* β (fator transformador de crescimento β).

Th 1. Abreviatura de T helper *cells* (células T auxiliares), em *cell*. **2.** Símbolo do tório.

Thal Alan P., cirurgião norte-americano, *1925. VER T. *procedure*.

♲ **thalam-.** Talam-. VER thalamo-.

thal·a·mec·to·my (thal - ã - mek′tō - mē). Talamectomia. VER chemothalamectomy. [thalamus + G. *ektomē*, excisão]

thal·a·men·ce·phal·ic (thal′ă-men-se-fal′ik). Talamoencefálico; relativo ao talamoencéfalo.

thal·a·men·ceph·a·lon (thal′ă-men-sef′ă-lon). Talamoencéfalo; a parte do diencéfalo que compreende o tálamo e suas estruturas associadas. [thalamus + G. *enkephalos*, cérebro]

tha·lam·ic (tha-lam′ik). Talâmico; relativo ao tálamo.

thal·a·mo-, thalam-. Tálamo-, talam-. O tálamo. [G. *thalamos*, quarto (tálamo)]

thal·a·mo·cor·ti·cal (thal′ă-mō-kōr′ti-kăl). Talamocortical; relativo às conexões eferentes do tálamo com o córtex cerebral.

thal·a·mo·len·tic·u·lar (thal′ă-mō-len-tik′oo-lăr). Talamolenticular; relativo ao tálamo, geralmente o tálamo dorsal, e ao núcleo lentiforme (putame e globo pálido).

thal·a·mot·o·my (thal-ă-mot′ō-mē). Talamotomia; destruição de uma parte selecionada do tálamo por estereotaxia para alívio da dor, movimentos involuntários, epilepsia e, raramente, distúrbios emocionais; produz poucos déficits neurológicos ou alterações indesejáveis da personalidade (ou nenhum). [thalamus + G. *tomē*, incisão]

thal·a·mus, pl. **thal·a·mi** (thal′ă-mŭs, -mī) [TA]. Tálamo; a grande massa ovóide de substância cinzenta que forma a subdivisão dorsal maior do diencéfalo; situado medialmente à cápsula interna e ao corpo e à cauda do núcleo caudado. Sua face medial forma a metade dorsal da parede lateral do terceiro ventrículo; sua superfície dorsal pode ser subdividida em um triângulo lateral que forma o assoalho do corpo (parte central) do ventrículo lateral e num triângulo medial, recoberto pelo *velum interpositum;* sua parte caudal, semelhante a uma cauda, curva-se ventralmente ao redor da face póstero-lateral do pedúnculo cerebral e termina no corpo geniculado lateral. O t. é composto de grande número de grupos celulares ou núcleos distintos do ponto de vista anatômico e funcional, geralmente classificados em 1) núcleos de transmissão sensitivos (núcleo ventral posterior e corpo geniculado lateral e medial), recebendo, cada um, um sistema de condução sensorial modalmente específico e, por sua vez, projetando-se, cada um, para a área sensorial primária correspondente do córtex; 2) núcleos de transmissão "secundários" (núcleo ventral intermédio e núcleo ventral anterior), que recebem fibras do segmento medial do globo pálido, dos núcleos cerebelares profundos contralaterais (isto é, fibras cerebelotalâmicas) e da parte reticulada da substância negra, que se projetam para várias regiões do córtex motor; 3) um núcleo associado ao sistema límbico: o núcleo anterior composto que recebe o trato mamilotalâmico e que se projeta até o giro fornicado; 4) núcleos de associação (núcleo medial dorsal, núcleo lateral incluindo o grande pulvinar), que se projetam, cada um, para uma grande expansão específica do córtex de associação; 5) a linha mediana e núcleos intralaminares ou núcleos "inespecíficos" (núcleo centro-mediano, núcleo lateral central, núcleo paracentral, núcleo reuniens). VER TAMBÉM dorsal t. [G. *thalamos*, leito, quarto]

dorsal t., t. dorsal; a grande parte do diencéfalo localizada dorsalmente ao hipotálamo e excluindo o subtálamo e os corpos geniculados medial e lateral (algumas vezes, os dois últimos são coletivamente denominados metatálamo); o tálamo dorsal inclui os núcleos motores principais e de transmissão somatossensoriais, núcleos que se projetam para áreas de associação e os núcleos intralaminares. VER TAMBÉM thalamus.

ventral t., t. ventral. SIN subthalamus.

thal·as·se·mia, thal·as·sa·ne·mia (thal-ă-sē′mē-ă, thă-las-ă-nē′mē-ă). Talassemia; qualquer um de um grupo de distúrbios hereditários do metabolismo da hemoglobina, caracterizado por comprometimento na síntese de uma ou mais das cadeias polipeptídicas de globina; existem vários tipos genéticos, e o quadro clínico correspondente pode variar desde anormalidades hematológicas dificilmente detectáveis até anemia grave e fatal. [G. *thalassa*, o mar, + *haima*, sangue]

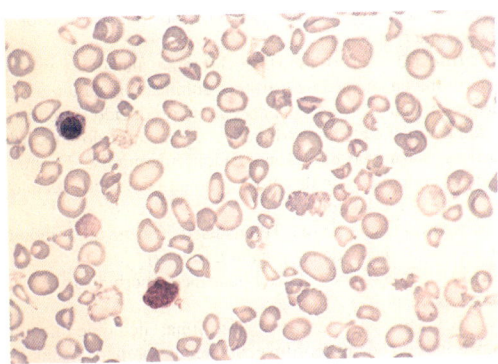

talassemia: esfregaço de paciente com β-talassemia homozigota, mostrando hipocromia, anisocitose e poiquilocitose (aumento original 250 ×; coloração de Wright-Giemsa)

α **t.,** α-talassemia; t. produzida por um de dois ou mais genes que deprimem (intensa ou moderadamente) a síntese de cadeias α-globina pelo cromossoma com o gene anormal. Estado heterozigoto: tipo grave, t. minor com 5-15% de Hb Barts ao nascimento, apenas traços de Hb Barts no adulto; tipo leve, 1-2% de Hb Barts ao nascimento, que se torna indetectável no adulto. Estado homozigoto: tipo grave, eritroblastose fetal e morte fetal, presença de apenas Hb Barts e Hb H; tipo leve não clinicamente definido. VER TAMBÉM *hemoglobin* H.

A_2 **t.,** talassemia A_2; β-talassemia, estado heterozigoto.

β **t.,** β-talassemia; t. produzida por um de dois ou mais genes que deprimem (parcial ou totalmente) a síntese de cadeias de β-globina pelo cromossoma que possui o gene anormal. Estado heterozigoto (t. A_2): t. minor com aumento da Hb A_2, Hb F normal ou variavelmente aumentada, Hb A normal ou ligeiramente reduzida. Estado homozigoto: t. major com redução da Hb A para níveis muito baixos, porém variáveis, nível muito alto de Hb F.

β-δ **t.,** β-δ-talassemia; t. produzida por um gene que deprime a síntese das cadeias β- e δ-globina pelo cromossoma que possui o gene anormal. Estado heterozigoto: t. minor, em que a Hb F representa 5-30% da hemoglobina normal, porém com distribuição desigual entre as células, Hb A_2 reduzida ou normal. Estado homozigoto: anemia moderada com presença de apenas Hb F e ausência de Hb A ou Hb A_2. SIN F t.

F t., talassemia F. SIN β-δ t.

t. interme'dia, t. intermédia; variante clínica da t. caracterizada por grau intermediário de gravidade. Esses pacientes apresentam anemia grave, mas geralmente não necessitam de transfusões sangüíneas regulares. Os distúrbios intermediários representam um grupo heterogêneo de distúrbios genéticos e podem incluir casos com anormalidades homozigota ou heterozigota no gene da cadeia de β-globina.

α **t. interme'dia,** α-talassemia intermédia. VER *hemoglobin* H.

Lepore t. [MIM*142000.0020 e outros], síndrome de t. devida à produção de hemoglobina Lepore de estrutura anormal. Estado heterozigoto: t. minor com cerca de 10% de Hb Lepore, aumento moderado da Hb F, Hb A_2 normal. Estado homozigoto: t. major com produção de apenas Hb F e Hb Lepore, sem Hb A ou Hb A_2.

t. ma'jor [MIM*141800-142310 passim], a síndrome de anemia grave que resulta do estado homozigoto de um dos genes da t. ou de um dos genes da hemoglobina Lepore, com início, na lactância ou na infância, de palidez, icterícia, fraqueza, esplenomegalia, cardiomegalia, adelgaçamento das tábuas interna e externa do crânio, anemia microcítica hipocrômica com poiquilocitose, anisocitose, células com pontilhado, células-alvo e eritrócitos nucleados. Os tipos de hemoglobina são variáveis e dependem do gene envolvido. SIN Cooley anemia, primary erythroblastic anemia.

t. mi'nor [MIM*141800-142310 passim], t. minor; o estado heterozigoto de um gene da talassemia ou de um gene da hemoglobina Lepore; em geral, assintomática e hematologicamente muito variável, com células-alvo, microcitose hipocrômica leve e, com freqüência, níveis ligeiramente reduzidos de hemoglobina com ligeiro aumento da contagem de eritrócitos; os tipos de hemoglobina são variáveis e dependem do gene envolvido.

tha·las·so·pho·bia (thal′ă-sō-fō′bē-ă, thă-las′ō). Talassofobia, medo mórbido de mar. [G. *thalassa*, o mar, + *phobos*, medo]

tha·las·so·po·sia (thal′ă-sō-pō′zē-ă, thă-las′ō-). Talassoposia; SIN mariposia. [G. *thalassa*, o mar, + *posis*, bebida]

tha·las·so·ther·a·py (thal′ă-sō-ther′ă-pē). Talassoterapia; tratamento de doença através de exposição ao ar marinho, banho de mar ou viagem pelo mar. [G. *thalassa*, o mar]

tha·lid·o·mide (thă-lid′ō-mīd). Talidomida; agente hipnótico que, quando utilizado no início da gravidez, pode levar ao nascimento de fetos com focomelia e outros defeitos; encontra-se em uso experimental para tratamento da hanseníase e como imunomodulador na infecção por HIV e em reações enxerto vs. hospedeiro.

thal·lic (thal′lik). Tálico; designa conídios produzidos sem aumento ou crescimento após delimitação por septos nas hifas (talo); toda a célula original torna-se um artroconídio.

thal·li·um (Tl) (thal′ē-ŭm). Tálio; elemento metálico branco, de número atômico 81, peso atômico 204.3833; o Tl[201] (meia-vida de 3,038 dias) é utilizado para cintilografia do miocárdio. [G. *thallos*, broto verde (produz uma linha verde no espectro)]

t.-201 ([201]**Tl**), o radioisótopo do t. utilizado amplamente para cintigrafia do miocárdio; é também captado por determinados tumores.

Thal·lo·phy·ta (thă-lof′i-tă). Em sistemas de classificação mais antigos, uma divisão primária do reino vegetal cujos membros, com poucas exceções, eram desprovidos de raízes, caules e folhas verdadeiras; incluía bactérias, fungos e algas. [G. *thallos*, broto verde, + *phyton*, planta]

thal·lo·phyte (thal′ō-fīt). Talófito; membro da divisão Thallophyta.

thal·lo·tox·i·co·sis (thal′ō-tok-si-kō′sis). Talotoxicose; envenenamento por tálio; caracterizada por estomatite, gastroenterite, neurite periférica e retrobulbar, distúrbios endócrinos e alopecia. [thallium + G. *toxikon*, veneno, + *-osis*, condição]

tha·lus (thal'ŭs). Talo; corpo vegetal ou fúngico simples, desprovido de raízes, caules e folhas. Crescimento vegetativo de um fungo. [G. *thallos*, broto novo]

♻ **thanato-.** Tanato-. Morte. VER TAMBÉM necro-. [G. *thanatos*, morte]

than·a·to·bi·o·log·ic (than'ă-tō-bī-ō-loj'ik). Tanatobiológico; relativo aos processos envolvidos na vida e na morte. [thanato- + G. *bios*, vida, + *logos*, estudo]

than·a·to·gno·mon·ic (than'ă-tō-nō-mon'ik). Tanatognomônico; de prognóstico fatal, indicando a proximidade da morte. [thanato- + G. *gnōmē*, um sinal]

than·a·tog·ra·phy (than-ă-tog'ră-fē). Tanatografia. 1. Descrição dos sintomas e pensamentos de um indivíduo enquanto está morrendo. 2. Tratado sobre a morte. [thanato- + G. *graphē*, escrito]

than·a·toid (than'ă-toyd). Tanatóide. 1. Semelhante à morte. 2. Mortal. [thanato- + G. *eidos*, semelhança]

than·a·tol·o·gy (than-ă-tol'ō-jē). Tanatologia; ramo da ciência que trata do estudo da morte e de seu processo. [thanato- + G. *logos*, estudo]

than·a·to·ma·nia (than'ă-tō-mā'nē-ă). Tanatomania; doença ou morte resultante da crença na eficácia da magia; fenômeno observado em sociedades primitivas ou pessoas analfabetas e supersticiosas que acreditam no poder de espíritos do mal, encantamentos, pragas, e de indivíduos sobre os processos corporais de alguém, sendo essa crença e medo resultante manifestados na forma de doença psicossomática e até mesmo morte. [thanato- + G. *mania*, frenesi]

than·a·to·phid·ia (than'ă-tō-fid'ē-ă). Tanatofídios; serpentes venenosas. [thanato- + G. *ophidion*, dim. de *ophis*, serpente]

than·a·to·pho·bia (than'ă-tō-fō'bē-ă). Tanatofobia; medo mórbido da morte. [thanato- + G. *phobos*, medo]

than·a·to·phor·ic (than'ă-tō-fōr'ik). Tanatofórico; que leva à morte. [thanato- + G. *phoros*, que conduz]

than·a·tos (than'ă-tos). Tánatos; em psicanálise, o princípio da morte, representando todas as tendências instintivas em direção à senescência e à morte. Ver também subentradas em instinct. Cf. eros. [G. morte]

Thane, Sir George D., anatomista inglês, 1850–1930. VER T. *method*.

thau·mat·ro·py (thaw-mat'rō-pē). Taumatropia; a transformação de uma forma de tecido em outra. [G. *thauma (thaumat-)*, milagre, + *tropē*, volta]

Thayer, James D. VER T.-Martin *medium, agar*.

THC Abreviatura de tetrahidrocannabinol (tetra-hidrocanabinol).

Thd Símbolo de ribothymidine (ribotimidina).

thea (thē-ă). Chá. SIN tea. [L. Mod.]

the·a·ism (thē'ă-izm). Teísmo. SIN theinism.

the·a·ter (thē'ă-ter). Anfiteatro. 1. Grande sala para palestras e demonstrações; algumas vezes, termo aplicado a uma sala de cirurgia equipada para observação por outras pessoas além da equipe cirúrgica. 2. Qualquer sala de operação ou conjunto dessas salas. [G. *theatron*, lugar para ver, teatro, de *theomai*, olhar]

the·ba·ic (thē-bā'ik). Tebaico; relativo a ou derivado do ópio. [L. *Thebaicus*, relativo a Tebas, lugar onde o ópio era antigamente obtido]

the·ba·ine (thē-bā'ēn, -in). Tebaína; alcalóide obtido do ópio (0,3-1,5%), assemelha-se à estricnina em sua ação, causando convulsões tetânicas. SIN paramorphine.

Thebesius, Adam C., médico alemão, 1686–1732. VER thebesian *foramina*, em *foramen*, thebesian *valve*, thebesian *veins*, em *vein*.

the·ca, pl. **the·cae** (thē'kă, thē'sē). Teca; bainha ou cápsula. [G. *thēkē*, caixa]

t. cor'dis, pericárdio. SIN pericardium.
t. exter'na, t. externa. SIN tunica externa thecae folliculi.
t. follic'uli, t. do folículo; a parede de um folículo ovariano vesicular. VER TAMBÉM tunica externa, tunica interna thecae folliculi.
t. inter'na, t. interna. SIN tunica interna thecae folliculi.
t. ten'dinis, t. tendínea. SIN synovial tendon *sheath*.
t. vertebra'lis, dura-máter espinal. SIN spinal *dura mater*.

the·cal (thē'kăl). Tecal; relativo a uma bainha, especialmente uma bainha tendínea. [ver theca]

thec·o·dont (thē'kō-dont). Tecodonte; que possui os dentes inseridos em alvéolos. [G. *thēkē*, caixa, + *odous (odont-)*, dente]

the·co·ma (thē-kō'mă). Tecoma; neoplasia derivada do mesênquima ovariano, que consiste principalmente em células fusiformes que freqüentemente contêm pequenas gotículas de gordura; em geral, as características macroscópicas assemelham-se às de um tumor de células granulosas, isto é, massa encapsulada, firme e amarela, habitualmente com cerca de 10 cm ou menos de diâmetro, mas que tende a ser menos maligna; pode formar quantidades consideráveis de estrogênios, resultando, assim, no desenvolvimento precoce dos caracteres sexuais secundários em meninas pré-puberais ou em hiperplasia do endométrio em pacientes idosas. SIN theca cell tumor. [G. *thēkē*, caixa (theca), + *-oma*, tumor]

the·co·ma·to·sis (thē'kō-mă-tō'sis). Tecomatose; hiperplasia do estroma ou aumento no número de elementos de tecido conjuntivo de um ovário.

Theden, Johann C.A., cirurgião alemão, 1714–1797. VER T. *method*.

Theile, Friedrich W., anatomista alemão, 1801–1879. VER T. *canal, glands,* em *gland, muscle*.

Theiler, Max, microbiologista sul-africano nos Estados Unidos e ganhador do Prêmio Nobel, 1899–1972. VER T. *virus*.

Thei·le·ri·i·dae (thī-lē'rē-i-dē). Família de protozoários esporozoários que, juntamente com a família Babesiidae, compreeende a ordem Piroplasmida; constituída de um gênero reconhecido, *Theileria,* transmitido por carrapatos ixodídeos.

the·in (thē'in, tē'in). Cafeína. SIN caffeine.

the·in·ism, the·ism (thē'i-nizm; thē'izm, tē'-). Teinismo, teísmo; intoxicação crônica resultante da ingestão exagerada de chá, caracterizada por palpitação, insônia, nervosismo, cefaléia e dispepsia. SIN theaism. [L. mod. *thea,* chá]

♻ **thel-.** Tel-. VER thelo-.

the·lar·che (thē-lar'kē). Telarca; o início do desenvolvimento das mamas na mulher. [thel- + G. *archē,* início]

The·la·zia (thē-lā'zē-ă). Os vermes oculares, um gênero de nematódeos espiruróides que habitam os ductos lacrimais e a superfície dos olhos de vários animais domésticos e selvagens, mas raramente dos seres humanos; foram relatadas diversas espécies em aves selvagens. Ocorre desenvolvimento cíclico em moscas muscóides; as larvas infectantes emergem das partes bucais da mosca, enquanto esta se alimenta sobre os olhos do hospedeiro ou próximo a eles. [G. *thēlazō,* sugar]

T. californien'sis, espécie de nematódeo que ocorre nos ductos lacrimais, no saco conjuntival e sobre a membrana nictante de cães, coiotes, ursos negros, ovinos, cervos, lebre, gatos e, por vezes, seres humanos no Oeste e Sudoeste dos Estados Unidos; as infecções maciças causam fotofobia, lacrimejamento, edema das pálpebras, conjuntivite e até mesmo cegueira.

T. callipae'da, espécie descrita em seres humanos no Sudeste da Ásia e na Califórnia; o verme, imerso num tumor subconjuntival ou nadando no humor aquoso após penetrar no limbo corneoescleral, provoca dor, fotofobia e lacrimejamento.

thel·a·zi·a·sis (thē-lă-zī'ă-sis, thel-ă-). Telazíase; infecção por nematódeos do gênero *Thelazia*.

the·le (thē'lē). Mamilo. SIN nipple. [G.]

the·li·um, pl. **the·lia** (thē'lē-ŭm, -lē-ă). Télio. 1. Estrutura semelhante a um mamilo. 2. Camada celular. 3. Mamilo. SIN nipple. [L. Mod., do G. *thēlē,* mamilo]

♻ **thelo-, thel-.** Telo-, tel-. Os mamilos. Cf. mamil-. [G. *thēlē*]

the·lor·rha·gia (thē-lō-rā'jē-ă). Telorragia; sangramento do mamilo. [thelo- + G. *rhēgnymi,* irromper]

the·nad (thē'nad). Em direção à face tenar ou lateral da palma da mão. [G. *thenar,* a palma da mão, + L. *ad,* para]

the·nal (thē'năl). Tenar. SIN thenar.

the·nal·dine (thē-nal'dēn). Tenaldina; agente anti-histamínico e antipruriginoso (como o tartarato).

the·nar (thē'nar) [TA] Tenar; termo aplicado a qualquer estrutura relacionada com a base do polegar ou seus componentes coletivos subjacentes. SIN thenal. VER thenar *eminence*. [G. a palma da mão]

the·nen (thē'nen). Relativo apenas à palma da mão, especificamente ao lado radial. [G. *thenar,* palma + *en,* dentro]

then·yl (then'il). Tenil; o radical do 2-metiltiofeno $(SC_4H_3)CH_2$–. Cf. thienyl.

then·yl·di·a·mine hy·dro·chlo·ride (then-il-dī'ă-mēn). Cloridrato de tenildiamina; um anti-histamínico.

Theobald Smith. VER Smith.

the·o·bro·ma (thē-ō-brō'mă). Teobroma. SIN cacao. [G. *theos,* deus + *brōma,* alimento]

t. oil, óleo de teobroma; a gordura obtida da semente triturada de *Theobroma cacao* (família Sterculiaceae); contém os glicerídios dos ácidos esteárico, palmítico, oléico, ariquídico e linoleico; utilizado como base para supositórios e pomadas e, em odontologia cirúrgica, como lubrificante protetor. SIN cacao butter, cocoa butter, cacao oil.

the·o·bro·mine (thē-ō-brō'men). Teobromina; alcalóide semelhante à cafeína e à teofilina na sua ação e estrutura química, preparado a partir da semente madura e seca do *Theobroma cacao* ou produzido sinteticamente; outrora utilizada amplamente como diurético, estimulante do miocárdio, dilatador das artérias coronárias e relaxante da musculatura lisa. Foram relacionados compostos com gliconato de cálcio, salicilato de cálcio, acetato de sódio, lactato de sódio e salicilato de sódio.

the·o·ma·nia (thē-ō-mā'nē-ă). Teomania; delírio em que o indivíduo acredita que é Deus. [G. *theos,* deus, + *mania,* frenesi]

the·o·pho·bia (thē-ō-fō'bē-ă). Teofobia; medo mórbido de Deus. [G. *theos,* deus, + *phobos,* medo]

the·o·phyl·line (thē-of'i-lēn, -lin). Teofilina; alcalóide encontrado com cafeína nas folhas de chá (a teofilina comercial é preparada sinteticamente); relaxante da musculatura lisa, diurético, estimulante cardíaco e vasodilatador; utilizada na asma brônquica e em outras formas de doença pulmonar obstrutiva crônica como broncodilatador e estimulante dos músculos respiratórios.

Além disso, acredita-se que aumenta o impulso respiratório, de modo que é algumas vezes utilizada em síndromes de hipoventilação. Compartilha propriedades químicas e farmacológicas com a cafeína e a teobromina.

t. ethylenediamine, etilenodiamina de teofilina. SIN aminophylline.

t. sodium glycinate, glicinato sódico de teofilina; mistura em equilíbrio contendo teofilina sódica e glicina em proporções aproximadamente moleculares, tamponada com um mol adicional de glicina; com ação e usos semelhantes aos da aminofilina, porém mais estável no ar e menos irritante para a mucosa gástrica.

the·o·rem (thē′ō-rem). Teorema; proposição que pode ser testada e estabelecida como lei ou princípio. VER TAMBÉM law, principle, rule.

Bayes t., t. de Bayes; os impactos de novos dados sobre os méritos evidenciais de hipóteses científicas competitivas são comparados ao se computar cada produto da plausibilidade antecedente (a probabilidade prévia) e a probabilidade dos dados atuais dessa hipótese (a probabilidade condicional) e ao se reescaloná-los, de modo que seu total corresponda à unidade (sendo os valores reescalonados as probabilidades posteriores). VER TAMBÉM diagnostic *sensitivity,* diagnostic *specificity,* predictive *value.*

Bernoulli t., t. de Bernoulli. SIN Bernoulli law.

central limit t., t. do limite central; a soma (ou média) de n realizações do mesmo processo, contanto que possua uma variação finita, aproxima-se da distribuição gaussiana quando n se torna indefinidamente grande. Essa teoria proporciona um amplo fundamento para o uso da teoria normal, mesmo para dados não-gaussianos. Na forma apresentada aqui, constitui a versão clássica; as versões mais gerais permitem um notável afrouxamento das pressuposições usuais.

Gibbs t., t. de Gibbs; substâncias que reduzem a tensão superficial do meio de dispersão puro tendem a acumular-se em sua superfície, enquanto as substâncias que elevam a tensão superficial tendem a permanecer fora da película superficial.

THEORY

the·o·ry (thē′ōr-ē). Teoria; explicação ponderada de fatos ou fenômenos conhecidos, que serve como base de investigação para chegar à verdade. VER TAMBÉM hypothesis, postulate. [G. *theōria,* contemplação, especulação, teoria, de *theōros,* espectador]

adsorption t. of narcosis, t. de adsorção da narcose; t. segundo a qual uma droga torna-se concentrada na superfície da célula em consequência da adsorção e, assim, altera a permeabilidade e o metabolismo.

aerodynamic t., t. aerodinâmica; t. geralmente aceita segundo a qual a vibração das pregas vocais na fonação é produzida pelo fluxo do ar expirado passando pelas pregas vocais ligeiramente aproximadas; oposta ao atual conceito inalcançável de que o movimento das pregas vocais na fonação resulta da contração dos músculos intrínsecos da laringe na freqüência da vibração das pregas vocais.

Altmann t., t. de Altmann; t. segundo a qual o protoplasma consiste em partículas granulares (denominadas bioblastos) que estão agrupadas e circundadas por matéria indiferente.

Arrhenius-Madsen t., t. de Arrhenius-Madsen; t. segundo a qual a reação de um antígeno com seu anticorpo é uma reação reversível, sendo o equilíbrio determinado de acordo com a lei de ação da massa pelas concentrações das substâncias reagentes.

atomic t., t. atômica; t. segundo a qual os compostos clínicos são formados pela união de átomos em determinadas proporções definidas; em sua forma moderna, desenvolvida pela primeira vez por John Dalton, em 1803.

Baeyer t., t. de Baeyer; teoria de que as ligações de carbono são estabelecidas em ângulos fixos (109° 28′) e que os anéis de carbono mais estáveis são os que menos distorcem esses ângulos; por essa razão, os anéis planares compostos de 5 ou 6 átomos de carbono (p. ex., ciclopentano, benzeno) são mais comuns do que os que contêm menos de 5 ou mais de 6 átomos de carbono.

balance t., t. do equilíbrio; em psicologia social, teoria que supõe que os estados de equilíbrio e de desequilíbrio podem ser especificados para unidades cognitivas (p. ex., num indivíduo e suas atitudes ou atos), e que essas unidades tendem a buscar estados de equilíbrio; p. ex., existe equilíbrio quando ambas as partes de uma unidade mostram-se iguais, enquanto surge desequilíbrio quando as duas partes não são equivalentes, levando a uma reavaliação cognitiva das partes ou à sua segregação. VER TAMBÉM cognitive dissonance t., consistency *principle.*

beta-oxidation-condensation t., t. de β-oxidação-condensação, t. segundo a qual os fragmentos de dois carbonos clivados da molécula de ácido graxo por beta-oxidação são convertidos em ácido acético e, a seguir, condensados a ácido acetoacético.

Bohr t., t. de Bohr; t. segundo a qual as linhas do espectro são produzidas 1) pela emissão quantizada de energia radiante quando elétrons caem de uma órbita de um maior nível de energia para um de menor energia, ou 2) por absorção da radiação quando um elétron eleva-se de um nível de energia menor para um maior.

Brønsted t., t. de Brønsted; t. segundo a qual um ácido é uma substância, com carga ou sem carga, que libera íons hidrogênio em solução, enquanto uma base é uma substância que os remove da solução (p. ex., NH_4^+, CH_3COOH e HSO_4^- são ácidos; NH_3, CH_3COO^- e SO_4^- são bases); útil no conceito de eletrólitos fracos e tampões. Cf. Brønsted *acid,* Brønsted *base.*

Burn and Rand t., t. de Burn e Rand; t. segundo a qual a estimulação de fibras simpáticas resulta inicialmente na produção de acetilcolina nas terminações nervosas pós-ganglionares, que então liberam norepinefrina para atuar sobre o local ativo da célula efetora.

Cannon t., t. de Cannon. SIN emergency t.

Cannon-Bard t., t. de Cannon-Bard; a visão de que o aspecto sentimental da emoção e o padrão de comportamento emocional são controlados pelo hipotálamo.

catastrophe t., t. da catástrofe; ramo da matemática que trata de grandes alterações que ocorrem no sistema total, as quais podem resultar de uma pequena mudança numa variável crítica do sistema; um exemplo é fornecido pela mudança nas propriedades físicas da H_2O quando à temperatura 0 ou 100°C; muitas aplicações da teoria da catástrofe são observadas na medicina clínica e na epidemiologia.

cellular immune t., t. imunológica celular; conceito, emitido por Elie Metchnikoff, de que as células, e não os anticorpos, são responsáveis pela resposta imune de um organismo.

celomic metaplasia t. of endometriosis, t. da metaplasia celômica da endometriose; t. segundo a qual o tecido endometrial origina-se diretamente do mesotélio peritoneal.

chaos t., t. do caos; ramo da matemática que trata de eventos e processos que não podem ser previstos com exatidão, baseando-se em teorias ou leis matemáticas convencionais; alguns processos biológicos, como, por exemplo, a disseminação de doença maligna, parecem confirmar a teoria do caos, pelo menos em alguns casos.

chemiosmotic t., t. quimiosmótica; hipótese propondo que os processos que exigem energia celular, como a síntese de ATP e o bombeamento de íons, podem ser impulsionados por um gradiente de pH ou de potencial de membrana; formulada por Peter Mitchell, em 1961.

cloacal t., t. cloacal; a crença algumas vezes mantida por adultos neuróticos ou crianças de que uma criança nasce, quando as fezes são eliminadas, de uma abertura comum.

clonal deletion t., t. da deleção clonal; a eliminação de determinadas populações de células T no timo que possuem receptores para auto-antígenos (clones proibidos). VER immunologic *tolerance.*

clonal selection t., t. da seleção clonal; t. que afirma que cada linfócito possui receptores de imunoglobulina ligados à membrana, específicos para determinado antígeno, e que, uma vez o receptor ocupado, ocorre proliferação da célula, produzindo um clone de células formadoras de anticorpos (plasmócitos).

cognitive dissonance t., t. da dissonância cognitiva; t. da formação de atitudes e comportamento descrevendo um estado motivacional que existe quando os elementos cognitivos de um indivíduo (atitudes, comportamentos percebidos etc.) são incoerentes entre si, como a aceitação dos Dez Mandamentos com a crença simultânea de que não há problema em sonegar impostos; teoria que indica que as pessoas procuram alcançar a coerência (consonância) e evitar a dissonância que, quando surge, pode ser enfrentada pela modificação das atitudes, racionalização, percepção seletiva e outros meios. VER TAMBÉM balance t., consistency *principle.*

colloid t. of narcosis, t. colóide na narcose; t. segundo a qual a coagulação ou floculação de proteína causa desidratação e redução do metabolismo.

darwinian t., teoria de Darwin; a t. da origem das espécies e do desenvolvimento dos organismos superiores a partir de formas inferiores por meio da seleção natural (sobrevida do mais capaz na luta pela existência) e da evolução dos seres humanos e dos macacos a partir de um ancestral comum.

decay t., t. da desintegração; t. do esquecimento baseada na premissa de que um engrama ou traço de memória dissipa-se progressivamente com o tempo durante o intervalo em que não é ativado.

dipole t., t. do dipolo; t. em que a corrente de ativação do coração é concebida como um único dipolo móvel final, a derivação do pólo positivo.

duplicity t. of vision, t. da duplicidade da visão; t. segundo a qual os cones da retina funcionam na luz intensa, enquanto os bastões funcionam na penumbra.

Ehrlich t., t. de Ehrlich. VER side-chain t.

t. of electrolytic dissociation, t. da dissociação eletrolítica. VER Arrhenius *doctrine.*

emergency t., t. da emergência; t. das emoções, formulada por W.B. Cannon, segundo a qual os animais e seres humanos respondem a situações de emergência através de um aumento da atividade do sistema nervoso simpático, incluindo aumento na produção de catecolaminas, com elevações associadas da pressão arterial, freqüências cardíaca e respiratória e fluxo sangüíneo do músculo esquelético. VER TAMBÉM relaxation *response.* SIN Cannon t.

enzyme inhibition t. of narcosis, t. de inibição enzimática da narcose; t. segundo a qual os narcóticos inibem as enzimas respiratórias ao suprimirem a formação de ligações de fosfato de alta energia no interior da célula.

Flourens t., t. de Flourens; t. antiga segundo a qual o pensamento é um processo que depende da ação de todo o cérebro.

Frerichs t., t. de Frerichs; t. segundo a qual a uremia representa uma condição tóxica causada por carbonato de amônio, que se forma em consequência da ação de uma enzima plasmática sobre as quantidades aumentadas de uréia.

Freud t., t. de Freud; t. abrangente sobre o processo de formação e desenvolvimento da personalidade em indivíduos normais e emocionalmente perturbados; p. ex., afirma que um ataque de histeria de conversão se deve a um traumatismo psíquico ao qual o indivíduo não reagiu adequadamente no momento em que ocorreu, persistindo como lembrança afetiva. VER TAMBÉM psychoanalysis.

game t., t. do jogo; ramo da lógica matemática que trata da amplitude de reações possíveis a determinada estratégia; cada reação pode estar associada a uma probabilidade e cada uma delas pode levar a uma contra-reação pelo "adversário" no jogo. A teoria do jogo, utilizada principalmente na análise de sistemas, tem algumas implicações na vigilância e no controle das doenças; constitui uma das teorias subjacentes na análise de decisões clínicas.

gastrea t., t. da gástrea. SIN Haeckel gastrea t.

gate-control t., t. de regulação-controle; t. formulada para explicar o mecanismo da dor; os estímulos aferentes de pequenas fibras, sobretudo a dor, que penetram na substância gelatinosa podem ser modulados por estímulos aferentes de grandes fibras e vias espinais descendentes, de modo que a sua transmissão para vias espinais ascendentes é bloqueada (regulada). SIN gate-control hypothesis.

germ t., t. do germe; a t., que hoje em dia é uma doutrina, segundo a qual as doenças infecciosas são causadas pela presença e atividade funcional de microrganismos no corpo.

germ layer t., t. da camada germinativa; o conceito de que os embriões jovens diferenciam três camadas germinativas primárias (ectoderma, mesoderma e endoderma), tendo, cada uma delas, a potencialidade de formar diferentes estruturas e órgãos característicos no corpo em desenvolvimento.

gestalt t., t. da gestalt. VER gestaltism.

Haeckel gastrea t., t. da gástrea de Haeckel; t. segundo a qual a gástrula de dois folhetos é a forma ancestral de todos os animais multicelulares. SIN gastrea t.

Helmholtz t. of accommodation, t. de Helmholtz da acomodação; t. segundo a qual o músculo ciliar relaxa a visão para perto e permite que a face anterior da lente se torne mais convexa.

Helmholtz t. of color vision, t. de Helmholtz da visão para cores. SIN Young-Helmholtz t. of color vision.

Helmholtz-Gibbs t., t. de Helmholtz-Gibbs. VER Gibbs-Helmholtz *equation*.

Helmholtz t. of hearing, t. de Helmholtz da audição. SIN resonance t. of hearing.

Hering t. of color vision, t. de Hering da visão para cores; t. segundo a qual existem três processos visuais oponentes: azul-amarelo, vermelho-verde e branco-preto.

humoral t., t. humoral. VER humoral *doctrine*.

hydrate microcrystal t. of anesthesia, t. do microcristal hidratado da anestesia; t. da narcose relativa a agentes sem ligação de hidrogênio; postula a interação das moléculas da droga anestésica com moléculas de água no cérebro. SIN Pauling t.

implantation t. of the production of endometriosis, t. de implantação na produção da endometriose; t. segundo a qual, no momento da menstruação, as células da mucosa uterina atravessam a tuba uterina e escapam para a cavidade pélvica, onde se implantam sobre o peritônio.

incasement t., t. da pré-formação. SIN preformation t.

information t., t. da informação; na ciência do comportamento, um sistema para estudo do processo de comunicação através da análise detalhada, freqüentemente matemática, de todos os aspectos do processo, incluindo a codificação, a transmissão e a decodificação de sinais; não relacionada, em qualquer sentido direto, com o significado de uma mensagem.

instructive t., t. da instrução; teoria segundo a qual o anticorpo aprende ou adquire a sua especificidade após contato com determinado antígeno.

kern-plasma relation t., t. da relação núcleo-plasma; t. enunciada por Hertwig (1903) segundo a qual existe normalmente uma relação definida quanto ao tamanho entre a massa de material nuclear e a do protoplasma. [Al. *kern*, semente, núcleo]

Knoop t., t. de Knoop; t. segundo a qual o metabolismo dos ácidos graxos ocorre em estágios, havendo, em cada um deles, uma perda de dois átomos de carbono em consequência da oxidação no átomo de carbono β; p. ex.,

$$C_6H_5-\overset{\beta}{CH_2}-\overset{\alpha}{CH_2}-COOH \rightarrow C_6H_5-COOH.$$

Ladd-Franklin t., t. de Ladd-Franklin. SIN molecular dissociation t.

lamarckian t., t. de Lamarck; t. segundo a qual as características adquiridas podem ser transmitidas aos descendentes, e a experiência, e não apenas a biologia, pode modificar e, portanto, influenciar a transmissão genética.

learning t., t. do aprendizado; qualquer uma de várias teorias proeminentes formuladas para explicar o aprendizado, especialmente aquelas promulgadas por Pavlov, Thorndike, Guthrie, Hull, Kohler, Spence, Miller, Skinner e seus seguidores modernos. VER TAMBÉM conditioning.

libido t., t. da libido; t. de Freud de que a vida psíquica de uma pessoa resulta principalmente de necessidades instintivas ou libidinosas e da busca para satisfazê-las.

Liebig t., t. de Liebig; t. segundo a qual os hidrocarbonetos que oxidam facilmente e queimam são alimentos que produzem a maior quantidade de calor animal.

lipoid t. of narcosis, t. lipóide da narcose; t. segundo a qual a eficiência da narcose acompanha o coeficiente de partição entre óleo e água, e os lipóides na célula e sobre a membrana celular absorvem a droga em virtude dessa afinidade. SIN Meyer-Overton t. of narcosis.

mass action t., t. de ação da massa; t. segundo a qual grandes áreas de tecido cerebral funcionam como um todo na ação aprendida ou inteligente.

t. of medicine, t. da medicina; a ciência, distinta da arte, ou prática, da medicina.

membrane expansion t., t. de expansão da membrana; t. segundo a qual a adsorção de anestésicos às membranas altera o volume e/ou a configuração da membrana a ponto de a sua função ser afetada, com conseqüente produção de anestesia.

Metchnikoff t., t. de Metchnikoff; a t. fagocítica de que o corpo é protegido contra infecções pelos leucócitos e outras células que ingerem e destroem os microrganismos invasores.

Meyer-Overton t. of narcosis, t. de Meyer-Overton da narcose. SIN lipoid t. of narcosis.

miasma t., t. do miasma; explicação da origem das epidemias, baseada na falsa noção de que eram causadas pelo ar de má qualidade, p. ex., emanação de vegetação e decomposição em pântanos.

Miller chemicoparasitic t., t. químico-parasitária de Miller; t. segundo a qual a cárie dentária é causada por microrganismos da boca que fermentam os carboidratos da dieta e produzem ácidos que desmineralizam os dentes.

mnemic t., t. mnêmica. SIN mnemic hypothesis.

molecular dissociation t., t. de dissociação molecular; t. relativa à visão para cores, de que o cinza é a primeira das sensações de cores, da qual derivam, por modificação molecular, duas substâncias pares, que, respectivamente, detectam o amarelo e o azul, e de que o amarelo origina substâncias pares para detecção do vermelho e do verde. SIN Ladd-Franklin t.

monophyletic t., t. monofilética. SIN monophyletism.

myoelastic t., t. mioelástica; t. que afirma que o som da voz humana é produzido por vibrações das cordas vocais resultantes do pregueamento para cima em virtude da pressão do ar abaixo e do subseqüente movimento para baixo, em virtude da tensão elástica das cordas.

neurochronaxic t., t. neurocronáxica; t. que afirma que as variações na freqüência da voz humana são causadas por alterações na taxa de contração dos músculos laríngeos; não é mais considerada verdadeira.

Ollier t., t. de Ollier; t. do crescimento compensatório; após ressecção da extremidade articular de um osso, a cartilagem articular do outro osso que entra na estrutura da articulação apresenta maior crescimento.

omega-oxidation t., t. da ômega-oxidação; t. segundo a qual a oxidação de ácidos graxos começa no grupo CH_3, isto é, o grupamento terminal ou ômega; a seguir, a beta-oxidação prossegue em ambas as extremidades da cadeia de ácido graxo.

overproduction t., t. da superprodução. SIN Weigert *law*.

oxygen deprivation t. of narcosis, t. de privação de oxigênio da narcose; t. segundo a qual os narcóticos inibem a oxidação, causando narcotização da célula.

Pauling t., t. de Pauling. SIN hydrate microcrystal t. of anesthesia.

permeability t. of narcosis, t. de permeabilidade da narcose; t. segundo a qual a permeabilidade da membrana celular é reduzida por concentrações narcóticas de depressores alifáticos e outros depressores do sistema nervoso central.

phlogiston t., t. do flogisto. VER phlogiston.

pithecoid t., t. pitecóide; t. de que o homem descende, juntamente com o macaco, de um ancestral comum. VER TAMBÉM darwinian t.

place t., t. do lugar; t. de percepção do timbre que afirma que a região da membrana basilar da cóclea que é colocada em vibração depende da freqüência do som. VER TAMBÉM resonance t. of hearing.

Planck t. t. de Planck. SIN quantum t.

polyphyletic t., t. polifilética. SIN polyphyletism.

preformation t., t. da pré-formação; t. arcaica de que o embrião estava totalmente formado em miniatura dentro de um gameta por ocasião da concepção. VER TAMBÉM homunculus; Cf. epigenesis. SIN emboitement, incasement t.

quantum t., t. do *quantum*; t. segundo a qual a energia pode ser emitida, transmitida e absorvida apenas em quantidades bem-definidas (quanta), de modo que os átomos e as partículas subatômicas só podem existir em determinados estados de energia. SIN Planck t.

recapitulation t., t. da recapitulação; t. formulada por E.H. Haeckel de que os indivíduos, em seu desenvolvimento embrionário, atravessam estágios semelhantes, no plano estrutural geral, aos estágios pelos quais suas espécies passaram em seu processo de evolução; expressa de maneira mais técnica, a t. segundo a qual a ontogenia é uma recapitulação abreviada da filogenia. SIN biogenetic law, law of biogenesis, Haeckel law, law of recapitulation.

Reed-Frost t. of epidemics, t. de Reed-Frost das epidemias; t. matemática para explicar como as epidemias se originam e continuam.

reed instrument t., t. do instrumento de sopro; t. não mais sustentável de que, na produção da voz humana, a laringe funciona de forma semelhante a um instrumento musical de sopro.

reentry t., t. da reentrada; t. segundo a qual as extra-sístoles são decorrentes da reentrada de um impulso iniciado pelo impulso sinusal ou juncional AV, ao qual a extra-sístole está acoplada, no foco ectópico.

resonance t. of hearing, t. da ressonância da audição; t. segundo a qual a membrana basilar da cóclea atua como uma estrutura de ressonância, ativada com tons de baixa freqüência na volta apical e com tons de alta freqüência na volta basal. Não é mais considerada correta; suplantada pela t. da onda de von Bekesy. SIN Helmholtz t. of hearing.

scientific t., t. científica; t. que pode ser testada e potencialmente excluída; a impossibilidade de refutá-la ou excluí-la aumenta a sua confiabilidade, embora não possa ser considerada provada.

Semon-Hering t., t. de Semon-Hering. SIN mnemic *hypothesis.*

sensorimotor t., t. sensorimotora; na t. do desenvolvimento de Piaget, a suposição de que, durante os primeiros 18 meses de vida, ocorre uma transformação de ação no pensamento; a princípio, observa-se deslocamento gradual do comportamento inato para o comportamento adquirido, a seguir, da atividade centrada no corpo para a atividade centrada no objeto, permitindo, finalmente, o comportamento intencional e o pensamento inventivo.

side-chain t., t. da cadeia lateral; Ehrlich postulou que as células continham extensões superficiais ou cadeias laterais (haptóforos) que se ligam aos determinantes antigênicos de uma toxina (toxóforos); após estimulação de uma célula, os haptóforos são liberados na circulação e transformam-se em anticorpos. VER TAMBÉM receptor. SIN Ehrlich postulate.

somatic mutation t. of cancer, t. da mutação somática do câncer; t. segundo a qual o câncer é causado por uma mutação ou mutações nas células do corpo (em contraposição às células germinativas), especialmente mutações não-letais associadas a aumento da proliferação das células mutantes.

Spitzer t., t. de Spitzer; interpretação da divisão do coração de embriões de mamíferos baseando-se, primariamente, em recapitulações do padrão estrutural do adulto de formas inferiores; mais freqüentemente citada em relação à divisão do tronco arterial para formar a aorta ascendente e o tronco pulmonar, que é obtida pelo desenvolvimento pilogenético dos pulmões.

stringed instrument t., t. do instrumento de cordas; t. não mais sustentável que afirma que, na produção da voz humana, as cordas vocais funcionam de modo semelhante às cordas de um instrumento musical de cordas.

surface tension t. of narcosis, t. de tensão superficial da narcose; t. segundo a qual as substâncias que reduzem a tensão superficial da água penetram mais facilmente na célula e causam narcose ao diminuírem o metabolismo.

telephone t., t. do telefone; t. da percepção do timbre que afirma que a cóclea não possui a faculdade de análise do som, mas que a freqüência dos impulsos transmitidos sobre as fibras nervosas auditivas corresponde à freqüência das vibrações sonoras, constituindo a única base para discriminação do timbre; t. não mais sustentável. VER TAMBÉM traveling wave t.

thermodynamic t. of narcosis, t. termodinâmica da narcose; t. segundo a qual a interposição de moléculas de narcóticos na fase celular não-aquosa causa alterações que interferem na facilitação da troca iônica.

traveling wave t., t. da onda propagada; t. geralmente aceita segundo a qual uma onda se propaga da base até o ápice da membrana basilar da cóclea em resposta à estimulação acústica, e o local de deslocamento máximo da membrana basilar depende da freqüência do tom estimulante, em que as freqüências mais altas causam deslocamento máximo próximo à base e as freqüências mais baixas, deslocamento máximo próximo ao ápice.

van't Hoff t., t. de van't Hoff; t. segundo a qual substâncias em solução diluída obedecem às leis dos gases. Cf. van't Hoff *law.*

Warburg t., t. de Warburg; t. segundo a qual o desenvolvimento de câncer é devido a uma lesão irreversível do mecanismo respiratório das células, levando à multiplicação seletiva de células com aumento do metabolismo glicolítico, tanto aeróbico quanto anaeróbico.

Wollaston t., t. de Wollaston; t. segundo a qual a semidecussação dos nervos ópticos no quiasma é comprovada pela hemianopsia homônima observada em lesões cerebrais.

Young-Helmholtz t. of color vision, t. de Young-Helmholtz da visão para cores; t. segundo a qual existem três elementos de percepção da cor na retina: vermelho, verde e azul. A percepção de outras cores origina-se da estimulação combinada desses elementos; a deficiência ou ausência de qualquer um desses elementos resulta na incapacidade de perceber aquela cor e numa percepção incorreta de qualquer outra cor da qual faz parte. SIN Helmholtz t. of color vision.

the·o·ther·a·py (thē-ō-thār'ă-pē). Teoterapia; tratamento de doença por oração ou exercícios religiosos. [G. *theos,* deus, + *therapeia,* terapia]

thèque (tek). Teca; ninho ou agregação de nevócitos na epiderme. [Fr. pequena caixa]

ther·a·peu·sis (thār-ă-pū'sis). Terapêutica, terapia **1.** SIN therapeutics. **2.** SIN therapy.

ther·a·peu·tic (ther-ă-pū'tik). Terapêutico; relativo à terapêutica ou ao tratamento ou cura de um distúrbio ou doença. [G. *therapeutikos*]

ther·a·peu·tics (thār-ă-pū'tiks). Terapêutica; o ramo prático da medicina relacionado ao tratamento de doença ou distúrbio. SIN therapeusis (1), therapia (2). [G. *therapeutikē,* prática médica]

 ray t., radioterapia; termo obsoleto para radiotherapy.

 suggestive t., t. sugestiva; tratamento de doença ou distúrbio por meio da sugestão.

ther·a·peu·tist (thār-ă-pū'tist). Terapeuta; termo antigo para referir-se a um especialista em terapêutica.

the·ra·pia (thā-ră-pē'ă). Terapia. **1.** SIN therapy. **2.** SIN therapeutics. [L. do G. *therapeia,* terapia]

 t. mag'na sterili'sans, t. esterilizante maciça; conceito de Ehrlich de que uma doença infecciosa, especialmente causada por protozoários, pode ser curada por uma grande dose de um remédio apropriado, grande o suficiente para esterilizar todos os tecidos e destruir os microrganismos neles contidos.

ther·a·pist (thār'ă-pist). Terapeuta; indivíduo profissionalmente treinado e/ou capacitado na prática de um tipo específico de terapia.

THERAPY

ther·a·py (ther-ă-pē). Terapia. **1.** O tratamento de doença ou distúrbio por qualquer método. VER TAMBÉM therapeutics. **2.** Em psiquiatria e psicologia clínica, forma abreviada para psicoterapia. VER TAMBÉM psychotherapy, psychiatry, psychology, psychoanalysis. SIN therapeusis (2), therapia (1). [G. *therapeia,* tratamento médico]

 alkali t., t. com álcalis. VER alkalitherapy.

 analytic t., t. analítica; abreviatura de psychoanalytic t. (t. psicanalítica).

 anticoagulant t., t. anticoagulante; o uso de agentes anticoagulantes para reduzir ou impedir a coagulação intravascular ou intracardíaca.

 antisense t., t. com DNA anti-sentido; uso do DNA anti-sentido para inibição da transcrição ou tradução de um gene ou produto gênico específico para fins terapêuticos.

 autoserum t., t. com auto-soro; t. com soro obtido do próprio sangue do paciente.

 aversion t., t. de aversão; forma de t. comportamental que associa um estímulo desagradável a comportamento(s) indesejável(is) de modo que o paciente aprende a evitá-lo(s). VER TAMBÉM aversive *training.*

 behavior t., t. comportamental; ramo da psicoterapia que envolve o uso de procedimentos e técnicas associados à pesquisa nos campos do condicionamento e do aprendizado para o tratamento de várias condições psicológicas; distinta da psicoterapia, visto que sintomas específicos (p. ex., fobia, enurese, pressão arterial elevada) são selecionados como alvo para modificação, empregando-se então intervenções planejadas ou etapas de t. para extinguir ou modificar esses sinais e sintomas, com monitorização contínua e quantitativa do progresso das mudanças. VER systematic *desensitization.* SIN conditioning t.

 client-centered t., t. centrada no cliente; sistema de psicoterapia não-diretiva baseada na suposição de que o cliente (paciente) possui os recursos internos para melhorar e encontra-se na melhor posição para resolver sua própria disfunção de personalidade, contanto que o terapeuta consiga estabelecer uma atmosfera permissiva, de aceitação genuína, em que o cliente se sente livre para discutir problemas e obter uma compreensão para atingir a auto-realização.

 cognitive t., t. cognitiva; qualquer uma de várias técnicas em psicoterapia que utiliza a autodescoberta orientada, imageamento, auto-instrução, modelagem simbólica e formas relacionadas de cognições explicitamente produzidas como principal forma de tratamento.

 collapse t., t. de colapso; o t. cirúrgico da tuberculose pulmonar, em que o pulmão doente é colocado, total ou parcialmente, temporária ou permanentemente, num estado respiratório não-funcional de retração e imobilização. Hoje em dia, raramente utilizada.

 conditioning t., t. do condicionamento. SIN behavior t.

 conjoint t., t. conjunta; tipo de t. em que o terapeuta vê os dois parceiros juntos ou os pais e a criança ou outros parceiros em sessões conjuntas.

 convulsive t., t. convulsiva. SIN electroshock t.

 cytoreductive t., t. citorredutora; t. com a intenção de reduzir o número de células numa lesão, geralmente maligna.

 depot t., t. de depósito; injeção de uma droga juntamente com uma substância que retarda a liberação e prolonga a ação da droga.

diathermic t., t. diatérmica; tratamento de várias lesões por diatermia.
directly observed t., t. diretamente observada; monitorização visual, por um profissional de saúde, da ingestão de medicações pelo paciente para garantir a sua adesão ao tratamento em esquemas difíceis ou a longo prazo, como no tratamento oral da tuberculose; aspecto controverso de alguns programas da OMS.
electroconvulsive t. (ECT), t. eletroconvulsiva. SIN electroshock t.
electroshock t. (ECT), t. por eletrochoque; forma de t. de transtornos mentais em que são produzidas convulsões pela passagem de uma corrente elétrica através do cérebro. SIN convulsive t., electroconvulsive t.
electrotherapeutic sleep t., t. do sono eletroterapêutico; tratamento mediante indução do sono através de estimulação elétrica não-convulsiva do cérebro.

estrogen replacement t., t. de reposição com estrogênio; administração de hormônios sexuais após menopausa ou ooforectomia. SIN hormone replacement t.

A administração de estrogênio após a menopausa natural ou cirúrgica reverte a vaginite atrófica, alivia a instabilidade vasomotora ("fogachos"), reduz os níveis de LDL-colesterol, eleva o HDL-colesterol, diminui o risco de osteoporose e câncer colorretal e pode retardar o início e a progressão do parkinsonismo, da demência de Alzheimer e do diabetes melito tipo 2. Estudos de observação constataram taxas mais baixas de coronariopatia em mulheres após a menopausa em uso de estrogênio; todavia, os estudos clínicos realizados não confirmaram esse efeito. Um grande estudo clínico aleatorizado de mulheres pós-menopáusicas com coronariopatia estabelecida não mostrou nenhuma diferença entre mulheres em uso de estrogênio-progestogênio e controles quanto à incidência de infarto do miocárdio fatal e não-fatal, insuficiência cardíaca congestiva, acidente vascular cerebral e taxa total de mortalidade. Em estudos limitados, o estrogênio reduziu a massa ventricular esquerda mais significativamente do que o placebo em mulheres pós-menopáusicas hipertensas submetidas a terapia anti-hipertensiva convencional. A opinião médica quanto à segurança da reposição de estrogênio permanece dividida. Embora alguns estudos tenham indicado um aumento na incidência de câncer de mama, a maioria das evidências não corrobora essa conclusão. Entretanto, a administração de estrogênio aumenta efetivamente o risco de câncer endometrial. A administração combinada cíclica de progestogênio com estrogênio diariamente provavelmente reduz esse risco (além de restabelecer os ciclos menstruais), porém desconhece-se a segurança do tratamento combinado a longo prazo com estrogênio e progestogênio em mulheres pós-menopáusicas. As mulheres mais jovens que tomam essa combinação em doses mais altas (em anticoncepcionais orais) correm risco aumentado de hipertensão e doença tromboembólica. Alguns progestogênios podem anular os efeitos favoráveis do estrogênio sobre as lipoproteínas. O raloxifeno, um modulador seletivo dos receptores de estrogênio (SERM, *selective estrogen receptor modulator*), provavelmente não aumenta o risco de câncer endometrial, mas também não alivia os fogachos, nem inibe a atividade osteoclástica ou controla o colesterol, bem como o estrogênio. Como alternativa para a via oral, o estrogênio pode ser administrado na forma de discos transdérmicos, isoladamente ou em combinação com progestogênio.

extended family t., t. familiar ampliada; tipo de t. familiar que envolve membros da família fora do núcleo familiar e que estão estreitamente associados a ela e a afetam.
family t., t. familiar; tipo de psicoterapia em grupo em que uma família em conflito encontra-se como um grupo com o terapeuta e explora suas relações e processos; concentra-se na resolução de interações atuais entre membros, mais do que em cada membro individualmente.
fast-neutron radiation t., t. de radiação com nêutrons rápidos; radioterapia utilizando nêutrons de alta energia de ciclotrons ou aceleradores de prótons.
fever t., t. por febre. VER pyrotherapy.
foreign protein t., t. com proteína estranha. SIN protein shock t.
functional orthodontic t., t. ortodôntica funcional. SIN functional jaw *orthopedics*.

gene t., t. gênica; alteração do DNA somático ou de linhagem germinativa para correção ou prevenção de doenças; o processo de introduzir um gene artificialmente no genoma de um organismo para corrigir um defeito genético ou de acrescentar uma nova propriedade ou função biológica com potencial terapêutico.

Na terapia gênica somática, são introduzidas seqüências funcionais de DNA em células que carecem de um gene específico ou que possuem uma versão defeituosa dele. Os vetores incluem vírus de replicação deficiente, lipossomas e plasmídios. Para transferência de material genético por infecção viral (denominada transdução), os vírus são particularmente apropriados como vetores, visto que seu RNA, convertido em DNA pela transcriptase reversa, torna-se parte do genoma da célula infectada. São também utilizados adenovírus e herpesvírus. Foram feitos progressos no tratamento de diversos distúrbios hereditários, incluindo doença por imunodeficiência combinada grave, fibrose cística e hemofilia B. A terapia gênica possui várias aplicações em oncologia, incluindo transdução, nas células tumorais malignas, de genes que codificam citocinas ou fatores de co-ativação para aumentar as respostas antitumorais do hospedeiro, e transferência de genes supressores tumorais, em particular o p53 (o gene que mais comumente sofre mutação em cânceres humanos), com o objetivo de aumentar a sensibilidade das células malignas a agentes quimioterápicos. A terapia de linhagem germinativa introduz genes específicos diretamente no DNA do espermatozóide, ovo ou embrião, produzindo alterações hereditárias do genoma. Já foram criadas quimeras através da introdução de DNA humano em células germinativas de porcos, camundongos e outros animais de laboratório, porém os experimentos com células germinativas humanas estão sob interdição federal.

geriatric t., t. geriátrica. SIN gerontotherapy.
gestalt t., terapia gestáltica; tipo de psicoterapia utilizada com indivíduos ou grupos que enfatiza o tratamento da pessoa como um todo: as partes do componente biológico do indivíduo e seu funcionamento orgânico, configuração perceptiva e inter-relações com o mundo externo; concentra-se na consciência sensorial das experiências imediatas da pessoa, mais do que em lembranças do passado ou expectativas do futuro, empregando a dramatização e outras técnicas para promover o crescimento e o desenvolvimento do indivíduo em seu pleno potencial.
heterovaccine t., t. com heterovacina; t. com vacina obtida de organismos não diretamente relacionados com o distúrbio que está sendo tratado.
hormone replacement t. (HRT), t. de reposição hormonal. SIN estrogen replacement t.
hyperbaric oxygen t., t. com oxigênio hiperbárico; t. em que o oxigênio é fornecido em uma câmara hermeticamente fechada numa pressão ambiental maior do que 1 atmosfera. VER TAMBÉM hyperbaric *oxygenation*.
implosive t., t. implosiva; tipo de t. comportamental que utiliza implosão.
individual t., t. individual. SIN dyadic *psychotherapy*.
inhalation t., inaloterapia; uso terapêutico de gases ou aerossóis por inalação.
insulin coma t., t. do coma insulínico. VER insulin coma *treatment*.
interstitial t., t. intersticial; radioterapia por meio de sementes ou agulhas radioativas implantadas diretamente nos tecidos a serem irradiados.
intralesional t., t. intralesional; t. por injeção diretamente numa lesão, como as injeções de corticosteróides em lesões cutâneas.
maintenance drug t., farmacoterapia de manutenção; em quimioterapia, administração sistemática em um nível que mantém a proteção contra a exacerbação.
marital t., t. conjugal. SIN marriage t.
marriage t., t. do casamento; tipo de t. familiar que envolve marido e mulher e concentra-se na relação conjugal, na medida em que afeta as personalidades, os comportamentos e as psicopatologias individuais dos parceiros; o fundamento lógico desse método é a suposição de que os processos emocionais ou psicopatológicos dentro da estrutura familiar e na matriz social do casamento perpetuam estruturas da personalidade patológica individual, que encontram expressão no casamento conturbado e são agravadas por retroalimentação entre parceiros. SIN marital t.
microwave t., t. por microondas. SIN microkymatotherapy.
milieu t., t. ambiental; t. psiquiátrica que emprega a manipulação do ambiente social para o benefício do paciente; p. ex., uso das experiências diárias de vida dos pacientes numa enfermaria como estímulos para discussão e mudança terapêutica.
myofunctional t., t. miofuncional; terapia da maloclusão e de outros distúrbios dentários e da fala, que utiliza exercícios musculares da língua e dos lábios; com mais freqüência, tem por objetivo alterar um padrão de deglutição impulsionado pela língua.
nonspecific t., t. inespecífica; t. que não está relacionada diretamente com a causa; p. ex., a injeção de uma proteína estranha, vacina tifóide etc., para induzir febre no tratamento de determinadas doenças, especialmente aquelas de natureza parassifilítica. SIN phlogotherapy.
occupational t. (OT), t. ocupacional; uso terapêutico de auto-assistência, trabalho e atividades recreativas para aumentar a função independente, estimular o desenvolvimento e evitar a incapacidade; pode incluir a adaptação de tarefas ou do ambiente para obter uma independência máxima e qualidade de vida ótima.
orthodontic t., t. ortodôntica. VER orthodontics.
orthomolecular t., t. ortomolecular; t. que tem por objetivo remediar deficiências em qualquer um dos constituintes químicos normais do organismo.
oxygen t., oxigenioterapia; t. em que é fornecida uma concentração aumentada de oxigênio para respiração através de cateter nasal, tenda, câmara ou máscara.
parenteral t., t. parenteral; t. introduzida habitualmente por agulha através de alguma via diferente do canal alimentar.

photodynamic t., t. fotodinâmica. SIN photoradiation.
photoradiation t., t. fotorradioterapia. SIN photoradiation.
physical t. (PT), fisioterapia; **(1)** t. da dor, da doença ou de lesões por meios físicos. SIN physiotherapy. **(2)** a profissão relacionada com a promoção da saúde, com a prevenção de incapacidades físicas, com a avaliação e reabilitação de indivíduos incapacitados por dor, doença ou lesão, e com o tratamento por medidas de fisioterapia, em oposição a medidas clínicas, cirúrgicas ou radiológicas.
plasma t., t. plasmática; tratamento com plasma.
play t., ludoterapia, tipo de terapia utilizada em crianças, em que elas podem expressar ou revelar seus problemas e suas fantasias brincando com bonecas ou outros brinquedos, desenhando etc.
proliferation t., t. de proliferação; reabilitação de uma estrutura incompetente (ligamento ou tendão) por proliferação induzida de novas células; efetuada através da injeção de uma substância irritante no ligamento frouxo ou tendão, com conseqüente formação de cicatriz e contratura, que servem para retesar o ligamento ou tendão à medida que o tecido cicatricial prolifera; raramente utilizada.
protein shock t., t. do choque protéico; injeção de proteína estranha para induzir febre como meio de tratamento de determinadas doenças. SIN foreign protein t.
psychedelic t., t. psicodélica; terapia psiquiátrica que utiliza drogas psicodélicas.
psychoanalytic t., t. psicanalítica. SIN psychoanalysis (1).
pulse t., t. em pulsos; curso intenso e de curta duração de farmacoterapia, geralmente administrada a intervalos semanais ou mensais; freqüentemente utilizada na quimioterapia de processos malignos.
quadrangular t., t. quadrangular; terapia do casamento envolvendo o marido e a mulher e seus respectivos terapeutas.
radiation t., radioterapia; tratamento com raios X ou radionuclídios. VER radiation *oncology*.
radium beam t., t. com feixe de rádio. SIN teleradium t.
rational t., t. racional; procedimentos terapêuticos introduzidos por Albert Ellis e baseados na premissa de que a ausência de informação ou padrões de pensamento ilógico constituem causas básicas das dificuldades de um paciente; pressupõe-se que o paciente possa ser assistido para superar seus problemas através de uma abordagem direta, prescritiva e de aconselhamento pelo terapeuta.
reflex t., t. reflexa; t. de alguma condição mórbida pela excitação de uma ação reflexa, como no tratamento domiciliar da epistaxe mediante aplicação de um pedaço de gelo à coluna cervical. SIN reflexotherapy.
replacement t., t. de reposição; t. que tem por objetivo compensar uma ausência ou deficiência como resultado de nutrição inadequada, determinadas disfunções (p. ex., hipossecreção glandular) ou perdas (p. ex., hemorragia); a reposição pode ser fisiológica ou pode incluir a administração de um substituto (p. ex., estrogênio sintético no lugar do estradiol).
respiratory t., t. respiratória; **(1)** t. de várias condições relacionadas às vias respiratórias, como aumento das secreções e broncospasmo; **(2)** a profissão especializada na administração de qualquer uma das terapias relacionadas com o sistema respiratório e a respiração.
root canal t., tratamento de canal; tratamento dentário para lesão da polpa mediante remoção da polpa e esterilização e preenchimento do canal radicular.
rotation t., terapia de rotação; teleterapia em que se obtém uma distribuição de uma dose de radiação desejável ao se submeter o paciente a rotação ou através de uma máquina em torno de um eixo passando pelo centro do tumor.
salvage t., t. de salvamento. SIN salvage *chemotherapy.*
sclerosing t., t. esclerosante. SIN sclerotherapy.
serum t., soroterapia. SIN serotherapy.
shock t., t. por choque. VER shock *treatment.*
social t., t. social; t. de reabilitação psiquiátrica para melhorar o funcionamento social de um paciente.
social network t., t. de estrutura social; tipo de t. que envolve a reunião de todas as pessoas emocional e funcionalmente importantes para o paciente com o propósito de efetuar uma mudança comportamental no paciente.
solar t., t. solar; tratamento de doença por exposição à luz solar. SIN solar treatment.
specific t., t. específica; t. orientada para a(s) causa(s) de um processo mórbido, em oposição à terapia sintomática.
substitution t., t. de substituição; t. de reposição, sobretudo quando a reposição não é fisiológica, mas inclui a administração de um substituto.
substitutive t., t. substitutiva. SIN allopathy.
teleradium t., t. com telerrádio; uso terapêutico de raios de rádio, cuja origem consiste numa determinada quantidade de rádio situada a uma distância do paciente. SIN radium beam t.
thrombolytic t., t. trombolítica; administração intravenosa de um agente com a finalidade de dissolver um coágulo que está causando isquemia aguda, como no infarto do miocárdio, no acidente vascular cerebral e na trombose venosa

ou arterial periférica. Os agentes trombolíticos degradam os coágulos de fibrina ao ativarem o plasminogênio, um modulador de ocorrência natural dos processos hemostáticos e trombóticos. O plasminogênio, que é sintetizado pelo fígado, está presente no sangue circulante e liga-se às plaquetas, ao endotélio e à fibrina. Nos locais de lesão vascular com formação de trombo, o ativador do plasminogênio tecidual (TPA), produzido pelas células endoteliais, também liga-se à fibrina e converte o plasminogênio ligado à fibrina em plasmina através da clivagem da ligação arginina-valina na posição 560–561 do plasminogênio. A conseqüente lise do coágulo resulta da degradação dos filamentos de fibrina, bem como das glicoproteínas necessárias para a adesão e agregação plaquetárias. Os agentes trombolíticos de uso atual imitam os efeitos do TPA natural. Estes incluem a alteplase, um TPA produzido pela tecnologia do DNA recombinante; a reteplase, uma variante da molécula de TPA, também obtida por engenharia genética; a uroquinase, uma proteína tecidual derivada de culturas de células renais humanas; a estreptoquinase, um produto derivado de estreptococos β-hemolíticos que catalisa a conversão do plasminogênio em plasmina; e a anistreplase, uma forma inativa de plasminogênio que se liga à estreptoquinase e sofre desacilação após a sua administração, resultando em ativação persistente do plasminogênio. Os dois últimos produtos são potencialmente antigênicos e podem causar reações de hipersensibilidade sistêmicas. VER TAMBÉM tissue plasminogen *activator*.

A t. trombolítica reduz a taxa de mortalidade hospitalar e de 1 ano do infarto agudo do miocárdio (IAM) em 20–40% quando administrada em tempo hábil (isto é, nos primeiros 100 minutos); pode-se obter algum benefício até mesmo após 6–12 horas. Cerca da metade dos indivíduos tratados para IAM com agente trombolítico apresenta desobstrução das artérias coronárias após 90 minutos. A angioplastia coronária transluminal percutânea de emergência pode proporcionar melhores índices de sobrevida, mas só pode ser efetuada em situações nas quais a derivação da artéria coronária de emergência é possível em caso de fracasso. Algumas vezes, a estreptoquinase tem sido preferida ao TPA no IAM, em virtude de seu menor custo. Todavia, uma análise exaustiva mostrou que o uso do TPA é custo-efetivo, sobretudo no IAM de parede anterior. O fato de os agentes trombolíticos ativarem as plaquetas anula parcialmente sua efetividade. Em estudos clínicos preliminares, a combinação de heparina e do inibidor plaquetário abciximab com TPA aumentou bastante a sua capacidade de restaurar a perviedade arterial no IAM. No acidente vascular cerebral (AVC) isquêmico, foi constatado que a administração de TPA nas primeiras 3 horas melhora o resultado global em 90 dias. A utilidade da t. trombolítica no AVC é limitada pela dificuldade de excluir a possibilidade de acidente vascular cerebral hemorrágico e o risco de hemorragia como efeito colateral da terapia. Dos cinco estudos clínicos realizados para avaliar o uso dos agentes trombolíticos em pacientes com AVC, quatro foram interrompidos prematuramente decorrente da excessiva mortalidade nos grupos de tratamento. Apenas o TPA é atualmente recomendado no tratamento do acidente vascular cerebral. Além do AVC e do infarto do miocárdio, a terapia trombolítica tem sido utilizada na embolia pulmonar, na trombose venosa profunda e na oclusão arterial periférica. A terapia trombolítica na oclusão aguda de uma artéria do membro inferior (ou enxerto com derivação arterial) pode evitar a necessidade de cirurgia em muitos pacientes, sem aumentar a taxa de mortalidade ou de amputação. Ocorre recanalização em até 80% dos pacientes. A ocorrência de hemorragia significativa constitui o principal risco da terapia trombolítica. A terapia trombolítica está contra-indicada na presença de hemorragia ativa ou recente, cirurgia recente, neoplasia intracraniana ou traumatismo cranioencefálico recente, dissecção da aorta, pericardite aguda, reanimação cardiopulmonar prolongada ou traumática, gravidez ou sensibilidade ao agente específico.

thyroid t., t. tireóidea; tratamento do hipotireoidismo.
Time-Line t., técnica baseada nos princípios de programação neurolingüística para liberar emoções negativas e rever decisões limitadoras, que orientam o cliente, no estado dissociado, a retornar a eventos passados significativos com novos recursos, de modo que as emoções negativas possam ser liberadas ou as decisões limitadoras reavaliadas. VER TAMBÉM dissociation (4).
total push t., terapia de *push* total; aplicação de todas as terapias disponíveis no tratamento de um paciente psiquiátrico em hospital.
ultrasonic t., t. ultra-sônica; tratamento para doença musculoesquelética que utiliza ondas de ultra-som para produzir calor.
viral t., t. viral; uso de partículas virais geneticamente alteradas para introduzir genes em locais específicos com propósito terapêutico.
x-ray t., t. com raios X; radioterapia que utiliza raios X; termo algumas vezes empregado ironicamente para referir-se ao uso excessivo de radiação diagnóstica.

ther·en·ceph·a·lous (thēr′en-sef′ă-lŭs, ther-). Terencéfalo; designa um crânio em que o ângulo no hórmio, formado por linhas que convergem a partir do ínio e do násio, mede 116°-129°. [G. *thēr*, animal selvagem, + *enkephalos*, cérebro]

the·ri·a·ca (thē-rī'a-ka). Teríaca; mistura que contém grande número de ingredientes, utilizada na Idade Média, e que se acreditava possuir poderes antídotos e curativos em grau quase milagroso. [L. antídoto para picada de cobra, do G. *thēriakos*, relativo a animais selvagens]

△ **therio-.** Terio-. Animais. [G. *thēr, thērion*, animal]

the·ri·o·mor·phism (thēr'ē-ō-mōr'fizm). Teriomorfismo; atribuição de características animais a seres humanos. Cf. anthropomorphism. [therio- + *morphē*, forma]

therm. Therm; unidade de calor utilizada indiscriminadamente para: 1) uma pequena caloria, 2) uma grande caloria, 3) 1.000 grandes calorias, 4) 100.000 unidades térmicas britânicas. [G. *thermē*, calor]

△ **therm-.** Term-. VER thermo-.

ther·ma·co·gen·e·sis (ther'ma-kō-jen'ē-sis). Termacogênese; elevação da temperatura corporal por ação farmacológica. [G. *thermē*, calor, + *pharmakon*, droga, + *genesis*, produção]

ther·mal (ther'mal). Termal; relativo a calor.

ther·mal·ge·sia (ther-mal-jē'zē-a). Termalgesia; elevada sensibilidade ao calor; dor causada por leve grau de calor. SIN thermoalgesia. [therm- + G. *algēsis*, sensação de dor]

ther·mal·gia (ther-mal'jē-a). Termalgia; dor em queimação. VER TAMBÉM causalgia. [therm- + G. *algos*, dor]

therm·an·al·ge·sia (therm'an-al-jē'zē-a). Termanalgesia. SIN thermoanesthesia. [therm- + analgesia]

therm·an·es·the·sia (therm'an-es-thē'zē-a). Termanestesia. SIN thermoanesthesia.

ther·ma·tol·o·gy (ther-ma-tol'ō-jē). Termatologia; o ramo da terapêutica relacionado com a aplicação de calor. VER TAMBÉM thermotherapy. [therm- + G. *logos*, estudo]

ther·me·lom·e·ter (ther-mē-lom'ē-ter). Termelômetro; termômetro elétrico, especialmente utilizado para registro de pequenas variações de temperatura. [therm- + electric + G. *metron*, medida]

therm·es·the·sia (therm-es-thē'zē-a). Termestesia. SIN thermoesthesia.

therm·es·the·si·om·e·ter (therm'es-thē-zē-om'ē-ter). Termestesiômetro. SIN thermoesthesiometer.

therm·is·tor (ther'mis-ter, -tōr). Termistor; dispositivo para determinar a temperatura; pode ser também utilizado para monitorizar o controle da temperatura. [G. *thermē*, calor]

△ **thermo-, therm-.** Termo-, term-. Calor. [G. *thermē*, calor; *thermos*, morno ou quente]

ther·mo·ac·id·o·philes (ther'mō-as-id-ō-filz). Termoacidófilos; Archaebacteria que crescem em fontes sulfurosas quentes em pH baixo.

ther·mo·al·ge·sia (ther'mō-al-jē'zē-a). Termoalgesia. SIN thermalgesia.

ther·mo·an·al·ge·sia (ther'mō-an'al-jē'zē-a). Termoanalgesia. SIN thermoanesthesia.

ther·mo·an·es·the·sia (ther'mō-an-es-thē'zē-a). Termoanestesia; perda da sensação de temperatura ou da capacidade de distinguir entre calor e frio; insensibilidade ao calor ou a mudanças de temperatura. SIN thermanalgesia, thermanesthesia, thermoanalgesia. [thermo- + G. *an-*, priv. + *aisthēsis*, sensação]

ther·mo·cau·ter·ec·to·my (ther'mō-kaw-ter-ek'tō-mē). Termocauterectomia; remoção de tecido por termocautério. [thermocautery + G. *ektomē*, excisão]

ther·mo·cau·tery (ther'mō-kaw'ter-ē). Termocautério; uso de cautério, como um eletrocautério. [thermo- + G. *kautērion*, ferro aquecido (cautério)]

ther·mo·chem·is·try (ther-mō-kem'is-trē). Termoquímica; a inter-relação da ação química e do calor.

ther·mo·chro·ic (ther-mō-krō'ik). Termocróico. 1. Relativo a termocrose. 2. Que exerce uma ação seletiva sobre os raios de calor.

ther·moch·ro·ism (ther-mok'rō-izm). Termocroísmo. SIN thermochrosis.

ther·mo·chrose (ther'mō-krōz). Termocrose; a propriedade que possui os raios térmicos de reflexão, refração e absorção, semelhante à dos raios luminosos. SIN thermochrosy. [thermo- + G. *chrōsis*, que colore]

ther·mo·chro·sis (ther-mō-krō'sis). Termocrose; a ação seletiva de determinadas substâncias sobre o calor radiante, absorvendo alguns dos raios, refletindo ou transmitindo outros. SIN thermochroism. [thermo- + G. *chrōsis*, que colore]

ther·moch·ro·sy (ther-mok'rō-sē). Termocrosia. SIN thermochrose.

ther·mo·co·ag·u·la·tion (ther'mō-kō-ag-ū-lā'shŭn). Termocoagulação; o processo de converter um tecido em gel pelo calor. SIN endocoagulation.

ther·mo·cou·ple (ther-mō-kŭp'l). Termopar; dispositivo para medir pequenas mudanças de temperatura, que consiste em dois fios de metais diferentes, sendo um fio mantido em determinada temperatura baixa, estando o outro no tecido ou em outro material cuja temperatura deve ser medida; estabelece-se uma corrente termoelétrica que é medida por um potenciômetro. SIN thermojunction.

ther·mo·cur·rent (ther-mō-ker'ent). Termocorrente; corrente de termoeletricidade.

ther·mo·dif·fu·sion (ther'mō-di-fū'zhŭn). Termodifusão; difusão de fluidos, gasosos ou líquidos, influenciada pela temperatura do fluido.

ther·mo·di·lu·tion (ther'mō-di-loo'shŭn). Termodiluição; redução da temperatura num líquido que ocorre quando este é introduzido em um líquido mais frio; o volume deste último líquido pode ser calculado a partir do grau de elevação de sua temperatura.

ther·mo·du·ric (ther-mō-doo'rik). Termodúrico; resistente aos efeitos da exposição a altas temperaturas. Termo empregado especialmente para referir-se a microrganismos. [thermo- + L. *durus*, duro, resistente]

ther·mo·dy·nam·ics (ther'mō-dī-nam'iks). Termodinâmica. 1. Ramo da ciência físico-química relacionado com o calor e a energia e suas interconversões envolvendo o trabalho mecânico. 2. O estudo do fluxo de calor. [thermo- + G. *dynamis*, força]

ther·mo·e·lec·tric (ther'mō-ē-lek'trik). Termoelétrico; relativo à termoeletricidade.

ther·mo·e·lec·tric·i·ty (ther'mō-ē-lek-tris'i-tē). Termoeletricidade; corrente elétrica gerada por uma termopilha.

ther·mo·es·the·sia (ther'mō-es-thē'zē-a). Termoestesia; capacidade de distinguir diferenças de temperatura. SIN temperature sense, thermal sense, thermic sense, thermesthesia. [thermo- + G. *aisthēsis*, sensação]

ther·mo·es·the·si·om·e·ter (ther'mō-es-thē'zē-om'ē-ter). Termoestesiômetro; instrumento para testar a sensação térmica, que consiste em um disco metálico com termômetro fixado, através do qual pode ser conhecida a temperatura exata do disco no momento da aplicação. SIN thermesthesiometer. [thermo- + G. *aisthēsis*, sensação, + *metron*, medida]

ther·mo·ex·ci·to·ry (ther'mō-ek-sī'tō-rē). Termoexcitatório; que estimula a produção de calor.

ther·mo·gen·e·sis (ther-mō-jen'ē-sis). Termogênese; a produção de calor; especificamente, o processo fisiológico de produção de calor no organismo. [thermo- + G. *genesis*, produção]

nonshivering t., t. sem tremor; t. resultante dos efeitos dos neurotransmissores do sistema nervoso simpático, epinefrina e norepinefrina, que atuam ao aumentar o metabolismo celular nos músculos esqueléticos e em outros tecidos, com conseqüente aumento da produção de calor. Numa forma especializada de tecido adiposo, a gordura marrom, o efeito dos neurotransmissores simpáticos consiste em aumentar a taxa de fosforilação oxidativa não-acoplada pelas mitocôndrias, resultando em produção de calor sem formação de ATP.

shivering t., t. com tremor; t. resultante do aumento do metabolismo dos músculos esqueléticos em conseqüência de tremor.

ther·mo·ge·net·ic, ther·mo·gen·ic (ther'mō-je-net'ik, -jen'ik). Termogenético, termogênico. 1. Relativo à termogênese. SIN thermogenous. 2. SIN calorigenic (2).

ther·mo·gen·ics (ther-mō-jen'iks). Termogênica; a ciência da produção de calor.

ther·mo·gen·in (ther-mō-jen'in). Termogenina; proteína encontrada no tecido adiposo marrom que atua como proteína de desacoplamento termogênica da fosforilação oxidativa; permite a termogênese nesse tipo de tecido.

ther·mog·e·nous (ther-moj'ē-nŭs). Termogênico. SIN thermogenetic (1).

ther·mo·gram (ther'mō-gram). Termograma. 1. Mapa da temperatura regional da superfície de uma parte do corpo, obtido por dispositivo sensível a infravermelho; mede o calor radiante e, portanto, o fluxo sangüíneo subcutâneo se o ambiente for constante. 2. Registro feito por um termógrafo. [thermo- + G. *gramma*, escrito]

ther·mo·graph (ther'mō-graf). Termógrafo; instrumento ou aparelho utilizado na produção de um termograma. [thermo- + G. *graphō*, escrever]

ther·mog·ra·phy (ther-mog'ra-fē). Termografia; a técnica de realização de um termograma.

infrared t., t. por infravermelho; medida da temperatura cutânea regional com dispositivo sensível a infravermelho.

liquid crystal t., t. por cristal líquido; medida da temperatura cutânea regional por contato com uma placa flexível contendo cristais líquidos que mudam de cor com as mudanças de temperatura.

ther·mo·hy·per·al·ge·sia (ther'mō-hī'per-al-jē'zē-a). Termoiperalgesia; termalgesia excessiva. [thermo- + G. *hyper*, excesso, + *algēsis*, percepção de dor]

ther·mo·hy·per·es·the·sia (ther'mō-hī'per-es-thē'zē-a). Termoiperestesia; termoestesia ou percepção de temperatura muito aguda; percepção exagerada de calor e de frio. [thermo- + G. *hyper*, excesso, + *aisthēsis*, sensação]

ther·mo·hyp·es·the·sia (ther-mō-hip'es-thē'zē-a, -hī'pes-thē'zē-a). Termoipestesia; percepção diminuída de diferenças de temperatura. SIN thermohypoesthesia. [thermo- + G. *hypo*, sob, + *aisthēsis*, sensação]

ther·mo·hy·po·es·the·sia (ther-mō-hī'pō-es-thē'zē-a). Termoipoestesia. SIN thermohypesthesia.

ther·mo·in·hib·i·to·ry (ther'mō-in-hib'i-tōr-ē). Termoinibitório; que inibe ou interrompe a termogênese.

ther·mo·in·te·gra·tor (ther-mō-in'tĕ-grā-ter, -tōr). Termointegrador; qualquer aparelho para avaliar o aquecimento ou resfriamento adequado de um ambiente, como poderia ser experimentado por um organismo vivo, levando em consideração a radiação e a convecção, bem como a condução. Concebido como modelo térmico de um organismo, o aparelho geralmente consiste num objeto padronizado (p. ex., esfera, cilindro), cuja temperatura superficial é medida enquanto está sendo aquecido internamente numa taxa padronizada.

ther·mo·junc·tion (ther - mō - jŭngk'shŭn). Termojunção. SIN thermocouple.

ther·mo·ker·a·to·plas·ty (ther - mō - ker'ă - tō - plas - tē). Termoceratoplastia; procedimento em que a aplicação de calor produz retração do colágeno do estroma da córnea e achatamento da córnea na área de aplicação do calor. Tende a tornar o olho menos miópico. VER refractive *keratoplasty*. [thermo- + G. *keras*, corno + *plassō*, formar]

ther·mo·la·bile (ther - mō - lā'bil, - bil). Termolábil; sujeito a alteração ou destruição pelo calor. [thermo- + L. *labilis*, perecível]

ther·mol·o·gy (ther - mol'ō - jē). Termologia; a ciência do calor. SIN thermotics. [thermo- + G. *logos*, estudo]

ther·mol·y·sis (ther - mol'i - sis). Termólise. **1.** Perda de calor corporal por evaporação, radiação etc. **2.** Decomposição química pelo calor. [thermo- + G. *lysis*, dissolução]

ther·mo·lyt·ic (ther - mō - lit'ik). Termolítico. **1.** Relativo à termólise. **2.** Agente que promove a dissipação de calor.

ther·mo·mas·sage (ther'mō - mă - sahzh'). Termomassagem; combinação de calor e massagem em fisioterapia.

ther·mom·e·ter (ther - mom'ĕ - ter). Termômetro; instrumento para indicar a temperatura de qualquer substância; com freqüência, consiste num tubo a vácuo hermeticamente fechado que contém mercúrio, que se expande com o calor e se contrai com o frio, produzindo conseqüentemente uma elevação ou queda de seu nível no tubo, cujo grau exato de variação é indicado por uma escala, ou, mais recentemente, dispositivo com sensor eletrônico que fornece a temperatura sem o uso de mercúrio. VER TAMBÉM scale. [thermo- + G. *metron*, medida]

 air t., t. de ar. VER gas t.
 axilla t., t. axilar; t. colocado no oco axilar, com o braço mantido firmemente de lado. SIN axillary t.
 axillary t., t. axilar. SIN axilla t.
 clinical t., t. clínico; pequeno t. auto-registrador, que consiste num tubo de vidro com escala simples contendo mercúrio, utilizado para medir a temperatura do corpo.
 differential t., t. diferencial. SIN thermoscope.
 gas t., t. gasoso; t. preenchido com ar seco ou com um gás, cuja expansão ou aumento de pressão indica o grau de calor; utilizado para medir temperaturas elevadas.
 resistance t., t. de resistência; aparelho que mede a temperatura pela mudança da resistência elétrica de um fio metálico. SIN resistance pyrometer.
 self-registering t., t. auto-registrador; t. em que a temperatura máxima ou mínima, durante o período de observação, é registrada por meio de um aparelho especial; no t. clínico, apenas a temperatura máxima é registrada, geralmente por uma barra de aço acima da coluna de mercúrio ou por um segmento do mercúrio separado da coluna principal por uma bolha de ar; após o registro da temperatura máxima, a barra ou segmento de mercúrio permanece no lugar à medida que a coluna de mercúrio se contrai.
 spirit t., t. de álcool; t. preenchido com álcool, utilizado para medir graus extremos de frio.
 surface t., t. de superfície; t. na forma de disco ou fita que indica a temperatura da parte da pele à qual é aplicado.
 wet and dry bulb t., t. de bulbo úmido e seco. SIN psychrometer.

ther·mo·met·ric (ther - mō - met'rik). Termométrico; relativo à termometria ou a uma leitura do t.

ther·mom·e·try (ther - mom'ĕ - trē). Termometria; a medida da temperatura. [thermo- + G. *metron*, medida]

ther·mo·neu·ro·sis (ther'mō - noo - rō'sis). Termoneurose; elevação da temperatura do corpo devido à influência emocional.

ther·mo·nu·cle·ar (ther - mō - noo'klē - er). Termonuclear; relativo a reações nucleares produzidas por fusão nuclear (por exemplo, a fusão do hidrogênio ao hélio em temperaturas acima de 100.000.000°C; a reação na "bomba de hidrogênio").

ther·mo·pen·e·tra·tion (ther'mō - pen - ĕ - trā'shŭn). Termopenetração. SIN medical *diathermy*.

ther·mo·phile, ther·mo·phil (ther'mō - fil, - fil). Termófilo; organismo que se desenvolve numa temperatura de 50°C ou mais. [thermo- + G. *phileō*, amar]

ther·mo·phil·ic (ther - mō - fil'ik). Termofílico; relativo a um termófilo.

ther·mo·pho·bia (ther - mō - fō'bē - ă). Termofobia; medo mórbido de calor. [thermo- + G. *phobos*, medo]

ther·mo·phore (ther'mō - fōr). Termóforo. **1.** Arranjo para a aplicação de calor a uma parte; consiste num aquecedor de água, num tubo que conduz a água para uma espiral e outro tubo que conduz de volta ao aquecedor. **2.** Bolsa plana contendo determinados sais que produzem calor quando umedecidos; utilizada como substituto da bolsa de água quente. [thermo- + G. *phoros*, que conduz]

ther·mo·phy·lic (ther - mō - fī'lik). Termofílico; resistente ao calor, designando determinados microrganismos. [thermo- + G. *phylaxis*, proteção]

ther·mo·pile (ther'mō - pīl). Termopilha; bipilha termoelétrica que consiste geralmente numa série de barras de antimônio e bismuto unidas, gerando uma corrente termoelétrica quando as junções são aquecidas; utilizada como termoscópio. SIN thermoelectric pile. [thermo- + pilha]

ther·mo·plac·en·tog·ra·phy (ther'mō - plă - sen - tog'ră - fē). Termoplacentografia; método obsoleto de determinação da posição da placenta mediante detecção de raios infravermelhos a partir das grandes quantidades de sangue que fluem através da placenta [thermo- + L. *placenta*, placenta, + G. *graphō*, escrever]

Ther·mo·plas·ma (ther'mō - plaz'mă). *Thermoplasma*. Gênero de bactérias (ordem Mycoplasmatales) que possuem as mesmas características que os microrganismos do gênero *Mycoplasma*, exceto que os termoplasmas não necessitam de esterol para o seu crescimento, possuem uma temperatura ideal de 55-59°C, apresentam pH ótimo de 1,0-2,0 e reproduzem-se por brotamento. A espécie-tipo é *T. acidophilum*. [thermo- + G. *plasma*, algo formado]
 T. acidoph'ilum, espécie encontrada numa pilha de refundição do carvão que havia sofrido auto-aquecimento; também encontrado em fontes quentes ácidas; trata-se da espécie-tipo do gênero *T*.

ther·mo·plas·ma, pl. **ther·mo·plas·ma·ta** (ther'mō - plaz'mă, - plaz'mah - tă). Termoplasma; termo vernacular utilizado para referir-se a qualquer membro do gênero *Thermoplasma*.

ther·mo·plas·tic (ther - mō - plas'tik). Termoplástico; classificação para materiais que podem tornar-se moles pela aplicação de calor e endurecer com o resfriamento.

ther·mo·ple·gia (ther - mō - plē'jē - ă). Termoplegia; termo raramente utilizado para insolação. [thermo- + G. *plēgē*, golpe]

ther·mo·re·cep·tor (ther'mō - rē - sep'ter, - tor). Termorreceptor; receptor sensível ao calor.

ther·mo·reg·u·la·tion (ther'mō - reg - ū - lā'shŭn). Termorregulação; controle da temperatura, como por um termostato.

ther·mo·reg·u·la·tor (ther - mō - reg'ū - lā - ter, - tor). Termorregulador. SIN thermostat.

ther·mo·scope (ther'mō - skōp). Termoscópio; instrumento para indicar pequenas diferenças de temperatura, sem registrá-las. SIN differential thermometer. [thermo- + G. *skopeō*, ver]

ther·mo·set (ther'mō - set). Termofixo; classificação para materiais que se tornam endurecidos ou curados pela aplicação de calor.

ther·mo·sta·bile, ther·mo·sta·ble (ther - mō - stā'bil, - stā'bl). Termostável; não facilmente sujeito a alteração ou destruição pelo calor. SIN heatstable. [thermo- + L. *stabilis*, estável]

ther·mo·stat (ther'mō - stat). Termostato; aparelho para regulação automática do calor, como numa incubadora. SIN thermoregulator. [thermo- + G. *statos*, parado]

ther·mo·ste·re·sis (ther - mō - stē - rē'sis). Termosterese; a abstração ou privação de calor. [thermo- + G. *sterēsis*, privação, perda]

ther·mo·stro·muhr (ther - mō - strom'oor). Aparelho que consiste num elemento de aquecimento entre dois termopares, que são aplicados à parte externa de um vaso; o fluxo sangüíneo é calculado a partir da diferença nas temperaturas registradas pelos termopares proximal e distal.

ther·mo·sys·tal·tic (ther'mō - sis - tal'tik). Termossistáltico; relativo ao termossistaltismo. [thermo- + G. *systaltikos*, contrátil]

ther·mo·sys·tal·tism (ther - mō - sis'tal - tizm). Termossistaltismo; contração, como a dos músculos, sob a influência do calor. [ver thermosystaltic]

ther·mo·tac·tic, ther·mo·tax·ic (ther - mō - tak'tik, tak'sik). Termotático, termotáxico; relativo à termotaxia.

ther·mo·tax·is (ther - mō - tak'sis). Termotaxia. **1.** Reação do protoplasma vivo ao estímulo térmico. Cf. thermotropism. **2.** Regulação da temperatura do corpo. [thermo- + G. *taxis*, arranjo ordenado]
 negative t., t. negativa; repulsão de uma planta ou de um animal pelo calor.
 positive t., t. positiva; atração de uma planta ou de um animal pelo calor.

ther·mo·ther·a·py (ther'mō - thār'ă - pē). Termoterapia. Tratamento de doença pela aplicação terapêutica de calor. [thermo- + G. *therapeia*, tratamento]

ther·mot·ic (ther - mot'ik). Termótico; relativo à termótica.

ther·mot·ics (ther - mot'iks). Termótica. SIN thermology. [G. *thermotēs*, calor]

ther·mo·to·nom·e·ter (ther - mō - tō - nom'ĕ - ter). Termotonômetro; instrumento para medir o grau de termossistaltismo ou contração muscular sob a influência do calor. [thermo- + G. *tonos*, tônus, tensão, + *metron*, medida]

ther·mot·ro·pism (ther - mot'rō - pizm). Termotropismo; o movimento por uma parte de um organismo (por exemplo, folhas ou caules) aproximando-se ou afastando-se de uma fonte de calor. Cf. thermotaxis. [thermo- + G. *tropē*, uma volta]

the·roid (thē'royd). Teróide; semelhante a um animal quanto aos instintos ou tendências. [G. *thēr*, animal selvagem, + *eidos*, semelhança]

the·rol·o·gy (thē - rol'ō - jē). Terologia; o estudo dos mamíferos. [G. *thēr*, animal selvagem, + *logos*, estudo]

the·sau·ris·mo·sis (thē-saw-riz-mō'sis). Tesaurismose; termo raramente empregado para referir-se a um distúrbio metabólico em que uma substância se acumula ou é armazenada em determinadas células, geralmente em grandes quantidades. [G. *thēsauros*, armazém, depósito, + G. *-osis,* condição]

the·sau·ris·mot·ic (thē'saw-riz-mot'ik). Tesaurismótico; relativo à tesaurismose.

the·sau·ro·sis (thē-saw-rō'sis). Tesaurose; armazenamento anormal ou excessivo de substâncias normais ou estranhas no corpo. [G. *thēsauros*, armazém, depósito]

the·sis, pl. **the·ses** (thē'sis, -sēz). Tese. **1.** Qualquer teoria ou hipótese formulada como base para discussão. **2.** Proposição apresentada pelo candidato para grau de doutorado em algumas universidades, que deve ser corroborada por argumentos contra quaisquer objeções oferecidas. **3.** Ensaio sobre um tópico médico preparado pelo estudante de graduação. [G. colocação, posição, tese]

the·ta (θ, Θ) (thā'ta). Teta. **1.** A oitava letra do alfabeto grego, θ. **2.** O oitavo numa série; indica a posição de um substituinte localizado no oitavo átomo a partir do grupo carboxila ou outro grupo funcional. **3.** Símbolo de ângulo.

the·tins (thē'tinz). Tetinas; compostos de sulfônio metílico, abundantes nas algas marinhas, em que o grupo *S*-metil é "ativo", atuando, portanto, como doadores de metila em algumas plantas; por exemplo, dimetilpropriotetina, $(CH_3)_2S^+\text{–}CH_2\text{–}CH_2\text{–}COO^-$.

THF Abreviatura de tetrahydrofolate (tetraidrofolato). VER 5,6,7,8-tetrahydrofolate dehydrogenase, tetrahydrofolate methyltransferase.

△ **thia-.** Tia-; substituição do carbono por enxofre num anel ou numa cadeia. Cf. thio-. [G. *theion*]

thi·a·ben·da·zole (thī-ă-ben'dă-zōl). Tiabendazol; anti-helmíntico de amplo espectro, especialmente útil contra infecção por *Strongyloides stercoralis* e, com corticosteróides, contra a infecção por *Trichinella*.

thi·a·bu·ta·zide (thī-ă-bū'tă-zīd). Tiabutazida. SIN buthiazide.

thi·a·cet·a·zone (thī-ă-set'ă-zōn, -ă-se'tă-zōn). Tiacetazona. SIN amithiozone.

thi·al·bar·bi·tal (thī-al-bar'bi-tawl). Tialbarbital; tiobarbitúrico de ação ultracurta para indução de anestesia geral por injeção intravenosa; utilizado na forma de sal sódico.

thi·am·bu·to·sine (thī-am-bū'tō-sēn). Tiambutosina; agente anti-hanseníase.

thi·a·min (thī'ă-min). Tiamina; vitamina termolábil e hidrossolúvel presente no leite, na levedura e no germe e casca de cereais; também sintetizada artificialmente; essencial para o crescimento; a deficiência de tiamina está associada ao beribéri e à síndrome de Wernicke-Korsakoff. SIN aneurine, antiberiberi factor, antiberiberi vitamin, antineuritic factor, antineuritic vitamin, thiamine, vitamina B₁. [*thia-* + vitamina]

t. hydrochloride, cloridrato de t.; coenzima utilizada na prevenção do beribéri e de outras condições associadas a uma deficiência de tiamina na dieta. SIN aneurine hydrochloride.

t. mononitrate, mononitrato de t.; possui ação idêntica à do cloridrato de tiamina.

t. pyridinylase, t. piridinilase; enzima que catalisa a transferência de uma piridina ou outras bases na posição da pirimidina na tiamina; por exemplo, a tiamina reagindo com piridina produz heteropiritiamina e 4-metil-5-(2'-hidroxietil)tiazol. SIN pyrimidine transferase, thiaminase I.

t. pyrophosphate (TPP), pirofosfato de t.; o éster difosfórico da tiamina, uma coenzima de várias (des)carboxilases, transcetolases e α-oxoácido desidrogenases. SIN aneurine pyrophosphate, cocarboxylase, diphosphothiamin.

thi·a·mi·nase (thī-am'i-nās). Tiaminase. **1.** Enzima presente na carne de peixe crua que destrói a tiamina e que pode produzir deficiência de tiamina em animais com dieta composta, em grande parte, de peixe cru. **2.** Hidrolase que cliva a tiamina em pirimidina (isto é, 2-metil-4-amino-5-hidroximetilpirimidina) e tiazol (isto é, 4-metil-5-(2'-hidroxietil)tiazol); o componente pirimidina pode aparecer na urina na forma de piramina. SIN t. II.

t. I, t. I. SIN *thiamin* pyridinylase.

t. II, t. II. SIN thiaminase (2).

thi·a·mine (thī'ă-min, -mēn). Tiamina. SIN thiamin.

thi·am·phen·i·col (thī-am-fen'i-kol). Tianfenicol. Antibiótico com usos e toxicidades semelhantes aos do cloranfenicol. SIN thiophenicol.

thi·am·y·lal so·di·um (thī-am'i-lawl). Tiamilal sódico. Barbitúrico de ação curta, preparado como mistura com bicarbonato de sódio, utilizado por via intravenosa para produzir anestesia.

Thi·a·ra (thī-ah'ră). *Thiara.* Gênero disseminado de caramujos operculados (família Thiaridae, subclasse Prosobranchiata) encontrados em águas doces e salobras, principalmente na África tropical e subtropical e na Ásia. O *T. tuberculata* é um dos hospedeiros intermediários iniciais do trematódeo pulmonar humano, *Paragonimus westermani,* e de vários trematódeos heterofídeos transmitidos por peixes de seres humanos e mamíferos que se alimentam de peixe.

thi·a·zides (thī'ă-zīdz). Tiazidas. Forma abreviada de benzothiadiazides.

thi·a·zin (thī'ă-zin). Tiazina; substância original de uma família de corantes azuis biológicos; por exemplo, azul-de-metileno, tionina, azul de toluidina.

thiazolidinediones (thī'ă-zol'ī-dīn-dī-ōnz). Tiazolidinedionas. SIN glitazones.

thi·a·zol·sul·fone (thī-ă-zol-sŭl'fōn). Tiazolsulfona. Possui os mesmos usos que a glicossulfona sódica, porém é menos tóxica e também menos eficaz no tratamento da hanseníase.

thick·ness (thik'nes). Espessura. **1.** A medida da profundidade de algo, em oposição ao seu comprimento ou largura. **2.** Uma camada ou estrato.

Breslow t., t. de Breslow; espessura máxima de um melanoma cutâneo primário medido em cortes histológicos a partir do topo da camada granulosa da epiderme ou a partir da base da úlcera (se o tumor for ulcerado), até a parte inferior do tumor; as taxas de metástases correlacionam-se estreitamente com a espessura do tumor.

thi·el. Tiel. SIN sulfhydryl.

thi·e·mia (thī-ē'mē-ă). Tiemia; presença de enxofre no sangue circulante. [G. *theion,* enxofre, + *haima,* sangue]

thi·e·na·my·cin (thī'en-ă-mī'sin). Tienamicina; o primeiro membro de uma família de antibióticos com núcleo destiacarbapenem, que apresentam uma cadeia lateral tioetilamina na porção enamina do anel de 5 membros fundido.

thi·e·nyl (thī'en-il). Tienil; o radical do tiofeno, $SC_4H_3\text{-}$. Cf. thenyl.

thi·e·nyl·al·a·nine (thī'ē-nil-al'ă-nēn). Tienilalanina. Composto estruturalmente semelhante à fenilalanina, que inibe o crescimento de *Escherichia coli,* presumivelmente por inibição competitiva de enzimas cujo substrato é a L-fenilalanina.

Thier, Carl Jörg, médico alemão. VER Weyers-T. *syndrome.*

Thiers, Joseph, médico francês, *1885. VER Achard-T. *syndrome.*

Thiersch, Karl, cirurgião alemão, 1822–1895. VER T. *graft, canaliculi,* em *canaliculus;* Ollier-T. *graft.*

thi·eth·yl·per·a·zine ma·le·ate (thī-eth'il-per'ă-zēn). Maleato de tietilperazina; agente antiemético utilizado para controlar as náuseas e os vômitos associados à vertigem, à administração de anestésicos gerais e a várias outras condições clínicas; possui também fraca ação hipotensora, espasmolítica, anti-histamínica e hipotérmica.

thigh (thī). [TA]. Coxa; a parte do membro inferior entre o quadril e o joelho. SIN femur (1) [TA], os femoris*, thigh bone*.

Heilbronner t., c. de Heilbronner; em casos de paralisia orgânica, achatamento e alargamento da coxa quando o paciente está em decúbito dorsal sobre um colchão duro; ausente na paralisia histérica.

thig·mes·the·sia (thig-mes-thē'zē-ă). Tigmestesia; sensibilidade tátil. [G. *thigma,* toque, + *aisthēsis,* sensação]

thig·mo·tax·is (thig-mō-tak'sis). Tigmotaxia; forma de barotaxia; designa a reação do protoplasma vegetal ou animal ao contato com um corpo sólido. Cf. thigmotropism. [G. *thigma,* toque, + *taxis,* arranjo ordenado]

thig·mot·ro·pism (thig-mot'rō-pizm). Tigmotropismo; movimento de aproximação ou afastamento de um estímulo tátil sobre a parte de uma porção de um organismo, como folhas ou gavinhas. Cf. thigmotaxis. [G. *thigma,* toque, + *tropē,* uma volta]

thi·mer·o·sal (thī-mer'ō-săl). Timerosal; anti-séptico. SIN thiomersal, thiomersalate.

think·ing. Pensamento; o ato de raciocinar.

abstract t., p. abstrato; raciocínio em termos de conceitos e princípios gerais (por exemplo, perceber uma mesa e uma cadeira como móveis), em contraste com o pensamento concreto.

archaic-paralogical t., t. arcaico-paralógico. SIN prelogical t.

concrete t., pensamento concreto; raciocínio de objetos ou idéias como itens específicos, e não como uma representação abstrata de um conceito mais geral, em contraste com o pensamento abstrato (por exemplo, perceber uma cadeira e uma mesa como itens úteis individuais, e não como membros de uma classe geral, os móveis).

creative t., pensamento criativo; pensamento produtivo, com elementos e resultados novos, e não rotineiros.

magical t., pensamento mágico; a equação irracional do pensamento com a realização.

prelogical t., pensamento pré-lógico; tipo concreto de pensamento, característico de crianças e povos primitivos, para os quais se diz, algumas vezes, que as pessoas esquizofrênicas regridem. SIN archaic-paralogical t., prelogical mind.

t. through, pensamento reflexivo; o processo psicológico da compreensão, através de percepção, do próprio comportamento.

thin·ning (thin'ing). Adelgaçamento; que provoca uma redução da viscosidade por diluição, incluindo por meios químicos, como através da adição de um solvente, ou por meios mecânicos, como no adelgaçamento por cisalhamento.

shear t., a. por cisalhamento; diminuição da viscosidade de um polímero ou macromolécula ou gel através de um aumento na taxa de cisalhamento; não constitui habitualmente uma função do tempo. VER TAMBÉM thixotropy.

△ **thio-.** Tio-; prefixo que designa a substituição de oxigênio por enxofre num composto. Cf. thia-. [G. *theion,* açúcar]

thi·o·ac·id (thī-ō-as'id). Tioácido; ácido orgânico em que um ou mais átomos de oxigênio foram substituídos por átomos de enxofre; por exemplo, ácido tiossulfúrico. SIN sulfacid, sulfoacid (1).

thi·o·al·co·hol (thī-ō-al′kō-hol). Tioálcool. SIN mercaptan (1).
thi·o·am·ide (thī-ō-am′īd). Tioamida. Uma amida em que o S substitui o O.
thi·o·ate (thī′ō-āt). Tioato; sal ou éster de um ácido -tióico.
thi·o·bar·bi·tu·rates (thī′ō-bar-bich′ur-āts). Tiobarbitúricos; hipnóticos do grupo dos barbitúricos, como, por exemplo, tiopental, em que o átomo de oxigênio no carbono 2 é substituído por enxofre.
thi·o·car·bam·ide (thī-ō-kar′ba-mīd). Tiocarbamida. SIN thiourea.
thi·o·car·lide (thī-ō-kar′līd). Tiocarlida; composto sintético cuja molécula contém os três grupos antituberculose: ácido p-aminosalicílico, p-aminobenzaldeído tiosemicarbazona e o grupo tiocarbamida; agente antituberculose.
thi·o·chrome (thī′ō-krōm). Tiocromo; composto fluorescente produzido pela oxidação da tiamina; utilizado em métodos para detecção e determinação da tiamina.
thi·oc·tic ac·id (thī-ok′tik). Ácido tióctico. SIN lipoic acid.
thi·o·cy·a·nate (thī-ō-sī′a-nāt). Tiocianato; sal do ácido tiociânico. SIN rhodanate, sulfocyanate.
thi·o·cy·an·ic ac·id (thī-ō-sī-an′ik). Ácido tiociânico; HS-CN; tiocianato de hidrogênio. SIN rhodanic acid, sulfocyanic acid.
thi·o·dep·si·pep·tide (thī-ō-dep′-sē-pep′tīd). Tiodepsipeptídio; peptídios que também contêm um ou mais grupos tióis acilados (por exemplo, de cisteína). [thio- + G. *depseō*, ligar, misturar, + peptídio]
thi·o·di·phen·yl·a·mine (thī′ō-dī-fen′il-am′ēn). Tiodifenilamina. SIN phenothiazine.
thi·o·es·ter (thī-ō-es′ter). Tioéster; tiol acilado; RCOSR′; por exemplo, acetil-CoA. SIN acylmercaptan.
thi·o·es·ter·ase (thī-ō-es-ter-ās). Tioesterase; enzima que hidrolisa tioésteres; por exemplo, a atividade de desacilação no final da biossíntese de ácidos graxos que libera palmitato. SIN thiolesterase.
thi·o·es·ters (thī′ō-es′-terz). Tioésteres; em enzimologia, um éster em que o oxigênio que liga o substrato ou o produto carbonil carbono e a enzima é substituído por um enxofre (geralmente através de um resíduo Cys); intermediário de alta energia em muitas enzimas.
thi·o·eth·a·nol·a·mine ace·tyl·trans·fer·ase (thī′ō-eth-ā-nol′ā-mēn). Tioetanolamina aceltiltransferase; enzima que transfere o acetil da acetil-CoA para o átomo de enxofre da tioetanolamina, com conseqüente produção de coenzima A e de S-acetiltioetanolamina. SIN thiotransacetylase B.
thi·o·e·ther (thī-ō-ē′ther). Tioéter; sulfeto orgânico; um éter em que o oxigênio é substituído por enxofre; R–S–R′.
thi·o·fla·vine S (thī-ō-flā′vin) [C.I. 49010]. Tioflavina S; derivado metilado e sulfonado da primulina; corante amarelado utilizado em microscopia de fluorescência como corante vital.
thi·o·fla·vin T (thī-ō-flā′vin) [C.I. 49005]. Tioflavina T; corante tiazol amarelo, utilizado em histopatologia como fluorocromo para hialina e amilóide.
thi·o·fu·ran (thī′ō-foor′an). Tiofurano. SIN thiophene.
thi·o·glu·co·si·dase (thī-ō-gloo′kō-si-dās). Tioglicosidase; enzima presente na semente da mostarda que converte tioglicosídios em tióis mais açúcares. SIN myrosinase, sinigrase, sinigrinase.
thi·o·glyc·er·ol (thī-ō-glis′er-ol). Tioglicerol. SIN monothioglycerol.
thi·o·gly·co·late, thi·o·gly·col·late (thī-ō-glī′kō-lāt). Tioglicolato; sal ou éster do ácido tioglicólico; freqüentemente utilizado em meios bacterianos para reduzir o conteúdo de oxigênio, de modo a criar condições favoráveis para o crescimento de anaeróbios; o tioglicolato também inativa qualquer mercurial passível de ser transportado com o inóculo.
thi·o·gly·col·ic ac·id (thī′ō-glī-kol′ik). Ácido tioglicólico; utilizado como reagente para detecção de metais, como ferro, molibdênio, prata e estanho; os sais de amônio e de sódio são utilizados em permanentes de uso caseiro, o sal de cálcio, como depilatório. SIN mercaptoacetic acid.
thi·o·gua·nine (thī-ō-gwah′nēn). Tioguanina; agente antineoplásico utilizado em leucemias e nefrose.
-thioic ac·id. Ácido -tióico; sufixo que designa o radical –C(S)OH ou –C(O)SH, o análogo sulfúrico de um ácido carboxílico, isto é, um ácido tiocarboxílico.
thi·o·ki·nase (thī-ō-kī′nās). Tiocinase; termo de grupo para enzimas que formam compostos de acil-CoA a partir dos ácidos graxos correspondentes e CoA; a ligação ocorre através do átomo de enxofre da CoA.
thi·ol (thī′ol). Tiol. **1.** O radical monovalente –SH quando fixado ao carbono; hidrossulfeto; mercaptano. **2.** Mistura de óleos de petróleo sulfurados e sulfonados, purificados com amônia; utilizada no tratamento de doenças cutâneas.
thi·o·lase (thī′ō-lās). Tiolase. SIN acetyl-CoA acetyltransferase.
thi·ole (thī′ōl). Tiol. SIN thiophene.
thi·ol·es·ter·ase (thī′ol-es′ter-āz). Tiolesterase. SIN thioesterase.
thi·ol·his·ti·dyl·be·ta·ine (thī′ol-his′ti-dil-bē′ta-ēn). Tiolistildilbetaína. SIN ergothioneine.
thi·ol·trans·a·cet·y·lase A (thī-ol-trans-ā-set′i-lās). Tioltransacetilase A. SIN dihydrolipoamide S-acetyltransferase.
thi·ol·y·sis (thī-ol′i-sis). Tiólise; a clivagem de uma ligação química com a adição de coenzima A a uma parte; análoga à hidrólise e fosforólise.

thi·o·mer·sal (thī-ō-mer′sal). Tiomersal. SIN thimerosal.
thi·o·mer·sa·late (thī-ō-mer′sa-lāt). Tiomersalato. SIN thimerosal.
thi·o·meth·yl·a·den·o·sine (thī′ō-meth′il-ā-den′ō-sēn). Tiometiladenosina. SIN methylthioadenosine.
β-thi·o·nase (thī′ō-nās). β-tionase. SIN cystathionine β-synthase.
-thione. -Tiona; sufixo que designa o radical ≠ C≠ S, o análogo sulfúrico de uma cetona, isto é, um grupo tiocarbonil.
thi·o·nein (thī′ō-nēn). Tioneína; a apoproteína da metalotioneína.
thi·o·ne·ine (thī′ō-ne′in). Tioneína. SIN ergothioneine.
thi·on·ic (thī-on′ik). Tiônico; relativo ao tiônio.
thi·o·nine (thī′ō-nin) [C.I. 52000]. Tionina; amidofentiazina; pó verde-escuro que produz uma solução púrpura em água, útil como corante básico em histologia para cromatina e mucina, devido às suas propriedades metacromáticas. SIN Lauth violet.
thiono-. Tiono-; prefixo algumas vezes utilizado para thioxo-.
thi·o·pan·ic ac·id (thī-ō-pan′ik). Ácido tiopânico. SIN pantoyltaurine.
thi·o·pen·tal so·di·um (thī-ō-pen′tawl). Tiopental sódico; barbitúrico de ação ultracurta, administrado por via intravenosa ou por via retal para indução de anestesia.
thi·o·phene (thī′ō-fēn). Tiofeno; o composto do anel fundamental. SIN thiofuran, thiole.
thi·o·phe·ni·col (thī-ō-fen′i-kol). Tiofenicol. SIN tiamphenicol.
thi·o·pro·pa·zate hy·dro·chlo·ride (thī-ō-prō′pa-zāt). Cloridrato de tiopropazato; derivado da fenotiazina, relacionado, do ponto de vista químico e farmacológico, à proclorperazina e à perfenazina; agente antipsicótico.
thi·o·pro·per·a·zine (thī-ō-prō-per′a-zēn). Tioproperazina; agente antiemético e ansiolítico.
thi·o·re·dox·in (thī-ō-rē-doks′in). Tiorredoxina; proteína que participa em reações de oxidação-redução associadas à biossíntese de desoxirribonucleotídios.
t. reductase, t. redutase; flavoproteína que utiliza NADPH para reduzir novamente a t. na formação de desoxirribonucleotídios.
thi·o·rid·a·zine hy·dro·chlo·ride (thī-ō-rid′a-zēn). Cloridrato de tioridazina; agente antipsicótico com ação semelhante à da clorpromazina, porém com efeitos anticolinérgicos relativamente mais acentuados.
thi·o·sem·i·car·ba·zide (thī′ō-sem′e-kar′ba-zid). Tiosemicarbazida; uma das tiosemicarbazonas com ação tuberculostática; utilizada como reagente na detecção de metais.
thi·o·sem·i·car·ba·zone (thī′ō-sem′e-kar′ba-zōn). Tiosemicarbazona. **1.** Composto que contém o radical tiosemicarbazida, ≠ N—NH—C(S)—NH₂. **2.** Um entre um grupo de agentes tuberculostáticos que inclui a tiosemicarbazida, a benzaldeído tiosemisemicarbazona e 4-aminoacetilbenzaldeído tiosemicarbazona.
thi·o·sul·fate (thī-ō-sul′fāt). Tiossulfato. $S_2O_3^=$; o ânion do ácido tiossulfúrico; elevado em indivíduos com deficiência do co-fator molibdênio.
t. cyanide transsulfurase, t. cianeto transulfurase. SIN t. sulfurtransferase.
t. sulfurtransferase, t. sulfurtransferase; transferase que catalisa a formação do tiocianato e do sulfeto a partir do cianeto e do tiossulfato. SIN rhodanese, t. cyanide transsulfurase, t. thiotransferase.
t. thiotransferase, t. tiotransferase. SIN t. sulfurtransferase.
thi·o·sul·fur·ic ac·id (thī′ō-sul-fūr′ik). Ácido tiossulfúrico. $H_2S_2O_3$; ácido sulfúrico em que um átomo de oxigênio foi substituído por um de enxofre.
thi·o·te·pa (thī-ō-tep′a). Tiotepa. SIN triethylenethiophosphoramide.
thi·o·thix·ene (thī-ō-thik′sēn). Tiotixeno; antipsicótico.
thi·o·trans·a·cet·y·lase B (thī′ō-trans-ā-set′i-lās). Tiotransacetilase B. SIN thioethanolamine acetyltransferase.
2-thi·o·u·ra·cil (thī-ō-ūr′a-sil). 2-tiouracil. Componente raro dos RNA de transferência; derivado tioamida que inibe a síntese dos hormônios tireóideos; trata-se, portanto, de um bociógeno; semelhante ao propiltiouracil.
4-thi·o·u·ra·cil (thī-ō-ūr′a-sil). 4-tiouracil. Uracil com substituição do O por S na posição 4, isomérico com o 2-tiouracil; componente raro dos RNA de transferência.
thi·o·u·rea (thī′ō-ū-rē′a). Tiouréia; substância antitireóidea do grupo tioamida, com as mesmas ações e aplicações que o tiouracil. Vários derivados da tiouréia são úteis no tratamento da lepra. SIN thiocarbamide.
thi·o·xan·thene (thī-ō-zan′thēn). Tioxanteno; classe de compostos tricíclicos semelhantes à fenotiazina, porém com o nitrogênio do anel central substituído por um átomo de carbono; o uso atual enfatiza as propriedades antipsicóticas e antieméticas dessa classe.
thioxo-. Tioxo-; prefixo que indica ≠ S numa tiocetona.
thi·ox·o·lone (thī-ok′sō-lōn). Tioxolona; anti-seborréico.
THIP. THIP; agonista dos receptores de ácido γ-aminobutírico (GABA) tipo A. Ao contrário de outros agonistas desse tipo, o THIP, após administração sistêmica, penetra na barreira hematoencefálica; utilizado como recurso farmacológico para explorar a função dos receptores de GABA no cérebro e na medula espinal.
thi·phen·a·mil hy·dro·chlo·ride (thī-fen′a-mil). Cloridrato de tifenamil; agente anticolinérgico.

thirst (thurst). Sede; desejo de beber associado a sensações desconfortáveis na boca e na faringe. [A.S. *thurst*]

  false t., s. falsa; sede que não é satisfeita pela ingestão de água; sede associada a boca seca, mas não a uma necessidade orgânica de água. SIN pseudodipsia.

  insensible t., s. insensível. SIN hypodipsia.

  morbid t., s. mórbida. SIN dipsesis.

  subliminal t., s. subliminar. SIN hypodipsia.

  true t., s. verdadeira; sede que pode ser satisfeita pela ingestão de água.

Thiry, Ludwig, fisiologista austríaco, 1817–1897. VER T. *fistula;* T.-Vella *fistula.*

thix·o·la·bile (thik-sō-lā'bil, -bīl). Tixolábil; suscetível à tixotropia.

thix·o·tro·pic (thik-sō-trop'ik). Tixotrópico; relativo a ou caracterizado por tixotropia.

thix·ot·ro·py (thik-sot'rō-pē). A propriedade de determinados géis de se tornarem menos viscosos quando agitados ou submetidos a forças de cisalhamento e de readquirirem a viscosidade original em repouso (por exemplo, líquido sinovial, gel de hidróxido ferroso); característica de um sistema que apresenta uma redução da viscosidade com aumento na taxa de cisalhamento, geralmente uma função do tempo. SIN reclotting phenomenon. [G. *thixis,* um toque, + *tropē,* volta]

Tho·go·to·vi·ruses (thō-gō-tō-vī-rus-ez). Thogotovírus. Grupo de vírus não-classificados, semelhantes aos Orthovírus e que compartilham alguma homologia de aminoácidos.

Thoma, Richard, histologista alemão, 1847–1923. VER T. *ampulla, fixative, laws,* em *law.*

Thomas, Hugh Owen, cirurgião inglês, 1834–1891. VER T. *splint.*

Thompson, Sir Henry, cirurgião inglês, 1820–1904. VER T. *test.*

Thomsen, Asmus J., médico dinamarquês, 1815–1896. VER T. *disease.*

Thomson, Frederic H., médico inglês, 1867–1938. VER T. *sign.*

Thomson, Matthew Sidney, dermatologista inglês, 1894–1969. VER Rothmund-T. *syndrome.*

thon·zo·ni·um bro·mide (thon-zō'nē-ŭm). Brometo de tonzônio; agente tensoativo utilizado em gotas e aerossóis ópticos.

thon·zyl·a·mine hy·dro·chlo·ride (thon-zil'ă-mēn). Cloridrato de tonzilamina; anti-histamínico nos receptores H_1.

♻ **thorac-.** Torac-. VER thoraco-.

tho·ra·cal (thor'ă-kăl). Torácico. SIN thoracic.

tho·ra·cal·gia (thōr-ă-kal'jē-ă). Toracalgia; dor no tórax. SIN thoracodynia. [thoraco- + G. *algos,* dor]

tho·ra·cen·te·sis (thōr'ă-sen-tē'sis). Toracentese; paracentese da cavidade pleural. SIN pleuracentesis, pleural tap, pleurocentesis, thoracocentesis. [thoraco- + G. *kentēsis,* punção]

tho·rac·ic (thō-ras'ik). Torácico; relativo ao tórax. SIN thoracal.

♻ **thoracico-.** Torácico-. VER thoraco-.

tho·rac·i·co·ab·dom·i·nal (thō-ras'i-kō-ab-dom'i-năl). Torácico-abdominal. SIN thoracoabdominal.

tho·rac·i·co·a·cro·mi·al (thor-as'i-kō-ă-krō'mē-al). Torácico-acromial. SIN thoracoacromial.

tho·rac·i·co·hu·mer·al (thō-ras'i-kō-hū'mer-ăl). Torácico-humeral; relativo ao tórax e ao úmero.

♻ **thoraco-, thorac-, thoracico-.** Toraco-, torac-, torácico-. O tórax. [G. *thōrax*]

tho·ra·co·ab·dom·i·nal (thōr'ă-kō-ab-dom'i-năl). Toracoabdominal; relativo ao tórax e ao abdome. SIN thoracicoabdominal.

tho·ra·co·a·cro·mi·al (thōr'ă-kō-ă-krō'mē-ăl). Toracoacromial; relativo ao acrômio e ao tórax; designa especialmente a *artéria* tóraco-acromial. SIN acromiothoracic, thoracicoacromial.

tho·ra·co·ce·los·chi·sis (thōr'ă-kō-sē-los'ki-sis). Toracocelosquise; fissura congênita do tronco envolvendo as cavidades torácica e abdominal. SIN thoracogastroschisis. [thoraco- + G. *koilia,* ventre, + *schisis,* fissura]

tho·ra·co·cen·te·sis (thōr'ă-kō-sen-tē'sis). Toracocentese. SIN thoracentesis.

tho·ra·co·cyl·lo·sis (thōr'ă-kō-si-lō'sis). Toracocilose; deformidade do tórax. [thoraco- + G. *kyllōsis,* deformidade]

tho·ra·co·cyr·to·sis (thōr'ă-kō-ser-tō'sis). Toracocirtose; curvatuva anormalmente ampla da parede torácica. [thoraco- + G. *kyrtōsis,* sendo curvado]

tho·ra·co·del·phus (thōr'ă-kō-del'fŭs). Toracodelfo. SIN thoradelphus.

tho·ra·co·dor·sal (thor-ak-ō-dōr'sal). Toracodorsal; relativo à parede torácica posterior externa, designando especialmente uma artéria, veia e nervo.

tho·ra·co·dyn·ia (thōr'ă-kō-din'ē-ă). Toracodinia. SIN thoracalgia. [thoraco- + G. *odynē,* dor]

tho·ra·co·gas·tros·chi·sis (thōr'ă-kō-gas-tros'ki-sis). Toracogastrosquise. SIN thoracoceloschisis. [thoraco- + G. *gastēr,* ventre, + *schisis,* fissura]

tho·ra·co·lap·a·rot·o·my (thōr'ă-kō-lap-ă-rot'ō-mē). Toracolaparotomia. Exposição da região diafragmática por uma incisão que abre tanto o tórax quanto o abdome (incisão toracoabdominal). [thoraco- + laparotomy]

tho·ra·co·lum·bar (thōr'ă-kō-lŭm'bar). Toracolombar. **1.** Relativo às partes torácica e lombar da coluna vertebral. **2.** Relativo às origens da divisão simpática do sistema nervoso autônomo. VER autonomic *division* of nervous system.

tho·ra·col·y·sis (thōr-ă-kol'i-sis). Toracólise; ruptura de aderências pleurais. [thoraco- + G. *lysis,* dissolução]

tho·ra·com·e·lus (thōr-ă-kom'ē-lŭs). Toracômelo; gêmeos unidos desiguais, em que o parasita, freqüentemente constituído apenas de um braço ou uma perna, está fixado ao tórax do autósito. VER conjoined *twins,* em *twin.* [thoraco- + G. *melos,* membro]

tho·ra·com·e·ter (thōr-ă-kom'ē-ter). Toracômetro; instrumento para medir a circunferência do tórax ou suas variações na respiração. [thoraco- + G. *metron,* medida]

tho·ra·co·my·o·dyn·ia (thōr'ă-kō-mī-ō-din'ē-ă). Toracomiodinia; dor nos músculos da parede torácica. [thoraco- + G. *mys,* músculo, + *odynē,* dor]

tho·ra·cop·a·gus (thōr-ă-kop'ă-gŭs). Toracópago; gêmeos unidos com fusão na região torácica. VER conjoined *twins,* em *twin.* SIN synthorax. [thoraco- + G. *pagos,* algo fixado]

tho·ra·co·par·a·ceph·a·lus (thōr'ă-kō-par-ă-sef'ă-lŭs). Toracoparacéfalo; gêmeos unidos desiguais, em que uma cabeça parasita rudimentar está fixada ao tórax do autósito. VER conjoined *twins,* em *twin.* [thoraco- + G. *para,* ao lado, + *kephalē,* cabeça]

tho·ra·cop·a·thy (thōr-ă-kop'ă-thē). Toracopatia; termo raramente empregado. Qualquer doença dos órgãos ou tecidos torácicos. [thoraco- + G. *pathos,* sofrimento]

tho·ra·co·plas·ty (thōr'ă-kō-plas-tē). Toracoplastia; cirurgia que diminui o espaço intratorácico mediante remoção de partes da parede torácica rígida. [thoraco- + G. *plastos,* formado]

  conventional t., t. convencional; ressecção de costelas para permitir a retração interna da parede torácica, a fim de diminuir o tamanho do espaço pleural; pode ser utilizada no tratamento do empiema.

tho·ra·co·pneu·mo·plas·ty (thōr'ă-kō-noo'mō-plas-tē). Toracopneumoplastia. Cirurgia plástica do tórax em que o pulmão também está envolvido. [thoraco- + G. *pneumōn,* pulmão ,+ *plastos,* formado]

tho·ra·cos·chi·sis (thōr-ă-kos'ki-sis). Toracosquise; fissura congênita da parede torácica. [thoraco- + G. *schisis,* fissura]

tho·ra·co·scope (thō-rak'ō-skōp). Toracoscópio; endoscópio utilizado para visualização das estruturas intratorácicas; pode ser assistido por vídeo. [thoraco- + G. *skopeō,* ver]

ℹ **tho·ra·cos·co·py** (thōr-ă-kos'kō-pē). Toracoscopia; exame da cavidade pleural com endoscópio. SIN pleuroscopy. [thoraco- + G. *skopeō,* ver]

tho·ra·co·ste·no·sis (thōr'ă-kō-stē-nō'sis). Toracostenose; estreitamento do tórax. [thoraco- + G. *stenōsis,* estreitamento]

thoracosternotomy. Toracosternotomia; incisão do tórax combinando uma incisão intercostal e transecção do esterno.

  transverse t., t. transversa; incisão do tórax combinando uma incisão intercostal e transecção do esterno.

tho·ra·cos·to·my (thōr-ă-kos'tō-mē). Toracostomia; estabelecimento de uma abertura na cavidade torácica, como para a drenagem de empiema. [thoraco- + G. *stoma,* boca]

tho·ra·cot·o·my (thōr-ă-kot'ō-mē). Toracotomia; incisão através da parede torácica no espaço pleural. SIN pleurotomy. [thoraco- + G. *tomē,* incisão]

  anterior t., t. anterior; incisão anterior no tórax, geralmente submamária.

  axillary t., t. axilar; toracotomia lateral efetuada abaixo da linha axilar; pode ser transversa ou vertical.

  clamshell t., t. em concha de molusco. SIN clamshell *incision.*

  minithoracotomy, minitoracotomia. Qualquer toracotomia envolvendo menor divisão dos músculos do que a toracotomia póstero-lateral clássica [coloquial]

  muscle-sparing t., t. com preservação dos músculos; qualquer tipo de toracotomia que não envolve divisão significativa do latíssimo do dorso (*músculo*) e do serrátil anterior (*músculo*).

  posterolateral t., t. póstero-lateral; toracotomia envolvendo a divisão do latíssimo do dorso (*músculo*) e do serrátil (*músculo*).

tho·ra·del·phus (thōr-ă-del'fŭs). Toracodelfo; duplicidade posterior em que o indivíduo é duplicado do umbigo para baixo. VER conjoined *twins,* em *twin.* SIN thoracodelphus. [thoraco- + G. *adelphos,* irmão]

ℹ **tho·rax,** gen. **tho·ra·cis,** pl. **tho·ra·ces** (thō'raks, thō'ră-sis, -ră'sēz) [TA]. Tórax; a parte superior do tronco entre o pescoço e o abdome; formado pelas 12 vértebras torácicas, pelos 12 pares de costelas, pelo esterno e pelos músculos e fáscias fixados a eles; abaixo, é separado do abdome pelo diafragma; contém os principais órgãos dos sistemas circulatório e respiratório. [L. do G. *thōrax,* placa torácica, peito, de *thōressō,* armar]

  barrel-shaped t., t. em barril; aumento do diâmetro ântero-posterior do tórax, de modo que as dimensões lateral e ântero-posterior são aproximadamente iguais, devido à hiperinsuflação dos pulmões. Observado em pacientes com enfisema.

  Peyrot t., t. de Peyrot; deformidade obliquamente oval do tórax em casos de derrame pleural muito grande.

tho·ri·um (Th) (thōr'ē-ŭm). Tório; elemento metálico radioativo; número atômico 90, peso atômico 232,0381. O Th^{232}, o único nuclídio de ocorrência natural, com meia-vida de 14×10^9 anos, é utilizado na forma coloidal em microscopia eletrônica como corante para mucopolissacarídios ácidos. [*Thor*, deus nórdico do trovão]

Thormählen, Johann, médico alemão do século 19. VER T. *test.*

Thorn, George W., médico norte-americano, *1906. VER T. *test, syndrome.*

thorn (thōrn). Espinha, espinho; em anatomia, uma estrutura espinhosa.
  dendritic t.'s, espinhas dendríticas. SIN dendritic *spines,* em *spine.*

thorn·ap·ple. Estramônio. SIN *Datura stramonium.*

Thornwaldt, Gustavus Ludwig. VER Tornwaldt.

thought. Pensamento. **1.** A faculdade de raciocinar. **2.** O processo ou ato de pensar. **3.** O resultado de pensar.
  t. broadcasting, irradiação do pensamento; delírio de sentir os pensamentos, à medida que surgem, como se estivessem sendo transmitidos da cabeça da pessoa para o mundo externo, onde outras pessoas podem ouvi-los.
  t. insertion, inserção do pensamento; delírio de que os pensamentos não são realmente do próprio indivíduo, mas que estão colocados em sua mente por uma força externa.
  trend of t., direção do pensamento; pensamento com tendência voltada para ou centrada numa idéia específica, com determinado afeto.
  t. withdrawal, retirada do pensamento; delírio de que os pensamentos foram removidos da cabeça, resultando em número diminuído de pensamentos remanescentes.

Thr Símbolo da treonina ou de suas formas radicais.

thread (thred). Fio. **1.** Filamento fino de material de sutura. **2.** Estrutura filamentosa. [M.E., do A.S. *thraed*]
  terminal t., fio terminal. SIN terminal *filum.*

thread-worm (thred′werm). Nematódeo; nome comum para espécies do gênero *Strongyloides;* termo algumas vezes aplicado a qualquer um dos nematódeos parasitas menores.

thre·on·ic ac·id (thrē-on′ik). Ácido treônico; o ácido derivado por oxidação do grupo CHO da treose a COOH; produto da oxidação do ácido ascórbico por hipoiodeto.

thre·o·nine (T, Thr) (thrē′ō-nēn). Treonina; ácido 2-amino-3-hidroxibutírico; o L-isômero é um dos aminoácidos de ocorrência natural, presente na estrutura da maioria das proteínas e nutricionalmente essencial na dieta humana e de outros mamíferos.
  t. deaminase, t. desaminase. SIN t. dehydratase.
  t. dehydratase, t. desidratase; enzima que catalisa a desaminação anaeróbica da L-treonina em ácido 2-cetobutírico e amônia; etapa central no catabolismo da treonina. SIN serine deaminase, t. deaminase.

thre·ose (thrē′ōs). Treose. Uma aldotetrose; uma das duas aldoses (sendo a outra a eritrose) que contém quatro átomos de carbono.

thresh·old (thresh′ōld). Limiar. **1.** O ponto em que determinado estímulo começa a produzir uma sensação. **2.** O limite mais baixo de percepção de um estímulo. O estímulo mínimo capaz de produzir excitação de qualquer estrutura.; por exemplo, o estímulo mínimo que desencadeia uma resposta motora. SIN limen (2) [TA]. [A.S. *therxold*]
  absolute t., l. absoluto; o limite inferior de qualquer percepção. Cf. differential t. SIN stimulus t.
  achromatic t., l. acromático. SIN visual t.
  auditory t., l. auditivo; a intensidade de qualquer som dificilmente perceptível.
  brightness difference t., l. de diferença de brilho; a menor diferença que pode ser percebida como diferença no brilho. SIN light difference (2).
  t. of consciousness, l. de consciência; o ponto mais baixo em que é possível perceber a sensação de um estímulo.
  convulsant t., l. convulsivante; a menor quantidade de estimulação, corrente elétrica ou droga necessária para induzir uma convulsão.
  differential t., l. diferencial; o limite mais baixo em que dois estímulos podem ser diferenciados. SIN threshold differential.
  displacement t., l. de deslocamento; a menor ruptura distinguível no contorno de uma linha.
  double-point t., l. de duplo ponto; o menor grau de separação de dois pontos aplicados à superfície corporal que permite que sejam percebidos como dois pontos.
  erythema t., l. do eritema; a dose em que o eritema da pele é produzido por irradiação com raios ultravioleta, gama ou X.
  fibrillation t., l. de fibrilação; menor intensidade de um estímulo elétrico capaz de iniciar uma fibrilação.
  galvanic t., l. galvânico. SIN rheobase.
  t. of island of Reil, l. da ilha de Reil. SIN *limen* insulae.
  light differential t., l. diferencial luminoso; a menor diferença de intensidade luminosa que pode ser percebida.
  minimum light t., l. luminoso mínimo. SIN visual t.
  t. of nose, l. do nariz. SIN *limen* nasi.
  pain t., l. da dor; a menor intensidade de um estímulo doloroso em que o indivíduo percebe dor.
  phenotypic t., l. fenotípico; traço genético quantitativo com uma distribuição contínua denominada predisposição; pode produzir dois tipos de fenótipos, dependendo de a predisposição estar situada acima ou abaixo de algum limiar crítico em torno do qual ocorre uma mudança radical de comportamento. Por exemplo, o nível sangüíneo de ácido úrico constitui uma predisposição com distribuição aproximadamente gaussiana. Em determinado ponto crítico de saturação química (o limiar), ocorre cristalização, e o conseqüente desenvolvimento ou não-desenvolvimento de gota constitui um traço limiar.
  relational t., l. relacional; o menor grau de diferença entre dois estímulos que permite a sua percepção como diferentes.
  renal t., l. renal; concentração plasmática da substância acima da qual ela aparece na urina.
  speech awareness t., l. de consciência da fala; a menor intensidade sonora em que a fala pode ser detectada. SIN speech detection t.
  speech detection t., l. de detecção da fala. SIN speech awareness t.
  speech reception t., l. de recepção da fala; a intensidade em que a fala é reconhecida como símbolos significativos; em audiometria, trata-se do nível em decibéis em que 50% das palavras podem ser repetidas corretamente pelo indivíduo.
  stimulus t., l. do estímulo. SIN absolute t.
  swallowing t., l. de deglutição; (1) o momento de início do ato da deglutição após a mastigação do alimento; (2) o momento crítico da ação reflexa iniciada por estimulação mínima, antes do ato da deglutição.
  visual t., t. of visual sensation, l. visual, l. da sensação visual; a intensidade luminosa mínima que produz uma sensação visual. SIN achromatic t., minimum light t.

thrill. Frêmito; vibração que acompanha um sopro cardíaco ou vascular passível de ser palpado. VER TAMBÉM fremitus.
  diastolic t., f. diastólico; frêmito percebido sobre o precórdio ou sobre um vaso sangüíneo durante a diástole ventricular.
  hydatid t., f. hidático; a sensação peculiar de tremor ou de vibração percebida à palpação de um cisto hidático. SIN Blatin syndrome, hydatid fremitus.
  presystolic t., f. pré-sistólico; frêmito imediatamente anterior à contração ventricular, que algumas vezes é percebido à palpação sobre o ápice do coração, como na estenose mitral.
  systolic t., f. sistólico; frêmito percebido sobre o precórdio ou sobre um vaso sangüíneo durante a sístole ventricular.

thrix (thriks) [TA]. Cabelo. SIN hair. [G.]

throat (thrōt). Garganta. **1.** As fauces e a faringe. SIN gullet. **2.** A face anterior do pescoço. SIN jugulum. **3.** Qualquer entrada estreita numa parte oca. [A.S. *throtu*]
  sore t., faringite; condição caracterizada por dor ou desconforto à deglutição; pode ser devida a qualquer de várias inflamações das tonsilas, da faringe ou da laringe.

throb. 1. Pulsar. **2.** Batimento ou pulsação.

thromb-. Tromb-. VER thrombo-.

throm·base (throm′bās). Trombase. SIN thrombin.

throm·bas·the·nia (throm-bas-thē′nē-ă). Trombastenia; anormalidade das plaquetas característica da trombastenia de Glanzmann. VER TAMBÉM Bernard-Soulier *syndrome.* SIN thromboasthenia. [thromb- + G. *astheneia,* fraqueza]
  Glanzmann t. [MIM*273800], t. de Glanzmann; diátese hemorrágica caracterizada por tempo de sangramento normal ou prolongado, tempo de coagulação normal, deficiência da retração do coágulo, contagem plaquetária normal, porém com anormalidade morfológica ou funcional das plaquetas; foram descritos vários tipos diferentes de anormalidades plaquetárias; causada por um defeito no complexo de glicoproteína IIb-IIIa da membrana plaquetária; herança autossômica recessiva, causada por mutação no gene do complexo de glicoproteína IIb-IIIa (ITGA2B) da membrana plaquetária no cromossoma 17. SIN constitutional thrombopathy, Glanzmann disease, hereditary hemorrhagic t.
  hereditary hemorrhagic t., t. hemorrágica hereditária. SIN Glanzmann t.

throm·bec·to·my (throm-bek′tō-mē). Trombectomia; excisão de um trombo. [thromb- + G. *ektomē,* excisão]

throm·bi (throm′bī). Trombos; plural de thrombus.

throm·bin. Trombina. **1.** Enzima (proteinase) formada no sangue derramado, que converte o fibrinogênio em fibrina através da hidrólise de peptídios (e amidas e ésteres) de L-arginina; formada a partir da protrombina pela ação da protrombinase (fator Xa, outra proteinase). **2.** Substância protéica estéril preparada a partir da protrombina de origem bovina através da interação com tromboplastina na presença de cálcio; produz coagulação do sangue total, do plasma ou de uma solução de fibrinogênio; utilizada como agente hemostático tópico para o sangramento capilar com ou sem espuma de fibrina em procedimentos cirúrgicos gerais e plásticos. SIN factor IIa, fibrinogenase, thrombase, thrombosin.
  human t., t. humana; t. obtida do plasma humano por precipitação com sais e solventes orgânicos apropriados; tem os mesmos usos que a t.

throm·bin·o·gen (throm-bin′ō-jen). Trombinogênio. SIN prothrombin.

throm·bi·no·gen·e·sis (throm′bi-nō-jen′ē-sis). Trombinogênese. Produção de trombina.

thrombo-, thromb-. Trombo-, tromb-. Coágulo sangüíneo; coagulação; trombina. [G. *thrombos,* coágulo (trombo)]

throm·bo·an·gi·i·tis (throm'bō - an - ji - ī'tis). Tromboangeíte; inflamação da íntima de um vaso sangüíneo, com trombose. [thrombo- + G. *angeion*, vaso, + *-itis*, inflamação]

t. oblit'erans, t. obliterante; inflamação de toda a parede e tecido conjuntivo que circunda as artérias e veias de calibre médio, especialmente das pernas de homens jovens e de meia-idade; associada a oclusão trombótica, resultando comumente em gangrena. SIN Buerger disease, Winiwarter-Buerger disease.

throm·bo·ar·te·ri·tis (throm'bō - ar - ter - ī'tis). Tromboarterite; inflamação arterial com formação de trombo.

throm·bo·as·the·nia (throm'bō - as - thē'nē - ă). Trombastenia. SIN thrombasthenia.

throm·bo·blast (throm'bō - blast). Tromboblasto. SIN megakaryocyte. [thrombo- + G. *blastos*, germe]

throm·bo·clas·tic (throm - bō - klas'tik). Tromboclástico. SIN thrombolytic.

throm·bo·cyst, throm·bo·cys·tis (throm'bō - sist, - sis'tis). Trombocisto; saco membranoso que encerra um trombo. [thrombo- + G. *kystis*, vesícula]

throm·bo·cy·tas·the·nia (throm'bō - sī - tas - thē'nē - ă). Trombocitastenia; termo que designa um grupo de distúrbios hemorrágicos em que as plaquetas podem estar apenas ligeiramente reduzidas em número ou até mesmo dentro da faixa normal, porém são morfologicamente anormais ou carecem de fatores que são eficazes na coagulação do sangue. [thrombocyte + G. *astheneia*, fraqueza]

throm·bo·cyte (throm'bō - sīt). Trombócito. SIN platelet. [thrombo- + G. *kytos*, célula]

throm·bo·cy·the·mia (throm'bō - sī - thē'mē - ă). Trombocitemia. SIN thrombocytosis. [thrombocyte + G. *haima*, sangue]

throm·bo·cy·tin (throm - bō - sī'tin). Trombocitina. SIN serotonin.

throm·bo·cy·top·a·thy (throm'bō - sī - top'ă - thē). Trombocitopatia; termo geral para referir-se a qualquer distúrbio do mecanismo da coagulação que resulta de disfunção das plaquetas sangüíneas. [thrombocyte + G. *pathos*, sofrimento]

throm·bo·cy·to·pe·nia (throm'bō - sī - tō - pē'nē - ă). Trombocitopenia; condição caracterizada por um número anormalmente pequeno de plaquetas no sangue circulante. SIN thrombopenia. [thrombocyte + G. *penia*, escassez]

autoimmune neonatal t., t. auto-imune neonatal. SIN isoimmune neonatal t.

essential t., t. essencial; forma primária de trombocitopenia, em contraste com as formas secundárias que estão associadas a neoplasias metastáticas, tuberculose e leucemia acometendo a medula óssea ou à supressão direta da medula óssea em decorrência do uso de agentes químicos ou a outras condições.

immune t., t. imune; trombocitopenia associada a anticorpos antiplaquetários. VER isoimmune neonatal t.

isoimmune neonatal t., t. isoimune neonatal; trombocitopenia imune resultante de incompatibilidade plaquetária materno-fetal. SIN autoimmune neonatal t.

throm·bo·cy·to·poi·e·sis (throm'bō - sī - tō - poy - ē'sis). Trombocitopoese; o processo de formação de trombócitos ou plaquetas. [thrombocyte + G. *poiēsis*, fazer]

throm·bo·cy·to·sis (throm'bō - sī - tō'sis). Trombocitose; aumento do número de plaquetas no sangue circulante. SIN thrombocythemia. [thrombocyte + G. -*osis*, condição]

throm·bo·e·las·to·gram (throm'bō - ē - las'tō - gram). Tromboelastograma; registro do processo da coagulação por um tromboelastógrafo.

throm·bo·e·las·to·graph (throm'bō - ē - las'tō - graf). Tromboelastógrafo; aparelho para registrar variações elásticas de um trombo durante o processo da coagulação. [thromb- + G. *elastreō*, empurrar, + *graphō*, escrever]

throm·bo·em·bo·lec·to·my (throm'bō - em - bō - lek'tō - mē). Tromboembolectomia; extração de um trombo embólico. [thrombo- + G. *embolos*, êmbolo, + *ektomē*, excisão]

throm·bo·em·bo·lism (throm'bō - em'bō - lizm). Tromboembolia; embolia por um trombo. [thrombo- + G. *embolismos*, embolia]

throm·bo·end·ar·ter·ec·to·my (throm'bō - end - ar - ter - ek'tō - mē). Tromboendarterectomia; operação que consiste na abertura de uma artéria, remoção de um trombo oclusivo juntamente com a íntima e material ateromatoso e permanência de um plano limpo e fresco internamente à adventícia. [thrombo- + endarterectomy]

throm·bo·en·do·car·di·tis (throm'bō - en'dō - kar - dī'tis). Tromboendocardite. SIN non-bacterial thrombotic endocarditis.

throm·bo·gen (throm'bō - jen). Trombogênio. SIN prothrombin. [thrombo- + G. -*gen*, que produz]

throm·bo·gene (throm'bō - jēn). Trombogene. SIN factor V.

throm·bo·gen·ic (throm - bō - jen'ik). Trombogênico. **1.** Relativo ao trombogênio. **2.** Que causa trombose ou coagulação do sangue.

throm·boid (throm'boyd). Trombóide; semelhante a um trombo. [thrombo- + G. *eidos*, semelhança]

throm·bo·kat·i·ly·sin (throm'bō - kat - i - lī'sin). Trombocatilisina; termo obsoleto para o fator VIII.

throm·bo·ki·nase (throm - bō - kī'nās). Trombocinase. SIN thromboplastin.

throm·bol·ic (throm - bol'ik). Trombólico; relativo a um trômbolo.

throm·bo·lus (throm'bō - lŭs). Trômbolo; êmbolo composto principalmente de plaquetas aglutinadas. [thrombo- + G. *embolos*, êmbolo]

throm·bo·lym·phan·gi·tis (throm'bō - lim-fan - jī'tis). Trombolinfangite; inflamação de um vaso linfático, com formação de um coágulo de linfa.

throm·bol·y·sis (throm - bol'i - sis). Trombólise; fluidificação ou dissolução de um trombo. [thrombo- + G. *lysis*, dissolução]

throm·bo·lyt·ic (throm - bō - lit'ik). Trombolítico; que rompe ou dissolve um trombo. SIN thromboclastic.

throm·bo·mod·u·lin (throm'bō - mo - doo - lin). Trombomodulina; glicoproteína presente na membrana plasmática das células endoteliais que se liga à trombina; participa num mecanismo regulador adicional da coagulação. [thrombo- + modulate + -in]

throm·bon. Trômbon; termo abrangente que inclui os trombócitos (plaquetas sangüíneas) e as formas celulares a partir das quais se originam (tromboplastos ou megacariócitos). É análogo ao éritron e ao leucon dos eritrócitos e leucócitos, respectivamente.

throm·bo·ne·cro·sis (throm'bō - ne - krō'sis). Trombonecrose; necrose das paredes de um vaso, com trombose na luz.

throm·bop·a·thy (throm - bop'ă - thē). Trombopatia; termo inespecífico aplicado a distúrbios das plaquetas do sangue, resultando em deficiência de tromboplastina, sem alteração óbvia no aspecto ou no número de plaquetas. [thrombo- + G. *pathos*, doença]

constitutional t., t. constitucional. SIN Glanzmann *thrombasthenia*.

throm·bo·pe·nia (throm - bō - pē'nē - ă). Trombopenia. SIN thrombocytopenia.

throm·bo·phil·ia (throm - bō - fil'ē - ă). Trombofilia; distúrbio do sistema hematopoético em que existe uma tendência à ocorrência de trombose. [thrombo- + G. *philos*, amigo]

throm·bo·phle·bi·tis (throm'bō - flē - bī'tis). Tromboflebite; inflamação venosa com formação de trombo. [thrombo- + G. *phleps*, veia, + *-itis*, inflamação]

t. mi'grans, t. migratória; t. serpiginosa ou que avança lentamente, aparecendo primeiro em uma veia e, a seguir, em outra.

t. sal'tans, t. saltatória; t. que ocorre na mesma veia, porém distante da lesão original, ou que aparece subitamente numa veia distante.

throm·bo·plas·tid (throm - bō - plas'tid). Tromboplastídio. **1.** SIN platelet. **2.** Célula fusiforme nucleada no sangue de mamíferos inferiores. [thrombo- + G. *plastos*, formado]

throm·bo·plas·tin (throm - bō - plas'tin). Tromboplastina; substância presente nos tecidos, nas plaquetas e nos leucócitos, necessária para a coagulação do sangue; na presença de íons cálcio, a t. é necessária para conversão da protrombina em trombina, uma importante etapa na coagulação do sangue. Hoje em dia, acredita-se em geral que a atividade da t. pode ser desenvolvida através dos sistemas sangüíneo (intrínseco) ou tecidual (extrínseco). A t. tecidual (fator III) interage com o fator VII e com o cálcio para ativar o fator X; o fator X ativo combina-se com o fator V na presença de cálcio e fosfolipídio para produzir atividade da t. (também comumente denominada t.). SIN platelet tissue factor, thrombokinase, thrombozyme, tissue factor, zymoplastic substance.

throm·bo·plas·tin·o·gen (throm'bō - plas - tin'ō - jen). Tromboplastinogênio; termo obsoleto para o fator VIII.

throm·bo·poi·e·sis (throm'bō - poy - ē'sis). Trombopoese; precisamente, o processo de formação de um coágulo no sangue, porém geralmente utilizado para referir-se à formação das plaquetas sangüíneas (trombócitos). [thrombo- + G. *poiēsis*, produção]

thrombopoietin (throm'bō - poy'ē - tin). Trombopoetina; citocina que atua como regulador humoral da produção de plaquetas sangüíneas através de sua ação sobre o receptor c-mp1. SIN megakaryocyte growth and development factor, megapoietin. [thrombo- + G. *poiētēs*, que produz, + in]

throm·bosed (throm'bōsd). Trombosado. **1.** Coagulado. **2.** Designa um vaso sangüíneo que é o local de trombose.

throm·bo·ses (throm - bō'sēz). Tromboses; plural de thrombosis.

throm·bo·sin (throm'bō - sin). Trombosina. SIN thrombin.

throm·bo·sis, pl. **throm·bo·ses** (throm - bō'sis, - sēz). Trombose; formação ou presença de um trombo; coagulação dentro de um vaso sangüíneo que pode causar infarto dos tecidos irrigados pelo vaso. [G. *thrombōsis*, coagulação, de *thrombos*, coágulo]

atrophic t., t. atrófica; t. causada por debilidade da circulação, como no marasmo. SIN marantic t., marasmic t.

cerebral t., t. cerebral; coagulação do sangue num vaso cerebral.

compression t., t. por compressão; t. decorrente de interrupção da circulação num vaso por compressão, p. ex., por um tumor.

coronary t., t. coronária; oclusão coronária por formação de trombo, geralmente em conseqüência de alterações ateromatosas na parede arterial, resultando, em geral, em infarto do miocárdio.

creeping t., t. serpiginosa; t. que aumenta gradualmente e acomete uma secção de uma veia após outra em continuidade.

dilation t., t. por dilatação; t. devido a diminuição da velocidade da circulação em conseqüência da dilatação de uma veia.

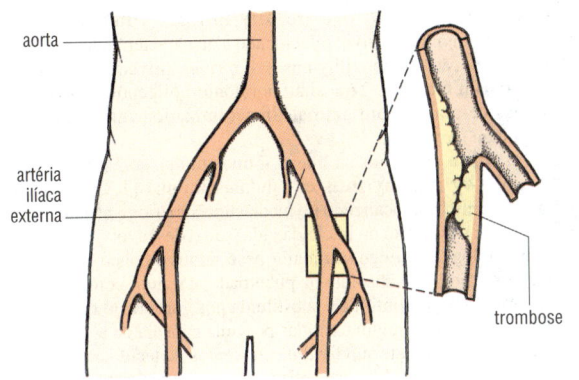

trombose na região iliofemoral

effort-induced t., t. induzida por esforço. SIN Paget-von Schrötter *syndrome.*
marantic t., marasmic t., t. marântica, t. marásmica. SIN atrophic t.
mural t., t. mural; a formação de um trombo em contato com o revestimento endocárdico de uma câmara cardíaca ou de vaso sangüíneo de grande calibre, se não for oclusivo.
placental t., t. placentária; t. das veias do útero no local da placenta.
plate t., platelet t., t. por placa, t. por plaquetas; t. causada por acúmulo anormal de plaquetas.
posttraumatic arterial t., posttraumatic venous t., t. arterial pós-traumática, t. venosa pós-traumática; coagulação intravascular devido a lesão da parede de um vaso.
throm·bo·sta·sis (throm-bos'tā-sis). Trombostasia; interrupção local da circulação por trombose. [thrombo- + G. *stasis,* parada]
throm·bo·sthe·nin (throm-bō-sthē'nin). Trombostenina. SIN platelet *actomyosin.*
throm·bot·ic (throm-bot'ik). Trombótico; relativo a, causado por ou caracterizado por trombose.
throm·bo·to·nin (throm-bō-tō'nin). Trombotonina. SIN serotonin.
throm·box·ane (throm-bok'sān). Tromboxano; a substância original formal dos tromboxanos; ácido prostanóico em que o –COOH foi reduzido a –CH$_3$, e foi inserido um átomo de oxigênio entre os carbonos 11 e 12.
throm·box·anes (throm'bok-zānz). Tromboxanos; grupo de compostos, pertencentes aos eicosanóides, formalmente baseados no t., mas com presença do grupamento COOH terminal; bioquimicamente relacionados às prostaglandinas e formados a partir delas através de uma série de etapas envolvendo a formação de um endoperóxido (uma ponte O–O entre os carbonos 9 e 11 nas prostaglandinas) por uma ciclooxigenase, seguida de rearranjo (catalisado pela tromboxano sintase), que insere um dos dois átomos de oxigênio entre os carbonos 11 e 12, deixando o outro ainda unindo os carbonos 9 e 11. Os t. são assim denominados em virtude de sua influência sobre a agregação plaquetária e a formação do anel de seis membros contendo oxigênio (pirano ou oxano). Como as prostaglandinas, os t. individuais (com abreviatura TX) são designados por letras (A, B, C etc.) e subscritos indicando características estruturais.
throm·bo·zyme (throm'bō-zīm). Trombozima. SIN thromboplastin.
throm·bus, pl. **throm·bi** (throm'bŭs, -bī). Trombo; coágulo presente no sistema cardiovascular, formado durante a vida a partir de constituintes do sangue; pode ser oclusivo ou fixado à parede do vaso ou do coração, sem obstruir a luz (trombomural). [L. do G. *thrombos,* coágulo]
agglutinative t., t. aglutinativo. SIN hyaline t.
agonal t., t. agônico; coágulo cardíaco formado durante o processo de morte após insuficiência cardíaca prolongada.
antemortem t., t. *antemortem;* coágulo formado na circulação durante a vida.
ball t., t. em bola; trombo *antemortem* esférico não-fixado, encontrado no átrio esquerdo ou direito, geralmente em determinados casos de estenose mitral.
ball-valve t., t. em válvula com bola; trombo esférico que causa oclusão intermitente do orifício mitral ou tricúspide.
bile t., t. biliar; depósito intracanalicular de bile, geralmente em conseqüência de obstrução da drenagem biliar.
currant jelly t., t. em geléia de groselha. SIN postmortem t.
fibrin t., t. de fibrina; trombo formado em conseqüência de depósitos repetidos de fibrina do sangue circulante; em geral, não produz oclusão completa do vaso.
globular t., t. globular; um dentre vários trombos de tamanho variável, desde uma ervilha até uma noz, no interior da cavidade cardíaca, conectados por uma delicada rede fibrinosa.
hyaline t., t. hialino; tampão incolor translúcido, que preenche parcial ou totalmente um capilar ou uma pequena artéria ou veia, formado por aglutinação de eritrócitos. SIN agglutinative t.
infective t., t. infeccioso; trombo formado na flebite séptica.
laminated t., t. laminado; trombo formado gradualmente por coagulação do sangue em camadas sucessivas.
marantic t., marasmic t., t. marântico, t. marásmico; trombo formado em casos de marasmo ou debilidade geral.
mixed t., t. misto; trombo laminado, sendo as camadas de diferentes idades de cor ou consistência diferentes. SIN stratified t.
mural t., t. mural; trombo formado sobre uma placa de endocárdio doente ou fixado a ela, mas não sobre uma valva ou uma face de um vaso sangüíneo de grande calibre. VER TAMBÉM parietal t.
obstructive t., t. obstrutivo; trombo formado em decorrência de obstrução do vaso por compressão ou por outra causa.
pale t., t. pálido. SIN white t.
parietal t., t. parietal; trombo arterial que adere a uma face da parede do vaso. VER TAMBÉM mural t.
postmortem t., t. *post-mortem;* coágulo formado dentro do coração ou em um vaso sangüíneo após a morte, constituído, em geral, principalmente de eritrócitos. SIN currant jelly t.
propagated t., t. propagado. VER creeping *thrombosis.*
red t., t. vermelho; trombo formado rapidamente pela coagulação do sangue estagnado, composto principalmente de eritrócitos, mais do que de plaquetas.
secondary t., t. secundário; trombo formado ao redor de um êmbolo, como um núcleo.
stratified t., t. estratificado. SIN mixed t.
valvular t., t. valvular; trombo parietal que se projeta na luz do vaso.
white t., t. branco; trombo branco opaco composto essencialmente de plaquetas sangüíneas. SIN pale t.
throughput (throo'pŭt). Termo aplicado a instrumentos analíticos, especificando o número de testes que podem ser realizados em determinado tempo.
thrush (thrŭsh). Candidíase oral; infecção dos tecidos orais por *Candida albicans;* com freqüência, infecção oportunista em seres humanos com AIDS/SIDA ou que padecem de outras condições que deprimem o sistema imune; também comum em lactentes normais que foram tratados com antibióticos. [do fungo do sapinho, *Candida albicans*]
thu·ja (thoo'jă, -yă). Tuia; as sumidades de *Thuja occidentalis* (família Pinaceae), uma conífera perene ornamental do leste da América do Norte, uma fonte de óleo de folha de cedro; tem sido utilizada internamente como expectorante, emenagogo e anti-helmíntico e externamente como contra-irritante suave. SIN thuya. [G. *thyia,* árvore africana com madeira de aroma doce]
t. oil, óleo de tuia. SIN cedar leaf oil.
thu·jol (thoo'jol). Tujol. SIN thujone.
thu·jone (thoo'jōn). Tujona; $C_{10}H_{16}O$; o principal constituinte do óleo de folha de cedro; estimulante e convulsivante semelhante à cânfora. SIN absinthol, tanacetol, tanacetone, thujol, thuyol, thuyone.
thu·li·um (Tm) (thoo'lē-ŭm). Túlio; elemento metálico da série dos lantanídeos, número atômico 69, peso atômico 168,93421. [L. *Thule,* o primeiro nome da Escandinávia]
thumb (thŭmb) [TA]. Polegar; o primeiro dedo na face radial da mão. SIN pollex [TA], digitus (manus) primus*, first finger. [A.S. *thuma*]
bifid t., p. bífido; malformação congênita do polegar em que a falange distal está dividida.
gamekeeper's t., p. de condeiro; subluxação radial crônica da articulação metacarpofalângica do polegar.
hitchhiker t., p. de carona; má posição do polegar que, em consequência do primeiro metacarpal curto, fica em ângulo reto com a borda radial da mão e no mesmo local; sinal característico de nanismo diastrófico.
tennis t., p. de tenista; tendinite com calcificação no tendão do músculo flexor longo do polegar causada por atrito e tensão, como no jogo de tênis, mas que também ocorre em outros exercícios nos quais o polegar está sujeito a repetida pressão ou tensão.
thumb·print·ing (thŭm'print-ing). Impressão de polegar; sinal radiográfico de isquemia intestinal associada à formação de hematoma e edema na parede intestinal; os tecidos espessados ou edemaciados invadem a luz preenchida de ar ou de contraste radiograficamente.
thumps (thŭmps). Soluços; contrações espasmódicas do diafragma, ou soluços, ocasionalmente observadas em animais.
thus (thŭs, thoos). Incenso. SIN olibanum. [L. incense]
thu·ya (thoo'yă). Tuia. SIN thuja.
thu·yol, thu·yone (thoo'yol, thoo'yōn). Tujol, tujona. SIN thujone.
Thy Abreviatura de thymine (timina).
Thygeson, Phillips, oftalmologista norte-americano, *1903. VER T. *disease.*
thym-. Tim-. VER thymo-.
thyme (tīm). Tomilho; as folhas secas e sumidades floridas do *Thymus vulgaris* (família Labiatae), utilizadas como condimento; contém um óleo volátil (óleo de t.) e constitui uma fonte de timol. [G. *thymon,* tomilho]
t. oil, oil of t., óleo de tomilho; óleo volátil destilado das plantas florescentes do *Thymus vulgaris* ou *T. zygis;* agente aromatizante.
thy·mec·to·my (thī-mek'tō-mē). Timectomia; remoção do timo. [thymus + G. *ektomē,* excisão]

extended t., t. extensa; t. efetuada através de esternotomia combinada e incisão cervical para permitir a remoção de todo o tecido tímico extraglandular. SIN maximal t.
maximal t., t. máxima. SIN extended t.
transcervical t., t. transcervical; t. efetuada através de uma incisão cervical apenas.

thy·mel·co·sis (thī - mel - kō'sis). Timelcose; termo obsoleto para supuração do timo. [thymus + G. *helkōsis,* ulceração]

△ **thymi-.** Timi-. VER thymo-.

△ **-thymia.** -Timia. Mente, alma, emoções. VER TAMBÉM thymo- (2). [G. *thymos,* a mente ou o coração como sede de emoções fortes ou da paixão.]

thy·mic (thī'mik). Tímico; relativo ao timo.

thy·mic ac·id. Ácido tímico. SIN thymol. [ver thyme]

thy·mi·co·lym·phat·ic (thī'mi - kō - lim - fat'ik). Timicolinfático; relativo ao timo e ao sistema linfático.

thy·mi·dine (dThd) (thī'mi - dēn). Timidina; 1-(2-desoxirribosil)timina; um dos quatro principais nucleosídios do DNA (sendo os outros desoxiadenosina, desoxicitidina e desoxiguanosina). SIN deoxythymidine, thymine deoxyribonucleoside.
t. phosphorylase, t. fosforilase; fosforilase que catalisa a fosforólise da timidina; isto é, a timidina e o P$_i$ reagem para formar timina e 2-desoxi-D-ribose 1-fosfato.
tritiated t., t. tritiatada; timidina que contém o radionuclídio de hidrogênio emissor de α, o trítio (H^3 ou hidrogênio-3); utilizada como marcador para medir e localizar por radioautografia a síntese de DNA, no qual é incorporada.

thy·mi·dine 5'-di·phos·phate (dTDP). Timidina 5'-difosfato; timidina esterificada em sua posição 5' com ácido difosfórico.

thy·mi·dine 5'-monophos·phate (dTMP). Timidina 5'- monofosfato. SIN thymidylic acid.

thy·mi·dine 5'-tri·phos·phate (dTTP). Timidina 5'-trifosfato; timidina esterificada em sua posição 5' com ácido trifosfórico; o precursor imediato do ácido timidílico no DNA.

thy·mi·dyl·ate syn·thase (thī - mi - dil'āt). Timidilato sintase; enzima que catalisa a conversão de desoxiuridina 5'-monofosfato em timidina 5'-monofosfato, em que o grupamento metil provém do N^5, N^{10}-metilenotetraidrofolato.

thy·mi·dyl·ic ac·id (thī'mi - dil'ik). Ácido timidílico; importante constituinte do DNA. SIN thymidine 5'-monophosphate, thymine nucleotide.

thy·min (thī'min). Timina. VER thymopoietin.

thy·mine (Thy) (thī'mēn, - min). Timina; 5-metiluracil; constituinte do ácido timidílico e do DNA; elevada na hiperuracil timinúria.
t. deoxyribonucleoside, t. desoxirribonucleosídio. SIN thymidine.
t. deoxyribonucleotide, t. desoxirribonucleotídio. SIN deoxythymidylic acid.
t. nucleotide, t. nucleotídio. SIN thymidylic acid.

thy·mi·nu·ria (thī - mēn - oor'ē - ă). Timinúria. VER hyperuracil thyminuria.

thy·mi·tis (thī - mī'tis). Timite; inflamação do timo.

△ **thymo-, thym-, thymi-.** Timo-, tim-, timi-. **1.** O timo. [G. *thymos*] **2.** Mente, alma, emoções. [G. *thymos,* a mente ou o coração como a sede de sentimentos fortes ou paixões.] **3.** Verruga, verrucoso. [G. *thymos, thymion*]

thy·mo·cyte (thī'mō - sīt). Timócito; célula que se desenvolve no timo, aparentemente a partir de uma célula-tronco da medula óssea e do fígado fetal, precursora do linfócito derivado do timo (linfócito T), responsável pela sensibilidade mediada por células (tipo tardio). [thymus + G. *kytos,* célula]

thy·mo·gen·ic (thī - mō - jen'ik). Timogênico; de origem afetiva. [G. *thymos,* mente + *genesis,* origem]

thy·mo·ki·net·ic (thī'mō - ki - net'ik). Timocinético; que ativa o timo. [thymus + G. *kinēsis,* movimento]

thy·mol (thī'mol). Timol; fenol presente no óleo volátil de *Thymus vulgaris* (timo), *Monarda punctata* (monarda) e outros óleos voláteis; utilizado externa e internamente como anti-séptico, como desodorizante de secreções fétidas e como específico da ancilostomíase. SIN thyme camphor, thymic acid.
t. blue [C.I. 52025], azul de timol; corante utilizado como indicador ácido-básico, com um valor de pK de 1,7 e outro de 8,9; vermelho em pH < 1,2, amarelo em pH entre 2,8 e 8,0 e azul acima de 9,6.
t. iodide, iodeto de timol; anti-séptico em pó seco; era usado como substituto do iodofórmio em doenças cutâneas, feridas, úlceras, rinite purulenta, otite etc.

thy·mo·ma (thī - mō'mă). Timoma; neoplasia no mediastino anterior, que se origina do tecido tímico, habitualmente benigna e, com freqüência, encapsulada; por vezes invasiva, embora as metástases sejam raras; histologicamente, consiste em qualquer tipo de célula epitelial tímica, bem como em linfócitos que, em geral, são abundantes. O linfoma maligno que acomete o timo, p. ex., doença de Hodgkin, não deve ser considerado timoma. [thymus + G. *-oma,* tumor]

thy·mo·nu·cle·ase (thī - mō - noo'klē - ās). Timonuclease. SIN *deoxyribonuclease* I.

thy·mo·poi·et·in (thī'mō - poy - ē'tin). Timopoetina; antigamente denominada timina; hormônio polipeptídico que induz a diferenciação dos linfócitos em timócitos. VER TAMBÉM thymic lymphopoietic *factor.*

thy·mo·pri·val, thy·mo·priv·ic, thy·mo·pri·vous (thī - mō - prī'văl, - priv'ik, - prī'vŭs). Timoprivo; relacionado a ou caracterizado por atrofia prematura ou remoção do timo. [thymus + L. *privus,* privado de]

thy·mo·sin (thī'mō - sin). Timosina; hormônio polipeptídico que restaura a função das células T num animal timectomizado. VER TAMBÉM thymic lymphopoietic *factor.*

thy·mox·a·mine (thī - mok'să - mēn). Timoxamina. SIN moxisylyte.

thy·mus, pl. **thy·mi, thy·mus·es** (thī'mŭs, thī'mī) [TA] [NA] Timo; órgão linfóide primário, localizado no mediastino superior e na parte inferior do pescoço, que é necessário no início da vida para o desenvolvimento normal da função imunológica. Atinge seu maior peso relativo pouco depois do nascimento e seu maior peso absoluto na puberdade; a seguir, começa a involuir, e grande parte do tecido linfóide é substituída por gordura. O timo consiste em duas partes de forma irregular, unidas por uma cápsula de tecido conjuntivo. Cada parte é parcialmente subdividida por septos de tecido conjuntivo em lóbulos, de 0,5 a 2 mm de diâmetro, que consistem numa porção medular interna, contínua com a medula dos lóbulos adjacentes, e numa porção cortical externa. É suprido pelas artérias tireóidea inferior e torácica interna, e seus nervos derivam dos nervos vago e simpático. SIN thymus gland. [G. *thymos,* excrescência, moleja]

△ **thyr-.** Tir-. VER thyro-.

△ **thyreo-.** Tireo-. VER thyro-.

△ **thyro-, thyr-.** Tiro-, tir-. A glândula tireóide. [ver thyroid]

thy·ro·a·ce·tic ac·id (thī'rō - ā - sē'tik). Ácido tireoacético; produto de degradação da tironina (cadeia lateral da alanina reduzida a ácido acético), que ele próprio é um produto de degradação (ou precursor da tiroxina).

thy·ro·ad·e·ni·tis (thī'rō - ad - ē - nī'tis). Tireoadenite. SIN thyroiditis. [thyro- + G. *adēn,* glândula, + *-itis,* inflamação]

thy·ro·a·pla·sia (thī'rō - ă - plā'zē - ă). Tireoaplasia; anomalias observadas em indivíduos com defeitos congênitos da glândula tireóide e deficiência de sua secreção. [thyro- + G. *a-* priv. + *plasis,* modelagem]

thy·ro·ar·y·te·noid (thī'rō - ar'ĭ - tē'noyd). Tireoaritenóideo; relativo às cartilagens tireóidea e aritenóidea. VER thyroarytenoid (*muscle*).

thy·ro·cal·ci·to·nin (thī'rō - kal - si - tō'nin). Tireocalcitonina. SIN calcitonin.

thy·ro·car·di·ac (thī - rō - kar'dē - ak). Tireocardíaco; que afeta o coração em conseqüência de hipo- ou hipertireoidismo.

thy·ro·cele (thī'rō - sēl). Tireocele; tumor da glândula tireóide, como o bócio. [thyro- + G. *kēlē,* tumor]

thy·ro·cer·vi·cal (thī - rō - ser'vi - kăl). Tireocervical; relativo à glândula tireóide e ao pescoço, designando um tronco arterial.

thy·ro·col·loid (thī - rō - kol'oyd). Tireocolóide; substância colóide na glândula tireóide.

thy·ro·ep·i·glot·tic (thī'rō - ep - i - glot'ik). Tireoepiglótico; relativo à cartilagem tireóidea e à epiglote.

thy·ro·fis·sure (thī'rō - fish'er). Tireofissura. SIN laryngofissure.

thy·ro·gen·ic, thy·rog·e·nous (thī - rō - jen'ik, - roj'e - nŭs). Tireogênico; tireógeno; que tem origem na glândula tireóide. [thyroid + G. *-gen,* que produz]

thy·ro·glob·u·lin (thī - rō - glob'ū - lin). Tireoglobulina. **1.** Proteína que contém precursores do hormônio tireóideo, geralmente armazenada no colóide, no interior dos folículos tireóideos; a biossíntese de hormônio tireóideo exige a iodação dos componentes L-tirosil dessa proteína e a combinação de duas iodotirosinas para formar a tiroxina, a tironina totalmente iodada; a secreção de hormônio tireóideo exige a degradação proteolítica da tireoglobulina, com conseqüente liberação do hormônio livre; a ocorrência de um defeito no metabolismo da tireoglobulina resulta em hipotireoidismo. SIN iodoglobulin, thyroprotein (1). **2.** Substância obtida pelo fracionamento de glândulas tireóides do porco, *Sus scrofa,* contendo não menos de 0,7% do iodo total; utilizada como hormônio tireóideo no tratamento do hipotireoidismo.

thy·ro·glos·sal (thī - rō - glos'ăl). Tireoglosso; relativo à glândula tireóide e à língua, designando especialmente um ducto embriológico. SIN thyrolingual.

thy·ro·hy·al (thī - rō - hī'ăl). O corno maior do osso hióide.

thy·ro·hy·oid (thī - rō - hī'oyd). Tíreo-hióideo; relativo à cartilagem tireóidea e ao osso hióide. VER thyrohyoid (*muscle*).

thy·roid (thī'royd). Tireóide. **1.** Semelhante a um escudo; designa uma glândula (glândula tireóide) e uma cartilagem da laringe (cartilagem tireóidea) que possuem essa forma. **2.** Glândula tireóide limpa, seca e pulverizada obtida de um dos animais domésticos usados como alimento e contendo 0,17-0,23% de iodo; outrora amplamente usada no tratamento do hipotireoidismo, do cretinismo e do mixedema, em determinados casos de obesidade e em distúrbios cutâneos. [G. *thyreoeidēs,* de *thyreos,* escudo oblongo, + *eidos,* forma]
accessory t., t. acessória. SIN accessory thyroid *gland.*

thy·roi·dea (thī - roy'dē - ă). Tireóide. SIN thyroid *gland.*
t. accesso'ria, t. i'ma, t. acessória. SIN accessory thyroid *gland.*

thy·roid·ec·to·my (thī - roy - dek'tō - mē). Tireoidectomia; remoção da glândula tireóide. [thyroid + G. *ektomē,* excisão]
"chemical" t., t. "química"; jargão para a redução da função tireóidea produzida pela administração de drogas antitireóideas. VER TAMBÉM radiothyroidectomy.

CORANTES

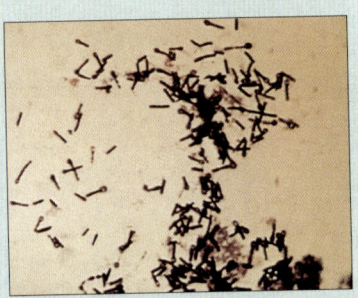
método de Gram: esporos característicos de *Clostridium tetani*

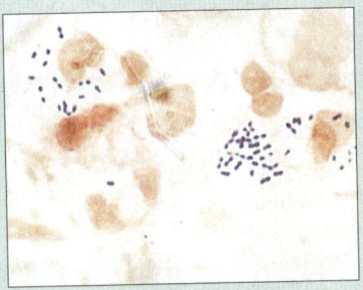
método de Gram: esfregaço de escarro purulento mostrando diplococos Gram-positivos, característicos de *Streptococcus pneumoniae*

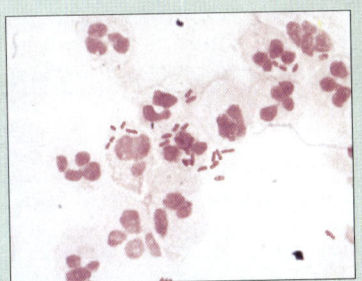
método de Gram: esfregaço de sedimento urinário de um caso de cistite aguda; observe os vários bacilos Gram-negativos (*Escherichia coli*)

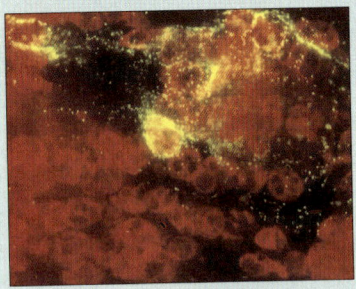
imunofluorescência: cervicite por *Chlamydia trachomatis*

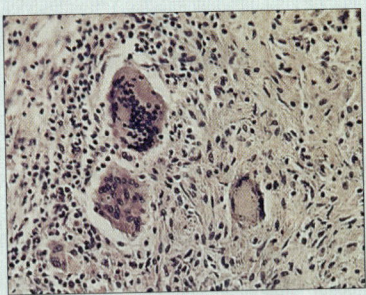
hematoxilina-eosina: corte de fígado através de um tuberculoma; observe as típicas células gigantes de Langhans

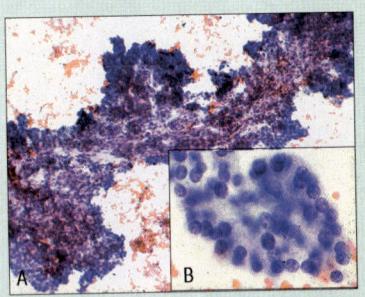
tecido acinar pancreático: (A) pequeno aumento, (B) grande aumento mostrando o padrão acinar

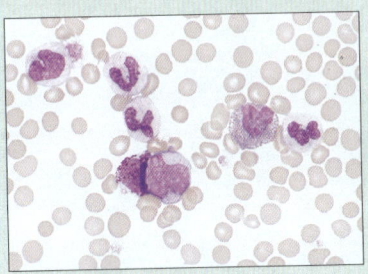
método de Wright-Giemsa: leucemia mielocítica crônica (LMC) com leucocitose; 250 ×

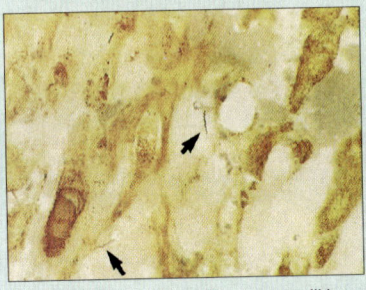
método de Warthin-Starry: *Treponema pallidum* na placenta de um caso de sífilis congênita; observe as espirais estreitas de espiroquetas (setas); 1.000 ×

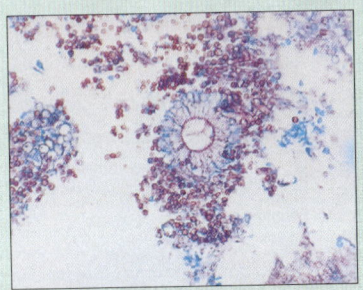
método do ácido periódico de Schiff (PAS): corpo frutificante de *Aspergillus* no aspirado de lesão do pulmão com bola de fungos

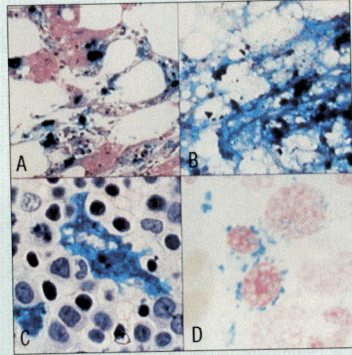
azul-da-Prússia: cortes de coágulo de medula óssea (A,B) e esfregaços (C,D) de um paciente com anemia refratária; o corante azul representa a hemossiderina

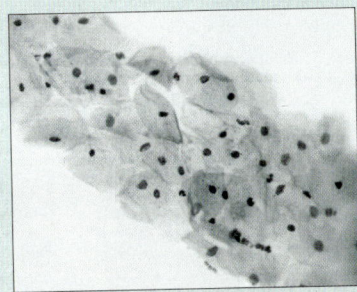
Papanicolaou: células epiteliais escamosas cervicais esfoliadas normais em esfregaço de Papanicolaou

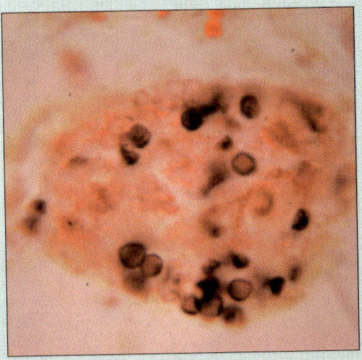
metenamina-prata: *Pneumocystis carinii* em tecido pulmonar; 1.000 ×

CÉLULAS DO SANGUE

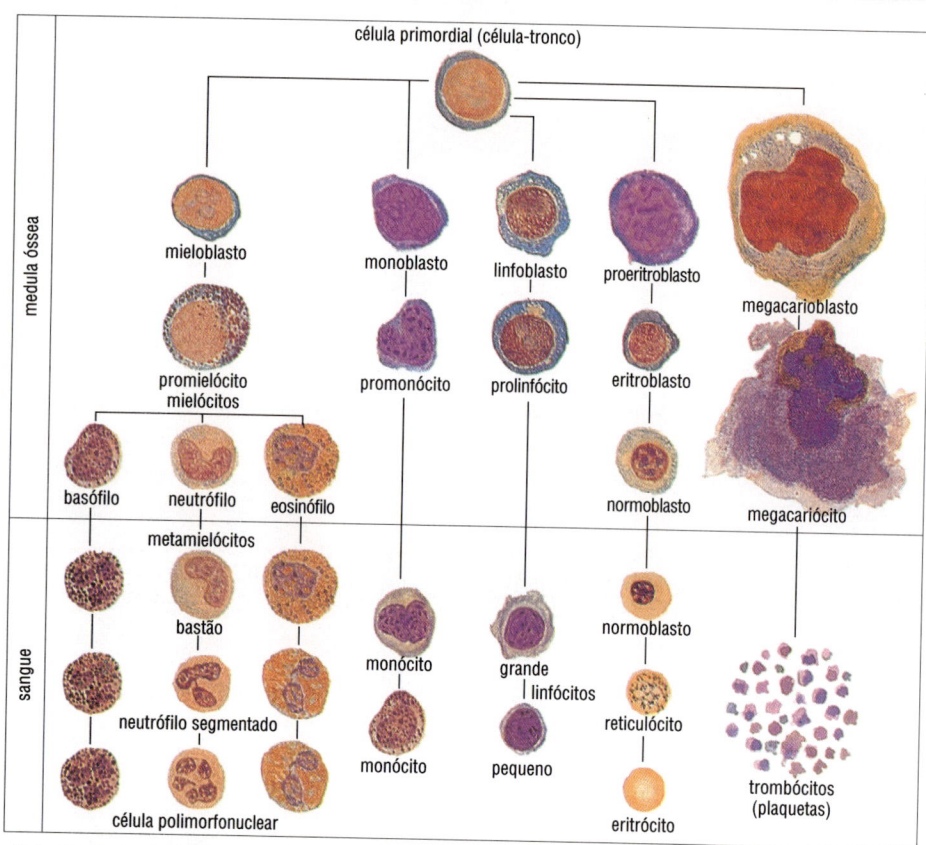

células do sangue: desenvolvimento (esquema simplificado)

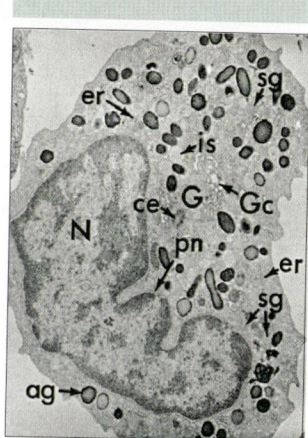

mielócito neutrofílico: coloração de peroxidase, 1.325 ×; (ag) grânulos azurófilos peroxidase-positivos; (sg) grânulos específicos; (is) grânulos específicos imaturos; (G) região de Golgi; (er) retículo endoplasmático rugoso; (pn) cisterna perinuclear; (Gc) cisterna de Golgi; (N) núcleo

os **eritrócitos** possuem uma região central pálida que representa a área mais fina do disco bicôncavo; os **neutrófilos** possuem citoplasma ligeiramente granular e núcleos lobulados (setas, à direita); os **eosinófilos** possuem grandes grânulos rosados e núcleos em forma de salsicha (seta); os **basófilos** caracterizam-se pelos seus grânulos escuros e densos; os **monócitos** caracterizam-se pelo seu grande núcleo reniforme excêntrico e ausência de grânulos específicos; os **linfócitos** são células pequenas com um único núcleo grande de localização excêntrica e uma estreita faixa de citoplasma azul claro

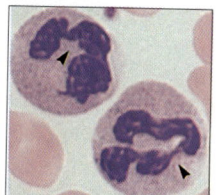

neutrófilo, 1.325 ×

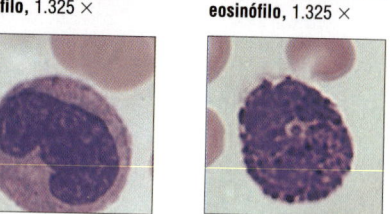

eosinófilo, 1.325 ×

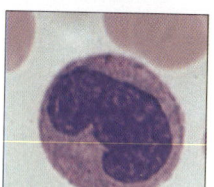

monócito, 1.325 ×

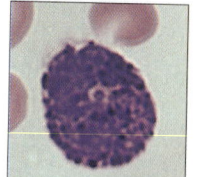

basófilo, 1.325 ×

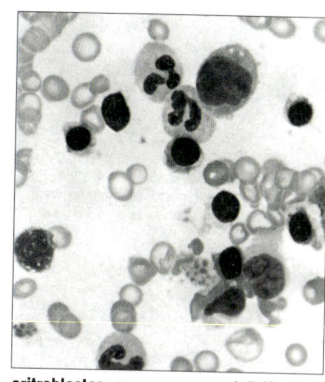

eritroblastos: em sangue com deficiência de ferro

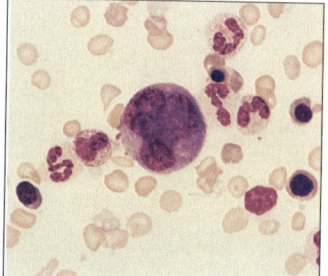

megacarioblasto

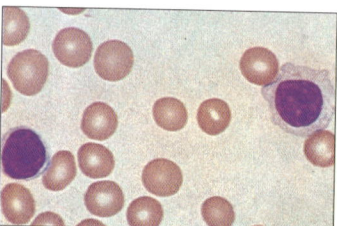

linfócitos: pequenos (à esquerda) e grandes (à direita) com eritrócitos em esfregaço corado de sangue normal

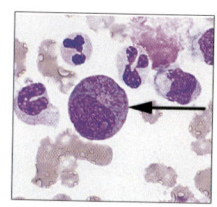

promielócito (seta): medula óssea, 250 ×, método de Wright-Giemsa

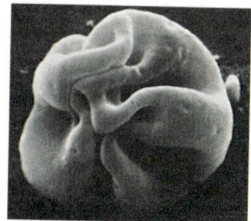

reticulócito: observado ao microscópio eletrônico de varredura

ANORMALIDADES DOS ERITRÓCITOS

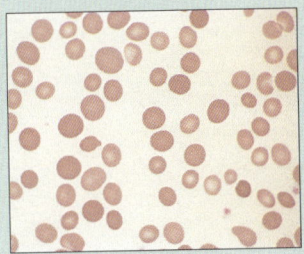
anisocitose: sangue periférico; 250 ×, método de Wright-Giemsa

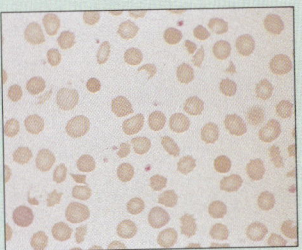
poiquilocitose: com vários tipos de eritrócitos; 250 ×; método de Wright-Giemsa

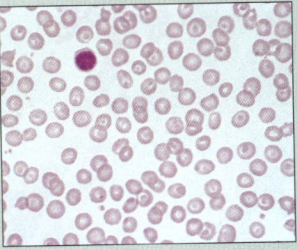
microcitose: observada na talassemia heterozigota (talassemia minor)

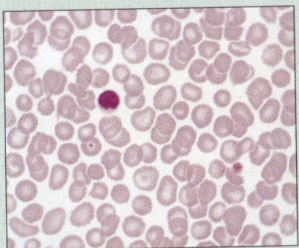
macrocitose: sangue periférico de recém-nascido; 250 ×; método de Wright-Giemsa

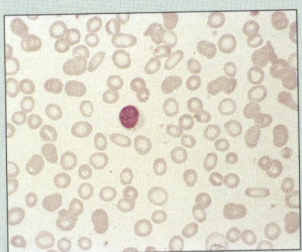
anemia microcítica hipocrômica: sangue periférico; 250 ×, método de Wright-Giemsa

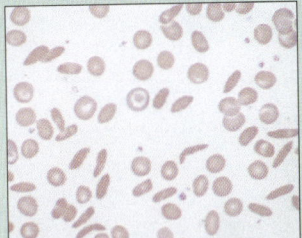
anemia falciforme: poiquilocitose; sangue periférico; 250 ×; método de Wright-Giemsa

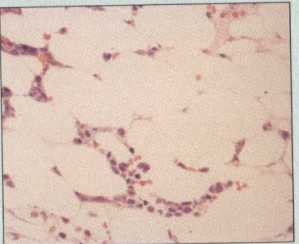
anemia aplásica: esfregaço de medula óssea mostrando os linfócitos e a ausência de precursores eritróides, leucocitários e plaquetários

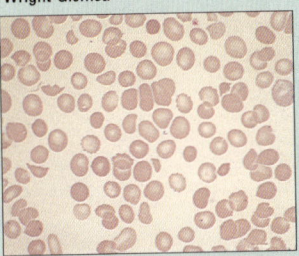
anemia hemolítica: poiquilocitose e ausência de plaquetas, porém sem sinais de hemólise

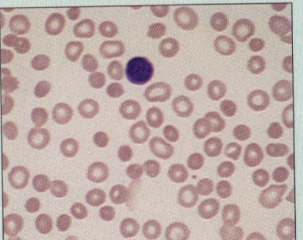
esferocitose: esfregaço sangüíneo; 250 ×, método de Wright-Giemsa

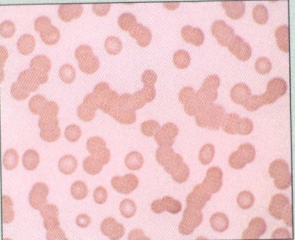
rouleaux: eritrócitos empilhados como moedas; paciente com mieloma múltiplo

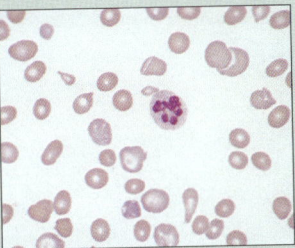
anemia perniciosa: esfregaço de sangue periférico mostrando macrócitos ovais e núcleo hipersegmentado de neutrófilo

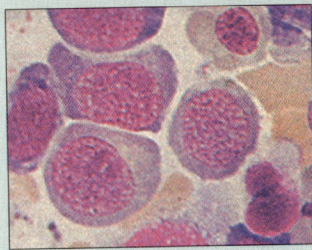
anemia perniciosa: medula óssea

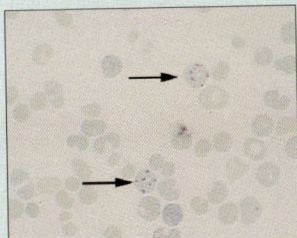
reticulócito (setas): coloração supravital com azul de cresil brilhante; sangue periférico, 250 ×

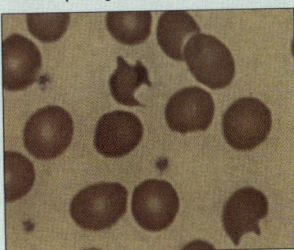
corpúsculos de Heinz: células "mordidas" observadas na hemólise mediada por corpúsculos de Heinz

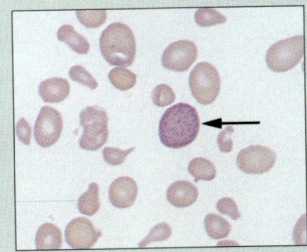
eritrócito com **pontilhado basófilo:** 250 ×, método de Wright-Giemsa

Doenças/Anormalidades

BACTÉRIAS E DOENÇAS BACTERIANAS

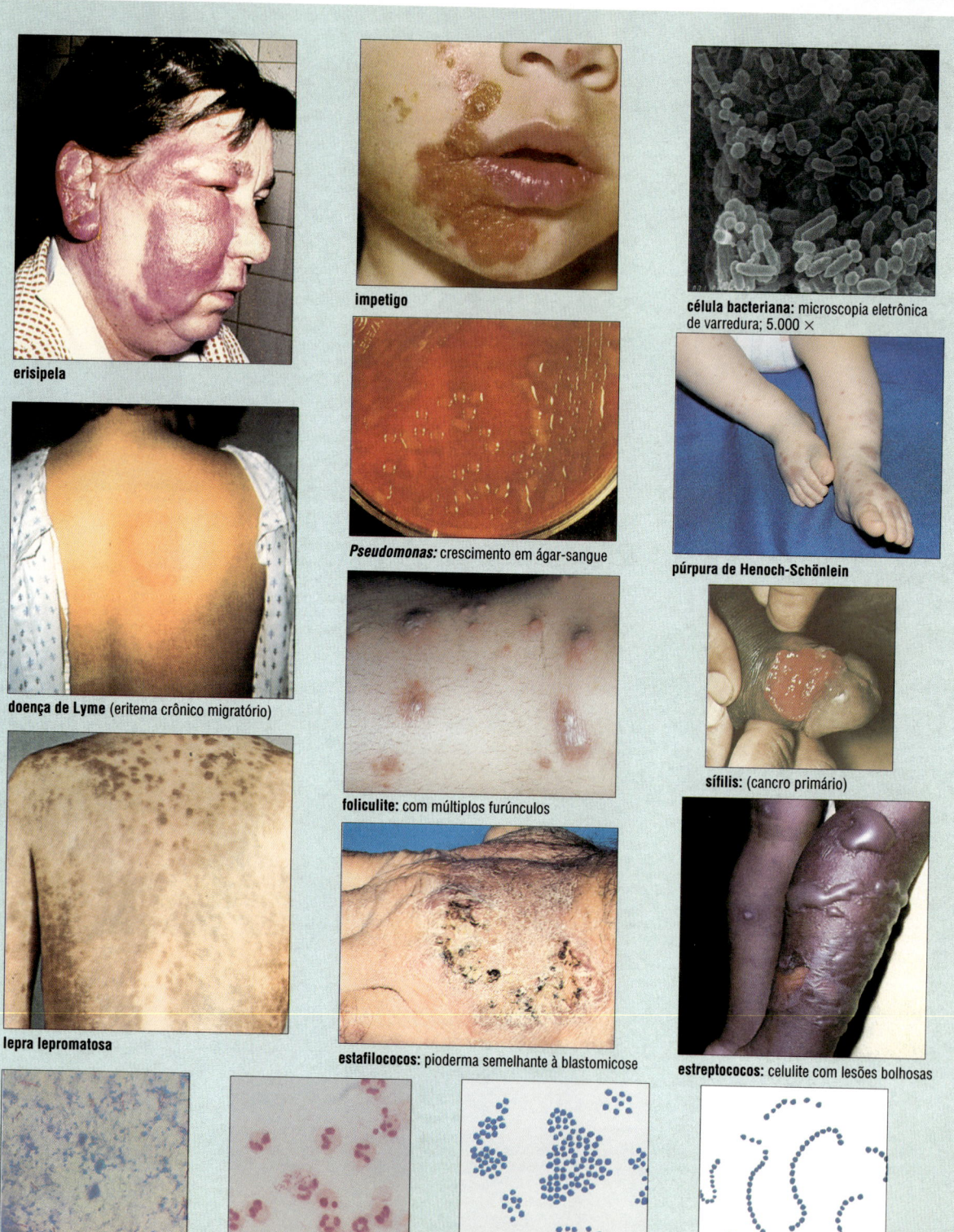

VÍRUS E DOENÇAS VIRAIS

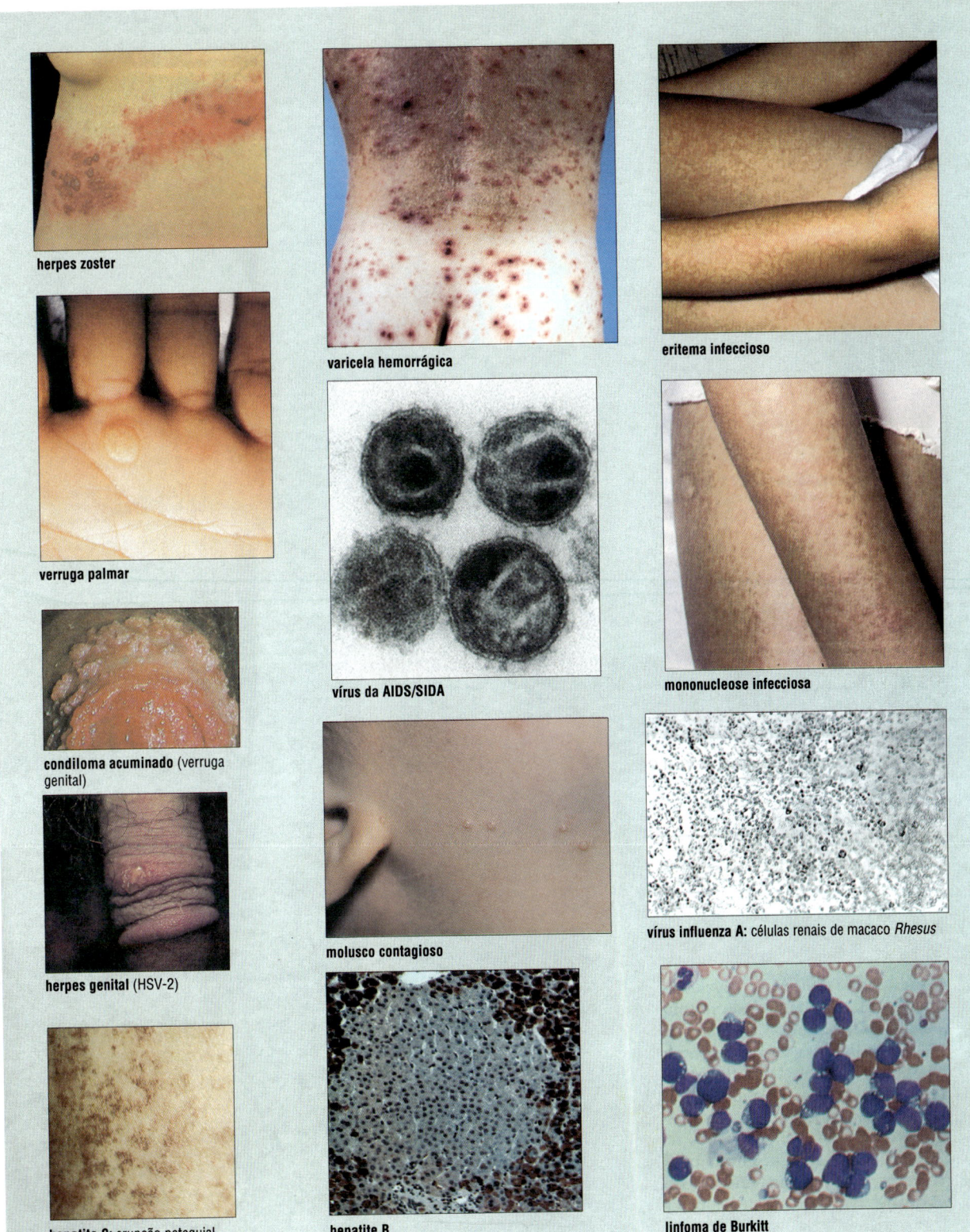

PARASITAS E DOENÇAS PARASITÁRIAS

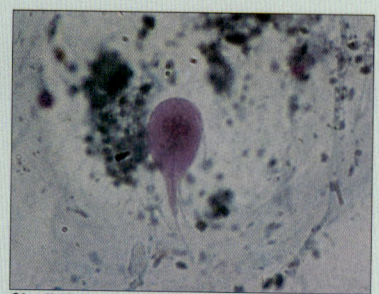
Giardia lamblia: trofozoíta; coloração tricrômica, 400 ×

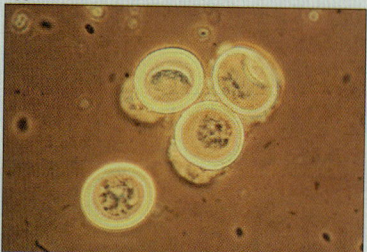
Taenia: microscopia de contraste de fase de quatro ovos

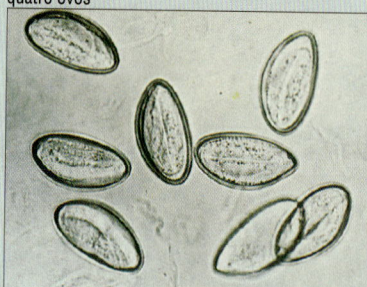
ovos de oxiúro: preparação em fita adesiva transparente

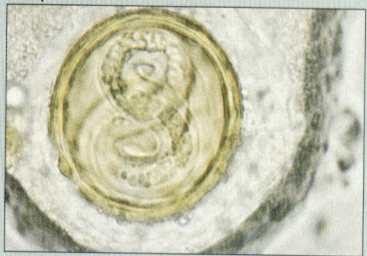
Ascaris lumbricoides: ovo contendo larvas

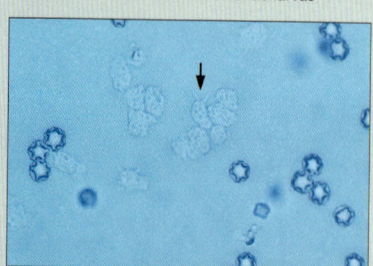
Acanthamoeba: trofozoítas (seta) e cistos; azul de tripan; 40 ×

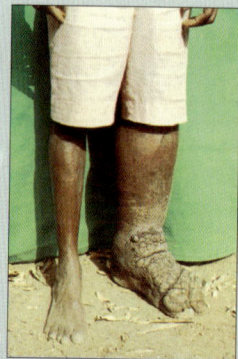
elefantíase: com hiperplasia verrucosa

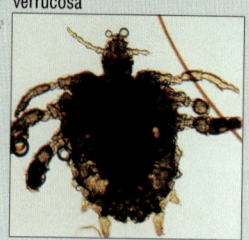
Pthirus pubis (fêmea adulta)

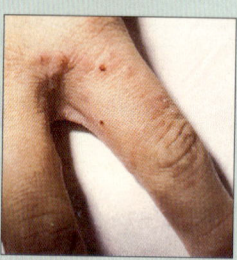
escabiose: lesões pruriginosas

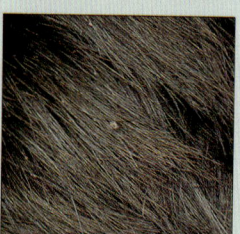
pediculose do couro cabeludo (piolhos da cabeça)

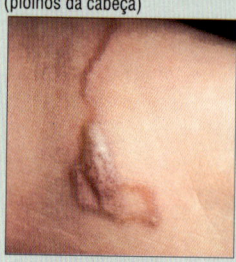
larva migrans cutânea: trajeto serpiginoso com formação de bolha na região plantar

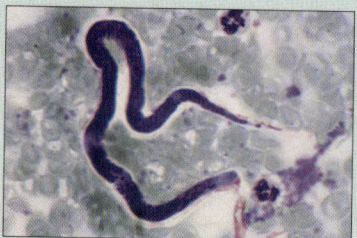
Brugia malayi: microfilária; 300 ×

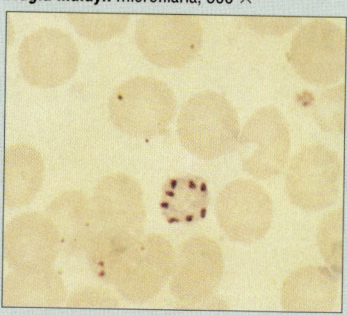
Plasmodium malariae: esquizonte com menos de 13 segmentos no interior de um eritrócito

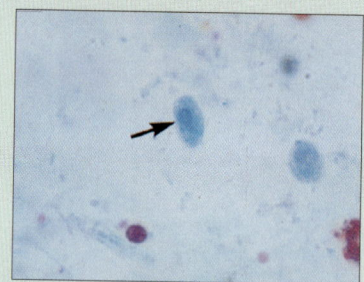
Trichomonas hominis: esfregaço de fezes, coloração tricrômica, 400 ×

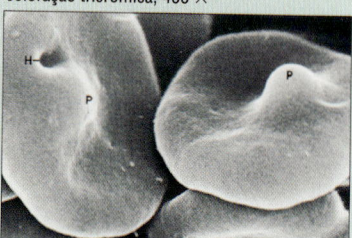
babesia: dois eritrócitos infectados; (H) perfuração, (P) protrusão

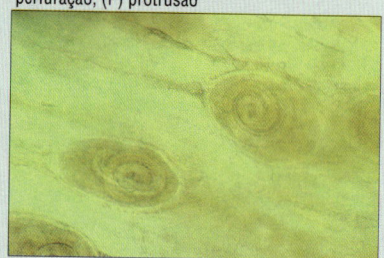
Trichinella: larvas espiraladas em camundongo de laboratório; não-corado; 160 ×

FUNGOS E DOENÇAS FÚNGICAS

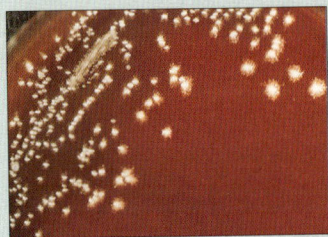

Candida albicans: extensões pediformes das colônias sobre a superfície de ágar-sangue de carneiro a 5%

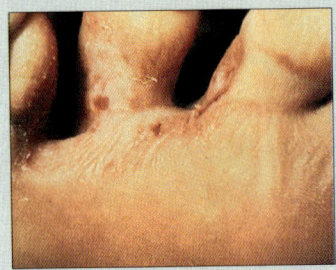

tinha do pé: infecção interdigital por *Trichophyton mentagrophytes*

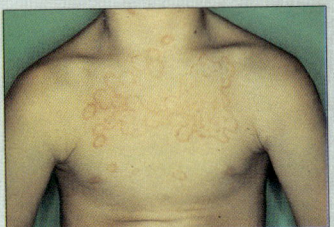

tinha do corpo

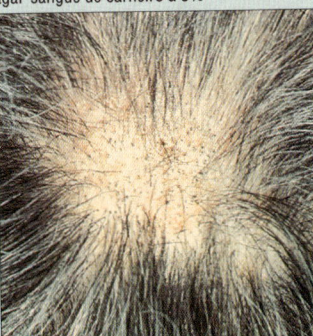

tinha do couro cabeludo: tipo de pontos negros; causada por *Trichophyton tonsurans*

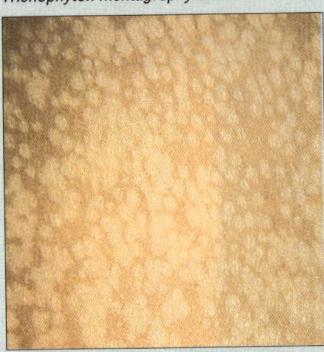

tinha versicolor: vista de perto de máculas hipopigmentadas nas costas

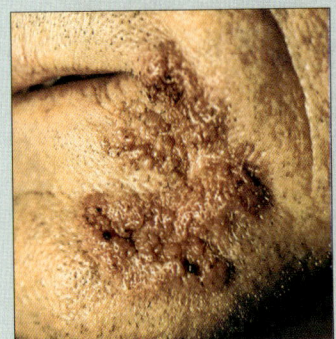

Cryptococcus: blastomicose disseminada; grande placa eritematosa

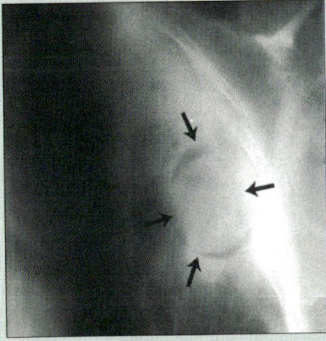

aspergiloma: tomograma de infecção fúngica numa cavidade pulmonar tuberculosa

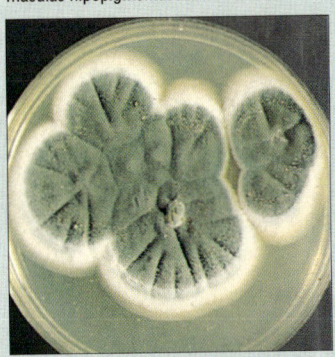

Alternaria (*Penicillium*): depois de 6 dias de crescimento

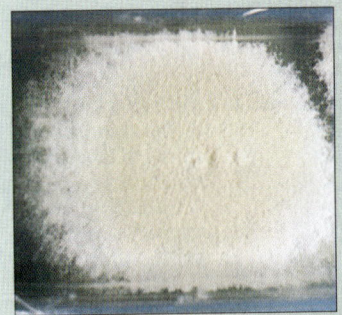

Microsporum gypseum: após 6 dias de incubação

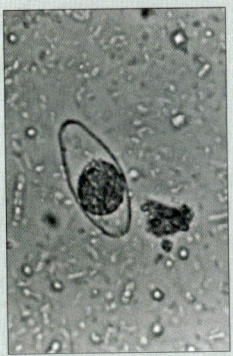

Isospora belli: oocisto imaturo

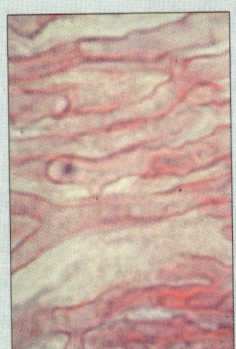

Aspergillus hyphae: em tecido; coloração pelo ácido periódico de Schiff

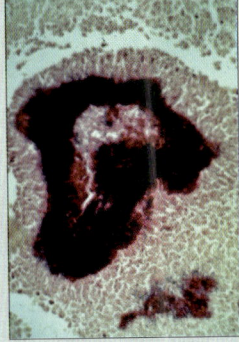

grânulo de micetoma: em tecido; método de Brown e Brenn

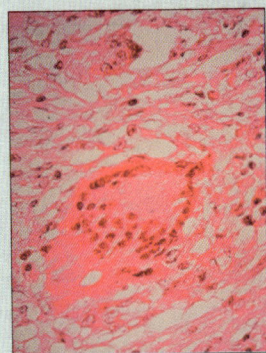

histoplasmose: célula gigante multinucleada no pulmão de paciente com histoplasmose

Doenças/Anormalidades

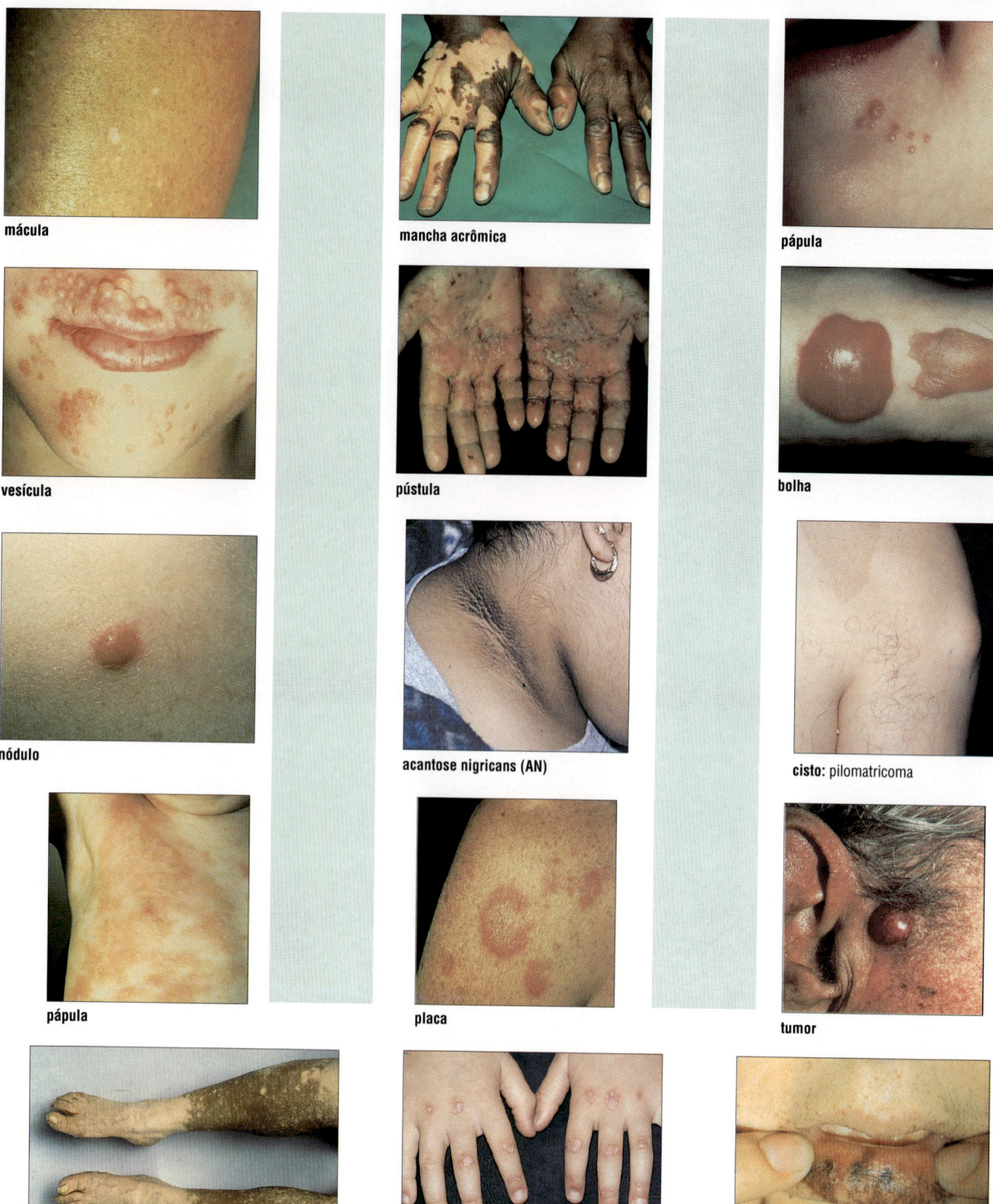

LESÕES SECUNDÁRIAS E VASCULARES

lesões secundárias

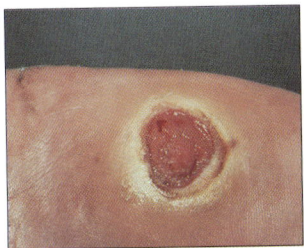
úlcera

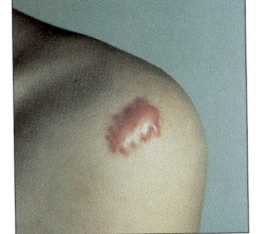
quelóide

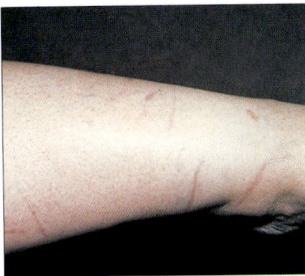
escoriação: arranhaduras de gato em paciente com líquen plano

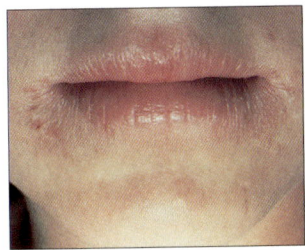
fissura

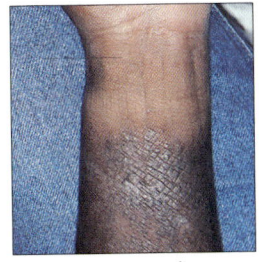
liquenificação: dermatite eczematosa (DE) crônica

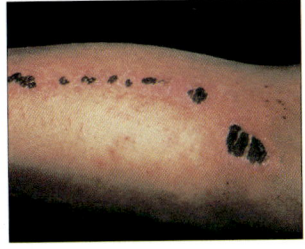
crosta

lesões vasculares

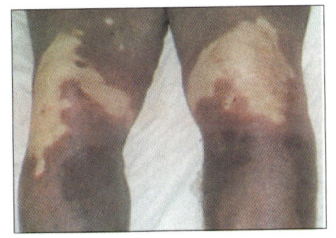
púrpura fulminante

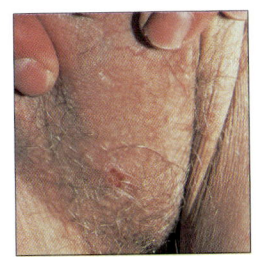
erosão

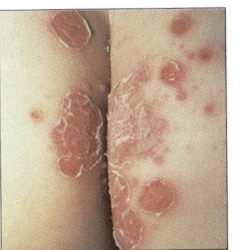
escama

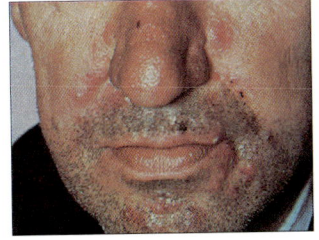
rosácea

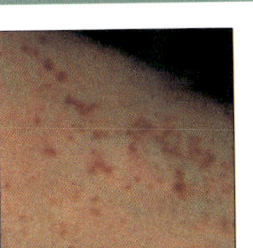
petéquias

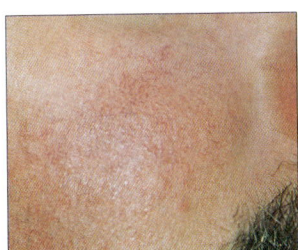
telangiectasia

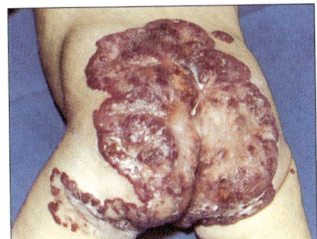
hemangioma cavernoso

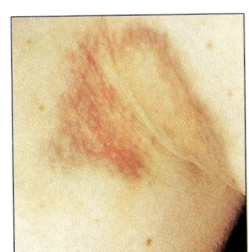
equimose

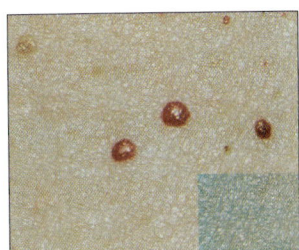
angioma em cereja

Doenças/Anormalidades

LESÕES ORAIS

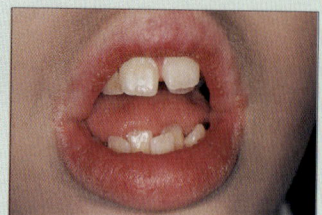
queilite esfoliativa

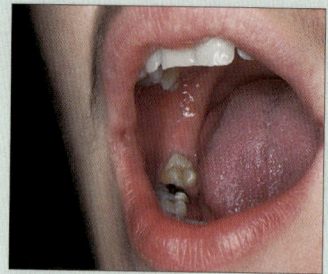
depressões comissurais

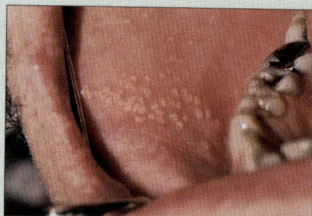
grânulos de Fordyce

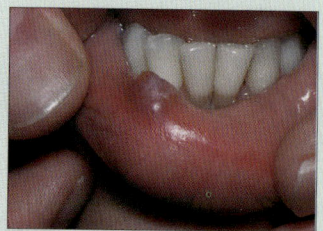
mucocele

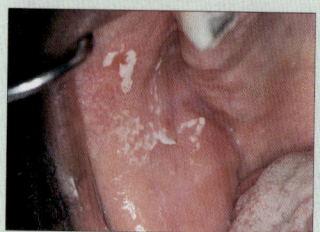
candidíase

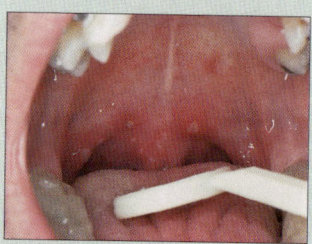
herpangina (vírus Coxsackie)

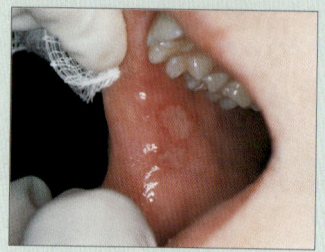
doença de Behçet

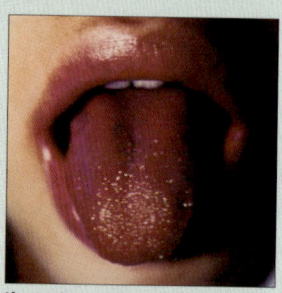
língua de morango: associada a doença de Kawasaki

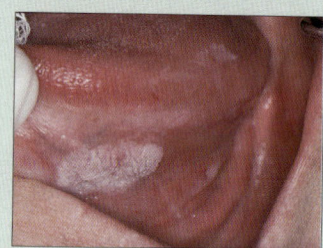
leucoplaquia: com leve displasia epitelial

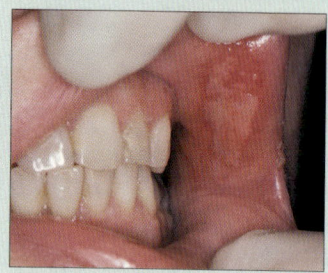
estomatite de contato: devido a acrílico

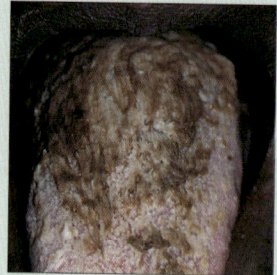
língua pilosa (glossotriquia)

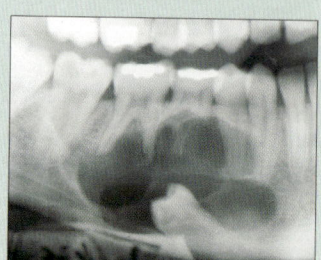
ameloblastoma: grande lesão multilocular ("em bolha de sabão") da mandíbula

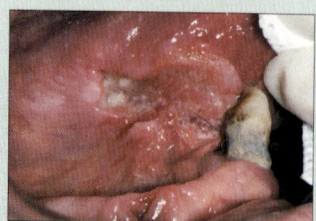
carcinoma de células escamosas

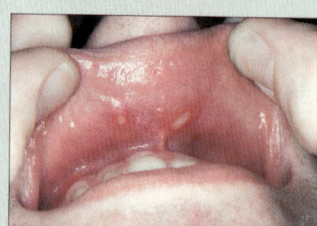
ulcerações aftosas

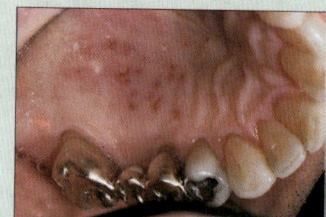
estomatite herpética recorrente

REAÇÕES ALÉRGICAS E DE SENSIBILIDADE

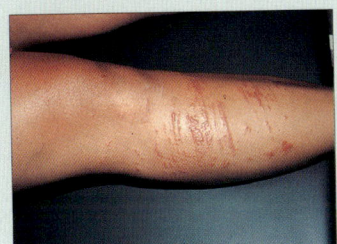

dermatite de contato (hera venenosa)

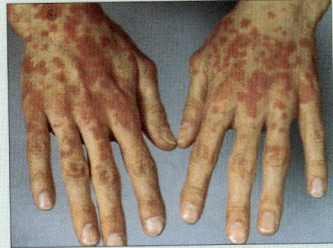

fotodermatose polimórfica

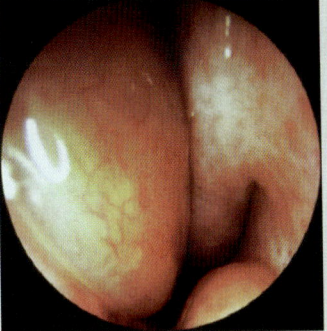

pólipos nasais: associados a alergia nasal crônica; vista com iluminador nasal

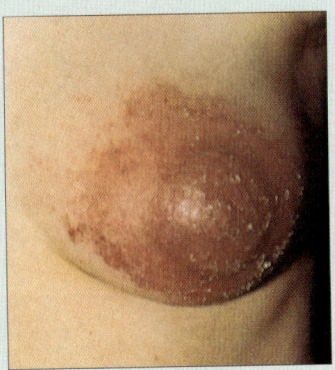

dermatite de contato alérgica aguda: doença de Paget do mamilo

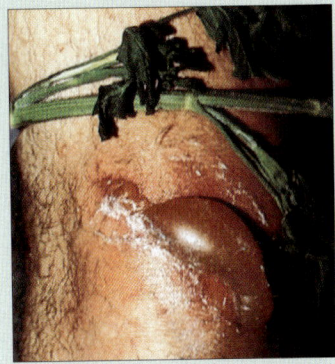

fotodermatite aguda: (fitofotodermatite, tipo fototóxico); lesão bolhosa formada após esfregar ambrósia americana (planta mostrada) contra a pele, que foi em seguida exposta à luz solar

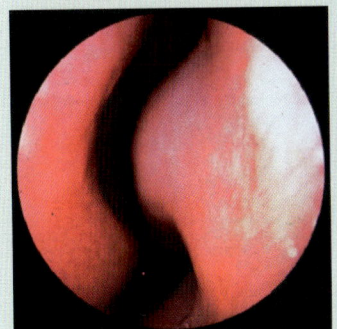

rinite alérgica (vista de rinoscópio)

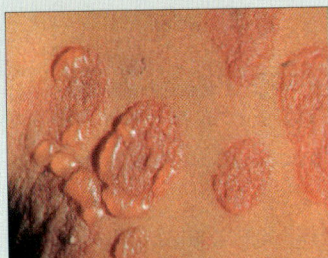

dermatite herpetiforme

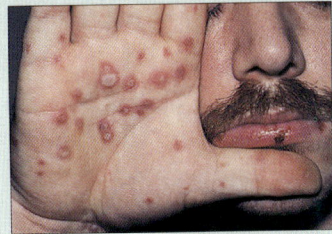

eritema multiforme minor: em paciente com infecção recorrente pelo vírus herpes simples (HSV)

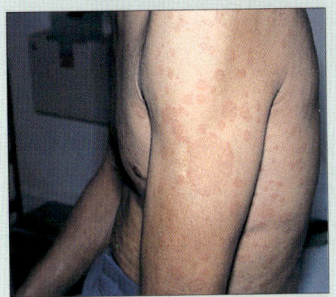

erupção medicamentosa urticariforme

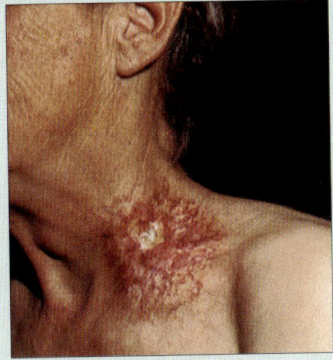

radiodermatite: ulceração crônica

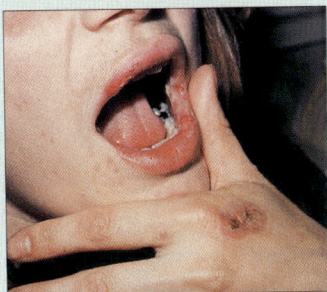

síndrome de Stevens-Johnson (eritema multiforme major)

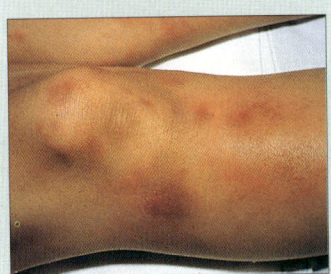

eritema nodoso (EN)

Doenças/Anormalidades

NEOPLASIAS — FOTOGRAFIAS CLÍNICAS

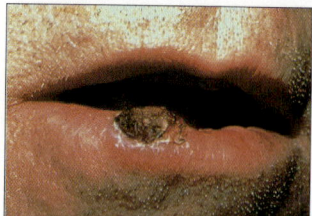
carcinoma de células escamosas (lábio)

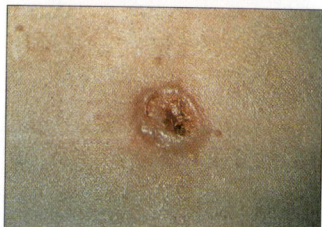
carcinoma basocelular

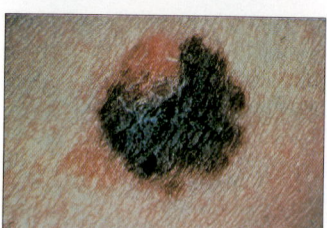
melanoma maligno

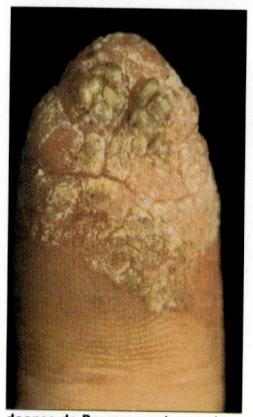
doença de Bowen: carcinoma de células escamosa *in situ* na ponta de um dedo da mão

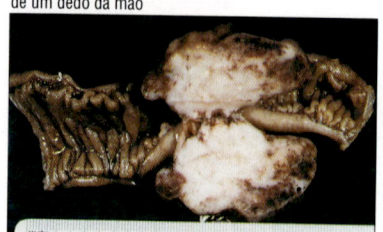
tumor de estroma: tumor maligno do intestino

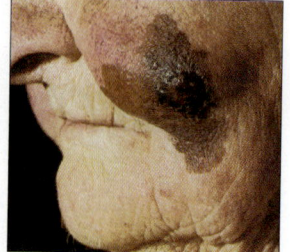
lentigo maligno-melanoma

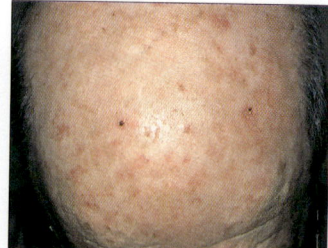
ceratose actínica: numerosas ceratoses no couro cabeludo induzidas por exposição crônica aos raios ultravioleta

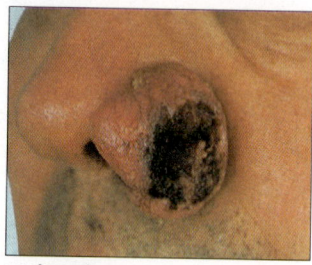
ceratoacantoma

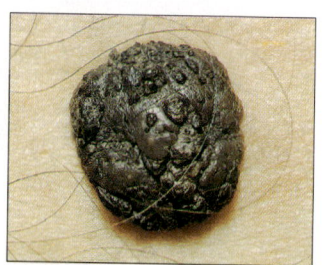
ceratose seborréica

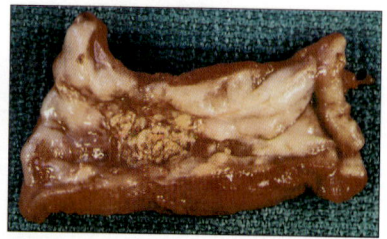
carcinoma ulcerativo de células escamosas: esôfago

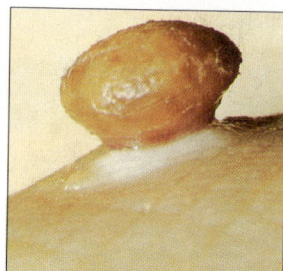
granuloma piogênico

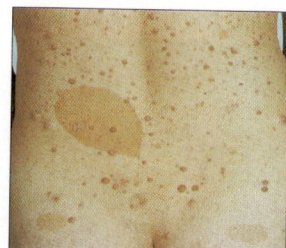
neurofibromatose

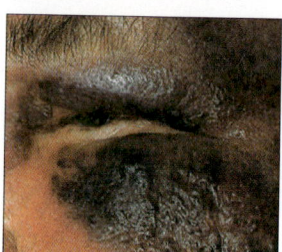
angiossarcoma: lado esquerdo da face

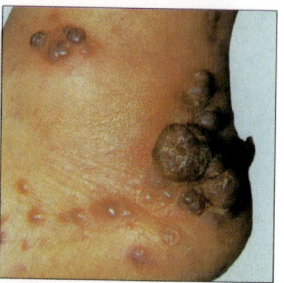
sarcoma de Kaposi

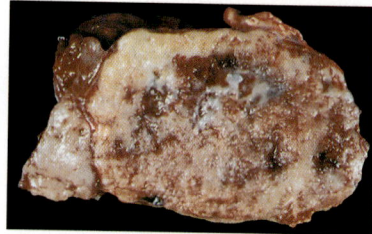
tumor benigno do estômago

NEOPLASIAS — IMAGENS HISTOLÓGICAS

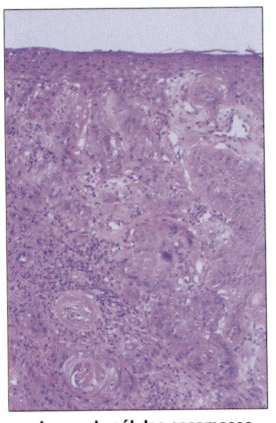
carcinoma de células escamosas

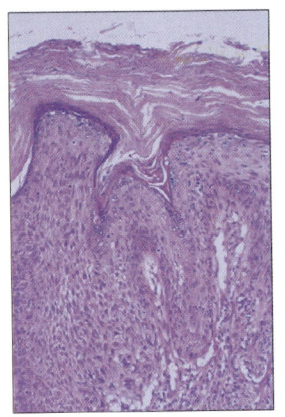
doença de Bowen

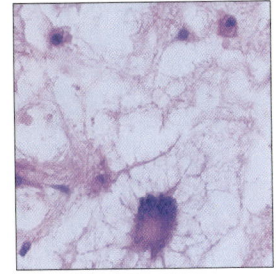
lipossarcoma

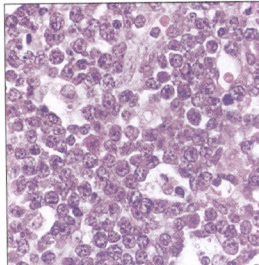
linfoma

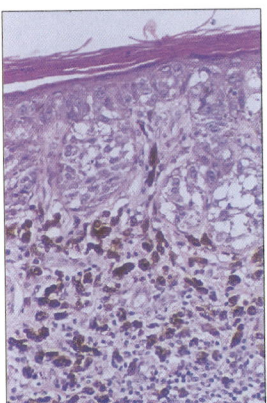
melanoma nodular

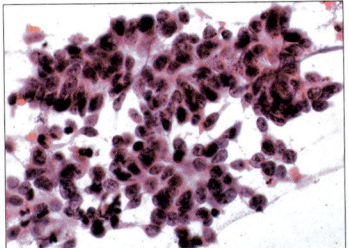
ependimoma: grande aumento

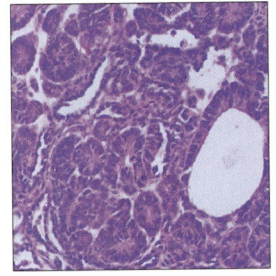
tumor de Wilms

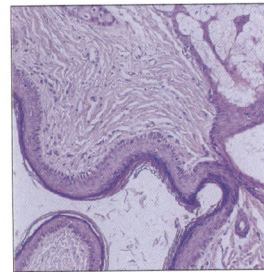
teratoma

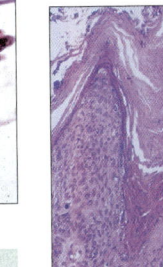
ceratose actínica

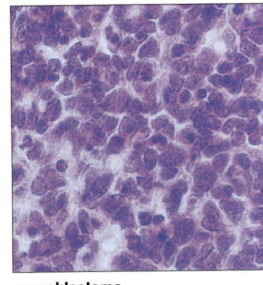
neuroblastoma

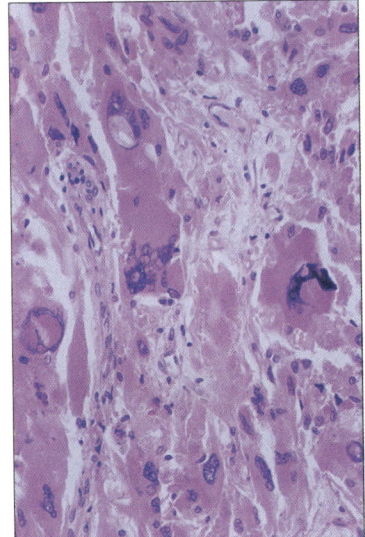
glioblastoma multiforme

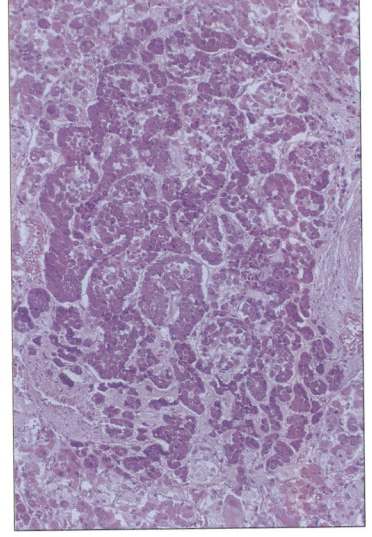
adenoma hipofisário: microadenoma

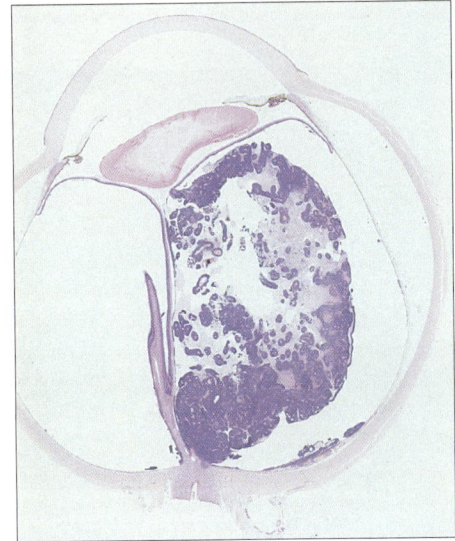
retinoblastoma

NEOPLASIA — IMAGENS DIAGNÓSTICAS

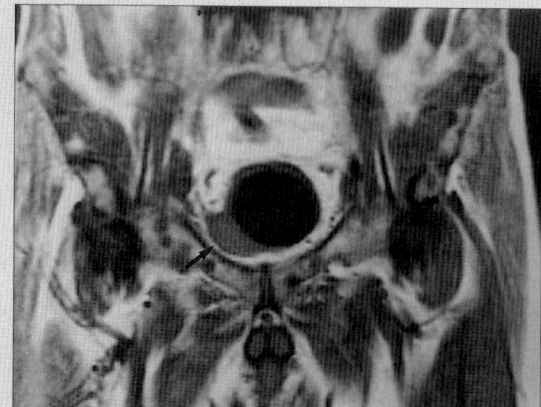

carcinoma de próstata: RM coronal, ponderada em T1, mostrando uma massa (seta) invadindo o assoalho da bexiga do lado direito

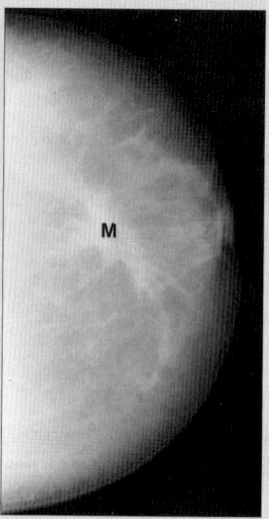

carcinoma de mama: mamografia revelando carcinoma de localização profunda (M)

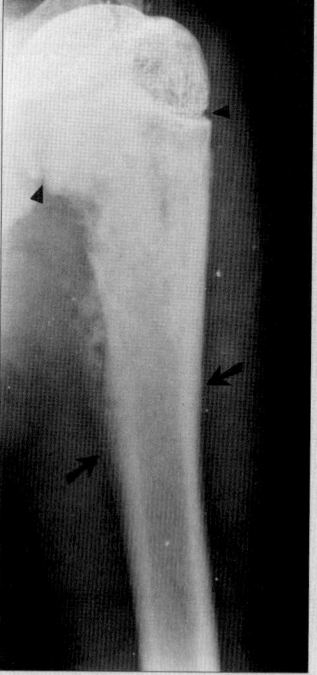

tumor de Ewing: parte proximal do úmero; observe a reação periósteа laminada interrompida (setas)

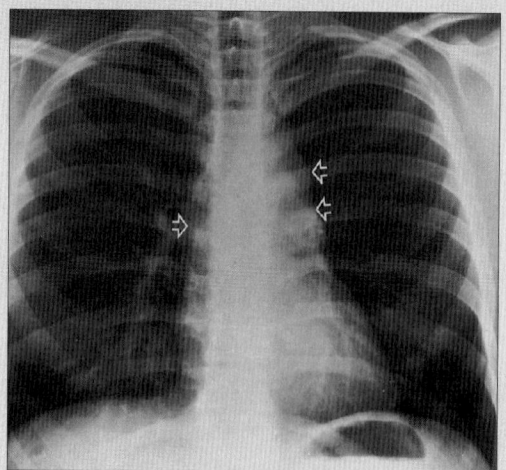

linfoma: radiografia frontal mostrando uma massa lobular no mediastino (setas)

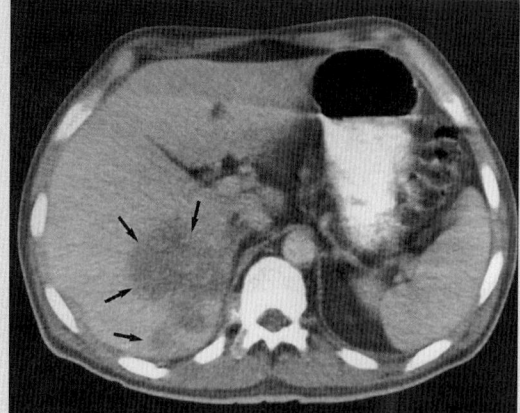

metástases hepáticas: TC de paciente com carcinoma renal, mostrando várias áreas mais claras intra-hepáticas (setas)

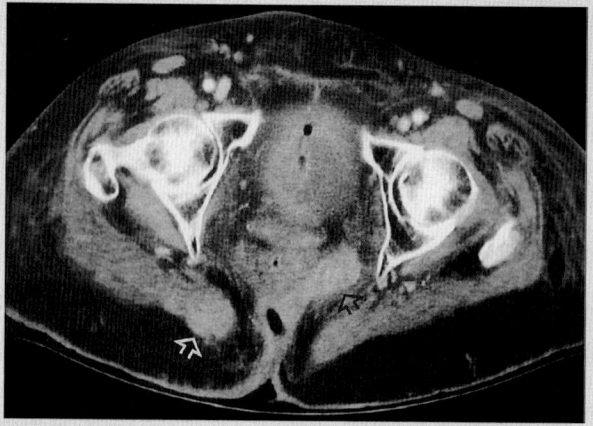

carcinoma de colo: TC da pelve mostrando massas peri-retais recorrentes (setas)

DIAGNÓSTICO FÍSICO

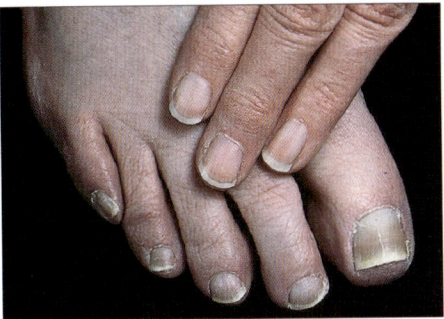

cianose: coloração azulada visível nos leitos ungueais

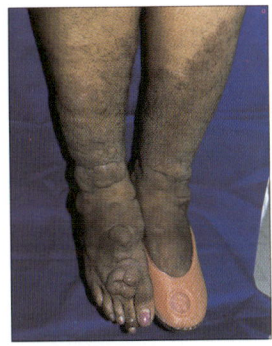

mixedema pré-tibial

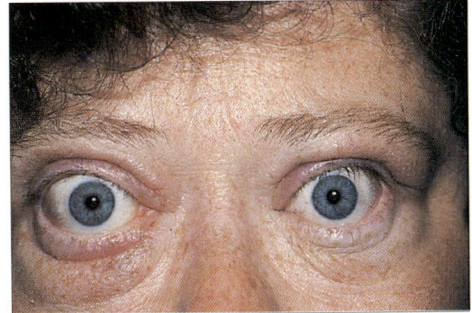

exoftalmia

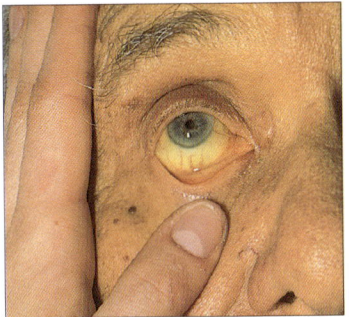

icterícia: observe a cor amarela da pele do paciente em comparação com a mão do examinador

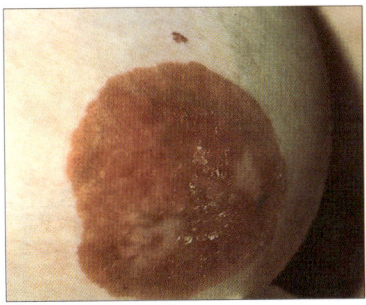

doença de Paget: mamilo

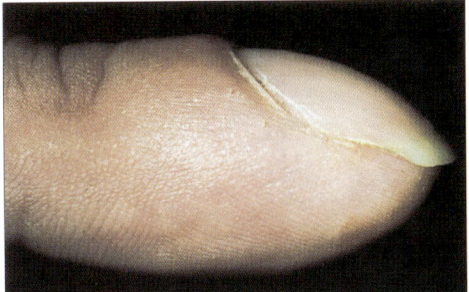

baqueteamento digital

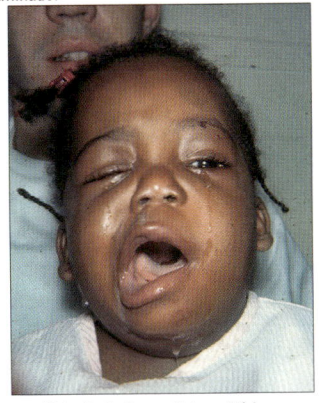

paralisia de Bell: paralisia periférica (neurônio motor inferior) do nervo facial

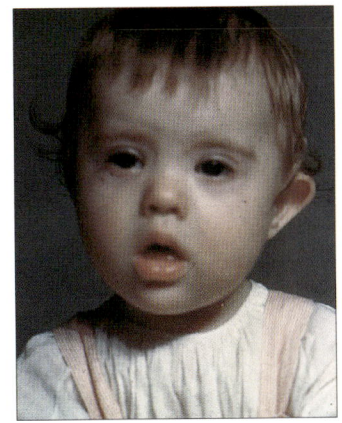

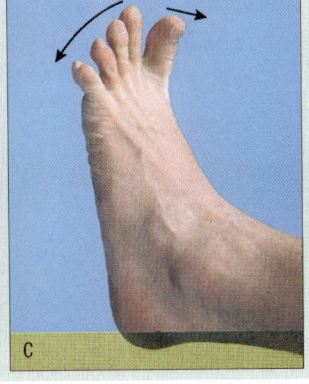

síndrome de Down (trissomia do 21): (à esquerda) traços faciais típicos, incluindo cabeça pequena e arredondada, ponte nasal achatada e língua relativamente grande;
manchas de Brushfield: (em cima) sugerem fortemente a síndrome de Down

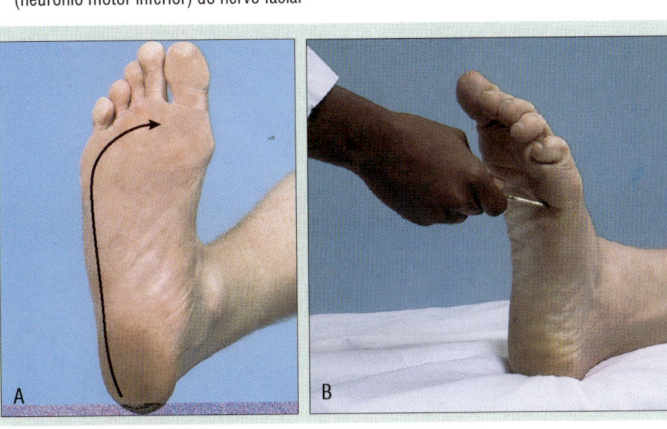

resposta de Babinski (plantar extensora) (A) a face lateral da planta do pé é estimulada com um objeto pontiagudo desde o calcanhar até o antepé; (B) a flexão de todos os dedos do pé é a resposta normal; (C) a extensão do hálux, freqüentemente com abertura dos outros dedos, constitui o sinal de Babinski; com freqüência, indica uma lesão do córtex motor ou de um trato piramidal (corticospinal).

Doenças/Anormalidades

MICROSCOPIA CLÍNICA

exame microscópico de urina

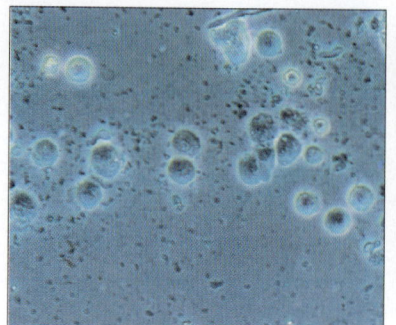
leucócitos

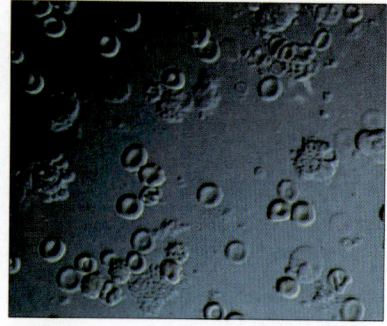
hemácias

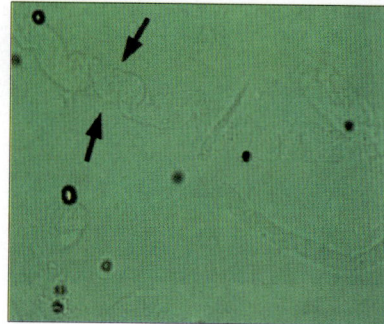
cilindro hialino

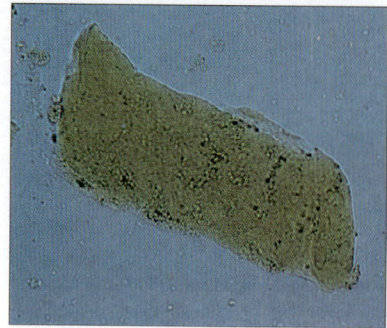
cilindro céreo

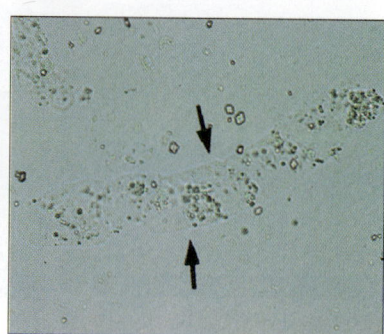
cilindro granuloso

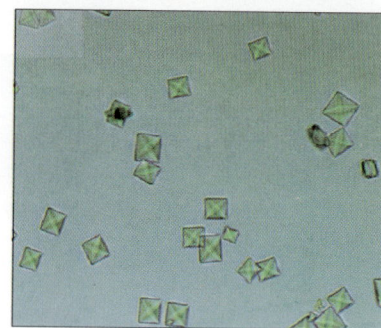
cristais de oxalato de cálcio

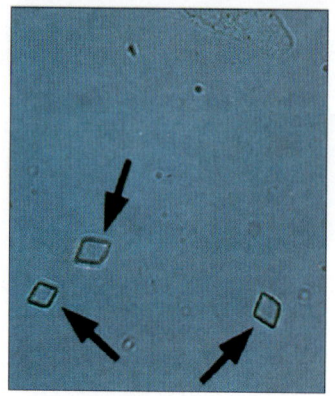
cristais de ácido úrico

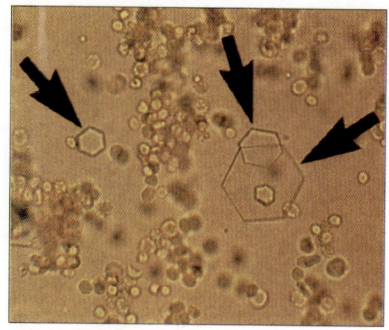
cristais de cistina

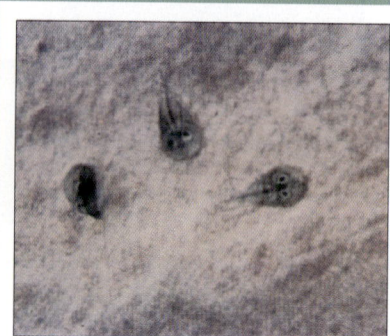
Giardia lamblia em esfregaço fecal

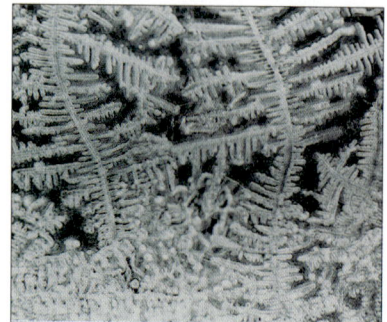
padrão em samambaia do muco cervical

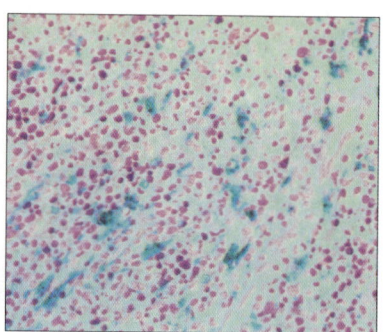
aspirado de medula óssea mostrando as reservas de ferro

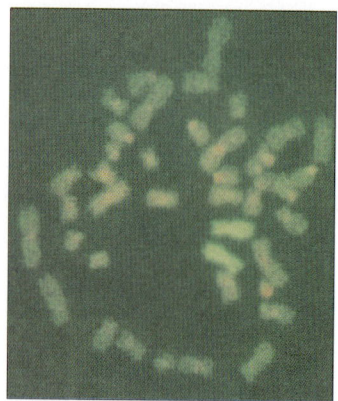
sonda cromossômica integral

near-total t., t. quase total; remoção de quase todos os lobos da tireóide, deixando apenas uma pequena parte da glândula adjacente à entrada do nervo laríngeo recorrente na laringe.
subtotal t., t. subtotal; remoção de pelo menos um lobo da tireóide, até uma tireoidectomia quase total.
thy·roid·ism (thī'roy-dizm). Tireoidismo; designação obsoleta para: **1.** SIN hyperthyroidism. **2.** Intoxicação por superdoses de extrato tireóideo.
thy·roid·i·tis (thī-roy-dī'tis). Tireoidite; inflamação da glândula tireóide. SIN thyroadenitis. [thyroid + G. -itis, inflamação]
autoimmune t., t. auto-imune. SIN Hashimoto t.
chronic atrophic t., t. atrófica crônica; substituição da glândula tireóide por tecido fibroso; é a causa mais comum de mixedema em indivíduos idosos.
chronic fibrous t., t. fibrosa crônica. SIN Riedel t.
chronic lymphadenoid t., t. linfadenóide crônica. SIN Hashimoto t.
chronic lymphocytic t., t. linfocítica crônica. SIN Hashimoto t.
de Quervain t, t. de Quervain. SIN subacute granulomatous t.
focal lymphocytic t., t. linfocítica focal; infiltração focal da tireóide por linfócitos e plasmócitos. VER TAMBÉM Hashimoto t.
giant cell t., t. de células gigantes. SIN subacute granulomatous t.
giant follicular t., t. folicular gigante; variante da t. de Hashimoto, em que o infiltrado linfocítico na tireóide formou-se no interior de folículos gigantes.
Hashimoto t., t. de Hashimoto; infiltração difusa da glândula tireóide por linfócitos, resultando em bócio difuso, destruição progressiva do parênquima e hipotireoidismo. SIN autoimmune t., chronic lymphadenoid t., chronic lymphocytic t., Hashimoto disease, Hashimoto struma, lymphocytic t., struma lymphomatosa.
ligneous t., t. lenhosa. SIN Riedel t.
lymphocytic t., t. linfocítica. SIN Hashimoto t.
parasitic t., t. parasítica; tripanossomíase sul-americana crônica com comprometimento da tireóide, causando mixedema.
Riedel t., t. de Riedel; induração fibrosa rara da glândula tireóide, com aderência a estruturas adjacentes, podendo causar compressão da traquéia. SIN chronic fibrous t., ligneous struma, ligneous t., Riedel disease, Riedel struma.
subacute granulomatous t., t. granulomatosa subaguda; t. com infiltração de células redondas (geralmente linfócitos), destruição de células da tireóide, proliferação de células gigantes epiteliais e evidência de regeneração; considerada por alguns um reflexo de infecção sistêmica, e não um exemplo de tireoidite crônica verdadeira. SIN de Quervain t., giant cell t.
subacute lymphocyte t., t. linfocítica subaguda; variante subaguda da t. de Hashimoto.
thy·roi·dol·o·gy (thī-roy-dol'ō-jē). Tireoidologia; o estudo da glândula tireóide, tanto normal quanto patológica. [thyroid + G. logos, estudo]
thy·roid·o·to·my (thī'roy-dot'ō-mē). Tireoidotomia. SIN laryngofissure. [thyroid + G. tomē, incisão]
thy·ro·in·tox·i·ca·tion. Tireointoxicação. SIN hyperthyroidism.
thy·ro·la·ryn·ge·al (thī'rō-là-rin'jē-ăl). Tireolaríngeo; relativo à glândula ou cartilagem tireóidea e à laringe.
thy·ro·lib·er·in (thī-rō-lib'er-in). Tireoliberina; hormônio tripeptídico do hipotálamo, que estimula a adeno-hipófise a liberar tireotropina; L-piroglutamil-L-histidil-L-prolinamida. SIN thyroid-stimulating hormone-releasing factor, thyrotropin-releasing hormone. [thyrotropin + L. libero, liberar, + -in]
thy·ro·lin·gual (thī'rō-ling'gwăl). Tireolingual. SIN thyroglossal. [thyro- + L. lingua, língua]
thy·ro·lyt·ic (thī-rō-lit'ik). Tireolítico; que causa destruição das células da glândula tireóide. [thyro- + G. lytikos, dissolução]
thy·ro·meg·a·ly (thī-rō-meg'a-lē). Tireomegalia; aumento da glândula tireóide. [thyro- + G. megas, grande]
thy·ro·nine (thī'rō-nēn, -nin). Tironina; aminoácido com grupamento éter difenil na cadeia lateral; ocorre em proteínas apenas na forma de derivados iodados (iodotironinas), como a tiroxina.
thy·ro·pal·a·tine (thī-rō-pal'ă-tīn). Tireopalatino; designa o músculo palatofaríngeo.
thy·ro·par·a·thy·roid·ec·to·my (thī'rō-par-ă-thī'roy-dek'tō-mē). Tireoparatireoidectomia; excisão das glândulas tireóide e paratireóides.
thy·rop·a·thy (thī-rop'ă-thē). Tireopatia; distúrbio da glândula tireóide. [thyro- + G. pathos, sofrimento]
thy·ro·per·ox·i·dase (thī-rō-per-oks'i-dās). Tireoperoxidase; proteína que participa do metabolismo do iodo no folículo da tireóide e no espaço folicular; utiliza H_2O_2 para produzir I^+.
thy·ro·pha·ryn·ge·al (thī-rō-fă-rin'jē-ăl). Tireofaríngeo; designa a parte tireofaríngea do músculo constritor inferior da faringe.
thy·ro·plas·ty. Tireoplastia; método cirúrgico para restaurar a qualidade vocal ao alterar a geometria da cartilagem tireóidea. [thyro- + G. plastos, formado]
thy·ro·pri·val (thī-rō-prī'văl). Tireoprivo; relativo à tireoprivia, referindo-se ao hipotireoidismo produzido por doença ou por tireoidectomia. SIN thyroprivic, thyroprivous. [thyro- + L. privus, privado de]
thy·ro·priv·ia (thī-rō-priv'ē-ă). Tireoprivia; estado caracterizado por redução da atividade da tireóide.

thy·ro·priv·ic, thy·ro·pri·vous (thī-rō-priv'ik, -priv'ŭs). Tireoprivo. SIN thyroprival.
thy·ro·pro·tein (thī-rō-prō'tēn). Tireoproteína. **1.** SIN thyroglobulin (1). **2.** Proteína iodada, geralmente caseína, que possui atividade de tiroxina.
thy·rop·to·sis (thī-rop-tō'sis). Tireoptose; deslocamento da glândula tireóide para baixo. [thyro- + G. ptōsis, queda]
thy·rot·o·my (thī-rot'ō-mē). Tireotomia. **1.** Qualquer operação de corte na glândula tireóide. **2.** SIN laryngofissure. [thyro- + G. tomē, corte]
thy·ro·tox·ic (thī-rō-tok'sik). Tireotóxico; referente à tireotoxicose.
thy·ro·tox·i·co·sis (thī'rō-tok-si-kō'sis). Tireotoxicose; o estado produzido por quantidades excessivas de hormônio tireóideo endógeno ou exógeno. [thyro- + G. toxikon, veneno, + -osis, condição]
apathetic t., t. apática; t. crônica que se manifesta na forma de doença cardíaca ou síndrome de debilitação, com fraqueza dos músculos proximais e depressão, porém com poucas das manifestações clínicas mais típicas da t.
t. medicamento'sa, t. medicamentosa; estado de hipertireoidismo resultante de doses excessivas de preparação de hormônio tireóideo.
thy·ro·tox·in (thī-rō-tok'sin). Tireotoxina. **1.** Substância hipotética outrora considerada um produto anormal de glândulas tireóides com hiperplasia difusa em indivíduos com doença de Graves; acredita-se que seja a causa dos sinais e sintomas característicos dessa condição (em contraste com o hipertireoidismo simples). **2.** Fator antigênico fixador de complemento associado a determinadas doenças da glândula tireóide. **3.** Termo raramente utilizado para referir-se a qualquer material tóxico para o tecido tireóideo.
thy·ro·troph (thī'rō-trof). Tireotrofo; célula da adeno-hipófise que produz tireotropina.
thy·ro·tro·phic (thī-rō-trof'ik). Tireotrófico. SIN thyrotropic. [thyro- + G. trophē, nutrição]
thy·rot·ro·phin (thī-rot'rō-fin, thī-rō-trō'fin). Tireotrofina. SIN thyrotropin.
thy·ro·tro·pic (thī-rō-trop'ik). Tireotrópico; que estimula ou nutre a glândula tireóide. SIN thyrotrophic. [thyro- + G. trophē, uma volta]
thy·rot·ro·pin (thī-rot'rō-pin, thī-rō-trō'pin). Tireotropina; hormônio glicoprotéico produzido pela adeno-hipófise que estimula o crescimento e a função da glândula tireóide; também utilizada em teste diagnóstico para diferenciar o hipotireoidismo primário do secundário. SIN thyroid-stimulating hormone, thyrotrophin, thyrotropic hormone. [em lugar de thyrotrophin, de thyro- + G. throphē, nutrição; corrompido para -tropin e reanalisado como do G. tropē, volta]
thy·rox·ine (T_4), thy·rox·in (thī-rok'sēn, -sin). Tirotoxina; o L-isômero é o composto de iodo ativo que existe normalmente na glândula tireóide e é extraído dela na forma cristalina para uso terapêutico; também preparada sinteticamente; utilizada para alívio do hipotireoidismo, do cretinismo e do mixedema.
labeled t., t. marcada. SIN radioactive t.
radioactive t., t. radioativa; t. a qual um radioisótopo do iodo (I^{125} ou I^{131}) é incorporado; utilizada em experimentos que estudam o metabolismo da tiroxina. SIN labeled t., radiolabeled t., radiothyroxin.
radiolabeled t., t. radiomarcada. SIN radioactive t.
t. sodium, t. sódica; preparação obtida pela ação de uma quantidade limitada de carbonato de sódio sobre a tiroxina; contém entre 61 e 65% de iodo. VER sodium levothyroxine, sodium liothyronine.
Thys·a·no·so·ma ac·ti·noi·des (this-ă-nō-sō'mă ak-ti-noyd'ez). Tênia fimbriada do carneiro, um verme relativamente curto e espesso (família Anocephalidae) cujas bordas posteriores das proglotes são fimbriadas. Habita o intestino delgado, porém invade freqüentemente os ductos biliares e faz com que muitos fígados sejam condenados para consumo humano. É essencialmente não-patogênica e comum em países pecuaristas, onde infecta uma grande variedade de ruminantes; os ácaros oribatídeos são provavelmente os vetores.
TI O tempo de demora entre o pulso invertido e o pulso "lido" no experimento de recuperação de inversão, no imageamento por ressonância magnética.
Ti Símbolo de titanium (titânio).
TIA Abreviatura de transient ischemic attack (ataque isquêmico transitório).
tib·ia, gen. e pl. **tib·i·ae** (tib'ē-ă, tib'ē-ē) [TA]. Tíbia; o medial e maior dos dois ossos da perna, que se articula com o fêmur, a fíbula e o tálus. SIN shin bone. [L. o grande osso da canela]
saber t., t. em sabre; deformidade da t. que ocorre na sífilis terciária ou bouba, exibindo o osso uma acentuada convexidade anterior em decorrência da formação de gomas e periostite.
t. val'ga, t. valga. SIN genu valgum.
t. va'ra, t. vara. SIN genu varum.
tib·i·ad (tib'ē-ad). Em direção à tíbia. [tibia + L. ad, para]
tib·i·al (tib'ē-ăl) [TA]. Tibial; relativo à tíbia ou a qualquer estrutura denominada a partir dela; designa também a face medial ou tibial do membro inferior. SIN tibialis [TA]. [L. tibialis]
tib·i·a·le pos·ti·cum (tib-ē-ā'lē pos-tī'kŭm). Osso tibial posterior (sesamóide). SIN os tibiale posterius.
tib·i·a·lis (tib-ē-ā'lis) [TA]. Tibial. SIN tibial. [L.]

tibio-. Tibio-. A tíbia. [L. *tibia,* o osso da canela]
  tib·i·o·cal·ca·ne·an (tib′ē-ō-kal-kā′nē-an). Tibiocalcâneo; relativo à tíbia e ao calcâneo.
  tib·i·o·fas·ci·a·lis (tib-ē-ō-fas-ē-ā′lis). Tibiofascial. Ver subentradas em musculus tibiofascialis.
  tib·i·o·fem·o·ral (tib-ē-ō-fem′ō-ral). Tibiofemoral; relativo à tíbia e ao fêmur.
  tib·i·o·fib·u·lar (tib-ē-ō-fib′u-lar). Tibiofibular; relativo à tíbia e à fíbula; designa especialmente as articulações e ligamentos entre os dois ossos. SIN peroneotibial, tibioperoneal.
  tib·i·o·na·vic·u·lar (tib-ē-ō-na-vik′u-lar). Tibionavicular; relativo à tíbia e ao osso navicular do tarso. SIN tibioscaphoid.
  tib·i·o·per·o·ne·al (tib′ē-ō-per′ō-nē′al). Tibiofibular. SIN tibiofibular.
  tib·i·o·scaph·oid (tib′ē-ō-skaf′oyd). Tibionavicular. SIN tibionavicular.
  tib·i·o·tar·sal (tib-ē-ō-tar′sal). Tibiotarsal; relativo aos ossos do tarso e à tíbia. SIN tarsotibial.
tic (tik). Tique; contração repetida habitual de determinados músculos, resultando em ações individualizadas estereotipadas que podem ser voluntariamente suprimidas durante apenas um breve período de tempo, como, por exemplo, limpar a garganta, fungar, enrugar os lábios, piscar excessivamente; especialmente proeminente quando o indivíduo está sob estresse; não existe nenhum substrato patológico conhecido. VER TAMBÉM spasm. SIN Brissaud disease, habit chorea, habit spasm. [Fr.]
  convulsive t., t. facial. SIN facial t.
  t. de pensée, t. de pensamento; termo raramente empregado para descrever o hábito de expressar involuntariamente qualquer pensamento que venha à mente. [Fr. de pensamento]
  t. douloureux, neuralgia do trigêmeo. SIN trigeminal neuralgia. [Fr. doloroso]
  facial t., t. facial; contração involuntária dos músculos faciais, algumas vezes unilateral. SIN Bell spasm, convulsive t., facial spasm, palmus (1).
  glossopharyngeal t., neuralgia do glossofaríngeo. SIN glossopharyngeal neuralgia.
  habit t., t. habitual; repetição habitual de alguma careta, encolher dos ombros, contração ou espasmo da cabeça ou outros hábitos semelhantes.
  local t., t. local; tique de extensão muito limitada, como o piscar de um olho ou a contração de um dedo da mão.
  psychic t., t. psíquico; gesto ou exclamação feito sob a influência de um impulso mórbido irresistível.
  rotatory t., torcicolo espasmódico. SIN spasmodic torticollis.
  spasmodic t., t. espasmódico; distúrbio em que movimentos coordenados espasmódicos súbitos de determinados músculos ou grupos de músculos fisiologicamente relacionados ocorrem a intervalos regulares. SIN Henoch chorea.
ti·car·cil·lin di·so·di·um (tī-kar-sil′in). Ticarcilina dissódica; o sal dissódico do ácido 6-(α-carboxi-α-tieno-3-ylacetamido)penicilânico; antibiótico bactericida útil no tratamento de infecções por *Pseudomonas aeruginosa*, cujo efeito é semelhante ao da carbenicilina dissódica.
tick (tik). Carrapato; acarino das famílias Ixodidae (carrapatos rígidos) ou Argasidae (carrapatos moles), que contêm numerosas espécies hematófagas que constituem importantes pragas dos seres humanos e aves e mamíferos domésticos, que provavelmente excedem todos os outros artrópodes no número e na variedade de agentes patogênicos que transmitem. Os c. são diferenciados dos ácaros verdadeiros, muito menores, por possuírem um hipóstomo armado e um par de aberturas espiraculares traqueais localizadas atrás do segmento basal do terceiro ou quarto par de pernas; a larva possui seis patas e, após a muda, surge como ninfa de oito patas. Alguns dos carrapatos importantes são: *Amblyomma americanum* (carrapato da estrela solitária) e *A. hebraeum* (carrapatos sul-africanos); *Argas persicus* (carrapato do barro, das galinhas ou persa) e *A. reflexus* (carrapato do pombo); *Boophilus* (carrapatos do gado bovino); *Dermacentor albopictus* (carrapato do cavalo ou do inverno), *D. andersoni* (carrapato da febre maculosa das Montanhas Rochosas ou da madeira), *D. nitens* (carrapato do cavalo tropical), *D. occidentalis* (carrapato do Pacífico ou da madeira) e *D. variabilis* (carrapato do cão americano); *Haemaphysalis chordeilis* (carrapato das aves) e *H. laporis-palustris* (carrapato do coelho); *Ixodes pacificus* (carrapato de patas pretas da Califórnia), *I. pilosus* (carrapato da paralisia), *I. ricinus* (carrapato da mamona) e *I. scapularis* (carrapato de patas pretas ou do ombro); *Ornithodoros coriaceus* (carrapato pajaroello) e *O. moubata* (carrapato da febre recidivante africana ou tampão) e *Rhipicephalus everti* (carrapato vermelho africano), *R. sanguineus* (carrapato marrom do cão) e *R. simus* (carrapato de foceta preta).
  tick·ling (tik′ling). Cócegas; designa um prurido peculiar ou sensação de formigamento causado pela excitação de nervos superficiais, como ocorre na pele com leve estimulação.
ticolubant (tī-kol′oo-bant). Ticolubante, antagonista dos receptores de leucotrieno B₄ utilizado como antipsoriático.
t.i.d. Abreviatura do L. *ter in die*, três vezes ao dia.
tid·al (tī′dal). Corrente; relativo a ou semelhante às marés, que aumenta e diminui alternadamente.

tide (tīd). Maré; elevação e queda alternada, fluxo e refluxo ou aumento ou diminuição. [A.S. *tīd*, tempo]
  acid t., maré ácida; aumento temporário da acidez da urina que ocorre durante o jejum. SIN acid wave.
  alkaline t., maré alcalina; período de neutralidade da urina ou até mesmo de alcalinidade após as refeições, devido à retirada do íon hidrogênio com a finalidade de produzir a secreção de suco gástrico altamente ácido. SIN alkaline wave.
  fat t., onda de gordura; aumento do conteúdo de gordura do sangue e da linfa após uma refeição.
  red t., maré vermelha; fenômeno natural produzido por concentrações mais altas do que o normal da alga microscópica *Gymnodinium breve* na água do mar. [quando o microrganismo responsável está extremamente concentrado, a água do mar pode adquirir uma cor castanho-avermelhada]
Tiedemann, Friedrich, anatomista alemão, 1781–1861. VER T. *gland, nerve.*
Tietze, Alexander, cirurgião alemão, 1864–1927. VER T. *syndrome.*
tig·late (tig′lāt). Tiglato; sal ou éster do ácido tíglico.
tig·li·an (tig′lē-an). Nome trivial original da forma saturada do forbol. [de *Croton tiglium* (Euphorbiaceae)]
tig·lic ac·id (tig′lik). Ácido tíglico; ácido graxo insaturado presente em glicerídios no óleo de cróton.
ti·glyl-CoA (tig′lil). Tiglil-CoA; intermediário na degradação da L-isoleucina. SIN tiglyl-coenzyme A.
ti·glyl-coen·zyme A. Tiglil-coenzima A. SIN tiglyl-CoA.
ti·groid (tī′groyd). Tigróide. VER chromophil *substance*. [G. *tigroeidēs*, de *tigris*, tigre, + *eidos*, aparência]
ti·grol·y·sis (tī-grol′i-sis). Tigrólise. SIN chromatolysis. [tigroid + G. *lysis*, dissolução]
TIL. Abreviatura de tumor-infiltrating *lymphocytes* (linfócitos infiltrantes de tumor), em *lymphocyte*.
Tillaux, Paul Jules, cirurgião francês, 1834–1904. VER *spiral* of T.
til·or·one (til′or-ōn). Tilorona; pequena molécula sintética utilizada para induzir o interferon em camundongos.
TILS Abreviatura de tumor-infiltrating *lymphocytes* (linfócitos infiltrantes de tumor), em *lymphocyte*.
tilt (tilt). Inclinação.
  pantoscopic t., t. pantoscópica; astigmatismo oblíquo causado por inclinação de uma lente esférica, de modo que os raios luminosos incidem na lente num ângulo não-perpendicular, alterando o poder de refração esférica e cilíndrica da lente.
tim·bre (tam′br, tim′br). Timbre; a qualidade distintiva de um som, pela qual se pode determinar a sua fonte, baseando-se principalmente na distribuição de sons harmônicos. SIN tone color. [Fr.]
time (t) (tīm). Tempo. **1.** A relação de eventos expressa pelos termos passado, presente e futuro, e medida por unidades, como minutos, horas, dias, meses ou anos. **2.** Determinado período durante o qual se efetua algo definido ou determinado. SIN tempus (2). [A.S. *tīma*]
  activated clotting t. (ACT), t. de coagulação ativada; o teste mais comum utilizado para o tempo de coagulação em cirurgia cardiovascular.
  activated partial thromboplastin t. (aPTT), t. de tromboplastina parcial ativada (TTPa); o t. necessário para que o plasma forme um coágulo de fibrina após a adição de cálcio e de um reagente fosfolipídico; utilizado para avaliar o sistema intrínseco da coagulação.
  AH conduction t., t. de condução AH. VER atrioventricular *conduction*.
  association t., t. de associação; t. decorrido entre um estímulo e a resposta verbalizada a ele.
  biologic t., t. biológico; o conceito de que nossa apreciação do tempo varia com a idade e é determinado pela organização neural do indivíduo; obedece a uma lei logarítmica, em vez de aritmética.
  bleeding t., t. de sangramento; o intervalo entre o aparecimento da primeira gota de sangue e a remoção da última após punção do lóbulo da orelha ou do dedo, geralmente de 1-3 min; fornece uma avaliação global porém imprecisa da função plaquetária e capilar.
  circulation t., t. de circulação; o t. necessário para o sangue passar por um determinado circuito do sistema vascular, p. ex., a circulação pulmonar ou sistêmica, de um braço até o outro, do braço até a língua ou do braço até o pulmão; e medido pela injeção, numa veia do braço, de uma substância, como desidrocolato de sódio, éter, fluoresceína, histamina ou sal de rádio, que pode ser detectada quando atinge outro ponto do sistema vascular.
  clot retraction t., t. de retração do coágulo; o t. necessário para que um coágulo sanguíneo se separe da parede do tubo de ensaio e libere soro, geralmente concluído em 18-24 horas, porém retardado ou ausente em indivíduos com púrpura trombocitopênica.
  clotting t., t. de coagulação. SIN coagulation t.
  coagulation t., t. de coagulação; o t. necessário para a ocorrência de coagulação do sangue. SIN clotting t.
  doubling t., tempo de duplicação; t. levado para a duplicação do número de células numa neoplasia, em que os tempos de duplicação mais curtos indicam crescimento mais rápido.

euglobulin clot lysis t., t. de lise do coágulo de euglobulina; medida da capacidade dos ativadores do plasminogênio e da plasmina de lisar um coágulo; normalmente, a lise do coágulo é determinada pelo equilíbrio de fatores que ativam a fibrinólise (ativadores do plasminogênio e plasmina) e daqueles que inibem a lise; em determinadas condições (p. ex., carcinoma ou insuficiência hepática), os efeitos de ativação predominam e podem ser medidos ao observar o tempo necessário para a ocorrência de coagulação da fração euglobulina do plasma (excluindo os inibidores da fibrinólise).

fading t., t. de desvanecimento; o t. necessário para a cessação de um estímulo constante aplicado a uma área fixa do campo visual periférico.

t. of flight, t. de vôo; t. levado por um fóton criado por anilação de um par de pósitron-elétron para alcançar um detector; como os fótons por aniilação são criados em pares e percorrem direções opostas em cerca de 3×10^{10} cm/s, a medida da diferença no tempo de chegada nos detectores, com resolução de subnanossegundo, permite o cálculo da localização do evento; a física básica da tomografia com emissão de pósitrons.

forced expiratory t. (FET), t. expiratório forçado (TEF); o t. decorrido para expirar um determinado volume ou determinada fração da capacidade vital durante a medida da capacidade vital forçada; os subscritos especificam os parâmetros exatos medidos.

half-t., meia-vida. VER half-time.

HR conduction t., t. de condução HR. VER intraventricular *conduction*.

HV conduction t., t. de condução HV. VER intraventricular *conduction*.

inertia t., t. de inércia; o intervalo decorrido entre a recepção do estímulo de um nervo e a contração do músculo.

interatrial conduction t., t. de condução interatrial. SIN intraatrial conduction t. (2).

intraatrial conduction t., t. de condução intra-atrial; (1) a duração total da atividade elétrica dos átrios em um ciclo cardíaco; (2) o t. decorrido entre a ativação do átrio direito e o esquerdo. SIN interatrial conduction t.

left ventricular ejection t. (LVET), t. de ejeção do ventrículo esquerdo (TEVE); o t. medido clinicamente desde o início até a incisura do pulso carótico ou outro pulso; para ser correto, o t. de ejeção do sangue do ventrículo esquerdo começando com a abertura da valva aórtica e terminando com o seu fechamento.

PA conduction t., t. de condução PA. VER atrioventricular *conduction*.

partial thromboplastin t. (PTT), t. de tromboplastina parcial (TTP). VER activated partial thromboplastin t.

PH conduction t., t. de condução PH. VER atrioventricular *conduction*.

prothrombin t. (PT), t. de protrombina (TP); o t. necessário para a coagulação após a adição de tromboplastina e cálcio em quantidades ideais ao sangue com conteúdo normal de fibrinogênio; se protrombina estiver diminuída, o t. de coagulação aumenta; utilizado para avaliar o sistema extrínseco da coagulação. VER TAMBÉM prothrombin *test*.

reaction t., t. de reação; o intervalo entre a apresentação de um estímulo e a reação de resposta a ele.

recognition t., t. de reconhecimento; o intervalo entre a aplicação de determinado estímulo e o reconhecimento de sua natureza.

relaxation t. (τ), t. de relaxamento; o t. necessário para que o substrato numa reação enzimática ou química sofra uma queda para 1/e de seu valor inicial.

repetition t. (TR), t. de repetição (TR); em ressonância magnética, o intervalo de t. entre repetições da seqüência de pulsos.

rise t., tempo de ascensão; (1) o t. necessário para que um pulso ou eco se eleve de seu início até sua amplitude máxima; (2) o t. necessário para que um pulso ou eco se eleve de 10-90% de sua amplitude máxima.

running t., t. de curso; o t. durante o qual ocorre determinada atividade (p. ex., desenvolvimento da cromatografia).

Russell's viper venom clotting t., t. de coagulação com veneno da víbora de Russell; determinação do t. de coagulação efetuada em plasma citratado pobre em plaquetas, utilizando o veneno (*venom*) da víbora de Russell como agente ativador. Isso permite a ativação do fator X diretamente, sem a necessidade de outros fatores da coagulação; utilizado para confirmar defeitos do fator X. VER TAMBÉM Stypven time *test*.

sensation t., t. de sensação; o t. mínimo em que uma imagem visual deve ser exposta para ser percebida.

sinoatrial conduction t. (SACT), t. de condução sinoatrial (TCSA); o t. necessário para que um impulso se desloque do nó sinusal até o átrio; estimado indiretamente durante o período de reajuste do nó sinoatrial, dividindo-se por dois o intervalo médio entre o batimento prematuro e o batimento sinusal normal seguinte do átrio.

sinoatrial recovery t. (SART), t. de recuperação sinoatrial (TRSA); intervalo entre a última onda P e a primeira onda P espontânea subseqüente (após 2-5 min de estimulação do átrio direito a 120-140 batimentos por minuto, e, quando expresso como percentagem da duração do ciclo de controle, varia normalmente de 115-159%).

survival t., t. de sobrevida; (1) o período de t. decorrido entre a conclusão ou a instituição de qualquer procedimento e a morte; (2) o período de vida de eritrócitos ou outras células biológicas ou fisicamente marcados.

thrombin t., t. de trombina; o t. necessário para a formação de um coágulo de fibrina após a adição de trombina ao plasma citratado; observa-se um prolongamento do t. de trombina em pacientes submetidos a heparinoterapia.

tissue thromboplastin inhibition t., t. de inibição da tromboplastina tecidual; teste utilizado para identificar o anticoagulante lúpico; a fonte de tromboplastina usada no teste de protrombina é diluída para aumentar a sensibilidade a inibidores.

utilization t., t. de utilização; a duração mínima de um estímulo de potência reobásica, que é apenas suficiente para produzir excitação. SIN temps utile.

TIMI Acrônimo de *t*hrombolysis *i*n *m*yocardial *i*nfarction (trombólise no infarto do miocárdio); grande estudo clínico controlado multicêntrico.

tim·no·don·ic ac·id (tim-nō-don′ok). Ácido timnodônico; ácido graxo de 20 carbonos com cinco ligações duplas *cis* localizadas nos carbonos 5, 8, 11, 14 e 17; importante componente de óleos de peixe; precursor das prostaglandinas de série 3, p. ex., PGE_3.

ti·mo·lol ma·le·ate (tī′mō-lōl). Maleato de timolol; agente bloqueador β-adrenérgico utilizado no tratamento da hipertensão e como colírio no tratamento do glaucoma de ângulo aberto crônico.

tin (Sn) (tin). Estanho; elemento metálico de número 50, peso atômico 118,710. SIN stannum. [A.S. tin]

t. oxide, óxido de estanho. SIN stannic oxide.

tin-113 (^{113}Sn). Estanho-113; radioisótopo do estanho com meia-vida física de 115,1 dias; utilizado na fabricação de geradores de radionuclídios para a produção de índio-113m.

tinct. Abreviatura do L. *tinctura*, tintura.

tinc·ta·ble (tingk′tă-bl). Tingível; corável.

tinc·tion (tingk′shŭn). Tintura. 1. Corante; preparação para coloração. 2. O ato de corar. [L. *tingo*, pp. *tinctus*, corar]

tinc·to·ri·al (tingk-tōr′ē-ăl). Tintorial; relativo a coloração. [L. *tinctorius*, de *tingo*, corar]

tinc·tu·ra, gen. e pl. **tinc·tu·rae** (tingk-too′ră, -rē). Tintura. SIN tincture. [L. tintura, de *tingo*, pp. *tinctus*, corar]

tinc·ture (tingk′choor). Tintura; solução alcoólica ou hidroalcoólica preparada a partir de materiais vegetais ou de substâncias químicas; a maioria das tinturas é preparada por percolação ou por maceração. As proporções da droga representadas nas diferentes tinturas não são uniformes, mas variam de acordo com os padrões estabelecidos para cada uma delas. As t. de drogas potentes representam essencialmente a atividade de 10 g da droga em cada 100 mL de tintura, sendo a potência ajustada após ensaio; a maioria das outras tinturas representa 20 g da droga em cada 100 mL de tintura. As tinturas compostas são produzidas de acordo com fórmulas estabelecidas há muito tempo. SIN tinctura.

alcoholic t., t. alcoólica; t. produzida com álcool não-diluído.

ammoniated t., t. amoniacada; t. produzida com álcool amoniacado.

belladonna t., t. de beladona; líquido móvel hidroalcoólico verde contendo os alcalóides atropina e escopolamina e outras substâncias extraídos das folhas de *Atropa belladonna,* a fonte vegetal desses agentes anticolinérgicos. A t. permite uma titulação gradual da dose ao contar as gotas da preparação ingerida. Já foi muito utilizada no tratamento de úlceras ou no tratamento sintomático da diarréia, isoladamente ou em combinação com antiácidos e argilas insolúveis.

digitalis t., t. digitálica; solução hidroalcoólica contendo os glicosídios das folhas da dedaleira (digital), *Digitalis purpurea* ou *D. lanata.* Embora as preparações digitálicas sejam muito utilizadas, são hoje em dia usadas na forma dos glicosídios puros, digoxina e digitoxina. A t. já foi muito utilizada, porém foi padronizada por bioensaio utilizando rãs, gatos ou pombos.

ethereal t., t. etérea; classe de preparações que consiste em percolações a 10% de drogas em um solvente de éter (1) e álcool (2).

glycerinated t., t. glicerinada; t. produzida com álcool diluído ao qual se adiciona glicerina para facilitar a extração ou para preservar a preparação.

green soap t., t. de sabão verde; preparação líquida contendo sabões de potássio e álcool; freqüentemente recomendada na limpeza de pele, sobretudo após exposição a toxinas vegetais, como sumagre venenoso.

hydroalcoholic t., t. hidroalcoólica; t. produzida com álcool diluído em várias proporções com água.

tine (tīn). Dente; ponta. 1. Em odontologia, a extremidade delgada e pontiaguda de um explorador. 2. Instrumento utilizado para introduzir antígeno, como a tuberculina na pele, contendo habitualmente várias pontas individuais. [A.S. *tind,* ponta]

tin·ea (tin′ē-ă). Tinha; infecção fúngica (dermatofitose) do componente de ceratina dos cabelos, da pele ou das unhas. Os gêneros de fungos que causam essa infecção são *Microsporum, Trichophyton* e *Epidermophyton.* SIN ringworm, serpigo (1). [L. verme, traça]

t. bar′bae, t. da barba; infecção fúngica da barba, que ocorre na forma de infecção folicular ou lesão granulomatosa; as lesões primárias consistem em pápulas e pústulas. SIN barber itch, folliculitis barbae, ringworm of beard, t. sycosis.

t. cap′itis, t. da cabeça; forma comum de infecção fúngica do couro cabeludo causada por várias espécies de *Microsporum* e *Trichophyton,* sobre ou no inte-

rior da haste do pêlo, que ocorre mais comumente em crianças; caracterizada por placas de calvície aparente, de localização irregular e tamanho variável, devido à quebra dos cabelos na superfície do couro cabeludo, descamação, pontos negros (ver black-dot *ringworm*) e, ocasionalmente, eritema e piodermatite. SIN ringworm of scalp.
  t. circina'ta, t. circinada. SIN t. corporis.
  t. cor'poris, t. do corpo; erupção macular descamativa e bem-definida de dermatofitose, que freqüentemente forma lesões anulares e pode surgir em qualquer parte do corpo. SIN ringworm of body, t. circinata.
  t. favo'sa, t. favosa. SIN favus.
  t. glabro'sa, t. glabrosa; tinha ou infecção fúngica da pele glabra.
  t. imbrica'ta, t. imbricada; erupção que consiste em diversos anéis concêntricos de escamas superpostas, formando placas papuloescamosas espalhadas pelo corpo; ocorre em climas tropicais e é causada pelo fungo *Trichophyton concentricum.* SIN Oriental ringworm, scaly ringworm, Tokelau ringworm.
  t. ke'rion, t. quérion; infecção fúngica inflamatória do couro cabeludo e da barba, caracterizada por pústulas e infiltração congestionada das partes circundantes; mais comumente causada por *Microscoporum audouinii.*
  t. ma'nus, t. da mão; t. que acomete a mão, referindo-se, em geral, a infecções da superfície palmar. VER TAMBÉM t. corporis.
  t. ni'gra, t. negra; infecção fúngica causada por *Exophiala werneckii,* caracterizada por lesões escuras que conferem uma aparência salpicada e que ocorrem mais comumente nas palmas das mãos. SIN pityriasis nigra.
  t. pe'dis, t. do pé; dermatofitose do pé, especialmente da pele interdigital, causada por um dos dermatófitos, geralmente uma espécie de *Trichophyton* ou *Epidermophyton*; a doença consiste em pequenas vesículas, fissuras, descamação, maceração e áreas erodidas entre os dedos dos pés e na superfície plantar do pé; pode haver comprometimento de outras áreas cutâneas. SIN athlete's foot, dermatomycosis pedis, ringworm of foot.
  t. profun'da, t. profunda. SIN Majocchi *granulomas,* em *granuloma.*
  t. syco'sis, t. da barba. SIN t. barbae.
  t. tonsu'rans, t. tonsurante; t. da cabeça ou do corpo, causada pelo fungo *Trichophyton tonsurans;* caracterizada por pequenas placas e menor número de fios de cabelo quebrados do que na t. da cabeça causada por outras espécies.
  t. un'guium, t. ungueal; t. das unhas causada por dermatófitos.
  t. versic'olor, t. versicolor; erupção de placas castanho-amareladas ou castanhas na pele do tronco, que freqüentemente parecem brancas, em contraste com a pele hiperpigmentada após exposição ao sol de verão; causada pelo crescimento do fungo *Malassezia furfur* no estrato córneo, com reação inflamatória mínima. SIN pityriasis versicolor.
Tinel, Jules, neurologista francês, 1879–1952. VER T. *sign.*
tin·foil (tin'foyl). Folha de estanho. **1.** Estanho laminado em folhas extremamente finas. **2.** Base de lâmina metálica utilizada como material de separação, como entre o molde e o material da base da dentadura durante procedimentos de moldagem e cura.
tin·gi·bil·i·ty (tin'ji-bil'i-tē) Tingibilidade; a propriedade de ser tingível.
tin·gi·ble (tin'ji-bl). Tingível; capaz de ser corado. [L. *tingo,* corar]
tin·gle (ting'gl). Formigar; experimentar uma sensação peculiar de picada.
tin·gling (ting'ling). Formigamento; tipo de parestesia.
  distal t. on percussion (DTP), formigamento distal à percussão. SIN Tinel *sign.*
ti·nid·a·zole (ti-nid'ā-zōl). Tinidazol; agente antiprotozoário.
tin·ni·tus (ti-nī'tŭs). Tinido, zumbido; ruídos (repique, sibilo, silvo, bramido, estrondo etc.) nas orelhas. [L. um tinido, de *tinnio,* pp. *tinnitus,* tinir]
  t. au'rium, t. auditivo; sensação de som em uma ou ambas as orelhas, geralmente associada a doença da orelha média, orelha interna ou vias auditivas centrais. SIN syrigmus.
  t. cere'bri, t. cerebral; sensação subjetiva de ruído na cabeça, em vez de nas orelhas.
  clicking t., t. de estalido; som de estalido objetivo na orelha em casos de otite média catarral crônica; pode ser audível pelo observador, bem como pelo paciente, e acredita-se que seja devido à abertura e ao fechamento do óstio da tuba auditiva ou a um espasmo rítmico do véu palatino.
  Leudet t., t. de Leudet; estalido espasmódico seco, também audível através do otoscópio, ouvido na inflamação catarral da tuba auditiva; causado por espasmo reflexo do músculo tensor do palato.
tint. Tonalidade, matiz; tonalidade de cor que varia de acordo com a quantidade de branco misturado com o pigmento. [L. *tingo,* pp. *tinctus,* corar]
ti·o·con·a·zole (ti-ō-kon'ā-zōl). Tioconazol; agente antifúngico.
tip. Ponta, ápice. **1.** Uma ponta; uma extremidade mais ou menos pontiaguda. **2.** Pedaço separado, porém fixo, da mesma estrutura ou de outra estrutura, formando a extremidade de uma parte.
  t. of auricle, ápice da orelha. SIN *apex* of auricle.
  t. of ear, ápice da orelha; *termo oficial alternativo para *apex* of auricle.
  t. of elbow, olécrano. SIN olecranon.
  t. of nose, ápice do nariz; *termo oficial alternativo para *apex* of nose.
  t. of posterior horn, ápice do corno posterior. SIN *apex* of posterior horn.
  root t., ápice da raiz. SIN root *apex.*
  t. of tongue, ápice da língua; *termo oficial alternativo para *apex* of tongue.
  t. of tooth root, ápice da raiz do dente. SIN root *apex.*
  Woolner t., ponta de Woolner. SIN *apex* of auricle.
tip·ping. Movimento do dente, em que a angulação do eixo longo do dente é alterada.
ti·pren·o·lol hy·dro·chlo·ride (tip-ren'ō-lol). Cloridrato de tiprenolol; bloqueador dos receptores β.
TIPS Acrônimo de transjugular intrahepatic portosystemic *shunt* (derivação porto-sistêmica intra-hepática transjugular).
Tiselius, Arne W.K., bioquímico sueco e ganhador do Prêmio Nobel, 1902–1971. VER T. *apparatus,* electrophoresis *cell.*
Tis·si·er·la prae·acuta. SIN Bacteroides praeacutus.
Tissot, Jules, fisiologista francês do início do século 20. VER T. *spirometer.*
tis·sue (tish'ū). Tecido; conjunto de células semelhantes e das substâncias intercelulares que as circundam. Existem quatro tecidos básicos no corpo: 1) epitélio; 2) tecidos conjuntivos, incluindo sangue, osso e cartilagem; 3) t. muscular e 4) t. nervoso. [Fr. *tissu,* tecido, entrelaçado, do L. *texo,* tecer]
  adenoid t., t. adenóide. SIN lymphatic t.
  adipose t., t. adiposo; t. conjuntivo que consiste principalmente em células adiposas (adipócitos) circundadas por fibras reticulares e dispostas em grupos lobulares ou ao longo do trajeto de um dos menores vasos sangüíneos. SIN fat (1), fatty t. (1), white fat (1).
  areolar t., t. areolar; t. conjuntivo frouxo irregularmente disposto, que consiste em fibras colágenas e elásticas, uma substância fundamental de polissacarídios e proteínas e células do tecido conjuntivo (fibroblastos, macrófagos, mastócitos e, algumas vezes, adipócitos, plasmócitos, leucócitos e células pigmentadas).
  bone t., t. ósseo. SIN osseous t.
  bronchus-associated lymphoid t. (BALT), t. linfóide associado aos brônquios; placas de tecido linfóide, compostas principalmente de linfócitos B e T, que se estendem pelas vias aéreas brônquicas do pulmão.
  brown adipose t., t. adiposo castanho. SIN brown *fat.*
  cancellous t., t. esponjoso; t. ósseo reticular ou esponjoso.
  cardiac muscle t., t. muscular cardíaco. VER cardiac *muscle.*
  cartilaginous t., t. cartilaginoso. VER cartilage.
  cavernous t., t. cavernoso. SIN erectile t.
  chondroid t., t. condróide; **(1)** no adulto, t. semelhante à cartilagem; SIN fibrohyaline t., pseudocartilage; **(2)** no embrião, estágio inicial na formação da cartilagem.
  chromaffin t., t. cromafim; t. celular, vascularizado e bem suprido por nervos, constituído principalmente de células cromafins; é encontrado na medula das glândulas supra-renais e, em menores coleções, nos paragânglios.
  connective t., t. conjuntivo; o t. de sustentação do corpo dos animais, formado de substância fibrosa ou fundamental, com células mais ou menos numerosas de vários tipos; é derivado do mesênquima, e este, por sua vez, do mesoderma; os tipos de t. conjuntivo são os seguintes: areolar ou frouxo; adiposo; fibroso branco denso, regular ou irregular; elástico; mucoso; linfóide; cartilagem e osso; o sangue e a linfa podem ser considerados tecidos conjuntivos cuja substância fundamental é líquida. SIN interstitial t., tela conjuntiva.
  dartoic t., t. dartóico; tecido semelhante à túnica dartos.
  elastic t., t. elástico; forma de t. conjuntivo em que as fibras elásticas predominam; constitui os ligamentos amarelos das vértebras e o ligamento da nuca, especialmente de quadrúpedes; ocorre também nas paredes das artérias e da árvore brônquica e conecta as cartilagens da laringe. SIN elastica (2), tela elastica.
  epithelial t., t. epitelial. VER epithelium.
  erectile t., t. erétil; t. com numerosos espaços vasculares que podem ser ingurgitados por sangue. SIN cavernous t.
  fatty t., t. adiposo. **(1)** SIN adipose t.; **(2)** em alguns animais, a gordura castanha (brown *fat*).
  fibrohyaline t., t. fibro-hialino. SIN chondroid t. (1).
  fibrous t., t. fibroso; t. composto de feixes de fibras brancas colágenas entre as quais existem fileiras de células de tecido conjuntivo; os tendões, os ligamentos, as aponeuroses e algumas das membranas, como a dura-máter.
  Gamgee t., t. de Gamgee; camada espessa de algodão absorvente entre duas camadas de gaze absorvente, utilizada em curativos cirúrgicos.
  gelatinous t., t. gelatinoso. SIN mucous connective t.
  gingival t.'s, tecidos gengivais. VER gingiva.
  granulation t., t. de granulação; t. conjuntivo vascular que forma projeções granulares na superfície de uma ferida, úlcera ou tecido inflamado em processo de cicatrização. VER TAMBÉM granulation.
  gut-associated lymphoid t. (GALT), t. linfóide associado ao intestino; t. linfóide da mucosa gastrintestinal que contém células B e T. Esse tecido é responsável pela imunidade localizada a patógenos como bactérias, vírus e parasitas.
  Haller vascular t., t. vascular de Haller. SIN vascular *lamina* of choroid.
  hard t., t. duro; **(1)** que se tornou mineralizado; **(2)** t. com substância intercelular firme, p. ex., cartilagem e osso.
  hemopoietic t., t. hemopoético; t. em que ocorre desenvolvimento de células do sangue ou outros elementos figurados.

indifferent t., t. indiferente; t. embrionário, não-especializado e indiferenciado.
interstitial t., t. intersticial. SIN connective t.
investing t.'s, tecidos de revestimento; os tecidos que recobrem ou encerram uma estrutura.
islet t., t. das ilhotas. SIN islets of Langerhans, em islet.
lymphatic t., lymphoid t., t. linfático, t. linfóide; rede tridimensional de fibras reticulares e células cujas redes são ocupadas por linfócitos em graus variáveis de densidade; o tecido linfático pode ser nodular, difuso e frouxo. SIN adenoid t.
mesenchymal t., t. mesenquimatoso; t. conjuntivo embrionário. VER mesenchyme.
mesonephric t., t. mesonéfrico; mesoderma intermediário situado nas regiões torácica e lombar do embrião ou do feto; transforma-se no mesonefro e nas estruturas associadas.
metanephrogenic t., t. metanefrogênico; t. derivado do mesoderma intermediário caudal aos níveis mesonéfricos e relacionado à formação dos néfrons do metanefro.
mucosa-associated lymphoid t. (MALT), t. linfóide associado à mucosa; classe de t. linfóide que compreende agregados nodulares encontrados em associação às superfícies mucosas úmidas do corpo, como as dos sistemas respiratório, digestório e urinário.
mucous connective t., t. conjuntivo mucoso; tipo de t. conjuntivo pouco diferenciado além do estágio mesenquimatoso; sua substância fundamental de glicoproteínas é abundante e contém fibras de colágeno finas e fibroblastos; em sua forma mais característica, aparece no cordão umbilical como geléia de Wharton. SIN gelatinous t.
multilocular adipose t., t. adiposo multilocular. SIN brown fat.
muscular t., t. muscular; t. caracterizado pela capacidade de contrair-se em resposta à estimulação; suas três variedades são: esquelético, cardíaco e liso. VER muscle. SIN flesh (2).
myeloid t., t. mielóide; medula óssea que consiste nos estágios em desenvolvimento e adulto dos eritrócitos, granulócitos e megacariócitos num estroma de células e fibras reticulares, com canais vasculares sinusoidais.
nasion soft t., t. mole do násio; o ponto externo de interseção entre a linha násio-sela e o perfil do t. mole.
nephrogenic t., t. nefrogênico; tecido a partir do qual se desenvolvem o pronefro, o mesonefro e o metanefro.
nervous t., t. nervoso; t. muito diferenciado composto de células nervosas, fibras nervosas, dendritos e um tecido de sustentação (neuróglia).
nodal t., t. nodal. VER atrioventricular node, sinuatrial node.
osseous t., t. ósseo; conjuntivo cuja matriz consiste em fibras de colágeno e substância fundamental e no qual se depositam sais de cálcio (fosfato, carbonato e algum fluoreto) na forma de apatita. SIN bone t.
osteogenic t., t. osteogênico; t. conjuntivo com a propriedade de formar tecido ósseo.
osteoid t., t. osteóide; t. ósseo antes da calcificação.
periapical t., t. periapical; as estruturas adjacentes ao ápice de uma raiz, particularmente o ligamento periodontal e o osso.
reticular t., retiform t., t. reticular, t. retiforme; t. em que as fibras de colágeno argirófilas formam uma rede e que habitualmente possui uma rede de células reticulares associadas às fibras.
rubber t., t. de borracha; delgada lâmina de borracha utilizada como protetor em curativos cirúrgicos.
skeletal muscle t., t. muscular esquelético. VER skeletal muscle.
smooth muscle t., t. muscular liso. VER smooth muscle.
subcutaneous t. [TA], t. subcutâneo; camada irregular de t. conjuntivo frouxo imediatamente abaixo da pele e superficial à fáscia profunda que em geral consiste primariamente numa camada adiposa [TA] (panículo adiposo [TA]), que também pode incluir uma camada muscular [TA] (estrato muscular [TA]) e/ou uma camada fibrosa [TA] (estrato fibroso [TA]), ou que pode ocorrer apenas como camada membranosa [TA] (estrato membranáceo [TA]), quase desprovido de gordura (como nas orelhas, pálpebras, escroto e pênis); é penetrado e sustentado por ligamentos cutâneos [TA] (retináculos da pele [TA]) que se estendem entre a derme e a fáscia profunda; os nervos cutâneos e os vasos superficiais seguem o seu trajeto no interior do tecido subcutâneo, e apenas seus ramos terminais estendem-se até a pele; dos revestimentos do corpo, essa camada é a que exibe maior variação entre os sexos e em diferentes estados nutricionais. A Terminologia Anatômica [TA] recomendou que os termos "fáscia superficial" e "fáscia profunda" não sejam utilizados genericamente de modo não-qualificado, em virtude da variação internacional de seu significado. Os termos recomendados são "tecido subcutâneo [TA] (tela subcutânea [TA])" para a fáscia superficial e "fáscia muscular" ou "fáscia visceral" em lugar de fáscia profunda. SIN tela subcutanea [TA], hypodermis*, fascia superficialis, hypoderm, stratum subcutaneum, subcutis, superficial fascia.
subcutaneous t. of penis [TA], fáscia do pênis; camada superficial contínua com o t. perineal superficial. SIN fascia penis superficialis, superficial fascia of penis.
subcutaneous t. of perineum [TA], fáscia do períneo; a camada membranácea do tecido subcutâneo na região urogenital que se fixa posteriormente à borda do diafragma urogenital, nos lados dos ramos isquiopúbicos, continuando anteriormente na parede abdominal. SIN Colles fascia, Cruveilhier fascia, fascia perinei superficialis, membranous layer of superficial fascia of perineum (1), membranous layer of superficial fascia (1), superficial fascia of perineum.
trabecular t. of sclera [TA], t. trabecular da esclera; a rede de fibras (retículo trabecular) no ângulo iridocorneal entre a câmara anterior do olho e o seio venoso da esclera; contém espaços entre as fibras que estão envolvidos na drenagem do humor aquoso; composto de duas porções: a parte corneoescleral (parte fixada à esclera) e a parte uveal (parte fixada à íris). SIN reticulum trabeculare sclerae [TA], Gerlach valvula, Hueck ligament, ligamentum anulare bulbi, pectinate ligaments of iridocorneal angle, pillar of iris, trabecular meshwork, trabecular network, trabecular reticulum, trabecular zone.
tis·sue-trim·ming. Modelagem de tecido. SIN border molding.
tis·su·lar (tish′u-lär). Tecidual; relativo a ou pertinente a um tecido.
ti·ta·ni·um (Ti) (tī-tā′nē-ŭm). Titânio; elemento metálico, de número atômico 22, peso anatômico 47,88. [*Titans,* na mit. G., filhos da Terra]
   t. dioxide, dióxido de titânio, TiO_2; contém não menos de 99,0% e não mais de 100,5% de TiO_2, calculado com base na substância seca; utilizado em cremes e pós como protetor contra irritações externas e raios solares.
ti·ter (tī′ter). Título; o padrão de concentração de uma solução de teste volumétrica; o valor de ensaio de uma medida desconhecida por meios volumétricos. [Fr. *titre,* padrão]
TITh Abreviatura de 3,5,3′-triiodothyronine (3,5,3′-triiodotironina).
tit·il·la·tion (tit-i-lā′shŭn). Titilação; o ato ou a sensação de cócegas. [L. *titillatio,* de *titillo,* pp. *-atus,* sentir cócegas]
ti·tin (tī′tin). Titina; proteína fibrosa muito grande que liga filamentos de miosina espessos aos discos Z no sarcômero.
ti·trant (tī′trant). Titulante; em química, a solução que é adicionada (titulada com) numa titulação.
ti·trate (tī′trāt). Titular; analisar volumetricamente por meio de uma solução (o titulante) de concentração conhecida até um ponto final.
ti·tra·tion (tī-trā′shŭn). Titulação; análise volumétrica por meio da adição de quantidades definidas de uma solução de teste a uma solução da substância que está sendo analisada. [Fr. *titre,* padrão]
   colorimetric t., t. colorimétrica; t. em que o ponto final é determinado por uma modificação da cor.
   formol t., t. com formol; método de t. dos grupamentos amino dos aminoácidos mediante adição de formaldeído à solução neutra; o formaldeído reage com o grupo NH_3^+, liberando uma quantidade equivalente de H^+, que pode ser então estimada por titulação com NaOH.
   potentiometric t., t. potenciométrica; t. durante a qual o pH é continuamente medido, com algum valor de pH servindo como ponto final.
tit·u·ba·tion (tit-u-bā′shŭn). Titubeação. **1.** Cambaleio ou vacilação ao tentar caminhar. **2.** Tremor ou agitação da cabeça de origem cerebelar. [L. *titubo,* pp. *-atus,* cambalear]
Tizzoni, Guido, médico italiano, 1853–1932. VER Tizzoni *stain.*
Tl Símbolo do thallium (tálio).
²⁰¹Tl Abreviatura de *thallium*-201 (tálio-201).
TLC Abreviatura de thin-layer *chromatography* (cromatografia de camada fina); total lung *capacity* (capacidade pulmonar total).
TLE Abreviatura de thin-layer *electrophoresis* (eletroforese de camada fina).
TLV Abreviatura de threshold limit *value* (valor limítrofe).
TM Abreviatura de transcendental meditation (meditação transcendental).
Tm Símbolo do thulium (túlio); transport *maximum* (transporte máximo) ou tubular *maximum* (máximo tubular).
TMD Abreviatura de temporomandibular joint *dysfunction* (disfunção da articulação temporomandibular).
TMJ Abreviatura coloquial de temporomandibular joint *dysfunction* (disfunção da articulação temporomandibular).
TM-mode Modo M. SIN M-mode.
TMP Abreviatura de ribothymidylic acid (ácido ribotimidílico); trimethoprim (trimetoprim); algumas vezes de deoxyribothymidylic acid (ácido desoxirribotimidílico).
T-my·co·plas·ma. SIN Ureaplasma.
Tn Abreviatura de ocular *tension* (tensão ocular).
TNF Abreviatura de tumor necrosis *factor* (fator de necrose tumoral).
TNM Acrônimo de Tumor-Node-Metastasis (Tumor-Linfonodo-Metástase). VER TNM *staging.*
TNP-470. Inibidor da angiogênese utilizado no tratamento do câncer para reduzir a formação de vasos sangüíneos em tumores.
TNT Abreviatura de trinitrotoluene (trinitrotolueno).

to·bac·co (tō-bak′ō). Tabaco; erva sul-americana, *Nicotiana tabacum,* que possui grandes folhas ovaladas ou lanceoladas e grupos terminais de flores tubulares brancas ou rosadas. As folhas do t. contêm 2-8% de nicotina e constituem a fonte do t. para fumar e para mascar. A fumaça do t. contém nicotina, monóxido de carbono (4%), óxido nítrico e numerosos hidrocarbonetos aromáticos e outras substâncias que são comprovadamente carcinógenas, incluindo benzo[a]pireno, β-naftilamina e nitrosaminas.

O fumo de cigarros é a principal causa de doença e morte passíveis de prevenção nos Estados Unidos, sendo responsável por cerca de 434.000 mortes (20% de todas as mortes) anualmente. O fumo de 2 maços de cigarros por dia reduz o tempo de vida em 8,3 anos. O fumo de t. em suas diversas formas (cigarros, charutos, cachimbo) representa um forte fator de risco independente de aterosclerose, infarto agudo do miocárdio, angina instável, acidente vascular cerebral (AVC) e morte súbita. É responsável por 45% de todas as mortes por coronariopatia em homens com menos de 65 anos de idade e por mais de 50% de todos os casos de AVC em ambos os sexos antes dos 65 anos. O fumo diminui os níveis de HDL-colesterol e eleva os níveis de LDL-colesterol e VLDL-colesterol, aumentando o risco de claudicação intermitente e aneurisma de aorta. Pode causar um aumento de até 30 vezes no risco de doença tromboembólica em mulheres em uso de anticoncepcionais orais. O tabagismo é responsável por 100.000 mortes anualmente por câncer de pulmão; além disso, aumenta acentuadamente o risco de outros cânceres, particularmente os da cavidade oral, laringe, esôfago, rim, bexiga, colo uterino e pâncreas. O fumo de cigarros é a principal causa de bronquite crônica e enfisema. O fumo passivo (inalação por não-fumantes de fumaça indireta ou de jatos secundários) causa 53.000 mortes por ano, das quais 37.000 são por coronariopatia. O tabagismo materno durante a gravidez está associado a um risco aumentado de aborto, natimorto e baixo peso ao nascimento. Os filhos de fumantes correm risco aumentado de síndrome de morte súbita do lactente e meningite meningocócica. O uso de t. sem fumaça (tabaco para mascar, rapé) aumenta acentuadamente o risco de câncer e de lesões pré-malignas da cavidade oral. O uso da nicotina é poderosamente viciante, resultando em hábito, tolerância e dependência. Nos Estados Unidos, 90% dos fumantes adquirem o hábito do tabaco antes dos 20 anos de idade; 3.000 crianças começam a fumar a cada dia. A probabilidade de tornar-se um fumante e assim permanecer aumenta em proporção inversa ao número de anos de escolaridade. A interrupção do hábito de fumar diminui o risco de morte de todas as causas em 30%. Estratégias efetivas para a interrupção do fumo incluem terapia de modificação comportamental, substituição da nicotina (goma de mascar, adesivos cutâneos, inalador), hipnose e farmacoterapia (bupropiona); todavia, a taxa de recidiva nos 3 meses após a interrupção é de 60%.

wild t., t. selvagem. SIN lobelia.
to·bra·my·cin (tō-bra-mī′sin). Tobramicina; antibiótico aminoglicosídio produzido por *Streptomyces tenebrarius*, que exerce efeitos bactericidas e é utilizado principalmente no tratamento de infecções por *Pseudomonas*.
to·cai·nide hy·dro·chlo·ride (tō-kā′nid). Cloridrato de tocainida; agente antiarrítmico oral, com ação semelhante à lidocaína, utilizado no tratamento de arritmias ventriculares.
toco-. Toco-; parto. [G. *tokos*, nascimento]
to·co·chro·ma·nol-3 (tō′kō-krō′mă-nol). Tococromanol-3; α-tocotrienol. VER tocotrienol.
toc·o·dy·na·graph (tō-kō-dī′nă-graf, tok-ō-). Tocodinágrafo; registro da força das contrações uterinas. SIN tocograph. [toco- + G. *dynamis*, força, + *graphē*, escrito]
toc·o·dy·na·mom·e·ter (tō′kō-dī-nă-mom′ĕ-ter, tok′ō-). Tocodinamômetro; instrumento para medir a força das contrações uterinas. SIN tocometer. [toco- + G. *dynamis*, força, + *metron*, medida]
toc·o·graph (tō′kō-graf). Tocógrafo. SIN tocodynagraph.
to·cog·ra·phy (tō-kog′ră-fē). Tocografia; o processo de registrar as contrações uterinas. [toco- + G. *graphō*, escrever]
to·col (tō′kol). Tocol; unidade fundamental dos tocoferóis; a 6-fitil-hidroquinona está em equilíbrio, na forma de cromanol, com o 2-metil-2-(4,8,12-trimetiltridecil)croman-6-ol.
to·col·o·gy (tō-kol′o-jē). Tocologia. SIN obstetrics. [toco- + G. *logos*, estudo]
to·co·lyt·ic (tō-kō-lit′ik). Tocolítico; designa qualquer agente farmacológico utilizado para interromper as contrações uterinas; freqüentemente utilizado numa tentativa de interromper as contrações do trabalho de parto prematuro, p. ex., ritodrina ou terbutalina. [G. *tokos*, nascimento, trabalho de parto, + *lysis*, afrouxamento]
to·com·e·ter (tō-kom′ĕ-ter). Tocômetro. SIN tocodynamometer.
to·coph·er·ol (T) (tō-kof′er-ōl). Tocoferol. **1.** Nome dado à vitamina E pelo seu descobridor; atualmente, termo genérico para designar vitamina E e compostos quimicamente relacionados a ela, com ou sem atividade biológica; possui estrutura química e propriedades semelhantes às da vitamina K e da coenzima Q. **2.** Tocol metilado ou tocotrienol metilado.
mixed t.'s concentrate, concentrado de tocoferóis mistos; fonte de vitamina E, obtida por destilação a vácuo de óleos vegetais comestíveis ou seus subprodutos.

α-to·coph·er·ol (α-T). α-tocoferol; 5,7,8-trimetiltocol; líquido oleoso amarelo-claro, viscoso e inodoro, que deteriora com a exposição à luz, obtido do óleo de germe de trigo ou por síntese; biologicamente, apresenta a maior atividade de vitamina E dos α-tocoferóis, atuando como antioxidante para retardar o ranço ao interferir na auto-oxidação das gorduras. Preparado a partir do fitol natural, é denominado 2-*ambo*-α-tocoferol; a partir do fitol sintético, *all-rac*-α-tocoferol ou *synt*-α-tocoferol; são também disponíveis o acetato de *d*-α-tocoferil, o acetato de *dl*-α-tocoferil, o succinato ácido *d*-α-tocoferil e o concentrado de acetato de *d*-α-tocoferil. Uma das várias formas de vitamina E. SIN vitamin E (1).
β-to·coph·er·ol (β-T). β-tocoferol; homólogo inferior do α-tocoferol, que contém um grupamento metil a menos no núcleo aromático e é biologicamente menos ativo; acompanha o α-tocoferol e o γ-β-tocoferol.
γ-to·coph·er·ol (γ-T). γ-tocoferol; forma biologicamente menos ativa do que o α-γ-tocoferol.
to·coph·er·ol·qui·none (TQ) (tō-kof′er-ol-kwī′nōn). Tocoferolquinona; tocoferol oxidado, formado a partir do 2-metil-2-fitil-6-cromenol isomérico, com grupamentos metil em uma ou mais posições 5, 7 e 8, por migração de um átomo de H do 6-OH para o C-4, produzindo uma 1,4-benzoquinona. Abreviada como TQ e precedida de α-, β- etc., como nos tocoferóis, para indicar o grau de metilação. SIN tocopherylquinone.
to·coph·er·yl·qui·none (tō-kof′er-il-kwī′nōn). Tocoferilquinona. SIN tocopherolquinone.
toc·o·pho·bia (tō′kō-fō′bē-ă, tok′ō-). Tocofobia; medo mórbido de parto. [toco- + G. *phobos*, medo]
to·co·qui·none (tō-kō-kwī′nōn). Tocoquinona; nome de uma classe para as 2,3,5-trimetil-6-multiprenil-1,4-benzoquinonas.
to·co·tri·en·ol (tō-kō-trī′en-ol). Tocotrienol; tocol com três ligações duplas na cadeia lateral, isto é, com três ligações duplas adicionais na cadeia fitil. Os produtos naturais possuem metilas em uma ou mais das posições 5, 7 e 8 do cromanol e, portanto, são idênticos, exceto pela insaturação na cadeia lateral semelhante ao fitil, aos tocoferóis; também análogas são a ciclização para formar um derivado cromanol e a oxidação para formar as tocotrienolquinonas (ou cromenóis). Abreviado como T-*n* (forma hidroquinona) ou TQ-*n* (forma quinona) e precedido de α-, β- etc. como nos tocoferóis, para indicar o grau de metilação (o *n* indica o número de unidades intactas de isopreno ou prenil remanescentes na forma cromanol ou cromenol). A terminologia t. é utilizada para indicar relações com os tocóis e tocoenóis (semelhantes à vitamina E), e a terminologia cromanol, para indicar a relação com os compostos isoprenóides das séries da vitamina K e da coenzima Q.
to·co·tri·en·ol·qui·none (tō-kō-trī′en-ol-kwī′nōn). Tocotrienolquinona; tocotrienol em que a hidroquinona foi oxidada a quinona (o cromanol tornou-se um cromenol); as tocotrienolquinonas apresentam prefixos α, β, γ e δ de acordo com o grau de metilação, da mesma forma que os tocotrienóis.
TOCP Abreviatura de triorthocresyl phosphate (triortocresilfosfato).
Tod, David, cirurgião inglês, 1794–1856. VER T. *muscle*.
Todaro, Francesco, anatomista italiano, 1839–1918. VER T. *tendon*.
Todd, Robert B., médico inglês, 1809–1860. VER T. *paralysis*, postepileptic *paralysis*.
toe (tō) [TA]. Dedo do pé; um dos dedos dos pés. SIN digitus pedis [TA], digits of foot*. [A.S. *ta*]
fourth t. [IV] [TA], quarto dedo do pé. SIN digitus (pedis) quartus [IV] [TA].
great t. I [TA], hálux; o primeiro dedo do pé. SIN hallux [TA], digitus pedis primus I*, hallex, hallus, pollex pedis, primary digit of foot.
hammer t., d. em martelo; flexão permanente na articulação falângica média de um ou mais dedos dos pés.
little t. [V] [TA], dedo mínimo; quinto dedo do pé. SIN digitus (pedis) minimus [V] [TA], digitus (pedis) quintus [V]*.
Morton t., d. de Morton; forma particular de metatarsalgia causada por aumento do nervo digital. Cf. Morton *syndrome*.
painful t., d. doloroso. SIN hallux dolorosus.
second t. [II] [TA], segundo dedo do pé. SIN digitus (pedis) secundus [II] [TA].
stiff t., d. rígido. SIN hallux rigidus.
third t. [III] [TA], terceiro dedo do pé. SIN digitus (pedis) tertius [III] [Ta].
webbed t.'s, dedos palmados; sindactilia afetando os dedos dos pés.
toe-drop (tō′drop). Dedo caído; incapacidade de dorsiflexão dos dedos do pé, geralmente devido à paralisia dos músculos extensores dos dedos dos pés.
toe-nail (tō′nāl). Unha do dedo do pé. VER nail.
ingrowing t., unha encravada. SIN ingrown *nail*.
to·fen·a·cin hy·dro·chlo·ride (tō-fen′ă-sin). Cloridrato de tofenacina; agente anticolinérgico.
To·ga·vir·i·dae (tō-gă-vir′i-dē). Família de vírus que inclui dois gêneros: Alphavirus, que inclui os vírus da encefalite eqüina do leste, encefalite eqüina do oeste e encefalite eqüina venezuelana, e Rubivirus, o vírus da rubéola. Os víriões têm 70 nm de diâmetro, possuem envoltório e são sensíveis ao éter; o capsídio possui simetria icosaédrica, contendo RNA de sentido positivo de filamento único.
to·ga·vi·rus (tō′gă-vī′rus). Togavírus; qualquer vírus da família Togaviridae. [L. *toga*, roupa, + vírus]

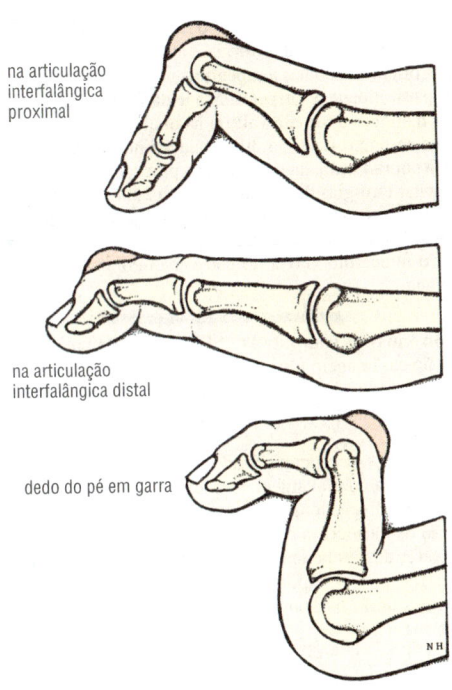

na articulação interfalângica proximal

na articulação interfalângica distal

dedo do pé em garra

dedo do pé em martelo

toi·let (toy-let'). **1.** Limpeza da paciente após o parto. **2.** Limpeza da superfície de uma ferida após uma cirurgia no preparo para a aplicação do curativo. **3.** Em odontologia, desbridamento da cavidade, a etapa final antes de colocar uma restauração num dente cuja cavidade é limpa, com remoção de todos os resíduos. [Fr. *toilette*]
  pulmonary t., toalete pulmonar; procedimento para remover o muco e as secreções da traquéia e da árvore brônquica através de exercícios respiratórios, mucocinéticos, drenagem postural e percussão.
Toison, J., histologista francês, 1858–1950. VER T. *stain.*
Toker, Cyril, patologista norte-americano, *1930. VER T. *cell.*
toko-. Toco-. VER toco-.
to·laz·a·mide (tō-laz'a-mīd). Tolazamida; agente hipoglicemiante oral de uso semelhante ao da tolbutamida.
to·laz·o·line hy·dro·chlo·ride (tō-laz'ō-lēn). Cloridrato de tolazolina; bloqueador dos receptores α-adrenérgicos utilizado para aumentar o fluxo sangüíneo em distúrbios vasculares periféricos.
tol·bu·ta·mide (tol-bū'ta-mīd). Tolbutamida; agente hipoglicemiante ativo por via oral, utilizado no tratamento do diabetes melito do adulto; parece estimular a síntese e a liberação de insulina endógena pelas ilhotas funcionais; disponível na forma de tolbutamida sódica para injeção.
tol·cy·cla·mide (tol-sī'klă-mīd). Tolciclamida. SIN glycyclamide.
Toldt, Karl, anatomista austríaco, 1840–1920. VER T. *fascia, membrane;* white *line* of T.
tol·er·ance (tol'er-ăns). Tolerância. **1.** A capacidade de resistir ou de responder menos a determinado estímulo, especialmente durante um período de exposição contínua. **2.** A capacidade de resistir à ação de um veneno ou à administração de uma droga continuamente ou em grandes doses, sem efeitos prejudiciais. [L. *tolero,* pp. *-atus,* resistir]
  acoustic t., t. acústica; o nível máximo de pressão sonora que pode ser experimentado sem produzir dor ou desvio permanente do limiar da audição num indivíduo normal.
  cross t., t. cruzada; a resistência a um ou vários efeitos de um composto, em decorrência da t. desenvolvida a um composto farmacologicamente semelhante.
  frustration t., t. à frustração; o nível de capacidade de um indivíduo de resistir à frustração sem desenvolver formas inadequadas de resposta, como descontrolar-se emocionalmente.
  high dose t., t. a altas doses; a indução de t. através de exposição a altas doses de antígeno.
  immunologic t., t. imunológica; ausência de resposta imune a um antígeno. As teorias de indução da t. incluem deleção e anergia clonais. Na deleção clonal, o verdadeiro clone de células é eliminado, enquanto na anergia clonal as células estão presentes, porém não são funcionais. SIN immunotolerance, nonresponder t.
  immunologic high dose t., t. imunológica a altas doses; indução de t. através de exposição a grandes quantidades de antígenos protéicos.
  impaired glucose t., t. à glicose comprometida; desenvolvimento de níveis excessivos de glicemia após uma refeição rica em carboidratos ou dose-teste de glicose (em geral, 75 g). Não é necessariamente diagnóstica de diabetes melito.
  individual t., t. individual; t. a uma droga que o indivíduo nunca recebeu anteriormente.
  nonresponder t., t. imunológica. SIN immunologic t.
  pain t., t. à dor; a maior intensidade de estimulação dolorosa capaz de ser tolerada por um indivíduo.
  species t., t. de espécie; a insensibilidade a determinada droga exibida por determinada espécie.
  split t., t. dividida; reação a um (ou mais) antígeno numa superfície celular, porém sem reação a outros. SIN immune deviation.
  vibration t., t. à vibração; os movimentos vibratórios ou oscilatórios máximos que um indivíduo pode experimentar e suportar sem dor; o limite de t. é uma função da amplitude e da freqüência da vibração e varia com a direção da aplicação.
tol·er·ant (tol'er-ănt). Tolerante; que possui a propriedade da tolerância.
tol·er·ize (tol'er-īz). Induzir tolerância.
tol·er·o·gen (tol'er-ō-jen). Tolerógeno; substância que produz tolerância imunológica.
tol·er·o·gen·ic (tol'er-ō-jen'ik). Tolerogênico; que produz tolerância imunológica.
tol·hex·a·mide (tol-hek'să-mīd). Tolexamida. SIN glycyclamide.
tol·met·in (tol'met-in). Tolmetina; agente antiinflamatório utilizado no tratamento da artrite reumatóide.
tol·naf·tate (tol-naf'tāt). Tolnaftato; agente antifúngico tópico.
to·lo·ni·um chlo·ride (tō-lō'nē-ŭm). Cloreto de tolônio; o grau medicinal do azul de toluidina O, utilizado como composto anti-heparina.
Tolosa, Eduardo, neurocirurgião espanhol do século 20. VER T.-Hunt *syndrome.*
tol·pro·pa·mine (tol-prō'pă-mēn). Tolpropamina; agente antipruriginoso tópico.
tol·u·ene (tol'ū-ēn). Tolueno; líquido incolor obtido por destilação seca do tolu e de outros corpos resinosos e também derivado do alcatrão; suas propriedades físicas e químicas assemelham-se às do benzeno. Utilizado em explosivos e corantes e como solvente na extração de vários princípios vegetais. SIN methylbenzene, toluol.
to·lu·ic ac·id (tō-loo'ik). Ácido tolúico; ácido metilbenzóico; produto de oxidação do xileno.
to·lu·i·dine (tō-loo'i-dēn, -din). Toluidina; aminotolueno; uma das três substâncias isoméricas, derivadas do tolueno.
  alkaline t. blue O, azul de tolueno O alcalino; azul de tolueno O em solução de bórax, utilizado com calor sobre cortes de espessura média de tecidos imersos em epóxi.
  t. blue O [C.I. 52040], azul de toluidina O, corante básico azul, utilizado como agente antibacteriano, como corante nuclear e para coloração metacromática de determinadas estruturas (p. ex., os grânulos dos mastócitos que se acredita contenham heparina e matriz cartilaginosa rica em sulfato de condroitina) e na eletroforese para corar RNA, RNase e mucopolissacarídios; antagoniza também a ação anticoagulante da heparina. VER TAMBÉM tolonium chloride.
tol·u·ol (tol'oo-ol). Toluol. SIN toluene.
tol·u·o·yl (tol-oo'ō-il). Toluoil; $CH_3C_6H_4CO-$; o radical do ácido tolúico.
tol·u·yl·ene red (tol-oo'i-lēn). Vermelho de toluileno. SIN neutral red.
tol·yl (tol'il). Tolil; $CH_3C_6H_4-$; o radical univalente do tolueno.
Toma sign. Sinal de Toma. Ver em sign.
-tome. -Tomo. **1.** Instrumento de corte, em que o primeiro elemento no termo geralmente indica a parte que o instrumento deve cortar. **2.** Segmento, parte, secção. **3.** Tomografia. **4.** Cirurgia. [G. *tomos,* cortante, pontiagudo; um corte (secção ou segmento)]
to·men·tum, to·men·tum ce·re·bri (tō-men'tŭm, tō-men'tŭm ser'ē-brī). Os numerosos pequenos vasos sangüíneos que passam entre a superfície cerebral da pia-máter e o córtex do cérebro. [L. enchimento para almofadas]
Tomes, Sir Charles S., dentista inglês, 1846–1928. VER T. *processes,* em *process.*
Tomes, Sir John, dentista e anatomista inglês, 1815–1895. VER T. *fibers,* em *fiber,* granular *layer.*
Tommaselli, Salvatore, médico italiano, 1834–1906. VER T. *disease.*
to·mo·gram (tō'mō-gram). Tomograma; radiografia obtida por tomógrafo. [G. *tomos,* corte (secção) + *gramma,* escrito]
to·mo·graph (tō'mō-graf). Tomógrafo; o equipamento radiográfico utilizado na tomografia. [G. *tomos,* corte (secção), + *graphō,* escrever]
to·mog·ra·phy (tō-mog'ră-fē). Tomografia; obtenção de imagem radiográfica de um plano selecionado através de movimento linear ou curvo recíproco do tubo de raios X e do filme; as imagens de todos os outros planos ficam borradas (fora de foco) ao serem relativamente deslocadas no filme. SIN conventional t., planigraphy, planography, sectional radiography, stratigraphy.
  computed t. (CT), t. computadorizada (TC); método de imagem que fornece dados anatômicos a partir de um plano transversal do corpo, sendo cada ima-

gem gerada por uma síntese computadorizada dos dados de transmissão de raios X obtidos em muitas direções diferentes em determinado plano. SIN computerized axial t.

computerized axial t. (CAT), t. computadorizada axial (TCA). SIN computed t.

conventional t., t. convencional. SIN tomography.

dynamic computed t., t. computadorizada dinâmica; t. computadorizada com rápida injeção de contraste, geralmente com varreduras seqüenciais em apenas um ou alguns níveis; utilizada para intensificar o compartimento vascular. SIN dynamic CT.

electron beam t. (EBT), t. de feixe de elétrons; t. computadorizada em que o movimento circular do tubo de raios X é substituído por rápido posicionamento eletrônico do raio catodo ao redor de um anodo circular, permitindo varreduras completas em dezenas de milissegundos.

helical computed t., t. computadorizada helicoidal. SIN spiral computed t.

high-resolution computed t. (HRCT), t. computadorizada de alta resolução; t. computadorizada com colimação estreita para reduzir a média do volume e um algoritmo de reconstrução de realce de borda para tornar a imagem mais precisa, algumas vezes com campo restrito de visão para minimizar o tamanho dos *pixels* na região; utilizada sobretudo na obtenção de imagens do pulmão.

hypocycloidal t., t. hypocicloidal; radiografia de secção do corpo utilizando um filme complexo e movimento do tubo com padrão semelhante a um trevo de três folhas.

nuclear magnetic resonance t., t. por ressonância magnética nuclear. SIN magnetic resonance *imaging.*

positron emission t. (PET), t. por emissão de pósitrons; criação de imagens tomográficas que revelam determinadas propriedades bioquímicas do tecido por análise computadorizada de pósitrons emitidos quando substâncias marcadas com isótopo radioativo são incorporadas no tecido. Os traçadores radioativos utilizados na PET são análogos de agentes fisiológicos ou farmacêuticos aos quais foram incorporados isótopos emissores de pósitrons com meias-vidas curtas (2-110 min). Os radioisótopos são produzidos artificialmente por bombardeio de um composto estável com um feixe de prótons gerado por um cíclotron. A captação e o metabolismo desses emissores de pósitrons imitam, pelo menos em parte, os das substâncias naturais radioestáveis das quais são análogos. Concentrando-se em determinados órgãos ou tecidos e incorporando-se em processos metabólicos, podem refletir a função bioquímica ou a existência de disfunção. O análogo da glicose 2-(flúor-18)fluoro-2-desoxi-D-glicose (FDG) é amplamente utilizado para localizar zonas de metabolismo energético aumentado. Quando um pósitron emitido por um marcador radioativo colide com um elétron, ocorre aniilação das partículas, e 2 raios gama são liberados em direções opostas (a 180°). Após a administração intravenosa do marcador radioativo, o indivíduo é colocado num *scanner,* que consiste num anel de cristais de cintilação que convertem os raios gama em *flashes* de luz visível. Esses *flashes* são detectados e registrados eletronicamente, e um programa de computador reúne os dados numa imagem tridimensional, codificada por cores para refletir a densidade de concentração.

Ao contrário de outros métodos de imagem, a PET avalia mais a atividade metabólica e a função fisiológica do que a estrutura anatômica. Como as meias-vidas dos radionuclídeos são curtas e o equipamento é dispendioso, a PET não tem sido, até agora, muito utilizada em serviços clínicos. Entretanto, desde o seu desenvolvimento em meados da década de 1970, provou ser o instrumento mais importante até hoje projetado para investigação experimental do cérebro vivo, tanto sadio quanto traumatizado ou doente. Além de fornecer importantes informações diagnósticas na demência de Alzheimer e em outras demências, no parkinsonismo e na doença de Huntington, a PET pode localizar focos epilépticos na preparação para intervenção cirúrgica, avaliar neoplasias intracranianas e ajudar a orientar escolhas terapêuticas no acidente vascular cerebral agudo. A sensibilidade e a especificidade da PET na determinação de neoplasias malignas a tornam valiosa na oncologia em evitar biopsias para tumores de baixo grau, na diferenciação não-invasiva entre tumores e necrose por radiação, na modificação precoce da quimioterapia ineficaz e em evitar cirurgias diagnósticas e terapêuticas desnecessárias. A PET tem sido empregada em cardiologia para rastreamento de coronariopatia, para avaliar as velocidades de fluxo e a reserva de fluxo e para distinguir o miocárdio viável do não-viável em candidatos a derivação e transplante.

single photon emission computed t. (SPECT), t. computadorizada por emissão fotônica única; imagem tomográfica das funções metabólicas e fisiológicas nos tecidos, sendo a imagem formada por síntese computadorizada de fótons de energia única emitidos por radionuclídios administrados de modo apropriado ao paciente.

spiral computed t., t. computadorizada espiral; t. computadorizada em que o tubo de raios X gira continuamente em torno do paciente, que é simultaneamente movido em direção longitudinal; a interpolação do computador permite a reconstrução de varreduras ou imagens transversais padronizadas em qualquer plano preferido. SIN helical computed t., helical CT, spiral CT.

trispiral t., t. triespiral; t. hipocicloidal que permite um plano de foco muito mais fino e mais uniforme; outrora utilizado especialmente para tomografia da orelha interna.

to·mo·lev·el (tō′mō-lev-el). Nível de corte; termo obsoleto para o nível em que a tomografia é realizada.

to·mo·ma·nia (tō-mō-mā′nē-ā). Tomomania; desejo irracional de um médico ou paciente de utilizar procedimentos cirúrgicos. [G. *tomos,* corte, + *mania,* frenesi]

-tomy. -Tomia; operação de corte. VER TAMBÉM -ectomy. [G. *tomē,* incisão]

ton·a·pha·sia (tōn-ā-fā′zē-ā). Tonafasia; perda, em decorrência de lesão cerebral, da capacidade de lembrar tons. [G. *tonos,* tom, + *a-* priv., + *phasis,* fala]

tone (tōn). **1.** Tom; som musical. **2.** Tonalidade; inflexão; o caráter da voz ao expressar uma emoção. **3.** Tônus; a tensão presente em músculos em repouso. **4.** Tonicidade; firmeza dos tecidos; funcionamento normal de todos os órgãos. **5.** Afinar. [G. *tonos,* tônus, ou tom]

affective t., emotional t., tom afetivo, tom emocional. SIN feeling t.

feeling t., tom sentimental; o estado mental (prazer, repugnância etc.) que acompanha cada ato ou pensamento. SIN affective t., emotional t., affectivity.

fundamental t., tom fundamental; o componente de menor freqüência num som complexo.

heart t.'s, bulhas cardíacas. SIN heart *sounds,* em *sound.*

Traube double t., tom duplo de Traube; som duplo ouvido à ausculta sobre os vasos femorais em casos de insuficiência aórtica e tricúspide.

ton·er (tō′ner). **1.** Toner; em processo eletrostático de máquina copiadora de documentos, o material que forma a imagem (desenhos, letras, algarismos etc.). **2.** Solução de cloreto de ouro. VER toning.

tongue (tŭng) [TA]. Língua. **1.** Massa móvel de tecido muscular coberta por uma mucosa, ocupando a cavidade oral e formando parte do seu assoalho, constituindo também, através de sua parte posterior, a parede anterior da faringe. Possui botões gustativos e auxilia na mastigação, na deglutição e na articulação dos sons. SIN glossa, lingua (1). **2.** Estrutura semelhante a uma língua. SIN lingua (2). [A.S. *tunge*]

baked t., l. tostada; língua seca e enegrecida observada quando pacientes com febre tifóide ou outros distúrbios sofrem desidratação.

revestimentos da língua		
doença subjacente	**sinais e sintomas clínicos**	**outros achados**
infecção inespecífica da boca	revestimento esbranquiçado (escamas)	associado à redução da ingestão de nutrientes (na gastrite e enterite) e febre
candidíase oral	placas membranáceas esbranquiçadas; remoção difícil, com bordas vermelhas	evidência de *Candida albicans* em esfregaços
escarlatina	revestimento branco opaco com vermelhidão na ponta e nas margens da língua	faringite, exantema, evidência de estreptococos β-hemolíticos em cultura de amostra de orofaringe
difteria	revestimento membranáceo branco-acinzentado, odor nauseante adocicado	revestimento difícil de remover, sangramento fácil sob a camada; manifestações generalizadas
febre tifóide	língua branco-acinzentada com margens vermelho-vivas	infecção por *Salmonella typhi;* manifestações generalizadas
uremia	revestimento castanho granuloso sobre a língua	insuficiência renal

bald t., l. calva, glossite atrófica. SIN atrophic *glossitis.*
beet-t., l. de beterraba; aspecto da língua na pelagra: surge eritema intenso, a princípio no ápice e, a seguir, ao longo das margens e, por fim, no dorso; pode haver dor e aumento da elevação; o aspecto brilhante resulta de edema, e não de atrofia, exceto na pelagra crônica.
bifid t., l. bífida; defeito estrutural da língua, cuja extremidade é dividida longitudinalmente por uma maior ou menor distância. VER diglossia. SIN cleft t.
black t., l. negra; (1) nos caninos, distúrbio associado a deficiência de ácido nicotínico; (2) coloração negra a castanho-amarelada do dorso da língua, devido a coloração por material exógeno, como componentes do tabaco; em geral, superposta à língua pilosa. SIN black hairy t., lingua nigra, melanoglossia, nigrites linguae.
black hairy t., l. negra pilosa. SIN black t.
burning t., glossodinia. SIN glossodynia.
t. of cerebellum, lígula do cerebelo. SIN lingula of cerebellum.
cleft t., l. fendida. SIN bifid t.
coated t., l. saburrosa; língua com camada esbranquiçada em sua superfície superior, composta de resíduos epiteliais, partículas alimentares e bactérias; constitui freqüentemente um indício de indigestão ou de febre. SIN furred t.
tongue crib, suporte para l.; dispositivo utilizado para controlar a deglutição visceral (do lactente) e o impulso da língua e para incentivar a postura e a função maduras ou somáticas da língua.
dotted t., l. pontilhada; l. em que cada papila separada é recoberta por um depósito esbranquiçado. SIN stippled t.
fissured t., l. fissurada; condição indolor da l., caracterizada por numerosos sulcos ou fissuras na superfície dorsal. SIN grooved t., lingua fissurata, lingua plicata, scrotal t.
furred t., l. saburrosa. SIN coated t.
geographic t., l. geográfica; máculas circinadas eritematosas assintomáticas e idiopáticas, muitas vezes circundadas, perifericamente, por uma faixa branca, em conseqüência de atrofia das papilas filiformes; com o decorrer do tempo, as lesões regridem, coalescem e modificam-se quanto à sua distribuição; freqüentemente associada a língua fissurada. SIN benign migratory glossitis, glossitis areata exfoliativa, pityriasis linguae.
grooved t., l. sulcada. SIN fissured t.
hairy t., l. pilosa; língua com alongamento anormal das papilas filiformes, resultando em aparência peluda e espessada. SIN glossotrichia, trichoglossia.
hobnail t., l. em cravo de ferradura; glossite intersticial com hipertrofia e alterações verrucosas nas papilas; observada em alguns casos de sífilis adquirida tardia.
magenta t., l. magenta; coloração vermelho-púrpura da língua, com edema e achatamento das papilas filiformes, que ocorre na deficiência de riboflavina. Cf. cyanosis.
mandibular t., lígula da mandíbula. SIN lingula of mandible.
raspberry t., l. em framboesa; l. em morango de cor vermelho-escura.
red strawberry t., l. em morango vermelho; manifestação clínica da doença de Kawasaki.
scrotal t., l. escrotal. SIN fissured t.
smoker's t., l. de fumante; designação para leucoplaquia.
stippled t., l. pontilhada. SIN dotted t.
strawberry t., l. em morango; l. com revestimento esbranquiçado através do qual as papilas fungiformes aumentadas projetam-se como pontos vermelhos; característica da escarlatina e da síndrome de linfonodos mucocutâneos.
tongue-swallowing, deglutição da língua; deslizamento da língua para trás, contra a faringe, causando sufocação.
tongue thrust, impulso da l.; o padrão do lactente do movimento de sucção-deglutição, em que a língua é colocada entre os dentes incisivos ou as cristas alveolares durante o estágio inicial da deglutição, resultando, algumas vezes, em mordida aberta anterior.
tongue-tie, "língua presa", encurtamento do frênulo da língua. SIN ankyloglossia.
ton·ic (ton'ik). Tônico. **1.** Num estado de ação contínua ininterrupta; refere-se, especialmente, a uma contração muscular prolongada. **2.** Revigorante; que aumenta o tônus ou a força física ou mental. **3.** Remédio com o propósito de restabelecer a função debilitada e promover o vigor e um sentido de bem-estar; os tônicos são qualificados, de acordo com o órgão ou o sistema sobre o qual supostamente atuam, em cardíacos, digestivos, hemáticos, vasculares, nervinos, uterinos, gerais etc. [G. *tonikos,* de *tonos,* tônus]
bitter t., t. amargo; tônico de sabor amargo, como a quinina, a genciana, a quássia etc., que atua principalmente por estimulação do apetite e melhora da digestão.
to·nic·i·ty (tō-nis'i-tē). Tonicidade. **1.** Estado de tensão normal nos tecidos, de modo que as partes são mantidas em forma, alerta e prontas para funcionar em resposta ao estímulo apropriado. No caso do músculo, refere-se a um estado de atividade contínua ou tensão além daquela relacionada com as propriedades físicas; isto é, resistência ativa ao estiramento; no músculo esquelético, depende da inervação eferente. SIN tonus. **2.** A pressão ou tensão osmótica de uma solução, geralmente em relação à do sangue. VER TAMBÉM isotonicity. [G. *tonos,* tônus].
ton·i·co·clon·ic (ton-i-kō-klon'ik). Tônico-clônico; tanto tônico quanto clônico, referindo-se a contrações musculares repetidas. SIN tonoclonic.

to·nin (tō'nin). Tonina; enzima que converte a angiotensina I em angiotensina II, semelhante ou idêntica, portanto, à enzima conversora de angiotensina.
ton·ing (tōn'ing). A substituição de um depósito de prata por um de ouro num corte histológico impregnado mediante tratamento com uma solução de cloreto de ouro.
ton·i·tro·pho·bia (tō'ni-trō-fō'bē-ă). Tonitrofobia. SIN brontophobia. [L. *tonitrus,* trovão, + G. *phobos,* medo]
tono-. Tono-. Tônus, tensão, pressão. [G. *tonos*]
ton·o·clon·ic (ton-ō-klon'ik). Tonoclônico. SIN tonicoclonic.
ton·o·fi·bril (ton-ō-fī'bril). Tonofibrila; uma dentre um sistema de fibras encontradas no citoplasma de células epiteliais. VER cytoskeleton, tonofilament. SIN epitheliofibril, tenofibril.
ton·o·fil·a·ment (ton-ō-fil'ă-ment). Tonofilamento; proteína citoplasmática estrutural, de uma classe conhecida como filamentos intermediários, cujos feixes formam juntos uma tonofibrila; o tonofilamento é constituído por um número variável de proteínas relacionadas, ceratinas, e é encontrado em todas as células epiteliais, porém está particularmente bem desenvolvido na epiderme.
ton·o·graph (ton'ō-graf, tō'nō-). Tonógrafo; tonômetro registrador. [tono- + G. *graphō,* escrever]
to·nog·ra·phy (tō-nog'ră-fē). Tonografia; medição contínua da pressão intra-ocular por meio de um tonômetro registrador, para determinar a facilidade do fluxo aquoso de saída.
to·nom·e·ter (tō-nom'e-ter). Tonômetro. **1.** Instrumento para determinar a pressão ou tensão, especialmente um instrumento para determinar a tensão ocular. **2.** Vaso para equilibrar um líquido (p. ex., sangue) com um gás, geralmente numa temperatura controlada; a princípio, assim denominado por ser usado com uma relação gás/sangue muito pequena para permitir que o gás se aproximasse da tensão de oxigênio do sangue, servindo, assim, como medida dessa tensão; hoje em dia, é comumente utilizado com uma relação gás-sangue muito grande para ajustar o sangue à pressão de oxigênio do gás. SIN aerotonometer (2). [tono- + G. *metron,* medida]
applanation t., t. de aplanação; instrumento para determinar a tensão ocular por aplicação de um pequeno disco plano à córnea.
Gärtner t., t. de Gärtner; aparelho para estimar a pressão arterial ao observar a força, expressa pela altura de uma coluna de mercúrio, necessária para interromper a pulsação em um dedo da mão circundado por um anel compressivo.
Goldmann applanation t., t. de aplanação de Goldmann; t. de aplanação que achata apenas 3 mm² de córnea, utilizado com lâmpada de fenda.
Mackay-Marg t., t. de Mackay-Marg; t. de aplanação eletrônico registrador.
Mueller electronic t., t. eletrônico de Mueller; t. de tipo de Schiøtz que indica eletronicamente a extensão da indentação da córnea; pode ser também um registrador acoplado para leituras contínuas da pressão (tonografia).
pneumatic t., t. pneumático; t. de aplanação registrador operado por gás comprimido.
Schiøtz t., t. de Schiøtz; instrumento que mede a tensão ocular indicando a facilidade com que a córnea é indentada.

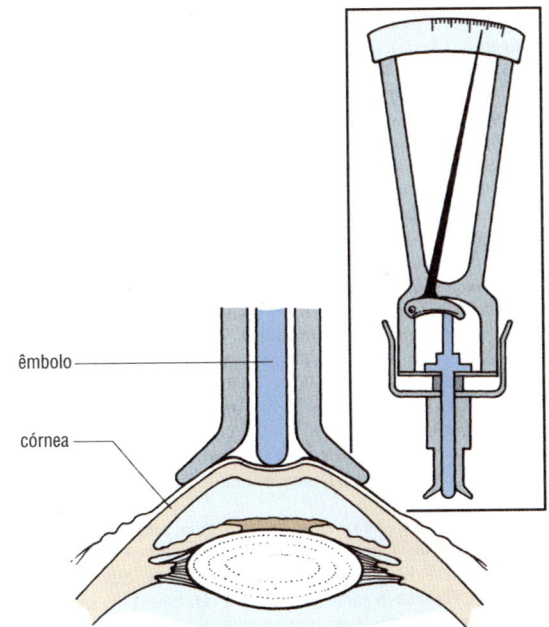

tonômetro de Schiøtz: indentação da córnea anestesiada pelo êmbolo (aqui exagerada) para medir a tensão ocular; (detalhe) tonômetro completo.

to·nom·e·try (tō-nom′ĕ-trē). Tonometria. **1.** Medida da tensão de uma parte, p. ex., tensão intravascular ou pressão arterial. **2.** Medida da tensão ocular.
ton·o·phant (tŏn′ō-fant, tŏn′ō-). Tonofanto; instrumento para visualização das ondas sonoras. [tono- + G. *phainō*, aparecer]
ton·o·plast (tō′nō-plast, tŏn′ō-). Tonoplasto; estrutura ou vacúolo intracelular. [tono- + G. *plastos*, formado]
to·nos·cil·lo·graph (tō-nos′i-lō-graf). Tonoscilógrafo; instrumento que produz registros gráficos das pressões arterial e capilar, bem como das características individuais do pulso. [tono- + L. *oscillo*, oscilar + G. *graphō*, escrever]
to·no·top·ic (tō-nō-top′ik). Tonotópico; designa um arranjo espacial de estruturas que servem a várias freqüências, como na via auditiva. [tono- + G. *topos*, lugar]
to·no·tro·pic (tō-nō-trop′ik). Tonotrópico; designa o encurtamento do comprimento de um músculo em repouso. [G. *tonikos*, *tonos*, tônus, + *tropos*, uma volta]
ton·sil (ton′sil). Tonsila; amígdala. **1.** Coleção intra-epitelial de linfócitos formando um anel linfoepitelial na faringe. **2.** SIN palatine t. [L. *tonsilla*, uma estaca, no pl. as tonsilas]
  cerebellar t., t. do cerebelo. SIN t. of cerebellum.
  t. of cerebellum [TA], t. do cerebelo; lóbulo arredondado na superfície inferior de cada hemisfério cerebelar, medialmente contínuo com a úvula do verme do cerebelo. SIN tonsilla cerebelli [TA], cerebellar t.
  eustachian t., t. tubária. SIN tubal t.
  faucial t., t. palatina. SIN palatine t.
  Gerlach t., t. de Gerlach. SIN tubal t.
  laryngeal t.'s, tonsilas laríngeas. SIN laryngeal lymphoid *nodules*, em *nodule*.
  lingual t. [TA], t. lingual; coleção de folículos linfóides na parte posterior ou faríngea do dorso da língua. SIN tonsilla lingualis [TA].
  Luschka t., t. de Luschka. SIN pharyngeal t.
  palatine t. [TA], t. palatina; grande massa oval de tecido linfóide imersa na parede lateral da orofaringe em cada lado, entre os pilares das fauces. SIN tonsilla palatina [TA], faucial t., tonsil (2), tonsilla.
  pharyngeal t. [TA], t. faríngea; coleção de nódulos linfóides mais ou menos estreitamente agregados na parede posterior e no teto da nasofaringe, cuja hipertrofia constitui a condição mórbida denominada adenóides. SIN tonsilla pharyngealis [TA], Luschka gland (1), Luschka t., third t., tonsilla adenoidea.
  submerged t., t. submersa; t. palatina que é plana e situa-se abaixo do nível dos pilares das fauces.
  third t., t. faríngea. SIN pharyngeal t.
  tubal t. [TA], t. tubária; coleção de nódulos linfóides próximo à abertura faríngea da tuba auditiva. SIN tonsilla tubaria [TA], eustachian t., Gerlach t.
ton·sil·la, pl. **ton·sil·lae** (ton-sil′ă, -ē). Tonsila. SIN palatine *tonsil*. [L. (ver tonsil)]
  t. adenoi'dea, t. faríngea. SIN pharyngeal *tonsil*.
  t. cerebel'li [TA], t. do cerebelo. SIN *tonsil* of cerebellum.
  t. intestina'lis, t. intestinal. VER aggregated lymphoid *nodules* of small intestine, em *nodule*.
  t. lingua'lis [TA], t. lingual. SIN lingual *tonsil*.
  t. palati'na [TA], t. palatina. SIN palatine *tonsil*.
  t. pharyngea'lis [TA], t. faríngea. SIN pharyngeal *tonsil*.
  t. tuba'ria [TA], t. tubária. SIN tubal *tonsil*.
ton·si·lar, ton·sil·lary (ton′si-lăr, ton′si-lă-rē). Tonsilar; amigdaliano. Relativo a uma tonsila, especialmente a tonsila palatina. SIN amygdaline (3).
ton·sil·lec·to·my (ton′si-lek′tō-mē). Tonsilectomia; remoção de toda a tonsila. [tonsil + G. *ektomē*, excisão]
ton·sil·li·tis (ton′si-lī′tis). Tonsilite; inflamação de uma tonsila, especialmente da tonsila palatina. [tonsil + G. *-itis*, inflamação]
  lacunar t., t. lacunar; inflamação da mucosa que reveste as criptas tonsilares.
  Vincent t., t. de Vincent; angina limitada principalmente às tonsilas, causada por microrganismos de Vincent (bacilo e espirilo).
tonsillo-. Tonsilo-. Tonsila. [L. *tonsilla*]
ton·sil·lo·lith (ton-sil′ō-lith). Tonsilólito; concreção calcárea numa cripta tonsilar distendida. SIN tonsillar calculus, tonsilolith. [tonsillo- + G. *lithos*, pedra]
ton·sil·lop·a·thy (ton′si-lop′ă-thē). Tonsilopatia; doença da tonsila. [tonsillo- + G. *pathos*, que sofre]
ton·sil·lo·tome (ton-sil′ō-tōm). Tonsilótomo; instrumento, algumas vezes modelado como uma guilhotina, para uso na tonsilectomia. [tonsillo- + G. *tomos*, corte]
ton·sil·lot·o·my (ton′si-lot′ō-mē). Tonsilotomia; remoção de uma parte ou de toda uma tonsila das fauces hipertrofiadas. [tonsillo- + G. *tomē*, incisão]
ton·sil·o·lith (ton′si-lith). Tonsilólito. SIN tonsillolith.
to·nus (tō′nŭs). Tônus. SIN tonicity (1). [L., do G. *tonos*]
  baseline t., t. basal; pressão intra-uterina entre as contrações durante o trabalho de parto.
  myogenic t., miogênico; contração de um músculo causada pelas propriedades intrínsecas do músculo e pela sua inervação intrínseca.
  neurogenic t., t. neurogênico; contração de um músculo causada pela influência de sua inervação intrínseca.
Tooth, Howard H., médico inglês, 1856–1925. VER Charcot-Marie-T. *disease*.

TOOTH

tooth, pl. **teeth** (tooth, tēth). [TA]. Dente; uma das estruturas cônicas duras situadas nos alvéolos da maxila e mandíbula, utilizadas na mastigação e que auxiliam a articulação. O dente é uma estrutura dérmica composta de dentina e revestida por cemento na raiz anatômica e por esmalte na coroa anatômica. Consiste numa raiz mergulhada no alvéolo, um colo recoberto pela gengiva e uma coroa, a parte exposta. No centro encontra-se a cavidade bulbar preenchida com retículo de tecido conjuntivo contendo uma substância gelatinosa (polpa do dente) e vasos sanguíneos e nervos que penetram através de uma abertura ou aberturas no ápice da raiz. Os 20 dentes decíduos ou dentes primários surgem entre o sexto e o nono e o vigésimo quarto mês de vida; sofrem esfoliação e são substituídos pelos 32 dentes permanentes, que aparecem entre o quinto e sétimo e entre o décimo sétimo e vigésimo terceiro anos. Existem quatro tipos de dentes: incisivo, canino, pré-molar e molar. SIN dens (1) [TA]. [A.S. *tōth*]

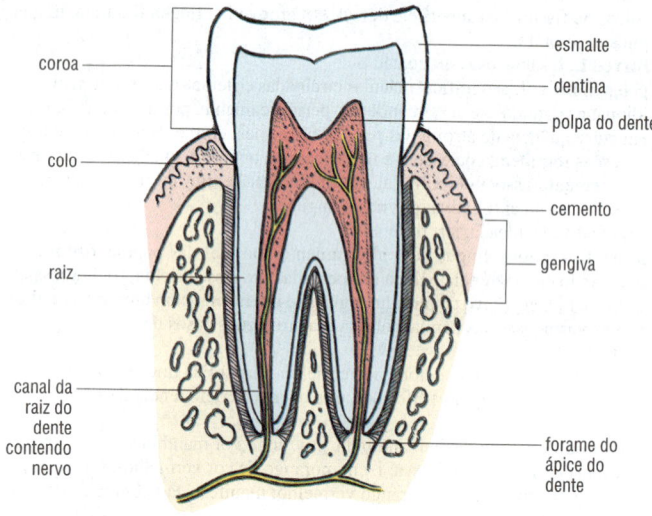

dente e tecidos de sustentação

  acrylic resin t., d. de resina acrílica; d. feito de resina acrílica.
  anatomic t., d. anatômico; d. artificial que duplica a forma anatômica de um d. natural.
  ankylosed t., d. ancilosado. VER dental *ankylosis*.
  anterior t., d. anterior; d. incisivo central, incisivo lateral ou canino. Compreendem os órgãos para incisão e localizam-se na parte frontal dos arcos dentais. SIN oral teeth.
  t. arrangement, arranjo dos dentes; **(1)** colocação de dentes numa base de dentadura com objetivos definidos; **(2)** colocação de dentes em bases temporárias.
  auditory teeth, dentes acústicos. SIN acoustic *teeth*.
  baby t., dente-de-leite. SIN deciduous t.
  back t., d. posterior; dente posterior aos caninos.
  bicuspid t., d. pré-molar. SIN premolar t.
  buck t., d. saliente; d. anterior em labioversão.
  canine t. [TA], d. canino; d. com uma coroa de forma cônica espessa e longa raiz cônica ligeiramente achatada; existem dois dentes caninos em cada maxila, um de cada lado adjacente à superfície distal dos incisivos laterais, tanto na dentição decídua quanto na permanente. SIN dens caninus [TA], canine (3), cuspid t., cuspidate t., cuspid (2), dens angularis, dens cuspidatus, eye t.
  carnassial t., **(1)** dente adaptado para cortar carne; **(2)** o último pré-molar superior ou o primeiro molar inferior de determinados carnívoros.
  cheek t., d. molar. SIN molar t.
  Corti auditory teeth, dentes auditivos de Corti. SIN acoustic *teeth*.
  crossbite t., d. de mordida cruzada; dente posterior destinado a permitir que a cúspide modificada do dente superior seja posicionada nas fossas do dente inferior.

cuspid t., cuspidate t., d. canino. SIN canine t.
cuspless t., d. sem cúspide; (1) dente desprovido de formação de cúspide; (2) abrasão acentuada de uma superfície oclusiva; (3) tipo de dente de dentadura artificial.
cutting teeth, dentes de corte; os dentes anteriores da maxila e da mandíbula.
dead t., d. morto; termo incorreto para pulpless t. (d. sem polpa).
deciduous t. [TA], d. decíduo; d. da primeira série de dentes, compreendendo ao todo 20, que irrompem entre 6 e 24 meses de vida, em média. SIN dens deciduus [TA], baby t., deciduous dentition, dens lacteus, first dentition, milk t., primary dentition, primary t., temporary t.
devitalized t., d. desvitalizado; termo incorreto para pulpless t. (d. sem polpa).
extruded teeth, dentes extrudados. VER *extrusion* of a tooth.
eye t., d. canino. SIN canine t.
fluoridated t., d. fluorado; d. exposto a sais de flúor durante a odontogênese.
fused teeth, dentes fundidos; dentes unidos por dentina em decorrência de fusão embriológica ou justaposição de dois germes dentários adjacentes.
geminated teeth, dentes geminados; anomalia de desenvolvimento que surge da tentativa de divisão de um broto dentário, resultando na formação incompleta de dois dentes, que se manifesta, em geral, na forma de coroa bífida sobre uma raiz única.
ghost t., d.-fantasma; d. com radiodensidade reduzida observado na odontodisplasia regional.
green t., d. verde; coloração verde a castanha dos dentes primários, associada à eritroblastose fetal e causada pela deposição de pigmentos de hemoglobina nos dentes em desenvolvimento.
Horner teeth, dentes de Horner; dentes incisivos com um sulco hipoplásico horizontal.
Huschke auditory teeth, dentes acústicos de Huschke. SIN acoustic *teeth.*
Hutchinson teeth, dentes de Hutchinson; os dentes do portador de sífilis congênita cuja borda incisiva é chanfrada e mais estreita do que a área cervical. VER TAMBÉM Hutchinson crescentic *notch.* SIN Hutchinson incisors, notched teeth, screwdriver teeth, syphilitic teeth.

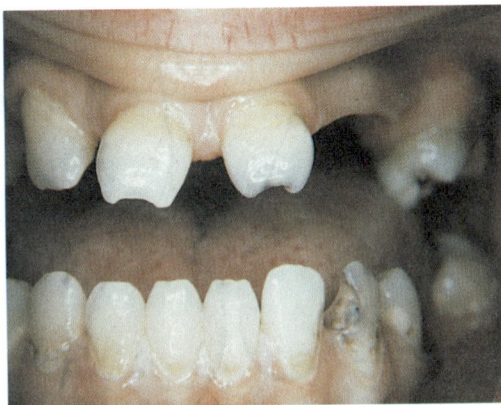

incisivos de Hutchinson: na sífilis congênita

impacted t., d. impactado; (1) d. cuja erupção normal é impedida por dentes ou osso adjacentes; (2) d. que foi direcionado para o processo alveolar ou tecido circundante em consequência de traumatismo.
incisor t. [TA], d. incisivo; d. com coroa em forma de cinzel e uma única raiz cônica afilada; existem quatro desses dentes na parte anterior da maxila e da mandíbula, tanto na dentição decídua quanto na permanente. SIN dens incisivus [TA], incisor.
metal insert teeth, dentes com inserção metálica; dentes protéticos contendo superfícies de corte metálicas nas superfícies oclusais.
migrating teeth, dentes migratórios; dentes que mudam de posição sob forças naturais.
milk t., dente-de-leite. SIN deciduous t.
molar t. [TA], d. molar; d. com coroa ligeiramente quadrangular com quatro ou cinco cúspides na superfície de trituração; a raiz é bífida na mandíbula, mas existem três raízes cônicas na maxila; existem seis molares em cada arco dental, três de cada lado atrás dos pré-molares na dentição permanente; na dentição decídua, existem quatro molares em cada arco dental, dois de cada lado atrás dos caninos. SIN dens molaris [TA], cheek t., molar (2), multicuspid t.
mottled t., d. mosqueado. VER mottled *enamel.*
multicuspid t., d. multicúspide. SIN molar t.
natal t., d. natal; d. supranumerário pré-decíduo presente ao nascimento.
neonatal t., d. neonatal; d. que surge até 30 dias após o nascimento.

nonanatomic teeth, dentes não-atômicos; (1) dentes com superfícies oclusais não baseadas em formas anatômicas; (2) dentes artificiais projetados de tal modo que as superfícies oclusais não são copiadas das formas naturais, mas recebem formas que, na opinião do projetista, parecem atender melhor às exigências de mastigação, tolerância tecidual etc.
nonvital t., d. não-vital; dente com polpa não-vital.
normally posed t., d. posicionado normalmente; d. em relação espacial correta com seu antagonista.
notched teeth, dentes chanfrados. SIN Hutchinson teeth.
oral teeth, dentes anteriores. SIN anterior t.
pegged t., d. em cavilha; d. cônico cujos lados convergem da região cervical para a incisiva.
permanent t. [TA], d. permanente; um dos 32 dentes pertencentes à segunda dentição ou dentição permanente; a erupção dos dentes permanentes começa do quinto ao sétimo ano e só se completa entre 17 e 23 anos de idade, quando aparece o último dos três molares. SIN dens permanens [TA], dens succedaneus, second t., secondary dentition, succedaneous dentition, succedaneous t.
perpetually growing t., d. com crescimento contínuo; fenômeno fisiológico em que o d. cresce contínua ou constantemente, calcifica e irrompe; p. ex., o dente incisivo do rato. SIN persistently growing t.
persistently growing t., d. com crescimento persistente. SIN perpetually growing t.
plastic teeth, dentes de plástico; dentes artificiais construídos com resinas sintéticas.
posterior t., d. posterior; d. bicúspide ou molar; esses dentes constituem os órgãos da mastigação e localizam-se na parte posterior dos arcos dentais.
premolar t. [TA], d. pré-molar; d. que habitualmente possui dois tubérculos ou cúspides na superfície de trituração e uma raiz achatada, única no arco dental mandibular e no segundo pré-molar superior, e sulcada no primeiro pré-molar superior. Existem quatro pré-molares em cada arco dental, dois de cada lado, entre o canino e os molares; não existem dentes pré-molares na dentição decídua. SIN dens premolaris [TA], bicuspid t., dens bicuspidus.
primary t., d. primário. SIN deciduous t.
protruding teeth, dentes protrusos; dentes que vão além do contorno normal dos arcos dentais; geralmente numa direção anterior.
pulpless t., d. sem polpa; d. com polpa não-vital ou necrótica ou cuja polpa foi extirpada.
sclerotic teeth, dentes escleróticos; dentes que naturalmente são duros e resistentes a cáries.
screwdriver teeth, dentes em chave de fenda. SIN Hutchinson teeth.
second t., segundo d. SIN permanent t.
spaced teeth, dentes espaçados; dentes que se separaram e perderam o contato proximal com dentes adjacentes.
stomach t., d. do estômago; um dos dentes caninos inferiores.
succedaneous t., d. sucedâneo. SIN permanent t.
syphilitic teeth, dentes sifilíticos. SIN Hutchinson teeth.
temporary t., d. temporário. SIN deciduous t.
third-year molar t. [TA], terceiro d. molar; oitavo d. permanente nos arcos dentais de cada lado, tornando-o o d. mais posterior nos seres humanos; em geral, irrompe entre 17 e 23 anos de idade; as raízes são freqüentemente fundidas, sendo a separação marcada apenas por sulcos; como tende a irromper em direção ântero-superior, o terceiro molar inferior muitas vezes torna-se impactado contra o segundo molar inferior; é comum que um ou mais dos terceiros molares não se desenvolvam. SIN dens molaris tertius [TA], dens serotinus*, dens sapientiae, third molar, wisdom t.
tricuspid t., d. tricúspide; d. que possui uma coroa com três cúspides.
tube t., d. em tubo; d. artificial com uma abertura cilíndrica vertical, que se estende do centro da base até o corpo do dente, dentro da qual pode ser colocado um pino ou cilindro para fixação do dente a uma base de dentadura.
Turner t., d. de Turner; hipoplasia do esmalte afetando um d. permanente solitário; relacionada à infecção no d. primário que o precedia ou a traumatismo durante a odontogênese.
unerupted t., d. não-irrompido; (1) d. antes de emergir; (2) d. incapaz de irromper ou de emergir dos tecidos alveolares dentários na cavidade oral.
vital t., d. vital; d. com polpa viva.
wisdom t., d. do siso. SIN third-year molar t.
zero degree teeth, dentes de zero grau; dentes protéticos que não possuem ângulos de cúspide em relação do eixo horizontal.

tooth·ache (tooth'āk). Odontalgia; dor de dente decorrente das condições da polpa ou do ligamento periodontal (cáries, infecção ou traumatismo). SIN dentalgia, odontalgia, odontodynia.
tooth-borne. Termo utilizado para descrever uma prótese ou parte de uma prótese que depende totalmente dos dentes contíguos para suporte.
top-. Top-. VER topo-.
top·ag·no·sis (top - ag - nō'sis). Topagnose; incapacidade de localizar sensações táteis. SIN topoanesthesia. [top- + G. *a-* priv., + *gnōsis*, reconhecimento]

top·es·the·sia (top′es-thē′zē-ā). Topestesia; a capacidade de localizar um toque leve aplicado a qualquer parte da pele. [top- + G. *aisthēsis*, sensação]

to·pha·ceous (tō-fā′shŭs). Tofáceo; arenoso; relativo a ou que manifesta as características de um tofo. [L. *tophaceus*]

to·phi (tō′fī). Tofos; plural de tophus.

to·phus, pl. **to·phi** (tō′fŭs, tō′fī). **1.** Tofo. VER gouty t. **2.** Cálculo salivar ou tártaro. SIN gouty pearl. [L. depósito calcáreo de nascentes, tufo calcáreo]
gouty t., t. gotoso; depósito de ácido úrico e uratos no tecido fibroso periarticular, na cartilagem da orelha externa ou no rim, na gota. SIN arthritic calculus, uratoma.

top·i·ca (top′i-kā). Tópicos; remédios para uso externo local. [neut. pl. do L. Mod. *topicus*, local]

top·i·cal (top′i-kăl). Tópico; relativo a um local ou localidade definidos; local. [G. *topikos*, de *topos*, lugar]

Topinard, Paul, antropologista francês, 1830–1911. VER T. facial *angle, line.*

to·pis·tic (tō-pis′tik). Topístico; designa uma região anatomicamente definida no sistema nervoso. [G. *topos*, lugar]

♻ **topo-, top-.** Topo-, top-. Lugar, tópico. [G. *topos*]

top·o·an·es·the·sia (top′ō-an-es-thē′zē-ā, tō′pō-). Topoanestesia. SIN topagnosis. [topo- + anesthesia]

top·og·no·sis, top·og·no·sia (top-og-nō′sis, -nō′zē-ā). Topognose, topognosia; reconhecimento da localização de uma sensação; no caso do tato, topestesia. [topo- + G. *gnōsis*, conhecimento]

top·o·gom·e·ter (top-ō-gom′e-ter). Topogômetro; alvo de fixação móvel preso diante de um ceratômetro, usado no ajuste de lentes de contato para medir as curvaturas da córnea em suas zonas periféricas. [topo- + G. *gonia*, ângulo, + *metron*, medida]

to·pog·ra·phy (tō-pog′ră-fē). Topografia; em anatomia, a descrição de qualquer parte do corpo, especialmente em relação a uma área definida e limitada da superfície. [topo- + G. *graphē*, escrito]

to·po·i·so·mer·ase (tō′pō-i-som′er-ās). Topoisomerase; tipo de enzima que converte (isomeriza) uma versão topológica do DNA em outra; atua ao catalisar a ruptura e nova formação de ligações fosfodiéster do DNA. [topo- + isomerase]

Topolanski, Alfred, oftalmologista austríaco, 1861–1960. VER T. *sign*.

to·pol·o·gy (tō-pol′ō-jē). Topologia. **1.** SIN regional anatomy. **2.** O estudo das dimensões da personalidade. [topo- + G. *logos*, estudo]

top·o·nar·co·sis (top′ō-nar-kō′sis). Toponarcose; anestesia cutânea localizada. [topo- + narcosis]

top·o·nym (top′ō-nim). Topônimo; nome próprio de uma região; designa uma região distinta do nome de uma estrutura, sistema ou órgão. [topo- + G. *onyma*, nome]

to·pon·y·my (tō-pon′i-mē). Toponimia; nomenclatura tópica ou regional, distinta da organonimia. [topo- + G. *onyma*, nome]

top·o·path·o·gen·e·sis (tō′pō-path-ō-jen′ē-sis). Topopatogenia; topografia de lesões relacionadas à sua patogenia. [topo- + pathogenesis]

top·o·pho·bia (tō-pō-fō′bē-ā). Topofobia; medo neurótico de ou relacionado a determinado local ou localidade. [topo- + G. *phobos*, medo]

top·o·phy·lax·is (tō′pō-fi-lak′sis). Topofilaxia; prevenção de choque causado por arsfenamina mediante aplicação de um torniquete ao membro acima do local de injeção e sua liberação lenta em cinco ou seis minutos. [topo- + G. *phylaxis*, proteção]

topotecan (tō-pō-tek′an). Topotecana; inibidor da topoisomerase I com atividade antitumoral, utilizada no tratamento do câncer ovariano.

TORCH Acrônimo de *t*oxoplasmose, *o*utras infecções, *r*ubéola, infecção por *c*itomegalovírus e *h*erpes simples (*t*oxoplasmosis, *o*ther infections, *r*ubella, *c*ytomegalovirus infection e *h*erpes simplex). VER TORCH *syndrome*.

tor·cu·lar he·roph·i·li (tōr′kŭ-lăr hĕ-rof′i-lī). Torcular de Herófilo; termo arcaico para a confluência dos seios da dura-máter (*confluence of sinuses*). [L. prensa de lagar de *Herophilus*, de *torqueo*, torcer]

Torek, Franz J. A., cirurgião norte-americano, 1861–1938. VER T. *operation*.

to·ric (tō′rik). Tórico; relativo a ou que possui a curvatura de um toro.

Torkildsen, Arne, neurocirurgião norueguês. 1899–1968. VER T. *shunt*.

Tornwaldt, Gustavus Ludwig, médico alemão, 1843–1910. VER T. *abscess, cyst, disease, syndrome*.

to·rose, to·rous (tō′rōs, -rŭs). Toroso; protuberante, nodos. [L. *torosus*, carnoso, de *torus*, nó, protuberância]

To·ro·vi·rus (tō-rō-vī-rus). Gênero da família Coronaviridae que causa infecções entéricas em animais.

tor·pent (tōr′pent). Torpente. **1.** Entorpecido. SIN torpid. **2.** Agente que entorpece. [L. *torpeo*, pres. p. *-ens*, estar lento]

tor·pid (tōr′pid). Tórpido; inativo; lento. SIN torpent (1). [L. *torpidus*, de *torpeo*, estar lento]

tor·pid·i·ty (tōr-pid′i-tē). Entorpecimento, torpor, estupor. SIN torpor.

tor·por (tōr′per, pōr). Torpor; inatividade, lentidão. SIN torpidity. [L. lentidão, dormência]

torque (T) (tōrk). Torque. **1.** Força rotatória. **2.** Em odontologia, uma força de torção aplicada a um dente para produzir ou manter o movimento da coroa ou da raiz. [L. *torqueo*, torcer]

torr (tōr). Torr; unidade de pressão suficiente para suportar uma coluna de mercúrio de 1 mm a 0°C contra a aceleração padrão da gravidade a 45° de latitude norte (980,621 cm/s²); equivalente a 1333,224 dinas/cm², 1.333,224 milibares, 1,35951 cm de H_2O, 133,3224 newtons/m² (ou Pa); 1 atm é igual a 760 Torr. [Evangelista *Torricelli*]

Torre, Douglas, dermatologista norte-americano, *1919. VER T. *syndrome*; Muir-Torre *syndrome*.

tor·re·fac·tion (tōr-ē-fak′shŭn). Torrefação; crestamento ou secagem pelo calor; operação farmacêutica para tornar drogas friáveis. [L. *torre-facio*, pp. *-factus*, tornar seco pelo calor, de *torreo*, crestar]

tor·re·fy (tōr′ē-fī). Torrefazer, torrificar; crestar.

Torricelli, Evangelista, cientista italiano, 1608–1647. VER torr.

tor·sade de pointes (tōr-săd dĕ pwant′). *Torsade de pointes;* forma de taquicardia ventricular quase sempre devida a medicações e caracterizada por longo intervalo QT e seqüência "curto-longo-curto" no batimento precedendo seu início. Os complexos QRS durante esse ritmo tendem a exibir uma série de complexos com pontas para cima, seguida de complexos de pontas para baixo, freqüentemente com um estreito intervalo de permeio e sem ondas T definidas; outrora denominada "cardiac ballet". [Fr. *torsade*, franja, torção, espiral, + *pointe*, ponta, extremidade (eufônico de "salva de ondas")]

tor·sion (tōr′shŭn). Torção. **1.** Torção ou rotação de uma parte sobre o seu eixo longitudinal ou seu mesentério; freqüentemente associada a comprometimento do suprimento sangüíneo. **2.** Torção da extremidade seccionada de uma artéria para interromper a hemorragia. **3.** Rotação do olho ao redor de seu eixo ântero-posterior. VER TAMBÉM intorsion, extorsion, dextrotorsion, levotorsion. [L. *torsio*, de *torqueo*, torcer]
t. of appendage, t. do apêndice; t. do apêndice do testículo ou do epidídimo.
extravaginal t., t. extravaginal; t. alta acima da inserção da túnica vaginal; tende a ocorrer no período neonatal.
intravaginal t., t. intravaginal; t. abaixo da inserção da túnica vaginal, que constitui o tipo mais comum de torção testicular. VER bell clapper *deformity*.
perinatal t., t. perinatal; t. que tende a ser do tipo extravaginal.
🛈 **t. of testis,** t. do testículo; rotação do cordão espermático, produzindo isquemia do testículo.

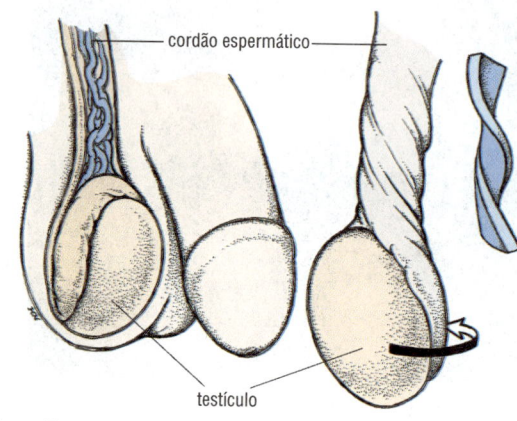

torção do cordão espermático

t. of a tooth, t. de um dente; rotação de um dente em seu alvéolo.

tor·sion·om·e·ter (tōr-shŭn-om′e-ter). Torcionômetro; dispositivo para medir o grau de rotação da coluna espinal.

tor·si·ver·sion (tōr-si-ver′shŭn). Torsiversão; má posição de um dente, que sofre rotação sobre o seu eixo longitudinal. SIN torsive occlusion, torsoclusion (2).

tor·so (tōr′sō). Torso; o tronco; o corpo sem relação com a cabeça ou com os membros. [It.]

tor·so·clu·sion (tōr′sō-kloo-zhŭn). Torsoclusão. **1.** Termo obsoleto para referir-se à acupressão realizada introduzindo-se uma agulha nos tecidos paralela à artéria, fazendo-a girar em seguida, de modo que atravesse a artéria transversalmente, e introduzindo-a nos tecidos do lado oposto do vaso. **2.** SIN torsiversion. [L. *torqueo*, torcer, + *claudo* ou *cludo*, fechar]

tor·ti·col·lar (tōr-ti-kol′ăr). Torcicolar; relativo a ou caracterizado por torcicolo.

tor·ti·col·lis (tōr-ti-kol′is). Torcicolo; contração ou encurtamento dos músculos do pescoço, principalmente aqueles supridos pelo nervo acessório espinal; a cabeça inclina-se para um lado e, em geral, sofre rotação, de modo que o queixo aponta para o outro lado. VER TAMBÉM dystonia. SIN wry neck, wryneck. [L. *tortus*, torcido, + *collum*, pescoço]

benign paroxysmal t. of infancy, t. paroxístico benigno do lactente; episódios recorrentes intermitentes de inclinação da cabeça e t., habitualmente associados a vômitos; em geral, o distúrbio aparece entre 2 e 8 meses de idade e regride aos 3 anos.
congenital t., t. congênito; t. devido a tumor fibroso unilateral no músculo esternocleidomastóideo, presente ao nascimento na forma de tumefação, que pode regredir ou pode levar ao t. por encurtamento do músculo. SIN muscular t.
dermatogenic t., t. dermatogênico; rigidez dolorosa do pescoço, com limitação da mobilidade, devido a lesões cutâneas extensas na área.
dystonic t., t. distônico. SIN spasmodic t.
fixed t., t. fixo; contratura persistente dos músculos cervicais de um lado.
hysterical t., t. histérico; t. que se acredita seja de etiologia psicossomática. VER hysteria.
labyrinthine t., t. labiríntico; t. devido a distúrbio vestibular.
muscular t., t. congênito. SIN congenital t.
ocular t., t. ocular; t. que acompanha a paralisia de um músculo extra-ocular, especialmente o músculo oblíquo.
psychogenic t., t. psicogênico; contrações espasmódicas dos músculos do pescoço, de origem psicossomática. VER TAMBÉM spasmodic t.
spasmodic t., t. espasmódico; distúrbio de causa desconhecida, manifestado na forma de distonia restrita, localizada em alguns dos músculos do pescoço, especialmente o esternomastóideo e o trapézio; ocorre em adultos e tende a progredir lentamente; os movimentos da cabeça aumentam com a posição ortostática e o caminhar e diminuem com estímulos contratuais, como, por exemplo, tocar o queixo ou o pescoço. SIN dystonic t., rotatory tic.
tor·ti·pel·vis (tōr-ti-pel'vis). Torcipelve; pelve torcida.
tor·tu·ous (tōr'choo-ŭs). Tortuoso; que possui muitas curvas; cheio de voltas e torções. [L. *tortuosus,* de *torqueo,* torcer]
Tor·u·lop·sis (tōr-oo-lop'sis). Gênero de leveduras com blastoconídios menores (2-4 nm), apresentando ampla fixação à célula-mãe; *T. glabrata,* atualmente denominado *Candida glabrata,* é uma causa de candidíase em seres humanos.
tor·u·lus, pl. **tor·u·li** (tōr'ū-lŭs, -lī). Tórulo; pequena elevação ou papila. [L. dim. de *torus,* protuberância, tumefação]
tor'uli tact'iles [TA], tórulos tácteis. SIN tactile elevations, em elevation.
to·rus, pl. **to·ri** (tō'rŭs, tō'rī) [TA]. Toro **1.** [TA]. Tumefação arredondada, como aquela causada por um músculo em contração. SIN elevation [TA]. **2.** Figura geométrica formada pela revolução de um círculo ao redor da base de qualquer um de seus arcos, como a moldagem convexa na base de um pilar. [L. tumefação, nó, protuberância]
t. fronta'lis, t. frontal; proeminência discreta no osso frontal, na raiz do nariz.
t. levator'ius [TA], t. do levantador; a protuberância na parede lateral da nasofaringe, abaixo da abertura da tuba auditiva, produzida pelo músculo levantador do véu palatino. SIN elevation of levator palati, levator cushion, levator swelling.
mandibular t., t. mandibula'ris, t. mandibular; exostose que se projeta da face lingual da mandíbula, geralmente oposta aos dentes pré-molares.
t. ma'nus, t. da mão; termo arcaico para os ossos do carpo.
t. occipita'lis, protuberância occipital; crista ocasional próxima à linha nucal superior do osso occipital.
palatine t., t. palati'nus, t. palatino; exostose que se projeta da linha média do palato duro.
t. tuba'rius [TA], t. tubário; crista na parede nasofaríngea posterior à abertura da tuba auditiva, causada pela projeção da parte cartilaginosa dessa tuba. SIN eustachian cushion, tubal prominence.
t. ureter'icus, prega interuretérica. SIN interureteric crest.
t. uteri'nus, t. uterino; crista transversal na parte posterior do colo do útero, formado pela junção das pregas retouterinas.
TOS Abreviatura de thoracic outlet *syndrome* (síndrome do desfiladeiro torácico).
tos·yl (tō'sil). Tosil; radical toluenossulfonil, amplamente utilizado para bloquear grupamentos amino durante a síntese orgânica de drogas e de outros compostos biologicamente ativos.
tos·yl·ate (tō'si-lāt). Tosilato; contração aprovada pela USAN para *p*-toluenossulfonato.
to·tem (tō'tem). Totem; objeto (geralmente animal ou vegetal) que serve como emblema de uma família ou clã e freqüentemente como lembrança de seus ancestrais; algo que serve como símbolo venerado. [Indígena americano]
to·tem·ism (tō'tem-izm). Totemismo; crença em um parentesco com ou numa relação mística entre um grupo ou indivíduo e um totem.
to·tem·is·tic (tō-tem-is'tik). Totemístico; relativo ao totemismo.
to·tip·o·ten·cy, to·tip·o·tence (tō-ti-pō'ten-sē, tō-tip'ō-tens). Totipotência; a capacidade de uma célula se diferenciar em qualquer tipo de célula e, portanto, formar um novo organismo ou regenerar qualquer parte de um organismo; p. ex., um ovo fertilizado ou uma pequena parte excisada de uma *Planaria,* que tem a capacidade de regenerar um novo organismo completo. [L. *totus,* todo, + *potentia,* poder]

to·tip·o·tent, to·ti·po·ten·tial (tō-tip'ō-tent, tō'ti-pō-ten'shăl). Totipotente, totipotencial; relativo à totipotência.
touch (tŭch). Toque. **1.** O sentido pelo qual se percebe um contato leve com a pele ou com as mucosas. SIN tactile sense. **2.** Exame digital. [Fr. *toucher*]
royal t., t. real; t. de um paciente pelo rei, que se acreditava fosse curativo; em geral, aplicado a pacientes com escrófula, mas também efetuado em pacientes com linfonodos aumentados (bubões) da peste.
Toupet, A., cirurgião francês. VER T. *fundoplication.*
Tourette. VER Gilles de la Tourette.
Tournay, Auguste, oftalmologista francês, 1878–1969. VER T. *sign.*
tour·ni·quet (toor'ni-ket). Torniquete; instrumento para interromper temporariamente o fluxo de sangue para uma parte distal ou a partir dela mediante aplicação de pressão com um dispositivo circundante. [Fr. de *tourner,* girar]
Dupuytren t., t. de Dupuytren; instrumento para compressão da aorta abdominal.
Esmarch t., t. de Esmarch; t. de borracha enrolado num membro em direção proximal antes de se iniciar um procedimento cirúrgico para exsangüinar o membro antes da inflação de um torniquete pneumático colocado proximalmente. SIN Esmarch bandage.
Rummel t., t. de Rummel; t. adaptado ao passar uma fita umbilical ao redor de um vaso e ao juntar ambas as extremidades através de um cateter de borracha vermelha curto. O t. pode ser apertado e fixado com um hemostato colocado perpendicularmente na extremidade do cateter mais distante do vaso.
Tourtual, Kaspar, anatomista prussiano, 1802–1865. VER T. *membrane, sinus.*
Touton, Karl, dermatologista alemão, *1858. VER T. *giant cell.*
Tovell, Ralph M., anestesiologista norte-americano, 1901–1967. VER T. *tube.*
Towne, E.B., otolaringologista norte-americano, 1883–1957. VER T. *projection, projection radiograph, view.*
tox-. Tox-. VER toxico-.
tox·al·bu·mins (toks-al-bū'minz). Toxoalbuminas; fitotoxinas que inibem a síntese de proteínas.
tox·a·ne·mia (tok-să-nē'mē-ă). Toxanemia; anemia resultante dos efeitos de um veneno hemolítico. [G. *toxikon,* veneno, + anemia]
tox·a·phene (tok'să-fēn). Toxafeno; inseticida hidrocarboneto clorado.
Tox·as·ca·ris le·o·ni·na (tok-sas'kă-ris lē-ō-nī'nă). Nematódeo ascarídeo do cão, que difere do *Toxocara* pelo fato de as larvas não migrarem através dos pulmões; todo o ciclo de desenvolvimento ocorre no intestino. Esse parasita foi encontrado nos seres humanos em alguns poucos casos e constitui uma causa de larva migrans visceral em crianças, embora seja menos freqüentemente implicado do que o *Toxocara canis.* [G. *toxon,* curva, + *Ascaris*]
tox·e·mia (tok-sē'mē-ă). Toxemia. **1.** Manifestações clínicas observadas durante determinadas doenças infecciosas, supostamente causadas por toxinas e outras substâncias nocivas elaboradas pelo agente infeccioso; em determinadas infecções por bactérias Gram-negativas, as endotoxinas provavelmente desempenham um papel quando a parede da célula bacteriana se rompe, liberando um lipopolissacarídio complexo; todavia, o papel de outras substâncias bacterianas permanece incerto, exceto no caso das exotoxinas específicas, como as da difteria e do tétano. **2.** A síndrome clínica causada por substâncias tóxicas no sangue. **3.** Termo leigo que se refere aos distúrbios de hipertensão da gravidez. SIN toxicemia. [G. *toxikon,* veneno, + *haima,* sangue]
tox·e·mic (tok-sē'mik). Toxêmico; relativo a, afetado por ou que manifesta as características de toxemia.
toxi-. Toxi-. VER toxico-.
tox·ic (tok'sik). Tóxico. **1.** Venenoso. SIN poisonous. **2.** Relativo a uma toxina. [G. *toxikon,* veneno de seta]
tox·i·cant (tok'si-kant). Tóxico. **1.** Venenoso. SIN poisonous. **2.** Qualquer agente venenoso, especificamente um veneno alcoólico ou outro veneno, que causa sintomas popularmente conhecidos como intoxicação.
tox·i·ce·mia (tok-si-sē'mē-ă). Toxicemia. SIN toxemia.
tox·ic·i·ty (tok-sis'i-tē). Toxicidade; o estado de ser tóxico, venenoso.
oxygen t., t. do oxigênio; **(1)** distúrbio orgânico resultante da respiração de altas pressões parciais de oxigênio; caracterizada por anormalidades visuais e auditivas, fadiga incomum durante a respiração, torção muscular, ansiedade, confusão, incoordenação e convulsões; pode ocorrer quando são administradas quantidades excessivas de oxigênio a pacientes (como a síndrome de angústia respiratória do adulto), resultando em agravamento dos infiltrados pulmonares e deterioração clínica; apesar de o mecanismo de desenvolvimento da condição ser obscuro, é provável o comprometimento da atividade enzimática, talvez em consequência da formação de radicais livres. Cf. retrolental *fibroplasia;* **(2)** a exposição dos pulmões a mais de 60% de oxigênio por períodos que ultrapassam 24-48 horas pode resultar em fibrose pulmonar irreversível grave. SIN oxygen poisoning.
toxico-, tox-, toxi-, toxo-. Toxico-, tox-, toxi-, toxo-. Veneno, toxina. [G. *toxikon,* arco, daí veneno (de seta)]
Tox·i·co·den·dron (tok'si-kō-den'dron). Gênero de plantas venenosas (família Anacardiaceae), também conhecido como *Rhus,* com frutas lisas e folhagem que contém urushiol, que produz dermatite de contato (dermatite por *Rhus*); as espécies incluem a hera venenosa (*T. radicans*), o carvalho veneno-

so (*T. diversilobum*) e o sumagre venenoso (*T. vernix*) [toxico- + G. *dendron*, árvore]

tox·i·co·gen·ic (tok′si-kō-jen′ik). Toxicogênico. **1.** Que produz um veneno. **2.** Causado por um veneno. [toxico- + G. *-gen*, que produz]

tox·i·coid (tok′si-koyd). Toxicóide; que possui ação semelhante a um veneno; temporariamente venenoso. [toxico- + G. *eidos*, semelhança]

tox·i·co·log·ic (tok′si-kō-loj′ik). Toxicológico; relativo à toxicologia.

tox·i·col·o·gist (tok-si-kol′ō-jist). Toxicologista; especialista em toxicologia.

tox·i·col·o·gy (tok-si-kol′ō-jē). Toxicologia; a ciência dos venenos, incluindo sua origem, composição química, ação, testes e antídotos. [toxico- + G. *logos*, estudo]

tox·i·co·path·ic (tok′si-kō-path′ik). Toxicopático; designa qualquer estado mórbido causado pela ação de um veneno.

tox·i·co·pho·bia (tok′si-kō-fō′bē-ā). Toxicofobia; medo mórbido de ser envenenado. SIN toxiphobia. [toxico- + G. *phobos*, medo]

tox·i·co·sis (tok-si-kō′sis). Toxicose; qualquer doença de origem tóxica. SIN systemic poisoning. [toxico- + G. *-osis*, condição]

endogenic t., t. endógena. SIN autointoxication.

exogenic t., t. exógena; qualquer doença causada por um veneno introduzido do meio externo e não produzido no interior do corpo.

thyroid t., t. tireóidea. SIN triiodothyronine t.

triiodothyronine t., T₃ t., t. por triiodotironina, t. por T₃; hipertireoidismo resultante do excesso de 3,5,3′-triiodotironina circulante. SIN thyroid t.

tox·if·er·ines (tok-sif′er-ēnz). Toxiferinas; o grupo mais potente dos alcalóides do curare; a principal fonte é *Strychnos toxifera*.

tox·if·er·ous (tok-sif′er-ŭs). Toxífero. SIN poisonous. [toxi- + L. *fero*, conduzir]

tox·i·gen·ic (tok-si-jen′ik). Toxigênico. SIN toxinogenic.

tox·i·ge·nic·i·ty (tok′si-jĕ-nis′i-tē). Toxigenicidade. SIN toxinogenicity.

tox·il·ic ac·id (tok-sil′ik). Ácido toxílico. SIN maleic acid.

tox·in (tok′sin). Toxina; substância nociva ou venenosa formada ou elaborada como parte integrante da célula ou do tecido, como um produto extracelular (exotoxina), ou como combinação dos dois, durante o metabolismo e o crescimento de determinados microrganismos e de algumas espécies superiores de vegetais e animais. [G. *toxikon*, veneno]

animal t., t. animal. SIN zootoxin.

anthrax t., t. do antraz; filtrado de cultura de *Bacillus anthracis* que contém uma exotoxina com pelo menos três componentes antigenicamente distintos: o fator do edema, o fator letal e o antígeno protetor. SIN *Bacillus anthracis* t.

Bacillus anthracis t., t. do *Bacillus anthracis*. SIN anthrax t.

bacterial t., t. bacteriana; qualquer t. intracelular ou extracelular formada no interior de células bacterianas ou elaborada por elas.

bee t., t. de abelha; a t. liberada pela ferroada de uma abelha; contém três princípios ativos: aminas biogênicas, peptídios ativos e certas enzimas hidrolíticas.

botulinus t., t. botulínica; potente exotoxina do *Clostridium botulinum*, que é altamente neurotóxica. SIN botulin, botulismotoxin.

cholera t., t. do cólera. VER *Vibrio cholerae*.

***Clostridium perfringens* alpha t.**, t. alfa de *Clostridium perfringens*; fosfolipase produzida por *Clostridium perfringens*, que aumenta a permeabilidade vascular e provoca necrose.

***Clostridium perfringens* beta t.**, t. beta de *Clostridium perfringens*; substância produzida por *Clostridium perfringens* que causa necrose e induz hipertensão ao provocar a liberação de catecolaminas.

***Clostridium perfringens* epsilon t.**, t. epsilon de *Clostridium perfringens*; t. produzida por *Clostridium perfringens* que aumenta a permeabilidade da parede gastrintestinal.

***Clostridium perfringens* iota t.**, t. iota de *Clostridium perfringens*; t. binária produzida por *Clostridium perfringens* responsável pela ocorrência de necrose e aumento da permeabilidade vascular.

cobra t., t. de *naja*. SIN cobrotoxin.

***Crotalus* t.**, t. de *Crotalus*; a toxina da cascavel.

diagnostic diphtheria t., t. diftérica diagnóstica. SIN Schick test t.

Dick test t., t. do teste de Dick. SIN streptococcus erythrogenic t.

dinoflagellate t., t. de dinoflagelados; potente neurotoxina cujo mecanismo de ação se acredita ser semelhante à toxina botulínica ao comprometer a síntese ou a liberação de acetilcolina. Responsável pela perda de mariscos devido à "maré vermelha".

diphtheria t., t. diftérica. VER *Corynebacterium diphtheriae*.

erythrogenic t., t. eritrogênica. SIN streptococcus erythrogenic t.

extracellular t., exotoxina. SIN exotoxin.

intracellular t., endotoxina. SIN endotoxin.

normal t., t. normal; solução de t. que contém exatamente 100 doses letais em 1 mL.

plant t., fitotoxina. SIN phytotoxin.

scarlet fever erythrogenic t., t. eritrogênica da escarlatina. SIN streptococcus erythrogenic t.

Schick test t., t. do teste de Schick; t. de *Corynebacterium diphtheriae* diluída, de modo que a dose inoculada (0,1 ou 0,2 mL) contém 1/50 de uma dose letal mínima para cobaia. VER TAMBÉM Schick *test*. SIN diagnostic diphtheria t.

Shiga t., t. de Shiga; a endotoxina formada por *Shigella dysenteriae* tipo 1.

Shigalike t., t. semelhante à Shiga. SIN vero cytotoxin.

streptococcus erythrogenic t., t. eritrogênica estreptocócica; filtrado de cultura de cepas lisogenizadas de estreptococos β-hemolíticos do grupo A, eritrogênica quando inoculada na pele de indivíduos suscetíveis e neutralizada por anticorpos que aparecem durante a convalescença da escarlatina; são reconhecidos três tipos imunológicos (A, B e C). SIN Dick test t., erythrogenic t., scarlet fever erythrogenic t.

tetanus t., t. tetânica; a exotoxina neurotrópica e termolábil do *Clostridium tetani* e a causa do tétano; foi isolada como proteína cristalina (PM = 67.000); trata-se de uma das substâncias mais venenosas conhecidas e parece funcionar bloqueando os impulsos sinápticos inibitórios. SIN tetanotoxin.

tox·in·ic (tok-sin′ik). Toxínico; relativo a uma toxina.

tox·i·no·gen·ic (tok′si-nō-jen′ik). Toxinogênico; que produz uma toxina, referindo-se a um organismo. SIN toxigenic. [toxin + G. *-gen*, que produz]

tox·i·no·ge·nic·i·ty (tok′si-nō-jĕ-nis′i-tē). Toxinogenicidade; a capacidade de produzir toxina. SIN toxigenicity.

tox·i·nol·o·gy (tok′si-nol′ō-jē). Toxinologia; o estudo das toxinas, em sentido restrito, com referência às substâncias proteináceas relativamente instáveis de origem microbiana, vegetal ou animal. [toxin + G. *logos*, estudo]

tox·i·no·sis (tok-si-nō′sis). Toxinose; qualquer doença ou lesão causada pela ação de uma toxina. SIN toxonosis. [toxin + G. *-osis*, condição]

tox·i·pho·bia (tok-si-fō′bē-ā). Toxifobia. SIN toxicophobia.

tox·is·ter·ol (tok-sis′ter-ol). Toxisterol; substância tóxica formada por irradiação excessiva de ergosterol ou calciferol.

♻ **toxo-.** Toxo-. VER toxico-.

Tox·o·ca·ra (tok′sō-kar′ā). Gênero de nematódeos ascarídeos, encontrado principalmente em carnívoros, que provoca a toxocaríase. [G. *toxon*, arco, + *kara*, cabeça]

T. ca′nis, a espécie de ascarídeo comum no intestino delgado do cão, cuja infecção pré-natal é uma forma comum de infecção de filhotes; também descrita em gatos, lobos, raposas, coiotes e texugos; a larva do segundo estágio é a causa mais freqüente de larva migrans visceral no fígado de crianças.

T. mys′tax, espécie de ascarídeo comum de gatos, cuja presença porém não foi relatada em cães; não ocorre infecção pré-natal de filhotes, sendo a infecção por ovos, que eclodem no intestino, liberando larvas do segundo estágio, que então migram através do coração, dos pulmões, da traquéia, da boca e do intestino, como o *Ascaris lumbricoides* no homem; os camundongos e outros vertebrados, bem como alguns invertebrados (p. ex., minhocas, baratas), podem servir como hospedeiros de transporte, no interior dos quais as larvas em migração encistam-se nos tecidos.

tox·o·ca·ri·a·sis (tok′sō-kā-rī′ā-sis). Toxocaríase; infecção por nematódeos do gênero *Toxocara*; as larvas em migração parenteral, principalmente de *Toxocara canis*, podem causar larva migrans visceral; o comprometimento ocular resulta em granuloma solitário na retina, massas inflamatórias periféricas ou endoftalmite crônica.

tox·oid (tok′soyd). Toxóide; toxina que foi tratada (comumente com formaldeído), de modo a destruir sua propriedade tóxica, porém preservar sua antigenicidade, isto é, a sua capacidade de estimular a produção de anticorpos antitoxina e, assim, produzir imunidade ativa. Para toxóides específicos, ver as subentradas em vaccine. SIN anatoxin. [toxin + G. *eidos*, semelhança]

tox·on, tox·one (tok′son, tok′sōn). Toxona; suposto produto bacteriano de toxicidade fraca e pequena afinidade por antitoxina.

tox·o·neme (tok′sō-nēm). Toxonema. SIN rhoptry. [G. *toxon*, arco, + *nema*, filamento]

tox·o·no·sis (tok-sō-nō′sis). Toxonose. SIN toxinosis. [toxo- + G. *nosos*, doença]

tox·o·phil, tox·o·phile (tok′sō-fil, -fīl). Toxófilo; suscetível à ação de um veneno; que possui afinidade por toxinas. [toxo- + G. *philos*, amigo]

tox·o·phore (tok′sō-fōr). Toxóforo; designa o grupo anatômico da molécula de toxina que contém o princípio venenoso. [toxo- + G. *phoros*, que conduz]

tox·oph·o·rous (tok-sof′ar-ŭs). Toxóforo; relativo ao grupamento toxóforo da molécula de toxina.

Tox·o·plas·ma gon·di·i (tok-sō-plaz′mă gon′dē-ī). Espécie de esporozoário (família Toxoplasmatidae) abundante e disseminada que é parasita intracelular sem hospedeiro específico de uma grande variedade de vertebrados. Desenvolve seu ciclo sexual, levando à produção de oocistos, exclusivamente em gatos e outros felídeos; os estágios proliferativos (taquizoítas) e cistos teciduais (contendo bradizoítas) desenvolvem-se numa grande variedade de espécies de animais, que contraem a infecção a partir da ingestão de oocistos, cistos teciduais em carne infectada, transplante de órgãos ou por migração transplacentária, resultando em infecção *in utero*. [G. *toxon*, arco, + *plasma*, algo formado]

Tox·o·plas·mat·i·dae (tok′sō-plaz-mat′i-dē). Família de esporozoários coccídeos que inclui os gêneros *Toxoplasma* e *Frankelia*, caracterizados por endodiogenia e pela presença de cistos (algumas vezes denominados pseudocistos) que contêm bradizoítas em células parenterais do hospedeiro; os esquizontes e os gamontes são produzidos em células intestinais, e estes últimos dão origem a oocistos. Os hospedeiros finais de *Toxoplasma* são gatos e outros felídeos; os hospedeiros finais de *Frankelia* não são conhecidos.

tox·o·plas·mo·sis (tok′sō-plaz-mō′sis). Toxoplasmose; doença causada pelo parasita protozoário *Toxoplasma gondii*, que pode produzir aborto em ovelhas, encefalite no bisão e inúmeras síndromes nos seres humanos. A infecção humana adquirida no período pré-natal pode resultar em anormalidades, como microcefalia ou hidrocefalia ao nascimento, desenvolvimento de icterícia com hepatoesplenomegalia ou meningoencefalite no início da infância, ou aparecimento tardio de lesões oculares, como coriorretinite no final da infância. As infecções humanas adquiridas no período pós-natal tipicamente permanecem subclínicas; se houver doença clínica, os sinais e sintomas consistem em febre, linfadenopatia, cefaléia, mialgia e fadiga, com recuperação final, exceto no paciente imunocomprometido, no qual é freqüente o desenvolvimento de encefalite fatal.

acquired t. in adults, t. adquirida em adultos; forma de t. que pode resultar em febre, encefalomielite, coriorretinopatia, exantema maculopapular, artralgia, mialgia, miocardite e pneumonite; uma forma linfadenopática parece ser mais prevalente em adultos, que podem manifestar febre, linfadenopatia, mal-estar e cefaléia, constituindo uma forma freqüentemente encontrada em pacientes com AIDS/SIDA.

congenital t., t. congênita; t. que aparentemente resulta de parasitas numa mãe infectada, transmitidos *in utero* ao feto; observada na forma de três síndromes: 1) aguda: a maioria dos órgãos contêm focos de necrose em associação a febre, icterícia, hidrocefalia, encefalomielite, pneumonite, erupção cutânea, lesões oftálmicas, hepatomegalia e esplenomegalia; 2) subaguda: a maioria das lesões encontra-se parcialmente cicatrizada ou calcificada, enquanto as situadas no cérebro e no olho parecem permanecer ativas; coriorretinite é encontrada em mais de 80% dos lactentes acometidos; 3) crônica: em geral, não é reconhecida durante o período neonatal; entretanto, podem-se detectar coriorretinite e lesões cerebrais semanas a anos depois.

tox·o·py·rim·i·dine (toks′ō-pi-rim′i-dēn). Toxopirimidina; um dos produtos resultantes da hidrólise da tiamina pela tiaminase, que aparecem na urina; inibidor competitivo do piridoxal. SIN pyramin, pyramine.

Toynbee, Joseph, otologista inglês, 1815–1866. VER T. *corpuscles,* em *corpuscle, muscle, tube.*

TPA, tPA Abreviaturas de tissue plasminogen *activator* (ativador do plasminogênio tecidual).

TPN Abreviatura de total parenteral *nutrition* (nutrição parenteral total).

TPP Abreviatura de *thiamin* pyrophosphate (pirofosfato de tiamina).

TPR Abreviatura de total peripheral *resistance* (resistência periférica total).

TQ Abreviatura de tocopherolquinone (tocoferolquinona).

TR Abreviatura de repetition *time* (tempo de repetição) na ressonância magnética.

tr. Abreviatura de L. *tinctura,* ou tincture (tintura).

tra·bec·u·la, gen. e pl. **tra·bec·u·lae** (tră-bek′ū-lă, -lē). [TA]. **1.** Trabécula; um dos feixes de sustentação de fibras que atravessam a substância de uma estrutura, geralmente derivado da cápsula ou de um dos septos fibrosos. **2.** Trabécula; pequeno pedaço da substância esponjosa do osso geralmente interconectado com outros pedaços semelhantes. **3.** Em histopatologia, faixa de tecido neoplásico com duas ou mais células de largura. [L. dim. de *trabs,* feixe]

anterior chamber t., t. da câmara anterior, tecido no ângulo da câmara anterior através do qual o humor aquoso sai do olho.

arachnoid t. [TA], t. aracnóidea; filamentos delicados e finos compostos de fibroblasto e colágeno extracelular que atravessam o espaço subaracnóideo entre a aracnóide-máter, que se fixam à dura e à pia-máter, aderente à superfície do cérebro. SIN trabeculae arachnoideae [TA].

trabeculae arachnoideae [TA], trabéculas aracnóideas. SIN arachnoid t.

trabec′ulae car′neae (of right and left ventricles) [TA], trabéculas cárneas (dos ventrículos direito e esquerdo); feixes musculares sobre as paredes de revestimento dos ventrículos do coração. SIN columnae carneae, Rathke bundles, trabeculae carneae ventriculorum dextri et sinistri.

trabeculae carneae ventriculorum dextri et sinistri, trabéculas cárneas dos ventrículos direito e esquerdo. SIN trabeculae carneae (of right and left ventricles)

trabeculae of corpora cavernosa [TA], trabéculas dos corpos cavernosos; faixas e cordões fibromusculares emitidos dos envoltórios fibrosos e do septo dos corpos cavernosos do pênis e que separam as veias cavernosas. SIN trabeculae corporum cavernosorum [TA].

trabec′ulae cor′poris spongi′osi pe′nis [TA], trabéculas do corpo esponjoso do pênis. SIN trabeculae of corpus spongiosum.

trabec′ulae cor′porum cavernoso′rum [TA], trabéculas dos corpos cavernosos. SIN trabeculae of corpora cavernosa.

trabeculae of corpus spongiosum [TA], trabéculas do corpo esponjoso; as faixas fibrosas entrelaçadas entre os espaços vasculares do corpo esponjoso e da glande do pênis. SIN trabeculae corporis spongiosi penis [TA].

trabec′ulae cra′nii, trabéculas do crânio; um par de centros de condrificação na base do neurocrânio cartilaginoso embrionário, localizados na frente da hipófise em desenvolvimento; transformam-se na sela turca.

trabec′ulae lie′nis, trabéculas esplênicas; *termo oficial alternativo para splenic trabeculae.

trabeculae of lymph node [TA], trabéculas esplênicas; feixes de sustentação de tecido conjuntivo que atravessam a substância do baço, derivados da cápsula do baço. SIN trabeculae nodi lymphoidei [TA].

trabeculae nodi lymphoidei [TA], trabéculas dos linfonodos. SIN trabeculae of lymph node.

septomarginal t. [TA], t. septomarginal; uma das trabéculas cárneas no ventrículo direito do coração; conduz parte do ramo direito do feixe AV do septo até o músculo papilar anterior na parede oposta do ventrículo. SIN t. septomarginalis [TA], moderator band, Reil band (1).

t. septomargina′lis [TA], t. septomarginal. SIN septomarginal t.

trabeculae of spleen, trabéculas esplênicas. SIN splenic trabeculae.

splenic trabeculae [TA], trabéculas esplênicas; pequenas faixas fibrosas emitidas da cápsula do baço e que constituem o arcabouço desse órgão. SIN trabeculae splenicae [TA], trabeculae lienis*, trabeculae of spleen.

trabec′ulae sple′nicae [TA], trabéculas esplênicas. SIN splenic trabeculae.

t. tes′tis, séptulos do testículo. SIN *septula* of testis, em *septulum.*

tra·bec·u·lar (tră-bek′ū-lăr). Trabecular; relativo a ou que contém trabéculas. SIN trabeculate.

tra·bec·u·late (tră-bek′ū-lāt). Trabeculado. SIN trabecular.

tra·bec·u·la·tion (tră-bek′ū-lā′shŭn). Trabeculação. **1.** A ocorrência de trabéculas nas paredes de um órgão ou parte dele. **2.** O processo de formação de trabéculas, como no osso esponjoso.

tra·bec·u·lec·to·my (tră-bek′ū-lek′tō-mē). Trabeculectomia; operação de filtração para glaucoma através da criação de uma fístula entre a câmara anterior do olho e o espaço subconjuntival, através de uma excisão subescleral de parte da rede trabecular. [trabekula + G. *ektomē,* excisão]

tra·bec·u·lo·plas·ty (tră-bek′ū-lō-plas-tē). Trabeculoplastia; fotocoagulação da rede trabecular do olho utilizando laser no tratamento do glaucoma.

laser t. (LTP), t. por laser; cirurgia para glaucoma em que a energia do laser é aplicada à rede trabecular.

> As investigações no tratamento do glaucoma de ângulo aberto com laser começaram no início da década de 1970, porém foi somente no final da década de 1980 que a LTP foi adotada como tratamento padrão para a condição. Nesse procedimento, utiliza-se um laser (geralmente argônio) para criar pequenas aberturas na rede trabecular, no ângulo de drenagem ocular, a fim de melhorar a drenagem do humor aquoso e aliviar a pressão intra-ocular. Algumas vezes, efetua-se ao mesmo tempo uma iridotomia com laser. A LTP diminui a probabilidade de infecção e hemorragia pós-operatórias e pode ser realizada numa base ambulatorial. Essa técnica obteve um índice de sucesso de 2 anos de mais de 70% (caindo para 59% depois de 5 anos), porém tem sido efetiva apenas em determinados tipos de glaucoma (especialmente os glaucomas capsular e pigmentar).

tra·bec·u·lot·o·my (tră-bek-ū-lot′ō-mē). Trabeculotomia; abertura cirúrgica do seio venoso da esclera (canal de Schlemm) para tratamento do glaucoma. [trabekula + G. *tomē,* incisão]

trace (trās). Traço. **1.** Evidências da existência, influência ou ação anteriores de um objeto, fenômeno ou evento. **2.** Quantidade extremamente pequena ou indicação dificilmente discernível de alguma coisa.

trac·er (trā′ser). Traçador, marcador. **1.** Elemento ou composto que contém átomos que podem ser distinguidos de seus equivalentes normais por meios físicos (p. ex., ensaio de radioatividade ou espectrografia de massa) e que, portanto, podem ser utilizados para acompanhar (traçar) o metabolismo das substâncias normais. **2.** Substância colorida ou radioativa que pode ser injetada na região de um tumor (melanoma, mama etc.) para mapear o fluxo de linfa do tumor para a sua bacia nodal mais próxima; utilizada na detecção de linfonodos sentinelas. **3.** Substância colorida (p. ex., corante) utilizada como traçador para acompanhar o fluxo de água. **4.** Instrumento usado na dissecção de nervos e vasos sangüíneos. **5.** Dispositivo mecânico com um ponto de marcação fixado a uma mandíbula e uma placa gráfica ou placa de traçado à outra; utilizado para registrar a digestão e a extensão dos movimentos da mandíbula. VER TAMBÉM tracing (2). [Rastro, do Fr. O. *tracier,* abrir caminho, do L. *traho,* pp. *tractum,* traçar, + *-er,* sufixo agente]

trache-. Traque-. VER tracheo-.

tra·chea, pl. **tra·che·ae** (trā′kē-ă, -kē-ē) [TA]. Traquéia; o tubo de ar que se estende da laringe até o tórax (nível da quinta ou sexta vértebra torácica), onde se bifurca nos brônquios principais direito e esquerdo. A traquéia é composta de 16-20 anéis de cartilagem hialina, conectados por uma membrana (ligamento anular); posteriormente, os anéis são deficientes em um quinto a um terço de sua circunferência, sendo o intervalo que forma a parede membranácea fechado por uma membrana fibrosa que contém fibras musculares lisas. Internamente, a mucosa é composta de epitélio colunar cilíndrico pseudo-estratificado, com células caliciformes mucosas; ocorrem numerosas glândulas serosas e mucosas mistas pequenas, cujos ductos se abrem na superfície do epitélio. SIN windpipe. [G. *tracheia artēria*, artéria rugosa]

saber-sheath t., t. em bainha de sabre; tipo de colapso da traquéia observado na doença pulmonar obstrutiva crônica, em que há um aumento na dimensão traqueal posterior externa com estreitamento látero-lateral envolvendo os dois terços inferiores da traquéia.

scabbard t., t. em bainha de espada; deformidade da traquéia causada por achatamento e aproximação das paredes laterais, produzindo estenose mais ou menos pronunciada.

tra·che·al (trā′kē-al). Traqueal; relativo à traquéia.

tra·che·al·gia (trā-kē-al′jē-a). Traquealgia; dor na traquéia. [trachea + G. *algos*, dor]

tra·che·a·lis. Traqueal. VER trachealis (*muscle*).

tra·che·i·tis (trā-kē-i′tis). Traqueíte; inflamação da membrana mucosa da traquéia. SIN trachitis. [trachea + G. *-itis*, inflamação]

trachel-. Traquel-. VER trachelo-.

trach·e·la·lis (trak-ē-lā′lis). Músculo longuíssimo da cabeça; termo arcaico para longissimus capitis (*muscle*).

trach·e·lec·to·my (trak-ē-lek′tō-mē). Traquelectomia. SIN cervicectomy. [trachel- + G. *ektomē*, excisão]

trach·e·le·ma·to·ma (trak′e-lē-ma-tō′ma). Traquelematoma; hematoma do pescoço. [trachel- + hematoma]

trach·e·li·an (trā-kē′lē-an). Traqueliano; termo arcaico para cervical. [G. *trachēlos*, pescoço]

trach·e·lism, trach·e·lis·mus (trak′e-lizm, -liz′mŭs). Traquelismo; inclinação do pescoço para trás, como a que algumas vezes precede um ataque epiléptico. [G. *trachēlismos*, captura pela garganta]

trach·e·li·tis (trak-ē-lī′tis). Traquelite. SIN cervicitis.

trachelo-, trachel-. Traquelo-, traquel-. Pescoço. [G. *trachēlos*]

trach·e·lo·cele (trak′e-lō-sēl). Traquelocele. SIN tracheocele. [trachelo- + G. *kēlē*, tumor, hérnia]

trach·e·lo·mas·toid (trak′e-lō-mas′toyd). Traquelomastóideo; termo arcaico para longissimus capitis (*muscle*).

trach·e·lo·oc·cip·i·ta·lis (trak′e-lō-ok-sip′i-tā′lis). Traqueloccipital; termo arcaico para semispinalis capitis (*muscle*).

trach·e·lo·pa·nus (trak′e-lō-pā′nŭs). Traquelopano. **1.** Tumefação dos vasos linfáticos do pescoço. **2.** Ingurgitamento linfático do colo do útero. [trachelo- + L. *panus*, tumor, tumefação]

trach·e·lo·pex·ia, trach·e·lo·pexy (trak′e-lō-pek′sē-a, -pek-sē). Traquelopexia; fixação cirúrgica do colo do útero. [trachelo- + G. *pēxis*, fixação]

trach·e·lo·plas·ty (trak′e-lō-plas-tē). Traqueloplastia; termo raramente utilizado para cirurgia plástica do colo do útero. [trachelo- + G. *plastos*, formado]

trach·e·lor·rha·phy (trak-ē-lōr′a-fē). Traquelorrafia; reparo por sutura de uma laceração do colo do útero. SIN Emmet operation. [trachelo- + G. *rhaphē*, sutura]

trach·e·los (trak′e-los). Traquelo; termo arcaico para colo. [G. *trachēlos*]

trach·e·los·chi·sis (trak-ē-los′ki-sis). Traquelosquise; fissura congênita no pescoço. [trachelo- + G. *schisis*, fissura]

trach·e·lot·o·my (trak-ē-lot′ō-mē). Traquelotomia. SIN cervicotomy. [trachelo- + G. *tomē*, incisão]

tracheo-, trache-. Traqueo-, traque-. A traquéia. [ver trachea]

tra·che·o·aer·o·cele (trā′kē-ō-ar′ō-sēl). Traqueoaerocele; cisto de ar no pescoço causado por distensão de uma traqueocele. [tracheo- + G. *aēr*, ar, + *kēlē*, hérnia]

tra·che·o·bil·i·ary (trā′kē-ō-bil′ē-ār-ē). Traqueobiliar; relativo à traquéia ou aos brônquios e ao sistema de ductos biliares.

tra·che·o·bron·che·o·pa·thia os·te·o·plas·ti·ca. Traqueobronqueopatia osteoplásica; tumor submucóide benigno ou série de tumores que ossificam próximo às paredes da traquéia.

tra·che·o·bron·chi·al (trā′kē-ō-brong′kē-al). Traqueobrônquico; relativo à traquéia e aos brônquios, referindo-se especialmente a um conjunto de linfonodos.

tra·che·o·bron·chi·tis (trā′kē-ō-brong-kī′tis). Traqueobronquite; inflamação da mucosa da traquéia e dos brônquios.

tra·che·o·bron·cho·meg·a·ly (trā′kē-ō-brong′kō-meg′a-lē). Traqueobroncomegalia; alargamento visível da traquéia e dos brônquios principais, geralmente congênito. SIN Mounier-Kuhn syndrome. [tracheo- + bronchus + G. *megas*, grande]

tra·che·o·bron·chos·co·py (trā′kē-ō-brong-kos′kō-pē). Traqueobroncoscopia; inspeção da luz da traquéia e dos brônquios. [tracheo- + bronchus, + G. *skopeō*, ver]

tra·che·o·cele (trā′kē-ō-sēl). Traqueocele; protrusão da mucosa através de um defeito na parede da traquéia. SIN trachelocele. [tracheo- + G. *kēlē*, hérnia]

tra·che·o·e·soph·a·ge·al (trā′kē-ō-ē-sof′a-jē′al). Traqueoesofágico; relativo à traquéia e ao esôfago.

tra·che·o·la·ryn·ge·al (trā′kē-ō-lā-rin′jē′al). Traqueolaríngeo; relativo à traquéia e à laringe.

tra·che·o·ma·la·cia (trā′kē-ō-mā-lā′shē-a). Traqueomalacia; amolecimento das cartilagens da traquéia. [tracheo- + G. *malakia*, amolecimento]

tra·che·o·meg·a·ly (trā′kē-ō-meg′a-lē). Traqueomegalia; dilatação anormal da traquéia que pode, à semelhança da bronquiectasia, resultar de infecção ou de ventilação com pressão positiva prolongada. [tracheo- + G. *megas* (*megal-*), grande]

tra·che·o·path·ia, tra·che·op·a·thy (trā′kē-ō-path′ē-a, -op′a-thē). Traqueopatia; qualquer doença da traquéia. [tracheo- + G. *pathos*, doença]

t. osteoplas′tica, t. osteoplásica; doença rara caracterizada por crescimentos cartilaginosos e ósseos na traquéia e nos brônquios, que produzem pólipos sésseis e placas que se projetam para a luz, obstruindo-a parcialmente.

tra·che·o·pha·ryn·ge·al (trā′kē-ō-fā-rin′jē-al). Traqueofaríngeo; relativo à traquéia e à faringe; designa uma faixa ocasional de fibras musculares que se estendem do músculo constritor inferior da faringe até a traquéia.

tra·che·o·pho·ne·sis (trā′kē-ō-fō-nē′sis). Traqueofonese; ausculta dos ruídos cardíacos na incisura esternal. [tracheo- + G. *phōnēsis*, som]

tra·che·oph·o·ny (trā-kē-of′ō-nē). Traqueofonia; o som vocal oco à ausculta sobre a traquéia. VER TAMBÉM bronchophony. [tracheo- + G. *phōnē*, voz]

tra·che·o·plas·ty (trā′kē-ō-plas-tē). Traqueoplastia; cirurgia plástica da traquéia. [tracheo- + G. *plastos*, formado]

slide t., t. deslizante; operação para reparo de estenose longa da traquéia, em que retalhos deslizantes anteriores e posteriores da parede da traquéia são suturados para reconstruir a luz da traquéia.

tra·che·or·rha·gia (trā-kē-ō-rā′jē-a). Traqueorragia; hemorragia da mucosa da traquéia. [tracheo- + G. *rhēgnymi*, irromper]

tra·che·os·chi·sis (trā-kē-os′ki-sis). Traqueósquise; fissura na traquéia. [tracheo- + G. *schisis*, fissura]

tra·che·o·scope (trā′kē-ō-skōp). Traqueoscópio; instrumento utilizado em traqueoscopia.

tra·che·o·scop·ic (trā-kē-ō-skop′ik). Traqueoscópico; relativo à traqueoscopia.

tra·che·os·co·py (trā-kē-os′kō-pē). Traqueoscopia; inspeção no interior da traquéia. [tracheo- + G. *skopeō*, examinar]

tra·che·o·ste·no·sis (trā′kē-ō-stē-nō′sis). Traqueostenose; estreitamento da luz da traquéia. [tracheo- + G. *stenōsis*, constrição]

tra·che·os·to·ma (trā′kē-os′tō-ma). Traqueostoma; abertura permanente na traquéia através do pescoço; refere-se também à abertura após laringectomia permanente. [tracheo- + G. *stoma*, boca]

tra·che·os·to·my (trā′kē-os′tō-mē). Traqueostomia; operação para fazer uma abertura na traquéia. VER TAMBÉM tracheotomy. [tracheo- + G. *stoma*, boca]

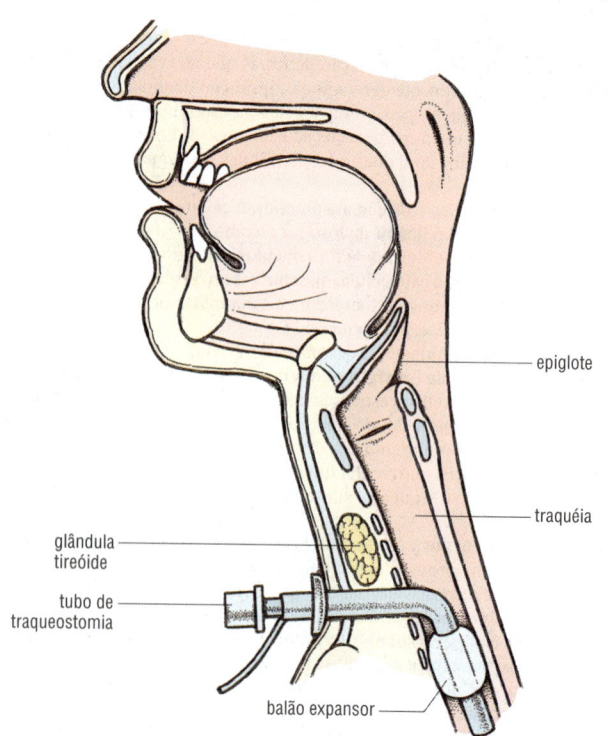

traqueostomia

tra·che·o·tome (tra̅′ke̅-o̅-to̅m). Traqueótomo; bisturi utilizado na operação de traqueotomia.

tra·che·ot·o·my (tra̅-ke̅-ot′o̅-me̅). Traqueotomia; a operação de abertura da traquéia, geralmente temporária. VER TAMBÉM tracheostomy. [tracheo- + G. *tome̅*, incisão]

Tra·chi·pleis·toph·ora (tra̅-ke̅-pli̅-stof′er-ă). Gênero de microsporídios que podem infectar seres humanos e causar miosite, ceratoconjuntivite e sinusite no indivíduo imunocomprometido.

tra·chi·tis (tra̅-ki̅′tis). Traqueíte. SIN tracheitis.

tra·cho·ma (tră-ko̅′mă). Tracoma; inflamação microbiana contagiosa crônica, com hipertrofia da conjuntiva, caracterizada pela formação de pequenos grânulos translúcidos acinzentados ou amarelados, causada por *Chlamydia trachomatis*. SIN Egyptian ophthalmia, granular lids, granular ophthalmia. [G. *tracho̅ma*, de *trachys*, rugoso]

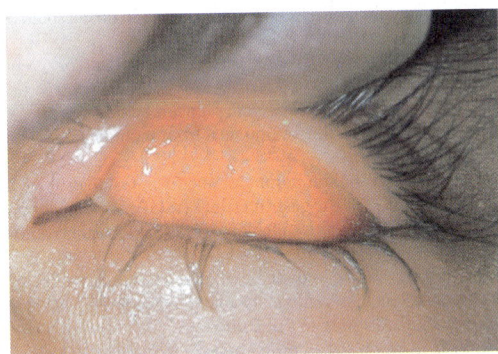

tracoma: observar os folículos esbranquiçados na superfície interna da pálpebra

follicular t., t. folicular; a forma comum de t. caracterizada pela presença de granulações sobre a conjuntiva. SIN granular t.

granular t., t. granular. SIN follicular t.

tra·chom·a·tous (tră-ko̅′mă-tŭs). Tracomatoso; relativo a ou que sofre de tracoma.

tra·chy·chro·mat·ic (trak-i-kro̅-mat′ik). Traquicromático; designa um núcleo com cromatina de coloração muito intensa. [G. *trachys*, rugoso, + *chro̅matikos*, cromático]

tra·chy·o·nych·ia (trak′e̅-o̅-nik′e̅-ă). Traquioníquia; unhas de superfície rugosa. [G. *trachys*, rugoso, + *onyx, onychos*, unha, + sufixo *-ia*, condição]

tra·chy·pho·nia (trak′e̅-fo̅′ne̅-ă). Traquifonia; aspereza da voz. [G. *trachys*, rugoso, + *pho̅ne̅*, voz]

trac·ing (tra̅s′ing). Traçado. **1.** Qualquer representação gráfica de eventos cardiovasculares elétricos ou mecânicos, como, por exemplo, eletrocardiograma, flebograma. VER TAMBÉM curve. **2.** Em odontologia, linha ou linhas inscritas num painel ou placa por um instrumento pontiagudo, representando um registro de movimentos da mandíbula; pode ser extra-oral (realizado fora da cavidade oral) ou intra-oral (realizado dentro da cavidade oral).

arrow point t., t. em ponta de seta. SIN needle point t.

cephalometric t., t. cefalométrico; desenho ou traçado sobreposto dos dentes, ossos da face e marcos antropométricos efetuado diretamente a partir de uma radiografia cefalométrica e utilizado como base para análise cefalométrica.

Gothic arch t., t. em arco gótico. SIN needle point t.

needle point t., t. em ponta de agulha; t. dos movimentos mandibulares efetuado por meio de um dispositivo fixado aos arcos opostos; sua forma assemelha-se a uma cabeça de seta ou arco gótico; quando a ponta de marcação do instrumento encontra-se no ápice do arco, considera-se que as mandíbulas estão em relação cêntrica. SIN arrow point t., Gothic arch t., Gothic arch, stylus t.

stylus t., t. em estilete. SIN needle point t.

TRACT

tract (trakt). Trato; área alongada, p. ex., via, trajeto, caminho. VER TAMBÉM fascicle. SIN tractus. [L. *tractus*, estender, extrair]

alimentary t., t. alimentar. SIN digestive t.

anterior corticospinal t., t. corticospinal anterior; fibras não-cruzadas que formam um pequeno feixe no funículo anterior da medula espinal. VER pyramidal t; VER TAMBÉM corticospinal t. SIN tractus corticospinalis anterior [TA], anterior pyramidal fasciculus, anterior pyramidal t., direct pyramidal t., fasciculus corticospinalis anterior, fasciculus pyramidalis anterior, tractus pyramidalis anterior, Türck bundle, Türck column, Türck t.

anterior pyramidal t., t. piramidal anterior. SIN anterior corticospinal t.

anterior raphespinal t. [TA], t. rafespinal anterior; grupo de axônios que se originam nos núcleos da rafe, primariamente da medula oblonga e ponte caudal, e que descem no funículo anterior. SIN tractus raphespinalis anterior [TA], ventral raphespinal t. [TA].

anterior spinocerebellar t. [TA], t. espinocerebelar anterior; feixe de fibras que se origina na base do corno posterior e zona intermédia em todos os segmentos lombossacros da medula espinal, cruzando para o lado oposto e ascendendo numa posição periférica na metade ventral do funículo lateral. Em sua ascensão através do robencéfalo, o trato curva-se agudamente em sentido dorsal ao longo da borda rostral do núcleo motor do nervo trigêmeo, entrando no cerebelo em direção caudal sobre a superfície dorsal do pedúnculo cerebelar superior e terminando como fibras musgosas na camada granular do córtex do verme do cerebelo. O feixe transmite informações proprioceptivas e exteroceptivas oriundas sobretudo do membro inferior oposto, apesar de algumas de suas fibras cruzarem novamente no cerebelo. SIN tractus spinocerebellaris anterior [TA], ventral spinocerebellar t.*, Gowers column, Gowers t.

anterior spinothalamic t. [TA], t. espinotalâmico anterior; a parte mais anterior ou ventral do feixe composto, o feixe ântero-lateral, formado pelos tratos espinotalâmicos anterior e lateral. Essas fibras específicas estão envolvidas na sensibilidade tátil. VER spinothalamic t; VER TAMBÉM anterolateral *system*. SIN tractus spinothalamicus anterior [TA], ventral spinothalamic t.

anterior trigeminothalamic t. [TA], t. trigeminotalâmico anterior; fibras que se originam do núcleo espinal do nervo trigêmeo, cruzam a linha mediana e ascendem no lado contralateral para terminar no núcleo póstero-medial ventral (PMV). Esse t. também contém, na ponte rostral e no mesencéfalo, fibras que se originam no núcleo sensitivo principal contralateral e que também terminam no PMV. SIN tractus trigeminothalamicus anterior [TA], ventral trigeminothalamic t. [TA].

anterolateral t., t. ântero-lateral. SIN anterolateral *system*.

Arnold t., t. de Arnold. SIN temporopontine t.

association t., t. de associação. VER association *system*.

auditory t., t. auditivo. SIN lateral *lemniscus*.

bulboreticulospinal t. [TA], t. bulboreticulospinal; t. que se origina do núcleo reticular gigantocelular da medula oblonga, desce primariamente como t. não-cruzado e termina principalmente nas lâminas espinais VII e VIII. SIN lateral reticulospinal t. [TA], medullary reticulospinal t. [TA], tractus bulboreticulospinalis [TA].

Burdach t., t. de Burdach. SIN cuneate *fasciculus*.

caerulospinal t. [TA], t. ceruleoespinal; conjunto de axônios que se originam do núcleo cerúleo e área subcerúlea e que se projetam bilateralmente para a substância cinza da medula espinal em todos os níveis espinais; constituem uma importante fonte de estímulo noradrenérgico para a medula espinal. SIN tractus caeruleospinalis [TA].

central tegmental t. [TA], t. tegmental central; grande feixe de fibras que segue longitudinalmente através do tegmento do mesencéfalo central e tegmento da ponte, distinto dos grupos longitudinais adjacentes de fibras-fascículos da formação reticular por uma composição mais compacta. Em cortes transversais do mesencéfalo, o feixe ocupa uma grande área triangular lateral ao fascículo longitudinal medial; mais caudalmente, sofre expansão em sentido ventral e, por fim, passa sobre a face lateral do núcleo olivar (inferior), tornando-se parte da cápsula de fibras desse último. O feixe contém fibras do tegmento do mesencéfalo e de regiões que circundam a substância cinzenta central descendo até o núcleo olivar; inclui também numerosas fibras que ascendem a partir da formação reticular da medula, ponte e mesencéfalo até o tálamo e região do subtálamo. SIN tractus tegmentalis centralis [TA], central tegmental fasciculus.

cerebellorubral t., t. cerebelorubral; componente do pedúnculo cerebelar superior que distribui fibras no interior do núcleo rubro do lado oposto. SIN tractus cerebellorubralis.

cerebellothalamic t., t. cerebelotalâmico; componente do pedúnculo cerebelar superior que se origina nos núcleos cerebelares, cruza completamente na decussação dos braços conjuntivos, desvia-se do núcleo rubro e termina em partes dos núcleos ventral anterior, ventral intermédio, ventral póstero-lateral e lateral central do tálamo. SIN dentatothalamic t., tractus cerebellothalamicus.

Collier t., t. de Collier. SIN medial longitudinal *fasciculus*.

comma t. of Schultze, t. em vírgula de Schultze. SIN semilunar *fasciculus*.

corticobulbar t., t. corticobulbar. VER corticonuclear *fibers*, em *fiber*. SIN tractus corticobulbaris.

corticopontine t., t. corticopontino; designação coletiva da multidão de fibras que, originando-se em todas as principais subdivisões do córtex cerebral, descem na cápsula interna e no pedúnculo cerebral para terminar nos núcleos da parte basilar da ponte. Os componentes individuais desse grande sistema de fibras estão indicados, de acordo com a sua origem no córtex cerebral, como fibras frontopontinas [TA], fibras parietopontinas [TA], fibras occipitopontinas [TA] e fibras temporopontinas [TA]. SIN tractus corticopontinus [TA].

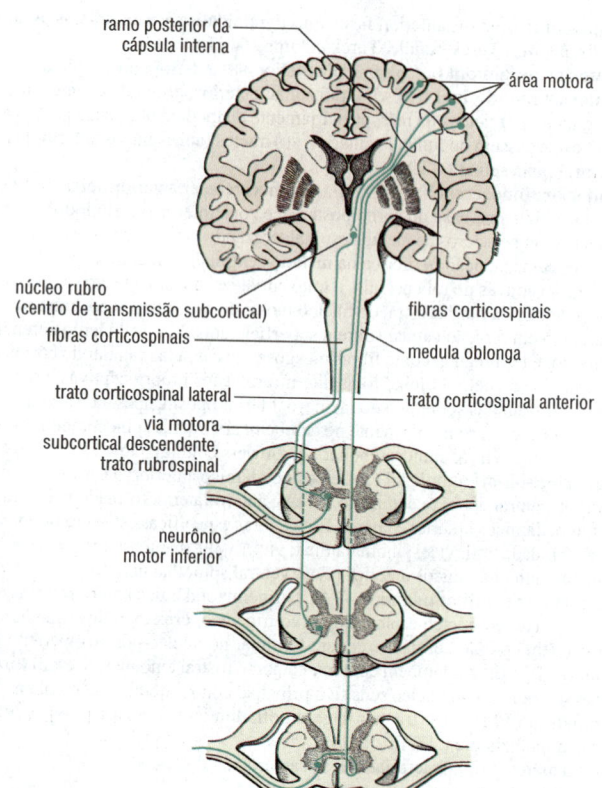

representação diagramática de vias motoras para a medula espinal através de uma via direta (**trato corticospinal**) e através de uma estação de transmissão subcortical (trato rubrospinal); a existência de uma decussação significa que um lado do cérebro controla a musculatura esquelética no lado oposto do corpo

corticospinal t., t. corticospinal; um composto de fibras corticospinais [TA] que descem na medula oblonga e através dela para formar o t. corticospinal lateral [TA] e o t. corticospinal anterior [TA]. Esse grande feixe de fibras origina-se das células piramidais de vários tamanhos na quinta camada da área motora pré-central (área 4), área pré-motora (área 6) e, em menor grau, do giro pós-central. As células que se originam na área 4 incluem as células gigantopiramidais de Betz. As fibras dessas regiões corticais descem através da cápsula interna, terço médio do pedúnculo cerebral e parte ventral da ponte para emergir na superfície ventral da medula oblonga, como a pirâmide. Continuando a direção caudal, a maioria das fibras cruza para o lado oposto na decussação da pirâmide e desce na metade dorsal do funículo lateral da medula espinal como t. corticospinal lateral, que distribui suas fibras por toda a extensão da medula espinal até interneurônios da zona intermédia da substância cinzenta espinal. Nas dilatações da medula espinal (relacionados com os membros), as fibras também seguem diretamente para grupos de neurônios motores que inervam os músculos distais dos membros, servindo para movimentos específicos da mão e dos dedos ou do pé e dedos do pé. As fibras não-cruzadas formam um pequeno feixe, o t. corticospinal anterior, que desce no funículo anterior da medula espinal e termina em contato sináptico com interneurônios na metade medial do corno anterior em ambos os lados da medula espinal. A interrupção das fibras corticospinais em sua origem cortical ou abaixo dela provoca comprometimento dos movimentos da metade oposta do corpo, grave sobretudo no braço e na perna; caracteriza-se por fraqueza muscular, espasticidade e hiper-reflexia, bem como perda de movimentos isolados dos dedos e da mão. O sinal de Babinski está associado a essa condição de hemiplegia. SIN pyramidal t. [TA], tractus pyramidalis [TA], tractus corticospinalis.
crossed pyramidal t., t. corticospinal lateral. SIN lateral corticospinal t.
cuneocerebellar t., fibras cuneocerebelares; o sistema de fibras nervosas que se origina do núcleo cuneiforme acessório e que penetra no cerebelo como componente do corpo restiforme, a parte maior do pedúnculo cerebelar inferior. SIN cuneocerebellar fibers [TA], fibrae cuneocerebellares [TA].
dead t.'s, tratos mortos; áreas de dentina caracterizadas por prolongamentos odontoblásticos degenerados; podem resultar de lesão causada por cárie, atrito, erosão ou preparo de cavidade.
deiterospinal t., t. vestibulospinal lateral. SIN lateral vestibulospinal t.
dentatothalamic t., t. dentatotalâmico. SIN cerebellothalamic t.
descending t. of trigeminal nerve, t. descendente do nervo trigêmeo. SIN spinal t. of trigeminal nerve.

digestive t., t. digestório; a passagem que leva da boca até o ânus, através da faringe, esôfago, estômago e intestino. SIN alimentary canal, alimentary t., digestive tube, tubus digestorius.
direct pyramidal t., t. corticospinal anterior. SIN anterior corticospinal t.
dorsal spinocerebellar t., t. espinocerebelar posterior; *termo oficial alternativo para posterior spinocerebellar t.
dorsal trigeminothalamic t. [TA], t. trigeminotalâmico posterior. SIN posterior trigeminothalamic t.
dorsolateral t., t. dorsolateral; *termo oficial alternativo para dorsolateral fasciculus.
fastigiobulbar t., t. fastigiobulbar; feixe de fibras que se origina no núcleo fastigial (núcleo do teto) de ambos os lados, saindo do cerebelo na parte medial do pedúnculo cerebelar inferior (corpo justa-restiforme) e distribuindo suas fibras para os núcleos vestibulares e outros grupos celulares na medula oblonga. Fibras cruzadas proeminentes formam uma alça sobre a superfície dorsal do pedúnculo cerebelar superior, antes de fazer uma volta ventralmente, formando o feixe uncinado de Russell ou feixe uncinado do cerebelo. SIN tractus fastigiobulbaris.
fastigiospinal t. [TA], t. fastigiospinal. VER fastigiospinal fibers, em fiber. SIN tractus fastigiospinalis [TA].
Flechsig t., t. de Flechsig. SIN posterior spinocerebellar t.
frontopontine t. [TA], t. frontopontino. VER frontopontine fibers, em fiber. SIN tractus frontopontinus.
frontotemporal t., t. frontotemporal. SIN unciform fasciculus.
gastrointestinal t., (G.I. t.) t. gastrintestinal (t. GI); o estômago, o intestino delgado e o intestino grosso; freqüentemente utilizado como sinônimo de t. digestório.
geniculocalcarine t., radiação óptica. SIN optic radiation.
genital t., t. genital; as vias genitais do aparelho urogenital. SIN genital duct.
t. of Goll, t. de Goll. SIN gracile fasciculus.
Gowers t., t. de Gowers. SIN anterior spinocerebellar t.
habenulointerpeduncular t., habenulopeduncular t. [TA], t. habenulointerpeduncular. SIN retroflex fasciculus.
Hoche t., t. de Hoche. VER semilunar fasciculus.
hypothalamohypophysial t. [TA], t. supra-óptico hipofisial. SIN supraopticohypophysial t.
iliopubic t. [TA], t. iliopúbico; margem inferior espessada da fáscia transversal vista como um feixe fibroso seguindo paralela e posteriormente (profundamente) ao ligamento inguinal, contribuindo para a parede posterior do canal inguinal quando liga os vasos ilíacos externos femorais do arco iliopectíneo ao ramo púbico superior. Marca a borda inferior do anel inguinal profundo e a margem medial do canal femoral. Observado apenas quando a região inguinal é vista de sua face interna; constitui um marcador útil na laparoscopia dessa região, p. ex., para reparo de hérnias inguinais. SIN tractus iliopubics [TA], deep crural arch, Thompson ligament.
iliotibial t. [TA], t. iliotibial; reforço fibroso da fáscia lata na superfície lateral da coxa, que se estende da crista ilíaca (especialmente o tubérculo da crista) até a face ântero-lateral do côndilo lateral da tíbia (tubérculo de Gerdy). SIN tractus iliotibialis [TA], iliotibial band, Maissiat band.
interpositospinal t. [TA], t. interpositospinal; grupo de axônios que se originam nos núcleos emboliforme e globoso do cerebelo, primariamente nesse último, e que desce até a medula espinal. SIN tractus interpositospinalis [TA].
interstitiospinal t. [TA], t. intersticiospinal; grupo de axônios que se originam no núcleo intersticial do mesencéfalo, desce ipsilateralmente e terminam primariamente nas lâminas espinais VII, VIII de Rexed. SIN tractus interstitiospinalis [TA].
James t.'s, fibras de James. SIN James fibers, em fiber.
lateral corticospinal t. [TA], t. corticospinal lateral; as fibras que cruzam para o lado oposto na decussação das pirâmides e descem na metade dorsal do funículo lateral da medula espinal; distribuem-se por toda a extensão da medula espinal até interneurônios da zona intermédia da substância cinzenta anterior, até alguns dos núcleos do corno posterior e até grupos de interneurônios do corno anterior. VER TAMBÉM corticospinal t. SIN tractus corticospinalis lateralis [TA], crossed pyramidal t., fasciculus corticospinalis lateralis, fasciculus pyramidalis lateralis, lateral pyramidal fasciculus, lateral pyramidal t., tractus pyramidalis lateralis.
lateral pyramidal t., t. corticospinal lateral. SIN lateral corticospinal t.
lateral raphespinal t. [TA], t. rafespinal lateral; grupo de axônios que surgem no núcleo magno da rafe, descem na parte posterior do funículo lateral e terminam primariamente no corno posterior (dorsal). Essas fibras serotoninérgicas estão envolvidas na transmissão de informações nociceptivas através do corno dorsal. SIN tractus raphespinalis lateralis [TA].
lateral reticulospinal t. [TA], t. reticulospinal lateral. SIN bulboreticulospinal t.
lateral spinothalamic t. [TA], t. espinotalâmico lateral; a parte mais dorsal ou dorsolateral do feixe composto, o sistema ântero-lateral, formado pelos tratos espinotalâmicos lateral e anterior; essas fibras específicas transmitem impulsos associados à sensação de dor e de temperatura. VER spinothalamic t. SIN tractus spinothalamicus lateralis [TA].

lateral vestibulospinal t., t. vestibulospinal lateral; feixe de fibras organizado somatopicamente, que se origina do núcleo vestibular lateral (núcleo de Deiters), que desce sem cruzar até o funículo anterior da medula espinal, lateralmente à fissura mediana anterior; o trato estende-se por toda a extensão da medula espinal, distribuindo fibras em todos os níveis até a parte medial do corno anterior. Os impulsos excitatórios conduzidos pelo t. vestibulospinal aumentam o tônus muscular extensor. SIN tractus vestibulospinalis lateralis [TA], deiterospinal t., tractus vestibulospinalis.
Lissauer t., t. de Lissauer. SIN dorsolateral *fasciculus.*
Loewenthal t., t. de Loewenthal. SIN tectospinal t.
mamillothalamic t., fascículo mamilotalâmico. SIN mammillothalamic *fasciculus.*
Marchi t., t. de Marchi. SIN tectospinal t.
medial reticulospinal t. [TA], t. pontoreticulospinal. SIN pontoreticulospinal t.
medial vestibulospinal t. [TA], t. vestibulospinal medial; fibras que se originam do núcleo vestibular medial e descem na medula espinal como componente do fascículo longitudinal medial. SIN tractus vestibulospinalis medialis [TA], tractus vestibulospinalis medialis [TA].
medullary reticulospinal t. [TA], t. bulboreticulospinal. SIN bulboreticulospinal t.
mesencephalic t. of trigeminal nerve [TA], t. mesencefálico do nervo trigêmeo; localizado ao longo da substância central do mesencéfalo e composto de fibras sensitivas primárias, cujas células de origem compõem o núcleo mesencefálico do trigêmeo. SIN tractus mesencephalicus nervi trigemini [TA].
Monakow t., t. de Monakow. SIN rubrospinal t.
t. of Münzer and Wiener, t. de Münzer e Wiener. SIN tectopontine t.
nerve t., t. nervoso; feixe ou grupo de fibras nervosas no cérebro ou na medula espinal.
occipitocollicular t., fibras occipitotetais. SIN occipitotectal t.
occipitopontine t., fibras occipitopontinas. VER occipitopontine *fibers,* em *fiber.* SIN tractus occipitopontinus.
occipitotectal t., fibras occipitotetais. VER occipitotectal *fibers,* em *fiber.* SIN occipitocollicular t.
olfactory t. [TA], t. olfatório; faixa branca, semelhante a um nervo, composta primariamente de fibras nervosas que se originam das células mitrais e células em tufo do bulbo olfatório, mas que também contém as células dispersas do núcleo olfatório anterior. O t. está estreitamente aplicado à superfície ventral do lobo frontal e fixa-se à base do hemisfério cerebral, no trígono olfatório, além do qual se estende na forma das estrias olfatórias que distribuem suas fibras para o tubérculo olfatório e, em maior número, para o córtex olfatório, sobre e ao redor do unco do giro para-hipocampal. VER TAMBÉM olfactory *nerves* [CN I], em *nerve.* SIN tractus olfactorius [TA], olfactory peduncle.
olivocerebellar t. [TA], t. olivocerebelar; grande grupo de fascículos de fibras frouxamente dispostos, que emerge do hilo do núcleo olivar, cruzando para o lado oposto da medula oblonga, através dos lemniscos do estrato interolivar e da oliva contralateral, e unindo-se ao corpo restiforme, a parte maior do pedúnculo cerebelar inferior contralateral; suas fibras terminam em todas as partes do córtex cerebelar como fibras ascendentes e nos núcleos cerebelares; todas as projeções olivocerebelares são cruzadas. SIN tractus olivocerebellaris [TA].
olivocochlear t. [TA], t. olivoclear; fibras que se originam dos núcleos perilivares bilateralmente, saem do tronco encefálico no nervo vestibular, unem-se ao nervo coclear na orelha interna e terminam nas células pilosas externas. SIN tractus olivocochlearis [TA], bundle of Rasmussen.
olivospinal t., fibras olivospinais. VER olivospinal *fibers,* em *fiber.* SIN Helweg bundle.
optic t. [TA], t. óptico; a continuação das fibras do nervo óptico além (atrás) da hemidecussação no quiasma óptico; cada um dos dois tratos ópticos simétricos é composto de fibras que se originam da metade temporal da retina do olho ipsilateral e de um número quase igual de fibras da metade nasal da retina contralateral; forma uma faixa de fibras compacta e ligeiramente achatada, que segue em direção caudolateral ao longo da base do hipotálamo e sobre a superfície basal dos pilares do cérebro; a maior parte de suas fibras termina no corpo geniculado lateral; um número menor de fibras entra no braço do colículo superior para terminar no colículo superior e na região pré-tetal. SIN tractus opticus.
parietopontine t., fibras parietopontinas. VER parietopontine *fibers,* em *fiber.* SIN tractus parietopontinus.
pontoreticulospinal t. [TA], t. pontoreticulospinal; t. que se origina dos núcleos reticulares rostral da ponte e caudal da ponte, desce bilateralmente, porém com preponderância ipsilateral, e termina principalmente nas lâminas espinais VII e VIII. SIN medial reticulospinal t. [TA], tractus pontoreticulospinalis [TA].
posterior spinocerebellar t. [TA], t. espinocerebelar posterior; feixe compacto de fibras espessas intensamente mielinizadas na periferia da metade dorsal do funículo lateral da medula espinal, que se originam no núcleo torácico ipsilateral (coluna de Clarke) e ascendem através do pedúnculo cerebelar inferior. As terminações terminam como fibras musgosas na camada granulosa do córtex do verme do cerebelo e, através de colaterais, nos núcleos cerebelares. O feixe conduz informações principalmente proprioceptivas, que se originam das terminações nervosas anulospirais que circundam os fusos musculares e dos órgãos tendíneos de Golgi. SIN tractus spinocerebellaris posterior [TA], dorsal spinocerebellar t.*, Flechsig t.
posterior trigeminothalamic t. [TA], t. trigeminotalâmico posterior; fibras que se originam primariamente na parte dorsomedial do núcleo sensitivo principal e que ascendem do mesmo lado e terminam no núcleo ventral pósteromedial. SIN dorsal trigeminothalamic t. [TA], tractus trigeminothalamicus posterior [TA].
posterolateral t. [TA], t. póstero-lateral. SIN dorsolateral *fasciculus.*
prepyramidal t., t. rubrospinal. SIN rubrospinal t.
pyramidal t. [TA], t. corticospinal. SIN corticospinal t.
respiratory t., t. respiratório; as vias respiratórias desde o nariz até os alvéolos pulmonares, passando pela faringe, laringe, traquéia e brônquios.
reticulospinal t., t. reticulospinal; designação coletiva de vários tratos de fibras que descem até a medula espinal, a partir da formação reticular da ponte e medula oblonga. Parte dessas fibras conduz impulsos dos mecanismos neurais que regulam funções autônomas para os neurônios motores somáticos e viscerais correspondentes da medula espinal; outras formam ligações em mecanismos motores não-piramidais que afetam o tônus muscular, a atividade reflexa e o movimento somático. VER TAMBÉM bulboreticulospinal t., pontoreticulospinal t. SIN tractus reticulospinalis.
rubrobulbar t. [TA], t. rubrobulbar; (1) componente do t. rubrospinal que distribui suas fibras para as partes laterais do tegmento do mesencéfalo, e não da medula espinal; (2) fibras rubroolivares não-cruzadas. SIN tractus rubrobulbaris [TA], tractus rubrobulbaris.
rubropontine t. [TA], t. rubropontino; axônios que surgem em células do núcleo rubro do mesencéfalo e terminam nos núcleos pontinos da ponte basilar. SIN tractus rubropontinus [TA].
rubroreticular t., t. rubroreticular; fibras que passam do núcleo rubro até a formação reticular da ponte e medula oblonga.
rubrospinal t. [TA], t. rubrospinal; feixe de fibras organizado somatotopicamente, relativamente pequeno nos seres humanos, que se origina do núcleo rubro, cruzando imediatamente na decussação tegmental ventral, desce próximo à superfície lateral do tronco encefálico no funículo lateral da medula espinal, na borda ventral do t. piramidal lateral. Termina na zona intermédia da medula espinal, onde sua distribuição coincide com a do t. piramidal lateral; em contraste com esse último, parece não possuir conexões diretas com neurônios motores espinais. Os impulsos conduzidos por esse trato aumentam indiretamente o tônus dos músculos flexores. SIN tractus rubrospinalis [TA], Monakow bundle, Monakow t., prepyramidal t.

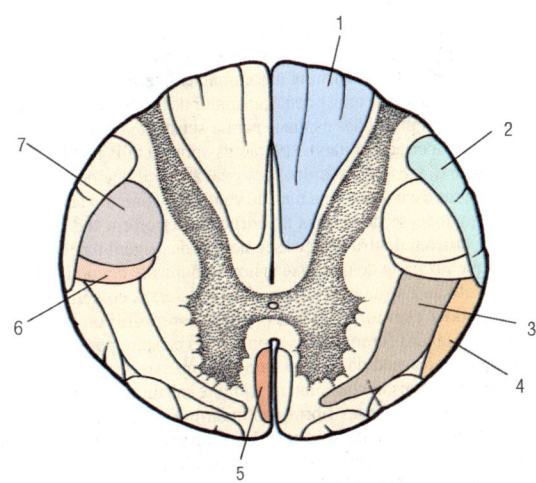

(1) colunas posteriores: percepção muscular consciente, toque preciso
(2) trato espinocerebelar posterior: percepção muscular inconsciente
(3) sistema ântero-lateral: dor, temperatura e toque leve
(4) trato espinocerebelar anterior: percepção muscular inconsciente
(5) trato corticospinal anterior: controle voluntário da musculatura esquelética
(6) trato rubrospinal: controle da musculatura esquelética
(7) trato corticospinal lateral: controle voluntário da musculatura esquelética

representação diagramática em corte transversal da medula espinal, mostrando suas principais vias; todos os **tratos** são bilaterais; os tratos ascendentes são numerados à direita, os descendentes, à esquerda

t. of Schütz, t. de Schütz. SIN dorsal longitudinal *fasciculus.*
sensory t., t. sensitivo. VER lemniscus.

septomarginal t., fascículo septomarginal. VER semilunar *fasciculus.*

solitariospinal t. [TA], t. solitariospinal; grupo de axônios que surgem no núcleo solitário e descem bilateralmente, sobretudo nas regiões dorsais do funículo lateral. SIN tractus solitariospinalis [TA].

solitary t. [TA], t. solitário; feixe de fibras compacto e delgado que se estende longitudinalmente através da região dorsolateral do tegmento medular, circundado pelo núcleo do t. solitário, abaixo do óbex que decussa sobre o canal central, e que desce até os segmentos cervicais superiores da medula espinal. É composto de fibras sensitivas primárias que entram com os nervos vago, glossofaríngeo e facial e, em parte, conduzem as informações provenientes de receptores de estiramento e quimiorreceptores nas paredes dos tratos cardiovascular, respiratório e intestinal; nas partes rostrais do trato, os impulsos são gerados pelas células receptoras dos botões gustativos na mucosa da língua. Suas fibras distribuem-se para o núcleo do t. solitário. SIN tractus solitarius [TA], fasciculus rotundus, fasciculus solitarius, funiculus solitarius, Gierke respiratory bundle, Krause respiratory bundle, round fasciculus, solitary bundle, solitary fasciculus.

sphincteroid t. of ileum, esfíncter basal. SIN basal *sphincter.*

spinal t., t. espinal; qualquer um de inúmeros fascículos de fibras que ascendem ou descem na medula espinal.

spinal t. of trigeminal nerve [TA], t. espinal do nervo trigêmeo; feixe de fibras compacto, em forma de vírgula em corte transversal, composto de fibras sensitivas primárias da parte principal do nervo trigêmeo, que desce do nível da entrada do trigêmeo na ponte superior através da região dorsolateral do tegmento do rombencéfalo ao longo da face lateral do núcleo espinal do nervo trigêmeo, emergindo na superfície dorsolateral da parte inferior da medula oblonga como tubérculo cinéreo e continuando até o segundo segmento cervical da medula espinal. Suas fibras distribuem-se para o núcleo espinal do trigêmeo. SIN tractus spinalis nervi trigemini [TA], descending t. of trigeminal nerve, tractus descendens nervi trigemini.

spinocerebellar t.'s, tratos espinocerebelares. VER anterior spinocerebellar t., posterior spinocerebellar t.

spinocervical t. [TA], t. espinocervical; t. composto de axônios que se originam das lâminas III-V e ascendem ipsolateralmente até o núcleo cervical lateral (NCL), onde fazem sinapse; os neurônios NCL projetam-se para o tálamo contralateral através do lemnisco medial. SIN tractus spinocervicalis [TA], spinocervicothalamic t., tractus spinocervicalis.

spinocervicothalamic t., t. espinocervicotalâmico. SIN spinocervical t.

spinoolivary t. [TA], t. espinoolivar; múltiplos tratos espinais que terminam nos núcleos olivares acessórios dorsal e medial. VER TAMBÉM olivospinal t. SIN tractus spinoolivaris [NA].

spinoolivary t. [TA], t. espinoolivar. Conjunto de axônios, que na realidade compreendem vários feixes, que se originam da substância cinzenta espinal e ascendem do mesmo lado, terminando nos núcleos olivares acessórios. SIN tractus spinoolivaris [TA].

spinoreticular t. [TA], t. espinorreticular. SIN spinoreticular *fibers,* em *fiber.*

spinotectal t. [TA], t. espinotetal; o componente relativamente pequeno do sistema ântero-lateral que termina nas camadas intermediária e profunda do colículo superior; parte de uma população maior de fibras espinomesencefálicas que também inclui projeções espinais para a substância cinzenta periaquedutal (fibras espinoperiaquedutais). SIN tractus spinotectalis [TA].

spinothalamic t., espinotalâmico; designação geral que descreve um grande feixe de fibras ascendentes na metade ventral do funículo lateral da medula espinal, originando-se de células no corno posterior em todos os níveis da medula, que cruzam dentro de seus segmentos de origem na comissura branca. Esse t., que faz parte de um feixe maior comumente denominado lemnisco espinal ou trato ântero-lateral (sistema ântero-lateral), contém fibras espinotalâmicas, fibras espinorreticulares, fibras espino-hipotalâmicas, fibras espinomesencefálicas (como fibras espinotetais e espinoperiaquedutais) e algumas projeções da medula espinal para o complexo olivar inferior (espinoolivar). Em sua ascensão contralateral, o feixe mistura-se com numerosas fibras intersegmentares. Essas fibras continuam desde a medula espinal até o tronco encefálico, ocupando uma posição ventrolateral e emitindo numerosas fibras para a formação reticular rombencefálica e mesencefálica (fibras espinorreticulares), para as fibras dos núcleos olivares acessórios (espinoolivares), para a parte lateral da substância cinzenta central do mesencéfalo (fibras espinoperiaquedutais) e para as camadas profunda e intermediária do colículo superior (fibras espinotetais); o número relativamente pequeno de fibras (10-20%) que permanecem consiste nas fibras espinotalâmicas que entram no diencéfalo e terminam no núcleo ventral posterior (parte caudal) e núcleos intralaminares do tálamo. Em sua ascensão na medula espinal, esse trato foi originalmente descrito como composto de uma parte dorsal, o trato espinotalâmico lateral, que conduz impulsos associados à sensação de dor e de temperatura, e uma parte mais ventral, o trato espinotalâmico anterior, envolvida na sensibilidade tátil. Hoje em dia, sabe-se que essa divisão não é tão óbvia quanto se acreditava a princípio. SIN lemniscus spinalis [TA], spinal lemniscus [TA], tractus spinothalamicus.

spinovestibular t. [TA], t. espinovestibular; grupo de axônios que se originam de neurônios primariamente em níveis lombossacros, ascendem do mesmo lado e em estreita aposição ao trato espinocerebelar posterior e terminam nos núcleos vestibulares lateral, medial e espinal. Alguns desses axônios podem ser colaterais de fibras espinocerebelares posteriores. SIN tractus spinovestibularis [TA].

spiral foraminous t., t. espiral foraminoso. SIN *tractus* spiralis foraminosus.

Spitzka marginal t., t. marginal de Spitzka. SIN dorsolateral *fasciculus.*

sulcomarginal t., t. sulcomarginal; designação coletiva dos tratos de fibras que descem no funículo anterior da medula espinal, ao longo da parede da fissura mediana anterior: t. tetospinal, fascículo longitudinal medial e t. piramidal anterior.

supraopticohypophysial t. [TA], t. supra-óptico-hipofisial; feixes de fibras não-mielinizadas que se originam de todas as células do núcleo supra-óptico e de cerca de 20% das do núcleo paraventricular do hipotálamo, que se estendem através do infundíbulo e do pedículo hipofisário até suas terminações no lobo posterior da hipófise; as fibras conduzem substâncias neurossecretoras, vasopressina e oxitocina, que são armazenadas (e podem ser liberadas no sangue circulante) em suas terminações. VER TAMBÉM pituitary *gland,* neurosecretion. SIN hipothalamohypophysial t. [TA], tractus supraopticohypophysialis [TA].

tectobulbar t. [TA], t. tetobulbar; fibras que se originam nas camadas profundas do colículo superior e que acompanham o trato tetospinal, mas que, ao contrário desse último, terminam nas regiões mediais dos tegmentos da ponte e do mesencéfalo. SIN tractus tectobulbaris [TA].

tectopontine t. [TA], t. tetopontino; feixe de fibras que se origina no colículo superior, segue em direção caudoventral do mesmo lado, ao longo da face medial do lemnisco lateral, enviando fibras que terminam na zona lateral do tegmento do mesencéfalo e terminando na parte lateral da substância cinzenta da parte ventral da ponte. SIN tractus tectopontinus [TA], t. of Münzer and Wiener.

tectospinal t. [TA], t. tetospinal; feixe de fibras espessas e intensamente mielinizadas, que se origina nas camadas profundas do colículo superior, cruzando para o lado oposto na decussação tegmentar dorsal, descendendo ao longo do plano mediano, entre o fascículo longitudinal medial dorsalmente, e o lemnisco medial ventralmente, para o funículo anterior da medula espinal. O trato termina na região medial do corno anterior da medula espinal cervical e parece estar envolvido nos movimentos da cabeça durante o rastreamento visual e auditivo. Em todo seu trajeto no tronco encefálico, é acompanhado por fibras do t. tetobulbar. SIN tractus tectospinalis [TA], Held bundle, Loewenthal bundle, Loewenthal t., Marchi t., predorsal bundle.

temporofrontal t., t. temporofrontal. SIN unciform *fasciculus.*

temporopontine t., t. temporopontino. VER temporopontine *fibers,* em *fiber.* SIN Arnold bundle, Arnold t., tractus temporopontinus.

trigeminospinal t. [TA], t. trigeminospinal; axônios que se originam de neurônios no núcleo espinal do nervo trigêmeo e descem para a medula espinal primariamente no lado ipsilateral. SIN tractus trigeminospinalis [TA].

trigeminothalamic t., t. trigeminotalâmico; designação geral para projeções dos núcleos espinal do nervo trigêmeo e principal do nervo trigêmeo para o tálamo. VER TAMBÉM trigeminal *lemniscus.*

tuberoinfundibular t., t. tuberoinfundibular; sistema de fibras não-mielinizadas finas que aparentemente se originam de núcleos de pequenas células do túber cinéreo, especialmente do núcleo arqueado, e que terminam na eminência mediana do infundíbulo, em contato com células ependimárias modificadas e com os tufos capilares a partir dos quais se originam as veias porta hipotalâmico-hipofisárias. VER TAMBÉM pituitary *gland,* neurosecretion. SIN tractus tuberoinfundibularis.

Türck t., t. de Türck. SIN anterior corticospinal t.

ℹ urinary t., t. urinário; a passagem da pelve renal para o meato urinário através dos ureteres, da bexiga e da uretra.

uveal t., t. uveal. SIN vascular *layer* of eyeball.

ventral raphespinal t. [TA], t. rafespinal anterior. SIN anterior raphespinal t.

ventral spinocerebellar t., t. espinocerebelar anterior; *termo oficial alternativo para anterior spinocerebellar t.

ventral spinothalamic t., t. espinotalâmico anterior. SIN anterior spinothalamic t.

ventral trigeminothalamic t. [TA], t. trigeminotalâmico anterior. SIN anterior trigeminothalamic t.

vestibulospinal t.'s, tratos vestibulospinais. VER medial vestibulospinal t.

vocal t., t. vocal; as passagens de ar acima da glote (incluindo a faringe, as cavidades oral e nasal e os seios paranasais) que contribuem para a qualidade da voz.

Waldeyer t., t. de Waldeyer. SIN dorsolateral *fasciculus.*

trac·tel·lum, pl. **trac·tel·la** (trak - tel'ŭm, - ă). Tratelo; flagelo locomotor anterior de um protozoário. [L. Mod. dim. do L. *tractus*]

trac·tion (trak'shŭn). Tração. **1.** O ato de tracionar ou puxar, como por uma força elástica ou por mola. **2.** Força de tração ou arrastamento exercida sobre um membro em direção distal. [L. *tractio,* de *traho,* pp. *tractus,* puxar, tracionar]

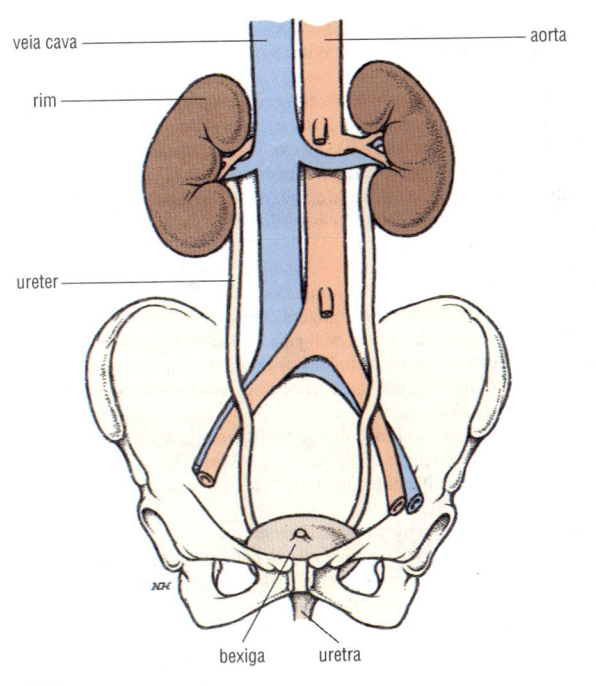

trato urinário

axis t., t. axial; procedimento raramente utilizado para aplicar tração à cabeça do feto na linha do canal de parto por meio de fórceps de t. axial.
Bryant t., t. de Bryant; t. do membro inferior colocado verticalmente, empregada especialmente para fraturas de fêmur em crianças.
Buck t., t. de Buck; aparelho para aplicar t. cutânea longitudinal à perna através do contato entre a pele e um esparadrapo; a fricção entre o esparadrapo e a pele permite a aplicação de força através de uma corda sobre uma polia, suspendendo um peso; a elevação do pé da cama permite ao corpo atuar como contrapeso. SIN Buck extension.
external t., t. externa; força de t. criada através do uso de ancoragem fixa (p. ex., um capacete ou estrado de cama) fora da cavidade oral; utilizada principalmente no tratamento de fraturas mesofaciais.
halo t., t. em halo; aplicação de t. óssea à cabeça por meio de um dispositivo em halo.
intermaxillary t., t. intermaxilar. SIN maxillomandibular t.
internal t., t. interna; força de t. criada através do uso de um dos ossos cranianos, acima do ponto de fratura, para ancoragem.
isometric t., t. isométrica; t. em que o comprimento do membro não se altera.
isotonic t., t. isotônica; t. em que a quantidade de força não se altera.
maxillomandibular t., t. maxilomandibular; força de t. desenvolvida através do uso de ligaduras elásticas ou com arame e fios ou imobilizações interdentárias ou ambos. SIN intermaxillary t.
Russell t., t. de Russell; aprimoramento da extensão de Buck que permite alterar o vetor resultante da força de tração aplicada; para fraturas do fêmur.
skeletal t., t. óssea; t. sobre uma estrutura óssea mediada através de um pino ou fio metálico inserido no osso para reduzir uma fratura de ossos longos. SIN skeletal extension.
skin t., t. cutânea; t. sobre um membro por meio de esparadrapo ou outros tipos de fitas aplicados ao membro.
trac·tor (trak′ter, tōr). Trator; instrumento para exercer tração sobre um órgão ou uma estrutura. [L. Mod. gaveta, ver traction]
Lowsley t., t. de Lowsley; instrumento curvo delgado com lâminas flexíveis em sua ponta, que pode ser aberto ou fechado por rotação na extremidade proximal do t.; é introduzido pela uretra até a bexiga e utilizado para retração da próstata para baixo no campo cirúrgico nos estágios iniciais da prostatectomia perineal.
Syms t., t. de Syms; bolsa de borracha colabável fixada à extremidade de um tubo; o tubo é introduzido na bexiga através da ferida perineal, e a bolsa é inflada; a tração produzida leva a próstata aumentada para a ferida, onde se torna mais acessível.
Young prostatic t., t. prostático de Young; instrumento tubular reto e curto com lâminas em sua ponta, que pode ser submetido a rotação, aberto e fechado; é introduzido na uretra prostática através de uma incisão de prostatotomia realizada durante os estágios finais da prostatectomia perineal a céu aberto, com sua ponta dentro da bexiga; a tração direta sobre um instrumento traz a próstata até o campo cirúrgico, onde a enucleação pode ser efetuada com mais facilidade.

trac·tot·o·my (trak - tot′o - me). Tratotomia; interrupção de um trato nervoso no tronco encefálico ou na medula espinal. [L. *tractus*, trato, + G. *tomē*, incisão]
anterolateral t., t. ântero-lateral. SIN anterolateral *cordotomy*.
intramedullary t., t. intramedular. SIN trigeminal t.
pyramidal t., t. piramidal; pode ser mesencefálica (pedunculotomia ou crusotomia), medular (piramidotomia medular) ou espinal (piramidotomia espinal).
Schwartz t., t. de Schwartz; tratotomia espinotalâmica medular.
Sjöqvist t., t. de Sjöqvist. SIN trigeminal t.
spinal t., t. espinal. SIN anterolateral *cordotomy*.
spinothalamic t., t. espinotalâmica; pode ser espinal (cordotomia), medular (t. de Schwartz) ou mesencefálica (t. de Walker).
trigeminal t., t. do trigêmeo; divisão das fibras descendentes do trato trigêmeo na medula. SIN intramedullary t., Sjöqvist t.
Walker t., t. de Walker; tratotomia espinotalâmica mesencefálica.

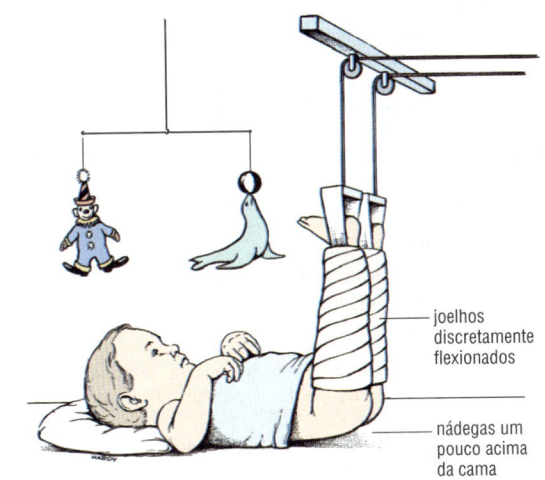

tração de Bryant

TRACTUS

trac·tus (trak′tūs). Trato. SIN tract. [L. puxada, extração, extensão, trato, de *traho*, pp. *tractus*, puxar]
t. anterolaterales, tratos ântero-laterais. SIN anterolateral *system*.
t. bulboreticulospinalis [TA], t. bulboreticulospinal. SIN bulboreticulospinal *tract*.
t. caeruleospinalis [TA], t. ceruleospinal. SIN caerulospinal *tract*.
t. cerebellorubra′lis, t. cerebelorrubral. SIN cerebellorubral *tract*.
t. cerebellothalam′icus, t. cerebelotalâmico. SIN cerebellothalamic *tract*.
t. corticobulba′ris, t. corticobulbar. SIN corticobulbar *tract*.
t. corticoponti′nus [TA], t. corticopontino. SIN corticopontine *tract*.
t. corticospina′lis, t. corticospinal. SIN corticospinal *tract*.
t. corticospina′lis ante′rior [TA], t. corticospinal anterior. SIN anterior corticospinal *tract*.
t. corticospina′lis latera′lis [TA], t. corticospinal lateral. SIN lateral corticospinal *tract*.
t. descen′dens ner′vi trigem′ini, t. espinal do nervo trigêmeo. SIN spinal *tract* of trigeminal nerve.
t. dorsolatera′lis [TA], t. dorsolateral. SIN dorsolateral *fasciculus*.
t. fastigiobulba′ris [TA], t. fastigiobulbar. SIN fastigiobulbar *tract*.
t. fastigiospinalis [TA], t. fastigiospinal. SIN fastigiospinal *tract*. VER fastigiospinal *fibers*, em *fiber*.
t. frontoponti′nus, t. frontopontino. SIN frontopontine *tract*.
t. habenulointerpeduncula′ris [TA], t. habenulointerpeduncular. SIN retroflex *fasciculus*.
t. iliopubicus [TA], t. iliopúbico. SIN iliopubic *tract*.
t. iliotibia′lis [TA], t. iliotibial. SIN iliotibial *tract*.
t. interpositospinalis [TA], t. interpositospinal. SIN interpositospinal *tract*.
t. interstitiospinalis [TA], t. interstiospinal. SIN interstitiospinal *tract*.
t. mesencephal′icus ner′vi trigem′ini [TA], t. mesencefálico do nervo trigêmeo. SIN mesencephalic *tract* of trigeminal nerve.
t. occipitoponti′nus, t. occipitopontino. SIN occipitopontine *tract*.

tractus

t. olfacto'rius [TA], t. olfatório. SIN olfactory tract.
t. olivocerebella'ris [TA], t. olivocerebelar. SIN olivocerebellar tract.
t. olivocochlearis [TA], t. olivococlear. SIN olivocochlear tract. VER olivocochlear bundle.
t. op'ticus, t. óptico. SIN optic tract.
t. parietoponti'nus, t. parietopontino. SIN parietopontine tract.
t. pontoreticulospinalis [TA], t. pontoreticulospinal. SIN pontoreticulospinal tract.
t. posterolateralis [TA], t. póstero-lateral. SIN dorsolateral fasciculus.
t. pyramida'lis [TA], t. corticospinal. SIN corticospinal tract.
t. pyramida'lis ante'rior, t. corticospinal anterior. SIN anterior corticospinal tract.
t. pyramida'lis latera'lis, t. corticospinal lateral. SIN lateral corticospinal tract.
t. raphespinalis anterior [TA], t. rafespinal anterior. SIN anterior raphespinal tract.
t. raphespinalis lateralis [TA], t. rafespinal lateral. SIN lateral raphespinal tract.
t. reticulospina'lis, t. reticulospinal. SIN reticulospinal tract.
t. rubrobulbaris, t. rubrobulbar. SIN rubrobulbar tract.
t. rubrobulbaris [TA], t. rubrobulbar. SIN rubrobulbar tract.
t. rubropontinus [TA], t. rubropontino. SIN rubropontine tract.
t. rubrospina'lis [TA], t. rubrospinal. SIN rubrospinal tract.
t. solitariospinalis [TA], t. solitariospinal. SIN solitariospinal tract.
t. solita'rius [TA], t. solitário. SIN solitary tract.
t. spina'lis ner'vi trigem'ini [TA], t. espinal do nervo trigêmeo. SIN spinal tract of trigeminal nerve.
t. spinocerebella'ris ante'rior [TA], t. espinocerebelar anterior. SIN anterior spinocerebellar tract.
t. spinocerebella'ris poste'rior [TA], t. espinocerebelar posterior. SIN posterior spinocerebellar tract.
t. spinocervicalis [TA], t. espinocervical. SIN spinocervical tract.
t. spinocervicalis, t. espinocervical. SIN spinocervical tract.
t. spinoolivaris [NA], t. espinolivar. SIN spinoolivary tract.
t. spinoolivaris [TA], t. espinolivar. SIN spinoolivary tract.
t. spinotecta'lis [TA], t. espinotetal. SIN spinotectal tract.
t. spinothalam'icus, t. espinotalâmico. SIN spinothalamic tract.
t. spinothalam'icus ante'rior [TA], t. espinotalâmico anterior. SIN anterior spinothalamic tract.
t. spinothalam'icus latera'lis [TA], t. espinotalâmico lateral. SIN lateral spinothalamic tract.
t. spinovestibularis [TA], t. espinovestibular. SIN spinovestibular tract.
t. spira'lis foramino'sus [TA], t. espiral foraminoso; aberturas na área coclear do fundo do meato acústico interno através das quais as fibras do nervo coclear deixam o labirinto ósseo para entrar na cavidade craniana. SIN spiral foraminous tract.
t. supraopticohypophysia'lis [TA], t. supra-óptico-hipofisário. SIN supraopticohypophysial tract.
t. tectobulba'ris [TA], t. tetobulbar. SIN tectobulbar tract.
t. tectoponti'nus [TA], t. tetopontino. SIN tectopontine tract.
t. tectospina'lis [TA], t. tetospinal. SIN tectospinal tract.
t. tegmenta'lis centra'lis [TA], t. tegmental central. SIN central tegmental tract.
t. temporoponti'nus, t. temporopontino. SIN temporopontine tract.
t. trigeminospinalis [TA], t. trigeminospinal. SIN trigeminospinal tract.
t. trigeminothalamicus anterior [TA], t. trigeminotalâmico anterior. SIN anterior trigeminothalamic tract.
t. trigeminothalamicus posterior [TA], t. trigeminotalâmico posterior. SIN posterior trigeminothalamic tract.
t. tuberoinfundibula'ris, t. tuberoinfundibular. SIN tuberoinfundibular tract.
t. vestibulospina'lis, t. vestibulospinal. SIN lateral vestibulospinal tract.
t. vestibulospinalis lateralis [TA], t. vestibulospinal lateral. SIN lateral vestibulospinal tract.
t. vestibulospinalis medialis [TA], t. vestibulospinal medial. SIN medial vestibulospinal tract.

traf·fick·ing (traf'ik-ing). Trânsito. SIN processing (1). VER targeting.
trag·a·canth, trag·a·can·tha (trag'a-kanth, -kan'tha; -santh). Tragacanto; exsudação resinosa de espécies de *Astragalus,* incluindo *A. gummifer,* arbustos do extremo leste do Mediterrâneo; ocorre como faixas ou cordões de uma substância resinosa resistente, formando uma mucilagem semelhante a gelatina com 50 partes de água; utilizado como demulcente e excipiente em emulsões e suspensões. [G. *tragakantha,* arbusto produtor de resina, de *tragos,* cabra, + *akanthos,* espinho]
tra·gal (trā'gãl). Tragal; relativo ao trago.
tra·gi (trā'jī). Tragos. **1.** Plural de tragus. **2.** [NA]. Os pêlos que crescem na entrada do meato acústico externo.
tra·gi·cus. Trágico. VER tragicus (*muscle*).
trag·i·on (trā'je-on). Trágio; ponto cefalométrico na incisura imediatamente acima do trago da orelha; situa-se 1-2 mm abaixo da espinha da hélice, que pode ser palpada.

trait

trag·o·mas·chal·ia (trag-ō-mas-kal'ē-ă). Tragomascalia; bromidrose das axilas. [G. *tragomaschalos,* com axilas fétidas, de *tragos,* cabra, + *maschalē,* axila]
trag·o·pho·nia, tra·goph·o·ny (trag'ō-fō'nē-ă, tră-gof'ō-nē). Tragofonia. SIN egophony. [G. *tragos,* cabra, + *phōnē,* voz]
tra·gus, pl. **tra·gi** (trā'gus, -jī). Trago. **1.** [NA]. Projeção semelhante a uma língua da cartilagem da orelha na frente da abertura do meato acústico externo e contínua com a cartilagem desse canal. SIN antilobium, hircus (3). **2.** VER tragi (2). [G. *tragos,* cabra, em alusão aos pêlos que crescem em uma parte, como um cavanhaque]
accessory t., t. acessório; pequenos nódulos presentes ao nascimento, anteriormente ao trago, derivados dos remanescentes do primeiro arco branquial e que freqüentemente contêm cartilagem central.
TRAIL. Um membro da família de ligantes do fator de necrose tumoral que induz rápida apoptose em várias linhagens celulares transformadas. SIN apo-2L.
train·ing (trān'ing). Treinamento; sistema organizado de educação, instrução ou disciplina.
assertive t., t. assertivo; forma de modificação ou terapia do comportamento, em que um cliente é ensinado a sentir-se livre para fazer pedidos e recusas legítimos em situações que previamente produziram respostas desconfiadas. SIN assertive conditioning.
aversive t., t. aversivo; forma de t. ou modificação do comportamento em que se utiliza um evento nocivo para punir ou extinguir um comportamento indesejável. VER TAMBÉM aversion therapy. SIN aversive conditioning.
avoidance t., t. de evitação. SIN avoidance conditioning.
escape t., t. de escape. VER escape conditioning.
toilet t., t. higiênico; t. direcionado para ensinar a uma criança o controle apropriado das funções vesical e intestinal; a teoria da personalidade psicanalítica acredita que as atitudes dos pais e da criança em relação a esse treinamento podem ter importantes implicações psicológicas para o desenvolvimento posterior da criança.

trait (trāt). Traço; caráter, característica qualitativa; atributo distinto, em contraste com caráter métrico. Um t. é acessível à análise de segregação, mais do que à análise quantitativa; é um atributo do fenótipo, e não do genótipo. [Fr. do L. *tractus,* tração, extensão]
Bombay t., t. de Bombay. VER Bombay phenomenon.
categorical t., t. categórico; em genética, uma característica que pode ser analisada de forma conveniente e efetiva por meio de separação em classes, visto que não existe nenhuma maneira satisfatória de medi-la (como os grupos sangüíneos) ou visto que recai em classes naturais, de modo que a variação entre classes excede de longe a existente dentro das classes (por exemplo, os efeitos fenotípicos de muitos polimorfismos enzimáticos); a existência de categorias sugere mas não prova a atuação de uma causa subjacente importante e simples. SIN qualitative t.
chromosomal t., t. cromossômico; t. que depende de uma aberração cromossômica recorrente.
codominant t., t. co-dominante. VER codominant.
dominant t., t. dominante; característica física ou mental proeminente. VER *dominance* of traits.
dominant lethal t., t. dominante letal; t. expresso no fenótipo que, quando presente no genótipo, impede a produção de descendentes. Todos esses casos são necessariamente esporádicos e devem representar novas mutações, visto que os métodos habituais da genética clássica não proporcionam nenhuma forma de demonstrar qualquer componente genético, à exceção de argumentos tênues, como idade paterna avançada. A biologia molecular pode ser útil, embora os métodos empregados possam ser tediosos; se houver um gene epistático passível de mascarar o t., a lógica é mais fácil, ainda que complexa.
galtonian t., t. galtoniano; t. genético quantitativo devido a contribuições de muito mais *loci* menos igualmente importantes, que se assemelha a um t. contínuo.
intermediate t., t. intermediário; t. mensurável em que há alguma evidência da operação de uma causa importante simples, porém em que a variação dentro das supostas categorias é tal que produz superposição e, portanto, ambigüidade na classificação de qualquer leitura específica.
liminal t., t. liminar. SIN threshold t.
marker t., t. marcador; t. que pode ser de pouca importância em si, mas que, em associação, ligação ou outros meios, facilita a detecção, a antecipação ou a compreensão de uma doença ou (para doenças genéticas) a localização do gene causador no cariótipo.
mendelian t., t. mendeliano; t. de categoria que segrega de acordo com um sistema genético de único *locus*.
nonpenetrant t., t. não-penetrante; t. genético que não se manifesta fenotipicamente em virtude de fatores não-genéticos; por conseguinte, não inclui recessividade, epistasia, hipostasia ou parastasia, porém inclui fatores ambientais e efeitos aleatórios puros, como lionização.
penetrant t., t. penetrante; t. que nos genótipos apropriados se manifesta fenotipicamente; estritamente falando, é o t. que é penetrante, e não o gene. VER penetrance.

qualitative t., t. qualitativo. SIN categorical t.
recessive t., t. recessivo. VER *dominance* of traits.
sickle cell t., t. falciforme; o estado heterozigoto do gene para a hemoglobina S na anemia falciforme.
threshold t., t. liminar; t. que cai em grupos naturais que não se originam em causas categoricamente distintas, mas no fato de o resultado atingir ou não valores críticos; p. ex., os cálculos biliares podem resultar de uma causa categórica ou de níveis incomuns de fatores causais que, por si próprios, não exibem evidências de agrupamento. SIN liminal t.

tra·jec·tor (tra-jek'ter, -tōr). Instrumento raramente utilizado para localizar o trajeto de uma bala em uma ferida. [L. de *tra-jicio,* pp. *-jectus,* lançar sobre ou através]

tram·a·dol (trăʹmă-dol). Tramadol; analgésico cujo mecanismo de ação é incomum, visto que um isômero óptico exerce efeitos típicos de opióides, enquanto outro isômero interage com a recaptação e/ou a liberação de norepinefrina e serotonina nas terminações nervosas.

tra·maz·o·line hy·dro·chlo·ride (tră-mazʹō-lēn). Cloridrato de tramazolina; agente adrenérgico e simpatomimético utilizado como descongestionante nasal.

trance (trans). Transe; estado alterado da consciência, como na hipnose, catalepsia ou êxtase. [L. *transeo,* cruzar, atravessar]
death t., t. de morte; condição de suspensão da animação, caracterizada por inconsciência e respiração e ação cardíaca dificilmente perceptíveis.
induced t., t. induzido; o estado artificialmente induzido de hipnose ou transe sonambulístico.
somnambulistic t., t. sonambulístico; estado de sonambulismo, paralisia, anestesia ou catalepsia induzido por sugestão na hipnose maior.

tran·ex·am·ic ac·id (tran-eks-amʹik). Ácido tranexâmico; inibidor competitivo da ativação do plasminogênio e da plasmina; utilizado na hemofilia para reduzir ou evitar hemorragia.

tran·quil·iz·er (trangʹkwi-lī-zer). Tranqüilizante; droga que promove tranqüilidade ao acalmar, confortar, aquietar ou apaziguar, com efeitos sedativos ou depressores mínimos
major t., agente antipsicótico. SIN antipsychotic *agent.*
minor t., agente ansiolítico. SIN antianxiety *agent.*

trans-. Trans-. **1.** Prefixo (em itálico) que significa através, além; oposto de *cis-*. **2.** Em genética, prefixo que designa a localização de dois genes em cromossomas opostos de um par homólogo. **3.** Em química orgânica (em itálico), forma de isomerismo geométrico em que os átomos fixados a dois átomos de carbono, unidos por ligações duplas, estão localizados em lados opostos da molécula. **4.** Em bioquímica, prefixo a um nome do grupo no nome de uma enzima ou de uma reação que designa a transferência desse grupo de um composto para outro; por exemplo, transformilase (transfere um grupo formil), transpeptidação. [L. *trans,* através]

trans·a·cet·y·lase (trans-ă-setʹi-lās). Transacetilase. SIN acetyltransferase.
trans·a·cet·y·la·tion (transʹă-set-i-lāʹshŭn). Transacetilação; transferência de um grupamento acetil (CH$_3$CO–) de um composto para outro; essas reações, que habitualmente envolvem a formação de acetil-CoA, ocorrem notavelmente no início do ciclo do ácido tricarboxílico pela transferência de um grupo acetil ao oxaloacetato para formar citrato.

trans·ac·tion (tranz-akʹshŭn). Transação. **1.** Interação originada do encontro de duas ou mais pessoas. **2.** Em análise transacional, a unidade de análise que envolve um estímulo social e uma resposta.

trans·ac·yl·as·es (trans-asʹi-lā-sez). Transacilases. SIN acyltransferases.
trans·ac·yl·a·tion (trans-asʹil-āʹshŭn). Transacilação; a transferência reversível de grupos acil.

trans·al·dol·ase (trans-alʹdō-lās). Transaldolase; transferase que efetua a interconversão da sedo-heptulose 7-fosfato e D-gliceraldeído 3-fosfato em D-eritrose 4-fosfato e D-frutose 6-fosfato; faz parte da via de pentose fosfato. VER TAMBÉM transketolase.

trans·al·do·la·tion (transʹal-dō-lāʹshŭn). Transaldolação; reação que envolve a transferência de um grupamento aldol (CH$_2$OH–CO–CHOH–) de um composto para outro; em geral, essas reações envolvem os fosfatos de açúcar e ocorrem na via de oxidação do fosfogliconato do catabolismo dos carboidratos.

trans·a·mi·da·tion (trans-amʹi-dāʹshŭn). Transamidação; a transferência de NH$_2$ de um componente amida (p. ex., da glutamina) para outra molécula.

trans·a·mi·di·nas·es (trans-amʹi-di-nās-ez). Transamidinases. SIN amidinotransferases.

trans·am·i·di·na·tion (trans-amʹi-di-nāʹshŭn). Transamidinação; reação que envolve a transferência de um grupamento amidina (NH$_2$C≠ NH) de um composto para outro; o doador da amidina é, em geral, L-arginina, e a reação é importante na biossíntese da creatina.

trans·am·i·nas·es (trans-amʹi-nās-ez). Transaminases. SIN aminotransferases.

trans·am·i·na·tion (trans-amʹi-nāʹshŭn). Transaminação; a reação entre um aminoácido e um α-cetoácido através da qual o grupamento amino é transferido do primeiro para o segundo; em determinados casos, a reação pode ocorrer entre um aminoácido e um aldeído (p. ex., glutamato com glutamato semialdeído através da ornitina transaminase)

trans·au·di·ent (trans-awʹdē-ent). Transaudiente; permeável às ondas sonoras. [trans- + L. *audio,* pres. p. *audiens,* ouvir]

trans·ca·lent (trans-kāʹlent). Diatérmico. SIN diathermanous. [trans- + L. *caleo,* ser aquecido]

trans·cap·si·da·tion (trans-kap-si-dāʹshŭn). Transcapsidação; o fenômeno pelo qual o capsídio do adenovírus SV40 "híbrido" é substituído pelo capsídio de outro adenovírus; ampliado para incluir um fenômeno semelhante em outros vírus.

trans·car·bam·o·y·las·es (trans-kar-bamʹō-i-lā-sez). Transcarbamoilases. SIN carbamoyltransferases.

trans·car·bam·o·yl·a·tion (trans-kar-bamʹō-il-āʹshŭn). Transcarbamoilação; a transferência de um componente carbamoil de uma molécula para outra; p. ex., a reação catalisada pela ornitina transcarbamoilase no ciclo da uréia.

trans·car·box·yl·as·es (trans-kar-boksʹi-lās-ez). Transcarboxilases. SIN carboxyltransferases.

tran·scen·den·tal med·i·ta·tion (TM) (tranzʹen-den-tal medʹi-tā-shŭn). Meditação transcendental (MT); forma de meditação praticada há mais de 2.500 anos nas culturas orientais e que recentemente se tornou popular no Ocidente através do Maharishi Mahesh Yogi como meio de ajudar a aumentar a energia, reduzir o estresse e ter um efeito positivo sobre a saúde mental e física; a pessoa permanece sentada durante 20 min, com os olhos fechados, e diz silenciosamente um mantra (palavra-chave de estímulo utilizada exclusivamente para cada indivíduo para retornar ao estado de meditação) sempre que o pensamento ocorrer.

trans·co·bal·a·mins (trans-kō-balʹăminz). Transcobalaminas; substâncias incluídas no "ligador R", o nome dado a uma família de proteínas de ligação da cobalamina; sua deficiência tem sido associada a baixos níveis séricos de cobalamina, podendo resultar em anemia megaloblástica.

trans·con·dy·lar (trans-konʹdi-lar). Transcondilar; através dos côndilos; designa a linha de incisão do osso na amputação de Carden.

trans·cor·ti·cal (tranz-kōrʹti-kăl). Transcortical. **1.** Através do córtex do cérebro, ovário, rim ou outro órgão. **2.** De uma parte do córtex cerebral para outra; designa os vários tratos de associação.

trans·cor·tin (trans-kōrʹtin). Transcortina; α$_2$-globulina no sangue, que se liga ao cortisol e à corticosterona; a principal proteína de ligação dos corticosteróides no plasma. SIN corticosteroid-binding globulin, corticosteroid-binding protein.

tran·scrip·tase (tran-skripʹtās). Transcriptase; polimerase associada ao processo de transcrição; pode ser RNA-dependente ou DNA-dependente. [L. *transcribo,* pp. *transcriptum,* copiar, + -ase]
reverse t., t. reversa; DNA polimerase RNA-dependente, presente em virions de vírus tumorais de RNA (retrovírus).

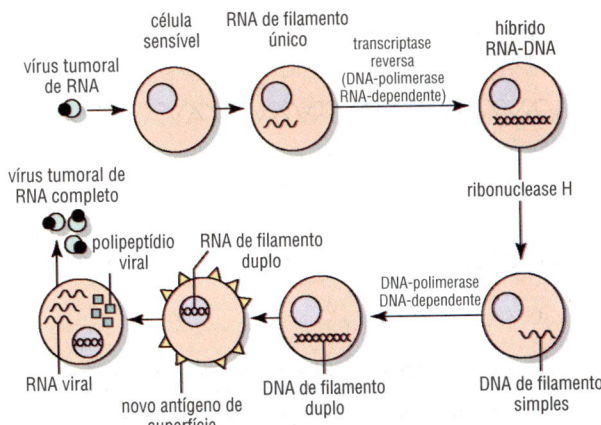

transcriptase reversa: integração do vírus tumoral de RNA no DNA da célula

tran·scrip·tion (tran-skripʹshŭn). Transcrição; transferência de informações do código genético de um tipo de ácido nucléico para outro, especialmente no que concerne ao processo pelo qual uma seqüência básica de RNA-mensageiro é sintetizada (por uma RNA polimerase) sobre um modelo de DNA complementar.
reverse t., t. reversa; reversão do padrão normal de t. (do DNA para o RNA); o meio efetivo é a enzima viral transcriptase reversa.

trans·cu·ta·ne·ous (trans-kū-tāʹnē-us). Transcutâneo. SIN percutaneous.

trans·cy·to·sis (trans-si-tōʹsis). Transcitose; mecanismo para o transporte transcelular, em que uma célula encerra material extracelular numa invaginação da membrana celular para formar uma vesícula (endocitose), que em seguida desloca a vesícula através da célula para expulsar o material através da membrana celular oposta pelo processo inverso (exocitose). O mecanismo de transporte pelo qual a maioria das proteínas alcança o aparelho de Golgi ou a membrana plasmática; as vesículas cujo destino são lisossomas e grânulos de armazenamento secretores parecem ser recobertas com clatrina. SIN cytopempsis, vesicular transport.

trans·der·mic (trans-der′mik). Transdérmico, percutâneo. SIN percutaneous.
trans·duce (trans-doos′). Transduzir; efetuar transdução.
trans·duc·er (trans-doo′ser). Transdutor; dispositivo projetado para converter a energia de uma forma para outra. VER TAMBÉM transduction.
   piezoelectric t., t. piezoelétrico; t. que converte energia elétrica em mecânica e vice-versa, utilizado no diagnóstico ou terapia com ultra-som.
   ultrasound t., t. de ultra-som; t. piezoelétrico utilizado na ultra-sonografia diagnóstica.
trans·duc·in (trans-doo′sin). Transducina; proteína que se liga a nucleotídios guanina (isto é, uma proteína G), encontrada em bastonetes e cones da retina, que desempenha importante papel na transdução de sinais; nos bastonetes de vertebrados, atua como ligação entre a fotólise da rodopsina e a ativação da cGMP fosfodiesterase.
trans·duc·tant (trans-dŭk′tănt). Transdutante; célula que adquiriu um novo caráter por meio da transdução; pode ser *completa,* com integração do fragmento genético transferido em seu genoma, ou *abortiva,* caso em que o fragmento genético não é integrado e passa apenas para uma das duas células filhas na divisão.
trans·duc·tion (trans-dŭk′shŭn). Transdução. **1.** Transferência de material genético (e de sua expressão fenotípica) de uma célula para outra através de infecção viral. **2.** Forma de recombinação genética nas bactérias. **3.** Conversão de energia de uma forma para outra. [trans- + L. *duco,* pp. *ductus,* levar através]
   abortive t., t. abortiva; t. em que o fragmento genético da bactéria doadora não se integra ao genoma da bactéria receptora e, quando esta última se divide, é transmitido apenas a uma das células filhas.
   complete t., t. completa; t. em que o fragmento genético transferido é totalmente integrado ao genoma da bactéria receptora.
   Davis battery model of t., modelo de bateria de t. de Davis; conceito em que o potencial endococlear positivo e o potencial intracelular negativo das células ciliadas proporcionam a força eletromotriz para a passagem de corrente através da lâmina reticular do órgão de Corti.
   general t., t. geral; t. em que o bacteriófago transdutor é capaz de transferir qualquer gene da bactéria doadora.

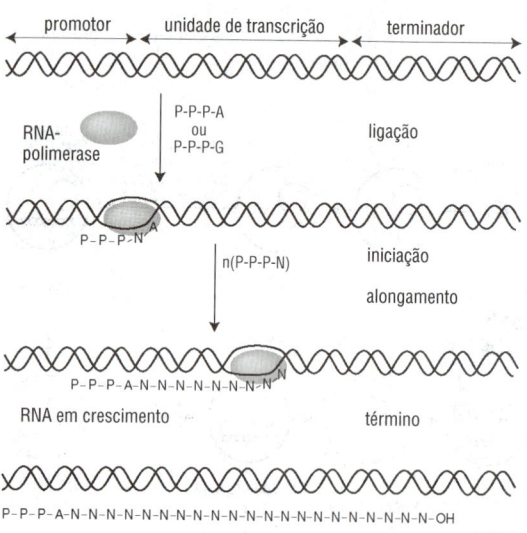

transcrição; representação esquemática: P-P-P-A = ATP; P-P-P-G = GTP; P-P-P-N = qualquer nucleosídio trifosfato.

   high-frequency t., t. de alta freqüência; t. especializada em que a bactéria doadora contém não apenas o pró-bacteriófago transdutor defeituoso, mas também o profago não-defeituoso que serve como vírus "auxiliar", permitindo que a maioria das partículas do profago defeituoso se desenvolva o suficiente para funcionar como agentes transdutores.
   low-frequency t., t. de baixa freqüência; t. especializada em que apenas uma pequena parte das partículas do profago, em virtude de seu defeito, é capaz de desenvolver-se o suficiente para servir como agentes transdutores eficazes.
   mechanoelectric t., t. mecanoelétrica; a conversão da energia mecânica em energia elétrica por células sensoriais, como células ciliadas auditivas e vestibulares.
   specialized t., t. especializada; t. em que a cepa do bacteriófago é capaz de transferir apenas alguns ou somente um dos genes da bactéria doadora. SIN specific t.
   specific t., t. específica. SIN specialized t.
tran·sec·tion (tran-sek′shŭn). Transecção. **1.** Secção transversal. **2.** Cortar transversalmente. SIN transsection. [trans- + L. *seco,* pp. *sectus,* cortar]
trans·eth·moi·dal (trans′eth-moy′dăl). Transetmoidal; através do osso etmóide.
trans·fec·tion (trans-fek′shŭn). Transfecção; método de transferência de genes que utiliza a infecção de uma célula por ácido nucléico (como no caso de um retrovírus), resultando em replicação viral subseqüente na célula transfectada. [trans- + in*fection*]
trans·fer. Transferência. **1.** Processo de remoção ou transferência. **2.** Condição em que o aprendizado numa situação influencia o aprendizado em outra situação; um transporte de aprendizado que pode ter efeito positivo, como quando o aprendizado de um comportamento facilita o aprendizado de outra coisa, ou que pode ser negativo, como quando um hábito interfere na aquisição de um posterior. SIN transmission (1). [L. *trans-fero,* conduzir através]
   embryo t., t. de embrião; após inseminação artificial *in vitro,* o ovo fertilizado é transferido no estágio de blastocisto para o útero ou oviduto receptor.
   Fourier t., t. de Fourier. SIN Fourier *analysis.*
   gamete intrafallopian t. (GIFT), t. intratubária de gametas; colocação do oócito e do esperma na ampola da tuba uterina; forma de reprodução assistida.
   group t., t. de grupo; a transferência de um componente funcional de uma molécula para outra.
   Jones t., t. de Jones; procedimento cirúrgico para tratamento de deformidades do hálux em garra, em que o tendão do músculo extensor longo do hálux é transferido para o colo do metatarso; pode ser também utilizada para corrigir deformidades em garra dos outros dedos do pé.
   linear energy t. (LET), t. de energia linear; a energia depositada por radiação por unidade de comprimento de percurso, expressa em keV por mícron; os prótons, os nêutrons e as partículas α possuem LET muito maior que os raios gama ou X. Uma propriedade da radiação que é levada em conta na proteção contra a radiação. VER relative biologic *effectiveness.*
trans·fer·as·es (trans′fer-ās-ez). Transferases; enzimas (EC classe 2) que transferem: grupamentos de um carbono (2.1, incluindo metiltransferases, 2.1.1; formiltransferases, 2.1.2; carboxil- e carbamoiltransferases, 2.1.3; e amidinotransferases, 2.1.4); resíduos acil (aciltransferases, 2.3); resíduos glicosil (glicosiltransferases, 2.4; incluindo hexosiltransferases, 2.4.1, e pentosiltransferases, 2.4.2); grupamentos alquil ou aril (2.5); grupos nitrogenados (2.6); grupos contendo fósforo (2.7, fosfotransferases); e grupos contendo enxofre (2.8, incluindo sulfurtransferases, 2.8.1; sulfotransferases, 2.8.2; e CoA-transferases 2.8.3). SIN transferring enzymes.
   terminal t., t. terminais; enzimas que adicionam covalentemente nucleotídios à extremidade 3' de ácidos polinucléicos; p. ex., DNA-nucleotidilexotransferase.
   terminal deoxynucleotidyl t. (TdT), desoxinucleotidil transferase terminal; DNA-polimerase especializada, expressa em células linfóides pré-B, pré-T imaturas e em células de linfoma/leucemia linfoblástica aguda.
trans·fer·ence (trans-fer′ens). Transferência. **1.** Transporte de um objeto de um lugar para outro. **2.** Deslocamento de sintomas de um lado do corpo para o outro, conforme observado em determinados casos de histeria de conversão. **3.** Deslocamento do afeto de uma pessoa ou uma idéia para outra; em psicanálise, aplica-se geralmente à projeção de sentimentos, pensamentos e desejos para o analista, que passou a representar alguma pessoa do passado do paciente.
   counter t., t. contratransferência. VER countertransference.
   extrasensory thought t., t. de pensamento extra-sensorial. SIN telepathy.
   t. love, amor de t.; amor expresso pelo paciente ao psicanalista como manifestação de t. (3).
   negative t., t. negativa; t. caracterizada por sentimentos predominantemente hostis por parte do paciente em relação ao analista.
   passive t., t. passiva; a passagem de imunidade ou suscetibilidade alérgica pela injeção de soro de um animal ou indivíduo que adquiriu imunidade ativa contra a doença.
   positive t., t. positiva; t. caracterizada por sentimentos predominantemente amistosos, respeitosos e positivos por parte do paciente em relação ao analista.
trans·fer·rin (trans-fer′in). Transferrina. **1.** β$_1$-globulina não-hêmica do plasma, que tem a capacidade de associar-se de modo reversível com até 1,25 μg de ferro por grama e que atua, portanto, como proteína de transporte do ferro. **2.** Glicoproteína encontrada no leite de mamíferos (lactoferrina) e na clara do ovo (conalbumina, ovotransferrina), que se liga ao ferro (Fe^{3+}) e o transporta. [trans- + L. *ferrum,* ferro, + -ia]
trans·fer-RNA. RNA de transferência. Ver subentradas em ribonucleic acid.

trans·fix (trans′fiks). Transfixar; perfurar com instrumento pontiagudo. [L. *trans-figo*, pp. *-fixus*, perfurar através, de *figo*, fixar]

trans·fix·ion (trans-fik′shun). Transfixação; manobra em amputação, em que o bisturi é passado de um lado a outro através das partes moles, próximo ao osso, e os músculos então divididos de dentro para fora. [L. *transfixio* (ver transfix)]

transform. Transformada.
   Fourier t., t. de Fourier. SIN Fourier *analysis.*

trans·form·ant (trans-fōr′mant). Transformante; bactéria que recebeu material genético (e sua expressão fenotípica) de outra bactéria por meio de transformação.

trans·for·ma·tion (trans-for-mā′shun). Transformação. 1. SIN metamorphosis. 2. Modificação de um tecido em outro, como a cartilagem em osso. 3. Em metais, alteração nas propriedades de fase e físicas no estado sólido, causada por tratamento térmico. 4. Em genética microbiana, transferência de informação genética entre bactérias por meio de fragmentos de DNA intracelulares "desnudos", derivados de células bacterianas doadoras e incorporados a uma célula receptora competente. [L. *trans-formo*, pp. *-atus*, transformar]
   cavernous t. of portal vein, t. cavernosa da veia porta; substituição da veia porta por diversos canais colaterais, em consequência de trombose.
   cell t., t. celular; alterações morfológicas e fisiológicas, incluindo perda da inibição de contato em decorrência da infecção de uma célula animal por vírus oncogênico.
   Haldane t., t. de Haldane; a multiplicação da concentração de oxigênio inspirado pela relação das concentrações de nitrogênio expirado e inspirado no cálculo do consumo de oxigênio ou quociente respiratório pelo método de circuito aberto.
   Lobry de Bruyn-van Ekenstein t., t. de Lobry de Bruyn-van Ekenstein; a conversão da glicose em frutose e manose em álcali diluído por enolização adjacente ao grupo carbonil para formar um enediol, uma reação análoga a determinadas transformações bioquímicas.
   logit t., t. de logit; método para linearizar curvas de dose-resposta para técnicas de radioimunoensaio; isto é, logit B (ligado)/B_o (ligação inicial) = log (B/B_o/1 − B/B_o).
   lymphocyte t., t. linfocítica; transformação em grandes formas semelhantes a blastos (imunoblastos), que ocorre quando linfócitos são expostos a antígenos histoincompatíveis (cultura de linfócitos mistos) ou mitógenos. VER TAMBÉM mixed lymphocyte culture *test*.
   nodular t. of the liver, t. nodular do fígado; condição rara em que surgem nódulos de hepatócitos hiperplásicos sem fibrose ou perda geral da arquitetura lobular. SIN nodular regenerative hyperplasia.

trans·fuse (trans-fūz′). Transfundir; realizar uma transfusão.

trans·fu·sion (trans-fū′zhun). Transfusão; transferência de sangue ou de hemoderivados de um indivíduo (doador) para outro (receptor). [L. *transfundo*, pp. *-fusus*, passar de um recipiente para outro]
   drip t., t. por gotejamento; t. lenta o suficiente para ser medida em gotas.
   exchange t., exsangüineotransfusão; remoção da maior parte do sangue de um paciente, seguida da introdução de uma quantidade igual proveniente de doadores. SIN exsanguination t., substitution t., total t.
   exsanguination t., exsangüineotransfusão. SIN exchange t.
   fetomaternal t., t. fetomaterna; passagem de sangue fetal para a circulação materna.
   indirect t., t. indireta; t. de sangue previamente obtido de um doador e armazenado em condições apropriadas. SIN mediate t.
   intramedullary t., t. intramedular; t., efetuada mais comumente em lactentes, na cavidade medular de um osso longo, geralmente o fêmur ou a tíbia.
   intrauterine t., t. intra-uterina; para tratamento da eritroblastose fetal, administração de sangue Rh-negativo na cavidade peritoneal do feto.
   mediate t., t. mediata. SIN indirect t.
   placental t., t. placentária; retorno de parte do sangue placentário fetal ao recém-nascido através dos vasos umbilicais.
   reciprocal t., t. recíproca; tentativa de conferir imunidade através da transfusão de sangue obtido de um doador para um receptor que padece da mesma afecção, sendo o equilíbrio mantido pela transfusão de uma quantidade igual do receptor para o doador.
   subcutaneous t., t. subcutânea; infusão de soluções absorvíveis sob a pele.
   substitution t., t. de substituição. SIN exchange t.
   total t., t. total. SIN exchange t.
   twin-twin t., t. gêmeo-gêmeo; anastomose vascular direta, arterial ou venosa, entre a circulação placentária de gêmeos.

trans·gene (trans′gēn). Transgene; gene recém-introduzido.

trans·gen·e·sis (tranz-jen′e-sis). Transgênese; reprodução envolvendo a introdução de DNA de espécie estranha num ovo.

trans·gen·ic (tranz-jen′ik). Transgênico; refere-se a um organismo no qual foi introduzido novo DNA nas células germinativas através de injeção no núcleo do ovo.

trans·glot·tic (trans-glot′ik). Transglótico; cruzamento vertical da glote, como na disseminação de carcinoma da área supraglótica para a infraglótica.

trans·glu·co·syl·ase (trans-gloo′kō-si-lās). Transglicosilase. SIN glucosyltransferase.

trans·glu·ta·min·ase (trans-gloo-ta′min-ās). Transglutaminase; grupo de enzimas que catalisam a reação de transferência de acil cálcio-dependente, em que a amida de resíduos de glutaminil ligados a peptídio serve como doador de acil; uma transglutaminase específica efetua ligações cruzadas covalentes de moléculas de fibrina entre a glutamina e o grupo ϵ de um resíduo de lisil, produzindo, assim, um coágulo de fibrina mais estável; outra transglutaminase participa na formação do envoltório quimicamente resistente do estrato córneo durante a diferenciação terminal dos ceratinócitos.

trans·gly·co·si·da·tion (trans-glī-ko-sid′ā-shun). Transglicosidação; transferência de um açúcar de ligação glicosídica para outra molécula.

trans·gly·co·syl·ase (trans-glī′kō-si-lās). Transglicosilase. SIN glycosyltransferase.

trans·hi·a·tal (trans-hī-ā′tal). Trans-hiatal; através de um hiato; por exemplo, esofagectomia trans-hiatal efetuada parcialmente através do hiato esofágico.

tran·sient (trans′shent, -sē-ent). Transitório. 1. De vida curta; passageiro; não-permanente; diz-se de uma doença ou ataque. 2. Som cardíaco de curta duração (menos de 0,12 s), distinto de um sopro; por exemplo, a primeira, segunda, terceira e quarta bulhas cardíacas, cliques e estalidos de abertura. [L. *transeo*, pres. p. *transiens*, atravessar, passar por cima]

trans·il·i·ac (trans-sil′ē-ak). Transilíaco; que se estende de um ílio ou crista ou espinha ilíaca até a outra.

tran·sil·i·ent (tran-sil′yent, -zil-). Descontínuo; que salta através, que passa sobre; relativo às fibras de associação corticais no cérebro que passam de uma convulsão para outra não-adjacente. [L. *transilio*, saltar através de, de *salio*, saltar]

trans·il·lu·mi·na·tion (trans-i-loo′mi-nā′shun). Transiluminação; método de exame pela passagem de luz através dos tecidos ou de uma cavidade corporal. [trans- + L. *illumino*, pp. *-atus*, iluminar]

trans·in·su·lar (tranz-in′soo-lar). Transinsular; através da ínsula ou da ilha de Reil.

trans·is·chi·ac (trans-is′kē-ak). Transiquiático; que se estende de um ísquio ao outro.

trans·isth·mi·an (trans-is′mē-an). Transístmico; através de qualquer istmo; especificamente, através do istmo do giro fornicado, designando o giro transitivo.

tran·si·tion (tran-sish′un, -zish′un). Transição. 1. Passagem de uma condição ou de uma parte para outra. 2. No ácido polinucléico, substituição de uma base purina por outra base purina ou pirimidina por uma pirimidina diferente. [L. *transitio*, de *transeo*, pp. *-itus*, atravessar]
   cervicothoracic t., t. cervicotorácica; a junção entre a última vértebra cervical e a primeira vértebra torácica.
   isomeric t., t. isomérica; transição de um isômero nuclear para um estado de quantum inferior; por exemplo, $Xe^{131m} \rightarrow Xe^{131m} + \gamma$.

tran·si·tion·al (tran-sish′un-al, -zish-). Transicional; relativo a ou caracterizado por uma transição; transitório.

trans·ke·tol·ase (trans-kē′tō-lās). Transcetolase; transferase que realiza a interconversão reversível da sedo-heptulose 7-fosfato e D-gliceraldeído 3-fosfato para produzir D-ribose 5-fosfato e D-xilulose 5-fosfato, bem como outras reações semelhantes, como hidroxipiruvato e um aldeído em CO_2 e hidroxipiruvato estendido; parte da fase não-oxidativa da via de pentose fosfato. VER TAMBÉM transaldolase. SIN glycolaldehydetransferase.

trans·ke·to·la·tion (trans′kē-tō-lā′shun). Transcetolação; reação que envolve a transferência de um grupo cetol ($HOCH_2CO-$) de um composto para outro.

trans·la·tion (trans-lā′shun). Tradução; translação. 1. Alteração ou conversão em outra forma. 2. O processo bastante complexo pelo qual o RNA-mensageiro, o RNA de transferência e os ribossomas realizam a produção de proteínas a partir dos aminoácidos, sendo a especificidade da síntese controlada pelas seqüências de bases do RNA-mensageiro. 3. Em odontologia, o movimento de um dente através do osso alveolar, sem modificação da inclinação axial. [L. *translatio*, transferência, de *transfero* pp. *-latus*, conduzir através]
   nick t., t. de clivagem; técnica em que uma DNA-polimerase bacteriana é utilizada para degradar um único filamento de DNA que foi clivado e, a seguir, ressintetizar o filamento, freqüentemente com nucleosídios trifosfatos marcados.

trans·lo·ca·tion (trans-lō-kā′shun). Translocação. 1. Transposição de dois segmentos entre cromossomas não-homólogos, em consequência de ruptura anormal e refusão dos segmentos recíprocos. 2. Transporte de um metabólito através de uma membrana biológica. [trans- + L. *location*, colocação, de *loco*, colocar]
   bacterial t., t. bacteriana; o movimento de bactérias ou produtos bacterianos através da membrana intestinal que aparecem nos vasos linfáticos ou na circulação visceral.
   balanced t., t. equilibrada; translocação do braço longo de um cromossoma acrocêntrico para outro cromossoma; um indivíduo com translocação equili-

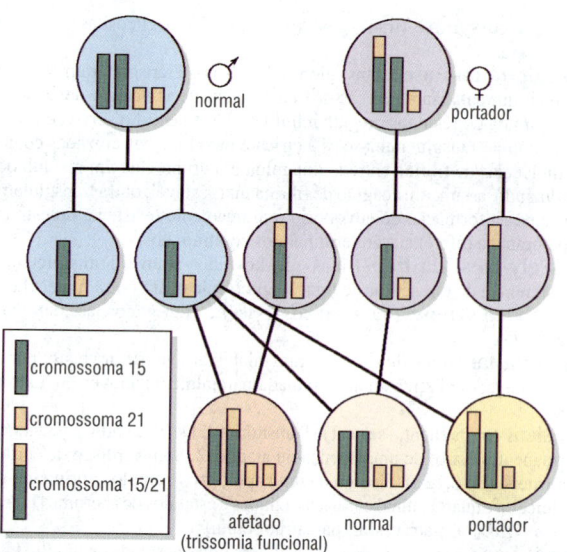

herança de trissomia por translocação

brada possui um genoma diplóide normal e é clinicamente normal, porém apresenta uma contagem de 45 cromossomas e, em conseqüência da meiose assimétrica, pode ter filhos que carecem dos genes do segmento translocado ou que os apresentam em trissomia.
group t., t. de grupo; forma de transporte ativo através de uma membrana biológica em que a molécula de transporte é alterada no curso do transporte.
reciprocal t., t. recíproca; translocação sem perda demonstrável de material genético.
robertsonian t., t. robertsoniana; translocação em que os centrômeros de dois cromossomas acrocêntricos parecem ter sofrido fusão, formando um cromossoma anormal que consiste nos braços longos de dois cromossomas diferentes, com perda dos braços curtos. O portador de uma translocação robertsoniana equilibrada possui apenas 45 cromossomas, porém um complemento cromossômico quase normal e fenótipo clinicamente normal; entretanto, corre risco de ter um filho com complemento cromossômico desequilibrado. O indivíduo com translocação robertsoniana desequilibrada apresenta trissomia para o braço longo do cromossoma. SIN centric fusion. [W.R.B. *Robertson,* geneticista norte-americano, *1881]
unbalanced t., t. desequilibrada; condição resultante da fertilização de um gameta contendo um cromossoma translocado por um gameta normal; se essa anormalidade for compatível com a vida, o indivíduo terá 46 cromossomas, porém um segmento do cromossoma translocado será representado três vezes em cada célula, existindo um estado trissômico parcial ou completo.
trans·lu·cent (trans-loo′sent). Translúcido; parcialmente transparente, que permite a passagem da luz difusamente. [L. *translucens,* de trans- + *luceo,* brilhar através de]
trans·mem·brane (trans-mem′brān). Transmembrana; através de ou cruzando uma membrana.
trans·meth·yl·ase (trans-meth′i-lās). Transmetilase. SIN methyltransferase.
trans·meth·yl·a·tion (trans′meth-i-lā′shŭn). Transmetilação; transferência de um grupamento metil de um composto para outro; p. ex., a L-homocisteína é convertida em L-metionina mediante transferência de um grupamento metil para a última. VER *methionine* synthase.
trans·mi·gra·tion (trans-mi-grā′shŭn). Transmigração; movimento de um lugar para outro; pode implicar atravessar alguma barreira geralmente limitada, como a passagem de células sangüíneas através das paredes dos vasos (diapedese). [L. *transmigro,* pp. *-atus,* remover de um lugar para outro]
  ovular t., t. ovular; passagem de um óvulo de um ovário na tuba uterina do outro lado; ocorre **t. ovular externa, t. ovular direta** quando o óvulo atravessa a cavidade pélvica; ocorre **t. ovular interna, t. ovular indireta** quando o óvulo atravessa a cavidade uterina e, assim, penetra na tuba do lado oposto.
trans·mis·si·ble (trans-mis′i-bl). Transmissível; capaz de ser transmitido (conduzido através) de uma pessoa para outra, como uma doença transmissível, uma doença infecciosa ou contagiosa.
trans·mis·sion (trans-mish′ŭn). Transmissão. **1.** Transferência. transfer. **2.** A transferência de uma doença de uma pessoa para outra. **3.** A passagem de um impulso nervoso através de uma fenda anatômica, como nas sinapses dos sistemas nervosos central ou autônomo e das junções neuromusculares, por ativação de um mediador químico específico que estimula ou inibe a estrutura através da sinapse. VER neurohumoral t. **4.** Em geral, passagem de energia através de um material. [L. *transmissio,* envio através de]

duplex t., t. dupla; a passagem de impulsos em ambas as direções através de um tronco nervoso.
horizontal t., t. horizontal; transmissão de agentes infecciosos de um indivíduo infectado para outro indivíduo suscetível, em contraposição com a t. vertical.
iatrogenic t., t. iatrogênica; t. de agentes infecciosos devido a interferência médica (por exemplo, através de agulhas contaminadas]
neurohumoral t., t. neuro-humoral; processo pelo qual uma célula pré-sináptica, ao sofrer excitação, libera um agente químico específico (um neurotransmissor) para atravessar uma sinapse a fim de estimular ou de inibir a célula pós-sináptica. SIN neurotransmission.
transovarial t., t. transovariana; passagem de parasitas ou agentes infecciosos do corpo materno para ovos dentro dos ovários, comumente utilizada para descrever determinados artrópodes, para explicar a capacidade de larvas da geração seguinte de transmitir patógenos, como a infecção de ácaros larvários ou carrapatos por riquétsias ou vírus.
transstadial t., t. transestadial; passagem de um parasita microbiano, como um vírus ou uma riquétsia, de um estágio (estádio) de desenvolvimento do hospedeiro para seu estágio ou estágios subseqüentes, conforme observado particularmente em ácaros. VER TAMBÉM transovarial t.
vertical t., t. vertical; **(1)** transmissão de um vírus (p. ex., vírus tumoral de RNA) por meio do aparelho genético de uma célula ao qual o genoma viral está integrado; **(2)** para agentes infecciosos em geral, refere-se à transmissão de um agente de um indivíduo para sua prole, isto é, de uma geração para a subseqüente. Cf. horizontal t.
trans·mu·ral (trans-mū′răl). Transmural; através de qualquer parede, como a do corpo ou de um cisto ou de qualquer estrutura oca. [trans- + L. *murus,* parede]
trans·mu·ta·tion (trans-mū-tā′shŭn). Transmutação; mudança; transformação. SIN conversion (1). [L. *transmuto,* pp. *-atus,* mudar, transmutar]
trans·oc·u·lar (trans-ok′ū-lăr). Transocular; através do olho.
tran·so·nance (trans′ō-nans). Transonância; transmissão de um som que se origina num órgão através de outro. [trans- + L. *sonans,* ressonância]
tran·son·ic (tran-son′ik). Transônico; na ultra-sonografia, descreve uma região de um meio relativamente não-atenuante. Deve-se fazer uma distinção entre uma região transônica e um eco acústico. [trans- + sonic]
trans·pa·ri·e·tal (trans-pă-rī′e-tăl). Transparietal; através de ou cruzando uma região, área ou estrutura parietal.
trans·pep·ti·dase (trans-pep′ti-dās). Transpeptidase; enzima que catalisa uma reação de transpeptidação; muitas enzimas proteolíticas (p. ex., tripsina, papaína) atuam como transpeptidase no decorrer da proteólise, formando uma enzima acilada como intermediário no processo; p. ex., γ-glutamil transpeptidase.
trans·pep·ti·da·tion (trans′pep-ti-dā′shŭn). Transpeptidação; reação que envolve a transferência de um ou mais aminoácidos de uma cadeia peptídica para outra, como por ação da transpeptidase, ou da própria cadeia peptídica, como na síntese da parede celular bacteriana.
trans·per·i·to·ne·al (trans′per-i-tō-nē′al). Transperitoneal; através do peritônio; p. ex., referindo-se a uma nefrectomia efetuada por secção abdominal.
trans·phos·pha·tas·es (trans-fos′fă-tās-ez). Transfosfatases. SIN phosphotransferases.
trans·phos·pho·ryl·as·es (trans-fos-fōr′i-lā-sez). Transfosforilases. VER phosphotransferases, phosphorylases, kinase.
trans·phos·pho·ryl·a·tion (trans′fos-fōr-i-lā′shŭn). Transfosforilação; reação que envolve a transferência de um grupamento fosfórico de um composto para outro, freqüentemente com a participação do ATP, como na ação de uma fosfotransferase ou cinase.
tran·spir·a·ble (trans-pī′ră-bl). Transpirável; capaz de transpirar ou ser transpirado.
tran·spi·ra·tion (trans-pi-rā′shŭn). Transpiração; passagem de vapor d'água através da pele ou de qualquer membrana. VER TAMBÉM insensible *perspiration.* [trans- + L. *spiro,* pp. *-atus,* respirar]
  pulmonary t., t. pulmonar; a passagem de vapor d'água do sangue para o ar através do trato respiratório.
tran·spire (trans-pīr′). Transpirar; exalar vapor pela pele ou mucosa respiratória. [trans- + L. *spiro,* respirar]
trans·pla·cen·tal (tranz-pla-sen′tăl). Transplacentário; que atravessa a placenta.
trans·plant (tranz′plant). Transplantar, transplante. **1.** Transferir de uma parte para outra, como no enxerto ou no transplante. **2.** O tecido ou órgão no enxerto e no transplante. VER TAMBÉM graft. [trans- + L. *planto,* plantar]
  Gallie t., t. de Gallie; faixas estreitas da fáscia lata femoral utilizadas para material de sutura.
  hair t., t. piloso; auto-enxertos de biopsias por punção de pele não-glabra, como couro cabeludo occipital, no couro cabeludo frontal na alopecia de padrão masculino.
trans·plan·tar (trans-plan′tar). Transplantar; através da planta do pé; designa determinadas fibras musculares ou estruturas ligamentares.

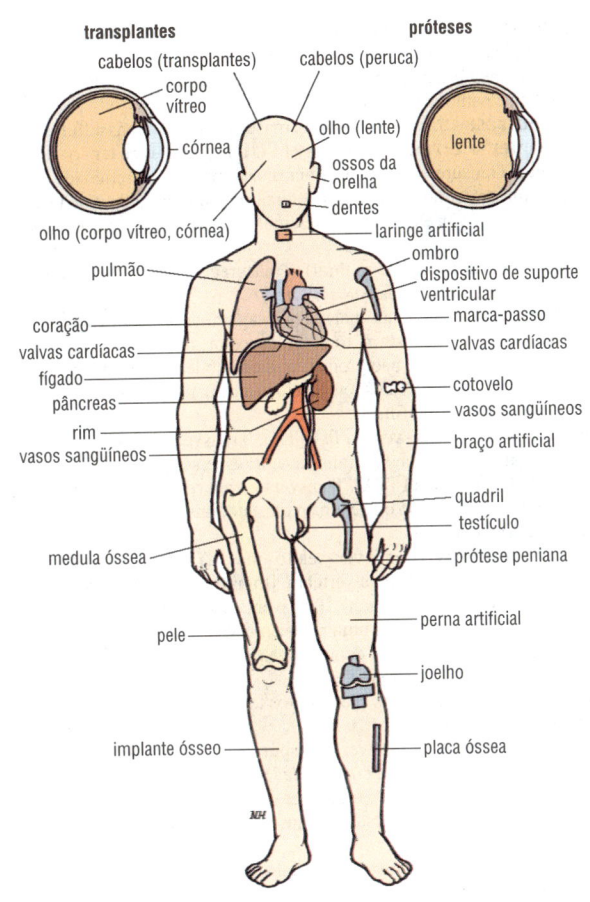

transplantes e próteses

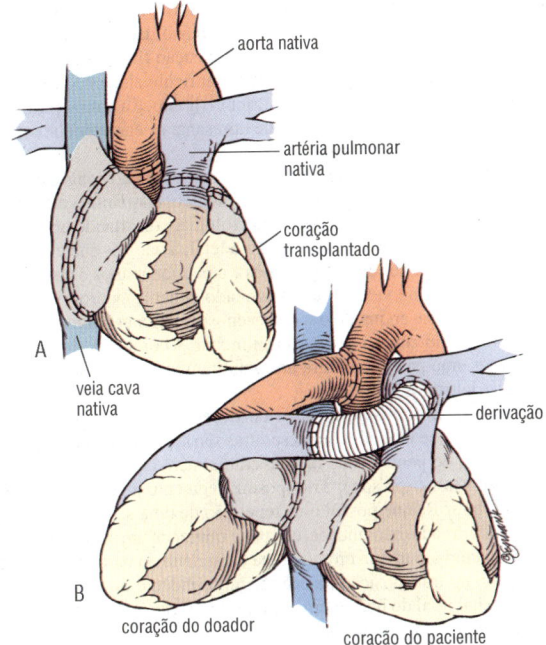

transplante cardíaco: (A) método ortotópico, (B) método heterotópico

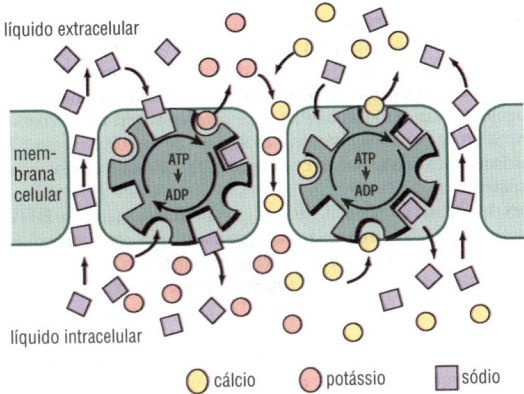

transporte ativo: o sódio difunde-se para dentro da célula através de poros na membrana celular e é ativamente bombeado para fora da célula por um sistema transportador; o cálcio e o potássio difundem-se para fora da célula e são ativamente bombeados de volta à célula; a energia para esse transporte é obtida do ATP

trans·plan·ta·tion (tranz-plan-tā'shŭn). Transplante; implante numa parte de tecido ou órgão retirado de outra parte ou de outro indivíduo. VER TAMBÉM graft. [L. *transplanto*, pp. *-atus*, transplantar]
bone marrow t., t. de medula óssea; enxerto de tecido de medula óssea; utilizado na anemia aplásica, na imunodeficiência primária, na leucemia aguda (após irradiação corporal total) e em pacientes com câncer (p. ex., de mama) submetidos a quimioterapia extensa que leva à destruição da medula óssea.
cardiopulmonary t., t. cardiopulmonar. SIN heart-lung t.
t. of cornea, t. de córnea. SIN keratoplasty.
corneal t., t. de córnea. SIN keratoplasty.
heart t., t. cardíaco; substituição de um coração gravemente lesado por um coração normal de um doador com morte cerebral.
heart-lung t., t. de coração-pulmão; transplante simultâneo do coração e de ambos os pulmões. SIN cardiopulmonary t.
pancreaticoduodenal t., t. pancreaticoduodenal; transplante tecnicamente possível, incluindo tanto o duodeno quanto o pâncreas.
renal t., t. renal; transplante de um rim de doador compatível para restabelecer a função renal num receptor que sofre de insuficiência renal.
tendon t., t. de tendão; (1) introdução de uma fita do tendão de um músculo sadio no tendão de um músculo paralisado; (2) substituição de parte do tendão por um enxerto livre.
tooth t., t. dentário; transferência de um dente de um alvéolo para outro.
trans·pleu·ral (trans-ploo'ral). Transpleural; através da pleura ou da cavidade pleural; do outro lado da pleura.
trans·port (trans'pōrt). Transporte; o movimento ou a transferência de substâncias bioquímicas em sistemas biológicos. [L. *transporto*, conduzir, transportar, de trans- + *porto*, transportar]
active t., t. ativo; a passagem de íons ou moléculas através de uma membrana celular, não por difusão passiva, mas por um processo que consome energia à custa de processos catabólicos que ocorrem na célula; no transporte ativo, o movimento ocorre contra um gradiente eletroquímico.
axoplasmic t., t. axoplásmico; t. através do fluxo de axoplasma em direção ao corpo da célula (retrógrado) ou em direção à terminação axonal (anterógrado).
facilitated t., t. facilitado; t. de um composto mediado por proteína através de uma membrana biológica que não é impulsionada por íons; sistema de transporte saturável. SIN passive t.
hydrogen t., t. de hidrogênio; a transferência de hidrogênio de um metabólito (doador de hidrogênio) para outro (aceptor de hidrogênio) através da ação de um sistema enzimático; o doador é, assim, oxidado, e o aceptor, reduzido.
paracellular t., t. paracelular; movimento de solvente através de uma camada de células epiteliais através das zônulas entre células. Cf. transcellular t.
passive t., t. passivo. SIN facilitated t.
transcellular t., t. transcelular; movimento de soluto através de uma camada de células epiteliais através das células. Cf. paracellular t.
vesicular t., t. vesicular. SIN transcytosis.
trans·pos·ase (tranz-pōz'ās). Transposase; enzima necessária para o transporte de segmentos de DNA. [L. *trans-pono*, pp. *transpositum*, colocar através, transferir, + -ase]
trans·pose (tranz-pōz). Transpor; transferir um tecido ou órgão para o lugar de outro e vice-versa. [L. *trans-pono*, pp. *-positus*, colocar através, transferir]
trans·po·si·tion (tranz-pō-zish'ŭn). Transposição. 1. Remoção de um lugar para outro; metátese. 2. A condição de estar no lugar ou no lado errado do corpo, como na transposição das vísceras, em que as vísceras estão localizadas em lugar oposto à sua posição normal; por exemplo, o fígado do lado esquerdo, o ápice do coração à direita. 3. Posicionamento dos dentes fora de sua seqüência normal em um arco.
t. of arterial stems, t. dos grandes vasos. SIN t. of the great vessels.
corrected t. of the great vessels, t. corrigida dos grandes vasos; má posição anatômica ou fisiologicamente corrigida das grandes artérias. Na transposição

anatomicamente corrigida, originam-se dos ventrículos corretos, porém possuem uma relação anormal entre si (trata-se, na realidade, de uma má posição, mais do que de uma transposição). Na transposição fisiológica ou funcionalmente corrigida, a aorta origina-se de um ventrículo sistêmico que possui as características morfológicas de um ventrículo direito, e a artéria pulmonar origina-se de um ventrículo "venoso", que apresenta as características morfológicas de um ventrículo esquerdo.

t. of the great vessels, t. dos grandes vasos; malformação congênita em que a aorta origina-se do ventrículo direito morfológico, enquanto a artéria pulmonar origina-se do ventrículo esquerdo morfológico, resultando em duas circulações separadas e paralelas. A condição é letal, a não ser que exista alguma comunicação entre a circulação sistêmica e a pulmonar após o nascimento; de outro modo, o sangue venoso não-oxigenado penetra inapropriadamente na circulação sistêmica, enquanto o sangue venoso pulmonar oxigenado é inapropriadamente dirigido para a circulação pulmonar. A comunicação para que haja vida pode ser uma passagem intra-arterial ou um canal arterial desobstruído. SIN t. of arterial stems.

penoscrotal t., t. penoscrotal; erro de desenvolvimento observado com hipospadias, em que unidades hemiescrotais são separadas e situam-se lateralmente ao corpo do pênis ou até mesmo cranialmente.

trans·po·son (trans-pō'son). Transposon; segmento de DNA (por exemplo, um gene do fator R) que possui uma repetição de uma seqüência de inserção de elementos em cada extremidade, que pode migrar de um plasmídio para outro na mesma bactéria, para um cromossoma bacteriano ou para um bacteriófago; o mecanismo de transposição parece ser independente do mecanismo de recombinação habitual do hospedeiro. VER jumping *gene,* transposable *element.* [L. *transpono,* pp. *transpositum,* transferir, + *-on*]

trans·sec·tion (trans-sek'shŭn). Transecção. SIN transection.

trans·seg·men·tal (trans-seg-men'tăl). Transegmentar; através de um segmento.

trans·sep·tal (trans-sep'tăl). Transeptal; através de um septo; no outro lado de um septo.

trans·sex·u·al (trans-sek'shoo-ăl). Transexual. **1.** Pessoa com genitália externa e características sexuais secundárias de um sexo, mas cuja identificação pessoal e configuração psicossocial são do sexo oposto; um estudo da estrutura morfológica, genética e gonadal pode ser genitalmente congruente ou incongruente. **2.** Que designa ou está relacionado com uma pessoa desse tipo. **3.** Relativo a procedimentos clínicos e cirúrgicos desenvolvidos para alterar as características sexuais externas de um paciente, de modo que se assemelhem às do sexo oposto.

trans·sex·u·al·ism (tranz-sek'shoo-ă-lizm). Transexualismo. **1.** O estado de ser transexual. **2.** O desejo de modificar as características sexuais anatômicas para ajustar-se fisicamente à própria percepção como membro do sexo oposto, juntamente com desejo de viver completamente o papel do sexo oposto.

trans·sphe·noi·dal (trans-sfē-noy'dăl). Transesfenoidal; através do osso esfenóide.

trans·splic·ing (trans-splīs'ing). Transjunção; formação de produtos de junção contendo porções de duas transcrições diferentes.

trans·sul·fu·rase (trans-sŭl'fer-ās). Transulfurase; termo descritivo aplicado às enzimas que catalisam, entre outras, as seguintes reações envolvendo compostos contendo enxofre: 1) cistationina → cisteína + α-cetobutirato + NH₃ (cistationina γ-liase); 2) cistationina → homocisteína + piruvato + NH₃ (cistationina β-liase); 3) cistina → tiocisteína + piruvato + NH₃ (cistationina γ-liase); 4) cistationina → serina + homocisteína (cistationina sintase). SIN transulfurase.

trans·sul·fu·ra·tion (trans-sŭl'fer-ā'shŭn). Transulfuração; a troca de enxofre ou componente contendo enxofre entre dois compostos diferentes.

trans·syn·ap·tic (trans-si-nap'tik). Transináptico; que indica a transmissão de um impulso nervoso através de uma sinapse.

trans·ten·to·ri·al (trans-ten-tōr'ē-ăl). Transtentorial; que passa através da incisura do tentório ou do tentório do cerebelo.

trans·tha·lam·ic (trans-tha-lam'ik). Transtalâmico; que atravessa o tálamo.

trans·ther·mia (trans-ther'mē-ă). Transtermia. SIN diathermy. [trans- + G. *thermē,* calor]

trans·tho·rac·ic (trans-thōr-as'ik). Transtorácico; que atravessa a cavidade torácica.

trans·tho·ra·cot·o·my (trans-thōr'ă-kot'ō-mē). Transtoracotomia; procedimento cirúrgico realizado através de uma incisão na parede torácica. [trans- + thorax + G. *tomē,* incisão]

trans·thy·ret·in (trans-thī'rĕ-tin). Transtiretina. SIN prealbumin (1).

tran·su·date (tran'soo-dāt). Transudato; qualquer líquido (solvente e soluto) que atravessou uma membrana presumivelmente normal, como a parede capilar, em conseqüência de desequilíbrio das forças hidrostática e osmótica; tipicamente pobre em proteínas, a não ser que tenha ocorrido concentração secundária. Cf. exudate. SIN transudation (2). [trans- + L. *sudo,* pp. *-atus,* suar]

tran·su·da·tion (tran-soo-dā'shŭn). Transudação. **1.** Passagem de um líquido ou soluto através de uma membrana por um gradiente de pressão hidrostática ou osmótica. VER transudate. **2.** SIN transudate.

tran·sude (tran-sood'). Transudar; em geral, vazamento ou passagem de um líquido gradualmente através de uma membrana, mais especificamente, através de uma membrana normal, em conseqüência de desequilíbrio das forças hidrostática e osmótica. [ver transudate]

tran·sul·fu·rase (tran-sŭl'fer-ās). Transulfurase. SIN transsulfurase.

trans·u·re·ter·o·u·re·ter·os·to·my (TUU) (tranz-ū-rē'ter-ō-ū-rē-ter-os'tō-mē). Transureteroureterostomia; anastomose da extremidade transeccionada de um ureter no ureter contralateral intacto através de uma técnica término-lateral direta ou elíptica. VER ureteroureterostomy. SIN transureteroureteral anastomosis.

trans·u·re·thral (trans-ū-rē'thrăl). Transuretral; através da uretra.

trans·vaa·lin. Transvaalina. SIN *scillaren A.*

trans·vag·i·nal (trans-vaj'i-năl). Transvaginal; através da vagina.

trans·vec·tor (trans-vek'tor, tor). Transvector; animal que transmite uma substância tóxica que ele não produz, mas que pode ser acumulada a partir de fontes animais (dinoflagelados) ou vegetais (algas); por exemplo, moluscos que se alimentam através de filtros.

trans·ver·sa·lis (trans-ver-sā'lis) [TA]. Transversal; transverso, designa especialmente uma fáscia. SIN transverse, transverse. [L.]

trans·verse (trans-vers') [TA]. Transverso; localizado através do eixo longitudinal do corpo ou de uma parte. SIN transversalis [TA], transversus [TA]. [L. *transversus*]

trans·ver·sec·to·my (trans-ver-sek'tō-mē). Transversectomia; ressecção do processo transverso de uma vértebra. [transverse + G. *ektomē,* excisão]

trans·ver·sion (trans-ver'zhŭn). Transversão. **1.** Substituição, no DNA e no RNA, de uma pirimidina por uma purina, ou vice-versa, por mutação. **2.** Em odontologia, a erupção de um dente numa posição normalmente ocupada por outro; transposição de um dente.

trans·ver·so·cos·tal (trans-ver'sō-kos'tăl). Transversocostal. SIN costotransverse.

transversospinales (tranz-ver-sō-spin-al'es). Transverso-espinais. SIN transversospinales *(muscles),* em *muscle.*

trans·ver·so·u·re·thra·lis (trans-ver-sō-ū-rē-thrā'lis). Transversouretral; designa as fibras transversais do músculo esfíncter da uretra, que se originam do arco púbico.

trans·ver·sus (trans-ver'sŭs) [TA]. Transverso. SIN transverse. [L. de *trans,* através, + *verto,* pp. *versus,* voltar]

trans·ves·tism (trans-ves'tizm). Transvestismo, travestismo; a prática de vestir-se ou mascarar-se com roupas do sexo oposto; especialmente a adoção de maneiras e costumes femininos por um homem. SIN transvestitism. [trans- + L. *vestio,* vestir]

trans·ves·tite (trans-ves'tīt). Travestido; pessoa que pratica o transvestismo.

trans·ves·ti·tism (trans-ves'ti-tizm). Transvestismo, travestismo. SIN transvestism.

Trantas, Alexios, oftalmologista grego, 1867–1960. VER T. *dots,* em *dot;* Horner-T. *dots,* em *dot.*

tran·yl·cyp·ro·mine sul·fate (tran-il-sip'rō-mēn). Sulfato de tranilcipromina; inibidor da monoamina oxidase; antidepressivo utilizado no tratamento da depressão mental grave. Interage com muitos alimentos e drogas, produzindo crise hipertensiva.

TRAP Abreviatura de twin reversed arterial perfusion (perfusão arterial inversa dupla).

tra·pe·zi·al (tra-pē'zē-ăl). Trapezial; relativo a qualquer trapézio.

tra·pe·zi·form (tra-pē'zi-form). Trapeziforme. SIN trapezoid (1).

tra·pe·zi·o·met·a·car·pal (tra-pē'zē-ō-met'ă-kar'păl). Trapeziometacarpal; relativo ao trapézio e ao metacarpo.

tra·pe·zi·um, pl. **tra·pe·zia, tra·pe·zi·ums** (tra-pē'zē-ŭm, -ă). Trapézio. **1.** Figura geométrica de quatro lados, que não tem dois lados paralelos. **2.** SIN trapezium *bone.* [G. *trapezion,* mesa ou balcão, um trapézio, dim. de *trapeza,* mesa, de *tra-* (= *tetra-*), quatro, + *pous* (*pod-*), pé]

tra·pe·zi·us (tra-pē'zē-us). Trapézio. SIN trapezius *(muscle).*

trap·e·zoid (trap'ĕ-zoyd) [TA]. Trapezóide. **1.** Que se assemelha a um trapézio. SIN trapeziform. **2.** Figura geométrica semelhante a um trapézio, exceto pelo fato de que dois de seus lados opostos são paralelos. **3.** SIN trapezoid (*bone*). **4.** SIN trapezoid *body.* [G. *trapeza,* mesa, + *eidos,* semelhança]

trap·i·dil (trap'ī-dil). Trapidil; antagonista e inibidor seletivo da síntese de tromboxano A₂; utilizado na prevenção do vasoespasmo cerebral.

Trapp. Julius, farmacêutico russo, 1815–1908. VER T. *formula;* T.-Häser *formula.*

Traube, Ludwig, médico e patologista alemão, 1818–1876. VER T. *bruit, corpuscle, dyspnea, plugs,* em *plug,* semilunar *space, sign,* double *tone;* T.-Hering *curves,* em *curve, waves,* em *wave.*

Traugott, Carl, internista alemão, *1885. VER Staub-T. *effect.*

△ **traum-.** Traum-. VER traumato-.

trau·ma, pl. **trau·ma·ta, trau·mas** (traw'mă, -mă-tă). Traumatismo; trauma; lesão física ou mental. SIN traumatism. [G. ferida]

birth t., t. ao nascimento; t. do nascimento; **(1)** lesão física de um lactente durante o parto; **(2)** suposta lesão emocional, produzida por eventos ocorridos ao nascimento, a um lactente que supostamente se apresenta em forma simbólica em pacientes com doença mental.

t. from occlusion, t. por oclusão; lesão reversível no periodonto causada pelo movimento excessivo dos dentes.

occlusal t., t. oclusal; estresses oclusais anormais capazes de produzir ou que produziram alterações patológicas no dente e em suas estruturas adjacentes.

psychic t., t. psíquico; experiência perturbadora que precipita ou que agrava um distúrbio emocional ou mental.

trau·ma·ta (traw′mă-tă). Traumatismos; plural de trauma.

trau·mat·ic (traw-mat′ik). Traumático; relativo a ou causado por traumatismo. [G. *traumatikos*]

trau·ma·tism (traw′mă-tizm). Traumatismo. SIN trauma.

trau·ma·tize (traw′mă-tīz). Traumatizar; causar ou infligir traumatismo. [G. *traumatizō*, ferir]

traumato-, traumat-, traum-. Traumato-, traumat-, traum-. Ferida, lesão. [G. *trauma*]

trau·ma·tol·o·gy (traw-mă-tol′ō-jē). Traumatologia; o ramo da cirurgia que trata dos lesados. [traumato- + G. *logos*, estudo]

trau·ma·to·ne·sis (traw′mă-tō-nē′sis, -ton′ē-sis). Traumatonose; reparo cirúrgico de uma ferida acidental. [traumato- + G. *nēsis*, fiação]

trau·ma·top·a·thy (traw-mă-top′ă-thē). Traumatopatia; qualquer condição patológica resultante de violência ou ferimentos. [traumato- + G. *pathos*, sofrimento]

trau·ma·top·nea (traw′mă-top-nē′ă). Traumatopnéia; entrada e saída de ar através de uma ferida da parede torácica. [traumato- + G. *pnoē*, respiração]

trau·ma·to·py·ra (traw′mă-tō-pī′ră). Traumatopira; sinônimo obsoleto de febre traumática (traumatic *fever*). [traumato- + G. *pyr*, fogo, febre]

trau·ma·to·sep·sis (traw′mă-tō-sep′sis). Traumatosepse; infecção de ferida; septicemia após um ferimento. [traumato- + G. *sēpsis*, putrefação]

trau·ma·to·ther·a·py (traw′mă-tō-thār′ă-pē). Traumatoterapia; tratamento de traumatismo ou do resultado da lesão.

Trautmann, Moritz F., otologista alemão, 1832–1902. VER T. triangular *space*.

tra·verse (trav′ers). Em tomografia computadorizada, movimento linear completo do *gantry* através do objeto que está sendo escaneado, como ocorre nas máquinas originais de TC de translação e rotação. [M.E., do Fr. Ant., do L.L. *transverso*, de L. *trans-verto*, girar através]

tray (trā). Bandeja; receptáculo plano com bordas elevadas.

acrylic resin t., b. de resina acrílica; bandeja de impressão plástica utilizada em odontologia; em geral, elaborada para um dado paciente a partir de uma resina acrílica autopolimerizante.

annealing t., b. de recozimento; dispositivo aquecido eletricamente e de controle termostático, utilizado para retirar a cobertura protetora de gás NH_3 da superfície de uma lâmina de ouro coesiva.

impression t., b. de impressão; receptáculo utilizado para transportar e guardar material de impressão plástico ao se efetuar uma impressão das estruturas orais.

traz·o·done hy·dro·chlo·ride (traz′ō-dōn). Cloridrato de trazodona; antidepressivo estruturalmente não-relacionado a outros agentes antidepressivos.

Trea·cher Collins, Edward, oftalmologista inglês, 1862–1919. VER Treacher Collins *syndrome*.

trea·cle (trē′kl). Teriaga. **1.** Melado, xarope viscoso que drena de moldes de refinamento do açúcar. **2.** Sacarina líquida. **3.** Antigamente, remédio contra veneno, portanto, qualquer remédio eficaz. VER TAMBÉM theriaca. [M.E. *triacle*, antídoto, do L. *theriaca*, antídoto para picada de cobra, do G. *trēriakos*, relativo a animais selvagens]

treat (trēt). Tratar; tratar de uma doença por meios medicinais, cirúrgicos ou outros meios; tratar de um paciente clínica ou cirurgicamente. [Fr. *traiter*, do L. *tracto*, arrastar, manipular, realizar]

treat·ment (trēt′ment). Tratamento; tratamento clínico ou cirúrgico de um paciente. VER TAMBÉM therapy, therapeutics. [Fr. *traitement* (ver treat)]

active t., t. ativo; substância ou curso terapêutico destinado a melhorar o problema básico da doença, em oposição ao tratamento de suporte ou paliativo. Cf. causal t.

Carrel t., t. de Carrel; tratamento de superfícies feridas por irrigação intermitente com solução de Dakin. SIN Dakin-Carrel t.

causal t., t. causal; tratamento destinado a reverter o fator causal numa doença.

conservative t., t. conservador; curso de ação terapêutica destinado a evitar qualquer prejuízo, com menor possibilidade de benefício em comparação com ações perigosas.

Dakin-Carrel t., t. de Dakin-Carrel. SIN Carrel t.

dietetic t., t. dietético; t. de uma condição clínica através de dieta específica.

empiric t., t. empírico; t. baseado na experiência, geralmente sem dados adequados para apoiar o seu uso.

endodontic t., t. endodôntico. SIN root canal t.

Goeckerman t., t. de Goeckerman; t. para psoríase; as áreas acometidas são pintadas com uma solução de alcatrão ou cobertas com pomada de alcatrão e, subseqüentemente, irradiadas com ultravioleta (UVB).

heat t., t. térmico; em odontologia, método de manipulação de metais sob temperatura controlada, de modo a modificar a estrutura microscópica e, portanto, as propriedades físicas. VER TAMBÉM temper, anneal.

insulin coma t., t. por coma insulínico; tratamento antigamente utilizado para doença mental grave através de coma hipoglicêmico induzido por insulina. SIN insulin shock t.

insulin shock t., t. por choque insulínico. SIN insulin coma t.

isoserum t., t. com isossoro; uso terapêutico de soro obtido de uma pessoa que é ou foi portadora da mesma doença que o paciente em tratamento.

Kenny t., t. de Kenny; método obsoleto para o t. da poliomielite anterior; as partes acometidas são envolvidas em roupas de lã retiradas de água quente; após o término do estágio agudo da doença, os membros eram exercitados passivamente para reeducar os músculos paralisados.

light t., fototerapia. SIN phototherapy.

medical t., t. clínico; t. de doença através de medidas higiênicas e farmacológicas, distinto dos procedimentos cirúrgicos invasivos.

Mitchell t., t. de Mitchell; t. de doença mental por repouso, dieta nutritiva e mudança de ambiente. SIN Weir Mitchell t.

moral t., t. moral; tipo de terapia utilizado no século 19, enfatizando a doutrina religiosa e a orientação benevolente em atividades da vida diária; como tal, representou uma forma de psicoterapia em oposição às terapias somáticas, como flebotomia e purgação.

Nauheim t., t. de Nauheim; terapia de determinadas afecções cardíacas por banhos em água, através da qual borbulha o gás ácido carbônico, seguidos de exercícios de resistência. SIN Nauheim bath, Schott t. [*Bad Nauheim*, Alemanha Ocidental]

palliative t., t. paliativo; t. para alívio dos sintomas, sem curar a doença.

preventive t., t. preventivo. SIN prophylactic t.

prophylactic t., t. profilático; a instituição de medidas destinadas a proteger o indivíduo de um ataque de doença ao qual ele foi ou é propenso a ser exposto. SIN preventive t.

root canal t., t. de canal; **(1)** meio pelo qual dentes dolorosos ou doentes, cuja polpa está acometida, são restaurados a um estado saudável; **(2)** remoção de uma polpa normal, doente ou morta por meios bioquímicos e mecânicos, aumento e esterilização do canal radicular, seguidos de preenchimento do canal para efetuar a cicatrização dos tecidos periapicais doentes; **(3)** diagnóstico e t. de doenças da polpa e suas seqüelas. SIN endodontic t.

Schott t., t. de Schott. SIN Nauheim t.

shock t., t. de choque. VER electroshock *therapy*.

solar t., t. solar. SIN solar *therapy*.

symptomatic t., t. sintomático; terapia cujo objetivo é aliviar os sintomas, sem afetar necessariamente a(s) causa(s) subjacente(s) básica(s) dos sintomas.

Tallerman t., t. de Tallerman; uso de aparelho especial para administração de calor seco a distúrbios reumáticos, entorses traumáticas etc.

thymus t., t. com timo; tratamento de doença através da administração de extratos do timo.

Tweed edgewise t., t. de perfil de Tweed. VER edgewise *appliance*.

Weir Mitchell t., t. de Weir Mitchell. SIN Mitchell t.

tre·ha·la (trē-hah′lă). Treala; substância da sacarina contendo trealose e semelhante ao manar, excretada por um besouro parasita, *Larinus maculatus*. [Fr. do Turq. *tigala*, do Pers. *tīghāl*]

tre·ha·lase (trē-hă′lās). Trealase; glicosidase secretada no duodeno que hidrolisa ligações 1,1 α-glicosídicas; a ausência ou deficiência dessa enzima resulta em digestão deficiente de trealose (herança autossômica recessiva).

tre·ha·lose (trē′hă-lōs). Trealose; dissacarídio não-redutor (α-D-glucosido)-α-D-glicose, contido na treala; também encontrada em fungos, como *Amanita muscaria*; presença de níveis elevados em indivíduos com deficiência de trealase. SIN mycose.

Treitz, Wenzel, patologista da Boêmia, 1819–1872. VER T. *arch, fascia, fossa, hernia, ligament, muscle*.

Trélat, Ulysse, cirurgião francês, 1828–1890. VER T. *stools*, em *stool*; Leser-T. *sign*.

tre·ma (trē′mă). Orifício. **1.** SIN foramen. **2.** SIN vulva. [G. *trēma*, orifício]

tre·ma·camra (trē-ma-kam′ra). Tremacamra; parte extracelular da molécula de adesão de superfície celular ICAM-1 envolvida na fixação do rinovírus a células da mucosa.

Trem·a·to·da (trem′ă-tō′dă). Classe do filo Platyhelminthes (platelmintos), que consiste em trematódeos com corpo em forma de folha e duas ventosas musculares, com cavidade corporal preenchida por parênquima acelomado. Não há sistema circulatório nem órgãos do sentido, porém há um canal alimentar incompleto (sem ânus). Os trematódeos de interesse para a medicina ou a veterinária são membros da ordem Digenea, com ciclos de vida completos envolvendo a multiplicação embrionária em um molusco como primeiro hospedeiro intermediário. A outra ordem, Monogenea, consiste principalmente em parasitas de peixes, que apresentam um padrão mais simples de desenvolvimento direto em um único hospedeiro. [G. *trēmatōdēs*, cheio de orifícios, de *trēma*, orifício, + *eidos*, aparência]

trem·a·tode, trem·a·toid (trem′ă-tōd, trem′ă-toyd). Trematódeo. **1.** Nome comum de um verme da classe Trematoda. **2.** Relativo a um verme da classe Trematoda.
trem·bles (trem′blz). Paralisia agitante; intoxicação do gado bovino causada pela ingestão da serpentária branca, *Eupatorium urticaefolium,* ou da vara-de-ouro sem raios; o agente ativo é um álcool superior, o tremetol, que as vacas intoxicadas eliminam em seu leite, causando a doença do leite quando ingerido pelo homem. [L. *tremulus,* trêmulo, de *tremo,* tremer]
trem·bling (trem′bling). Tremor; a agitação de um tremor.
trem·el·loid, trem·el·lose (trem′ĕ-loyd, -lōs). Tremelóide, tremelose; semelhante à gelatina. [L. *tremulus,* trêmulo]
trem·o·gram (trem′ō-gram). Tremograma; a representação gráfica de um tumor obtida por meio do tremógrafo ou simógrafo. SIN tremorgram.
trem·o·graph (trem′ō-graf). Tremógrafo; aparelho para fazer um registro gráfico de um tremor. [L. *tremor,* tremor, + G. *graphō,* escrever]
trem·o·la·bile (trem-ō-lā′bil, -bil). Tremolábil; inativado ou destruído por tremor. [L. *tremor,* tremor, + *labilis,* perecível]
trem·o·pho·bia (trem-ō-fō′bē-ă). Medo mórbido de tremor. [L. *tremor,* tremor, + G. *phobos,* medo]
trem·or (trem′er, -ōr). Tremor. **1.** Movimentos oscilatórios repetitivos, freqüentemente regulares, causados pela contração alternada ou sincrônica, porém irregular, de grupos musculares opostos; geralmente involuntários. **2.** Pequeno movimento ocular que ocorre durante a fixação em um objeto. [L. tremor]
  action t., t. de ação. SIN intention t.
  alcoholic withdrawal t., t. da abstinência alcoólica; t. de intenção observado no período de abstinência de um de dois tipos: 1) t. de mais de 8 Hz, com atividade contínua do músculo antagonista, e 2) t. de menos de 8 Hz, com atividade espontânea intermitente do músculo antagonista.
  alternating t., t. alternante; forma de hipercinesia caracterizada por movimentos de vaivém regulares e simétricos (cerca de 4 por segundo), que são produzidos pela contração padronizada alternante dos músculos e seus antagonistas.
  alternative t., t. alternativo; t. patológico grosseiro, de baixa freqüência (3-8 Hz), produzido pela contração alternante de músculos e seus antagonistas; observado na doença de Parkinson e no tremor de ação predominante cinético.
  benign essential t., t. essencial benigno. SIN heredofamilial t.
  coarse t., t. grosseiro; t. cuja amplitude é grande, com oscilações habitualmente irregulares e lentas.
  continuous t., t. contínuo. SIN persistent t.
  essential t., t. essencial; t. de ação de freqüência de 4-8 Hz que habitualmente começa no início da vida adulta e se limita aos membros superiores e à cabeça; denominado familiar quando aparece em vários membros da família.
  familial t., t. familiar. SIN heredofamilial t.
  fine t., t. fino; t. de amplitude pequena e freqüência geralmente superior a 12 Hz.
  flapping t., t. agitante. SIN asterixis.
  head t.'s, tremores da cabeça. SIN head-nodding.
  heredofamilial t. [MIM*190300], t. heredofamiliar; t. benigno herdado como caráter dominante; pode ser uma oscilação rápida semelhante àquela observada na tireotoxicose, t. grosseiro durante o repouso e inibido por um esforço voluntário, ou aquele que só aparece durante o movimento; de herança autossômica dominante. SIN benign essential t., familial t.
  hysterical t., t. histérico; t. habitualmente intermitente, grosseiro e irregular, limitado a um membro. SIN psychogenic t.
  intention t., t. de intenção; t. que ocorre durante o desempenho de movimentos voluntários precisos, causado por distúrbios do cerebelo ou de suas conexões. SIN action t., kinetic t., volitional t. (2).
  kinetic t., t. cinético. SIN intention t.
  passive t., t. passivo. SIN resting t.
  persistent t., t. persistente; t. constante, esteja o indivíduo em repouso ou em movimento. SIN continuous t.
  physiologic t., t. fisiológico; t. fino, com freqüência de 8-13 Hz, que é um fenômeno normal.
  pill-rolling t., t. de rolar pílulas; t. em repouso do polegar e dos dedos observado na doença de Parkinson.
  postural t., t. postural; t. presente quando os membros ou o tronco são mantidos em determinadas posições e quando são movidos ativamente, geralmente devido a surtos rítmicos quase sincrônicos nos grupos musculares opostos. SIN static t.
  progressive cerebellar t., t. cerebelar progressivo. SIN Hunt *syndrome* (1).
  psychogenic t., t. psicogênico. SIN hysterical t.
  resting t., t. de repouso; t. rítmico grosseiro, com freqüência de 3-5 Hz, geralmente limitado às mãos e aos antebraços, que aparece quando os membros estão relaxados e desaparece com movimentos ativos dos membros. Característico da doença de Parkinson. SIN passive t.
  senile t., t. senil; t. essencial que se torna sintomático em adultos idosos.
  static t., t. estático. SIN postural t.
  volitional t., t. volitivo; **(1)** t. que pode ser interrompido por um forte esforço de vontade; **(2)** SIN intention t.
  wing-beating t., t. em bater de asas; t. grosseiro e irregular que é mais proeminente quando os membros são mantidos estendidos, lembrando o bater das asas de um pássaro; devido a excursão para cima e para baixo do braço com o ombro em abdução. Observado principalmente na doença de Wilson.
trem·or·gram (trem′ōr-gram). Tremograma. SIN tremogram.
trem·or·ine (trem′er-ēn). Tremorina; substância química que, no laboratório, produz tremor semelhante ao tremor parkinsoniano; utilizada para produzir parkinsonismo experimental.
trem·o·sta·ble (trem-ō-stā′bl). Tremostável; não sujeito a alteração ou destruição por sofrer tremor. [L. *tremor,* tremor, + *stabilis,* estável]
trem·u·lor (trem′ū-ler, -lōr). Instrumento para produzir massagem vibratória.
trem·u·lous (trem′ū-lŭs). Trêmulo; caracterizado por tremor.
Trenaunay, Paul, médico francês, *1875. VER Klippel-T.-Weber *syndrome.*
Trendelenburg, Friedrich, cirurgião alemão, 1844–1924. VER T. *operation, position;* reverse T. *position;* T. *sign, symptom, test;* Trendelenburg *gait.*
trep·a·na·tion (trep-ă-nā′shŭn). Trepanação. SIN trephination.
  corneal t., t. of cornea, t. da córnea. SIN keratoplasty.
treph·i·na·tion (tref-i-nā′shŭn). Trepanação; remoção de um fragmento circular ("botão") de crânio por um trépano. SIN trepanation.
tre·phine (trē-fīn′, -fēn′). **1.** Trépano. SIN perforator. **2.** Trepanação; remover um disco do osso ou outro tecido por meio de trépano. [criado do L. *tres fines,* três pontas]
treph·o·cyte (tref′ō-sīt). Trefócito. SIN trophocyte. [G. *trephō,* nutrir, + *kytos,* célula]
trep·i·da·tio cor·dis (trep-i-dā′shē-ō kōr′dis). Palpitação. SIN palpitation.
trep·i·da·tion (trep-i-dā′shŭn). Trepidação; agitação. [L. *trepidatio,* de *trepido,* tremer, ser agitado]
Trep·o·ne·ma (trep-ō-nē′mă). Gênero de bactérias anaeróbicas (ordem Spirochaetales), que consistem em células de 3-8 μm de comprimento, com espirais agudas, regulares ou irregulares e sem estrutura protoplasmática óbvia. Pode haver um filamento terminal. Coram-se com dificuldade, exceto pelo método de Giemsa ou de impregnação pela prata. Algumas espécies são patogênicas e parasitárias para seres humanos e outros animais, produzindo, em geral, lesões locais nos tecidos. A espécie-tipo é *T. pallidum.* [G. *trepō,* voltar, + *nēma,* fio]
  T. cara′teum, espécie bacteriana que provoca pinta ou carate.
  T. cunic′uli, espécie bacteriana que causa espiroquetose em coelhos.
  T. dentico′la, espécie bacteriana cultivável que não fermenta carboidratos e que pode ser isolada da cavidade oral de seres humanos.
  T. genita′lis, espécie não-patogênica encontrada na genitália de seres humanos.
  T. hyodysente′riae, espécie enteropatogênica que provoca disenteria suína.
  T. muco′sum, espécie bacteriana encontrada na piorréia alveolar; possui propriedades piogênicas.
  T. pal′lidum, espécie bacteriana que causa sífilis no homem; esse microrganismo pode ser experimentalmente transmitido para macacos antropóides e para coelhos; trata-se da espécie-tipo do gênero *T.*
  T. perten′ue, espécie que causa bouba; os pacientes com essa doença apresentam resultados positivos nos testes de triagem sorológica para sífilis.
trep·o·ne·ma·to·sis (trep′ō-nē-mă-tō′sis). Treponematose. SIN treponemiasis.
trep·o·neme (trep′ō-nēm). Treponema; termo vernacular utilizado para referir-se a qualquer membro do gênero *Treponema.*
trep·o·ne·mi·a·sis (trep′ō-nē-mī′ă-sis). Treponemíase; infecção causada por *Treponema.* SIN treponematosis.
trep·o·ne·mi·ci·dal (trep′ō-nē′mi-sī′dăl). Treponemicida; destrutivo para qualquer espécie de *Treponema,* mas referindo-se habitualmente ao *T. pallidum,* o microrganismo responsável pela sífilis. SIN antitreponemal. [*Treponema* + L. *caedo,* matar]
trep·pe (trep′eh). Fenômeno no músculo cardíaco observado pela primeira vez por H.P. Bowditch; se diversos estímulos da mesma intensidade foram enviados para o músculo depois de um período quiescente, as primeiras contrações da série exibem um aumento sucessivo de amplitude (força). SIN staircase phenomenon. [Al. *Treppe,* escada]
Tresilian, Frederick J., médico inglês, 1862–1926. VER T. *sign.*
tre·sis (trē′sis). Perfuração. SIN perforation. [G. *trēsis,* perfuração]
tret·i·noin (tret′i-nō-in). Tretinoína; agente ceratolítico. VER retinoic acid.
Treves, Sir Frederick, cirurgião inglês, 1853–1923. VER T. *fold.*
Treves, Norman, cirurgião norte-americano, 1894–1964. VER Stewart-T. *syndrome.*
Trevor, David, cirurgião ortopédico inglês do século 20. VER T. *disease.*
TRF Abreviatura de thyrotropin-releasing *factor* (fator de liberação da tireotropina).
TRH Abreviatura de thyrotropin-releasing *hormone* (hormônio de liberação da tireotropina).
♲ **tri-.** Tri-. Três. Cf. tris-. [L e G.]
tri·a·ce·tic ac·id (trī-ă-sē′tik). Ácido triacético; formado por condensação de acetil e malonil CoA durante a síntese de ácidos graxos.

tri·ac·e·tin (trī-as′ē-tin). Triacetina; utilizada como solvente de corantes básicos, como fixador em perfumaria e como agente antifúngico tópico. SIN glyceryl triacetate, triacetylglycerol.

tri·a·ce·tyl·glyc·er·ol (trī-as′i-til-glis′er-ol). Triacetilglicerol. SIN triacetin.

tri·a·ce·tyl·o·le·an·do·my·cin (trī-as′ē-til-ō′lē-an-dō-mī′sin). Triacetiloleandomicina. SIN troleandomycin.

tri·ac·yl·glyc·er·ol (trī-as′il-glis′er-ol). Triacilglicerol; glicerol esterificado em cada um de seus três grupos hidroxila por um ácido graxo (alifático); por exemplo, tristearoilglicerol. SIN triglyceride.

t. lipase, t. lipase; a enzima de decomposição da gordura no suco pancreático; hidrolisa o t., produzindo um diacilglicerol e ânion de ácido graxo; a deficiência da enzima hepática resulta em hipercolesterolemia e hipertrigliceridemia. SIN lipase (2), steapsin, tributyrase, tributyrinase.

tri·ad (trī′ad). Tríade. **1.** Um conjunto de três coisas que possuem algo em comum. **2.** O túbulo transverso e as cisternas terminais de cada lado nas fibras musculares esqueléticas. **3.** SIN portal t. **4.** A relação entre pai, mãe e filho experimentada projetivamente na psicoterapia de grupo. [G. *trias (triad-),* o número 3, de *treis,* três.

acute compression t., t. de compressão aguda; elevação da pressão venosa, queda da pressão arterial e diminuição dos ruídos cardíacos do tamponamento pericárdico. SIN Beck t.

Beck t., t. de Beck. SIN acute compression t.

Charcot t., t. de Charcot; **(1)** na esclerose múltipla (disseminada), os três sinais e sintomas: nistagmo, tremor e fala escandida; **(2)** combinação de icterícia, febre e dor na parte superior do abdome, que ocorre em conseqüência de colangite.

Fallot t., t. de Fallot. SIN *trilogy of Fallot.*

hepatic t., t. hepática. SIN portal t.

Hull t., t. de Hull; a associação de galope diastólico, anasarca e pequena pressão diferencial.

Hutchinson t., t. de Hutchinson; ceratite parenquimatosa, doença do labirinto e dentes de Hutchinson, indicando sífilis congênita.

Kartagener t., t. de Kartagener. SIN Kartagener *syndrome.*

portal t., t. porta; ramos da veia porta, da artéria hepática e ductos biliares reunidos na cápsula fibrosa perivascular ou trato porta à medida que se ramificam dentro da substância hepática. SIN hepatic t., triad (3).

Saint t., t. de Saint; presença concomitante de hérnia de hiato, diverticulose e colelitíase.

tri·age (trē′ahzh). Triagem. **1.** Triagem médica de pacientes para determinar sua prioridade relativa para tratamento. **2.** A separação de um grande número de casos, na assistência médica em desastres militares ou civis, em três grupos: 1) aqueles que não se pode esperar que sobrevivam, mesmo com tratamento; 2) aqueles que irão se recuperar sem tratamento; e 3) o maior grupo de prioridade, aqueles que não irão sobreviver sem tratamento. [Fr. triagem]

tri·al. Estudo clínico; ensaio; teste ou experimento, geralmente conduzido em condições específicas.

clinical t., estudo clínico; experimento controlado envolvendo um conjunto definido de indivíduos, apresentando um evento clínico como medida de resultado, destinado a obter informações cientificamente válidas acerca da eficácia ou segurança de um fármaco, vacina, teste diagnóstico, procedimento cirúrgico ou outra forma de intervenção médica.

> Distinguem-se quatro fases no estudo clínico. Os estudos clínicos de Fase I envolvem, em geral, menos de 100 voluntários sadios, que são expostos a uma nova droga ou vacina. Esses estudos procuram estabelecer a melhor dose e via de administração e detectar as reações adversas. Os estudos de Fase II geralmente envolvem 200-500 voluntários que são distribuídos de forma aleatória em grupos de controle e grupos de estudo. Trata-se dos estudos pilotos de eficácia, com ênfase na imunogenicidade no caso de vacinas e na eficácia e segurança relativas no caso de drogas. Os estudos de Fase III, que são freqüentemente multicêntricos, envolvem milhares de voluntários, distribuídos aleatoriamente em grupos de controle e grupos de estudo. O objetivo é obter dados estatisticamente relevantes. Os estudos de Fase IV são conduzidos após a aprovação, por uma autoridade nacional de registro de drogas (nos Estados Unidos, a Food and Drug Administration), de um agente para distribuição ou venda. Podem explorar efeitos farmacológicos específicos, reações adversas ou efeitos a longo prazo.

randomized controlled t. (RCT), estudo clínico controlado randomizado; experimento epidemiológico em que os indivíduos numa população são distribuídos aleatoriamente em grupos, denominados grupos "experimental" ou "de estudo" e "de controle", para receber ou não receber um esquema terapêutico ou preventivo experimental, procedimento, manobra ou intervenção.

tri·al and er·ror. Tentativa e erro; a atividade exploratória aparentemente aleatória, desenvolvida sem planejamento, que freqüentemente precede a aquisição de novas informações ou ajustes; pode ser aberta, como um rato que corre num labirinto, ou encoberta (vicária), como quando se pensa de diversas maneiras para enfrentar uma determinada situação.

tri·am·cin·o·lone (trī-am-sin′ō-lōn). Triancinolona; glicocorticóide com ações e usos semelhantes aos da prednisolona.

t. acetonide, acetonido de t.; potente glicocorticóide para tratamento tópico de dermatoses.

t. diacetate, diacetato de t.; agente antiinflamatório e antialérgico para uso parenteral.

tri·a·me·lia (trī′ă-mē′lē-ă). Triamelia; ausência de três membros. [tri- + G. *a-,* priv. + *melos,* membro]

tri·am·ter·ene (trī-am′ter-ēn). Triantereno; agente diurético poupador de potássio, freqüentemente associado a hidroclorotiazida.

TRIANGLE

tri·an·gle (trī′ang-gl) [TA]. Triângulo, trígono; em anatomia e cirurgia, uma área de três lados com limites arbitrários ou naturais. VER TAMBÉM trigonum, region. [L. *triangulum,* de *tri-,* três, + *angulus,* ângulo]

anal t. [TA], região anal; a porção posterior da região perineal através da qual se abre o canal anal; delimitada por uma linha através de ambas as tuberosidades isquiáticas, os ligamentos sacrotuberais e o cóccix. SIN regio analis [TA], anal region.

anterior t. of neck, trígono anterior do pescoço; *termo oficial alternativo para anterior cervical *region.*

Assézat t., triângulo de Assézat; triângulo formado por linhas que conectam o násio com o ponto alveolar e o ponto nasal; utilizado para indicar prognatismo em craniologia comparativa.

auricular t., triângulo da orelha; triângulo formado pela base da orelha e por linhas traçadas a partir do verdadeiro ápice da orelha até as extremidades da base.

auscultatory t. [TA], triângulo auscultatório; espaço delimitado pela borda inferior do trapézio, latíssimo do dorso e margem medial da escápula, onde a ausência de musculatura permite que os sons respiratórios sejam claramente ouvidos com um estetoscópio. SIN trigonum auscultationis [TA], t. of auscultation*.

t. of auscultation, triângulo auscultatório; *termo oficial alternativo para ausculatory t.

axillary t., triângulo axilar; área triangular que compreende a face medial do braço, a axila e a região peitoral, que é um dos locais prediletos da erupção petequial inicial da varíola. VER TAMBÉM axillary *region.*

Béclard t., triângulo de Béclard; área delimitada pela borda posterior do músculo hioglosso, ventre posterior do digástrico e corno maior do osso hióide.

Bonwill t., triângulo de Bonwill; triângulo eqüilátero formado por linhas a partir dos pontos de contato dos incisivos centrais inferiores ou linha medial da crista residual da mandíbula até o côndilo de cada lado e de um côndilo ao outro.

Burger t., triângulo de Burger; triângulo escaleno que representa as derivações eletrocardiográficas de plano frontal, comparável ao triângulo de Einthoven, porém mais acurado. VER Einthoven t.

Burow t., triângulo de Burow; triângulo de pele e gordura subcutânea excisado de forma que um retalho possa ser avançado sem deformar o tecido adjacente.

Calot t. [TA], triângulo de Calot. SIN cystohepatic t.

cardiohepatic t., triângulo cárdio-hepático. SIN cardiohepatic *angle.*

carotid t. [TA], trígono carótico; espaço delimitado pelo ventre superior do músculo omo-hióideo, pela borda anterior do músculo esternocleidomastóideo e pelo ventre posterior do digástrico; contém a bifurcação da artéria carótida comum. SIN trigonum caroticum [TA], fossa carotica, Gerdy hyoid fossa; Malgaigne fossa, Malgaigne t., superior carotid t.

cephalic t., triângulo cefálico; triângulo sobre o crânio formado por linhas que conectam o metópio, o pogônio e o ponto occipital.

cervical t., trígono cervical; qualquer um dos triângulos do pescoço.

clavipectoral t. [TA], trígono clavipeitoral; área da região torácica anterior delimitada superiormente pela clavícula, ínfero-medialmente pelo (músculo) peitoral maior e súpero-lateralmente pelo (músculo) deltóide; tipicamente, a veia cefálica passa de um curso superficial para um trajeto profundo, e o ramo peitoral do tronco (arterial) toracoacromial emerge aqui. SIN trigonum clavipectorale [TA], trigonum deltopectorale*, deltoideopectoral t., deltopectoral t., trigonum deltoideopectorale.

Codman t., triângulo de Codman; em radiologia, a interface entre o tumor ósseo em crescimento e o osso normal, apresentando-se como um triângulo incompleto formado por periósteo.

crural t., triângulo crural; área de predileção da erupção petequial inicial da varíola; ocupa as regiões abdominal inferior, inguinal e genital e as faces internas das coxas, atravessando a base do triângulo, o umbigo.

cystohepatic t. [TA], trígono cisto-hepático; área delimitada pela artéria cística, ducto cístico e ducto hepático (comum) — estruturas importantes a identificar na realização de colecistectomia laparoscópica. SIN Calot t. [TA], trigonum cystohepaticum [TA].
deltoideopectoral t., trígono clavipeitoral. SIN clavipectoral t.
deltopectoral t., trígono clavipeitoral. SIN clavipectoral t.
digastric t., triângulo digástrico. SIN submandibular t.
Einthoven t., triângulo de Einthoven; t. eqüilátero imaginário que tem o coração em seu centro, em que os lados iguais representam as três derivações padrões dos membros do eletrocardiograma.
Elaut t., triângulo de Elaut; triângulo formado pelas artérias ilíacas e pelo promontório do sacro.
t. of elbow, triângulo do cotovelo. SIN cubital fossa.
facial t., triângulo facial; triângulo formado por linhas que conectam o básio, o próstio e o násio.
Farabeuf t., triângulo de Farabeuf; triângulo formado pelas veias jugular interna e facial e pelo nervo hipoglosso.
femoral t. [TA], trígono femoral; espaço triangular na parte superior da coxa, limitado pelos músculos sartório e adutor longo e pelo ligamento inguinal, sendo o assoalho formado lateralmente pelo músculo iliopsoas e medialmente pelo músculo pectíneo; os ramos do nervo femoral distribuem-se dentro do trígono femoral; é bisseccionado pelos vasos femorais, que penetram no canal adutor no ápice do trígono. SIN trigonum femorale [TA], trigonum femoris*, fossa scarpae major, Scarpa t., subinguinal t.
t. of fillet, trígono do lemnisco lateral. SIN trigone of lateral lemniscus.
frontal t., triângulo frontal; triângulo limitado acima pelo diâmetro frontal máximo e lateralmente por linhas que unem as extremidades desse diâmetro com a glabela.
Garland t., triângulo de Garland; área triangular de ressonância relativa na região lombar próximo à coluna, encontrada no mesmo lado de um derrame pleural.
Gombault t., triângulo de Gombault. VER semilunar *fasciculus*.
Grocco t., triângulo de Grocco; área triangular de macicez na base do tórax, ao longo da coluna vertebral, do lado oposto de um derrame pleural. SIN paravertebral t.
Grynfeltt t., triângulo de Grynfeltt; espaço triangular limitado, acima, pela extremidade da última costela e pelo músculo serrátil posterior inferior, anteriormente pelo músculo oblíquo interno e posteriormente pelo músculo quadrado lombar; ocorre hérnia lombar nesse espaço. SIN Lesshaft t.
Hesselbach t., triângulo de Hesselbach. SIN inguinal t.
inferior carotid t., trígono muscular. SIN muscular t. (of neck).
inferior lumbar t. [TA], trígono lombar inferior; área na parede abdominal posterior limitada pelas bordas dos músculos latíssimo do dorso e oblíquo externo e pela crista ilíaca; por vezes, ocorrem herniações nesse local. SIN trigonum lumbale inferius [TA], lumbar t., Petit lumbar t.
inferior occipital t., trígono occipital inferior; triângulo com ápice na protuberância occipital externa; sua base é formada por uma linha que une os dois processos mastóideos.
infraclavicular t., fossa infraclavicular. SIN infraclavicular *fossa*.
inguinal t. [TA], trígono inguinal; área triangular na parede abdominal inferior limitada inferiormente pelo ligamento inguinal (externamente) ou trato iliopúbico (internamente), borda do reto do abdome medialmente e vasos epigástricos inferiores (dobra umbilical lateral) lateralmente. Constitui o local de hérnia inguinal direta. SIN trigonum inguinale [TA], Hesselbach t., inguinal trigone.
interscalene t., triângulo interescaleno. SIN scalene *hiatus*.
Killian t., triângulo de Killian; área do esôfago cervical em forma triangular, ladeada pelas fibras oblíquas do músculo constritor inferior da faringe e fibras transversas do músculo cricofaríngeo através do qual ocorre o divertículo de Zenker.
Koch t., triângulo de Koch; área triangular da parede do átrio direito do coração que marca a posição aproximada do nó atrioventricular.
Labbé t., triângulo de Labbé; área limitada, abaixo, por uma linha horizontal que toca a borda inferior da cartilagem da nona costela esquerda, lateralmente pela linha das falsas costelas e do lado direito pelo fígado; nesse local, o estômago está normalmente em contato com a parede abdominal.
Langenbeck t., triângulo de Langenbeck; triângulo formado por linhas traçadas da espinha ilíaca ântero-superior até a superfície do trocanter maior e até o colo cirúrgico do fêmur; a ocorrência de ferida penetrante nessa área provavelmente acomete a articulação.
lateral pelvic wall t. [TA], trígono parietal lateral da pelve; área da parede lateral da pelve coberta pela porção do músculo obturador interno e fáscia superior até o arco tendíneo do (músculo) levantador do ânus, anteriormente à incisura isquiática e inferiormente à linha arqueada do ílio. SIN trigonum parietale laterale pelvis [TA].
Lesser t., triângulo de Lesser; o espaço entre os ventres do músculo digástrico e o nervo hipoglosso.
Lesshaft t., triângulo de Lesshaft. SIN Grynfeltt t.

Lieutaud t., triângulo de Lieutaud. SIN *trigone* of bladder.
lumbar t., trígono lombar. SIN inferior lumbar t.
lumbocostal t. of diaphragm [TA], trígono lombocostal do diafragma; área triangular no diafragma entre suas partes lombar e costal e superiormente ao ligamento arqueado lateral que é desprovida de fibras musculares; é coberta pela pleura superiormente e pelo peritônio inferiormente; quando há falha congênita de sua formação (defeito de fechamento do hiato pleuroperitoneal fetal), o conseqüente forame de Bochdalek constitui o local mais comum de hérnia diafragmática das vísceras abdominais. SIN trigonum lumbocostale diaphragmatis [TA], Bochdalek gap, vertebrocostal trigone.
lumbocostoabdominal t., trígono lombocostoabdominal; área irregular limitada pelos músculos serrátil posterior inferior, oblíquo externo, oblíquo interno e eretor da espinha.
Macewen t., triângulo de Macewen. SIN suprameatal t.
Malgaigne t., triângulo de Malgaigne. SIN carotid t.
Marcille t., triângulo de Marcille; área limitada pela borda medial do psoas maior, pela margem lateral da coluna vertebral e pelo ligamento iliolombar abaixo; é cruzada pelo nervo obturador.
muscular t. (of neck) [TA], trígono muscular (do pescoço); triângulo limitado pelo músculo esternocleidomastóideo, pelo ventre superior do músculo omo-hióideo e pela linha mediana anterior do pescoço; os músculos infra-hióideos ocupam a maior parte do triângulo. SIN trigonum musculare (regionis cervicalis anterioris) [TA], omotracheal t.*, trigonum omotracheale*, inferior carotid t., tracheal t.
occipital t., trígono occipital; triângulo do pescoço limitado pelos músculos trapézio, esternocleidomastóideo e omo-hióideo. VER TAMBÉM inferior occipital t.
omoclavicular t. [TA], trígono omoclavicular. SIN supraclavicular t.
omotracheal t., trígono omotraqueal; *termo oficial alternativo para muscular t. (of neck).
palatal t., trígono palatal; área triangular limitada pelo diâmetro transverso maior do palato e por linhas que convergem de suas extremidades até o ponto alveolar. SIN trigonum palati.
paravertebral t., trígono paravertebral. SIN Grocco t.
Petit lumbar t., trígono lombar de Petit. SIN inferior lumbar t.
Philippe t., triângulo de Philippe. VER semilunar *fasciculus*.
Pirogoff t., triângulo de Pirogoff; triângulo formado pelo tendão intermediário do músculo digástrico, pela borda posterior do músculo milo-hióideo e pelo nervo hipoglosso.
posterior t. of neck, triângulo posterior do pescoço; *termo oficial alternativo para lateral cervical *region*.
pubourethral t., trígono pubouretral; triângulo no períneo limitado pelos músculos transverso do períneo, isquiocavernoso e bulbo cavernoso.
Reil t., triângulo de Reil. SIN *trigone* of lateral lemniscus.
retromolar t. [TA], trígono retromolar; área triangular posterior ao terceiro dente molar mandibular. SIN trigonum retromolare [TA].
sacral t., triângulo sacral; área superficial sobre o sacro.
t. of safety, triângulo de segurança; a área na borda esternal esquerda inferior onde o pericárdio não é recoberto pelo pulmão (incisura pericárdica); local preferido para a aspiração de líquido pericárdico.
Scarpa t., triângulo de Scarpa. SIN femoral t.
sternocostal t., trígono esternocostal. SIN *trigonum* sternocostale.
sternocostal t. (of diaphragm) [TA], trígono esternocostal (do diafragma); área fibrosa (não-muscular) do diafragma entre as tiras musculares da parte esternal do diafragma e a parte costal; quando ocorre falha congênita de formação, o conseqüente forame de Morgagni pode permitir a herniação de vísceras abdominais no tórax. SIN trigonum sternocostale diaphragmatis [TA].
subclavian t., trígono subclávio; *termo oficial alternativo para supraclavicular t.
subinguinal t., trígono femoral. SIN femoral t.
submandibular t. [TA], trígono submandibular; triângulo do pescoço limitado pela mandíbula e pelos dois ventres do músculo digástrico; contém a glândula submandibular. SIN trigonum submandibulare [TA], digastric t., submaxillary t.
submaxillary t., trígono submandibular. SIN submandibular t.
submental t. [TA], trígono submentual; triângulo limitado pelo ventre anterior dos músculos digástricos, osso hióide e linha mediana; o músculo milo-hióide forma o seu assoalho. SIN trigonum submentale [TA].
suboccipital t., trígono suboccipital; triângulo profundo limitado pelos músculos oblíquo inferior da cabeça, oblíquo superior da cabeça e reto posterior maior da cabeça.
superior carotid t., trígono carótico superior. SIN carotid t.
supraclavicular t. [TA], trígono omoclavicular; triângulo limitado pela clavícula, músculo omo-hióideo e músculo esternocleidomastóideo; contém a artéria e a veia subclávia. SIN omoclavicular t. [TA], trigonum omoclaviculare [TA], subclavian t.*.
suprameatal t. [TA], trígono supraméatico; triângulo formado pela raiz do arco zigomático, pela parede posterior do meato acústico externo ósseo e por uma

triangle   1665   **trichinization**

linha imaginária que conecta as extremidades das duas primeiras linhas; a espinha suprameática localiza-se em suas margens anteriores; utilizado como orientação em cirurgias do mastóide, visto que constitui a parede lateral do antro mastóideo. SIN foveola suprameatica [TA], foveola suprameatalis, Macewen t., mastoid fossa, fossa mastoidea, suprameastoid fossa, suprameatal pit.

tracheal t., trígono muscular. SIN muscular t. (of neck).

Tweed t., triângulo de Tweed; triângulo definido por limites faciais e dentários numa imagem cefalométrica lateral, utilizando o plano horizontal de Frankfort como base e projetado para uso como orientação na avaliação e planejamento do tratamento ortodôntico.

umbilicomammillary t., trígono umbilicomamilar; triângulo com ápice no umbigo e base na linha que une os mamilos.

urogenital t. [TA], região urogenital; a porção anterior da região perineal contendo as aberturas da uretra e da vagina na mulher e a uretra e as estruturas da raiz do pênis no homem. SIN regio urogenitalis [TA], urogenital region.

t. of vertebral artery, trígono da artéria vertebral; área triangular na raiz do pescoço, limitada lateralmente pelo músculo escaleno anterior e medialmente pelo músculo longo do pescoço; os dois músculos encontram-se no ápice do triângulo, formado pelo tubérculo anterior (carótico) do processo transverso da vértebra C6; a artéria vertebral origina-se da artéria subclávia na base do triângulo, bisseccionando o triângulo quando ascende para o ápice, entrando no forame transverso da vértebra C6.

vesical t., trígono da bexiga. SIN trigone of bladder.

Ward t., triângulo de Ward; área de densidade diminuída no padrão trabecular do colo do fêmur, observada por raios X, bem como por inspeção direta.

Weber t., triângulo de Weber; na região plantar uma área indicada pelas cabeças do primeiro e quinto ossos metatarsais e centro da superfície plantar do calcanhar.

Wilde t., triângulo de Wilde. SIN light reflex (3).

tri·an·gu·la·ris. Triangular. VER triangular muscle. [L. triangular]

tri·an·gu·lum (trī-ang'goo-lŭm). Triângulo. VER triangle. [L.]

Tri·at·o·ma (trī-ă-tō'mă). Gênero de inseto (subfamília Triatominae, família Reduviidae), que inclui vetores importantes do *Trypanosoma cruzi*, como *T. dimidiata*, *T. infestans* e *T. maculata*.

Tri·a·tom·i·nae (trī-ă-tō'mi-nē). Subfamília de insetos (família Reduviidae, subordem Heteroptera) que são hematófagos de vertebrados e incluem importantes vetores de doenças, como *Panstrongylus*, *Rhodnius* e *Triatoma*; são comumente denominados conenose ou barbeiros.

tri·a·zo·lam (trī-ā'zō-lam). Triazolam; derivado benzodiazepínico de ação curta, utilizado como sedativo e hipnótico.

tri·az·o·lo·gua·nine (trī'ă-zol-ō-gwah'nēn). Triazologuanina. SIN 8-azaguanine.

tri·ba·sic (trī-bā'sik). Tribásico; que possui três átomos de hidrogênio tituláveis; designa um ácido com basicidade de 3.

tri·bas·i·lar (trī-bas'i-lăr). Tribasilar; que possui três bases.

tribe (trīb). Tribo; na classificação biológica, uma divisão ocasionalmente utilizada entre família e gênero; com freqüência, sinônimo de subfamília. [L. *tribus*]

tri·bol·o·gy (trī-bol'ō-jē). Tribologia; o estudo da fricção e de seus efeitos em sistemas biológicos, especialmente em relação às superfícies articuladas do esqueleto. [G. *tribō*, friccionar, + *logos*, estudo]

tri·bo·lu·mi·nes·cence (trib'ō-loo-mi-nes'ens). Triboluminescência; luminosidade produzida por fricção. [G. *tribō*, friccionar, + luminescence]

tri·bra·chia (trī-brā'kē-ă). Tribraquia; condição observada em gêmeos unidos, em que existem apenas três braços para dois corpos. VER conjoined twins, em twin. [tri- + G. *brachion*, braço]

tri·bra·chi·us (trī-brā'kē-ŭs). Tribráquio; gêmeos unidos que apresentam tribraquia.

tri·brom·sa·lan (trī-brom'să-lan). Tribromsalan; desinfetante utilizado em sabões.

tri·bu·ty·rase (trī-bū'ti-rās). Tributirase. SIN triacylglycerol lipase.

tri·bu·tyr·in (trī-bū'ti-rin). Tributirina; substrato sintético para ensaios de lipase. SIN glyceryl tributyrate, tributyrylglycerol.

tri·bu·tyr·in·ase (trī-bū'ti-ri-nās). Tributirinase. SIN triacylglycerol lipase.

tri·bu·tyr·yl·glyc·er·ol (trī-bū'ti-ril-glis'er-ol). Tributirilglicerol. SIN tributyrin.

TRIC Acrônimo para *trachoma and inclusion conjunctivitis* (tracoma e conjuntivite de inclusão). VER TRIC agents, em agent.

tri·cal·ci·um phos·phate (trī-kal'sē-ŭm). Fosfato tricálcico. SIN tribasic calcium phosphate.

tri·ceph·a·lus (trī-sef'ă-lŭs). Tricéfalo; feto com três cabeças. [tri- + G. *kephalē*, cabeça]

tri·ceps (trī'seps). Tríceps; que possui três cabeças; designa especialmente dois músculos: o tríceps braquial e o tríceps sural. VER muscle. [L. de *tri-*, três, + *caput*, cabeça]

trich-. Tric-. VER tricho-.

trich·al·gia (trik-al'jē-ă). Tricalgia; dor produzida ao tocar o cabelo; cabelo doloroso, como pode ocorrer na angina atípica. SIN trichodynia. [trich- + G. *algos*, dor]

trich·an·gi·on (trik-an'jē-on). Tricângio. SIN telangion. [trich- + G. *angeion*, vaso]

trich·a·tro·phia (trik-ă-trō'fē-ă). Tricatrofia; atrofia dos bulbos dos pêlos, com cabelos quebradiços e queda dos cabelos. [trich- + G. *atrophia*, atrofia]

trich·aux·is (trik-awk'sis). Tricauxe; crescimento excessivo dos pêlos em comprimento e quantidade. [trich- + G. *auxis*, aumento]

trichi-. Triqui-. VER tricho-.

-trichia. -Triquia. Condição ou tipo de cabelo. [G. *thrix* (*trich-*), cabelo, + *-ia*, condição]

tri·chi·a·sis (trī-kī'ă-sis). Triquíase; condição em que o pêlo adjacente a um orifício natural volta-se para dentro e provoca irritação; p. ex., na inversão de uma pálpebra (entrópio), os cílios irritam o olho. SIN trichoma, trichomatosis. [trich- + G. *-iasis*, condição]

trich·i·lem·mo·ma (trik'i-le-mō'mă). Triquilemoma; tumor benigno derivado do epitélio da bainha radicular externa de um folículo piloso, que consiste em células com citoplasma de coloração pálida contendo glicogênio; são observados múltiplos triquilemomas na face na doença de Cowden. SIN tricholemmoma. [trichi- + G. *lemma*, casca, + *-oma*, tumor]

Tri·chi·na (tri-kī'nă). Designação antiga de um gênero de vermes nematódeos, corretamente denominado *Trichinella*.

tri·chi·na, pl. **tri·chi·nae** (tri-kī'nă, -nē). Triquina; larva do verme do gênero *Trichinella*; a forma infectante no porco. [L. Mod. do G. *thrix* (*trich-*), pêlo]

Trich·i·nel·la (trik'i-nel'ă). Gênero de nematódeos no grupo dos afasmídeos, que causa triquinose nos seres humanos e em carnívoros. [L. Mod. de *trichina* + sufixo dim. *ella*]

T. pseudospiralis, espécie de nematódeo com ciclo de vida normal em pequenos predadores; os seres humanos representam um hospedeiro acidental.

T. spira'lis, o verme do porco ou triquina, espécie de parasitas que causam a triquinose, encontrado na maioria das regiões do mundo, porém mais freqüentemente no Hemisfério Norte; ocorre transmissão em conseqüência da ingestão de carne crua ou inadequadamente cozida (principalmente de porco), que contém larvas encistadas que se transformam em adultos, os quais sobrevivem no jejuno e no íleo durante cerca de 6 semanas; a fêmea é vivípara e transporta cerca de 1.500 larvas embrionárias, que são depositadas profundamente na mucosa, de modo que são capturadas nos capilares da submucosa e transportadas através do fígado para o coração, os pulmões e a circulação sistêmica; por fim, as larvas saem dos capilares, penetram numa fibra muscular, espiralam-se e encistam-se, induzindo, assim, a acentuada sensibilização, dor, febre, edema e reação eosinofílica característica da triquinose.

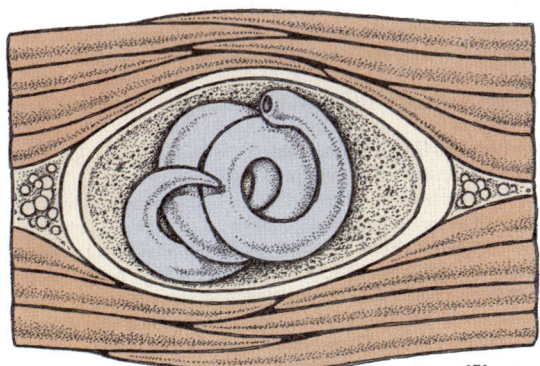

Trichinella spiralis: larva encistada no músculo humano

trich·i·nel·li·a·sis (trik'i-nel-ī'ă-sis). Triquinelíase. SIN trichinosis.

Trich·i·nel·li·cae (tri-ki-nel'i-kē). SIN Trichinelloidea.

Trich·i·nel·loi·dea (trik'i-nel-oy'dē-ă). Superfamília de nematódeos, incluindo os seguintes parasitas no homem: *Trichinella spiralis*, o verme triquina (família Trichinellidae); *Trichuris trichiura;* o parasita do intestino humano; *Capillaria hepatica*, o verme do capilar hepático; e *C. philippinensis* (família Trichuridae). SIN Trichinellicae.

trich·i·nel·lo·sis (trik'i-nel-ō'sis). Triquinelose. SIN trichinosis.

trich·i·ni·a·sis (trik-i-nī'ă-sis). Triquiníase. SIN trichinosis.

trich·i·nif·er·ous (trik-i-nif'e-rŭs). Triquinífero; que contém vermes triquina.

trich·i·ni·za·tion (trik'i-ni-zā'shŭn). Triquinização; infecção por vermes triquina.

tri·chi·no·scope (trik′i-nō-skōp). Triquinoscópio; lente de aumento utilizada no exame de carne com suspeita de triquinose. [trichina + G. *skopeō*, ver]

trich·i·no·sis (trik-i-nō′sis). Triquinose; a doença resultante da ingestão de carne de porco crua ou inadequadamente cozida (ou de carne de urso ou de morsa) que contém larvas encistadas do nematódeo parasita *Trichinella spiralis*. Os sinais e sintomas iniciais da doença humana consistem em dor abdominal, cólica e diarréia, associados ao desenvolvimento dos parasitas no intestino delgado. Quando os parasitas larvares resultantes migram para o tecido muscular e o invadem, surge um segundo grupo de manifestações clínicas, incluindo edema facial e periorbitário, mialgia, febre, prurido, urticária, conjuntivite e sinais de miocardite. SIN trichinelliasis, trichinellosis, trichiniasis. [*Trichinella* (trichina) + G. *-osis*, condição]

tri·chi·nous (trik′i-nŭs). Triquinoso; infectado por vermes triquina.

trich·i·on (trik′ē-on). Tríquio; ponto cefalométrico situado no ponto médio da linha de implantação dos cabelos no topo da fronte. [G. *thrix*, pêlo]

trich·ite (trik′īt). Triquite. SIN trichocyst.

tri·chlo·ral (trī-klōr′al). Tricloral. SIN m-chloral.

tri·chlor·fon (trī-klōr′fon). Triclorfon; composto organofosforado eficaz contra os estágios imaturos e maduros de *Schistosoma haematobium*, porém que não é efetivo contra outras espécies de *Schistosoma* nos seres humanos. SIN metrifonate.

tri·chlo·ride (trī-klōr′īd). Tricloreto; cloreto que possui três átomos de cloro na molécula; p. ex., PCl_3.

tri·chlor·me·thi·a·zide (trī-klōr-me-thī′a-zīd). Triclormetiazida; diurético benzotiazídico e agente anti-hipertensivo eficaz por via oral.

tri·chlor·meth·ine (trī-klōr-meth′ēn). Triclormetina; mostarda nitrogenada utilizada no tratamento da leucemia.

tri·chlo·ro·a·ce·tic ac·id (trī-klōr′ō-a-sē′tik). Ácido tricloroacético; utilizado como anti-séptico adstringente em solução a 1–5% ou como escarótico para verrugas venéreas e outras verrugas; precipitante de proteínas amplamente utilizado.

tri·chlo·ro·eth·ane (trī-klōr-ō-eth′ān). Tricloroetano; solvente industrial com acentuada atividade anestésica por inalação. SIN methylchloroform.

tri·chlo·ro·eth·a·nol (trī-klōr-ō-eth′a-nol). Tricloroetanol; hipnótico e sedativo; como metabólito do hidrato de cloral, contribui para a atividade depressora do hidrato de cloral. SIN trichloroethyl alcohol.

tri·chlo·ro·eth·ene (trī-klōr-ō-eth′ēn). Tricloroeteno. SIN trichloroethylene.

tri·chlo·ro·eth·yl al·co·hol (trī-klōr-ō-eth′il). Álcool tricloroetílico. SIN trichloroethanol.

tri·chlo·ro·eth·yl·ene (trī-klōr-ō-eth′i-lēn). Tricloroetileno; analgésico e anestésico inalatório utilizado em cirurgias de pequeno porte e na prática obstétrica; sua administração exige apenas o uso de circuitos unidirecionais, devido à toxicidade do dicloroacetileno resultante da interação do t. com cal sodada. SIN ethinyl trichloride, trichloroethene.

tri·chlo·ro·flu·o·ro·meth·ane (trī-klōr′ō-flōr-ō-meth′ān). Triclorofluorometano; propelente utilizado em aerossol; possui atividade anestésica e arritmogênica quando inalado em alta concentração. SIN trichloromonofluoromethane.

tri·chlo·ro·meth·ane (trī-klōr-ō-meth′ān). Triclorometano. SIN chloroform.

tri·chlo·ro·mon·o·flu·o·ro·meth·ane (trī-klōr-ō-mon′ō-flōr-ō-meth′ān). Triclormonofluorometano. SIN trichlorofluoromethane.

tri·chlo·ro·phe·nol (trī-klōr-ō-fē′nol). Triclorofenol; utilizado como anti-séptico, desinfetante e fungicida.

(2,4,5-tri·chlo·ro·phen·oxy)ace·tic ac·id (2,4,5-T) (trī-klōr-ō-fe-nok′sē-a-sē-tik). Ácido (2,4,5-triclorofenoxi) acético; herbicida e desfoliante sintetizado por condensação do ácido cloroacético e 2,4,5-triclorofenol, utilizado como principal constituinte do Agent Orange (agente laranja).

tricho-, trich-, trichi-. Trico-, tric-, triqui-. O pêlo, cabelo; estrutura semelhante a um pêlo. [G. *thrix* (*trich*-)]

Trich·o·ceph·a·lus (trik-ō-sef′a-lŭs). Nome incorreto de *Trichuris*. [tricho- + G. *kephalē*, cabeça]

trich·o·chrome (trī′kō-krōm). Tricromo; pigmentos naturais amarelo-alaranjados e violeta relacionados com as melaninas; em parte responsáveis pela cor vermelha e castanho-avermelhada do cabelo humano. [tricho- + G. *chrōma*, cor]

trich·o·cyst (trik′ō-sist). Tricocisto; uma de várias estruturas, na forma de pequenos cistos alongados, dispostos radialmente ao redor da periferia de uma célula de protozoário e contendo líquido que, quando eliminado, serve para agressão ou defesa; encontrado em ciliados, tais como espécies de *Paramecium*. SIN trichite. [tricho- + G. *kystis*, bexiga]

Trich·o·dec·tes (trik-ō-dek′tēz). Gênero de piolho que pica, incluindo a espécie *T. canis* (*T. latus*), o piolho dos cães que comumente serve de hospedeiro intermediário para a tênia do cão, *Dipylidium caninum*, bem como as espécies *T. climax* (*Bovicola caprae*), *T. parumpilosus* (*B. equi*), *T. scalaris* (*B. bovis*) e *T. sphaerocephalus* (*B. ovis*). VER TAMBÉM *Bovicola*, *Damalinia*. [tricho- + G. *dektēs*, mendigo]

Trich·o·der·ma (trik-ō-der′mă). Gênero de fungos no solo que fornece o antibiótico gliotoxina. Produz infecções oportunistas raras. [tricho- + G. *derma*, pele]

trich·o·dis·co·ma (trik′ō-dis-kō′mă). Tricodiscoma; hamartomas mesenquimatosos parafoliculares elípticos de herança dominante ou não-familiares.

trich·o·dyn·ia (trik-ō-din′ē-a). Tricodinia. SIN trichalgia. [tricho- + G. *odynē*, dor]

trich·o·dys·tro·phy (trik′ō-dis-trō-fē). Tricodistrofia; nutrição ou crescimento deficientes dos cabelos, culminando freqüentemente em alopecia. Pode ser adquirida ou congênita; esta última ocorre freqüentemente com defeitos metabólicos ou outros defeitos congênitos. [tricho- + prefixo G. *dys-*, anormal, + *trophē*, crescimento]

trich·o·ep·i·the·li·o·ma (trik′ō-ep-i-thē-lē-ō′mă) [MIM*132700]. Tricoepitelioma; múltiplos nódulos benignos e pequenos, que ocorrem principalmente na pele da face, derivados de células basais de folículos pilosos que encerram pequenos cistos de ceratina; herança autossômica dominante. SIN Brooke tumor, epithelioma adenoides cysticum, hereditary multiple t. [tricho- + epithelioma]

desmoplastic t., t. desmoplásico; pápula solitária, dura, anular, com depressão central, que ocorre habitualmente em mulheres na face; consiste em filamentos dérmicos de células basalóides e pequenos cistos ceratinosos no interior do estroma desmoplásico esclerótico.

hereditary multiple t., t. múltiplo hereditário. SIN trichoepithelioma.

trich·o·es·the·sia (trik′ō-es-thē′zē-a). Tricoestesia. **1.** A sensação percebida quando se toca um cabelo. **2.** Forma de parestesia em que existe uma sensação de pêlo sobre a pele, a mucosa da boca ou a conjuntiva. [tricho- + G. *aisthēsis*, sensação]

trich·o·fol·lic·u·lo·ma (trik′ō-fol-ik-ū-lō′mă). Tricofoliculoma; tumor ou hamartoma habitualmente solitário, em que múltiplos folículos pilosos abortivos se abrem num cisto ou espaço central, que se abre na superfície da pele. [tricho- + L. *folliculus*, fonte, + G. *-oma*, tumor]

trich·o·gen (trik′o-jen). Tricógeno; agente que promove o crescimento do pêlo. [tricho- + G. *-gen*, que produz]

trich·o·glos·sia (trik-ō-glos′ē-a). Tricoglossia. SIN hairy tongue. [tricho- + G. *glōssa*, língua]

trich·o·hy·a·lin (trik-ō-hī′a-lin). Tricoialina; substância da natureza da ceratoialina, encontrada na bainha radicular interna em desenvolvimento do folículo piloso.

trich·oid (trik′oyd). Tricóide; semelhante a um pêlo. [tricho- + G. *eidos*, semelhança]

trich·o·lem·mo·ma (trik′ō-le-mō′mă). Tricolemoma. SIN trichilemmoma.

trich·o·lo·gia (trik-ō-lō′jē-a). Hábito nervoso de arrancar o cabelo. SIN trichology (2). [G. *trichologeō*, arrancar os cabelos, de tricho- + *legō*, puxar, reunir]

tri·chol·o·gy (tri-kol′o-jē). **1.** Tricologia; o estudo da anatomia, do crescimento e das doenças do pêlo ou cabelo. [tricho- + G. *logos*, estudo] **2.** SIN trichologia. [G. *trichologeo*, de tricho- + *legō*, arrancar]

tri·cho·ma (tri-kō′mă). Tricoma. SIN trichiasis. [tricho- + G. *-oma*, tumor]

tri·cho·ma·to·sis (tri-kō′mă-tō′sis). Tricomatose. SIN trichiasis.

trich·o·meg·a·ly (trik′ō-meg′a-lē). Tricomegalia; condição congênita caracterizada por cílios anormalmente longos; associada a nanismo. [tricho- + G. *megas*, grande]

trich·o·mo·na·cide (trik-ō-mō′nă-sīd). Tricomonacida; agente que destrói *Trichomonas*.

trich·o·mon·ad (trik-ō-mō′nad). Tricomônade; nome comum para membros da família Trichomonadidae.

Trich·o·mo·nad·i·dae (trik′ō-mō-nad′i-dē). Família de protozoários flagelados que inclui o gênero *Trichomonas*.

Trich·o·mon·as (trik-ō-mō′nas). Gênero de protozoários flagelados parasitas (subfamília Trichomonidinae, família Trichomonadidae) que causa tricomoníase nos seres humanos, outros primatas e aves. A especificidade é mais pronunciada para seu micro-hábitat preciso do que para as espécies de hospedeiro. O gênero foi dividido em vários gêneros: *Trichomonas*, *Pentatrichomonas*, *Tetratrichomonas* e *Tritrichomonas*. [tricho- + G. *monas*, único (unidade)]

***T. bucca′lis*,** SIN *T. tenax*.

***T. foe′tus*,** designação antiga de *Tritrichomonas foetus*.

***T. gallina′rum*,** designação antiga de *Tetratrichomonas gallinarum*.

***T. hom′inis*,** designação antiga de *Pentatrichomonas hominis*.

***T. o′vis*,** designação antiga de *Tetratrichomonas ovis*.

***T. su′is*,** designação antiga de *Tritrichomonas suis*.

***T. te′nax*,** espécie que vive como comensal na boca dos seres humanos e de outros primatas, especialmente no tártaro ao redor dos dentes ou nos defeitos de dentes cariados; não há evidências de patogenia direta, porém está freqüentemente associada a microrganismos piogênicos em alvéolos dentários ou na base dos dentes. SIN *T. buccalis*.

***T. vagina′lis*,** espécie freqüentemente encontrada na vagina e na uretra de mulheres (nas quais provoca vaginite por tricomoníase) e na uretra e próstata dos homens (os únicos hospedeiros naturais conhecidos); existem consideráveis diferenças na patogenia entre várias cepas dessa espécie.

trich·o·mo·ni·a·sis (trik′ō - mō - nī′ă - sis). Tricomoníase; doença causada por infecção por uma espécie de protozoário do gênero *Trichomonas* ou gêneros correlatos.

t. vagini'tis, vaginite ou uretrite agudas causadas pela infecção por *Trichomonas vaginalis,* que não invade a mucosa nem o tecido, mas provoca uma reação inflamatória; a infecção é de transmissão venérea ou por outras formas de contato; a infecção disseminada em populações humanas é habitualmente assintomática, mas pode provocar vaginite, com prurido vaginal e vulvar, leucorréia com corrimento aquoso espumoso e (raramente) uretrite purulenta nos homens.

trich·o·my·ce·to·sis (trik′ō - mī - sē - tō′sis). Tricomicetose. SIN trichomycosis.

trich·o·my·co·sis (trik′ō - mī - kō′sis). Tricomicose; termo outrora utilizado para designar qualquer doença dos pêlos ou cabelos causada por um fungo; atualmente sinônimo de triconocardiose ou t. axilar. Em seu uso atual, o termo tricomicose é uma designação incorreta, visto que o agente etiológico da doença é uma *Nocardia* (entidade intermediária entre fungo e bactéria) ou *Corynebacterium,* e não um verdadeiro fungo. SIN trichomycetosis. [tricho- + G. *mykēs,* fungo, + G. *-osis,* condição]

t. axilla'ris, t. axilar; infecção dos pêlos axilares e púbicos por *Corynebacterium,* com desenvolvimento de concreções amarelas (flava), pretas (nigra) ou vermelhas (rubra) ao redor das hastes dos pêlos; freqüentemente assintomática. SIN lepothrix, trichonodosis.

trich·o·no·do·sis (trik - o - no - dō'sis). Triconodose. SIN *trichomycosis axillaris.* [tricho- + L. *nodus,* nódulo (tumefação), + G. *-osis,* condição]

trich·o·no·sis (trik′ō - nō′sis). Triconose. SIN trichopathy.

trich·o·path·ic (trik - ō - path′ik). Tricopático; relativo a qualquer doença dos pêlos ou cabelos.

trich·o·path·o·pho·bia (trik′ō - path - ō - fō′bē - ă). Tricopatofobia; preocupação excessiva em relação a doenças dos cabelos, sua cor ou anormalidades de seu crescimento. [tricho- + G. *pathos,* sofrimento + *phobos,* medo]

tri·chop·a·thy (tri - kop′ă - thē). Tricopatia; qualquer doença dos pêlos ou cabelos. SIN trinchonosis, trichosis. [tricho- + G. *pathos,* sofrimento]

trich·o·pha·gia (tri - kō - fāj′ē - a). Tricofagia; hábito de comer cabelos ou lã.

tri·choph·a·gy (tri - kof′ă - jē). Tricofagia; hábito de morder os cabelos. [tricho- + G. *phagein,* comer]

trich·o·pho·bia (trik - ō - fō′bē - ă). Tricofobia; repugnância mórbida causada pela visão de fios de cabelos sobre a roupa ou em outro local. [tricho- + G. *phobos,* medo]

trich·o·phyt·ic (trik - ō - fit′ik). Tricofítico; relativo à tricofitose.

trich·o·phy·to·be·zoar (trik′ō - fī′tō - bē′zōr). Tricofitobezoar; bola de pêlos e alimentos misturados, que consiste em fibras vegetais, sementes e cascas de frutas e pêlos animais misturados para formar uma bola no estômago de seres humanos ou outros animais, especialmente ruminantes. SIN phytotrichobezoar. [tricho- + G. *phyton,* planta, + bezoar]

Trich·o·phy·ton (tri - kof′i - ton). Gênero de fungos patogênicos que causam dermatofitose em seres humanos e animais; as espécies podem ser antropofílicas, zoofílicas ou geofílicas e atacam os pêlos, a pele e as unhas e caracterizam-se por seu crescimento nos pêlos. As espécies endotrix crescem da pele para o folículo piloso, penetram na haste e crescem em seu interior, produzindo fileiras de artroconídios com septação das hifas; não há crescimento sobre a superfície externa da haste. As espécies ectotrix são de dois tipos, com grandes esporos e pequenos esporos. Em ambas, o fungo cresce para o folículo piloso, circunda a haste do pêlo e penetra nela, mas continua a crescer tanto dentro quanto fora da haste do pêlo, produzindo artroconídios externamente. [tricho- + G. *phyton,* planta]

T. concen'tricum, espécie de fungo antropofílica, agente etiológico da tinha imbricada; assemelha-se bastante ao micélio ramificado de *T. schoenleinii.*

T. equi'num, espécie de fungo zoofílica que causa infecções ectotrix dos pêlos em cavalos, a partir dos quais os seres humanos também podem ser infectados; exige ácido nicotínico para o seu crescimento.

T. megnin'ii, espécie ectotrix antrofílica de dermatófito com esporos em cadeias, que causa infecção em seres humanos; exige histidina, o que a diferencia do *Microsporum gallinae.*

T. mentagrophy'tes, espécie ectotrix zoofílica de pequenos esporos que causa infecção dos pêlos, da pele e das unhas; trata-se de uma causa de tinha em cães, cavalos, coelhos, camundongos, ratos, chinchilas, raposas e seres humanos (especialmente tinha do pé com grave inflamação e tinha crural).

T. ru'brum, espécie antropofílica amplamente distribuída, que causa infecções persistentes na pele, especialmente tinha do pé e tinha crural, bem como nas unhas, que são especialmente resistentes ao tratamento; raramente invade os pêlos, nos quais é de natureza ectotrix; foram relatados casos ocasionais de infecções subcutâneas e sistêmicas.

T. schoenlei'nii, espécie endotrix antropofílica de dermatófito que causa tinha favosa em seres humanos; é endêmica em toda a Eurásia e África e, por causa do aumento de viagens internacionais, está sendo observada mais freqüentemente no Hemisfério Ocidental; produz túneis dentro da haste do pêlo, que são preenchidos por bolhas de ar após a desintegração das hifas.

T. sim'ii, espécie zoofílica de fungos que provoca infecções em macacos rhesus, cães e seres humanos; a maioria das infecções teve a sua origem na Índia.

T. ton'surans, espécie endotrix antrofílica que causa dermatofitose epidêmica na Europa, na América do Sul e nos Estados Unidos; infecta alguns animais e exige tiamina para o seu crescimento. Trata-se da causa mais comum de tinha da cabeça nos Estados Unidos, formando pontos negros onde o fio de cabelo se quebra na superfície da pele.

T. verrucos'um, espécie zoofílica que causa tinha no gado bovino, a partir do qual os seres humanos podem tornar-se infectados.

T. viola'ceum, espécie antropofílica que causa tinha do couro cabeludo de pontos negros ou infecção favosa do couro cabeludo; a infecção dos pêlos é do tipo endotrix; habitualmente encontrada na América do Sul, Europa, Ásia e África.

trich·o·phy·to·sis (trik′ō - fi - tō′sis). Tricofitose; infecção fúngica superficial causada por espécies de *Trichophyton.* [tricho- + G. *phyton,* planta, + -osis, condição]

Trich·o·pleu·ris (trik′ō - ploo′ris). Gênero de piolhos que picam e infestam ruminantes, p. ex., *T. lipeuroides* e *T. parallelus* em cervídeos americanos; considerado por alguns um subgênero de *Damalinia.* [tricho- + G. *pleura,* costela, lado]

tri·chop·o·li·o·dys·tro·phy. Tricopoliodistrofia. SIN kinky-hair *disease.*

trich·o·po·li·o·sis (trik′ō - pō - lē - ō′sis). Tricopoliose. SIN poliosis. [tricho- + G. *polios,* cinza, + -osis, condição]

Tri·chop·ter·a (tri - kop′ter - ă). Ordem de insetos cujas larvas aquáticas (friganas) constroem um casulo protetor (fio de lã) a partir de fragmentos de material submerso numa forma altamente específica; comumente encontradas fixadas sob pedras em correntes de água doce. As friganas adultas, que possuem asas peludas, eliminam seus pêlos e epitélios, causando sintomas semelhantes aos de febre do feno (alérgicos) em indivíduos sensíveis. [tricho- + G. *pteron,* asa]

trich·o·pti·lo·sis (trik′ō - ti - lō′sis, tri - kop - ti - lō′sis). Tricoptilose; condição de divisão da haste do pêlo, produzindo uma aparência de pena. [tricho- + G. *ptilosis,* plumagem, + -osis, condição]

trich·or·rhex·is (trik - ō - rek′sis). Tricorrexe; condição em que os pêlos tendem a romper ou quebrar facilmente. [tricho- + G. *rhēxis,* ruptura]

t. invagina'ta, t. invaginada. SIN bamboo *hair.*

t. nodo'sa, t. nodosa; condição congênita ou adquirida caracterizada pela formação de pequenos nodos nas hastes do pêlo; podem ocorrer divisão e ruptura, completa ou incompleta, nesses pontos ou nodos.

tri·chos·chi·sis (tri - kos′ki - sis). Tricosquise; presença de pêlos quebrados ou divididos. VER TAMBÉM trichorrhexis. [tricho- + G. *schisis,* clivagem]

tri·cho·sis (tri - kō′sis). Tricose. SIN trichopathy. [tricho- + G. *-osis,* condição]

t. carun'culae, t. caruncular; crescimento de pêlo na carúncula lacrimal.

t. sensiti'va, t. sensitiva; hiperestesia de partes pilosas.

t. seto'sa, t. cerdosa; engrossamento dos pêlos.

trich·o·so·ma·tous (trik - ō - sō′mă - tŭs). Tricosomatoso; que possui flagelos com um pequeno corpo; designa certos protozoários. VER *Trichomonas.* [tricho- + G. *sōma,* corpo]

Tri·cho·spo·ron (tri - kos′pō - ron, trik - ō - spor′on). Gênero de fungos imperfeitos que possuem hifas septadas ramificadas com artroconídios e blastoconídios; esses organismos fazem parte da flora normal do trato intestinal de seres humanos. *T. beigelii* é o agente etiológico da piedra branca ou tricosporonose e fungiemia fatal em pacientes imunocomprometidos. [tricho- + G. *sporos,* semente (esporo)]

trich·o·spor·o·no·sis (trik′ō - spor - o - nō - sis). Tricosporonose; infecção sistêmica por *Trichosporan beigelii;* caracterizada por febre ou pneumonia com alta taxa de mortalidade; observada em pacientes neutropênicos. A infecção localizada por *T. beigelii* é denominada piedra branca, também conhecida como tricosporose.

trich·o·spo·ro·sis (trik′ō - spō - rō′sis). Tricosporose; infecção por *Trichosporon beigelii.* [*Trichosporon* + G. *-osis,* condição]

trich·o·sta·sis spi·nu·lo·sa (tri - kos′tă - sis, spī′noo - lō′să). Tricostase espinhosa; condição em que os folículos pilosos são bloqueados por um tampão de ceratina contendo múltiplos pêlos lanuginosos, formando pápulas pruriginosas. [tricho- + G. *stasis,* permanência; L. *spinulosus,* espinhoso]

trich·o·stron·gyle (trik - ō - stron′jil). Tricostrôngilo; designação comum de membros da família Trichostrongylidae.

Trich·o·stron·gyl·i·dae (trik′ō - stron - jil′i - dē). Família de nematódeos (ordem Strongylida ou, na terminologia antiga, Strongylata); inclui os gêneros importantes *Cooperia, Ostertagia, Haemonchus, Trichostrongylus, Nematodirus* e *Hippostrongylus.* VER *Trichostrongylus.*

trich·o·stron·gy·lo·sis (trik′ō - stron - ji - lō′sis). Tricostrongilose; infecção por nematódeos do gênero *Trichostrongylus.*

Trich·o·stron·gy·lus (trik - ō - stron′ji - lŭs). Gênero economicamente importante (cerca de 30 espécies) de pequenos nematódeos delgados (família

Trichostrongylidae) que habitam o intestino delgado, em alguns casos o estômago, de vários animais herbívoros e aves galináceas. Escondem-se na mucosa e são hematófagos; em grande número, provocam lesão grave, especialmente em hospedeiros jovens. [tricho- + G. *strongylos,* redondo]

T. ax'ei, a espécie mais comum no gado bovino, que também ocorre no abomaso de carneiros, cavalos, antílopes, bisões, lhamas e cervos, bem como no estômago de porcos e cavalos.

T. capric'ola, espécie que ocorre no intestino delgado e no abomaso de carneiros, cabras, cervos e antilocaprídeos.

T. colubrifor'mis, espécie encontrada nas porções anteriores do intestino delgado e, algumas vezes, no abomaso de carneiros, cabras, bois, camelos e alguns ruminantes selvagens, bem como no estômago de primatas (incluindo seres humanos), coelhos e esquilos; possui distribuição mundial e é comum nos Estados Unidos, especialmente em carneiros.

T. longispicula'ris, espécie encontrada no intestino delgado de bois, carneiros e cabras; possui distribuição mundial, porém é raro nos Estados Unidos.

T. ten'uis, espécie que é parasita patogênico disseminado no ceco e intestino delgado de aves domésticas, incluindo patos, gansos, perus, faisões e perdizes.

T. vitri'nus, espécie que é um importante patógeno de cordeiros, encontrado principalmente no duodeno de carneiros, camelos, coelhos e cabras, mas também relatado no homem e em porcos.

Trich·o·the·ci·um (tri-kō-thē'sē-ŭm). Gênero de fungos imperfeitos, geralmente considerado saprófita comum.

trich·o·thi·o·dys·tro·phy (trik'ō-thī'ō-dis'trō-fē). [MIM*234050]. Tricotiodistrofia; anormalidade congênita caracterizada por cabelos e pêlos quebradiços em decorrência do baixo conteúdo de aminoácido contendo enxofre (cisteína), algumas vezes associada a comprometimento mental e baixa estatura; herança autossômica recessiva. [tricho- + thio- + G. *dys,* mau, + *trophē,* nutrição]

trich·o·til·lo·ma·nia (trik'ō-til-ō-mā'nē-ă). Tricotilomania; compulsão a arrancar o próprio cabelo. [tricho- + G. *tillo,* arrancar, + *mania,* insanidade]

tri·chot·o·my (tri-kot'ō-mē). Tricotomia; divisão em três partes. [G. *trichia,* três vezes, + *tomē,* corte]

trich·o·tox·in (trik'ō-tok'sin). Tricotoxina; citotoxina que possui efeito prejudicial, especificamente para o epitélio ciliado.

tri·chot·ro·phy (tri-kot'rō-fē). Tricotrofia; nutrição do pêlo ou cabelo. [tricho- + G. *trophē,* nutrição]

tri·chro·ic (trī-krō'ik). Tricróico; relativo a ou caracterizado por tricroísmo.

tri·chro·ism (trī'krō-izm). Tricroísmo; a propriedade que possuem alguns cristais birrefringentes e biaxiais de emitir diferentes cores em três direções diferentes. [G. *trichroos,* de três cores, de tri + *chroa,* cor]

tri·chro·mat (trī-krō'mat). Tricrômato; indivíduo que vê as três cores primárias; por conseguinte, indivíduo com visão para cores normal. [tri- + G. *chrōma,* cor]

tri·chro·mat·ic (trī-krō-mat'ik). Tricromático. **1.** Que possui ou se relaciona às três cores primárias: vermelho, verde e azul. **2.** Capaz de perceber as três cores primárias; que possui visão normal para cores. SIN trichromic.

tri·chro·ma·tism (trī-krō'mă-tizm). Tricromatismo; o estado de ser tricromático. [tri- + G. *chrōma,* cor]

anomalous t., t. anômalo; defeito na percepção das cores em que parece haver uma anormalidade ou deficiência de um dos três pigmentos primários dos cones da retina. VER protanomaly, deuteranomaly, tritanomaly.

tri·chro·ma·top·sia (trī-krō'mă-top'sē-ă). Tricromatopsia; visão normal para cores; a capacidade de perceber as três cores primárias. [tri- + G. *chrōma,* cor, + *opsis,* visão]

tri·chro·mic (trī-krō'mik). Tricrômico. SIN trichromatic.

trich·ter·brust (tricht'er-broost). Tórax em funil, peito escavado. SIN *pectus excavatum.* [Alemão *Trichterbrust,* tórax em funil]

trich·u·ri·a·sis (tri-koo-rī'ă-sis). Tricuríase; infecção por nematódeos do gênero *Trichuris.* Nos seres humanos, o parasitismo intestinal por *T. trichiura* é habitualmente assintomático e não está associado a eosinofilia periférica; nas infecções maciças, induz freqüentemente diarréia ou prolapso retal.

Trich·u·ris (tri-koo'ris). Gênero de nematódeos afasmídeos (algumas vezes inadequadamente denominados *Trichocephalus*), relacionados ao verme *Trichinella spiralis:* possuem um corpo com uma porção anterior alongada e delgada, que penetra na mucosa do cólon ou do intestino grosso do hospedeiro, e uma porção posterior espessa que carrega os órgãos reprodutivos e seus produtos. T. contém cerca de 70 espécies, todas elas encontradas em mamíferos. [tricho- + *oura,* cauda]

T. suis, espécie de nematódeo encontrada no porco; os vermes adultos já foram encontrados em seres humanos.

T. trichiu'ra, espécie que causa tricuríase; o corpo é filiforme e delgado nos três quintos anteriores e mais robusto posteriormente; as fêmeas têm 4 ou 5 cm de comprimento, e os machos são mais curtos (com extremidade caudal espiralada e uma única espícula eversível); os ovos possuem a forma de barril, têm 50-56 μm por 20-22 μm, com casca dupla e protuberâncias translúcidas em cada um dos dois pólos; os seres humanos são os únicos hospedeiros suscetíveis e, em geral, adquirem a infecção por contato direto dos dedos da mão com a boca ou por ingestão de solo, água ou alimento contendo ovos com larvas (o desenvolvimento no solo leva 3-6 semanas em condições apropriadas de calor e umidade, explicando a distribuição principalmente tropical do verme); as larvas saem dos ovos no íleo, amadurecem em cerca de um mês e, a seguir, passam diretamente para o ceco sem sofrer migração parenteral, como ocorre com o *Ascaris lumbricoides;* os adultos podem persistir durante 2-7 anos.

T. vulpis, espécie de nematódeo encontrada no cão; o verme adulto sexualmente maduro já foi encontrado no apêndice de seres humanos.

tri·cip·i·tal (trī-sip'i-tăl). Tricipital; que possui três cabeças; designa um músculo tríceps.

tri·clo·bi·so·ni·um chlo·ride (trī'klō-bi-sō-nē-ŭm). Cloreto de triclobisônio; composto de amônio biquaternário utilizado topicamente no tratamento de infecções superficiais da pele e da vagina; anti-séptico catiônico efetivo contra microrganismos Gram-negativos e Gram-positivos. É inativado por sabão e por alterações do pH.

tri·clo·fen·ol pi·per·a·zine (trī-klō'fen-ol). Triclofenol piperazina; anti-helmíntico.

tri·clo·fos (trī'klō-fōs). Triclofos; derivado fosforilado do hidrato de cloral, hidrolisado a hidrato de cloral no organismo, e que produz propriedades sedativo-hipnóticas características.

tri·corn (trī'kōrn). **1.** Um dos ventrículos laterais do cérebro. **2.** Tricorne. SIN tricornute. [tri- + L. *cornu,* corno]

tri·cor·nute (trī-kōr'noot). Tricorne; que possui três cornos. SIN tricorn (2). [tri- + L. *cornutus,* cornudo, de *cornu,* corno]

tri·cre·sol (trī-krē'sol). Tricresol. SIN cresol.

tri·crot·ic (trī-krot'ik). Tricrótico; que bate três vezes; caracterizado por três ondas no traçado do pulso arterial. SIN tricrotous. [tri- + G. *krotos,* batimento]

tri·cro·tism (trī'krō-tizm). Tricrotismo; condição de ser tricrótico.

tri·cro·tous (trī'krō-tŭs). Tricroto. SIN tricrotic.

Tric·u·la (trik'ū-lă). Gênero de caramujos operculados de água doce relacionado a *Oncomelania* (os hospedeiros intermediários do *Schistosoma japonicum*) da subfamília Triculinae, família Hydrobiidae, subclasse Prosobranchiata; inclui *T. aperta,* hospedeiro intermediário do *Schistosoma mekongi.*

tri·cus·pid, tri·cus·pi·dal, tri·cus·pi·date (trī-kŭs'pid, -kŭs'pi-dăl, -kŭs'pi-dāt). Tricúspide. **1.** Que possui três pontas, saliências ou cúspides, como a valva tricúspide do coração. **2.** Que possui três tubérculos ou cúspides, como o segundo dente molar superior (ocasionalmente) e o terceiro molar superior (habitualmente). SIN trituberculuar.

tri·cy·cla·mol chlo·ride (trī-sī'klă-mol). Cloreto de triciclamol. SIN procyclidine methochloride.

tri·dac·ty·lous (trī-dak'ti-lŭs). Tridáctilo, tridátilo. SIN tridigitate.

tri·dent (trī'dent). Tridente, tridentado. SIN tridentate.

tri·den·tate (trī-den'tāt). Tridentado; tridenteado; com três dentes; três saliências. SIN trident. [tri- + L. *dentatus,* denteado]

tri·der·mic (trī-der'mik). Tridérmico; relativo a ou derivado das três camadas germinativas primárias do embrião: ectoderma, endoderma e mesoderma. [tri- + G. *derma,* pele]

tri·der·mo·ma (trī-der-mō'mă). Tridermoma. SIN triphyllomatous teratoma. [tri- + G. *derma,* pele, + *-oma,* tumor]

tri·dig·i·tate (trī-dij'i-tāt). Tridáctilo; que possui três dedos das mãos ou dos pés em uma mão ou pé. SIN tridactylous. [tri- + L. *digitus,* dedo]

tri·di·hex·eth·yl chlo·ride (trī'dī-heks-eth'il). Cloreto de tridi-hexetil; agente anticolinérgico.

trid·y·mite (trid'i-mīt). Tridimita; forma de sílica empregada no revestimento de modelo dentário. [do G. *tridymos,* três vezes]

trid·y·mus (trid'i-mŭs). Trídimo. SIN triplet (1). [L. do G. *tridymos,* três vezes]

tri·el·con (trī-el'kon). Trielcon; pinça longa de três pontas para extração de corpos estranhos de feridas ou canais. [tri- + G. *helkō,* retirar]

tri·en·tine hy·dro·chlo·ride (trī'en-tēn). Cloridrato de trientina; agente quelante utilizado para remover o excesso de cobre do organismo na doença de Wilson. SIN triethylenetetramine dihydrochloride.

tri·eth·a·nol·a·mine (trī'eth-ă-nol'ă-mēn). Trietanolamina; mistura de mono-, di- e trietanolamina utilizada como agente emulsificante no preparo de pomadas e loções medicamentosas e como auxiliar na absorção desses medicamentos através da pele.

tri·eth·yl·ene gly·col (trī-eth'i-lēn). Trietilenoglicol; utilizado no estado de vapor como agente esterilizante do ar; tóxico para bactérias, fungos e vírus em concentrações muito baixas no ar; as variações na umidade do ar limitam a efetividade germicida.

tri·eth·yl·ene·mel·a·mine (TEM) (trī-eth'i-lēn-mel'ă-mēn). Trietilenomelamina; agente antineoplásico quimicamente relacionado com as mostardas nitrogenadas; utilizado no tratamento da leucemia.

tri·eth·yl·ene·phos·phor·a·mide (TEPA) (trī-eth'i-lēn-fos-fōr'ă-mīd). Trietilenofosforamida; droga com as mesmas ações e usos que a trietilenomelamina no tratamento das leucemias.

tri·eth·yl·ene·tet·ra·mine di·hy·dro·chlo·ride (trī-eth′i-lēn-tet′ră-am′ēn). Dicloridrato de trietilenotetramina. SIN trientine hydrochloride.

tri·eth·yl·ene·thi·o·phos·phor·a·mide (trī-eth′i-lēn-thī′ō-fos-fōr′ă-mīd). Trietilenotiofosforamida; agente alquilante utilizado no tratamento paliativo de doenças malignas como leucemia, linfoma e carcinoma. SIN thiotepa.

tri·fa·cial (trī-fā′shăl). Trifacial; designa o quinto par de nervos cranianos, o nervo trigêmeo. [tri- + L. *facies,* face]

tri·fid (trī′fid). Trífido, trigêmino; dividido em três. [L. *trifidus,* com três fendas]

tri·flu·o·per·a·zine hy·dro·chlo·ride (trī′floo-ō-per′ă-zēn). Cloridrato de trifluoperazina; agente antipsicótico do tipo fenotiazínico.

tri·flu·o·ro·ace·tyl (trī-flur′ō-as′ē-til). Trifluoroacetil; grupamento utilizado para proteger os componentes amino de aminoácidos e peptídios durante a síntese de peptídios.

2,2,2-tri·flu·o·ro·ethyl·vi·nyl (trī-flōr-ō-eth′il). 2,2,2-trifluoroetilvinil. SIN fluroxene.

5-tri·flu·o·ro·meth·yl·de·ox·y·u·ri·dine (trī-flōr′ō-meth′il-dē-ok-si-ū′ri-dēn). 5-trifluorometildesoxiuridina; análogo da pirimidina utilizado topicamente no tratamento da ceratite do herpes simples.

tri·flu·per·i·dol hy·dro·chlo·ride (trī-floo-per′i-dol). Cloridrato de trifluperidol; tranqüilizante.

tri·flu·pro·ma·zine hy·dro·chlo·ride (trī-floo-prō′mă-zēn). Cloridrato de triflupromazina; antipsicótico estreitamente relacionado dos pontos de vista químico e farmacológico à clorpromazina.

tri·flur·i·dine (trī-floor′i-dēn). Trifluridina; agente antiviral utilizado na forma de colírio para tratamento do herpes simples ocular.

tri·fo·cal (trī′fō-kăl). Trifocal; que possui três focos. VER trifocal *lens.*

tri·fur·ca·tion (trī-fur-kā′shŭn). Trifurcação. 1. Divisão em três ramos. 2. A área onde a raiz do dente se divide em três porções distintas. [tri- + L. *furca,* garfo]

tri·gas·tric (trī-gas′trik). Trigástrico; que possui três ventres; designa um músculo com duas interrupções tendíneas. [tri- + G. *gastēr,* ventre]

tri·gem·i·nal (trī-jem′i-năl). Trigeminal; relativo ao quinto nervo craniano ou nervo trigêmeo. SIN trigeminus. [L. *trigeminus,* três vezes]

tri·gem·i·nus (trī-jem′i-nŭs). Trigêmeo. SIN trigeminal. [L. três vezes, de tri- + *geminus,* gêmeo]

tri·gem·i·ny (trī-jem′i-nē). Trigeminismo. SIN trigeminal *rhythm.* [L. *trigeminus,* três vezes]

trig·e·nol·line (trig-ĕ-nol′ēn). Trigenolina. SIN trigonelline.

trig·ger (trig′er). Deflagrador; termo que descreve um sistema em que um estímulo relativamente pequeno transforma-se numa resposta relativamente grande, cuja magnitude não está relacionada com a magnitude do estímulo.
ECG t., d. ECG; uso do eletrocardiograma, geralmente a onda R, para controlar eletronicamente algum aparelho de registro ou imagem. VER cardiac *gating.* SIN EKG t.
EKG t., d. ECG. SIN ECG t.

tri·glyc·er·ide (trī-glis′er-īd). Triglicerídio. SIN triacylglycerol.

tri·go·na (trī-gō′nă). Trígonos; plural de trigonum. [L.]

trig·o·nal (trig′ō-năl). Trigonal; triangular; relativo a um trígono.

tri·gone (trī′gōn). Trígono. 1. SIN trigonum. 2. As três primeiras cúspides dominantes (protocone, paracone e metacone), consideradas coletivamente, de um dente molar superior. [L. *trigonum,* do G. *trigōnon,* triângulo]
t. of auditory nerve, t. do nervo vestibulococlear; discreta proeminência do assoalho do recesso lateral do quarto ventrículo, que corresponde aos núcleos coclear e vestibular subjacentes. SIN acoustic tubercle, trigonum nervi acustici.
t. of bladder [TA], t. da bexiga; área lisa triangular na base da bexiga, entre as aberturas dos dois ureteres e a da uretra. SIN trigonum vesicae [TA], Lieutaud body, Lieutaud triangle, Lieutaud t., vesical triangle.
cerebral t., fórnice. SIN fornix.
collateral t. [TA], t. colateral; proeminência triangular do assoalho do ventrículo lateral, na transição entre o corno occipital e o corno temporal, contínua rostralmente com a eminência colateral e, como esta última, causada pela penetração profunda do sulco colateral a partir da superfície ventral do lobo temporal. SIN trigonum collaterale [TA], t. of lateral ventricle, trigonum ventriculi, ventricular t.
deltoideopectoral t., t. clavipeitoral. SIN clavipectoral *triangle.*
fibrous t.'s of heart, trígonos fibrosos do coração. SIN right fibrous t. (of heart), left fibrous t. (of heart).
t. of fillet, t. do lemnisco lateral. SIN t. of lateral lemniscus.
t. of habenula, t. habenular. SIN habenular t.
habenular t. [TA], t. habenular; pequena área triangular na superfície dorsomedial do tálamo, na extremidade caudal da estria medular, correspondente à habênula subjacente. SIN trigonum habenulae [TA], t. of habenula.
hypoglossal t. [TA], t. do nervo hipoglosso; ligeira elevação no assoalho do recesso inferior do quarto ventrículo, sob a qual está o núcleo de origem do décimo segundo nervo craniano. SIN trigonum nervi hypoglossi [TA], t. of hypoglossal nerve*, eminentia hypoglossi; hypoglossal eminence, trigonum hypoglossi, tuberculum hypoglossi.
t. of hypoglossal nerve, t. do nervo hipoglosso; *termo oficial alternativo para hypoglossal t.
inguinal t., t. inguinal. SIN inguinal *triangle.*
t. of lateral lemniscus [TA], t. do lemnisco lateral; área triangular na superfície lateral da metade caudal do mesencéfalo, limitada caudalmente pela discreta proeminência do lemnisco lateral, dorsalmente pela base do colículo inferior e braço do colículo superior e ventralmente pelo pilar do cérebro. SIN lemniscal t., Reil triangle, triangle of fillet, t. of fillet.
t. of lateral ventricle, t. do ventrículo lateral. SIN collateral t.
left fibrous t. (of heart), t. fibroso esquerdo (do coração); a parte do esqueleto fibroso do coração localizada no intervalo entre o lado esquerdo do anel atrioventricular esquerdo e o anel aórtico. SIN trigonum fibrosum sinistrum.
lemniscal t., t. do lemnisco lateral. SIN t. of lateral lemniscus.
Lieutaud t., t. de Lieutaud. SIN t. of bladder.
Müller t., t. de Müller; o assoalho do recesso supra-óptico do terceiro ventrículo.
olfactory t. [TA], t. olfatório; área triangular acinzentada que corresponde à fixação do pedúnculo olfatório ("nervo olfatório" ou trato olfatório) à base do cérebro, na borda anterior da substância perfurada anterior. SIN trigonum olfactorium [TA].
right fibrous t. (of heart) [TA], t. fibroso direito (do coração); parte do esqueleto fibroso do coração, localizada entre o anel fibroso aórtico e os anéis que circundam os óstios atrioventriculares direito e esquerdo. SIN trigonum fibrosum dextrum.
vagal (nerve) t. [TA], t. do nervo vago; proeminência no assoalho da fóvea inferior do quarto ventrículo, sobrejacente ao núcleo motor dorsal do vago. SIN trigonum nervi vagi [TA], t. of vagus nerve*, trigonum vagale*, ala cinerea, ashen wing, gray wing, vagi eminentia.
t. of vagus nerve, t. do nervo vago; * termo oficial alternativo para vagal (nerve) t.
ventricular t., t. colateral. SIN collateral t.
vertebrocostal t., t. lombocostal do diafragma. SIN lumbocostal *triangle* of diaphragm.

trig·o·nel·line (trig-ō-nel′ēn). Trigonelina; a metil betaína do ácido nicotínico; produto do metabolismo do ácido nicotínico; excretada na urina. SIN caffearine, trigenolline.

tri·go·nid (trī-gon′id, -gō′nid). Trigônide; as três primeiras cúspides dominantes, consideradas em conjunto, de um dente molar inferior. VER TAMBÉM trigone.

tri·go·ni·tis (trī′gō-nī′tis). Trigonite; inflamação da bexiga, localizada no trígono. [trigone + G. *-itis,* inflamação]

trig·o·no·ce·phal·ic (trig′ō-nō-se-fal′ik). Trigonocefálico; relativo à trigonocefalia.

trig·o·no·ceph·a·ly (trig′ō-nō-sef′ă-lē, trī′gō-nō-). Trigonocefalia; malformação caracterizada por uma configuração triangular do crânio, decorrente, em parte, de sinostose prematura dos ossos do crânio, com compressão dos hemisférios cerebrais. [trigone + G. *kephalē,* cabeça]

tri·go·num, pl. **tri·go·na** (trī-gō′nŭm, -nă). [TA]. Trígono; qualquer área triangular. VER triangle. SIN trigone (1) [TA]. [L., do G. *trigōnon,* triângulo]
t. auscultationis [TA], triângulo auscultatório. SIN auscultatory *triangle.*
t. carot′icum [TA], t. carótico. SIN carotid *triangle.*
t. cerebra′le, fórnice. SIN fornix (2).
t. cervica′le, t. cervical; qualquer um dos triângulos do pescoço. SIN t. colli.
t. cervica′le ante′rius, t. cervical anterior; *termo oficial alternativo para anterior cervical *region.*
t. cervica′le poste′rius, t. cervical posterior; *termo oficial alternativo para lateral cervical *region.*
t. clavipectorale [TA], t. clavipeitoral. SIN clavipectoral *triangle.*
t. collatera′le [TA], t. colateral. SIN collateral *trigone.*
t. col′li, t. cervical. SIN t. cervicale.
t. colli anterius, t. cervical anterior; *termo oficial alternativo para anterior cervical *region.*
t. colli laterale, t. cervical lateral; *termo oficial alternativo para lateral cervical *region.*
t. cystohepaticum [TA], triângulo cisto-hepático. SIN cystohepatic *triangle.*
t. deltoideopectora′le [TA], t. clavipeitoral. SIN clavipectoral *triangle.*
t. deltopectorale, t. clavipeitoral; *termo oficial alternativo para clavipectoral *triangle.*
t. femora′le [TA], t. femoral. SIN femoral *triangle.*
t. femoris, t. femoral; *termo oficial alternativo para femoral *triangle.*
trigo′na fibro′sa cor′dis, trígonos fibrosos do coração. VER right fibrous *trigone* (of heart), left fibrous *trigone* (of heart).
t. fibro′sum dex′trum, t. fibroso direito (do coração). SIN right fibrous *trigone* (of heart).
t. fibro′sum sinis′trum, t. fibroso esquerdo (do coração). SIN left fibrous *trigone* (of heart).
t. haben′ulae [TA], t. habenular. SIN habenular *trigone.*
t. hypoglos′si, t. do nervo hipoglosso. SIN hypoglossal *trigone.*

t. inguina'le [TA], t. inguinal. SIN inguinal triangle.
t. lemnis'ci lateralis [TA], t. do lemnisco lateral. SIN trigone of lateral lemniscus.
t. lumba'le inferius [TA], t. lombar. SIN inferior lumbar triangle.
t. lumbocosta'le diaphragmatis [TA], t. lombocostal do diafragma. SIN lumbocostal triangle of diaphragm.
t. muscula're (regionis cervicalis anterioris) [TA], t. muscular (região cervical anterior). SIN muscular triangle (of neck).
t. nervi acus'tici, t. do nervo vestibulococlear (VIII). SIN trigone of auditory nerve.
t. ner'vi hypoglos'si [TA], t. do nervo hipoglosso. SIN hypoglossal trigone.
t. ner'vi va'gi [TA], t. do nervo vago. SIN vagal (nerve) trigone.
t. olfacto'rium [TA], t. olfatório. SIN olfactory trigone.
t. omoclavicula're [TA], t. omoclavicular. SIN supraclavicular triangle.
t. omotrachea'le, t. omotraqueal; *termo oficial alternativo para muscular triangle (of neck).
t. pala'ti, t. do palato. SIN palatal triangle.
t. parietale laterale pelvis [TA], t. parietal lateral da pelve. SIN lateral pelvic wall triangle.
t. retromolare [TA], t. retromolar. SIN retromolar triangle.
t. sternocosta'le, t. esternocostal; defeito muscular no diafragma entre as porções costal e esternal. SIN Larrey cleft, sternocostal triangle.
t. sternocostale diaphragmatis [TA], t. esternocostal do diafragma. SIN sternocostal triangle (of diaphragm).
t. submandibula're [TA], t. submandibular. SIN submandibular triangle.
t. submenta'le [TA], t. submentual. SIN submental triangle.
t. vagale, t. do nervo vago; *termo oficial alternativo para vagal (nerve) trigone.
t. ventric'uli, t. colateral. SIN collateral trigone.
t. vesi'cae [TA], t. da bexiga. SIN trigone of bladder.
tri·hex·o·syl·cer·a·mide. Triexosilceramida. SIN globotriaosylceramide.
tri·hex·y·phen·i·dyl hy·dro·chlo·ride (trī-heks′ē-fen′ĭ-dil). Cloridrato de triexifenil; agente anticolinérgico sintético que se acredita exerça maior grau de atividade anticolinérgica no cérebro em comparação com as junções neuroefetoras parassimpáticas periféricas. Amplamente utilizado no tratamento do parkinsonismo secundário a parkinsonismo idiopático ou induzido por neurolépticos.
tri·hy·brid (trī-hī′brid). Tri-híbrido; a prole de pais que diferem em três caracteres mendelianos. [tri- + L. hybrida, híbrido]
tri·hy·dric (trī-hī′drik). Tri-hídrico; designa um composto químico que contém três átomos de hidrogênio substituíveis.
tri·hy·drox·y·es·trin (trī′hī-drok′sē-es′trin). Tri-hidroxiestrina. SIN estriol.
tri·in·i·od·y·mus (trī-in′i-od′i-mŭs). Triiniódimo; feto flagrantemente malformado com três cabeças unidas no occipúcio e um único corpo. [tri- + G. inion, nuca do pescoço, + didymos, gêmeo]
tri·i·o·dide (trī-ī′ō-dīd, -dĭd). Triiodeto; iodeto com três átomos de iodo na molécula; p. ex., KI₃.
tri·i·o·do·meth·ane (trī-ī′ō-dō-meth′ān). Triiodometano. SIN iodoform.
3,5,3′-tri·i·o·do·thy·ro·nine (TITh, T₃) (trī-ī′ō-dō-thī′rō-nēn). 3,5,3′-triiodotironina (TITh, T₃); hormônio tireóideo normalmente sintetizado em menores quantidades do que a tiroxina; presente no sangue e na glândula tireóide, exerce os mesmos efeitos biológicos que a tiroxina, porém, numa base molecular, é mais potente, com início mais rápido dos efeitos.
tri·ke·to·hy·drin·dene hy·drate (trī-kē-tō-hī′drin-dēn). Hidrato de tricetoidrindeno; designação antiga da ninidrina.
tri·ke·to·pu·rine (trī-kē-tō-pūr′ēn). Tricetopurina. SIN uric acid.
tri·labe (trī′lāb). Trilábio; pinça de três dentes para remoção de corpos estranhos da bexiga. [tri- + G. labē, cabo]
tri·lam·i·nar (trī-lam′i-nar). Trilaminar; que possui três lâminas.
tri·lat·er·al (trī-lat′ĕ-răl). Trilateral; que possui três lados.
tri·lo·bate, tri·lobed (trī-lō′bāt, trī′bobd). Trilobado; que possui três lobos.
tri·loc·u·lar (trī-lok′ū-lăr). Trilocular; que possui três cavidades ou células.
tril·o·gy (tril′ō-jē). Trilogia; tríade de entidades relacionadas. [G. trilogia, de tri- + logos, estudo, discurso]
t. of Fallot, t. de Fallot; conjunto de defeitos congênitos incluindo estenose pulmonar, defeito do septo interatrial e hipertrofia do ventrículo direito. SIN Fallot triad.
tri·lo·stane (trī′lō-stān). Trilostano; inibidor dos esteróides supra-renais utilizado para melhorar a hiperfunção supra-renal na síndrome de Cushing.
tri·mas·ti·gote (trī-mas′ti-gōt). Trimastigota; que possui três flagelos, conforme observado em determinados protozoários. [tri- + G. mastix, chicote]
tri·mep·ra·zine tar·trate (trī-mep′ra-zēn). Tartarato de trimeprazina; composto fenotiazínico relacionado, dos pontos de vista químico e farmacológico, com a promazina, porém com ação antagonista da histamina mais pronunciada; utilizado para alívio sintomático do prurido.
trim·er (trī′mer). Trímero; composto, complexo ou estrutura constituído de três componentes.
tri·mes·ter (trī′mes-ter, trī-mes′ter); Trimestre; período de 3 meses; um terço da duração de uma gravidez. [L. trimestris, de três meses de duração]

tri·met·a·phan cam·sy·late (trī-met′ă-fan). Cansilato de trimetafano. SIN trimethaphan camsylate.
tri·me·taz·i·dine (trī-me-taz′i-dēn). Trimetazidina; vasodilatador coronariano.
tri·meth·a·di·one (trī′meth-ă-dī′ōn). Trimetadiona; anticonvulsivante que está caindo em desuso, empregado no tratamento das crises de ausência (pequeno mal) e epilepsia psicomotora. SIN troxidone.
tri·meth·a·phan cam·sy·late (trī-meth′ă-fan). Cansilato de trimetafano; agente bloqueador ganglionar que provoca vasodilatação fugaz; utilizado em cirurgia, sobretudo neurocirurgia, para produzir um campo operatório relativamente sem sangue (hipotensão controlada). SIN trimetaphan camsylate.
tri·meth·i·di·um meth·o·sul·fate (trī-me-thid′ē-ŭm meth-ō-sŭl′fat). Metossulfato de trimetídio; composto de amônio quaternário que bloqueia a transmissão ganglionar nos gânglios simpáticos e parassimpáticos; utilizado no tratamento da hipertensão grave.
tri·meth·o·benz·a·mide hy·dro·chlo·ride (trī′meth-ō-ben′ză-mīd). Cloridrato de trimetobenzamida; antiemético.
tri·meth·o·prim (trī-meth′ō-prim). Trimetoprima; agente antimicrobiano que potencializa o efeito das sulfonamidas e sulfonas; em geral associado a sulfametoxazol.
tri·meth·o·prim-sul·fa·meth·ox·a·zole. Trimetoprima-sulfametoxazol; combinação farmacológica que consiste num inibidor da diidrofolato redutase (trimetoprima) e um agente antibacteriano sulfonamida (sulfametoxazol). A combinação é sinérgica, visto que os fármacos interferem em duas etapas sucessivas na formação/utilização do ácido fólico por microrganismos. Combinação utilizada no tratamento de muitas doenças infecciosas.
tri·meth·yl·a·mine (trī-meth′il-am′ēn). Trimetilamina; produto de decomposição, freqüentemente por putrefação, de substâncias vegetais e animais nitrogenadas, como resíduos do açúcar de beterraba ou arenque em salmoura; no corpo, resulta provavelmente da decomposição da colina.
tri·meth·yl·am·i·nur·ia (trī-meth′il-am-i-noor′ē-ă). Trimetilaminúria; aumento da excreção de trimetilamina na urina e no suor, com característico odor corporal de peixe fétido.
tri·meth·yl·car·bin·ol (trī-meth′il-kar′bin-ol). Trimetilcarbinol; álcool butílico terciário. VER butyl alcohol.
tri·meth·yl·ene (trī-meth′il-ēn). Trimetileno. SIN cyclopropane.
tri·meth·yl·eth·yl·ene (trī-meth-il-eth′il-ēn). Trimetiletileno. SIN amylene.
N^ε-**tri·meth·yl·ly·sine** (trī-meth-il-lī-sēn). N^ε-trimetilisina; resíduo aminoácido encontrado em diversas proteínas pela ação da S-adenosil-L-metionina sobre resíduos de L-lisil; com liberação por proteólise, a N^ε-trimetilisina torna-se o precursor da carnitina.
tri·meth·y·lo·mel·a·mine (trī′meth-i-lō-mel′ă-mēn). Trimetilomelamina; agente antineoplásico.
tri·met·o·zine (trī-met′ō-zēn). Trimetozina; agente ansiolítico.
tri·me·trex·ate (trī-me-treks′āt). Trimetrexato; agente antineoplásico e droga órfão antiprotozoário utilizado no tratamento da pneumonia por *Pneumocystis carinii* em pacientes com AIDS–SIDA.
tri·mip·ra·mine (trī-mip′ra-mēn). Trimipramina; antidepressivo.
tri·mor·phic (trī-mōr′fik). Trimórfico. SIN trimorphous.
tri·mor·phism (trī-mōr′fizm). Trimorfismo; existência em três formas, como nos insetos holometabólicos que passam pelos estágios de larva, pupa e imago. [tri- + G. morphē, forma]
tri·mor·phous (trī-mōr′fŭs). Trimórfico; que existe em três formas; caracterizado por trimorfismo. SIN trimorphic.
tri·ni·tro·cel·lu·lose (trī′nī-trō-sel′ū-lōs). Trinitrocelulose; constituinte do algodão-pólvora solúvel; utilizada no preparo de colódio e de piroxilina.
tri·ni·tro·glyc·er·in (trī′nī-trō-glis′ĕ-rin). Trinitroglicerina. SIN nitroglycerin.
tri·ni·tro·tol·u·ene (TNT) (trī′nī-trō-tol′ū-ēn). Trinitrotolueno; explosivo produzido por nitrificação do tolueno; causa distúrbios gástricos e intestinais e dermatite em trabalhadores de fábricas de munição. SIN trinitrotoluol.
tri·ni·tro·tol·u·ol (trī′nī-trō-tol′ū-ol). Trinitrotoluol. SIN trinitrotoluene.
tri·nu·cle·o·tide (trī-noo′klē-ō-tīd). Trinucleotídio; combinação de três nucleotídios adjacentes, livres ou numa molécula de polinucleotídio ou de ácido nucléico; termo freqüentemente utilizado com referência específica à unidade (códon ou anticódon) que especifica um determinado aminoácido na expressão do código genético.
tri·o·ki·nase (trī-ō-kī′nās). Triocinase; fosfotransferase que catalisa a fosforilação do D-gliceraldeído pelo ATP para produzir D-gliceraldeído 3-fosfato e ADP; participa numa etapa do metabolismo da D-frutose. SIN triosekinase.
tri·ol (trī-ol). Triol; composto que contém três grupamentos hidroxila; p. ex., glicerol.
tri·o·le·in (trī-ō′lē-in). Trioleína. SIN olein.
tri·oph·thal·mos (trī-of-thal′mos). Trioftalmo; gêmeos unidos com fusão na região facial, de modo que existe um olho comum nos lados unidos; uma variedade de ofodídimo. VER conjoined twins, em twin. [tri- + G. ophthalmos, olho]

tri·or·chism (trī-ōr′kizm). Triorquismo; condição de possuir três testículos (triórquido).

tri·orth·o·cres·yl phos·phate (TOCP) (trī′-ōr-thō-kres′il). Triortocresil fosfato; triaril fosfato; produz neurotoxicidade tardia. Ocorreu um incidente notório quando apareceu como adulterante no gengibre-da-jamaica e foi responsável por milhares de casos de paralisia durante o período da Lei Seca.

tri·ose (trī′ōs). Triose; monossacarídio com três carbonos; p. ex., gliceraldeído e diidroxiacetona.

tri·ose ki·nase (trī′ōs-kī′nās). Triosecinase. SIN triokinase.

tri·ose phos·phate isom·er·ase (trī′ōs-fos′fāt). Triose fosfato isomerase; enzima isomerizante que catalisa a interconversão reversível do D-gliceraldeído 3-fosfato e do diidroxiacetona fosfato, uma importante reação na glicólise e gliconeogênese; a deficiência dessa enzima resulta em anemia hemolítica e graves déficits neurológicos. SIN phosphotriose isomerase.

tri·o·tus (trī-ō′tŭs). Trioto; diprosopo que apresenta três orelhas. [tri- + G. *ous*, orelha]

tri·ox·ide (trī-oks′īd). Trióxido; molécula que contém três átomos de oxigênio. SIN teroxide.

tri·ox·sa·len (trī-ok′sa-len). Trioxsaleno; agente fotossensibilizante de pigmentação efetivo; utilizado como bronzeador e no tratamento do vitiligo.

tri·ox·y·meth·yl·ene (trī′ok-sē-meth′i-lēn). Trioximetileno. SIN paraformaldehyde.

tri·pal·mi·tin (trī-pal′mi-tin). Tripalmitina. SIN palmitin.

tri·par·a·nol (trī-par′a-nol). Triparanol; outrora utilizado como inibidor da biossíntese de colesterol, porém retirado do mercado norte-americano pela sua capacidade de promover a formação de cataratas.

tri·pel·en·na·mine hy·dro·chlo·ride (trī-pĕ-len′a-mēn). Cloridrato de tripelenamina; anti-histamínico. O citrato cloridrato de tripelenamina é também disponível, com as mesmas ações; é menos amargo do que o sal cloridrato e, portanto, é utilizado como elixir.

tri·pep·tid·ases (trī-pep′ti-dās-es). Tripeptidases; classe de enzimas com diferentes especificidades que catalisa a hidrólise de tripeptídios, produzindo um dipeptídio e um aminoácido.

tri·pep·tide (trī-pep′tīd). Tripeptídio; composto que contém três aminoácidos unidos por ligações peptídicas.

tri·pha·lan·gia (trī-fā-lan′jē-ā). Tripalangia; malformação em que existem três falanges no polegar ou no hálux. [tri- + phalanx]

Tripier, Léon, cirurgião francês, 1842–1891. VER T. *amputation.*

tri·plant (trī′plant). Implante tríplice. Ver triplant *implant.*

tri·ple·gia (trī-plē′jē-ā). Triplegia. **1.** Paralisia de três membros, com ambas as extremidades de um lado e um do outro lado. **2.** Paralisia de um membro superior e inferior e da face. [tri- + G. *plēgē*, golpe]

trip·let. Trípleto. **1.** Uma das três crianças nascidas no mesmo parto. SIN tridymus. **2.** Conjunto de três objetos semelhantes, como uma lente composta num microscópio, formada de três lentes planoconvexas. **3.** SIN codon.
nonsense t., t. sem sentido; **(1)** trinucleotídio (códon) em que uma alteração de base num códon de terminação resulta na interrupção prematura da cadeia polipeptídica em crescimento e, consequentemente, em moléculas incompletas de proteína; **(2)** códon de terminação.

trip·lo·blas·tic (trip-lō-blas′tik). Triploblástico; formado pelas três camadas germinativas primárias (ectoderma, mesoderma, endoderma) ou que contém tecido derivado de todas as três camadas. [G. *triploos*, três vezes, + *blastos*, germe]

trip·loid (trip′loyd). Triplóide; relativo a ou característico de triploidia. [tri- + -ploid]

trip·loi·dy (trip′loy-dē). Triploidia; a presença de três conjuntos haplóides de cromossomas, em lugar de dois, em todas as células; resulta em morte fetal ou neonatal.

trip·lo·pia (trip-lō′pē-ā). Triplopia; defeito visual em que são vistas três imagens do mesmo objeto. SIN triple vision. [G. *triploos*, triplo, + *opsis*, visão]

tri·pod (trī′pod). Trípode. **1.** Que possui três pernas. **2.** Banco que possui três pernas ou suportes. [G. *tripous*, de tri- + *pous*, pé]
Haller t., t. de Haller. SIN celiac (arterial) *trunk.*
vital t., t. vital; o cérebro, o coração e os pulmões, considerados os três órgãos essenciais à vida.

tri·po·dia (trī-pō′dē-ā). Tripodia; condição observada em gêmeos unidos em que os membros inferiores dos lados unidos formam um único pé, de modo que existem apenas três pés para os dois corpos. VER conjoined *twins,* em *twin.* [tri- + G. *pous*, pé]

tri·prol·i·dine hy·dro·chlo·ride (trī-prol′i-dēn). Cloridrato de triprolidina; anti-histamínico H₁ utilizado no tratamento de condições alérgicas e pruriginosas.

tri·pro·so·pus (trī′prō-sō′pŭs). Triprosopo; feto com três cabeças unidas, deixando apenas partes de três faces. [tri- + G. *prosōpon*, face]

trip·sis (trip′sis). Tripse. **1.** SIN trituration (1). **2.** SIN massage. [G. fricção]

tri·que·trous (trī-kwē′trŭs, -kwet-). Tríquetro, triangular, que tem três ângulos. [L. *triquetrus*, que possui três cantos]

tri·que·trum (trī-kwē′trŭm, -kwet-) [TA]. Piramidal; osso do lado medial (ulnar) da fileira proximal do carpo que se articula com os ossos semilunar, fisiforme e hamato. SIN os triquetrum [TA], cubital bone, os pyramidale, os triangulare, pyramidal bone, pyramidale, three-cornered bone, triquetrum bone. [L. *triquetrus*, que possui três cantos]

tri·ra·di·al, tri·ra·di·ate (trī-rā′dē-ăl, trī-rā′dē-āt). Trirradiado; que se irradia em três direções.

tri·ra·di·us (trī-rā′dē-ŭs). Trirrádio; em dermatoglifos, a figura na base de cada dedo da palma da mão, produzida por fileiras de papilas que correm em três direções, formando um ângulo. SIN Galton delta (2).

Tris Abreviatura de tris(hydroxymethyl)aminomethane (tris(hidroximetil)aminometano) e tris(hydroxymethyl)methylamine (tris(hidroximetil)metilamina); utilizado como nome trivial.

tris-. Tris-; prefixo químico que indica três dos substituintes que se seguem, ligados independentemente. Cf. tri-.

tri·sac·cha·ride (trī-sak′a-rīd). Trissacarídio; carboidrato que contém três resíduos de monossacarídio, p. ex., rafinose.

tris(hy·drox·y·meth·yl)a·mi·no·meth·ane (Tris). Tris(hidroximetil)aminometano. SIN tromethamine.

tris(hy·drox·y·meth·yl)meth·yl·a·mine (Tris). Tris(hidroximetil)metilamina. SIN tromethamine.

tris·kai·dek·a·pho·bia (tris′kī-dek-ā-fō′bē-ā). Triscaidecafobia; medo supersticioso do número 13. [G. *triskaideka*, treze, + *phobos*, medo]

tris·mic (triz′mik). Trísmico; relativo a ou caracterizado por trismo.

tris·moid (triz′moyd). **1.** Trismóide; semelhante ao trismo. **2.** Trismo do recém-nascido, outrora considerado uma variedade distinta, devido à pressão exercida sobre o occipúcio durante o parto. [trismus + G. *eidos*, semelhança]

tris·mus (triz′mŭs). Trismo; contração persistente dos músculos masseter, devido à falha de inibição central; com frequência, é a manifestação inicial do tétano generalizado. SIN *Ankylostoma* (2), lock-jaw, lockjaw. [L. do G. *trismos*, rangido, som irritante]
t. capistra′tus, t. amordaçado; aderência congênita das bochechas às gengivas.
t. nascen′tium, t. neonatal; rigidez dos músculos da mandíbula em recém-nascidos, geralmente como início de tétano neonatal. SIN t. neonatorium.
t. neonato′rum, t. neonatal. SIN t. nascentium.
t. sardon′icus, t. sardônico. SIN *risus caninus.*

tri·so·mic (trī-sō′mik). Trissômico; relativo à trissomia.

tri·so·my (trī′sō-mē). Trissomia; o estado de um indivíduo ou célula com um cromossoma extra, em lugar do par normal de cromossomas homólogos; nos seres humanos, o estado de uma célula que contém 47 cromossomas normais. Para os vários tipos de síndrome de trissomia, ver em *syndrome*. [tri- + (chromo)some]

tri·splanch·nic (trī-splangk′nik). Trisplâncnico; relativo às três cavidades viscerais: crânio, tórax e abdome. [tri- + G. *splanchnon*, víscera]

tri·ste·a·rin (trī-stē′a-rin). Tristearina. SIN stearin.

tri·stich·ia (trī-stik′ē-ā). Tristíquia; presença de três fileiras de cílios. [G. *tristichos*, em três fileiras, de *tri-*, três, + *stichos*, fileira]

tri·sul·cate (trī-sŭl′kāt). Trissulcado; marcado por três sulcos.

tri·ta·nom·a·ly (trī-tā-nom′a-lē). Tritanomalia; tipo de deficiência parcial para cores, devido a deficiência ou anormalidade dos cones retinianos sensíveis ao azul. [G. *tritos*, terceiro, + *anōmalia*, irregularidade]

trit·an·o·pia (trī′tā-nō′pē-ā). Tritanopia; percepção deficiente das cores, em que há ausência do pigmento sensível ao azul nos cones da retina. [G. *tritos*, terceiro, + *an-* priv. + *ōps*, olho]

tri·ter·penes (trī-ter′penz). Triterpenos; hidrocarbonetos e seus derivados formados pela condensação de seis unidades de isopreno (equivalente a três unidades de terpeno) e contendo, portanto, 30 átomos de carbono; p. ex., esqualeno, determinados esteróides, glicosídeos cardíacos.

trit·i·at·ed (trit′ē-ā-ted). Tritiado; que contém átomos de trítio (hidrogênio-3) na molécula.

ti·ti·ce·o·glos·sus (tri-tish′ē-ō-glos′ŭs). Triticeoglosso. VER *musculus* triticeoglossus. [L. *triticeum*, + G. *glossa*, língua]

tri·ti·ceous (tri-tish′ŭs). Tritíceo; semelhante a ou que possui forma semelhante a um grão de trigo. [L. *triticeus*, de *triticum*, grão de trigo]

tri·tic·e·um (tri-tish′ē-ŭm). Tritíceo. SIN triticeal *cartilage.* [L. *triticeus*, tritíceo, semelhante a um grão de trigo]

trit·i·um (T, t) (trit′ē-ŭm, trish′-). Trítio. SIN hydrogen-3.

Tri·trich·o·mon·as (trī′trik-ō-mō′nas). Gênero de protozoários flagelados parasitas que outrora faziam parte do gênero *Trichomonas* mas que são agora separados como gênero distinto pela ausência de um escudo e a presença de três flagelos anteriores. As espécies incluem *T. foetus*, que causa tricomoníase bovina, e *T. suis*, que ocorre nas vias nasais, no estômago, ceco e colo de porcos. VER TAMBÉM *Trichomonas*. [G. *tri-*, três, + *Trichomonas*]

tri·tu·ber·cu·lar (trī-too-ber′kū-lar). Tritubercular. SIN tricuspid (2).

trit·u·ra·ble (trit′ū-ra-bl). Triturável; capaz de ser triturado.

trit·u·rate (trit′ū-rāt). **1.** Triturar; realizar a trituração. **2.** Substância triturada.

tri·tu·ra·tion (trit-ū-rā'shŭn). Trituração. **1.** O ato de reduzir uma droga a um pó fino e incorporá-la totalmente com lactose por meio de atrito das duas num pilão. SIN tripsis (1). **2.** Mistura de amálgama dentário em um pilão ou com dispositivo mecânico. [L. *trituratio*, de *trituro*, triturar, de *tero*, pp. *tritus*, desgastar]

tri·tyl (trī'til). Tritil; o radical trifenilmetil, Ph₃C-.

tri·va·lence, tri·va·len·cy (trī-vā'lens, -len-sē). Trivalência; a propriedade de ser trivalente.

tri·va·lent (trī-vā'lent). Trivalente; que possui o poder de combinação (valência) de 3.

tri·valve (trī'valv). Trivalvar; que possui três valvas, como um espéculo com três lâminas divergentes.

triv·i·al name. Nome comum; o nome de uma substância química, do qual nenhuma parte é necessariamente utilizada num sentido sistemático, isto é, fornece pouca ou nenhuma indicação quanto à estrutura química. Esses nomes são comuns para drogas, hormônios, proteínas e outros produtos biológicos e são utilizados pelo público em geral. Podem não ser oficialmente sancionados, em contraste com os nomes não-comerciais, mas podem ser adotados como nomes não-comerciais oficiais em consequência de seu uso disseminado. Os exemplos incluem: água, aspirina, clorofila, heme, metotrexato, ácido fólico, cafeína, tiroxina, adrenalina, barbital etc.; são também comuns abreviaturas para substâncias quimicamente definidas, como ACTH, MSH, BAL, DDT, que são ditas como tais, e não em termos das palavras que representam. Raramente efetua-se uma distinção entre nomes comuns e semicomuns; assim, o tetraidrofolato, a metilglicina, a glicosamina etc. são freqüentemente denominados nomes comuns, embora cada um contenha uma parte sistemática que é utilizada no sentido sistemático correto (tetraidro para quatro átomos de hidrogênio, metil para um grupo –CH₃, amina para –NH₂ nos exemplos anteriormente citados). Os nomes comuns são freqüentemente atribuídos de forma arbitrária a compostos químicos, principalmente de fontes naturais, antes que as estruturas químicas e, portanto, os nomes sistemáticos possam ser determinados. Além disso, proporcionam uma simplificação útil de longos nomes sistemáticos, mesmo quando esses podem ser estabelecidos (embora a maioria dessas reduções se torne semi-sistemática, visto que incorporam alguma parte do nome sistemático).

tri·zon·al (trī-zō'năl). Trizonal; que possui ou é disposto em três zonas ou camadas.

tRNA. Abreviatura de transfer RNA (RNA de transferência).

tro·car (trō'kar). Trocarte; instrumento para a retirada de líquido de uma cavidade ou para uso em paracentese; consiste num tubo de metal (cânula) ao qual se encaixa um obturador com uma ponta de três arestas agudas, que é retirado após o instrumento penetrar na cavidade; o nome t. é habitualmente aplicado apenas ao obturador, sendo todo o instrumento designado por t. e cânula. [Fr. *trocart*, de *trois*, três, + *carre*, lado (de uma lâmina de espada)]
  Hasson t., t. de Hasson; t. rombo inserido na cavidade peritoneal após a realização de pequena celiotomia; utilizado para insuflação e introdução de um laparoscópio.

troch Abreviatura de trochiscus (trocisco).

tro·chan·ter (trō-kan'ter). Trocanter; uma das proeminências ósseas desenvolvida a partir de centros ósseos independentes próximos da extremidade superior do fêmur; existem dois trocanteres nos seres humanos e três no cavalo. [G. *trochantēr*, corredor, de *trechō*, correr]
  greater t. [TA], t. maior; forte processo na parte proximal e lateral da diáfise do fêmur, projetando-se na raiz do colo; proporciona uma inserção para os músculos glúteo médio e mínimo, piriforme, obturadores interno e externo e gêmeos. SIN t. major [TA].
  lesser t. [TA], t. menor; processo piramidal que se projeta da parte medial e proximal da diáfise do fêmur, na linha de junção da diáfise com o colo; recebe a inserção dos músculos psoas maior e ilíaco (iliopsoas). SIN t. minor [TA], small t., trochantin.
  t. ma'jor [TA], t. maior. SIN greater t.
  t. mi'nor [TA], t. menor. SIN lesser t.
  small t., t. menor. SIN lesser t.
  t. tertius [TA], t. terceiro. SIN third t.
  third t. [TA], t. terceiro; processo ocasional na extremidade proximal do lábio lateral da linha áspera do fêmur, aproximadamente no nível do trocanter menor, proporcionando a inserção para a parte maior do músculo glúteo máximo. VER TAMBÉM gluteal *tuberosity.* SIN t. tertius [TA].

tro·chan·ter·i·an, tro·chan·ter·ic (trō-kan-ter'ē-an, -ter'ik). Trocantérico; relativo a um trocanter; especialmente o trocanter maior.

tro·chan·ter·plas·ty (trō-kan'ter-plas-tē). Trocanterplastia; cirurgia plástica dos trocanteres e do colo do fêmur. [trochanter + G. *plastos*, formado]

tro·chan·tin (trō-kan'tin). Trocanter menor. SIN lesser *trochanter.*

tro·chan·tin·i·an (trō-kan-tin'ē-an). Relativo ao trocanter menor.

tro·che (trōk, trō'kē). Trocisco, pastilha; pequeno corpo discóide ou romboide composto de pasta solidificante que contém uma droga adstringente, antiséptica ou demulcente, utilizada para tratamento local da boca ou da orofaringe, sendo o trocisco mantido na boca até dissolver. O veículo ou a base do t. é habitualmente açúcar, tornado adesivo pela mistura com acácia ou tragacanto, pasta de fruta, feita de groselha preta ou vermelha, confeito de rosa ou bálsamo de tolu. SIN lozenge, morsulus, pastil (2), pastille trochiscus. [L. *trochiscus*, do G. *trochiskos*, pequena roda, de *trochos*, roda]

tro·chis·cus (troch), pl. **tro·chis·ci** (trō-kis'kŭs). Trocisco. SIN troche. [L., do G. *trochiskos*, pequena roda, pastilha, de *trochos*, roda]

troch·lea, pl. **troch·le·ae** (trook'lē-ă, -lē-ē) [TA]. Tróclea. **1.** Estrutura que serve como roldana. **2.** Superfície (face) articular lisa do osso sobre a qual outro desliza. [L. roldana, do G. *trochileia*, roldana, de *trechō*, correr]
  t. fem'oris, patelar do fêmur. SIN patellar *surface* of femur.
  fibular t. of calcaneus [TA], t. fibular do calcâneo; projeção da face lateral do calcâneo entre os tendões dos músculos fibulares longo e curto. SIN t. fibularis calcanei [TA], peroneal t. of calcaneus*, t. peronealis*, peroneal pulley, processus trochlearis, spina peronealis, trochlear process.
  t. fibula'ris calca'nei [TA], t. fibular do calcâneo. SIN fibular t. of calcaneus.
  t. hu'meri [TA], t. do úmero. SIN t. of humerus.
  t. of humerus [TA], t. do úmero; a superfície sulcada na extremidade inferior do úmero que se articula com a incisura troclear da ulna. SIN t. humeri [TA], pulley of humerus.
  muscular t. [TA], t. muscular; alça fibrosa através da qual passa o tendão de um músculo; o tendão intermediário dos músculos digástrico e omo-hióideo passa através dessa tróclea. SIN t. muscularis [TA], muscular pulley.
  t. muscula'ris [TA], t. muscular. SIN muscular t.
  t. musculi obliqui superioris bulbi, t. do músculo oblíquo superior do bulbo do olho. SIN t. of superior oblique (muscle).
  peroneal t. of calcaneus, t. fibular do calcâneo; *termo oficial alternativo para fibular t. of calcaneus.
  t. peronea'lis, t. fibular; *termo oficial alternativo para fibular t. of calcaneus.
  trochleae of phalanges of hand and foot, trócleas das falanges da mão e do pé; face palmar ou plantar do sulco intercondilar das cabeças das falanges que acomodam os tendões do flexor longo. SIN t. phalangis (manus et pedis).
  t. phalan'gis (manus et pedis), t. das falanges (mão e pé). SIN trochleae of phalanges of hand and foot.
  t. of superior oblique (muscle), t. do (músculo) oblíquo superior; alça fibrosa na órbita, próximo ao processo nasal do osso frontal, através da qual passa o tendão do músculo oblíquo superior do olho. SIN t. musculi obliqui superioris bulbi.
  t. ta'li [TA], t. do tálus. SIN t. of the talus.
  t. of the talus [TA], t. do tálus; a superfície articular superior arredondada do tálus que se articula com as extremidades distais da tíbia e da fíbula. SIN t. tali [TA], pulley of talus.

troch·le·ar (trok'lē-ar). Troclear. **1.** Relativo a uma tróclea, especialmente a tróclea do músculo oblíquo superior do olho. SIN trochlearis (1). **2.** Trocleiforme. SIN trochleiform.

troch·le·ar·i·form (trok-lē-ar'i-fōrm). Trocleiforme. SIN trochleiform.

troch·le·ar·is (trok-lē-ā'ris). Troclear. **1.** SIN trochlear (1). **2.** SIN trochleiform. [L.]

troch·le·i·form (trok'lē-i-fōrm). Trocleiforme; em forma de tróclea ou roldana. SIN trochlear (2), trochleariform, trochlearis (2).

troch·o·car·dia (trok-ō-kar'dē-ă). Trococardia; deslocamento rotatório do coração ao redor do seu eixo. [G. *trochos*, roda, + *kardia*, coração]

tro·choid (trō'koyd). Trocóide; que gira; que faz rotação; designa uma articulação que faz rotação ou semelhante a uma roda. [G. *trochōdēs*, de *trochos*, roda, + *eidos*, semelhança]

tro·chor·i·zo·car·dia (trō-kōr-ī'zō-kar'dē-ă). Trocorizocardia; trocardia e horizocardia combinadas.

troglitazone (trō-gli'ta-zon). Troglitazona; sensibilizador à insulina associado a sulfoniluréia ou insulina para melhorar o controle da glicemia.

Trog·lo·tre·ma sal·min·co·la (trog-lō-trē'mă sal-mingk'ō-lă). SIN *Nanophyetus salmincola.*

Troisier, Charles Émile, médico francês, 1844–1919. VER T. *ganglion, node.*

tro·la·mine (trō'lă-mēn). Trolamina; contração aprovada pela USAN para trietanolamina, N(CH₂CH₂OH)₃.

Troland, L.T., físico norte-americano, 1889–1932. VER troland.

tro·land (trō'land). Troland; unidade de estimulação visual na retina igual à iluminação por milímetro quadrado de pupila recebida de uma superfície com iluminação de 1 lux.

Trolard, Paulin, anatomista francês, 1842–1910. VER T. *vein.*

tro·le·an·do·my·cin (trō'lē-an-dō-mī'sin). Troleandomicina; o éster triacetil da oleandomicina, um antibiótico macrolídio com potência não inferior a 760 μg por mg; antibiótico efetivo por via oral para infecções causadas por bactérias Gram-positivas resistentes à penicilina. SIN triacetyloleandomycin.

trol·ni·trate phos·phate (trol-nī'trāt). Fosfato de trolnitrato; nitrato orgânico com ação vasodilatadora leve, porém persistente, sobre o músculo liso dos vasos menores de leitos vasculares pós-arteriolares; utilizado para a prevenção de ataques de angina de peito.

Tröltsch, Anton F. von, otologista alemão, 1829–1890. VER T. *corpuscles,* em *corpuscle, pockets,* em *pocket, recesses,* em *recess.*

Trom·bic·u·la (trom-bik′ū-lă). O ácaro micuim, um gênero de ácaros (família Trombiculidae) cujas larvas (micuins, percevejos vermelhos) incluem pragas do homem e de outros animais e vetores de riquetsioses.
  T. akamu'shi. SIN Leptotrombidium akamushi.
  T. alfredduge'si, espécie comum em áreas de vegetação secundária e de cerrado das Américas; as larvas atacam o homem (bem como répteis, aves e mamíferos selvagens e domésticos), causando dermatite intensamente pruriginosa.
  T. delien'sis. VER Leptotrombidium akamushi.
trom·bic·u·li·a·sis (trom-bik-ū-lī′ă-sis). Trombiculíase; infestação por ácaros do gênero *Trombicula*.
trom·bic·u·lid (trom-bik′ū-lid). Trombiculídeo; nome comum dos membros da família Trombiculidae.
Trom·bic·u·li·dae (trom-bik-oo-lī′dē). Família de ácaros cujas larvas (percevejos vermelhos, ácaros do cerrado ou micuins) são parasitas de vertebrados e cujas ninfas e adultos são de cor vermelho-viva e de vida livre, sendo encontrados em ovos de insetos ou em pequenos organismos no solo. As larvas de seis patas são parasitas de cor vermelha ou laranja dificilmente visíveis, que se fixam à pele durante alguns dias a um mês, produzindo uma reação extremamente irritante. No Oriente, os micuins trombiculídeos do gênero *Leptotrombidium* transmitem a doença tsutsugamushi, causada por *Rickettsia tsutsugamushi*, que é transmitida por via transovariana nesses ácaros.
Trom·bi·di·i·dae (trom-bi-dī′i-dē). Família de ácaros que outrora incluía a subfamília Trombiculinae, atualmente elevada à família Trombiculidae (incluindo os vetores da doença tsutsugamushi). As larvas de Trombidiidae são tipicamente parasitas de insetos, e não de vertebrados, como as larvas de Trombiculidae.
tro·meth·a·mine (tro-meth′ă-mēn). Trometamina; composto fracamente básico utilizado como agente alcalinizante e como tampão em reações enzimáticas. SIN tris(hydroxymethyl)aminomethane, tris(hydroxymethyl)methylamine.
Trömner, Ernest, L.O., neurologista alemão, *1868. VER T. *reflex*.
tro·na (tro′nă). Trona; carbonato de sódio natural.
tro·pa·ic ac·id (tro-pā′ik). Ácido tropaico. SIN tropic acid.
tro·pane (tro′pān). Tropano. 1. Hidrocarboneto bicíclico, que constitui a estrutura fundamental da tropina, da atropina e de outras substâncias fisiologicamente ativas. 2. No plural, classe de alcalóides contendo a estrutura do tropano (1).
tro·pate (tro′pāt). Tropato; um sal ou éster do ácido trópico.
tro·pe·ic ac·id (tro-pē′ik). Ácido tropéico. SIN tropic acid.
tro·pe·ine (tro′pē-in). Tropeína; éster da tropina; alcalóide de ocorrência natural ou preparado sinteticamente.
tro·pen·tane (tro-pen′tān). Tropentano; antiespasmódico com propriedades anticolinérgicas.
tro·pe·o·lins (tro-pē′o-linz). Tropeolinas; grupo de corantes azo utilizados como indicadores; p. ex., metil orange. [G. *tropaios*, relativo a uma volta ou alteração, de *tropē*, uma volta]
⟳ **troph-.** Trof-. VER tropho-.
troph·ec·to·derm (trof-ek′tō-derm). Trofectoderma; camada mais externa de células na vesícula blastodérmica de mamíferos, que irá estabelecer contato com o endométrio e participará no estabelecimento dos meios pelos quais o embrião receberá nutrição; a camada celular a partir da qual se diferencia o trofoblasto. [troph- + ectoderm]
Tropheryma whippelii. Microrganismo não-cultivável não-classificado, cujo nome foi dado em 1992, identificado por microscopia eletrônica e definido por tecnologias de amplificação do DNA; foi constatado ser o agente infeccioso responsável pela doença de Whipple.
tro·phic (trof′ik, tro′fik). Trófico. 1. Relativo a ou que depende de nutrição. 2. Resultante de interrupção da inervação. [G. *trophē*, nutrição]
⟳ **-trophic.** -Trófico. Nutrição. Cf. -tropic. [G. *trophē*, nutrição]
tro·phic·i·ty (tro-fis′i-tē). Troficidade; influência ou condição trófica. SIN trophism (1).
tro·phism (trof′izm). Trofismo. 1. SIN trophicity. 2. SIN nutrition (1). [G. *trophē*, nutrição]
⟳ **tropho-, troph-.** Trofo-, trof-. Alimento, nutrição. [G. *trophē*, nutrição]
troph·o·blast (trof′ō-blast, tro′fō-blast). Trofoblasto; a camada celular mesoectodérmica que recobre o blastocisto que erode a mucosa uterina e através da qual o embrião recebe nutrição da mãe; as células não entram na formação do embrião propriamente dito, mas contribuem na formação da placenta. O trofoblasto desenvolve processos que mais tarde recebem um centro de mesoderma vascular e passam a ser conhecidos como vilosidades coriônicas; o trofoblasto adquire logo duas camadas, diferenciando-se no sinciciotrofoblasto, uma camada externa constituída por uma massa protoplasmática multinucleada (sincício), e o citotrofoblasto, a camada interna próxima ao mesoderma, na qual as células mantêm as suas membranas. SIN chorionic ectoderm. [tropho- + G. *blastos*, germe]
  plasmodial t., sinciciotrofoblasto. SIN syncytiotrophoblast.
  syncytial t., sinciciotrofoblasto. SIN syncytiotrophoblast.

troph·o·blas·tic (tro-fō-blas′tik). Trofoblástico; relativo ao trofoblasto.
tro·pho·blas·tin (tro-fō-blas′tin). Trofoblastina. SIN interferon-tau.
troph·o·chro·ma·tin (trof-ō-krō′mă-tin). Trofocromatina. SIN trophochromidia. [tropho- + G. *chrōma*, cor]
troph·o·chro·mid·ia (trof′ō-krō-mid′ē-ă). Trofocromídios; massas extranucleares não-germinativas ou vegetativas de cromatina, encontradas em determinados protozoários; p. ex., o macronúcleo de determinados ciliados, como *Paramecium*. SIN trophochromatin.
troph·o·cyte (trof′ō-sit). Trofócito; célula que fornece nutrição; por exemplo, as células de Sertoli nos túbulos seminíferos. SIN trephocyte. [tropho- + G. *kytos*, célula]
troph·o·derm (trof′ō-derm). Trofoderma; o trofoectoderma ou trofoblasto, juntamente com a camada mesodérmica vascular subjacente. VER TAMBÉM serosa (2). [tropho- + G. *derma*, pele]
troph·o·der·ma·to·neu·ro·sis (trof′ō-der′mă-tō-noo-rō′sis). Trofodermatoneurose; alterações tróficas cutâneas causadas por comprometimento neural.
troph·o·dy·nam·ics (trof′ō-dī-nam′iks). Trofodinâmica; a dinâmica da nutrição ou do metabolismo. SIN nutritional energy. [tropho- + G. *dynamis*, força]
troph·o·neu·ro·sis (trof′ō-noo-rō′sis). Trofoneurose; distúrbio trófico, com atrofia, hipertrofia ou erupção cutânea, que ocorre em consequência de doença ou lesão dos nervos da parte. [tropho- + G. *neuron*, nervo, + *-osis*, condição]
troph·o·neu·rot·ic (trof-ō-noo-rot′ik). Trofoneurótico; relativo a uma trofoneurose.
troph·o·nu·cle·us (trof-ō-noo′klē-ŭs). Trofonúcleo. SIN macronucleus (2).
troph·o·plast (trof′ō-plast). Trofoplasto. SIN plastid (1). [tropho- + G. *plastos*, formado]
troph·o·spon·gia (trof′ō-spon′jē-ă). Trofospongia. 1. Estruturas canaliculares descritas por A.F. Holmgren no protoplasma de determinadas células. 2. Endométrio vascular do útero entre o miométrio e o trofoblasto. [tropho- + G. *spongia*, esponja]
troph·o·tax·is (trof-ō-tak′sis). Trofotaxia. SIN trophotropism. [tropho- + G. *taxis*, arranjo]
troph·o·tro·pic (trof-ō-trō′pik). Trofotrópico; relativo ao trofotropismo.
troph·o·tro·pism (tro-fot′rō-pizm). Trofotropismo; quimiotaxia de células vivas em relação ao material nutritivo; pode ser positivo (em direção ao material nutritivo) ou negativo (afastando-se do material nutritivo). SIN trophotaxis. [tropho- + G. *tropē*, uma volta]
troph·o·zo·ite (trof-ō-zō′it). Trofozoíta; a forma amebóide, vegetativa e assexuada de determinados Sporozoea, como o esquizonte dos plasmódios da malária e parasitas relacionados. [tropho- + G. *zōon*, animal]
⟳ **-trophy.** -Trofia. Alimento, nutrição. [G. *trophē*, nutrição]
tro·pia (tro′pē-ă). Tropia; desvio anormal do olho. VER strabismus. [G. *tropē*, uma volta]
⟳ **-tropic.** -Trópico. Uma volta em direção a, que possui afinidade por. Cf. -trophic. [G. *tropē*, uma volta]
tro·pic ac·id (trop′ik). Ácido trópico; constituinte da atropina e da escopolamina, nas quais é esterificado através de seu COOH ao 3-CHOH da tropina. SIN tropaic acid, tropeic acid.
tro·pic·a·mide (tro-pik′ă-mid). Tropicamida; agente anticolinérgico utilizado para produzir midríase rápida e de curta duração para exames oculares.
tro·pine (tro′pēn). Tropina; o principal constituinte da atropina e da escopolamina, das quais é obtida por hidrólise.
  t. mandelate, homatropina. SIN homatropine.
  t. tropate, atropina. SIN atropine.
tro·pism (tro′pizm). Tropismo; o fenômeno, observado em organismos vivos, de aproximar-se (**t. positivo**) ou afastar-se (**t. negativo**) de um foco de luz, calor ou outro estímulo; em geral, aplica-se ao movimento de uma parte do organismo, em contraste com a taxia, o movimento de todo um organismo. [G. *tropē*, uma volta]
  viral t., t. viral; a especificidade de um vírus por um tecido específico do hospedeiro, determinada, em parte, pela interação de estruturas da superfície viral com receptores de superfície da célula do hospedeiro.
trop·o·col·la·gen (trō-pō-kol′ă-jen, trop′ō-). Tropocolágeno; as unidades fundamentais das fibrilas de colágeno, que consistem em três cadeias polipeptídicas dispostas de forma helicoidal.
trop·o·e·las·tin (trō-pō-e-las′tin). Tropoelastina; o precursor da elastina; a tropoelastina não contém ligações cruzadas de desmosina ou isodesmosina.
tro·pom·e·ter (trō-pom′e-ter). Trôpômetro; qualquer instrumento para medir o grau de rotação ou torção, como a do bulbo do olho ou da diáfise de um osso longo. [G. *tropē*, uma volta, + *metron*, medida]
tro·po·my·o·sin (trō-pō-mī′ō-sin). Tropomiosina; proteína fibrosa extraível do músculo; algumas vezes especificada como tropomiosina B para distingui-la da tropomiosina A (paramiosina) proeminente em moluscos.
tro·po·nin (trō′pō-nin). Troponina; proteína globular do músculo que se liga à tropomiosina e possui considerável afinidade por íons cálcio; uma proteína

reguladora central da contração muscular. A troponina T liga-se à tropomiosina; a troponina I inibe as interações actina F-miosina; a troponina C é uma proteína de ligação do cálcio que desempenha um papel-chave na contração muscular.

trough (trawf). Canal, orifício; depressão ou canal longo, estreito e superficial.
  gingival t., depressão gengival; a formação de uma cratera em consequência da destruição de tecidos interdentários, de modo que existe, com efeito, uma cortina labial e lingual da gengiva sem conexão interproximal.
  Langmuir t., cuba de Langmuir; cuba com barreira superficial móvel para estudo da compressão de películas superficiais.
  synaptic t., depressão sináptica; a depressão da superfície da fibra muscular estriada que acomoda a placa terminal motora.

Trousseau, Armand, médico francês, 1801–1867. VER T. *point, sign, spot, syndrome;* T.-Lallemand *bodies,* em *body.*

trox·e·ru·tin (troks'ē-roo-tin). Troxerutina; utilizada no tratamento de distúrbios venosos.

trox·i·done (trok'si-dōn). Troxidona. SIN trimethadione.

Trp Símbolo de tryptophan (triptofano) e seus radicais.

trun·cal (trŭng'kal). Troncular, troncal; relativo ao tronco do corpo ou a qualquer tronco arterial ou nervoso etc.

trun·cate (trŭng'kāt). Truncado; seccionado transversalmente em ângulos retos ao eixo longo ou que parece ter sido cortado (mutilado) dessa maneira. [L. *trunco,* pp. *-atus,* amputar, cortar]

trun·cus, gen. e pl. **trun·ci** (trŭn'kŭs, -kī) [TA]. Tronco. SIN trunk. [L. caule, tronco]
  t. arterio'sus, t. arterial; o tronco arterial comum que parte de ambos os ventrículos no início da vida fetal, destinado posteriormente a dividir-se em aorta e artéria pulmonar em consequência do desenvolvimento do septo espiral.
  t. arterio'sus commu'nis, t. arterial comum. VER t. arteriosus.
  t. brachiocepha'licus [TA], t. braquiocefálico. SIN brachiocephalic (arterial) trunk.
  t. celi'acus [TA], t. celíaco. SIN celiac (arterial) trunk.
  t. cor'poris callo'si [TA], t. do corpo caloso. SIN trunk of corpus callosum.
  t. costocervica'lis [TA], t. costocervical. SIN costocervical (arterial) trunk.
  t. encephali [TA], t. encefálico. SIN brainstem.
  t. fascicula'ris atrioventricula'ris, t. do feixe atrioventricular. SIN atrioventricular *bundle;* VER TAMBÉM conducting *system* of heart.
  t. infe'rior plex'us brachia'lis [TA], t. inferior do plexo braquial. SIN inferior trunk of brachial plexus.
  t. linguofacia'lis [TA], t. linguofacial. SIN linguofacial (arterial) trunk.
  t. lum'bosacra'lis [TA], t. lombossacral. SIN lumbosacral (nerve) trunk.
  trun'ci (lymphatici) intestina'les [TA], troncos intestinais (linfáticos). SIN intestinal (lymphatic) trunks, em trunk.
  trun'ci (lymphatici) lumba'les [TA], troncos lombares (linfáticos). SIN lumbar (lymphatic) trunks, em trunk.
  t. (lymphaticus) bronchiomediastina'lis [TA], t. bronquiomediastinal (linfático). SIN bronchomediastinal (lymphatic) trunk.
  t. (lymphaticus) jugula'ris [TA], t. jugular (linfático). SIN jugular lymphatic trunk.
  t. me'dius plex'us brachia'lis [TA], t. médio do plexo braquial. SIN middle trunk of brachial plexus.
  t. nervi accessorii [TA], t. do nervo acessório. SIN accessory nerve trunk.
  persistent t. arterio'sus, persistência do canal arterial; anomalia cardiovascular congênita resultante da falha de desenvolvimento do septo espiral; consiste num tronco arterial comum que sai de ambos os ventrículos, sendo as artérias pulmonares emitidas do tronco comum ascendente.
  trun'ci plex'us brachia'lis [TA], troncos do plexo braquial. SIN trunks of brachial plexus, em trunk.
  t. pulmona'lis [TA], t. pulmonar. SIN pulmonary trunk.
  t. subcla'vius [TA], t. subclávio. SIN subclavian lymphatic trunk.
  t. supe'rior plex'us brachia'lis [TA], t. superior do plexo braquial. SIN superior trunk of brachial plexus.
  t. sympath'icus [TA], t. simpático. SIN sympathetic trunk.
  t. thyrocervica'lis [TA], t. tireocervical. SIN thyrocervical (arterial) trunk.
  t. vaga'lis, t. vagal. SIN vagal (nerve) trunk.

Trunecek, Karel, médico tchecoslovaco, *1865. VER T. *sign.*

trunk (trŭnk) [TA]. Tronco. **1.** O corpo (tronco), excluindo a cabeça e os membros. **2.** Um nervo, vaso ou coleção de tecido antes de sua divisão. **3.** Grande vaso linfático coletor. SIN truncus [TA]. [L. *truncus*]
  accessory nerve t. [TA], t. do nervo acessório; parte do nervo acessório formado dentro da cavidade craniana pela união das raízes craniana e espinal; a seguir, divide-se no forame jugular em ramos interno e externo, unindo-se o primeiro com o vago, enquanto o segundo abandona o forame com ramo independente, que é comumente considerado nervo acessório. SIN truncus nervi accessorii [TA].
  t. of atrioventricular bundle, t. do feixe atrioventricular. SIN atrioventricular *bundle.*
  t.'s of brachial plexus [TA], troncos do plexo braquial; os troncos superior, médio e inferior; dividem-se distalmente para formar os cordões (fascículos) do plexo. SIN trunci plexus brachialis [TA].
  brachiocephalic (arterial) t. [TA], t. braquiocefálico (arterial); *origem,* arco da aorta; *ramos,* artérias subclávia direita e carótida comum direita; por vezes, emite a artéria tireóidea íntima. SIN truncus brachiocephalicus [TA].
  bronchomediastinal (lymphatic) t. [TA], t. bronquiomediastinal (linfático); vaso linfático que se origina da união dos linfáticos eferentes dos linfonodos traqueobrônquicos e mediastinais de cada lado. À esquerda, pode ser substituído, em grande parte, por drenagem direta no ducto torácico. SIN truncus (lymphaticus) bronchiomediastinalis [TA].
  celiac (arterial) t. [TA], t. celíaco (arterial); *origem,* aorta abdominal imediatamente abaixo do diafragma; *ramos,* gástrica esquerda, hepática comum, esplênica. SIN truncus celiacus [TA], arteria celiaca, celiac artery, celiac axis, Haller tripod.
  t. of corpus callosum [TA], t. do corpo caloso; a principal parte arqueada do corpo caloso. SIN truncus corporis callosi [TA], body of corpus callosum*.
  costocervical (arterial) t. [TA], t. costocervical (arterial); artéria curta que se origina da artéria subclávia de cada lado e se divide em ramos cervical profundo e intercostal superior, dividindo-se este último habitualmente para formar a primeira e segunda artérias intercostais posteriores. SIN truncus costocervicalis [TA], costocervical artery.
  inferior t. of brachial plexus [TA], t. inferior do plexo braquial; o feixe de nervos formado pela união dos ramos ventrais do oitavo nervo cervical e primeiro nervo torácico; emite fibras para os cordões (fascículos) posterior e medial do plexo braquial. SIN truncus inferior plexus brachialis [TA].
  intestinal (lymphatic) t.'s [TA], troncos intestinais (linfáticos); os vasos que transportam a linfa da parte inferior do fígado, estômago, baço, pâncreas e intestino delgado; drenam na cisterna do quilo e, algumas vezes, são duplicados. SIN trunci (lymphatici) intestinalis [TA].
  jugular lymphatic t. [TA], t. jugular linfático; vaso linfático de cada lado, que transporta linfa da cabeça e do pescoço; o vaso do lado direito drena para o ducto linfático direito, e o do lado esquerdo, para o ducto torácico. SIN truncus (lymphaticus) jugularis [TA], jugular duct.
  linguofacial (arterial) t. [TA], t. linguofacial (arterial); o tronco comum pelo qual as artérias lingual e facial originam-se freqüentemente da artéria carótida externa. SIN truncus linguofacialis [TA].
  lumbar (lymphatic) t.'s [TA], troncos lombares (linfáticos); dois ductos linfáticos que transportam a linfa dos membros inferiores, das vísceras e paredes pélvicas, do intestino grosso, dos rins e das glândulas supra-renais; drenam para a cisterna do quilo. SIN trunci (lymphatici) lumbales [TA].
  lumbosacral (nerve) t. [TA], t. lombossacral (nervoso); grande nervo, formado pela união do quinto nervo lombar e primeiro nervo sacral com um ramo proveniente do quarto nervo lombar, que entra na formação do plexo sacral. SIN truncus lumbosacralis [TA].
  middle t. of brachial plexus [TA], t. médio do plexo braquial; a continuação do ramo ventral do sétimo nervo cervical; fornece fibras para os cordões (fascículos) posterior e lateral do plexo braquial. SIN truncus medius plexus brachialis [TA].
  nerve t., t. nervoso; uma coleção de funículos ou feixes de fibras nervosas encerradas numa bainha de tecido conjuntivo, o epineuro.
  pulmonary t. [TA], t. pulmonar; *origem,* ventrículo direito do coração; *distribuição,* divide-se na artéria pulmonar direita e na artéria pulmonar esquerda, que entram nos pulmões correspondentes e se ramificam juntamente com os brônquios segmentares. SIN truncus pulmonalis [TA], arteria pulmonalis, pulmonary artery, venous artery.
  subclavian lymphatic t. [TA], t. subclávio linfático; formado pela união dos vasos que drenam os linfonodos dos membros superiores, desaguando no ducto torácico, na raiz do pescoço, à esquerda, ou no ducto linfático direito. SIN truncus subclavius [TA], subclavian duct.
  superior t. of brachial plexus [TA], t. superior do plexo braquial; o feixe de nervos formado pela união dos ramos ventrais dos quinto e sexto nervos cervicais e algumas fibras do quarto; fornece fibras para os cordões (fascículos) posterior e lateral do plexo braquial. SIN truncus superior plexus brachialis [TA].
  sympathetic t. [TA], t. simpático; um dos dois filamentos nervosos ganglionados extensos ao longo da coluna vertebral, que se estendem da base do crânio até o cóccix; estão conectados a cada nervo espinal através de ramos cinzentos e recebem fibras da medula espinal através dos ramos brancos, que se conectam com os nervos espinais torácico e lombar superior. SIN truncus sympathicus [TA], gangliated cord, ganglionic chain.
  thoracoacromial t., t. toracoacromial. SIN thoracoacromial *artery.*
  thyrocervical (arterial) t. [TA], t. tireocervical (arterial); tronco arterial curto que se origina da artéria subclávia, dando origem à supra-escapular (que também pode surgir diretamente da artéria subclávia) e terminando através de sua divisão nas artérias cervical ascendente e tireóidea inferior. SIN truncus thyrocervicalis [TA], thyroid axis.
  vagal (nerve) t., t. vagal (nervoso); um dos dois feixes nervosos, anterior e posterior, no qual o plexo esofágico continua quando atravessa o diafragma. SIN truncus vagalis.

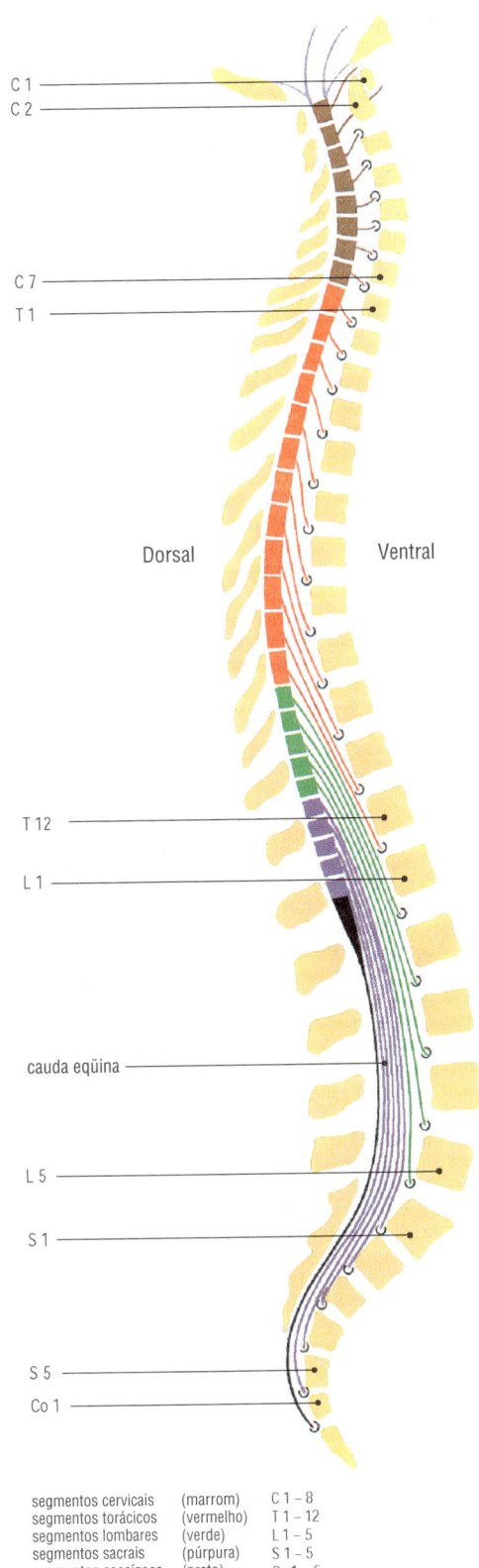
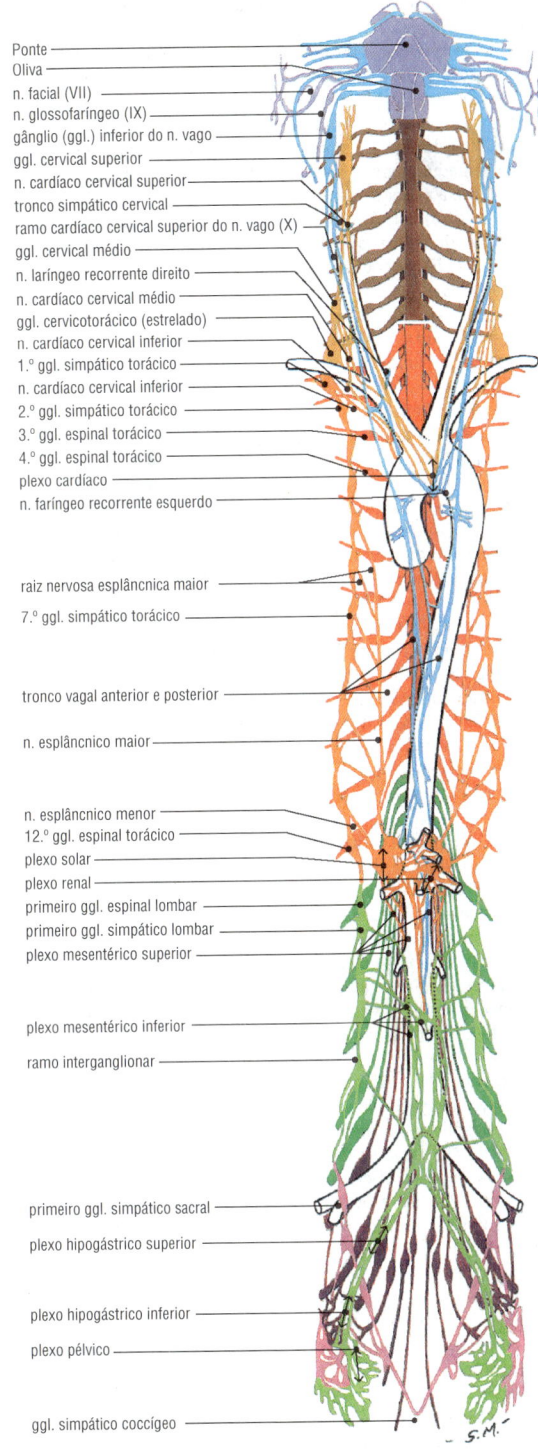

medula espinal: à esquerda, a medula espinal na coluna vertebral, com código de cores mostrando a relação entre segmentos neurais e vértebras; à direita, o código de cores mostra a relação do tronco simpático com os nervos e ramos espinais

tru·sion (troo′zhŭn). Trusão; deslocamento de um corpo, como, por exemplo, um dente, de sua posição inicial. [L. *trudo,* pp. *trusus,* empurrar]

truss (trŭs). Funda; dispositivo para evitar o retorno de uma hérnia reduzida ou o aumento de tamanho de uma hérnia; consiste numa almofada fixada a um cinto e mantida no lugar por um elástico ou alças. [Fr. *trousser,* amarrar, apertar]

Try Abreviatura antiga de tryptophan (triptofano).

try·in (trī′in). Inserção preliminar de um molde de dentadura completa (dentadura de prova), de dentadura parcial ou de restauração concluída para determinar o ajuste, a estética, a relação maxilomandibular etc.

try·pan blue (trī′pan, trip′) [C.I. 23850]. Azul de tripano; corante azo ácido, utilizado para coloração vital do sistema reticuloendotelial, túbulos uriníferos e células em cultura de tecido, e como teratógeno experimental; antigamente utilizado como tripanocida.

try·pan·i·ci·dal (tri - pan - i - sī′dăl). Tripanicida. SIN trypanocidal.

try·pan·i·cide (tri - pan′i - sīd). Tripanicida. SIN trypanocide.

tryp·a·nid (trip′a - nid). Tripanide. SIN trypanosomatid.

try·pan·o·ci·dal (tri - pan′o - sī′dăl, trip′a - nō-). Tripanocida; destrutivo para tripanossomas. SIN trypanicidal.

try·pan·o·cide (tri - pan′ō - sīd, trip′a - nō-). Tripanocida; agente que mata tripanossomas. SIN trypanicide, trypanosomicide. [trypanosome + L. *caedo,* matar]

Try·pan·o·plas·ma (tri - pan - ō - plaz′mă, trip′a - nō-). Gênero de Protozoa flagelados (família Cryptobiidae), cujos membros possuem corpo de forma variável, com membrana ondulante e um flagelo que se projeta de uma extremidade; parasita no sangue de peixes. [G. *trypanon,* escavador, + *plasma,* algo formado]

Try·pan·o·so·ma (tri - pan′ō - sō′mă, trip′a - nō-). Gênero de protozoários flagelados digenéticos assexuados (família Trypanosomatidae) que possuem corpo fusiforme com uma membrana ondulante em um dos lados, um único flagelo anterior e um cinetoplasta; são parasitas no plasma sangüíneo de muitos vertebrados (sendo apenas alguns patogênicos) e, via de regra, possuem um hospedeiro intermediário, um invertebrado hematófago, como sanguessuga, carrapato ou inseto; as espécies patogênicas causam tripanossomíase no homem e várias outras doenças em animais domésticos. [G. *trypanon,* escavador, + *soma,* corpo]

T. a′vium, espécie que ocorre em corujas, corvos e outras aves; vários artrópodes hematófagos são vetores, incluindo mosquitos, moscas negras e hipoboscídios; essa espécie foi descrita sob um grande número de nomes, hoje em dia considerados cepas fisiológicas da espécie.

T. bru′cei, espécie atualmente dividida em três subespécies: *T. brucei brucei, T. brucei rhodesiense* e *T. brucei gambiense.*

T. bru′cei bru′cei, subespécie que causa nagana na África; provoca doença fatal em camelos, doença aguda em eqüinos, cães e gatos, e doença crônica em suínos, gado bovino, carneiros e cabras; transmitido primariamente por moscas tsé-tsé do gênero *Glossina.* Nos ungulados africanos selvagens, a infecção é disseminada, porém raramente fatal.

T. bru′cei gambien′se, subespécie causadora da tripanossomíase gambiense nos seres humanos; transmitido por moscas tsé-tsé, especialmente *Glossina palpalis.* SIN *T. gambiense, T. hominis, T. ugandense.*

T. bru′cei rhodesien′se, subespécie causadora da tripanossomíase rodesiense; transmitido por moscas tsé-tsé, especialmente por *Glossina morsitans* nos seres humanos; vários animais de caça podem atuar como hospedeiros reservatórios. SIN *t. rhodesiense.*

T. cru′zi, espécie que causa a tripanossomíase sul-americana, endêmica no México e em vários países das Américas Central e do Sul; a transmissão e a infecção são comuns apenas quando o percevejo triatomíneo vetor defeca enquanto se alimenta de sangue, visto que as fezes do percevejo contêm os agentes infecciosos que são introduzidos na pele ou colocados em contato com as mucosas quando o indivíduo se coça. Os tripomastigotas são encontrados no sangue, enquanto os amastigotas ocorrem no meio intracelular, em grupos ou colônias nos tecidos; as fibras musculares cardíacas e as células de muitos outros órgãos são atacadas, e os organismos não ficam restritos aos macrófagos, como na leishmaniose visceral; os seres humanos, os cães, gatos, ratos domésticos, tatus, morcegos, determinados macacos e gambás são os hospedeiros vertebrais habituais; os vetores são membros da família Triatominae. Também conhecido como *Schizotrypanum cruzi,* uma designação genérica distinta amplamente utilizada nas regiões endêmicas. SIN *T. escomelis, T. triatomae.*

T. dimor′phon, espécie africana encontrada em cavalos, gado bovino, carneiros, cabras, porcos e cães, outrora considerada igual ao *T. congolense,* mas atualmente reconhecida como espécie distinta e mais patogênica no gado, em carneiros e cães; transmitido por moscas tsé-tsé através da África central.

T. escome′lis. SIN *T. cruzi.*

T. gambien′se. SIN *T. brucei gambiense.*

T. hom′inis. SIN *T. brucei gambiense.*

T. igno′tum, nome antigo do *T. simiae.*

T. lew′isi, espécie que é parasita não-patogênico mundial no sangue de ratos, amplamente utilizada para estudo laboratorial; transmitido pela pulga do rato, *Nosopsyllus fasciatus.*

T. melopha′gium, espécie não-patogênica (relacionada com *T. theileri*) encontrada em carneiros em todo o mundo e provavelmente também em cabras; o vetor é *Melophagus ovinus.*

T. range′li, espécie que parasita uma grande variedade de mamíferos, incluindo o homem, na América do Sul, sendo transmitida pelos percevejos triatomídeos *Rhodnius prolixus* e *Tiratoma dimidiata* e provavelmente outros; aparentemente, não é patogênico, mas pode ser patogênico no percevejo hospedeiro.

T. rhodesien′se. SIN *T. brucei rhodesiense.*

T. thei′leri, grande espécie relativamente não-patogênica, encontrada em antílopes africanos e no gado bovino em muitas partes do mundo; os parasitas são transmitidos por mutucas tabanídeas hematófagas.

T. triatom′ae. SIN *T. cruzi.*

T. uganden′se. SIN *T. brucei gambiense.*

try·pan·o·so·mat·id (tri - pan′o - sō - mat′id). Tripanossomatídeo; designação comum a um membro da família Trypanosomatidae. SIN trypanid.

Try·pan·o·so·mat·i·dae (tri - pan′o - sō - mat′i - dē). Família de protozoários hemoflagelados (ordem Kinetoplastida, classe Zoomastigophorea, subfilo Mastigophora); parasitas assexuados do sangue e/ou dos tecidos de sanguessugas, insetos e vertebrados e habitantes da seiva das plantas, caracterizados por uma forma arredondada ou alongada, um único núcleo, uma mitocôndria alongada (cuja posição em relação ao núcleo constitui uma característica de cada gênero) e um único flagelo de direção anterior (em alguns gêneros, ladeia uma membrana ondulante). A família T. inclui os gêneros *Crithidia, Herpetomonas, Leptomonas* e *Bastocrithidia,* todos monogenéticos e encontrados em insetos, e *Phytomonas* (encontrado em plantas), *Endotrypanum, Leishmania* e *Trypanosoma,* todos digenéticos; *Leishmania* e *Trypanosoma* incluem importantes patógenos dos seres humanos e de animais. Muitos tripanossomas passam por estágios de desenvolvimento ou do ciclo biológico semelhantes às formas do corpo características dos gêneros; essas formas incluem: amastigota, coanomastigota, opistomastigota, promastigota, epimastigota e tripomastigota.

try·pan·o·some (tri - pan′ō - sōm, trip′a - nō-). Tripanossoma; designação comum de qualquer membro do gênero *Trypanosoma* ou da família Trypanosomatidae. [G. *trypanon,* escavador, + *soma,* corpo]

try·pan·o·so·mi·a·sis (tri - pan′o - sō - mī′a - sis, trip′a - nō-). Tripanossomíase; qualquer doença causada por tripanossoma. SIN trypanosomosis.

acute t., t. aguda. SIN Rhodesian t.

African t., t. africana; doença endêmica grave na África tropical, de dois tipos: t. gambiense ou da África Ocidental e t. rodesiense ou da África Oriental.

American t., t. americana. VER South American t.

chronic t., t. crônica. SIN Gambian t.

Cruz t., t. de Cruz. SIN South American t.

East African t., t. da África Oriental. SIN Rhodesian t.

Gambian t., t. gambiense; doença crônica de seres humanos causada por *Trypanosoma brucei gambiense* no norte e na região subsaariana da África, do leste do Senegal até o Sudão e Uganda; caracterizada por esplenomegalia, sonolência e urgência incontrolável de dormir e desenvolvimento de alterações psicóticas; o comprometimento dos gânglios da base e do cerebelo leva comumente a coréia e atetose; a fase terminal da doença caracteriza-se por debilitação, anorexia e emagrecimento que gradualmente levam ao coma e à morte, geralmente por infecção intercorrente. SIN chronic African sleeping sickness, chronic t., West African sleeping sickness, West African t.

Rhodesian t., t. rodesiense; doença humana causada por *Trypanosoma brucei rhodesiense,* na África Oriental, desde a Etiópia e sul de Uganda até Zimbábue; assemelha-se clinicamente à tripanossomíase gambiense, porém é de menor duração e mais aguda; os pacientes sofrem episódios repetidos de pirexemia, tornam-se anêmicos e morrem comumente por insuficiência cardíaca. SIN acute African sleeping sickness, acute t., East African sleeping sickness, East African t.

South American t., t. sul-americana; tripanossomíase causada pelo *Trypanosoma* (ou *Schizotrypanum*) *cruzi* e transmitida por determinadas espécies de percevejos reduvídeos (triatomíneos). Na sua forma aguda, é observada mais freqüentemente em crianças de pouca idade, com edema da pele no local de entrada, mais comumente na face, e aumento dos linfonodos regionais; em sua forma crônica, pode assumir vários aspectos, em geral com miocardiopatia, embora ocorram também megacólon e megaesôfago; os reservatórios naturais incluem cães, tatus, roedores e outros mamíferos domésticos, domiciliados e selvagens. SIN Chagas disease, Chagas-Cruz disease, Cruz t.

West African t., t. da África Ocidental. SIN Gambian t.

try·pan·o·so·mic (tri - pan - ō - sō′mik, trip′a - nō-). Tripanossômico; relativo a tripanossomas, referindo-se especialmente à infecção por esses organismos.

try·pan·o·so·mi·cide (tri - pan′ō - sō′mi - sīd). Tripanossomicida. SIN trypanocide.

try·pan·o·so·mid (tri - pan′ō - sō - mid). Tripanossomide; lesão cutânea resultante de alterações imunológicas da doença por tripanossoma. [trypanosome + G. *-id* (1)]

trypanosomosis (trip′an - ō - sō - mō′sis, tri - pan′). Tripanossomose. SIN trypanosomiasis.

try·pan red (trī′pan, trip′) [C.I. 22850]. Vermelho tripano; corante azo utilizado antigamente no tratamento da tripanossomíase.

tryp·ar·sa·mide (trī - par′sa - mid). Triparsamida; utilizada no tratamento de infecções tripanossômicas e por espiroquetas, especialmente neurossífilis, e nos estágios tardios da doença do sono africana.

tryp·o·mas·ti·gote (trip - ō - mas′ti - gōt). Tripomastigota; termo para substituir a antiga designação "estágio tripanossoma", que era freqüentemente confundido com o gênero *Trypanosoma*. Designa o estágio (estágio infectante para a tripanossomíase sul-americana e a tripanossomíase africana, e o único estágio encontrado no homem nessa última doença), em que o flagelo se origina de um cinetoplasto de localização posterior e emerge do lado do corpo, com uma membrana ondulante correndo ao longo do comprimento do corpo. [G. *trypanon*, escavador, + *mastix*, chicote]

tryp·sin (trip′sin). Tripsina; enzima proteolítica formada no intestino delgado a partir do tripsinogênio através da ação da enteropeptidase; serina proteinase que hidrolisa peptídios, amidas, ésteres etc. em ligações dos grupos carboxila de resíduos de L-arginil ou L-lisil; produz também as meromiosinas.
   crystallized t., t. cristalizada; preparação purificada da enzima pancreática; utilizada como adjuvante da cirurgia para debridamento de feridas necróticas e úlceras.

tryp·sin·o·gen, tryp·so·gen (trip - sin′ō - jen, trip′sō - jen). Tripsinogênio; proteína inativa secretada pelo pâncreas, que é convertida em tripsina pela ação da enteropeptidase. SIN protrypsin.

trypt·a·mine (trip′ta - mēn, - min). Triptamina; produto de descarboxilação do L-triptofano que ocorre em vegetais e determinados alimentos (p. ex., queijo). Eleva a pressão arterial através de uma ação vasoconstritora, pela liberação de norepinefrina nas terminações nervosas simpáticas pós-ganglionares, e acredita-se que seja um dos agentes responsáveis por episódios hipertensivos após terapia com inibidores da monoamina oxidase (p. ex., cloridrato de pargilina).

trypt·a·mine-stro·phan·thi·din (trip′ta - mēn - strō - fan′thi - din). Triptamina-estrofantidina. Glicosídio cardíaco semi-sintético que é um produto da condensação da estrofantidina e triptamina; administrado por via oral, possui início rápido e curta duração de ação cardíaca.

tryp·tic (trip′tik). Tríptico; relativo à tripsina, como a digestão tríptica.

tryp·tone (trip′tōn). Triptona; peptona produzida por digestão proteolítica com tripsina.

tryp·to·ne·mia (trip - tō - nē′mē - ă). Triptonemia; presença de triptona no sangue circulante.

tryp·to·phan (Trp, W) (trip′tō - fan). Triptofano; ácido 2-amino-3-(3-indolil)-propiônico; o isômero L é um componente de proteínas; aminoácido nutricionalmente essencial.
   t. decarboxylase, t. descarboxilase. SIN aromatic D-amino acid decarboxylase.
   t. desmolase, t. desmolase. SIN t. synthase.
   t. 2,3-dioxygenase, t. 2,3-dioxigenase; óxido redutase que catalisa a reação do L-triptofano e O_2 para produzir L-*N*-formilcinurenina; enzima adaptativa, cujo nível (no fígado) é controlado por hormônios supra-renais; uma etapa no metabolismo do triptofano; além disso, uma etapa na síntese de NAD^+ a partir do triptofano. SIN pyrrolase, t. oxygenase, t. pyrrolase, tryptophanase (1).
   t. oxygenase, t. oxigenase. SIN t. 2,3-dioxygenase.
   t. pyrrolase, t. pirrolase. SIN t. 2,3-dioxygenase.
   t. synthase, t. sintase; hidroliase não encontrada em mamíferos que condensa a L-serina indol-3-glicerol fosfato para produzir L-triptofano e gliceraldeído fosfato; é necessária a presença de piridoxal fosfato; atua também na reação da L-serina com indol. SIN t. desmolase, t. synthetase.
   t. synthetase, t. sintetase. SIN t. synthase.

tryp·to·pha·nase (trip′to - fă - nās). Triptofanase. **1.** SIN *tryptophan* 2,3-dioxygenase. **2.** Enzima encontrada em bactérias que catalisa a clivagem do L-triptofano em indol, ácido pirúvico e amônia; o piridoxal fosfato é uma coenzima.

tryp·to·pha·nu·ria (trip′tō - fă - noo′rē - ă). Triptofanúria; aumento da excreção urinária de triptofano.
   t. with dwarfism [MIM*276100], t. com nanismo; síndrome de nanismo, defeito mental, fotossensibilidade cutânea e distúrbio da marcha associado a t.; herança autossômica recessiva.

tset·se (tset′sē, tsē′tsē). Tsé-tsé. VER *Glossina*. [nome nativo da África do Sul]

TSH Abreviatura de thyroid-stimulating *hormone* (hormônio tireoestimulante).

TSH-RF Abreviatura de thyroid-stimulating hormone-releasing *factor* (fator liberador do hormônio tireoestimulante).

TSI Abreviatura de thyroid-stimulating *immunoglobulins* (imunoglobulinas estimuladoras da tireóide), em *immunoglobulin*.

TSS Abreviatura de toxic shock *syndrome* (síndrome do choque tóxico).

TSTA Abreviatura de tumor-specific transplantation *antigens* (antígenos de transplante tumor-específicos), em *antigen*.

TTP Abreviatura de ribothymidine 5′-triphosphate (ribotimidina 5′-trifosfato).

TTP-HUS Abreviatura de thrombotic thrombocytopenic purpura and hemolytic uremic syndrome (púrpura trombocitopênica trombótica e síndrome hemolítico-urêmica). VER thrombotic thrombocytopenic *purpura,* hemolytic uremic *syndrome*.

TTX Abreviatura de tetrodotoxin (tetrodotoxina).

T.U. Abreviatura de toxic *unit* (unidade tóxica) ou toxin *unit* (unidade de toxina).

tu·a·mi·no·hep·tane (too′am - i - nō - hep′tān). Tuamino-heptano; amina volátil simpatomimética, utilizada por inalação como descongestionante nasal; também disponível como sulfato de tuamino-heptano, com as mesmas ações, e mais potente do que a efedrina como vasoconstritor.

tu·ba, gen. e pl. **tu·bae** (too′bă, too′bē) [TA]. Tuba; trompa. SIN tube. [L. uma trompa reta]
   t. acus′tica, tuba auditiva. SIN pharyngotympanic (auditory) *tube*.
   t. auditi′va [TA], tuba auditiva. SIN pharyngotympanic (auditory) *tube*.
   t. audito′ria, tuba auditiva, *termo oficial alternativo para pharyngotympanic (auditory) *tube,* pharyngotympanic (auditory) *tube*.
   t. eustachia′na, t. eusta′chii, trompa de Eustáquio. SIN pharyngotympanic (auditory) *tube*.
   t. fallopia′na, t. fallo′pii, trompa de Falópio. SIN uterine *tube*.
   t. uteri′na [TA], tuba uterina. SIN uterine *tube*.

tub·age (too′baj). Tubagem; introdução de um tubo em um canal. VER TAMBÉM intubation.

tub·al (too′băl). Tubário; relativo a uma tuba, especialmente a tuba uterina.

tu·ba·tor·sion (too - bă - tor′shŭn). Tubotorção. SIN tubotorsion.

TUBE

tube (toob) [TA], Tubo, tuba. **1.** Estrutura ou canal cilíndrico oco. **2.** Cilindro ou cano oco. SIN tuba [TA]. [L. *tubus*]
   Abbott t., t. de Abbott. SIN Miller-Abbott t.
   air t., vias respiratórias; traquéia, brônquios ou qualquer um de seus ramos que conduzem ar para os pulmões.
   auditory t., tuba auditiva; *termo oficial alternativo para pharyngotympanic (auditory) t.
   Babcock t., t. de Babcock; tubo em que o leite, após tratamento com ácido sulfúrico, é centrifugado, sendo o seu teor de gordura então determinado num colo graduado.
   Bouchut t., t. de Bouchut; tubo cilíndrico curto utilizado na intubação da laringe.
   bronchial t.'s, brônquios. SIN bronchia.
   Cantor t., t. de Cantor; tubo intestinal longo, de luz única, com uma extremidade provida de uma bolsa de borracha preenchida por mercúrio e hermeticamente fechada; utilizado para descomprimir e/ou manter a desobstrução do intestino delgado.
   cardiac t., t. cardíaco; o coração tubular primitivo no embrião, antes de sua divisão em câmaras.
   Carlen t., t. de Carlen; tubo endobrônquico flexível de dupla luz, utilizado em broncoespirometria, para isolamento de um pulmão a fim de evitar a contaminação ou secreções do pulmão contralateral, ou para ventilação de um pulmão.
   cathode ray t. (CRT), t. de raios catódicos; tubo evacuado contendo um feixe de elétrons, que podem ser defletidos para várias partes de uma tela fluorescente; utilizado no osciloscópio de raios catódicos.
   Celestin t., t. de Celestin; tubo de plástico introduzido através de um tumor no esôfago; permite a deglutição de determinadas substâncias.
   Coolidge t., t. de Coolidge; tubos de raios X em que o catodo consiste num fio espiralado de tungstênio circundado por uma taça de focalização; a espiral de tungstênio é aquecida por uma corrente elétrica; a quantidade e a qualidade dos raios X assim gerados são reguladas pela variação da temperatura do catodo e pela voltagem entre o catodo e o anodo.
   Crookes-Hittorf t., t. de Crookes-Hittorf; tubo evacuado simples contendo um catodo, que emitia raios X do envoltório de vidro quando se aplicava uma corrente; o tipo utilizado por Roentgen na descoberta dos raios X.
   digestive t., trato digestório. SIN digestive *tract*.
   drainage t., t. de drenagem; tubo introduzido em uma ferida ou cavidade para facilitar a remoção de um líquido.
   Durham t., t. de Durham; tubo de traqueotomia articulado.
   empyema t., tubo para empiema; cateter utilizado para drenagem de empiema.
   endobronchial t., t. endobrônquico; tubo de luz única ou dupla com balonete (*cuff*) inflável na extremidade distal que, após ser introduzido pela faringe e traquéia, é posicionado de modo a restringir a ventilação a um pulmão; o tubo de luz única é colocado no brônquio principal do pulmão; o de luz dupla é posicionado na carina da traquéia para permitir a ventilação de um ou de ambos os pulmões.
   endotracheal t., t. endotraqueal; tubo flexível inserido na traquéia por via nasal, oral ou através de traqueotomia, a fim de assegurar uma via aérea, como na intubação traqueal. SIN intratracheal t., tracheal t.

eustachian t., trompa de Eustáquio, tuba auditiva. SIN pharyngotympanic (auditory) t.
fallopian t., trompa de Falópio, tuba uterina. SIN uterine t.
feeding t., t. para alimentação; tubo flexível introduzido pelo nariz e no trato alimentar, através do qual se administra alimento líquido.
Ferrein t., túbulo de Ferrein. SIN convoluted tubule of kidney.
field emission t., tubo de emissão de campo; tubo de raios X que utiliza um catodo frio, que depende da voltagem do tubo para extrair dele elétrons para o anodo.
Geiger-Müller t., t. de Geiger-Müller. VER Geiger-Müller *counter.*
germ t., t. germinativo; hifa jovem que cresce a partir de uma célula de levedura ou esporo, o início de um micélio; também utilizado como rápido teste para diferenciar *Candida albicans* de outras espécies de *Candida*.
Haldane t., t. de Haldane; tubo para obter amostras de ar alveolar humano; consiste num tubo flexível estreito com bocal no qual se fixa um tubo para retirada do ar expirado no final de uma expiração máxima súbita.
intratracheal t., t. intratraqueal. SIN endotracheal t.
Levin t., t. de Levin; tubo flexível introduzido através do nariz até o trato alimentar superior para facilitar a descompressão gástrica.
Martin t., t. de Martin; tubo de drenagem com peça transversal próximo à extremidade para impedir que deslize para fora de uma cavidade.
medullary t., t. neural. SIN neural t.
Miescher t.'s, tubos de Miescher; corpos cilíndricos ou fusiformes alongados que formam o estágio intramuscular cístico encapsulado do protozoário *Sarcocystis*.
Miller-Abbott t., t. de Miller-Abbott; tubo com duas luzes, em que uma delas termina num pequeno balão colabável enquanto a outra termina numa ponta metálica com numerosas perfurações; utilizada para descompressão e desobstrução do intestino delgado. SIN Abbott t.
molybdenum target t., t. de molibdênio; tubo de raios X com superfície de anodo feita de molibdênio em lugar de tungstênio, utilizado em mamografia.
Moss t., t. de Moss; (1) tubo nasogástrico de luz tripla para alimentação e descompressão que utiliza um balão gástrico para ocluir a junção cardioesofágica, com aspiração esofágica e alimentação intragástrica simultâneas; (2) tubo de luz dupla para lavagem gástrica, que permite a administração contínua de solução salina através de um pequeno calibre, com aspiração simultânea de líquido e algumas partículas através de um grande calibre.
nasogastric t., t. nasogástrico; tubo flexível introduzido pelo nariz em direção ao estômago para descomprimi-lo.
nasotracheal t., t. nasotraqueal; tubo traqueal inserido através das vias nasais.
nephrostomy t., t. de nefrostomia; tubo colocado no sistema coletor renal para drenagem, testes diagnósticos ou remoção de cálculos. Pode ser colocado através de via percutânea ou durante uma cirurgia aberta.
neural t., t. neural; o tubo epitelial formado a partir do neuroectoderma do embrião inicial pelo fechamento do sulco neural; através de complexos processos de proliferação e organização celulares, o t. neural transforma-se na medula espinal e no cérebro. SIN medullary t.
O'Dwyer t., t. de O'Dwyer; tubo metálico antigamente utilizado para intubação da laringe na difteria.
orotracheal t., t. orotraqueal; tubo traqueal inserido através da boca.
otopharyngeal t., tuba auditiva. SIN pharyngotympanic (auditory) t.
pharyngotympanic (auditory) t. [TA], tuba auditiva; tubo que se estende da cavidade timpânica até a nasofaringe; consiste numa parte óssea (póstero-lateral) na extremidade timpânica e numa parte fibrocartilaginosa (ântero-medial) na extremidade faríngea; no local onde as duas partes se unem, na região da fissura esfenopetrosa, encontra-se a parte mais estreita da tuba (istmo); a tuba auditiva permite a equalização da pressão no interior da cavidade timpânica com a pressão do ar ambiente, descrita comumente como "estalido dos ouvidos". SIN tuba auditiva [TA], auditory t.*, tuba auditoria*, eustachian t., guttural duct, otopharyngeal t., otosalpinx, tuba acustica, tuba eustachiana, tuba eustachii.
photomultiplier t., t. fotomultiplicador; detector que amplifica um sinal (em até 10^6) de radiação eletromagnética por uma aceleração de elétrons emitidos de um fotocatodo através de uma série de dinodos; à medida que cada elétron incide num estágio dinodo, 3-4 elétrons são liberados e acelerados para o dinodo subseqüente.
Pitot t., t. de Pitot; tubo estacionário em forma de L introduzido numa corrente de líquido, com a sua abertura voltada contra a corrente; utilizado para medir a velocidade do movimento do líquido nesse ponto em termos da pressão desenvolvida no tubo pelo líquido colidindo nele, em comparação com um segundo tubo que se abre lateralmente ou a jusante.
pus t., trompa de Falópio com pus. SIN pyosalpinx.
rectifier t., t. retificador; tubo eletrônico utilizado em transformadores de raios X para converter a corrente alternada em direta.
Rehfuss stomach t., t. gástrico de Rehfuss; tubo com uma seringa calibrada, utilizado antigamente para aspiração do conteúdo gástrico na análise gástrica; substituído por tubos gástricos de plástico descartáveis.
Robertshaw t., t. de Robertshaw; variação do tubo de Carlen que elimina algumas desvantagens mecânicas do último.

roll t., t. de rolo; modificação da cultura em placas; coloca-se um meio semeado contendo ágar num tubo de ensaio, que é rolado horizontalmente até ocorrer solidificação uniforme do meio no interior do tubo.
rotating anode t., tubo de anodo rotatório; tubo moderno de raios X, em que o calor produzido distribui-se através de um maior volume por rotação do alvo.
Ruysch t., t. de Ruysch; pequena cavidade tubular que se abre na parte inferior e anterior de cada superfície do septo nasal; mais bem observada no período fetal inicial, quando está associada ao órgão vomeronasal (órgão de Jacobson).
Ryle t., t. de Ryle; tubo fino de borracha, com a luz correspondente aproximadamente a um cateter número 8 e extremidade em oliva, utilizado na administração de uma refeição de teste.
Sengstaken-Blakemore t., t. de Sengstaken-Blakemore; tubo com três luzes, uma para drenagem do estômago e duas para inflação de balões gástrico e esofágico fixados; utilizado para o tratamento de emergência de varizes esofágicas hemorrágicas.
Southey t.'s, tubos de Southey; cânulas obsoletas de pequeno calibre, quase capilar, impelidas por um trocarte nos tecidos subcutâneos para drenar o líquido de anasarca.
speaking t., t. acústico; tubo com fone de ouvido em uma extremidade e um cone na outra para amplificar a fala no fone.
stomach t., t. gástrico; tubo flexível introduzido no estômago para lavagem ou para alimentação.
T t., t. em T; tubo em forma de T cujo ápice é colocado no interior de uma estrutura tubular, como o ducto colédoco, e a haste através da pele; utilizado para descompressão.
test t., t. de ensaio; tubo de vidro fino fechado em uma extremidade, utilizado no exame de urina e outras operações químicas, para culturas bacterianas etc.
thoracostomy t., t. de toracostomia; tubo colocado através da parede torácica que drena o espaço pleural.
Tovell t., t. de Tovell; tubo endotraqueal com uma espiral de metal encerrada na parede para evitar a obstrução da luz quando o tubo é comprimido e torcido ou quando o tubo é curvado em ângulo agudo.
Toynbee t., t. de Toynbee; tubo pelo qual se pode ouvir os sons na orelha do paciente durante politzerização.
tracheal t., t. traqueal. SIN endotracheal t.
tracheostomy t., t. de traqueostomia; tubo curvo utilizado para manter a abertura livre após traqueotomia; pode ser de metal ou de plástico. SIN tracheotomy t.
tracheotomy t., t. de traqueotomia. SIN tracheostomy t.
tympanostomy t., t. de timpanostomia; pequeno tubo introduzido através da membrana timpânica após miringotomia para ventilar a orelha média; freqüentemente utilizado para derrame da orelha média.
uterine t. [TA], tuba uterina; uma das tubas que se estende de cada lado da extremidade superior ou externa do ovário, em grande parte envolvida pelo seu infundíbulo expandido, até o fundo do útero; proporciona a via pela qual o óvulo segue o seu trajeto do ovário até o útero onde, se for fertilizado na tuba, irá se implantar como zigoto; consiste no infundíbulo, na ampola, no istmo e nas partes uterinas. SIN tuba uterina [TA], salpinx*, fallopian t., gonaduct (2), oviduct, salpinx uterina, tuba fallopiana, tuba fallopii.

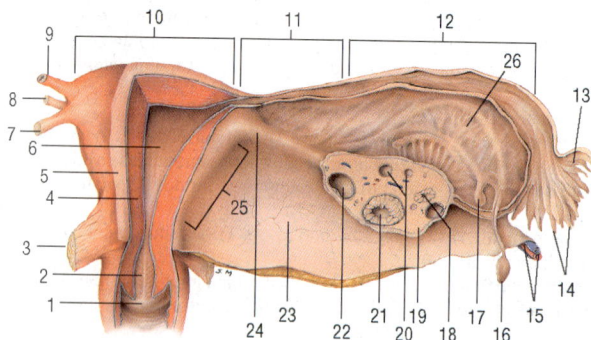

trato genital feminino: vista dorsal com apêndices esticados e útero aberto, vagina e tuba uterina direita, estando o ovário direito em corte frontal

1. colo do útero
2. canal do colo do útero
3. ligamento sacrouterino
4. miométrio
5. perimétrio
6. cavidade uterina, endométrio
7. ligamento ovariano
8. ligamento redondo
9. tuba uterina
10. fundo do útero
11. istmo da tuba uterina
12. ampola da tuba uterina
13. infundíbulo da tuba uterina
14. fímbrias da tuba uterina
15. veia e artéria ovarianas
16. hidátide pedunculada
17. fímbrias ovaricas
18. corpo albicante
19. estroma do ovário
20. folículos ovarianos primários
21. corpo lúteo
22. folículo ovariano vesicular
23. ligamento largo
24. ligamento ovariano
25. corpo do útero
25. epoóforo

vacuum t., t. a vácuo; tubo de vidro do qual foi removido o ar, contendo dois ou mais eletrodos, entre os quais passa uma corrente ou descarga elétrica; utilizado na produção de raios X ou para controlar circuitos. Outrora muito utilizado, o tubo a vácuo foi suplantado por transistores em circuitos eletrônicos.
Venturi t., t. de Venturi; tubo com uma constrição especialmente aerodinâmica para minimizar as perdas de energia no líquido que flui através dele, enquanto maximiza a queda da pressão na constrição, de acordo com a lei de Bernoulli; a base do venturímetro.
Wangensteen t., t. de Wangensteen. SIN Wangensteen suction.
x-ray t., t. de raios X. VER x-ray.

tu·bec·to·my (too-bek′tō-mē). Tubectomia, salpingectomia. SIN salpingectomy. [L. *tuba*, tubo, + G. *ektomē*, excisão]
tu·ber, pl. **tu·bera** (too′ber, too′ber-ă). Túber; tuberosidade. **1.** [TA] Tumefação localizada; protuberância. **2.** Caule subterrâneo curto, carnoso e espesso de plantas, como a batata. [L. protuberância, tumefação]
t. ante′rius, túber cinéreo. SIN t. cinereum.
ashen t., túber cinéreo. SIN t. cinereum.
calcaneal t., tuberosidade do calcâneo. SIN calcaneal tuberosity.
t. calca′nei [TA], tuberosidade do calcâneo. SIN calcaneal tuberosity.
t. cal′cis, tuberosidade do calcâneo. SIN calcaneal tuberosity.
t. cine′reum [TA], túber cinéreo; proeminência da base do hipotálamo, limitada caudalmente pelos corpos mamilares, rostralmente pelo quiasma óptico e lateralmente pelo trato óptico, estendendo-se ventralmente até o infundíbulo e o pedúnculo hipofisário. SIN ashen t., gray t., t. anterius.
t. coch′leae, promontório da cavidade timpânica. SIN promontory of tympanic cavity.
t. cor′poris callo′si, esplênio do corpo caloso. SIN splenium of corpus callosum.
t. dorsa′le, túber do verme. SIN t. vermis.
eustachian t., tuberosidade de Eustáquio; ligeira projeção da parede do labirinto da orelha média, abaixo da janela do vestíbulo (oval).
frontal t. [TA], túber frontal; a parte mais proeminente do osso frontal de cada lado. SIN t. frontale [TA], eminentia frontalis*, frontal eminence*.
t. fronta′le [TA], túber frontal. SIN frontal t.
gray t., túber cinéreo. SIN t. cinereum.
t. ischiad′icum [TA], túber isquiático. SIN ischial tuberosity.
t. of ischium, túber isquiático. SIN ischial tuberosity.
t. maxil′lae [TA], túber da maxila. SIN maxillary tuberosity.
omental t., túber omental do pâncreas. SIN omental eminence of pancreas.
t. omentale hepatis [TA], túber omental do fígado. SIN omental tuberosity of liver.
t. omentale pancreatis [TA], túber omental do pâncreas. SIN omental eminence of pancreas.
parietal t. [TA], túber parietal; porção proeminente do osso parietal, um pouco acima do centro de sua superfície externa, que corresponde habitualmente ao ponto de largura máxima da cabeça. SIN t. parietale [TA], eminentia parietalis*, parietal eminence*.
t. parieta′le [TA], túber parietal. SIN parietal t.
t. ra′dii, tuberosidade do rádio. SIN radial tuberosity.
t. val′vulae, túber do verme. SIN t. vermis.
t. of vermis, túber do verme. SIN t. vermis.
t. ver′mis, túber do verme; a divisão posterior do verme inferior do cerebelo, localizada entre a folha e a pirâmide. SIN t. dorsale, t. of vermis, t. valvulae.
t. zygomat′icum, tubérculo articular do (osso) temporal. SIN articular tubercle of temporal bone.

tu·ber·cle (too′ber-kl). Tubérculo. **1.** Nódulo, especialmente em sentido anatômico, e não patológico. **2.** Elevação sólida, arredondada e circunscrita na pele, mucosa ou superfície de um órgão. **3.** Pequena elevação na superfície de um osso, proporcionando fixação para um músculo ou ligamento. **4.** Em odontologia, pequena elevação que surge na superfície de um dente. **5.** Lesão granulomatosa causada pela infecção por *Mycobacterium tuberculosis*. Embora um pouco variáveis quanto ao tamanho (0,5-2 ou 3 mm de diâmetro) e às proporções de vários componentes histológicos, os tubérculos tendem a ser lesões firmes esferoidais bem-circunscritas, que habitualmente consistem em três zonas de contorno irregular, porém moderadamente distintas: 1) um foco interno de necrose, a princípio coagulativa e, a seguir, caseosa; 2) uma zona média, que consiste num acúmulo bastante denso de grandes fagócitos mononucleares (macrófagos), freqüentemente dispostos de modo um tanto radial (em relação ao material necrótico), assemelhando-se a um epitélio e, portanto, denominados células epiteliódes; pode haver também células gigantes multinucleadas do tipo de Langhans; 3) uma zona externa de numerosos linfócitos e alguns monócitos e plasmócitos. Em casos em que a cicatrização já começou, uma quarta zona de tecido fibroso pode formar-se na periferia. Podem ocorrer lesões morfologicamente indistinguíveis em doenças causadas por outros agentes; muitos observadores utilizam o termo de modo inespecífico, isto é, com referência a qualquer desses granulomas; outros utilizam o termo "tubérculo" para referir-se apenas a lesões tuberculosas e designam aquelas de causas indeterminadas como granulomas de células epitelióides. SIN tuberculum [TA]. [L. *tuberculum*, dim. de *tuber*, protuberância, tumefação, tumor]
accessory t., processo acessório. SIN accessory process of lumbar vertebra.
acoustic t., tubérculo acústico. SIN trigone of auditory nerve.
adductor t. of femur [TA], tubérculo do adutor; proeminência acima do epicôndilo medial do fêmur à qual se fixa o tendão do músculo adutor magno. SIN tuberculum adductorium femoris [TA].
amygdaloid t., tubérculo amigdalóide; projeção do teto da parte terminal anterior do corno temporal do ventrículo lateral, marcando a localização do núcleo amigdalóide.
anatomic t., t. anatômico. SIN postmortem wart.
anterior t. of atlas [TA], tubérculo anterior do atlas; protuberância cônica sobre a superfície anterior do arco do atlas. SIN tuberculum anterius atlantis [TA].
anterior t. of cervical vertebrae [TA], tubérculo anterior das vértebras cervicais; a projeção anterior do processo transverso. SIN tuberculum anterius vertebrarum cervicalium [TA].
t. of anterior scalene muscle, tubérculo do músculo escaleno anterior. SIN scalene t.
anterior thalamic t. [TA], tubérculo anterior do tálamo; proeminência na extremidade anterior do tálamo que corresponde aos núcleos anteriores. SIN tuberculum anterius thalami [TA], anterior t. of thalamus.
anterior t. of thalamus, tubérculo anterior do tálamo. SIN anterior thalamic t.
areolar t.'s [TA], tubérculos areolares; pequenas elevações na aréola da mama feminina, especialmente proeminentes durante a gravidez e a lactação, que consistem numa manifestação superficial das glândulas areolares subjacentes. SIN tubercula areolae [TA].
articular t. of temporal bone [TA], tubérculo articular do (osso) temporal; eminência articular do osso temporal que limita a fossa mandibular anteriormente; forma a raiz anterior do processo zigomático; é encerrado pela cápsula articular da articulação temporomandibular com a fossa articular; a cabeça da mandíbula (e disco articular interveniente) move-se sobre o tubérculo articular, permitindo a depressão total da mandíbula (abertura da boca). SIN tuberculum articulare ossis temporalis [TA], articular eminence of temporal bone, eminentia articularis ossis temporalis, tuber zygomaticum.
ashen t., túber cinéreo. SIN tuberculum cinereum.
auricular t. [TA], t. da orelha; pequena projeção inconstante da extremidade superior da parte posterior da margem livre curva da hélice da orelha. SIN tuberculum auriculae [TA], darwinian t., tuberculum superius.
calcaneal t. [TA], t. do calcâneo; projeção, freqüentemente dupla, na face inferior do calcâneo na extremidade anterior da área para fixação do ligamento plantar longo. SIN tuberculum calcanei [TA].
Carabelli t., t. de Carabelli; pequeno t. semelhante a uma cúspide supranumerária, encontrado por vezes sobre a superfície lingual da cúspide mesiolingual de um primeiro molar maxilar permanente.
carotid t. [TA], t. carótico; o t. anterior do processo transverso da sexta vértebra cervical, contra o qual a artéria carótida pode ser comprimida pelo dedo. SIN tuberculum caroticum [TA], Chassaignac t.
caseous t., t. caseoso. SIN soft t.
Chassaignac t., t. de Chassaignac. SIN carotid t.
conoid t. (of clavicle) [TA], t. conóide (da clavícula); a proeminência próxima à extremidade lateral da superfície inferior da clavícula que fornece fixação ao ligamento conóide. SIN tuberculum conoideum (claviculare) [TA], conoid process.
corniculate t. [TA], t. corniculado; a menor e mais medial das duas eminências arredondadas na parte posterior da prega ariepiglótica, formadas pelas cartilagens corniculadas subjacentes. SIN tuberculum corniculatum [TA], Santorini t.
crown t., t. da coroa. SIN dental t.
cuneate t., t. cuneiforme; a extremidade rostral bulbosa do fascículo cuneiforme, que corresponde à posição do núcleo cuneiforme, situado lateralmente à clava e separado do túber cinéreo em sua face lateral pelo sulco lateral posterior. SIN tuberculum cuneatum, wedge-shaped t.
cuneiform t. [TA], t. cuneiforme; a maior e mais lateralmente localizada das duas eminências arredondadas na parte superior da prega ariepiglótica, formada pela cartilagem cuneiforme subjacente. SIN tuberculum cuneiforme [TA], Wrisberg t.
darwinian t., tubérculo de Darwin. SIN auricular t.
deltoid t. (of spine of scapula) [TA], t. deltóide (da escápula); proeminência no dorso da espinha da escápula, lateralmente a raiz da espinha, à qual se fixa um tendão triangular plano da parte mais inferior da parte média do (músculo) trapézio. SIN tuberculum deltoideum (spinae scapulae) [TA].
dental t. [TA], t. do dente; pequena elevação em algumas porções de uma coroa, produzida por uma formação adicional de esmalte. SIN tuberculum dentis [TA], crown t., t. of tooth, tuberculum coronae.
dorsal t. of radius [TA], t. dorsal do rádio; pequena proeminência na face dorsal da extremidade distal do rádio, lateralmente ao sulco para o tendão do extensor longo do polegar; serve como tróclea ou roldana para o tendão. SIN tuberculum dorsale radii [TA], Lister t.

epiglottic t. [TA], t. epiglótico; convexidade na parte inferior da epiglote na parte superior do ligamento tireoepiglótico. SIN tuberculum epiglotticum [TA], cushion of epiglottis.

fibrous t., t. fibroso; t. em que os fibroblastos proliferam ao redor da periferia (e dentro das zonas celulares), resultando finalmente numa borda ou parede de tecido fibroso celular ou material colagenoso em torno do tubérculo.

genial t., espinal geniana. SIN mental spine.

genital t., t. genital; a elevação mediana cefálica ao orifício urogenital de um embrião; trata-se do primórdio do pênis no sexo masculino e do clitóris no sexo feminino. SIN phallic t.

Gerdy t., t. de Gerdy; t. na face ântero-lateral da extremidade superior da tíbia, que fornece fixação ao trato iliotibial e a algumas fibras do músculo tibial anterior.

Ghon t., t. de Ghon; calcificação observada no parênquima pulmonar (em geral, no meio do pulmão) resultante de tuberculose anterior, geralmente na infância; algumas vezes confundido com uma combinação de lesão parenquimatosa e linfonodo calcificado, que é apropriadamente denominada complexo de Ranke. SIN Ghon complex, Ghon focus, Ghon primary lesion.

gracile t., t. grácil; a extremidade superior um tanto expandida do fascículo grácil, que corresponde à posição do núcleo grácil. SIN clava, tuberculum gracile.

gray t., t. trigeminal. SIN trigeminal t.

greater t. (of humerus) [TA], t. maior (do úmero); o maior dos dois tubérculos próximos à cabeça do úmero; proporciona inserção aos músculos supra-espinal, infra-espinal e redondo menor. SIN tuberculum majus (humeri) [TA], greater tuberosity of humerus.

hard t., t. duro; t. sem necrose.

hyaline t., t. hialino; forma de t. fibroso em que o tecido fibroso celular e as fibras colágenas são alterados e fundidos numa massa firme bastante homogênea, acelular e intensamente acidofílica.

iliac t., t. ilíaco. SIN t. of iliac crest.

t. of iliac crest [TA], t. ilíaco; proeminência no lábio externo da crista ilíaca, cerca de 5 cm posterior à espinha ilíaca ântero-superior. SIN tuberculum iliacum [TA], iliac t.

inferior thyroid t. [TA], t. tireóideo inferior; pequena projeção lateral da margem inferior da lâmina da cartilagem tireóidea de cada lado, na extremidade inferior da linha oblíqua. SIN tuberculum thyroideum inferius [TA].

infraglenoid t. (of scapula) [TA], t. infraglenoidal (da escápula); superfície rugosa abaixo da cavidade glenoidal da escápula que fornece fixação ao tendão longo do tríceps. SIN tuberculum infraglenoidale (scapulae) [TA], infraglenoid tuberosity.

intercolumnar t., t. intercolunar. VER subfornical organ.

intercondylar t. [TA], t. intercondilar; uma de duas projeções, medial e lateral, que surgem do lábio central de cada superfície articular da tíbia, de cada lado da eminência intercondilar. SIN tuberculum intercondylare (mediale et laterale) [TA].

intervenous t. (of right atrium) [TA], t. intervenoso (do átrio direito); pequena projeção da parede do átrio direito, entre os óstios das veias cavas. SIN tuberculum intervenosum (atrii dextri) [TA], Lower t.

jugular t. of occipital bone [TA], t. jugular do osso occipital; elevação oval na superfície cerebral da junção das partes lateral e basal do osso occipital, de cada lado do forame magno medialmente à borda inferior e ântero-superiormente à abertura do canal hipoglosso. SIN tuberculum jugulare ossis occipitalis [TA].

labial t., t. do lábio. SIN t. of upper lip.

lateral t. (of posterior process) of talus [TA], t. lateral (do processo posterior) do tálus; a proeminência lateral ao sulco para o tendão flexor longo do hálux. SIN tuberculum laterale (processus posterioris) tali [TA].

lesser t. (of humerus) [TA], t. menor do úmero; o tubérculo anterior dos dois tubérculos do colo do úmero sobre o qual está inserido o subescapular. SIN tuberculum minus (humeri) [TA], lesser tuberosity of humerus.

Lisfranc t., t. de Lisfranc. SIN scalene t.

Lister t., t. de Lister. SIN dorsal t. of radius.

Lower t., t. de Lower. SIN intervenous t. (of right atrium).

mammillary t., processo mamilar. SIN mammillary process of lumbar vertebra.

mammillary t. of hypothalamus, corpo mamilar do hipotálamo. SIN mammillary body.

marginal t., t. marginal. SIN marginal t. (of zygomatic bone).

marginal t. (of zygomatic bone) [TA], t. marginal (do osso zigomático); proeminência inconstante sobre a borda temporal do osso zigomático à qual se fixa a fáscia temporal. SIN tuberculum marginale (ossis zygomatici) [TA], marginal t.

medial t. (of posterior process) of talus [TA], t. medial (do processo posterior) do tálus; a eminência medial ou sulco para o tendão do flexor longo do hálux. SIN tuberculum mediale (processus posterioris) tali [TA].

mental t. (of mandible) [TA], t. mentual (da mandíbula); par de eminências sobre a protuberância mentual da mandíbula. SIN tuberculum mentale (mandibulae) [TA], eminentia symphysis.

molar t. [TA], t. molar; proeminência não-oclusiva ocasional de tamanho variável na coroa de um dente molar. SIN tuberculum molare [TA].

Montgomery t.'s, tubérculos de Montgomery; glândulas areolares avermelhadas elevadas, habitualmente associadas à gravidez.

Morgagni t., t. de Morgagni. SIN cuneiform cartilage.

Müller t., t. de Müller; protuberância mediana que se projeta para o seio urogenital embrionário a partir de sua parede dorsal; é formado pelas extremidades caudais fundidas dos ductos paramesonéfricos e constitui a primeira evidência de útero e vagina embrionários. SIN sinus t.

nuchal t., vértebra proeminente (sétima cervical). SIN vertebra prominens.

obturator t. [TA], t. obturatório; um dos dois processos, anterior e posterior, na margem da parte púbica do forame obturatório, delimitando a terminação do sulco obturatório. O t. obturatório posterior é inconstante. SIN tuberculum obturatorium [TA].

olfactory t., t. olfatório; pequena área oval na base do hemisfério cerebral, entre as estrias olfatórias medial e lateral divergentes, na parte ântero-medial da substância perfurada anterior; é formado por uma pequena área do alocórtex, caracterizada pela presença das ilhas de Calleja. Correspondendo a uma estrutura muito mais proeminente nos mamíferos não-primatas (especialmente roedores e insetívoros), o tubérculo olfatório recebe fibras do bulbo olfatório através da estria olfatória intermediária; possui conexões eferentes com o hipotálamo e o núcleo médio dorsal do tálamo. SIN tuberculum olfactorium [TA].

orbital t. (of zygomatic bone) [TA], t. orbital (do osso zigomático); pequena elevação na superfície orbital do osso zigomático, imediatamente dentro da margem orbital, cerca de 1 cm abaixo da sutura zigomaticofrontal; fornece fixação ao ligamento controlador lateral, ao ligamento palpebral lateral e ao ligamento suspensor do bulbo do olho. SIN tuberculum orbitale ossis zygomatici [TA], eminentia orbitalis (ossis zygomatici), orbital eminence of zygomatic bone, Whitnall t.

phallic t., t. fálico. SIN genital t.

pharyngeal t. (of basilar part of occipital bone) [TA], t. faríngeo (da parte basilar do osso occipital); projeção da superfície inferior da parte basilar do osso occipital que fornece fixação à rafe fibrosa da faringe. SIN tuberculum pharyngeum (partis basilaris ossis occipitalis) [TA].

posterior t. of atlas [TA], t. posterior do atlas; protuberância da extremidade posterior do arco do atlas, um rudimento do processo espinhoso que fornece inserção ao músculo reto posterior menor da cabeça. SIN tuberculum posterius atlantis [TA].

posterior t. of cervical vertebrae [TA], t. posterior das vértebras cervicais; projeção posterior dos processos transversos. SIN tuberculum posterius vertebrarum cervicalium [TA].

Princeteau t., t. de Princeteau; discreta proeminência no osso temporal, próximo ao ápice da parte petrosa, onde começa o seio petroso superior.

pterygoid t., processo pterigóide; discreta proeminência na superfície posterior da lâmina medial, inferior e no lado medial do canal pterigóideo.

pubic t. [TA], t. púbico; pequena projeção palpável na extremidade anterior da crista do púbis, cerca de 2 cm da sínfise; local de inserção do ligamento inguinal. SIN tuberculum pubicum [TA], pubic spine, spina pubis.

t. of rib [TA], t. da costela; a proeminência na superfície posterior de uma costela, na junção de seu colo e corpo, que se articula com o processo transverso da vértebra e que corresponde, quanto ao número, à costela, formando uma articulação costotransversa. SIN tuberculum costae [TA].

Rolando t., t. de Rolando. SIN trigeminal t.

t. of saddle, t. da sela. SIN tuberculum sellae.

Santorini t., t. de Santorini. SIN corniculate t.

scalene t. [TA], t. do músculo escaleno anterior; pequena espinha na borda interna da primeira costela, fornecendo inserção ao músculo escaleno anterior, situada entre os sulcos para a artéria subclávia (anteriormente) e veia subclávia (posteriormente), demarcando-os. SIN tuberculum musculi scaleni anterioris [TA], Lisfranc t., scalene t. of Lisfranc, t. of anterior scalene muscle.

scalene t. of Lisfranc, t. escaleno de Lisfranc. SIN scalene t.

t. of scaphoid (bone) [TA], t. do (osso) escafóide; projeção no ângulo lateral inferior do osso escafóide; pode ser percebido na raiz do polegar; fornece fixação ao ligamento transverso do carpo (retináculo dos flexores). SIN tuberculum ossis scaphoidei [TA].

sinus t., t. de Müller. SIN Müller t.

soft t., tubérculo caseoso; t. que apresenta necrose caseosa. SIN caseous t.

superior thyroid t. [TA], t. tireóideo superior; projeção lateral romba sobre a face externa da lâmina da cartilagem tireóidea, de cada lado na extremidade superior da linha oblíqua. SIN tuberculum thyroideum superius [TA].

supraglenoid t. (of scapula) [TA], t. supraglenoidal (da escápula); superfície rugosa acima da cavidade glenoidal da escápula que fornece inserção ao tendão da cabeça longa do bíceps dentro da cavidade articular da articulação do ombro. SIN tuberculum supraglenoidale (scapulae) [TA].

supratragic t. [TA], t. supratrágico; pequena elevação inconstante, freqüentemente presente na borda do trago superior. SIN tuberculum supratragicum [TA].

t. of tooth, t. do dente. SIN dental t.
t. of trapezium (bone), t. do (osso) trapézio. SIN *tuberculum* of trapezium bone.
trigeminal t. [TA], t. trigeminal; proeminência longitudinal na superfície dorsolateral da medula oblonga ao longo da borda lateral do tubérculo cuneiforme; é o perfil superficial do trato espinal do nervo trigêmeo, que se continua caudalmente com o fascículo dorsolateral (trato de Lissauer). SIN tuberculum trigeminale [TA], gray t., Rolando t.
t. of upper lip [TA], t. do lábio superior; pequena projeção na borda livre do centro do lábio superior na extensão inferior do filtro. SIN tuberculum labii superioris [TA], labial t., procheilon, prochilon.
wedge-shaped t., t. cuneiforme. SIN cuneate t.
Whitnall t., t. de Whitnall. SIN orbital t. (of zygomatic bone).
Wrisberg t., t. de Wrisberg. SIN cuneiform t.

tubercul-. Tubercul-. VER tuberculo-.
tu·ber·cu·la (too-ber′kū-lă). Tubérculos; plural de tuberculum.
tu·ber·cu·lar, tu·ber·cu·lat·ed (too-ber′kū-lăr, -lāt-ed). Tubercular, tuberculado; relativo a ou caracterizado por tubérculos ou pequenos nódulos. Cf. tuberculous.
tu·ber·cu·la·tion (too-ber-kū-lā′shŭn). Tuberculação; a disposição de tubérculos ou nódulos numa parte.
tu·ber·cu·lid (too-ber′kū-lid). Tubercúlide; lesão da pele ou da mucosa em decorrência de hipersensibilidade a antígenos micobacterianos disseminados a partir de um local distante de tuberculose ativa. [tubercul- + G. -id (1)]
  nodular t., eritema indurado. SIN *erythema* induratum.
  papular t., líquen escrofuloso. SIN *lichen* scrofulosorum.
  papulonecrotic t., t. papulonecrótica; pápulas vermelho-escuras seguidas de formação de crosta e ulceração com alterações vasculares não-granulomatosas primariamente nos membros, com ocorrência predominante em adultos jovens com foco profundo de tuberculose ou história de infecção prévia. SIN tuberculosis papulonecrotica.
  rosacea-like t., rosácea granulomatosa. SIN granulomatous *rosacea.*
tu·ber·cu·lin (too-ber′kū-lin). Tuberculina. **1.** Cultura de *Mycobacterium tuberculosis* em caldo de glicerina evaporado a volume 1/10 a 100°C e filtrado; introduzida por Robert Koch para o tratamento da tuberculose, mas agora utilizada principalmente para testes diagnósticos; originalmente conhecida como tuberculina velha de Koch (OT) ou tuberculina original de Koch. **2.** Um ou outro de um número relativamente grande de extratos de culturas de *Mycobacterium tuberculosis,* diferente da OT e atualmente obsoleto.
  Koch old t. (OT), t. velha de Koch. VER tuberculin (1).
  purified protein derivative of t. (PPD), derivado protéico purificado de tuberculina (PPD); tuberculina purificada contendo a fração protéica ativa; a tuberculina a partir da qual é preparada difere da tuberculina (1) principalmente pelo fato de as bactérias serem cultivadas em meio sintético, e não em caldo.
tu·ber·cu·li·tis (too-ber-kū-lī′tis). Tuberculite; inflamação de qualquer tubérculo. [tubercul- + G. *-itis,* inflamação]
tuberculo-, tubercul-. Tuberculo-, tuberculose. [L. *tuberculum,* tubérculo]
tu·ber·cu·lo·cele (too-ber′kū-lō-sēl). Tuberculocele; tuberculose dos testículos. [tuberculo- + G. *kēlē,* tumor, hérnia]
tu·ber·cu·lo·che·mo·ther·a·peu·tic (too-ber′kū-lō-ke′mō-ther-ă-pū′tik). Tuberculoquimioterápico; relativo ao tratamento da tuberculose por drogas tuberculostáticas ou tuberculocidas.
tu·ber·cu·lo·ci·dal (too-ber′kū-lō-sī′dăl). Tuberculocida; destrutivo para o bacilo da tuberculose.
tu·ber·cu·lo·der·ma (too-ber′kū-lō-der′mă). Tuberculoderma. **1.** Qualquer processo tubercular da pele. **2.** A manifestação cutânea da tuberculose.
tu·ber·cu·lo·fi·broid (too-ber′kū-lō-fī′broyd). Tuberculofibróide; nódulo encapsulado, distinto, bem-circunscrito, habitualmente esferóide, de consistência moderada a extremamente firme, que se forma durante o processo de cicatrização em um foco de inflamação granulomatosa tubercular.
tu·ber·cu·loid (too-ber′kū-loyd). Tuberculóide; que se assemelha à tuberculose ou a um tubérculo. [tuberculo- + G. *eidos,* semelhança]
tu·ber·cu·lo·ma (too-ber-kū-lō′mă). Tuberculoma; massa arredondada, semelhante a tumor, porém não-neoplásica, habitualmente nos pulmões ou no cérebro, devido a infecção tuberculosa localizada. [tuberculo- + G. *-oma,* tumor]
tu·ber·cu·lo·pro·tein (too-ber′kū-lō-prō′tēn). Tuberculoproteína; qualquer uma ou uma mistura de qualquer uma ou de todas as proteínas presentes no corpo do bacilo da tuberculose, todas as quais possuem certas propriedades de tuberculina.
tu·ber·cu·lo·sis (TB) (tū-ber′kyū-lō′sis). Tuberculose (TB); doença específica causada pela infecção por *Mycobacterium tuberculosis,* o bacilo da tuberculose, que pode afetar quase qualquer tecido ou órgão do corpo, sendo os pulmões o local mais comum da doença. A t. primária é tipicamente uma infecção pulmonar local leve ou assintomática. Pode ocorrer comprometimento dos linfonodos regionais; todavia, em pessoas sadias sob os demais aspectos, a doença generalizada não se desenvolve imediatamente. Uma resposta imune celular detém a disseminação dos microrganismos e isola a zona de infecção. Por fim, os tecidos e linfonodos infectados sofrem calcificação. O teste cutâneo da tuberculina torna-se positivo em algumas semanas e assim permanece durante toda a vida. Os microrganismos numa lesão primária permanecem viáveis e podem sofrer reativação dentro de meses ou anos, iniciando a tuberculose secundária. A progressão para o estágio secundário acaba ocorrendo em 10–15% dos indivíduos que tiveram t. primária. O risco de reativação é aumentado pela coexistência de diabetes melito, infecção por HIV, silicose e várias condições sistêmicas ou malignas, bem como em alcoólatras, usuários de drogas IV, residentes em asilos e indivíduos submetidos a terapia imunossupressora ou com esteróides córtico-supra-renais. A t. secundária ou de reativação geralmente resulta em infecção pulmonar disseminada denominada crônica, que afeta mais freqüentemente os lobos superiores. Verifica-se o desenvolvimento de granulomas (tubérculos) minúsculos, malvisíveis a olho nu, no tecido pulmonar afetado; cada um deles consiste numa zona de necrose de caseificação, circundada por células inflamatórias crônicas (histiócitos epitelióides e células gigantes). Essas lesões, que deram à doença o seu nome, são também encontradas em outros tecidos (linfonodos, intestino, rim, pele) para os quais a doença pode disseminar-se. Raramente a reativação resulta em disseminação generalizada de tubérculos por todo o corpo (t. miliar). Os sinais e sintomas da tuberculose pulmonar ativa consistem em fadiga, anorexia, perda de peso, febre baixa, sudorese noturna, tosse crônica e hemoptise. Os sintomas locais dependem das partes afetadas. A tuberculose pulmonar ativa é inexoravelmente crônica e, se não for tratada, leva à destruição progressiva do tecido pulmonar. Formam-se cavidades nos pulmões, e a erosão dos vasos sangüíneos pulmonares pode resultar em hemorragia potencialmente fatal. A deterioração gradual do estado nutricional e da saúde geral culmina em morte devido a consunção, infecção ou falência de múltiplos órgãos. Diversas síndromes (linfadenite tuberculosa em crianças, doença sistêmica grave em indivíduos com AIDS/SIDA) são causadas por microrganismos do complexo *Mycobacterium avium-intracellulare.* [tuberculo- + G. *-osis,* condição]

Em 1993, a Organização Mundial de Saúde (OMS) declarou ser a tuberculose uma emergência global. Um terço da população mundial possui TB. Numa escala global, a TB ocupa o primeiro lugar entre as doenças infecciosas como causa de morte. Dois terços de todos os casos no mundo inteiro concentram-se na Ásia, porém a doença também é endêmica em partes da África e outras regiões. A guerra e as revoluções sociais são fatores na propagação da tuberculose além das zonas endêmicas; a prevalência da infecção é maior entre refugiados e imigrantes. Nos Estados Unidos, um terço de todos os indivíduos com tuberculose nasceu em outro país. Entre a década de 1950, quando os antibióticos começaram a ser utilizados no tratamento da tuberculose, e a década de 1980, tanto a incidência quanto a taxa de mortalidade da doença declinaram ininterruptamente nos Estados Unidos. Durante a década de 1980, a incidência começou a aumentar, devido a muitos casos novos em pessoas com AIDS/SIDA e devido à prevalência crescente de cepas de *M. tuberculosis* multidroga-resistentes (MDR). Desde 1993, os números voltaram a declinar, principalmente como resultado de progressos nos programas de prevenção e controle da tuberculose nos departamentos de saúde tanto locais quanto estaduais, devido a um aumento das verbas fornecidas pelo governo dos Estados Unidos aos estados. Pelo menos um terço dos indivíduos com AIDS/SIDA contrai a tuberculose, e a tuberculose é a causa de morte de um terço dos pacientes que morrem de AIDS/SIDA. Como a resistência do *M. tuberculosis* a antibióticos tem sido um problema crescente há anos, os esquemas de multidrogas, incluindo geralmente isoniazida, rifampicina e pirazinamida, tornaram-se padronizados. Outros fármacos, como etambutol, estreptomicina, canamicina e capreomicina, podem ser acrescentados ou substituir outros fármacos. O sucesso do tratamento é limitado não apenas pela resistência dos microrganismos a vários agentes, mas também pelo risco dos efeitos tóxicos graves observados com todos os agentes padrões. Em contraste com a maioria das infecções tratadas com antibióticos, a tuberculose não necessita de dias ou semanas de tratamento, mas de meses e até anos. A adesão a longo prazo ao tratamento tende a ser precária entre pessoas que se deslocam de um local para outro, indigentes e incultas. De acordo com a OMS, a principal causa da disseminação de cepas de *M. tuberculosis* MDR consiste na administração não-efetiva dos programas de controle da tuberculose, particularmente nos países do Terceiro Mundo. Um curso de quimioterapia inapropriado ou incompleto não apenas deixa o paciente ainda mais doente e contagioso como também favorece a seleção de bactérias resistentes. Estima-se que 50 milhões de casos de tuberculose no mundo inteiro envolvam bacilos da tuberculose MDR. Atualmente, a OMS recomenda com insistência que os programas de tuberculose no mundo inteiro adotem a prática da terapia de observação direta (TOD), em que um profissional de saúde deve observar cada paciente tomando cada dose do medicamento. Em um estudo realizado em diversos centros nos Estados Unidos, foi constatado que a TOD para a tuberculose é custo-efetiva quando o custo envolvido nas recidivas e fracassos do tratamento foi somado ao custo da terapia auto-administrada, embora o custo bruto da TOD fosse maior. As autoridades sanitárias dos Estados Unidos estabeleceram como meta nacional a eliminação da TB (definida como uma incidência de < 1 caso por milhão da população) até 2010.

adult t., t. do adulto. SIN secondary t.
aerogenic t., t. aerogênica; infecção por *Mycobacterium tuberculosis* transmitido por inalação de perdigotos infectados.
anthracotic t., pneumoconiose. SIN pneumoconiosis.
arrested t., t. inativa. SIN inactive t.
attenuated t., t. atenuada; forma crônica leve caracterizada por tubérculos caseosos da pele e pela ocorrência de abscessos frios.
basal t., t. basal; tuberculose das partes basilares dos pulmões.
cerebral t., t. cerebral. (1) SIN tuberculous meningitis; (2) tuberculoma cerebral.
childhood t., t. infantil; infecção inicial (primária) por *Mycobacterium tuberculosis*, caracterizada por lesões pulmonares nas partes médias dos pulmões, raramente cavitárias, com rápida disseminação para os linfonodos hilares e paratraqueais; mais freqüentemente observada na infância, embora o padrão não seja limitado a crianças.
childhood type t., t. do tipo infantil. SIN primary t.
cutaneous t., t. cutânea; lesões patológicas da pele causadas por *Mycobacterium tuberculosis*. SIN t. cutis.
t. cu'tis, t. cutânea. SIN cutaneous t.
t. cu'tis orificia'lis, t. cutânea orificial; qualquer lesão tuberculosa na boca ou no ânus ou em torno deles.
t. cu'tis verruco'sa, t. cutânea verrucosa; lesão cutânea tuberculosa com superfície verrucosa e base inflamatória crônica, observada nas mãos em adultos e nos membros inferiores em crianças, com acentuada hipersensibilidade a antígenos tuberculosos. VER TAMBÉM postmortem *wart*. SIN tuberculous wart.
disseminated t., t. disseminada. SIN miliary t.
enteric t., t. entérica; complicação da tuberculose pulmonar cavitária que habitualmente resulta da expectoração e deglutição dos bacilos, que passam a infectar áreas do trato digestório, onde há estase relativa ou tecido linfóide abundante; pode ser causada pela ingestão de microrganismos da tuberculose bovina no leite infectado, atualmente rara. VER TAMBÉM tuberculous enteritis.
exudative t., t. exsudativa; estágio da infecção por *Mycobacterium tuberculosis* que causa edema grave e reação inflamatória celular sem muita necrose ou fibrose.
generalized t., t. generalizada. SIN miliary t.
healed t., t. cicatrizada; cicatriz ou nódulo calcificado, fibroso ou caseoso na pleura pulmonar, em linfonodos e outros órgãos, resultante de tuberculose prévia que regrediu. Quando verdadeiramente cicatrizada, não há nenhum microrganismo, e não é possível a ocorrência de reativação.
inactive t., t. inativa; área fibrosa ou nodular de tuberculose previamente ativa que regrediu, permanecendo a lesão estável por um longo período de tempo; pode ser calcificada; é possível haver reativação. SIN arrested t.
miliary t., t. miliar; disseminação generalizada de bacilos da tuberculose no sangue, resultando na formação de tubérculos miliares em vários órgãos e tecidos e, por vezes, produzindo sintomas de toxemia profunda. SIN disseminated t., generalized t.
open t., t. aberta; tuberculose pulmonar, ulceração tuberculosa ou outra forma na qual existem bacilos da tuberculose nas excreções ou secreções; no pulmão, constitui habitualmente o resultado da formação de cavidades.
t. papulonecrot'ica, t. papulonecrótica. SIN papulonecrotic tuberculid.
postprimary t., t. secundária. SIN secondary t.
primary t., t. primária; primeira infecção por *Mycobacterium tuberculosis*, tipicamente observada em crianças, mas que também ocorre em adultos, caracterizada pela formação de um complexo primário nos pulmões, que consiste num pequeno foco pulmonar periférico com disseminação para os linfonodos hilares ou paratraqueais; pode sofrer cavitação ou cicatrizar com fibrose ou pode progredir. SIN childhood type t.
pulmonary t., t. pulmonar; t. dos pulmões.
reactivation t., t. de reativação. SIN secondary t.
reinfection t., t. por reinfecção. SIN secondary t.
secondary t., t. secundária; t. observada em adultos e caracterizada por lesões próximas ao ápice de um lobo superior, que podem sofrer cavitação ou cicatrizar com fibrose, sem disseminação para os linfonodos; teoricamente, a t. secundária deve-se à reinfecção exógena ou à reativação de uma infecção endógena latente. SIN adult t., postprimary t., reactivation t., reinfection t.
tu·ber·cu·lo·stat (too-ber′kū-lō-stat). Tuberculostato; agente tuberculostático.
tu·ber·cu·lo·stat·ic (too-ber′kū-lō-stat′ik). Tuberculostático; relativo a um agente que inibe o crescimento dos bacilos da tuberculose. [tuberculo- + G. *statikos*, que causa uma parada]
tu·ber·cu·lous (too-ber′kū-lŭs). Tuberculoso; relativo a ou afetado por tuberculose. Cf. tubercular.

TUBERCULUM

tu·ber·cu·lum, pl. **tu·ber·cu·la** (too-ber′kū-lŭm,-lă) [TA]. Tubérculo. SIN tubercle. [L. dim. de *tuber*, protuberância, tumefação, tumor]
t. adducto'rium femoris [TA], t. do adutor do fêmur. SIN adductor tubercle of femur.
t. ante'rius atlan'tis [TA], t. anterior do atlas. SIN anterior tubercle of atlas.
t. ante'rius thal'ami [TA], t. anterior do tálamo. SIN anterior thalamic tubercle.
t. ante'rius vertebra'rum cervica'lium [TA], t. anterior das vértebras cervicais. SIN anterior tubercle of cervical vertebrae.
tubercula areolae [TA], tubérculos areolares. SIN areolar tubercles, em tubercle.
t. arthrit'icum, (1) nódulos de Heberden. SIN Heberden nodes, em node; (2) qualquer concreção gotosa dentro ou ao redor de uma articulação.
t. articula're os'sis tempora'lis [TA], t. articular do temporal. SIN articular tubercle of temporal bone.
t. auric'ulae [TA], t. da orelha. SIN auricular tubercle.
t. calca'nei [TA], t. do calcâneo. SIN calcaneal tubercle.
t. carot'icum [TA], t. carótico. SIN carotid tubercle.
t. cine'reum, túber cinéreo; proeminência longitudinal na superfície dorsolateral da medula oblonga ao longo da borda lateral do tubérculo cuneiforme; constitui o perfil superficial do trato espinal do nervo trigêmeo, que se continua caudalmente com o fascículo dorsolateral (trato de Lissauer).
t. conoi'deum (claviculare) [TA], t. conóide (da clavícula). SIN conoid tubercle (of clavicle).
t. cornicula'tum [TA], t. corniculado. SIN corniculate tubercle.
t. coro'nae, t. do dente. SIN dental tubercle.
t. cos'tae [TA], t. da costela. SIN tubercle of rib.
t. cunea'tum, t. cuneiforme. SIN cuneate tubercle.
t. cuneifor'me [TA], t. cuneiforme. SIN cuneiform tubercle.
t. deltoideum (spinae scapulae) [TA], t. deltóide (da escápula). SIN deltoid tubercle (of spine of scapula).
t. den'tis [TA], t. do dente. SIN dental tubercle.
t. dorsa'le radii [TA], t. dorsal do rádio. SIN dorsal tubercle of radius.
t. epiglot'ticum [TA], t. epiglótico. SIN epiglottic tubercle.
t. grac'ile, t. grácil do bulbo. SIN gracile tubercle.
t. hypoglos'si, t. do hipoglosso. SIN hypoglossal trigone.
t. ili'acum [TA], t. ilíaco. SIN tubercle of iliac crest.
t. im'par, t. ímpar; pequena protuberância mediana no assoalho da cavidade oral do embrião, entre os arcos mandibular e hióideo, que desempenha um pequeno papel no desenvolvimento da língua. SIN median tongue bud.
t. infraglenoida'le (scapulae) [TA], t. infraglenoidal. SIN infraglenoid tubercle (of scapula).
t. intercondyla're (mediale et laterale) [TA], t. intercondilar (medial e lateral). SIN intercondylar tubercle.
t. interveno'sum (atrii dextri) [TA], t. intervenoso (átrio direito). SIN intervenous tubercle (of right atrium).
t. jugula're ossis occipitalis [TA], t. jugular do osso occipital. SIN jugular tubercle of occipital bone.
t. la'bii superio'ris [TA], t. do lábio superior. SIN tubercle of upper lip.
t. latera'le (proces'sus posterio'ris) ta'li [TA], t. lateral (processo posterior) do tálus. SIN lateral tubercle (of posterior process) of talus.
t. ma'jus (hu'meri) [TA], t. maior (do úmero). SIN greater tubercle (of humerus).
t. mal'lei, t. do martelo. SIN lateral process of malleus.
t. margina'le (os'sis zygomat'ici) [TA], t. marginal (do osso zigomático). SIN marginal tubercle (of zygomatic bone).
t. media'le (proces'sus posterio'ris) ta'li [TA], t. medial (processo posterior) do tálus. SIN medial tubercle (of posterior process) of talus.
t. menta'le (mandibulae) [TA], t. mental. SIN mental tubercle (of mandible).
t. mi'nus (hu'meri) [TA], t. menor (do úmero). SIN lesser tubercle (of humerus).
t. molare [TA], t. molar. SIN molar tubercle.
t. mus'culi scale'ni anterio'ris [TA], t. do músculo escaleno anterior. SIN scalene tubercle.
t. obturato'rium [TA], t. obturatório. SIN obturator tubercle.
t. olfacto'rium [TA], t. olfatório. SIN olfactory tubercle.
t. orbitale ossis zygomatici [TA], t. orbital (do osso zigomático). SIN orbital tubercle (of zygomatic bone).
t. os'sis scaphoi'dei [TA], t. do escafóide. SIN tubercle of scaphoid (bone).
t. os'sis trape'zii [TA], t. do trapézio. SIN t. of trapezium bone.
t. pharyn'geum (partis basilaris ossis occipitalis) [TA], t. faríngeo (da parte basilar do osso occipital). SIN pharyngeal tubercle (of basilar part of occipital bone).
t. poste'rius atlan'tis [TA], t. posterior (do atlas). SIN posterior tubercle of atlas.
t. poste'rius vertebra'rum cervica'lium [TA], t. posterior das vértebras cervicais. SIN posterior tubercle of cervical vertebrae.

t. pu'bicum [TA], t. púbico. SIN pubic tubercle.
t. sel'lae [TA], t. da sela; pequena elevação na frente da fossa hipofisária (sela turca) sobre o corpo do osso esfenóide. SIN tubercle of saddle.
t. sep'ti na'rium, t. do septo do nariz; elevação plana sobre o septo de cada narina em oposição à extremidade anterior da concha média; resulta de uma agregação de glândulas.
t. supe'rius, t. superior. SIN auricular tubercle.
t. supraglenoida'le (scapulae) [TA], t. supraglenoidal (da escápula). SIN supraglenoid tubercle (of scapula).
t. supratra'gicum [TA], t. supratrágico. SIN supratragic tubercle.
t. thyroi'deum infe'rius [TA], t. tireóideo inferior. SIN inferior thyroid tubercle.
t. thyroi'deum supe'rius [TA], t. tireóideo superior. SIN superior thyroid tubercle.
t. of trapezium bone [TA], t. do trapézio; crista proeminente do trapézio formando a borda lateral do sulco no qual corre o tendão do flexor radial do carpo e ao qual está fixada parte do ligamento transverso do carpo (retináculo dos flexores). SIN t. ossis trapezii [TA], oblique ridge of trapezium, tubercle of trapezium (bone).
t. trigeminale [TA], t. trigeminal. SIN trigeminal tubercle.

tu·ber·if·er·ous (too-ber-if′er-ŭs). Tuberífero. SIN tuberous. [tuber + L. *ferro*, transportar]
tu·ber·ose (too′ber-ōs). Tuberoso. SIN tuberous.
tu·ber·os·i·tas (too′ber-os′i-tas) [TA]. Tuberosidade. SIN tuberosity. [LL., do L. *tuberosus*, cheio de nodulações, de *tuber*, protuberância]
t. coracoi'dea, t. dos ligamentos coracoclaviculares. SIN tuberosity for coracoclavicular ligament.
t. costa'lis, t. impressão do ligamento costoclavicular. SIN impression for costoclavicular ligament.
t. deltoi'dea (humeri) [TA], t. deltóidea (do úmero). SIN deltoid tuberosity (of humerus).
t. glu'tea [TA], t. glútea. SIN gluteal tuberosity.
t. ili'aca [TA], t. ilíaca. SIN iliac tuberosity.
t. ligamenti coracoclavicularis [TA], t. dos ligamentos coracoclaviculares. SIN tuberosity for coracoclavicular ligament.
t. masseter'ica [TA], t. massetérico. SIN masseteric tuberosity.
t. mus'culi serra'ti anterio'ris [TA], t. para o músculo serrátil anterior. SIN tuberosity for serratus anterior (muscle).
t. os'sis cuboi'dei [TA], t. do cubóide. SIN tuberosity of cuboid (bone).
t. os'sis metatarsa'lis pri'mi [I], t. do primeiro metatarsal [I]. SIN tuberosity of first metatarsal (bone) [I].
t. os'sis metatarsa'lis quin'ti [V] [TA], t. do quinto metatarsal [V]. SIN tuberosity of fifth metatarsal (bone) [V].
t. os'sis navicula'ris [TA], t. do osso navicular. SIN tuberosity of navicular bone.
t. phalan'gis dista'lis (manus et pedis) [TA], t. da falange distal (da mão e do pé). SIN tuberosity of distal phalanx (of hand and foot).
t. pronatoria [TA], t. para o músculo pronador. SIN pronator tuberosity.
t. pterygoi'dea (mandibulae) [TA], t. pterigóidea (da mandíbula). SIN pterygoid tuberosity (of mandible).
t. ra'dii [TA], t. do rádio. SIN radial tuberosity.
t. sacra'lis [TA], t. sacral. SIN sacral tuberosity.
t. tib'iae [TA], t. da tíbia. SIN tibial tuberosity.
t. ul'nae [TA], t. da ulna. SIN tuberosity of ulna.
t. unguicula'ris, t. da falange distal. SIN tuberosity of distal phalanx (of hand and foot).
tu·ber·os·i·ty (too′ber-os′i-tē) [TA]. Tuberosidade; grande tubérculo ou elevação arredondada, especialmente da superfície de um osso. SIN tuberositas [TA].
bicipital t., t. do rádio. SIN radial t.
calcaneal t. [TA], t. do calcâneo; a extremidade posterior do calcâneo ou osso do calcâneo, formando a projeção do calcanhar. SIN tuber calcanei [TA], calcaneal tuber, tuber calcis.
t. for coracoclavicular ligament [TA], t. dos ligamentos coracoclaviculares; o tubérculo conóide e a linha trapezóidea do processo coracóide da escápula, fornecendo fixação às duas partes do ligamento coracoclavicular: os ligamentos conóide e trapezóide. SIN tuberositas ligamenti coracoclavicularis [TA], coracoid t., tuberositas coracoidea.
coracoid t., t. dos ligamentos coracoclaviculares. SIN t. for coracoclavicular ligament.
costal t., t. costal. SIN impression for costoclavicular ligament.
t. of cuboid (bone) [TA], t. do (osso) cubóide; pequena eminência na superfície lateral do osso cubóide, tem uma face articular para um osso sesamóide no tendão do músculo fibular longo. SIN tuberositas ossis cuboidis [TA].
deltoid t. (of humerus) [TA], t. para o músculo deltóide; elevação rugosa próximo ao meio da face lateral da diáfise do úmero, proporcionando inserção ao músculo deltóide. SIN tuberositas deltoidea (humeri) [TA], deltoid crest, deltoid eminence, deltoid impression.
t. of distal phalanx (of hand and foot) [TA], t. da falange distal (da mão e do pé); superfície elevada e rugosa em forma de ferradura na superfície palmar da extremidade distal da falange terminal ou ungueal de cada dedo da mão e do pé que serve para sustentar a polpa do dedo. SIN tuberositas phalangis distalis (manus et pedis) [TA], tuberositas unguicularis, ungual t.
t. of fifth metatarsal (bone) [V] [TA], t. do quinto (osso) metatarsal [V]; tubérculo na base desse osso, em cuja parte posterior está fixado o tendão do músculo fibular curto. SIN tuberositas ossis metatarsalis quinti [V] [TA].
t. of first metatarsal (bone) [I] [TA], t. do primeiro (osso) metatarsal [I]; tubérculo na base do osso ao qual está fixado o tendão do músculo fibular longo. SIN tuberositas ossis metatarsalis primi [I].
gluteal t. [TA], t. glútea; área rugosa de inserção na parte superior da diáfise do fêmur da parte profunda menor do músculo glúteo máximo; quando acentuadamente desenvolvida, essa tuberosidade é denominada terceiro trocanter. VER TAMBÉM third *trochanter*. SIN tuberositas glutea [TA], crista glutea, gluteal crest, gluteal ridge.
greater t. of humerus, tubérculo maior do úmero. SIN greater tubercle (of humerus).
iliac t. [TA], t. ilíaca; área rugosa acima da superfície auricular na face medial da asa do ílio, proporcionando inserção ao ligamento sacroilíaco posterior. SIN tuberositas iliaca [TA].
infraglenoid t., t. infraglenoidal. SIN infraglenoid tubercle (of scapula).
ischial t. [TA], túber isquiático; a projeção óssea rugosa na junção da extremidade inferior do corpo do ísquio e seu ramo; trata-se de um ponto de sustentação do peso na posição sentada; proporciona inserção ao ligamento sacrotuberal e constitui o local de origem dos músculos posteriores da coxa. SIN tuber ischiadicum [TA], tuber of ischium.
lateral femoral t., epicôndilo lateral do fêmur. SIN lateral epicondyle of femur.
lesser t. of humerus, tubérculo menor do úmero. SIN lesser tubercle (of humerus).
masseteric t. [TA], t. massetérica; superfície rugosa sobre a face externa do ângulo da mandíbula, fornecendo inserção às fibras do músculo masseter. SIN tuberositas masseterica [TA].
maxillary t. [TA], túber da maxila; a extremidade inferior protuberante da superfície posterior do corpo da maxila, atrás da raiz do último dente molar. SIN tuber maxillae [TA], eminentia maxillae, maxillary eminence.
medial femoral t., epicôndilo medial do fêmur. SIN medial epicondyle of femur.
t. of navicular bone [TA], t. do osso navicular; eminência arredondada sobre a superfície medial do osso navicular, proporcionando inserção a uma parte do tendão do músculo tibial posterior. SIN tuberositas ossis navicularis [TA], scaphoid t.
omental t. of liver [TA], túber omental do fígado; eminência na superfície visceral do lobo hepático esquerdo até a esquerda da fossa para o ducto venoso. SIN tuber omentale hepatis [TA].
pronator t. [TA], t. para o músculo pronador; pequena área rugosa no meio da face lateral convexa da diáfise do rádio, à qual se fixa (insere) o (músculo) pronador redondo. SIN tuberositas pronatoria [TA].
pterygoid t. (of mandible) [TA], t. pterigóidea (da mandíbula); área rugosa sobre a face interna da mandíbula, fornecendo inserção a fibras do músculo pterigóideo medial. SIN tuberositas pterygoidea (mandibulae) [TA].
radial t. [TA], t. do rádio; projeção oval da superfície medial do rádio, imediatamente distal ao colo, fornecendo fixação (inserção), em sua metade posterior, ao tendão do bíceps. SIN tuberositas radii [TA], bicipital t., tuber radii, t. of radius.
t. of radius, t. do rádio. SIN radial t.
sacral t. [TA], t. sacral; proeminência rugosa na superfície lateral do sacro, posteriormente à superfície auricular, para inserção dos ligamentos sacroilíacos posteriores. SIN tuberositas sacralis [TA].
scaphoid t., tubérculo do escafóide. SIN t. of navicular bone.
t. for serratus anterior (muscle) [TA], t. para o (músculo) serrátil anterior; área oval rugosa, aproximadamente no meio da superfície externa e borda inferior da segunda costela [II], para fixação do músculo serrátil anterior. SIN tuberositas musculi serrati anterioris [TA].
tibial t. [TA], t. da tíbia; elevação oval sobre a superfície anterior da tíbia, cerca de 3 cm distalmente à superfície articular, proporcionando inserção, em sua parte distal, ao ligamento da patela. SIN tuberositas tibiae [TA].
t. of ulna, t. da ulna; proeminência na borda inferior da superfície anterior do processo coronóide, fornecendo fixação (inserção) ao músculo braquial. SIN tuberositas ulnae [TA].
ungual t., t. da falange distal. SIN t. of distal phalanx (of hand and foot).
tu·ber·ous (too′ber-ŭs). Tuberoso; protuberante, nodoso ou nodular; que apresenta muitas tuberosidades. SIN tuberiferous, tuberose. [L. *tuberosus*]
tubo-. Tubo-. Tubular, um tubo. VER TAMBÉM salpingo-. [L. *tubus, tuba,* tubo]
tu·bo·ab·dom·i·nal (too′bō-ab-dom′i-nal). Tuboabdominal; relativo a uma tuba uterina e ao abdome.
tu·bo·cu·ra·rine chlo·ride (too′bō-koor-ar′ēn). Cloreto de tubocurarina; alcalóide (obtido dos caules do *Chondodendron,* particularmente do *C.*

tomentosum) que bloqueia a ação da acetilcolina na junção mioneural ao ocupar os receptores de modo competitivo; bloqueia também a transmissão ganglionar e libera histamina; utilizado para produzir relaxamento muscular durante cirurgias.

tu·bo·lig·a·men·tous (too′bō - lig - ă - men′tŭs). Tuboligamentoso; relativo à tuba uterina e ao ligamento largo do útero.

tu·bo-o·var·i·an (too′bō - ō - vā′rē - an). Tubovárico; relativo à tuba uterina e ao ovário.

tu·bo-o·var·i·ec·to·my (too′bō - ō - var - ē - ek′to - mī). Salpingo-ooforectomia. SIN salpingo-oophorectomy.

tu·bo-o·va·ri·tis (too′bō - ō - va - rī′tis). Salpingo-ooforite. SIN salpingo-oophoritis.

tu·bo·per·i·to·ne·al (too′bō - per - i - tō - nē′al). Tuboperitoneal; relativo às tubas uterinas e ao peritônio.

tu·bo·plas·ty (too′bō - plas′tē). Tuboplastia, salpingoplastia. SIN salpingoplasty.

tu·bo·tor·sion (too′bō - tōr - shŭn). Tubotorção; rotação de uma estrutura tubular, como um oviduto. SIN tubatorsion. [tubo- + L. *torsio*, torção].

tu·bo·tym·pan·ic, tu·bo·tym·pa·nal (too′bō - tim - pan′ik, - tim′pă - năl). Tubotimpânico; relativo à tuba auditiva e à cavidade timpânica da orelha.

tu·bo·u·ter·ine (too′bō - oo′ter - in). Tubouterino; relativo a uma tuba uterina e ao útero.

tu·bo·vag·i·nal (too - bō - vaj′i - năl). Tubovaginal; relativo a uma tuba uterina e à vagina.

tu·bu·lar (too′bū - lăr). Tubular; relativo a ou que possui a forma de um tubo ou túbulo. SIN tubuliform.

tu·bu·la·ture (tu′bū - lă - choor). Tubuladura; o gargalo curto de uma retorta ou vaso.

tu·bule (too′bŭl) [TA]. Túbulo. Pequeno tubo. SIN tubulus [TA]. [L. *tubulus*, dim. de *tubus*, tubo]

Albarran y Dominguez t.'s, túbulos de Albarran e Dominguez. SIN Albarran glands, em gland.

connecting t., t. conector; t. arqueado estreito do rim que se une ao túbulo contornado distal e ao túbulo coletor.

convoluted t. of kidney, t. contornado do rim; os segmentos altamente contornados do néfron no labirinto renal que compreende o túbulo contornado proximal, que se estende da cápsula de Bowman até o ramo descendente da alça de Henle, e o túbulo contornado distal, que se estende do ramo ascendente da alça de Henle até o tubo coletor. SIN Ferrein tube, tubuli contorti (1), tubulus renalis contortus.

convoluted seminiferous t., t. seminífero contorcido. SIN seminiferous t.'s.

dental t.'s, túbulos dentários. SIN canaliculi dentales, em canaliculus.

dentinal t.'s, túbulos dentinários. SIN canaliculi dentales, em canaliculus.

discharging t., t. de excreção; túbulo urinário formado pela união de vários túbulos coletores e que termina como ducto papilar.

Henle t.'s, túbulos de Henle; as porções retas dos túbulos urinários que formam a alça de Henle, distintos dos túbulos descendente e ascendente de Henle.

Kobelt t.'s, túbulos de Kobelt; remanescentes dos túbulos mesonéfricos no sexo feminino, contidos no epoóforo. SIN wolffian t.'s.

malpighian t.'s, túbulos de Malpighi; nos insetos, estruturas excretoras delgadas tubulares ou semelhantes a cabelos que se originam do canal alimentar entre o mesêntero (intestino médio) e o proctodeo (intestino posterior), numa região freqüentemente denominada piloro; variam de 1 a mais de 100 e podem ser dispostos em feixes de tamanho igual em alguns insetos.

mesonephric t., túbulo mesonéfrico; túbulo excretor do mesonefro. SIN segmental t.

metanephric t., t. metanéfrico; unidade excretora do metanefro ou rim permanente.

paragenital t.'s, túbulos paragenitais; remanescentes dos túbulos mesonéfricos embrionários, alguns dos quais formam o paradídimo.

pronephric t., t. pronéfrico; unidade excretora do pronefro, presente apenas em forma vestigial nos embriões humanos.

segmental t., t. segmentar. SIN mesonephric t.

seminiferous t.'s, túbulos seminíferos; um de dois ou três túbulos curvos torcidos em cada lóbulo do testículo, onde ocorre a espermatogênese. SIN tubuli seminiferi recti [TA], convoluted seminiferous t., tubuli contorti (2).

Skene t.'s, túbulos de Skene; as glândulas uretrais embrionárias que são o homólogo feminino da próstata.

spiral t., t. espiral; o segmento do túbulo urinário logo após o túbulo contornado proximal.

straight t., t. reto; um dos túbulos retos do rim, presente na medula e na parte radial do córtex.

straight seminiferous t., t. seminífero reto; *termo oficial alternativo para straight t. of testis.

straight t. of testis [TA], t. seminífero reto; a continuação do túbulo seminífero contorcido, que se torna reto pouco antes de entrar no mediastino para formar a rede testicular. SIN tubuli seminiferi recti testi [TA], straight seminiferous t.*, tubulus rectus.

T t., t. em T. SIN *tubulus* transversus.

uriniferous t., t. urinífero; a unidade funcional do rim, composta de uma parte contornada longa (néfron) e de um ducto coletor intra-renal.

wolffian t.'s, túbulos de Wolff. SIN Kobelt t.'s.

tu·bu·li (too′bū - lī). Túbulos; plural de tubulus.

tu·bu·li·form (too′bū - li - fōrm). Tubuliforme. SIN tubular.

tu·bu·lin (too′bū - lin). Tubulina; subunidade protéica de microtúbulos; trata-se de um dímero composto de dois polipeptídios globulares, a α-tubulina e a β-tubulina. VER TAMBÉM dynein.

t.-tyrosine ligase, tubulina-tirosina ligase; enzima que liga de forma covalente uma tirosina ao resíduo glutamil C-terminal da tubulina, acoplada à hidrólise de ATP em ADP e ortofosfato; trata-se de uma modificação pós-tradução peculiar, que pode ser importante no transporte, no arranjo e na estabilidade do citoesqueleto.

tu·bu·li·za·tion (too′bū - li - zā′shŭn). Tubulização; inclusão das extremidades unidas de um nervo seccionado, após neurorrafia, num cilindro de parafina ou em algum material lentamente absorvível para evitar que os tecidos adjacentes empurrem e impeçam a união.

tu·bu·lo·cyst (too′bū - lō - sist). Tubulocisto; cisto formado pela dilatação de qualquer canal ou tubo ocluído. SIN tubular cyst.

tu·bu·lo·der·moid (too′bū - lō - der′moyd). Tubulodermóide; cisto dermóide que se origina de uma estrutura tubular embrionária persistente.

tu·bu·lo·neo·gen·e·sis (too - bū - lō - nē′ō - jen′ē - sis). Tubuloneogênese; a formação de novos túbulos; em geral, refere-se à proliferação de túbulos em tumores renais, como tumor de Wilms ou nefroma mesoblástico. [tubule + neogenesis]

tu·bu·lo·rac·e·mose (too′bū - lō - ras′ē - mōs). Tubulorracemoso; designa uma glândula de estrutura tubular e racemosa combinada.

tu·bu·lor·rhex·is (too′bū - lō - rek′sis). Tubulorrexe; processo patológico caracterizado por necrose do revestimento epitelial em segmentos localizados dos túbulos renais, com ruptura focal ou perda da membrana basal. [tubule + G. *rhēxis*, ruptura]

tu·bu·lose, tu·bu·lous (too′bū - lōs, - lŭs). Tubuloso; que possui muitos túbulos.

tu·bu·lus, pl. **tu·bu·li** (too′bū - lŭs, - lī) [TA]. Túbulo. SIN tubule. [L. dim. de *tubus*, tubo]

tu'buli bilif'eri, ductos bilíferos. SIN biliary *ductules*, em *ductule*.

tubuli contor'ti, túbulos contornados; **(1)** SIN convoluted *tubule* of kidney; **(2)** SIN seminiferous *tubules*, em *tubule*.

tu'buli denta'les, túbulos dentários. SIN canaliculi dentales, em canaliculus.

tu'buli epoöph'ori, dúctulos do epoóforo. SIN transverse *ductules* of epoöphoron, em *ductule*.

tu'buli galactoph'ori, ductos lactíferos. SIN lactiferous *ducts*, em *duct*.

tu'buli lactif'eri, ductos lactíferos. SIN lactiferous *ducts*, em *duct*.

tu'buli paroöph'ori, dúctulos do para-oóforo. SIN *ductuli* paroöphori, em *ductulus*.

t. rec'tus, t. reto. SIN straight *tubule* of testis.

t. rena'lis contor'tus, t. contornado do rim. SIN convoluted *tubule* of kidney.

tubuli semi'niferi recti [TA], túbulos seminíferos retos. SIN seminiferous *tubules*, em *tubule*.

tubuli semi'niferi rec'ti testi [TA], túbulos seminíferos retos. SIN straight *tubule* of testis.

t. transver'sus, t. transverso, t. T; invaginação tubular do sarcolema das fibras musculares esqueléticas ou cardíacas que circunda miofibrilas como elemento intermediário da tríade; envolvido na transmissão do potencial de ação do sarcolema para o interior da miofibrila. SIN T. tubule.

tu·bus, pl. **tu·bi** (too′bŭs, - bī). Tubo ou canal. [L.]

t. digesto'rius, trato digestório. SIN digestive *tract*.

t. medulla'ris, canal central da medula espinal. SIN central *canal*.

t. vertebra'lis, canal vertebral. SIN vertebral *canal*.

Tucker, Ervin Alden, obstetra norte-americano, 1862–1902. VER T.-McLean *forceps*.

tuft (tŭft). Tufo; aglomerado, massa ou cacho, como de cabelos.

enamel t., t. de esmalte; grupo de estruturas que representam defeitos na mineralização do dente que se estendem da junção dentino-esmalte para dentro do esmalte até aproximadamente metade de sua espessura.

malpighian t., t. de Malphighi. SIN glomerulus (2).

synovial t.'s, vilosidades sinoviais. SIN synovial *villi*, em *villus*.

tuft·sin (tuf′sin). Tuftsina; tetrapeptídio derivado da região Fc de uma imunoglobulina. A tuftsina potencializa as funções dos macrófagos. [*Tufts* University + -in]

tug, tug·ging (tŭg, tŭg′ing). Tração, arranco, puxão; movimento ou sensação de tração ou de arrastamento.

tracheal t., tração da traquéia; **(1)** tração da traquéia para baixo, que se manifesta por um movimento descendente da cartilagem tireóidea, sincrônico com a ação do coração e sintomático de aneurisma do arco aórtico; o sinal é mais facilmente produzido pela tração da cartilagem cricóidea para cima com o polegar e o indicador, enquanto o paciente está sentado com a cabeça inclinada para trás e a boca fechada; (2) tipo espasmódico de inspiração observado quando os músculos intercostais e as partes esternocostais do diafragma são paralisados por anestesia geral profunda ou relaxantes musculares; causado pela ação sem oposição dos pilares tracionando a cúpula do diafragma e, portanto, o pericárdio, as raízes pulmonares e a árvore traqueobrônquica durante cada inspiração.

tu·la·re·mia (too - lā - rē′mē - ă). Tularemia; doença causada por *Francisella tularensis* e transmitida por roedores aos seres humanos através da picada da mosca *Chrysops discalis* e outros insetos hematófagos; pode ser também adquirida diretamente através da mordida de um animal infectado ou através do manuseio de carcaça de um animal infectado; os sinais e sintomas, que se assemelham aos da febre ondulante e da peste, consistem em febre prolongada intermitente ou remitente e, com freqüência, edema e supuração dos linfonodos que drenam o local de infecção; os coelhos representam um hospedeiro reservatório importante. SIN deer-fly disease, deer-fly fever, Pahvant Valley fever, Pahvan Valley plague, rabbit fever. [*Tulare,* Lago e Condado, CA, + G. *haima,* sangue]
glandular t., t. glandular; t. com infecção predominante de linfonodos como principal manifestação.
pulmonary t., t. pulmonar; t. que afeta os pulmões; pneumonia tularêmica (tularemic *pneumonia*). SIN pulmonic t.
pulmonic t., t. pulmonar. SIN pulmonary t.

tulle gras (tool grä′). Curativo para ferimentos, utilizado principalmente na França, constituído de filó de malha aberta cortado em quadrados e impregnado com parafina mole (98 partes), bálsamo-do-peru (1 parte) e azeite de oliva (1 parte). [Fr. filó oleoso]
Tulp (Tulpius), Nicholas (Nicolaus), anatomista holandês, 1593–1674. VER T. *valve.*
tu·me·fa·cient (too - mĕ - fā′shent). Tumefaciente; que causa ou que tende a causar tumefação. [L. *tume-facio,* causar tumefação, de *tumeo,* tumefazer]
tu·me·fac·tion (too - mĕ - fak′shŭn). Tumefação. **1.** Inchação. SIN tumentia. **2.** Tumescência, intumescência. SIN tumescence. [ver tumefacient]
tu·me·fy (too′mĕ - fī). Tumefazer; inchar ou causar inchação.
tu·men·tia (too - men′shē - ă). Tumefação. SIN tumefaction (1). [L. de *tumeo,* inchar]
tu·mes·cence (too - mes′ens). Tumescência; a condição de ser ou de tornar-se tumefeito. SIN tumefaction (2), turgescence. [L. *tumesco,* começar a inchar]
tu·mes·cent (too - mes′ent). Tumescente; referente a tumescência. SIN turgescent.
tu·mid (too′mid). Túmido; inchado, como por congestão, edema, hiperemia. SIN turgid. [L. *tumidus*]

TUMOR

tu·mor (too′mŏr). Tumor. **1.** Qualquer inchação ou tumefação. **2.** Neoplasia. SIN neoplasm. **3.** Um dos quatro sinais de inflamação (tumor, calor, dor, rubor) enunciados por Celsus. [L. *tumor,* inchação]
acinar cell t., t. de células acinares; t. sólido e cístico do pâncreas, que ocorre em mulheres jovens; as células tumorais contêm grânulos de zimogênio.
acoustic t., t. do acústico. SIN vestibular *schwannoma.*
acute splenic t., t. esplênico agudo; esplenite aguda, aumento e amolecimento do baço, geralmente devido a bacteriemia ou toxemia bacteriana grave.
adenoid t., t. adenóide; adenoma ou neoplasia com espaços semelhantes a glândulas.
adenomatoid t., t. adenomatóide; pequeno t. benigno do epidídimo masculino e do trato genital feminino que consiste em tecido fibroso ou músculo liso envolvendo espaços semelhantes a glândulas que se anastomosam, contendo mucopolissacarídio ácido, revestidos por células achatadas que possuem características ultra-estruturais de células mesoteliais. SIN benign mesothelioma of genital tract.
adenomatoid odontogenic t., t. adenomatóide odontogênico; t. odontogênico epitelial benigno, que é visto como lesão radiotransparente-radiopaca bem-circunscrita, que geralmente circunda a coroa de um dente impactado em adolescente ou adulto jovem; caracterizado histologicamente por células colunares organizadas numa configuração semelhante a um ducto, interpostas com células fusiformes e deposição de tipo amilóide que gradualmente sofre calcificação distrófica. SIN adenoameloblastoma, ameloblastic adenomatoid t.
adipose t., lipoma. SIN lipoma.
ameloblastic adenomatoid t., t. adenomatóide ameloblástico. SIN adenomatoid odontogenic t.
amyloid t., amiloidose nodular. SIN nodular *amyloidosis.*
aortic body t., t. do corpo aórtico. SIN chemodectoma.
Bednar t., t. de Bednar. SIN pigmented *dermatofibrosarcoma protuberans.*
benign t., t. benigno; t. que não forma metástases e que não invade nem destrói o tecido normal adjacente. SIN innocent t.
blood t., t. sangüíneo; termo algumas vezes utilizado para designar um aneurisma, cisto hemorrágico ou hematoma.
borderline ovarian t., t. ovariano limítrofe; t. epitelial da superfície do ovário cujo padrão de crescimento é intermediário entre benigno e maligno; inclui tumores mucinoso, seroso, endometrióide e de Brenner do ovário; altamente curável, embora possa sofrer recidiva após remoção cirúrgica. SIN low malignant potential t.
Brenner t., t. de Brenner; neoplasia benigna relativamente rara do ovário, que consiste principalmente em tecido fibroso que contém ninhos de células semelhantes ao epitélio do tipo transicional, bem como estruturas semelhantes a glândulas que contêm mucina; a origem é controvertida; todavia, pode originar-se dos restos celulares de Walthard; habitualmente encontrado de modo incidental em ovários removidos por outras razões, especialmente após a menopausa.
Brooke t., t. de Brooke. SIN trichoepithelioma.
brown t., t. marrom; massa de tecido fibroso que contém macrófagos pigmentados com hemossiderina e células gigantes multinucleadas, substituindo e expandindo parte de um osso no hiperparatireoidismo primário.
t. burden, carga tumoral; a massa total de tecido tumoral apresentada por um paciente com processo maligno.
calcifying epithelial odontogenic t., t. odontogênico epitelial calcificado; neoplasia odontogênica epitelial benigna derivada do estrato intermédio do órgão do esmalte; lesão radiotransparente-radiopaca mista, indolor e de crescimento lento, caracterizada, do ponto de vista histológico, por cordões de células epiteliais poliédricas, depósitos de amilóide e calcificações esféricas. SIN Pindborg t.
carcinoid t., t. carcinóide; neoplasia de crescimento lento, geralmente pequena, composta de ilhas de células arredondadas, oxifílicas ou fusiformes de tamanho médio, com núcleos vesiculares moderadamente pequenos, recobertas por mucosa intacta com superfície de corte amarela; as células neoplásicas apresentam-se freqüentemente em paliçada na periferia dos pequenos grupos, e estes últimos têm tendência a infiltrar o tecido circundante. Essas neoplasias ocorrem em qualquer parte do trato gastrintestinal (bem como nos pulmões e em outros locais), com cerca de 90% dos casos no apêndice, e o restante principalmente no íleo, mas também no estômago, em outras partes do intestino delgado, no colo e no reto; as neoplasias do apêndice e os pequenos tumores raramente metastatizam, porém as incidências relatadas de metástases de outros locais primários e de tumores com mais de 2,0 cm de diâmetro variam de 25-75%; os linfonodos no abdome e no fígado podem estar nitidamente afetados, porém as metástases acima do diafragma são raras. VER TAMBÉM carcinoid *syndrome.*
carotid body t., t. do corpo carótico. SIN chemodectoma.
cellular t., t. celular; t. composto principalmente de células bem "acondicionadas".
cerebellopontine angle t., t. do ângulo cerebelopontino. SIN vestibular *schwannoma.*
chromaffin t., cromafinoma. SIN chromaffinoma.
Codman t., t. de Codman; condroblastoma da parte proximal do úmero.
collision t., t. de colisão; dois tumores originalmente separados, em particular um carcinoma e um sarcoma, que parecem ter-se desenvolvido por acaso em estreita proximidade, resultando numa área de mistura. VER TAMBÉM carcinosarcoma.
connective t., t. conjuntivo; qualquer tumor do grupo do tecido conjuntivo, como osteoma, fibroma, sarcoma.
dermal duct t., t. do ducto dérmico; pequeno t. benigno derivado da parte intradérmica dos ductos das glândulas sudoríparas écrinas, que ocorre freqüentemente na cabeça e no pescoço.
dermoid t., cisto dermóide. SIN dermoid *cyst.*
desmoid t., desmóide. SIN desmoid (2).
desmoplastic small cell t., t. desmoplásico de células pequenas; t. maligno de alto grau encontrado mais freqüentemente no abdome de adolescentes do sexo masculino; tipicamente, as células tumorais contêm desmina e ceratina, isto é, exibem características híbridas como as células mesoteliais fetais; a natureza exata dessas células permanece desconhecida.
dysembryoplastic neuroepithelial t., t. neuroepitelial disembrioplástico; neoplasia de baixo grau rara, observada mais freqüentemente em crianças e associada a convulsões e displasia cortical; o t. multicístico freqüentemente multinodular é composto de células de tipo oligodendroglial, com neurônios associados.
eighth nerve t., t. do oitavo nervo. SIN vestibular *schwannoma.*
embryonal t., embryonic t., t. embrionário; neoplasia habitualmente maligna, que surge durante o desenvolvimento intra-uterino ou pós-natal inicial a partir de um órgão rudimentar ou tecido imaturo; forma estruturas imaturas características da parte da qual se origina e pode formar também outros tecidos. O termo inclui o neuroblastoma e o t. de Wilms, mas também é utilizado para incluir determinadas neoplasias que surgem posteriormente durante a vida,

sendo esse uso baseado na crença de que esses tumores originam-se de restos embrionários. VER TAMBÉM teratoma. SIN embryoma.
embryonal t. of ciliary body, t. embrionário do corpo ciliar. SIN embryonal medulloepithelioma.
endocervical sinus t., t. do seio endocervical; t. maligno de células germinativas comumente encontrado no ovário. O tumor origina-se de células germinativas primitivas e desenvolve-se em tecido extra-embrionário semelhante ao saco vitelino. SIN yolk sac carcinoma.
endodermal sinus t., t. do seio endodérmico, t. do saco vitelínico; neoplasia maligna que ocorre nas gônadas, em teratomas sacrococcígeos e no mediastino; produz α-fetoproteína, e acredita-se que seja derivado de células endodérmicas primitivas. SIN yolk sac t.
endometrioid t., t. endometrióide; t. do ovário que contém elementos epiteliais ou do estroma, semelhante aos tumores do endométrio.
Erdheim t., tumor de Erdheim. SIN craniopharyngioma.
Ewing t., t. de Ewing; neoplasia maligna que ocorre habitualmente antes dos 20 anos de idade, cerca de duas vezes mais freqüentemente em homens, afetando os ossos dos membros em 75% dos pacientes, incluindo o cíngulo do membro superior, com predileção pela metáfise; histologicamente, são observados focos conspícuos de necrose em associação a massas irregulares de pequenas células regulares, arredondadas ou ovóides (2-3 vezes o diâmetro dos eritrócitos), com citoplasma muito escasso. SIN endothelial myeloma, Ewing sarcoma.
fecal t., fecaloma. SIN fecaloma.
fibroid t., t. fibróide; designação antiga para determinados fibromas e leiomiomas.
gastrointestinal autonomic nerve t., t. de nervo autônomo gastrintestinal; t. benigno ou maligno do estômago e do intestino delgado, histogeneticamente relacionado ao plexo mioentérico; pode ser familiar e relacionado a displasia neuronal gastrintestinal.
gastrointestinal stromal t., t. estromal gastrintestinal; t. benigno ou maligno composto de células fusiformes não-classificáveis; imuno-histoquimicamente distinto dos tumores do músculo liso e das células de Schwann.
giant cell t. of bone, t. de células gigantes do osso; t. osteolítico mole, castanho-avermelhado, algumas vezes maligno, composto de células gigantes multinucleadas e células ovóides ou fusiformes, que ocorrem mais freqüentemente numa extremidade de um osso tubular longo em adultos jovens. SIN giant cell myeloma, osteoclastoma.
giant cell t. of tendon sheath, t. de células gigantes da bainha tendínea; nódulo, possivelmente de natureza inflamatória, que surge comumente da bainha flexora dos dedos da mão e do polegar; composto de tecido fibroso, macrófagos contendo lipídios e hemossiderina e células gigantes multinucleadas. SIN localized nodular tenosynovitis.
glomus t. [MIM*138000], t. glômico; neoplasia vascular composta de pericitos especializados (algumas vezes denominados células glômicas), habitualmente em massas nodulares encapsuladas únicas, que podem ter vários milímetros de diâmetro e que ocorrem quase exclusivamente na pele, muitas vezes de localização subungueal no membro superior; é extremamente hipersensível e pode ser doloroso a ponto de os pacientes imobilizarem voluntariamente um membro, levando, algumas vezes, à atrofia dos músculos; ocorrem múltiplos tumores glômicos, algumas vezes com herança autossômica dominante. Os tumores com espaços cavernosos revestidos por células glômicas são denominados glomangiomas (*glomangiomas*).
glomus jugulare t., glômico jugular; t. que se origina do glomo jugular; em geral, manifesta-se inicialmente na porção mais baixa da cavidade timpânica.
glomus tympanicum t., t. glômico timpânico; tumor glômico que se origina na parede medial da orelha média.
Godwin t., t. de Godwin. SIN benign lymphoepithelial *lesion*.
granular cell t., t. de células granulares; t. geralmente benigno, microscopicamente específico, que muitas vezes afeta os nervos periféricos na pele, mucosa ou tecido conjuntivo, derivado das células de Schwann; o citoplasma abundante contém grânulos lisossomais, as células infiltram-se entre os tecidos adjacentes, embora o crescimento seja lento, e o epitélio da superfície adjacente pode exibir hiperplasia.
granulosa cell t., t. de células granulosas; t. benigno ou maligno do ovário, que se origina da membrana granulosa do folículo ovariano vesicular (de de Graaf) e freqüentemente secretor de estrogênio; é mole, sólido, branco ou amarelo, e consiste em pequenas células redondas algumas vezes encerrando corpúsculos de Call-Exner; pode haver células maiores contendo lipídios. SIN folliculoma (1).
Grawitz t., t. de Grawitz; epônimo antigo para o adenocarcinoma renal (renal *adenocarcinoma*).
heterologous t., t. heterólogo; t. composto de tecido diferente daquele do qual se origina.
hilar cell t. of ovary, t. de células hilares do ovário. SIN steroid cell t.
histoid t., t. históide; termo antigo para descrever um t. composto de um único tipo de tecido diferenciado.
homologous t., t. homólogo; t. composto do mesmo tecido do qual se originou.

innocent t., t. inocente, t. benigno. SIN benign t.
interstitial cell t. of testis, t. de células intersticiais do testículo. SIN Leydig cell t.
islet cell t., t. de células das ilhotas; t. endócrino composto de células equivalentes ou relacionadas àquelas encontradas nas ilhotas normais de Langerhans; pode ser benigno ou maligno; em geral, hormonalmente ativo; inclui insulinomas, glucagonomas, vipomas, somatostatinomas, gastrinomas, t. pancreático secretor de polipeptídio e tumores de células das ilhotas pancreáticas multihormonais ou hormonalmente inativos.
juxtaglomerular cell t., t. de células justaglomerulares; t. de origem de células justaglomerulares que habitualmente apresenta sintomas de aldosteronismo secundário, incluindo hipertensão diastólica grave, que parece ser devida à renina produzida pelo tumor. O aspecto histológico lembra um hemangiopericitoma.
Klatskin t., t. de Klatskin; adenocarcinoma localizado na bifurcação do ducto hepático comum.
Krukenberg t., t. de Krukenberg; carcinoma metastático do ovário, habitualmente bilateral e secundário a um carcinoma da mucosa gástrica, que contém células em anel de sinete repletas de muco.
Landschutz t., t. de Landschutz; neoplasia transplantável, possivelmente isoantigênica e altamente virulenta, que pode ser cultivada em qualquer cepa de camundongos; o hospedeiro é morto em poucos dias, aparentemente por um carcinoma anaplásico.
Leydig cell t., t. de células de Leydig; neoplasia testicular e, com menos freqüência, ovariana, composta de células de Leydig, habitualmente benigna, embora possa ser maligna; pode secretar androgênios ou estrogênios. SIN interstitial cell t. of testis.
Lindau t., t. de Lindau. SIN hemangioblastoma.
low malignant potential t., t. de baixo potencial maligno. SIN borderline ovarian t.
malignant t., t. maligno; t. que invade tecidos adjacentes, habitualmente capaz de produzir metástases, que pode sofrer recidiva após tentativa de remoção e que tende a causar a morte do hospedeiro, a não ser que seja tratado adequadamente. VER TAMBÉM cancer.
malignant mixed müllerian t. (MMMT), t. mülleriano misto maligno. SIN mixed mesodermal t.
melanotic neuroectodermal t. of infancy, t. neuroectodérmico melanótico do lactente; neoplasia benigna de origem neuroectodérmica que acomete mais freqüentemente a porção anterior da maxila no primeiro ano de vida. Manifesta-se clinicamente como lesão negro-azulada de rápido crescimento, que produz uma radiotransparência destrutiva; do ponto de vista histológico, caracteriza-se por pequenas células tumorais redondas e indiferenciadas, intercaladas com células poliédricas maiores produtoras de melanina, dispostas numa configuração alveolar. SIN melanoameloblastoma, pigmented ameloblastoma, pigmented epulis, progonoma of jaw, retinal anlage t.
Merkel cell t., t. de células de Merkel; t. cutâneo maligno raro, observado na pele exposta ao sol de pacientes idosos, composto de nódulos dérmicos de pequenas células redondas, com citoplasma escasso num padrão trabecular; as células tumorais contêm grânulos citoplasmáticos de centro denso, semelhantes aos grânulos neurossecretores observados nas células de Merkel. SIN primary neuroendocrine carcinoma of the skin, trabecular carcinoma.
mesonephroid t., t. mesonefróide. SIN mesonephroma.
mixed t., t. misto; tumor composto de duas ou mais variedades de tecido.
mixed mesodermal t., t. mesodérmico misto; sarcoma do corpo do útero que surge em mulheres idosas, composto de mais de um tecido mesenquimatoso, incluindo especialmente células musculares estriadas. SIN malignant mixed müllerian t.
mixed t. of salivary gland, t. misto da glândula salivar; t. composto de epitélio das glândulas salivares e tecido fibroso, com áreas mucóides ou cartilaginosas. SIN pleomorphic adenoma.
mixed t. of skin, siringoma condróide. SIN chondroid *syringoma*.
mucoepidermoid t., carcinoma mucoepidermóide. SIN mucoepidermoid *carcinoma*.
Nelson t., t. de Nelson; t. hipofisário que causa os sinais e sintomas da síndrome de Nelson (Nelson *syndrome*).
oil t., lipogranuloma. SIN lipogranuloma.
oncocytic hepatocellular t., t. hepatocelular oncocítico. SIN fibrolamellar liver cell *carcinoma*.
organoid t., t. organóide; t. de estrutura complexa, de origem glandular, contendo epitélio, tecido conjuntivo etc.
Pancoast t., t. de Pancoast; qualquer carcinoma do ápice pulmonar que causa síndrome de Pancoast por invasão ou compressão do plexo braquial e gânglio estrelado. SIN superior pulmonary sulcus t.
papillary t., papiloma. SIN papilloma.
paraffin t., parafinoma. SIN paraffinoma.
phantom t., t. fantasma; acúmulo de líquido nos espaços interlobares do pulmão, secundariamente a insuficiência cardíaca congestiva, simulando, radiologicamente, uma neoplasia.

tumor

phyllodes t., t. filodes; espectro de neoplasias que consistem numa mistura de epitélio benigno e estroma, com celularidade variável e anormalidades citológicas, incluindo desde o tumor filodes benigno até o cistossarcoma filodes; afeta mais freqüentemente a mama.
pilar t. of scalp, tumor solitário do couro cabeludo em mulheres idosas que pode ulcerar; microscopicamente, assemelha-se ao carcinoma de células escamosas composto de células claras ricas em glicogênio, porém benigno. SIN proliferating tricholemmal cyst.
Pindborg t., t. de Pindborg. SIN calcifying epithelial odontogenic t.
Pinkus t., t. de Pinkus. SIN fibroepithelioma.
placental site trophoblastic t., t. trofoblástico de local placentário; tumor que habitualmente surge no útero de mulheres multíparas durante os anos férteis. Histologicamente, o tumor consiste em predomínio de células trofoblásticas intermediárias, com material fibrinóide e invasão vascular.
pontine angle t., t. do ângulo pontino; t. no ângulo formado pelo cerebelo e pela porção lateral da ponte, referindo-se freqüentemente a um schwannoma do acústico.
potato t. of neck, t. do pescoço em batata; massa nodular firme no pescoço, geralmente um tumor do corpo carótico (quimiodectoma).
pregnancy t., t. da gravidez. SIN granuloma gravidarum.
primitive neuroectodermal t., t. neuroectodérmico primitivo; designação utilizada para referir-se a um grupo de neoplasias embrionárias morfologicamente semelhantes, que se originam em locais intracranianos e periféricos do sistema nervoso, podendo exibir vários graus de diferenciação celular; inclui o meduloblastoma, o pineoblastoma etc.
ranine t., rânula. SIN ranula (2).
Rathke pouch t., t. da bolsa de Rathke. SIN craniopharyngioma.
retinal anlage t., t. do primórdio da retina. SIN melanotic neuroctodermal t. of infancy.
Rous t., sarcoma de Rous. SIN Rous sarcoma.
sand t., t. arenoso. SIN psammomatous meningioma.
t. cell t., tumor de células t.; t. do testículo ou do ovário composto de células de Sertoli, mais freqüentemente benigno, embora possa ser maligno.
Sertoli-Leydig cell t., t. de células de Sertoli-Leydig; t. ovariano composto de células de Sertoli e células de Leydig; pode secretar androgênios. SIN arrhenoblastoma, gynandroblastoma (1).
Sertoli-stromal cell t., t. de células de Sertoli-estroma; termo genérico para o t. dos cordões sexuais ovarianos compostos de células de Sertoli, células de Leydig e células que se assemelham às células epiteliais da rede do testículo, numa forma pura ou como mistura desses tipos celulares.
solitary fibrous t., t. fibroso solitário; t. benigno de tecido fibroso que habitualmente surge no espaço pleural ou em outros locais. SIN benign mesothelioma.
squamous odontogenic t., t. odontogênico escamoso; t. odontogênico epitelial benigno cuja provável origem é nos restos de células epiteliais de Malassez; aparece clinicamente como lesão radiotransparente, estreitamente associada à raiz do dente, e histologicamente como ilhotas de epitélio escamoso envolto por uma camada periférica de células achatadas.
steroid cell t., t. de células esteróides; termo coletivo empregado para os tumores ovarianos compostos de células que se assemelham às células luteínicas secretoras de esteróides; inclui vários tumores, como luteoma do estroma, t. de células de Leydig, tumor de células esteróides sem outra especificação; hormonalmente ativo; pode ser benigno ou maligno. SIN hilar cell t. of ovary.
sugar t., t. benigno de células claras do pulmão que contém glicogênio em quantidades abundantes.
superior pulmonary sulcus t., t. do sulco pulmonar superior. SIN Pancoast t.
teratoid t., teratoma. SIN teratoma.
theca cell t., t. de células da teca. SIN thecoma.
triton t., t. de tritão; t. de nervo periférico com diferenciação de músculo estriado, observado mais freqüentemente na neurofibromatose; assim denominado em homenagem à teoria de Masson da transformação de fibras nervosas motoras em músculo em salamandras-tritão.
turban t., t. em turbante; cilindromas múltiplos do couro cabeludo que, quando crescem em excesso, assemelham-se a um turbante.
villous t., t. viloso. SIN villous papilloma.
Warthin t., t. de Warthin. SIN adenolymphoma.
Wilms t., t. de Wilms; t. renal maligno de crianças pequenas, composto de pequenas células fusiformes e de vários outros tipos de tecido, incluindo túbulos e, em alguns casos, estruturas semelhantes aos glomérulos fetais, músculo estriado e cartilagem. Com freqüência, herdado como caráter autossômico dominante [MIM*194070, *194080, *194090]. SIN nephroblastoma.
yolk sac t., t. do saco vitelino. SIN endodermal sinus t.
Zollinger-Ellison t., t. de Zollinger-Ellison; t. de células não-beta das ilhotas pancreáticas que causa a síndrome de Zollinger-Ellison.

tu·mor·i·ci·dal (too′mŏr - i - sī′dăl). Tumoricida; designa um agente destrutivo para tumores. [tumor + L. *caedo,* matar]

tu·mor·i·gen·e·sis (too′mŏr - i - jen′ĕ - sis). Tumorigênese; produção de novo crescimento ou crescimentos. [tumor + G. *genesis,* origem]
  foreign body t., t. por corpo estranho; indução de tumores malignos em tecidos por material sólido inviável e não-absorvível, que se ignora contenha algum carcinógeno químico.
tu·mor·i·gen·ic (too′mŏr - i - jen′ik). Tumorigênico; que causa ou produz tumores.
tu·mor·lets (too′mŏr - lets). Pequenos tumores; diminutos focos de hiperplasia epitelial bronquiolar atípica que são multifocais; embora sejam atualmente considerados benignos, acreditava-se outrora que fossem precursores de carcinoma.
tu·mor·ous (too′mŏr - ŭs). Tumefeito, inchado; semelhante a um tumor; protuberante.
tu·mul·tus cor·dis (too - mŭl′tŭs kŏr′dis). Palpitação e atividade irregular do coração.
TUNEL Abreviatura de terminal deoxynucleotidyl transferasemediated dUTP-biotin end labeling of fragmented DNA; esse método utiliza a imuno-histoquímica para identificar a fragmentação do DNA em núcleos de células em processo de apoptose.
Tun·ga pen·e·trans (tŭng′ă pen′ĕ - tranz). Membro da família das pulgas, Tungidae, comumente conhecido como bicho-de-pé, pulga-da-areia ou tunga; a minúscula fêmea penetra na pele, freqüentemente sob as unhas dos dedos dos pés; quando se distende com ovos até o tamanho de uma ervilha, surge uma úlcera dolorosa com inflamação no local. SIN *Sarcopsylla penetrans.*
tun·gi·a·sis (tŭng - ī′ă - sis). Tungíase; infestação por pulgas-da-areia (*Tunga penetrans*).
Tung·i·dae (tŭng′i - dē). Família de pulgas incluindo a espécie bicho-de-pé ou tunga, *Tunga penetrans.*
tung·state (tŭng′stāt). Tungstato; forma aniônica do tungstênio.
  calcium t., t. de cálcio; substância fosforescente com alto poder de interrupção dos raios X, que outrora era muito utilizado em telas fluoroscópicas e telas de intensificação para radiografia.
tung·sten (W) (tŭng′sten). Tungstênio; elemento metálico, de número atômico 74, peso atômico 183,85. SIN wolfram, wolframium. [Sueco *tung,* pesado, + *sten,* pedra]
  t. carbide, carbureto (carbonato, carbeto) de tungstênio; um dos materiais mais duros conhecidos, utilizado como abrasivo e na fabricação de instrumentos dentários de corte.
tu·nic (too′nik). Túnica; revestimento ou cobertura; uma das camadas de revestimento de uma parte, especialmente um dos revestimentos de um vaso sangüíneo ou outra estrutura tubular. VER TAMBÉM layer. SIN tunica. [L. *tunica*]
  Bichat t., t. de Bichat; a túnica íntima dos vasos sangüíneos.
  Brücke t., t. de Brücke. SIN tunica nervea.
  fibrous t. of corpus spongiosum, t. albugínea do corpo esponjoso. SIN tunica albuginea of corpus spongiosum.
  fibrous t. of eye, t. fibrosa do bulbo do olho. SIN fibrous layer of eyeball.
  mucosal t.'s, mucous t.'s, túnicas mucosas. SIN mucosa.
  muscular t.'s, túnicas musculares. VER muscular layer.
  muscular t. of gallbladder, t. muscular da vesícula biliar. SIN muscular layer of gallbladder.
  nervous t. of eyeball, t. interna do bulbo do olho. SIN inner layer of eyeball.
  serous t., t. serosa. SIN serosa.
  vascular t. of eye, t. vascular do bulbo do olho. SIN vascular layer of eyeball.

TUNICA

tu·ni·ca, pl. tu·ni·cae (too′ni - kă, - kē). Túnica; cápsula. SIN tunic. [L. casaco, capa]
  t. adventi′tia, t. adventícia. SIN adventitia.
  t. albugin′ea, t. albugínea; túnica colagenosa branca e densa que circunda uma estrutura.
  t. albuginea of corpora cavernosa [TA], t. albugínea dos corpos cavernosos; membrana fibrosa forte que envolve os corpos cavernosos do pênis. SIN t. albuginea corporum cavernosorum [TA].
  t. albugin′ea cor′poris spongio′si [TA], t. albugínea do corpo esponjoso. SIN t. albuginea of corpus spongiosum.
  t. albugin′ea cor′porum cavernoso′rum [TA], t. albugínea dos corpos cavernosos. SIN t. albuginea of corpora cavernosa.
  t. albuginea of corpus spongiosum [TA], t. albugínea do corpo esponjoso; camada espessa de tecido fibroso que circunda o corpo esponjoso do pênis; é mais fina do que a camada correspondente ao redor de cada corpo cavernoso. SIN t. albuginea corporis spongiosi [TA], fibrous tunic of corpus spongiosum.
  t. albugin′ea oc′uli, esclera. SIN sclera.
  t. albuginea ovarii [TA], t. albugínea do ovário. SIN t. albuginea of ovary.

t. albuginea of ovary [TA], t. albugínea do ovário; cápsula fina do ovário profundamente ao epitélio germinativo. SIN t. albuginea ovarii [TA].
t. albugin'ea tes'tis [TA], t. albugínea do testículo. SIN t. albuginea of testis.
t. albuginea of testis [TA], t. albugínea do testículo; membrana fibrosa branca e espessa que forma o revestimento externo ou cápsula do testículo. SIN t. albuginea testis [TA], peridídymis.
t. car'nea, t. dartos. SIN dartos fascia.
t. conjuncti'va [TA], t. conjuntiva. SIN conjunctiva.
t. conjuncti'va bul'bi [TA], t. conjuntiva do bulbo. SIN bulbar conjunctiva.
t. conjuncti'va palpebra'rum [TA], t. conjuntiva da pálpebra. SIN palpebral conjunctiva.
t. dar'tos [TA], t. dartos. SIN dartos fascia. VER dartos muliebris.
t. elas'tica, t. elástica; túnica média das grandes artérias.
t. exter'na [TA], t. externa; (1) a túnica externa de duas ou mais camadas de revestimento de qualquer estrutura; (2) especificamente, o revestimento fibroelástico externo de um vaso sangüíneo ou linfático. SIN t. extima [TA].
t. exter'na oc'uli, t. fibrosa do bulbo do olho. SIN fibrous layer of eyeball.
t. exter'na the'cae follic'uli, t. externa da teca do folículo; a camada fibrosa externa da teca de um folículo ovariano vesicular bem-desenvolvido; as células e as fibras estão dispostas de modo concêntrico. SIN theca externa.
t. ex'tima [TA], t. externa. SIN t. externa.
t. fibromusculocartilaginea bronchi [TA], t. fibromusculocartilagínea dos brônquios. SIN fibromusculocartilagenous layer of bronchi.
t. fibro'sa [TA], t. fibrosa. SIN fibrous capsule.
t. fibro'sa bul'bi [TA], t. fibrosa do bulbo do olho. SIN fibrous layer of eyeball.
t. fibro'sa hep'atis [TA], t. fibrosa do fígado. SIN fibrous capsule of liver (2).
t. fibro'sa lie'nis, cápsula do baço. SIN fibrous capsule of spleen.
t. fibro'sa re'nis, cápsula fibrosa do rim. SIN fibrous capsule of kidney.
t. fibro'sa sple'nis, cápsula fibrosa do baço; *termo oficial alternativo para fibrous capsule of spleen.
tu'nicae funic'uli spermat'ici, túnicas do funículo espermático. SIN coverings of spermatic cord, em covering.
Haller t. vasculosa, t. vascular de Haller. SIN vascular layer of eyeball.
t. interna bulbi [TA], t. interna do bulbo. SIN inner layer of eyeball.
t. inter'na the'cae follic'uli, t. interna da teca do folículo; a camada celular e vascular interna do folículo ovariano vesicular; há evidências de que as células epitelióides produzem estrogênio e contribuem para a formação do corpo lúteo após a ovulação. SIN theca interna.
t. in'tima [TA], t. íntima; a camada mais interna de um vaso sangüíneo ou linfático; consiste em endotélio, geralmente uma camada subendotelial fibroelástica fina, e em uma membrana elástica interna ou fibras longitudinais.
t. me'dia [TA], t. média; a camada média, habitualmente muscular, de uma artéria ou outra estrutura tubular. SIN media (1).
t. muco'sa [TA], t. mucosa. SIN mucosa.
t. muco'sa bronchi [TA], t. mucosa dos brônquios. SIN mucosa of bronchi.
t. muco'sa cavita'tis tym'pani [TA], t. mucosa da cavidade timpânica. SIN mucosa of tympanic cavity.
t. muco'sa co'li, t. mucosa do colo. SIN mucosa of colon.
t. muco'sa duc'tus deferen'tis [TA], t. mucosa do ducto deferente. SIN mucosa of ductus deferens.
t. muco'sa esoph'agi [TA], t. mucosa do esôfago. SIN mucosa of esophagus.
t. muco'sa gas'trica [TA], t. mucosa do estômago. SIN mucosa of stomach.
t. mucosa intestini crassi [TA], t. mucosa do intestino grosso. SIN mucosa of large intestine.
t. muco'sa intesti'ni ten'uis [TA], t. mucosa do intestino delgado. SIN mucosa of small intestine.
t. muco'sa laryn'gis [TA], t. mucosa da laringe. SIN mucosa of larynx.
t. muco'sa lin'guae [TA], t. mucosa da língua. SIN mucosa of tongue.
t. muco'sa na'si [TA], t. mucosa do nariz. SIN mucosa of nose.
t. muco'sa o'ris [TA], t. mucosa da boca. SIN mucosa of mouth.
t. mucosa pelvis renalis [TA], t. mucosa da pelve renal. SIN mucosa of renal pelvis.
t. muco'sa pharyn'gis [TA], t. mucosa da faringe. SIN mucosa of pharynx.
t. muco'sa tra'cheae [TA], t. mucosa da traquéia. SIN mucosa of trachea.
t. muco'sa tu'bae auditi'vae [TA], t. mucosa da tuba auditiva. SIN mucosa of pharyngotympanic (auditory) tube.
t. mucosa tubae auditoriae [TA], t. mucosa da tuba auditiva. SIN mucosa of pharyngotympanic (auditory) tube.
t. muco'sa tu'bae uteri'nae [TA], t. mucosa da tuba uterina. SIN mucosa of uterine tube.
t. muco'sa ure'teris [TA], t. mucosa do ureter. SIN mucosa of ureter.
t. muco'sa ure'thrae femini'nae [TA], t. mucosa da uretra feminina. SIN mucosa of female urethra.
t. muco'sa u'teri [TA], endométrio. SIN endometrium.
t. muco'sa vagi'nae [TA], t. mucosa da vagina. SIN mucosa of vagina.
t. muco'sa vesi'cae bilia'ris [TA], t. mucosa da vesícula biliar. SIN mucosa of gallbladder.
t. muco'sa vesi'cae fel'leae, t. mucosa da vesícula biliar; *termo oficial alternativo para mucosa of gallbladder.
t. muco'sa vesi'cae urina'riae [TA], t. mucosa da bexiga. SIN mucosa of (urinary) bladder.
t. muco'sa vesic'ulae semina'lis, t. mucosa da vesícula seminal; *termo oficial alternativo para mucosa of seminal gland.
t. muscula'ris [TA], t. muscular. SIN muscular layer.
t. muscula'ris bronchio'rum [TA], t. muscular dos brônquios. SIN muscular layer of bronchi.
t. muscula'ris co'li [TA], t. muscular de colo. SIN muscular layer of colon.
t. muscula'ris duc'tus deferen'tis [TA], t. muscular do ducto deferente. SIN muscular layer of ductus deferens.
t. muscula'ris esoph'agi [TA], t. muscular do esôfago. SIN muscular layer of esophagus.
t. muscula'ris gas'trica [TA], t. muscular do estômago. SIN muscular layer of stomach.
t. muscularis glandulae vesiculosae [TA], t. muscular da glândula seminal. SIN muscular layer of seminal gland.
t. muscularis intestini crassi [TA], t. muscular do intestino grosso. SIN muscular layer of large intestine.
t. muscula'ris intesti'ni ten'uis [TA], t. muscular do intestino delgado. SIN muscular layer of small intestine.
t. muscularis partis intermediae urethrae masculinae [TA], t. muscular da parte intermédia da uretra masculina. SIN muscular layer of intermediate part of (male) urethra.
t. muscularis partis prostaticae urethrae masculinae [TA], t. muscular da parte prostática da uretra masculina. SIN muscular layer of prostatic urethra.
t. muscularis partis spongiosae urethrae masculinae [TA], t. muscular da parte esponjosa da uretra masculina. SIN muscular layer of spongy (male) urethra.
t. muscularis pelvis renalis [TA], t. muscular da pelve renal. SIN muscular layer of renal pelvis.
t. muscula'ris pharyn'gis [TA], t. muscular da faringe. SIN muscular layer of pharynx.
t. muscula'ris rec'ti [TA], t. muscular do reto. SIN muscular layer of rectum.
t. muscula'ris tra'cheae [TA], t. muscular da traquéia. SIN muscular layer of trachea.
t. muscula'ris tu'bae uteri'nae [TA], t. muscular da tuba uterina. SIN muscular layer of uterine tube.
t. muscula'ris ure'teris [TA], t. muscular do ureter. SIN muscular layer of ureter.
t. muscula'ris ure'thrae femini'nae [TA], t. muscular da uretra feminina. SIN muscular layer of female urethra.
t. muscula'ris urethrae masculinae [TA], t. muscular da uretra masculina. SIN muscular layer of male urethra.
t. muscula'ris u'teri [TA], t. muscular do útero. SIN myometrium.
t. muscularis vagi'nae [TA], t. muscular da vagina. SIN muscular layer of vagina.
t. muscula'ris ventric'uli, t. muscular do ventrículo. SIN muscular layer of stomach.
t. muscula'ris vesi'cae bilia'ris [TA], t. muscular da vesícula biliar. SIN muscular layer of gallbladder.
t. muscula'ris vesi'cae fel'leae, t. muscular da vesícula biliar; *termo oficial alternativo para muscular layer of gallbladder.
t. muscula'ris vesi'cae urina'riae [TA], t. muscular da bexiga. SIN muscular layer of urinary bladder.
t. ner'vea, termo antigo, outrora utilizado para designar a retina separada da camada de bastonetes e cones. SIN Brücke tunic.
t. pro'pria, t. própria; o envoltório especial de uma parte, distinta do revestimento peritoneal ou outro revestimento comum a várias partes.
t. pro'pria co'rii, t. própria do cório. SIN stratum reticulare corii.
t. pro'pria lie'nis, t. própria do baço. SIN fibrous capsule of spleen.
t. reflex'a, t. reflexa; a camada refletida da túnica vascular do testículo que reveste o escroto.
t. sclerot'ica, esclera. SIN sclera.
t. sero'sa [TA], t. serosa. SIN serosa.
t. sero'sa co'li, t. serosa do colo. SIN serosa of large intestine.
t. serosa esophagi [TA], t. serosa do esôfago. SIN serosa of esophagus.
t. sero'sa gas'tricae [TA], t. serosa do estômago. SIN serosa of stomach.
t. sero'sa hep'atis [TA], t. serosa do fígado. SIN serosa of liver.
t. serosa intestini crassi [TA], t. serosa do intestino grosso. SIN serosa of large intestine.
t. sero'sa intesti'ni ten'uis [TA], t. serosa do intestino delgado. SIN serosa of small intestine.
t. serosa pericardii serosi [TA], t. serosa do pericárdio seroso. SIN serosa of serous pericardium.
t. sero'sa peritone'i [TA], t. serosa do peritônio. SIN serosa of peritoneum.
t. serosa pleurae parietalis [TA], t. serosa da pleura parietal. SIN serosa of parietal pleura.

t. serosa pleurae visceralis [TA], t. serosa da pleura visceral. SIN *serosa* of visceral pleura.
t. serosa splenis [TA], t. serosa do baço. SIN *serosa* of the spleen.
t. sero·sa tu'bae uteri'nae [TA], t. serosa da tuba uterina. SIN *serosa* of uterine tube.
t. sero·sa u'teri [TA], t. serosa do útero. SIN *perimetrium, serosa* of uterus.
t. sero·sa ventric'uli, t. serosa do ventrículo. SIN *serosa* of stomach.
t. sero·sa vesi'cae bilia'ris [TA], t. serosa da vesícula biliar. SIN *serosa* of gallbladder.
t. sero·sa vesi'cae fel'leae, t. serosa da vesícula biliar; *termo oficial alternativo para *serosa* of gallbladder.
t. sero·sa vesi'cae (urina'riae) [TA], t. serosa da bexiga. SIN *serosa* of (urinary) bladder.
t. spongiosa urethrae femininae [TA], t. esponjosa da uretra feminina. SIN spongy *layer* of female urethra.
t. spongiosa vaginae [TA], t. esponjosa da vagina. SIN spongy *layer* of vagina.
t. submuco'sa, t. submucosa. SIN submucosa.
t. urethrae masculinae [TA], t. mucosa da uretra masculina. SIN *mucosa* of male urethra.
t. vagina'lis commu'nis, fáscia espermática interna. SIN internal spermatic *fascia*.
t. vagina'lis tes'tis, t. vaginal do testículo; bainha serosa do testículo e do epidídimo, derivada do peritônio; consiste em uma camada serosa parietal externa e uma camada serosa visceral interna.
t. vasculo'sa, t. vascular; qualquer camada vascular.
t. vasculo'sa bul'bi [TA], t. vascular do bulbo do olho. SIN vascular *layer* of eyeball.
t. vasculo'sa len'tis, t. vascular da lente; camada vascular nutriente que envolve a lente do olho no feto.
t. vasculo'sa oc'uli, t. vascular do bulbo do olho. SIN vascular *layer* of eyeball.
t. vasculo'sa tes'tis, t. vascular do testículo; a camada vascular que envolve o testículo abaixo da túnica albugínea.
t. vasculosa testis [TA], t. vascular do testículo. SIN vascular *layer* of testis.
t. vit'rea, lâmina limitante posterior da córnea. SIN posterior limiting *lamina* of cornea.

tun·nel (tŭn'el). Túnel, canal; passagem alongada, geralmente aberta em ambas as extremidades.
aortico-left ventricular t., t. aórtico-ventricular esquerdo; conexão congênita entre a aorta acima da saída das artérias coronárias e o ventrículo esquerdo.
carpal t. [TA], t. do carpo; a passagem profundamente ao ligamento transverso do carpo entre os tubérculos dos ossos escafóide e trapezóide no lado radial e o pisiforme e o hâmulo do hamato no lado ulnar, através da qual passam o nervo mediano e os tendões flexores dos dedos e do polegar; nesse local, pode ocorrer compressão do nervo mediano (síndrome do túnel do carpo). SIN canalis carpi [TA], carpal canal (1).

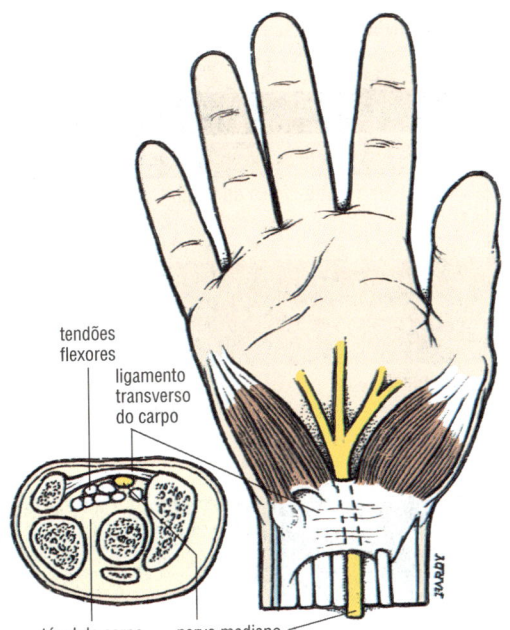

túnel do carpo: contém o nervo mediano e os tendões flexores dos dedos da mão e do polegar

Corti t., t. de Corti; o canal espiral no órgão de Corti, formado pelas células pilares externas e internas ou bastonetes de Corti; é preenchido por líquido e, por vezes, atravessado por fibras nervosas amielínicas. SIN Corti canal.
Tuohy, Edward B., anestesiologista norte-americano do século 20. VER T. *needle*.
tu·ran·ose (toor'ā-nōs). Turanose; dissacarídio redutor.
Tur·ba·trix (ter-bā'triks). Gênero de nematódeos de vida livre da família Cephalobidae. [L. *turbare*, perturbar]
T. aceti, espécie encontrada no vinagre velho ou em frutas e vegetais podres e, por vezes, como contaminante em soluções de laboratório. SIN vinegar eel.
tur·bid (ter'bid). Turvo, túrbido, em consequência da presença de sedimento ou matéria insolúvel numa solução. [L. *turbidus*, confuso, desordenado]
tur·bi·dim·e·ter (ter-bi-dim'e-ter). Turbidímetro; instrumento para medir a turvação (turbidez).
tur·bi·di·met·ric (ter'bid-i-met'rik). Turbidimétrico; relativo à medida da turvação.
tur·bi·dim·e·try (ter-bi-dim'e-trē). Turbidimetria; método para determinar a concentração de uma substância numa solução pelo grau de turvação que causa ou pelo grau de clarificação que induz em uma solução turva. [turbidity + G. *metron*, medida]
tur·bid·i·ty (ter-bid'i-tē). Turbidez, a qualidade de ser turvo, de perder a transparência em virtude da presença de sedimento ou matéria insolúvel. [L. *turbiditas*, de *turbidus*, turvo]
tur·bi·nal (ter'bi-nal). Turbinal. SIN turbinated *body* (1).
tur·bi·nate (ter'bi-nāt). Osso com forma semelhante a uma concha, referindo-se especialmente às conchas nasais. VER inferior nasal *concha*, middle nasal *concha*, superior nasal *concha*, supreme nasal *concha*.
tur·bi·nat·ed (ter'bi-nāt-ed). Turbinado, em forma de um cone invertido. [L. *turbinatus*, forma semelhante a uma concha]
tur·bi·nec·to·my (ter'bi-nek'tō-mē). Turbinectomia; remoção cirúrgica de uma concha nasal. [turbinate + G. *ektomē*, excisão]
tur·bi·no·tome (ter'bi-nō-tōm). Turbinótomo; instrumento para uso na turbinotomia ou turbinectomia.
tur·bi·not·o·my (ter'bi-not'ō-mē). Turbinotomia; incisão ou excisão de uma concha nasal. [turbinate + G. *tomē*, incisão]
tur·bu·lence. Turbulência, agitação, perturbação da ordem normal.
heart rate t., t. da frequência cardíaca; flutuações da duração do ciclo eletrocardiográfico após uma contração ventricular prematura.
Türck, Ludwig, neurologista austríaco, 1810–1868. VER T. *bundle, column, degeneration, tract*.
Turcot syn·drome. Síndrome de Turcot. Ver em syndrome.
tur·ges·cence (ter-jes'ens). Turgescência. SIN tumescence. [L. *turgesco*, começar a inchar, de *turgeo*, inchar]
tur·ges·cent (ter-jes'ent). Turgescente. SIN tumescent.
tur·gid (ter'jid). Túrgido, túmido. SIN tumid. [L. *turgidus*, inchado, de *turgeo*, inchar]
tur·gor (ter'gōr). Turgor; plenitude. [L., de *turgeo*, intumescer]
t. vita'lis, t. vital; a plenitude normal dos capilares.
tu·ris·ta (too-rēs'ta). Designação de origem mexicana para a diarréia do viajante (traveller's *diarrhea*). [do espanhol, turista]
Türk, Siegmund, oftalmologista suíço do século 20. VER Ehrlich-T. *line*.
Türk, Wilhelm, hematologista austríaco, 1871–1916. VER T. *cell, leukocyte*.
tur·key red (ter'kē). Vermelho-alaranjado. SIN madder.
tur·mer·ic (ter'mer-ik). Açafrão-da-índia; açafrão-da-terra (*Curcuma longa*).
turn (tern). Girar; dar uma volta ou causar uma rotação; especificamente, mudar a posição do feto dentro do útero para converter uma apresentação imprópria numa apresentação para permitir o parto normal. [A.S. *tyrnan*]
Turner, George Grey, cirurgião inglês, 1877–1951. VER Grey T. *sign*.
Turner, Henry H., endocrinologista norte-americano, 1892–1970. VER T. *syndrome*.
Turner, Joseph G., dentista inglês, †1955. VER T. *tooth*.
Turner, Sir William, anatomista inglês, 1832–1916. VER intraparietal *sulcus* of Turner, Turner *sulcus*.
turn·o·ver (tern'ō-ver). Renovação; a quantidade de um material metabolizado ou processado, geralmente em determinado período de tempo.
tur·pen·tine (ter'pen-tin). Terebintina; oleorresina extraída do *Pinus palustris* e de outras espécies de *Pinus;* fonte do óleo de terebintina e constituinte de pomadas estimulantes. [G. *terebinthinos*, relativo a *terebinthos*, a árvore da terebintina]
Canada t., bálsamo-do-canadá. SIN Canada *balsam*.
Chian t., t.-de-quio; exsudação de *Pistacia terebinthus*, uma pequena árvore de Quio (ilha grega no mar Egeu) e regiões ao leste; com exposição ao ar, torna-se espessa e forma massas amarelas transparentes semelhantes à almécega (mástica).
larch t., t. de lárix; líquido espesso, amarelado e transparente, a oleorresina obtida de *Larix europaea* (família Pinaceae). SIN Venice t.
Venice t., t.-de-veneza. SIN larch t.
white t., t. branca; t. do *Pinus palustris*.

tur·pen·tine oil. Óleo de terebintina; óleo volátil, destilado da terebintina, que era usado como diurético, carminativo, vermífugo, expectorante, rubefaciente e contra-irritante. SIN oleum terebinthinae, turpentine spirit.
   rectified t. o., óleo de terebintina retificado; obtido por tratamento do óleo de terebintina com hidróxido de sódio e redestilação; utilizado externamente como contra-irritante.

tur·pen·tine spir·it. Espírito de terebintina. SIN turpentine oil.

turps (terps). Aguarrás; nome popular do óleo de terebintina.

tur·ri·ceph·a·ly (toor-i-sef´a-le). Turricefalia. SIN oxycephaly. [L. *turris*, torre, + G. *kephale*, cabeça]

tu·run·da, pl. **tu·run·dae** (too-run´da, -de). Tenda cirúrgica, dreno de gaze ou tampão. [L.]

tus·sal (tŭs´al). Tussivo. SIN tussive.

tus·sic·u·lar (tŭ-sik´u-lar). Tussicular. SIN tussive. [L. *tussicularis*, de *tussicula*, pequena tosse, dim. de *tussis*, tosse]

tus·sic·u·la·tion (tŭ-sik´u-la´shŭn). Tosse seca.

tus·si·gen·ic (tŭs´i-jen´ik). Tussígeno; que causa tosse. [L. *tussis*, tosse + *-gen*, que produz]

tus·sis (tŭs´is). Tosse. [L.]

tus·sive (tŭs´siv). Relativo a tosse. SIN tussal, tussicular. [L. *tussis*, tosse]

tu·ta·men, pl. **tu·ta·mi·na** (too-ta´men, -ta´mi-na). Qualquer estrutura de defesa ou protetora. [L. proteção]
   tuta'mina cer'ebri, o couro cabeludo, o crânio e as meninges do cérebro.
   tuta'mina oc'uli, as sobrancelhas, as pálpebras e os cílios.

Tuttle, James P., cirurgião norte-americano, 1857–1913. VER T. *proctoscope*.

TUU Abreviatura de transureteroureterostomy (transureteroureterostomia).

TVG Abreviatura de time-varied *gain* (ganho variado de tempo).

TWAR SIN *Chlamydia pneumoniae*. [a partir das designações laboratoriais dos dois primeiros microrganismos isolados, TW-83 e AR-39].

Tweed, Charles H., ortodontista norte-americano, 1895–1970. VER T. edgewise *treatment, triangle*.

tweez·ers (twe´zerz). Tenazes, pinças; instrumento com tenazes que são comprimidas para segurar ou extrair estruturas delicadas. [A.S. *twisel*, garfo]

twig. Râmulo, ramúsculo; um dos ramos terminais mais finos de uma artéria; pequeno ramo. [A.S.]

twi·light (twi´lit). Crepúsculo. **1.** Figurativamente, luz fraca. **2.** Relativo à percepção mental fraca ou indistinta, como no estado crepuscular (twilight *state*). [A.S. *twi-*, dois]

twin. Gêmeo. **1.** Uma das duas crianças nascidas no mesmo parto. **2.** Duplo, que cresce em pares. [A.S. *getwin*, duplo]
   allantoidoangiopagous t.'s, gêmeos alantoidoangiópagos; gêmeos monocoriais desiguais com fusão dos vasos alantóicos intraplacentários; o gêmeo menor é essencialmente um parasita na circulação placentária do gêmeo maior.
   conjoined t.'s, gêmeos unidos; gêmeos monozigóticos com extensão variável de união e diferentes graus de duplicação residual. Os vários tipos de união são designados pelo uso de um prefixo que indica a região que está unida, acrescentando o sufixo *-pago*, que significa unido (p. ex., craniópago, toracópago); os vários tipos de duplicação residual são indicados pela designação das partes duplicadas, acrescentando-se o sufixo *-dídimo* ou *-dimo*, que significa gêmeo (p. ex., cefalodídimo, cefalódimo).
   conjoined asymmetric t.'s, gêmeos assimétricos unidos. SIN conjoined unequal t.'s.
   conjoined equal t.'s, gêmeos iguais unidos; gêmeos unidos em que ambos os membros têm quase o mesmo tamanho e são quase normais, exceto pelas áreas de união. SIN conjoined symmetric t.'s.
   conjoined symmetric t.'s, gêmeos simétricos unidos. SIN conjoined equal t.'s.
   conjoined unequal t.'s, gêmeos desiguais unidos, gêmeos unidos em que um membro é quase normal (hospedeiro ou autósito), enquanto o outro (parasita) é pequeno, incompleto e dependente do membro mais próximo do normal para sua nutrição. SIN conjoined asymmetric t.'s.
   dichorial t.'s, gêmeos dicoriais. SIN dizygotic t.'s.
   diovular t.'s, gêmeos diovulares. SIN dizygotic t.'s.
   dizygotic t.'s, gêmeos dizigóticos; gêmeos derivados de dois zigotos separados. SIN dichorial t.'s, diovular t.'s, fraternal t.'s, heterologous t.'s.
   enzygotic t.'s, gêmeos enzigóticos. SIN monozygotic t.'s.
   fraternal t.'s, gêmeos fraternos. SIN dizygotic t.'s.
   heterologous t.'s, gêmeos heterólogos. SIN dizygotic t.'s.
   identical t.'s, gêmeos idênticos. SIN monozygotic t.'s.
   incomplete conjoined t.'s, gêmeos unidos incompletos, gêmeos unidos, em que os dois componentes são iguais entre si, porém menores do que indivíduos completos.
   locked t.'s, gêmeos engatados; forma de má apresentação em que um gêmeo com apresentação de nádegas e outro gêmeo com apresentação de vértice ficam engatados no queixo durante o trabalho de parto e a tentativa de parto.
   monoamniotic t.'s, gêmeos monoamnióticos; gêmeos com um âmnio comum; esses gêmeos têm origem monovular e podem ser unidos.
   monochorial t.'s, gêmeos monocoriais. SIN monozygotic t.'s.
   monovular t.'s, gêmeos monovolares. SIN monozygotic t.'s.
   monozygotic t.'s, gêmeos monozigóticos; gêmeos resultantes de um único óvulo fertilizado que, num estágio inicial de desenvolvimento, é separado em agregações celulares de crescimento independente, originando dois indivíduos do mesmo sexo e constituição genética idêntica. SIN enzygotic t.'s, identical t.'s, monochorial t.'s, monovular t.'s, uniovular t.'s.
   parasitic t., gêmeo parasita; o menor de gêmeos unidos desiguais.
   placental parasitic t., gêmeo parasita placentário. SIN omphalosite.
   polyzygotic t.'s, gêmeos polizigóticos; gêmeos resultantes da fertilização de mais de dois óvulos que foram eliminados num único ciclo ovulatório.
   Siamese t.'s, gêmeos siameses; originalmente, um par unido de gêmeos muito divulgados (xifópagos) do Sião no século 19; desde então, o termo passou a ser utilizado por leigos para designar qualquer tipo de gêmeos unidos, apesar de ser incorreto.
   uniovular t.'s, gêmeos uniovulares. SIN monozygotic t.'s.

twinge (twinj). Pontada; ferroada; dor aguda súbita e momentânea.

twin·ning. Geminação; produção de estruturas equivalentes por divisão; a tendência de partes divididas a assumir relações simétricas.

twitch. 1. Contrair espasmodicamente. **2.** Contração espasmódica momentânea de uma fibra muscular. [A.S. *twiccian*]

Twort, Frederick W., bacteriologista inglês, 1877–1950. VER T. *phenomenon*; T.-d'Herelle *phenomenon*.

TX Abreviatura dos tromboxanos individuais, designados por letras maiúsculas com subscritos indicando características estruturais.

classificação dos gêmeos unidos		
terato catadídimo	**terato anadídimo**	**terato anacatadídimo**
unidos pela parte inferior do corpo, ou gêmeos com parte inferior única e duplicidade superior	parte superior única e duplicidade na parte inferior, ou unidos por alguma parte do corpo	unidos num ponto médio do corpo
a) pigópago unidos pelas costas, no cóccix e sacro	a) cefalópago unidos na abóbada craniana	a) toracópago ligados ao longo de parte da parede torácica; os órgãos torácicos e abdominais podem ser anormais
b) isquiópago fusão das partes inferiores do cóccix e do sacro; colunas vertebrais separadas e no mesmo eixo	b) sincéfalo unidos na face; podem estar também unidos pelo tórax (cefalotoracópago)	b) onfalópago unidos desde o umbigo até a cartilagem xifóide
c) dicéfalo duas cabeças separadas num único corpo	c) dípigo cabeça, tórax e/ou abdome únicos; duplicação da pelve, genitália externa e membros	c) raquípago unidos na coluna vertebral acima do sacro
d) diprosopo duas faces com uma cabeça e um corpo		

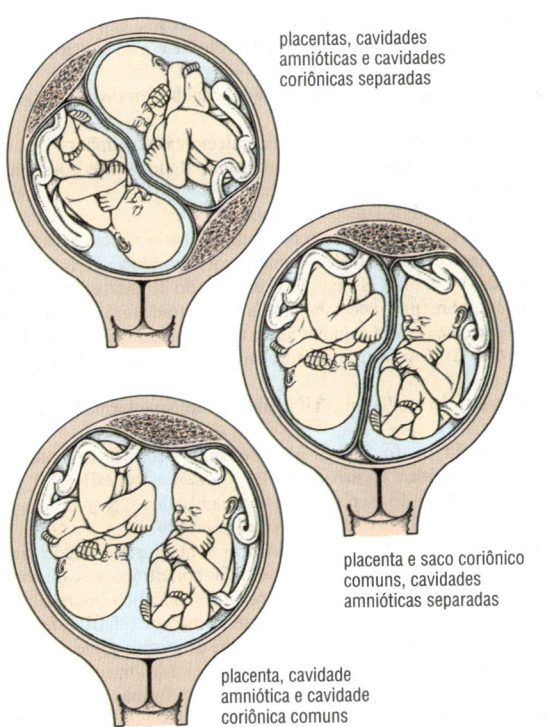

gêmeos: diagramas esquemáticos mostrando as possíveis relações das membranas fetais em gêmeos monozigóticos

- placentas, cavidades amnióticas e cavidades coriônicas separadas
- placenta e saco coriônico comuns, cavidades amnióticas separadas
- placenta, cavidade amniótica e cavidade coriônica comuns

ty·ba·mate (tī'bă-māt). Tibamato; tranqüilizante relacionado com o meprobamato.

ty·lec·to·my (tī-lek'tō-mē). Tilectomia; remoção cirúrgica de uma tumefação ou tumor localizado. VER TAMBÉM lumpectomy. [G. *tylē*, tumoração, + *ektomē*, excisão]

tyl·i·on, pl. **tyl·i·a** (til'ē-on, -lē-ă; tī'lē-on). Tílio; ponto craniométrico no meio da borda anterior do sulco quiasmático. [G. pequeno alfinete, dim. de *tylē*, tumoração]

ty·lo·ma (tī-lō'mă). Tiloma. SIN callosity. [G. um calo]
  t. conjuncti'vae, t. conjuntival; queratinização localizada na conjuntiva, que ocorre na xerose da conjuntiva.

ty·lo·sis, pl. **ty·lo·ses** (tī-lō'sis, -sēz). Tilose; formação de calosidades (tilomas). [G. que se torna caloso]
  t. cilia'ris, t. ciliar. SIN pachyblepharon.
  t. ling'uae, t. lingual; leucoplaquia da língua.
  t. palma'ris et planta'ris, t. palmar e plantar. SIN palmoplantar keratoderma.

ty·lox·a·pol (tī-lok'să-pol). Tiloxapol; detergente e agente mucolítico utilizado como aerossol para liquefazer o escarro.

ty·maz·o·line (tī-maz'ō-lēn). Timazolina; descongestionante nasal.

tympan-. Timpan-. VER tympano-.

tym·pa·nal (tim'pă-năl). **1.** Timpânico, timpanal. SIN tympanic (1). **2.** Ressonante. **3.** Timpânico. SIN tympanitic (2).

tym·pa·nec·to·my (tim'pă-nek'tō-mē). Timpanectomia; excisão da membrana timpânica. [tympan- + G. *ektomē*, excisão]

tym·pan·ia (tim-pan'ē-ă). Timpania. SIN tympanites.

tym·pan·ic (tim-pan'ik). Timpânico. **1.** Relativo à cavidade ou membrana timpânica. SIN tympanal (1). **2.** Ressoante. **3.** SIN tympanitic (2).

tym·pan·i·chord (tim-pan'i-kōrd). Corda do tímpano. SIN *chorda tympani.*

tym·pan·i·chor·dal (tim-pan-i-kōr'dăl). Relativo à corda do tímpano.

tym·pa·nic·i·ty (tim'pă-nis'i-tē). Timpanicidade; a qualidade de ser timpânico ou de possuir um tom semelhante ao do tímpano (tambor).

tym·pa·nism (tim'pă-nizm). Timpanismo. SIN tympanites.

tym·pa·ni·tes (tim-pă-nī'tēz). Timpanismo; distensão do abdome causada por gás na cavidade intestinal ou peritoneal. SIN meteorism, tympania, tympanism. [L. do G. *tympanitēs*, distensão que faz o ventre semelhante a um tambor, *tympanon*]
  uterine t., t. uterina. SIN physometra.

tym·pa·nit·ic (tim-pă-nit'ik). **1.** Timpanítico; referente à timpanite. SIN tympanous. **2.** Timpânico; designa a qualidade de som produzida por percussão do intestino inflado ou de uma grande cavidade pulmonar. SIN tympanal (3), tympanic (3).

tym·pa·ni·tis (tim-pă-nī'tis). Timpanite. SIN myringitis.

tympano-, tympan-, tympani-. Tímpano-, timpan-, timpani-; tímpano, timpanite. [G. *tympanon*, tímpano]

tym·pa·no·cen·te·sis (tim'pă-nō-sen-tē'sis). Timpanocentese; punção da membrana timpânica com uma agulha para aspirar o líquido da orelha média. [tympano- + G. *kentēsis*, punção]

tym·pa·no·eu·sta·chian (tim'pă-nō-oo-stā'shun, -stā'kē-an). Timpanoeustaquiano; relativo à cavidade timpânica e à tuba auditiva.

tym·pan·o·gram (tim'pah-nō-gram). Timpanograma; impressão de uma ponte de impedância mostrando a rigidez ou a complacência das estruturas da orelha média à medida que varia com mudanças na pressão dentro do meato acústico externo.

tym·pa·no·hy·al (tim'pă-nō-hī'ăl). Designa a relação entre a cavidade timpânica e o arco hióideo.

tym·pa·no·mal·le·al (tim'pă-nō-malē-ăl). Relativo à membrana timpânica e ao martelo.

tym·pa·no·man·dib·u·lar (tim'pă-nō-man-dib'ū-lăr). Timpanomandibular; relativo à cavidade timpânica e à mandíbula.

tym·pa·no·mas·toid (tim'pă-nō-mas'toyd). Timpanomastóideo; relativo à cavidade timpânica e ao processo mastóideo.

tympanomastoidectomy. Timpanomastoidectomia. SIN radical *mastoidectomy.*

tym·pa·no·mas·toid·i·tis (tim'pă-nō-mas-toy-dī'tis). Timpanomastoidite; inflamação da orelha média e das células mastóideas.

tym·pan·om·e·try (tim-pan-om'et-rē). Timpanometria; técnica que mede a complacência da membrana timpânica em vários níveis de pressão do ar; útil no diagnóstico de derrame na orelha média, função da tuba auditiva e otite média.

tym·pa·no·pho·nia, tym·pa·noph·o·ny (tim'pă-nō-fō'nē-ă, tim'pă-nof'ō-nē). Timpanofonia. SIN autophony. [tympano- + G. *phōnē*, som]

tym·pa·no·plas·ty (tim'pă-nō-plas-tē). Timpanoplastia; correção cirúrgica de lesão da orelha média. [tympano- + G. *plassō*, formar]

tym·pan·o·scler·o·sis (tim'pan-ō-skler-ō'sis). Timpanosclerose; a formação de tecido conjuntivo denso na orelha média, resultando freqüentemente em perda da audição quando há comprometimento dos ossículos.

tym·pa·no·squa·mo·sal (tim'pă-nō-skwā-mō'săl). Timpanoescamoso; relativo às partes timpânica e escamosa do osso temporal. SIN squamotympanic.

tym·pa·no·sta·pe·di·al (tim'pă-nō-stā-pē'dē-ăl). Timpanostapédico; relativo à cavidade timpânica e ao estribo.

tym·pan·os·to·my (tim-pan-os'tō-mē). Timpanostomia; cirurgia para efetuar uma abertura na membrana timpânica. VER TAMBÉM myringotomy. [tympano- + G. *ostium*, boca]

tym·pa·no·tem·po·ral (tim'pă-nō-tem'pō-răl). Timpanotemporal; relativo à membrana timpânica ou à região ou osso temporal.

tym·pa·not·o·my (tim'pă-not'ō-mē). Timpanotomia. SIN myringotomy. [tympano- + G. *tomē*, incisão]

tym·pa·nous (tim'pă-nŭs). Timpânico. SIN tympanitic (1).

tym·pa·num, pl. **tym·pa·na, tym·pa·nums** (tim'pă-nŭm, tim'pă-nă). Tímpano. SIN eardrum. [L. do G. *tympanon*, tímpano]

tym·pa·ny (tim'pă-nē). Timpanismo; som de timbre baixo, ressonante e semelhante ao de um tímpano (tambor), obtido por percussão da superfície de um grande espaço contendo ar, como o abdome distendido ou o tórax com ou sem pneumotórax. SIN tympanitic resonance.
  Skoda t., t. de Skoda. SIN skodaic *resonance.*

Tyndall, John, médico inglês, 1820–1893. VER T. *effect;* tyndallization; T. *phenomenon.*

tyn·dal·li·za·tion (tin'dăl-i-zā'shun). Tindalização. SIN fractional *sterilization.* [John *Tyndall*]

type (tīp). Tipo. **1.** A forma habitual ou uma forma composta à qual todas as outras da classe assemelham-se mais ou menos estreitamente; um modelo, referindo-se particularmente a uma doença ou complexo sintomático que é característico de uma classe. VER TAMBÉM constitution, habitus, personality. **2.** Em química, substância cuja disposição dos átomos numa molécula pode ser considerada representativa de outras substâncias dessa classe. **3.** Variação específica de uma estrutura. SIN typus, variation (2). [G. *typos*, marca, modelo]

  ampullary t. of renal pelvis [TA], tipo ampular de pelve renal; pelve renal de formato sacular, em que os cálices se abrem numa pelve dilatada comum. SIN typus ampullaris pelvis renalis [TA].

  basic personality t., t. básico de personalidade; **(1)** as tendências da personalidade peculiares, ocultas ou subjacentes de um indivíduo, independentemente de serem manifestas ou ocultas em termos de comportamento; **(2)** características de personalidade de um indivíduo, que são também compartilhadas pela maioria dos outros membros de um grupo social.

  blood t., t. sangüíneo. VER blood type.

  branching t. of renal pelvis [TA], tipo ramificado de pelve renal; pelve renal em que não há uma pelve comum, expandida e sacular; nesse tipo, os cálices principais simplesmente fundem-se e formam o ureter. SIN typus dendriticus pelvis renalis [TA].

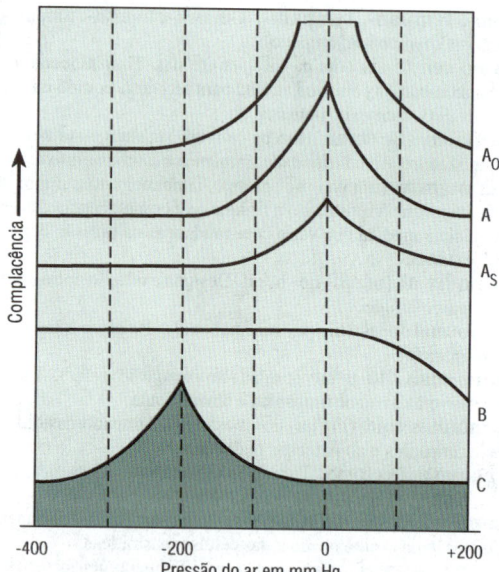

timpanograma: cinco timpanogramas ilustrando várias condições da orelha média: o tipo A é típico da orelha média normal; o tipo A_S está associado a rigidez do estribo; o tipo A_O está associado a interrupções na cadeia de ossículos ou a flacidez da membrana timpânica; o tipo B sugere a presença de líquido na orelha média; o tipo C sugere que a pressão dentro da orelha média é inferior à pressão atmosférica

buffalo t., giba de búfalo; termo utilizado para descrever a distribuição de um depósito de gordura observado posteriormente sobre a coluna torácica superior; observado no hiperadrenocorticalismo (síndrome de Cushing [Cushing *syndrome*]). SIN buffalo hump.
nomenclatural t., t. de nomenclatura; o elemento constituinte de um táxon ao qual está permanentemente ligado; o tipo de uma espécie é preferencialmente uma cepa (em casos especiais, pode ser uma descrição, uma amostra preservada ou preparação ou uma ilustração); o tipo de um gênero é uma espécie; e o tipo de uma ordem, família ou tribo é o gênero em cujo nome se baseia o nome do taxon superior.
test t., t. de teste. VER test types.
wild t., t. selvagem; gene, fenótipo ou genótipo que é extremamente comum entre aqueles possíveis em um *locus* de interesse, que representa a característica padrão; por conseguinte, presumivelmente não é prejudicial.
ty·phin·ia (tī-fin'ē-ă). Tifínia. SIN relapsing *fever*. [G. *typhos,* fumaça, torpor que se origina de febre]
△ **typhl-.** Tifl-. VER typhlo-.
typh·lec·ta·sis (tif-lek'tă-sis). Tiflectasia; dilatação do ceco. [G. *typhlon,* ceco, + *ektasis,* distensão]
typh·lec·to·my (tif-lek'tō-mē). Tiflectomia. SIN cecectomy.
typh·len·ter·i·tis (tif'len-ter-ī'tis). Tiflenterite. SIN cecitis.
typh·li·tis (tif'lī'tis). Tiflite; inflamação do ceco. SIN cecitis.
△ **typhlo-, typhl-.** Tiflo-, tifl-. **1.** O ceco. VER TAMBÉM ceco-. [G. cecum]. **2.** Cegueira. [G. *typhlos,* cego]
typh·lo·dic·li·di·tis (tif-lō-dik-li-dī'tis). Tiflodiclidite; inflamação da válvula ileocecal. [G. *typhlon,* ceco, + *diklis (diklid-),* dupla dobradiça (de portas), + *-itis,* inflamação]
typh·lo·em·py·e·ma (tif'lō-em-pī-ē'mă). Tiflopempiema; abscesso após tiflite. [G. *typhlon,* ceco, + *empyēma,* abscesso]
typh·lo·en·ter·i·tis (tif'lō-en-ter-ī'tis). Tifloenterite. SIN cecitis.
typh·lo·li·thi·a·sis (tif'lō-li-thī'ă-sis). Tiflolitíase; presença de concreções fecais no ceco. [G. *typhlon,* ceco, + *lithos,* pedra]
typh·lo·meg·a·ly (tif'lō-meg'ă-lē). Tiflomegalia; termo antigo para referir-se ao aumento do ceco. [G. *typhlon,* ceco,+*megas (megal-),* grande]
typh·lon (tif'lon). Ceco. SIN cecum (1). [G.]
typh·lo·pexy, typh·lo·pex·ia (tif'lō-pek-sē, tif-lō-pek'sē-ă). Tiflopexia. SIN cecopexy.
typh·lor·rha·phy (tif-lōr'ă-fē). Tiflorrafia. SIN cecorrhaphy.
typh·lo·sis (tif-lō'sis). Tiflose, cegueira. SIN blindness. [G. *typhlos,* cego]
typh·los·to·my (tif-los'tō-mē). Tiflostomia. SIN cecostomy.
typh·lot·o·my (tif-lot'ō-mē). Tiflotomia. SIN cecotomy.
△ **typho-.** Tifo-; tifo, tifóide. [G. *typhos,* fumaça, embotamento]
ty·phoid (tī'foyd). **1.** Tifóide, tifoso, tifóideo; semelhante ao tifo; torporoso em consequência de febre. **2.** Febre tifóide. SIN typhoid *fever.* [typhus + G. *eidos,* semelhança]
abdominal t., febre tifóide. SIN typhoid *fever.*
ambulatory t., febre tifóide deambulatória. SIN walking t.
apyretic t., febre tifóide apirética; febre tifóide em que a temperatura não se eleva mais do que um ou dois graus.
bilious t. of Griesinger, febre tifóide biliosa de Griesinger. SIN relapsing *fever.*
fowl t., febre tifóide aviária; doença septicêmica de galinhas e perus, causada por *Salmonella gallinarum;* foram relatadas algumas infecções humanas por esse microrganismo.
latent t., febre tifóide latente. SIN walking t.
provocation t., febre tifóide por provocação; início acelerado de febre tifóide; algumas vezes de intensidade incomum, em decorrência de vacinação tifóide-paratifóide A e B (T.A.B.) tardia (já no período de incubação da doença).
walking t., febre tifóide deambulatória; febre tifóide sem muita prostração, estando o paciente de pé e algumas vezes trabalhando. SIN ambulatory t., latent t.
ty·phoi·dal (tī-foyd'ăl). Tifóide; relativo a ou que se assemelha à febre tifóide.
ty·phol·y·sin (tī-fol'i-sin). Tifolisina; hemolisina formada por *Salmonella typhi.*
ty·pho·ma·nia (tī-fō-mā'nē-ă). Tifomania; delírio sussurrante característico da febre tifóide e do tifo. [typho- + G. *mania,* frenesi]
ty·pho·sep·sis (tī-fō-sep'sis). Septicemia tifóidea. SIN typhoid septicemia.
ty·phous (tī'fŭs). Tifoso, tifóideo; relativo ao tifo.
ty·phus (tī'foos). Tifo; grupo de doenças contagiosas e infecciosas agudas, causadas por riquétsias, que são transmitidas por artrópodes e que ocorrem em duas formas principais: tifo epidêmico e tifo endêmico (murino); os sinais e sintomas típicos incluem: cefaléia intensa, tremores e calafrios, febre alta, mal-estar e exantema. Também denominada febre de prisões, febre de acampamento ou febre do navio. SIN jail fever, ship fever. [G. *typhos,* fumaça, torpor]
Australian tick t., tifo do carrapato australiano; forma raramente fatal de tifo causada por *Rickettsia australis,* observada no leste da Austrália, transmitida por picada de carrapato e caracterizada por cefaléia intensa e conjuntivite. Reservatório em roedores e marsupiais. SIN Queensland tick t.
endemic t., t. endêmico. SIN murine t.
epidemic t., t. epidêmico; t. causado por *Rickettsia prowazekii* e transmitido por piolhos do corpo; caracterizado por febre alta, depressão mental e física e erupção macular e papular; dura cerca de 2 semanas e ocorre quando são reunidas grandes multidões e a higiene pessoal é precária; podem ocorrer recrudescências. SIN European t., hospital fever, louse-borne t., prison fever t.
European t., t. da Europa. SIN epidemic t.
exanthematous t., t. exantematoso; febre associada às lesões cutâneas petequiais habituais do tifo.
flea-borne t., t. murino. SIN murine t.
Indian tick t., febre maculosa do Mediterrâneo. SIN Mediterranean spotted *fever.*
louse-borne t., t. epidêmico. SIN epidemic t.
Manchurian t., t. da Manchúria; infecção por *Rickettsia sibirica* transmitido por carrapato. VER TAMBÉM Korean hemorrhagic *fever.*
Mexican t., t. mexicano; infecção por *Rickettsia typhi (mooseri),* que causa uma síndrome semelhante ao tifo epidêmico, porém transmitida de ratos para seres humanos pela pulga do rato (*Xenopsylla (Polyplax) cheopis*). A transmissão de rato para rato é feita pelo piolho do rato (*Polyplax spinulosa*). Forma mais comum de t. nos Estados Unidos. Tem vários nomes geográficos, de acordo com a região em que foi observado.
mite t., t. do ácaro. SIN tsutsugamushi *disease.*
mite-born t., t. transmitido por ácaros. SIN rickettsialpox.
t. mit'ior, t. mais leve; t. leve ou abortivo.
murine t., t. murino; forma mais leve de t. epidêmico causado por *Rickettsia typhi* e transmitido aos seres humanos por pulgas de rato ou de camundongo. SIN Congolian red fever, endemic t., flea-borne t., red fever, red fever of the Congo.
North Queensland tick t., t. do carrapato de North Queensland; tifo causado por *Rickettsia australis.*
prison fever t., t. epidêmico. SIN epidemic t.
Queensland tick t., t. do carrapato de Queensland. SIN Australian tick t.
recrudescent t., t. recrudescente. SIN Brill-Zinsser *disease.*
Sao Paulo t., t. de São Paulo; infecção por *Rickettsia rickettsii;* transmitida pela picada do carrapato. VER TAMBÉM Rocky Mountain spotted *fever.*
scrub t., t. rural. SIN tsutsugamushi *disease.*
shop t., t. urbano; forma leve de tifo que ocorre em áreas urbanas; relatado em áreas do Mediterrâneo. SIN urban t.
Siberian tick t., t. do carrapato da Sibéria; riquetsiose transmitida por carrapato, causada pela infecção por *Rickettsia sibirica.*
tick t., t. do carrapato. SIN Mediterranean spotted *fever.*
tropical t., t. tropical. SIN tsutsugamushi *disease.*
urban t., t. urbano. SIN shop t.
typ·ing (tīp'ing). Tipagem; classificação de acordo com o tipo. [ver type]
bacteriophage t., t. por bacteriófagos; procedimento microbiológico de importância epidemiológica para distinguir tipos de uma espécie ou cepa de bac-

téria aparentemente homogênea através do uso de bacteriófago tipo-específico.

HLA t., t. HLA; testes realizados para determinar se um paciente possui anticorpos contra os antígenos HLA de um doador potencial. A presença de anticorpos significa a rápida rejeição de um dado enxerto. Também utilizada para estabelecer paternidade e na medicina forense.

typus. Tipo. SIN type (3).
   typus ampullaris pelvis renalis [TA], tipo ampular de pelve renal. SIN ampullary *type* of renal pelvis.
   typus dendriticus pelvis renalis [TA], tipo dendrítico de pelve renal. SIN branching *type* of renal pelvis.

Tyr Símbolo de tyrosine (tirosina) e tyrosyl (tirosil).

ty·ra·mi·nase (tī′ră-mi-nās, tir′ā-). Tiraminase. SIN amine oxidase (flavin-containing).

ty·ra·mine (tī′ră-mēn, tir′ā-). Tiramina; tirosina descarboxilada, amina simpatomimética que possui ação semelhante, em alguns aspectos, à da epinefrina; presente no esporão do centeio, no visco, no queijo maduro, em cervejas, vinhos tintos e matéria animal putrefeita; elevada em indivíduos com tirosinemia tipo II.
   t. oxidase, t. oxidase. SIN amine oxidase (flavin-containing).

tyr·an·nism (tir′ă-nizm). Tiranismo; forma de sadismo que se caracteriza por um desejo de dominação e crueldade, com humilhação subseqüente do parceiro. [G. *tyrannos,* tirano]

ty·rem·e·sis (tī-rem′ē-sis). Tirêmese; vômito de material caseoso por lactentes. SIN tyrosis (1). [G. *tyros,* queijo, + *emesis,* vômito]

ty·ro·ci·din, ty·ro·ci·dine (tī-rō-sī′din). Tirocidina; ciclopeptídio antibacteriano obtido do *Bacillus brevis.* VER TAMBÉM tyrothricin.

Tyrode, Maurice V., farmacologista norte-americano, 1878–1930. VER T. *solution.*

ty·rog·e·nous (tī-roj′ē-nŭs). Tirógeno; produzido por ou que se origina no queijo. [G. *tyros,* queijo, + G. *-gen,* que produz]

Ty·rog·ly·phus lon·gi·or (tī-rog′li-fŭs lon′gē-ōr, tī′rō-glif′ŭs). SIN *Tyrophagus putrescentiae.* [G. *tyros,* queijo, + *glyphē,* entalhe]

ty·roid (tī′royd). Tiróide; semelhante a queijo; caseoso. [G. *tyrōdēs,* de *tyros,* queijo, + *eidos,* semelhança]

ty·ro·ke·to·nu·ri·a (tī′rō-kē-tō-noo′rē-ă). Tirocetonúria; a excreção urinária de metabólitos cetônicos da tirosina, como o ácido *p*-hidroxifenilpirúvico.

ty·ro·ma (tī-rō′mă). Tiroma; tumor caseoso. [G. *tyros,* queijo, + *-oma,* tumor]

ty·ro·pa·no·ate so·di·um (tī′rō-pă-nō′āt sō′dē-ŭm). Tiropanoato sódico; contraste oral para colecistografia.

Ty·roph·a·gus pu·tres·cen·ti·ae (tī-rof′ă-gŭs pū′tre-sen′tē-ē). Uma das espécies de ácaros de cereais que causa várias formas de dermatite em conseqüência da infestação de alimentos e derivados de cereais por ácaros, produzindo sensibilização e dermatite nas pessoas que trabalham no seu armazenamento e manuseio. SIN *Tyroglyphus longior.* [G. *tyros,* queijo, + *phagō,* comer]

ty·ro·sin·ase (tī′rō-si-nās, tir′ō-). Tirocinase, tiroquinase. SIN monophenol monooxygenase (1).

β-ty·ro·sin·ase. β-tirocinase, β-tiroquinase. SIN tyrosine phenol-lyase.

ty·ro·sine (Tyr, Y) (tī′rō-sēn, -sin). Tirosina; ácido 2-amino-3-(4-hidroxifenil) propiônico; 3-(4-hidroxifenil) alanina; o isômero L é um α-aminoácido presente na maioria das proteínas.
   t. aminotransferase, t. aminotransferase; enzima que catalisa a reação reversível da L-tirosina e α-cetoglutarato, produzindo *p*-hidroxifenilpiruvato e L-glutamato; essa enzima catalisa uma etapa no catabolismo da L-fenilalanina e L-tirosina; a deficiência dessa enzima está associada a tirosinemia II. SIN t. transaminase.
   t. iodinase, t. iodinase; suposta enzima na tireóide que catalisa a iodação da tirosina, uma reação importante na biossíntese final da tiroxina. VER TAMBÉM peroxidases.
   t. kinase, t. cinase, t. quinase; enzima que fosforila resíduos de tirosil em determinadas proteínas; muitas são produtos de oncogenes virais; diversos receptores (p. ex., receptores do fator de crescimento epidérmico, da insulina etc.) exibem essa atividade enzimática; trata-se de uma designação incorreta, visto que o substrato fisiológico não é a tirosina, porém resíduos de tirosil numa proteína.
   t. phenol-lyase, t. fenol-liase; enzima que catalisa a hidrólise da L-tirosina a fenol, piruvato e NH_3. SIN β-tyrosinase.
   t. transaminase, t. transaminase. SIN t. aminotransferase.

ty·ro·si·ne·mia (tī′rō-si-nē′mē-ă). [MIM*276600, *276700 e *276710]. Tirosinemia; grupo de distúrbios do metabolismo da tirosina, de herança autossômica recessiva, associados a concentrações sangüíneas elevadas de tirosina e aumento da excreção urinária de tirosina e compostos tirosil. A t. tipo I, causada pela deficiência de fumarilacetoacetase (FAH), caracteriza-se por esplenomegalia, cirrose hepática nodular, múltiplos defeitos de reabsorção tubular renal e raquitismo resistente à vitamina D; causada pela mutação no gene FAH no cromossoma 15q. A t. tipo II, produzida pela deficiência de tirosina aminotransferase (TAT), caracteriza-se por úlceras da córnea e ceratose dos dedos, das palmas das mãos e plantas dos pés; causada por mutação no gene TAT no cromossoma 16q. A t. tipo III está associada a ataxia intermitente e sonolência sem disfunção hepática; é causada pela deficiência de 4-hidroxifenilpiruvato dioxigenase (4HPPD). SIN hypertyrosinemia. [tyrosine + G. *haima,* sangue]

ty·ro·si·no·sis (tī′rō-si-nō′sis) [MIM*276800]. Tirosinose; distúrbio muito raro, possivelmente hereditário, do metabolismo da tirosina, que pode ser causado pela formação deficiente de ácido *p*-hidroxifenilpirúvico oxidase e de tirosina transaminase; caracterizada por excreção urinária aumentada de ácido *p*-hidroxifenilpirúvico e de outros metabólitos tirosil após a ingestão de tirosina ou de proteínas contendo esse aminoácido; herança autossômica recessiva. [tyrosine + G. *-osis,* condição]

ty·ro·si·nu·ria (tī′rō-si-noo′rē-ă). Tirosinúria; excreção de tirosina na urina. [tyrosine + G. *ouron,* urina]

ty·ro·sis (tī-rō′sis). Tirose. **1.** SIN tyremesis. **2.** SIN caseation. [G. *tyros,* queijo]

ty·ro·sy·lu·ria (tī′rō-si-loo′rē-ă). Tirosilúria; aumento da excreção urinária de determinados metabólitos da tirosina, como ácido *p*-hidroxifenilpirúvico; presente na tirosinose, no escorbuto, na anemia perniciosa e em outras doenças.

ty·ro·thri·cin (tī-rō-thrī′sin). Tirotricina; mistura antibacteriana obtida de culturas do *Bacillus brevis* em peptona; bactericida e bacteriostática, ativa contra bactérias Gram-positivas. Produz os agentes antibacterianos cristalinos gramicidina e tirocidina; o componente gramicidina é um polipeptídio que contém L-triptofano, D-leucina, D-valina, L-valina, L-alanina, glicina e um aminoetanol; o componente tirocidina é um ciclopolipeptídio que contém tirosina, ornitina e vários outros aminoácidos.

ty·ro·tox·ism (tī-rō-tok′sizm). Tirotoxismo; intoxicação por queijo ou por qualquer laticínio. [G. *tyros,* queijo, + *toxikon,* veneno]

Tyrrell, Frederick, anatomista e cirurgião inglês, 1797–1843. VER T. *fascia.*

Tyson, Edward, anatomista inglês, 1649–1708. VER T. *glands,* em *gland.*

Tyz·ze·ria (tī-zē′rē-ă). Gênero de coccídeos (família Eimeriidae) cujo oocisto contém oito esporozoítas nus. As espécies importantes são *T. anseris,* uma espécie relativamente não-patogênica encontrada no intestino delgado de gansos domésticos e selvagens, cisnes e alguns patos selvagens, e *T. perniciosa,* que ocorre no intestino delgado dos patos domésticos na América do Norte e na Europa e é patogênica em patos jovens.

Tzanck, Arnault, dermatologista russo, 1886–1954. VER T. *cells,* em *cell, test.*

U

υ 1. Ípsilon, 20ª letra do alfabeto grego. **2.** Símbolo de kinematic *viscosity* (viscosidade cinemática).
U 1. Abreviatura de unidade. **2.** Símbolo de quilurano; urânio; uridina em polímeros; uracil; concentração urinária, seguida por subscritos indicando localização e espécie química.
U Símbolo de internal *energy* (energia interna).
ubi·hy·dro·qui·none (ū′bi - hī - drō - quī′nōn). Ubiidroquinona. SIN ubiquinol.
ubi·qui·nol (QH$_2$, H$_2$Q) (ū′bi - kwī′nol, ū - bik′wi - nol). Ubiquinol; a produção da redução de uma ubiquinona. SIN ubihydroquinone.
ubi·qui·none (ū′bi - kwī′nōn, ū - bik′wi - nōn). Ubiquinona; uma 2,3-dimetoxi-5-metil-1,4-benzoquinona com uma cadeia lateral multiprenil; um componente móvel do transporte de elétrons. VER TAMBÉM coenzyme Q.
ubi·qui·none-6 (-Q$_6$). Ubiquinona-6; ubiquinona-30; coenzima Q$_6$; 2,3-dimetoxi-5-metil-6-hexaprenil-1,4-benzoquinona.
ubi·qui·none-10 (-Q$_{10}$). Ubiquinona-10; ubiquinona-50; coenzima Q$_{10}$; 2,3-dimetoxi-5-metil-6-decaprenil-1,4-benzoquinona.
ubiq·ui·tin (oo - bik′kwi - tin). Ubiquitina; uma proteína pequena (76 resíduos amino acil) encontrada em todas as células de organismos superiores e cuja estrutura sofreu modificação mínima durante a história evolutiva; envolvida em, pelo menos, dois processos: modificação da histona e decomposição da proteína intracelular.
UDP Abreviatura de *uridine* 5′-*diphosphate*.
UDP-*N*-ace·tyl·glu·co·sam·ine:ly·so·som·a len·zyme *N*-ace·tyl·-glu·co·sam·in·yl-1-phos·pho·trans·fer·ase. UDP-*N*-acetilglucosamina:enzima lisossômica *N*-acetilglicosaminil-1-fosfotransferase; uma enzima que participa da modificação pós-tradução de várias proteínas lisossômicas; uma deficiência ou defeito nessa enzima resulta em duas formas de mucolipidoses, doença da célula I e pseudopolidistrofia de Hurler.
UDPG Abreviatura de uridina difosfoglicose (uridine diphosphoglucose).
UDPGal Abreviatura de uridina difosfogalactose (uridine diphosphogalactose).
UDPga·lac·tose. UDP galactose; uridina difosfogalactose (uridine diphosphogalactose).
UDPga·lac·tose 4-ep·i·mer·ase. UDPgalactose 4-epimerase. SIN UDPglucose 4-epimerase.
UDPGlc Abreviatura de uridina difosfoglicose (uridine diphosphoglucose).
UDP-GlcUA. Abreviatura do ácido uridina difosfoglicurônico (uridine diphosphoglucuronic acid).
UDPglu·cose. UDPglicose. SIN uridine diphosphoglucose.
UDPglu·cose 4-ep·i·mer·ase. UDPglicose 4-epimerase; enzima que catalisa a inversão de Walden reversível de UDPglicose em UDPgalactose; a deficiência dessa enzima está associada a um tipo de galactosemia. SIN UDPgalactose 4-epimerase, uridine diphosphoglucose 4-epimerase.
UDPglu·cose-hex·ose-1-phos·phate uri·dyl·yl·trans·fer·ase. UDPglicose-hexose-1-fosfato uridililtransferase; enzima que catalisa a reação reversível da α-D-glicose 1-fosfato UDPgalactose para produzir UDPglicose e α-D-galactose 1-fosfato. VER TAMBÉM UDPglucose 4-epimerase. SIN hexose-1-phosphate uridylyltransferase, phosphogalactoisomerase.
UDPglu·cur·o·nate-bil·i·ru·bin glu·cu·ron·o·side glu·cu·ron·o·syl·trans·fer·ase. UDPglicuronato-bilirrubina glicuronosídio glicuronosil transferase. SIN UDPglucuronate-bilirubin glucuronosyltransferase.
UDPglu·cur·o·nate-bil·i·ru·bin glu·cu·ron·o·syl·trans·fer·ase. UDPglicuronato-bilirrubina glicuronosil transferase; transferases hepáticas que catalisam a transferência da porção glicurônica do ácido UDP-glicurônico em bilirrubina ou glicuronídio de bilirrubina, assim produzindo UDP e bilirrubina-glicuronosídio ou bilirrubina bisglicuronosídio, respectivamente; esses conjugados biliares são então secretados para a bile. SIN UDPglucuronate-bilirubinglucuronoside glucuronosyltransferase.
UDP·xy·lose. UDPxilose; um derivado açúcar no qual um grupamento pirofosfato liga a posição 5′ da uridina e a posição 1 da D-xilose; formada pela descarboxilação do ácido UDPglicurônico; necessária para a síntese de proteoglicanos; inibe a UDPglicose desidrogenase.
Uehlinger, E., patologista suíço, *1899. VER Meyenburg-Altherr-U. *syndrome*.
UFA Abreviatura de unesterified free *fatty acid* (ácido graxo livre não-esterificado).
Uffelmann, Jules A.C., médico alemão, 1837–1894. VER U. *reagent*.
UGI Abreviatura de upper gastrointestinal series (seriografia esôfago-estômago-duodeno).
Uhl, Henry S.M., clínico norte-americano, *1921. VER U. *anomaly*.
Uhthoff, Wilhelm, oftalmologista alemão, 1853–1927. VER U. *sign*; Uhthoff *symptom*.
UIP Abreviatura de usual interstitial *pneumonia* of Liebow (pneumonia intersticial habitual de Liebow).
ukam·bin (oo-kam′bin). Ucambina; um veneno africano para flechas derivado de plantas da família Apocynaceae; veneno cardíaco com ação semelhante à do digital ou estrofanto.

ULCER

ul·cer (ŭl′ser). Úlcera; uma lesão através da pele ou mucosa resultante da perda de tecido, geralmente com inflamação. VER erosion. SIN ulcus. [L. *ulcus* (*ulcer-*), uma úlcera]
  acute decubitus u., ú. de decúbito aguda; uma forma grave de úlcera, de origem neurotrófica, que ocorre na hemiplegia ou paraplegia.
  anastomotic u., ú. anastomótica; uma ú. do jejuno, após gastroenterostomia.
  Buruli u., ú. de Buruli; ú. da pele, com necrose ampla do tecido adiposo subcutâneo, devido à infecção por *Mycobacterium ulcerans*; ocorre em Uganda em pessoas que vivem sobre os bancos de areia do Rio Nilo. [*Buruli*, distrito de Uganda]
  chrome u., ú. por cromo; ú. dos membros ou do septo nasal produzida por exposição aos compostos do cromo. SIN tanner's u.
  chronic u., ú. crônica; ú. de longa data com tecido cicatricial fibroso no seu assoalho.
  stress u., ú. de estresse; ú. do duodeno em um paciente com extensas queimaduras superficiais, lesões intracranianas ou lesão corporal grave. SIN Curling u.
  decubitus u., ú. de decúbito; ú. crônica que surge em áreas de compressão da pele sobre uma proeminência óssea em pacientes debilitados confinados ao leito ou imobilizados, devido a um defeito circulatório. SIN bedsore, decubital gangrene, hospital gangrene, pressure gangrene, pressure sore, pressure u.
  dendritic corneal u., ú. de córnea dendrítica; ceratite causada pelo vírus herpes simples.
  dental u., ú. dentária; ú. da mucosa oral causada por mordedura ou pelo atrito contra a borda de um dente quebrado.
  diphtheritic u., ú. diftérica; ú. recoberta por uma membrana aderente cinza, causada por *Corynebacterium diphtheriae*.
  distention u., ú. de distensão; ú. do intestino na parte dilatada acima de um estreitamento.
  elusive u., úlcera de Hunner. SIN Hunner u.
  fascicular u., ú. fascicular; vascularização localizada da córnea no local de uma ú. da córnea.
  Fenwick-Hunner u., ú. de Fenwick-Hunner; SIN Hunner u.
  Gaboon u., ú. de Gaboon; uma forma de ú. tropical que afeta os residentes nessa região; assemelha-se a uma ú. sifilítica, principalmente pelo aspecto de sua cicatriz. [*Gaboon*, uma região da África]
  gastric u., ú. gástrica; uma ú. do estômago.
  gravitational u., ú. postural; ú. crônica da perna que não cicatriza devido à posição pendente do membro e à incompetência das válvulas no sistema venoso profundo da perna e da coxa; o retorno venoso pára e causa hipoxemia. VER TAMBÉM varicose u.
  gummatous u., ú. gomatosa; ú. gomosa; lesão da pele que ocorre na sífilis tardia.
  hard. u., cancro. SIN chancre.

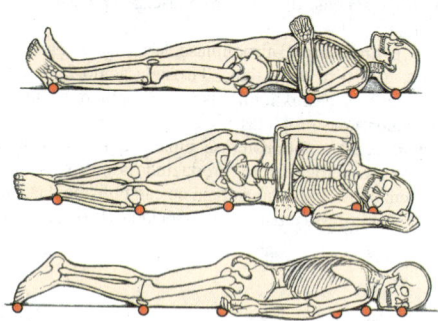

úlcera de decúbito: locais mais comuns devido à proximidade entre o osso e a pele

---

△ Formas Combinantes ☆ Termo oficial alternativo para a *Terminologia Anatomica*
Indica que o termo é ilustrado, ver Índice de Ilustrações
SIN Sinônimo [MIM] Mendelian Inheritance in Man
Cf. Comparar, confrontar I.C. Índice de Corantes
[NA] *Nomina Anatomica*
[TA] *Terminologia Anatomica* Termo de Alta Importância

1694

healed u., ú. cicatrizada; ú. recoberta por regeneração epitelial, sob a qual pode haver fibrose e ausência de glândulas ou anexos.
herpetic u., ú. herpética; ú. causada pelo vírus herpes simples.
Hunner u., ú. de Hunner; uma lesão focal e freqüentemente múltipla envolvendo todas as camadas da parede vesical na cistite intersticial crônica; o epitélio superficial é destruído por inflamação e a lesão inicialmente pálida se rompe e sangra, com distensão da bexiga. SIN elusive u., Fenwick-Hunner u.
hypopyon u., ú. de hipópio; (1) ú. supurativa central progressiva da córnea; VER TAMBÉM hypopyon; (2) ú. da córnea com pus na câmara anterior.
indolent u., ú. indolente; ú. crônica, com bordas elevadas duras e pouca ou nenhuma granulação, não mostrando tendência a cicatrizar.
inflamed u., ú. inflamada; ú. com secreção purulenta e bordas inflamadas.
Mann-Williamson u., ú. de Mann-Williamson. VER Mann-Williamson *operation*.
marginal ring u. of cornea, ú. anular marginal da córnea; ú. intermitente de evolução lenta, que envolve a circunferência da margem da córnea.
Marjolin u., ú. de Marjolin; carcinoma de células escamosas bem diferenciado, mas agressivo, observado no tecido cicatricial na borda epidérmica de um seio que drena a osteomielite subjacente.
Meleney u., ú. de Meleney; ú. escavada da pele e dos tecidos subcutâneos, causada por infecção sinérgica por estreptococos não-hemolíticos microaerófilos e estafilococos hemolíticos aeróbicos. SIN Meleney gangrene, progressive bacterial synergistic gangrene.
Mooren u., ú. de Mooren; inflamação crônica da periferia da córnea que evolui lentamente no centro com adelgaçamento da córnea e, algumas vezes, perfuração.
Oriental u., ú. oriental; a lesão que ocorre na leishmaniose cutânea.
penetrating u., ú. penetrante; ú. que se estende para os tecidos mais profundos de um órgão.
peptic u., ú. péptica; ú. da mucosa alimentar, geralmente no estômago ou duodeno, exposta à secreção de ácido gástrico.
perforated u., ú. perfurada; ú. que se estende através da parede de um órgão.
perforating u. of foot, ú. perfurante do pé; ú. trófica, profunda e redonda, na região plantar, após doença ou lesão em qualquer parte do trajeto do centro até a periferia do nervo que supre a parte.
phagedenic u., ú. fagedênica; ú. que se dissemina rapidamente acompanhada pela formação de descamação extensa. SIN sloughing u.
phlegmonous u., ú. flegmonosa; ú. acompanhada por inflamação dos tecidos vizinhos.
pressure u., ú. por compressão. SIN decubitus u.
recurrent aphthous u.'s, úlceras aftosas recorrentes. SIN aphtha (2).
ring u. of cornea, ú. anular da córnea; inflamação total ou da maior parte da periferia da córnea.
rodent u., ú. corrosiva; designação histórica para um carcinoma basocelular ulcerado de crescimento lento, geralmente na face.
Saemisch u., ú. de Saemisch; uma forma de ceratite serpiginosa, freqüentemente acompanhada por hipópio.
serpent u. of cornea, ú. serpiginosa da córnea. SIN serpiginous *keratitis*.
serpiginous u., ú. serpiginosa; ú. que se estende de um lado enquanto cicatriza na borda oposta, formando uma margem ondulada.
serpiginous corneal u., ú. serpiginosa da córnea; ulceração serpiginosa da córnea causada por infecção, mais freqüentemente por *Streptococcus pneumoniae*.
simple u., ú. simples; ú. local, não-constitucional, que não se acompanha de dor ou inflamação acentuada.
sloughing u., úlcera necrosada. SIN phagedenic u.
soft u., cancro mole. SIN chancroid.
stasis u., ú. de estase. SIN varicose u.
stercoral u., ú. estercoral; ú. do cólon devida à compressão e irritação pela massa fecal retida.
stomal u., ú. de estoma; ú. intestinal que ocorre após gastrojejunostomia na mucosa jejunal próxima da abertura (estoma) entre o estômago e o jejuno.
Curling u., ú. de Curling. SIN stress u.
Sutton u., ú. de Sutton; uma ú. solitária, profunda e dolorosa na mucosa oral ou genital.
syphilitic u., ú. sifilítica; (1) cancro; SIN chancre; (2) qualquer ulceração causada por uma infecção sifilítica.
Syriac u., Syrian u., nomes antigos da difteria.
tanner's u., ú. dos curtidores. SIN chrome u.
trophic u., ú. trófica; ú. resultante de desnervação sensorial cutânea. VER TAMBÉM perforating u. of foot. SIN trophic gangrene.
tropical u., ú. tropical; (1) a lesão que ocorre na leishmaniose cutânea; SIN tropical sore. VER TAMBÉM cutaneous *leishmaniasis*; (2) ulceração fagedênica tropical causada por vários microrganismos, incluindo micobactérias; comum no norte da Nigéria.
undermining u., ú. solapada; ú. cutânea crônica com margens salientes; causada por estreptococos hemolíticos, bacilos da tuberculose ou outras bactérias.
varicose u., ú. varicosa; a perda de superfície cutânea na área de drenagem de uma veia varicosa, na perna, resultante de estase e infecção. VER TAMBÉM gravitational u. SIN stasis u., venous u.
venereal u., ú. venérea. SIN chancroid.
venous u., ú. venosa. SIN varicose u.
Zambesi u., ú. de Zambesi; ú., geralmente única, com cerca de 3 cm de diâmetro, no pé ou na perna, que ocorre em trabalhadores no delta do rio Zambesi; possui uma superfície descamativa, mas não se dissemina e não provoca sintomas constitucionais ou aumento glandular; está associada à presença de um espirilo e de um grande bacilo fusiforme; uma crise parece conferir imunidade parcial.

ul·cer·ate (ŭl′ser-āt). Ulcerar; formar uma úlcera.
ul·cer·at·ed (ŭl′ser-āt-ed). Ulcerado; que sofreu ulceração.
ul·cer·a·tion (ŭl-ser-ā′shŭn). Ulceração. 1. A formação de uma úlcera. 2. Uma úlcera ou agregação de úlceras.
  tracheal u., u. traqueal; erosão da mucosa traqueal, em alguns casos com exposição dos anéis cartilaginosos, no local em que foi inserido um tubo de traqueostomia com balonete durante algum tempo.
ul·cer·a·tive (ŭl′ser-ă-tiv). Ulcerativo; relativo a, causador de ou caracterizado por uma úlcera ou úlceras.
ul·cer·o·gen·ic (ŭl′ser-ō-jen′ik). Ulcerogênico; causador de úlcera.
ul·cer·o·glan·du·lar (ŭl′ser-ō-gland′ū-lăr). Ulceroglandular; designa uma ulceração local em uma área de infecção seguida por linfadenopatia regional ou generalizada.
ul·cer·o·mem·bra·nous (ŭl′ser-ō-mem′bră-nŭs). Ulceromembranoso; relativo a ou caracterizado por ulceração e formação de uma falsa membrana.
ul·cus, pl. **ul·ce·ra** (ŭl′kŭs, ŭl′ser-ă). Úlcera. SIN ulcer. [L.]
ule-. VER ulo-.
ule·gy·ri·a (ū′lē-jī′rē-ă). Ulegiria; defeito do córtex cerebral caracterizado por giros estreitos e distorcidos; pode ser congênito ou resultar de cicatrizes. [G. *oulē*, cicatriz, + *gyros*, anel]
uler·y·the·ma (oo″ler-i-thē′mă). Uleritema; fibrose com eritema. [G. *oulē*, cicatriz, + *erythēma*, rubor da pele]
  u. ophryog′enes, u. ofriógeno; foliculite das sobrancelhas resultando em fibrose e alopecia.
u·lex eu·ro·pae·us (oo-leks oor′o-pā-ŭs). Ulex européia; uma lectina que reage especificamente com a α-L-fucose, usada como marcador de células endoteliais em cortes de parafina.
Ullmann, Emerich, cirurgião húngaro, 1861–1937. VER U. *line, syndrome*.
Ullrich, Otto, médico alemão, 1894–1957. VER Morquio-U. *disease*.
ul·na, gen. e pl. **ul·nae** (ŭl′nă, ŭl′nē) [TA]. Ulna; o medial e maior dos dois ossos do antebraço. SIN cubitus (2) [TA]. [L. cotovelo, braço, do G. ōlenē]
ul·nad (ŭl′nad). Ulnar; na direção da ulna. [ulna + L. *ad*, para]
ul·nar (ŭl′năr) [TA]. Ulnar; referente à ulna ou a qualquer das estruturas (p. ex., artéria, nervo) cujo nome dela deriva; relativo à face ulnar ou medial do membro superior. SIN ulnaris [TA]
ul·na·ris (ŭl′nă ris) [TA]. Ulnar. SIN ulnar. [L. Mod.]
ul·nen (ŭl′nen). Relativo à ulna independente de outras estruturas. [ulna + G. *en*, em]
ul·no·car·pal (ŭl′nō-kar′păl). Ulnocarpal; relativo à ulna e ao carpo, ou à face ulnar do punho.
ul·no·ra·di·al (ŭl′nō-rā′dē-ăl). Ulnorradial; relativo à ulna e ao rádio; designa as duas articulações, ligamentos, etc., entre eles.
ulo-, ule-. 1. Cicatriz, fibrose. [G. *oulē*] 2. As gengivas. VER TAMBÉM gingivo-. [G. *oulon*] 3. Crespo. [G. *oulo-, ouli-,* lanoso]
uloid (ū′loyd). Ulóide. 1. Semelhante a uma cicatriz. 2. Lesão semelhante a uma cicatriz causada por um processo degenerativo em camadas mais profundas da pele. [G. *oulē*, cicatriz + *eidos*, semelhança]
ulot·ri·chous (ū-lot′ri-kŭs). Ulótrico; que possui cabelo crespo. Cf. leiotrichous. [G. *oulotrichos*, cabelo crespo, de *oulos*, lanoso, + *thrix (trich-)*, cabelo]
ul·ti·mo·bran·chi·al (ŭl′ti-mō-brang′kē-ăl). Ultimobranquial; em embriologia, relativo à bolsa faríngea mais caudal. [L. *ultimus*, último, + G. *branchia*, guelras]
ul·ti·mum mo·ri·ens (ŭl′ti-mŭm mōr′ĭ-enz). O átrio direito do coração, citado como aquele que se contrai após parada do resto do coração. [L. o último a morrer]
ultra-. Ultra-; excesso, exagero, além. [L. além]
ul·tra·brach·y·ce·phal·ic (ŭl-trā-brak-ē-se-fal′ik). Ultrabraquicefálico; designa um crânio extremamente curto, com um índice de, pelo menos, 90.
ul·tra·cen·tri·fu·ga·tion (ŭl-trā-sen′tri-fū-gā-shŭn). Ultracentrifugação; o processo de submeter a uma ultracentrífuga.
ul·tra·cen·tri·fuge (ŭl-trā-sen′tri-fūj). Ultracentrífuga; uma centrífuga de alta velocidade (até 100.000 rpm) por meio da qual grandes moléculas, como, p. ex., de proteína ou ácidos nucleicos, são levadas a sedimentar em velocidades viáveis; usada para determinações de pesos moleculares, separação de grandes moléculas, critérios de homogeneidade de grandes moléculas, estudos de conformação, etc.

ul·tra·cy·to·stome (ŭl-tră-sī'tō-stōm). Ultracitóstomo; designação antiga de microporo. [ultra- + G. *kytos*, célula, + *stoma*, boca]

ul·tra·di·an (ŭl-trā'dē-ăn). Ultradiano; relativo a variações ou ritmos biológicos que ocorrem em ciclos mais freqüentes que a cada 24 horas. Cf. circadian, infradian. [ultra- + L. *dies*, dia]

ul·tra·dol·i·cho·ce·phal·ic (ŭl-trā-dol-i-kō-se-fal'ik). Ultradolicocefálico; designa um crânio muito longo, com um índice cefálico menor que 65.

ul·tra·fil·ter (ŭl'tră-fil-ter). Ultrafiltro; uma membrana semipermeável (colódio, bexiga de peixe ou papel de filtro impregnado com géis) usada como filtro para separar colóides e grandes moléculas da água e pequenas moléculas, que a atravessam.

ul·tra·fil·tra·tion (ŭl'tră-fil-trā'shŭn). Ultrafiltração; filtração através de uma membrana semipermeável ou de qualquer filtro que separa soluções colóides de cristalóides ou que separa partículas de tamanhos diferentes em uma mistura colóide.

ul·tra·li·ga·tion (ŭl-tră-lī-gā'shŭn). Ultraligadura; ligadura de um vaso sangüíneo além do ponto onde emite um ramo.

ul·tra·mi·cro·scope (ŭl-tră-mī'krō-skōp). Ultramicroscópio; microscópio que utiliza luz refratada para visualizar objetos não-visíveis com o microscópio comum quando se usa luz direta.

ul·tra·mi·cro·scop·ic (ŭl'tră-mī-krō-skop'ik). Ultramicroscópico. SIN submicroscopic.

ul·tra·mi·cro·tome (ŭl-tră-mī'krō-tōm). Ultramicrótomo; micrótomo usado na realização de cortes ≤ 0,1 μm de espessura para microscopia eletrônica.

ul·tra·mi·crot·o·my (ŭl'tră-mī-krot'o-mē). Ultramicrotomia; a realização de cortes ultrafinos para microscopia eletrônica por meio de um ultramicrótomo.

ul·tra·son·ic (ŭl-tră-son'ik). Ultra-sônico; relativo a ondas de energia semelhantes às ondas sonoras, mas de maiores freqüências (> 30.000 Hz). [ultra- + L. *sonus*, som]

ul·tra·son·ics (ŭl-tră-son'iks). Ultra-acústica; a ciência e a tecnologia do ultra-som, suas características e fenômenos.

ul·tra·son·o·gram (ŭl-tră-son'ō-gram). Ultra-sonograma; ecograma; sonograma; a imagem obtida por ultra-sonografia. VER TAMBÉM echogram. SIN sonogram.

ul·tra·son·o·graph (ŭl'tră-son'ō-graf). Ultra-sonógrafo; ecógrafo; sonógrafo; instrumento computadorizado usado para criar uma imagem utilizando ultra-som. SIN sonograph. [ultra- + L. *sonus*, som, + G. *graphō*, escrever]

ul·tra·so·nog·ra·pher (ŭl'tră-sō-nog'ră-fer). Ultra-sonografista; ecografista; sonografista; pessoa que realiza e/ou interpreta exames de ultra-sonografia. SIN ecographer, sonographer.

ul·tra·so·nog·ra·phy (ŭl'tră-sō-nog'ră-fē). Ultra-sonografia; ecografia; sonografia; a localização, medida ou delineação de estruturas profundas através da medida da reflexão ou transmissão de ondas de alta freqüência ou ultra-sônicas. O cálculo computadorizado da distância até a superfície que reflete ou absorve o som somado à orientação conhecida do feixe de som produz uma imagem bidimensional. VER TAMBÉM ultrasound. SIN echography, sonography. [ultra- + L. *sonus*, som, + G. *graphō*, escrever]

Doppler u., u. Doppler; aplicação do efeito Doppler ao ultra-som para detectar movimento de alvos dispersos (geralmente hemácias) pela análise da mudança na freqüência dos ecos que retornam.

> Em muitas situações, o ultra-som superou a radiografia como método de escolha para estudo por imagens, porque não representa risco conhecido para os pacientes, não é invasivo e seu custo é moderado. O ultra-som Doppler torna possível a visualização em tempo real dos tecidos, do fluxo sangüíneo e de órgãos que não podem ser observados por qualquer outro método. É particularmente útil em cardiologia e obstetrícia.

duplex u., u. dúplex; a combinação de u. em tempo real e Doppler.

endovaginal u., u. intravaginal; u. pélvica utilizando um transdutor introduzido na vagina.

gray-scale u., u. de escala cinza; a exibição da amplitude do eco do ultra-som ou da intensidade do sinal como diferentes tons de cinza, melhorando a qualidade da imagem em comparação com a apresentação obsoleta em preto-e-branco.

real-time u., u. em tempo real; imagens de ultra-som seriadas rápidas, produzidas utilizando-se um sistema de fases ou transdutor; produz uma imagem em vídeo do movimento do órgão, como o movimento de uma válvula cardíaca ou o movimento fetal.

ul·tra·son·o·sur·gery (ŭl'tră-son-ō-ser'jer-ē). Ultra-sonocirurgia; uso de técnicas de ultra-som para romper células, tecidos ou tratos, sobretudo no sistema nervoso central.

ul·tra·sound (ŭl'tră-sownd). Ultra-som; som que possui uma freqüência > 30.000 Hz.

diagnostic u., u. diagnóstico; o uso do u. para obter imagens para fins de diagnóstico clínico, empregando freqüências que variam de 1,6 a, aproximadamente, 10 MHz.

obstetric u., u. obstétrica; uso de u. diagnóstica durante a gravidez.

ul·tra·struc·ture (ŭl-tră-strŭk'choor). Ultra-estrutura; estruturas ou partículas observadas ao microscópio eletrônico. SIN fine structure.

ul·tra·therm (ŭl'tră-therm). Ultratermo; máquina diatérmica de ondas curtas. [ultra- + G. *thermē*, calor]

ul·tra·vi·o·let (ŭl-tră-vī'o-let). Ultravioleta; designa raios eletromagnéticos de freqüência mais elevada que a extremidade violeta do espectro visível.

u. A (UVA), u. A (UVA); radiação u. de 320 a 400 nm que causa bronzeamento da pele, mas com capacidade muito pequena de provocar queimaduras solares e câncer.

u. B (UVB), u. B (UVB); radiação u. de 290 a 320 nm que provoca mais efetivamente queimadura solar e bronzeamento; a exposição excessiva ao UVB é uma causa de câncer em pessoas de pele clara.

u. C, u. C; radiação u. de 200 a 290 nm; a radiação UVC na luz solar não alcança a superfície da terra; lâmpadas germicidas e de mercúrio podem causar queimadura solar e fotoceratite.

extravital u., u. extravital; que possui comprimentos de onda de 2.900 a 1.850 Å.

intravital u., u. intravital; que possui comprimentos de onda de 3.900 a 3.200 Å.

ul·tro·mo·tiv·i·ty (ŭl'trō-mō-tiv'i-tē). Ultramotividade; capacidade de movimento espontâneo. [L. *ultro*, além, espontâneo, + L. *motio*, movimento]

ulu·la·tion (oo-loo-lā'shŭn). Ululação; termo raramente empregado para designar o choro desarticulado de pessoas emocionalmente perturbadas. [L. *ululo*, pp. *-atus*, uivo]

Ulysses, forma latina do personagem mitológico grego. VER Ulysses *syndrome*.

um·bil·i·cal (ŭm-bil'i-kăl). Umbilical; onfálico; relativo ao umbigo. SIN omphalic.

um·bil·i·cate, um·bil·i·cat·ed (ŭm-bil'i-kāt,-kāt-ed). Umbilicado; em forma de umbigo; deprimido; escavado. [L. *umbilicatus*]

um·bil·i·ca·tion (ŭm-bil-i-kā'shŭn). Umbilicação. **1.** Uma depressão em forma de umbigo. **2.** Formação de uma depressão no ápice de uma pápula, vesícula ou pústula.

um·bil·i·cus, pl. **um·bil·i·ci** (ŭm-bil'i-kŭs, ŭm-bi-lī-kŭs; -i-sī, -lī'kī). Umbigo; ônfalo; a depressão no centro da parede abdominal que marca o ponto de entrada do cordão umbilical no feto. SIN belly button, navel. [L. *umbigo*]

um·bo, gen. **um·bo·nis**, pl. **um·bo·nes** (ŭm'bō, -bō-nis, -bō-nēs) [TA]. Umbigo. **1.** [NA]. Um ponto que se projeta de uma superfície. **2.** SIN u. of tympanic membrane. [L. bossa em um anteparo, protuberância]

u. membra'nae tym'pani [TA], umbigo da membrana do tímpano. SIN u. of tympanic membrane.

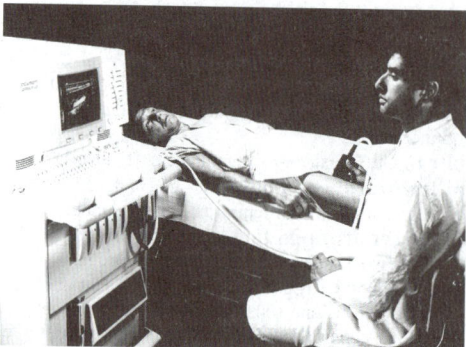
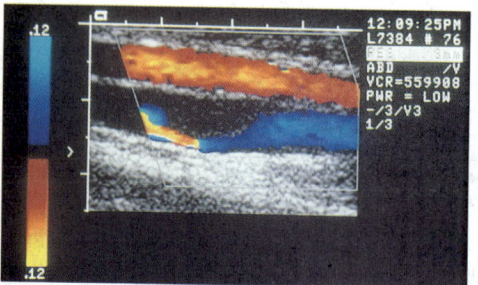

ultra-sonografia Doppler: (A) estudo vascular por imagens; (b) Doppler de fluxo colorido mostrando trombo na veia femoral

u. of tympanic membrane [TA], umbigo da membrana do tímpano; a projeção da superfície interna da membrana timpânica na extremidade do manúbrio do martelo; isso corresponde ao ponto mais deprimido da membrana, visto de lado, que é comumente denominado umbigo. SIN u. membranae tympani [TA], umbo (2) [TA].

UMP Abreviatura de *uridine* 5′-monophosphate.

UMP syn·thase. UMP sintase. SIN uridylic acid.

un-. 1. Prefixo de negação, semelhante ao L. *in-* e ao G. *a-, an-*. 2. Inversão, remoção, liberação, privação. 3. Uma ação intensiva [I. M.]

un·cal (ŭng′kăl). Uncal; relativo ao unco.

un·ci (ŭn′sī). Plural de unco.

un·cia (ŭn′sē-ă). Uma onça. [L. décima segunda parte, uma onça]

un·ci·form (ŭn′si-fōrm). Unciforme; uncinado. SIN uncinate. [L. *uncus*, gancho, + *forma*, forma]

un·ci·for·me (ŭn-si-fōr′me). Unciforme; osso hamato. SIN hamate (*bone*). [L. Mod. unciform]

Un·ci·nar·ia (ŭn-si-nar′ē-ă). Gênero de nematódeos que infestam vários mamíferos. As espécies incluem *U. stenocephala*, o nematódeo europeu de cães, gatos e vários carnívoros selvagens, também encontrado na América do Norte, onde é muito menos comum que o *Ancylostoma caninum*, embora tenha sido implicado na larva migrans cutânea. [LL. *uncinus*, gancho]

un·ci·na·ri·a·sis (ŭn′si-nă-rī′ă-sis). Uncinaríase; ancilostomíase. SIN ancylostomiasis.

un·ci·nate (ŭn′si-nāt). Uncinado; unciforme. 1. Em forma de ou semelhante a um gancho. 2. Relativo a um unco ou, especificamente, ao giro uncinado (2) ou a um processo do pâncreas ou de uma vértebra. SIN unciform. [L. *uncinatus*]

un·ci·na·tum (ŭn-si-nă′tŭm). Uncinado. SIN hamate (*bone*).

un·ci·pres·sure (ŭn′si-presh-ŭr). Uncipressão; interrupção da hemorragia de uma artéria seccionada por compressão com um gancho rombo. [L. *uncus*, gancho]

un·com·ple·ment·ed (ŭn-kom′plē-men-ted). Acomplementado; não unido por complemento e, portanto, inativo.

un·con·scious (ŭn-kon′shŭs). Inconsciente. 1. Não-consciente. 2. Em psicanálise, a estrutura psíquica que compreende os impulsos e sentimentos dos quais o indivíduo não tem consciência. SIN insensible (1).
  collective u., i. coletivo; na psicologia jungiana, os engramas combinados ou potenciais de memória herdados do passado filogenético de um indivíduo.

un·con·scious·ness (ŭn-kon′shŭs-ness). Inconsciência; termo impreciso para designar um estado de comprometimento acentuado da percepção de si mesmo e do ambiente ao seu redor; usado, na maioria das vezes, como sinônimo de coma e ausência de responsividade.

un·co·os·si·fied (ŭn-kō-os′i-fīd). Não co-ossificado; que não se encontra unido a um osso.

un·cou·plers (ŭn-kŭp′lerz). Desacopladores; substâncias como o dinitrofenol que permitem o prosseguimento da oxidação em mitocôndrias sem a fosforilação concomitante habitual para produzir ATP; assim, esses venenos "desacoplam" a oxidação e a fosforilação. SIN uncoupling factors.

un·co·ver·te·bral (ŭn-kō-ver′te-bral). Uncovertebral; relativo a, ou que afeta, o processo uncinado de uma vértebra.

unc·tion (ŭngk′shŭn). Unção; o ato de ungir ou untar com pomada ou óleo. [L. *unctio*, de *ungo*, pp. *unctus*, untar]

unc·tu·ous (ŭngk′shoo-ŭs, -choo-ŭs). Untuoso; gorduroso; oleoso. [L. *unctuosus*, de *unctio*, unção]

unc·ture (ŭnk′choor). Untura; ungüento; pomada. SIN ointment.

un·cus, pl. **un·ci** (ŭn′kŭs, ŭn′sī) [TA]. Unco; giro uncinado; gancho do giro para-hipocampal. 1. Qualquer processo ou estrutura em forma de gancho. 2. A extremidade anterior, em forma de gancho, do giro para-hipocampal na superfície basomedial do lobo temporal; a face anterior do u. corresponde ao córtex olfatório, sua superfície ventral à área entorrinal; profundamente ao u. está a amígdala (corpo amigdalóide). SIN uncinate gyrus, u. gyri parahippocampalis. [L. um gancho, do G. *onkos*]
  u. gy′ri parahippocampa′lis, gancho do giro para-hipocampal. SIN uncus (2).

un·dec·e·no·ic ac·id (ŭn′des-ē-nō′ik). Ácido undecenóico; ácido undecilênico. SIN undecylenic acid.

un·de·co·yl·i·um chlo·ride (ŭn-de-kō-il′ē-ŭm). Cloreto de undecoílio; um anti-séptico tópico.

un·de·co·yl·i·um chlo·ride-io·dine. Cloreto iodado de undecoílio; um complexo de iodo com cloreto de undecoílio; um detergente catiônico usado topicamente como agente germicida.

un·dec·y·len·ate (ŭn-des′i-li-nāt). Undecilenato; um sal do ácido undecilênico.

un·dec·y·len·ic ac·id (ŭn-des-i-len′ik). Ácido undecilênico; ácido undecenóico; um ácido presente em pequenas quantidades no suor; usado com seu sal zíncico em pomadas, ou como pó no tratamento de doenças fúngicas da pele, psoríase e algumas outras afecções cutâneas. SIN undecenoic acid.

un·der·a·chieve·ment (ŭn′der-ă-chēv′ment). Incapacidade de realizar aquilo que o potencial de um indivíduo parece permitir.

un·der·a·chiev·er (ŭn′der-ă-chēv′er). Pessoa que não consegue realizar aquilo que seu potencial parece permitir.

un·der·bite (ŭn′der-bīt). Termo não-técnico aplicado ao subdesenvolvimento mandibular ou ao desenvolvimento maxilar excessivo.

un·der·cut (ŭn′der-kŭt). Rebaixo; subcorte. 1. A parte do dente situada entre a linha de delineamento (altura do contorno) e a gengiva. 2. O contorno de um corte transversal de uma crista residual ou arcada dentária que impediria a inserção de uma prótese dentária. 3. O contorno de uma caixa de moldar que se fecha de forma a impedir a separação das partes.

un·der·drive pac·ing (ŭn′der-drīv pās′ing). Estimulação elétrica do coração em uma freqüência menor que a de uma taquicardia existente; designada para capturar o coração entre os batimentos, isto é, interromper uma via de reentrada a fim de interromper a bradicardia.

un·der·nu·tri·tion (ŭn′der-noo-tri′shŭn). Subnutrição; uma forma de desnutrição resultante de redução do suprimento de alimentos ou da incapacidade de digerir, assimilar e utilizar os nutrientes necessários.

un·der·sens·ing (ŭn′der-sen′sing). Subpercepção; não-percepção do sinal de despolarização intracardíaco atrial ou ventricular por um marcapasso.

un·der·shoot (ŭn′der-shoot). Subimpulso; redução temporária abaixo do valor do estado de equilíbrio final que pode ocorrer imediatamente após a retirada de uma influência que estava elevando aquele valor, ou seja, impulso excessivo em uma direção negativa.

un·der·stain (ŭn′der-stān). Subcorar; corar menos profundamente que o habitual.

un·der·ven·ti·la·tion (ŭn′der-ven-ti-lā′shŭn). Hipoventilação. SIN hypoventilation.

un·der·wind·ing (ŭn′der-wīnd′ing). Subenovelamento; o efeito da superespiralação negativa em uma estrutura de DNA.

un·dif·fer·en·ti·at·ed (ŭn′dif-er-en′shē-ā-ted). Indiferenciado; não-diferenciado; p. ex., primitivo, embrionário, imaturo, ou que não possui estrutura ou função especial.

un·dine (ŭn′dēn, -dīn). Undina; pequeno recipiente de vidro usado na irrigação da conjuntiva. [L. Mod. *undina*, do L. *unda*, onda]

un·di·ver·sion (ŭn-di-ver′shŭn). Reversão de uma derivação; restauração cirúrgica da continuidade de qualquer sistema orgânico cujo fluxo havia sido previamente desviado; p. ex., entre as vias urinárias superiores e a bexiga após derivação urinária supravesical.

un·do·ing (ŭn-doo′ing). Anulação; em psicologia e psiquiatria, um mecanismo de defesa inconsciente pelo qual uma pessoa reverte simbolicamente uma conduta inaceitável anterior.

un·du·late (ŭn′doo-lāt). Ondulado; que possui uma borda irregular, ondulada; designa o formato de uma colônia de bactérias. [L. Mod. *undula*, dim. de *unda*, onda]

un·du·li·po·di·um, pl. **un·du·li·po·dia** (ŭn′doo-li-pō′dē-um, -ă). Ondulipódio; extensão intracelular flexível, semelhante a um chicote, de muitas células eucarióticas, com uma característica simetria de nove pregas, um arranjo de nove pares de microtúbulos periféricos e um par central, freqüentemente denominada simetria 9 + 2; parece crescer a partir de um corpúsculo basal (cinetossoma) na célula e é um componente fundamental da célula eucariótica. Tanto o cílio quanto o flagelo eucariótico (não o flagelo bacteriano, que não possui o padrão 9 + 2) são considerados ondulipódios. [LL. *undulo*, mover em ondas, do L. *unda*, onda, + L. Mod. *podium*, do G. *podion*, dim. de *pous*, pé]

ung Abreviatura do L. *unguentum*, pomada.

un·gual (ŭng′gwăl). Ungueal; relativo a uma unha ou às unhas. SIN unguinal. [L. *unguis*, unha]

un·guent (ŭng′gwent). Ungüento; pomada. SIN ointment. [L. *unguentum*]

un·gues (ŭng′gwēz). Plural de unguis (unha).

Un·guic·u·la·ta (ŭng-gwik-ū-lā′tă). Ungüiculados; divisão dos mamíferos na qual se incluem todos os mamíferos que possuem unhas ou garras, que diferem dos Ungulata (ungulados). [L. *unguiculus*, unha ou garra]

un·guic·u·late (ŭng-gwik′ū-lāt). Ungüiculado; que possui unhas ou garras, diferente daqueles com cascos.

un·guic·u·lus (ŭn-gwik′ū-lŭs). Ungüícula; pequena unha ou garra. [L. dim. de *unguis*, unha]

un·gui·nal (ŭng′gwi-năl). Ungüinal, ungueal. SIN ungual.

un·guis, pl. **un·gues** (ŭng′gwis, -gwēz) [TA]. Unha; placa ungueal. SIN nail (1). [L.]
  u. adun′cus, u. encravada, onixe. SIN ingrown nail.
  u. a′vis, u. de ave. SIN calcarine *spur*.
  Haller u., u. de Haller. SIN calcarine *spur*.
  u. incarna′tus, u. encravada. SIN ingrown nail.

Un·gu·la·ta (ŭng-gū-lā′tă). Ungulados; divisão dos mamíferos que compreende os que possuem cascos, diferente dos Unguiculata (ungüiculados).

un·gu·late (ŭng′gū-lāt). Ungulado; que possui cascos. [L. *ungulatus*, de *ungula*, casco].

un·gu·li·grade (ŭng′gū-li-grād). Unguligrado; que anda sobre cascos, como os cavalos, porcos e ruminantes. [L. *ungula*, casco, + *gradus*, passo].

uni-. Prefixo que indica um, único, ímpar; corresponde ao G. mono- [L. *unus*]

u·ni·ar·tic·u·lar (ū-nē-ar-tik′ū-lăr). Uniarticular; monoarticular. SIN monarticular.

uni·ax·i·al (oo-nē-ak′sē-ăl). Uniaxial; que possui apenas um eixo; que cresce principalmente em uma direção.

uni·bas·al (ū-ni-bā′săl). Unibasal; que possui apenas uma base.

Un·i·blue A (ū′nē-bloo) [C.I. 14553]. Coloração proteica utilizada em eletroforese.

uni·cam·er·al, uni·cam·er·ate (oo-nē-kam′ĕ-răl, -kam′ĕ-rāt). Unicameral. SIN monolocular.

uni·cel·lu·lar (ū-ni-sel′ū-lăr). Unicelular; composto apenas de uma célula, como nos protozoários; para esses microrganismos u. capazes de realizar processos vitais independentemente de outras células, também é usado o termo acelular.

u·ni·cen·tral (ū-ni-sen′trăl). Unicentral; que possui um único centro, como de crescimento ou de ossificação.

uni·corn (ū′nē-kōrn). Unicorne. SIN unicornous.

uni·cor·nous (ū′ni-kōr′nŭs). Unicórneo, unicorne; que possui um corno. SIN unicorn. [L. *unicornis*, de uni- + *cornu*-, corno]

uni·cus·pid, uni·cus·pi·date (ū-ni-kŭs′pid, -kŭs′pi-dāt). Unicúspide; que possui apenas uma cúspide, como um dente canino.

uni·fa·mil·i·al (ū′nē-fa-mil′ē-ăl). Unifamilial; relativo a, ou que ocorre, em uma única família; designa particularmente uma doença nervosa que acomete várias crianças na mesma família, sem traço hereditário evidente.

uni·fla·gel·late (ū-ni-flaj′ĕ-lāt). Uniflagelado. SIN monotrichous.

uni·fo·rate (oo-ni-fō′rāt). Que só possui um forame, poro ou abertura de qualquer tipo.

uni·form (oo′ni-fōrm). Uniforme. 1. Que possui apenas uma forma; cuja forma é invariável. 2. Da mesma forma que outra estrutura ou objeto. [L. *uniformis*, de uni- + *forma*, forma]

uni·ger·mi·nal (ū-ni-jer′mi-năl). Unigerminal; unigerminativo; monogerminal; relativo a um único germe ou ovo; p. ex., monozigótico. SIN monogerminal, monozygotic, monozygous.

uni·glan·du·lar (oo-ni-glan′doo-lăr). Uniglandular; que envolve, relacionado a ou que contém apenas uma glândula.

uni·lam·i·nar, uni·lam·i·nate (oo-ni-lam′i-năr, -lam′i-nāt). Unilaminar; unilaminado; que possui apenas uma camada ou lâmina.

uni·lat·e·ral (oo-ni-lat′ĕ-răl). Unilateral; restrito a um lado apenas.

uni·lo·bar (oo-ni-lō′băr). Unilobar; que possui um lobo apenas.

uni·lo·cal (ū-ni-lō′kăl). Unilocal; em sentido estrito, designa um traço no qual o componente genético provém exclusivamente de um *locus*; na prática, qualquer traço no qual a contribuição de um *locus* é tão grande que os dados são facilmente interpretados como mendelianos.

uni·loc·u·lar (oo-ni-lok′ū-lăr). Unilocular; que possui apenas um compartimento ou cavidade, como em um adipócito. [uni- + L. *loculus*, compartimento]

uni·mo·lec·u·lar (ū′ni-mō-lek′ū-lăr). Unimolecular; monomolecular; designa uma única molécula. VER TAMBÉM molecularity. SIN monomolecular (1).

uni·nu·cle·ar, uni·nu·cle·ate (oo-ni-noo′klē-ăr, -noo′klē-āt). Uninuclear; uninucleado; que possui apenas um núcleo. Cf. mononuclear.

uni·oc·u·lar (ū-ni-ok′ū-lăr). Uniocular. 1. Relativo a um olho apenas. 2. Que tem visão em um olho apenas.

un·ion (ūn′yŭn). União. 1. Junção ou amalgamação de dois ou mais corpos. 2. Adesão estrutural ou crescimento conjunto das bordas de uma ferida. 3. Consolidação de uma fratura representada pelo desenvolvimento de continuidade entre fragmentos fraturados. [L. *unus*, um]

autogenous u., u. autógena; em odontologia, a união de dois pedaços de metal sem solda.

faulty u., u. falha; consolidação defeituosa. SIN fibrous u.

fibrous u., u. fibrosa; consolidação fibrosa; u. de fratura por tecido fibroso. VER nonunion. SIN faulty u.

primary u., u. primária. SIN healing by first intention.

secondary u., u. secundária. SIN healing by second intention.

vicious u., u. viciosa. SIN malunion.

uni·o·val, uni·ov·u·lar (ū-nē-ō′val, -ov′ū-lăr). Unioval; uniovular; relativo a, ou formado a partir de, um único óvulo.

uni·pen·nate (ū-ni-pen′āt). Unipenado; monopenado. *Termo alternativo oficial para semipennate. [uni- + L. *penna*, pena]

uni·po·lar (oo-ni-pō′lăr). Unipolar. 1. Que possui um só pólo; indica uma célula nervosa a partir da qual se projetam ramos apenas de um lado. 2. Situado apenas em uma extremidade de uma célula.

uni·port (ū′ni-pōrt). Uniporte; transporte de uma molécula ou íon através de uma membrana, por um mecanismo carreador (uniportador), sem acoplamento conhecido com qualquer outro transporte de moléculas ou íons. Cf. antiport, symport. [uni- + L. *porto*, carregar]

uni·port·er (ū′ni-pōrt-er). Uniportador; uma proteína que medeia o transporte de uma molécula ou íon através de uma membrana sem acoplamento conhecido ao transporte de qualquer outra molécula ou íon.

uni·po·tent (ū′ni-pō′tent). Unipotente; referente àquelas células que produzem um único tipo de célula-filha; p. ex., uma célula-tronco (primordial) u. Cf. pluripotent *cells*, em *cell*.

uni·sep·tate (oo-ni-sep′tāt). Unisseptado; que possui apenas um septo ou divisão.

UNIDADE

unit (U) (ū′nit). Unidade. 1. Um; uma única pessoa ou objeto. 2. Um padrão de medida, peso ou qualquer outra qualidade, por multiplicações ou frações, com os quais é formada uma escala ou sistema. 3. Um grupo de pessoas ou objetos considerados como um todo devido a atividades ou funções mútuas. VER TAMBÉM international u. [L. *unus*, um]

absolute u., u. absoluta; uma u. cujo valor é constante, independentemente do lugar ou tempo, e não derivada, ou dependente, de gravitação.

alexin u., u. alexínica. SIN complement u.

Allen-Doisy u., u. de Allen-Doisy; a menor quantidade de estrogênio capaz de produzir, em uma fêmea de camundongo castrada, uma alteração característica do epitélio vaginal, a saber, desaparecimento de leucócitos e surgimento de células cornificadas, conforme determinado por um esfregaço vaginal; igual a, aproximadamente, metade de uma u. estrona. SIN mouse u.

alpha u.'s, unidades alfa; grânulos citoplasmáticos de glicogênio dispostos em rosetas.

amboceptor u., u. de amboceptor. SIN hemolysin u.

androgen u. (international), u. de androgênio (internacional); a atividade androgênica de 100 μg (0,1 mg) de androsterona cristalina conforme analisado pela resposta de crescimento da crista em capões.

Ångström u. (Å), u. Ångström. VER Ångström.

antigen u., u. de antígeno; a menor quantidade de antígeno que, na presença de anti-soro específico, fixará 1 u. de complemento.

antitoxin u., u. de antitoxina; uma u. que expressa a potência ou a atividade de uma antitoxina; em geral, determinada em referência a uma preparação padrão preservada de antitoxina. VER TAMBÉM L. *doses*, em *dose*.

antivenene u., u. de antiveneno; a quantidade de antiveneno que, injetada na veia da orelha, protegerá 1 g de peso de coelho contra uma dose fatal de veneno de cobra.

atomic mass u. (amu), u. de massa atômica (uma); uma u. de massa, por definição, igual a 1/12 da massa de um átomo de carbono-12, que é igual a $1,6605402 \times 10^{-27}$ kg; em termos de energia, 1 uma é igual a 931,49432 MeV. Cf. dalton.

base u.'s, unidades básicas; as unidades fundamentais de comprimento, massa, tempo, corrente elétrica, temperatura termodinâmica, quantidade de substância e intensidade luminosa no Sistema Internacional de Unidades (SI); os nomes e símbolos das unidades para essas quantidades são metro (m), quilograma (kg), segundo (s), ampère (A), kelvin (K), mol (mol) e candela (cd). VER TAMBÉM International System of Units.

Bethesda u., u. de Bethesda; uma medida de atividade inibidora; a quantidade de inibidor que inativará 50% ou 0,5 u. de um fator da coagulação durante o período de incubação. [*Bethesda*, MD]

biological standard u., u. padrão biológica; uma quantidade específica de material de referência biologicamente ativo (antibiótico, antitoxina, enzima, hormônio, vitamina, etc.).

bird u., u. aviária; uma u. de atividade da prolactina; a quantidade mínima do hormônio que produzirá um certo aumento do peso da glândula do papo de pombos.

Bodansky u., u. de Bodansky; aquela quantidade de fosfatase que libera 1 mg de fósforo sob a forma de fosfato inorgânico durante a primeira hora de incubação com um substrato tamponado contendo β-glicerofosfato de sódio.

British thermal u. (BTU), u. térmica britânica (UTB); a quantidade de calor necessária para elevar a temperatura de uma libra de água de 3,9°C para 4,4°C; igual a 251,996 calorias ou 1.055,056 J. SIN u. of heat (2).

capon u., u. de capão; quantidade de androgênio necessária para produzir um aumento de 20% da superfície da crista de um capão. SIN capon-comb u.

capon-comb u., u. da crista do capão. SIN capon u.

cat u., a dose de uma droga (por quilograma de peso corporal do gato) suficiente para matar um gato quando administrada por via intravenosa; foi aplicada na padronização de digitálicos.

centimeter-gram-second u., CGS u., cgs u., u. centímetro-grama-segundo; uma u. absoluta do sistema centímetro-grama-segundo.

chlorophyll u., u. de clorofila; o número de moléculas de clorofila necessário para reduzir uma molécula de dióxido de carbono por fotossíntese.
chorionic gonadotropin u. (international), u. de gonadotrofina coriônica (internacional); a atividade gonadotrófica específica de 0,1 mg da preparação padrão de gonadotrofina coriônica obtida da urina ou das placentas de gestantes.
Clauberg u., u. de Clauberg. VER Clauberg *test*.
colony-forming u., u. formadora de colônias (UFC); uma u. de células na medula óssea capazes de gerar ou aumentar a proliferação de novas células do sangue.
complement u., u. de complemento; a menor quantidade (maior diluição) de complemento que causará lise de uma u. de hemácias na presença de uma u. de hemolisina. SIN alexin u.
Corner-Allen u., u. de Corner-Allen; uma u. de atividade progestacional, medida em coelhos, cuja dose mínima, dividida em cinco porções diárias iguais, produz, no sexto dia, as alterações uterinas características do oitavo dia da gravidez normal; a u. tem aproximadamente a mesma potência que a u. internacional.
coronary care u. (CCU), u. coronariana; um grupo de leitos em um setor do hospital separado para o tratamento de pacientes com infarto do miocárdio real ou suspeito.
corpus luteum hormone u., u. do hormônio do corpo lúteo. SIN progesterone u.
critical care u. (CCU), u. de terapia intensiva (UTI). SIN intensive care u.
CT u., u. TC; uma u. de atenuação dos raios X em cada elemento da imagem de TC. VER Hounsfield u.
Dam u., u. de Dam; u. de atividade da vitamina K; a menor quantidade de vitamina K, por grama de pinto por dia, capaz de produzir coagulabilidade normal no sangue de pintos com avitaminose K após 3 dias de administração oral.
digitalis u. (international), u. de digitálico (internacional); a atividade de 0,1 g do digitálico padrão internacional em pó.
diphtheria antitoxin u., u. de antitoxina diftérica; a atividade antitoxina de 0,0628 mg de antitoxina diftérica padrão.
dog u., a quantidade de extrato do córtex supra-renal por quilograma de peso corporal que, administrada diariamente, manterá um cão adrenalectomizado em boas condições por 7–10 dias.
electromagnetic u. (emu), u. eletromagnética (uem); a u. em um sistema absoluto (CGS) de unidades utilizando os efeitos magnéticos da corrente; p. ex., abampère, abfarad, abhenry, abohm, abvolt.
electrostatic u. (esu), u. eletrostática (ues); a u. em um sistema absoluto (CGS) de unidades utilizando eletricidade estática; p. ex., statampère, statcoulomb, statfarad, stathenry, statvolt.
u. of energy, u. de energia. **(1)** sistema CGS: erg, joule; **(2)** sistema MKS: newton-metro (joule); **(3)** sistema FPS: pé-*poundal*; **(4)** u. gravitacional: grama-centímetro, grama-metro, quilograma-metro, pé-libra; **(5)** SI: joule.
epidermal-melanin u., u. de melanina epidérmica; uma associação de um melanócito com vários queratinócitos epidérmicos adjacentes, provavelmente favorecendo a transferência de grânulos de melanina do melanócito para os queratinócitos.
equine gonadotropin u. (international), u. de gonadotrofina eqüina (internacional); a atividade gonadotrófica específica de 0,25 mg de preparação padrão do princípio gonadotrófico do soro de éguas grávidas.
estradiol benzoate u. (international), u. de benzoato de estradiol (internacional); a atividade estrogênica de 0,1 μg de uma preparação padrão de benzoato de estradiol.
estrone u. (international), u. de estrona; a atividade estrogênica de 0,1 μg (0,0001 mg) de uma preparação padrão de estrona cristalina.
Fishman-Lerner u., u. de Fishman-Lerner; uma u. de atividade da fosfatase ácida sérica baseada na medida da quantidade de fenol liberada de um substrato fenilfosfato.
Florey u., u. de Florey. SIN Oxford u.
foot-pound-second u., FPS u., fps u., pé-libra-segundo; uma u. absoluta do sistema pé-libra-segundo.
u. of force, u. de força; **(1)** sistema CGS: dina; **(2)** sistema FPS; poundal; **(3)** sistema MKS e SI: newton.
gravitational u.'s (G), unidades gravitacionais; de energia: grama-centímetro, grama-metro, quilograma-metro e pé-libra.
G u. of streptomycin, u. G. de estreptomicina. VER streptomycin u.'s.
u. of heat, u. de calor; **(1)** caloria (grama-caloria; quilocaloria); **(2)** SIN British thermal u.; **(3)** SIN joule.
hemolysin u., hemolytic u., u. de hemolisina; u. hemolítica; u. de amboceptor; a menor quantidade (maior diluição) de soro imune inativado (hemolisina) que sensibilizará a suspensão padrão de eritrócitos de forma que o complemento padrão causará hemólise completa. SIN amboceptor u.
heparin u., u. de heparina; u. de Howell; a quantidade de heparina necessária para manter 1 ml de sangue de gato fluido por 24 horas a 0°C; é equivalente a cerca de 0,002 mg de heparina pura. SIN Howell u.
Holzknecht u. (H), u. de Holzknecht; uma u. obsoleta de dosagem de raios X igual a um quinto da dose de eritema.
Hounsfield u., u. Hounsfield; um índice normalizado de atenuação de raios X baseado em uma escala de −1.000 (ar) a +1.000 (osso), sendo a água 0; usada em TC.

Howell u., u. de Howell. SIN heparin u.
insulin u. (international), u. de insulina (internacional); a atividade contida em 1/22 mg do padrão internacional de cristais de insulina zíncica.
intensive care u. (ICU), u. de terapia intensiva (UTI); unidade hospitalar para tratamento intensivo médico e de enfermagem de pacientes em estado grave, caracterizada por alta qualidade e supervisão contínua médica e de enfermagem e pelo uso de sofisticados equipamentos de monitorização e reanimação; pode ser organizada para o tratamento de grupos específicos de pacientes, p. ex., UTI neonatal, UTI neurológica, UTI pulmonar. SIN critical care u.
u. of intermedin, u. de intermedina; u. baseada na ação do hormônio na produção de expansão dos melanóforos em uma rã hipofisectomizada; igual a 1 μg de Padrão de Referência da Hipófise Posterior USP sob tratamento alcalino.
international u. (IU), u. internacional; a quantidade de uma substância, como uma droga, hormônio, vitamina, enzima, etc., que produz um efeito específico definido por um órgão internacional e aceito internacionalmente; p. ex., para uma enzima é micromoles de produto formado (ou substrato consumido) por minuto.
International System of U.'s, Sistema Internacional de Unidades. VER International System of Units.
Jenner-Kay u., u. de Jenner-Kay; quantidade de fosfatase que libera 1 mg de fósforo; cerca de 2 unidades de Bodansky ou 1 u. de King.
Karmen u., u. de Karmen; u. enzimática utilizada anteriormente para medir a atividade da aminotransferase; uma modificação de 0,001 na absorbância de NADH/min.
Kienböck u. (X), u. de Kienböck; u. obsoleta de dose de raios X equivalente a 1/10 da dose de eritema.
King u., u. de King; u. de King-Armstrong; a quantidade de fosfatase que, agindo sobre o excesso de fenilfosfato dissódico, em pH 9 por 30 minutos, libera 1 mg de fenol. SIN King-Armstrong u.
King-Armstrong u., u. de King-Armstrong. SIN King u.
u. of length, u. de comprimento; **(1)** sistema métrico e SI: metro; **(2)** sistema CGS: centímetro; **(3)** variável no sistema inglês: polegada para curtas distâncias, pé para distâncias moderadas e para elevação, milha para longas distâncias.
u. of light, u. luminosa. VER candela, lux.
L u. of streptomycin, u. L de estreptomicina. VER streptomycin u.'s.
u. of luminous flux, u. de fluxo luminoso. VER lumen.
u. of luminous intensity, u. de intensidade luminosa. VER candela.
lung u., u. pulmonar; **(1)** um bronquíolo respiratório, juntamente com os ductos e sacos alveolares e alvéolos pulmonares para os quais ele conduz; **(2)** alguns consideram que inclui o bronquíolo terminal e suas subdivisões, e denomina-se *ácino* pulmonar.
u. of luteinizing activity (international), u. de atividade luteinizante (internacional). SIN progesterone u.
u. of magnetic field intensity, u. de intensidade do campo magnético. VER gauss, tesla.
u. of magnetic flux intensity, u. de intensidade do fluxo magnético. VER gauss, tesla.
u. of mass, u. de massa. **(1)** sistema métrico: grama; **(2)** SI: quilograma; **(3)** sistema inglês: libra.
meter-kilogram-second u., MKS u., mks u., u. absoluta do sistema metro-quilograma-segundo.
Montevideo u.'s, unidades de Montevidéo; uma medida da intensidade da contração uterina no trabalho de parto expressa como a soma da intensidade de cada contração em um período de 10 minutos, com a intensidade definida como a pressão máxima obtida pela contração menos o tônus basal. [de Montevideo, Argentina, onde foi desenvolvida]
motor u., u. motora; um único neurônio motor somático e o grupo de fibras musculares por ele inervadas.
mouse u. (m.u.), SIN Allen-Doisy u.
u. of ocular convergence, u. de convergência ocular. SIN meter *angle*.
ostiomeatal u., u. ostiomeatal. SIN ostiomeatal *complex*.
Oxford u., u. Oxford; u. de Florey; a quantidade mínima de penicilina que impedirá o crescimento de *Staphylococcus aureus* sobre uma área de 26 mm de diâmetro em um meio de cultura padrão; 1 u. é igual a 0,6 μg do sal sódico cristalino de penicilina. SIN Florey u.
u. of oxytocin, u. de ocitocina; a atividade ocitócica de 0,5 mg do Padrão de Referência da Hipófise Posterior USP; 1 mg de ocitocina sintética corresponde a 500 UI.
u. of penicillin (international), u. de penicilina (internacional); a atividade de 0,6 μg de penicilina G.
phosphatase u., u. de fosfatase. VER Bodansky u., King u.
physiologic u., u. fisiológica; **(1)** a u. vital final (hipotética) de protoplasma, concebida por Spencer; **(2)** a menor divisão de um órgão que realizará sua função; p. ex., o túbulo urinífero.
practical u.'s, unidades práticas; unidades de magnitudes convenientes para uso nas aplicações práticas de eletricidade; segundo a definição original, eram unidades absolutas (múltiplos de unidades eletromagnéticas do CGS); incluem o ampère, coulomb, farad, henry, joule, ohm, volt e watt.

u. of progestational activity (international), u. de atividade progestacional (internacional). VER progesterone u.
progesterone u. (international), u. de progesterona; a atividade progestacional de 1 mg de u. de atividade progestacional (internacional); preparação padrão de progesterona pura. VER TAMBÉM Clauberg *test,* Corner-Allen u. SIN corpus luteum hormone u., u. of luteinizing activity.
prolactin u. (international), u. de prolactina (internacional); a atividade lactogênica específica contida em 0,1 mg da preparação padrão da substância lactogênica da hipófise anterior.
u. of radioactivity, u. de radioatividade. VER Becquerel.
riboflavin u., u. de riboflavina; u. de vitamina B_2; potência geralmente expressa em termos de peso de riboflavina pura. VER TAMBÉM Sherman-Bourquin u. of vitamin B_2. SIN vitamin B_2 u.
roentgen u., u. roentgen. VER Roentgen.
Schwann cell u., u. da célula de Schwann; uma única célula de Schwann e todos os axônios situados em depressões entalhando sua superfície; essa u. é considerada como uma fibra não-mielinizada no sistema nervoso periférico.
Sherman u., u. de Sherman; u. de vitamina C, dose protetora mínima; a quantidade de vitamina C que, administrada diariamente, protegerá uma cobaia de 300 g do escorbuto por 90 dias; equivalente a 0,5–0,6 mg de ácido ascórbico.
Sherman-Bourquin u. of vitamin B_2, u. de Sherman-Bourquin de vitamina B_2; a quantidade de vitamina B_2 necessária na dieta diária para manter um ganho semanal médio de 3 g durante 8 semanas em ratos de teste padronizados; uma u. equivale a 1–7 µg (0,001–0,007 mg) de riboflavina, dependendo da deficiência da dieta usada na análise supracitada.
Sherman-Munsell u., u. de Sherman-Munsell; u. de crescimento do rato; a quantidade diária de vitamina A que mantém um índice de ganho de 3 g por semana em ratos de teste padronizados.
SI u.'s, unidades SI. VER base u.'s, International System of Units.
Somogyi u., u. Somogyi; uma medida do nível de atividade da amilase no soro, analisada por meio do método de Somogyi (o procedimento mais usado); uma u. é equivalente a 1 mg de açúcar reduzido liberado como glicose por 100 ml de soro, quando uma alíquota de glicose é misturada a um substrato amido padrão (mais cloreto de sódio para ativação máxima) e incubada por um tempo padronizado; a faixa normal é de 80–150 unidades, mas os valores geralmente não são considerados clinicamente significativos, exceto se forem maiores que 200.
S u. of streptomycin, u. S de estreptomicina. VER streptomycin u.'s.
Steenbock u., u. de Steenbock; uma u. de vitamina D; a quantidade total de vitamina D que produzirá, em 10 dias, uma linha estreita de depósito de cálcio nas metáfises raquíticas das extremidades distais dos rádios e ulnas de ratos raquíticos padronizados.
streptomycin u.'s, unidades de estreptomicina; **(1)** u. G: igual a 1 g de material cristalino ou aproximadamente 1.000.000 unidades S; **(2)** u. L: igual a 1.000 unidades S; **(3)** u. S: a quantidade de estreptomicina que inibirá o crescimento de uma cepa padrão de *Escherichia coli* em 1 ml de caldo nutriente ou outro meio adequado.
Svedberg u. (S), u. Svedberg; constante de sedimentação de 1×10^{-13} s.
terminal respiratory u., u. respiratória terminal; todos os alvéolos e ductos alveolares além do bronquíolo respiratório mais proximal; contém cerca de 100 ductos alveolares e 2.000 alvéolos.
tetanus antitoxin u., u. de antitoxina tetânica; a atividade antitoxina de 0,3094 mg de antitoxina tetânica padronizada.
thiamin chloride u., u. de cloreto de tiamina; u. de cloridrato de tiamina (internacional).
thiamin hydrochloride u. (international), u. de cloridrato de tiamina (internacional); a atividade antineurítica de 0,003 mg de cloridrato de vitamina B_1 cristalino padrão. SIN vitamin B_1 hydrochloride u.
u. of thyrotrophic activity, u. de atividade tireotrófica; a atividade de uma quantidade de um extrato do lobo anterior da hipófise que, administrado diariamente durante 5 dias, fará com que a tireóide de uma cobaia (pesando 200 g) alcance um peso de 600 mg.
Todd u., u. de Todd; a u. na qual são expressos os resultados do teste para antiestreptolisina O (ASO). Designa o recíproco da maior diluição do soro de teste no qual continua a haver neutralização de uma preparação padronizada da enzima estreptocócica estreptolisina O.
toxic u. (T.U.), u. tóxica; u. de toxina; uma u. que já foi sinônimo de dose letal mínima em cobaia, mas que, devido à instabilidade de toxinas, agora é medida em termos de quantidade de antitoxina padrão com a qual a toxina se combina. VER TAMBÉM L *doses,* em *dose,* minimal lethal *dose.* SIN toxin u.
toxin u. (T.U.), u. de toxina. SIN toxic u.
USP u., u. USP; u. definida e adotada pela *United States Pharmacopeia.*
u. of vasopressin, u. de vasopressina; a atividade pressora de 0,5 mg do Padrão de Referência da Hipófise Posterior USP; 1 mg de vasopressina sintética corresponde a 600 UI.
vitamin A u. (international), u. de vitamina A (internacional); a atividade biológica específica de 0,3 µg de vitamina A (forma alcoólica). VER TAMBÉM Sherman-Munsell u.
vitamin B_2 u., u. de vitamina B_2; u. de riboflavina. SIN riboflavin u.
vitamin B_6 u., u. de vitamina B_6; potência expressa em termos de peso de piridoxina cristalina pura.
vitamin B_1 hydrochloride u., u. de cloridrato de vitamina B_1; u. de cloridrato de tiamina. SIN thiamin hydrochloride u.
vitamin C u. (international), u. de vitamina C (internacional); a atividade de vitamina C de 0,05 mg do ácido levoascórbico cristalino padrão; 1 mg de vitamina C cristalina fornece 20 unidades USP. VER TAMBÉM Sherman u.
vitamin D u. (international), u. de vitamina D (internacional); a atividade antiraquítica contida em 0,025 µg de uma preparação de vitamina D_3 cristalina (7-desidrocolesterol ativado). VER TAMBÉM Steenbock u.
vitamin E u., u. de vitamina E; potência geralmente expressa em termos de peso de α-tocoferol puro.
vitamin K u., u. de vitamina K. VER Dam u.
volume u. (VU), u. de volume; u. de uma escala logarítmica para expressar o nível de potência de um complexo sinal elétrico de audiofreqüência, como aquele que transmite música ou a fala; a potência nas unidades de volume é igual aos decibéis de potência acima de um nível de referência de 1 miliwatt, determinado com um medidor apropriado.
u. of wavelength, u. de comprimento de onda. VER Ångström, nanometer.
u. of weight, u. de peso. VER u. of mass.
Wood u.'s, unidades de Wood; uma medida simplificada da resistência vascular pulmonar que usa pressões em vez de unidades mais complicadas, que são medidas subtraindo-se a pressão capilar pulmonar (encunhada) da pressão arterial pulmonar média, e dividindo-se pelo débito cardíaco em litros por minuto.
u. of work, u. de trabalho. VER u. of energy.

Uni·ted States Adopt·ed Names (USAN). Designação dos nomes não-comerciais (para drogas) adotado pelo USAN Council em cooperação com os fabricantes; a designação USAN só pode ser aplicada a nomes não-comerciais cunhados a partir de junho de 1961.
Uni·ted States Phar·ma·co·pe·ia (USP). VER Pharmacopeia.
Uni·ted States Pub·lic Health Ser·vice (USPHS). Serviço de Saúde Pública dos EUA; órgão do Department of Health and Human Services, servido por um corpo de médicos presididos pelo Cirurgião Geral, relacionado a pesquisa científica, quarentena doméstica e insular, administração de hospitais do governo, publicação de laudos sanitários e estatísticos; estão associados a ele o National Institutes of Health, Centers for Disease Control and Prevention, bem como outras unidades.
uni·va·lence, uni·va·len·cy (ū - ni - vā′lens, - vā′len - sē). Univalência. SIN monovalence.
uni·va·lent (ū - ni - vā′lent). Univalente. SIN monovalent (1).

Universal Precautions. (na íntegra, Universal Blood and Body Fluid Precautions). Precauções Universais (na íntegra, Precauções Universais com Sangue e Líquidos Corporais). Um conjunto de diretrizes e orientações de procedimentos publicado em agosto de 1987 pelo Centers for Disease Control and Prevention (CDC) (como *Recommendations for Prevention of HIV Transmission in Health-Care Settings*) para evitar exposições parenterais, mucosas e da pele não-intacta de profissionais da área de saúde a patógenos presentes no sangue. Em dezembro de 1991, a Occupational Safety and Health Administration (OSHA) promulgou seu *Occupational Exposure to Bloodborne Pathogens Standard*, incorporando precauções universais e impondo exigências detalhadas aos empregadores dos trabalhadores da área de saúde, incluindo controles de engenharia, fornecimento de protetores de barreira, identificação padronizada de riscos biológicos, treinamento obrigatório dos empregados em Precauções Universais, tratamento de acidentes com exposição parenteral acidental e imunização dos empregados contra hepatite B.

O princípio subjacente às precauções universais é que o sangue e alguns outros líquidos corporais de todos os pacientes devem ser considerados potencialmente infectados pelo vírus da imunodeficiência humana (HIV), vírus da hepatite B (HBV) e outros patógenos transmitidos pelo sangue. As precauções universais se aplicam ao sangue, tecidos não-fixados (exceto a pele íntegra), líquido cefalorraquidiano, líquido sinovial, líquido pleural, líquido peritoneal, líquido pericárdico, líquido amniótico, sêmen e secreções vaginais, mas não a fezes, secreções nasais, escarro, suor, lágrimas, urina ou vômito, exceto se esses materiais contiverem sangue visível. Precauções específicas são prescritas em relação à reanimação boca-a-boca, cirurgia, procedimentos diagnósticos invasivos, obstetrícia, diálise renal, odontologia, laboratórios de análises clínicas, necrotérios e serviços funerários. Em determinadas circunstâncias são necessários dispositivos de barreira, como luvas, capotes, aventais à prova d'água, máscaras e óculos de proteção, para evitar exposição ao sangue e a outros materiais biologicamente perigosos. O padrão da OSHA exige o uso de luvas para flebotomia e exames e manipulações intra-orais. Também são impostos padrões para lavanderia, limpeza de superfícies e descarte de lixo contaminado. São recomendadas precauções especiais para o manuseio de agulhas, bisturis e outros instrumentos ou dispositivos cortantes após o uso. A imunização com vacina HBV é recomendada como um importante adjunto às precauções universais para profissionais de saúde expostos ao sangue. As precauções universais têm por objetivo suplementar, e não substituir, as recomendações para controle rotineiro das infecções, como lavagem das mãos e uso de luvas para evitar contaminação flagrante das mãos. A implementação das precauções universais não elimina a necessidade de outras precauções de isolamento específicas para a categoria ou para a doença, como precauções entéricas na diarréia infecciosa ou isolamento na tuberculose pulmonar.

un·med·ul·lat·ed (ŭn - med′oo - lā - ted). Desmielinizado. SIN unmyelinated.

un·my·e·li·nat·ed (ŭn - mī′e - li - nā - ted). Amielinizado; amielínico; designa fibras nervosas (axônios) que não possuem uma bainha de mielina. SIN amyelinated, amyelinic, nonmedullated, nonmyelinated, unmedullated.

Unna, Paul G., dermatologista e especialista em coloração alemão, 1850–1929. VER U. *disease;* Unna *nevus;* U. *stain;* U.-Pappenheim *stain;* U.-Taenzer *stain;* Unna-Thost *syndrome.*

un·of·fi·cial (ŭn - ō - fish′ăl). Não-oficial; refere-se a uma droga que não está relacionada na *United States Pharmacopeia* ou no *National Formulary.*

un·phys·i·o·log·ic (ŭn - fis′ē - ō - loj′ik). Não-fisiológico; refere-se a condições no organismo que são anormais; pode ser usado para referir-se à submissão do corpo a quantidades anormais de substâncias normalmente presentes.

un·san·i·tary (ŭn - san′i - tār - ē). Não-sanitário. SIN insanitary.

un·sat·u·rat·ed (ŭn - sach′ur - āt - ed). Insaturado. **1.** Não-saturado; designa uma solução na qual o solvente é capaz de dissolver mais soluto. **2.** Designa uma substância química cujas afinidades não foram totalmente satisfeitas, de forma que ainda podem ser acrescentados outros átomos ou radicais a ela. **3.** Em química orgânica, designa substâncias contendo ligações duplas e/ou triplas ou uma estrutura anular.

un·sex (ŭn′seks). Castrar; privar das gônadas.

un·stri·at·ed (ŭn - strī′āt - ed). Não-estriado; sem estriações; designa a estrutura dos músculos lisos ou involuntários.

un·thrifty (ŭn - thrif′tē). Impróspero; em animais, designa ausência de crescimento ou desenvolvimento normais em virtude de doença.

Unverricht, Heinrich, médico alemão, 1853–1912. VER U. *disease.*

UPJ Abreviatura de ureteropelvic *junction.*

up·reg·u·la·tion. Supra-regulação; oposto de infra-regulação (down-regulation).

up·si·loid (ŭp′si - loyd). Ipsilóide. SIN hypsiloid.

up·si·lon (ŭp′si - lon). Ípsilon; a 20ª letra do alfabeto grego, Ψ.

up·stream (ŭp′strēm). Contra a corrente; refere-se às seqüências básicas de ácido nucléico que prosseguem na direção oposta da expressão.

up·take (ŭp′tāk). Captação; absorção; a absorção por um tecido de alguma substância, alimento, mineral, etc., e sua retenção permanente ou temporária.

Ura Abreviatura de uracil.

ura·chal (ūr′ă - kăl). Uracal; referente ao úraco.

ura·chus (ūr′ă - kŭs). Úraco; aquela parte do pedículo alantóico reduzido entre o ápice da bexiga e o umbigo; no período pós-natal, o u. normalmente é apenas um cordão fibroso, o ligamento umbilical mediano, mas, ocasionalmente, a antiga luz alantóica pode persistir como uma fístula vesicoumbilical. [G. *ourachos,* o canal urinário de um feto]

ura·cil (Ura, U) (ūr′ă - sil). Uracil; 2,4-dioxopirimidina; uma pirimidina (base) presente no ácido ribonucléico.

 u. dehydrogenase, u. desidrogenase; u. oxidase; uma oxidorredutase que catalisa a oxidação de uracil em ácido barbitúrico; também oxida a timina. SIN u. oxidase.

 u. mustard, u. de mostarda; uramustina; um agente antineoplásico alquilante. SIN uramustine.

 u. oxidase, u. desidrogenase. SIN u. dehydrogenase.

 u. phosphoribosyltransferase, u. fosforribosiltransferase. VER phosphoribosyltransferase.

ura·cil-6-car·box·yl·ic ac·id. Ácido uracil-6-carboxílico. SIN orotic acid.

Ur·a·go·ga (ūr′ă - gō - ga). Gênero de plantas tropicais (família Rubiaceae). *U. ipecacuanha (Cephaelis ipecacuanha)* é a fonte da ipeca do Rio ou Brasil; *U. acuminata (C. acuminata)* é a fonte da ipeca de Cartagena, Nicarágua ou Panamá. SIN *Cephaelis.*

ur·a·mus·tine (ūr - ă - mŭs′tēn). Uramustina. SIN uracil mustard.

ura·nin (ū′ră - nin). Uranina. SIN fluorescein sodium.

ura·ni·nite (ū - ran′i - nīt). Uraninita. SIN pitchblende.

uranisco-. VER urano-.

ura·nis·co·chasm (ū′ră - nis′kō - kazm). SIN uranoschisis. [uranisco- + G. *chasma,* fenda]

ura·nis·co·ni·tis (ū′ră - nis - kō - nī′tis). Uranisconite. SIN palatitis.

ura·nis·co·plas·ty (ū′ră - nis′kō - plas - tē). Uranisconiplastia; uranoplastia. SIN palatoplasty. [uranisco- + G. *plassō,* formar]

ura·nis·cor·rha·phy (ū′ră - nis - kor′ă - fē). Uraniscorrafia. SIN palatorrhaphy. [uranisco- + G. *rhaphē,* sutura]

ura·nis·cus (ū′ră - nis′kŭs). Uranisco. SIN palate. [G. *ouraniskos,* teto da boca, dim. de *ouranos,* céu]

ura·ni·um (U) (ū - rā′nē - ŭm). Urânio; um elemento metálico radioativo, nº atômico 92, peso atômico 238,0289, que ocorre principalmente no pecheblende e notável por seus dois isótopos: U^{238} e U^{235} (99,2745% e 0,720%, respectivamente, com o restante constituído por U^{234}), U^{235} sendo a primeira substância capaz de manter uma reação em cadeia auto-sustentada. [G. personagem da mitologia, *Uranus*]

urano-, uranisco-. Formas combinantes relativas ao palato duro. [G. *ouranos,* abóbada celeste, *ouraniskos,* teto da boca (palato)]

ura·no·plas·ty (ū′ră - nō - plas - tē). Uranoplastia. SIN palatoplasty.

ura·nor·rha·phy (ū′ră - nōr′ă - fē). Uranorrafia. SIN palatorrhaphy. [urano- + G. *rhaphē,* sutura]

ura·nos·chi·sis (ū′ră - nos′ki - sis). Uranosquise; fenda do palato duro. SIN uraniscochasm. [urano- + G. *schisis,* fissura]

ura·no·staph·y·lo·plas·ty (ū′ră - nō - staf′i - lō - plas - tē). Uranostafiloplastia; reparo de uma fenda dos palatos duro e mole. SIN uranostaphylorrhaphy. [urano- + G. *staphylē,* úvula, + *plassō,* formar]

ura·no·staph·y·lor·rha·phy (ū′ră - nō - staf - i - lōr′ă - fē). Uranostafilorrafia. SIN uranostaphyloplasty.

ura·no·staph·y·los·chi·sis (ū′ră - nō - staf′i - los′ki - sis). Uranostafilosquise; fenda dos palatos mole e duro. SIN uranoveloschisis. [urano- + G. *staphylē,* úvula, + *schisis,* fissura]

ura·no·ve·los·chi·sis (ū′ră - nō - vĕ - los′ki - sis). Uranovelosquise. SIN uranostaphyloschisis.

ura·nyl (ū′ră - nil). Uranil; uranila; o íon, UO_2^{2+}, geralmente encontrado em sais como o nitrato de uranil, $UO_2(NO_3)_2$; o acetato de uranil, $UO_2(CH_3COO)_2$, é usado em microscopia eletrônica.

urap·i·dil (oo′ră′pī - dil). Urapidil; um agente anti-hipertensivo que atua influenciando os receptores de serotonina.

ura·ro·ma (ū′ră - rō′mă). Uraroma; termo obsoleto para descrever um odor aromático e condimentado da urina. [G. *ouron,* urina, + *arōma,* condimento]

urar·thri·tis (ū - rar - thrī′tis). Urartrite; inflamação gotosa de uma articulação. [urate + arthritis]

urate (ū′rāt). Urato; um sal do ácido úrico.

 u. oxidase, u. oxidase; uma oxirredutase que contém cobre, exige oxigênio e oxida o ácido úrico; usada no diagnóstico clínico de níveis aumentados de ácido úrico. SIN uricase.

ura·te·mia (ū - ră - tē′mē - ă). Uratemia; presença de uratos, principalmente urato de sódio, no sangue. [urate + G. *haima,* sangue]

ur·ate·ri·bo·nu·cle·o·tide phos·pho·ryl·ase (ūr′āt - rī - bō - noo′klē - ō - tīd). Urateribonucleotídio fosforilase; uma ribosiltransferase que causa reação do urato D-ribonucleotídio com o ortofosfato para produzir urato mais D-ribose 1-fosfato.

urat·ic (ū - rat′ik). Urático; relativo a um urato ou uratos.

ura·tol·y·sis (ū - ră - tol′i - sis). Uratólise; a decomposição ou solução de uratos. [urate + G. *lysis,* solução]

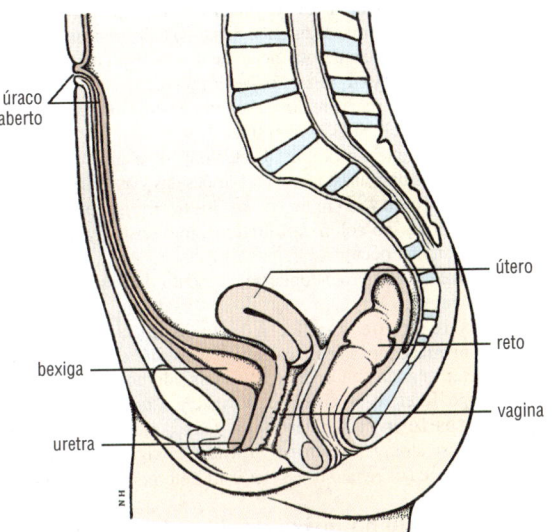

úraco aberto

ura·to·ly·tic (ū′rā-tō-lit′ik). Uratolítico; que causa a decomposição, ou solução e remoção de uratos, dos tecidos.

ura·to·ma (ū-rā-tō′mā). Uratoma. SIN gouty *tophus*. [urate + G. *-oma*, tumor]

ura·to·sis (ū-rā-tō′sis). Uratose; qualquer condição mórbida devida à presença de uratos no sangue ou tecidos.

ura·tu·ria (ū-rā-too′rē-ā). Uratúria; a eliminação de uma quantidade aumentada de uratos na urina. [urate + G. *ouron*, urina]

Urbach, Erich, dermatologista norte-americano, 1893–1946. VER U.-Wiethe *disease*.

Urban, Jerome A., cirurgião norte-americano, *1914. VER U. *operation*.

ur·ce·i·form (ūr-sē′i-fōrm). Urceiforme; urceolado; em forma de ânfora. SIN urceolate. [L. *urceus*, ânfora, + *forma*, forma]

ur·ce·o·late (ūr′sē-ō-lāt). Urceolado. SIN urceiform. [L. *urceolus*, dim. de *urceus*, ânfora]

Urd Abreviatura de uridina.

ur·de·fens·es (oor′dē-fens-ez). Termo raramente usado para defesas primitivas. [Al. *ur-*, primitivo, primeiro, + defenses]

△ **ure-, urea-, ureo-.** Uréia; urina. VER TAMBÉM urin-, uro-. [G. *ouron*, urina]

urea (ū-rē′ā). Uréia; o principal produto final do metabolismo do nitrogênio em mamíferos, formado no fígado por meio do ciclo de Krebs-Henseleit e excretado na urina humana adulta normal na quantidade de aproximadamente 32 g por dia (cerca de 6/7 do nitrogênio excretado do corpo). Pode ser obtida artificialmente aquecendo-se uma solução de cianato de amônio. Ocorre na forma de cristais prismáticos incolores ou brancos, sem odor, mas com um sabor salino refrescante; é solúvel em água e forma sais com ácidos; foi usada como diurético em provas de função renal e, topicamente, para várias dermatites. [G. *ouron*, urina]

u. peroxide, peróxido de u., uma substância cristalina branca usada em uma solução aquosa como colutório oxidante.

u. stibamine, u. estibamina; um derivado ureico do ácido estibanílico, sendo usado no tratamento do calazar e de algumas outras doenças tropicais.

ure·a·gen·e·sis (ū-rē-ā-jen′ē-sis). Ureagênese; formação de uréia, geralmente referindo-se ao metabolismo de aminoácidos em uréia. SIN ureapoiesis. [urea + G. *genesis*, produção]

ure·al (ū-rē′al). Ureico; relativo a, ou contendo, uréia. SIN ureic.

Ure·a·plas·ma (ū-rē′ā-plaz′mā). Gênero de bactérias imóveis microaerófilas e anaeróbicas (família Mycoplasmataceae) sem paredes celulares. Gram-negativos, são elementos predominantemente cocóides a cocobacilares, com cerca de 0,3 μm de diâmetro, que freqüentemente crescem em filamentos curtos; as colônias geralmente são pequenas, com 20–30 μm de diâmetro, e podem não possuir zonas de crescimento superficial. Esses microrganismos hidrolisam a uréia com produção de amônia, e são encontrados no trato genitourinário humano, ocasionalmente na faringe e no reto. Em homens, estão associados à uretrite não-gonocócica e prostatite; em mulheres, a infecções genitourinárias e infertilidade; em recém-nascidos, podem causar pneumonia ou meningite. A espécie típica é *U. urealyticum*. SIN T-mycoplasma.

U. urealy′ticum, uma espécie que foi isolada do trato respiratório e do sistema nervoso central de recém-nascidos. Causa infecções genitourinárias, sobretudo uretrite; acredita-se que a transmissão seja por contato sexual e da mãe para o lactente. O diagnóstico laboratorial é simplificado pelo uso de ágar contendo uréia, permitindo a detecção das minúsculas colônias.

ure·a·poi·e·sis (ū-rē′ā-poy-ē′sis). Ureopoiese. SIN ureagenesis. [urea + G. *poiēsis*, produção]

ure·ase (ūr′ē-ās). Urease; uma enzima que catalisa a hidrólise da uréia em dióxido de carbono e amônia; usada como enzima antitumoral; é encontrada nas bactérias intestinais, sendo responsável pela maior parte da amônia produzida a partir da uréia em mamíferos.

ure·de·ma (ū-re-dē′mā). Uredema; edema devido à infiltração dos tecidos subcutâneos por urina. [G. *ouron*, urina, + *oidēma*, edema]

ure·ic (ūr-ē′ik). Ureico. SIN ureal.

ure·ide (ūr′ē-īd). Ureído; qualquer composto da uréia no qual um ou mais de seus átomos de hidrogênio foram substituídos por radicais ácidos.

3-ure·i·do·hy·dan·to·in (u-rē′i-dō-hī′dan-tō-in). 3-ureidoidantoína. SIN allantoin.

3-ure·i·do·i·so·bu·tyr·ic acid (ū-rē′i-dō-ī′sō-bū-tir′ik). Ácido 3-ureidoisobutírico; um intermediário no catabolismo da timina.

3-ure·i·do·pro·pi·on·ic acid (ū-rē′i-dō-prō-pi-on′ik). Ácido 3-ureidopropiônico; um intermediário do catabolismo do uracil.

ure·i·do·suc·cin·ic acid (ū-rē′i-dō-suk-sin′ik). Ácido ureidossuccínico; um precursor das pirimidinas. SIN *N*-carbamoylaspartic acid.

urel·co·sis (ū-rel-kō′sis). Urelcose; designação obsoleta para ulceração de qualquer parte das vias urinárias. [G. *ouron*, urina, + *helkōsis*, ulceração]

ure·mia (ū-rē′mē-ā). Uremia. **1.** Excesso de uréia e outras escórias nitrogenadas no sangue. **2.** O complexo de sintomas devido à insuficiência renal persistente grave que pode ser aliviado por diálise. [G. *ouron*, urina, + *haima*, sangue]

hypercalcemic u., u. hipercalcêmica; u. devida à insuficiência renal causada por hipercalcemia com nefrocalcinose.

ure·mic (ū-rē′mik). Urêmico; relativo à uremia.

ure·mi·gen·ic (ū-rē-mi-jen′ik). Uremigênico. **1.** De origem ou causa urêmica. **2.** Que causa ou resulta em uremia.

△ **ureo-.** VER ure-.

ure·o·tele (ū′rē-ō-tēl). Ureotelo; um organismo que é ureotélico; p. ex., primatas.

ure·o·tel·ia (ū′rē-ō-tēl′ē-a). Ureotelia; o processo ou tipo de excreção de nitrogênio no qual a uréia é o produto final primário. [urea + G. *telos*, final, resultado, + *-ia*]

ure·o·tel·ic (ū′rē-ō-tel′ik). Ureotélico; que excreta nitrogênio basicamente na forma de uréia. [ureo- + G. *telos*, fim]

ur·er·y·thrin (ūr-er′i-thrin). Ureritrina. SIN uroerythrin.

ure·si·es·the·sia (ū-rē′si-es-thē′zē-a). Uresiestesia; o desejo de urinar. SIN uriesthesia. [G. *ourēsis*, micção, + *aisthēsis*, sensação].

ure·sis (ū-rē′sis). Urese. SIN urination. [G. *ourēsis*]

ure·ter (ū-rē′ter, ū′rē-ter) [TA]. Ureter; o tubo que conduz a urina da pelve renal até a bexiga; consiste em uma parte abdominal e uma parte pélvica, é revestido por epitélio de transição circundado por músculo liso, tanto circular como longitudinal, e é recoberto externamente por uma túnica adventícia. [G. *ourētēr*, canal urinário]

curlicue u., u. em arabesco; termo dado ao aspecto radiológico de um u. opacificado, herniado através do forame ciático; uma condição muito rara.

ectopic u., u. ectópico; aquele que se abre em outro lugar que não a parede vesical.

ileal u., u. ileal. SIN ureteroileoneocystostomy.

postcaval u., u. pós-cava; defeito congênito onde o u. direito passa profundamente à veia cava inferior em sua descida até a bexiga.

retrocaval u., u. retrocava; na urografia, o desvio medial do u. direito na rara circunstância em que passa atrás da veia cava inferior antes de entrar na pelve.

retroiliac u., u. retroilíaco; defeito congênito no qual o u. passa profundamente à artéria ilíaca.

ure·ter·al (ū-rē′te-ral). Ureteral; relativo ao ureter. SIN ureteric.

ure·ter·al·gia (ū-rē-ter-al′jē-a). Ureteralgia; dor no ureter. [ureter + G. *algos*, dor]

ure·ter·cys·to·scope (ū-rē′ter-sis′tō-skōp). Ureterocistoscópio. SIN ureterocystoscope.

ure·ter·ec·ta·sia (ū-rē′ter-ek-tā′zē-a). Ureterectasia; hidroureter; megaloureter; dilatação de um ureter. SIN hydroureter, megaloureter. [ureter + G. *ektasis*, distensão]

ure·ter·ec·to·my (ū-rē-ter-ek′tō-mē). Ureterectomia; excisão de um segmento ou de todo o ureter. [ureter + G. *ektomē*, excisão]

ure·ter·ic (ū-rē-ter′ik). Uretérico. SIN ureteral.

ure·ter·i·tis (ū-rē-ter-ī′tis). Ureterite; inflamação de um ureter.

△ **uretero-.** O ureter. [G. *ourētēr*, canal urinário]

ure·ter·o·cal·i·cos·to·my (ū-rē′ter-kal-ī-kos′tō-mē). Ureterocalicostomia; anastomose do ureter ao sistema coletor do pólo inferior do rim após amputação de uma porção do parênquima do pólo inferior. [uretero- + G. *kalyx*, cálice de uma flor, + *stoma*, boca]

ure·ter·o·cele (ū-rē′ter-ō-sēl). Ureterocele; dilatação sacular da porção terminal do ureter que se projeta para a luz da bexiga, provavelmente devido a estenose congênita do meato ureteral. [uretero- + G. *kēlē*, hérnia]

ectopic u., u. ectópica; u. que se estende distal ao colo vesical.

orthotopic u., u. ortotópica; u. totalmente dentro da bexiga.

ure·ter·o·ce·lor·ra·phy (ū-rē′ter-ō-se-lōr′a-fē). Ureterocelorrafia; excisão e sutura de uma ureterocele realizada através de uma incisão de cistostomia a céu aberto. [ureterocele + G. *raphē*, sutura]

ure·ter·o·col·ic (ū-rē′ter-ō-kol′ik). Ureterocólico; relativo ao ureter e ao cólon, particularmente a uma anastomose para lesões das vias urinárias inferiores.

ure·ter·o·co·los·to·my (ū-rē′ter-ō-kō-los′tō-mē). Ureterocolostomia; implantação do ureter no cólon. SIN ureterosigmoidostomy. [uretero- + G. *kolon*, cólon, + *stoma*, boca]

ureterocystoplasty. Ureterocistoplastia; aumento da bexiga utilizando um ureter dilatado nativo.

ure·ter·o·cys·to·scope (ū-rē′ter-ō-sis′tō-skōp). Ureterocistoscópio; cistoscópio com uma conexão para cateterismo dos ureteres; o cateter é introduzido no ureter quando seu orifício é visualizado com o cistoscópio. SIN uretercystoscope. [uretero- + G. *kystis*, bexiga, + *skopeō*, ver]

ure·ter·o·cys·tos·to·my (ū-rē′ter-ō-sis-tos′tō-mē). Ureterocistostomia. SIN ureteroneocystostomy. [uretero- + G. *kystis*, bexiga, + *stoma*, boca]

ure·ter·o·en·ter·ic (ū-rē′ter-ō-en-ter′ik). Ureteroentérico; relativo a um ureter e ao intestino.

ure·ter·o·en·ter·os·to·my (ū-rē′ter-ō-en-ter-os′tō-mē). Ureteroenterostomia; formação de uma abertura entre um ureter e o intestino. [uretero- + G. *enteron*, intestino, + *stoma*, boca]

ure·ter·og·ra·phy (ū-rē′ter-og′ră-fē). Ureterografia; radiografia do ureter após a injeção direta de contraste. [Uretero- + G. *graphē*, escrita]

ure·ter·o·hy·dro·ne·phro·sis (ū-rē′ter-ō-hī′drō-nef-rō′sis). Ureteroidronefrose; hidronefrose que também envolve os ureteres. SIN hydroureteronephrosis, nephroureterectasis.

ure·ter·o·il·e·o·ne·o·cys·tos·to·my (ū-rē′ter-ō-il′ē-ō-nē′ō-sis-tos′tō-mē). Ureteroileoneocistostomia; restauração da continuidade das vias urinárias por anastomose do segmento superior de um ureter parcialmente destruído a um segmento do íleo, cuja extremidade inferior é então implantada na bexiga. SIN ileal ureter. [uretero- + ileum + G. *neos*, novo, + *hystis*, bexiga, + *stoma*, boca]

ure·ter·o·il·e·os·to·my (ū-rē′ter-ō-il-ē-os′tō-mē). Ureteroileostomia; implantação de um ureter em um segmento isolado do íleo que drena através de um estoma abdominal. [uretero- + ileum + G. *stoma*, boca]

ure·ter·o·li·thi·a·sis (ū-rē′ter-ō-li-thī′ă-sis). Ureterolitíase; a formação ou presença de um cálculo ou cálculos em um ou ambos os ureteres. [ureterolith + G. *-iasis*, condição]

ure·ter·o·li·thot·o·my (ū-rē′ter-ō-li-thot′ō-mē). Ureterolitotomia; remoção de um cálculo alojado em um ureter. [ureterolith + G. *tomē*, incisão]

ure·ter·ol·y·sis (ū′rē-ter-ol′i-sis). Ureterólise; liberação cirúrgica do ureter de doença ou aderências adjacentes. [uretero- + G. *lysis*, afrouxamento]

ure·ter·o·ne·o·cys·tos·to·my (ū-rē′ter-ō-nē′ō-sis-tos′tō-mē). Ureteroneocistostomia; ureterocistostomia; cirurgia na qual um ureter é implantado na bexiga. VER TAMBÉM detrusorrhaphy. SIN neocystostomy, ureteral reimplantation, ureterocystostomy, ureterovesicostomy. [uretero- + G. *neos*, novo, + *kystis*, bexiga, + *stoma*, boca]

ure·ter·o·ne·phrec·to·my (ū-rē′ter-ō-nĕ-frek′tō-mē). Ureteronefrectomia. SIN nephroureterectomy. [uretero- + G. *nephros*, rim, + *ektomē*, excisão]

ure·ter·op·a·thy (ū-rē′ter-op′ă-thē). Ureteropatia; doença do ureter. [uretero- + G. *pathos*, sofrimento]

ure·ter·o·plas·ty (ū-rē′ter-ō-plas-tē). Ureteroplastia; reconstrução cirúrgica dos ureteres. [uretero- + G. *plastos*, formado]

ure·ter·o·proc·tos·to·my (ū-rē′ter-ō-prok-tos′tō-mē). Ureteroproctostomia; estabelecimento de uma abertura entre um ureter e o reto. SIN ureterorectostomy. [uretero- + G. *prōktos*, reto, + *stoma*, boca]

ure·ter·o·py·e·li·tis (ū-rē′ter-ō-pī-ĕ-lī′tis). Ureteropielite; inflamação da pelve de um rim e seu ureter. [uretero- + G. *pyelos*, pelve, + *-itis*, inflamação]

ure·ter·o·py·e·log·ra·phy (ū-rē′ter-ō-pī′ĕ-log′ră-fē). Ureteropielografia. SIN pyelography.

ure·ter·o·py·e·lo·plas·ty (ū-rē′ter-ō-pī′ĕ-lō-plas-tē). Ureteropieloplastia; reconstrução cirúrgica do ureter e da pelve renal, geralmente para obstrução congênita da junção ureteropélvica. [uretero- + G. *pyelos*, pelve, + *plastos*, formado]

ure·ter·o·py·e·los·to·my (ū-rē′ter-ō-pī-ĕ-los′tō-mē). Ureteropielostomia; junção cirúrgica do ureter com a pelve renal. [uretero- + pelvis + *stoma*, boca]

ure·ter·o·py·o·sis (ū-rē′ter-ō-pī-ō′sis). Ureteropiose; acúmulo de pus no ureter. [uretero- + G. *pyōsis*, supuração]

ure·ter·o·rec·to·my (ū-rē′ter-ō-rek-tos′tō-mē). Ureterorretostomia. SIN ureteroproctostomy.

ure·ter·or·rha·gia (ū-rē′ter-ō-rā′jē-ă). Ureterorragia; hemorragia de um ureter. [uretero- + G. *rhēgnymi*, expelir]

ure·ter·or·rha·phy (ū-rē-ter-ōr′ă-fē). Ureterorrafia; sutura de um ureter. [uretero- + G. *rhaphē*, sutura]

ure·ter·o·scope (ū-rē′ter-o-skōp). Ureteroscópio; dispositivo óptico introduzido retrogradamente através da bexiga até o ureter, para inspecionar a luz ureteral e o sistema coletor renal.

ure·ter·o·sig·moid (ū-rē′ter-ō-sig′moyd). Ureterossigmóide; relativo ao ureter e ao cólon sigmóide, sobretudo a uma anastomose entre os dois.

ure·ter·o·sig·moi·dos·to·my (ū-rē′ter-ō-sig-moy-dos′tō-mē). Ureterossigmoidostomia. SIN ureterocolostomy.

ure·ter·o·sten·o·sis (ū-rē′ter-ō-ste-nō′sis). Ureteroestenose; estreitamento de um ureter. [uretero- + G. *stenōsis*, estreitamento]

ure·ter·os·to·my (ū-rē-ter-os′tō-mē). Ureterostomia; estabelecimento de uma abertura externa para o ureter. [uretero- + G. *stoma*, boca]

   cutaneous u., u. cutânea; um estoma construído com o ureter ao nível da pele para drenagem de urina. Este pode ser um estoma terminal ou um estoma em alça. Geralmente realizado devido à obstrução distal. SIN cutaneous loop u.

   cutaneous loop u., u. cutâneo em alça. SIN cutaneous u.

ure·ter·ot·o·my (ū-rē-ter-ot′ō-mē). Ureterotomia; incisão de um ureter. [uretero- + G. *tomē*, incisão]

ure·ter·o·tri·go·no·en·ter·os·to·my (ū-rē′ter-ō-tri-gō′nō-en-ter-os′tō-mē). Ureterotrigonoenterostomia; implantação de um ureter e sua porção do trígono vesical no intestino. [uretero- + trigone (da bexiga) + enterostomy]

ure·ter·o·u·re·ter·al (ū-rē′ter-ō-ū′re′ter-al). Ureteroureteral; relativo a dois segmentos do mesmo ureter ou de ambos os ureteres, principalmente uma anastomose artificial entre eles.

ure·ter·o·u·re·ter·os·to·my (ū-rē′ter-ō-ū-rē′ter-os′tō-mē). Ureteroureterostomia; estabelecimento de uma anastomose entre os dois ureteres ou entre dois segmentos do mesmo ureter. VER transureteroureterostomy.

ure·ter·o·ves·i·cal (ū-rē′ter-ō-ves′i-kăl). Ureterovesical; relativo ao ureter e à bexiga, especificamente à junção do ureter com a bexiga.

ure·ter·o·ves·i·cos·to·my (ū-rē′ter-ō-ves-i-kos′tō-mē). Ureterovesicostomia. SIN ureteroneocystostomy. [uretero- + L. *vesica*, bexiga, + *stoma*, boca]

ure·than, ure·thane (ū′rē-than, -thān). Uretana; uretano; possui atividade antimitótica; já foi usado clinicamente como hipnótico, mas agora é usado com maior freqüência como anestésico em animais de laboratório. SIN ethyl carbamate.

♲ **urethr-.** VER urethro-.

ure·thra (ū-rē′thră) [TA]. Uretra; o canal que sai da bexiga, eliminando a urina para o meio externo. [G. *ourēthra*]

   anterior u., u. anterior; a porção da u. distal ao diafragma urogenital (esfíncter externo).

   female u. [TA], u. feminina; um canal com cerca de 4 cm de comprimento que vai da bexiga, em íntima relação com a parede anterior da vagina, e possui um eixo longitudinal paralelo à vagina, abrindo-se no vestíbulo da vagina posterior ao clitóris e anterior ao orifício vaginal. SIN u. feminina [TA], u. muliebris.

   u. femini′na [TA], u. feminina. SIN female u.

   male u. [TA], u. masculina; um canal com cerca de 20 cm de comprimento que se abre na extremidade da glande peniana; exceto pelas porções intramural e prostática superior, dá passagem ao líquido espermático e também à urina; os componentes incluem as uretras intramural, prostática, intermediária e esponjosa. SIN u. masculina [TA], u. virilis.

   u. mascu1i′na [TA], u. masculina. SIN male u.

   membranous u., u. membranosa;*termo alternativo oficial para intermediate part of male urethra.

   u. mulie′bris, u. feminina. SIN female u.

   penile u., u. peniana; SIN spongy u.

   posterior u., u. posterior; a porção da u. posterior ao diafragma urogenital (esfíncter externo).

   prostatic u. [TA], u. prostática; a parte prostática da u. masculina, com cerca de 2,5 cm de comprimento, que atravessa a próstata; inclui o colículo seminal, e os ductos ejaculatório e prostático abrem-se nela. SIN pars prostatica urethrae [TA].

   spongy u. [TA], u. esponjosa; a porção da u. masculina, com cerca de 15 cm de comprimento, que atravessa o corpo esponjoso. SIN pars spongiosa urethrae masculinae [TA], pars cavernosa, penile u., spongy part of the male urethra.

   u. viri′lis, u. masculina. SIN male u.

ure·thral (ū-rē′thrăl). Uretral; relativo à uretra.

ure·thral·gia (ū-rē-thral′jē-ă). Uretralgia; dor na uretra. SIN urethrodynia. [urethr- + G. *algos*, dor]

ure·threc·to·my (ūr-ē-threk′tō-mē). Uretrectomia; excisão parcial ou total da uretra. [urethr- + G. *ektomē*, excisão]

ure·threm·or·rha·gia (ū-rē′threm-or-rā′jē-ă). Uretremorragia; uretrorragia. SIN urethrorrhagia. [urethr- + G. *haima*, sangue, + *rhēgnymi*, impelir]

ure·thrism, ure·thris·mus (ū′rē-thrizm, -thriz′mus). Uretrismo; uretrospasmo; irritabilidade ou estreitamento espasmódico da uretra. SIN urethrospasm.

ure·thri·tis (ū-rē-thrī′tis). Uretrite; inflamação da uretra. [ureth- + G. *-itis*, inflamação]

   anterior u., u. anterior; inflamação da porção da uretra anterior ao ligamento triangular.

   follicular u., u. folicular; u. crônica com infiltrações linfocíticas nodulares na mucosa. SIN granular u.

   gonorrheal u., u. gonorreica; infecção da uretra, geralmente associada a corrimento purulento, causada por *Neisseria gonorrhoeae*.

   granular u., u. granular. SIN follicular u.

   nongonococcal u., u. não-gonocócica; u. não resultante de infecção gonocócica; *Chlamydia trachomatis* transmitida sexualmente é a causa mais comum.

   nonspecific u., u. inespecífica; u. não causada por gonococo, clamídia ou outros agentes infecciosos específicos. SIN simple u.

   u. petrif′icans, u. petrificante; u., algumas vezes de origem gotosa, na qual há um depósito de material calcário na parede da uretra.

   posterior u., u. posterior; inflamação das porções membranosa e prostática da uretra.

   simple u., u. simples. SIN nonspecific u.

♲ **urethro-, urethr-.** A uretra. [G. *ourēthra*]

ure·thro·bul·bar (ū-rē′thrō-bul′băr). Uretrobulbar. SIN bulbourethral.

ure·thro·cele (ū-rē′thrō-sēl). Uretrocele; prolapso da uretra feminina. [urethro- + G. *kēlē*, tumor, hérnia]

ure·thro·cys·to·me·trog·ra·phy (ū-rē′thrō-sis′tō-me-trog′ră-fē). Uretrocistometrografia. SIN urethrocystometry. [urethro- + G. *kystis*, bexiga, + *metron*, medir, + *skopeō*, ver]

ure·thro·cys·tom·e·try (ū-rē′thrō-sis-tom′ĕ-trē). Uretrocistometria; procedimento que mede simultaneamente as pressões na bexiga e uretra. SIN urethrocystometrography. [urethro- + G. *kystis*, bexiga, + *metron*, medir]

ure·thro·cys·to·pexy (ū - rē′thrō - sis′tō - pek - sē). Uretrocistopexia; fixação da uretra e da bexiga na incontinência de esforço. SIN urethropexy. [urethro- + G. *kystis*, bexiga, + *pēxis*, fixação]

ure·thro·dyn·ia (ū - rē - thrō - din′ē - ā). Uretrodinia. SIN urethralgia. [urethro- + G. *odynē*, dor]

ure·throg·ra·phy (ū - rē - throg′ră - fē). Uretrografia; radiografia contrastada da uretra masculina ou feminina, por injeção retrógrada ou durante a passagem de contraste na bexiga (cistouretrograma). [urethro + G. *graphō*, escrever]

ure·throm·e·ter (ū - rē - throm′e - ter). Uretrômetro; instrumento para medir o calibre da uretra. [urethro- + G. *metron*, medir]

ure·thro·pe·nile (ū - rē′thrō - pē′nīl). Uretropeniano; relativo à uretra e ao pênis.

ure·thro·per·i·ne·al (ū - rē′thrō - pe - ri - nē′al). Uretroperineal; relativo à uretra e ao períneo.

ureth·ro·per·i·ne·o·scro·tal (ū - rē′thrō - pe - ri - nē - ō - skrō′tal). Uretroperineoescrotal; relativo à uretra, ao períneo e ao escroto.

ure·thro·pexy (ū - rē′thrō - pek - sē). Uretropexia. SIN urethrocystopexy. [urethro- + G. *pēxis*, fixação]

ure·thro·plasty (ū - rē′thrō - plas - tē). Uretroplastia; reconstrução cirúrgica da uretra. [urethro- + G. *plastos*, formado]
  Cecil u., u. de Cecil; um procedimento de reconstrução uretral em estágios, no qual a porção uretral do pênis é deixada sepultada no escroto, após o primeiro estágio da u., devido ao revestimento cutâneo ventral inadequado.

ure·thro·pros·ta·tic (ū - rē′thrō - pros - tat′ik). Uretroprostático; relativo à uretra e à próstata.

ure·thro·rec·tal (ū - rē′thrō - rek′tal). Uretrorretal; relativo à uretra e ao reto.

ure·thror·rha·gia (ū - rē - thrō - rā′jē - ā). Uretrorragia; hemorragia uretral. SIN urethremorrhagia.

ure·thror·rha·phy (ū - rē - thrōr′ă - fē). Uretrorrafia; sutura da uretra. [urethro- + G. *rhaphē*, sutura]

ure·thror·rhea (ū - rē - thrō - rē′ă). Uretrorréia; corrimento anormal da uretra. [urethro- + G. *rhoia*, fluxo]

ure·thro·scope (ū - rē′thrō - skōp). Uretroscópio; instrumento para visualizar o interior da uretra. [urethro- + G. *skopeō*, ver]

ure·thro·scop·ic (ū - rē - thrō - skop′ik). Uretroscópico; relativo ao uretroscópio ou à uretroscopia.

ure·thros·co·py (ū - rē - thros′kŏ - pē). Uretroscopia; inspeção da uretra com um uretroscópio.

ure·thro·spasm (ū - rē′thrō - spazm). Uretrospasmo. SIN urethrism.

ure·thro·stax·is (ū - rē′thrō - stak′sis). Uretrostaxe; gotejamento de sangue da uretra. [urethro- + G. *staxis*, gotejamento]

ure·thro·ste·no·sis (ū - rē′thrō - ste - nō′sis). Uretroestenose; estreitamento da uretra. [urethro- + G. *stenōsis*, estreitamento]

ure·thros·to·my (ū - rē - thros′tō - mē). Uretrostomia; formação cirúrgica de uma abertura permanente entre a uretra e a pele. [urethro- + G. *stoma*, boca]
  perineal u., u. perineal; formação de uma abertura permanente para a porção bulbar da uretra através de uma incisão cutânea perineal.

ure·thro·tome (ū - rē′thrō - tōm). Uretrótomo; instrumento para seccionar uma estenose da uretra. [urethro- + G. *tomos*, cortante]

ure·throt·o·my (ū - rē - throt′ō - mē). Uretrotomia; incisão cirúrgica de uma estenose da uretra. [urethro- + G. *tomē*, incisão]
  external u., u. externa; u. através de uma abertura externa na pele do períneo ou do pênis. SIN perineal u.
  internal u., u. interna; u. por meio de um instrumento introduzido na uretra.
  perineal u., u. perineal. SIN external u.

ure·thro·vag·i·nal (ū - rē′thrō - vaj′i - nal). Uretrovaginal; relativo à uretra e à vagina.

ure·thro·ves·i·cal (ū - rē′thrō - ves′i - kăl). Uretrovesical; relativo à uretra e à bexiga.

ure·thro·ves·i·co·pexy (ū - rē′thrō - ves′i - kō - pek - sē). Uretrovesicopexia; suspensão cirúrgica da uretra e da base vesical pela superfície posterior da sínfise púbica (ou parede abdominal anterior ou ligamento de Cooper) para correção de incontinência de esforço. [urethro- + L. *vesica*, bexiga, + G. *pexis*, fixação]

-uretic. Urina. [G. *ourētikos*, relativo à urina]

URF Abreviatura de unidentified *reading frame*.

ur·gen·cy (er′jen - sē). Urgência; forte desejo de urinar.
  motor u., u. motora; u. decorrente de função hiperativa do detrusor.
  sensory u., u. sensorial; u. devida à hipersensibilidade vesicouretral.

ur·gi·nea (er - jin′ē - ă). Urgínea; os bulbos da *Urginea indica* (cebola-albarrã indiana) e *Urginea maritima* (cebola-albarrã branca ou do Mediterrâneo); fonte da cila. [L. *urgeo*, comprimir, relativo ao formato das sementes]

uri-, uric-, urico-. Ácido úrico. [G. *ouron*, urina]

uri·an (ū′rē - ăn). SIN urochrome.

uric (ū′rik). Úrico; referente à urina.

uric ac·id. Ácido úrico; 2,6,8-trioxipurina; cristais brancos, pouco solúveis, contidos em solução na urina de mamíferos e na forma sólida na urina de aves e répteis; algumas vezes solidificado em pequenas massas como cálculos ou cristais, ou em concreções maiores como cálculos; com o sódio e outras bases, forma uratos; níveis elevados estão associados à presença de gota. SIN lithic acid, triketopurine.
  u. a. oxidase, a. u. oxidase. VER *urate* oxidase.

uri·case (ū′ri - kās). Uricase. SIN urate oxidase.

urico-. VER uri-.

uri·col·y·sis (ūr - i - kol′i - sis). Uricólise; decomposição de ácido úrico. [urico- + G. *lysis*, afrouxamento]

uri·co·lyt·ic (ūr′i - kō - lit′ik). Uricolítico; relativo a, ou que efetua a, hidrólise do ácido úrico.

uri·cos·o·me (ūr - ik′ō - sōm). Uricossoma; um microcorpo rico em urato oxidase.

uri·co·su·ria (ū′ri - kō - soo′rē - ă). Uricosúria; quantidades excessivas de ácido úrico na urina. [urico- + G. *ouron*, urina]

uri·co·su·ric (ū′ri - kō - soo′rik). Uricosúrico; que tende a aumentar a excreção de ácido úrico.

uri·co·tele (oor′ik - ō - tēl). Uricotelo; organismo que é uricotélico; p. ex., aves e répteis que vivem na terra.

uri·co·tel·ia (ūr′ik′ō - tēl - ē - ă). Uricotelia; o processo ou tipo de excreção de nitrogênio no qual o ácido úrico é o principal produto excretado. [uric (acid) + G. *telos*, fim, resultado, + -ia]

uri·co·tel·ic (ūr′i - kō - tel′ik). Uricotélico; que produz ácido úrico como o principal produto excretor do metabolismo do nitrogênio. [urico- + G. *telos*, fim]

uri·dine (Urd) (ūr′i - dēn). Uridina; uracil ribonucleosídeo; um dos principais nucleosídios nos RNA; como o pirofosfato (UDP, UDPG, etc.), a u. é ativa no metabolismo do açúcar. SIN 1-β-D-ribofuranosyluracil.
  cyclic u. 3′,5′-monophosphate (cUMP), 3′,5′-monofosfato cíclico de u. (UMPc); um nucleotídio cíclico envolvido na regulação metabólica; inibe o crescimento de alguns tumores.
  u. 5′-diphosphate (UDP), 5′-difosfato de u. (UDP); 5′-pirofosfato de uridina; um produto da condensação da uridina e do ácido pirofosfórico.
  u. 5′monophosphate (UMP), 5′-monofosfato de u. (UMP). SIN uridylic acid.
  u. phosphorylase, u. fosforilase; uma ribosiltransferase que catalisa a reação da uridina com ortofosfato para produzir uracil e α-D-ribose 1-fosfato.
  u. 5′-triphosphate (UTP), 5′-trifosfato de u.; u. esterificada com ácido trifosfórico em sua posição 5′; o precursor imediato de resíduos do ácido uridílico no RNA.

uri·dine di·phos·pho·ga·lac·tose (UDPGal) (ūr′i - dēn - dī - fos′fō - gă - lak′tōs). Uridina difosfogalactose; um grupamento pirofosfato liga a posição 5′ da uridina e a posição 1 da D-galactose.
  u. d. 4-epimerase, u.d. 4-epimerase. VER UDPglucose 4-epimerase.

uri·dine di·phos·pho·glu·cose (UDPG, UDPGlc) (ūr′i - dēn - dī - fos′fō - gloo′kōs). Uridina difosfoglicose; UDP glicose; um grupamento pirofosfato liga a posição 5′ da uridina e a posição 1 da D-glicose; um intermediário na biossíntese do glicogênio. SIN UDPglucose.
  u. d. 4-epimerase, u. d. 4-epimerase. SIN UDPglucose 4-epimerase.

uri·dine di·phos·pho·glu·cu·ron·ic ac·id (UDP-GlcUA) (ūr′i - dēn - dī - fos′fō - gloo - koo - ron′ik). Ácido uridinodifosfoglicurônico; uridina difosfoglicose na qual o 6-CH₂OH da glicose foi oxidado em COOH (assim, tornou-se um resíduo glicuronil); participa da formação de conjugados de bilirrubina ou fármacos como o ácido acetilsalicílico.

uri·dine di·phos·pho·xylose. Uridina difosfoxilose. SIN xylose.

uri·dro·sis (ū - ri - drō′sis). Uridrose; a excreção de uréia ou ácido úrico no suor. [uri- + G. *hidrōs*, suor]
  u. crystalli′na, u. cristalina. SIN urea *frost*.

uri·dyl·ic ac·id (ūr - i - dil′ik). Ácido uridílico; uridina esterificada por ácido fosfórico em um ou mais grupamentos hidroxila açúcar; a UMP é tipicamente 5′-monofosfato de uridina; também ocorrem derivados 2′ e 3′; precursor da biossíntese de outros nucleotídeos pirimidina. SIN UMP synthase, uridine 5′-monophosphate.
  u. a. synthase, a. u. sintase; uma enzima bifuncional que contém as atividades tanto da orotato fosforribosiltransferase como da orotidina-5′-monofosfato descarboxilase; catalisa uma etapa fundamental na biossíntese da pirimidina; uma deficiência dessa enzima leva à acidúria orótica.

uri·dyl·trans·fer·ase (ūr′i - dil - trans′fer - ās). Uridiltransferase; UDPglicose-hexose 1-fosfato; uridililtransferase.

uri·es·the·sia (ūri - es - thē′zē - ă). Uriestesia. SIN uresiesthesia.

urin-, urino-. Urina. VER TAMBÉM ure-, uro-. [G. *ouron*]

uri·nal (ū′rin - ăl). Urinol; vaso para receber a urina.

uri·nal·y·sis (ū - ri - nal′i - sis). Urinálise; análise da urina.

uri·nary (ūr′i - nār′ē). Urinário; relativo à urina.

uri·nate (ūr′i - nāt). Urinar; eliminar urina. SIN micturate.

uri·na·tion (ūr′i - nā′shŭn). Micção; a eliminação de urina. SIN miction, micturition (1), uresis.

stuttering u., u. intermitente; a eliminação de urina em jatos causados por contração espasmódica intermitente da bexiga.

urine (ūr'in). Urina; o líquido e as substâncias dissolvidas excretadas pelo rim. [L. *urina*; G. *ouron*]
  ammoniacal u., u. amoniacal. SIN ammoniuria.
  black u., u. negra; a u. escura da melanúria ou hemoglobinúria.
  chylous u., u. quilosa; u. de aparência leitosa, contendo quilo. SIN milky u.
  cloudy u., u. turva; u. com aspecto turvo, geralmente devido à presença de pus, cristais, bactérias, sangue ou glóbulos de gordura livres. SIN nebulous u.
  crude u., u. pálida de baixa densidade específica, com muito pouco sedimento.
  febrile u., u. febril; u. escura, concentrada e de odor forte, eliminada por uma pessoa com febre. SIN feverish u.
  feverish u., u. febril. SIN febrile u.
  gouty u., u. gotosa; u. de cor forte contendo excesso de ácido úrico.
  honey u., u. melosa; designação obsoleta do diabetes melito (*diabetes* mellitus).
  maple syrup u., u. em xarope de bordo. VER maple syrup urine *disease*.
  milky u., u. leitosa. SIN chylous u.
  nebulous u., u. turva. SIN cloudy u.
  residual u., u. residual; u. que permanece na bexiga ao fim da micção em casos de obstrução prostática, atonia vesical, etc.

u·rin·if·er·ous (ūr-i-nif'ē-rŭs). Uriniífero; que conduz urina; designa os túbulos renais. [urine + L. *fero*, conduzir]

u·ri·nif·ic (oor-i-nif'ik). Urinífico. SIN uriniparous. [urine + L. *facio*, fazer]

u·ri·nip·a·rous (oor-i-nip'a-rŭs). Uriníparo; que produz ou excreta urina; designa os corpúsculos de Malpighi e alguns túbulos no córtex renal. SIN urinific. [urine + L. *pario*, produzir]

urino-. VER urin-.

u·ri·no·gen·i·tal (ūr'i-nō-jen'i-tăl). Urinogenital; urogenital. SIN genitourinary.

u·ri·nog·e·nous (ūr-i-noj'ĕ-nŭs). Urinógeno. **1.** Que produz ou excreta urina. **2.** De origem urinária. SIN urogenous.

u·ri·no·ma (ūr'i-nō'mă). Urinoma; uma coleção de urina extravasada. SIN urinary cyst.

u·ri·nom·e·ter (ūr-i-nom'ē-ter). Urinômetro; um hidrômetro para determinar a densidade específica da urina. SIN urogravimeter, urometer. [urine + G. *metron*, medida]

u·ri·nom·e·try (ūr-i-nom'ē-trē). Urinometria; a determinação da densidade específica da urina.

u·ri·nos·co·py (ūr-i-nos'kō-pē). Urinoscopia. SIN uroscopy.
u·ri·no·sex·u·al (ūr-i-nō-sek'shoo-ăl). Urinossexual. SIN genitourinary.
u·ri·nous (ūr'i-nŭs). Urinoso; relativo à ou da natureza da urina.
u·ri·po·sia (ūr-i-pō'sē-ă). Uriposia; ato de beber urina. [urine + G. *posis*, bebida]

uro-. Urina. VER TAMBÉM ure-, urin-. [G. *ouron*]

u·ro·am·mo·ni·ac (ū-rō-ă-mo'nē-ak). Uroamoníaco; relativo ao ácido úrico e amônia; designa um tipo de cálculo urinário.

u·ro·an·the·lone (ūr-ō-an'thē-lōn). Uroantelona. SIN urogastrone.

u·ro·bi·lin (ūr-ō-bī'lin, -bil'in). Urobilina; uma uroporfirina; um tetrapirrol acíclico que é um dos produtos da degradação natural do heme através da coleglobina, verdoemocromo, biliverdina, bilirrubina e *d*-urobilinogênio; um pigmento urinário que provoca coloração laranja-avermelhado variável da urina, de acordo com seu grau de oxidação. SIN urohematin, urohematoporphyrin.

u·ro·bi·lin IXα, urobilina IXα. SIN mesobilene.

u·ro·bi·li·ne·mia (ū'rō-bil-i-nē'mē-ă). Urobilinemia; a presença de urobilina no sangue.

u·ro·bi·lin·o·gen (ūr-ō-bī-lin'ō-jen). Urobilinogênio; precursor da urobilina.

u·ro·bi·lin·o·gen IXα. Urobilinogênio IXα. SIN mesobilane.

u·ro·bi·lin·u·ria (ū'rō-bil-i-noo'rē-ă). Urobilinúria; a presença na urina de urobilinas em quantidades excessivas, formadas principalmente a partir da hemoglobina.

u·ro·can·ase (ū'rō-kă-nās). Urocanase. SIN urocanate hydratase.

ur·o·can·ate (ūr'ō-kă-nāt). Urocanate; um sal ou éster de ácido urocânico.
  u. hydratase, u. hidratase; uma enzima que catalisa a reação da água com ácido urocânico para produzir ácido 4-imidazolona-5-propiônico, uma etapa no catabolismo da L-histidina; essa enzima está ausente em casos de acidúria urocânica. SIN urocanase.

u·ro·can·ic ac·id (ūr-ō-kan'ik). Ácido urocânico; ácido 4-imidazolacrílico; um ácido derivado da desaminação oxidativa da L-histidina; encontrado no suor e na urina do cachorro; são observados níveis elevados em casos de deficiência de urocanato hidratase. A forma *cis*, resultante da exposição à radiação UV, ativa células T supressoras.

u·ro·can·ic ac·i·du·ria (oor'ō-kan'ik-as'id-ūr'ē-a). Acidúria urocânica; níveis elevados de ácido urocânico na urina.

u·ro·can·i·case (ūr-ō-kan'i-kās). Urocanicase; uma dentre um grupo de pelo menos três enzimas que convertem o ácido urocânico em ácido glutâmico.

urina			
em geral		**componentes orgânicos (em mg/24 h, exceto observação contrária)**	
volume (em ml/24 h)	500 – 2.000	corpos cetônicos	10 – 100
densidade	1,010 – 1,025	aminoácidos, total (g/24 h)	1,3 – 3,2
matéria sólida (g/24 h, 100% de resíduo seco)	40 – 60	aminoácidos, livres (g/24 h)	0,35 – 1,20
depressão do ponto de congelamento (°C)	0,1 – 2,5	aminoácido N	40 – 130
osmolalidade (mosm/l)	50 – 1.400	creatina ♂	10 – 190
pH	4,8 – 7,5	creatina ♀	10 – 270
acidez total (mval/24 h)	50 – 60	creatinina	500 – 2.500
acidez (por titulação)	20 – 60	corpos diazo	traços
nitrogênio total (g/24 h)	7 – 17	ácidos graxos	8 – 50
aminoácido–N (% do total)	< 2	bilirrubina	0,02 – 1,9
amônia (NH$_4^+$)–N	4,6	urobilinogênio	0,05 – 2,5
creatinina–N	3,7	ácido biliar (g/24 h, como ácido glico e taurocólico)	5 – 10
ácido úrico–N	1,6	ácido glucurônico	200 – 600
uréia–N	82,7	ácido úrico	80 – 1.000
componentes inorgânicos (em mg/24 h, exceto observação contrária)		uréia (g/24 h)	12 – 30
amônia	0,3 – 1,2	ácido hipúrico (g/24 h)	1,0 – 2,5
cálcio	130 – 330	ácido hidroxiindolacético	1,0 – 14,7
cloreto (g/24 h)	4,3 – 8,5	indican	4,0 – 20,0
ferro	0,4 – 0,15	ácido indoxilsulfúrico	15 – 100
iodo	0,02 – 0,5	ácido lático	100 – 600
potássio (g/24 h)	1,4 – 3,1	ácido oxálico	10 – 25
cobre	0,03 – 0,07	ácido aminolevulínico	1,5 – 7,0
magnésio	60,7 – 200	coproporfirina	0,02 – 0,2
sódio (g/24 h)	2,8 – 5,0	porfobilinogênio	0,4 – 2,4
fósforo, total (g/24 h)	0,8 – 2,5	uroporfirina	0,004 – 0,02
enxofre, total (g/24 h)	1,24 – 1,50	proteínas	10 – 100
enxofre, inorgânico (g/24 h)	1,07 – 1,30	bases purina (g/24 h)	0,2 – 0,5
enxofre, neutro (g/24 g)	0,05 – 0,08	ácido cítrico	150 – 1.200
enxofre, esterizado (g/24 h)	0,08 – 0,10	açúcar (substâncias redutoras)	500 – 1.500
zinco	0,14 – 0,70	galactose	3 – 25
		glicose	15 – 130
		lactose	0 – 90

uro·cele (ū′rō-sēl). Urocele; extravasamento de urina para o saco escrotal. [uro- + G. *kēlē*, hérnia]

uroch·er·as (ū-rok′er-as). Uroquera; uropsamo. **1.** SIN gravel. **2.** SIN uropsammus (2). [uro- + G. *cheras*, sedimento (uma forma incorreta de *cherados*, sedimento)]

uro·che·sia (ū-rō-kē′zē-ă). Uroquesia; eliminação de urina pelo ânus. [uro- + G. *chezō*, defecar]

uro·chrome (ūr′ō-krōm). Urocromo; o principal pigmento da urina, um composto de urobilina e um peptídio de estrutura desconhecida. SIN urian.

uro·chro·mo·gen (ūr-ō-krō′mō-jen). Urocromogênio; originalmente, um corpo na urina que, ao captar oxigênio, formava urocromo; agora, provavelmente urobilinogênio.

uro·cris·ia (ū-rō-kris′ē-ă, -kriz′ē-ă). Urocrise. **1.** SIN urocrisis. **2.** Termo obsoleto para diagnóstico baseado nos resultados de um exame de urina. [uro- + G. *krinō*, separar, julgar]

uro·cri·sis (ū′rō-krī′sis). Urocrise. **1.** Termo obsoleto para o estágio crítico de uma doença acompanhada por emissão abundante de urina. **2.** Dor intensa em qualquer dos órgãos ou das vias urinárias, que ocorre na tabes dorsal. SIN urocrisia (1). [uro- + G. *krisis*, uma substância azul]

uro·cy·a·nin (ū′rō-sī′ă-nin). Urocianina; uroglaucina; um pigmento azul índigo observado algumas vezes na urina em determinadas doenças, principalmente na escarlatina. [uro- + G. *kyanos*, uma substância azul]

uro·cy·an·o·gen (ū-rō-sī-an′ō-jen). Urocianogênio; um pigmento azul observado algumas vezes na urina em casos de cólera.

uro·cy·a·no·sis (ū′rō-sī-ă-nō′sis). Urocianose; coloração azulada da urina na indicanúria.

uro·cyst (ū′rō-sist). Urocisto. SIN urinary bladder. [uro- + G. *kystis*, bexiga]

uro·cys·tic (ū′rō-sis′tik). Urocístico; relativo à bexiga.

uro·cys·tis (ū′rō-sis′tis). Urocisto. SIN urinary bladder.

uro·dy·na·mics (ū′rō-dī-nam′iks). Urodinâmica; o estudo do armazenamento de urina no interior, e o fluxo de urina através e proveniente, das vias urinárias. [uro- + G. *dynamis*, força]

uro·dyn·ia (ū-rō-din′ē-ă). Urodinia; dor à micção. [uro- + G. *odynē*, dor]

uro·en·ter·one (ūr-ō-en′ter-ōn). Uroenterona. SIN urogastrone.

uro·er·y·thrin (ū-rō-er′i-thrin). Uroeritrina; ureritrina; pigmento urinário que confere uma coloração rósea aos depósitos de uratos; provavelmente derivada da melanina. SIN purpurin (1), urerythrin.

uro·fla·vin (ūr-ō-flā′vin). Uroflavina; produto fluorescente do catabolismo da riboflavina, ou talvez da própria riboflavina, encontrado na urina e nas fezes de mamíferos.

uro·flow·me·ter (ū-rō′flō-mē-ter). Urofluxômetro; dispositivo que mede as velocidades de fluxo urinário durante a micção, incluindo esses parâmetros; velocidade máxima de fluxo, velocidade média de fluxo, volume eliminado e tempo de micção.

ur·o·fol·li·tro·pin (ūr-ō-fol′i-trō-pin). Urofolitropina; uma preparação de gonadotrofina extraída da urina de mulheres pós-menopausa, usada em conjunto com a gonadotrofina coriônica humana para induzir ovulação. VER TAMBÉM menotropins.

uro·fus·co·hem·a·tin (ū-rō-fūs-kō-hē′mă-tin). Urofuscoematina; pigmento vermelho-acastanhado encontrado na urina em determinadas doenças, como a hanseníase.

uro·gas·trone (ūr-ō-gas′trōn). Urogastrona; pigmento fluorescente extraído da urina; um inibidor da secreção e da motilidade gástrica. Cf. enterogastrone. SIN anthelone U, anthelone, uroanthelone, uroenterone.

uro·gen·i·tal (ū′rō-jen′i-tăl). Urogenital. SIN genitourinary.

urog·e·nous (ū-roj′ē-nŭs). Urógeno. SIN urinogenous.

uro·glau·cin (ū-rō-glaw′sin). Uroglaucina. SIN urocyanin. [uro- + G. *glaukos*, cinza-azulado]

ur·o·go·nad·o·tro·pin (ūr′ō-gō-nad-ō-trō′pin). Urogonadotrofina. VER human menopausal *gonadotropin*.

uro·graf·fin (ūr-ō-graf′fin). Nome comercial de uma mistura de sais de ácido diatrizóico usada para formar gradientes de densidade.

uro·gram (ūr′ō-gram). Urograma; o registro radiológico obtido por urografia.

urog·ra·phy (ū-rog′ră-fē). Urografia; radiografia de qualquer parte (rins, ureteres ou bexiga) das vias urinárias. VER TAMBÉM pyelography. [uro- + G. *graphō*, escrever]

antegrade u., u. anterógrada; radiografia após injeção intravenosa ou percutânea de contraste com uma agulha ou cateter nos cálices renais ou na pelve renal (pielografia anterógrada) ou na bexiga (cistografia anterógrada).

cystoscopic u., u. cistoscópica. SIN retrograde u.

intravenous u., excretory u., u. intravenosa, u. excretora; radiografia dos rins, ureteres e bexiga após injeção de contraste em uma veia periférica.

retrograde u., u. retrógrada; radiografia das vias urinárias após injeção de contraste diretamente na uretra, bexiga, ureter ou pelve renal. SIN cystoscopic u.

uro·gra·vim·e·ter (ūr′ō-gră-vim′ē-ter). Urogravímetro. SIN urinometer. [uro- + L. *gravis*, pesado, + G. *metron*, medida]

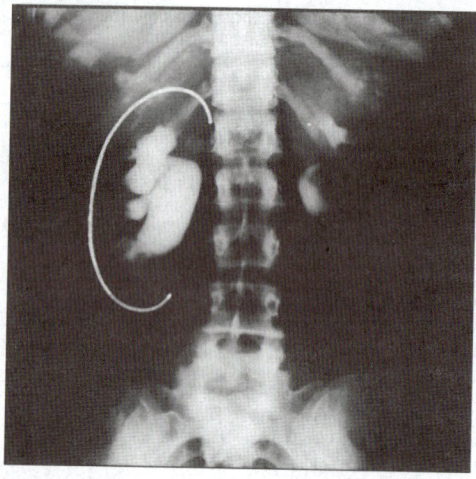

urografia: urografia intravenosa mostrando retenção de uma grande quantidade de contraste na pelve renal direita, indicando hidronefrose causada por obstrução ureteral

uro·hem·a·tin (ūr-ō-hem′ă-tin). Uroematina. SIN urobilin.

uro·hem·a·to·por·phy·rin (ūr′ō-hēm′ă-tō-pōr′fi-rin). Uroematoporfirina. SIN urobilin.

uro·hep·a·rin (ūr-ō-hep′ă-rin). Uroeparina; uma forma inativa de heparina excretada na urina.

uro·hy·per·ten·sin (ūr′ō-hī-per-ten′sin). Uroipertensina; substância pressora derivada da urina.

uro·ki·na·se (ūr-ō-kī′nās). Uroquinase; urocinase. SIN plasminogen *activator*.

uro·lag·nia (ūr-ō-lag′nē-ă). Urolagnia; estimulação sexual ocasionada pela observação de uma pessoa urinando. [uro- + G. *lagneia*, prazer]

uro·leu·cin·ic ac·id, uro·leu·cic ac·id (ū′rō-loo-sin′ik, ū-rō-loo′sik). Ácido uroleucínico; ácido uroleúcico; uma substância aromática excretada na urina de pessoas com alcaptonúria.

uro·lith (ū′rō-lith). Urólito. SIN urinary calculus. [uro- + G. *lithos*, cálculo]

uro·li·thi·a·sis (ū-rō-li-thī′ă-sis). Urolitíase; presença de cálculos no sistema urinário.

uro·lith·ic (ū-rō-lith′ik). Urolítico; relativo a cálculos urinários.

uro·li·thol·o·gy (ū′rō-li-thol′ō-jē). Urolitologia; o ramo da medicina relacionado à formação, composição, efeitos e remoção dos cálculos urinários. [uro- + G. *lithos*, cálculo, + *logus*, estudo]

uro·log·ic, uro·log·i·cal (ū-rō-loj′ik, i-kăl). Urológico; relativo à urologia.

urol·o·gist (ū-rol′ō-jist). Urologista; especialista em urologia. SIN genitourinary surgeon.

urol·o·gy (ū-rol′ō-jē). Urologia; a especialidade médica relacionada ao estudo, diagnóstico e tratamento de doenças das vias genitourinárias. [uro- + G. *logos*, estudo]

uro·lu·te·in (ū-rō-loo′tē-in). Uroluteína; nome dado ao pigmento amarelo na urina. VER urochrome, uroporphyrin (1).

uro·mel·a·nin (ū-rō-mel′ă-nin). Uromelanina; um pigmento preto ocasionalmente encontrado na urina, possivelmente um produto da decomposição do urocromo.

urom·e·ter (ū-rom′ē-ter). Urômetro. SIN urinometer.

uron·cus (ū-rong′kŭs). Uronco; cisto urinário; uma área circunscrita de extravasamento de urina. [uro- + G. *onkos*, massa (tumor)]

uron·ic ac·ids (ū-ron′ik). Ácidos urônicos; ácidos derivados de monossacarídeos por oxidação do grupamento álcool primário ($-CH_2OH$) removido do grupo carbonil para um grupo carboxila ($-COOH$); p. ex., ácido glicurônico.

uro·nos·co·py (ū-rō-nos′kō-pē). Uronoscopia; uroscopia. SIN uroscopy.

urop·a·thy (ū-rop′ă-thē). Uropatia; qualquer distúrbio que envolva as vias urinárias. [uro- + G. *pathos*, sofrimento]

obstructive u., u. obstrutiva; qualquer patologia, anatômica ou funcional, das vias urinárias causada por obstrução.

uro·phan·ic (ūr-ō-fan′ik). Urofânico; que aparece na urina; designa qualquer constituinte, normal ou patológico, da urina. [uro- + G. *phainō*, aparecer]

uro·phe·in (ū-rō-fē′in). Urofeína; pigmento acinzentado ocasionalmente encontrado na urina, possivelmente idêntico à urobilina. [uro- + G. *phaios*, cinza]

uro·poi·e·sis (ū′rō-poy-ē′sis). Uropoese; a produção ou secreção e excreção de urina. [uro- + G. *poiēsis*, produção]

uro·poi·e·tic (ū′rō-poy-et′ik). Uropoético; relativo ou pertinente à uropoese.

uro·por·phy·rin (ūr - ō - pōr′fi - rin). Uroporfirina. **1.** Porfirina excretada na urina na porfirinúria; p. ex., urobilina. **2.** Nome genérico de todas as porfirinas que contêm 4 grupamentos de ácido acético e 4 grupamentos de ácido propiônico nas posições 1 a 8. VER TAMBÉM porphyrinogens.
u. I, u. I; porfina-1,3,5,7-ácido tetraacético-2,4,6,8-ácido tetrapropiônico; formada pela ação da luz sobre o uroporfirinogênio I; níveis elevados são encontrados em determinadas porfirias.
u. III, u. III; porfina-1,3,5,8-ácido tetraacético-2,4,6,7-ácido tetrapropiônico; formada pela ação da luz sobre o uroporfirinogênio III; em determinadas porfirias são encontrados níveis elevados.
ur·o·por·phy·rin·o·gen (ūr′ō - pōr - fi - rin′ō - jen). Uroporfirinogênio. VER porphyrinogens.
u. decarboxylase, u. descarboxilase; enzima que participa da biossíntese do heme; catalisa a descarboxilação da uroporfirina III para produzir coproporfirinogênio III; também atua sobre a uroporfirina I; a deficiência dessa enzima resultará em porfiria cutânea tardia ou em porfiria hepatoeritropoética.
u. III cosynthase, u. III co-sintase; enzima da biossíntese do heme que participa da formação de u. III; uma deficiência dessa proteína resulta em porfiria eritropoética congênita.
uro·psam·mus (ū - rō - sam′ŭs). Uropsamo. **1.** SIN gravel. **2.** Qualquer sedimento urinário inorgânico ou urático. SIN urocheras (2). [uro- + G. *psammos*, areia]
urop·ter·in (ū - rop′ter - in). Uropterina. SIN urothion.
uro·pur·pur·in (ūr - ō - pŭr′poor - in). Uropurpurina; pigmento púrpura na urina.
u·o·ra·di·ol·o·gy (ū′rō - rā - dē - ol′ō - jē). Urorradiologia; o estudo da radiologia das vias urinárias.
uro·rec·tal (ū′rō - rek′tal). Urorretal; relativo às vias urinárias e ao reto.
uro·ro·se·in (ūr - ō - rō′zē - in). Urorroseína; um cromógeno na urina que adquire uma cor vermelha com o acréscimo de ácido nítrico; normalmente existe em quantidades muito pequenas, mas está aumentada na tuberculose e em outras doenças consuptivas, e está relacionada à ingestão de compostos indólicos.
uro·ru·bin (ūr - ō - roo′bin). Urorrubina; pigmento vermelho na urina que se torna mais visível por tratamento com ácido clorídrico.
uro·ru·bro·hem·a·tin (ūr′ō - roo - brō - hē′mă - tin). Urorrubroematina; um pigmento avermelhado presente ocasionalmente na urina em várias doenças crônicas.
uros·che·sis (ū - ros′kē - sis). Urosquese. **1.** Retenção de urina. **2.** Supressão de urina. [uro- + G. *schesis*, retenção]
uro·scop·ic (ūr - ō - skop′ik). Uroscópico; relativo à uroscopia.
uros·co·py (ū - ros′kŏ - pē). Uroscopia; exame da urina, geralmente por meio de um microscópio. SIN urinoscopy, uronoscopy. [uro- + G. *skopeō*, ver]
uro·sem·i·ol·o·gy (ū′rō - sem - ē - ol′ō - jē). Urossemiologia; estudo da urina como auxílio ao diagnóstico. [uro- + G. *sēmeion*, um sinal, + *logos*, estudo]
uro·sep·sin (ūr - ō - sep′sin). Urossepsina; designação obsoleta de uma substância formada pela decomposição da urina, supostamente a causa da intoxicação séptica após extravasamento urinário.
uro·sep·sis (ūr - ō - sep′sis). Urossépsis; urossepse. **1.** Sépsis resultante da infecção de urina extravasada. **2.** Sépsis por obstrução de urina infectada. [uro- + G. *sēpsis*, decomposição]
uro·spec·trin (ūr - ō - spek′trin). Uroespectrina; pigmento encontrado na urina, possivelmente o mesmo que urobilina.
u·ro·the·li·um (ū - rō - thē′lē - ŭm). Urotélio; o revestimento epitelial das vias urinárias. [uro- + epithelium]
ur·o·thi·on (ūr - ō - thī′on). Urotion; uropterina; um derivado da pteridina, contendo enxofre. SIN uropterin.
ur·o·thor·ax (ūr - ō - thōr′aks). Urotórax; a presença de urina na cavidade torácica, geralmente após lesões complexas de múltiplos órgãos.
urox·an·thin (ūr - ō - zan′thin). Uroxantina. SIN indican (2).
urox·in (ū - rok′sin). Uroxina. SIN alloxantin.
ursodeoxycholic acid. Ácido ursodesoxicólico. SIN ursodiol.
ursodiol (er - sō - dī′ol). Ursodiol; um ácido biliar usado para facilitar a dissolução de cálculos biliares nos pacientes; uma possível alternativa à colecistectomia. SIN ursodeoxycholic acid.
ur·ti·ca (er - tī′kă, er′ti-). Urtiga; a erva *Urtica dioica* (família Urticaceae); erva daninha cujas folhas produzem uma sensação de picada ao tocar a pele. Tem sido usada como diurético e hemostático na metrorragia, epistaxe e hematêmese. SIN nettle. [L. *urtiga*, de *uro*, pp. *ustus*, queimar]
ur·ti·cant (er′ti - kant). Urticante; que provoca uma pápula ou outro agente pruriginoso semelhante. [L. *urtica*, urtiga; ver urtica]
ur·ti·car·ia (er′ti - kar′ē - ă). Urticária; erupção de pápulas pruriginosas, geralmente de origem sistêmica; pode ser devida a um estado de hipersensibilidade a alimentos ou drogas, focos de infecção, agentes físicos (calor, frio, luz, atrito) ou estímulos físicos. SIN hives (1), urtication (2). [L. *urtica*]
  acute u., u. aguda. SIN febrile u.
  u. bullo′sa, u. bolhosa; erupção de pápulas recobertas por vesículas subepidérmicas. SIN u. vesiculosa.
  cholinergic u., u. colinérgica; uma forma de u. física ou não-alérgica iniciada por calor (p. ex., banhos quentes, exercício físico, pirexia, exposição ao sol ou a um ambiente quente) ou por excitação; as lesões bastante distintas consistem em áreas pruriginosas com 1–2 mm de diâmetro circundadas por máculas vermelho-brilhantes. SIN heat u.
  chronic u., u. crônica; uma forma de u. na qual as pápulas recorrem freqüentemente, ou persistem. SIN u. chronica.
  u. chron′ica, u. crônica. SIN chronic u.
  cold u., u. do frio; u. do congelamento; formação de pápula após exposição a baixas temperaturas, com ou sem anticorpos de transferência passiva demonstráveis.
  u. endem′ica, u. epidem′ica, u. endêmica; u. epidêmica; u. causada pelas cerdas urticantes de certas lagartas.
  factitious u., u. factícia. SIN dermatographism.
  febrile u., u. febril; u. acompanhada por febre leve. SIN acute u.
  giant u., u. gigante. SIN angioedema.
  heat u., u. do calor. SIN cholinergic u.
  u. hemorrhag′ica, u. hemorrágica; u. bolhosa na qual o exsudato seroso contém sangue.
  u. maculo′sa, u. maculosa; forma crônica de u. com lesões vermelhas e pouco edema.
  u. medicamento′sa, u. medicamentosa; forma de urticária por alergia a medicamentos.
  papular u., u. papular; reação de sensibilidade a picadas de insetos, sobretudo pulgas humanas e de animais domésticos, observada sobretudo em crianças pequenas como vergões seguidos por pápulas em áreas expostas.
  u. per′stans, u. persistente; forma de u. crônica na qual as pápulas persistem inalteradas por longos períodos; inclui a vasculite urticariácea.
  u. pigmento′sa, u. pigmentosa; mastocitose cutânea resultante de excesso de mastócitos na derme superficial, provocando uma erupção crônica caracterizada por pápulas acastanhadas planas ou um pouco elevadas, que causam urticação quando tocadas. A doença em crianças costuma involuir espontaneamente, enquanto a resolução é rara quando começa na idade adulta, e pode haver lesões sistêmicas. VER TAMBÉM diffuse cutaneous *mastocytosis*.
  pressure u., u. de pressão; u. de etiologia desconhecida que ocorre após compressão local da pele.
  solar u., u. solar; forma de u. resultante da exposição à luz solar; alguns pacientes apresentam anticorpos de transferência passiva e outros não.
  u. subcuta′nea, u. subcutânea; u. na qual há prurido sem pápulas.
  u. vesiculo′sa, u. vesiculosa. SIN u. bullosa.
  vibratory u., u. vibratória; forma de u. que ocorre em resposta a estímulos vibratórios.
ur·ti·car·i·al (er - ti - kar′ē - ăl). Urticariáceo; relativo a ou caracterizado por urticária.
ur·ti·cate (er′ti - kāt). Urticar. **1.** Realizar urticação. **2.** Caracterizado pela presença de pápulas. [L. *urticatus*]
ur·ti·ca·tion (er - ti - kā′shŭn). Urticação. **1.** Sensação de queimação semelhante à produzida por urticária ou resultante de envenenamento por urtiga. **2.** SIN urticaria. [L. *urticatio*]
uru·shi·ol (oo′roo - shē - ol). Urushiol; mistura de hidrocarbonetos não-voláteis, derivados de catecol com cadeias laterais C_{15} ou C_{17} insaturadas, constituindo o alérgeno ativo do óleo irritante da hera venenosa, *Toxicodendron radicans*, do carvalho venenoso, *T. diversilobum*, e da árvore da laca asiática, *T. verniciferum*. [Jap. *urushi*, lago, + L. *oleum*, óleo]
  u. oxidase, u. oxidase. SIN laccase.
USAN Abreviatura de United States Adopted Names (Nomes Adotados nos Estados Unidos).
Usher, Charles Howard, oftalmologista inglês, 1865–1942. VER U. *syndrome*.
Usher, Barney D., dermatologista canadense, 1899–1978. VER Senear-U. *disease, syndrome*.
USP Abreviatura de United States Pharmacopeia (Farmacopéia dos Estados Unidos). VER Pharmacopeia.
USPHS Abreviatura de United States Public Health Service (Serviço de Saúde Pública dos Estados Unidos).
us·ti·lag·i·nism (ŭs - ti - laj′i - nizm). Ustilaginismo; intoxicação por *Ustilago maydis* (ferrugem do milho), que produz queimação, prurido, hiperemia, acrocianose e edema dos membros; assemelha-se ao ergotismo, pelagra ou acrocinia do lactente.
Us·ti·la·go (ŭs - ti - lā′gō). Gênero de fungos (ordem Ustilaginales). [L. um tipo de cardo, de *ustio*, queimação]
  U. may′dis, uma espécie de fungo que se assemelha ao esporão-do-centeio em sua ação metabólica; seus esporos negros nas espigas de milho são dispersos pelo vento e podem causar contaminação de culturas laboratoriais. SIN corn ergot, corn smut, *U. zeae*.
  U. ze′ae, SIN *U. maydis*.
us·tu·la·tion (ŭs - tū - lā′shŭn). Ustulação. **1.** Separação de compostos pelo calor, como no processo de purificar minérios do enxofre por chamuscamento.

ustulation 1708 **uterus**

2. Secagem de um composto pelo calor para prepará-lo para pulverização. [L. *ustulo*, pp. *-atus*, chamuscar]

usur·pa·tion (ū'sĕr - pā'shŭn). Usurpação; tomada da função marcapasso do coração por um foco subsidiário em virtude de seu próprio aumento da automaticidade; p. ex., marcapasso juncional acelerado assume o comando quando ultrapassa a frequência sinusal. [L. *usurpo*, pp. *-atus*, agarrar]

uta (oo'tä). Uta; forma leve de leishmaniose cutânea do Novo Mundo ou americana causada por *Leishmania peruana*, que ocorre nos altos vales andinos do Peru e da Bolívia, caracterizada por numerosas e pequenas lesões dérmicas observadas quase exclusivamente nas superfícies cutâneas expostas; o cachorro é um reservatório importante. Ao contrário de todas as outras formas de leishmaniose cutânea americana, essa doença é encontrada em grandes altitudes (2.000–2.500 m) em regiões abertas, e não em florestas tropicais baixas. [Sp.]

uter-. VER utero-.

uter·ine (ū'tĕr - in, ū'tĕr - īn). Uterino; relativo ao útero.

in utero (in ū'tĕr - ō). *In utero*; intra-uterino; dentro do útero; ainda não nascido. [L.]

utero-, uter-. O útero. VER TAMBÉM hystero- (1), metr-. [L. *uterus*]

uter·o·ab·dom·i·nal (ū'tĕr - ō - ab - dom'i - năl). Uteroabdominal; relativo ao útero e ao abdome. SIN uteroventral.

uter·o·cer·vi·cal (ū'tĕr - ō - ser'vi - kăl). Uterocervical; relativo ao colo do útero.

uter·o·cys·tos·to·my (ū'tĕr - ō - sis - tos'tō - mē). Uterocistostomia; formação de uma comunicação entre o útero (colo) e a bexiga. [utero- + G. *kystis*, bexiga, + *stoma*, boca]

uter·o·fix·a·tion (ū'tĕr - ō - fik - sā'shŭn). Histeropexia. SIN hysteropexy.

uteroglobin. Uteroglobina; proteína secretada homodimérica, evolutivamente conservada, indutível por esteróides, com muitas atividades biológicas, incluindo um efeito pró-inflamatório, inibição de lipoproteína-lipase A_2 solúvel e quimiotaxia de neutrófilos e monócitos. Liga-se a vários supostos receptores em vários tipos celulares e inibe a invasão celular da matriz extracelular. É encontrada no sangue e na urina, no útero e em numerosos outros tecidos, mas não nos rins. Em camundongos, foi demonstrado que a uteroglobina se liga à fibronectina (Fn), evitando auto-agregação da Fn e subsequente deposição tecidual anormal, principalmente nos glomérulos. É essencial para manter a função renal normal em camundongos. SIN bastokinin.

uteroglobin-adducin. Uteroglobina-aducina; uma proteína α/β heterodimérica encontrada nas células tubulares renais, considerada reguladora do transporte iônico através de canais no citoesqueleto de actina. Foi encontrado um alelo mutante, em alguns pacientes hipertensos, que estaria associado à forma de hipertensão essencial sensível ao sal.

uter·o·lith (ū'tĕr - ō - lith). Uterólito. SIN uterine calculus. [utero- + G. *lithos*, cálculo]

uter·om·e·ter (ū - tĕr - om'ĕ - tĕr). Uterômetro. SIN hysterometer.

uter·o·o·var·i·an (ū'tĕr - ō - ō - văr'ē - an). Útero-ovariano; relativo ao útero e a um ovário.

uter·o·pa·ri·e·tal (ū'tĕr - ō - pa - rī'ĕ - tăl). Uteroparietal; relativo ao útero e à parede abdominal.

uter·o·pel·vic (ū'tĕr - ō - pel'vik). Uteropélvico; relativo ao útero e à pelve.

uter·o·pexy (ū'tĕr - ō - pek - sē). Uteropexia. SIN hysteropexy.

uter·o·pla·cen·tal (ū'tĕr - ō - pla - sen'tăl). Uteroplacentário; relativo ao útero e à placenta.

uter·o·plas·ty (ū'tĕr - ō - plas - tē). Uteroplastia; cirurgia plástica do útero. SIN hysteroplasty, metroplasty. [utero- + G. *plastos*, formado]

uter·o·sa·cral (ū'tĕr - ō - sā'krăl). Uterossacral; relativo ao útero e ao sacro.

uter·o·sal·pin·gog·ra·phy (ū'tĕr - ō - sal - pin - gog'ră - fē). Uterossalpingografia. SIN hysterosalpingography.

uter·o·scope (ū'tĕr - ō - skōp). Uteroscópio. SIN hysteroscope.

uter·os·co·py (ū - tĕr - os'kō - pē). Uteroscopia. SIN hysteroscopy.

uter·ot·o·my (ū - tĕr - ot'ō - mē). Uterotomia. SIN hysterotomy.

uter·o·ton·ic (ū'tĕr - ō - ton'ik). Uterotônico. **1.** Que confere tônus ao músculo uterino. **2.** Um agente que supera o relaxamento da parede muscular do útero. [utero- + G. *tonos*, tônus, tensão]

uter·o·tro·pic (ū'tĕr - ō - trō'pik). Uterotrópico; que tem um efeito sobre o útero.

uter·o·tub·al (ū'tĕr - ō - too'băl). Uterotubário; relativo ao útero e às tubas uterinas.

uter·o·tu·bog·ra·phy (ū'tĕr - ō - too - bog'ră - fē). Uterotubografia. SIN hysterosalpingography.

uter·o·vag·i·nal (ū - tĕr - ō - vaj'i - năl). Uterovaginal; relativo ao útero e à vagina.

uter·o·ven·tral (ū'tĕr - ō - ven'trăl). Uteroventral. SIN uteroabdominal. [utero- + L. *venter*, ventre]

uter·o·ver·dine (ū'tĕr - ō - ver'din). Uteroverdina; biliverdina da placenta de cachorro.

uter·o·ves·i·cal (ū'tĕr - ō - ves'i - kăl). Uterovesical; relativo ao útero e à bexiga.

uter·us, pl. **uteri** (ū'tĕr - ŭs, ū'tĕr - ī) [TA]. Útero; órgão muscular oco no qual o óvulo fecundado se desenvolve; tem cerca de 7,5 cm de comprimento na mulher não-grávida, e consiste em uma porção principal (corpo) com uma parte inferior alongada (cérvice) em cuja extremidade se situa a abertura (óstio externo). A porção arredondada superior do u., oposta ao óstio, é o fundo, em cada extremidade do qual está o corno, marcando a parte onde a tuba uterina se une ao u. e através da qual o óvulo chega à cavidade uterina após deixar o ovário. O órgão é sustentado passivamente na cavidade pélvica pelos ligamentos cardinais e pela anteflexão e anteversão do útero normal, que coloca sua massa superior à bexiga; é sustentado ativamente pela contração tônica e fásica dos músculos do assoalho pélvico. SIN metra, womb. [L.]

u. acol'lis, u. acólico; u. com atresia ou ausência do colo.

anomalous u., u. anômalo; u. malformado causado por desenvolvimento anormal ou fusão dos ductos paramesonéfricos.

arcuate u., u. arqueado; u. com uma depressão no fundo; um u. bífido incompleto. SIN u. arcuatus.

u. arcua'tus, u. arqueado. SIN arcuate u.

bicornate u., u. bicorne; u. bífido; u. que é mais ou menos completamente dividido em dois cornos laterais em virtude da união imperfeita dos ductos paramesonéfricos; difere do u. septado por não haver uma marca externa de separação; no u. bicorne, a cérvice pode ser única (u. bicornis unicollis) ou dupla (u. bicornis bicollis). SIN bifid u., u. bicornis, u. bifidus.

u. bicor'nis, u. bicorne. SIN bicornate u.

u. bicornis bicollis, u. bicorne bicervical. VER bicornate u.

u. bicornis unicollis, u. bicorne unicervical. VER bicornate u.

bifid u., u. bífido. SIN bicornate u.

u. bi'fidus, u. bífido. SIN bicornate u.

biforate u., u. bífore; u. com dupla entrada; u. septado no qual o colo é dividido em dois por um septo. SIN double-mouthed u., u. biforis.

u. bifor'is, u. bífore. SIN biforate u.

u. bilocula'ris, u. bilocular. SIN septate u.

bipartite u., u. bipartido. SIN septate u.

u. biparti'tus, u. bipartido. SIN septate u.

cordiform u., u. cordiforme; um u. bicorne incompleto com uma depressão cuneiforme no fundo. SIN heart-shaped u., u. cordiformis.

u. cordiform'is, u. cordiforme. SIN cordiform u.

Couvelaire u., u. de Couvelaire; extravasamento de sangue para a musculatura uterina e sob o peritônio uterino associado a formas graves de descolamento prematuro da placenta. SIN uteroplacental apoplexy.

u. didel'phys, u. didelfo; u. duplo com colo duplo e vagina dupla; devido à falha de união dos ductos paramesonéfricos. [G. *di-*, dois, + *delphys*, útero]

double-mouthed u., u. com dupla entrada. SIN biforate u.

duplex u., u. duplo; qualquer u. com luz dupla (u. didelfo, u. bicorne bicervical ou u. septado). SIN u. duplex.

u. du'plex, u. duplo. SIN duplex u.

gravid u., u. grávido; a condição do u. na gravidez.

heart-shaped u., u. em forma de coração. SIN cordiform u.

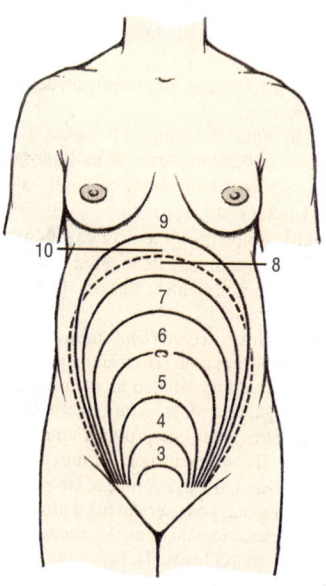

útero: alterações no tamanho durante a gravidez

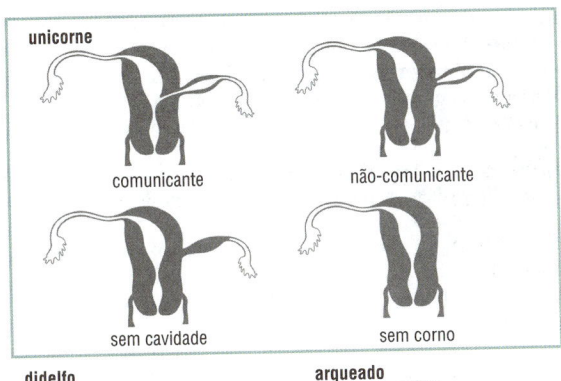
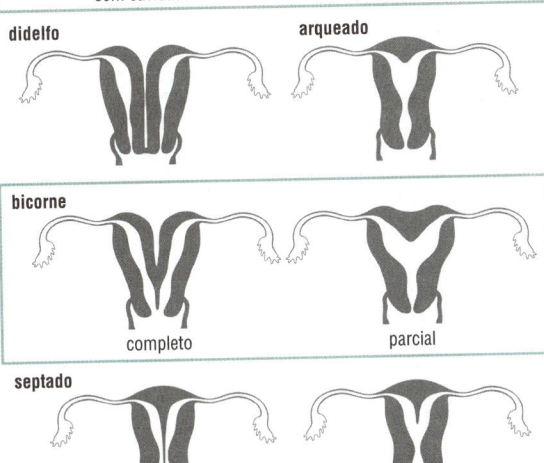

anomalias do desenvolvimento do útero

incudiform u., u. triangular; u. bicorne no qual o fundo entre os dois cornos é largo e plano. SIN triangular u., u. incudiformis, u. triangularis.
u. incudiform'is, u. triangular. SIN incudiform u.
masculine u., utrículo prostático. SIN prostatic utricle.
u. masculi'nus, utrículo prostático. SIN prostatic utricle.
one-horned u., designação obsoleta de unicorn u.
u. parvicol'lis, u. parvicólico; u. de tamanho normal com um colo anormal, desproporcionalmente pequeno.
septate u., u. septado; u. dividido em duas cavidades por um septo ântero-posterior. SIN bipartite u., u. bilocularis, u. bipartitus, u. septus.
u. sep'tus, u. septado. SIN septate u.
subseptate u., u. subseptado; um septo u. incompleto. SIN u. subseptus.
u. subsep'tus, u. subseptado. SIN subseptate u.
triangular u., u. triangular. SIN incudiform u.
u. triangula'ris, u. triangular. SIN incudiform u.
unicorn u., u. unicorne; u. em qual existe apenas uma metade lateral, sendo a outra metade subdesenvolvida ou ausente. SIN u. unicornis.
u. unicor'nis, u. unicorne. SIN unicorn u.
UTI Abreviatura de urinary tract infection (infecção das vias urinárias).
util·i·ty. Utilidade; em ética biomédica e na análise de decisões clínicas, a satisfação ou vantagem econômica obtida com os resultados de uma determinada decisão.
UTP Abreviatura de uridine 5′-triphosphate (5′-trifosfato de uridina).
utri·cle (oo'tri·kl) [TA]. Utrículo. SIN utriculus [TA], sacculus communis.
prostatic u. [TA], u. prostático; uma bolsa diminuta na próstata, que se abre no topo do colículo seminal, o análogo do útero e da vagina na mulher, sendo o remanescente das extremidades caudais fundidas dos ductos paramesonéfricos. SIN utriculus prostaticus [TA], masculine uterus, Morgagni sinus (2), sinus pocularis, uterus masculinus, vagina masculina, vesica prostatica, Weber organ.
u. of vestibular labyrinth [TA], u. do labirinto vestibular; o maior dos dois sacos membranosos no vestíbulo do labirinto, situado no recesso elíptico; dele se originam os ductos semicirculares.
utric·u·lar (ū-trik′ū-lar). Utricular; relativo, ou semelhante, a um utrículo.
utric·u·li (oo-trik′ū-lī). Plural de utriculus.
utric·u·li·tis (ū-trik-ū-lī′tis). Utriculite; inflamação do ouvido interno. [utriculus + G. -itis, inflamação]

utric·u·lo·sac·cu·lar (ū-trik′ū-lō-sak′ū-lar). Utriculossacular; relativo ao utrículo e ao sáculo do labirinto, designando particularmente um ducto que une as duas estruturas.
utric·u·lus, pl. **utric·u·li** (oo′trik′ū-lŭs, -lī) [TA]. Utrículo. SIN utricle. VER TAMBÉM vestibular labyrinth. [L. dim. de uter; bolsa de couro]
u. prostat'icus [TA], u. prostático. SIN prostatic utricle.
utri·form (ū′tri-fōrm). Utriforme; em forma de garrafa de couro (odre de vinho). [L. uter, bolsa de pele, + forma, forma]
UV, uv. Abreviatura de ultraviolet.
UVA Abreviatura de ultraviolet A.
uvae·for·mis (ū-vē-fōr′mis). Uviforme. SIN vascular lamina of choroid. [L. uva, uva, + forma, forma]
uva ur·si (oo′vă er′sī). Uva-ursina; as folhas secas de Arctostaphylos uva-ursi (família Ericaceae), uva-ursina, uma planta comum na região temperada do norte; contém glicosídios anti-sépticos, arbutina, metilarbutina e taninos; tem sido usada em inflamações crônicas das vias urinárias. [L. uva, uva + ursus, urso]
UVB Abreviatura de ultraviolet B.
uvea (oo′vē-ă). Úvea. SIN vascular layer of eyeball. [L. uva, uva]
uve·al (oo′vē-ăl). Uveal; relativo à úvea.
uve·it·ic (ū-vē-it′ik). Uveítico; relativo à úvea.
uve·i·ti·des (ū-vē-it′i-dēz). Plural de uveitis; uveítes.
uve·i·tis, pl. **uve·i·ti·des** (ū-vē-ī′tis, -it′ī-dēz). Uveíte; inflamação do trato uveal: íris, corpo ciliar e coróide. [uvea + G. -itis, inflamação]
anterior u., u. anterior; inflamação envolvendo o corpo ciliar e a íris.
Förster u., u. de Förster; inflamação sifilítica, com nódulos difusos envolvendo a coróide e vasculite retiniana.
Fuchs u., u. de Fuchs. SIN heterochromic u.
heterochromic u., u. heterocrômica; uveíte anterior e despigmentação da íris. SIN Fuchs u.
intermediate u., u. intermediária; uma u. que não é anterior nem posterior, mas tende a envolver a porção plana e o corpo ciliar.
lens-induced u., u. induzida pelo cristalino. SIN phacoanaphylactic u.
phacoanaphylactic u., u. facoanafilática; inflamação intra-ocular que ocorre após extração de catarata extracapsular; provavelmente uma reação imune às proteínas lenticulares liberadas pelo paciente. SIN lens-induced u.
phacogenic u., u. facogênica; u. secundária à catarata hipermadura.
posterior u., u. posterior. SIN choroiditis.
sympathetic u., u. simpática; inflamação bilateral do trato uveal causada por uma ferida perfurante de um olho que lesa a úvea.
uve·o·en·ceph·a·li·tis (ū′vē-ō-en-sef-ă-lī′tis). Uveoencefalite. SIN Harada syndrome.
uve·o·scle·ri·tis (ū′vē-ō-sklē-rī′tis). Uveoesclerite; inflamação da esclerótica envolvida por extensão a partir da úvea.
uvi·form (oo′vi-fōrm). Uviforme. SIN botryoid. [L. uva, uva, + forma, forma]
uvi·o·fast (ū′vē-ō-fast). Uviorresistente; não enfraquecido ou destruído pela radiação ultravioleta. SIN uvioresistant. [uviol (ultraviolet), + fast]
uvi·ol (ū′vē-ol). Uviol; um tipo especial de vidro mais transparente que o habitual aos raios ultravioleta ou actínicos, p. ex., quartzo cristalino. [ultra-violet]
uvi·om·e·ter (ū-vē-om′e-ter). Uviômetro; instrumento para medida da radiação ultravioleta. [uviol (ultraviolet) + meter]
uvi·o·re·sis·tant (ū′vē-ō-rē-zis′tant). Uviorresistente. SIN uviofast.
uvi·o·sen·si·tive (ū′vē-ō-sen′si-tiv). Uviossensível; sensível aos raios ultravioleta. [uviol (ultraviolet) + sensitive]
uvitex 2B. Uvitex 2B; um corante fluorescente que reage com a quitina; útil no diagnóstico de infecções por microsporídios ou criptosporídios.
uvo·mor·u·lin (ū-vō-mō′roo-lin). Uvomorulina; uma proteína transmembrana que une as membranas plasmáticas de células adjacentes de forma Ca^{2+}-dependente; ajuda a manter a rigidez da camada celular. SIN E-cadherin. [L. uva, cacho de uvas, + L. Mod. morula, dim. do L. morum, do G. moron, amora, + -in]
uvul-. VER uvulo-.
uvu·la, pl. **uvu·li** (ū-vū-lă, -lī) [TA]. Úvula; uma massa carnosa pendente; estrutura que possui semelhança imaginária com a u. palatina. [L. Mod. dim. de L. uva, uva, a úvula]
bifid u., u. bífica; bifurcação da u., constituindo uma fenda parcial do palato mole.
u. of bladder [TA], u. da bexiga; uma pequena projeção para a cavidade da bexiga, geralmente mais proeminente em homens idosos, logo atrás da abertura uretral, marcando a localização do lobo médio da próstata. SIN u. vesicae [TA], Lieutaud u.
u. cerebel'li, u. do cerebelo. SIN uvula [TA] of cerebellum.
uvula [TA] of cerebellum, u. do cerebelo; uma elevação triangular do verme do cerebelo, situada entre as duas amígdalas anteriores à pirâmide. SIN u. cerebelli, u. vermis.
Lieutaud u., u. de Lieutaud. SIN u. of bladder.
u. palati'na [TA], u. palatina. SIN u. of soft palate.

palatine u., u. palatina. SIN u. of soft palate.
u. of soft palate [TA], u. do palato mole; uma projeção cônica da borda posterior do meio do palato mole, composta de tecido conjuntivo contendo várias glândulas racemosas e algumas fibras musculares (músculo da úvula). SIN u. palatina [TA], palatine u., pendulous palate.
u. ver'mis, u. do verme. SIN uvula [TA] of cerebellum.
u. vesi'cae [TA]. u. vesical. SIN u. of bladder.
uvu·lap·to·sis (ū′vū - lap - tō′sis). Uvuloptose. SIN uvuloptosis.
uvu·lar (ū′vū - lăr). Uvular; relativo à úvula.
uvu·la·ris (ū′vū - lā′ris). Uvular. SIN muscle of uvula.
uvu·la·tome (ū′vū - lā - tōm). Uvulótomo. SIN uvulotome.
uvu·lec·to·my (ū - vū′lek′tō - mē). Uvulectomia; excisão da úvula. SIN staphylectomy. [uvula + G. *ektomē*, excisão]

uvu·li·tis (ū - vū - lī′tis). Uvulite; inflamação da úvula.
uvulo-, uvul-. A úvula. VER TAMBÉM staphylo-. [L. *uvula*]
uvu·lo·pal·a·to·pha·ryn·go·plas·ty (ū′vū - lō - pal′ă - tō - fa - rin′gō - plas - tē). Uvulopalatofaringoplastia. SIN palatopharyngoplasty.
uvu·lo·pal·a·to·plas·ty (ū′vū - lō - pal′ă - tō - plas - tē). Uvulopalatoplastia. SIN palatoplasty.
uvu·lop·to·sis (ū′vū - lop - tō′sis). Uvuloptose; relaxamento ou alongamento da úvula. SIN falling palate, staphylodialysis, staphyloptosis, uvulaptosis. [uvulo- + G. *ptōsis*, queda]
uvu·lo·tome (ū′vū - lō - tōm). Uvulótomo; instrumento para secção da úvula. SIN uvulatome.
uvu·lot·o·my (ū′vū - lot′ō - mē). Uvulotomia; qualquer cirurgia de secção da úvula. [uvulo- + G. *tomē*, corte]

V

V 1. Abreviatura para vision ou visual *acuity* (visão ou acuidade visual) volt; com subscrito 1, 2, 3, etc., a abreviatura para as derivações eletrocardiográficas unipolares. **2.** Símbolo de vanadium (vanádio); valine (valina); valyl (valil); volume (volume), freqüentemente com os subscritos indicando a localização, espécie química e/ou condições.
V̇ 1. Símbolo para o fluxo de gás, freqüentemente com os subscritos indicando a localização e a espécie química. VER flow (3). **2.** Símbolo para ventilation (3) (ventilação), freqüentemente com um subscrito. Ver entradas em ventilation (3). [volume + um ponto indicando o derivado do tempo]
V$_D$. Símbolo para physiologic dead *space* (espaço morto fisiológico).
V$_T$. Símbolo para tidal *volume* (volume corrente).
V̇$_{O_2}$. Símbolo para oxygen *consumption* (consumo de oxigênio).
V̇$_A$. Símbolo para alveolar *ventilation* (ventilação alveolar).
V̇$_{CO_2}$. Símbolo para carbon dioxide *elimination* (eliminação de dióxido de carbono).
V Abreviatura para volume (volume).
V$_{max}$ Símbolo para maximum *velocity* (velocidade máxima).
v 1. Abreviatura para volt (volt); initial rate velocity (velocidade inicial); velocity (velocidade); vel [L. ou]. **2.** Como um subscrito, refere-se ao venous *blood* (sangue venoso).
v̄. Como um subscrito, refere-se ao sangue venoso misto (arterial pulmonar).
VA Abreviatura para ventriculoatrial (ventriculoatrial).
VAC Abreviatura para ventriculoatrial *conduction* (condução ventriculoatrial).
vac·cen·ic ac·id (vak-sen′ik). Ácido vacênico; um ácido graxo insaturado cujos isômeros *cis* e *trans* são encontrados na manteiga e em outras gorduras animais.
vac·ci·na (vak-sin′ă). Vacina. SIN vaccinia.
vac·ci·nal (vak′si-năl). Vacinal; relativo à vacina ou vacinação.
vac·ci·nate (vak′si-nāt). Vacinar; administrar uma vacina.
vac·ci·na·tion (vak′si-nā′shŭn). Vacinação; o ato de administrar uma vacina.
vac·ci·na·tor (vak′si-nā-tŏr). Vacinador. **1.** Uma pessoa que vacina. SIN vaccinist. **2.** Um escarificador ou outro instrumento utilizado na vacinação.

VACCINE

vac·cine (vak′sēn, vak-sēn′). Vacina; originalmente, a v. de vírus vivo (vacínia) inoculada na pele como profilaxia contra a varíola e obtida a partir da pele de bezerros inoculados com vírus. O uso estendeu o significado para incluir essencialmente qualquer preparação destinada a profilaxia imunológica ativa; p.ex., as preparações de micróbios mortos de cepas virulentas ou de micróbios vivos de cepas atenuadas (variantes ou mutantes); ou produtos ou derivados de micróbios, de fungos, de vegetais, de protozoários ou de metazoários. O método de administração varia de acordo com a v., sendo a inoculação o mais comum, porém com a ingestão sendo preferida em alguns casos e o *spray* nasal sendo empregado ocasionalmente. SIN vaccinum. [L. *vaccinus*, relativo a uma vaca]
adjuvant v., v. adjuvante; uma v. que contém um adjuvante; o antígeno (imunógeno) é incluído em uma emulsão de água-em-óleo (adjuvante do tipo incompleto de Freund), ou adsorvido em um gel inorgânico (alume, fosfato ou hidróxido de alumínio) ou misturado a outro material para evitar a eliminação rápida pelo hospedeiro.
aqueous v., v. aquosa; uma v. que possui um veículo líquido (p.ex., solução salina fisiológica), diferente de uma emulsão.
attenuated v., v. atenuada; os patógenos vivos que perderam sua virulência mas ainda são capazes de induzir uma resposta imune protetora para as formas virulentas do patógeno, p.ex., Sabin para a pólio.
autogenous v., v. autógena; uma v. feita a partir dos microrganismos do próprio paciente.
bacillus Calmette-Guérin v., v. do bacilo de Calmette-Guérin. SIN BCG v.
BCG v., v. BCG; uma suspensão de uma cepa atenuada (bacilo de Calmette-Guérin) do *Mycobacterium tuberculosis*, tipo bovino, que é inoculada na pele para a profilaxia da tuberculose. SIN bacillus Calmette-Guérin v., Calmette-Guérin v., tuberculosis v.
brucella strain 19 v., v. contra a cepa 19 da brucela; uma v. de bactérias vivas preparadas a partir de uma cepa variante atenuada da *Brucella abortus* (cepa 19); usada para vacinar o gado contra a brucelose.
Calmette-Guérin v., v. de Calmette-Guérin. SIN BCG v.
cholera v., v. anticólera; uma suspensão inativada das cepas Inaba e Ogawa do *Vibrio cholerae* desenvolvida em ágar ou em caldo de cultura e preservada com fenol.
crystal violet v., v. de violeta cristal. VER hog cholera v.'s.
diphtheria toxoid, tetanus toxoid, and pertussis v. (DTP), v. antidiftérica, antitetânica e antipertussis; uma v. disponível em três formas: 1) toxóides diftérico e tetânico mais v. antipertussis (DTP); 2) toxóides tetânico e diftérico, do tipo adulto (Td); e 3) toxóide tetânico (T); usada para a imunização ativa contra difteria, tétano e coqueluche (pertussis).
duck embryo origin v. (DEV), v. anti-rábica. VER rabies v.
Flury strain v., v. contra a cepa Flury. VER rabies v., Flury strain egg-passage.
foot-and-mouth disease virus v.'s, vacinas antiaftosa; vacinas de vírus inativado a partir do epitélio da língua do gado infectado ou, mais recentemente, de vírus vivo atenuado por passagem em ovo embrionado ou camundongo e propagado em cultura de tecido.
***Haemophilus influenzae* type B v.,** v. contra *Haemophilus influenzae* do tipo B; um conjugado de oligossacarídeos do antígeno capsular do *H. influenzae* do tipo B e proteína CRM da difteria. SIN Hib v.
Haffkine v., v. de Haffkine; **(1)** uma cultura morta de *Vibrio cholerae* em duas potências: uma mais fraca, para a inoculação inicial, e uma mais forte, para a segunda inoculação 7 a 10 dias depois da primeira; **(2)** uma v. do bacilo da peste (*Yersinia pestis*) morto.
hepatitis B v., v. contra hepatite B; originalmente, uma v. inativada em formalina preparada a partir do antígeno de superfície (HBsAg) do vírus da hepatite B; o antígeno foi originalmente obtido a partir do plasma de portadores humanos do vírus; hoje em dia, nos Estados Unidos, o HBsAg purificado é preparado principalmente por tecnologia com DNA recombinante e, atualmente, é usado quase exclusivamente para imunização.
heterogenous v., v. heterógena; a v. que não é autógena, podendo ser preparada a partir de outras espécies de bactérias.
Hib v., v. contra Hib. SIN *Haemophilus influenzae* type B v.
high-egg-passage v., HEP v., v. anti-rábica. VER rabies v., Flury strain egg-passage.
hog cholera v.'s, vacinas anticólera suínas; vacinas do vírus do sangue de suíno infectado, inativado com cristal violeta, ou vírus vivo atenuado em coelhos ou cultura de tecido e freqüentemente utilizado em conjunto com o anti-soro do vírus da cólera suína.
human diploid cell v. (HDCV), v. anti-rábica preparada em célula diplóide humana; uma v. anti-rábica de vírus fixado usada para a proteção contra a raiva e preparada na célula diplóide humana WI-38. SIN human diploid cell rabies v.
human diploid cell rabies v. (HDCV), v. anti-rábica preparada em célula diplóide humana. SIN human diploid cell v.
inactivated poliovirus v. (IPV), v. de poliovírus inativado. VER poliovirus v.'s (2).
influenza virus v.'s, vacinas de vírus influenza; o vírus influenza desenvolvido em ovos embrionados e inativado, usualmente pela adição de formalina; são empregadas tanto preparações de vírus total como de subunidade viral, contendo hemaglutininas e neuraminidase; por causa da variação antigênica acentuada e progressiva dos vírus influenza, as cepas incluídas mudam regularmente após vários surtos de *influenza*, de modo a incluir as cepas epidêmicas de vírus influenza dos tipos A e B isoladas mais recentemente.
live v., v. viva; v. preparada a partir de microrganismos vivos e atenuados.
live oral poliovirus v., v. de poliovírus vivo oral. VER poliovirus v.'s (2).
low-egg-passage v., LEP v., v. com baixa passagem por ovo. VER rabies v., Flury strain egg-passage.
measles, mumps, and rubella v. (MMR), v. anti-sarampo, anticaxumba e anti-rubéola; uma combinação de vírus vivos atenuados do sarampo, caxumba e rubéola em uma suspensão aquosa; usada para a imunização contra as respectivas doenças.
measles virus v., v. anti-sarampo; a v. que contém cepas vivas atenuadas do vírus do sarampo em cultura de células de embrião de pinto. VER measles, mumps, and rubella v.
multivalent v., v. multivalente. SIN polyvalent v.
mumps virus v., v. anticaxumba; v. que contém vírus vivo e atenuado da caxumba preparada em culturas de células de embrião de pinto. VER measles, mumps, and rubella v.
oil v., v. adjuvante. VER adjuvant v.

△ Formas Combinantes
🗒 Indica que o termo é ilustrado, ver Índice de Ilustrações
SIN Sinônimo
Cf. Comparar, confrontar
[NA] *Nomina Anatomica*
[TA] *Terminologia Anatomica*

☆ Termo oficial alternativo para a *Terminologia Anatomica*
[MIM] Mendelian Inheritance in Man
I.C. Índice de Corantes

Termo de Alta Importância

oral poliovirus v. (OPV), v. oral contra poliovírus. VER poliovirus v.'s (2).
Pasteur v., v. anti-rábica. VER rabies v.
pertussis v., v. antipertussis. VER diphtheria toxoid, tetanus toxoid, and pertussis v.
plague v., v. contra a peste; v. (liberada para uso nos Estados Unidos) preparada a partir de culturas da *Yersinia pestis*, inativada com formaldeído e preservada com fenol a 0,5%; as injeções são administradas por via intramuscular, sendo as inoculações de reforço recomendadas a cada 6–12 meses, enquanto os indivíduos permanecerem em uma área de risco; também existem vacinas obtidas por fracionamento químico e com bactérias vivas atenuadas.
pneumococcal v., v. pneumocócica; a v. composta de antígeno polissacarídico capsular purificado a partir de 23 tipos de *Streptococcus pneumoniae* (representando aqueles tipos responsáveis pela maioria das doenças pneumocócicas notificadas nos Estados Unidos); alguns tipos foram conjugados com proteína para se tornarem antigênicos para crianças com menos de 2 anos de idade.
poliomyelitis v.'s, vacinas contra a poliomielite. SIN poliovirus v.'s.
poliovirus v.'s, vacinas contra poliovírus; (1) v. com poliovírus inativado (IPV), uma suspensão aquosa de cepas inativadas do vírus da poliomielite (tipos 1, 2 e 3) usada por injeção; foi substituída em grande parte pela v. oral. VER Salk v.; (2) v. oral contra poliovírus (OPV), uma suspensão aquosa de cepas vivas atenuadas de vírus da poliomielite (tipos 1, 2 e 3) fornecida por via oral para a imunização ativa contra a poliomielite. VER Sabin v. SIN poliomyelitis v.'s.
polysaccharide conjugated v., v. de polissacarídeo conjugado; uma v. feita de polissacarídeo capsular do microrganismo conjugado com uma proteína, como a vacina para o *Haemophilus influenzae* do tipo B contra a meningite.
polyvalent v., v. polivalente; uma v. preparada a partir de culturas de duas ou mais cepas da mesma espécie ou microrganismo. SIN multivalent v.
rabies v., v. anti-rábica; uma v. introduzida por Pasteur como um método de tratamento para uma mordida de um animal raivoso: eram fornecidas injeções diárias (14–21) de vírus que aumentavam em série, desde o vírus "fixo" não-infeccioso até o totalmente infeccioso, de modo a tornar o sistema nervoso central refratário à infecção pelo vírus virulento; essa v., com uma modificação apenas discreta (p.ex., v. Semple), foi empregada durante muitos anos, mas tinha o grave defeito de que a grande quantidade de tecido nervoso heterólogo inoculado junto com o vírus originava, ocasionalmente, desmielinização alérgica (imunológica). Ela foi substituída, no caso dos seres humanos, pela vacina anti-rábica originária do embrião de pato (DEV), preparada a partir de ovos de pato embrionados infectados por vírus "fixo" e inativada com β-propiolactona. Atualmente, a DEV foi substituída pela v. preparada em células diplóides humanas (HDCV), que é desenvolvida em células WI-38, ou v. anti-rábica adsorvida (RVA), que é desenvolvida em células de feto de macaco *Rhesus*. Elas são inativadas e possuem uma baixa incidência de reações adversas, exigindo um menor número de injeções.
rabies v., Flury strain egg-passage, v. anti-rábica, da cepa Flury com passagem em ovo; (1) v. com alta passagem por ovo (HEP): o vírus vivo da raiva da cepa Flury entre o 180.º e o 190.º níveis de passagem em ovo (ovos embrionados), usado para a vacinação do gado e de gatos; (2) v. com baixa passagem por ovo (LEP): entre o 40.º e o 50.º níveis de passagem, contendo 10^3–10^4 LD$_{50}$ em camundongo; não-patogênica em cães, mas retém alguma patogenicidade para gado bovino e gatos.
rickettsia v., attenuated, v. anti-riquétsia atenuada. VER typhus v.
Rocky Mountain spotted fever v., v. contra a febre maculosa das Montanhas Rochosas; suspensão de *Rickettsia rickettsii* preparada por meio do crescimento de riquétsias em saco vitelino embrionado de ovos de aves.
rubella virus v., live, v. de vírus de rubéola vivo; uma v. de vírus vivo originalmente preparada a partir de embriões de pato (HPV77), mas atualmente preparada a partir de culturas de células diplóides humanas infectadas pelo vírus da rubéola (RA27/3); administrada como uma injeção subcutânea única. VER measles, mumps, and rubella v.
Sabin v., v. Sabin; uma v. administrada por via oral, contendo cepas de poliovírus vivos atenuados. VER poliovirus v.'s.
Salk v., v. Salk; a v. contra poliovírus original, composta de vírus propagado em cultura de tecido de macaco *Rhesus* e inativado. VER poliovirus v.'s.
Semple v., v. Semple; uma modificação da v. anti-rábica original (Pasteur) outrora amplamente utilizada nos Estados Unidos, preparada a partir do tecido nervoso de coelho, inativada com fenol e administrada em 14 a 21 injeções diárias; possui potência variável e está associada a uma alta incidência de desmielinização pós-vacinal.
smallpox v., v. antivariólica; v. de suspensões de vírus de vacínia preparada a partir de lesões cutâneas de vacínia de bezerros (linfa de bezerros) ou originária de embrião de pinto; atualmente não é usada por causa da erradicação mundial da varíola.
split-virus v., v. de subunidade. VER subunit v.
staphylococcus v., v. estafilocócica; uma suspensão de microrganismos a partir de culturas de uma ou mais cepas de *Staphylococcus*; usada para furunculose, acne e outras condições supurativas.
stock v., v. preparada a partir de uma cepa microbiana estocada, diferente da v. autógena.

subunit v., v. de subunidade; uma v. que, através de extração química, não tem ácido nucleico viral e contém apenas subunidades específicas de determinado vírus; essas vacinas são relativamente livres de reações adversas (p.ex., vírus influenza) associadas às vacinas que contêm o vírion total.
T.A.B. v., v. contra febres tifóide-paratifóide A e B. SIN typhoid-paratyphoid A e B v.
tetanus v., v. antitetânica. VER diphtheria toxoid, tetanus toxoid, and pertussis v.
tuberculosis v., v. contra tuberculose. SIN BCG v.
typhoid v., v. contra febre tifóide; uma suspensão de *Salmonella typhi* inativada por calor ou por substância química (acetona) com adição de conservante; nos Estados Unidos, as vacinas tifóide e paratifóide A e B combinadas foram substituídas, em grande parte, pela v. tifóide monovalente por causa da falta de evidências de efetividade dos ingredientes paratifóide A e B.
typhoid-paratyphoid A and B v., v. contra febres tifóide-paratifóide A e B; uma suspensão de bacilos tifóide e paratifóide A e B mortos. VER TAMBÉM typhoid v. SIN T.A.B. v.
typhus v., v. do tifo; uma suspensão de *Rickettsia prowazekii* inativada em formaldeído desenvolvida em ovos embrionados; efetiva contra o tifo transmitido por piolho (epidêmico); a imunização primária consiste em duas injeções subcutâneas com intervalo de 4 ou mais semanas; as doses de reforço são necessárias a cada 6 a 12 meses, enquanto existir a possibilidade de exposição. Uma v. que contém riquétsias vivas de uma cepa atenuada de *R. prowazekii* também tem sido utilizada.
whooping-cough v., v. antipertussis. VER diphtheria toxoid, tetanus toxoid, and pertussis v.
yellow fever v., v. contra a febre amarela; (1) uma cepa viva e atenuada (17D) de vírus da febre amarela em ovos de aves embrionados; (2) uma suspensão de cérebro seco de camundongo infectado com a cepa neurotrópica francesa (Dakar) do vírus da febre amarela, administrada topicamente pelo método da escarificação; não recomendada oficialmente nos Estados Unidos por causa das reações meningoencefalíticas.

vac·cin·i·a (vak-sin′ē-ă). Vacínia; uma infecção, principalmente local e limitada ao local da inoculação, induzida em seres humanos através da inoculação com o vírus da v., a espécie típica no gênero Orthopoxvirus (família Poxviridae), a fim de conferir resistência à varíola. Em torno do terceiro dia depois dessa vacinação, formam-se pápulas no local da inoculação, que se transformam em vesículas umbilicadas e, mais adiante, em pústulas; em seguida, elas secam e a crosta se desprende em torno do 21.º dia, deixando uma cicatriz deprimida; em alguns casos, existem distúrbios constitucionais mais ou menos acentuados. Por causa da erradicação global da varíola, a vacinação de rotina não é atualmente praticada. SIN primary reaction, vaccina, variola vaccine, variola vaccinia. [L. *vaccinus*, relativo a uma vaca, de *vacca*, uma vaca.]
v. gangreno′sa, v. gangrenosa. SIN progressive v.
generalized v., v. generalizada; lesões secundárias da pele após a vacinação, que podem ocorrer em pessoas com pele previamente saudável; contudo, são mais comuns no caso de pele traumatizada, especialmente no caso de eczema (*eczema vaccinatum*). No último caso, a v. generalizada pode resultar do simples contato com uma pessoa vacinada. As lesões secundárias da vacínia também podem ocorrer após a transferência do vírus do local da vacinação para outro local através dos dedos das mãos.
progressive v., v. progressiva; uma forma grave ou, até mesmo, fatal de v. que acontece principalmente nas pessoas com deficiência imunológica ou discrasia, sendo caracterizada por aumento progressivo das lesões iniciais e, também, das lesões secundárias. SIN v. gangrenosa.
variola v., vacínia. SIN vaccinia.
vac·cin·i·al (vak-sin′ē-ăl). Vacinial; relativo à vacínia.
vac·cin·i·form (vak-sin′i-fōrm). Vaciniforme; que se assemelha à vacínia.
vac·ci·nist (vak′si-nist). Vacinador. SIN vaccinator (1).
vac·cin·i·za·tion (vak′sin-i-zā′shŭn). Vacinização; vacinação repetida em intervalos curtos até que não seja mais necessária.
vac·cin·o·gen (vak-sin′ō-jen). Vacinógeno; uma fonte de vacina, como uma novilha inoculada.
vac·ci·nog·e·nous (vak-si-noj′ē-nŭs). Vacinógeno; que produz vacina ou relativo à produção de vacina.
vac·ci·noid (vak′si-noyd). Vacinóide; que se assemelha à vacínia.
vac·ci·no·style (vak′si-nō-stīl). Vacinostilo; um instrumento pontiagudo utilizado na vacinação.
vac·ci·num (vak′si-nŭm). Vacina. SIN vaccine. [L.]
vac·u·o·lar (vak-oo-ō′lăr). Vacuolar; relativo ou semelhante a um vacúolo.
vac·u·o·late, vac·u·o·lat·ed (vak′oo-ō-lāt, -lāt′ed). Vacuolado; que possui vacúolos.
vac·u·o·la·tion (vak′oo-ō-lā′shŭn). Vacuolação. **1.** Formação de vacúolos. **2.** A condição de possuir vacúolos. SIN vacuolization.
vac·u·ole (vak′oo-ōl). Vacúolo. **1.** Um espaço diminuto em qualquer tecido. **2.** Um espaço claro na substância de uma célula, por vezes de caráter degenerativo, por vezes circundando um corpo estranho englobado e servindo como

um estômago temporário da célula para a digestão do corpo. [L. mod. *vacuolum*, dim. do L. *vacuum*, um espaço vazio]

autophagic v., v. autofágico. SIN cytolysosome.

contractile v., v. contrátil; uma cavidade formada pelo acúmulo de líquido no ectoplasma de um protozoário; depois de aumentar durante um tempo, ele se esvazia externamente por uma contração súbita; funciona como um mecanismo osmorregulador para o equilíbrio hídrico, especialmente nos protozoários de água doce.

digestive v., v. digestivo. SIN secondary lysosomes, em lysosome.

parasitophorous v., v. parasitóforo; um v. formado por camadas do retículo endoplasmático ao redor de um parasita intracelular, o qual pode servir para isolar o parasita e englobá-lo para o ataque lisossomal.

vac·u·o·li·za·tion (vak′oo-o-li-zā′shŭn). Vacuolização. SIN vacuolation.

vac·u·ome (vak′oo-ōm). Vacuoma; um sistema de vacúolos que podem ser corados com vermelho neutro na célula viva. [vacuole + G. *-oma*, tumor]

vac·u·um (vak′oom). Vácuo; um espaço vazio, aquele praticamente sem ar ou gás. [L. neut. de *vacuus*, vazio]

va·dum (vā′dŭm). Uma elevação ocasional a partir do fundo de um sulco cerebral, quase obliterando-o por uma curta distância. [L. uma eminência]

va·gal (vā′găl). Vagal; relativo ao nervo vago.

va·gec·to·my (va-jek′tō-mē). Vagectomia; remoção cirúrgica de segmento de um nervo vago.

va·gi (vā′gī, -jī). Vagos; plural de vagus.

vagin-. VER vagino-.

va·gi·na, gen. e pl. **va·gi·nae** (vă-jī′nă, -nē). Vagina. **1.** Bainha. SIN sheath (1). **2** [TA]. O canal genital na mulher, estendendo-se do útero até a vulva. [L. bainha, a vagina]

bipartite v., b. bipartida. SIN septate v.

v. bul′bi [TA], b. do bulbo do olho. SIN fascial sheath of eyeball.

v. carot′ica [TA], b. carótica. SIN carotid sheath.

v. cellulo′sa, b. celulosa; a b. de tecido conjuntivo de um nervo ou músculo (perineuro ou perimísio, respectivamente).

v. communis ten′dinum musculo′rum fibularium commu′nis [TA], b. comum dos tendões dos músculos fibulares. SIN common peroneal tendon sheath.

v. commu′nis tendinum musculo′rum flexo′rum (manus) [TA], b. comum dos tendões dos músculos flexores (da mão). SIN common flexor sheath (of hand).

v. exter′na ner′vi op′tici [TA], b. externa do nervo óptico. SIN outer sheath of optic nerve.

vagi′nae fibro′sae digito′rum ma′nus [TA], bainhas fibrosas dos dedos da mão. SIN fibrous sheaths of digits of hand, em sheath. VER anular part of fibrous digital sheath of digits of hand and foot, cruciform part of fibrous digital sheath.

vagi′nae fibro′sae digito′rum pe′dis [TA], bainhas fibrosas dos dedos do pé. SIN fibrous digital sheaths of toes, em sheath. VER anular part of fibrous digital sheath of digits of hand and foot, cruciform part of fibrous digital sheath.

v. fibro′sa ten′dinis, b. fibrosa do tendão. SIN fibrous tendon sheath.

v. inter′na ner′vi op′tici [TA], b. interna do nervo óptico. SIN inner sheath of optic nerve.

v. masculi′na, utrículo prostático. SIN prostatic utricle.

v. muco′sa ten′dinis, b. do tendão sinovial. SIN synovial tendon sheath.

v. mus′culi rec′ti abdo′minis [TA], b. do músculo reto do abdome. SIN rectus sheath.

vagi′nae ner′vi op′tici, bainhas do nervo óptico; as bainhas do nervo óptico, formadas por extensões das meninges centrais. VER inner sheath of optic nerve, external sheath of optic nerve.

v. oc′uli, b. do bulbo do olho. SIN fascial sheath of eyeball.

v. proces′sus styloi′dei [TA], b. do processo estilóide. SIN sheath of styloid process.

septate v., b. septada; uma b. bipartida causada pela presença de um septo longitudinal mais ou menos completo. SIN bipartite v.

vagi′nae synovia′les digito′rum ma′nus [TA], bainhas sinoviais dos dedos da mão. SIN synovial sheaths of digits of hand, em sheath.

v. synovia′lis [TA], b. sinovial. SIN synovial sheath.

v. synovia′lis ten′dinis [TA], b. sinovial tendínea. SIN synovial tendon sheath.

v. synovia′lis troch′leae, b. tendínea do músculo oblíquo superior. SIN tendinous sheath of superior oblique muscle.

vaginae tendinum carpalium [TA], bainhas dos tendões do carpo. SIN carpal tendinous sheaths, em sheath.

vaginae tendinum carpalium dorsalium [TA], bainhas dos tendões dorsais do carpo. SIN dorsal carpal tendinous sheaths, em sheath.

v. ten′dinis intertubercula′ris [TA], b. tendínea intertubercular. SIN intertubercular tendon sheath.

v. ten′dinis mus′culi extenso′ris car′pi ulna′ris [TA], b. dos tendões dos músculos extensores radiais do carpo. SIN tendinous sheath of extensor carpi ulnaris muscle.

v. ten′dinis mus′culi extenso′ris dig′iti min′imi [TA], b. do tendão do músculo extensor do dedo mínimo. SIN tendinous sheath of extensor digiti minimi muscle.

v. ten′dinis mus′culi extenso′ris hal′lucis lon′gi [TA], b. do tendão do músculo extensor longo do hálux. SIN tendinous sheath of extensor hallucis longus muscle.

v. ten′dinis mus′culi extenso′ris pol′licis lon′gi [TA], b. do tendão do músculo extensor longo do polegar. SIN tendinous sheath of extensor pollicis longus muscle.

v. tendinis musculi fibularis longi plantaris [TA], b. do tendão plantar do músculo fibular longo. SIN plantar tendon sheath of fibularis longus muscle.

v. ten′dinis mus′culi flexo′ris car′pi radia′lis [TA], b. do tendão do músculo flexor radial do carpo. SIN tendinous sheath of flexor carpi radialis muscle.

v. ten′dinis mus′culi flexo′ris hal′lucis lon′gi [TA], b. do tendão do músculo flexor longo do hálux. SIN tendinous sheath of flexor hallucis longus muscle.

v. ten′dinis mus′culi flexo′ris pol′licis lon′gi [TA], b. do tendão do músculo flexor longo do polegar. SIN tendinous sheath of flexor pollicis longus muscle.

v. ten′dinis mus′culi obli′qui superio′ris [TA], b. tendínea do músculo oblíquo superior. SIN tendinous sheath of superior oblique muscle.

v. ten′dinis mus′culi perone′i lon′gi planta′ris, b. do tendão plantar do músculo fibular longo; *termo oficial alternativo para plantar tendon sheath of fibularis longus muscle.

v. ten′dinis mus′culi tibia′lis anterio′ris [TA], b. do tendão do músculo tibial anterior. SIN tendinous sheath of tibialis anterior muscle.

v. ten′dinis mus′culi tibia′lis posterio′ris [TA], b. do tendão do músculo tibial posterior. SIN tendinous sheath of tibialis posterior muscle.

vaginae tendinum carpales palmares [TA], bainhas dos tendões palmares do carpo. SIN palmar carpal tendinous sheaths, em sheath.

vagi′nae tendinum digito′rum pe′dis [TA], bainhas dos tendões dos dedos dos pé. SIN synovial sheaths of toes, em sheath.

v. ten′dinum mus′culi extenso′ris digito′rum pe′dis lon′gi [TA], b. do tendão do músculo extensor longo dos dedos do pé. SIN tendinous sheath of extensor digitorum longus muscle of foot.

v. ten′dinum mus′culi flexo′ris digito′rum pe′dis lon′gi [TA], b. do tendão do músculo flexor longo dos dedos do pé. SIN tendinous sheath of flexor digitorum longus muscle (of foot).

v. ten′dinum musculo′rum abducto′ris lon′gi et extenso′ris bre′vis pol′licis [TA], b. dos tendões dos músculos abdutor longo e extensor curto do polegar. SIN tendinous sheath of abductor pollicis longus and extensor pollicis brevis muscles.

v. ten′dinum musculo′rum extenso′ris digitor′um et extenso′ris in′dicis [TA], b. dos tendões dos músculos extensor dos dedos e extensor do indicador. SIN tendinous sheath of extensor digitorum and extensor indicis muscles.

v. ten′dinum musculo′rum extenso′rum car′pi radia′lium [TA], b. do tendão dos músculos extensores radiais do carpo. SIN tendinous sheath of extensor carpi radialis muscles.

v. ten′dinum musculo′rum fibula′rium commu′nis, b. comum dos músculos fibulares. SIN common peroneal tendon sheath.

v. tendinum musculo′rum peroneo′rum commu′nis, b. comum do tendão dos músculos fibulares. SIN common peroneal tendon sheath.

vaginae ten′dinum tarsa′les ante′riores [TA], bainhas dos tendões anteriores do tarso. SIN anterior tarsal tendinous sheaths, em sheath.

vaginae ten′dinum tarsa′les fibula′res [TA], bainhas dos tendões fibulares do tarso. SIN fibular tarsal tendinous sheaths, em sheath.

vaginae ten′dinum tarsa′les tibia′lis [TA], bainhas dos tendões tibiais do tarso. SIN tibial tarsal tendinous sheaths, em sheath.

vagi′nae vaso′rum, bainhas vasculares. SIN vascular sheaths, em sheath.

vag·i·nal (vaj′i-năl). Vaginal; relativo à vagina ou a qualquer bainha. [L. mod. *vaginalis*]

va·gi·na·pexy (va-jī′nă-pek-sē). Vaginopexia. SIN vaginofixation.

vag·i·nate (vaj′i-nāt). Invaginar. **1.** Embainhar; envolver em uma bainha. **2.** Embainhado; provido com uma bainha.

vag·i·nec·to·my (vaj-i-nek′tō-mē). Vaginectomia; excisão da vagina ou de um segmento desta. SIN colpectomy. [vagina + G. *ektomē*, excisão]

vag·i·nism (vaj′i-nizm). Vaginismo. SIN vaginismus.

vag·i·nis·mus (vaj-i-niz′mŭs). Vaginismo; espasmo doloroso da vagina que impede a relação sexual. SIN vaginism, vulvismus. [vagina + L. *-ismus*, ação, condição]

posterior v., v. posterior; estenose espasmódica da vagina causada por contração do músculo elevador do ânus.

vag·i·ni·tis, pl. **vag·i·ni·ti·des** (vaj-i-nī′tis, -nī′ti-dēz). Vaginite; inflamação da vagina. [vagina + G. *-itis*, inflamação]

v. adhesi′va, v. adesiva. SIN adhesive v.

adhesive v., v. adesiva; inflamação da mucosa vaginal com aderências das paredes vaginais entre elas. SIN v. adhesiva.

amebic v., v. amebiana; v. causada por *Entamoeba histolytica*.

atrophic v., v. atrófica; adelgaçamento e atrofia do epitélio vaginal resultando comumente da redução da estimulação por estrogênio: comum após a menopausa.

v. cys′tica, v. cística. SIN v. emphysematosa.

desquamative inflammatory v., v. inflamatória descamativa; inflamação aguda da vagina de etiologia desconhecida, caracterizada por pseudomembrana acinzentada, corrimento e sangramento fácil perante o traumatismo; o corrimento contém pus e células epiteliais imaturas, embora os níveis de estrogênio sejam normais.
v. emphysemato'sa, v. enfisematosa; v. caracterizada por acúmulo de gás nos pequenos espaços do tecido conjuntivo revestidos por células gigantes do tipo corpo estranho. SIN pachyvaginitis cystica, v. cystica.
***Gardnerella* v.,** v. por *Gardnerella*. SIN bacterial *vaginosis*.
nonspecific v., v. inespecífica. SIN bacterial *vaginosis*.
pinworm v., v. por oxiúro; v. causada por *Enterobius vermicularis*.
senile v., v. senil; v. atrófica resultante da retirada da estimulação da mucosa por estrogênio, assumindo, com freqüência, a forma de v. adesiva. SIN v. senilis.
v. seni'lis, v. senil. SIN senile v.

♻ **vagino-, vagin-.** Formas combinantes que designam a vagina. VER TAMBÉM colpo-. [L. *vagina*, bainha]
vag·i·no·ab·dom·i·nal (vaj'i-nō-ab-dom'i-nǎl). Vaginoabdominal; relativo à vagina e ao abdome.
vag·i·no·cele (vaj'i-nō-sēl). Vaginocele. SIN colpocele (1).
vag·i·no·dyn·ia (vaj'i-nō-din'ē-ǎ). Vaginodinia; dor vaginal. SIN colpodynia.
vag·i·no·fix·a·tion (vaj'i-nō-fik-sā'shŭn). Vaginofixação; a sutura de uma vagina relaxada ou prolapsada à parede abdominal. SIN colpopexy, vaginapexy, vaginopexy.
vag·i·no·hys·ter·ec·to·my (vaj'i-nō-his-ter-ek'tō-mē). Vagino-histerectomia. SIN vaginal hysterectomy.
vag·i·no·la·bi·al (vaj'i-nō-lā'bē-ǎl). Vaginolabial; relativo à vagina e aos lábios do pudendo.
vag·i·no·my·co·sis (vaj'i-nō-mī-kō'sis). Vaginomicose; infecção vaginal provocada por um fungo. SIN colpomycosis.
vag·i·nop·a·thy (vaj-i-nop'ǎ-thē). Vaginopatia; qualquer condição patológica da vagina. [vagino- + G. *pathos*, sofrimento]
vag·i·no·per·i·ne·al (vaj'i-nō-per-i-nē'ǎl). Vaginoperineal; relativo a ou que envolve a vagina e o períneo.
vag·i·no·per·i·ne·o·plas·ty (vaj'i-nō-per-i-nē'ō-plas-tē). Vaginoperineoplastia; a cirurgia plástica do períneo que envolve a vagina. SIN colpoperineoplasty. [vagino- + perineum, + G. *plastos*, formado]
vag·i·no·per·i·ne·or·rha·phy (vaj'i-nō-per-i-nē-ōr'ǎ-fē). Vaginoperineorrafia; reparação de vagina e períneo lacerados. SIN colpoperineorrhaphy. [vagino- + perineum, + G. *rhaphē*, sutura]
vag·i·no·per·i·ne·ot·o·my (vaj'i-nō-per-i-nē-ot'ō-mē). Vaginoperineotomia. SIN episiotomy. [vagino- + perineum, + G. *tomē*, incisão]
vag·i·no·per·i·to·ne·al (vaj'i-nō-per-i-tō-nē'ǎl). Vaginoperitoneal; relativo à vagina e ao peritônio.
vag·i·no·pexy (vaj'i-nō-pek-sē). Vaginopexia. SIN vaginofixation.
vag·i·no·plas·ty (vaj'i-nō-plas-tē). Vaginoplastia; cirurgia plástica da vagina. SIN colpoplasty. [vagino- + G. *plastos*, formado]
vag·i·nos·co·py (vaj-i-nos'kŏ-pē). Vaginoscopia; inspeção da vagina, comumente por meio de um instrumento.
vag·in·o·sis (vǎ'jin-ō'sis). Vaginose; doença da vagina.
bacterial v., v. bacteriana; a infecção da vagina humana que pode ser causada por bactérias anaeróbicas, especialmente por espécies de *Mobiluncus* ou por *Gardnerella vaginalis*. Caracterizada por corrimento excessivo, por vezes fétido. SIN *Gardnerella* vaginitis, nonspecific vaginitis.
vag·i·not·o·my (vaj-i-not'ō-mē). Vaginotomia. SIN colpotomy.
vag·i·no·ves·i·cal (vaj'i-nō-ves'i-kǎl). Vaginovesical; relativo à vagina e à bexiga urinária.
vag·i·no·vul·var (vaj'i-nō-vŭl'vǎr). Vaginovulvar; relativo à vagina e à vulva.
Va·gin·u·lus ple·be·i·us (vaj-i-noo'lŭs plē'bē-ē-ŭs). O molusco vetor do *Angiostrongylus costaricensis*.
va·gi·tus uter·i·nus (va-jī'tŭs ū-ter-ī'nŭs). Vagido uterino; o choro do feto quando ainda dentro do útero, possível quando as membranas foram rompidas e o ar penetrou na cavidade uterina. [L. de *vagio*, vagir; L. de *uterus*, útero]
vago-. Forma combinante relativa ao nervo vago. [L. *vagus*]
♻ **va·go·ac·ces·so·ri·us** (vā-gō-ak-ses-sō'rē-ŭs). Vagoacessório; o nervo vago e a raiz craniana (porção acessória) do nervo acessório, considerados como um só nervo. VER accessory *nerve* [CN XI].
va·go·glos·so·pha·ryn·ge·al (vā-gō-glos'ō-fǎ-rin'jē-ǎl). Vagoglossofaríngeo; relativo aos nervos vago e glossofaríngeo; indica seus núcleos contínuos ou comuns de origem e terminação e as regiões inervadas por ambos os nervos, como a musculatura da faringe.
va·gol·y·sis (vā-gol'i-sis). Vagólise; destruição cirúrgica do nervo vago. [vago- + G. *lysis*, uma desintegração]
va·go·lyt·ic (vā-gō-lit'ik). Vagolítico. **1.** Pertinente a ou que causa vagólise. **2.** Um agente terapêutico ou químico que apresenta efeitos inibitórios sobre o nervo vago. **3.** Indica um agente que possui esses efeitos.

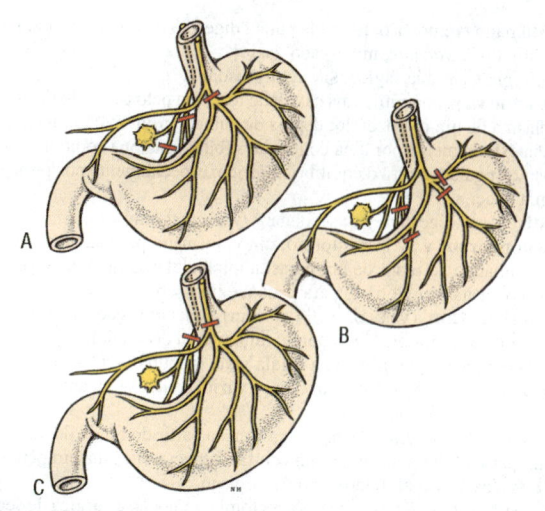

vagotomia: (A) gástrica seletiva, (B) proximal seletiva, (C) troncular

va·go·mi·met·ic (vā'gō-mi-met'ik). Vagomimético; que imita a ação das fibras eferentes do nervo vago.
ℹ **va·got·o·my** (vā-got'ō-mē). Vagotomia; divisão do nervo vago. [vago- + G. *tomē*, incisão]
va·go·to·nia (vā-gō-tō'nē-ǎ). Vagotonia; designação obsoleta para uma condição em que o sistema nervoso parassimpático está supostamente hiperativo. SIN parasympathotonia, sympathetic imbalance. [vago- + G. *tonos*, tensão]
va·go·ton·ic (vā-gō-ton'ik). Vagotônico; relativo a ou marcado por vagotonia.
va·go·tro·pic (vā-gō-trop'ik). Vagotrópico; atraído pelo nervo vago, atuando sobre ele. [vago- + G. *tropos*, volta]
va·go·va·gal (vā'gō-vā'gǎl). Vagovagal; pertinente a um processo que utiliza as fibras vagais aferentes e eferentes.
va·gus, gen. e pl. **va·gi** (vā'gŭs; vā'gī, -jī). Vago. SIN vagus *nerve* [CN X]. [L. vaguear, assim chamado por causa da ampla distribuição do nervo]
Val Símbolo para valine (valina) e valyl (valil).
va·lence, va·len·cy (vā'lens, -len-sē). Valência; o poder de combinação de um átomo de um elemento (ou radical), sendo a valência do átomo de hidrogênio usada como unidade de comparação, determinado pelo número de elétrons na camada externa do átomo (elétrons de v.); p.ex., no HCl, o cloro é monovalente; no H_2O, o oxigênio é bivalente; no NH_3, o nitrogênio é trivalente. [L. *valentia*, força]
negative v., v. negativa; o número de elétrons de v. que um átomo consegue captar.
positive v., v. positiva; o número de elétrons de v. que um átomo pode ceder.
va·lent (vā'lent). Valente; que possui valência.
Valentin, Gabriel G., fisiologista alemão-suíço, 1810–1883. VER V. *corpuscles*, em *corpuscle, ganglion, nerve*.
Valentine, Ferdinand C., cirurgião norte-americano, 1851–1909. VER V. *position, test*.
va·lep·o·tri·ates (val'ē-pō'trē-āts). Valepotriatos; uma classe de alcalóides iridóides oriundos de *Valeriana* sp. e *Kentranthus* sp.; p.ex., a substância valtrato é um membro dessa classe.
val·er·ate (val'ē-rāt). Valerato; um sal do ácido valérico; alguns são usados na medicina moderna. SIN valerianate.
va·le·ri·an (vā-lēr'ē-an). Valeriana. **1.** O rizoma e as raízes da *Valeriana officinalis* (família Valerianaceae), uma planta nativa do sul da Europa e norte da Ásia, cultivada também na Grã-Bretanha e nos Estados Unidos; tem sido empregada como sedativo na histeria e na menopausa. **2.** Que se refere a uma classe de alcalóides terpenos obtidos a partir da v. (1). SIN vandal root.
va·le·ri·a·nate (va-lēr'ē-ǎ-nāt). Valerianato. SIN valerate.
va·le·ric ac·id (vā-lēr'ik, vǎ-ler'ik). Ácido valérico; ácido alifático normal, destilado a partir da valeriana; alguns de seus sais são utilizados em medicina; encontrado no colo humano. SIN pentanoic acid.
va·leth·a·mate bro·mide (vā-leth'ǎ-māt). Brometo de valetamato; um agente anticolinérgico.
val·e·tu·di·nar·i·an (val'ē-too-di-nār'ē-an). Valetudinário. **1.** Uma pessoa inválida ou com a saúde cronicamente deficiente. **2.** Aquele cuja principal preocupação é com sua invalidez ou saúde deficiente. [L. *valetudinarius*, doentio]
val·e·tu·di·nar·i·an·ism (val'ē-too-di-nār'ē-an-izm). Valetudinarianismo; um estado fraco ou enfermo devido à invalidez.

val·goid (val'goyd). Valgóide; relativo ao valgo; que tem joelho valgo; que sofre de talipe valgo. [L. *valgus*, com arqueamento das pernas, + G. *eidos*, semelhança]

val·gus (val'gŭs). Valgo; curvo ou rodado para fora a partir da linha média do corpo; o uso moderno aceito, particularmente em ortopedia, transpõe erroneamente o significado de varo para v., como no *genu* valgum (joelho valgo). [L. mod. virado para fora, do L. com as pernas arqueadas]

val·id. Válido; efetivo; que produz o resultado desejado; verificavelmente correto. [L. *valeo*, ser forte]

val·i·da·tion (val-i-dā'shŭn). Validação; o ato ou processo de tornar válido.
   consensual v., v. consensual; a confirmação da experiência ou julgamento de uma pessoa por outra.

va·lid·i·ty (vă-lid'i-tē). Validade; um índice de quão bem um teste ou procedimento mede, realmente, aquilo que ele se propõe a medir; um índice objetivo através do qual se descreve como é válido um teste ou procedimento.
   concurrent v., v. concomitante; um índice de v. relacionado ao critério usado para predizer o desempenho em uma situação de vida real, fornecido aproximadamente junto como um teste ou procedimento; a extensão em que o índice de um teste se correlaciona com aquele de um teste ou índice diferente; p.ex., quão bem um escore em um teste de aptidão se correlaciona com o escore em um teste de inteligência.
   construct v., v. construída; a extensão com que um teste ou procedimento parece medir uma ordem superior, construção teórica inferida ou traço, em contraste com a medição de uma dimensão específica mais limitada.
   content v., v. de conteúdo; a extensão em que os itens de um teste ou procedimento constituem, na realidade, uma amostra representativa daquilo que deve ser medido; p.ex., os itens que se relacionam com a capacidade em aritmética e na definição das palavras formam o conteúdo apropriado para um teste de inteligência.
   criterion-related v., v. relacionada ao critério; o grau de efetividade com o qual o desempenho em um teste ou procedimento prediz o desempenho em uma situação de vida real; p.ex., uma boa correlação entre um escore em um teste de inteligência, como o Scholastic Aptitude Test e a média de pontos dos 4 anos de faculdade de uma pessoa.
   face v., v. superficial; a extensão em que os itens de um teste ou procedimento parecem gerar uma amostra superficial daquilo que deve ser medido.
   predictive v., v. preditiva; a v. relacionada a um critério usada para predizer o desempenho em uma tarefa da vida real em dado momento futuro. VER construct v., criterion-related v.

va·line (Val, V) (val'in). Valina; ácido 2-amino-3-metilbutanóico; o L-isômero é um constituinte da maioria das proteínas; um aminoácido nutricionalmente essencial.

va·lin·o·myc·in (val'i-nō-mī-sin). Valinomicina; antibiótico ionóforo ciclododecadepsipeptídeo derivado do *Streptomyces fulvissius*; uma estrutura anelar com 36 membros, consistindo em 3 mol de cada de L-valina, ácido D-α-hidroxi-isovalérico, D-valina e ácido L-láctico ligados de maneira alternada. O material é utilizado como inseticida e nematocida.

val·la (val'ă). Plural de vallum.

val·late (val'āt). Valado; limitado por uma elevação, como uma estrutura em forma de cúpula; indica especialmente determinadas papilas linguais. VER TAMBÉM circumvallate. [L. *vallo*, pp. *-atus*, circundar com, de *vallum*, muralha]

val·lec·u·la, pl. val·lec·u·lae (vă-lek'ū-lă, -lē) [TA]. Valécula; uma fenda ou depressão em qualquer superfície, principalmente os espaços entre a epiglote e a base da língua, direita e esquerda. SIN valley. [L. dim. de *vallis*, vale]
   v. cerebel'li [TA], v. do cerebelo; uma cavidade profunda na superfície inferior do cerebelo, entre os hemisférios, contendo o mielencéfalo e a foice do cérebro. SIN v. of cerebellum [TA], vallis.
   v. of cerebellum [TA], v. do cerebelo. SIN v. cerebelli.
   epiglottic v. [TA], v. epiglótica; uma depressão imediatamente posterior à raiz da língua, entre as pregas glossoepiglóticas mediana e lateral em ambos os lados. SIN v. epiglottica.
   v. epiglot'tica [TA], v. epiglótica. SIN epiglottic v.
   v. syl'vii, v. de Sylvius. SIN lateral cerebral fossa.
   v. un'guis, v. ungueal. SIN sulcus matricis unguis.

Valleix, François L. I., médico francês, 1807–1855. VER V. *points*, em *point*.

val·ley (val'ē). Valécula. SIN vallecula.

val·lis (val'is). Valécula. SIN *vallecula* cerebelli. [L. vale]

val·lum, pl. val·la (val'ŭm, -ă). **1** [NA]. Vale; qualquer crista elevada, mais ou menos circular. **2.** A parede externa discretamente elevada da depressão circular, ou fossa, que circunda uma papila circunvalada da língua. [L. uma vala, de *vallus*, uma trincheira]
   v. un'guis [TA], vale da unha. SIN nail wall.

val·meth·a·mide (val-meth'ă-mīd). Valmetamida. SIN valnoctamide.

val·noc·ta·mide (val-nok'tă-mīd). Valnoctamida; um agente ansiolítico. SIN valmethamide.

val·oid (val'oyd). Valóide. SIN equivalent *extract*. [L. *valeo*, ficar forte]

val·pro·ic ac·id (val-prō'ik). Ácido valpróico; um anticonvulsivante usado para tratar os distúrbios convulsivos; também empregado como um sal sódico, valproato de sódio.

Valsalva, Antonio M., anatomista italiano, 1666–1723. VER *aneurysm* of sinus of V.; V. *antrum*, *ligaments*, em *ligament*, *maneuver*, *muscle*, *sinus*; *teniae* of V., em *tenia*; V. *test*.

val·ue (val'ū). Valor; uma determinação quantitativa específica. Para os valores não arrolados adiante, ver o nome específico. VER TAMBÉM index, number. [I. m., do Fr. ant., do L. *valeo*, ter valor]
   acetyl v., v. de acetil; os miligramas de KOH necessários para neutralizar o ácido acético produzido pela hidrólise de 1 g de gordura acetilada; uma medida dos hidroxi-ácidos presentes em glicerídeos; notadamente alto no óleo de rícino.
   buffer v., v. tampão; a potência de uma substância em solução para absorver o ácido ou base sem mudar o pH; este é o mais elevado em um valor de pH igual ao valor do pK_a do ácido do par tampão. VER TAMBÉM buffer *capacity*. SIN buffer index.
   buffer v. of the blood, v. tampão do sangue; a capacidade do sangue de compensar adições de ácido ou base sem distúrbio do pH.
   C v., v. C; a quantidade total de DNA em um genoma haplóide.
   caloric v., v. calórico; o calor produzido por um alimento quando queimado ou metabolizado.
   Hehner v., v. de Hehner. SIN Hehner *number*.
   homing v., v. residente; em um sistema cibernético como a homeostasia, aquele v. de um traço ou interesse em que as forças de restauração são direcionadas no sentido da manutenção.
   iodine v., v. do iodo. SIN iodine *number*.
   maturation v., v. de maturação; um indicador do nível de maturação atingido pelo epitélio vaginal e usado como um fator na avaliação cito-hormonal a partir do índice de maturação, atribuindo-se às células parabasais 0,0, às células intermediárias 0,5 e às células superficiais 1,0; para pesquisas especiais, os subtipos de uma célula principal podem receber valores diferentes.
   normal v.'s, valores normais; um conjunto de valores de exames laboratoriais usados para caracterizar indivíduos aparentemente saudáveis; atualmente substituído pelos valores de referência.
   pH v., v. de pH. VER pH.
   phenotypic v., v. fenotípico; na genética quantitativa, a quantidade métrica de algum traço associado a determinado fenótipo.
   predictive v., v. preditivo; uma expressão da probabilidade que o resultado de determinado teste correlaciona com a presença ou ausência da doença. Um v. preditivo positivo é a proporção dos pacientes com a doença com testes positivos em toda a população dos indivíduos com resultados de teste positivos; um v. preditivo negativo é a proporção dos pacientes sem a doença com testes negativos na população de indivíduos com um teste negativo.
   R_f v., v. R_f. VER R_f.
   reference v.'s, v. de referência; um grupo de valores de exames laboratoriais obtido a partir de um indivíduo ou grupo em um estado definido de saúde; esse termo substitui os valores normais, pois baseia-se em um estado definido de saúde, em lugar da saúde aparente.
   thiocyanogen v., v. de tiocianogênio. SIN thiocyanogen *number*.
   threshold limit v. (TLV), v. limítrofe; a concentração máxima de uma substância química recomendada pela American Conference of Government Industrial Hygienists para a exposição repetida sem efeitos de saúde adversos sobre os trabalhadores.

val·va, pl. val·vae (val'vă, -vē) [TA]. Valva, válvula. SIN valve. [L. uma folha de uma porta dupla]
   v. aor'tae [TA], valva da aorta. SIN aortic *valve*.
   v. atrioventricula'ris dex'tra [TA], v. atrioventricular direita. SIN tricuspid *valve*.
   v. atrioventricula'ris sinis'tra [TA], v. atrioventricular esquerda. SIN mitral *valve*.
   v. ileoceca'lis [TA], papila ileal. SIN ileal *papilla*.
   v. mitra'lis, v. atrioventricular esquerda; *termo oficial alternativo para mitral *valve*.
   v. tricuspida'lis, v. atrioventricular direita; *termo oficial alternativo para tricuspid *valve*.
   v. trun'ci pulmona'lis [TA], valva do tronco pulmonar. SIN pulmonary *valve*.

val·val, val·var (val'văl, val'văr). Valvar; relativo a uma valva.

val·vate (val'vāt). Valvado; relativo a ou provido com uma válvula. SIN valvular.

valve (valv) [TA]. Valva, válvula. **1.** Uma prega da membrana de revestimento de um canal ou outro órgão oco que serve para retardar ou impedir um refluxo de líquido. **2.** Qualquer formação ou reduplicação do tecido, ou estrutura em forma de retalho, que se assemelha a ou funciona como uma v. VER TAMBÉM valvule, plica. SIN valva [TA]. [L. *valva*]
   Amussat v., válvula de Amussat, prega espiral. SIN spiral *fold* of cystic duct.
   anal v.'s [TA], válvulas anais; pregas delicadas da mucosa que passam entre as extremidades inferiores das colunas anais adjacentes; a pequena bolsa assim formada é um seio anal. SIN valvulae anales [TA], Morgagni v.'s.

valve

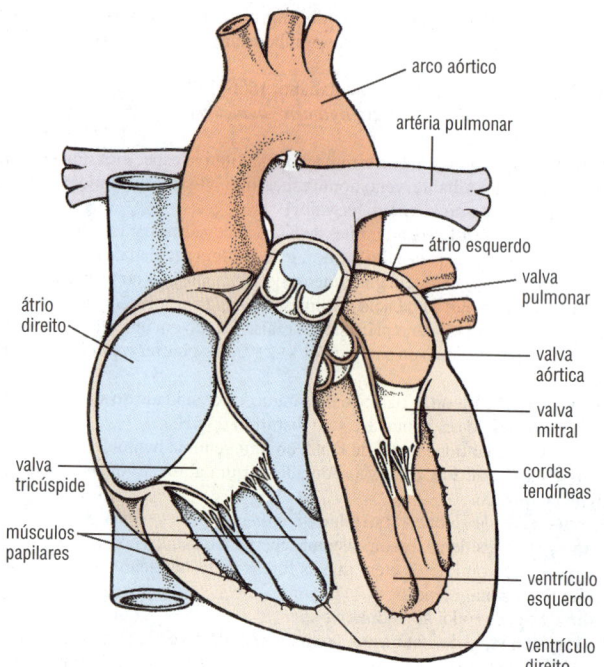

valvas cardíacas: aórtica, pulmonar, tricúspide e mitral

anterior urethral v., válvula uretral anterior; uma prega horizontal em crescente na uretra esponjosa proximal.
aortic v. [TA], v. da aorta; a v. entre o ventrículo esquerdo e a aorta ascendente, consistindo em três válvulas semilunares fibrosas, localizada, no adulto, nas posições anterior, posterior direita e posterior esquerda; no entanto, elas são nomeadas de acordo com sua derivação embrionária na qual a válvula anteriormente localizada é a válvula direita (acima da qual se origina a artéria coronária direita), a válvula esquerda posicionada posteriormente é designada válvula esquerda (acima da qual se origina a artéria coronária esquerda) e a válvula direita posicionada posteriormente é designada válvula posterior ou não-coronária. SIN valva aortae [TA].
atrioventricular v.'s, valvas atrioventriculares. VER tricuspid v., mitral v.
A-V v.'s, valvas A-V; abreviatura para as valvas atrioventriculares cardíacas; as valvas mitral e tricúspide.
ball v., válvula esférica; qualquer uma dentre inúmeras próteses valvulares cardíacas que contenham uma esfera dentro de uma estrutura de retenção afixada ao orifício; quando de tamanho apropriado, usada na posição aórtica, mitral ou tricúspide.
Bauhin v., válvula de Bauhin. SIN ileal *papilla.*
Béraud v., válvula de Béraud; uma pequena prega no saco lacrimal em sua junção com o duto lacrimal. SIN Krause v.
bicuspid v., valva bicúspide. SIN mitral v.
bi-leaflet v., uma valva cardíaca mecânica de baixo perfil que exibe menor obstrução ao efluxo, especialmente em tamanho pequeno.
biologic v., valva biológica. SIN tissue v.
Björk-Shiley v., valva de Björk-Shiley; uma valva cardíaca mecânica de baixo perfil, por inclinação de disco.
Blom-Singer v., valva de Blom-Singer; uma prótese para manter a permeabilidade de uma punção traqueoesofágica para a reabilitação vocal depois de laringectomia.
Bochdalek v., valva de Bochdalek; uma prega da mucosa no canalículo lacrimal no ponto lacrimal. SIN Foltz valvule.
Braune v., v. de Braune; uma prega da mucosa na junção do esôfago com o estômago.
Carpentier-Edwards v., valva de Carpentier-Edwards; uma bioprótese valvar feita a partir de valvas aórticas suínas preservadas.
caval v., válvula da veia cava inferior. SIN v. of inferior vena cava.
congenital v., v. congênita; uma prega de revestimento anormal que obstrui uma passagem; p.ex., de uma mucosa na uretra.
coronary v., válvula do seio coronariano. SIN v. of coronary sinus.
v. of coronary sinus [TA], válvula do seio coronário; uma delicada prega do endocárdio na abertura do seio coronário para dentro do átrio direito. SIN valvula sinus coronarii [TA], coronary v., thebesian v.
eustachian v., válvula de Eustáquio. SIN v. of inferior vena cava.

v. of foramen ovale [TA], válvula do forame oval; uma prega que se projeta para dentro do átrio esquerdo a partir da margem do forame oval no feto; quando, com o início da inspiração, a pressão arterial dentro do átrio esquerdo aumenta, a v. se fecha e suas bordas aderem à margem do forame oval, ocluindo-o. SIN valvula foraminis ovalis [TA], falx septi, v. of oval foramen.
Gerlach v., válvula de Gerlach. SIN v. of vermiform appendix.
Guérin v., válvula de Guérin. SIN v. of navicular fossa.
Heister v., válvula de Heister. SIN spiral *fold* of cystic duct.
Heyer-Pudenz v., válvula de Heyer-Pudenz; uma v. usada no procedimento de desvio para a hidrocefalia; consiste em um sistema de cateter–válvula em que o cateter ventricular leva o líquido cefalorraquidiano em uma bomba unidirecional, através da qual o líquido cefalorraquidiano percorre o cateter distal até chegar ao átrio direito do coração.
Hoboken v.'s, válvulas de Hoboken; as protrusões em forma de flanges para a luz das artérias umbilicais, onde são torcidas ou dobradas em seu trajeto através do cordão umbilical.
Huschke v., válvula de Huschke. SIN lacrimal *fold.*
ileocecal v., papila ileal. SIN ileal *papilla.*
ileocolic v., papila ileal. SIN ileal *papilla.*
v. of inferior vena cava [TA], válvula da veia cava inferior; uma prega endocárdica que se estende da margem ântero-inferior da veia cava inferior até a parte anterior do limbo da fossa oval. SIN valvula venae cavae inferioris [TA], caval v., eustachian v., sylvian v.
Kerckring v.'s, válvulas de Kerckring. SIN circular *folds* of small intestine, em *fold.*
Krause v., válvula de Krause. SIN Béraud v.
left atrioventricular v., v. atrioventricular esquerda; *termo oficial alternativo para mitral v.
Mercier v., válvula de Mercier; uma prega ocasional da mucosa da bexiga que oclui parcialmente o orifício uretral.
mitral v. [TA], valva atrioventricular esquerda; a valva que fecha o orifício entre o átrio esquerdo e o ventrículo esquerdo do coração; seus dois folhetos são chamados anterior e posterior. SIN valva atrioventricularis sinistra [TA], left atrioventricular v.*, valva mitralis*, bicuspid v., valvula bicuspidalis.
Morgagni v.'s, válvulas de Morgagni. SIN anal v.'s
nasal v., válvula nasal; a abertura variável entre o septo nasal e a margem caudal da cartilagem nasal lateral superior.
v. of navicular fossa [TA], válvula da fossa navicular; uma prega inconstante de mucosa por vezes encontrada na raiz da fossa navicular da uretra. SIN valvula fossae navicularis [TA], Guérin fold, Guérin v.
nonrebreathing v., válvula unidirecional; um tipo de v. que impede a mistura dos gases inspirados e expirados.
O'Beirne v., v. de O'Beirne. SIN rectosigmoid *sphincter.*
v. of oval foramen, válvula do forame oval. SIN v. of foramen ovale.
parachute mitral v., valva mitral em pára-quedas; anormalidade congênita da v. mitral caracterizada por um único músculo papilar, a partir do qual se dividem as cordas tendíneas dos folhetos valvares; daí a semelhança com um pára-quedas; com freqüência, a condição provoca estenose como resultado combinado da ação da tração forte das cordas tendíneas sobre os folhetos e o subseqüente estreitamento entre eles. SIN parachute deformity.
porcine v., valva suína; a valva oriunda de suínos para enxerto heterólogo.
posterior urethral v.'s, válvulas uretrais posteriores; pregas anômalas que ocorrem no nível do colículo seminal. SIN Amussat valvula.
prosthetic v.'s, próteses valvares; as valvas usadas para substituir as valvas humanas. Elas são divididas em valvas mecânicas e teciduais. As teciduais são divididas em homoenxertos e heteroenxertos.
pulmonary v. [TA], valva do tronco pulmonar; a valva na entrada do tronco pulmonar a partir do ventrículo direito; consiste em válvulas semilunares, as quais, no adulto, estão dispostas nas posições anterior direita, anterior esquerda e posterior; entretanto, elas são denominadas de acordo com sua derivação embrionária; assim, a válvula posterior é designada válvula esquerda, a válvula anterior direita é designada válvula direita, e a válvula anterior esquerda é denominada válvula anterior. SIN valva trunci pulmonalis [TA], pulmonic v., v. of pulmonary trunk.
v. of pulmonary trunk, valva do tronco pulmonar. SIN pulmonary v.
pulmonic v., valva pulmonar. SIN pulmonary v.
rectal v.'s, pregas transversas do reto. SIN transverse *folds* of rectum, em *fold.*
reducing v., válvula redutora; uma válvula designada para diminuir a pressão de um gás proveniente de um cilindro que contém gás comprimido sob alta pressão.
right atrioventricular v., valva atrioventricular direita; *termo oficial alternativo para tricuspid v.
Rosenmüller v., válvula de Rosenmüller. SIN lacrimal *fold.*
semilunar v. [TA], valva semilunar; uma valva cardíaca composta de um conjunto de três válvulas semilunares; portanto, as valvas da aorta e do tronco pulmonar são valvas semilunares. SIN valvula semilunaris [TA].
spiral v. of cystic duct, prega espiral. SIN spiral *fold* of cystic duct.
Starr-Edwards v., valva de Starr-Edwards; uma valva cardíaca artificial com um arcabouço e uma esfera com alta durabilidade e confiabilidade.

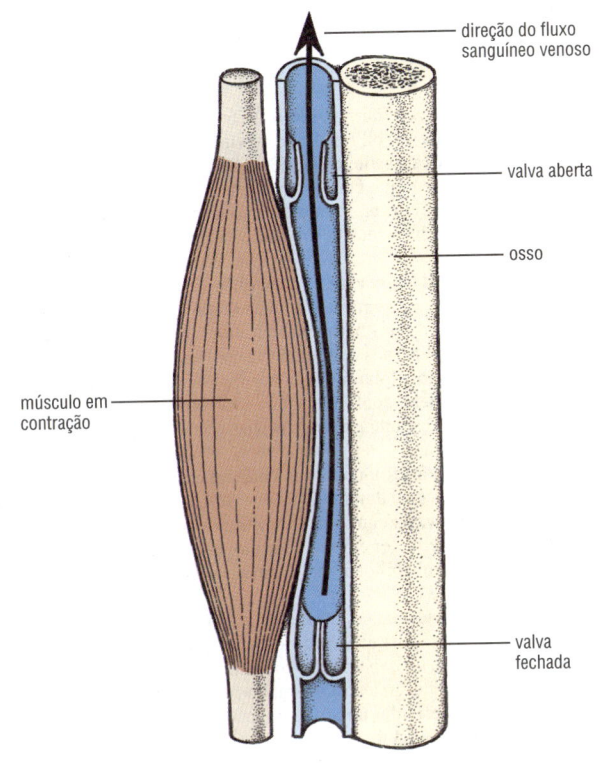

valvas venosas: princípio de fluxo sanguíneo venoso

sylvian v., válvula de Sylvius. SIN v. of inferior vena cava.
Tarin v., válvula de Tarin. SIN inferior medullary *velum*.
Terrien v., válvula de Terrien; uma prega semelhante a uma válvula entre a vesícula biliar e o canal cístico; a primeira crista da prega espiral do canal cístico.
thebesian v., válvula de Thebesius. SIN v. of coronary sinus.
tilting disk v., valva de disco inclinado; uma variedade de prótese valvar cardíaca composta de um disco envolto por um arcabouço.
tissue v., v. tecidual; uma prótese valvar cardíaca derivada do coração de porco, pericárdio bovino ou outra fonte biológica. VER TAMBÉM prosthesis. SIN biologic v.
tricuspid v. [TA], valva atrioventricular direita; a valva que fecha o orifício entre o átrio direito e o ventrículo direito do coração; suas três válvulas são chamadas de anterior, posterior e septal. SIN valva atrioventricularis dextra [TA], right atrioventricular v.*, valva tricuspidalis*, valvula tricuspidalis.
Tulp v., Tulpius v., válvula de Tulp, válvula de Tulpius. SIN ileal *papilla*.
urethral v.'s, válvulas uretrais; as pregas na mucosa da uretra. VER TAMBÉM anterior urethral v., posterior urethral v.'s.
v. of Varolius, válvula de Varolius. SIN ileal *papilla*.
venous v. [TA], valva venosa; as pregas da camada de revestimento de uma veia para impedir o refluxo do sangue. SIN valvula venosa (2) [TA].
v. of vermiform appendix, válvula do apêndice vermiforme; uma prega de mucosa, simulando uma válvula, por vezes encontrada na origem do apêndice vermiforme. SIN Gerlach v., valvula processus vermiformis.
vesicoureteral v., válvula vesicoureteral; um mecanismo de travamento na parede da porção intravesical do ureter que, normalmente, impede o refluxo urinário.
v. of Vieussens, válvula de Vieussens; uma válvula proeminente na veia cardíaca maior, onde ela gira ao redor da margem obtusa para se transformar no seio coronário.
Vieussens v., válvula de Vieussens. SIN superior medullary *velum*.
valve·less (valv'les). Desvalvulado; sem válvulas; indica determinadas veias, como a veia porta, que não têm válvulas como as existentes na maioria das veias.
val·vi·form (val'vi-fōrm). Valviforme; com o formato de válvula.
val·vo·plas·ty (val'vō-plas-tē). Valvoplastia; reconstrução cirúrgica de uma valva cardíaca deformada, para alívio da estenose ou incompetência. SIN valvuloplasty. [valve + G. *plastos*, formado]
val·vot·o·my (val-vot'ō-mē). Valvotomia. **1.** Incisão através de uma valva cardíaca estenosada para aliviar a obstrução. SIN valvulotomy. **2.** Incisão de uma estrutura valvar. [valve + G. *tomē*, incisão]

mitral v., v. mitral; a incisão deliberada ou ampliação por meio da inserção de um dedo da mão na valva mitral estenótica.
rectal v., v. retal; a incisão através das pregas retais que são muito rígidas ou grandes.
val·vu·la, pl. **val·vu·lae** (val'vū-lã, -lē) [TA]. Válvula. SIN valvule. [L. mod. dim. de *valva*]
Amussat v., v. de Amussat. SIN posterior urethral *valves*, em *valve*.
val'vulae ana'les [TA], válvulas anais. SIN anal *valves*, em *valve*.
v. bicuspida'lis, valva bicúspide, valva atrioventricular esquerda. SIN mitral *valve*.
val'vulae conniven'tes, pregas circulares. SIN circular *folds* of small intestine, em *fold*.
v. fora'minis ova'lis [TA], válvula do forame oval. SIN *valve* of foramen ovale.
v. fos'sae navicula'ris [TA], válvula da fossa navicular. SIN *valve* of navicular fossa.
Gerlach v., válvula de Gerlach. SIN trabecular *tissue* of sclera.
v. lymphat'ica [TA], válvula linfática. SIN lymphatic *valvule*.
v. proces'sus vermifor'mis, válvula do apêndice vermiforme. SIN *valve* of vermiform appendix.
v. semiluna'ris [TA], válvula semilunar. SIN semilunar *valve*.
v. semiluna'ris ante'rior val'vae trun'ci pulmona'lis, válvula semilunar anterior da valva do tronco pulmonar; a válvula semilunar anterior da valva pulmonar.
v. semiluna'ris dex'tra val'vae aor'tae, válvula semilunar direita da valva aórtica; a válvula semilunar direita da valva aórtica.
v. semiluna'ris dex'tra val'vae trun'ci pulmona'lis, válvula semilunar direita da valva do tronco pulmonar; a válvula semilunar direita da valva pulmonar.
v. semiluna'ris poste'rior val'vae aor'tae, válvula semilunar posterior da valva aórtica; a válvula semilunar posterior da valva aórtica.
v. semiluna'ris sinis'tra val'vae aor'tae, válvula semilunar esquerda da valva aórtica; a válvula semilunar esquerda da valva aórtica.
v. semiluna'ris sinis'tra val'vae trun'ci pulmona'lis, válvula semilunar esquerda da valva do tronco pulmonar; a válvula semilunar esquerda da valva pulmonar.
v. semiluna'ris tari'ni, válvula semilunar de Tarin. SIN inferior medullary *velum*.
v. si'nus corona'rii [TA], válvula do seio coronário. SIN *valve* of coronary sinus.
v. spiral'is, prega espiral. SIN spiral *fold* of cystic duct.
v. tricuspida'lis, valva tricúspide. SIN tricuspid *valve*.
v. ve'nae ca'vae inferio'ris [TA], válvula da veia cava inferior. SIN *valve* of inferior vena cava.
v. veno'sa [TA], válvula venosa; **(1)** no embrião, uma válvula do par de válvulas na abertura do seio venoso para dentro do átrio direito; **(2)** [NA] SIN venous *valve*.
v. vestib'uli, válvula vestibular; termo obsoleto para v. venosa (1).
val·vu·lar (val'vū-lăr). Valvular. SIN valvate.
val·vule (val'vūl) [TA]. Válvula; uma válvula, especialmente aquela de pequeno tamanho. SIN valvula [TA]. [L. *valvula*]
Foltz v., v. de Foltz. SIN Bochdalek *valve*.
lymphatic v. [TA], v. linfática; uma das delicadas válvulas semilunares encontradas nos vasos linfáticos; elas são geralmente pareadas e de estrutura similar às válvulas venosas e ocorrem a intervalos próximos ao longo da parede vascular. SIN valvula lymphatica [TA].
val·vu·li·tis (val-vū-lī'tis). Valvulite; a inflamação de uma válvula, principalmente de uma valva cardíaca. [L. mod. *valvula*, válvula, + G. *-itis*, inflamação]
rheumatic v., v. reumática; valvulite caracterizada, no estágio agudo, por pequenas vegetações de fibrina ao longo das linhas de fechamento e por corpúsculos de Aschoff nas válvulas; no estágio crônico, caracteriza-se por fibrose, aderência das comissuras e estenose e/ou regurgitação.
val·vu·lo·plas·ty (val'vū-lō-plas'tē). Valvuloplastia. SIN valvoplasty.
val·vu·lo·tome (val'vū-lō-tōm). Valvulótomo; instrumento para seccionar uma válvula.
val·vu·lot·o·my (val-vū-lot'ō-mē). Valvulotomia. SIN valvotomy (1).
val·yl (Val, V) (val'il). Valil; o radical da valina.
Van, van. Alguns termos com esse prefixo não são encontrados adiante; ver então a parte principal do termo.
van·a·date (van'ā-dāt). Vanadato; um sal do ácido vanádico.
va·na·dic ac·id (vă-nad'ik). Ácido vanádico; um ácido, H_3VO_4, derivado do vanádio, formando sais com diversas bases.
va·na·di·um (V) (vă-nā'dē-ŭm). Vanádio; um elemento metálico, n.º atômico 23, peso atômico 50,9415; um bioelemento, cuja deficiência pode resultar em crescimento ósseo anormal e elevação nos níveis de colesterol e de triacilglicerol. [*Vanadis*, deusa escandinava]
v. group, grupo do vanádio; aqueles elementos que se assemelham ao vanádio em propriedades químicas e metalúrgicas; incluídos com o vanádio estão o nióbio e o tântalo.

van Bogaert, Ludo, neurologista belga do século XX. VER Canavan-v. B.-Bertrand *disease*; v. B. *encephalitis*.

van Buchem, Francis Steven Peter, clínico holandês, *1897. VER Van B. *syndrome*.

van Buren, William H., cirurgião norte-americano, 1819–1883. VER van B. *sound, disease*.

van·co·my·cin (van-kō-mī'sin). Vancomicina; um antibiótico isolado a partir de culturas de *Nocardia orientalis*, bactericida e bacteriostático contra microrganismos Gram-positivos; disponível como cloridrato.

van Creveld, S., pediatra holandês, *1894. VER Ellis-van C. *syndrome*.

van·dal root (van'dăl). Valeriana. SIN valerian.

van Deen, Izaak A., fisiologista holandês, 1804–1869. VER van D. *test*.

van den Bergh, A.A.H., médico holandês, 1869–1943. VER van den B. *test*.

van der Kolk, Jacobus L.C.S., médico holandês, 1797–1862.

van der Spieghel. VER Spigelius.

van der Velden, Reinhardt, médico alemão, 1851–1903. VER van der V.'s *test*.

van der Waals, Johannes D., físico holandês e laureado com o Prêmio Nobel, 1837–1923. VER van der W. *forces*, em *force*.

van Ekenstein, W.A., cientista do século XIX. VER Lobry de Bruyn-van E. *transformation*.

van Ermengen, Emile P., bacteriologista belga, 1851–1932. VER van E. *stain*.

van Gieson, Ira, histologista e bacteriologista norte-americano, 1865–1913. VER van G. *stain*.

van Helmont, Jean B., médico e químico francês, 1577–1644. VER van H. *mirror*.

van Horne (Hoorne, Hoorn, Heurenius), Jan (Johannes), anatomista holandês, 1621–1670. VER van H. *canal*.

va·nil·la (vă-nĭl'ă). Baunilha; o fruto verde, curado e completamente crescido da *Vanila planifolia* (b. mexicana ou de Bourbon) ou da *V. tahitensis* (b. do Taiti), orquídeas (família Orchidaceae) oriundas do México e cultivadas em outros países tropicais; um agente flavorizante. [Esp. *vainilla*, pequena vagem]

va·nil·late (vă-nĭl'āt). Vanilato; um composto do ácido vanílico; $C_8H_8O_4$.

va·nil·lic ac·id (vă-nĭl'ik). Ácido vanílico; um agente flavorizante.

va·nil·lin (vă-nĭl'in). Vanilina; obtida da baunilha e também preparada de forma sintética; um agente flavorizante; usada para detectar ornitina, álcoois de açúcar, fenóis e determinados esteróis.

va·nil·lism (vă-nĭl'izm). Vanilismo. 1. Os sinais e sintomas de irritação da pele, mucosa nasal e conjuntiva sofridos, por vezes, por algumas pessoas que trabalham com a baunilha. 2. Infestação da pele pelos ácaros sarcoptiformes encontrados nas vagens da baunilha.

va·nil·lyl·man·del·ic ac·id (VMA) (van'i-lil-man-del'ik, vă-nĭl'il-). Ácido vanilmandélico; nome errôneo para o ácido 4-hidroxi-3-metoximandélico (ácido α,3-diidroxi-2-metoxibenzenoacético); o principal metabólito urinário das catecolaminas supra-renais e simpáticas (p.ex., a partir da epinefrina e norepinefrina); elevado na maioria dos pacientes com feocromocitoma.

Van Slyke, Donald D., bioquímico norte-americano, 1883–1971. VER slyke; Van S. *apparatus, formula*.

van't Hoff, Jacobus, químico holandês e laureado com o Prêmio Nobel, 1852–1911. VER van't H. *equation, law, theory*; Le Bel-van't H. *rule*.

va·por (vā'per). Vapor. 1. Moléculas na fase gasosa de uma substância sólida ou líquida exposta a um gás. 2. Uma emanação visível de partículas finas de um líquido. 3. Uma preparação medicinal a ser administrada por inalação. [L. vapor]

   anesthetic v., v. anestésico; a fase gasosa de um anestésico líquido com pressão parcial suficiente, na temperatura ambiente, para produzir a anestesia geral, quando inalada.

va·por·i·za·tion (vā-pŏr-i-zā'shŭn). Vaporização. 1. A alteração de um sólido ou líquido para um estado de vapor. 2. A aplicação terapêutica de um vapor.

va·por·ize (vā'-per-īz). Vaporizar. 1. Converter um sólido ou líquido em um vapor. 2. Aplicar um vapor com fim terapêutico.

va·por·iz·er (vā'per-īz-er). Vaporizador. 1. Um aparelho para diminuir os medicamentos líquidos para um estado de vapor apropriado para a inalação ou aplicação em mucosas acessíveis. VER TAMBÉM nebulizer, atomizer. 2. Um aparelho para volatilizar os anestésicos líquidos.

   flow-over v., v. de hiperfluxo; um aparelho para a vaporização de um anestésico líquido ao fazer com que os gases passem sobre o anestésico ou sobre o material saturado com o anestésico.

   temperature-compensated v., v. de temperatura compensada; um v. de anestésicos líquidos com ajustes graduados calibrados para liberar uma concentração constante conhecida de um anestésico específico, apesar das alterações no volume de influxo e apesar do resfriamento provocado por vaporização.

va·por·tho·rax (văp-er-thō'raks). Vaportórax; a existência de grandes bolhas de vapor d'água no espaço pleural entre os pulmões e a parede torácica em uma pessoa desprotegida exposta a altitudes superiores a 19.000 m, onde a pressão barométrica é inferior a 47 mm Hg e onde a água na temperatura corporal vaporiza a partir do estado líquido.

va·po·ther·a·py (vā'pō-thār'ă-pē). Vapoterapia; o tratamento da doença por meio do vapor ou aerossol.

V̇a/Q̇ Abreviatura para ventilation/perfusion *ratio* (relação ventilação/perfusão).

Vaquez, Louis H., médico frânces, 1860–1936. VER V. *disease*.

var·i·a·bil·i·ty (var'ē-ă-bil'i-tē). Variabilidade. 1. A capacidade de ser variável. 2. Em genética, as diferenças potenciais ou reais, quer quantitativas, quer qualitativas, no fenótipo entre os indivíduos.

   baseline v. of fetal heart rate, v. basal da freqüência cardíaca fetal; as alterações na freqüência cardíaca fetal de um batimento para outro, conforme registrado em um gráfico.

   beat-to-beat v. of fetal heart rate, v. da freqüência cardíaca fetal de um batimento para outro; a v. na freqüência cardíaca fetal medida em alterações no intervalo QRS–QRS de um batimento cardíaco para outro; medida com monitores eletrônicos internos de freqüência cardíaca fetal.

var·i·a·ble (var'ē-ă-bl). Variável. 1. Aquilo que é inconstante, que pode alterar-se ou que se altera, conforme contrastado com uma constante. 2. Que se desvia do padrão em estrutura, forma, fisiologia ou comportamento. [L. *vario, variar, mudar, diferir*]

   continuous v., v. contínua; uma v. que pode refletir qualquer valor em um intervalo ou intervalos (seu domínio).

   continuous random v., v. contínua aleatória; a v. contínua que pode assumir, ao acaso, qualquer valor em seu domínio, mas determinado valor qualquer não apresenta probabilidade de ocorrência, apenas uma densidade de probabilidade.

   dependent v., v. dependente; em experiências, uma v. que é influenciada por ou dependente de alterações na v. independente; p.ex., a quantidade de uma passagem escrita retida (v. dependente) como uma função de um número diferente de minutos (v. independente) permitido para estudar a passagem.

   discrete v., v. bem definida; uma v. que pode assumir apenas um número mensurável (geralmente finito) de valores.

   discrete random v., v. aleatória bem definida; uma v. aleatória que pode assumir um número mensurável de valores, cada qual com uma probabilidade estritamente maior que zero.

   independent v., v. independente; uma característica que está sendo medida ou observada para a qual se faz a hipótese de influenciar outro evento ou manifestação (a v. dependente) dentro de uma área definida de relações sob estudo; isto é, a v. independente não é influenciada nem pelo evento, nem pela manifestação, mas pode causá-los ou contribuir para sua variação. VER dependent v.

   intermediate v., v. intermediária; uma v., em uma via causal, que provoca variação na v. dependente e, por si própria, sabe-se que varia pela v. independente.

   intervening v., v. interveniente; um evento, como uma atitude ou emoção, que se deduz que ocorra dentro de um organismo entre a estimulação e a resposta, de tal modo a influenciar ou determinar a resposta.

   mixed discrete-continuous random v., v. aleatória contínua-bem definida mista; uma v. que pode assumir alguns valores com probabilidades e outros com densidades de probabilidade. Por exemplo, em um homem de 35 anos de idade com polipose familial do colo, a distribuição do tempo, até que a doença maligna ocorra, consiste em uma probabilidade de que ele já tenha câncer (que seria designada como momento 0), uma densidade de probabilidade de desenvolvê-lo no futuro e uma probabilidade de que ele morrerá por alguma outra causa antes que o câncer se desenvolva.

   moderator v., v. moderadora; uma v. que interage por ser antecedente ou intermediária na via causal.

   random v., v. aleatória; uma v. que pode assumir um conjunto de valores, cada qual com probabilidades fixas ou densidades de probabilidade (sua distribuição), de tal modo que a probabilidade total destinada à distribuição é a unidade; a variável ao acaso pode ser discreta, contínua ou contínuo-discreta mista.

var·i·ance (var'ē-ans). Variância. 1. O estado de ser variável, diferente, divergente ou desviado; um grau de desvio. 2. Uma medida da variação mostrada por um conjunto de observações, definida como o somatório dos quadrados dos desvios da média, dividido pelo número de graus de liberdade no conjunto das observações.

   ball v., v. da esfera; edema e alterações na forma e consistência da esfera em uma prótese de válvula-esfera, especialmente para se substituir a valva aórtica.

var·i·ant (var'ē-ant). Variante. 1. Aquilo ou aquele que é variável. 2. Ter a tendência de alterar ou mudar, exibir a variedade ou diversidade, não se conformar com, ou diferir do tipo.

   inherited albumin v.'s [MIM*103600], variantes da albumina hereditária; os tipos de albumina sérica humana, diferenciados por padrões de mobilidade característicos na eletroforese; cada tipo é devido a uma mutação de um gene que controla a síntese de albumina; os genes mutantes são co-dominantes com o gene normal para a albumina A, e o grupo forma um sistema de polimorfismo genético; os tipos incluem: albumina b (lenta), encontrada ocasionalmente nas pessoas de ascendência européia; albumina Ghent (rápida), encontrada primeiramente em Ghent, Bélgica; albumina México (lenta), encontrada em indígenas do México e no sudoeste dos Estados Unidos; albumina Naskapi (rápida), encontrada nos indígenas Naskapi e em outros indígenas do norte da América do Norte; e albumina Reading (rápida), encontrada primeiramente em Reading, England.

L-phase v.'s, variantes da fase L; as variantes bacterianas que não possuem paredes celulares rígidas, mas que podem conter quantidades variadas de material da parede celular; elas têm forma esférica ou cocobacilar e variam em tamanho desde pequenos corpos que atravessam filtros, que retêm bactérias, até corpos maiores que a forma bacteriana; são Gram-negativas e resistentes à penicilina. As variantes diferem muito das células bacterianas originais quanto ao modo de reprodução, fisiologia, requisitos de crescimento e morfologia individual e colonial; geralmente são consideradas não-patogênicas, mesmo quando derivadas de uma bactéria patogênica. [L. de Lister Institute]

var·i·ate (var′ē-āt). Variável; uma quantidade mensurável capaz de levar em consideração inúmeros valores; pode ser binária (isto é, capaz de considerar dois valores em determinado intervalo de valores), contínua (isto é, capaz de considerar todos os valores em determinado intervalo de valores reais), ou bem definida (isto é, capaz de considerar um número limitado de valores em determinado intervalo de valores reais).

var·i·a·tion (var-ē-ā′shŭn). Variação. **1.** Desvio do tipo, especialmente do tipo original, em estrutura, forma, fisiologia ou comportamento. **2.** SIN type (3). [L. *variatio,* de *vario,* mudar, variar]

continuous v., v. contínua; uma série de variações muito discretas.

var·i·ca·tion (var-i-kā′shŭn). Varicação; formação ou existência de varizes.

var·i·ce·al (var-ī-sē′ăl, vă-ris′ē-ăl). Varicoso; de ou pertinente a uma variz.

var·i·cel·la (var-i-sel′ă). Varicela, catapora; uma doença contagiosa aguda, que usualmente ocorre em crianças, causada pelo vírus varicela-zoster do gênero Varicellovirus, um membro da família Herpesviridae, e caracterizada por erupção esparsa de pápulas, que se tornam vesículas e, em seguida, pústulas, como as da varíola, embora menos graves e em estágios variados, comumente com sintomas constitucionais brandos; o período de incubação é de cerca de 14 a 17 dias. VER TAMBÉM *herpes* zoster. SIN chickenpox. [L. mod. dim. de *variola*]

v. gangreno′sa, v. gangrenosa; ulceração gangrenosa de lesões da varicela com ou sem infecção secundária, ocorrendo principalmente em crianças com doença subjacente grave.

var·i·cel·la·tion (var-i-se-lā′shŭn). Varicelação; a inoculação com o vírus da varicela como um meio de proteção contra a catapora.

var·i·cel·li·form (var-i-sel′i-form). Variceliforme; que se assemelha à varicela. SIN varicelloid.

var·i·cel·loid (var-ī-sel′oyd). Varicelóide. SIN varicelliform.

Var·i·cel·lo·vi·rus (var-ē-sel′ō-vī′rŭs). SIN varicella-zoster *virus.*

va·ri·ces (var′i-sēz). Varizes; plural of varix (variz).

var·i·ci·form (var′ī-si-form, vă-ris′ī-form). Variciforme; que se assemelha a uma variz. SIN cirsoid, varicoid.

varico-. Forma combinante que designa variz, varicoso e varicosidade. [L. *varix,* uma veia dilatada]

var·i·co·bleph·a·ron (var′i-kō-blef′ă-ron). Varicobléfaro; uma varicosidade da pálpebra. [varico- + G. *blepharon,* pálpebra]

var·i·co·cele (var′i-kō-sēl). Varicocele; uma condição manifestada por dilatação anormal das veias do cordão espermático, causada por válvulas incompetentes na veia espermática interna e resultando na drenagem comprometida para as veias do cordão espermático, quando o paciente fica de pé. SIN pampinocele. [varico- + G. *kēlē,* tumor, hérnia]

ovarian v., v. ovariana; uma condição varicosa do plexo pampiniforme no ligamento largo do útero. SIN tubo-ovarian v., utero-ovarian v.

symptomatic v., v. sintomática; uma v. causada por obstrução da veia espermática interna, usualmente no nível da veia renal e, em geral, devido a carcinoma invasivo de células renais, caracterizado pela incapacidade de as veias dilatadas no cordão espermático se esvaziarem quando o paciente se deita.

tubo-ovarian v., v. tubovariana. SIN ovarian v.

utero-ovarian v., v. uterovariana. SIN ovarian v.

var·i·co·ce·lec·to·my (var′i-kō-se-lek′tō-mē). Varicocelectomia; cirurgia para a correção de uma varicocele por laqueadura e excisão e por laqueadura apenas das veias dilatadas. [varicocele + G. *ektomē,* excisão]

var·i·cog·ra·phy (var′i-kog′ră-fē). Varicografia; a radiografia das veias depois da injeção de contraste nas veias varicosas. [varico- + G. *graphō,* escrever]

var·i·coid (var′i-koyd). Varicóide. SIN variciform.

var·i·com·pha·lus (var-i-kom′fă-lŭs). Varicônfalo; tumefação formada por veias varicosas no umbigo. [varico- + G. *omphalos,* umbigo]

var·i·co·phle·bi·tis (var′i-kō-flē-bī′tis). Varicoflebite; inflamação de veias varicosas. [varico- + G. *phleps,* veia, + *-itis,* inflamação]

var·i·cose (var′i-kōs). Varicoso; relativo a, afetado ou caracterizado por varizes ou varicose.

var·i·co·sis, pl. **var·i·cos·es** (var-i-kō′sis, -sēz). Varicose; um estado dilatado ou varicoso de uma veia ou veias. [varico- + G. *-osis,* condição]

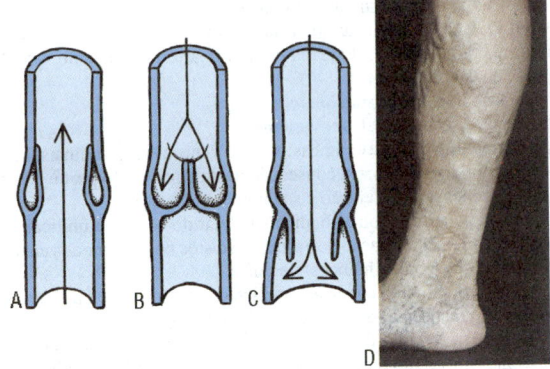

varicose: em uma veia saudável, as valvas permitem que o sangue flua para o coração (A), enquanto impede que o sangue reflua do coração (B); as valvas nas veias varicosas (C) não mais funcionam adequadamente, permitindo, assim, que o sangue reflua para os membros, (D) fotografia da perna com veias varicosas

var·i·cos·i·ty (var-i-kos′i-tē). Varicosidade; uma variz ou condição varicosa.

var·i·cot·o·my (var-i-kot′ō-mē). Varicotomia; cirurgia para as veias varicosas por meio de incisão subcutânea. [varico- + G. *tomē,* um corte]

va·ric·u·la (vă-rik′ū-lă). Varícula; condição varicosa das veias da conjuntiva. SIN conjunctival varix. [L. dim. de *varix*]

var·i·cule (var′i-kūl). Varícula; uma pequena veia varicosa comumente observada na pele; pode estar associada a estrelas venosas, lagos venosos ou a veias varicosas maiores. [L. *varicula,* dim. de *varix*]

va·ri·eg·a·tion (ver′ē-a-gā′shŭn). Variegação; a diversificação ou alteração de um fenótipo produzido por uma alteração no genótipo durante o desenvolvimento somático.

va·ri·o·la (vă-rī′ō-lă). Varíola. SIN smallpox. [L. med. dim. do L. *varius,* manchado]

v. benig′na, v. benigna, v. modificada. SIN varioloid (2).

v. hemorrha′gica, v. hemorrágica. SIN hemorrhagic *smallpox.*

v. ma′jor, v. major. SIN smallpox.

v. malig′na, v. maligna; varíola maligna, usualmente da forma hemorrágica. SIN malignant smallpox.

v. milia′ris, v. miliar; uma forma de variolóide cuja erupção consiste em vesículas miliares sem a formação de pústulas.

v. mi′nor, v. menor. SIN alastrim.

v. pemphigo′sa, v. penfigosa; uma forma de varíola cuja erupção consiste em bolhas semelhantes ao pênfigo.

v. si′ne erupcio′ne, v. sem erupção; uma forma abortiva de varíola em que a doença desaparece sem o aparecimento de qualquer erupção ou, no máximo, algumas pápulas que nunca evoluem para pústula.

v. vaccine, variola v., vacina de varíola. SIN vaccinia.

v. ve′ra, v. verdadeira; varíola de gravidade habitual no não-vacinado.

v. verruco′sa, v. verrucosa; uma forma branda ou abortiva de variolóide cuja erupção consiste, principalmente, em pápulas, com vesículas diminutas ocasionalmente nos ápices, que persistem por algum tempo como lesões verrucosas. SIN wartpox.

va·ri·o·lar (vă-rī′ō-lăr). Variolar; relativo à varíola. SIN variolic, variolous.

var·i·o·late (var′ē-ō-lāt). **1.** Inocular com varíola. **2.** Com cicatrizes ou marcas, como se tivesse varíola.

var·i·o·la·tion (var′ē-ō-lā′shŭn). Variolação; o processo obsoleto de inocular uma pessoa suscetível com o material originário de uma vesícula de um paciente com varíola. SIN variolization.

var·i·ol·ic (var-ē-ol′ik). Variólico. SIN variolar.

var·i·ol·i·form (vă-rī′ō-li-form, var-ē-ō′li-form). Varioliforme. SIN varioloid (1). [variola + L. *forma,* forma]

var·i·o·li·za·tion (var′ē-ō-li-zā′shŭn). Variolização. SIN variolation.

va·ri·o·loid (var′ē-ō-loyd). Variolóide. **1.** Que se assemelha à varíola. SIN varioliform. **2.** Uma forma branda de varíola que ocorre em pessoas que são relativamente resistentes, geralmente em decorrência de vacinação prévia. SIN modified smallpox, varicelloid smallpox, variola benigna. [variola + G. *eidos,* semelhança]

va·ri·o·lous (vă-rī′ō-lŭs). Varioloso. SIN variolar.

va·ri·o·lo·vac·cine (vă-rī′ō-lō-vak′sēn). Variolovacina; uma vacina obtida a partir da erupção após a inoculação de uma novilha com varíola obtida de um ser humano.

var·ix, pl. **va·ri·ces** (var′iks, var′i-sēz). Variz, varizes. **1.** Uma veia dilatada. **2.** Uma veia, artéria ou vaso linfático aumentado de calibre e tortuoso. [L. *varix* (*varic-*), uma veia dilatada]

v. anastomot'icus, v. anastomótica. SIN aneurysmal v.
aneurysmal v., v. aneurismática; dilatação e tortuosidade de uma veia resultantes de uma comunicação adquirida com uma artéria adjacente. SIN Pott aneurysm, v. anastomoticus.
cirsoid v., v. cirsóide. SIN cirsoid aneurysm.
conjunctival v., v. conjuntival. SIN varicula.
esophageal varices, varizes esofágicas; varizes venosas longitudinais, na extremidade inferior do esôfago, em consequência da hipertensão porta; elas são superficiais e propensas a ulceração e sangramento maciço.
gelatinous v., v. gelatinosa; uma condição nodular do cordão umbilical.
lymph v., v. linfática; a formação de varizes ou cistos nos linfonodos em consequência da obstrução nos linfáticos eferentes.
turbinal v., v. turbinal; uma condição de dilatação permanente das veias dos corpos turbinados, especialmente do turbinado inferior.

var·nish (den·tal). Verniz (dentário); soluções de resinas e gomas naturais em um solvente solúvel, do qual um fino revestimento é aplicado sobre as superfícies de preparações cavitárias antes da colocação das restaurações, usado como um agente protetor para o dente contra os constituintes de materiais de restauração. SIN cavity liner, vernix.

Varolius (Varolio), Constantius (Costanzio), anatomista e médico italiano, 1543–1575. VER ileal *sphincter; valve* of V.; *pons* varolii.

var·us (va'rŭs). Varo; curvatura ou torção para dentro, em direção à linha média do membro ou corpo; o uso moderno aceito, principalmente em ortopedia, transpõe erroneamente o significado de valgo para v., como no *genu* varum (joelho varo). [L. mod. curvado para dentro, do L. cambaio]

vas, gen. **va·'sis,** pl. **va·sa,** gen. e pl. **va·so·rum** (vas, vā'sis, vā'sa, vā-sō'rum) [TA]. Vaso; um ducto ou canal que conduz qualquer líquido, como sangue, linfa, quilo ou sêmen. VER TAMBÉM vessel. [L. um vaso, prato]
v. aber'rans hep'atis, pl. **va'sa aberran'tia hep'atis,** v. aberrante hepático; resquícios de ductos biliares atróficos e/ou cegos no apêndice fibroso e na cápsula do fígado nas margens do lobo esquerdo e no sulco para a veia cava inferior.
v. aberrans of Roth, v. aberrante de Roth; um divertículo ocasional da rede testicular ou dos dúctulos eferentes do testículo.
va'sa aberran'tia, dúctulos aberrantes. SIN aberrant ductules, em ductule.
v. af'ferens, pl. **va'sa afferen'tia,** vasos aferentes. SIN afferent glomerular arteriole.
v. anastomot'icum [TA], v. anastomótico. SIN anastomotic vessel.
va'sa bre'via, vasos curtos. SIN short gastric arteries, em artery.
v. capilla're [TA], v. capilar. SIN capillary (2). VER blood *capillary,* lymph *capillary.*
va'sa chylif'era, vasos quilíferos. VER lacteal (2).
v. collatera'le, v. colateral. SIN collateral vessel.
v. def'erens, pl. **va'sa deferen'tia,** ducto deferente. SIN ductus deferens.
v. ef'ferens, pl. **va'sa efferen'tia,** v. eferente; (1) uma veia que transporta o sangue para longe de uma região. SIN efferent lymphatic, v. lymphaticum efferens; (2) arteríola glomerular eferente. SIN efferent glomerular *arteriole;* (3) dúctulos eferentes do testículo. SIN efferent *ductules* of testis, em *ductule.*
Ferrein vasa aberrantia, vasos aberrantes de Ferrein; canalículos biliares que não estão ligados aos lóbulos hepáticos.
Haller v. aberrans, vaso aberrante de Haller. SIN inferior aberrant *ductule.*
va'sa lymphat'ica, vasos linfáticos. SIN lymph *vessels,* em *vessel.*
v. lympha'ticum, v. linfático. SIN lymphatic (3).
v. lympha'ticum af'ferens, v. linfático aferente. SIN afferent *lymphatic.*
v. lympha'ticum ef'ferens, v. linfático eferente. SIN v. efferens (1).
v. lympha'ticum profun'dum [TA], v. linfático profundo. SIN deep lymph *vessel.*
v. lympha'ticum superficia'le [TA], v. linfático superficial. SIN superficial lymph *vessel.*
va'sa nervor'um, vasos dos nervos; os vasos sanguíneos que irrigam os nervos.
va'sa pre'via, os vasos umbilicais que precedem a cabeça fetal, geralmente atravessando as membranas e cruzando o óstio cervical interno.
v. prom'inens duc'tus cochlea'ris, v. proeminente do canal coclear; um vaso sanguíneo na substância da proeminência espiral do ducto coclear.
va'sa rec'ta, vasos retos; os vasos retos nos quais a arteríola eferente dos glomérulos justaglomerulares desemboca; eles formam um entrelaçado de vasos que, originando-se nas bases das pirâmides, correm através da medula renal em direção ao ápice de cada pirâmide, mudando, então, a direção em uma rotação semelhante a um grampo de cabelo, e dirigem-se em linha reta novamente para trás, no sentido da base da pirâmide, como veias retas.
va'sa recta renis [TA], vasos retos renais; as artérias que penetram e irrigam a medula renal (pirâmides). SIN arteriolae rectae [TA], straight arteries*.
va'sa sanguinea aur'is inter'nae [TA], vasos sanguíneos da orelha interna. SIN vessels of internal ear, em *vessel.*
vasa sanguinea choroideae [TA], vasos sanguíneos da coróide. SIN choroid blood vessels, em blood vessel.
vasa sanguinea intrapulmonalia [TA], vasos sanguíneos intrapulmonares. SIN intrapulmonary blood vessel, em blood vessel.
va'sa sanguin'ea ret'inae [TA], vasos sanguíneos da retina. SIN retinal blood vessels, em blood vessel.
v. sanguineum [TA], v. sanguíneo. SIN blood vessel.
v. spira'le, v. espiral; um vaso sanguíneo, maior que seus companheiros, que corre na camada timpânica da membrana basilar, logo abaixo do túnel de Corti.
va'sa vaso'rum [TA], vasos dos vasos; pequenas artérias distribuídas para as camadas externa e média de vasos sanguíneos maiores, e suas veias correspondentes. SIN vessels of vessels.
va'sa vortico'sa, veias vorticosas. SIN vorticose veins, em vein.

♲ **vas-.** Forma combinante que indica um vaso sanguíneo. VER TAMBÉM vasculo-, vaso-. [L. *vas*]

va·sa (vā'să). Vasos; plural de vas (vaso).
va·sal (vā'săl). Vasal; relativo a um ou mais vasos.
vas·cu·lar (vas'kŭ-lăr). Vascular; relativo a ou que contém vasos sanguíneos. [L. *vasculum,* um pequeno vaso, dim. de *vas*]
vas·cu·lar·i·ty (vas-kŭ-lar'i-tē). Vascularidade; a condição de ser vascular.
vas·cu·lar·i·za·tion (vas'kŭ-lăr-i-zā'shŭn). Vascularização; a formação de novos vasos sanguíneos em uma região. SIN arterialization (3).
vas·cu·lar·ized (vas-kŭ-lăr-īzd). Vascularizado; tornado vascular pela formação de novos vasos.
vas·cu·la·ture (vas'kŭ-lă-choor). Vasculatura; a rede vascular de um órgão.
vas·cu·li·tis (vas-kŭ-lī'tis). Vasculite. SIN angiitis.
 cutaneous v., v. cutânea; uma forma aguda de v. que pode afetar apenas a pele, mas também pode envolver outros órgãos, com infiltrado polimorfonuclear nas paredes e circundando os pequenos vasos (dérmicos). Fragmentos nucleares são formados por cariorrexe dos neutrófilos. VER TAMBÉM leukocytoclastic v. SIN hypersensitivity v.
 hypersensitivity v., v. por hipersensibilidade. SIN cutaneous v.
 hypocomplementemic v., v. hipocomplementêmica. SIN urticarial v.
 leukocytoclastic v., v. leucocitoclástica; v. cutânea aguda clinicamente caracterizada por púrpura palpável, especialmente nas pernas, e, do ponto de vista histológico, por exsudação de neutrófilos e, por vezes, fibrina ao redor das vênulas dérmicas, com poeira nuclear e extravasamento de eritrócitos; pode ser limitada à pele ou envolver outros tecidos como na purpura de Henoch-Schönlein. VER TAMBÉM cutaneous v. [G. *leukos,* branco, + *kytos,* célula, + *klastos,* rompido, de *klao,* romper]
 livedo v., v. em livedo; degeneração hialina das paredes dos pequenos vasos sanguíneos dérmicos com oclusão trombótica, observada na crioglobulinemia ou na *atrophie blanche.* Não se observa necrose.
 nodular v., v. nodular; lesões nodulares crônicas ou recorrentes do tecido subcutâneo, especialmente nas pernas de mulheres idosas, com paniculite lobular, inflamação granulomatosa com células gigantes multinucleadas, necrose focal e inflamação obliterativa dos pequenos vasos sanguíneos, assemelhando-se ao eritema endurado, mas sem evidências de tuberculose associada.
 urticarial v., v. urticariforme; lesões cutâneas dolorosas e purpúricas que se assemelham à urticária, mas que duram mais de 24 horas, com achados de biopsia da v. leucocitoclástica e alterações sistêmicas variáveis, freqüentemente com hipocomplementemia. SIN hypocomplementemic v.

♲ **vasculo-.** Forma combinante que indica um vaso sanguíneo. VER TAMBÉM vas-, vaso-. [L. *vasculum,* um pequeno vaso, dim. de *vas*]

vas·cu·lo·car·di·ac (vas'kŭ-lō-kar'dē-ak). Vasculocardíaco. SIN cardiovascular.
vas·cu·lo·gen·e·sis (vas'kŭ-lō-jen'ē-sis). Vasculogênese; formação do sistema vascular. [vasculo- + G. *genesis,* produção]
vas·cu·lo·mo·tor (vas'koo-lō-mō'ter). Vasculomotor. SIN vasomotor.
vas·cu·lo·my·e·li·nop·a·thy (vas'kŭ-lō-mī-ē-li-nop'ă-thē). Vasculomielinopatia; vasculopatia dos pequenos vasos cerebrais com subsequente desmielinização perivascular, presumivelmente causada por imunocomplexos circulantes.
vas·cu·lop·a·thy (vas-kŭ-lop'ă-thē). Vasculopatia; qualquer doença dos vasos sanguíneos. [vasculo- + G. *pathos,* doença]
vas·cu·lum, pl. **vas·cu·la** (vas'kŭ-lŭm, -lă). Vásculo; um pequeno vaso. [L. dim. de *vas,* um vaso]

ⓘ **va·sec·to·my** (va-sek'tō-mē). Vasectomia; excisão de um segmento do ducto deferente, realizada em associação à prostatectomia ou para produzir esterilidade. [vas- + G. *ektomē,* excisão]
vas·i·fac·tion (vas-i-fak'shŭn). Vasiformação. SIN angiopoiesis.
vas·i·fac·tive (vas-i-fak'tiv). Vasiformador. SIN angiopoietic.
vas·i·form (vas'i-fōrm). Vasiforme; que tem a forma de um vaso ou estrutura tubular.
vas·i·tis (va-sī'tis). Vasite. SIN deferentitis.
 v. nodo'sa (va-sī'tis nō-dō'sa), v. nodosa; uma condição inflamatória do ducto deferente caracterizada por inúmeros espaços revestidos por epitélio, com as camadas muscular e adventícia contendo freqüentemente espermatozóides;

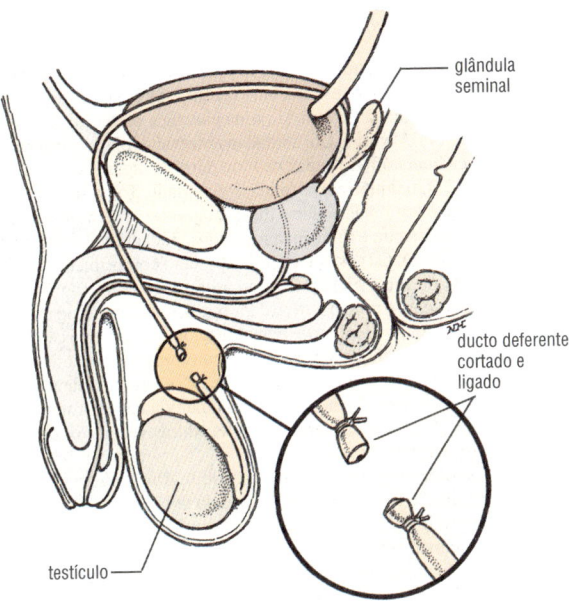

vasectomia

geralmente observada depois da vasectomia e pode, do ponto de vista clínico e microscópico, mimetizar o adenocarcinoma. VER TAMBÉM *vas* deferens.

vaso-. Forma combinante que significa vaso, vaso sanguíneo. VER TAMBÉM vas-, vasculo-. [L. *vas*, um vaso]

va·so·ac·tive (vā-sō-ak′tiv, vas-ō-). Vasoativo; que influencia o tônus e o calibre dos vasos sanguíneos.

va·so·con·stric·tion (vā′sō-kon-strik′shŭn, vas′ō-). Vasoconstrição; estreitamento dos vasos sanguíneos.
 active v., v. ativa; calibre reduzido de um vaso causado por tônus aumentado na musculatura lisa em suas paredes.
 passive v., v. passiva; o calibre reduzido de um vaso causado por pressão intraluminal diminuída.

va·so·con·stric·tive (vā′sō-kon-strik′tiv, vas′ō-). Vasoconstritivo. **1.** Que provoca o estreitamento dos vasos sanguíneos. **2.** SIN vasoconstrictor (1).

va·so·con·stric·tor (vā′sō-kon-strik′ter, vas′ō-). Vasoconstritor. **1.** Um agente que causa estreitamento dos vasos sanguíneos. SIN vasoconstrictive (2). **2.** Um nervo cuja estimulação provoca constrição vascular.

va·so·den·tin (vā-sō-den′tin, vas-ō-). Vasodentina; a dentina em que os capilares primitivos permaneceram sem calcificação e, dessa maneira, são suficientemente amplos para permitir a passagem dos elementos formados do sangue. SIN vascular dentin.

va·so·de·pres·sion (vā′sō-dē-presh′ŭn, vas′ō). Vasodepressão; redução do tônus nos vasos sanguíneos com vasodilatação e resultando em pressão arterial diminuída.

va·so·de·pres·sor (vā′sō-dē-pres′er, vas′ō). Vasodepressor. **1.** Que provoca vasodepressão. **2.** SIN depressor (4).

va·so·di·la·ta·tion (vā′sō-dil-ā-tā′shŭn, vas′ō-). Vasodilatação. SIN vasodilation.

va·so·di·la·tion (vā′sō-dī-lā′shŭn, vas-ō-). Vasodilatação; alargamento da luz dos vasos sanguíneos. SIN vasodilatation.
 active v., v. ativa; a v. causada por diminuição no tônus da musculatura lisa na parede de um vaso.
 passive v., v. passiva; v. relacionada com a pressão aumentada na luz de um vaso.

va·so·di·la·tive (vā′sō-dī-lā′tiv, vas′ō-). Vasodilatador. **1.** Que causa dilatação dos vasos sanguíneos. **2.** SIN vasodilator (1).

va·so·di·la·tor (vā′sō-dī-lā′ter, vas′ō-). Vasodilatador. **1.** Um agente que causa dilatação dos vasos sanguíneos. SIN vasodilative (2). **2.** Um nervo cuja estimulação resulta em dilatação dos vasos sanguíneos.

va·so·ep·i·did·y·mos·to·my (vā′sō-ep-i-did-i-mos′tō-mē, vas′ō-). Vasoepididimostomia; a anastomose cirúrgica dos ductos deferentes ao epidídimo, para evitar uma obstrução ao nível da porção média ou distal do epidídimo ou do vaso proximal. [vaso- + epididymis + G. *stoma*, boca]

va·so·fac·tive (vā-sō-fak′tiv, vas-ō-). Vasoformador. SIN angiopoietic.

va·so·for·ma·tion (vā-sō-fōr-mā′shŭn, vas-ō-). Vasoformação. SIN angiopoiesis.

va·so·for·ma·tive (vā-sō-fōr′mā-tiv, vas-ō-). Vasoformador. SIN angiopoietic.

va·so·gan·gli·on (vā-sō-gang′glē-on, vas-ō-). Vasogânglio; uma massa de vasos sanguíneos.

va·sog·ra·phy (vā-sog′ră-fē). Vasografia; radiografia dos ductos deferentes para determinar a permeabilidade, ao se injetar o contraste em sua luz, quer por via transuretral, quer por vasotomia a céu aberto. [vas + G. *graphō*, escrever]

va·so·in·hib·i·tor (vā′sō-in-hib′i-ter, vas′ō-). Vasoinibidor; um agente que restringe ou evita o funcionamento dos nervos vasomotores.

va·so·in·hib·i·to·ry (vā′sō-in-hib′i-tōr-ē, vas′ō-). Vasoinibitório; que restringe a ação vasomotora.

va·so·la·bile (vā-sō-lā′bil, -bil, vas-ō-). Vasolábil; que caracteriza a condição em que existe labilidade ou vasomotricidade ativa dos vasos sanguíneos.

va·so·li·ga·tion (vā′sō-li-gā′shŭn, vas′ō-). Vasoligadura; ligadura do ducto deferente, usualmente depois de sua divisão.

va·so·mo·tion (vā-sō-mō′shŭn, vas-ō-). Vasomotricidade; alteração no calibre de um vaso sanguíneo.

va·so·mo·tor (vā-sō-mō′ter, vas-ō-). Vasomotor. **1.** Que causa dilatação ou constrição dos vasos sanguíneos. **2.** Indica os nervos que possuem essa ação. SIN vasculomotor.

va·so·neu·rop·a·thy (vā′sō-noo-rop′ă-thē, vas′ō-). Vasoneuropatia; qualquer doença que envolve os nervos e os vasos sanguíneos. [vaso- + G. *neuron*, nervo, + *pathos*, sofrimento]

va·so-or·chi·dos·to·my (vā′sō-ōr-ki-dos′tō-mē, vas′ō-). Vasorquidostomia; restabelecimento dos ductos seminíferos interrompidos ao unir os túbulos do epidídimo ou da rede testicular à extremidade dividida do ducto deferente. [vaso- + G. *orchis*, testículo, + *stoma*, boca]

va·so·pa·ral·y·sis (vā′sō-pă-ral′i-sis, vas′ō-). Vasoparalisia; paralisia, atonia ou hipotonia dos vasos sanguíneos. SIN angiohypotonia, angioparalysis.

va·so·pa·re·sis (vā′sō-pă-rē′sis, -par′ē-sis, vas′ō-). Vasoparesia; vasoparalisia discreta. SIN angioparesis, vasomotor paralysis. [vaso- + G. *paresis*, fraqueza]

va·so·pres·sin (VP) (vā-sō-pres′in, vas-ō-). Vasopressina; um hormônio neuro-hipofisário nonapeptídico relacionado com a ocitocina e vasotocina; preparado sinteticamente ou obtido a partir do lobo posterior da hipófise de animais domésticos saudáveis. Em doses farmacológicas, a v. provoca a contração da musculatura lisa, notadamente aquela de todos os vasos sanguíneos; as grandes doses podem produzir espasmos de artérias cerebrais ou coronarianos. SIN antidiuretic hormone, Pitressin. [vaso- + L. *premo*, pp. *pressum*, pressionar, + -in)
 arginine v. (AVP), arginina vasopressina; a v. que contém um resíduo arginil na posição 8 (como em galinhas e na maioria dos mamíferos, inclusive nos seres humanos); a v. suína possui um resíduo lisil na posição 8. Todas são vasopressoras. SIN argipressin.

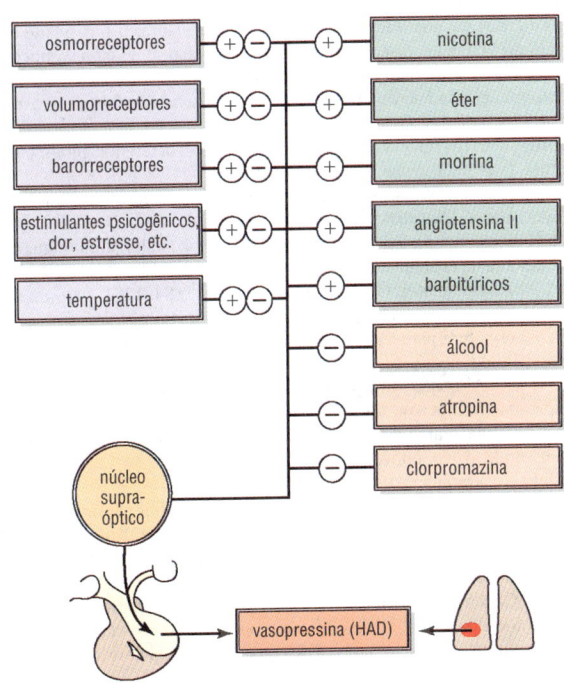

vasopressina: regulação da secreção do HAD; os efeitos de vários fatores neurais e mecânicos no núcleo supra-óptico (+ = estimulação, − = inibição); observe que algumas neoplasias malignas (p.ex., carcinoma broncogênico) também podem secretar HAD

va·so·pres·sor (vā-sō-pres′er, vas-ō-). Vasopressor. **1.** Que provoca vasoconstrição e um aumento na pressão arterial, geralmente compreendida como pressão arterial sistêmica, exceto quando especificado em contrário. **2.** Um agente que apresenta esse efeito.

va·so·punc·ture (vā-sō-pŭnk′choor, vas-ō-). Vasopunção; o ato de puncionar um vaso com uma agulha.

va·so·re·flex (vā-sō-rē′fleks, vas′ō-). Vasorreflexo; reflexo que influencia o calibre dos vasos sanguíneos.

va·so·re·lax·a·tion (vā′sō-rē-lak-sā′shŭn, vas-ō). Vasorrelaxamento; redução na tensão das paredes dos vasos sanguíneos.

va·so·sec·tion (vā-sō-sek′shŭn, vas-ō-). Vasotomia. SIN vasotomy.

va·so·sen·so·ry (vā-sō-sen′ser-ē, vas-ō-). Vasossensorial. **1.** Relativo à sensibilidade nos vasos sanguíneos. **2.** Indica fibras nervosas sensoriais que inervam os vasos sanguíneos.

va·so·spasm (vā′sō-spazm, vas′ō-). Vasoespasmo; a contração ou hipertonia das camadas musculares dos vasos sanguíneos. SIN angiohypertonia, angiospasm.

va·so·spas·tic (vā-sō-spas′tik, vas-ō-). Vasoespástico; relativo a, ou caracterizado por, vasoespasmo. SIN angiospastic.

va·so·stim·u·lant (va-sō-stim′ū-lant). Vasoestimulante. **1.** Que excita a ação vasomotora. **2.** Um agente que leva os nervos vasomotores à ação. **3.** SIN vasotonic (2).

va·sos·to·my (vā-sos′tō-mē). Vasostomia; estabelecimento de uma abertura no ducto deferente. [vaso- + G. *stoma*, boca]

va·so·throm·bin (vā-sō-throm′bin, vas-ō-). Vasotrombina; trombina derivada das células de revestimento dos vasos sanguíneos.

va·so·to·cin (vā-sō-tō′sin, vas-ō-). Vasotocina; um hormônio nonapeptídeo da neuro-hipófise dos subvertebrados, com atividades similares àquelas da vasopressina e ocitocina; quimicamente idêntica à vasopressina humana, exceto por um resíduo isoleucil na posição 3; dessa maneira, [3-isoleucina]vasopressina ou [Ile³]vasopressina. [*vaso*, pressin + oxy*tocin*]

arginine v., arginina v.; v. com resíduo arginil na posição 8 (idêntico à arginina ocitocina). VER TAMBÉM arginine *vasopressin*.

va·sot·o·my (vā-sot′ō-mē). Vasotomia; incisão no ou divisão do ducto deferente. SIN vasosection. [vaso- + G. *tomē*, incisão]

va·so·to·nia (vā-sō-tō′nē-ă, vas-ō-). Vasotonia; o tônus dos vasos sanguíneos, principalmente das arteríolas. [vaso- + G. *tonos*, tônus]

va·so·ton·ic (vā-sō-ton′ik, vas-ō-). Vasotônico. **1.** Relativo ao tônus vascular. **2.** Um agente que aumenta a tensão vascular. SIN vasostimulant (3).

va·so·tro·phic (vā-sō-trof′ik, vas-ō-). Vasotrófico; relativo à nutrição dos vasos sanguíneos ou dos linfáticos. [vaso- + G. *trophē*, nutrição]

va·so·tro·pic (vā-sō-trō′pik, vas-ō-). Vasotrópico; que tende a atuar sobre os vasos sanguíneos. [vaso- + G. *tropē*, uma volta]

va·so·va·gal (vā-sō-vā′gal, vas-ō-). Vasovagal; relativo à ação do nervo vago sobre os vasos sanguíneos.

va·so·va·sos·to·my (vā′sō-vă-sos′tō-mē, vas′ō-). Vasovasostomia; anastomose cirúrgica dos ductos deferentes, para restaurar a fertilidade em um homem previamente vasectomizado. [vaso- + vaso- + G. *stoma*, boca]

va·so·ve·sic·u·lec·to·my (vā′sō-vĕ-sik-ū-lek′tō-mē, vas′ō-). Vasovesiculectomia; excisão do ducto deferente e das vesículas seminais. [vaso- + L. *vesicula*, vesícula, + G. *ektomē*, excisão]

vas·tomy (vas′tō-mē). Vastomia; secção do ducto deferente, geralmente com ligadura. [vas + G. *tomē*, um corte]

vas·tus (vas′tŭs). Vasto; grande. VER vastus intermedius (*muscle*), vastus lateralis (*muscle*), vastus medialis (*muscle*). [L.]

VATER Acrônimo para defeitos *v*ertebrais, *a*tresia *a*nal, fístula *t*raqueoesofágica com atresia *e*sofágica e anomalias *r*adiais e renais. VER VATER *complex*.

Vater, Abraham, anatomista e botânico alemão, 1684–1751. VER *ampulla* of Vater; V. *corpuscles*, em *corpuscle, fold*; V.-Pacini *corpuscles*, em *corpuscle*.

VATS Abreviatura para video-assisted thoracic *surgery* (cirurgia torácica vídeo-assistida).

vault (vawlt). Abóbada; uma parte que se assemelha ao teto arqueado ou cúpula, p.ex., a a. faríngea ou fórnice, a parte superior não-muscular da nasofaringe; a. palatina, o arco do palato; a. da vagina, fórnice da vagina. [Através do Fr. ant., do L. *volvo*, pp. *volutus*, girar]

cranial v., a. craniana. SIN neurocranium.

v. of pharynx [TA], a. faríngea; a extremidade superior não-muscular e não-colapsante da nasofaringe, onde a mucosa faríngea está firmemente aplicada ao corpo do osso esfenóide e à fáscia faringobasilar. SIN fornix pharyngis [TA], pharyngeal fornix.

V-bends. Ganchos em forma de V incorporados em um freio dentário, usualmente colocados mesial ou distalmente aos caninos (cúspides) e usados como uma área "morta" do freio, através dos quais podem ser colocados os ganchos de torção.

VC Abreviatura de colored *vision* (visão em cores); vital *capacity* (capacidade vital).

VCUG Abreviatura de voiding *cystourethrogram* (uretrocistografia miccional).

VDRL Abreviatura para Venereal Disease Research Laboratories. VER VDRL *test*.

vec·tion (vek′shŭn). Vecção; transferência dos agentes da doença de um indivíduo infectado para um não-infectado por um vetor. [L. *vectio*, condução]

vec·tis (vek′tis). Alavanca; um instrumento que se assemelha a uma das lâminas de um fórceps obstétrico, usado como um auxiliar no parto ao fazer a elevação da parte apresentada do feto. [L. uma alavanca ou barra]

vec·tor (vek′ter, tōr). Vetor. **1.** Um animal invertebrado (p.ex., carrapato, ácaro, mosquito, mosca hematófaga) capaz de transmitir um agente infeccioso entre os vertebrados. **2.** Qualquer coisa (p.ex., velocidade, força mecânica, força eletromotiva) que possui magnitude e direção; pode ser representada por uma linha reta de comprimento e direção apropriados. **3.** O eixo elétrico resultante de qualquer onda do ECG (geralmente o QRS), cujo comprimento é proporcional à magnitude da força elétrica, a direção fornece a direção da força e a extremidade representa o pólo positivo da força. **4.** O DNA, como um cromossoma ou plasmídeo, que se replica de maneira autônoma em uma célula na qual outro segmento de DNA pode ser inserido e auto-replicar-se, como na clonagem. **5.** SIN recombinant v. **6.** Os sistemas de DNA recombinantes especialmente adaptados para a produção de grandes quantidades de proteínas específicas em sistemas de células bacterianas, de leveduras, de insetos ou de mamíferos. [L. *vector*, um transportador]

biologic v., v. biológico; um v., como o mosquito *Anopheles* para os agentes da malária ou a mosca tsé-tsé para os agentes da doença do sono africana, em que o agente se multiplica antes de ser transmitido para outro hospedeiro.

cloning v., v. de clonagem; um plasmídeo ou fago de replicação autônoma com regiões que não são essenciais para sua propagação nas bactérias e no qual pode ser inserido DNA estranho; esse DNA estranho é replicado e propagado como se fosse um componente normal do v.

expression v., v. de expressão; um v. (plasmídeo, levedura ou genoma de vírus animal) usado experimentalmente para introduzir o material genético estranho em uma célula hospedeira propagável, a fim de replicar e amplificar as seqüências de DNA estranho como uma molécula recombinante (clonagem de seqüências de DNA recombinante).

instantaneous v., v. instantâneo; o v. resultante das correntes de ação cardíaca em determinado momento, geralmente representado como uma seta de direção e magnitude apropriadas.

manifest v., v. manifesto; projeção de um v. cardíaco espacial em um único plano.

mean v., v. médio; um v. cardíaco único que representa a média de todos os vetores presentes durante determinado intervalo de tempo. SIN mean manifest v.

mean manifest v., v. médio. SIN mean v.

mechanical v., v. mecânico; um v. que conduz patógenos para um indivíduo suscetível sem o desenvolvimento biológico essencial dos patógenos no v., como na transferência de organismos sépticos nos pés ou boca da mosca doméstica.

recombinant v., v. recombinante; um v. em que um DNA estranho foi inserido. SIN vector (5).

retroviral v., v. retroviral; um retrovírus especialmente construído que contém um ou mais genes para corrigir determinados distúrbios genéticos.

shuttle v., v. de transporte; um v. (4) que contém sinais de replicação bacteriana e eucariótica; dessa forma, a replicação pode acontecer nos dois tipos de células.

spatial v., v. espacial; um v. cardíaco representado em mais de um plano de maneira simultânea; a orientação bi- ou tridimensional de um v.

vec·tor-borne (vek′ter-bōrn). Transmitido por vetor; indica uma doença ou infecção que é transmitida por um vetor invertebrado.

vec·tor·car·di·o·gram (vek′tōr-kar′dē-ō-gram). Vetorcardiograma; uma representação gráfica da magnitude e direção das correntes de ação do coração a cada instante na forma de alças de vetor.

vec·tor·car·di·og·ra·phy. Vetorcardiografia; a integração dos registros eletrocardiográficos em dois ou três planos para produzir um vetorcardiograma, consistindo nas alças divididas por um mecanismo de regulação para todas as ondas do eletrocardiograma.

spatial vectorcardiography, vetorcardiografia espacial; a vetorcardiografia tridimensional em que as alças dos vetores são inscritas nos planos frontal, sagital e horizontal.

vec·to·ri·al (vek-tōr′ē-ăl). Vetorial; relativo, de qualquer forma, a um vetor.

ve·cu·ro·ni·um bro·mide (ve-kū-rō′nē-ŭm). Brometo de vecurônio; um relaxante neuromuscular despolarizante com duração de ação relativamente curta; um homólogo não-quaternário do pancurônio.

VEE Abreviatura para Venezuelan equine *encephalomyelitis* (encefalomielite eqüina venezuelana).

veg·an (veg′an). Um vegetariano estrito; ou seja, aquele que não consome produtos de animais ou laticínios de qualquer tipo. Cf. vegetarian.

veg·e·ta·ble (vej′tă-bl, vej′ē-tă-bl). Vegetal. **1.** Uma planta, especificamente aquela utilizada como alimento. **2.** Relativo a plantas, conforme diferenciado de animais ou minerais. SIN vegetal (1). [I. m. do L. *vegetabilis* (ver vegetation)]

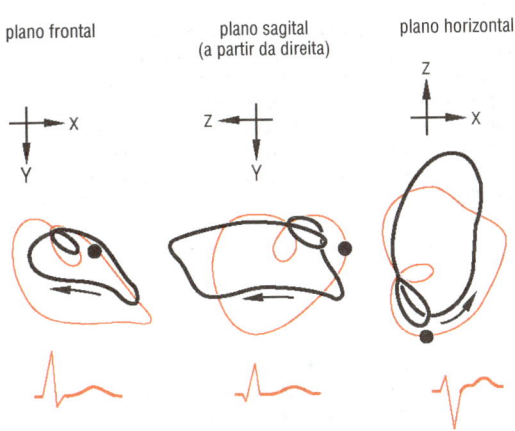

vetorcardiograma: as derivações do ECG em escala normal, bem como as alças de vetor de QRS e T em um vetorcardiograma (linha preta = adulto; linha vermelha = criança; linha espessa = vetor 0,02 s após o início da estimulação ventricular)

veg·e·tal (vej′ĕ-tăl). Vegetal. **1.** SIN vegetable (2). **2.** Indica as funções vitais comuns a vegetais e animais, como respiração, metabolismo, crescimento, geração, etc., diferenciadas daquelas peculiares aos animais, como a sensação consciente e as faculdades mentais.

veg·e·tal·i·ty (vej-ĕ-tal′i-tē). Vegetalidade; o agregado das funções vitais comuns a vegetais e animais.

veg·e·tar·i·an (vej-ĕ-tār′ē-ăn). Vegetariano; aquele cuja dieta é restrita aos alimentos de origem vegetal, excluindo principalmente as carnes de animais. Cf. vegan.

lacto-ovo-v., v. de leite e ovos; um v. que consome laticínios e ovos, mas não ingere carne animal.

ovo-v., um v. que consome ovos, mas não consome laticínios, nem carne animal.

semi-v., semivegetariano; um v. que consome laticínios, ovos, galinha e peixe, mas não consome carne de outro animal.

veg·e·tar·i·an·ism (vej-ĕ-tār′ē-ăn-izm). Vegetarianismo; a prática dietética de um vegetariano.

veg·e·ta·tion (vej-ĕ-tā′shŭn). Vegetação. **1.** O processo de crescimento em plantas. **2.** A condição de lentidão, comparável à inatividade da vida vegetal. **3.** Um crescimento ou excrescência de qualquer tipo. **4.** Especificamente, um coágulo, composto em grande parte de plaquetas sanguíneas fundidas, fibrina e, por vezes, microrganismos, aderente a um orifício ou valva cardíaca enferma, sendo freqüentemente iniciado por infecção das estruturas envolvidas. (L. mod. *vegetatio*, crescimento]

bacterial v.'s, vegetações bacterianas; as lesões da endocardite bacteriana que se formam em qualquer ponto no endocárdio, mas, preferencialmente, nas áreas lesionadas e de maior pressão e principalmente nas valvas. Elas também podem aparecer na camada íntima das artérias e em um canal arterial persistente, assim como em outras áreas de *shunt* dentro e fora do coração.

verrucous v.'s, vegetações verrucosas; as vegetações semelhantes a verruga, por vezes devido a endocardite, também relacionada com as alterações degenerativas nas valvas e na amiloidose.

veg·e·ta·tive (vej′ĕ-tā-tiv). Vegetativo. **1.** Crescer ou funcionar de maneira involuntária ou inconsciente, como se supõe ser a maneira da vida vegetal; indica especialmente um estado de consciência macroscopicamente comprometida, como depois do traumatismo craniano ou doença cerebral grave, em que um indivíduo é incapaz de atos voluntários ou propositados e apenas responde de maneira reflexa aos estímulos dolorosos. **2.** Repouso; inativo; indica o estágio de uma célula ou de seu núcleo em que o processo de cariocinese é quiescente. VER TAMBÉM vegetation.

veg·e·to·an·i·mal (vej′ĕ-tō-an′i-măl). Vegetoanimal; relativo aos vegetais e animais.

ve·hi·cle (vē′hi-kl). Veículo. **1.** Um excipiente ou solvente; uma substância, geralmente sem ação terapêutica, usada como um meio para dar volume à administração de medicamentos. **2.** Uma substância inanimada (p.ex., alimento, leite, poeira, roupa, instrumento) pela qual ou na qual um agente infeccioso passa de um hospedeiro infectado para um suscetível; por conseguinte, os veículos agem como fontes importantes de infecção. [L. *vehiculum*, um conduto, de *veho*, carregar]

veil (vāl). Véu. **1.** SIN velum (1). **2.** Âmnio. SIN caul (1). [L. *velum*]

aqueduct v., v. do aqueduto; uma membrana que obstrui o aqueduto de Sylvius, gerando uma hidrocefalia não-comunicante.

Jackson v., v. de Jackson. SIN Jackson *membrane*.

Sattler v., v. de Sattler; edema difuso do epitélio córneo que pode desenvolver-se depois do uso de lentes de contato.

Veil·lo·nel·la (vā′yō-nel′ă). Um gênero de bactérias anaeróbicas imóveis e não-formadoras de esporos (família Veillonellaceae) contendo pequenos cocos Gram-negativos (0,3 a 0,5 μm de diâmetro) que ocorrem como curtas cadeias de diplococos e em massas. O dióxido de carbono é necessário para o crescimento, e os carboidratos não são fermentados. Esses microrganismos são parasitas na boca e nos tratos respiratório e intestinal de seres humanos e de outros animais; essas bactérias produzem endotoxinas sorologicamente específicas (lipopolissacarídeos) que induzem pirogenicidade e o fenômeno de Schwarzman em coelhos; nos seres humanos, elas foram associadas a infecções por mordedura humana e como um componente de abscessos polimicrobianos. A espécie típica é *V. parvula*. [Adrien *Veillon*, bacteriologista francês, 1864–1931]

V. alcales'cens subsp. *alcales'cens*, uma subespécie bacteriana encontrada principalmente na boca dos seres humanos, mas, ocasionalmente, na cavidade bucal de coelhos e ratos; é a subespécie típica da espécie *V. alcalescens*.

V. alcales'cens subsp. *dis'par*, uma subespécie encontrada na boca e no trato respiratório de seres humanos.

V. alcales'ens, uma espécie bacteriana encontrada na saliva de seres humanos e de outros animais.

V. aty'pica, SIN *V. parvula* subsp. *atypica*.

V. par'vula, uma espécie bacteriana encontrada normalmente como um parasita inócuo nas cavidades naturais, especialmente na boca e no trato digestivo de seres humanos e de outros animais, é a espécie típica do gênero *V*.

V. par'vula subsp. *atyp'ica*, uma subespécie bacteriana encontrada na cavidade bucal de ratos e de seres humanos. SIN *V. atypica*.

V. par'vula subsp. *par'vula*, uma subespécie bacteriana encontrada na boca ou no trato intestinal ou respiratório de seres humanos; é a subespécie típica da espécie *V. parvula*.

V. par'vula subsp. *roden'tium*, uma subespécie bacteriana encontrada na cavidade bucal e no trato intestinal de *hamsters*, ratos e coelhos. SIN *V. rodentium*.

V. roden'tium, SIN *V. parvula* subsp. *rodentium*.

Veil·lo·nel·la·ce·ae (vā′yō-ne-lā′sē-ē). Uma família de bactérias anaeróbicas imóveis e não-formadoras de esporos (ordem Eubacteriales) contendo cocos Gram-negativos (com tendência para resistir à descoloração), os quais variam em diâmetro de pequenos (0,3–0,5 μm) a grandes (2,5 μm). De maneira característica, elas ocorrem em pares; células isoladas, massas ou cadeias também podem ocorrer, mas as cadeias podem mostrar hiatos que ilustram a disposição básica em diplococos. Esses microrganismos são quimio-organotróficos; podem ou não fermentar carboidratos; são parasitas de animais homotérmicos, como seres humanos, ruminantes, roedores e porcos, sendo encontrados principalmente no trato alimentar. O gênero típico é *Veillonella*.

VEIN

vein (vān) [TA]. Veia; um vaso sanguíneo que conduz o sangue em direção ao coração; no período pós-natal, todas as veias conduzem sangue não-oxigenado, com exceção da pulmonar. SIN vena [TA]. [L. *veia*]

accessory cephalic v. [TA], v. cefálica acessória; uma v. variável que passa ao longo da borda radial do antebraço para se unir à veia cefálica próximo ao cotovelo. SIN vena cephalica accessoria [TA].

accessory hemiazygos v. [TA], v. hemiázigo acessória; formada pela união da quarta à sétima veias intercostais posteriores esquerdas, passa ao longo do lado dos corpos da quinta, sexta e sétima vértebras torácicas, cruza a seguir a linha média atrás da aorta, esôfago e ducto torácico, indo desembocar na v. ázigo, por vezes junto com a v. hemiázigo. SIN vena hemiazygos accessoria [TA], vena azygos minor superior.

accessory saphenous v. [TA], v. safena acessória; uma v. ocasional, localizada na coxa, que corre em paralelo com a v. safena magna, a qual se une pouco antes que a última desemboque na v. femoral. SIN vena saphena accessoria [TA].

accessory vertebral v. [TA], v. vertebral acessória; v. que acompanha a veia vertebral, mas atravessa o forame do processo transverso da sétima vértebra cervical e deságua independentemente na v. braquiocefálica. SIN vena vertebralis accessoria [TA].

accompanying v., v. acompanhante. SIN *vena comitans*.

accompanying v. of hypoglossal nerve, v. acompanhante do nervo hipoglosso. SIN *vena comitans of hypoglossal nerve*.

anastomotic v.'s, veias anastomóticas. VER inferior anastomotic v., superior anastomotic v.

angular v. [TA], v. angular; uma v. curta, localizada no ângulo medial do olho, formada pelas veias supra-orbitária e supratroclear e que continua como a v. facial. SIN vena angularis [TA].

anonymous v.'s, veias anônimas; termo obsoleto para as veias braquiocefálicas (esquerda e direita).

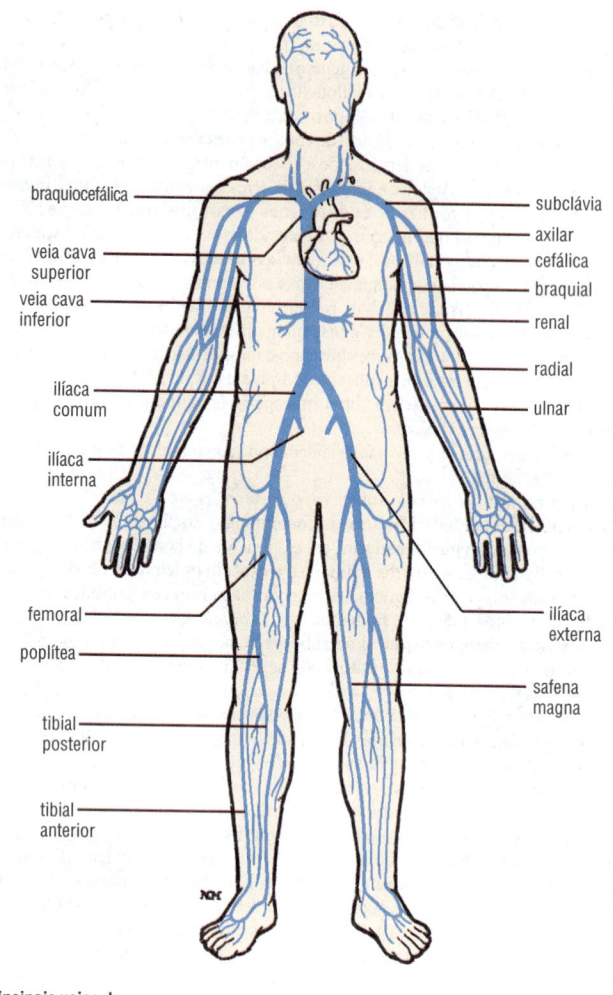

principais veias do corpo

anterior auricular v. [TA], v. auricular anterior; uma das diversas veias que drenam a orelha e o meato acústico e desembocam na v. retromandibular. SIN vena auricularis anterior, vena preauricularis.
anterior basal v. [TA], v. basilar anterior. SIN vena basalis anterior [TA], anterior basal branch of superior basal vein (of right and left inferior pulmonary veins)*, ramus basalis anterior venae basalis superioris*.
anterior cardiac v.'s [TA], veias cardíacas anteriores; duas ou três pequenas veias, localizadas na parede anterior do ventrículo direito, que se abrem diretamente para dentro do átrio direito, de forma independente do seio coronário. SIN venae cardiacae anteriores [TA].
anterior cerebral v.'s [TA], veias cerebrais anteriores; pequenas veias que fazem trajeto em paralelo com a artéria cerebral anterior e que drenam para a v. basal. SIN venae anteriores cerebri [TA].
anterior ciliary v.'s [TA], veias ciliares anteriores; diversas veias pequenas, anteriores e posteriores, que se originam do corpo ciliar. SIN venae ciliares anteriores [TA].
anterior circumflex humeral v. [TA], v. circunflexa anterior do úmero; v. que acompanha a artéria de mesmo nome, passando anteriormente ao colo cirúrgico do úmero para penetrar na v. axilar. SIN vena circumflexa humeri anterior [TA].
anterior facial v., v. facial anterior. SIN facial v.
anterior intercostal v.'s [TA], veias intercostais anteriores; as tributárias para as veias musculofrênicas ou torácicas internas a partir das porções anteriores dos espaços intercostais. SIN venae intercostales anteriores [TA].
anterior jugular v. [TA], v. jugular anterior; origina-se abaixo do queixo, a partir das veias que drenam o lábio inferior e a região mentoniana, desce pela porção anterior do pescoço, superficial ou profundamente à fáscia de investidura cervical, terminando na v. jugular externa, na borda lateral do músculo escaleno anterior. SIN vena jugularis anterior [TA].
anterior labial v.'s [TA], veias labiais anteriores; as tributárias das veias femoral ou pudenda externa que drenam o monte do púbis e a porção anterior dos grandes lábios do pudendo. SIN venae labiales anteriores [TA].

anterior pontomesencephalic v., v. pontomesencefálica anterior; uma v. localizada na linha média da fossa interpeduncular, nas faces superior e anterior da ponte; comunica-se com a v. basal, superiormente, e com a v. petrosa, inferiormente. SIN vena pontomesencephalica anterior.
(anterior and posterior) vestibular v.'s [TA], veias vestibulares (anterior e posterior); as veias que drenam o sáculo e o utrículo; são tributárias das veias do labirinto e da v. do aqueduto vestibular. SIN venae vestibulares (anterius et posterius) [TA].
anterior scrotal v.'s [TA], veias escrotais anteriores; tributárias da veia femoral ou da veia pudenda externa que drenam a face anterior do escroto e a pele e a túnica dartos do corpo e da base do pênis. SIN venae scrotales anteriores [TA].
anterior v. of septum pellucidum [TA], v. anterior do septo pelúcido; a v. que drena a parte anterior do septo transparente; ela desemboca na v. tálamo-estriada superior. SIN vena anterior septi pellucidi [TA].
anterior tibial v.'s [TA], veias tibiais anteriores; as veias acompanhantes da artéria tibial anterior que desembocam na v. poplítea. SIN venae tibiales anteriores [TA].
anterior vertebral v. [TA], v. vertebral anterior; a pequena v. que acompanha a artéria cervical ascendente; ela desemboca na v. vertebral. SIN vena vertebralis anterior [TA].
apical v. [TA], v. apical. SIN vena apicalis [TA], apical branch of right superior pulmonary vein*, ramus apicalis venae pulmonalis dextrae superioris*.
apicoposterior v. [TA], v. apicoposterior; drena o segmento broncopulmonar apicoposterior do lobo superior do pulmão esquerdo. SIN vena apicoposterior [TA], apicoposterior branch of left superior pulmonary vein*, ramus apicoposterior venae pulmonalis sinistrae superioris*.
appendicular v. [TA], v. apendicular; a tributária da v. ileocólica que acompanha a artéria apendicular. SIN vena appendicularis [TA].
aqueous v., v. aquosa; uma tributária da v. ciliar anterior que recebe o humor aquoso a partir do seio venoso da esclerótica.
arciform v.'s of kidney, veias arqueadas do rim. SIN arcuate v.'s of kidney.
arcuate v.'s of kidney, veias arqueadas do rim; veias cujo trajeto é paralelo ao das artérias arqueadas, recebem sangue das veias interlobulares e das vênulas retas, terminando nas veias interlobares. SIN arciform v.'s of kidney, venae arcuatae renis.
arterial v., v. arterial; assim chamada porque se ramifica como uma artéria (v. porta) ou porque, embora saindo do coração como uma artéria, contém sangue não-oxigenado, como uma v. (artéria pulmonar). SIN vena arteriosa.
ascending lumbar v. [TA], v. lombar ascendente; v. vertical, pareada, da parede abdominal posterior, adjacente e paralela à coluna vertebral, posterior à origem do músculo psoas maior; une-se às veias ilíaca comum, iliolombar e lombar na linha paravertebral, a v. direita une-se à v. subcostal direita para formar a v. ázigos, e a v. esquerda une-se à v. subcostal esquerda para formar a v. hemiázigos. SIN vena lumbalis ascendens [TA].
auricular v.'s, veias auriculares. VER anterior auricular v., posterior auricular v.
axillary v. [TA], v. axilar; uma continuação das veias basílica e braquial a partir da borda inferior do músculo redondo maior até a borda externa da primeira costela, onde se transforma na v. subclávia. SIN vena axillaris [TA].
azygos v. [TA], v. ázigo; origina-se da fusão da v. lombar ascendente direita com a v. subcostal direita e, com freqüência, de uma comunicação com a veia cava inferior; ascende através do hiato aórtico do diafragma ou de sua cruz direita; corre ao longo do lado direito dos corpos vertebrais torácicos, no mediastino posterior, e termina por arquear-se anteriormente sobre a raiz do pulmão direito para penetrar na face posterior da v. cava superior. SIN vena azygos [TA], azygos (2), vena azygos major.
basal v., uma grande v. que se origina da confluência das veias oriundas do córtex cerebral (veias cerebrais anteriores [TA]) e da área do córtex insular [veia cerebral média profunda [TA] (vena media profunda cerebri [TA]), veias insulares [TA] (venae insulares [TA])], passando, caudal e dorsalmente, ao longo da superfície medial do lobo temporal, indo desembocar mais adiante, na veia cerebral magna. A v. basal recebe tributárias das estruturas encontradas ao longo de seu trajeto; estas incluem a v. do giro olfatório [TA] (vena gyri olfactori [TA]), veias tálamo-estriadas inferiores [TA] (venae thalamostriatae inferiores [TA]), v. ventricular inferior [TA] (vena ventricularis inferior [TA]), v. coroidea inferior [TA] (vena choroidea inferior [TA]) e veias pedunculares [TA] (venae pedunculares [TA]). VER TAMBÉM common basal v., inferior basal v., superior basal v. SIN vena basalis [TA], basal. of Rosenthal, Rosenthal v.
basal v. of Rosenthal, v. basilar de Rosenthal. SIN basal v.
basilic v. [TA], v. basílica; origina-se do lado ulnar da rede venosa dorsal da mão; faz curva ao redor do lado medial do antebraço (como a veia basílica do antebraço), comunica-se com a v. cefálica por meio da v. intermédia do cotovelo e dirige-se para cima, no lado medial do braço, até se unir à v. axilar. SIN vena basilica [TA].
basivertebral v.'s [TA], veias basivertebrais; as veias localizadas na substância esponjosa dos corpos das vértebras e que desembocam no plexo venoso vertebral interno anterior. SIN venae basivertebrales [TA].

Baumgarten v.'s, veias de Baumgarten; resquícios não-obliterados da veia umbilical.
Boyd communicating perforation v., v. comunicante perfurante de Boyd; uma v. que conecta os sistemas venosos superficial e profundo na porção anteromedial da panturrilha.
brachial v.'s [TA], veias braquiais; as veias acompanhantes da artéria braquial que desembocam na v. axilar. SIN venae brachiales [TA].
Breschet v., v. de Breschet, v. diplóica. SIN diploic v.
bronchial v.'s [TA], veias brônquicas; o conjunto de veias que correm à frente e atrás dos brônquios e que se unem em troncos principais, os quais desembocam no lado direito da v. ázigos, à esquerda na v. hemiázigos acessória ou na intercostal superior esquerda. SIN venae bronchiales [TA].
Browning v., v. de Browning, v. anastomótica inferior. SIN inferior anastomotic v.
v. of bulb of penis [TA], v. do bulbo do pênis; uma tributária da v. pudenda interna que drena o bulbo do pênis. SIN vena bulbi penis [TA].
v. of bulb of vestibule [TA], v. do bulbo do vestíbulo; a v. que drena o bulbo do vestíbulo; uma tributária da v. pudenda interna. SIN vena bulbi vestibuli [TA], v. of vestibular bulb.
Burow v., v. de Burow; (1) uma v. ocasional que se origina na v. epigástrica inferior, por vezes recebendo uma tributária da bexiga urinária, que desemboca na v. porta; (2) uma das veias renais.
capillary v., vênula. SIN venule.
cardiac v.'s, v. cardíaca. VER anterior cardiac v.'s, great cardiac v., middle cardiac v., smallest cardiac v.'s.
cardinal v.'s, veias cardinais; os principais canais venosos sistêmicos nos vertebrados primitivos adultos e nos embriões dos vertebrados superiores; as **veias cardinais anteriores** são os principais canais de drenagem a partir da porção cefálica do corpo, e as **veias cardinais posteriores**, a partir da porção caudal; as **veias cardinais comuns**, formadas pela anastomose das veias cardinais anteriores e posteriores, são os principais canais de retorno sistêmico para o coração; na literatura antiga, por vezes chamadas de ductos de Cuvier.
v.'s of caudate nucleus [TA], veias do núcleo caudado; pequenas veias, originárias do núcleo caudado, que drenam para a v. tálamo-estriada superior. SIN venae nuclei caudati [TA].
cavernous v.'s of penis [TA], veias cavernosas do pênis; os espaços venosos cavernosos no tecido erétil do pênis. SIN venae cavernosae penis [TA].
central v.'s of liver [TA], veias centrais do fígado; a v. inicial do sistema venoso hepático, localizada no centro do lóbulo hepático conceitual, que recebe o sangue dos seios e drena para as veias coletoras, que se transformam em veias hepáticas. SIN Krukenberg v.'s, venae centrales hepatis.
central retinal v. [TA], v. central da retina; a v. formada por união das veias retinianas; acompanha a artéria de mesmo nome no nervo óptico. SIN vena centralis retinae [TA].
central v. of suprarenal gland [TA], v. central da glândula supra-renal; a única veia que drena a glândula; recebe inúmeras veias medulares; no lado direito, desemboca diretamente na v. cava inferior e, à esquerda, na v. renal esquerda. SIN vena centralis glandulae suprarenalis [TA].
cephalic v. [TA], v. cefálica; v. subcutânea que se origina na borda radial da rede venosa dorsal da mão, dirige-se para cima à frente do cotovelo e ao longo do lado lateral do braço; desemboca na parte superior da v. axilar. SIN vena cephalica [TA].
cephalic v. of forearm [TA], v. cefálica do antebraço; a porção da veia cefálica entre a rede venosa dorsal da mão e a região do cotovelo (cubital). SIN vena cephalica antebrachii [TA].
cerebellar v.'s [TA], veias cerebelares; as veias que drenam o cerebelo. VER inferior v.'s of cerebellar hemisphere, superior v.'s of cerebellar hemisphere, petrosal v., precentral cerebellar v., inferior v. of vermis, superior v. of vermis. SIN venae cerebelli [TA], v.'s of cerebellum.
v.'s of cerebellum, veias cerebelares. SIN cerebellar v.'s.
cerebral v.'s, veias cerebrais. VER anterior cerebral v.'s, deep middle cerebral v., great cerebral v., superficial middle cerebral v.
cervical v., v. cervical. VER deep cervical v.
choroid v., v. coróidea. VER inferior choroid v., superior choroid v.
choroid v.'s of eye, veias vorticosas. SIN vorticose v.'s.
circumflex v.'s, veias circunflexas. VER anterior circumflex humeral v., circumflex scapular v., deep circumflex iliac v., lateral circumflex femoral v.'s, medial circumflex femoral v.'s, posterior circumflex humeral v., superficial circumflex iliac v.
circumflex scapular v. [TA], v. circunflexa da escápula; a v. que acompanha a artéria de mesmo nome que drena as estruturas da fossa infra-espinhosa ao redor do lado lateral da escápula para dentro da v. subescapular.
v. of cochlear aqueduct, v. do aqueduto da cóclea. SIN v. of cochlear caniliculus.
v. of cochlear canaliculus, v. do aqueduto da cóclea; a v. que drena a volta basal da cóclea, o sáculo e parte do utrículo, desembocando no bulbo superior da v. jugular ao acompanhar o ducto perilinfático (aqueduto da cóclea) através do canalículo da cóclea. SIN v. of cochlear aqueduct, vena aqueductus cochleae, vena canaliculi cochleae.
v. of cochlear window [TA], v. da janela da cóclea; a v. da orelha interna que drena a região da janela redonda; desemboca na v. vestibulococlear. SIN vena fenestrae cochleae [TA].
Cockett communicating perforating v.'s, veias comunicantes perfurantes de Cockett; as veias perfurantes da porção média da coxa que conectam os sistemas venosos superficial e profundo.
colic v.'s, veias cólicas. VER right colic v., middle colic v., left colic v.
common basal v. [TA], v. basilar comum; uma tributária da v. pulmonar inferior (direita e esquerda) que recebe o sangue das veias basais superior e inferior. SIN vena basalis communis [TA].
common cardinal v.'s, veias cardinais comuns. VER cardinal v.'s.
common facial v., v. facial comum; um vaso curto, formado pela união da v. facial e v. retromandibular, que desemboca na v. jugular; considerada como continuação da v. facial na NA. SIN vena facialis communis.
common iliac v. [TA], v. ilíaca comum; formada pela união das veias ilíacas externa e interna na borda da pelve, e passa para cima, por trás da artéria ilíaca interna, até o lado direito do corpo da quinta vértebra lombar, onde ela se une com sua congênere do lado oposto para formar a veia cava inferior; a v. ilíaca comum esquerda é submetida a compressão pulsátil pela artéria ilíaca comum direita contra a coluna vertebral, o que pode resultar em obstrução parcial da v. SIN vena iliaca communis [TA].
common modiolar v. [TA], v. comum do modíolo; a v. que faz um trajeto espiralado no modíolo da cóclea; é tributária para a v. do labirinto e para a v. do aqueduto da cóclea. SIN vena modioli communis [TA], spiral v. of modiolus, vena spiralis modioli.
companion v.'s, veias acompanhantes. SIN venae comitantes, em vena.
condylar emissary v. [TA], v. emissária condilar; uma v. que conecta o seio sigmóide e os plexos venosos vertebrais externos através do canal condilar do osso occipital. SIN vena emissaria condylaris [TA], emissarium condyloideum.
conjunctival v.'s [TA], veias conjuntivais; as veias da conjuntiva que drenam principalmente para as veias oftálmicas. SIN venae conjunctivales [TA].
coronary v., v. gástrica esquerda. SIN left gastric v.
v. of corpus striatum, v. tálamo-estriada superior. SIN superior thalamostriate v.
costoaxillary v., v. costoaxilar; uma das inúmeras veias anastomóticas que unem as veias intercostais do primeiro ao sétimo espaços intercostais com a v. torácica lateral ou a v. tóraco-epigástrica.
cutaneous v., v. superficial. SIN superficial v.
Cuvier v.'s, veias de Cuvier; as veias cardinais comuns do embrião. VER cardinal v.'s.
cystic v.'s [TA], v. cística; as veias, usualmente anterior e posterior, que drenam o colo da vesícula biliar e o ducto cístico, ao longo do qual elas passam para entrar no ramo direito da v. porta; elas comunicam-se abundantemente com as veias circunvizinhas do estômago, duodeno e pâncreas. SIN vena cystica [TA].
deep cerebral v.'s [TA], veias cerebrais profundas; as inúmeras veias que drenam as estruturas profundas dos hemisférios cerebrais; elas desembocam nas tributárias da v. cerebral magna. SIN venae profundae cerebri [TA].
deep cervical v. [TA], v. cervical profunda; a grande v. que corre com a artéria de mesmo nome entre os músculos semi-espinhal da cabeça e o semi-espinhal do pescoço, drenando os músculos profundos na parte posterior do pescoço e desembocando na v. braquiocefálica ou na v. vertebral. SIN vena cervicalis profunda [TA], vena colli profunda*.
deep circumflex iliac v. [TA], v. ilíaca circunflexa profunda; corresponde à artéria de mesmo nome, avança medialmente, paralela ao ligamento inguinal, e desemboca próximo à v. epigástrica inferior ou em um tronco comum com esta, dentro da v. ilíaca externa. SIN vena circumflexa iliaca profunda [TA].
deep v.'s of clitoris [TA], veias profundas do clitóris; as veias que passam do dorso do clitóris para formar o plexo vesical. SIN venae profundae clitoridis [TA].
deep dorsal v. of clitoris [TA], v. dorsal profunda do clitóris; uma tributária do plexo venoso vesical; faz um trajeto profundamente à fáscia no dorso do clitóris. SIN vena dorsalis clitoridis profunda [TA].
deep dorsal v. of penis [TA], v. dorsal profunda do pênis; uma v. no dorso do pênis profundamente à fáscia do pênis; é uma tributária do plexo venoso prostático. SIN vena dorsalis penis profunda [TA].
deep epigastric v., v. epigástrica profunda. SIN inferior epigastric v.
deep facial v. [TA], v. facial profunda; a v. comunicante que passa do plexo venoso pterigóide da fossa infratemporal até a v. facial; é desprovida de válvulas. SIN vena faciei profunda [TA].
deep femoral v., v. femoral profunda. SIN profunda femoris v.
deep lingual v. [TA], v. lingual profunda; a principal v. da língua que acompanha a artéria lingual profunda e se une à v. lingual. Drena o corpo e o ápice da língua, correndo posteriormente, próximo ao plano mediano; freqüentemente visível através da mucosa no lado inferior da língua, em cada lado do freio. SIN vena profunda linguae [TA].

deep middle cerebral v. [TA], v. cerebral profunda média; a v. que acompanha a artéria cerebral média na porção profunda do sulco lateral e desemboca na v. basal de Rosenthal. SIN vena media profunda cerebri [TA].

deep v.'s of penis [TA], veias profundas do pênis; as veias profundas à fáscia do pênis que drenam, por meio da veia pudenda interna, para a veia ilíaca interna. SIN venae profundae penis.

deep temporal v.'s [TA], veias temporais profundas; as veias que correspondem às artérias de mesmo nome; elas desembocam no plexo venoso pterigóide. SIN venae temporales profundae [TA].

deep v. of thigh, v. femoral profunda; *termo oficial alternativo para profunda femoris v.

digital v.'s, veias digitais. VER dorsal digital v.'s of foot, palmar digital v.'s, plantar digital v.'s.

diploic v. [TA], v. diplóica; uma das veias na díploe dos ossos cranianos, conectadas aos seios cerebrais por veias emissárias; as principais veias diplóicas são frontal, temporal anterior, temporal posterior e occipital. SIN vena diploica [TA], Breschet v., Dupuytren canal.

direct lateral v.'s [TA], veias laterais diretas; uma ou mais veias que exibem um trajeto subependimário em um plano coronal sobre o tálamo, terminando na veia cerebral interna. SIN venae directae laterales [TA], surface thalamic v.'s.

dorsal callosal v., v. posterior do corpo caloso. SIN posterior v. of corpus callosum.

dorsal v.'s of clitoris, veias dorsais do clitóris. VER deep dorsal v. of clitoris, superficial dorsal v.'s of clitoris.

dorsal v. of corpus callosum [TA], v. posterior do corpo caloso. SIN posterior v. of corpus callosum.

dorsal digital v.'s of foot [TA], veias digitais dorsais do pé; recebem as veias intercapitulares oriundas do arco venoso plantar, unem-se para formar as quatro veias digitais dorsais do pé e terminam no arco venoso dorsal. SIN venae digitales dorsales pedis [TA], dorsal digital v.'s of toes.

dorsal digital v.'s of toes, veias digitais dorsais dos pés. SIN dorsal digital v.'s of foot.

dorsal lingual v. [TA], v. dorsal da língua; as múltiplas tributárias da v. lingual que drenam o dorso da língua, tornando-se cada vez maiores no sentido da raiz da língua. SIN venae dorsales linguae [TA].

dorsal metacarpal v.'s [TA], veias metacarpais dorsais; três veias no dorso da mão que drenam o sangue dos quatro dedos mediais para a rede venosa dorsal da mão. SIN venae metacarpeae dorsales [TA].

dorsal metatarsal v.'s [TA], veias metatarsais dorsais; as veias que se originam das veias digitais dorsais que formam o arco venoso dorsal do pé. SIN venae metatarseae dorsales [TA].

dorsal v.'s of penis, veias dorsais do pênis. VER deep dorsal v. of penis, superficial dorsal v.'s of penis.

dorsal scapular v. [TA], v. dorsal da escápula; a veia acompanhante da artéria escapular descendente; é uma tributária da v. subclávia ou da v. jugular externa. SIN vena scapularis dorsalis [TA].

dorsispinal v.'s, veias espinais posteriores; as veias que formam um plexo ao redor dos arcos neurais e processos das vértebras.

emissary v. [TA], v. emissária; um dos canais de comunicação entre os seios venosos da dura-máter e as veias da díploe e do couro cabeludo. VER TAMBÉM condylar emissary v., mastoid emissary v., occipital emissary v., parietal emissary v. SIN vena emissaria [TA], emissarium, emissary (2).

epigastric v.'s, veias epigástricas. VER inferior epigastric v., superficial epigastric v., superior epigastric v.'s.

episcleral v.'s [TA], veias esclerais; uma série de pequenas vênulas na esclerótica, próximo à margem da córnea, que desembocam nas veias ciliares anteriores. SIN venae episclerales [TA].

esophageal v.'s [TA], veias esôfágicas; série de veias que drenam o plexo venoso submucoso do esôfago; dirigindo-se inferiormente a partir da porção cervical do esôfago, elas drenam para a v. tireóidea inferior, veias intercostais superiores e veias ázigos, hemiázigo acessória e hemiázigo, as quais, sem exceção, são tributárias da v. cava superior; as veias esofágicas mais inferiores, oriundas da cárdia do esôfago, drenam por meio dos ramos esofágicos da v. gástrica esquerda, uma tributária da v. porta. Dessa maneira, as veias da submucosa do esôfago inferior formam uma anastomose portocava e estão sujeitas à formação de varicosidades na hipertensão porta. SIN venae esophageae [TA].

ethmoidal v.'s [TA], veias etmoidais; as veias que acompanham as artérias etmoidais anterior e posterior e penetram na v. oftálmica superior; elas drenam os seios etmoidais. SIN venae ethmoidales [TA].

external iliac v. [TA], v. ilíaca externa; uma continuação direta da v. femoral acima do ligamento inguinal, unindo-se com a veia ilíaca interna para formar a v. ilíaca comum. SIN vena iliaca externa [TA].

external jugular v. [TA], v. jugular externa; a v. superficial formada abaixo da glândula parótida por meio da junção da v. auricular posterior e da v. retromandibular, e que passa por baixo, pelo lado do pescoço, cruzando o músculo esternocleidomastóideo verticalmente para desembocar na v. subclávia. SIN vena jugularis externa [TA].

external nasal v.'s [TA], veias nasais externas; vários vasos que drenam a parte externa do nariz, desembocando na v. angular ou facial. SIN venae nasales externae [TA].

external palatine v. [TA], v. palatina externa; drena as regiões palatinas e desemboca na v. facial. SIN vena palatina externa [TA].

external pudendal v.'s [TA], veias pudendas externas; estas correspondem às artérias de mesmo nome; elas desembocam na v. safena magna, ou diretamente na v. femoral, e recebem a v. dorsal superficial do pênis (ou do clitóris) e as veias escrotais (ou labiais) anteriores. SIN vena pudendae externae [TA].

v.'s of eyelids, veias palpebrais. SIN palpebral v.'s.

facial v. [TA], v. facial; uma continuação da v. angular no ângulo medial do olho; dirige-se para baixo e para fora, no sentido diagonal, unindo-se com a v. retromandibular abaixo da borda da mandíbula inferior antes de desembocar dentro da v. jugular interna. SIN vena facialis [TA], anterior facial v., vena facialis anterior.

femoral v. [TA], v. femoral; é uma continuação da v. poplítea e acompanha a artéria femoral através do canal adutor e no triângulo femoral, onde se situa dentro da bainha femoral; transforma-se na v. ilíaca externa, quando passa profundamente ao ligamento inguinal. SIN vena femoralis [TA].

fibular v.'s [TA], veias fibulares; veias acompanhantes da artéria fibular; unem-se às veias tibiais posteriores para penetrar na v. poplítea. SIN venae fibulares [TA], peroneal v.'s*, venae peroneae*.

frontal v.'s, (1) veias frontais; as veias superficiais que drenam o córtex frontal e desembocam no seio sagital superior; (2) veias supratrocleares. SIN supratrochlear v.'s.

v.'s of Galen, veias de Galeno; (1) veias cerebrais internas. SIN internal cerebral v.'s; (2) VER great cerebral v.

gastric v.'s, veias gástricas. VER short gastric v.'s, right gastric v., left gastric v.

gastroepiploic v.'s, veias gastroepiplóicas. VER right gastroomental v., left gastroomental v.

genicular v.'s [TA], veias geniculares; as veias que acompanham as artérias geniculares; drenam o sangue das estruturas ao redor do joelho, terminando na v. poplítea. SIN venae geniculares [TA], v.'s of knee.

gluteal v.'s, veias glúteas. VER inferior gluteal v.'s, superior gluteal v.'s.

great cardiac v. [TA], v. cardíaca magna; começa no ápice do coração (onde se anastomosa com a v. cardíaca média), faz trajeto primeiramente com a artéria interventricular anterior, à medida que esta ascende ao sulco interventricular anterior; em seguida, vira para a esquerda, à medida que se aproxima do sulco coronário ou o alcança, indo fazer trajeto com o ramo circunflexo da artéria coronária esquerda; funde-se com a v. oblíqua do átrio esquerdo para formar o seio coronário. SIN vena cordis magna [TA], left coronary v., vena cardiaca magna.

great cerebral v. [TA], v. cerebral magna. SIN great cerebral v. of Galen.

great cerebral v. of Galen, v. cerebral magna de Galeno; uma grande v. isolada, formada pela junção das duas veias cerebrais internas na porção caudal da tela coróide do terceiro ventrículo; passa caudalmente entre o esplênio do corpo caloso e a glândula pineal, curvando-se dorsalmente para se fundir com o seio sagital inferior e formar o seio reto. SIN great cerebral v. [TA], vena magna cerebri [TA], great v. of Galen.

great v. of Galen, v. magna de Galeno. SIN great cerebral v. of Galen.

great saphenous v. [TA], v. safena magna; formada pela união da v. dorsal do primeiro artelho com o arco venoso dorsal do pé; ascende à frente do maléolo medial, atrás do côndilo medial do fêmur, e atravessa o hiato safeno na fáscia lata para desembocar na v. femoral, na parte superior do triângulo femoral. SIN vena saphena magna [TA], large saphenous v., long saphenous v.

v.'s of heart [TA], veias cardíacas; termo coletivo para todas as estruturas venosas do coração, incluindo o seio coronário e todas as veias cardíacas. SIN venae cordis [TA].

hemiazygos v. [TA], v. hemiázigo; formada pela união da v. lombar ascendente esquerda com a v. subcostal esquerda, ou uma comunicação oriunda da veia cava inferior, ela perfura o pilar esquerdo do diafragma, ascende ao longo do lado esquerdo dos corpos das vértebras torácicas inferiores, oposto à oitava vértebra, cruza a linha média por trás da aorta, ducto torácico e esôfago, e desemboca na v. ázigo, por vezes em comum com a v. hemiázigo acessória. SIN vena hemiazygos [TA], inferior hemiazygos v., vena azygos minor inferior.

hemorrhoidal v.'s, veias hemorroidárias; termo obsoleto para as veias retais. VER inferior rectal v.'s, middle rectal v.'s, superior rectal v.

hepatic v.'s [TA], veias hepáticas; as veias que drenam o fígado; coletam o sangue a partir das veias centrais e terminam em três grandes veias que desembocam na veia cava inferior, abaixo do diafragma, e em diversas veias pequenas e inconstantes, que penetram na v. cava em níveis mais inferiores. SIN venae hepaticae [TA].

hepatic portal v. [TA], v. porta do fígado; uma veia curta e calibrosa formada pela confluência das veias mesentérica superior e esplênica posteriormente ao colo do pâncreas, ascendendo anteriormente à v. cava inferior e dividindo-se na extremidade direita da porta do fígado em ramos direito e esquerdo, que se ramificam no parênquima hepático. SIN vena portal hepatis [TA], portal v., vena portalis.

highest intercostal v., v. intercostal suprema. SIN supreme intercostal v.
hypogastric v., v. hipogástrica; termo obsoleto para a v. ilíaca interna.
ileal v.'s, veias ileais. VER jejunal and ileal v.'s.
ileocolic v. [TA], v. ileocólica; uma grande tributária da v. mesentérica superior que faz trajeto em paralelo com a artéria ileocólica e drena o íleo terminal, apêndice, ceco e porção inferior do colo ascendente. SIN vena ileocolica [TA].
iliac v.'s, veias ilíacas. VER common iliac v., external iliac v., internal iliac v., deep circumflex iliac v., superficial circumflex iliac v.
iliolumbar v. [TA], v. iliolombar; acompanhando a artéria de mesmo nome, faz anastomose com as veias lombar e ilíaca circunflexa profunda, desembocando na v. ilíaca interna. SIN vena iliolumbalis [TA].
inferior anastomotic v. [TA], v. anastomótica inferior; uma v. inconstante que se origina da v. vertebral média superficial posteriormente, sobre a face lateral do lobo temporal, para penetrar no seio transverso. SIN vena anastomotica inferior [TA], Browning v., Labbé v.
inferior basal v. [TA], v. basal inferior; tributária da v. basal comum que drena as partes medial e posterior do lobo inferior em cada pulmão. SIN vena basalis inferior [TA].
inferior cardiac v., v. interventricular posterior. SIN middle cardiac v.
inferior v.'s of cerebellar hemisphere [TA], veias inferiores do hemisfério cerebelar; várias veias que drenam a porção inferior dos hemisférios cerebelares; terminam na v. petrosa. SIN venae inferiores cerebelli [TA].
inferior cerebral v.'s [TA], veias cerebrais inferiores; inúmeras veias cerebrais que drenam a superfície inferior dos hemisférios cerebrais e desembocam nos seios cavernoso e transverso. Dessas veias fazem parte os ramos nomeados que servem ao giro uncinado (veia do giro uncinado [TA], vena uncalis [TA]), córtex orbitário (veias orbitárias [TA], venae orbitae [TA]) e lobo temporal (veias temporais [TA], venae temporales [TA]). SIN venae inferiores cerebri [TA].
inferior choroid v. [TA], v. coróidea inferior; uma pequena v. que drena a porção inferior do plexo coróide do ventrículo lateral para a v. basal. VER TAMBÉM basal v. SIN vena choroidea inferior [TA], vena choroidea inferior [TA].
inferior epigastric v. [TA], v. epigástrica inferior; corresponde à artéria de mesmo nome e desemboca na v. ilíaca externa, exatamente proximal ao ligamento inguinal. SIN vena epigastrica inferior [TA], deep epigastric v.
v.'s of inferior eyelid, veias da pálpebra inferior. SIN inferior palpebral v.'s.
inferior gluteal v.'s [TA], veias glúteas inferiores; as veias que acompanham a artéria glútea inferior unindo-se, no forame isquiático, para formar um tronco comum que desemboca na v. ilíaca interna. SIN venae gluteae inferiores [TA].
inferior hemiazygos v., v. hemiázigo. SIN hemiazygos v.
inferior hemorrhoidal v.'s, veias hemorroidárias inferiores; termo obsoleto para as veias retais inferiores.
inferior labial v. [TA], v. labial inferior; uma tributária da v. facial que drena o lábio inferior. SIN vena labialis inferior [TA].
inferior laryngeal v. [TA], v. laríngea inferior; a v. que se origina da parte inferior da laringe até o plexo tireóideo único. SIN vena laryngea inferior [TA].
inferior mesenteric v. [TA], v. mesentérica inferior; uma continuação da v. retal superior na borda da pelve, ascendendo à esquerda da aorta, por trás do peritônio, e desembocando na v. esplênica ou na v. mesentérica superior ou, raramente, no ângulo entre essas veias. SIN vena mesenterica inferior [TA].
inferior ophthalmic v. [TA], v. oftálmica inferior; origina-se das veias palpebral inferior e lacrimal e divide-se em dois ramos terminais, um dos quais corre para o plexo pterigóide, enquanto o outro vai até a veia oftálmica superior ou desemboca no seio cavernoso. SIN vena ophthalmica inferior [TA].
inferior palpebral v.'s [TA], veias palpebrais inferiores; as veias da pálpebra inferior; as veias que se originam da pálpebra inferior e desembocam na v. angular. SIN venae palpebrales inferiores [TA], v.'s of inferior eyelid.
inferior phrenic v. [TA], v. frênica inferior; a v. que drena a substância do diafragma e desemboca à direita, na veia cava inferior, e à esquerda, na v. supra-renal esquerda; com freqüência, uma segunda v. no lado esquerdo atravessa o diafragma, anterior ao hiato esofágico, indo penetrar na veia cava inferior. SIN vena phrenica inferior [TA].
inferior rectal v.'s [TA], veias retais inferiores; as veias que passam até a v. pudenda interna a partir do plexo venoso retal inferior ao redor do canal anal. SIN venae rectales inferiores [TA].
inferior thalamostriate v.'s [TA], veias talamoestriadas inferiores; as veias que drenam o tálamo e o corpo estriado, saindo da substância perfurada anterior; tributária para a v. basal. VER TAMBÉM basal v. SIN venae thalamostriatae inferiores [TA], striate v.'s, venae striatae.
inferior thyroid v. [TA], v. tireóidea inferior; v. não-pareada formada por veias oriundas do istmo e do lobo lateral da glândula tireóide e do plexo tireóideo ímpar; termina na v. braquiocefálica esquerda. SIN vena thyroidea inferior [TA], vena thyroidea ima.
inferior ventricular v. [TA], v. ventricular inferior; a veia que drena a substância branca profunda das porções superior e lateral do lobo temporal; começa no corpo do ventrículo lateral e sai da fissura corióidea do corno inferior, onde se une à v. basal. VER TAMBÉM basal v. SIN vena ventricularis inferior [TA].

inferior v. of vermis [TA], v. inferior do verme; uma v. que drena parte da porção inferior do cerebelo; avança sobre a superfície inferior do verme e termina no seio reto. SIN vena inferior vermis [TA].
infrasegmental v.'s, parte infra-segmentar das veias pulmonares. VER intersegmental v.
innominate v.'s, veias inominadas; termo obsoleto para as veias braquiocefálicas (esquerda e direita).
innominate cardiac v.'s, veias cardíacas inominadas; as pequenas veias superficiais do coração. SIN Vieussens v.'s.
insular v.'s [TA], veias insulares. SIN venae insulares, em vena.
intercapitular v.'s [TA], veias intercapitulares; as veias que unem as veias dorsais e palmares na mão, ou as veias dorsais e plantares no pé. SIN venae intercapitulares.
intercostal v.'s, veias intercostais. VER anterior intercostal v.'s, posterior intercostal v.'s, supreme intercostal v., left superior intercostal v.
interlobar v.'s of kidney [TA], veias interlobares do rim; as veias no rim que ficam em paralelo com as artérias interlobares, recebendo sangue das veias arqueadas, e terminam na v. renal. SIN venae interlobares renis [TA].
interlobular v.'s of kidney [TA], veias interlobulares do rim; as veias que ficam em paralelo com as artérias interlobulares e drenam o plexo capilar peritubular, desembocando nas veias arqueadas. SIN venae interlobulares renis [TA].
interlobular v.'s of liver [TA], veias interlobulares do fígado; os ramos terminais da v. porta que avançam nos canais porta entre os lóbulos hepáticos conceituais e desembocam nos sinusóides hepáticos. SIN venae interlobulares hepatis [TA].
intermediate antebrachial v., v. intermédia do antebraço. SIN median antebrachial v.
intermediate basilic v. [TA], v. basílica do antebraço; o ramo medial da v. intermédia do antebraço que se une à v. basílica, substituindo freqüentemente uma veia intermédia do cotovelo. SIN vena intermedia basilica [TA], median basilic v., vena mediana basilica.
intermediate cephalic v. [TA], v. cefálica do antebraço; o ramo lateral da v. intermédia do antebraço que se une à veia cefálica próximo ao cotovelo, substituindo com freqüência uma v. intermédia do cotovelo. SIN vena intermedia cephalica [TA], median cephalic v., vena mediana cephalica.
intermediate cubital v., v. intermédia do cotovelo. SIN median cubital v.
intermediate v. of forearm, v. intermédia do antebraço. SIN median antebrachial v.
intermediate hepatic v.'s [TA], veias hepáticas intermédias; as veias que drenam a porção central do fígado (os lados esquerdos do segmento ântero-superior [VIII]), o segmento ântero-inferior [V] do fígado (parte) direito e o lado direito do segmento medial [IV] do fígado esquerdo (parto do), formando um tronco que se une com o tronco das veias hepáticas esquerdas em cerca de 90% dos casos, antes de penetrarem no lado esquerdo da veia cava inferior. SIN venae hepaticae intermediae [TA], venae hepaticae mediae [TA], middle hepatic v.'s.
internal auditory v.'s, veias do labirinto. SIN labyrinthine v.'s.
internal cerebral v.'s [TA], veias cerebrais internas; veias pareadas que passam caudalmente próximo à linha média na tela corióidea do terceiro ventrículo, formada pela união da v. corióidea, v. tálamo-estriada (terminal) e v. do septo pelúcido, e que se une caudalmente, de modo a formar a v. cerebral magna. SIN venae internae cerebri [TA], v.'s of Galen (1).
internal iliac v. [TA], v. ilíaca interna; as veias que avançam na pelve menor, a partir da borda superior da incisura isquiática maior até a borda da pelve, onde se une à v. ilíaca externa para formar a v. ilíaca comum; drena a maior parte do território irrigado pela artéria ilíaca interna. SIN vena iliaca interna [TA].
internal jugular v. [TA], v. jugular interna; a principal estrutura venosa do pescoço, formada como uma continuação do seio sigmóide da dura-máter, contida dentro da bainha carotídea, à medida que ela desce no pescoço, unindo-se, por trás da articulação esternoclavicular, com a veia subclávia para formar a v. braquiocefálica. SIN vena jugularis interna [TA].
internal pudendal v. [TA], v. pudenda interna; uma tributária da v. ilíaca interna que acompanha a artéria pudenda interna como um vaso único ou duplo; drena o períneo. SIN vena pudenda interna [TA].
interna thoracic v. [TA], v. torácica interna; veias acompanhantes de cada artéria de mesmo nome, fundindo-se na porção superior do tórax e desembocando na v. braquiocefálica do mesmo lado; recebe a drenagem da parede anterior do tórax. SIN vena thoracica interna [TA].
intersegmental v., parte intersegmentar da v. pulmonar; uma v. que recebe sangue dos segmentos broncopulmonares adjacentes; emerge da margem inferior de um segmento para se transformar em tributária de um ramo de uma v. pulmonar. SIN intersegmental part of pulmonary vein [TA], partes intersegmentales venarum pulmonum [TA], infrasegmental part.
intervertebral v. [TA], v. intervertebral; uma das inúmeras veias que acompanham os nervos espinais através dos forames intervertebrais, drenando a medula espinal e os plexos venosos vertebrais, e desembocando no pescoço, na v. vertebral; no tórax, nas veias intercostais; e nas regiões lombar e sacral, nas veias lombares e sacral. SIN vena intervertebralis [TA].

intrasegmental v.'s, parte intra-segmentar da v. pulmonar. SIN intrasegmental part of pulmonary veins.
jejunal and ileal v.'s [TA], veias jejunais e ileais; as veias que drenam o jejuno e o íleo; terminam na v. mesentérica superior. SIN venae jejunales et ilei [TA].
jugular v.'s, veias jugulares. VER anterior jugular v., external jugular v., internal jugular v. VER TAMBÉM posterior anterior jugular v., jugular venous arch.
key v., uma v. dilatada, profundamente situada, que gera uma "aranha vascular" na superfície.
v.'s of kidney [TA], veias do rim; as tributárias da v. renal que drenam o rim; fazem trajeto paralelo às artérias no rim e consistem nas veias interlobulares, arqueadas e interlobares.
v.'s of knee, veias geniculares. SIN genicular v.'s.
Krukenberg v.'s, veias de Krukenberg. SIN central v.'s of liver.
Labbé v., v. de Labbé. SIN inferior anastomotic v.
labial v.'s, veias labiais. VER anterior labial v.'s, posterior labial v.'s, inferior labial v., superior labial v.
labyrinthine v.'s [TA], veias do labirinto; uma ou mais veias que acompanham a artéria do labirinto; drenam a orelha interna, atravessam o meato acústico interno e desembocam no seio transverso ou no seio petroso inferior. SIN venae labyrinthi [TA], internal auditory v.'s.
lacrimal v. [TA], v. lacrimal; pequena v. que drena a glândula lacrimal, passando posteriormente através da órbita com a artéria lacrimal, desembocando na v. oftálmica superior. SIN vena lacrimalis [TA].
large v., grande v.; uma v., como a veia cava inferior, caracterizada por ter uma túnica média reduzida ou ausente e uma camada adventícia com grandes feixes de músculo liso dispostos longitudinalmente.
large saphenous v., v. safena magna. SIN great saphenous v.
laryngeal v.'s, veias laríngeas. VER inferior laryngeal v., superior laryngeal v.
Latarget v., v. de Latarget, v. pré-pilórica. SIN prepyloric v.
lateral atrial v., v. lateral do ventrículo lateral. SIN lateral v. of lateral ventricle.
lateral circumflex femoral v.'s [TA], veias circunflexas femorais laterais; as veias que acompanham a artéria circunflexa femoral lateral, terminando geralmente na v. femoral. SIN venae circumflexae femoris laterales [TA].
lateral direct v.'s [TA], veias diretas laterais; uma ou mais veias que exibem um trajeto subependimário em um plano coronal sobre o tálamo, terminando na veia cerebral interna.
lateral v. of lateral ventricle [TA], v. lateral do ventrículo lateral; uma v. que drena as porções profundas dos lobos temporal e parietal; avança na parede lateral do ventrículo lateral para terminar na v. tálamo-estriada superior. SIN vena lateralis ventriculi lateralis [TA], lateral atrial v., vena atrii lateralis.
v. of lateral recess of fourth ventricle [TA], v. do recesso lateral do quarto ventrículo; uma pequena veia que se origina na tonsila do cerebelo, avançando pelo recesso lateral do quarto ventrículo para terminar na v. petrosa. SIN vena recessus lateralis ventriculi quarti [TA].
lateral sacral v.'s [TA], veias sacrais laterais; as diversas veias que recebem a drenagem do plexo venoso sacral e das veias intervertebrais sacrais, acompanhando, então, a artéria correspondente e desembocando na v. ilíaca interna em cada lado. SIN venae sacrales laterales [TA].
lateral thoracic v. [TA], v. torácica lateral; uma tributária da v. axilar que drena a parede torácica lateral e comunica-se com as veias toracoepigástricas e intercostais. SIN vena thoracica lateralis [TA].
left colic v. [TA], v. cólica esquerda; uma tributária da v. mesentérica inferior que acompanha a artéria cólica esquerda e drena a flexura esquerda e o colo descendente. SIN vena colica sinistra [TA].
left coronary v., v. cardíaca magna. SIN great cardiac v.
left gastric v. [TA], v. gástrica esquerda; origina-se da união de veias a partir de ambas as superfícies da cárdia do estômago e de uma tributária esofágica a partir da porção da cárdia do esôfago; faz trajeto no omento menor e desemboca na v. porta. VER TAMBÉM esophageal v.'s. SIN vena gástrica sinistra [TA], coronary v., vena coronaria ventriculi.
left gastroepiploic v., v. gastro-omental esquerda; *termo oficial alternativo para left gastroomental v.
left gastroomental v. [TA], v. gastro-omental esquerda; a v. que acompanha a artéria gastroepiplóica esquerda ao longo da curvatura maior do estômago; desemboca na v. esplênica. SIN left gastroepiploic v.*, vena gastro-omentalis sinistra.
left hepatic v. [TA], v. hepática esquerda; v. que drena o segmento medial [IV] e os segmentos laterais esquerdos [II e III] do fígado, um tronco único ou pareado de tamanho variável que geralmente (90% das vezes) se une com a v. hepática intermédia antes de penetrar na porção terminal da veia cava superior. SIN venae hepaticae sinistrae [TA].
left inferior pulmonary v. [TA], v. pulmonar esquerda inferior; a v. que retorna o sangue oxigenado do lobo inferior do pulmão esquerdo para o átrio esquerdo; as tributárias incluem as veias basilares superior e comum (ramos) oriundas do lobo inferior. SIN vena pulmonalis inferior sinistra [TA].
left ovarian v. [TA], v. ovárica esquerda; começa como o plexo pampiniforme no hilo do ovário e desemboca na v. renal esquerda. SIN vena ovarica sinistra [TA].

(left and right) brachiocephalic v.'s [TA], veias braquiocefálicas (esquerda e direita); formadas pela união das veias jugular interna e subclávia; as outras tributárias da v. braquiocefálica direita são as veias vertebral direita e torácica interna, bem como o ducto linfático direito; as outras tributárias da v. braquiocefálica esquerda são as veias vertebral esquerda, torácica interna, intercostal superior, tireóidea ima e diversas veias mediastinais, brônquicas e pericárdicas anteriores, além do ducto torácico. SIN venae brachiocephalicae (dextrae et sinistrae) [TA].
left superior intercostal v. [TA], v. intercostal superior esquerda; a v. formada pela união da segunda, terceira e quarta veias intercostais esquerdas; passa para diante, através do arco da aorta, indo desembocar na v. braquiocefálica esquerda, e, com freqüência, comunica-se também com a v. hemiázigo acessória. SIN vena intercostalis superior sinistra [TA].
left superior pulmonary v. [TA], v. pulmonar esquerda superior; a v. que retorna o sangue oxigenado do lobo superior esquerdo do pulmão para o átrio esquerdo; as tributárias incluem as veias apicoposterior, anterior e lingular (ramos) a partir do lobo superior. SIN vena pulmonalis superior sinistra [TA].
left suprarenal v. [TA], v. supra-renal esquerda; a v. a partir do hilo da glândula supra-renal esquerda que se dirige para baixo até desembocar na v. renal esquerda; geralmente se une à v. frênica inferior esquerda. SIN vena suprarenalis sinistra [TA].
left testicular v. [TA], v. testicular esquerda; a v. que conduz o sangue oriundo do testículo esquerdo, originando-se como o plexo pampiniforme e entrando na v. renal esquerda. SIN vena testicularis sinistra [TA].
left umbilical v., umbilical esquerda; a v. que retorna o sangue da placenta para o feto; avançando dentro do cordão umbilical, penetra no corpo do feto no umbigo, seguindo daí para dentro do fígado, onde se une à v. porta; então, seu sangue flui, através do ducto venoso e da veia cava inferior, até o átrio direito. SIN vena umbilicalis [TA].
levoatrio-cardinal v., v. levoatriocardinal; a comunicação de uma v. sistêmica com o átrio esquerdo, diferente de uma veia cava superior esquerda ou do seio coronário; pode ser a veia cava superior direita.
lingual v. [TA], v. lingual; a v. que recebe o sangue da língua, das glândulas sublinguais e submandibulares e dos músculos do assoalho da boca; desemboca na v. jugular interna ou na v. facial. SIN vena lingualis.
lingular v. [TA], v. lingular; o ramo lingular da v. pulmonar superior esquerda. SIN ramus lingularis venae pulmonis sinistrae superioris*, vena lingularis.
long saphenous v., v. safena magna. SIN great saphenous v.
long thoracic v., termo incorreto para a v. torácica lateral.
v.'s of lower limb [TA], veias do membro inferior; todas as veias, superficiais e profundas, que drenam o sangue proveniente do membro inferior. SIN venae membri inferioris [TA].
lumbar v.'s [TA], veias lombares; em número de cinco, essas veias acompanham as artérias lombares, drenam a parede posterior do corpo e os plexos venosos vertebrais lombares, indo terminar anteriormente da seguinte maneira: a primeira e a segunda, na v. lombar ascendente; a terceira e a quarta, na veia cava inferior; e a quinta, na v. iliolombar; todas se comunicam por meio das veias lombares ascendentes. SIN venae lumbales [TA].
Marshall oblique v., v. oblíqua de Marshall. SIN oblique v. of left atrium.
masseteric v.'s, veias massetéricas; veias plexiformes que acompanham a artéria massetérica, desembocando no plexo venoso pterigóide.
mastoid emissary v. [TA], v. emissária mastóidea; a v. que conecta o seio sigmóide com a v. occipital ou uma das tributárias da v. jugular externa por meio do forame mastóide. SIN vena emissaria mastoidea [TA], emissarium mastoideum.
maxillary v. [TA], v. maxilar; a continuação posterior do plexo pterigóideo; une-se à v. temporal superficial para formar a v. retromandibular. SIN vena maxillaris [TA].
Mayo v., v. de Mayo. SIN prepyloric v.
medial atrial v., v. medial do ventrículo lateral. SIN medial v. of lateral ventricle.
medial circumflex femoral v.'s [TA], veias circunflexas femorais mediais; as veias acompanhantes que são paralelas à artéria circunflexa femoral medial. SIN venae circumflexae femoris mediales [TA].
medial v. of lateral ventricle [TA], v. medial do ventrículo lateral; uma v. que drena as porções profundas dos lobos parietal e occipital; corre na parede medial do ventrículo lateral para desembocar na v. da cápsula interna ou na v. cerebral magna. SIN vena medialis ventriculi lateralis [TA], medial atrial v., vena atrii medialis.
median antebrachial v. [TA], v. intermédia do antebraço; começa na base do dorso do polegar, faz curva ao redor do lado radial, ascende no meio do antebraço e, exatamente abaixo da flexura do cotovelo, divide-se nas veias basílica do antebraço e cefálica do cotovelo; por vezes divide-se mais abaixo, com um ramo indo para a veia basílica e o outro para a v. intermédia do cotovelo. SIN vena mediana antebrachii [TA], median v. of forearm*, intermediate antebrachial v., intermediate v. of forearm, vena intermedia antebrachii.
median basilic v., v. basílica intermédia. SIN intermediate basilic v.
median cephalic v., v. cefálica do antebraço. SIN intermediate cephalic v.

median cubital v. [TA], v. intermédia do cotovelo; uma v. que passa através da face anterior do cotovelo a partir da v. cefálica até a v. basílica; comumente, essa v. é substituída pelas veias basílica do antebraço e cefálica. A v. intermédia do cotovelo é freqüentemente utilizada para a punção venosa. SIN vena mediana cubiti [TA], intermediate cubital v., vena intermedia cubiti.
median v. of forearm, v. intermédia do antebraço; *termo oficial alternativo para median antebrachial v.
median v. of neck, veia mediana do pescoço; uma veia ocasionalmente presente devido à fusão das duas veias jugulares anteriores.
median sacral v. [TA], v. sacral mediana; uma v. ímpar que acompanha a artéria sacral mediana, recebendo o sangue do plexo venoso sacral e desembocando na v. ilíaca comum esquerda. SIN vena sacralis mediana [TA].
mediastinal v.'s [TA], veias mediastinais; várias pequenas veias, oriundas do mediastino, que desembocam nas veias braquiocefálicas ou na v. cava superior. SIN venae mediastinales [TA].
medium v., v. média; uma v. caracterizada por ter uma parede mais fina e luz maior que sua artéria correspondente, e por uma camada média com pequenos feixes de músculo circular separados por tecido conjuntivo considerável; válvulas também estão presentes.
v.'s of medulla oblongata, veias do bulbo; as diversas veias que drenam o bulbo; são tributárias principalmente das veias espinal anterior e petrosa. As veias do bulbo são a veia ântero-mediana do bulbo [TA] (vena medullaris anteromediana [TA]), veia ântero-lateral do bulbo [TA] (vena medullaris anteromedialis [TA]), veias transversas do bulbo [TA] (venae medullares transversae [TA]), veias dorsais do bulbo [TA] (venae medullares dorsales [TA]) e v. póstero-mediana do bulbo [TA] (vena medullaris posteromediana [TA]). SIN venae medullae oblongatae [TA].
meningeal v.'s [TA], veias meníngeas; as veias que acompanham as artérias meníngeas; comunicam-se com os seios venosos e veias diplóicas e drenam para as veias regionais fora da calota craniana. SIN venae meningeae [TA].
mesencephalic v.'s, veias mesencefálicas; as várias veias que drenam o mesencéfalo; as posteriores são tributárias para a v. cerebral magna; as laterais são tributárias para a v. basilar. As principais veias são: v. pontomesencefálica [TA] (vena pontomesencephalica [TA]), veias interpedunculares [TA] (venae interpedunculares [TA]), v. intercondilar [TA] (vena intercollicularis [TA]) e a v. mesencefálica lateral [TA] (vena mesencephalica lateralis [TA]). SIN venae mesencephalicae.
mesenteric v.'s, veias mesentéricas. VER inferior mesenteric v., superior mesenteric v.
metacarpal v.'s, veias metacarpais. VER dorsal metacarpal v.'s, palmar metacarpal v.'s.
middle cardiac v. [TA], v. interventricular posterior; a v. que começa no ápice do coração (onde se anastomosa com a v. cardíaca magna) e sobe dentro do sulco interventricular posterior até o seio coronário. SIN vena cordis media [TA], inferior cardiac v.
middle colic v. [TA], v. cólica média; a tributária da v. mesentérica superior que carrega a drenagem do colo transverso e acompanha a artéria cólica média. SIN vena colica media [TA].
middle hemorrhoidal v.'s, termo obsoleto para as veias retais médias. VER middle rectal v.'s.
middle hepatic v.'s, veias hepáticas intermédias. SIN intermediate hepatic v.'s.
middle lobe v. [TA], v. do lobo médio; o ramo do lobo médio da 1) artéria pulmonar direita (arteriae pulmonalis dextrae [NA]); 2) v. pulmonar direita superior (venae pulmonalis dextrae superior [NA]). SIN vena lobi medii [TA], middle lobe branch of right superior pulmonary vein, ramus lobi medii venae pulmonalis dextrae superioris.
middle meningeal v.'s [TA], veias meníngeas médias; as veias acompanhantes da artéria meníngea média que desembocam no plexo pterigóide. SIN venae meningeae mediae [TA].
middle rectal v.'s [TA], veias retais médias; várias veias que passam do plexo venoso retal (no qual elas se anastomosam com as veias retais superiores) até a v. ilíaca interna, que, por fim, drena para a v. cava inferior. Como as veias retais superiores drenam por fim para a v. porta, as veias retais médias participam em uma anastomose portocava, sendo o plexo venoso retal sujeito às varicosidades (hemorróides), embora elas comumente ocorram na ausência de hipertensão porta. SIN venae rectales mediae [TA].
middle temporal v. [TA], v. temporal média; a v. que se origina próximo ao ângulo lateral do olho e se une às veias temporais superficiais para formar a v. retromandibular. SIN vena temporalis media [TA].
middle thyroid v. [TA], v. tireóidea média; a v. que passa da glândula tireóide através da artéria carótida comum (geralmente em paralelo com esta, mas separadamente), com as artérias tireóideas inferiores desembocando na v. jugular interna. SIN vena thyroidea media [TA].
musculophrenic v.'s [TA], veias musculofrênicas; as veias que acompanham a artéria musculofrênica e drenam o sangue da parede abdominal superior e porções anteriores dos espaços intercostais inferiores e do diafragma. SIN venae musculophrenicae [TA].

nasofrontal v. [TA], v. nasofrontal; a v. localizada na parte medial anterior da órbita que conecta a v. oftálmica superior com a v. angular. SIN vena nasofrontalis [TA].
oblique v. of left atrium [TA], v. oblíqua do átrio esquerdo; uma pequena v., localizada na parede posterior do átrio esquerdo, que se funde com a veia cardíaca magna para formar o seio coronário; é desenvolvida a partir da v. cardinal comum esquerda e, ocasionalmente, persiste como uma veia cava superior esquerda. SIN vena obliqua atrii sinistri [TA], Marshall oblique v.
obturator v.'s [TA], veias obturatórias; formadas pela união das tributárias que drenam a articulação do quadril e os músculos obturadores e adutores da coxa; entram na pelve, através do canal obturatório, como veias acompanhantes da artéria obturatória e desembocam na v. ilíaca interna. SIN vena obturatoria [TA].
occipital v. [TA], v. occipital; a v. que drena a região occipital e desemboca na v. jugular interna ou no plexo suboccipital. SIN venae occipitalis [TA].
occipital cerebral v.'s, veias occipitais; as veias cerebrais superiores que drenam o córtex occipital e desembocam no seio sagital superior e no seio transverso. SIN venae encephali occipitales [TA].
occipital emissary v. [TA], v. emissária occipital; um vaso inconstante que perfura as lâminas do osso occipital para conectar as veias occipitais com a confluência dos seios. SIN vena emissaria occipitalis [TA], emissarium occipitale.
v. of olfactory gyrus [TA], v. do giro olfatório; uma tributária da v. basilar que drena as estrias olfatórias mediais. VER TAMBÉM basal v. SIN vena gyri olfactorii [TA].
ophthalmic v.'s, veias oftálmicas. VER inferior ophthalmic v., superior ophthalmic v.
ovarian v.'s, veias ováricas. VER right ovarian v., left ovarian v.
palmar digital v.'s [TA], veias digitais palmares; veias pareadas acompanhantes das artérias digital comum e própria que desembocam no arco venoso palmar superficial. SIN venae digitales palmares [TA].
palmar metacarpal v.'s [TA], veias metacarpais palmares; as veias que desembocam no arco venoso profundo, a partir do qual se originam as veias radiais e ulnares. SIN venae metacarpeae palmares [TA].
palpebral v.'s [TA], veias palpebrais; as veias que drenam a pálpebra superior, posteriormente, como tributárias da v. oftálmica superior. SIN venae palpebrales [TA], v.'s of eyelids.
pancreatic v.'s [TA], veias pancreáticas; as veias que drenam o pâncreas, desembocando na v. esplênica e na v. mesentérica superior. SIN venae pancreaticae [TA].
pancreaticoduodenal v.'s [TA], veias pancreaticoduodenais; veias que acompanham as artérias pancreaticoduodenais superior e inferior, que deságuam na v. mesentérica superior ou porta. SIN venae pancreaticoduodenales [TA].
paraumbilical v.'s [TA], veias paraumbilicais; inúmeras pequenas veias que se originam de veias cutâneas ao redor do umbigo, correndo ao longo do ligamento redondo do fígado e terminando como veia porta acessória no parênquima hepático; constituem uma anastomose portocava e estão sujeitas à varicosidade durante a hipertensão porta; as veias paraumbilicais varicosas formam a "cabeça de medusa". SIN venae paraumbilicales [TA], Sappey v.'s.
parietal v.'s [TA], veias parietais; as veias superficiais que drenam o córtex cerebral parietal e desembocam no seio sagital superior. SIN venae parietales.
parietal emissary v. [TA], v. emissária parietal; a v. que conecta o seio sagital superior com as tributárias da v. temporal superficial e de outras veias do couro cabeludo. SIN vena emissaria parietalis [TA], emissarium parietale, Santorini v.
parotid v.'s [TA], veias parotídeas; os ramos que drenam parte da glândula parótida e desembocam na v. retromandibular. SIN venae parotideae [TA], posterior parotid v.'s.
pectoral v.'s [TA], veias peitorais; as veias que drenam os músculos peitorais e desembocam diretamente na v. subclávia. SIN venae pectorales [TA].
peduncular v.'s [TA], veias pedunculares; pequenas tributárias da veia basal oriundas do pedúnculo cerebral. VER TAMBÉM basal v. SIN venae pedunculares [TA].
perforating v.'s [TA], veias perfurantes; (1) as veias que acompanham as artérias perfurantes a partir da artéria femoral profunda; drenam o sangue dos músculos vasto lateral e do jarrete e terminam na v. femoral profunda; (2) veias comunicantes valvuladas que drenam as veias superficiais — especialmente aquelas do membro inferior — para as veias profundas (subfasciais), de modo que a bomba musculovenosa possa impulsionar o sangue venoso para o coração contra a gravidade. SIN venae perforantes [TA].
pericardiacophrenic v.'s [TA], veias pericardicofrênicas; as veias que acompanham a artéria pericardiofrênica e desembocam nas veias braquiocefálicas ou na v. cava superior. SIN venae pericardiacophrenicae [TA].
pericardial v.'s [TA], veias pericárdicas; diversas pequenas veias, oriundas do pericárdio, que deságuam diretamente nas veias braquiocefálicas ou na v. cava superior. SIN venae pericardiacae [TA].
peroneal v.'s, veias fibulares; *termo oficial alternativo para fibular v.'s.

petrosal v. [TA], v. petrosa; uma tributária do seio petroso superior que recebe os canais venosos a partir do mesencéfalo, ponte e porções laterais do lobo anterior do cerebelo.

pharyngeal v.'s [TA], veias faríngeas; diversas veias, oriundas do plexo venoso faríngeo, que desembocam na v. jugular interna. SIN venae pharyngeae [TA].

phrenic v.'s, veias frênicas. VER inferior phrenic v., superior phrenic v.'s.

plantar digital v.'s [TA], veias digitais plantares; as veias que drenam as faces plantar e dorsal distal (leitos ungueais) dos artelhos, dirigindo-se para trás para formar as quatro veias metatarsais, as quais, por sua vez, desembocam no arco venoso plantar. SIN venae digitales plantares [TA].

plantar metatarsal v.'s [TA], veias metatarsais plantares; as veias que recebem as veias digitais plantares e desembocam, por sua vez, no arco venoso plantar profundo, que deságua nas veias plantares medial e lateral. SIN venae metatarseae plantares [TA].

v.'s of pons, veias da ponte. SIN pontine v.'s.

pontine v.'s, veias da ponte; diversas veias que correm no sentido transversal ou oblíquo sobre a ponte para se unirem à v. petrosa; as principais veias da ponte são: a v. ântero-mediana da ponte [TA] (vena pontis anteromediana [TA]), v. ântero-lateral da ponte [TA] (vena pontis anterolateralis [TA]), veias transversas da ponte [TA] (venae pontis transversae [TA]) e a v. lateral da ponte [TA] (vena pontis lateralis [TA]). SIN venae pontis [TA], v.'s of pons.

pontomesencephalic v., v. pontomesencefálica. VER anterior pontomesencephalic v.

popliteal v. [TA], v. poplítea; formada na borda inferior do músculo poplíteo pela união das veias tibiais anterior e posterior, ascende através do espaço poplíteo, onde recebe a v. safena parva e passa através do hiato adutor, penetrando no canal adutor como a v. femoral. SIN vena poplitea [TA].

portal v., v. porta do fígado. SIN hepatic portal v.

posterior anterior jugular v., v. jugular ântero-posterior; uma tributária variável da v. jugular externa que se origina na parte póstero-superior do pescoço.

posterior auricular v. [TA], v. auricular posterior; a v. que drena a região posterior à orelha e, em seguida, une-se à v. retromandibular para formar a v. jugular externa. SIN vena auricularis posterior [TA].

posterior cardinal v.'s, veias cardinais posteriores. VER cardinal v.'s.

posterior circumflex humeral v. [TA], v. circunflexa posterior do úmero; a veia que acompanha a artéria de mesmo nome, passando posteriormente ao colo cirúrgico do úmero e através do espaço quadrangular para entrar na v. axilar. SIN vena circumflexa humeri posterior [TA].

posterior v. of corpus callosum [TA], v. posterior do corpo caloso; origina-se na superfície superior do corpo caloso e corre posteriormente, indo terminar na v. cerebral magna. SIN dorsal v. of corpus callosum [TA], vena posterior corporis callosi [TA], vena dorsalis corporis callosi*, dorsal callosal v., posterior marginal v., posterior pericallosal v.

posterior facial v., v. retromandibular. SIN retromandibular v.

v. of posterior horn, v. do corno posterior; uma pequena v. que drena a região superficial do corno posterior do ventrículo lateral; é uma tributária para a v. cerebral magna. SIN vena cornus posterioris [TA].

posterior intercostal v.'s [TA], veias intercostais posteriores; as veias que drenam os espaços intercostais posteriormente; as do primeiro espaço 1–C drenam para as veias braquiocefálicas; a partir dos espaços 2–3, elas drenam para as veias intercostais superiores direita e esquerda; do 4.º ao 11.º espaços à direita, elas são tributárias da v. ázigo; à esquerda, elas deságuam nas veias hemiázigo ou hemiázigo acessória. SIN venae intercostales posteriores [TA].

posterior labial v.'s [TA], veias labiais posteriores; as veias que passam posteriormente, oriundas dos lábios maior e menor do pudendo para as veias pudendas internas. SIN venae labiales posteriores [TA].

posterior marginal v., v. posterior do corpo caloso. SIN posterior v. of corpus callosum.

posterior parotid v.'s, veias parotídeas. SIN parotid v.'s.

posterior pericallosal v., v. posterior do corpo caloso. SIN posterior v. of corpus callosum.

posterior scrotal v.'s [TA], v. escrotais posteriores; veias oriundas da face posterior do escroto para as veias pudendas internas. SIN venae scrotales posteriores [TA].

posterior v. of septum pellucidum [TA], v. posterior do septo pelúcido; v. que drena a parte posterior do septo pelúcido; desemboca na v. tálamo-estriada superior. SIN vena posterior septi pellucidi [TA].

posterior v.(s) of left ventricle [TA], v. posterior do ventrículo esquerdo; origina-se na superfície diafragmática do coração próximo ao ápice, corre para a esquerda e em paralelo com o sulco interventricular posterior, indo desembocar no seio coronário. SIN vena(e) posterior(es) ventriculi sinistri.

posterior tibial v.'s [TA], veias tibiais posteriores; veias acompanhantes da artéria tibial posterior que se unem àquelas da artéria tibial anterior para formar a v. poplítea. SIN venae tibiales posteriores [TA].

precentral cerebellar v. [TA], v. cerebelar pré-central; uma v. ímpar que se origina na fissura cerebelar pré-central, passando anterior e superior ao cúlmen em seu trajeto, para terminar na v. cerebral magna. SIN vena precentralis cerebelli [TA].

prefrontal v.'s, veias pré-frontais; as veias superficiais que drenam o córtex cerebral pré-frontal e desembocam no seio sagital superior. SIN venae prefrontales [TA].

prepyloric v. [TA], v. pré-pilórica; uma tributária da v. gástrica direita que passa anterior ao piloro em sua junção com o duodeno. SIN vena prepylorica [TA], Latarget v., Mayo v.

profunda femoris v. [TA], v. femoral profunda; a v. que acompanha a artéria femoral profunda, recebendo as veias perfurantes oriundas das faces lateral e posterior da coxa. Une-se à v. femoral no triângulo femoral, usualmente em conjunto com as veias circunflexas femorais medial e lateral. SIN vena profunda femoris [TA], deep v. of thigh*, deep femoral v.

v. of pterygoid canal [TA], v. do canal pterigóideo; uma v. que acompanha o nervo e a artéria através do canal pterigóideo e desemboca no plexo venoso faríngeo. SIN vena canalis pterygoidei [TA], vidian v.

pudendal v.'s, veias pudendas. VER external pudendal v.'s, internal pudendal v.

pulmonary v.'s [TA], veias pulmonares; quatro veias, duas de cada lado, que conduzem o sangue oxigenado dos pulmões para o átrio esquerdo do coração. As veias pulmonares esquerdas e a v. pulmonar direita inferior são veias lobares, cada uma drenando um único lobo com o nome correspondente; a v. pulmonar direita superior drena os lobos superior e médio do pulmão direito. VER TAMBÉM left inferior pulmonary v., left superior pulmonary v., right inferior pulmonary v., right superior pulmonary v. SIN venae pulmonales [TA].

pyloric v., v. gástrica direita. SIN right gastric v.

radial v.'s [TA], veias radiais; as veias acompanhantes da artéria radial que são a continuação das veias da face radial do arco palmar profundo, drenando para as veias acompanhantes da artéria braquial na fossa cubital. SIN venae radiales [TA].

renal v.'s [TA], veias renais; grandes veias formadas no hilo renal pela união das veias segmentares anteriormente às artérias correspondentes; elas se abrem em ângulos retos na v. cava inferior, no nível da segunda vértebra lombar. A v. renal esquerda recebe a v. supra-renal esquerda e a v. gonadal esquerda, e passa através do ângulo entre a aorta abdominal e a artéria mesentérica superior, podendo aí ser comprimida. SIN venae renales.

retromandibular v. [TA], v. formada pela união das veias temporal superficial e maxilar na frente do ouvido; corre posterior ao ramo da mandíbula, através da glândula parótida, unindo-se com a v. auricular posterior para formar a v. jugular externa; em geral, possui um grande ramo comunicante com a v. facial. SIN vena retromandibularis [TA], posterior facial v., temporomaxillary v., vena facialis posterior.

retroperitoneal v.'s, veias retroperitoneais; anastomoses portocavas formadas a partir das veias nas paredes das vísceras retroperitoneais, como os colos ascendente e descendente, passando para as tributárias da v. cava inferior na parede corporal posterior, em lugar daquelas da v. porta. SIN Retzius v.'s, Ruysch v.'s, venae retroperitoneales.

Retzius v.'s, veias de Retzius. SIN retroperitoneal v.'s.

right colic v. [TA], v. cólica direita; a v. paralela à artéria cólica direita que drena o sangue oriundo do colo ascendente e flexura direita do colo. SIN vena colica dextra [TA].

right gastric v. [TA], v. gástrica direita; recebe as veias de ambas as superfícies da porção superior do estômago, corre para a direita, ao longo da curvatura menor do estômago, e desemboca na v. porta. SIN vena gastrica dextra [TA], pyloric v.

right gastroepiploic v., v. gastro-omental direita; *termo oficial alternativo para right gastroomental v.

right gastroomental v. [TA], v. gastro-omental direita; uma tributária da v. mesentérica superior que acompanha a artéria gastro-omental direita ao longo da curvatura maior do estômago. SIN vena gastro-omentalis dextra [TA], right gastroepiploic v. *.

right hepatic v.'s [TA], veias hepáticas direitas; as veias que drenam grande parte do lobo direito do fígado (segmento lateral posterior [VI] e segmento lateral anterior direito [VI] e as partes laterais dos segmentos mediais anteriores posterior e inferior [V e VII]) que se unem para formar um único tronco ou, por vezes, duplo, drenando para o lado direito da porção supra-hepática da veia cava inferior (entre a superfície superior do fígado e o diafragma); quando única, é a maior v. do fígado. SIN venae hepaticae dextrae [TA].

right inferior pulmonary v. [TA], v. pulmonar direita inferior; a v. que retorna o sangue oxigenado oriundo do lobo inferior do pulmão direito para o átrio esquerdo; as tributárias incluem a v. superior e a veia basilar comum a partir do lobo inferior direito. SIN vena pulmonalis inferior dextra [TA].

right ovarian v. [TA], v. ovárica direita; começa como o plexo pampiniforme no hilo do ovário e abre-se na v. cava inferior. SIN vena ovarica dextra [TA].

right superior intercostal v. [TA], v. intercostal superior direita; uma tributária da v. ázigo formada pela união da segunda, terceira e quarta veias intercostais posteriores direitas. SIN vena intercostalis superior dextra [TA].

right superior pulmonary v. [TA], v. pulmonar direita superior; a v. que retorna o sangue oxigenado oriundo dos lobos superior e médio do pulmão direito para o átrio esquerdo; as tributárias incluem as veias apical, anterior e posterior (ramos), oriundas do lobo superior direito, e a v. do lobo médio. SIN vena pulmonalis superior dextra [TA].

right suprarenal v. [TA], v. supra-renal direita; a v. curta que vai do hilo da supra-renal direita até a v. cava inferior. SIN vena suprarenalis dextra [TA].

right testicular v. [TA], v. testicular direita; começa como o plexo pampiniforme e ascende para se unir à veia cava inferior. SIN vena testicularis dextra [TA].

Rosenthal v., v. de Rosenthal. SIN basal v.

Ruysch v.'s, veias de Ruysch. SIN retroperitoneal v.'s.

sacral v.'s, veias sacrais. VER lateral sacral v.'s, median sacral v.

Santorini v., v. de Santorini. SIN parietal emissary v.

saphenous v.'s, veias safenas. VER accessory saphenous v., great saphenous v., small saphenous v.

Sappey v.'s, veias de Sappey. SIN paraumbilical v.'s.

v. of scala tympani [TA], v. da rampa do tímpano; tributária da v. comum do modíolo que drena a rampa do tímpano da cóclea. SIN vena scalae tympani [TA].

v. of scala vestibuli [TA], v. da rampa do vestíbulo; tributária da v. comum do modíolo que drena a rampa do tímpano da cóclea. SIN vena scalae vestibuli [TA].

scleral v.'s [TA], veias esclerais; pequenas veias que drenam a esclerótica; são tributárias das veias ciliares anteriores. SIN venae sclerales [TA].

scrotal v.'s, veias escrotais. VER anterior scrotal v.'s, posterior scrotal v.'s.

v.'s of semicircular ducts [TA], veias dos ductos semicirculares; as veias que drenam os ductos semicirculares, especialmente das partes ampulares, para a v. do aqueduto do vestíbulo. SIN venae ductuum semicircularium [TA].

v. of septum pellucidum, v. do septo pelúcido. VER anterior v. of septum pellucidum, posterior v. of septum pellucidum.

short gastric v.'s [TA], veias gástricas curtas; pequenos vasos que drenam o fundo e a porção esquerda da parede do estômago e desembocam na v. esplênica. SIN venae gastricae breves [TA].

short saphenous v., v. safena parva. SIN small saphenous v.

sigmoid v.'s [TA], veias sigmóideas; as várias tributárias da v. mesentérica inferior que drenam o colo sigmóide. SIN venae sigmoideae [TA].

small v., v. pequena; uma v. em que as três túnicas são mal definidas e finas; existem redes elásticas longitudinais, e a musculatura lisa da camada média, que é disposta de maneira circular, pode estar incompleta ou em uma ou duas camadas.

small cardiac v. [TA], v. cardíaca parva; um vaso inconstante, que acompanha a artéria coronária direita no sulco coronário, a partir da margem direita do ventrículo direito, desembocando no seio coronário ou na v. interventricular posterior. SIN vena cordis parva [TA].

smallest cardiac v.'s [TA], veias cardíacas mínimas; inúmeros canais venosos pequenos e sem válvula que se abrem diretamente nos compartimentos do coração oriundos do leito capilar na parede cardíaca, possibilitando uma forma de circulação colateral própria do coração. SIN venae cardiacae minimae [TA], venae cordis minimae*, thebesian v.'s.

small saphenous v. [TA], v. safena parva; origina-se na face lateral do pé a partir de uma união da v. digital dorsal com o arco venoso dorsal, ascende por trás do maléolo lateral, ao longo da borda lateral do tendão do calcâneo e, em seguida, através do meio da panturrilha até a porção inferior do espaço poplíteo, onde desemboca na v. poplítea. SIN vena saphena parva [TA], short saphenous v.

spermatic v., v. testicular. VER right testicular v., left testicular v.

spinal v.'s [TA], veias espinais; as veias que drenam a medula espinal; formam um plexo na superfície da medula espinal, de onde as veias passam ao longo das raízes espinais até o plexo venoso vertebral interno e, em seguida, para as veias segmentares regionais, p.ex., as veias intercostais posteriores na região torácica. SIN venae spinales [TA].

v.'s of spinal cord [TA], veias da medula espinal; as veias espinais anteriores e posteriores que se situam na superfície da medula espinal. SIN venae medullae spinalis [TA].

spiral v. of modiolus, v. comum do modíolo. SIN common modiolar v.

splenic v. [TA], v. esplênica; origina-se pela união de várias pequenas veias no hilo na superfície anterior do baço com as veias gástricas curtas e gastromental esquerda; passa para trás, através do ligamento esplenorrenal até o rim esquerdo, corre, em seguida, por trás da borda superior do pâncreas até o colo do pâncreas, onde se une à v. mesentérica superior para formar a v. porta. SIN vena splenica [TA], vena lienalis.

stellate v.'s, veias estelares. SIN *venulae* stellatae, em *venula*.

Stensen v.'s, veias de Stensen. SIN vorticose v.'s.

sternocleidomastoid v. [TA], v. esternocleidomastóidea; origina-se no músculo esternocleidomastóide e acompanha o ramo esternocleidomastóideo da artéria occipital; drena para a v. jugular interna ou tireóidea superior. SIN vena sternocleidomastoidea [TA].

striate v.'s, veias tálamo-estriadas inferiores. SIN inferior thalamostriate v.'s.

stylomastoid v. [TA], v. estilomastóidea; drena a cavidade timpânica, atravessa o canal facial, saindo através do forame estilomastóideo, e desemboca na v. retromandibular. SIN vena stylomastoidea [TA].

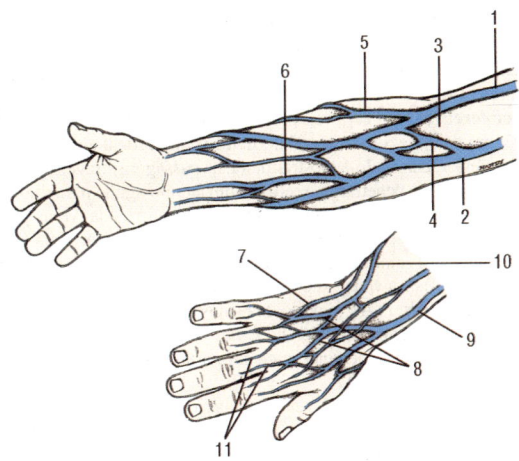

veias superficiais da mão e do antebraço: mostrando os locais para a inserção de agulhas ou cateteres intravenosos para a administração parenteral de líquidos, medicamentos ou hemoderivados; (1) veia cefálica, (2) veia basílica, (3) fossa antecubital, (4) veia intermédia do cotovelo, (5) veia cefálica acessória, (6) veia intermédia do antebraço, (7) rede venosa dorsal, (8) veias metacarpais, (9) veia cefálica, (10) veia basílica, (11) veias digitais

subclavian v. [TA], v. subclávia; a continuação direta da v. axilar na borda lateral da primeira costela; passa medialmente para se unir à v. jugular interna e formar a v. braquiocefálica em cada lado. SIN vena subclavia [TA].

subcutaneous v.'s of abdomen, veias subcutâneas do abdome; a rede de veias superficiais da parede abdominal que desembocam nas veias toracoepigástricas, epigástrica superficial ou epigástrica superior e formam anastomoses portocavas através de suas comunicações com as veias paraumbilicais. SIN venae subcutaneae abdominis.

sublingual v. [TA], v. sublingual; a v. que acompanha a artéria sublingual no assoalho da boca, lateral ao nervo hipoglosso; pode unir-se à v. lingual profunda para formar a v. lingual ou unir-se às veias acompanhantes do nervo hipoglosso. SIN vena sublingualis [TA].

submental v. [TA], v. submentual; uma v. situada sob o queixo, fazendo anastomose com a v. sublingual, que se une com a v. jugular anterior e desemboca na v. facial. SIN vena submentalis [TA].

superficial v. [TA], v. superficial; uma das inúmeras veias existentes no tecido subcutâneo e que deságuam nas veias profundas; formam sistemas proeminentes de vasos nos membros e, em geral, não são acompanhadas por artérias. SIN vena superficialis [TA], cutaneous v., vena cutanea.

superficial cerebral v.'s [TA], veias cerebrais superficiais; as veias na superfície dos hemisférios cerebrais; compreendem três grupos: superior, médio e inferior. SIN venae superficiales cerebri [TA].

superficial circumflex iliac v. [TA], v. circunflexa ilíaca superficial; correspondendo à artéria de mesmo nome, desemboca geralmente na v. safena magna ou, por vezes, na v. femoral. SIN vena circumflexa iliaca superficialis [TA].

superficial dorsal v.'s of clitoris, veias dorsais superficiais do clitóris; um par de veias no dorso do clitóris, tributárias à v. pudenda externa em ambos os lados. SIN venae dorsales clitoridis superficiales [TA].

superficial dorsal v.'s of penis [TA], veias dorsais superficiais do pênis; um par de veias no dorso do pênis superficiais à fáscia do pênis; são tributárias das veias pudendas externas em cada lado. SIN venae dorsales penis superficiales [TA].

superficial epigastric v. [TA], v. epigástrica superficial; drena as partes inferior e medial da parede abdominal anterior e desemboca na v. safena magna. SIN vena epigastrica superficialis [TA].

superficial middle cerebral v. [TA], v. cerebral superficial média; uma grande v. que avança ao longo da linha da fissura de Sylvius para se unir ao seio cavernoso; comunica-se com o seio sagital superior e com o seio transverso através das veias anastomóticas superior e inferior, respectivamente. SIN vena media superficialis cerebri.

superficial temporal v.'s [TA], veias temporais superficiais; as veias que passam da região temporal para se unirem com a v. maxilar, formando a v. retromandibular. SIN venae temporales superficiales [TA].

superior anastomotic v. [TA], v. anastomótica superior; uma grande v. comunicante entre a v. cerebral superficial média e o seio sagital superior; ascende a partir do sulco lateral, seguindo, com freqüência, a linha do sulco central (fissura de Rolando). SIN vena anastomotica superior [TA], Trolard v.

superior basal v. [TA], v. basilar superior; tributária para a v. basilar comum que drena as porções lateral e anterior do lobo inferior de cada pulmão. SIN vena basalis superior [TA].

superior v.'s of cerebellar hemisphere [TA], veias cerebelares superiores; várias veias que drenam a parte superior dos hemisférios cerebelares; elas terminam no seio petroso superior ou na v. petrosa. SIN venae hemispherii cerebelli superiores [TA].

superior cerebral v.'s [TA], veias cerebrais superiores; numerosas (8–10) veias que drenam a convexidade dorsal do hemisfério cortical e deságuam no seio sagital superior, curvando-se rostralmente na passagem através do espaço subdural, de modo que penetram no seio em um ângulo agudo para diante; podem ser divididas em 5 grupos gerais com base na área irrigada: veias pré-frontais [TA], veias frontais [TA] (venae frontales [TA]), veias parietais [TA], veias temporais [TA] (venae temporales [TA]) e veias occipitais [TA] (venae occipitales [TA]). SIN venae superiores cerebri [TA].

superior choroid v. [TA], v. corióidea superior; uma v. tortuosa que segue o plexo corióide do ventrículo lateral e se une com a v. tálamo-estriada superior e à v. anterior do septo pelúcido para formar as veias cerebrais internas. SIN vena choroidea superior [TA].

superior epigastric v.'s [TA], veias epigástricas superiores; as veias acompanhantes da artéria de mesmo nome, tributárias das veias torácicas internas. SIN venae epigastricae superiores [TA].

v.'s of superior eyelid, veias palpebrais superiores. SIN superior palpebral v.'s.

superior gluteal v.'s [TA], veias glúteas superiores; as veias que acompanham a artéria glútea superior, entrando na pelve como duas veias que se unem e desembocam na v. ilíaca interna. SIN venae gluteae superiores [TA].

superior hemorrhoidal v., termo obsoleto para v. retal superior. VER superior rectal v.

superior intercostal v., v. intercostal superior. VER left superior intercostal v., right superior intercostal v.

superior labial v. [TA], v. labial superior; as veias que captam o sangue do lábio superior e desembocam na v. facial. SIN vena labialis superior [TA].

superior laryngeal v. [TA], v. laríngea superior; a v. que acompanha a artéria laríngea superior e deságua na v. tireóidea superior. SIN vena laryngea superior [TA].

superior mesenteric v. [TA], v. mesentérica superior; começa no íleo na fossa ilíaca direita, ascende na raiz do mesentério, unindo-se por trás do pâncreas com a v. esplênica para formar a v. porta do fígado. SIN vena mesenterica superior [TA].

superior ophthalmic v. [TA], v. oftálmica superior; começa anteriormente a partir da v. nasofrontal, passa ao longo da parte superior da parede medial da órbita, atravessa a fissura orbitária superior, para desembocar no seio cavernoso. SIN vena ophthalmica superior [TA].

superior palpebral v.'s [TA], veias palpebrais superiores; as veias que drenam a pálpebra superior anteriormente para a v. angular. SIN venae palpebrales superiores [TA], v.'s of superior eyelid.

superior phrenic v.'s [TA], veias frênicas superiores; pequenas veias que drenam a superfície superior do diafragma; são tributárias das veias ázigo e hemiázigo. SIN venae phrenicae superiores [TA].

superior rectal v. [TA], v. retal superior; drena a maior parte do plexo venoso retal e ascende entre as camadas do mesorreto até a borda da pelve, onde se torna a v. mesentérica inferior. Como tributária da v. porta, forma uma anastomose portocava com as veias retais média e inferior (tributárias cavas) por meio do plexo venoso retal. SIN vena rectalis superior [TA].

superior thalamostriate v. [TA], v. tálamo-estriada superior; uma longa v. que passa para diante, no sulco entre o tálamo e o núcleo caudado, coberta pela lâmina afixa, recebendo as veias transversas do núcleo caudado ao longo de seu lado lateral, e unindo-se à parede caudal do forame de Monro com a v. coroidal e a v. do septo pelúcido, indo formar a v. cerebral interna. SIN vena thalamostriata superior [TA], terminal v. *, vena terminalis*, v. of corpus striatum.

superior thyroid v. [TA], v. tireóidea superior; recebe o sangue da parte superior da glândula tireóide e da laringe, acompanha a artéria de mesmo nome e deságua na v. jugular interna. SIN vena thyroidea superior [TA].

superior v. of vermis [TA], v. superior do verme; uma v. que drena parte da porção superior do cerebelo; corre sobre a superfície do verme para terminar nas veias cerebrais internas. SIN vena superior vermis [TA].

supraorbital v. [TA], v. supra-orbital; drena a parte frontal do couro cabeludo e une-se às veias supratrocleares para formar a v. angular. SIN vena supraorbitalis [TA].

suprarenal v.'s, veias supra-renais. VER right suprarenal v., left suprarenal v.

suprascapular v. [TA], v. supra-escapular; v. que acompanha a artéria supraescapular e desemboca na v. jugular externa. SIN vena suprascapularis [TA], transverse v. of scapula, vena transversa scapulae.

supratrochlear v.'s [TA], veias supratrocleares; diversas veias que drenam a parte frontal do couro cabeludo, unindo-se à v. supra-orbital para formar a v. angular. SIN venae supratrochleares [TA], frontal v.'s (2), venae frontales.

supreme intercostal v. [TA], v. intercostal suprema; a v. que drena o primeiro espaço intercostal para a v. vertebral ou para a v. braquiocefálica. SIN vena intercostalis suprema [TA], highest intercostal v.

surface thalamic v.'s, veias diretas laterais. SIN direct lateral v.'s.

temporal v.'s, veias temporais. VER middle temporal v., deep temporal v.'s, superficial temporal v.'s.

v.'s of temporomandibular joint, veias da articulação temporomandibular; várias pequenas tributárias para a v. retromandibular a partir da articulação temporomandibular. SIN venae articulares temporomandibulares.

temporomaxillary v., v. retromandibular. SIN retromandibular v.

terminal v., v. tálamo-estriada superior; *termo oficial alternativo para superior thalamostriate v.

testicular v.'s, veias testiculares. VER right testicular v., left testicular v.

thalamostriate v.'s, veias tálamo-estriadas. VER inferior thalamostriate v.'s, superior thalamostriate v.

thebesian v.'s, veias de Thebesius. SIN smallest cardiac v.'s.

thoracic v.'s, veias torácicas. VER internal thoracic v., lateral thoracic v.

thoracoacromial v. [TA], v. toracoacromial; v. que corresponde à artéria do mesmo nome, desembocando na v. axilar, por vezes por um tronco comum com a v. cefálica. SIN vena thoracoacromialis [TA], thoracic axis (2).

thoracoepigastric v. [TA], v. toracoepigástrica; uma das duas veias, por vezes uma única v., que se originam da região da v. epigástrica superficial e que se abrem na v. axilar ou na v. torácica lateral, formando, dessa maneira, uma via anastomótica ou colateral entre as tributárias das veias cava inferior e superior. SIN vena thoracoepigastrica [TA].

thymic v.'s [TA], veias tímicas; inúmeras pequenas veias, oriundas do timo, que desembocam na v. braquiocefálica esquerda. SIN venae thymicae [TA].

thyroid v.'s, veias tireóideas. VER inferior thyroid v., middle thyroid v., superior thyroid v., *plexus* venosus thyroideus impar.

tracheal v.'s [TA], veias traqueais; vários pequenos troncos venosos, oriundas da traquéia, que desembocam nas veias braquiocefálicas ou na v. cava superior. SIN venae tracheales [TA].

transverse cervical v.'s [TA], veias cervicais transversas; as veias acompanhantes das artérias correspondentes, desaguando na v. jugular externa ou, por vezes, na v. subclávia. SIN venae transversae cervicis [TA], venae transversae colli*, transverse v.'s of neck.

transverse v. of face, v. facial transversa. SIN transverse facial v.

transverse facial v. [TA], v. facial transversa; uma tributária das veias temporais superficiais ou da veia retromandibular que se anastomosa com a v. facial. SIN vena transversa faciei [TA], transverse v. of face.

transverse v.'s of neck, veias cervicais transversas. SIN transverse cervical v.'s.

transverse v. of scapula, v. supra-escapular. SIN suprascapular v.

Trolard v., v. de Trolard. SIN superior anastomotic v.

tympanic v.'s [TA], veias timpânicas; as veias que saem da cavidade timpânica através da fissura petrotimpânica com a corda do tímpano e que desembocam na v. retromandibular. SIN venae tympanicae [TA].

ulnar v.'s [TA], veias ulnares; as veias acompanhantes da artéria ulnar, que são a continuação daquelas do arco palmar superficial e que se unem àquelas da artéria radial para formar as veias braquiais na fossa cubital. SIN venae ulnares [TA].

umbilical v. [TA], v. umbilical. VER left umbilical v.

v. of uncus [TA], v. do unco. SIN vena uncalis.

v.'s of upper limb [TA], veias do membro superior; todas as veias, superficiais e profundas, que drenam o sangue do membro superior. SIN venae membri superioris [TA].

uterine v.'s [TA], veias uterinas; duas veias em cada lado que se originam do plexo venoso uterino, atravessam uma parte do ligamento largo do útero e, em seguida, atravessam uma prega peritoneal, desembocando na v. ilíaca interna. SIN venae uterinae [TA].

varicose v.'s, veias varicosas; dilatação permanente e tortuosidade das veias; mais comumente observadas nas pernas, provavelmente em consequência de válvulas congenitamente incompletas; as pessoas cujas profissões exigem longos períodos em pé e as gestantes apresentam predisposição para as veias varicosas.

vertebral v. [TA], v. vertebral; uma v. derivada de tributárias (veias acompanhantes) que avançam através dos forames nos processos transversos das seis primeiras vértebras cervicais, formando um plexo ao redor da artéria vertebral; desemboca como um tronco único nas veias braquiocefálicas. SIN vena vertebralis [TA].

v.'s of vertebral column [TA], veias da coluna vertebral; incluem os plexos venosos vertebrais interno e externo, as veias basivertebrais e as veias espinais anteriores e posteriores. SIN venae columnae vertebralis [TA].

Vesalius v., v. de Vesalius; a v. emissária que passa através do forame venoso.

vesical v.'s [TA], veias vesicais; as veias que drenam o plexo venoso vesical; unem-se às veias ilíacas internas. SIN venae vesicales [TA].

v. of vestibular aqueduct [TA], v. do aqueduto do vestíbulo; uma pequena v. que acompanha o ducto endolinfático; drena grande parte da porção vestibular do labirinto e termina no seio petroso inferior. SIN vena aqueductus vestibuli [TA].

v. of vestibular bulb, v. do bulbo do vestíbulo. SIN v. of bulb of vestibule.

vidian v., v. do canal pterigóideo. SIN v. of pterygoid canal.
Vieussens v.'s, veias de Vieussens. SIN innominate cardiac v.'s.
vitelline v., v. vitelina; uma v. que retorna o sangue do saco vitelino para o embrião. SIN vena vitellina.
vortex v.'s, veias vorticosas. SIN vorticose v.'s.
vorticose v.'s [TA], veias vorticosas; várias veias (geralmente quatro) oriundas da túnica vascular formada pelas veias que acompanham as artérias ciliares posteriores e o corpo ciliar; em seguida, drenam para a v. oftálmica superior ou inferior. SIN venae vorticosae [TA], choroid v.'s of eye, Stensen v.'s, vasa vorticosa, venae choroideae oculi, vortex v.'s.

---

veined (vānd). Venado; marcado por veias ou linhas que se assemelham às veias na superfície.
vein·let (vān'let). Vênula. SIN venule.
Ve·jo·vis (vē - jō'vis). Um gênero de escorpiões (os chamados escorpiões-do-diabo da América do Norte), incluindo V. spinigerus, o escorpião-do-diabo com cauda listrada; V. carolinianus, o escorpião-do-diabo do sul; e V. flavus, o escorpião-do-diabo delgado.
vel (vel). Numa prescrição médica significa "ou". [L. ou]
ve·la (vē'lă). Véus; plural de velum.
ve·la·men, pl. **ve·lam·i·na** (vĕ - lā'men, vĕ - lam'i - nă). Velame. SIN velum (1). [L. um véu]
  v. vul'vae, v. da vulva; termo obsoleto para a hipertrofia dos lábios menores do pudendo.
vel·a·men·tous (vel - ă - men'tŭs). Velamentoso; expandido na forma de uma lâmina ou véu. SIN veliform.
vel·a·men·tum, pl. **vel·a·men·ta** (vel'ă - men'tŭm, - tă). Velame. SIN velum (1). [L. uma cobertura]
ve·lam·i·na (vĕ - lam'i - nă). Velames; plural de velamen.
ve·lar (vē'lăr). Velar; relativo a qualquer véu, especialmente ao véu palatino (palato mole).
ve·li·form (vel'i - fōrm). Veliforme. SIN velamentous. [L. velum, véu, + forma, forma]
Vella, Luigi, fisiologista italiano, 1825–1886. VER V. fistula; Thiry-V. fistula.
vel·li·cate (vel'i - kāt). Estremecer; contrair de forma voluntária ou espasmódica; diz-se especialmente dos espasmos musculares fibrilares. [L. vellico, pp. -atus, contrair, estrangular, de vello, privar de ar, estrangular]
vel·li·ca·tion (vel'i - kā'shŭn). Estremecimento; um espasmo muscular fibrilar.
vel·lus (vel'ŭs). Velo. **1.** Pêlo fino não-pigmentado que cobre a maior parte do corpo. **2.** Uma estrutura que tem aparência macia ou felpuda e delicada. [L. velocino]
  v. oli'vae inferio'ris, v. da oliva inferior; um estrato de fibras nervosas que circunda a oliva inferior.
ve·loc·i·ty (v) (vĕ - los'i - tē). Velocidade; a velocidade de movimento; especificamente, a distância percorrida ou convertida por unidade de tempo em determinada direção. Cf. speed. [L. velocitas, de velox (veloc-), rápido, veloz]
  initial v., v. inicial; a velocidade de uma reação, p.ex., uma reação catalisada por enzima, nos estágios iniciais da reação de tal modo que as concentrações do(s) produto(s) não aumentem até um nível que afete, de maneira significativa, a velocidade observável; tipicamente, as velocidades iniciais são observadas quando ocorreu uma fração de menos de 10% da totalidade da reação no sentido do equilíbrio. SIN initial rate.
  maximum v. ($V_{máx}$), v. máxima; **(1)** a velocidade máxima de uma reação catabolizada por enzima que pode ser alcançada pelo aumento progressivo da concentração de substrato em uma determinada concentração da enzima; nos casos de inibição de substrato, a $V_{máx}$ é um valor extrapolado na ausência dessa inibição. Cf. Michaelis-Menten equation; **(2)** a velocidade inicial máxima de encurtamento de uma fibra miocárdica que pode ser obtida sem carga; usada para avaliar a contratilidade da fibra.
  nerve conduction v., v. de condução nervosa; a velocidade de condução do impulso em um nervo periférico ou em suas várias fibras componentes, geralmente expressa em metros por segundo.
  PSA v., v. de PSA; uma medida da rapidez da mudança em um nível de PSA (antígeno próstata-específico) de uma pessoa.
  sedimentation v., v. de sedimentação; a velocidade de movimento de um substrato, tipicamente uma macromolécula, na centrifugação; esses estudos de centrifugação fornecem dados sobre a estrutura da macromolécula.
  steady-state v., v. uniforme; a v. de uma reação catalisada por enzima na qual, durante o intervalo de tempo do estudo, a concentração de qualquer espécie de intermediária é constante (isto é, para um complexo binário enzima–substrato, ES, $d[ES]/dt \cong 0$; para que isso seja verdadeiro, a concentração enzimática total deve ser muito menor que a concentração inicial de substrato. SIN steady-state rate.
vel·o·gen·ic (vel - ō - jen'ik). Indica a virulência de um vírus capaz de induzir, depois de um breve período de incubação, uma doença fulminante e, com freqüência, letal em hospedeiros embrionários, imaturos e adultos; usado na caracterização do vírus da doença de Newcastle. [L. velox, rápido, + G. -gen, que produz]
vel·o·pha·ryn·ge·al (vē'lō - fă - rin'jē - ăl). Velofaríngeo; pertinente ao palato mole (véu palatino) e às paredes faríngeas.
ve·lo·syn·the·sis (vē'lō - sin'thĕ - sis). Palatorrafia. SIN palatorrhaphy.
Velpeau, Alfred A.L.M., cirurgião francês, 1795–1867. VER V. bandage, canal, fossa, hernia.
ve·lum, pl. **ve·la** (vē'lŭm, - lă). **1.** Véu; qualquer estrutura semelhante a um véu ou cortina. SIN veil (1), velamen, velamentum. **2.** Âmnio. SIN caul (1). **3.** Omento maior. SIN greater omentum. **4.** Qualquer membrana serosa, envelope ou revestimento membranoso. [L. véu, vela]
  anterior medullary v., v. medular superior. SIN superior medullary v.
  inferior medullary v. [TA], v. medular inferior; uma fina lâmina de substância branca, oculto pela tonsila cerebelar, fixado ao longo do pedúnculo do flóculo e, na linha média ou próximo a ela, até o nódulo do verme; é contínuo caudalmente com a lâmina epitelial e plexo coróide do quarto ventrículo. SIN v. medullare inferius [TA], posterior medullary v., Tarin valve, valvula semilunaris tarini, v. semilunare, v. tarini.
  v. interpos'itum, tela corióidea do terceiro ventrículo. SIN tela choroidea of third ventricle.
  v. medulla're infe'rius [TA], v. medular inferior. SIN inferior medullary v.
  v. medulla're supe'rius [TA], v. medular superior. SIN superior medullary v.
  v. palati'num, palato mole; *termo oficial alternativo para soft palate.
  v. pen'dulum pala'ti, palato mole. SIN soft palate.
  posterior medullary v., v. medular inferior. SIN inferior medullary v.
  v. semiluna're, v. medular inferior. SIN inferior medullary v.
  superior medullary v. [TA], v. medular superior; a fina camada de substância branca que se estende entre os dois pedúnculos cerebelares superiores, formando o teto do recesso superior do quarto ventrículo. SIN v. medullare superius [TA], anterior medullary v., Vieussens valve.
  v. tari'ni, v. de Tarinus. SIN inferior medullary v.
  v. termina'le, lâmina terminal. SIN lamina terminalis of cerebrum.
  transverse v., v. transverso; uma prega na parede dorsal do cérebro embrionário, no limite entre o telencéfalo e o diencéfalo. SIN v. transversum.
  v. transver'sum, v. transverso. SIN transverse v.
  v. triangula're, tela corióidea do terceiro ventrículo. SIN tela choroidea of third ventricle.

VENA

ve·na, gen. e pl. **ve·nae** (vē'nă, - nē) [TA]. Veia. SIN vein. [L.]
  v. ad'vehens, pl. **ve'nae advehen'tes**, v. aferente hepática; termo coletivo para uma série de canais ramificantes no embrião inicial que recebem o sangue do sistema venoso umbilical e/ou vitelino e que conduzem o sangue misto até os sinusóides do fígado; tornam-se ramos terminais da veia porta do fígado. SIN v. afferens hepatis.
  v. af'ferens hep'atis, v. aferente hepática. SIN v. advehens.
  v. anastomot'ica infe'rior [TA], v. anastomótica inferior. SIN inferior anastomotic vein.
  v. anastomot'ica supe'rior [TA], v. anastomótica superior. SIN superior anastomotic vein.
  v. angula'ris [TA], v. angular. SIN angular vein.
  venae ante'riores cer'ebri [TA], veias cerebrais anteriores. SIN anterior cerebral veins, em vein.
  v. ante'rior sep'ti pellu'cidi [TA], v. anterior do septo pelúcido. SIN anterior vein of septum pellucidum.
  v. apicalis [TA], v. apical. SIN apical vein.
  v. apicoposterior [TA], v. apicoposterior. SIN apicoposterior vein.
  v. appendicula'ris [TA], v. apendicular. SIN appendicular vein.
  v. aqueduc'tus coch'leae, v. do aqueduto da cóclea. SIN vein of cochlear canaliculi.
  v. aqueduc'tus vestib'uli [TA], v. do aqueduto do vestíbulo. SIN vein of vestibular aqueduct.
  ve'nae arcua'tae re'nis, veias arqueadas do rim. SIN arcuate veins of kidney, em vein.
  v. arterio'sa, v. arterial. SIN arterial vein.
  ve'nae articula'res temporomandibula'res, veias articulares temporomandibulares. SIN veins of temporomandibular joint, em vein.
  v. atrii lateralis, v. lateral do átrio. SIN lateral vein of lateral ventricle.
  v. atrii medialis, v. medial do átrio. SIN medial vein of lateral ventricle.
  v. auricula'ris ante'rior, v. auricular anterior. SIN anterior auricular vein.
  v. auricula'ris poste'rior [TA], v. auricular posterior. SIN posterior auricular vein.
  v. axilla'ris [TA], v. axilar. SIN axillary vein.

vena

v. az′ygos [TA], v. ázigo. SIN azygos vein.
v. az′ygos ma′jor, v. ázigo. SIN azygos vein.
v. az′ygos mi′nor infe′rior, v. hemiázigo. SIN hemiazygos vein.
v. az′ygos mi′nor supe′rior, v. hemiázigo acessória. SIN accessory hemiazygos vein.
v. basa′lis [TA], v. basilar. SIN basal vein.
v. basalis anterior [TA], v. basilar anterior. SIN anterior basal vein.
v. basa′lis commu′nis [TA], v. basilar comum. SIN common basal vein.
v. basa′lis infe′rior [TA], v. basilar inferior. SIN inferior basal vein.
v. basa′lis supe′rior [TA], v. basilar superior. SIN superior basal vein.
v. basil′ica [TA], v. basílica. SIN basilic vein.
venae basivertebra′les [TA], veias basivertebrais. SIN basivertebral veins, em vein.
Billroth venae cavernosae, veias cavernosas de Billroth. SIN venae cavernosae of spleen.
ve′nae brachia′les [TA], veias braquiais. SIN brachial veins, em vein.
ve′nae brachiocephal′icae (dextrae et sinistrae) [TA], veias braquiocefálicas (direita e esquerda). SIN (left and right) brachiocephalic veins, em vein.
ve′nae bronchia′les [TA], veias bronquiais. SIN bronchial veins, em vein.
v. bul′bi pe′nis [TA], v. do bulbo do pênis. SIN vein of bulb of penis.
v. bul′bi vestib′uli [TA], v. do bulbo do vestíbulo. SIN vein of bulb of vestibule.
v. canalic′uli coch′leae, v. do aqueduto da cóclea. SIN vein of cochlear canaliculus.
v. cana′lis pterygoi′dei [TA], v. do canal pterigóideo. SIN vein of pterygoid canal.
ve′nae cardiacae anterio′res [TA], veias anteriores do ventrículo direito. SIN anterior cardiac veins, em vein.
venae cardiacae minimae [TA], veias cardíacas mínimas. SIN smallest cardiac veins, em vein.
v. cardi′aca mag′na, v. cardíaca magna. SIN great cardiac vein.
v. ca′va infe′rior [TA], v. cava inferior. SIN inferior v. cava.
v. ca′va supe′rior [TA], v. cava superior. SIN superior v. cava.
ve′nae caverno′sae pe′nis [TA], veias cavernosas do pênis. SIN cavernous veins of penis, em vein.
ve′nae centra′les hep′atis, veias centrais do fígado. SIN central veins of liver, em vein.
v. centra′lis glan′dulae suprarena′lis [TA], v. central da glândula supra-renal. SIN central vein of suprarenal gland.
v. centra′lis ret′inae [TA], v. central da retina. SIN central retinal vein.
v. cephal′ica [TA], v. cefálica. SIN cephalic vein.
v. cephal′ica accesso′ria [TA], v. cefálica acessória. SIN accessory cephalic vein.
v. cephalica antebrachii [TA], v. cefálica do antebraço. SIN cephalic vein of forearm.
ve′nae cerebel′li [TA], veias cerebelares. SIN cerebellar veins, em vein.
v. cervica′lis profun′da [TA], v. cervical profunda. SIN deep cervical vein.
ve′nae choroi′deae oc′uli, veias vorticosas. SIN vorticose veins, em vein.
v. choroidea inferior [TA], v. coróidea inferior. SIN inferior choroid vein. VER basal vein.
v. choroi′dea supe′rior [TA], v. coróidea superior. SIN superior choroid vein.
ve′nae cilia′res anteriores [TA], veias ciliares anteriores. SIN anterior ciliary veins, em vein.
ve′nae circumflex′ae fem′oris latera′les [TA], veias circunflexas femorais laterais. SIN lateral circumflex femoral veins, em vein.
ve′nae circumflex′ae fem′oris media′les [TA], veias femorais circunflexas mediais. SIN medial circumflex femoral veins, em vein.
v. circumflexa humeri anterior [TA], v. circunflexa anterior do úmero. SIN anterior circumflex humeral vein.
v. circumflexa humeri posterior [TA], v. circunflexa posterior do úmero. SIN anterior circumflex humeral vein.
v. circumflex′a ili′aca profun′da [TA], v. circunflexa ilíaca profunda. SIN deep circumflex iliac vein.
v. circumflex′a ili′aca superficia′lis [TA], v. circunflexa ilíaca superficial. SIN superficial circumflex iliac vein.
v. col′ica dex′tra [TA], v. cólica direita. SIN right colic vein.
v. col′ica me′dia [TA], v. cólica média. SIN middle colic vein.
v. col′ica sinis′tra [TA], v. cólica esquerda. SIN left colic vein.
v. colli profunda, v. cervical profunda; *termo oficial alternativo para deep cervical vein.
ve′nae colum′nae vertebra′lis [TA], veias da coluna vertebral. SIN veins of vertebral column, em vein.
v. com′itans, v. acompanhante; uma veia que acompanha outra estrutura. SIN accompanying vein.
v. comitans of hypoglossal nerve [TA], v. acompanhante do nervo hipoglosso; corre com o nervo hipoglosso abaixo do músculo hioglosso e lateralmente a este, desembocando geralmente na veia lingual. SIN v. comitans nervi hypoglossi [TA], accompanying vein of hypoglossal nerve.

v. com′itans ner′vi hypoglos′si [TA], v. acompanhante do nervo hipoglosso. SIN v. comitans of hypoglossal nerve.
ve′nae comitan′tes [TA], veias acompanhantes; duas ou mais veias que acompanham de perto uma artéria, de tal modo que as pulsações desta auxiliam o retorno venoso. SIN companion veins.
ve′nae conjunctiva′les [TA], veias conjuntivais. SIN conjunctival veins, em vein.
venae cordis [TA], veias cardíacas. SIN veins of heart, em vein.
v. cor′dis mag′na [TA], v. cardíaca magna. SIN great cardiac vein.
v. cor′dis me′dia [TA], v. interventricular posterior. SIN middle cardiac vein.
ve′nae cor′dis min′imae, veias cardíacas mínimas; *termo oficial alternativo para smallest cardiac veins, em vein.
v. cor′dis par′va [TA], v. cardíaca parva. SIN small cardiac vein.
v. cor′nus posterio′ris [TA], v. do corno posterior. SIN vein of posterior horn.
v. corona′ria ventric′uli, v. gástrica esquerda. SIN left gastric vein.
v. cuta′nea, v. cutânea. SIN superficial vein.
v. cys′tica [TA], v. cística. SIN cystic veins, em vein.
ve′nae digita′les dorsa′les pe′dis [TA], veias digitais dorsais do pé. SIN dorsal digital veins of foot, em vein.
ve′nae digita′les palma′res [TA], veias digitais palmares. SIN palmar digital veins, em vein.
ve′nae digita′les planta′res [TA], v. digitais plantares. SIN plantar digital veins, em vein.
v. diplo′ica [TA], v. diplóica. SIN diploic vein.
ve′nae direc′tae latera′les [TA], veias diretas laterais. SIN direct lateral veins, em vein.
ve′nae dorsa′les clitor′idis superficia′les [TA], veias dorsais superficiais do clítoris. SIN superficial dorsal veins of clitoris, em vein.
venae dorsa′les lin′guae [TA], veias dorsais da língua. SIN dorsal lingual vein.
ve′nae dorsa′les pe′nis superficia′les [TA], veias dorsais superficiais do pênis. SIN superficial dorsal veins of penis, em vein.
v. dorsa′lis clitor′idis profun′da [TA], v. dorsal profunda do clítoris. SIN deep dorsal vein of clitoris.
v. dorsa′lis cor′poris callo′si, v. posterior do corpo caloso; *termo oficial alternativo para posterior vein of corpus callosum.
v. dorsa′lis pe′nis profun′da [TA], v. dorsal profunda do pênis. SIN deep dorsal vein of penis.
venae ductuum semicircularium [TA], veias dos ductos semicirculares. SIN veins of semicircular ducts, em vein.
v. emissa′ria, pl. ve′nae emissa′riae [TA], v. emissária. SIN emissary vein.
v. emissa′ria condyla′ris [TA], v. emissária condilar. SIN condylar emissary vein.
v. emissa′ria mastoi′dea [TA], v. emissária mastóidea. SIN mastoid emissary vein.
v. emissa′ria occipita′lis [TA], v. emissária occipital. SIN occipital emissary vein.
v. emissa′ria parieta′lis [TA], v. emissária parietal. SIN parietal emissary vein.
ve′nae encephali occipita′les [TA], veias occipitais. SIN occipital cerebral veins, em vein.
ve′nae epigas′tricae superio′res [TA], veias epigástricas superiores. SIN superior epigastric veins, em vein.
v. epigas′trica infe′rior [TA], v. epigástrica inferior. SIN inferior epigastric vein.
v. epigas′trica superficia′lis [TA], v. epigástrica superficial. SIN superficial epigastric vein.
ve′nae episclera′les [TA], veias esclerais. SIN episcleral veins, em vein.
ve′nae esopha′geae [TA], veias esofágicas. SIN esophageal veins, em vein.
ve′nae ethmoida′les [TA], veias etmoidais. SIN ethmoidal veins, em vein.
v. facia′lis [TA], veia facial. SIN facial vein.
v. facia′lis ante′rior, v. facial. SIN facial vein.
v. facia′lis commu′nis, v. facial comum. SIN common facial vein.
v. facia′lis poste′rior, v. retromandibular. SIN retromandibular vein.
v. facie′i profun′da [TA], v. facial profunda. SIN deep facial vein.
v. femora′lis [TA], v. femoral. SIN femoral vein.
v. fenestrae cochleae [TA], v. da janela da cóclea. SIN vein of cochlear window.
ve′nae fibula′res [TA], veias fibulares. SIN fibular veins, em vein.
ve′nae fronta′les [NA], veias frontais. SIN supratrochlear veins, em vein.
v. gas′trica dex′tra [TA], v. gástrica direita. SIN right gastric vein.
ve′nae gas′tricae bre′ves [TA], veias gástricas curtas. SIN short gastric veins, em vein.
v. gas′trica sinis′tra [TA], v. gástrica esquerda. SIN left gastric vein.
v. gastro-omenta′lis dex′tra [TA], v. gastro-omental direita. SIN right gastroomental vein.
v. gastro-omenta′lis sinis′tra, v. gastro-omental esquerda. SIN left gastroomental vein.
ve′nae geniculares [TA], veias geniculares. SIN genicular veins, em vein.
ve′nae glu′teae inferio′res [TA], veias glúteas inferiores. SIN inferior gluteal veins, em vein.

ve'nae glu'teae superio'res [TA], veias glúteas superiores. SIN superior gluteal veins, em vein.
v. gyri olfactorii [TA], v. do giro olfatório. SIN vein of olfactory gyrus. VER basal vein.
v. hemiaz'ygos [TA], v. hemiázigo. SIN hemiazygos vein.
v. hemiaz'ygos accesso'ria [TA], v. hemiázigo acessória. SIN accessory hemiazygos vein.
ve'nae hemisphe'rii cerebel'li superio'res [TA], veias cerebelares superiores. SIN superior veins of cerebellar hemisphere, em vein.
ve'nae hemorrhoida'les inferio'res, veias retais inferiores; termo obsoleto para inferior rectal veins, em vein.
ve'nae hemorrhoida'les me'diae, veias retais médias; termo obsoleto para middle rectal veins, em vein.
v. hemorrhoida'lis supe'rior, v. retal superior; termo obsoleto para superior rectal vein.
ve'nae hepat'icae [TA], veias hepáticas. SIN hepatic veins, em vein.
ve'nae hepat'icae dex'trae [TA], veias hepáticas direitas. SIN right hepatic veins, em vein.
venae hepaticae intermediae [TA], veias hepáticas intermédias. SIN intermediate hepatic veins, em vein.
ve'nae hepat'icae me'diae [TA], veias hepáticas intermédias. SIN intermediate hepatic veins, em vein.
ve'nae hepat'icae sinis'trae [TA], veias hepáticas esquerdas. SIN left hepatic vein.
v. hypogas'trica, v. ilíaca interna; termo obsoleto para internal iliac vein.
v. ileocol'ica [TA], v. ileocólica. SIN ileocolic vein.
v. ili'aca commu'nis [TA], v. ilíaca comum. SIN common iliac vein.
v. ili'aca exter'na [TA], v. ilíaca externa. SIN external iliac vein.
v. ili'aca inter'na [TA], v. ilíaca interna. SIN internal iliac vein.
v. iliolumba'lis [TA], v. iliolombar. SIN iliolumbar vein.
inferior v. cava (VCI) [TA], v. cava inferior; a v. que recebe o sangue dos membros inferiores e da maior parte dos órgãos pélvicos e abdominais; ela começa no nível da quinta vértebra lombar, no lado direito, pela união das veias ilíacas comuns esquerda e direita, perfura o diafragma no nível da oitava vértebra torácica, desembocando na face póstero-inferior do átrio direito do coração. SIN v. cava inferior [TA], postcava.
ve'nae inferio'res cerebel'li [TA], veias cerebelares inferiores. SIN inferior veins of cerebellar hemisphere, em vein.
ve'nae inferio'res cer'ebri [TA], veias cerebrais inferiores. SIN inferior cerebral veins, em vein.
v. infe'rior ver'mis [TA], v. inferior do verme. SIN inferior vein of vermis.
v. innomina'ta, v. braquiocefálica; termo obsoleto para left and right brachiocephalic veins, em vein.
ve'nae insula'res [TA], veias insulares; as veias que drenam o córtex da ínsula, tributárias para a veia média profunda do cérebro. SIN insular veins [TA].
ve'nae intercapitulares, veias intercapitulares. SIN intercapitular veins, em vein.
ve'nae intercosta'les anterio'res [TA], veias intercostais anteriores. SIN anterior intercostal veins, em vein.
ve'nae intercosta'les posterio'res [TA], veias intercostais posteriores. SIN posterior intercostal veins, em vein.
v. intercosta'lis supe'rior dex'tra [TA], v. intercostal superior direita. SIN right superior intercostal vein.
v. intercosta'lis supe'rior sinis'tra [TA], v. intercostal superior esquerda. SIN left superior intercostal vein.
v. intercosta'lis supre'ma [TA], v. intercostal suprema. SIN supreme intercostal vein.
ve'nae interloba'res re'nis [TA], veias interlobares renais. SIN interlobar veins of kidney, em vein.
ve'nae interlobula'res hep'atis [TA], veias interlobulares do fígado. SIN interlobular veins of liver, em vein.
ve'nae interlobula'res re'nis [TA], veias interlobulares do rim. SIN interlobular veins of kidney, em vein.
v. interme'dia antebra'chii, v. intermédia do antebraço. SIN median antebrachial vein.
v. interme'dia basil'ica, v. basílica do antebraço. SIN intermediate basilic vein.
v. interme'dia cephal'ica, v. cefálica do antebraço. SIN intermediate cephalic vein.
v. interme'dia cu'biti, v. intermédia do cotovelo. SIN median cubital vein.
ve'nae inter'nae cer'ebri [TA], veias cerebrais internas. SIN internal cerebral veins, em vein.
v. intervertebra'lis [TA], v. intervertebral. SIN intervertebral vein.
ve'nae jejuna'les et il'ei [TA], veias jejunais e ileais. SIN jejunal and ileal veins, em vein.
v. jugula'ris ante'rior [TA], v. jugular anterior. SIN anterior jugular vein.
v. jugula'ris exter'na [TA], v. jugular externa. SIN external jugular vein.
v. jugula'ris inter'na [TA], v. jugular interna. SIN internal jugular vein.

ve'nae labia'les anterio'res [TA], veias labiais anteriores. SIN anterior labial veins, em vein.
ve'nae labia'les posterio'res [TA], veias labiais posteriores. SIN posterior labial veins, em vein.
v. labia'lis infe'rior [TA], v. labial inferior. SIN inferior labial vein.
v. labia'lis supe'rior [TA], v. labial superior. SIN superior labial vein.
ve'nae labyrin'thi [TA], veias do labirinto. SIN labyrinthine veins, em vein.
v. lacrima'lis [TA], v. lacrimal. SIN lacrimal vein.
v. laryn'gea infe'rior [TA], v. laríngea inferior. SIN inferior laryngeal vein.
v. laryn'gea supe'rior [TA], v. laríngea superior. SIN superior laryngeal vein.
v. latera'lis ventric'uli latera'lis [TA], v. lateral do ventrículo lateral. SIN lateral vein of lateral ventricle.
v. liena'lis, v. esplênica. SIN splenic vein.
v. lingualis, v. lingual. SIN lingual vein.
v. lingula'ris, v. lingular. SIN lingular vein.
v. lobi medii [TA], v. do lobo médio. SIN middle lobe vein.
ve'nae lumba'les [TA], veias lombares. SIN lumbar veins, em vein.
v. lumba'lis ascen'dens [TA], v. lombar ascendente. SIN ascending lumbar vein.
v. mag'na cer'ebri [TA], v. cerebral magna. SIN great cerebral vein of Galen.
v. mamma'ria inter'na, v. torácica interna; termo obsoleto para internal thoracic vein.
v. maxilla'ris, pl. **ve'nae maxilla'res** [TA], v. maxilar. SIN maxillary vein.
v. media'lis ventric'uli latera'lis [TA], v. medial do ventrículo lateral. SIN medial vein of lateral ventricle.
v. media'na antebra'chii [TA], v. intermédia do antebraço. SIN median antebrachial vein.
v. media'na basil'ica, v. basílica intermédia. SIN intermediate basilic vein.
v. media'na cephal'ica, v. cefálica intermédia. SIN intermediate cephalic vein.
v. media'na cu'biti [TA], v. intermédia do cotovelo. SIN median cubital vein.
v. me'dia profun'da cer'ebri [TA], v. cerebral profunda média. SIN deep middle cerebral vein.
ve'nae mediastina'les [TA], veias mediastinais. SIN mediastinal veins, em vein.
v. me'dia superficia'lis cer'ebri, v. cerebral superficial média. SIN superficial middle cerebral vein.
ve'nae medul'lae oblonga'tae [TA], veias do bulbo. SIN veins of medulla oblongata, em vein.
venae medullae spinalis [TA], veias da medula espinal. SIN veins of spinal cord, em vein.
venae membri inferioris [TA], veias do membro inferior. SIN veins of lower limb, em vein.
venae membri superioris [TA], veias do membro superior. SIN veins of upper limb, em vein.
ve'nae menin'geae [TA], veias meníngeas. SIN meningeal veins, em vein.
ve'nae menin'geae me'diae [TA], veias meníngeas médias. SIN middle meningeal veins, em vein.
ve'nae mesencephal'icae, veias mesencefálicas. SIN mesencephalic veins, em vein.
v. mesenter'ica infe'rior [TA], v. mesentérica inferior. SIN inferior mesenteric vein.
v. mesenter'ica supe'rior [TA], v. mesentérica superior. SIN superior mesenteric vein.
ve'nae metacar'peae dorsa'les [TA], veias metacarpais dorsais. SIN dorsal metacarpal veins, em vein.
ve'nae metacar'peae palma'res [TA], veias metacarpais palmares. SIN palmar metacarpal veins, em vein.
ve'nae metatar'seae dorsa'les [TA], veias metatarsais dorsais. SIN dorsal metatarsal veins, em vein.
ve'nae metatar'seae planta'res [TA], veias metatarsais plantares. SIN plantar metatarsal veins, em vein.
v. modioli communis [TA], v. comum do modíolo. SIN common modiolar vein.
ve'nae mus'culophren'icae [TA], veias musculofrênicas. SIN musculophrenic veins, em vein.
ve'nae nasa'les exter'nae [TA], veias nasais externas. SIN external nasal veins, em vein.
v. nasofronta'lis [TA], v. nasofrontal. SIN nasofrontal vein.
ve'nae nu'clei cauda'ti [TA], veias do núcleo caudado. SIN veins of caudate nucleus, em vein.
v. obli'qua a'trii sinis'tri [TA], v. oblíqua do átrio esquerdo. SIN oblique vein of left atrium.
v. obturato'ria, pl. **ve'nae obturato'riae** [TA], v. obturatória. SIN obturator veins, em vein.
v. occipita'lis [TA], v. occipital. SIN occipital vein.
v. ophthal'mica infe'rior [TA], v. oftálmica inferior. SIN inferior ophthalmic vein.
v. ophthal'mica supe'rior [TA], v. oftálmica superior. SIN superior ophthalmic vein.
v. ova'rica dex'tra [TA], v. ovárica direita. SIN right ovarian vein.
v. ova'rica sinis'tra [TA], v. ovárica esquerda. SIN left ovarian vein.

v. palati'na externa [TA], v. palatina externa. SIN external palatine vein.
ve'nae palpebra'les [TA], veias palpebrais. SIN palpebral veins, em vein.
ve'nae palpebra'les inferio'res [TA], veias palpebrais inferiores. SIN inferior palpebral veins, em vein.
ve'nae palpebra'les superio'res [TA], veias palpebrais superiores. SIN superior palpebral veins, em vein.
ve'nae pancreat'icae [TA], veias pancreáticas. SIN pancreatic veins, em vein.
ve'nae pancreat'icoduodena'les [TA], veias pancreaticoduodenais. SIN pancreaticoduodenal veins, em vein.
ve'nae paraumbilica'les [TA], veias paraumbilicais. SIN paraumbilical veins, em vein.
ve'nae parieta'les, veias parietais. SIN parietal veins, em vein.
ve'nae parotid'eae [TA], veias parotídeas. SIN parotid veins, em vein.
ve'nae pectora'les [TA], veias peitorais. SIN pectoral veins, em vein.
ve'nae pedunculares [TA], veias pedunculares. SIN peduncular veins, em vein. VER basal vein.
ve'nae perforan'tes [TA], veias perfurantes. SIN perforating veins, em vein.
ve'nae pericardi'acae [TA], veias pericárdicas. SIN pericardial veins, em vein.
ve'nae pericardiacophren'icae [TA], veias pericardicofrênicas. SIN pericardiacophrenic veins, em vein.
ve'nae perone'ae, veias fibulares; *termo oficial alternativo para fibular veins, em vein.
v. petro'sa [TA], v. petrosa. VER petrosal vein.
ve'nae pharyn'geae [TA], veias faríngeas. SIN pharyngeal veins, em vein.
ve'nae phren'icae superio'res [TA], veias frênicas superiores. SIN superior phrenic veins, em vein.
v. phren'ica infe'rior [TA], v. frênica inferior. SIN inferior phrenic vein.
ve'nae pon'tis [TA], veias da ponte. SIN pontine veins, em vein.
v. pontomesencephalica [TA], v. pontomesencefálica. VER anterior pontomesencephalic vein.
v. pontomesencephal'ica ante'rior, v. pontomesencefálica anterior. SIN anterior pontomesencephalic vein.
v. poplit'ea [TA], v. poplítea. SIN popliteal vein.
v. por'tae hep'atis [TA], v. porta do fígado. SIN hepatic portal vein.
v. porta'lis, v. porta do fígado. SIN hepatic portal vein.
v. posterior corporis callosi [TA], v. posterior do corpo caloso. SIN posterior vein of corpus callosum.
v. poste'rior sep'ti pellu'cidi [TA], v. posterior do septo pelúcido. SIN posterior vein of septum pellucidum.
v.(e) poste'rior(es) ventric'uli sinis'tri, v.(s) posterior(es) do ventrículo esquerdo. SIN posterior vein(s) of left ventricle.
v. preauricula'ris, v. auricular anterior. SIN anterior auricular vein.
v. precentra'lis cerebel'li [TA], v. cerebelar pré-central. SIN precentral cerebellar vein.
ve'nae prefronta'les [TA], veias pré-frontais. SIN prefrontal veins, em vein.
v. prepylo'rica [TA], v. pré-pilórica. SIN prepyloric vein.
ve'nae profun'dae cer'ebri [TA], v. cerebrais profundas. SIN deep cerebral veins, em vein.
ve'nae profun'dae clitor'idis [TA], veias profundas do clitóris. SIN deep veins of clitoris, em vein.
venae profun'dae pe'nis, veias profundas do pênis. SIN deep veins of penis, em vein.
v. profun'da fem'oris [TA], v. femoral profunda. SIN profunda femoris vein.
v. profun'da lin'guae [TA], v. profunda da língua. SIN deep lingual vein.
ve'nae puden'dae exter'nae [TA], veias pudendas externas. SIN external pudendal veins, em vein.
v. puden'da inter'na [TA], v. pudenda interna. SIN internal pudendal vein.
ve'nae pulmona'les [TA], veias pulmonares. SIN pulmonary veins, em vein.
v. pulmona'lis infe'rior dex'tra [TA], v. pulmonar direita inferior. SIN right inferior pulmonary vein.
v. pulmona'lis infe'rior sinis'tra [TA], v. pulmonar esquerda inferior. SIN left inferior pulmonary vein.
v. pulmona'lis supe'rior dex'tra [TA], v. pulmonar direita superior. SIN right superior pulmonary vein.
v. pulmona'lis supe'rior sinis'tra [TA], v. pulmonar esquerda superior. SIN left superior pulmonary vein.
ve'nae radia'les [TA], veias radiais. SIN radial veins, em vein.
v. reces'sus latera'lis ventric'uli quar'ti [TA], v. do recesso lateral do quarto ventrículo. SIN vein of lateral recess of fourth ventricle.
ve'nae rec'tae, veias retas; os ramos ascendentes dos vasos retos na medula renal.
ve'nae recta'les inferio'res [TA], veias retais inferiores. SIN inferior rectal veins, em vein.
ve'nae recta'les me'diae [TA], veias retais médias. SIN middle rectal veins, em vein.
v. recta'lis supe'rior [TA], v. retal superior. SIN superior rectal vein.
ve'nae rena'les, veias renais. SIN renal veins, em vein.
v. retromandibula'ris [TA], v. retromandibular. SIN retromandibular vein.
venae retroperitoneales, veias retroperitoneais. SIN retroperitoneal veins, em vein.
v. re'vehens, pl. **ve'nae revehen'tes**, v. reveente; as veias que, no embrião, fazem trajeto desde os vasos sinusóides, no fígado, até a v. cava inferior, desenvolvendo-se nas veias hepáticas.
ve'nae sacra'les latera'les [TA], veias sacrais laterais. SIN lateral sacral veins, em vein.
v. sacra'lis media'na [TA], v. sacral mediana. SIN median sacral vein.
v. saphe'na accesso'ria [TA], v. safena acessória. SIN accessory saphenous vein.
v. saphe'na mag'na [TA], v. safena magna. SIN great saphenous vein.
v. saphe'na par'va [TA], v. safena parva. SIN small saphenous vein.
v. scalae tympani [TA], v. da rampa do tímpano. SIN vein of scala tympani.
v. scalae vestibuli [TA], v. da rampa do vestíbulo. SIN vein of scala vestibuli.
v. scapula'ris dorsa'lis [TA], v. dorsal da escápula. SIN dorsal scapular vein.
ve'nae sclera'les [TA], veias esclerais. SIN scleral veins, em vein.
ve'nae scrota'les anterio'res [TA], veias escrotais anteriores. SIN anterior scrotal veins, em vein.
ve'nae scrota'les posterio'res [TA], veias escrotais posteriores. SIN posterior scrotal veins, em vein.
ve'nae sigmoi'deae [TA], veias sigmóideas. SIN sigmoid veins, em vein.
ve'nae spina'les [TA], veias espinais. SIN spinal veins, em vein.
v. spira'lis modi'oli, v. comum do modíolo. SIN common modiolar vein.
venae cavernosae of spleen, veias cavernosas do baço; pequenas tributárias da veia esplênica na polpa do baço. SIN Billroth venae cavernosae.
v. sple'nica [TA], v. esplênica. SIN splenic vein.
ve'nae stella'tae, veias estelares. SIN venulae stellatae, em venula.
v. sternocleidomastoi'dea [TA], v. esternocleidomastóidea. SIN sternocleidomastoid vein.
ve'nae stria'tae, veias tálamo-estriadas inferiores. SIN inferior thalamostriate veins, em vein.
v. stylomastoi'dea [TA], v. estilomastóidea. SIN stylomastoid vein.
v. subcla'via [TA], v. subclávia. SIN subclavian vein.
ve'nae subcuta'neae abdom'inis, veias subcutâneas do abdome. SIN subcutaneous veins of abdomen, em vein.
v. sublingua'lis [TA], v. sublingual. SIN sublingual vein.
v. submenta'lis [TA], v. submentual. SIN submental vein.
ve'nae superficia'les cer'ebri [TA], veias cerebrais superficiais. SIN superficial cerebral veins, em vein.
v. superficialis [TA], v. superficial. SIN superficial vein.
superior v. cava [TA], v. cava superior; retorna o sangue da cabeça e do pescoço, dos membros superiores e do tórax para a face póstero-superior do átrio direito; formada no mediastino superior pela união das duas veias braquiocefálicas. SIN v. cava superior; precava.
ve'nae superio'res cerebel'li [TA], veias cerebelares superiores. SIN superior veins of cerebellar hemisphere, em vein.
ve'nae superio'res cer'ebri [TA], veias cerebrais superiores. SIN superior cerebral veins, em vein.
v. supe'rior ver'mis [TA], v. superior do verme. SIN superior vein of vermis.
v. supraorbita'lis [TA], v. supra-orbital. SIN supraorbital vein.
v. suprarena'lis dex'tra [TA], v. supra-renal direita. SIN right suprarenal vein.
v. suprarena'lis sinis'tra [TA], v. supra-renal esquerda. SIN left suprarenal vein.
v. suprascapula'ris [TA], v. supra-escapular. SIN suprascapular vein.
ve'nae supratrochlea'res [TA], veias supratrocleares. SIN supratrochlear veins, em vein.
ve'nae tempora'les profun'dae [TA], veias temporais profundas. SIN deep temporal veins, em vein.
ve'nae tempora'les superficia'les [TA], veias temporais superficiais. SIN superficial temporal veins, em vein.
v. tempora'lis me'dia [TA], v. temporal média. SIN middle temporal vein.
v. termina'lis, v. tálamo-estriada superior; *termo oficial alternativo para superior thalamostriate vein.
v. testicula'ris dex'tra [TA], v. testicular direita. SIN right testicular vein.
v. testicula'ris sinis'tra [TA], v. testicular esquerda. SIN left testicular vein.
ve'nae thalamostria'tae inferio'res [TA], veias tálamo-estriadas inferiores. SIN inferior thalamostriate veins, em vein.
v. thalamostria'ta supe'rior [TA], v. tálamo-estriada superior. SIN superior thalamostriate vein.
v. thora'cica inter'na [TA], v. torácica interna. SIN internal thoracic vein.
v. thora'cica latera'lis [TA], v. torácica lateral. SIN lateral thoracic vein.
v. thoracoacromia'lis [TA], v. toracoacromial. SIN thoracoacromial vein.
v. thoracoepigas'trica [TA], v. toracoepigástrica. SIN thoracoepigastric vein.
ve'nae thy'micae [TA], veias tímicas. SIN thymic veins, em vein.
v. thyroi'dea i'ma, v. tireóidea inferior. SIN inferior thyroid vein.
v. thyroi'dea infe'rior [TA], v. tireóidea inferior. SIN inferior thyroid vein.
v. thyroi'dea me'dia [TA], v. tireóidea média. SIN middle thyroid vein.
v. thyroi'dea supe'rior [TA], v. tireóidea superior. SIN superior thyroid vein.
ve'nae tibia'les anterio'res [TA], veias tibiais anteriores. SIN anterior tibial veins, em vein.

ve′nae tibia′les posterio′res [TA], veias tibiais posteriores. SIN posterior tibial veins, em vein.
ve′nae trachea′les [TA], veias traqueais. SIN tracheal veins, em vein.
venae transversae cervicis [TA], veias cervicais transversas. SIN transverse cervical veins, em vein.
ve′nae transver′sae col′li, veias cervicais transversas; *termo oficial alternativo para transverse cervical veins, em vein.
v. transver′sa facie′i [TA], v. facial transversa. SIN transverse facial vein.
v. transver′sa scap′ulae, v. supra-escapular. SIN suprascapular vein.
ve′nae tympan′icae [TA], veias timpânicas. SIN tympanic veins, em vein.
ve′nae ulna′res [TA], veias ulnares. SIN ulnar veins, em vein.
v. umbilica′lis [TA], v. umbilical. SIN left umbilical vein.
v. un′calis [TA], v. do unco; uma veia que drena o unco para a veia cerebral inferior do mesmo lado. SIN vein of uncus [TA].
ve′nae uteri′nae [TA], veias uterinas. SIN uterine veins, em vein.
v. ventricularis inferior [TA], v. ventricular inferior. SIN inferior ventricular vein. VER basal vein.
v. vertebra′lis [TA], v. vertebral. SIN vertebral vein.
v. vertebra′lis accesso′ria [TA], v. vertebral acessória. SIN accessory vertebral vein.
v. vertebra′lis ante′rior [TA], v. vertebral anterior. SIN anterior vertebral vein.
ve′nae vesica′les [TA], veias vesicais. SIN vesical veins, em vein.
ve′nae vestibula′res (anterius et posterius) [TA], veias vestibulares (anterior e posterior). SIN (anterior and posterior) vestibular veins, em vein.
v. vitelli′na, v. vitelina. SIN vitelline vein.
ve′nae vortico′sae [TA], veias vorticosas. SIN vorticose veins, em vein.

ve·na·ca·vog·ra·phy (vē′nă - kā - vog′ră - fē). Venocavografia; angiografia de uma veia cava. SIN cavography.
ve·na·tion (vē - nā′shŭn). Venação, nervação; o arranjo e a distribuição das veias. [L. *vena*, veia]
♻ **vene-. 1.** Forma combinante que indica as veias, venoso. VER TAMBÉM veno-. [L. *vena*, veia] **2.** Forma combinante relativa ao veneno. [L. *venenum*, veneno]
ve·nec·ta·sia (ve - nek - tā′sē - ă). Flebectasia, varizes. SIN phlebectasia.
ve·nec·to·my (ve - nek′tō - mē). Flebectomia. SIN phlebectomy.
🛈 **ve·neer** (vĕ - nēr′). Verniz. **1.** Uma fina camada superficial disposta sobre uma base do material comum. **2.** Em odontologia, uma camada de material da cor do dente, usualmente de porcelana ou resina composta, presa e que reveste a superfície de uma coroa metálica ou a estrutura dentária natural. [Fr. *fournir*, fornecer]
ven·e·na·tion (ven - ĕ - nā′shŭn, vē - nĕ-). Envenenamento, como por uma picada ou mordida. [L. *veneno*, pp. *-atus*, envenenar, de *venenum*, veneno]
ven·e·nif·er·ous (ven - ĕ - nif′ĕ - rŭs). Venenoso; que conduz veneno, como através de uma picada ou mordida. [L. *venenifer*, de *venenum*, veneno, + *fero*, transportar]
ven·e·no·sal·i·vary (venĕ - nō - sal′i - var- ē). Venenossalivar; que secreta uma saliva venenosa; diz-se dos répteis venenosos. SIN venomosalivary.
ven·e·nos·i·ty (ven - ĕ - nos′i - tē). Venenosidade; propriedade ou atributo daquilo que tem veneno ou é venenoso. [L. *venenosus*, venenoso]
ven·e·nous (venĕ - nŭs). Venenoso. SIN poisonous. [L. *venenosus*]
ve·ne·re·al (ve - nēr′ē - ăl). Venéreo; relativo a ou que resulta da relação sexual. [L. *Venus* (*vener-*), deusa do amor]
ve·ne·re·ol·o·gy (ve - nēr - ē - ol′ō - jē). Venereologia; o estudo da doença venérea. [venérea (doença) + G. *logos*, estudo]
ve·ne·re·o·pho·bi·a (ve - nēr′ē - ō - fō′bē - ă). Venereofobia; medo mórbido da doença venérea. [venérea (doença) + G. *phobos*, medo]
ven·e·sec·tion (ven - ĕ - sek′shŭn). Venissecção, flebotomia. SIN phlebotomy. [L. *vena*, veia, + *sectio*, um corte]
♻ **veni-.** VER veno-.
ven·in (ven′in). Venina; qualquer substância venenosa encontrada no veneno de cobra. [ver venom]
ven·i·punc·ture (ven′i - pŭnk - choor, vē′ni-). Venipuntura; a punção de uma veia, usualmente para coletar sangue ou injetar uma solução.
Venn, John, filósofo e lógico inglês, 1834–1923. VER Venn *diagram*.
♻ **veno-, veni-.** Formas combinantes que indicam veia. VER TAMBÉM vene- (1). [L. *vena*]
ve·no·cly·sis (vē - nok′li - sis). Venóclise, flebóclise. SIN phleboclysis. [veno- + G. *klysis*, cortar]
ve·no·fi·bro·sis (vē′nō - fī - brō′sis). Venofibrose, flebosclerose. SIN phlebosclerosis.
ve·no·gram (vē′nō - gram). Venograma. **1.** Radiografia de veias opacificadas. **2.** Flebograma. SIN phlebogram. [veno- + G. *gramma*, algo escrito]
ve·nog·ra·phy (vē - nog′ră - fē). Venografia; demonstração radiográfica de uma veia depois da injeção de um contraste. SIN phlebography (2). [veno- + G. *graphō*, escrever]
splenic portal v., esplenoportografia. SIN splenoportography.
transosseous v., v. transóssea; demonstração radiográfica das veias que drenam a medula de um osso, através da injeção de contraste na medula em um ponto apropriado, como na v. vertebral ou azigografia por injeção costal.

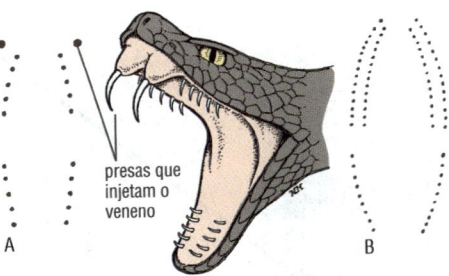

veneno: as marcas dentárias de uma cobra venenosa (A) quando comparadas com aquelas de uma cobra não-venenosa (B)

vertebral v., v. vertebral; demonstração radiográfica do plexo venoso epidural por injeção de contraste no processo espinhoso da vértebra.
🛈 **ven·om** (ven′ŏm). Veneno; um fluido venenoso secretado por cobras, aranhas, escorpiões, etc. [I. med. ou Fr. ant. *venim*, do L. *venenum*, veneno]
kokoi v., uma potente neurotoxina encontrada na rã *Phyllobates bicolor*; é um composto não-proteico, com peso molecular de aproximadamente 400, e é letal na quantidade de microgramas.
Russell's viper v., v. da víbora de Russell; um v. derivado da víbora de Russell (*Vipera russelli*), que age como uma tromboplastina intrínseca; usado na avaliação laboratorial das deficiências de fator X ou topicamente para deter a hemorragia local na hemofilia.
ven·o·mo·sal·i·vary (ven′ō - mō - sal′i - var- ē). Venenossalivar. SIN venenosalivary.
ve·no·mo·tor (vē′nō - mō′ter). Venomotor; que causa alteração no calibre de uma veia. [veno- + L. *motor*, motor]
ve·no·per·i·to·ne·os·to·my (vē′nō - per - i - tō - nē - os′tō - mē). Venoperitoneostomia; uma cirurgia obsoleta que envolve a inserção da extremidade seccionada da veia safena na cavidade peritoneal nos casos de ascite; a veia é invertida, de modo que suas válvulas evitam a regurgitação do sangue para a cavidade, enquanto o líquido ascítico flui para a veia. [veno- + peritoneum + G. *stoma*, boca]
ve·no·pres·sor (vē - nō - pres′er). Venopressor; relativo à pressão sanguínea venosa e, por conseguinte, ao volume do suprimento venoso para o lado direito do coração.
ve·no·scle·ro·sis (vē′nō - skle - rō′sis). Venosclerose, flebosclerose. SIN phlebosclerosis.
ve·nose (vē′nōs). Venoso; que possui veias. [L. *venosus*]
ve·no·si·nal (vē′nō - sī′nal). Venossinusal; pertinente à veia cava e ao seio atrial do coração.
ve·nos·i·ty (vē - nos′i - tē). Venosidade. **1.** Um estado venoso; uma condição em que a maior parte do sangue está nas veias à custa das artérias. **2.** A condição não-oxigenada do sangue oxigenado ou do sangue arterial hipoxêmico.
ve·nos·ta·sis (vē - nō - stā′sis, vē - nos′tă - sis). Venostase, flebostase. SIN phlebostasis. [veno- + G. *stasis*, uma parada]
ve·no·stat (vē′nō - stat). Venostato; qualquer instrumento para conter o sangramento venoso. [veno- + G. *statos*, parada, estacionário]
ve·nos·to·my (vē - nos′tō - mē). Venostomia. SIN cutdown.
ve·not·o·my (vē - not′ō - mē). Venotomia, flebotomia. SIN phlebotomy.
ve·nous (vē′nŭs). Venoso; relativo a uma veia ou veias. SIN phleboid (2). [L. *venosus*]
ve·no·ve·nos·to·my (vē′nō - vē - nos′tō - mē). Venovenostomia; a formação de uma anastomose entre duas veias. SIN phlebophlebostomy. [veno- + veno- + G. *stoma*, boca]
vent. Fenda; uma abertura para dentro de uma cavidade ou canal, principalmente aquela através da qual o conteúdo dessa cavidade é liberado, como o ânus. [Fr. ant. *fente*, uma fenda, abertura]
ven·ter (ven′ter) [TA]. **1.** Abdome. SIN abdomen. **2** [NA]. Ventre. SIN belly (2). **3.** Uma das grandes cavidades do corpo. **4.** O útero. [L. *venter* (*ventr-*), ventre]
v. ante′rior mus′culi digas′trici [TA], ventre anterior do músculo digástrico. SIN anterior *belly* of digastric muscle.
v. fronta′lis mus′culi occipitofronta′lis [TA], v. frontal do músculo occipitofrontal. SIN frontal *belly* of occipitofrontalis muscle.
v. infe′rior mus′culi omohyoi′dei [TA], v. inferior do músculo omo-hióideo. SIN inferior *belly* of omohyoid *muscle*.
v. occipita′lis mus′culi occipitofron′talis [TA], v. occipital do músculo occipitofrontal. SIN occipital *belly* of occipitofrontalis muscle.
v. poste′rior mus′culi digas′trici [TA], v. posterior do músculo digástrico. SIN posterior belly of digastric muscle.
v. supe′rior mus′culi omohyoi′dei [TA], v. superior do músculo omo-hióideo. SIN superior *belly* of omohyoid muscle.

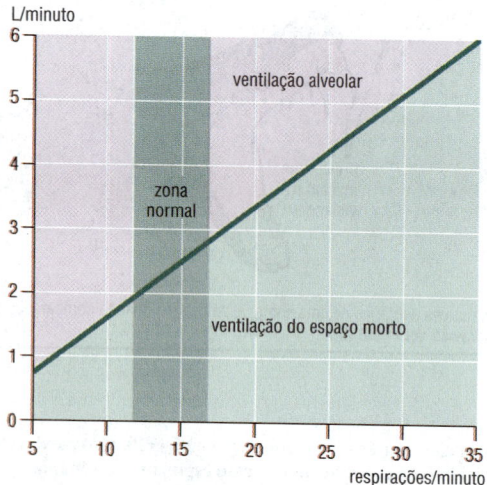

ventilação alveolar e do espaço morto: dependendo do número de respirações realizadas (freqüência respiratória), com um volume corrente constante de 6 l

ven·ti·late (ven′ti-lāt). Ventilar; aerar ou oxigenar o sangue nos capilares pulmonares. SIN air (2). [L. *ventilo*, pp. *-atus*, ventilar, de *ventus*, o vento]

ven·ti·la·tion (ven-ti-lā′shŭn). Ventilação. **1.** A substituição, em um espaço, do ar ou de outro gás por ar ou gás fresco. **2.** Movimento de gás(es) para dentro e para fora dos pulmões. SIN oxidative metabolism, respiration (2). **3 (V).** Em fisiologia, a troca corrente do ar entre os pulmões e a atmosfera que acontece na respiração. VER TAMBÉM respiration. [ver ventilate]

airway pressure release v., v. com liberação da pressão da via aérea; a v. mecânica em que os pacientes que estão sendo tratados com pressão positiva contínua nas vias aéreas apresentam diminuições intermitentes, em vez de aumentos, da pressão e do volume das vias aéreas.

alveolar v. (V_A), v. alveolar; o volume de gás expirado pelos alvéolos para fora do corpo por minuto; calculado como a freqüência respiratória (f) multiplicada pela diferença entre o volume corrente e o espaço morto ($V_T - V_D$); unidades: ml/min (gás na temperatura corporal, na pressão ambiente e saturado com vapor d'água).

artificial v., v. artificial; qualquer meio de produção de troca gasosa por meios mecânicos ou manuais entre os pulmões e o ar circunvizinho, que não seja realizado inteiramente pelo próprio sistema respiratório da pessoa. SIN artificial respiration.

assist-control v., v. assistocontrolada; a v. com pressão positiva artificial por máquina, na qual uma respiração completa é produzida de maneira automática, após um esforço inspiratório natural do paciente. No caso de o paciente não iniciar esse esforço, a máquina proporcionará uma freqüência respiratória basal ou de suporte (*backup*).

assisted v., v. assistida; a aplicação de pressão positiva gerada por meios mecânicos ou manuais ao(s) gás(es) dentro ou em torno das vias aéreas durante a inspiração, como um meio de aumentar o movimento dos gases para dentro dos pulmões. SIN assisted respiration.

bag v., v. manual. SIN manual v.

continuous positive pressure v. (CPPV), v. com pressão positiva contínua. SIN controlled mechanical v.

controlled v., v. controlada; aplicação intermitente de pressão positiva, gerada por meios mecânicos ou manuais, ao(s) gás(es) dentro ou ao redor das vias aéreas como um meio de forçar os gases para dentro dos pulmões quando não há esforço ventilatório espontâneo. SIN controlled respiration.

controlled mechanical v. (CMV), v. mecânica controlada; v. artificial em que todas as inspirações são fornecidas por pressão positiva aplicada às vias aéreas, independentemente dos esforços respiratórios do paciente. Na prática clínica atual, essa modalidade quase nunca é utilizada. SIN continuous positive pressure v., intermittent positive pressure v.

high-frequency v., v. de alta freqüência; v. mecânica usando a administração de "jatos" de ar em freqüências entre 300–3.000 incursões por minuto para evitar algumas complicações da v. mais convencional.

intermittent mandatory v. (IMV), v. mandatória intermitente (VMI); aplicação mecânica de pressão positiva às vias aéreas em uma freqüência predeterminada, entremeada com a respiração natural do paciente através do circuito do respirador. Não é feita nenhuma tentativa para sincronizar a ventilação imposta pela máquina com a do paciente.

intermittent positive pressure v. (IPPV), v. com pressão positiva intermitente. SIN controlled mechanical v.

inverse-ratio v., v. com proporção invertida; v. mecânica em que o tempo conferido pela máquina para a inspiração é maior do que o da expiração, o que é oposto à situação em modalidades mais padronizadas de v.

liquid v., v. com líquido; um meio experimental de ventilar os pulmões que sofreram lesão grave, através do uso de O_2 e CO_2 dissolvido em perfluorocarbonetos em um líquido, diminuindo assim (teoricamente) a incidência de atelectasia e de outros problemas.

mandatory minute v., v.-minuto mandatória; a v. mecânica em que o respirador é configurado para garantir determinado volume-minuto, mas somente quando é necessário.

manual v., v. manual; a compressão manual intermitente de uma bolsa-reservatório cheia de gás para forçar o gás para dentro dos pulmões do paciente e, dessa maneira, manter a oxigenação e a eliminação de dióxido de carbono durante a apnéia ou hipoventilação. SIN bag v.

maximum voluntary v. (MVV), v. voluntária máxima; o volume de ar respirado quando uma pessoa respira, da forma mais profunda e rápida possível, durante determinado intervalo de tempo (p.ex., 15 s). Geralmente extrapolado para o que poderia ser respirado durante 1 minuto. SIN maximum breathing capacity.

mechanical v., v. mecânica; qualquer respiração assistida mecanicamente, empregando aparelhos com pressão positiva ou negativa. Alguns aparelhos com pressão positiva exigem intubação da traquéia, e outros exigem apenas uma máscara aplicada à boca ou ao nariz. Nas últimas décadas, o modo padronizado de ventilar mecanicamente um paciente com insuficiência respiratória envolvia a intubação da traquéia e a aplicação de pressão positiva limitada por pressão ou volume aos pulmões através do tubo endotraqueal; atualmente, a necessidade de intubação em todos os casos está sendo questionada, e muitos pacientes com insuficiência respiratória crônica podem ser adequadamente ventilados por aparelhos não-invasivos.

negative pressure v., v. com pressão negativa; v. mecânica em que são usados diversos aparelhos em torno do tórax de tal modo que o desenvolvimento da pressão negativa ou subatmosférica possa provocar expansão torácica e, assim, inspiração; a liberação da pressão negativa permite que o tórax relaxe e, dessa forma, ocorre a expiração. Esse tipo de v. tornou-se famoso por causa do "pulmão de ferro", usado em grande número de pacientes com poliomielite. Outros respiradores desse tipo incluem a couraça e o colete corporal.

noninvasive positive pressure v., v. não-invasiva com pressão positiva; a aplicação de pressão positiva através de uma máscara nasal ou facial completa, englobando o nariz e a boca, que é ciclada de uma maneira similar às modalidades de v. em que foi alcançado o controle mais direto das vias aéreas ou da traquéia do paciente. Esse tipo de v. é freqüentemente utilizado como medida contemporizadora, enquanto se trata o paciente, a fim de evitar a intubação endotraqueal.

permissive hypercapnic v., v. hipercápnica permissiva; v. mecânica em que se permite que o nível de dióxido de carbono no sangue aumente bem acima dos valores normais, de modo a minimizar o suporte mecânico fornecido ao paciente e, assim, diminuir as complicações desse suporte, como o barotrauma. Essa modalidade de v. é comumente empregada em pacientes asmáticos graves, nos quais uma ventilação de maneira mais tradicional geraria enormes pressões em suas vias aéreas, com resultante pneumotórax.

pressure-controlled v., v. controlada pela pressão; v. mecânica independente da respiração espontânea do paciente, mas que emprega a pressão como a principal variável determinante, juntamente com a freqüência e o tempo, de quanto ar o paciente recebe.

pressure-support v., v. com suporte pressórico; suporte ventilatório mecânico no qual cada incursão respiratória deflagra certo suporte limitado por pressão. O respirador apenas fornece o suporte de cada respiração até um volume predeterminado de pressão; assim sendo, o volume respirado pode diferir de uma incursão respiratória para outra.

proportional assist v., v. assistida proporcional; v. mecânica em que o respirador, em sincronia com a respiração do paciente, fornece o suporte proporcional ao esforço gerado pelo paciente. Essa modalidade permite que o paciente determine por completo quanto de suporte é fornecido pela máquina.

pulmonary v., v. pulmonar; o volume-minuto respiratório, ou seja, o volume total de gás inspirado (V_I) ou expirado (V_E) por minuto, expresso em litros por minuto; difere da v. alveolar por incluir a troca de gás do espaço morto.

synchronized intermittent mandatory v. (SIMV), v. mandatória intermitente sincronizada; v. mandatória intermitente iniciada espontaneamente pelo paciente para aumentar o volume corrente até um volume predeterminado e, depois, sincronizada com o ciclo respiratório do paciente; quando o paciente não empreende esforço respiratório, a máquina libera automaticamente um número predeterminado de ventilações.

wasted v., v. desperdiçado; aquela parte da v. pulmonar que não é efetiva na troca de oxigênio e dióxido de carbono com o sangue capilar pulmonar; calculado como o espaço morto fisiológico multiplicado pela freqüência respiratória.

ven·ti·la·tion/per·fu·sion mis·match. Desequilíbrio ventilação/perfusão; desequilíbrio entre a ventilação alveolar e o fluxo sanguíneo capilar pulmonar.

ventilator (ven′til-ā-tōr). Respirador. SIN respirator. [L. *ventilo*, ventilar, de *ventus*, vento, + *-ator*, sufixo de agente]

cuirass v., r. de couraça; a placa mamária rígida que se adapta sobre a porção anterior do tórax e, através da aplicação e liberação de pressão negativa, movimenta a parede torácica, "respirando", assim, para o paciente.

vent·plant. Um implante endosteal, geralmente constituído de titânio, utilizado para dar suporte e fixação a uma prótese dentária por meio de projeções através da mucosa; termo também utilizado para designar uma família de implantes.

ven·trad (ven′trad). Em direção à face ventral; oposto a dorsad. [L. *venter*, ventre, + *-ad*, para]

ven·tral (ven′trăl) [TA]. Ventral. **1.** Pertinente ao abdome ou a qualquer ventre. **2.** SIN *anterior (1).* **3.** Em anatomia veterinária, a superfície inferior de um animal; frequentemente usado para indicar a posição de uma estrutura em relação a outra, isto é, situada mais próximo à superfície inferior do corpo. [L. *ventralis*]

ven·tra·lis (ven-trā′lis) [TA]. Ventral, anterior. SIN *anterior (1).* [L.]

ventral paraflocculus. Paraflóculo ventral; uma pequena porção hemisférica do lobo posterior do cerebelo (lóbulo IX) que está estruturalmente associada à tonsila do cerebelo (também conhecida como lóbulo H IX) e à úvula (lóbulo IX do verme). SIN *paraflocculus ventralis.*

ven·tri·cle (ven′tri-kl) [TA]. Ventrículo; uma cavidade normal, como do cérebro ou do coração. SIN *ventriculus (2)* [TA]. [L. *ventriculus*, dim. de *venter*, ventre]

Arantius v., v. de Arantius. SIN *calamus scriptorius.*
cerebral v.'s, ventrículos cerebrais. VER lateral v., fourth v., third v., *cavity of septum pellucidum.*
v. of cerebral hemisphere, v. lateral. SIN *lateral v.*
v. of diencephalon, terceiro v. SIN *third v.*
double outlet right v., v. direito com dupla saída; uma categoria heterogênea de anormalidades congênitas, embora não sejam assim classificadas. Basicamente, as duas grandes artérias originam-se, completa ou parcialmente, do v. direito ou de um compartimento infundibular. Quase sempre existe defeito do septo interventricular (comunicação interventricular).
Duncan v., v. de Duncan. SIN *cavity of septum pellucidum.*
fifth v., cavidade de septo pelúcido. SIN *cavity of septum pellucidum.*
fourth v. [TA], quarto ventrículo; uma cavidade de formato irregular, semelhante a uma tenda, que se estende desde o óbex, rostralmente, até sua comunicação com o aqueduto de Silvius, contido entre o cerebelo, dorsalmente, e o tegmento rombencefálico, ventralmente; tem um assoalho em forma rombóide (fossa rombóide) e um teto semelhante a uma tenda, que, em sua parte caudal, é formado pela tela corióidea e véu medular posterior, em sua parte média pela substância branca do cerebelo, e em sua parte rostral estreitada (recesso superior), pelo véu medular anterior. O quarto ventrículo alcança sua maior largura na transição pontobulbar, onde se expande lateralmente, por trás dos pedúnculos cerebelares, para dentro do recesso lateral, semelhante a um bico, e atinge sua maior altura no recesso fastigial, que chega até a substância branca cerebelar. A comunicação direta do sistema ventricular do cérebro e com o espaço subaracnóide é estabelecida, no nível do quarto ventrículo, por uma abertura mediana na tela corióidea, a abertura medial do forame de Magendie, que se abre para a cisterna cerebelobulbar, e, em ambos os lados, pela abertura lateral ou forame de Luschka, que conecta o recesso lateral com a cisterna interpeduncular. SIN *ventriculus quartus* [TA], *v. of rhombencephalon.*
laryngeal v. [TA], v. da laringe; o recesso em cada parede lateral da laringe, entre as pregas vestibular e vocal, dentro do qual desemboca o sáculo laríngeo. SIN *ventriculus laryngis* [TA], *laryngeal sinus, Morgagni sinus (3), Morgagni v., sinus laryngeus.*
lateral v. [TA], v. lateral; uma cavidade com formato que lembra uma ferradura em conformidade com o formato geral do hemisfério; cada v. lateral comunica-se com o terceiro v. através do forame interventricular de Monro, expandindo-se então, a partir desse ponto, para diante (para o lobo frontal) como o corno anterior, bem como caudalmente (sobre o tálamo) como o corpo ou a parte central, que, por trás do tálamo, curva-se ventral e lateralmente, e então para diante (para o lobo temporal) como o corno inferior; a partir do ápice da curva, um corno posterior de tamanho variável estende-se para trás, para a substância branca do lobo occipital. O grande plexo corióideo do v. lateral invade a parte central do v. lateral e o corno inferior (mas não os cornos anterior e posterior) a partir do lado medial. SIN *ventriculus lateralis* [TA], *v. of cerebral hemisphere.*
left v. [TA], v. esquerdo do coração; a câmara inferior no lado esquerdo do coração que recebe o sangue arterial proveniente do átrio esquerdo e direciona-o, através da contração de suas paredes, para a aorta. SIN *ventriculus sinister* [TA].
Morgagni v., v. de Morgagni. SIN *laryngeal v.*
parchment right v., v. direito apergaminhado. SIN *Uhl anomaly.*
v. of rhombencephalon, quarto v. SIN *fourth v.*
right v. [TA], v. direito do coração; o compartimento inferior no lado direito do coração que recebe o sangue venoso oriundo do átrio direito e o direciona, através da contração de suas paredes, para a artéria pulmonar. SIN *ventriculus dexter* [TA].
(right/left) v.'s of heart, ventrículos (direito/esquerdo) do coração; uma das duas câmaras inferiores do coração. SIN *ventriculus cordis dexter/sinister.*
single v., v. único; ausência congênita ou ausência quase total do septo ventricular.
sixth v., v. de Verga. SIN *Verga v.*
sylvian v., v. de Silvius. SIN *cavity of septum pellucidum.*
v. of Sylvius, v. de Silvius. SIN *cavity of septum pellucidum.*
terminal v. [TA], v. terminal; uma dilatação do canal central da medula espinal na extremidade do cone medular. SIN *ventriculus terminalis* [TA].
third v. [TA], terceiro ventrículo; uma cavidade estreita, verticalmente orientada, com forma de um quadrilátero irregular no plano médio, que se estende desde a lâmina terminal até a abertura rostral do aqueduto do mesencéfalo. Esse v. comunica-se, em seu canto rostrodorsal, com cada um dos dois ventrículos laterais através dos forames interventriculares de Monro esquerdo e direito. Seu teto estreito é formado pela tela corióidea, que se insere em ambos os lados na tênia do tálamo; sua parede lateral é formada pela superfície medial do tálamo e, abaixo do sulco hipotalâmico, pelo hipotálamo, que também forma seu assoalho. No perfil lateral, o terceiro v. exibe inúmeros recessos: em seu assoalho, da frente para trás: 1) o recesso pré-óptico, no ângulo agudo entre a base da lâmina terminal e o dorso do quiasma óptico; 2) o recesso infundibular, que se estende ventralmente para o infundíbulo, mas (nos seres humanos) não para o pedúnculo hipofisário; e 3) o recesso mamilar ou inframamilar, causado pela protrusão dos corpos mamilares para o v. A partir de seu canto dorsocaudal, o recesso pineal estende-se caudalmente para o pedúnculo pineal. SIN *ventriculus tertius* [TA], *v. of diencephalon.*
Verga v., v. de Verga; um espaço inconstante, horizontal, semelhante a uma fenda, entre o terço posterior do corpo caloso e o fórnice da comissura subjacente (comissura do hipocampo), resultando da falha dessas duas placas comissurais em se fundir por completo durante o desenvolvimento fetal; como a cavidade do septo pelúcido, o espaço não constitui um v. verdadeiro porque não se desenvolveu a partir do canal central do tubo neural. SIN *cavum psalterii, cavum vergae, sixth v.*
Vieussens v., v. de Vieussens. SIN *cavity of septum pellucidum.*
Wenzel v., v. de Wenzel. SIN *cavity of septum pellucidum.*

ven·tri·cose (ven′tri-kōs). Ventricoso; abaulamento ou inchação em um lado ou de forma desigual.

ven·tric·u·lar (ven-trik′ū-lăr). Ventricular; relativo a um ventrículo, em qualquer sentido. SIN *ventricularis (1).*

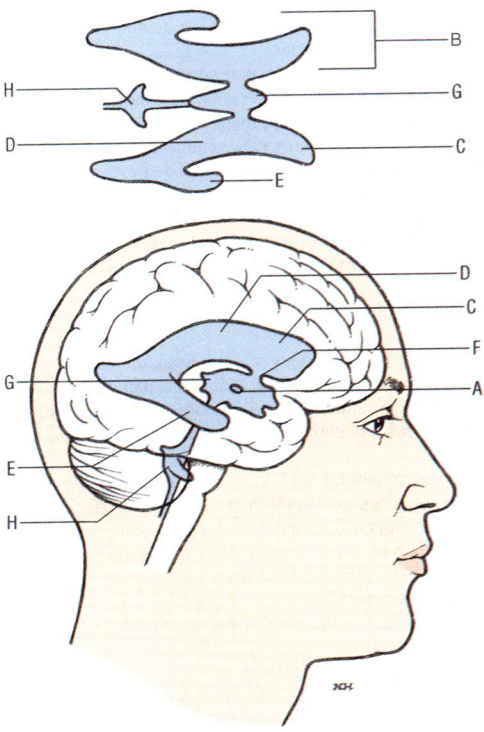

ventrículos do cérebro (incidências superior e lateral): (A) massa intermédia, (B) ventrículo esquerdo, (C) corno anterior do ventrículo lateral direito, (D) parte central do ventrículo lateral direito, (E) corno inferior do ventrículo lateral direito, (F) forame interventricular, (G) terceiro ventrículo, (H) quarto ventrículo

ven·tric·u·lar·is (ven-trik′u-la′ris). **1.** Ventricular. SIN ventricular. **2.** Parte tireoepiglótica do músculo tireoaritenóideo. SIN thyroepiglottic part of thyroarytenoid (muscle). [L. mod. do L. *ventriculus*]

ven·tric·u·lar·i·za·tion (ven-trik′u-lar-i-za′shun). Ventricularização; a transformação de um fenômeno atrial para estimular um ventricular, especialmente do traçado de pulso atrial (ou venoso) na regurgitação tricúspide.

ven·tric·u·lar pon·der·ance (ven-trik′u-lar pon′der-ans). Ponderância ventricular; um termo eletrocardiográfico semi-obsoleto sugerindo que um ventrículo é maior ou mais espesso que o outro.

ventriculectomy. Ventriculectomia.
   partial left v., v. esquerda parcial. SIN left ventricular volume reduction surgery.

ven·tric·u·li·tis (ven-trik-u-li′tis). Ventriculite; inflamação dos ventrículos do cérebro. [ventrículo + G. *-itis*, inflamação]

ventriculo-. Forma combinante relativa a um ventrículo. [L. *ventriculus*]

ven·tric·u·lo·a·tri·al (VA) (ven-trik′u-lo-a′tre-al). Ventriculoatrial; relativo a ambos os ventrículos e átrios, especialmente para descrever a passagem seqüencial da condução na direção retrógrada do ventrículo para o átrio.

ven·tric·u·lo·cis·ter·nos·to·my (ven-trik′u-lo-sis′ter-nos′to-me). Ventriculocisternostomia; uma abertura artificial entre os ventrículos do cérebro e a cisterna magna. VER TAMBÉM shunt (2). [ventriculo- + L. *cisterna*, cisterna, + G. *stoma*, boca]

ven·tric·u·log·ra·phy (ven-trik-u-log′ra-fe). Ventriculografia. **1.** Demonstração radiográfica dos ventrículos cerebrais por injeção direta de ar ou contraste; desenvolvida e descrita por Dandy em 1918. Cf. pneumoencephalography. **2.** Demonstração da contratilidade dos ventrículos cardíacos através do registro seriado da distribuição do radionuclídeo injetado por via intravenosa ou de contraste radiográfico injetado através de um cateter intracardíaco. [ventriculo- + G. *graphe*, escrita]
   radionuclide v., v. com radionuclídeo. SIN radionuclide angiocardiography.

ven·tric·u·lo·mas·toi·dos·to·my (ven-trik′u-lo-mas′toy-dos′to-me). Ventriculomastoidostomia; cirurgia para criar uma comunicação entre o ventrículo cerebral lateral e o antro da mastóide por meio de um tubo de politeno para o alívio da hidrocefalia. VER TAMBÉM shunt (2). [ventriculo- + mastoid, + G. *stoma*, boca]

ven·tric·u·lo·nec·tor (ven-trik′oo-lo-nek′ter, -tor). Feixe atrioventricular. SIN atrioventricular bundle. [ventriculo- + L. *necto*, unir]

ven·tric·u·lo·pha·sic (ven-trik′u-lo-fa′zik). Ventriculofásico; influenciado pela contração ventricular; aplicado ao ritmo atrial quando este é modificado por contração ventricular; na arritmia sinusal ventriculofásica no bloqueio AV completo, o impulso sinusal, imediatamente após uma contração ventricular, aparece, em geral, mais precocemente que o esperado.

ven·tric·u·lo·plas·ty (ven-trik′u-lo-plas-te). Ventriculoplastia; qualquer procedimento cirúrgico para reparar um defeito de um dos ventrículos do coração. [ventriculo- + G. *plastos*, formado]
   reduction left v., v. esquerda redutora. SIN left ventricular volume reduction surgery.

ven·tric·u·lo·punc·ture (ven-trik′u-lo-pŭnk′choor). Ventriculopuntura; a inserção de uma agulha em um ventrículo.

ven·tric·u·los·co·py (ven-trik-u-los′ko-pe). Ventriculoscopia; a inspeção direta de um ventrículo com um endoscópio. [ventriculo- + G. *skopeo*, visualizar]

ven·tric·u·los·to·my (ven-trik-u-los′to-me). Ventriculostomia; criação de uma abertura em um ventrículo, usualmente através do assoalho do terceiro ventrículo para o espaço subaracnóide, visando aliviar hidrocefalia. VER TAMBÉM shunt (2). [ventriculo- + G. *stoma*, boca]
   third v., v. do terceiro ventrículo; uma cirurgia para criar uma abertura no terceiro ventrículo para as cisternas pré-quiasmática e interpeduncular (operação de Stookey-Scarff) ou do terceiro ventrículo para a cisterna interpeduncular (cirurgia de Dandy).

ven·tric·u·lo·sub·a·rach·noid (ven-trik′u-lo-sub-ă-rak′noyd). Ventriculossubaracnóideo; relativo ao espaço ocupado pelo líquido cefalorraquidiano ou cerebroespinal. [ventriculo- + subarachnoid]

ven·tric·u·lot·o·my (ven-trik-u-lot′o-me). Ventriculotomia; incisão em um ventrículo; p.ex., no terceiro ventrículo cerebral, para o alívio da hidrocefalia, ou em um ventrículo cardíaco, para corrigir cirurgicamente uma anormalidade. [ventriculo- + G. *tome*, incisão]

ven·tric·u·lus, pl. **ven·tric·u·li** (ven-trik′u-lŭs, -li) [TA]. **1.** Estômago. SIN stomach. **2.** Ventrículo. SIN ventricle. **3.** A porção posterior dilatada do mesêntero do canal alimentar do inseto, na qual ocorre a digestão. [L. dim. de *venter*, ventre]
   v. cor′dis dexter/sinister, v. direito/esquerdo do coração. SIN (right/left) ventricles of heart, em ventricle.
   v. dex′ter [TA], v. direito do coração. SIN right ventricle.
   v. laryn′gis [TA], v. da laringe. SIN laryngeal ventricle.
   v. latera′lis [TA], v. lateral. SIN lateral ventricle.
   v. quar′tus [TA], quarto v. SIN fourth ventricle.
   v. quin′tus, cavidade do septo pelúcido. SIN cavity of septum pellucidum.
   v. sinis′ter [TA], v. esquerdo do coração. SIN left ventricle.
   v. termina′lis [TA], v. terminal. SIN terminal ventricle.
   v. ter′tius [TA], terceiro v. SIN third ventricle.

ven·tri·duct (ven′tri-dŭkt). Trazer em direção ao abdome. [L. *venter*, ventre, + *duco*, pp. *ductus*, levar]

ven·tri·duc·tion (ven-tri-dŭk′shŭn). Ventridução; trazer em direção ao abdome ou à parede abdominal.

ventro-. Forma combinante que significa ventral. [L. *venter*, ventre]

ven·tro·cys·tor·rha·phy (ven′tro-sis-tor′a-fe). Cistopexia. SIN cystopexy. [ventro- + G. *kystis*, cyst, + *rhaphe*, sutura]

ven·tro·dor·sad (ven-tro-dor′sad). Ventrodorsal; em uma direção do ventre para o dorso.

ven·tro·in·gui·nal (ven′tro-ing′gwi-nal). Ventroinguinal; relativo ao abdome e à virilha.

ven·tro·lat·er·al (ven-tro-lat′e-ral). Ventrolateral; tanto ventral quanto lateral, ou seja, para a frente e para o lado.

ven·tro·me·di·an (ven-tro-me′de-an). Ventromediano; relativo à linha média da superfície ventral.

ven·trop·to·sis, ven·trop·to·sia (ven-tro-to′sis, -to′se-a). Gastroptose. SIN gastroptosis. [ventro- + G. *ptosis*, uma queda]

ven·tros·co·py (ven-tros′ko-pe). Peritoneoscopia. SIN peritoneoscopy. [ventro- + G. *skopeo*, visualizar]

ven·trot·o·my (ven-trot′o-me). Celiotomia. SIN celiotomy. [ventro- + G. *tome*, incisão]

Venturi, Giovanni B., físico italiano, 1746–1822. VER V. *effect*, *meter*, *tube*.

ven·u·la, pl. **ven·u·lae** (ven′oo-la, -le) [TA]. Vênula. SIN venule. [L. dim. de *vena*, veia]
   v. macula′ris infe′rior [TA], v. macular inferior. SIN inferior macular venule.
   v. macula′ris supe′rior [TA], v. macular superior. SIN superior macular venule.
   v. media′lis ret′inae [TA], v. medial da retina. SIN medial venule of retina.
   v. nasa′lis ret′inae infe′rior [TA], v. nasal inferior da retina. SIN inferior nasal retinal venule.
   v. nasa′lis ret′inae supe′rior [TA], v. nasal superior da retina. SIN superior nasal retinal venule.
   venulae rectae of kidney [TA], vênulas retas do rim; as vênulas que drenam as pirâmides medulares do rim; desembocam nas veias arqueadas. SIN venulae rectae renis [TA], straight venules of kidney.
   ven′ulae rec′tae re′nis [TA], vênulas retas do rim. SIN venulae rectae of kidney.
   ven′ulae stella′tae, veias estelares; os grupos de vênulas em formato de estrela no córtex renal. SIN stellate veins, stellate venules, stellulae verheyenii, venae stellatae, Verheyen stars.
   v. tempora′lis ret′inae infe′rior [TA], v. temporal inferior da retina. SIN inferior temporal retinal venule.
   v. tempora′lis ret′inae supe′rior [TA], v. temporal superior da retina. SIN superior temporal retinal venule.

ven·u·lar (ven′oo-lar). Venular; pertinente às vênulas. SIN venulous.

ven·ule (ven′ool, ve′nool) [TA]. Vênula; uma radícula venosa contínua com um capilar. SIN venula [TA], cappillary vein, veinlet.
   high endothelial postcapillary v.'s, vênulas pós-capilares endoteliais altas; as vênulas nos linfonodos, tonsilas e placas de Peyer que apresentam um endotélio com parede alta através da qual os linfócitos sanguíneos migram do sangue para o parênquima linfático.
   inferior macular v. [TA], v. macular inferior; uma pequena tributária da veia central da retina que drena a parte inferior da mácula. SIN venula macularis inferior [TA].
   inferior nasal v. of retina, v. nasal inferior da retina. SIN inferior nasal retinal v.
   inferior nasal retinal v. [TA], v. nasal inferior da retina; a pequena veia que passa da parte medial inferior (nasal) da retina para se unir à veia central. SIN venula nasalis retinae inferior [TA], inferior nasal v. of retina.
   inferior temporal v. of retina, v. temporal inferior da retina. SIN inferior temporal retinal v.
   inferior temporal retinal v. [TA], v. temporal inferior da retina; a pequena veia que vai desde a parte lateral inferior (temporal) da retina até a veia central. SIN venula temporalis retinae inferior [TA], inferior temporal v. of retina.
   medial v. of retina [TA], v. medial da retina; a pequena veia que vai desde a parte da retina entre a mácula e o disco óptico até se unir à veia central. SIN venula medialis retinae [TA].
   nasal v.'s of retina, vênulas nasais da retina. VER inferior nasal retinal v., superior nasal retinal v.
   pericytic v.'s, vênulas pós-capilares. SIN postcapillary v.'s.
   postcapillary v.'s, vênulas pós-capilares; a microvasculatura imediatamente após os capilares, variando de tamanho de 10 a 50 μm, e que se caracteriza por seu envoltório de células pericapilares; constituem o local de extravasamento das células sanguíneas, são muito sensíveis à histamina, e acredita-se que são importantes nas trocas de líquido entre o sangue e o interstício. SIN pericytic v.'s.
   stellate v.'s, veias estelares. SIN venulae stellate, em venula.

straight v.'s of kidney, vênulas retas do rim. SIN *venulae rectae of kidney,* em *venula.*

superior macular v. [TA], v. macular superior; uma pequena tributária da veia central da retina que drena a parte superior da mácula. SIN venula macularis superior [TA].

superior nasal v. of retina, v. nasal superior da retina. SIN superior nasal retinal v.

superior nasal retinal v. [TA], v. nasal superior da retina; a pequena veia que drena o sangue da parte medial superior (nasal) da retina; une-se à veia central. SIN venula nasalis retinae superior [TA], superior nasal v. of retina.

superior temporal v. of retina, v. temporal superior da retina. SIN superior temporal retinal v.

superior temporal retinal v. [TA], v. temporal superior da retina; a v. que passa da parte lateral superior (temporal) da retina para se unir à veia central. SIN venula temporalis retinae superior [TA], superior temporal v. of retina.

temporal v.'s of retina, vênulas temporais da retina. SIN inferior temporal retinal v., superior temporal retinal v.

ven·u·lous (ven'oo-lŭs). Venuloso. SIN venular.

VER Abreviatura para visual evoked response (resposta visual evocada). VER evoked *response.*

ve·rap·a·mil (ver-ap'ă-mil). Verapamil; um agente bloqueador do canal de cálcio usado para tratar arritmias cardíacas e angina de peito. SIN iproveratril.

ve·rat·ric ac·id (vē-rat'rik). Ácido verátrico; obtido pela metilação e subseqüente oxidação do ácido protocatecóico; presente nas sementes da *Schoenocaulon officinale (Sabadilla officinarum).*

ver·a·tri·dine (ver-ă-trī'dĕn). Veratridina; um alcalóide derivado do *Veratrum viridae* e do *V. album.* Provavelmente responsável pelas propriedades anti-hipertensivas dessa classe de alcalóides.

ver·a·trine (ver'ă-trēn, -trin). Veratrina; uma mistura de alcalóides obtida das sementes de *Schoenocaulon officinale (Sabadilla officinarum)* (família Liliaceae), incluindo cevina, cevadina, cevadilina, sabadina e veratridina; um pó com sabor acre, intensamente irritante para a mucosa nasal, que tem sido utilizado como contra-irritante anódino nas neuralgias e artrite.

Ve·ra·trum (vē-rā'trŭm). Um gênero de plantas liliáceas tóxicas. [L. helébero]
V. al'bum, o rizoma apresenta ações emetizantes e catárticas.
V. vir'ide, o rizoma seco e as raízes contêm alcalóides terapeuticamente importantes (cevadina, veratridina, jervina, pseudojervina, rubijervina e diversos ésteres de alcalóides da base germina) usados no tratamento de distúrbios hipertensivos.

ver·big·er·a·tion (ver-bij-er-ā'shŭn). Verbigeração; repetição constante de palavras ou frases sem significado; observada na esquizofrenia. SIN oral stereotypy. [L. *verbum,* palavra, + *gero,* levar]

ver·bo·ma·nia (ver-bō-mā'nē-ă). Verbomania; um termo raramente utilizado para a loquacidade anormal; um fluxo psicótico da fala. [L. *verbum,* palavra, + G. *mania,* mania]

ver·di·gris (ver'di-grēs, -gris, -grē). Verdete, acetato cúprico, azinhavre. [Fr. ant. *verd,* verde, *de,* de, *Gris,* gregos]

ver·dine (ver'dīn). Biliverdina. SIN biliverdin.

ver·do·glo·bin (ver-dō-glō-bin). Verdoglobina; termo obsoleto para choleglobin (coleglobina).

ver·do·he·mo·chrome (ver-dō-hē'mō-krōm). Hemocromo verde; um estágio intermediário na degradação da hemoglobina para produzir pigmentos biliares, ou seja, a hemoglobina fornece a coleglobina (hemoglobina verde) e a perda da globina deixa o hemocromo verde, o precursor da biliverdina.

ver·do·he·mo·glo·bin (ver'dō-hē-mō-glō'bin). Coleglobina. SIN choleglobin.

ver·do·per·ox·i·dase (ver'dō-per-oks'i-dās). Verdeperoxidase; uma peroxidase, que ocorre nos leucócitos, contendo um ferriheme esverdeado; responsável pela atividade da peroxidase do pus.

Verga, Andrea, neurologista italiano, 1811–1895. VER V. *ventricle; cavum vergae.*

verge (verj). Uma borda ou margem.
anal v., b. anal; a zona de transição entre a pele úmida, sem pêlos e modificada do canal anal, e a pele perianal.

ver·gence (ver'jens). Vergência; um movimento não-conjugado dos olhos no qual os eixos de fixação não são paralelos, como na convergência ou divergência. [L. *vergo,* inclinar, voltar]
v. of lens, v. da lente; o inverso da distância focal principal usado como uma medida da divergência ou convergência dos raios paralelos.

Verheyen, Philippe, anatomista flamengo, 1648–1710. VER V. *stars,* em *star; stellulae* verheyenii, em *stellula.*

Verhoeff, Frederick H., oftalmologista norte-americano, 1874–1968. VER V. elastic tissue *stain.*

Ver·mes (ver'mēz). Designação arcaica para um sub-reino do reino animal contendo vermes e organismos semelhantes a vermes; uma divisão artificial que não é mais usada em taxonomia. [L. *vermis,* verme]

⚠ **vermi-.** Forma combinante que indica um verme, semelhante a um verme. [L. *vermis*]

ver·mi·ci·dal (ver'mi-sī'dăl). Vermicida; destrutivo para os vermes; especificamente, destrutivo para os vermes parasitas intestinais. [vermi- + L. *caedo,* matar]

ver·mi·cide (ver'mi-sīd). Vermicida; um agente que mata os vermes parasitas intestinais. [vermi- + L. *caedo,* matar]

ver·mic·u·lar (ver-mik'oo-lăr). Vermicular; relativo ou semelhante a um verme ou que se move como este. [L. *vermiculus,* dim. de *vermis,* verme]

ver·mic·u·la·tion (ver-mik-ū-lā'shŭn). Vermiculação; um movimento semelhante ao de um verme, como na peristalse.

ver·mi·cule (ver'mi-kool). Vermículo. **1.** Um pequeno verme, ou organismo ou estrutura semelhante a um verme. **2.** SIN ookinete. [L. *vermiculus,* um pequeno verme]

ver·mic·u·lose, ver·mic·u·lous (ver-mik'ū-lōs, -lŭs). Vermículo. **1.** Infectado por vermes ou larvas. **2.** Semelhante ao verme. VER TAMBÉM vermiform.

ver·mic·u·lus (ver-mik'ū-lŭs). Vermículo. VER vermicule. [L. dim. de *vermis,* verme]

ver·mi·form (ver'mi-fōrm). Vermiforme; com formato de verme; que se assemelha a um verme na forma, indicando especialmente o apêndice do ceco. VER TAMBÉM lumbricoid, scolecoid (2). [vermi- + L. *forma,* forma]

ver·mif·u·gal (ver-mif'ū-găl). Vermífugo, anti-helmíntico. SIN anthelmintic (2). [vermi- + L. *fugo,* expulsar]

ver·mi·fuge (ver'mi-fooj). Vermífugo, anti-helmíntico. SIN anthelmintic (1). [vermi- + L. *fugo,* expulsar]

ver·mil·ion (ver-mil'yon) [C.I. 77766]. Vermelhão; um pigmento vermelho feito de cinábrio ou sulfeto mercúrico vermelho.

ver·mil·ion·ec·to·my (ver-mil-yon-ek'tō-mē). Vermilionectomia; excisão da borda vermelha do lábio. [borda do vermelhão + G. *ektomē,* excisão]

ver·min (ver'min). Insetos parasitas, como piolho e percevejos. [L. *vermis,* um verme]

ver·mi·nal (ver'mi-năl). Verminoso, verminado. SIN verminous.

ver·mi·na·tion (ver-mi-nā'shŭn). Verminação. **1.** A produção ou reprodução por vermes ou larvas. **2.** Infestação por insetos parasitas.

ver·min·ous (ver'mi-nŭs). Verminoso; relativo a, causado por ou infestado por vermes ou larvas. SIN verminal. [L. *verminosus,* verminal]

ver·mis, pl. **ver·mes** (ver'mis, -mēz). Verme. **1.** Verme; qualquer estrutura ou parte que se assemelha a um verme no formato. **2** [TA]. Verme do cerebelo, a estreita zona média entre os dois hemisférios do cerebelo; a porção que se projeta acima do nível dos hemisférios na superfície superior é chamada de v. superior; a porção inferior, afundada entre os dois hemisférios e formando o assoalho da valécula, é o v. inferior. [L. verme]

ver·mix (ver'miks). Apêndice vermiforme. SIN appendix (2).

Verner, John, clínico norte-americano, *1927. VER V.-Morrison *syndrome.*

Vernet, Maurice, neurologista francês, 1887–1974. VER V. *syndrome.*

Vernier, Pierre, matemático francês, 1580–1637. VER V. *acuity.*

ver·nix (ver'niks). Verniz. SIN varnish (dental). [L. mod.]
v. caseo'sa, v. caseoso; a substância gordurosa, consistindo em células epiteliais descamadas, lanugem e material sebáceo, que reveste a pele do feto.

Verocay, José, patologista tchecoeslovaco, 1876–1927. VER V. *bodies,* em *body.*

Ver·on·al (ver'ō-nal). Nome comercial do barbital. SIN barbital.

ver·ru·ca, pl. **ver·ru·cae** (vĕ-roo'kă, -kē). Verruga; um crescimento da cor da pele caracterizado por hipertrofia circunscrita das papilas do cório, com espessamento das camadas de Malpighi, granular e de queratina da epiderme, causada por papilomavírus humano; termo também aplicado aos tumores verrucosos epidérmicos de etiologia não-viral. SIN verruga, wart. [L.]
v. digita'ta, v. digitada; uma v. em que as papilas se projetam como dedos; ocorrem em grupos, freqüentemente no couro cabeludo. SIN digitate wart.
v. filifor'mis, v. filiforme; uma v. composta de uma ou muitas papilas bastante alongadas; aparece mais amiúde na face e no pescoço. SIN filiform wart.
v. perua'na, v. peruvia'na, v. peruana. SIN *verruga* peruana.
v. pla'na, v. plana; uma v. lisa, plana, cor da pele, pequena, que ocorre em grupos, observada especialmente na face do jovem; com freqüência associada a verrugas comuns nas mãos, causadas por papilomavírus humano, comumente dos tipos 3 e 10. SIN flat wart, plane wart, v. plana juvenilis.
v. pla'na juveni'lis, v. plana juvenil. SIN v. plana.
v. pla'na seni'lis, v. plana senil, ceratose actínica. SIN actinic *keratosis.*
v. planta'ris, v. plantar. SIN plantar *wart.*
seborrheic v., ceratose seborreica. SIN seborrheic *keratosis.*
v. seni'lis, v. senil. SIN actinic *keratosis.*
v. sim'plex, v. simples. SIN v. vulgaris.
v. vulga'ris, v. vulgar; um papiloma ceratótico da epiderme que acontece com maior freqüência nas pessoas jovens em consequência da infecção localizada pelo papilomavírus humano, usualmente dos tipos 2 e 4; as lesões têm duração variável, sofrendo, mais adiante, regressão espontânea, e são exofíticas e endofíticas, com hiperqueratose, paraqueratose, hipergranulose, coilocitose e papilomatose. SIN common wart, infectious wart, v. simplex, viral wart.

ver·ru·ci·form (vĕ-roo'si-form). Verruciforme; em forma de verruga. [L. *verruca,* wart, + *forma,* forma]

ver·ru·cose (vĕ-roo'kōs). Verrucoso; que se assemelha a uma verruga; indica elevações semelhantes a verruga. SIN verrucous. [L. *verrucosus*]

ver·ru·co·sis (ver-oo-kō'sis). Verrucose; uma condição caracterizada pelo aparecimento de múltiplas verrugas. [L. *verruca*, wart, + G. *-osis*, condição]
lymphostatic v., v. linfostática. SIN mossy foot.
ver·ru·cous (vĕ-roo'kŭs). Verrucoso. SIN verrucose.
ver·ru·ga (vĕ-roo'gă). Verruga. SIN verruca. [Sp.]
  v. perua'na, v. peruana; estágio tardio e eruptivo da bartonelose; caracterizada por pápulas vasculares pedunculadas ou cônicas macias, em qualquer ponto na pele ou mucosas, com tamanho miliar até vários centímetros, resolvendo sem cicatriz depois de alguns meses. SIN Peruvian wart, verruca peruana, verruca peruviana.
ver·si·col·or (ver-si-kŏl'ŏr). Versicolor, variegado; caracterizado por várias cores. [L. multicolorido, de *verso*, virar, torcer, + *color*, cor]
ver·sion (ver'zhŭn, -shŭn). Versão. **1.** Deslocamento do útero, com a inclinação de todo o órgão sem a inclinação de si próprio; esse deslocamento pode ser anteversão, retroversão ou lateroversão. **2.** Alteração da posição do feto no útero, que acontece espontaneamente ou efetuada por manipulação. **3.** SIN inclination. **4.** Rotação conjugada dos olhos na mesma direção; essa rotação pode ser dextroversão, levoversão, supraversão ou infraversão. [L. *verto*, pp. *versus*, virar]
  bimanual v., v. bimanual; a rotação do feto no útero, realizada com as mãos que agem sobre as duas extremidades do feto; pode ser v. externa ou v. combinada. SIN bipolar v.
  bipolar v., v. bipolar. SIN bimanual v.
  cephalic v., v. cefálica; v. em que o feto é virado de modo que a cabeça se apresenta; pode ser v. cefálica externa ou v. cefálica interna. VER TAMBÉM external cephalic v., internal cephalic v.
  combined v., v. combinada; a v. bipolar com uma das mãos na vagina e a outra sobre a parede abdominal.
  external cephalic v., v. cefálica externa; v. realizada inteiramente por manipulação externa. VER TAMBÉM cephalic v.
  internal cephalic v., v. cefálica interna; a v. realizada com uma das mãos dentro do útero. VER TAMBÉM cephalic v.
  internal podalic v., v. podálica interna; manobra para liberar o feto na qual uma mão é inserida na cavidade uterina, segurando um ou ambos os pés, e puxando-os através do colo uterino; raramente indicada em nossos dias, exceto para o delivramento de um segundo gemelar. SIN podalic v.
  pelvic v., v. pélvica; v. por meio da qual uma apresentação transversa ou oblíqua é convertida em uma apresentação pélvica através da manipulação das nádegas do feto.
  podalic v., v. podálica. SIN internal podalic v.
  postural v., v. postural; v. não-manual obtida graças à mudança da posição da mãe.
  Potter v., v. de Potter; termo obsoleto para uma v. em que os dois pés do feto são liberados antes das nádegas, sendo as costas então rodadas para uma posição anterior, com os braços e os ombros liberados por movimentos de torção e tração para baixo.
  spontaneous v., v. espontânea; a rotação do feto efetuada pela contração não-auxiliada da musculatura uterina.
  Wright v., v. de Wright; uma v. cefálica empregada nos casos de apresentação de ombro quando os ombros são empurrados para cima, enquanto as ná-

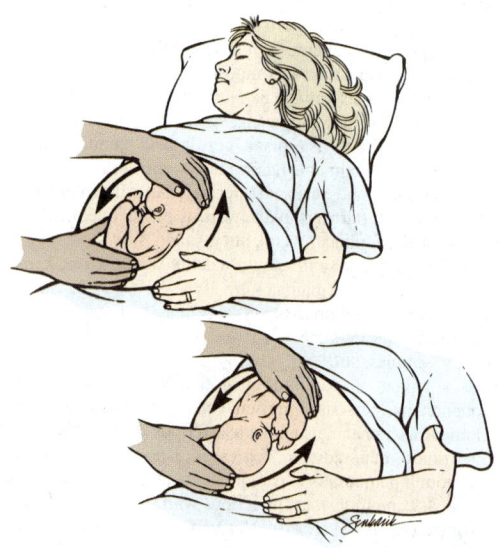

versão cefálica externa: o feto é rodado por pressão externa para uma apresentação cefálica

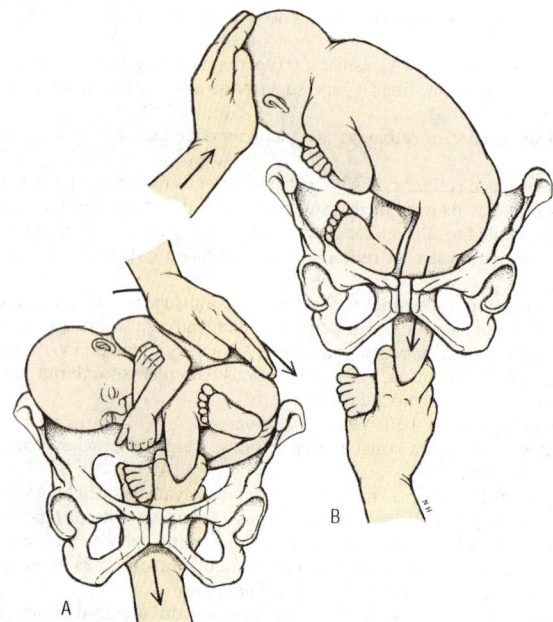

versão podálica interna: a conversão da apresentação transversa dorsoposterior para a de nádegas: (A) a mão direita do obstetra segura o pé fetal dentro do útero, enquanto a mão esquerda aplica pressão externamente para rodar a nádega em direção à entrada pélvica; (B) o obstetra manobra o feto para a orientação longitudinal aplicando tração ao pé, enquanto, externamente, direciona a cabeça para o fundo do útero, de modo que o parto possa prosseguir como na apresentação de nádegas

degas são movidas para o centro do útero pela outra mão; em seguida, a cabeça é guiada para a pelve.
ver·te·bra, gen. e pl. **ver·te·brae** (ver'tĕ-bră, -brē) [TA]. Vértebra; um dos segmentos da coluna vertebral; nos seres humanos, geralmente existem 33 vértebras: 7 cervicais, 12 torácicas, 5 lombares, 5 sacrais (fundidas em um osso, o sacro) e 4 coccígeas (fundidas em um osso, o cóccix). [L. articulação, de *verto*, virar]
  basilar v., a v. lombar mais baixa.
  block vertebrae, vértebras em bloco; corpos vertebrais hipoplásicos e congenitamente fundidos que, nas radiografias, são vistos como uma massa óssea mais ou menos sólida. VER Klippel-Feil *syndrome*.
  butterfly v., v. em borboleta; uma hemivértebra ou v. sagitalmente fendida que apresenta uma configuração de asa de borboleta nas radiografias frontais; de origem congênita.
  v. C1, v. C1; *termo oficial alternativo para atlas.
  v. C2, v. C2; *termo oficial alternativo para axis (5).
  caudal vertebrae, vértebras caudais; as vértebras que formam o esqueleto da cauda.
  cervical vertebrae [C1–C7] [TA], vértebras cervicais; os sete segmentos da coluna vertebral localizados no pescoço. SIN vertebrae cervicales [C1–C7].
  ver'tebrae cervica'les [C1–C7], vértebras cervicais. SIN cervical vertebrae [C1–C7].
  ver'tebrae coccyg'eae [Co1–Co4] [TA], vértebras coccígeas. SIN coccygeal vertebrae [Co1–Co4].
  coccygeal vertebrae [Co1–Co4] [TA], vértebras coccígeas; os quatro segmentos terminais da coluna vertebral, usualmente fundidos para formar o cóccix. SIN vertebrae coccygeae [Co1–Co4] [TA], tail vertebrae.
  codfish vertebrae, vértebras de bacalhau; o exagero da concavidade das placas terminais superior e inferior das vértebras, como se vê em radiografias de vários tipos de osteopenia.
  cranial v., v. craniana; um segmento do crânio considerado como homólogo a um segmento da coluna vertebral.
  v. denta'ta, áxis. SIN axis (5).
  dorsal vertebrae, vértebras dorsais; [L1–L4] um termo arcaico para as vértebras torácicas.
  false vertebrae, vértebras falsas; os segmentos vertebrais fundidos do sacro e do cóccix. SIN vertebrae spuriae.
  first cervical v., primeira vértebra cervical. SIN atlas.
  hourglass vertebrae, vértebras em ampulheta; o aspecto radiográfico de algumas vértebras na osteogênese imperfeita tardia.
  H-shape vertebrae, vértebras em forma de H; depressão bem delimitada da porção central das placas terminais das vértebras, produzindo uma forma de

"H" grosso nas radiografias, como na anemia falciforme.
ivory v., v. ebúrnea; uma v. radiograficamente densa, geralmente decorrente da doença metastática, especialmente o linfoma, quando solitário.
ver'tebrae lumba'les [L1–L5], vértebras lombares [L1–L5]. SIN lumbar vertebrae [L1–L5].
lumbar vertebrae [L1–L5], vértebras lombares; as vértebras, usualmente em número de cinco, localizadas na região lombar. SIN vertebrae lumbales [L1–L5].
v. mag'na, sacro. SIN sacrum.
odontoid v., áxis. SIN axis (5).
picture frame v., v. em porta-retrato; densidade radiograficamente diminuída do osso trabecular com relativa preservação do córtex, um sinal de osteopenia.
v. pla'na, v. plana; espondilite com redução do corpo vertebral para um disco fino.
v. prom'inens [TA], v. proeminente; a v., na região cervicotorácica, que possui o processo espinhoso mais proeminente (sétima v. cervical em 70% dos casos, sexta em 20% e primeira v. torácica em 10%). SIN nuchal tubercle.
rugger jersey v., v. em camisa de rúgbi; aspecto de um corpo vertebral com faixas escleróticas horizontais adjacentes às placas terminais; associada à osteodistrofia renal.
ver'tebrae sacra'les [S1–S5], vértebras sacrais [S1–S5]. SIN sacral vertebrae [S1–S5].
sacral vertebrae [S1–S5], vértebras sacrais; os segmentos da coluna vertebral, usualmente em número de cinco, que se fundem para formar o sacro. SIN vertebrae sacrales [S1–S5].
second cervical v., segunda v. cervical. SIN axis (5).
ver'tebrae spu'riae, vértebras falsas. SIN false vertebrae.
tail vertebrae, vértebras coccígeas. SIN coccygeal vertebrae [Co1–Co4].
ver'tebrae thora'cicae [T1–T12], vértebras torácicas. SIN thoracic vertebrae [T1–T12].
thoracic vertebrae [T1–T12] [TA], vértebras torácicas; os segmentos da coluna vertebral, usualmente 12, que se articulam com as costelas para formar parte do gradil torácico. SIN vertebrae thoracicae [T1–T12].
toothed v., áxis. SIN axis (5).
true v., v. verdadeira; qualquer uma das vértebras cervicais, torácicas ou lombares. SIN v. vera.
v. ve'ra, v. verdadeira. SIN true v.
ver·te·bral (ver'tĕ - brăl). Vertebral; relativo a uma vértebra ou às vértebras.
ver·te·bra·ri·um (ver - tĕ - bra'rē - ŭm). Coluna vertebral. SIN vertebral column. [L. mod.]
Ver·te·bra·ta (ver - tĕ - brah'tă, - bra'tă). Os vertebrados, uma importante divisão do filo Chordata, consistindo naqueles animais com uma medula espinal dorsal oca envolta por uma coluna vertebral cartilaginosa ou óssea; inclui várias classes de peixes, anfíbios, répteis, pássaros e mamíferos. SIN Craniata. [L. *vertebratus*, articulado]
ver·te·brate (ver'tĕ - brāt). Vertebrado. **1.** Ter uma coluna vertebral. **2.** Um animal que possui vértebras.
ver·te·brat·ed (ver'tĕ - brāt - ed). Vertebrado; articulado; composto de segmentos dispostos longitudinalmente como em determinados instrumentos.
ver·te·brec·to·my (ver'tĕ - brek'tō - mē). Vertebrectomia; ressecção de um corpo vertebral. [vertebra + G. *ektomē*, excisão]
△ **vertebro-.** Forma combinante que indica uma vértebra, vertebral. [L. *vertebra*]
ver·te·bro·ar·te·ri·al (ver'tĕ - brō - ar - tēr'ē - ăl). Vertebroarterial; relativo a uma vértebra e uma artéria, ou à artéria vertebral.
ver·te·bro·chon·dral (ver'tĕ - brō - kon'drăl). Vertebrocondral; que indica as três costelas falsas (oitava, nona e décima), as quais estão conectadas com as vértebras em uma extremidade e com as cartilagens costais na outra; essas cartilagens não se articulam diretamente com o esterno. SIN vertebrocostal (2). [vertebro- + G. *chondros*, cartilagem]
ver·te·bro·cos·tal (ver'tĕ - brō - kos'tăl). Vertebrocostal. **1.** SIN costovertebral. **2.** SIN vertebrochondral. [vertebro- + L. *costa*, costela]
ver·te·bro·fem·o·ral (ver - tĕ - brō - fem'ō - răl). Vertebrofemoral; relativo às vértebras e ao fêmur.
ver·te·bro·il·i·ac (ver'tĕ - brō - il'ē - ak). Vertebroilíaco; relativo às vértebras e ao osso ilíaco.
ver·te·bro·sa·cral (ver - tĕ - brō - sā'krăl). Vertebrossacral; relativo às vértebras e ao sacro.
ver·te·bro·ster·nal (ver'tĕ - brō - ster'năl). Vertebrossacral. SIN sternovertebral.
ver·tex, pl. **ver·ti·ces** (ver'teks, ver'ti - sēz) [TA]. Vértice. **1** [NA]. Ápice, o ponto mais elevado da calota do crânio, um marco em craniometria. **2.** Em obstetrícia, a porção da cabeça fetal limitada pelos planos dos diâmetros traquelobregmático e biparietal, com a fontanela posterior no ápice. [L. *vórtice*, turbilhão]
v. cor'dis, v. cardíaco. SIN *apex* of heart.
v. of cornea, v. da córnea. SIN corneal v.
v. cor'neae [TA], v. da córnea. SIN corneal v.
corneal v. [TA], v. da córnea; a parte central da córnea, um pouco mais fina que a parte periférica. SIN v. corneae [TA], v. of cornea.

ver·ti·cal (ver'ti - kăl) [TA]. Vertical. **1.** Relativo ao vértice ou coroa da cabeça. **2.** Perpendicular. **3.** Indica qualquer plano ou linha que passe longitudinalmente através do corpo na posição anatômica. SIN verticalis [TA].
ver·ti·ca·lis (ver - ti - kā'lis) [TA]. Vertical. SIN vertical. [L.]
ver·ti·ces (ver'ti - sēz). Vértices; plural de vertex.
ver·ti·cil (ver'ti - sil). Verticilo; uma coleção de partes similares que se irradiam a partir de um eixo comum. SIN vortex (1) whorl (4). [L. *verticillus*, o giro de um fuso, dim. de *vertex*, um giro]
ver·ti·cil·late (ver'ti - sil'āt). Verticilado; disposto na forma de um verticilo.
Ver·ti·cil·li·um (ver - ti - sil'ē - ŭm). Um gênero de fungos hifomicetos freqüentemente encontrados em amostras clínicas como contaminantes. São ocasionalmente encontrados no meato acústico nos casos de otite externa, mas são de patogenicidade duvidosa. [L. *verticillus*, um giro de um fuso]
ver·ti·co·men·tal (ver - ti - kō - men'tăl). Verticomentual; relativo à coroa da cabeça e ao queixo; indica um diâmetro em craniometria.
ver·tig·i·nous (ver - tij'i - nŭs). Vertiginoso; relativo a ou que sofre de vertigem.
ver·ti·go (ver'ti - gō, ver - tī'gō). Vertigem. **1.** Sensação de movimento de rotação ou giro. A v. implica uma sensação definida de rotação da pessoa (v. subjetiva) ou dos objetos ao redor da pessoa (v. objetiva) em qualquer plano. **2.** Usada de forma imprecisa como um termo geral para descrever a tonteira. [L. *vertigo* (*vertigin*-), tonteira, de *verto*, virar]
aural v., v. aural; **(1)** v. causada por doença do ouvido interno ou pressão do cerume sobre a membrana timpânica; **(2)** termo inespecífico para a v. causada por distúrbios do labirinto.
benign paroxysmal positional v., v. posicional paroxística benigna; uma forma breve e recorrente da v. posicional que ocorre em salvas; acredita-se que resulte de resquícios deslocados de otocônios utriculares. SIN cupulolithiasis.
benign positional v., v. posicional benigna; crises breves de v. paroxística e nistagmo que acontecem unicamente com determinados movimentos ou posições cranianas, p.ex., com a extensão do pescoço; decorrente de disfunção do labirinto. SIN positional v. of Bárány, postural v. (1).
Charcot v., v. de Charcot. SIN tussive *syncope*.
chronic v., v. crônica. SIN *status* vertiginosus.
endemic paralytic v., v. paralítica endêmica. SIN vestibular *neuronitis*.
epidemic v., v. epidêmica. SIN vestibular *neuronitis*.
height v., v. das alturas; tonteira experimentada quando se olha para baixo de uma grande altura, ou ao se olhar para cima em um prédio ou encosta alta. SIN vertical v. (1).
horizontal v., v. horizontal; tonteira experimentada ao se deitar.
hysterical v., v. histérica; sensação de tonteira, como aquela decorrente de um movimento de giro, cuja etiologia é psicossomática.
laryngeal v., v. laríngea. SIN tussive *syncope*.
lateral v., v. lateral; tonteira causada por observar fileiras de objetos verticais (p.ex., postes telegráficos, árvores e cercas) da janela de um veículo em movimento rápido.
mechanical v., v. mecânica; v. causada pela rotação ou vibração contínua do corpo.
nocturnal v., v. noturna; sensação de queda quando se adormece.
ocular v., v. ocular; tonteira atribuída a erros de refração ou desequilíbrio dos músculos extrínsecos.
organic v., v. orgânica; v. decorrente de lesão cerebral.
paralyzing v., neuronite vestibular. SIN vestibular *neuronitis*.
physiologic v., v. fisiológica. SIN space *sickness*.
positional v., v. posicional; a v. que ocorre com uma alteração na posição corporal.
positional v. of Bárány, v. posicional de Bárány. SIN benign positional v.
postural v., v. postural; **(1)** SIN benign positional v.; **(2)** tonteira que aparece principalmente nas pessoas idosas com a alteração da posição, geralmente da posição deitada ou sentada para a ortostática; decorrente de hipotensão ortostática.
sham-movement v., v. do movimento simulado; a tonteira que é acompanhada por uma impressão de que o corpo está rodando ou que os objetos estão rodando em torno do corpo.
vertical v., v. vertical; **(1)** SIN height v.; **(2)** tonteira experimentada em posição ortostática.
visual v., v. visual; v. induzida por estímulos visuais.
ver·tom·e·ter (ver - tom'ĕ - ter). Lensômetro. SIN lensometer. [vertex + G. *metron*, medida]
ver·u·mon·ta·num (ver - oo - mon - tā'nŭm). Colículo seminal. SIN seminal *colliculus*. [L. *veru*, ponta, + *montanus*, montanhoso]
ve·sa·li·a·num (ve - sā'lē - ā'nŭm). Vesaliano. SIN *os vesalianum*.
Vesalius (Wesal, Vesal), Andreas (Andre), anatomista flamengo, 1514–1564. VER V. *bone, foramen, vein.*
△ **vesic-.** VER vesico-.
ve·si·ca, gen. e pl. **ve·si·cae** (vĕ - sī'kă, vĕ - sī'sē; - kē) [TA]. **1** [NA]. Bexiga urinária. SIN urinary *bladder*. **2.** Vesícula; qualquer estrutura ou saco oco, normal ou patológico, que contenha um líquido seroso. [L.]

v. bilia'ris [TA], vesícula biliar. SIN gallbladder.
v. fel'lea, vesícula biliar; *termo oficial alternativo para gallbladder.
v. prostat'ica, utrículo prostático. SIN prostatic utricle.
v. urina'ria [TA], bexiga urinária. SIN urinary bladder.
ves·i·cal (ves'i-kăl). Vesical; relativo a qualquer vesícula, mas, em geral, à bexiga urinária.
ves·i·cant (ves'i-kănt). Vesicante; um agente que produz uma vesícula.
ves·i·cate (ves'i-kāt). Vesicar; formar uma vesícula.
ves·i·ca·tion (ves-i-kā'shŭn). Vesicação. SIN vesiculation (1).
ves·i·cle (ves'i-kl) [TA]. Vesícula. **1.** SIN vesicula. **2.** Uma elevação pequena (<1,0 cm de diâmetro) e circunscrita da pele contendo líquido. VER TAMBÉM bleb, blister, bulla. **3.** Um pequeno saco que contém líquido ou gás. **4.** Uma estrutura fechada circundada por uma membrana única. [L. *vesicula*, uma bolha, dim. de *vesica*, vesícula]
acoustic v., v. acústica. SIN otic v.
acrosomal v., v. acrossômica; v. derivada do aparelho de Golgi durante a espermatogênese, cuja membrana limitante adere ao envelope nuclear; em conjunto com o grânulo acrossômico interno, dissemina-se em uma camada fina, sobre o pólo do núcleo, para formar o capuz acrossômico.
air v.'s, alvéolos pulmonares. SIN pulmonary *alveolus*.
allantoic v., v. alantóica; a porção oca do alantóide.
amniocardiac v., v. amniocardíaca; a porção rostral do celoma intra-embrionário mais primitivo.
auditory v., v. auditiva. SIN otic v.
blastodermic v., v. blastodérmica. SIN blastocyst.
cerebral v., v. cerebral; cada uma das três divisões do cérebro embrionário inicial (prosencéfalo, mesencéfalo e rombencéfalo). SIN encephalic v., primary brain v.
cervical v., v. cervical; um vestígio do seio cervical ou de seus sulcos branquiais associados que persiste de forma anormal.
coated v., v. revestida; uma v. que apresenta sua biomembrana revestida com a proteína clatrina. É envolvida no transporte de proteínas de um sítio da membrana para outro.
encephalic v., v. encefálica. SIN cerebral v.
forebrain v., prosencéfalo; *termo oficial alternativo para prosencephalon.
germinal v., v. germinativa; termo obsoleto para o núcleo do ovo.
hindbrain v., rombencéfalo; *termo oficial alternativo para rhombencephalon.
lens v., v. da lente; no embrião, a invaginação ectodérmica que se forma em oposição à papila óptica; é o primórdio da lente do olho. SIN lenticular v.
lenticular v., da lente. SIN lens v.
malpighian v.'s, vesículas de Malpighi; as diminutas vesículas cheias de ar na superfície de um pulmão expandido.
matrix v.'s, vesículas da matriz; vesículas envoltas por membrana, contendo hidroxiapatita, secretadas por odontoblastos e alguns condrócitos; acredita-se que atuem como centros de nucleação para o processo de mineralização na dentina e na cartilagem calcificada.
midbrain v., mesencéfalo; *termo oficial alternativo para mesencephalon.
ocular v., v. ocular. SIN optic v.
ophthalmic v., v. oftálmica. SIN optic v.
optic v., v. óptica; no embrião, uma das invaginações pareadas das paredes ventrolaterais do prosencéfalo, a partir das quais as camadas sensorial e pigmentar da retina se desenvolvem. SIN ocular v., ophthalmic v., vesicula ophthalmica.
otic v., v. auditiva; um dos sacos pareados do ectoderma invaginado que se desenvolvem para dentro do labirinto membranoso do ouvido interno. SIN acoustic v., auditory v.
pinocytotic v., v. pinocitótica; uma v. com uma fração de 1 micrômetro de diâmetro, contendo líquido ou soluto que é "ingerido" dentro de uma célula por endocitose. VER TAMBÉM pinocytosis.
primary brain v., v. cerebral primária. SIN cerebral v.
seminal v., v. seminal; *termo oficial alternativo para seminal *gland*.
synaptic v.'s, vesículas sinápticas; as pequenas vesículas intracelulares (diâmetro médio de 30 nm), limitadas por membrana, próximo à membrana pré-sináptica de uma junção sináptica, contendo a substância transmissora que, nas sinapses químicas, medeia a passagem dos impulsos nervosos através da junção. VER TAMBÉM synapse.
telencephalic v., v. telencefálica; divertículos pareados que se originam do prosencéfalo, a partir dos quais se desenvolve o prosencéfalo.
umbilical v., saco vitelínico. SIN yolk *sac*.
vesico-, vesic-. Formas combinantes que indicam uma vesícula. VER TAMBÉM vesiculo-. [L. *vesica*, vesícula]
ves·i·co·ab·dom·i·nal (ves'i-kō-ab-dom'i-năl). Vesicoabdominal; relativo à bexiga urinária e à parede abdominal.
ves·i·co·bul·lous (ves'i-kō-bŭl'ŭs). Vesicobolhosa; indica uma erupção de lesões de tamanhos variados que contêm líquido.
ves·i·co·cele (ves'i-kō-sēl). Cistocele. SIN cystocele.
ves·i·co·cer·vi·cal (ves'i-kō-ser'vi-kăl). Vesicocervical; relativo à bexiga urinária e ao colo do útero.

ves·i·coc·ly·sis (ves'i-kok'li-sis). Vesicoclise; depuração ou lavagem da bexiga urinária. [vesico- + G. *klysis*, uma lavagem]
ves·i·co·in·tes·ti·nal (ves'i-kō-in-tes'ti-năl). Vesicointestinal; relativo à bexiga urinária e ao intestino; p.ex., fístula vesicointestinal.
ves·i·co·li·thi·a·sis (ves'i-kō-li-thī-ā-sis). Cistolitíase. SIN cystolithiasis. [vesico- + G. *lithos*, pedra, + *-iasis*, condição]
ves·i·co·pros·ta·tic (ves'i-kō-pros-tat'ik). Vesicoprostático; relativo à bexiga e à próstata.
ves·i·co·pu·bic (ves'i-kō-pū'bik). Vesicopúbico; relativo à bexiga e ao osso púbis.
ves·i·co·pus·tu·lar (ves'i-kō-pŭs'tū-lăr). Vesicopustular; pertinente a uma vesicopústula.
ves·i·co·pus·tule (ves'i-kō-pŭs'tūl). Vesicopústula; uma vesícula que está desenvolvendo a formação de pus.
ves·i·co·rec·tal (ves'i-kō-rek'tăl). Vesicorretal; relativo à bexiga e ao reto.
ves·i·co·rec·tos·to·my (ves'i-kō-rek-tos'tō-mē). Vesicorretostomia; desvio cirúrgico do trato urinário por anastomose da parede vesical posterior com o reto. [vesico- + *rectum* + G. *stoma*, boca]
ves·i·co·sig·moid (ves'i-kō-sig'moyd). Vesicossigmóide; relativo à bexiga e ao colo sigmóide.
ves·i·co·sig·moi·dos·to·my (ves'i-kō-sig-moy-dos'tō-mē). Vesicossigmoidostomia; formação operatória de uma comunicação entre a bexiga e o colo sigmóide. [vesico- + *sigmoid* + G. *stoma*, boca]
ves·i·co·spi·nal (ves'i-kō-spī-năl). Vesicoespinal; relativo à bexiga urinária e à medula espinal; indica os mecanismos neurais que controlam a retenção e a eliminação da urina pela bexiga, localizada na segunda vértebra lombar e segundo segmento sacral, respectivamente, da medula espinal.
ves·i·cos·to·my (ves'i-kos'tō-mē). Vesicostomia, cistostomia. SIN cystostomy. [vesico- + G. *stoma*, boca]
ves·i·cot·o·my (ves'i-kot'ō-mē). Vesicotomia, cistotomia. SIN cystotomy.
ves·i·co·um·bi·li·cal (ves'i-kō-ŭm-bil'i-kăl). Vesicoumbilical; relativo à bexiga urinária e ao umbigo. SIN omphalovesical.
ves·i·co·u·re·ter·al (ves'i-kō-ū-rē'ter-ăl). Vesicoureteral; relativo à bexiga e aos ureteres.
ves·i·co·u·re·thral (ves'i-kō-ū-rē'thrăl). Vesicouretral; relativo à bexiga e à uretra.
ves·i·co·u·ter·ine (ves'i-kō-ū-ter-in). Vesicouterino; relativo à bexiga e ao útero.
ves·i·co·u·ter·o·vag·i·nal (ves'i-kō-ū'ter-ō-vaj'i-năl). Vesicouterovaginal; relativo à bexiga, útero e vagina.
ves·i·co·vag·i·nal (ves-i-kō-vaj'i-năl). Vesicovaginal; relativo à bexiga e à vagina.
ves·i·co·vag·i·no·rec·tal (ves'i-kō-vaj'i-nō-rek'tăl). Vesicovaginorretal; relativo à bexiga, vagina e reto.
ves·i·co·vis·cer·al (ves'i-kō-vis'er-ăl). Vesicovisceral; relativo à bexiga urinária e a qualquer outro órgão ou víscera adjacente.
ve·sic·u·la, gen. e pl. **ve·sic·u·lae** (vĕ-sik'ŭ-lă, -lē). Vesícula; uma pequena bexiga ou estrutura semelhante à bexiga. SIN vesicle (1) [TA]. [L. bolha, vesícula, dim. de *vesica*, bexiga]
v. fel'lis, v. biliar. SIN gallbladder.
v. ophthal'mica, v. oftálmica. SIN optic *vesicle*.
v. semina'lis, glândula seminal; *termo oficial alternativo para seminal *gland*.
v. umbilica'lis, v. umbilical. SIN yolk *sac*.
ve·sic·u·lar (vĕ-sik'ŭ-lăr). Vesicular. **1.** Relativo a uma vesícula. **2.** Caracterizado por ou que contém vesículas. SIN vesiculate (2).
ve·sic·u·late (vĕ-sik'ŭ-lāt). Vesiculado. **1.** Transformar em vesícula. **2.** SIN vesicular (2).
ve·sic·u·la·tion (vĕ-sik'ŭ-lā'shŭn). Vesiculação. **1.** A formação de vesículas. SIN blistering, vesication. **2.** Presença de inúmeras vesículas.
ve·sic·u·lec·to·my (vĕ-sik'ŭ-lek'tō-mē). Vesiculectomia; ressecção de uma parte ou da totalidade de cada uma das glândulas seminais. [L. *vesicula*, vesícula, + G. *ektomē*, excisão]
ve·sic·u·li·tis (vĕ-sik-ū-lī'tis). Vesiculite; inflamação de qualquer vesícula; especialmente de uma glândula seminal. [L. *vesicula*, vesícula, + G. *-itis*, inflamação]
vesiculo-. Forma combinante que indica uma vesícula. [L. *vesicula*, vesícula, dim. de *vesica*, bexiga]
ve·sic·u·lo·bron·chi·al (vĕ-sik'ŭ-lō-brong'kē-ăl). Vesiculobrônquico; indica um som auscultatório que possui as características vesicular e brônquica.
ve·sic·u·lo·cav·ern·ous (vĕ-sik'ŭ-lō-kav'er-nŭs). Vesiculocavernoso; tanto vesicular squanto cavernoso; indica: **1.** Um som da ausculta que possui as características vesicular e cavernosa. **2.** A estrutura de determinadas neoplasias.
ve·sic·u·log·ra·phy (vĕ-sik-ū-log'ră-fi). Vesiculografia; estudo das glândulas seminais com contraste radiográfico. [vesiculo- + G. *graphō*, escrever]
ve·sic·u·lo·pap·u·lar (vĕ-sik'ŭ-lō-pap'ū-lăr). Vesiculopapular; pertinente a ou que consiste em uma combinação de vesículas e pápulas, ou de pápulas

ve·sic·u·lo·pros·ta·ti·tis (vĕ-sik′u-lō-pros′ta-tī′tis). Vesiculoprostatite; inflamação da bexiga e da próstata. [vesiculo- + prostate + G. -itis, inflamação]

ve·sic·u·lot·o·my (vĕ-sik-u-lot′o-mē). Vesiculotomia; incisão cirúrgica das glândulas seminais. [vesiculo- + G. tomē, incisão]

ve·sic·u·lo·tu·bu·lar (vĕ-sik′u-lō-too′bū-ler). Vesiculotubular; indica um som de ausculta com características vesicular e tubular.

ve·sic·u·lo·tym·pan·ic (vĕ-sik′u-lō-tim-pan′ik). Vesiculotimpânica; indica um som de percussão com características vesicular e timpânica.

Ve·si·cu·lo·vi·rus (vĕ-sik′u-lō-vī′rus). Um gênero de vírus (família Rhabdoviridae) que inclui o vírus da estomatite vesicular (do gado) e vírus correlatos.

vesp (ves′per). Abreviatura para L. vesper, noite. [L. noite]

ves·sel (ves′el). [TA]. Vaso, ducto; uma estrutura que conduz ou contém um fluido, principalmente um líquido. VER TAMBÉM vas. [Fr. ant. do L. vascellum, dim. de vas]

   absorbent v.'s, vasos linfáticos. SIN lymph v.'s.
   afferent v., v. aferente; (1) qualquer artéria que conduz sangue para uma região; (2) arteríola glomerular aferente. SIN afferent glomerular arteriole; (3) linfático aferente. SIN afferent lymphatic.
   anastomosing v., v. anastomótico. SIN anastomotic v.
   anastomotic v. [TA], v. anastomótico; um v. que estabelece uma conexão entre artérias, entre veias ou entre vasos linfáticos. SIN vas anastomoticum [TA], anastomosing v.
   blood v., v. sanguíneo. VER blood vessel.
   capillary v., v. capilar. SIN capillary (2). VER blood capillary, lymph capillary.
   chyle v., ducto quiloso. SIN lacteal (2).
   collateral v., v. colateral; (1) um ramo de uma artéria que corre em paralelo com o tronco principal; (2) um v. que corre em paralelo com outro v., nervo ou outra estrutura longa. SIN vas collaterale.
   corkscrew v.'s, vasos em saca-rolhas, vasos em grampo de cabelo. SIN hairpin v.'s.
   deep lymph v. [TA], v. linfático profundo; um dos vasos que drenam linfa a partir de estruturas profundas do corpo; tendem a acompanhar os vasos sanguíneos para alcançar os linfonodos regionais. SIN vas lymphaticum profundum [TA].
   efferent v., v. eferente. SIN efferent glomerular arteriole.
   hairpin v.'s, vasos em grampo de cabelo; vasos sanguíneos atípicos que se dobram sobre si mesmos, observados na colposcopia do colo; sua presença indica câncer cervical invasivo inicial. SIN corkscrew v.'s.
   v.'s of internal ear [TA], vasos da orelha interna; os vasos sanguíneos da orelha interna, consistindo na artéria do labirinto e seus ramos e nas veias do labirinto e suas tributárias. SIN vasa sanguinea auris internae [TA].
   lacteal v., ducto lactífero. SIN lacteal (1).
   lymph v.'s [TA], vasos linfáticos; os vasos que conduzem a linfa; anastomosam-se livremente entre si. SIN lymphatic v.'s [TA], absorbent v.'s, lymphatics, vasa lymphatica.
   lymphatic v.'s [TA], vasos linfáticos. SIN lymph v.'s.
   nutrient v., artéria nutrícia. SIN nutrient artery.
   superficial lymph v. [TA], vasos linfáticos superficiais; um dos vasos linfáticos que se situam na pele e nos tecidos subcutâneos; unem-se aos vasos linfáticos profundos. SIN vas lymphaticum superficiale [TA].
   v.'s of vessels, vasos dos vasos. SIN vasa vasorum, em vas.
   vitelline v.'s, vasos vitelinos. VER vitelline artery, vitelline vein.

ves·tib·u·la (ves-tib′u-lā). Vestíbulos; plural de vestibulum.

ves·tib·u·lar (ves-tib′u-lar). Vestibular; relativo a um vestíbulo, principalmente ao vestíbulo do ouvido. SIN vestibularis.

ves·ti·bu·la·ris (ves-tib-u-lā′ris). Vestibular. SIN vestibular. [L.]

ves·tib·u·late (ves-tib′u-lāt). Vestibulado; que possui um vestíbulo.

ves·ti·bule (ves′ti-bool) [TA]. Vestíbulo. **1.** Uma pequena cavidade ou um espaço na entrada de um canal. **2.** Especificamente, a cavidade central, algo ovóide, do labirinto ósseo que se comunica com os canais semicirculares, posteriormente, e com a cóclea, anteriormente. SIN vestibulum [TA]. [L. vestibulum]

   aortic v., v. da aorta; a porção ântero-posterior do ventrículo esquerdo do coração logo abaixo do orifício aórtico, que possui paredes fibrosas e confere espaço para os segmentos da válvula aórtica fechada. SIN vestibulum aortae [TA], Sibson aortic v.
   buccal v., aquela parte do vestíbulo da boca relacionada com a bochecha.
   esophagogastric v., v. gastroesofágico. SIN gastroesophageal v.
   gastroesophageal v., v. gastroesofágico; a porção aboral dilatada do esôfago, logo acima do orifício da cárdia; geralmente corresponde à luz da parte abdominal do esôfago, embora sua relação com o diafragma seja variável. SIN esophagogastric v.
   labial v., aquela parte do vestíbulo da boca relacionada com os lábios.
   v. of larynx [TA], v. da laringe; a parte superior da cavidade laríngea desde a abertura superior até as pregas vestibulares ou rima vestibular, limitada anteriormente pela epiglote, lateralmente pela mucosa suprajacente às membranas quadrangulares e posteriormente pela mucosa suprajacente às cartilagens aritenóides e músculo aritenóide. SIN vestibulum laryngis [TA], atrium glottidis, superior laryngeal cavity.
   v. of mouth, v. da boca. SIN oral v.
   nasal v. [TA], v. do nariz; a parte anterior da cavidade nasal, especialmente aquela encerrada por cartilagem. SIN vestibulum nasi [TA], v. of nose.
   v. of nose, v. do nariz. SIN nasal v.
   v. of omental bursa [TA], v. da bolsa omental; a parte superior da bolsa omental, exatamente dentro do forame epiplóico (de Winslow), atrás do lobo caudado do fígado. SIN vestibulum bursae omentalis [TA].
   oral v. [TA], v. da boca; a parte da boca limitada anterior e lateralmente pelos lábios e bochechas, posterior e medialmente por dentes e/ou gengivas, e acima e abaixo pelas reflexões da mucosa desde os lábios e bochechas até as gengivas. SIN vestibulum oris [TA], buccal cavity, v. of mouth.
   Sibson aortic v., v. aórtico de Sibson. SIN aortic v.
   v. of vagina [TA], v. da vagina; o espaço posterior à glande do clitóris e entre os lábios menores do pudendo, contendo as aberturas da vagina, uretra e ductos das glândulas vestibulares maiores. SIN vestibulum vaginae [TA], vaginal introitus, vestibulum pudendi.

ves·tib·u·li·tis. Vestibulite; inflamação do vestíbulo vulvar e do estroma periglandular e subepitelial caracterizada por sensação de queimação e coito doloroso.

vestibulo-. Forma combinante que indica vestíbulo. [L. vestibulum]

ves·tib·u·lo·cer·e·bel·lum (ves-tib′u-lō-ser-e-bel′um). [TA]. Arquicerebelo; as regiões do córtex cerebelar cujas fibras aferentes predominantes originam-se do gânglio vestibular e dos núcleos vestibulares; as estruturas designadas por esse termo são o nódulo, o flóculo, as partes ventrais da úvula e as pequenas partes ventrais da língua. SIN archeocerebellum. [vestibulo- + L. cerebellum]

ves·tib·u·lo·co·chle·ar (ves-tib′u-lō-kok′lē-ar). Vestibulococlear. **1.** Relativo ao vestíbulo e à cóclea do ouvido. **2.** SIN statoacoustic.

ves·tib·u·lop·a·thy (ves-tib′u-lop′a-thē). Vestibulopatia; qualquer anormalidade do aparelho vestibular, p.ex., doença de Ménière.

   idiopathic bilateral v., v. idiopática bilateral; distúrbio lentamente progressivo que afeta adultos jovens e de meia-idade, manifestado como instabilidade da marcha (principalmente quando não há indícios visuais) e oscilopsia, não sendo acompanhado por vertigem nem por perda da audição.
   migraine-related v., v. relacionada à enxaqueca; transtorno caracterizado por desequilíbrio associado ao movimento, instabilidade, desconforto associado a espaço e movimento, e vertigem antes do início da cefaléia.

ves·tib·u·lo·plas·ty (ves-tib′u-lō-plas-tē). Vestibuloplastia; qualquer um de uma série de procedimentos cirúrgicos idealizados para restaurar a altura da crista alveolar através de rebaixamento dos músculos que se inserem nas faces bucal, labial e lingual das mandíbulas. [vestibulo- + G. plassō, formar]

ves·tib·u·lo·spi·nal (ves-tib′u-lō-spī′nal). Vestibuloespinal. VER lateral vestibulospinal tract.

ves·tib·u·lot·o·my (ves-tib′u-lot′o-mē). Vestibulotomia; a cirurgia para criar uma abertura para o vestíbulo do labirinto. [vestibulo- + G. tomē, incisão]

ves·tib·u·lo·u·re·thral (ves-tib′u-lō-oo-rē′thral). Vestibulouretral; relativo ao vestíbulo da vagina e à uretra.

ves·tib·u·lum, pl. **ves·tib·u·la** (ves-tib′u-lum, -lā).[TA]. Vestíbulo. SIN vestibule. [L. antecâmara, ante-sala]

   v. aor′tae [TA], v. da aorta. SIN aortic vestibule.
   v. bur′sae omenta′lis [TA], v. da bolsa omental. SIN vestibule of omental bursa.
   v. laryn′gis [TA], v. da laringe. SIN vestibule of larynx.
   v. na′si [TA], v. do nariz. SIN nasal vestibule.
   v. o′ris [TA], v. da boca. SIN oral vestibule.
   v. puden′di, v. da vagina. SIN vestibule of vagina.
   v. vagi′nae [TA], v. da vagina. SIN vestibule of vagina.

ves·tige (ves′tij). [TA]. Vestígio; uma estrutura residual ou rudimentar; os resquícios degenerados de qualquer estrutura que ocorre como uma entidade no embrião ou no feto. SIN vestigium [TA]. [L. vestigium]

   v. of ductus deferens [TA], v. do ducto deferente; resquício, em uma mulher, da porção do ducto mesonéfrico embrionário que evolui para ducto deferente nos homens.
   v. of processus vaginalis [TA], v. do processo vaginal; os resquícios obliterados de maneira incompleta do processo vaginal do peritônio que persistem no funículo espermático. SIN vestigium processus vaginalis [TA], v. of vaginal process.
   v. of vaginal process, v. do processo vaginal. SIN v. of processus vaginalis.

ves·tig·i·al (ves-tij′ē-al). Vestigial; relativo a um vestígio.

ves·tig·i·um, pl. **ves·tig·ia** (ves-tij′ē-um, -a) [TA]. Vestígio. SIN vestige. [L. pegada (traço), de vestigo, rastrear, traçar]

   v. proces′sus vagina′lis [TA], v. do processo vaginal. SIN vestige of processus vaginalis.

ve·su·vin (vĕ-soo′vin) [C.I. 21000]. Vesuvina. SIN Bismarck brown Y. [Vesuvius, vulcão na Itália]

vet·er·i·nar·i·an (vet′e-rin-ār′e-ăn). Veterinário; uma pessoa que possui um grau acadêmico em medicina veterinária; um profissional licenciado em medicina veterinária. [ver veterinary]

vet·er·i·nary (vet′e-rin-ār-e). Veterinário; relativo às doenças dos animais. [L. *veterinarius*, de *veterina*, burro de carga]

via, pl. **vi·ae** (vi′a, vi′e; ve′a). Via; qualquer passagem no corpo, como o intestino, a vagina, etc. [L. caminho, trajeto]

vi·a·bil·i·ty (vi-ă-bil′i-te). Viabilidade; capacidade de viver; o estado de ser viável; usualmente conota um feto que alcançou 500 g de peso e idade gestacional de 20 semanas. [Fr. *viabilité*, do L. *vita*, vida]

vi·a·ble (vi′ă-bl). Viável; capaz de viver; indica um feto suficientemente desenvolvido para viver fora do útero. [Fr. de *vie*, vida, do L. *vita*]

vi·al (vi′ăl). Frasco; uma pequena garrafa ou receptáculo para armazenar líquidos, inclusive medicamentos. SIN phial. [G. *phiale*, uma taça]

vi·bes·ate (vi′bĕ-sāt). Vibesato; uma mistura de polvinato e malrosinol em solvente orgânico e um propelente; um plástico de polivinila modificado usado como *spray* tópico para feridas.

vi·bra·tion (vi-brā′shŭn). Vibração. **1.** Uma sacudidela. **2.** Um movimento de vaivém, como na oscilação. [L. *vibratio*, de *vibro*, pp. *-atus*, sacudir, oscilar].

vi·bra·tive (vi′brā-tiv). Vibratório. SIN vibratory.

vi·bra·tor (vi′brā-ter, tor). Vibrador; um instrumento usado para produzir vibrações.

vi·bra·to·ry (vi′brā-tor-e). Vibratório; caracterizado por vibrações. SIN vibrative.

Vib·rio (vib′re-o). Um gênero de bactérias Gram-negativas, móveis (ocasionalmente imóveis), não-formadoras de esporos, aeróbicas a facultativamente anaeróbicas (família Spirillaceae), contendo bastonetes curtos (0,5–3,0 μm), curvos ou retos, que ocorrem isoladamente ou que estão ocasionalmente unidos em forma de S ou espirais. As células móveis contêm um único flagelo polar; em algumas espécies, dois ou mais flagelos ocorrem em um tufo polar. Alguns desses microrganismos são saprófitas em água salgada e água doce, bem como no solo; outros são parasitas ou patógenos. A espécie típica é *V. cholerae*. [L. *vibro*, *vibrar*]
 V. alginolyt′icus, uma espécie bacteriana associada a infecções de ferida e orelha, e bacteremia em pacientes imunocomprometidos e pacientes queimados.
 V. chol′erae, uma espécie bacteriana que produz uma exotoxina solúvel, é a causa da cólera em seres humanos; é a espécie típica do gênero *V*. SIN cholera bacillus, comma bacillus.
 V. fe′tus, nome original do *Campylobacter fetus*.
 V. fluvia′lis, uma espécie bacteriana similar às cepas de *Aeromonas*, associada à doença diarreica em seres humanos.
 V. furnis′sii, uma cepa aerogênica de bactérias, similar a *V. fluvialis*, associada à doença diarreica e a surtos de gastrenterite.
 V. hol′isae, uma espécie bacteriana que pode causar disenteria em seres humanos.
 V. metschniko′vii, uma espécie bacteriana que causa doença entérica aguda em galinhas e outras espécies de aves; também isolada a partir das fezes humanas.
 V. mim′icus, uma cepa bacteriana sacarose-negativa, similar a *V. cholerae*, isolada a partir das fezes humanas na doença diarreica e a partir de infecções otológicas em seres humanos.
 V. parahaemolyt′icus, uma espécie bacteriana marinha que causa gastrenterite e diarréia sanguinolenta, usualmente após ingestão de mariscos contaminados.
 V. sputo′rum, nome original para *Campylobacter sputorum*.
 V. vulnif′icus, uma espécie capaz de causar gastrenterite e lesões cutâneas que podem resultar em septicemia fatal, sobretudo em paciente cirrótico ou imunocomprometido; usualmente contraído de ostras contaminadas; também causa infecções de feridas, especialmente aquelas associadas ao manuseio de crustáceos.

vib·rio (vib′re-o). Vibrião; um membro do gênero *Vibrio*.
 El Tor v., v. El Tor; uma bactéria considerada como biovariante do *Vibrio cholerae*. Foi originalmente isolado de seis peregrinos que morreram de disenteria ou gangrena do colo na estação de quarentena Tor, na Península do Sinai.
 Nasik v., v. Nasik; um microrganismo que difere do *V. cholerae*, sendo mais curto e mais espesso, e menos semelhante a uma vírgula; suas culturas são muito tóxicas para os animais de laboratório em injeções intravenosas.

Vib·ri·on sep·tique (ve-bre-on′ sep-tēk′). *Vibrio septicum*. SIN *Clostridium septicum*. [Fr. vibrião séptico]

vib·ri·o·sis, pl. **vib·ri·o·ses** (vib-re-o′sis). Vibriose; infecção causada por espécies de bactérias do gênero *Vibrio*.

vi·bris·sa, pl. e gen. **vi·bris·sae** (vi-bris′a, vi-bris′e) [TA]. Vibrissa. SIN hairs of vestibule of nose, em *hair*. [L. encontrado apenas no pl. *vibrissae*, de *vibro*, sacudir]

vi·bris·sal (vib-ris′ăl). Vibrissal; relativo às vibrissas.

vi·bro·car·di·o·gram (vi′bro-kar′de-o-gram). Vibrocardiograma; um registro gráfico das vibrações torácicas produzidas por eventos hemodinâmicos do ciclo cardíaco; o registro fornece uma medição indireta, registrada externamente, da contração isovolumétrica e dos tempos de ejeção. [L. *vibro*, sacudir, + G. *kardia*, coração, + *gramma*, um desenho]

vi·bro·mas·seur (vi′bro-ma-ser′). Vibromassageador; um tipo de vibrador para fornecer a massagem vibratória.

vi·bro·ther·a·peu·tics (vi′bro-thăr-ă-pu′tiks). Vibroterapêutica. SIN vibratory *massage*.

Vi·bur·num pru·ni·fo·li·um (vii-bur′num proo-′ni-fo′le-um). Viburno, espinheiro-preto; medicação derivada da casca da raiz do *Viburnum prunifolium* (família Caprifoliaceae); contém viburnina; resina amarga; tanino; açúcar; ácidos cítrico, málico, oxálico e valérico. Originalmente utilizado como relaxante da musculatura lisa/antiespasmódico (uterino).

vi·car·i·ous (vi-ker′e-ŭs). Vicariante; que atua como substituto; que ocorre em uma situação anormal. [L. *vicarius*, de *vicis*, que toma o lugar de]

vi·cine (vi′sen). Vicina; um glicosídeo de ocorrência em uma erva daninha que contamina o *Lathyrus sativus*, bem como na ervilhaca (*Vicia sativa*), uma planta cujo fruto substitui as lentilhas vermelhas; alguns acreditam que seja responsável pelos sintomas de latirismo. [*Vicia* (nome do gênero) + *-ine*]

Vicq d'Azyr, Félix, anatomista francês, 1748–1794. VER V. d'*bundle*, *centrum semiovale*, *foramen*.

Vic·to·ria blue. Azul-vitória; qualquer um dos diversos derivados azuis do difenilnaftilmetano; usado como corante em histologia. [Rainha *Victoria*]

Vic·to·ria or·ange. Laranja-vitória; um sal alcalino do dinitrocresol; um corante amarelo-avermelhado originalmente utilizado em histologia.

vi·dar·a·bine (vi-der′ă-bēn). Vidarabina; um nucleosídeo purínico obtido a partir de culturas de fermentação do *Streptomyces antibioticus* e usado para tratar as infecções por herpes simples.

vid·e·o·en·do·scope (vid′e-o-end′o-skop). Videoendoscópio; um endoscópio adaptado com uma câmera de vídeo.

vid·e·o·en·dos·co·py (vid′e-o-en-dos′ka-pe). Videoendoscopia; endoscopia realizada com um endoscópio adaptado com uma câmera de vídeo.

vid·e·o·ker·a·to·scope (vid′e-o-ker′ah-to-skop). Videoceratoscópio; um ceratoscópio adaptado com uma câmera de vídeo.

vid·i·an (vid′e-an). Vidiano; descrito por Vidius ou derivado de seu nome.

Vidius (Vidus), Guidi (Guido), médico e anatomista italiano, 1500–1569. VER vidian *artery*, vidian *canal*, vidian *nerve*, vidian *vein*.

Vierra, J.P., dermatologista brasileiro do século XX. VER V. *sign*.

Vieussens, Raymond de, anatomista francês, 1641–1715. VER V. *anulus*, *ansa*, *centrum*, *foramina*, em *foramen*, *ganglia*, em *ganglion*, *isthmus*, *limbus*, *loop*, *ring*; *valve* of V.; V. *valve*, *veins*, em *vein*, *ventricle*.

view (vu). Incidência. SIN projection.
 axial v., i. axial. SIN axial *projection*.
 base v., i. submentovértice. SIN submentovertex *radiograph*.
 Caldwell v., i. de Caldwell. SIN Caldwell *projection*.
 half axial v., i. mesoaxial. SIN Towne *projection*.
 Judet v., i. de Judet; consiste em duas incidências radiográficas oblíquas centradas no quadril em questão, inclinado 45° medial ou lateralmente a partir de uma direção ântero-posterior verdadeira; útil para as fraturas ou deformidades do acetábulo.
 long axis v., i. do eixo pulmonar; em ecocardiografia ou nas imagens do coração por ressonância magnética, uma i. paralela ao eixo ventricular e perpendicular ao eixo do septo interventricular do coração; i. de quatro câmaras.
 Stenvers v., i. de Stenvers. SIN Stenvers *projection*.
 Towne v., i. de Towne. SIN Towne *projection*.
 verticosubmental v., i. axial. SIN axial *projection*.
 Waters v., i. de Waters. SIN Waters *projection*.

vig·a·bat·rin (vi-gă′bă-trin). Vigabatrina; um inibidor irreversível da transaminase do ácido γ-aminobutírico, uma enzima que degrada o ácido γ-aminobutírico (GABA), o neurotransmissor inibitório; intensifica os efeitos do GABA e, dessa maneira, a inibição do sistema nervoso central; usado como agente antiepiléptico.

vig·il (vij′il). Vigília; um estado de alerta ou insônia. [L. *vigilia*, alerta, vigília; de *vigeo*, estar ativo, despertar]
 coma v., coma vigil. SIN akinetic *mutism*.

vig·il·am·bu·lism (vij-i-lam′bū-lizm). Vigilambulismo; um termo antigo para uma condição de olhar sem tomar consciência dos arredores, com automatismo; assemelha-se ao sonambulismo, mas ocorre no estado de vigília. [L. *vigil*, acordado, alerta, + *ambulo*, caminhar]

vig·i·lance (vij′i-lans). Vigilância; atenção, alerta ou observação para tudo que possa ocorrer. [L. *vigilantia*, vigília]

vil·li (vil′i). Vilos; plural de villus.

vil·lin (vil′in). Vilina; uma proteína de fixação de actina que, em baixas concentrações de íon cálcio, comanda a polimerização dos filamentos de actina; o Ca^{2+} micromolar faz com que a vilina seccione os filamentos de actina em fragmentos curtos.

vil·li·tis. Vilite, vilosite. SIN villositis.

vil·lose (vil′ōs). Viloso. SIN villous (2).

vil·lo·si·tis (vil-ō-sī′tis). Vilosite; inflamação da superfície da vilosidade coriônica da placenta. SIN villitis. [villous + G. *-itis*, inflamação]

vil·los·i·ty (vi-los′i-tē). Vilosidade; emaranhado; um agregado de vilosidades.

vil·lous (vil′ŭs). Viloso. **1.** Relativo às vilosidades. **2.** Emaranhado; coberto por vilosidades. SIN villose.

vil·lus, pl. **vil·li** (vil′ŭs, vil′ī). Vilo; vilosidade. **1.** Uma projeção a partir da superfície, especialmente de uma mucosa. Quando a projeção é diminuta, como a partir de uma superfície celular, ela é denominada microvilosidade. **2.** Uma papila dérmica alongada que se projeta para dentro de uma vesícula ou fenda intra-epitelial. VER festooning. [L. pêlos emaranhados (de feras)]
  anchoring v., v. de fixação; uma v. coriônica que está fixada à decídua basal.
  arachnoid villi, vilosidades aracnóides; prolongamentos em tufos da pia-aracnóide através da camada meníngea da dura-máter, possuindo uma membrana limitante fina; as coleções de v. aracnóide formam granulações aracnóides que se situam nas lacunas venosas na margem do seio sagital superior; o tecido esponjoso da v. aracnóide contém túbulos que servem como válvulas unidirecionais para a transferência de líquido cefalorraquidiano do espaço subaracnóide para o sistema venoso. Tanto as vilosidades aracnóides como as granulações formadas a partir delas são os principais locais de transferência de líquido. VER TAMBÉM arachnoid *granulations*, em *granulation*.
  chorionic villi, vilosidades coriônicas; os processos vasculares do córion do embrião que entram na formação da placenta.
  floating v., v. flutuante, v. livre. SIN free v.
  free v., v. livre; uma v. coriônica que não está fixada à decídua basal, mas está "livre" no sangue materno dos espaços intervilosos. SIN floating v.
  intestinal villi [TA], vilosidades intestinais; projeções (0,5–1,5 mm de comprimento) da mucosa do intestino delgado; têm formato de folha no duodeno e tornam-se mais curtas, mais digitiformes e mais escassas no íleo. SIN villi intestinales [TA].
  vil′li intestina′les [TA], vilosidades intestinais. SIN intestinal villi.
  vil′li pericardi′aci [TA], vilosidades pericárdicas. SIN pericardial villi.
  pericardial villi [TA], vilosidades pericárdicas; diminutas projeções filiformes (vilosidades sinoviais) a partir da superfície do pericárdio seroso. SIN villi pericardiaci [TA].
  peritoneal villi [TA], vilosidades peritoneais; vilosidades sinoviais na superfície do peritônio. SIN villi peritoneales [TA].
  vil′li peritonea′les [TA], vilosidades peritoneais. SIN peritoneal villi.
  pleural villi [TA], vilosidades pleurais; apêndices emaranhados (vilosidades sinoviais) na pleura nas vizinhanças do seio costomediastinal. SIN villi pleurales [TA].
  vil′li pleura′les [TA], vilosidades pleurais. SIN pleural villi.
  primary v., v. primária; o primeiro estágio do desenvolvimento da v. coriônica, com as colunas de células citotrofoblásticas cobertas por sinciciotrofoblasto.
  secondary v., v. secundária; um estágio intermediário do desenvolvimento da v. coriônica após a invasão por um cerne de tecido conjuntivo.
  synovial villi [TA], vilosidades sinoviais; pequenos processos vasculares que partem de uma membrana sinovial. SIN villi synoviales [TA], synovial fringe, synovial tufts.
  vil′li synovia′les [TA], vilosidades sinoviais. SIN synovial villi.
  tertiary v., v. terciária; a v. coriônica definitiva com um cerne vascular separado do sangue por tecido conjuntivo, citotrofoblasto e sinciciotrofoblasto.

vi·men·tin (vī-men′tin). Vimentina; o principal polipeptídeo que se copolimeriza com outras subunidades para formar o citoesqueleto filamentar intermediário das células mesenquimatosas; participariam na manutenção da organização interna de determinadas células. VER TAMBÉM desmina.

vin·blas·tine sul·fate (vin-blas′tēn). Sulfato de vimblastina; um alcalóide dimérico obtido a partir da *Vinca rosea*; pára a mitose na metáfase (embora a vincristina seja mais ativa nesse sentido) e exibe maior atividade antimetabólica que a vincristina; usada no tratamento da doença de Hodgkin, coriocarcinoma, leucemias agudas e crônicas e em outras doenças neoplásicas; bloqueia o agrupamento de microtúbulos. SIN vincaleucoblastine.

vin·ca·leu·co·blas·tine (ving′kă-loo-kō-blas′tēn). Vincaleucoblastina. SIN vinblastine sulfate.

Vin·ca ro·sea (ving′kă rō′zē-ă). Pervinca; uma espécie de murta (família Myrtaceae) usada em várias partes do mundo como remédio caseiro; dois alcalóides diméricos ativos, obtidos a partir dessa planta, são a vimblastina e a vincristina. SIN periwinkle.

Vincent, Henri, médico frances, 1862–1950. VER V. *angina, bacillus, disease, infection, spirillum, tonsillitis.*

vin·cris·tine sul·fate (vin-kris′tēn). Sulfato de vincristina; um alcalóide dimérico obtido a partir da *Vinca rosea*; sua atividade antineoplásica é similar à da vimblastina, mas não surge resistência cruzada entre esses dois agentes, sendo mais útil que a vimblastina no linfossarcoma linfocítico e na leucemia aguda. SIN leurocristine.

vin·cu·lin (ving′koo-lin). Vinculina; uma proteína associada aos microfilamentos da actina; encontrada nos discos intercalados do músculo cardíaco e nas placas de adesão focal; pode ter um papel em como um vírus tumoral causa efeitos pleotrópicos de transformação. [L. *vinculum*, ligação, de *vincio*, ligar + *-in*]

vin·cu·lum, pl. **vin·cu·la** (ving′koo-lŭm, -lă) [TA]. Vínculo, frênulo; freio ou ligamento. [L. grilhão, de *vincio*, ligar]
  v. bre′ve digitorum manus [TA], v. curto dos dedos das mãos. SIN v. breve of fingers. VER TAMBÉM vincula tendinea of digits of hand and foot.
  v. breve of fingers [TA], v. curto dos dedos das mãos; uma faixa triangular que se estende a partir da superfície dorsal de cada um dos tendões flexores de um dedo até a cápsula da articulação interfalângica próxima e até a falange proximal à inserção do tendão. SIN v. breve digitorum manus [TA], short v.
  v. lin′guae, frênulo da língua. SIN frenulum of tongue.
  vin′cula lin′gulae cerebell′i, frênulos da língua do cerebelo; pequenos prolongamentos laterais da língua do verme do cerebelo que repousam sobre a superfície dorsal do pedúnculo cerebelar superior.
  long v., v. longo. SIN v. longum of fingers.
  v. lon′gum digitorum manus [TA], v. longo dos dedos das mãos. SIN v. longum of fingers. VER TAMBÉM vincula tendinea of digits of hand and foot.
  v. longum of fingers [TA], v. longo dos dedos das mãos; uma faixa longa e filiforme que se estende da superfície dorsal de cada um dos tendões flexores de um dedo até a falange proximal. SIN v. longum digitorum manus [TA], long v.
  v. prepu′tii, frênulo do prepúcio. SIN frenulum of prepuce.
  short v., v. curto. SIN v. breve of fingers.
  vincula tendinea of digits of hand and foot [TA], vínculos tendíneos dos dedos das mãos e dos pés; feixes fibrosos que se estendem desde os tendões flexores dos dedos e dos artelhos até as cápsulas das articulações interfalângicas e falanges; conduzem pequenos vasos até os tendões. SIN synovial frena, synovial frenula, vincula of tendons, vincula tendinum digitorum manus et pedis.
  vin′cula ten′dinum digitorum manus et pedis, vínculos tendíneos dos dedos das mãos e dos pés. SIN vincula tendinea of digits of hand and foot. VER TAMBÉM v. breve of fingers, v. longum of fingers.
  vincula of tendons, vínculos tendíneos. SIN vincula tendinea of digits of hand and foot.

vin·de·sine (vin′dĕ-sēn). Vindesina; derivado sintético da vimblastina com a qual compartilha propriedades antineoplásicas. Usada no tratamento da leucemia linfocítica da infância.

Vineberg, Arthur M., cirurgião torácico canadense, 1903–1988. VER V. *procedure.*

vin·e·gar (vin′ē-găr). Vinagre; ácido acético diluído impuro, feito a partir de vinho, cidra, malte, etc. SIN acetum. [Fr. *vinaigre*, de *vin*, vinho, + *aigre*, azedo]
  mother of v., borra de vinagre; no vinagre, o fungo da fermentação acetosa que aparece como um sedimento viscoso. [A.S. *modder*, lama]
  pyroligneous v., v. pirolenhoso. SIN wood v.
  wood v., v. da madeira; o ácido acético impuro produzido pela destilação destrutiva da madeira e do alcatrão do pinheiro. SIN pyroligneous v.

vi·nic (vī′nik). Vínico; relativo, pertencente a ou extraído do vinho. [L. *vinum*, vinho]

vi·nous (vī′nŭs). Vinhoso, vinoso; relativo a, que contém ou da natureza do vinho.

Vinson, Porter P., cirurgião norte-americano, 1890–1959. VER Plummer-V. *syndrome.*

vi·nyl (vī′nil). Vinil, vinila; o radical hidrocarboneto, $CH_2=CH-$. SIN ethenyl.
  v. carbinol, carbinol vinílico. SIN allyl alcohol.
  v. chloride, cloreto vinílico; uma substância utilizada na indústria de plásticos e suspeita de ser um potente carcinógeno em seres humanos. SIN chloroethylene.

vi·nyl ben·ze·ne (vī′nil-ben′zēn). Vinilbenzeno. SIN styrene.

vi·nyl·ene (vī′nil-ēn). Vinileno; o radical bivalente, $-CH=CH-$. SIN ethenylene.

vi·nyl·i·dene (vī-nil′i-dēn). Vinilideno; o radical bivalente, $H_2C=C=$.

vi·o·la·ceous (vī-ō-lā′shŭs). Violáceo; de coloração púrpura, usualmente a pele. [L. *viola*, violeta]

vi·o·let (vī′ō-let). Violeta; a cor produzida por comprimentos de onda do espectro visível menores que 450 nm. Para os corantes violeta individuais, ver o nome específico. [L. *viola*]
  Hoffman v., v. de Hoffman; dália.
  visual v., v. visual, iodopsina. SIN iodopsin.

vi·o·my·cin (vī-ō-mī′sin). Viomicina; um agente antibiótico obtido de *Streptomyces puniceus* var. *floridae*; ativa contra bactérias álcool-ácido-resistentes, incluindo as cepas do bacilo da tuberculose resistentes à estreptomicina; pode causar lesão vestibular e surdez.

vi·os·ter·ol (vī-os′ter-ōl). Viosterol. SIN ergocalciferol.

VIP Abreviatura para vasoactive intestinal *polypeptide* (polipeptídeo intestinal vasoativo).

vi·per (vī′per). Víbora; um membro da família de cobras Viperidae. [L. *vipera*, serpente, cobra]
  Russell's v., v. de Russell; cobra extremamente venenosa (*Vipera russellii*), com marcas características, do Sudeste asiático. O veneno tem ação coagulante

e é usado localmente, em uma solução de 1:10.000, para conter a hemorragia na hemofilia.

Vi·per·i·dae (vī-per′i-dē). Uma família de cobras venenosas do Velho Mundo, as víboras verdadeiras, composta de cerca de 50 espécies e caracterizada por duas presas caniculadas relativamente longas na frente da mandíbula superior, as quais estão inseridas em ossos móveis, permitindo que fiquem eretas durante a picada, quando a boca está aberta, e dobradas para dentro de uma prega cutânea do palato, quando as mandíbulas estão fechadas. [L. *vipera*, víbora]

VI·Po·ma (vi-pō′mă). Vipoma; um tumor endócrino, originado usualmente no pâncreas e produtor de um polipeptídeo intestinal vasoativo tido como responsável por alterações eletrolíticas e cardiovasculares profundas, com hipotensão vasodilatadora, diarréia aquosa, hipopotassemia e desidratação. [*v*asoactive *i*ntestinal *p*olypeptide + G. *-ōma*, tumor]

Vipond, médico francês. VER V. *sign.*

vip·ryn·i·um em·bo·nate (vip-rin′ē-ŭm em′bō-nāt). Embonato de viprínio. SIN pyrvinium pamoate.

vir·a·gin·i·ty (vir′ă-jin′i-tē). Viraginidade; um termo raramente utilizado para descrever qualidades psicológicas masculinas pronunciadas em uma mulher. [L. *virago* (*viragin-*), uma mulher guerreira]

vi·ral (vī′răl). Viral, virótico; de, pertinente a ou causado por um vírus.

Virchow, Rudolf L.K., político e patologista alemão, 1821–1902. VER V. *angle, cells,* em *cell, corpuscles,* em *corpuscle,* em *crystal, disease, node, psammoma;* V.-Holder *angle;* V.-Hassall *bodies,* em *body;* V.-Robin *space.*

vi·re·mia (vi-rē′mē-ă). Viremia; a presença de vírus na corrente sanguínea. [virus + G. *haima*, sangue]

vi·res (vī′rēz). Forças; energias; plural de vis.

vir·ga (vir′gă). Verga. SIN penis. [L. um bastão]

vir·gin (ver′jin). Virgem. 1. Uma pessoa que nunca teve uma relação sexual. 2. Puro; não-utilizado; não-contaminado. SIN virginal (2). [L. *virgo* (*virgin-*), donzela]

vir·gin·al (ver′ji-năl). Virginal. 1. Relativo a uma virgem. 2. Puro. SIN virgin (2). [L. *virginalis*]

vir·gin·i·ty (ver-jin′i-tē). Virgindade; estado ou atributo do que é virgem. [L. *virginitas*]

vir·go·phre·nia (ver-gō-frē′nē-ă). Virgofrenia; um termo raramente usado para a mente receptiva, capaz e retentora do jovem. [L. *virgo*, donzela, + G. *phrēn*, mente]

vir·i·ci·dal (vī-ri-sī′dă). Viricida, virucida. SIN virucidal.

vir·i·cide (vī′ri-sīd). Viricida, virucida. SIN virucide.

△ **-viridae.** Sufixo que indica uma família de vírus. [L. *virus*, veneno]

vir·ile (vir′il). Viril. 1. Relativo ao sexo masculino. 2. Másculo, forte, masculino. 3. Que possui traços masculinos. [L. *virilis*, masculino, de *vir*, um homem]

vir·i·les·cence (vir-i-les′ens). Virilescência; um termo raramente empregado para a adoção de características masculinas pela mulher.

vi·ril·ia (vi-ril′ē-ă). Os órgãos sexuais masculinos. [L. pl. neut. de *virilis*, viril]

vir·i·lism (vir′i-lizm). Virilismo; a posse de características somáticas masculinas maduras por uma menina, mulher ou homem pré-púbere; pode existir ao nascimento ou pode aparecer mais adiante, dependendo de sua causa; pode ser relativamente leve (p.ex., hirsutismo) ou grave e, comumente, resulta de disfunção gonadal ou adrenocortical, ou de terapia androgênica. [L. *virilis*, masculino] **adrenal v.,** v. adrenal, v. supra-renal; v. produzido por padrões secretores excessivos ou anormais dos esteróides adrenocorticais. SIN adrenal virilizing syndrome.

vi·ril·i·ty (vi-ril′i-tē). Virilidade; a condição ou qualidade de ser viril. [L. *virilitas*, masculinidade, de *vir*, homem]

vir·i·li·za·tion (vir′i-li-zā′shŭn). Virilização; produção ou aquisição do virilismo.

vir·i·liz·ing (vir′i-līz-ing). Virilizante; que causa virilismo.

△ **-virinae.** Terminação que indica uma subfamília de vírus.

vi·ri·on (vī′rē-on, vir′ē-on). Vírion; a partícula viral completa que está estruturalmente intacta e é infecciosa.

vi·rip·o·tent (vir-i-pō′tent, vī-rip′ō-tent). Viripotente; termo obsoleto que indica um macho sexualmente maduro. [L. *viripotens*, de *vir*, homem, + *potens*, que tem força]

vi·roid (vī′royd). Viróide; um patógeno infeccioso dos vegetais que é menor que um vírus (PM 75.000-100.000) e difere deste por consistir apenas de RNA circular fechado de filamento único, sem revestimento proteico (capsídeo); a replicação não depende de um vírus auxiliar, mas é mediada por enzimas da célula do hospedeiro. [virus + G. *eidos*, semelhança]

vi·rol·o·gist (vī′rol′ō-jist). Virologista; um especialista em virologia.

vi·rol·o·gy (vi-rol′ō-jē, vi-). Virologia; o estudo dos vírus e da doença viral. [virus + G. *logos*, estudo]

vi·ro·pex·is (vī-rō-pek′sis). Viropexia; a ligação do vírus a uma célula e subseqüente absorção (engolfamento) das partículas virais por esta célula. [viro- + G. *pēxis*, fixação]

vi·ru·ci·dal (vī-rū-sī′dăl). Virucida, viricida; que extermina vírus. SIN viricidal.

vi·ru·ci·de (vī-rū-sīd). Virucida, viricida; um agente ativo contra as infecções virais. SIN viricide. [vírus + L. *caedo*, matar]

vi·ru·co·pria (vī-rū-kō′prē-ă). Virucopria; presença de vírus nas fezes. [vírus + G. *kopros*, fezes]

vir·u·lence (vir′oo-lens). Virulência; a capacidade de provocar doença de um patógeno; numericamente expresso como a relação entre o número de casos de infecção franca e o número total de infectados, conforme determinado por imunoensaio. [L. *virulentia*, de *virulentus*, venenoso]

vir·u·lent (vir′oo-lent). Virulento; extremamente tóxico, indicando um microrganismo muito patogênico. [L. *virulentus*, venenoso]

vir·u·lif·er·ous (vī-rū-lif′er-ŭs). Virulífero; que conduz vírus.

vir·u·ria (vī-roo′rē-ă). Virúria; a presença de vírus na urina. [virus + G. *ouron*, urina]

VIRUS

vi·rus, pl. **vi·rus·es** (vī′rŭs). Vírus. 1. Originalmente, o agente específico de uma doença infecciosa. 2. Especificamente, um termo para um grupo de agentes infecciosos, os quais, com poucas exceções, são capazes de atravessar filtros com microporos que retêm a maioria das bactérias; geralmente não são visíveis à microscopia óptica, não têm metabolismo independente e são incapazes de crescer ou de se reproduzir fora de células vivas. Possuem um aparelho genético procariótico, mas diferem muito das bactérias em outros aspectos. Em geral, a partícula completa contém DNA ou RNA, e não ambos, e está comumente revestida por uma "concha" proteína ou capsídeo, que protege o ácido nucleico. Variam de tamanho, desde 15 nanômetros a várias centenas de nanômetros. A classificação dos vírus depende das características fisioquímicas dos víons, bem como da modalidade de transmissão, gama de hospedeiros, sintomatologia e outros fatores. Para os vírus não arrolados adiante, ver nome específico. SIN filtrable v. 3. Relacionado a ou causado por um v., como uma doença viral. 4. (Uso obsoleto) Antes da era da bacteriologia, qualquer agente que provocasse doença, incluindo uma substância química, como uma enzima ("fermento") semelhante ao veneno de cobra; sinônimo, outrora, de "veneno". [L. veneno]

Abelson murine leukemia v., da leucemia murina de Abelson; um retrovírus que pertence à subfamília do grupo do retrovírus do tipo C, família Retroviridae, que está associado à leucemia e induz transformação *in vitro* de determinadas células de camundongo.

adeno-associated v. (AAV), v. adeno-associado. SIN Dependovirus.
adenoidal-pharyngeal-cojunctival v., v. adenovírus. SIN adenovirus.
adenosatellite v., v. adeno-satélite. SIN Dependovirus.
AIDS-related v., v. ligado à AIDS; termo obsoleto para o vírus da imunodeficiência humana (HIV).
Akabane v., Akabane, um v. do gênero Bunyavirus, família Bunyaviridae, que provoca aborto no gado e artrogripose congênita e hidranencefalia nos fetos bovinos em Israel, no Japão e na Austrália; é transmitido por mosquitos.
amphotropic v., v. anfotrópico; um v. usualmente associado aos retrovírus que pode não produzir doença em seu hospedeiro natural, mas que se replica nas células de cultura de tecidos da espécie hospedeira, bem como em células de outras espécies.
Andes v., v. Andes; uma espécie de Hantavirus na Argentina que provoca síndrome pulmonar.
animal viruses, vírus animais; os vírus que ocorrem em seres humanos e em outros animais, causando infecção inaparente ou produzindo doença.
A-P-C v., adenovírus. SIN adenovirus.
Argentine hemorrhagic fever v., v. da febre hemorrágica da Argentina; um membro da família Arenaviridae.
attenuated v., v. atenuado; uma cepa variante de um v. patogênico, modificada de modo a provocar a produção de anticorpos protetores, mas sem produzir a doença específica.
Aujeszky disease v., v. da doença de Aujeszky. SIN pseudorabies v.
Australian X disease v., v. da doença X australiana. SIN Murray Valley encephalitis v.
avian encephalomyelitis v., v. da encefalomielite aviária; um v. do gênero Enterovirus, família Picornaviridae, que provoca a encefalomielite infecciosa aviária em pintos.
avian influenza v., v. da *influenza* das aves; um v. influenza do tipo A que provoca a peste aviária.
avian lymphomatosis v., v. da neurolinfomatose aviária. SIN avian neurolymphomatosis v.
avian neurolymphomatosis v., v. da neurolinfomatose aviária; o herpesvírus que causa a linfomatose aviária (doença de Marek); é diferente daqueles que causam outras formas de leucose. SIN avian lymphomatosis v., Marek disease v.

embriopatia viral

infecções virais durante a gravidez e suas possíveis conseqüências para a criança (embriopatia, fetopatia, infecção perinetal)

vírus	sintomas de infecção durante a 1.ª à 14.ª semana de gestação	sintomas de infecção a partir da 15.ª semana até o nascimento	sintomas de infecção logo antes do nascimento, ou perinatais
citomegalovírus	aborto, microcefalia	encefalite, hepatoesplenomegalia, coriorretinite, nascimento prematuro, trombocitopenia, lesão cerebral mínima	citomegalia
rubéola	aborto, defeitos cardíacos, catarata, microftalmia, deficiência auditiva, etc.	encefalite, hepatoesplenomegalia, trombocitopenia, nascimento prematuro	—
sarampo	microcefalia, defeitos cardíacos, atresia anal, etc.	morte fetal, nascimento prematuro	sarampo
herpes simples I e II	casos isolados: microftalmia, microcefalia coriorretinite	—	infecção generalizada por herpes, encefalite fatal
varicela-zoster	casos isolados: deformidade ocular, lesão cerebral	encefalite, exantema, nascimento prematuro	varicela generalizada
Coxsackie B	—	—	encefalite, miocardite, hepatite
caxumba	casos isolados: aborto	—	—
coriomeningite linfocítica	aborto (?)	casos isolados: encefalite, coriorretinite	—
hepatite B	—	—	hepatite (parcialmente crônica)
hepatite C	—	—	hepatite
poliomielite	aborto	morte fetal, nascimento prematuro	poliomielite

avian pneumoencephalitis v., v. da pneumoencefalite aviária. SIN Newcastle disease v.
avian viral arthritis v., v. da artrite aviária; um v. do gênero Reovirus, família Reoviridae, que causa tenossinovite e artrite em galinhas.
B v., v. B. SIN cercopithecrine *herpesvirus.* SIN monkey B v.
B 19 v., v. B19; um parvovírus humano associado à artrite e à artralgia e a inúmeras entidades clínicas específicas, incluindo eritema infeccioso e crise aplásica na vigência de anemia hemolítica.
bacterial v., um v. que "infecta" as bactérias; um bacteriófago.
Barmah Forest v., v. da Floresta de Barmah; uma espécie de Alphavirus que provocou surtos de poliartrite em seres humanos na Austrália; transmitido por mosquitos. [o vírus foi isolado pela primeira vez em mosquitos coletados na Floresta de Barmah, no sudeste da Austrália, em 1974]
Bayou v., v. Bayou; uma espécie de Hantavirus nos Estados Unidos que causa síndrome pulmonar; transmitido pelo rato-do-mato (gênero Oryzomys).
Bittner v. (bit′ner). v. Bittner. SIN mammary tumor v. of mice.
BK v., v. BK; um poliomavírus humano, da família Papovaviridae, de distribuição mundial, que provoca infecções renais usualmente subclínicas em pessoas imunocompetentes. [iniciais do paciente no qual foi isolado pela primeira vez]
Black Creek Canal v., v. do canal de Black Creek; uma espécie de Hantavirus nos Estados Unidos que provoca síndrome pulmonar; transmitido pelo rato do algodão. [Canal de Black Creek, na Flórida, onde foram capturados os ratos do algodão nos quais o vírus foi isolado pela primeira vez]
bluetongue v., v. da língua azul; um v. do gênero Orbivirus, da família Reoviridae; o agente da língua azul em carneiros.
Bolivian hemorrhagic fever v., v. da febre hemorrágica boliviana; um membro do grupo Arenavirus de vírus com filamento único de RNA, também conhecidos como v. Machupo; o principal reservatório está nos roedores; produz múltiplas anormalidades no sistema de coagulação, incluindo síndrome de extravasamento capilar disseminado, que pode ser fatal.
Borna disease v., v. da doença de Borna; um v. RNA de filamento único, com sentido negativo, não-classificado, que é a causa da doença de Borna, uma doença grave de eqüinos que envolve a infecção do sistema nervoso central. SIN enzootic encephalomyelitis v.
Bornholm disease v., v. da doença de Bornholm. SIN epidemic pleurodynia v.
bovine leukemia v. (BLV), v. da leucemia bovina; retrovírus BLV-HTLV, da família Retroviridae, que infecta comumente o gado bovino, especialmente as vacas leiteiras; em uma pequena proporção do gado infectado, provocará leucose bovina enzoótica. SIN bovine leukosis v.
bovine leukosis v., v. da leucose bovina. SIN bovine leukemia v.

bovine papular stomatitis v., v. da estomatite papular bovina; um poxvírus do gênero Parapoxvirus, relatado na América do Norte, África e Europa, causando estomatite papular bovina.
bovine virus diarrhea v., v. da diarréia viral bovina; um v. do gênero Pestivirus, da família Flaviviridae, causando diarréia viral bovina; são reconhecidas as cepas New York, Oregon e Indiana do v. SIN mucosal disease v.
Bunyamwera v., v. Bunyamwera; um grupo sorológico do gênero Bunyavirus, composto por mais de 150 tipos de v. da família Bunyaviridae. [*Bunyamwera*, Uganda, onde foi isolado pela primeira vez]
Bwamba v., v. Bwamba; uma espécie de Bunyavirus da família Bunyaviridae; associado a casos de febre Bwamba em Uganda. [*Bwamba*, floresta em Uganda onde foi isolado pela primeira vez]
CA v., v. CA; abreviatura para croup-associated v. (v. associado ao crupe).
California v., v. Califórnia; um grupo sorológico do gênero Bunyavirus, compreendendo cerca de 14 cepas, incluindo os v. La Crosse e Tahyna e a cepa típica, o v. Califórnia, que provoca encefalite, principalmente no grupo etário de 4–14 anos.
canine distemper v., v. da cinomose; um v. RNA do gênero Morbillivirus, um membro da família Paramyxoviridae, que causa a cinomose. SIN dog distemper v.
Capim viruses, vírus Capim; um grupo sorológico do gênero Bunyavirus, cuja espécie típica é o v. Capim.
Caraparu v., v. Caraparu; uma espécie de Bunyavirus do grupo C e um agente de encefalite.
Catu v., v. Catu; um arbovírus do gênero Bunyavirus, da família Bunyaviridae; um agente de encefalite.
CELO v., v. CELO; um v. no gênero Aviadenovirus e similar ao v. da bronquite da codorna. SIN chicken embryo lethal orphan v.
Central European tick-borne encephalitis v., v. da encefalite centro-européia transmitida por carrapato; um dos vírus do complexo de arbovírus do grupo B (gênero Flavivirus) transmitido por carrapato; o agente causal da encefalite transmitida por carrapato (subtipo centro-europeu).
C group viruses, vírus do grupo C; um grupo sorológico do gênero Bunyavirus (originalmente denominados arbovírus do grupo C), composto de cerca de 14 espécies, incluindo os v. Caraparu, Murutucu e Oriboca.
Chagres v., v. Chagres; um v. no gênero Phlebovirus, família Bunyaviridae, um agente de encefalite.
chicken embryo lethal orphan v., v. órfão letal do embrião de galinha. SIN CELO v.
chickenpox v., v. da varicela. SIN varicella-zoster v.
chikungunya v., v. chikungunya; um arbovírus do gênero Alphavirus, família Togaviridae, transmitido por mosquito, encontrado em regiões da África e na

Índia, Tailândia e Malásia; causa uma doença febril semelhante ao dengue, com dores articulares. [denominado segundo a posição "encurvada" das pessoas por ele infectadas]

Coe v., v. Coe; nome obsoleto para a cepa A-21 do vírus Coxsackie; a causa de uma doença semelhante ao resfriado comum em recrutas militares.

cold v., v. do resfriado. SIN common cold v.

Colorado tick fever v., v. da febre do carrapato do Colorado; um v. do gênero Coltivirus, da família Reoviridae, encontrado na região das Montanhas Rochosas dos Estados Unidos e transmitido pelo carrapato *Dermacentor andersoni*; provoca a febre do carrapato do Colorado.

Columbia S. K. v., v. Columbia S. K.; uma cepa do v. da encefalomiocardite.

common cold v., v. do resfriado comum; qualquer uma das inúmeras cepas de v. etiologicamente associados ao resfriado comum, principalmente os rinovírus, mas também a cepas de adenovírus, vírus Coxsackie, vírus ECHO e v. parainfluenza. SIN cold v.

contagious ecthyma (pustular dermatitis) v. of sheep, v. da ectima contagiosa (dermatite pustular) do carneiro; o poxvírus do gênero Parapoxvirus que provoca a ectima contagiosa (dermatite pustular) do carneiro. SIN soremouth v.

contagious pustular stomatitis v., v. da estomatite pustular contagiosa; **(1)** SIN horsepox v.; **(2)** SIN orf v.

Côte-d'Ivoire virus, v. da Costa do Marfim; uma variante do vírus Ebola. SIN Ebola v. Côte-d'Ivoire.

cowpox v., v. da vacínia; um v. do gênero Orthopoxvirus que provoca a vacínia.

coxsackie v., vírus Coxsackie. VER coxsackievirus.

Crimean-Congo hemorrhagic fever v., v. da febre hemorrágica da Criméia-Congo; um v. do gênero Nairovirus, família Bunyaviridae, oriundo da África e transmitido por carrapatos (Hyalomma e Amblyomma), sendo encontrado no sangue humano; a causa da febre hemorrágica da Criméia-Congo.

croup-associated v. (CA v.), v. associado a crupe (v. CA); v. parainfluenza dos tipos 1 e 2. VER parainfluenza viruses.

cytopathogenic v., v. citopatogênico; um v. cuja multiplicação leva a alterações degenerativas na célula hospedeira. VER TAMBÉM cytopathic *effect*.

defective v., v. defeituoso; uma partícula viral que não contém ácido nucleico suficiente para produzir todos os componentes virais essenciais; por conseguinte, não é produzido v. infeccioso, exceto em determinadas situações (p.ex., quando a célula hospedeira também é infectada por um v. "auxiliar").

delta v., v. delta. SIN hepatitis D v.

dengue v., v. do dengue; um v. do gênero Flavivirus, com cerca de 50 nm de diâmetro; o agente etiológico do dengue em seres humanos e que também ocorre em macacos e chimpanzés, usualmente como uma infecção inaparente; quatro sorotipos são reconhecidos; a transmissão é efetuada por mosquitos do gênero *Aedes*.

distemper v., v. da cinomose. VER canine distemper v.

DNA v., v. DNA; um importante grupo de vírus animais cujo cerne consiste em ácido desoxirribonucleico (DNA); inclui parvovírus, papovavírus, adenovírus, herpesvírus, poxvírus e outros vírus DNA não classificados. SIN deoxyribovirus.

dog distemper v., v. da cinomose. SIN canine distemper v.

duck hepatitis v., v. da hepatite do pato; um v. DNA do gênero Hepadnavirus, da família Hepadnaviridae, causando a hepatite viral dos patos.

duck influenza v., v. da influenza do pato; um v. influenza A, um membro da família Orthomyxoviridae, diferente das cepas do vírus influenza A humano com base na inibição da hemaglutinação.

duck plague v., v. da peste do pato; um herpesvírus que causa a peste do pato.

Duvenhage v., v. Duvenhage; uma espécie de Lyssavirus que provoca uma doença semelhante à raiva, em seres humanos, na África; transmitido pela picada de morcegos insetívoros. [o vírus foi denominado em homenagem à sua primeira vítima, um homem infectado próximo à Pretória, na África do Sul]

eastern equine encephalomyelitis v., v. da encefalomielite eqüina do leste; um v. do gênero Alphavirus (originalmente arbovírus do grupo A), da família Togaviridae, que ocorre no leste dos Estados Unidos; normalmente é encontrado em determinados pássaros selvagens e pequenos roedores como uma infecção inaparente, mas é capaz de provocar a encefalomielite eqüina do leste, em cavalos e seres humanos, após a transferência pelas picadas de mosquitos culicídeos. SIN EEE v.

EB v., v. EB. SIN Epstein-Barr v.

Ebola v., v. Ebola; um v. da família Filoviridae, morfologicamente similar, mas antigenicamente diferente, ao v. Marburg; a causa da febre Ebola (febre hemorrágica viral). A transmissão é parenteral, não-oral, sexual ou por inalação. Após um período de incubação de aproximadamente 1 semana, a doença aparece de maneira aguda, com febre, cefaléia, vômitos e diarréia, fraqueza e erupção maculopapular. O sangramento gastrointestinal e outras manifestações hemorrágicas, inclusive coagulação intravascular disseminada, surgem em um alto percentual de casos e, com freqüência, são fatais. A taxa de fatalidade por caso aproxima-se de 80%. Não há prevenção nem tratamento específicos.

O vírus Ebola foi manchete em 1995, quando um surto repentino e devastador ocorreu em Kikwit, Zaire. Nesse grupo, que envolveu inúmeros profissionais de saúde, 315 pessoas foram infectadas, das quais 243 morreram (77%). A maioria dos casos no surto de Kikwit foi atribuída à reutilização, em clínicas e hospitais, de equipamentos médicos e cirúrgicos não-esterilizados, contaminados com sangue, vômitos, fezes e urina dos pacientes. No ano seguinte, dois grandes surtos aconteceram no Gabão. Os estudos sorológicos dos pacientes no Gabão sugeriram que a sobrevida depende da formação precoce de anticorpo IgG contra a proteína da cápsula viral. Apesar dos relatos sensacionalistas e exagerados pelos meios de comunicação, epidemias da doença pelo vírus Ebola e outras febres hemorrágicas virais não ocorrem quando são empregadas as medidas de controle de infecção padronizadas. As futuras epidemias ocorrerão nos países do Terceiro Mundo, enquanto a pobreza e a ignorância levarem a práticas inseguras de cuidados de saúde, mas a doença não representa risco de disseminação epidêmica nos países desenvolvidos.

Ebola v. Côte-d'Ivoire, v. Ebola da Costa do Marfim. SIN Côte-d'Ivoire virus.

Ebola v. Reston, v. Ebola Reston. SIN Reston v.

Ebola v. Sudan, v. Ebola do Sudão. SIN Sudan v.

Ebola v. Zaire, v. Ebola do Zaire. SIN Zaire v.

ECHO v., v. ECHO; um enterovírus de um grande grupo de vírus não-correlatos que pertence à família Picornaviridae, isolado de seres humanos; embora existam muitas infecções inaparentes, parte dos vários sorotipos estão associados à febre e à meningite asséptica, e alguns parecem causar doença respiratória branda. SIN echovirus, enteric cytopathogenic human orphan v.

ECMO v., v. ECMO; picornavírus de símios isolados de células renais e fezes de macaco. SIN enteric cytopathogenic monkey orphan v.

ecotropic v., v. ecotrópico; um retrovírus que não produz doença em seu hospedeiro natural, mas se replica em células de cultura de tecidos derivadas da espécie de hospedeiro.

vírus tumorais que contêm DNA representativos

vírus	hospedeiro de origem	tumores naturais (hospedeiro de origem)
papovavírus		
polioma	camundongo	não
SV40	macaco	não
BK, JC	ser humano	não
papiloma humano	ser humano	sim
coelho	coelho	sim
bovino	vaca	sim
adenovírus		
humano (vários tipos)	humano	não
símio (alguns)	macaco	não
herpesvírus		
ser humano		
herpes simples do tipo 2	ser humano	
vírus Epstein-Barr	ser humano	sim
citomegalovírus	ser humano	
macaco	macaco	não
aves (Marek)	galinha	sim
rã (Lucké)	rã	sim
Hepadnavírus		
hepatite B humana	ser humano	sim
hepatite da marmota	marmota	sim
poxvírus		
molusco contagioso	ser humano	sim
Yaba	macaco	sim
fibroma-mixoma	coelho, cervo	sim

ECSO v., v. ECSO; um picornavírus isolado de surtos de enterite em suínos, mas não se sabe se constitui um patógeno natural. SIN enteric cytopathogenic swine orphan v.

ectromelia v., v. da ectromelia. SIN infectious ectromelia v.

EEE v., v. EEE. SIN eastern equine encephalomyelitis v.

EMC v., v. EMC. SIN encephalomyocarditis v.

emerging viruses, vírus emergentes; em epidemiologia, uma classe de vírus que há muito tempo infecta seres humanos ou animais, porém agora tem a oportunidade de atingir proporções epidêmicas devido à entrada de seres humanos em florestas tropicais, aumento das viagens internacionais, crescimento das populações em países menos desenvolvidos e, possivelmente, mutações. Inúmeros vírus têm sido denominados emergentes, inclusive vírus hemorrágicos, como Ebola, Marburg e Hantaan; vírus Mokola e Duvenhage semelhantes ao vírus da raiva; vírus Junin e Lassa transmitidos por roedores; e dengue, transmitido por mosquito. Os virologistas especulam que a cepa de HIV que causa AIDS/SIDA também pode situar-se nessa categoria, tendo acometido os seres humanos através do contato com os macacos na África Central, tendo possivelmente existido entre as populações de macacos há cerca de 50.000 anos.

encephalitis v., v. da encefalite; qualquer um de vários vírus que causam encefalite.

encephalomyocarditis v., v. da encefalomiocardite; um Cardiovirus na família Picornaviridae, usualmente oriundo de roedores, isolado do sangue e das fezes de seres humanos, outros primatas, porcos e coelhos; ocasionalmente causa doença febril, com envolvimento do sistema nervoso central em seres humanos, e uma miocardite freqüentemente fatal em chimpanzés, macacos e porcos; as cepas desse v. incluem v. Columbia S. K. e v. Mengo. SIN EMC v.

enteric viruses, vírus entéricos; os vírus do gênero Enterovirus.

enteric cytopathogenic human orphan v., v. órfão enterocitopatogênico humano. SIN ECHO v.

enteric cytopathogenic monkey orphan v., v. órfão enterocitopatogênico do macaco. SIN ECMO v.

enteric cytopathogenic swine orphan v., v. órfão enterocitopatogênico suíno. SIN ECSO v.

enteric orphan viruses, vírus órfãos entéricos; enterovírus isolados de seres humanos e outros animais; o termo "órfão" implica a carência de associação conhecida com a doença quando isolado; muitos vírus do grupo são agora conhecidos como sendo patogênicos; eles incluem vírus ECBO, vírus ECHO e vírus ECSO.

enzootic encephalomyelitis v., v. da encefalomielite enzoótica. SIN Borna disease v.

ephemeral fever v., v. da febre transitória; um rhabdovírus que causa a febre transitória do gado.

epidemic gastroenteritis v., v. da gastrenterite epidêmica; um v. RNA, com cerca de 27 nm de diâmetro, que ainda não foi cultivado *in vitro*; é a causa de gastrenterite não-bacteriana epidêmica; pelo menos cinco sorotipos antigenicamente distintos já foram reconhecidos, incluindo o agente Norwalk. Esses vírus são classificados com os Calicivírus na família Caliciviridae. SIN gastroenteritis v. type A.

epidemic keratoconjunctivitis v., v. da ceratoconjuntivite epidêmica; um adenovírus (tipo 8) que causa ceratoconjuntivite epidêmica, especialmente entre trabalhadores de estaleiros, estando também associada a surtos de conjuntivite em piscinas. SIN shipyard eye.

epidemic myalgia v., v. da mialgia epidêmica. SIN epidemic pleurodynia v.

epidemic parotitis v., v. da parotidite epidêmica. SIN mumps v.

epidemic pleurodynia v., v. da pleurodinia epidêmica; vírus Coxsackie do tipo B (Enterovirus), da família Picornaviridae, que causa a pleurodinia epidêmica. SIN Bornholm disease v., epidemic myalgia v.

Epstein-Barr v. (EBV), v. Epstein-Barr; um herpesvírus do gênero Lymphocryptovirus que causa mononucleose infecciosa e também é encontrado em culturas de células do linfoma de Burkitt; associado ao carcinoma nasofaríngeo. SIN EB v., human herpesvirus 4.

FA v., v. FA; uma cepa do v. da encefalomielite do camundongo.

fibrous bacterial viruses, vírus bacterianos fibrosos. SIN filamentous bacterial viruses.

filamentous bacterial viruses, vírus bacterianos filamentosos; desoxirribonucleoproteínas que "infectam" bactérias Gram-negativas e nelas se replicam; possuem fímbrias (*pili*) sexuais e, diferentemente do bacteriófago, desprendem-se das bactérias infectadas sem lesionar a célula; parecem ser de dois tipos, um dos quais apresenta especificidade por *pili* F e o outro por *pili* I. SIN fibrous bacterial viruses.

filtrable v., v. filtráveis. SIN virus (2).

fixed v., v. fixo; v. da raiva cuja virulência em coelhos foi estabilizada por numerosas passagens através desse hospedeiro experimental. VER TAMBÉM street v.

Flury strain rabies v., v. da raiva da cepa Flury. VER rabies v., Flury strain.

FMD v., v. FMD. SIN foot-and-mouth disease v.

foamy viruses, vírus espumosos; retrovírus do gênero Spumavirus, família Retroviridae, encontrados em primatas e outros mamíferos; assim denominados por causa das alterações reticulares produzidas nas células renais do macaco; também são produzidos sincícios. SIN foamy agents.

foot-and-mouth disease v., v. da febre aftosa; um picornavírus do gênero Aphthovirus, família Picornaviridae, que causa a febre aftosa no gado bovino, em suíno, em carneiros, em cabras e em ruminantes selvagens; apresenta ampla distribuição por toda a África e Ásia, gerando graves perdas econômicas; o v. é disseminado por contaminação do ambiente animal com saliva e excrementos infectados. SIN FMD v.

Four Corners v., v. Four Corners. SIN Sin Nombre v. [oriundo da região dos Estados Unidos onde os estados do Novo México, Colorado, Utah e Arizona fazem fronteira, sendo o local de maior ocorrência]

Friend v., v. Friend; uma cepa do grupo esplênico dos vírus da leucemia do camundongo, relacionado com os vírus Moloney e Rauscher. SIN Friend leukemia v., Swiss mouse leukemia v.

Friend leukemia v., v. da leucemia de Friend. SIN Friend v.

GAL v., v. GAL; um v. com características de adenovírus, que não se sabe se está associado a doença natural. SIN gallus adenolike v.

gallus adenolike v., v. GAL, vírus de galináceos, semelhante ao adenovírus. SIN GAL v.

gastroenteritis v. type A, v. da gastrenterite do tipo A. SIN epidemic gastroenteritis v.

gastroenteritis v. type B, v. da gastrenterite do tipo B. SIN rotavirus.

GB viruses, vírus GB; membros da família Flaviviridae; GBV-A e GBV-B foram isolados a partir de saguis infectados por agentes virais humanos; GBV-C é um patógeno humano relacionado ao vírus da hepatite G.

German measles v., v. da rubéola. SIN rubella v.

Germiston v., v. Germiston; um vírus do gênero Bunyavirus, família Bunyaviridae.

goatpox v., v. da varíola caprina; um v. do gênero Capripoxvirus; a causa da varíola caprina.

Graffi v., v. de Graffi; v. da mieloleucemia do tipo C do camundongo isolado em filtrados de tumores transplantáveis; possivelmente relacionados ao v. Gross.

green monkey v., v. do macaco verde. SIN Marburg v.

Gross v., v. Gross; a primeira cepa isolada do v. da leucemia do camundongo. SIN Gross leukemia v.

vírus associados à gastrenterite aguda em seres humanos			
vírus	**tamanho (nm)**	**epidemiologia**
Rotavírus grupo A	70	causa isolada mais importante (viral ou endêmica) de doença diarreica grave endêmica em lactentes e crianças pequenas em todo o mundo (nos meses mais frios nos climas temperados)
grupo B	70	surtos de doença diarreica em adultos e crianças na China
grupo C	70	casos esporádicos e surtos ocasionais de doença diarreica em crianças
Adenovírus entérico	70–80	segundo agente viral mais importante de doença diarreica endêmica dos lactentes e crianças pequenas em todo o mundo
Vírus Norwalk e vírus Norwalk-símiles	27–32	causa importante de surtos de vômitos e doença diarreica em crianças com mais idade e adultos nas famílias, comunidades e instituições, freqüentemente associados à ingestão de alimento
Calicivírus	28–40	casos esporádicos e surtos ocasionais de doença diarreica em lactentes, crianças pequenas e idosos
Astrovírus	28	casos esporádicos e surtos ocasionais de doença diarreica em lactentes, crianças pequenas e idosos

Gross leukemia v., v. da leucemia de Gross. SIN Gross v.
Guama v., v. de Guama; um grupo sorológico do gênero Bunyavirus, composto de 6 espécies, incluindo o v. Catu e a cepa típica, o v. Guama.
Guanarito v., v. Guanarito; uma espécie de Arenavirus que causa a febre hemorrágica venezuelana. [recebeu esse nome por causa do município, na Venezuela, onde todos os casos iniciais da febre hemorrágica venezuelana foram confirmados]
Guaroa v., v. Guaroa; um v. do grupo Bunyamwera do gênero Bunyavirus e um agente de encefalite.
HA1 v., v. HA1. SIN hemadsorption v. type 1. VER parainfluenza viruses.
HA2 v., v. HA2. SIN hemadsorption v. type 2. VER parainfluenza viruses.
hand-foot-and-mouth disease v., v. da doença mão-pé-boca; o v. que causa a doença da mão-pé-boca; principalmente do tipo A16, mas também por Enterovirus Coxsackie dos tipos A4, A5, A7, A9 ou A10.
Hantaan v., v. Hantaan; um Hantavirus da família Bunyaviridae que causa a febre hemorrágica da Coréia, com síndrome renal.
helper v., v. auxiliar; um v. cuja replicação possibilita que um v. defeituoso ou um virusóide (também presente na célula hospedeira) se desenvolva em um agente plenamente infeccioso.
hemadsorption v. type 1, v. de hemadsorção do tipo 1; v. parainfluenza do tipo 3. VER parainfluenza viruses. SIN HA1 v.
hemadsorption v. type 2, v. de hemadsorção do tipo 2; v. parainfluenza do tipo 1. VER parainfluenza viruses. SIN HA2 v.
Hendra v., v. Hendra. SIN equine *Morbillivirus.* [recebeu o nome de Hendra, o subúrbio de Brisbane, Austrália, onde foi isolado pela primeira vez]
hepatitis A v. (HAV), v. da hepatite A; um vírus RNA, gênero Hepatovirus, da família Picornaviridae; o agente causal da hepatite viral do tipo A. SIN infectious hepatitis v.
hepatitis B v. (HBV), v. da hepatite B; um vírus DNA do gênero Orthohepadnavirus, família Hepadnaviridae; o agente causal da hepatite viral do tipo B. SIN serum hepatitis v.
hepatitis C v. (HCV), v. da hepatite C; um v. RNA não-A, não-B, que causa hepatite pós-transfusão; é um membro da família Flaviviridae. Existem novos testes para detectar a infecção por hepatite C.
hepatitis D v., v. da hepatite D; um pequeno v. RNA "defeituoso", similar aos viróides e virusóides, que exige a presença do v. da hepatite B para a replicação. A evolução clínica é variável, mas, em geral, é mais grave que outras hepatites. SIN delta agent, delta antigen, delta v., hepatitis delta v.
hepatitis delta v. (HDV), v. da hepatite delta. SIN hepatitis D v.
hepatitis E v. (HEV), v. da hepatite E; um v. RNA, possivelmente um Calicivirus, que é a principal causa de hepatite não-A, não-B transmitida entericamente, pela água ou epidêmica, que ocorre principalmente na Ásia e na África.
hepatitis G v. (HGV), v. da hepatite G; um v. RNA relacionado com o v. da hepatite C e que pode causar co-infecção com esse agente.
herpes v., herpesvírus. VER herpesvirus.
herpes simplex v. (HSV), v. do herpes simples. VER *herpes* simplex.
herpes zoster v., v. do herpes zoster. SIN varicella-zoster v.
hog cholera v., v. da cólera suína; um vírus RNA do gênero Pestivirus, da família Flaviviridae, que causa a cólera suína. SIN swine fever v.
horsepox v., v. da varíola eqüina; o poxvírus que causa a varíola eqüina. SIN contagious pustular stomatitis v. (1).
human immunodeficiency v. (HIV), v. da imunodeficiência humana; v. linfotrópico da célula T humana do tipo III; um retrovírus citopático, do gênero Lentivirus, família Retroviridae, que tem 100–120 nm de diâmetro, possui um envelope lipídico e apresenta um característico nucleóide cilíndrico denso que contém as proteínas do cerne e o RNA genômico. Atualmente, existem dois tipos: o HIV-1 infecta apenas seres humanos e chimpanzés, e é mais virulento que o HIV-2, que está mais relacionado aos vírus dos símios ou macacos. O HIV-2 é encontrado principalmente na África Ocidental e não está tão disseminado quanto o HIV-1. Além do gene usual associado aos retrovírus, o HIV-1 apresenta pelo menos 6 genes que regulam sua replicação. É o agente etiológico da síndrome da imunodeficiência humana adquirida (AIDS/SIDA). Originalmente conhecido como v. da linfadenopatia (LAV) ou v. linfotrópico da célula T humana do tipo III (HTLV-III). Identificado em 1984 por Luc Montagnier e colaboradores. SIN lymphadenopathy-associated v.
human immunodeficiency v.-2, v. da imunodeficiência humana do tipo 2 (HIV-2); um v., encontrado principalmente na África Ocidental, que causa uma forma menos virulenta de AIDS e está mais intimamente relacionado com as cepas de vírus dos macacos.
human T-cell lymphoma/leukemia v. (HTLV), v. da leucemia/linfoma de células T humanas; um grupo de vírus do gênero de retrovírus BLTV-HTLV, família Retroviridae, que são linfotrópicos com uma afinidade seletiva pelo subgrupo de células auxiliares/indutoras dos linfócitos T e que estão associados à leucemia da célula T adulta e à paraparesia espástica tropical. SIN human T-cell lymphotropic v.
human T-cell lymphotropic v., v. linfotrópico da célula T humana. SIN human T-cell lymphoma/leukemia v.

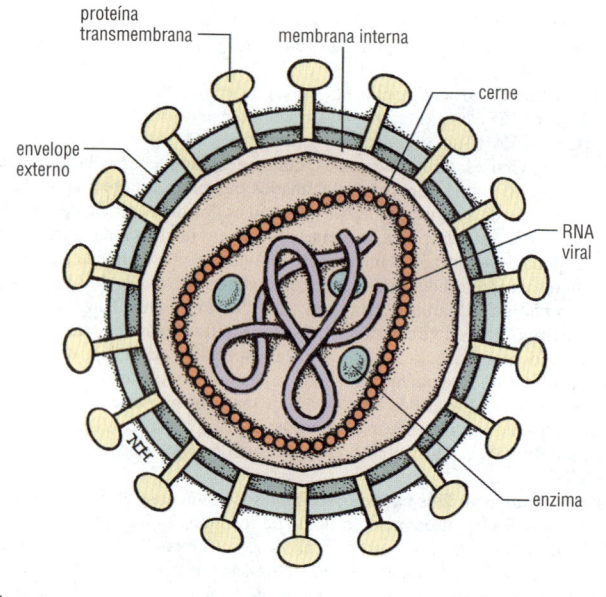

HIV

human T lymphotrophic v., v. linfotrófico T humano; um vírus que apresenta uma predileção pelas células linfóides humanas.
v. III of rabbits, v. III dos coelhos; nome obsoleto para uma infecção latente do coelho por herpesvírus. [a terceira cepa isolada, utilizada para estudo]
Ilhéus v., v. Ilhéus; um v. do gênero Flavivirus (arbovírus do grupo B) isolado pela primeira vez no Brasil, depois encontrado na Colômbia, na América Central e no Caribe; a causa da encefalite de Ilhéus e da febre de Ilhéus.
inclusion conjunctivitis viruses, v. da conjuntivite de inclusão; nome original da *Chlamydia trachomatis.*
infantile gastroenteritis v., v. da gastrenterite infantil. SIN rotavirus.
infectious ectromelia v., v. da ectromelia infantil; um v. que pertence à família Poxviridae, morfologicamente similar ao v. da vacínia, ocorrendo como uma infecção latente em camundongos de laboratório, mas que pode ser ativado por estresses como irradiação e transporte e causar doença; a inoculação no coxim adiposo da pata do camundongo resulta em edema e necrose. SIN ectromelia v., mousepox v., pseudolymphocytic choriomeningitis v.
infectious hepatitis v., v. da hepatite A. SIN hepatitis A v.
infectious papilloma v., papilomavírus humano. SIN human papillomavirus.
infectious porcine encephalomyelitis v., v. da encefalomielite suína infecciosa. SIN Teschen disease v.
influenza viruses, vírus influenza; vírus da família Orthomyxoviridae que causa *influenza* e infecções semelhantes a *influenza* em seres humanos e em outros animais. Esses vírus contêm RNA com filamento único, que é segmentado, contribuindo em parte para sua disseminação epidêmica. Os vírus incluídos são os v. influenza do tipo A e B do gênero Influenzavirus, causando, respectivamente, *influenza* A e B, e Influenzavirus C, que pertence a um gênero separado e provoca a *influenza* C.
insect viruses, vírus de insetos; vírus patogênicos para os insetos.
iridescent v., v. iridescente; um vírus de inseto da família Iridoviridae.
Jamestown Canyon v., v. Jamestown Canyon; um membro do grupo Califórnia dos arbovírus, família Bunyaviridae, que foi associado a uma doença febril branda em seres humanos na América do Norte.
Japanese B encephalitis v., v. da encefalite B japonesa; um v. do gênero Flavivirus (arbovírus do grupo B) que ocorre principalmente no Japão, mas provavelmente disseminado por todo o Sudeste asiático; o v. está normalmente presente em seres humanos, especialmente em crianças, como uma infecção inaparente, mas pode causar resposta febril e, por vezes, encefalite; pode provocar encefalite em cavalos e aborto em porcos; os pássaros selvagens são, provavelmente, os hospedeiros naturais, e os mosquitos culicídeos, os vetores. SIN Russian autumn encephalitis v.
JC v., v. JC; um poliomavírus humano, família Papovaviridae, de distribuição mundial, produzindo infecções que são usualmente subclínicas nos indivíduos imunocompetentes, mas está associado à leucoencefalopatia multifocal progressiva em indivíduos imunossuprimidos. [iniciais do paciente no qual foi isolado pela primeira vez]
Junin v., v. Junin; um v. do complexo Tacaribe dos arbovírus, gênero Arenavirus, e a causa da febre hemorrágica argentina; também isolado em ácaros e roedores.
K v., v. K; um poliomavírus, família Papovaviridae, que causa pneumonia em camundongos jovens por várias vias de inoculação.

Kasokero v., v. Kasokero; um v. da família Bunyaviridae que causa, em seres humanos, uma doença febril caracterizada por cefaléia, dor abdominal, diarréia, mialgia intensa e artralgia. [recebeu o nome da caverna Kasokero em Uganda, onde o vírus foi isolado pela primeira vez em morcegos]

Kelev strain rabies v., v. da raiva da cepa Kelev. VER rabies v., Kelev strain.

Kilham rat v., v. do rato de Kilham; um v. do gênero Parvovirus que provoca infecção inaparente em ratos; também pode ser isolado de tumores em ratos. SIN latent rat v.

Koongol viruses, vírus Koongol; um grupo sorológico do gênero Bunyavirus, compreendendo duas espécies: Koongol (espécie típica) e v. Wongal.

Korean hemorrhagic fever v., v. da febre hemorrágica da Coréia. VER Hantavirus.

Kyasanur Forest disease v., v. da doença da floresta de Kyasanur; um arbovírus do grupo B, na família Flaviviridae, isolado de macacos na Índia e capaz de provocar a doença da floresta de Kyasanur em seres humanos; o v. é disseminado por macacos e pássaros que apresentam infecções brandas; os vetores são, provavelmente, espécies do carrapato *Haemaphysalis*.

La Crosse v., v. La Crosse; um bunyavírus do grupo Califórnia, família Bunyaviridae, e um agente de encefalite.

lactate dehydrogenase v., v. lactato desidrogenase; um arterivírus presente, talvez como "passageiro", em vários tumores transplantáveis de camundongo; o v. pode provocar uma infecção por toda a vida e é reconhecido pela elevação da lactato desidrogenase plasmática. SIN LDH agent.

Lassa v., v. Lassa; um arenavírus, família Arenaviridae, que provoca a febre Lassa, uma doença febril aguda com elevada taxa de mortalidade.

latent rat v., v. latente do rato. SIN Kilham rat v.

LCM v., v. LCM. SIN lymphocytic choriomeningitis v.

louping-ill v., um v. do gênero Flavivirus que causa a encefalomielite denominada *louping ill*; é transmitido pelo carrapato *Ixodes ricinus*.

Lucké v., v. Lucké; um herpesvírus associado ao carcinoma de Lucké.

Lunyo v., v. Lunyo; uma cepa atípica do v. da febre do vale Rift.

lymphadenopathy-associated v. (LAV), v. associado à linfadenopatia. SIN human immunodeficiency v.

lymphocytic choriomeningitis v., v. da coriomeningite linfocítica; um vírus RNA da família Arenaviridae que infecta camundongos, seres humanos, macacos, cães e cobaias; causa a coriomeningite linfocítica; no ser humano, a infecção pode ser inaparente, mas, por vezes, o v. causa doença semelhante a *influenza*, meningite ou, raramente, meningoencefalite; as infecções *in utero* de camundongo estabelecem um tipo de tolerância imunológica. SIN LCM v.

lymphogranuloma venereum v., v. do linfogranuloma venéreo; nome original da *Chlamydia trachomatis*.

Machupo v., v. Machupo; um v. do complexo Tacaribe (gênero Arenavirus, família Arenaviridae); a causa da febre hemorrágica boliviana.

malignant catarrhal fever v., v. da febre catarral maligna; um herpesvírus de ampla distribuição que causa a febre catarral maligna do gado; carneiros e animais silvestres têm infecções inaparentes e podem transmitir o v. para o gado bovino.

mammary cancer v. of mice, v. do câncer mamário do camundongo. SIN mammary tumor v. of mice.

mammary tumor v. of mice, v. do tumor mamário do camundongo; um dos retrovírus do tipo B de mamíferos, antigenicamente diferenciado do complexo de leucemia–sarcoma murino, que está associado a tumores adenocarcinomatosos da glândula mamária, comumente latente em camundongos selvagens e de laboratório; causa o câncer apenas em cepas geneticamente suscetíveis sob determinadas influências hormonais. SIN Bittner agent, Bittner milk factor, Bittner v., mammary cancer v. of mice, milk factor, mouse mammary tumor v.

Marburg v., v. Marburg; um v. contendo RNA, gênero Filovirus, família Filoviridae, reconhecido pela primeira vez na Marburg University (Alemanha), onde foi a causa de uma febre hemorrágica extremamente fatal em trabalhadores de laboratório e tratadores de macacos verdes. SIN green monkey v.

Marek disease v., v. da doença de Marek. SIN avian neurolymphomatosis v.

marmoset v., v. do sagüi; um herpesvírus obtido repetidamente a partir de *swabs* de orofaringe e tecidos de macacos do Novo Mundo.

masked v., v. mascarado; um v. que ocorre comumente no hospedeiro em um estado não-infeccioso, mas que pode ser ativado e demonstrado por procedimentos especiais, como a passagem às cegas em animais experimentais.

Mason-Pfizer v., v. Mason-Pfizer; um membro do gênero retrovírus do tipo D, família Retroviridae, que foi isolado do carcinoma mamário de um macaco Rhesus.

Mayaro v., v. Mayaro; um v. do gênero Alphavirus, família Togaviridae, causando epidemias de febre do tipo indiferenciado na América do Sul.

measles v., v. do sarampo; um v. RNA do gênero Morbillivirus, família Paramyxoviridae, que causa o sarampo em seres humanos e é transmitido através do trato respiratório; possui propriedades hemaglutinantes, hemadsorventes e hemolisantes. SIN rubeola v.

Menangle v., v. Menangle; um v. da família Paramyxoviridae causador de infecção em porcos, seres humanos e morcegos que se alimentam de frutas na Austrália; a infecção humana resultou em uma doença semelhante a *influenza*, com erupção cutânea. [recebeu o nome do local na Austrália onde ficava o laboratório no qual foi isolado pela primeira vez]

Mengo v., v. Mengo; uma cepa do v. da encefalomiocardite.

milker´s nodule v., v. do nódulo do ordenhador; um v. da família Poxviridae.

mink enteritis v., v. da enterite da marta; um parvovírus que provoca a enterite da marta.

MM v., v. MM; uma cepa do v. da encefalomiocardite.

Mokola v., v. Mokola; um v. do gênero Lyssavirus, família Rhabdoviridae, relacionado com a raiva, primeiramente isolado do musaranho (Crocidura spp.) na Nigéria, que causou uma doença neurológica fatal em seres humanos e em gatos na África.

molluscum contagiosum v., v. do molusco contagioso; o poxvírus que causa o molusco contagioso em seres humanos.

Moloney v., v. Moloney; um retrovírus da leucemia linfóide do camundongo, da família Retroviridae, isolado originalmente durante a propagação do sarcoma S 37 do camundongo.

monkey B v., v. B do macaco. SIN B v.

monkeypox v., v. da varíola do macaco; um v. do gênero Orthopoxvirus que causa a varíola do macaco.

mouse encephalomyelitis v., v. da encefalomielite do camundongo; um v. do gênero Enterovirus, família Picornavirus, normalmente associado a infecções inaparentes e encontrado nos tratos intestinais de camundongos infectados, por vezes causando a encefalomielite em camundongos suscetíveis experimentalmente inoculados. SIN mouse poliomyelitis v., Theiler v.

mouse hepatitis v., v. hepatite do camundongo; um coronavírus, família Coronaviridae, que, na presença de *Eperythrozoon coccoides*, causa hepatite fatal em camundongos recém-desmamados; caso contrário, provoca infecção inaparente.

mouse leukemia viruses, vírus da leucemia de camundongos, retrovírus do complexo leucemia–sarcoma murino que provocam leucemia e, por vezes, linfossarcomas em camundongos, incluindo as cepas Abelson, Gross, Moloney, Friend e Rauscher do v.; foram isolados de camundongos resultantes de procriação consanguínea que possuem uma alta incidência de leucemia linfóide espontânea.

mouse mammary tumor v., v. do tumor mamário do camundongo. SIN mammary tumor v. of mice.

mouse parotid tumor v., v. do tumor parotídeo do camundongo. SIN polyoma v.

mouse poliomyelitis v., v. da poliomielite do camundongo. SIN mouse encephalomyelitis v.

mousepox v., v. da ectromelia infecciosa. SIN infectious ectromelia v.

mouse thymic v., v. tímico do camundongo; um membro éter-sensível da família Herpesviridae que causa necrose do timo em camundongos jovens.

mucosal disease v., v. da doença das mucosas. SIN bovine virus diarrhea v.

mumps v., v. da caxumba; um v. do gênero Rubulavirus, família Paramyxoviridae, que causa parotidite em seres humanos, por vezes com complicações de orquite, ooforite, pancreatite, meningoencefalite e outras, sendo transmitido por secreções salivares infecciosas. SIN epidemic parotitis v.

murine sarcoma v., v. do sarcoma murino; um retrovírus aparentemente defeituoso que provoca sarcoma em camundongos quando cresce na presença de um v. "auxiliar"; p.ex., v. da leucemia do camundongo.

Murray Valley encephalitis v., v. da encefalite do Vale Murray; um arbovírus do grupo B do gênero Flavivirus que causa a encefalite do Vale Murray; é transmitido por mosquitos *Culex* e também infecta pássaros e cavalos. SIN Australian X disease v., MVE v.

Murutucu v., v. Murutucu; um v. do grupo C do gênero Bunyavirus, transmitido por mosquito, que causou febre do tipo indiferenciado no Brasil e na Guiana Francesa.

MVE v., v. MVE. SIN Murray Valley encephalitis v.

myxomatosis v., v. da mixomatose. SIN rabbit myxoma v.

naked v., v. desnudo; um v. que consiste apenas em um nucleocapsídeo; ou seja, aquele que não possui um envelope de revestimento.

ND v., v. ND. SIN Newcastle disease v.

negative strand v., v. do filamento negativo; um v. cujo genoma é um filamento de RNA que é complementar ao RNA mensageiro; os vírus de filamento negativo também carregam RNA polimerases necessárias para a síntese do RNA mensageiro.

Negishi v., v. Negishi; um dos arbovírus do grupo B (gênero Flavivirus) do complexo de encefalites transmitidos por carrapato, isolado de infecções fatais no Japão.

neonatal calf diarrhea v., v. da diarréia neonatal do bezerro; um dos dois vírus que causam diarréia neonatal do bezerro; um rotavírus-símile está associado à doença em bezerros recém-nascidos, e um coronavírus está associado à doença nos bezerros com mais de 5 dias de idade.

neurotropic v., v. neurotrópico; um v. que apresenta afinidade pelo tecido nervoso, p.ex., v. da poliomielite, v. neurotrópico variante da febre amarela e o v. "fixo" da raiva.

Newcastle disease v., v. da doença de Newcastle; um v. do gênero Rubulavirus, família Paranexoviridae, que provoca a doença de Newcastle em galinhas e, em menor grau, em perus e outros pássaros; ocasionalmente infecta laboratoristas e tratadores de aves, provocando conjuntivite e linfadenite. SIN avian pneumoencephalitis v., ND v.

New York v., v. New York; uma espécie de Hantavirus nos Estados Unidos que causa síndrome pulmonar.

Nipah v., v. Nipah; um paramixovírus que pode causar doença fatal em seres humanos, com manifestações de encefalite e meningite; o v. dissemina-se dos suínos para os seres humanos. [Nipah, Malásia, onde o primeiro caso humano foi detectado, 1999]

non-A, non-B hepatitis v., v. da hepatite não-A, não-B; termo usado para designar qualquer um dos inúmeros vírus, diferentes do A ou B, que causem a hepatite em seres humanos.

nonoccluded v., v. não-ocluído; um v. que não está contido em um corpúsculo de inclusão, usualmente com referência a um v. de inseto.

Norwalk v., v. Norwalk; um v. associado a gastrenterite viral aguda e que pertence ao grupo Calicivirus.

occluded v., v. ocluído; um v. contido por um corpúsculo de inclusão, usualmente com referência a um v. de inseto.

Omsk hemorrhagic fever v., v. da febre hemorrágica de Omsk; um v. do gênero Flavivirus, transmitido por carrapato, que causa a febre hemorrágica de Omsk.

oncogenic v., v. oncogênico; qualquer v. capaz de induzir tumores. Os vírus tumorais RNA (família Retroviridae), que são bem definidos e algo homogêneos, ou vírus DNA, que contêm inúmeros vírus capazes de induzir tumores, inclusive poxvírus, herpesvírus, papilomavírus e poliomavírus. SIN tumor v.

o'nyong-nyong v., v. o'nyong-nyong; um v. do gênero Alphavirus, família Togaviridae, encontrado em Uganda, Quênia e Congo, que causa a febre o'nyong-nyong.

orf v., v. da estomatite pustular contagiosa; um parapoxivírus que causa estomatite pustular contagiosa em carneiros e cabras e, por vezes, em seres humanos. SIN contagious pustular dermatitis, contagious pustular stomatitis v. (2).

Oriboca v., v. Oriboca; um v. do grupo C do gênero Bunyavirus e um agente de encefalite.

ornithosis v., v. da ornitose; nome antigo da *Chlamydia psittaci*.

orphan viruses, vírus órfãos; vírus, como os vírus órfãos entéricos, que, quando originalmente encontrados, não foram especificamente associados à doença; desde então, demonstrou-se que inúmeros são patogênicos e foram subseqüentemente reclassificados.

Pacheco parrot disease v., v. da doença do papagaio de Pacheco; um v. da família Herpesviridae, possivelmente relacionado ao v. da laringotraqueíte infecciosa. SIN parrot v. (2).

pantropic v., v. pantrópico; a cepa comum do v. da febre amarela, diferente da cepa neurotrópica; possui afinidade por diferentes tecidos.

papilloma v., papilomavírus. SIN Papillomavirus.

pappataci fever viruses, vírus da febre pappataci. SIN phlebotomus fever viruses.

parainfluenza viruses, vírus parainfluenza; vírus do gênero Paramyxovirus, de quatro tipos: o tipo 1 (v. da hemadsorção do tipo 2), que inclui o v. sendai, causa laringotraqueíte aguda em crianças e, ocasionalmente, em adultos; o tipo 2 (v. associado à crupe) está associado especialmente a laringotraqueíte aguda ou crupe em crianças pequenas e a infecções pouco importantes do trato respiratório superior em adultos; o tipo 3 (v. de hemadsorção do tipo 1; v. da febre do embarque) foi isolado em crianças pequenas com faringite, bronquiolite e pneumonia, e causa infecção respiratória ocasional em adultos; as cepas bovinas foram isoladas em gado bovino com febre do embarque, e o v. também foi isolado em carneiros; o tipo 4 foi isolado em pouquíssimas crianças com doença respiratória branda.

paravaccinia v., v. da paravacínia. SIN pseudocowpox v.

parrot v., v. do papagaio; (1) termo obsoleto da *Chlamydia psittaci*; (2) SIN Pacheco parrot disease v.

Patois v., v. Patois; um grupo sorológico do gênero Bunyavirus, compreendendo 4 espécies.

pharyngoconjunctival fever v., v. da febre faringoconjuntival; um dentre vários tipos de adenovírus associados a surtos de febre e faringite, por vezes com conjuntivite, especialmente em recrutas militares e pessoas em internatos.

phlebotomus fever viruses, vírus da febre do flebótomo; um grupo de pelo menos 5 vírus da família Bunyaviridae, mas antigenicamente não-relacionados, transmitidos por *Phlebotomus papatasii* (mosquito-pólvora) e que causam a febre do flebótomo. SIN pappataci fever viruses, sandfly fever viruses.

plant viruses, vírus vegetais; vírus patogênicos para vegetais superiores.

pneumonia v. of mice, v. da pneumonia do camundongo; um v. RNA do gênero Pneumovirus, família Paramyxoviridae, que ocorre normalmente como uma infecção latente em camundongos de laboratório, mas capaz de ativação por passagem intranasal seriada e que causa pneumonia. SIN PVM v.

poliomyelitis v., v. da poliomielite; um pequeno v. RNA de filamento único, do gênero Enterovirus, família Picornaviridae, que causa poliomielite em seres humanos; a via de infecção é o trato alimentar, mas o v. pode entrar na corrente sanguínea e no sistema nervoso, por vezes causando paralisia dos membros e, raramente, encefalite; muitas infecções são inaparentes; os tipos sorológicos 1, 2 e 3 são reconhecidos, sendo o tipo 1 responsável pela maioria dos casos de poliomielite paralítica e pela maioria das epidemias. SIN poliovirus hominis.

polyoma v., poliomavírus; um pequeno v. desnudo com DNA circular de filamento duplo (gênero Polyomavirus, família Papovaviridae) que normalmente ocorre em infecções inaparentes em camundongos selvagens e de laboratório, mas, após crescimento em cultura de tecido, é capaz de produzir tumores parotídeos em camundongos e sarcomas em *hamsters*, bem como tumores em outros animais de laboratório. SIN mouse parotid tumor v.

porcine hemagglutinating encephalomyelitis v., v. da encefalomielite hemaglutinante suína; um Coronavirus que causa vômitos, emaciação e encefalomielite em porcos jovens.

Powassan v., v. Powassan; um v. do gênero Flavivirus, família Flaviviridae, transmitido por carrapatos ixodídeos e que causa a encefalite Powassan em

vírus oncogênicos

família do vírus	vírus	hospedeiro de origem	tumores associados
Herpesviridae	rã, herpesvírus	rã leopardo	adenocarcinomas
	vírus da doença Marek	galinha	neurolinfomatose (célula T)
	herpesvírus	macacos	linfoma, leucemia
	vírus Epstein-Barr (EBV)	ser humano	linfoma de Burkitt, carcinoma nasofaríngeo
	herpes simples (tipo 2)	ser humano	neoplasia cervical
	herpes simples do tipo 8 (HHV8)	ser humano	sarcoma de Kaposi
Poxviridae	fibroma de Shope	coelho	fibroma
	vírus Yaba	macaco	hiperplasia fibromatosa nodular
	molusco contagioso	ser humano	hiperplasia epidérmica nodular
Hepadnaviridae	hepatite do grupo B	seres humanos, macacos, roedores, patos	carcinoma hepatocelular
Papovaviridae	polioma	camundongo	vários carcinomas e sarcomas
	SV40	macaco	sarcoma (em roedores)
	BK e JC	ser humano	nenhum em seres humanos; tumores neurais em roedores e macacos
	papiloma	ser humano	verrugas genitais, laríngeas e cutâneas; pode progredir para carcinoma cervical, carcinoma laríngeo, carcinoma de pele
		gado bovino	verrugas genitais, alimentares, cutâneas; pode progredir para carcinoma do trato alimentar, carcinoma cutâneo
		outros mamíferos	papilomas: pode progredir para carcinomas

crianças; também capaz de produzir meningoencefalomielite em coelhos e crianças. [*Powassan*, Canadá, onde foi isolado pela primeira vez]

pseudocowpox v., v. da pseudovacínia; um v. do gênero Parapoxvirus que causa pseudovacínia em seres humanos e no gado bovino; está intimamente relacionado ao v. da estomatite pustular contagiosa e ao v. da estomatite papular. SIN paravaccinia v.

pseudolymphocytic choriomeningitis v., v. da coriomeningite pseudolinfocítica. SIN infectious ectromelia v.

pseudorabies v., v. da pseudo-raiva; um herpesvírus, família Herpesviridae, que causa a pseudo-raiva em suínos. SIN Aujeszky disease v.

psittacosis v., v. da psitacose; nome original da *Chlamydia psittaci*.

Puumala v., v. Puumala; uma espécie de Hantavirus encontrada na Europa que provoca febre hemorrágica com síndrome renal.

PVM v., v. PVM. SIN pneumonia v. of mice.

quail bronchitis v., v. da bronquite da codorna; um v. do gênero Aviadenovirus, relacionado antigenicamente ao v. CELO.

Quaranfil v., v. Quaranfil; um arbovírus não-classificado isolado no sangue humano e de garças.

rabbit fibroma v., v. do fibroma do coelho; um poxvírus do gênero Leporipoxvirus, família Poxviridae, intimamente relacionado com os vírus da vacínia e do mixoma, que causa o fibroma de Shope. SIN Shope fibroma v.

rabbit myxoma v., v. do mixoma do coelho; o poxvírus do gênero Leporipoxvirus que causa a mixomatose de coelhos. SIN myxomatosis v.

rabbitpox v., v. da varíola do coelho; um Orthopoxvirus que causa epidemia de varíola em coelhos de laboratório; imunologicamente, apresenta grande correlação com o v. da vacínia, mas é mais virulento em coelhos.

rabies v., v. da raiva; um grande v. RNA de filamento único, com formato de bala, do gênero Lyssavirus, família Rhabdoviridae; é o agente causal da raiva.

rabies v., Flury strain, v. da raiva, cepa Flury; um v. isolado no cérebro humano, atenuado (fixo) por propagação seriada em hospedeiros não-mamíferos e, subseqüentemente, estabelecido na cultura de embrião de pinto.

rabies v., Kelev strain, v. da raiva, estirpe (cepa) Kelev, uma estirpe atenuada, embrionada, com passagem em aves domésticas.

Rauscher v., v. Rauscher. SIN Rauscher leukemia v.

Rauscher leukemia v., v. da leucemia de Rauscher; um retrovírus RNA associado a leucemia em roedores; similar ao v. Friend. SIN Rauscher v.

REO v., v. REO. SIN respiratory enteric orphan v.

respiratory enteric orphan v., v. órfão entérico respiratório; um vírus icosaédrico não-envelopado com um capsídeo de dupla camada, cujo genoma consiste em múltiplos segmentos de RNA de duplo filamento, pertencendo à família Reoviridae, freqüentemente encontrado nos tratos respiratório e entérico. SIN REO v.

respiratory sincytial v. (RSV), v. sincicial respiratório; um v. RNA do gênero Pneumovirus, família Paramyxoviridae, com uma tendência a formar sincícios na cultura de tecidos, causando infecção respiratória branda, com rinite e tosse em adultos, mas é capaz de provocar bronquite grave e broncopneumonia em crianças pequenas; isolado primeiramente em chimpanzés com doença respiratória. SIN chimpanzee coryza agent, Rs v.

Reston v., v. Reston; uma variante do v. Ebola. SIN Ebola v. Reston.

Rida v., v. Rida; uma variante do agente do *scrapie*.

Rift Valley fever v., v. da febre do vale Rift; um v. do gênero Phlebovirus (família Bunyaviridae) que ocorre nas regiões central e sul da África em carneiros, cabras e no gado, provocando abortos e doença febril grave, em especial nos cordeiros jovens; os seres humanos, principalmente pastores e veterinários, podem ser infectados através do contato próximo com animais infectados, desenvolvendo uma doença semelhante ao dengue; o v. também infecta búfalos, camelos e antílopes; é transmitido por mosquitos, mas, provavelmente, também infecta por contato e pelo trato respiratório.

RNA v., v. RNA; um grupo de vírus em que o cerne consiste em RNA; um grupo importante de vírus animais que engloba as famílias Picornaviridae, Reoviridae, Togaviridae, Flaviviridae, Bunyaviridae, Arenaviridae, Paramyxoviridae, Retroviridae, Coronaviridae, Orthomyxoviridae e Rhabdoviridae. SIN ribovirus.

principais grupos de vírus

vírus DNA família do vírus	envelope presente	simetria do capsídeo	tamanho da partícula (nm)	estrutura do DNA*	vírus clinicamente importantes
Parvoviridae	não	icosaédrico	22	ss, linear	vírus B19
Papovaviridae	não	icosaédrico	55	ds circular, superespiralado	papilomavírus, poliomavírus (JC, BK)
Adenoviridae	não	icosaédrico	75	ds linear	adenovírus
Hepadnaviridae	sim	icosaédrico	42	ds circular incompleto	vírus da hepatite B
Herpesviridae	sim	icosaédrico	100**	ds, linear	vírus herpes simples, vírus varicela-zoster, citomegalovírus, vírus Epstein-Barr
Poxviridae	sim	complexa	250 × 400	ds, linear	vírus da varíola, vírus da vacínia

vírus RNA família do vírus	envelope presente	simetria do capsídeo	tamanho da partícula (nm)	estrutura do RNA†	vírus clinicamente importantes
Picornaviridae	não	icosaédrico	28	ss, linear, não-segmentado, sentido +	poliovírus, rinovírus, vírus da hepatite A, enterovírus
Reoviridae	não	icosaédrico	75	ds, linear, 10 segmentos	reovírus, rotavírus, vírus da febre do carrapato do Colorado
Togaviridae	sim	icosaédrico	40–70	ss, linear, não-segmentado, sentido +	vírus da rubéola, vírus da febre amarela
Retroviridae	sim	icosaédrico	100	ss, linear, 2 segmentos, sentido +	HIV, vírus linfotrópico da célula T humana (HTLV)
Coronaviridae	sim	helicoidal	100	ss, linear, não-segmentado sentido +	coronavírus
Caliciviridae	não	icosaédrico	35–40	RNA de filamento único com sentido +	agente Norwalk
Orthomyxoviridae	sim	helicoidal	80–120	ss, linear, 8 segmentos, sentido −	vírus influenza
Paramyxoviridae	sim	helicoidal	150	ss, linear, não-segmentado, sentido +	vírus do sarampo, caxumba, parainfluenza, sincicial respiratório
Rhabdoviridae	sim	helicoidal	75 × 180	ss, linear, não-segmentado, sentido −	vírus da raiva
Arenaviridae	sim	helicoidal	80–130	ss, circular, 2 segmentos com terminações coesivas, sentido −	vírus da coriomeningite linfocítica
Bunyaviridae	sim	helicoidal	100	ss, circular, 3 segmentos com terminações coesivas, sentido −	vírus da encefalite da Califórnia e da febre do flebótomo
Filoviridae	sim	complexa	80 × (800–900)	RNA, ss, sentido −	vírus Marburg, Ebola

* ss, filamento único; ds, filamento duplo; +, positivo; −, negativo
**o nucleocapsídeo do herpesvírus tem 100 nm, mas o envelope varia de tamanho; o vírus inteiro pode chegar a 200 nm de diâmetro
†O retrovírus RNA contém 2 moléculas idênticas de peso molecular de $3,5 \times 10^6$

RNA tumor viruses, vírus RNA tumorais; vírus RNA da família Retroviridae que provocam tumores.
Ross River v., v. do rio Ross; um alfavírus, família Togaviridae, transmitido por mosquito e causador de poliartrite epidêmica.
Rous-associated v. (RAV), v. associado de Rous; um v. de leucemia dos retrovírus do tipo C das aves (complexo leucose–sarcoma), família Retroviridae, que, por mistura fenotípica com uma cepa defeituosa (não-infecciosa) do sarcoma de Rous, efetua a produção de v. do sarcoma infeccioso com a antigenicidade do envelope do RAV.
Rous sarcoma v. (RSV), v. do sarcoma de Rous; um v. produtor de sarcoma dos retrovírus do tipo C das aves (complexo de leucose–sarcoma), família Retroviridae, identificado por Rous em 1911.
Rs v., v. Rs. SIN respiratory syncytial v.
Rubarth disease v., v. da doença de Rubarth. SIN canine *adenovirus* 1.
rubella v., v. da rubéola; um v. RNA do gênero Rubivirus, família Togaviridae; o agente causal da rubéola nos seres humanos. SIN German measles v.
rubeola v., v. do sarampo. SIN measles v.
Russian autumn encephalitis v., v. da encefalite russa do outono. SIN Japanese B encephalitis v.
Russian spring-summer encephalitis v., v. da encefalite russa da primavera-verão. SIN tick-borne encephalitis v.
Sabia v., v. Sabia; um arenavírus associado à febre hemolítica.
Salisbury common cold viruses, vírus do resfriado comum de Salisbury; cepas de rinovírus de interesse histórico por causa dos estudos iniciais que estabeleceram a etiologia viral dos resfriados comuns.
salivary v., herpesvírus humano 5. SIN human *herpesvirus* 5.
salivary gland v., herpesvírus humano 5. SIN human *herpesvirus* 5.
sandfly fever viruses, vírus da febre do flebótomo. SIN phlebotomus fever viruses.
San Miguel sea lion v., v. do leão marinho de São Miguel; um calicivírus, família Caliciviridae, isolado pela primeira vez em leões-marinhos de São Miguel, ilha da costa da Califórnia, que é indistinguível do exantema vesicular do v. suíno, tanto biofísica quanto clinicamente, em termos da síndrome da doença vesicular que produz em suínos.
Semliki Forest v., v. da floresta Semliki; um alfavírus, família Togaviridae, raramente associado à doença humana.
Sendai v., v. Sendai; um v. parainfluenza do tipo 1 reportado como causa de infecção inaparente em muitos animais; também é muito empregado para efetuar fusão celular em cultura de tecidos.
Seoul v., v. Seoul; uma espécie de Hantavirus no Extremo Oriente que causa febre hemorrágica com síndrome renal. [o vírus recebeu esse nome por causa de Seul, na Coréia do Sul, a cidade onde foi isolado pela primeira vez.]
serum hepatitis v., v. da hepatite sérica. SIN hepatitis B v.
sheep-pox v., v. da varíola do carneiro; um poxvírus do gênero Capripoxvirus que causa a varíola dos carneiros.
shipping fever v., v. da febre do embarque; uma cepa bovina do v. parainfluenza do tipo 3. VER parainfluenza viruses.
Shope fibroma v., v. do fibroma de Shope. SIN rabbit fibroma v.
Shope papilloma v., v. do papiloma de Shope; um papilomavírus que infecta lebres selvagens. VER Shope *papilloma*.
Simbu v., v. Simbu; um grupo sorológico do gênero Bunyavirus, compreendendo inúmeras espécies, incluindo a cepa típica, v. Simbu.
simian v. (SV), v. de símio; qualquer um de inúmeros vírus, pertencentes a várias famílias, isolados em macacos ou culturas de células de macacos. SIN vacuolating v.
simian v. 40, v. de símio 40. SIN simian vacuolating v. No. 40.
simian vacuolating v. No. 40 (SV40), v. de símio vacuolizante n.º 40; um pequeno v. DNA (40–45 nm) do gênero Polyomavirus, família Papoviridae; a causa de infecções aparentemente inaparentes em macacos, especialmente o Rhesus, e um contaminante comum de culturas de células de macaco; o v. pode causar infecção inaparente em seres humanos e ser excretado nas fezes de crianças durante várias semanas; pode provocar fibrossarcoma em *hamsters* recém-nascidos, podendo a transformação ocorrer em células diplóides humanas; também pode formar v. "híbrido" em células também infectadas por determinados adenovírus. SIN simian v. 40.
Sindbis v., v. Sindbis; a espécie típica do gênero Alphavirus, família Togaviridae, comumente transmitido por mosquitos do gênero *Culex*; é agente causal da febre Sindbis. [vila no Egito onde foi isolado pela primeira vez]
Sin Nombre v., v. Sin Nombre; uma espécie de Hantavirus, encontrada na América do Norte, que causa síndrome pulmonar. SIN Four Corners v. [Espanhol, sem nome]
slow v., v. lento; um v. ou um agente vírus-símile, etiologicamente associado a uma doença que possui um longo período de incubação de meses a anos com estabelecimento gradual, freqüentemente terminando em doença grave e/ou morte.
smallpox v., v. da varíola. SIN variola v.
snowshoe hare v., v. da lebre-da-neve; um membro do grupo Califórnia dos arbovírus, gênero Bunyavirus, família Bunyaviridae, que causa febre, cefaléia grave e náuseas em seres humanos na América do Norte.

soremouth v., v. da dermatite pustular de carneiros. SIN contagious ecthyma (pustular dermatitis) v. of sheep.
Spondweni v., v. Spondweni; um arbovírus do gênero Flavivirus isolado em mosquitos na África; pode causar doença em seres humanos.
St. Louis encephalitis v., v. da encefalite de St. Louis; um arbovírus do grupo B, gênero Flavivirus, família Flaviviridae, que ocorre nos Estados Unidos, Trinidad e Panamá; normalmente presente como infecção inaparente em seres humanos, mas, por vezes, uma causa de encefalite; foi isolado em pássaros no Panamá e em diversas espécies de mosquito, especialmente *Psorophora*.
street v., um v. da raiva isolado em um animal doméstico naturalmente infectado.
Sudan v., v. Sudan; uma variante do v. Ebola. SIN Ebola v. Sudan.
swine encephalitis v., v. da encefalite suína; um coronavírus, família Coronaviridae, que causa a encefalite suína.
swine fever v., v. da febre suína. SIN hog cholera v.
swine influenza viruses, vírus influenza suínos; cepas de v. influenza do tipo A que causam *influenza* em suínos e podem infectar os seres humanos.
swinepox v., v. da varíola suína; um poxvírus do gênero Suipoxvirus diferente do v. da vacínia e a causa da varíola suína; o piolho do porco é importante na transmissão.
Swiss mouse leukemia v., v. Friend. SIN Friend v.
Tacaribe v., v. Tacaribe; o v. típico do complexo Tacaribe dos vírus do gênero Arenavirus, tendo sido isolado em morcegos e mosquitos em Trinidad.
Tahyna v., v. Tahyna; um arbovírus do grupo Califórnia do gênero Bunyavirus, família Bunyaviridae, oriundo da Europa Central, que, sabidamente, infecta seres humanos.
Taiwan Dobrava-Belgrade v., v. Taiwan Dobrava-Belgrado; uma espécie de Hantavirus nos Balcãs que causa febre hemorrágica com síndrome renal. [de Dobrava, Eslovênia (onde foi isolado pela primeira vez em camundongos silvestres) e de Belgrado, antiga Iugoslávia (onde foi isolado pela primeira vez em seres humanos)]
temperate v., um fago que não lisa seu hospedeiro imediatamente, mas que pode persistir na forma latente e, mais adiante, lisar seu hospedeiro. VER lysogeny.
Teschen disease v., v. da doença de Teschen; um picornavírus que causa a doença de Teschen dos porcos; o v. é, em geral, um habitante inócuo do trato intestinal, mas as cepas virulentas causam epidemias. SIN infectious porcine encephalomyelitis v.
Tete viruses, vírus Tete; um grupo sorológico do gênero Bunyavirus, compreendendo inúmeros tipos.
TGE v., v. TGE. SIN transmissible gastroenteritis v. of swine.
Theiler v., v. Theiler. SIN mouse encephalomyelitis v.
Theiler mouse encephalomyelitis v., v. da encefalomielite do camundongo de Theiler; um vírus do gênero Cardiovirus, família Picornaviridae. SIN Theiler original v.
Theiler original v., v. original de Theiler. SIN Theiler mouse encephalomyelitis v.
tick-borne v., v. transmitido por carrapato. SIN tick-borne encephalitis v.
tick-borne encephalitis v., v. da encefalite transmitido por carrapato; arbovírus do gênero Flavivirus que ocorrem na Europa Central e Rússia em múltiplos subtipos, causando duas formas de encefalite em seres humanos: encefalite transmitida por carrapato (subtipo da Europa Central) e encefalite transmitida por carrapato (subtipo do leste); os vetores são carrapatos do gênero *Ixodes*. SIN Russian spring-summer encephalitis v., tick-borne v.
TO v., v. TO; v. original de Theiler. VER mouse encephalomyelitis v.
Topografov v., v. de Topografov; uma espécie de Hantavirus encontrada na Sibéria.
trachoma v., v. do tracoma; nome antigo da *Chlamydia trachomatis*.
transmissible gastroenteritis v. of swine, v. da gastrenterite transmissível do suíno; um v. do gênero Coronavirus que causa a gastrenterite transmissível do suíno. SIN TGE v.
tumor v., v. tumoral. SIN oncogenic v.
Turlock v., v. Turlock; um grupo sorológico não-classificado de arbovírus do gênero Bunyavirus, mas antigenicamente não relacionado a ele.
Umbre v., v. Umbre; um Bunyavirus relacionado sorologicamente ao v. Turlock.
vaccine v., v. da vacínia. VER vaccine.
vaccinia v., v. da vacínia; o poxvírus (gênero Orthopoxvirus) usado na imunização de pessoas contra a varíola, causando, em geral, uma reação local, mas, por vezes, vacínia generalizada, especialmente em crianças; o v. apresenta significativa correlação sorológica com os vírus da varíola e da vacínia, mas certas diferenças foram demonstradas, as quais indicam que talvez sejam cepas distintas, porém intimamente relacionadas, de um complexo varíola-vacínia-varíola bovina; a linhagem do v. da vacínia é incerta e é muito improvável que descenda do v. original de Jenner. SIN poxvirus officinalis.
vacuolating v., v. vacuolizante. SIN simian v.
varicella-zoster v., v. varicela-zoster; um herpesvírus, morfologicamente idêntico ao v. herpes simples, que causa a varicela (catapora) e o herpes zoster em

crianças; também capaz de produzir meningoencefalomielite em coelhos e crianças. [*Powassan*, Canadá, onde foi isolado pela primeira vez]

pseudocowpox v., v. da pseudovacínia; um v. do gênero Parapoxvirus que causa pseudovacínia em seres humanos e no gado bovino; está intimamente relacionado ao v. da estomatite pustular contagiosa e ao v. da estomatite papular. SIN paravaccinia v.

pseudolymphocytic choriomeningitis v., v. da coriomeningite pseudolinfocítica. SIN infectious ectromelia v.

pseudorabies v., v. da pseudo-raiva; um herpesvírus, família Herpesviridae, que causa a pseudo-raiva em suínos. SIN Aujeszky disease v.

psittacosis v., v. da psitacose; nome original da *Chlamydia psittaci*.

Puumala v., v. Puumala; uma espécie de Hantavirus encontrada na Europa que provoca febre hemorrágica com síndrome renal.

PVM v., v. PVM. SIN pneumonia v. of mice.

quail bronchitis v., v. da bronquite da codorna; um v. do gênero Aviadenovirus, relacionado antigenicamente ao v. CELO.

Quaranfil v., v. Quaranfil; um arbovírus não-classificado isolado no sangue humano e de garças.

rabbit fibroma v., v. do fibroma do coelho; um poxvírus do gênero Leporipoxvirus, família Poxviridae, intimamente relacionado com os vírus da vacínia e do mixoma, que causa o fibroma de Shope. SIN Shope fibroma v.

rabbit myxoma v., v. do mixoma do coelho; o poxvírus do gênero Leporipoxvirus que causa a mixomatose de coelhos. SIN myxomatosis v.

rabbitpox v., v. da varíola do coelho; um Orthopoxvirus que causa epidemia de varíola em coelhos de laboratório; imunologicamente, apresenta grande correlação com o v. da vacínia, mas é mais virulento em coelhos.

rabies v., v. da raiva; um grande v. RNA de filamento único, com formato de bala, do gênero Lyssavirus, família Rhabdoviridae; é o agente causal da raiva.

rabies v., Flury strain, v. da raiva, cepa Flury; um v. isolado no cérebro humano, atenuado (fixo) por propagação seriada em hospedeiros não-mamíferos e, subseqüentemente, estabelecido na cultura de embrião de pinto.

rabies v., Kelev strain, v. da raiva, estirpe (cepa) Kelev, uma estirpe atenuada, embrionada, com passagem em aves domésticas.

Rauscher v., v. Rauscher. SIN Rauscher leukemia v.

Rauscher leukemia v., v. da leucemia de Rauscher; um retrovírus RNA associado a leucemia em roedores; similar ao v. Friend. SIN Rauscher v.

REO v., v. REO. SIN respiratory enteric orphan v.

respiratory enteric orphan v., v. órfão entérico respiratório; um vírus icosaédrico não-envelopado com um capsídeo de dupla camada, cujo genoma consiste em múltiplos segmentos de RNA de duplo filamento, pertencendo à família Reoviridae, freqüentemente encontrado nos tratos respiratório e entérico. SIN REO v.

respiratory sincytial v. (RSV), v. sincicial respiratório; um v. RNA do gênero Pneumovirus, família Paramyxoviridae, com uma tendência a formar sincícios na cultura de tecidos, causando infecção respiratória branda, com rinite e tosse em adultos, mas é capaz de provocar bronquite grave e broncopneumonia em crianças pequenas; isolado primeiramente em chimpanzés com doença respiratória. SIN chimpanzee coryza agent, Rs v.

Reston v., v. Reston; uma variante do v. Ebola. SIN Ebola v. Reston.

Rida v., v. Rida; uma variante do agente do *scrapie*.

Rift Valley fever v., v. da febre do vale Rift; um v. do gênero Phlebovirus (família Bunyaviridae) que ocorre nas regiões central e sul da África em carneiros, cabras e no gado, provocando abortos e doença febril grave, em especial nos cordeiros jovens; os seres humanos, principalmente pastores e veterinários, podem ser infectados através do contato próximo com animais infectados, desenvolvendo uma doença semelhante ao dengue; o v. também infecta búfalos, camelos e antílopes; é transmitido por mosquitos, mas, provavelmente, também infecta por contato e pelo trato respiratório.

RNA v., v. RNA; um grupo de vírus em que o cerne consiste em RNA; um grupo importante de vírus animais que engloba as famílias Picornaviridae, Reoviridae, Togaviridae, Flaviviridae, Bunyaviridae, Arenaviridae, Paramyxoviridae, Retroviridae, Coronaviridae, Orthomyxoviridae e Rhabdoviridae. SIN ribovirus.

principais grupos de vírus

vírus DNA família do vírus	envelope presente	simetria do capsídeo	tamanho da partícula (nm)	estrutura do DNA*	vírus clinicamente importantes
Parvoviridae	não	icosaédrico	22	ss, linear	vírus B19
Papovaviridae	não	icosaédrico	55	ds circular, superespiralado	papilomavírus, poliomavírus (JC, BK)
Adenoviridae	não	icosaédrico	75	ds linear	adenovírus
Hepadnaviridae	sim	icosaédrico	42	ds circular incompleto	vírus da hepatite B
Herpesviridae	sim	icosaédrico	100**	ds, linear	vírus herpes simples, vírus varicela-zoster, citomegalovírus, vírus Epstein-Barr
Poxviridae	sim	complexa	250 × 400	ds, linear	vírus da varíola, vírus da vacínia
vírus RNA família do vírus	**envelope presente**	**simetria do capsídeo**	**tamanho da partícula (nm)**	**estrutura do RNA†**	**vírus clinicamente importantes**
Picornaviridae	não	icosaédrico	28	ss, linear, não-segmentado, sentido +	poliovírus, rinovírus, vírus da hepatite A, enterovírus
Reoviridae	não	icosaédrico	75	ds, linear, 10 segmentos	reovírus, rotavírus, vírus da febre do carrapato do Colorado
Togaviridae	sim	icosaédrico	40–70	ss, linear, não-segmentado, sentido +	vírus da rubéola, vírus da febre amarela
Retroviridae	sim	icosaédrico	100	ss, linear, 2 segmentos, sentido +	HIV, vírus linfotrópico da célula T humana (HTLV)
Coronaviridae	sim	helicoidal	100	ss, linear, não-segmentado sentido +	coronavírus
Caliciviridae	não	icosaédrico	35–40	RNA de filamento único com sentido +	agente Norwalk
Orthomyxoviridae	sim	helicoidal	80–120	ss, linear, 8 segmentos, sentido −	vírus influenza
Paramyxoviridae	sim	helicoidal	150	ss, linear, não-segmentado, sentido +	vírus do sarampo, caxumba, parainfluenza, sincicial respiratório
Rhabdoviridae	sim	helicoidal	75 × 180	ss, linear, não-segmentado, sentido −	vírus da raiva
Arenaviridae	sim	helicoidal	80–130	ss, circular, 2 segmentos com terminações coesivas, sentido −	vírus da coriomeningite linfocítica
Bunyaviridae	sim	helicoidal	100	ss, circular, 3 segmentos com terminações coesivas, sentido −	vírus da encefalite da Califórnia e da febre do flebótomo
Filoviridae	sim	complexa	80 × (800–900)	RNA, ss, sentido −	vírus Marburg, Ebola

* ss, filamento único; ds, filamento duplo; +, positivo; −, negativo
**o nucleocapsídeo do herpesvírus tem 100 nm, mas o envelope varia de tamanho; o vírus inteiro pode chegar a 200 nm de diâmetro
†O retrovírus RNA contém 2 moléculas idênticas de peso molecular de $3,5 \times 10^6$

RNA tumor viruses, vírus RNA tumorais; vírus RNA da família Retroviridae que provocam tumores.
Ross River v., v. do rio Ross; um alfavírus, família Togaviridae, transmitido por mosquito e causador de poliartrite epidêmica.
Rous-associated v. (RAV), v. associado de Rous; um v. de leucemia dos retrovírus do tipo C das aves (complexo leucose–sarcoma), família Retroviridae, que, por mistura fenotípica com uma cepa defeituosa (não-infecciosa) do sarcoma de Rous, efetua a produção de v. do sarcoma infeccioso com a antigenicidade do envelope do RAV.
Rous sarcoma v. (RSV), v. do sarcoma de Rous; um v. produtor de sarcoma dos retrovírus do tipo C das aves (complexo de leucose–sarcoma), família Retroviridae, identificado por Rous em 1911.
Rs v., v. Rs. SIN respiratory syncytial v.
Rubarth disease v., v. da doença de Rubarth. SIN canine *adenovirus* 1.
rubella v., v. da rubéola; um v. RNA do gênero Rubivirus, família Togaviridae; o agente causal da rubéola nos seres humanos. SIN German measles v.
rubeola v., v. do sarampo. SIN measles v.
Russian autumn encephalitis v., v. da encefalite russa do outono. SIN Japanese B encephalitis v.
Russian spring-summer encephalitis v., v. da encefalite russa da primavera-verão. SIN tick-borne encephalitis v.
Sabia v., v. Sabia; um arenavírus associado à febre hemolítica.
Salisbury common cold viruses, vírus do resfriado comum de Salisbury; cepas de rinovírus de interesse histórico por causa dos estudos iniciais que estabeleceram a etiologia viral dos resfriados comuns.
salivary v., herpesvírus humano 5. SIN human *herpesvirus* 5.
salivary gland v., herpesvírus humano 5. SIN human *herpesvirus* 5.
sandfly fever viruses, vírus da febre do flebótomo. SIN phlebotomus fever viruses.
San Miguel sea lion v., v. do leão marinho de São Miguel; um calicivírus, família Caliciviridae, isolado pela primeira vez em leões-marinhos de São Miguel, ilha da costa da Califórnia, que é indistinguível do exantema vesicular do v. suíno, tanto biofísica quanto clinicamente, em termos da síndrome da doença vesicular que produz em suínos.
Semliki Forest v., v. da floresta Semliki; um alfavírus, família Togaviridae, raramente associado a doença humana.
Sendai v., v. Sendai; um v. parainfluenza do tipo 1 reportado como causa de infecção inaparente em muitos animais; também é muito empregado para efetuar fusão celular em cultura de tecidos.
Seoul v., v. Seoul; uma espécie de Hantavirus no Extremo Oriente que causa febre hemorrágica com síndrome renal. [o vírus recebeu esse nome por causa de Seul, na Coréia do Sul, a cidade onde foi isolado pela primeira vez.]
serum hepatitis v., v. da hepatite sérica. SIN hepatitis B v.
sheep-pox v., v. da varíola do carneiro; um poxvírus do gênero Capripoxvirus que causa a varíola dos carneiros.
shipping fever v., v. da febre do embarque; uma cepa bovina do v. parainfluenza do tipo 3. VER parainfluenza viruses.
Shope fibroma v., v. do fibroma de Shope. SIN rabbit fibroma v.
Shope papilloma v., v. do papiloma de Shope; um papilomavírus que infecta lebres selvagens. VER Shope *papilloma*.
Simbu v., v. Simbu; um grupo sorológico do gênero Bunyavirus, compreendendo inúmeras espécies, incluindo a cepa típica, v. Simbu.
simian v. (SV), v. de símio; qualquer um de inúmeros vírus, pertencentes a várias famílias, isolados em macacos ou culturas de células de macacos. SIN vacuolating v.
simian v. 40, v. de símio 40. SIN simian vacuolating v. No. 40.
simian vacuolating v. No. 40 (SV40), v. de símio vacuolizante n.° 40; um pequeno v. DNA (40–45 nm) do gênero Polyomavirus, família Papovaviridae; a causa de infecções aparentemente inaparentes em macacos, especialmente o Rhesus, e um contaminante comum de culturas de células de macaco; o v. pode causar infecção inaparente em seres humanos e ser excretado nas fezes de crianças durante várias semanas; pode provocar fibrossarcoma em *hamsters* recém-nascidos, podendo a transformação ocorrer em células diplóides humanas; também pode formar v. "híbrido" em células também infectadas por determinados adenovírus. SIN simian v. 40.
Sindbis v., v. Sindbis; a espécie típica do gênero Alphavirus, família Togaviridae, comumente transmitido por mosquitos do gênero *Culex*; é agente causal da febre Sindbis. [vila no Egito onde foi isolado pela primeira vez]
Sin Nombre v., v. Sin Nombre; uma espécie de Hantavirus, encontrada na América do Norte, que causa síndrome pulmonar. SIN Four Corners v. [Espanhol, sem nome]
slow v., v. lento; um v. ou um agente vírus-símile, etiologicamente associado a uma doença que possui um longo período de incubação de meses a anos com estabelecimento gradual, freqüentemente terminando em doença grave e/ou morte.
smallpox v., v. da varíola. SIN variola v.
snowshoe hare v., v. da lebre-da-neve; um membro do grupo Califórnia dos arbovírus, gênero Bunyavirus, família Bunyaviridae, que causa febre, cefaléia grave e náuseas em seres humanos na América do Norte.
soremouth v., v. da dermatite pustular de carneiros. SIN contagious ecthyma (pustular dermatitis) v. of sheep.
Spondweni v., v. Spondweni; um arbovírus do gênero Flavivirus isolado em mosquitos na África; pode causar doença em seres humanos.
St. Louis encephalitis v., v. da encefalite de St. Louis; um arbovírus do grupo B, gênero Flavivirus, família Flaviviridae, que ocorre nos Estados Unidos, Trinidad e Panamá; normalmente presente como infecção inaparente em seres humanos, mas, por vezes, uma causa de encefalite; foi isolado em pássaros no Panamá e em diversas espécies de mosquito, especialmente *Psorophora*.
street v., um v. da raiva isolado em um animal doméstico naturalmente infectado.
Sudan v., v. Sudan; uma variante do v. Ebola. SIN Ebola v. Sudan.
swine encephalitis v., v. da encefalite suína; um coronavírus, família Coronaviridae, que causa a encefalite suína.
swine fever v., v. da febre suína. SIN hog cholera v.
swine influenza viruses, vírus influenza suínos; cepas de v. influenza do tipo A que causam *influenza* em suínos e podem infectar os seres humanos.
swinepox v., v. da varíola suína; um poxvírus do gênero Suipoxvirus diferente do v. da vacínia e a causa da varíola suína; o piolho do porco é importante na transmissão.
Swiss mouse leukemia v., v. Friend. SIN Friend v.
Tacaribe v., v. Tacaribe; o v. típico do complexo Tacaribe dos vírus do gênero Arenavirus, tendo sido isolado em morcegos e mosquitos em Trinidad.
Tahyna v., v. Tahyna; um arbovírus do grupo Califórnia do gênero Bunyavirus, família Bunyaviridae, oriundo da Europa Central, que, sabidamente, infecta seres humanos.
Taiwan Dobrava-Belgrade v., v. Taiwan Dobrava-Belgrado; uma espécie de Hantavirus nos Balcãs que causa febre hemorrágica com síndrome renal. [de Dobrava, Eslovênia (onde foi isolado pela primeira vez em camundongos silvestres) e de Belgrado, antiga Iugoslávia (onde foi isolado pela primeira vez em seres humanos)]
temperate v., um fago que não lisa seu hospedeiro imediatamente, mas que pode persistir na forma latente e, mais adiante, lisar seu hospedeiro. VER lysogeny.
Teschen disease v., v. da doença de Teschen; um picornavírus que causa a doença de Teschen dos porcos; o v. é, em geral, um habitante inócuo do trato intestinal, mas as cepas virulentas causam epidemias. SIN infectious porcine encephalomyelitis v.
Tete viruses, vírus Tete; um grupo sorológico do gênero Bunyavirus, compreendendo inúmeros tipos.
TGE v., v. TGE. SIN transmissible gastroenteritis v. of swine.
Theiler v., v. Theiler. SIN mouse encephalomyelitis v.
Theiler mouse encephalomyelitis v., v. da encefalomielite do camundongo de Theiler; um vírus do gênero Cardiovirus, família Picornaviridae. SIN Theiler original v.
Theiler original v., v. original de Theiler. SIN Theiler mouse encephalomyelitis v.
tick-borne v., v. transmitido por carrapato. SIN tick-borne encephalitis v.
tick-borne encephalitis v., v. da encefalite transmitido por carrapato; arbovírus do gênero Flavivirus que ocorrem na Europa Central e Rússia em múltiplos subtipos, causando duas formas de encefalite em seres humanos: encefalite transmitida por carrapato (subtipo da Europa Central) e encefalite transmitida por carrapato (subtipo do leste); os vetores são carrapatos do gênero *Ixodes*. SIN Russian spring-summer encephalitis v., tick-borne v.
TO v., v. TO; v. original de Theiler. VER mouse encephalomyelitis v.
Topografov v., v. de Topografov; uma espécie de Hantavirus encontrada na Sibéria.
trachoma v., v. do tracoma; nome antigo da *Chlamydia trachomatis*.
transmissible gastroenteritis v. of swine, v. da gastrenterite transmissível do suíno; um v. do gênero Coronavirus que causa a gastrenterite transmissível do suíno. SIN TGE v.
tumor v., v. tumoral. SIN oncogenic v.
Turlock v., v. Turlock; um grupo sorológico não-classificado de arbovírus do gênero Bunyavirus, mas antigenicamente não relacionado a ele.
Umbre v., v. Umbre; um Bunyavirus relacionado sorologicamente ao v. Turlock.
vaccine v., v. da vacínia. VER vaccine.
vaccinia v., v. da vacínia; o poxvírus (gênero Orthopoxvirus) usado na imunização de pessoas contra a varíola, causando, em geral, uma reação local, mas, por vezes, vacínia generalizada, especialmente em crianças; o v. apresenta significativa correlação sorológica com os vírus da varíola e da vacínia, mas certas diferenças foram demonstradas, as quais indicam que talvez sejam cepas distintas, porém intimamente relacionadas, de um complexo varíola-vacínia-varíola bovina; a linhagem do v. da vacínia é incerta e é muito improvável que descenda do v. original de Jenner. SIN poxvirus officinalis.
vacuolating v., v. vacuolizante. SIN simian v.
varicella-zoster v., v. varicela-zoster; um herpesvírus, morfologicamente idêntico ao v. herpes simples, que causa a varicela (catapora) e o herpes zoster em

vi·tal red [C.I. 23570]. Vermelho vital; sal trissódico de um corante diazo sulfonado (um grupamento ditolil diazotizado em resíduos aminonaftaleno sulfonados), usado como corante vital. SIN brilliant vital red.

vi·tals (vīt′ălz). Vísceras. SIN viscera.

vi·ta·mer (vī′tă - mer). Um de dois ou mais compostos similares capazes de preencher uma função vitamínica específica no corpo; p.ex., niacina, niacinamida.

VITAMIN

vi·ta·min (vīt′ă - min). Vitamina; uma de um grupo de substâncias orgânicas, presentes em quantidades diminutas nos alimentos naturais, que são essenciais para o metabolismo normal; quantidades insuficientes na dieta podem provocar doenças. [L. *vita*, vida, + *amine*]

v. A, v. A; **(1)** qualquer derivado β-ionona, exceto os carotenóides pró-vitamina A, que possuem, qualitativamente, a atividade biológica do retinol; a deficiência interfere com a produção e síntese de nova rodopsina, gerando, por conseguinte, a cegueira noturna, além de produzir metaplasia queratinizante das células epiteliais, a qual pode resultar em xeroftalmia, ceratose, suscetibilidade às infecções e retardo do crescimento; **(2)** a v. A original, atualmente conhecida como retinol. SIN axerophthol.

v. A_1, v. A_1, retinol. SIN retinol.

v. A_2, v. A_2, desidrorretinol. SIN dehydroretinol.

v. A_1 acid, v. A_1 ácida, ácido retinóico. SIN retinoic acid.

v. A_1 alcohol, v. A_1 alcoólica, retinol. SIN retinol.

v. A aldehyde, retinaldeído. SIN retinaldehyde.

v. A_2 aldehyde, desidrorretinaldeído. SIN dehydroretinaldehyde.

antiberiberi v., tiamina. SIN thiamin.

antihemorrhagic v., v. K. SIN v. K.

antineuritic v., tiamina. SIN thiamin.

antirachitic v.'s, vitaminas anti-raquitismo; ergocalciferol (v. D_2) e colecalciferol (v. D_3).

antiscorbutic v., ácido ascórbico. SIN ascorbic acid.

antisterility v., v. E (2). SIN v. E (2).

v. B, v. B; um grupo de substâncias hidrossolúveis originalmente consideradas como uma única v.

v. B_1, v. B_1, tiamina. SIN thiamin.

v. B_2, v. B_2; **(1)** SIN riboflavin; **(2)** termo obsoleto para um complexo de ácido fólico, ácido nicotínico, nicotinamida, ácido pantotênico e riboflavina.

v. B_3, v. B_3; **(1)** termo obsoleto para nicotinamida e/ou ácido nicotínico; **(2)** termo obsoleto para ácido pantotênico.

v. B_4, v. B_4; **(1)** outrora acreditava-se que era um fator necessário para a nutrição do pinto, atualmente identificada apenas como determinados aminoácidos essenciais e/ou adenina; **(2)** termo obsoleto para adenina.

v. B_5, v. B_5; termo outrora utilizado para descrever atividades biológicas agora atribuídas ao ácido pantotênico ou ao ácido nicotínico.

v. B_6, v. B_6; a piridoxina e os compostos correlatos (piridoxal; piridoxamina).

v. B_{12}, v. B_{12}; termo geral para os compostos que exibem a atividade biológica da cianocobalamina (cianocob(III)alamina); o fator antianemia do extrato hepático que contém cobalto, um grupamento ciano e corrina em uma estrutura cobamida. Várias substâncias com fórmulas similares e ação hematínica característica foram isoladas e designadas: $B12_a$, hidroxicobalamina; B_{12b}, aqua-

vitaminas e minerais: fontes, etc.

vitamina/mineral	fontes	benefícios	deficiência	cotas dietéticas recomendadas (CDR)
vitamina A*	batatas doces, cenoura, leite	resistência cutânea melhorada à infecção; boa visão noturna	cegueira noturna, xeroftalmia	equivalentes a 1.000 µg de retinol (5.000 UI)
vitamina D*	luz solar, laticínios	fortalece o desenvolvimento ósseo	raquitismo	5–10 µg (1.000–1.200 UI)
vitamina E*	vegetais verdes folhosos, amêndoas, grãos integrais, germe de trigo	proteção oxidativa dos eritrócitos	anemia	8–10 mg (30 UI)
vitamina K*	vegetais verdes folhosos, tomates	cascata da coagulação sanguínea	diáteses hemorrágicas	70–140 µg
vitamina B_1† (tiamina)	grãos integrais, vegetais, amêndoas, germe de trigo	metabolismo de carboidratos	beribéri	1–1,5 mg
vitamina B_2† (riboflavina)	produtos animais, cogumelos, brócolis	metabolismo de proteína, protetor cutâneo e ocular	estomatite angular/blefarite	1,2–1,5 mg
vitamina B_6† (piridoxina)	levedo de cerveja, grãos integrais, amêndoas, carne	ajuda a regular o sistema nervoso central	neuropatia periférica convulsões	1,7–2 mg
vitamina B_{12}†	produtos animais, peixe, soja	formação de eritrócitos	alterações do estado mental	3 µg
ácido fólico	vegetais verdes folhosos, fígado, levedo	proteger contra os defeitos do nascimento, produção de eritrócitos	anemia	0,4 mg (ou 400 µg)
vitamina C†	brócolis, tomates, couve de Bruxelas, frutas cítricas	resistência ao estresse; higiene oral; cura de feridas	escorbuto	60 mg
niacina†	amêndoas, carne de aves, peixe	agente redutor do colesterol, coenzimas em oxidações, reduções	pelagra	13–16 mg
cálcio	laticínios	crescimento ósseo; nervo, músculo, função	raquitismo, osteomalacia, osteoporose	800 mg
potássio	tomates, frutas cítricas	função celular	íleo paralítico, fraqueza muscular	1,8–6 g
sódio	maioria dos alimentos	função celular	fraqueza, confusão	1–3,3 g
fósforo	cereais, laticínios	função celular	alterações do estado mental, osteomalacia	800 mg
ferro	vegetais verdes folhosos, frutas secas, carne, germe de trigo	formação do eritrócito	anemia	10–18 mg
iodo	alguns produtos lácteos, frutos do mar, sal iodado	função tireóidea normal, anti-séptico tópico	bócio	150 µg

* lipossolúvel
† hidrossolúvel

cobalamina; B_{12c}, nitritocobalamina; B_{12r}, cob(II)alamina; B_{12s}, cob(I)alamina; B_{12III}, fatores A e V_{1a} (ácido cobírico) e pseudovitamina B_{12}. Sabe-se que as vitaminas B_{12a} e B_{12b} são compostos tautoméricos; a B_{12b} foi obtida de culturas de *Streptomyces aureofaciens*; a B_{12c} foi obtida de culturas de *Streptomyces griseus* e é diferenciada da B_{12} por seu espectro de absorção. As coenzimas da v. B_{12} fisiologicamente ativas são metilcobalamina e desoxiadenosinocobalamina. Uma deficiência de v. B_{12} está freqüentemente associada a determinadas acidúrias metilmalônicas. SIN animal protein factor, antianemic factor, antipernicious anemia factor (1), erythrocyte maturation factor, maturation factor, methylcobalamin.

v. B_T, v. B_T, carnitina. SIN carnitine.

v. B_x, v. B_x, ácido *p*-aminobenzóico. SIN p-aminobenzoic acid.

v. B complex, complexo da v. B; um termo farmacêutico aplicado aos produtos que contêm uma mistura das vitaminas B, usualmente B_1, B_2, B_3, B_5 e B_6.

v. B_c conjugase, v. B_c conjugase; uma enzima que catalisa a hidrólise dos ácidos pteroilpoliglutâmicos em ácido pteroilmonoglutâmico, com conseqüente aumento da atividade da vitamina; v. B_c é um termo obsoleto para ácido fólico.

v. B_{12} with intrinsic factor concentrate, v. B_{12} com concentrado de fator intrínseco; uma combinação de v. B_{12} com preparações adequadas da mucosa do estômago ou intestino de animais domésticos usada como alimento pelos seres humanos.

v. C, v. C, ácido ascórbico. SIN ascorbic acid.

coagulation v., v. da coagulação; termo obsoleto para v. K.

v. D, v. D; termo genérico para todos os esteróides que exibem a atividade biológica do ergocalciferol ou colecalciferol, as vitaminas anti-raquitismo popularmente denominadas de "vitaminas dos raios solares". Elas promovem a utilização apropriada do cálcio e fósforo, promovendo assim o crescimento, juntamente com a formação apropriada de ossos e dentes, em crianças pequenas; o sulfato, um conjugado hidrossolúvel, é encontrado na fase aquosa do leite humano; a v. D_1 é uma mistura de lumisterol e v. D_2.

v. D_2, v. D_2, ergocalciferol. SIN ergocalciferol.

v. D_3, v. D_3, colecalciferol. SIN cholecalciferol.

v. E, v. E; (1) SIN α-tocopherol; (2) termo genérico dos derivados tocol e tocotrienol que possuem a atividade biológica do α-tocoferol; contido em vários óleos (germe de trigo, semente de algodão, azeite de dendê, arroz) e em cereais integrais, onde constitui a fração não-saponificável; também contido em tecido animal (fígado, pâncreas, coração) e na alface; a deficiência produz reabsorção ou absorção em ratos fêmeas e esterilidade nos machos. SIN antisterility factor, antisterility v., fertility v.

v. F, v. F; termo por vezes aplicado a ácidos graxos essenciais insaturados, ácidos linoleico, linolênico e araquidônico.

fat-soluble v.'s, vitaminas lipossolúveis; as vitaminas solúveis em solventes lipídicos (solventes não-polares) e relativamente insolúveis em água, cuja estrutura química é caracterizada pela presença de grandes parcelas de hidrocarboneto na molécula; p.ex., vitaminas A, D, E, K.

fertility v., v. E (2). SIN v. E (2).

v. G, v. G; termo obsoleto para riboflavina.

v. H, v. H, biotina. SIN biotin. [Alem., H de *Haut*, pele]

v. K, v. K; termo genérico para os compostos com a atividade biológica da filoquinona; compostos lipossolúveis e termoestáveis encontrados na alfafa, fígado de porco, carne de peixe e óleos vegetais, essenciais para a formação de quantidades normais de protrombina. SIN antihemorrhagic factor, antihemorrhagic v.

v. K_1, v. K_1(20), v. K_1, filoquinona. SIN phylloquinone.

v. K_2, v. K_2 (30), v. K_2, menaquinona-6. SIN menaquinone-6.

v. K_3, v. K_3, menadiona. SIN menadione.

v. K_4, v. K_4, diacetato de menadiol. SIN menadiol diacetate.

v. K_5, v. K_5; uma v. anti-hemorrágica.

v. K_2(35), v. K_2(35), menaquinona-7. SIN menaquinone-7.

microbial v., v. microbiana; uma substância necessária para o crescimento de determinados microrganismos, p.ex., biotina, ácido *p-aminobenzóico*.

v. P, v. P; uma mistura de bioflavonóides extraída de vegetais (principalmente das frutas cítricas). Reduz a permeabilidade e a fragilidade dos capilares e é útil no tratamento de determinados casos de púrpura que são resistentes à terapia com v. C. VER TAMBÉM hesperidin, quercetin, rutin. SIN capillary permeability factor, citrin, permeability v.

permeability v., v. P. SIN v. P.

v. PP, v. PP, ácido nicotínico. SIN nicotinic acid.

v. U, v. U; termo dado a um fator no suco de couve fresca que encoraja a cura da úlcera péptica (cloreto de 3-amino-3-carboxipropil)-dimetilsulfônio, um derivado metionina.

vi·tel·lar·i·um (vit′ĕl-lar′ē-ŭm). Vitelário; nos cestódeos e trematódeos, um compartimento comum que recebe material vitelino (gema) dos dois ductos vitelínicos; o material da gema passa, então, para dentro do oótipo para circundar o ovo com grânulos vitelínicos nutritivos que são envoltos por uma casca de ovo formada de forma característica. SIN vitelline reservoir.

vi·tel·li·form (vī-tel′i-form) Viteliforme; relativo a ou que se assemelha a gema de ovo.

vi·tel·lin (vī-tel′in). Vitelina; uma lipofosfoproteína combinada à lecitina na gema do ovo. SIN lipovitellin, ovovitellin.

vi·tel·line (vī-tel′in, -ēn) Vitelino; relativo ao vitelo. VER yolk *sac*.

vi·tel·lo·gen·e·sis (vī-tel′lō-jen′ē-sis, vī′tĕ-lō-). Vitelogênese; formação da gema e seu acúmulo no saco vitelino. [L. *vitellus*, gema, + G. *genesis*, produção]

vi·tel·lo·gen·in (vī′tel-ō-jen′in). Vitelogenina; uma proteína precursora da gema de ovo; a produção é estimulada por estrogênios. [L. *vitellus*, gema de ovo, + *-gen*, + *-in*]

vi·tel·lo·lu·te·in (vī-tel-ō-loo′tē-in). Viteloluteína; a luteína da gema do ovo.

vitel·lo·ru·bin (vī-tel-ō-roo′bin). Vitelorrubina; um pigmento avermelhado obtido da gema do ovo.

vi·tel·lose (vī-tel′ōs). Um fragmento proteico da vitelina.

vi·tel·lus (vī-tel′ŭs). Vitelo. SIN yolk (1). [L.]

v. o′vi, v. do ovo; gema do ovo; usado em farmácia para a emulsificação de óleos e cânforas.

vi·ti·a·tion (vish-ē-ā′shŭn). Contaminação; uma alteração que compromete a utilidade ou reduz a eficiência. [L. *vitiatio*, de *vitio*, pp. *vitiatus*, corromper, de *vitium*, vício]

vit·i·lig·i·nes (vit-i-lij′i-nēz). Vitiligos; plural de vitiligo.

vit·i·lig·i·nous (vit-i-lij-i-nŭs). Vitiliginoso; relativo a ou caracterizado por vitiligo.

vit·i·li·go, pl. **vit·i·lig·i·nes** (vit-i-lī′gō, vit-i-lij′i-nēz). Vitiligo; o aparecimento, na pele normal, de placas esbranquiçadas não-pigmentadas de tamanhos variados, freqüentemente com distribuição simétrica e, em geral, limitada por áreas hiperpigmentadas; os pêlos nas áreas afetadas são usualmente esbranquiçados. Os melanócitos epidérmicos desaparecem por completo nas áreas despigmentadas por um processo auto-imune. SIN acquired leukoderma. [L. uma erupção cutânea, de *vitium*, vício, defeito]

v. i′ridis, v. da íris; pequenas placas esbranquiçadas na íris castanha.

vit·rec·to·my (vi-trek′tō-mē). Vitrectomia; a remoção do humor vítreo por meio de um instrumento que remove simultaneamente o humor vítreo por aspiração e incisão, substituindo-o por soro fisiológico ou algum outro líquido. [vitreous + G. *ektomē*, excisão]

anterior v., v. anterior; remoção do gel vítreo central.

posterior v., v. posterior; a remoção do humor vítreo cortical posterior; por vezes, as membranas pré-retinianas são removidas.

vit·re·in (vit′rē-in). Vitreína; uma proteína semelhante ao colágeno que, com o ácido hialurônico, contribui para o estado de gel do humor vítreo. SIN vitrosin.

vit·re·i·tis (vit-rē-ī′tis). Vitreíte; a inflamação do corpo vítreo. SIN hyalitis. [L. *vitreus*, vítreo, + G. *-itis*, inflamação]

vitreo-. Forma combinante que indica o humor vítreo. [L. *vitreus*, vítreo]

vit·re·o·den·tin (vit′rē-ō-den′tin). Vitreodentina; a dentina especialmente quebradiça.

vit·re·o·ret·i·nal (vit′rē-ō-ret′i-năl). Vitreorretinal; pertinente à retina e ao corpo vítreo.

vit·re·o·ret·i·nop·a·thy (vit′rē-ō-ret′i-nop′ă-thē). Vitreorretinopatia; retinopatia com complicações de v.

exudative v. [MIM*193220], v. exsudativa; uma doença ocular familial, lentamente progressiva, caracterizada por descolamento do humor vítreo posterior, membranas vítreas, heterotopia da mácula, descolamento da retina, neovascularização e hemorragia recorrente.

vit·re·ous (vit′rē-ŭs). Vítreo. **1.** Vítreo; que se assemelha ao vidro. **2.** SIN vitreous *body*. [L. *vitreus*, vítreo, de *vitrum*, vidro]

persistent anterior hyperplastic primary v., v. primário hiperplásico anterior persistente; uma anormalidade congênita unilateral que ocorre em neonatos a termo; caracterizada por uma membrana fibrovascular retrolenticular formada por v. primário persistente com resquícios da artéria hialóide e da túnica vascular da lente do olho; associado a leucocoria, microftalmia, câmara anterior rasa e processos ciliares alongados.

persistent posterior hyperplastic primary v., v. primário hiperplásico posterior persistente; uma anomalia congênita unilateral em neonatos a termo; associado a uma prega retiniana congênita e um pedículo membranoso do v. que contém os resquícios da artéria hialóide.

primary v., v. primário; o primeiro v. formado no embrião entre o cálice óptico e a vesícula do cristalino e, mais adiante, vascularizado pela artéria hialóide e seus ramos.

secondary v., v. secundário; o v. avascular formado ao redor do v. primário.

tertiary v., v. terciário; as fibrilas do v. derivado a partir do neuroepitélio do corpo ciliar e que forma a zônula ciliar.

vit·re·um (vit′rē-ŭm). Corpo vítreo. SIN vitreous *body*. [L. neut. de *vitreus*, vítreo]

vit·ri·fi·ca·tion (vit′ri-fi-kā′shŭn). Vitrificação; a conversão da porcelana dentária (frita) em uma substância vítrea por calor e fusão. [L. *vitrium*, vítreo, + *facio*, tornar]

vit·ri·ol (vit′rē-ol). Vitriol; qualquer um dos diversos sais de ácido sulfúrico, p.ex., v. azul (sulfato cúprico), v. verde (sulfato ferroso), v. branco (sulfato de zinco). [L. *vitreolus*, vítreo]

vitronectin (vit′rō-nek′tin). Vitronectina; uma glicoproteína plasmática envolvida nas reações inflamatórias e de reparo nos locais de lesão tecidual.

vit·ro·sin (vit′rō-sin). Vitrosina, vitreína. SIN vitrein.

Vit·ta·for·ma (vē-ta-for′ma). Um gênero de microsporídeos que podem infectar os seres humanos e provocar ceratite no imunocompetente e infecção disseminada no imunocomprometido; originalmente *Nosema*.

vi·var·i·um, pl. **vi·var·ia** (vī-var′ē-ŭm, -ă). Viveiro; compartimentos em que os animais são alojados, principalmente os animais usados em pesquisa médica. [L. *vivarius*, pertinente às criaturas vivas]

vivi-. Forma combinante que significa vivo. [L. *vivus*, vivo]

viv·i·di·al·y·sis (viv′i-dī-al′i-sis). Vividiálise; a remoção por diálise, como pela lavagem da cavidade peritoneal.

viv·i·dif·fu·sion (viv′i-di-fū′zhŭn). Vividifusão; termo arcaico para um método pelo qual o sangue circulante pode ser submetido a diálise fora do corpo e retornado para a circulação sem exposição ao ar ou a qualquer influência nociva; o princípio utilizado no desempenho da diálise renal com o rim artificial. [vivi- + diffusion]

viv·i·fi·ca·tion (viv′i-fi-kā′shŭn). Vivificação. SIN revivification (2). [L. *vivifico*, pp. *-atus*, de *vivus*, vivo, + *facio*, fazer]

viv·i·par·i·ty (viv′i-păr′i-tē). Viviparidade; a qualidade ou estado de ser vivíparo, ou seja, que produz prole que é viva no momento do nascimento. SIN zoogony.

vi·vip·a·rous (vī′vip′ă-rŭs). Vivíparo; que dá à luz filhotes vivos, diferente dos ovíparos, que põem ovos. SIN zoogonous. [vivi- + L. *pario*, dar à luz]

viv·i·per·cep·tion (viv′i-per-sep′shŭn). Vivipercepção; observação dos processos vitais no organismo sem o auxílio da vivissecção. [vivi- + perception]

viv·i·sect (viv-i-sekt′). Vivisseccionar; praticar vivissecção.

viv·i·sec·tion (viv-i-sek′shŭn). Vivissecção; qualquer cirurgia de incisão em um animal vivo para fins de experimentação; termo freqüentemente ampliado para indicar qualquer forma da experimentação animal. [vivi- + section]

viv·i·sec·tion·ist, viv·i·sec·tor (vi-vi-sek′shŭn-ist, -tŏr; vi-vi-sek′tŏr). Vivisseccionista, vivissector; aquele que pratica a vivissecção.

Vladimiroff, Vladimir D., cirurgião russo, 1837–1903. VER Mikulicz-V *amputation*; V.-Mikulicz *amputation*.

VLDL Abreviatura para very low density lipoprotein (lipoproteína de densidade de muito baixa). VER lipoprotein.

VMA Abreviatura de vanillylmandelic acid (ácido vanililmandélico).

V-max. V. máx. VER $V_{máx}$.

VMC Abreviatura para void metal composite (composto metálico vazio).

V-MI Abreviatura para Volpe-Manhold *Index* (Índice de Volpe-Manhold).

vo·cal (vō-kăl). Vocal; pertinente à voz ou aos órgãos da fala. [L. *vocalis*]

vo·cal fry (vō′kal frī). Voz glotalizada; fonação em uma freqüência artificialmente baixa, resultando em sons de estalido e tique-taque. SIN glottalization.

Vogel law. Lei de Vogel. VER em law.

Voges, Otto, médico alemão,*1867. VER V.-Proskauer *reaction*.

Vogt, Alfred, oftalmologista suíço, 1879–1943. VER V.-Koyanagi *syndrome*.

Vogt, Cécile, neurologista alemã, 1875–1962. VER V. *syndrome*.

Vogt, Heinrich W., neurologista alemão, *1875. VER Spielmeyer-V. *disease*.

Vogt, Karl C., fisiologista alemão, 1817–1895. VER V. *angle*.

Vogt, Oskar, neurologista alemão, 1870–1959. VER V. *syndrome*.

Vogt ceph·a·lo·dac·ty·ly. Cefalodactilia de Vogt. SIN type II acrocephalosyndactyly.

Vohwinkel, H. H., dermatologista alemão do século XX. VER Vohwinkel *syndrome*.

voice (voys). Voz; o som feito por vibração das pregas vocais causada pela passagem de ar através da laringe e do trato respiratório superior, sendo aproximadas as pregas vocais. SIN vox. [L. *vox*]

amphoric v., v. anfórica; um som vocal que tem caráter oco, soprado, ouvido sobre uma cavidade pulmonar quando o paciente fala ou sussurra. SIN amphorophony.

bronchial v., broncofonia. SIN bronchophony.

cavernous v., v. cavernosa; o som vocal oco ou metálico ouvido sobre uma cavidade pulmonar.

epigastric v., v. epigástrica; a ilusão de uma v. que provém do epigástrio.

eunuchoid v., v. eunucóide; v. em tom agudo de um homem adulto que se assemelha à v. de um menino; usualmente de origem funcional.

myxedema v., v. mixedematosa; a v. forçada, rouca e áspera de pessoas com mixedema, provavelmente devido ao espessamento mixedematoso das pregas vocais.

void (voyd). Eliminar urina ou fezes.

flow v., vazio de fluxo; na ressonância magnética, a ausência de sinal a partir do sangue, cujos prótons ativados deixam uma região antes de sua magnetização ser medida. VER TAMBÉM signal v.

signal v., vazio de sinal; na ressonância magnética, uma região que não emite sinal de radiofreqüência devido à ausência de prótons ativados na mesma (como o sangue fluindo), a um elemento diferente que predomina, principalmente o cálcio, ou à defasagem descompensada, como acontece nas interfaces ar–tecido no pulmão.

void met·al com·pos·ite (VMC). Composto metálico vazio; uma estrutura metálica porosa que possibilita o crescimento de tecido nas aberturas para estabelecer uma ligação de longo prazo entre a prótese e o tecido.

vol. Abreviatura para [L.] volatilis, volátil.

vo·la (vō′lă). Palma da mão ou da sola do pé. [L.]

vo·lar (vō′lăr) [TA]. Volar; indica a palma da mão ou a planta do pé. SIN volaris [TA].

vo·la·ris (vō-lā′ris) [TA]. Volar. SIN volar.

vol·a·tile (vol.) (vol′ă-til). Volátil. **1.** Que tende a evaporar rapidamente. **2.** Que tende à violência, explosividade ou alteração rápida. [L. *volatilis*, de *volo*, voar]

vol·a·til·i·za·tion (vol′ă-til-i-zā′shŭn). Volatilização. SIN evaporation. [do L. *volatilis*, volátil, de *volo*, pp. *volatus*, voar]

vol·a·til·ize (vol′ă-til-īz). Volatilizar. SIN evaporate.

Volhard, Franz, médico alemão, 1872–1950. VER V. *test*.

vo·li·tion (vō-lish′ŭn). Volição; o impulso consciente para realizar qualquer ato ou abster-se de seu desempenho; ação voluntária. [L. *volo*, desejar]

vo·li·tion·al (vō-lish′ŭn-ăl). Volicional; feito por um ato voluntário; relativo à volição.

Volkmann, Alfred W., fisiologista alemão, 1800–1877. VER V. *canals*, em canal.

Volkmann, Richard, cirurgião alemão, 1830–1889. VER V. *cheilitis*, *contracture*, *spoon*.

vol·ley (vol′ē). Salva; um grupo sincrônico de impulsos induzidos simultaneamente por estimulação artificial das fibras nervosas ou fibras musculares. [Fr. *volée*, do L. *volo*, voar]

Vollmer, Herman, pediatra norte-americano, 1896–1959. VER V. *test*.

Volpe, Anthony R., odontólogo norte-americano, *1932. VER V.-Manhold *Index*.

vol·sel·la (vol-sel′ă). Vulsela. SIN vulsella *forceps*. [ver vulsella]

volt (v, V) (vōlt). Volt; a unidade de força eletromotiva; a força eletromotiva que produzirá uma corrente de 1 A em um circuito que possui uma resistência de 1 ohm, ou seja, joule por coulomb. [Alessandro *Volta*, físico italiano, 1745–1827]

volt·age (vōl′tej). Voltagem; força, pressão ou potencial eletromotivo expresso em volts.

vol·ta·ic (vōl-tā′ik). Voltaico. SIN galvanic.

vol·ta·ism (vōl′tă-izm). Voltaísmo. SIN galvanism.

volt·am·e·ter (vōl-tam′ē-ter). Voltâmetro; um aparelho para medir a força de uma corrente galvânica por sua ação eletrolítica. [volt + G. *metron*, medida]

volt·am·pere (vōlt-am-pēr). Voltampère; uma unidade de força elétrica; o produto de 1 V por 1 A; equivalente a 1 W ou 1/1.000 kW.

volt·me·ter (vōlt′mē-ter). Voltímetro; um aparelho para medir a força eletromotiva ou diferença de potencial.

Voltolini, Friedrich E.R., laringologista alemão, 1819–1889. VER V. *disease*.

vol·ume (V, V) (vol′yŭm). Volume; o espaço ocupado por matéria, expresso usualmente em milímetros cúbicos, centímetros cúbicos, litros, etc. VER water. VER TAMBÉM capacity. [L. *volumen*, algo envolvido, de *volvo*, enrolar]

atomic v., v. atômico; o peso atômico de um elemento dividido por sua densidade no estado sólido; o v. do peso atômico em gramas de um elemento sólido.

v. averaging, ponderação do volume; em tomografia computadorizada ou ressonância magnética, o efeito de expressar a densidade média de um voxel como um pixel na imagem; quanto maior a espessura do corte, maior será a ponderação necessária, com perda da resolução da densidade.

closing v. (CV), v. de fechamento; o v. pulmonar em que o fluxo oriundo das partes inferiores dos pulmões se torna bastante reduzido ou cessa durante a expiração, presumivelmente por causa do fechamento das vias aéreas; medido por um aumento agudo na concentração expiratória de um gás marcador inspirado no início de uma respiração que se iniciou a partir do volume residual.

distribution v., v. de distribuição; o v. em que uma substância marcadora adicionada parece ter sido uniformemente distribuída por todo ele, calculado ao se dividir a quantidade do marcador adicionado por sua concentração depois do equilíbrio.

end-diastolic v., v. diastólico final; a capacidade ou o volume de sangue no ventrículo imediatamente antes que se inicie uma contração cardíaca; uma medida do enchimento cardíaco entre os batimentos, relacionada com a função diastólica.

end-systolic v., v. sistólico final; a capacidade ou o volume de sangue no ventrículo ao término do período de ejeção ventricular e imediatamente anterior ao início do relaxamento ventricular; uma medida da adequação do esvaziamento cardíaco, relacionada com a função sistólica.

expiratory reserve v. (ERV), v. de reserva expiratória; o v. máximo de ar (cerca de 1.000 ml) que pode ser expelido dos pulmões após uma expiração normal. SIN reserve air, supplemental air.

volume (V, V)

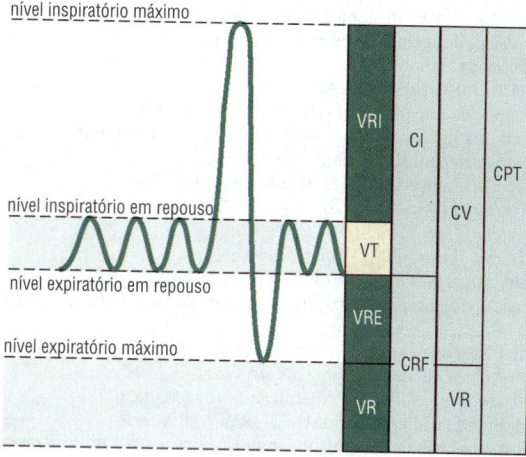

compartimentos e subdivisões do volume pulmonar: (baseado em um espirograma de volume–tempo) **VRE:** volume de reserva expiratória; o volume máximo de ar que pode ser expirado a partir da posição de volume corrente em repouso (posição expiratória final). **CRF:** capacidade residual funcional; o volume de ar nos pulmões do volume corrente na posição expiratória final, ou a soma de VR e VRE. **CI:** capacidade inspiratória; o volume máximo de ar que pode ser inalado a partir do volume corrente na posição expiratória final, ou a soma de VRI e VT. Em geral, essa capacidade constitui 60–70% da capacidade vital nos indivíduos saudáveis. **VRI:** volume de reserva inspiratória; o volume máximo de ar inspirado a partir da posição inspiratória final. **VR:** volume residual; o volume de ar que resta nos pulmões após expiração máxima, ou CPT – CV. **CPT:** capacidade pulmonar total; o somatório de todos os compartimentos de volume ou o volume de ar nos pulmões após inspiração máxima. **VT:** volume corrente; o volume de ar inspirado ou expirado a cada respiração durante a respiração tranqüila. **CV:** capacidade vital; o volume máximo de ar expirado a partir do ponto da inspiração máxima. CV também pode ser descrita como o somatório da VT, VRI e VRE. Em indivíduos saudáveis, a CV constitui cerca de 70% do volume pulmonar total.

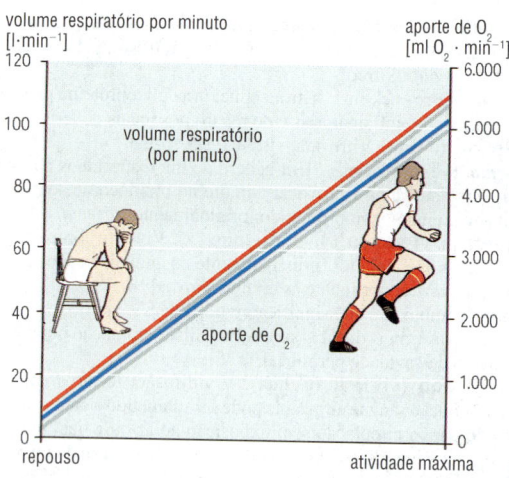

volume respiratório (por minuto): aporte de oxigênio e volume respiratório por minuto de um homem de 70 kg, em repouso e na atividade máxima

extracellular fluid v. (ECFV), v. de líquido extracelular (VLEC); a fração de água corporal que não está nas células, cerca de 25% do peso corporal; consiste em água plasmática (4,5% do peso corporal), água entre as células (linfa-água intersticial, 11,5% de peso corporal), água no tecido ósseo denso e no tecido conjuntivo (7,5% do peso corporal), e secreções aquosas. Ver entradas em água. VER TAMBÉM intracellular *fluid*.
forced expiratory v. (FEV), v. expiratório forçado (VEF); o v. máximo que pode ser expirado em um intervalo de tempo específico quando se inicia a partir da inspiração máxima. Uma anotação em subscrito normalmente indica o número de segundos que o paciente ficou expirando, p.ex., VEF_{30-60}.
inspiratory reserve v. (IRV), v. de reserva inspiratória (VRI); o v. máximo de ar que pode ser inspirado após uma inspiração normal; a capacidade inspiratória menos o v. corrente. SIN complemental air.
mean corpuscular v. (MCV), v. corpuscular médio; o v. médio dos eritrócitos, calculado a partir do hematócrito e contagem de eritrócitos nos índices eritrocitários.
minute v., v. minuto; o v. de qualquer gás ou líquido movido por minuto; p.ex., débito cardíaco ou o v. minuto respiratório.
packed cell v., v. globular; o v. de células sanguíneas em uma amostra de sangue depois que ela foi centrifugada no hematócrito; normalmente, perfaz 45% da amostra sanguínea.
partial v., v. parcial; o v. real ocupado por uma espécie de molécula ou partícula em uma solução; o inverso da densidade da molécula.
residual v. (RV), v. residual; o v. de ar que permanece nos pulmões após um esforço expiratório máximo. SIN residual air, residual capacity.
respiratory minute v. (RMV), v. minuto respiratório; o v. minuto da respiração; o produto do v. corrente vezes a freqüência respiratória. VER pulmonary *ventilation*.
resting tidal v., v. corrente em repouso; o v. corrente em condições normais, ou seja, na ausência de exercício ou outras condições que estimulam a respiração.
standard v., v. padrão; o v. de um gás ideal em temperatura e pressão padronizadas, aproximadamente 22,414 l.
stroke v., v. sistólico; o v. bombeado de um ventrículo do coração em um único batimento. SIN stroke output.
tidal v. (V_T), v. corrente; o v. de ar que é inspirado ou expirado em uma respiração única durante a respiração regular. SIN tidal air.
vol·ume·nom·e·ter (vol'ū - mĕ - nom'ĕ - ter). Volumenômetro; um aparelho para determinar o volume de um sólido por medir o volume de líquido que ele desloca. SIN volumometer. [volume + G. *metron*, medida]
vol·u·met·ric (vol - ū - met'rik). Volumétrico; relativo à medida por volume.
vol·u·mom·e·ter (vol - ū - mom'ĕ - ter). Volumômetro. SIN volumenometer.

vol·un·tary (vol'ŭn - tār - ē). Voluntário; relativo a ou que atua em obediência à vontade; não-obrigatório. [L. *voluntarius*, de *voluntas*, desejo, de *volo*, desejar]
vo·lup·tu·ous (vō - lŭp'tū - ŭs). Voluptuoso; que causa ou é causado por prazer sensual; determinado pela gratificação dos sentidos. [L. *voluptuosus*, de *voluptas*, prazer]
vo·lute (vō - loot). Voluto; enrolado; convoluto. [L. *voluta*, um giro, de *volvo*, pp. *volutus*, enrolar]
vol·u·tin (vol'oo - tin). Volutina; uma nucleoproteína complexa encontrada como grânulos citoplasmáticos em determinadas bactérias, leveduras e protozoários (como os flagelados tripanossomas), que servem como reservas alimentares. SIN volutin granules.
Vol·vox (vol'voks). Um gênero de flagelados esverdeados em colônias muito organizadas da classe Phytomastigophorea. [L. *volvo*, enrolar]
vol·vu·lo·sis (vol - voo - lō'sis). Oncocercose. SIN onchocerciasis.
vol·vu·lus (vol'vū - lŭs). Vólvulo; torção do intestino que causa obstrução; quando permanece sem tratamento, pode resultar em comprometimento vascular do intestino envolvido. [L. *volvo*, enrolar]
cecal v., v. cecal; rotação e torção do ceco em direção ao quadrante superior esquerdo, com obstrução do colo ascendente; associado a um ceco em um mesentério longo.
gastric v., v. gástrico; torção do estômago que pode resultar em obstrução e comprometimento do suprimento sanguíneo para o órgão; pode ocorrer na hérnia paraesofágica e, ocasionalmente, na eventração do diafragma. VER organoaxial.
mesenteroaxial v., v. mesenteroaxial; um tipo de v. gástrico em que o eixo de torção é paralelo à linha do mesentério gástrico. VER TAMBÉM organoaxial.
sigmoid v., v. sigmóide; localização relativamente comum do v., com obstrução, quer proximal, quer distal ao segmento sigmóide.
vo·mer, gen. vo·me·ris (vō'mer, vō'mer - is). [TA]. Vômer; um osso chato, de formato trapezóide, que forma a porção inferior e posterior do septo nasal; articula-se com o esfenóide, etmóide, com as duas maxilas e com os dois ossos palatinos. [L. relha do arado]
v. cartilagin'eus, v. cartilaginoso. SIN vomeronasal *cartilage*.
vo·mer·ine (vō'mer - ēn). Vomeriano; relativo ao vômer.
vom·er·o·bas·i·lar (vō'mer - ō - bas'i - lār). Vomerobasilar; relativo ao vômer e à base do crânio.
vom·er·o·na·sal (vō'mer - ō - nā'sal). Vomeronasal; relativo ao vômer e ao osso nasal.
vom·it (vom'it). **1.** Vomitar; ejetar o conteúdo do estômago através da boca. **2.** Vômito; o material assim ejetado. SIN vomitus (2). [L. *vomo*, pp. *vomitus*, vomitar]
Barcoo v., vômito de Barcoo; crises de náuseas e vômitos acompanhadas por bulimia que afetam aqueles que vivem no interior da região sul da Austrália.
bilious v., vômito bilioso; v. que contém bastante bile, sugestivo de obstrução intestinal distal à papila de Vater.
black v., vômito negro; o material com coloração de borra de café que é vomitado, especificamente, na febre amarela grave. VER TAMBÉM coffee-ground v. SIN vomitus niger.
coffee-ground v., vômito em borra de café; v. que consiste em sangue fresco ou coagulado. VER TAMBÉM black v.
vom·it·ing (vom'i - ting). Vômito; a ejeção de material do estômago, de forma retrógrada, através do esôfago e da boca. SIN emesis (1), vomition, vomitus (1).

causas de vômitos

causas funcionais
psicogênica, gravidez, doença esofágica funcional

causas orgânicas
esôfago: tumores, infecções, estenoses, divertículos, tumores mediastinais, inclusive carcinoma broncogênico

estômago: gastrite aguda, úlcera, estenose por fibrose ou tumores (atonia gástrica pós-operatória), piloroespasmo (em crianças)

intestinos delgado e grosso: gastroenterite aguda, íleo paralítico mecânico, obstrução

fígado, vesícula biliar, pâncreas: infecções, cálculos biliares, tumores; peritônio: peritonite aguda (difusa e local)

doenças extra-abdominais
cerebral: meningite, encefalite, doença de Ménière, cefaléia enxaqueca, glaucoma, tumores, lesão craniencefálica, sangramento, crise hipertensiva

distúrbios do metabolismo: pré-coma diabético, acidose láctica, uremia, tireotoxicose, doença de Addison

causas exógenas
numerosos medicamentos (digitálicos, antibióticos, opiáceos, etc.)

intoxicações (intoxicação por cogumelo, álcool, alimento estragado, etc.)

---

cerebral v., v. cerebral; v. decorrente de doença intracraniana, especialmente a pressão intracraniana elevada.

cyclic v., v. cíclico; uma síndrome de surtos recorrentes de v. observada principalmente em crianças pré-verbais; muitas crianças afetadas desenvolvem, mais adiante, enxaquecas típicas.

dry v., v. seco. SIN retching.

epidemic v., v. epidêmico; v. causado pelo vírus Norwalk, um vírus RNA com 27 nm, família Caliciviridae, que freqüentemente ocorre em um grupo de pessoas (p.ex., em uma escola ou comunidade pequena) de forma súbita e sem doença ou indisposição prodrômica; é intenso enquanto dura, mas cessa de forma repentina após 24–48 horas; os sintomas são cefaléia, dor abdominal, lipotímia e diarréia na maioria dos casos, com prostração extrema em cerca de 75%. SIN epidemic nausea.

fecal v., v. fecal; o vômito com aspecto e/ou odor de fezes, sugestivo de obstrução colônica ou da porção distal do intestino delgado de longa duração. SIN copremesis, stercoraceous v.

morning v., v. matinal; v. que ocorre ao acordar ou imediatamente depois do café da manhã em algumas mulheres durante o início da gestação. SIN morning sickness.

pernicious v., v. pernicioso; v. incontrolável.

v. of pregnancy, v. da gravidez; v. que ocorre nos primeiros meses de gestação.

projectile v., v. em jato; expulsão do conteúdo do estômago com grande força.

psychogenic v., v. psicogênico; v. associado a angústia emocional e ansiedade.

retention v., v. de retenção; v. devido à obstrução mecânica, usualmente horas após a ingestão de uma refeição.

stercoraceous v., v. estercoráceo. SIN fecal v.

vo·mi·tion (vō-mish′ŭn). Vomitação. SIN vomiting. [L. *vomitio*, de *vomo*, vomitar]

vom·i·tu·ri·tion (vom′i-too-rish′ŭn). Ânsia de vômito. SIN retching.

vom·i·tus (vom′i-tŭs). Vômito. **1.** SIN vomiting. **2.** SIN vomit (2). [L. um vômito, vomitação]

v. cruen′tes, hematêmese. SIN hematemesis.

v. mari′nus, enjôo causado pelo balanço do navio. SIN seasickness.

v. ni′ger, v. negro. SIN black vomit.

von. Freqüentemente abreviado para v. Para os nomes com esse prefixo que não forem encontrados aqui, ver sob a parte principal do nome.

von Bruns. VER Bruns.

von Ebner, Victor, histologista austríaco, 1842–1925. VER Ebner *glands*, em *gland*; Ebner *reticulum*; imbrication *lines* of von E., em *line*; incremental *lines* of von E. em *line*.

von Economo, Constantin F., neurologista austríaco, 1876–1931. VER von E. *disease*.

von Hansemann, D. P., patologista alemão, 1858–1920. VER Hansemann *macrophage*.

von Hippel, Eugen, oftalmologista alemão, 1867–1939. VER von H.-Lindau *syndrome*.

von Kossa, Julius, patologista austro-húngaro do século XIX. VER von K. *stain*.

von Linné. VER Linné.

von Meyenburg. VER Meyenburg.

von Recklinghausen. VER von Recklinghausen *disease*. VER Recklinghausen.

von Schrötter, Leopold, laringologista austríaco, 1837–1908. VER Paget-von S. *syndrome*.

von Willebrand, E. A., médico finlandês, 1870–1949. VER von W. *disease*.

Voorhoeve, N., radiologista holandês, 1879–1927. VER V. *disease*.

vor·tex, pl. **vor·ti·ces** (vōr′teks, vōr′ti-sēz). Vórtice. **1.** SIN verticil. **2.** SIN whorl (5). **3.** Vértice da lente. SIN v. lentis. [L. whirlpool, whorl, de *verto* ou *vorto*, turbilhão]

v. coccy′geus, v. coccígeo; um arranjo espiral de pêlos grossos, por vezes sobre a região do cóccix. SIN coccygeal whorl.

v. cor′dis [TA], v. do coração. SIN v. of heart.

Fleischer v., v. de Fleischer. SIN cornea verticillata.

v. of heart [TA], v. do coração; um arranjo espiral de fibras musculares no ápice do coração. SIN v. cordis [TA], whorl (2).

v. len′tis, v. da lente; uma das figuras estreladas do olho. SIN vortex (3).

vor′tices pilo′rum [TA], vórtices pilosos. SIN hair whorls, em whorl.

Vor·ti·cel·la (vōr′ti-sel′ă). Um gênero de Ciliata da ordem Peritrichida, em formato de sino e com uma espiral de cílios ao redor da zona adoral; várias espécies de vida livre foram encontradas por vezes nas fezes, urina e secreções mucosas. [L. mod. dim. do L. *vortex*, um turbilhão]

vor·ti·ces (vōr′ti-sēz). Vórtices; plural de vortex.

vor·ti·cose (vōr′ti-kōs) Vorticoso; arranjado em um turbilhão. [L. *vorticosus*, de *vortex*, um turbilhão]

Vossius, Adolf, patologista alemão, 1855–1925. VER V. lenticular *ring*.

vox (voks). Voz. SIN voice. [L.]

v. cholera′ica, v. colérica; uma voz peculiar, áspera, quase inaudível, do paciente no estágio terminal da cólera asiática.

vox·el (vok′sel). Uma contração de elemento de volume, que é a unidade básica da reconstrução por TC ou RM; representada como um pixel nas imagens por TC ou RM.

voy·eur (vwah-yer′). *Voyer*; aquele que pratica o voyeurismo.

voy·eur·ism (vwah-yer′izm). Voyeurismo; a prática de obter o prazer sexual por contemplação, especialmente do corpo no ou de órgãos genitais de outra pessoa ou em atos eróticos entre outras pessoas. SIN scopophilia. [Fr. *voir*, ver]

VP Abreviatura para vasopressin (vasopressina); variegate *porphyria* (porfiria variegada).

VR Abreviatura para vocal *resonance* (ressonância vocal).

VS Abreviatura de volumetric *solution*.

VU Abreviatura para volume *unit* (unidade de volume).

vul·ga·ris (vŭl-gā′ris). Vulgar; comum; do tipo usual. [L. de *vulgus*, uma multidão]

Vulpian, Edme F. A., médico francês, 1826–1887. VER V. *atrophy*.

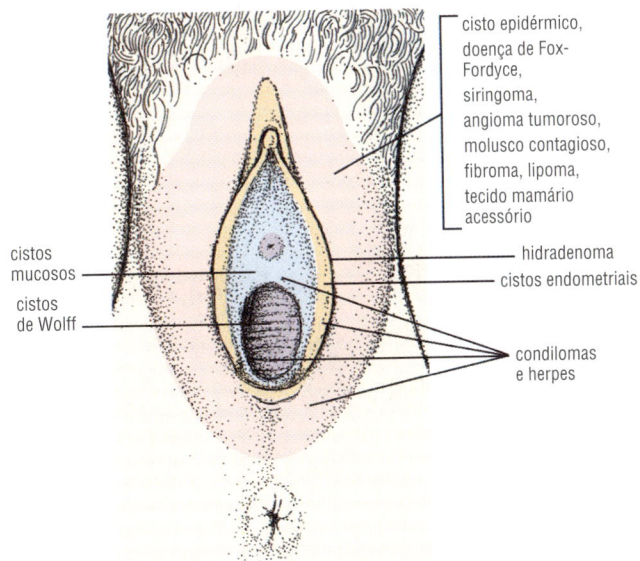

diferenciação dos tumores e cistos da **vulva**: de acordo com a localização, (púrpura) vagina e uretra, (azul) vestíbulo, (amarelo) lábios menores do pudendo, (róseo) lábios maiores do pudendo

vul·sel·la, vul·sel·lum (vŭl-selʹă, -lŭm). Vulsela. SIN vulsella *forceps*. [L. pinças, de *vello*, pp. *vulsus*, apanhar]

vul·va, pl. **vulʹ·vae** (vŭlʹvă). Vulva; [NA] a genitália externa da mulher, composta do monte pubiano, lábios maiores e menores do pudendo, clitóris, vestíbulo da vagina e sua glande, e abertura da uretra e da vagina. SIN cunnus, pudendum femininum, trema (2). [L. uma coberta ou manta, revestimento, de *volvo*, enrolar]

vul·var, vul·val (vŭlʹvar, vŭlʹvăl). Vulvar; relativo à vulva.

vul·vec·to·my (vŭl-vekʹtō-mē). Vulvectomia; excisão (parcial, completa ou radical) da vulva. [vulva + G. *ektomē*, excisão]

vul·vis·mus (vŭl-vizʹmŭs). Vulvismo. SIN vaginismus.

vul·vi·tis (vŭl-vīʹtis). Vulvite; inflamação da vulva. [vulva + G. *-itis*, inflamação]

    chronic atrophic v., v. atrófica crônica; inflamação da pele vulvar atrófica, usualmente com prurido intenso.

    chronic hypertrophic v., v. hipertrófica crônica; termo obsoleto para a inchação dos tecidos vulvares devido à obstrução linfática; em alguns casos, pode ser causada por filaríase, com induração ou ulceração da pele. SIN elephantiasis vulvae.

    follicular v., v. folicular; inflamação dos folículos pilosos vulvares.

vulvo-. Forma combinante que significa a vulva. [L. *vulva*]

vul·vo·cru·ral (vŭlʹvō-krooʹrăl). Vulvocrural; relativo à vulva e ao clitóris.

vul·vo·dyn·ia. Vulvodinia; desconforto vulvar crônico com queixas de queimação e irritação superficial.

vul·vo·u·ter·ine (vŭl-vō-ūʹter-in). Vulvouterino; relativo à vulva e ao útero.

vul·vo·vag·i·nal (vŭlʹvō-vajʹi-năl). Vulvovaginal; relativo à vulva e à vagina.

vul·vo·vag·i·ni·tis (vŭlʹvō-vaj-i-nīʹtis). Vulvovaginite; inflamação da vulva e da vagina.

Vve·den·skii. Sobrenome alternativo de Wedenski, Nikolai I.

V-Y plas·ty. V-Y-plastia. SIN V-Y *flap*.

W

W Símbolo do tungstênio; watt; triptofano; triptofanil.
Waage, P., químico norueguês, 1833–1900. VER Guldberg-W. *law*.
Waaler, Erik, biólogo norueguês, *1903. VER Rose-W. *test*.
Waardenburg, Petrus Johannes, oftalmologista holandês, 1886–1979. VER W. *syndrome*.
Wachendorf, Eberhard J., botânico e anatomista alemão, 1702–1758. VER W. *membrane*.
Wachstein, Max, histologista e patologista norte-americano, 1905–1965. VER W.-Meissel *stain* for calcium-magnesium-ATPase.
Wächter, Herman J.G., patologista alemão, *1878. VER Bracht-W. *lesion*.
Wada, Juhn A., neurologista nipo-canadense do século XX. VER W. *test*.
wad·ding (wahd′ing). Chumaço, algodão em rama. **1.** Algodão cardado ou lã em folhas, usado para curativos cirúrgicos. **2.** Material fibroso que faz parte da cápsula das espingardas de caça; freqüentemente encontrado na ferida se a lesão foi a curta distância.
Waddington, Conrad H., embriologista e geneticista inglês, 1905–1975. VER waddingtonian *homeostasis*.
wad·dle (wod′l). Andar bambolendo. SIN waddling *gait*.
wa·fer (wā′fer). Hóstia; fina lâmina de massa de farinha seca, usada para encerrar um pó, sendo a lâmina umedecida e dobrada sobre a droga, de forma que esta possa ser engolida sem que se perceba o sabor. [I.M., do Fr. ant. *waufre*, do Alemão]
Wagner, Hans, oftalmologista suíço, *1905. VER W. *disease, syndrome*.
Wagstaffe, William, cirurgião inglês, 1843–1910.
waist (wāst). Cintura; parte do tronco localizada entre as costelas e a pelve. [A.S. *waext*]
Walcher, Gustav A., obstetra alemão, 1856–1935. VER W. *position*.
Waldenström, Jan G., médico sueco, *1906. VER W. *macroglobulinemia, purpura, syndrome, test*.
Waldeyer (Waldeyer-Hartz), Heinrich W.G. von, anatomista e patologista alemão, 1836–1921. VER W. *fossae*, em *fossa, glands*, em *gland*, zonal *layer*, throat *ring, sheath, space, tract*.
walk. Caminhar; andar. **1.** Deslocar-se sobre os pés. **2.** A forma característica como uma pessoa caminha. VER TAMBÉM *gait*. [I.M. *walken*, do I. Ant. *wealcen*, rolar]
Walker, Arthur Earl, neurologista norte-americano, *1907. VER W. *tractotomy*; Dandy-W. *syndrome*.
Walker, J.T. Ainslie, químico inglês, 1868–1930. VER Rideal-W. *coefficient, method*.
Walker, James, ginecologista inglês, *1916. VER W. *chart*.
wall (wawl) [TA]. Parede; uma parte que encerra uma cavidade como o tórax ou o abdome, ou que cobre uma célula ou qualquer unidade anatômica. Uma parede, como a parede torácica, abdominal ou de qualquer órgão oco. SIN paries [TA]. [L. *vallum*].
anterior w. of middle ear, p. anterior do ouvido médio. SIN carotid w. of tympanic cavity.
anterior w. of stomach [TA], p. anterior do estômago; a parte da p. gástrica voltada para a cavidade peritoneal. SIN paries anterior gastris [TA]
anterior w. of tympanic cavity, p. anterior da cavidade timpânica. SIN carotid w. of tympanic cavity.
anterior w. of vagina [TA], p. anterior da vagina; um pouco mais curta que a p. posterior e em sua extremidade superior é penetrada pelo colo uterino. SIN paries anterior vaginae [TA]
axial w.'s of the pulp chambers, paredes axiais das câmaras pulpares; as paredes paralelas ao eixo longitudinal de um dente: as paredes medial, distal, bucal e lingual.
carotid w. of middle ear, p. carótica do ouvido médio. SIN carotid w. of tympanic cavity.
carotid w. of tympanic cavity [TA], p. carótica da cavidade timpânica; contém o canal carotídeo e a abertura da tuba auditiva. SIN paries caroticus cavi tympani [TA], anterior w. of middle ear, anterior w. of tympanic cavity, carotid w. of middle ear.
cavity w., p. cavitária; uma das superfícies que limitam uma cavidade.
cell w., p. celular; **(1)** a camada externa ou membrana de algumas células animais e vegetais; nestas últimas, é composta principalmente de celulose. **(2)** em bactérias, a estrutura rígida, geralmente contendo uma camada de peptidoglicanos, que proporciona proteção osmótica e define o formato bacteriano e as propriedades tintoriais.
chest w., p. torácica; em fisiologia respiratória, o sistema total de estruturas fora dos pulmões que se movimentam durante a respiração; inclui a caixa torácica, o diafragma, a parede abdominal e o conteúdo abdominal. SIN thoracic w.
enamel w., p. de esmalte; em odontologia, a parte da p. de uma cavidade que consiste em esmalte.
external w. of cochlear duct, p. externa do ducto coclear. SIN external surface of cochlear duct.
inferior w. of orbit, p. inferior da órbita. SIN floor of orbit.

inferior w. of tympanic cavity, p. inferior da cavidade timpânica. SIN jugular w. of middle ear.
jugular w. of middle ear [TA], p. jugular do ouvido médio; o assoalho da cavidade timpânica; uma fina lâmina de osso que separa a cavidade timpânica da fossa jugular. SIN paries jugularis cavi tympani [TA], floor of tympanic cavity*, fundus tympani, inferior w. of tympanic cavity.
labyrinthine w. of middle ear, SIN labyrinthine w. of tympanic cavity.
labyrinthine w. of tympanic cavity [TA], p. labiríntica do ouvido médio; uma camada óssea que separa o ouvido médio do ouvido interno ou labirinto; contém a janela vestibular e a janela coclear. SIN paries labyrinthicus cavi tympani [TA], medial w. of tympanic cavity*, labyrinthine w. of middle ear, medial w. of middle ear.
lateral w. of middle ear, p. lateral do ouvido médio. SIN membranous w. of tympanic cavity.
lateral w. of orbit [TA], p. lateral da órbita; uma p. triangular da órbita formada pelo osso zigomático, pela asa maior do osso esfenóide e por uma pequena parte do osso frontal; posteriormente é limitada pelas fissuras orbitais superior e inferior. SIN paries lateralis orbitae [TA].
lateral w. of tympanic cavity, *p. lateral da cavidade timpânica; termo oficial alternativo para membranous w. of tympanic cavity.
mastoid w. of middle ear, p. mastóidea do ouvido médio. SIN mastoid w. of tympanic cavity.
mastoid w. of tympanic cavity [TA], p. mastóidea da cavidade timpânica; contém a abertura para o antro mastóideo. SIN paries mastoideus cavi tympani [TA], posterior w. of tympanic cavity*, mastoid w. of middle ear, posterior w. of middle ear.
medial w. of middle ear, p. medial do ouvido médio. SIN labyrinthine w. of tympanic cavity.
medial w. of orbit [TA], p. medial da órbita; a p. fina e retangular da órbita formada pela lâmina orbital dos ossos etmóide, lacrimal, frontal e por uma pequena parte dos ossos esfenóides; a fossa para o saco lacrimal está situada em seu limite anterior. SIN paries medialis orbitae [TA].
medial w. of tympanic cavity, *p. medial da cavidade timpânica; termo oficial alternativo para labyrinthine w. of tympanic cavity.
membranous w. of middle ear, p. membranosa do ouvido médio. SIN membranous w. of tympanic cavity.
membranous w. of trachea [TA], p. membranosa da traquéia; a parte posterior da parede traqueal que não é reforçada por cartilagens traqueais. SIN paries membranaceus tracheae [TA].
membranous w. of tympanic cavity [TA], p. membranosa da cavidade timpânica; parede formada principalmente pela membrana timpânica. SIN paries membranaceus cavi tympani [TA], lateral w. of tympanic cavity*, lateral w. of middle ear, membranous w. of middle ear.
nail w. [TA], p. ungueal; a prega cutânea superposta às margens lateral e proximal da unha. SIN vallum unguis [TA], nail fold.
parietal w., p. parietal; a p. do corpo ou a somatopleura a partir da qual ela é formada.
posterior w. of middle ear, p. posterior do ouvido médio. SIN mastoid w. of tympanic cavity.
posterior w. of stomach [TA], p. posterior do estômago; aquela parte da p. gástrica que fica voltada para a bursa omental. SIN paries posterior gastris [TA].
posterior w. of tympanic cavity, p. posterior da cavidade timpânica; *termo oficial alternativo para mastoid w. of tympanic cavity.
posterior w. of vagina [TA], p. posterior da vagina; é mais longa que a p. anterior e tem uma crista baixa na linha média na maior parte de sua extensão. SIN paries posterior vaginae [TA].
pulpal w., p. pulpar; **(1)** uma das paredes da cavidade pulpar; **(2)** a p. de uma cavidade adjacente ao espaço pulpar; p. ex., p.pulpar mesial.
splanchnic w., p. esplâncnica; a p. de uma das vísceras ou a esplancnopleura a partir da qual é formada.
superior w. of orbit, p. superior da órbita. SIN roof of orbit.
tegmental w. of middle ear, p. tegmental do ouvido médio. SIN tegmental w. of tympanic cavity.
tegmental w. of tympanic cavity [TA], p. tegmental da cavidade timpânica; a parede superior, ou teto, da cavidade timpânica, formada pelo tegmento

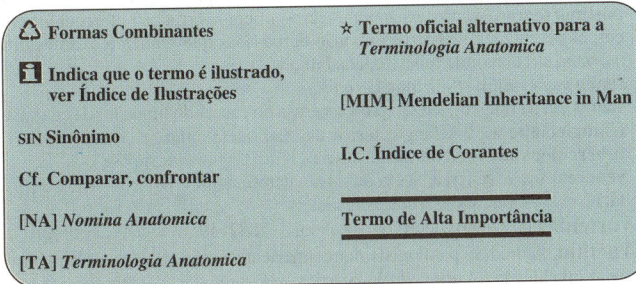

♻ Formas Combinantes	⋆ Termo oficial alternativo para a *Terminologia Anatomica*
🔍 Indica que o termo é ilustrado, ver Índice de Ilustrações	[MIM] Mendelian Inheritance in Man
SIN Sinônimo	I.C. Índice de Corantes
Cf. Comparar, confrontar	
[NA] *Nomina Anatomica*	Termo de Alta Importância
[TA] *Terminologia Anatomica*	

do tímpano do osso temporal. SIN paries tegmentalis cavi tympani [TA], tegmental root of tympanic cavity*, roof of tympanic cavity, tegmental w. of middle ear.

thoracic w., p. torácica. SIN chest w.

tympanic w. of cochlear duct, p. timpânica do ducto coclear. SIN tympanic surface of cochlear duct.

vestibular w. of cochlear duct, p. vestibular do ducto coclear. SIN vestibular surface of cochlear duct.

Wallenberg, Adolf, médico alemão, 1862–1949. VER W. *syndrome.*

Waller, Augustus V., fisiologista inglês, 1816–1870. VER wallerian *degeneration,* wallerian *law.*

wal·le·ri·an (waw-ler′ē-an). Walleriano; relativo a ou descrito por A.V. Waller.

wall-eye (wawl′ī). Exotropia. **1.** SIN exotropia. **2.** Ausência de cor na íris, ou leucoma da córnea.

Walsh, Patrick Craig, urologista norte-americano, *1938. VER neurovascular *bundle* of Walsh, Walsh *procedure.*

Walthard, Max, ginecologista suíço, 1867–1933. VER W. cell *rest.*

Walther, August F., anatomista alemão, 1688–1746. VER W. *dilator, canals,* em *canal, ducts,* em *duct, ganglion, plexus.*

wan·der·ing (wahn′der-ing). Errante; não-fixado; peregrino; anormalmente móvel. [A.S. *wandrian,* vagar]

Wang, Chung Yik, patologista chinês, 1889–1931. VER W. *test.*

Wangensteen, Owen H., cirurgião norte-americano, 1898–1981. VER W. *drainage, suction, tube.*

Wang·i·el·la (wang-gē-el′ă). Gênero dematiáceo de fungos caracterizado por fiálides, sem colaretes, por uma colônia leveduriforme preta com tais formas e, mais tarde, por hifas; os fungos crescem bem a 40°C. A *W. (Exophiala) dermatitidis* é um agente etiológico da cromoblastomicose.

Warburg, Otto H., bioquímico alemão e Prêmio Nobel, 1883–1970. VER W. *apparatus,* respiratory *enzyme,* old yellow *enzyme, theory;* W.-Lipmann-Dickens-Horecker *shunt;* Barcroft-W. *apparatus, technique.*

Ward, Frederick O., osteologista inglês, 1818–1877. VER w.W. *triangle.*

Ward, Owen C., pediatra do século XX. VER Romano-W. *syndrome.*

ward (wōrd). Enfermaria; uma grande sala ou corredor em um hospital contendo vários leitos. VER TAMBÉM unit. [A.S. *weard*]

Wardrop, James, cirurgião inglês, 1782–1869. VER W. *method.*

war·fa·rin so·di·um (war′fă-rin). Warfarin sódico; um anticoagulante com a mesma ação do dicumarol; também usado como rodenticida; também disponível como o sal de potássio, com as mesmas ações e usos. [*W*isconsin *A*lumni *R*esearch *F*oundation + coum*arin*]

warm-blood·ed (wȧrm′blŭd-ed). Homeotérmico. SIN homeothermic.

Warren, Dean, cirurgião norte-americano, 1924–1989. VER W. *shunt.*

wart (wōrt). Verruga. SIN verruca.
  anatomic w., v. anatômica. SIN postmortem w.
  asbestos w., v. do asbesto. SIN asbestos *corn.*
  common w., v. comum. SIN *verruca* vulgaris.
  digitate w., v. digitiforme. SIN *verruca* digitata.
  filiform w., v. filiforme. SIN *verruca* filiformis.
  flat w., v. plana. SIN *verruca* plana.
  fugitive w., v. fugaz; uma v. transitória; que não persiste.
  genital w., v. genital. SIN *condyloma* acuminatum.
  Henle w.'s, verrugas de Henle. SIN Hassall-Henle *bodies,* em *body.*
  infectious w., v. infecciosa. SIN *verruca* vulgaris.
  mosaic w., v. em mosaico; crescimento plantar de numerosas verrugas intimamente agregadas formando um aspecto em mosaico, freqüentemente causado por papilomavírus humano (HPV) tipo 2.
  Peruvian w., v. peruana. SIN *verruga* peruana.
  pitch w., v. do piche; um tumor epidérmico ceratótico pré-canceroso, comum em trabalhadores que lidam com piche e derivados do alcatrão. VER pitch-worker's *cancer.*
  plane w., v. plana. SIN *verruca* plana.
  plantar w., v. plantar; uma v. freqüentemente dolorosa na região plantar, em geral causada por papilomavírus humano (HPV) tipo 1. SIN verruca plantaris.
  postmortem w., v. *post mortem;* um crescimento verrucoso tuberculoso (tuberculose cutânea verrucosa) na mão de pessoas que realizam exames *post mortem.* SIN anatomic tubercle, anatomic w.
  senile w., v. senil. SIN actinic *keratosis.*
  soot w., v. da fuligem; a lesão pré-cancerosa do câncer do limpador de chaminé.
  telangiectatic w., v. telangiectásica. SIN angiokeratoma.
  tuberculous w., v. tuberculosa. SIN *tuberculosis* cutis verrucosa.
  venereal w., v. venérea. SIN *condyloma* acuminatum.
  viral w., v. viral. SIN *verruca* vulgaris.

Wartenberg, Robert, neurologista alemão, 1887–1956. VER W. *symptom.*

Warthin, Aldred S., patologista norte-americano, 1866–1931. VER W. *tumor;* W.-Finkeldey *cells,* em *cell;* W.-Starry silver *stain.*

wart·pox (wōrt′poks). Varíola verrucosa. SIN *variola* verrucosa.

warty (wōrt′ē). Verrucoso; relativo a, ou coberto por, verrugas.

wash (wosh). Loção; uma solução usada para limpar ou banhar uma parte. Quanto aos tipos de loções, ver o termo específico; p. ex., eyewash, mouthwash.

Wasmann, Adolphus, anatomista alemão do século XIX. VER W. *glands,* em *gland.*

Wassermann, August P. von, bacteriologista alemão, 1866–1925. VER W. *antibody, reaction, test;* provocative W. *test.*

Wassermann-fast. Wassermann-resistente; termo usado para designar um caso no qual a reação de Wassermann permanece positiva apesar de todo o tratamento.

wast·ing (wāst′ing). Definhamento; emaciação. **1.** SIN emaciation. **2.** Designa uma doença caracterizada por emaciação.
  salt w., perda de sal; excreção renal impropriamente alta de sal apesar da aparente necessidade do corpo de retê-lo.

wa·ter (wah′ter). Água. **1.** H_2O; um líquido incolor, inodoro, que se solidifica a 32°F (0°C, 0°R) e ferve a 212°F (100°C, 80°R), existente em todos os tecidos animais e vegetais, e que dissolve mais substâncias que qualquer outro líquido. VER volume. **2.** Eufemismo para designar urina. **3.** Uma preparação da farmacopéia de uma solução aquosa saturada clara (exceto especificação em contrário) de óleos voláteis, ou outras substâncias aromáticas ou voláteis, preparada por processos que envolvem destilação ou solução (agitação seguida por filtração). SIN aromatic w. [A.S. *waeter*]
  w. of adhesion, a. de adesão; água mantida por atração molecular em contato com superfícies sólidas, mas que não é parte essencial de sua constituição.
  alkaline w., a. alcalina; a. que contém quantidades consideráveis dos bicarbonatos de cálcio, lítio, potássio ou sódio.
  aromatic w., a. aromática. SIN water (3).
  baryta w., a. de barita; solução aquosa saturada de hidróxido de bário; usada como reagente alcalino.
  bitter w., a. amarga; uma a. mineral natural contendo sal de Epsom.
  bound w., a. ligada; água ligada a colóides e outras substâncias e não removida por filtração simples.
  bromine w., a. de bromo; água contendo os brometos de magnésio, potássio ou sódio em quantidades terapêuticas.
  calcic w., a. cálcica; a. que contém quantidades consideráveis de sais de cálcio em solução.
  carbonated w., carbonic w., a. carbonatada; a. carbônica; água que contém uma quantidade considerável de ácido carbônico em solução.
  carbon dioxide-free w., a. isenta de dióxido de carbono; água purificada que foi fervida vigorosamente por 5 minutos ou mais.
  chalybeate w., a. calibeada ou ferruginosa; a. que contém sais de ferro em quantidades consideráveis.
  chlorine w., a. clorada; água que contém os cloretos de sódio, potássio, cálcio e magnésio em quantidades variadas.
  w. of combustion, a. de combustão. SIN a. of metabolism.
  w. of constitution, a. de constituição; água mantida por uma unidade de estrutura como uma parte essencial de sua constituição, embora não seja um ingrediente de suas moléculas. VER w. of crystallization.
  w. of crystallization, a. de cristalização; água de constituição que se une a determinados sais e é essencial para seu arranjo na forma cristalina; p. ex., $CuSO_4 \cdot 5H_2O$.
  deionized w., a. desionizada; água purificada através da passagem por colunas de troca iônica.
  distilled w., a. destilada; água purificada por destilação.
  earthy w., a. terrosa; água que contém uma grande quantidade de substâncias minerais, principalmente sulfato, em solução.
  free w., a. livre; a. no corpo que pode ser removida por ultrafiltração e na qual as substâncias podem ser dissolvidas.
  gentian aniline w., a. de genciana-anilina; violeta genciana com a. de anilina saturada, uma coloração mais efetiva que a violeta de genciana simples.
  hard w., a. dura; a. contendo íons, como Mg^{2+} e Ca^{2+}, que formam sais insolúveis com ácidos graxos, de modo que o sabão comum nela não forma espuma.
  heavy w., a. pesada; óxido de deutério; D_2O; a. na qual os átomos de hidrogênio consistem em deutério, ou hidrogênio pesado (H^2), com propriedades físicas que diferem notavelmente daquelas da a. comum; volumes elevados promoverão diminuição da atividade metabólica; usada como moderador em reatores nucleares devido à sua capacidade de absorver neutrons. SIN deuterium oxide.
  indifferent w., a. indiferente; a. mineral contendo apenas uma pequena quantidade de material salino.
  w. for injection, a. para injeção; a. purificada por destilação e destinada ao preparo de produtos para uso parenteral.
  intracellular w., a. intracelular. SIN intracellular *fluid.*
  lime w., a. de cal; solução de hidróxido de cálcio; uma solução saturada preparada pela mistura de 3 g de hidróxido de cálcio a 1.000 ml de a. fria purificada. Deixa-se o hidróxido de cálcio não-dissolvido precipitar, e a solução é aviada sem agitação; a a. de cal é um ingrediente comum em loções, sendo muito usada internamente em medicina veterinária.
  w. of metabolism, a. do metabolismo; a. formada no corpo por oxidação do hidrogênio dos alimentos, sendo a maior quantidade produzida no meta-

water

bolismo da gordura (cerca de 117 g por 100 g de gordura). SIN w. of combustion.

mineral w., a. mineral; a. que contém quantidades consideráveis de determinados sais, que lhe conferem propriedades terapêuticas.

potable w., a. potável; a. adequada para beber, sendo livre de contaminação e não contendo uma quantidade suficiente de material salino para ser considerada a. mineral.

purified w., a. purificada; a. obtida por destilação ou desionização.

saline w., a. salina; a. que contém sais neutros (cloretos, brometos, iodetos, sulfatos) em quantidades consideráveis.

Selters w., Seltzer w., a. de Selters; a. de Seltzer; a. mineral contendo carbonatos de sódio, cálcio e magnésio, e cloreto de sódio. [Nieder *Selters*, uma fonte mineral na Prússia]

soft w., a. mole; a. que não possui íons, como Mg^{2+} e Ca^{2+}, que formam sais insolúveis com ácidos graxos, de modo que o sabão comum nela forma espuma facilmente.

sulfate w., a. sulfatada; a. que mantém em solução quantidades consideráveis dos sulfatos de cálcio, magnésio ou sódio.

sulfur w., a. sulfurada; a. contendo sulfeto de hidrogênio ou sulfetos metálicos.

total body w. (TBW), a. corporal total; a soma da a. intracelular e a. extracelular (volume); cerca de 60% do peso corporal.

transcellular w., a. transcelular; a fração de a. extracelular nas secreções cefalorraquidianas, digestivas, epiteliais, intra-oculares, pleurais, sudoríparas e sinoviais; cerca de 1,5% do peso corporal.

wa·ter·fall (wah'ter-fawl). Queda d'água; termo usado para descrever o fluxo nos leitos vasculares nos quais a pressão lateral que tende a colabar os vasos é muito maior que a pressão venosa. O fluxo é independente da pressão venosa e ocorre apenas quando a pressão arterial é maior que a pressão lateral; semelhante ao fluxo que gera uma queda d'água a partir de um dique ou vertedouro sobre uma represa, com a pressão arterial sendo a altura da água atrás da represa, a pressão lateral a altura do vertedouro e a pressão venosa a altura da água atrás da represa. SIN sluice.

Waterhouse, Rupert, médico inglês, 1873–1958. VER W.-Friderichsen *syndrome*.

Waters, Charles Alexander, radiologista norte-americano, 1885–1961. VER W. view *radiography*.

Waters, Edward G., ginecologista e obstetra norte-americano, *1898. VER W. operation*.

wa·ters (wah'ters). Águas; termo coloquial para designar o líquido amniótico; amnionic *fluid*.

bag of w., bolsa das águas. VER *bag* of waters.

false w., falsas águas; extravasamento de líquido antes ou no início do trabalho de parto, antes da ruptura do âmnio.

wa·ter·shed. Divisor de águas; limite. **1.** A área de fluxo sanguíneo marginal na periferia extrema de um leito vascular. **2.** Declives na cavidade abdominal, formados por projeções das vértebras lombares e da margem pélvica, que determinam a direção em que um derrame livre se depositará quando o corpo estiver em decúbito dorsal.

Waterston, David J., cirurgião torácico e pediátrico inglês, *1910. VER W. *operation, shunt*.

Watson, Cecil J., médico norte-americano, 1901–1983. VER Watson-Schwartz *test*.

Watson, James Dewey, geneticista norte-americano e Prêmio Nobel, *1928. VER W.-Crick *helix*.

watt (W) (waht). A unidade SI da energia elétrica; a energia disponível quando a corrente é de 1 ampère e a força eletromotriz é de 1 volt; igual a 1 joule (10^7 ergs) por segundo ou 1 voltampère. [James *Watt*, engenheiro escocês, 1736–1819]

wave (wāv). Onda. **1.** Um movimento de partículas em um corpo elástico, seja sólido ou líquido, no qual é produzida uma série progressiva de elevações e depressões alternadas, ou rarefações e condensações. **2.** A elevação do pulso, percebida pelo dedo da mão, ou representada na linha curva do esfigmógrafo. **3.** O ciclo completo de alterações no nível de uma fonte de energia que varia repetitivamente em relação ao tempo; no eletrocardiograma e no eletroencefalograma, a onda é essencialmente um gráfico que relaciona voltagem e tempo. VER TAMBÉM rhythm. [A.S. *wafian*, flutuar]

A w., o. A; **(1)** a deflexão negativa inicial na eletrorretinografia, provavelmente refletindo atividade fotorreceptora retiniana; **(2)** uma deflexão atrial em um eletrograma registrado no interior do átrio cardíaco; **(3)** a primeira deflexão positiva dos pulsos atrial e venoso devido à sístole atrial.

acid w., o. ácida. SIN acid *tide*.

alkaline w., o. alcalina. SIN alkaline *tide*.

alpha w., o. alfa. SIN alpha *rhythm*.

arterial w., o. arterial; uma onda no flebograma jugular devida à transmissão da pulsação da artéria carótida.

B w., o. B; a deflexão positiva inicial no eletrorretinograma, possivelmente originada da camada nuclear interna da retina.

beta w., o. beta. SIN beta *rhythm*.

brain w., termo coloquial para designar o eletroencefalograma.

C w., o. C; **(1)** uma deflexão positiva monofásica no eletrorretinograma originada no epitélio pigmentar da retina. **(2)** onda nos pulsos venoso e atrial, que ocorre durante a contração ventricular isovolumétrica na qual as válvulas atrioventriculares fechadas (mitral e tricúspide) são abruptamente deslocadas para dentro dos átrios com a criação de uma pressão transitória.

cannon w., o. em canhão; uma onda A exagerada no pulso jugular causada por contração do átrio direito que ocorre após a contração ventricular ter fechado a válvula tricúspide, como nas extra-sístoles ventriculares e no bloqueio AV completo.

D w., o. D; uma deflexão positiva ou negativa no eletrorretinograma, que ocorre quando se retira um estímulo luminoso (resposta de retirada).

delta w., o. delta; uma ascensão prematura do complexo QRS devido a uma via anômala atrioventricular como na síndrome WPW.

dicrotic w., o. dicrótica; a segunda ascensão no traçado de um pulso dicrótico. SIN recoil w.

electrocardiographic w., o. eletrocardiográfica; uma deflexão de formato e extensão especiais no eletrocardiograma, representando a atividade elétrica de uma parte do músculo cardíaco.

epsilon w., o. epsilon; onda R tardia (na derivação V_1) da ativação ventricular direita tardia na displasia arritmogênica do ventrículo direito.

excitation w., o. de excitação; uma o. de condições elétricas alteradas que é propagada ao longo de uma fibra muscular no preparo para sua contração.

F w.'s, ondas F; as ondas do *flutter* atrial que, geralmente, são mais bem observadas em DII, DIII e AVF do ECG. (Uma onda f pequena indica fibrilação atrial).

f w., ff w.'s, onda f ou ondas ff; o. da fibrilação atrial. SIN fibrillary w.'s, fibrillatory w.'s, flutter-fibrillation w.'s.

fibrillary w.'s, ondas fibrilares. SIN f w.

fibrillatory w.'s, ondas fibrilatórias. SIN f w.

flat top w.'s, ondas em platô; atividade no eletroencefalograma que possui um padrão sugestivo de um platô; essas ondas freqüentemente são encontradas em descargas do lobo temporal.

fluid w., o. líquida; sinal do piparote; um sinal de líquido livre na cavidade abdominal; a percussão em um lado do abdome transmite uma onda que é sentida do lado oposto.

flutter-fibrillation w.'s, ondas de flutter-fibrilação. SIN f w.

microelectric w.'s, ondas microelétricas. SIN microwaves.

mucosal w., o. mucosa; o movimento da mucosa da corda vocal durante a fonação.

overflow w., a o. descendente do esfigmograma desde o ápice até a primeira interrupção anacrótica.

P w., o. P; o primeiro complexo do eletrocardiograma, durante ritmos sinusais e atriais, representando a despolarização dos átrios; se a o. P for retrógrada ou ectópica em eixo ou forma, é denominada P'.

percussion w., o. de percussão; a principal o. positiva de um traçado do pulso arterial.

postextrasystolic T w., o. T pós-extra-sístole; a o. T modificada do batimento imediatamente após uma extra-sístole.

pulse w., o. de pulso; a expansão progressiva das artérias que ocorre a cada contração do ventrículo esquerdo.

Q w., o. Q; a deflexão inicial do complexo QRS quando essa deflexão é negativa (para baixo).

R w., o. R; a primeira deflexão positiva (para cima) do complexo QRS no eletrocardiograma; deflexões positivas sucessivas no mesmo complexo QRS são designadas R', R'', etc.

random w.'s, ondas aleatórias; ondas no eletroencefalograma que ocorrem de forma paroxística e assincrônica.

recoil w., o. dicrótica. SIN dicrotic w.

retrograde P w., o. P retrógrada; o padrão de o. P no eletrocardiograma que representa despolarização retrógrada dos átrios, o impulso que se propaga para cima a partir da junção AV ou da parte inferior do átrio.

S w., o. S; uma deflexão negativa (para baixo) do complexo QRS após uma o. R; deflexões negativas sucessivas no mesmo complexo QRS são designadas S', S'', etc.

sonic w.'s, ondas sônicas; ondas sonoras audíveis, diferentes das ondas ultra-sônicas.

supersonic w.'s, ondas supersônicas; ondas sonoras de maior freqüência que o nível de audibilidade.

T w., o. T; a próxima deflexão no eletrocardiograma após o complexo QRS; representa a repolarização ventricular.

theta w., o. teta. SIN theta *rhythm*.

tidal w., o. de maré; a o. situada entre a o. de percussão e a o. dicrótica no ramo descendente do traçado do pulso arterial.

Traube-Hering w.'s, ondas de Traube-Hering. SIN Traube-Hering *curves*, em *curve*.

U w., o. U; uma o. positiva após uma o. T positiva do eletrocardiograma. É negativa após uma onda T invertida.

ultrasonic w.'s, ondas ultra-sônicas; a configuração periódica de energia produzida pelo som que possui uma freqüência maior que 30.000 Hz.

V w., o. V; uma grande o. de pressão visível em registros realizados no átrio ou nas veias aferentes, normalmente produzida por retorno venoso, mas apa-

wave

rentemente tornando-se muito grande quando há regurgitação de sangue através da válvula AV além da câmara onde é feito o registro. Essa onda regurgitante não é uma o. V verdadeira, que é uma onda passiva (de enchimento).

x w., o. x, colapso x; a o. negativa nas curvas de pulso atrial e venoso produzidas quando a ejeção ventricular desloca os assoalhos atriais em direção aos ápices ventriculares.

y w., o. y, colapso y; a o. negativa nas curvas atrial e de pulso venoso refletindo o enchimento rápido dos ventrículos logo após a abertura das válvulas atrioventriculares.

waveform. Forma de onda, perfil de onda; a forma de um pulso; p. ex., uma onda de pressão arterial ou deslocamento; ou do pulso do marcapasso conforme demonstrado ao osciloscópio sob uma carga específica.

pressure w., o. de pressão; a representação gráfica da pressão intravascular ou intracardíaca relacionada a fases do ciclo cardíaco, exibida em um monitor osciloscópico ou impressa em papel.

wave·length (Λ) (wāv'length). Comprimento de onda; a distância de um ponto em uma onda (freqüentemente com o formato de uma curva sinusal) até o próximo ponto na mesma fase; isto é, de pico a pico ou de depressão a depressão.

wave·num·ber (σ) (wāv'num - ber). Número de ondas; o número de ondas por centímetro (cm^{-1}), usado para simplificar os números grandes e de difícil manuseio antes utilizados para designar freqüência.

wave·shape (wāv'shāp). Contorno de onda. SIN waveform.

wax (waks). Cera. 1. Uma substância espessa, viscosa, plástica em temperatura ambiente, secretada por abelhas para a construção da colméia. SIN beeswax, cera. 2. Qualquer substância com propriedades físicas semelhantes às da cera de abelhas, de origem animal, vegetal ou mineral (óleos, lipídios ou gorduras sólidos na temperatura ambiente). 3. Ésteres de ácidos graxos de alto peso molecular com álcoois monoídricos ou diídricos (alifáticos ou cíclicos), que são sólidos em temperatura ambiente. Freqüentemente acompanhados por ácidos graxos livres. [A.S. weax]

animal w., c. animal; cera de abelhas, espermacete e qualquer cera derivada do reino animal.

baseplate w., c. da placa básica; uma cera rósea de consistência dura usada em odontologia para fazer bordas oclusivas.

bleached w., c. branqueada. SIN white w.

bone w., c. óssea; uma mistura de agentes anti-sépticos, óleo e cera usada para interromper hemorragias mediante o tamponamento das cavidades ósseas ou dos canais de Havers. SIN Horsley bone w.

boxing w., c. utilizada para analisar impressões. VER TAMBÉM boxing.

Brazil w., c. do Brasil. SIN carnauba w.

carnauba w., c. de carnaúba; cera obtida da palmeira brasileira *Copernica cerifera*; usada em farmácias para revestir medicamentos em preparações de liberação prolongada e superfícies de comprimidos; usada em ceras para madeira e metal. SIN Brazil w., palm w.

casting w., c. de molde; qualquer cera sólida e macia usada em odontologia para padrões de todos os tipos e para muitos outros fins; constituída, em sua maior parte, de parafina, mas modificada por adição de resina, c. de carnaúba, ou outros ingredientes para várias finalidades. SIN inlay w.

Chinese w., c. chinesa; **(1)** uma c. vegetal; **(2)** uma c. secretada por um inseto, *Coccus ceriferus* ou *C. pela*, e depositada nos galhos de uma espécie de freixo; usada na China para fazer velas e, também, medicinalmente.

ear w., c. do ouvido. SIN cerumen.

earth w., c. mineral. SIN ceresin.

emulsifying w., c. emulsificante; uma base lavável para pomadas que consiste em uma mistura de álcool cetoestearil, laurilsulfato de sódio e água.

grave w., SIN adipocere.

Horsley bone w., c. óssea de Horsley. SIN bone w.

inlay w., SIN casting w.

Japan w., c. do Japão; uma cera vegetal derivada da *Rhus succedanea* e *Toxicodendron verniciferum*.

mineral w., c. mineral; **(1)** SIN paraffin w.; **(2)** SIN ceresin; **(3)** uma substância mineral cujas propriedades físicas são semelhantes às da cera.

montan w., c. da montanha; c. mineral extraída do linhito. [L. *montanus*, de uma montanha, de *mons*, montanha]

palm w., c. de palmeira. SIN carnauba w.

paraffin w., c. parafínica; uma c. derivada do petróleo. SIN mineral w. (1)

vegetable w., c. vegetal; c. de palmeira ou qualquer c. derivada de plantas como a árvore-da-cera.

white w., c. branca; c. amarela branqueada pela produção de lâminas muito finas e exposição à luz e ao ar, ou branqueada por oxidantes químicos; mesmos empregos que a c. amarela. SIN bleached w., white beeswax.

wool w., c. de lã. SIN adeps lanae.

yellow w., c. amarela; substância amarelada, sólida, quebradiça preparada a partir da colméia da abelha, *Apis mellifera*; o principal constituinte é a miricina (palmitato de miricil); outros são o ácido cerótico (cerina), o ácido melíssico, o heptacosano e o hentriacontano; usada no preparo de pomadas, ceratos, emplastros e supositórios.

wax·ing, wax·ing-up (wak'sing). O contorno de um molde em cera, geralmente aplicado ao molde em cera dos contornos de uma dentadura ou uma coroa, antes da modelagem em metal.

weight

Wb Símbolo de weber.

WBC Abreviatura de white blood *cell* (leucócito).

weak·ness (wēk'nes). Fraqueza. 1. Ausência de força ou potência. 2. Incapacidade de atuar normalmente.

directional w., f. direcional; diminuição à direita ou esquerda do nistagmo, calculada a partir das respostas para o teste calórico bitérmico, biauricular.

wean (wēn). Desmamar; realizar o desmame. [A.S. *wenian*]

wean·ing (wēn'ing). Desmame. 1. Privação permanente do leite materno e início da nutrição com outros alimentos. 2. Retirada gradual de um paciente da dependência de um sistema de manutenção da vida ou de outra forma de tratamento.

wean·ling (wēn'ling). Desmamado; animal jovem que se adaptou a outro alimento que não o leite materno.

wear (wār). Desgaste; desgaste ou deterioração causada por atrito.

occlusal w., d. oclusivo; perda de substância por atrito ao se oporem unidades ou superfícies oclusivas. VER TAMBÉM abrasion (3).

web (web). Teia; tecido; membrana; um tecido ou membrana que une um espaço. VER TAMBÉM tela. [A.S.]

esophageal w., membrana esofágica; uma formação cribriforme ou membrana no esôfago causada por atrofia irregular.

w. of fingers/toes, membrana interdigital; uma das pregas cutâneas, ou membrana rudimentar entre os dedos das mãos e artelhos. SIN interdigital folds, plica interdigitalis.

laryngeal w., membrana laríngea; anomalia congênita que consiste em tecido conjuntivo coberto de mucosa entre as cordas vocais, localizado ventralmente e que se estende dorsalmente por uma distância variável; causa obstrução das vias aéreas e choro rouco no recém-nascido.

terminal w., rede terminal; rede de filamentos de actina na extremidade apical das células epiteliais cilíndricas que se fixam na zônula de adesão.

web·bing (web'ing). Condição congênita aparente quando estruturas adjacentes são unidas por uma faixa larga de tecido, que normalmente não existe nesse grau.

Weber, Rainer, patologista norte-americano do século XX. VER W. *stain*.

Weber, Ernst Heinrich, fisiologista e anatomista alemão, 1795–1878. VER W. *glands*, em *gland, law, paradox, test* for hearing; Fechner-Weber *law*; W-Fechner *law*.

Weber, Frederick Parkes, médico inglês, 1863–1962. VER W.-Christian *disease*; W.-Cockayne *syndrome*; Rendu-Osler-W. *syndrome*; Sturge-Kalischer-W. *syndrome*; Sturge-W. *disease, syndrome*; Klippel-Trenaunay-W. *syndrome*.

Weber, Moritz Ignaz, anatomista alemão, 1795–1875. VER W. *organ*.

Weber, Sir Hermann, médico inglês, 1823–1918. VER Weber *sign*; Weber *syndrome*.

Weber, Wilhelm E., físico alemão, 1804–1891. VER W. *point, triangle*.

we·ber (Wb) (web'er). Unidade SI de fluxo magnético, igual a volt-segundos (V.s) [Wilhelm E. Weber, 1804–1891]

WEBINO Acrônimo para wall-eyed bilateral internuclear *ophthalmoplegia* (oftalmoplegia internuclear bilateral com exotropia).

Webster, John C., ginecologista norte-americano, 1863–1950.

Webster, John, químico inglês, 1878–1927. VER W. *test*.

Wechsler, David, psicólogo norte-americano, *1896. VER W. intelligence *scales*, em *scale*; W.-Bellevue *scale*.

wed·del·lite (hwed'del - īte). Weddellita; um diidrato de oxalato de cálcio; encontrado em cálculos renais. Cf. whewellite. [para *Weddell* Sea, por causa de James Weddell, navegador inglês (1787–1834), + -ite]

Wedensky (Vve-den-skii), Nikolai I., neurofisiologista russo, 1852–1922. VER W. *effect, facilitation, inhibition*.

wedge (wej). Cunha; corpo sólido que possui o formato de um prisma triangular de ângulo agudo. [A.S. *weeg*]

dental w., c. dentária; plano inclinado duplo usado para separar os dentes, mantendo a separação já obtida, ou segurando uma matriz no lugar.

WEE Abreviatura de western equine *encephalomyelitis* (encefalomielite eqüina ocidental).

Weeks, John E., oftalmologista norte-americano, 1853–1949. VER W. *bacillus*; Koch-W. *bacillus*.

Weeksella (wēk - sel'a). Gênero de bacilos Gram-negativos, aeróbicos, não-oxidativos.

w. zoohelcum, bactéria causadora de infecções em mordeduras ou arranhaduras por cães ou gatos.

Wegener, Friedrich, patologista alemão, 1907–1990. VER W. *granulomatosis*.

Wegner, Friedrich R.G., patologista alemão, 1843–1917. VER W. *disease, line*.

Weibel, Ewald R., médico suíço, *1929. VER W.-Palade *bodies*, em *body*.

Weichselbaum, Antom, patologista austríaco, 1845–1920. VER W. *coccus*.

Weidel, Hugo, químico austríaco, 1849–1899. VER W. *reaction*.

Weigert, Carl, patologista alemão, 1845–1904. VER W. *law*, iodine *solution*. Ver entradas em stain.

weight (wāt). Peso; o produto da força da gravidade, definida internacionalmente como 9,80665 m/s², multiplicado pela massa do corpo. [A.S. *gewiht*]

apothecaries w., peso farmacêutico; sistema obsoleto de pesos baseado no peso de um grão de trigo. Foi usado durante séculos para pesar medicamentos e metais preciosos (medida Troy). Algumas substâncias, existentes há muito tempo, ainda são freqüentemente designadas como grãos (p. ex., 5 grãos de ácido acetilsalicílico, 1/2 grão de codeína, 1/100 grão de nitroglicerina). Esse sistema de peso foi amplamente superado pelo sistema métrico (baseado em gramas). Um grão equivale a 64,8 miligramas. Um escrópulo contém 20 grãos; um dracma contém 60 grãos; uma onça farmacêutica contém 8 dracmas (480 grãos); 1 libra farmacêutica contém 12 onças (5.760 grãos).
atomic w. (at. wt., AW), a massa em gramas de 1 mol ($6{,}02 \times 10^{23}$ átomos) de uma espécie atômica; a massa de um átomo de um elemento químico em relação à massa de um átomo de carbono-12 (C^{12}), que é igual a 12.000, sendo assim uma razão e, portanto, sem dimensão (embora a massa real, numericamente igual, algumas vezes seja expressa em daltons); não necessariamente, o peso de qualquer átomo individual de um elemento, pois a maioria dos elementos são constituídos de vários isótopos de diferentes massas; p. ex., o peso atômico do cloro é 35,4527, porque é composto de Cl^{35} e Cl^{37} em proporções que produzem uma média de 35,4527. VER TAMBÉM molecular w.
birth w., peso ao nascimento; nos seres humanos, o primeiro peso de um recém-nascido determinado antes de completar 60 minutos de vida; um recém-nascido de peso normal pesa 2.500 g ou mais, enquanto o de baixo peso tem menos de 2.500 g; o recém-nascido de peso muito baixo tem menos de 1.500 g, e o de peso extremamente baixo tem menos de 1.000 g.
combining w., p. equivalente. SIN gram *equivalent.*
dry w., p. seco; o peso do material após retirar a água (p. ex., após aquecimento acima de 100°C).
equivalent w., p. equivalente. SIN gram *equivalent.*
gram-atomic w., átomo-grama; p. atômico expresso em gramas. Cf. mole.
gram-molecular w., relativo a molécula-grama; p. molecular expresso em gramas. Cf. mole.
molecular w. (mol wt, MW), p. molecular (PM); a soma dos pesos atômicos de todos os átomos que formam uma molécula; a massa de uma molécula em relação à massa de um átomo padrão, agora C^{12} (considerada como 12,000). A massa molecular relativa (M_r) é a massa relativa ao dalton e não tem unidades. VER TAMBÉM atomic w. SIN molecular mass, molecular weight ratio, relative molecular mass.

weight·less·ness (wāt′les - nes). Imponderabilidade; o efeito psicofisiológico da gravidade zero, experimentado por uma pessoa em queda livre no vácuo (p. ex., astronautas em uma órbita estável). Pode ser atingido um estado temporário de imponderabilidade simulada durante um vôo a propulsão na atmosfera terrestre, atravessando-se uma curva parabólica invertida onde o empuxo gravitacional e a força centrífuga se neutralizam mutuamente.
Weil, Adolf, médico alemão, 1848–1916. VER W. *disease.*
Weil, Edmund, médico austríaco, 1880–1922. VER W.-Felix *reaction, test.*
Weil, Ludwig A., dentista alemão, 1849–1895. VER W. basal *layer,* basal *zone.*
Weill, Georges J., oftalmologista francês, 1866–1952. VER W.-Marchesani *syndrome.*
Weill, Jean A., médico francês, *1903. VER Leri-W. *disease, syndrome.*
Weinberg, Michel, patologista francês, 1868–1940. VER W. *reaction.*
Weinberg, Wilhelm, médico alemão, 1862–1937. VER Hardy-W. *equilibrium, law.*
Weingrow re·flex. Reflexo de Weingrow. Ver *reflex.*
Weir Mitchell, Silas, neurologista, poeta e novelista norte-americano, 1829–1914. VER Mitchell *treatment;* Gerhardt-Mitchell *disease;* W. M. *treatment.*
Weisbach, Albin, antropologista austríaco, 1837–1914. VER W. *angle.*
Weismann, August Friedrich Leopold, biólogo alemão, 1834–1914. VER weismannism.
weis·mann·ism (vīs′ man - izm). Weismanismo; teoria da não-herança de características adquiridas.
Weiss, Nathan, médico austríaco, 1851–1883. VER W. *sign.*
Weiss, Soma, médico norte-americano, 1898–1942. VER Charcot-W.-Baker *syndrome;* Mallory-W. *lesion, syndrome, tear.*
Weitbrecht, Josias, anatomista alemão-russo em St. Petersburg, 1702–1747. VER W. *cartilage, cord, fibers,* em *fiber, foramen, ligament; apparatus* ligamentosus weitbrechti.
Welander, Lisa, neurologista sueca, *1909. VER Kugelberg-W. *disease;* Wohlfart-Kugelberg-W. *disease.*
Welch, William H., patologista norte-americano, 1850–1934. VER W. *bacillus.*
Welcker, Hermann, antropologista e anatomista alemão, 1822–1898. ver W. *angle.*

well·ness (wel′nĕs). Bem-estar; uma filosofia de vida e higiene pessoal que considera a saúde não apenas como a ausência de doença, mas a realização completa do potencial físico e mental de uma pessoa, alcançada através de atitudes positivas, treinamento físico, dieta pobre em gordura e rica em fibras e afastamento de práticas prejudiciais à saúde (tabagismo, abuso de drogas e álcool, ingestão excessiva de alimentos). Programas de bem-estar são amplamente oferecidos por empregadores, programas de seguro-saúde e agências de serviço social. Os programas formais tipicamente incluem medidas preventivas (p. ex., imunizações contra pneumonia pneumocócica e gripe para os idosos) e supervisão de doenças comuns (p. ex., hipertensão, diabetes melito e câncer de mama e cólon). Esses programas tendem a atrair pessoas já integradas a atitudes e práticas saudáveis. Há poucas evidências clínicas que apóiem sua utilidade ou justifiquem seu custo.

Wells, G.C., dermatologista inglês do século XX. VER W. *syndrome.*
Wells, Michael Vernon, médico inglês do século XX. VER Muckle-W. *syndrome.*
welt (wĕlt). Vergão. SIN wheal [I. ant. *waelt*]
wen (wĕn). Cisto sebáceo; termo antigo de pilar *cyst.* [A.S.]
Wenckebach, Karel F., clínico holandês, 1864–1940. VER W. *block, period, phenomenon.*
Wenzel, Joseph, anatomista e fisiologista alemão, 1768–1808. VER W. *ventricle.*
Wepfer, Johann J., 1620–1695. VER W. *glands,* em *gland.*
Werdnig, Guido, neurologista austríaco, 1862–1919. VER W.-Hoffmann *disease;* Werdnig-Hoffmann muscular *atrophy.*
Werlhof, Paul G., médico alemão, 1699–1767. VER Werlhof *disease.*
Wermer, Paul L., clínico norte-americano, 1898–1975. VER Wermer *syndrome.*
Wernekinck (Werneking), Friedrich C.G., anatomista e médico alemão, 1798–1835. VER W. *commissure, decussation.*
Werner, F.F., químico alemão do início do século XX. VER W. *test.*
Werner, Otto, médico alemão, *1879. VER W. *syndrome.*
Wernicke, Karl, neurologista alemão, 1848–1905. VER W. *aphasia, area, center, disease, encephalopathy, field, radiation, reaction, region, sign, syndrome, zone;* W.-Korsakoff *encephalopathy, syndrome.*
Wertheim, Ernst, ginecologista austríaco, 1864–1920. VER W. *operation.*
Werther, J., médico alemão do século XX. VER W. *disease.*
West, Charles, médico inglês, 1816–1898. VER W. *syndrome.*
West, John B., fisiologista pulmonar australiano-norte-americano, *1928.
Westberg, Friedrich, médico alemão do século XIX. VER W. *space.*
Westergren, Alf, médico sueco, *1891. VER W. *method.*
West·ern blot, West·ern blot·ting. SIN Western blot *analysis.*
Westphal, Karl F.O., neurologista alemão, 1833–1890. VER W. pupillary *reflex;* W.-Piltz *phenomenon;* Edinger-W. *nucleus.*
Wetzel, Norman C., pediatra norte-americano, *1897. VER W. *grid.*
Wever, Ernest Glen, psicólogo norte-americano, *1902. VER W.-Bray *phenomenon.*
Weyers, Helmut, pediatra alemão do século XX. VER W.-Thier *syndrome.*
WF Abreviatura de Working Formulation for Clinical Usage.
Wharton, Thomas, anatomista e médico inglês, 1614–1673. VER W. *duct, jelly.*
wheal (hwēl). Vergão; pápula; uma pápula evanescente e circunscrita ou placa irregular de edema cutâneo, parecendo uma urticária, algo avermelhada, que freqüentemente muda de tamanho e formato e estende-se para áreas adjacentes, em geral acompanhada por prurido intenso; produzida por injeção ou teste intradérmico, ou por exposição a substâncias alergênicas em pessoas suscetíveis; também encontrada na dermatite herpetiforme (Sinal de Darier). SIN hives (2), welt. [A.S. *hwēle*]
wheat germ oil (hwēt jerm). Óleo de germe de trigo; óleo obtido por expressão do germe da semente do trigo, *Triticum aestivum* (família Gramineae); uma das fontes mais ricas de vitamina E natural; usado como suplemento nutricional.
Wheatstone, Charles, físico inglês, 1802–1875. VER W. *bridge.*
wheel (hwēl). Roda; disco; uma estrutura circular ou disco designado para girar em torno de um eixo.
Burlew w., disco de Burlew. SIN Burlew *disk.*
Wheeler, Henry Lord, químico norte-americano, 1867–1914. VER Wheeler-Johnson *test.*
Wheeler, John M., oftalmologista norte-americano, 1879–1938. VER W. *method.*
wheeze (hwēz). Sibilo. **1.** Sibilar; respirar com dificuldade e ruidosamente. **2.** Um som sibilante, rangido, musical ou soprado produzido durante a expiração pelo ar que atravessa as fauces, a glote ou vias aéreas traqueobrônquicas estreitadas. [A.S. *hwēsan*]
asthmatoid w., sibilo asmatóide; ruído soprado ou musical ouvido à expiração na frente da boca aberta do paciente em um caso de corpo estranho na traquéia ou brônquio.
whe·wel·lite (hwa′wel - īt). Whewellita; um monoidrato de oxalato de cálcio; encontrado em cálculos renais. Cf. weddellite. [William *Whewell,* filósofo inglês (1794–1866), + -ite]
whey (hwā). Soro; a parte aquosa do leite que permanece após a separação da caseína. SIN serum lactis. [A.S. *hwaeg*]
alum w., s. de alume; soro produzido pela coagulação do leite por meio do acréscimo de alume em pó.

whey

w. protein, proteína do soro. VER whey *protein*.
whip·lash (hwip′lash). Chicote. VER whiplash *injury*.
Whipple, Allen O., cirurgião norte-americano, 1881–1963. VER W. *operation*.
Whipple, George H., patologista norte-americano e Prêmio Nobel, 1878–1976. VER W. *disease*.
whip·worm (hwip′werm). VER *Trichuris trichiura*.
whis·ky, whis·key (hwis′kē). Uísque; líquido alcoólico obtido pela destilação da mistura de malte fermentada de grãos de cereais total ou parcialmente maltados, contendo 47 a 53% por volume de C_2H_5OH, a 15,56°C; tem de ser armazenado em barris de madeira durante pelo menos 2 anos. Os vários grãos usados na fabricação do uísque são cevada, milho, centeio e trigo. [Gael, *usquebaugh*, água da vida]
whis·per (hwis′per). Sussurrar; cochichar; falar sem fonação, p. ex., com uma parte posterior da glote aberta. [A.S. *hwisprian*]
whis·tle (hwis′l). Sibilo. **1.** Som produzido forçando a passagem do ar através de uma abertura estreita. **2.** Instrumento para produzir um sibilo. [A.S. *hwistle*]
  Galton w., sibilador de Galton; sibilador cilíndrico fixado a um bulbo compressível, com uma fixação por rosca que modifica a freqüência; usado para testar a audição.
Whitaker, Robert, cirurgião inglês, *1939. VER W. *test*.
White, Paul Dudley, cardiologista norte-americano, 1886–1973. VER Lee-W. *method*; Wolff-Parkinson-W. *syndrome*.
white (hwīt). Branco; a cor que resulta da combinação de todos os raios do espectro; a cor do giz ou da neve. SIN albicans (1). [A.S. *hwīt*]
  w. of eye, branco do olho; a porção visível da esclerótica.
Whitehead, Walter, cirurgião inglês, 1840–1913. VER W. *deformity, operation*.
white·head (hwīt′hed). **1.** SIN milium. **2.** SIN closed comedo.
white·pox (hwīt′poks). Alastrim. SIN alastrim.
whites (hwīts). Termo coloquial que indica leucorréia ou blenorréia.
whit·ing (hwīt′ing). Giz ($CaCO_3$) usado para polir metais ou limpar objetos plásticos.
whit·loc·kite (hwīt′lok - īt). SIN tribasic calcium phosphate. [Herbert P. *Whitlock*, mineralogista Am. (*1868), + -ite]
whit·low (hwīt′lō). Panarício; paroníquia; infecção purulenta através de uma prega perioníquia causando um abscesso da extremidade distal bulbar de um dedo da mão. SIN felon. [I.M. *whitflawe*]
  herpetic w., p. herpético; infecção dolorosa, pelo vírus herpes simples, de um dedo da mão por inoculação direta da prega perioníquia desprotegida, freqüentemente acompanhada por linfangite e adenopatia regional, com duração de até várias semanas; mais comum em médicos, dentistas e enfermeiros em virtude da exposição ao vírus na boca dos pacientes.
  thecal w., p. tecal; lesão supurativa da falange distal; pode envolver a bainha do tendão e o osso.
Whitman, Royal, cirurgião norte-americano, 1857–1946. VER W. *frame*.
Whitmore, Alfred, cirurgião inglês, 1876–1946. VER W. *disease*.
Whitnall, Samuel E., anatomista inglês, 1876–1952. VER W. *tubercle*.
WHO Abreviatura de World Health Organization (Organização Mundial de Saúde).
whoop (hoop). Estridor; guincho; inspiração sonora alta na coqueluche com a qual termina o paroxismo da tosse, devido ao espasmo da laringe (glote).
  systolic w., e. sistólico. SIN systolic honk.
whorl (hwerl). Vórtice; turbilhão. **1.** Uma volta da espiral da cóclea do ouvido. **2.** SIN vortex of heart. **3.** Uma volta de uma concha nasal. **4.** SIN verticil. **5.** Uma área de crescimento radial do cabelo, sugerindo um turbilhão ou redemoinho. SIN vortex (2). VER hair w.'s. **6.** Um dos padrões distintos que constituem o sistema de Galton de classificação das impressões digitais. SIN digital w.
  coccygeal w., v. coccígeo. SIN vortex coccygeus.
  digital w., v. digital. SIN whorl (6)
  hair w.'s [TA], vórtices do cabelo; um arranjo espiral do cabelo, como na coroa da cabeça. SIN vortices pilorum [TA].
whorled (hwerld). Verticilado; espiralado; caracterizado por, ou disposto em, espirais. VER TAMBÉM vorticose, turbinate, convoluted, verticillate.
Wickham, Louis-Frédéric, dermatologista francês, 1860–1913. VER W. *striae*, em *stria*.
Widal, George F.I., médico francês, 1862–1929. VER W. *reaction, syndrome*; Gruber-W. *reaction*; Hayem-W. *syndrome*.
wide·band (wīd - band). Banda larga; uma ampla faixa de freqüências sonoras, em oposição a uma faixa estreita de freqüências.
wid·ow's peak. Bico-de-viúva; ponta bem definida de crescimento do cabelo na linha média da margem anterior do couro cabeludo, geralmente resultante do recuo do cabelo nas regiões temporais, ou que ocorre como configuração congênita do cabelo.
width (width, with). Largura; a distância de um lado de um objeto ou área ao outro.
  orbital w., l. orbital; a distância entre o dácrio e o ponto mais distante na margem anterior da borda externa da órbita (Broca), ou entre esse último ponto e a junção da sutura frontolacrimal e a margem posterior do sulco lacrimal.

window

window w., l. da janela; a faixa de números de TC (em unidades Hounsfield) compreendidos na exibição em vídeo da faixa de escala cinza da imagem de TC, variando de 1 a 2.000 ou 3.000, dependendo do tipo de aparelho. Também a faixa de energias eletromagnéticas passadas por um módulo de rastreamento eletrônico de um dispositivo de imagem, como por uma câmera de cintilação. VER TAMBÉM window *level*.
Wiedemann, Hans Rudolf, pediatra alemão, *1915. VER Beckwith-W. *syndrome*.
Wiener, H. VER *tract* of Münzer and W.
Wigand, Justus Heinrich, obstetra e ginecologista alemão, 1769–1817. VER W. *maneuver*.
Wilde, Sir William R. W., oculista e otologista irlandês, 1815–1876. VER W. *cords*, em *cord, triangle*.
Wilder, Helenor C., cientista norte-americana do século XX. VER W. *stain* for reticulum.
Wilder, Joseph F., neuropsiquiatra norte-americano, 1895–1976.
Wilder, William H., oftalmologista norte-americano, 1860–1935. VER W. *sign*.
Wildermuth, Hermann A., psiquiatra alemão, 1852–1907. VER W. *ear*.
Wildervanck, L.S., geneticista holandês do século XX. VER W. *syndrome*.
wild·fire (wīld′fīr). Fogo selvagem. SIN fogo selvagem.
Wilhelmy, Ludwig F., cientista alemão, 1812–1864. VER W. *balance*.
Wilkie, David P.D., cirurgião escocês, 1882–1938. VER W. *artery, disease*.
Wilkinson, Daryl Sheldon, dermatologista inglês do século XX. VER Sneddon-W. *disease*.
Willebrand, E.A., von. VER von Willebrand.
Willett, J. Abernethy, obstetra inglês, †1932. VER W. *forceps*.
Willi, Heinrich, pediatra suíço do século XX. VER Prader-W. *syndrome*.
Williams, Anna W., bacteriologista norte-americana, 1863–1955. VER W. *stain*; Park-W. *fixative*.
Williams, J.C.P., cardiologista neozelandês do século XX. VER W. *syndrome*.
Williamson, Carl S., cirurgião norte-americano, 1896–1952. VER Mann-W. *operation, ulcer*.
Willis, Thomas, médico inglês, 1621–1675. VER W. *centrum* nervosum, *cords*, em *cord, pancreas, paracusis, pouch; circle* of W.; *accessorius* willisii; *chordae* willisii, em *chorda*.
Williston, Samuel Wendell, paleontologista norte-americano, 1852–1918. VER W. *law*.
wil·low (wil′ō). Salgueiro; árvore do gênero *Salix*; a casca de várias espécies, principalmente *S. fragilis*, é uma fonte de salicina. [A.S. *welig*]
Wilms, Max, cirurgião alemão, 1867–1918. VER W. *tumor*.
Wilson, Clifford, médico inglês, *1906. VER Kimmelstiel-W. *disease, syndrome*.
Wilson, James, anatomista, fisiologista e cirurgião inglês, 1765–1821. VER W. *muscle*.
Wilson, Miriam G., pediatra norte-americana, *1922. VER W.-Mikity *syndrome*.
Wilson, Samuel A. Kinnier, neurologista inglês, 1878–1937. VER W. *disease*.
Wilson, Sir William J.E., dermatologista inglês, 1809–1884. VER W. *disease*.
Wilson meth·od. Método de Wilson. VER em method.
wind·age (win′dej). Deslocamento de ar; lesão interna sem lesão superficial, causada por colisão com a pressão de ar comprimido ou com um objeto propelido por ar comprimido.
wind·burn (wind′bern). Dermatite pelo vento; eritema da face causado pela exposição ao vento.
win·dow (win′dō) [TA]. Janela. **1.** SIN fenestra. **2.** Qualquer abertura no espaço ou tempo. **3.** *Radiologia*. Uma incidência especialmente inventada para acentuar o contraste tecidual.
  aortic w., j. aórtica; termo obsoleto para designar uma região abaixo do arco aórtico em uma radiografia oblíqua anterior esquerda do tórax, formada pela bifurcação da traquéia e cruzada pela artéria pulmonar esquerda.
  aorticopulmonary w., j. aortopulmonar. SIN aortic septal *defect*.
  aortic-pulmonic w., j. aortopulmonar. SIN aortopulmonary w.
  aortopulmonary w., j. aortopulmonar; o entalhe no lado esquerdo do mediastino pelo pulmão parcialmente interposto entre o arco aórtico e a artéria pulmonar esquerda, observada em radiografias frontais do tórax. SIN aorticpulmonic w.
  cochlear w., j. coclear. SIN round w.
  lung w., j. pulmonar; ajustes de TC do nível e largura da j. apropriados para mostrar detalhes pulmonares.
  mediastinal w., j. mediastinal; ajustes de TC de nível e largura da janela apropriados para mostrar estruturas de tecidos moles. SIN soft tissue w.
  oval w. [TA], j. oval; uma abertura oval na parede medial da cavidade timpânica que leva ao vestíbulo, fechada em vida pelo pé do estribo. SIN fenestra vestibuli [TA], fenestra of the vestibule, fenestra ovalis, vestibular w.
  round w. [TA], j. redonda; abertura na parede medial do ouvido médio que leva até a cóclea, fechada em vida pela membrana timpânica secundária. SIN fenestra cochleae [TA], cochlear w., fenestra of the cochlea, fenestra rotunda.
  soft tissue w., j. dos tecidos moles. SIN mediastinal w.

tachycardia w., j. taquicárdica; na taquicardia paroxística do tipo reentrada, o intervalo de tempo (a janela) entre a primeira e a última ativações prematuras que podem excitar o paroxismo.
vestibular w., j. vestibular. SIN oval w.
wind·pipe (wind′pīp). Traquéia. SIN trachea.
wine (wīn). Vinho. **1.** Suco fermentado de uva. SIN vinous liquor. **2.** Um grupo de preparações que consistem em uma solução de uma ou mais substâncias medicinais no vinho, geralmente o vinho branco, devido à sua relativa ausência de tanino. Não há vinhos autorizados pela Farmacopéia. [Fr. *vin*; L. *vinum*]
high w., v. forte; bebida alcoólica obtida por retificação ou redestilação de um v. fraco durante a fabricação de uísque.
low w., v. fraco; o primeiro destilado fraco obtido do malte no processo de fabricação do uísque.
red w., v. palhete; clarete; bebida alcoólica produzida pela fermentação de uvas, os frutos da *Vitis vinifera*, com suas cascas (que conferem cor); tem sido usado como tônico.
sherry w., xerez; vinho cor de âmbar, obtido originalmente em Jerez, Espanha, contendo cerca de 20% de álcool; usado no preparo de vinhos medicinais.
wing. Asa; o apêndice anterior de uma ave. SIN ala (1).
angel w., escápula alada; uma deformidade na qual as duas escápulas se projetam visivelmente. VER TAMBÉM winged *scapula*.
ashen w., a. cinérea, trígono do nervo vago. SIN vagal (nerve) *trigone*.
w. of central lobule [TA], a. do lóbulo central; a projeção lateral, semelhante a uma asa, do lóbulo central do cerebelo; constituída de uma parte inferior [TA], que é a porção lateral do lóbulo II (de Larsell), e uma parte superior [TA], que é a porção lateral do lóbulo III (de Larsell). SIN ala central lobule [TA], ala lobulis centralis [TA], ala cerebelli.
w. of crista galli, asa da crista etmoidal. SIN ala of crista galli.
gray w., a. cinérea. SIN vagal (nerve) *trigone*.
greater w. of sphenoid (bone) [TA], a. maior do osso esfenóide; fortes processos escamosos que se estendem em uma larga curva súpero-lateral a partir do corpo do osso esfenóide. A a. maior apresenta estas superfícies (faces): 1) superfície cerebral: forma o terço anterior do assoalho da porção lateral da fossa craniana média; 2) superfície temporal: forma a porção mais profunda da fossa temporal; 3) superfície infratemporal, forma o "teto" da fossa infratemporal; 4) superfície orbital: forma a parede póstero-lateral da órbita. A a. maior forma a borda inferior da fissura supra-orbital, sendo perfurada em sua raiz pelos forames redondo, oval e espinhoso e pelo canal pterigóide. SIN ala major ossis sphenoidalis [TA], ala temporalis.
w. of ilium, asa do ílio; *termo oficial alternativo para *ala* of ilium.
lesser w. of sphenoid (bone) [TA], a. menor do osso esfenóide; uma asa de um par bilateral de lâminas triangulares, pontudas, que se estendem ântero-lateral do corpo do osso esfenóide. Formando a porção mais posterior do assoalho da fossa anterior do crânio, sua borda posterior aguda forma a crista esfenoidal, que separa as fossas cranianas anterior e média. A extremidade medial da a. menor se fixa ao corpo por meio de dois pedículos, assim formando o canal óptico. A própria asa forma a margem superior da fissura supra-orbital. SIN ala minor ossis sphenoidalis [TA], ala orbitalis, Ingrassia process.
w. of nose, a. do nariz. SIN ala of nose.
w. of sacrum, a. do sacro; *termo oficial alternativo para *ala* of sacrum.
w. of vomer, a. do vômer. SIN ala of vomer.
Winiwarter, Felix von, cirurgião alemão, 1852–1931. VER W.-Buerger *disease*.
wink (wink). Piscar. SIN blink. [A.S. *wincian*]
Winslow, Jacques B., anatomista, físico e cirurgião dinamarquês que viveu em Paris, 1669–1760. VER *foramen* of W.; W. *ligament, pancreas, stars,* em *star*; *stellulae* winslowii, em *stellula*.
Winterbottom, Thomas Masterman, médico inglês, 1765–1859. VER W. *sign*.
win·ter·green oil (win′ter - grēn). Óleo de gaultéria. SIN methyl salicylate.
Winternitz, Wilhelm, médico austríaco, 1835–1917. VER W. *sound*.
Wintersteiner, Hugo, oftalmologista austríaco, 1865–1918. VER W. *rosettes*, em *rosette*.
wire (wīr). Arame; fio; bastão ou fio de metal delgado e flexível.
arch w., aparelho dentário. SIN archwire.
guide w., fio condutor. VER guidewire.
Kirschner w., fio de Kirschner; um aparelho para tração óssea de fraturas dos ossos longos ou para fixação da fratura. SIN Kirschner apparatus.
ligature w., fio de ligadura; um fio fino e flexível de aço inoxidável, usado em odontologia para fixar um aparelho dentário a sustentações ou colchetes.
separating w., fio de separação; fio, geralmente de latão flexível, usado para obter separação entre os dentes. VER TAMBÉM separation (2).
wrought w., fio forjado passando-se um molde através de um cubo para adquirir o formato e o tamanho desejados; usado em odontologia para dentaduras parciais e aparelhos ortodônticos.
wir·ing (wīr′ing). Fixação; unir as extremidades de um osso fraturado por fios metálicos.
circumferential w., f. circunferencial; fixação de fraturas da mandíbula pela passagem de fios ao redor de um corte de osso e tala intra-oral; isto é, fio circumandibular. VER TAMBÉM circumzygomatic w.
circumzygomatic w., f. circunzigomática; uma forma de fixação para fraturas mandibulares na qual a mandíbula é fixada aos arcos zigomáticos com fio.
continuous loop w., f. de alça contínua; a formação de alças de fio nos dentes maxilares e mandibulares, para a colocação de elásticos intermaxilares; usada na redução e fixação de fraturas. SIN Stout w.
craniofacial suspension w., f. de suspensão craniofacial; um método de f. utilizando áreas de ossos não-contíguas com a cavidade oral para a sustentação de segmentos mandibulares fraturados (p. ex., abertura piriforme, arco zigomático, processo zigomático do osso frontal).
Gilmer w., f. de Gilmer; um método de fixação intermaxilar no qual fios metálicos são passados em torno de dentes opostos e torcidos juntos.
Ivy loop w., f. por alça de Ivy; colocação de um fio ao redor de dois dentes adjacentes para proporcionar uma fixação para elásticos intermaxilares.
perialveolar w., f. perialveolar; fixação de uma tala à arcada maxilar pela passagem de um fio através do processo alveolar, desde a superfície bucal até a superfície lingual.
pyriform aperture w., f. da abertura piriforme; um método de f. da área da abertura piriforme para a estabilização de fraturas da mandíbula.
Stout w., f. de Stout. SIN continuous loop w.
Wirsung, Johann G., anatomista alemão em Pádua, 1589–1643. VER W. *canal, duct*.
wiry (wīr′ē). De arame; semelhante a um arame; filiforme e rígido; designa uma forma de pulso.
Wiskott, Arthur, pediatra alemão do século XX. VER W.-Aldrich *syndrome*.
Wissler, Hans, pediatra suíço, *1906. VER W. *syndrome*.
Wistar, Caspar, biólogo norte-americano, 1761–1818, em homenagem ao qual foi denominado o Wistar Institute. VER W. *rats*, em *rat*.
witch ha·zel (wich - hāz′l). Hamamélis. SIN hamamelis.
with·draw·al (with - draw′al). Supressão. **1.** O ato de remover ou retirar. **2.** Abstinência; uma síndrome psicológica e/ou física pela interrupção abrupta do uso de uma droga/fármaco em um indivíduo habituado. **3.** O processo terapêutico de interromper o uso de uma droga de forma a evitar os sintomas da abstinência (2). **4.** Um padrão de comportamento observado na esquizofrenia e na depressão, caracterizado por retraimento patológico do contato interpessoal e do envolvimento social, e levando à autopreocupação.
wit·kop (vit′kop). Um distúrbio favoso do couro cabeludo observado em sul-africanos.
wit·zel·sucht (vit′sel - zŭkht). Tendência mórbida a fazer trocadilhos, fazer piadas de mau gosto e contar histórias sem sentido, com os quais o indivíduo se diverte imensamente. [Al. *witzeln*, afetar a sagacidade + *Sucht*, mania]
wob·ble (wah′bl). Oscilação; balanço; em biologia molecular, o pareamento não-ortodoxo entre a base na extremidade 5′ de um anticódon e a base que faz par com esta (na posição 3′ do códon); assim, o anticódon 3′-UCU-5′ pode fazer par com 5′-AGA-3′ (pareamento normal ou de Watson-Crick) ou com 5′-AGG-3′ (*wobble*). Podem ocorrer pareamentos *wobble* entre a base inocumum hipoxantina e adenina, uracil ou citosina, entre uracil e guanina, e entre guanina e uracil, quando na posição 5′ de um anticódon. VER TAMBÉM wobble *base*.
Wohl·fahr·tia (vōl - far′tē - ă). Gênero de dípteros larvíparos (família Sarcophagidae), em que as larvas de algumas espécies reproduzem-se em superfícies ulceradas e ferimentos de seres humanos e animais. Espécies importantes incluem *W. magnifica*, uma mosca varejeira obrigatória de distribuição ampla, cujas larvas destruidoras de tecido invadem feridas ou cavidades na cabeça de animais domésticos e de seres humanos; *W. nuba*, uma mosca varejeira facultativa, encontrada no Velho Mundo, também encontrada em ferimentos ou cavidades na cabeça, mas não em úlceras dérmicas; e *W. vigil* (*W. opaca*), que produz míiase cutânea em lactentes humanos no norte dos Estados Unidos e sul do Canadá por larvas que penetram na pele e causam lesões infectadas, furunculares; filhotes de arminhos e raposas em fazendas de pele, e provavelmente, coelhos e roedores, são atacados por essa espécie. [P. *Wohlfahrt*, escritor médico alemão, † 1726]
wohl·fahr·ti·o·sis (vōl - far - tē - ō′sis). Infestação de animais e seres humanos por larvas de moscas do gênero *Wohlfahrtia*.
Wohlfart, Gunnar, neurologista sueco, 1910–1961. VER W.-Kugelberg-Welander *disease*.
Wolf, A., patologista norte-americano do século XX. VER W.-Orton *bodies*, em *body*.
Wolfe, John R., oftalmologista escocês, 1824–1904. VER W. *graft*; W.-Krause *graft*.
Wolff, Julius, anatomista alemão, 1836–1902. VER Wolff *law*.
Wolff, Kaspar F., embriologista alemão que viveu na Rússia, 1733–1794. VER wolffian *body*; wolffian *cyst*; wolffian *duct*; wolffian *rest*; wolffian *ridge*; wolffian *tubules*, em *tubule*.
Wolff, Louis, cardiologista norte-americano, 1898–1972. VER W.-Chaikoff *block, effect*; W.-Parkinson-White *syndrome*.
wolff·i·an (wulf′ē - an). Relativo a, ou descrito por, Kaspar Wolff.
Wölfler, Anton, cirurgião de Boêmia, 1850–1917. VER W. *gland*.

wolf·ram, wolf·ram·i·um (wulf′ram, wulf - ram′ē - ŭm). Volfrâmio. SIN tungsten. VER Wolfram *syndrome*. [reproduzido de *wolframite*]

Wolfring, Emilj F. von, oftalmologista polonês, 1832–1906. VER W. *glands*, em *gland*.

wolfs·bane (wulfs′bān). Acônito. VER aconite.

Wolinel·la (wō - li - nel′ah). Gênero de bactérias microaerófilas, Gram-negativas com células helicoidais a curvas; exibe motilidade por um único flagelo polar. Isolado do sulco gengival e de infecções do canal da raiz, em seres humanos, e do rúmen dos bovinos. A espécie típica é *Wolinella succinogenes*.

Wollaston, William H., médico e físico inglês, 1766–1828. VER W. *doublet, theory*.

Wolman, Moshe, neuropatologista israelense do século XX, *1914. VER W. *disease, xanthomatosis*.

womb (woom). Útero. SIN uterus. [A.S. o ventre]
  falling of the w., prolapso do útero. SIN *prolapse* of the uterus.

Wood, Paul. VER Wood *units*, em *unit*.

Wood, Robert, físico norte-americano, 1868–1955. VER W. *glass, lamp, light*.

wood al·co·hol (wud). Álcool metílico. SIN methyl *alcohol*.

wood wool. Lã de madeira; uma fibra de madeira especialmente preparada, não-comprimida, usada para curativos cirúrgicos.

wool (wul). Lã; o pêlo do carneiro; algumas vezes, quando desengordurado, é usado como curativo cirúrgico. SIN lana.
  w. alcohols, álcoois da cera de lã; preparados por saponificação da gordura da lã do carneiro e separação da fração que contém colesterol (não menos que 30%) e outros álcoois; usados no preparo de pomadas com lanolina.
  w. fat, lanolina; a substância gordurosa, anidra, purificada obtida da lã de carneiros. VER TAMBÉM *adeps* lanae.
  hydrous w. fat, lanolina hidratada. SIN *adeps lanae*.

Woolf, B., bioquímico inglês do século XX. VER W.-Lineweaver-Burk *plot*.

Woolner, Thomas, escultor inglês, 1826–1892. VER W. *tip*.

word sal·ad (werd sal′ăd). Salada de palavras; amontoado de palavras sem significado e não relacionadas emitidas por pessoas com determinados tipos de esquizofrenia.

Woringer, M.M.F., dermatologista francês do século XX. VER Woringer-Kolopp *disease*.

work (work). Trabalho. **1.** Esforço físico e/ou mental para alcançar um resultado. **2.** Aquilo que é realizado quando uma força atua contra uma resistência para produzir movimento.

workaholic (werk-a-hawl′ik). Pessoa que apresenta uma necessidade compulsiva de trabalhar, mesmo à custa das responsabilidades familiares, vida social e saúde. [por analogia com *alcoholic*]

> Embora seja cada vez mais reconhecida como causa de angústia emocional, disfunção social e doença física, a necessidade patológica de algumas pessoas de investir toda a sua energia em trabalho intensivo e com um objetivo não foi estudada profundamente, nem é citada ou definida no Diagnostic and Statistical Manual of Mental Disorders (DSM-IV). O *workaholic* pode realizar trabalho físico ou mental ou uma combinação dos dois, e pode trabalhar para uma pessoa ou uma empresa, ser autônomo, ou mesmo realizar atividades voluntárias não-remuneradas. O *workaholic* típico parece ser incapaz de relaxar e usa o trabalho não apenas como sustento, mas também como forma de recreação, substituindo a diversão como socialização, passatempos, esportes e atividades artísticas e culturais. Nesse contexto, o trabalho torna-se uma droga que vicia. Os *workaholics* tendem a adiar as refeições ou a não fazê-las, permanecer no trabalho após os outros terem ido para casa, e até mesmo continuar trabalhando até tarde da noite, fazer horas extras em excesso (algumas vezes não reclamando o devido pagamento) e abusar de nicotina, cafeína, etanol e outros agentes para aliviar o estresse e resistir à fadiga. O estilo de vida *workaholic* é uma característica comum de vários distúrbios da personalidade, incluindo uma compulsão em atingir o sucesso, reconhecimento ou avanço no campo de empenho escolhido; um interesse mórbido na aquisição de riqueza e uma necessidade de mergulhar no trabalho para se afastar dos estresses ou insatisfações da vida diária. Parte do comportamento *workaholic* é estimulado por expectativas familiares, sociais ou culturais. Muitos *workaholics* manifestam uma compulsão para trabalhar mesmo na infância; alguns parecem ser influenciados pelo exemplo ativo e bem-sucedido de um pai, parente, amigo da família ou figura pública. No Japão, a morte por excesso de trabalho (*karoshi*) é formalmente reconhecida como uma forma indenizável de distúrbio ocupacional. Os tribunais japoneses determinaram que mortes por insuficiência cardíaca, acidente vascular cerebral e até mesmo suicídio são exemplos de *karoshi*.

Working Formulation for Clinical Usage (WF). Classificação de linfomas malignos introduzida pelo National Cancer Institute em 1982, baseada na correlação de características clínicas e histopatológicas de vários linfomas; amplamente usada na prática clínica.

work·ing·out (werk′ing). Elaboração; em psicanálise, o estado no processo de tratamento em que são reveladas a história pessoal e a psicodinâmica do paciente.

work·ing through. Perlaboração; em psicanálise, o processo de obtenção de uma perspectiva adicional e alterações da personalidade em um paciente através de exame repetido e variado de um conflito ou problema; as interações entre livre associação, resistência, interpretação e elaboração constituem as facetas fundamentais desse processo.

work·sta·tion (werk′stā′shŭn). Estação de trabalho; um monitor de computador ou televisão com controles para estudo e manipulação de imagens gráficas ou clínicas.

World Health Or·ga·ni·za·tion (WHO). Organização Mundial de Saúde (OMS); uma unidade das Nações Unidas dedicada aos problemas internacionais na área de saúde.

Worm, Ole, anatomista dinamarquês, 1588–1654. VER wormian *bones*, em *bone*.

worm (werm). Verme. **1.** Em anatomia, qualquer estrutura semelhante a um verme, p. ex., a parte mediana do cerebelo nas formas de "vermis" e "lumbrical". **2.** Termo usado antigamente para designar qualquer membro do grupo invertebrado ou do antigo sub-reino Vermes, um termo coletivo não mais usado em taxonomia; agora comumente usado para designar qualquer membro dos distintos filos Annelida (os vermes segmentados ou verdadeiros), Nematoda (nematódeos) e Platyhelminthes (platelmintos). Entre as espécies importantes estão *Dracunculus medinensis, Enterobius vermicularis* (oxiúro), *Loa loa* (v. ocular africano), *Moniliformis* (filo Acanthocephala), *Oxyspirura mansoni, Pentastomida, Strongylus, Thelazia* (v. ocular) e *Trichinella spiralis*. Quanto a alguns tipos de vermes não relacionados como subentradas aqui (porque geralmente são escritos com uma só palavra), ver o nome completo. [A.S. *wyrm*]

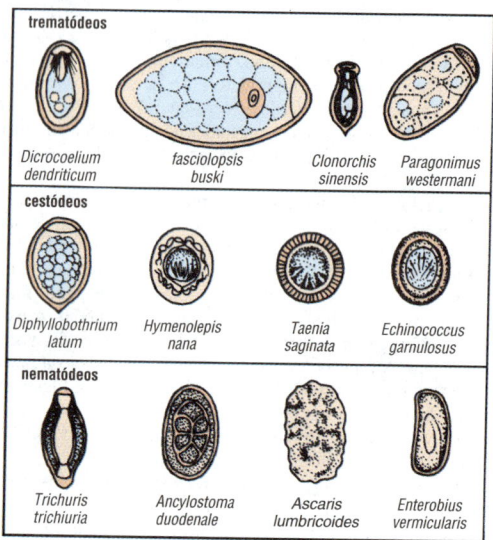

vermes: ovos de várias espécies

caddis w., larva aquática de insetos da ordem Trichoptera.

Manson eye w. SIN *Oxyspirura mansoni*.

meal w., v. da farinha; larva de besouros do gênero *Tenebrio*; tanto as larvas quanto os adultos são pestes importantes, destruindo farinhas de trigo, de milho e outros cereais; também são hospedeiros intermediários de nematódeos do gênero Gongylonema, e de várias tênias do gênero *Hymenolepis*.

worm bark. Andira. SIN *andira*.

wor·mi·an (werm′ē - an). Relativo a, ou descrito por, Ole Worm.

Wormley, Theodore G., químico norte-americano, 1826–1897. VER W. *test*.

worm·seed (werm′sēd). Erva-de-santa-maria; santônica, santonina. **1.** Santônica. **2.** SIN chenopodium.

worm·wood (werm′wud). Absinto; losna. SIN *absinthium*.

wort (wōrt). Planta; erva. **1.** Sufixo nos nomes populares de muitas plantas, tais como liverwort, lungwort, woundwort, etc. **2.** Uma infusão de malte. [A.S. *wyrt*, uma planta]

St. John's w., erva-de-são-joão; hipérico; uma planta perene, cheia de arbustos (*Hypericum perforatum*) com muitas flores amarelo-alaranjadas, cujas pétalas podem ter pontos pretos ao longo de suas margens; uma erva antidepressiva comparada favoravelmente com psicofármacos sintéticos padronizados para o tratamento da depressão leve a moderada.

Na medicina popular medieval, essa erva, tradicionalmente colhida na véspera da festa de São João Batista (24 de junho), foi usada no tratamento de várias doenças, incluindo histeria e epilepsia, e também contra feitiços e possessão diabólica. Na Europa, é amplamente prescrita para o tratamento da depressão. Em estudos controlados com placebo, a erva mostrou reduzir a depressão, a ansiedade, a apatia, os distúrbios do sono, a insônia, a anorexia e sentimentos de inutilidade. Estudos eletroencefalográficos mostraram que melhora a intensidade do sono sem aumentar a duração total do sono ou interferir com o sono REM. Em comparações clínicas foi apenas um pouco inferior aos agentes tricíclicos imipramina, amitriptilina e desipramina na supressão dos sintomas depressivos. Além disso, a memória e outras funções mentais podem melhorar em vez de serem embotadas, como ocorre com o uso de fármacos antidepressivos. Não foram publicados estudos controlados comparando a eficácia da erva-de-são-joão com a dos inibidores seletivos da recaptação de serotonina. Menos de 3% das pessoas em provas clínicas observaram efeitos colaterais. Os efeitos colaterais mais freqüentes foram irritação gastrointestinal, reações alérgicas, fadiga, agitação e fotodermatite. Acredita-se que o princípio ativo mais importante da erva-de-são-joão seja a hipericina, que mostrou inibir *in vitro* a captação ou a biodegradação de vários neurotransmissores, incluindo serotonina, noradrenalina e dopamina. Também se liga aos receptores do ácido γ-aminobutírico nos neurônios do SNC e melhora o sinal produzido pela serotonina após a ligação aos seus receptores. Estudos que estão sendo realizados procuram definir mais precisamente o potencial psicofarmacêutico desse agente e confirmar a segurança de seu uso. Como inibe a monoamina oxidase, ao menos *in vitro*, não se recomenda sua associação a outros antidepressivos. Não é considerada apropriada durante a gravidez ou no tratamento da depressão grave com sério risco de suicídio ou de depressão acompanhada por psicose.

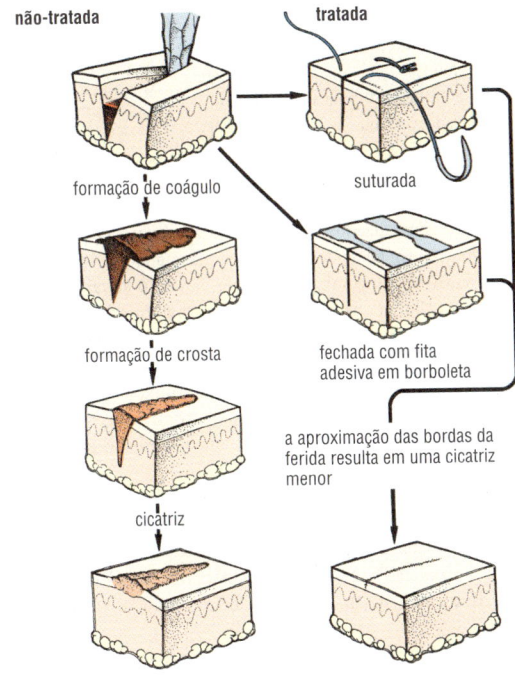

cicatrização de feridas

Worth, Claud A., oftalmologista britânico, 1869–1936. VER W. *amblyoscope*.
Woulfe, Peter, químico inglês, 1727–1803. VER W. *bottle*.
wound (woond). Ferida; ferimento. **1.** Traumatismo de qualquer tecido do corpo, principalmente causado por meios físicos e com soluções da continuidade. **2.** Uma incisão cirúrgica. [I. ant. *wund*]
  abraded w., abrasão. SIN abrasion (1).
  avulsed w., f. causada por, ou resultante de, avulsão.
  crease w., ferimento de raspão. SIN gutter w.
  glancing w., SIN gutter w.
  gunshot w., ferimento por arma de fogo; ferimento produzido por uma bala ou outro projétil de arma de fogo.
  gutter w., ferimento tangencial que produz um sulco sem perfurar a pele. SIN crease w., glancing w.
  incised w., f. incisa; uma ferida de bordas regulares, como a feita por um instrumento cortante.
  nonpenetrating w., f. não-penetrante; lesão, principalmente no tórax ou abdome, produzida sem ruptura da superfície do corpo.
  open w., f. aberta; f. na qual os tecidos são expostos ao ar.
  penetrating w., f. penetrante; f. com ruptura da superfície do corpo que se estende até o tecido subjacente ou até uma cavidade.
  perforating w., f. perfurante; uma f. com orifícios de entrada e saída.
  puncture w., f. punctiforme; uma f. na qual a abertura é relativamente pequena em comparação com a profundidade, como a produzida por um objeto estreito e pontiagudo.
  septic w., f. séptica; uma f. que foi infectada.
  seton w., f. em sedenho; f. perfurante tangencial, estando os orifícios de entrada e saída do mesmo lado do corpo, cabeça ou membro envolvido.
  stab w., f. punctória produzida pelo movimento pérfuro-cortante de uma faca ou objeto semelhante.
  subcutaneous w., f. subcutânea; uma lesão ou ferida que se estende abaixo da pele até o tecido subcutâneo, mas que não afeta ossos ou órgãos subjacentes.
  sucking chest w., f. torácica aspirativa. SIN open *pneumothorax*.
  tangential w., f. tangencial; uma f. perfurante ou f. em sedenho que envolve apenas uma face da parte lesada.
W-plas·ty. W-plastia; cirurgia para evitar a contratura de uma cicatriz em linha reta; as bordas da ferida são recortadas no formato de um W, ou uma série de W, e fechadas em ziguezague.
W.r. Abreviatura de Wassermann *reaction* (reação de Wassermann).
Wrª Abreviatura de Wright *antigens* (antígenos de Wright), em *antigen*. Ver grupos sanguíneos de baixa freqüência no apêndice Grupos Sanguíneos.
  wrap (rap). Cobertor; uma cobertura, particularmente a que embrulha ou envolve.
    cardiac muscle w., miocardioplastia. SIN cardiomyoplasty.
  wreath (rēth). Grinalda; coroa; estrutura semelhante a uma fita torcida ou trançada ou uma grinalda. [A.S. *wraeth*, uma bandagem]

  ciliary w., coroa ciliar. SIN corona ciliaris.
Wright, Basil Martin, médico britânico do século XX. VER W. *respirometer*.
Wright, James Homer, patologista norte-americano, 1869–1928. VER W. *stain*.
Wright, Marmaduke Burr, obstetra norte-americano, 1803–1879. VER W. *version*.
wright·ine (rīt′en). Wrightina. SIN conessine.
wrin·kle (ring′kl). Ruga; um sulco, dobra ou prega na pele, que tem ocorrência particularmente crescente com a exposição solar ou, na pele perioral, com o tabagismo; associada à degeneração do tecido elástico dérmico.
Wrisberg, Heinrich A., anatomista e ginecologista alemão, 1739–1808. VER W. *cartilage*, *ganglia*, em *ganglion*, *ligament*, *nerve*, *tubercle*.
wrist (rist) [TA]. Punho; o segmento proximal da mão que consiste nos ossos do carpo e nas partes moles associadas. SIN carpus (1) [TA]. [A.S. articulação do punho, articulação do tornozelo]
  w.-drop, punho caído; mão caída; carpoptosia; carpoptose; paralisia dos extensores do punho e dos dedos da mão; causada na maioria das vezes por lesão do nervo radial. SIN carpoptosis, carpoptosia, drop hand.
wry·neck (rī′nek). Torcicolo. SIN torticollis.
Wuch·er·e·ri·a (voo - ker - e′rē - ā). Gênero de nematódeos filarianos (família Onchocercidae, superfamília Filarioidea) caracterizados por formas adultas que vivem principalmente nos vasos linfáticos e produzem numerosos embriões ou microfilárias que circulam na corrente sanguínea (microfilaremia), freqüentemente aparecendo no sangue periférico a intervalos regulares. A forma extrema desta infecção (wuchereriasis ou filariasis) é a elefantíase ou paquidermia.
  W. brancrof′ti, a filária de Bancroft, uma espécie endêmica nas ilhas do Sul do Pacífico, costa da China, Índia e Burma, e em toda a África tropical e nordeste da América do Sul (incluindo algumas ilhas do Caribe); transmitida aos seres humanos (aparentemente o único hospedeiro definitivo) por mosquitos, particularmente *Culex quinquefasciatus* e *Aedes pseudoscutellaris*, também por várias outras espécies de *Culex*, *Aedes*, *Anopheles* e *Mansonia*, dependendo da área geográfica específica; os adultos são vermes filiformes, cilindróides, brancos, medindo 40–100 mm, e as microfilárias são embainhadas, com extremidade anterior arredondada e cauda afilada e não nucleada; os vermes adultos habitam os vasos linfáticos maiores (p. ex., nos membros (principalmente inferiores), as mamas, o cordão espermático e os tecidos retroperitoneais) e os seios dos linfonodos (p. ex., os grupos poplíteo, femoral e inguinal, e também os linfonodos epitrocleares e axilares), onde algumas vezes causam obstrução temporária do fluxo de linfa e inflamação leve ou moderada.
  W. mala′yi, nome antigo da *Brugia malayi*.
wu·cher·e·ri·a·sis (voo′ ker - ē - rī′ā - sis). Wuchereríase; infestação por vermes do gênero *Wuchereria*. VER TAMBÉM filariasis.
Wurster, Casimir, químico alemão, 1856–1913. VER W. *reagent*, *test*.
Wyburn-Mason, Roger, médico britânico. VER Wyburn-Mason *syndrome*.
Wyman, Jeffries, bioquímico norte-americano, 1901–1995. VER Monod-Wyman-Changeux *model*.

X

X Símbolo da unidade de Kienböck (Kienböck *unit*); xantosina; átomo de halogênio; aminoácido não-especificado.
X Símbolo de reatância.
Xaa Símbolo de aminoácido não-especificado.
Xan Abreviatura de xantina.
⟡ **xanth-.** VER xantho-.
xan·the·las·ma (zan - thē - laz′mă). Xantelasma. SIN x. palpebrarum. [xanth- + G. *elasma*, placa de metal batido]
  generalized x., x. generalizado; xantoma plano do pescoço, do tronco, dos membros e das pálpebras em pacientes com níveis plasmáticos normais de lipídios.
  x. palpebra′rum, x. palpebral; placas moles amarelo-alaranjadas nas pálpebras e no canto medial; a forma mais comum de xantoma; pode estar associado a lipoproteínas de baixa densidade (LDL), especialmente em adultos jovens. SIN xanthelasma, xanthoma palpebrarum.
xan·them·a·tin (zan - thĕm′ă - tin). Xantematina; uma substância amarela derivada da hematina por tratamento com ácido nítrico.
xan·the·mia (zan - thē′mē - ă). Xantemia. SIN carotenemia. [xanth- + G. *haima*, sangue]
xan·thene (zan′thēn). Xanteno. **1.** A estrutura básica de muitos produtos naturais, drogas, corantes (p. ex., fluoresceína, pironina, eosinas), indicadores, pesticidas, antibióticos, etc. **2.** Uma classe de moléculas baseadas no x. (1).
xan·thic (zan′thik). Xântico. **1.** Amarelo ou amarelado. **2.** Relacionado à xantina.
xan·thi·dy·lic ac·id (zan′thi-dil-ik). Ácido xantidílico. SIN xanthosine 5′-monophosphate.
xan·thine (Xan) (zan′thēn). Xantina; 2,6-disoxopurina; 2,6-(1*H*,3*H*)-purinediona; produto da oxidação da guanina e hipoxantina, precursor do ácido úrico; presente em muitos órgãos e na urina, ocasionalmente formando cálculos urinários; elevada na deficiência do co-fator molibdênio e na xantinúria.
  x. dehydrogenase, x. desidrogenase; uma oxidorredutase que oxida a x. a urato com NAD$^+$ como oxidante; menor atividade em indivíduos com deficiência de co-fator molibdênio.
  x. nucleotide, nucleotídeo da x. SIN xanthosine 5′-monophosphate.
  x. oxidase, x. oxidase; uma flavoproteína que contém molibdênio; uma oxidorredutase que catalisa a reação de x., O_2 e H_2O para produzir urato e superóxido; também oxida hipoxantina, algumas outras purinas e pterinas, bem como aldeídos. Uma menor atividade é observada na deficiência do co-fator molibdênio. SIN hypoxanthine oxidase, Schardinger enzyme.
  x. ribonucleoside, ribonucleosídeo da x.. SIN xanthosine.
xan·thi·nol ni·a·cin·ate, xan·thi·nol nic·o·tin·ate (zan′thi - nōl). Xantinol niacinato, xantinol nicotinato; um vasodilatador periférico.
xan·thi·nu·ria (zan - thi - noo′rē - ă). Xantinúria. **1.** Excreção de quantidades anormalmente grandes de xantina na urina. **2.** Um distúrbio [MIM*278300] caracterizado por excreção urinária de xantina no lugar do ácido úrico, hipouricemia e, ocasionalmente, formação de cálculos renais de xantina. Há dois tipos: o tipo I é causado por deficiência de xantina desidrogenase (XDH), e o tipo II é devido a deficiências da xantina desidrogenase assim como da aldeído oxidase. Herança autossômica recessiva, causada por mutação do gene XDH no cromossomo 2p em alguns casos. SIN xanthiuria, xanthuria. [xanthine + G. *ouron*, urina]
xan·thism (zan′thizm) [MIM*278400]. Xantismo; uma anomalia pigmentar de negros, caracterizada por cabelo de cor vermelha ou amarelo-avermelhada, pele vermelho-cobre e, freqüentemente, diluição do pigmento da íris; herança autossômica recessiva causada por mutação no gene 1 da proteína relacionada à tirosinase (TYRP1) no cromossoma 9. SIN rufous albinism. [G. *xanthos*, amarelado]
xan·thi·u·ria (zan - thē - ū′rē - ă). Xantiúria. SIN xanthinuria.
⟡ **xantho-, xanth-.** Amarelo, amarelado. [G. *xanthos*]
xan·tho·as·tro·cy·to·ma (zan′thrō - as′trō - sī - tō - mă). Xantoastrocitoma. SIN pleomorphic x. [xantho + astrocytoma]
  pleomorphic x., x. pleomórfico; uma forma rara de astrocitoma que geralmente se apresenta no início da vida com convulsões. O tumor é superficial e composto por células gliais pleomórficas, astrócitos lipidizados e linfócitos perivasculares. SIN xanthoastrocytoma.
xan·tho·chro·mat·ic (zan′thō - krō - mat′ik). Xantocromático; amarelado. SIN xanthochromic.
xan·tho·chro·mia (zan - thō - krō′mē - ă). Xantocromia; a ocorrência de placas de cor amarela na pele, semelhantes ao xantoma, mas sem os nódulos ou placas. SIN xanthoderma (1), yellow disease, yellow skin (1). [xantho- + G. *chrōma*, cor]
xan·tho·chro·mic (zan - thō - krō′mik). Xantocrômico. SIN xanthochromatic.

xan·tho·der·ma (zan - thō - der′mă). Xantoderma, xantodermia. **1.** SIN xanthochromia. **2.** Qualquer coloração amarela da pele. SIN yellow skin (2). [xantho- + G. *derma*, pele]
xan·tho·dont (zan′thō - dont). Xantodonte; aquele que possui dentes amarelos. [xantho- + G. *odous*, dente]
xan·tho·gran·u·lo·ma (zan′thō - gran′ū - lō′mă). Xantogranuloma; uma infiltração peculiar do tecido retroperitoneal por macrófagos lipídicos, sendo mais comum em mulheres.
  juvenile x., x. juvenil; pápulas ou nódulos avermelhados a amarelos, únicos ou múltiplos, geralmente encontrados em crianças pequenas, que consistem em infiltração dérmica por histiócitos e células gigantes de Touton, com fibrose progressiva. SIN nevoxanthoendothelioma.
  necrobiotic x., x. necrobiótico; x. cutâneo e subcutâneo com necrose focal, que se apresenta como múltiplos nódulos granulomatosos vermelhos a amarelos, grandes, algumas vezes ulcerados com células gigantes (freqüentemente ao redor dos olhos) associados a paraproteinemia (geralmente gamopatia monoclonal).
xan·tho·gran·u·lo·ma·tous (zan′thō - gran′ū - lō′mă - tŭs). Xantogranulomatoso; relativo a, da natureza de ou afetado por xantogranuloma.
xan·tho·ma (zan - thō′mă). Xantoma; um nódulo ou placa amarela, principalmente da pele, composta de histiócitos repletos de lipídios. [xantho- + G. -*oma*, tumor]
  x. diabetico′rum, x. diabético; x. eruptivo associado ao diabetes melito grave.
  x. dissemina′tum, x. disseminado; um distúrbio normolipêmico benigno raro de adultos com xantomas cutâneos coalescentes compostos de histiócitos não-X nas superfícies flexurais, freqüentemente com diabetes insípido leve.
  eruptive x., x. eruptivo; o surgimento súbito de grupos de pápulas céreas amarelas ou castanho-amareladas de 1–4 mm, com um halo eritematoso, principalmente sobre as superfícies extensoras dos cotovelos e joelhos, e no dorso e nas nádegas de pacientes com hiperlipemia grave, freqüentemente familiar ou, mais raramente, no diabetes melito grave.
  fibrous x., x. fibroso. VER fibroxanthoma.
  x. mul′tiplex, x. múltiplo. SIN xanthomatosis.
  x. palpebra′rum, x. palpebral. SIN xanthelasma palpebrarum.
  x. pla′num, x. plano; uma forma caracterizada pela ocorrência de faixas amarelas planas ou placas retangulares minimamente palpáveis no cório, normolipêmico ou associado à hiperlipoproteinemia do tipo IIa ou III.
  tendinous x., x. tendinoso; x. envolvendo tendões, ligamentos e fáscia, formando nódulos profundos, lisos e algumas vezes dolorosos sob a pele livremente móvel e de aspecto normal dos membros; associado a metabolismo lipídico anormal, comumente lipoproteínas β aumentadas familiares, ou hepatopatia obstrutiva.
  x. tubero′sum, x. tuberoso; xantomatose associada à hiperlipoproteinemia familiar do tipo II e, ocasionalmente, do tipo III. SIN x. tuberosum simplex.
  x. tubero′sum sim′plex, x. tuberoso simples. SIN x. tuberosum.
  verrucous x., x. verrucoso; histiocitose Y; um papiloma da mucosa oral e da pele no qual o epitélio de células escamosas recobre as papilas de tecido conjuntivo cheias de grandes histiócitos espumosos. SIN histiocytosis Y.
xan·tho·ma·to·sis (zan - thō - mă - tō′sis). Xantomatose; xantomas disseminados, principalmente nos cotovelos e joelhos, que algumas vezes afetam as mucosas e podem estar associados a distúrbios metabólicos. SIN lipid granulomatosis, lipoid granulomatosis, xanthoma multiplex.
  biliary x., x. biliar; x. com hipercolesterolemia, resultante de cirrose biliar. SIN Rayer disease.
  x. bul′bi, x. bulbar; degeneração gordurosa ulcerativa da córnea após lesão.
  cerebrotendinous x. [MIM*213700], x. cerebrotendinosa; um distúrbio metabólico associado à deposição de colestanol e colesterol no cérebro e outros tecidos; o nível plasmático de colestanol é alto, mas o nível plasmático de co-

---

⟡ Formas Combinantes	☆ Termo oficial alternativo para a *Terminologia Anatomica*
▣ Indica que o termo é ilustrado, ver Índice de Ilustrações	
SIN Sinônimo	[MIM] Mendelian Inheritance in Man
Cf. Comparar, confrontar	I.C. Índice de Corantes
[NA] *Nomina Anatomica*	
[TA] *Terminologia Anatomica*	Termo de Alta Importância

xanthomatosis

lesterol é normal; caracterizado por ataxia cerebelar progressiva que se inicia após a puberdade, catarata, envolvimento da medula espinhal, aterosclerose prematura e xantomas tendinosos ou tuberosos; devido a um defeito da esterol 27-hidroxilase mitocondrial hepática na biossíntese de ácido biliar; herança autossômica recessiva, causada por mutação no gene envolvido no citocromo P-450 na posição C27 (CYP27) no cromossoma 2q.

chronic idiopathic x., x. idiopática crônica; termo vago ou indefinido para anormalidades hereditárias do metabolismo lipídico, levando à formação de xantoma (p. ex., xantomatose familiar primária).

familial hypercholesteremic x., x. hipercolesterêmica familiar. VER type II familial *hyperlipoproteinemia*.

generalized plane x., x. plana generalizada; x. disseminada associada ao mieloma múltiplo (multiple *myeloma*), hiperlipoproteinemia familiar (familial *hyperlipoproteinemia*) ou, menos comumente, à cirrose biliar primária (primary biliary *cirrhosis*) ou sem doença subjacente.

normal cholesteremic x., x. colesterêmica normal. SIN Hand-Schüller-Christian disease.

Wolman x., x. de Wolman. SIN cholesterol ester storage *disease*.

Xan·tho·mo·nas (zan - thō - mō'as). Gênero da família Pseudomonadaceae; bacilos retos, aeróbicos, Gram-negativos, quimioorganotróficos e que exibem motilidade por flagelos. A espécie típica é *Xanthomonas campestris*.

X. maltophil'ia, uma espécie encontrada basicamente em amostras clínicas, mas também na água, no leite e nos alimentos congelados; causa freqüente de infecção em seres humanos hospitalizados e imunodeprimidos, é resistente a muitos antibióticos comumente usados; antes denominada *Pseudomonas maltophilia*. VER *Stenotrophomonas maltophilia*.

xan·tho·phyll (zan'thō - fil). Xantofila; derivado oxigenado do caroteno; um pigmento vegetal amarelo, presente também na gema de ovo e no corpo lúteo. SIN lutein (2), luteol, luteole.

xan·tho·pro·te·ic (zan - thō - prō'tē - ik). Xantoproteico; relativo à xantoproteína.

xan·tho·pro·te·ic ac·id. Ácido xantoproteico; uma substância amarela não-cristalizável, derivada das proteínas após tratamento com ácido nítrico.

xan·tho·pro·tein (zan - thō - prō'tēn). Xantoproteína; o produto amarelo formado após tratamento da proteína com ácido nítrico quente, provavelmente pela nitrificação dos grupamentos fenílicos.

xan·thop·sia (zan - thop'sē - ā). Xantopsia; uma condição na qual os objetos parecem amarelos; pode ocorrer no envenenamento por ácido pícrico e santonina, na icterícia e na intoxicação digitálica. SIN yellow vision. [xantho- + G. *opsis*, visão]

xan·tho·puc·cine (zan - thō - pŭk'sēn). Xantopucina. SIN canadine.

xan·tho·sine (X, Xao) (zan'thō - sēn, - sin). Xantosina; 9-β-D-ribosilxantina; o produto da desaminação da guanosina (O substituindo –NH$_2$). SIN xanthine ribonucleoside.

x. 5'-monophosphate (XMP), 5'-monofosfato de x.; o éster monofosfórico da x.; um intermediário na biossíntese de GMP. SIN xanthidylic acid, xanthine nucleotide, xanthylic acid.

x. 5'-triphosphate (XTP), 5'-trifosfato de x.; x. com um ácido trifosfórico esterificado em sua posição 5'.

xan·tho·sis (zan - thō'sis). Xantose; coloração amarelada dos tecidos em degeneração, observada principalmente em neoplasias malignas. [xantho- + G. *-osis*, condição]

xan·thous (zan'thŭs). Xantoso amarelado; amarelo. [G. *xanthos*, amarelo]

xanth·u·ren·ic ac·id (zan - thoo - rēn'ik). Ácido xanturênico; os cristais amarelo-enxofre formam um composto vermelho com o reagente de Millon, ou um intensamente verde com o sulfato ferroso; excretado na urina de animais com deficiência de piridoxina, após a ingestão de triptofano, e de ratos alimentados quase exclusivamente com fibrina.

xan·thu·ria (zan - thoo'rē - ā). Xantúria. SIN xanthinuria.

xan·thyl (zan'thil). Xantil; xantila; um radical que consiste em xantina menos um átomo de hidrogênio.

xan·thyl·ic (zan-thil'ik). Xantílico; relativo à xantina.

xan·thyl·ic ac·id. Ácido xantílico. SIN *xanthosine* 5'-monophosphate.

Xao Símbolo de xantosina.

Xe Símbolo do xenônio.

^{133}Xe Símbolo do xenônio-133 (Xe^{133}).

xemilofiban (zem - il - of'ī - ban). Xemilofibam; um novo agente antiplaquetário que bloqueia a ligação do fibrinogênio a receptores integrina GPIIb/IIIa específicos da membrana, impedindo assim a agregação plaquetária induzida por qualquer agonista plaquetário conhecido.

xeno-. Xeno-; estranho; material estranho; parasita. VER hetero-, allo-. [G. *xenos*, visitante, hóspede, estranho, forasteiro]

xen·o·bi·ot·ic (zen'ō - bī - ot'ik). Xenobiótico. **1.** Uma substância farmacológica, endocrinológica ou toxicologicamente ativa, não produzida endogenamente e, portanto, estranha ao organismo. **2.** Relativo à associação de duas espécies animais, geralmente insetos, na ausência de uma relação de dependência, em oposição ao parasitismo. [xeno- + G. *bios*, vida + -ic]

xen·o·di·ag·no·sis (zen'ō - dī - ag - nō'sis). Xenodiagnóstico. **1.** Um método de diagnosticar infestação por *Trypanosoma cruzi* aguda ou incipiente (doença de Chagas) em seres humanos. Insetos da família Reduviidae (triatomíneos) não-infestados (criados em laboratório) são alimentados com amostras de tecido da pessoa suspeita, e o tripanossoma é identificado por exame microscópico do conteúdo intestinal do inseto (barbeiro) após um período de incubação adequado. **2.** Um método semelhante de diagnóstico biológico baseado na exposição experimental de um hospedeiro normal sem parasitas capaz de permitir que o organismo em questão se multiplique, sendo assim detectado com maior facilidade e fidedignidade.

xen·o·gen·e·ic (zen'ō - jĕ - nē'ik). Xenogênico; xenogenético; heterólogo, em relação a enxertos teciduais, principalmente quando doador e receptor pertencem a espécies muito distintas. SIN xenogenic (2), xenogenous (2). [xeno- + G. *–gen*, que produz]

xen·o·gen·ic (zen - ō - jen'ik). Xenogênico. **1.** Originado fora do organismo, ou de uma substância estranha que foi introduzida no organismo. SIN xenogenous (1). **2.** SIN xenogeneic. [xeno- + G. *-gen*, que produz]

xe·nog·e·nous (zē - noj'ĕ - nŭs). Xenógeno. **1.** SIN xenogenic (1). **2.** SIN xenogeneic.

xen·o·graft (zen'ō - graft). Xenoenxerto; um enxerto transferido de um animal de uma espécie para um animal de outra espécie. SIN heterograft, heterologous graft, heteroplastic graft, xenogeneic graft.

xe·non (Xe) (zē'non). Xenônio; um elemento gasoso, número atômico 54, peso atômico 131,29; presente em percentual mínimo (0,087 ppm) na atmosfera seca; produz anestesia geral em concentrações de 70 vol.%. [G. *xenos*, estranho]

xe·non-133 (^{133}Xe). Xenônio-133 (Xe^{133}); um radioisótopo do xenônio com uma emissão gama de 81 keV e uma meia-vida física de 5,243 dias; usado no estudo da função pulmonar e do fluxo sanguíneo dos órgãos.

xen·o·par·a·site (zen - ō - par'ă - sīt). Xenoparasita; um ecoparasita que se torna patogênico em consequência do enfraquecimento da resistência de seu hospedeiro.

xen·o·pho·bia (zen - ō - fō'bē - ā). Xenofobia; medo mórbido de estrangeiros. [xeno- + G. *phobos*, medo]

xen·o·pho·nia (zen - ō - fō'nē - ā). Xenofonia; um defeito da fala caracterizado por alteração do acento (tonicidade) e da entonação. [xeno- + G. *phōnē*, voz]

Xen·o·psyl·la (zen - op - sil'ă). A pulga do rato; um gênero de pulgas parasitas do rato e envolvidas na transmissão da peste bubônica. A espécie *X. cheopis* serve como potente vetor da *Yersinia pestis*, principalmente porque seu intestino é "bloqueado" por uma massa de células de *Y. pestis* que impede que a pulga se alimente normalmente, de forma que tende a atacar seres humanos e outros hospedeiros; é uma importante fonte de infecção em áreas epidêmicas tradicionais, como a Índia. *X. astia* e *X. braziliensis* também são eficientes vetores da peste. [xeno- + G. *psylla*, pulga]

xen.yl (zen'il). Xenil; xenila; um radical que consiste em bifenil menos um átomo de hidrogênio.

xe·ran·sis (zē - ran'sis). Dessecação; perda gradual da umidade nos tecidos. [G. *xēransis*, de *xēros*, seco]

xe·ran·tic (zē - ran'tik). Xerântico; dessecante; secativo.

xe·ra·sia (zē - rā'zē - ā). Xerasia; uma condição dos pêlos caracterizada por ressecamento e encrespação. [G. *xērasia*, de *xēros*, seco]

xero-. Seco. [G. *xeros*]

xer·o·chi·lia (zēr - ō - kī'lē - ā). Xeroquilia; xeroqueilia; ressecamento dos lábios. [xero- + G. *cheilos*, lábio]

xe·ro·der·ma (zēr'ō - der'mă). Xerodermia, xeroderma; forma leve de ictiose caracterizada por ressecamento excessivo da pele devido a pequeno aumento da camada córnea e diminuição do conteúdo de água do estrato córneo por diminuição da transpiração, vento ou baixa umidade; observada no envelhecimento, dermatite atópica, deficiência de vitamina A, etc. [xero- + G. *derma*, pele]

x. pigmento'sum [MIM*278700], x. pigmentosa; uma erupção da pele exposta que ocorre na infância, caracterizada por fotossensibilidade com queimadura solar grave na lactância e pelo desenvolvimento de numerosas manchas pigmentadas semelhantes a efélides, lesões atróficas maiores, que acabam resultando em adelgaçamento branco brilhante da pele, circundadas por telangiectasias, e múltiplas ceratoses solares que sofrem alteração maligna em pessoas jovens; resulta de alguns grupamentos de complementação autossômica recessiva raros nos quais os processos de reparo do DNA são defeituosos, de forma que são mais sensíveis a quebras cromossomiais e degeneração cancerosa quando expostos à luz ultravioleta. Também são encontradas anormalidades oftálmicas e neurológicas graves. VER TAMBÉM De Sanctis-Cacchione *syndrome*.

xe·ro·gram (zē′rō - gram). Xerograma. SIN xeroradiograph.

xe·rog·ra·phy (zēr - og′rā - fē). Xerografia. SIN xeroradiography.

xe·ro·ma (zē - rō′mă). Xeroma. SIN xerophthalmia.

xe·ro·mam·mog·ra·phy (zēr′ō - mam - og′rā - fē). Xeromamografia; exame da mama por xerorradiografia.

xe·ro·me·nia (zēr - ō - mē′nē - ă). Xeromenia; designação obsoleta para a ocorrência dos sinais e sintomas constitucionais habituais no período menstrual sem sangramento. [xero- + G. *mēniaia*, menstruação]

xe·ro·myc·te·ria (zēr′ō - mik - tēr′ē - ă). Xeromicteria; ressecamento extremo da mucosa nasal. [xero- + G. *myktēr*, o nariz]

xe·ro·pha·gia, xe·roph·a·gy (zēr - ō - fā′jē - ă, zēr - of′ă - jē). Xerofagia; ingestão de alimentos secos; subsistir com uma dieta seca. [xero- + G. *phagō*, comer]

xe·roph·thal·mia (zēr - of - thal′mē - ă). Xeroftalmia; ressecamento excessivo da conjuntiva e córnea, que perdem seu brilho e tornam-se queratinizadas; pode ser devida a doença local ou a uma deficiência sistêmica de vitamina A. SIN conjunctivitis arida, xeroma, xerophthalmus. [xero- + G. *ophthalmos*, olho]

xe·roph·thal·mus (zēr′of - thal′mŭs). Xeroftalmia. SIN xerophthalmia.

xe·ro·ra·di·o·graph (zē - rō - rā′dē - ō - graf). Xerorradiograma; o registro permanente feito por xerorradiografia. SIN xerogram.

xe·ro·ra·di·og·ra·phy (zē′rō - rā′dē - og′rā - fē). Xerorradiografia; radiografia utilizando uma placa carregada especialmente revestida em vez de filme de raios X, revelada com um pó seco em vez de substâncias químicas líquidas, e transferindo a imagem no pó para o papel para um registro permanente; o realce da borda é inerente. SIN xerography.

xe·ro·sis (zē - rō′sis). Xerose; ressecamento patológico da pele (xerodermia), da conjuntiva (xeroftalmia) ou das mucosas. [xero- + G. *-osis*, condição]

x. parenchymato′sus, x. parenquimatosa; ressecamento superficial da conjuntiva devido a fibrose difusa, com fechamento das aberturas das glândulas lacrimais.

xe·ro·sto·mia (zēr′o - stō′mē - ă). Xerostomia; ressecamento da boca, de etiologia variada, resultante de diminuição ou interrupção da secreção salivar, ou assialia. [xero- + G. *stoma*, boca]

xe·rot·ic (zē - rot′ik). Xerótico; seco; afetado por xerose.

xe·ro·trip·sis (zēr - ō - trip′sis). Xerotripsia; fricção seca. [xero- + G. *tripsis*, atrito, de *tribō*, atritar]

Xg blood group. Grupo sanguíneo Xg. Ver apêndice Grupos Sanguíneos.

X-in·ac·ti·va·tion. Inativação do X. SIN lyonization.

△ **xiph-.** VER xipho-.

xiph·i·ster·nal (zif - i - ster′năl). Xifoesternal; relativo ao processo xifóide.

xiph·i·ster·num (zif′i - ster′nŭm). Xifoesterno. SIN xiphoid *process*. [xiphoid + G. *sternon*, tórax]

△ **xipho-, xiph-, xiphi-.** Xifóide, geralmente o processo xifóide. [G. *xiphos*, espada]

xiph·o·cos·tal (zif′ō - kos′tăl). Xifocostal; relativo ao processo xifóide e às costelas. [xipho- + L. *costa*, costela]

xiph·o·dyn·ia (zif - ō - din′ē - ă). Xifodinia; dor de caráter nevrálgico na região da cartilagem xifóide. VER TAMBÉM hypersensitive xiphoid *syndrome*. SIN xiphoidalgia. [xipho- + G. *odynē*, dor]

xi·phoid (zi′foyd) [TA]. Xifóide; em forma de espada; aplicado especialmente ao processo xifóide. SIN ensiform, gladiate, mucronate. [xipho- + G. *eidos*, aparência]

xi·phoi·dal·gia (zif - oy - dal′jē - ă). Xifoidalgia. SIN xiphodynia. [xiphoid + G. *algos*, dor]

xi·phoi·di·tis (zif′oy - dī′tis). Xifoidite; inflamação do processo xifóide do esterno. [xiphoid + G. *-itis*, inflamação]

xi·phop·a·gus (zi - fop′ă - gŭs). Xifópago; gêmeos unidos na região do processo xifóide do esterno. VER conjoined *twins*, em *twin*. [xipho- + G. *pagos*, algo fixo]

X-linked. Ligado ao X; relativo a genes situados no cromossoma X. Comumente, mas erroneamente, usado como sinônimo de ligado ao sexo, que também compreenderia traços ligados ao Y.

XMP Abreviatura de 5′-monofosfato de xantosina (*xanthosine* 5′-*monophosphate*).

x-o·mat (eks′ō - mat). Um nome comercial (da Kodak) que se tornou designação genérica de uma processadora automática para filmes de raios X.

x-ra·di·a·tion. Radiação X; energia radiante de um tubo de raios X. VER TAMBÉM x-ray.

x-ray. Raio X. 1. A radiação eletromagnética ionizante emitida de um tubo altamente evacuado, resultante da excitação dos elétrons orbitais internos pelo bombardeio do anodo alvo com uma corrente de elétrons de um catodo aquecido. SIN roentgen ray. Cf. glass *rays*, em *ray*, indirect *rays*, em *ray*. 2. Radiação eletromagnética ionizante produzida pela excitação dos elétrons orbitais internos de um átomo por outros processos, como retardo nuclear e suas seqüelas. 3. SIN radiograph.

XTP Abreviatura de 5′-trifosfato de xantosina (*xanthosine* 5′-*triphosphate*).

Xy Abreviatura de xilose (*xylose*).

Xyl Abreviatura de xilose (*xylose*).

△ **xyl-, xylo-.** Madeira; de madeira; xilose; xileno. [G. *xylon*]

xy·la·zine (zī′la - zēn). Xilazina; um sedativo/hipnótico/anestésico amplamente usado em medicina veterinária e em animais de laboratório.

xy·lene (zī′lēn). Xileno. SIN xylol.

x. cyanol FF [C.I. 43535], x. cianol FF; um corante trifenilmetano ácido usado para coloração histoquímica da hemoglobina peroxidase e como corante de rastreamento de seqüências de DNA na eletroforese.

xy·le·nol (zī′lē - nol). Xilenol; que ocorre em seis formas isoméricas; usado na fabricação de desinfetantes de alcatrão e resinas sintéticas. SIN dimethylphenol.

xy·li·dine (zī′li - dēn). Xilidina; aminodimetilbenzeno; usado como reagente e na fabricação de corantes.

xy·li·tol (zī′li - tol). Xilitol; um álcool de açúcar opticamente inativo; freqüentemente usado como substituto do açúcar em dietas para diabéticos; a síntese de x. a partir da L-xilulose é bloqueada em pessoas com pentosúria idiopática.

xy·li·tol de·hy·dro·gen·ase. Xilitol desidrogenase. SIN *xylulose* reductase.

△ **xylo-.** VER xyl-.

xy·lo·bi·ose (zī′lō - bī′ōs). Xilobiose; um dissacarídio de dois resíduos xilose ligados β1→4, ambos em anéis piranose.

xy·loi·din (zī - loy′din). Xiloidina. SIN pyroxylin.

xy·lo·ke·tose (zī - lō - kē′tōs). Xilocetose. SIN xylulose.

xy·lol (zī′lol). Xilol; um líquido volátil, obtido do alcatrão, que possui propriedades físicas e químicas semelhantes às do benzeno; ocorre como três isômeros: *m-, o-* e *p-*xilol; usado como solvente, na fabricação de substâncias químicas e fibras sintéticas, e em histologia como agente clareador. SIN dimethylbenzene, xylene.

xy·lo·met·az·o·line hy·dro·chlo·ride (zī′lō - mě - taz′ō - lēn). Cloridrato de xilometazolina; um agente simpaticomimético usado como descongestionante nasal.

xy·lon·ic ac·id (zī′lon-ik). Ácido xilônico; um produto da oxidação leve da xilose.

xy·lo·py·ra·nose (zī - lō - pir′ă - nōs). Xilopiranose; xilose na forma piranose.

xy·lose (Xy, Xyl) (zī′lōs). Xilose; uma aldopentose, isômera da ribose, obtida por fermentação ou hidrólise de carboidratos naturais; p. ex., na fibra da madeira. Um componente alimentar importante para herbívoros. O isômero D também é conhecido como açúcar da madeira ou faia. SIN uridine diphosphoxylose.

xy·lu·lose (zī′loo - lōs). Xilulose; *threo*-pentulose; uma 2-cetopentose. A L-xilulose aparece na urina em casos de pentosúria essencial; também é um intermediário na via do glucuronato. SIN xyloketose.

x. 5-phosphate, x. 5-fosfato; o isômero D é um intermediário na via da pentose fosfato e na transcetolização.

x. reductase, x. redutase; uma enzima que converte reversivelmente a x. em xilitol utilizando NADH (D-x. redutase) ou NADPH (L-x. redutase); é observada uma deficiência da forma L em pessoas com pentosúria essencial. SIN xylitol dehydrogenase.

L-xy·lu·lo·su·ria (zī′loo - lō - soo′rē - ă). L-xilulosúria. SIN essential *pentosuria*.

xy·lyl (zī′lil). Xilil; o radical consiste em xileno (xilol) menos um átomo de hidrogênio.

x. bromide, brometo de x., as formas *o-, m-* e *p-* são potentes lacrimogênios.

xy·lyl·ene (zī′li - lēn). Xilileno; o radical que consiste em xileno (xilol) menos dois átomos de hidrogênio.

xys·ma (ziz′mă). Xisma; fragmentos membranosos nas fezes. [G. tiras, raspas, de *xyō*, raspar]

Y

Y Símbolo de ítrio; tirosina; nucleosídio de pirimidina.

y⁺ VER system (5).

YAC Abreviatura de cromossomas artificiais de levedura (yeast artificial *chromosomes*, em *chromosome*).

YAG Abreviatura de ítrio-alumínio-granada.

yang (yang). VER yin-yang.

yang·go·na (yang′gō - na). Iangona. SIN yaqona.

ya·qo·na (ya′kōna). Iacona; cava; uma bebida fijiana feita com a raiz pulverizada do *Piper methysticum* (família Piperaceae); sua ingestão excessiva causa um estado de hiperexcitabilidade e perda da força muscular nas pernas; a intoxicação crônica induz aspereza da pele e um estado de debilidade. VER TAMBÉM methysticum. SIN kava (2), yanggona. [nome fijiano]

yaw (yau). Framboesioma; lesão individual da erupção da framboesia ou bouba.
mother y., bouba-mãe; framboesioma; uma grande lesão granulomatosa, considerada a lesão primária por inoculação na bouba, mais comum na mão, perna ou pé. SIN buba madre, frambesioma, protopianoma.

yawn (yaun). **1.** Bocejar. **2.** Uma abertura involuntária da boca, geralmente acompanhada por inspiração; pode ser um sinal de sonolência ou de depressão dos sinais vitais, como após hemorragia, mas freqüentemente é causado por sugestão. [A.S. *gānian*]

yawn·ing. Bocejo; oscitação; o ato de produzir um bocejo. SIN oscitation.

yaws (yawz). Framboesia; bouba; uma doença infecciosa tropical causada por *Treponema pertenue* e caracterizada pelo desenvolvimento de úlceras granulomatosas crostosas nos membros; pode envolver os ossos, mas, ao contrário da sífilis, não acomete o sistema nervoso central nem o cardiovascular. VER TAMBÉM nonvenereal *syphilis*. SIN boubas, frambesia tropica, granuloma tropicum, mycosis framboesioides, pian, zymotic papilloma. [de origem caribenha; semelhante à yaya do Calinago, a doença]
bosch y., bouba do bosque. SIN *pian bois.*
bush y., bouba do bosque. SIN *pian* bois.
foot y., bouba do pé; bouba dos pés com ceratodermia das regiões palmares e plantares e formação de úlcera.

Yb Símbolo do itérbio.

year.
disability-adjusted life y.'s (DALYs), anos de vida ajustados para a incapacidade; uma medida do ônus da doença em uma população definida, baseada no ajuste da expectativa de vida para considerar a incapacidade prolongada estimada pelas estatísticas oficiais. VER TAMBÉM global *burden* of disease. [Desenvolvido em 1990 por C.L. Murray e A. Lopez para o estudo Harvard University/WHO Global Burden of Disease.]
y.'s of potential life lost (YPLL), anos de vida potencial perdidos; medida do impacto relativo de várias doenças e forças letais sobre a sociedade, calculado pela estimativa dos anos que as pessoas teriam vivido se não tivessem morrido prematuramente por traumatismo, câncer, cardiopatia ou outras causas.

yeast (yēst). Levedura; um termo geral que designa fungos verdadeiros da família Saccharomycetaceae amplamente distribuídos em substratos que contêm açúcares (como frutas) e no solo, em excrementos de animais, partes vegetativas de plantas, etc. Devido à sua capacidade de fermentar carboidratos, algumas leveduras são importantes para as indústrias de bebidas fermentadas e de panificação. [A.S. *gyst*]
brewers' y., levedo de cerveja; l. produzida por *Saccharomyces cerevisiae;* um produto intermediário da fermentação da cerveja.
compressed y., l. comprimida; as células vivas úmidas do *Saccharomyces cerevisiae* combinadas a uma base de amido ou absorvente.
cultivated y., l. cultivada; uma forma de l. propagada por cultura e usada em panificação, cervejaria, etc.
dried y., l. seca; as células secas de uma cepa adequada de *Saccharomyces cerevisiae;* l. seca dos cervejeiros, levedura seca dos cervejeiros sem sabor amargo, ou levedura seca primária são as fontes de l. seca; contém não menos que 45% de proteínas, e, em 1 g, não menos de 0,3 mg de ácido nitocínico, 0,04 mg de riboflavina e 0,12 mg de cloridrato de tiamina; usado como suplemento alimentar.
primary dried y., l. seca primária; uma fonte de l. seca; obtida de cepas adequadas de *Saccharomyces cerevisiae* cultivadas em outros meios além daqueles necessários para a produção de cerveja.
wild y., l. selvagem; qualquer das formas não-cultivadas de leveduras, inúteis como fermentos e algumas vezes patogênicas.

yel·low (yel′ō). Amarelo; uma cor que ocupa uma posição no espectro entre verde e laranja. Quanto a corantes amarelos individuais, veja o nome específico. [A.S. *geolu*]
corralin y., a. coralino; o sal sódico do ácido rosólico.
indicator y., a. indicador; uma substância formada no clareamento da rodopsina pela luz; apresenta-se como a. cromo em pH 3,3–4,0 e a. pálido em pH 9,0–10,0.
tumeric y., a. tumérico. SIN curcumin.
visual y., a. visual. SIN all-*trans*-retinal.

yel·low root. Hidraste, raiz-amarela. SIN hydrastis.

yer·ba san·ta (yer′bä san′tä). Erva-santa, bálsamo-da-montanha. SIN eriodictyon. [Esp. erva sagrada]

Yer·sin·ia (yer - sin′ē - ä). Um gênero de bactérias móveis e imóveis, não-formadoras de esporos (família Enterobacteriaceae) contendo células ovóides a baciliformes, não-encapsuladas, Gram-negativas; as *Y.* são imóveis a 37°C, mas algumas espécies são móveis em temperaturas abaixo de 30°C; as células móveis são peritríquias; o citrato não é usado como única fonte de carbono; esses microrganismos são parasitas de seres humanos e outros animais; a espécie típica é a *Y. pestis.* [A.J.E. *Yersin,* bacteriologista suíço, 1862–1943]
Y. enterocolit'ica, uma espécie bacteriana que causa iersiniose no homem; é encontrada nas fezes e nos linfonodos de animais doentes e saudáveis, incluindo seres humanos, em material provavelmente contaminado por fezes e em cadáveres de bois, coelhos, lebres, cães, cobaias, cavalos, macacos, porcos e carneiros; replica-se nas temperaturas atingidas em refrigerador e foi associada à contaminação de sangue e hemoderivados.
Y. frederikse'nii, diferenciada da *Y. enterocolitica;* causa rara de enterocolite no homem.
Y. interme'dia, diferenciada da *Y. enterocolitica;* causa rara de enterocolite no homem.
Y. kristense'nii, diferenciada da *Y. enterocolitica;* patogenicidade incerta.
Y. pes'tis, uma espécie bacteriana causadora de peste em seres humanos, roedores e em muitas outras espécies de mamíferos, sendo transmitida de rato para rato e de rato para seres humanos pela pulga do rato, *Xenopsylla;* é a espécie típica do gênero *Y.* SIN Kitasato bacillus, *Pasteurella pestis,* plague bacillus.
Y. pseudotuberculo'sis, uma espécie bacteriana causadora de pseudotuberculose em aves, roedores e, raramente, em seres humanos. SIN *Pasteurella pseudotuberculosis.*

yer·sin·i·o·sis (yer - sin- ē - ō′sis). Iersiniose; uma doença infecciosa humana comum causada pela *Yersinia enterocolitica* e caracterizada por diarréia, enterite, pseudoapendicite, ileíte, eritema nodoso e, algumas vezes, septicemia ou artrite aguda.
pseudotubercular y., y. pseudotubercular. SIN pseudotuberculosis.

yield (yēld). Rendimento; produtividade; a quantidade produzida ou devolvida, freqüentemente medida como uma percentagem do material inicial; p. ex., o rendimento de uma preparação enzimática é igual às unidades de atividade enzimática recuperadas ao fim da preparação divididas pelo total de unidades observadas no material inicial.
quantum y. (φ), rendimento quântico; o número de moléculas transformadas (p. ex., através de uma reação) por *quantum* de luz absorvido; o inverso da exigência quântica. SIN quantum efficiency.

yin-yang (yin′yang). Yin-yang; no pensamento chinês antigo, o conceito de duas influências complementares e opostas, Yin e Yang, que fundamentam e

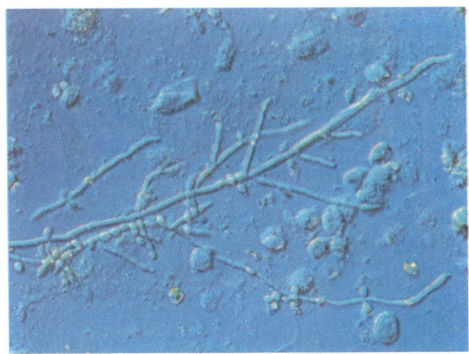

levedura

⌂ Formas Combinantes	★ Termo oficial alternativo para a *Terminologia Anatomica*
Indica que o termo é ilustrado, ver Índice de Ilustrações	[MIM] Mendelian Inheritance in Man
SIN Sinônimo	
Cf. Comparar, confrontar	I.C. Índice de Corantes
[NA] *Nomina Anatomica*	
[TA] *Terminologia Anatomica*	**Termo de Alta Importância**

controlam toda a natureza, sendo o objetivo da medicina chinesa produzir equilíbrio apropriado entre elas. Usado atualmente para caracterizar qualquer sistema de controle recíproco e dualista no qual uma influência tende a promover coisas que a influência oposta tende a inibir, e vice-versa; p. ex., a hipótese yin-yang de controle biológico na qual se supõe que o GMP cíclico e o AMP cíclico atuam de forma recíproca e dualista no controle das funções celulares.

-yl. –Il; sufixo químico que indica que a substância é um radical por perda de um átomo H (p. ex., alquil, metil, fenil) ou grupamento OH (p. ex., acil, acetil, carbamoil).

-ylene. –Ileno; sufixo químico que designa um radical hidrocarboneto bivalente (p. ex., metileno, -CH$_2$-) ou que possui uma ligação dupla (p. ex., etileno, CH$_2$=CH$_2$).

yl·ides (il'idz). Ilídios; uma classe de substâncias nas quais um elemento negativo positivamente carregado do grupo V ou VI da tabela periódica (p. ex., N, O, S, P) é ligado a um átomo de carbono que possui um par de elétrons não-compartilhado; os ilídios foram observados em várias reações catalisadas por enzimas.

Y-link·age. Ligação ao X; o estado de um fator genético (gene) carreado pelo cromossoma Y. Essa idéia é análoga à ligação ao X, mas, como o cromossoma Y não participa completamente da formação do quiasma e da recombinação, não é sensível à análise por métodos de ligação convencionais. Sabe-se pouco sobre seu conteúdo. Há um gene para o antígeno H-Y, e provas indiretas sugerem haver um princípio que determina a formação do testículo e a masculinização do feto, mas sua localização, embora estreitando os limites, ainda não foi determinada.

yo·gurt, yo·ghurt (yō'gert). Iogurte; leite integral fermentado, parcialmente evaporado, preparado por sua manutenção a 50°C por 12 horas após a adição de uma cultura mista de *Lactobacillus bulgaricus*, *L. acidophilus* e *Streptococcus lactis*; usado como alimento. [Turco]

yo·him·bine (yō-him'bēn). Ioimbina; um alcalóide, o princípio ativo da ioimbé, a casca da *Corynanthe yohimbi* (família Rubiaceae); promove bloqueio competitivo, de duração limitada, de receptores α-adrenérgicos; também tem sido usada em virtude de suas supostas propriedades afrodisíacas.

yoke (yōk). [TA]. Jugo; canga. SIN jugum (1). [A.S. geoc]

alveolar y.'s [TA], jugos alveolares; uma das eminências na superfície externa do processo alveolar do maxilar ou da mandíbula, formado pelas raízes dos dentes incisivos. SIN juga alveolaria [TA].

sphenoidal y., jugo esfenoidal; *termo oficial alternativo para *jugum sphenoidale*.

yolk (yōk, yōlk). **1.** Vitelo; gema de ovo; um dos tipos de material nutritivo armazenado no ovo para a nutrição do embrião; é particularmente abundante e visível em ovos de aves. SIN vitellus. **2.** Material gorduroso encontrado na lã de carneiros; quando extraído e purificado, torna-se lanolina. [A.S. *geolca; geolu*, amarelo]

white y., v. branco; v. que consiste em partículas muito mais finas que aquelas do v. amarelo; finas camadas deste situam-se entre as zonas de v. amarelo e formam a látebra.

yellow y., v. amarelo; o principal constituinte do v. em um ovo de ave; consiste em partículas relativamente grosseiras de substâncias nutrientes armazenadas e está depositado em zonas concêntricas com finas camadas de v. branco interpostas.

Yorke au·to·lyt·ic re·ac·tion. Reação autolítica de Yorke; ver em *reaction*.

Young, Hugh H., urologista norte-americano, 1870–1945. VER Y. prostatic *tractor*.

Young, William John, bioquímico australiano do século XX. VER Harden-Y. *ester*.

Young, Thomas, médico e físico inglês, 1773–1829. VER Y. *modulus, rule*; Y.-Helmholtz *theory* of color vision.

YPLL. Abreviatura de *years* of potential life lost, em *year*.

yp·sil·i·form (ip'si-li-fōrm). Ipsiliforme. SIN hypsiloid. [G. *ypsilon, upsilon*, a letra u ou y, + L. *forma*, forma]

yt·ter·bi·um (Yb) (i-ter'bē-ŭm). Itérbio; elemento metálico do grupo lantanídeo; número atômico 70, peso atômico 173,04. Yb^{169}, com meia-vida de 32,03 dias, tem sido usado em cisternografia e em cintigrafias cerebrais. [*Ytterby*, povoado na Suécia]

yt·tri·um (Y) (it'rē-ŭm). Ítrio; um elemento metálico, número atômico 39, peso atômico 88,90585. [*Ytterby*, um povoado na Suécia]

yt·tri·um-90. Ítrio-90 (Y^{90}) isótopo radioativo artificial com uma meia-vida física de 2,67 dias, que decai com a emissão de uma partícula β de 2,282 MeV; usado como implante na ablação hipofisária.

Yvon, Paul, médico e químico francês, 1848–1913. VER Y. *test*.

Z

Z Abreviatura de benziloxicarbonil (carbobenzoxi-); símbolo de um aminoácido que pode ser o ácido glutâmico, glutamina ou uma substância que produza ácido glutâmico durante a hidrólise ácida de peptídios (p. ex., 4-carboxiglutamato ou 5-oxoprolina); carbobenzoxi; em itálico, zusammen.

Z Abreviatura de atomic *number* (número atômico).

z Abreviatura de zepto-.

Zaffaroni, Alejandro, químico e bioquímico uruguaio-norte-americano, *1923. VER Zaffaroni *system*.

zafirlukast (za-fir-loo′kast). Zafirlukast; um bloqueador dos leucotrienos D_4 e E_4 (LTD_4 e LTE_4), componentes de uma substância de reação lenta da anafilaxia (SRSA); usado na profilaxia dos ataques de asma.

Zaglas, John, assistente de anatomia do século XIX em Edimburgo. VER Z. *ligament*.

Zahn, Friedrich W., patologista alemão, 1845–1904. VER Z. *infarct; lines* of Z., em *line; striae* of Z., em *stria*.

Zambusch, Leo von, médico alemão do século XX. VER generalized pustular *psoriasis* of Z.

zanamivir (zan - am′ĭ - vir). Zanamivir; um agente que inibe a neuraminidase do vírus influenza.

Zappert, Julius, médico austríaco, 1867–1942. VER Z. counting *chamber*.

Zavanelli, William, obstetra norte-americano do século XX. VER Z. *maneuver*.

zea (zē′ă). Estilos e estigmas de *Zea mays* (família Gramineae), milho; usado antigamente como diurético e antiespasmódico. SIN cornsilk. [L. Mod. maize]

ze·a·ral·e·none (zē′ă - ral - en - ōn). Uma das lactonas do ácido resorcílico; usada em medicina veterinária como anabólico.

ze·a·tin (zē′ă - tin). Zeatina; uma citocina isolada pela primeira vez dos grãos do milho doce. SIN maize factor.

ze·a·xan·thin (zē′ă - zan′thin). Zeaxantina; caroteno encontrado no milho, nas frutas, nas sementes e na gema de ovo; isomérico em relação à xantofila. SIN zeaxanthol. [L. Mod. *Zea*, milho, do L. *zea*, grão + G. *xanthos*, amarelo, + -in]

ze·ax·an·thol (zē - ă - za - thol). Zeaxantol. SIN zeaxanthin.

Zeeman, Pieter, físico holandês e Prêmio Nobel, 1865–1943. VER Z. *effect*.

ZEEP Abreviatura de zero end-expiratory *pressure* (pressão expiratória final zero).

ze·in (zē′in). Zeína; uma prolamina presente no milho; não possui principalmente os aminoácidos L-triptofano e L-lisina, e também tem baixo conteúdo de cisteína. É a principal proteína de armazenamento no milho.

Zeis, Eduard, oftalmologista de Dresden, 1807–1868. VER Z. *glands*, em *gland*; zeisian *sty*.

zeis·i·an (zīs′ē - ăn). Relativo a, ou descrito por, Eduard Zeis.

Zeit·geist (zīt′gīst). Em psicologia, a atmosfera de opinião, convenções de pensamento, influências ocultas e suposições não-questionadas que estão implícitas em uma determinada cultura, nas artes ou na ciência em qualquer período, e no qual o indivíduo atua e, assim, é influenciado. [Al. *zeit*, tempo, + *geist*, espírito]

Zellweger, Hans U., pediatra norte-americano, 1909–1990. VER Z. *syndrome*.

ze·lo·pho·bia (zē - lō - fō′bē - ă). Zelofobia; medo mórbido do ciúme. [G. *zēlos*, zelo, + *phobos*, medo]

ze·lo·typ·ia (zē - lō - tip′ē - ă). Zelotipia; zelo excessivo, levado até o ponto da morbidade, na defesa de qualquer causa. [G. *zēlotypia;* rivalidade, inveja, de *zēlos*, zelo, + *typtō*, bater]

Zenker, Friedrich A., patologista alemão, 1825–1898. VER Z. *degeneration, diverticulum, fixative, paralysis*; formol-Z. *fixative*.

ze·o·lite (zē′ō - līt). Zeolita; um silicato sódico de alumínio hidratado, $Na_2O.Al_2O_3.(SiO_2)_x.(H_2O)_x$, usado para abrandamento da água dura (calcária) através da troca de seu Na^+ pelo Ca^{2+} da água; assim a zeolita é um trocador iônico. Alguns trocadores iônicos sintéticos são denominados zeolitas sintéticas, embora não haja relação química.

ze·o·scope (zē′ō - skōp). Zeoscópio; dispositivo para determinar o conteúdo alcoólico de um líquido através da determinação de seu ponto exato de fervura. [G. *zeō*, ferver, + *skopeō*, examinar]

zep·to- (z). Prefixo usado nos sistemas SI e métrico que significa submúltiplos de 10^{-21}.

ze·ro (zē′rō). Zero. **1.** O número 0, indicando a ausência de magnitude, ou nada. **2.** Em termometria, o ponto a partir do qual os números na escala iniciam-se em uma ou outra direção; nas escalas Celsius e Réaumur, o zero indica o ponto de congelamento da água destilada; na escala Fahrenheit, está 32° abaixo do ponto de congelamento da água. [Esp. do Ar. *sifr*, cifra]

absolute z., z. absoluto; a menor temperatura possível, na qual a forma de movimento de translação que constitui o calor supostamente não existe mais, determinada −273,15°C ou 0° Kelvin.

ze·ro grav·i·ty (zē - rō - grav′i - tē). Gravidade zero; estado físico existente no espaço ou em um momento no vôo quando a força centrífuga de uma curva parabólica neutraliza exatamente a força da gravidade.

ze·ta (zāt′ă). Zeta. **1.** A sexta letra do alfabeto grego, ζ. **2.** Em química, designa o sexto em uma série, p. ex., o sexto carbono de um grupamento funcional. **3.** Símbolo de potencial eletrocinético.

ze·ta·crit (zā′tă - krit). Zetácrito; o volume de células produzido por centrifugação vertical do sangue em tubos capilares, permitindo compactação controlada e dispersão das hemácias; ler com um hematócrito para obter o índice de sedimentação zeta.

ze·ta·pro·tein. Zetaproteína. SIN fibronectins.

zeug·ma·tog·ra·phy (zoog - mă - tog′ră - fē). Zeumatografia; termo cunhado por Lauterbur em 1972 para a união de um campo magnético e gradientes de campo de radiofreqüência definidos espacialmente a fim de gerar uma imagem bidimensional dos tempos de densidade protônica e relaxamento nos tecidos, a primeira imagem de ressonância magnética nuclear. [G. *zeugma*, o que se une]

zi·do·vu·dine (zī - dō′voo - dēn). Zidovudina; um análogo da timidina que é um inibidor da replicação *in vitro* do HIV, o agente causador da AIDS/SIDA e do complexo relacionado à AIDS/SIDA, sendo usada no tratamento dessas doenças. SIN azidothymidine.

Ziegler, Samuel L., oftalmologista norte-americano, 1861–1926.

Ziehen, Georg T., psiquiatra alemão, 1862–1950. VER Z.-Oppenheim *disease*.

Ziehl, Franz, bacteriologista alemão, 1857–1926. VER Z. *stain;* Z.-Neelsen *stain*.

Ziemann, Hans R.P., patologista alemão, 1865–1939. VER Z. *dots*, em *dot, stippling*.

Zieve, Leslie, médico norte-americano, *1915. VER Z. *syndrome*.

Zimmerlin, Franz, médico suíço, 1858–1932. VER Z. *atrophy*.

Zimmermann, Karl W., histologista alemão, 1861–1935. VER Z. *corpuscle, granule*, elementary *particle;* polkissen of Z.

Zimmermann, Wilhelm, médico alemão, *1910. VER Z. *reaction, test*.

zinc (Zn) (zingk). Zinco; um elemento metálico, número atômico 30, peso atômico 65,39; um bioelemento essencial; vários sais de zinco são usados na medicina; um co-fator em muitas proteínas. [Al. *Zink*]

z. acetate, acetato de z.; emético, hemostático e adstringente.

z. caprylate, caprilato de z.; antifúngico tópico.

z. chloride, cloreto de zinco; $ZnCl_2$; anteriormente usado como cáustico para a remoção de cânceres cutâneos, nevos, etc., e em solução fraca no tratamento da gonorréia e conjuntivite. SIN butter of zinc.

z. gelatin, gelatina de z.; óxido de z., gelatina, glicerina e água purificada; usada topicamente como protetor.

z. iodide, iodeto de z.; ZnI_2; foi usado como anti-séptico e adstringente.

medicinal z. peroxide, peróxido de z. medicinal; uma mistura de peróxido de z., carbonato de z. e hidróxido de z.; um desinfetante tópico, adstringente e desodorante.

z. oxide, óxido de z.; ZnO; usado como protetor em pomadas, como pó secante; também usado em tintas como substituto do carbonato de chumbo. SIN flowers of zinc, z. white.

z. oxide and eugenol, óxido de z. e eugenol; usado como material de base sob restaurações dentárias metálicas e como material de enchimento temporário ou material de impressão; a fixação e o endurecimento resultam de reações complexas entre o pó e o eugenol.

z. permanganate, permanganato de z.; tem ação semelhante à do permanganato de potássio, porém mais adstringente; usado na uretrite, por injeção ou ducha em uma solução 1:4.000.

z. peroxide, peróxido de z.; ZnO_2; pó branco amarelado, insolúvel em água e decomposto por ácidos; usado em preparações farmacêuticas. SIN z. superoxide.

z. phenolsulfonate, fenolsulfonato de z.; usado como anti-séptico intestinal e localmente como adstringente na inflamação crônica das mucosas. SIN z. sulfocarbolate.

z. phosphide, fosfeto de z.; Zn_3P_2; usado como veneno (isca) para exterminar ratos e camundongos.

△ Formas Combinantes	☆ Termo oficial alternativo para a *Terminologia Anatomica*
🅸 Indica que o termo é ilustrado, ver Índice de Ilustrações	
	[MIM] Mendelian Inheritance in Man
SIN Sinônimo	
Cf. Comparar, confrontar	I.C. Índice de Corantes
[NA] *Nomina Anatomica*	
[TA] *Terminologia Anatomica*	Termo de Alta Importância

z. stearate, estearato de z.; composto zíncico com proporções variáveis de ácidos esteárico e palmítico; um agente protetor, que repele a água, usado em pós e pomadas no tratamento de eczema, acne e outras doenças cutâneas.
z. sulfate, sulfato de z.; usado como adstringente local no tratamento de gonorréia, úlceras indolentes, conjuntivite e várias doenças cutâneas, e internamente como emético.
z. sulfocarbolate, sulfocarbolato de z. SIN z. phenolsulfonate.
z. superoxide, superóxido de z. SIN z. peroxide.
z. undecylenate, z. undecenoate, undecilenato de z.; undecenoato de z.; o sal zíncico do ácido undecilênico; usado no tratamento de micoses e de outras afecções da pele, incluindo psoríase.
z. white, branco de z. SIN z. oxide.
zinc-65 (^{65}**Zn**). Zinco 65 (Zn^{65}); um radioisótopo do zinco que decai principalmente por captura de K com uma meia-vida de 243,8 dias; usado como marcador em estudos do metabolismo do zinco.
zinc·if·er·ous (zing - kif′er - ŭs). Zincífero; que contém zinco.
zinc·oid (zing′koyd). Zincóide; relativo ou semelhante ao zinco. [G. *eidos*, semelhança]
zin·gi·ber (zin′ji - ber). Gengibre. SIN ginger.
Zinn, Johann G., anatomista alemão, 1727–1759. VER Z. *artery,* vascular *circle, corona, ligament, membrane, ring, tendon, zonule.*
Zinsser, Hans, bacteriologista e imunologista norte-americano, 1878–1940. VER Brill-Z. *disease.*
zir·co·ni·um (Zr) (zir - kō′nē - ŭm). Zircônio; elemento metálico, número atômico 40, peso atômico 91,224; amplamente distribuído na natureza, mas nunca encontrado em quantidade em um único lugar. [*zircon*, um mineral, do Ár. *zarkūn*, cinábrio, Pers., *zargun*, semelhante ao ouro]
zir·co·ni·um ox·ide. Óxido de zircônio; usado como revestimento para a pele nos fármacos dermatológicos e como pigmento em tintas.
zm Abreviatura de zeptometer (zeptômetro).
Zn Símbolo do zinco.
^{65}Zn Zn^{65}; abreviatura de zinco-65.
Zo$_2$ Símbolo de microlitros de oxigênio captados por hora por 10^8 espermatozóides; pode variar em função da temperatura.
zo-. VER zoo-.
zo·an·throp·ic (zō - an - throp′ik). Zoantrópico; relativo a, ou caracterizado por, zoantropia.
zo·an·thro·py (zō - an′ - thrō - pē). Zoantropia; delírio de que alguém é um animal, como um cão. [G. *zōon*, animal, + *anthorōpos*, homem]
zo·et·ic (zō - et′ik). Zoético; relativo à vida. [G. *zōē*, vida]
zo·ic (zō′ik). Zóico; relativo às coisas vivas; que possui vida. [G. *zōikos*, relativo a um animal]
zo·ite (zō′īt). Zoíta. SIN sporozoite. [G. *zōon*, animal]
Zollinger, Robert M., cirurgião norte-americano, *1903. VER Z.-Ellison *syndrome, tumor.*
Zöllner, Johann F., físico alemão, 1834–1882. VER Z. *lines,* em *line.*
zol·pi·dem (zol′pē - dem). Zolpidem; sedativo/hipnótico útil para tratamento da ansiedade e semelhante aos benzodiazepínicos em sua farmacologia, mas um pouco diferente na estrutura química. Ao contrário dos benzodiazepínicos, o zolpidem não possui propriedades anticonvulsivantes proeminentes, e pode surgir menos tolerância com seu uso.
zo·me·pir·ac so·di·um (zō - mē - pir′ak). Zomepirac sódico; um analgésico antiinflamatório, não mais comercializado.
zo·na, pl. **zo·nae** (zō′nă, zō′nē). [TA]. Zona. **1.** SIN zone. **2.** SIN herpes zoster. [L. do G. *zōnē*, uma circunferência, uma das zonas da esfera]
z. arcua′ta, z. arqueada. SIN arcuate zone.
z. cilia′ris, z. ciliar. SIN ciliary zone.
z. coro′na, z. corona. SIN costal fringe.
z. dermat′ica, z. dermática; crista de pele espessa que circunda a protrusão na espinha bífida.
z. epitheliosero′sa, z. epitheliosserosa; o anel membranoso, dentro da z. dermática, que circunda a protrusão da espinha bífida.
z. externa medullae renalis [TA], z. externa da medula renal. SIN outer zone of renal medulla.
z. fascicula′ta, z. fasciculada; a camada de cordões celulares dispostos radialmente na porção cortical da glândula supra-renal, entre a z. glomerulosa e a z. reticular; secreta cortisol e desidroepiandrosterona.
z. glomerulo′sa, z. glomerulosa; a camada externa do córtex da glândula supra-renal logo abaixo da cápsula; secreta aldosterona.
z. hemorrhoida′lis, z. hemorroidária. SIN hemorrhoidal zone.
zonae hypothalamicae [TA], zonas hipotalâmicas. SIN zones of hypothalamus, em *zone.*
z. incer′ta [TA], z. incerta do subtálamo; uma lâmina plana, disposta obliquamente, de substância cinzenta na região subtalâmica situada entre o fascículo talâmico (campo tegmentar H$_1$ de Forel) e o fascículo lenticular (campo tegmentar H$_2$). Medialmente, as células desse núcleo são adjacentes à área pré-rubra (campo tegmentar H) e, lateralmente, são contínuas com o núcleo reticular do tálamo. A z. incerta é um derivado do tálamo ventral; recebe aferentes do córtex motor pré-central e do cerebelo.
z. interna medullae renalis [TA], z. interna da medula renal. SIN inner zone of renal medulla.
z. lateralis [TA], z. lateral. SIN lateral zone. VER *zones* of hypothalamus, em *zone.*
z. medialis [TA], z. medial. SIN medial zone. VER *zones* of hypothalamus, em *zone.*
z. medullovasculo′sa, z. medulovascular; o segmento fissurado da medula espinhal que fecha dorsalmente o saco na mielomeningocele.
z. ophthal′mica, z. oftálmica; herpes zoster na distribuição do nervo oftálmico.
z. orbicula′ris (articulationis coxae) [TA], z. orbicular; faixa anular; ligamento anular; fibras da cápsula articular do quadril circundando o colo do fêmur. SIN orbicular zone of hip joint, ring ligament, zonular band.
z. pectina′ta, z. pectínea. SIN pectinate zone.
z. pellu′cida, z. pelúcida; uma camada extracelular, rica em glicoproteínas, que circunda o ovócito; contém microvilosidades do ovócito e processos celulares de células foliculares e apresenta-se homogênea e translúcida à microscopia óptica. SIN pellucid zone.
z. perfora′ta, z. perfurada. SIN foramina nervosa, em *foramen.*
z. periventricularis [TA], z. periventricular. SIN periventricular zone. VER *zones* of hypothalamus, em *zone.*
z. pupilla′ris, z. pupilar. SIN pupillary zone.
z. radia′ta, z. radiada. SIN z. striata.
z. reticula′ris, z. reticular; a camada interna do córtex da glândula supra-renal, onde os cordões celulares se anastomosam como uma rede.
z. stria′ta, z. estriada; a membrana celular espessada do óvulo em formas, como determinados anfíbios, nos quais aparece radialmente estriada à microscopia óptica; à microscopia eletrônica, pode-se ver que as estriações são microvilosidades. SIN membrana striata, striated membrane, z. radiata.
z. tec′ta, SIN arcuate zone.
z. transitionalis analis [TA], z. de transição anal. SIN anal transitional zone.
z. vasculo′sa, z. vascular. SIN vascular zone.
zon·al (zō′năl). Zonal; relativo a uma zona.
zo·na·ry (zō′nar - ē). Zonar; relativo a, ou que possui a forma de, uma zona ou cinto.
zon·ate (zō′nāt). Zonado; anelado; que possui camadas concêntricas de diferente textura ou pigmentação.

ZONE

zone (zōn). [TA]. Zona; um segmento; qualquer estrutura circundante ou semelhante a um cinto, externa ou interna, longitudinal ou transversal. VER TAMBÉM area, band, region, space, spot. SIN zona (1) [TA]. [L. *zona*]
abdominal z.'s, zonas abdominais. SIN abdominal regions, em *region.*
anal transitional z. [TA], z. anal de transição; região do canal anal na qual há mudança do epitélio cilíndrico simples de uma mucosa para o epitélio escamoso estratificado da pele anal; essa região é suscetível a vários carcinomas. SIN zona transitionalis analis [TA].
androgenic z., z. androgênica; **(1)** SIN X z. (1); **(2)** SIN fetal reticularis (2). SIN fetal adrenal *cortex*. [Assim designada por se acreditar (ainda não comprovado) que as células nessa zona secretam andrógenos.]
arcuate z., z. arqueada; o terço interno da membrana basilar do ducto coclear, que se estende do lábio timpânico da lâmina espiral óssea até a célula pilar externa do órgão espiral (de Corti). SIN zona arcuata, zona tecta.
Barnes z., z. de Barnes; o quarto inferior do útero grávido, podendo a fixação da placenta a qualquer parte do mesmo causar perigosa hemorragia. SIN cervical z.
cervical z., z. cervical. SIN Barnes z.
cervical z. of tooth, z. cervical do dente. SIN neck of tooth.
ciliary z., z. ciliar; a z. externa, mais larga da superfície anterior da íris, separada da z. pupilar pela prega da íris. SIN zona ciliaris.
comfort z., z. de conforto; faixa de temperatura entre 28°C e 30°C na qual o corpo nu é capaz de manter o equilíbrio térmico sem calafrios ou sudorese; no corpo vestido a faixa é de 13°C a 21°C.
z.'s of discontinuity, zonas de descontinuidade; zonas concêntricas de densidade óptica variável no cristalino, observadas à biomicroscopia por lâmpada de fenda.
dolorogenic z., z. dolorogênica. SIN trigger *point.*
entry z., z. de entrada; a área do funículo dorsal da medula espinhal, medial à ponta do corno posterior, na qual as fibras de entrada da raiz nervosa posterior dividem-se em ramos ascendentes e descendentes.

ependymal z., z. ependimária. SIN ependymal layer.
epileptogenic z., z. epileptogênica; uma região cortical que, à estimulação, reproduz a convulsão espontânea do paciente ou aura.
equivalence z., z. de equivalência; em uma reação de precipitina, a z. na qual não há excesso de anticorpo nem de antígeno. VER TAMBÉM precipitation. SIN equivalence point.
erogenous z.'s, erotogenic z.'s, zonas erógenas; zonas erotogênicas; áreas do corpo, como os órgãos genitais e os mamilos, que causam excitação sexual quando estimuladas.
fetal z., z. fetal. SIN fetal adrenal cortex.
gingival z., z. gengival; a porção da mucosa oral que circunda os dentes e está firmemente fixada ao osso alveolar subjacente.
Golgi z., z. de Golgi; (1) parte do citoplasma ocupada pelo aparelho de Golgi; (2) nas células secretoras das glândulas exócrinas, uma z. entre o núcleo e a superfície luminal.
grenz z., z. limítrofe; em histopatologia, uma camada estreita sob a epiderme que não é infiltrada nem envolvida da mesma forma que as camadas inferiores da derme. [Al. *Grenze*, limítrofe, limite]
Head z.'s, zonas de Head. SIN Head lines, em line.
hemorrhoidal z., z. hemorroidária; a parte do canal anal que contém o plexo venoso retal. SIN anulus hemorrhoidalis, zona hemorrhoidalis.
z.'s of hypothalamus [TA], zonas do hipotálamo; regiões do hipotálamo com orientação rostrocaudal caracterizadas por sua posição e grupos celulares. A z. periventricular [TA] (zona periventricularis [TA]) é um folheto fino de pequenos neurônios localizados na parede do terceiro ventrículo. A z. medial [TA] (zona medialis [TA]) situa-se entre a z. periventricular e uma linha rostrocaudal traçada entre o trato mamilotalâmico e o fórnice pós-comissural, e consiste em regiões supra-óptica, tuberal e mamilar. A z. lateral [TA] (zona lateralis [TA]) situa-se lateral às zonas mediais, e contém os núcleos tuberais e as fibras do feixe prosencefálico medial. SIN zonae hypothalamicae [TA].
inner z. of renal medulla [TA], z. interna da medula renal; porção apical das pirâmides renais, incluindo papila renal. SIN zona interna medullae renalis [TA].
intermediate z. [TA], z. intermediária. SIN intermediate column.
intermediate z. of iliac crest [TA], z. intermediária da crista ilíaca; a linha na crista do ílio entre os lábios externo e interno, para a origem do músculo oblíquo interno. SIN linea intermedia cristae iliacae [TA], intermediate line of iliac crest.
interpalpebral z., z. interpalpebral; a área exposta da córnea e da esclerótica entre as pálpebras do olho aberto.
intertubular z., z. intertubular; a matriz da dentina localizada entre zonas de dentina peritubular; é menos calcificada e contém fibras de colágeno maiores que a dentina peritubular.
isoelectric z., z. isoelétrica; a faixa de concentração de íons H+ (pH) na qual ocorre precipitação isoelétrica.
isopycnic z., z. isopícnica; a região que, na centrifugação com gradiente de densidade, possui a mesma densidade que a densidade de flutuação da macromolécula.
language z., z. de linguagem; uma grande área do córtex cerebral, no lado esquerdo (em pessoas destras), que alguns supõem envolver todos os centros de memórias e associações relacionados à linguagem.
latent z., z. latente; a porção do córtex cerebral, cuja estimulação não produz movimento e cuja lesão não causa sintomas; principalmente as áreas mais anteriores dos lobos frontais.
lateral z. [TA], z. lateral. VER z.'s of hypothalamus. SIN zona lateralis [TA].
Lissauer marginal z., z. marginal de Lissauer. SIN dorsolateral fasciculus.
Looser z.'s, zonas de Looser. SIN Looser lines, em line.
mantle z., z. do manto; (1) SIN mantle layer; (2) uma camada de pequenos linfócitos B circundando os centros germinativos de coloração mais clara dos tecidos linfóides.
Marchant z., z. de Marchant; a área nos ossos esfenóide e occipital na base do crânio, da qual a dura-máter é facilmente destacada.
marginal z., z. marginal; (1) uma z. situada entre as polpas vermelha e branca do baço, contendo numerosos macrófagos e um plexo rico de sinusóides supridos por arteríolas da polpa branca que transportam antígenos veiculados pelo sangue. (2) SIN marginal layer.
medial z. [TA], z. medial. VER z.'s of hypothalamus. SIN zona medialis [TA].
motor z., z. motora; a porção do córtex cerebral, basicamente a região posterior do lobo frontal, próxima do sulco central, que, quando estimulada, produz um movimento e, quando lesada, produz espasticidade ou paralisia.
neutral z., z. neutra; em odontologia, o espaço virtual entre os lábios e as bochechas de um lado e a língua do outro; dentes naturais ou artificiais nessa z. estão sujeitos a forças iguais e opostas da musculatura adjacente.
nucleolar z., z. nucleolar. SIN nucleolar organizer.
Obersteiner-Redlich z., z. de Obersteiner-Redlich; a linha estreita ao longo do trajeto de um nervo (ou raiz nervosa) onde as células de Schwann e o tecido conjuntivo que sustentam seus axônios são substituídos por células da glia. A z. marca o limite verdadeiro entre os sistemas nervosos central e periférico. Geralmente localizada na superfície da medula espinhal ou do tronco cerebral, ou próxima desta, pode estender-se (p. ex., no oitavo nervo) alguns milímetros ao longo do nervo. SIN Obersteiner-Redlich line.

orbicular z. of hip joint, z. orbicular da articulação do quadril. SIN zona orbicularis (articulationis coxae).
outer z. of renal medulla [TA], z. externa da medula renal; porção basal da pirâmide renal. SIN zona externa medullae renalis [TA].
pectinate z., z. pectínea; os dois terços externos da membrana basilar do ducto coclear. SIN zona pectinata.
pellucid z., z. pelúcida. SIN zona pellucida.
peritubular z., z. peritubular; a matriz de dentina que circunda o processo odontoblástico; é mais calcificada e contém fibras de colágeno mais finas que o restante da matriz da dentina.
periventricular z. [TA], z. periventricular. VER z.'s of hypothalamus. SIN zona periventricularis [TA].
polar z., z. polar; a região adjacente a um eletrodo aplicado ao corpo. VER TAMBÉM electrotonus.
protective z., z. de proteção; o período no ciclo cardíaco, imediatamente após o período vulnerável, durante o qual um segundo estímulo impedirá o início de fibrilação ventricular por um estímulo prévio aplicado durante o período vulnerável, provavelmente através do bloqueio de uma via de reentrada.
pupillary z., z. pupilar; a região central da superfície anterior da íris localizada entre a prega da íris e a margem pupilar. SIN zona pupillaris.
reflexogenic z., z. reflexogênica; a área ou z. onde a estimulação causará um determinado reflexo.
secondary X z., z. X secundária; uma z. do córtex supra-renal, situada na zona fasciculada interna, que aparece após gonadectomia pós-puberal em alguns roedores do sexo masculino, mais notavelmente o camundongo; acredita-se que o desenvolvimento dessa z. seja estimulado por gonadotrofinas hipofisárias.
segmental z., z. segmentar; placa segmentar; em um embrião jovem, a porção dorsal espessada do mesoderma paraxial indiferenciado que se divide metamericamente para formar os somitos mesodérmicos. SIN segmental plate.
Spitzka marginal z., z. marginal de Spitzka. SIN dorsolateral fasciculus.
subplasmalemmal dense z., z. densa suplasmalêmica. SIN corneocyte envelope.
sudanophobic z., z. sudanofóbica; uma z. de células, na periferia da zona fasciculada do córtex supra-renal do rato, que não é corada por corantes de Sudan.
tender z.'s, zonas dolorosas. SIN Head lines, em line.
thymus-dependent z., z. timo-dependente. SIN paracortex.
trabecular z., z. trabecular. SIN trabecular tissue of sclera.
transformation z., z. de transformação; z. do colo uterino na qual o epitélio escamoso e o epitélio cilíndrico se encontram; muda de localização em resposta ao estado hormonal da mulher.
transitional z., z. de transição; (1) a região equatorial do cristalino onde as células epiteliais anteriores se transformam nas fibras do cristalino; (2) aquela porção de uma lente de contato escleral entre as seções corneana e escleral.
transitional z. of lips [TA], z. de transição dos lábios; pele fina, glabra, que começa na borda do vermelhão labial; parece vermelha devido ao leito capilar subjacente.
trigger z., zona-gatilho. SIN trigger point.
trophotropic z. of Hess, z. trofotrópica de Hess; uma área no hipotálamo relacionada às sensações corporais de gratificação.
vascular z., z. vascular; uma área no meato acústico externo onde penetram vários pequenos vasos sanguíneos provenientes do osso mastóide. SIN spongy spot, zona vasculosa.
vermilion z., vermilion transitional z., z. do vermelhão; z. transicional do vermelhão. SIN vermilion border.
Weil basal z., z. basal de Weil. SIN Weil basal layer.
Wernicke z., z. de Wernicke. SIN Wernicke center.
z. 1, 2, 3, 4 of West, z. 1, 2, 3, 4 de West; em fisiologia pulmonar, define os níveis em um pulmão vertical de acordo com as relações de pressão dos gases alveolares, pressão sanguínea capilar e pressão venosa pulmonar.
X z., z. X; (1) uma z. transitória do córtex supra-renal, presente em alguns roedores ao nascimento, mais notavelmente em camundongos, situada entre a zona reticular e a medula supra-renal; degenera nos machos com a secreção na puberdade e nas fêmeas durante a primeira gravidez; aumenta lentamente em fêmeas não-acasaladas após a puberdade e não degenera antes da meia-idade; a z. X parece não secretar hormônio. SIN androgenic z. (1). (2) nome errado do córtex supra-renal fetal (fetal adrenal cortex) de primatas. SIN fetal reticularis (3).

zo·nes·the·sia (zōn - es - the′zē - ă). Zonestesia; sensação como se fosse passado um cordão ao redor do corpo, constringindo-o. SIN girdle sensation, strangalesthesia. [G. *zōnē*, cintura, + *aisthēsis*, sensação]

zon·ing (zō′ing). Zonagem; a ocorrência de uma reação mais forte em uma menor quantidade de soro suspeito, observada algumas vezes em testes sorológicos usados no diagnóstico de sífilis, provavelmente resultante de elevado título de anticorpos.

zon·og·ra·phy (zō - nog′ră - fē). Zonografia; forma de tomografia com um plano de foco relativamente espesso; usada particularmente em radiografia renal. [zone + G. *graphō*, escrever]

zo·no·skel·e·ton (zō′nō - skel′ĕ - tŏn). Zonoesqueleto; os segmentos ósseos proximais dos membros, isto é, escápula, clavícula, osso do quadril (hip *bone*). [L. *zona*, zone, + skeleton]

zo·nu·la, pl. **zo·nu·lae** (zō′nū-lă, zon′ū; -lē). Zônula. SIN zonule. [L. dim. de *zona*, zona]
  z. adhe'rens, z. de adesão; uma fixação desmossômica semelhante a um cinto entre células epiteliais colunares, na qual se fixam os filamentos. SIN intermediate junction.
  z. cilia'ris [TA], z. ciliar. SIN ciliary *zonule*.
  z. occlu'dens, z. de oclusão; junções firmes formadas pela fusão de proteínas integrais das membranas celulares laterais de células epiteliais adjacentes, limitando a permeabilidade transepitelial. SIN impermeable junction, tight junction.

zo·nu·lar (zō′nū-lăr, zon′ū-). Zonular; relativo a uma zônula.

zon·ule (zō′nŭl, zon′ūl). Zônula; uma pequena zona. SIN zonula.
  ciliary z. [TA], z. ciliar; uma série de delicadas fibras meridionais originadas na superfície interna do orbículo ciliar, que seguem em feixes entre e, em uma camada muito fina, sobre os processos ciliares; na borda interna da coroa, as fibras divergem em dois grupos que se fixam à cápsula nas superfícies anterior e posterior do cristalino próximo do equador; os espaços entre essas duas camadas de fibras são preenchidos por humor aquoso. SIN zonula ciliaris [TA], apparatus suspensorius lentis, suspensory ligament of lens, Zinn z.
  Zinn z., z. de Zinn. SIN ciliary z.

zo·nu·li·tis (zō-nū-lī′tis). Zonulite; suposta inflamação da zônula de Zinn, ou ligamento suspensor do cristalino. [zonule + G. –*itis*, inflamação]

zo·nu·lol·y·sis, zo·nu·ly·sis (zō′nū-lol′i-sis, -lī′sis). Zonulólise; dissolução da zônula ciliar por enzimas (α-quimiotripsina) para facilitar a remoção cirúrgica de uma catarata. SIN Barraquer method. [zonule + G. *lysis*, dissolução]

△ **zoo-, zo.** Animal, vida animal. [G. *zōon*]

zo·o·an·thro·po·no·sis (zō′ō-an′thrō-pō-nō′sis). Zooantroponose; uma zoonose normalmente mantida por seres humanos, mas que pode ser transmitida para outros vertebrados (p. ex., amebíase para cães, tuberculose). Cf. anthropozoonosis, amphixenosis. [zoo- + G. *anthrōpos*, homem, + *nosos*, doença]

zo·o·blast (zō′-ō-blast). Zooblasto; uma célula animal. [zoo- + G. *blastos*, germe]

zo·o·chrome (zō′ō-krōm). Zoocromo; pigmento animal de ocorrência natural; inclui pigmentos humanos.

zo·o·der·mic (zō-ō-der′mik). Zoodérmico; relativo à pele de um animal. [zoo- + G. *derma*, pele]

zo·o·e·ras·tia (zō′ō-ē-ras′tē-ă). Zooerastia. SIN zoophilia. [zoo- + G. *erastēs*, amante]

zo·o·ful·vin (zō′ō-fŭl′vin). Zoofulvina; pigmento amarelo obtido das penas de certos pássaros.

zo·o·gen·e·sis (zō-ō-jen′ĕ-sis). Zoogênese; a doutrina de produção ou geração animal. [zoo- + G. *genesis*, origem]

zo·o·ge·og·ra·phy (zō′ō-jē-og′ră-fē). Zoogeografia; a geografia dos animais; o estudo da distribuição dos animais na superfície da Terra.

zo·o·glea (zō-og′lē-ă, zō′ō-glē′ă). Zoogléia; em bacteriologia, um termo antigo para designar uma massa de bactérias mantidas juntas por uma substância gelatinosa transparente. [zoo- + G. *glia*, cola]

zo·og·o·nous (zō-oj′ō-nŭs). Zoógono. SIN viviparous.

zo·og·o·ny (zō-oj′ō-nē). Zoogonia. SIN viviparity.

zo·o·graft (zō′ō-graft). Zooenxerto; enxerto de tecido de um animal em um ser humano. SIN animal graft, zooplastic graft.

zo·o·graft·ing (zō-ō-graft′ing). Zooenxerto. SIN zooplasty.

zo·oid (zō′oyd). Zoóide. **1.** Semelhante a um animal; um organismo ou objeto com aspecto semelhante ao de um animal. **2.** Uma célula animal capaz de existência ou movimento independente, como o óvulo ou um espermatozóide, ou o segmento de uma tênia. **3.** Um indivíduo de uma colônia de invertebrados, como um coral. [G. *zōodēs*, de *zōon*, animal, + *eidos*, semelhança]

zo·o·lag·nia (zō-ō-lag′nē-ă). Zoolagnia; termo antigo para designar atração sexual por animais. [zoo- + G. *lagneia*, luxúria]

zo·o·lite, zo·o·lith (zō′ō-līt, zō-ō-lith). Zoolito; um animal petrificado. [zoo- + G. *lithos*, pedra]

zo·ol·o·gist (zō-ol′ō-jist). Zoologista; zoólogo; aquele que se especializa em zoologia.

zo·ol·o·gy (zō-ol′ō-jē). Zoologia; o ramo da biologia que estuda os animais. [zoo- + G. *logos*, estudo]

zoom (zoom). Zoom; zum; a ação de um sistema de lentes de vários focos em uma câmara ou microscópio que mantém um objeto em foco enquanto se aproxima ou afasta dele; esse efeito pode ser obtido movendo-se dois ou mais dos componentes da lente em velocidades que guardam uma relação linear entre si.

zo·o·ma·nia (zō-ō-mā′nē-ă). Zoomania; amor excessivo, anormal, pelos animais. [zoo- + G. *mania*, mania]

zo·o·mar·ic ac·id (zō′ō-mer-ik). Ácido zoomárico. SIN palmitoleic acid.

Zo·o·mas·tig·i·na (zō′ō-mas-ti-jī′nă). SIN Zoomastigophorea. [zoo- + G. *mastix*, chicote, flagelo]

Zo·o·mas·ti·go·pho·ras·i·da (zō′ō-mas-ti-gō-fō-ras′i-dă). SIN Zoomastigophorea.

Zo·o·mas·ti·go·pho·rea (zō′ō-mas-ti-gō-fō′rē-ă). Classe de flagelados (superclasse Mastigophora) no filo Sarcomastigophora (protozoários flagelados e amebóides), com características semelhantes a animais em oposição às vegetais. Não há cromatóforos; são encontrados um a muitos flagelos, embora estes possam estar ausentes nas formas amebóides; a sexualidade é conhecida em alguns grupos. Inclui muitos parasitas humanos como os tripanossomas e tricomonas, bem como várias outras formas parasitárias e simbióticas. SIN Zoomastigina, Zoomastigophorasida. [zoo- + G. *mastix*, flagelo, + *phoros*, que carrega]

zo·o·no·sis (zō-ō-nō′sis). Zoonose; uma infecção ou infestação compartilhada na natureza pelos seres humanos e outros animais. VER TAMBÉM anthropozoonosis, cyclozoonosis, metazoonosis, saprozoonosis, zooanthroponosis. [zoo- + G. *nosos*, doença]
  direct z., z. direta; z. transmitida entre seres humanos e outros animais, de um hospedeiro infectado para um suscetível por contato, por gotículas respiratórias, por pequenas partículas das secreções respiratórias, ou por algum veículo de transmissão; o agente exige um único hospedeiro vertebrado para completar seu ciclo vital e não desenvolve nem mostra alteração significativa durante a transmissão; pode incluir antropozoonoses (raiva), zooantroponoses (amebíase) e anfixenoses (algumas estreptococoses).

zo·o·not·ic (zō′ō-not′ik). Zoonótico; relativo a uma zoonose.

zo·o·par·a·site (zō-ō-par′ă-sīt). Zooparasita; um parasita animal; um animal que existe como parasita.

zo·o·pa·thol·o·gy (zō-ō-pă-thol′ō-jē). Zoopatologia; o estudo ou ciência das doenças dos animais inferiores.

zo·oph·a·gous (zō-of′ă-gŭs). Zoófago. SIN carnivorous. [G. *zōophagos*, de *zōon*, animal, + *phagein*, comer]

zo·o·phile (zō′ō-fīl). Zoófilo. **1.** Um amante dos animais; particularmente aquele que prefere os animais aos seres humanos. **2.** Aquele que é contrário a qualquer experiência com animais; um antivivisseccionista. [zoo- + G. *philos*, amigo]

zo·o·phil·ia (zō-ō-fil′ē-ă). Zoofilia; uma parafilia na qual a excitação sexual e o orgasmo são facilitados por atividades sexuais com animais. SIN bestiality, zooerastia.

zo·o·phil·ic (zō-ō-fil′ik). Zoofílico. **1.** Relativo a ou que exibe zoofilismo. **2.** Que busca ou prefere animais; designa a preferência de um parasita por um hospedeiro animal, em lugar do homem. [zoo- + G. *philos*, amigo, amante]

zo·oph·i·lism (zō-of′i-lizm). Zoofilismo; amor por animais, particularmente um amor extravagante por eles.
  erotic z., z. erótico; obtenção de prazer sexual pelo ato de afagar ou bater em animais. VER TAMBÉM zoophilia, bestiality.

zo·o·pho·bia (zō-ō-fō′bē-ă). Zoofobia; medo mórbido de animais. [zoo- + G. *phobos*, medo]

zo·o·phyte (zō′ō-fit). Zoófito; animal que se assemelha a um vegetal, como as esponjas ou as anêmonas do mar. [zoo + G. *phyton*, vegetal]

zo·o·plas·ty (zō′ō-plas-tē). Zooplastia; zooenxerto; enxerto de tecido de um animal em um ser humano. SIN zoografting.

zo·o·sa·dism (zō-ō-sā′dizm). Zoossadismo; prazer sexual obtido com o tratamento cruel de animais.

zo·os·mo·sis (zō-os-mō′sis). Zoosmose; o processo de osmose em tecidos vivos. [G. *zōos*, vivo, + -osmosis]

zo·o·sperm·ia (zō-ō-sper′mē-ă). Zoospermia; a presença de espermatozóides vivos no sêmen ejaculado. [G. *zoon*, vivo, + -*sperma*, semente, + -ia]

zo·o·ster·ol (zō′ō-ster′ol). Zoosterol; um esterol animal.

zo·o·tech·nics (zō-ō-tek′niks). Zootecnia; a arte de tratar de animais domésticos ou cativos, incluindo manejo, reprodução e guarda. [zoo- + G. *technē*, arte]

zo·ot·ic (zō-ot′ik). Zoótico; pertinente a outros animais além do ser humano.

zo·o·tox·in (zō-ōtok′sin). Zootoxina; toxina animal; substância, semelhante às toxinas bacterianas em suas propriedades antigênicas, encontrada nos líquidos corporais de determinados animais; p. ex., no veneno de cobra, nas secreções de insetos venenosos, no sangue de enguia. SIN animal toxin.

zo·o·tro·phic (zō-ō-trof′ik). Zootrófico; relativo a, ou que serve para, nutrição dos animais inferiores. [zoo- + Gr. *trophē*, nutrição]

zor·ub·i·cin (zō-roo-bī-sin). Zorrubicina; derivado semi-sintético da daunorrubicina; também é semelhante à doxorrubicina. Como esses agentes, a zorrubicina exerce toxicidade miocárdica significativa. Usada como antineoplásico no câncer de mama.

zos·ter (zos′ter). Zoster. SIN herpes zoster. [G. *zōstēr*, cintura]
  geniculate z. (jen-i′kyu-lāt zos′ter). Zoster geniculado. SIN herpes zoster oticus.

ℹ **zos·ter·i·form** (zos-ter′i-form). Zosteriforme. SIN zosteroid.

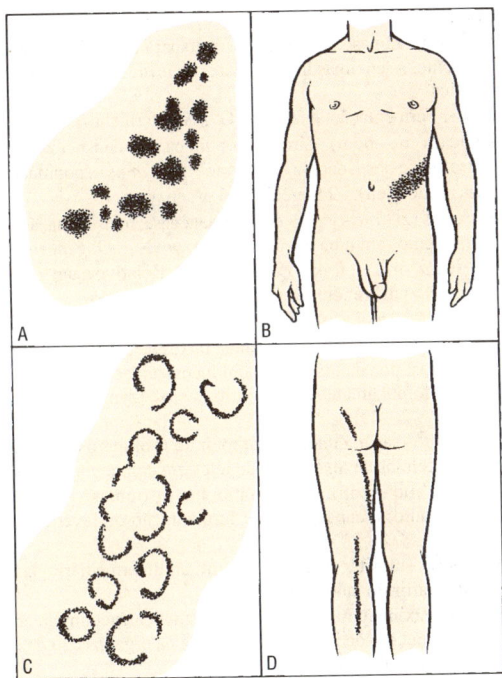

diferentes configurações das lesões cutâneas: (A) agrupadas; (B) zosteriforme; (C) anular (circular) e arciforme (arco); (D) linear

zos·ter·oid (zos′ter - oyd). Zosteróide; semelhante ao herpes zoster. SIN zosteriform. [zoster + G. *eidos*, semelhança]

zox·a·zo·la·mine (zok - să - zō′lă - mēn). Zoxazolamina; um relaxante muscular esquelético de ação central, não mais usado devido à sua toxicidade hepática.

Z-plas·ty. Z-plastia; zetaplastia; técnica para alongar uma cicatriz contraída ou para rodar a tensão em 90°; a linha média de uma incisão em forma de Z é feita ao longo da linha de maior tensão de contração, e retalhos triangulares são levantados em lados opostos das duas extremidades e transpostos.

Zr Símbolo do zircônio.

Zsigmondy, Richard A., químico austríaco-alemão e Prêmio Nobel, 1865–1929. VER Z. *test*; brownian-Z. *movement*.

ZSR Abreviatura de zeta sedimentation *ratio*.

Zuckerkandl, Emil, anatomista austríaco, 1849–1910. VER Z. *bodies*, em *body*, *convolution, fascia; organs* of Z., em *organ*.

zu·sam·men (Z) (zu-sam′men). 1. SIN cis- (4). 2. Uma forma de isomerismo geométrico em relação às ligações duplas carbono-carbono nas quais todas as quatro porções fixadas aos carbonos são diferentes. Se os substitutos com a posição mais alta (baseada nas regras estabelecidas) estiverem do mesmo lado da ligação dupla, é usado Z. VER entgegen. [Al. *junto*]

zwie·back (zwī′bak). Pão adocicado assado duas vezes, preferido para alimentação de lactentes durante o nascimento dos dentes. [Al., assado duas vezes]

Zwis·chen·fer·ment (tsvish′en-fer-ment′). SIN glucose-6-phosphate dehydrogenase. [Al. *zwischen*, entre, + *Fermen*, fermentação]

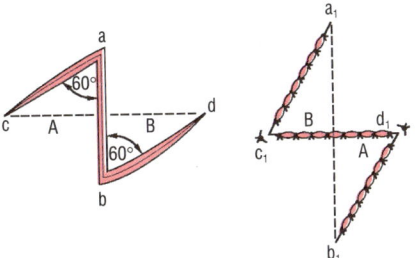

z-plastia: retalhos triangulares (A) e (B) são transpostos para rodar a linha de tensão 90° (de c- -d para a¹- -b¹)

zwit·ter·gents (tsvit′er-jents). Detergentes que são íons dipolares; freqüentemente usados como surfactantes e na liberação de proteínas das biomembranas. SIN switterionic detergent. [*zwitter*ion + deter*gent*]

zwit·ter·i·on·ic (tsvit′er - ī - on′ik). Íon dipolar; que possui tanto carga elétrica positiva como negativa; designa uma substância com as propriedades de um zwitterion; p. ex., em pH de 6,11, a alanina é um íon dipolar.

zwit·ter·i·ons (tsvit′er - ī - onz). Zwitterions. SIN dipolar *ions*, em *ion*. VER TAMBÉM zwitter *hypothesis*. [Al. *Zwitter*, hermafrodita, híbrido + íon]

zyg-. VER zygo-.

zy·gal (zī′găl). Zigal; relativo a, ou que possui o formato de, um jugo; em formato de H.

zyg·a·poph·y·si·al, zyg·a·poph·y·se·al (zī′ga - pō - fiz′ē - ăl, zī - gă - pof′i - se′ăl). Zigapofisário; relativo a uma zigapófise ou processo articular de uma vértebra.

zyg·a·poph·y·sis, pl. **zyg·a·poph·y·ses** (zī′gă - pof′i - sis, -sēz). Zigapófise ou processo articular. SIN articular *process*, articular *process*. [G. *zygon*, jugu, + *apophysis*, protuberância]
 z. inferior [TA], z. inferior. SIN inferior articular *process*.
 z. superior [TA], z. superior. SIN superior articular *process*.

zyg·i·on (zig′ē - on). Zígio; em cefalometria e craniometria, o ponto mais lateral do arco zigomático. [G. uma forma tardia de *zygon*, jugo]

zygo-, zyg-. Um jugo, uma união. [G. *zygon*, jugo, *zygōsis*, união]

zy·go·ma (zī - gō′mă). Zigoma. 1. SIN zygomatic *bone*. 2. SIN zygomatic *arch*. [G. barra, virote, ponto jugal, de *zygon*, jugo]

zy·go·mat·ic (zī′gō - mat′ik). Zigomático; relativo ao osso zigomático.

zygomatico-. Zigomático; relativo geralmente ao osso zigomático. VER zygo-. [G. *zygōma*]

zy·go·mat·i·co·au·ric·u·lar (zī′gō - mat′i - kō - aw - rik′ū - lăr). Zigomaticoauricular; relativo ao osso zigomático e à orelha.

zy·go·mat·i·co·au·ri·cu·la·ris (zī′gō - mat′i - kō - aw - rik′ū - lār′is). Zigomaticoauricular. SIN auricularis anterior (*muscle*).

zy·go·mat·i·co·fa·cial (zī′gō - mat′ikō - fā′shăl). Zigomaticofacial; relativo ao osso zigomático e à face.

zy·go·mat·i·co·fron·tal (zī′gō - mat′i - kō - fron′tăl). Zigomaticofrontal; relativo aos ossos zigomático e frontal.

zy·go·mat·i·co·max·il·lary (zī′gō - mat′i - kō - mak′si - lār - ē). Zigomaticomaxilar; relativo ao osso zigomático e ao maxilar.

zy·go·mat·i·co-or·bi·tal (zī′gō - mat′i - kō - ōr′bi - tăl). Zigomaticoorbital; relativo ao osso zigomático e à órbita.

zy·go·mat·i·co·sphe·noid (zī′gō - mat′i - kō - sfē′noyd). Zigomaticoesfenóide; relativo aos ossos zigomático e esfenóide.

zy·go·mat·i·co·tem·po·ral (zī′gō - mat′i - kō - tem′pō - răl). Zigomaticotemporal; relativo aos ossos zigomático e temporal.

zy·go·max·il·la·re (zī′gō - mak - si - lā′rē). Zigomaxilar; ponto zigomaxilar; um ponto craniométrico localizado externamente na extensão mais baixa da sutura zigomaticomaxilar. SIN key ridge, zygomaxillary point.

zy·go·max·il·lary (zī′gō - mak′si - lār - ē). Zigomaxilar; relativo ao osso zigomático e ao maxilar.

Zy·go·my·ce·tes (zī′gō - mī - sē′tēz). Zigomicetos; ficomicetos; uma classe de fungos caracterizada por reprodução sexual, resultando na formação de um zigosporo, e reprodução assexuada através de esporos imóveis denominados esporangiosporos ou conídios. SIN Phycomycetes. [zygo- + G. *mykēs* (*mykēt-*), fungo]

zy·go·my·co·sis (zī′gō - mī - kō′sis). Zigomicose; um termo amplo que inclui mucormicose e entamoftaromicose; geralmente aplicado quando não há cultura disponível e a condição clínica não é clara. SIN phycomycetosis, phycomycosis.

zy·gon (zī′gon). Zígon; a linha curta que une os ramos de uma fissura zigal. [G. canga, jugo]

zy·go·ne·ma (zī - g - ō - nē′mă). Zigonema. SIN zygotene. [zygo- + G. *nēma*, fio]

zy·go·po·di·um (zī - gō - pō′dē - um). Zigopódio; o segmento intermediário distal do esqueleto do membro, isto é, rádio e ulna, tíbia e fíbula. [zygo- + G. *podion*, pequeno pé]

zy·go·sis (zī - gō′sis). Zigose; conjugação verdadeira ou união sexual de dois microrganismos unicelulares, que consiste principalmente na fusão dos núcleos das duas células. [G. uma união]

zy·gos·i·ty (zī - gos′i - tē). Zigosidade; a natureza dos zigotos dos quais são derivados os indivíduos; p. ex., seja por separação da divisão de um zigoto (monozigóticos), caso em que serão geneticamente idênticos, ou de dois óvulos fertilizados distintos (dizigóticos).

zy·go·sperm (zī′gō - sperm). Zigosperma. SIN zygospore. [zygo- + G. *sperma*, semente]

zy·go·spore (zī′gō - spōr). Zigosporo; entre os Phycomycetes, um esporo sexual de parede espessa originado da fusão de duas estruturas morfologicamente idênticas, geralmente extremidades de hifas, que possuem núcleos de tipos de acasalamento opostos (gametangia). SIN zygosperm.

zygosyndactyly (zī - gō - sin- dak′til - ē). Zigossindactilia; união dos dedos das mãos ou dos pés por membrana completa ou incompleta. [zygo- + syndactyly]

zy·gote (zī′gōt). Zigoto. **1.** A célula diplóide resultante da união de um espermatozóide e um óvulo. Cf. conceptus. **2.** O indivíduo que se desenvolve a partir de um óvulo fertilizado. [G. *zygōtos*, conjugado]

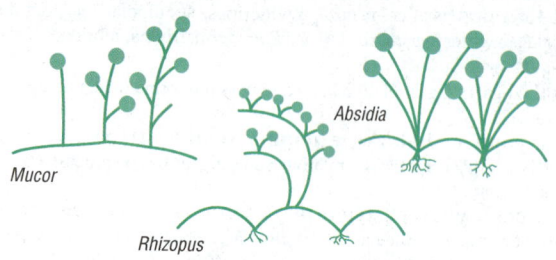

Zigomicetos: aspectos diferenciais de três gêneros

zy·go·tene (zī′gō - tēn). Zigóteno; o estágio de prófase na meiose em que começa o ponto exato para pareamento dos cromossomas homólogos. SIN zygonema. [zygo- + G. *tainia* (L. *taenia*), faixa]

zy·got·ic (zī - got′ik). Zigótico; relativo a um zigoto ou à zigose.

zy·go·to·blast (zī - gō′tō - blast). Zigotoblasto. SIN sporozoite. [G. *zygōtos*, conjugado, + *blastos*, germe]

zy·go·to·mere (zī - gō′tō - mēr). Zigotômero. SIN sporoblast. [G. *zygōtos*, conjugado, + *meros*, parte]

zym-. VER zymo-.

zy·mase (zī′mās). Zimase. **1.** Termo obsoleto para uma mistura de enzimas. **2.** Especificamente, as enzimas intracelulares de levedura que promove fermentação alcoólica.

zymo-, zym-. Fermentação, enzimas. [G. *zymē*, fermento]

zy·mo·deme (zī′mō - dēm). Zimódemo; um padrão de isoenzima, identificado por eletroforese das isoenzimas. [zymo- + G. *dēmos*, população]

zy·mo·gen (zī′mō - jen). Zimogênio. SIN proenzyme.

zy·mo·gen·e·sis (zī - mō - jen′ē - sis). Zimogênese; transformação de uma pró-enzima (zimogênio) em uma enzima ativa. [zymo- + G. *genesis*, produção]

zy·mo·gen·ic (zī - mō - jen′ik). Zimogênico. **1.** Relativo a um zimogênio ou à zimogênese. SIN zymogenous. **2.** Que causa fermentação.

zy·mog·e·nous (zī - moj′ē - nŭs). Zimógeno. SIN zymogenic (1).

zy·mo·gram (zī′mō - gram). Zimograma; faixas de papel, géis, etc., nas quais são demonstradas, por métodos histoquímicos, as localizações das enzimas, separadas eletroforeticamente ou por outros meios. [zymo- + G. *gramma*, algo escrito]

zy·mo·san (zī′mō - san). Zimosan; carboidrato (polímero da glicose), obtido das paredes de células de levedura, que interfere com o complemento.

zy·mo·scope (zī′mō - skōp). Zimoscópio; um instrumento que mede o CO_2 liberado e, portanto, a capacidade de fermentação da levedura. [zymo- + G. *skopeō*, ver]

zy·mos·ter·ol (zī - mos′ter - ol). Zimosterol; um intermediário na biossíntese do colesterol a partir do lanosterol.

zy·xin (ziks′in). Zixina; uma proteína citoplasmática encontrada em vários tipos distintos de junções de adesão; participaria na organização de fixações do citoesqueleto da membrana.

ZZ VER ZZ genotype.

CONTEÚDO DOS APÊNDICES

Formas Combinantes na Linguagem Médica 1786

Abreviaturas Médicas Comuns 1789

Símbolos 1795

Quadros de Anatomia 1799

Tabela de Elementos e Seus Pesos Atômicos 1839

Escalas Comparativas de Temperatura 1841

Temperaturas Equivalentes 1842

Pesos e Medidas 1843

Valores de Referência em Laboratório 1847

Grupos Sangüíneos 1861

Grupos de Diagnósticos Correlatos 1863

FORMAS COMBINANTES NA LINGUAGEM MÉDICA

Prefixos, Sufixos e Formas Combinantes em Medicina

a- não, sem, menos
ab- a partir de, distante de, afastado
abs- a partir de, distante de, afastado
acantho- espinho
acou- audição
acro- extremidade
acu- audição
ad- aumento, aderência, movimento no sentido de; muito
-ad no sentido de, na direção de
adeno- glândula
adip- gordura
adipo- gordura
-agog- agogo, promotor, estimulador
aidoio- genitais
-al pertinente a
alb- branco
albo- branco
alge- dor
algesi- dor
algio- dor
algo- dor
allo- outro, diferente
ambi- ao redor de, nos (ambos) lados, em todos os lados, ambos
ambly- embotamento
amblyo- embotamento
amyl- amido, polissacarídeo
amylo- amido, polissacarídeo
an- não, sem
ana- para cima, no sentido de, separado
andro- masculino
angi- vaso
angio- vaso
ankylo- rígido
ante- antes
anthraco- carvão, carbono
anti- 1 contra, oposto; 2 curativo; 3 anticorpo
apo- separado de, derivado de
aque- água
aqueo- água
-ar pertinente a
-arche início
arteri- artéria
arterio- artéria
arthr- articulação
arthro- articulação
-ary pertinente a
-ase uma enzima
-ate um sal ou éster de um ácido ("-ic")
athero- pastoso, gorduroso
atto- um quintilionésimo (10^{-18})
audi- audição
audio- audição
aur- ouvido
auri- ouvido
auro- ouvido
aut- próprio, idêntico
auto- próprio, idêntico
bacteri- bactéria
bacterio- bactéria
balano- glande do pênis
bi- duas vezes, duplo
bio- vida
blasto- brotamento por células ou tecido
blephar- pálpebra
blepharo- pálpebra
brachi- braço
brachio- braço
brachy- curto
bronch- brônquio

bronchi- brônquio
broncho- brônquio
carcin- câncer
carcino- câncer
cardi- 1 coração; 2 abertura do estômago para o esôfago (cárdia)
cardio- 1 coração; 2 abertura do estômago para o esôfago (cárdia)
carpo- punho
cata- baixo
caud- cauda, parte inferior do corpo
caudo- cauda, parte inferior do corpo
-cele hérnia, tumefação
celio- abdome
-centesis punção cirúrgica
centi- um centésimo (10^{-2})
cephal- a cabeça
cephalo- a cabeça
cervic- 1 pescoço; 2 colo uterino
cervico- 1 pescoço; 2 colo uterino
cheil- lábio
cheilo- lábio
cheir- mão
cheiro- mão
chem- 1 química; 2 medicamento
chemo- 1 química; 2 medicamento
chir- mão
chiro- mão
chlor- 1 verde; 2 cloro
chloro- 1 verde; 2 cloro
chol- bile
chondrio- 1 cartilagem; 2 granular; 3 arenoso
chondro- 1 cartilagem; 2 granular; 3 arenoso
chrom- cor
chromat- cor
chromo- cor
chron- tempo
chrono- tempo
-cidal que mata, que destrói
-cide que mata, que destrói
cis- neste lado, no lado próximo
-clast que rompe, degrada, fragmenta
-clysis que lava
co- com, junto, em associação a, muito, completo
col- com, junto, em associação a, muito, completo
colp- vagina
colpo- vagina
com- com, junto, em associação a, muito, completo
con- com, junto, em associação a, muito, completo
conio- poeira
cor- com, junto, em associação a, muito, completo
coreo- pupila
cost- costela
costo- costela
crani- crânio
cranio- crânio
-crine secreção
cry- frio
cryo- frio
crypt- oculto
crypto- oculto
culdo- fundo-de-saco
cyan- 1 azul; 2 cianeto
cyano- 1 azul; 2 cianeto

cycl- 1 círculo, ciclo; 2 corpo ciliar
cyst- 1 bexiga; 2 cisto; 3 ducto cístico
cysti- 1 bexiga; 2 cisto; 3 ducto cístico
cysto- 1 bexiga; 2 cisto; 3 ducto cístico
cyt- célula
-cyte célula
cyto- célula
dacry- lágrimas
dacryo- lágrimas
dactyl- dedo da mão ou do pé
dactylo- dedo da mão ou do pé
de- longe de, cessação
deca- dez
deci- um décimo (10^{-1})
deka- dez
dent- dente
denti- dente
derm- pele
derma- pele
dermat- pele
dermato- pele
dermo- pele
-desis ligação
dextr- direito, no sentido de ou no lado direito
dextro- direito, no sentido de ou no lado direito
di- separação, afastamento, reversão, não
dif- separação, afastamento, reversão, não
dipso- sede
dir- separação, afastamento, reversão, não
dis- separação, afastamento, reversão, não
duo- dois
duodeno- duodeno
-dynia dor
dynamo- força, energia
dys- ruim, difícil
ect- externo, no lado de fora
-ectasia dilatação, alongamento
-ectasis dilatação, alongamento
ecto- externo, no lado de fora
-ectomy excisão
-emphraxis obstrução
encephal- cérebro
encephalo- cérebro
end- dentro, interno
endo- dentro, interno
enter- intestino
entero- intestino
ent- interno, dentro
ento- interno, dentro
epi- sobre, após, subseqüente a
ergo- trabalho
erythr- vermelho, vermelhidão
erythro- vermelho, vermelhidão
eso- voltado para dentro
esthesio- sensação, percepção
eu- bom, bem
ex- fora de, a partir de, longe de
exo- exterior, externo, para fora
extra- sem, fora de
ferri- íon férrico (Fe^{3+})
ferro- 1 ferro metálico; 2 íon ferroso (Fe^{2+})
fibr- fibra
fibro- fibra
-form na forma ou formato de
galact- leite

galacto- leite
gastr- 1 estômago; 2 ventre
gastro- 1 estômago; 2 ventre
-gen 1 que produz, vir a ser; 2 precursor
gen- 1 que produz, vir a ser; 2 precursor
giga- um bilhão (10^9)
gingiv- gengiva
gingivo- gengiva
gloss- língua
glosso- língua
gluco- glicose
glyco- açúcares
gnath- mandíbula
gnatho- mandíbula
gon- semente, sêmen
gonio- ângulo
gono- semente, sêmen
-gram registro
granul- granular, grânulo
granulo- granular, grânulo
-graph instrumento de registro
gyn- mulher
gyne- mulher
gyneco- mulher
gyno- mulher
hecto- uma centena (10^2)
hem- sangue
hema- sangue
hemat- sangue
hemato- sangue
hemi- metade
hemo- sangue
hepat- fígado
hepatico- fígado
hepato- fígado
hept- sete
hepta- sete
hidr- suor
hidro- suor
hist- tecido
histio- tecido
histo- tecido
homeo- igual, constante
hydr- água; hidrogênio
hydro- água; hidrogênio
hyper- excessivo, acima do normal
hypo- abaixo de; diminuição, deficiência; o menor
hyster- 1 útero; histeria; 2 tardio, após
hystero- 1 útero; histeria; 2 tardio, após
-ia condição
-iasis condição, estado
-ic pertinente a
-ics conhecimento organizado, prática, tratamento
ileo- fleo
ilio- flio
in- 1 dentro; 2 não
-in sufixo químico
-ine sufixo químico
infra- abaixo de
inguino- virilha, inguinal
inter- entre, no meio de
intra- dentro
intro- dentro
irid- íris
irido- íris
ischi- ísquio
ischio- ísquio

FORMAS COMBINANTES NA LINGUAGEM MÉDICA

-ism 1 condição, doença; 2 prática, doutrina
-ismus espasmo, contração
iso- 1 igual, semelhante; 2 isômero; 3 igualdade
-ite a natureza de, que se assemelha
-ites semelhante
-itides plural de -itis (ite)
-itis inflamação
kal- potássio
kali- potássio
karyo- núcleo
kerat- córnea
kerato- córnea
kilo- mil (10^3)
kin- movimento
kine- movimento
kinesi- movimento
kinesio- movimento
kineso- movimento
kino- movimento
labio- lábio
lacrim- lágrimas
lacrimo- lágrimas
lact- leite
lacti- leite
lacto- leite
laparo- abdome, parede abdominal
laryng- laringe
laryngo- laringe
lateri- lateral, de um lado, lado
latero- lateral, de um lado, lado
-lepsis convulsão
-lepsy convulsão
lepto- leve, magro, fino, frágil
leuk- branco
leuko- branco
linguo- língua
lip- gordura, lipídeo
lipo- gordura, lipídeo
lith- pedra, cálculo, calcificação
litho- pedra, cálculo, calcificação
-log fala, palavras
log- fala, palavras
logo- fala, palavras
-logy 1 estudo de; 2 que coleta
lymph- linfa
lympho- linfa
lys- lise, dissolução
lyso- lise, dissolução
macr- grande; longo
macro- grande; longo
mal- ruim, deficiente
-malacia amolecimento
mamm- mama
mamma- mama
mammo- mama
mast- mama
masto- mama
meg- grande, com tamanho excessivo
mega- 1 grande, com tamanho excessivo; 2 um milhão (10^6)
megal- grande
megalo- grande
-megaly aumento
melan- preto
melano- preto
men- menstruação
mening- meninges
meningo- meninges
meno- menstruação
ment- queixo
mento- queixo
-mer membro de uma série
mes- 1 meio, média, intermediário; 2 que se prende à membrana
meso- 1 meio, média, intermediário; 2 que se prende à membrana

meta- 1 depois, atrás; 2 ação articular, compartilhamento
-meter medida, aparelho de mensuração
metr- útero
metro- útero
micr- 1 pequeno, microscópico; 2 um milionésimo (10^{-6})
micro- 1 pequeno, microscópico; 2 um milionésimo (10^{-6})
milli- um milésimo (10^{-3})
mon- único
mono- único
morph- forma, formato, estrutura
morpho- forma, formato, estrutura
my- músculo
myo- músculo
myel- 1 medula óssea; 2 medula espinal
myelo- 1 medula óssea; 2 medula espinal
myring- membrana timpânica
myringo- membrana timpânica
myx- muco
myxo- muco
nano- 1 anão; 2 um bilionésimo (10^{-9})
nas- nariz
naso- nariz
natr- sódio
natri- sódio
necr- morte, necrose
necro- morte, necrose
neo- novo
nephr- rim
nephro- rim
neur- nervo, sistema nervoso
neuri- nervo, sistema nervoso
neuro- nervo, sistema nervoso
norm- normal
normo- normal
octo- oito
oculo- olho, ocular
odont- dente
odonto- dente
odyn- dor
odyno- dor
-oid semelhante a
olig- pouco, pequeno
oligo- pouco, pequeno
-oma tumor, neoplasia
-omata plural de -oma
oncho- onco-
onco- tumor, massa, volume
-one cetona (grupamento —CO—)
onych- unha da mão e/ou do pé
onycho- unha da mão e/ou do pé
oo- ovo, ovário
oophor- ovário
oophoro- ovário
ophthalm- olho
ophthalmo- olho
-opia visão
-opsia visão
or- boca
orchi- testículo
orchido- testículo
orchio- testículo
ori- boca
oro- boca
-ose açúcar
-oses plural de -osis
-osis processo, condição, estado
ossi- osso
osseo- ósseo
ost- osso
oste- osso
osteo- osso
ovari- ovário

ovario- ovário
ovi- ovo
ovo- ovo
oxa- oxigênio
oxo- oxigênio
oxy- 1 pungente, ácido; 2 agudo, penetrante, rápido; 3 oxigênio
pachy- espesso
pan- todo, inteiro
pant- todo, inteiro
panto- todo, inteiro
para- 1 anormal; 2 envolvimento de duas partes semelhantes
pari- igual
path- doença
patho- doença
-pathy doença
ped- 1 criança; 2 pé
pedi- 1 criança; 2 pé
pedo- 1 criança; 2 pé
-penia deficiência
penta- cinco
per- através de, completamente, intensamente
peri- ao redor de, em torno de
-pexy fixação, geralmente cirúrgica
phaco- lente
-phage comer, devorar
-phagia comer, devorar
phago- comer, devorar
-phagy comer, devorar
phako- lente
phanero- visível, evidente
pharmaco- medicamentos, remédios
pharyng- faringe
pharyngo- faringe
phil- 1 atração; 2 afinidade química
-philia 1 atração; 2 afinidade química
philo- 1 atração; 2 afinidade química
phleb- veia
phlebo- veia
-phobia medo
phon- som, fala
phono- som, fala
phor- que carrega, que suporta
phoro- que carrega, que suporta
phos- luz
phot- luz
photo- luz
phren- 1 diafragma; 2 mente; 3 frênico
phreni- 1 diafragma; 2 mente; 3 frênico
-phrenia da mente
phrenico- 1 diafragma; 2 mente; 3 frênico
phreno- 1 diafragma; 2 mente; 3 frênico
-phylaxis proteção
phyll- folha
phyllo- folha
physi- 1 físico; 2 natural
physio- 1 físico; 2 natural
physo- 1 tumefação, insuflação; 2 ar, gás
phyt- vegetais
phyto- vegetais
pico- um trilionésimo (10^{-12})
plan- plano
plani- plano
plano- plano
-plasia formação
plasma- plasma
plasmat- plasma
plasmato- plasma
plasmo- plasma
platy- amplo, plano
-plegia paralisia

pleo- mais
plesio- próximo, similar
pleur- costela, lado, pleura
pleura- costela, lado, pleura
pleuro- costela, lado, pleura
pluri- vários, mais
-pnea respiração
pneo- respiração
pneum- 1 ar, gás; 2 pulmão; 3 respiração
pneuma- 1 ar, gás; 2 pulmão; 3 respiração
pneumat- 1 ar, gás; 2 pulmão; 3 respiração
pneumato- 1 ar, gás; 2 pulmão; 3 respiração
pod- pé, em formato de pé
-pod pé, em formato de pé
podo- pé, em formato de pé
-poiesis produção
poikilo- irregular, variável
polio- cinza
poly- 1 multiplicidade; 2 polímero
post- depois, atrás, posterior
pre- anterior, antes
presby- antigo, velho
pro- 1 antes, dianteiro; 2 precursor
proct- ânus, reto
procto- ânus, reto
prot- primeiro
proto- primeiro
pseud- falso
pseudo- falso
psych- mente
psyche- mente
psycho- mente
-ptosis que pende, que cai
pyel- pelve (renal)
pyelo- pelve (renal)
pykn- denso, compacto
pykno- denso, compacto
pyo- supuração, pus
pyreto- febre
pyro- fogo, calor, febre
quadr- quatro
quadri- quatro
rachi- coluna vertebral
rachio- coluna vertebral
radio- 1 radiação, raios X; 2 rádio
re- novamente, para trás
rect- reto
recto- reto
ren- rim
reno- rim
retro- para trás, atrás
rhin- nariz
rhino- nariz
-rrhagia corrimento
-rrhaphy sutura cirúrgica
-rrhea fluxo
-rrhexis ruptura
salping- tuba
salpingo- tuba
sarco- carne, músculo
schisto- divisão, fenda
schiz- divisão, fenda
schizo- divisão, fenda
scler- endurecimento (induração), esclerose, esclera do bulbo do olho
sclero- endurecimento (induração), esclerose, esclera do bulbo do olho
scolio- torto, recurvado
-scope instrumento para visualização
-scopy a visualização
scot- sombra, escuridão
scoto- sombra, escuridão

semi- metade; parcialmente
sept- 1 sete; **2** septo; **3** sepse, infecção
septi- sete
septo- 1 sete; **2** septo; **3** sepse, infecção
sial- saliva, glândula salivar
sialo- saliva, glândula salivar
sider- ferro
sidero- ferro
sigmoid- 1 em forma de S; **2** colo sigmóide
sigmoido- 1 em forma de S; **2** colo sigmóide
sin- seio
sino- seio
sinu- seio
sito- alimento, grão
somat- corpo, corpóreo
somato- corpo, corpóreo
somatico- corpo, corpóreo
somno- sono
son- 1 som; **2** ultra-som
sono- 1 som; **2** ultra-som
spasmo- espasmo
spermato- sêmen, espermatozóide
spermo- sêmen, espermatozóide
sperma- sêmen, espermatozóide
sphygmo- pulso
spir- respiração
spiro- respiração
splanchn- vísceras

splanchni- vísceras
splanchno- vísceras
splen- baço
spleno- baço
staphyl- uva, cacho de uvas; estafilococos
staphylo- uva, cacho de uvas; estafilococos
-stasis parada
-stat que paralisa a alteração ou movimento
steno- estreito, constrição
stereo- sólido
stheno- vigor, força, potência
stom- boca
stoma- boca
stomat- boca
stomato- boca
sub- sob, menos que o normal, inferior
super- em excesso, acima, superior, na parte superior
supra- acima de
sy- junto
syl- junto
sym- junto
syn- junto
sys- junto
tachy- rápido
tel- distante
tele- distante
ten- tendão

tendin- tendão
teno- tendão
tenont- tendão
tenonto- tendão
tera- um quatrilhão (10^{15})
tetra- quatro
thel- mamilo
thelo- mamilo
therm calor
thermo- calor
thorac- tórax
thoracico- tórax
thoraco- tórax
thromb- coágulo sangüíneo
thrombo- coágulo sangüíneo
thyr- glândula tireóide
thyro- glândula tireóide
toco- parto
-tome 1 instrumento de corte; **2** segmento, seção
-tomy cirurgia de corte
tono- tônus, tensão, pressão
top- local, tópico
topo- local, tópico
tox- toxina, veneno
toxi- toxina, veneno
toxico- toxina, veneno
toxo- toxina, veneno
trache- traquéia
tracheo- traquéia
trans- através, além de
tri- três

trich- cabelo
trichi- cabelo
-trichia cabelo
tricho- cabelo
tris- três
-trophic alimento, nutrição
tropho- alimento, nutrição
-trophy alimento, nutrição
-tropia virado para
-tropic que se vira em direção a, afinidade por
ultra- além de
uni- um, único
uri- ácido úrico
-uria urina, micção
uric- ácido úrico
úrico- ácido úrico
uro- 1 urina; **2** trato urinário
vas- ducto, vaso sangüíneo
vasculo- vaso sangüíneo
vaso- ducto, vaso sangüíneo
vesic- bexiga urinária, vesícula
vesico- bexiga urinária, vesícula
xanth- amarelo, amarelado
xantho- amarelo, amarelado
xero- seco
zo- 1 animal; **2** vida
zoo- 1 animal; **2** vida
zym- fermentação, enzimas
zymo- fermentação, enzimas

ABREVIATURAS MÉDICAS COMUNS

α alfa; coeficiente de solubilidade de Bunsen; primeiro em uma série; termo de rotação específica; classe de cadeia pesada correspondendo à IgA

a (específico) absorção (coeficiente) (USUALMENTE EM ITÁLICO); acidez (total); área; (sangue) arterial (sistêmico) (SUBSCRITO); assimétrico; atto-

A absorvência

A adenosina (ou ácido adenílico); gás alveolar (SUBSCRITO); ampère

Å angstrom; unidade Ångström

a͞a [G.] um de cada (USADO em prescrições)

AA aminoácido; aminoacil

AB aborto

Ab anticorpo

ABG gasometria arterial

abl vírus da leucemia murina de Abelson

ABLB (teste do) equilíbrio da intensidade binaural alternada

ABO sistema de grupo sangüíneo

ABR (teste de) Bang (rastreamento de brucelose); resposta auditiva do tronco encefálico (audiometria)

abs. feb. [L.] *absente febre*, quando não há febre

γ-Abu ácido γ-aminobutírico

ABVD Adriamycin (doxorrubicina), bleomicina, vimblastina e dacarbazina

ac acetil; [L.] *ante cibum*, antes de uma refeição

aC arabinosilcitosina

Ac acetil; actínio

AC acetato; acromioclavicular; atriocarótico

AC/A (relação) convergência de acomodação-acomodação

ACE enzima conversora de angiotensina

ACEI inibidor da enzima conversora de angiotensina

ac-g globulina aceleradora, fator V da coagulação

AcG globulina aceleradora, fator V da coagulação

Ach acetilcolina

aCL anticardiolipina (anticorpo)

ACP proteína transportadora de acil

ACTH hormônio adrenocorticotrópico (corticotropina)

AD [L.] *auris dextra*, orelha direita; doença de Alzheimer

add. [L.] *adde*, acrescentar

Ade adenina

ADH hormônio antidiurético

adhib. [L.] *adhibendus*, para ser administrado

ADL atividades cotidianas

ad lib [L.] *ad libitum*, livremente, quando desejado

admov. [L.] *admove*, aplicar

Ado adenosina

ADP 5´-difosfato de adenosina

ad sat. [L.] *ad saturatum, ad saturandum*, até a saturação

adst. feb. [L.] *adstante febre*, quando há febre

ad us. ext. [L.] *ad usum externum*, para uso externo

adv. [L.] *adversum*, contra

A-E acima do cotovelo (amputação)

AFB bacilo álcool-ácido-resistente (BAAR)

AFORMED falha intermitente da resposta mecânica à despolarização elétrica

AFP α-fetoproteína

Ag antígeno; [L.] *argentum*, prata

A/G R relação albumina/globulina

AHF fator anti-hemofílico

AHG globulina anti-hemofílica

AID doador de inseminação artificial

AIDS síndrome da imunodeficiência adquirida

AIH inseminação artificial pelo marido; inseminação artificial, homóloga

A-K acima do joelho (amputação)

Al alumínio

Ala alanina (ou seu mono- ou dirradical)

ALA ácido δ-aminolevulínico

ALD adrenoleucodistrofia

ALL leucemia linfocítica aguda

ALS soro antilinfócito; suporte de vida avançado

ALT alanina aminotransferase

alt. hor. [L.] *alternis horis*, em horas alternadas (p. ex., às 08:00h, 10:00h, 12:00h, 14:00h)

Am amerício

AML leucemia mielógena aguda

AMP monofosfato de adenosina (ácido adenílico)

amu unidade de massa atômica

ANA anticorpo antinuclear

ANF fator antinuclear

ANOVA análise de variância

ANS sistema nervoso autônomo

ANUG gengivite ulcerativa necrotizante aguda

APA (fator) antianemia perniciosa

APC célula apresentadora de antígeno

A-P-C (vírus) adenóideo-faríngeo-conjuntival

aPS síndrome do anticorpo antifosfolipídeo

APTT tempo de tromboplastina parcial ativada

Ar argônio

araC arabinosilcitosina (citarabina)

ARDS síndrome de angústia respiratória do adulto

ARF insuficiência renal aguda; febre reumática aguda

Arg arginina (ou seu mono- ou dirradical)

As arsênico

AS [L.] *auris sinistra*, orelha esquerda

ASA ácido acetilsalicílico (aspirina)

ASCUS células escamosas anormais de importância indeterminada

ASHD cardiopatia arteriosclerótica

Asn asparagina (ou seu mono- ou dirradical)

ASO antiestreptolisina O

Asp ácido aspártico (ou seus radicais)

AST aspartato aminotransferase

At astatina

ATFL ligamento talofibular anterior

ATL leucemia de células T do adulto; linfoma de células T do adulto

atm atmosfera (padrão)

ATP 5´-trifosfato de adenosina

ATPase adenosina trifosfatase

ATPD temperatura e pressão ambientes, ar seco

ATPS temperatura e pressão ambientes, ar saturado (com vapor d'água)

at. wt. peso atômico

Au [L.] *aurum*, ouro

AU [L.] *auris utraque*, cada orelha, as duas orelhas

AV arteriovenoso

A-V arteriovenoso; atrioventricular

AVN nó atrioventricular

AVP proteína antiviral

AW peso atômico

ax. eixo

AZT azidotimidina (zidovudina)

b segundo em uma série

b sangue (SUBSCRITO)

B (pressão) barométrica (SUBSCRITO); boro

Ba bário

BADL atividades cotidianas básicas

BAER resposta auditiva evocada no tronco encefálico

BAL dimercaprol; lavado broncoalveolar

BALB (teste do) equilíbrio de intensidade binaural alternada

BBB barreira hematoencefálica

BCG bacilo de Calmette-Guérin (vacina)

BE enema baritado

Be berílio

B-E abaixo do cotovelo (amputação)

Bi bismuto

bib. [L.] *bibe*, beber

b.i.d. [L.] *bis in die*, duas vezes ao dia

BIDS (síndrome) cabelo quebradiço, comprometimento da inteligência, diminuição da fertilidade e baixa estatura

BIPAP pressão positiva nas vias aéreas em dois níveis

Bk berquélio

BM evacuação, defecação

BMI índice de massa corporal

bp par de base

BP pressão arterial; ponto de ebulição; *British Pharmacopoeia*

BPF fístula broncopleural

BPH hiperplasia prostática benigna

Bq bequerel (unidade do SI da atividade de radionuclídeo)

Br bromo

BRAT (dieta) banana, cereal de arroz, suco de maçã, torrada

BSA área de superfície corporal

BSER resposta evocada do tronco encefálico (audiometria)

BT tempo de sangramento

BTPS temperatura corporal, pressão ambiente, ar saturado (com vapor d'água)

BTU unidade térmica britânica

BUN uréia sangüínea

BUS glândulas de Bartholin, uretra, glândulas de Skene

C caloria (quilocaloria); carbono; Celsius; centígrado; depuração (taxa, renal) (seguido por SUBSCRITO); complacência; concentração; (lente) cilíndrica; citidina

c caloria (gramacaloria); capilar (sangue) (SUBSCRITO); centi-

ca. [L.] *circa*, cerca de, aproximadamente

c-a cardioarterial

Ca cálcio; catódico; catódio

CA câncer; carcinoma; parada cardíaca; idade cronológica; (vírus) associado ao crupe; citosina arabinosídeo

CABG enxerto em artéria coronária

cal caloria (gramacaloria)

Cal caloria (quilocaloria)

cAMP AMP cíclico (monofosfato de adenosina)

CAP proteína ativadora do catabólito (gene)

CAPD diálise peritoneal ambulatorial contínua

CAT tomografia axial computadorizada

CBC hemograma completo

CBG globulina fixadora de corticosteróide

Cbz carbobenzoxi (cloreto)

cc, c.c. centímetro cúbico

C.C. queixa principal

CCK colecistocinina

CCNU cloroetilcicloexilnitrosuréia (lomustina)

CCU unidade coronariana; unidade de terapia intensiva

cd candela

Cd cádmio

CDC Centers for Disease Control and Prevention

cDNA DNA complementar

CDP 5´-difosfato de citidina

Ce cério

CEA antígeno carcinoembrionário

CELO (vírus) órfão letal do embrião de galinha

CEP porfiria eritropoética congênita

Cf califórnio

CF fixação de complemento; fibrose cística; fator de acoplamento

CG gonadotrofina coriônica

CGA ativador do gene do catabólito

cGMP GMP cíclico

cgs, CGS centímetro-grama-segundo (sistema, unidade)

Ch[1] (cromossoma) Christchurch

CHF insuficiência cardíaca congestiva

CHO carboidrato

μCi microcurie

Ci curie

CI índice de corantes; *Colour Index*

CIB [L.] *cibus*, alimento

CIQ quociente de lateralidade cognitiva

CJD doença de Creutzfeldt-Jakob

CK creatinocinase, creatinoquinase

Apêndices

Cl cloro
CL cardiolipina
CLIA Clinical Laboratory Improvement Amendments
CLL leucemia linfocítica crônica
cm centímetro
cM centimorgan
Cm cúrio
CMA Certified Medical Assistant
CMC carpometacarpal
CMI imunidade celular
CML leucemia miélogena crônica
CMP 5´-fosfato de citidina (ou qualquer monofosfato de citidina)
CMT Certified Medical Transcriptionist
CMV ventilação mecânica controlada; citomegalovírus
CNM Certified Nurse Midwife
CNS sistema nervoso central
Co cobalto
c/o queixa-se de
CoA coenzima A
COG centro de gravidade
conA concanavalina A
cont. rem. [L.] *continuetur remedium*, mantenha a medicação
COPD doença pulmonar obstrutiva crônica
CP paralisia cerebral; costofrênico
CPAP pressão positiva contínua (ou constante) nas vias aéreas
CPD desproporção céfalo-pélvica
CPM mobilização passiva contínua
CPPB ventilação com pressão positiva contínua (ou constante)
CPPV ventilação com pressão positiva contínua
CPR reanimação cardiopulmonar
cps ciclos por segundo
Cr cromo; creatinina
CR reflexo condicionado; vértice-tornozelo (comprimento)
CRD doença respiratória crônica
CRH hormônio liberador de corticotropina
CRL comprimento vértice-tornozelo
CRNA Certified Registered Nurse Anesthetist
CRP proteína de reação cruzada
CRST (síndrome) calcinose cutânea, fenômeno de Raynaud, esclerodactilia e telangiectasia
Cs césio
C&S cultura e antibiograma
CSD doença da arranhadura do gato
CSF líquido cefalorraquidiano
CT tomografia computadorizada
CTP 5´-trifosfato de citidina
CTR relação cardiotorácica
Cu [L.] *cuprum*, cobre
CV cardiovascular
CVA acidente vascular cerebral
CVP pressão venosa central
CXR radiografia de tórax
Cyd citidina
cyl cilindro; cilíndrica (lente)
CYP citocromo P-450 (enzima)
Cys cisteína
Cyt citosina
δ delta; classe de cadeia pesada correspondendo à IgD
Δ delta; alteração; calor
d deci-
d deutério
d- dextrorrotatório
D espaço morto (gás) (SUBSCRITO); decíduo; deutério; difusão (capacidade de); diidrouridina (em ácidos nucléicos); dioptria; [L.] *dexter*, direito (oposto ao esquerdo); potência da vitamina D do óleo de fígado de bacalhau
D- prefixo que indica que uma molécula é estericamente análoga ao D-gliceraldeído
da deca-
dA desoxiadenosina
Da dalton
DA idade de desenvolvimento
dAdo desoxiadenosina
dAMP ácido desoxiadenílico
DANS ácido 1-dimetilaminonafta-leno-5-sulfônico
db decibel
dB decibel
DC Dental Corps; Doctor of Chiropractic
D & C dilatação e curetagem
DCG dacriocistografia
DCI dicloroisoproterenol
dCMP ácido desoxicitidílico
DDS Doctor of Dental Surgery
DDT diclorodifenil-tricloroetano (clorofenotano)
D & E dilatação e evacuação
def cariado, extraído ou obturado (dentes decíduos)
DEF cariado, extraído ou obturado (dentes permanentes)
deglut. [L.] *degluttiatur*, deixar ser engolido
DES dietilestilbestrol
det. [L.] *detur*, deixar ser administrado
DET dietiltriptamina
DEV vacina de embrião de pato; vírus do embrião de pato
DEXA absorptiometria de raio X de energia dual
df cariado e obturado (dentes decíduos)
Df deficiência (ausência ou inativação de um gene)
DF cariado e obturado (dentes permanentes)
dGMP monofosfato de desoxiguanosina (ácido desoxiguanílico)
DHEA desidro-3-epiandrosterona
DIC coagulação intravascular disseminada
dieb. alt. [L.] *diebus alternis*, em dias alternados
dil. [L.] *dilue*, diluir
dim. [L.] *dimidius*, metade
DIP pneumonia intersticial descamativa; (articulação) interfalângica distal
dir. prop. [L.] *directione propria*, com orientação apropriada
div. in par. aeq. [L.] *divide in partes aequales*, dividir em partes iguais
DJD doença articular degenerativa
dk deca-
dM decimorgan
DMD Doctor of Dental Medicine; distrofia muscular de Duchenne
dmf cariado, ausente ou obturado (dentes decíduos)
DMF cariado, ausente ou obturado (dentes permanentes)
DMSO dimetil-sulfóxido
DMT *N, N*-dimetiltriptamina
DN número de dibucaína
DNA ácido desoxirribonucléico
DNAase nuclease do ácido desoxirribonucléico
DNase desoxirribonuclease
DNAse desoxirribonuclease
DNP desoxirribonucleoproteína; 2,4-dinitrofenol
DNR não reanimar
DNS Director of Nursing Service(s)
DO Doctor of Osteopathy
DOA morto ao chegar
DOC ácido desoxicólico
DOC desoxicorticosterona
DOM 2,5-dimetoxi-4-metilanfetamina
Dp duplicação de um gene ou segmento cromossomial
DP Doctor of Podiatry
2,3-DPG 2,3-difosfoglicerato
DPH Doctor of Public Health; Doctor of Public Hygiene
DPI inalador de pó (seco)
DPM Doctor of Physical Medicine; Doctor of Podiatric Medicine
DPN difosfopiridina nucleotídeo
DPT dipropiltriptamina; difteria, coqueluche e tétano (vacinas)
dr dracma
DR reação de degeneração
DRG grupo de diagnóstico correlato
DrPH Doctor of Public Health; Doctor of Public Hygiene
DRVVT teste com veneno da víbora de Russell (diluído)
D-S Doerfler-Stewart (teste)
DSA angiografia de subtração digital
dsDNA DNA com filamento duplo
dT desoxitimidina
DT *delirium tremens*; duração da tetania
dTDP 5-difosfato de desoxitimidina
dThd timidina
DTIC dimetiltrizenoimidazol carboxamida (dacarbazina)
dTMP ácido desoxitimidílico
DTP toxóides tetânico e diftérico e vacina de coqueluche; formigamento distal à percussão (sinal de Tinel)
DTPA ácido dietilenotriamina pentacético
DTR reflexo tendinoso profundo
dTTP 5´-trifosfato de desoxitimidina
dur. dol. [L.] *durante dolore*, enquanto perdurar a dor
DVM Doctor of Veterinary Medicine
Dx diagnóstico
Dy disprósio
ε épsilon; coeficiente de absorção molar; classe de cadeia pesada correspondendo à IgE
E exa-; extração (relação)
EB (vírus) Epstein-Barr
EBV vírus Epstein-Barr
ECF líquido extracelular
ECF-A fator quimiotáxico eosinofílico da anafilaxia
ECG eletrocardiograma
ECHO (vírus) órfão humano enterocitopatogênico
ECM eritema migratório crônico
ECMO oxigenação por membrana extracorpórea
ECS silêncio eletrocerebral
ECT terapia eletroconvulsiva
ED dose efetiva
EDTA ácido etilenodiaminotetracético (edatamil, ácido edético)
EEG eletroencefalograma
EENT olho, ouvido, nariz e garganta
EIA imunoensaio enzimático
EKG [Alemão] *Elektrokardiogramme*, eletrocardiograma
EKY eletroquimograma
ELISA ensaio imunossorvente ligado à enzima
EMC (vírus) encefalomiocardite
EMF força eletromotora
EMG eletromiografia; exonfalia, macroglossia e gigantismo (síndrome)
emp. [L.] *emplastrum, plaster; ex modo praescripto*, da maneira prescrita
ENG eletronistagmografia
ENT ouvido, nariz e garganta
EOG eletrooculografia
EPAP pressão expiratória positiva nas vias aéreas
Er érbio
ER retículo endoplasmático; sala de emergência
ERBF fluxo sangüíneo renal efetivo
ERCP colangiopancreatografia retrógrada endoscópica
ERG eletrorretinografia
ERPF fluxo plasmático renal efetivo
ERV volume de reserva expiratória
Es einstênio
ESEP potencial somatossensorial evocado extremo
ESP percepção extra-sensorial
ESR ressonância com densidade *spin*; velocidade de hemossedimentação
ESRD doença renal em estágio terminal
EtOH álcool etílico
Eu európio
ev elétron-volt
eV elétron-volt
f femto-; freqüência (respiratória)
F Fahrenheit; faraday (constante); fertilidade (fator); campo (de visão); flúor; força; fracionada (concentração); livre (energia)
F1.2 fragmento 1,2 (protrombina)
F₁ primeira geração de filhos
Fab fragmento da molécula de anticorpo envolvida na ligação do antígeno
FAD flavina-adenina dinucleotídeo; doença de Alzheimer familial
FANA anticorpo antinuclear fluorescente (teste)
FB corpo estranho
FBS glicemia em jejum
Fc fragmento constante de uma molécula de anticorpo
FDA Food and Drug Administration
Fe [L.] *ferrum*, ferro
FEF fluxo expiratório forçado
FET tempo expiratório forçado
FEV volume expiratório forçado
FF fração de filtração
FFD distância foco-filme
FHR freqüência cardíaca fetal
FHT batimentos cardíacos fetais
FIA imunoensaio fluorescente

FIGLU formiminoglutâmico (ácido)
FISH hibridização *in situ* fluorescente
Fm férmio
FMN flavina mononucleotídeo
fps, FPS pé-libra-segundo (sistema, unidade)
Fr frâncio; French (calibre, escala)
FRC capacidade residual funcional (dos pulmões)
FRF fator liberador do hormônio folículo-estimulante
FRS sintoma de primeira ordem
Fru frutose
FSH hormônio folículo-estimulante
FSH-RF fator liberador do hormônio folículo-estimulante
FSH-RH hormônio liberador do hormônio folículo-estimulante
ft. [L] *fiat*, deixar fazer
FTA-ABS absorção de anticorpo fluorescente antitreponêmico (teste)
FU fluorouracil
FUO febre de origem indeterminada
FVC capacidade vital forçada
Fw onda F (onda fibrilar, onda de flutter)
Fx fratura
γ gama; coeficiente de solubilidade de Ostwald; o terceiro em uma série; classe de cadeia pesada que corresponde à IgG
μg micrograma
g grama
G giga-; glicose; gravidade (constante newtoniana de); resíduos guanosina (ou ácido guanílico) em polinucleotídeos; grávida (história obstétrica)
G 1 intervalo 1
G 2 intervalo 2
G6P glicose-6-fosfato
Ga gálio
GABA ácido γ-aminobutírico
GABHS estreptococo β-hemolítico do grupo A
Gal galactose
GC gonococo, gonorréia
Gd gadolínio
GDP manose-1-fosfato guanililtransferase
Ge germânio
GERD doença do refluxo gastroesofágico
GFR taxa de filtração glomerular
GGT γ-glutamil transferase
GH glenoumeral; hormônio do crescimento
GHB γ-hidroxibutirato
GHRF fator liberador do hormônio do crescimento
GH-RF fator liberador do hormônio do crescimento
GHRH hormônio liberador do hormônio do crescimento
GH-RH hormônio liberador do hormônio do crescimento
GI gastrintestinal; Índice Gengival
GIP polipeptídeo inibidor gástrico
GLC cromatografia em gás-líquido
Gln glutamina; glutaminil
Glu ácido glutâmico; glutamil
Gly glicina; glicil
GMP monofosfato de guanosina (ácido guanílico)
GMS (corante) metenamina prata de Gomori (ou Grocott)
GnRH hormônio liberador de gonadotropina

GOT transaminase glutâmico-oxalacética (aspartato aminotransferase)
GPI Índice Gengivo-Periodontal
GPT transaminase glutâmico-pirúvica (alanina aminotransferase)
gr grão
grad. [L.] *gradatim*, gradualmente
GSH glutationa reduzida
GSR resposta cutânea galvânica
GSSG glutationa oxidada
gt. [L.] *gutta*, uma gota
GTP 5´-trifosfato de guanosina
gtt. [L.] *guttae*, gotas
GTT teste de tolerância à glicose
GU genitourinário
Guo guanosina
guttat. [L.] *guttatim*, gota a gota
GVHD doença enxerto-versus-hospedeiro
Gy gray (unidade de dose absorvida de radiação ionizante)
GYN ginecologia
h hecto-
h constante de Planck
α-h a forma helicoidal orientada para a direita adotada por muitas proteínas
H henry; hidrogênio; hiperopia; hiperópico
¹H hidrogênio-1 (prótio, hidrogênio leve)
²H hidrogênio-2 (deutério, hidrogênio pesado)
³H hidrogênio-3 (trítio, hidrogênio radioativo)
H⁺ íon hidrogênio
Ha hânio
HA ácido hialurônico; hemaglutinina
HAV vírus da hepatite A
Hb hemoglobina
HbA hemoglobina do adulto
HbA₁ principal componente da hemoglobina do adulto
HbA₂ fração menor da hemoglobina do adulto
HbAS heterozigosidade para a hemoglobina A e hemoglobina S (traço falciforme)
HB_cAg antígeno do cerne da hepatite B
HbCO carboxiemoglobina
HB_eAg antígeno inicial da hepatite B
HB_eAb anticorpo inicial da hepatite B
HB_eAg antígeno inicial da hepatite B
HBIG imunoglobulina da hepatite B
HbF hemoglobina fetal
HbO₂ oxiemoglobina, hemoglobina oxigenada
HbS hemoglobina falciforme
HB_sAb anticorpo de superfície da hepatite B
HB_sAg antígeno de superfície da hepatite B
HBV vírus da hepatite B
HCFA Health Care Financing Administration
HCG gonadotropina coriônica humana
HCS somatomamotropina coriônica humana (lactogênio placentário humano)
Hct hematócrito

h. d. [L.] *hora decubitus*, ao deitar
HDL lipoproteína de alta densidade
HDRV vacina diplóide humana (cepa celular) anti-rábica
He hélio
H&E hematoxilina e eosina
HEMPAS multinuclearidade eritroblástica hereditária associada a soro acidificado positivo
Hf háfnio
HFJV ventilação com jato de alta freqüência
HFOV ventilação oscilatória de alta freqüência
HFPPV ventilação com pressão positiva de alta freqüência
HFV ventilação de alta freqüência
Hg [L.] *hydrargyrum*, mercúrio
HGE erliquiose granulocítica humana
HGH hormônio de crescimento humano (hipofisário)
HGSIL lesão escamosa intra-epitelial de alto grau
HI inibição da hemaglutinação (teste, título)
His histidina
His- histidil
-His histidino
HIV vírus da imunodeficiência humana
HI hiperopia, latente
HLA antígeno linfocitário humano
Hm hiperopia, manifesta (hipermetropia)
HME erliquiose monocítica humana
HMG gonadotropina humana da menopausa
HMG CoA-3-hidroxi-3-metilglutaril coenzima A
HMO Health Maintenance Organization
HMWK cininogênio de alto peso molecular (fator Fletcher)
Ho hólmio
hor. decub. [L.] *hora decubitus*, ao deitar
hor. som. [L.] *hora somni*, ao deitar
HPF campo de grande aumento
HPI história da doença atual
HPL lactogênio placentário humano
HPLC cromatografia líquida de alta performance
HPV papilomavírus humano
h. s., HS [L.] *hora somni*, ao deitar
HSV herpesvírus simples
Ht hiperopia, total
5-HT 5-hidroxitriptamina (serotonina)
HTLV vírus linfocitotrófico da célula T humana; vírus da leucemia/linfoma da célula T humana
HVL camada de valor médio
Hx história (clínica)
Hyp hidroxiprolina
Hz hertz
I inspirado (gás) (SUBSCRITO); iodo
¹²³I iodo-123 (radioisótopo)
¹²⁵I iodo-125
¹³¹I iodo-131
IADL atividades instrumentais de vida diária
IAP porfiria aguda intermitente
ICD *International Classification of Diseases of the World Health Organization*

ICDA *International Classification of Diseases, Adapted for Use in the United States*
ICF líquido intracelular
ICP pressão intracraniana
ICSH hormônio estimulador da célula intersticial
ICU unidade de terapia intensiva
ID dose infecciosa
I&D incisão e drenagem
IDU idoxuridina
IF fator de iniciação; fator intrínseco
IFN interferon
Ig imunoglobulina
IGF fator de crescimento insulina-símile
IH hepatite infecciosa
IL interleucina
ILA atividade insulina-símile
Ile isoleucina
IM medicina interna; intramuscular (por via); mononucleose infecciosa
IMP monofosfato de inosina (ácido inosínico)
IMV ventilação mandatória intermitente
in d. [L.] *in dies*, diariamente
In índio
Ino inosina
INR relação normalizada internacional
int. cib. [L.] *inter cibos*, entre as refeições
I&O balanço hídrico
IOML linha infra-orbitomeatal
IP interfalângica; intraperitoneal (por via)
IPAP pressão positiva inspiratória nas vias aéreas
IPPB respiração com pressão positiva intermitente
IPPV ventilação com pressão positiva intermitente
IPV vacina de poliovírus inativado
IQ quociente de inteligência
Ir irídio
IRV volume de reserva inspiratória
ISI Índice Internacional de Sensibilidade
ITP purpura trombocitopênica idiopática; 5´-trifosfato de inosina
IU Unidade Internacional
IUCD dispositivo contraceptivo intra-uterino
IUD dispositivo intra-uterino
IV intravenoso, por via intravenosa; intraventricular
J joule
J fluxo (densidade)
K quilo-
K [L. Moderno] *kalium*, potássio; kelvin
K_M constante de Michaelis
kat catal
kb quilobase
kc quilociclo
kcal quilocaloria
KCT tempo de coagulação com caolin
kDa quilodalton
kg quilograma
KJ reflexo patelar
Kr criptônio
KS sarcoma de Kaposi
17-KS 17-cetosteróides
kv quilovolt

Apêndices

kVp quilovolt máximo
KW Kimmelstiel-Wilson (doença); Keith-Wagener (alterações retinianas)
μl, μL microlitro
l litro
L indutância; esquerda; [L.] *limes*, limite; litro
L- prefixo que indica que uma molécula é estericamente análoga ao L-gliceraldeído
La lantânio
LA anticoagulante lúpico
LAP leucina aminopeptidase
LATS estimulador tireóideo de ação prolongada
LBT teste lúpico
LC concentração letal
LCAT lecitina-colesterol aciltransferase
LCM coriomeningite linfocítica (vírus)
LD dose letal
LDH lactato desidrogenase, desidrogenase láctica
LDL lipoproteína de baixa densidade
LE olho esquerdo; lúpus eritematoso
LEEP procedimento de excisão eletrocirúrgica em alça
LES esfíncter esofágico inferior
LETS sensível à grande transformação externa (fibronectina)
Leu leucina
LFA frontoanterior esquerdo (posição fetal)
LFP frontoposterior esquerdo (posição fetal)
LFT frontotransversa esquerda (posição fetal)
LGSIL lesão escamosa intra-epitelial de baixo grau
LGV linfogranuloma venéreo
LH hormônio luteinizante
LH/FSH-RF hormônio luteinizante/ fator liberador do hormônio folículo-estimulante
LH-RF fator liberador do hormônio luteinizante
LH-RH hormônio liberador do hormônio luteinizante
Li lítio
LLQ quadrante inferior esquerdo
LM Licentiate in Midwifery
LMA mentoanterior esquerda (posição fetal)
LMP mentoposterior esquerda (posição fetal)
LMT mentotransversa esquerda (posição fetal)
LNPF fator de permeabilidade ganglionar
LOA occipitoanterior esquerda (posição fetal)
LOP occipitoposterior esquerda (posição fetal)
LOT occipitotransversa esquerda (posição fetal)
LPF campo de pequeno aumento
LPH hormônio hipofisário lipotrópico (lipotropina)
LPN Licensed Practical Nurse
Lr laurêncio
LRH hormônio liberador do hormônio luteinizante
LSA sacroanterior esquerda (posição fetal)
LSD dietilamida do ácido lisérgico
LSP sacroposterior esquerda (posição fetal)

L/S R relação lecitina/esfingomielina
LST sacrotransversa esquerda (posição fetal)
LTH hormônio luteotrópico
LTM memória de longo prazo
LTR repetição terminal longa
Lu lutécio
LUQ quadrante superior esquerdo
LVET tempo de ejeção do ventrículo esquerdo
LVH hipertrofia ventricular esquerda
LVN Licensed Visiting Nurse; Licensed Vocational Nurse
Lw (símbolo antigo para) laurêncio (atualmente Lr)
Lys lisina (ou seus radicais nos peptídeos)
μ mu; micro-; classe de cadeia pesada que corresponde à IgM
m massa; metro; milimínimo; molar
m- *meta-*
M mega-, meg-; molar; moles (por litro); morgan; miópico; miopia
M molar; moles (por litro)
m moles (por litro)
μμ micromicro-
μm micrômetro
mμ milimícron
mA miliampère
MA idade mental
MAA albumina macroagregada
M + Am astigmatismo miópico composto
MAC complexo *Mycobacterium avium*
MAI *Mycobacterium avium intracellulare*
man. pr. [L.] *mane primo*, de manhã cedo, primeira coisa ao acordar
MAO monoamina oxidase
MAOI inibidor da monoamina oxidase
MAP pílula do dia seguinte
mA-S miliampère-segundo
Mb mioglobina
MBC capacidade respiratória máxima
MbCO mioglobina com carbono monoxidado
MbO$_2$ oximioglobina
MC Medical Corps
MCH hemoglobina corpuscular média
MCHC concentração da hemoglobina corpuscular média
mCi milicurie
MCP metacarpofalângica
MCV volume corpuscular médio
Md mendelévio
MD [L.] *Medicinae Doctor*, Doutor em Medicina
MDF fator depressor do miocárdio
MDI inalador com dosímetro
Me metila
MEDLARS Medical Literature Analysis and Retrieval System
MEP pressão expiratória máxima
meq, mEq miliequivalente
Met metionina
MET equivalente metabólico da tarefa
metHb metemoglobina
metMb metemioglobina
MEV milhão de elétron-volts (10^6 ev)
mg miligrama

Mg magnésio
MHC complexo de histocompatibilidade principal
mho unidade siemens
MHz megahertz
MI infarto do miocárdio
MID dose infectante mínima
MIP pressão inspiratória máxima
MK menaquinona (vitamina K$_2$)
mks, MKS metro-quilograma-segundo (sistema, unidade)
ml, mL mililitro
MLC cultura mista de linfócitos (teste)
MLD dose letal mínima
mm milímetro
mmol milimol
MMPI Minnesota Multiphasic Personality Inventory
MMR sarampo-caxumba-rubéola (vacina)
Mn manganês
Mo molibdênio
MO Medical Officer; óleo mineral
mol mol
mol wt peso molecular
MOM Leite de Magnésia
MOPP Mustargen (cloridrato de mecloretamina), Oncovin (sulfato de vincristina), cloridrato de procarbazina e prednisona
mor. dict. [L.] *more dicto*, da maneira determinada
mor. sol. [L.] *more solito*, da forma habitual
MPD dose máxima permissível
MPS sistema de fagócitos mononucleares
MR anel de leite (teste)
M$_r$ relação molecular (peso)
mrd, MRD dose reagente mínima
MRI ressonância magnética
mRNA RNA mensageiro
ms milissegundo
MS esclerose múltipla; sulfato de morfina
msec milissegundo
MSG glutamato monossódico
MSH hormônio estimulante de melanócitos
mtDNA DNA mitocondrial
MTP metatarsofalângica (articulação)
Mu unidade Mache
MUGA aquisição com regulação múltipla (técnica de imagem)
mV milivolt
Mv mendelévio
MVE encefalite do vale Murray (vírus)
MVV ventilação voluntária máxima
MW peso molecular
My miopia
ν nu; viscosidade cinemática
n índice de refração; nano-
N newton; nitrogênio; normal (concentração)
N normal (letra MINÚSCULA)
Na [L. Moderno] *natrium*, sódio
NAD nicotinamida adenina dinucleotídeo; sem doença aguda
NAD$^+$ nicotinamida adenina dinucleotídeo (forma oxidada)
NADH nicotinamida adenina dinucleotídeo (forma reduzida)
NADP nicotinamida adenina dinucleotídeo fosfato
NADP$^+$ nicotinamida adenina dinucleotídeo fosfato (forma oxidada)

NADPH nicotinamida adenina dinucleotídeo fosfato (forma reduzida)
NAME nevos, mixoma atrial, neurofibromas mixóides e efélides (síndrome)
Nb nióbio
NCV velocidade de condução nervosa
Nd neodímio
Ne neon
NE norepinefrina; não examinado
NEEP pressão expiratória terminal negativa
NF National Formulary
ng nanograma
NGF fator de crescimento de nervos (antígeno)
Ni níquel
NIH National Institutes of Health
NK natural killer (célula), destruidora natural
NKA nenhuma alergia conhecida
NLM National Library of Medicine
nm nanômetro
NMN nicotinamida mononucleotídeo
No nobélio
noc. maneq. [L.] *nocte maneque*, à noite e pela manhã
Np netúnio
NREM sem movimento ocular rápido (sono)
nRNA RNA nuclear
NS soro fisiológico
NSAID agente antiinflamatório não-esteróide
NSR ritmo sinusal normal
NUG gengivite ulcerativa necrotizante
Ω ômega; ohm
o- *orto-*
O [L.] *oculus*, olho; abertura (nas fórmulas para reações elétricas); oxigênio
OAV oculoauriculovertebral (displasia, síndrome)
OB obstetrícia
OB/GYN obstetrícia (e) ginecologia
OBS síndrome cerebral orgânica
OC contraceptivo oral
OCD distúrbio obsessivo-compulsivo
OD Doctor of Optometry; [L.] *oculus dexter*, olho direito; overdose
ODD oculodentodigital (displasia, síndrome)
Oe oersted (unidade centímetro-grama-segundo de força do campo magnético)
OFD orofaciodigital (disostose, síndrome)
OKT (célula) T de Ortho-Kung
OML linha orbitomeatal
OMM (displasia, síndrome) oftalmomandibulomélica
omn. hor. [L.] *omni hora*, de hora em hora
OMS síndrome mental orgânica
OP pressão osmótica; paciente ambulatorial
O&P ovos e parasitas
OPV vacina oral com poliovírus
OR sala de cirurgia
ORD dispersão rotatória óptica
Orn ornitina (ou seu radical)

Oro orotato; ácido orótico
Os ósmio
OS [L.] *oculus sinister*, olho esquerdo
OSHA Occupational Safety and Health Administration
OT terapia ocupacional; tuberculina velha de Koch
OTC venda livre (medicamento vendido sem receita médica)
OU [L.] *oculus uterque*, cada olho (ambos os olhos)
OXT ocitocina
oz onça
p pico-; pupila
p- para-
P parcial (pressão); peta-; fósforo, fosfórico (resíduo); plasma (concentração); pressão; para (história obstétrica)
^{32}**P** fósforo-32
P$_1$ primeira geração parental
Pa Pascal; protactínio
PA Physician's Assistant
PABA ácido para-aminobenzóico
PAF fator agregador (ou ativador) de plaqueta
PAH para-amino-hipúrico (ácido)
PAO$_2$ pressão parcial de oxigênio arterial
part. aeq. [L.] *partes aequales*, partes iguais (quantidades)
part. vic. [L.] *partes vicibus*, em doses divididas
PAS para-aminossalicílico (ácido), ácido periódico de Schiff (reagente)
PASA ácido para-aminossalicílico
PAT taquicardia atrial paroxística
Pb [L.] *plumbum*, chumbo
PBG porfobilinogênio
pc [L.] *post cibum*, após uma refeição
PCB bifenil policlorado
Pco$_2$ pressão parcial de dióxido de carbono
PCP fenciclidina
Pd paládio
PD dioptria do prisma
PDGF fator de crescimento derivado da plaqueta
PDLL linfoma linfocítico pouco diferenciado
PEEP pressão expiratória terminal positiva
PEG polietilenoglicol
PET tomografia com emissão de pósitrons
PF$_4$ fator 4 plaquetário
PFT prova de função pulmonar
pg picograma
PG prostaglandina
PGA prostaglandina A
PGB prostaglandina B
PGE prostaglandina E
PGF prostaglandina F
pH concentração de íon hidrogênio; log decádico negativo da [H$^+$]
Ph fenil
Ph^1 Filadélfia (cromossoma)
PHA fitoemaglutinina (antígeno)
Pharm D [L.] *Pharmaciae Doctor*, Doutor em Farmácia
PhD [L.] *Philosophiae Doctor*, Doutor em Filosofia
Phe fenilalanina (ou seu radical)
PhG Graduado em Farmácia
PhG [L.] *Pharmacopoeia Germanica*, Farmacopéia Germânica

PICC cateter central com inserção periférica
PID doença inflamatória pélvica
PIF fator inibitório da prolactina
PIP (articulação) interfalângica proximal
pK logaritmo negativo da constante de ionização (K$_a$) de um ácido
PK piruvatoquinase, piruvatocinase
PKU fenilcetonúria
pm picômetro
Pm prométio
PM *post mortem*
PMN polimorfonuclear (leucócito)
PMS síndrome pré-menstrual
PND dispnéia paroxística noturna; gotejamento pós-nasal
PNP procedimento de neutralização de plaquetas
PNPB ventilação com pressão positiva-negativa
Po polônio
PO [L.] *per os*, por via oral
PO$_2$, Po$_2$ pressão parcial de oxigênio
POEMS polineuropatia, organomegalia, endocrinopatia, proteína monoclonal e alterações cutâneas (síndrome)
POMP prednisona, Oncovin (sulfato de vincristina), metotrexato e Purinethol (6-mercaptopurina)
POR prontuário orientado por problema
PP pirofosfato
PPCA pró-acelerador da conversão da protrombina sérica
PPD derivado protéico purificado (da tuberculina)
PPLO microrganismo semelhante à pleuropneumonia
ppm partes por milhão
PPO 2,5-difeniloxazol
PPPPP dor, palidez, ausência de pulso, parestesia, paralisia
PPPPPP dor, palidez, ausência de pulso, parestesia, paralisia, prostração
PPV ventilação com pressão positiva
Pr praseodímio; presbiopia
PRA atividade da renina plasmática
PRF fator liberador de prolactina
PRL prolactina
prn [L.] *pro re nata*, quando necessário, SOS
PRN [L.] *pro re nata*, quando necessário, SOS
pro rat. aet. [L.] *pro ratione aetatis*, de acordo com a idade (do paciente)
Pro prolina (ou seus radicais)
psi libras por polegada quadrada
PSV ventilação mantida por pressão
Pt platina
PT fisioterapia; tempo de protrombina
PTA antecessor da tromboplastina plasmática; ácido fosfotúngstico; antes da internação
PTAH hematoxilina e ácido fosfotúngstico
PTCA angioplastia coronária transluminal percutânea

PTH paratormônio
PTU propiltiouracil
Pu plutônio
PUO febre (pirexia) de origem indeterminada
PUPPP pápulas e placas urticariformes pruriginosas da gravidez
PUVA (administração oral de) psoraleno (e subseqüente exposição ao) comprimento de onda A da luz ultravioleta (UV-A)
PVC cloreto de polivinila; contração ventricular prematura
PVP polivinilpirrolidona (povidona)
Q volume de fluxo sangüíneo
Q coulomb
Qco$_2$ microlitros de CO$_2$ retirados por miligrama de peso seco de tecido por hora
qd [L.] *quaque die*, a cada dia
qh [L.] *quaque hora*, a cada hora
qid [L.] *quater in die*, quatro vezes ao dia
q. l. [L.] *quantum libet*, tanto quanto for desejado
QNS quantidade insuficiente
Qo consumo de oxigênio
Qo$_2$ consumo de oxigênio
q. s. [L.] *quantum satis*, quanto for suficiente; [L.] *quantum sufficiat*, quanto pode ser suficiente; quantidade suficiente
r racêmico, roentgen
R constante gasosa (8,315 joules); radical (orgânico); Réamur (escala); [L.] *recipe*, tomar; resistência determinante (plasmídeo); resistência (elétrica); resistência (unidade) (no sistema cardiovascular); resolução; respiração; respiratória (razão de troca); roentgen
Ra rádio
RA artrite reumatóide
rad radiano
RAS sistema ativador reticular
RAST teste radioalergossorvente
RAV vírus Rous-associado
RAW resistência, vias aéreas
Rb rubídio
rbc eritrócito; contagem de hemácias
RBC eritrócito; contagem de hemácias
RBF fluxo sangüíneo renal
RD reação de degeneração; reação de desnervação; Registered Dietician
RDA cota diária recomendada
rDNA DNA ribossomial
RDH Registered Dental Hygienist
RDS síndrome de angústia respiratória
RDW índice de anisocitose
Re rênio
RE orelha direita; olho direito
rem roentgen-equivalente, homem
REM movimento ocular rápido (sono); mucinose eritematosa reticular
rep roentgen-equivalente, físico
RF fator liberador; fator reumatóide
RFA frontoanterior direita (posição fetal)
RFLP polimorfismo do comprimento do fragmento de restrição
RFP frontoposterior direita (posição fetal)
RFT frontotransversa direita (posição fetal)

Rh Rhesus (grupo sangüíneo Rh); ródio
RH hormônio liberador
RIA radioimunoensaio
Rib ribose
RLL lobo inferior direito
RLQ quadrante inferior direito
RMA mentoanterior direita (posição fetal)
RML lobo médio direito
RMP mentoposterior direita (posição fetal)
RMT mentotransversa esquerda (posição fetal)
Rn radônio
RN Registered Nurse
RNA ácido ribonucléico
RNase ribonuclease
RNP ribonucleoproteína
ROA occipitoanterior direita (posição fetal)
ROM amplitude de movimento
ROP occipitoposterior direita (posição fetal)
ROT occipitotransversa direita (posição fetal)
RP retinite pigmentosa
RPF fluxo plasmático renal
RPh Registered Pharmacist
rpm rotações por minuto
RPR reagente plasmático rápido (teste)
RQ quociente respiratório
rRNA RNA ribossomial
Rs resolução
RS sincicial respiratório (vírus)
RSA sacroanterior direita (posição fetal)
RSP sacroposterior direita (posição fetal)
RST sacrotransversa direita (posição fetal)
RSV vírus do sarcoma de Rous; vírus sincicial respiratório
rTMP ácido ribotimidílico
Ru rutênio
RUL lobo superior direito
RUQ quadrante superior direito
RV volume residual
RVH hipertrofia ventricular direita
℞ [L.] *recipe* (a primeira palavra em uma prescrição), tomar; prescrição; tratamento
σ sigma; coeficiente de reflexão; desvio-padrão; 1 milissegundo (0,001 s)
s [L.] *semis*, metade; estado de equilíbrio dinâmico (SUBSCRITO); [L.] *sinister*, esquerdo
S [L.] *sinister*, esquerdo; saturação da hemoglobina (porcentagem de) (seguido pelo subscrito o$_2$ ou co$_2$); siemens; esférico; esférica (lente); enxofre; Svedberg (unidade)
S$_1$ primeira geração própria
S-A sinoatrial
SaO$_2$ saturação arterial de oxigênio (oxiemoglobina)
sat. saturado
sat. sol. solução saturada
Sb [L.] *stibium*, antimônio
SBE endocardite bacteriana subaguda
sc subcutânea (por via)
Sc escândio
SC esternoclavicular; subcutânea (por via)
SCID imunodeficiência combinada grave

SD desvio-padrão; estreptodornase
SDA ação dinâmica específica
Se selênio
Ser serina
Sf flutuação de Svedberg (constante, unidade)
SGOT transaminase glutâmico-oxalacética sérica (aspartato aminotransferase)
SGPT transaminase glutâmico-pirúvica sérica (alanina aminotransferase)
SH hepatite sérica
Si silício
SI [Francês] Système International d'Unités; International System of Units
SID distância fonte-imagem (receptor)
SIDS síndrome da morte súbita infantil
sig. [L.] *signa*, afixar um rótulo, inscrever
SIMV ventilação mandatória intermitente espontânea; ventilação mandatória intermitente sincronizada
SIRD distância fonte-imagem-receptor
SISI (teste) índice de sensibilidade de pequeno aumento (ou aumento curto)
SK estreptoquinase
SLE lúpus eritematoso sistêmico
SLR levantamento da perna reta
Sm samário
Sn [L.] *stannum*, estanho
SOAP dados subjetivos, dados objetivos, avaliação e plano (prontuário orientado por problema)
SOB dispnéia
sol. solução
soln. solução
s.o.s. [L.] *si opus sit*, se necessário
sp. espécie
SPCA acelerador da conversão da protrombina sérica (fator VII)
SPECT tomografia computadorizada com emissão fotônica única
SPF fator de proteção solar
sp. gr. densidade
sph esférica (lente)
spm supressão e mutação
spp. espécies (plural)
SQ subcutânea
Sr estrôncio
SRF fator liberador de somatotropina
SRF-A fator de anafilaxia de liberação lenta
SRIF fator inibidor da liberação de somatotropina
sRNA RNA solúvel
SRS substância de reação lenta (da anafilaxia)
SRS-A substância de reação lenta da anafilaxia
ssDNA DNA de filamento único
ssp. subespécie

SSRI inibidor seletivo da recaptação de serotonina
ST escapulotorácico
stat [L.] *statim*, imediatamente, de imediato
STD doença sexualmente transmitida
STEL limite de exposição de curto prazo
STH hormônio somatotrópico
STM memória de curto prazo
STPD temperatura padrão (0°C) e pressão (760 mm Hg absoluto), ar seco
Sv sievert (unidade)
SV sievert (unidade)
SVT taquicardia supraventricular
t tonelada métrica
t temperatura (Celsius); trítio
α-T α-tocoferol
T temperatura, absoluta (Kelvin); tensão (intra-ocular); tera-; tesla; tétano (toxóide); corrente (volume) (SUBSCRITO); tocoferol; transverso (túbulo); trítio; tumor (antígeno)
T temperatura absoluta (Kelvin)
T₃ 3,5,5′-triiodotironina
T₄ tetraiodotironina (tiroxina)
T! tensão diminuída (pressão)
T+ tensão aumentada (pressão)
Ta tântalo
TA *Terminologia Anatomica*
TAD dermatose acantolítica transitória
TAF fator de angiogênese tumoral
TAR trombocitopenia associada a ausência do rádio (síndrome)
TAT teste de apreciação temática
Tb térbio
TB tuberculose
TBP proteína fixadora de tiroxina
TBV volume sangüíneo total
Tc tecnécio
⁹⁹ᵐTc tecnécio-99m
T&C tipagem e prova cruzada
TCA ácido tricarboxílico; ácido tricloroacético
TCN talocalcaneonavicular (articulação)
Td tetânico-diftérico (toxóides, tipo adulto)
TDP 5′-difosfato de ribotimidina
Te telúrio
TEDD diâmetro diastólico terminal total
TEN necrólise epidérmica tóxica
TESD diâmetro sistólico terminal total
Th tório
THC tetraidrocanabinol
Thr treonina (ou seus radicais)
t/t_tot ciclo de responsabilidade
Ti titânio
TIA crise isquêmica transitória
t.i.d. *ter in die*, três vezes ao dia
tinct. tintura
TITh 3,5,3′-triiodotironina
TKO manter (cateter de infusão venosa)

Tl tálio
TLC cromatografia em camada fina; capacidade pulmonar total; atendimento delicado, carinhoso
TLV valor limítrofe
t_m temperatura de ponto médio (Celsius)
Tm túlio; tubular máxima (capacidade excretora do rim)
T_m temperatura em ponto médio (Kelvin)
TM transporte máximo
TMJ articulação temporomandibular
TMP 5′-monofosfato de ribotimidina
TMT tarsometatarsal
TMV vírus do mosaico do tabaco
Tn tensão (ocular); tensão normal (intra-ocular)
TNF fator de necrose tumoral
TNM tumor, linfonodo, metástase (estagiamento tumoral)
TORCH toxoplasmose, outra, rubéola, citomegalovírus e herpes simples (infecções maternas)
t-PA, TPA ativador do plasminogênio tecidual
TPHA hemaglutinação do *Treponema pallidum* (teste)
TPI imobilização do *Treponema pallidum* (teste)
TPN nutrição parenteral total
TPR temperatura, pulso e pressão
tr. tintura
TRH hormônio liberador de tireotropina (teste de estimulação)
TRIC conjuntivite de inclusão do tracoma (microrganismo)
tRNA RNA de transferência
Trp triptofano (e seus radicais)
TSH hormônio tireoestimulante
TSS síndrome do choque tóxico
TSTA antígeno de transplante tumor-específico
TTP púrpura trombocitopênica idiopática
TU unidade tóxica; unidade de toxina
Tyr tirosina (e seus radicais)
U unidade; urânio; uridina (em polímeros); urinária (concentração)
UA exame de urina
UDP difosfato de uridina
UDPG UDP-glicose
UGIS seriografia esôfago-estômago-duodeno
UMP monofosfato de uridina (ácido uridílico)
ung. [L.] *unguentum*, pomada
u-PA uroquinase
Urd uridina
URI infecção respiratória alta
USAN United States Adopted Names (Council)
USP *United States Phamacopoeia*
USPHS United States Public Health Service
UTI infecção do trato urinário
UTP trifosfato de uridina
UV ultravioleta
v venoso (sangue); volt

V vanádio; visão; visual (acuidade); volt; volume (freqüentemente com subscritos indicando localização, espécie química e condições)
V̇ ventilação; fluxo de gás (freqüentemente com subscritos indicando a localização e a espécie química); ventilação
V₁CV₆ derivações torácicas do eletrocardiograma precordial unipolar
VA antígeno viral
V_A ventilação alveolar
V-A ventriculoatrial
Val valina (e seus radicais)
Va/Q relação ventilação/perfusão
VATER defeitos vertebrais, ânus imperfurado, fístula traqueoesofágica com atresia de esôfago, e displasia radial e renal (complexo)
VC visão, em cores; capacidade vital
VCE vagina, (ecto)cérvice, canal endocervical
V_D espaço morto (fisiológico)
VDRL Venereal Disease Research Laboratory (teste)
VHDL lipoproteína de densidade muito alta
VIP polipeptídeo intestinal vasoativo
VLDL lipoproteína de densidade muito baixa
VMA ácido vanililmandélico (teste)
V_max velocidade máxima
VP vasopressina
VR ressonância vocal
VS solução volumétrica
V_T volume corrente
W watt; [Alemão] *Wolfram*, tungstênio
Wb weber
WBC contagem de leucócitos; leucograma
WD bem-desenvolvido
WDLL linfoma linfocítico (ou linfático) bem-diferenciado
WHO World Health Organization
WN bem-nutrido
X xantosina
Xao xantosina
Xe xenônio
¹³³Xe xenônio-133
XU urografia excretora
Y ítrio
YAG ítrio-alumínio-granada (laser)
Yb itérbio
Z carbobenzoxi (cloreto)
ZEEP pressão expiratória terminal zero
ZES síndrome de Zollinger-Ellison
Zn zinco
⁶⁵Zn zinco-65
Zr zircônio
ZSR velocidade de sedimentação zeta

SÍMBOLOS

Ângulos, Triângulos e Círculos

∧   acima • pressão arterial diastólica (registros anestésicos) • elevado • aumentado • melhorado • crescido • superior (posição) • acima

∨   abaixo • diminuído • deficiência • déficit • deprimido • deteriorado • reduzido • abaixado • inferior (posição) • mais baixo • pressão arterial sistólica (registros anestésicos)

>   causa • demonstra • distal • seguido por • derivado de • maior que • indica • leva a • mais grave que • produz • irradia-se para • irradiando-se até • resulta em • revela • mostra • para • no sentido de • pior que • produz

<   causado por • derivado de • menos grave que • menor que • produzido por • proximal

∠   ângulo • flexão • flexor

∠E   ângulo de entrada

∠X   ângulo de saída

⌞   produto fatorial • quadrante inferior direito

⌜   quadrante superior direito

⌐   quadrante superior esquerdo

⌟   quadrante inferior esquerdo

Δ   intervalo aniônico • prisma central • alteração • intervalo delta • calor • acréscimo • triângulo occipital • dioptria do prisma • temperatura (registros anestésicos)

Δ+   intervalo de tempo

Δ A   alteração na absorvência

Δ dB   diferença em decibéis

Δ P   alteração na pressão (intra-ocular)

Δ pH   alteração no pH

Δ t   intervalo de tempo

ΔH, HΔ   triângulo de Hesselbach

○   respiração (registros anestésicos)

♀   mulher • sexo feminino

♂   homem • sexo masculino

Ⓐ, ⓐx   axilar (temperatura)

Ⓗ, ⓗ   hipodérmico • por via hipodérmica

ⒾⓂ   intramuscular • por via intramuscular

Ⓘ︎Ⓥ   intravenoso • por via intravenosa

Ⓛ   esquerda

Ⓜ   sopro

ⓜ   por via oral • bucal (temperatura) • sopro

√ⓜ   sopro artificial

Ⓞ   pela boca • oral • por via oral

Ⓡ   retal • por via retal • retal (temperatura) • direita

Ⓧ   término da anestesia (registro anestésico) • término da cirurgia

Setas

↑   acima • elevado • elevação • alargado • gás • maior que • melhorado • aumento • aumentado • aumenta • maior que • crescente • superior (posição) • para cima • superior

↑g   aumentando • crescente

↑V   aumento devido a efeito *in vivo* (lab)

↓   abaixo • diminuir • diminuído • deficiência • déficit • deprimido • depressão • deteriorado • deteriorando • abaixado • diminuição • para baixo • caindo • inferior (posição) • menor que • mais baixo que • reflexo plantar normal • precipitado • precipita

↓g   decrescente • diminuindo • caindo • abaixando

↓V   diminuição devido a efeito *in vivo* (lab)

↗   desviado • deslocado • crescendo

↘   diminuindo

→   aproxima-se do limite de • demonstra as causas • direção do fluxo ou reação • distal • devido a • seguido por • indica • leva a • produz • irradiando-se para • resulta em • revela • mostra • para • para a direita • no sentido de • fornece

←   causado por • derivado de • direção do fluxo ou reação • devido a • produzido por • proximal • resultando de • secundário a • para a esquerda

↑↑   resposta extensora (sinal de Babinski) • Babinski positivo • testículos ectópicos

↓↓   para baixo bilateralmente • resposta plantar (sinal de Babinski) • testículos tópicos

↓↑   reação reversível • para cima e para baixo

⇆, ⇌   reação reversível (química)

Símbolos Genéticos

☐	masculino		■●	probando (primeiro membro da família afetado que procura cuidados médicos)
○	feminino			
◇	sexo não-especificado		☐	profissionalmente examinado • normal para o traço
☐○	indivíduos normais		☐	não examinado • relato duvidoso de que é portador do traço
■●◆	indivíduo afetado (com ≥ 2 condições, o símbolo é dividido e sombreado com um enchimento diferente definido em uma chave ou legenda)		☐	não examinado • relato confiável de que é portador do traço
			◧ ◐	heterozigotos para traço autossômico recessivo
⑤ ⑤ ⑤	múltiplos indivíduos, número conhecido (número de filhos escrito dentro do símbolo)		⊙	portador de traço recessivo ligado ao sexo
ⓝ ⓝ ⓝ	múltiplos indivíduos, número desconhecido ("n" usado no lugar do número específico)		⊘ ∅	morte
			(SB 28, SB 30, SB 34 semanas)	natimorto (SB)
☐—○	cruzamento			
☐=○	consangüinidade		(LMP 7/1/94, P 20 semanas, P)	gestação (P); idade gestacional e cariótipo (se conhecido) abaixo do símbolo
(+)	modalidade de herança incomum ou incerta			
I ☐○ / II ☐○	pais e descendentes, em gerações		↗☐ ↗○	consultante (indivíduo que procura aconselhamento genético/teste)
☐∧○	gêmeos dizigóticos		△ △ △ (masculino, feminino, ECT)	aborto espontâneo (SAB); ECT abaixo do símbolo indica prenhez ectópica
☐∧○	gêmeos monozigóticos			
④ ③	número de crianças do sexo indicado		▲ ▲ ▲ (masculino, feminino, 16 semanas)	SAB afetado (idade gestacional, quando conhecida, abaixo do símbolo, e chave ou legenda usada para definir o sombreamento)
☐ ○	indivíduos adotados			
⚰ ⚰	indivíduo morto sem deixar prole		△ △ △ (masculino, feminino)	término da gestação (TOP)
☐○	sem filhos			
■●	indivíduos afetados		▲ ▲ ▲ (masculino, feminino)	TOP afetado (chave ou legenda usada para definir o sombreamento)

Fonte: Os símbolos genéticos são de domínio público; reconhecemos o *American Journal of Human Genetics* (56:746–747, 1995) como nossa fonte para esses símbolos.
LMP = data da última menstruação.

Números

0	completamente ausente (pulso) sem resposta (reflexos)
+1, 1+	bastante comprometido (pulso)
1+	normal baixo ou um tanto diminuído (reflexos) reação leve ou residual (exames laboratoriais)
+2, 2+	moderadamente comprometido (pulso)
2+	média ou normais (reflexos) reação perceptível ou residual (exames laboratoriais)
+3, 3+	ligeiramente comprometido (pulso)
3+	reação moderada (exames laboratoriais) mais brusco que a média (reflexos)
+4, 4+	normal (pulso)
4+	hiperativos (reflexos) grande quantidade (exames laboratoriais) reação pronunciada (exames laboratoriais)
•	muito vigoroso (reflexos)
$\bar{1}$	defecação (o numeral indica o número de evacuações em um determinado período)
1×	único uma vez
2×, ×2	duplo duas vezes
3×, ×3	três vezes etc.

SÍMBOLOS

Arábico	Romano
0	
1	I,
2	II, ii
3	III, iii
4	IV, iv
5	V, v
6	VI, vi
7	VII, vii
8	VIII, viii
9	IX, ix
10	X, x
11	XI, xi
12	XII, xii
13	XIII, xiii
14	XIV, xiv
15	XV
16	XVI
17	XVII
18	XVIII
19	XIX
20	XX
30	XXX
40	XL
50	L
60	LX
70	LXX
80	LXXX
90	XC
100	C
1.000	M
5.000	$\overline{V}$
10.000	$\overline{X}$
100.000	$\overline{C}$
1.000.000	$\overline{M}$

Sinais Positivos, Negativos e Equivalências

Símbolo	Significado
+	ácida (reação) • adicionado a • lente convexa • diminuído ou deprimido (reflexos) • excesso • menos que 50% • inibição de • hemólise (Wassermann) • normal baixo (reflexos) • bastante comprometido (pulso) • leve (gravidade) • mais • positivo (exames laboratoriais) • presente • reação discreta ou residual (exames laboratoriais) • lentos (reflexos) • um tanto diminuído (reflexos)
(+)	significativo
(+)ive	positivo
+ a ++	dor discreta
++	médio (reflexos) • inibição de 50% da hemólise (Wassermann) • moderada (dor, gravidade) • moderadamente comprometido (pulso) • normalmente ativo (reflexos) • reação perceptível ou residual (exames laboratoriais)
+++	reflexos aumentados • inibição de 75% da hemólise (Wassermann) • quantidade moderada • reação moderada (exames laboratoriais) • moderadamente hiperativo (reflexos) • moderadamente grave (dor, gravidade) • mais vigoroso que a média (reflexos) • pouco comprometido (pulso)
++++	inibição completa da hemólise (Wassermann) • grande quantidade (exames laboratoriais) • bastante hiperativo (reflexos) • moderadamente grave (dor, gravidade) • normal (pulso) • reação pronunciada (exames laboratoriais) • muito vigoroso (reflexos)
−	ausente • alcalina (reação) • lente côncava • deficiência • deficiente • menos • negativo (exame laboratorial) • nenhum • subtrair • sem
(−)	insignificante
±	duvidoso • positivo ou negativo • duvidoso (reflexos, exames qualitativos) • adejantes (reflexos) • indefinido • mais ou menos • possivelmente significativo • questionável • sugestivo • variável • muito discreto (reação, gravidade, resíduo) • com ou sem
(±)	possivelmente significativo
± a +	dor mínima
∓	menos ou mais
‡	moderada (gravidade) • normalmente ativo (reflexos)
#	fratura • calibre • número • libra(s) • peso
∼	cerca de • aproximado • aproximadamente • proporcional a
≈	aproximadamente igual a
=	igual a
±	diferente de
○	combinado a
⇌	equivalente
≄	não equivalente a
≡	idêntico • idêntico a
≢	não idêntico • não idêntico a
≒	quase igual a
÷	aproximadamente igual a
≅	aproximadamente • aproximadamente igual • congruente com
≐	aproxima-se
⊥	equilateral
△	equiangular
>	maior que
≥	não maior que
<	menor que
≤	não menor que
≥, ⩾	maior ou igual a
≤, ⩽	menor ou igual a

Primos, Marcas, Pontos, Raízes e Outros Símbolos

?	duvidoso • equívoco (reflexos) • adejante (reflexos) • não testado (gravidade) • possível • questionável • dúvida • sugerido • sugestivo (gravidade) • desconhecido	$\sqrt{}$qs	eliminado volume suficiente
!	produto fatorial	$\sqrt{}$	raiz
†	morte • falecido	$\sqrt[2]{}$	raiz quadrada
/	dividido por • duplo significado • extensão • fração dos extensores • de • por • para	$\sqrt[3]{}$	raiz cúbica
′	pé • hora • univalente	*	nascimento • sinal de multiplicação • (genética) • não verificado • presumido • suposto
″	bivalente • idem • polegada • minuto • segundo (1/60 graus)	°	grau • medição (1/360 do círculo) • gravidade (queimaduras, feridas) • temperatura • tempo (hora)
‴	linha (0,2 mm) • trivalente	:	está para • relação
$\sqrt{}$	verificação • observar • urina • micção (urina)	...	nenhum dado (em determinada categoria)
$\sqrt{}$.	urina e defecação • micções e evacuações realizadas	∴	portanto
$\sqrt{\overline{c}}$	verificar com	∵	porque • como
$\sqrt{}$**d**	verificado • observado	::	como • igualdade entre relações • proporção • proporcional a
$\sqrt{}$**g**, $\sqrt{}$**ing**	verificando		

Símbolos Estatísticos

α	probabilidade de erro do Tipo I / nível de significância	s	desvio-padrão da amostra
β	probabilidade de erro do Tipo II	s^2	variância da amostra
$1-\beta$	eficácia do teste estatístico	SE	erro padrão da estimativa
$n^C k; \binom{n}{k}$	coeficiente do binômio / número de combinações de n coisas a partir de k em um período	σ	desvio-padrão da população
		σ^2	variância da população
χ^2	estatística do qui-quadrado	$\sigma_{diff.}$	erro padrão da diferença entre os resultados
E	freqüência esperada na célula do quadro de contingências	$\sigma_{est.}$	erro padrão da estimativa
$E(X)$	valor esperado da variável X aleatória	$\sigma_{meas.}$	erro padrão da medida
F	estatística F (relação de variância)	$\sum_{i=1}^{n} x_i, \sum_i^n x_i$	$x_1 + x_2 + \ldots + x_n$
f	freqüência	t	estatística t de Student / variável do teste de Student
H_0	hipótese nula		
H_1	hipótese alternativa	θ	traço latente
μ	população média	U	estatística do somatório de classificação de Mann-Whitney
N	tamanho da população	W	estatística do somatório da classificação de Wilcoxon
n	tamanho da amostra	$\overline{X}$	média da amostra
$n!$	fatorial	$|x|$	valor absoluto de x
O	freqüência observada em um quadro de contingência	$\sqrt{x}$	raiz quadrada de x
ϕ	coeficiente phi do continuum de capacidade	z	escore padrão
P	probabilidade	=	igual
p	probabilidade de sucesso em tentativas independentes	≠	desigual
$P(A)$	probabilidade de que um evento A ocorra	≈	aproximadamente igual
$P(A\backslash B)$	probabilidade condicionada de que A ocorra desde que B tenha ocorrido	>	maior que
		≥	não maior que
r	coeficiente de correlação da amostra, geralmente a correlação de momento-produto de Pearson	<	menor que
		≤	não menor que
r^2	coeficiente de determinação	≥, ⩾	maior ou igual a
r_s	classificação de Spearman correlação coeficiente	≤, ⩽	menor ou igual a
		∞	infinito
ρ	coeficiente de correlação populacional		

ARTÉRIAS DO CORPO HUMANO

Artéria/Artérias	Origem	Trajeto	Ramos/Distribuição
Alveolar inferior	1.ª parte da artéria maxilar	Desce posterior ao nervo de mesmo nome entre o músculo pterigóideo medial e o ramo da mandíbula para entrar no canal mandibular através do forame mandibular	Ramos: ramo milo-hióideo, ramos dentais, ramo mental; nutre os músculos do assoalho da boca, mandíbula e dentes inferiores, tecidos moles do queixo
Alveolar superior anterior	Artéria infra-orbital	Surge dentro do canal infra-orbital e ascende através dos canais alveolares anteriores	Irriga a mucosa do seio maxilar, e os dentes incisivos e caninos da maxila
Alveolar superior posterior	3.ª parte da artéria maxilar	Sai a partir da fossa pterigopalatina por meio da fissura pterigomaxilar; ramifica-se e penetra na superfície infratemporal da maxila, com alguns ramos entrando nos canais alveolares e outros continuando sobre o processo alveolar	Nutre a mucosa do seio maxilar, dentes molares e pré-molares maxilares, e gengiva adjacente
Angular	Ramo terminal da artéria facial	Passa para o ângulo medial (canto) do olho	Parte superior da bochecha e pálpebra inferior
Apendicular	Artéria ileocólica	Passa entre as camadas do mesoapêndice	Apêndice vermiforme
Arco da aorta	Continuação da parte ascendente da aorta	Arqueia-se posteriormente no lado esquerdo da traquéia e esôfago e superior à raiz do pulmão esquerdo	Tronco braquiocefálico, artéria carótida comum esquerda, artéria subclávia esquerda
Arco palmar profundo	Continuação direta da artéria radial, completada no lado medial pelo ramo profundo da artéria ulnar	Curva-se medialmente, sob os tendões flexores longos em contato com as bases dos metacarpais	Ramos: artérias metacarpais palmares
Arco palmar superficial	Continuação direta da artéria ulnar; o arco é completado no lado lateral pelo ramo superficial da artéria radial ou outro de seus ramos	Curva-se lateralmente sob a aponeurose palmar e superficial aos tendões dos flexores longos; a curva do arco situa-se através da região palmar no nível da borda distal do polegar estendido	Ramos: três artérias digitais palmares comuns
Arco plantar profundo	Continuação da artéria plantar lateral	Corre ântero-medialmente entre a 3.ª e a 4.ª camada dos músculos da planta do pé; anastomosa-se com a artéria dorsal do pé por meio da artéria plantar profunda entre a 1.ª e 2.ª bases dos metatarsais	Ramos: artérias metatarsais plantares
Arqueada (do pé)	Continuação da dorsal do pé	Passa lateralmente, dorsal às bases dos metatarsais	2.ª, 3.ª e 4.ª artérias metatarsais dorsais
Artéria braquial profunda	Artéria braquial próximo à sua origem	Acompanha o nervo radial através do sulco radial no úmero; os ramos terminais fazem parte da anastomose ao redor da articulação do cotovelo	Ramos: ramos deltóide, muscular (para a cabeça do tríceps) e nutrício (para o úmero) Ramos terminais: artérias colaterais média e radial
Artéria central da retina	Artéria oftálmica	Corre na bainha dural do nervo óptico e perfura o nervo próximo ao globo ocular; ramifica-se a partir do centro do disco óptico nas arteríolas retinianas	Irriga a parte óptica da retina (exceto cones e bastonetes); ramos: arteríolas macular, retiniana nasal e temporal
Artéria circunflexa da escápula	Ramo terminal (com a artéria toracodorsal) da artéria subescapular	Curva-se ao redor da borda axilar da escápula e entra na fossa infra-espinal	Irriga os músculos subescapular e infra-espinal; une-se à anastomose colateral do ombro ao redor da escápula
Artéria do bulbo do pênis ou do vestíbulo da vagina	Artéria pudenda interna	Perfura a membrana perineal para alcançar o bulbo do pênis ou o vestíbulo da vagina	Irriga o bulbo do pênis ou o vestíbulo e a glândula bulbouretral (masculino) e a glândula vestibular maior (feminino)
Artéria do canal pterigóideo	3.ª parte da artéria maxilar ou a partir da artéria palatina maior	Passa posteriormente através do canal pterigóideo	Mucosa da porção mais superior da faringe (recesso faríngeo), tuba auditiva e cavidade timpânica
Artéria do ducto deferente	Vesical inferior (ou superior)	Avança pelo retroperitônio até o ducto deferente	Ducto deferente
Artéria dorsal do pênis ou do clitóris	Ramo terminal da artéria pudenda interna	Perfura a membrana perineal e atravessa o ligamento suspensor do pênis ou do clitóris para correr no dorso do pênis ou clitóris	Pele do pênis e tecido erétil do pênis ou clitóris

Artéria/Artérias	Origem	Trajeto	Ramos/Distribuição
Artéria femoral profunda	Artéria femoral no trígono femoral (cerca de 4 cm distal ao ligamento inguinal)	Passa inferiormente no septo intermuscular medial, profundamente ao músculo adutor longo	Os ramos perfurantes atravessam o músculo adutor magno até as partes posterior e lateral dos compartimentos anteriores da coxa
Artéria hepática própria	Tronco celíaco	Passa pelo espaço retroperitoneal para alcançar o ligamento hepatoduodenal e passa entre suas camadas até a porta hepática; bifurca-se nas artérias hepáticas direita e esquerda	Ramos: (gástrica direita, supraduodenal), artérias hepáticas direita e esquerda; nutre o fígado e a vesícula biliar (estômago, pâncreas, duodeno)
Artéria marginal (do colo)	Formada por anastomoses (arcadas) entre as artérias cólicas direita, média e esquerda e sigmóide	Canal anastomótico raramente interrompido que avança paralelo ao colo em sua borda mesentérica	Ramos que passam para as faces anterior e posterior do colo
Artéria profunda do pênis ou do clitóris	Ramo terminal da artéria pudenda interna	Perfura a membrana perineal até alcançar os corpos eréteis do clitóris ou do pênis (corpos cavernosos)	Terminações (artérias helicinas) se desenrolam para ingurgitar os seios eréteis com sangue arterial
Artérias digitais dorsais (dos artelhos)	Artérias metatarsais dorsais	Correm distalmente nas faces póstero-laterais de uma e meia falanges proximais	Nutrem as faces dorsais de uma e meia falanges proximais dos dedos dos pés
Artérias digitais dorsais (dos dedos)	Artérias metacarpais dorsais	Correm distalmente sobre as faces póstero-laterais de uma e meia falanges proximais	Inervam as faces dorsais de uma e meia falanges proximais dos dedos das mãos
Artérias digitais plantares comuns	Porções terminais das artérias metatarsais plantares	Segmentos curtos distais à porção transversa do músculo adutor do hálux proximal às membranas interdigitais dos pés	Ramos terminais: artérias digitais plantares próprias
Artérias segmentares do fígado (anterior direita, posterior direita, medial esquerda e lateral esquerda)	Ramos esquerdo e direito da artéria hepática própria	Originam-se dentro do fígado; os ramos direito e esquerdo correm horizontalmente, o ramo direito origina as artérias segmentares anterior e posterior, o esquerdo as artérias segmentares medial e lateral	Cada artéria segmentar irriga uma divisão do fígado que, exceto pela divisão medial, é subdividida em dois segmentos hepáticos; os ramos direito e esquerdo da artéria hepática enviam uma artéria para o lobo caudado
Artérias segmentares do pulmão	Artérias lobares	Originam-se no pulmão como ramos terciários das artérias pulmonares direita e esquerda	Cada artéria segmentar serve a um segmento broncopulmonar do pulmão
Artérias segmentares do rim (superior, anterior superior, anterior inferior, inferior e posterior)	Divisões anterior e posterior (ou diretamente a partir das) das artérias renais	Originam-se no hilo, atravessam o tecido adiposo perirrenal do seio renal ao redor da pelve renal para alcançar o segmento renal	Segmento renal (as artérias segmentares são artérias terminais. Não há anastomoses significativas entre os segmentos)
Auricular posterior	Artéria carótida externa	Corre posteriormente, profundamente à parótida, ao longo do processo estilóide entre o processo mastóideo e a orelha	Couro cabeludo posterior à orelha e orelha
Auricular profunda	1.ª parte da artéria maxilar	Ascende na glândula parótida posterior à articulação temporomandibular, perfurando a parede do meato acústico externo	Nutre a articulação temporomandibular e a pele do meato acústico externo e a membrana timpânica
Axilar	Continuação da artéria subclávia depois de cruzar a 1.ª costela	Corre ínfero-lateralmente através da fossa axilar, transformando-se na artéria braquial quando cruza a borda inferior do músculo redondo maior; as partes são medial (1.ª), posterior (2.ª) e lateral (3.ª) até o músculo peitoral menor	1.ª parte: artéria torácica superior 2.ª parte: artérias tóraco-acromial e torácica lateral 3.ª parte: artérias subclávia e circunflexas anterior e posterior do úmero
Basilar	Formada pela união intracraniana das artérias vertebrais	Ascende ao clivo na cisterna da ponte; termina por se bifurcar nas artérias cerebrais posteriores	Ramos: artérias cerebelar inferior anterior, do labirinto, pontina, mesencefálica e cerebelar superior
Braquial	Continuação da artéria axilar depois da borda inferior do músculo redondo maior	Acompanha o nervo mediano no septo intermuscular medial; termina por bifurcar-se nas artérias radial e ulnar na fossa cubital	Principal artéria do braço: artéria braquial profunda, ramos musculares e nutrientes, colaterais ulnares superior e inferior
Braquiocefálica (tronco)	1.º e maior ramo do arco da aorta	Ascende póstero-lateralmente para a direita, correndo anterior e, em seguida, à direita da traquéia; profundamente à articulação esternoclavicular, bifurca-se em ramos terminais	Artérias carótida comum direita e subclávia direita

ARTÉRIAS DO CORPO HUMANO

Artéria/Artérias	Origem	Trajeto	Ramos/Distribuição
Brônquicas (1–2 ramos)	Face anterior da 1.ª parte da aorta torácica ou 3.ª artéria intercostal posterior direita	Corre sobre as faces posteriores dos brônquios principais e segue a árvore traqueobrônquica	Tecido brônquico e peribrônquico, pleura visceral
Bucal	Artéria maxilar	Corre ântero-lateralmente com o nervo bucal, emergindo por baixo da borda anterior do ramo da mandíbula	Irriga o músculo bucinador, a pele suprajacente e a mucosa oral subjacente; anastomosa-se com os ramos das artérias facial e infra-orbital
Carótida comum, esquerda e direita	Esquerda: 2.º ramo do arco da aorta. Direita: ramo terminal (com a artéria subclávia direita) do tronco braquiocefálico	Ascende a partir de/passa profundamente à articulação esternoclavicular na bainha carótica sob a cobertura do músculo esternocleidomastóideo no nível da vértebra C4 (ou osso hióide)	Ramos terminais: artérias carótidas interna e externa
Carótida externa	Artéria carótida comum na borda superior da cartilagem tireóidea	Ascende algo anteriormente e, em seguida, inclina-se posterior e lateralmente, passando entre o processo mastóideo e a mandíbula; penetra na substância da glândula parótida, bifurcando-se nos ramos terminais profundamente ao colo da mandíbula	Ramos anteriores: artérias tireóidea superior, facial e lingual. Ramos posteriores: artérias occipital e auricular posterior. Ramo medial: faríngea ascendente. Ramos terminais: artérias maxilar e temporal superficial
Carótida interna	Artéria carótida comum na borda superior da cartilagem tireóidea	Ascende verticalmente no pescoço para penetrar no canal carotídeo, torna-se horizontal e corre ântero-medialmente através do seio cavernoso, faz uma curva de 180° sob o processo clinóide anterior, bifurca-se nas artérias cerebrais anterior e média	Fornece ramos para as paredes do seio cavernoso, a hipófise e o gânglio trigêmeo; fornece o aporte sangüíneo primário para a órbita/globo ocular, cavidade nasal superior/nariz e cérebro
Cerebelar inferior anterior	Parte inferior (inicial) da artéria basilar	Corre póstero-lateralmente, freqüentemente formando uma alça para dentro e para fora do meato acústico interno	Irriga a face inferior dos lobos laterais do cerebelo, parte ínfero-lateral da ponte e plexo corióideo no ângulo pontocerebelar; geralmente dá origem à artéria do labirinto
Cerebelar inferior posterior	Porção intracraniana da artéria vertebral	Passa posteriormente ao redor do lado da medula oblonga para alcançar a face inferior do cerebelo	Nutre a porção medial da face inferior do cerebelo (tonsila cerebelar e núcleo dentado), porção póstero-lateral da medula oblonga e plexo corióideo do quarto ventrículo
Cerebelar superior	Parte superior (terminal) da artéria basilar	Curva-se ao redor do pedúnculo cerebral	Nutre a face superior do cerebelo, colículo e maioria dos núcleos cerebelares; ponte, corpo da pineal; véu medular superior; e plexo corióide do terceiro ventrículo
Cerebral anterior	Ramo terminal (com a artéria cerebral média) da artéria carótida interna	Corre anteriormente, contorna o joelho do corpo caloso, em seguida dirige-se posteriormente na fissura inter-hemisférica	Parte pré-comunicante: tálamo e corpo estriado. Parte pós-comunicante: córtex das faces mediais dos lobos frontal e parietal
Cerebral média	Maior ramo terminal (com a artéria cerebral anterior) da artéria carótida interna	Corre no sulco cerebral lateral, em seguida póstero-superiormente sobre a ínsula	Ínsula e maior parte da superfície lateral dos hemisférios cerebrais
Cerebral posterior	Ramo terminal da artéria basilar	Passa lateralmente, curvando-se ao redor do pedúnculo cerebral para alcançar a superfície do tentório cerebral	Face inferior do lobo temporal e lobo occipital do cérebro
Cervical ascendente	Ramo terminal (com a artéria tireóidea inferior) do tronco tireocervical	Ascende na fáscia pré-vertebral	Irriga os músculos pré-vertebrais anteriores; anastomosa-se amplamente com outras artérias do pescoço
Cervical profunda	Tronco costocervical	Passa posteriormente entre o processo transverso de C7 e o colo da 1.ª costela e ascende entre os músculos semiespinais da cabeça e do pescoço até o nível de C2	Supre os músculos posteriores profundos do pescoço e se anastomosa com o ramo descendente da artéria occipital e ramos da artéria vertebral
Cervical superficial (variante, substituindo o ramo superficial da artéria cervical transversa)	Tronco tireocervical	Passa lateralmente entre os músculos esternocleidomastóideo e escaleno anterior, através do plexo braquial e do triângulo posterior do pescoço, para se bifurcar e correr com o nervo acessório sobre a face profunda do trapézio	Músculo escaleno anterior, músculo esternocleidomastóideo, plexo braquial, músculos do trígono posterior do pescoço e — principalmente — o músculo trapézio

Artéria/Artérias	Origem	Trajeto	Ramos/Distribuição
Cervical transversa (variante: pode ser substituída pelas artérias cervical transversa e dorsal da escápula)	Tronco tireocervical	Corre através do escaleno anterior, plexo braquial e trígono posterior do pescoço e passa profundamente ao músculo trapézio, dividindo-se nos ramos profundo e superficial	O ramo superficial bifurca-se nos ramos ascendente e descendente que correm com o nervo acessório sobre o lado inferior do músculo trapézio; o ramo profundo corre com o nervo escapular dorsal, profundamente aos músculos rombóides
Ciliares anteriores	Ramos musculares (retos) da artéria oftálmica	Perfura a esclera nas inserções dos músculos retos e forma rede na íris e no corpo ciliar	Íris e corpo ciliar
Ciliares posteriores curtas	Artéria oftálmica	Perfuram a esclera na periferia do nervo óptico para nutrir a corióide, que, por sua vez, nutre os cones e bastonetes da retina óptica	Perfuram a esclera na periferia do nervo óptico para nutrir a corióide, que, por sua vez, nutre os cones e bastonetes da retina óptica
Ciliares posteriores longas	Artéria oftálmica	Perfura a esclera para nutrir o corpo ciliar e a íris	Perfura a esclera para nutrir o corpo ciliar e a íris
Circunflexa (ramo)	Artéria coronária esquerda	Passa para a esquerda no sulco atrioventricular e avança até a superfície posterior do coração	Principalmente átrio esquerdo e ventrículo esquerdo; ramos: ventricular esquerdo, atrial e marginal
Circunflexa femoral lateral	Artéria profunda da coxa; pode originar-se da artéria femoral	Dirige-se lateral e profundamente aos músculos sartório e reto femoral e se divide em três ramos	O ramo ascendente supre a parte anterior da região glútea; o ramo transverso curva-se ao redor do fêmur; o ramo descendente desce até o joelho e se une às anastomoses geniculares
Circunflexa femoral medial	Artéria profunda da coxa; pode originar-se da artéria femoral	Passa medial e posteriormente entre os músculos pectíneo e iliopsoas, penetra na região glútea e divide-se em dois ramos	Fornece a maior parte do sangue para a cabeça e o colo do fêmur; o ramo transverso toma parte na anastomose cruzada da coxa; o ramo ascendente une-se à artéria glútea inferior
Circunflexas anterior e posterior do úmero	Terceira parte da artéria axilar, tipicamente oposta à origem da artéria subescapular	Essas artérias anastomosam-se para formar um círculo ao redor do colo cirúrgico do úmero; a artéria circunflexa posterior do úmero, maior, atravessa o espaço quadrangular com o nervo axilar	Irriga a articulação do ombro e os músculos proximais do braço: deltóide, redondos maior e menor e as cabeças longa e lateral do tríceps
Cística	Artéria hepática direita	Surge no ligamento hepatoduodenal	Vesícula biliar e ducto cístico
Colateral média	Artéria braquial profunda	Desce para se anastomosar com a artéria interóssea recorrente	Parte da via colateral ao redor do cotovelo; nutre as cabeças lateral e medial do tríceps
Colateral radial	Ramo terminal (com a artéria colateral média) da artéria braquial profunda	Perfura o septo intermuscular lateral com o nervo radial, corre entre os músculos braquial e braquiorradial para se anastomosar com a artéria recorrente radial, anterior ao epicôndilo lateral do úmero	Forma parte da anastomose cubital; nutre a parte superior dos músculos braquial e braquiorradial, e a face ântero-lateral da articulação do cotovelo
Colateral ulnar (superior e inferior)	A artéria colateral ulnar superior origina-se da artéria braquial próximo ao meio do braço; a artéria colateral ulnar inferior origina-se a partir da artéria braquial exatamente superior ao cotovelo	A artéria colateral ulnar superior acompanha o nervo ulnar até a face posterior do cotovelo; a artéria colateral ulnar inferior divide-se nos ramos anterior e posterior; as duas artérias colaterais ulnares tomam parte na anastomose ao redor da articulação do cotovelo	Anastomosam-se distalmente com as artérias recorrentes ulnares anterior e posterior
Cólica direita	Artéria mesentérica superior	Passa pelo espaço retroperitoneal para alcançar o colo ascendente	Colo ascendente
Cólica esquerda	Artéria mesentérica inferior	Passa pelo espaço retroperitoneal para a esquerda até o colo descendente	Colo descendente
Cólica média	Artéria mesentérica superior	Ascende retroperitonealmente e corre entre as camadas do mesocolo transverso	Colo transverso
Comunicante anterior	Artéria cerebral anterior	Conecta as artérias cerebrais anteriores na cisterna pré-quiasmática, para completar o círculo arterial cerebral	Artérias comunicantes centrais ântero-mediais

Artéria/Artérias	Origem	Trajeto	Ramos/Distribuição
Comunicante posterior	Anastomose entre as artérias carótida interna e cerebral posterior	Passa superiormente ao nervo oculomotor (NC III)	Trato óptico, pedúnculo cerebral, cápsula interna e tálamo
Coronária direita	Seio aórtico direito	Segue o sulco coronário (AV) entre os átrios e ventrículos	Átrio direito, nós SA e AV, e parte posterior do septo IV
Coronária esquerda	Seio aórtico esquerdo	Corre no sulco AV e emite ramos interventricular anterior e circunflexo	Maior parte do átrio e ventrículo esquerdos, septo IV e feixes AV; pode suprir o nó AV
Costocervical (tronco)	2.ª parte da artéria subclávia	Artéria muito curta que passa posterior e superiormente à parte cervical da pleura até o colo da 1.ª costela e se bifurca em seus ramos terminais	Ramos terminais: artérias intercostal suprema e cervical profunda
Cremastérica	Epigástrica inferior	Acompanha o cordão espermático através do canal inguinal e para dentro da bolsa escrotal	Nutre o músculo cremaster e outros revestimentos do cordão nos homens; ligamento redondo no sexo feminino
Descendente do joelho	Artéria femoral, no canal adutor	Desce no músculo vasto medial, exatamente anterior ao tendão do adutor magno, para se anastomosar com a artéria genicular superior medial	Ramos: ramo safeno, que acompanha o nervo safeno até a pele medial da perna; ramos musculares para os músculos vasto medial e adutor magno
Digitais palmares próprias	Artérias digitais palmares comuns	Correm ao longo dos lados do 2.º–5.º dedos; na base da falange média, originam o ramo dorsal, que substitui as artérias digitais dorsais	Todas as porções palmares e distais (inclusive os leitos ungueais) da face dorsal dos dedos das mãos
Digital palmar comum	Arco palmar superficial	Passa distalmente anterior às lumbricais para se bifurcar proximal aos espaços interdigitais	Recebe as artérias metacarpais palmares a partir do arco palmar profundo; ramos terminais: artérias digitais palmares próprias
Divisão anterior da artéria ilíaca interna	Ilíaca interna	Passa anteriormente ao longo da parede lateral da pelve menor na bainha hipogástrica e se divide nos ramos visceral e parietal	Ramo parietal: artéria obturatória Ramos viscerais: artéria umbilical, vesical inferior, uterina, vaginal, retal média e pudenda
Divisão posterior da artéria ilíaca interna	Ilíaca interna	Passa posteriormente e origina os ramos parietais	Parede pélvica e região glútea
Do joelho (superior lateral e medial, inferior lateral e medial, e média)	Poplítea	Originam-se e correm para os "quatro cantos" da articulação do joelho (visto anteriormente) ao redor da patela e dos côndilos femoral e tibial; a artéria média do joelho perfura o ligamento poplíteo oblíquo no centro posterior da cápsula articular	Formam, com participação também da artéria descendente do joelho, do ramo descendente da circunflexa femoral lateral e das artérias circunflexa fibular e recorrente tibial, a anastomose da articulação do joelho
Do labirinto	Basilar ou através de um tronco comum com a artéria cerebelar anterior inferior	Sai da cavidade craniana através do meato acústico interno; entra no labirinto ósseo	Labirinto membranáceo
Do nó atrioventricular (AV) (ramo)	Artéria coronária direita próximo à origem da artéria IV posterior	Corre anteriormente na parte mais superior do septo interventricular até o nó AV	Nó AV
Dorsal da escápula (variação — 1/3 das vezes é substituída por um ramo profundo da a. cervical transversa)	3.ª (ou 2.ª) parte da artéria subclávia	Passa lateralmente através do plexo braquial, em seguida profundamente ao músculo levantador da escápula; une-se ao nervo dorsal da escápula, correndo ao longo da borda vertebral da escápula, profundamente aos músculos rombóides	Emite ramos para os músculos trapézio, rombóides, latíssimo do dorso; participa nas anastomoses ao redor da escápula (ombro)
Dorsal do nariz	Artéria oftálmica	Corre ao longo da face dorsal do nariz e nutre sua superfície	Corre ao longo da face dorsal do nariz e nutre sua superfície
Dorsal do pé	Continuação da artéria tibial anterior distal à porção inferior do retináculo dos músculos extensores	Desce ântero-medialmente ao primeiro espaço interósseo e se divide nas artérias plantar e arqueada	Músculos no dorso do pé; perfura o primeiro músculo interósseo dorsal como a artéria plantar profunda para contribuir para a formação do arco plantar

Artéria/Artérias	Origem	Trajeto	Ramos/Distribuição
Epigástrica inferior	Artéria ilíaca externa	Corre superiormente e penetra na bainha dos músculos retos; corre profundamente ao músculo reto do abdome	Reto do abdome e parte medial da parede abdominal ântero-lateral
Epigástrica superficial	Artéria femoral	Corre na fáscia superficial para o umbigo	Tecido subcutâneo e pele sobre a região suprapúbica
Epigástrica superior	Artéria torácica interna	Desce na bainha dos músculos retos, profundamente ao reto abdominal	Músculo reto do abdome e parte superior da parede abdominal ântero-lateral
Escrotal posterior ou labial posterior	Ramos terminais da artéria perineal	Corre na fáscia superficial da parte posterior da bolsa escrotal ou dos lábios maiores do pudendo	Pele da bolsa escrotal ou dos lábios maiores do pudendo
Esfenopalatina	3.ª parte da artéria maxilar	Passa medialmente através do forame esfenopalatino, dividindo-se imediatamente nas artérias nasal septal e lateral posterior	Mucosa da metade póstero-inferior da cavidade nasal, células etmoidais e seios paranasais maxilar e esfenoidal
Esofágica (4–5 ramos)	Face anterior da aorta torácica	Corre anteriormente ao esôfago	Esôfago
Espinal anterior	Superiormente, por fusão dos ramos intracranianos, um de cada artéria vertebral; continua inferiormente por bifurcações das artérias medulares segmentares anteriores em vários níveis	Forma uma cadeia anastomótica contínua que desce por todo o comprimento da medula espinal na entrada até a fissura mediana anterior	Irriga a porção anterior da medula espinal por meio de ramos sulcais, os quais se estendem para dentro da fissura mediana anterior, e o plexo pial, que se ramifica sobre a superfície da medula espinal
Espinal posterior	Superiormente, a partir de um ramo intracraniano da artéria vertebral; continua inferiormente por bifurcações das artérias medulares segmentares posteriores em vários níveis	Forma uma cadeia anastomótica contínua que desce no comprimento da medula espinal no sulco póstero-lateral, adjacente às raízes dorsais emergentes (radículas) dos nervos espinais	Nutre a face póstero-lateral da medula espinal, através do plexo pial e de seus ramos periféricos
Esplênica	Tronco celíaco	Corre pelo retroperitoneal ao longo da borda superior do pâncreas; em seguida, passa entre as camadas do ligamento esplenorrenal até o hilo do baço	Corpo do pâncreas, baço e curvatura maior do estômago
Estilomastóidea	Auricular posterior	Entra no forame estilomastóideo e ascende o canal facial, correndo com (e suprindo) o nervo facial	Ramos: artéria timpânica posterior (para a membrana timpânica); ramos mastóideo (para as células mastóideas) e estapédio (para o estapédio, estribo e membrana timpânica secundária)
Etmoidal anterior	Artéria oftálmica	Atravessa o forame etmoidal até a fossa craniana anterior e para dentro da cavidade nasal, emitindo ramos para a pele do nariz	Irriga as células etmoidais anterior e média, dura-máter da fossa craniana anterior, cavidade nasal ântero-superior e pele no dorso do nariz
Etmoidal posterior	Artéria oftálmica	Passa através do forame etmoidal posterior até as células etmoidais posteriores	Passa através do forame etmoidal posterior até as células etmoidais posteriores
Facial	Artéria carótida externa	Ascende profundamente à glândula submandibular, curva-se ao redor da borda inferior da mandíbula e penetra na face, ascendendo obliquamente através da bochecha e lateral ao nariz até o ângulo medial do olho	Ramos: palatina ascendente, tonsilar, glandular, submentual, labiais inferior e superior e lateral do nariz Ramo terminal (continuação): artéria angular
Facial transversa	Artéria temporal superficial no interior da glândula parótida	Cruza a face superficial ao músculo masseter e inferior ao arco zigomático	Glândula e ducto parotídeo, músculos e pele da face
Faríngea ascendente	Face medial da artéria carótida externa	Ascende entre a artéria carótida interna e a faringe até à base do crânio, emitindo ramos através do forame jugular e do canal hipoglosso	Irriga a parede faríngea, tonsila palatina, palato mole e dura-máter da fossa craniana posterior

Artéria/Artérias	Origem	Trajeto	Ramos/Distribuição
Femoral	Continuação da artéria ilíaca externa distal ao ligamento inguinal	Desce através do trígono femoral, atravessa o canal adutor e muda de nome para "poplítea" no hiato adutor	Nutre as superfícies anterior e ântero-medial da coxa
Fibular	Tibial posterior	Desce no compartimento posterior adjacente ao septo intermuscular posterior	Compartimento posterior da perna: ramos perfurantes nutrem o compartimento lateral da perna
Frênica inferior	Como 1.os ramos da aorta abdominal (por vezes através de um vaso comum, ou a partir do tronco celíaco)	Ascende o pilar até a face inferior das cúpulas; os ramos mediais se anastomosam e fazem anastomoses com as artérias pericardiofrênicas; os ramos laterais aproximam-se da parede torácica, anastomosam-se com as artérias intercostal posterior e musculofrênica	Ramos: artérias supra-renais superiores Nutre: diafragma, veia cava inferior (ramo direito), esôfago (ramo esquerdo), glândulas supra-renais
Frênicas superiores (variam em número)	Face anterior da aorta torácica	Originam-se no hiato aórtico e passam para a face superior do diafragma	Nutrem o diafragma e as partes diafragmáticas do pericárdio e da pleura parietal
Gástrica direita	Artéria hepática	Corre entre as camadas do ligamento hepatogástrico	Porção direita da curvatura menor do estômago
Gástrica esquerda	Tronco celíaco	Ascende pelo espaço retroperitoneal até o hiato esofágico, onde passa entre as camadas do ligamento hepatogástrico	Porção distal do esôfago e curvatura menor do estômago
Gástrica posterior	Artéria esplênica	Ascende pelo espaço retroperitoneal (na parede posterior da bolsa omental) e corre até o fundo gástrico através da prega gastrofrênica (ligamento)	Parede posterior do estômago
Gástricas curtas (n = 4–5)	Artéria esplênica no hilo do baço	Passa entre as camadas do ligamento gastroesplênico para o fundo do estômago	Fundo do estômago
Gastroduodenal	Artéria hepática	Desce pelo espaço retroperitoneal, posterior à junção gastroduodenal	Estômago, pâncreas, primeira parte do duodeno e parte distal do ducto biliar
Gastromental direita (gastroepiplóica)	Artéria gastroduodenal	Passa entre as camadas do omento maior para a curvatura maior do estômago	Porção direita da curvatura maior do estômago
Gastromental esquerda (gastroepiplóica)	Artéria esplênica no hilo do baço	Passa entre as camadas do ligamento gastroesplênico até a curvatura maior do estômago	Porção esquerda da curvatura maior do estômago
Glútea superior	Divisão posterior da artéria ilíaca interna	Entra na região glútea através do forame isquiático maior superior ao músculo piriforme e se divide nos ramos superficial e profundo; anastomosa-se com as artérias glútea inferior e circunflexa femoral medial (não mostrada acima)	Músculo piriforme Ramo superficial: nutre o glúteo máximo Ramo profundo: corre entre os músculos glúteo médio e mínimo, nutrindo ambos, bem como o músculo tensor da fáscia lata
Glútea inferior	Divisão anterior da ilíaca interna	Deixa a pelve para entrar na região glútea através do forame isquiático maior inferior ao piriforme e desce sobre o lado medial do nervo isquiático; anastomosa-se com a artéria glútea superior e participa na anastomose cruzada da coxa, envolvendo a primeira artéria perfurante das artérias femoral profunda e circunflexas femorais medial e lateral	Diafragma pélvico (músculos pubococcígeo e levantador do ânus), músculo piriforme, quadrado femoral, parte mais superior dos músculos da face posterior da coxa, músculo glúteo máximo, nervo isquiático
Hepática comum	Ramo terminal (com a artéria esplênica) do tronco celíaco	Passa para a direita ao longo da borda superior do pâncreas, correndo anterior à veia porta	Ramos terminais: artéria própria e artéria gastroduodenal
Ileocólica	Ramo terminal da artéria mesentérica superior	Corre ao longo da raiz do mesentério e se divide nos ramos ileal e cólico	Íleo, ceco e colo ascendente
Ilíaca circunflexa profunda	Artéria ilíaca externa	Corre na face profunda da parede abdominal anterior, em paralelo com o ligamento inguinal	Irriga o músculo ilíaco e a parte inferior da parede abdominal ântero-lateral
Ilíaca circunflexa superficial	Artéria femoral	Corre na fáscia superficial ao longo do ligamento longitudinal	Tecido subcutâneo e pele sobre a parte inferior da parede abdominal ântero-lateral

Artéria/Artérias	Origem	Trajeto	Ramos/Distribuição
Ilíaca comum, esquerda e direita	Ramos terminais da parte abdominal da aorta	Começa anterior ao corpo vertebral L4, separando-se à medida que descem para terminar no nível de L5/S1, anterior às articulações sacroilíacas	Ramos terminais: artérias ilíacas externa e interna
Ilíaca interna	Ilíaca comum	Passa sobre a borda pélvica até atingir a cavidade pélvica	Principal suprimento sangüíneo para os órgãos pélvicos, músculos glúteos e períneo
Iliolombar	Divisão posterior da artéria ilíaca interna	Ascende anterior à articulação sacroilíaca e posterior aos vasos ilíacos comuns e ao músculo psoas maior	Psoas maior, músculos ilíaco e quadrado lombar, cauda eqüina no canal vertebral
Infra-orbital	Terceira parte da artéria maxilar	Passa ao longo do sulco infra-orbital e forame para a face	Nutre os músculos reto inferior e oblíquo, a pálpebra inferior, o saco lacrimal, o seio maxilar, os dentes incisivos e caninos maxilares e a parte anterior da bochecha
Intercostais anteriores (ramos)	Artérias torácica interna (espaços intercostais 1–6) e musculofrênica (espaços intercostais 7–9)	Passam entre os músculos internos e intercostais mais internos	Músculos intercostais, pele suprajacente e pleura parietal subjacente
Intercostais posteriores	Artéria intercostal superior (espaços intercostais 1 e 2) e parte torácica da aorta (espaços intercostais restantes)	Passam entre os músculos intercostais internos e profundos	Músculos intercostais e pele suprajacente, pleura parietal
Intercostal posterior	Face posterior da parte torácica da aorta	Corre lateral e, em seguida, anteriormente em paralelo com as costelas	Ramos cutâneos lateral e anterior
Intercostal suprema	Tronco costocervical	Desce entre a pleura e os colos das duas primeiras costelas; anastomosa-se com a 3.ª artéria intercostal posterior	Ramos: 1.ª e 2.ª artérias intercostais posteriores, para os músculos e costelas que limitam os 1.º e 2.º espaços intercostais
Interóssea comum	Artéria ulnar, exatamente distal à bifurcação da artéria braquial na fossa cubital	Passa profundamente para se bifurcar nos ramos terminais depois de um trajeto muito curto	Ramos terminais: artérias interósseas anterior e posterior
Interósseas, anterior e posterior	Artéria interóssea comum	Passa para os lados anterior e posterior da membrana interóssea	Compartimentos anterior e posterior do antebraço; a artéria interóssea anterior nutre os compartimentos anterior e posterior na parte distal do antebraço; a artéria interóssea posterior emite a artéria interóssea recorrente, que participa nas anastomoses arteriais ao redor do cotovelo
Interventricular (IV) posterior	Artéria coronária direita	Corre a partir do sulco IV posterior até o ápice do coração	Ventrículos direito e esquerdo e septo IV
Interventricular anterior (ramo)	Artéria coronária esquerda	Passa ao longo do sulco IV anterior até o ápice do coração	Paredes dos ventrículos direito e esquerdo, incluindo a maior parte do septo IV e feixe atrioventricular e ramos (tecido de condução) contidos
Intestinal (n = 15–18)	Artéria mesentérica superior	Passa entre as duas camadas de mesentério	Jejuno e íleo
Labial inferior	Artéria facial próximo ao ângulo da boca	Corre medialmente no lábio inferior	Lábio inferior e queixo
Labial superior	Artéria facial próximo ao ângulo da boca	Corre medialmente no lábio superior	Lábio superior e asa (lado) e septo do nariz
Lacrimal	Artéria oftálmica	Passa ao longo da borda superior do músculo reto lateral para nutrir as glândulas lacrimais, as conjuntivas e as pálpebras	Passa ao longo da borda superior do músculo reto lateral para nutrir as glândulas lacrimais, a conjuntiva e as pálpebras
Laríngea superior	Tireóidea superior	Corre profundamente ao músculo tíreo-hióideo para perfurar a membrana tíreo-hióidea com o nervo laríngeo interno	Nutre a laringe

ARTÉRIAS DO CORPO HUMANO

Artéria/Artérias	Origem	Trajeto	Ramos/Distribuição
Lingual	Artéria carótida externa	Forma uma alça sobre o corno maior do hióide, passa medialmente ao hioglosso e ascende para correr ao longo do lado da língua	Ramos: ramo supra-hióideo, artérias dorsais da língua e artéria sublingual; continua como a artéria lingual profunda
Lingual profunda	Continuação (terceira parte) da artéria lingual	Vira-se superiormente próximo à borda anterior do músculo hioglosso e, em seguida, passa anteriormente, flanqueando o frênulo da língua, profundamente à mucosa	Nutre o músculo genioglosso, o músculo longitudinal inferior e a mucosa da face inferior da língua, ponta da língua
Lingular, inferior e superior	Artéria lobar superior (do pulmão esquerdo), na fissura oblíqua	Desce anteriormente à língula	Divisão lingular (segmentos broncopulmonar superior [S4] e inferior [S5]) do pulmão esquerdo
Lombar	Parte abdominal da aorta	Seu trajeto é horizontal, correndo posteriormente ao redor dos lados das vértebras lombares e, em seguida, lateralmente na parede abdominal posterior	Ramos: dorsal, para os músculos profundos das costas e da pele suprajacente; espinal, para as vértebras, conteúdo do canal vertebral, raízes e alguns (como artérias medulares segmentais) para a medula espinal
Marginal direita	Artéria coronária direita	Passa para a margem inferior do coração e para o ápice	Ventrículo direito e ápice do coração
Marginal esquerda (ramo)	Ramo circunflexo	Segue a borda esquerda do coração	Ventrículo esquerdo
Massetérica	2.ª parte da artéria maxilar	Passa posterior ao tendão temporal que acompanha o nervo massetérico através da incisura mandibular	Nutre o masseter e a articulação temporomandibular; anastomosa-se com as artérias facial e facial transversa
Maxilar	Ramo terminal (com a artéria temporal superficial) da carótida externa	Passa posterior e medialmente ao colo da mandíbula (1.ª parte), superficial ou profunda à cabeça inferior do músculo pterigóideo lateral (2.ª parte) e dentro da fossa pterigopalatina (3.ª parte)	1.ª parte: auricular profunda, timpânica anterior, meníngea média, meníngea acessória, alveolar inferior 2.ª parte: temporal profunda, pterigóideo (ramos), massetérica, bucal 3.ª parte: alveolar superior posterior, palatina descendente, artéria do canal pterigóideo, faríngea, esfenopalatina, infra-orbital
Medular segmentar, anterior e posterior	Ramos espinais das artérias segmentares (artérias vertebral, intercostal posterior, lombar e sacral)	Fazem trajeto ao longo das raízes anterior e posterior dos nervos espinais, e continuam medialmente para se anastomosar com as artérias espinais longitudinais anterior e posterior	Raízes dorsal e ventral de determinados nervos espinais, e a medula espinal; a artéria medular segmentar anterior maior (Adamkiewicz) é a maior, ocorrendo na porção torácica inferior, lombar superior, no lado esquerdo, em 65% das vezes
Meníngea média	1.ª parte da artéria maxilar	Ascende verticalmente através do forame espinhoso para dentro da fossa craniana média; corre lateralmente, dividindo-se nos ramos frontal e parietal, os quais, por sua vez, ramificam-se, ascendendo as paredes laterais na dura-máter craniana	Ramos: ramos ganglionares, ramos petrosos, artéria timpânica superior, ramos temporais, ramo anastomótico para a artéria lacrimal; a maior parte do sangue distribui-se para o periósteo, os ossos e a medula óssea
Mentual (ramo)	Ramo terminal da artéria alveolar inferior	Emerge do forame mentual e se dirige para o queixo	Músculos faciais e pele do queixo
Mesentérica inferior	Parte abdominal da aorta	Desce pelo espaço retroperitoneal para a esquerda da parte abdominal da aorta	Nutre parte do trato gastrintestinal derivado do intestino posterior
Mesentérica superior	Parte abdominal da aorta	Corre na raiz do mesentério até a junção ileocecal	Parte do trato gastrintestinal derivada do intestino médio
Metacarpal dorsal	Ramo carpal dorsal	Correm sobre o 2.º–4.º interósseos dorsais	Bifurcam-se nas artérias digitais dorsais; nutrem a pele, o músculo e o osso do dorso da mão e os dedos até o centro da falange média
Metacarpal palmar	Arco palmar profundo (a partir da artéria radial)	Corre distalmente no plano entre os músculos adutor do polegar e interósseo	Anastomosa-se distalmente com as artérias digitais palmares comuns
Metatarsais plantares	1.ª: junção entre as artérias plantar lateral e dorsal do pé 2.ª–4.ª: arco plantar profundo	Estendem-se distalmente entre os ossos metatarsais na face plantar dos músculos interósseos	Ramos: ramos perfurantes, artérias digitais plantares comuns

Artéria/Artérias	Origem	Trajeto	Ramos/Distribuição
Metatarsal dorsal	1.ª: terminação da dorsal do pé; 2.ª, 3.ª e 4.ª: artéria arqueada	Corre distalmente sobre a face superficial dos músculos interósseos dorsais correspondentes	Ramos: artérias digitais dorsais (dos dedos dos pés)
Milo-hióidea (ramo)	Alveolar inferior (antes que penetre no forame mandibular)	Perfura o ligamento esfenomandibular para correr ântero-inferiormente com o nervo no sulco na face medial do ramo da mandíbula	Músculos do assoalho da boca; anastomosa-se com a artéria submentual
Musculofrênica	Ramo terminal (com a artéria epigástrica superior) da artéria torácica interna	Originando-se no 6.º espaço intercostal, desce ínfero-lateralmente, acompanhando a margem costal	Ramos: artérias intercostais anteriores do 7.º–9.º espaços intercostais; também nutre os músculos abdominais superiores e o pericárdio
Nasal lateral	Artéria facial à medida que ela ascende ao lado do nariz	Dirige-se para as asas do nariz	Pele das asas e dorso do nariz
Nasal lateral posterior	Artéria esfenopalatina	Ramifica-se sobre as conchas e meatos; anastomosa-se com os ramos nasais das artérias etmoidal e palatina maior	Nutre as paredes laterais da cavidade nasal póstero-inferior, contribuindo também para nutrir as células etmoidais e os seios paranasais maxilar e esfenoidal
Nó sinoatrial (SA)	Artéria coronária direita próximo à sua origem (em 60%); ramo circunflexo da coronária esquerda (em 40%)	Curva-se ao redor do lado direito (60%) ou esquerdo (40%) da aorta ascendente e ascende até o nó SA	Átrio esquerdo e nó SA
Obturatória	Divisão anterior da ilíaca interna	Corre ântero-inferiormente na parede pélvica lateral para sair da pelve por meio do canal obturatório	Músculos pélvicos, artéria nutriente para o ílio, cabeça do fêmur, músculos do compartimento medial da coxa
Occipital	Artéria carótida externa	Passa medialmente até o ventre posterior do músculo digástrico e processo mastóideo; acompanha o nervo occipital na região occipital	Couro cabeludo da parte posterior da cabeça, até o vértice
Oftálmica	Artéria carótida interna	Atravessa o forame óptico para alcançar a cavidade orbital	Atravessa o forame óptico para alcançar a cavidade orbital
Ovárica	Aorta abdominal, inferior às artérias renais	Corre ínfero-lateralmente sobre o músculo psoas maior, em seguida dirige-se medialmente para cruzar a borda pélvica e desce no ligamento suspensor do ovário	Ramos: uretérica, tubária (para as tubas uterinas) e ovárica; as duas últimas anastomosam-se com ramos da artéria uterina de mesmo nome
Palatina ascendente	Artéria facial	Ascende ao longo e cruza a borda superior do músculo constritor superior da faringe para atingir o palato mole e a fossa tonsilar	Irriga a parede lateral da faringe, as tonsilas, a tuba auditiva e o palato mole
Palatina descendente	3.ª parte da artéria maxilar	Surge na fossa pterigopalatina; desce no canal palatino	Ramos: artérias palatinas maior e menor
Palatina menor	Palatina descendente	Desce ínfero-posteriormente através do forame palatino menor	Nutre o palato mole
Pancreática dorsal	Artéria esplênica	Desce posterior ao pâncreas, dividindo-se nos ramos direito e esquerdo	Nutre a porção média do pâncreas
Pancreática magna	Artéria esplênica	Penetra na porção esquerda do pâncreas, dividindo-se nos ramos direito e esquerdo, que fazem trajeto em paralelo com o ducto pancreático	Anastomoses com outros ramos pancreáticos; supre, em sua maioria, a cauda do pâncreas e o ducto contido
Pancreaticoduodenais inferiores, anterior e posterior	Artéria mesentérica superior	Ascende pelo espaço retroperitoneal sobre a cabeça do pâncreas	Porção distal do duodeno e cabeça inferior e processo uncinado do pâncreas
Pancreaticoduodenal superior, anterior e posterior	Artéria gastroduodenal	Desce sobre a cabeça do pâncreas	Porção proximal do duodeno e cabeça do pâncreas
Parte abdominal da aorta	Continuação da parte torácica da aorta	Corre sobre a face anterior dos corpos das vértebras lombares	Ramos viscerais: artérias, mesentéricas superior e inferior, renal, supra-renal média, ovárica e testicular, tronco celíaco. Ramos parietais: artérias lombares, sacral mediana

Artéria/Artérias	Origem	Trajeto	Ramos/Distribuição
Parte ascendente da aorta	Orifício aórtico do ventrículo esquerdo	Ascende aproximadamente 5 cm até o nível do ângulo esternal, onde se transforma no arco da aorta	Artérias coronárias direita e esquerda
Parte torácica da aorta	Continuação do arco da aorta	Desce no mediastino posterior à esquerda da coluna vertebral; desloca-se gradualmente para a direita para se localizar no plano mediano no hiato aórtico	Artérias intercostais posteriores, subcostal, algumas artérias frênicas e ramos viscerais (traqueal e esofágica)
Pericardicofrênica	Artéria torácica interna	Desce em paralelo com o nervo frênico, entre a pleura parietal mediastinal e o pericárdio	Nutre a parte mediastinal da pleura parietal e o pericárdio; anastomosa-se com as artérias frênica e musculofrênica
Perineal	Artéria pudenda interna	Deixa o canal pudendo e penetra no espaço perineal superficial	Nutre os músculos perineais superficiais e a bolsa escrotal ou os lábios maiores do pudendo
Plantar lateral	Ramo terminal (com a artéria plantar medial) da artéria tibial posterior	Forma-se medialmente ao calcâneo, avança ântero-lateralmente entre a 1.ª e 2.ª camadas musculares da planta do pé até a base do 5.º metatarsal, em seguida dirige-se ântero-medialmente entre a 3.ª e 4.ª camadas como o arco plantar profundo	Ramos: musculares, para os músculos da 1.ª e 2.ª camadas; superficiais, para a pele e o tecido subcutâneo da parte lateral da planta; anastomóticos, com as artérias arqueada e tarsal lateral; e calcâneo, para o calcâneo
Plantar medial	Ramo terminal (com a artéria plantar lateral) da artéria tibial posterior	Origina-se medialmente ao calcâneo, passa distalmente ao longo do lado medial do pé entre a 1.ª e 2.ª camadas dos músculos plantares	Ramos: muscular, para os músculos flexor curto do hálux e abdutor do hálux; superficial, para a pele e tecido subcutâneo da planta medial; e digital superficial, que se une à 1.ª–3.ª metatarsais plantares
Poplítea	Continuação da artéria femoral no hiato adutor no adutor magno	Passa através da fossa poplítea até a perna; termina na borda inferior do músculo poplíteo dividindo-se nas artérias tibiais anterior e posterior	Artérias superior, média e inferior do joelho para as faces lateral e medial do joelho
Principal do polegar	Artéria radial quando se curva para dentro da região palmar	Desce na face palmar do primeiro metacarpal e se divide na base da falange proximal em dois ramos que correm ao longo dos lados do polegar	Polegar
Prostático (ramos)	Artéria vesical inferior	Desce na face póstero-lateral da próstata	Próstata
Pudenda externa, ramos superficial e profundo	Artéria femoral	Passa medialmente através da coxa até alcançar a bolsa escrotal ou os lábios maiores do pudendo	Pele do monte do púbis e da porção anterior dos lábios do pudendo (feminino); ou da raiz do pênis e porção anterior da bolsa escrotal (masculino)
Pudenda interna	Divisão anterior da artéria ilíaca interna	Deixa a pelve através do forame isquiático maior; circunda a espinha isquiática e penetra no períneo por meio do forame isquiático menor e corre no canal pudendo até o trígono urogenital (UG)	Principal artéria para o períneo, incluindo os músculos e a pele dos trígonos anal e urogenital; corpos eréteis (não emite ramos para a região glútea)
Pulmonar direita	Tronco pulmonar	Passa abaixo do arco da aorta para se unir ao brônquio direito e veias pulmonares para formar a raiz do pulmão direito; desce no pulmão	Nutre o pulmão direito; Ramos: artérias lobares superior, média e inferior (que por sua vez originam as artérias segmentares)
Pulmonar esquerda	Tronco pulmonar	Une-se ao brônquio esquerdo e às veias pulmonares para formar a raiz do pulmão esquerdo; desce no pulmão	Nutre o pulmão esquerdo; Ramos: (canal arterial no feto), artérias lobares superior e inferior (por sua vez, emitem as artérias segmentares)
Radial	Divisão terminal menor (com a artéria ulnar) da artéria braquial na fossa cubital	Corre ínfero-lateralmente sob a cobertura do músculo braquiorradial e distalmente se situa lateral ao tendão do flexor radial do carpo; curva-se ao redor da face lateral do rádio e cruza o assoalho da tabaqueira anatômica para perfurar a fáscia; termina por formar o arco palmar profundo	Nutre os músculos das porções laterais dos compartimentos anterior e posterior do antebraço, face lateral do punho, pele do dorso da mão e porções proximais dos dedos, músculos profundos da palma da mão
Radial do indicador	Artéria radial, mas pode originar-se da artéria principal do polegar	Passa ao longo do lado lateral do dedo indicador até sua extremidade distal	Toda a porção palmar lateral e parte distal (incluindo o leito ungueal) da face dorsal do dedo indicador

Artéria/Artérias	Origem	Trajeto	Ramos/Distribuição
Radiculares, anterior e posterior	Ramos espinais das artérias segmentares (artérias vertebral, intercostal posterior, lombar e sacral)	Faz trajeto ao longo das raízes anterior e posterior dos nervos espinhais, terminando antes de alcançar as artérias espinais longitudinais anterior e posterior	Nutre as raízes anterior e posterior dos nervos espinais e revestimentos (bainhas durais e aracnóide)
Ramo carpal dorsal	Artérias radial e ulnar	Ramo na fáscia no dorso da mão	Ramos: artérias metacarpais dorsais
Ramos carpais, dorsais e palmares	Artérias radial e ulnar no nível do punho	Anastomosam-se com os ramos correspondentes da artéria oposta (ulnar) ou para formar os arcos carpais dorsal e palmar	Fornecem a circulação colateral no punho
Recorrente radial	Lado lateral da artéria radial, exatamente distal à sua origem	Ascende sobre o músculo supinador e, em seguida, passa entre os músculos braquiorradial e braquial para se anastomosar com a artéria colateral radial, anterior ao epicôndilo lateral do úmero	Forma parte da anastomose cubital; nutre o supinador, a parte inferior dos músculos braquial e braquiorradial e a face ântero-lateral da articulação do cotovelo
Recorrentes ulnares, anterior e posterior	Artéria ulnar, exatamente distal à articulação do cotovelo	A artéria recorrente ulnar anterior passa superiormente e a artéria colateral ulnar posterior passa posteriormente	Anastomosam-se com as artérias colaterais ulnares anterior e posterior
Renais, esquerda e direita	Face póstero-lateral da parte abdominal da aorta, usualmente no nível vertebral L2	Corre horizontalmente e lateralmente através do pilar do diafragma e do músculo psoas maior, situando-se posterior à veia renal, bifurcando-se nas divisões anterior e posterior, ou ramificando-se nas artérias segmentares próximo ao hilo renal	Fonte de sangue para os rins; ramos: supra-renal inferior, ramos capsulares, uma divisão anterior originando as artérias superior, superior anterior, inferior anterior e segmentar inferior; a divisão posterior se torna artéria segmentar posterior
Retal inferior	Artéria pudenda interna	Deixa o canal pudendo e cruza a fossa isquioanal até o canal anal	Porção distal do canal anal (principalmente inferior à linha pectínea)
Retal média	Divisão anterior da artéria ilíaca interna	Desce na pelve até a parte inferior do reto	Vesículas seminais e parte inferior do reto
Retal superior	Ramo terminal (continuação da) da artéria mesentérica inferior	Cruza os vasos ilíacos comuns esquerdos e desce para a pelve entre as camadas do mesocolo sigmóide	Parte superior do reto; anastomosa-se com as artérias retais média e inferior
Retroduodenal	Artéria gastroduodenal	Origina-se e corre posterior à primeira parte do duodeno	Nutre a primeira parte do duodeno, o ducto colédoco e a cabeça do pâncreas
Sacral lateral (superior e inferior)	Divisão posterior da ilíaca interna	Corre na face ântero-medial do músculo piriforme para emitir ramos para os forames sacrais pélvicos	Piriforme, estruturas no canal sacral, músculo eretor da espinha e pele suprajacente
Sacral mediana	Face posterior da aorta abdominal	Desce na linha mediana sobre as vértebras L4 e L5 e o sacro e cóccix	Vértebras lombares inferiores, sacro e cóccix
Septal posterior	Artéria esfenopalatina	Cruza a superfície inferior do corpo do esfenóide até alcançar o septo nasal, corre ântero-inferiormente sobre o vômer até os canais dos incisivos	Nutre o septo nasal; anastomosa-se com a artéria palatina maior e o ramo septal da artéria labial superior
Sigmóideas (n = 3–4)	Artéria mesentérica inferior	Passa pelo espaço retroperitoneal para a esquerda para o colo descendente	Colos descendente e sigmóide
Subclávia	Esquerda: arco aórtico Direita: tronco braquiocefálico	Origina-se — ou passa — posterior à articulação esternoclavicular, arqueia-se sobre a pleura cervical anterior ao ápice do pulmão, e cruza a primeira costela posterior ao escaleno anterior, transformando-se na artéria axilar na borda externa da costela	Ramos: 1.ª parte: vertebral, torácico interno, tireocervical (e costocervical no lado direito) 2.ª parte: escapular dorsal (e costocervical no lado esquerdo) [Partes: medial (1.ª), posterior (2.ª) e lateral (3.ª) para o músculo escaleno anterior]
Subcostal	Parte torácica da aorta	Corre ao longo da borda inferior da 12.ª costela	Músculos da parede abdominal ântero-lateral
Subescapular	Terceira parte da artéria axilar	Maior ramo (porém curto — 4 cm) da artéria axilar, desce ao longo da borda lateral do músculo subescapular e da borda axilar da escápula para se bifurcar no nível do ângulo inferior	Através de seus ramos terminais, as artérias circunflexa da escápula e toracodorsal, nutre os músculos dos dois lados da escápula, o músculo latíssimo do dorso e a parede torácica posterior

Artéria/Artérias	Origem	Trajeto	Ramos/Distribuição
Sublingual	Ramo terminal (com a artéria lingual profunda) da artéria lingual	Corre no músculo genioglosso superior ao músculo milo-hióideo	Nutre os músculos e a mucosa do assoalho da boca, e a gengiva lingual anterior
Submentual	Artéria facial, distal à glândula submandibular no trígono submentual	Corre ao longo da face inferior do músculo milo-hióideo, adjacente à sua inserção na mandíbula, até a sínfise mandibular	Nutre o músculo milo-hióideo, ventre anterior do músculo digástrico, linfonodos submentuais e, através de suas anastomoses com as artérias labial inferior e mentual, o lábio inferior
Supraduodenal	Artérias gastroduodenal, hepática, gástrica direita ou retroduodenal	Freqüentemente duplas, passam superiormente à 1.ª parte do duodeno	Nutre a porção superior proximal da parte superior do duodeno
Supra-escapular	Tronco tireocervical	Passa ínfero-lateralmente sobre o músculo escaleno anterior e o nervo frênico, cruza a artéria subclávia e o plexo braquial e corre látero-posteriormente e em paralelo à clavícula; em seguida, passa superiormente ao ligamento escapular transverso para dentro da fossa supra-espinal e, em seguida, sob o acrômio para a fossa infra-espinal	Nutre os músculos supra-espinal e infra-espinal e participa na anastomose ao redor da escápula
Supra-orbital	Ramo terminal da artéria oftálmica	Passa superior e posteriormente a partir do forame supra-orbital até a fronte e o couro cabeludo	Nutre os músculos e a pele da maior parte da fronte e couro cabeludo anterior (até o vértice)
Supra-renal inferior	Renal	Ascende verticalmente até a glândula supra-renal	Faces posterior e inferior da glândula supra-renal
Supra-renal média	Parte abdominal da aorta	Surge no nível da artéria mesentérica superior; seu trajeto é muito curto sobre o pilar do diafragma	Nutre as glândulas supra-renais; faz anastomose com os ramos supra-renais das artérias frênica inferior e renal
Supra-renal superior	Frênica inferior	Múltiplos ramos curtos que se originam dos troncos das artérias frênicas inferiores, à medida que elas ascendem a cruz diafragmática, correndo ao longo da face súpero-medial da glândula	Parte superior das glândulas supra-renais
Supratroclear	Ramo terminal (com a artéria supra-orbital) da artéria oftálmica	Passa desde a incisura supratroclear até a parte medial da fronte e o couro cabeludo anterior	Pele e músculos da parte medial da fronte e do couro cabeludo adjacente
Surais, direita e esquerda	Poplítea	Grandes ramos originados no nível dos côndilos do fêmur e passam diretamente para as cabeças do gastrocnêmio, enviando ramos para o sóleo	Nutrem as cabeças lateral e medial do músculo gastrocnêmio, músculos plantar e sóleo
Temporal profunda, anterior e posterior	2.ª parte da artéria maxilar	Ascende entre o osso temporal e o osso da fossa temporal	Nutre o músculo temporal, o periósteo e o osso
Temporal superficial	Menor ramo terminal da artéria carótida externa	Ascende anteriormente à orelha na região temporal e termina no couro cabeludo	Músculos faciais e pele das regiões frontal e temporal
Testiculares	Aorta abdominal, inferior às artérias renais	Descem ínfero-lateralmente através dos músculos psoas, atravessam o canal inguinal como parte do cordão espermático e alcançam o testículo na bolsa escrotal	A parte abdominal fornece ramos/sangue arterial para os ureteres, linfonodos ilíacos; a parte inguinal/escrotal nutre o músculo cremaster e outros revestimentos do cordão espermático e testículo
Tibial anterior	Ramo terminal (com a tibial posterior) da artéria poplítea	Passa entre a tíbia e a fíbula para dentro do compartimento anterior, através do hiato na parte superior da membrana interóssea e desce nessa membrana, entre o tibial anterior e o extensor longo dos dedos	Compartimento anterior da perna
Tibial posterior	Poplítea	Atravessa o compartimento posterior da perna e termina distal ao retináculo flexor ao se dividir nas artérias plantares medial e lateral	Compartimentos posterior e lateral da perna; ramo circunflexo fibular une-se às anastomoses ao redor do joelho; artéria nutrícia passa para a tíbia
Tireóidea ima	Tronco braquiocefálico ou arco da aorta	Ascende na face anterior da traquéia até a glândula tireóide	Nutre a face medial de ambos os lobos da tireóide

Artéria/Artérias	Origem	Trajeto	Ramos/Distribuição
Tireóidea inferior	Ramo terminal (com a artéria cervical ascendente) do tronco tireocervical	Ascende anteriormente ao músculo escaleno anterior, vira-se medialmente, passando entre os vasos vertebrais e a bainha carótica, em seguida desce sobre o músculo longo do pescoço até a borda inferior da glândula tireóide	Ramos: artéria laríngea inferior; ramos faríngeo, traqueal, esofágico e glandulares inferior e ascendente (último para as glândulas paratireóides); principal artéria visceral do pescoço
Tireóidea superior	1.º ramo da face anterior da artéria carótida externa	Passa no sentido ínfero-medial, profundamente aos músculos infra-hióideos, até o pólo superior da glândula tireóide; sua anastomose com a artéria tireóidea inferior fornece uma importante via colateral entre as artérias carótida externa e subclávia	Ramos: artéria laríngea superior, e ramos infra-hióideo, esternocleidomastóideo, cricotireóideo e ramos glandulares anterior, posterior e lateral
Torácica interna	Superfície inferior da artéria subclávia	Desce, inclinando-se ântero-medialmente, posterior à extremidade esternal da clavícula e cartilagens costais, lateral ao esterno e anterior aos revestimentos do transverso do tórax; divide-se no nível da 6.ª cartilagem costal nas artérias epigástrica superior e musculofrênica	Esterno e pele anterior a ele; por meio das artérias intercostais anteriores chega aos espaços intercostais 1–6; por meio das artérias perfurantes, para a face medial da mama
Torácica lateral	Segunda parte da artéria axilar	Desce ao longo da borda axilar do músculo peitoral menor e o segue sobre a parede torácica	Parede torácica lateral (músculos peitorais, serrátil anterior, intercostais) e mama
Torácica superior	Ramo único da primeira parte da artéria axilar	Corre ântero-medialmente ao longo da borda superior do músculo peitoral menor e, em seguida, passa entre ele e o músculo peitoral maior para a parede torácica	Ajuda a nutrir o 1.º e 2.º espaços intercostais e a parte superior do músculo serrátil anterior
Toracoacromial	Segunda parte da artéria axilar profundamente ao músculo peitoral menor	Enrola-se ao redor da borda súpero-medial do peitoral menor, perfura a fáscia clavipeitoral e divide-se em quatro ramos	Ramos: acromial, clavicular, peitoral e deltóide
Toracodorsal	Artéria subescapular	Continua o trajeto da artéria subescapular e acompanha o nervo toracodorsal até o latíssimo do dorso	Músculo latíssimo do dorso
Tronco celíaco	Parte abdominal da aorta algo distal ao hiato aórtico do diafragma	Percorre um curto trajeto (1,25 cm), dando origem à artéria gástrica esquerda e bifurcando-se nas artérias esplênica e hepática comum	Irriga a parte mais inferior do esôfago, estômago, duodeno (proximal ao ducto biliar), fígado e aparelho biliar e pâncreas
Tronco tireocervical	Face anterior da primeira parte da artéria subclávia	Ascende como um tronco curto e largo próximo à borda medial do escaleno anterior e posterior à bainha carótica	Ramos a partir do tronco: cervical transverso (ou cervical superficial) e supra-escapular; ramos terminais: artérias cervical ascendente e tireóidea inferior
Ulnar	Maior ramo terminal da artéria braquial na fossa cubital	Passa ínfero-medialmente e, em seguida, diretamente inferiormente, profundamente aos músculos pronador redondo, palmar longo e flexor superficial dos dedos para atingir o lado medial do antebraço; passa superficial ao retináculo dos músculos flexores no punho e emite um ramo palmar profundo para o arco profundo e continua como o arco palmar superficial	Nutre a parte medial (ulnar) do compartimento anterior do antebraço, punho e mão; nutre as estruturas superficiais da porção central da região palmar, e a maior parte das faces palmar e dorsal distal dos dedos
Umbilical	Divisão anterior da artéria ilíaca interna	Oblitera-se para se transformar no ligamento umbilical medial depois de fazer um curto trajeto pélvico, durante o qual origina as artérias vesicais superiores	Face superior da bexiga urinária (através das artérias vesicais superiores); ocasionalmente artérias para o ducto deferente (masculino)
Uterina	Divisão anterior da ilíaca interna	Corre medialmente na base do ligamento largo superior ao ligamento cardinal, cruzando superiormente ao ureter, para os lados do útero	Útero, ligamentos uterinos, tuba uterina e vagina
Vaginal	Artéria uterina	Origina-se lateral ao ureter e desce inferiormente a ele até a face lateral da vagina	Vagina; ramos para a parte inferior da bexiga urinária e término do ureter

Artéria/Artérias	Origem	Trajeto	Ramos/Distribuição
Vertebral	1.ª parte da artéria subclávia	Ascende verticalmente através dos forames transversos das vértebras C6–C2, passa lateralmente para atravessar os forames de C1, em seguida corre horizontal e medialmente e penetra no forame magno; no nível intracraniano, funde-se com a artéria contralateral para formar a artéria basilar	Ramos cervicais: espinais (dando origem às artérias radiculares e medular segmentar) e musculares (para os músculos suboccipitais) Ramos intracranianos: meníngeo, espinais anterior e posterior, cerebelar inferior posterior, medulares medial e lateral
Vesical inferior (masculino)	Divisão anterior da artéria ilíaca interna	Passa pelo espaço retroperitoneal até a face inferior da bexiga urinária masculina	Face inferior da bexiga urinária, ducto deferente, vesícula seminal e próstata
Vesical superior	Parte permeável (proximal) da artéria umbilical	Em geral múltiplas, essas artérias passam para a face superior da bexiga urinária	Face superior da bexiga urinária, porção pélvica do ureter

MÚSCULOS DO CORPO HUMANO

Músculo(s)	Origem	Inserção	Inervação	Ação(ões) Principal(is)
Abdutor curto do polegar	Retináculo dos músculos flexores e tubérculos do escafóide e trapézio	Lado lateral da base da falange proximal do polegar	Ramo recorrente do nervo mediano (C8 e T1)	Abduz o polegar e ajuda a fazer sua oposição
Abdutor do dedo mínimo da mão	Pisiforme, ligamento piso-hamato, retináculo dos músculos flexores	Lado medial da base da falange proximal do dedo mínimo da mão	Ramo profundo do nervo ulnar (C8 e T1)	Abduz o 5.º dedo da mão
Abdutor do dedo mínimo do pé	Tubérculos medial e lateral da tuberosidade do calcâneo, aponeurose plantar e septos intermusculares	Lado lateral da base da falange proximal do 5.º dedo do pé	Nervo plantar lateral (S2 e S3)	Abduz e flexiona o 5.º dedo do pé
Abdutor do hálux	Tubérculo medial da tuberosidade do calcâneo, retináculo dos músculos flexores e aponeurose plantar	Lado medial da base da falange proximal do 1.º dedo	Nervo plantar medial (S2 e S3)	Abduz e flexiona o 1.º dedo (polegar, hálux)
Abdutor longo do polegar	Superfícies posteriores da ulna, rádio e membrana interóssea	Base do 1.º metacarpal	Nervo interósseo posterior (C7 e C8), a continuação do ramo profundo do nervo radial	Abduz o polegar e o estica na articulação carpometacarpal
Adutor curto	Corpo e ramo inferior do púbis	Linha pectínea e a parte proximal da linha áspera do fêmur	Nervo obturatório (L2, L3 e L4), ramo da divisão anterior	Aduz a coxa e, em alguma extensão, a flexiona
Adutor do hálux	Cabeça oblíqua: bases do 2.º–4.º metatarsais Cabeça transversa: ligamentos plantares das articulações metatarsofalângicas	Tendões de ambas as cabeças inserem-se no lado lateral da base da falange proximal do 1.º dedo	Ramo profundo do nervo plantar lateral (S2 e S3)	Aduz o 1.º dedo; auxilia na manutenção do arco transverso do pé
Adutor do polegar	Cabeça oblíqua: bases do 2.º e 3.º metacarpais, capitato e carpais adjacentes; Cabeça transversa: superfície anterior do corpo do 3.º metacarpal	Lado medial da base da falange proximal do polegar	Ramo profundo do nervo ulnar (C8 e T1)	Aduz o polegar em direção ao dedo médio
Adutor longo	Corpo do púbis inferior à crista púbica	Terço médio da linha áspera do fêmur	Nervo obturatório, ramo da divisão anterior (L2, L3 e L4)	Aduz a coxa
Adutor magno	Parte adutora: ramo inferior do púbis, ramo do ísquio; Parte dos músculos isquiotibiais: tuberosidade isquiática	Parte adutora: tuberosidade glútea, linha áspera, linha supracondilar medial; Parte dos músculos isquiotibiais: tubérculo adutor do fêmur	Parte adutora: nervo obturatório (L2, L3 e L4), ramos da divisão posterior; Parte dos músculos isquiotibiais: parte tibial do nervo isquiático (L4)	Aduz a coxa; Parte adutora: flexiona a coxa; Parte dos músculos isquiotibiais: estica a coxa
Adutor mínimo	Ramo púbico inferior	Lábio medial, porção mais superior da linha áspera do fêmur	Nervo obturatório (L2, 3 & 4)	Aduz e roda lateralmente a coxa
Ancôneo	Epicôndilo lateral do úmero	Superfície lateral do olécrano e parte superior da superfície posterior da ulna	Nervo radial (C7, C8 e T1)	Auxilia o tríceps na extensão do antebraço; estabiliza a articulação do cotovelo; abduz a ulna durante a pronação
Aritenóides, transverso e oblíquo	Borda póstero-lateral de uma cartilagem aritenóidea	Borda póstero-lateral da cartilagem aritenóidea oposta	Nervo laríngeo recorrente (ramo do vago (NC X))	Fecha a porção intercartilagínea da rima glótica
Articular do cotovelo	Porção distal da face posterior da diáfise do úmero	Cápsula fibrosa posterior da articulação do cotovelo	Nervo radial (C7 e C8)	Retrai a cápsula articular posterior durante a extensão do cotovelo
Articular do joelho	Porção distal da face anterior da diáfise do fêmur	Membrana sinovial da bolsa suprapatelar da articulação do joelho	Nervo femoral (L2–L4)	Retrai a membrana sinovial durante a extensão do joelho

MÚSCULOS DO CORPO HUMANO

Músculo(s)	Origem	Inserção	Inervação	Ação(ões) Principal(is)
Auriculares anterior, posterior e superior	Aponeurose epicraniana e parte mastóide do osso temporal	Orelha (ouvido externo)	Nervo facial (NC VII)	Protração, retração e elevação da orelha no lado da cabeça
Bíceps braquial	Cabeça curta: extremidade do processo coracóide da escápula; Cabeça longa: tubérculo supraglenóide da escápula	Tuberosidade do rádio e fáscia do antebraço por meio da aponeurose bicipital	Nervo musculocutâneo (C5 e C6)	Supina o antebraço e, quando está em posição supinada, flexiona o antebraço
Bíceps femoral	Cabeça longa: tuberosidade isquiática Cabeça curta: linha áspera e linha supracondilar lateral do fêmur	Lado lateral da cabeça da fíbula; o tendão desdobra-se nesse local através do ligamento colateral fibular do joelho	Cabeça longa: divisão tibial do nervo isquiático (L5, S1 e S2) Cabeça curta: divisão fibular comum do nervo isquiático (L5, S1 e S2)	Flexiona a perna e a roda lateralmente quando o joelho é flexionado; estende a coxa (p.ex., quando começa a caminhar)
Braquial	Metade distal da superfície anterior do úmero	Processo coronóide e tuberosidade da ulna	Nervo musculocutâneo (C5 e C6)	Flexiona o antebraço em todas as posições
Braquirradial	Dois terços proximais da crista supracondilar do úmero	Superfície lateral da extremidade distal do rádio	Nervo radial (C5, C6 e C7)	Flexiona o antebraço
Bucinador	Mandíbula, rafe pterigomandibular e processos alveolares da maxila e mandíbula	Ângulo da boca	Nervo facial (NC VII)	Pressiona a bochecha contra os dentes molares, auxiliando, portanto, a mastigação; expele o ar da cavidade oral como ao tocar um instrumento de sopro; desvia a boca para um lado quando age unilateralmente
Bulboesponjoso	Masculino: rafe mediana, superfície ventral do bulbo do pênis e corpo perineal Feminino: corpo perineal	Masculino: corpos esponjosos e cavernosos e fáscia do bulbo do pênis Feminino: fáscia do corpo cavernoso	Ramo profundo do nervo perineal, um ramo do nervo pudendo (S2, 3 e 4)	Funciona com o esfíncter anal externo para apoiar/fixar o corpo perineal; Masculino: comprime o bulbo do pênis para expulsar as últimas gotas de urina/sêmen; auxilia a ereção empurrando o sangue para dentro do corpo do pênis e comprimindo as veias de efluxo; Feminino: "esfíncter" da vagina e auxilia na ereção do clitóris
Ciliar	Esporão da esclera	Fibras meridionais, radiais e circulares são intrínsecas ao corpo ciliar	Fibras parassimpáticas do nervo oculomotor e gânglio ciliar	Alivia a tensão sobre a lente do olho, permitindo que ela se torne mais convexa para a visão de perto
Coccígeo (isquiococcígeo)	Espinha isquiática	Extremidade inferior do sacro	Ramos dos nervos S4 e S5	Forma uma pequena parte do diafragma pélvico que suporta as vísceras pélvicas; flexiona o cóccix
Constritor inferior da faringe	Linha oblíqua da cartilagem tireóidea e lado da cartilagem cricóidea	Rafe mediana da faringe	Raiz craniana do nervo acessório (NC XI) conforme acima, mais ramos de nervos laríngeos externo e recorrente do vago (NC X)	Contrai a parede da faringe durante a deglutição
Constritor médio da faringe	Ligamento estilo-hióideo e cornos superior (maior) e inferior (menor) do osso hióide	Rafe mediana da faringe	Raiz craniana do nervo acessório (NC XI) mais ramos dos nervos laríngeos externo e recorrente do vago (NC X)	Contrai a parede da faringe durante a deglutição
Constritor superior da faringe	Hâmulo pterigóideo, rafe pterigomandibular, extremidade posterior da linha milo-hióidea da mandíbula e lado da língua	Rafe mediana da faringe e tubérculo faríngeo na porção basilar do osso occipital	Raiz craniana do nervo acessório através do ramo faríngeo do vago e plexo faríngeo	Contrai a parede da faringe durante a deglutição

Apêndices

Músculo(s)	Origem	Inserção	Inervação	Ação(ões) Principal(is)
Coracobraquial	Extremidade do processo coracóide da escápula	Terço médio da superfície medial do úmero	Nervo musculocutâneo (C5, C6 e C7)	Ajuda a flexionar e aduzir o braço
Corrugador do supercílio	Extremidade medial do arco superciliar do osso frontal	Pele acima do meio da sobrancelha	Nervo facial (NC VII)	Puxa medial e inferiormente as sobrancelhas, produzindo rugas verticais acima do nariz
Cremaster	Músculo oblíquo interno e ligamento inguinal	Cordão espermático e túnica vaginal	Ramo genital do nervo genitofemoral (L1–L2)	Elevação do testículo
Cricoaritenóide lateral	Arco da cartilagem cricóidea	Processo muscular da cartilagem aritenóidea	Nervo laríngeo recorrente (ramo do vago (NC X))	Aduz a prega vocal (porção interligamentosa)
Cricoaritenóide posterior	Superfície posterior das lâminas da cartilagem cricóidea	Processo muscular da cartilagem aritenóidea	Nervo laríngeo recorrente (ramo do vago (NC X))	Abduz a prega vocal
Cricofaríngeo	Cartilagem cricóidea póstero-lateral em um lado	Cartilagem cricóidea póstero-lateral do outro lado	Vago (NC X)	Serve como esfíncter esofágico superior
Cricotireóideo	Parte ântero-lateral da cartilagem cricóidea	Margem inferior e corno inferior da cartilagem tireóidea	Nervo laríngeo externo	Alonga e tensiona a prega vocal
Deltóide	Terço lateral da clavícula, acrômio e espinha da escápula	Tuberosidade deltóide do úmero	Nervo axilar (C5 e C6)	Parte anterior: flexiona e roda medialmente o braço; Parte medial: abduz o braço; Parte posterior: estica e roda lateralmente o braço
Depressor do lábio inferior/ângulo da boca	Face ântero-lateral do corpo da mandíbula	Lábio inferior/ângulo da boca	Ramo mandibular marginal do nervo facial (NC VII)	Deprime e/ou everte o lábio inferior/puxa inferiormente o ângulo da boca e o modíolo
Depressor do septo nasal	Fossa incisiva da maxila	Parte móvel do septo nasal	Nervo facial	Ajuda a dilatar as narinas durante a inspiração profunda e deprime o septo nasal
Diafragma	Processo xifóide; 6 cartilagens costais inferiores e costelas associadas; ligamentos arqueados; ligamentos longitudinais anteriores e corpos e discos das vértebras lombares 1–3	Tendão central do diafragma	Nervo frênico (C3–C5)	Rebaixa o diafragma, diminuindo a pressão intratorácica e resultando em inspiração, além de auxiliar o retorno do sangue venoso para o coração
Digástrico	Ventre anterior: fossa digástrica da mandíbula Ventre posterior: incisura mastóidea do osso temporal	Tendão intermediário para o corpo e corno maior do osso hióide	Ventre anterior: nervo milo-hióideo, um ramo do nervo alveolar inferior Ventre posterior: nervo facial (NC VII)	Deprime a mandíbula; eleva o osso hióide e o estabiliza durante a deglutição e a fala
Eretor da espinha	Origina-se por um largo tendão a partir da parte posterior da crista ilíaca, superfície posterior do sacro, processos espinhosos sacral e lombar inferior e ligamento supra-espinal	Iliocostal — lombar, torácica e cervical: as fibras correm superiormente até os ângulos das costelas inferiores e os processos transversos cervicais Longuíssimo — torácica, cervical e craniana: as fibras correm superiormente até as costelas entre tubérculos e ângulos, até os processos transversos nas regiões torácica e cervical e até o processo mastóide do osso temporal Espinal — torácica, cervical e craniana: as fibras correm superiormente até os processos espinhosos na região torácica superior e até o crânio	Ramos posteriores dos nervos espinais	Agindo bilateralmente, esticam a coluna vertebral e a cabeça; quando as costas são flexionadas, eles controlam o movimento graças ao alongamento gradual de suas fibras; agindo unilateralmente, eles curvam a coluna vertebral para os lados

Músculo(s)	Origem	Inserção	Inervação	Ação(ões) Principal(is)
Escaleno anterior	Processos transversos das vértebras C4–C6	1.ª costela	Nervos espinais cervicais de C4, C5 e C6	Eleva a 1.ª costela; flexiona lateralmente e roda o pescoço
Escaleno médio	Tubérculos posteriores dos processos transversos das vértebras C4–C6	Superfície superior da 1.ª costela, sulco posterior para a artéria subclávia	Ramos anteriores dos nervos espinais cervicais	Flexiona o pescoço lateralmente; eleva a 1.ª costela durante a inspiração forçada
Escaleno posterior	Tubérculos posteriores dos processos transversos das vértebras C4–C6	Borda externa da 2.ª costela	Ramos anteriores dos nervos espinais cervicais C7 e C8	Flexiona lateralmente o pescoço; eleva a 2.ª costela durante a inspiração forçada
Esfíncter anal externo	Pele e fáscia que circundam o ânus e o cóccix por meio do ligamento anococcígeo	Corpo perineal	Nervo anal inferior	Fecha o canal anal; "trabalha" com o músculo bulboesponjoso para apoiar e fixar o corpo perineal
Esfíncter uretral externo	Superfície interna do ramo ísquio-púbico e tuberosidade isquiática	Circunda a uretra; nos homens também ascende a face anterior da próstata; no sexo feminino, algumas fibras também envolvem a vagina (esfíncter uretrovaginal)	Ramo profundo do nervo perineal, um ramo do nervo pudendo (S2, 3 e 4)	Comprime a uretra para manter a continência urinária; no sexo feminino, a porção do esfíncter uretrovaginal também comprime a vagina
Esplênio da cabeça e do pescoço	Origina-se da metade inferior do ligamento nucal e processos espinhosos das vértebras C7–T3 ou T4	Esplênio da cabeça: as fibras correm súpero-lateralmente até o processo mastóideo do osso temporal e terço lateral da linha nucal superior do osso occipital. Esplênio do pescoço: tubérculos posteriores dos processos transversos das vértebras C1–C3 ou C4	Ramos posteriores dos nervos espinhais	Atuando isoladamente, curvam lateralmente e rodam a cabeça para o lado dos músculos ativos; atuando em conjunto, eles estendem a cabeça e o pescoço
Estapédio	Paredes internas da eminência piramidal da parede posterior da cavidade timpânica	Colo do estribo	Nervo facial (NC VII)	Amortece as vibrações do estribo por reflexo, em resposta ao ruído alto
Esternocleidomastóideo	Superfície lateral do processo mastóideo do osso temporal e metade lateral da linha nucal superior	Cabeça esternal: superfície anterior do manúbrio do esterno. Cabeça clavicular: superfície superior do terço medial da clavícula	Raiz espinal do nervo acessório (motor) e nervos C2 e C3 (dor e propriocepção)	Inclina a cabeça para um lado, ou seja, lateralmente; flexiona o pescoço e o roda, de modo que a face fica virada superiormente no sentido do lado oposto; atuando em conjunto, os dois músculos flexionam o pescoço, de modo que o queixo é empurrado para diante
Esterno-hióideo	Manúbrio do esterno e extremidade medial da clavícula	Corpo do osso hióide	C1–C3 por um ramo da alça cervical	Deprime o osso hióide depois que foi elevado durante a deglutição
Esternotireóideo	Superfície posterior do manúbrio do esterno	Linha oblíqua da cartilagem tireóidea	C2 e C3 por um ramo da alça cervical	Deprime o osso hióide e a laringe
Estilofaríngeo	Processo estilóide do osso temporal	Bordas posterior e superior da cartilagem tireóidea com o palatofaríngeo	Nervo glossofaríngeo (NC IX)	Eleva (encurta e alarga) a faringe e a laringe durante a deglutição e a fala
Estiloglosso	Processo estilóide e ligamento estilo-hióideo	Lado e face inferior da língua	Nervo hipoglosso (NC XII)	Retrai a língua e a puxa para cima para criar uma depressão para a deglutição
Estilo-hióideo	Processo estilóide do osso temporal	Corpo do osso hióide	Ramo cervical do nervo facial (NC VII)	Eleva e retrai o osso hióide, alongando, assim, o assoalho da boca
Extensor curto do hálux	Porção mais anterior da superfície superior do calcâneo	Face dorsal da base da falange proximal do hálux	Nervo fibular profundo (L5 e S1)	Estica o hálux
Extensor curto do polegar	Superfície posterior do rádio e membrana interóssea	Base da falange proximal do polegar	Nervo interósseo posterior (C7 e C8), a continuação do ramo profundo do nervo radial	Estende a falange proximal do polegar na articulação carpometacarpal

Músculo(s)	Origem	Inserção	Inervação	Ação(ões) Principal(is)
Extensor curto dos dedos	Porções mais anteriores das superfícies lateral e superior do calcâneo	Lado lateral dos tendões do extensor longo, com fibras até as falanges proximais do 2.º–4.º artelhos	Nervo fibular profundo (L5 e S1)	Auxilia na extensão dos três artelhos médios
Extensor do dedo mínimo	Epicôndilo lateral do úmero	Expansão do extensor do 5.º dedo	Nervo interósseo posterior (C7 e C8), a continuação do ramo profundo do nervo radial	Estende o 5.º dedo nas articulações metacarpofalângicas e interfalângicas
Extensor do indicador	Superfície posterior da ulna e membrana interóssea	Expansão do extensor do 2.º dedo	Nervo interósseo posterior (C7 e C8), a continuação do ramo profundo do nervo radial	Estende o 2.º dedo e ajuda a esticar a mão
Extensor dos dedos	Epicôndilo lateral do úmero	Expansões extensoras dos quatro dedos mediais	Nervo interósseo posterior (C7 e C8), a continuação do ramo profundo do nervo radial	Estende os quatro dedos mediais nas articulações metacarpofalângicas; estende a mão na articulação do punho
Extensor longo do hálux	Parte média da superfície anterior da fíbula e membrana interóssea	Face dorsal da base da falange distal do hálux	Nervo fibular profundo (L5 e S1)	Estende o hálux e dorsiflete o tornozelo
Extensor longo do polegar	Superfície posterior do terço médio da ulna e membrana interóssea	Base da falange distal do polegar	Nervo interósseo posterior (C7 e C8), a continuação do ramo profundo do nervo radial	Estende a falange distal do polegar nas articulações metacarpofalângicas e interfalângicas
Extensor longo dos dedos	Côndilo lateral da tíbia e três quartos superiores da superfície medial da fíbula e da membrana interóssea	Falanges média e distal dos quatro dedos laterais	Nervo fibular profundo (L5 e S1)	Estica os quatro dedos laterais e dorsiflete o tornozelo
Extensor radial curto do carpo	Epicôndilo lateral do úmero	Base do 3.º osso metacarpal	Ramo profundo do nervo radial (C7 e C8)	Estica e abduz a mão na articulação do punho
Extensor radial longo do carpo	Crista supracondilar lateral do úmero	Base do 2.º osso metacarpal	Nervo radial (C6 e C7)	Estende e abduz a mão na articulação do punho
Extensor ulnar do carpo	Epicôndilo lateral do úmero e borda posterior da ulna	Base do 5.º osso metacarpal	Nervo interósseo posterior (C7 e C8), a continuação do ramo profundo do nervo radial	Estende e aduz a mão na articulação do punho
Fibular curto	Dois terços inferiores da superfície lateral da fíbula	Superfície dorsal da tuberosidade no lado lateral da base do 5.º metatarsal	Nervo fibular superficial (L5, S1 e S2)	Everte o pé e faz flexão plantar fraca do tornozelo
Fibular longo	Cabeça e dois terços superiores da superfície lateral da fíbula	Base do 1.º metatarsal e cuneiforme medial	Nervo fibular superficial (L5, S1 e S2)	Everte o pé e faz a flexão plantar fraca do tornozelo
Fibular terceiro	Terço inferior da superfície anterior da fíbula e membrana interóssea	Dorso da base do 5.º metatarsal	Nervo fibular profundo (L5 e S1)	Dorsiflete o tornozelo e auxilia na eversão do pé
Flexor curto do dedo mínimo da mão	Hâmulo do osso hamato e retináculo dos músculos flexores	Lado medial da base da falange proximal do dedo mínimo	Ramo profundo do nervo ulnar (C8 e T1)	Flete a falange proximal do 5.º dedo
Flexor curto do dedo mínimo do pé	Base do 5.º metatarsal	Base da falange proximal do 5.º dedo	Ramo superficial do nervo plantar lateral (S2 e S3)	Flete a falange proximal do 5.º dedo, auxiliando, assim, em sua flexão
Flexor curto do hálux	Superfícies plantares do cubóide e dos cuneiformes laterais	Ambos os lados da base da falange proximal do 1.º dedo	Nervo plantar medial (S2 e S3)	Flexiona a falange proximal do 1.º dedo
Flexor curto do polegar	Retináculo dos músculos flexores e tubérculos do escafóide e trapézio	Lado lateral da base da falange proximal do polegar	Ramo recorrente do nervo mediano (C8 e T1)	Flexiona o polegar
Flexor curto dos dedos	Tubérculo medial da tuberosidade do calcâneo, aponeurose plantar e septos intermusculares	Ambos os lados das falanges médias dos quatro dedos laterais	Nervo plantar medial (S2 e S3)	Flexiona os quatro dedos laterais

Músculo(s)	Origem	Inserção	Inervação	Ação(ões) Principal(is)
Flexor longo do hálux	Dois terços inferiores da superfície posterior da fíbula e parte inferior da membrana interóssea	Base da falange distal do hálux	Nervo tibial (S2 e S3)	Flexiona o hálux em todas as articulações e faz a flexão plantar fraca do tornozelo; sustenta os arcos longitudinais mediais do pé
Flexor longo do polegar	Superfície anterior do rádio e membrana interóssea adjacente	Base da falange distal do polegar	Nervo interósseo anterior a partir do mediano (C8 e T1)	Flexiona as falanges do 1.º dedo (polegar)
Flexor longo dos dedos	Parte medial da superfície posterior da tíbia, inferior à linha solear e por um amplo tendão para a fíbula	Bases das falanges distais dos quatro dedos laterais	Nervo tibial (S2 e S3)	Flexiona os quatro dedos laterais e faz a flexão plantar do tornozelo; sustenta os arcos longitudinais do pé
Flexor profundo dos dedos	Três quartos proximais das superfícies medial e anterior da ulna e membrana interóssea	Bases das falanges distais dos quatro dedos mediais	Parte medial: nervo ulnar (C8 e T1); Parte lateral: nervo mediano (C8 e T1)	Flexiona as falanges distais nas articulações interfalângicas distais dos quatro dedos mediais; auxilia com a flexão da mão
Flexor radial do carpo	Epicôndilo medial do úmero	Base do 2.º osso metacarpal	Nervo mediano (C6 e C7)	Flexiona e abduz a mão (no punho)
Flexor superficial dos dedos	Cabeça úmero-ulnar: epicôndilo medial do úmero, ligamento colateral ulnar e processo coronóide da ulna. Cabeça radial: metade superior da borda anterior do rádio	Corpos das falanges médias dos quatro dedos mediais	Nervo mediano (C7, C8 e T1)	Flexiona as falanges médias nas articulações interfalângicas proximais dos quatro dedos mediais; atuando com maior vigor, também flexiona as falanges proximais nas articulações metacarpofalângicas e a mão no punho
Flexor ulnar do carpo	Cabeça umeral: epicôndilo medial do úmero. Cabeça ulnar: olécrano e borda posterior da ulna	Osso pisiforme, músculo do osso hamato e 5.º osso metacarpal	Nervo ulnar (C7 e C8)	Flexiona e aduz a mão (no punho)
Gastrocnêmio	Cabeça lateral: face lateral do côndilo lateral do fêmur. Cabeça medial: superfície poplítea do fêmur, superior ao côndilo medial	Superfície posterior do calcâneo através do tendão do calcâneo	Nervo tibial (S1 e S2)	Faz a flexão plantar do tornozelo quando o joelho está esticado. Eleva o calcanhar durante a marcha e flexiona a perna na articulação do joelho
Gêmeos superior e inferior	Superior: espinha isquiática. Inferior: tuberosidade isquiática	Superfície medial do trocanter maior (fossa trocantérica) do fêmur	Gêmeo superior: nervo para o músculo obturatório interno (L5 e S1); Gêmeo inferior: nervo para o músculo quadrado femoral (L5 e S1)	Roda lateralmente a coxa esticada e abduz a coxa flexionada; estabiliza a cabeça do fêmur no acetábulo
Genioglosso	Parte superior da espinha geniana da mandíbula	Dorso da língua e corpo do osso hióide	Nervo hipoglosso (NC XII)	Deprime a língua; sua parte posterior puxa anteriormente a língua para a protrusão
Genio-hióideo	Espinha geniana inferior da mandíbula	Corpo do osso hióide	C1 através do nervo hipoglosso	Puxa o osso hióide ântero-superiormente, encurta o assoalho da boca e alarga a faringe
Glúteo máximo	Ílio posterior até a linha glútea posterior, superfície dorsal do sacro e cóccix, e ligamento sacrotuberoso	A maioria das fibras termina no trato iliotibial que se insere no côndilo lateral da tíbia; algumas fibras inserem-se na tuberosidade maior do fêmur	Nervo glúteo inferior (L5, S1 e S2)	Estica a coxa (especialmente a partir da posição fletida) e auxilia em sua rotação lateral; equilibra a coxa e auxilia na elevação a partir da posição sentada
Glúteo médio	Superfície externa do ílio entre as linhas glúteas anterior e posterior	Superfície lateral do trocanter maior do fêmur	Nervo glúteo superior (L5 e S1)	Abduz e roda medialmente a coxa; mantém a pelve nivelada quando a perna oposta é levantada do solo
Glúteo mínimo	Superfície externa do ílio entre as linhas glúteas anterior e inferior	Superfície anterior do trocanter maior do fêmur	Nervo glúteo superior (L5 e S1)	Abduz e roda medialmente a coxa; mantém a pelve nivelada quando a perna oposta é levantada do solo

Músculo(s)	Origem	Inserção	Inervação	Ação(ões) Principal(is)
Grácil	Corpo e ramo inferior do púbis	Parte superior da superfície medial da tíbia	Nervo obturatório (L2 e L3)	Aduz a coxa, flexiona a perna e ajuda a rodá-la medialmente
Hioglosso	Corpo e corno maior do osso hióide	Lado e face inferior da língua	Nervo hipoglosso (NC XII)	Deprime e retrai a língua
Ilíaco	Crista ilíaca, dois terços superiores da fossa ilíaca, asa do sacro e ligamentos sacroilíacos anteriores	Trocanter menor do fêmur e diáfise inferior a ele, e para o tendão do músculo psoas maior	Nervo femoral (L2–L4)	Flexiona a coxa e estabiliza a articulação do quadril; atua com o músculo psoas maior
Infra-espinal	Fossa infra-espinal da escápula	Face média no tubérculo maior do úmero	Nervo supra-escapular (C5 e C6)	Roda lateralmente o braço; ajuda a manter a cabeça do úmero na cavidade glenoidal da escápula
Intercostais mais internos	Borda inferior das costelas	Borda superior das costelas abaixo	Nervos intercostais	Provavelmente eleva as costelas
Intercostais mais internos	Superfície interna das costelas, desde os ângulos até a junção costocondral	Borda superior das costelas abaixo	Nervos intercostais	Provavelmente deprime as costelas
Intercostal externo	Borda inferior das costelas, desde o tubérculo até a junção costocondral	Borda superior das costelas abaixo	Nervos intercostais	Eleva as costelas (quando as costelas superiores são fixadas pelos músculos escaleno e esternocleidomastóideo)
Intercostal interno	Superfície interna das costelas, desde os ângulos até o esterno	Borda superior das costelas abaixo	Nervos intercostais	A porção intercondral eleva as costelas (quando as costelas superiores estão fixas), a porção interóssea deprime as costelas (quando as costelas inferiores estão fixas)
Interespinais	Superfícies superiores dos processos espinhosos das vértebras cervicais e lombares	Superfícies internas dos processos espinhosos das vértebras superiores às vértebras de origem	Ramos posteriores dos nervos espinais	Auxiliam na extensão e rotação da coluna vertebral
Interósseos dorsais (quatro músculos) do pé	Lados adjacentes dos metatarsais 1–5	Primeiro: lado medial da falange proximal do 2.º dedo; Segundo ao quarto: lados laterais do 2.º ao 4.º dedos	Nervo plantar lateral (S2 e S3)	Abduz os dedos (2–4) e flexiona as articulações metatarsofalângicas
Interósseos dorsais 1–4 da mão	Lados adjacentes dos dois metacarpais (músculos bipenados)	Expansões extensoras e bases das falanges proximais dos dedos 2–4	Ramo profundo do nervo ulnar (C8 e T1)	Abduz os dedos a partir da linha axial e atua com os músculos lumbricais para flexionar as articulações metacarpofalângicas e esticar as articulações interfalângicas
Interósseos palmares 1–3	Superfícies palmares do 2.º, 4.º e 5.º metacarpais (músculos unipenados)	Expansões extensoras dos dedos e bases das falanges proximais dos dedos 2, 4 e 5	Ramo profundo do nervo ulnar (C8 e T1)	Aduz os dedos em direção à linha axial e auxilia os músculos lumbricais na flexão das articulações metacarpofalângicas e na extensão das articulações interfalângicas
Interósseos plantares 1–3	Bases e lados mediais dos metatarsais 3–5	Lados mediais das bases das falanges proximais do 3.º ao 5.º dedos	Nervo plantar lateral (S2 e S3)	Aduz os dedos (2–4) e flexiona as articulações metatarsofalângicas
Intertransversários	Processos transversos das vértebras cervicais e lombares	Processos transversais das vértebras adjacentes	Ramos posterior e anterior dos nervos espinais	Auxiliam na curvatura lateral da coluna vertebral; agindo bilateralmente, estabilizam a coluna vertebral
Isquiocavernoso	Superfície interna do ramo isquiopúbico e tuberosidade isquiática	Ramo do pênis ou ramo do clitóris	Ramo profundo do nervo fibular, um ramo do nervo pudendo (S2, 3 e 4)	Mantém a ereção do pênis ou clitóris comprimindo as veias de efluxo e empurrando o sangue para o corpo do pênis ou clitóris

Músculo(s)	Origem	Inserção	Inervação	Ação(ões) Principal(is)
Latíssimo do dorso	Processos espinhosos das 6 vértebras torácicas inferiores, fáscia tóraco-lombar, crista ilíaca e 3 ou 4 costelas inferiores	Assoalho do sulco intertubercular do úmero	Nervo tóraco-dorsal (C6, C7 e C8)	Estende, aduz e roda medialmente o úmero; eleva o corpo em direção aos braços durante a escalada
Levantador da escápula	Tubérculos posteriores dos processos transversos das vértebras C1–C4	Parte superior da borda medial da escápula	Nervos dorsal da escápula (C5) e cervical (C3 e C4)	Eleva a escápula e inclina sua cavidade glenoidal inferiormente rodando a escápula
Levantador da pálpebra superior	Asa menor do osso esfenóide, superior e anterior ao canal óptico	Tarso e pele da pálpebra superior	Nervo óculo-motor (NC III); a camada profunda (músculo tarsal superior) é suprida por fibras simpáticas	Eleva a pálpebra superior
Levantador do ângulo da boca	Fossa canina da maxila	Orbicular da boca e pele no ângulo da boca	Nervo facial (NC VII)	Eleva o ângulo da boca, como no sorriso
Levantador do ânus (pubococcígeo, puborretal e iliococcígeo)	Corpo do púbis, arco tendinoso da fáscia obturatória e espinha isquiática	Corpo perineal, cóccix, ligamento anococcígeo, paredes da próstata ou vagina, reto e canal anal	Nervo para o músculo levantador do ânus (ramos de S4) e nervo anal (retal) inferior e plexo coccígeo	Ajuda a sustentar as vísceras pélvicas e resiste aos aumentos da pressão intra-abdominal
Levantador do lábio superior	Processo frontal da maxila e da região infra-orbital	Pele do lábio superior e cartilagem alar do nariz	Nervo facial (NC VII)	Eleva o lábio, dilata as narinas e eleva o ângulo da boca
Levantador do véu palatino	Cartilagem da tuba auditiva e porção petrosa do osso temporal	Aponeurose palatina	Parte craniana do NC XI através do ramo faríngeo do nervo vago (NC X) por meio do plexo faríngeo	Eleva o palato mole durante a deglutição e o bocejo
Levantadores das costelas	Extremidades dos processos transversos das vértebras C7 e T1–T11	Passam ínfero-lateralmente e se inserem na costela subjacente entre seu tubérculo e o ângulo	Ramos posteriores dos nervos espinhais C8–T11	Elevam as costelas, auxiliando a inspiração; ajudam na inclinação lateral da coluna vertebral
Longo da cabeça	Parte basilar do osso occipital	Tubérculos anteriores dos processos transversos de C3–C6	Ramos anteriores dos nervos espinais de C1–C3	Flexiona a cabeça
Longo do pescoço	Tubérculo anterior da vértebra C1 (atlas); corpos de C1–C3 e processos transversos das vértebras C3–C6	Corpos das vértebras C5–T3, processo transverso das vértebras C3–C5	Ramos anteriores dos nervos espinais C2–C6	Flexiona o pescoço com rotação (torção) para o lado oposto, quando atua unilateralmente
Lumbricais 1 e 2 da mão	Dois tendões laterais do flexor profundo dos dedos (músculos unipenados)	Faces laterais das expansões extensoras dos dedos 2 e 3	Nervo mediano (C8 e T1)	Flexionam os dedos nas articulações metacarpofalângicas e esticam as articulações interfalângicas
Lumbricais 3 e 4 da mão	Três tendões mediais do flexor profundo dos dedos (músculos bipenados)	Lados laterais das expansões extensoras dos dedos 4 e 5	Ramo profundo do nervo ulnar (C8 e T1)	Flexionam os dedos nas articulações metacarpofalângicas e esticam as articulações interfalângicas
Masseter	Borda inferior e superfície medial do arco zigomático	Superfície lateral do ramo da mandíbula e seu processo coronóide	Nervo mandibular (NC V3) através do nervo massetérico, que penetra sua superfície profunda	Eleva e faz a protrusão da mandíbula, fechando, assim, a mesma; as fibras profundas a retraem
Mentual	Fossa incisiva da mandíbula	Pele do queixo	Nervo facial (NC VII)	Eleva e projeta o lábio inferior para a frente
Milo-hióideo	Linha milo-hióidea da mandíbula	Rafe e corpo do osso hióide	Nervo milo-hióideo, um ramo do nervo alveolar inferior do NC V3	Eleva o osso hióide, o assoalho da boca e a língua durante a deglutição e a fala
Músculo longitudinal inferior da língua	Raiz da língua e corpo do osso hióide	Ápice da língua	Nervo hipoglosso (NC XII)	Enrola inferiormente a ponta da língua e encurta a língua
Músculo longitudinal superior da língua	Camada fibrosa submucosa e septo fibroso mediano	Margens da língua e mucosa	Nervo hipoglosso (NC XII)	Enrola a extremidade e os lados da língua superiormente e encurta a língua

Músculo(s)	Origem	Inserção	Inervação	Ação(ões) Principal(is)
Músculo transverso da língua	Septo fibroso mediano	Tecido fibroso nas margens da língua	Nervo hipoglosso (NC XII)	Estreita e alonga a língua Age simultaneamente para fazer a protrusão da língua
Músculo transverso profundo do períneo	Superfície interna do ramo ísquio-púbico e a tuberosidade isquiática	Rafe mediana, corpo perineal e esfíncter anal externo	Ramo profundo do nervo perineal, um ramo do nervo pudendo (S2, 3 e 4)	Suportam e fixam o corpo perineal (assoalho pélvico) para sustentar as vísceras abdominopélvicas e resistem à pressão intra-abdominal aumentada
Músculo transverso superficial do períneo	(Apenas a porção compressora da uretra)	Corpo perineal	Ramo profundo do nervo perineal, um ramo do nervo pudendo (S2, 3 e 4)	Sustenta e fixa o corpo perineal (assoalho pélvico) para apoiar as vísceras abdominopélvicas e resistir à pressão intra-abdominal aumentada
Músculo vertical da língua	Superfície superior das bordas da língua	Superfície inferior das bordas da língua	Nervo hipoglosso (NC XII)	Retifica e alarga a língua Age simultaneamente para fazer a protrusão da língua
Músculos da úvula	Espinha nasal posterior e aponeurose palatina	Mucosa da úvula	Parte craniana do NC XI através do ramo faríngeo do nervo vago (NC X) por meio do plexo faríngeo	Encurta a úvula e a puxa para cima
Músculos lumbricais do pé	Tendões do flexor longo dos dedos	Face medial da expansão sobre os quatro dedos laterais	Um medial: nervo plantar medial (S2 e S3) Três laterais: nervo plantar lateral (S2 e S3)	Flexiona as falanges proximais e estica as falanges média e distal dos quatro dedos laterais
Nasal	Parte superior da crista canina da maxila	Cartilagens nasais	Nervo facial (NC VII)	Puxa as asas do nariz em direção ao septo nasal
Oblíquo externo	Superfícies externas da 5.ª–2.ª costelas	Linha alba, tubérculo púbico e metade anterior da crista ilíaca	Nervos toracoabdominais (6 nervos torácicos inferiores) e nervo subcostal	Comprime e sustenta as vísceras abdominais, flexiona e roda o tronco
Oblíquo inferior	Parte anterior do assoalho da órbita	Esclerótica profundamente ao músculo reto lateral	Nervo oculomotor (NC III)	Abduz, eleva e roda lateralmente o bulbo do olho
Oblíquo inferior da cabeça	Processo espinhoso do áxis (vértebra C2)	Processo transverso do atlas (vértebra C1)	Nervo suboccipital	Rotação da cabeça na articulação atlantoaxial
Oblíquo interno	Fáscia toracolombar, dois terços anteriores da crista ilíaca e metade lateral do ligamento inguinal	Bordas inferiores da 10.ª–12.ª costelas, linha alba e linha pectínea do púbis através do tendão comum	Nervos toracoabdominal (ramos anteriores dos 6 torácicos inferiores) e primeiros nervos lombares	Comprime e sustenta as vísceras abdominais e flexiona e roda o tronco
Oblíquo superior	Corpo do osso esfenóide	Seu tendão passa através de um anel fibroso ou tróclea, muda sua direção e se insere na esclera, profundamente ao músculo reto superior	Nervo troclear (NC IV)	Abduz, deprime e roda medialmente o bulbo do olho
Oblíquo superior da cabeça	Processo espinhoso do atlas (vértebra C1)	Terço lateral da linha nucal inferior do osso occipital	Nervo suboccipital	Rotação da cabeça na articulação atlantoaxial
Obturador externo	Margens do forame obturado e da membrana obturadora	Fossa trocantérica do fêmur	Nervo obturatório (L3 e L4)	Roda lateralmente a coxa; estabiliza a cabeça do fêmur no acetábulo
Obturador interno	Superfície pélvica da membrana obturadora e ossos circunvizinhos	Superfície medial do trocanter maior (fossa trocantérica) do fêmur	Nervo para o músculo obturador interno (L5 e S1)	Roda lateralmente a coxa esticada e abduz a coxa fletida; estabiliza a cabeça do fêmur no acetábulo
Occipitofrontal (ventre occipital/ventre frontal)	2/3 laterais da linha nucal superior e osso temporal e mastóide/aponeurose epicraniana	Aponeurose epicraniana/pele da fronte e sobrancelhas	Ramo posterior/ramo temporal do nervo facial (NC VII)	Retrai o couro cabeludo/eleva as sobrancelhas e a pele da fronte
Omo-hióideo	Borda superior da escápula próximo à incisura supra-escapular	Borda inferior do osso hióide	C1–C3 (inervação por um ramo da alça cervical)	Deprime, retrai e equilibra o osso hióide

Músculo(s)	Origem	Inserção	Inervação	Ação(ões) Principal(is)
Oponente do dedo mínimo	Hâmulo do osso hamato e retináculo dos músculos flexores	Borda medial do 5.º metacarpal	Ramo profundo do nervo ulnar (C8 e T1)	Puxa anteriormente o 5.º metacarpal e o roda, colocando o 5.º dedo em oposição com o polegar
Oponente do polegar	Retináculo dos músculos flexores e tubérculos dos ossos escafóide e trapézio	Face lateral do 1.º metacarpal	Ramo recorrente do nervo mediano (C8 e T1)	Puxa lateralmente o 1.º osso metacarpal para se opor ao polegar em direção ao centro da região palmar e roda-o medialmente
Orbicular da boca	Algumas fibras originam-se próximo ao plano mediano da maxila superiormente e da mandíbula inferiormente; outras fibras originam-se da superfície profunda da pele	Mucosa dos lábios	Nervo facial (NC VII)	Como esfíncter da abertura oral, comprime e projeta os lábios para a frente (p.ex., enruga os lábios ao assobiar ou sugar)
Orbicular do olho	Margem orbital medial, ligamento palpebral medial e osso lacrimal	Pele ao redor da margem da órbita; placa tarsal	Nervo facial (NC VII)	Fecha as pálpebras; a parte palpebral fecha suavemente as pálpebras; a parte orbital as fecha bem
Palatofaríngeo	Palato duro e aponeurose palatina	Parede lateral da faringe	Parte craniana do nervo acessório (NC XI) através do ramo faríngeo do nervo vago (NC X) por meio do plexo faríngeo	Tensiona o palato mole e puxa as paredes da faringe para cima, para a frente e medialmente durante a deglutição
Palatoglosso	Aponeurose palatina	Lado da língua	Parte craniana do nervo acessório (NC XI) através do ramo faríngeo do nervo vago (NC X) por meio do plexo faríngeo	Eleva a parte posterior da língua e "puxa" o palato mole em direção à língua
Palmar curto	Face ulnar da porção central da aponeurose palmar	Pele do lado ulnar da mão	Nervo ulnar superficial (T1)	Enruga a pele no lado palmar da mão
Palmar longo	Epicôndilo medial do úmero	Metade distal do retináculo dos músculos flexores e aponeurose palmar	Nervo mediano (C7 e C8)	Flexiona a mão (no punho) e retesa a aponeurose palmar
Pectíneo	Ramo superior do púbis	Linha pectínea do fêmur, logo embaixo do trocanter menor	Nervo femoral (L2 e L3); pode receber um ramo do nervo obturatório	Aduz e flexiona a coxa; auxilia na rotação medial da coxa
Peitoral maior	Cabeça clavicular: superfície anterior da metade medial da clavícula; Cabeça esternocostal: superfície anterior do esterno, seis cartilagens costais superiores e aponeurose do músculo oblíquo externo	Lábio lateral do sulco intertubercular do úmero	Nervos peitorais lateral e medial; cabeça clavicular (C5 e C6), cabeça esternocostal (C7, C8 e T1)	Aduz e roda medialmente o úmero; puxa a escápula anteriormente e inferiormente Atuando sozinho: a cabeça clavicular flexiona o úmero, e a cabeça esternocostal o estica
Peitoral menor	3.ª a 5.ª costelas próximo às suas cartilagens costais	Borda medial e superfície superior do processo coracóide da escápula	Nervo peitoral medial (C8 e T1)	Estabiliza a escápula ao puxá-la inferior e anteriormente contra a parede torácica
Piramidal	Crista do púbis	Porção inferior da linha alba	Nervo subcostal	Tensiona a linha alba
Piriforme	Superfície anterior do sacro e ligamento sacrotuberoso	Borda superior do trocanter maior do fêmur	Ramos dos ramos anteriores de S1 e S2	Roda lateralmente a coxa esticada e abduz a coxa fletida; estabiliza a cabeça do fêmur no acetábulo
Plantar	Extremidade inferior da linha supracondilar lateral do fêmur e ligamento poplíteo oblíquo	Superfície posterior do calcâneo através do tendão do calcâneo	Nervo tibial (S1 e S2)	Auxilia fracamente o músculo gastrocnêmio na flexão plantar do tornozelo e na flexão do joelho
Platisma	Fáscia superficial das regiões deltóide e peitoral	Mandíbula, pele da bochecha, ângulo da boca e orbicular do olho	Nervo facial (NC VII)	Deprime a mandíbula e tensiona a pele da parte inferior da face e do pescoço

Músculo(s)	Origem	Inserção	Inervação	Ação(ões) Principal(is)
Poplíteo	Superfície lateral do côndilo lateral do fêmur e do menisco lateral	Superfície posterior da tíbia, superior à linha soleal	Nervo tibial (L4, L5 e S1)	Flexiona fracamente o joelho e o "destrava"
Prócero	Aponeurose que reveste a crista do nariz	Pele da parte inferior da fronte entre as sobrancelhas	Nervo facial (NC VII)	Deprime a extremidade medial da sobrancelha; produz rugas transversais sobre a crista do nariz; produz o olhar de concentração
Pronador quadrado	Quarto distal da superfície anterior da ulna	Quarto distal da superfície anterior do rádio	Nervo interósseo anterior a partir do nervo mediano (C8 e T1)	Faz a pronação do antebraço; as fibras profundas unem o rádio e a ulna entre si
Pronador redondo	Epicôndilo medial do úmero e processo coronóide da ulna	Meio da superfície lateral do rádio	Nervo mediano (C6 e C7)	Pronação e flexão do antebraço (no cotovelo)
Psoas maior	Lados das vértebras T12–L5 e os discos entre elas; processos transversos de todas as vértebras lombares	Trocanter menor do fêmur	Ramos anteriores dos nervos lombares (L1, L2 e L3)	Flexiona e roda a coxa lateralmente na articulação do quadril; quando a coxa está fixa, flexiona as vértebras lombares anterior e lateralmente
Psoas menor	Lados das vértebras T12–L1 e discos intervertebrais	Linha pectínea, eminência iliopectínea através do arco iliopectíneo	Ramos anteriores dos nervos lombares (L1 e L2)	Age em conjunto com o músculo psoas maior na flexão da coxa na articulação do quadril e na estabilização dessa articulação
Pterigóide lateral	Cabeça superior: superfície infratemporal e crista infratemporal da asa maior do osso esfenóide Cabeça inferior: superfície lateral da lâmina pterigóide lateral	Colo da mandíbula (fóvea pterigóidea); disco e cápsula articular da articulação temporomandibular	Nervo mandibular (NC V3) através do nervo pterigóide lateral a partir do tronco anterior, que entra sua superfície profunda	Atuando em conjunto, projetam a mandíbula para a frente e abaixam o queixo; atuando isoladamente ou de forma alternada, promovem movimentos da mandíbula de um lado para outro
Pterigóide medial	Cabeça profunda: superfície medial da placa pterigóide lateral e processo piramidal do osso palatino Cabeça superficial: tuberosidade da maxila	Superfície medial do ramo da mandíbula, inferior ao forame mandibular	Nervo mandibular (NC V3) através do nervo pterigóideo medial	Atuando bilateralmente, eleva a mandíbula, cerrando-a; auxilia na protrusão da mandíbula; atuando isoladamente, auxilia na protrusão do mesmo lado da mandíbula; atuando de forma alternada, produz um movimento de trituração
Quadrado do lombo	Metade medial da borda inferior da 12.ª costela e extremidades dos processos transversos lombares	Ligamento iliolombar e extremidade interna da crista ilíaca	Ramos ventrais dos nervos T12 e L1–L4	Estica e flexiona lateralmente a coluna vertebral; fixa a 12.ª costela durante a inspiração
Quadrado femoral	Borda lateral da tuberosidade isquiática	Tubérculo quadrado na crista intertrocantérica do fêmur e área inferior a ela	Nervo para o quadrado do fêmur (L5 e S1)	Roda lateralmente a coxa; equilibra a cabeça do fêmur no acetábulo
Quadrado plantar	Superfície medial e margem lateral da superfície plantar do calcâneo	Margem posterolateral do tendão do flexor longo dos dedos	Nervo plantar lateral (S2 e S3)	Auxilia o flexor longo dos dedos na flexão dos quatro dedos laterais
Redondo maior	Superfície dorsal do ângulo inferior da escápula	Lábio medial do sulco intertubercular do úmero	Nervo subescapular inferior (C6 e C7)	Aduz e roda medialmente o braço
Redondo menor	Parte superior da borda lateral da escápula	Faceta inferior sobre o tubérculo maior do úmero	Nervo axilar (C5 e C6)	Roda lateralmente o braço; ajuda a manter a cabeça do úmero na cavidade glenoidal da escápula
Reto anterior da cabeça	Superfície anterior da massa lateral da vértebra C1 (atlas)	Base do crânio, exatamente anterior ao côndilo occipital	Ramos a partir da alça entre os nervos espinais C1 e C2	Flexiona a cabeça na articulação atlanto-occipital

Músculo(s)	Origem	Inserção	Inervação	Ação(ões) Principal(is)
Reto do abdome	Sínfise púbica e crista púbica	Processo xifóide e 5.ª–7.ª cartilagens costais	Nervos toracoabdominais (ramos anteriores dos seis nervos torácicos inferiores)	Flexiona o tronco (vértebras lombares) e comprime as vísceras abdominais (opondo-se indiretamente ao diafragma)
Reto femoral	Espinha ilíaca ântero-inferior e ílio superior ao acetábulo	Base da patela e por ligamento patelar para a tuberosidade tibial	Nervo femoral (L2, L3 e L4)	Estica a perna na articulação do joelho; o músculo reto femoral também estabiliza a articulação do quadril e ajuda o músculo iliopsoas a flexionar a coxa
Reto inferior	Anel tendinoso comum	Esclerótica exatamente posterior à córnea	Nervo oculomotor (NC III)	Deprime, aduz e roda medialmente o bulbo do olho
Reto lateral	Anel tendinoso comum	Esclera exatamente posterior à córnea	Nervo abducente (NC VI)	Abduz o bulbo do olho
Reto lateral da cabeça	Processo transverso da vértebra C1 (atlas)	Processo jugular do osso occipital	Ramos a partir da alça entre os nervos espinais C1 e C2	Flexiona a cabeça e ajuda a estabilizá-la
Reto medial	Anel tendinoso comum	Esclera exatamente posterior à córnea	Nervo oculomotor (NC III)	Aduz o bulbo do olho
Reto posterior maior da cabeça	Processo espinhoso do áxis (vértebra C2)	Meio da linha nucal inferior do osso occipital	Nervo suboccipital	Estica a cabeça na altura da articulação atlanto-occipital
Reto posterior menor da cabeça	Tubérculo dorsal do atlas (vértebra C1)	Terço medial da linha nucal inferior do osso occipital	Nervo suboccipital	Estica a cabeça na articulação atlanto-occipital
Reto superior	Anel tendinoso comum	Esclera exatamente posterior à córnea	Nervo oculomotor (NC III)	Eleva, aduz e roda medialmente o bulbo do olho
Risório	Platisma e fáscia do músculo masseter	Orbicular do olho, pele do canto da boca, modíolo	Nervo facial (NC VII)	Retrai o ângulo da boca, alongando a rima oral
Rombóides menor e maior	Menor: ligamento nucal e processos espinhosos das vértebras C7 e T1 Maior: processos espinhosos das vértebras T2–T5	Borda medial da escápula desde o nível da coluna vertebral até o ângulo inferior	Nervo dorsal da escápula (C4 e C5)	Retrai a escápula e a roda para abaixar a cavidade glenoidal; fixa a escápula à parede torácica
Salpingofaríngeo	Porção cartilaginosa da tuba auditiva	Mistura-se com o músculo palatofaríngeo	Raiz craniana do nervo acessório através do ramo faríngeo do vago e plexo faríngeo	Eleva (encurta e alarga) a faringe e a laringe durante a deglutição e a fala
Sartório	Espinha ilíaca ântero-superior e porção superior da incisura inferior a ela	Parte superior da superfície medial da tíbia	Nervo femoral (L2 e L3)	Flexiona, abduz e roda lateralmente a coxa na articulação coxofemoral; flexiona a perna na articulação do quadril
Semimembranáceo	Tuberosidade isquiática	Parte posterior do côndilo medial da tíbia; a inserção refletida forma o ligamento poplíteo oblíquo (para o côndilo femoral lateral)	Divisão tibial do nervo isquiático (L5, S1 e S2)	Estende a coxa; flexiona a perna e, quando o joelho é flexionado, roda-o medialmente; quando o quadril é flexionado e o joelho é estendido, pode elevar o tronco contra a gravidade
Semitendinoso	Tuberosidade isquiática	Superfície medial da parte superior da tíbia	Divisão tibial do nervo isquiático (L5, S1 e S2)	Estica a coxa; flexiona a perna e, quando o joelho é flexionado, a roda medialmente; quando o quadril é flexionado e o joelho é esticado, pode elevar o tronco contra a gravidade
Serrátil anterior	Superfície externa das partes laterais da 1.ª à 8.ª costela	Superfície anterior da borda medial da escápula	Nervo torácico longo (C5, C6 e C7)	Faz a protração da escápula e a mantém contra a parede torácica; roda a escápula
Serrátil posterior inferior	Processos espinhosos das vértebras T11 a L2	Bordas inferiores da 8.ª à 12.ª costela próximo a seus ângulos	Ramos anteriores do 9.º ao 12.º nervos espinais torácicos	Deprime as costelas

Músculo(s)	Origem	Inserção	Inervação	Ação(ões) Principal(is)
Serrátil posterior superior	Ligamento nucal, processos espinhosos das vértebras C7 a T3	Bordas superiores da 2.ª à 4.ª costela	2.º ao 5.º nervos intercostais	Eleva as costelas
Sóleo	Face posterior da cabeça da fíbula, quarto superior da superfície posterior da fíbula, linha solear e borda medial da tíbia	Superior posterior do calcâneo através do tendão do calcâneo	Nervo tibial (S1 e S2)	Faz a flexão plantar do tornozelo, independente da posição do joelho, e estabiliza a perna sobre o pé
Subclávio	Junção da 1.ª costela e sua cartilagem costal	Superfície inferior do terço médio da clavícula	Nervo para o subclávio (C5 e C6)	Ancora e deprime a clavícula
Subcostal	Superfície interna das costelas inferiores próximo a seus ângulos	Bordas superiores de duas ou três costelas abaixo	Nervos intercostais	Eleva as costelas
Subescapular	Fossa subescapular	Tubérculo menor do úmero	Nervos subescapulares superior e inferior (C5, C6 e C7)	Roda medialmente o braço e o aduz; ajuda a manter a cabeça do úmero na cavidade glenoidal
Supinador	Epicôndilo lateral do úmero, ligamentos colateral radial e anular, fossa supinadora e crista da ulna	Superfícies lateral, posterior e anterior do terço proximal do rádio	Ramo profundo do nervo radial (C5 e C6)	Supina o antebraço (i.e., roda o rádio para virar a região palmar para a frente)
Supra-espinal	Fossa supra-espinal da escápula	Faceta superior no tubérculo maior do úmero	Nervo supra-escapular (C4, C5 e C6)	Inicia e auxilia o músculo deltóide na abdução do braço e age com os músculos do manguito rotador
Temporal	Assoalho da fossa temporal e superfície profunda da fáscia temporal	Extremidade e superfície medial do processo coronóide e borda anterior do ramo da mandíbula	Ramos temporais profundos do nervo mandibular (NC V3)	Eleva a mandíbula, fechando as mandíbulas; suas fibras posteriores retraem a mandíbula depois da protrusão
Tensor da fáscia lata	Espinha ilíaca ântero-superior e parte anterior da crista ilíaca	Trato iliotibial que se insere no côndilo lateral da tíbia	Glúteo superior (L4 e L5)	Abduz, roda medialmente e flexiona a coxa; ajuda a manter o joelho esticado; equilibra o tronco sobre a coxa
Tensor do tímpano	Canal para o tensor do tímpano da porção petrosa do osso temporal e cartilagem da tuba auditiva	Manúbrio do martelo	Ramo do nervo mandibular (NC V3) através do gânglio ótico	Tensiona a membrana timpânica para amortecer a vibração excessiva causada pelo ruído alto
Tensor do véu palatino	Fossa escafóide da placa pterigóide medial, espinha do osso esfenóide e cartilagem da tuba auditiva	Aponeurose palatina	Nervo pterigóide medial (um ramo do nervo mandibular — NC V3) através do gânglio ótico	Tensiona o palato mole e abre o orifício da tuba auditiva durante a deglutição e o bocejo
Tibial anterior	Côndilo lateral e metade superior da superfície lateral da tíbia e membrana interóssea	Superfícies medial e inferior do cuneiforme medial e base do 1.º metatarsal	Nervo fibular profundo (L4 e L5)	Dorsiflexão do tornozelo e inversão do pé
Tibial posterior	Membrana interóssea, superfície posterior da tíbia inferior à linha solear e superfície posterior da fíbula	Tuberosidade do navicular, cuneiforme e cubóide e bases do 2.º, 3.º e 4.º metatarsais	Nervo tibial (L4 e L5)	Faz a flexão plantar do tornozelo e a inversão do pé
Tireoaritenóideo	Superfície posterior da cartilagem tireóidea	Processo muscular da cartilagem aritenóidea	Nervo laríngeo recorrente	Relaxa a prega vocal
Tireo-hióideo	Linha oblíqua da cartilagem tireóidea	Borda inferior do corpo e corno maior do osso hióide	C1 através do nervo hipoglosso	Deprime o osso hióide e eleva a laringe
Transverso do abdome	Superfícies internas da 7.ª–12.ª cartilagens costais, fáscia toracolombar, crista ilíaca e terço lateral do ligamento inguinal	Linha alba com a aponeurose do músculo oblíquo interno, crista púbica e linha pectínea do púbis por meio do tendão conjunto	Tóraco-abdominal (ramos anteriores dos 6 nervos torácicos inferiores) e primeiros nervos lombares	Comprime e sustenta as vísceras abdominais

Músculo(s)	Origem	Inserção	Inervação	Ação(ões) Principal(is)
Transverso do tórax	Superfície posterior da parte inferior do esterno	Superfície interna das cartilagens costais 2–6	Nervos intercostais	Deprime as costelas
Transverso-espinais	Processos transversos: O músculo semi-espinal origina-se dos processos transversos das vértebras C4–T12 O músculo multífido origina-se do sacro e do ílio, processos transversos de T1–T3 e processos articulares de C4–C7 Os músculos rotadores originam-se dos processos transversos das vértebras; são mais bem desenvolvidos na região torácica	Processos espinhosos: Semi-espinal — do tórax, do pescoço e da cabeça: as fibras correm no sentido súpero-medial para o osso occipital e os processos espinhosos nas regiões torácica e cervical, englobando 4–6 segmentos; Multífido: as fibras correm no sentido súpero-medial para os processos espinhosos das vértebras acima, englobando 2–4 segmentos; Rotadores: correm no sentido súpero-medial para se inserir na junção da lâmina e processo transverso, ou processo espinhoso, das vértebras acima de suas origens, englobando 1–2 segmentos	Ramos posteriores dos nervos espinais	Esticam a cabeça e as regiões torácica e cervical da coluna vertebral e as rodam no sentido contralateral; Estabilizam as vértebras durante os movimentos locais da coluna vertebral; Estabilizam as vértebras e auxiliam com a extensão local e os movimentos rotatórios da coluna vertebral; podem funcionar como órgãos da propriocepção
Trapézio	Terço medial da linha nucal superior; protuberância occipital externa, ligamento nucal e processos espinhosos das vértebras C7–T12	Terço lateral da clavícula, acrômio e espinha da escápula	Raiz espinal do nervo acessório (NC XI) (motor) e nervos cervicais (C3 e C4) (dor e propriocepção)	Eleva, retrai e roda a escápula; as fibras superiores elevam, as fibras médias retraem, e as fibras inferiores deprimem a escápula; as fibras superiores e inferiores agem em conjunto na rotação superior da escápula
Tríceps braquial	Cabeça longa: tubérculo infraglenoidal da escápula Cabeça lateral: superfície posterior do úmero, superior ao sulco radial Cabeça medial: superfície posterior do úmero, inferior ao sulco radial	Extremidade proximal do olécrano da ulna e fáscia do antebraço	Nervo radial (C6, C7 e C8)	Principal extensor do antebraço no cotovelo; a cabeça longa estabiliza a cabeça do úmero abduzido
Vasto intermédio	Superfícies anterior e lateral do corpo do fêmur	Base da patela e por meio do ligamento patelar na tuberosidade tibial	Nervo femoral (L2, L3 e L4)	Estica a perna na articulação do joelho; o músculo reto femoral também estabiliza a articulação do quadril e ajuda o músculo iliopsoas a flexionar a coxa
Vasto lateral	Trocanter maior e lábio lateral da linha áspera do fêmur	Base da patela e por meio do ligamento patelar na tuberosidade tibial	Nervo femoral (L2, L3 e L4)	Estica a perna na articulação do joelho; o músculo reto femoral também estabiliza a articulação do quadril e ajuda o músculo iliopsoas a flexionar a coxa
Vasto medial	Linha intertrocantérica e lábio medial da linha áspera do fêmur	Base da patela e, através do ligamento patelar, na tuberosidade tibial	Nervo femoral (L2, L3 e L4)	Estica a perna na articulação do joelho; o reto femoral também estabiliza a articulação do quadril e ajuda o iliopsoas a flexionar a coxa
Vocal	Processo vocal da cartilagem aritenóidea	Ligamentos vocais	Nervo laríngeo recorrente (ramo do vago (NC X))	Relaxa o ligamento vocal posterior enquanto mantém (ou aumenta) a tensão da parte anterior
Zigomáticos maior/menor	Osso zigomático anterior/posterior à sutura temporozigomática	Músculos no ângulo da boca/orbicular da boca do lábio superior	Nervo facial (NC VII)	Eleva e everte o lábio superior

NERVOS DO CORPO HUMANO

Nervo(s)/Ramo(s) do(s) Nervo(s)	Origem	Trajeto	Estruturas Inervadas
Abducente (NC VI)	Ponte	Torna-se intradural no clivo: atravessa o seio cavernoso e a fissura orbital superior para penetrar na órbita	Motor: reto lateral
Acessório (NC XI)	Raiz craniana: medula oblonga Raiz espinal: medula espinal cervical	A raiz espinal ascende dentro da cavidade craniana através do forame magno; sai através do forame jugular; atravessa o trígono posterior do pescoço	Motor: esternocleidomastóideo e trapézio
Alça cervical	Raiz superior: nervo hipoglosso (fibras de C1 e C2) Raiz inferior: plexos cervical (fibras de C2 e C3)	Desce sobre a superfície externa da bainha carótica	Motor: omo-hióideo, esterno-hióideo e esternotireóideo
Alveolar inferior	Como ramo terminal (com o nervo lingual) do tronco posterior do nervo mandibular (NC V3)	Desce entre os músculos pterigóides lateral e medial da fossa infratemporal para entrar no canal mandibular da mandíbula	Sensorial: dentes inferiores, periodonto, periósteo e gengiva da mandíbula inferior. VER TAMBÉM: nervo milo-hióideo, nervo mentual
Alveolar superior	Nervo maxilar (NC V2) ou sua continuação como o nervo infra-orbital	Posterior: emerge da fissura pterigomaxilar para dentro da fossa infratemporal; perfura a face posterior da maxila Médio e anterior: originam-se do nervo infra-orbital no teto do seio maxilar, descem as paredes do seio	Sensorial: mucosa do seio maxilar, dentes maxilares e gengiva
Anal (retal) inferior	Nervo pudendo (fibras de S2-S4)	Origina-se na entrada do canal pudendo (espinha isquiática), corre medialmente através do coxim adiposo isquioanal até o canal anal	Motor: esfíncter anal externo Sensorial: derme anal, pele perianal
Auricular magno	Plexo cervical (fibras de C2 e C3)	Ascende verticalmente sobre o músculo esternocleidomastóideo, anterior e em paralelo à veia jugular externa	Sensorial: pele da orelha, couro cabeludo adjacente e sobre o ângulo da mandíbula; bainha parotídea
Auricular posterior	Como primeiro ramo extracraniano do nervo facial (NC VII)	Passa posterior à orelha, emitindo ramo para a região occipital	Motor: músculo auricular posterior e músculos auriculares intrínsecos, ventre occipital do músculo occipitofrontal (epicrânio)
Auriculotemporal	Nervo mandibular (NC V3)	A partir da divisão posterior do NC V3 passa entre o colo da mandíbula e o meato acústico externo para acompanhar a artéria temporal superficial	Sensorial: pele anterior à aurícula e região temporal posterior, trago e parte da hélice da orelha, e teto do meato acústico externo e parte superior da membrana timpânica
Axilar	Ramo terminal do cordão posterior do plexo braquial (fibras de C5 e C6)	Passa para a face posterior do braço através do espaço quadrangular em companhia com a artéria circunflexa posterior do úmero e, em seguida, curva-se ao redor do colo cirúrgico do úmero; dá origem ao nervo cutâneo lateral do braço	Motor: redondo menor e deltóide Sensorial: articulação do ombro e pele sobre a parte inferior do músculo deltóide
Bucal	Nervo mandibular (NC V3)	A partir da divisão anterior do NC V3 na fossa infratemporal, passa anteriormente para alcançar a bochecha	Sensorial: pele e mucosa da bochecha, gengiva bucal adjacente ao 2.º e 3.º dentes molares
Ciliares (longo, curto)	Ciliar longo: nervo nasociliar (NC V1) Ciliar curto: gânglio ciliar	Passa para a face posterior do globo ocular	Sensorial: córnea, conjuntiva Motor: corpo ciliar e íris
Clúnios (superior, médio e inferior)	Superior: ramos posteriores de L1, 2 e 3 Médio: ramos posteriores de S1, 2 e 3 Inferior: nervo cutâneo posterior da coxa	Nervos superiores cruzam a crista ilíaca; os nervos médios saem através dos forames sacrais posteriores e entram na região glútea; os nervos inferiores curvam-se ao redor da borda inferior do glúteo máximo	Sensorial: pele da nádega ou região glútea até o trocanter maior

Nervo(s)/Ramo(s) do(s) Nervo(s)	Origem	Trajeto	Estruturas Inervadas
Coccígeo (Co)	Cone medular da medula espinal	Ramos anteriores e posteriores de S4 e S5; ramos anteriores formam o plexo coccígeo, que origina o nervo anococcígeo	Sensorial: pele sobre o cóccix
Corda do tímpano	Nervo facial (NC VII) dentro do canal facial	Atravessa a cavidade timpânica, passando entre a bigorna e o martelo; sai do osso temporal através da fissura petrotimpânica para entrar na fossa infratemporal, onde se mistura com o nervo lingual	Motor: glândulas submandibular e sublingual (salivares) Sensorial: paladar nos 2/3 anteriores da língua
Cutâneo femoral anterior	Nervo femoral (fibras de L2 e L3)	Surge no trígono femoral e perfura a fáscia lata da coxa ao longo do trajeto do músculo sartório	Sensorial: pele nas faces medial e anterior da coxa
Dorsal da escápula	Ramo anterior de C5 com uma freqüente contribuição de C4	Perfura o músculo escaleno médio, desce profundamente ao músculo levantador da escápula e penetra profundamente à superfície dos músculos rombóides	Motor: rombóides e inerva, ocasionalmente, o levantador da escápula
Esplâncnico (porção abdominopélvica)	Segmentos torácico inferior e lombar do tronco simpático	Passa medial e inferiormente ao gânglio pré-vertebral do plexo para-aórtico	Motor: simpáticos pré-sinápticos para a inervação dos vasos sangüíneos e vísceras abdominopélvicas
Esplâncnico (porção cardiopulmonar)	Gânglios cervicais e torácicos superiores do tronco simpático	Desce ântero-medialmente para os plexos cardíaco, pulmonar e esofágico	Motor: conduz as fibras simpáticas pós-sinápticas para os plexos nervosos das vísceras torácicas
Esplâncnico (porção cervical)	Gânglios cervicais do tronco simpático	Passa medial e inferiormente para os plexos cardíaco e pulmonar	Tecido de condução (nós SA e AV) e artérias coronárias
Esplâncnico (porção pélvica)	Plexo sacral (fibras de S2–S4)	Corre anterior e inferiormente para se misturar com o plexo hipogástrico inferior	Motor: fibras parassimpáticas pré-sinápticas para as vísceras pélvicas, colos descendente e sigmóide Sensorial: fibras aferentes viscerais oriundas das vísceras pélvicas subperitoneais (colo do útero e parte superior da vagina, assoalho da bexiga, reto e porção superior do canal anal; próstata)
Esplâncnico (porção torácica)	Gânglios torácicos do tronco simpático	Passa ântero-medialmente sobre os corpos das vértebras torácicas como nervos esplâncnicos cardiopulmonares menores para os plexos autônomos torácicos (cardíaco, pulmonar e esofágico) e como nervos esplâncnicos abdominopélvicos superiores para os gânglios pré-vertebrais do plexo para-órtico	Motor: nervos esplâncnicos a partir do 1.º ao 5.º gânglios torácicos que conduzem as fibras simpáticas pós-sinápticas para o coração, pulmões e esôfago; aquelas a partir do 6.º ao 12.º gânglios torácicos (i.e., os nervos esplâncnicos maior, menor e mínimo) conduzem as fibras simpáticas pré-sinápticas para os gânglios pré-vertebrais
Esplâncnico lombar	Gânglios lombares dos troncos simpáticos	Passa ântero-medialmente nos corpos das vértebras lombares para os gânglios pré-vertebrais do plexo para-aórtico	Motor: fibras simpáticas pré-sinápticas para as vísceras abdominais inferiores e pélvicas Sensoriais: aferentes viscerais a partir das mesmas
Esplâncnico maior	Gânglios simpáticos torácicos do 5.º–6.º até 9.º–10.º	Nervo esplâncnico abdominopélvico mais alto; passa ântero-medialmente sobre os corpos das vértebras torácicas, perfurando o diafragma para convergir na raiz do tronco celíaco	Motor: conduz as fibras simpáticas pré-sinápticas para os gânglios celíacos para a inervação das artérias celíacas e derivados e da porção do intestino que elas inervam
Esplâncnico menor	10.º e 11.º gânglios torácicos do tronco simpático	Desce ântero-medialmente para perfurar o diafragma até atingir o gânglio aórtico-renal	Motor: fibras simpáticas pré-sinápticas para os gânglios pré-vertebrais Sensoriais: aferentes viscerais a partir do trato GI superior
Esplâncnico mínimo	12.º (mais baixo) gânglio torácico do tronco simpático	Atravessa o diafragma com o tronco simpático e termina no plexo renal	Motor: fibras simpáticas pré-sinápticas para as artérias renais e derivadas
Etmoidal anterior	Nervo nasociliar (NC V1)	Nasce na órbita, passa através do forame etmoidal anterior para a cavidade craniana, em seguida atravessa a lâmina cribriforme do etmóide para a cavidade nasal	Sensorial: dura-máter da fossa craniana anterior; mucosas do seio esfenoidal, células etmoidais e cavidade nasal superior

Nervo(s)/Ramo(s) do(s) Nervo(s)	Origem	Trajeto	Estruturas Inervadas
Etmoidal posterior	Nasociliar	Deixa a órbita através do forame etmoidal posterior	Inerva os seios paranasais etmoidal e esfenoidal
Facial (VII)	Borda posterior da ponte	Corre através do meato acústico interno e canal facial da porção petrosa do osso temporal, saindo através do forame estilomastóideo; o tronco principal forma o plexo intraparotídeo	Motor: estapédio, ventre posterior do digástrico, estilo-hióideo, músculos facial e do couro cabeludo Sensorial: parte da pele do meato acústico externo VER TAMBÉM: nervo intermédio
Faríngeo	Gânglio pterigopalatino	Passa posteriormente através do canal palatovaginal	Inerva a mucosa da nasofaringe posterior às tubas auditivas
Femoral	Plexo lombar (fibras de L2–L4)	Passa profundamente ao ponto médio do ligamento inguinal, lateral aos vasos femorais, e divide-se nos ramos musculares e cutâneos	Motor: músculos da região anterior da coxa Sensorial: articulações do quadril e do joelho; pele no lado ântero-medial da coxa e da perna
Fibular comum	Ramo terminal (com o nervo tibial) do nervo isquiático (fibras L4–S2)	Começa no ápice da fossa poplítea; segue a borda medial do músculo bíceps femoral para a face posterior da cabeça da fíbula; bifurca-se nos nervos fibulares superficial e profundo quando se curva ao redor do colo da fíbula	Sensorial: pele na parte lateral da face posterior da perna através de seu ramo, o nervo cutâneo sural lateral; articulação do joelho através de seu ramo articular Motor: cabeça curta do músculo bíceps femoral
Fibular profundo	Nervo fibular comum	Origina-se entre o fibular longo e colo da fíbula; passa através do extensor longo dos dedos e desce sobre a membrana interóssea; passa profundamente ao retináculo dos músculos extensores, cruza a extremidade distal da tíbia e penetra no dorso do pé	Motor: músculos do compartimento anterior da perna e dorso do pé Sensorial: pele da primeira fenda interdigital (i.e., pele sobre os lados adjacentes do 1.º e 2.ª artelhos); e envia os ramos articulares para as articulações que ele cruza
Fibular superficial	Nervo fibular comum	Origina-se entre o músculo fibular longo e o colo da fíbula e desce no compartimento lateral da perna; perfura a fáscia profunda no terço distal da perna para tornar-se cutâneo e emitir ramos para o pé e para os dedos	Motor: fibulares longo e curto Sensorial: pele sobre o terço distal da superfície anterior da perna e dorso do pé e todos os dedos, exceto o lado lateral do 5.º e os lados adjacentes do 1.º e 2.º dedos
Frênico	Plexo cervical (fibras de C3–C5)	Passa através da abertura torácica superior e corre entre a pleura mediastinal e o pericárdio	Motor: diafragma Sensorial: saco pericárdico, pleura mediastinal e diafragmática e peritônio diafragmático
Frontal	Nervo oftálmico (NC V1)	Cruza a órbita na face superior do músculo levantador da pálpebra superior; divide-se nos ramos supra-orbital e supratroclear	Sensorial: pele da fronte, couro cabeludo, pálpebra superior e nariz; conjuntiva da pálpebra superior e mucosa do seio frontal
Genitofemoral	Plexo lombar (fibras de L1 e L2)	Desce na superfície anterior do psoas maior e se divide nos ramos genital e femoral	Sensorial: o ramo femoral inerva a pele sobre o trígono femoral; o ramo genital inerva a bolsa escrotal ou os lábios maiores do pudendo Motor: ramo genital para o músculo cremaster
Glossofaríngeo (NC IX)	Extremidade rostral da medula	Sai do crânio por meio do forame jugular, passa entre os músculos constritores superior e médio da faringe até a fossa tonsilar, penetra no terço posterior da língua	Motor: somático para o estilofaríngeo; visceral (parassimpático pré-sináptico) para a glândula parótida Sensorial: 2/3 posteriores da língua (inclusive paladar), faringe, cavidade timpânica, tuba auditiva, corpo e seio caróticos
Glúteo inferior	Plexo sacral (fibras L5–S2)	Deixa a pelve através do forame isquiático maior inferior ao piriforme e se divide em vários ramos	Motor: glúteo máximo
Glúteo superior	Plexo sacral (fibras de L4–S1)	Deixa a pelve através do forame isquiático maior, superior ao piriforme, e corre entre os músculos glúteos médio e mínimo	Motor: glúteo médio, glúteo mínimo e tensor da fáscia lata
Hipogástrico	Como continuação do plexo hipogástrico superior para a pelve	Faz trajeto anterior ao sacro dentro da bainha hipogástrica para se misturar com os nervos esplâncnicos pélvicos no plexo hipogástrico inferior	Motor: conduz as fibras simpáticas pré- e pós-sinápticas destinadas às vísceras pélvicas Sensoriais: conduz as fibras de dor das vísceras pélvicas infraperitoneais (p.ex., fundo/corpo do útero)

Nervo(s)/Ramo(s) do(s) Nervo(s)	Origem	Trajeto	Estruturas Inervadas
Hipoglosso (NC XII)	Entre a pirâmide e a oliva do miencéfalo	Atravessa o canal do hipoglosso, em seguida corre inferior e anteriormente, avançando medialmente ao ângulo da mandíbula e entre os músculos milo-hióideo e hioglosso até atingir os músculos da língua	Motor: músculos intrínsecos e extrínsecos da língua (exceção: palatoglosso)
Ílio-hipogástrico	Plexo lombar (fibras de L1)	Seu trajeto é paralelo à crista ilíaca; perfura o músculo transverso do abdome; os ramos perfuram a aponeurose do músculo oblíquo externo para alcançar as regiões inguinal e púbica	Motor: músculos oblíquo interno e transverso do abdome Sensorial: ramo cutâneo lateral supre o quadrante súpero-lateral da nádega; pele sobre a crista ilíaca e da região hipogástrica
Ilioinguinal	Plexo lombar (fibras de L1)	Passa entre a 2.ª e 3.ª camadas dos músculos abdominais, atravessa o canal inguinal e se divide nos ramos femoral e escrotal ou labial	Motor: parte mais interna dos músculos oblíquo interno e transverso do abdome Sensorial: o ramo femoral inerva a pele sobre o triângulo femoral; o ramo genital supre o monte do púbis e a pele adjacente dos grandes lábios ou bolsa escrotal
Infra-orbital	Ramo terminal do nervo maxilar (NC V2)	Corre no assoalho da órbita e emerge no forame infra-orbital	Sensorial: pele da bochecha, lábio inferior, lado lateral do nariz e septo inferior e lábio superior, incisivos pré-molares superiores e dentes caninos; mucosa do seio maxilar e lábio superior
Infratroclear	Nervo nasociliar (NC V1)	Segue a parede medial da órbita até a pálpebra superior	Sensorial: pele/conjuntiva (revestimento) da pálpebra superior
Intercostais	Ramos anteriores dos nervos T1 a T11	Correm nos espaços intercostais entre as camadas interna e mais interna dos músculos intercostais	Motor: músculos intercostais; os nervos inferiores inervam os músculos da parede abdominal ântero-lateral Sensorial: pele suprajacente e pleura/peritônio profundamente aos músculos inervados
Intermédio	Desde a ponte como uma raiz menor do nervo facial (NC VII)	Atravessa o meato acústico interno misturando-se, em sua extremidade distal, com o (raiz do) nervo facial maior	Motor: fibras parassimpáticas pré-sinápticas para os gânglios pterigopalatino e submandibular através do nervo petroso maior e da corda do tímpano, respectivamente Sensorial: paladar a partir dos 2/3 anteriores da língua e do palato mole
Interósseo anterior	Nervo mediano na parte distal da fossa cubital	Passa inferiormente sobre a membrana interóssea	Motor: flexor profundo dos dedos, flexor longo do polegar e pronador quadrado
Interósseo posterior	Ramo terminal do ramo profundo do nervo radial (continuação do nervo radial profundo depois de emergir do músculo supinador)	Corre entre as camadas superficial e profunda do antebraço posterior, em seguida passa entre o extensor longo do polegar e membrana interóssea	Motor: extensor ulnar do carpo, extensores dos dedos (incluindo o polegar) e abdutor longo do polegar
Isquiático	Plexo sacral (fibras de L4–S3)	Entra na região glútea através do forame isquiático maior, inferior ao músculo piriforme, desce ao longo da face posterior da coxa e se divide proximalmente ao joelho nos nervos tibial e fibular comum	Motor: jarrete por sua divisão tibial (exceto para a cabeça curta do bíceps femoral, que é inervado por sua divisão fibular comum) Sensorial: fornece ramos articulares para as articulações do quadril e do joelho
Labial posterior	Nervo perineal	Emerge do canal pudendo e ramifica-se no tecido subcutâneo	Pele da porção posterior dos lábios maiores do pudendo
Lacrimal	Nervo oftálmico (NC V1)	Passa através da fáscia palpebral da pálpebra superior próximo ao ângulo lateral (canto) do olho	Sensorial: uma pequena área da pele e conjuntiva da parte lateral da pálpebra superior
Laríngeo recorrente	Nervo vago (NC X)	Contorna a subclávia à direita; à esquerda, corre ao redor do arco da aorta e ascende no sulco traqueoesofágico	Motor: músculos intrínsecos da laringe (exceto o cricotireóideo) Sensorial: inferior ao nível das pregas vocais
Laríngeo superior	Vago (NC X)	Desce no espaço parafaríngeo; lateral à cartilagem tireóidea, divide-se nos nervos laríngeos interno e externo; o primeiro perfura a membrana tireo-hióidea; o último corre ínfero-medialmente até o intervalo entre as cartilagens cricóidea e tireóidea	Motor: músculo cricotireóideo (nervo laríngeo externo) Sensorial: supraglótico

Nervo(s)/Ramo(s) do(s) Nervo(s)	Origem	Trajeto	Estruturas Inervadas
Lingual	Ramo terminal (com o nervo alveolar inferior) do tronco posterior do nervo mandibular (NC V3)	Unido pela corda do tímpano na fossa infratemporal; passa ântero-inferiormente entre os músculos pterigóideos lateral e medial e acima do músculo milo-hióideo para entrar na cavidade oral	Motor: fibras parassimpáticas pré-sinápticas para o gânglio submandibular para as glândulas salivares submandibulares e sublinguais Sensorial: 2/3 anteriores da língua, assoalho da boca e gengiva mandibular lingual
Mandibular (NC V3)	Gânglio trigeminal (raiz motora a partir da ponte)	Desce através do forame oval para dentro da fossa infratemporal; divide-se nos troncos anterior e posterior, com o primeiro ramificando-se imediatamente para vários ramos menores e o último bifurcando-se para os nervos lingual e alveolar inferior	Motor: músculos da mastigação, milo-hióideo, ventre anterior do digástrico, tensor do tímpano e tensor do véu palatino Sensorial: pele suprajacente à mandíbula (exceto o ângulo), metade inferior da boca (incluindo dentes, gengiva, mucosa do assoalho e vestíbulo e 2/3 anteriores da língua) e articulação temporomandibular
Massetérico	Tronco anterior do nervo mandibular (NC V3)	Passa lateralmente através da incisura mandibular	Motor: masseter Sensorial: articulação temporomandibular
Maxilar (NC V2)	Gânglio trigêmeo	Corre anteriormente através do forame redondo para dentro da fossa pterigopalatina, enviando raízes sensoriais para o gânglio pterigopalatino (ramos do gânglio são considerados ramos do nervo maxilar); o tronco principal continua anteriormente através da fissura infra-orbital como nervo infra-orbital	Motor: nenhuma fibra motora inicialmente; ramos do gânglio pterigopalatino distribuem fibras parassimpáticas pós-sinápticas para a glândula lacrimal e glândulas mucosas da cavidade nasal, palato e porção superior da faringe Sensorial: pele suprajacente à maxila, mucosa da cavidade nasal póstero-inferior e seio maxilar; metade superior da boca (inclusive dentes, gengiva e mucosa do palato, vestíbulo e bochecha)
Mediano	Apresenta duas raízes, uma oriunda do cordão lateral do plexo braquial (fibras de C6 e C7) e outra do cordão medial (fibras de C8 e T1); as raízes unem-se lateralmente à artéria axilar	Ao longo do braço, cruza para o lado medial da artéria braquial; sai da fossa cubital entre as cabeças do músculo pronador redondo, correndo entre as camadas intermediária e profunda do compartimento anterior do antebraço; torna-se superficial proximal ao punho e passa profundamente ao retináculo dos músculos flexores (ligamento transverso do carpo), à medida que ele atravessa o túnel carpal em direção à mão	Motor: músculos flexores no antebraço (exceto flexor ulnar do carpo, metade ulnar do flexor profundo dos dedos); músculos tenares (exceto o adutor do polegar e a cabeça profunda do flexor curto do polegar), lumbricais laterais (para os dedos 2 e 3) Sensorial: pele das faces dorsal distal e palmar dos 3 1/2 dedos laterais (radiais) e região palmar adjacente
Mentual	Ramo terminal do nervo alveolar inferior (NC V3)	Emerge do canal mandibular no forame mentual	Sensorial: pele do queixo; pele e mucosa do lábio inferior
Musculocutâneo	Cordão lateral do plexo braquial (fibras de C5–C7)	Penetra profundamente no músculo coracobraquial e desce entre os músculos bíceps braquial e braquial	Motor: músculos flexores do braço (coracobraquial, bíceps braquial e braquial) Sensorial: continua como o nervo cutâneo lateral do antebraço
Nasal externo	Nervo etmoidal anterior (NC V1)	Corre na cavidade nasal e emerge na face entre o osso nasal e a cartilagem nasal lateral	Sensorial: pele no dorso do nariz, incluindo a extremidade do nariz
Nasal póstero-inferior	Palatino maior	Origina-se no canal palatino maior, perfura a placa perpendicular do osso palatino	Mucosa da concha nasal inferior e paredes dos meatos nasais inferior e médio
Nasociliar	Nervo oftálmico (NC V1)	Origina-se na fissura orbital superior, passa ântero-medialmente através da porção retrobulbar do olho, proporcionando a raiz sensorial para o gânglio ciliar e terminando como o nervo infratroclear e ramos nasais	Motor: nenhuma fibra motora inicialmente; ramos do gânglio ciliar (nervos ciliares curtos) conduzem as fibras simpáticas pós-sinápticas e as parassimpáticas para o corpo ciliar e a íris Sensorial: sensibilidade tátil do bulbo do olho (conjuntiva e córnea); mucosa das células etmoidais e cavidade nasal ântero-superior; pele da raiz, dorso e ápice do nariz
Nasopalatino	Gânglio pterigopalatino (nervo maxilar — NC V2)	Sai da fossa pterigopalatina através do forame esfenopalatino; cruzando e, em seguida, correndo ântero-inferiormente através do septo nasal; passa através do forame incisivo para o palato	Motor: fibras parassimpáticas pós-sinápticas para as glândulas mucosas do septo nasal Sensorial: mucosa do septo nasal, parte mais anterior do palato duro

Nervo(s)/Ramo(s) do(s) Nervo(s)	Origem	Trajeto	Estruturas Inervadas
Nervo coclear	Como uma divisão do nervo vestibulococlear (NC VIII)	Atravessa o meato acústico interno, entrando no modíolo com os gânglios espirais e processos periféricos na lâmina espiral	Sensorial: órgão espiral (para a audição)
Nervo cutâneo dorsal medial	Nervo fibular superficial	Desce através do tornozelo, correndo anteriormente para a face medial do dorso do pé	Inerva a maior parte da pele do dorso do pé e da porção proximal dos artelhos, exceto pela membrana entre o hálux e o 2.º artelho
Nervo cutâneo lateral da coxa	Plexo lombar (fibras de L2 e L3)	Passa profundamente ao ligamento inguinal, 2–3 cm medial à espinha ilíaca ântero-superior	Sensorial: pele sobre as faces anterior e lateral da coxa
Nervo cutâneo lateral do antebraço	Continuação do nervo musculocutâneo (fibras C6 e C7)	Desce ao longo da borda lateral do antebraço até o punho	Sensorial: pele da face lateral do antebraço
Nervo cutâneo medial da perna	Nervo safeno	Desce no lado medial da perna com a veia safena magna	Pele do lado ântero-medial da perna e lado medial do pé
Nervo cutâneo medial do antebraço	Cordão medial do plexo braquial (fibras de C8 e T1)	Corre entre a artéria e a veia axilares	Sensorial: pele sobre o lado medial do antebraço
Nervo cutâneo medial do braço	Cordão medial do plexo braquial (fibras de C8 e T1)	Corre ao longo do lado medial da veia axilar e se comunica com o nervo intercostobraquial	Sensorial: pele no lado medial do braço
Nervo cutâneo posterior da coxa	Plexo sacral (fibras de S1–S3)	Deixa a pelve através do forame isquiático maior inferior ao músculo piriforme, corre profundamente ao músculo glúteo máximo e emerge de sua borda inferior	Sensorial: pele da nádega através dos ramos clúneos inferiores e pele sobre a face posterior da coxa e da panturrilha; porção lateral do períneo, porção medial superior da coxa através do ramo perineal
Nervo cutâneo posterior do antebraço	Origina-se no braço a partir do nervo radial (fibras de C5–C8)	Perfura a cabeça lateral do músculo tríceps e desce ao longo do lado lateral do braço e face posterior do antebraço até o punho	Sensorial: pele da parte posterior distal do braço, face posterior do antebraço
Nervo cutâneo posterior do braço	Nervo radial (fibras de C5–C8)	Emerge por baixo da borda posterior do músculo deltóide, entre as cabeças longa e lateral do músculo tríceps braquial	Sensorial: pele da face posterior do braço
Nervo milo-hióideo	Nervo alveolar inferior	Origina-se a partir da face posterior do nervo alveolar inferior imediatamente fora do forame mandibular; desce no sulco ósseo sobre a face medial do ramo da mandíbula	Motor: milo-hióideo e ventre anterior do músculo digástrico
Nervo para o canal pterigóideo	Formado pela fusão dos nervos petrosos maior e profundo	Atravessa o canal pterigóideo para atingir o gânglio pterigopalatino na fossa pterigopalatina	Motor: conduz as fibras simpáticas pós-sinápticas e parassimpáticas pré-sinápticas para o gânglio pterigopalatino
Nervo para o músculo estapédio	Nervo facial (NC VII)	Origina-se como nervo facial, desce posterior ao músculo no canal facial	Motor: estapédio
Nervo para o músculo quadrado femoral	Plexo sacral (L5, S1 e S2)	Deixa a pelve através do forame isquiático maior profundamente ao nervo isquiático	Motor: gêmeo inferior e quadrado femoral Sensorial: articulação do quadril
Nervo para o obturador interno	Plexo sacral (L5, S1 e S2)	Penetra a região glútea através do forame isquiático maior inferior ao piriforme; desce posteriormente para a espinha isquiática; entra no forame isquiático menor e passa para o músculo obturador interno	Motor: gêmeo superior e obturador interno
Nervo para o tensor do tímpano	Gânglio ótico (nervo mandibular — NC V3)	Corre ao longo da porção cartilaginosa da tuba auditiva para o hemicanal para o tensor do tímpano	Motor: tensor do tímpano
Nervo para o tensor do véu palatino	Tronco anterior do nervo mandibular — NC V3	Origina-se como um ramo do nervo para o músculo pterigóideo medial	Motor: tensor do véu palatino

Nervo(s)/Ramo(s) do(s) Nervo(s)	Origem	Trajeto	Estruturas Inervadas
Nervo subclávio	Tronco superior do plexo braquial (C5–C6; com freqüência, também C4)	Desce posterior à clavícula e anterior ao plexo braquial e à artéria subclávia	Motor: subclávio Sensorial: articulação esternoclavicular
Nervos cavernosos	Fibras parassimpáticas do plexo nervoso prostático	Perfura a membrana perineal para alcançar os corpos eréteis do pênis	Motor: artérias helicinas dos corpos cavernosos; a estimulação promove ingurgitamento à pressão arterial (ereção)
Nervos para os pterigóideos lateral/medial	Tronco anterior do nervo mandibular (NC V3)	Originam-se na fossa infratemporal imediatamente inferior ao forame oval	Motor: músculos pterigóideos lateral e medial
Obturatório	Plexo lombar (fibras de L2–L4)	Penetra na coxa através do forame obturado e divide-se; seu ramo anterior desce entre os músculos adutor longo e adutor curto; seu ramo posterior desce entre os músculos adutor curto e adutor magno	Motor: o ramo anterior inerva os músculos adutor longo, adutor curto, grácil e pectíneo; o ramo posterior inerva os músculos obturador externo e adutor magno Sensorial: pele da parte medial da coxa acima do joelho
Occipital maior	Como ramo medial do ramo posterior do nervo espinal C2	Perfura os músculos profundos do pescoço e trapézio para ascender no couro cabeludo até o vértice	Motor: multífido cervical, semi-espinal da cabeça Sensorial: parte posterior do couro cabeludo
Occipital menor	Plexo cervical (fibras de C2 e C3)	Ascende póstero-superiormente, em paralelo com a borda ântero-superior do esternocleidomastóideo	Sensorial: pele da superfície posterior da orelha e couro cabeludo adjacente
Oculomotor (NC III)	Fossa interpeduncular do mesencéfalo	Perfura a dura-máter lateral ao processo clinóide posterior, corre na parede lateral do seio cavernoso, penetra na órbita através da fissura orbital superior e se divide nos ramos superior e inferior	Motor: somático: todos os músculos extra-oculares, exceto o oblíquo superior e o reto lateral; as fibras parassimpáticas pré-sinápticas para o gânglio ciliar para o corpo ciliar e esfíncter pupilar
Oftálmico (NC V1)	Gânglio trigêmeo	Passa anteriormente na parede lateral do seio cavernoso para entrar na órbita através do tecido orbital superior, ramificando-se nos nervos frontal, nasociliar e lacrimal	Sensorial: sensibilidade geral oriunda no bulbo do olho (conjuntiva e córnea); mucosa das células etmoidais e seio frontal, dura-máter da fossa craniana anterior, foice do cérebro e tentório do cerebelo, cavidade nasal ântero-superior; pele da fronte, lábio superior, raiz, dorso e ápice do nariz
Olfatório (NC I)	Células olfatórias no epitélio olfatório (mucosa) do teto da cavidade nasal	Aproximadamente 20 fascículos de fibras nervosas ascendem através dos forames da placa cribriforme do etmóide até atingirem os bulbos olfatórios (fossa craniana anterior)	Sensorial: mucosa olfatória (olfato)
Óptico (NC II)	Estrato ganglionar da retina	Sai da órbita através dos canais ópticos; as fibras oriundas da metade nasal da retina cruzam para o lado contralateral no quiasma; as fibras passam através dos tratos ópticos até os corpos geniculados, colículo superior e pré-tecto	Sensorial: visão a partir da retina
Palatino maior	Ramo do gânglio pterigopalatino	Passa inferiormente através do canal e forame palatino maior	Motor: parassimpáticas pós-sinápticas para as glândulas palatinas Sensoriais: mucosa do palato duro
Palatino menor	Gânglio pterigopalatino (nervo maxilar — NC V2)	Passa inferiormente através do canal palatino e forame palatino menor	Motor: fibras parassimpáticas pós-sinápticas para as glândulas do palato mole Sensorial: mucosa do palato mole
Palmares digitais comuns	Mediano e ramo superficial do nervo ulnar	Correm distalmente entre os tendões do flexor longo da região palmar, bifurcando-se na região distal da palma da mão	Ramos: nervos palmares digitais próprios, que inervam a pele e as articulações das faces palmar e dorsal distal dos dedos das mãos
Peitoral lateral	Cordão lateral do plexo braquial (fibras C5–C7)	Perfura a fáscia clavipeitoral para atingir a superfície profunda dos músculos peitorais	Motor: principalmente peitoral maior, mas envia uma alça para o nervo peitoral medial que inerva o músculo peitoral menor
Peitoral medial	Cordão medial do plexo braquial (fibras de C8 e T1)	Passa entre a artéria e a veia axilares e entra na superfície profunda do peitoral menor	Motor: peitoral menor e parte do peitoral maior

Nervo(s)/Ramo(s) do(s) Nervo(s)	Origem	Trajeto	Estruturas Inervadas
Perineal	Ramo terminal (com o nervo dorsal do pênis/clitóris) do nervo pudendo (fibras S2–S4)	Separa-se do nervo pudendo na saída do canal pudendo; corre para o períneo superficial, dividindo-se em um ramo cutâneo superficial (parte posterior dos lábios maiores do pudendo/bolsa escrotal) e um ramo motor profundo	Motor: músculos do trígono urogenital (músculos perineais superficial e profundo) Sensorial: pele do trígono urogenital posterior (porção posterior dos lábios maior e menor do pudendo, vestíbulo da vagina; face posterior da bolsa escrotal)
Petroso maior	Joelho do nervo facial (NC VII)	Sai do canal facial através do hiato para o nervo petroso maior; atravessa o tegme timpânico e passa através da cartilagem do forame lacerado para se unir ao nervo petroso profundo na abertura do canal pterigóideo	Motor: parassimpáticos pré-sinápticos para o gânglio pterigopalatino para a inervação das glândulas lacrimal e nasal, palatino e da mucosa da parte superior da faringe
Petroso menor	Plexo timpânico (nervo glossofaríngeo — NC IX)	Perfura o tegme do tímpano para sair da cavidade timpânica para dentro da fossa craniana média; corre anteriormente para descer através da fissura esfenopetrosa ou forame oval	Motor: conduz fibras parassimpáticas pré-sinápticas até o gânglio ótico para a inervação secretomotora da glândula parótida
Petroso profundo	Plexo carotídeo interno	Atravessa a cartilagem do forame lácero para se unir ao nervo petroso maior na entrada do canal pterigóideo	Conduz as fibras simpáticas pós-sinápticas destinadas à glândula lacrimal e à mucosa da cavidade nasal, palato e faringe superior
Plantar lateral	Ramo terminal menor do nervo tibial (fibras S1–S2)	Passa lateralmente no pé, entre os músculos quadrado plantar e flexor curto dos dedos, e se divide nos ramos superficial e profundo	Motor: quadrado plantar, abdutor do dedo mínimo e flexor curto do dedo mínimo; o ramo profundo inerva os interósseos plantares e dorsais, três lumbricais laterais e adutor do hálux Sensorial: pele na parte lateral da região plantar até uma linha que divide o 4.º dedo
Plantar medial	Ramo terminal maior do nervo tibial (fibras de L4 e L5)	Passa distalmente no pé, entre o abdutor do hálux e o flexor curto dos dedos, e se divide nos ramos muscular e cutâneo	Motor: abdutor do hálux, flexor curto dos dedos, flexor curto do hálux e primeiro lumbrical Sensorial: pele do lado medial da planta do pé e lados dos três primeiros dedos
Plantares digitais comuns	Nervos plantares medial e lateral	Correm anteriormente na planta do pé entre os tendões flexores, bifurcando-se na parte distal da planta	Ramos: nervos plantares digitais próprios, inervando a pele e as articulações das faces plantar e dorsal distal dos artelhos
Plexo cardíaco	Ramos cervical e cardíaco do nervo vago e nervos esplâncnicos cardiopulmonares a partir do tronco simpático	A partir do arco da aorta e superfície posterior do coração, as fibras estendem-se ao longo das artérias coronárias e para o nó SA	Tecido do nó SA e artérias coronárias; as fibras parassimpáticas alentecem a freqüência cardíaca, reduzem a força do batimento cardíaco e contraem as artérias; as fibras simpáticas exercem efeito oposto
Plexo esofágico	Nervo vago, gânglios simpáticos, nervo esplâncnico maior	Distal à bifurcação da traquéia, o vago e os nervos simpáticos formam um plexo ao redor do esôfago	Fibras vagais (parassimpáticas) e simpáticas para a musculatura lisa e glândulas dos dois terços inferiores do esôfago
Plexo pulmonar	Nervo vago e nervos esplâncnicos cardiopulmonares a partir do tronco simpático	Forma-se sobre os brônquios principais e se estende ao longo da raiz do pulmão e subdivisões brônquicas	Motor: as fibras parassimpáticas contraem os bronquíolos; as fibras simpáticas os dilatam
Pudendo	Plexo sacral (S2–S4)	Penetra na região glútea através do forame isquiático maior inferior em direção ao músculo piriforme; desce posterior ao ligamento sacroespinal; penetra no períneo através do forame isquiático menor	Fornece a maior parte da inervação motora e sensorial para o períneo (não inerva estruturas na região glútea)
Radial	Ramo terminal do cordão posterior do plexo braquial (fibras de C5–C8 e T1)	Desce posteriormente à artéria axilar; entra no sulco radial com a artéria braquial profunda para passar entre as cabeças longa e medial do músculo tríceps, bifurca-se na fossa cubital nos nervos radiais superficial e profundo	Motor: proximal à bifurcação, inerva os músculos tríceps braquial, ancôneo, braquiorradial e extensor radial longo do carpo Sensorial: pele na face posterior do braço e antebraço através dos nervos cutâneos posteriores do braço e antebraço
Ramo cutâneo palmar do nervo mediano	Origina-se do nervo mediano proximal ao retináculo dos músculos flexores	Passa entre os tendões dos músculos palmar longo e flexor radial do carpo e corre superficial ao retináculo dos músculos flexores	Sensorial: pele da região central da palma da mão

Nervo(s)/Ramo(s) do(s) Nervo(s)	Origem	Trajeto	Estruturas Inervadas
Ramo cutâneo palmar do nervo ulnar	Origina-se do nervo ulnar próximo ao meio do antebraço	Desce sobre a artéria ulnar e perfura a fáscia profunda no terço distal do antebraço	Sensorial: pele na base da região medial da palma da mão, suprajacente aos carpais mediais
Ramo dorsal do nervo ulnar	Nervo ulnar cerca de 5 cm proximalmente ao retináculo dos músculos flexores	Passa distalmente profundamente ao flexor ulnar do carpo, em seguida perfura dorsalmente a fáscia profunda e corre ao longo do lado medial do dorso da mão, dividindo-se em 2 a 3 nervos digitais dorsais	Sensorial: pele da face medial do dorso da mão e porções proximais do dedo mínimo e metade medial do dedo anelar (ocasionalmente também os lados adjacentes das porções proximais dos dedos anelar e médio)
Ramo lateral do nervo mediano	Nervo mediano quando ele penetra na palma da mão	Corre lateralmente à porção palmar do polegar e lado radial do dedo indicador	Motor: 1.º lumbrical Sensorial: pele das faces palmar e dorsal distal do polegar e metade radial do dedo indicador
Ramo medial do nervo mediano	Nervo mediano quando entra na palma da mão	Corre medialmente para os lados adjacentes dos dedos indicador, médio e anelar	Motor: 2.º lumbrical Sensorial: pele das faces palmar e dorsal distal dos lados adjacentes dos dedos indicador, médio e anelar
Ramo profundo do nervo radial	Nervo radial exatamente distal ao cotovelo	Curva-se ao redor do colo do rádio no músculo supinador; entra no compartimento posterior do antebraço, transformando-se no nervo interósseo posterior	Motor: extensor radial curto do carpo e supinador
Ramo profundo do nervo ulnar	Nervo ulnar no punho à medida que passa entre os ossos pisiforme e hamato (fibras de T1)	Passa profundamente entre os músculos da eminência hipotenar, em seguida através da região palmar com o arco palmar profundo (arterial)	Motor: músculos hipotenares (abdutor, flexor e oponente do dedo mínimo), lumbricais dos dedos 4 e 5, todos os interósseos, adutor do polegar e cabeça profunda do flexor curto do polegar
Ramo recorrente (tenar) do nervo mediano	Nervo mediano imediatamente distal ao retináculo flexor	Forma alças ao redor da borda distal do retináculo flexor e entra nos músculos tenares	Motor: abdutor curto do polegar, oponente do polegar e cabeça superficial do flexor curto do polegar
Ramo superficial do nervo radial	Continuação do nervo radial depois da emissão do ramo profundo na fossa cubital	Passa distalmente, anterior ao músculo pronador redondo e profundamente ao músculo braquiorradial; emergindo para perfurar a fáscia profunda no punho e correr no dorso da mão	Sensorial: pele da metade lateral (radial) do dorso da mão e polegar, as porções proximais das faces dorsais dos dedos 2 e 3, e da metade lateral (radial) do 4.º dedo
Ramo superficial do nervo ulnar	Origina-se do nervo ulnar no punho à medida que passa entre os ossos pisiforme e hamato	Passa o palmar curto e divide-se nos dois nervos palmares digitais comuns	Motor: palmar curto Sensorial: pele das faces palmar e dorsal distal do 5.º dedo e do lado medial (ulnar) do 4.º dedo e porção proximal da região palmar
Ramos calcâneos	Nervos tibial e sural	Passa desde a parte distal da face posterior da perna até a pele sobre o calcanhar	Sensorial: pele do calcanhar
Safeno	Nervo femoral	Desce com os vasos femorais através do trígono femoral e canal adutor e, em seguida, desce com a veia safena magna	Sensorial: pele no lado medial da perna e do pé
Subcostal	Ramo anterior do nervo espinhal T12	Corre ao longo da borda inferior da 12.ª costela da mesma maneira que os nervos intercostais	Motor: músculos da parede abdominal ântero-lateral Sensorial: o ramo cutâneo lateral inerva a pele inferior à crista ilíaca anterior
Subescapular inferior	Cordão posterior do plexo braquial (fibras de C5 e C6)	Passa ínfero-lateralmente, profundamente à artéria e veia subescapulares, para o subescapular e o redondo maior	Motor: porção inferior do músculo subescapular e músculo redondo maior
Subescapular superior	Ramo do cordão posterior do plexo braquial (fibras de C5 e C6)	Passa posteriormente e penetra no subescapular	Motor: porção superior do subescapular
Suboccipital	Ramo posterior do nervo espinal C1	Emerge entre o osso occipital e o atlas, inferior à porção transversa da artéria vertebral, para dentro do trígono suboccipital; comunica-se com o nervo occipital (C2)	Motor: músculos suboccipitais (retos maior e menor da cabeça, oblíquos inferior e superior da cabeça)

Nervo(s)/Ramo(s) do(s) Nervo(s)	Origem	Trajeto	Estruturas Inervadas
Supraclavicular (lateral, intermediário, medial)	Plexo cervical (fibras de C3 e C4)	Originam-se através de um tronco comum que emerge no centro da borda posterior do músculo esternocleidomastóideo; espalham-se à medida que descem sobre a parte inferior do pescoço, tórax superior e ombro	Sensorial: pele da porção ântero-lateral inferior do pescoço, porção mais superior do tórax e ombro
Supra-escapular	Tronco superior do plexo braquial (C5–C6; freqüentemente também C4)	Passa lateralmente através do trígono posterior do pescoço, através da incisura escapular sob o ligamento transverso superior da escápula	Motor: músculos supra-espinhoso, infra-espinhoso Sensorial: articulação glenoumeral superior e posterior (ombro)
Supra-orbital	Continuação do nervo frontal (NC V1)	Emerge através da incisura supra-orbital, ou forame, e divide-se em pequenos ramos	Sensorial: mucosa do seio frontal e conjuntiva (revestimento) da pálpebra superior; pele da fronte até o vértice
Supratroclear	Nervo frontal (NC V1)	Passa superiormente sobre a face medial do nervo supratroclear e se divide em dois ou mais ramos	Sensorial: pele na metade da fronte até a linha de implantação capilar
Sural	Geralmente origina-se da mistura dos nervos cutâneos surais medial e lateral (a partir dos nervos tibial e fibular comum, respectivamente)	Desce entre as cabeças do músculo gastrocnêmio e se torna superficial na metade da perna; desce com a veia safena pequena e passa posterior ao maléolo lateral para o lado lateral do pé	Sensorial: pele sobre as faces posterior e lateral e o lado lateral do pé
Temporal profundo	Nervo mandibular (NC V3)	Ascende a fossa temporal profundamente ao músculo temporal	Motor: temporal Sensorial: periósteo da fossa temporal
Tentorial	Porção intracraniana do nervo oftálmico (NC V1)	Origina-se como o ramo recorrente que passa abruptamente e posteriormente ao redor das margens da incisura tentorial e face superior do tentório do cerebelo e ascende no ramo posterior da foice do cérebro	Sensorial: dura-máter supratentorial (face superior do tentório cerebral e da foice do cérebro)
Tibial	Nervo isquiático (fibras L4–S3)	Forma-se como isquiático, bifurca-se no ápice da fossa poplítea; desce através da fossa poplítea e situa-se sobre o poplíteo; corre inferiormente sobre o tibial posterior com os vasos tibiais posteriores; termina abaixo do retináculo dos músculos flexores ao se dividir nos nervos plantares medial e lateral	Motor: músculos do compartimento posterior da coxa (exceto a cabeça curta do bíceps), fossa poplítea, compartimento posterior da perna e planta do pé Sensorial: articulação do joelho; pele da perna (através do sural medial) e planta do pé (através dos nervos plantares medial e lateral)
Timpânico	Como primeiro ramo extracraniano do nervo glossofaríngeo (NC IX), a partir do gânglio glossofaríngeo inferior (petroso)	Passa de maneira recorrente para dentro do canalículo timpânico, entrando na cavidade timpânica e ramificando-se sobre o promontório da parede do labirinto como o plexo timpânico	Motor: conduz as fibras parassimpáticas pré-sinápticas que alcançarão o gânglio ótico para a inervação secretomotora da glândula parótida Sensorial: mucosa da cavidade timpânica, células da mastóide e tuba auditiva
Torácico longo	Ramos anteriores de C5–C7	Desce posterior aos ramos C8 e T1 e passa distalmente na superfície externa do músculo serrátil anterior	Motor: músculo serrátil anterior
Toracoabdominal	Continuação dos nervos intercostais inferiores (T7–T11)	Cruza a margem costal para correr entre a 2.ª e a 3.ª camadas dos músculos abdominais	Motor: músculos abdominais ântero-laterais Sensorial: pele suprajacente, peritônio subjacente e periferia do diafragma
Toracodorsal	Cordão posterior do plexo braquial (fibras de C6–C8)	Origina-se entre os nervos subescapular superior e inferior e corre ínfero-lateralmente ao longo da parede axilar posterior até o músculo latíssimo do dorso	Motor: latíssimo do dorso
Transverso do pescoço	Plexo cervical (fibras de C2 e C3)	Emerge do meio da borda posterior do músculo esternocleidomastóideo; corre anteriormente através do músculo	Sensorial: pele sobre o trígono anterior do pescoço

Nervo(s)/Ramo(s) do(s) Nervo(s)	Origem	Trajeto	Estruturas Inervadas
Trigêmeo (NC V)	Superfície lateral da ponte por duas raízes: motora e sensorial	As raízes cruzam a parte medial da crista da porção petrosa do osso temporal, entrando na cavidade do trigêmeo da dura-máter lateral ao corpo do esfenóide e seio cavernoso; a raiz sensorial leva ao gânglio trigêmeo; a raiz motora desvia-se do gânglio, tornando-se parte do nervo mandibular (NC V3)	Motor: somático: músculos da mastigação, milo-hióideo, ventre anterior do músculo digástrico, tensor do tímpano e tensor do véu palatino; visceral: distribui as fibras parassimpáticas pós-sinápticas da cabeça para suas destinações Sensorial: dura-máter das fossas craniana anterior e média. Pele da face, dentes, gengivas, mucosa da cavidade nasal, seios paranasais e boca
Troclear (NC IV)	Face dorsolateral do mesencéfalo abaixo do colículo inferior (único nervo craniano a emergir da face dorsal do tronco encefálico)	Faz o mais longo trajeto intracraniano, passando ao redor do tronco cerebral para entrar na dura-máter na borda livre do tentório, próximo ao processo clinóide posterior; corre na parede lateral do seio cavernoso, entrando na órbita através da fissura orbital superior	Motor: músculo oblíquo superior
Ulnar	Ramo terminal do cordão medial do plexo braquial (fibras de C8 e T1; freqüentemente também recebe fibras de C7)	Desce pelo braço, por trás do epicôndilo medial do úmero e pela face ulnar do compartimento anterior do antebraço até a mão	Motor: maioria dos músculos intrínsecos da mão (hipotenar, interósseo, adutor do polegar e cabeça profunda do flexor curto do polegar, mais os lumbricais mediais [para os dedos 4 e 5]) Sensorial: pele das faces palmar e dorsal distal dos 1 1/2 dedos mediais (ulnares) e região palmar adjacente
Vago (NC X)	Através de 8 a 10 radículas a partir da medula do tronco cerebral	Entra no mediastino superior posterior à articulação esternoclavicular e veia braquiocefálica; origina o nervo laríngeo recorrente; continua dentro do abdome	Motor: musculatura voluntária da laringe e esôfago superior; musculatura involuntária e glândulas da árvore traqueobrônquica, intestino (até a flexura cólica esquerda) e coração através do plexo pulmonar, plexo esofágico e plexo cardíaco Sensorial: faringe, laringe, aferentes reflexos oriundas das mesmas áreas mencionadas antes
Vestibular	Como uma divisão do nervo vestibulococlear (NC VIII)	Atravessa o meato acústico interno para atingir o gânglio vestibular no fundo; os ramos passam para o vestíbulo do labirinto ósseo	Sensorial: cristas das ampolas dos ductos semicirculares, máculas do sáculo e utrículo (para a sensação do equilíbrio)
Vestibulococlear (NC VIII)	Sulco entre a ponte e o miencéfalo	Atravessa o meato acústico interno, dividindo-se nos nervos coclear e vestibular	Sensorial: órgão espiral (audição) e cristas das ampolas dos ductos semicirculares, máculas do sáculo e utrículo (equilíbrio)
Zigomático	Nervo maxilar (NC V2)	Origina-se no assoalho da órbita, divide-se nos ramos zigomaticofacial e zigomaticotemporal, que atravessam os forames de mesmo nome; os ramos comunicantes unem-se ao nervo lacrimal	Sensorial: pele sobre o arco zigomático e a região temporal anterior Motor: conduz fibras parassimpáticas pós-sinápticas secretoras do gânglio pterigopalatino para a glândula lacrimal

TABELA DE ELEMENTOS E SEUS PESOS ATÔMICOS

(Ordem Alfabética)

Elemento	Símbolo	Número Atômico	Peso Atômico	Elemento	Símbolo	Número Atômico	Peso Atômico
Actínio	Ac	89	227,0278*	Lutécio	Lu	71	174,967
Alumínio	Al	13	26,981539	Magnésio	Mg	12	24,3050
Amerício	Am	95	243,0614*	Manganês	Mn	25	54,93805
Antimônio	Sb	51	121,760	Mendelévio	Md	101	258,10*
Argônio	Ar	18	39,948	Mercúrio	Hg	80	200,59
Arsênico	As	33	74,92159	Molibdênio	Mo	42	95,94
Astatínio	At	85	209,9871*	Neodímio	Nd	60	144,24
Bário	Ba	56	137,327	Neônio	Ne	10	20,1797
Berílio	Be	4	9,012182	Netúnio	Np	93	237,0482*
Berquélio	Bk	97	247,0703*	Nióbio	Nb	41	92,90638
Bismuto	Bi	83	208,98037	Níquel	Ni	28	58,6934
Boro	B	5	10,811	Nitrogênio	N	7	14,00674
Bromo	Br	35	79,904	Nobélio	No	102	259,1009*
Cádmio	Cd	48	112,411	Ósmio	Os	76	190,23
Cálcio	Ca	20	40,078	Ouro	Au	79	196,96654
Califórnio	Cf	98	251,0796*	Oxigênio	O	8	15,9994
Carbono	C	6	12,011	Paládio	Pd	46	106,42
Cério	Ce	58	140,115	Platina	Pt	78	195,08
Césio	Cs	55	132,90543	Plutônio	Pu	94	244,0642*
Chumbo	Pb	82	207,2	Polônio	Po	84	208,9824*
Cloro	Cl	17	35,4527	Potássio	K	19	39,0983
Cobalto	Co	27	58,93320	Praseodímio	Pr	59	140,90765
Cobre	Cu	29	63,546	Prata	Ag	47	107,8682
Criptônio	Kr	36	83,80	Prométio	Pm	61	144,9127*
Cromo	Cr	24	51,9961	Protactínio	Pa	91	231,0388*
Cúrio	Cm	96	247,0703*	Rádio	Ra	88	226,0254*
Disprósio	Dy	66	162,50	Radônio	Rn	86	222,0176*
Einstênio	Es	99	252,083*	Rênio	Re	75	186,207
Enxofre	S	16	32,066	Ródio	Rh	45	102,90550
Érbio	Er	68	167,26	Rubídio	Rb	37	85,4678
Escândio	Sc	21	44,955910	Rutênio	Ru	44	101,07
Estanho	Sn	50	118,710	Samário	Sm	62	150,36
Estrôncio	Sr	38	87,62	Selênio	Se	34	78,96
Európio	Eu	63	151,965	Silício	Si	14	28,0855
Férmio	Fm	100	257,0951*	Sódio	Na	11	22,989768
Ferro	Fe	26	55,845	Tálio	Tl	81	204,3833
Flúor	F	9	18,9984032	Tântalo	Ta	73	180,9479
Fósforo	P	15	30,973762	Tecnécio	Tc	43	97,9072*
Frâncio	Fr	87	223,0197*	Telúrio	Te	52	127,60
Gadolínio	Gd	64	157,25	Térbio	Tb	65	158,92534
Gálio	Ga	31	69,723	Titânio	Ti	22	47,867
Germânio	Ge	32	72,61	Tório	Th	90	232,0381
Háfnio	Hf	72	178,49	Túlio	Tm	69	168,93421
Hélio	He	2	4,002602	Tungstênio	W	74	183,84
Hidrogênio	H	1	1,00794	Uniléxio	Unh	106	263,118*
Hólmio	Ho	67	164,93032	Unilpêntio	Unp	105	262,114*
Índio	In	49	114,818	Unilquádio	Unq	104	261,11*
Iodo	I	53	126,90447	Unilséptio	Uns	107	262,12*
Irídio	Ir	77	192,217	Urânio	U	92	238,0289
Itérbio	Yb	70	173,04	Vanádio	V	23	50,9415
Ítrio	Y	39	88,90585	Xenônio	Xe	54	131,29
Lantânio	La	57	138,9055	Zinco	Zn	30	65,39
Laurêncio	Lr	103	262,11*	Zircônio	Zr	40	91,224
Lítio	Li	3	6,941				

Baseado em 1993 IUPAC Table of Standard Atomic Weights of the Elements.
*Massa atômica relativa do isótopo daquele elemento com a maior meia-vida conhecida.

TABELA DE ELEMENTOS E SEUS PESOS ATÔMICOS

(Ordem de Número Atômico)

Número Atômico	Elemento	Símbolo	Peso Atômico	Número Atômico	Elemento	Símbolo	Peso Atômico
1	Hidrogênio	H	1,00794	55	Césio	Cs	132,90543
2	Hélio	He	4,002602	56	Bário	Ba	137,327
3	Lítio	Li	6,941	57	Lantânio	La	138,9055
4	Berílio	Be	9,012182	58	Cério	Ce	140,115
5	Boro	B	10,811	59	Praseodímio	Pr	140,90765
6	Carbono	C	12,011	60	Neodímio	Nd	144,24
7	Nitrogênio	N	14,00674	61	Prométio	Pm	144,9127*
8	Oxigênio	O	15,9994	62	Samário	Sm	150,36
9	Flúor	F	18,9984032	63	Európio	Eu	151,965
10	Neônio	Ne	20,1797	64	Gadolínio	Gd	157,25
11	Sódio	Na	22,989768	65	Térbio	Tb	158,92534
12	Magnésio	Mg	24,3050	66	Disprósio	Dy	162,50
13	Alumínio	Al	26,981539	67	Hólmio	Ho	164,93032
14	Silício	Si	28,0855	68	Érbio	Er	167,26
15	Fósforo	P	30,973762	69	Túlio	Tm	168,93421
16	Enxofre	S	32,066	70	Itérbio	Yb	173,04
17	Cloro	Cl	35,4527	71	Lutécio	Lu	174,967
18	Argônio	Ar	39,948	72	Háfnio	Hf	178,49
19	Potássio	K	39,0983	73	Tântalo	Ta	180,9479
20	Cálcio	Ca	40,078	74	Tungstênio	W	183,84
21	Escândio	Sc	44,955910	75	Rênio	Re	186,207
22	Titânio	Ti	47,867	76	Ósmio	Os	190,23
23	Vanádio	V	50,9415	77	Irídio	Ir	192,217
24	Cromo	Cr	51,9961	78	Platina	Pt	195,08
25	Manganês	Mn	54,93805	79	Ouro	Au	196,96654
26	Ferro	Fe	55,845	80	Mercúrio	Hg	200,59
27	Cobalto	Co	58,93320	81	Tálio	Tl	204,3833
28	Níquel	Ni	58,6934	82	Chumbo	Pb	207,2
29	Cobre	Cu	63,546	83	Bismuto	Bi	208,98037
30	Zinco	Zn	65,39	84	Polônio	Po	208,9824*
31	Gálio	Ga	69,723	85	Astatínio	At	209,9871*
32	Germânio	Ge	72,61	86	Radônio	Rn	222,0176*
33	Arsênico	As	74,92159	87	Frâncio	Fr	223,0197*
34	Selênio	Se	78,96	88	Rádio	Ra	226,0254*
35	Bromo	Br	79,904	89	Actínio	Ac	227,0278*
36	Criptônio	Kr	83,80	90	Tório	Th	232,0381*
37	Rubídio	Rb	85,4678	91	Protactínio	Pa	231,0388*
38	Estrôncio	Sr	87,62	92	Urânio	U	238,0289
39	Ítrio	Y	88,90585	93	Netúnio	Np	237,0482*
40	Zircônio	Zr	91,224	94	Plutônio	Pu	244,0642*
41	Nióbio	Nb	92,90638	95	Amerício	Am	243,0614*
42	Molibdênio	Mo	95,94	96	Cúrio	Cm	247,0703*
43	Tecnécio	Te	97,9072*	97	Berquélio	Bk	247,0703*
44	Rutênio	Ru	101,07	98	Califórnio	Cf	251,0796*
45	Ródio	Rh	102,90550	99	Einstênio	Es	252,083*
46	Paládio	Pd	106,42	100	Férmio	Fm	257,0951*
47	Prata	Ag	107,8682	101	Mendelévio	Md	258,10*
48	Cádmio	Cd	112,411	102	Nobélio	No	259,1009*
49	Índio	In	114,818	103	Laurêncio	Lr	262,11*
50	Estanho	Sn	118,710	104	Unilquádio	Unq	261,11*
51	Antimônio	Sb	121,760	105	Unilpêntio	Unp	262,114*
52	Telúrio	Te	127,60	106	Uniléxio	Unh	263,118*
53	Iodo	I	126,90447	107	Unilséptio	Uns	262,12*
54	Xenônio	Xe	131,29				

The Merck Index: An Encyclopedia of Chemicals, Drugs, and Biologicals, Twelfth Edition, Susan Budavari, Maryadele J. O'Neil, Ann Smith, Patricia E. Heckelman, Joanne F. Kinneary, Eds. (Merck & Co., Inc., Whitehouse Station, NJ, USA, 1996).

ESCALAS COMPARATIVAS DE TEMPERATURA

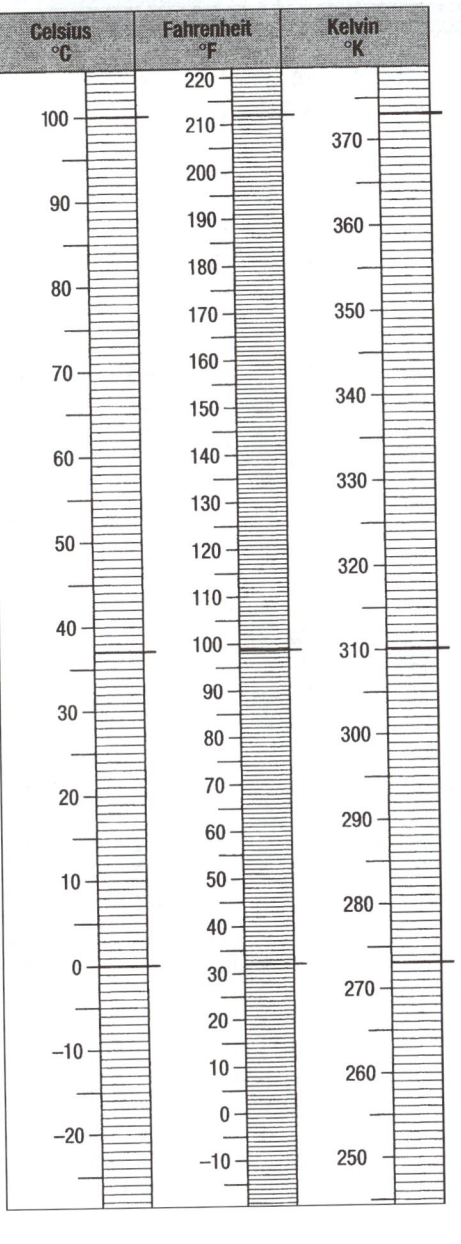

Para converter Celsius ou Fahrenheit em Kelvin:

C para K: acrescentar 273,16
10°C para K: 10 + 273,16 = 283,16 K

F para K: converter para C, acrescentar 273,16
63° F = 17,2°C + 273,16 = 290,36 K

Para converter de Fahrenheit para Celsius, Celsius para Fahrenheit:

Acima de 0°C ou 32°F

F para C: subtrair 32, multiplicar por 5, dividir por 9
63°F para C: 63 − 32 = 31 × 5 = 155 ÷ 9 = 17,2°C

C para F: multiplicar por 9, dividir por 5, acrescentar 32
37°C para F: 37 × 9 = 333 ÷ 5 = 66,6 + 32 = 98,6°F

TEMPERATURAS EQUIVALENTES

Celsius para Fahrenheit / Fahrenheit para Celsius

°C	°F	°C	°F	°F	°C	°F	°C	°F	°C
−50	−58,0	49	120,0	−50	−46,7	99	37,2	157	69,4
−40	−40,0	50	122,0	−40	−40,0	100	37,7	158	70,0
−35	−31,0	51	123,8	−35	−37,2	101	38,3	159	70,5
−30	−22,0	52	125,6	−30	−34,4	102	38,8	160	71,1
−25	−13,0	53	127,4	−25	−31,7	103	39,4	161	71,6
−20	−4,0	54	129,2	−20	−28,9	104	40,0	162	72,2
−15	−5,0	55	131,0	−15	−26,6	105	40,5	163	72,7
−10	−14,0	56	132,8	−10	−23,3	106	41,1	164	73,3
−5	−23,0	57	134,6	−5	−20,6	107	41,6	165	73,8
0	**32,0**	58	136,4	0	−17,7	108	42,2	166	74,4
1	33,8	59	138,2	1	−17,2	109	42,7	167	75,0
2	35,6	60	140,0	5	−15,0	110	43,3	168	75,5
3	37,4	61	141,8	10	−12,2	111	43,8	169	76,1
4	39,2	62	143,6	15	−9,4	112	44,4	170	76,6
5	41,0	63	145,4	20	−6,6	113	45,0	171	77,2
6	42,8	64	147,2	25	−3,8	114	45,5	172	77,7
7	44,6	65	149,0	30	−1,1	115	46,1	173	78,3
8	46,4	66	150,8	31	−0,5	116	46,6	174	78,8
9	48,2	67	152,6	**32**	**0**	117	47,2	175	79,4
10	50,0	68	154,4	33	0,5	118	47,7	176	80,0
11	51,8	69	156,2	34	1,1	119	48,3	177	80,5
12	53,6	70	158,0	35	1,6	120	48,8	178	81,1
13	55,4	71	159,8	36	2,2	121	49,4	179	81,6
14	57,2	72	161,6	37	2,7	122	50,0	180	82,2
15	59,0	73	163,4	38	3,3	123	50,5	181	82,7
16	60,8	74	165,2	39	3,8	124	51,1	182	83,3
17	62,6	75	167,0	40	4,4	125	51,6	183	83,8
18	64,4	76	168,8	41	5,0	126	52,2	184	84,4
19	66,2	77	170,6	42	5,5	127	52,7	185	85,0
20	68,0	78	172,4	43	6,1	128	53,3	186	85,5
21	69,8	79	174,2	44	6,6	129	53,8	187	86,1
22	71,6	80	176,0	45	7,2	130	54,4	188	86,6
23	73,4	81	177,8	46	7,7	131	55,0	189	87,2
24	75,2	82	179,6	47	8,3	132	55,5	190	87,7
25	77,0	83	181,4	48	8,8	133	56,1	191	88,3
26	78,8	84	183,2	49	9,4	134	56,6	192	88,8
27	80,6	85	185,0	50	10,0	135	57,2	193	89,4
28	82,4	86	186,8	55	12,7	136	57,7	194	90,0
29	84,2	87	188,6	60	15,5	137	58,3	195	90,5
30	86,0	88	190,4	65	18,3	138	58,8	196	91,1
31	87,8	89	192,2	70	21,1	139	59,4	197	91,6
32	89,6	90	194,0	75	23,8	140	60,0	198	92,2
33	91,4	91	195,8	80	26,6	141	60,5	199	92,7
34	93,2	92	197,6	85	29,4	142	61,1	200	93,3
35	95,0	93	199,4	86	30,0	143	61,6	201	93,8
36	96,8	94	201,2	87	30,5	144	62,2	202	94,4
37	**98,6**	95	203,0	88	31,0	145	62,7	203	95,0
38	100,4	96	204,8	89	31,6	146	63,3	204	95,5
39	102,2	97	206,6	90	32,2	147	63,8	205	96,1
40	104,0	98	208,4	91	32,7	148	64,4	206	96,6
41	105,8	99	210,2	92	33,3	149	65,0	207	97,2
42	107,6	**100**	**212,0**	93	33,8	150	65,5	208	97,7
43	109,4	101	213,8	94	34,4	151	66,1	209	98,3
44	111,2	102	215,6	95	35,0	152	66,6	210	98,8
45	113,0	103	217,4	96	35,5	153	67,2	211	99,4
46	114,8	104	219,2	97	36,1	154	67,7	**212**	**100,0**
47	116,6	105	221,0	98	36,6	155	68,3	213	100,5
48	118,4	106	222,8	**98,6**	**37,0**	156	68,8	214	101,1

PESOS E MEDIDAS

Escala do Sistema Métrico e SI

Prefixo	Símbolo	Potência
iota-	Y	10^{24}
zeta-	Z	10^{21}
exa-	E	10^{18}
peta-	P	10^{15}
tera-	T	10^{12}
giga-	G	10^{9}
mega-	M	10^{6}
quilo-	k	10^{3}
hecto-	h	10^{2}
deca-	da	10^{1}
UNIDADE		
deci-	d	10^{-1}
centi-	c	10^{-2}
mili-	m	10^{-3}
micro-	μ	10^{-6}
nano-	n	10^{-9}
pico-	p	10^{-12}
fento-	f	10^{-15}
ato-	a	10^{-18}
zepto-	z	10^{-21}
iocto-	y	10^{-24}

Unidades Básicas SI

Quantidade	Nome	Símbolo
comprimento	metro	m
massa*	quilograma†	kg
tempo	segundo	s
corrente elétrica	ampère	a
temperatura termodinâmica	kelvin‡	K
intensidade luminosa	candela	cd
quantidade de substância	mol	mol

*No uso comercial e cotidiano, "peso" geralmente significa massa; p. ex., quando se fala do peso de uma pessoa, a quantidade referida é a massa.
†Por motivos históricos, o quilograma é a única unidade de base com um prefixo. Múltiplos e submúltiplos do quilograma são formados pela junção do prefixo adequado à palavra-tronco "grama" (p. ex., miligrama) e o símbolo do prefixo adequado ao símbolo "g" (p. ex., mg).
‡O grau Celsius (°C) ainda é o uso amplamente aceito para expressar a temperatura e os intervalos de temperatura. A *temperatura* Celsius (antes centígrado) é convertida na temperatura termodinâmica kelvin (K) através do acréscimo de 273,16 à escala Celsius. Para o *intervalo de temperatura*, 1°C equivale a K.

Algumas Unidades Derivadas do SI Expressas em Termos das Unidades Básicas

Quantidade	Nome	Símbolo
área	metro quadrado	m^2
volume*	metro cúbico	m^3
volume específico	metro cúbico por quilograma	m^3/kg
velocidade	metro por segundo	m/s
aceleração	metro por segundo quadrado	m/s^2
densidade de massa	quilograma por metro cúbico	kg/m^3
concentração	mol por metro cúbico	mol/m^3
luminância	candela por metro quadrado	cd/m^2

*Litro (L, l). 10^{-3} m^3, é considerado um nome especial para o decímetro cúbico.

Algumas Unidades Derivadas do SI com Nomes Especiais

Quantidade	Nome	Símbolo	Expressão
Freqüência	hertz	Hz	s^{-1}
força	newton	N	$m\ kg\ s^{-2}$
pressão, estresse	pascal	Pa	$m^{-1}\ kg\ s^{-2}$
energia	joule	J	$m^2\ kg\ s^{-2}$
potência	watt	W	$m^2\ kg\ s^{-3}$
quantidade de eletricidade, carga elétrica	coulomb	C	s A
potencial elétrico, força eletromotiva	volt	V	$m^2\ kg\ s^{-3}\ A^{-1}$
capacitância	farad	F	$m^{-2}\ kg^{-1}\ s^4\ A^2$
resistência elétrica	ohm	Ω	$m^2\ kg^{-2}\ A^{-2}$
condutância elétrica	siemens	S	$m^{-2}\ kg\ s^{-2}\ A^{-1}$
fluxo magnético	weber	Wb	$m^2\ kg\ s^{-2}\ A^{-1}$
densidade de fluxo magnético	tesla	T	$kg\ s^{-2}\ A^{-1}$
atividade de radionuclídeo	becquerel*	Bq	s^{-1}
dose de radiação absorvida	gray†	Gy	$m^2\ s^{-2}$
exposição (radiação x e γ)	coulomb por quilograma‡	C kg	$kg^{-1}\ s\ A$

*Substituindo o curie (Ci), $3,7 \times 10^{10}\ s^{-1}$.

†Substituindo o rad (rad), $10^{-2}\ J\ kg^{-1}$.

‡Substituindo o roentgen (R), $2,58 \times 10^{-4}\ C\ kg^{-1}$.

Medidas de Comprimento

Micrômetros	Milímetros	Centímetros	Metros	Quilômetros	Milhas	Jardas	Pés	Polegadas
1	0,001	10^{-4}						0,000039
10^3	1	10^{-1}					0,00328	0,03937
10^4	10	1	0,01			0,0109	0,03281	0,3937
254.000	25,4	2,54	0,0254			0,0278	0,0833	1
	304,8	30,48	0,3048			0,333	1	12
10^6	10^3	10^2	1	0,001	0,0006213	1,0936	3,2808	39,37
914.400	914,40	91,44	0,9144	0,009	0,0005681	1	3	36
10^9	10^6	10^5	10^3	1	0,6215	1093,6121	3280,8	
			1609,0	1,609	1	1760,0	5280,0	

Para converter:

Milímetros em polegadas: dividir por 25,4
Polegadas em milímetros: multiplicar por 25,4

Centímetros em pés: dividir por 30,7
Pés em centímetros: multiplicar por 30,7

Metros em jardas: multiplicar por 1,09375
Jardas em metros: multiplicar por 0,9143

Quilômetros em milhas: multiplicar por 0,625
Milhas em quilômetros: multiplicar por 1,6

Medidas de Massa (Peso)

Pesos Avoirdupois

				Equivalentes Métricos		
Grãos	Dracmas	Onças	Libras	Miligramas	Gramas	Quilogramas
1	0,0366	0,0023	0,00014	64,8	0,0648	0,000065
27,34	1	0,0625	0,0039		1,772	0,001772
437,5	16	1	0,0625		28,350	0,028350
7.000	256	16	1		453,5924	0,453592
0,0154				1	0,001	
15,4324	0,5648	0,0353	0,002205	1000	1	0,001
15.432,358	564,32	35,27	2,2046		1000	1

Para converter (aproximadamente):

Quilogramas em libras: multiplicar por 2,2
Libras em quilogramas: multiplicar por 0,454

Gramas em onças: multiplicar por 0,03527
Onças em gramas: multiplicar por 28,35

Pesos Farmacêuticos

Grãos	Escrópulos	Dracmas	Onças	Libras	Miligramas	Equivalentes Métricos Gramas	Quilogramas
1	0,05	0,0167	0,0021	0,00017	64,8	0,0648	0,000065
20	1	0,333	0,042	0,0035		1,296	0,001296
60	3	1	0,125	0,0104		3,888	0,000389
480	24	8	1	0,0833		31,103	0,031103
5.760	288	96	12	1		373,2418	0,373242
0,0154					1	0,001	
15,4324		0,2572	0,0322	0,0027	1000	1	0,001
15.432,358		257,2	32,15	2,6792		1000	1

Medidas de Capacidade

Medidas Farmacêuticas

Mínimos	Dracmas Líquidas	Onças Líquidas	Quartilho	Quartos	Galões	Equivalentes Métricos Litros	Mililitros
1	0,0166	0,002	0,00013			0,0006	0,06161
60	1	0,125	0,0078	0,0039		0,0037	3,6967
480	8	1	0,0625	0,0312	0,0078	0,0296	29,5737
7.680	128	16	1	0,5	0,125	0,4732	473,166
15.360	256	32	2	1	0,25	0,9464	946,358
61.440	1024	128	8	4	1	3,7854	3785,434
16.230	270,52	33,8418	2,1134	1,0567	0,2642	1	1000
16,23	0,2705	0,0338	0,00212	0,00106	0,000265	0,001	1

Para converter (aproximadamente):

1 galão imperial britânico = 1,201 galão norte-americano
1 galão norte-americano = 0,8327 galão imperial britânico

litros em galões: multiplicar por 0,264
galões em litros: multiplicar por 3,788

litros em quartilhos: multiplicar por 2,1
quartilhos em litros: multiplicar por 0,4762

Medidas e Pesos Domiciliares Aproximados*

Colher de Chá	Colher de Sopa	Copos ou Xícaras**	Dracmas	Onças Líquidas	Mililitros	Gramas
1			1	0,125	5	5
3	1		4	0,50	15	15
48	16***	1	64	8	237	240

*Uma gota é uma medida de quantidade incerta, dependendo da natureza do líquido, assim como do formato do recipiente e da abertura a partir da qual o líquido cai. Uma gota de água equivale aproximadamente a 1 mínimo.

**Um copo geralmente significa 8 onças líquidas (237 ml).

***Para medidas secas, 12 colheres de chá equivalem a 1 xícara.

VALORES DE REFERÊNCIA EM LABORATÓRIO

Show-Hong Duh, PhD, DABCC, Department of Pathology,
University of Maryland School of Medicine
Janine Denis Cook, PhD, Department of Medical and Research Technology,
University of Maryland School of Medicine

Os valores dos intervalos de referência são para indivíduos aparentemente saudáveis, e, com freqüência, existe uma superposição significativa com os valores de pessoas doentes. Os valores reais podem variar muito em decorrência das metodologias do ensaio e da padronização. As instituições também podem estabelecer seus próprios intervalos de referência com base nas populações atendidas, portanto, podem existir diferenças regionais. Por conseguinte, os valores reportados por laboratórios individuais podem diferir dos arrolados neste apêndice.

Todos os valores são fornecidos em unidades convencionais e unidades do SI. Entretanto, onde as unidades SI não foram amplamente aceitas, as unidades convencionais são utilizadas. Por causa da natureza heterogênea dos materiais medidos ou da incerteza do peso molecular exato dos compostos, o SI não pode ser usado, e a massa por volume é utilizada como unidade de concentração.

Abreviaturas:

ACD, ácido-citrato-dextrose; **ICC**, insuficiência cardíaca congestiva; **Cit**, citrato; **SNC**, sistema nervoso central; **LCR**, líquido cefalorraquidiano; **AMP cíclico**, fosfato cíclico de 3´-5´-adenosina; **EDTA**, ácido etilenodiaminotetracético; **HDL**, lipoproteína de alta densidade; **Hep**, heparina; **LDL-C**, colesterol-lipoproteína de baixa densidade; **Ox**, oxalato; **RIA**, radioimunoensaio; **DP**, desvio-padrão

Referências:

Reference Intervals. In Tietz Textbook of Clinical Chemistry. 3rd ed., C. A. Burtis and E. R. Ashwood, Ed. Philadelphia, W. B. Saunders Co., 1998.

Hematologic Values. In Clinical Hematology and Fundamentals of Hemostasis. 2nd ed., D. M. Harmening, Ed. Philadelphia, F. A. Davis Co., 1992.

National Cholesterol Education Program: Report of the expert panel on detection, evaluation, and treatment of high blood cholesterol in adults. Arch. Intern. Med. 1988; 148:36-69.

Clinical Chemistry Laboratory: Reference Range Values in Clinical Chemistry. Professional services manual. Baltimore, Department of Pathology, University of Maryland Medical System, 1999.

Triglyceride, High Density Lipoprotein, and Coronary Heart Disease. National Institute of Health Consensus Statement, NIH Consensus Development Conference, 1992, Volume 10, Number 2.

Testes	Unidades Convencionais	Unidades SI
Acetaminofeno, soro ou plasma (Hep ou EDTA)		
Terapêutico	10–30 µg/mL	66–199 µmol/L
Tóxico	>200 µg/mL	>1324 µmol/L
Acetona		
Soro		
Qualitativo	Negativo	Negativo
Quantitativo	0,3–2,0 mg/dL	0,05–0,34 mmol/L
Urina		
Qualitativo	Negativo	Negativo
Ácido δ-aminolevulínico, urina	1,3–7,0 mg/24 h	10–53 µmol/24 h
Ácido β-hidroxibutírico, soro, plasma	0,21–2,81 mg/dL	20–270 µmol/L
Ácido 5-hidroxindolacético, urina		
Qualitativo	Negativo	Negativo
Quantitativo	2–7 mg/24 h	10,4–36,6 µmol/24 h
Ácido ascórbico, plasma (Ox, Hep, EDTA)	0,4–1,5 mg/dL	23–85 µmol/L
Ácido homogentísico, urina, qualitativo	Negativo	Negativo
*Ácido úrico		
Soro, enzimático		
Homem	4,5–8,0 mg/dL	0,27–0,47 mmol/L
Mulher	2,5–6,2 mg/dL	0,15–0,37 mmol/L
Criança	2,0–5,5 mg/dL	0,12–0,32 mmol/L
Urina	250–750 mg/24 h (com dieta normal)	1,48–4,43 mmol/24 h (com dieta normal)
Ácido valpróico, soro ou plasma (Hep ou EDTA); valor mínimo		
Terapêutico	50–100 µg/mL	347–693 µmol/L
Tóxico	>100 µg/mL	>693 µmol/L
Ácido vanilmandélico (VMA), urina (ácido 4-hidróxi-3-metoximandélico)	1,4–6,5 mg/24 h	7–33 µmol/dia
§Ácidos graxos, total, soro	190–420 mg/dL	7–15 mmol/L
Não-esterificados, soro	8–25 mg/dL	0,28–0,89 mmol/L
Adrenocorticotropina (ACTH), plasma		
08:00 h	<120 pg/mL	<26 pmol/L
Meia-noite (decúbito dorsal)	<10 pg/mL	<2,2 pmol/L
*Alanina Aminotransferase (ALT, TGP), sérica		
Homem	13–40 U/L (37°C)	0,22–0,68 µkat/L (37°C)
Mulher	10–28 U/L (37°C)	0,17–0,48 µkat/L (37°C)
Albumina		
Soro		
Adulto	3,5–5,2 g/dL	35–52 g/L
>60 anos	3,2–4,6 g/dL	32–46 g/L
	Em média 0,3 g/dL mais alta quando o indivíduo está de pé	Em média 0,3 g/dL mais alta quando o indivíduo está de pé
Urina		
Qualitativo	Negativo	Negativo
Quantitativo	50–80 mg/24 h	50–80 mg/24 h
LCR	10–30 mg/dL	100–300 mg/L
*Aldolase, soro	1,0–7,5 U/L (30°C)	0,02–0,13 µkat/L (30°C)
Aldosterona		
Soro		
Decúbito dorsal	3–16 ng/dL	0,08–0,44 nmol/L
De pé	7–30 ng/dL	0,19–0,83 nmol/L
Urina	3–19 µg/24 h	8–51 nmol/24 h
Amicacina, soro ou plasma (EDTA)		
Terapêutico		
Máximo	25–35 µg/mL	43–60 µmol/L
Mínimo		
Infecção menos grave	1–4 µg/mL	1,7–6,8 µmol/L
Infecção com risco de vida	4–8 µg/mL	6,8–13,7 µmol/L

*Os valores são método-dependentes.

§O termo "ácidos graxos" inclui uma mistura de ácidos alifáticos diferentes de vários pesos moleculares variáveis; um peso molecular médio de 284 daltons foi presumido.

VALORES DE REFERÊNCIA EM LABORATÓRIO

Testes	Unidades Convencionais	Unidades SI
Tóxico		
Máximo	>35–40 µg/mL	>60–68 µmol/L
Mínimo	>10–15 µg/mL	>17–26 µmol/L
*Amilase		
Soro	27–131 U/L	0,46–2,23 µkat/L
Urina	1–17 U/h	0,017–0,29 µkat/h
Amilase/depuração de creatinina	1–4%	0,01–0,04
Amitriptilina, soro ou plasma (Hep ou EDTA); valor mínimo (≥12 h após a dose)		
Terapêutico	80–250 ng/mL	289–903 nmol/L
Tóxico	>500 ng/mL	>1805 nmol/L
Amônia		
Plasma (Hep)	9–33 µmol/L	9–33 µmol/L
AMP cíclico		
Plasma (EDTA)		
Homem	4,6–8,6 ng/mL	14–26 nmol/L
Mulher	4,3–7,6 ng/mL	13–23 nmol/L
Urina, 24 h	0,3–3,6 mg/dia ou 0,29–2,1 mg/g de creatinina	1,0–10,9 µmol/d ou 100–723 µmol/ml de creatinina
Androstenediona, soro		
Homem	75–205 ng/dL	2,6–7,2 nmol/L
Mulher	85–275 ng/dL	3,0–9,6 nmol/L
*Antígeno prostático-específico (PSA), soro		
Homem	<4,0 ng/mL	<4,0 µg/L
α_1-Antitripsina, soro	78–200 mg/dL	0,78–2,00 g/L
Apolipoproteína A-1		
Homem	94–178 mg/dL	0,94–1,78 g/L
Mulher	101–199 mg/L	1,01–1,99 g/L
Apolipoproteína B		
Homem	63–133 mg/dL	0,63–1,33 g/L
Mulher	60–126 mg/dL	0,60–1,26 g/L
Arsênico		
Sangue total (Hep)	0,2–2,3 µg/dL	0,03–0,31 µmol/L
Intoxicação crônica	10–50 µg/dL	1,33–6,65 µmol/L
Intoxicação aguda	60–930 µg/dL	7,98–124 µmol/L
Urina, 24 h	5–50 µg/d	0,07–0,67 µmol/d
*Aspartato aminotransferase (AST, TGO), soro	10–59 U/L (37°C)	0,17–1,00 −2 a +3 kat/L (37°C)
Bicarbonato, soro (venoso)	22–29 mEq/L	22–29 mmol/L
*Bilirrubina		
Soro		
Adulto		
Conjugada	0,0–0,3 mg/dL	0–5 µmol/L
Não-conjugada	0,1–1,1 mg/dL	1,7–19 µmol/L
Delta	0–0,2 mg/dL	0–3 µmol/L
Total	0,2–1,3 mg/dL	3–22 µmol/L
Neonatos		
Conjugada	0–0,6 mg/dL	0–10 µmol/L
Não-conjugada	0,6–10,5 mg/dL	10–180 µmol/L
Total	1,5–12 mg/dL	1,7–180 µmol/L
Urina, qualitativa	Negativa	Negativa
CA 125, soro	<35 U/mL	<35 kU/L
CA 15–3, soro	<30 U/mL	<30 kU/L
CA 19–9, soro	<37 U/mL	<37 kU/L
Cádmio, sangue total (Hep)	0,1–0,5 µg/dL	8,9–44,5 nmol/L
Tóxico	10–300 µg/dL	0,89–26,70 µmol/L
Cádmio, urina, 24 h	<15 µg/d	<0,13 µmol/d
Cálcio, ionizado, soro	4,64–5,28 mg/dL	1,16–1,32 mmol/L
Cálcio, sérico	8,6–10,0 mg/dl (Um pouco mais elevado em crianças)	2,15–2,50 mmol/L (Um pouco mais elevado em crianças)

*Os valores são método-dependentes.

Testes	Unidades Convencionais	Unidades SI
Cálcio, urina		
Dieta pobre em cálcio	50–150 mg/24 h	1,25–3,75 mmol/24 h
Dieta habitual; valor mínimo	100–300 mg/24 h	2,50–7,50 mmol/24 h
Calcitonina, soro ou plasma (Hep, EDTA)		
Homem	≤100 pg/mL	≤100 ng/L
Mulher	≤30 pg/mL	≤30 ng/L
Capacidade de fixação do ferro, soro, total (TIBC)	250–425 µg/dL	44,8–71,6 µmol/L
Carbamazepina, sérica ou plasmática (Hep ou EDTA), valor mínimo		
Terapêutico	4–12 µg/mL	17–51 µmol/L
Tóxico	>15 µg/mL	>63 µmol/L
Caroteno, soro	10–85 µg/dL	0,19–1,58 µmol/L
Catecolaminas, plasma (EDTA)		
Dopamina	<30 pg/mL	<196 pmol/L
Epinefrina	<140 pg/mL	<764 pmol/L
Norepinefrina	<1700 pg/mL	<10.047 pmol/L
Catecolaminas, urina		
Dopamina	65–400 µg/24 h	425–2.610 nmol/24 h
Epinefrina	0–20 µg/24 h	0–109 nmol/24 h
Norepinefrina	15–80 µg/24 h	89–473 nmol/24 h
CEA, soro		
Não-fumantes	<5,0 ng/mL	<5,0 µg/L
Células, LCR	0–10 linfócitos/mm^3	0–10 linfócitos/mm^3
	0 eritrócitos/mm^3	0 eritrócitos/mm^3
Ceruloplasmina, soro	20–60 mg/dL	0,2–0,6 g/L
17–Cetosteróides, urina		
Homem	10–25 mg/24 h	38–87 µmol/24 h
Mulher	6–14 mg/24 h (diminui com a idade)	21–52 µmol/24 h (diminui com a idade)
Chumbo		
Sangue total (Hep)	<10 µg/dL	<0,48 µmol/L
Urina, 24 h	<80 µg/dia	<0,39 µmol/dia
Cianeto		
Soro		
Não-fumantes	0,004 mg/L	0,15 µmol/L
Fumantes	0,006 mg/L	0,23 µmol/L
Terapia com nitroprussiato	0,01–0,06 mg/L	0,38–2,30 µmol/L
Tóxico	>0,1 mg/L	>3,84 µmol/L
Sangue total (Ox)		
Não-fumantes	0,016 mg/L	0,61 µmol/L
Fumantes	0,041 mg/L	1,57 µmol/L
Terapia com nitroprussiato	0,05–0,5 mg/L	1,92–19,20 µmol/L
Tóxico	>1 mg/L	>38,40 µmol/L
*,#Ciclosporina, sangue total		
Terapêutico, mínimo	100–200 ng/mL	83–166 nmol/L
Cistina ou cisteína, urina, qualitativa	Negativa	Negativa
Clonazepam, soro ou plasma (Hep ou EDTA); valor mínimo		
Terapêutico	15–60 ng/mL	48–190 nmol/L
Tóxico	>80 ng/mL	>254 nmol/L
Cloranfenicol, soro ou plasma (Hep ou EDTA); valor mínimo		
Terapêutico	10–25 µg/mL	31–77 µmol/L
Tóxico	>25 µg/mL	>77 µmol/L
Cloreto		
Sérico ou plasmático (Hep)	98–107 mmol/L	98–107 mmol/L
Suor		
Normal	5–35 mmol/L	5–35 mmol/L
Fibrose cística	60–200 mmol/L	60–200 mmol/L

*Os valores são método-dependentes.
#O intervalo terapêutico real deve ser ajustado para cada paciente.

Testes	Unidades Convencionais	Unidades SI
Urina, 24 h (varia muito com o consumo de Cl)		
Lactente	2–10 mmol/24 h	2–10 mmol/24 h
Criança	15–40 mmol/24 h	15–40 mmol/24 h
Adulto	110–250 mmol/24 h	110–250 mmol/24 h
LCR	118–132 mmol/L (20 mmol/L mais elevado que no soro)	118–132 mmol/L (20 mmol/L mais elevado que no soro)
Coagulograma		
Antitrombina III (substrato sintético)	80–120% do normal	0,8–1,2 do normal
Tempo de sangramento (Duke)	0–6 min	0–6 min
Tempo de sangramento (Ivy)	1–6 min	1–6 min
Tempo de sangramento (padrão)	2,3–9,5 min	2,3–9,5 min
Retração do coágulo, qualitativa	50–100% em 2 h	0,5–1,0/2 h
Cobre		
Soro		
Homem	70–140 µg/dL	11–22 µmol/L
Mulher	80–155 µg/dL	13–24 µmol/L
Urina	3–35 µg/24 h	0,05–0,55 µmol/24 h
Colesterol, soro		
Adulto Desejável	<200 mg/dL	<5,2 mmol/L
Limítrofe	200–239 mg/dL	5,2–6,2 mmol/L
Alto risco	≥240 mg/dL	≥6,2 mmol/L
*Colinesterase, soro	4,9–11,9 U/mL	4,9–11,9 kU/L
Inibição com dibucaína	79–84%	0,79–0,84
Inibição com fluoreto	58–64%	0,58–0,64
Componentes do complemento		
Atividade hemolítica total do complemento, plasma (EDTA)	75–160 U/mL	75–160 kU/L
Taxa de decaimento do complemento total (funcional), plasma (EDTA)	10–20% Deficiência: >50%	Taxa de decaimento fracional: 0,10–0,20 >0,50
C1q, soro	14,9–22,1 mg/dL	149–221 mg/L
C1r, soro	2,5–10,0 mg/dL	25–100 mg/L
C1s (C1 esterase), soro	5,0–10,0 mg/dL	50–100 mg/L
C2, soro	1,6–3,6 mg/dL	16–36 mg/L
C3, soro	90–180 mg/dL	0,9–1,8 g/L
C4, soro	10–40 mg/dL	0,1–0,4 g/L
C5, soro	5,5–11,3 mg/dL	55–113 mg/L
C6, soro	17,9–23,9 mg/dL	179–239 mg/L
C7, soro	2,7–7,4 mg/dL	27–74 mg/L
C8, soro	4,9–10,6 mg/dL	49–106 mg/L
C9, soro	3,3–9,5 mg/dL	33–95 mg/L
Consumo de protrombina	>20 s	>20 s
Cortisol, soro		
Plasma (Hep, EDTA, Ox)		
08:00 h	5–23 µg/dL	138–635 nmol/L
16:00 h	3–16 µg/dL	83–441 nmol/L
22:00 h	<50% do valor às 08:00 h	<0,5 do valor às 08:00 h
Livre, urina	<50 µg/24 h	<138 mmol/24 h
*Creatinina		
Soro ou plasma, adulto		
Homem	0,7–1,3 mg/dL	62–115 µmol/L
Mulher	0,6–1,1 mg/dL	53–97 µmol/L
Urina		
Homem	14–26 mg/kg de peso corporal/24 h	124–230 µmol/kg de peso corporal/24 h
Mulher	11–20 mg/kg de peso corporal/24 h	97–177 µmol/kg de peso corporal/24 h
*[†]Creatinoquinase (CK), sérica		
Homem	15–105 U/L (30°C)	0,26–1,79 µkat/L (30°C)
Mulher	10–80 U/L (30°C)	0,17–1,36 µkat/L (30°C)
Nota: O exercício extenuante ou injeções intramusculares podem causar a elevação transitória da CK.		
*Creatinoquinase, isoenzima B, soro	0–7 ng/mL	0–7 µg/L

*Os valores são método-dependentes.
[†]Os valores são raça-dependentes.

Testes	Unidades Convencionais	Unidades SI
Crioglobulinas, soro	0	0
Densidade, urina	1,002–1,030	1,002–1,030
*Depuração da creatinina, soro ou plasma e urina		
Homem	94–140 mL/min/1,73 m²	0,91–1,35 mL/s/m²
Mulher	72–110 mL/min/1,73 m²	0,69–1,06 mL/s/m²
Desidroepiandrosterona (DHEA), soro		
Homem	180–1250 ng/dL	6,2–43,3 nmol/L
Mulher	130–980 ng/dL	4,5–34,0 nmol/L
Desipramina, soro ou plasma (Hep ou EDTA); valor mínimo (12 h depois da dose)		
Terapêutico	75–300 ng/mL	281–1.125 nmol/L
Tóxico	>400 ng/mL	>1500 nmol/L
Diazepam, soro ou plasma (Hep ou EDTA); valor mínimo		
Terapêutico	100–1000 ng/mL	0,35–3,51 µmol/L
Tóxico	>5000 ng/mL	>17,55 µmol/L
Digitoxina, soro ou plasma (Hep ou EDTA) 7,8 h depois da dose		
Terapêutico	20–35 ng/mL	26–46 nmol/L
Tóxico	>45 ng/mL	>59 nmol/L
Digoxina, soro ou plasma (Hep ou EDTA); ≥12 h após a dose		
Terapêutico		
ICC	0,8–1,5 ng/mL	1,0–1,9 nmol/L
Arritmias	1,5–2,0 ng/mL	1,9–2,6 nmol/L
Tóxico		
Adulto	>2,5 ng/mL	>3,2 nmol/L
Criança	>3,0 ng/mL	>3,8 nmol/L
Dióxido de carbono (PCO_2), sangue arterial	Homem 35–48 mm Hg	4,66–6,38 kPa
	Mulher 32–45 mm Hg	4,26–5,99 kPa
Dióxido de carbono, total, soro/plasma (Hep)	22–28 mmol/L	22–28 mmol/L
Disopiramida, soro ou plasma (Hep ou EDTA); valor mínimo		
Terapêuticos		
Arritmias		
Atriais	2,8–3,2 µg/mL	8,3–9,4 µmol/L
Ventriculares	3,3–7,5 µg/mL	9,7–22 µmol/L
Tóxico	>7 µg/mL	>20,7 µmol/L
Doxepina, soro ou plasma (Hep ou EDTA); valor mínimo (≥12 h depois da dose)		
Terapêutico	150–250 ng/mL	537–895 nmol/L
Tóxico	>500 ng/mL	>1790 nmol/L
Eletroforese de hemoglobina, sangue total (EDTA, Cit ou Hep)		
HbA	>95%	Fração de Hb >0,95
HbA$_2$	1,5–3,7%	Fração de Hb de 0,015–0,037
HbF	<2%	Fração de Hb <0,02
*Estradiol, soro		
Adulto		
Homem	10–50 pg/mL	37–184 pmol/L
Mulher	Varia com o ciclo menstrual	
Etanol, sangue total (Ox) ou soro		
Depressão do SNC	>100 mg/dL	>21,7 mmol/L
Mortes notificadas	>400 mg/dL	>86,8 mmol/L
Etossuximida, sérica ou plasmática (Hep ou EDTA); valor mínimo		
Terapêutico	40–100 µg/mL	283–708 µmol/L
Tóxico	>150 µg/mL	>1062 µmol/L
Excesso de base, sangue (Hep)	−2 a +3 mEq/L	−2 a +3 mmol/L
Excreção de fenolsulfonoftaleína (PSP), urina	28–51% em 15 min	0,28–0,51 em 15 min
	13–24% em 30 min	0,13–0,24 em 30 min

*Os valores são método-dependentes.

Testes	Unidades Convencionais	Unidades SI
	9–17% em 60 min	0,09–0,17 em 60 min
	3–10% em 2 h	0,03–0,10 em 2 h
	(Após injeção IV de 1 mL de PSP)	(Após injeção IV de 1 mL de PSP)
Fenacetina, plasma (EDTA)		
Terapêutico	1–30 µg/mL	6–167 µmol/L
Tóxico	50–250 µg/mL	279–1395 µmol/L
Fenilalanina, soro	0,8–1,8 mg/dL	48–109 µmol/L
Fenitoína, soro ou plasma (Hep ou EDTA);		
valor mínimo		
Terapêutico	10–20 µg/mL	40–79 µmol/L
Tóxico	>20 µg/mL	>79 µmol/L
Fenobarbital, soro ou plasma (Hep ou EDTA);		
valor mínimo		
Terapêutico	15–40 µg/mL	65–172 µmol/L
Tóxico		
Lentidão, ataxia, nistagmo	35–80 µg/mL	151–345 µmol/L
Coma com reflexos	65–117 µg/mL	280–504 µmol/L
Coma sem reflexos	>100 µg/mL	>430 µmol/L
Ferritina, soro		
Homem	20–250 ng/mL	20–250 µg/L
Mulher	10–120 ng/mL	10–120 µg/L
Valores da ferritina <20 ng/mL (20 µg/L) foram relatados como estando geralmente associados a reservas de ferro depletadas		
*Ferro, soro		
Homens	65–175 µg/dL	11,6–31,3 µmol/L
Mulheres	50–170 µg/dL	9,0–30,4 µmol/L
α-Fetoproteína (AFP), soro	<15 ng/mL	<15 µg/L
*Fibrinogênio, plasma (NaCit)	200–400 mg/dL	2–4 g/L
Fluoreto		
Plasma (Hep)	0,01–0,2 µg/mL	0,5–10,5 µmol/L
Urina	0,2–3,2 µg/mL	10,5–168 µmol/L
Urina, exposição ocupacional	<8 µg/mL	<421 µmol/L
*Folato Soro	3–20 ng/mL	7–45 nmol/L
Eritrócitos	140–628 ng/mL de eritrócitos	317–1422 nmol/L de eritrócitos
*Fosfatase ácida, prostática, soro (RIA)	<3,0 ng/mL	<3,0 µg/L
*Fosfatase, alcalina, total, soro	38–126 U/L (37°C)	0,65–2,14 µkat/L
Fosfatidilglicerol (PG), líquido amniótico		
Imaturidade pulmonar fetal	Ausente	Ausente
Maturidade pulmonar fetal	Presente	Presente
Fosfato, inorgânico, soro		
Adultos	2,7–4,5 mg/dL	0,87–1,45 mmol/L
Crianças	4,5–5,5 mg/dL	1,45–1,78 mmol/L
Fosfolipídios, soro	125–275 mg/dL	1,25–2,75 g/L
Fósforo, urina	0,4–1,3 g/24 h	12,9–42 mmol/24 h
Fragilidade osmótica dos eritrócitos	Começa em NaCl 0,45–0,39%	Começa em 77–67 mmol/L NaCl
	Completo em 0,33–0,30% NaCl	Completo em 56–51 mmol/L NaCl
Gastrina, soro	<100 pg/mL	<100 ng/L
Gentamicina, soro ou plasma (EDTA)		
Terapêutico		
Máximo		
Infecção menos grave	5–8 µg/mL	10,4–16,7 µmol
Infecção grave	8–10 µg/mL	16,7–20,9 µmol/L
Mínimo		
Infecção menos grave	<1 µg/mL	<2,1 µmol/L
Infecção moderada	<2 µg/mL	<4,2 µmol/L
Infecção grave	<2–4 µg/mL	<4,2–8,4 µmol/L
Tóxico		
Máximo	>10–12 µg/mL	>21–25 µmol/L
Mínimo	>2–4 µg/mL	>4,2–8,4 µmol/L
Glicose (jejum)		
Sangue	65–95 mg/dL	3,5–5,3 mmol/L
Plasma ou soro	74–106 mg/dL	4,1–5,9 mmol/L

*Os valores são método-dependentes.

Testes	Unidades Convencionais		Unidades SI
Glicose, 2 h pós-prandial, soro	<120 mg/dL		<6,7 mmol/L
Glicose, LCR	40–70 mg/dL		2,2–3,9 mmol/L
Glicose, urina			
Quantitativa	<500 mg/24 h		<2,8 mmol/24 h
Qualitativa	Negativa		Negativa
*Glicose-6-fosfato desidrogenase (G-6-PD) em eritrócitos, sangue total (ACD, EDTA ou Hep)	12,1 ± 2,1 U/g Hb (DP) 351 ± 60,6 U/10^{12} hemácias 4,11 ± 0,71 U/mL hemácias		0,78 ± 0,13 mU/mol Hb 0,35 ± 0,06 nU/hemácia 4,11 ± 0,71 kU/L hemácia
Globulina fixadora de tiroxina (TBG), soro	1,2–3,0 mg/dL		12–30 mg/L
γ-Glutamiltransferase (GGT), soro			
Homem	2–30 U/L (37°C)		0,03–0,51 μkat/L (37°C)
Mulher	1–24 U/L (37°C)		0,02–0,41 μkat/L (37°C)
Glutetimida, soro			
Terapêutico	2–6 μg/mL		9–28 μmol/L
Tóxico	>5 μg/mL		>23 μmol/L
*Gonadotropina coriônica, intacta			
Soro ou plasma (EDTA)			
Homem e mulher não-grávida	<5,0 mUI/mL		<5,0 UI/L
Gestante	Varia com a idade gestacional		
Urina, qualitativa			
Homem e mulher não-grávida	Negativa		Negativa
Gestante	Positiva		Positiva
Haptoglobina, sérica	30–200 mg/dL		0,3–2,0 g/L
HDL-colesterol (HDL-C), soro ou plasma (EDTA)			
Adulto Desejável	>40 mg/dL		>1,04 mmol/L
Limítrofe	35–40 mg/dL		0,78–1,04 mmol/L
Alto risco	<35 mg/dL		<0,78 mmol/L
Hematócrito			
Homem	42–52%		0,42–0,52
Mulher	37–47%		0,37–0,47
Neonato	53–65%		0,53–0,65
Crianças (varia com a idade)	30–43%		0,30–0,43
Hemoglobina (Hb)			
Homem	14,0–18,0 g/dL		2,17–2,79 mmol/L
Mulher	12,0–16,0 g/dL		1,86–2,48 mmol/L
Neonato	17,0–23,0 g/dL		2,64–3,57 mmol/L
Crianças (varia com a idade)	11,2–16,5 g/dL		1,74–2,56 mmol/L
Hemoglobina e mioglobina, urina, qualitativa	Negativa		Negativa
Hemoglobina glicosilada (Hemoglobina A1c), sangue total (EDTA)	4,2%–5,9%		0,042–0,059
Hemoglobina, fetal	≥1 ano de idade: <2% da Hb total		≥1 ano de idade: <0,02% da Hb total
Hemoglobina, plasma	<3 mg/dL		<0,47 μmol/L
*Hemograma, adulto			
Eritrócitos Homem	4,7–6,1 × 10^6/μL		4,7–6,1 × 10^{12}/L
Mulher	4,2–5,4 × 10^6/μL		4,2–5,4 × 10^{12}/L
Leucócitos			
Total	4,8–10,8 × 10^3/μL		4,8–10,8 × 10^6/L
Diferencial	Percentual	Absoluta	Absoluta (SI)
Mielócitos	0	0/μL	0/L
Neutrófilos			
Bastões	3–5	150–400/μL	150–400 × 10^6/L
Segmentados	54–62	3.000–5.800/μL	3.000–5.800 × 10^6/L
Linfócitos	20,5–51,1	1,2–3,4 × 10^3/μL	1,2–3,4 × 10^9/L
Monócitos	1,7–9,3	0,11–0,59 × 10^3/μL	0,11–0,59 × 10^9/L
Granulócitos	42,2–75,2	1,4–6,5 × 10^3/μL	1,4–6,5 × 10^9/L
Eosinófilos		0–0,7 × 10^3/μL	0–0,7 × 10^9/L
Basófilos		0–0,2 × 10^3/μL	0–0,2 × 10^9/L
Plaquetas	130–400 × 10^3/μL		130–400 × 10^9/L
Reticulócitos	0,5–1,5% dos eritrócitos 24.000–84.000/μL		0,005–0,015 dos eritrócitos 24–84 × 10^9/L

*Os valores são método-dependentes.

Testes	Unidades Convencionais	Unidades SI
Valores corpusculares dos eritrócitos (os valores são para adultos; em crianças, os valores variam com a idade)		
Hemoglobina corpuscular média (HCM)	27–31 pg	0,42–0,48 fmol
Concentração da hemoglobina corpuscular média (CHCM)	33–37 g/dL	330–370 g/L
Volume corpuscular médio (VCM)	Homem 80–94 µ³	80–94 fL
	Mulher 81–99 µ³	81–99 fL
17-Hidroxicorticosteróides		
Urina		
Homens	3–10 mg/24 h	8,3–27,6 µmol/24 h (como cortisol)
Mulheres	2–8 mg/24 h	5,5–22 µmol/24 h (como cortisol)
Hormônio do crescimento, soro		
Homem	<5 ng/mL	<5 µg/L
Mulher	<10 ng/mL	<10 µg/L
*Hormônio folículo-estimulante (FSH), soro e plasma (Hep)		
Homem	1,4–15,4 mUI/mL	1,4–15,4 UI/L
Mulher		
Fase folicular	1–10 mUI/mL	1–10 UI/L
Metade do ciclo	6–17 mUI/mL	6–17 UI/L
Fase lútea	1–9 mUI/mL	1–9 UI/L
Pós-menopausa	19–100 mUI/mL	19–100 UI/L
*Hormônio luteinizante (LH), soro ou plasma (Hep)		
Homem	1,24–7,8 mUI/mL	1,24–7,8 UI/L
Mulher		
Fase folicular	1,68–15,0 mUI/mL	1,68–15,0 UI/L
Pico no meio do ciclo	21,9–56,6 mUI/mL	21,9–56,6 UI/L
Fase luteínica	0,61–16,3 mUI/mL	0,61–16,3 UI/L
Pós-menopausa	14,2–52,5 mUI/mL	14,2–52,3 UI/L
*Hormônio tireoestimulante (TSH), soro	0,4–4,2 µU/mL	0,4–4,2 mU/L
Imipramina, soro ou plasma (Hep ou EDTA); valor mínimo (≥12 h depois da dose)		
Terapêutico	150–250 ng/mL	536–893 nmol/L
Tóxico	>500 ng/mL	>1785 nmol/L
Imunoglobulina G (IgG), LCR	0,5–6,1 mg/dL	0,5–6,1 g/L
Imunoglobulinas, soro		
IgG	700–1600 mg/dL	7–16 g/L
IgA	70–400 mg/dL	0,7–4,0 g/L
IgM	40–230 mg/dL	0,4–2,3 g/L
IgD	0–8 mg/dL	0–80 mg/L
IgE	3–423 UI/mL	3–423 kUI/L
*Índice de Tiroxina Livre (FTI), soro	4,2–13	4,2–13
Insulina, plasma (jejum)	2–25 µU/mL	13–174 pmol/L
Intervalo aniônico		
(Na–(Cl + HCO$_3$))	7–16 mEq/L	7–16 mmol/L
((Na + K) – (Cl + HCO$_3$))	10–20 mEq/L	10–20 mmol/L
*Lactato desidrogenase ou desidrogenase láctica (LDH)		
Total (L → P), 37°C, soro		
Neonato	170–580 U/L	170–580 U/L
Lactente	180–430 U/L	3,1–7,3 µkat/L
Criança	110–295 U/L	1,9–5 µkat/L
Adulto	100–190 U/L	1,7–3,2 µkat/L
>60 anos	110–210 U/L	1,9–3,6 µkat/L
*Isoenzimas, soro por eletroforese em gel de agarose		
Fração 1	14–26% do total	Fração de 0,14–0,26 do total
Fração 2	29–39% do total	Fração de 0,29–0,39 do total
Fração 3	20–26% do total	Fração de 0,20–0,26 do total
Fração 4	8–16% do total	Fração de 0,08–0,16 do total
Fração 5	6–16% do total	Fração de 0,06–0,16 do total
*Lactato desidrogenase ou desidrogenase láctica, LCR	10% do valor sérico	Fração de 0,10 do valor sérico

*Os valores são método-dependentes.

Testes	Unidades Convencionais	Unidades SI
LDL-colesterol (LDL-C), soro ou plasma (EDTA)		
Adulto		
Desejável	<130 mg/dL	<3,37 mmol/L
Limítrofe	130–159 mg/dL	3,37–4,12 mmol/L
Alto risco	≥160 mg/dL	≥4,13 mmol/L
Lidocaína, soro ou plasma (Hep ou EDTA); 45 min após dose IV		
Terapêutico	1,5–6,0 µg/mL	6,4–26 µmol/L
Tóxico		
SNC, depressão cardiovascular	6–8 µg/mL	26–34,2 µmol/L
Convulsões, obnubilação, débito cardíaco diminuído	>8 µg/mL	>34,2 µmol/L
*Lipase, soro	23–300 U/L (37°C)	0,39–5,1 µkat/L (37°C)
Lipídios, fecais, F, 72 h		
Lactente (aleitamento materno)	<1 g/dia	<1 g/dia
0–6 anos	<2 g/dia	<2 g/dia
Adulto	<7 g/dia	<7 g/dia
Adulto (dieta sem lipídios)	<4 g/dia	<4 g/dia
Lise da euglobina	Nenhuma lise em 2 h	Nenhuma lise em 2 h
Lítio, soro ou plasma (Hep ou EDTA); 12 h após a última dose		
Terapêutico	0,6–1,2 mEq/L	0,6–1,2 mmol/L
Tóxico	>2 mEq/L	>2 mmol/L
L-Lactato		
Plasma (NaF)		
Venoso	4,5–19,8 mg/dL	0,5–2,2 mmol/L
Arterial	4,5–14,4 mg/dL	0,5–1,6 mmol/L
Sangue total (Hep), em repouso no leito		
Venoso	8,1–15,3 mg/dL	0,9–1,7 mmol/L
Arterial	<11,3 mg/dL	<1,3 mmol/L
Urina, 24 h	496–1982 mg/dia	5,5–22 mmol/dia
LCR	10–22 mg/dL	1,1–2,4 mmol/L
Lorazepam, soro ou plasma (Hep ou EDTA), terapêutico	50–240 ng/mL	156–746 nmol/L
Magnésio		
Soro	1,3–2,1 mEq/L	0,65–1,07 mmol/L
	1,6–2,6 mg/dL	16–26 mg/L
Urina	6,0–10,0 mEq/24 h	3,0–5,0 mmol/24 h
Medula óssea, contagem diferencial de células		
Adulto		
Células indiferenciadas	0–1%	0–0,01
Mieloblasto	0–2%	0–0,02
Pró-mielócito	0–4%	0–0,04
Mielócitos		
Neutrofílicos	5–20%	0,05–0,20
Eosinofílicos	0–3%	0–0,03
Basofílicos	0–1%	0–0,01
Metamielócitos e bastões		
Neutrofílicos	5–35%	0,05–0,35
Eosinofílicos	0–5%	0–0,05
Basofílicos	0–1%	0–0,01
Neutrófilos segmentados	5–15%	0,05–0,15
Pró-normoblastos	0–1,5%	0–0,015
Normoblasto basofílico	0–5%	0–0,05
Normoblasto policromatofílico	5–30%	0,05–0,30
Normoblasto ortocromático	5–10%	0,05–0,10
Linfócitos	10–20%	0,10–0,20
Plasmócitos	0–2%	0–0,02
Monócitos	0–5%	0–0,05
Mercúrio		
Sangue total (EDTA)	0,6–59 µg/L	<0,29 µmol/L
Urina, 24 h	<20 µg/dia	<0,1 µmol/dia
Tóxico	>150 µg/dia	>0,75 µmol/dia

*Os valores são método-dependentes.

Testes	Unidades Convencionais	Unidades SI
Metanefrinas, total, urina	0,1–1,6 mg/24 h	0,5–8,1 µmol/24 h
Metemoglobina (MetHb, hemoglobina), sangue total (EDTA, Hep ou ACD)	0,06–0,24 g/dL ou 0,78 ± 0,37% da Hb total (DP)	9,3–37,2 µmol/L ou Fração da massa total de Hb: 0,008 ± 0,0037 (DP)
Metotrexato, soro ou plasma (Hep ou EDTA)		
Terapêutico	Variável	Variável
Tóxico		
1–2 semanas após terapia com dose baixa	≥0,02 µmol/L	≥0,02 µmol/L
pós-infusão IV 24 h	≥5 µmol/L	≥5 µmol/L
48 h	≥0,5 µmol/L	≥0,5 µmol/L
72 h	≥0,05 µmol/L	≥0,05 µmol/L
Mioglobina, soro	<85 ng/mL	<85 µg/L
Monóxido de carbono como carboxiemoglobina (HbCO), sangue total (EDTA)		
Não-fumantes	0,5–1,5% da Hb total	Fração de HbCO de 0,005–0,015
Fumantes		
1–2 maços/dia	4–5% da Hb total	Fração de HbCO de 0,04–0,05
>2 maços/dia	8–9% da Hb total	Fração de HbCO de 0,08–0,09
Tóxico	>20% da Hb total	Fração de HbCO >0,20
Letal	>50% da Hb total	Fração de HbCO >0,5
N-Acetilprocainamida, soro ou plasma (Hep ou EDTA); valor mínimo		
Terapêutico	5–30 µg/mL	18–108 µmol/L
Tóxico	>40 µg/mL	>144 µmol/L
Nortriptilina, soro ou plasma (Hep ou EDTA); valor mínimo (≥12 h após a dose)		
Terapêutico	50–150 ng/mL	190–570 nmol/L
Tóxico	>500 ng/mL	>1900 nmol/L
*5′-Nucleotidase, soro	2–17 U/L	0,034–0,29 µkat/L
Osmolalidade		
Soro	275–295 mOsm/kg de água do soro	275–295 mmol/kg de água do soro
Urina	50–1.200 mOsm/kg de água	50–1.200 mmol/kg de água
Relação, urina/soro	1,0–3,0, 3,0–4,7 após 12 h de restrição hídrica	1,0–3,0, 3,0–4,7 após 12 h de restrição hídrica
Oxazepam, soro ou plasma (Hep ou EDTA), terapêutico	0,2–1,4 µg/mL	0,70–4,9 µmol/L
Oxigênio, sangue		
Capacidade	16–24% vol (varia com a hemoglobina)	7,14–10,7 mmol/L (varia com a hemoglobina)
Conteúdo		
Arterial	15–23 vol%	6,69–10,3 mmol/L
Venoso	10–16 vol%	4,46–7,14 mmol/L
Saturação		
Arterial e capilar	95–98% da capacidade	0,95–0,98 da capacidade
Venoso	60–85% da capacidade	0,60–0,85 da capacidade
Pressão		
pO_2 arterial e capilar	83–108 mm Hg	11,1–14,4 kPa
Venosa	35–45 mm Hg	4,6–6,0 kPa
P50, sangue	25–29 mm Hg (ajustado ao pH 7,4)	3,33–3,86 kPa
Pentobarbital, soro ou plasma (Hep ou EDTA); valor mínimo		
Terapêutico		
Hipnótico	1–5 µg/mL	4–22 µmol/L
Coma terapêutico	20–50 µg/mL	88–221 µmol/L
Tóxico	>10 µg/mL	>44 µmol/L
*Peptídio C, sérico	0,78–1,89 ng/mL	0,26–0,62 nmol/L
pH		
Sangue, arterial	7,35–7,45	7,35–7,45
Urina	4,6–8,0 (depende da dieta)	4,6–8,0 (depende da dieta)
Piruvato, sangue	0,3–0,9 mg/dL	34–103 µmol/L

*Os valores são método-dependentes.

Testes	Unidades Convencionais	Unidades SI
Porfirinas, urina		
Coproporfirina	34–230 µg/24 h	52–351 nmol/24 h
Uroporfirina	27–52 µg/24 h	32–63 nmol/24 h
Porfobilinogênio, urina		
Qualitativo	Negativo	Negativo
Quantitativo	<2,0 mg/24 h	<9 µmol/24 h
Potássio		
Soro		
Prematuro		
Cordão umbilical	5,0–10,2 mEq/L	5,0–10,2 mmol/L
48 h	3,0–6,0 mEq/L	3,0–6,0 mmol/L
Neonato, cordão umbilical	5,6–12,0 mEq/L	5,6–12,0 mmol/L
Neonato	3,7–5,9 mEq/L	3,7–5,9 mmol/L
Lactente	4,1–5,3 mEq/L	4,1–5,3 mmol/L
Criança	3,4–4,7 mEq/L	3,4–4,7 mmol/L
Adulto	3,5–5,1 mEq/L	3,5–5,1 mmol/L
Urina, 24 h	25–125 mEq/dia, varia com a dieta	25–125 mmol/dia; varia com a dieta
LCR	70% do nível plasmático ou 2,5–3,2 mEq/L; aumenta com a hiperosmolalidade plasmática	0,70 do nível plasmático ou 2,5–3,2 mmol/L; aumenta com a hiperosmolalidade plasmática
Potássio, plasma (Hep)		
Homem	3,5–4,5 mEq/L	3,5–4,5 mmol/L
Mulher	3,4–4,4 mEq/L	3,4–4,4 mmol/L
Pré-albumina (Transtiretina), soro	10–40 mg/dL	100–400 mg/L
Primidona, soro ou plasma (Hep ou EDTA); valor mínimo		
Terapêutico	5–12 µg/mL	23–55 µmol/L
Tóxico	>15 µg/mL	>69 µmol/L
Procainamida, soro ou plasma (Hep ou EDTA); valor mínimo		
Terapêutico	4–10 µg/mL	17–42 µmol/L
Tóxico (também considerar o efeito do metabólito (NAPA))	>10–12 µg/mL	>42–51 µmol/L
Produtos da degradação da fibrina	<10 µg/mL	<10 mg/L
*Progesterona, soro		
Adulto		
Homem	13–97 ng/dL	0,4–3,1 nmol/L
Mulher		
Fase folicular	15–70 ng/dL	0,5–2,2 nmol/L
Fase luteínica	200–2500 ng/dL	6,4–79,5 nmol/L
Gravidez	Varia com a idade gestacional	
*Prolactina, soro		
Homem	2,5–15,0 ng/mL	2,5–15,0 µg/L
Mulher	2,5–19,0 ng/mL	2,5–19,0 µg/L
Propoxifeno, plasma (EDTA)		
Terapêutico	0,1–0,4 µg/mL	0,3–1,2 µmol/L
Tóxico	>0,5 µg/mL	>1,5 µmol/L
Propranolol, soro ou plasma (Hep ou EDTA); valor mínimo		
Terapêutico	50–100 ng/mL	193–386 nmol/L
Proteína básica da mielina, LCR	<2,5 ng/mL	<2,5 µg/L
Proteína C reativa, sérica	<0,5 mg/dL	<5 mg/L
*Proteína, soro		
Total	6,4–8,3 g/dL	64–83 g/L
Albumina	3,9–5,1 g/dL	39–51 g/L
Globulina		
α_1	0,2–0,4 g/dL	2–4 g/L
α_2	0,4–0,8 g/dL	4–8 g/L
β	0,5–1,0 g/dL	5–10 g/L
γ	0,6–1,3 g/dL	6–13 g/L
Urina		
Qualitativo	Negativo	Negativo
Quantitativo	50–80 mg/24 h (em repouso)	50–80 mg/24 h (em repouso)
LCR, total	8–32 mg/dL	80–320 mg/dL

*Os valores são método-dependentes.

Testes	Unidades Convencionais	Unidades SI
Protoporfirina, total, sangue total	<60 µg/dL	<600 µg/L
Quinidina, soro ou plasma (Hep ou EDTA); valor mínimo		
Terapêutico	2–5 µg/mL	6–15 µmol/L
Tóxico	>6 µg/mL	>18 µmol/L
Relação lecitina-esfingomielina (L/S), líquido amniótico	2,0–5,0 indica provável maturidade pulmonar fetal; >3,5 em diabéticos	2,0–5,0 indica provável maturidade pulmonar fetal; >3,5 em diabéticos
Relação uréia/creatinina, soro	12:1 a 20:1	Relação de 48–80 moles uréia/creatinina
Salicilatos, soro ou plasma (Hep ou EDTA); valor mínimo		
Terapêutico	150–300 µg/mL	1,09–2,17 mmol/L
Tóxico	>500 µg/mL	>3,62 mmol/L
Sangue oculto, fezes, amostra aleatória	Negativo (<2 ml de sangue/150 g de fezes/dia)	Negativo (<13,3 ml de sangue/kg de fezes/dia)
Qualitativa, urina, amostra aleatória	Negativo	Negativo
Saturação de ferro, soro		
Homem	20–50%	0,2–0,5
Mulher	15–50%	0,15–0,5
Sódio		
Soro ou plasma (Hep)		
Prematuro		
Cordão umbilical	116–140 mEq/L	116–140 mmol/L
48 h	128–148 mEq/L	128–148 mmol/L
Neonato, cordão umbilical	126–166 mEq/L	126–166 mmol/L
Neonato	133–146 mEq/L	133–146 mmol/L
Lactente	139–146 mEq/L	139–146 mmol/L
Criança	138–145 mEq/L	138–145 mmol/L
Adulto	136–145 mEq/L	136–145 mmol/L
Urina, 24 h	40–220 mEq/dia (dependente da dieta)	40–220 mmol/dia (dependente da dieta)
Suor		
Normal	10–40 mEq/L	10–40 mmol/L
Fibrose cística	70–190 mEq/L	70–190 mmol/L
Sulfato de desidroepiandrosterona (DHEAS), soro ou plasma (Hep, EDTA)		
Homem	59–452 µg/mL	1,6–12,2 µmol/L
Mulher		
Pré-menopausa	12–379 µg/mL	0,8–10,2 µmol/L
Pós-menopausa	30–260 µg/mL	0,8–7,1 µmol/L
Tempo de coagulação (Lee-White)	5–15 min (tubos de vidro)	5–15 min (tubos de vidro)
	19–60 min (tubos siliconizados)	19–60 min (tubos siliconizados)
*Tempo de protrombina	12–14 s	12–14 s
Tempo de tromboplastina parcial, ativado (TTPa)	<35 s	<35 s
Teofilina, soro ou plasma (Hep ou EDTA)		
Terapêutico		
Broncodilatador	8–20 µg/mL	44–111 µmol/L
Apnéia prematura	6–13 µg/mL	33–72 µmol/L
Tóxico	>20 µg/mL	>110 µmol/L
Teste de Coombs		
Direto	Negativo	Negativo
Indireto	Negativo	Negativo
Teste de crioemolisina (Donath-Landsteiner)	Nenhuma hemólise	Nenhuma hemólise
Teste de hemólise ácida (Ham)	<5% de lise	Fração lisada <0,05
*Testosterona, soro		
Homem	280–1100 ng/dL	0,52–38,17 nmol/L
Mulher	15–70 ng/dL	0,52–2,43 nmol/L
Gravidez	3–4 × normal	3–4 × normal
Pós-menopausa	8–35 ng/dL	0,28–1,22 nmol/L
Tiocianato		
Soro ou plasma (EDTA)		
Não-fumante	1–4 µg/mL	17–69 µmol/L
Fumante	3–12 µg/mL	52–206 µmol/L
Terapêutico após infusão de nitroprussiato	6–29 µg/mL	103–499 µmol/L

*Os valores são método-dependentes.

Testes	Unidades Convencionais	Unidades SI
Urina		
Não-fumante	1–4 mg/dia	17–69 µmol/dia
Fumante	7–17 mg/dia	120–292 µmol/dia
Tiopental, soro ou plasma (Hep ou EDTA); valor mínimo		
Hipnótico	1,0–5,0 µg/mL	4,1–20,7 µmol/L
Coma	30–100 µg/mL	124–413 µmol/L
Anestesia	7–130 µg/mL	29–536 µmol/L
Concentração tóxica	>10 µg/mL	>41 µmol/L
Tiroxina (T_4), soro	5–12 µg/dL (varia com a idade, mais elevada em crianças e gestantes)	65–155 nmol/L (varia com a idade, mais elevada em crianças e gestantes)
*Tiroxina, livre, soro	0,8–2,7 ng/dL	10,3–35 pmol/L
Tobramicina, soro ou plasma (Hep ou EDTA)		
Terapêutico		
Máximo		
Infecção menos grave	5–8 µg/mL	11–17 µmol/L
Infecção grave	8–10 µg/mL	17–21 µmol/L
Mínimo		
Infecção menos grave	<1 µg/mL	<2 µmol/L
Infecção moderada	<2 µg/mL	<4 µmol/L
Infecção grave	<2–4 µg/mL	<4–9 µmol/L
Tóxico		
Máximo	>10–12 µg/mL	>21–26 µmol/L
Mínimo	>2–4 µg/mL	>4–9 µmol/L
Transferrina, soro		
Neonato	130–275 mg/dL	1,30–2,75 g/L
Adulto	212–360 mg/dL	2,12–3,60 g/L
>60 anos	190–375 mg/dL	1,9–3,75 g/L
Triglicerídeos, soro, jejum		
Desejável	<250 mg/dL	<2,83 mmol/L
Limítrofe alto	250–500 mg/dL	2,83–5,67 mmol/L
Hipertrigliceridêmico	>500 mg/dL	>5,65 mmol/L
*Triiodotironina, total (T_3), soro	45–137 ng/dL	0,69–2,1 nmol/L
*Troponina-I, cardíaca, soro	Indetectável	Indetectável
Troponina-T, cardíaca, soro	Indetectável	Indetectável
Uréia, soro	6–20 mg/dL	2,1–7,1 mmol uréia/L
Urobilinogênio, urina	0,1–0,8 unidade Ehrlich/2 h	0,1–0,8 unidade Ehrlich/2h
	0,5–4,0 mg/24 h	0,5–4,0 mg/24 h
Vancomicina, soro ou plasma (Hep ou EDTA)		
Terapêutico		
Máximo	20–40 µg/mL	14–28 µmol/L
Mínimo	5–10 µg/mL	3–7 µmol/L
Tóxico	>80–100 µg/mL	>55–69 µmol/L
Velocidade de hemossedimentação		
Wintrobe		
Homem	0–10 mm em 1 h	0–10 mm/h
Mulher	0–20 mm em 1 h	0–20 mm/h
Westergren		
Homens (<50 anos de idade)	0–15 mm em 1 h	0–15 mm/h
Mulheres (<50 anos de idade)	0–20 mm em 1 h	0–20 mm/h
Viscosidade, soro	1,00–1,24 cP	1,00–1,24 cP
Vitamina A, soro	30–80 µg/dL	1,05–2,8 µmol/L
Vitamina B_{12}, soro	110–800 pg/mL	81–590 pmol/L
Vitamina E, soro		
Normal	5–18 µg/mL	12–42 µmol/L
Terapêutico	30–50 µg/mL	69,6–116 µmol/L
Zinco, soro	70–120 µg/dL	10,7–18,4 µmol/L

*Os valores são método-dependentes.

GRUPOS SANGÜÍNEOS

Linda A. Smith, PhD, CLS(NCA), Associate Professor and Graduate Program Director, Department of Clinical Laboratory Sciences, University of Texas Health Science Center, San Antonio, TX.

Neste apêndice, e nos termos correlatos definidos no próprio dicionário, grupo sangüíneo designa um sistema inteiro, consistindo em antígenos herdáveis, cuja especificidade é controlada por uma série de genes alelos. Tradicionalmente, o termo grupo sangüíneo é empregado em referência aos antígenos eritrocitários; contudo, muitos componentes sangüíneos, incluindo eritrócitos, leucócitos e plaquetas, possuem antígenos herdáveis identificados como pertencentes a sistemas. O termo tipo ou fenótipo sangüíneo é usado para referir-se a um padrão de reação específico para testar anti-soros dentro de um sistema. O termo fator de grupo sangüíneo é utilizado para referir-se a um antígeno específico de um sistema; entretanto, esse uso não é universal. Deve-se perceber que, na literatura atual, um sistema único pode ser referido no plural (i.e., grupos sangüíneos ABO), e o termo grupo sangüíneo pode ser atribuído a um único fenótipo (i.e., grupo sangüíneo A).

Cada grupo sangüíneo é definido em termos da reação aos anti-soros originais com os quais o sistema foi descoberto. Os acréscimos e modificações em um sistema ocorrem através da descoberta de anti-soros adicionais que, comprovadamente, estão relacionados com o mesmo sistema. Um antígeno ou fator de um novo grupo sangüíneo pode ser definido através da demonstração de que é detectado por um anti-soro com reações diferentes daquelas dos anti-soros previamente conhecidos. Quando se demonstra que o novo antígeno é geneticamente independente dos sistemas de grupos sangüíneos conhecidos, ele pode qualificar-se como um antígeno-protótipo para um novo grupo sangüíneo. Por outro lado, se pode ser demonstrado que o novo antígeno é controlado por um gene alélico para um dos genes de grupo sangüíneo conhecido, ele é designado para o sistema de grupo sangüíneo de seus alelos.

Nas definições de grupo sangüíneo, a ênfase foi dada à identificação dos símbolos para os genes, antígenos, anti-soros e fenótipos. Aqui se segue a convenção geral de que os símbolos para os produtos genéticos e genótipos são estabelecidos em itálico, enquanto os símbolos para os produtos genéticos ou antígenos, anti-soros e fenótipos são estabelecidos no tipo redondo. Na terminologia Rh-Hr para o grupo sangüíneo Rh, o tipo redondo é usado para designar as substâncias antigênicas, e o negrito é usado para designar os fatores sorológicos e seus anticorpos correspondentes. Esses parâmetros têm uso amplo, mas não são seguidos de maneira consistente por todos os autores.

Nomenclatura

A designação dos sistemas e antígenos de grupo sangüíneo baseou-se na designação alfabética dos nomes ou iniciais do primeiro produto de anticorpo, origem do eritrócito reativo ou não-reativo, ou derivação do nome, localização ou instituição que descobriu. A International Society of Blood Transfusion (ISBT) desenvolveu uma Working Party on Terminology of Red Cell Surface Antigens para estabelecer uma nomenclatura uniforme, embora não tenha modificado as designações e orientações históricas. Parte do encargo do grupo de trabalho (Working Party) é rever periodicamente os dados disponíveis e reportar adições, alterações ou deleções para os antígenos de grupo sangüíneo considerados extintos. Além disso, o Working Party desenvolveu um sistema de codificação da nomenclatura baseado na ordem de descoberta dos sistemas de grupos sangüíneos, para auxiliar a computação dos dados. Os relatos do Working Party e as atualizações são publicados no Vox Sanguinis (1990; 58:152–169, 1993; 65:77–80, 1995; 69:265–279, 1996; 71:246–248).

A ISBT classifica todos os antígenos em uma das quatro classificações: sistemas, coleções, antígenos de alta incidência e de baixa incidência. Atualmente, existem 23 sistemas de grupos sangüíneos. Comprova-se, por meios sorológicos, imunoquímicos e genéticos, que cada sistema é formado por produtos de genes nitidamente independentes. Embora tenham sido identificados 52 antígenos Rh, alguns foram retirados do sistema por causa da identificação inicial, e o sistema possui, atualmente, 45 antígenos. Outros sistemas (i.e., sistemas P, Xg, Hh e Kx) possuem apenas um antígeno associado ao sistema. O Quadro 1 lista os nomes aprovados do sistema, símbolos abreviados e designação numérica desenvolvida pela ISBT. Para considerações clínicas, o ABO e o Rh são da maior importância; outros são úteis para a ligação genética ou estudos de proteínas da membrana eritrocitária.

Além do sistema de grupo sangüíneo definido, existem outros antígenos de grupo sangüíneo que não se "encaixam" com os critérios do sistema. Alguns estão relacionados geneticamente ou estão associados de forma inconsistente por reatividade sorológica e imunoquímica, mas existem dados insuficientes para classificá-los como um sistema. Daí, são denominados coleções. Atualmente, existem cinco coleções reconhecidas pela ISBT (Quadro 2).

As classificações restantes de antígenos de alta incidência e de baixa incidência contêm antígenos que não podem ser incluídos em um sistema ou coleção. Os antígenos cuja incidência é alta na população aleatória são coletivamente denominados antígenos de alta incidência ou públicos. Estes ocorrem em quase todos os indivíduos, mas estão ausentes em alguns. Anticorpos contra esses antígenos têm sido encontrados geralmente no soro de pacientes sem o antígeno incitador mas que foram imunizados por transfusão ou gravidez. Existem 12 antígenos de alta incidência distintos, e alguns dos símbolos aplicados aos antígenos públicos incluem Vel, Lan, Ata, Jra e JMH.

Outros antígenos eritrocitários são incomuns e podem ser encontrados apenas em membros de pouquíssimas famílias. Por causa de sua raridade, são freqüentemente denominados antígenos particulares ou de baixa incidência. Anticorpos contra esses antígenos geralmente têm sido encontrados no soro de pacientes transfundidos ou em mulheres com filho com a doença hemolítica do recém-nascido. Com freqüência, recebem o nome da família em que foram descobertos pela primeira vez. Existem 34 antígenos de baixa incidência distintos, e alguns símbolos atribuídos aos antígenos particulares são: By, Swa, Bi, NFLD, RASM, HJK e ELO.

Quadro 1. Designação dos Sistemas de Grupo Sangüíneo

No.	Nome do Sistema	Símbolo do Sistema	Nome do Gene
001	ABO	ABO	*ABO*
002	MNS	MNS	*GYPA, GYPB, GYPE*
003	P	P1	*P1*
004	Rh	RH	*RHD, RHCE*
005	Lutheran	LU	*LU*
006	Kell	KEL	*KEL*
007	Lewis	LE	*FUT3*
008	Duffy	FY	*FY*
009	Kidd	JK	*JK*
010	Diego	DI	*AE1*
011	Yt	YT	*ACHE*
012	Xg	XG	*XG*
013	Scianna	SC	*SC*
014	Dombrock	DO	*DO*
015	Colton	CO	*AQPI*
016	Landsteiner-Wiener	LW	*LW*
017	Chido/Rodgers	CH/RG	*C4A, C4B*
018	Hh	H	*FUT1*
019	Kx	XK	*XK*
020	Gerbich	GE	*GYPC*
021	Cromer	CROM	*DAF*
022	Knops	KN	*CRI*
023	Indian	IN	*CD44*

Quadro 2. Designação das Coleções

Coleção			Antígeno		
No.	Nome	Símbolo	No.	Símbolo	Incidência %
205	Cost	COST	205001	Cs^a	95
			205002	Cs^b	34
207	Ii	I	207001	I	>99
			207002	i	*
208	Er	ER	208001	Er^a	>99
			208002	Er^b	<1
209		GLOB	209001	P	>99
			209002	P^k	*
			209003	LKE	98
210			210001	Le^c	1
			210002	Le^d	6

Adaptado de: Daniels, GL, Anstee, DJ, Cartron, JP et al. Blood Group Terminology 1995. *Vex Sang* 1995; 69:265–279.

GRUPOS DE DIAGNÓSTICOS CORRELATOS (GDC)

GDC	Descrição do GDC
1.	Craniotomia, Idade Superior a 17 Anos, Exceto por Traumatismo
2.	Craniotomia por Traumatismo, Idade Superior a 17 anos
3.	Craniotomia, Idade 0–17 anos
4.	Procedimentos Vertebrais
5.	Procedimentos Vasculares Extracranianos
6.	Liberação do Túnel do Carpo
7.	Procedimentos em Nervos Cranianos e Periféricos e Outros Locais do Sistema Nervoso com Complicações e Co-morbidades
8.	Procedimentos em Nervos Cranianos e Periféricos e Outros Locais do Sistema Nervoso sem Complicações e Co-morbidades
9.	Lesões e Distúrbios Vertebrais
10.	Neoplasias do Sistema Nervoso com Complicações e Co-morbidades
11.	Neoplasias do Sistema Nervoso sem Complicações e Co-morbidades
12.	Distúrbios Degenerativos do Sistema Nervoso
13.	Esclerose Múltipla e Ataxia Cerebelar
14.	Distúrbios Vasculares Cerebrais Específicos Exceto o Ataque Isquêmico Transitório
15.	Ataque Isquêmico Transitório e Oclusões Pré-Cerebrais
16.	Distúrbios Vasculares Cerebrais Inespecíficos com Complicações e Co-morbidades
17.	Distúrbios Vasculares Cerebrais Inespecíficos sem Complicações e Co-morbidades
18.	Distúrbios dos Nervos Cranianos e Periféricos com Complicações e Co-morbidades
19.	Distúrbios dos Nervos Cranianos e Periféricos sem Complicações e Co-morbidades
20.	Infecção do Sistema Nervoso, Exceto Meningite Viral
21.	Meningite Viral
22.	Encefalopatia Hipertensiva
23.	Torpor e Coma Não-traumático
24.	Convulsão e Cefaléia, Idade Superior a 17 Anos com Complicações e Co-morbidades
25.	Convulsão e Cefaléia, Idade Superior a 17 Anos sem Complicações e Co-morbidades
26.	Convulsão e Cefaléia, Idade 0–17 Anos
27.	Torpor e Coma Traumático, Coma por Mais de Uma Hora
28.	Torpor e Coma Traumático, Coma Há Menos de Uma Hora, Idade Superior a 17 Anos com Complicações e Co-morbidades
29.	Estupor e Coma Traumático, Coma por Menos de Uma Hora, Maior que 17 Anos sem Complicações e Co-morbidades
30.	Torpor e Coma Traumático, Coma Há Menos de Uma Hora, Idade 0–17 Anos
31.	Concussão, Idade Superior a 17 Anos com Complicações e Co-morbidades
32.	Concussão, Idade Superior a 17 Anos sem Complicações e Co-morbidades
33.	Concussão, Idade 0–17 Anos
34.	Outros Distúrbios do Sistema Nervoso com Complicações e Co-morbidades
35.	Outros Distúrbios do Sistema Nervoso sem Complicações e Co-morbidades
36.	Procedimentos Retinianos
37.	Procedimentos Orbitais
38.	Procedimentos Primários da Íris
39.	Procedimentos da Lente, com ou sem Vitrectomia
40.	Procedimentos Extra-oculares Exceto na Órbita, Idade Superior a 17 Anos
41.	Procedimentos Extra-oculares Exceto a Órbita, Idade 0–17 Anos
42.	Procedimentos Intra-oculares Exceto Retina, Íris e Lente
43.	Hifema
44.	Infecções Oculares Agudas Importantes
45.	Distúrbios Oculares Neurológicos
46.	Outros Distúrbios do Olho, Idade Superior a 17 Anos com Complicações e Co-morbidades
47.	Outros Distúrbios do Olho, Idade Superior a 17 Anos sem Complicações e Co-morbidades
48.	Outros Distúrbios do Olho, Idade de 0–17 Anos
49.	Procedimentos Importantes de Cabeça e Pescoço
50.	Sialoadenectomia
51.	Procedimentos da Glândula Salivar, Exceto Sialoadenectomia
52.	Reparação de Fenda Labial e Palatina
53.	Procedimentos em Seios Paranasais e Mastóides, Idade Superior a 17 Anos
54.	Procedimentos em Seios Paranasais e Mastóides, Idade de 0–17 Anos
55.	Procedimentos Mistos de Orelha, Nariz e Garganta
56.	Rinoplastia
57.	Procedimentos em Tonsilas e Adenóides Exceto Apenas Tonsilectomia e/ou Adenoidectomia, Idade Superior a 17 Anos
58.	Procedimentos em Tonsilas e Adenóides Exceto Apenas Tonsilectomia e/ou Adenoidectomia, Idade 0–17 Anos
59.	Apenas Tonsilectomia e/ou Adenoidectomia, Idade Superior a 17 Anos
60.	Apenas Tonsilectomia e/ou Adenoidectomia, Idade 0–17 Anos
61.	Miringotomia com Inserção de Tubo de Ventilação, Idade Superior a 17 Anos
62.	Miringotomia com Inserção de Tubo de Ventilação, Idade 0–17 Anos
63.	Outros Procedimentos em Orelha, Nariz, Boca e Garganta
64.	Malignidade de Orelha, Nariz, Boca e Garganta
65.	Desequilíbrio
66.	Epistaxe
67.	Epiglotite
68.	Otite Média e Infecções de Vias Respiratórias Altas, Idade Superior a 17 Anos com Complicações e Co-morbidades
69.	Otite Média e Infecções de Vias Respiratórias Altas, Idade Superior a 17 Anos sem Complicações e Co-morbidades
70.	Otite Média e Infecções de Vias Respiratórias Altas, Idade 0–17 Anos
71.	Laringotraqueíte
72.	Trauma e Deformidade Nasal
73.	Outros Diagnósticos de Orelha, Nariz, Boca e Garganta, Idade Superior a 17 Anos
74.	Outros Diagnósticos de Orelha, Nariz, Boca e Garganta, Idade de 0–17 Anos
75.	Procedimentos Torácicos Importantes
76.	Outros Procedimentos em Sistema Respiratório em Centro Cirúrgico com Complicações e Co-morbidades
77.	Outros Procedimentos em Sistema Respiratório em Centro Cirúrgico sem Complicações e Co-morbidades
78.	Embolia Pulmonar
79.	Infecções e Inflamações Respiratórias, Idade Superior a 17 Anos com Complicações e Co-morbidades
80.	Infecções e Inflamações Respiratórias, Idade Superior a 17 Anos sem Complicações e Co-morbidades
81.	Infecções e Inflamações Respiratórias, Idade de 0–17 Anos
82.	Neoplasias Respiratórias
83.	Traumatismo Torácico Importante com Complicações e Co-morbidades
84.	Traumatismo Torácico Importante sem Complicações e Co-morbidades
85.	Derrame Pleural com Complicações e Co-morbidades
86.	Derrame Pleural sem Complicações e Co-morbidades
87.	Edema Pulmonar e Insuficiência Respiratória

GDC	Descrição do GDC
88.	Doença Pulmonar Obstrutiva Crônica
89.	Pneumonia Simples e Pleurisia, Idade Superior a 17 Anos com Complicações e Co-morbidades
90.	Pneumonia Simples e Pleurisia, Idade Superior a 17 Anos sem Complicações e Co-morbidades
91.	Pneumonia Simples e Pleurisia, Idade de 0–17 Anos
92.	Doença Pulmonar Intersticial com Complicações e Co-morbidades
93.	Doença Pulmonar Intersticial sem Complicações e Co-morbidades
94.	Pneumotórax com Complicações e Co-morbidades
95.	Pneumotórax sem Complicações e Co-morbidades
96.	Bronquite e Asma, Idade Superior a 17 Anos com Complicações e Co-morbidades
97.	Bronquite e Asma, Idade Superior a 17 Anos sem Complicações e Co-morbidades
98.	Bronquite e Asma, Idade de 0–17 Anos
99.	Sinais e Sintomas Respiratórios com Complicações e Co-morbidades
100.	Sinais e Sintomas Respiratórios sem Complicações e Co-morbidades
101.	Outros Diagnósticos do Sistema Respiratório com Complicações e Co-morbidades
102.	Outros Diagnósticos do Sistema Respiratório sem Complicações e Co-morbidades
103.	Transplante Cardíaco
104.	Procedimentos em Valvas Cardíacas e Outros Procedimentos Cardiotorácicos Importantes com Cateterismo Cardíaco
105.	Procedimentos em Valvas Cardíacas e Outros Procedimentos Cardiotorácicos Importantes sem Cateterismo Cardíaco
106.	Revascularização Miocárdica por Angioplastia Coronária Transluminal Percutânea
107.	Revascularização Miocárdica com Cateterismo Cardíaco
108.	Outros Procedimentos Cardiotorácicos
109.	Revascularização sem Cateterismo Cardíaco
110.	Procedimentos Cardiovasculares Importantes com Complicações e Co-morbidades
111.	Procedimentos Cardiovasculares Importantes sem Complicações e Co-morbidades
112.	Procedimentos Cardiovasculares Percutâneos
113.	Amputação por Distúrbios do Sistema Circulatório Exceto do Membro Superior e Dedos dos Pés
114.	Amputação de Membro Superior e Dedos dos Pés por Distúrbios do Sistema Circulatório
115.	Implante de Marca-passo Cardíaco Permanente na Vigência de Infarto Agudo do Miocárdio, Insuficiência Cardíaca ou Choque ou Implantação de Desfibrilador-Cardioversor Automático ou Procedimento Geral
116.	Outros Implantes de Marca-passos Cardíacos Permanentes ou Angioplastia Coronária Transluminal Percutânea com *Stent* Coronariano
117.	Revisão de Marca-passo Cardíaco Exceto a Substituição do Aparelho
118.	Substituição de Marca-passo Cardíaco
119.	Desnudamento e Ligadura Venosa
120.	Outros Procedimentos do Sistema Circulatório em Centro Cirúrgico
121.	Distúrbios Circulatórios com Infarto Agudo do Miocárdio com Complicação Cardiovascular Importante, Alta com Vida
122.	Distúrbios Circulatórios com Infarto Agudo do Miocárdio sem Complicação Cardiovascular Importante, Alta com Vida
123.	Distúrbios Circulatórios com Infarto Agudo do Miocárdio, Falecido
124.	Distúrbios Circulatórios Exceto o Infarto Agudo do Miocárdio com Cateterismo Cardíaco e Diagnóstico Complexo
125.	Distúrbios Circulatórios Exceto o Infarto Agudo do Miocárdio com Cateterismo Cardíaco sem Diagnóstico Complexo
126.	Endocardite Aguda e Subaguda
127.	Insuficiência Cardíaca e Choque
128.	Tromboflebite Venosa Profunda
129.	Parada Cardíaca, Inexplicada
130.	Distúrbios Vasculares Periféricos com Complicações e Co-morbidades
131.	Distúrbios Vasculares Periféricos sem Complicações e Co-morbidades
132.	Aterosclerose com Complicações e Co-morbidades
133.	Aterosclerose sem Complicações e Co-morbidades
134.	Hipertensão Arterial
135.	Distúrbios Cardíacos e Valvares Congênitos, Idade Superior a 17 Anos com Complicações e Co-morbidades
136.	Distúrbios Cardíacos e Valvares Congênitos, Idade Superior a 17 Anos sem Complicações e Co-morbidades
137.	Distúrbios Cardíacos e Valvares Congênitos, Idade 0–17 Anos
138.	Arritmia Cardíaca e Distúrbios de Condução com Complicações e Co-morbidades
139.	Arritmia Cardíaca e Distúrbios de Condução sem Complicações e Co-morbidades
140.	Angina de Peito
141.	Síncope e Colapso com Complicações e Co-morbidades
142.	Síncope e Colapso sem Complicações e Co-morbidades
143.	Dor Torácica
144.	Outros Diagnósticos do Sistema Circulatório com Complicações e Co-morbidades
145.	Outros Diagnósticos do Sistema Circulatório sem Complicações e Co-morbidades
146.	Ressecção Retal com Complicações e Co-morbidades
147.	Ressecção Retal sem Complicações e Co-morbidades
148.	Procedimentos Importantes nos Intestinos Delgado e Grosso com Complicações e Co-morbidades
149.	Procedimentos Importantes nos Intestinos Delgado e Grosso sem Complicações e Co-morbidades
150.	Adesiólise Peritoneal com Complicações e Co-morbidades
151.	Adesiólise Peritoneal sem Complicações e Co-morbidades
152.	Procedimentos de Pequeno Porte nos Intestinos Delgado e Grosso com Complicações e Co-morbidades
153.	Procedimentos de Pequeno Porte nos Intestinos Delgado e Grosso sem Complicações e Co-morbidades
154.	Procedimentos em Estômago, Esôfago e Duodeno, Idade Superior a 17 Anos com Complicações e Co-morbidades
155.	Procedimentos do Estômago, Esôfago e Duodeno, Idade Superior a 17 Anos sem Complicações e Co-morbidades
156.	Procedimentos em Estômago, Esôfago e Duodeno, Idade 0–17 Anos
157.	Procedimentos Estomais e Anais com Complicações e Co-morbidades
158.	Procedimentos Estomais e Anais sem Complicações e Co-morbidades
159.	Procedimentos em Hérnias Exceto Inguinais e Femorais, Idade Superior a 17 Anos com Complicações e Co-morbidades
160.	Procedimentos em Hérnias Exceto Inguinais e Femorais, Idade Superior a 17 Anos sem Complicações e Co-morbidades
161.	Procedimentos em Hérnias Inguinal e Femoral, Idade Superior a 17 Anos com Complicações e Co-morbidades
162.	Procedimentos em Hérnias Inguinal e Femoral, Idade Superior a 17 Anos sem Complicações e Co-morbidades
163.	Procedimentos em Hérnia, Idade 0–17 Anos
164.	Apendicectomia com Diagnóstico Principal Complicado com Complicações e Co-morbidades
165.	Apendicectomia com Diagnóstico Principal Complicado sem Complicações e Co-morbidades
166.	Apendicectomia sem Diagnóstico Principal Complicado com Complicações e Co-morbidades.
167.	Apendicectomia sem Diagnóstico Principal Complicado sem Complicações e Co-morbidades
168.	Procedimentos na Boca com Complicações e Co-morbidades
169.	Procedimentos na Boca sem Complicações e Co-morbidades

GDC	Descrição do GDC
170.	Outros Procedimentos em Centro Cirúrgico no Sistema Digestivo com Complicações e Co-morbidades
171.	Outros Procedimentos no Sistema Digestivo em Centro Cirúrgico sem Complicações e Co-morbidades
172.	Malignidade Digestiva com Complicações e Co-morbidades
173.	Malignidade Digestiva sem Complicações e Co-morbidades
174.	Hemorragia GI com Complicações e Co-morbidades
175.	Hemorragia GI sem Complicações e Co-morbidades
176.	Úlcera Péptica Complicada
177.	Úlcera Péptica Não-Complicada com Complicações e Co-morbidades
178.	Úlcera Péptica Não-Complicada sem Complicações e Co-morbidades
179.	Doença Intestinal Inflamatória
180.	Obstrução GI com Complicações e Co-morbidades
181.	Obstrução GI sem Complicações e Co-morbidades
182.	Esofagite, Gastrenterite e Distúrbios Digestivos Mistos, Idade Superior a 17 Anos com Complicações e Co-morbidades
183.	Esofagite, Gastrenterite e Distúrbios Digestivos Mistos, Idade Superior a 17 Anos sem Complicações e Co-morbidades
184.	Esofagite, Gastrenterite e Distúrbios Digestivos Mistos, Idade 0–17 Anos
185.	Doenças Dentárias e Orais Exceto Extrações e Restaurações, Idade Superior a 17 Anos
186.	Doenças Dentárias e Orais Exceto Extrações e Restaurações, Idade 0–17 Anos
187.	Extrações e Restaurações Dentárias
188.	Outros Diagnósticos do Sistema Digestivo, Idade Superior a 17 Anos com Complicações e Co-morbidades
189.	Outros Diagnósticos do Sistema Digestivo, Idade Superior a 17 Anos sem Complicações e Co-morbidades
190.	Outros Diagnósticos do Sistema Digestivo, Idade 0–17 Anos
191.	Procedimentos em Pâncreas, Fígado e Derivação com Complicações e Co-morbidades
192.	Procedimentos em Pâncreas, Fígado e Derivação sem Complicações e Co-morbidades
193.	Procedimentos no Trato Biliar Exceto Apenas Colecistectomia com ou sem Exploração do Ducto Colédoco com Complicações e Co-morbidades
194.	Procedimentos no Trato Biliar Exceto Apenas Colecistectomia com ou sem Exploração do Ducto Colédoco sem Complicações e Co-morbidades
195.	Colecistectomia com Exploração do Ducto Colédoco com Complicações e Co-morbidades
196.	Colecistectomia com Exploração do Ducto Colédoco sem Complicações e Co-morbidades
197.	Colecistectomia Exceto por Laparoscópio sem Exploração do Ducto Colédoco com Complicações e Co-morbidades
198.	Colecistectomia Exceto por Laparoscópio sem Exploração do Ducto Colédoco sem Complicações e Co-morbidades
199.	Procedimento Diagnóstico Hepatobiliar para Malignidade
200.	Procedimento Diagnóstico Hepatobiliar para Não-Malignidade
201.	Outros Procedimentos Hepatobiliares e Pancreáticos em Centro Cirúrgico
202.	Cirrose e Hepatite Alcoólica
203.	Malignidade do Sistema Hepatobiliar ou Pâncreas
204.	Distúrbios do Pâncreas Exceto Malignidade
205.	Distúrbios do Fígado Exceto Malignidade, Cirrose e Hepatite Alcoólica com Complicações e Co-morbidades
206.	Distúrbios do Fígado Exceto Malignidade, Cirrose e Hepatite Alcoólica sem Complicações e Co-morbidades
207.	Distúrbios do Trato Biliar com Complicações e Co-morbidades
208.	Distúrbios do Trato Biliar sem Complicações e Co-morbidades
209.	Procedimentos em Grandes Articulações e de Reinserção de Membro Inferior
210.	Procedimentos em Quadril e Fêmur Exceto em Grandes Articulações, Idade Superior a 17 Anos com Complicações e Co-morbidades
211.	Procedimentos de Quadril e Fêmur Exceto em Grandes Articulações, Idade Superior a 17 Anos sem Complicações e Co-morbidades
212.	Procedimentos de Quadril e Fêmur Exceto em Grandes Articulações, Idade 0–17 Anos
213.	Amputação para Distúrbios do Sistema Musculoesquelético e do Tecido Conjuntivo
214.	Não É Mais Válido
215.	Não É Mais Válido
216.	Biópsias do Sistema Musculoesquelético e do Tecido Conjuntivo
217.	Debridamento de Ferida e Enxerto Cutâneo Exceto em Mão por Causa de Distúrbios Musculoesqueléticos e do Tecido Conjuntivo
218.	Procedimentos em Membro Inferior e Úmero, Exceto Quadril, Pé e Fêmur, Idade Maior que 17 Anos com Complicações e Co-morbidades
219.	Procedimentos do Membro Inferior e Úmero, Exceto do Quadril, Pé e Fêmur, Idade Superior a 17 Anos sem Complicações e Co-morbidades
220.	Procedimentos em Membro Inferior e Úmero, Exceto Quadril, Pé e Fêmur, Idade 0–17 Anos
221.	Não É Mais Válido
222.	Não É Mais Válido
223.	Procedimentos Importantes em Ombro/Cotovelo ou Outros Procedimentos em Membro Superior com Complicações e Co-morbidades
224.	Procedimentos Importantes do Ombro/Cotovelo ou Outros Procedimentos do Membro Superior sem Complicações e Co-morbidades
225.	Procedimentos no Pé
226.	Procedimentos nos Tecidos Moles com Complicações e Co-morbidades
227.	Procedimentos nos Tecidos Moles sem Complicações e Co-morbidades
228.	Procedimentos Importantes no Polegar ou em Articulações ou Outros Procedimentos da Mão ou do Punho com Complicações e Co-morbidades
229.	Procedimentos da Mão ou do Punho, Exceto Procedimentos em Grandes Articulações sem Complicações e Co-morbidades
230.	Excisão Local e Remoção de Aparelhos de Fixação Interna do Quadril ou do Fêmur
231.	Excisão Local e Remoção de Aparelhos de Fixação Interna Exceto Quadril e Fêmur
232.	Artroscopia
233.	Outros Procedimentos em Sistema Musculoesquelético e Tecido Conjuntivo em Centro Cirúrgico com Complicações e Co-morbidades
234.	Outros Procedimentos em Sistema Musculoesquelético e Tecido Conjuntivo em Centro Cirúrgico sem Complicações e Co-morbidades
235.	Fraturas do Fêmur
236.	Fraturas do Quadril e da Pelve
237.	Entorses, Distensões e Luxações do Quadril, da Pelve e da Coxa
238.	Osteomielite
239.	Fraturas Patológicas e Malignidades Musculoesqueléticas e do Tecido Conjuntivo
240.	Distúrbios do Tecido Conjuntivo com Complicações e Co-morbidades
241.	Distúrbios do Tecido Conjuntivo sem Complicações e Co-morbidades
242.	Artrite Séptica
243.	Problemas Clínicos nas Costas
244.	Doenças Ósseas e Artropatias Específicas com Complicações e Co-morbidades
245.	Doenças Ósseas e Artropatias Específicas sem Complicações e Co-morbidades
246.	Artropatias Inespecíficas
247.	Sinais e Sintomas do Sistema Musculoesquelético e do Tecido Conjuntivo

GDC	Descrição do GDC
248.	Tendinite, Miosite e Bursite
249.	Pós-Cuidado, Sistema Musculoesquelético e Tecido Conjuntivo
250.	Fraturas, Entorses, Distensões e Luxações de Antebraço, Mão e Pé, Idade Superior a 17 Anos com Complicações e Co-morbidades
251.	Fraturas, Entorses, Distensões e Luxações de Antebraço, Mão e Pé, Idade Superior a 17 Anos sem Complicações e Co-morbidades
252.	Fraturas, Entorses, Distensões e Luxações de Antebraço, Mão e Pé, Idade 0–17 Anos
253.	Fraturas, Entorses, Distensões e Luxações de Braço e Perna, Exceto Pé, Idade Superior a 17 Anos com Complicações e Co-morbidades
254.	Fraturas, Entorses, Distensões e Luxações do Braço e Perna, Exceto Pé, Idade Superior a 17 Anos sem Complicações e Co-morbidades
255.	Fraturas, Entorses, Distensões e Luxações do Braço e Perna, Exceto Pé, Idade 0–17 Anos
256.	Outros Diagnósticos do Sistema Musculoesquelético e do Tecido Conjuntivo
257.	Mastectomia Total para Malignidade com Complicações e Co-morbidades
258.	Mastectomia Total para Malignidade sem Complicações e Co-morbidades
259.	Mastectomia Subtotal para Malignidade com Complicações e Co-morbidades
260.	Mastectomia Subtotal para Malignidade sem Complicações e Co-morbidades
261.	Procedimento Mamário para Não-Malignidade Exceto Biopsia e Excisão Local
262.	Biopsia Mamária e Excisão Local para Não-Malignidade
263.	Enxerto Cutâneo e/ou Debridamento para Úlcera Cutânea ou Celulite com Complicações e Co-morbidades
264.	Enxerto Cutâneo e/ou Debridamento para Úlcera Cutânea ou Celulite sem Complicações e Co-morbidades
265.	Enxerto Cutâneo e/ou Debridamento Exceto para Úlcera Cutânea ou Celulite com Complicações e Co-morbidades
266.	Enxerto Cutâneo e/ou Debridamento Exceto para Úlcera Cutânea ou Celulite sem Complicações e Co-morbidades
267.	Procedimentos Perianal e Pilonidal
268.	Procedimentos Plásticos Cutâneos em Tecido Subcutâneo e Mamas
269.	Outros Procedimentos Cutâneos em Tecido Subcutâneo e Mamas com Complicações e Co-morbidades
270.	Outros Procedimentos Cutâneos em Tecido Subcutâneo e Mamas sem Complicações e Co-morbidades
271.	Úlceras Cutâneas
272.	Distúrbios Cutâneos Importantes com Complicações e Co-morbidades
273.	Distúrbios Cutâneos Importantes sem Complicações e Co-morbidades
274.	Distúrbios Mamários Malignos com Complicações e Co-morbidades
275.	Distúrbios Mamários Malignos sem Complicações e Co-morbidades
276.	Distúrbios Mamários Não-Malignos
277.	Celulite, Idade Superior a 17 Anos com Complicações e Co-morbidades
278.	Celulite, Idade Superior a 17 Anos sem Complicações e Co-morbidades
279.	Celulite, Idade de 0–17 Anos
280.	Trauma de Pele, Tecido Subcutâneo e Mama, Idade Superior a 17 Anos com Complicações e Co-morbidades
281.	Traumatismo de Pele, Tecido Subcutâneo e Mama, Idade Superior a 17 Anos sem Complicações e Co-morbidades
282.	Traumatismo de Pele, Tecido Subcutâneo e Mama, Idade 0–17 Anos
283.	Distúrbios Cutâneos de Pequeno Porte com Complicações e Co-morbidades
284.	Distúrbios Cutâneos de Pequeno Porte sem Complicações e Co-morbidades
285.	Amputação de Membro Inferior por Distúrbios Endócrinos, Nutricionais e Metabólicos
286.	Procedimentos Hipofisários e Supra-Renais
287.	Enxertos Cutâneos e Debridamento de Ferida Causada por Distúrbios Endócrinos, Nutricionais e Metabólicos
288.	Procedimentos para Obesidade em Centro Cirúrgico
289.	Procedimentos em Paratireóides
290.	Procedimentos em Tireóide
291.	Procedimentos Tireoglossos
292.	Outros Procedimentos Endócrinos, Nutricionais e Metabólicos em Centro Cirúrgico com Complicações e Co-morbidades
293.	Outros Procedimentos Endócrinos, Nutricionais e Metabólicos em Centro Cirúrgico sem Complicações e Co-morbidades
294.	Diabetes Melito, Idade Superior a 35 Anos
295.	Diabetes Melito, 0–35 Anos
296.	Distúrbios Nutricionais e Metabólicos Mistos, Idade Superior a 17 Anos com Complicações e Co-morbidades
297.	Distúrbios Nutricionais e Metabólicos Mistos, Idade Superior a 17 Anos sem Complicações e Co-morbidades
298.	Distúrbios Nutricionais e Metabólicos Mistos, Idade 0–17 Anos
299.	Erros Inatos do Metabolismo
300.	Distúrbios Endócrinos com Complicações e Co-morbidades
301.	Distúrbios Endócrinos sem Complicações e Co-morbidades
302.	Transplante Renal
303.	Procedimentos Importantes em Rim, Ureter e Bexiga para Neoplasia
304.	Procedimentos Importantes em Rim, Ureter e Bexiga para Não-Neoplasia com Complicações e Co-morbidades
305.	Procedimentos Importantes do Rim, Ureter e Bexiga para Condições Outras que Não Neoplasias sem Complicações e Co-morbidades
306.	Prostatectomia com Complicações e Co-morbidades
307.	Prostatectomia sem Complicações e Co-morbidades
308.	Procedimentos Vesicais de Pequeno Porte com Complicações e Co-morbidades
309.	Procedimentos Vesicais de Pequeno Porte sem Complicações e Co-morbidades
310.	Procedimentos Transuretrais com Complicações e Co-morbidades
311.	Procedimentos Transuretrais sem Complicações e Co-morbidades
312.	Procedimentos Uretrais, Idade Superior a 17 Anos com Complicações e Co-morbidades
313.	Procedimentos Uretrais, Idade Superior a 17 Anos sem Complicações e Co-morbidades
314.	Procedimentos Uretrais, Idade 0–17 Anos
315.	Outros Procedimentos Renais e do Trato Urinário em Centro Cirúrgico
316.	Insuficiência Renal
317.	Internação para Diálise Renal
318.	Neoplasias do Rim e Trato Urinário com Complicações e Co-morbidades
319.	Neoplasias do Rim e Trato Urinário sem Complicações e Co-morbidades
320.	Infecções Renais e do Trato Urinário, Idade Superior a 17 Anos com Complicações e Co-morbidades
321.	Infecções Renais e do Trato Urinário, Idade Superior a 17 Anos sem Complicações e Co-morbidades
322.	Infecções Renais e do Trato Urinário, Idade 0–17 Anos
323.	Cálculos Urinários com Complicações e Co-morbidades e/ou Litotripsia por Ondas Sonoras Extracorpóreas
324.	Cálculos Urinários sem Complicações e Co-morbidades
325.	Sinais e Sintomas Renais e do Trato Urinário, Idade Superior a 17 Anos com Complicações e Co-morbidades
326.	Sinais e Sintomas Renais e do Trato Urinário, Idade Superior a 17 Anos sem Complicações e Co-morbidades
327.	Sinais e Sintomas Renais e do Trato Urinário, Idade 0–17 Anos
328.	Estenose Uretral, Idade Superior a 17 Anos com Complicações e Co-morbidades

GDC	Descrição do GDC
329.	Estenose Uretral, Idade Superior a 17 Anos sem Complicações e Co-morbidades
330.	Estenose Uretral, Idade 0–17 Anos
331.	Outros Diagnósticos Renais e Urinários, Idade Superior a 17 Anos com Complicações e Co-morbidades
332.	Outros Diagnósticos Renais e Urinários, Idade Superior a 17 Anos sem Complicações e Co-morbidades
333.	Outros Diagnósticos Renais e Urinários, Idade 0–17 Anos
334.	Procedimentos Pélvicos Masculinos Importantes com Complicações e Co-morbidades
335.	Procedimentos Pélvicos Masculinos Importantes sem Complicações e Co-morbidades
336.	Prostatectomia Transuretral com Complicações e Co-morbidades
337.	Prostatectomia Transuretral sem Complicações e Co-morbidades
338.	Procedimentos Testiculares, para Malignidade
339.	Procedimentos Testiculares, para Não-Malignidade, Idade Superior a 17 Anos
340.	Procedimentos Testiculares, para Não-Malignidade, Idade de 0–17 Anos
341.	Procedimentos Penianos
342.	Circuncisão, Idade Superior a 17 Anos
343.	Circuncisão, Idade 0–17 Anos
344.	Outros Procedimentos em Sistema Reprodutor Masculino em Centro Cirúrgico para Malignidade
345.	Outros Procedimentos do Sistema Reprodutor Masculino em Centro Cirúrgico Exceto para Malignidade
346.	Malignidade do Sistema Reprodutor Masculino com Complicações e Co-morbidades
347.	Malignidade do Sistema Reprodutor Masculino sem Complicações e Co-morbidades
348.	Hipertrofia Prostática Benigna com Complicações e Co-morbidades
349.	Hipertrofia Prostática Benigna sem Complicações e Co-morbidades
350.	Inflamação do Sistema Reprodutor Masculino
351.	Esterilização, Masculina
352.	Outros Diagnósticos do Sistema Reprodutor Masculino
353.	Evisceração Pélvica, Histerectomia Radical e Vulvectomia Radical
354.	Procedimentos Uterinos e Anexiais para Malignidade Não-ovárica/Anexial com Complicações e Co-morbidades
355.	Procedimentos Uterinos e Anexiais para Malignidade Não-ovárica/Anexial sem Complicações e Co-morbidades
356.	Procedimentos Reconstrutores do Sistema Reprodutor Feminino
357.	Procedimentos Uterinos e Anexiais para Malignidade Ovárica ou Anexial
358.	Procedimentos Uterinos e Anexiais para Não-Malignidade com Complicações e Co-morbidades
359.	Procedimentos Uterinos e Anexiais para Não-Malignidade sem Complicações e Co-morbidades
360.	Procedimentos em Vagina, Colo e Vulva
361.	Laparoscopia e Interrupção Tubária Incisional
362.	Interrupção Tubária Endoscópica
363.	Dilatação e Curetagem, Conização e Radioimplante para Malignidade
364.	Dilatação e Curetagem, Conização Exceto para Malignidade
365.	Outros Procedimentos em Sistema Reprodutor Feminino em Sala de Cirurgia
366.	Malignidade do Sistema Reprodutor Feminino com Complicações e Co-morbidades
367.	Malignidade do Sistema Reprodutor Feminino sem Complicações e Co-morbidades
368.	Infecções do Sistema Reprodutor Feminino
369.	Distúrbios Menstruais e Outros Distúrbios do Sistema Reprodutor Feminino
370.	Cesariana com Complicações e Co-morbidades
371.	Cesariana sem Complicações e Co-morbidades
372.	Parto Vaginal com Diagnósticos Complicadores
373.	Parto Vaginal sem Diagnósticos Complicadores
374.	Parto Vaginal com Esterilização e/ou Dilatação e Curetagem
375.	Parto Vaginal com Procedimentos em Centro Cirúrgico Exceto Esterilização e/ou Dilatação e Curetagem
376.	Diagnósticos Pós-Parto e Pós-Aborto sem Procedimentos em Centro Cirúrgico
377.	Diagnósticos Pós-Parto e Pós-Aborto com Procedimentos em Centro Cirúrgico
378.	Gravidez Ectópica
379.	Ameaça de Aborto
380.	Aborto sem Dilatação e Curetagem
381.	Aborto com Dilatação e Curetagem, Curetagem por Aspiração ou Histerotomia
382.	Falso Trabalho de Parto
383.	Outros Diagnósticos Pré-Parto com Complicações Clínicas
384.	Outros Diagnósticos Pré-Parto sem Complicações Clínicas
385.	Neonatos, Mortos ou Transferidos para Outra Instituição de Cuidados Agudos
386.	Imaturidade Extrema ou Síndrome de Angústia Respiratória do Neonato
387.	Prematuridade com Problemas Importantes
388.	Prematuridade sem Problemas Importantes
389.	Neonato a Termo com Problemas Importantes
390.	Neonato com Outros Problemas Significativos
391.	Neonato Normal
392.	Esplenectomia, Idade Superior a 17 Anos
393.	Esplenectomia, Idade de 0–17 Anos
394.	Outros Procedimentos Relacionados a Sangue e Órgãos Formadores de Sangue em Centro Cirúrgico
395.	Distúrbios Eritrocitários, Idade Superior a 17 Anos
396.	Distúrbios Eritrocitários, Idade 0–17 Anos
397.	Distúrbios da Coagulação
398.	Distúrbios Reticuloendoteliais e da Imunidade com Complicações e Co-morbidades
399.	Distúrbios Reticuloendoteliais e da Imunidade sem Complicações e Co-morbidades
400.	Linfoma e Leucemia com Procedimento Importante em Centro Cirúrgico
401.	Linfoma e Leucemia Não-Aguda com Outro Procedimento em Centro Cirúrgico com Complicações e Co-morbidades
402.	Linfoma e Leucemia Não-Aguda com Outro Procedimento em Centro Cirúrgico sem Complicações e Co-morbidades
403.	Linfoma e Leucemia Não-Aguda com Complicações e Co-morbidades
404.	Linfoma e Leucemia Não-Aguda sem Complicações e Co-morbidades
405.	Leucemia Aguda sem Procedimento Importante em Centro Cirúrgico, Idade 0–17 Anos
406.	Distúrbios Mieloproliferativos ou Neoplasias Pouco Diferenciadas com Procedimentos Importantes em Centro Cirúrgico com Complicações e Co-morbidades
407.	Distúrbios Mieloproliferativos ou Neoplasias Pouco Diferenciadas com Procedimentos Importantes em Centro Cirúrgico sem Complicações e Co-morbidades
408.	Distúrbios Mieloproliferativos ou Neoplasias Pouco Diferenciadas com Outros Procedimentos em Centro Cirúrgico
409.	Radioterapia
410.	Quimioterapia sem Leucemia Aguda como Diagnóstico Secundário
411.	História de Malignidade sem Endoscopia
412.	História de Malignidade com Endoscopia
413.	Outros Distúrbios Mieloproliferativos ou Diagnósticos de Neoplasia Pouco Diferenciada com Complicações e Co-morbidades

GDC	Descrição do GDC
414.	Outros Distúrbios Mieloproliferativos ou Diagnósticos de Neoplasia Pouco Diferenciada sem Complicações e Co-morbidades
415.	Procedimentos em Centro Cirúrgico para Infecções e Doenças Parasitárias
416.	Septicemia, Idade Superior a 17 Anos
417.	Septicemia, Idade 0–17 Anos
418.	Infecções Pós-Operatórias e Pós-Traumáticas
419.	Febre de Origem Indeterminada, Idade Superior a 17 Anos com Complicações e Co-morbidades
420.	Febre de Origem Indeterminada, Idade Superior a 17 Anos sem Complicações e Co-morbidades
421.	Doença Viral, Idade Superior a 17 Anos
422.	Doença Viral e Febre de Origem Indeterminada, Idade 0–17 Anos
423.	Outros Diagnósticos de Doenças Infecciosas e Parasitárias
424.	Procedimento em Centro Cirúrgico com Diagnósticos Principais de Doença Mental
425.	Reações Agudas de Ajuste e Distúrbios da Disfunção Psicossocial
426.	Neuroses Depressivas
427.	Neuroses, Exceto a Depressiva
428.	Distúrbios da Personalidade e Controle de Impulsos
429.	Distúrbios Orgânicos e Retardo Mental
430.	Psicoses
431.	Distúrbios Mentais da Infância
432.	Outros Diagnósticos de Distúrbio Mental
433.	Vício ou Dependência em Álcool/Drogas, Abandono Contra Conselho Médico
434.	Vício ou Dependência de Álcool/Drogas, Detoxificação ou Outro Tratamento Sintomático com Complicações e Co-morbidades
435.	Vício ou Dependência de Álcool/Drogas, Detoxificação ou Outro Tratamento Sintomático sem Complicações e Co-morbidades
436.	Vício ou Dependência de Álcool/Drogas com Reabilitação
437.	Vício ou Dependência de Álcool/Drogas com Reabilitação e Detoxificação Combinada
438.	Não É Mais Válido
439.	Enxertos Cutâneos para Lesões
440.	Debridamento de Feridas para Lesões
441.	Procedimentos Manuais para Lesões
442.	Outros Procedimentos em Centro Cirúrgico para Lesões com Complicações e Co-morbidades
443.	Outros Procedimentos em Centro Cirúrgico para Lesões sem Complicações e Co-morbidades
444.	Lesão Traumática, Idade Superior a 17 Anos com Complicações e Co-morbidades
445.	Lesão Traumática, Idade Superior a 17 Anos sem Complicações e Co-morbidades
446.	Lesão Traumática, Idade 0–17 Anos
447.	Reações Alérgicas, Idade Superior a 17 Anos
448.	Reações Alérgicas, Idade 0–17 Anos
449.	Intoxicação e Efeitos Tóxicos de Medicamentos, Idade Superior a 17 Anos com Complicações e Co-morbidades
450.	Intoxicação e Efeitos Tóxicos de Medicamentos, Idade Superior a 17 Anos sem Complicações e Co-morbidades
451.	Intoxicação e Efeitos Tóxicos de Medicamentos, Idade 0–17 Anos
452.	Complicações do Tratamento com Complicações e Co-morbidades
453.	Complicações do Tratamento sem Complicações e Co-morbidades
454.	Outras Lesões, Intoxicações e Diagnósticos de Efeitos Tóxicos com Complicações e Co-morbidades
455.	Outras Lesões, Intoxicações e Diagnósticos de Efeitos Tóxicos sem Complicações e Co-morbidades
456.	Não É Mais Válido
457.	Não É Mais Válido

GDC	Descrição do GDC
458.	Não É Mais Válido
459.	Não É Mais Válido
460.	Não É Mais Válido
461.	Procedimentos em Centro Cirúrgico com Diagnósticos de Outro Contato com Serviços de Saúde
462.	Reabilitação
463.	Sinais e Sintomas com Complicações e Co-morbidades
464.	Sinais e Sintomas sem Complicações e Co-morbidades
465.	Pós-Cuidado com História de Malignidade como Diagnóstico Secundário
466.	Pós-Cuidado sem História de Malignidade como Diagnóstico Secundário
467.	Outros Fatores que Influenciam o Estado de Saúde
468.	Procedimento de Grande Porte em Centro Cirúrgico Não-Relacionado ao Diagnóstico Principal
469.	Diagnóstico Principal Inválido como Diagnóstico de Alta
470.	Não-agrupável
471.	Procedimentos Articulares Importantes Bilaterais ou Múltiplos no Membro Inferior
472.	Não É Mais Válido
473.	Leucemia Aguda sem Procedimento Importante em Centro Cirúrgico, Idade Superior a 17 Anos
474.	Não É Mais Válido
475.	Diagnóstico do Sistema Respiratório com Suporte Ventilatório
476.	Procedimento Prostático em Centro Cirúrgico Não-Relacionado com o Diagnóstico Principal
477.	Procedimento Sucinto em Centro Cirúrgico Não-Relacionado com o Diagnóstico Principal
478.	Outros Procedimentos Vasculares com Complicações e Co-morbidades
479.	Outros Procedimentos Vasculares sem Complicações e Co-morbidades
480.	Transplante Hepático
481.	Transplante de Medula Óssea
482.	Traqueostomia para Diagnósticos de Face, Boca e Pescoço
483.	Traqueostomia Exceto para Diagnósticos de Face, Boca e Pescoço
484.	Craniotomia para Politraumatismo Significativo
485.	Reinserção de Membro, Procedimentos de Quadril e Fêmur para Politraumatismo Significativo
486.	Outros Procedimentos em Centro Cirúrgico para Politraumatismo Significativo
487.	Outros Politraumatismos Significativos
488.	HIV com Procedimento de Grande Porte em Centro Cirúrgico
489.	HIV com Condição Importante Correlata
490.	HIV com ou sem Outra Condição Correlata
491.	Procedimentos Articulares Importantes e de Reinserção de Membro Superior
492.	Quimioterapia com Leucemia Aguda como Diagnóstico Secundário
493.	Colecistectomia Laparoscópica sem Exploração do Ducto Comum com Complicações e Co-morbidades
494.	Colecistectomia Laparoscópica sem Exploração do Ducto Colédoco e sem Complicações e Co-morbidades
495.	Transplante Pulmonar
496.	Fusão Vertebral Anterior/Posterior Combinada
497.	Fusão Vertebral com Complicações e Co-morbidades
498.	Fusão Vertebral sem Complicações e Co-morbidades
499.	Procedimentos em Dorso e Pescoço Exceto Fusão Vertebral com Complicações e Co-morbidades
500.	Procedimentos em Dorso e Pescoço Exceto Fusão Vertebral sem Complicações e Co-morbidades
501.	Procedimentos em Joelho com Sinais de Infecção com Complicações e Co-morbidades

GDC	Descrição do GDC
502.	Procedimentos em Joelho com Sinais de Infecção sem Complicações e Co-morbidades
503.	Procedimentos em Joelho sem Sinais de Infecção
504.	Queimadura de 3.º Grau Extensa com Enxerto Cutâneo
505.	Queimadura de 3.º Grau Extensa sem Enxerto Cutâneo
506.	Queimadura de Espessura Total com Enxerto Cutâneo ou Lesões Internas com Complicações e Co-morbidades ou Traumatismo Significativo
507.	Queimadura de Espessura Total com Enxerto Cutâneo ou Lesões Internas sem Complicações e Co-morbidades ou Traumatismo Significativo
508.	Queimadura de Espessura Total sem Enxerto Cutâneo ou Lesões Internas com Complicações e Co-morbidades ou Traumatismo Significativo
509.	Queimadura de Espessura Total sem Enxerto Cutâneo ou Lesões Internas sem Complicações e Co-morbidades ou Traumatismo Significativo
510.	Queimaduras Não-Extensas com Complicações e Co-morbidades ou Traumatismo Significativo
511.	Queimaduras Não-Extensas sem Complicações e Co-morbidades ou Traumatismo Significativo

GLOSSÁRIO

A

Abacaxi: pineapple
Abampère: abampere
Abapical: abapical
Abarognosia: abarognosis
Abasia: abasia
Abasia-astasia: abasia-astasia
Abásico: abasic, abatic
Abatimento: dejection
Abaxial: abaxial, abaxile
Abcoulomb: abcoulomb
Abdome: abdomen, venter
Abdominal: abdominal
Abdominocentese: abdominocentesis
Abdominociese: abdominocyesis
Abdominocístico: abdominocystic
Abdominoescrotal: abdominoscrotal
Abdominogenital: abdominogenital
Abdominopélvico: abdominopelvic
Abdominoperineal: abdominoperineal
Abdominoplastia: abdominoplasty
Abdominoscopia: abdominoscopy
Abdominotorácico: abdominothoracic
Abdominovaginal: abdominovaginal
Abdominovesical: abdominovesical
Abdução: abduction
Abducente: abducens, abducent
Abdutor: abductor
Abduzir: abduce, abduct
Abelha: bee
Abembriônico: abembryonic
Abentérico: abenteric
Aberração: aberration
Aberrante: aberrant
Aberrômetro: aberrometer
Aberto: open, patulous
Abertura: apertura, pl. aperturae; aperture, opening, outlet
Abetalipoproteinemia: abetalipoproteinemia
Abfarad: abfarad
Abhenry: abhenry
Abiótico: abiotic
Abiotrofia: abiotrophy
Abirritação: abirritation
Ablação: ablation
Ablastêmico: ablastemic
Ablastina: ablastin
Ablefaria: ablepharia
Ablução: ablution
Abluente: abluent
Abneural: abnerval, abneural
Abóbada: cope, vault
Abohm: abohm
Aboral: aborad, aboral
Abordagem: approach
Abortado: abortive
Abortamento: miscarriage
Abortar: abort, miscarry
Aborteiro: abortionist
Abortifaciente: aborticide, abortient, abortifacient, abortigenic
Aborto: abortion, abortus
Abraquia: abrachia
Abraquiocefalia: abrachiocephaly, abrachiocephalia
Abrasão: abrasion
Abrasividade: abrasiveness
Abrasivo: abrasive
Ab-reação: abreaction
Ab-reagir: abreact
Abrina: abrin
Abscesso gengival: gumboil
Abscesso: abscess
Abscissa: abscissa
Abscissão: abscission
Absconso: absconsio
Absídeos: *Absidia*
Absintina: absinthin
Absinto: absinthium, wormwood
Absintol: absinthol
Absoluto: absolute
Absorção: absorption, insorption
Absortivo: absorptive
Absorvência: absorbance (*A*, A), absorbancy, absorbency
Absorvente: absorbefacient, absorbent
Absorver: absorb
Absorvibilidade: absorptivity (*a*)
Abstinência: abstinence
Abstração: abstraction
Abstrição: abstriction
Abulia: aboulia, abulia
Abúlico: abulic
Abundância: abundance
Abuso: abuse
Abvolt: abvolt
Acácia: acacia
Açafrão: saffron
Açafrão-da-índia: turmeric
Açafroa: safflower
Acalasia: achalasia
Acalculia: acalculia
Acampsia: acampsia
Acantameba: *Acanthamoeba*
Acantamebíase: acanthamebiasis
Acantela: acanthella
Acantestesia: acanthesthesia
Acantião: acanthion, akanthion
Acantocefalíase: acanthocephaliasis
Acantocéfalos: Acanthocephala
Acantócito: acanthocyte
Acantocitose: acanthocytosis
Acantóide: acanthoid
Acantólise: acantholysis
Acantoma: acanthoma
Acantópodes: acanthopodia
Acântor: acanthor
Acantose: acanthosis
Acantótico: acanthotic
Acantrócito: acanthrocyte
Acantrocitose: acanthrocytosis
Ação: action
Acapnia: acapnia
Acarbose: acarbose
Acardia: acardia
Acardíaco: acardiac
Acárdio: acardius
Acaríase: acariasis
Acaricida: acaricide, miticidal, miticide
Acarídeos: Acaridae
Acarino: acarine
Acariócito: acaryote, akaryocyte
Acariota: akaryote
Ácaro: acarid, acaridan, mite
Ácaro trombiculídeo: chigger
Acarodermatite: acarodermatitis
Acarofobia: acarophobia
Acaróide: acaroid
Acarologia: acarology
Acasalamento: mating
Acatalasia: acatalasia
Acatalassemia: acatalasemia
Acatético: acathectic
Acatexia: acathexia
Acatisia: acathisia, akathisia
Acaudado: acaudal, acaudate
Acavalgamento: overriding
Acebutolol: acebutolol
Aceclidina: aceclidine
Acedapsona: acedapsone
Acedia: acedia
Acefalia: acephalia, acephalism, acephaly
Acefalina: acephaline
Acéfalo: acephalous, acephalus
Acefalobraquia: acephalobrachia
Acefalocardia: acephalocardia
Acefalocisto: acephalocyst
Acefalogastria: acephalogasteria
Acefalopodia: acephalopodia
Acefaloquiria: acephalocheiria, acephalochiria
Acefalorraquia: acephalorrhachia
Acefalotoracia: acephalothoracia
Aceleração: acceleration
Acelerador: accelerator
Acelerina: accelerin
Acelerômetro: accelerometer
Aceloma: acelom
Acelomado: acelomate, acelomatous
Acelular: acellular
Acenocumarina: acenocoumarin
Acenocumarol: acenocoumarol
Acêntrico: acentric
Acentuador: accentuator
Aceptor: acceptor
Acérvulo: acervulus
Acesso: access
Acessório: accessorius, accessory
Acessulfamo: acesulfame
Acestoma: acestoma
Acetabular: acetabular
Acetabulectomia: acetabulectomy
Acetábulo: acetabulum, **pl.** acetabula
Acetabuloplastia: acetabuloplasty
Acetal: acetal
Acetaldeído: acetaldehyde
Acetamida: acetamide
Acetamidobenzoato de deanol: deanol acetamidobenzoate
2-acetamidofluoreno: 2-acetamidofluorene (AAF)
Acetaminofeno: acetaminophen
Acetaminosalol: acetaminosalol
Acetaminossalol: phenetsal
Acetarsol: acetarsol
Acetarsona: acetarsone
Acetato: acetate
Acetato-CoA ligase: acetate-CoA ligase
Acetato de anagestona: anagestone acetate
Acetato de bizoxatina: bisoxatin acetate
Acetato de ciproterona: cyproterone acetate
Acetato de clogestona: clogestone acetate
Acetato de clomegestona: clomegestone acetate
Acetato de clormadinona: chlormadinone acetate
Acetato de cobre: cupric acetate, cupric acetate normal

Acetato de cresil violeta: cresyl violet acetate
Acetato de criptenamina, tanato de criptenamina: cryptenamine acetates, cryptenamine tannates
Acetato de dequalínio: dequalinium acetate
Acetato de flecainida: flecainide acetate
Acetato de fludrocortisona: fludrocortisone acetate
Acetato de 9α-fluoro-hidrocortisona: 9α-fluorohydrocortisone acetate
Acetato de fluperolona: fluperolone acetate
Acetato de flurogestona: flurogestone acetate
Acetato de guanabenzo: guanabenz acetate
Acetato de leuprolida: leuprolide acetate
Acetato de medroxiprogesterona: medroxyprogesterone acetate
Acetato de megestrol: megestrol acetate
Acetato de melengestrol: melengestrol acetate
Acetato de menadiol: menadiol diacetate
Acetato de mepazina: mepazine acetate
Acetato de oxifenisatina: oxyphenisatin acetate
Acetato de quingestanol: quingestanol acetate
Acetato de saralasina: saralasin acetate
13-acetato de 12-O-tetradecanoilforbol: 12-O-tetradecanoylphorbol 13-acetate (TPA, tPA)
Acetato fenilmercúrico: phenylmercuric acetate
Acetazolamida: acetazolamide
Acetenil: acetenyl
Acético: acetic
Aceticoceptor: aceticoceptor
Acetificar: acetify
Acetil: acetyl (Ac)
Acetil-CoA: acetyl-CoA
Acetil sulfisoxazol: acetyl sulfisoxazole
Acetilação: acetylation
Acetiladenilato: acetyladenylate
2-acetilaminofluoreno: 2-acetylaminofluorene (AAF)
Acetilase: acetylase
Acetilcarbromal: acetylcarbromal
Acetilcisteína: acetylcysteine
Acetilcoenzima A: acetyl-coenzyme A
Acetilcolina: acetylcholine (ACH, Ach)
Acetilcolina: Ach
Acetilcolinesterase: acetylcholinesterase
Acetildigitoxina: acetyldigitoxin
Acetildigoxina: acetyldigoxin
α-N-acetilgalactosaminidase: α-N-acetylgalactosaminidase
α-N-acetilglicosaminidase: α-N-acetylglucosaminidase
Acetilmetadol: acetylmethadol
Acetilornitina desacetilase: acetylornithine deacetylase
3-acetilpiridina: 3-acetylpyridine
Acetiltransferase: acetyltransferase
Acetímetro: acetimeter
Acetoacetato: acetoacetate
Acetoacetil-CoA: acetoacetyl-CoA
Acetoacetil coenzima A: acetoacetyl-coenzyme A
Acetoclareamento: acetowhitening
Acetoexamida: acetohexamide
Acetofenetidina: acetophenetidin
Acetofenida de alfasona: alphasone acetophenide
Acetofenida de algestona: algestone acetophenide
Acetoína: acetoin
Acetol: acetol
Acetólise: acetolysis
Acetomenaftona: acetomenaphthone
Acetômetro: acetometer
Acetona: acetone
Acetonemia: acetonemia
Acetonêmico: acetonemic
Acetonida de fluocinolona: fluocinolone acetonide
Acetonitrilo: acetonitrile
Acetonúria: acetonuria
Acetoso: acetous
Acetossulfona sódica: acetosulfone sodium
Acetrizoato sódico: acetrizoate sodium
Aceturato: aceturate
Achado: finding
Acianótico: acyanotic
Acíclico: acyclic
Acicloguanosina: acycloguanosine
Aciclovir: acyclovir
Acicular: acicular
Acidemia: acidemia
Acidemia fumárica: fumaric acidemia
Acidemia isovalérica: isovaleric acidemia
Acidemia metilmalônica: methylmalonic acidemia
Acidemia propiônica: propionic acidemia
Acidente: accident
Acidente vascular cerebral: stroke
Acidez: acidity
Acidificar: acidify
Ácido: acid
Ácido (2,4-diclorofenoxi)acético: (2,4-dichlorophenoxy)acetic acid (2,4-D)
Ácido (2,4,5-triclorofenoxi)acético: (2,4,5-trichlorophenoxy)acetic acid (2,4,5-T)
Ácido 2-cetoadípico: 2-ketoadipic acid
Ácido 2-oxo-5-guanidovalérico: 2-oxo-5-guanidovaleric acid
Ácido 2-oxoglutárico: 2-oxoglutaric acid
Ácido 3-hidroxi-2-pirrolidinocarboxílico: 3-hydroxy-2-pyrrolidinecarboxylic acid
Ácido 3-hidroxiantranílico: 3-hydroxyanthranilic acid
Ácido 3-hidroxibutanóico: 3-hydroxybutanoic acid
Ácido 3-hidroxibutírico: 3-hydroxybutyric acid
Ácido 3-hidroxiglutárico: 3-hydroxyglutaric acid
Ácido 3-metoxi-4-hidroximandélico: 3-methoxy-4-hydroxymandelic acid
Ácido 3-ureidoisobutírico: 3-ureidoisobutyric acid
Ácido 3-ureidopropiônico: 3-ureidopropionic acid
Ácido 4-carboxiglutâmico: 4-carboxyglutamic acid (Gla)
Ácido 4-metoxibenzóico: 4-methoxybenzoic acid
Ácido 4-piridóxico: 4-pyridoxic acid
Ácido 5,5-dietilbarbitúrico: 5,5-diethylbarbituric acid
Ácido 5-pirrolidona-2-carboxílico: 5-pyrrolidone-2-carboxylic acid
Ácido 6-amino-penicilânico: 6-aminopenicillanic acid (6-APS)
Ácido 7,8-diidrofólico: 7,8-dihydrofolic acid
Ácido 9-eicosenóico: 9-eicosenoic acid
Ácido α-acetoláctico: α-acetolactic acid
Ácido α-aminoadípico: α-aminoadipic acid (Aad)
Ácido α-amino-β-cetoadípico: α-amino-β-ketoadipic acid
Ácido α-aminoisobutírico: α-aminoisobutyric acid
Ácido α-aminovalérico: norvaline (Nva)
Ácido α-cetoglutarâmico: α-ketoglutaramic acid
Ácido α-cetossuccinâmico: α-ketosuccinamic acid
Ácido acético: acetic acid
Ácido acetilsalicílico (AAS): acetylsalicylic acid
Ácido acetiltânico: acetyltannic acid
Ácido acetoacético: acetoacetic acid
Ácido acetoidroxâmico: acetohydroxamic acid
Ácido adenílico: adenylic acid
Ácido adenililsuccínico: adenylylosuccinic acid
Ácido adenilsuccínico: adenylosuccinic acid (sAMP)
Ácido adípico: adipic acid
Ácido agárico: agaric acid
Ácido alantóico: allantoic acid
Ácido aldárico: aldaric acid
Ácido aldobiurônico: aldobiuronic acid
Ácido alodesoxicólico: allodeoxycholic acid
Ácido alofânico: allophanic acid
Ácido ametriodínico: ametriodinic acid
Ácido aminocapróico: aminocaproic acid
Ácido aminopropiônico: aminopropionic acid
Ácido anísico: anisic acid
Ácido antranílico: anthranilic acid
Ácido apirimidínico: apyrimidinic acid
Ácido apurínico: apurinic acid
Ácido arábico: arabic acid
Ácido aráquico: arachic acid
Ácido araquídico: arachidic acid
Ácido araquidônico: arachidonic acid
Ácido argininossuccínico: argininosuccinic acid
Ácido arilarsônico: arylarsonic acid
Ácido aristolóquico: aristolochic acid
Ácido arsenioso: arsenous acid
Ácido arsônico: arsonic acid
Ácido ascórbico: ascorbic acid, sorbic acid
Ácido aspártico: aspartic acid (Asp)
Ácido aspergílico: aspergillic acid
Ácido atractílico: atractylic acid
Ácido atractossilídico: atractosylidic acid
Ácido aureólico: aureolic acid
Ácido aurintricarboxílico: aurintricarboxylic acid
Ácido β-aminoisobutírico: β-aminoisobutyric acid
Ácido β-hidroxibutírico: β-hydroxybutyric acid
Ácido β-hidroxiisobutírico: β-hydroxyisobutyric acid
Ácido β-hidroxipropiônico: β-hydroxypropionic acid
Ácido β-sulfinilpirúvico: β-sulfinylpyruvic acid
Ácido barbitúrico: barbituric acid
Ácido behênico: behenic acid
Ácido benzóico: benzoic acid
Ácido bórico: boracic acid, boric acid
Ácido butanóico: butanoic acid
Ácido butírico: butyric acid
Ácido cacodílico: cacodylic acid
Ácido caínico: kainic acid

Glossário

Ácido cantarídico: cantharidic acid
Ácido caprílico: caprylic acid
Ácido carbâmico: carbamic acid
Ácido carbamoilcarbâmico: carbamoylcarbamic acid
Ácido carbazótico: carbazotic acid
Ácido carbólico: carbolic acid
Ácido carbônico: carbonic acid
Ácido carboxílico: carboxylic acid
Ácido carmínico: carminic acid
Ácido catéquico: catechuic acid
Ácido catequínico: catechinic acid
Ácido cefalosporânico: cephalosporanic acid
Ácido celulósico: cellulosic acid
Ácido cerebrônico: cerebronic acid
Ácido cerotínico: cerotinic acid
Ácido cetopantóico: ketopantoic acid
Ácido cetossuccínico: ketosuccinic acid
Ácido cevitâmico: cevitamic acid
Ácido cianúrico: cyanuric acid
Ácido ciclâmico: cyclamic acid
Ácido cicloexanossulfâmico: cyclohexanesulfamic acid
Ácido cicloexilsulfâmico: cyclohexylsulfamic acid
Ácido cinâmico: cinnamic acid
Ácido cinamílico: cinnamylic acid
Ácido *cis*-aconítico: *cis*-aconitic acid
Ácido cisteico: cysteic acid
Ácido cisteinossulfínico: cysteine sulfinic acid
Ácido citidílico: cytidylic acid
Ácido-citrato-dextrose: acid-citrate-dextrose (ACD)
Ácido cítrico: citric acid
Ácido clavulânico: clavulanic acid
Ácido clórico: chloric acid
Ácido clorídrico: hydrochloric acid
Ácido cloroacético: chloracetic acid, chloroacetic acid
Ácido cloroso: chlorous acid
Ácido clupanodônico: clupanodonic acid
Ácido cobírico: cobyric acid
Ácido cobirínico: cobyrinic acid
Ácido cójico: kojic acid
Ácido colaico: cholaic acid
Ácido colálico: cholalic acid
Ácido colânico: cholanic acid
Ácido cólico: cholic acid
Ácido colomínico: colominic acid
Ácido crômico: chromic acid
Ácido cromotrópico: chromotropic acid

Ácido δ-aminobutírico aminotransferase: δ-aminobutyric acid amino transferase
Ácido δ-aminolevulínico: δ-aminolevulinic acid (ALA)
Ácido desidroacético: dehydroacetic acid
Ácido desidrocólico: dehydrocholic acid
Ácido desidrorretinóico: dehydroretinoic acid
Ácido desoxiadenílico: deoxyadenylic acid (dAMP)
Ácido desoxicitidílico: deoxycytidylic acid (dCMP)
Ácido desoxicólico: deoxycholic acid
Ácido desoxiguanílico: deoxyguanylic acid (dGMP)
Ácido desoxirribonucleico: deoxyribonucleic acid (DNA)
Ácido desoxitimidílico: deoxythymidylic acid (dTMP)
Ácido D-galacturônico: D-galacturonic acid
Ácido diacetiltânico: diacetyltannic acid
Ácido dietanossulfônico de piperazina: piperazine diethanesulfonic acid (PIPES)
Ácido dietilenotriamina pentacético: diethylenetriamine pentaacetic acid (DTPA)
Ácido difenoxílico: difenoxylic acid
Ácido diidroascórbico: dihydroascorbic acid
Ácido diidrolipóico: dihydrolipoic acid
Ácido diidropteróico: dihydropteroic acid
Ácido diisopropil iminodiacético: diisopropyl iminodiacetic acid (DISIDA)
Ácido dimercaptossuccínico-Tc99m: 99mTc-dimercaptosuccinic acid
Ácido dimetil iminodiacético: dimethyl iminodiacetic acid (HIDA)
Ácido dimetilarsínico: dimethylarsinic acid
Ácido djencólico: djenkolic acid
Ácido edético: edetic acid
Ácido elaídico: elaidic acid
Ácido eleosteárico: eleostearic acid
Ácido erúcico: erucic acid
Ácido esteárico: stearic acid
Ácido etacrínico: ethacrynic acid
Ácido etanóico: ethanoic acid
Ácido etidrônico: etidronic acid
Ácido etilenodiaminotetracético: ethylenediaminetetraacetic acid (EDTA)
Ácido eugênico: eugenic acid

Ácido fenacetúrico: phenaceturic acid
Ácido fenilacético: phenylacetic acid
Ácido fenilacetúrico: phenylaceturic acid
Ácido fenilacrílico: phenylacrylic acid
Ácido fenilático: phenyllactic acid
Ácido feniletilbarbitúrico: phenylethylbarbituric acid
Ácido fenilglicólico: phenylglycolic acid
Ácido fenilpirúvico: phenylpyruvic acid
Ácido fitânico: phytanic acid
Ácido fítico: phytic acid
Ácido flaviânico: flavianic acid
Ácido flufenâmico: flufenamic acid
Ácido fluorídrico: hydrofluoric acid
Ácido fólico: folic acid
Ácido folínico: folinic acid
Ácido fórmico: formic acid
Ácido formiminoglutâmico: formiminoglutamic acid (FIGLU)
Ácido fosfâmico: phosphamic acid
Ácido fosfatídico: phosphatidic acid
Ácido fosfo*enol*pirúvico: phospho*enol*pyruvic acid
Ácido fosfoglicérico: phosphoglyceric acid
Ácido fosfórico: phosphoric acid
Ácido fosforoso: phosphorous acid
Ácido fosfotúngstico: phosphotungstic acid (PTA)
Ácido frangúlico: frangulic acid
Ácido frenosínico: phrenosinic acid
Ácido ftálico: phthalic acid
Ácido fumárico: fumaric acid
Ácido fusídico: fusidic acid
Ácido G: G acid
Ácido gadoléico: gadoleic acid
Ácido gálico: gallic acid
Ácido γ-aminobutírico: γ-aminobutyric acid (GABA, γ-Abu)
Ácido γ-poliglutâmico: poly(γ-glutamic acid)
Ácido gentísico: gentisic acid
Ácido giberélico: gibberellic acid
Ácido glicérico: glyceric acid
Ácido glicerofosfórico: glycerophosphoric acid
Ácido glicoascórbico: glucoascorbic acid
Ácido glicocólico: glycocholic acid
Ácido glicólico: glycolic acid
Ácido glicônico: gluconic acid
Ácido glicurônico: glucuronic acid, glycuronic acid
Ácido glioxílico: glyoxylic acid

Ácido glutacônico: glutaconic acid
Ácido glutâmico: glutamic acid (E, Glu)
Ácido glutárico: glutaric acid
Ácido graxo: fatty acid
Ácido guanílico: guanylic acid (GMP)
Ácido heparínico: heparinic acid
Ácido hexacosanóico: hexacosanoic acid
Ácido hexadecanóico: hexadecanoic acid
Ácido hexônico: hexonic acid
Ácido hexurônico: hexuronic acid
Ácido hialobiurônico: hyalobiuronic acid
Ácido hialurônico: hyaluronic acid
Ácido hidrobrômico: hydrobromic acid
Ácido hidrociânico: hydrocyanic acid
Ácido hidroxiacético: hydroxyacetic acid
Ácido hidroxigraxo: hydroxyfatty acid
Ácido hidroxinervônico: hydroxynervonic acid
Ácido hidroxitoluico: hydroxytoluic acid
Ácido hígrico: hygric acid
Ácido hipobromoso: hypobromous acid
Ácido hipocloroso: hypochlorous acid
Ácido hipofosforoso: hypophosphorous acid
Ácido hipúrico: hippuric acid
Ácido homogentísico: homogentisic acid
Ácido homoprotocatequínico: homoprotocatechuic acid
Ácido homovanílico: homovanillic acid (HVA)
Ácido ibotênico: ibotenic acid
Ácido idurônico: iduronic acid
Ácido inosínico: inosinic acid
Ácido iobenzâmico: iobenzamic acid
Ácido iocetâmico: iocetamic acid
Ácido iódico: iodic acid
Ácido iodoalfiônico: iodoalphionic acid
Ácido iodogorgóico: iodogorgoic acid
Ácido iodopanóico: iodopanoic acid
Ácido iofenóico: iophenoic acid
Ácido iofenóxico: iophenoxic acid
Ácido ioglicâmico: ioglycamic acid
Ácido iopanóico: iopanoic acid
Ácido iotalâmico: iothalamic acid
Ácido isetiônico: isethionic acid
Ácido isobutírico: isobutyric acid

Ácido isociânico: isocyanic acid
Ácido isocítrico: isocitric acid
Ácido isonicotínico: isonicotinic acid
Ácido isossuccínico: isosuccinic acid
Ácido isovalérico: isovaleric acid
Ácido itacônico: itaconic acid
Ácido L-desidroascórbico: L-dehydroascorbic acid
Ácido L-gulônico: L-gulonic acid
Ácido lactobacílico: lactobacillic acid
Ácido lático: lactic acid
Ácido láurico: lauric acid
Ácido levúlico: levulic acid
Ácido levulínico: levulinic acid
Ácido lignocérico: lignoceric acid
Ácido linoleico: linoleic acid
Ácido linolênico: linolenic acid
Ácido linólico: linolic acid
Ácido lipóico: lipoic acid, ovoprotogen, protogen, protogen A
Ácido lisérgico: lysergic acid
Ácido lisofosfatídico: lysophosphatidic acid
Ácido lítico: lithic acid
Ácido litocólico: lithocholic acid
Ácido maleico: maleic acid
Ácido málico: malic acid
Ácido málico desidrogenase: malic acid dehydrogenase
Ácido malônico: malonic acid
Ácido mandélico: mandelic acid
Ácido manurônico: mannuronic acid
Ácido meclofenâmico: meclofenamic acid
Ácido mecônico: meconic acid
Ácido mefenâmico: mefenamic acid
Ácido melíssico: melissic acid
Ácido mercaptoacético: mercaptoacetic acid
Ácido mercaptúrico: mercapturic acid
Ácido metacrílico: methacrylic acid
Ácido metafosfórico: metaphosphoric acid
Ácido metaperiódico: metaperiodic acid
Ácido metilacrílico: methylacrylic acid
Ácido metilenossuccínico: methylenesuccinic acid
Ácido metilmalônico: methylmalonic acid
Ácido mevalônico: mevalonic acid
Ácido mirístico: myristic acid
Ácido miristoleico: myristoleic acid
Ácido molíbdico: molybdic acid
Ácido monoidroxissuccínico: monohydroxysuccinic acid
Ácido montânico: montanic acid

Ácido murâmico: muramic acid (Mur)
Ácido N-acetilneuramínico: N-acetylneuraminic acid (NeuAc)
Ácido n-acilamino: n-acylamino acid
Ácido n-cáprico: n-capric acid
Ácido n-capróico: n-caproic acid
Ácido N-carbamoilaspártico: N-carbamoylaspartic acid
Ácido N-carbamoilglutâmico: N-carbamoylglutamic acid
Ácido n-decanóico: n-decanoic acid
Ácido n-docosanóico: n-docosanoic acid
Ácido n-dodecanóico: n-dodecanoic acid
Ácido n-eicosanóico: n-eicosanoic acid
Ácido n-hexanóico: n-hexanoic acid
Ácido n-icosanóico: n-icosanoic acid
Ácido N^5,N^{10}-meteniltetraidrofólico: N^5,N^{10}-methenyltetrahydrofolic acid
Ácido N-metil D-aspártico: N-methyl D-aspartic acid
Ácido n-nonanóico: n-nonanoic acid
Ácido N-succiniladenílico: N-succinyladenylic acid
Ácido n-tetracosanóico: n-tetracosanoic acid
Ácido nalidíxico: nalidixic acid
Ácido nervônico: nervonic acid
Ácido neuramínico: neuraminic acid
Ácido nicotínico: nicotinic acid
Ácido nítrico: nitric acid
Ácido nitrimuriático: nitrimuriatic acid
Ácido nitroclorídrico: nitrohydrochloric acid
Ácido nitroso: nitrous acid
Ácido nitroxântico: nitroxanthic acid
Ácido noroftálmico: norophthalmic acid
Ácido nucleico: nucleic acid
Ácido o-aminobenzóico: o-aminobenzoic acid
Ácido octacosanóico: octacosanoic acid
Ácido octanodióico: octandioic acid
Ácido octanóico: octanoic acid
Ácido octulossônico: octulosonic acid
Ácido oftálmico: ophthalmic acid
Ácido oleico: oleic acid
Ácido orótico: orotic acid (Oro)
Ácido orotidílico: orotidylic acid (OMP)
Ácido ortofosfórico: orthophosphoric acid
Ácido ósmico: osmic acid
Ácido oxálico: oxalic acid

Ácido oxaloacético: oxaloacetic acid
Ácido oxalossuccínico: oxalosuccinic acid
Ácido oxalúrico: oxaluric acid
Ácido oxoacético: oxoacetic acid
Ácido oxolínico: oxolinic acid
Ácido oxossuccínico: oxosuccinic acid
Ácido p-aminobenzóico: p-aminobenzoic acid (PABA)
Ácido p-amino-hipúrico: p-aminohippuric acid (PAH)
Ácido p-aminossalicílico: p-aminosalicylic acid (PAS, PASA)
Ácido p-rosólico: p-rosolic acid
Ácido palmítico: palmitic acid
Ácido palmitoleico: palmitoleic acid
Ácido pantóico: pantoic acid
Ácido pantotênico: pantothenic acid
Ácido para-aminobenzóico: paraaminobenzoic acid
Ácido parabânico: parabanic acid
Ácido péctico: pectic acid
Ácido pelargônico: pelargonic acid
Ácido penicilânico: penicillanic acid
Ácido penicílico: penicillic acid
Ácido penicilóico: penicilloic acid
Ácido pentanóico: pentanoic acid
Ácido pentético: pentetic acid
Ácido perfórmico: performic acid
Ácido periódico: periodic acid
Ácido permangânico: permanganic acid
Ácido peroxi: peroxy acid
Ácido peroxifórmico: peroxyformic acid
Ácido persulfúrico: persulfuric acid
Ácido picolínico: picolinic acid
Ácido picolinúrico: picolinuric acid
Ácido picrâmico: picramic acid
Ácido pícrico: picric acid
Ácido pimélico: pimelic acid
Ácido pipecólico: pipecolic acid
Ácido pipecolínico: pipecolinic acid
Ácido pirobórico: pyroboric acid
Ácido pirofosfórico: pyrophosphoric acid
Ácido pirogálico: pyrogallic acid
Ácido piroglutâmico: pyroglutamic acid (Pyr)
Ácido pirúvico: pyruvic acid
Ácido plasmênico: plasmenic acid
Ácido poliadenílico (poli(A)): poly(adenylic acid) (poly(A))

Ácido poliglicólico: poly(glycolic acid)
Ácido poliglutâmico: poly(glutamic acid)
Ácido poliuridílico (poli(U)): poly(uridylic acid) (poly(U))
Ácido prefênico: prephenic acid
Ácido pré-hematamínico: prehemataminic acid
Ácido propanodióico: propanedioic acid
Ácido propanóico: propanoic acid
Ácido propiônico: propionic acid
Ácido prostanóico: prostanoic acid
Ácido protocatecóico: protocatechuic acid
Ácido prússico: prussic acid
Ácido pteróico: pteroic acid
Ácido pteroilmonoglutâmico: pteroylmonoglutamic acid
Ácido pteroiltriglutâmico: pteroyltriglutamic acid
Ácido quenodesoxicólico: chenodeoxycholic acid
Ácido quináldico: quinaldic acid
Ácido quinaldínico: quinaldinic acid
Ácido quínico: kinic acid, quinic acid
Ácido quinolínico: quinolinic acid
Ácido quinurênico: kynurenic acid
Ácido quisquálico: quisqualic acid
Ácido redútico: reductic acid
Ácido retinóico: retinoic acid
Ácido ribonucléico (RNA): ribonucleic acid (RNA)
Ácido ribotimidílico: ribothymidylic acid (rTMP, TMP)
Ácido ricinoléico: ricinoleic acid
Ácido rodânico: rhodanic acid
Ácido rubeânico: rubeanic acid
Ácido sacárico: saccharic acid
Ácido salicílico: salicylic acid
Ácido salicilsalicílico: salicylsalicylic acid
Ácido salicilsulfônico: salicylsulfonic acid
Ácido salicilúrico: salicyluric acid
Ácido senecióico: senecioic acid
Ácido silícico: silicic acid
Ácido subérico: suberic acid
Ácido succínico: succinic acid
Ácido sulfindigótico: sulfindigotic acid
Ácido sulfociânico: sulfocyanic acid
Ácido sulfônico: sulfonic acid
Ácido sulfossalicílico: sulfosalicylic acid
Ácido sulfúrico: oil of vitriol, sulfuric acid
Ácido sulfuroso: sulfurous acid
Ácido tânico: tannic acid

Ácido tarírico: tariric acid
Ácido tartárico: tartaric acid
Ácido taurocólico: taurocholic acid
Ácido tetrabórico: tetraboric acid
Ácido tetradecanóico: tetradecanoic acid
Ácido tetraidrofólico: tetrahydrofolic acid (FH$_4$)
Ácido tíglico: tiglic acid
Ácido tímico: thymic acid
Ácido timidílico: thymidylic acid
Ácido timnodônico: timnodonic acid
Ácido tiociânico: thiocyanic acid
Ácido tióctico: thioctic acid
Ácido tioglicólico: thioglycolic acid
Ácido tiopânico: thiopanic acid
Ácido tiossulfúrico: thiosulfuric acid
Ácido tireoacético: thyroacetic acid
Ácido tolúico: toluic acid
Ácido toxílico: toxilic acid
Ácido tranexâmico: tranexamic acid
Ácido treônico: threonic acid
Ácido triacético: triacetic acid
Ácido tricloroacético: trichloroacetic acid
Ácido tropaico: tropaic acid
Ácido tropéico: tropeic acid
Ácido trópico: tropic acid
Ácido undecenóico: undecenoic acid
Ácido undecilênico: undecylenic acid
Ácido uracil-6-carboxílico: uracil-6-carboxylic acid
Ácido ureidossuccínico: ureidosuccinic acid
Ácido úrico: uric acid
Ácido uridílico: uridylic acid
Ácido uridinodifosfoglicurônico: uridine diphosphoglucuronic acid (UDP-GlcUA)
Ácido urocânico: urocanic acid
Ácido uroleucínico; ácido urolêucico: uroleucinic acid, uroleucic acid
Ácido ursodesoxicólico: ursodeoxycholic acid
Ácido vacênico: vaccenic acid
Ácido valérico: valeric acid
Ácido valpróico: valproic acid
Ácido vanádico: vanadic acid
Ácido vanílico: vanillic acid
Ácido vanililmandélico: vanillylmandelic acid (VMA)
Ácido verátrico: veratric acid
Ácido xantidílico: xanthidylic acid
Ácido xantílico: xanthylic acid
Ácido xantoproteico: xanthoproteic acid
Ácido xanturênico: xanthurenic acid
Ácido xilônico: xylonic acid
Ácido zoomárico: zoomaric acid
Acidofílico: acidophilic
Acidófilo: acidophil, acidophile
Ácidos acrílicos: acrylic acids
Ácidos alcoólicos: alcohol acids
Ácidos aldônicos: aldonic acids
Ácidos coleicos: choleic acids
Ácidos crisântemo-carboxílicos: chrysanthemum-carboxylic acids
Ácidos de açúcar: sugar acids
Ácidos fíbricos: fibric acids
Ácidos glicônicos: glyconic acids
Ácidos hidroxâmicos: hydroxamic acids
Ácidos indólicos: indolic acids
Ácidos micólicos: mycolic acids
Ácidos pectínicos: pectinic acids
Ácidos penílicos: penillic acids
Ácidos poliênicos: polyenic acids
Ácidos polienóicos: polyenoic acids
Ácidos resínicos: resin acids, resinic acids
Ácidos siálicos: sialic acids (Sia)
Ácidos teicóicos: teichoic acids
Ácidos urônicos: uronic acids
Acidose: acidosis
Acidótico: acidotic
Acidúria: aciduria
Acidúria β-hidroxipropiônica: β-hydroxypropionic aciduria
Acidúria D-glicérica: D-glyceric aciduria
Acidúria glicólica: glycolic aciduria
Acidúria L-glicérica: L-glyceric aciduria
Acidúria metilmalônica: methylmalonic aciduria
Acidúria orótica: orotic aciduria
Acidúria urocânica: urocanic aciduria
Acidúrico: aciduric
Acil-ACP desidrogenase ou redutase: acyl-ACP dehydrogenase, acyl-ACP reductase
Acil-CoA: acyl-CoA
Acil-CoA desidrogenase de cadeia longa: long-chain acyl-CoA dehydrogenase
Acil-coenzima A: acyl-coenzyme A
Acil: acyl
Acilação: acylation
Acilcarnitina: acylcarnitine
Acildenilato: acyladenylate
1-acilglicerol-3-fosfato aciltransferase: 1-acylglycerol-3-phosphate acyltransferase
Acilmalonil ACP sintase: acyl-malonyl-ACP synthase
Acilmercaptano: acylmercaptan
Acinar: acinar, acinic
Acinese: akinesis
Acinesia: akinesia
Acinésico: akinesic
Acinestesia: akinesthesia
Acinético: akinetic
Aciniforme: aciniform
Ácino: acinus, **gen. e pl.** acini
Acinoso: acinose, acinous
Acistia: acystia
Áclase: aclasia, aclasis
Aclimação: acclimation
Aclimatação: acclimatization
Aclomida: aklomide
Acloridria: achlorhydria
Aclorófilo: achlorophyllous
Acme: acme
Acne: acne
Acneiforme: acneform, acneiform
Acnemia: acnemia, aknemia
Acocantera: acokanthera
Acolia: acholia
Acólico: acholic
Ácolo: acolous
Acolúria: acholuria
Acolúrico: acholuric
Acomodação: accommodation
Acomodativo: accommodative
Acompanhante: chaperone, comes, **pl.** comites
Acomplementado: uncomplemented
Acondrogênese: achondrogenesis
Acondroplasia: achondroplasia
Acondroplásico: achondroplastic
Aconitase: aconitase
Aconitato hidratase: aconitate hydratase
Aconitina: aconitine
Acônito: aconite, monkshood, wolfsbane
Aconselhamento: counseling
Acoplamento: coupling
Acordal: achordate, achordal
Acoréia: acorea
Acorese: achoresis
Acotovelado: elbowed
ACP-acetiltransferase: ACP-acetyltransferase
ACP-maloniltransferase: ACP-malonyltransferase
Acral: acral
Acrania: acrania
Acranial: acranial
Acrânio: acranius
Acraniotas: Acrania
Acre: acrid
Acreção: accrementition, accretion
Acribômetro: acribometer
Acridina: acridine
Acriflavina: acriflavine
Acrilato: acrylate
Acrílico: acrylic
Acrimonia: acrimonia
Acrimônia: acrimony
Acrisorcina: acrisorcin
Acrítico: acritical
Acroácito: achroacyte
Acroagnose: acroagnosis
Acroanestesia: acroanesthesia
Acroartrite: acroarthritis
Acroasfixia: acroasphyxia
Acroataxia: acroataxia
Acroblasto: acroblast
Acrobraquicefalia: acrobrachycephaly
Acrocefalia: acrocephalia, acrocephaly
Acrocefálico: acrocephalic
Acrocéfalo: acrocephalous
Acrocefalopolissindactilia: acrocephalopolysyndactyly
Acrocefalossindactilia: acrocephalosyndactyly (ACPS)
Acrocêntrico: acrocentric
Acroceratoelastoidose: acrokeratoelastoidosis
Acroceratose: acrokeratosis
Acrocianose: acrocyanosis
Acrocianótico: acrocyanotic
Acrocinesia, acrocinese: acrocinesia, acrocinesis, acrokinesia
Acrocontratura: acrocontracture
Acrocórdone: acrochordon
Acrodermatite: acrodermatitis
Acrodermatose: acrodermatosis
Acrodextrina: achrodextrin
Acrodinia: acrodynia
Acrodisestesia: acrodysesthesia
Acrodisostose: acrodysostosis
Acrodontia: acrodont
Acroesclerose: acrosclerosis
Acroestesia: acroesthesia
Acrofobia: acrophobia
Acrógeno: acrogenous
Acrogeria: acrogeria
Acrognose: acrognosis
Acro-hiperceratose: acrohyperkeratosis
Acro-hiperidrose: acrohyperhidrosis
Acromácito: achromacyte
Acromasia: achromasia
Acromático: achromatic
Acromatina: achromatin
Acromatínico: achromatinic
Acromatismo: achromatism
Acromatócito: achromatocyte
Acromatofilia: achromatophilia
Acromatófilo: achromatophil
Acromatólise: achromatolysis
Acromatope: achromat
Acromatopsia: achromatopsia, achromatopsy
Acromatose: achromatosis
Acromatoso: achromatous
Acromatúria: achromaturia
Acromegalia: acromegalia, acromegaly
Acromegálico: acromegalic
Acromegalogigantismo: acromegalogigantism
Acromegaloidismo: acromegaloidism
Acromelalgia: acromelalgia
Acromelia: acromelia
Acromélico: acromelic
Acromesomelia: acromesomelia
Acrometagênese: acrometagenesis

Acromia: achromia
Acromial: acromial
Acrômico: achromic
Acromicria: acromicria
Acrômio: acromion
Acromioclavicular: acromioclavicular, scapuloclavicular
Acromiocorácóide: acromiocoracoid
Acromioplastia: acromioplasty
Acromioscapular: acromioscapular
Acromiotonia: acromyotonia
Acromiotônus: acromyotonus
Acromiotorácico: acromiothoracic
Acromioumeral: acromiohumeral
Acromócito: achromocyte
Acromofílico, acromófilo: achromophilic, achromophil, achromophilous
Acromotriquia: achromotrichia
Acrônfalo: acromphalus
Acroodextrina: achroodextrin
Acropaquia: acropachy
Acropaquidermia: acropachyderma
Acroparestesia: acroparesthesia
Acrópeto: acropetal
Acropigmentação: acropigmentation
Acropleurógeno: acropleurogenous
Acropustulose: acropustulosis
Acrosclerodermia: acroscleroderma
Acrosina: acrosin
Acrospiroma: acrospiroma
Acrossomina: acrosomin
Acrossomo: acrosome
Acrosteólise: acroosteolysis
Acrotérico: acroteric
Acrótico: acrotic
Acrotismo: acrotism
Acrotrofodinia: acrotrophodynia
Acrotrofoneurose: acrotrophoneurosis
Actina: actin
Actina F: F-actin
Actina G: G-actin
Actínico: actinic
Actinídios: actinides
α-actinina: α-actinin
Actínio: actinium (Ac)
Actinobacilos: *Actinobacillus*
Actinobacilose: actinobacillosis
Actinoematina: actinohematin
Actinófago: actinophage
Actinofitose: actinophytosis
Actinomicelial: actinomycelial
Actinomicetales: Actinomycetales
Actinomicetoma: actinomycetoma
Actinomicetos: actinomycetes
Actinomicina: actinomycin
Actinomicose: actinomycosis
Actinomicótico: actinomycotic

Actinópodes: Actinopoda
Actinosina: actinosin
Actinoterapia: actinotherapy
Actomiosina: actomyosin
Açúcar: saccharum, sugar
Açúcar de óleo: oleosaccharum, **pl.** oleosaccharа
Açúcares: sugars
Açúcares de nucleosídeo difosfato: nucleoside diphosphate sugars
Acuidade: acuity
Aculeado: aculeate
Acumentina: acumentin
Acuminado: acuminate
Acuologia: acuology
Acupressão: acupressure
Acupuntura: acupuncture
Acurácia: accuracy
Acusia: acusis
Acústica: acoustics
Acústico: acoustic
Acusticofobia: acousticophobia
Adacria: adacrya
Adáctilo: adactylous
Adamantino: adamantine
Adamantinoma: adamantinoma
Adaptação: adaptation
Adaptador: adapter, adaptor, conformer
Adaptômetro: adaptometer
Adaxial: adaxial
Adejar: flicks
Adelgaçamento: thinning
Adelomorfo: adelomorphous
Adenalgia: adenalgia
Adêndrico: adendric
Adendrítico: adendritic
Adenectomia: adenectomy
Adenectopia: adenectopia
Adenenfraxia: adenemphraxis
Adeniforme: adeniform
Adenil: adenyl
Adenil ciclase: adenyl cyclase
Adenil succinase: adenylosuccinase
Adenilato: adenylate
Adenilil: adenylyl
Adenililsuccinato liase: adenylosuccinate lyase, adenylylosuccinate lyase
Adenililsuccinato sintase: adenylylosuccinate synthase
Adenililsulfato cinase: adenylylsulfate kinase
Adenilsuccinato sintase: adenylosuccinate synthase
Adenina: adenine (A, Ade)
Adenite: adenitis
Adenização: adenization
Adenoacantoma: adenoacanthoma
Adenoameloblastoma: adenoameloblastoma
Adenoblasto: adenoblast
Adenocarcinoma: adenocarcinoma
Adenocistoma: adenocystoma
Adenócito: adenocyte
Adenodiastase: adenodiastasis
Adenodinia: adenodynia

Adenofibroma: adenofibroma
Adenofibrose: adenofibrosis
Adenofleimão: adenophlegmon
Adenoforasídeos: Adenophorasida
Adenógeno: adenogenous
Adeno-hipofisário: adenohypophysial
Adeno-hipófise: adenohypophysis
Adeno-hipofisite: adenohypophysitis
Adenóide: adenoid
Adenoidectomia: adenoidectomy
Adenóides: adenoids
Adenoidite: adenoiditis
Adenolinfocele: adenolymphocele
Adenolinfoma: adenolymphoma
Adenolipoma: adenolipoma
Adenolipomatose: adenolipomatosis
Adenoma: adenoma
Adenomatóide: adenomatoid
Adenomatose: adenomatosis
Adenomatoso: adenomatous
Adenomegalia: adenomegaly
Adenômero: adenomere
Adenomioma: adenomyoma
Adenomiose: adenomyosis
Adenopatia: adenopathy
Adenose: adenosis
Adenosil: adenosyl
Adenosilcobalamina: adenosylcobalamin
Adenosina: adenosine (Ado)
Adenosina trifosfatase: adenosine triphosphatase (ATPase)
Adenoso: adenose
Adenossalpingite: adenosalpingitis
Adenossarcoma: adenosarcoma
Adenotomia: adenotomy
Adenotonsilectomia: adenotonsillectomy
Adenovírus: adenovirus
Adequação: goodness of fit
Aderência: adherence
Adermia: adermia
Adesão: adhesio, adhesion, **pl.** adhesiones
Adesinas: adhesins
Adesiólise: adhesiolysis
Adesiotomia: adhesiotomy
Adesivo: adhesive
Adiabático: adiabatic
Adiadococinesia, adiadocinese: adiadochocinesia, dysdiadochokinesis, adiadochocinesis, adiadochokinesis
Adiaforese: adiaphoresis
Adiaforético: adiaphoretic
Adiaforia: adiaphoria
Adiaspiromicose: adiaspiromycosis
Adiásporo: adiaspore
Adiástole: adiastole

Adiatermância: adiathermancy
Adicção: addiction
Adicto: addict
Adiemórrise: adiemorrhysis
Adinamia: adynamia
Adinâmico: adynamic
Adipiodona: adipiodone
Adipocelular: adipocellular
Adipocera: adipocere
Adipoceratoso: adipoceratous
Adipocinético: adipokinetic
Adipocinina: adipokinin
Adipócito: adipocyte
Adipogênese: adipogenesis
Adipogênico: adipogenic, adipogenous
Adipóide: adipoid
Adipômetro: adipometer
Adiponecrose: adiponecrosis
Adiposalgia: adiposalgia
Adipose: adiposis
Adiposidade: adiposity
Adiposo: adipose
Adiposúria: adiposuria
Adipsia: adipsia, adipsy
Adissoniano: addisonian
Aditivo: additive
Ádito: aditus
Adjuvante: adjuvant
Adleriano: adlerian
Admediano: admedial, admedian
Adminículo: adminiculum, **pl.** adminicula
Administração: management
Admitância: admittance
Adneural: adnerval, adneural
Adnexectomia: adnexectomy
Adnexite: adnexitis
Adnexo: adnexa, **sing.** adnexum; adnexal
Adnexopexia: adnexopexy
Adolescência: adolescence
Adolescente: adolescent
Adonitol: adonitol
Adoral: orad
Adornado: ornate
ADPase: ADPase
Adquirido: acquired
Adrenal: adrenal, adrenic
Adrenalectomia: adrenalectomy
Adrenalina: adrenaline
Adrenalismo: adrenalism
Adrenalite: adrenalitis
Adrenalona: adrenalone
Adrenarca: adrenarche
Adrenérgico: adrenergic
Adrenoceptivo: adrenoceptive
Adrenoceptor: adrenoceptor
Adrenocortical: adrenocortical
Adrenocorticóide: adrenocorticoid
Adrenocorticomimético: adrenocorticomimetic
Adrenocorticotrópico, adrenocorticotrófico: adrenocorticotropic, adrenocorticotrophic
Adrenocorticotropina: adrenocorticotropin

Adrenogênico, adrenogenoso: adrenogenic, adrenogenous
Adrenoleucodistrofia: adrenoleukodystrophy (ALD)
Adrenolítico: adrenolytic
Adrenomegalia: adrenomegaly
Adrenomieloneuropatia: adrenomyeloneuropathy
Adrenomimético: adrenomimetic
Adrenopatia: adrenalopathy, adrenopathy
Adrenopausa: adrenopause
Adrenoprivo: adrenoprival
Adrenorreativo: adrenoreactive
Adrenorreceptores: adrenoreceptors
Adrenosterona: adrenosterone
Adrenotoxina: adrenotoxin
Adrenotrópico, adrenotrófico: adrenotropic, adrenotrophic
Adrenotropina: adrenotropin
Adressina: addressin
Adsorbato: adsorbate
Adsorção: adsorption
Adsorvente: adsorbent
Adsorver: adsorb
Adstringente: astringent
Adução: adduction
Aducente: adducent
Adulteração: adulteration
Adulterante: adulterant
Adulto: adult
Adultomorfismo: adultomorphism
Adutor: adductor
Aduzir: adduct
Adventícia: adventitia
Adventício: adventitial, adventitious
Aerar: aerate
Aerendocardia: aerendocardia
Aeróbico: aerobic
Aeróbio: aerobe
Aerobiologia: aerobiology
Aerobioscópio: aerobioscope
Aerobiose: aerobiosis
Aerobiótico: aerobiotic
Aerocele: aerocele
Aerococo: *Aerococcus*
Aerocolpo: aerocolpos
Aerodermectasia: aerodermectasia
Aerodinâmica: aerodynamics
Aerodontalgia: aerodontalgia, aero-odontalgia, aero-odontodynia
Aerodontia: aerodontia
Aerofagia: aerophagia, aerophagy
Aerofilia, aerofílico: aerophil, aerophile, aerophilic, aerophilous
Aerofobia: aerophobia
Aerogastria: aerogastria
Aerogênese: aerogenesis
Aerogênico, aerógeno: aerogenic, aerogen, aerogenous
Aeromedicina: aeromedicine
Aeromônada: aeromonad
Aeropausa: aeropause

Aeropiesoterapia: aeropiesotherapy
Aeroplâncton: aeroplankton
Aerose: aerosis
Aerossialofagia: aerosialophagy
Aerossinusite: aerosinusitis
Aerossol: aerosol
Aerossolização: aerosolization
Aeroterapia: aerotherapeutics, aerotherapy
Aerotite média: aerotitis media
Aerotonômetro: aerotonometer
Afagia: aphagia
Afalangia: aphalangia
Afalgesia: haphalgesia
Afaquia: aphakia
Afasia: aphasia
Afásico: aphasiac, aphasic
Afasiologia: aphasiology
Afasiologista: aphasiologist
Afasmídio: aphasmid
Afasmídios: Aphasmidia
Afebril: afebrile
Afeição: affection
Afeliotropismo: apheliotropism
Aferente: afferent, esodic
Aférese: apheresis
Afetal: afetal
Afetividade: affectivity
Afetivo: affective
Afeto: affect
Afetomotor: affectomotor
Afibrilar: afibrillar
Afibrinogenemia: afibrinogenemia
Afilático: aphylactic
Afilaxia: aphylaxis
Afilofonia: aphilopony
Afim: affinous
Afinidade: affinity
Afirmação: affirmation
Aflatoxicose: aflatoxicosis
Aflatoxina: aflatoxin
Afogamento: drowning
Afoiçamento: sickling
Afonia: aphonia
Afônico: aphonic, aphonous
Afotestesia: aphotesthesia
Afrasia: aphrasia
Afrodisia: aphrodisia
Afrodisíaco: aphrodisiac
Afrodisiomania: aphrodisiomania
Afta: aphtha, **pl.** aphthae
Aftóide: aphthoid
Aftose: aphthosis
Aftoso: aphthous
Afundamento: subsidence
Afusão: affusion
Agalácteo: agalactous
Agalactia: agalactia, agalactosis
Agalactorréia: agalactorrhea
Agamaglobulinemia: agammaglobulinemia
Agameta: agamete
Agâmico: agamic, agamous
Agamocitogenia: agamocytogeny
Agamogênese: agamogenesis
Agamogenético: agamogenetic
Agamogonia: agamogony

Aganglônico: aganglionic
Aganglionose: aganglionosis
Agapismo: agapism
Ágar: agar
Agárico: agaric, amadou
Agaropectina: agaropectin
Agarose: agarose
Agástrico: agastric
Agastroneuria: agastroneuria
Agenesia: agenesis
Agenitalismo: agenitalism
Agenossomia: agenosomia
Agente: agent
Agente Laranja: Agent Orange
Agerasia: agerasia
Ageusia: ageusia
Ageustia: ageustia
Agiria: agyria
Agitar: jar
Agitofasia: agitophasia
Agitolalia: agitolalia
Aglicona: aglycon, aglycone, **pl.** aglyca
Aglicosúria: aglycosuria
Aglicosúrico: aglycosuric
Aglomeração: agglomeration, aggregation
Aglomerado: agglomerate, agglomerated
Aglomerular: aglomerular
Aglossia: aglossia
Aglossostomia: aglossostomia
Aglucona: aglucon
Aglutição: aglutition
Aglutinação: agglutination, clumping
Aglutinante: agglutinant
Aglutinar: agglutinate
Aglutinativo: agglutinative
Aglutinina: agglutinin
Aglutinofílico: agglutinophilic
Aglutinogênico: agglutinogenic
Aglutinogênio: agglutinogen
Aglutogênico: agglutogenic
Aglutogênio: agglutogen
Agnatia: agnathia
Ágnato: agnathous
Agnogênico: agnogenic
Agnosia: agnea, agnosia
Agnosia tátil: stereoagnosis, stereoanesthesia
Agonádico: agonadal
Agonfo: agomphious
Agonfose: agomphosis, agomphiasis
Agonia: agony
Agônico: agonal
Agonista: agonist
Agorafobia: agoraphobia
Agorafóbico: agoraphobic
Agrafe: agraffe
Agrafia: agraphia
Agráfico: agraphic
Agramatismo: agrammatica, agrammatism
Agramatologia: agrammatologia
Agranulócito: agranulocyte
Agranulocitose: agranulocytosis
Agranuloplásico: agranuloplastic
Agrecano: aggrecan

Agregado: aggregated (adjetivo), aggregate (substantivo)
Agregar: aggregate
Agregatopo: agretope
Agregômetro: aggregometer
Agressão: aggression
Agressina: aggressin
Agressivo: aggressive
Agrupamento: assortment
Água: aqua, **gen. e pl.** aquae; water, **pl.** waters
Aguarrás: turps
Agudo: acute, exquisite
Agulha: needle
Agulha de Gillmore: Gillmore needle
Aguti: *agouti*
AIDS/SIDA: AIDS
Ainhum: ainhum
Ajmalina: ajmaline
Ajustamento: adjustment
Akembe: onyalai
Alacrimia: alacrima
Alalia: alalia
Alálico: alalic
Alanil: alanyl
Alanina: alanine (A, Ala)
β-alanina: β-alanine
β-alanina-piruvato aminotransferase: β-alanine-pyruvate aminotransferase
Alanina aminotransferase: alanine aminotransferase (ALT)
Alanina-glioxilato aminotransferase: alanine-glyoxylate aminotransferase
Alanina-oxomalonato aminotransferase: alanine-oxomalonate aminotransferase
Alanina racemase: alanine racemase
Alanina transaminase: alanine transaminase
Alanosina: alanosine
Alantina: alantin
Alantoato desiminase: allantoate deiminase
Alantocório: allantochorion
Alantogênese: allantogenesis
Alantóico: allantoic
Alantóide: allantoid, allantois
Alantoidoangiópago: allantoidoangiopagus
Alantoína: allantoin
Alantoinase: allantoinase
Alantoinúria: allantoinuria
Alantol: alantol
Alaquestesia: allachesthesia
Alar: alar
Alargador: reamer
Alarmona: alarmone
Alastrim: alastrim, milkpox, whitepox
Alavanca: lever, vectis
Albedo: albedo
Álbido: albidus
Albino: albino
Albinúria: albiduria, albinuria
Albocinério: albocinereous

Albugínea: albuginea
Albugíneo: albugineous
Albugineotomia: albugineotomy
Albume: albumen
Albumina: albumin
Albuminato: albuminate
Albuminatúria: albuminaturia
Albuminífero: albuminiferous
Albumíniparo: albuminiparous
Albuminógeno: albuminogenous
Albuminóide: albuminoid
Albuminólise: albuminolysis
Albuminoptise: albuminoptysis
Albuminorréia: albuminorrhea
Albuminoso: albuminous
Albuminúria: albuminuria
Albuminúrico: albuminuric
Albuterol: albuterol
Alc-1-enil: alk-1-enyl
Alça: ansa, **gen e pl.** ansae; loop, snare
Alcaçuz: licorice, liquorice
Alcadieno: alkadiene
Alçado: ansate
Alcalemia: alkalemia
Álcali: alkali, **pl.** alkalies
Alcalinidade: alkalinity
Alcalinização: alkalinization
Alcalino: alkaline
Alcalinúria: alkalinuria
Alcaliterapia: alkalitherapy
Alcalização: alkalization
Alcalizador: alkalizer
Alcalóide: alkaloid
Alcalóides da dibenzilisoquinolina: bisbenzylisoquinoline alkaloids
Alcalóides de Catharanthus: Catharanthus alkaloids
Alcalose: alkalosis
Alcalótico: alkalotic
Alcalúria: alkaluria
Alcanan: alkannan
Alcaneto: alkanet
Alcanina: alkannin
Alcano: alkane
Alcaptona: alcapton, alkapton
Alcaptonúria: alcaptonuria, alkaptonuria
Alcaptonúrico: alcaptonuric, alkaptonuric
Alcatrão: coal tar, tar
Alcatrão da bétula: birch tar
Alcatrão de faia: beechwood tar
Alcatrieno: alkatriene
Alcavervir: alkavervir
Alce-1-enilglicerofosfolipídeo: alk-1-enylglycerophospholipid
Alcenil: alkenyl
Alclofenaco: alclofenac
Alclometasona: alclometasone
Alcogel: alcogel
Álcool: alcohol
Álcool-ácido-resistente: acid-fast
Álcool cetoestearílico: cetostearyl alcohol
Álcool cetônico: ketone alcohol
Álcool cinâmico: cinnamic alcohol
Álcool de farneseno: farnesene alcohol

Álcool desidrogenase: alcohol dehydrogenase (ADH)
Álcool desidrogenase (aceptor): alcohol dehydrogenase (acceptor)
Álcool desidrogenase (NADP$^+$): alcohol dehydrogenase (NADP$^+$)
Álcool dicloroisopropílico: dichloroisopropyl alcohol
Álcool do açúcar: sugar alcohol
Álcool esteárilico: stearyl alcohol
Álcool fenetílico: phenethyl alcohol
Álcool feniletílico: phenylethyl alcohol
Álcool fitílico: phytyl alcohol
Álcool isopropílico: isopropyl alcohol
Álcool metílico: wood alcohol
Álcool nicotínico: nicotinic alcohol
Álcool nicotinílico: nicotinyl alcohol
Álcool oleílico: oleyl alcohol
Álcool palmitílico: palmityl alcohol
Álcool polivinílico: polyvinyl alcohol
Álcool tricloroetílico: trichloroethyl alcohol
Alcoolato: alcoholate
Alcoolato de cloral: chloral alcoholate
Alcoólico: alcoholic, spirituous
Alcoólise: alcoholysis
Alcoolismo: alcoholism
Alcoolização: alcoholization
Alcoolofobia: alcoholophobia
Aldadieno: aldadiene
Aldeído: aldehyde
Aldeído acético: acetic aldehyde
Aldeído benzóico: benzoic aldehyde
Aldeído betaínico desidrogenase: betaine-aldehyde dehydrogenase
Aldeído cinâmico: cinnamic aldehyde
Aldeído de açúcar: sugar aldehyde
Aldeído desidrogenase (acetilante): aldehyde dehydrogenase (acylating)
Aldeído desidrogenase (NAD$^+$): aldehyde dehydrogenase (NAD$^+$)
Aldeído desidrogenase (NAD(P)$^+$): aldehyde dehydrogenase (NAD(P)$^+$)
Aldeído fórmico: formic aldehyde
Aldeído glicérico: glyceric aldehyde
Aldeído liases: aldehyde-lyases
Aldeído pirúvico: pyruvic aldehyde
Aldeído salicílico: salicylic aldehyde

Aldeol: aldehol
Aldimina: aldimine
Alditol: alditol
Aldocetomutase: aldoketomutase
Aldocortina: aldocortin
Aldo-hexose: aldohexose
Aldol: aldol
Aldolase: aldolase
Aldopentose: aldopentose
Aldose: aldose
Aldose 1-epimerase: aldose 1-epimerase
Aldosídeo: aldoside
Aldosterona: aldosterone
Aldosteronismo: aldosteronism
Aldosteronogênese: aldosteronogenesis
Aldotetrose: aldotetrose
Aldotriose: aldotriose
Aldoxima: aldoxime
Aldrin: aldrin
Aleatório: random
Alecítico: alecithal
Alelismo: allelism
Alelo: allele
Alelo amorfo: amorph
Alelocatálise: allelocatalysis
Alelocatalítico: allelocatalytic
Alelomórfico: allelomorphic
Alelomorfismo: allelomorphism
Alelomorfo: allelomorph
Aleloquímicos: allelochemicals
Alelotaxia: allelotaxis, allelotaxy
Alergênico: allergenic
Alérgeno: allergen
Alergia: allergy
Alérgico: allergic
Alergista: allergist
Alergização: allergization
Alergizado: allergized
Alergologia: allergology
Alergose: allergosis
Alestesia: allesthesia, alloesthesia
Aletrina: allethrins
Aletrolona: allethrolone
Aleucemia: aleukemia
Aleucêmico: aleukemic
Aleucemóide: aleukemoid
Aleucia: aleukia
Aleucocítico: aleukocytic
Aleucocitose: aleukocytosis
Aleurioconídio: aleurioconidium
Aleuriósporo: aleuriospore
Aleurona: aleuron
Aleuronato: aleuronate
Aleuronóide: aleuronoid
Alexia: alexia
Aléxico: alexic
Alexina: alexin
Alexitimia: alexithymia
Alfa: alpha
Alfa-amilase: alpha amylase
Alfabeto dactilológico: finger spelling
Alfabeto manual: handshapes
Alfacalcidol: alfacalcidol
Alfadiona: alphadione
Alfaprodina: alphaprodine
Alforra: smut

Algal: algal
Algas: algae
Algesia: algesia, algesthesia, algesthesis
Algésico: algesic
Algesímetro: algesimeter, algesiometer
Algesiogênico: algesiogenic
Algesocronômetro: algesichronometer
Algético: algetic
Algicida: algicide
Álgido: algid
Algina: algin
Alginato: alginate
Algiomotor: algiomotor
Algodão: cotton
Algodistrofia: algodystrophy
Algoespasmo: algospasm
Algofilia: algophilia
Algofobia: algophobia
Algogenesia: algogenesis, algogenesia
Algogênico: algogenic
Algolagnia: algolagnia
Algologia: algology
Algometria: algometry
Algômetro: algometer
Algomotor: algiomuscular
Algoritmo: algorithm
Algoscopia: algoscopy
Algovascular: algiovascular, algovascular
Alho: allium, garlic
Alíbil: alible
Alicíclico: alicyclic
Alienação: alienation
Alienia: alienia
Alifático: aliphatic
Aliforme: aliform
Alilamina: allylamine
Alilestrenol: allylestrenol
Alilmercaptometilpenicilina: allylmercaptomethylpenicillin
Alilo: allyl
Alimentação: alimentation, feeding
Alimentar: alimentary
Alimento: aliment, food, nourishment
Alinasal: alinasal
Alinfia: alymphia
Alinfocitose: alymphocytosis
Alinfoplasia: alymphoplasia
Alinhamento: alignment, alinement
Alipóide: alipoid
Alipotrópico: alipotropic
Alíquota: aliquot
Alisfenóide: alisphenoid
Alisinas: allysines
Aliteração: alliteration
Aliviar: relieve
Alívio: relief
Alizarina: alizarin
Alma: anima
Almíscar: moschus
Almofariz: mortar
Aloalbuminemia: alloalbuminemia
Aloanticorpo: alloantibody

Aloantígeno: alloantigen
Alobarbital: allobarbital
Alocêntrico: allocentric
Aloceratoplastia: allokeratoplasty
Alocinesia: allokinesis
Alocolesterol: allocholesterol
Alocórtex: allocortex
α-alocortol: α-allocortol
β-alocortol: β-allocortol
α-alocortolona: α-allocortolone
β-alocortolona: β-allocortolone
Alocróico: allochroic
Alocroísmo: allochroism
Alodinia: allodynia
Alodiplóide: allodiploid
Aloé: aloe
Aloé-emodina: aloe-emodin
Aloenxerto: allograft
Aloerotismo: alloerotism
Aloetina: aloetin
Alofasia: allophasis
Alofênico: allophenic
Alóforo: allophore
Aloftalmia: allophthalmia
Alogamia: allogamy
Alogenação: halogenation
Alogênico: allogenic, allogeneic
Alógeno: halogen
Alogenoderma: halogenoderma
Alogia: alogia
Alogotrofia: allogotrophia
Alogrupo: allogroup
Alo-hexaplóide: allohexaploid
Alo-hidroxilisina: allohydroxylysine (aHyl)
Aloimune: alloimmune
Aloína: aloin
Aloisoleucina: alloisoleucine (alle)
Aloisômero: alloisomer
Alojamento conjunto: rooming-in
Alolactose: allolactose
Alolalia: allolalia
Alomerismo: allomerism
Alometria: allometron
Alômetro: halometer
Alomonas: allomones
Alomorfismo: allomorphism
Alongamento: allongement, elongation
Alopata: allopath, allopathist
Alopatia: allopathy
Alopático: allopathic
Alopecia: alopecia
Alopécico: alopecic
Alopentaplóide: allopentaploid
Alópilo: halophil, halophile, halophilic
Aloplasia: alloplasia
Aloplastia: alloplasty
Aloplasto: alloplast
Aloplóide: alloploid
Aloploidia: alloploidy
Alopoliplóide: allopolyploid
Alopoliploidia: allopolyploidy
α-alopregnanediol: α-allopregnanediol
β-alopregnanediol: β-allopregnanediol

Alopregnano: allopregnane
Alopsíquico: allopsychic
Alopurinol: allopurinol
Aloquiria: allochiria, allocheiria
Alorritmia: allorhythmia
Alorrítmico: allorhythmic
Alose: allose
Alossensibilização: allosensitization
Alossoma: allosome
Alosterese: halosteresis
Alosteria: allosterism, allostery
Alostérico: allosteric
Alotetraplóide: allotetraploid
Alotípico: allotypic
Alótipo: allotype
Alotopia: allotopia
Alótopo: allotope
Alotransplante: allotransplantation
Alotreoninas: allothreonines (aThr)
Alotriodontia: allotriodontia
Alotriosmia: allotriosmia
Alotriplóide: allotriploid
Alotrófico: allotrophic
Alotrópico: allotropic
Alotropismo: allotropism, allotropy
Alótropo: allotrope
Aloxana: alloxan
Aloxantina: alloxantin
Aloxuremia: alloxuremia
Aloxúria: alloxuria
Alpidem: alpidem
Alprazolam: alprazolam
Alprostadil: alprostadil
Alqueno: alkene
Alquila: alkide, alkyl
Alquilação: alkylation
Alquilamina: alkylamine
Alseroxilona: alseroxylon
Altéia: althea
Alteração: alteration
Alternação: alternation
Alternador: alternator
Alternância: alternans
Alternocular: alternocular
Altitudinal: altitudinal
D-*altro*-2-heptulose: D-*altro*-2-heptulose
Altrose: altrose
Altura: height (h)
Alucinação: hallucination
Alucinogênese: hallucinogenesis
Alucinogênico: hallucinogenic
Alucinógeno: hallucinogen
Alucinose: hallucinosis
Alume: alum
Alume-hematoxilina: alum-hematoxylin
Alumina: alumina
Aluminado: aluminated
Alumínio: aluminum (Al)
Aluminose: aluminosis
Álveo: alveus, **pl.** alvei
Alveoalgia: alveoalgia
Alveolado: alveolate
Alveolalgia: alveolalgia
Alveolar: alveolar
Alveolectomia: alveolectomy

Alveolingual: alveolingual
Alveolite: alveolitis
Alvéolo: alveolus, **gen. e pl.** alveoli; socket
Alveoloclasia: alveoloclasia
Alveolodental: alveolodental
Alveololabial: alveololabial, alveololabialis
Alveololingual: alveololingual
Alveolopalatal: alveolopalatal
Alveoloplastia: alveoloplasty, alveoplasty
Alveolosquise: alveoloschisis
Alveolotomia: alveolotomy
Alvo: target
Alzima: alzyme
Amácrina: amacrine
Amadurecer: maturate
Amálgama: amalgam
Amalgamação: amalgamation
Amalgamador: amalgamator
Amalgamar: amalgamate
Amamentar: nurse, suckle
α-amanitina: α-amanitin
Amanteigado: butyroid
Amaranto: amaranth, amaranthum
Amarelamento: flavedo
Amarelo: yellow
Amarelo acridina: acridine yellow
Amarelo brilhante: brilliant yellow
Amarelo-cromo: chrome yellow
Amarelo de cromo: lemon yellow
Amarelo de hidrazina: hydrazine yellow
Amarelo de Leipzig: Leipzig yellow
Amarelo de Martius: martius yellow
Amarelo de metanila: metanil yellow
Amarelo de metila: butter yellow, methyl yellow
Amargo: amarum
Amargos: amara
Amarina: amarine
Amaroidal: amaroidal
Amaróide: amaroid
Amassamento: pétrissage
Amastia: amastia
Amastigota: amastigote
Amatofobia: amathophobia
Amatoxina: amatoxin
Amaurose: amaurosis
Amaurótico: amaurotic
Amaxofobia: amaxophobia
Ambageusia: ambageusia
Âmbar: amber
Âmbar-gris: ambergris
Ambiceptor: amboceptor
Ambidestrismo: ambidexterity, ambidextrism
Ambidestro: ambidextrous
Ambiente: ambient, surround
Ambigüidade: ambiguity
Ambíguo: ambiguous
Ambilateral: ambilateral

Ambílevo: ambilevous, ambisinister, ambisinistrous
Ambissexual: ambisexual
Ambivalência: ambivalence
Ambivalente: ambivalent
Ambivertido: ambivert
Ambligeustia: amblygeustia
Ambliogênico: amblyogenic
Ambliopia: amblyopia
Ambliópico: amblyopic
Amblioscópio: amblyoscope
Ambomalear: ambomalleal
Ambrosina: ambrosin
Ambucetamida: ambucetamide
Ambufilina: ambuphylline
Ambulância: ambulance
Ambulatorial, ambulante: ambulatory, ambulant
Ameba: ameba, **pl.** amebae, amebas
Amebaporo: amoebapore
Amebíase: amebiasis
Amebicida: amebacide, amebicidal, amebicide
Amébico: amebic
Amebiforme: amebiform
Amebócito: amebocyte
Amebóide: ameboid
Ameboidicidade: ameboididity
Ameboísmo: amebaism
Ameboma: ameboma
Amébula: amebula, **pl.** amebulae, amebule
Amebúria: ameburia
Ameixa seca: prune
Amelanótico: amelanotic
Amelia: amelia
Ameloblasto: ameloblast, enameloblast, ganoblast
Ameloblastoma: ameloblastoma
Amelodentinário: amelodentinal, dentinoenamel
Amelogênese: amelogenesis, enamelogenesis
Amelogeninas: amelogenins
Amência: amentia
Amencial: amential
Amenia: amenia
Amenorréia: amenorrhea
Amenorreico: amenorrheal, amenorrheic
Amerício: americium (Am)
Amerismo: amerism
Amerístico: ameristic
Ametopterina: amethopterin
Ametria: ametria
Ametropia: ametropia
Ametrópico: ametropic
Amiantáceo: amiantaceous
Amiantóide: amianthoid
Amicofobia: amychophobia
Amicrobiano: amicrobic
Amicroscópico: amicroscopic
Amida: amide
Amida acética: acetic amide
Amida da angiotensina: angiotensin amide
Amida do ácido nicotínico: nicotinic acid amide
Amidase: amidase
Amidases: amidases

Amidina: amidine
Amidinoidrolases: amidinohydrolases
Amidinotransferases: amidinotransferases
Amido: amylum, starch
Amidoidrolases: amidohydrolases
Amidopirina: amidopyrine
Amidoxil: amidoxyl
Amidoximas: amidoximes
Amielencefalia: amyelencephalia
Amielencefálico, amielencéfalo: amyelencephalic, amyelencephalous
Amielia: amyelia
Amiélico: amyelic, amyelous
Amielínico: amyelinic
Amielinização: amyelination
Amielinizado: amyelinated, unmyelinated
Amielóico: amyeloic, amyelonic
Amígdala: amygdala, **gen. e pl.** amygdalae
Amigdalase: amygdalase
Amigdalina: amygdalin, amygdaline
Amigdalóide: amygdaloid
Amigdalose: amygdalose
Amigdalosídeo: amygdaloside
Amil valerato: apple oil
Amila: amyl
Amiláceo: amylaceous
Amilase: amylase
α-amilase: α-amylase
β-amilase: β-amylase
γ-amilase: γ-amylase
Amilase do sacarogênio: saccharogen amylase
Amilasúria: amylasuria
Amilemia: amylemia
Amileno: amylene
Amilina: amylin
Amilo-1,4:1,6-glicanotransferase: amylo-1,4:1,6-glucantransferase
Amilo-(1,4→1,6)-transglicosidase ou transglicosilase: amylo-(1,4→1,6)-transglucosidase, amylo-(1,4→1,6)-transglucosylase
Amilo-1,6-glicosidase: amylo-1,6-glucosidase
Amilodextrina: amylodextrin
Amilofagia: amylophagia, starch-eating
Amilogênese: amylogenesis
Amilogênico: amylogenic
Amiloglicosidase: amyloglucosidase
Amilóide: amyloid
Amiloidoma: amyloidoma
Amiloidose: amyloidosis
Amilólise: amylolysis
Amilolítico: amylolytic
Amilomaltase: amylomaltase
Amilopectina: amylopectin
Amilopectina 1,6-glicosidase: amylopectin 1,6-glucosidase
Amilopectina 6-glicanoidrolase: amylopectin 6-glucanohydrolase
Amilopectinose: amylopectinosis
Amiloplasto: amyloplast
Amilopsina: amylopsin
Amilorréia: amylorrhea
Amilose: amylose
Amilosúria: amylosuria
Amilúria: amyluria
Amimia: amimia
Amina: amine
Aminação: amination
Aminar: aminate
Aminase fumárica: fumaric aminase
Aminérgico: aminergic
Aminoacetato de diidroxialumínio: dihydroxyaluminum aminoacetate
Aminoacidemia: aminoacidemia
Aminoácido: amino acid (AA, aa)
α-aminoácido: α-amino acid
Aminoácido-ARNt ligases: aminoacid-tRNA ligases
D-aminoácido aromático descarboxilase: aromatic D-amino acid decarboxylase
Aminoacidúria: aminoaciduria
Aminoacila: aminoacyl (AA, aa)
Aminoaciladenilato: aminoacyl adenylate
Aminoacil-ARNt: aminoacyl-tRNA
Aminoacilase: aminoacylase
9-aminoacridina: 9-aminoacridine
Aminobenzeno: aminobenzene
D(-)-α-aminobenzilpenicilina: D(-)-α-aminobenzylpenicillin
Aminocarbonil: aminocarbonyl
2-amino-2-desoxi-D-galactose: 2-amino-2-deoxy-D-galactose
Aminofenazona: aminophenazone
Aminofilina: aminophylline
Aminoglicosídeo: aminoglycoside
Aminoglutetimida: aminoglutethimide
5-aminoimidazol ribose 5′-fosfato: 5-aminoimidazole ribose 5′-phosphate (AIR)
5-aminoimidazol ribotídeo: 5-aminoimidazole ribotide (AIR)
5-aminoimidazol-4-N-succinocarboxamida ribonucleotídeo: 5-aminoimidazole-4-N-succinocarboxamide ribonucleotide
β-aminoisobutirato:piruvato aminotransferase: β-aminoisobutyrate:pyruvate aminotransferase
δ-aminolevulinato desidratase: δ-aminolevulinate dehydratase
Aminólise: aminolysis
Aminometradina: aminometradine
Aminometramida: aminometramide
Aminopenicilinas: aminopenicillins
Aminopeptidase (citosol): aminopeptidase (cytosol)
Aminopeptidase (microssomial): aminopeptidase (microsomal)
Aminopeptidases: aminopeptidases
4-aminopiridina: 4-aminopyridine
Aminopirina: aminopyrine
Aminopromazina: aminopromazine
Aminopterina: aminopterin
6-aminopurina: 6-aminopurine
Aminorex: aminorex
Aminoterminal: amino-terminal
Aminotransferases: aminotransferases
Aminotriazol: aminotriazole
Aminotripeptidase: aminotripeptidase
Aminúria: aminuria
Amioestesia: amyoesthesia, amyoesthesis
Amioplasia: amyoplasia
Amiostasia: amyostasia
Amiostático: amyostatic
Amiostenia: amyosthenia
Amiostênico: amyosthenic
Amiotaxia: amyotaxy, amyotaxia
Amiotonia: amyotonia
Amiotrofia: amyotrophia, amyotrophy
Amitiozona: amithiozone
Amitose: amitosis
Amitótico: amitotic
Amitrol: amitrole
Amixorréia: amyxorrhea
Amlodipina: amlodipine
Amnésia: amnesia
Amnésico: amnesiac, amnesic, amnestic
Âmnio: amnion
Amniocele: amniocele
Amniocentese: amniocentesis
Amniocorial: amniochorial, amniochorionic
Amniogênese: amniogenesis
Amniografia: amniography
Amnioinfusão: amnioinfusion
Amnioma: amnioma
Amniônico: amnionic
Amnionite: amnionitis
Amniorréia: amniorrhea
Amniorrexe: amniorrhexis
Amnioscopia: amnioscopy
Amnioscópio: amnioscope
Amniótico: amniotic
Amniotomia: amniotomy
Amniótomo: amniotome
Amobarbital: amobarbital
Amolecimento: mollities
Amonemia: ammonemia, ammoniemia
Amônia: ammonia
Amônia liases: ammonia-lyases
Amoníaca: ammoniac
Amoniacado: ammoniated
Amoniacal: ammoniacal
Amônio: ammonium
Amoniólise: ammonolysis
Amoniotelia: ammonotelia
Amoniotélico: ammonotelic
Amoniotelismo: ammonotelism
Amoniúria: ammoniuria
Amoque: amok, amuck
Amor próprio: self-love
Amorfagnosia: amorphagnosia
Amorfia: amorphia, amorphism
Amorfo: amorphous, amorphus
Amorfossíntese: amorphosynthesis
Amortecedor de tensão: stress breaker
Amortecimento: damping
Amostra: sample, specimen
Amostragem: sampling
Amoxapina: amoxapine
Amoxicilina: amoxicillin
AMP cíclico: cyclic AMP
3′,5′-AMP cíclico sintetase: 3′,5′-cyclic AMP synthetase
AMP desaminase: AMP deaminase
AMPc fosfodiesterase: cAMP phosphodiesterase
Amperagem: amperage
Ampere: ampere (A)
Amperimetria: amperometry
Amperômetro: ammeter (am)
Ampicilina: ampicillin
Amplexo: amplexus
Ampliação: amplification, magnification
Amplificador: amplifier
Amplitude: amplitude, span
Amplo espectro: broad-spectrum
Ampola: ampoule, ampule, ampul, ampulla, **gen. e pl.** ampullae
Ampular: ampullar
Ampulite: ampullitis
Amputação: amputation
Amputado: amputee
Amusia: amusia
Anabiose: anabiosis
Anabiótico: anabiotic
Anabólico: anabolic
Anabolismo: anabolism
Anabolito: anabolite
Anacamptômetro: anacamptometer
Anacatadídimo: anakatadidymus, anacatadidymus
Anacatestesia: anacatesthesia
Anacidez: anacidity
Anáclase: anaclasis
Anaclítico: anaclitic
Anacmese: anakmesis
Anacré: anákhré
Anacrótico: anacrotic
Anacrotismo: anacrotism
Anacusia: anacusis, anakusis

Glossário

Anadenia: anadenia
Anadicrótico: anadicrotic
Anadicrotismo: anadicrotism
Anadídimo: anadidymus
Anadipsia: anadipsia
Anadrenalismo: anadrenalism
Anádromo: anadromous
Anaeróbico: anaerobic
Anaeróbio: anaerobe
Anaerobiose: anaerobiosis
Anaerófito: anaerophyte
Anaerogênico: anaerogenic
Anaeroplastia: anaeroplasty
Anáfase: anaphase
Anafia: anaphia, anhaphia
Anafilactogênese: anaphylactogenesis
Anafilactogênico: anaphylactogenic
Anafilactógeno: anaphylactogen
Anafilactóide: anaphylactoid
Anafilático: anaphylactic
Anafilatoxina: anaphylatoxin
Anafilaxia: anaphylaxis
Anafilotoxina: anaphylotoxin
Anaforese: anaphoresis
Anaforético: anaphoretic
Anafrodisíaco: anaphrodisiac
Anagênese: anagenesis
Anagenético: anagenetic
Anágeno: anagen
Anagogia: anagogy
Anal: anal
Analbuminemia: analbuminemia
Analéptico: analeptic
Analérgico: anallergic
Analfalipoproteinemia: analphalipoproteinemia
Analgesia: analgesia
Analgésico: analgesic
Analgesímetro: analgesimeter
Analgético: analgetic
Analidade: anality
Analisado: analyte
Analisador: analyzer, analyzor
Analisando: analysand
Análise: analysis, **pl.** analyses; assay
Análise de Grunstein-Hogness: Grunstein-Hogness assay
Analista: analyst
Analítico: analytic, analytical
Análogo: analog, analogous, analogue
Anamnese: anamnesis
Anamnéstico: anamnestic
Anamniônico, anamniótico: anamnionic, anamniotic
Anamorfo: anamorph
Anamorfose: anamorphosis
Ananastasia: ananastasia
Anancasma: anancasm
Anancastia: anancastia
Anancástico: anancastic
Anandria: anandria
Anangioplasia: anangioplasia
Anangioplásico: anangioplastic
Anão: dwarf
Anaplasia: anaplasia
Anaplástico: anaplastic

Anaplastologia: anaplastology
Anaplerose: anaplerosis
Anaplerótico: anaplerotic
Anapófise: anapophysis
Anáptico: anaptic
Anarritmia: anarithmia
Anartria: anarthria
Anasarca: anasarca
Anasarco: anasarcous
Anastigmata: anastigmats
Anastigmático: anastigmatic
Anástole: anastole
Anastomosar: anastomose
Anastomose: anastomosis, **pl.** anastomoses
Anastomótico: anastomotic
Anastral: anastral
Anatomia: anatomy
Anatômico: anatomical
Anatomista: anatomist
Anatomocirúrgico: anatomicosurgical
Anatomomédico: anatomicomedical
Anatomopatológico: anatomicopathologic
Anatopismo: anatopism
Anatóxico: anatoxic
Anatoxina: anatoxin
Anatricrótico: anatricrotic
Anatricrotismo: anatricrotism
Anatripsia: anatripsis
Anatríptico: anatriptic
Anaxônio: anaxon, anaxone
Anazotúria: anazoturia
Ancestral: ancestor
Ancilobléfaro: ankyloblepharon
Ancilodactilia, anquilodactilia: ankylodactyly, ankylodactylia
Anciloglossia: ankyloglossia
Ancilômelo: ankylomele
Ancilosado: ankylosed
Ancilose: ankylosis
Ancilostomático: ancylostomatic
Ancilostomatídeo: hookworm
Ancilostomíase: ancylostomiasis, ankylostomiasis
Ancilóstomo: *Ancylostoma*
Ancilótico: ankylotic
Ancinonida: amcinonide
Ancipital: ancipital, ancipitate, ancipitous
Ancirina: ankyrin
Anciróide: ancyroid, ankyroid
Ancôneo: anconad, anconal, anconeal, anconeus
Anconóide: anconoid
Ancoragem: anchorage
Ancorina: anchorin
Ancusina: anchusin
Andira: andira, worm bark
Andrenosterona: andrenosterone
Andriatria: andriatrics, andriatry
Androfobia: androphobia
Androgênese: androgenesis
Androgênico: androgenic
Androgênio: androgen

Andrógeno: androgenous
Androginia: androgyny
Androginismo: androgynism
Andrógino: androgynous
Androginóide: androgynoid
Andróide: android, andromorphus
Andrologia: andrology
Andromedotoxina: andromedotoxin
Andropatia: andropathy
Andropausa: andropause
Androstanediol: androstanediol
Androstanediona: androstanedione
Androstano: androstane
Androstenediol: androstenediol
Androstenediona: androstenedione
Androsteno: androstene
Androstenol: androstenol
Androstenolona: androstenolone
Androsterona: androsterone
Anecóico: anechoic, echo-free
Anedonia: anhedonia
Anéfrico: anephric
Anel: anulus, **pl.** anuli; ring
Aneletrotônico: anelectrotonic
Aneletrotônus: anelectrotonus
Anelídeo: annellide
Anelídios: annelids
Aneloconídio: annelloconidium
Anemia: anemia
Anêmico: anemic
Anemofobia: anemophobia
Anemômetro: anemometer
Anemonol: anemonol
Anemotrofia: anemotrophy
Anencefalia: anencephalia, anencephaly
Anencefálico: anencephalic
Anencéfalo: anencephalous
Anêntero: anenterous
Anenzimia: anenzymia
Anepiplóico: anepiploic
Anergia: anergia, anergy
Anérgico: anergic
Aneritroplasia: anerythroplasia
Aneritroplástico: anerythroplastic
Aneritrorregenerativo: anerythroregenerative
Aneróide: aneroid
Anestecinesia: anesthecinesia, anesthekinesia
Anestesia: anesthesia
Anestesiação: anesthetization
Anestesiar: anesthetize
Anestésico: anesthetic
Anestesiologia: anesthesiology
Anestesiologista: anesthesiologist
Anestesista: anesthetist
Anestro: anestrum, anestrus
Anetodermia: anetoderma
Anetopata: anethopath
Aneuplóide: aneuploid
Aneuploidia: aneuploidy
Aneurina: aneurine
Aneurisma: aneurysm

Aneurismático: aneurysmal, aneurysmatic
Aneurismectomia: aneurysmectomy
Aneurismoplastia: aneurysmoplasty
Aneurismorrafia: aneurysmorrhaphy
Aneurismotomia: aneurysmotomy
Aneurolêmico: aneurolemmic
Anexal: annexal
Anexinas: annexins
Anexos: annexa
Anfetamina: amphetamine
Anfiartrodial: amphiarthrodial
Anfiartrose: amphiarthrosis
Anfiáster: amphiaster
Anfibólico: amphibolic
Anficário: amphikaryon
Anficelo: amphicelous
Anficêntrico: amphicentric
Anfícito: amphicyte
Anficlexe: amphiclexis
Anficróico: amphichroic
Anficromático: amphichromatic
Anficromatófilo: amphochromatophil, amphochromatophile
Anficromófilo: amphochromophil, amphochromophile
Anfídio: amphid
Anfidiplóide: amphidiploid
Anfifílico: amphiphilic
Anfifóbico: amphiphobic
Anfileucêmico: amphileukemic
Anfimicróbio: amphimicrobe
Anfimítico: amphimictic
Anfimixia: amphimixis
Anfinucléolo: amphinucleolus
Anfioxo: Amphioxus
Anfipático: amphipathic
Anfístoma: amphistome
Anfiteatro: theater
Anfitipia: amphitypy
Anfítrico: amphitrichate, amphitrichous
Anfixenose: amphixenosis
Anfócito: amphocyte
Anfofílico: amphophilic, amphophilous
Anfófilo: amphophil, amphophile
Anfolito: ampholyte
Anfomicina: amphomycin
Anfórico: amphoric
Anforilóquia: amphoriloquy
Anforofonia: amphorophony
Anfotericina, anfotericina B: amphotericin, amphotericin B
Anfotérico: amphoteric
Angelim branco: cabbage tree
Angiectasia: angiectasia, angiectasis
Angiectático: angiectatic
Angiectopia: angiectopia
Angiite: angiitis, angitis
Angina: angina
Anginiforme: anginiform
Anginofobia: anginophobia

Anginóide: anginoid
Anginoso: anginal, anginose, anginous
Angioarquitetura: angioarchitecture
Angioblasto: angioblast
Angioblastoma: angioblastoma
Angiocardiocinético: angiocardiokinetic, angiocardiocinetic
Angiocardiografia: angiocardiography
Angiocardiopatia: angiocardiopathy
Angioceratoma: angiokeratoma
Angioceratose: angiokeratosis
Angiocisto: angiocyst
Angiocolite: angiocholitis
Angioderma: angioderm
Angiodisplasia: angiodysplasia
Angiodistrofia: angiodystrophy, angiodystrophia
Angioedema: angioedema
Angioelefantíase: angioelephantiasis
Angioendoteliomatose: angioendotheliomatosis
Angiofacomatose: angiophacomatosis, angiophakomatosis
Angiofibrolipoma: angiofibrolipoma
Angiofibroma: angiofibroma
Angiofibrose: angiofibrosis
Angiogênese: angiogenesis
Angiogênico: angiogenic
Angioglioma: angioglioma
Angiogliomatose: angiogliomatosis
Angiogliose: angiogliosis
Angiografia: angiography
Angiográfico: angiographic
Angiograma: angiogram
Angioialinose: angiohyalinosis
Angióide: angioid
Angioinvasivo: angioinvasive
Angioipertonia: angiohypertonia
Angioipotonia: angiohypotonia
Angioleiomioma: angioleiomyoma
Angiolipofibroma: angiolipofibroma
Angiolipoma: angiolipoma
Angiólise: angiolysis
Angiolítico: angiolithic
Angiolito: angiolith
Angiologia: angiologia, angiology
Angioma: angioma
Angiomatóide: angiomatoid
Angiomatose: angiomatosis
Angiomatoso: angiomatous
Angiomegalia: angiomegaly
Angiomiocárdico: angiomyocardiac
Angiomiofibroma: angiomyofibroma
Angiomiolipoma: angiomyolipoma
Angiomioma: angiomyoma

Angiomiopatia: angiomyopathy
Angiomiossarcoma: angiomyosarcoma
Angiomixoma: angiomyxoma
Angioneurectomia: angioneurectomy
Angioneuropatia: angioneuropathy
Angioneurótico: angioneurotic
Angioneurotomia: angioneurotomy
Angioparalisia: angioparalysis
Angioparesia: angioparesis
Angiopatia: angiopathy
Angiopático: angiopathic
Angioplania: angioplany
Angioplastia: angioplasty
Angiopoese: angiopoiesis
Angiopoético: angiopoietic
Angiorrafia: angiorrhaphy
Angioscopia: angioscopy
Angioscópio: angioscope
Angioscotoma: angioscotoma
Angioscotometria: angioscotometry
Angiose: angiosis
Angiospasmo: angiospasm
Angiospástico: angiospastic
Angiossarcoma: angiosarcoma
Angiossoma: angiosome
Angiostenose: angiostenosis
Angiostrongilose: angiostrongylosis
Angiotelectasia: angiotelectasis, angiotelectasia
Angiotensina: angiotensin
Angiotensina I: angiotensin I
Angiotensina II: angiotensin II
Angiotensina III: angiotensin III
Angiotensinase: angiotensinase
Angiotensinogenase: angiotensinogenase
Angiotensinogênio: angiotensinogen
Angiotomia: angiotomy
Angulação: angulation
Ângulo: angle (θ), angulus, **gen. e pl.** anguli
Aniacinamidose: aniacinamidosis
Aniacinose: aniacinosis
Anictérico: anicteric
Anídeo: anidean, anideus, anidous
Anidrase: anhydrase
Anidratação: anhydration
Anidrido: anhydride
Anidrido carbônico: carbonic anhydride
Anidrido cumárico: coumaric anhydride
Anidrido silícico: silicic anhydride
Anidroaçúcares: anhydrosugars
3,6-anidrogalactose: 3,6-anhydrogalactose
Anidrogitalina: anhydrogitalin
Anidroleucovorina: anhydroleucovorin
Anidrose: anhidrosis
Anidroso: anhydrous

Anidrótico: anhidrotic
Anileridina: anileridine
Anilida: anilide
Anilina: aniline
Anilina azul: aniline blue
Anilíngua: anilinction, anilinctus, anilingus
Anilinófilo: anilinophil, anilinophile, anilinophilous
Anilismo: anilinism, anilism
Animação: animation
Animal: animal
Animálculo: animalcule
Animatismo: animatism
Animismo: animism
Ânimo: animus
Ânion: anion (A^-)
Aniônico: anionic
Anionotropia: anionotropy
Aniridia: aniridia
Anis: anise
Anis estrelado ou anis chinês: illicium
Anisado: anisate
Anisaquíase: anisakiasis
Anísico: anisic
Anisindiona: anisindione
Anisoacomodação: anisoaccommodation
Anisocariose: anisokaryosis
Anisocitose: anisocytosis
Anisoconia: aniseikonia
Anisocoria: anisocoria
Anisocromasia: anisochromasia
Anisocromático: anisochromatic
Anisodactilia: anisodactyly
Anisodáctilo: anisodactylous
Anisogamia: anisogamy
Anisognato: anisognathous
Anisol: anisole
Anisomastia: anisomastia
Anisomelia: anisomelia
Anisometropia: anisometropia
Anisometrópico: anisometropic
Anisopiese: anisopiesis
Anisorritmia: anisorrhythmia
Anisosfigmia: anisosphygmia
Anisostênico: anisosthenic
Anisotônico: anisotonic
Anisotrópico: anisotropic
Anístico: anhistic, anhistous
Anociassociação: anociassociation
Anococcígeo: anococcygeal
Anocromasia: anochromasia
Anoderma: anoderm
Anódico: anodal, anodic, anodyne
Anódio: anode
Anodontia: anodontia, anodontism
Anoespinal: anospinal
Anoético: anoetic
Anofelicida: anophelicide
Anofelífugo: anophelifuge
Anofelino: anopheline
Anofelinos: Anophelini
Anofelismo: anophelism
Anoftalmia: anophthalmia, anophthalmos
Anogenital: anogenital

Anomalia: anomalad, anomaly
Anomaloscópio: anomaloscope
Anômero: anomer
Anomia: anomia, anomie
Anoníquia: anonychia, anonychosis
Anoplastia: anoplasty
Anorético: anorectic, anoretic, anorexic
Anorexia: anorexia
Anorexiante: anorexiant
Anorexigênico: anorexigenic
Anorgasmia: anorgasmy, anorgasmia
Anormal: abnormal
Anormalidade: abnormality
Anorquia: anorchia, anorchism
Anorretal: anorectal
Anoscópio: anoscope
Anosmia: anosmia
Anósmico: anosmic
Anosodiaforia: anosodiaphoria
Anosognosia: anosognosia
Anosognósico: anosognosic
Anossigmoidoscopia: anosigmoidoscopy
Anosteoplasia: anosteoplasia
Anostose: anostosis
Anotia: anotia
Anoto: annotto
Anovesical: anovesical
Anovulação: anovulation
Anovulatório: anovular, anovulatory
Anoxemia: anoxemia
Anoxia: anoxia
Anóxico: anoxic
Anserino: anserine
Ânsia de vômito: gag, retch, retching, vomiturition
Ansiedade: anxiety
Ansiforme: ansiform
Ansiolítico: anxiolytic
Ansotomia: ansotomy
Antagonismo: antagonism
Antagonista: antagonist
Antalgesia: antalgesia
Antálgico: antalgic
Antebraço: antebrachium, antibrachium, forearm
Antebraquial: antebrachial, antibrachial
Antecedente: antecedent
Antecipação: anticipation
Antecipar: anticipate
Antecubital: antecubital
Antefletir: anteflex
Anteflexão: anteflexion
Antélice: anthelix, antihelix
Antelona: anthelone
Anteparto: antepartum
Antepirético: antepyretic
Anteposição: anteposition
Anterídio: antheridium
Anterior: anterior
Ântero-externo: anteroexternal
Anterógrado: antegrade, anterograde
Ântero-inferior: anteroinferior
Ântero-interno: anterointernal
Ântero-lateral: anterolateral

Glossário

Anteromedial: anteromedial
Anteromediano: anteromedian
Ântero-posterior: anteroposterior
Ântero-superior: anterosuperior
Ante-sístole: antesystole
Anteversão: anteversion
Antevertido: anteverted
Antiácido: antacid, antiacid
Antiadrenérgico: antiadrenergic
Antiafrodisíaco: antaphrodisiac, antaphroditic
Antiaglutinina: antiagglutinin
Antialcalino: antalkaline
Antialérgico: antiallergic
Antialexina: antialexin
Antianafilaxia: antianaphylaxis
Antiandrogênio: antiandrogen
Antianêmico: antianemic
Antianticorpo: antiantibody
Antiantígeno: isoantigen
Antiantitoxina: antiantitoxin
Antiaracnolisina: antiarachnolysin
Antiarrítmico: antiarrhythmic, antidysrhythmic
Antiartrítico: antarthritic, antiarthritic
Antiasmático: antasthmatic, antiasthmatic
Antiastênico: antasthenic
Antiatrófico: antatrophic
Antiautolisina: antiautolysin
Antibacteriano: antibacterial
Antibionte: antibiont
Antibiose: antibiosis
Antibiótico: antibiotic
Antibiótico-resistente: antibiotic-resistant
Antibiotina: antibiotin
Antiblenorrágico: antiblennorrhagic
Antibrômico: antibromic
Anticalculoso: anticalculous
Anticarioso: anticarious
Anticatexia: anticathexis
Anticefalálgico: anticephalalgic
Anticetogênese: antiketogenesis
Anticetogênico: antiketogenic
Anticitotoxina: anticytotoxin
Anticlinal: anticlinal
Anticoagulante: anticoagulant
Anticódon: anticodon
Anticolagogo: anticholagogue
Anticolinérgico: anticholinergic
Anticolinesterase: anticholinesterase
Anticomplementar: anticomplementary
Anticomplemento: anticomplement
Anticontagioso: anticontagious
Anticonvulsivante: anticonvulsant
Anticonvulsivo: anticonvulsive
Anticorpo (Ac): antibody (Ab)
Anticorpo catalítico: abzyme
Anticurare: anticurare
Antidepressivo: antidepressant
Antidiabético: antidiabetic

Antidiarreico: antidiarrheal, antidiarrhetic
Antidisentérico: antidysenteric
Antidisúrico: antidysuric
Antidiurese: antidiuresis
Antidiurético: antidiuretic
Antidotal: antidotal
Antídoto: antidote
Antidrômico: antidromic
Antiemético: antiemetic
Antienérgico: antienergic
Antienzima: antienzyme
Antiepiléptico: antiepileptic
Antierótico: anterotic
Antiescorbútico: antiscorbutic
Antiespasmódico: antispasmodic
Antiestafilocócico: antistaphylococcic
Antiestafilolisina: antistaphylolysin
Antiesteapsina: antisteapsin
Antiestreptocinase: antistreptokinase
Antiestreptocócico: antistreptococcic
Antiestreptolisina: antistreptolysin
Antiestrogênio: antiestrogen
Antifagocítico: antiphagocytic
Antifebril: antefebrile, antifebrile
Antifibrilatório: antifibrillatory
Antifibrinolisina: antifibrinolysin
Antifibrinolítico: antifibrinolytic
Antiflogístico: antiphlogistic
Antifóbico: antiphobic
Antifólico: antifolic
Antifúngico: antifungal
Antigenemia: antigenemia
Antigenicidade: antigenicity
Antigênico: antigenic
Antígeno (Ag): antigen (Ag)
Antígeno de Gerbich: Gerbich antigen
Antigenoma: antigenome
Antigonorreico: antigonorrheic
Antigravidade: antigravity
Anti-HB$_c$: anti-HB$_c$
Anti-HB$_e$: anti-HB$_e$
Anti-HB$_s$: anti-HB$_s$
Anti-helmíntico: anthelminthic, anthelmintic, antihelminthic
Anti-hemaglutinina: antihemagglutinin
Anti-hemolisina: antihemolysin
Anti-hemolítico: antihemolytic
Anti-hemorrágico: antihemorrhagic
Anti-hidrópico: antihydropic
Anti-higiênico: insanitary
Anti-hipertensivo: antihypertensive
Anti-hipnótico: antihypnotic
Anti-hipotensivo: antihypotensive
Anti-histaminas: antihistamines
Anti-histamínico: antihistaminic
Anti-hormônios: antihormones

Antiictérico: anti-icteric
Antiinflamatório: antiinflammatory
Antiinsulina: anti-insulin
Antileucocidina: antileukocidin
Antileucotoxina: antileukotoxin
Antileucotrieno: antileukotriene
Antilipotrópico: antilipotropic
Antilisina: antilysin
Antilítico: antilithic
Antiluteogênico: antiluteogenic
Antimalárico: antimalarial
Antímero: antimere
Antimesentérico: antimesenteric
Antimetabólito: antimetabolite
Antimetropia: antimetropia
Antimiastênico: antimyasthenic
Antimicótico: antimycotic
Antimicrobiano: antimicrobial
Antimitótico: antimitotic
Antimongolóide: antimongoloid
Antimonídio: antimonid
Antimonil: antimonyl
Antimônio: stibium
Antimônio (Sb): antimony (Sb)
Antimuscarínico: antimuscarinic
Antimutagênico: antimutagenic
Antimutágeno: antimutagen
Antinauseante: antinauseant
Antineoplásico: antineoplastic
Antineurotoxina: antineurotoxin
Antinial: antiniad, antinial
Antínio: antinion
Antinomia: antinomy
Antinuclear: antinuclear
Antiodontálgico: antiodontalgic
Antiolimina: anthiolimine
Antioncogene: antioncogene
Antioxidante: antioxidant
Antiparalelo: antiparallel
Antiparasitário: antiparasitic
Antipediculótico: antipediculotic
Antiperiódico: antiperiodic
Antiperistalse: antiperistalsis
Antiperistáltico: antiperistaltic
Antiperspirante: antiperspirant
Antipiogênico: antipyogenic
Antipirese: antipyresis
Antipirético: antipyretic
Antipirimidina: antipyrimidine
Antipirina: antipyrine
Antipirótico: antipyrotic
Antiplaquetário: antiplatelet
Antiplasmina: antiplasmin
Antipneumocócico: antipneumococcic
Antípoda: antipodal
Antípoda: antipode
Antiprecipitina: antiprecipitin
Antiprogestina: antiprogestin
Antiprotrombina: antiprothrombin
Antiprurítico: antipruritic
Antipsicótico: antipsychotic
Antipurina: antipurine
α_1-antiquimotripsina: α_1-antichymotrypsin
Anti-raquítico: antirachitic
Anti-reumático: antirheumatic

Anti-ricina: antiricin
Anti-ruminante: antiruminant
Anti-S: anti-S
Anti-seborreico: antiseborrheic
Anti-secretório: antisecretory
Anti-sentido: antisense
Anti-sepsia: antisepsis
Anti-séptico: antiseptic
Anti-sialagogo: antisialagogue
Anti-siderótico: antisideric
Anti-social: antisocial
Anti-soro: antiserum
Antitenar: antithenar
Antiterminal: antitermination
Antitetânico: antitetanic
Antitifóide: antityphoid
Antitireóideo: antithyroid
Antitônico: antitonic
Antitóxico: antitoxic
Antitoxígeno: antitoxigen
Antitoxina: antitoxin
Antitoxinogênio: antitoxinogen
Antitrago: antitragus
Antitreponêmico: antitreponemal
Antitripsina: antitrypsin
Antitríptico: antitrypsic, antitryptic
Antitrismo: antitrismus
Antitrombina: antithrombin
Antitrópico: antitropic
Antítropo: antitrope
Antitumorigênese: antitumorigenesis
Antitussígeno: antibechic
Antitussivo: antitussive
Antiveneno: antivenene
Antivenéreo: antivenereal
Antivenina: antivenin
Antiviral: antiviral
Antivitamina: antivitamin
Antivivissecção: antivivisection
Antixeroftálmico: antixerophthalmi
Antixerótico: antixerotic
Antocianinas: anthocyanins
Antracemia: anthracemia
Antraceno: anthracene
Antraciclina: anthracycline
Antrácico: anthracic
Antracina: anthracin
Antracose: anthracosis
Antracossilicose: anthracosilicosis
Antracótico: anthracotic
Antral: antral
Antralina: anthralin
Antramucina: anthramucin
Antraniloíla: anthraniloyl
Antrapurpurina: anthrapurpurin
9,10-antraquinona: 9,10-anthraquinone
Antraz: anthrax, charbon
Antrectomia: antrectomy
Antro: antrum, **gen.** antri, **pl.** antra
Antrofosia: antrophose
Antrona: anthrone
Antronasal: antronasal
Antropilórico: antropyloric

Antropobiologia: anthropobiology
Antropocêntrico: anthropocentric
Antropofílico: anthropophilic
Antropofobia: anthropophobia
Antropogênese: anthropogenesis
Antropogenia: anthropogeny
Antropogênico: anthropogenic, anthropogenetic
Antropogonia: anthropogony
Antropografia: anthropography
Antropóide: anthropoid
Antropologia: anthropology
Antropometria: anthropometry
Antropométrico: anthropometric
Antropômetro: anthropometer
Antropomorfismo: anthropomorphism
Antroponomia: anthroponomy
Antropopatia: anthropopathy
Antroposcopia: anthroposcopy
Antropossomatologia: anthroposomatology
Antropozoonose: anthropozoonosis
Antroscopia: antroscopy
Antroscópio: antroscope
Antrostomia: antrostomy
Antrotimpânico: antrotympanic
Antrotomia: antrotomy
Antrotonia: antrotonia
Anulação: undoing
Anular: annular, anular
Ânulo: annulus
Anuloplastia: annuloplasty
Anulorrafia: annulorrhaphy
Anúria: anuria
Anúrico: anuric
Ânus: anus, **gen. e pl.** ani
Aorta: aorta, **gen. e pl.** aortae
Aortalgia: aortalgia
Aortectasia: aortectasis, aortectasia
Aortectomia: aortectomy
Aórtico: aortal, aortic
Aórtico-pulmonar: pulmoaortic
Aortite: aortitis
Aortocoronário: aortocoronary
Aortoesclerose: aortosclerosis
Aortoestenose: aortostenosis
Aortografia: aortography
Aortograma: aortogram
Aortopatia: aortopathy
Aortopexia: aortopexy
Aortoplastia: aortoplasty
Aortoptose: aortoptosia, aortoptosis
Aortorrafia: aortorrhaphy
Aortorrenal: aorticorenal
Aortotomia: aortotomy
Apagamento: effacement
Apalestesia: apallesthesia
Apálico: apallic
Apancreático: apancreatic
Aparalítico: aparalytic
Aparatireoidismo: aparathyroidism
Aparatireose: aparathyreosis
Aparecimento: show

Aparelho: apparatus, splint
Aparelho auditivo: hearing aid
Aparelho de diatermia: dynatherm
Aparente: apparent
Apareunia: apareunia
Apatia: apathy
Apático: apathetic
Apatismo: apathism
Apatita: apatite
Apendalgia: appendalgia
Apendectomia: appendectomy
Apêndice: appendage, appendix, **gen.** appendicis, **pl.** appendices
Apêndice vermiforme: vermix
Apendicectasia: appendicectasis
Apendicectomia: appendicectomy
Apendicismo: appendicism
Apendicite: appendicitis
Apendicocele: appendicocele
Apendicólise: appendicolysis
Apendicolitíase: appendicolithiasis
Apendicolito: appendicolith
Apendicostomia: appendicostomy
Apendicovesicostomia: appendicovesicostomy
Apendicular: appendical, appendiceal, appendicular
Apepsinia: apepsinia
Apercepção: apperception
Aperceptivo: apperceptive
Aperiódico: aperiodic
Aperistalse: aperistalsis
Aperitivo: aperitive
Apersonação: appersonation, appersonification
Apertognatia: apertognathia
Apertômetro: apertometer
Apetite: appetite
Apexcardiografia: apexcardiography
Apexcardiograma: apexcardiogram
Apexígrafo: apexigraph
Apical: apical, apicalis
Ápice: apex, **gen** apicis, **pl.** apices
Apicectomia: apicoectomy, apicectomy
Apicificação: apexification
Apicnomorfo: apyknomorphous
Apicólise: apicolysis
Apicolocalizador: apicolocator
Apicostomia: apicostomy
Apicóstomo: apicostome
Apicotomia: apiceotomy, apicotomy
Apiculado: apiculate
Apículo: apiculus
Apicuretagem: apicurettage
Apifobia: apiphobia
Apinealismo: apinealism
Apinhamento: crowding
Apirase: apyrase
Apirético: apyretic, apyrexial
Apirexia: apyrexia
Apituitarismo: apituitarism

Aplacentário: aplacental
Aplainamento radicular: root planing
Aplanação: applanation
Aplanático: aplanatic
Aplanatismo: aplanatism
Aplanometria: applanometry
Aplasia: aplasia
Aplásico: aplastic
Apleuria: apleuria
Aplicador: applicator
Apnéia: apnea
Apneico: apneic
Apneumia: apneumia
Apneuse: apneusis
apo-2L: apo-2L
Apobiose: apobiosis
Apócrino: apocrine
Apocrústico: apocrustic
Ápode: apodal, apodous
Apodia: apodia, apody
Apodrecer: rot
Apoenzima: apoenzyme (apo)
Apoferritina: apoferritin
Apofilaxia: apophylaxis
Apofisário: apophysary, apophysial, apophyseal
Apófise: apophysis, **pl.** apophyses
Apofisite: apophysitis
Apogamia: apogamia, apogamy
Apogeu: apogee
Apoindutor: apoinducer
Apoio: backing
Apoio vital avançado: advanced life support
Apolar: apolar
Apolipoproteína: apolipoprotein (apo)
Apomixia: apomixia
Aponeurectomia: aponeurectomy
Aponeurorrafia: aponeurorrhaphy
Aponeurose: aponeurosis, **pl.** aponeuroses
Aponeurosite: aponeurositis
Aponeurótico: aponeurotic
Aponeurotomia: aponeurotomy
Aponeurótomo: aponeurotome
Apoplasmia: apoplasmia
Apoplectiforme: apoplectiform
Apoplético: apoplectic
Apoplexia: apoplexy
Apoproteína: apoprotein
Apoptose: apoptosis
Aporrepressor: aporepressor
Aposição: apposition
Apossoma: aposome
Apostaxia: apostaxis
Apostia: aposthia
Apostilb: apostilb
Apotanásia: apothanasia
Apótemo: apothem, apotheme
Apózema: apozem, apozema
Apractagnosia: apractagnosia
Apragmatismo: apragmatism
Apraxia: apraxia
Apráxico: apractic, apraxic
Aprendizado: learning
Apresentação: presentation

Apresentação anômala: malpresentation
Aproctia: aproctia
Aprofeno: aprofen, aprofene, aprophen
Aprosodia: aprosody
Aprosopia: aprosopia
Aprotinina: aprotinin
Aproximação: approximation
Aproximar: approximate
Aquacobalamina: aquacobalamin
Aquafobia: aquaphobia
Aquapuntura: aquapuncture
Aquático: aquatic
Aquecimento global: global warming
Aqueduto: aqueduct, aqueductus
Aquembe: akembe
Aquiles: Achilles
Aquilia: acheilia, achylia
Aquiloso: acheilous, achilous
Aquiria: acheiria
Aquiropodia: acheiropody, achiropody
Aquiroso: acheirous, achirous
Aquisição: acquisition
Aquocobalamina: aquocobalamin
Aquosidade: aquosity
Aquoso: aqueous
Arabana: araban
Arábico: arabic
Arabina: arabin
Arabinoadenosina: arabinoadenosine
Arabinocitidina: arabinocytidine
Arabinofuranosiladenina: arabinofuranosyladenine
Arabinofuranosilcitosina: arabinofuranosylcytosine
Arabinose: arabinose (Ara), arabinosis
Arabinosídeo: arabinoside
Arabinosiladenina: arabinosyladenine
Arabinosilcitosina: arabinosylcytosine (aC, araC)
Arabinosúria: arabinosuria
Arabitol: arabitol
Aracnídeos: Arachnida
Aracnidismo: arachnidism
Aracnodactilia: arachnodactyly
Aracnofobia: arachnephobia, arachnophobia
Aracnoidal: arachnoidal
Aracnóide-máter: arachnoid, arachnoidea mater, arachnoides
Aracnoidite: arachnoiditis
Aracnolisina: arachnolysin
Aralquila: aralkyl
Arame: wire
Aranha: spider
Araruta: arrowroot
Arborescente: arborescent
Arborização: arborization
Arborizar: arborize
Arboróide: arboroid
Arbovírus: arbovirus
Arcada: arcade

Arcaico: archaic
Arciforme: arciform
Arco: arc, arch, arcus, bow
Arco em dobradiça: hingebow
Arco facial: face-bow
Arctação: arctation
Arcual: arcual
Ardência: scalding
Ardor: ardor
Área: area (a), **pl.** areae
Arecaidina: arecaidine
Arecaína: arecaine
Arecolina: arecoline
Areia: sand
Arenáceo: arenaceous
Arenoso: psammous
Aréola: areola, **pl.** areolae
Areolar: areolar
Areômetro: areometer
Arganaz do campo: field-vole
Argasídeo: argasid
Argentação: argentation
Argentafim: argentaffin, argentaffine
Argêntico: argentic
Argentino: argentine
Argentófilo: argentophil, argentophile
Argentoso: argentous
Arginase: arginase
Arginil: arginyl
Arginina: arginine (Arg)
Argininossuccinase: argininosuccinase
Argininossuccinato liase: argininosuccinate lyase
Argininossuccinicacidúria: argininosuccinicaciduria
Argipressina: argipressin
Argiria: argyria
Argírico: argyric
Argirismo: argyrism
Argirófilo: argyrophil, argyrophile
Argirol: argyrol
Argônio (Ar): argon (Ar)
Argueiro: mote
Ariepiglótico: aryepiglottic
Aril: aryl
Arilamidase: arylamidase
Arilsulfatase: arylsulfatase
Aristotélico: aristotelian
Aritenoepiglótico: arytenoepiglottidean
Aritenóide: arytenoid
Aritenoidectomia: arytenoidectomy
Aritenóideo: arytenoideus
Aritenoidite: arytenoiditis
Aritenoidopexia: arytenoidopexy
Aritmomania: arithmomania
Armação: cradle
Armadura do caráter: character armor
Armazenamento: storage
Arnica: arnica, leopard's bane
Aroil: aroyl
Aromático: aromatic
Arotinóide: arotinoid
Arpão: harpoon

Arqueado: arcate, arcuate
Arqueamento: arcuation
Arqueísmo: archaeus, archeus
Arquêntero: archenteron
Arqueocinético: archeokinetic
Arqueótipo: archetype
Arquicerebelo: archaeocerebellum, archicerebellum, vestibulocerebellum
Arquicórtex: archicortex, archipallium
Arquitetônico: architectonics
Arquitetura óssea: bone architecture
Arrafia: arrhaphia
Arranjo tridimensional: stereotaxis
Arraque: arrack
Arrasto: drag
Arreflexia: areflexia
Arrênico: arrhenic
Arrenoblastoma: arrhenoblastoma
Arriboflavinose: ariboflavinosis
Arrinencefalia: arrhinencephaly, arrhinencephalia, arhinencephaly
Arrinia: arhinia, arrhinia
Arritmia: arrhythmia
Arrítmico: arrhythmic
Arritmogênico: arrhythmogenic
Arroto: ructus
Arroz: rice
Arsacetina: arsacetin
Arsenal: armamentarium
Arsenamida: arsenamide
Arseníase: arseniasis
Arseniato: arsenate
Arsenical: arsenical
Arsenicalismo: arsenicalism
Arsênico (As): arsenic (As), arsenic, arsenium, ratsbane
Arsênico-resistente: arsenic-fast
Arsenieto: arsenide, arseniuret
Arsenioso: arsenious, arsenous
Arsenito de cobre: cupric arsenite
Arsenoterapia: arsenotherapy
Arsenóxidos: arsenoxides
Arsfenamina: arsphenamine
Arsina: arsine
Arsônio: arsonium
Arstinol: arsthinol
Artefato: artefact, artifact
Artemetro: artemether
Artemisinina: artemisinin
Arterenol: arterenol
Artéria: arteria (a), **gen. e pl.** arteriae (aa); artery (a)
Artéria anastomótica de Kugel: Kugel anastomotic artery
Artéria de Abbott: Abbott artery
Arterial: arterial
Arterialização: arterialization
Arteriectasia: arteriectasis, arteriectasia
Arteriectomia: arteriectomy
Arterioatonia: arterioatony

Arteriocapilar: arteriocapillary
Arterioestenose: arteriostenosis
Arteriografia: arteriography
Arteriográfico: arteriographic
Arteriograma: arteriogram
Arteríola: arteriola, **pl.** arteriolae; arteriole
Arteriolar: arteriolar
Arteriolite: arteriolitis
Arteriólito: arteriolith
Arteriologia: arteriology
Arteriolonecrose: arteriolonecrosis
Arteriolonefrosclerose: arteriolonephrosclerosis
Arteriolosclerose: arteriolosclerosis
Arteriolovenoso: arteriolovenous
Arteriolovenular: arteriolovenular
Arteriomalacia: arteriomalacia
Arteriômetro: arteriometer
Arteriomiomatose: arteriomyomatosis
Arteriomotor: arteriomotor
Arterionefrosclerose: arterionephrosclerosis
Arteriopatia: arteriopathy
Arterioplania: arterioplania
Arterioplastia: arterioplasty
Arteriopressor: arteriopressor
Arteriorrafia: arteriorrhaphy
Arteriorrexia: arteriorrhexis
Arteriosclerose: arteriosclerosis
Arteriosclerótico: arteriosclerotic
Arteriospasmo: arteriospasm
Arteriotomia: arteriotomy
Arteriovenoso (AV): arteriovenous (AV)
Arterite: arteritis
Articulação: articulatio, **pl.** articulationes; articulation, articulus, joint, junctura, **pl.** juncturae
Articulação sinovial: perarticulation
Articulado: articulate, articulated
Articulador dentário: articulator
Articular: arthral, articular, articulare
Articulatório: articulatory
Articulostato: articulostat
Artificial: artifactitious, artifactual
Artralgia: arthralgia
Artrálgico: arthralgic
Artrectomia: arthrectomy
Artrestesia: arthresthesia
Artrite: arthritis, **pl.** arthritides
Artrítico: arthritic
Artrítide: arthritides
Artrocatadise: arthrokatadysis
Artrocentese: arthrocentesis
Artroclasia: arthroclasia
Artrocondrite: arthrochondritis
Artroconídio: arthroconidium
Artrodese: arthrodesis

Artródia: arthrodia
Artrodial: arthrodial
Artrodinia: arthrodynia
Artrodínico: arthrodynic
Artrodisplasia: arthrodysplasia
Artroendoscopia: arthroendoscopy
Artroftalmopatia: arthroophthalmopathy
Artrógeno: arthrogenous
Artrografia: arthrography
Artrograma: arthrogram
Artrogripose: arthrogryposis
Artrólise: arthrolysis
Artrolitíase: arthrolithiasis
Artrólito: arthrolith
Artrologia: arthrologia, arthrology
Artrometria: arthrometry
Artrômetro: arthrometer
Artropatia: arthropathy
Artropatia psoriática: arthropatia psoriatica
Artropatologia: arthropathology
Artropiose: arthropyosis
Artroplastia: arthroplasty
Artropneumorradiografia: arthropneumoradiography
Artropodíase: arthropodiasis
Artropódico: arthropodic, arthropodous
Artrópodo: arthropod
Artrorese: arthroereisis
Artrórise: arthrorisis
Artrosclerose: arthrosclerosis
Artroscopia: arthroscopy
Artroscópio: arthroscope
Artrósporo: arthrospore
Artrossinovite: arthrosynovitis
Artrostomia: arthrostomy
Artrotifóide: arthrotyphoid
Artrotomia: arthrotomy
Artrótomo: arthrotome
Artrotrópico: arthrotropic
Árvore: arbor, **pl.** arbores
Árvore de decisão: decision tree
Árvore genealógica: pedigree
Asa: ala, **gen. e pl.** alae; wing
Asbesto: asbestos
Asbestóide: asbestoid
Asbestose: asbestosis
Ascaríase: ascariasis
Ascaricida: ascaricide
Ascarídeo: ascarid
Ascaridida: Ascaridata, Ascarididea, Ascaridorida
Ascaridol: ascaridole
Ascaron: ascaron
Ascendente: ascendens
Ascensão: ascensus
Ascite: ascites
Ascítico: ascitic
Ascitógeno: ascitogenous
Asco: ascus, **pl.** asci
Ascocarpo: ascocarp
Ascógeno: ascogenous
Ascogônio: ascogonium
Ascomicetoso: ascomycetous
Ascorbase: ascorbase
Ascorbato: ascorbate
Ascósporo: ascospore

Asférico: aspheric
Asfigmia: asphygmia
Asfixia: asphyxia, asphyxiation
Asfixiante: asphyxiant, asphyxiating
Asfixiar: asphyxiate, choke
Asfíxico: asphyxial
Asilo: asylum, hospice
Asma: asthma
Asmático: asthmatic
Asmogênico: asthmogenic
Aspalassoma: aspalasoma
Asparaginase: asparaginase, asparagine (N, Asn)
Asparaginil: asparaginyl
Aspargo: Asparagus
Aspartame: aspartame
Aspartase: aspartase
Aspartato: aspartate
Aspartato 1-descarboxilase: aspartate 1-decarboxylase
Aspartato 4-descarboxilase: aspartate 4-decarboxylase
Aspartil: aspartyl
β-aspartil (acetilglicosamina): β-aspartyl (acetylglucosamine)
Aspartilglicosamina: aspartylglycosamine
Aspartilglicosaminidase: aspartylglycosaminidase
Aspartilglicosaminúria: aspartylglycosaminuria
Aspecto: aspect
Aspergilina: aspergillin
Aspergiloma: aspergilloma
Aspergilose: aspergillosis
Aspermatogênico: aspermatogenic
Aspermia: aspermia
Aspersão: aspersion
Aspidina: aspidin
Aspidinol: aspidinol
Aspídio: aspidium
Aspidosamina: aspidosamine
Aspidospermina: aspidospermine
Aspiração: aspiration
Aspirador: aspirator
Aspirar: aspirate
Asplenia: asplenia
Asplênico: asplenic
Ásporo: asporous
Asporogenoso: asporogenous
Asporulado: asporulate
Assa-fétida: asafetida
Assento: seat
Assepsia: asepsis
Asseptado: aseptate
Assepticismo: asepticism
Asséptico: aseptic
Assexual: asexual
Assialismo: asialism
Assialoglicoproteína: asialoglycoprotein
Assilabia: asyllabia
Assimbolia: asymbolia
Assimetria: asymmetry
Assimétrico: asymmetric (a)
Assimilação: assimilation
Assimilável: assimilable
Assimptótico: asymptotic

Assinclitismo: asynclitism
Assincrônico: desynchronous
Assinéquia: asynechia
Assinergia: asynergia, asynergy
Assinérgico: asynergic
Assinesia: asynesia, asynesis
Assintomático: asymptomatic
Assistemático: asystematic
Assistência: care
Assistolia: asystole, asystolia
Assistólico: asystolic
Assitia: asitia
Assoalho: floor
Associação: association
Associacionismo: associationism
Associado: associate
Associal: asocial
Assoma: asoma, pl. asomata
Astasia: astasia
Astasia-abasia: astasia-abasia
Astático: astatic
Astatínio: astatine (At)
Asteatose: asteatosis
Astemizol: astemizole
Astenia: asthenia
Astênico: asthenic
Astenopia: asthenopia
Astenópico: asthenopic
Astenospermia: asthenospermia
Astenozoospermia: asthenozoospermia
Áster: aster
Astério: asterion
Asteriossaponinas: asteriosaponins
Asteriotoxinas: asteriotoxins
Asterixe: asterixis
Asternal: asternal
Asternia: asternia
Asteróide: asteroid
Astigmático: astigmatic
Astigmatismo: astigmatism, astigmia
Astigmatometria: astigmatometry, astigmometry
Astomatoso: astomatous
Astomia: astomia
Astomoso: astomous
Astral: astral
Astrapofobia: astrapophobia
Astroblasto: astroblast
Astroblastoma: astroblastoma
Astrocele: astrocele
Astrocinético: astrokinetic
Astrócito: astrocyte
Astrocitoma: astrocytoma
Astrocitose: astrocytosis
Astroependimoma: astroependymoma
Astróglia: astroglia
Astróide: astroid
Astrosfera: astrosphere
Asverina: asverin
Atactilia: atactilia
Atadura: roller, spica, pl. spicae
Ataque: attack, seizure
Atarático: ataractic
Ataraxia: ataraxia
Ataráxico: ataraxic
Atávico: atavistic
Atavismo: atavism

Ataxia: ataxia, ataxy
Ataxiadinamia: ataxiadynamia
Ataxiafasia: ataxiaphasia
Ataxia-telangiectasia: ataxia-telangiectasia
Atáxico: ataxic
Ataxiofobia: ataxiophobia
Ataxiógrafo: ataxiagraph
Ataxiograma: ataxiagram
Ataxômetro: ataxiameter
Atelectasia: atelectasis
Atelectásico: atelectatic
Atelia: athelia
Ateliose: atelia, ateliosis
Ateliótico: ateliotic
Atelopitoxina: atelopidtoxin
Atenolol: atenolol
Atenuação: attenuation
Atenuador: attenuator
Atenuante: attenuant
Atenuar: attenuate
Aterectomia: atherectomy
Atermancia: athermancy
Atérmano: athermanous
Atermossistáltico: athermosystaltic
Ateroembolismo: atheroembolism
Aterogênese: atherogenesis
Aterogênico: atherogenic
Ateroma: atheroma
Ateromatoso: atheromatous
Aterosclerose: atherosclerosis
Aterosclerótico: atherosclerotic
Aterose: atherosis
Aterotrombose: atherothrombosis
Aterotrombótico: atherothrombotic
Atetóide: athetoid
Atetose: athetosis
Atetose pupilar: hippus
Atetósico: athetosic, athetotic
Ático: attic
Atimia: athymia, athymism
Atipia: atypia, atypism
Atípico: atypical
Atireóideo: athyrotic
Atireoidismo: athyroidism, athyrosis
Atitude: attitude
Atitudinal: attitudinal
Ativação: activation
Ativador: activator
Ativar: activate
Atividade mental: mentation
Ativina: activin
Ativo: quick
Atlantoaxial: atlantoaxial, atlantoepistrophic, atloaxoid
Atlantoccipital: atlanto-occipital, atlo-occipital
Atlantodídimo: atlantodidymus, atlodidymus
Atlanto-odontóide: atlanto-odontoid
Atlas: atlas
Atlóide: atlantal, atloid
Atmólise: atmolysis
Atmômetro: atmometer
Atmosfera: atmosphere

Atmosferização: atmospherization
Atômico: atomic
Atomismo: atomism
Atomístico: atomistic
Atomização: atomization
Atomizador: atomizer
Átomo: atom
Atonia: atonia, atonicity, atony
Atônico: atonic
Atópeno: atopen
Atopia: atopy
Atópico: atopic
Atopognosia: atopognosia, atopognosis
Atordoar: stun
Atóxico: atoxic
ATP-citrato liase: ATP citrate lyase
ATP-difosfatase: ATP-diphosphatase
ATP-sulfurilase: ATP sulfurylase
Atração: attraction
Atractiligenina: atractyligenin
Atractilina: atractylin
Atractina: attractin
Atraente: attrahens
Atrepsia: athrepsia, athrepsy, atrepsy
Atresia: atresia
Atrético: atresic, atretic
Atretoblefaria: atretoblepharia
Atretocistia: atretocystia
Atretogastria: atretogastria
Atretopsia: atretopsia
Atrial: atrial
Atricose: atrichosis
Átrio: atrium, pl. atria
Atriomegalia: atriomegaly
Atriopeptina: atriopeptin
Atriosseptoplastia: atrioseptoplasty
Atriosseptostomia: atrioseptostomy
Atriotomia: atriotomy
Atrioventricular: atrioventricular (AV)
Atriplicismo: atriplicism
Atriquia: atrichia
Atrito: attrition, rub
Atrocitose: athrocytosis
Atrofia: atrophia, atrophy
Atrofia branca: atrophie blanche
Atrofiado: atrophied
Atrófico: atrophic
Atrofodermatose: atrophodermatosis
Atrofodermia: atrophoderma
Atrombia: athrombia
Atropina: atropine
Atropínico: atropinic
Atropinismo: atropinism
Atropinização: atropinization
Atroscina: atroscine
Atrotoxina: atrotoxin
Aturdido: punchdrunk
Audição: audition, hearing
Audioanalgesia: audioanalgesia
Audiofone: earpiece

Audiogênico: audiogenic
Audiograma: audiogram
Audiologia: audiology
Audiólogo: audiologist
Audiometria: audiometry
Audiométrico: audiometric
Audiometrista: audiometrist
Audiômetro: audiometer
Audiovisual: audiovisual
Auditivo: audile, auditory
Auditoria: audit
Augnato: augnathus
Aumento: enlargement, increase
Aura: aura, **pl.** aurae
Aural: aural
Auramina: auramine O
Auranofina: auranofin
Auríase: auriasis
Áurico: auric
Aurícula: auricula, **pl.** auriculae
Auricular: auricular
Auriculocranial: auriculocranial
Auriculotemporal: auriculotemporal
Auriculoventricular: auriculoventricular
Áuride: aurid, **pl.** aurides
Auriforme: auriform
Aurina: aurin
Aurocromodermia: aurochromoderma
Auromercaptoacetanilida: auromercaptoacetanilid
Aurona: aurone
Auroterapia: aurotherapy
Aurotioglicanida: aurothioglycanide
Aurotioglicose: aurothioglucose
Ausculta: auscultation
Auscultar: auscultate, auscult
Auscultatório: auscultatory
Ausência: absence, excalation
Autacóide: autacoid
Autécico: autecic, autecious
Autemésia: autemesia
Autenticidade: authenticity
Autismo: autism
Autista: autistic
Auto-acusação: self-accusation
Auto-aglutinação: autoagglutination
Auto-aglutinina: autoagglutinin
Auto-alergia: autoallergy
Auto-alérgico: autoallergic
Auto-alergização: autoallergization
Auto-anafilaxia: autoanaphylaxis
Auto-analisador: autoanalyzer
Auto-análise: autoanalysis, self-analysis
Auto-anticomplemento: autoanticomplement
Auto-anticorpo: autoantibody
Auto-antígeno: autoantigen
Auto-ativação: autoactivation
Autoblasto: autoblast
Autocatálise: autocatalysis
Autocatalítico: autocatalytic
Autocateterismo: autocatheterization, autocatheterism
Autocentrismo: self-centeredness
Autoceratoplastia: autokeratoplasty
Autocinesia: autokinesia, autokinesis
Autocinético: autokinetic
Autocistoplastia: autoaugmentation, autocystoplasty
Autocitólise: autocytolysis
Autocitolisina: autocytolysin
Autocitotoxina: autocytotoxin
Autoclasia: autoclasis, autoclasia
Autoclave: autoclave
Autocóide: autocoid
Autoconhecimento: self-awareness, self-knowledge
Autocontrole: self-control
Autócrino: autocrine
Autóctone: autochthonous
Autodérmico: autodermic
Autodescoberta: self-discovery
Autodiferenciação: self-differentiation
Autodigestão: autodigestion
Autodiplóide: autodiploid
Autodrenagem: autodrainage
Auto-ecolalia: autoecholalia
Auto-eficácia: self-efficacy
Auto-ensaio: autoassay
Auto-envenenamento: self-poisoning
Auto-enxerto: autograft, autografting
Auto-eroticismo: autoeroticism
Auto-erótico: autoerotic
Auto-erotismo: autoerotism
Auto-estimulação: self-stimulation
Autofagia: autophagia, autophagy
Autofágico: autophagic
Autofagolisossoma: autophagolysosome
Autofertilização: self-fertilization
Autofluoroscópio: autofluoroscope
Autofobia: autophobia
Autofonia: autophony
Autogamia: autogamy
Autógamo: autogamous
Autogênese: autogenesis
Autogenético, autogênico: autogenetic, autogenic
Autógeno: autogenous
Autognose: autognosis
Autografismo: autographism
Autograma: autogram
Auto-hemaglutinação: autohemagglutination
Auto-hemólise: autohemolysis
Auto-hemolisina: autohemolysin
Auto-hexaplóide: autohexaploid
Auto-hipnose: autohypnosis, autohypnotism
Auto-hipnótico: autohypnotic
Auto-imune: autoimmune
Auto-imunidade: autoimmunity
Auto-imunização: autoimmunization
Auto-imunocitopenia: autoimmunocytopenia
Auto-infecção: autoinfection, self-infection
Auto-infusão: autoinfusion
Auto-inoculação: autoinoculation
Auto-inoculável: autoinoculable
Auto-internação: self-commitment
Auto-intoxicação: autointoxication
Auto-intoxicante: autointoxicant
Auto-isolisina: autoisolysin
Autolesão: autolesion
Autolimitado: self-limited
Autolisado: autolysate
Autolisar: autolyse, autolyze
Autólise: autolysis
Autolisina: autolysin
Autolítico: autolytic
Autólogo: autologous
Automatismo: automatism
Automatógrafo: automatograph
Automisofobia: automysophobia
Automixia: automixis
Automnésia: automnesia
Autonomia: autonomy
Autônomo: autonomic, autonomous
Autonomotrópico: autonomotropic
Auto-oxidação: auto-oxidation, autoxidation
Auto-oxidável: auto-oxidizable
Autopático: autopathic
Autopentaplóide: autopentaploid
Autopepsia: autopepsia
Autoplóide: autoploid
Autoploidia: autoploidy
Autópode: autopod, autopodium, **pl.** autopodia
Autopolimerização: autopolymerization
Autopolímero: autopolymer
Autopoliplóide: autopolyploid
Autopoliploidia: autopolyploidy
Auto-radiografia: autoradiograph, autoradiography
Auto-radiograma: autoradiogram
Auto-rafia: autorrhaphy
Auto-receptor: autoreceptor
Auto-regulação: autoregulation, self-regulation
Auto-reinfecção: autoreinfection
Auto-reprodução: autoreproduction
Auto-sensibilizar: autosensitize
Auto-septicemia: autosepticemia
Auto-sinóia: autosynnoia
Auto-síntese: autosynthesis
Autosito: autosite
Autosmia: autosmia
Auto-somatognose: autosomatognosis
Auto-somatognóstico: autosomatognostic
Auto-soro: autoserum
Auto-soroterapia: autoserotherapy
Autossoma: autosome
Autossômico: autosomal
Auto-sugestão: autosuggestion
Auto-sugestibilidade: autosuggestibility
Autotélico: autotelic
Autóteno: autotemnous
Autoterapia: autotherapy
Autotetraplóide: autotetraploid
Autotolerância: self-tolerance
Autotomia: autotomy
Autotopagnosia: autotopagnosia
Autotoxemia: autotoxemia
Autotóxico: autotoxic
Autotoxicose: autotoxicosis
Autotoxina: autotoxin
Autotransfusão: autotransfusion
Autotransplante: autotransplant, autotransplantation
Autotriplóide: autotriploid
Autotrofia: autotrophy
Autotrófico: autotrophic
Autótrofo: autotroph
Autovacinação: autovaccination
Autovenenoso: autopoisonous
Auxanografia: auxanography
Auxanográfico: auxanographic
Auxanograma: auxanogram
Auxanologia: auxanology
Auxese: auxesis
Auxiliar: auxiliary
Auxiliar médico: physician assistant (P.A.)
Auxiliomotor: auxiliomotor
Auxilítico: auxilytic
Auxocromo: auxochrome
Auxódromo: auxodrome
Auxofloro: auxoflore
Auxoglico: auxogluc
Auxotônico: auxotonic
Auxotóxico: auxotox
Auxotrófico: auxotrophic
Auxotrofo: auxotroph
Avaliação: assessment, evaluation
Avalvar: avalvular
Avançar: advance
Avascular: avascular
Avascularização: avascularization
Aveleira: hazelwort
Avenina: avenin
Avermectinas: avermectins
Aviar: dispense
Aviário: avian
Avidez: avidity
Avidina: avidin
Avirulento: avirulent
Avitaminose: avitaminosis
Avivamento: avivement

Avulsão: avulsion
Axênico: axenic
Axial: axial, axialis, axile
Axífugo: axifugal
Axila: armpit, axil, axilla, **gen. e pl.** axillae; maschale
Axilar: axillary
Axiobucal: axiobuccal
Axiobucogengival: axiobuccogingival
Axioclusal: axio-occlusal
Axioincisal: axioincisal
Axiolabial: axiolabial
Axiolabiolingual: axiolabiolingual
Axiolingual: axiolingual
Axiolinguocervical: axiolinguocervical
Axiolinguoclusal: axiolinguoclusal
Axiolinguogengival: axiolinguogingival
Axiomesial: axiomesial
Axiomesiocervical: axiomesiocervical
Axiomesiodistal: axiomesiodistal
Axiomesiogengival: axiomesiogingival
Axiomesioincisal: axiomesioincisal
Axioplasma: axioplasm
Axiopódio: axiopodium, **pl.** axiopodia
Axiopulpar: axiopulpal
Axioversão: axioversion
Axípeto: axipetal
Axirramificar: axiramificate
Axoaxônico: axoaxonic
Axodendrítica: axodendritic
Axofugo: axofugal
Axógrafo: axograph
Axolema: axolemma
Axólise: axolysis
Axonal: axonal
Axonema: axoneme
Axônio: axon
Axonografia: axonography
Axonopatia: axonopathy
Axonotmese: axonotmesis
Axópeto: axopetal
Axoplasma: axoplasm
Axópodo: axopodium, **pl.** axopodia
Axossomático: axosomatic
Axóstilo: axostyle
Axotomia: axotomy
Ayahuasca: ayahuasca
Azacrina: azacrine
9-azafluoreno: 9-azafluorene
8-azaguanina: 8-azaguanine
Azaperona: azaperone
Azapironas: azapirones
Azaribina: azaribine
Azaspirodecanodiona: azaspirodecanedione
Azasserina: azaserine
6-azatimina: 6-azathymine
Azatioprina: azathioprine
6-azauridina: 6-azauridine (AZUR)

Azeite de oliva: olive oil
Azeotrópico: azeotropic
Azeótropo: azeotrope
Azida: azide
Azidotimidina (AZT): azidothymidine (AZT)
Ázigo: azygos, azygous
Azigografia: azygography
Azigograma: azygogram
Azlocilina sódica: azlocillin sodium
Azobilirrubina: azobilirubin
Azocarmim: azocarmine
Azocarmim B, azocarmim G: azocarmine B, azocarmine G
Azofloxina: azophloxin
Azóico: azoic
Azol: azole
Azolitimina: azolitmin
Azoproteína: azoprotein
Azospermia: azoospermia
Azossulfamida: azosulfamide
Azotemia: azotemia
Azotêmico: azotemic
Azotermia: azothermia
Azotúria: azoturia
Aztreonam: aztreonam
Azul: blue
Azul alcião: Alcian blue
Azul brilhante de Coomassie R-250: Coomassie brilliant blue R-250
Azul cresil brilhante: brilliant cresyl blue
Azul da Prússia: Berlin blue
Azul de bromofenol: bromophenol blue, bromphenol blue
Azul de bromotimol: bromthymol blue
Azul de cresil: cresyl blue, cresyl blue brilliant
Azul de Evans: azovan blue, Evans blue
Azul de isamina: Isamine blue
Azul de isossulfano: isosulfan blue
Azul de metila: methyl blue
Azul de metileno: methylene blue
Azul de rodanila: rhodanile blue
Azul de tripano: trypan blue
Azul resistente ao luxol: Luxol fast blue
Azul-celeste B: celestine blue B
Azul-vitória: Victoria blue
Azur: azure
Azur de metileno: methylene azure
Azurofilia: azurophilia
Azurófilo: azurophil, azurophile
Azurresina: azuresin

B

Babar: dribble
Babesiose: babesiosis
Bacia: basin

Baciforme: baccate, bacciform
Bacilar: bacillar, bacillary
Bacilemia: bacillemia
Baciliforme: bacilliform
Bacilina: bacillin
Bacilo: bacillus, **pl.** bacilli
Bacilo de Calmette-Guérin: bacille Calmette-Guérin (BCG)
Bacilomixina: bacillomyxin
Bacilose: bacillosis
Bacilúria: bacilluria
Bacitracina: bacitracin
Baclofeno: baclofen
Baço: lien, spleen, splen
Baço acessório: lienculus, lienunculus
Bactéria: bacterium, **pl.** bacteria
Bacteriano: bacterial
Bactericida: bactericidal, bactericide, bacteriocidal, bacteriocide
Bactericólia: bactericholia
Bactéride: bacterid
Bacteriemia: bacteremia, bacteriemia
Bacterioaglutinina: bacterioagglutinin
Bacteriocidina: bacteriocidin
Bacteriocinas: bacteriocins
Bacteriocinógenos: bacteriocinogens
Bacterioclorina: bacteriochlorin
Bacterioclorofila: bacteriochlorophyll
Bacterioestase: bacteriostasis
Bacteriofagia: bacteriophagia
Bacteriófago: bacteriophage
Bacteriofagologia: bacteriophagology
Bacteriofeoforbina: bacteriopheophorbin
Bacteriofitoma: bacteriophytoma
Bacteriofluoresceína: bacteriofluorescin
Bacteriogênico: bacteriogenic
Bacteriógeno: bacteriogenous
Bacterióide: bacterioid
Bacteriolisar: bacteriolyze
Bacteriólise: bacteriolysis
Bacteriolisina: bacteriolysin
Bacteriolítico: bacteriolytic
Bacteriologia: bacteriology
Bacteriológico: bacteriologic, bacteriological
Bacteriologista: bacteriologist
Bacteriopexia: bacteriopexy
Bacterioproteína: bacterioprotein
Bacteriopsonina: bacteriopsonin
Bacteriose: bacteriosis
Bacteriospermia: bacteriospermia
Bacteriostático: bacteriostatic
Bacteriostato: bacteriostat
Bacteriotóxico: bacteriotoxic
Bacteriotripsina: bacteriotrypsin
Bacteriotrópico: bacteriotropic
Bacteriotropina: bacteriotropin
Bacteriúria: bacteriuria

Bacteróide: bacteroid
Bacteroidose: bacteroidosis
Baculiforme: baculiform
Baculovírus: baculovirus
Bagaço: marc
Bagaçose: bagassosis
Bailisascaríase: baylisascariasis
Baioneta: bayonet
Balança: balance
Balanço: balance
Balânico: balanic
Balanite: balanitis
Bálano: balanus
Balanoplastia: balanoplasty
Balanopostite: balanoposthitis
Balantidíase: balantidiasis
Balantidose: balantidosis
Balão: balloon
Balão de Florence: Florence flask
Balé cardíaco: cardiac ballet
Balismo: ballism, ballismus
Balistocardiografia: ballistocardiography
Balistocardiógrafo: ballistocardiograph (BCG)
Balistocardiograma: ballistocardiogram
Balistofobia: ballistophobia
Balneoterapia: balneotherapeutics, balneotherapy
Balsâmico: balsamic
Bálsamo: balm, balsam, ointment
Bamipina: bamipine
Banco de olhos: eyebank
Banco de sangue: blood bank
Bancroftíase, bancroftose: bancroftiasis, bancroftosis
Banda estreita: narrowband
Banda larga: wideband
Bandagem: bandage
Bandeamento C: C-banding
Bandeja: tray
Bando: herd
Banha: lard
Banho: bath
Banisterina: banisterine
Baptitoxina: baptitoxine
Baqueteamento digital: clubbing
Bar: bar
Baragnose: baragnosis
Barba: barba, beard
Barba de milho: cornsilk
Barbaloína: barbaloin
Barbeiro: barbiero
Barbital: barbital
Barbitúrico: barbiturate
Barbiturismo: barbiturism
Barbotagem: barbotage
Barestesia: baresthesia
Barestesiômetro: baresthesiometer
Bariatria: bariatrics
Bariátrico: bariatric
Baricidade: baricity
Bárico: baric
Bário: barium (Ba)
Barita: baryta

Glossário

Baritose: baritosis
Barn: barn (b)
Baroceptor: baroceptor
Barofílico: barophilic
Barognose: barognosis
Barógrafo: barograph
Barometrógrafo: barometrograph
Barorreceptor: baroreceptor
Barorreflexo: baroreflex
Baroscópio: baroscope
Barossinusite: barosinusitis
Barostato: barostat
Barotaxia: barotaxis
Barotite média: barotitis media
Barotrauma: barotrauma
Barotropismo: barotropism
Barreira: barrier
Barreira sanitária: cordon sanitaire
Barrilha: barilla
Bartolinite: bartholinitis
Bartonelose: bartonellosis
Barúria: baruria
Basal: basad, basal, basalis, basialis
Basalóide: basaloid
Base: background, base, basis
Base alveolar: basialveolar
Base do crânio: basicranium
Base do estribo: footplate, footplate
Basecranial: basicranial
Basedóide: basedoid
Basedoviano: basedowian
Basicidade: basicity
Básico: basic
Basídio: basidium, **pl.** basidia
Basidiobolos: *Basidiobolus*
Basidiomicetos: Basidiomycetes
Basidiosporo: basidiospore
Basifacial: basifacial
Basifobia: basiphobia
Basilar: basilar, basilaris
Basilateral: basilateral
Basilema: basilemma
Basílico: basilicus
Basinasal: basinasal
Básio: basion
Basioccipital: basioccipital, basiocciput
Basioglosso: basioglossus
Basípeto: basipetal
Basitemporal: basitemporal
Basivertebral: basivertebral
Basócito: basocyte
Basocitopenia: basocytopenia
Basocitose: basocytosis
Basoeritrócito: basoerythrocyte
Basoeritrocitose: basoerythrocytosis
Basoesfenóide: basisphenoid
Basofilia: basophilia, basophilism
Basofílico: basophilic
Basófilo: basophil, basophile
Basofilócito: basophilocyte
Basolateral: basolateral
Basometacromófilo: basometachromophil, basometachromophile

Basopenia: basopenia
Basoplasma: basoplasm
Bassorina: bassorin
Bastão de Esculápio: staff of Aesculapius
Bastocinina: bastokinin
Bastonete: rod
Bateria: battery
Batianestesia: bathyanesthesia
Baticardia: bathycardia
Batida: beat
Batiestesia: bathyesthesia
Batigastria: bathygastry
Bati-hiperestesia: bathyhyperesthesia
Bati-hipestesia: bathyhypesthesia
Batimento: knock, palmic
Batimento cardíaco: heartbeat
Batocrômico: bathochromic
Batofloro: bathoflore
Batofobia: bathophobia
Batracotoxina: batrachotoxin
Baunilha: vanilla
Bdelina: bdellin
Bebê: baby
Behaviorismo: behaviorism
Behaviorista: behaviorist
Bejel: bejel
Bel: bel
Bela indiferença: belle indifférence
Beladona: belladonna
Beladonina: belladonnine
Belemnóide: belemnoid
Belonefobia: belonephobia
bem: ben
Bemegrida: bemegride
Bem-estar: fitness, wellness
Bemperidol: benperidol
Bendazac: bendazac
Bendrofluazida: bendrofluazide
Bendroflumetiazida: bendroflumethiazide
Beneceptor: beneceptor
Beneficência: beneficence
Benigno: benign
Benoxaprofeno: benoxaprofen
Benserazida: benserazide
Bentiromida: bentiromide
Bentonita: bentonite
Benzalacetofenona: benzalacetophenone
Benzalcumaran-3-ona: benzalcoumaran-3-one
Benzaldeído: benzaldehyde
Benzantraceno: benz[a]anthracene
Benzantreno: benzanthrene
Benzeno: benzene
Benzenoamina: benzeneamine
Benzestrol: benzestrol
Benzidina: benzidine
Benzila: benzyl
Benzilato de quinuclidinil: quinuclidinyl benzilate (QNB)
Benzílico: benzylic
Benzilideno: benzylidene
Benzilisoquinolinas: benzylisoquinolines

Benziloxicarbonila: benzyloxycarbonyl (Z, Cbz)
Benzilpenicilina: benzylpenicillin
Benzimidazol: benzimidazole
Benzina: benzin, benzine
Benziodarona: benziodarone
Benzoatado: benzoated
Benzoato: benzoate
Benzoato de denatônio: denatonium benzoate
Benzoato de *p*-hidroxi mercúrio: *p*-hydroxymercuribenzoate
Benzocaína: benzocaine
Benzodiazepina: benzodiazepine
Benzóico: benzoic
Benzoil: benzoyl
Benzoilecgonina: benzoylecgonine
Benzoil-PAS-cálcio: benzoylpas calcium
Benzoína: benzoin
Benzol: benzol
Benzomorfan: benzomorphan
Benzonatato: benzonatate
Benzoperidol: benzperidol
Benzopireno: benzpyrene
Benzopurpurina 4B: benzopurpurin 4B
Benzoquinamida: benzquinamide
1,4-benzoquinona: 1,4-benzoquinone
Benzorresinol: benzoresinol
Benzossulfimida: benzosulfimide
Benzotiadiazidas: benzothiadiazides
Benzotiazida: benzthiazide
Benzoxilina: benzoxyline
Benzoxiquina: benzoxiquine
Bequerel: becquerel (Bq)
Berberina: berberine
Beribéri: beriberi, beri beri
Berílio: beryllium (Be)
Beriliose: berylliosis
Bernes: bots
Berquélio: berkelium (Bk)
Bertielose: bertiellosis
Besilato: besylate
Besilato de atracúrio: atracurium besylate
Besilato de mesoridazina: mesoridazine besylate
Bestialidade: bestiality, buggery
Beta: beta (β)
Betabloqueador: beta-blocker
Betacianina: betacyanin
Betacianinúria: beeturia, betacyaninuria
Betacismo: betacism
Betaína: betaine
Betalaínas: betalains
Betametasona: betamethasone
Betanina: betanin
Betatron: betatron
Betel: betel
Bétula: betula
Bexiga: bladder

Bexiga urinária: vesica, **gen. e pl.** vesicae
Bezerro: calf, **pl.** calves
Bezoar: bezoar
Biângulo: binangle
Biarticular: biarticular
Biasteriônico: biasterionic
Biauricular: biauricular
Biaxilar: bisaxillary
Bibliomania: bibliomania
Biblioteca: library
Biblioteca de genes: gene library
Bíbulo: bibulous
Bicameral: bicameral
Bicapsular: bicapsular
Bicarbonato: bicarbonate
Bicardiograma: bicardiogram
Bicéfalo: bicephalus
Bicelular: bicellular
Bíceps: biceps
Bicho: bicho
Bicho-do-pé: chigoe, jigger
Biciliado: biciliate
Bicipital: bicipital
Biclonal: biclonal
Biclonalidade: biclonality
Bico: beak, nib
Bico de Bunsen: Bunsen burner
Bico-de-viúva: widow's peak
Bicôncavo: biconcave
Biconvexo: biconvex
Bicorne, bicornado, bicórneo: bicornous, bicornuate, bicornate
Bicuculina: bicuculline
Bicunina: bikunin
Bicúspide: bicuspid
Bicuspidização: bicuspidization
Bidactilia: bidactyly
Bidé: bidet
Bidiscoidal: bidiscoidal
Bíduo: biduous
Biestefânico: bistephanic
Biesteróide: bisteroid
Biestratificado: bistratal
Bifascicular: bifascicular
Bifenil: biphenyl
Bifenotipia: biphenotypy
Bifenotípico: biphenotypic
Bífido: bifid
Bifocal: bifocal
1,3-bifosfoglicerato (1,3-P$_2$Gri): 1,3-bisphosphoglycerate (1,3-P$_2$Gri)
2,3-bifosfoglicerato (2,3-P$_2$Gri): 2,3-bisphosphoglycerate (2,3-P$_2$Gri)
Bifosfonatos: bisphosphonates
Bifuncional: bifunctional
Bifurado: biforate
Bifurcação: bifurcatio, bifurcation, furcation
Bifurcar, bifurcado: bifurcate, bifurcated
Bigêmeo: bigemina
Bigeminal: bigeminal
Bigeminismo: bigemini, bigeminum, bigeminy
Bigerminal: bigerminal
Bigitalina: bigitalin

Blefaroestenose: blepharostenosis
Blefarofimose: blepharophimosis
Blefaroplastia: blepharoplasty
Blefaroplástico: blepharoplastic
Blefaroplasto: blepharoplast
Blefaroplegia: blepharoplegia
Blefaroptose: blepharoptosis, blepharoptosia
Blefarossinéquia: blepharosynechia
Blefarostato: blepharostat
Blefarotomia: blepharotomy
Blenadenite: blennadenitis
Blenêmese: blennemesis
Blenoftalmia: blennophthalmia
Blenogênico: blennogenic
Blenógeno: blennogenous
Blenóide: blennoid
Blenorrágico: blennorrhagic, blennorrheal
Blenorréia: blennorrhea
Blenostase: blennostasis
Blenostático: blennostatic
Blenúria: blennuria
Bloqueador: blocker
Bloqueador alfa: alpha-blocker
Bloquear: block
Bloqueio: blockade, blocking
Bobierita: bobierrite
Boca: mouth
Boca de eclusa: sluiceway
Boca de tapir: bouche de tapir
Bocas: ora
Bocejar: oscitate, yawn
Bocejo: oscitation, yawning
Bochecha: bucca, **gen. e pl.** buccae, cheek
Bócio: goiter
Bociogênico: goitrogen, goitrogenic
Bocioso: goitrous
Bola: ball
Boldina: boldin
Boldo: boldo, boldus
Boldoglucina: boldoglucin
Bolha: bulla, **gen. e pl.** bullae
Bolhoso: bullous
Bolo: bolus (bol)
Bolômetro: bolometer
Bolsa: bag, bursa, **pl.** bursae; pocket, pouch, sac
Bolsa-das-águas: forewaters
Bolsite: pouchitis
Bomba: pump
Bombardeio: bombard
Bombesina: bombesin
Bondina: boldine
Boratado: borated
Borato: borate
Bórax: borax
Borboleta: butterfly
Borborigmo: borborygmus, **pl.** borborygmi; rugitus
Borismo: borism
Bornano: bornane
Boro: boron (B)
Boroglicerina: boroglycerin
Boroglicerol: boroglycerol
Borracha: rubber

Borracha de polissulfeto: polysulfide rubber
Borramento visual: lippitude, lippitudo
Borreliose: borreliosis
Bossa: boss
Bosselação: bosselation
Bosselado: bosselated
Bota: boot
Botão: bud, button
Botão de Biskra: bouton de Biskra
Boticário: apothecary, druggist
Botoeira: boutonnière, buttonhole
Botões de mescal: mescal buttons
Botriomicose: botryomycosis
Botriomicótico: botryomycotic
Bótrios: bothria
Botulina: botulin
Botulinogênico: botulinogenic
Botulismo: botulism
Botulismotoxina: botulismotoxin
Botulogênico: botulogenic
Bouba: boubas, pian
Bovino: bovine
Braço: arm, brachium, **pl.** brachia
Bradiarritmia: bradyarrhythmia
Bradiartria: bradyarthria
Bradicardia: bradycardia
Bradicardíaco: bradycardiac
Bradicárdico: bradycardic
Bradicina: bradykinin
Bradicinesia: bradykinesia, bradykinesia
Bradicinético: bradykinetic
Bradicininogênio: bradykininogen
Bradicrótico: bradycrotic
Bradidiástole: bradydiastole
Bradiestesia: bradyesthesia
Bradifagia: bradyphagia
Bradifasia: bradyphasia
Bradifemia: bradyphemia
Bradiglossia: bradyglossia
Bradilalia: bradylalia
Bradilexia: bradylexia
Bradilogia: bradylogia
Bradipepsia: bradypepsia
Bradipnéia: bradypnea
Bradipsiquia: bradypsychia
Bradirritmia: bradyrhythmia
Bradisfigmia: bradysphygmia
Bradispermatismo: bradyspermatism
Bradistalsia: bradystalsis
Braditeleocinese: bradyteleokinesis
Braditeleocinesia: bradyteleocinesia
Bradiúria: bradyuria
Bradizoíto: bradyzoite
Braile: braille
Branco: white
Branco de metileno: methylene white
Branquial: branchial

Brânquias: branchia, **pl.** branchiae
Branquiogênico: branchiogenic, branchiogenous
Branquiomerismo: branchiomerism
Branquiômero: branchiomere
Branquiomotor: branchiomotor
Braquial: brachial
Braquialgia: brachialgia
Braquibasia: brachybasia
Braquibasocamptodactilia: brachybasocamptodactyly
Braquibasofalangia: brachybasophalangia
Braquicardia: brachycardia
Braquicefalia: brachycephalia, brachycephaly
Braquicefálico: brachycephalic, brachycephalous
Braquicefalismo: brachycephalism
Braquicnêmico: brachycnemic
Braquicrânico: brachycranic
Braquicubital: brachiocubital
Braquidactilia: brachydactylia, brachydactyly
Braquidactílico: brachydactylic
Braquiesôfago: brachyesophagus
Braquifacial: brachyfacial
Braquifalangia: brachyphalangia
Braquiglosso: brachyglossal
Braquignatia: brachygnathia
Braquignato: brachygnathous
Braquimelia: brachymelia
Braquimesofalangia: brachymesophalangia
Braquimetacarpalia: brachymetacarpalia, brachymetacarpalism
Braquimetacarpia: brachymetacarpia
Braquimetapodia: brachymetapody
Braquimetatarsia: brachymetatarsia
Braquimórfico: brachymorphic
Braquiocefálico: brachiocephalic
Braquiocrural: brachiocrural
Braquiodôntico: brachyodont
Braquiograma: brachiogram
Braquioníquia: brachyonychia
Braquipélico: brachypellic
Braquipélvico: brachypelvic
Braquípode: brachypodous
Braquiprosópico: brachyprosopic
Braquiqueilia: brachycheilia, brachychilia
Braquiquérquico: brachykerkic
Braquirrinco: brachyrhynchus
Braquirrinia: brachyrhinia
Braquisquélico: brachyskelic
Braquissindactilia: brachysyndactyly
Braquistafilino: brachystaphyline

Braquitelefalangia: brachytelephalangia
Braquiterapia: brachytherapy
Brasileína: brazilein
Brasilina: brazilin
Bregma: bregma
Bregmático: bregmatic
Bretílio: bretylium
Breve: brevis
Brevetoxinas: brevetoxins (BTX)
Brevícolo: brevicollis
Brida: bridle
Broca: broach, bur
Brocresina: brocresine
Bromado: bromated, brominated
Bromato: bromate
Bromazepam: bromazepam
Bromelina: bromelain, bromelin
Brometo: bromide
Brometo de azametônio: azamethonium bromide
Brometo de benzoestigmina: benzstigminum bromidum
Brometo de benzopirínio: benzpyrinium bromide
Brometo de cetexônio: cethexonium bromide
Brometo de cetiltrimetilamônio: cetyltrimethylammonium bromide
Brometo de cetrimônio: cetrimonium bromide
Brometo de clidínio: clidinium bromide
Brometo de decametônio: decamethonium bromide
Brometo de demecário: demecarium bromide
Brometo de domifeno: domiphen bromide
Brometo de etídio: ethidium bromide
Brometo de hexafluorênio: hexafluorenium bromide
Brometo de homídio: homidium bromide
Brometo de mepenzolato: mepenzolate bromide
Brometo de metantelina: methantheline bromide
Brometo de metescopolamina: methscopolamine bromide
Brometo de metila: methyl bromide
Brometo de metilatropina: methylatropine bromide
Brometo de oxifenônio: oxyphenonium bromide
Brometo de pancurônio: pancuronium bromide
Brometo de pentionato: penthienate bromide
Brometo de perfluorooctil: perfluorooctyl bromide (PFOB)
Brometo de pipecurônio: pipecuronium bromide
Brometo de piridostigmina: pyridostigmine bromide

Biglicano: biglycan
Bigorna: anvil, incus, **gen.** incudis, **pl.** incudes
Bilateral: bilateral
Bilateralismo: bilateralism
Bile: bile, gall
Bilharzíase: bilharziasis
Bilharzioma: bilharzioma
Bilharziose: bilharziosis
Biliar: biliary
Bilífero: biliferous
Bilificação: bilifaction, bilification
Biligênese: biligenesis
Biligênico: biligenic
Bilina: bilin, biline
Biliosidade: biliousness
Bilioso: bilious
Bilirraquia: bilirachia
Bilirrubina: bilirubin
Bilirrubina glicuronosídeo glicuronosiltransferase: bilirubin-glucuronoside glucuronosyltransferase
Bilirrubinemia: bilirubinemia
Bilirrubinóides: bilirubinoids
Bilirrubinúria: bilirubinuria
Biliterapia: bilitherapy
Biliúria: biliuria
Biliverdina: biliverdin, biliverdine, verdine
Bilobado: bilobate, bilobed
Bilobectomia: bilobectomy
Bilobular: bilobular
Biloculado: bilocular, biloculate
Bimanual: bimanual
Bimastóide: bimastoid
Bimaxilar: bimaxillary
Bimodal: bimodal
Bimolecular: bimolecular
Binário: binary
Binauricular: binaural
Binocular: binocular
Binomial: binomial
Binótico: binotic
Binuclear, binucleado: binuclear, binucleate
Binucleolado: binucleolate
Bioacústica: bioacoustics
Bioastronáutica: bioastronautics
Bioativo: bioactive
Biocarga: bioburden
Biocatalisador: biocatalyst
Biocenose: biocenosis
Biocibernética: biocybernetics
Biocida: biocidal
Biocinética: biokinetics
Biocitina: biocytin
Biocitinase: biocytinase
Bioclimatologia: bioclimatology
Biocompatibilidade: biocompatibility
Biocromo: biochrome
Biodegradação: biodegradation
Biodegradável: biodegradable
Biodinâmica: biodynamic, biodynamics
Biodisponibilidade: bioavailability
Bioecologia: bioecology

Bioelemento: bioelement
Bioenergética: bioenergetics
Bioengenharia: bioengineering
Bioensaio: bioassay
Bioespectrometria: biospectrometry
Bioespectroscopia: biospectroscopy
Bioespeleologia: biospeleology
Bioestático: biostatics
Bioestatística: biostatistics
Biofagia: biophagy
Biofagismo: biophagism
Biófago: biophage, biophagous
Biofarmacêutica: biopharmaceutics
Biofilático: biophylactic
Biofilaxia: biophylaxis
Biofísica: biophysics
Bioflavonóides: bioflavonoids
Biogênese: biogenesis
Biogenética: biogenetic
Biogênico: biogenic
Biogeoquímica: biogeochemistry
Biogravimetria: biogravics
Bioinformática: bioinformatics
Bioinstrumento: bioinstrument
Biólise: biolysis
Biolítico: biolytic
Biologia: biology
Biológico: biologic, biological
Biólogo: biologist
Bioluminescência: bioluminescence
Bioma: biome
Biomacromolécula: biomacromolecule
Biomassa: biomass
Biomaterial: biomaterial
Biomecânica: biomechanics
Biomédico: biomedical
Biomembrana: biomembrane
Biômetra: biometrician
Biometria: biometry
Biômetro: biometer
Biomicroscopia: biomicroscopy
Biomicroscópio: biomicroscope
Bionecrose: bionecrosis
Biônica: bionics
Biônico: bionic
Bionomia: bionomics, bionomy
Biopatologia: pathobiology
Bioplasma: bioplasm
Bioplásmico: bioplasmic
Biopolímero: biopolymer
Biopsia: biopsy
Biopsicologia: biopsychology
Biopsicossocial: biopsychosocial
Biopterina: biopterin
Bioquímica: biochemistry
Bioquímico: biochemical
Bioquimórfico: biochemorphic
Biorbital: biorbital
Biorreologia: biorheology
Biorritmo: biorhythm
Biose: biosis
Biosfera: biosphere
Biossegurança: biosafety
Biossíntese: biosynthesis

Biossintético: biosynthetic
Biossistema: biosystem
Biossocial: biosocial
Biota: biota
Biotaxia: biotaxis
Biotecnologia: biotechnology
Biotelemetria: biotelemetry
Bioteste: biotest
Biótica: biotics
Biótico: biotic
Biotina: biotin
Biotinidas: biotinides
Biotinidase: biotinidase
Biotinilisina: biotinyllysine
Biótipo: biotype
Biótomo: bioptome
Biótopo: biotope
Biotoxicologia: biotoxicology
Biotoxina: biotoxin
Biotransformação: biotransformation
Biovular: biovular
Bipalatinóide: bipalatinoid
Biparietal: biparietal
Bíparo: biparous
Bipartite: bipartite
Bipedal: bipedal
Bípede: biped
Bipenado, bipeniforme: bipennate, bipenniform
Biperfurado: biperforate
Biperideno: biperiden
Bipolar: bipolar
Bipotencialidade: bipotentiality
Birramoso: biramous
Birrefringência: birefringence
Birrefringente: birefringent
Birrotação: birotation
Bisacodil: bisacodyl
Bisacromial: bisacromial
Bisalbuminemia: bisalbuminemia
1,4-bis(5-feniloxazol-2-il)benzeno: 1,4-bis(5-phenyloxazol-2-yl)benzene
2,5-bis(5-t-butilbenzoxazol-2-il)tiofeno (BBOT): 2,5-bis(5-t-butylbenzoxazol-2-yl)thiophene (BBOT)
Bisel: bevel
Bisel contrário: contrabevel
Bisférico: bisferious
Bisidroxicumarina: bishydroxycoumarin
Bisilíaco: bisiliac
Bismutila: bismuthyl
Bismuto: bismuth (Bi)
Bismutose: bismuthosis
Bissexual: bisexual
Bissinose: byssinosis
Bissulfato: bisulfate
Bissulfeto: bisulfide, bisulfite
Bisturi: bistoury, knife, **pl.** knives
Bisturi de Merrifield: Merrifield knife
Bitartarato: bitartrate
Bitartarato de metaraminol: metaraminol bitartrate
Bitemporal: bitemporal
Bitionol: bithionol

Bitrocantérico: bitrochanteric
Bitrópico: bitropic
Biureto: biuret
Bivalência: bivalence, bivalency
Bivalente: bivalent
Biventral: biventral
Biventre: biventer
Biventricular: biventricular
Bixina: bixin
Bizigomático: bizygomatic
Blastema: blastema
Blastêmico: blastemic
Blástico: blastic
Blasto: blast
Blastocele: blastocele, blastocoele
Blastocélico: blastocelic, blastocoelic
Blastocisto: blastocyst
Blastócito: blastocyte
Blastoconídio: blastoconidium
Blastoderma: blastoderm, blastoderma
Blastodérmico: blastodermal, blastodermic
Blastodisco: blastodisk
Blastóforo: blastophore
Blastogênese: blastogenesis
Blastogenético, blastogênico: blastogenetic, blastogenic
Blastólise: blastolysis
Blastolítico: blastolytic
Blastoma: blastoma
Blastômero: blastomere
Blastomerotomia: blastomerotomy
Blastomicina: blastomycin
Blastomicose: blastomycosis
Blastomogênico: blastomogenic
Blastoneuroporo: blastoneuropore
Blastóporo: blastopore
Blastosporo: blastospore
Blastotomia: blastotomy
Blástula: blastula
Blastulação: blastulation
Blastular: blastular
Blefarectomia: blepharectomy
Blefaredema: blepharedema
Blefário: blepharal
Blefarite: blepharitis
Blefaroadenite: blepharadenitis, blepharoadenitis
Blefaroadenoma: blepharoadenoma
Blefarocalasia: blepharochalasis
Blefaroceratoconjuntivite: blepharokeratoconjunctivitis
Blefaroclono: blepharoclonus
Blefarocoloboma: blepharocoloboma, filiform adnatum
Blefaroconjuntivite: blepharoconjunctivitis
Blefarodiastase: blepharodiastasis
Blefaroespasmo: blepharospasm, blepharospasmus

Glossário

Brometo de propantelina: propantheline bromide
Brometo de tonzônio: thonzonium bromide
Brometo de valetamato: valethamate bromide
Brometo de vecurônio: vecuronium bromide
Brômico: bromic
Bromidrato: hydrobromate
Bromidrato de dextrometorfano: dextromethorphan hydrobromide
Bromidrose: bromhidrosis, bromidrosis
Bromidrosifobia: bromidrosiphobia
Bromindiona: bromindione
Bromismo, brominismo: bromism, brominism
Bromo: bromine (Br)
Bromocriptina: bromocriptine
Bromoderma: bromoderma
Bromodesoxiuridina: bromodeoxyuridine (BrDu)
Bromoiperidrose: bromohyperhidrosis, bromohyperidrosis
Bromossulfoftaleína: bromosulfophthalein
Bromossulfoftaleína: bromsulfophthalein
5-bromouracil: 5-bromouracil
Broncatar: broncatar
Broncoalveolar: bronchoalveolar
Broncocavernoso: bronchocavernous
Broncocele: bronchocele
Broncoconstrição: bronchoconstriction
Broncoconstritor: bronchoconstrictor
Broncodilatação: bronchodilatation, bronchodilation
Broncodilatador: bronchodilator
Broncoedema: bronchoedema
Broncoesofagologia: bronchoesophagology
Broncoesofagoscopia: bronchoesophagoscopy
Broncoespasmo: bronchospasm
Broncoespasmolítico: bronchospasmolytic
Broncofibroscópio: bronchofiberscope
Broncofonia: bronchophony
Broncogênico: bronchiogenic, bronchogenic
Broncografia: bronchography
Broncograma: bronchogram
Broncolitíase: broncholithiasis
Broncolito: broncholith
Broncomalacia: bronchomalacia
Broncomicose: bronchomycosis
Broncomotor: bronchomotor
Broncoplastia: bronchoplasty
Broncopneumonia: bronchopneumonia
Broncopulmonar: bronchopulmonary
Broncorrafia: bronchorrhaphy
Broncorréia: bronchorrhea
Broncoscopia: bronchoscopy
Broncoscópio: bronchoscope
Broncospirografia: bronchospirography
Broncospirometria: bronchospirometry
Broncospirômetro: bronchospirometer
Broncospiroquetose: bronchospirochetosis
Broncostaxia: bronchostaxis
Broncostenose: bronchostenosis
Broncostomia: bronchostomy
Broncotomia: bronchotomy
Broncotraqueal: bronchotracheal
Broncovesicular: bronchovesicular
Brônquico: bronchial
Bronquiectasia: bronchiectasia, bronchiectasis
Bronquiectásico: bronchiectatic
Bronquiloquia: bronchiloquy
Brônquio, brônquios: bronchium, bronchus, **pl.** bronchi
Bronquiolectasia: bronchiolectasia, bronchiolectasis
Bronquiolite: bronchiolitis
Bronquíolo: bronchiole, bronchiolus, **pl.** bronchioli
Bronquiolopulmonar: bronchiolopulmonary
Bronquiostenose: bronchiostenosis
Bronquite: bronchitis
Bronquítico: bronchitic
Brontofobia: brontophobia
Brotamento: budding
Brotizolam: brotizolam
Broto: sprout
Browniano: brownian
Brucelergina: brucellergin
Brucelina: brucellin
Brucelose: brucellosis
Bruchita: brushite
Brucina: brucine
Bruxismo: bruxism
Bruxoleio: flicker
Buaque: buaki
Buba: bubas
Buba-mãe: buba madre
Bubão: bubo
Bubonalgia: bubonalgia
Bubônico: bubonic
Bubônulo: bubonulus
Bucal: buccal
Bucardia: bucardia
Bucho: buchu
Bucinador: buccinator
Buclosamida: buclosamide
Bucoaxial: buccoaxial
Bucoaxiocervical: buccoaxiocervical
Bucoaxiogengival: buccoaxiogingival
Bucocervical: buccocervical
Bucoclusal: buccoclusal
Bucodistal: buccodistal
Bucofaríngeo: buccopharyngeal
Bucogengival: buccogingival
Bucolabial: buccolabial
Bucolingual: buccolingual
Bucomesial: buccomesial
Bucopulpar: buccopulpal
Bucoversão: buccoversion
Bucrilato: bucrylate
Búcula: buccula
Bufadienolídeo: bufadienolide
Bufageninas: bufagenins
Bufaginas: bufagins
Bufanolídeo: bufanolide
Bufatrienolídeo: bufatrienolide
Bufenolídeo: bufenolide
Bufogeninas: bufogenins
Buformina: buformin
Bufotenina: bufotenine
Bufotoxinas: bufotoxins
Buftalmo, buftalmia: buphthalmia, buphthalmus, buphthalmos
Bugalho: oak apple
Bulbar: bulbar
Bulbite: bulbitis
Bulbo, bulbos: bulbus, gen. e pl. bulbi; bulb
Bulbo do olho: eyeball
Bulbo terminal: end-bulb
Bulbocapnina: bulbocapnine
Bulbocavernoso: bulbocavernosus
Bulbóide: bulboid
Bulbonuclear: bulbonuclear
Bulbopontino: bulbopontine
Bulbospinal: bulbospinal
Bulbossacral: bulbosacral
Bulbouretral: bulbourethral
Bulectomia: bullectomy
Bulimia: boulimia, bulimia
Bulímico: bulimic
Bumetanida: bumetanide
Bungarotoxinas: bungarotoxins
Bunodonte: bunodont
Bunolofodonte: bunolophodont
Bunosselenodonte: bunoselenodont
Bupivacaína: bupivacaine
Buquê: bouquet
Bureta: buret, burette
Bursectomia: bursectomy
Bursite: bursitis
Bursite aquiléia: achillobursitis
Busca: hunting
Bussulfam: busulfan, busulphan
Butabarbital: butabarbital
Butano: butane
Butanoil: butanoyl
Butanol: butanol
Butaperazina: butaperazine
Butaverina: butaverine
Butetamato: butethamate
Butiazida: buthiazide
Butil aminobenzoato: butamben
Butila: butyl
Butilparabeno: butylparaben
Butionina sulfoximina: buthionine sulfoximine
Butiráceo: butyraceous
Butirato: butyrate
Butirato-CoA ligase: butyrate-CoA ligase
Butírico: butyric
Butiril: butyryl
Butiril-CoA: butyryl-CoA
Butirilcolinesterase: butyrylcholine esterase
γ-butirobetaína: γ-butyrobetaine
Butirocolinesterase: butyrocholinesterase
Butirofenona: butyrophenone
Butirômetro: butyrometer
Butiroso: butyrous
Butopironoxil: butopyronoxyl

C

Caapi: caapi
Cabeça: caput, **gen.** capitis, **pl.** capita; head
Cabeçote de absorção: absorber head
Cabelo: thrix
Cabeludo: hairy
Cacau: cacao, cocoa
Cacho: forelock
Cacodilato: cacodylate
Cacodílico: cacodylic
Cacodilo: cacodyl
Cacogeusia: cacogeusia
Cacomelia: cacomelia
Cacoplástico: cacoplastic
Cacosmia: cacosmia
Cactinomicina: cactinomycin
Cacume, cacúmen: cacumen, **pl.** cacumina
Cacumial: cacuminal
Cadáver: cadaver, corpse
Cadavérico: cadaveric, cadaverous
Cadaverina: cadaverine
Cadeia: chain
Cadela: bitch
Caderina: cadherin
Cadinho: crucible
Cádmio: cadmium (Cd)
Caduca: caduca
Caduceu: caduceus
Cafearina: caffearine
Cafeína: caffeine, thein
Cafeinismo: caffeinism
Cafindo: kafindo
Cãibra: cramp
Cairomônios: kairomones
Caixa: box
Caixa ou recipiente: canister
Caixa torácica: compages thoracis
Cajeputol: cajeputol, cajuputol

Glossário

Cal: lime
Cal virgem: quicklime
Calafrio: chill
Calamina: calamine
Cálamo: calamus
Calasia: chalasia, chalasis
Calazar: kala azar
Calázio: chalaza, chalazion, **pl.** chalazia
Calça militar antichoque: military antishock trousers (MAST)
Calcâneo: calcaneal, calcanean, calcaneum, calcaneus, **gen. e pl.** calcanei
Calcaneoapofisite: calcaneoapophysitis
Calcaneocavo: calcaneocavus
Calcaneocubóide: calcaneocuboid
Calcaneodinia: calcaneodynia
Calcaneoescafóide: calcaneoscaphoid
Calcaneofibular: fibulocalcaneal
Calcaneonavicular: calcaneonavicular
Calcaneotibial: calcaneotibial
Calcaneovalgo: calcaneovalgus
Calcaneovalgocavo: calcaneovalgocavus
Calcaneovaro: calcaneovarus
Calcanhar: calx, **gen.** calcis, **pl.** calces; heel
Calcarino: calcarine
Calcário: calcareous
Calcariúria: calcariuria
Calcergia: calcergy
Cálcico: calcic
Calcicose: calcicosis
Calcidiol: calcidiol
Calcifediol: calcifediol
Calcífero: calciferous
Calciferol: calciferol
Calcificação: calcification
Calcificar: calcify
Calcifilaxia: calciphylaxis
Calcifilia: calciphilia
Calcígero: calcigerous
Calcinação: calcination
Calcinar: calcine
Calcineurina: calcineurin
Calcinose: calcinosis
Cálcio: calcium (Ca), **gen.** calcii
Cálcio-45 (Ca^{45}): calcium-45 (^{45}Ca)
Cálcio-47 (Ca^{47}): calcium-47 (^{47}Ca)
Calciocinesia: calciokinesis
Calciocinético: calciokinetic
Calciol: calciol
Calciorraquia: calciorrhachia
Calciostato: calciostat
Calciotraumático: calciotraumatic
Calcipéctico: calcipectic
Calcipenia: calcipenia
Calcipênico: calcipenic
Calcipexia: calcipexis, calcipexy
Calcipéxico: calcipexic
Calciprivia: calciprivia

Calciprívico: calciprivic
Calcita: calcite, calcspar
Calcite: chalkitis
Calcitetrol: calcitetrol
Calcitonina: calcitonin
Calcitriol: calcitriol
Calciúria: calciuria
Calcóforo: calcophorous
Calcona: chalcone
Calcose: chalcosis
Calcosferita: calcospherite
Cálculo: calculus, **gen. e pl.** calculi; stone
Cálculo biliar: gallstone
Calculose: calculosis
Caldesmona: caldesmon
Caldo: bouillon
Calefaciente: calefacient
Calemia: kalemia
Calibeado: chalybeate
Calibrador: calibrator, gauge, sizer
Calibragem: calibration
Calibrar: calibrate
Calibre: caliber
Cálice: calix, **pl.** calices; calyx, **pl.** calyces
Caliceal: calyceal
Calicectasia: calicectasis
Calicectomia: calicectomy
Calicial: caliceal
Caliciforme: caliciform, calyciform
Calicina: calycine
Calicino: calicine
Calicoplastia: calicoplasty
Calicose: chalicosis
Calicotomia: calicotomy
Calicreína: kallikrein
Calículo: caliculus, **pl.** caliculi; calycle, calyculus
Calidina: kallidin
Caliectasia: caliectasis
Califórnio (CF): californium (Cf)
Caliopenia: kaliopenia
Caliopênico: kaliopenic
Calioplastia: calioplasty
Caliorrafia: caliorrhaphy
Caliotomia: caliotomy
Calistenia: calisthenics
Caliurese: kaliuresis, kaluresis
Caliurético: kaliuretic, kaluretic
Calmante: calmative
Calmodulina: calmodulin
Calo: callus, corn
Calomelano: calomel
Calônio: chalone
Calor: calor, heat (q)
Caloria: calorie, calory
Calórico: caloric
Calorífero: calorigenic
Calorífico: calorific
Calorimetria: calorimetry
Calorimétrico: calorimetric
Calorímetro: calorimeter
Calorotrópico: caloritropic
Calose: callose
Calosidade: callosity
Caloso: callosal, callous
Calosomarginal: callosomarginal

Calota craniana: skullcap
Calpaínas: calpains
Calseqüestrina: calsequestrin
Calusterona: calusterone
Calvária: calvaria, **pl.** calvariae
Calvície: baldness, calvities
Calvo: bald
Camada: coat, shell
Câmara: camera, **pl.** camerae, cameras; chamber
Cambalear: stagger
Cambendazol: cambendazole
Cambiador contracorrente: countercurrent exchanger
Câmbio: cambium
Camecefálico: chamecephalic
Camecéfalo: chamecephalous
Cameprosópico: chameprosopic
Camerostoma: camerostome
Caminhar: walk
Camisa: chemise
Camisa-de-força: camisole, straitjacket
Camomila: comomile, chamomile, matricaria
Campilobacteriose: campylobacteriosis
Campilodactilia: camplodactyly
Campímetro: campimeter
Campo: field
Campo cirúrgico: drape
Campos de Forel: campi foreli
Campotecinas: campothecins
Camptocormia: camptocormia
Camptodactilia: camptodactyly, camptodactylia, streblodactyly
Camptoespasmo: camptospasm
Camptomelia: camptomelia
Camptomélico: camptomelic
Camptotecina: camptothecin
Camundongo: mouse
Canabidiol: cannabidiol
Canabinóides: cannabinoids
Canabinol: cannabinol
Canábis: cannabis
Canabismo: cannabism
Canadina: canadine
Canais: canales
Canal: canal, canalis, **pl.** canales; channel, trough
Canal gástrico: magenstrasse
Canalicular: canalicular
Canaliculite: canaliculitis
Canaliculização: canaliculization
Canalículo: canaliculus, **pl.** canaliculi
Canalização: canalization
Canavanase: canavanase
Canavanina: canavanine
Câncer: cancer (CA)
Cancerofobia: cancerophobia
Canceroso: cancerous
Cancriforme: cancriform, chancriform
Cancro: cancrum, **pl.** cancra; canker, chancre
Cancróide: cancroid, chancroid, chancroidal
Cancroso: chancrous
Candela: candela (cd)

Candicidina: candicidin
Candidemia: candidemia
Candidíase: candidiasis, candidosis
Candidíase oral: thrush
Canfano: camphene
Cânfora: camphor
Canforáceo: camphoraceous
Canforado: camphorated
Canície: canities
Caniemba: kanyemba
Caniniforme: caniniform
Canino: canine
Cansaço: defatigation
Cansilato de trimetafano: trimetaphan camsylate
Cantárida: cantharis, **gen.** cantharidis, **pl.** cantharides
Cantaridato: cantharidate
Cantarídico: cantharidal
Cantaridina: cantharidin
Cantectomia: canthectomy
Cantite: canthitis
Canto: canthus, **pl.** canthi
Cantólise: cantholysis
Cantoplastia: canthoplasty
Cantorrafia: canthorrhaphy
Cantotomia: canthotomy
Cânula: cannula
Cânula de Karman: Karman cannula
Canulação: cannulation, cannulization
Caolim: kaolin
Caolinose: kaolinosis
Caos: chaos
Caotrópico: chaotropic
Caotropismo: chaotropism
Capacidade: ability, capacity
Capacismo: kappacism
Capacitação: capacitation
Capacitância: capacitance
Capacitor: capacitor
Capactinas: capactins
Capeamento: capping
Capilar: capillary
Capilarectasia: capillarectasia
Capilaríase: capillariasis
Capilaridade: capillarity
Capilariomotor: capillariomotor
Capilarioscopia: capillarioscopy
Capilarite: capillaritis
Capilaropatia: capillaropathy
Capilaroscopia: capillaroscopy
Capitação: capitation
Capitato: capitate, magnum
Capitopodálico: capitopedal
Capitular: capitular
Capítulo: capitellum, capitulum, **pl.** capitula
Capnógrafo: capnograph
Capnograma: capnogram
Capnometria: capnometry
Caprato: caprate
Caprilato: caprylate
Capriloquismo: capriloquism
Caprina: caprin
Caprino: caprine
Caprizante: caprizant
Caproato: caproate
Caproíla: caproyl

Caproilato: caproylate
Capsaicina: capsaicin
Capsicina: capsicin
Cápsico: capsicum
Capsídeo: capsid
Capsômero: capsomer, capsomere
Cápsula: capsula, gen. e pl. capsulae; capsule
Cápsula da lente: phacocyst
Capsular: capsular
Capsulectomia: capsulectomy
Capsulite: capsulitis
Capsulolenticular: capsulolenticular
Capsuloplastia: capsuloplasty
Capsulorrafia: capsulorrhaphy
Capsulorrexe: capsulorrhexis
Capsulotomia: capsulotomy
Capsulótomo: capsulotome
Captação: uptake
Captopril: captopril
Captura: capture
Capuz: hood
Caquético: cachectic
Caquetina: cachectin
Caquexia: cachexia
Caquinação: cachinnation
Característica: characteristic
Características: features
Caracterização: characterization
Caramelo: caramel
Caramujo: snail
Caranguejo: crab
Carate: carate
Caráter: character
Caravela: man-of-war
Carbacol: carbachol
Carbadox: carbadox
Carbamato: carbamate
Carbamazepina: carbamazepine
Carbamida: carbamide
Carbamilação: carbamylation
Carbaminoemoglobina: carbaminohemoglobin
Carbamoato: carbamoate
Carbamoil: carbamoyl, carbamyl
Carbamoil fosfato: carbamoyl phosphate
Carbamoilação: carbamoylation
Carbamoilaspartato desidrase: carbamoylaspartate dehydrase
Carbamoiltransferases: carbamoyltransferases
Carbamoiluréia: carbamoylurea
Carbanion: carbanion
Carbapenêmicos: carbapenems
Carbaril: carbaril, carbaryl
Carbarsona: carbarsone
Carbazidas: carbazides
Carbazol: carbazole
Carbenicilina dissódica: carbenicillin disodium
Carbênio: carbenium
Carbidopa: carbidopa
Carbimazol: carbimazole
Carbinol: carbinol
Carbocátion: carbocation

Carboemoglobina: carbhemoglobin, carbohemoglobin
Carbogênio: carbogen
Carboidratos: carbohydrates
Carboidratúria: carbohydraturia
Carboidrazidas: carbohydrazides
Carbolfucsina: carbolfuchsin
Carbólico: carbolate
Carbolizado: carbolated
Carbolizar: carbolize
Carbolúria: carboluria
Carbômero: carbomer
Carbometria: carbometry
Carbomicina: carbomycin
Carbonato: carbonate
Carbonato de amônio: hartshorn
Carbonato sódico de diidroxialumínio: dihydroxyaluminum sodium carbonate
Carboneto: carbide
Carbônico: carbonic
Carbonila: carbonyl
Carbônio: carbonium
Carbono: carbon (C)
Carbono-11 (C^{11}): carbon-11 (^{11}C)
Carbono-12 (C^{12}): carbon-12 (^{12}C)
Carbono-13 (C^{13}): carbon-13 (^{13}C)
Carbono-14 (C^{14}): carbon-14 (^{14}C)
Carbonometria: carbonometry
Carbonômetro: carbonometer
Carbonúria: carbonuria
Carboplatina: carboplatin
Carboprost-trometamina: carboprost tromethamine
Carboxamida: carboxamide
Carboxicatepsina: carboxycathepsin
Carboxidismutase: carboxydismutase
Carboxiemoglobina: carboxyhemoglobin (HbCO)
Carboxiemoglobinemia: carboxyhemoglobinemia
Carboxila: carboxyl
Carboxilação: carboxylation
Carboxilase: carboxylase
Carboxilase pirúvico-málica: pyruvic-malic carboxylase
Carboxiltransferases: carboxyltransferases
Carboximetilcelulose: carboxymethylcellulose
Carboximida: carboximide
Carboxipeptidase: carboxypeptidase
Carboxipeptidase A: carboxypeptidase A
Carboxipeptidase B: carboxypeptidase B
Carboxipeptidase C: carboxypeptidase C

Carboxipeptidase G: carboxypeptidase G
Carbromal: carbromal
Carbúnculo: carbuncle
Carbureto: carburet
Carbutamida: carbutamide
Carcaça: carcass
Carcinoembrionário: carcinoembryonic
Carcinoestático: carcinostatic
Carcinofobia: carcinophobia
Carcinogênese: carcinogenesis
Carcinogenicidade: carcinogenicity
Carcinogênico: carcinogenic
Carcinógeno: carcinogen
Carcinóide: carcinoid
Carcinolítico: carcinolytic
Carcinoma: carcinoma (CA), **pl.** carcinomas, carcinomata
Carcinoma ex-adenoma pleomórfico: carcinoma ex pleomorphic adenoma
Carcinomatose: carcinomatosis
Carcinomatoso: carcinomatous
Carcinossarcoma: carcinosarcoma
Carcoma: carcoma
Cardagem: carding
Cardamomo: cardamom
Cardenolídeo: cardenolide
Cárdia: cardia, gastric cardia
Cardíaco: cardiac
Cardialgia: cardialgia
Cardiectasia: cardiectasia
Cardiectomia: cardiectomy
Cardiectopia: cardiectopia
Cardinal: cardinal
Cardioacelerador: cardioaccelerator
Cardioangiografia: cardioangiography
Cardioaórtico: cardioaortic
Cardioarterial: cardioarterial
Cardioativo: cardioactive
Cardiocalásia: cardiochalasia
Cardiocele: cardiocele
Cardiocimografia: cardiokymography
Cardiocimógrafo: cardiokymograph
Cardiocimograma: cardiokymogram
Cardiodinâmica: cardiodynamics
Cardiodinia: cardiodynia
Cardiodiose: cardiodiosis
Cardioemotrombo: cardiohemothrombus
Cardioesfigmógrafo: cardiosphygmograph
Cardioesofágico: cardioesophageal
Cardioespasmo: cardiospasm
Cardiofobia: cardiophobia
Cardiofonia: cardiophony
Cardiófono: cardiophone
Cardiofrenia: cardiophrenia
Cardiogênese: cardiogenesis
Cardiogênico: cardiogenic
Cardiografia: cardiography

Cardiógrafo: cardiograph
Cardiograma: cardiogram
Cárdio-hepático: cardiohepatic
Cárdio-hepatomegalia: cardiohepatomegaly
Cardióide: cardioid
Cardioinibidor: cardioinhibitory
Cardiolipina: cardiolipin
Cardiólise: cardiolysis
Cardiologia: cardiology
Cardiologista: cardiologist
Cardiomalacia: cardiomalacia
Cardiomegalia: cardiomegaly
Cardiometria: cardiometry
Cardiomotilidade: cardiomotility
Cardiomuscular: cardiomuscular
Cardionatrina: cardionatrin
Cardionecrose: cardionecrosis
Cardionector: cardionector
Cardionéfrico: cardionephric
Cardioneural: cardioneural
Cardioneurose: cardioneurosis
Cardioomentopexia: cardioomentopexy
Cardiopaludismo: cardiopaludism
Cardiopata: cardiopath
Cardiopatia: cardiopathy
Cardiopatia negra: cardiopathia nigra
Cardiopilórico: cardiopyloric
Cardioplastia: cardioplasty
Cardioplegia: cardioplegia
Cardioplégico: cardioplegic
Cardioptose: cardioptosia
Cardiopulmonar: cardiopulmonary, pneumocardial
Cardiorrafia: cardiorrhaphy
Cardiorrenal: cardiorenal
Cardiorrexe: cardiorrhexis
Cardioscópio: cardioscope
Cardiosseletividade: cardioselectivity
Cardiosseletivo: cardioselective
Cardiotacômetro: cardiotachometer
Cardiotaxia: cardiataxia
Cardiotelia: cardiatelia
Cardiotireotoxicose: cardiothyrotoxicosis
Cardiotomia: cardiotomy
Cardiotônico: cardiotonic
Cardiotóxico: cardiotoxic
Cardiotoxina: cardiotoxin
Cardiotrombo: cardiothrombus
Cardiovalvite: cardiovalvulitis
Cardiovascular: cardiovascular (CV), cardiovasculare
Cardiovasculorrenal: cardiovasculorenal
Cardioversão: cardioversion
Cardioversor: cardioverter
Cardioverter: cardiovert
Cardite: carditis
Carfologia: floccillation
Carga: burden
Carga de corpo: body burden
Cariado: carious

Caribe: caribi
Cárie: caries
Carina: carina, **pl.** carinae
Carinado: carinate
Cariócito: karyocyte
Carioclase: karyoclasis
Cariocroma: karyochrome
Cariófago: karyophage
Cariófilo: caryophyllus, caryophyllum
Cariogamia: karyogamy
Cariogâmico: karyogamic, cariogenesis
Cariogênese: cariogenesis, karyogenesis
Cariogenicidade: cariogenicity
Cariogênico: cariogenic, karyogenic
Cariogônada: karyogonad
Cariograma: karyogram
Cariolinfa: karyolymph
Cariólise: karyolysis
Cariolítico: karyolytic
Cariologia: cariology, karyology
Cariômero: karyomere
Cariomicrossoma: karyomicrosome
Cariomitoma: karyomitome
Cariomorfismo: karyomorphism
Cárion: karyon
Cariopicnose: karyopyknosis
Cariopicnótico: karyopyknotic
Carioplasma: karyoplasm
Carioplasmólise: karyoplasmolysis
Carioplastina: karyoplastin
Carioplasto: karyoplast
Cariorrexe: karyorrhexis
Cariossoma: karyosome
Cariostase: karyostasis
Cariostático: cariostatic
Carioteca: caryotheca, karyotheca
Cariótipo: karyotype
Cariozóico: karyozoic
Carisoprodol: carisoprodate, carisoprodol
Carissina: carisin
Carmalume: carmalum
Carmim: carmine
Carminado: carminate
Carminativo: carminative
Carminófilo: carminophil, carminophile, carminophilous
Carmustina: BCNU, carmustine
Carne: caro, **gen.** carnis, **pl.** carnes
Carniceiro: carnassial
Carnificação: carnification
Carnitina: carnitine
Carnívoro: carnivore, carnivorous
Carnosidade: carnosity
Carnosina: carnosine
Carnosinase: carnosinase
Carnosinemia: carnosinemia
Carnoso: carneous
Carotenase: carotenase
Carotenemia: carotenemia
Caroteno: carotene

β-caroteno 15,15′-dioxigenase: β-carotene 15,15′-dioxygenase
Carotenodermia: carotenoderma
Carotenóide: carotenoid
Carotenóides: carotenoids
Carotenoproteína: carotenoprotein
Carotenose cutânea: carotenosis cutis, carotinosis cutis
Carótico: carotic
Caroticotimpânico: caroticotympanic
Carotídeo: carotid
Carotidinia: carotidynia
Carotinemia: carotinemia
Carotodinia: carotodynia
Carpal: carpal
Carpectomia: carpectomy
Carpocarpal: carpocarpal
Carpometacarpal: carpometacarpal
Carpopodal: carpopedal
Carpoptose: carpoptosis, carpoptosia
Carragena: carrageen, carragheen
Carragenina: carrageenan, carrageenin
Carrapato: tick
Cártamo: carthamus
Cartesiano: cartesian
Cartilagem: cartilage, cartilago, **pl.** cartilagines; chondrus, gristle
Cartilagem costal: costicartilage
Cartilaginóide: cartilaginoid
Cartilaginoso: cartilaginous
Carúncula: caruncle, caruncula, **pl.** carunculae
Carvacrol: carvacrol
Carvão: carbo, charcoal
Carvão animal: animal black, bone black
Carvedilol: carvedilol
Casaminoácidos: casamino acids
Casca: bark
Casca de canela: cassia bark
Casca de cereira: bayberry bark
Casca de kurchi: kurchi bark
Casca de laranja: peau d'orange
Casca de ovo: eggshell
Casca-de-honduras: Honduras bark
Cáscara: cascara
Cascata: cascade
Cascata do ácido araquidônico: arachidonic acid cascade
Cascavel: rattlesnake
Caseificação: caseation
Caseína: casein
Caseinato: caseinate
Caseinogênio: caseinogen
Caseose: caseose
Caseoso: caseous
Caso: case
Caspa: dandruff, scurf
Cassete: cassette
Cássia imperial: cassia fistula

Cássia purgativa: purging cassia
Castanho de Bismarck R: Bismarck brown R
Castanho de Bismarck Y: Bismarck brown Y
Castração: castration
Castrar: castrate, spay, unsex
Casualidade: casualty
Catabasial: catabasial
Catabiótico: catabiotic
Catabólico: catabolic
Catabolismo: catabolism
Catabólito: catabolite
Catacronobiologia: catachronobiology
Catacrótico: catacrotic
Catacrotismo: catacrotism
Catadicrótico: catadicrotic
Catadicrotismo: catadicrotism
Catadídimo: catadidymus
Catadióptrico: catadioptric
Catádromo: catadromous
Cataforese: cataphoresis
Cataforético: cataphoretic
Catagênese: catagenesis
Catágeno: catagen
Catal: katal (kat)
Catalase: catalase
Catalepsia: catalepsy
Catalépico: cataleptic
Cataleptóide: cataleptoid
Catalisador: catalyst, catalyzer
Catalisar: catalyze
Catálise: catalysis
Catalítico: catalytic
Catamnese: catamnesis
Catamnésico: catamnestic
Catapasma: catapasm
Cataplasia: cataplasia, cataplasis
Cataplasma: cataplasm, poultice
Catapléctico: cataplectic
Cataplexia: cataplexy
Catarata: cataract, cataracta
Cataratogênese: cataractogenesis
Cataratogênico: cataractogenic
Cataratoso: cataractous
Catária: cataria, catnep, catnip
Catarral: catarrhal
Catarse: catharsis
Catártico: cathartic
Catastalse: catastalsis
Catastáltico: catastaltic
Catástase: catastasis
Catatermômetro: katathermometer
Catatonia: catatonia
Catatônico: catatonic, catatoniac
Catatricrótico: catatricrotic
Catatricrotismo: catatricrotism
Catatriquia: catatrichy
Catecase: catechase
Catechu: catechu nigrum, cutch
Catecol: catechol
Catecol 1,2-dioxigenase: catechol 1,2-dioxygenase
Catecol 2,3-dioxigenase: catechol 2,3-dioxygenase
Catecolaminas: catecholamines
Categute: catgut

Cateletrotônus: catelectrotonus
Catemoglobina: cathemoglobin
Catenina: catenin
Catenóide: catenoid
Catenulado: catenulate
Catepsina: cathepsin
Catequina: catechin
Cateter: cathether
Cateterização: catheterization
Cateterizar: catheterize
Cateterostato: catheterostat
Catético: cathectic
Catexia: cathexis, kathexis
Cátion: cation
Catiônico: cationic
Cationógeno: cationogen
Catlin: catlin, catling
Catódico: cathodal (C), cathodic
Catodo: cathode (Ca, C)
Católise: catholysis
Catóptrico: catoptric
Cauda: cauda, **pl.** caudae; tail
Caudado: caudate, caudatum
Caudal: caudad, caudal, caudalis
Caudatolenticular: caudatolenticular
Caudocefálico: caudocephalad
Caudolenticular: caudolenticular
Causa: cause
Causalgia: causalgia
Causalidade: causality
Cáustico: caustic
Cautério: cautery
Cauterização: cauterization
Cauterizador: cauterant
Cauterizar: cauterize
Cava: cava, caval
Cava-cava: kava
Cavagrama: cavagram
Cavalo-vapor: horsepower
Cavéola: caveola, **pl.** caveolae
Caverna: cave, cavern, caverna, **pl.** cavernae
Caverniloquia: caverniloquy
Cavernite: cavernitis
Cavernosite: cavernositis
Cavernoso: cavernous
Cavidade: cavea, cavitas, **pl.** cavitates; cavity
Cavitação: cavitation
Cavitário: cavitary
Cavite: cavitis
Cavo: cavum, **pl.** cava
Cavografia: cavography
Cavograma: cavogram
Cavossuperficial: cavosurface
Caxumba: mumps
Cebocefalia: cebocephaly
Cecal: cecal
Cecectomia: cecectomy
Ceceio: lisping
Cecite: cecitis
Ceco: caecum, cecum, **pl.** ceca; typhlon
Cecocolostomia: cecocolostomy
Cecofixação: cecofixation
Cecoileostomia: cecoileostomy
Cecopexia: cecopexy
Cecoplicatura: cecoplication
Cecorrafia: cecorrhaphy

Cecossigmoidostomia: cecosigmoidostomy
Cecostomia: cecostomy
Cecotomia: cecotomy
Cecoureterocele: cecoureterocele
Cecropinas: cecropins
Cefaclor: cefaclor
Cefadroxil: cefadroxil
Cefaelina: cephaeline
Cefalalgia: cephalalgia
Cefaledema: cephaledema
Cefaléia: headache
Cefalematocele: cephalhematocele
Cefalematoma: cephalhematoma
Cefalemia: cephalemia
Cefalemômetro: cephalohemometer
Cefalexina: cephalexin
Cefálico: cephalic
Cefalina: cephalin, cephaline, kephalin
Cefalite: cephalitis
Cefalização: cephalization
Cefalocaudal: cephalocaudal
Cefalocele: cephalocele
Cefalocentese: cephalocentesis
Cefalocórdio: cephalochord
Cefalodactilia de Vogt: Vogt cephalodactyly
Cefalodídimo: cephalodidymus
Cefalodinia: cephalodynia
Cefalodiprosopo: cephalodiprosopus
Cefaloematocele: cephalohematocele
Cefaloematoma: cephalohematoma
Cefalofaríngeo: cephalopharyngeus
Cefalogênese: cephalogenesis
Cefalogírico: cephalogyric
Cefaloglicina: cephaloglycin
Cefalograma: cephalogram
Cefaloidrocele: cephalhydrocele
Cefalomegalia: cephalomegaly
Cefalômelo: cephalomelus
Cefalomeningite: cephalomeningitis
Cefalometria: cephalometrics, cephalometry
Cefalômetro: cephalometer
Cefalomotor: cephalomotor
Cefalonte: cephalont
Cefalópago: cephalopagus
Cefalopélvico: cephalopelvic
Cefalopelvimetria: cephalopelvimetry
Cefaloridina: cephaloridine
Cefalorraquidiano: cephalorrhachidian
Cefalosporina: cephalosporin
Cefalosporinase: cephalosporinase
Cefalostato: cephalostat
Cefalotina: cephalothin
Cefalotomia: cephalotomy
Cefalótomo: cephalotome
Cefalotorácico: cephalothoracic
Cefalotoracópago: cephalothoracopagus
Cefalotoxina: cephalotoxin
Cefalótribo: cephalotribe
Cefamicina: cephamycins
Cefapirina sódica: cephapirin sodium
Cefazolina: cefazolin
Cefonicida dissódica: cefonicid disodium
Cefoperazona sódica: cefoperazone sodium
Ceforanida: ceforanide
Cefotaxima sódica: cefotaxime sodium
Cefotetan dissódico: cefotetan disodium
Cefoxitina sódica: cefoxitin sodium
Cefradina: cephradine
Ceftazidima sódica: ceftazidime sodium
Ceftizoxima sódica: ceftizoxime sodium
Ceftriaxona dissódica: ceftriaxone disodium
Cego: blind
Cegueira: blindness
Cel: cel
Celenterados: coelenterate
Celêntero: celenteron
Celíaco: celiac
Celiagra: celiagra
Celícola: cellicolous
Celiocentese: celiocentesis
Celiomialgia: celiomyalgia
Celiomiosite: celiomyositis
Celioparacentese: celioparacentesis
Celiopatia: celiopathy
Celiorrafia: celiorrhaphy
Celioscopia: celioscopy
Celiotomia: celiotomy, ventrotomy
Celite: celitis
Celobiase: cellobiase
Celobiose: cellobiose
Celoexose: cellohexose
Celoflebite: celophlebitis
Celoidina: celloidin
Celoma: celom, celoma, coelom
Celômico: celomic
Celoscopia: celoscopy
Celoscópio: celoscope
Celossomia: celosomia
Celozóico: celozoic
Célula: cell, cellula, **gen. e pl.** cellulae; cellule
Célula falciforme: meniscocyte
Célula oxifílica: oxyphil, oxyphile
Celular: cellular
Celularidade: cellularity
Células de Berger: Berger cells
Celulase: cellulase
Celulicida: cellulicidal
Celulífugo: cellulifugal
Celulina: cellulin
Celulípeto: cellulipetal
Celulite: cellulite, cellulitis
Celulose: cellulose
Cem: centum
Cementificação: cementification
Cemento: cement, cementum
Cementoblasto: cementoblast
Cementoblastoma: cementoblastoma
Cementócito: cementocyte
Cementoclasia: cementoclasia
Cementoclasto: cementoclast
Cementodentário: cementodentinal
Cementogênese: cementogenesis
Cementoma: cementoma
Cena: scene
Cenestesia: cenesthesia, coenesthesia
Cenestésico: cenesthesic, cenesthetic
Cenocítico: cenocytic, coenocytic
Cenócito: cenocyte, coenocyte
Cenósito: cenosite
Cenótropo: cenotrope
Censo: census
Censor: censor
Centese: centesis
Centibar: centibar
Centígrado: centigrade (C)
Centigrama: centigram
Centil: centile
Centilitro: centiliter
Centímetro: centimeter (cm)
Centimorgan (cM): centimorgan (cM)
Centinormal: centinormal
Centípode: centipede
Centipoise: centipoise
Centragem: centrage
Central: centralis
Centrencefálico: centrencephalic
Centricipúcio: centriciput
Cêntrico: centric
Centrífuga: centrifuge
Centrifugação: centrifugalization, centrifugation
Centrifugar: centrifugalize
Centrífugo: centrifugal
Centrilobular: centrilobular
Centríolo: centriole
Centrípeto: centripetal
Centro: center, centrum, **pl.** centra
Centro de saúde: health center
Centro mediano de Luys: centre médian de Luys
Centroblasto: centroblast
Centrocinesia: centrokinesia
Centrocinético: centrokinetic
Centrócito: centrocyte
Centrolécito: centrolecithal
Centrômero: centromere
Centroplasma: centroplasm
Centrosfera: centrosphere
Centrossoma: centrosome
Centrostáltico: centrostaltic
Cenuro: cenuris, coenuris
Cenurose: cenurosis, cenuriasis, coenurosis
Cepa: strain
Cera: cera, wax
Cera de abelha: beeswax
Ceráceo: ceraceous
Ceramida: ceramide
Ceramidase: ceramidase
Cerasina: cerasin, kerasin
Ceratectomia: keratectomy
Cerateína: keratein
Ceratina: ceratin
Ceratinócito: keratinocyte
Ceratinofílico: keratinophilic
Ceratinoso: keratinous
Ceratinossoma: keratinosome
Ceratite: keratitis
Cerato: cerate
Ceratoacantoma: keratoacanthoma
Ceratoangioma: keratoangioma
Ceratocele: keratocele
Ceratocisto: keratocyst
Ceratócito: keratocyte
Ceratocone: keratoconus
Ceratoconjuntivite: keratoconjunctivitis
Ceratocricóide: ceratocricoid, keratocricoid
Ceratoderma: keratoderma
Ceratodermatite: keratodermatitis
Ceratoectasia: keratectasia, keratoectasia
Ceratoelastoidose: keratoelastoidosis
Ceratoepitelioplastia: keratoepithelioplasty
Ceratoesclerite: keratoscleritis
Ceratofaquia: keratophakia
Ceratogênese: keratogenesis
Ceratogenético: keratogenetic
Ceratógeno: keratogenous
Ceratoglobo: keratoglobus
Ceratografia: keratography
Ceratoialino: keratohyalin
Ceratóide: keratoid
Ceratoióide: ceratohyal, keratohyal
Ceratoleptinse: keratoleptynsis
Ceratoleucoma: keratoleukoma
Ceratólise: keratolysis
Ceratolítico: keratolytic
Ceratoma: keratoma
Ceratomalacia: keratomalacia
Ceratometria: keratometry
Ceratômetro: keratometer
Ceratomicose: keratomycosis
Ceratomileuse: keratomileusis
Ceratonose: keratonosis
Ceratopaquidermia: keratopachyderma
Ceratopatia: keratopathia, keratopathy
Ceratoplasia: keratoplasia
Ceratoplastia: keratoplasty
Ceratoprótese: keratoprosthesis
Ceratoro: keratorus
Ceratorrexe: keratorhexis, keratorrhexis
Ceratoscopia: keratoscopy
Ceratoscópio: keratoscope

Glossário

Ceratose: keratosis, pl. keratoses
Ceratossulfato: keratosulfate
Ceratotomia: keratotomy
Ceratótomo: keratome, keratotome
Ceraunofobia: keraunophobia
Cercária: cercaria, pl. cercariae
Cerclagem: cerclage
Cerco: cercus, gen. e pl. cerci
Cercocisto: cercocystis
Cercômero: cercomer
Cercomonídeos: cercomonad
Cercos: cerci
Cerda: chaeta, seta, pl. setae
Cerebelar: cerebellar
Cerebelina: cerebellin
Cerebelite: cerebellitis
Cerebelo: cerebellum, pl. cerebella
Cerebelobulbar: cerebellomedullary
Cerebelolenticular: cerebellolental
Cerebelo-olivar: cerebello-olivary
Cerebelopontino: cerebellopontine
Cerebelorrubro: cerebellorubral
Cerebração: cerebration
Cerebral: cerebral
Cerebriforme: cerebriform
Cerebrite: cerebritis
Cérebro: brain, cerebrum, pl. cerebra, cerebrums
Cérebro isolado: cerveau isolé, encéphale isolé
Cerebrocupreína: cerebrocuprein
Cerebroespinal: cerebrospinal
Cerebrofisiologia: cerebrophysiology
Cerebroma: cerebroma
Cerebromalacia: cerebromalacia
Cerebromeningite: cerebromeningitis
Cerebrona: cerebron
Cerebropatia: cerebropathia, cerebropathy
Cerebrosclerose: cerebrosclerosis
Cerebrosídeo: cerebroside
Cerebrosidose: cerebrosidosis
Cerebrosterol: cerebrosterol
Cerebrotomia: cerebrotomy
Cerebrovascular: cerebrovascular
Ceresina: ceresin
Cerila: ceryl
Cerina: cerin
Cério: cerium (Ce)
Cerne: kernel
Ceróide: ceroid
Ceroplastia: ceroplasty
Cerosina: cerosin
Certificação: certification
Ceruleína: cerulein
Cerúleo: cerulean
Ceruloplasmina: ceruloplasmin
Cerume: cerumen, earwax

Ceruminolítico: ceruminolytic
Ceruminoma: ceruminoma
Ceruminose: ceruminosis
Ceruminoso: ceruminal, ceruminous
Cerusa: ceruse
Cervical: cervical, cervicalis
Cérvice: cervix, gen. cervicis, pl. cervices
Cervicectomia: cervicectomy
Cervicite: cervicitis
Cervicobraquial: cervicobrachial
Cervicobucal: cervicobuccal
Cervicodinia: cervicodynia
Cervicofacial: cervicofacial
Cervicografia: cervicography
Cervicolabial: cervicolabial
Cervicolingual: cervicolingual
Cervicolinguoaxial: cervicolinguoaxial
Cervico-occipital: cervico-occipital
Cervicoplastia: cervicoplasty
Cervicoscopia: cervicoscopy
Cervicotomia: cervicotomy
Cervicotorácico: cervicothoracic
Cervicovesical: cervicovesical
Cervilaxina: cervilaxin
Cesariana: cesarean, C-section
Césio: cesium (Cs)
Cestódeo: cestode, cestoid
Cestodíase: cestodiasis
Cetal: ketal
Cetamina: ketamine
Cetanserina: ketanserin
Ceteno: ketene
Cetila: cetyl
Cetimina: ketimine
Cetoacidemia: ketoacidemia
Cetoácido: keto acid, oxo acid
3-cetoácido-CoA transferase: 3-ketoacid-CoA transferase
Cetoacidose: ketoacidosis
Cetoacidúria: ketoaciduria
β-cetoacil-ACP redutase: β-ketoacyl-ACP reductase
β-cetoacil-ACP sintase: β-ketoacyl-ACP synthase
3-cetoacil-CoA tiolase: 3-ketoacyl-CoA thiolase
2-cetoadípico acidemia: 2-ketoadipic acidemia
Cetoconazol: ketoconazole
α-cetodescarboxilase: α-ketodecarboxylase
Cetoeptose: ketoheptose
Cetoexose: ketohexose
Cetogênese: ketogenesis
Cetogênico: ketogenic
α-cetoglutarato: α-ketoglutarate
β-cetoidrogenase: β-ketohydrogenase
Cetoidroxiestrina: ketohydroxyestrin
Cetol: ketol, ketole
Cetolítico: ketolytic
Cetona: ketone
Cetona-aldeído mutase: ketone-aldehyde mutase

Cetonemia: ketonemia
Cetônico: ketonic
Cetonização: ketonization
Cetonúria: ketonuria
Cetopentose: ketopentose
Cetorolaco: ketorolac
β-cetorredutase: β-ketoreductase
Cetose: ketose, ketosis
Cetose-1-fosfato aldolase: ketose-1-phosphate aldolase
Cetose redutase: ketose reductase
17-cetosteróides: 17-ketosteroids (17-KS)
Cetosúria: ketosuria
Cetotetrose: ketotetrose
Cetótico: ketotic
β-cetotiolase: β-ketothiolase
Cetotriose: ketotriose
Cetrária: cetraria
Cevadilha: cevadilla, sabadilla
Cevadina: cevadine
Chá: tea, thea
Chagoma: chagoma
Chance: odds
Chanfrado: notched
Chanfradura: nick, nicking
Chanfro: chamfer
Charlatanismo: charlatanism, quackery
Charlatão: charlatan, quack
Cheirar: smell
Chicle: chicle
Chicote: whiplash
Chimpanzé: chimpanzee
Chinchona: Jesuits bark
Choque: shock
Chumaço: wadding
Chumbo: lead (Pb), plumbum
Chumbo tetraetila: tetraethyllead
Ciagnófilo: cyanophilous
Cianamida: cyanamide
Cianato: cyanate
Cianemia: cyanemia
Cianeto: cyanide
Cianeto de bromobenzila: bromobenzylcyanide (BBC)
Cianidenona: cyanidenon
Cianidol: cyanidol
Cianoálcoois: cyanalcohols
Cianocobalamina: cyanocobalamin
Cianocróico: cyanochroic, cyanochrous
Cianofíceas: Cyanophyceae
Cianófilo: cyanophil, cyanophile
Cianogênico: cyanogenic
Cianogênio: cyanogen
Cianoidrinas: cyanohydrins
Cianometemoglobina: cyanmethemoglobin
Cianopia: cyanopia
Cianopsia: cyanopsia
Cianose: cyanosis
Cianótico: cyanosed, cyanotic
Cianúria: cyanuria
Ciática: sciatica
Ciático: sciatic
Ciatóstoma: *Cyathostoma*

Cíbalo; coprólito: scybalum, pl. scybala
Cibaloso: scybalous
Cibernética: cybernetics
Cibofobia: cibophobia
Cíbrido: cybrid
Cicatrectomia: cicatrectomy
Cicatricial: cicatricial
Cicatricotomia: cicatricotomy, cicatrisotomy
Cicatriz: cicatrix, pl. cicatrices; scar
Cicatrização: cicatrization
Cicatrizante: cicatrizant
Ciclamato: cyclamate
Ciclamida: cyclamide
Ciclandelato: cyclandelate
Ciclartrodial: cyclarthrodial
Ciclartrose: cyclarthrosis
Ciclase: cyclase
Ciclectomia: cyclectomy
Cíclico: cyclic
Ciclina D: cyclin D
Ciclite: cyclitis
Ciclo: cycle
Ciclocefalia: cyclocephaly, cyclocephalia
Ciclocoroidite: cyclochoroiditis
Ciclocrioterapia: cyclocryotherapy
Ciclocumarol: cyclocumarol
Ciclodestrutivo: cyclodestructive
Ciclodiálise: cyclodialysis
Ciclodiatermia: cyclodiathermy
Ciclodução: cycloduction
Cicloencefalia: cyclencephaly, cyclencephalia
Cicloeximida: cycloheximide
Cicloforases: cyclophorases
Cicloforia: cyclophoria
Ciclofosfamida: cyclophosphamide
Ciclofotocoagulação: cyclophotocoagulation
Ciclóide: cycloid
Ciclol: cyclol
Ciclonamina: cyclonamine
Ciclooxigenase: cyclooxygenase
Ciclope: cyclops
Ciclopenta[a]fenantreno: cyclopenta[a]phenanthrene
Ciclopentano: cyclopentane
Ciclopentiazida: cyclopenthiazide
Ciclopeptídeo: cyclopeptide
Ciclopia: cyclopea, cyclopia
Ciclópico: cyclopean, cyclopian
Ciclopiroxolamina: ciclopiroxolamine
Cicloplegia: cycloplegia
Cicloplégico: cycloplegic
Ciclopropano: cyclopropane
Ciclos por segundo: cycles per second (cps)
Ciclose: cyclosis
Ciclosporina: cyclosporine
Ciclosporina A: cyclosporin A
Ciclosserina: cycloserine
Ciclotiazida: cyclothiazide
Ciclotimia: cyclothymia

Ciclotímico: cyclothymiac, cyclothymic
Ciclotomia: cyclotomy
Ciclotorção: cyclotorsion
Ciclótron: cyclotron
Ciclotropia: cyclotropia
Ciclozoonose: cyclozoonosis
Cicuta: conium, hemlock
Cicutoxina: cicutoxin
Ciência: science
Ciências comportamentais: behavioral sciences
Cientimetria: scientometrics
Ciese: cyesis
Cifióideo: scyphiform, scyphoid
Cifo: kyphos
Cifoescoliose: kyphoscoliosis
Cifose: kyphosis
Cifótico: kyphotic
Ciguatera: ciguatera, siguatera
Ciguatoxina: ciguatoxin
Cila: scilla, squill
Cilareno: scillaren
Cilaricida: scillaricide
Cilastatina sódica: cilastatin sodium
Ciliado: ciliated
Ciliados: Ciliata, ciliates
Ciliar: ciliary
Ciliectomia: ciliectomy
Cilíndrico: cylindrical
Cilindro: cylinder (cyl., C)
Cilindroadenoma: cylindroadenoma
Cilindro-eixo: cylindraxis
Cilindróide: cylindroid
Cilindroma: cylindroma
Cilindrúria: cylindruria
Cílio: cilium, **pl.** cilia; eyelash
Ciliocitoftoria: ciliocytophthoria
Cilioescleral: cilioscleral
Cilioespinhal: ciliospinal
Cilióforos: Ciliophora
Ciliogênese: ciliogenesis
Ciliorretiniano: cilioretinal
Ciliostático: ciliastatic
Ciliotoxicidade: ciliotoxicity
Cilirosídeo: scilliroside
Cilobactéria: *Cillobacterium*
Cilossoma: cyllosoma
Cimarina: cymarin
Cimbocefalia: cymbocephaly
Cimbocefálico: cymbocephalic, cymbocephalous
Cimentação: cementation
Cimentículo: cementicle
Cimetidina: cimetidine
Cinamaldeído: cinnamaldehyde
Cinamato: cinnamate
Cinameína: cinnamein
Cinameno: cinnamene
Cinâmico: cinnamic
Cinamomo: cinnamon
Cinanestesia: cinanesthesia, kinanesthesia
Cinantropia: cynanthropy
Cinarizina: cinnarizine
Cinase: kinase
Cinase II: kinase II
Cinchofeno: cinchophen
Cinchona: cinchona, Peruvian bark
Cinchônico: cinchonic
Cinchonina: cinchonine
Cinchonismo: cinchonism
Cínclise: cinclisis
Cincol: cinchol
Cineangiocardiografia: cineangiocardiography
Cinefluorografia: cinefluorography
Cinefluoroscopia: cinefluoroscopy
Cinefotomicrografia: cinephotomicrography
Cinegastroscopia: cinegastroscopy
Cinemática: cinematics, kinematics
Cinemômetro: kinemometer
Cineol: cineole, cineol
Cineplástica: cineplastics
Cinéreo: cinerea, cinereal
Cinerício: cineritious
Cinerradiografia: cineradiography, cineroentgenography
Cinese: kinesis
Cinesia: kinesics
Cinesiatria: kinesiatrics
Cinesímetro: kinesimeter
Cinesina: kinesin
Cinesiofobia: kinesophobia
Cinesiologia: kinesiology
Cinesiômetro: kinesiometer
Cinesiopatista: kinesipathist
Cinesioterapia: kinesitherapy
Cinessismografia: cineseismography
Cinestesia: kinesthesia, kinesthesis
Cinestésico: kinesthetic
Cinestesiômetro: kinesthesiometer
Cinética: kinetics
Cinético: kinetic
Cinetocardiógrafo: kinetocardiograph
Cinetocardiograma: kinetocardiogram
Cinetócoro: kinetochore
Cinetócoros: kinetochores
Cinetogênico: kinetogenic
Cinetoplasma: cinetoplasm, cinetoplasma, kinetoplasm
Cinetoplasto: kinetoplast
Cinetoscópio: kinetoscope
Cinetossoma: kinetosome
Cingulado: cingulate
Cingulectomia: cingulectomy
Cíngulo: cingulum, **gen.** cinguli, **pl.** cingula
Cingulotomia: cingulotomy
Cinina: kinin
Cininogenase: kininogenase
Cininogenina: kininogenin
Cininogênio: kininogen
Cinipirina: cinnipirine
Cinocefalia: cynocephaly
Cinocentro: cinocentrum, kinocentrum
Cinocílio: kinocilium
Cinodonte: cynodont
Cinofobia: cynophobia
Cinomômetro: kinomometer
Cinoplasma: kinoplasm
Cinoplásmico: kinoplasmic
Cinoxacina: cinoxacin
Cinoxato: cinoxate
Cinticisternografia: scinticisternography
Cintilação: scintilation
Cintilador: scintillator
Cintilascópio: scintillascope
Cintilofotografia: scintiphotograph, scintiphotography
Cintilografia: scintigraphy, scintography
Cintilográfico: scintigraphic
Cintilógrafo: scintiscanner
Cintilograma: scintigram, scintiscan
Cintilomamografia: scintimammography
Cintilômetro: scintillometer
Cintura: waist
Cinturão: girdle
Cinzel: chisel
Cinzento: griseus
Cíon: cion
Cipridofobia: cypridophobia
Cirantina: cirantin
Circadiano: circadian
Circelo: circellus
Circinado: circinate
Circorário: circhoral
Circuito: circuit
Circulação: circulation
Circulatório: circulatory
Círculo: circle, circulus, **gen. e pl.** circuli
Circum-anal: circumanal
Circumandibular: circummandibular
Circum-articular: circumarticular
Circum-axilar: circumaxillary
Circumbulbar: circumbulbar
Circum-intestinal: circumintestinal
Circum-ocular: circumocular
Circum-oral: circumoral
Circum-orbitário: circumorbital
Circuncidado: apellous
Circuncisão: circumcision
Circuncisar: circumcise
Circuncórneo: circumcorneal
Circundução: circumductio, circumduction
Circunferência: circumference (c), circumferentia
Circunflexo: circumflex
Circungemal: circumgemmal
Circunlenticular: circumlental
Circunrenal: circumrenal
Circunscrito: circumscribed, circumscriptus
Circunstancialidade: circumstantiality
Circunuclear: circumnuclear
Circunvalado: circumvallate
Circunvascular: circumvascular
Circunventricular: circumventricular
Circunvoluto: circumvolute
Cirro: cirrus, **pl.** cirri; scirrhus
Cirrogênico: cirrhogenous, cirrhogenic
Cirronose: cirrhonosus
Cirrose: cirrhosis
Cirrosidade: scirrhosity
Cirroso: cirrose, cirrous, scirrhous
Cirrótico: cirrhotic
Cirsoftalmia: cirsophthalmia
Cirsóide: cirsoid
Cirsônfalo: cirsomphalos
Cirurgia: surgery
Cirurgião: surgeon
Cirúrgico: surgical
Cisalhamento: shear
Cisplatina: cisplatin
11-*cis*-retinal: 11-*cis*-retinal
11-*cis*-retinol: 11-*cis*-retinol
Cissão: scission
Cissiparidade: scissiparity
Cissura: scissura, **pl.** scissurae; scissure
Cistacanto: cystacanth
Cistadenocarcinoma: cystadenocarcinoma
Cistadenoma: cystadenoma
Cistalgia: cystalgia
Cistamina: cystamine
Cistationase: cystathionase
β-cistationase: β-cystathionase
γ-cistationase: γ-cystathionase
Cistationina: cystathionine
Cistationina β-liase: cystathionine β-lyase
Cistationina β-sintase: cystathionine β-synthase
Cistationina γ-liase: cystathionine γ-lyase
Cistationina γ-sintase: cystathionine γ-synthase
Cistationinúria: cystathioninuria
Cisteamina: cysteamine
Cistectomia: cystectomy
Cisteína: cysteine (C, Cys)
Cisteinil: cysteinyl
Cisterna: cistern, cisterna, **gen. e pl.** cisternae
Cisternografia: cisternography
Cisticerco: cysticercus, **pl.** cysticerci
Cisticercóide: cysticercoid
Cisticercose: cysticercosis
Cístico: cystic
Cistiforme: cystiform
Cistilaminopeptidase: cystyl-aminopeptidase
Cistina: cystine
Cistinemia: cystinemia
Cistinil: cystinyl
Cistinose: cystinosis
Cistinúria: cystinuria
Cististaxe: cystistaxis
Cistite: cystitis
Cisto: cyst, cystis, **pl.** cystides
Cisto sebáceo: wen
Cistoadenoma: cystoadenoma

Glossário

Cistocarcinoma: cystocarcinoma
Cistocele: cystocele, vesicocele
Cistocromoscopia: cystochromoscopy
Cistoduodenostomia: cystoduodenostomy
Cistoenterocele: cystoenterocele
Cistoenterostomia: cystoenterostomy
Cistoepiplocele: cystoepiplocele
Cistoespasmo: cystospasm
Cistofibroma: cystofibroma
Cistofotografia: cystophotography
Cistogastrostomia: cystogastrostomy
Cistografia: cystography
Cistograma: cystogram
Cistóide: cystoid
Cistojejunostomia: cystojejunostomy
Cistolitíase: cystolithiasis, vesicolithiasis
Cistolítico: cystolithic
Cistólito: cystolith
Cistolitolapaxia: cystolitholapaxy
Cistolitotomia: cystolithotomy
Cistoma: cystoma
Cistometria: cystometry
Cistômetro: cystometer
Cistometrografia: cystometrography
Cistometrograma (CMG): cystometrogram (CMG)
Cistomioma: cystomyoma
Cistomixoadenoma: cystomyxoadenoma
Cistomixoma: cystomyxoma
Cistomorfo: cystomorphous
Cistopanendoscopia: cystopanendoscopy
Cistoparalisia: cystoparalysis
Cistopexia: cystopexy, ventrocystorrhaphy
Cistopielite: cystopyelitis
Cistopielonefrite: cystopyelonephritis
Cistoplastia: cystoplasty
Cistoplegia: cystoplegia
Cistoprostatectomia: cystoprostatectomy
Cistorrafia: cystorrhaphy
Cistorréia: cystorrhea
Cistoscopia: cystoscopy
Cistoscópio: cystoscope
Cistossarcoma: cystosarcoma
Cistostomia: cystostomy
Cistotomia: cystotomy
Cistótomo: cystotome
Cistoureterite: cystoureteritis
Cistoureterografia: cystoureterography
Cistoureterograma: cystoureterogram
Cistouretrite: cystourethritis
Cistouretrocele: cystourethrocele

Cistouretrografia: cystourethrography
Cistouretrograma: cystourethrogram
Cistouretroscópio: cystourethroscope
Cístron: cistron
Cisvestismo: cisvestism, cisvestitism
Citaférese: cytapheresis
Citarabina: cytarabine
Citase: cytase
Citidina: cytidine (C, Cyd)
Citidina difosfoaçúcar (CAP- açúcar): cytidine diphosphosugar (CDP-sugar)
Citidina difosfocolina (CDP-colina): cytidine diphosphocholine (CDP-choline)
Citidina difosfoglicerídeo (CDP-glicerídeo): cytidine diphosphoglyceride (CDP-glyceride)
Citisina: cytisine
Citoanalisador: cytoanalyzer
Citoarquitetônico: cytoarchitectural
Citoarquitetura: cytoarchitectonics, cytoarchitecture
Citobiologia: cytobiology
Citobiotaxia: cytobiotaxis
Citocalasinas: cytochalasins
Citocentro: cytocentrum
Citocida: cytocidal, cytocide
Citocina: cytokine
Citocinese: cytokinesis
Citocisto: cytocyst
Citoclasia: cytoclasis
Citoclástico: cytoclastic
Citoclese: cytoclesis
Citocromo: cytochrome
Citocromo aa_3: cytochrome aa_3
Citocromo b: cytochrome b
Citocromo b_5: cytochrome b_5
Citocromo b_5 redutase: cytochrome b_5 reductase
Citocromo c: cytochrome c
Citocromo c oxidase: cytochrome c oxidase
Citocromo c redutase: cytochrome c reductase
Citocromo c_2 redutase: cytochrome c_2 reductase
Citocromo c_3 hidrogenase: cytochrome c_3 hydrogenase
Citocromo cd: cytochrome cd
Citocromo férrico: ferricytochrome
Citocromo ferroso: ferrocytochrome
Citocromo oxidase: cytochrome oxidase (*Pseudomonas*)
Citocromo P-450: cytochrome $P-450_{scc}$
Citocromo peroxidase: cytochrome peroxidase
Citocromo redutase: cytochrome reductase

Citocupreína: cytocuprein
Citodiagnóstico: cytodiagnosis
Citodiérese: cytodieresis
Citoesqueleto: cytoskeleton
Citoestoma: cytostome
Citofagia: cytophagy
Citofânero: cytophanere
Citofaringe: cytopharynx
Citofilático: cytophylactic
Citofilaxia: cytophylaxis
Citofilético: cytophyletic
Citófilo: cytophilic
Citofotometria: cytophotometry
Citogene: cytogene
Citogênese: cytogenesis
Citogenética: cytogenetics
Citogeneticista: cytogeneticist
Citogênico: cytogenic
Citógeno: cytogenous
Citoglicopenia: cytoglucopenia
Citóide: cytoid
Citolema: cytolemma
Citolipina: cytolipin
Citólise: cytolysis
Citolisina: cytolysin
Citolisossoma: cytolysosome
Citolítico: cytolytic
Citologia: cytology
Citológico: cytologic
Citologista: cytologist
Citomatriz: cytomatrix
Citomegálico: cytomegalic
Citomegalovírus (CMV): Cytomegalovirus (CMV)
Citomembrana: cytomembrane
Citômero: cytomere
Citometria: cytometry
Citômetro: cytometer
Citomicrossoma: cytomicrosome
Citomorfologia: cytomorphology
Citomorfose: cytomorphosis
Citopatia: cytopathy
Citopático: cytopathic
Citopatogênico: cytopathogenic
Citopatologia: cytopathology
Citopatológico: cytopathologic, cytopathological
Citopatologista: cytopathologist
Citopempese: cytopempsis
Citopenia: cytopenia
Citopígio: cytopyge
Citopipeta: cytopipette
Citoplasma: cytoplasm
Citoplasmático: cytoplasmic
Citoplasto: cytoplast
Citopoese: cytopoiesis
Citopreparação: cytopreparation
Citoqueratina: cytokeratin
Citoquilema: cytochylema
Citoquímica: cytochemistry
Citorictes: cytoryctes, cytorrhyctes
Citose: cytosis
Citosídeos: cytosides
Citosina: cytosine (Cyt)
Citosol: cytosol
Citosólico: cytosolic
Citossoma: cytosome

Citostase: cytostasis
Citostático: cytostatic
Citotático: cytotactic
Citotaxia: cytotaxis, cytotaxia
Citotecnólogo: cytoscreener, cytotechnologist
Citotese: cythothesis
Citotoxicidade: cytotoxicity
Citotóxico: cytotoxic
Citotoxina: cytotoxin
Citotrofoblasto: cytotrophoblast
Citotrópico: cytotropic
Citotropismo: cytotropism
Citozóico: cytozoic
Citozoon: cytozoon
Citral: citral
Citrase, citratase: citrase, citratase
Citratado: citrated
Citrato: citrate
Citrato de carbetapentano: carbetapentane citrate
Citrato de clomifeno: clomiphene citrate
Citrato de cloroteno: chlorothen citrate
Citrato de cobre: cupric citrate
Citrato de deptropina: deptropine citrate
Citrato de dibenzetropina: dibenzheptropine citrate
Citrato de dietilcarbamazina: diethylcarbamazine citrate
Citrato de etoeptazina: ethoheptazine citrate
Citrato de fentanila: fentanyl citrate
Citrato de orfenadrina: orphenadrine citrate
Citrato de sufentanil: sufentanil citrate
Citrato de tamoxifeno: tamoxifen citrate
Citrato férrico de amônio: ferric ammonium citrate
Citrato férrico de amônio, verde: ferric ammonium citrate, green
Citrato ferroso: ferrous citrate
Citrina: citrin
Citronela: citronella
Citronelal: citronellal
Citrulina: citrulline
Citrulinemia: citrullinemia
Citrulinúria: citrullinuria
Citúria: cyturia
Cladiose: cladiosis
Cladosporiose: cladosporiosis
Clamídia: chlamydia, pl. chlamydiae
Clamidial: chlamydial
Clamidiose: chlamydiosis
Clamidoconídio: chlamydoconidium
Clarificação: clarification, lucidification
Clarificante: clarificant, clearer
Clarividência: clairvoyance
Claro: lucent
Clasmatócito: clasmatocyte

Clasmatose: clasmatosis
Classe: class
Classificação: classification
Classificação de Lukes-Collins: Lukes-Collins classification
Clástico: clastic
Clastogênico: clastogenic
Clastógeno: clastogen
Clatrato: clathrate
Clatrina: clathrin
Claudicação: claudication, limp
Claudicatório: claudicatory
Claustral: claustral
Claustro: claustrum, **pl.** claustra
Claustrofobia: claustrophobia
Claustrofóbico: claustrophobic
Cláusula Delaney: Delaney clause
Clausura: clausura
Clava: clava
Claval: claval
Clavícula: clavicle, clavicula, **pl.** claviculae
Clavicular: clavicular
Clavículo: claviculus, **pl.** claviculi
Claviforme: clavate
Clemastina: clemastine
Cleóide: cleoid
Cleptofobia: kleptophobia
Cleptomania: kleptomania
Cleptomaníaco: kleptomaniac
Cleptoparasita: cleptoparasite
Clidagra: cleidagra, clidagra
Clidal: cleidal, clidal
Clidocostal: cleidocostal, clidocostal
Clidocranial: cleidocranial, clidocranial
Clidotomia: cleidotomy
Climacofobia: climacophobia
Climatério: climacteric, climacterium
Climatologia: climatology
Climatoterapia: climatotherapy
Clímax: climax
Climograma: climograph
Clindamicina: clindamycin
Cline: cline
Clínica: clinic, sanitarium
Clínica de repouso: nursing home
Clínica de tratamento parcial: halfway house
Clínico: clinical
Clínico-cirúrgico: medicochirurgical
Clinicopatológico: clinicopathologic
Clinocefalia: clinocephaly
Clinocefálico: clinocephalic, clinocephalous
Clinodactilia: clinodactyly
Clinografia: clinography
Clinóide: clinoid
Clioquinol: clioquinol
Clioxanida: clioxanide
Clique: click
Clise: clysis
Clister: clyster
Clistotécio: cleistothecium

Clítio: clition
Clitoridectomia: clitoridectomy
Clitoridiano: clitoridean
Clitoridite: clitoriditis
Clítóris: clitoris, **pl.** clitorides
Clitorismo: clitorism
Clitorite: clitoritis
Clitoromegalia: clitoromegaly
Clitoroplastia: clitoroplasty
Clitrofobia: clithrophobia
Clivagem: cleavage
Clival: clival
Clivo: clivus, **pl.** clivi
Cloaca: cloaca
Cloacal: cloacal
Cloasma: chloasma
Clobazam: clobazam
Clocortolona: clocortolone
Clofazimina: clofazimine
Clofenamida: clofenamide
Clofibrate: clofibrate
Clonagem: cloning
Clonal: clonal
Clonazepam: clonazepam
Clone: clone
Clonicidade: clonicity
Clônico: clonic
Clonicotônico: clonicotonic
Clonismo: clonism
Clonogênico: clonogenic
Clonógrafo: clonograph
Clonorquíase: clonorchiasis
Clonorquiose: clonorchiosis
Clônus: clonus
Clopamida: clopamide
Cloracne: chloracne
Clorado: chlorinated
Cloral: chloral
Cloralismo: chloralism
α-cloralose: α-chloralose
Clorambucil: chlorambucil, chloroambucil
Cloramifeno: chloramiphene
Cloramina B: chloramine B
Cloramina T: chloramine T
Cloraminofeno: chloraminophene
Cloranfenicol: chloramphenicol
Clorato: chlorate
Clorazanil: chlorazanil
Clorazeno: chlorazene
Clorazepato: clorazepate
Clorazol negro E: chlorazol black E
Clorbenzoxamina: chlorbenzoxamine
Clorbenzoxietamina: chlorbenzoxyethamine
Clorbetamida: chlorbetamide
Clorbutol: chlorbutol
Clordano: chlordane
Clordantoína: chlordantoin
Cloremia: chloremia
Cloremina: chlorohemin
Cloreto: chloride
Cloreto cobaltoso: cobaltous chloride
Cloreto de alcurônio: alcuronium chloride

Cloreto de ambenônio: ambenonium chloride
Cloreto de benzalcônio: benzalkonium chloride
Cloreto de (γ)-benzeno: (γ)-benzene hexachloride
Cloreto de benzetônio: benzethonium chloride
Cloreto de benzoquinônio: benzoquinonium chloride
Cloreto de betanecol: bethanechol chloride
Cloreto de bisdequalínio: bisdequalinium chloride
Cloreto de cetalcônio: cetalkonium chloride
Cloreto de cetilpiridínio: cetylpyridinium chloride
Cloreto de clorisondamina: chlorisondamine chloride
Cloreto de cobre: cupric chloride
Cloreto de dequalínio: dequalinium chloride
Cloreto de dimetil *d*-tubocurarina: dimethyl tubocurarine chloride
Cloreto de dodecarbônio: dodecarbonium chloride
Cloreto de doxacúrio: doxacurium chloride
Cloreto de edrofônio: edrophonium chloride
Cloreto de fenacridana: phenacridane chloride
Cloreto de metacolina: methacholine chloride
Cloreto de metilbenzetônio: methylbenzethonium chloride
Cloreto de metileno: methylene chloride
Cloreto de metilrosanilina: methylrosaniline chloride
Cloreto de obidoxima: obidoxime chloride
Cloreto de oxibutinina: oxybutynin chloride
Cloreto de pralidoxima: pralidoxime chloride
Cloreto de tetraetilamônio: tetraethylammonium chloride
Cloreto de tolônio: tolonium chloride
Cloreto de triciclamol: tricyclamol chloride
Cloreto de triclobisônio: triclobisonium chloride
Cloreto de tridi-hexetil: tridihexethyl chloride
Cloreto de tubocurarina: tubocurarine chloride
Cloreto de undecoílio: undecoylium chloride
Cloreto estânico: stannic chloride
Cloreto férrico: ferric chloride
Cloreto iodado de undecoílio: undecoylium chloride-iodine
Cloreto mercúrico: mercuric chloride

Cloreto mercuroso: mercurous chloride
Cloreto polivinílico: polyvinyl chloride (PVC)
Clorfenesina: chlorphenesin
Clorfenindiona: chlorphenindione
Clorfenoxamina: chlorphenoxamine
Cloridimetria: chloridimetry
Cloridômetro: chloridometer
Cloridrato: hydrochloride
Cloridrato de 5 ou 9-aminoacridina: 5-aminoacridine hydrochloride, 9-aminoacridine hydrochloride
Cloridrato de adifenina: adiphenine hydrochloride
Cloridrato de alfentanil: alfentanil hydrochloride
Cloridrato de alprenolol: alprenolol hydrochloride
Cloridrato de amantadina: amantadine hydrochloride
Cloridrato de amilorida: amiloride hydrochloride
Cloridrato de aminacrina: aminacrine hydrochloride
Cloridrato de amiodarona: amiodarone hydrochloride
Cloridrato de amitriptilina: amitriptyline hydrochloride
Cloridrato de amodiaquina: amodiaquine hydrochloride
Cloridrato de antazolina: antazoline hydrochloride
Cloridrato de apomorfina: apomorphine hydrochloride
Cloridrato de atabrina: atabrine hydrochloride
Cloridrato de azaciclonol: azacyclonol hydrochloride
Cloridrato de bacampicilina: bacampicillin hydrochloride
Cloridrato de bamifilina: bamifylline hydrochloride
Cloridrato de becantona: becanthone hydrochloride
Cloridrato de benactizina: benactyzine hydrochloride
Cloridrato de benzidamina: benzydamine hydrochloride
Cloridrato de benzindamina: benzindamine hydrochloride
Cloridrato de benzofetamina: benzphetamine hydrochloride
Cloridrato de beta-histamina: betahistine hydrochloride
Cloridrato de betaxolol: betaxolol hydrochloride
Cloridrato de betazol: betazole hydrochloride
Cloridrato de bifenamina: biphenamine hydrochloride
Cloridrato de bromazina: bromazine hydrochloride
Cloridrato de bromexina: bromhexine hydrochloride
Cloridrato de bromodifenidramina:

Glossário

bromodiphenhydramine hydrochloride
Cloridrato de buclizina: buclizine hydrochloride
Cloridrato de bunamidina: bunamidine hydrochloride
Cloridrato de bunolol: bunolol hydrochloride
Cloridrato de buprenorfina: buprenorphine hydrochloride
Cloridrato de bupropiona: bupropion hydrochloride
Cloridrato de buspirona: buspirone hydrochloride
Cloridrato de butetamina: buthetamine hydrochloride
Cloridrato de butoxamina: butoxamine hydrochloride
Cloridrato de butriptilina: butriptyline hydrochloride
Cloridrato de camoxiquina: clamoxyquin hydrochloride
Cloridrato de caramifeno: caramiphen hydrochloride
Cloridrato de carbuterol: carbuterol hydrochloride
Cloridrato de ciclizina: cyclizine hydrochloride
Cloridrato de ciclobenzaprina: cyclobenzaprine hydrochloride
Cloridrato de ciclofenazina: cyclophenazine hydrochloride
Cloridrato de ciclopentamina: cyclopentamine hydrochloride
Cloridrato de ciclopentolato: cyclopentolate hydrochloride
Cloridrato de cinanserina: cinanserin hydrochloride
Cloridrato de ciproeptadina: cyproheptadine hydrochloride
Cloridrato de ciprofloxacina: ciprofloxacin hydrochloride
Cloridrato de clofedianol: chlophedianol hydrochloride
Cloridrato de clomipramina: clomipramine hydrochloride
Cloridrato de clonidina: clonidine hydrochloride
Cloridrato de clorciclizina: chlorcyclizine hydrochloride
Cloridrato de clordiazepóxido: chlordiazepoxide hydrochloride
Cloridrato de clorexidina: chlorhexidine hydrochloride
Cloridrato de clorfentermina: chlorphentermine hydrochloride
Cloridrato de clorguanida: chlorguanide hydrochloride
Cloridrato de cloroguanida: chloroguanide hydrochloride
Cloridrato de cloroprocaína: chloroprocaine hydrochloride
Cloridrato de clorprenalina: clorprenaline hydrochloride
Cloridrato de clorproguanil: chlorproguanil hydrochloride
Cloridrato de desipramina: desipramine hydrochloride
Cloridrato de dextropropoxifeno: dextropropoxyphene hydrochloride
Cloridrato de diafeno: diaphen hydrochloride
Cloridrato de dibenzepina: dibenzepin hydrochloride
Cloridrato de dibucaína: dibucaine hydrochloride
Cloridrato de diciclomina: dicyclomine hydrochloride
Cloridrato de diclonina: dyclonine hydrochloride
Cloridrato de diclorofenarsina: dichlorophenarsine hydrochloride
Cloridrato de dietilpropiona: diethylpropion hydrochloride
Cloridrato de difenidramina: diphenhydramine hydrochloride
Cloridrato de difenilpiralina: diphenylpyraline hydrochloride
Cloridrato de difenoxilato: diphenoxylate hydrochloride
Cloridrato de diidromorfinona: dihydromorphinone hydrochloride
Cloridrato de diltiazem: diltiazem hydrochloride
Cloridrato de dimetoxanato: dimethoxanate hydrochloride
Cloridrato de dipivefrina: dipivefrin hydrochloride
Cloridrato de doxapram: doxapram hydrochloride
Cloridrato de doxepina: doxepin hydrochloride
Cloridrato de eflornitina: eflornithine hydrochloride
Cloridrato de encainida: encainide hydrochloride
Cloridrato de esmolol: esmolol hydrochloride
Cloridrato de espectinomicina: spectinomycin hydrochloride
Cloridrato de etafedrina: etafedrine hydrochloride
Cloridrato de etambutol: ethambutol hydrochloride
Cloridrato de etaverina: ethaverine hydrochloride
Cloridrato de etilefrina: etilefrine hydrochloride
Cloridrato de etilfenilefrina: ethylphenylephrine hydrochloride
Cloridrato de etilmorfina: ethylmorphine hydrochloride
Cloridrato de etilpapaverina: ethylpapaverine hydrochloride
Cloridrato de etopropazina: ethopropazine hydrochloride
Cloridrato de etoxazeno: ethoxazene hydrochloride
Cloridrato de eucatropina: eucatropine hydrochloride
Cloridrato de euprocina: euprocin hydrochloride
Cloridrato de famotina: famotine hydrochloride
Cloridrato de fenacaína: phenacaine hydrochloride
Cloridrato de fenazolina: phenazoline hydrochloride
Cloridrato de fenazopiridina: phenazopyridine hydrochloride
Cloridrato de fenetilina: fenethylline hydrochloride
Cloridrato de fenfluramina: fenfluramine hydrochloride
Cloridrato de fenformina: phenformin hydrochloride
Cloridrato de fenglutarimida: phenglutarimide hydrochloride
Cloridrato de fenilefrina: phenylephrine hydrochloride
Cloridrato de feniramidol: phenyramidol hydrochloride
Cloridrato de fenmetrazina: phenmetrazine hydrochloride
Cloridrato de fenoxibenzamina: phenoxybenzamine hydrochloride
Cloridrato de fentolamina: phentolamine hydrochloride
Cloridrato de flavoxato: flavoxate hydrochloride
Cloridrato de fluoxetina: fluoxetine hydrochloride
Cloridrato de flurazepam: flurazepam hydrochloride
Cloridrato de gonadorrelina: gonadorelin hydrochloride
Cloridrato de hidralazina: hydralazine hydrochloride
Cloridrato de hidrocortamato: hydrocortamate hydrochloride
Cloridrato de hidromorfona: hydromorphone hydrochloride
Cloridrato de imipramina: imipramine hydrochloride
Cloridrato de isoprenalina: isoprenaline hydrochloride
Cloridrato de isoprofenamina: isoprophenamine hydrochloride
Cloridrato de isopropilarterenol: isopropylarterenol hydrochloride
Cloridrato de isoproterenol: isoproterenol hydrochloride
Cloridrato de isoxuprina: isoxsuprine hydrochloride
Cloridrato de labetalol: labetalol hydrochloride
Cloridrato de lidocaína: lidocaine hydrochloride
Cloridrato de loperamida: loperamide hydrochloride
Cloridrato de lucantona: lucanthone hydrochloride
Cloridrato de mebeverina: mebeverine hydrochloride
Cloridrato de mecamilamina: mecamylamine hydrochloride
Cloridrato de meclizina: meclizine hydrochloride
Cloridrato de mecloretamina: mechlorethamine hydrochloride
Cloridrato de meclozina: meclozine hydrochloride
Cloridrato de medazepam: medazepam hydrochloride
Cloridrato de mefenorex: mefenorex hydrochloride
Cloridrato de melitraceno: melitracen hydrochloride
Cloridrato de mepacrina: mepacrine hydrochloride
Cloridrato de meperidina: meperidine hydrochloride
Cloridrato de mepivacaína: mepivacaine hydrochloride
Cloridrato de metaciclina: methacycline hydrochloride
Cloridrato de metadona: methadone hydrochloride
Cloridrato de metanfetamina: methamphetamine hydrochloride
Cloridrato de metidilazina: methdilazine hydrochloride
Cloridrato de metilanfetamina: methylamphetamine hydrochloride
Cloridrato de metilfenidato: methylphenidate hydrochloride
Cloridrato de metixeno: methixene hydrochloride
Cloridrato de metoclopramida: metoclopramide hydrochloride
Cloridrato de metoxamina: methoxamine hydrochloride
Cloridrato de metoxifenamina: methoxyphenamine hydrochloride
Cloridrato de mexiletina: mexiletine hydrochloride
Cloridrato de mianserina: mianserin hydrochloride
Cloridrato de midazolam: midazolam hydrochloride
Cloridrato de mitoxantrona: mitoxantrone hydrochloride
Cloridrato de molindona: molindone hydrochloride
Cloridrato de mustina: mustine hydrochloride
Cloridrato de nafazolina: naphazoline hydrochloride
Cloridrato de naftazolina: naphthazoline hydrochloride
Cloridrato de naftifina: naftifine hydrochloride
Cloridrato de nalbufina: nalbuphine hydrochloride
Cloridrato de naloxona: naloxone hydrochloride
Cloridrato de natrexona: natrexone hydrochloride
Cloridrato de nefopam: nefopam hydrochloride
Cloridrato de nilidrina: nylidrin hydrochloride
Cloridrato de nordefrina: nordefrin hydrochloride
Cloridrato de nortriptilina: nortriptyline hydrochloride

Cloridrato de opipramol: opipramol hydrochloride
Cloridrato de orfenadrina: orphenadrine hydrochloride
Cloridrato de oxifenciclimina: oxyphencyclimine hydrochloride
Cloridrato de oximetazolina: oxymetazoline hydrochloride
Cloridrato de oximorfona: oxymorphone hydrochloride
Cloridrato de oxiprenolol: oxprenolol hydrochloride
Cloridrato de oxofenarsina: oxophenarsine hydrochloride
Cloridrato de pargilina: pargyline hydrochloride
Cloridrato de piperidolato: piperidolate hydrochloride
Cloridrato de piperocaína: piperocaine hydrochloride
Cloridrato de piperoxano: Fourneau 933, piperoxan hydrochloride
Cloridrato de pipradrol: pipradrol hydrochloride
Cloridrato de piratiazina: pyrathiazine hydrochloride
Cloridrato de pramoxina: pramoxine hydrochloride
Cloridrato de prazosin: prazosin hydrochloride
Cloridrato de prilocaína: prilocaine hydrochloride
Cloridrato de procaína: procaine hydrochloride
Cloridrato de procainamida: procainamide hydrochloride
Cloridrato de procarbazina: procarbazine hydrochloride
Cloridrato de prociclidina: procyclidine hydrochloride
Cloridrato de α-prodina: α-prodine hydrochloride
Cloridrato de profenamina: profenamine hydrochloride
Cloridrato de proguanila: proguanil hydrochloride
Cloridrato de prometazina: promethazine hydrochloride
Cloridrato de proparacaína: proparacaine hydrochloride
Cloridrato de propitocaína: propitocaine hydrochloride
Cloridrato de propoxifeno: propoxyphene hydrochloride
Cloridrato de propranolol: propranolol hydrochloride
Cloridrato de protoquilol: protokylol hydrochloride
Cloridrato de protriptilina: protriptyline hydrochloride
Cloridrato de proximetacaína: proxymetacaine hydrochloride
Cloridrato de pseudo-efedrina: pseudoephedrine hydrochloride
Cloridrato de quinacrina: quinacrine hydrochloride
Cloridrato de quinocida: quinocide hydrochloride
Cloridrato de racefedrina: racephedrine hydrochloride
Cloridrato de sotalol: sotalol hydrochloride
Cloridrato de tenildiamina: thenyldiamine hydrochloride
Cloridrato de terazosina: terazosin hydrochloride
Cloridrato de tetracaína: tetracaine hydrochloride
Cloridrato de tetraidrozolina: tetrahydrozoline hydrochloride
Cloridrato de tifenamil: thiphenamil hydrochloride
Cloridrato de tiopropazato: thiopropazate hydrochloride
Cloridrato de tioridazina: thioridazine hydrochloride
Cloridrato de tiprenolol: tiprenolol hydrochloride
Cloridrato de tocainida: tocainide hydrochloride
Cloridrato de tofenacina: tofenacin hydrochloride
Cloridrato de tolazolina: tolazoline hydrochloride
Cloridrato de tonzilamina: thonzylamine hydrochloride
Cloridrato de tramazolina: tramazoline hydrochloride
Cloridrato de trazodona: trazodone hydrochloride
Cloridrato de trientina: trientine hydrochloride
Cloridrato de triexifenidil: trihexyphenidyl hydrochloride
Cloridrato de trifluoperazina: trifluoperazine hydrochloride
Cloridrato de trifluperidol: trifluperidol hydrochloride
Cloridrato de triflupromazina: triflupromazine hydrochloride
Cloridrato de trimetobenzamida: trimethobenzamide hydrochloride
Cloridrato de tripelenamina: tripelennamine hydrochloride
Cloridrato de triprolidina: triprolidine hydrochloride
Cloridrato de xilometazolina: xylometazoline hydrochloride
Cloridria: chlorhydria
Cloridúria: chloriduria
Clorina: chlorin
Clorindanol: chlorindanol
Cloriodoquina: chloriodoquin
Clorito: chlorite
Clormerodrina: chlormerodrin
Clormezanona: chlormezanone
Cloro: chlorine (Cl)
Cloroacetofenona: chloroacetophenone
Cloroanemia: chloroanemia
Cloroazodina: chloroazodin
Clorobutanol: chlorobutanol
Clorocresol: chlorocresol
Clorocruorina: chlorocruorin
Cloroetano: chloroethane
Cloroetileno: chloroethylene
Clorofenol: chlorophenol
Clorofenotano: chlorophenothane
Clorofila: chlorophyll
Clorofilase: chlorophyllase
Clorofilídeo: chlorophyllide, chlorophyllid
Clorofórmio: chloroform
Cloroformismo: chloroformism
Cloroiodado: chloriodized
Cloroma: chloroma
Clorometano: chloromethane
Clorometria: chlorometry
Cloropenia: chloropenia
Cloropercha: chloropercha
Cloropicrina: chloropicrin
Cloropiramina: chloropyramine
Cloroplasto: chloroplast
Cloroprednisona: chloroprednisone
Cloropsia: chloropsia
Cloroquina: chloroquine
Clorose: chlorosis
Cloroso: chlorous
Clorotiazida: chlorothiazide
Clorótico: chlorotic
Clorotimol: chlorothymol
Clorotrianiseno: chlorotrianisene
β-clorovinildiclorarsina: β-chlorovinyldichloroarsine
Clorozotocina: chlorozotocin
Clorpromazina: chlorpromazine
Clorpropamida: chlorpropamide
Clorprotixeno: chlorprothixene
Clorquinaldol: chlorquinaldol
Clortalidona: chlorthalidone
Clortenoxazina: chlorthenoxazin
Clortetraciclina: chlortetracycline
Clortimol: chlorthymol
Clorurese: chloruresis
Clorurético: chloruretic
Clorúria: chloruria
Clorzoxazona: chlorzoxazone
Closilato: closylate
Clostrídico: clostridial
Clostrídio: clostridium, **pl.** clostridia
Clostridiopeptidase A: clostridiopeptidase A
Clostridiopeptidase B: clostridiopeptidase B
Clostripaína: clostripain
Clotrimazol: clotrimazole
Cloxacilina sódica: cloxacillin sodium
Clozapina: clozapine
Cnêmio: cnemial
Cnismogênico: knismogenic
CoA transferases: CoA transferases
Coacervação: coacervation
Coacervato: coacervate
Coadaptação: coadaptation
Coaglutinação: coagglutination
Coagulação: coagulation
Coagulante: coagulant
Coagular: coagulate
Coagulativo: coagulative
Coagulável: coagulable
Coágulo: clot, coagulum, **pl.** coagula; curd
Coagulopatia: coagulopathy
Co-alcóolatra: co-alcoholic
Co-alcoolismo: co-alcoholism
Coalescência: coalescence
Coalescentes: confertus
Coalho: rennet
Coana: postnaris
Coanado: choanate
Coanal: choanal
Cóano: choanae
Coanoflagelado: choanoflagellate
Coanóide: choanoid
Coanomastigoto: choanomastigote
Coaptação: coaptation, knitting
Coaptar: coapt
Coarctação: coarctation
Coarctar: coarct, coarctate
Coarctectomia: coarctectomy
Coarctotomia: coarctotomy
Cobalamina: cobalamin (Cbl)
Cobalto: cobalt (Co)
Cobalto-57 (Co^{57}): cobalt-57 (^{57}Co)
Cobalto-58 (Co^{58}): cobalt-58 (^{58}Co)
Cobalto-60 (Co^{60}): cobalt-60 (^{60}Co)
Cobertor: blanket, wrap
Cobertura: coating, coping, coverage, covering
Cobirinamida: cobyrinamide
Cobra: adder
Cobre: copper (Cu)
Cobre-64 (Cu^{64}): copper-64 (^{64}Cu)
Cobre-67 (Cu^{67}): copper-67 (^{67}Cu)
Cobrotoxina: cobrotoxin
Cocaína: cocaine
Cocainização: cocainization
Cocarboxilase: cocarboxylase
Cocarcinógeno: cocarcinogen
Coccicefalia: coccycephaly
Coccídico: coccidial
Coccidinia: coccydynia
Coccídio: coccidium, **pl.** coccidia
Coccidióidico: coccidioidal
Coccidioidina: coccidioidin
Coccidioidoma: coccidioidoma
Coccidioidomicose: coccidioidomycosis
Coccidiose: coccidiosis
Coccidiostático: coccidiostat
Coccigectomia: coccygectomy
Coccígeo: coccygeal (Co), coccygeus
Coccigodinia: coccygodynia
Coccigotomia: coccygotomy
Cocciodinia: coccyodynia
Cóccix: coccyx, **gen.** coccygis, **pl.** coccyges
Cócegas: tickling
Cochonilha: coccinella, cochineal

Cochonilina: coccinellin
Cocilana: cocillana
Cóclea: cochlea, **pl.** cochleae
Cocleado: cochleate
Coclear: cochlear
Cocleariforme: cochleariform
Cocleíte: cochleitis
Cocleossaculotomia: cochleosacculotomy
Cocleotópico: cochleotopic
Cocleovestibular: cochleovestibular
Coco: coccus, **pl.** cocci
Cocobacilar: coccobacillary
Cocobacilo: coccobacillus
Cocóide: coccal, coccoid
Co-consciência: coconsciousness
Co-conversão: coconversion
Coctoestável: coctostabile, coctostable
Coctolábil: coctolabile
Coculina: cocculin
Codeína: codeine
Codificação: coding, encoding
Código: code
Codogênico: codogenic
Co-dominante: codominant
Códon: codon
Coeficiente: coefficient
Coenzima: coenzyme
Coenzima A: coenzyme A (CoA)
Coenzima F: coenzyme F
Coenzima Q: coenzyme Q (CoQ, Q)
Coenzima R: coenzyme R
Coesão: cohesion
Co-específico: conspecific
Coevolução: coevolution
Co-fator: cofactor
Cognição: cognition
Cognitivo: cognitive
Coifa: galea
Coilócito: koilocyte
Coilocitose: koilocytosis
Coiloníquia: koilonychia
Coilosternia: koilosternia
Co-integrada: cointegrate
Coito: coition, coitus, pareunia
Coitofobia: coitophobia
Cola de peixe: isinglass
Cola: cola, kola
Colaboração: collaboration
Colacina: collacin
Colagenação: collagenation
Colagenase: collagenase
Colagenase A, colagenase I: collagenase A, collagenase I
Colagênico: collagenic
Colagenização: collagenization
Colágeno: collagen, ossein, osseine
Colagenolítico: collagenolytic
Colagenose: collagenosis
Colagenoso: collagenous
Colagogo: cholagogic, cholagogue
Colanerese: cholaneresis
Colangectasia: cholangiectasis
Colangeíte: cholangeitis

Colangiocarcinoma: cholangiocarcinoma
Colangioenterostomia: cholangioenterostomy
Colangiofibrose: cholangiofibrosis
Colangiogastrostomia: cholangiogastrostomy
Colangiografia: cholangiography
Colangiograma: cholangiogram
Colangiolite: cholangiolitis
Colangíolo: cholangiole
Colangioma: cholangioma
Colangiopancreatografia: cholangiopancreatography
Colangioscopia: cholangioscopy
Colangiostomia: cholangiostomy
Colangiotomia: cholangiotomy
Colangite: cholangitis
Colano, 5β-colano: cholane, 5β-cholane
Colanopoese: cholanopoiesis
Colanopoético: cholanopoietic
Colantreno: cholanthrene
Colapso: collapse
Colar: collar, necklace
Colarete: collarette
Colasco: cholascos
Colastina: collastin
Colateral: collateral
Colato: cholate
Colchicina: colchicine
Colecalciferol: cholecalciferol
Colecintigrafia: cholescintigraphy
Colecistagógico: cholecystagogic
Colecistagogo: cholecystagogue
Colecistatonia: cholecystatony
Colecistectasia: cholecystectasia
Colecistectomia: cholecystectomy
Colecistenterostomia: cholecystenterostomy
Colecistenterotomia: cholecystenterotomy
Colecístico: cholecystic
Colecistite: cholecystitis
Colecistocinase: cholecystokinase
Colecistocinético: cholecystokinetic
Colecistocinina: cholecystokinin (CCK)
Colecistoduodenostomia: cholecystoduodenostomy
Colecistogastrostomia: cholecystogastrostomy
Colecistografia: cholecystography
Colecistograma: cholecystogram
Colecistoileostomia: cholecystoileostomy
Colecistojejunostomia: cholecystojejunostomy
Colecistolitíase: cholecystolithiasis

Colecistolitotripsia: cholecystolithotripsy
Colecistomia: cholecystomy
Colecistopatia: cholecystopathy
Colecistopexia: cholecystopexy
Colecistorrafia: cholecystorrhaphy
Colecistossonografia: cholecystosonography
Colecistostomia: cholecystostomy
Colecistotomia: cholecystotomy
Colecromopoese: cholechromopoiesis
Colectasia: colectasia
Colectinas: collectins
Colectomia: colectomy
Coledocectomia: choledochectomy
Colédoco: choledoch, choledochus
Coledococoledocostomia: choledochocholedochostomy
Coledocoduodenostomia: choledochoduodenostomy
Coledocoenterostomia: choledochoenterostomy
Coledocojejunostomia: choledochojejunostomy
Coledocolitíase: choledocholithiasis
Coledocólito: choledocholith
Coledocolitotomia: choledocholithotomy
Coledocolitotripsia: choledocholithotripsy
Coledocolitotritia: choledocholithotrity
Coledocoplastia: choledochoplasty
Coledocorrafia: choledochorrhaphy
Coledocostomia: choledochostomy
Coledocotomia: choledochotomy
Coledoquendise: choledochendysis
Coledoquiartia: choledochiarctia
Coledoquite: choledochitis
Coleglobina: choleglobin, verdohemoglobin
Coleico: choleic
Colelitíase: cholelithiasis, chololithiasis
Colélito: cholelith
Colelitotomia: cholelithotomy
Colelitotripsia: cholelithotripsy
Colelitotrotia: cholelithotrity
Colematina: cholehematin
Colêmese: cholemesis
Colemia: cholehemia, cholemia
Colêmico: cholemic
Coleoptose: coleoptosis
Coleotomia: coleotomy
Colepatia: cholepathia
Coleperitonite: choleperitonitis
Colepoese: cholepoiesis
Colepoético: cholepoietic
Cólera: cholera

Coleráfago: choleraphage
Colerágeno: choleragen
Colerese: choleresis
Colerético: choleretic
Colérico: choleraic, choleric
Coleriforme: choleriform
Colerigênico: cholerigenic, cholerigenous
Colerina: cholerine
Coleróide: choleroid
Colerragia: cholerrhagia
Colerrágico: cholerrhagic
Colerreico: cholerheic
Colestano: cholestane
Colestanol: cholestanol
Colestanona: cholestanone
Colestase: cholestasia, cholestasis
Colestático: cholestatic
Colesteatoma: cholesteatoma
Colesteatomatoso: cholesteatomatous
Colestenona: cholestenone
Colesteremia: cholesteremia
Colesterinemia: cholesterinemia
Colesterinose: cholesterinosis
Colesterinúria: cholesterinuria
Colesterol: cholesterol
Colesterolemia: cholesterolemia
Colesterologênese: cholesterologenesis
Colesterolose: cholesterolosis
Colesterolúria: cholesteroluria
Colestipol: colestipol
Colestiramina: cholestyramine
Colete: jacket
Coletes: braces
Coleúria: choleuria
Colher: spoon
Colher de chá: teaspoon
Colher de sopa: tablespoon
Colibacilo: colibacillus, **pl.** colibacilli
Colibacilose: colibacillosis
Cólica: colica
Colicativo: colicky
Colicele: cholicele
Colicina: colicin
Colicinogenia: colicinogeny
Cólico: cholic, colic
Colicoplegia: colicoplegia
Coliculectomia: colliculectomy
Colículo: colliculus, **pl.** colliculi
Colículo seminal: verumontanum
Colífago: coliphage
Coligação: colligation
Coligativo: colligative
Colil-coenzima A: cholyl-coenzyme A
Colimação: collimation
Colimador: collimator
Colimicina: colimycin
Colina: choline
Colinearidade: colinearity
Colinérgico: cholinergic
Colinéster: cholinester
Colinesterase: cholinesterase
Colinoceptivo: cholinoceptive
Colinolítico: cholinolytic

Colinomimético: cholinomimetic
Colinorreativo: cholinoreactive
Colinorreceptores: cholinoreceptors
Coliotomia: colliotomy
Colipase: colipase
Colipéptico: colypeptic
Coliplicatura: coliplication
Colipunctura: colipuncture
Coliquação: colliquation
Coliquativo: colliquative
Colírio: collyrium, eyewash
Colistimetato sódico: colistimethate sodium
Colistina: colistin
Colite: colitis
Colítico: kolytic
Colitose: colitose
Colo: collum, **pl.** colla
Coloboma: coloboma
Colocentese: colocentesis
Colocinto: bitter apple
Colocistoplastia: colocystoplasty
Colocólico: colocolic
Colocolostomia: colocolostomy
Colódio: collodion, collodium
Coloenterite: coloenteritis
Colofônia: rosin
Colofônio: colophony
Colo-hepatopexia: colohepatopexy
Coloidal: colloidal
Colóide: colloid
Colóide de ouro radiológico: [198]Au colloid
Coloidina: colloidin
Coloidoclasia: colloidoclasia, colloidoclasis
Coloidoclástico: colloidoclastic
Coloidógeno: colloidogen
Coloíla: choloyl
Colólise: cololysis
Cólon: colon
Colonalgia: colonalgia
Colônia: colony
Colônico: colonic
Colonização: colonization, innidiation
Colonograma: colonogram
Colonômetro: colonometer
Colonopatia: colonopathy
Colonorragia: colonorrhagia
Colonorréia: colonorrhea
Colonoscopia: colonoscopy
Colonoscópio: colonoscope
Colopatia: colopathy
Colopexia: colopexy
Colopexostomia: colopexostomy
Colopexotomia: colopexotomy
Coloplania: choloplania
Coloplicatura: coloplication
Colopoese: cholopoiesis
Coloproctite: coloproctitis
Coloproctostomia: coloproctostomy
Coloptose: coloptosis, coloptosia
Colopunctura: colopuncture
Coloquíntida: colocynth

Coloração: staining
Coloração com fluorocromo: fluorochroming
Coloração de banda G: G-banding
Coloração de Dane: Dane stain
Coloração de Gordon e Sweet: Gordon and Sweet stain
Coloração de Hirsch-Peiffer: Hirsch-Peiffer stain
Colorações de Rambourg: Rambourg stains
Colorimetria: colorimetry
Colorimétrico: colorimetric
Colorímetro: colorimeter
Colorrafia: colorrhaphy
Colorragia: colorrhagia
Colorréia: cholorrhea, colorrhea
Colorretal: colorectal
Colorretite: colorectitis
Colorretostomia: colorectostomy
Coloscopia: choloscopy, coloscopy
Colossigmoidostomia: colosigmoidostomy
Colostomia: colostomy
Colostro: colostrum, foremilk
Colostrorréia: colostrorrhea
Colostroso: colostrous
Colotomia: colotomy
Colotórax: cholothorax
Coloxilina: colloxylin
Colpatresia: colpatresia
Colpectasia: colpectasis, colpectasia
Colpectomia: colpectomy
Colpocele: colpocele
Colpocistoplastia: colpocystoplasty
Colpocistotomia: colpocystotomy
Colpocistoureterotomia: colpocystoureterotomy
Colpoclise: colpocleisis
Colpodinia: colpodynia
Colpo-histerectomia: colpohysterectomy
Colpo-histeropexia: colpohysteropexy
Colpo-histerotomia: colpohysterotomy
Colpomicose: colpomycosis
Colpomicroscopia: colpomicroscopy
Colpomicroscópio: colpomicroscope
Colpomiomectomia: colpomyomectomy
Colpoperineoplastia: colpoperineoplasty
Colpoperioneorrafia: colpoperineorrhaphy
Colpopexia: colpopexy
Colpoplastia: colpoplasty
Colpopoese: colpopoiesis
Colpoptose: colpoptosis, colpoptosia
Colporrafia: colporrhaphy
Colporretopexia: colporectopexy

Colporrexe: colporrhexis
Colposcopia: colposcopy
Colposcópio: colposcope
Colpospasmo: colpospasm
Colpossuspensão: colposuspension
Colpostato: colpostat
Colpostenose: colpostenosis
Colpostenotomia: colpostenotomy
Colpotomia: colpotomy
Colpoureterotomia: colpoureterotomy
Colpoxerose: colpoxerosis
Columbina: calumbin
Colúmbio: columbium (Cb)
Columbo: calumba
Columela: columella, **pl.** columellae; columnella, **pl.** columnellae
Coluna: column, columna, **gen. e pl.** columnae
Coluna vertebral: backbone, vertebrarium
Colúria: choluria
Colutório: collutorium, collutory, mouthwash
Com: cum
Coma: coma
Comatoso: comatose
Combinação: combination
Combinatório: combinatorial
Combustão: combustion
Combustível: combustible
Comedão: comedo, **pl.** comedos, comedones
Comedocarcinoma: comedocarcinoma
Comedogênico: comedogenic
Comedonecrose: comedonecrosis
Comensal: commensal
Comensalismo: commensalism
Comer: eat
Cominuição: comminution
Cominutivo: comminuted
Comissão de Enzimas: Enzyme Commission
Comissura: commissura, **gen. e pl.** commissurae; commissure
Comissural: commissural
Comissurotomia: commissurotomy
Comitância: comitance
Comitante: comitant
Comitê: board
Comoção: commotio
Co-morbidade: comorbidity
Comparoscópio: comparascope
Compartimentalização: compartmentation
Compartimento ou célula: cella, **gen. e pl.** cellae; compartimentum, compartment
Compasso de calibre: calipers
Compatibilidade: compatibility
Compatível: compatible
Compensação: compensation
Compensatório: compensatory
Competência: competence

Competição: competition
Complacência: compliance
Compleição: complexion
Complementação: complementation
Complementaridade: complementarity
Complemento: complement
Complexidade: complexity
Complexo: complex, complexus
Complexo bilirrubina-globulina: bilirubinglobulin
Complexo polivinilpirrolidona-iodo: polyvinylpyrrolidone-iodine complex
Complicação: complication
Complicado: complicated
Componente: component
Comporta: sluice
Comportamental: behavioral
Comportamento: behavior
Composição: composition
Composto: composite, compound
Composto metálico vazio: void metal composite (VMC)
Compreensão: comprehension
Compressa: compress, pad, pledget, splenium, **pl.** splenia; stupe
Compressa de gelo: ice pack
Compressão: compression, sarmassation
Compressor: compressor, compressorium
Comprimento: length(l)
Comprimento de onda: wavelength (Λ)
Comprimido ou pastilha medicinal: tabella, **pl.** tabellae
Comprometimento: impairment
Comprometimento da audição, perda de audição: hearing impairment, hearing loss
Compulsão: compulsion
Compulsão à repetição: repetition-compulsion
Compulsivo: compulsive
Computador: computer
Comunicação: communication
Comunicante: communicans, **pl.** communicantes
Comunidade: community
Conação: conation
Conalbumina: conalbumin
Conanina: conanine
Conário: conarium
Conativo: conative
Concameração: concameration
Concanavalina A: concanavalin A (conA, con A)
Concatenado: catenating, concatenate
Concatenar: catenate
Concavidade: concavity
Côncavo: concave
Côncavo-côncavo: concavoconcave
Côncavo-convexo: concavoconvex

Glossário

Conceito: conception
Conceitual: conceptual
Concentração: concentration (c)
Concepto: conceptus, **pl.** concepti
Concha: concha, **pl.** conchae
Concha nasal suprema: supraturbinal
Concoidal: conchoidal
Concomitância: concomitance
Concomitante: concomitant
Concordância: concordance
Concordante: concordant
Concreção: concrement, concretion
Concrecionar: sinter
Concrescência: concrescence
Concretização: concretization
Concussão: concussion
Condensação: condensation
Condensador: condenser
Condensar: condense
Condicionamento: conditioning
Condicionar: condition
Condilar: condylar
Condilartrose: condylarthrosis
Condilectomia: condylectomy
Condílio: condylion
Côndilo: condyle, condylus
Condilóide: condyloid
Condiloma: condyloma, **pl.** condylomata
Condilomatoso: condylomatous
Condilotomia: condylotomy
Condral: chondral
Condraloplasia: chondralloplasia
Condrectomia: chondrectomy
Condrificação: chondrification
Condrificar: chondrify
Condrite: chondritis
Condroblasto: chondroblast
Condroblastoma: chondroblastoma
Condrocalcina: chondrocalcin
Condrocalcinose: chondrocalcinosis
Condrócito: chondrocyte
Condroclasto: chondroclast
Condrocostal: chondrocostal
Condrocrânio: chondrocranium
Condrodermatite nodular crônica da hélice: chondrodermatitis nodularis chronica helicis
Condrodisplasia: chondrodysplasia
Condrodistrofia: chondrodystrophy
Condroectodérmico: chondroectodermal
Condroesqueleto: chondroskeleton
Condroesternal: chondrosternal
Condroesternoplastia: chondrosternoplasty
Condrofaríngeo: chondropharyngeus
Condrofibroma: chondrofibroma

Condrófito: chondrophyte
Condrogênese: chondrogenesis
Condroglosso: chondroglossus
Condróide: chondroid
Condroitina: chondroitin
Condrólise: chondrolysis
Condrologia: chondrology
Condroma: chondroma
Condromalacia: chondromalacia
Condromatose: chondromatosis
Condromatoso: chondromatous
Condrômero: chondromere
Condromixoma: chondromyxoma
Condronectina: chondronectin
Condro-osteodistrofia: chondro-osteodystrophy
Condropatia: chondropathy
Condroplastia: chondroplasty
Condroplasto: chondroplast
Condroporose: chondroporosis
Condrosina: chondrosin, chondrosine
Condrossarcoma: chondrosarcoma
Condrósseo: chondro-osseous
Condrotomia: chondrotomy
Condrótomo: chondrotome
Condrotrófico: chondrotrophic
Condroxifóide: chondroxiphoid
Condução: conduction
Condução óssea: osteophony
Conduplicado: conduplicate
Condurango: condurango
Condutância: conductance
Condutividade: conductivity
Conduto: conduit
Condutor: conductor
Cone: cone, conus, **pl.** coni
Cone l: l-cone
Cone m: m-cone
Cone S: s-cone
Conectinas: connectins
Conector: bar, connector
Conessi: conessi
Conessina: conessine
Conexão: attachment, bearing, conexus, **pl.** conexus; connection, connexus
Conexina 26: connexin 26
Conexinas, conexonas: connexins, connexons
Confabulação: confabulation, fabrication
Confiabilidade: reliability
Configuração: configuration
Confinamento: confinement, containment
Conflito: conflict
Confluência: confluence, confluens
Confluente: confluent
Confocal: confocal
Conformação: conformation
Confrontação: confrontation
Confusão: confusion
Confusional: confusional
Congelamento: freezing, frost
Congelamento-dessecação: freeze-drying

Congênere: congener
Congêneres: congenerous
Congênico: congenic
Congênito: congenital, congenitus
Congestão: congestion
Congestão sangüínea: bloodshot
Congestionado: congested, engorged
Congestivo: congestive
Conglobação: conglobation
Conglobado: conglobate
Conglomerado: conglomerate
Conglutinação: conglutination
Conglutinante: conglutinant
Conglutinina: conglutinin
Congofílico: congophilic
Conhaque: brandy
Cônico: conic, conical, conular
Conidial: conidial
Conídio: conidium, **pl.** conidia
Conidióforo: conidiophore
Conidiógeno: conidiogenous
Coniina: coniine
Coniocórtex: koniocortex
Coniófago: coniophage
Coniofibrose: coniofibrosis
Coniolinfoestase: coniolymphstasis
Coniômetro: coniometer
Coniose: coniosis
Coniotomia: coniotomy
Conização: conization
Conjugação: conjugation
Conjugado: conjugate, conjugated
Conjugante: conjugant
Conjuntival: conjunctival
Conjuntivite: conjunctivitis
Conjuntivite contagïosa aguda: pinkeye
Conjuntivo: conjunctive
Conjuntivocalásia: conjunctivochalasis
Conjuntivodacriocistorrinostomia: conjunctivodacryocystorhinostomy
Conjuntivodacriocistostomia: conjunctivodacryocystostomy
Conjuntivoplastia: conjunctiviplasty, conjunctivoplasty
Conjuntivorrinostomia: conjunctivorhinostomy
Conjunto: set
Conóide: conoid
Conomioidina: conomyoidin
Conquinina: conquinine
Consangüíneo: consanguineous
Consangüinidade: consanguinity
Consciência: consciousness
Consciência da realidade: reality awareness
Consciente: conscious
Consensual: consensual
Conservação: conservation
Conservador: conservative
Conservante: preservative
Consolidação: consolidation

Consolidação viciosa: malunion
Consolidante: consolidant
Conspicuidade: conspicuity
Constância: constancy
Constante: constant
Constante de flutuação: negative S, Svedberg of flotation
Constelação: constellation
Constipação: constipation, costiveness
Constipado: constipated
Constipante: costive
Constipar: constipate
Constitucional: constitutional
Constituição: constitution, habitus
Constitutivo: constitutive
Constrição: constrictio, constriction
Constritor: constrictor
Consulente: consultand
Consultor: consultant
Consumido: consumptive
Consumo: consumption
Contactante: contactant
Contador: counter
Contagem: count
Contagem sangüínea: blood count
Contágio: contagion
Contagiosidade: contagiousness
Contagioso: contagious
Conta-gotas: dropper
Contaminação: contamination, vitiation
Contaminante: contaminant
Contaminar: contaminate
Contato: contact
Contenção: restraint
Conteúdo: content
Contigüidade: contiguity
Contíguo: contiguous
Continência: continence
Continente: continent
Continuidade: continuity
Contínuo: continued
Contorno: contour
Contorno de onda: waveshape
Contra-abertura: contraaperture, counteropening
Contra-ângulo: contraangle
Contrabalanceamento: counterbalancing
Contração: contraction (C)
Contracepção: contraception
Contraceptivo: contraceptive
Contrachoque: countershock
Contracondicionamento: counterconditioning
Contracorante: conterstain
Contracorrente: countercurrent
Contra-extensão: counterextension
Contrafissura: contrafissura
Contrafóbico: counterphobic
Contragolpe: contrecoup
Contraimunoeletroforese: counterimmunoelectrophoresis
Contra-incisão: counterincision

Contra-indicação: contraindication
Contra-indicante: contraindicant
Contra-investimento: counterinvestment
Contrair: contract
Contra-irritação: counterirritation
Contra-irritante: counterirritant
Contralateral: contralateral
Contramolde: counterdie
Contrapulsação: counterpulsation
Contrapunção: counterpuncture
Contraste: contrast
Contrátil: contractile
Contratilidade: contractility
Contratilidade farádica: faradocontractility
Contratração: countertraction
Contratransferência: countertransference
Contratransportador: antiporter
Contratransporte: antiport, countertransport
Contratura: contracture
Controlar: control
Controle de qualidade: quality assurance
Contusão: bruise, contusion
Convalária: convallaria
Convalescença: convalescence
Convalescente: convalescent
Convecção: convection
Convenção de Genebra: Geneva Convention
Convergência: convergence
Convergente: convergent
Conversão: conversion
Convertase: convertase
Convertina: convertin
Convexidade: convexity
Convexo: convex
Convexobasia: convexobasia
Convexo-côncavo: convexoconcave
Convexo-convexo: convexoconvex
Convolução: convolution
Convoluto: convolute, convoluted
Convulsão: convulsion
Convulsivante: convulsant
Convulsivo: convulsive
Cooba: cohoba
Cooperatividade: cooperativity
Coordenação: coordination
Coordenada: coordinate
Coorte: cohort
Co-ossificação: co-ossification
Co-ossificar: co-ossify
Copaíba: copaiba
Copázio: beaker
Copépode: copepod
Copofobia: kopophobia
Copolímero: copolymer
Co-precipitação: coprecipitation
Coprêmese: copremesis

Coproanticorpos: coproantibodies
Coproestigmastano: coprostigmastane
Coprofagia: coprophagia, coprophagy
Coprófago: coprophagous
Coprofilia: coprophilia
Coprófilo: coprophil, coprophilic, coprophile
Coprofobia: coprophobia
Coprofrasia: coprophrasia
Coprolalia: coprolalia
Coprólito: coprolith
Coprologia: coprology
Coproma: coproma
Coproplanesia: coproplanesia
Coproporfiria: coproporphyria
Coproporfirina: coproporphyrin
Coproporfirinogênio: coproporphyrinogen
Coprostano: coprostane
3β-coprostanol: 3β-coprostanol
Coprostanona: coprostanone
Coprostase: coprostasis
Coprostenol: coprostenol
Coprosterol: coprosterol
Coprozoário: coprozoa
Coprozóico: coprozoic
Coptose: coptosis
Copulação: copulation
Copular: couple
Copulinas: copulines
Coqueluche: pertussis
Coquetel: cocktail
Cor: color
Cor rajada: brindle
Coração: coeur, cor, **gen.** cordis; heart
Coração blindado: panzerherz
Coracídio: coracidium
Coracoacromial: coracoacromial
Coracobraquial: coracobrachialis
Coracoclavicular: coracoclavicular
Coracóide: coracoid
Coracoumeral: coracohumeral
Coralina: corallin
Corante: dye
Corante azul de metileno-eosina de Mann: Mann methyl blue-eosin stain
Corante de Becker para espiroquetas: Becker stain for spirochetes
Corante de Berg: Berg stain
Corante de Dieterle: Dieterle stain
Corante de Hucker-Conn: Hucker-Conn stain
Corante de Maldonado-São José: Maldonado-San Jose stain
Corante de May-Grünwald: May-Grünwald stain
Corante prata-metenamina de Grocott-Gomori: Grocott-Gomori methenamine-silver stain

Corante rápido de Field: Field rapid stain
Corcunda: hump, humpback, hunchback
Corda: string
Corda, cordão: chorda, **pl.** chordae
Corda do tímpano: tympanichord
Corda mesodérmica: chorda-mesoderm
Cordado: chordate
Cordal: chordal
Cordão: cord
Cordão umbilical: funis
Cordectomia: cordectomy
Cordial: cordial, cordis
Cordianina: cordianine
Cordiforme: cordate, cordiform
Cordilobíase: cordylobiasis
Cordite: chorditis
Cordocentese: cordocentesis, funipuncture
Cordoesqueleto: chordoskeleton
Cordoma: chordoma
Cordopexia: cordopexy
Cordotomia: cordotomy
Co-receptor: co-receptor
Corectopia: corectopia
Coréia: chorea, jerks **(pl.)**
Coreico: choreal, choreic
Coreiforme: choreiform
Corélise: corelysis
Corêmio: coremium
Coreoatetóide: choreoathetoid
Coreoatetose: choreoathetosis
Coreóide: choreoid
Coreoplastia: coreoplasty
Corepexia: corepexy
Corepraxia: corepraxy
Co-repressor: corepressor
Coriandro: coriander
Corimbiforme: corymbiform
Coríndon: corundum
Corinebactéria: corynebacterium, **pl.** corynebacteria
Corinebacteriófago: corynebacteriophage
Corioadenoma: chorioadenoma
Corioalantóico: chorioallantoic
Corioalantóide: chorioallantois
Corioamnionite: chorioamnionitis
Corioangioma: chorioangioma
Corioangiomatose: chorioangiomatosis
Corioangiose: chorioangiosis
Coriocapilar: choriocapillaris
Coriocarcinoma: choriocarcinoma
Coriocele: choriocele
Corioepitelioma: chorioepithelioma
Coriogonadotrofina: choriogonadotropin
Coriomamotropina: choriomammotropin
Coriomeningite: choriomeningitis
Córion: chorion, corium, **pl.** coria

Coriônico: chorionic
Coriorretiniano: chorioretinal
Coriorretinite: chorioretinitis
Coriorretinopatia: chorioretinopathy
Coristo: chorista
Coristoblastoma: choristoblastoma
Coristoma: choristoma
Coriza: coryza
Cormo de *Colchicum*: Colchicum corm
Córnea: cornea
Corneano: corneal
Córneo: corneum, cornual, horny
Corneobléfaro: corneoblepharon
Corneócito: corneocyte
Corneoesclera: corneosclera
Corneoescleral: corneoscleral
Corniculado: corniculate
Cornículo: corniculum
Cornificação: cornification
Cornificado: cornified
Corno: cornu, **gen.** cornus, **pl.** cornua, horn
Coroa: cap, corona, **pl.** coronae; crown
Coroação: crowning
Coróide: choroid, choroidal, choroidea
Coroideremia: choroideremia
Coroidite: choroiditis
Coroidociclite: choroidocyclitis
Coroidopatia: choroidopathy
Coroidose: choroidosis
Coronal: coronal, coronale, coronalis
Coronária: coronaria,
Coronário: coronad, coronary
Coronarismo: coronarism
Coronarite: coronaritis
Coronavírus: coronavirus
Corônio: coronion, koronion
Coronóide: coronoid
Coronoidectomia: coronoidectomy
Corpo: body, corpus, **gen.** corporis, **pl.** corpora
Corpo do esterno: gladiolus
Corpo médico: medical corps
Corpo médio: midbody
Corpo vítreo: vitreum
Corpóreo: corporeal
Corporina: corporin
Corpulência: corpulence, corpulency
Corpulento: corpulent
Corpuscular: corpuscular
Corpúsculo: corpuscle, corpusculum, **pl.** corpuscula
Corpúsculo de Odland: Odland body
Corpúsculos escleróticos: copper pennies
Correção: correction
Correlação: correlation
Corrente: current, stream, tidal

Glossário

Corrente de ar: draught
Corrente final: end-tidal
Corrente sangüínea: bloodstream
Correspondência: correspondence
Correspondência de cores: color match
Corretivo: corrective, corrigent
Corrina: corrin
Corrinóide: corrinoid
Corroer: corrode
Corrosão: corrosion, fretting
Corrosivo: corrosive
Corrugador: corrugator
Cortar: lase
Corte: cut
Corte transversal: cross-section
Córtex: cortex, gen. corticis, pl. cortices
Córtex cerebral: pallium
Cortexolona: cortexolone
Cortexona: cortexone
Cortical: cortical
Corticalização: corticalization
Corticalosteotomia: corticalosteotomy
Corticectomia: corticectomy
Corticífugo: corticifugal, corticofugal
Corticípeto: corticipetal
Corticoaferente: corticoafferent
Corticobulbar: corticobulbar
Corticocerebelo: corticocerebellum
Corticoeferente: corticoefferent
Corticóide: corticoid
Corticomedial: corticomedial
Corticosteróide: corticosteroid, cortin
Corticosterona: corticosterone
Corticotalâmico: corticothalamic
Corticotrofina: corticotropin
β-corticotrofina: β-corticotropin
Corticotrofo: corticotroph
Cortilinfa: cortilymph
Cortina aórtica: aortic curtain
Cortisol: cortisol
Cortisona: cortisone
α-cortol: α-cortol
β-cortol: β-cortol
α-cortolona: α-cortolone
β-cortolona: β-cortolone
Cosintropina: cosyntropin
Cosmético: cosmetic, cosmetics
Cosmídio: cosmid
Cosmopolita: cosmopolitan
Costal: costal
Costalgia: costalgia
Costectomia: costectomy
Costela [I-XII]: costa, gen. e pl. costae; rib [I-XII]
Costiforme: costiform
Costocentral: costocentral
Costoclavicular: costoclavicular
Costocondral: costochondral
Costocondrite: costochondritis
Costocoracóide: costocoracoid

Costoescapular: costoscapular, costoscapularis
Costoesternal: costosternal
Costoesternoplastia: costosternoplasty
Costogênico: costogenic
Costoinferior: costoinferior
Costo-superior: costosuperior
Costotomia: costotomy
Costótomo: costotome
Costotransversectomia: costotransversectomy
Costotransverso: costotransverse
Costovertebral: costovertebral
Costoxifóide: costoxiphoid
Costumes: mores
Co-substrato: cosubstrate
Cota basal: basal ration
Cotarnina: cotarnine
Cotilédone: cotyledon
Cótilo: cotyle
Cotilóide: cotyloid
Cotinina: cotinine
Coto: stump
Cotovelo: ancon, cubitus, gen. e pl. cubiti; elbow
Co-transporte: cotransport
Coulomb: coulomb (C, Q)
Couraça: cuirass
Covalente: covalent
Covinha: dimple
Cowperiano: cowperian
Coxa: coxa, thigh
Coxalgia: coxalgia, coxodynia
Coxim: cushion
Coxim adiposo: fatpad
Coxite: coxitis
Coxofemoral: coxofemoral
Coxotuberculose: coxotuberculosis
Cranial: craniad, cranial, cranialis
Cranianfitomia: craniamphitomy
Craniectomia: craniectomy
Crânio: cranium, pl. crania; skull
Crânio em folha de trevo: kleeblattschädel
Cranioauricular: cranio-aural
Craniocele: craniocele
Craniocerebral: craniocerebral
Cranioclasia: cranioclasia, cranioclasis
Cranioclasto: cranioclast
Craniocleidodisostose: craniocleidodysostosis
Craniodídimo: craniodidymus
Cranioespinal: craniospinal
Cranioestenose: craniostenosis
Craniofacial: craniofacial
Craniofaríngeo: craniopharyngeal
Craniofaringioma: craniopharyngioma
Craniofenestria: craniofenestria
Craniófero: craniophore
Craniognomia: craniognomy
Craniografia: craniography
Craniógrafo: craniograph

Craniolacunia: craniolacunia
Craniolacunia com meningocele ou encefalocele: lückenschädel
Craniologia: craniology
Craniomalacia: craniomalacia
Craniomeningocele: craniomeningocele
Craniometria: craniometry
Craniométrico: craniometric
Craniômetro: craniometer
Craniópago: craniopagus
Craniopatia: craniopathy
Cranioplastia: cranioplasty
Craniopunção: craniopuncture
Craniorraquidiano: craniorrhachidian
Craniorraquisquise: craniorrhachischisis
Craniosclerose: craniosclerosis
Cranioscopia: cranioscopy
Craniosquise: cranioschisis
Craniossacral: craniosacral
Craniossinostose: craniosynostosis
Craniostose: craniostosis
Craniotabe: craniotabes
Craniotimpânico: craniotympanic
Craniotomia: craniotomy
Craniótomo: craniotome
Craniotonoscopia: craniotonoscopy
Craniotripese: craniotrypesis
Crápula: crapulent, crapulous
Cratera: crater
Crateriforme: crateriform
Craterização: saucerization
Craurose vulvar: kraurosis vulvae
Cravo, calo: clavus, pl. clavi
Creatina: creatine
Creatinase: creatinase
Creatinemia: creatinemia
Creatinina: creatinine (Cr)
Creatininase: creatininase
Creatinúria: creatinuria
Credenciamento: credentialing
Cremaster: cremaster
Cremastérico: cremasteric
Creme: cream
Cremnocele: cremnocele
Cremnofobia: cremnophobia
Crenação: crenation
Crenado: crenate, crenated
Crenócito: crenocyte
Crenocitose: crenocytosis
Creofagia: creophagy, creophagism
Creosol: creosol
Creosoto: creosote
Crepitação: crackling, crepitation, crepitus, decrepitation
Crepitações pleurais: pleural crackles
Crepitante: crepitant
Crepúsculo: twilight
Crescente: crescent
Crescêntico: crescentic
Crescimento: growth

Crescógrafo: crescograph
Cresil verdadeiro: cresyl echt, cresyl fast violet
Cresilato: cresylate
Cresol: cresol
Cresolase: cresolase
Creta: creta
Cretinismo: cretinism
Cretino: cretin
Cretinóide: cretinoid
Cretinoso: cretinistic, cretinous
Criador de tensão: stress riser
Crialgesia: cryalgesia
Crianestesia: cryanesthesia
Cribriforme: cribrate, cribriform, polyporous
Cricoaritenóideo: cricoarytenoid, cricoarytenoideus
Cricofaríngeo: cricopharyngeal
Cricóide: cricoid
Cricoidinia: cricoidynia
Cricotireóideo: cricothyroid, cricothyroideus
Cricotireoidotomia: cricothyroidotomy
Cricotirotomia: cricothyrotomy
Cricotomia: cricotomy
Criestesia: cryesthesia
Criminologia: criminology
Crimofilático: crymophylactic
Crimófilo: crymophilic
Crinina: crinin
Crinofagia: crinophagy
Crinogênico: crinogenic
Crioanestesia: cryoanesthesia
Criobiologia: cryobiology
Criocautério: cryocautery
Criocirurgia: cryosurgery
Crioconização: cryoconization
Crioextração: cryoextraction
Crioextrator: cryoextractor
Criofibrinogenemia: cryofibrinogenemia
Criofibrinogênio: cryofibrinogen
Criofilático: cryophylactic
Criofílico: cryophilic
Criofluorano: cryofluorane
Criofratura: cryofracture
Criogenia: cryogenics
Criogênico: cryogenic
Criógeno: cryogen
Crioglobulinas: cryoglobulins
Crioglobulinemia: cryoglobulinemia
Crioidrato: cryohydrate
Crioipofisectomia: cryohypophysectomy
Criólise: cryolysis
Criômetro: cryometer
Criopalidectomia: cryopallidectomy
Criopatia: cryopathy, frigorism
Criopexia: cryopexy
Crioprecipitação: cryoprecipitation
Crioprecipitado: cryoprecipitate
Criopreservação: cryopreservation

Crioprostatectomia: cryoprostatectomy
Crioproteína: cryoprotein
Criopulvinectomia: cryopulvinectomy
Crioscopia: cryoscopy
Crioscópio: cryoscope
Criospasmo: cryospasm
Criossonda: cryoprobe
Criostato: cryostat
Criotalamectomia: cryothalamectomy
Crioterapia: cryotherapy
Criotolerante: cryotolerant
Cripta: crypt, crypta, **pl.** cryptae
Criptectomia: cryptectomy
Críptico: cryptic
Criptite: cryptitis
Criptococoma: cryptococcoma
Criptococose: cryptococcosis
Criptocristalino: cryptocrystalline
Criptocromo: cryptochrome
Criptodídimo: cryptodidymus
Criptoftalmia: cryptophthalmus, cryptophthalmia
Criptogamia: Cryptogamia
Criptogênico: cryptogenic
Criptólito: cryptolith
Criptomenorréia: cryptomenorrhea
Criptônio: krypton (Kr)
Criptopirrol: cryptopyrrole
Criptopodia: cryptopodia
Criptorquidia: cryptorchidism, cryptorchism
Criptórquio: cryptorchid
Criptoscópio: cryptoscope
Criptosporidiose: cryptosporidiosis
Criptotia: cryptotia
Criptoxantina: cryptoxanthin
Criptozigoso: cryptozygous
Criptozoíta: cryptozoite
Crisarobina: chrysarobin
Crisazina: chrysazine
Crise: crisis, **pl.** crises
Crisíase: chrysiasis
Crisocianose: chrysocyanosis
Crisoidina: chrysoidin
Crisoterapia: chrysotherapy
Crispação: crispation
Crista: agger, **pl.** aggeres; crest, cresta, crista, **pl.** cristae; ridge
Cristal: crystal
Cristal violeta: crystal violet
Cristalina: crystallin
Cristalino: crystalline
Cristalização: crystallization
Cristalofobia: crystallophobia
Cristalografia: crystallography
Cristalograma: crystallogram
Cristalóide: crystalloid
Cristalúria: crystalluria
Critério: criterion, **pl.** criteria
Crítico: critical
Crivação: cribration
Croco: crocus
Cromafil: chromaphil
Cromafim: chromaffin
Cromafinoma: chromaffinoma
Cromafinopatia: chromaffinopathy
Cromano: chroman, chromane
Cromanol: chromanol
Cromático: chromatic
Cromátide: chromatid
Cromatina: chromatin
Cromatinólise: chromatinolysis
Cromatinorrexe: chromatinorrhexis
Cromatismo: chromatism
Cromato: chromate
Cromatocinesia: chromatokinesis
Cromatofilia: chromatophilia
Cromatofílico: chromatophil, chromatophilic, chromatophilous
Cromatofobia: chromatophobia
Cromatóforo: chromatophore
Cromatoforotrópico: chromatophorotropic
Cromatógeno: chromatogenous
Cromatografar: chromatograph
Cromatografia: chromatography
Cromatográfico: chromatographic
Cromatograma: chromatogram
Cromatóide: chromatoid
Cromatólise: chromatolysis
Cromatolítico: chromatolytic
Cromatômetro: chromatometer
Cromatopético: chromatopectic
Cromatopexia: chromatopexis
Cromatoplasma: chromatoplasm
Cromatopsia: chromatopsia
Cromatossoma: chromatosome
Cromatotropismo: chromatotropism
Cromatúria: chromaturia
Cromeno: chromene
Cromenol: chromenol
Cromestesia: chromesthesia
Cromidiação: chromidiation
Cromídio: chromidium, **pl.** chromidia
Cromidiose: chromidiosis
Cromidrose: chromhidrosis, chromidrosis
Cromo: chrome, chromium (Cr)
Cromoblasto: chromoblast
Cromoblastomicose: chromoblastomycosis
Cromocentro: chromocenter
Cromócito: chromocyte
Cromofilia: chromophilia
Cromofílico: chromophilic, chromophilous
Cromófilo: chromophil, chromophile
Cromofobia: chromophobia
Cromofóbico: chromophobic
Cromófobo: chromophobe
Cromofórico: chromophoric, chromophorous
Cromóforo: chromophore
Cromofototerapia: chromophototherapy
Cromogênese: chromogenesis
Cromogênico: chromogenic
Cromógeno: chromogen
Cromoglicato sódico: cromolyn sodium
Cromograninas: chromogranins
Cromoisomerismo: chromoisomerism
Cromolipídio: chromolipid
Cromólise: chromolysis
Cromômero: chromomere
Cromômetro: chromometer
Cromomicose: chromomycosis
Cromona: chromone
Cromonema: chromonema, **pl.** chromonemata
Cromoníquia: chromonychia
Cromopético: chromopectic
Cromopexia: chromopexis
Cromoplastídio: chromoplastid
Cromoplasto: chromoplast
Cromoproteína: chromoprotein
Cromossoma: chromosome
Cromossoma acessório: monosome
Cromossomas sexuais: gonosome
Cromossômico: chromosomal
Cromoterapia: chromotherapy
Cromotóxico: chromotoxic
Cromotriquia: chromotrichia
Cromotríquico: chromotrichial
Cromótropo: chromotrope
Cromótropo 2R: chromotrope 2R
Cronaxia: chronaxia, chronaxie, chronaxis, chronaxy
Cronaximetria: chronaximetry
Cronaxímetro: chronaximeter
Cronicidade: chronicity
Crônico: chronic
Cronobiologia: chronobiology
Cronofarmacologia: chronopharmacology
Cronofobia: chronophobia
Cronofotografia: chronophotograph
Cronognose: chronognosis
Cronógrafo: chronograph
Cronometria: chronometry
Cronooncologia: chrono-oncology
Cronotaraxia: chronotaraxis
Cronoterapia: chronotherapy
Cronotrópico: chronotropic
Cronotropismo: chronotropism
Crosta: crust, crusta, **pl.** crustae; scab, slough
Crotáfio: crotaphion
Crotalídeo: crotalid
Crotalina: crotalin
Crotalismo: crotalism
Crotamiton: crotamiton
Crotonase: crotonase
Crotonil-ACP redutase: crotonyl-ACP reductase
Crotoxina: crotoxin
Cruciforme: cruciate
Crufomato: crufomate
Cruor: cruor
Crupal: croupous, croupy
Crupe: croup
Crural: crural
Crusotomia: crusotomy
Cruz: cross, crux, **pl.** cruces
Cruz Vermelha: Red Cross
Cruzamento: intercross
Cruzamento linear: linebreeding
Cubeba: cubeb
Cubeta: cuvet, cuvette
Cubóide: cuboid, cuboidal
Culdocentese: culdocentesis
Culdoplastia: culdoplasty
Culdoscopia: culdoscopy
Culdoscópio: culdoscope
Culdotomia: culdotomy
Culicida: culicidal, culicide
Culicídeos: Culicidae
Culicífugo: culicifuge
Cúlmen: culmen, **pl.** culmina
Cultivo: cultivation
Culto: cult
Cultura: culture
Cumaranona: coumaranone
Cumarina: coumarin, cumarin
Cumetarol: coumetarol, cumetharol
Cumetoxetano: cumethoxaethane
Cúmplice: accomplice
Cumulativo: cumulative
Cúmulo: cumulus, **pl.** cumuli
Cuneiforme: cuneate, cuneiform
Cúneo: cuneus, **pl.** cunei
Cuneocubóide: cuneocuboid
Cuneoescafóide: cuneoscaphoid
Cuneonavicular: cuneonavicular
Cunha: wedge
Cunículo: cuniculus, **pl.** cuniculi
Cunilíngua: cunnilingus
Cúprico: cupric
Cupriurese: cupriuresis
Cúpula: cupola, cupula, **pl.** cupulae; dome
Cupular: cupular
Cupuliforme: cupulate, cupuliform
Cupulograma: cupulogram
Cupulolitíase: cupulolithiasis
Cura: curing, healing
Curagem: curage
Curar: cure, heal
Curare: curare
Curariforme: curariform
Curarimimético: curarimimetic
Curarina: curarine
Curarização: curarization
Curativo: curative, dressing
Curcumina: curcumin
Cureta: curet, curette, scoop
Curetagem: curettage, curettement
Curetagem subgengival: apoxesis
Curie: curie (C, c, Ci)
Cúrio: curium (Cm)
Curtose: kurtosis
Curva: curve

Curvatura: curvatura, **pl.** curvaturae; curvature
Cushingóide: cushingoid
Cuspidado: cuspid, cuspidate
Cuspidal: cuspal
Cúspide: cusp, cuspis, **pl.** cuspides
Cuspir: spitting
Cutâneo: cutaneous
Cutâneo-mucoso: cutaneomucosal
Cutelo: cleaver
Cutícula: cuticle, cuticula, **pl.** cuticulae; hangnail
Cutina: cutin
Cútis: cutis
Cutização: cutization
Cysticercus: bladderworm

D

Dacarbazina (DTIC): dacarbazine (DTIC)
Dácrio: dacryon
Dacrioadenite: dacryadenitis, dacryoadenitis
Dacrioblenorréia: dacryoblennorrhea
Dacriocele: dacryocele
Dacriocistalgia: dacryocystalgia
Dacriocistectomia: dacryocystectomy
Dacriocistite: dacryocystitis
Dacriocisto: dacryocyst
Dacriocistocele: dacryocystocele
Dacriocistograma: dacryocystogram
Dacriocistorrinostomia: dacryocystorhinostomy
Dacriocistotomia: dacryocystotomy
Dacrioemorréia: dacryohemorrhea
Dacrioestenose: dacryostenosis
Dacriolitíase: dacryolithiasis
Dacriólito: dacryolith
Dacriopiorréia: dacryopyorrhea
Dacriopo: dacryops
Dacriorréia: dacryorrhea
Dactilalgia: dactylalgia
Dactilite: dactylitis
Dáctilo: dactyl, dactylus, **pl.** dactyli
Dactilocampsia: dactylocampsis
Dactilocampsodinia: dactylocampsodynia
Dactilodinia: dactylodynia
Dactilogripose: dactylogryposis
Dactilologia: dactylology
Dactilomegalia: dactylomegaly
Dactiloscopia: dactyloscopy
Dactilospasmo: dactylospasm
Dactinomicina: dactinomycin
Dacurônio: dacuronium
Dado: datum
Dados: data
Dados de avaliação objetiva: objective assessment data

Daga: dagga
Dalina: dahlin
Dálton: dalton (Da)
Daltoniano: daltonian
Daltonismo: daltonism
Damar: dammar
Danazol: danazol
Dança: dance
Dansil: dansyl (Dns, DNS)
Dantroleno sódico: dantrolene sodium
Dantron: danthron
Dapsona: dapsone
Dartóico: dartoic, dartoid
Darwiniano: darwinian
Daturina: daturine
Daunomicina: daunomycin
Daunorrubicina: daunorubicin
De novo: de novo
DEAE-celulose: DEAE-cellulose
Dealbação: dealbation
Debilidade: debility
Debilitante: debilitant, debilitating
Débito: debt, output
Decagrama: decagram
Decalitro: decaliter
Decalvante: decalvant
Decâmetro: decameter
Decamina: decamine
Decanoína: decanoin
Decanormal: decanormal
Decantação: decantation
Decantar: decant
Decapagem: pickling
Decapeptídeo: decapeptide
Decapitação: decapitation
Decapitar: decapitate
Decepação: dedolation
Decibel: decibel (dB, db)
Decídua: decidua
Deciduação: deciduation
Deciduado: deciduate
Decidual: decidual
Deciduíte: deciduitis
Decíduo: deciduous
Deciduoma: deciduoma
Decigrama: decigram
Decilitro: deciliter
Decímetro: decimeter
Decimorgan: decimorgan
Decinormal: decinormal
Decisão: decision
Declinador: declinator
Declive: declive, declivis
Decocção: decoction
Decompor: decompose
Decomposição: decay, decomposition
Decorticação: decortication
Decrepitude: dotage
Decrudescência: decrudescence
Decúbito: decubital, decubitus
Decussação: crossway, decussatio, **pl.** decussationes, decussation
Decussar: decussate
Dedaleira: foxglove
Dedicação: attending
Dedo: digit, digitus, **pl.** digiti

Dedo caído: toe-drop
Dedo da mão: finger
Dedo do pé: toe
Dedo indicador: forefinger
Dedução: deduction
Defasagem: dephasing
Defecação: defecation
Defecar: defecate
Defecografia: defecography
Defeito: blemish, defect
Defeituoso: defective
Defensinas: defensins
Deferencial: deferential
Deferente: deferent
Deferentite: deferentitis
Defervescência: defervescence
Defesa: defense
Defesa muscular: guarding
Deficiência: deficiency
Déficit: deficit
Definhamento: wasting
Definição: definition, determination
Deflagrador: trigger
Deflexão: deflection, deflexion
Deflorescência: deflorescence
Deflúvio: defluvium
Defluxo: defluxion
Deformabilidade: deformability
Deformação: deformation
Deformante: deforming
Deformidade: deformity
Degeneração: degeneracy, degeneratio, degeneration
Degenerar: degenerate
Degenerativo: degenerative
Deglutição: deglutition
Deglutir: swallow
Deglutivo: deglutitive
Degradação: degradation
Degustação: degustation
Deiscência: dehiscence
Dejeto: dejecta
Delaminação: delamination
Deleção: deletion
Deletério: deleterious
Delfinina: delphinine
Delicado: delicate
Delimitação: delimitation
Delinqüente juvenil: juvenile delinquent
Deliqüescência: deliquescence
Deliqüescente: deliquescent
Deliqüescer: deliquesce
Delirante: delirious
Delírio: delirium, **pl.** deliria
Delitescência: delitescence
Delomorfo: delomorphous
Delta: delta (Δ)
Deltóide: deltoid
Demanda: demand
Demarcação: demarcation
Dematiáceas: Dematiaceae
Dematiáceo: dematiaceous
Demeclociclina: demeclocycline
Demecolcina: demecolcine
Demência: dementia, folie
Demente: demented
Demo: deme
Demografia: demography
Demoníaco: demoniac

Demonstrador: demonstrator
Demora: lag
Demulcente: demulcent
Dendriforme: dendriform
Dendrítico: dendritic
Dendrito: dendrite, dendron
Dendrograma: dendrogram
Dendróide: dendroid
Dengue: dengue
Denominador: denominator
Densidade: density
Densímetro: densimeter
Densitometria: densitometry
Densitômetro: densitometer
Dentadura: denture
Dental: dental
Dentalgia: dentalgia
Dentatectomia: dentatectomy
Dente: dens, **pl.** dentes; tine, tooth, **pl.** teeth
Denteado: dentate
Dentição: dentia, dentition, teething
Denticulado: denticulate, denticulated
Dentículo: denticle
Dentiforme: dentiform
Dentifrício: dentifrice
Dentígero: dentigerous
Dentilabial: dentilabial
Dentilingual: dentilingual
Dentina: dentin, dentine, dentinum
Dentinalgia: dentinalgia
Dentinário: dentinal
Dentinocementário: dentinocemental
Dentinogênese: dentinogenesis
Dentinóide: dentinoid
Dentinoma: dentinoma
Dentíparo: dentiparous
Dentista: dentist
Dentoalveolar: dentoalveolar
Dentodo: dentode
Dentóide: dentoid
Dentolegal: dentolegal
Deontologia: deontology
Dependência: dependence, dependency
Dependovírus: Dependovirus
Depilação: depilation
Depilar: depilate
Depilatório: depilatory
Depleção: depletion
Depósito: deposit
Depravação: depravation, depravity
Depravado: depraved
Deprenil: deprenyl
Depressão: blues, depression, pit
Depressivo: depressive
Depressões: dellen
Depressor: depressant, depressor
Deprimido: depressed
Depsipeptídeo: depsipeptide
Depuração: clearance, depuration
Depurante: depurant
Depurativo: depurative
Deradelfo: deradelphus

Deranencefalia: deranencephaly, deranencephalia
Dereísmo: dereism
Dereístico: dereistic
Derencefalia: derencephalia, derencephaly
Derencefalocele: derencephalocele
Derivação: lead
Derivado: derivative
Derivar ou desviar: shunt
Dermabrasão: dermabrasion
Dermabrasivo: dermabrader
Dermatalgia: dermatalgia
Dermatite: dermatitis, **pl.** dermatitides
Dermatite pelo vento: windburn
Dermatoartrite: dermatoarthritis
Dermatobíase: dermatobiasis
Dermatocalase: dermatochalasis
Dermatocelulite: dermatocellulitis
Dermatocisto: dermatocyst
Dermatoconiose: dermatoconiosis
Dermatodinia: dermatodynia
Dermatofibroma: dermatofibroma
Dermatofibrose lenticular disseminada: dermatofibrosis lenticularis disseminata
Dermatofibrossarcoma protuberante: dermatofibrosarcoma protuberans
Dermatofilaxia: dermatophylaxis
Dermatofilose: dermatophilosis
Dermatofítide: dermatophytid
Dermatófito: dermatophyte
Dermatofitose: dermatophytosis
Dermatofobia: dermatophobia
Dermatoglifo: dermatoglyphics
Dermatografismo: dermatographism, skin writing
Dermatógrafo: dermatograph
Dermatóide: dermatoid
Dermatólise: dermatolysis
Dermatologia: dermatology
Dermatologista: dermatologist
Dermatoma: dermatoma
Dermatomegalia: dermatomegaly
Dermatômero: dermatomere
Dermatomicose: dermatomycosis
Dermatomioma: dermatomyoma
Dermatomiosite: dermatomyositis
Dermátomo: dermatome
Dermatoneurose: dermatoneurosis
Dermatonosologia: dermatonosology
Dermatopatia: dermatopathia, dermatopathy
Dermatopatologia: dermatopathology

Dermatopolineurite: dermatopolyneuritis
Dermatorragia: dermatorrhagia
Dermatorréia: dermatorrhea
Dermatorrexe: dermatorrhexis
Dermatoscopia: dermatoscopy
Dermatose: dermatosis, **pl.** dermatoses
Dermatoterapia: dermatotherapy
Dermatotlasia: dermatothlasia
Dermatotrópico: dermatotropic
Dermatozoário: dermatozoon
Dermatozoonose: dermatozoonosis
Dermatrofia: dermatrophia, dermatrophy
Derme: dermis
Dermenquise: dermenchysis
Dérmico: dermal
Dermoblasto: dermoblast
Dermocima: dermocyma
Dermoesqueleto: dermoskeleton
Dermoestenose: dermostenosis
Dermoflebite: dermophlebitis
Dermóide: dermoid
Dermoidectomia: dermoidectomy
Dermólise: dermolysis
Dermonecrótico: dermonecrotic
Dermopatia: dermopathy
Dermotoxina: dermotoxin
Dermotrópico: dermotropic
Dermovascular: dermovascular
Derodídimo: derodidymus
Derramamento: spill
Desaceleração: deceleration
Desacidificação: deacidification
Desacilase: deacylase
Desacopladores: uncouplers
Desaferenciação: deafferentation
Desagregação: disaggregation
Desajustamento: maladjustment
Desalcoolização: dealcoholization
Desalergizar: deallergize
Desalinhamento: malalignment
Desalogenase: dehalogenase
Desamidação, desamidização: deamidation, deamidization
Desamidases: deamidases
Desamidizar: deamidize, desamidize
Desaminação, desaminização: deamination, deaminization
Desaminases: deaminases
Desaminizar: deaminize
Desamparo aprendido: learned helplessness
Desarmonia: disharmony
Desarticulação: disarticulation
Desassimilação: disassimilation
Desassociação: disassociation
Desativação: deactivation
Desbridamento: débridement, épluchage, freshening
Descalcificação: decalcification
Descalcificante: decalcifying
Descalcificar: decalcify
Descamação: desquamation

Descamar: desquamate
Descamativo: desquamative
Descanso: rest
Descanulização: decannulation
Descapacitação: decapacitation
Descapsulação: decapsulation
Descarbonização: decarbonization
Descarboxilação: decarboxylation
Descarboxilase: decarboxylase
Descarboxilase oxidativa do ácido lático: lactic acid oxidative decarboxylase
Descarrilamento: derailment
Descascar: peel
Descemetite: descemetitis
Descemetocele: descemetocele
Descendente: descendens, descending
Descentralização: decentration
Descerebração: decerebration
Descerebrar: decerebrate, decerebrize
Descida: descensus, descent
Descloretação: dechloruration
Desclorização: dechloridation, dechlorination
Descolamento: décollement, detachment, sublation
Descolesterolização: decholesterolization
Descolorar: stain
Descompensação: decompensation
Descompressão: decompression
Desconectar: debond
Desconexão: debanding
Descongestionante: decongestant
Descongestivo: decongestive
Desconjugado: disconjugate
Descontaminação: decontamination
Descontínuo: transilient
Descontrole: dyscontrol
Desconvolução: deconvolution
Desdentado: edentulous
Desdentição: dedentition
Desdiferenciação: dedifferentiation
Desdobramento: splitting
Deseferenciação: de-efferentation
Desejo: bulesis
Desembocadura: débouchement
Desembocar: debouch
Desenluvamento: degloving
Desenvolvimento: development
Desepicardialização: de-epicardialization
Desequilíbrio: disequilibrium, imbalance
Desequilíbrio ventilação/ perfusão: ventilation/perfusion mismatch
Deserpidina: deserpidine
Desfeminização: defemination
Desfibrilação: defibrillation
Desfibrilador: defibrillator
Desfibrinação: defibrination

Desfluoridização: defluoridation
Desflurano: desflurane
Desfosforilação: dephosphorylation
Desfurfuração: defurfuration
Desganglionar: deganglionate
Desgastar: abrade
Desgaste: grinding, wear
Desgaste corretivo intrabucal: grinding-in
Desgranulação: degranulation
Desidrase: dehydrase
Desidratação: dehydration
Desidratar: dehydrate
Desidratase: dehydratase
Desidremia: deshydremia
Desidro-3-epiandrosterona: dehydro-3-epiandrosterone (DHEA)
Desidroaçúcares: dehydrosugars
Desidrobilirrubina: dehydrobilirubin
Desidrocolato: dehydrocholate
7-desidrocolesterol: 7-dehydrocholesterol
24-desidrocolesterol: 24-dehydrocholesterol
11-desidrocorticosterona: 11-dehydrocorticosterone
Desidroemetina: dehydroemetine
Desidroepiandrosterona: dehydroepiandrosterone
Desidrogenação: dehydrogenation
Desidrogenar: dehydrogenate
Desidrogenase: dehydrogenase
Desidrogenase da acil-CoA de cadeia curta: short-chain acyl-CoA dehydrogenase
Desidrogenase da acil-CoA de cadeia média: medium-chain acyl-CoA dehydrogenase (MCAD)
Desidrogenase málica: malic dehydrogenase
Desidroisoandrosterona: dehydroisoandrosterone
Desidrorretinaldeído: dehydroretinaldehyde
Desidrorretinol: dehydroretinol
Desiminases: deiminases
Desinfecção: disinfection
Desinfestação: disinfestation
Desinfetante: disinfectant
Desinfetar: disinfect
Desinibição: disinhibition
Desinsetização: disinsection, disinsectization
Desinstitucionalização: deinstitutionalization
Desintegração: disintegration
Desintoxicar: detoxicate
Desionização: deionization
Desipnotizar: dehypnotize
Deslanosídeo: deslanoside
Deslizamento: glide
Deslocabilidade: displaceability
Deslocamento: creep, displacement
Deslocamento de ar: windage

Desmamado: weanling
Desmamar: wean
Desmame: weaning
Desmasculinizante: demasculinizing
Desmedular: emedullate
Desmembrar: dismember
Desmetilação: demethylation
Desmetilase: demethylase
Desmielinização: demyelination, demyelinization, dysmyelination
Desmielinizado: unmedullated
Desmina: desmin
Desmineralização: demineralization
Desmite: desmitis
Desmocrânio: desmocranium
Desmodente: desmodentium
Desmodonto: desmodontium
Desmógeno: desmogenous
Desmografia: desmography
Desmóide: desmoid
Desmolases: desmolases
Desmologia: desmology
Desmopatia: desmopathy
Desmoplasia: desmoplasia
Desmoplásico: desmoplastic
Desmopressina: desmopressin
Desmorfinização: demorphinization
Desmosina: desmosine
Desmossoma: desmosome
Desmosterol: desmosterol
Desmucosação: demucosation
Desnarcotizar: denarcotize
Desnaturação: denaturation
Desnaturado: denatured
Desnaturar: melt
Desnervação: denervation
Desnervar: denervate
Desnidação: denidation
Desnitração: denitration
Desnitrificação: denitrification
Desnitrificar: denitrify
Desnitrogenação: denitrogenation
Desnucleado: denucleated
Desnudação: denudation
Desnudar: denude
Desnutrição: malnutrition
Desobstrução: disobliteration, patency
Desodorante: deodorant
Desodorizante: deodorizer
Desodorizar: deodorize
Desonida: desonide
Desorganização: disorganization
Desorientação: disorientation
Desossificação: deossification
5′-desoxiadenosilcobalamina: 5′-deoxyadenosylcobalamin
Desoxiadenosina: deoxyadenosine (dA, dAdo)
Desoxiadenosina metilase: dam methylase, deoxyadenosine methylase
Desoxibarbiturato: deoxybarbiturate
Desoxicitidina: deoxycytidine

2-desoxicoformicina: 2-deoxycoformycin
Desoxicoformicina: deoxycoformycin
Desoxicolato: deoxycholate (DOC)
Desoxicorticosterona: deoxycorticosterone (DOC), desoxycorticosterone
Desoxicortona: deoxycortone, desoxycortone
Desoxidação: deoxidation
Desoxidar: deoxidize
Desoxiepinefrina: deoxyepinephrine
Desoxiexose: deoxyhexose
Desoxiguanosina: deoxyguanosine
Desoximetasona: desoximetasone
Desoxinucleosídeo: deoxynucleoside
Desoxinucleotídeo: deoxynucleotide
Desoxinucleotidil transferase terminal: terminal deoxynucleotidyltransferase
Desoxipentose: deoxypentose
Desoxirriboaldolase: deoxyriboaldolase
Desoxirribodipirimidina fotoliase: deoxyribodipyrimidine photolyase
Desoxirribonuclease: deoxyribonuclease (DNAse, DNAase, DNase)
Desoxirribonucleoproteína: deoxyribonucleoprotein (DNP, Dnp)
Desoxirribonucleosídeo: deoxyribonucleoside
Desoxirribonucleotídeo: deoxyribonucleotide
Desoxirribose: deoxyribose
Desoxirribosefosfato aldolase: deoxyribosephosphate aldolase
Desoxirribosídeo: deoxyriboside
Desoxirribosil: deoxyribosyl
Desoxirribosiltransferases: deoxyribosyltransferases
Desoxirribotídeo: deoxyribotide
Desoxirribovírus: deoxyribovirus
Desoxitimidina: deoxythymidine
Desoxiuridina: deoxyuridine
Desozonizar: deozonize
Despejar: dumping
Despersonalização: depersonalization
Despigmentação: depigmentation, dyspigmentation
Despiolhar: delouse
Despolarização: depolarization
Despolarizar: depolarize
Despolimerase: depolymerase
Desprendimento: disengagement
Desproporção: disproportion

Despulgação: depulization
Despumação: despumation
Desrealização: derealization
Desrepressão: derepression
Dessaturação: desaturation
Dessaturar: desaturate
Dessecação: desiccation, xeransis
Dessecador: desiccator
Dessecante: desiccant
Dessecar: desiccate
Dessecativo: desiccative
Dessensibilização: desensitization
Dessensibilizar: desensitize
Dessincronização: dischronation
Dessincronose: jet lag
Dessulfidrases: desulfhydrases
Dessulfinase: desulfinase
Dessulfurases: desulfurases
Destilação: distillation
Destilado: distillate
Destilar: distill
Destino: fate
Destiobiotina: desthiobiotin
Destoxificação: detoxication, detoxification
Destoxificar: detoxify
Destrímano: dextral, dextromanual, right-handed
Destrocular: right-eyed
Destropedal: right-footed
Destrudo: destrudo
Desumanização: dehumanization
Desvalvulado: valveless
Desvantagem: handicap
Desvascularização: devascularization
Desvio: bypass, deviance, drift, pl. drifts; skew
Desvio A-V: A-V shunt
Desviômetro: deviometer
Desvitalização: devitalization
Desvitalizado: devitalized
Desvitalizar: devitalize
Detecção: detection
Detector: detector
Detergente: detergent
Deterioração: deterioration
Determinação: ascertainment
Determinante: determinant
Determinismo: determinism
Detersivo: detersive
Detetor de mentira: lie detector
Detrito: detritus
Detrusor: detrusor
Detrussorrafia: detrusorrhaphy
Detumescência: detumescence
Deturgescência: deturgescence
Deutencéfalo: deutencephalon
Deuteranomalia: deuteranomaly
Deuterânope: deuteranope
Deuteranopia: deuteranopia
Deutério: deuterium (D)
Deuteromicetos: deuteromycetes
Dêuteron: deuteron, diplon
Deuteropatia: deuteropathy
Deuteropático: deuteropathic

Deuteroplasma: deuteroplasm
Deuteroporfirina: deuteroporphyrin
Deuterossoma: deuterosome
Deuterotocia: deuterotocia
Deuterotoquia: deuterotoky
Deutogênico: deutogenic
Deutomerito: deutomerite
Dêuton: deuton
Deutoninfa: deutonymph
Deutoplasma: deutoplasm
Deutoplásmico: deutoplasmic
Deutoplasmígeno: deutoplasmigenon
Deutoplasmólise: deutoplasmolysis
Dexametasona: dexamethasone
Dexanfetamina: dexamphetamine
Dexiocardia: dexiocardia
Dexpantenol: dexpanthenol
Dextralidade: dextrality
Dextrana: dextran
Dextranase: dextranase
Dextransacarase: dextransucrase
Dextrase: dextrase
Dextriferron: dextriferron
Dextrina: dextrin
Dextrina → dextrana transglucosidase: dextrin → dextran transglucosidase
Dextrina dextranase: dextrin dextranase
α-dextrina endo-1,6-α-glicosidase: α-dextrin endo-1,6-α-glucosidase
Dextrina 6-α-D-glucosidase: dextrin 6-α-D-glucosidase
Dextrina 6-glucosiltransferase: dextrin 6-glucosyltransferase
Dextrina glicosiltransferase: dextrin glycosyltransferase
Dextrina limite: dextrin limit
Dextrina transglicosilase: dextrin transglycosylase
Dextrinase: dextrinase
Dextrinogênico: dextrinogenic
Dextrinose: dextrinosis
Dextrinúria: dextrinuria
Dextro: dexter (D)
Dextrocardia: dextrocardia
Dextrocardiograma: dextrocardiogram
Dextrocerebral: dextrocerebral
Dextrociclodução: dextrocycloduction
Dextrocular: dextrocular
Dextrodução: dextroduction
Dextrogastria: dextrogastria
Dextroglicose: dextroglucose
Dextrograma: dextrogram
Dextropedal: dextropedal
Dextroposição: dextroposition
Dextrorrotação: dextrogyration, dextrorotation
Dextrorrotatório: dextrorotatory
Dextrose: dextrose
Dextrossinistro: dextrosinistral

Dextrotiroxina sódica: dextrothyroxine sodium
Dextrotorção: dextrotorsion
Dextrotrópico: dextrotropic
Dextroversão: dextroversion
Di(2-cloroetil)sulfeto: di(2-chloroethyl)sulfide
Diabetes: diabetes
Diabético: diabetic
Diabetogênico: diabetogenic
Diabetógeno: diabetogenous
Diabetologia: diabetology
Diacele: diacele
Diacetal: diacetal
Diacetato: diacetate
Diacetato de diflorasona: diflorasone diacetate
Diacetemia: diacetemia
Diacetil, diacetal: diacetyl, diacetal
Diacetilcolina: diacetylcholine
Diacetilmonoxima: diacetylmonoxime (DAM)
Diacetilmorfina: diacetylmorphine
Diacetonúria: diacetonuria
Diacetúria: diaceturia
Diácido: diacid
Diacilglicerol: diacylglycerol (DAG)
Diacinese: diakinesis
Diáclase: diaclasis, diaclasia
Diácrino: diacrinous
Diácrise: diacrisis
Diacrítico: diacritic, diacritical
Diacrônico: diachronic
Diactínico: diactinic
Díade: diad, dyad
Diadococinesia: diadochocinesia, diadochokinesia, diadochokinesis
Diadococinético: diadochokinetic
Diafanografia: diaphanography
Diafanoscopia: diaphanoscopy
Diafanoscópio: diaphanoscope
Diafemétrico: diaphemetric
Diafisário: diaphyseal, diaphysial
Diáfise: diaphysis, **pl.** diaphyses; shaft
Diafisectomia: diaphysectomy
Diafisite: diaphysitis
Diaforase: diaphorase
Diaforese: diaphoresis
Diaforético: diaphoretic
Diafragma: diaphragm, diaphragma, **pl.** diaphragmata; midriff, phren
Diafragmalgia: diaphragmalgia
Diafragmático: diaphragmatic
Diafragmatocele: diaphragmatocele
Diafragmodinia: diaphragmodynia
Diagnosticar: diagnose
Diagnosticista: diagnostician
Diagnóstico: diagnosis, diagnostic

Diagnóstico errado: misdiagnosis
Diagnóstico por DNA: DNA diagnostics
Diagrama: diagram
Diagrama de Dieuaide: Dieuaide diagram
Dialil: diallyl
Dialisado: dialysate
Dialisador: dialyzer
Dialisância: dialysance
Dialisar: dialyze
Diálise: dialysis
Diamagnético: diamagnetic
Diamagnetismo: diamagnetism
Diamelia: diamelia
Diâmetro: conjugata, diameter
Diamida: diamide
Diamidinas: diamidines
Diamina: diamine
Diamniótico: diamniotic
Diandria: diandry, diandria
Dianético: dianoetic
Diapausa: diapause
Diapedese: diapedesis
Diapirese: diapiresis
Diaplacentário: diaplacental
Diaplexo: diaplexus
Diapnóico, diapnótico: diapnoic, diapnotic
Diapófise: diapophysis
Diarréia: diarrhea
Diarreico: diarrheal, diarrheic, diarrhetic
Diarticular: diarthric, diarticular
Diartrose: diarthrosis, **pl.** diarthroses
Diascopia: diascopy
Diascópio: diascope
Diásquise: diaschisis
Diastalse: diastalsis
Diastáltico: diastaltic
Diástase: diastase, diastasis
Diastasúria: diastasuria
Diastático: diastatic
Diastema: diastema, **pl.** diastemata
Diastematocrania: diastematocrania
Diastematomielia: diastematomyelia
Diáster: diaster
Diastereoisômeros: diastereoisomers
Diástole: diastole
Diástole do coração: auxocardia
Diastólico: diastolic
Diastólico final: end-diastolic
Diastologia: diastology
Diastrofismo: diastrophism
Diataxia: diataxia
Diatela: diatela
Diatermância: diathermancy
Diatérmano: diathermanous
Diatermia: diathermy
Diatérmico: diathermal, diathermic, transcalent
Diatermocoagulação: diathermocoagulation
Diátese: diathesis
Diatético: diathetic

Diatomácea: diatom
Diatomáceo: diatomaceous
Diatômico: diatomic
Diatórico: diatoric
Diatrizoato: diatrizoate
Diazepam: diazepam
Diazinas: diazines
Diazinona: diazinon
Diazotar: diazotize
Diazóxido: diazoxide
Dibásico: dibasic
Dibenamina: dibenamine
Dibenzopiridina: dibenzopyridine
Dibenzotiazina: dibenzothiazine
Dibenzotiona: dibenzthione
Dibronsalam: dibromsalan
Dibucaína: dibucaine
Dicacodil: dicacodyl
Dicéfalo: dicephalous
Dicéfalos: dicephalus
Dicélico: dicelous
Dicêntrico: dicentric
2,3-diceto-L-gulonato: 2,3-diketo-L-gulonate
Dicetoidrindilideno-dicetoidrindamina: diketohydrindylidene-diketohydrindamine
Dicetona: diketone
Dicetopiperazinas: diketopiperazines
Dicisteína: dicysteine
Diclofenaco: diclofenac
Dicloramina-T: dichloramine-T
Dicloreto: dichloride
Diclorfenamida: dichlorphenamide
Dicloridrato de diantazol: diamthazole dihydrochloride
Dicloridrato de trietilenotetramina: triethylenetetramine dihydrochloride
Diclorisona: dichlorisone
Diclorobenzeno: dichlorobenzene
Diclorodifeniltricloroetano: dichlorodiphenyltrichloroethane (DDT)
Diclorodifluorometano: dichlorodifluoromethane
Diclorofeno: dichlorophen
2,6-diclorofenol-indofenol: 2,6-dichlorophenol-indophenol
Dicloroformoxima: dichloroformoxime
Dicloroidrina: dichlorohydrin
2,6-dicloroindofenol: 2,6-dichloroindophenol
Diclorovos: dichlorovos
Diclorvos: dichlorvos
Dicloxacilina sódica: dicloxacillin sodium
Dicófano: dicophane
Dicoria: dicoria
Dicoriônico: dichorial, dichorionic
Dicótico: dichotic
Dicotilédone: dicotyledon

Dicotomia: dichotomy
Dicotômico: dichotomous
Dicroceliose: dicrocoeliosis
Dicróico: dichroic
Dicroísmo: dichroism
Dicromático: dichromat, dichromatic
Dicromatismo: dichromatism
Dicromato: dichromate
Dicromatopsia: dichromatopsia
Dicrômico: dichromic
Dicromófilo: dichromophil, dichromophile
Dicrótico: dicrotic
Dicrotismo: dicrotism
Dictioma: dictyoma
Dictiossoma: dictyosome
Dictióteno: dictyotene
Dicumarol: dicumarol
Didactilismo: didactylism
Didático: didactic
Didélfico: didelphic
Didesoxiadenosina: dideoxyadenosine (DDA)
Didesoxicitidina: dideoxycytidine
Didesoxiinosina: dideoxyinosine (DDI)
Dídimo: didymus
Didrogesterona: dydrogesterone
Diécio: diecious
Dieldrina: dieldrin
Dieletrografia: dielectrography
Dieletrólise: dielectrolysis
Diencéfalo: diencephalon, **pl.** diencephala
Diencéfalo-hipofisário: diencephalohypophysial
Dienestrol: dienestrol
Diérese: dieresis
Dierético: dieretic
Diesterase: diesterase
Diéstrico: diestrous
Diestro: diestrus
Dieta: diet
Dieta de Giordano-Giovannetti: Giordano-Giovannetti diet
Dieta zero: NPO, n.p.o.
Dietadiona: diethadione
Dietanolamina: diethanolamine
Dietazina: diethazine
Dieterozigoto: diheterozygote
Dietética: dietetics
Dietético: dietary, dietetic
Dietil: diethyl
Dietileno glicol: diethylene glycol
Dietilenodiamina: diethylenediamine
Dietilestilbestrol: diethylstilbestrol (DES)
Dietilolamina: diethylolamine
Dietiltoluamida: diethyltoluamide
Dietiltriptamina: diethyltryptamine (DET)
Dietista: dietitian
Difalia: diphallus
Difásico: diphasic

Difemetoxidina: diphemethoxidine
Difenadiona: diphenadione
Difenano: diphenan
Difenidol: diphenidol
Difenil: diphenyl
Difenilcianoarsina: diphenylcyanoarsine
Difenilclorarsina: diphenylchlorarsine
Difenilenimina: diphenylenimine
Difenilidantoína: diphenylhydantoin
5,5-difenilidantoína: 5,5-diphenylhydantoin
2,5-difeniloxazol: 2,5-diphenyloxazole (PPO)
Difenol oxidase: diphenol oxidase
Difenoxina: difenoxin
Diferença: difference
Diferenciação: differentiation
Diferenciado: differentiated
Diferencial: differential
Difilina: dyphylline
Difilobotríase: bothriocephaliasis, diphyllobothriasis
Difiodonte: diphyodont
Diflucortolona: diflucortolone
Difluência: diffluence
Diflunisal: diflunisal
Difosfatase: diphosphatase
Difosfato: diphosphate
5'-difosfato de adenosina: adenosine 5'-diphosphate (ADP)
5'-difosfato de citidina: cytidine 5'-diphosphate (CDP)
5'-difosfato de guanosina: guanosine 5'-diphosphate (GDP)
Difosfato sódico de menadiol: menadiol sodium diphosphate
Difosfotiamina: diphosphothiamin
Difosgênio: diphosgene
Difração: diffraction
Difteria: diphtheria
Diftérico: diphtherial, diphtheritic, diphtheric
Difteróide: diphtheroid
Difterotoxina: diphtherotoxin
Difundido: diffusate
Difundir: diffuse
Difusão: diffusion
Difusível: diffusible
Difuso: effuse
Digamético: digametic
Digástrico: digastric, digastricus
Digenesia: digenesis
Digenético: digenetic
Digerir: digest
Digestão: digestion
Digestivo: digestant, digestive
Diginia: digyny, digynia
Digitação: digitation
Digitações do hipocampo: digitationes hippocampi
Digitado: digitate

Digital: digital
Digitalina: digitalin
Digitalismo: digitalism
Digitalização: digitalization
Digitina: digitin
Digitonina: digitonin
Digitoxigenina: digitoxigenin
Digitoxina: digitoxin
Digitoxose: digitoxose
D-digitoxose: D-digitoxose
Diglicerídeo lipase: diglyceride lipase
Diglossia: diglossia
Dignato: dignathus
Digoxigenina: digoxigenin
Digoxina: digoxin
Diíbrido: dihybrid
Diidralazina: dihydralazine
Diidrato: dihydrate
Diidrazona: dihydrazone
Diidrobiopterina: dihydrobiopterin
Diidrocloreto de dimazol: dimazole dihydrochloride
Diidrocodeinona: dihydrocodeinone
4,5α-diidrocortisol: 4,5α-dihydrocortisol
Diidrocortisona: dihydrocortisone
Diidroergocornina: dihydroergocornine
Diidroergocriptina: dihydroergocryptine
Diidroergocristina: dihydroergocristine
Diidroergotamina: dihydroergotamine
Diidroestreptomicina: dihydrostreptomycin
Diidrofolato redutase: dihydrofolate reductase (DHFR)
Diidrogênio: dihydrogen
Diidrolipoamida desidrogenase: dihydrolipoamide dehydrogenase
Diidrolipoamida S-acetiltransferase: dihydrolipoamide S-acetyltransferase
Diidro-orotase: dihydro-orotase
Diidro-orotato: dihydro-orotate
Diidropirimidina desidrogenase: dihydropyrimidine dehydrogenase
Diidropteridina redutase: dihydropteridine reductase
Diidrotaquisterol: dihydrotachysterol
Diidrotestosterona: dihydrotestosterone
Diidrouracil: dihydrouracil
Diidrouracil desidrogenase: dihydrouracil dehydrogenase
Diidrouridina: dihydrouridine (hU, hu, D)
Diidroxiacetona: dihydroxyacetone

2,8-diidroxiadenina: 2,8-dihydroxyadenine
1α,25-diidroxicolecalciferol: 1α,25-dihydroxycholecalciferol
1,25-diidroxiergocalciferol: 1,25-dihydroxyergocalciferol
3,4-diidroxifenilalanina: 3,4-dihydroxyphenylalanine
Diiodeto: diiodide
Diiodoidroxiquina: diiodohydroxyquin
Diiodotirosina: diiodotyrosine (DIT)
Diisopromina: diisopromine
2,6-diisopropil fenol: 2,6-diisopropyl phenol
Dilatação: dilatation, dilation
Dilatação e curetagem: dilation and curettage (D & C)
Dilatação e evacuação: dilation and evacuation (D & E)
Dilatador: dilatator, dilator
Dilatância: dilatancy
Dilatar: dilate
Dilema: dilemma
Diluente: diluent
Diluição: dilution
Diluir: dilute (dil.)
Dimazona: dimazon
Dimelia: dimelia
Dimenidrinato: dimenhydrinate
Dimensão: dimension
Dimensão aerodinâmica: aerodynamic size
Dimercaprol: antilewisite, dimercaprol
Dimercúrio: dimercurion
Dimérico: dimeric
Dímero: dimer, dimerous
Dímero d: d-dimer
Dimetadiona: dimethadione
Dimeticona: dimethicone
5,6-dimetilbenzimidazol: 5,6-dimethylbenzimidazole
β,β-dimetilcisteína: β,β-dimethylcysteine
Dimetil cetona: dimethyl ketone
Dimetil d-tubocurarina: dimethyl d-tubocurarine
Dimetil mercúrio: dimethyl mercury
Dimetilalilpirofosfato: dimethylallylpyrophosphate
Dimetilaminoazobenzeno: dimethylaminoazobenzene
Dimetilbenzeno: dimethylbenzene
Dimetilcarbinol: dimethylcarbinol
Dimetilfenilpiperazínio: dimethylphenylpiperazinium (DMPP)
Dimetilfenol: dimethylphenol
Dimetisterona: dimethisterone
Dimetoxianfetamina: dimethoxyamphetamine (DMA)
2,5-dimetoxi-4-metilanfetamina: 2,5-dimethoxy-4-methylamphetamine (DOM)

Dimetria: dimetria
Diminuição: decrement
Diminuição cruzada: cross-taper
Dimórfico: dimorphic, dimorphous
Dimorfismo: dimorphism
Dina: dyne
Dinâmica: dynamics
Dinamogênese: dynamogenesis
Dinamogenia: dynamogeny
Dinamogênico: dynamogenic
Dinamógrafo: dynamograph
Dinamômetro: dynamometer
Dinamoscopia: dynamoscopy
Dinamoscópio: dynamoscope
Dineína: dynein
Dinérico: dineric
Dinitrato de isossorbida: isosorbide dinitrate
Dinitrocelulose: dinitrocellulose
2,4-dinitrofenol: 2,4-dinitrophenol (DNP, Dnp)
4,6-dinitro-o-cresol: 4,6-dinitro-o-cresol
Dinoflagelado: dinoflagellate
Dinoprost: dinoprost
Dinoprostona: dinoprostone
Dinorfina: dynorphin
Dinucleotídeo: dinucleotide
Dioctofimíase: dioctophymiasis
Diodona: diodone
Diodoquina: diodoquin
Diolamina: diolamine
Dioptria: diopter (D)
Dióptrico: dioptrics
Dioscina: dioscin
Diose: diose
Diosgenina: diosgenin
Diótico: diotic
Diovular: diovular
Diovulatório: diovulatory
Dioxana: dioxane
Dioxibenzona: dioxybenzone
Dióxido: dioxide
Dióxido de 1,4-dietileno: 1,4-diethylene dioxide
Dióxido de silício: silicon dioxide
Dioxigenase: dioxygenase
Dioxina: dioxin
Dipeptidase: dipeptidase
Dipeptídeo: dipeptide
Dipeptidil carboxipeptidase: dipeptidylcarboxypeptidase
Dipeptidil peptidase: dipeptidyl peptidase
Dipeptidil transferase: dipeptidyl transferase
Dípigo: dipygus
Dipilidíase: dipylidiasis
Dipiproverina: dipiproverine
Dipiridamol: dypiridamole
Dipirimidina fotoliase: dipyrimidine photolyase
Dipirina: dipyrine
Dipirona: dipyrone
Diplacusia: diplacusis
Diplegia: diplegia
Diploalbuminúria: diploalbuminuria

Diplobacilo: diplobacillus
Diploblástico: diploblastic
Diplocardia: diplocardia
Diplocárion: diplokaryon
Diplocéfalo: diplocephalus
Diplococcemia: diplococcemia
Diplococcina: diplococcin
Diplococo: diplococcus, **pl.** diplococci
Diplocoria: diplocoria
Díploe: diploë
Diplogênese: diplogenesis
Diplóico: diploic
Diplóide: diploid
Diplomelitúria: diplomelituria
Diplomielia: diplomyelia
Diplonema: diplonema
Diploneural: diploneural
Diplópago: diplopagus
Diplopia: diplopia
Diplopodia: diplopodia
Diploquiria: diplocheiria, diplochiria
Diplossoma: diplosome
Diplossomia: diplosomia
Diplóteno: diplotene
Dipodia: dipodia
Dipolo: dipole
Diprenorfina: diprenorphine
Dipropiltriptamina: dipropyltryptamine
Dipropionato de beclometasona: beclomethasone dipropionate
Dipropionato de prometestrol: promethestrol dipropionate
Diprosopo: diprosopus
Dipsógeno: dipsogen
Dipsomania: dipsomania
Dipsose: dipsesis, dipsosis
Dipsoterapia: dipsotherapy
Diptérico: dipterous
Díptero: dipteran
Dique posterior: postdam
Diquelia: dicheilia, dichilia
Diqueria: dicheiria, dichiria
Diretor: director
Diretriz: directive, guideline
Dirofilária: heartworm
Dirofilaríase: dirofilariasis
Disacusia: dysacousia, dysacusia, dysacusis
Disafia: dysaphia
Disáfico: dysaphic
Disantigrafia: dysantigraphia
Disarteriotonia: dysarteriotony
Disartria: dysarthria
Disártrico: dysarthric
Disartrose: dysarthrosis
Disautonomia: dysautonomia
Disbarismo: dysbarism
Disbasia: dysbasia
Disbetalipoproteinemia: dysbetalipoproteinemia
Disbolismo: dysbolism
Disbulia: dysbulia
Disbúlico: dysbulic
Discalculia: dyscalculia
Discariose: dyskaryosis
Discariótico: dyskaryotic
Discectomia: discectomy

Discefalia: dyscephalia, dyscephaly
Disceratoma: dyskeratoma
Disceratose: dyskeratosis
Disceratótico: dyskeratotic
Disciforme: disciform
Discinesia: dyscinesia, dyskinesia, dyskinesis
Discinético: dyskinetic
Discissão: discission
Discite: discitis, diskitis
Disco: disc, discus, **pl.** disci; disk
Disco articular: fibroplate
Disco de Burlew: Burlew disk
Disco prolígero: ovigerus
Discoblástico: discoblastic
Discoblástula: discoblastula
Discogástrula: discogastrula
Discogênico: discogenic
Discografia: diskography
Discograma: diskogram
Discóide: discoid
Discondrogênese: dyschondrogenesis
Discondroplasia: dyschondroplasia
Discondrosteose: dyschondrosteosis
Discopatia: discopathy
Discoplacenta: discoplacenta
Discordância: discordance
Discoria: dyscoria
Discotomia: discotomy
Discrasia: dyscrasia
Discrasia de plasmócitos: plasma cell dyscrasia
Discrásico: dyscrasic, dyscratic
Discriminação: discrimination
Discromatopsia: dyschromatopsia
Discromatose: dyschromatosis
Discromia: dyschromia
Disdiaclasto: disdiaclast
Disdiadococinesia: dysdiadochokinesia, dysdiadochocinesia
Disematopoese: dyshematopoiesis
Disematopoético: dyshematopoietic
Disemia: dysemia
Disemopoese: dyshemopoiesis
Disemopoético: dyshemopoietic
Disencefalia esplancnocística: dysencephalia splanchnocystica
Disenteria: dysentery
Disentérico: dysenteric
Diseretismo: dyserethism
Disergia: dysergia
Disestesia: dysesthesia
Disfagia: dysphagia, dysphagy
Disfagocitose: dysphagocytosis
Disfasia: dysphasia
Disfemia: dysphemia
Disfibrinogenemia: dysfibrinogenemia
Disfonia: dysphonia
Disforia: dysphoria
Disfrasia: dysphrasia
Disfunção: dysfunction, malfunction

Disgamaglobulinemia: dysgammaglobulinemia
Disgenesia: dysgenesis
Disgênico: dysgenic
Disgerminoma: disgerminoma, dysgerminoma
Disgeusia: dysgeusia
Disgnatia: dysgnathia
Disgnático: dysgnathic
Disgnosia: dysgnosia
Disgônico: dysgonic
Disgrafia: dysgraphia
Disidria: dyshidria
Disidrose: dyshidrosis
Disjunção: disjunction, dysjunction
Dislexia: dyslexia
Disléxico: dyslexic
Dislogia: dyslogia
Dismasese: dysmasesis
Dismaturidade: dysmaturity
Dismaturo: dysmature
Dismelia: dysmelia
Dismenorréia: dysmenorrhea
Dismetria: dysmetria
Dismiotonia: dysmyotonia
Dismorfismo: dysmorphia, dysmorphism
Dismorfofobia: dysmorphophobia
Dismorfogênese: dysmorphogenesis
Dismorfologia: dysmorphology
Dismutação: dismutation
Dismutase: dismutase
Disnistaxe: dysnystaxis
Disodontíase: dysodontiasis
Disofenina: disofenin
Disontogênese: dysontogenesis
Disontogenético: dysontogenetic
Disopiramida: disopyramide
Disopromina: disopromine
Disorexia: dysorexia
Disosmia: dysosmia
Disosteogênese: dysosteogenesis
Disostose: dysostosis
Dispalia: dyspallia
Díspar: disparate
Dispareunia: dyspareunia
Disparidade: disparity
Dispensário: dispensary
Dispensatório: dispensatory
Dispepsia: dyspepsia
Dispéptico: dyspeptic
Dispermia: dispermy, dispermia
Dispersão: dispersal, dispersion, scatter
Dispersão de Compton: Compton scattering
Dispersar: disperse
Dispersidade: dispersity
Dispersóide: dispersoid
Dispinealismo: dyspinealism
Dispirema: dispireme
Dispituitarismo: dyspituitarism
Displasia: dysplasia
Displásico: dysplastic
Dispnéia: dyspnea
Dispneico: dyspneic
Dispondilismo: dysspondylism

Dispositivo: appliance, device
Dispraxia: dyspraxia
Disprósio: dysprosium (Dy)
Disproteinemia: dysproteinemia
Disproteinêmico: dysproteinemic
Disquezia: dyschezia
Disquiria: dyscheiria, dyschiria
Disrafismo, disrafia: dysraphism, dysraphia
Disritmia: dysrhythmia
Dissacaridases: disaccharidases
Dissacarídeo: disaccharide
Dissecar: dissect
Dissecção: cutdown, dissection
Dissector: prosector
Disseminado: disseminated
Dissilabia: dyssyllabia, syllable-stumbling
Dissimetria: dissymmetry
Dissimilação: dissimilation, dissimulation
Dissinergia: dyssynergia
Dissociação: dissociation
Dissolver: dissolve
Dissomia: disomy
Dissômico: disomic
Dissonância: dissonance
Dissonia: dyssomnia
Dissulfamida: disulfamide
Dissulfato: disulfate
Dissulfeto: disulfide
Dissulfeto de lipoamida: lipoamide disulfide
Dissulfeto de tetraetiltiuram: tetraethylthiuram disulfide
Dissulfiram: disulfiram
Distal: distad, distal, distalis
Distância: distance
Distância interarco: interarch
Distância no mapa: map distance
Distasia: dysstasia, dystasia
Distático: dysstatic
Distelefalangia: dystelephalangy
Distensão: distention, distension
Distensibilidade: distensibility
Distimia: dysthymia
Distímico: dysthymic
Distinto: discrete
Distiquíase: distichiasis
Distobucal: distobuccal
Distobucoclusal: distobucco-occlusal
Distobucopulpar: distobuccopulpal
Distocervical: distocervical
Distocia: dystocia
Distoclusal: distoclusal, disto-occlusal
Distoclusão: distoclusion, disto-occlusion
Distogengival: distogingival
Distoincisal: distoincisal
Distolabial: distolabial
Distolabiopulpar: distolabiopulpal
Distolingual: distolingual
Distolinguoclusal: distolinguo-occlusal

Distomíase, distomatose: distomiasis, distomatosis
Distomolar: distomolar
Distonia: dystonia
Distônico: dystonic
Distopia: dystopia
Distópico: dystopic
Distoposição: distoplacement
Distopulpar: distopulpal
Distorção: distortion
Distoversão: distoversion
Distração: distraction
Distribuição: distribution
Distribuição do nitrogênio: nitrogen distribution, nitrogen partition
Distriquia: distrix
Distriquíase: districhiasis
Distrofia: dystrophia, dystrophy
Distrofia de Favre: Favre dystrophy
Distrófico: dystrophic
Distrofina: dystrophin, dystropin
Distropia: dystropy
Distropina: distropin
Distúrbio: disturbance
Disúria: dysuria, dysury
Disúrico: dysuric
Diterpênicos: diterpenes
Ditiotreitol: dithiothreitol
Ditranol: dithranol
Diurese: diuresis
Diurético: diuretic
Diurno: diurnal
Divalência: divalence, divalency
Divalente: divalent
Divalproex sódico: divalproex sodium
Divaricação: divarication
Divergência: divergence
Divergente: deviant, divergent
Diversidade cultural: cultural diversity
Diverticular: diverticular
Diverticulectomia: diverticulectomy
Diverticulite: diverticulitis
Divertículo: diverticulum, **pl.** diverticula
Diverticuloma: diverticuloma
Diverticulopexia: diverticulopexy
Diverticulose: diverticulosis
Divicina: divicine
Divisão: divisio, division
Divisor de águas: watershed
Divulsão: divulsion
Divulsionar: divulse
Divulsor: divulsor
Dixirazina: dixyrazine
Dizigótico: dizygotic, dizygous
***dl*-hiosciamina:** *dl*-hyoscyamine
***dl*-narcotina:** *dl*-narcotine
Doador: donor
Dobutamina: dobutamine
Docusato cálcico: docusate calcium
Docusato sódico: docusate sodium
Dodecano: dodecane

Dodecanoil-CoA sintetase: dodecanoyl-CoA synthetase
Dodecil: dodecyl
Doença das alturas: puna
Doença de Bosin: Bosin disease
Doença do movimento: kinesia
Doença: disease, illness, maladie, malady, sickness
Doente: sick
Dogma: dogma
Dogmático: dogmatic
Dogmatista: dogmatist
Dol: dol
Dolicocefalia, dolicocefalismo: dolichocephaly, dolichocephalism
Dolicocefálico, dolicocéfalo: dolichocephalic, dolichocephalous
Dolicocólon: dolichocolon
Dolicocraniano: dolichocranial
Dolicoestenomelia: dolichostenomelia
Dolicofacial: dolichofacial
Dolicol: dolichol
Dolicopélvico: dolichopellic, dolichopelvic
Dolicoprosópico: dolichoprosopic, dolichoprosopous
Dolicourânico: dolichouranic, dolichuranic
Dolorífico: dolorific
Dolorimetria: dolorimetry
Dolorologia: dolorology
Domiciliado: domiciliated
Dominância: dominance
Dominante: dominant
Domínio: domain
Domiodol: domiodol
Domperidona: domperidone
Dopa: dopa, DOPA, Dopa
L-dopa: L-dopa
Dopamina: dopamine (DM)
Dopamina β-hidroxilase: dopamine β-hydroxylase
Dopamina β-monoxigenase: dopamine β-monooxygenase
Dopaminérgico: dopaminergic
Doping: doping
Dor: ache, dolor, pain
Dor aguda: pang
Dor de barriga: bellyache
Dor intermenstrual: midpain, mittelschmerz
Dorafobia: doraphobia
Dores pós-parto: afterpains
Dornase: dornase
Doromania: doromania
Dorsal: dorsad, dorsal, dorsalis
Dorsalgia: backache
Dorsiduzir: dorsiduct
Dorsiescapular: dorsiscapular
Dorsiespinal: dorsispinal
Dorsiflexão: dorsiflexion
Dorso: back, dorsum, **gen.** dorsi, **pl.** dorsa
Dorso do pé: instep
Dorsoabdominal: dorsabdominal
Dorsocefálico: dorsocephalad

Dorsolateral: dorsolateral
Dorsolombar: dorsolumbar
Dorsoventral: dorsoventrad
Dosagem: dosage
Dose: dose, draft
Dosimetria: dosimetry
Dosímetro: dosimeter
Doutor: doctor
Doutrina: doctrine
Doxazocina: doxazocin
Doxiciclina: doxycycline
Doxofilina: doxophylline
Doxorrubicina: doxorubicin
Dracma: drachm, dram (dr)
Dracma líquida: fluidrachm, fluidram
Dracunculíase: dracunculiasis, dracunculosis
Drágea: dragée
Dramatização: role-playing
Drenagem: drainage
Drenar: drain
Drepanídio: drepanidium
Drepanocítico: drepanocytic
Drepanócito: drepanocyte
Droga: drug
Dromomania: dromomania
Dronabinol: dronabinol
Droperidol: droperidol
Drusas: drusen
DT-diaforase: DT-diaphorase
dTDP-açúcares: dTDP-sugars
Dualismo: dualism
Dubleto: doublet
Duboisina: duboisine
Dução: duction
Ducha: douche
Ducha de ar de Politzer: politzerization
Ductal: ductal
Dúctil: ductile
Ducto: duct, ductus, **gen. e pl.** ductus
Ducto deferente: spermiduct
Ducto seminal: gonaduct
Ductular: ductular
Dúctulo: ductule, ductulus, **pl.** ductuli
Dulcina: dulcin
Dulcita, dulcitol, dulcose: dulcite, dulcitol, dulcose
Duocrinina: duocrinin
Duodenal: duodenal
Duodenectomia: duodenectomy
Duodenite: duodenitis
Duodeno: duodenum, **gen.** duodeni, **pl.** duodena
Duodenocistostomia: duodenocystostomy
Duodenocolangite: duodenocholangitis
Duodenocolecistostomia: duodenocholecystostomy
Duodenocoledocotomia: duodenocholedochotomy
Duodenoenterostomia: duodenoenterostomy
Duodenojejunostomia: duodenojejunostomy
Duodenólise: duodenolysis
Duodenorrafia: duodenorrhaphy

Duodenoscopia: duodenoscopy
Duodenostomia: duodenostomy
Duodenotomia: duodenotomy
Duovírus: duovirus
Dúplex: duplex
Duplicação: duplication
Duplicidade: duplicitas
Duração: duration (D)
Dura-encefalo-sinangiose: duraencephalosynangiosis
Dural: dural, duramatral
Dura-máter: dura, dura mater
Duraplastia: duraplasty
Durável: fast
Dureza: hardness

E

Eburnação: eburnation
Ebúrneo: eburneous
Eburnite: eburnitis
E-caderina: E-cadherrin
Ecbolina: ecboline
Ecciese: eccyesis
Ecdêmico: ecdemic
Ecdise: ecdysis
Ecdisiasmo: ecdysiasm
Ecdisita: ecdysist
Ecfima: ecphyma
Ecgonina: ecgonine
Eclábio: eclabium
Eclâmpsia: eclampsia
Eclâmptico: eclamptic
Eclamptogênico: eclamptogenic, eclamptogenous
Ecleticismo: eclecticism
Eclético: eclectic
Eco: echo
Ecoacusia: echoacousia
Ecoaortografia: echoaortography
Ecocardiografia: echocardiography
Ecocardiograma: echocardiogram
Ecoencefalografia: echoencephalography
Ecoendocrinologia: ecoendocrinology
Ecoespécies: ecospecies
Ecofonia: echophony, echophonia
Ecofrasia: echophrasia
Ecogênico: echogenic
Ecografia: echographia, echography
Ecografista: echographer
Ecograma: echogram
Ecolalia: echolalia
Ecolocalização: echolocation
Ecologia: ecology
Ecomotismo: echomotism
Econazol: econazole
Econdroma: ecchondroma
Econdrose: ecchondrosis
Economia: economy
Ecopatia: echopathy

Ecopraxia: echopraxia
Ecoscópio: echoscope
Ecossistema: ecosystem
Ecotaxia: ecotaxis
Écrino: eccrine
Ecrinologia: eccrinology
Écrise: eccrisis
Ecrítico: eccritic
Ectasia: ectasia, ectasis
Ectático: ectatic
Ectental: ectental
Ectetmóide: ectethmoid
Ectiluréia: ectylurea
Ectima: ecthyma
Ectipo: ectype
Ectíris: ectiris
Ectoantígeno: ectoantigen
Ectoblasto: ectoblast
Ectocardia: ectocardia
Ectocervical: ectocervical
Ectocisto: ectocyst
Ectocórnea: ectocornea
Ectocoróide: ectochoroidea
Ectócrino: ectocrine
Ectoderma: ectoderm
Ectodermatose: ectodermatosis
Ectodérmico: ectodermal, ectodermic
Ectodermose: ectodermosis
Ectoental: ectoental
Ectoenzima: ectoenzyme
Ectoetmóide: ectoethmoid
Ectófito: ectophyte
Ectógeno: ectogenous
Ectômero: ectomere
Ectomerogonia: ectomerogony
Ectomesênquima: ectomesenchyme
Ectomórfico: ectomorphic
Ectomorfo: ectomorph
Ectópago: ectopagus
Ectoparasita: ectoparasite
Ectoparasiticida: ectoparasiticide
Ectoparasitismo: ectoparasitism
Ectoperitonite: ectoperitonitis
Ectopia: ectopia, ectopy
Ectópico: ectopic
Ectoplacentário: ectoplacental
Ectoplasma: ectoplasm
Ectoplasmático, ectoplásmico, ectoplástico: ectoplasmatic, ektoplasmic, ektoplastic
Ectormônio: ectohormone
Ectorretina: ectoretina
Ectoscopia: ectoscopy
Ectossarco: ectosarc
Ectósteo: ectosteal
Ectostose: ectostosis
Ectotoxina: ectotoxin
Ectótrico: ectothrix
Ectozoário: ectozoon
Ectrodactilia: ectrodactyly, ectrodactylia, ectrodactylism
Ectrogenia: ectrogeny
Ectrogênico: ectrogenic
Ectromelia: ectromelia
Ectromélico: ectromelic
Ectrópio: ectropion, ectropium
Ectropodia: ectropody

Ectroquiria: ectrocheiry, ectrochiry
Ectrossindactilia: ectrosyndactyly
Ecurese: ecuresis
Eczema: eczema
Eczematização: eczematization
Eczematóide: eczematoid
Eczematoso: eczematous
Edatamil: edathamil
Edéia: edea
Edema: edema
Edematização: edematization
Edematoso: edematous
Edentado: edentate
Edestina: edestin
Edetato: edetate
Edetato de cálcio dissódico: edetate calcium disodium
Edipismo: oedipism
Edisilato: edisylate
Edulcorante: edulcorant
Edulcorar: edulcorate
Efapse: ephapse
Efáptico: ephaptic
Efébico: ephebic
Efebologia: ephebology
Éfedra: ephedra
Efedrina: ephedrine
Efeito: effect
Efeito colateral: side effect
Efeito secundário: aftereffect
Efélide: ephelis, **pl.** ephelides
Efeminação: effemination
Eferente: efferent
Efervescente: effervescent
Efervescer: effervesce
Efetividade: effectiveness
Efetor: effector
Eficácia: efficacy
Eficiência: efficiency
Eflorescente: efflorescent
Eflorescer: effloresce
Eflúvio: effluvium, **pl.** effluvia
Efusão: effusion
Egesta: egesta
Eglanduloso: eglandulous
Ego: ego
Egobroncofonia: egobronchophony
Egocentricidade: egocentricity
Egocêntrico: egocentric, egotropic
Egodistônico: ego-alien, ego-dystonic
Egofonia: egophony
Egofônico: egophonic
Egomania: egomania
Egossintônico: ego-syntonic
Eiconômetro: eikonometer
Eicosanóides: eicosanoids
Eidético: eidetic
Eilóide: eiloid
Einstein: einstein
Einstênio: einsteinium (Es)
Eisódico: eisodic
Eixo: axis (ax), **pl.** axes
Ejaculação: ejaculation
Ejacular: ejaculate
Ejaculatório: ejaculatory
Ejeção: ejection

Ejeto: ejecta
Ejetor: ejector
Elaboração: elaboration, workingout
Elação: elation
Elapídeo: elapid
Elastância: elastance
Elastase: elastase
Elástica: elastica
Elasticidade: elasticity
Elasticina: elasticin
Elástico: elastic
Elastina: elastin
Elastofibroma: elastofibroma
Elastoidina: elastoidin
Elastólise: elastolysis
Elastoma: elastoma
Elastômetro: elastometer
Elastomucina: elastomucin
Elastorrexe: elastorrhexis
Elastose: elastosis
Elaunina: elaunin
Electuário: confectio, **gen.** confectionis, **pl.** confectiones; confection
Eledoisina: eledoisin
Elefantíase: elephantiasis
Eleidina: eleidin
Elemento: element
Eleoma: eleoma
Eleômetro: eleometer
Eleopatia: elaiopathia, eleopathy
Eletroanalgesia: electroanalgesia
Eletroanálise: electroanalysis
Eletroanestesia: electroanesthesia
Eletroaxonografia: electroaxonography
Eletrobioscopia: electrobioscopy
Eletrocardiofonografia: electrocardiophonography
Eletrocardiofonograma: electrocardiophonogram
Eletrocardiografia: electrocardiography
Eletrocardiógrafo: electrocardiograph
Eletrocardiograma: electrocardiogram (ECG, EKG)
Eletrocautério: electrocautery
Eletrocauterização: electrocauterization
Eletrochoque: electroshock
Eletrocirurgia: electrosurgery
Eletrocisão: electroscission
Eletrocistografia: electrocystography
Eletrocoagulação: electrocoagulation
Eletrococleografia: electrocochleography
Eletrococleograma: electrocochleogram
Eletrocontratilidade: electrocontractility
Eletroconvulsivo: electroconvulsive

Eletrocorticografia: electrocorticography (ECoG)
Eletrocorticograma: electrocorticogram
Eletrocução: electrocution
Eletrocutar: electrocute
Eletrodérmico: electrodermal
Eletrodessecação: electrodesiccation
Eletrodiagnóstico: electrodiagnosis
Eletrodiálise: electrodialysis
Eletrodo: electrode
Eletroemostasia: electrohemostasis
Eletroencefalografia: electroencephalography (EEG)
Eletroencefalógrafo: electroencephalograph
Eletroencefalograma: electroencephalogram (EEG)
Eletroendosmose: electroendosmosis
Eletroespectrografia: electrospectrography
Eletroespinografia: electrospinography
Eletroespinograma: electrospinogram
Eletroestenólise: electrostenolysis
Eletroestetógrafo: electrostethograph
Eletroferograma: electropherogram
Eletrofílico: electrophilic
Eletrófilo: electrophil, electrophile
Eletrofisiologia: electrophysiology
Eletrofobia: electrophobia
Eletrofocalização: electrofocusing
Eletroforese: electrophoresis
Eletroforético: electrophoretic
Eletroforetograma: electrophoretogram
Eletrofrênico: electrophrenic
Eletrogastrografia: electrogastrography
Eletrogastrógrafo: electrogastrograph
Eletrogastrograma: electrogastrogram
Eletrograma: electrogram
Eletroimunodifusão: electroimmunodiffusion
Eletroisterógrafo: electrohysterograph
Eletrolisador: electrolyzer
Eletrolisar: electrolyze
Eletrólise: electrolysis
Eletrolítico: electrolytic
Eletrólito: electrolyte
Eletromagneto: electromagnet
Eletromassagem: electromassage
Eletromicção: electromicturation
Eletromiografia (EMG): electromyography

Glossário

Eletromiógrafo: electromyograph
Eletromiograma (EMG): electromyogram (EMG)
Eletromorfo: electromorph
Eletromotilidade: electromotility
Elétron: electron
Eletronarcose: electronarcosis
Eletronegativo: electronegative
Eletroneurografia: electroneurography
Eletroneurólise: electroneurolysis
Eletroneuromiografia: electroneuromyography
Eletrônico: electronic
Eletronistagmografia (ENG): electronystagmography (ENG)
Elétron-volt: electron-volt (eV, ev)
Eletrooculografia: electrooculography (EOG)
Eletrooculograma: electrooculogram
Eletroolfatograma: electroolfactogram (EOG)
Eletroosmose: electro-osmosis
Eletroparacentese: electroparacentesis
Eletroporação: electroporation
Eletropositivo: electropositive
Eletropunção: electropuncture
Eletroquímico: electrochemical
Eletroquimógrafo: electrokymograph
Eletroquimograma: electrokymogram (EKY)
Eletrorradiologia: electroradiology
Eletrorradiômetro: electroradiometer
Eletrorretinografia: electroretinography
Eletrorretinograma: electroretinogram (ERG)
Eletroscópio: electroscope
Eletrostrição: electrostriction
Eletrotanásia: electrothanasia
Eletrotaxia: electrotaxis
Eletroterapêutica, eletroterapia: electrotherapeutics, electrotherapy
Eletrotermo: electrotherm
Eletrotomia: electrotomy
Eletrótomo: electrotome
Eletrotônico: electrotonic
Eletrotônus: electrotonus
Eletrotropismo: electrotropism
Eletuário: conserve, electuary
Elevador: elevator
Elevando: attollens
Eliminação: elimination
Elinguação: elinguation
Elinina: elinin
Elipse: ellipsis
Elipsóide: ellipsoid
Eliptocitose: elliptocytosis
Elixir: elixir
Eluante: eluant

Eluato: eluate
Eluente: eluent, elutant
Eluição: elution, elutriation
Eluir: elute, elutriate
Em bloco: en bloc
Emaciação: emaciation
Emagrecedor: marcid
Emanação: emanation
Emanatório: emanatorium
Emancipação: emancipation
Emanoterapia: emanotherapy
Emaranhado: tangle
Emarginação: emargination
Emarginado: emarginate
Emasculação: emasculation
Embainhado: insheathed
Embainhamento: cuffing
Embalsamar: embalm
Embebição: imbibition
Embelina: embelin
Embocadura: embouchement
Emboçar: block-out
Embolectomia: embolectomy
Embolemia: embolemia
Embolia: embolism
Embólico: embolic
Emboliforme: emboliform
Embolização: embolization
Êmbolo: embolus, **pl.** emboli
Embolomicótico: embolomycotic
Emboloterapia: embolotherapy
Embonato de viprínio: viprynium embonate
Embriaguez: drunkenness, inebriety
Embrião: embryo
Embrioblasto: embryoblast
Embriocardia: embryocardia
Embrióforo: embryophore
Embriogênese: embryogenesis
Embriogenia: embryogeny
Embriogênico, embriogenético: embryogenic, embryogenetic
Embrióide: embryoid
Embriologia: embryology
Embriologista: embryologist
Embrioma: embryoma
Embriomorfo: embryomorphous
Embrionado: embryonate
Embrionário: embryonal
Embrionia: embryony
Embriônico: embryonic
Embrioniforme: embryoniform
Embrionização: embryonization
Embrionóide: embryonoid
Embriopatia: embryopathy
Embrioplásico: embryoplastic
Embriotomia: embryotomy
Embriotoxicidade: embryotoxicity
Embriotoxo: embryotoxon
Embriotrofia: embryotrophy
Embriotrófico: embryotrophic
Embriotrofo: embryotroph
Embrocação: embrocation
Emeiocitose: emeiocytosis
Emergência: emergence
Emergente: emergent
Êmese: emesis

Emético: emetic
Emetina: emetine
Emetocatártico: emetocathartic
Emetogenicidade: emetogenicity
Emetogênico: emetogenic
Emetropia: emmetropia
Emetrópico: emmetropic
Emetropização: emmetropization
Emigração: emigration
Emilcamato: emylcamate
Eminência: eminence, eminentia, **pl.** eminentiae
Emiocitose: emiocytosis
Emissão: emission
Emissário: emissary
Emissividade: emissivity
Emoção: emotion
Emocional: emotional
Emodina: archin, emodin
Emoliente: emollient
Emparelhamento: matching
Empasma: empasm, empasma
Empatia: empathy
Empático: empathic
Emperipolese: emperipolesis
Empiectomia: empyectomy
Empiema: empyema
Empiêmico: empyemic
Empiese: empyesis
Empilhamento: rouleau, **pl.** rouleaux
Empiocele: empyocele
Empireuma: empyreuma
Empírico: empiric, empirical
Empirismo: empiricism
Emplastro: plaster
Emporiatria: emporiatrics
Emprostótono: emprosthotonos
Emulgente: emulgent
Emulsão: emulsion
Emulsificador: emulsifier
Emulsificar: emulsify
Emulsina: emulsin
Emulsivo: emulsive
Emulsóide: emulsoid
Emurese: emuresis
Enalaprilato: enalaprilat
Enamelinas: enamelins
Enantal: enanthal
Enantato: enanthate
Enantema: enanthem, enanthema
Enantiomérico: enantiomeric
Enantiomerismo: enantiomerism
Enantiômero: enantiomer
Enantiomórfico: enantiomorphic, enantiomorphous
Enantiomorfismo: enantiomorphism
Enantiomorfo: enantiomorph
Enantol: oenanthal
Enartrodial: enarthrodial
Enartrose: enarthrosis
Encadeamento: chaining
Encaixamento: emboitement
Encaixe: mortise
Encaixotamento: boxing

Encapsulação: capsulation, encapsulation
Encapsulado: encapsulated, encapsuled
Encarcerado: incarcerated
Encarnante: incarnant
Encarnativo: incarnative
Encefalalgia: encephalalgia
Encefalemia: encephalemia
Encefálico: encephalic
Encefalinas: enkephalins
Encefalinérgico: enkephalinergic
Encefalite: encephalitis, **pl.** encephalitides
Encefalítico: encephalitic
Encefalitogênico: encephalitogenic
Encefalitógeno: encephalitogen
Encefalização: encephalization
Encéfalo: encephalon, **pl.** encephala
Encefalocele: encephalocele
Encefalocistocele: encephalocystocele
Encefalodinia: encephalodynia
Encefalodisplasia: encephalodysplasia
Encefaloduroarteriossinangiose: encephaloduroarteriosynangiosis
Encefaloespinal: encephalospinal
Encefalografia: encephalography
Encefalograma: encephalogram
Encefalóide: encephaloid
Encefalólito: encephalolith
Encefalologia: encephalology
Encefaloma: encephaloma
Encefalomalacia: encephalomalacia
Encefalomeningite: encephalomeningitis
Encefalomeningocele: encephalomeningocele
Encefalomeningopatia: encephalomeningopathy
Encefalômero: encephalomere
Encefalômetro: encephalometer
Encefalomielite: encephalomyelitis
Encefalomielocele: encephalomyelocele
Encefalomieloneuropatia: encephalomyeloneuropathy
Encefalomielopatia: encephalomyelopathy
Encefalomielorradiculite: encephalomyeloradiculitis
Encefalomielorradiculopatia: encephalomyeloradiculopathy
Encefalomiocardite: encephalomyocarditis
Encefalopatia: encephalopathia, encephalopathy
Encefalopiose: encephalopyosis
Encefalorraquidiano: encephalorrhachidian
Encefalosclerose: encephalosclerosis
Encefaloscopia: encephaloscopy

Encefaloscópio: encephaloscope
Encefalose: encephalosis
Encefalosquise: encephaloschisis
Encefalotomia: encephalotomy
Encefalótomo: encephalotome
Encelite: encelitis, enceliitis
Encher: pack
Encistado: encysted
Encistamento: encystment
Encondral: enchondral
Encondroma: enchondroma
Encondromatose: enchondromatosis
Encondromatoso: enchondromatous
Encoprese: encopresis
Encrânio: encranius
Encravamento: nailing
Encurvamento: incurvation
Endadelfo: endadelphos
Endangeíte: endangiitis, endangeitis
Endaortite: endaortitis
Endarterectomia: endarterectomy
Endarterite: endarteritis
Endaural: endaural
Endectocida: endectocide
Endemia: endemia
Endêmico: endemic
Endemoepidêmico: endemoepidemic
Endergônico: endergonic
Endérmico: endermic, endermatic
Endermose: endermosis
Endoabdominal: endoabdominal
Endoamilase: endoamylase
Endoaneurismoplastia: endoaneurysmoplasty
Endoaneurismorrafia: endoaneurysmorrhaphy
Endoangiíte: endoangiitis
Endoaortite: endo-aortitis
Endoapendicite: endoappendicitis
Endoarterite: endoarteritis
Endoausculta: endoauscultation
Endobásio: endobasion
Endobiótico: endobiotic
Endobrônquico: endobronchial
Endocardíaco: endocardiac, endocardial
Endocárdio: endocardium, **pl.** endocardia
Endocardiografia: endocardiography
Endocardite: encarditis, endocarditis
Endocardítico: endocarditic
Endocelíaco: endoceliac
Endocervical: endocervical
Endocérvice: endocervix
Endocervicite: endocervicitis
Endocíclico: endocyclic
Endocistite: endocystitis
Endocisto: endocyst
Endocitose: endocytosis

Endocoagulação: endocoagulation
Endocolite: endocolitis
Endocondral: endochondral
Endocranial: endocranial
Endocraniano: encranial
Endocrânio: endocranium
Endócrino: endocrine
Endocrinologia: endocrinology
Endocrinologista: endocrinologist
Endocrinoma: endocrinoma
Endocrinopatia: endocrinopathy
Endocrinopático: endocrinopathic
Endocrinoterapia: endocrinotherapy
Endoderma: endoderm
Endodiascopia: endodiascopy
Endodiascópio: endodiascope
Endodióciito: endoyocyte
Endodiogenia: endodyogeny
Endodontia: endodontia, endodontics
Endodontista: endodontist
Endodontologia: endodontology
Endodontologista: endodontologist
Endoenterite: endoenteritis
Endoenzima: endoenzyme
Endoesofagite: endoesophagitis
Endoesqueleto: endoskeleton
Endofaradismo: endofaradism
Endofítico: endophytic
Endófito: endophyte
Endoflebite: endophlebitis
Endoftalmite: endophthalmitis
Endoftalmodonese: endophthalmodonesis
Endogalvanismo: endogalvanism
Endogamia: endogamy, inbreeding
Endógamo: inbred
Endogástrico: endogastric
Endogastrite: endogastritis
Endógeno: endogenic, endogenous
Endogenota: endogenote
Endoglina: endoglin
Endognátio: endognathion
Endo-herniotomia: endoherniotomy
Endointoxicação: endointoxication
Endolaríngeo: endolaryngeal
Endolinfa: endolymph, endolympha
Endolínfico: endolymphic
Endólito: endolith
Endomerogonia: endomerogony
Endometrial: endometrial
Endométrio: endometrium, **pl.** endometria
Endometrióide: endometrioid
Endometrioma: endometrioma
Endometriose: endometriosis
Endometrite: endometritis
Endometrópico: endometropic
Endomiocárdico: endomyocardial

Endomiocardite: endomyocarditis
Endomiometrite: endomyometritis
Endomísio: endomysium
Endomitose: endomitosis
Endomórfico: endomorphic
Endomorfo: endomorph
Endomotorsonda: endomotorsonde
Endoneuro: endoneurium
Endonuclease: endonuclease
Endonuclease nuclear monofilamentar: endonuclease S_1 *Aspergillus*
Endonuclease *Serratia marcescens*: endonuclease *Serratia marcescens*
Endonucléolo: endonucleolus
Endoparasita: endoparasite
Endopeptidase: endopeptidase
Endoperiarterite: endoperiarteritis
Endopericardíaco: endopericardiac
Endoperimiocardite: endoperimyocarditis
Endoperitonite: endoperitonitis
Endoperóxido: endoperoxide
Endoplásico: endoplastic
Endoplasma: endoplasm
Endoplásmico: endoplasmic
Endoplasto: endoplast
Endopoligenia: endopolygeny
Endopoliplóide: endopolyploid
Endopoliploidia: endopolyploidy
Endorfinas: endorphins
Endorfinérgico: endorphinergic
Endorraque: endorrhachis
Endorreduplicação: endoreduplication
Endoscopia: endoscopy
Endoscópio: endoscope
Endoscopista: endoscopist
Endosperma: endosperm
Endósporo: endospore
Endossaco: endobag, endosac
Endossalpinge: endosalpinx
Endossalpingiose: endosalpingiosis
Endossalpingite: endosalpingitis
Endossarco: endosarc
Endossoma: endosome
Endossonografia: endosonography
Endossonoscopia: endosonoscopy
Endosteal: endosteal
Endosteíte: endosteitis, endostitis
Endósteo: endosteum
Endosteoma: endosteoma
Endostetoscópio: endostethoscope
Endostoma: endostoma
Endotelial: endothelial
Endotelina: endothelin
Endotélio: endothelium, **pl.** endothelia
Endotelióciito: endotheliocyte

Endotelióide: endothelioid
Endotelioma: endothelioma
Endoteliose: endotheliosis
Endotendíneo: endotendineum
Endotérmico: endothermic
Endotoxemia: endotoxemia
Endotóxico: endotoxic
Endotoxicose: endotoxicosis
Endotoxina: endotoxin
Endotraqueal: endotracheal
Endotrix: endothrix
Endourologia: endourology
Endovacinação: endovaccination
Endovasculite: endovasculitis
Endovenoso: endovenous
Enediol: enediol
Enema: enema
Enemador: enemator
Enemíase: enemiasis
Energética: energetics
Energia: energy
Enfermaria: ward
Enfermeira-obstetriz: certified nurse-midwife (C.N.M.)
Enfermidade: infirmity
Enfermo: infirm
Enfisema: emphysema
Enfisematoso: emphysematous
Enflurano: enflurane
Enfraxia: emphraxis
Engástrio: engastrius
Engenharia: engineering
Englobamento: englobement
Englobar: englobe
Engrafia: engraphia
Engrama: engram
Enguia: eel
Enjôo do mar: seasickness
Enoftalmia: enophthalmia, enophthalmos
Enoil: enoyl
Enoil hidrase: enoyl hydrase
Enoil-ACP redutase: enoyl-ACP reductase
Enoil-ACP redutase (NADPH): enoyl-ACP reductase (NADPH)
Enoil-CoA hidratase: enoyl-CoA hydratase
Enoil-CoA redutase: enoyl-CoA reductase
2-enoil-CoA redutase: 2-enoyl-CoA reductase
Enol: enol
Enol **piruvato:** *enol* pyruvate
Enolase: enolase
Enolização: enolization
Enorgânico: enorganic
Enostose: enostosis
Enrubescimento: erubescence
Ensaio de Bernoulli: Bernoulli trial
Ensiforme: ensiform
Ensisterno: ensisternum
Entactina: entactin
Entalhador: carver
Entalpia: enthalpy (H)
Entamebíase: entamebiasis
Enteral: enteral

Glossário

Enteralgia: enteralgia
Enteramina: enteramine
Enterectasia: enterectasis
Enterectomia: enterectomy
Enterelcose: enterelcosis
Entérico: enteric
Enterite: enteritis
Enteroanastomose: enteroanastomosis
Enteroantelona: enteroanthelone
Enterobactéria: enterobacterium, **pl.** enterobacteria
Enterobíase: enterobiasis
Enterocele: enterocele
Enterocentese: enterocentesis
Enterocida: enterocidal
Enterocinase: enterokinase
Enterocinese: enterokinesis
Enterocinético: enterokinetic
Enterocisto: enterocyst
Enterocistocele: enterocystocele
Enterocistoma: enterocystoma
Enterocleise: enterocleisis
Enteróclise: enteroclysis
Enterococcemia: enterococcemia
Enterococo: enterococcus, **pl.** enterococci
Enterocolecistostomia: enterocholecystostomy
Enterocolecistotomia: enterocholecystotomy
Enterocolite: enterocolitis
Enterocolostomia: enterocolostomy
Enterodinia: enterdynia, enterodynia
Enteroenterostomia: enteroenterostomy
Enteroepatite: enterohepatitis
Enteroepatocele: enterohepatocele
Enterogastrite: enterogastritis
Enterogastrona: enterogastrone
Enterógeno: enterogenous
Enterografia: enterography
Enterógrafo: enterograph
Enteróide: enteroidea
Enterólise: enterolysis
Enterolitíase: enterolithiasis
Enterólito: enterolith
Enterologia: enterology
Enteromegalia: enteromegaly, enteromegalia, megaloenteron
Enteromenia: enteromenia
Enteromerocele: enteromerocele
Enterômetro: enterometer
Enteromicose: enteromycosis
Enteroparesia: enteroparesis
Enteropatia: enteropathy
Enteropatogênico: enteropathogenic
Enteropatógeno: enteropathogen
Enteropeptidase: enteropeptidase
Enteropexia: enteropexy
Enteroplegia: enteroplegia

Enteroproctia: enteroproctia
Enteroptose: enteroptosis, enteroptosia
Enteroptótico: enteroptotic
Enterorrafia: enterorrhaphy
Enterorragia: enterorrhagia
Enterorrenal: enterorenal
Enterorrexe: enterorrhexis
Enteroscópio: enteroscope
Enterospasmo: enterospasm
Enterossépsis: enterosepsis
Enterostase: enterostasis
Enterostenose: enterostenosis
Enterostomia: enterostomy
Enterotomia: enterotomy
Enterótomo: enterotome
Enterotoxicação: enterotoxication
Enterotoxigênico: enterotoxigenic
Enterotoxina: enterotoxin
Enterotoxismo: enterotoxism
Enterotrópico: enterotropic
Enterozoário: enterozoon
Enterozóico: enterozoic
Entesite: enthesitis
Entesopatia: enthesopathy
Entesopático: enthesopathic
Entidade: entity
Entipia: entypy
Entlasia: enthlasis
Entoblasto: entoblast
Entocele: entocele
Entocone: entocone
Entoconídio: entoconid
Entocórnea: entocornea
Entocoróide: entochoroidea
Entocranial: entocranial
Entocrânio: entocranium
Entoderma: entoderm
Entômio: entomion
Entomofobia: entomophobia
Entomoftoramicose: entomophthoramycosis
Entomologia: entomology
Entópico: entopic
Entoplasma: entoplasm
Entóptico: entoptic
Entorpecente: dope
Entorpecimento: numbness, torpidity
Entorretina: entoretina
Entorse: sprain
Entossarco: entosarc
Entozoário: entozoal, entozoon, **pl.** entozoa
Entrada: inlet
Entranhas: entrails
Entrelaçamento do RNA: RNA splicing
Entrevista: interview
Entropia: entropy
Entrópio: entropion, entropium
Entropionizar: entropionize
Enucleação: enucleation
Enuclear: enucleate
Enurese: bed-wetting, enuresis
Envelhecimento: aging, ripening
Envenenamento: envenomation, poisoning
Envolver: infold

Enxadrezado: tessellated
Enxaguar: perifuse
Enxaqueca: migraine
Enxertar: grafting
Enxerto: graft
Enxofre: brimstone, sulfur (S)
Enxofre-35 (S^{35}): sulfur-35 (^{35}S)
Enzigótico: enzygotic
Enzima: enzyme
Enzima ramificadora da 1,4-α-D-glicana: 1,4-α-D-glucan-branching enzyme
Enzimático: enzymatic, enzymic
Enzimólise: enzymolysis
Enzimologia: enzymology
Enzimologista: enzymologist
Enzimopatia: enzymopathy
Enzoótico: enzootic
Eosina: eosin
Eosinócito: eosinocyte
Eosinofilia: eosinophilia
Eosinofílico: eosinophilic
Eosinófilo: eosinophil, eosinophile
Eosinofilúria: eosinophiluria
Eosinopenia: eosinopenia
Eosinotático: eosinotactic
Eosinotaxia: eosinotaxis
Eosofobia: eosophobia
Epacmástico: epimastical
Epactal: epactal
Epamniótico: epamniotic
Eparterial: eparterial
Epaxial: epaxial
Epêndima: endyma, ependyma
Ependimário: ependymal
Ependimite: ependymitis
Ependimoblasto: ependymoblast
Ependimoblastoma: ependymoblastoma
Ependimócito: ependymocyte
Ependimoma: ependymoma
Epiandrosterona: epiandrosterone
Epibatidina: epibatidine
Epiblástico: epiblastic
Epiblasto: epiblast
Epibléfaro: epiblepharon
Epibolia: epiboly, epibole
Epibulbar: epibulbar
Epicanto: epicanthus
Epicárdia: epicardia
Epicárdico: epicardial
Epicárdio: epicardium
Epiceratofaquia: epikeratophakia
Epiceratoprótese: epikeratoprosthesis
Epicilina: epicillin
Epicistite: epicystitis
Epícito: epicyte
Epícomo: epicomus
Epicondilalgia: epicondylalgia
Epicondiliano: epicondylian
Epicondílico: epicondylic
Epicondilite: epicondylitis
Epicôndilo: epicondyle, epicondylus, **pl.** epicondyli
epi-**coprostanol:** *epi*-coprostanol
epi-**coprosterol:** *epi*-coprosterol

Epicoracóide: epicoracoid
Epicórdico: epichordal
Epicrânico: epicranial, epicranius
Epicrânio: epicranium
Epicrise: epicrisis
Epicrítico: epicritic
Epidemia: epidemic
Epidemicidade: epidemicity
Epidemiografia: epidemiography
Epidemiologia: epidemiology
Epidemiologista: epidemiologist
Epidermalização: epidermalization
Epiderme: epiderm, epiderma, epidermis, **pl.** epidermides
Epidérmico: epidermal, epidermatic, epidermic
Epidermidose: epidermidosis
Epidermite: epidermitis
Epidermodisplasia: epidermodysplasia
Epidermóide: epidermoid
Epidermólise: epidermolysis
Epidermose: epidermosis
Epidermotropismo: epidermotropism
Epidiascópio: epidiascope
Epididimal: epididymal
Epididimectomia: epididymectomy
Epididimite: epididymitis, **pl.** epididymiditides
Epidídimo: epididymis, **gen.** epididymidis, **pl.** epididymides
Epididimoplastia: epididymoplasty
Epididimorquite: epididymo-orchitis
Epididimotomia: epididymotomy
Epididimovasectomia: epididymovasectomy
Epididimovasostomia: epididymovasostomy
Epidural: epidural
Epidurografia: epidurography
Epiespinal: epispinal
Epiestriol: epiestriol
Epifaringe: epipharynx
Epifascial: epifascial
Epifenômeno: epiphenomenom
Epifisário: epiphysial, epiphyseal
Epífise: epiphysis, **pl.** epiphyses
Epifisiodese: epiphysiodesis
Epifisiólise: epiphysiolysis
Epifisiopatia: epiphysiopathy
Epifisite: epiphysitis
Epífora: epiphora, tearing
Epifrênico: epiphrenic, epiphrenal
Epigastralgia: epigastralgia
Epigástrico: epigastric
Epigástrio: epigastrium
Epigástrios: epigastrius
Epigênese: epigenesis
Epigenético: epigenetic
Epiglote: epiglottis

Epiglótico: epiglottic, epiglottidean
Epiglotidectomia: epiglottidectomy
Epiglotidite: epiglottiditis
Epiglotite: epiglottitis
Epignatos: epignathus
Epiial: epihyal
Epiióide: epihyoid
Epilação: epilation
Epilamelar: epilamellar
Epilar: epilate
Epilatório: epilatory
Epilema: epilemma
Epilepidoma: epilepidoma
Epilepsia: epilepsia, epilepsy
Epiléptico: epileptic
Epileptiforme: epileptiform
Epileptogênico: epileptogenic, epileptogenous
Epileptóide: epileptoid
Epilóia: epiloia
Epimandibular: epimandibular
Epimastigota: epimastigote
Epimenorragia: epimenorrhagia
Epimenorréia: epimenorrhea
Epimerase: epimerase
Epimerito: epimerite
Epímero: epimer, epimere
Epimicroscópio: epimicroscope
Epimísio: epimysium
Epimisiotomia: epimysiotomy
Epimorfose: epimorphosis
Epinefrina: epinephrine
Epinefro: epinephros
Epineural: epineural, epineurial
Epineuro: epineurium
Epioníquio: epionychium
Epiótico: epiotic
Epipástico: epipastic
Epipericárdico: epipericardial
Epipial: epipial
Epípigo: epipygus
Epiplocele: epiplocele
Epiplóico: epiploic
Epíploo: epiploon
Epipodofilotoxina: epipodophyllotoxin
Epiptérico: epipteric
D-epirranose: D-epirhamnose
Episclera: episclera
Episcleral: episcleral
Episclerite: episcleritis
Episioestenose: episiostenosis
Episioperineorrafia: episioperineorrhaphy
Episioplastia: episioplasty
Episiorrafia: episiorrhaphy
Episiotomia: episiotomy
Episódio: episode
Epispádia: epispadias
Episplenite: episplenitis
Epissoma: episome
Epístase: epistasis
Epistase: epistasy
Epistático: epistatic
Epistaxe: epistaxis
Epistemofilia: epistemophilia
Epistemologia: epistemology
Episternal: episternal
Episterno: episternum
Epistrofeu: epistropheus
Epitálamo: epithalamus
Epitalaxia: epithalaxia
Epitarso: epitarsus
Epitaxia: epitaxy
Epitelial: epithelial
Epitélio: epithelium, **pl.** epithelia
Epiteliócito: epitheliocyte
Epiteliofibrila: epitheliofibril
Epitelioglandular: epithelioglandular
Epitelióide: epithelioid
Epiteliolítico: epitheliolytic
Epitelioma: epithelioma
Epiteliomatoso: epitheliomatous
Epiteliopatia: epitheliopathy
Epiteliose: epitheliosis
Epiteliotrópico: epitheliotropic
Epitelização: epithelialization, epithelization
Epitema: epithem
Epitendão: epitenon
Epitendíneo: epitendineum
17-epitestosterona: 17-epitestosterone
Epíteto: epithet
Epitiazida: epithiazide
Epitiflite: epityphlitis
Epitimpânico: epitympanic
Epitímpano: epitympanum
Epítopo: epitope
Epitoxóide: epitoxoid
Epitriquial: epitrichial
Epitríquio: epitrichium
Epitróclea: epitrochlea
Epitroclear: epitrochlear
Epituberculose: epituberculosis
Epizoário: epizoon, **pl.** epizoa
Epizóico: epizoic
Epizoologia: epizoology
Epizoótico: epizootic
Epizootiologia: epizootiology
Epoetina alfa: epoetin alfa
Eponímico: eponymic
Epônimo: eponym
Eponíquia: eponychia
Eponíquio: eponychium
Epoóforo: epoophoron
Epoprostenol, epoprostenol sódico: epoprostenol, epoprostenol sodium
Epornítico: epornitic
Epóxi: epoxy
2,3-epoxiesqualeno: 2,3-epoxysqualene
Épsilon: epsilon
Epúlide: epulis
Epulóide: epuloid
Equação: equation
Equador: equator
Equatorial: equatorial
Equiaxial: equiaxial
Equicalórico: equicaloric
Equilenina: equilenin
Equilibração: equilibration
Equilíbrio: balance, equilibrium
Equilina: equilin
Equimolar: equimolar
Equimolecular: equimolecular
Equimoma: ecchymoma
Equimose: ecchymosis
Equimótico: ecchymotic
Equinado: echinate, echinulate
Eqüino: equine
Equinócito: echinocyte
Equinococose: echinococciasis, echinococcosis
Equinose: echinosis
Equinostomíase: echinostomiasis
Eqüinovalgo: equinovalgus
Eqüinovaro: equinovarus
Equipe: staff
Equitóxico: equitoxic
Equivalência: equivalence, equivalency
Equivalente: equivalent (Eq, eq)
Equorina: aequorin
Érbio: erbium (Er)
Ercalcidiol: ercalcidiol
Ercalciol: ercalciol
Ercalcitriol: ercalcitriol
Ereção: erection
Eremofobia: eremophobia
Erétil: erectile
Eretor: arrector, **pl.** arrectores; erector
Ereutofobia: ereuthophobia
Ergasia: ergasia
Ergasiofobia: ergasiophobia
Ergastenia: ergasthenia
Ergastoplasma: ergastoplasm
Ergina: ergine
Ergobasina: ergobasine
Ergocalciferol: ergocalciferol
Ergocornina: ergocornine
Ergocriptina: ergocryptine
Ergocristina: ergocristine
Ergodinamógrafo: ergodynamograph
Ergoestesiógrafo: ergoesthesiograph
Ergogênico: ergogenic
Ergográfico: ergographic
Ergógrafo: ergograph
Ergolinas: ergolines
Ergometrina: ergometrine
Ergômetro: ergometer
Ergonomia: ergonomics
Ergonovina: ergonovine
Ergosina: ergosine
Ergosterina: ergosterin
Ergosterol: ergosterol
Ergostetrina: ergostetrine
Ergotamina: ergotamine
Ergotaminina: ergotaminine
Ergotioneína: ergothioneine
Ergotismo: ergotism
Ergotoxina: ergotoxine
Ergotrópico: ergotropic
Erisipela: erysipelas
Erisipelóide: erysipeloid
Erisipelotoxina: erysipelotoxin
Erisofaco: erisophake
Eritema: erythema
Eritematoso: erythematous
Eritermalgia: erythermalgia
Eritralgia: erythralgia
Eritrasma: erythrasma
Eritredema: erythredema
Eritremia: erythremia
Eritrita: erythrite
Eritritol: erythritol
Eritroblastemia: erythroblastemia
Eritroblasto: erythroblast
Eritroblastopenia: erythroblastopenia
Eritroblastose: erythroblastosis
Eritroblastótico: erythroblastotic
Eritrocatálise: erythrocatalysis
Eritroceratodermia: erythrokeratodermia
Eritrocianose: erythrocyanosis
Eritrocinética: erythrokinetics
Eritrocitemia: erythrocythemia
Eritrocítico: erythrocytic
Eritrócito: erythrocyte
Eritrocitoblasto: erythrocytoblast
Eritrocitólise: erythrocytolysis
Eritrocitolisina: erythrocytolysin
Eritrocitômetro: erythrocytometer
Eritrocitopenia: erythrocytopenia
Eritrocitopoese: erythrocytopoiesis
Eritrocitorrexia: erythrocytorrhexis
Eritrocitose: erythrocytosis
Eritrocitosquise: erythrocytoschisis
Eritrocitúria: erythrocyturia
Eritroclasia: erythroclasis
Eritroclástico: erythroclastic
Eritrocromia: erythrochromia
Eritrocupreína: erythrocuprein
Eritrodegenerativo: erythrodegenerative
Eritrodermatite: erythrodermatitis
Eritrodermia: erythroderma
Eritrodextrina: erythrodextrin
Eritrodontia: erythrodontia
Eritrofagia: erythrophagia
Eritrofagocitose: erythrophagocytosis
Eritrofílico: erythrophilic
Eritrófilo: erythrophil
Eritróforo: erythrophore
Eritrogênese imperfeita: erythrogenesis imperfecta
Eritrogênico: erythrogenic
Eritrogônia: erythrogonium, **pl.** erythrogonia
Eritróide: erythroid
Eritroidina: erythroidin
Eritrol: erythrol
Eritroleucemia: erythroleukemia
Eritroleucose: erythroleukosis
Eritrólise: erythrolysis
Eritrolisina: erythrolysin
Eritromelalgia: erythromelalgia
Eritromelia: erythromelia
Eritromicina: erythromycin
Éritron: erythron

Glossário

Eritroneocitose: erythroneocytosis
Eritropenia: erythropenia
Eritropicnose: erythropyknosis
Eritroplaquia: erythroplakia
Eritroplasia: erythroplasia
Eritropoese: erythropoiesis
Eritropoético: erythropoietic
Eritropoetina: erythropoietin
Eritroprosopalgia: erythroprosopalgia
Eritropsia: erythropsia
Eritrorrexia: erythrorrhexis
Eritrose: erythrose
Eritrosina B: erythrosin B
Eritroxilina: erythroxyline
Eritrulose: erythrulose
Eritrúria: erythruria
Erliquiose: ehrlichiosis
Erodir: erode
Erógeno: erogenous
Eros: eros
Erosão: erosion
Erosivo: erosive
Erótico: erotic
Erotismo: erotism, eroticism
Erotização: erotization
Erotofobia: erotophobia
Erotogênese: erotogenesis
Erotogênico: erotogenic
Erotomania: erotomania
Erotopatia: erotopathy
Erotopático: erotopathic
Erradicação: eradication
Errante: wandering
Errático: erratic
Erro: error
Ertacalciol: ertacalciol
Eructação: belching, eructation
Erupção: eruption, rash
Erupção cutânea: blotch
Eruptivo: eruptive
Erva-de-santa-maria: wormseed
Erva-mate: maté
Erva-santa: eriodictyon, yerba santa
Escabicida: scabicidal, scabicide
Escabiose: scabies
Escabrícia: scabrities
Escafa: scapha
Escafocefalia: scaphocephaly, tectocephaly
Escafocefálico: scaphocephalic, tectocephalic
Escafocefalismo: scaphocephalism
Escafocéfalo: scaphocephalous
Escafóide: scaphoid
Escafoidrocefalia: scaphohydrocephalus, scaphohydrocephaly
Escala: scala, **pl.** scalae; scale
Escala cinza: latitude
Escala de coma de Maryland: Maryland coma scale
Escala de coma de Glasgow: Glasgow coma scale
Escala de percepção do esforço: rating of perceived exertion
Escaldar: scald
Escalenectomia: scalenectomy
Escaleno: scalene, scalenus
Escalenotomia: scalenotomy
Escalpelo: scalpel
Escalpo: scalp
Escalpriforme: scalpriform
Escalpro: scalprum
Escama: furfur, **pl.** furfures; squama, **pl.** squamae; squame
Escamatização: squamatization
Escamoccipital: squamo-occipital
Escamocelular: squamocellular
Escamocolunar: squamocolumnar
Escamoesfenóide: sphenosquamosal, squamosphenoid
Escamofrontal: squamofrontal
Escamomastóide: squamomastoid
Escamônia: scammony
Escamoparietal: squamoparietal
Escamopetroso: squamopetrosal
Escamoso: scaly, squamosal, squamous
Escamotemporal: squamotemporal
Escamotimpânico: squamotympanic
Escamozigomático: squamozygomatic
Escândio: scandium (Sc)
Escaneador: scanner
Escanometria: scanogram
Escape: escape
Escapo: scapus, **pl.** scapi
Escápula: scapula, **gen. e pl.** scapulae; shoulder blade
Escapulalgia: scapulalgia
Escapular: scapular
Escapulário: scapulary
Escapulectomia: scapulectomy
Escapulodinia: scapulodynia
Escapulopexia: scapulopexy
Escapuloumeral: scapulohumeral
Escara: eschar
Escarectomia: escharectomy
Escarificação: scarification
Escarificar: scarify
Escarlate: scarlet
Escarlatina: scarlatina
Escarlatinela: scarlatinella
Escarlatiniforme: scarlatiniform
Escarlatinóide: scarlatinoid
Escarlatinoso: scarlatinal
Escarótico: escharotic
Escarotomia: escharotomy
Escatemia: scatemia
Escatofagia: scatophagy
Escatol: skatole
Escatologia: scatology
Escatológico: scatologic
Escatoma: scatoma
Escatoscopia: scatoscopy
Escatoxil: skatoxyl
Escátula: scatula
Escavação: burrow, cupping, drill-out, excavatio, excavation
Escavado: cupped
Escavador: excavator
Escelalgia: scelalgia
Esclera: sclera, **pl.** scleras, sclerae; sclerotica
Escleradenite: scleradenitis
Escleral: scleral
Escleratógeno: scleratogenous
Esclerectasia: sclerectasia
Esclerectomia: sclerectomy
Escleredema: scleredema
Esclerema: sclerema
Esclerencefalia: sclerencephaly, sclerencephalia
Esclerite: scleritis
Escleroatrofia: scleroatrophy
Escleroblastema: scleroblastema
Escleroceratite: sclerokeratitis
Escleroceratoirite: sclerokeratoiritis
Esclerócio: sclerotium, **pl.** sclerotia
Escleroconjuntival: scleroconjunctival
Esclerocorióide: sclerochoroidal
Esclerocorioidite: sclerochoroiditis
Esclerocórnea: sclerocornea
Esclerodactilia: sclerodactyly, sclerodactylia
Esclerodermatoso: sclerodermatous
Esclerodermia: scleroderma
Escleroftalmia: sclerophthalmia
Esclerógeno, esclerogênico: sclerogenous, sclerogenic
Escleróide: scleroid
Escleroirite: scleroiritis
Escleroma: scleroma
Escleromalacia: scleromalacia
Esclerômero: scleromere
Esclerômetro: sclerometer
Escleromixedema: scleromyxedema
Escleroniquia: scleronychia
Esclero-ooforite: sclero-oophoritis
Escleroplastia: scleroplasty
Escleroproteína: scleroprotein
Esclerosante: sclerosant
Esclerosar: sclerose
Esclerose: sclerosis, **pl.** scleroses
Escleroso: sclerosal, sclerous
Esclerostenose: sclerostenosis
Esclerostomia: sclerostomy
Escleroterapia: sclerotherapy
Esclerótico: sclerotic
Esclerotilose: sclerotylosis
Esclerotomia: sclerotomy
Esclerótomo: sclerotome
Esclerotriquia: sclerothrix, sclerotrichia
Escola: school
Escolecíase: scoleciasis
Escoleciforme: scoleciform
Escolecóide: scolecoid
Escolecologia: scolecology
Escólex, escólece: scolex, **pl.** scoleces, scolices
Escoliocifose: scoliokyphosis
Escoliômetro: scoliometer
Escoliose: scoliosis
Escoliótico: scoliotic
Escoliótono: scoliotone
Escopina: scopine
Escopofilia: scopophilia
Escopofobia: scopophobia
Escopolamina: scopolamine
Escopólia: scopolia
Escopolina: scopoline
Escopômetro: scopometer
Escorbútico: scorbutic
Escorbutigênico: scorbutigenic
Escorbuto: scorbutus, scurvy
Escorcina, escorcinol: escorcin, escorcinol
Escordinema: scordinema
Escore: score
Escoriação: excoriation
Escoriar: excoriate
Escorpião: scorpion
Escotocromógenos: scotochromogens
Escotofilia: scotophilia
Escotofobia: scotophobia
Escotógrafo: scotograph
Escotoma: scotoma, **pl.** scotomata
Escotomatoso: scotomatous
Escotometria: scotometry
Escotômetro: scotometer
Escotopia: scotopia
Escotópico: scotopic
Escotopsina: scotopsin
Escotoscopia: scotoscopy
Escova: brush
Escovilhão: écouvillon
Escrita em espelho: mirror-writing
Escrobiculado: scrobiculate
Escrófula: scrofula
Escrofulodermia: scrofuloderma
Escrofuloso: scrofulous
Escrópulo: scruple
Escrotal: oscheal, scrotal
Escrotectomia: scrotectomy
Escrotiforme: scrotiform
Escrotite: scrotitis
Escroto: scrotum, **pl.** scrota, scrotums
Escrotoplastia: scrotoplasty
Escudo: shield
Esculapiano: aesculapian, esculapian
Esculento: esculent
Esculina: esculin
Escuma: scum
Escutiforme: scutate, scutiform
Escútulo: scutulum, **pl.** scutula
Eseridina: eseridine
Eserina: eserine
Esfacelado: sphacelous
Esfacelamento: sphacelation
Esfacelar: sphacelate
Esfacelismo: sphacelism
Esfácelo: sphacelus
Esfênio: sphenion
Esfenobasilar: sphenobasilar, sphenoccipital, sphenooccipital
Esfenocefalia: sphenocephaly

Esfenoetmóide: sphenethmoid, sphenoethmoid
Esfenoetmoidectomia: sphenoethmoidectomy
Esfenofrontal: sphenofrontal
Esfenoidal: sphenoid, sphenoidal
Esfenoidite: sphenoiditis
Esfenoidostomia: sphenoidostomy
Esfenoidotomia: sphenoidotomy
Esfenomaxilar: sphenomaxillary
Esfenopalatino: sphenopalatine
Esfenoparietal: sphenoparietal
Esfenopetroso: sphenopetrosal
Esfenorbital: sphenorbital
Esfenossalpingostafilino: sphenosalpingostaphylinus
Esfenotemporal: sphenotemporal
Esfenótico: sphenotic
Esfenoturbinal: sphenoturbinal
Esfenovomerino: sphenovomerine
Esfenozigomático: sphenomalar, sphenozygomatic
Esfera: sphere
Esférico: spherical (sph.)
Esferócito: spherocyte
Esferocitose: spherocytosis
Esferofaquia: spherophakia
Esferóide: spheroid, spheroidal
Esferômetro: spherometer
Esferoplasto: spheroplast
Esferoprisma: spheroprism
Esferospermia: spherospermia
Esférula: spherule
Esfígmico: sphygmic
Esfigmocardiógrafo: sphygmocardiograph
Esfigmocardioscópio: sphygmocardioscope
Esfigmocronógrafo: sphygmochronograph
Esfigmofone: sphygmophone
Esfigmografia: sphygmography
Esfigmográfico: sphygmographic
Esfigmógrafo: sphygmograph
Esfigmograma: sphygmogram
Esfigmóide: sphygmoid
Esfigmomanometria: sphygmomanometry
Esfigmomanômetro: sphygmomanometer
Esfigmômetro: sphygmometer
Esfigmometroscópio: sphygmometroscope
Esfigmooscilômetro: sphygmo-oscillometer
Esfigmopalpação: sphygmopalpation
Esfigmoscopia: sphygmoscopy
Esfigmoscópio: sphygmoscope
Esfigmossístole: sphygmosystole
Esfigmotonógrafo: sphygmotonograph
Esfigmotonômetro: sphygmotonometer
Esfigmoviscosimetria: sphygmoviscosimetry
Esfíncter: sphincter
Esfincteralgia: sphincteralgia
Esfincterectomia: sphincterectomy
Esfincteriano: sphincteral, sphincterial, sphincteric
Esfincterismo: sphincterismus
Esfincterite: sphincteritis
Esfincteróide: sphincteroid
Esfincterólise: sphincterolysis
Esfincteroplastia: sphincteroplasty
Esfincteroscopia: sphincteroscopy
Esfincteroscópio: sphincteroscope
Esfincterotomia: sphincterotomy
Esfincterótomo: sphincterotome
Esfinganina: sphinganine
(4E)-esfingenina: (4E)-sphingenine
Esfingol: sphingol
Esfingolipídio: sphingolipid
Esfingolipidose: sphingolipidosis
Esfingolipodistrofia: sphingolipodystrophy
Esfingomielina fosfodiesterase: sphingomyelin phosphodiesterase
Esfingomielinas: sphingomyelins
Esfingomielinase: sphingomyelinase
Esfingosina: sphingosine
Esfoladura: chafe
Esfoliação: exfoliation
Esfoliativo: exfoliative
Esforço: conatus, effort
Esfregaço: smear
Esfregaço citológico: cytosmear
Esgotamento nervoso: nervous breakdown
Esilato: esylate
Esmagar: crush
Esmalte: enamel, enamelum
Esmegma: smegma
Esmegmólito: smegmalith
Esmeril: emery
Esodesvio: esodeviation
Esofagalgia: esophagalgia
Esofagectomia: esophagectomy
Esofágico: esophageal
Esofagismo: esophagism
Esofagite: esophagitis
Esôfago: esophagus, **pl.** esophagi
Esofagocardioplastia: esophagocardioplasty
Esofagocele: esophagocele
Esofagodinia: esophagodynia
Esofagoenterostomia: esophagoenterostomy
Esofagoespasmo: esophagospasm
Esofagoestenose: esophagostenosis
Esofagogastrectomia: esophagogastrectomy
Esofagogastroanastomose: esophagogastroanastomosis
Esofagogastroduodenoscopia: esophagogastroduodenoscopy (EGD)
Esofagogastromiotomia: esophagogastromyotomy
Esofagogastroplastia: esophagogastroplasty
Esofagogastrostomia: esophagogastrostomy
Esofagografia: esophagography
Esofagograma: esophagogram, esophagram
Esofagologia: esophagology
Esofagomalacia: esophagomalacia
Esofagomiotomia: esophagomyotomy
Esofagoplastia: esophagoplasty
Esofagoplicatura: esophagoplication
Esofagoptose: esophagoptosis, esophagoptosia
Esofagoscopia: esophagoscopy
Esofagoscópio: esophagoscope
Esofagostomia: esophagostomy
Esofagostomíase: esophagostomiasis, oesophagostomiasis
Esofagotomia: esophagotomy
Esoforia: esophoria
Esofórico: esophoric
Esotropia: esotropia
Esotrópico: esotropic
Espaçamento: spacing
Espacial: spatial
Espaço: space, spatium, **pl.** spatia
Espaço aéreo: airspace
Espagírico: spagyric
Espagirista: spagyrist
Espalhador: spreader
Espargano: sparganum
Esparganoma: sparganoma
Esparganose: sparganosis
Esparteína: sparteine
Espasmo: spasm, spasmus
Espasmo muscular: myopalmus
Espasmódico: spasmodic
Espasmofílico: spasmophilic
Espasmogênico: spasmogenic
Espasmógeno: spasmogen
Espasmólise: spasmolysis
Espasmolítico: spasmolytic
Espasticidade: spasticity
Espástico: spastic
Espátula: spatula
Espatulação: spatulation
Espatulado: spatulate, spatulated
Especiação: speciation
Especialidade: specialty
Especialista: specialist
Especialização: specialization
Especializar: specialize
Espécie: species, **pl.** species
Espécie-específico: species-specific
Especificidade: specificity
Específico: specific
Especilho: specillum, **pl.** specilla
Espectral: spectral
Espectrina: spectrin
Espectro: spectrum, **pl.** spectra, spectrums
Espectro de fortificação: telehopsias
Espectro de vida: lifespan
Espectrocolorímetro: spectrocolorimeter
Espectrofluorômetro: spectrofluorometer
Espectrofobia: spectrophobia
Espectrofotofluorimetria: spectrophotofluorimetry
Espectrofotometria: spectrophotometry
Espectrofotômetro: spectrophotometer
Espectrografia: spectrography
Espectrógrafo: spectrograph
Espectrograma: spectrogram
Espectrometria: spectrometry
Espectrômetro: spectrometer
Espectropolarímetro: spectropolarimeter
Espectroquímica: spectrochemistry
Espectroscopia: spectroscopy
Espectroscópico: spectroscopic
Espectroscópio: spectroscope
Espéculo: speculum, **pl.** specula
Espéculo de Pedersen: Pedersen speculum
Espelencefalia: spelencephaly
Espelho: mirror
Esperado: expected
Espermacete: cetaceum, spermaceti
Espermaglutinação: spermagglutination
Espermaster: sperm-aster
Espermaticida: spermatocidal, spermatocide
Espermático: spermatic
Espermátide: spermatid
Espermatina: spermatin
Espermatoblasto: spermatoblast
Espermatocele: spermatocele
Espermatocisto: spermatocyst
Espermatocitário: spermatocytal
Espermatócito: spermatocyte
Espermatocitogênese: spermatocytogenesis
Espermatofobia: spermatophobia
Espermatóforo: spermatophore
Espermatogênese: spermatogenesis
Espermatogenético: spermatogenetic
Espermatogenia: spermatogeny
Espermatogênico: spermatogenic
Espermatógeno: spermatogenous

Espermatogônia: spermatogone, spermatogonium
Espermatóide: spermatoid
Espermatólise: spermatolysis
Espermatolisina: spermatolysin
Espermatolítico: spermatolytic
Espermatologia: spermatology
Espermatopoético: spermatopoietic
Espermatorréia: spermatorrhea
Espermatoxina: spermatoxin, spermotoxin
Espermatozóico: spermatozoal, spermatozoan
Espermatozóide: sperm, spermatozoon, **pl.** spermatozoa
Espermatúria: semenuria, seminuria, spermaturia
Espermicida: spermicidal, spermicide
Espermidina: spermidine
Espermina: spermine
Espérmio: spermium, **pl.** spermia
Espermiogênese: spermiogenesis
Espermismo: spermism
Espermista: spermist
Espermólise: spermolysis
Espermólito: spermolith
Espessado: brawny
Espessamento: crassamentum
Espessidão: spissitude
Espessura: thickness
Espícula: spicule, spiculum, **pl.** spicula
Espicular: spicular
Espigeliano: spigelian
Espinal: spinal, spinalis
Espinha: spina, **gen. e pl.** spinae; spine, thorn
Espinheiro: buckthorn
Espinho: acantha
Espinhoso: spinate, spinose, spinous
Espinobulbar: spinobulbar
Espinocerebelo: spinocerebellum
Espinocolicular: spinocollicular
Espinocostal: spinocostalis
Espinoglenóide: spinoglenoid
Espinomuscular: spinomuscular
Espinoneural: spinoneural
Espinotectal: spinotectal
Espinotransverso: spinotransversarius
Espintariscópio: spintharicon, spinthariscope
Espiperona: spiperone
Espiráculo: spiracle
Espiradenoma: spiradenoma
Espiral: spiral
Espiramicina: spiramycin
Espirema: skein, spirem, spireme
Espirilar: spirillar
Espirilicida: spirillicidal
Espirilo: spirillum, **pl.** spirilla
Espirilose: spirillosis
Espírito de terebintina: turpentine spirit

Espirógrafo: spirograph
Espirograma: spirogram
Espirometria: spirometry
Espirômetro: spirometer
Espironolactona: spironolactone
Espiroqueta: spirochete
Espiroquetemia: spirochetemia
Espiroqueticida: spirocheticide
Espiroquético: spirochetal
Espiroquetólise: spirochetolysis
Espiroquetose: spirochetosis
Espiroquetótico: spirochetotic
Espiroscópio: spiroscope
Espirostano: spirostan
Espirrar: sneeze
Espirro: ptarmus
Espiruróide: spiruroid
Esplanalgia: splenalgia
Esplancnapofisário: splanchnapophysial, splanchnapophyseal
Esplancnapófise: splanchnapophysis
Esplancnectopia: splanchnectopia
Esplancnestesia: splanchnesthesia
Esplancnicectomia: splanchnicectomy
Esplâncnico: splanchnic
Esplancnicotomia: splanchnicotomy
Esplancnocele: splanchnocele
Esplancnocrânio: splanchnocranium
Esplancnoesquelético: splanchnoskeletal
Esplancnoesqueleto: splanchnoskeleton
Esplancnografia: splanchnography
Esplancnólito: splanchnolith
Esplancnologia: splanchnologia, splanchnology
Esplancnomegalia: splanchnomegaly
Esplancnomicria: splanchnomicria
Esplancnopatia: splanchnopathy
Esplancnopleura: splanchnopleure
Esplancnopleural: splanchnopleural, splanchnopleuric
Esplancnoptose: splanchnoptosis, splanchnoptosia
Esplancnosclerose: splanchnosclerosis
Esplancnossomático: splanchnosomatic
Esplancnotomia: splanchnotomy
Esplancnótribo: splanchnotribe
Esplenectomia: splenectomy
Esplenectopia: splenectopia, splenectopy
Esplenelcose: splenelcosis
Espleneólo: spleneolus
Esplenial: splenial

Esplênico: lienal, splenetic, splenic
Esplenículo: spleniculus
Espleniforme: spleniform
Esplênio: splenius
Espleniosserrátil: spleniserrate
Esplenite: splenitis
Esplenocele: splenocele
Esplenoclise: splenocleisis
Esplenocólico: splenocolic
Esplenodinia: splenodynia
Esplenofrênico: splenophrenic
Espleno-hepatomegalia, hepatoesplenomegalia: splenohepatomegaly, splenohepatomegalia
Esplenóide: splenoid
Esplenolinfático: splenolymphatic
Esplenoma: splenoma
Esplenomalacia: splenomalacia
Esplenomedular: splenomedullary
Esplenomegalia: megalosplenia, splenomegaly, splenomegalia
Esplenomielógeno: splenomyelogenous
Esplenomielomalacia: splenomyelomalacia
Esplenonéfrico: splenonephric
Esplenopancreático: splenopancreatic
Esplenopatia: splenopathy
Esplenopexia: splenopexy, splenopexia
Esplenoportografia: splenoportography
Esplenoportograma: splenoportogram
Esplenoptose: splenoptosis, splenoptosia
Esplenorrafia: splenorrhaphy
Esplenorragia: splenorrhagia
Esplenorrenal: splenorenal
Esplenose: splenosis
Esplenotomia: splenotomy
Esplenotoxina: splenotoxin
Esplênulo: splenule, splenulus, **pl.** splenuli
Esplenúnculo: splenunculus, **pl.** splenunculi
Espodóforo: spodophorous
Espodógeno: spodogenous
Espodografia: spodography
Espodograma: spodogram
Espondaico: spondaic
Espondeu: spondee
Espondilalgia: spondylalgia
Espondilartrite: spondylarthritis
Espondilite: spondylitis
Espondilítico: spondylitic
Espondilólise: spondylolysis
Espondilolistese: spondylolisthesis
Espondilolistético: spondylolisthetic
Espondilomalacia: spondylomalacia
Espondilopatia: spondylopathy
Espondilopiose: spondylopyosis
Espondiloptose: spondyloptosis

Espondilose: spondylosis
Espondiloso: spondylous
Espondilosquise: spondyloschisis
Espondilossíndese: spondylosyndesis
Espondilotorácico: spondylothoracic
Espongiforme: spongiform
Espongioblasto: spongioblast
Espongioblastoma: spongioblastoma
Espongiócito: spongiocyte
Espongióide: spongioid
Espongiose: spongiosis
Espongiosite: spongiositis
Esponja: sponge, spongia
Esponjoso: cancellated, cancellous, spongiose, spongy
Espontâneo: spontaneous
Esporádico: sporadic
Esporadina: sporadin
Esporângio: sporangium
Esporangióporo: sporangiophore
Esporão: calcar, spur
Esporão de Grunert: Grunert spur
Esporão do centeio: ergot, rye smut
Esporicida: sporicidal, sporicide
Esporídio: sporidium, **pl.** sporidia
Esporinha: larkspur
Esporo: spore
Esporoaglutinação: sporoagglutination
Esporoblasto: sporoblast
Esporocisto: sporocyst
Esporodóquio: sporodochium
Esporóforo: sporophore
Esporogênese: sporogenesis
Esporogenia: sporogeny
Esporógeno: sporogenous
Esporogonia: sporogony
Esporonte: sporont
Esporoplasma: sporoplasm
Esporoteca: sporotheca
Esporotricose: sporotrichosis
Esporozoário: sporozoan, sporozoon
Esporozoíto: sporozoite
Esporulação: sporulation
Esporular: sporular
Espórulo: sporule
Espremer: express
Espru: sprue
Espuma: foam
Espúndia: espundia
Espúrio: spurious
Esputo: sputum, **pl.** sputa
Esqualeno: squalene
Esquecimento: forgetting
Esquelético: skeletal
Esqueleto: skeleton
Esqueletologia: skeletology
Esquema: schedule, schema, **pl.** schemata; scheme
Esquemático: schematic

Esquematógrafo: schematograph
Esquemocromos: schemochromes
Esqueneite, esquenite: skeneitis, skenitis
Esqueneoscópio: skeneoscope
Esquinância: esquinancea
Esquindilese: schindylesis
Esquinência: quinsy
Esquistocelia: schistocelia
Esquistocisto: schistocystis
Esquistócito: schistocyte
Esquistocitose: schistocytosis
Esquistocormia: schistocormia
Esquistoglossia: schistoglossia
Esquistomelia: schistomelia
Esquistorraque: schistorrhachis
Esquistossoma: schistosome
Esquistossomia: schistosomia
Esquistossomose: schistosomiasis
Esquistossômulo: schistosomulum, **pl.** schistosomula
Esquistosternia: schistosternia
Esquistotórax: schistothorax
Esquizâmnio: schizamnion
Esquizaxônio: schizaxon
Esquizencefalia: schizencephaly
Esquizoafetivo: schizo-affective
Esquizócito: schizocyte
Esquizocitose: schizocytosis
Esquizofasia: schizophasia
Esquizofrenia: schizophrenia
Esquizofrênico: schizophrenic
Esquizogênese: schizogenesis
Esquizogiria: schizogyria
Esquizogonia: schizogony
Esquizóide: schizoid
Esquizoidismo: schizoidism
Esquizomicético: schizomycetic
Esquizomiceto: schizomycete
Esquizoniquia: schizonychia
Esquizonte: agamont, schizont
Esquizonticida: schizonticide
Esquizotonia: schizotonia
Esquizotriquia: schizotrichia
Esquizozoíta: schizozoite
Essência: essence
Essencial: essential
Estabilidade: stability
Estabilímetro: stabilimeter
Estabilização: stabilization
Estabilizador: stabilizer
Estação: season
Estação de trabalho: workstation
Estadiamento: staging
Estádio: stadium, **pl.** stadia
Estadiômetro: stadiometer
Estado: state, status
Estafilectomia: staphylectomy
Estafiledema: staphyledema
Estafilina: staphyline
Estafílio: staphylion
Estafilocinase: staphylokinase
Estafilococcemia: staphylococcemia
Estafilocócico: staphylococcal, staphylococcic

Estafilococo: staphylococcus, **pl.** staphylococci
Estafilococólise: staphylococcolysis
Estafilococolisina: staphylococcolysin
Estafilococose: staphylococcosis, **pl.** staphylococcoses
Estafilodiálise: staphylodialysis
Estafiloemia: staphylohemia
Estafiloemolisina: staphylohemolysin
Estafilofaringorrafia: staphylopharyngorrhaphy
Estafilolisina: staphylolysin
Estafiloma: staphyloma
Estafilomatoso: staphylomatous
Estafiloplastia: staphyloplasty
Estafiloptose: staphyloptosis
Estafilorrafia: staphylorrhaphy
Estafilotoxina: staphylotoxin
Estágio: stage
Estágio Tanner: Tanner stage
Estagnação: stagnation
Estalagmômetro: stactometer, stalagmometer
Estalido: snap
Estanho: stannum, tin (Sn)
Estanho-113: tin-113 (^{113}Sn)
Estanhoso: stannous
Estânico: stannic
Estanolona: stanolone
Estanozolol: stanozolol
Estapedectomia: stapedectomy
Estapédico: stapedial
Estapédio: stapedius, **pl.** stapedii
Estapediotenotomia: stapediotenotomy
Estapediovestibular: stapediovestibular
Estapedotomia: stapedotomy
Estaquibotriotoxicose: stachybotryotoxicosis
Estaquidrina: stachydrine
Estaquiose: stachyose
Estase: stasis, **pl.** stases
Estasimórfia: stasimorphia
Estatampère: statampere
Estatinas: statins
Estatística: statistics
Estatmocinese: stathmokinesis
Estatoacústico: statoacoustic
Estatocinética: statokinetic, statokinetics
Estatocônios: statoconia, **sing.** statoconium
Estatólitos: statoliths
Estatômetro: statometer
Estatosfera: statosphere
Estatura: stature
Estáurio: staurion
Estável: stabile, stable
Estazolam: estazolam
Esteapsina: steapsin
Estearal: stearal
Estearaldeído: stearaldehyde
Estearato: stearate
Estearato de polioxil 40: polyoxyl 40 stearate

Estearil-CoA, estearil-coenzima A: stearyl-CoA, stearyl-coenzyme A
Estearina: stearin
Estearréia: stearrhea
Esteatite: steatitis
Esteatito: steatite
Esteatocistoma: steatocystoma
Esteatogênese: steatogenesis
Esteatólise: steatolysis
Esteatolítico: steatolytic
Esteatonecrose: steatonecrosis
Esteatopígeo: steatopygous
Esteatopigia: steatopyga, steatopygia
Esteatorréia: steatorrhea
Esteatose: steatosis
Esteatozoário: steatozoon
Estefânico: stephanial
Estefânio: stephanion
Estegnose: stegnosis
Estegnótico: stegnotic
Estematologia: esthematology
Estender: extend
Estenia: sthenia
Estênico: sthenic
Estênio: stenion
Estenobregmático: stenobregmatic
Estenocardia: stenocardia
Estenocefalia: stenocephalia, stenocephaly
Estenocéfalo, estenocefálico: stenocephalous, stenocephalic
Estenocompressor: stenocompressor
Estenocoria: stenochoria
Estenocrotafia: stenocrotaphy, stenocrotaphia
Estenometria: sthenometry
Estenômetro: sthenometer
Estenopeico, estenopaico: stenopeic, stenopaic
Estenosado: stenosed
Estenose: stenosis, **pl.** stenoses
Estenose da aorta: aortarctia, aortartia
Estenostenose: stenostenosis
Estenostomia: stenostomia
Estenotérmico: stenothermal
Estenótico: stenosal, stenotic
Estenotórax: stenothorax
Estenoxênico: stenoxenous
Estequiologia: stoichiology
Estequiométrico: stoichiometric
Éster: ester
Esterano: sterane
Esterase: esterase
Estercobilina: stercobilin
Estercólito: stercolith
Estercoráceo: stercoraceous
Estercoral: stercoral
Estercorina: stercorin
Estercoroma: stercoroma
Estercoroso: stercorous
Estere: stere
Estereoartrólise: stereoarthrolysis
Estereocampímetro: stereocampimeter

Estereocílio: stereocilium, **pl.** stereocilia
Estereocinefluorografia: stereocinefluorography
Estereocolpograma: stereocolpogram
Estereocolposcópio: stereocolposcope
Estereoeletroencefalografia: stereoelectroencephalography
Estereoencefalometria: stereoencephalometry
Estereoespecífico: stereospecific
Estereoforômetro: stereophorometer
Estereofotomicrografia: stereophotomicrograph
Estereognose: astereognosis, stereognosis
Estereognóstico: stereognostic
Estereografia: stereography
Estereógrafo: stereograph
Estereograma: stereogram
Estereoisomérico: stereoisomeric
Estereoisomerismo: stereoisomerism
Estereoisômero: stereoisomer
Estereologia: stereology
Estereometria: stereometry
Estereômetro: stereometer
Estereopatia: stereopathy
Estereopsia: stereopsis
Estereoquímica: stereochemistry
Estereoquímico: stereochemical
Estereorradiografia: stereoradiography, stereoroentgenography
Estereortóptero: stereo-orthopter
Estereoscopia: stereoscopy
Estereoscópico: stereoscopic
Estereoscópio: stereoscope
Estereosseletivo: stereoselective
Estereotático, estereotáxico: stereotactic, stereotaxic
Estereotaxia: stereotaxy
Estereotipia: stereotypy
Estereotrópico: stereotropic
Estereotropismo: stereotropism
Estérico: steric
Esterídeo: sterid
Esterificação: esterification
Estigma: sterigma, **pl.** sterigmata
Estéril: barren, sterile
Esterilidade: sterility
Esterilização: sterilization
Esterilizador: sterilizer
Esterilizar: sterilize
Esternal: sternal, sternalis
Esternalgia: sternalgia
Estérnebra: sternebra, **pl.** sternebrae
Esterno: sternum, **gen.** sterni, **pl.** sterna
Esternoclavicular: sternoclavicular, sternoclavicularis
Esternocleido: sternocleidal

Glossário

Esternocleidomastóideo: sternocleidomastoid, sternocleidomastoideus
Esternocondroescapular: sternochondroscapularis
Esternocostal: sternocostal
Esternodinia: sternodynia
Esternofascial: sternofascialis
Esternoglosso: sternoglossal
Esterno-hióideo: sternohyoideus
Esternóide: sternoid
Esternomastóide: sternomastoid
Esternopagia: sternopagia
Esternopericárdico: sternopericardial
Esternosquise: sternoschisis
Esternotireóideo: sternothyroideus
Esternotomia: sternotomy
Esternotraqueal: sternotracheal
Esternotripese: sternotrypesis
Esternovertebral: sternovertebral
Esternutação: sternutation
Esternutatório: sternutator, sternutatory
Esteróide: steroid, steroidal
Esteróides: steroids
Esteroidogênese: steroidogenesis
Esterol: sterol
Esterorradiano: steradian (sr)
Estertor: crackle, rale, stertor
Estertor de morte: death-rattle
Estertoroso: stertorous
Estesia: esthesia
Estésico: esthesic
Estesiódico: esthesiodic
Estesiofisiologia: esthesiophysiology
Estesiogênese: esthesiogenesis
Estesiogênico: esthesiogenic
Estesiografia: esthesiography
Estesiologia: esthesiology
Estesiometria: esthesiometry
Estesiômetro: esthesiometer
Estesioneuroblastoma: esthesioneuroblastoma
Estesioneurocitoma: esthesioneurocytoma
Estesioscopia: esthesioscopy
Estesódico: esthesodic
Estetalgia: stethalgia
Estetarterite: stetharteritis
Estética: esthetics
Estético: esthetic
Estetógrafo: stethograph
Estetomiite: stethomyitis
Estetomiosite: stethomyositis
Estetoparalisia: stethoparalysis
Estetoscopia: stethoscopy
Estetoscópico: stethoscopic
Estetoscópio: stethoscope
Estetoscópio do tipo Bowles: Bowles type stethoscope
Estibenil: stibenyl
Estibiação: stibiation
Estibiado: stibiated
Estibialismo: stibialism
Estibocaptato: stibcaptate
Estibofeno: stibophen

Estibônio: stibonium
Esticromo: stichochrome
Estigma: stigma, **pl.** stigmas, stigmata
Estigmastano: stigmastane
Estigmático: stigmatic
Estigmatismo: stigmatism
Estigmatização: stigmatization
Estilbamidina: stilbamidine
Estilbeno: stilbene
Estilbestrol: stilbestrol
Estilete: stilet, stilette, style, stylet, stylette
Estiliforme: styliform
Estilo: stilus
Estilo de vida: life-style
Estiloauricular: styloauricularis
Estilofaríngeo: stylopharyngeus
Estiloglosso: styloglossus
Estilo-hióideo: stylohyal, stylohyoid
Estilóide: styloid
Estiloidite: styloiditis
Estilolaríngeo: stylolaryngeus
Estilomandibular: stylomandibular
Estilomastóide: stylomastoid
Estilomaxilar: stylomaxillary
Estilopódio: stylopodium
Estilostafilina: stylostaphyline
Estilosteófito: stylosteophyte
Estimador: estimator
Estimativa: estimate, estimation
Estimulação: stimulation
Estimulador: stimulator
Estimulante: stimulant
Estímulo: stimulus, **pl.** stimuli
Estíptico: styptic
Estiramato: styramate
Estireno: styrene
Estirol: styrol
Estirona: styrone
Estivação: estivation
Estival: aestival, estival
Estivo-outonal: estivoautumnal
Estolho: stolon
Estoma: stoma, **pl.** stomas, stomata
Estomacal: stomachal
Estomacalgia: stomachalgia
Estomacodinia: stomachodynia
Estômago: gaster, stomach, ventriculus, **pl.** ventriculi
Estomal: stomal
Estomáquico: stomachic
Estomatal: stomatal
Estomatalgia: stomatalgia
Estomático: stomatic
Estomatite: stomatitis
Estomatócito: stomatocyte
Estomatocitose: stomatocytosis
Estomatodinia: stomatodynia
Estomatodisodia: stomatodysodia
Estomatognático: stomatognathic
Estomatologia: stomatology
Estomatológico: stomatologic
Estomatologista: stomatologist
Estomatomalacia: stomatomalacia

Estomatomicose: stomatomycosis
Estomatonecrose: stomatonecrosis
Estomatopatia: stomatopathy
Estomatoplastia: stomatoplasty
Estomatorragia: stomatorrhagia
Estomatoscópio: stomatoscope
Estomatose: stomatosis
Estômio: stomion
Estomocéfalo: stomocephalus
Estomodeal: stomodeal
Estomodeu: stomatodeum, stomodeum
Estoquiometria: stoichiometry
Estoraque: storax, styrax
Estoriforme: storiform
Estrábico: strabismal, strabismic
Estrabismo: cross-eye, squint, strabismus
Estrabismologista: strabismologist
Estradiol: estradiol, oestradiol
Estramônio: Jamestown weed, jimson weed, stink weed, stramonium, thornapple
Estrangalaestesia: strangalesthesia
Estrangulado: strangulated
Estrangulamento: strangulation
Estrangular: strangle
Estrangúria: strangury
Estranho: extraneous
Estrano: estrane
Estratificação: stratification
Estratificado: stratified
Estrato: layer, stratum, **gen.** strati, **pl.** strata
Estrato compacto: compacta
Estratrieno: estratriene
Estrefossimbolia: strephosymbolia
Estreito: strait
Estrela: star, stella, **pl.** stellae
Estrelado: stellate
Estrelectomia: stellectomy
Estremecer: vellicate
Estremecimento: shudder, vellication
Estrépito: strepitus
Estreptavidina: streptavidin
Estrepticemia: strepticemia
Estreptidina: streptidine
Estreptobiosamina: streptobiosamine
Estreptobiose: streptobiose
Estreptocercíase: streptocerciasis
Estreptocinase: streptokinase (SK)
Estreptocinase-estreptodornase: streptokinase-streptodornase
Estreptococcemia: streptococcemia
Estreptocócico: streptococcal, streptococcic
Estreptococo: streptococcus, **pl.** streptococci
Estreptococose: streptococcosis

Estreptodornase: streptodornase (SD)
Estreptofuranose: streptofuranose
Estreptolisina: streptolysin
Estreptomiceto: streptomycete
Estreptomicina: streptomycin
Estreptomicina A: streptomycin A
Estreptomicose: streptomycosis
Estreptonivicina: streptonivicin
Estreptose: streptose
Estreptossepticemia: streptosepticemia
Estreptotricose: streptothrichosis, streptotrichosis
Estreptotriquíase: streptotrichiasis
Estreptozocina: streptozocin
Estreptozotocina: streptozotocin
Estresse: stress
Estria: streak, striation, stripe
Estriação: stria, **gen. e pl.** striae
Estriado: striate, striatum
Estriadonigral: striatonigral
Estribo: stapes, **pl.** stapes, stapedes, stirrup
Estricnina: strychnine
Estricninismo: strychninism
Estridente: strident
Estrídeos: oestrids
Estridor: stridor, whoop
Estriduloso: stridulous
Estrina: estrin
Estriol: estriol, folliculin hydrate, oestriol
Estro: estrus
Estróbilo: strobila, **pl.** strobilae
Estrobilocerco: strobilocercus
Estrobilóide: strobiloid
Estroboscopia: stroboscopy
Estroboscópico: stroboscopic
Estroboscópio: stroboscope
Estrodienol: estrodienol
Estrofantina: strophanthin
Estrofantina G: G-strophanthin
Estrofocefalia: strophocephaly
Estrofossomia: strophosomia
Estrogênico: estrogenic
Estrogênio: estrogen, oestrogen
Estroma: stroma, **pl.** stromata
Estromal: stromal, stromic
Estromatina: stromatin
Estromatólise: stromatolysis
Estrona: estrone (E_1), folliculin, oestrone
Estrôncio: strontium (Sr)
Estrôncio-85: strontium-85 (^{85}Sr)
Estrôncio-87: strontium-87m (^{87m}Sr)
Estrôncio-89: strontium-89 (^{89}Sr)
Estrôncio-90: strontium-90 (^{90}Sr)
Estrôngilo: strongyle
Estrongiloidíase: strongyloidiasis, strongyloidosis
Estrongilose: strongylosis
Estrose: oestrosis

Estrual: estrous, estrual
Estruma: struma, **pl.** strumae
Estrumoso: strumous
Estrutura: frame, framework, structura, structure
Estrutura de Foster: Foster frame
Estrutura ocular acessória: structurae oculi accessoriae
Estrutural: structural
Estruturalismo: structuralism
Estruvita: struvite
Estudo: study
Estudo clínico: trial
Estupor: stupor
Estuporoso: stuporous
Estupro: rape
Eta: eta
Etacrinato sódico: ethacrynate sodium
Etadiona: ethadione
Etafenona: etafenone
Etamivan: ethamivan
Etamoxitrifetol: ethamoxytriphetol
Etanal: ethanal
Etano: ethane
Etanodiamina: ethanediamine
Etanodissulfonato de caramifeno: caramiphen ethanedisulfonate
Etanol: ethanol
Etanolamina: ethanolamine
Etanolaminafosfotransferase: ethanolaminephosphotransferase
Etansilato: etamsylate, ethamsylate
Etenil: ethenyl
Etenilbenzeno: ethenylbenzene
Éter: ether
Éter de metil-*tert*-butil: methyl-*tert*-butyl ether (MTBE)
Éter dietílico: diethyl ether
Éter dimetílico de bondina: boldine dimethyl ether
Éter etílico: ethyl ether
Éter sulfúrico: sulfuric ether
Etéreo: ethereal
Eterificação: etherification
Eterização: etherization
Etiazida: ethiazide
Ética: ethics
Eticlorvinol: etchlorvynol
Ético: ethical
Etideno: ethidene
Etídio: ethidium
Etidocaína: etidocaine
Etidronato dissódico: etidronate disodium
Etila: ethyl (Et)
Etilato: ethylate
Etilbenzatropina: ethylbenztropine
Etilcelulose: ethylcellulose
Etildicloroarsina: ethyldichloroarsine (ED)
Etileno: ethylene
Etilenodiamina: ethylenediamine
Etilenodibrometo: ethylene dibromide
Etilenoglicol: ethylene glycol
Etilestibamina: ethylstibamine
Etilestrenol: ethylestrenol
Etilideno: ethylidene
Etilidina: ethylidyne
Etilnorepinefrina: ethylnorepinephrine (E.N.E., E.N.S.)
Etilparabeno: ethylparaben
Etimemazina: etymemazine
Etindrona: ethindrone
Etinil: ethinyl, ethynyl
Etinilestrenol: ethinylestrenol
Etinodiol: ethynodiol
Etiocolanolona: etiocholanolone
Etiogênico: etiogenic
Etiolado: etiolated
Etiolamento: etiolation
Etiologia: etiology
Etiológico: etiologic
Etionamida: ethionamide
Etionina: ethionine
Etiopático: etiopathic
Etiopatologia: etiopathology
Etioporfirina: etioporphyrin
Etiotrópico: etiotropic
Etisterona: ethisterone
Etmocraniano: ethmocranial
Etmoesfenóide: ethmosphenoid
Etmofrontal: ethmofrontal
Etmoidal: ethmoidal, ethmoidale
Etmóide: ethmoid
Etmoidectomia: ethmoidectomy
Etmoidite: ethmoiditis
Etmolacrimal: ethmolacrimal
Etmomaxilar: ethmomaxillary
Etmonasal: ethmonasal
Etmopalatino: ethmopalatal
Etmoturbinados: ethmoturbinals
Etmovomerino: ethmovomerine
Etnocentrismo: ethnocentrism
Etnofarmacologia: ethnopharmacology
Etnologia: ethnology
Etoexadiol: ethohexadiol
Etofamida: etofamide
Etofarmacologia: ethopharmacology
Etologia: ethology
Etologista: ethologist
Etomidato: etomidate
Etomoxano: ethomoxane
Etoposídeo: etoposide
Etorfina: etorphine
Etossuximida: ethosuximide
Etotoína: ethotoin
Etotrimeprazina: ethotrimeprazine
Etoxi: ethoxy
Etoxibutamoxano: ethoxybutamoxane
Etoxizolamida: ethoxyzolamide
Etozolina: etozolin
Etretinato: etretinate
Eualelos: eualleles
Eubiótica: eubiotics
Eucaína: eucaine
Eucalipto: eucalyptus
Eucaliptol: eucalyptol
Eucapnia: eucapnia
Eucariótico: eucaryotic, eukaryotic
Eucarioto: eucaryote, eukaryote
Eucariotos: Eukaryotae, Eucaryotae
Eucasina: eucasin
Eucinesia: eukinesia
Eucloridria: euchlorhydria
Eucolia: eucholia
Eucorticalismo: eucorticalism
Eucrasia: eucrasia
Eucromático: euchromatic
Eucromatina: euchromatin
Eucromossoma: euchromosome
Eucupina: eucupine
Eudiaforese: eudiaphoresis
Eudipsia: eudipsia
Eufenia: euphenics
Euforia: euphoria
Euforizante: euphoretic, euphoriant
Eugenia: eugenics
Eugênico: eugenic
Eugenismo: eugenism
Eugenol: eugenol
Euglicemia: euglycemia
Euglicêmico: euglycemic
Euglobulina: euglobulin
Eugnatia: eugnathia
Eugnosia: eugnosia
Eugônico: eugonic
Euidratação: euhydration
Eumelanina: eumelanin
Eumelanossoma: eumelanosome
Eumetria: eumetria
Eumicetoma: eumycetoma
Eumicetos: eumycetes
Eumicetozoários: Eumycetozoea
Eumorfismo: eumorphism
Eunuco: eunuch
Eunucóide: eunuchoid
Eunucoidismo: eunuchoidism
Eunuquismo: eunuchism
Euosmia: euosmia
Eupancreatismo: eupancreatism
Euparal: euparal
Eupaverina: eupaverin
Eupepsia: eupepsia
Eupéptico: eupeptic
Eupeptídeo: eupeptide
Euplasia: euplasia
Euplástico: euplastic
Eupdóide: euploid
Euploidia: euploidy
Eupnéia: eupnea
Eupraxia: eupraxia
Euqueratina: eukeratin
Euribléfaro: euryblepharon
Euricefálico, euricéfalo: eurycephalic, eurycephalous
Eurignático: eurygnathic
Eurignatismo: eurygnathism
Eurignato: eurygnathous
Êurio: euryon
Európico: euryopic
Eurissomático: eurysomatic
Európio: europium (Eu)
Eurritmia: eurhythmia
Euscópio: euscope
Eussistolia: eusystole
Eussistólico: eusystolic
Eustenia: eusthenia
Eustrongilóide: eustrongyloides
Eutanásia: euthanasia
Eutenia: euthenics
Euterapêutico: eutherapeutic
Eutérmico: euthermic
Eutético: eutectic
Eutimia: euthymia
Eutímico: euthymic
Eutireoidismo: euthyroidism
Eutiscopia: euthyscopy
Eutiscópio: euthyscope
Eutônico: eutonic
Eutricose: eutrichosis
Eutrofia: eutrophia, eutrophy
Eutrófico: eutrophic
Euvolia: euvolia
Evacuação: evacuation
Evacuação do intestino: stool
Evacuador: evacuator
Evacuante: eliminant, evacuant
Evacuar: evacuate
Evaginação: evagination
Evanescente: evanescent
Evaporação: evaporation
Evaporar: evaporate
Evasão: evasion
Evento: event
Eventração: eventration
Eversão: eversion
Everter: evert
Eviração: eviration
Evisceração: evisceration
Evisceroneurotomia: evisceroneurotomy
Evocação: evocation
Evocador: evocator
Evolução: evolution
Evulsão: evulsion
Exacerbação: exacerbation
Exalação: exhalation
Exalar: exhale
Exaltação: exaltation
Exame: examination
Examinador: examiner
Examinar (screen 5): screening
Exangue: exsanguine
Exantema: exanthem, exanthema
Exantematoso: exanthematous
Exantropia: exanthrope
Exantrópico: exanthropic
Exarterite: exarteritis
Exaustão: exhaustion
Excementose: excementosis
Excêntrico: eccentric, excentric
Excentrocondroplasia: eccentrochondroplasia
Excentropiese: eccentropiesis
Excesso: excess
Excicloducção: excycloduction
Excicloforia: excyclophoria
Exciclotorção: excyclotorsion
Exciclotropia: excyclotropia
Exciclovergência: excyclovergence
Excipiente: excipient
Excisão: excision
Excisar: excise

Glossário

Excistação: excystation
Excitabilidade: excitability
Excitação: excitation
Excitamento: excitement
Excitante: excitant, excitor
Excitatório: excitatory
Excitável: excitable
Excitoglandular: excitoglandular
Excitometabólico: excitometabolic
Excitomotor: excitomotor
Excitomuscular: excitomuscular
Excitossecretor: excitosecretory
Excitotóxico: excitotoxic
Excitotoxinas: excitotoxins
Exclusão: exclusion
Exconjugante: exconjugant
Excreção: excretion
Excreções: excreta
Excrementício: excrementitious
Excremento: excrement
Excrescência: excrescence
Excretar: excrete
Excretor: excretory
Excursão: excursion
Exdução: exduction
Exemia: exemia
Exencefalia: exencephalia, exencephaly
Exencefálico: exencephalic, exencephalous
Exencefalocele: exencephalocele
Exenteração: exenteration
Exenterite: exenteritis
Exercício: exercise
Exérese: exeresis
Exergônico: exergonic
Exflagelação: exflagellation, polymitus
Exibicionismo: exhibitionism
Exibicionista: exhibitionist
Existencial: existential
Exo-1,4-α-D-glicosidase: exo-1,4-α-D-glucosidase
Exoalavanca: exolever
Exoamilase: exoamylase
Exoantígeno: exoantigen
Exocardia: exocardia
Exocíclico: exocyclic
Exocitose: exocytosis
Exócrino: exocrine
Exodesvio: exodeviation
Exodontia: exodontia
Exodontista: exodontist
Exoenzima: exoenzyme
Exoesqueleto: exoskeleton
Exofítico: exophytic
Exófito: exophyte
Exoforia: exophoria
Exofórico: exophoric
Exoftalmia: exophthalmos, exophthalmus
Exoftálmico: exophthalmic
Exoftalmômetro: exophthalmometer
Exogamia: exogamy
Exogástrula: exogastrula
Exogenético: exogenetic
Exógeno: exogenous
Exogenoto: exogenote

Exon: exon
Exonfalia: exomphalos
Exonuclease: exonuclease
Exopeptidase: exopeptidase
Exoplasma: exoplasm
Exospório: exosporium
Exósporo: exospore
Exosserose: exoserosis
Exostectomia: exostectomy, exostosectomy
Exostose: exostosis, **pl.** exostoses
Exotérico: exoteric
Exotérmico: exothermic
Exotóxico: exotoxic
Exotoxina: exotoxin
Exotropia: exotropia, wall-eye
Expansão: expansion
Expansividade: expansiveness
Expectativa: expectation
Expectativa de vida: expectation of life
Expectoração: expectoration
Expectorante: expectorant
Expectorar: expectorate
Experiência: experience
Experimento: experiment
Expiração: expiration
Expirar: expire
Expiratório: expiratory
Explantação: explantation
Explante: explant
Exploração: exploration
Explorador: explorer, searcher
Exploratório: exploratory
Explosão: burst, explosion
Expoente de hidrogênio: hydrogen exponent
Expor: expose
Exposição: exposure
Expressão: expression
Expressividade: expressivity
Expressões de afeto: affect display
Expulsar: extrude
Expulsivo: expulsive
Exsangue: bloodless
Exsanguinação: exsanguination
Exsanguinar: exsanguinate
Exsicação: exsiccation
Exsicante: exsiccant
Exsicar: exsiccate
Exsomatizar: exsomatize
Exsorpção: exsorption
Exsudação: exudation
Exsudar: exude
Exsudativo: exudative
Exsudato: exudate
Êxtase das profundezas: rapture of the deep
Êxtase: ecstasy
Extasiado: ecstatic
Extensão: extension
Extensor: extensor
Exterior: exterior, superficies
Exteriorizar: exteriorize
Externo: ectal, extern, external, externus
Exteroceptivo: exteroceptive
Exteroceptor: exteroceptor
Extinção: extinction, quenching

Extinguir: extinguish
Extirpação: extirpation, stripping
Extra-articular: extra-articular
Extra-axial: extraaxial
Extrabucal: extrabuccal
Extrabulbar: extrabulbar
Extracalicial: extracaliceal
Extração: extraction
Extracapsular: extracapsular
Extracarpal: extracarpal
Extracelular: extracellular
Extracístico: extracystic
Extracorpóreo: extracorporeal
Extracorpuscular: extracorpuscular
Extracraniano: extracranial
Extracromossomial: extrachromosomal
Extradural: extradural
Extra-embrionário: extraembryonic
Extra-epifisário: extraepiphysial
Extrafisiológico: extraphysiologic
Extragenital: extragenital
Extra-hepático: extrahepatic
Extraligamentar: extraligamentous
Extramaléolo: extramalleolus
Extramedular: extramedullary
Extramitocondrial: extramitochondrial
Extramural: extramural
Extranuclear: extranuclear
Extra-ocular: extraocular
Extra-oral: extraoral
Extra-ovular: extraovular
Extrapapilar: extrapapillary
Extraparenquimatoso: extraparenchymal
Extraperineal: extraperineal
Extraperiosteal: extraperiosteal
Extraperitoneal: extraperitoneal
Extrapiramidal: extrapyramidal
Extraplacentário: extraplacental
Extraprostático: extraprostatic
Extrapsíquico: extrapsychic
Extrapulmonar: extrapulmonary
Extra-sensorial: extrasensory
Extra-seroso: extraserous
Extra-sístole: extrasystole
Extra-somático: extrasomatic
Extratarsal: extratarsal
Extrato: abstract, educt, extract, extractives
Extrato líquido: fluidextract
Extrator: extractant, extractor, stripper
Extratraqueal: extratracheal
Extratubário: extratubal
Extra-uterino: extrauterine
Extravaginal: extravaginal
Extravasamento: extravasation
Extravasar: extravasate
Extravascular: extravascular
Extraventricular: extraventricular
Extravisual: extravisual

Extremidade: extremitas, extremity
Extremidade cega: blunt-end
Extremo: extremital
Extrínseco: extrinsic
Extrofia: ecstrophe, exstrophy
Extrogastrulação: extrogastrulation
Extroversão: extraversion, extroversion
Extroverter: extravert
Extrovertido: extrovert
Extrusão: extrusion
Extubação: extubation
Extubar: extubate
Exuberante: exuberant
Exumbilicação: exumbilication

F

Fabela: fabella
Face, fóvea: face, facet, facette, facies, **pl.** facies; norma, **pl.** normae
Facetectomia: facetectomy
Facial: facial, facialis
Facilitação: facilitation
Faciolingual: faciolingual
Facioplastia: facioplasty
Facioplegia: facioplegia
Facoanafilaxia: phacoanaphylaxis
Facocele: phacocele
Facocistectomia: phacocystectomy
Facodonese: phacodonesis
Facoemulsificação: phacoemulsification
Facoérise: phacoerysis
Facofragmentação: phacofragmentation
Facóide: phacoid
Facólise: phacolysis
Facolítico: phacolytic
Facoma: phacoma, phakoma
Facomalacia: phacomalacia
Facomatose: phacomatosis, phakomatosis
Facoscópio: phacoscope
Factício: factitious
Faculdade: faculty
Facultativo: facultative
Fadiga: fatigue
Fadiga visual: eyestrain
Fagedena: phagedena
Fagedênico: phagedenic
Fago: phage
Fagocitar: phagocytize, phagocytose
Fagocítico: phagocytic
Fagocitina: phagocytin
Fagócito: phagocyte
Fagocitoblasto: phagocytoblast
Fagocitólise: phagocytolysis
Fagocitolítico: phagocytolytic
Fagocitose: phagocytosis
Fagodinamômetro: phagodynamometer

Fagofobia: phagophobia
Fagólise: phagolysis
Fagolisossoma: phagolysosome
Fagolítico: phagolytic
Fagossoma: phagosome
Fagotipo: phagotype
Faixa: band
Fala: speech
Falácia ecológica: ecological fallacy
Falalgia: phallalgia
Falange: phalanx, **gen.** phalangis, **pl.** phalanges
Falangectomia: phalangectomy
Falângico: phalangeal
Falcato: falcate
Falcemia: sicklemia
Falcial: falcial, falcine
Falciforme: falciform
Fálcula: falcula
Falcular: falcular
Falectomia: phallectomy
Falicismo: phallicism
Fálico: phallic
Faliforme: phalliform
Falismo: phallism
Falo: phallus, **pl.** phalli
Falocampse: phallocampsis
Falocripsia: phallocrypsis
Falodinia: phallodynia
Falóide: phalloid
Faloidina: phalloidin
Falolisina: phallolysin
Faloncose: phalloncus
Falopiano: fallopian
Faloplastia: phalloplasty
Falotomia: phallotomy
Falotoxinas: phallotoxins
Falsa dominância: quasidominance
Falsete: falsetto
Falsificação: falsification
Falso-negativo: false negative
Falso-positivo: false positive
Família: family
Familial: familial
Famotidina: famotidine
Fanerogênico: phanerogenic
Faneromania: phaneromania
Faneroscópio: phaneroscope
Fanerose: phanerosis
Fanerozoíto: phanerozoite
Fango: fango
Fanquona: phanquone
Fantasia: fantasy, phantasia
Fantasiar: phantomize
Fantasma: phantasm, phantom
Fantasmagoria: phantasmagoria
Fantasmologia: phantasmology
Fantasmoscopia: phantasmoscopia, phantasmoscopy
Farad: farad (F)
Faraday: faraday (*F*), Faraday
Faradismo: faradism
Faradização: faradization
Faradomuscular: faradomuscular

Faradopalpação: faradopalpation
Faradoterapia: faradotherapy
Farcinose: farcy
Fardo: fardel
Farelento: branny
Farelo: bran
Fárfara: farfara
Farináceo: farinaceous
Faringe: pharynx, **gen.** pharyngis, **pl.** pharynges
Faringectomia: pharyngectomy
Farmgeo: pharyngeal, pharyngeus
Faringismo: pharyngismus
Faringite: pharyngitis
Faringítico: pharyngitic
Faringocele: pharyngocele
Faringoepiglótico: pharyngoepiglottic, pharyngoepiglottidean
Faringoesofágico: pharyngoesophageal
Faringoesofagoplastia: pharyngoesophagoplasty
Faringoglosso: pharyngoglossal
Faringolaríngeo: pharyngolaryngeal
Faringolaringite: pharyngolaryngitis
Faringólito: pharyngolith
Faringomaxilar: pharyngomaxillary
Faringonasal: pharyngonasal
Faringopalatino: pharyngopalatine
Faringoplastia: pharyngoplasty
Faringoplegia: pharyngoplegia
Faringorrinoscopia: pharyngorhinoscopy
Faringoscopia: pharyngoscopy
Faringoscópio: pharyngoscope
Faringospasmo: pharyngospasm
Faringostenose: pharyngostenosis
Faringotomia: pharyngotomy
Faringotonsilite: pharyngotonsillitis
Farinha de alfarroba: algaroba, carob flour
Farmacêutico: pharmacal, pharmaceutic, pharmaceutical, pharmaceutist, pharmacist
Farmácia: pharmaceutics, pharmacy
Farmacocinética: pharmacokinetics
Farmacocinético: pharmacokinetic
Farmacodiagnóstico: pharmacodiagnosis
Farmacodinâmica: pharmacodynamics
Farmacodinâmico: pharmacodynamic
Farmacoendocrinologia: pharmacoendocrinology
Farmacoepidemiologia: pharmacoepidemiology
Farmacofilia: pharmacophilia
Farmacofobia: pharmacophobia

Farmacogenética: pharmacogenetics, pharmacogenomics
Farmacognosia: pharmacognosy
Farmacognosista: pharmacognosist
Farmacografia: pharmacography
Farmacologia: pharmacology
Farmacológico: pharmacologic, pharmacological
Farmacologista: pharmacologist
Farmacomania: pharmacomania
Farmacopéia: Pharmacopeia, Pharmacopoeia
Farmacopéia Britânica: British Pharmacopoeia (BP)
Farmacopeico: pharmacopeial
Farmacopsicose: pharmacopsychosis
Farmacoquímica: pharmacochemistry
Fármaco-resistente: drug-fast
Farmacoterapia: pharmacotherapy
α-farneseno: α-farnesene
β-farneseno: β-farnesene
Farnesol: farnesol
Farnoquinona: farnoquinone
Fas: Fas
Fáscia: fascia, **pl.** fasciae, fascias
Fáscia retossacral: mesoprocton
Fascial: fascial
Fasciculação: fasciculation
Fascicular, fasciculado: fascicular, fasciculate, fasciculated
Fascículo: bundle, fascicle, fasciculus, **gen. e pl.** fasciculi
Fasciectomia: fasciectomy
Fasciodese: fasciodesis
Fascíola: fasciola, **pl.** fasciolae
Fasciolar: fasciolar
Fasciolíase: fascioliasis
Fasciolídeo: fasciolid
Fasciolopsíase: fasciolopsiasis
Fasciorrafia: fasciorrhaphy
Fasciotomia: fasciotomy
Fascite: fasciitis, fascitis
Fase: phase
Fase de leitura: reading frame
Fasmídeo: phasmid
Fasmofobia: phasmophobia
Fastidioso: fastidious
Fastígio: fastigium
Fatal: fatal
Fatalidade: fatality
Fatigabilidade: fatigability
Fatigável: fatigable
Fator: factor
Fator agravante: overlay
Fator de Laki-Lorand: Laki-Lorand factor
Fatorial (n!): factorial
Faucal: faucial
Fauces: fauces, **gen.** faucium
Fauna: fauna
Fava de ordálio: ordeal bean
Fava dos pântanos: buckbean
Fava-de-calabar: Calabar bean
Faveolado: faveolate

Favéolo: faveolus, **pl.** faveoli
Fávide: favid
Favismo: fabism, favism
Favo: favus
Febre: febris, fever, fièvre
Febre aftosa: aftosa
Febre paratifóide: keel, paratyphoid
Febre sakushu: akiyami
Febricitante: febricant, febrifacient, febriferous, febrific
Febrícula: febricula
Febrífugo: febrifugal, febrifuge
Febril: febrile, feverish
Fecal: fecal
Fecalito: fecalith
Fecalóide: fecaloid
Fecaloma: fecaloma
Fecalúria: fecaluria
Fechamento: closure
Fécula de mandioca: cassava starch
Feculento: feculent
Fecundação: fecundation
Fecundar: fecundate
Fecundidade: fecundity
Fecundo: fecund
Fedor: fetor
Feijão: bean
Feixe atrioventricular: ventriculonector
Felação: fellatio, irrumation
Felbamato: felbamate
Felino: feline
Felipressina: felypressin
Felodipina: felodipine
Fembufeno: fenbufen
Fêmea: female
Feminização: feminization
Femoral: femoral
Femorocele: femorocele
Femorotibial: femorotibial
Fempipramida: fenpipramide
Femprobamato: phenprobamate
Fempropionato: phenpropionate
Fêmur: femur, **gen.** femoris, **pl.** femora
Fenacemida: phenacemide
Fenacetina: phenacetin (APC)
Fenacetolina: phenacetolin
Fenaciclamina: phenacyclamine
Fenaglicodol: phenaglycodol
Fenantreno: phenanthrene
Fenarsenamina: phenarsenamine
Fenato: phenate
Fenazocina: phenazocine
Fencamina: fencamine
Fenciclidina: phencyclidine (PCP)
Fenclofenaco: fenclofenac
Fenclonina: fenclonine
Fenda: cleft, crack, crevice, slit, vent
Fenestração: fenestration
Fenestrado: fenestrated
Fenetamina: phenetamine
Feneticilina potássica: phenethicillin potassium
Feneturida: pheneturide

Fengofobia: phengophobia
Fenicarbazida: phenicarbazide
Fenil: phenyl (Ph, Φ)
Fenil salicilato: salol
Fenilaceliluréia: phenylacetylurea
Fenilalanina: phenylalanine (Phe, F)
Fenilalaninase: phenylalaninase
Fenilamina: phenylamine
Fenilbenzeno: phenylbenzene
Fenilbutazona: phenylbutazone
Fenilcarbinol: phenylcarbinol
Fenilcetonúria: phenylketonuria (PKU)
Fenildicloroarsina: phenyldichloroarsine (PD)
Feniletanolamina N-metiltransferase: phenylethanolamine N-methyltransferase (PNMT)
Feniletilmalonamida: phenylethylmalonamide
Feniletilmaloniluréia: phenylethylmalonylurea
Fenilindanediona: phenylindanedione
Fenilisotiocianato: phenylisothiocyanate (PITC, PhNCS)
Fenilpropanolamina: phenylpropanolamine
Feniltiocarbamida: phenylthiocarbamide
Feniltiocarbamoil: phenylthiocarbamoyl (PTC)
Feniltioidantoína: phenylthiohydantoin (PTH)
Feniltiouréia: phenylthiourea
Feniltoloxamina: phenyltoloxamine
Feniltrimetilamônio: phenyltrimethylammonium (PTMA)
Fenindiona: phenindione
Fenitoína: phenytoin
Fenmetilol: phenmethylol
Fenobarbital: phenobarbital
Fenobutiodil: phenobutiodil
Fenocópia: phenocopy
Fenodina: phenodin
Feno-grego: fenugreek
Fenol: phenol
Fenolado: phenolated
Fenolase: phenolase
Fenolemia: phenolemia
Fenolftaleína: phenolphthalein
Fenologia: phenology
Fenolsulfonoftaleína: phenolsulfonphthalein (PSP)
Fenolúria: phenoluria
Fenômeno: phenomenon, **pl.** phenomena
Fenômeno crepuscular: sundowning
Fenomenologia: phenomenology
Fenoperidina: phenoperidine
Fenoprocumona: phenprocoumon

Fenoprofeno cálcico: fenoprofen calcium
Fenoterol: fenoterol
Fenotiazina: phenothiazine
Fenotípico: phenotypic
Fenótipo: phenotype
Fenoxazina: phenoxazine
Fenoxazona: phenoxazone
2-fenoxietanol: 2-phenoxyethanol
α-fenoxietilpenicilina potássica: α-phenoxyethylpenicillin potassium
Fenoximetilpenicilina: phenoxymethylpenicillin
α-fenoxipropilpenicilina potássica: α-phenoxypropylpenicillin potassium
Fenózigo: phenozygous
Fensuximida: phensuximide
Fentermina: phentermine
Fenticlor: fenticlor
Feocromo: pheochrome
Feocromoblasto: pheochromoblast
Feocromócito: pheochromocyte
Feocromocitoma: pheochromocytoma
Feoifomicose: phaeohyphomycosis
Feomelanina: pheomelanin
Feomelanogênese: pheomelanogenesis
Feomelanossoma: pheomelanosome
Ferese: pheresis
Ferida: sore, wound
Fermentação: fermentation
Fermentador: fermenter
Fermentar: ferment
Fermentativo: fermentative
Fermentável: fermentable
Férmio: fermium (Fm)
Feromônios: pheromones
Feroz: feral
Ferramenta: instrument
Ferratina: ferratin
Ferredoxinas: ferredoxins
Ferricianeto: ferricyanide
Férrico: ferric
Ferritina: ferritin
Ferro: iron (Fe)
Ferro-52 (Fe^{52}): iron-52 (^{52}Fe)
Ferro-55 (Fe^{55}): iron-55 (^{55}Fe)
Ferro-59 (Fe^{59}): iron-59 (^{59}Fe)
Ferrocianeto: ferrocyanide
Ferrocinética: ferrokinetics
Ferrocolinato: ferrocholinate
Ferroproteínas: ferroproteins
Ferroquelatase: ferrochelatase
Ferroso: ferrous
Ferrosoférrico: ferrosoferric
Ferroterapia: ferrotherapy
Ferrugem: rusts
Ferruginoso: ferruginous
Fértil: fertile
Fertilidade: fertility
Fertilização: fertilization
Fertilizina: fertilizin

Fervescência: fervescence
Festão: festoon
Festinação: festination
Festinante: festinant
Festonado: festooning
Fetação: fetation
Fetal: fetal
Fetalismo: fetalism
Fetiche: fetish
Fetichismo: fetishism
Feticida: feticide
Fétido: fetid
Feto: fetus, **pl.** fetuses
Fetoglobulinas: fetoglobulins
Fetografia: fetography
Fetologia: fetology
Fetometria: fetometry
Fetopatia: fetopathy
Fetoplacentário: fetoplacental
Fetoproteínas: fetoproteins
Fetoscopia: fetoscopy
Fetoscópio: fetoscope
Fetuína: fetuin
Fezes: feces, stercus
Fiálide: phialide
Fialoconídio: phialoconidium, **pl.** phialoconidia
Fibra: fiber, fibra, **pl.** fibrae; fibre
Fibra de Rosenthal: Rosenthal fiber
Fibras de algodão: lint
Fibratos: fibrates
Fibremia: fibremia
Fibrila: fibril, fibrilla, **pl.** fibrillae
Fibrilação: fibrillation
Fibrilar: fibrillar, fibrillary, fibrillate, fibrillated, filar
Fibrilina: fibrillin
Fibrilo-*flutter*: fibrilloflutter
Fibrilogênese: fibrillogenesis
Fibrina: fibrin
Fibrinase: fibrinase
Fibrinocelular: fibrinocellular
Fibrinocinase: fibrinokinase
Fibrinogenase: fibrinogenase
Fibrinogenemia: fibrinogenemia
Fibrinogênese: fibrinogenesis
Fibrinogênico: fibrinogenic, fibrinogenous
Fibrinogênio: fibrinogen
Fibrinogenólise: fibrinogenolysis
Fibrinogenopenia: fibrinogenopenia
Fibrinóide: fibrinoid
Fibrinólise: fibrinolysis
Fibrinolisina: fibrinolysin
Fibrinolisocinase: fibrinolysokinase
Fibrinolítico: fibrinolytic
Fibrinopeptídeo: fibrinopeptide
Fibrinopurulento: fibrinopurulent
Fibrinoscopia: fibrinoscopy
Fibrinoso: fibrinous
Fibrinúria: fibrinuria
Fibroadenoma: fibroadenoma
Fibroadiposo: fibroadipose, fibrofatty

Fibroareolar: fibroareolar
Fibroblástico: fibroblastic
Fibroblasto: fibroblast
Fibrocartilagem: fibrocartilage, fibrocartilago
Fibrocartilaginoso: fibrocartilaginous
Fibrocelular: fibrocellular
Fibrocístico: fibrocystic
Fibrócito: fibrocyte
Fibrocondrite: fibrochondritis
Fibrocondroma: fibrochondroma
Fibrocongestivo: fibrocongestive
Fibrodisplasia: fibrodysplasia
Fibroelástico: fibroelastic
Fibroelastose: fibroelastosis
Fibroepitelioma: fibroepithelioma
Fibrofoliculoma: fibrofolliculoma
Fibrogênese: fibrogenesis
Fibrogliose: fibrogliosis
Fibróide: fibroid
Fibroidectomia: fibroidectomy
Fibroína: fibroin
Fibroleiomioma: fibroleiomyoma
Fibrolipoma: fibrolipoma
Fibroma: fibroma
Fibromatóide: fibromatoid
Fibromatose: fibromatosis
Fibromatoso: fibromatous
Fibromectomia: fibromectomy
Fibrômetro: fibrometer
Fibromialgia: fibromyalgia
Fibromiectomia: fibromyectomy
Fibromioma: fibromyoma
Fibromiosite: fibromyositis
Fibromixoma: fibromyxoma
Fibromuscular: fibromuscular
Fibronectinas: fibronectins
Fibroneuroma: fibroneuroma
Fibroosteoma: fibro-osteoma
Fibropapiloma: fibropapilloma
Fibroplasia: fibroplasia
Fibroplásico: fibroplastic
Fibróptica: fiberoptics
Fibróptico: fiberoptic
Fibrorreticular: fibroreticulate
Fibrosar: fibrose
Fibroscópio: fiberscope
Fibrose: fibrosis
Fibrosite: fibrositis
Fibroso: fibrosa, fibrous
Fibrossarcoma: fibrosarcoma
Fibrosseroso: fibroserous
Fibrótico: fibrotic
Fibrotórax: fibrothorax
Fibroxantoma: fibroxanthoma
Fíbula: calf-bone, fibula, perone
Fibular: fibular, fibularis, peroneal
Ficaína: ficain
Ficina: ficin
Ficomicetose: phycomycetosis
Ficomicose: phycomycosis
Fígado: hepar, **gen.** hepatis, liver
Figo: fig

Figura: figure
Figura e fundo: figure and ground
Figurado: figuratus
Filacagógico: phylacagogic
Filagrina: filaggrin
Filamento: filament, filamentum, **pl.** filamenta; filum, **pl.** fila; strand
Filamentoso: filaceous, filamentous
Filamina: filamen, filamin
Filária: filaria, **pl.** filariae
Filariase: filariasis
Filaricida: filaricidal, filaricide
Filarióide: filariform
Filaxia: phylaxis
Filético: phyletic
Filha: daughter
Filial: filial
Filiforme: filiform
Filioparental: filioparental
Filitra: philiater
Filme: film
Filo: phylum, **pl.** phyla; filum, **pl.** fila
Filoanálise: phyloanalysis
Filódio: phyllode
Filogênese: phylogenesis
Filogenético, filogênico: phylogenetic, phylogenic
Filogenia: phylogeny
Filomimesia: philomimesia
Filópode: filopodium, **pl.** filopodia
Filopódios: filopodia
Filoprogenitivo: philoprogenitive
Filoquinona: phylloquinone (K), phylloquinone K
Filtração: filtration
Filtrado: filtrate
Filtrável: filtrable, filterable
Filtro: filter, filtrum, philtrum, **pl.** philtra
Fimatóide: phymatoid
Fimatorrisina: phymatorrhysin
Fímbria: fimbria, **pl.** fimbriae
Fimbriado: fimbriate, fimbriated
Fimbriectomia: fimbriectomy
Fimbrina: fimbrin
Fimbriocele: fimbriocele
Fimbrioplastia: fimbrioplasty
Fimose: phimosis, **pl.** phimoses
Fimótico: phimotic
Finasterida: finasteride
Fio: thread
Fio dental: floss
Fio para microssutura: microsuture
Fio-guia: glidewire, guidewire
Fisálide: physalis
Fisaliforme: physaliform
Fisalíforo: physaliferous, physaliphore, physaliphorous
Fisalopteríase: physalopteriasis
Fisário(a): physeal
Fise: physis
Fisiatra: physiatrician, physiatrist
Fisiatria: physiatrics, physiatry
Física: physics
Físico: physical, physique
Físico-químico: physicochemical
Fisiogênico: physiogenic
Fisiognomonia: physiognomy
Fisiognose: physiognosis
Fisiologia: physiology
Fisiológico: physiologic, physiological
Fisiológico-anatômico: physiologicoanatomical
Fisiologista: physiologist
Fisiopatologia: pathophysiology, physiopathology
Fisiopatológico: physiopathologic
Fisiopirexia: physiopyrexia
Fisiopsíquico: physiopsychic
Fisioterapeuta: physiotherapist
Fisioterapêutico: physiotherapeutic
Fisioterapia: physiotherapy
Fisocefalia: physocephaly
Fisocele: physocele
Fisometria: physometra
Fisopiossalpinge: physopyosalpinx
Fisostigma: physostigma
Fisostigmina: physostigmine
Fissão: fission
Fissiparidade: fissiparity
Fissíparo: fissiparous
Fissura: fissura, **pl.** fissurae, fissure
Fissura antitrago-helicina: antitragohelicine
Fissuração: crazing, fissuration
Fissurado: crevicular, chapped
Fissural: fissural
Fístula: fistula, **pl.** fistulae, fistulas
Fistulectomia: fistulectomy
Fistulização: fistulation, fistulization
Fistuloenterostomia: fistuloenterostomy
Fistuloso: fistulous
Fistulotomia: fistulotomy
Fistulótomo: fistulatome
Fita: ribbon, tape
Fitanato: phytanate
6-fitase: 6-phytase
Fitato: phytate
Fitil: phytyl
Fitina: phytin
Fitoaglutinina: phytoagglutinin
Fitobezoar: phytobezoar
Fitodermatite: phytodermatitis
Fitoemaglutinina: phytohemagglutinin (PHA)
Fitoesfingosina: phytosphingosine
Fitófago: phytophagous
Fitóide: phytoid
Fitol: phytol
Fitolectina: phytolectin
Fitomenadiona: phytomenadione
Fitomitógeno: phytomitogen
Fitonadiona: phytonadione
Fitopneumoconiose: phytopneumoconiosis
Fitoporfirina: phytoporphyrin
Fitoquímica: phytochemistry
Fitose: phytosis
Fitosterol: phytosterol
Fitosterolemia: phytosterolemia
Fitotóxico: phytotoxic
Fitotoxina: phytotoxin
Fitotricobezoar: phytotrichobezoar
Fixação: fixation, fixing, wiring
Fixador: fixative, fixator
Fixador de Newcomer: Newcomer fixative
Flacidez: flaccidity
Flácido: flaccid
Flagelação: flagellation
Flagelado: flagellate, flagellated
Flagelina: flagellin
Flagelo: flagellum, **pl.** flagella
Flanco: flank, loin
Flashback: flashback
Flato: flatus
Flatulência: flatulence
Flatulento: flatulent
Flavo: flavus
Flavocinase: flavokinase
Flavoenzima: flavoenzyme
Flavona: flavone
Flavonóides: flavonoids
Flavonol: flavonol
Flavoproteína: flavoprotein
Flebalgia: phlebalgia
Flebectasia: phlebectasia, venectasia
Flebectomia: phlebectomy, venectomy
Flebite: phlebitis
Flebítico: phlebitic
Flebóclise: phleboclysis
Flebodinâmica: phlebodynamics
Fleboflebostomia: phlebophlebostomy
Flebografia: phlebography
Flebógrafo: phlebograph
Flebograma: phlebogram
Flebóide: phleboid
Flebolitíase: phlebolithiasis
Flebólito: phlebolite, phlebolith
Flebologia: phlebology
Flebomanômetro: phlebomanometer
Flebometrite: phlebometritis
Flebomiomatose: phlebomyomatosis
Fleboplastia: phleboplasty
Fleborismo: phlebeurysm
Fleborrafia: phleborrhaphy
Flebosclerose: phlebosclerosis
Flebostase: phlebostasis
Flebostenose: phlebostenosis
Flebotomia: phlebotomy
Flebotomíneo: phlebotomine
Flebotomista: phlebotomist
Flebotomizar: phlebotomize
Flebotrombose: phlebothrombosis
Flegma: phlegm
Flegmasia: phlegmasia
Flegmático: phlegmatic
Flegmonoso: phlegmonous
Flexão: flexion
Flexibilidade cérea: cerea flexibilitas
Flexionar: flex
Flexor: flexor
Flexura: flexura, **pl.** flexurae; flexure
Flexural: flexural
Flictena: bleb
Flictênula: phlyctenula, **pl.** phlyctenulae; phlyctenule
Flictenular: phlyctenular
Flictenulose: phlyctenulosis
Floco: floc
Flocose: floccose
Flocosidade: flocculence
Flocoso: flocculent
Floculação: flocculation
Flocular: floccular, flocculate
Flóculo: floccule, flocculus, **pl.** flocculi
Floculonodular: flocculonodular
Flogisto: phlogiston
Flogosina: phlogosin
Flogoterapia: phlogotherapy
Flora: flora
Florantirona: florantyrone
Floridizina: phloridzin
Florizina: phlorizin
Floroglucina, floroglucinol, floroglucol: phloroglucin, phloroglucinol, phloroglucol
Flotação: flotation
Floxacilina: floxacillin
Floxina: phloxine
Floxuridina: floxuridine
Fluanisona: fluanisone
Flucitosina: flucytosine
Flucrilato: flucrylate
Fluência: fluency
Fluente: fluent
Flufenazina: fluphenazine
Fluidez: fluidity
Fluido: fluid
Flumazenil: flumazenil
Flúmen: flumen, **pl.** flumina
Flumetasona: flumethasone
Flumetiazida: flumethiazide
Flunarizina: flunarizine
Flunisolida: flunisolide
Flunitrazepam: flunitrazepam
Fluocinonida: fluocinonide
Fluocortolona: fluocortolone
Flúor: fluorine (F)
Fluoração: fluoridation, fluoridization
Fluorapatita: fluorapatite
9H-fluoreno: 9H-fluorene
Fluorescamina: fluorescamine
Fluoresceína: fluorescein
Fluorescência: fluorescence
Fluorescente: fluorescent
Fluorescer: fluoresce
Fluorescina: fluorescin
Fluoreto: fluoride
Fluoreto estanhoso: stannous fluoride
Fluoro-2,4-dinitrobenzeno: fluoro-2,4-dinitrobenzene

Glossário

(FDNB)
Fluorócito: fluorocyte
9α-fluorocortisol: 9α-fluorocortisol
Fluorocromo: fluorochrome
Fluorofosfato de diisopropil: diisopropyl fluorophosphate (DFP)
Fluorofotometria: fluorophotometry
Fluorografia: fluorography
Fluorometolona: fluorometholone
Fluorometria: fluorometry
Fluorômetro: fluorometer
Fluoroquinolona: fluoroquinolone
Fluoroquinolonas: fluoroquinolones
Fluoroscopia: fluoroscopy
Fluoroscópico: fluoroscopic
Fluoroscópio: fluoroscope
Fluorose: fluorosis
Fluorouracil: fluorouracil
Fluoximesterona: fluoxymesterone
Flupentixol: flupentixol
Fluprednisolona: fluprednisolone
Flurandrenolida: flurandrenolide
Flurbiprofeno: flurbiprofen
Flurotila: flurothyl
Fluroxeno: fluroxene
Flutamida: flutamide
Flutter-**fibrilação:** flitter, flutter-fibrillation
Flutuação: fluctuance, fluctuation
Flutuante: floater, floating
Flutuar: fluctuate
Fluxo: flow, fluence (H), streaming
Fluxo invertido: backflow
Fluxômetro: flowmeter
Fobia: phobia
Fóbico: phobic
Fobofobia: phobophobia
Focal: focal
Foco: focus, **pl.** foci
Focomelia: phocomelia, phocomely
Focômetro: focimeter
Fodrina: fodrin
Fogo selvagem: fogo selvagem, wildfire
Foice: falx, **pl.** falces
Folato: folate
Folcodina: pholcodine
Foledrina: pholedrine
Folha: folium, **pl.** folia
Folha de estanho: tinfoil
Folha de ouro: gold foil
Folha de platina: platinum foil
Folheto: leaflet
Foliáceo: foliaceous, foliate, foliose
Foliar: foliar
Folicular: follicular
Foliculite: folliculitis

Folículo: follicle, folliculus, **pl.** folliculi
Foliculose: folliculosis
Folinato: folinate
Folistatina: follistatin
Folitropina: follitropin
Fome: hunger
Fomentação: fomentation
Fomites: fomes, **pl.** fomites; fomite
Fon: phon
Fonação: phonation
Fonacoscopia: phonacoscopy
Fonacoscópio: phonacoscope
Fonarteriografia: phonarteriography
Fonarteriograma: phonarteriogram
Fonastenia: phonasthenia
Fonatório: phonatory
Fonema: phoneme
Fonêmico: phonemic
Fonendoscópio: phonendoscope
Fonética: phonetics
Fonético: phonetic
Foniatria: phoniatrics
Fônico: phonal, phonic
Fonoangiografia: phonoangiography
Fonocardiografia: phonocardiography
Fonocardiógrafo: phonocardiograph
Fonocardiograma: phonocardiogram
Fonocateter: phonocatheter
Fonocirurgia: phonosurgery
Fonofobia: phonophobia
Fonóforo: phonophore
Fonofotografia: phonophotography
Fonograma: phonogram
Fonologia: phonology
Fonomania: phonomania
Fonômetro: phonometer
Fonomioclônus: phonomyoclonus
Fonomiografia: phonomyography
Fonopatia: phonopathy
Fonopsia: phonopsia
Fonorreceptor: phonoreceptor
Fonoscopia: phonoscopy
Fonoscópio: phonoscope
Fonte pontual: point source
Fontículo: fontanelle, fonticulus, **pl.** fonticuli
Fora de fase: out of phase
Forame: foramen, **pl.** foramina
Foraminoso: foraminiferous
Forbina: phorbin
Forbol: phorbol
Força: force (F), strength, vis, **pl.** vires
Fórceps: forceps
Forcipressão: forcipressure
Forense: forensic
Forese: phoresis, phoresy
Foria: phoria
Forma: form

Forma de onda: waveform
Forma frustra: forme fruste, **pl.** formes frustes
Formação: formatio, **pl.** formationes, formation
Formaldeído: formaldehyde
Formaldeído de melamina: melamine formaldehyde
Formalina: formalin
Formamidase: formamidase
Formazana: formazan
Formiato: formate
Formicação: formication
Fórmico: formic
Formiga: ant
Formigamento: tingling
Formigar: tingle
Formila: formyl (f)
Formilase: formylase
Formilmetionil-RNAt: formylmethionyl-tRNA
Formina: formin
Formocresol: formocresol
Formol: formol
Formossulfatiazol: formosulfathiazole
Fórmula: formula, **pl.** formulas, formulae
Fórmula de Bernhardt: Bernhardt formula
Formulário: formulary
Formulário de consentimento: informed consent
Fornicação: fornication
Fornicar: fornicate
Fórnice: fornix, **gen.** fornicis, **pl.** fornices
Forno: furnace
Foróptero: Phoroptor
Forozoário: phorozoon
Forquilha: fork
Forscolina: forskolin
Foscarnet: foscarnet
Fosfagênico: phosphagenic
Fosfagênio: phosphagen
Fosfamidase: phosphamidase
Fosfatado: phosphated
Fosfatase: phosphatase
Fosfatemia: phosphatemia
Fosfático: phosphatic
Fosfatidal: phosphatidal
Fosfatidase: phosphatidase
Fosfatidato: phosphatidate
Fosfatídeo: phosphatide
Fosfatidil: phosphatidyl (Ptd)
Fosfatidilcolina: phosphatidylcholine (PtdCho)
Fosfatidiletanolamina: phosphatidylethanolamine (PtdEth)
Fosfatidilglicerol: phosphatidylglycerol
Fosfatidilinositol: phosphatidylinositol (PtdIns)
Fosfatidilserina: phosphatidylserine (PtdSer)
Fosfatidolipase: phosphatidolipase
Fosfato: phosphate
Fosfato acetiltransferase: phosphate acetyltransferase

3′-fosfato de adenosina: adenosine 3′-phosphate
5′-fosfato de adenosina: adenosine 5′-phosphate
Fosfato de amprotropina: amprotropine phosphate
Fosfato de azapetina: azapetine phosphate
Fosfato de clomacram: clomacran phosphate
Fosfato de *d*-anfetamina: *d*-amphetamine phosphate
Fosfato de dextroanfetamina: dextroamphetamine phosphate
Fosfato de dimetil-1-carbometoxi-1-propeno-2-il: dimethyl-1-carbomethoxy-1-propen-2-yl phosphate
Fosfato de dipotássio: dipotassium phosphate
Fosfato de nicotinamida adenina dinucleotídeo (NADP, NADP$^+$, NADPH): nicotinamide adenine dinucleotide phosphate (NADP, NADP$^+$, NADPH)
Fosfato de oleandomicina: oleandomycin phosphate
Fosfato de pirrobutamina: pyrrobutamine phosphate
Fosfato de poliestradiol: polyestradiol phosphate
Fosfato de primaquina: primaquine phosphate
Fosfato de retinila: retinyl phosphate
5′-fosfato de riboflavina: riboflavin 5′-phosphate
Fosfato de trolnitrato: trolnitrate phosphate
Fosfato férrico: ferric phosphate
3′-fosfato 5-fosfossulfato de adenosina (PAPS): adenosine 3′-phosphate 5′-phosphosulfate (PAPS)
Fosfato sódico de estramustina: estramustine phosphate sodium
Fosfato tribásico de cálcio: bone ash
Fosfato tricálcico: tricalcium phosphate
Fosfatúria: phosphaturia, phosphoruria, phosphuria
Fosfeno: phosphene
Fosfeto: phosphide
Fosfina: phosphine
Fosfito: phosphite
Fosfoacilase: phosphoacylase
Fosfoaçúcar: phosphosugar
3′-fosfoadenosina 5′-fosfato: 3′-phosphoadenosine 5′-phosphate (PAP)
3′-fosfoadenosina 5′-fosfossulfato: 3′-phosphoadenosine 5′-phosphosulfate (PAPS)
Fosfoamidas: phosphoamides
Fosfoamidase: phosphoamidase
Fosfoarginina: phosphoarginine
Fosfocolina: phosphocholine
Fosfocreatina: phosphocreatine

Fosfodiéster: phosphodiester
Fosfodiesterase de 3′,5′-fosfato cíclico de adenosina: adenosine 3′,5′-cyclic phosphate phosphodiesterase
Fosfodiesterases: phosphodiesterases
Fosfodismutase: phosphodismutase
Fosfo*enol*piruvato carboxiquinase: phospho*enol*pyruvate carboxykinase
Fosfoesfingosídeos: phosphosphingosides
Fosfoetanolamina: phosphoethanolamine
Fosfoexomutase: phosphohexomutase
Fosfoexoquinase: phosphohexokinase
Fosfoexose isomerase: phosphohexose isomerase
Fosfoforina: phosphophorin
1-fosfofrutaldolase: 1-phosphofructaldolase
1-fosfofrutocinase: 1-phosphofructokinase
6-fosfofrutocinase: 6-phosphofructokinase
Fosfogalactoisomerase: phosphogalactoisomerase
Fosfoglicerato quinase: phosphoglycerate kinase
Fosfoglicerídeos: phosphoglycerides
Fosfogliceromutase: phosphoglyceromutase
Fosfoglucomutase: phosphoglucomutase
6-fosfogluconolactonase: 6-phosphogluconolactonase
Fosfogluconato desidrogenase: phosphogluconate dehydrogenase
Fosfogluconato desidrogenase (descarboxilante): phosphogluconate dehydrogenase (decarboxylating)
6-fosfo-D-glucono-δ-lactona: 6-phospho-D-glucono-δ-lactone
Fosfoglucoquinase: phosphoglucokinase
Fosfoidrolases: phosphohydrolases
Fosfoinositídeo: phosphoinositide
Fosfolipase: phospholipase
Fosfolipídio: phospholipid
Fosfomutase: phosphomutase
Fosfonecrose: phosphonecrosis
Fosfônio: phosphonium
4′-fosfopanteteína: 4′-phosphopantetheine
Fosfopenia: phosphopenia, phosphorpenia
Fosfopentose epimerase: phosphopentose epimerase
Fosfopentose isomerase: phosphopentose isomerase

Fosfopiruvato hidratase: phosphopyruvate hydratase
Fosfoproteína: phosphoprotein
Fosfoquinase: phosphokinase
Fosforado: phosphorated
Fosforescência: phosphorescence
Fosforescente: phosphorescent
Fosforidrose: phosphorhidrosis, phosphoridrosis
Fosforila: phosphoryl
Fosforilação: phosphorylation
Fosforilase: phosphorylase
Fosforilases: phosphorylases
Fosforilcolina: phosphorylcholine
Fosforiletanolamina gliceridotransferase: phosphorylethanolamine glyceridetransferase
Fosforismo: phosphorism
Fosforizado: phosphorized
Fósforo: phosphor, phosphorous, phosphorus (P)
Fósforo-32: phosphorus-32 (^{32}P)
Fósforo-33: phosphorus-33 (^{33}P)
Fosforólise: phosphorolysis
Fosforriboisomerase: phosphoriboisomerase
5-fosforribose 1-difosfato: 5-phosphoribose 1-diphosphate
5-fosfo-α-D-ribosil-1-pirofosfato: 5-phospho-α-D-ribosyl-1-pyrophosphate (PPRibp, PPRP, PRPP)
5-fosforribosilamina: 5-phosphoribosylamine
Fosforribosilglicinamida sintetase: phosphoribosylglycineamide synthetase
Fosforribosiltransferase: phosphoribosyltransferase
Fosforribuloquinase: phosphoribulokinase
Fosforribulose epimerase: phosphoribulose epimerase
Fosfotransacetilase: phosphotransacetylase
Fosfotransferases: phosphotransferases
Fosfotriose isomerase: phosphotriose isomerase
Fosfovitina: phosphovitin
Fosfurese: phosphuresis
Fosgênio: phosgene (CG)
Fossa: fossa, **gen. e pl.** fossae
Fossa epigástrica: scrobiculus cordis
Fossa poplítea: ham, poples
Fóssula: fossette, fossula, **pl.** fossulae
Fossulado: fossulate
5′-fosfossulfato de adenosina: adenosine 5′-phosphosulfate (APS)
Fosvitina: phosvitin
Fot: phot
Fotalgia: photalgia
Fotaugiafobia: photaugiaphobia
Fotestesia: photesthesia

Fótico: photic
Fotismo: photism
Fotoablação: photoablation
Fotoactínico: photoactinic
Fotoalergia: photoallergy
Fotoautotrófico: photoautotrophic
Fotoautótrofo: photoautotroph
Fotobactéria: photobacterium, **pl.** photobacteria
Fotobiologia: photobiology
Fotobiótico: photobiotic
Fotocatalisador: photocatalyst
Fotoceratoscópio: photokeratoscope
Fotocimógrafo: photokymograph
Fotocinesia: photokinesis
Fotocinética: photokinetics
Fotocinético: photokinetic
Fotocintilografia photoscan
Fotoclareamento: photobleach
Fotocoagulação: photocoagulation
Fotocoagulador: photocoagulator
Fotocromógenos: photochromogens
Fotodermatite: photodermatitis
Fotodinâmico: photodynamic
Fotodinia: photodynia
Fotodisforia: photodysphoria
Fotodistribuição: photodistribution
Fotodromia: photodromy
Fotoelétrico: photoelectric
Fotoeletrômetro: photoelectrometer
Fotoelétron: photoelectron
Fotoenvelhecimento: photoaging
Fotoeritema: photoerythema
Fotoestável: photostable
Fotoestético: photoesthetic
Fotoestetoscópio: photostethoscope
Fotoestresse: photostress
Fotoeterotrófico: photoheterotrophic
Fotoeterótrofo: photoheterotroph
Fotofitodermatite: phytophotodermatitis
Fotofluorografia: fluororoentgenography, photofluorography
Fotofobia: photophobia
Fotofóbico: photophobic
Fotoforese: photophoresis
Fotóforo: photophore
Fotofosforilação: photophosphorylation
Fotoftalmia: photophthalmia
Fotogastroscópio: photogastroscope
Fotogênese: photogenesis
Fotogênico: photogenic, photogenous
Fotógeno: photogen
Foto-hemotacômetro: photohemotachometer

Fotoinativação: photoinactivation
Fotoliase: photolyase
Fotólise: photolysis
Fotolítico: photolytic
Fotólito: photolyte
Fotolitótrofo: photolithotroph
Fotoluminescente: photoluminescent
Fotomacrografia: photomacrography
Fotomania: photomania
Fotometria: photometry
Fotômetro: photometer
Fotomicrografar: photomicrograph
Fotomicrografia: photomicrography
Fotomioclônus: photomyoclonus
Fóton: photon ($h\nu, \gamma$)
Fotopatia: photopathy
Fotoperceptivo: photoperceptive
Fotoperiodismo: photoperiodism
Fotopia: photopia
Fotópico: photopeak, photopic
Fotopsia: photopsia, photopsy
Fotopsina: photopsin
Fotoquímica: photochemistry
Fotoquímico: photochemical
Fotoquimioterapia: photochemotherapy
Fotorradiação: photoradiation
Fotorreação: photoreaction
Fotorreativação: photoreactivation
Fotorreceptivo: photoreceptive
Fotorreceptor: photoceptor, photoreceptor
Fotorrespiração: photorespiration
Fotorretinite: photoretinitis
Fotorretinopatia: photoretinopathy
Fotossensibilidade: photosensitivity
Fotossensibilização: photosensitization
Fotossensível: photosensitive
Fotossensor: photosensor
Fotossíntese: photosynthesis
Fototaxia: phototaxis
Fototemporizador: phototimer
Fototerapia: phototherapy
Fototérmico: photothermal
Fototoxicidade: phototoxicity
Fototóxico: phototoxic
Fotótrofo: phototroph
Fototropismo: phototropism
Fotúria: photuria
Fóvea: fovea, **pl.** foveae
Fovéola: foveola, **pl.** foveolae
Foveolado: foveate, foveated, foveolate
Foveolar: foveolar
Fração: fraction
Fracionamento: fractionation
Fractais: fractals
Fragilidade: fragilitas, fragility
Fragilócito: fragilocyte

Fragilocitose: fragilocytosis
Fragmentação: fragmentation, spallation
Fragmento: fragment, spall
Fragmoplasto: phragmoplast
Fragrância: scent
Framboesia: yaws
Framboesia trópica: frambesia tropica
Framboesiforme: frambesiform
Framboesioma: yaw
Framboesoma: frambesioma
Frâncio: francium (Fr)
Franco: frank
Frângula: frangula
Frangulina: frangulin
Franja: fringe
Frankliniano: franklinic
Fraqueza: weakness
Frasco: bottle, flask, vial
Fratura: fracture
Freio: frenum, **pl.** frena, frenums
Freio dentário: archwire
Frêmito: fremitus, thrill
Frenal: frenal
Frenalgia: phrenalgia
Frenectomia: frenectomy, phrenectomy
Frenesi: frenzy
Frenético: phrenetic
Frenicectomia: phrenicectomy
Freniclasia: phrenemphraxis
Frênico: phrenic
Frenicoclasia: phreniclasia
Frenicocólico: phrenicocolic
Frenicoesplênico: phrenicosplenic
Frenicoexérese: phrenicoexeresis
Frenicogástrico: phrenicogastric
Frenicoglótico: phrenicoglottic
Freniconeurectomia: phreniconeurectomy
Frenicotomia: phrenicotomy
Frenicotripsia: phrenicotripsy
Frenocardia: phrenocardia
Frenocólico: phrenocolic
Frenoepático: phrenicohepatic, phrenohepatic
Frenogástrico: phrenogastric
Frenógrafo: phrenograph
Frenologia: phrenology
Frenologista: phrenologist
Frenoplastia: frenoplasty
Frenoplegia: phrenoplegia
Frenoptose: phrenoptosia
Frenosina: phrenosin
Frenospasmo: phrenospasm
Frenotomia: frenotomy
Frenotrópico: phrenotropic
Frênulo dos lábios menores do pudendo: fourchette
Frênulo: frenulum, **pl.** frenula
Freqüência: frequency (v)
Frese: fraise
Freudiano: freudian
Friável: friable
Fricativo: fricative
Fricção: friction, frottage
Frigidez: frigidity
Frígido: frigid
Frigorífico: frigorific
Frinoderma: phrynoderma
Frinolisina: phrynolysin
Frio: cold
Frita: frit
Frontal: frontal, frontalis
Fronte: forehead, frons, **gen.** frontis
Frontoccipital: frontooccipital
Frontomalar: frontomalar
Frontomaxilar: frontomaxillary
Frontonasal: frontonasal
Frontoparietal: frontoparietal
Frontotemporal: frontotemporal, frontotemporale
Frontozigomático: frontozygomatic
Frustração: frustration
Frutano: fructan
Frutocinase: fructokinase
Frutofuranose: fructofuranose
β-frutofuranosidase: β-fructofuranosidase
Frutólise: fructolysis
Frutosana: fructosan
Frutose: fructose (Fru)
Frutose-difosfatase: fructose-bisphosphatase
Frutose 1,6-difosfato: fructose 1,6-bisphosphate
Frutose 2,6-difosfato: fructose 2,6-bisphosphate
Frutose-difosfato aldolase: fructose-bisphosphate aldolase, fructose-diphosphate aldolase
Frutose férrica: ferric fructose
Frutose 1-fosfato: fructose 1-phosphate
Frutose 6-fosfato: fructose 6-phosphate
Frutosemia: fructosemia
Frutosídeo: fructoside
Frutosúria: fructosuria
Ftalato de butil: dibutyl phthalate
Ftalato de dimetila: dimethyl phthalate
Ftaleína: phthalein
Ftalil: phthalyl
Ftalilsulfacetamida: phthalylsulfacetamide
Ftalilsulfatiazol: phthalylsulfathiazole
Ftaloíla: phthaloyl
Ftiríase: pthiriasis
Fucose: fucose (Fuc)
α-fucosidase: α-fucosidase
Fucosidose: fucosidosis
Fucsina: fuchsin
Fucsinofilia: fuchsinophilia
Fucsinófilo: fuchsinophil, fuchsinophilic
Fuga da realidade: retreat from reality
Fuga: fugue
Fugacidade: fugacity (f)
Fugutoxina: fugutoxin
Fulcro: fulcrum, **pl.** fulcra, fulcrums

Fulguração: fulguration
Fulgurante: fulgurant, fulgurating
Fulminante: fulminant, fulminating
Fumarase: fumarase
Fumarato de pentapiperida: pentapiperide fumarate
Fumarato ferroso: ferrous fumarate
Fumarato hidratase: fumarate hydratase
Fumarato redutase: fumarate reductase (NADH)
Fumarilacetoacetato: fumarylacetoacetate
Fumegante: fuming
Fumigação: fumigation
Fumigante: fumigant
Fumigar: fumigate
Função: function
Funcho: fennel
Funcional: functional
Funcionalismo: functionalism
Funda: truss
Fundação: foundation
Fundador: founder
Fundamento: basement, fundament
Fundectomia: fundectomy, fundusectomy
Fúndico: fundic
Fundiforme: fundiform
Fundo: bas-fond, fundus, **pl.** fundi; solum
Fundo-de-saco: cul-de-sac, **pl.** culs-de-sac
Fundo do olho: eyegrounds
Fundoplicatura: fundoplication
Fundoscopia: funduscopy
Fundoscópio: funduscope
Fungicida: fungicidal, fungicide, mycocide
Fungicidina: fungicidin
Fungiemia: fungemia
Fungiforme: fungiform, fungilliform
Fungistático: fungistat, fungistatic
Fungo: fungus, **pl.** fungi
Fungo do milho: corn smut
Fungóide: fungoid
Fungos imperfeitos: Fungi Imperfecti
Fungoso: fungal, fungous
Funicular: funic, funicular
Funiculite: funiculitis
Funículo: funicle, funiculus, **pl.** funiculi
Funiforme: funiform
Funil: funnel
Funisite: funisitis
Furaltadona: furaltadone
Furano: furan
Furanose: furanose
Furazolidona: furazolidone
Furcado: furcal
Fúrcula: furcula
Furfuráceo: furfuraceous, pityroid
Furfural: furfural

Furfurila: furfuryl
Furfurol: furfurol
Furoato de diloxanida: diloxanide furoate
Furosemida: frusemide, furosemide
Furúnculo: boil, furuncle, furunculus, **pl.** furunculi
Furunculose: furunculosis
Fusão: fusion
Fusidato de sódio: fusidate sodium
Fusiforme: fusiform
Fusimotor: fusimotor
Fusina: fusin
Fuso: fuseau, spindle
Fusocelular: fusocellular
Fusoespiroquetal: fusospirochetal
Fusonuclear: nucleoospindle
Fustigação: fustigation

G

G positivo: positive G
G(u)estalt: gestalt
G(u)estaltismo: gestaltism
G negativa: negative G
Gadodiamida: gadodiamide
Gadolínio: gadolinium (Gd)
Gadopentetato: gadopentetate
Gadoteridol: gadoteridol
Gaiola: cage
Galactagogo: galactagogue
Galactanas: galactans
Galáctico: galactic
Galactidrose: galactidrosis
Galactitol: galactitol
Galactoblasto: galactoblast
Galactocele: galactocele
Galactocrasia: galactacrasia
Galactófago: galactophagous
Galactoforite: galactophoritis
Galactóforo: galactophore, galactophorous
Galactógeno: galactogen
Galactômetro: galactometer
Galactopiranose: galactopyranose
Galactopoese: galactopoiesis
Galactopoético: galactopoietic
Galactoquinase: galactokinase
Galactorréia: galactorrhea
Galactosamina: galactosamine
Galactosaminoglicana: galactosaminoglycan
Galactosanas: galactosans
Galactoscópio: galactoscope
Galactose: galactose (Gal), galactosis
Galactose-1-fosfato: galactose-1-phosphate
Galactose-6-sulfatase: galactose-6-sulfatase
Galactose-6-sulfurase: galactose-6-sulfurase
Galactosemia: galactosemia

β-galactosidase: β-galactosidase
α-D-galactosidase: α-D-galactosidase
β-D-galactosidase: β-D-galactosidase
Galactosídeo: galactoside
Galactosil: galactosyl
Galactosilceramida: galactosylceramide
β-galactosilceramidase: β-galactosylceramidase
Galactosúria: galactosuria
Galactoterapia: galactotherapy
Galacturonana: galacturonan
Galanga: galangal, galanga
Galantamina: galanthamine
Galão: gallon
Galeatomia: galeatomy
Galeína: gallein
Galena: galena
Galênico: galenic
Galênicos: galenicals
Galiformes: Galliformes
Galináceo: gallinaceous
Gálio (Ga): gallium (Ga)
Gálio-67 (Ga^{67}): gallium-67 (^{67}Ga)
Gálio-68 (Ga^{68}): gallium-68 (^{68}Ga)
Galocianina: gallocyanin, gallocyanine
Galope: gallop
Galtoniano: galtonian
Galvânico: galvanic
Galvanismo: galvanism
Galvanização: galvanization
Galvanocautério: galvanocautery
Galvanocirurgia: galvanosurgery
Galvanocontratilidade: galvanocontractility
Galvanofaradização: galvanofaradization
Galvanômetro: galvanometer
Galvanomuscular: galvanomuscular
Galvanopalpação: galvanopalpation
Galvanoscópio: galvanoscope
Galvanotaxia: galvanotaxis
Galvanoterapia: galvanotherapy
Galvanotônus: galvanotonus
Galvanotropismo: galvanotropism
Gama: gamma
Gamabufagina: gamabufagin
Gamabufogenina: gamabufogenin
Gamabufotalina: gamabufotalin
Gamacismo: gammacism
Gamagrama: gammagram
Gambir: gambir
Gameta: gamete
Gametângio: gametangium
Gametocida: gametocide
Gametocinético: gametokinetic
Gametocisto: gametocyst
Gametócito: gametocyte, gamont
Gametofagia: gametophagia
Gametogênese: gametogenesis
Gametogonia: gametogonia, gametogony
Gametóide: gametoid
Gâmico: gamic
Gamofagia: gamophagia
Gamofobia: gamophobia
Gamogênese: gamogenesis
Gamogonia: gamogony
Gamopatia: gammopathy
Gancho: hook
Gancho de conexão: clamp connection
Ganchos: hooklets
Ganciclovir: ganciclovir
Ganga: ganga
Gangliectomia: ganglionectomy
Gangliforme: gangliform, ganglioform
Gânglio: ganglion, pl. ganglia, ganglions
Gânglio ótico: otoganglion
Ganglioblasto: ganglioblast
Gangliócito: gangliocyte
Gangliocitoma: gangliocytoma
Ganglioglioma: ganglioglioma
Gangliólise: gangliolysis
Ganglioma: ganglioma
Ganglionado: gangliate, gangliated, ganglionated
Ganglionar: ganglial, ganglionic
Ganglioneuroblastoma: ganglioneuroblastoma
Ganglioneuroma: ganglioneuroma
Ganglioneuromatose: ganglioneuromatosis
Ganglionite: gangliitis, ganglionitis
Ganglioplégico: ganglioplegic
Gangliosialidose: gangliosialidosis
Gangliosídeo: ganglioside
Gangliosidose: gangliosidosis
Gangliostomia: ganglionostomy
Gangosa: gangosa
Gangrena: gangrene
Gangrenoso: gangrenous
Ganho: gain
Garança: madder
Garganta: gullet, jugulum, throat
Gargarejar: gargle
Garra: claw
Garra de macaco: monkey-paw
Gás: gas
Gasometria: gasometry
Gasométrico: gasometric
Gasômetro: gasometer
Gasoso: gaseous
Gasseriano: gasserian
Gastralgia: gastralgia
Gastrectasia: gastrectasis, gastrectasia
Gastrectomia: gastrectomy
Gástrico: gastric, gastricus
Gastricsina: gastricsin
Gastrinas: gastrins
Gastrinoma: gastrinoma
Gastrite: gastritis
Gastroacéfalo: gastroacephalus
Gastroalbuminorréia: gastroalbumorrhea
Gastroamorfo: gastroamorphus
Gastroanastomose: gastroanastomosis
Gastroatonia: gastroatonia
Gastroblenorréia: gastroblennorrhea
Gastrocardíaco: gastrocardiac
Gastrocele: gastrocele
Gastrocinesógrafo: gastrokinesograph
Gastrocistoplastia: gastrocystoplasty
Gastrocnêmio: gastrocnemius
Gastrocólico: gastrocolic
Gastrocolite: gastrocolitis
Gastrocoloptose: gastrocoloptosis
Gastrocolostomia: gastrocolostomy
Gastrocronorréia: gastrochronorrhea
Gastrodiálise: gastrodialysis
Gastrodinia: gastrodynia
Gastroduodenal: gastroduodenal
Gastroduodenite: gastroduodenitis
Gastroduodenoscopia: gastroduodenoscopy
Gastroduodenostomia: gastroduodenostomy
Gastroentérico: gastroenteric
Gastroenterite: gastroenteritis
Gastroenteroanastomose: gastroenteroanastomosis
Gastroenterocolite: gastroenterocolitis
Gastroenterocolostomia: gastroenterocolostomy
Gastroenterologia: gastroenterology
Gastroenterologista: gastroenterologist
Gastroenteropatia: gastroenteropathy
Gastroenteroplastia: gastroenteroplasty
Gastroenteroptose: gastroenteroptosis
Gastroenterostomia: gastroenterostomy
Gastroenterotomia: gastroenterotomy
Gastroepiplóico: gastroepiploic
Gastroesofágico: gastroesophageal
Gastroesofagite: gastroesophagitis
Gastroesofagostomia: gastroesophagostomy
Gastroespasmo: gastrospasm
Gastroesplênico: gastrolienal, gastrosplenic
Gastroestaxe: gastrostaxis
Gastroestenose: gastrostenosis
Gastrofrênico: gastrophrenic
Gastrogastrostomia: gastrogastrostomy
Gastrogênico: gastrogenic
Gastrógrafo: gastrograph
Gastro-hepático: gastrohepatic
Gastro-hidrorréia: gastrohydrorrhea
Gastroileíte: gastroileitis
Gastroileostomia: gastroileostomy
Gastrointestinal: gastrointestinal (GI)
Gastrojejunocólico: gastrojejunocolic
Gastrojejunostomia: gastrojejunostomy, gastronesteostomy
Gastrólise: gastrolysis
Gastrolitíase: gastrolithiasis
Gastrólito: gastrolith
Gastrologia: gastrology
Gastrologista: gastrologist
Gastromalacia: gastromalacia
Gastromegalia: gastromegaly
Gastrômelo: gastromelus
Gastromixorréia: gastromyxorrhea, myxorrhea gastrica
Gastrópago: gastropagus
Gastroparalisia: gastroparalysis
Gastroparasita: gastroparasitus
Gastroparesia: gastroparesis
Gastropatia: gastropathy
Gastropático: gastropathic
Gastropexia: gastropexy
Gastropilórico: gastropyloric
Gastroplastia: gastroplasty
Gastroplicatura: gastroplication, gastroptyxis
Gastropneumônico: gastropneumonic
Gastrópode: gastropod
Gastroptose: gastroptosis, gastroptosia, ventroptosis, ventroptosia
Gastropulmonar: gastropulmonary
Gastrorrafia: gastrorrhaphy
Gastrorragia: gastrorrhagia
Gastrorréia: gastrorrhea
Gastrorrexe: gastrorrhexis
Gastroscopia: gastroscopy
Gastroscópico: gastroscopic
Gastroscópio: gastroscope
Gastrosquise: gastroschisis
Gastrostolavagem: gastrostolavage
Gastrostomia: gastrostomy
Gastrotomia: gastrotomy
Gastrótomo: gastrotome
Gastrotonometria: gastrotonometry
Gastrotonômetro: gastrotonometer
Gastrotoracópagos: gastrothoracopagus
Gastrotóxico: gastrotoxic
Gastrotoxina: gastrotoxin
Gastrotrópico: gastrotropic
Gastroxia: gastroxia
Gastroxinse: gastroxynsis
Gástrula: gastrula
Gastrulação: gastrulation

Gaulterina: gaultherin
Gauss: gauss (G)
Gaussiano: gaussian
Gavagem: gastrogavage, gastrostogavage, gavage
Gaze: gauze
GDP manose fosforilase: GDP mannose phosphorylase
Gedoelstiose: gedoelstiosis
Gefirina: gephyrin
Gefirofobia: gephyrophobia
Gel: gel, gelatum
Gelação: gelation
Geladura: frostbite
Gelatina: gelatin
Gelatinase: gelatinase
Gelatinização: gelatinization
Gelatinizar: gelate, gelatinize
Gelatinóide: gelatinoid
Gelatinoso: gelatinous
Geléia: jelly
Gelo seco: dry ice
Gelose: gelosis
Gelsemina: gelsemine
Gelsolina: gelsolin
Gema: gemma
Gemação: gemmation
Gêmeo: gemellus, twin
Geminação: gemination, twinning
Geminado: geminate, geminous
Gemistócito: gemistocyte
Gemistocitoma: gemistocytoma
Gêmula: gemmule
Gena: gena
Genal: genal
Genciana: gentian, gentian root
Gencianófilo: gentianophil, gentianophile, gentianophilous
Gencianofóbico: gentianophobic
Genciobiase: gentiobiase
Genciobiose: gentiobiose
Gene: gene
Generalista: generalist
Generalização: generalization
Generalizado: generalized
Generativo: generative
Genérico: generic
Gênero: gender, genus, **pl.** genera
Gênese: genesis
Genésico: genesial
Genesiologia: genesiology
Genética: genetics
Geneticista: geneticist
Genético: genetic
Genfibrozila: gemfibrozil
Gengibre: ginger, zingiber
Gengiva: gingiva, **gen. e pl.** gingivae
Gengival: gingival
Gengivectomia: gingivectomy
Gengivite: gingivitis
Gengivite descamativa crônica: gingivosis
Gengivoaxial: gingivoaxial
Gengivoestomatite: gingivostomatitis
Gengivoglossite: gingivoglossitis
Gengivolabial: gingivolabial

Gengivolinguoaxial: gingivolinguoaxial
Gengivo-ósseo: gingivo-osseous
Gengivoplastia: gingivoplasty
Geniantro: genyantrum
Geniculado: geniculate, geniculated
Genicular: genicular, genual
Gênio: genion, genius
Genioglosso: genioglossus
Genioióideo: geniohyoid, geniohyoideus
Genioplastia: genioplasty
Genital: genital
Genitália: genitalia, genitals
Genitalidade: genitality
Genitocrural: genitocrural
Genitofemoral: genitofemoral
Genitor: parent
Genitourinário: genitourinary (GU)
Genoblasto: genoblast
Genocópia: genocopy
Genodermatologia: genodermatology
Genodermatose: genodermatosis
Genoespécie: genospecies
Genoma: genome
Genômica: genomics
Genômico: genomic
Genotípico: genotypic, genotypical
Genótipo: genotype
Genoto: genote
Genotóxico: genotoxic
Gentamicina: gentamicin
Geode: geode
Geofagia: dirt-eating, geophagia, geophagism, geophagy
Geófilo: geophilic
Geomedicina: geomedicine
Geopatologia: geopathology
Geotaxia: geotaxis
Geotricose: geotrichosis
Geotropismo: geotropism
Gepirona: gepirone
Geração: breeding, generation
Gerador: generator
Geraniol: geraniol
Gerar: generate
Geratologia: geratology
Geriatria: geriatrics
Geriátrico: geriatric
Germânio (Ge): germanium (Ge)
Germe: germ
Germicida: germicidal, germicide
Germina: germine
Germinal: germinal
Germinoma: germinoma
Gerodermia: geroderma
Gerodontia: gerodontics, gerodontology
Geromarasmo: geromarasmus
Gerôntico: gerontal
Gerontina: gerontine
Gerontofilia: gerontophilia
Gerontofobia: gerontophobia
Gerontologia: gerontology
Gerontologista: gerontologist

Gerontoterapêutica: gerontotherapeutics
Gerontoterapia: gerontotherapy
Gerotoxo: gerontoxon
Gestação: gestation
Gestagênico: gestagenic
Gestagênio: gestagen
Gestágeno: gestin
Gesto: gesture
Gestose: gestosis, **pl.** gestoses
Giardíase: giardiasis
Giba: gibbus
Gibão: gibbon
Giberelinas: gibberellins
Giboso: gibbous
Gigantismo: giantism, gigantism
Gigantomastia: gigantomastia
Gimnofobia: gymnophobia
Gimnotécio: gymnothecium
Ginandrismo: gynandrism
Ginandroblastoma: gynandroblastoma
Ginandróide: gynandroid
Ginandromorfismo: gynandromorphism
Ginandromorfo: gynandromorphous
Ginástica: gymnastics
Ginatresia: gynatresia
Ginecóide: gynecoid
Ginecologia: gynecology (GYN)
Ginecológico: gynecologic, gynecological
Ginecologista: gynecologist
Ginecomania: gynecomania
Ginecomastia: gynecomastia, gynecomasty
Gínglimo: ginglymus
Ginglimoartrodial: ginglymoarthrodial
Ginglimoidal: ginglyform, ginglymoid
Giniatria: gyniatrics, gyniatry
Ginofobia: gynephobia
Ginogênese: gynogenesis
Ginopatia: gynopathy
Ginoplastia: gynoplasty
Ginseng: ginseng
Gipso: gypsum
Girar: gyrate, turn
Girase: gyrase
Girectomia: gyrectomy
Girencefálico: gyrencephalic
Giro: gyration, gyrus, **gen. e pl.** gyri
Girocromo: gyrochrome
Girose: gyrose
Girospasmo: gyrospasm
Gitagismo: githagism
Gitalina: gitalin
Gitogenina: gitogenin
Gitonina: gitonin
Gitoxigenina: gitoxigenin
Gitoxina: gitoxin
Giz: chalk
Glabela: glabella
Glabro: glabrous, glabrate
Glafenina: glaphenine
Glande: glans, **pl.** glandes
Glandilema: glandilemma

Glândula: gland, glandula, **pl.** glandulae
Glândula pineal: pinus
Glândula salivar: sialaden
Glândula seminal: gonecyst, gonecystis
Glandular: glandular
Glândulas de Eglis: Eglis glands
Glanduloso: glandulous
Glarômetro: glarometer
Glaseriano: glaserian
Glaucina: glaucine
Glaucoma: glaucoma
Glaucomatociclítico: glaucomatocyclitic
Glaucomatoso: glaucomatous
Glaucosúria: glaucosuria
Glenóide: glenoid
Glenoumeral: glenohumeral
Glia: glia
Gliadina: gliadin
Glial: glial
Gliburida: glyburide
Glicação: glycation
Glical: glucal, glycal
Glicana: glucan, glycan
α-glicana fosforilase: α-glucan phosphorylase
1,4-α-D-glicano 6-α-D-glicosiltransferase: 1,4-α-D-glucan 6-α-D-glucosyltransferase
Glicano-hidrolases: glycanohydrolases
4-α-D-glicanotransferase: 4-α-D-glucanotransferase
Glicato: glycate
Glicemia: glycemia
Gliceptato: gluceptate
Gliceraldeído: glyceraldehyde
Gliceraldeído 3-fosfato: glyceraldehyde 3-phosphate
Gliceratos líquidos: fluidglycerates
Gliceridases: glyceridases
Glicerídeo: glyceride
Glicerila: glyceryl
Glicerina: glycerin
Glicerita: glycerite
Glicerocinase: glycerokinase
Glicerofosfato: glycerophosphate
Glicerofosfato férrico: ferric glycerophosphate
Glicerofosfocolina: glycerophosphocholine
Glicerofosforilcolina: glycerophosphorylcholine
Glicerogelatina: glycerogelatin
Glicerol: glycerol
Glicerol-3-fosfato aciltransferase: glycerol-3-phosphate acyltransferase
Glicerol-3-fosfato desidrogenase: glycerol-3-phosphate dehydrogenase (NAD^+)
Glicerona: glycerone
Glicerulose: glycerulose
Gliciclamida: glycyclamide

Glicíforo: gluciphore
Glicila: glycyl (Gly)
Glicina: glycine (G, Gly)
Glicinamida ribonucleotídeo: glycinamide ribonucleotide, glycineamide ribonucleotide
Glicinato: glycinate
Glicinina: glycinin
Glicínio: glycinium
Glicinúria: glycinuria
Glicirriza: glycyrrhiza
Gliclazida: gliclazide
Glicoamilase: glucoamylase
Glicobiarsol: glycobiarsol
Glicocálice: glycocalyx
β-glicocerebrosidase: β-glucocerebrosidase
Glicocerebrosídeo: glucocerebroside
Glicociamina: glucocyamine, glycocyamine
Glicocinase: glucokinase
Glicocinético: glucokinetic
Glicocolato: glycocholate
Glicoconjugados: glycoconjugates
Glicocorticóide: glucocorticoid, glycocorticoid
Glicocorticotrófico: glucocorticotrophic
Glicoesfingolipídio: glycosphingolipid
Glicofilia: glycophilia
Glicoforinas: glycophorins
Glicofuranose: glucofuranose
Glicogelatina: glycogelatin
Glicogenase: glycogenase
Glicogênese: glucogenesis, glycogenesis
Glicogênico: glucogenic, glycogenetic, glycogenic
D-glicogênico: D-glycogenous
Glicogênio: glycogen
Glicogenólise: glycogenolysis
Glicogenose: glycogenosis
Glicogeusia: glycogeusia
Glicoglicinúria: glycoglycinuria
Glico-histoquímica: glycohistochemistry
Glicoinvertase: glucoinvertase
Glicol: glycol
Glicolaldeído: glycolaldehyde
Glicolaldeidotransferase: glycolaldehydetransferase
Glicolato: glycolate
Glicoleucina: glycoleucine
Glicolila: glycolyl
Glicoliluréia: glycolylurea
Glicolipídio: glycolipid
Glicolipídios: glucolipids
Glicólise: glucolysis, glycolysis
Glicolítico: glycolytic
Gliconeogênese: gluconeogenesis, glyconeogenesis
Gliconolactonase: gluconolactonase
Glicopenia: glucopenia, glycopenia
Glicopeptídeo: glycopeptide

Glicopiranose: glucopyranose
Glicopirrolato: glycopyrrolate
Glicoplástico: glucoplastic
Glicoproteína: glucoprotein, glycoprotein
Glicoptialismo: glycoptyalism
Glicorraquia: glycorrhachia
Glicorréia: glycorrhea
Glicosamina: glucosamine
Glicosaminoglicana: glycosaminoglycan (GAG)
Glicosaminoglicanas: glucosaminoglycans
Glicosana: glucosan
D-glicose: D-glucose (G, Glc)
D-glicose 1,6-difosfato: D-glucose 1,6-bisphosphate
Glicose-6-fosfatase: glucose-6-phosphatase
D-glicose 1-fosfato: D-glucose 1-phosphate
Glicose 6-fosfato: glucose 6-phosphate
D-glicose 6-fosfato: D-glucose 6-phosphate
Glicose-1-fosfato cinase: glucose-1-phosphate kinase
Glicose-6-fosfato desidrogenase: glucose-6-phosphate dehydrogenase
Glicose-1-fosfato fosfodismutase: glucose-1-phosphate phosphodismutase
Glicose-fosfato isomerase: glucose-phosphate isomerase
Glicose-6-fosfato translocase: glucose-6-phosphate translocase
Glicose-1-fosfato uridililtransferase: glucose-1-phosphate uridylyltransferase
α-D-glicosidase: α-D-glucosidase
β-D-glicosidase: β-D-glucosidase
Glicosidases: glucosidases, glycosidases
Glicosídeo: glucoside, glycoside
Glicosídeo de estibamina: stibamine glucoside
Glicosídeos purpúricos A e B: purpurea glycosides A, purpurea glycosides B
Glicosídico: glycosidic
Glicosil: glucosyl
Glicosila: glycosyl
Glicosilação: glycosylation
Glicosilceramida: glucosylceramide
Glicosiltransferase: glucosyltransferase, glycosyltransferase
Glicosiltransferase ramificadora da α-glicana: α-glucan-branching glycosyltransferase
Glicosinolatos: glucosinolates
Glicosona: glucosone
Glicossecretor: glycosecretory
Glicossialia: glycosialia
Glicossialorréia: glycosialorrhea

Glicossulfona sódica: glucosulfone sodium
Glicostático: glycostatic
Glicosúria: glycosuria, glucosuria
Glicotrópico: glycotropic, glycotrophic
Glicurese: glycuresis
Glicurona: glucurone
Glicuronato: glucuronate, glycuronate
Glicuronidase: glycuronidase
β-D-glicuronidase: β-D-glucuronidase
Glicuronídeo: glucuronide, glycuronide
D-glicuronolactona: D-glucuronolactone
Glicuronosídeo: glucuronoside
Glicuronosiltransferase: glucuronosyltransferase
Glicuronúria: glycuronuria
Glioblasto: glioblast
Glioblastoma multiforme: glioblastoma multiforme
Glioblastose cerebral: glioblastosis cerebri
Gliócito: gliacyte
Glioma: glioma
Gliomatose: gliomatosis
Gliomatoso: gliomatous
Gliomixoma: gliomyxoma
Glioneuroma: glioneuroma
Gliose: gliosis
Gliossarcoma: gliosarcoma
Glioxal: glyoxal
Glioxalase: glyoxalase
Glioxilato transacetilase: glyoxylate transacetylase
Glioxildiureída: glyoxyldiureide
Glipizida: glipizide
Glissonite: glissonitis
Glitazonas: glitazones
Global: global
Globina: globin
Globo: globe, globus, **pl.** globi
Globosídeo: globoside
Globotriaosilceramida: globotriaosylceramide
Globulífero: globuliferous
Globulina: globulin
Globulinúria: globulinuria
Glóbulo: globule, globulus
Glomangioma: glomangioma
Glomangiose: glomangiosis
Glomectomia: glomectomy
Glomerular: glomerular, glomerulose
Glomerulite: glomerulitis
Glomérulo: glomerule, glomerulus, **pl.** glomeruli
Glomeruloesclerose: glomerulosclerosis
Glomerulonefrite: glomerulonephritis
Glomerulopatia: glomerulopathy
Glômico: glomal
Glomo: glome, glomus, **pl.** glomera

Glomos paraaórticos: glomera aortica
Glossa: glossa
Glossagra: glossagra
Glossalgia: glossalgia
Glossectomia: glossectomy, glossosteresis
Glóssico: glossal
Glossite: glossitis
Glossocele: glossocele
Glossocinestésico: glossocinesthetic, glossokinesthetic
Glossodinamômetro: glossodynamometer
Glossodinia: glossodynia
Glossodiniotropismo: glossodyniotropism
Glossodontotropismo: glossodontotropism
Glossoepiglótico: glossoepiglottic, glossoepiglottidean
Glossoespasmo: glossospasm
Glossofaríngeo: glossopharyngeal, glossopharyngeus
Glossógrafo: glossograph
Glossoial: glossohyal
Glossolalia: glossolalia
Glossologia: glossology
Glossoncose: glossoncus
Glossopalatino: glossopalatinus
Glossopatia: glossopathy
Glossopirose: glossopyrosis
Glossoplastia: glossoplasty
Glossoplegia: glossoplegia
Glossoptose: glossoptosis, glossoptosia
Glossorrafia: glossorrhaphy
Glossotomia: glossotomy
Glossotriquia: glossotrichia
Glotalização: glottalization
Glote: glottis, **pl.** glottides
Glótico: glottal, glottic
Glotidoespasmo: glottidospasm
Glotite: glottitis
Glotologia: glottology
Glucagon: glucagon
Glucagonoma: glucagonoma
Gluco-heptanato-Tc^{99m}: ^{99m}Tc-glucoheptanate
Gluconato ferroso: ferrous gluconate
Glusulase: glusulase
Glutamato: glutamate
γ-glutamato carboxipeptidase: γ-glutamate (glutamate γ-) carboxypeptidase
Glutamato monossódico: monosodium glutamate (MSG)
Glutamil: glutamyl (E, Glu, Glx)
γ-glutamil carboxilase: γ-glutamyl carboxylase
γ-glutamil hidrolase: γ-glutamyl hydrolase
γ-glutamil transferase: γ-glutamyltransferase
γ-glutamil transpeptidase: γ-glutamyl transpeptidase

γ-glutamilcisteína: γ-glutamylcysteine
Glutamina: glutamine (Gln, Q)
Glutaminase: glutaminase
Glutaminato: glutaminate
Glutaminil: glutaminyl (Gln, Glx, Q)
Glutamoil: glutamoyl
Glutaral: glutaral
Glutaraldeído: glutaraldehyde
Glutaril-CoA: glutaryl-CoA
Glutationa: glutathione (GSH)
Glutationúria: glutathionuria
Glutelinas: glutelins
Glúten: gluten
Glutenina: glutenin
Glúteo: cluneal, gluteal, gluteus
Glúteo médio: mesogluteus
Gluteofemoral: gluteofemoral
Gluteoinguinal: gluteoinguinal
Glutetimida: glutethimide
Glutinóide: glutinoid
Glutinoso: glutinous
Glutite: glutitis
GMP cíclico: cyclic GMP
Gnático: gnathic
Gnátio: gnathion
Gnatocéfalo: gnathocephalus
Gnatodinâmica: gnathodynamics
Gnatodinamômetro: gnathodynamometer
Gnatoestática: gnathostatics
Gnatografia: gnathography
Gnatologia: gnathology
Gnatológico: gnathological
Gnatosquise: gnathoschisis
Gnatostomíase: gnathostomiasis
Gnoscopina: gnoscopine
Gnosia: gnosia
Gnotobiologia: gnotobiology
Gnotobiota: gnotobiota
Gnotobiótico: gnotobiotic
Gnotobioto: gnotobiote
Goiva: gouge
Golgiocinese: golgiokinesis
Goma: gum, gumma, **pl.** gummata, gum-mas
Goma-laca: shellac
Gomelina: gommelin
Gomenol: gomenol
Gônada: gonad
Gonadal: gonadal
Gonadectomia: gonadectomy
Gonadoblastoma: gonadoblastoma
Gonadócrinos: gonadocrins
Gonadoliberina: gonadoliberin
Gonadopatia: gonadopathy
Gonadotrófico: gonadotrophic
Gonadotrofina: gonadotrophin
Gonadotrofina placentária: placentagonadotropin
Gonadotrofo: gonadotroph
Gonadotrópico: gonadotropic
Gonadotropina: gonadotropin
Gonalgia: gonalgia
Gonana: gonane
Gonartrite: gonarthritis
Gonfose: gomphosis

Gongilonemíase: gongylonemiasis
Gonicampse: gonycampsis
Gônio: gonion, **pl.** gonia
Goniocraniometria: goniocraniometry
Goniodisgenesia: goniodysgenesis
Goniômetro: fleximeter, goniometer
Goniopunção: goniopuncture
Gonioscopia: gonioscopy
Gonioscópio: gonioscope
Goniossinéquia: goniosynechia
Goniotomia: goniotomy
Gonócito: gonocyte
Gonococcemia: gonococcemia
Gonocócico: gonococcal, gonococcic
Gonococida: gonocide, gonococcicide
Gonococo: gonococcus, **pl.** gonococci
Gonocorismo: gonochorism, gonochorismus
Gonoemia: gonohemia
Gonóforo: gonophore, gonophorus
Gono-opsonina: gonoopsonin
Gonorréia: gonorrhea
Gonorreico: gonorrheal
Gonotil: gonotyl
Gonotoxemia: gonotoxemia
Gonotoxina: gonotoxin
Gorjal: gorget
Goserelina: goserelin
Gossipol: gossypol
Gosto secundário: aftertaste
Gota: gout, gutta (gt.), **pl.** guttae (gtt.)
Gotas: drops
Goteira: gutter
Gotejar: drip, drop
Gotícula: droplet
Gotoso: gouty
Grácil: gracilis
Grade: grid
Gradiente: gradient
Graduado: graduated
Grafanestesia: graphanesthesia
Grafestesia: graphesthesia
Gráfico: graph, plot
Grafite: graphite, plumbago
Grafofobia: graphophobia
Grafologia: graphology
Grafomania: graphomania
Grafomotor: graphomotor
Grafopatologia: graphopathology
Grafospasmo: graphospasm
Gram-negativo: Gram-negative
Gram-positivo: Gram-positive
Grama: gram (g, gm)
Grama-centímetro: gram-centimeter
Grama-metro: gram-meter
Gramicidina: gramicidin
Grampeamento: stapling
Grampo: clasp, clip, hairpin
Grandioso: grandiose

Granulação: granulatio, **pl.** granulationes, granulation
Granular: granular
Grânulo: granule
Granuloblasto: granuloblast
Granulócito: granulocyte
Granulocitopenia: granulocytopenia
Granulocitopoese: granulocytopoiesis
Granulocitopoético: granulocytopoietic
Granulocitose: granulocytosis
Granuloma: granuloma
Granulomatose: granulomatosis
Granulomatoso: granulomatous
Granulômero: granulomere
Granulopenia: granulopenia
Granuloplásico: granuloplastic
Granuloplasma: granuloplasm
Granulopoese: granulopoiesis
Granulopoético: granulopoietic
Granulosa: granulosa
Granulose: granulosis
Grão: grain
Grãos: grains, grana
Grasnada: honk
Grau: degree, grade
Grau de pureza: fineness
Gravela: gravel
Grávida: gravid, gravida, pregnant
Gravidade: gravity
Gravidade zero: zero gravity
Gravidez: gravidism, graviditas, pregnancy
Gravidez e parto: childbearing
Gravidez ovariana: oocyesis, ovariocyesis
Gravídico: gravidic
Gravimétrico: gravimetric
Gravímetro: gravimeter
Gravirreceptores: gravireceptors
Gravitação: gravitation
Gregalóide: gregaloid
Gregarino: gregarine
Gregarinose: gregarinosis
Grinalda: wreath
Grindélia: grindelia
Griocroma: gryochrome
Gripal: influenzal
Gripe: flu, grip, grippe
Gripose: gryposis
Griseofulvina: griseofulvin
Grisu: firedamp
Grumar: clump
Grumoso: grumous
Grupamento cetol: ketole group
Grupamento difarnesílico: difarnesyl group
Grupo: group
Grupo Bethesda-Ballerup: Bethesda-Ballerup Group
Grupo da platina: platinum group
Grupo de nitrogênio: nitrogen group
Grupo do alumínio: aluminum group
Grupo do cálcio: calcium group

Grupo do cloro: chlorine group
Grupo étnico: ethnic group
Grupo sangüíneo: blood group
Guaiacina: guaiacin
Guaiaco: guaiac
Guaiacol: guaiacol
Guaifenesina: guaifenesin
Guanase: guanase
Guanazol: guanazolo
Guanfacina: guanfacine
Guanidina: guanidine
Guanidínio: guanidinium
Guanidinoacetato: guanidinoacetate
Guanidinoacetato N-metiltransferase: guanidinoacetate N-methyltransferase
Guanila: guanyl
Guanilato ciclase: guanylate cyclase
Guanilila: guanylyl
Guanilorribonuclease: guanyloribonuclease
Guanina: guanine (Gua, G)
Guanosina: guanosine (G, Guo)
Guaraná: guarana
Guaranina: guaranine
Gubernáculo: gubernaculum
Guia: guidance, guide, pathfinder
Guilhotina: guillotine
L-gulono-γ-lactona: L-gulono-γ-lactone
L-gulonolactona: L-gulonolactone
Gulose: gulose
Gundu: gorondou, goundou
Gustação: gustation
Gustatório: gustatory
Gustoducina: gustducin
Guta-percha: gutta-percha
Gutural: guttural
Guturotetania: gutturotetany

H

Habena: habena, **pl.** habenae
Habenal: habenal, habenar
Habênula: habenula, **pl.** habenulae
Habenular: habenular
Hábito: habit
Habituação: habituation
Hafefobia: haphephobia
Hagioterapia: hagiotherapy
Hahnemanniano: hahnemannian
Halacromo: hallachrome
Halazona: halazone
Halifagia: haliphagia
Halisterese: halisteresis
Halisterético: halisteretic
Hálito: halitus
Halitose: halitosis
Halo: halation, halo
Haloalquilaminas: haloalkylamines

Halóide: halide
Halotano: halothane
Halucal: hallucal
Hálux: hallex, **pl.** hallices; hallus, hallux, **pl.** halluces
Hálux valgo: intoe
Hamamélis: hamamelis, witch hazel
Hamartia: hamartia
Hamartoblastoma: hamartoblastoma
Hamartocondromatose: hamartochondromatosis
Hamartofobia: hamartophobia
Hamartoma: hamartoma
Hamartomatoso: hamartomatous
Hamato: hamate, hamatum
Hamster: hamster
Hamular: hamular
Hâmulo: hamulus, **gen. e pl.** hamuli
Hapaloníquia: hapalonychia
Haplodonte: haplodont
Haplóide: haploid
Haplologia: haplology
Haploproteína: haploprotein
Haploscópico: haploscopic
Haploscópio: haploscope
Haplótipo: haplotype
Hapteno: hapten
Haptodisforia: haptodysphoria
Haptoglobina (HP): haptoglobin (HP)
Haptômetro: haptometer
Hardware: hardware
Harmalina: harmaline
Harmidina: harmidine
Harmina: harmine
Harmonia: harmony
Harmônico: harmonic
Harpaxofobia: harpaxophobia
Hasamiyami: hasamiyami
Hauch (H): Hauch (H)
Hausto: haustus
Haustório: haustorium, **pl.** haustoria
Haustração: haustration
Haustral: haustral
Haustro: haustrum, **pl.** haustra
Haversiano: haversian
Haxixe: hashish
Hebefrenia: hebephrenia
Hebefrênico: hebephrenic
Hebético: hebetic
Hebetude: hebetude
Hebiatria: hebiatrics
Hecatomérico: hecateromeric, hecatomeral, hecatomeric
Héctico: hectic
Hectograma: hectogram
Hectolitro: hectoliter
Hedenofobia: hedonophobia
Hedeoma: hedeoma
Hederiforme: hederiform
Hela: HeLa
Helcomenia: helcomenia
Heleborina: helleborin
Heleborismo: helleborism
Heléboro: hellebore
Heléboro-preto: helleborus
Heliantina: helianthine
Hélice: helix, **pl.** helices
Helicino: helicine
Helicoidal: helical
Helicóide: helicoid
Helicopodia: helicopodia
Helicotrema: helicotrema
Heliencefalite: heliencephalitis
Hélio: helium (He)
Hélio-3: helium-3
Hélio-4: helium-4
Helioaeroterapia: helioaerotherapy
Heliofobia: heliophobia
Heliopatia: heliopathy
Heliose: heliosis
Heliotaxia: heliotaxis
Heliotropismo: heliotropism
Helmintagogo: helminthagogue
Helmintêmese: helminthemesis
Helmintíase: helminthiasis
Helmíntico: helminthic, helmintic
Helmintismo: helminthism
Helminto: helminth
Helmintofobia: helminthophobia
Helmintóide: helminthoid
Helmintologia: helminthology
Helmintoma: helminthoma
Hemacromo: hemachrome
Hemadostenose: hemadostenosis
Hemadsorção: hemadsorption
Hemafeico: hemapheic
Hemafeína: hemaphein
Hemafeísmo: hemapheism
Hemaglutinação: hemagglutination
Hemaglutinina: hemagglutinin, hemoagglutinin
Hemagógico: hemagogic
Hemal: hemal
Hemalume: hemalum
Hemamebíase: hemamebiasis
Hemanálise: hemanalysis
Hemangiectasia: hemangiectasis, hemangiectasia
Hemangioblasto: hemangioblast
Hemangioblastoma: hemangioblastoma
Hemangioendotelioblastoma: hemangioendothelioblastoma
Hemangioendotelioma: hemangioendothelioma
Hemangiofibroma: hemangiofibroma
Hemangioma: hemangioma
Hemangiomatose: hemangiomatosis
Hemangiopericitoma: hemangiopericytoma
Hemangiossarcoma: hemangiosarcoma
Hemantitoxina: hemoantitoxin
Hemartrose: hemarthrosis
Hemastrôncio: hemastrontium
Hematacômetro: hematachometer
Hematapostema: hematapostema
Hemateína: hematein
Hematêmese: hematemesis
Hematencéfalo: hematencephalon
Hemático: hematic
Hemátide: hematid
Hematidrose: hematidrosis
Hematímetro: hematimeter
Hematina: hematin, oxyheme, oxyhemochromogen
Hematinemia: hematinemia
Hematínico: hematinic
Hematobilia: hematobilia
Hematóbio: hematobium
Hematoblasto: hematoblast
Hematocefalia: hematocephaly
Hematocele: hematocele
Hematocistia: hematocystis
Hematocisto: hematocyst
Hematócito: hematocyte
Hematocitoblasto: hematocytoblast
Hematocitólise: hematocytolysis
Hematocitômetro: hematocytometer
Hematoclorina: hematochlorin
Hematocolpia: hematocolpos
Hematocolpometria: hematocolpometra
Hematocômetro: hemotachometer
Hematócrito: hematocrit (Hct)
Hematodiscrasia: hematodyscrasia
Hematodistrofia: hematodystrophy
Hematofagia: hematophagia
Hematófago: hematophagous, hematophagus
Hematogênese: hematogenesis
Hematogênico: hematogenic, hematogenous
Hemato-histioblasto: hematohistioblast
Hemato-histona: hematohiston
Hematoidina: hematoidin
Hematolinfangioma: hematolymphangioma
Hematólise: hematolysis
Hematolítico: hematolytic
Hematologia: hematology, hemology
Hematologista: hematologist
Hematoma: hematoma
Hematometra: hematometra
Hematometria: hematometry
Hematomielia: hematomyelia
Hematomieloporo: hematomyelopore
Hematonfalocele: hematomphalocele
Hematônico: hematonic
Hematopatia: hematopathy
Hematopatologia: hematopathology
Hematopenia: hematopenia
Hematoplásico: hematoplastic
Hematopoese: hematopoiesis
Hematopoético: hematopoietic
Hematopoetina: hematopoietin
Hematoporfiria: hematoporphyria
Hematoporfirina: hematoporphyrin
Hematoporfirinemia: hematoporphyrinemia
Hematoporfirinúria: hematoporphyrinuria
Hematopsia: hematopsia
Hematoquezia: hematochezia
Hematoquilúria: hematochyluria
Hematorraquia: hematorrhachis
Hematose: hematosis
Hematosina: hematosin
Hematospectroscopia: hematospectroscopy
Hematospectroscópio: hematospectroscope
Hematospermatocele: hematospermatocele
Hematospermia: hematospermia
Hematossalpinge: hematosalpinx
Hematossepse: hematosepsis
Hematostático: hematostatic
Hematostaxia: hematostaxis
Hematósteo: hematosteon
Hematoterapia: hematherapy
Hematotímpano: hematotympanum
Hematotoxina: hematotoxin
Hematotrópico: hematotropic
Hematoxilina: hematoxylin
Hematoxina: hematoxin
Hematozoário: hematozoon
Hematozóico: hematozoic
Hematúria: hematuria
Heme: ferroheme, heme
Heme férrico: ferriheme
Hemeralopia: hemeralopia
Hemeranopia: hemeranopia
Hemeritrinas: hemerythrins
Hemiacárdio: hemicardius
Hemiacetal: hemiacetal
Hemiacrossomia: hemiacrosomia
Hemiageusia: hemiageusia, hemiageustia
Hemialgia: hemialgia
Hemianalgesia: hemianalgesia
Hemianencefalia: hemianencephaly
Hemianestesia: hemianesthesia
Hemianopia: hemianopia
Hemianópico: hemianopic
Hemianopsia: hemianopsia
Hemianosmia: hemianosmia
Hemiaplasia: hemiaplasia
Hemiapraxia: hemiapraxia
Hemiartroplastia: hemiarthroplasty
Hemiassinergia: hemiasynergia
Hemiataxia: hemiataxia
Hemiatetose: hemiathetosis
Hemiatrofia: hemiatrophy
Hemibalismo: hemiballism, hemiballismus
Hemibloqueio: hemiblock
Hemicardia: hemicardia

Glossário

Hemicario: hemikaryon
Hemicefalalgia: hemicephalalgia
Hemicefalia: hemicephalia
Hemicelulose: cellulosan, hemicellulose
Hemicentro: hemicentrum
Hemicérebro: hemicerebrum
Hemicetal: hemiketal
Hêmico: hemic
Hemicolectomia: hemicolectomy
Hemicolínio: hemicholinium
Hemicordado: Hemichorda
Hemicoréia: hemichorea
Hemicorporectomia: hemicorporectomy
Hemicrânia: hemicrania
Hemicraniectomia: hemicraniectomy
Hemicraniose: hemicraniosis
Hemicraniotomia: hemicraniotomy
Hemidesmossomas: hemidesmosomes
Hemidiaforese: hemidiaphoresis
Hemidisestesia: hemidysesthesia
Hemidistrofia: hemidystrophy
Hemidrose: hemidrosis
Hemiectromelia: hemiectromelia
Hemiesferectomia: hemispherectomy
Hemiespasmo: hemispasm
Hemifacial: hemifacial
Hemigastrectomia: hemigastrectomy
Hemigeusia: hemigeusia
Hemiglossectomia: hemiglossectomy
Hemiglossite: hemiglossitis
Hemignatia: hemignathia
Hemi-hepatectomia: hemihepatectomy
Hemi-hidranencefalia: hemihydranencephaly
Hemi-hidrose: hemihidrosis
Hemi-hipalgesia: hemihypalgesia
Hemi-hiperestesia: hemihyperesthesia
Hemi-hiper-hidrose: hemihyperhidrosis
Hemi-hipertonia: hemihypertonia
Hemi-hipertrofia: hemihypertrophy
Hemi-hipestesia: hemihypesthesia
Hemi-hipoestesia: hemihypoesthesia
Hemi-hipotonia: hemihypotonia
Hemilaminectomia: hemilaminectomy
Hemilaringectomia: hemilaryngectomy
Hemilateral: hemilateral
Hemilesão: hemilesion
Hemilingual: hemiglossal, hemilingual

Hemimacroglossia: hemimacroglossia
Hemimandibulectomia: hemimandibulectomy
Hemimelia: hemimelia
Hemimetábolo: hemimetabolous
Hemina: hemin
Heminstrumectomia: hemistrumectomy
Hemiopalgia: hemiopalgia
Hemípago: hemipagus
Hemipancreatectomia: hemipancreatectomy
Hemiparesia: hemiparesis
Hemipelvectomia: hemipelvectomy
Hemiplegia: hemiplegia
Hemiplégico: hemiplegic
Hemisfério: hemisphere, hemisphericum, hemispherium
Hemissecção: hemisection
Hemissensorial: hemisensory
Hemissepto: hemiseptum
Hemissíndrome: hemisyndrome
Hemissubstância: hemisubstance
Hemissulfato de proflavina: proflavine (hemi)sulfate
Hemitermoanestesia: hemithermoanesthesia
Hemiterpeno: hemiterpene
Hemitórax: hemithorax
Hemitremor: hemitremor
Hemitronco: hemitruncus
Hemivértebra: hemivertebra
Hemizigosidade: hemizygosity
Hemizigótico: hemizygotic, hemizygous
Hemizigoto: hemizygote
Hemoaglutinação: hemoagglutination
Hemobilia: hemobilia
Hemoblasto: hemoblast
Hemoblastose: hemoblastosis
Hemocatarse: hemocatharsis
Hemocaterese: hemocatheresis
Hemocaterético: hemocatheretic
Hemocele: hemocele
Hemocianina: hemocyanin
Hemócito: hemocyte
Hemocitoblasto: hemocytoblast
Hemocitocaterese: hemocytocatheresis
Hemocitólise: hemocytolysis
Hemocitometria: hemocytometry
Hemocitômetro: hemacytometer, hemocytometer
Hemocitotripsia: hemocytotripsis
Hemocitozoário: hemacytozoon, hemocytozoon
Hemoclasia: hemoclasis, hemoclasia
Hemoclástico: hemoclastic
Hemocolecistite: hemocholecystitis
Hemoconcentração: hemoconcentration
Hemoconia: blood dust

Hemocônia: hemoconia
Hemoconiose: hemoconiosis
Hemocrioscopia: hemocryoscopy
Hemocromatose: hemochromatosis
Hemocromo: hemochrome
Hemocromo verde: verdohemochrome
Hemocromogênio: hemochromogen
Hemocupreína: hemocuprein
Hemodiagnóstico: hemodiagnosis
Hemodialisador: hemodialyzer
Hemodiálise: hemodialysis
Hemodiastase: hemodiastase
Hemodiluição: hemodilution
Hemodinâmica: hemodynamics
Hemodinâmico: hemodynamic
Hemodiscrasia: hemodyscrasia
Hemodistrofia: hemodystrophy
Hemofagia: hemophagia
Hemofagocitose: hemophagocytosis
Hemofilia: hemophilia
Hemofílico: hemophiliac, hemophilic
Hemófilo: hemophil, hemophile
Hemofilose: hemophilosis
Hemofiltração: hemofiltration
Hemoflagelados: hemoflagellates
Hemofobia: hemophobia
Hemoforese: hemophoresis
Hemoftalmia: hemophthalmia, hemophthalmus
Hemofuscina: hemofuscin
Hemogênese: hemogenesis
Hemogênico: hemogenic
Hemoglobina (Hb): hemoglobin (Hb)
Hemoglobina férrica: ferrihemoglobin
Hemoglobinemia: hemoglobinemia
Hemoglobinocolia: hemoglobincholia
Hemoglobinofílico: hemoglobinophilic
Hemoglobinólise: hemoglobinolysis
Hemoglobinopatia: hemoglobinopathy
Hemoglobinopepsia: hemoglobinopepsia
Hemoglobinúria: hemoglobinuria
Hemoglobinúrico: hemoglobinuric
Hemograma: hemogram
Hemo-histioblasto: hemohistioblast
Hemolamela: hemolamella
Hemolinfa: hemolymph
Hemolipase: hemolipase
Hemolisado: hemolysate
Hemolisar: hemolyze
Hemólise: hemolysis
Hemolisina: hemolysin

Hemolisinogênio: hemolysinogen
Hemolítico: hemolytic
Hemólito: hemolith
Hemolização: hemolyzation
Hemomediastino: hemomediastinum
Hemometra: hemometra
Hemometria: hemometry
Hemopatia: hemopathy
Hemopatologia: hemopathology
Hemoperfusão: hemoperfusion
Hemopericárdio: hemopericardium
Hemoperitônio: hemoperitoneum
Hemopexina: hemopexin
Hemopielectasia: hemopyelectasis, hemopyelectasia
Hemoplásico: hemoplastic
Hemoplastia: hemoplasty
Hemopneumopericárdio: hemopneumopericardium, pneumohemopericardium
Hemopneumotórax: hemopneumothorax
Hemopoese: hemopoiesis
Hemopoético: hemafacient, hemopoietic
Hemopoetina: hemopoietin
Hemoporfirina: hemoporphyrin
Hemoprecipitina: hemoprecipitin
Hemoproteína: hemoprotein
Hemoptise: hemoptysis
Hemorragia: flood, flooding, hemorrhage
Hemorrágico: hemorrhagic
Hemorraginas: hemorrhagins
Hemorreologia: hemorheology
Hemorrepelente: hemorepellant
Hemorróida: hemorrhoid
Hemorroidário: hemorrhoidal
Hemorróidas: hemorrhoids, piles
Hemorroidectomia: hemorrhoidectomy
Hemospermia: hemospermia
Hemosporídio: hemosporidium
Hemosporinas: hemosporines
Hemossalpinge: hemosalpinx
Hemossialêmese: hemosialemesis
Hemossiderina: hemosiderin
Hemossiderose: hemosiderosis
Hemostasia: hemostasia, hemostasis
Hemostático: hemostatic
Hemostato: hemostat
Hemostíptico: hemostyptic
Hemotacograma: hemotachogram
Hemoterapia, hemoterapêutica: hemotherapy, hemotherapeutics
Hemotímpano: hemotympanum
Hemotísica: hemophthisis
Hemotocitozoário: hematocytozoon
Hemotórax: hemathorax, hemothorax

Hemotóxico, hematotóxico, hematóxico: hemotoxic, hematotoxic, hematoxic
Hemotoxina: hemotoxin
Hemotrofo: hemotroph, hemotrophe
Hemotrópico: hemotropic
Hemozoário: hemozoon
Hemozóico: hemozoic
Hena: henna
Henry (H): henry (H)
Heparana N-sulfatase: heparan N-sulfatase
Heparina: heparin
Heparinase: heparinase
Heparinemia: heparinemia
Heparinizar: heparinize
Hepatatrofia: hepatatrophia, hepatatrophy
Hepatectomia: hepatectomy
Hepático: hepatic
Hepatina: hepatin
Hepatite: hepatitis
Hepatítico: hepatitic
Hepatização: hepatization
Hepatoblastoma: hepatoblastoma
Hepatocarcinoma: hepatocarcinoma
Hepatocele: hepatocele
Hepatocístico: hepatocystic
Hepatócito: hepatocyte
Hepatocolangioenterostomia: hepatocholangioenterostomy
Hepatocolangiojejunostomia: hepatocholangiojejunostomy
Hepatocolangiostomia: hepatocholangiostomy
Hepatocolangite: hepatocholangitis
Hepatocupreína: hepatocuprein
Hepatodisenteria: hepatodysentery
Hepatodocotomia: hepaticodochotomy
Hepatoduodenostomia: hepaticoduodenostomy, hepatoduodenostomy
Hepatoemia: hepatohemia
Hepatoentérico: hepatoenteric
Hepatoenterostomia: hepaticoenterostomy
Hepatoesplenite: hepatosplenitis
Hepatoesplenografia: hepatosplenography
Hepatoesplenomegalia: hepatosplenomegaly
Hepatoesplenopatia: hepatosplenopathy
Hepatofima: hepatophyma
Hepatófugo: hepatofugal
Hepatogástrico: hepatogastric
Hepatogastrostomia: hepaticogastrostomy
Hepatogênico: hepatogenic, hepatogenous
Hepatografia: hepatography
Hepatóide: hepatoid
Hepatojugularômetro: hepatojugularometer

Hepatolienografia: hepatolienography
Hepatolienomegalia: hepatolienomegaly
Hepatolisina: hepatolysin
Hepatolitectomia: hepatolithectomy
Hepatolitíase: hepatolithiasis
Hepatólito: hepatolith
Hepatolitotomia: hepaticolithotomy
Hepatolitotripsia: hepaticolithotripsy
Hepatologia: hepatology
Hepatologista: hepatologist
Hepatoma: hepatoma
Hepatomalacia: hepatomalacia
Hepatomegalia: hepatomegaly, hepatomegalia
Hepatomelanose: hepatomelanosis
Hepatonecrose: hepatonecrosis
Hepatonéfrico: hepatonephric
Hepatonefromegalia: hepatonephromegaly
Hepatônfalo: hepatomphalos
Hepatonfalocele: hepatomphalocele
Hepatopatia: hepatopathy
Hepatopático: hepatopathic
Hepatoperitonite: hepatoperitonitis
Hepatópeto: hepatopetal
Hepatopexia: hepatopexy
Hepatopneumônico: hepatopneumonic
Hepatoporta: hepatoportal
Hepatoptose: hepatoptosis
Hepatopulmonar: hepaticopulmonary, hepatopulmonary
Hepatorrafia: hepatorrhaphy
Hepatorragia: hepatorrhagia
Hepatorrenal: hepatorenal
Hepatorrexe: hepatorrhexis
Hepatoscopia: hepatoscopy
Hepatostomia: hepaticostomy, hepatostomy
Hepatoterapia: hepatotherapy
Hepatotomia: hepaticotomy, hepatotomy
Hepatotoxemia: hepatotoxemia
Hepatotoxicidade: hepatotoxicity
Hepatotóxico: hepatotoxic
Hepatotoxina: hepatotoxin
Heptanal: heptanal
Heptapeptídeo: heptapeptide
Heptavalente: heptad
Heptoclor: heptachlor
Heptose: heptose
Heptulose: heptulose
Hera venenosa, carvalho venenoso, sumagre venenoso: poison ivy, poison oak, poison sumac
Herança: heritage, inheritance
Herbívoro: herbivorous
Hereditariedade: genealogy, heredity, heritability

Hereditário: hereditary, inherited
Heredopatia atáxica polineuritiforme: heredopathia atactica polyneuritiformis
Heredotaxia: heredotaxia
Hermafrodismo: hermaphrodism
Hermafrodita: hermaphrodite
Hermafroditismo: hermaphroditism
Hermético: hermetic
Hérnia: hernia, rupture
Hérnia abdominal: laparocele
Herniação: herniation
Herniado: herniated
Herniário: hernial
Hernioenterotomia: hernioenterotomy
Herniografia: herniography
Hernióide: hernioid
Herniolaparotomia: herniolaparotomy
Herniopunção: herniopuncture
Herniorrafia: herniorrhaphy
Herniotomia: herniotomy
Herniótomo: herniotome
Heróico: heroic
Heroína: heroin (H)
Herpangina: herpangina
Herpes: herpes
Herpes zoster: shingles
Herpesvírus: herpesvirus
Herpético: herpetic
Herpetiforme: herpetiform
Herpetologia: herpetology
Herpetologista: herpetologist
Herpetovírus: herpetovirus
Hertz: hertz (Hz)
Hertziano: hertzian
Hesitação: hesitancy
Hesitante: hesitant
Hesperidina: hesperidin
Hetamido: hetastarch
Heteradelfo: heteradelphus
Heterálio: heteralius
Heteraxial: heteraxial
Heterécio: heterecious
Heterecismo: heterecism
Heterestesia: heteresthesia
Heteroaglutinina: heteroagglutinin
Heteroalelos: heteroalleles
Heteroanticorpo: heteroantibody
Heteroanti-soro: heteroantiserum
Heteroátomo: heteroatom
Heteroblástico: heteroblastic
Heterocárion: heterokaryon
Heterocariótico: heterokaryotic
Heterocéfalo: heterocephalus
Heterocelular: heterocellular
Heterocêntrico: heterocentric
Heteroceratoplastia: heterokeratoplasty
Heterocinese: heterokinesis
Heterocinesia: heterokinesia
Heterocitotrópico: heterocytotropic
Heterocládico: heterocladic

Heterócrino: heterocrine
Heterocrise: heterocrisis
Heterocromático: heterochromatic
Heterocromatina: heterochromatin
Heterocromia: heterochromia
Heterocrômico: heterochromous
Heterocronia: heterochronia
Heterocrônico: heterochronic, heterochronous
Heterócrono: heterochron
Heteródimo: heterodymus
Heterodisperso: heterodisperse
Heterodonte: heterodont
Heterodrômico: heterodromous
Heteroduplex: heteroduplex
Heteroenxerto: heterograft
Heteroerotismo: heteroeroticism
Heterofagia: heterophagy
Heterofíase: heterophyiasis
Heterofíideo: heterophyid
Heterofiidíase: heterophyidiasis
Heterófilo: heterophil, heterophile
Heterofonia: heterophonia
Heteroforia: heterophoria
Heteroftalmia: heterophthalmus
Heteroftongia: heterophthongia
Heterogamético: heterogametic
Heterogamia: heterogamy
Heterogâmico: heterogamous
Heterogeneidade: heterogeneity
Heterogêneo: heterogeneous, heterogenous
Heterogênese: heterogenesis
Heterogenético: heterogenetic
Heterogênico: heterogenic, heterogeneic
Heterogenota: heterogenote
Heteroglicana: heteroglycan
Heterolateral: heterolateral
Heterolipídios: heterolipids
Heterólise: heterolysis
Heterolisina: heterolysin
Heteroliteral: heteroliteral
Heterolítico: heterolytic
Heterologia: heterology
Heterólogo: heterologous
Heteromastigota: heteromastigote
Heteromérico: heteromeral, heteromeric, heteromerous
Heterometábolo: heterometabolous
Heterometaplasia: heterometaplasia
Heterométrico: heterometric
Heterometropia: heterometropia
Heteromorfismo: heteromorphism
Heteromorfo: heteromorphous
Heteromorfose: heteromorphosis
Heterônimo: heteronymous
Heteronomia: heteronomy
Heterônomo: heteronomous
Heteronuclear: heteronuclear
Herópago: heteropagus
Heteropatia: heteropathy
Heteropicnose: heteropyknosis

Glossário

Heteropicnótico: heteropyknotic
Heteroplasia: heteroplasia
Heteroplásico: heteroplastic
Heteroplastídeo: heteroplastid
Heteroplóide: heteroploid
Heteroploidia: heteroploidy
Heteropolissacarídeo: heteropolysaccharide
Heteroproteose: heteroproteose
Heteroquiro: heterocheiral, heterochiral
Heterorreceptor: heteroreceptor
Heteroscedasticidade: heteroscedasticity
Heterose: heterosis
Heterosídeo: heteroside
Heterosmia: heterosmia
Heterospecífico: heterospecific
Heterossacarídeo: heterosaccharide
Heterossexual: heterosexual
Heterossexualidade: heterosexuality
Heterossoma: heterosome
Heterossugestão: heterosuggestion
Heterotálico: heterothallic
Heterotaxia: heterotaxia, heterotaxis, heterotaxy
Heterotáxico: heterotaxic
Heterotérmico: heterothermic
Heterotermo: heterotherm
Heterótico: heterotic
Heterotípico: heterotypic
Heterotonia: heterotonia
Heterotopia: heterotopia
Heterotópico: heterotopic
Heterótopo: heterotopous
Heterotransplante: heterotransplantation
Heterotricose: heterotrichosis
Heterotrofia: heterotrophy
Heterotrófico: heterotrophic
Heterótrofo: heterotroph
Heterotropia: heterotropia, heterotropy
Heteroxantina: heteroxanthine
Heteroxeno: heteroxenous
Heterozigosidade: heterozygosity, heterozygosis
Heterozigoto: heterozygote, heterozygous
Heterozóico: heterozoic
Hexacanto: hexacanth
Hexacloreto de gamabenzeno: gamma benzene hexachloride (GBH)
Hexaclorociclo-hexano: hexachlorocyclohexane
Hexaclorofano: hexachlorophane
Hexaclorofeno: hexachlorophene
Hexacosanol: hexacosanol
Hexacosil: hexacosyl
Hexadactilia: hexadactyly, hexadactylism
1-hexadecanol: 1-hexadecanol
Hexamérico: hexameric
Hexâmero: hexamer
Hexametazima [HMPAO]: hexametazime (HMPAO)
Hexametilpropilenamina oxima: hexamethylpropyleneamine oxime
Hexamina: hexamine
Hexano: hexane
Hexanoato: hexanoate
Hexanoil: hexanoyl
Hexapeptídeo: hexapeptide
Hexaploidia: hexaploidy
Hexavalente: sexivalent
Hexestrol: hexestrol
Hexil: hexyl
Hexilresorcinol: hexylresorcinol
Hexitol: hexitol
Hexocinase: hexokinase
Hexon: hexon
Hexosamina: hexosamine
Hexosaminidase: hexosaminidase
Hexosanos: hexosans
Hexose: hexose
Hexose difosfatase: hexosebisphosphatase, hexosediphosphatase
Hexose fosfatase: hexose phosphatase
Hexose fosfato isomerase: hexosephosphate isomerase
Hexose-1-fosfato uridililtransferase: hexose-1-phosphate uridylyltransferase
Hexulose: hexulose
Hialina: hyalin
Hialinização: hyalinization
Hialino: hyaline
Hialinose: hyalinosis
Hialinúria: hyalinuria
Hialite: hyalitis
Hialócito: hyalocyte
Hialofagia: hyalophagia, hyalophagy
Hialofobia: hyalophobia
Hialogênios: hyalogens
Hialo-hifomicose: hyalohyphomycosis
Hialóide: hyaloid
Hialômero: hyalomere
Hialoplasma: hyaloplasm, hyaloplasma
Hialose: hyalosis
Hialosserosite: hyaloserositis
Hialossoma: hyalosome
Hialurato: hyalurate
Hialuronato: hyaluronate
Hialuronidase: hyaluronidase
Hialuronoglicosaminidase: hyaluronoglucosaminidase
Hialuronoglicuronidase: hyaluronoglucuronidase
Hiatal: hiatal
Hiato: hiatus
Hibaroxia: hybaroxia
Hibenzato: hybenzate
Hibernação: hibernation
Hibernoma: hibernoma
Hibridismo: hybridism
Hibridização: crossbreeding, hybridization
Híbrido: crossbreed, hybrid
Hibridoma: hybridoma
Hiclato: hyclate
Hidantoína: hydantoin
Hidantoinato: hydantoinate
Hidátide: hydatid
Hidatidocele: hydatidocele
Hidatidose: hydatidosis
Hidatidostomia: hydatidostomy
Hidatiforme: hydatidiform
Hidatóide: hydatoid
Hidracetina: hydracetin
Hidradenite: hidradenitis, hydradenitis
Hidradenoma: hidradenoma, hydradenoma
Hidragogo: hydragogue
Hidralostano: hydrallostane
Hidrâmnio: hydramnios, hydramnion
Hidranencefalia: hydranencephaly
Hidrargiria: hydrargyria, hydrargyrism
Hidrargírio: hydrargyrum
Hidrartrodial: hydrarthrodial
Hidrartrose: hydrarthrosis
Hidrase: hydrase
Hidraste: hydrastis, jaundice root, yellow root
Hidraste-do-canadá (*Hydrastis canadensis*): golden seal
Hidrastina: hydrastine
Hidrastinina: hydrastinine
Hidratação: hydration
Hidratado: hydrated, hydrous
Hidratase: hydratase
Hidrato: hydrate
Hidrato de tricetoidrindeno: triketohydrindene hydrate
Hidrazida: hydrazide
Hidrazina: hydrazine
Hidrazinólise: hydrazinolysis
Hidrazona: hydrazone
Hidremia: hydremia, polyplasmia
Hidrencefalia: hydrencephalus
Hidrencefalocele: hydrencephalocele
Hidrencefalomeningocele: hydrencephalomeningocele
Hidreto: hydride
Hidreto de arsênico: arsenous hydride
Hidriático: hydriatric, hydriatic
Hídrico: hydric
Hidrindantina: hydrindantin
Hidroa: hidroa, hydroa
Hidroadipsia: hydroadipsia
Hidroapêndice: hydroappendix
Hidrobilirrubina: hydrobilirubin
Hidrocalicose: hydrocalycosis
Hidrocarboneto: hydrocarbon
Hidrocefalia: hydrocephalus, hydrocephaly
Hidrocefálico: hydrocephalic
Hidrocefalocele: hydrocephalocele
Hidrocefalóide: hydrocephaloid
Hidrocele: hydrocele
Hidrocelectomia: hydrocelectomy
Hidrocianismo: hydrocyanism
Hidrocinética: hydrokinetics
Hidrocinético: hydrokinetic
Hidrocisto: hydrocyst
Hidrocistoma: hidrocystoma, hydrocystoma
Hidroclorotiazida (HCTZ): hydrochlorothiazide
Hidrocodona: hydrocodone
Hidrocolecisto: hydrocholecystis
Hidrocolerese: hydrocholeresis
Hidrocolerético: hydrocholeretic
Hidrocolóide: hydrocolloid
Hidrocolpocele: hydrocolpocele, hydrocolpos
Hidrocortisona: hydrocortisone
Hidrocotarnina: hydrocotarnine
Hidrodinâmica: hydrodynamics
Hidrodipsia: hydrodipsia
Hidrodipsomania: hydrodipsomania
Hidrodiurese: hydrodiuresis
Hidroencefalocele: hydroencephalocele
Hidroesfigmógrafo: hydrosphygmograph
Hidrofilia: hydrophilia
Hidrofílico: hydrophilic
Hidrófilo: hydrophil, hydrophile, hydrophilous
Hidrofobia: hydrophobia
Hidrofóbico: hydrophobic
Hidroftalmia: hydrophthalmia, hydrophthalmos, hydrophthalmus
Hidrogel: hydrogel
Hidrogenação: hydrogenation
Hidrogenase: hydrogenase
Hidrogenase fumárica: fumaric hydrogenase
Hidrogênio: hydrogen (H)
Hidrogênio-1: hydrogen-1 (^{1}H)
Hidrogênio-2: hydrogen-2 (^{2}H)
Hidrogênio-3: hydrogen-3 (^{3}H)
Hidrogenliase: hydrogenlyase
Hidroiodeto-iodo de diglicocola: diglycocoll hydroiodide-iodine
Hidrolábil: hydrolabile
Hidrolabilidade: hydrolability
Hidrolases: hydrolases
Hidroliases: hydrolyases
Hidrolinfa: hydrolymph
Hidrolisado: hydrolysate
Hidrolisado de proteínas: protein hydrolysate
Hidrolisar: hydrolyze
Hidrólise: hydrolysis
Hidrolítico: hydrolytic
Hidroma: hydroma
Hidromassagem: hydromassage
Hidromeiose: hidromeiosis
Hidromeningocele: hydromeningocele
Hidrometria: hydrometra, hydrometry

Hidrométrico: hydrometric
Hidrômetro: hydrometer
Hidrometrocolpo: hydrometrocolpos
Hidromicrocefalia: hydromicrocephaly
Hidromielia: hydromyelia
Hidromielocele: hydromyelocele
Hidronefrose: hydronephrosis, pelvocaliectasis
Hidronefrótico: hydronephrotic
Hidrônfalo: hydromphalus
Hidrônio: hydronium
Hidroparassalpinge: hydroparasalpinx
Hidropatia: hydropathy
Hidropático: hydropathic
Hidropenia: hydropenia
Hidropênico: hydropenic
Hidropericárdio: hydropericardium
Hidroperiodeto de tetraglicina: tetraglycine hydroperiodine
Hidroperitônio: hydroperitoneum, hydroperitonia
Hidroperoxidases: hydroperoxidases
Hidroperóxido: hydroperoxide
Hidrópico: dropsical, hydropic
Hidropionefrose: hydropyonephrosis
Hidropisia: dropsy, hydrops
Hidropneumatose: hydropneumatosis
Hidropneumopericárdio: hydropneumopericardium
Hidropneumoperitônio: hydropneumoperitoneum
Hidropneumotórax: hydropneumothorax, pneumoserothorax
Hidropoese: hidropoiesis
Hidroposia: hydroposia
Hidroquinol: hydroquinol
Hidroquinona: hydroquinone
Hidrorquia: hydrorchis
Hidrorréia: hydrorrhea
Hidrorreostato: hydrorheostat
Hidrose: hidrosis
Hidrosquese: hidroschesis
Hidrossalpinge: hydrosalpinx
Hidrossarca: hydrosarca
Hidrossarcocele: hydrosarcocele
Hidrossiringomielia: hydrosyringomyelia
Hidrossol: hydrosol
Hidrossudopatia: hydrosudopathy
Hidrossudoterapia: hydrosudotherapy
Hidrostático: hydrostatic
Hidrostato: hydrostat
Hidrotaxia: hydrotaxis
Hidroterapêutica: hydrotherapeutics
Hidroterapêutico: hydrotherapeutic
Hidroterapia: hydrotherapy
Hidrotérmico: hydrothermal
Hidrótico: hidrotic
Hidrotionemia: hydrothionemia
Hidrotionúria: hydrothionuria
Hidrotomia: hydrotomy
Hidrotórax: hydrothorax
Hidrotropismo: hydrotropism
Hidrotubação: hydrotubation
Hidroureter: hydroureter
Hidroureteronefrose: hydroureteronephrosis
Hidrovário: hydrovarium
Hidroxiácido: hydroxy acid
3-hidroxiacil-CoA desidrogenase: 3-hydroxyacyl-CoA dehydrogenase
Hidroxiacilglutationa hidrolase: hydroxyacylglutathione hydrolase
Hidroxianisol butilado: butylated hydroxyanisole (BHA)
Hidroxiapatita: hydroxyapatite
γ-hidroxibutirato: γ-hydroxybutyrate (GHB)
4-hidroxibutirato: 4-hydroxybutyrate
4-hidroxibutiricacidúria: 4-hydroxybutyric aciduria
Hidroxicarbamida: hydroxycarbamide
3-L-hidroxicinurenina: 3-L-hydroxykynurenine
Hidroxicinureninúria: hydroxykynureninuria
25-hidroxicolecalciferol: 25-hydroxycholecalciferol (HCC)
7α-hidroxicolesterol: 7α-hydroxycholesterol
Hidroxicromano: hydroxychroman
Hidroxicromeno: hydroxychromene
Hidróxido: hydroxide
Hidróxido férrico: ferric hydroxide
Hidroxiefedrina: hydroxyephedrine
Hidroxiemina: hydroxyhemin
25-hidroxiergocalciferol: 25-hydroxyergocalciferol
3β-hidroxiesteróide sulfatase: 3β-hydroxysteroid sulfatase
α-hidroxietiltiamina pirofosfato: α-hydroxyethylthiamin pyrophosphate
Hidroxifenilúria: hydroxyphenyluria
Hidroxila: hydroxyl
Hidroxilação: hydroxylation
Hidroxilamina: hydroxylamine
Hidroxilamino: hydroxylamino
Hidroxilapatita: hydroxylapatite
Hidroxilases: hydroxylases
δ-hidroxilisina: δ-hydroxylysine
5-hidroxilisina: 5-hydroxylysine (5Hyl)
3-hidroxi-3-metilglutaril-CoA: 3-hydroxy-3-methylglutaryl-CoA
β-hidroxi-β-metilglutaril-CoA (HMG-CoA): β-hydroxy-β-methylglutaryl-CoA (HMG-CoA)
Hidroxinaftoato de befênio: bephenium hydroxynaphthoate
Hidroxinervona: hydroxynervone
3α-hidroxi-5α-pregnan-20-ona: 3α-hydroxy-5α-pregnan-20-one
17α-hidroxiprogesterona: 17α-hydroxyprogesterone
21-hidroxiprogesterona: 21-hydroxyprogesterone
3-hidroxiprolina: 3-hydroxyproline (3Hyp)
4-hidroxiprolina: 4-hydroxyproline (4Hyp, Hyp)
Hidroxiprolinemia: hydroxyprolinemia
15-hidroxiprostaglandina desidrogenase: 15-hydroxyprostaglandin dehydrogenase
6-hidroxipurina: 6-hydroxypurine
8-hidroxiquinolina: 8-hydroxyquinoline
3-hidroxitiramina: 3-hydroxytyramine
Hidroxitolueno butilado: butylated hydroxytoluene (BHT)
5-hidroxitriptamina: 5-hydroxytryptamine (5-HT)
Hidroxitriptofano descarboxilase: hydroxytryptophan decarboxylase
Hidroxiuréia: hydroxyurea
Hidroxizina: hydroxyzine
Hidroxocobalamina: hydroxocobalamin
Hidroxocobemina: hydroxocobemine
Hierarquia: hierarchy
Hierofobia: hierophobia
Hieroterapia: hierotherapy
Hifa: hypha, **pl.** hyphae
Hifema: hyphema
Hifemia: hyphemia
Hifomicose: hyphomycosis
Higiene: hygiene
Higiênico: hygienic
Higienista: hygieist, hygienist
Higiologia: hygieiology
Hígrico: hygric
Higrofobia: hygrophobia
Higroma: hygroma
Higrometria: hygrometry
Higrômetro: hygrometer
Higroscópico: hygroscopic
Higrostomia: hygrostomia
Hilar: hilar
Hilariante: exhilarant
Hilefobia: hylephobia
Hilite: hilitis
Hilo: hilum, hilus, **pl.** hila, hyla
Himantose: himantosis
Hímen: hymen
Himenal: hymenal
Himenectomia: hymenectomy
Himenite: hymenitis
Himenóide: hymenoid
Himenolepíase: hymenolepiasis
Himenolepidídeo: hymenolepidid
Himenologia: hymenology
Himenorrafia: hymenorrhaphy
Himenotomia: hymenotomy
Hioepiglótico: hyoepiglottic, hyoepiglottidean
Hiofaríngeo: hyopharyngeus
Hioglosso: hyoglossal, hyoglossus
Hióide: hyoid
Hiosciamina: hyoscyamine
Hioscíamo: hyoscyamus
Hioscina: hyoscine
Hiotireóideo: hyothyroid
Hipalgesia: hypalgesia
Hipalgésico: hypalgesic, hypalgetic
Hipâmnio: hypamnion, hypamnios
Hipanacinesia: hypanakinesia, hypanakinesis
Hiparterial: hyparterial
Hipaxial: hypaxial
Hipazotúria: hypazoturia
Hipencéfalo: hypencephalon
Hipengiofobia: hypengyophobia
Hiperabdução: hyperabduction
Hiperacidemia pipecólica: hyperpipecolic acidemia
Hiperacidez: hyperacidity
Hiperacidúria β-aminoisobutírica: hyper-β-aminoisobutyric aciduria
Hiperacusia: hyperacusis, hyperacusia
Hiperadenose: hyperadenosis
Hiperadiposidade: hyperadiposis, hyperadiposity
Hiperadrenocorticalismo: hyperadrenocorticalism
Hiperadrenocorticismo: hyperadrenalcorticalism
Hiperafia: hyperaphia
Hiperáfico: hyperaphic
Hiper-β-alaninemia: hyper-β-alaninemia
Hiperalaninemia: hyperalaninemia
Hiperalantoinúria: hyperallantoinuria
Hiperaldosteronismo: hyperaldosteronism
Hiperalfalipoproteinemia: hyperalphalipoproteinemia
Hiperalgesia: hyperalgesia
Hiperalgésico: hyperalgesic, hyperalgetic
Hiperalimentação: hyperalimentation

Hiperamilasemia: hyperamylasemia
Hiperaminoacidúria: hyperaminoaciduria
Hiperamonemia: hyperammonemia
Hiperanacinesia: hyperanacinesia, hyperanacinesis, hyperanakinesia, hyperanakinesis
Hiperaprendizado: overlearning
Hiperargininemia: hyperargininemia
Hiperatividade: hyperactivity
Hiperbárico: hyperbaric
Hiperbarismo: hyperbarism
Hiperbetalipoproteinemia: hyperbetalipoproteinemia
Hiperbilirrubinemia: hyperbilirubinemia
Hiperbraquicefalia: hyperbrachycephaly
Hipercalcemia: hypercalcemia
Hipercalcinúria: hypercalcinuria
Hipercalciúria: hypercalciuria
Hipercalcúria: hypercalcuria
Hipercaliemia: hyperkaliemia
Hipercaliurese: hyperkaluresis
Hipercapnia: hypercapnia
Hipercarbia: hypercarbia
Hipercardia: hypercardia
Hipercatabólico: hypercatabolic
Hipercatabolismo: hypercatabolism
Hipercatarse: hypercatharsis
Hipercatexe: hypercathexis
Hipercementose: hypercementosis
Hiperceratinização: hyperkeratinization
Hiperceratose: hyperkeratosis
Hipercetonemia: hyperketonemia
Hipercetonúria: hyperketonuria
Hipercianótico: hypercyanotic
Hiperciese: hypercyesis, hypercyesia
Hipercinemia: hyperkinemia
Hipercinese, hipercinesia: hypercinesis, hypercinesia, hyperkinesis, hyperkinesia
Hipercinético: hyperkinetic
Hipercitemia: hypercythemia
Hipercitocromia: hypercytochromia
Hipercitose: hypercytosis
Hipercloremia: hyperchloremia
Hipercloridria: hyperchlorhydria
Hiperclorúria: hyperchloruria
Hipercoagulabilidade: hypercoagulability
Hipercoagulável: hypercoagulable
Hipercolesterinemia: hypercholesterinemia
Hipercolesterolemia: hypercholesteremia, hypercholesterolemia

Hipercolesterolia: hypercholesterolia
Hipercolia: hypercholia
Hipercorreção: overcorrection
Hipercorticoidismo: hypercorticoidism
Hipercortisolismo: hypercortisolism
Hipercrialgesia: hypercryalgesia
Hipercriestesia: hypercryesthesia
Hipercromafinismo: hyperchromaffinism
Hipercromasia: hyperchromasia
Hipercromático: hyperchromatic
Hipercromatismo: hyperchromatism
Hipercromia: hyperchromia
Hipercrômico: hyperchromic
Hipercupremia: hypercupremia
Hiperdetecção: oversensing
Hiperdicrótico: hyperdicrotic
Hiperdicrotismo: hyperdicrotism
Hiperdiplóide: hyperdiploid
Hiperdipsia: hyperdipsia
Hiperdistensão: hyperdistention
Hiperecóico: hyperechoic
Hiperecplexia: hyperekplexia
Hiperedonia, hiperedonismo: hyperhedonia, hiperhedonism
Hiperêmese: hyperemesis
Hiperemético: hyperemetic
Hiperemia: hyperemia
Hiperêmico: hyperemic
Hiperencefalia: hyperencephaly
Hipereosinofilia: hypereosinophilia
Hiperergia: hyperergia
Hiperérgico: hyperergic
Hipereritrocitemia: hypererythrocythemia
Hiperesoforia: hyperesophoria
Hiperesplenismo: hypersplenism
Hiperesqueocitose: hyperskeocytosis
Hiperesteatose: hypersteatosis
Hiperestenia: hypersthenia
Hiperestênico: hypersthenic
Hiperestenúria: hypersthenuria
Hiperestesia: hyperesthesia
Hiperestésico: hyperesthetic
Hipereuriprosópico: hypereuryprosopic
Hiperexoforia: hyperexophoria
Hiperextensão: hyperextension, overextension
Hiperfagia: hyperphagia
Hiperfalangismo: hyperphalangism, polyphalangism
Hiperfenilalaninemia: hyperphenylalaninemia
Hiperferremia: hyperferremia
Hiperfibrinogenemia: hyperfibrinogenemia
Hiperfibrinólise: hyperfibrinolysis

Hiperflexão: hyperflexion
Hiperfonese: hyperphonesis
Hiperfonia: hyperphonia
Hiperforia: hyperphoria
Hiperfosfatasemia: hyperphosphatasemia
Hiperfosfatasia: hyperphosphatasia
Hiperfosfatemia: hyperphosphatemia
Hiperfosfatúria: hyperphosphaturia
Hiperfrenia: hyperphrenia
Hiperfrutosemia: hyperfructosemia
Hipergalactose: hypergalactosis
Hipergamaglobulinemia: hypergammaglobulinemia
Hiperganglionose: hyperganglionosis
Hipergênese: hypergenesis
Hipergenético: hypergenetic
Hipergenitalismo: hypergenitalism
Hipergeusia: hypergeusia
Hipergia: hypergia
Hipérgico: hypergic
Hiperginecosmia: hypergynecosmia
Hiperglandular: hyperglandular
Hiperglicemia: hyperglycemia
Hipergliceridemia: hyperglyceridemia
Hiperglicinemia: hyperglycinemia
Hiperglicinúria: hyperglycinuria
Hiperglicogenólise: hyperglycogenolysis
Hiperglicorraquia: hyperglycorrhachia
Hiperglicosemia: hyperglycosemia
Hiperglicosúria: hyperglycosuria
Hiperglioxilemia: hyperglyoxylemia
Hiperglobulia, hiperglobulismo: hyperglobulia, hyperglobulism
Hiperglobulinemia: hyperglobulinemia
Hipergnose: hypergnosis
Hipergonadismo: hypergonadism
Hipergonadotrópico: hypergonadotropic
Hipergranulose: hypergranulosis
Hiperguanidinemia: hyperguanidinemia
Hiper-hemoglobinemia: hyperhemoglobinemia
Hiper-heparinemia: hyperheparinemia
Hiperidratação: hyperhydration
Hiperidrocloria: hyperhydrochloria

Hiperidrocloridia: hyperhydrochloridia
Hiperidropexia: hyperhydropexy, hyperhydropexis
Hiperidrose: hyperhidrosis, sudorrhea
Hiperidroxiprolinemia: hyperhydroxyprolinemia
Hiperimidodipeptidúria: hyperimidodipeptiduria
Hiperimune: hyperimmune
Hiperimunidade: hyperimmunity
Hiperimunização: hyperimmunization
Hiperindicanemia: hyperindicanemia
Hiperinfecção: hyperinfection
Hiperinflação: hyperinflation
Hiperinose: hyperinosis
Hiperinosemia: hyperinosemia
Hiperinsulinemia: hyperinsulinemia
Hiperinsulinismo: hyperinsulinism
Hiperinvolução: hyperinvolution
Hiperisotônico: hyperisotonic
Hiperlactação: hyperlactation
Hiperleucocitose: hyperleukocytosis
Hiperlexia: hyperlexia
Hiperlipemia: hyperlipemia
Hiperlipidemia: hyperlipidemia
Hiperlipoidemia: hyperlipoidemia
Hiperlipoproteinemia: hyperlipoproteinemia
Hiperlipose: hyperliposis
Hiperlisinemia: hyperlysinemia
Hiperlisinúria: hyperlysinuria
Hiperlitúria: hyperlithuria
Hiperlogia: hyperlogia
Hiperlordose: hyperlordosis
Hipermagnesemia: hypermagnesemia
Hipermastia: hypermastia
Hipermenorréia: hypermenorrhea
Hipermetabolismo: hypermetabolism
Hipermetamorfose: hypermetamorphosis
Hipermetioninemia: hypermethioninemia
Hipermetria: hypermetria
Hipermétrope: hypermetrope
Hipermetropia: farsightedness, hypermetropia
Hipermiotrofia: hypermyotrophy
Hipermnésia: hypermnesia
Hipermobilidade: hypermobility
Hipermorfo: hypermorph
Hipernatremia: hypernatremia
Hipernefróide: hypernephroid
Hiperneocitose: hyperneocytosis
Hipernóia: hypernoia

Hipernômico: hypernomic
Hipernutrição: hypernutrition
Hiperoncótico: hyperoncotic
Hiperoníquia: hyperonychia
Hiperope: hyperope
Hiperopia: hyperopia (H)
Hiperópico: hyperopic (H)
Hiperoralidade: hyperorality
Hiperorexia: hyperorexia
Hiperornitinemia: hyperornithinemia
Hiperortocitose: hyperorthocytosis
Hiperosmia: hyperosmia
Hiperosmolalidade: hyperosmolality
Hiperosmolaridade: hyperosmolarity
Hiperosmótico: hyperosmotic
Hiperosteoidose: hyperosteoidosis
Hiperostose: hyperostosis
Hiperovarianismo: hyperovarianism
Hiperoxalúria: hyperoxaluria
Hiperoxia: hyperoxia
Hiperoxidação: hyperoxidation
Hiperpancreatismo: hyperpancreatism
Hiperparasita: hyperparasite
Hiperparasitismo: hyperparasitism
Hiperparatireoidismo: hyperparathyroidism
Hiperparotidismo: hyperparotidism
Hiperpatia: hyperpathia
Hiperpepsia: hyperpepsia
Hiperpepsinia: hyperpepsinia
Hiperperistaltismo: hyperperistalsis
Hiperpiese: hyperpiesis, hyperpiesia
Hiperpiético: hyperpietic
Hiperpigmentação: hyperpigmentation
Hiperpipecolatemia: hyperpipecolatemia
Hiperpirético: hyperpyretic, hyperpyrexial
Hiperpirexia: hyperpyrexia
Hiperpituitarismo: hyperpituitarism
Hiperplasia: hyperplasia
Hiperplásico: hyperplastic
Hiperpnéia: hyperpnea
Hiperpolarização: hyperpolarization
Hiperpotassemia: hyperkalemia, hyperpotassemia
Hiperpré-β-lipoproteinemia: hyperprebetalipoproteinemia
Hiperprocorese: hyperprochoresis
Hiperpró-insulinemia: hyperproinsulinemia
Hiperprolactinemia: hyperprolactinemia
Hiperprolinemia: hyperprolinemia

Hiperproteinemia: hyperproteinemia
Hiperproteose: hyperproteosis
Hiperquilia: hyperchylia
Hiperquilomicronemia: hyperchylomicronemia
Hiper-reflexia: hyperreflexia
Hiper-resposta: overresponse
Hiper-ressonância: hyperresonance
Hipersaliemia: hypersalemia
Hipersalino: hypersaline
Hipersalivação: hypersalivation
Hipersarcosinemia: hypersarcosinemia
Hipersecreção: hypersecretion
Hipersegmentação: hypersegmentation
Hipersensibilidade: hypersensitivity, tenderness
Hipersensibilização: hypersensitization
Hipersensível: tender
Hiperserotonemia: hyperserotonemia
Hipersístole: hypersystole
Hipersistólico: hypersystolic
Hipersomatotropismo: hypersomatotropism
Hipersonia: hypersomnia
Hipersônico: hypersonic
Hipersuscetibilidade: hypersusceptibility
Hipertecose: hyperthecosis
Hipertelia: hyperthelia
Hipertelorismo: hypertelorism
Hipertensão: hypertension
Hipertensina: hypertensin
Hipertensinogênio: hypertensinogen
Hipertensivo: hypertensive
Hipertensor: hypertensor
Hipertermalgesia: hyperthermalgesia
Hipertermia: hyperthermia
Hipertermoestesia: hyperthermoesthesia
Hipertestoidismo: hypertestoidism
Hipertimia: hyperthymia
Hipertímico: hyperthymic
Hipertimismo: hyperthymism
Hipertimização: hyperthymization
Hipertireoidismo: hyperthyroidism
Hipertireose: hyperthyrea
Hipertirosinemia: hypertyrosinemia
Hipertiroxinemia: hyperthyroxinemia
Hipertonia: hypertonia
Hipertonicidade: hypertonicity
Hipertônico: hypertonic
Hipertransparente: hyperlucent
Hipertricofridia: hypertrichophrydia
Hipertricose: hypertrichosis
Hipertrigliceridemia: hypertriglyceridemia

Hipertriquíase: hypertrichiasis
Hipertrofia: hypertrophia, hypertrophy
Hipertrofia muscular: myopachynsis
Hipertrófico: hypertrophic
Hipertrofo: hypertroph
Hipertrombinemia: hyperthrombinemia
Hipertropia: hypertropia
Hiperuracil timinúria: hyperuracil thyminuria
Hiperuricemia: hyperuricemia
Hiperuricêmico: hyperuricemic
Hiperuricúria: hyperuricuria
Hipervacinação: hypervaccination
Hipervalinemia: hypervalinemia
Hipervascular: hypervascular
Hiperventilação: hyperventilation, overventilation
Hipervitaminose: hypervitaminosis
Hipervolemia: hypervolemia, repletion
Hipervolêmico: hypervolemic
Hipervolia: hypervolia
Hipestesia: hypesthesia
Hipnagógico: hypnagogic
Hipnoanálise: hypnoanalysis
Hipnoanalítico: hypnoanalytic
Hipnocatarse: hypnocatharsis
Hipnocisto: hypnocyst
Hipnofobia: hypnophobia
Hipnogênese: hypnogenesis
Hipnogênico: hypnogenic, hypnogenous
Hipnoidal: hypnoidal
Hipnóide: hypnoid
Hipnopômpico: hypnopompic
Hipnose: hypnosis
Hipnoterapia: hypnotherapy
Hipnótico: hypnotic
Hipnotismo: hypnotism, somnolism
Hipnotizador: hypnotist
Hipnotizar: hypnotize
Hipnozoíta: hypnozoite
Hipoacidez: hypoacidity
Hipoacusia: hypacusia, hypacusis, hypoacusis
Hipoadenia: hypoadenia
Hipoadrenalismo: hypoadrenalism
Hipoalbuminemia: hypalbuminemia, hypoalbuminemia
Hipoaldosteronismo: hypoaldosteronism
Hipoaldosteronúria: hypoaldosteronuria
Hipoalgesia: hypoalgesia
Hipoalimentação: hypoalimentation
Hipoazotúria: hypoazoturia
Hipobaria: hypobaria
Hipobárico: hypobaric
Hipobarismo: hypobarism
Hipobaropatia: hypobaropathy

Hipobetalipoproteinemia: hypobetalipoproteinemia
Hipoblástico: hypoblastic
Hipoblasto: hypoblast
Hipobranquial: hypobranchial
Hipobrometo: hypobromite
Hipocalcemia: hypocalcemia
Hipocalcificação: hypocalcification
Hipocaliemia: hypokalemia
Hipocampal: hippocampal
Hipocampo: hippocampus
Hipocapnia: hypocapnia
Hipocarbia: hypocarbia
Hipoceloma: hypocelom
Hipocicloidal: hypocycloidal
Hipocinemia: hypokinemia
Hipocinese, hipocinesia: hypocinesis, hypocinesia, hypokinesis, hypokinesia
Hipocinético: hypokinetic
Hipocistotomia: hypocystotomy
Hipocitemia: hypocythemia
Hipocitose: hypocytosis
Hipocitratúria: hypocitraturia
Hipocloremia: hypochloremia
Hipoclorêmico: hypochloremic
Hipocloreto: hypochlorite
Hipocloridria: hypochlorhydria
Hipoclorúria: hypochloruria
Hipocolesteremia: hypocholesteremia
Hipocolesterinemia: hypocholesterinemia
Hipocolesterolemia: hypocholesterolemia
Hipocolia: hypocholia
Hipocomplementemia: hypocomplementemia
Hipocondria: hypochondria, hypochondriasis
Hipocondríaco: hypochondriac, hypochondriacal
Hipocôndrio: hypochondrium, **pl.** hypochondria
Hipocondroplasia: hypochondroplasia
Hipocone: hypocone
Hipoconide: hypoconid
Hipocônule: hypoconule
Hipoconulídeo: hypoconulid
Hipocordal: hypochordal
Hipocorticoidismo: hypocorticoidism
Hipocrático: hippocratic
Hipocratismo: hippocratism
Hipocromasia: hypochromasia
Hipocromático: hypochromatic
Hipocromatismo: hypochromatism
Hipocromia: hypochromia
Hipocrômico: hypochromic
Hipocrose: hypochrosis
Hipocupremia: hypocupremia
Hipodactilia: hypodactyly, hypodactylia, hypodactylism
Hipodermatóclise: hypodermatoclysis
Hipodermatomia: hypodermatomy
Hipodermatose: hypodermatosis

Glossário

Hipoderme: hypoderm, hypodermis
Hipodérmico: hypodermic
Hipodermóclise: hypodermoclysis
Hipodinamia: hypodynamia
Hipodinâmico: hypodynamic
Hipodipisia: hypodipsia
Hipodontia: hypodontia
Hipoecóico: hypoechoic
Hipoecrisia: hypoeccrisis
Hipoecrítico: hypoeccritic
Hipoeosinofilia: hypoeosinophilia
Hipoepatia: hypohepatia
Hipoesclerótico: hyposcleral
Hipoesoforia: hypoesophoria
Hipoesplenismo: hyposplenism
Hipoesqueocitose: hyposkeocytosis
Hipoestesia: hypoesthesia
Hipoexoforia: hypoexophoria
Hipofalangismo: hypophalangism
Hipofaringe: hypopharynx
Hipoferremia: hypoferremia
Hipofibrinogenemia: hypofibrinogenemia
Hipofisário: hypophyseal, hypophysial
Hipófise: hypophysis
Hipofisectomia: hypophysectomy
Hipofisectomizar: hypophysectomize
Hipofisina: hypophysin
Hipofisiotrópico: hypophysiotropic
Hipofisite: hypophysitis
Hipofisoprivo: hypophyseoprivic, hypophysioprivic
Hipofisotrópico: hypophyseotropic
Hipofonese: hypophonesis
Hipofonia: hypophonia
Hipoforia: hypophoria
Hipofosfatasemia: hypophosphatasemia
Hipofosfatasia: hypophosphatasia
Hipofosfatemia: hypophosphatemia
Hipofosfatúria: hypophosphaturia
Hipofrasia: hypophrasia
Hipofrontalidade: hypofrontality
Hipofunção: hypofunction
Hipogalácteo: hypogalactous
Hipogalactia: hypogalactia
Hipogamaglobinemia: hypogammaglobinemia
Hipogamaglobulinemia: hypogammaglobulinemia
Hipoganglionose: hypoganglionosis
Hipogástrico: hypogastric
Hipogástrio: hypogastrium
Hipogastrocele: hypogastrocele
Hipogastrópago: hypogastropagus
Hipogastrosquise: hypogastroschisis
Hipogênese: hypogenesis
Hipogenético: hypogenetic
Hipogenitalismo: hypogenitalism
Hipogeusia: hypogeusia
Hipoglicemia: hypoglycemia
Hipoglicêmico: hypoglycemic
Hipoglicogenólise: hypoglycogenolysis
Hipoglicorraquia: hypoglycorrhachia
Hipoglobulia: hypoglobulia
Hipoglosse: hypoglossis
Hipoglosso: hypoglossal, hypoglossus
Hipoglote: hypoglottis
Hipognato: hypognathous, hypognathus
Hipogonadismo: hypogonnadism
Hipogonadotrópico: hypogonadotropic
Hipogranulocitose: hypogranulocytosis
Hipo-hedonismo: hyphedonia
Hipoidremia: hypohydremia
Hipoidrocloria: hypohydrochloria
Hipoidrose: hypohidrosis
Hipoisotônico: hypoisotonic
Hipoleidigismo: hypoleydigism
Hipoleucemia: hypoleukemia
Hipolinfemia: hypolymphemia
Hipolipoproteinemia: hypolipoproteinemia
Hipolipose: hypoliposis
Hipologia: hypologia
Hipomagnesemia: hypomagnesemia
Hipomania: hypomania
Hipomastia: hypomastia
Hipomelancolia: hypomelancholia
Hipomelanose: hypomelanosis
Hipomelia: hypomelia
Hipomenorréia: hypomenorrhea
Hipômero: hypomere
Hipometabolismo: hypometabolism
Hipometria: hypometria
Hipomielinização: hypomyelination, hypomyelinogenesis
Hipomiotonia: hypomyotonia
Hipomixia: hypomyxia
Hipomnésia: hypomnesia
Hipomorfo: hypomorph
Hipomotilidade: hypomotility
Hiponatremia: hyponatremia
Hiponeocitose: hyponeocytosis
Hiponiquial: hyponychial
Hiponíquio: hyponychium, hyponychon
Hiponóia: hyponoia
Hipooncótico: hypooncotic
Hipopancreatismo: hypopancreatism
Hipopancreorréia: hypopancreorrhea
Hipoparatireoidismo: hypoparathyroidism
Hipoperistaltismo: hypoperistalsis
Hipopesia: hypopepsia
Hipopiese: hypopiesis
Hipopigmentação: hypopigmentation
Hipópio: hypopyon
Hipopituitarismo: hypopituitarism
Hipoplasia: hypoplasia
Hipoplásico: hypoplastic
Hipopnéia: hypopnea
Hipoposia: hypoposia
Hipopotassemia: hypopotassemia
Hipoproacelerinemia: hypoproaccelerinemia
Hipoproconvertinemia: hypoproconvertinemia
Hipoproteinemia: hypoproteinemia
Hipoproteinose: hypoproteinosis
Hipoprotrombinemia: hypoprothrombinemia
Hipoptialismo: hypoptyalism
Hipoquilia: hypochylia
Hiporreflexia: hyporeflexia
Hiporreninemia: hyporeninemia
Hiporreninêmico: hyporeninemic
Hiporriboflavinose: hyporiboflavinosis
Hiportocitose: hypoorthocytosis
Hiposfigmia: hyposphygmia
Hiposmia: hyposmia
Hiposmose: hyposmosis
Hiposmótico: hyposmotic
Hipospádia: hypospadias
Hipospadíaco: hypospadiac
Hiposqueotomia: hyposcheotomy
Hipossalivação: hyposalivation
Hipossensibilidade: hyposensitivity
Hipossensibilização: hyposensitization
Hipossístole: hyposystole
Hipossomatotropismo: hyposomatotropism
Hipossomia: hyposomia
Hipossoníaco: hyposomniac
Hipossupradrenalismo: hyposupradrenalism
Hipóstase: hypostasis
Hipostático: hypostatic
Hipostenúria: hyposthenuria
Hipostomia: hypostomia
Hipóstomo: hypostome
Hipostose: hypostosis
Hipotálamo: hypothalamus
Hipotálamo-hipofisário: hypothalamohypophysial
Hipotelorismo: hypotelorism
Hipotenar: hypothenar
Hipotensão: hypotension
Hipotensivo: hypotensive
Hipotensor: hypotensor
Hipotermia: hypothermia
Hipotérmico: hypothermal
Hipótese: hypothesis
Hipotimia: hypothymia
Hipotímico: hypothymic
Hipotimismo: hypothymism
Hipotímpano: hypotympanum
Hipotimpanotomia: hypotympanotomy
Hipotireóideo: hypothyroid
Hipotireoidismo: athyrea, hypothyroidism
Hipotiroxinemia: hypothyroxinemia
Hipotonia: hypotonia, hypotonus, hypotony
Hipotonicidade: hypotonicity
Hipotônico: hypotonic
Hipotricose: hypotrichosis
Hipotriquíase: hypotrichiasis
Hipotrombinemia: hypothrombinemia
Hipotromboplastinemia: hypothromboplastinemia
Hipotropia: hypotropia
Hipourese: hypouresis
Hipouricemia: hypouricemia
Hipouricúria: hypouricuria
Hipovarianismo: hypoovarianism, hypovarianism
Hipoventilação: hypoventilation, underventilation
Hipovitaminose: hypovitaminosis
Hipovolemia: hypovolemia
Hipovolêmico: hypovolemic
Hipovolia: hypovolia
Hipoxantina: hypoxanthine (Hyp)
Hipoxantinosina: hypoxanthinosine
Hipoxemia: hypoxemia
Hipoxia: hypoxia
Hipóxico: hypoxic
Hipsarritmia: hypsarhythmia, hypsarrhythmia
Hipsilóide: hypsiloid
Hipsistafilia: hypsistaphylia
Hipsistenocefálico: hypsistenocephalic
Hipsobraquicefálico: hypsibrachycephalic
Hipsocefalia: hypsicephaly, hypsocephaly
Hipsoconcho: hypsiconchous
Hipsocrômico: hypsochromic
Hipsodonte: hypsodont
Hipurato: hippurate
Hipurgia: hypurgia
Hipúria: hippuria
Hipuricase: hippuricase
Hircismo: hircismus
Hirco: hircus, **gen. e pl.** hirci
Hirsutismo: hirsuties, hirsutism
Hirsuto: hirsute

Hirteloso: hirtellous
Hirudicida: hirudicide
Hirudina: hirudin
Hirudiníase: hirudiniasis
Hirudinização: hirudinization
Histamina: histamine (H)
Histamina-resistente: histamine-fast
Histaminase: histaminase
Histaminemia: histaminemia
Histaminúria: histaminuria
Histângico: histangic
Histeralgia: hysteralgia
Histeratresia: hysteratresia
Histerectomia: hysterectomy
Histerectomia abdominal: abdominohysterectomy
Histerese: hysteresis
Histeria: hysteria
Histérico: hysteric, hysterical, hysterics
Histerocatalepsia: hysterocatalepsy
Histerocele: hysterocele
Histerocistopexia: hysterocystopexy
Histeroclise: hysterocleisis
Histerocolposcópio: hysterocolposcope
Histerodinia: hysterodynia
Histerogênico: hysterogenic, hysterogenous
Histerografia: hysterography
Histerógrafo: hysterograph
Histerograma: hysterogram
Histeróide: hysteroid
Histerólise: hysterolysis
Histerômetro: hysterometer
Histeromiomectomia: hysteromyomectomy
Histeromiotomia: hysteromyotomy
Histerooforectomia: hystero-oophorectomy
Histeropatia: hysteropathy
Histeropexia: hysteropexy, uterofixation
Histeroplastia: hysteroplasty
Histerorrafia: hysterorrhaphy
Histeroscopia: hysteroscopy
Histeroscópio: hysteroscope
Histerospasmo: hysterospasm
Histerossalpingectomia: hysterosalpingectomy
Histerossalpingoforectomia: hysterosalpingo-oophorectomy
Histerossalpingografia: hysterosalpingography
Histerossalpingostomia: hysterosalpingostomy
Histerossístole: hysterosystole
Histerotermometria: hysterothermometry
Histerotomia: hysterotomy
Histerotomia abdominal: abdominohysterotomy
Histerotraquelectomia: hysterotrachelectomy
Histerotraqueloplastia: hysterotracheloplasty

Histerotraquelorrafia: hysterotrachelorrhaphy
Histerotraquelotomia: hysterotrachelotomy
Histerotubografia: hysterotubography
Histidase: histidase
Histidil: histidyl (His–)
Histidina: histidine (H, His)
Histidinal: histidinal
Histidinase: histidinase
Histidinemia: histidinemia
Histidino: histidino (–His)
Histidinol: histidinol
Histidinúria: histidinuria
Histioblasto: histioblast
Histiócito: histiocyte, histocyte
Histiocitoma: histiocytoma
Histiocitose: histiocytosis, histocytosis
Histiogênico: histiogenic
Histióide: histioid
Histioma: histioma
Histiônico: histionic
Histoângico: histoangic
Histoblasto: histoblast
Histocompatibilidade: histocompatibility
Histodiferenciação: histodifferentiation
Histofisiologia: histophysiology
Histofluorescência: histofluorescence
Histogênese: histogenesis
Histogenético: histogenetic
Histogenia: histogeny
Histogênico: histogenous
Histograma: histogram
Históide: histoid
Histoincompatibilidade: histoincompatibility
Histólise: histolysis
Histologia: histology
Histológico: histologic, histological
Histologista: histologist
Histoma: histoma
Histometaplásico: histometaplastic
Histomorfometria: histomorphometry
Histona: histone (H)
Histonectomia: histonectomy
Histoneurologia: histoneurology
Histonomia: histonomy
Histonúria: histonuria
Histopatogênese: histopathogenesis
Histopatologia: histopathology
Histoplasmina: histoplasmin
Histoplasmoma: histoplasmoma
Histoplasmose: histoplasmosis
Histoquímica: histochemistry
Historradiografia: historadiography
Historrexe: historrhexis
Histotomia: histotomy
Histótomo: histotome
Histótopo: histotope
Histotóxico: histotoxic
Histotrófico: histotrophic

Histotrofo: histotroph
Histotrópico: histotropic
Histozima: histozyme
Histozóico: histozoic
Hodofobia: hodophobia
Hodoneurômero: hodoneuromere
Holândrico: holandric
Holartrite: holarthritis
Holartrítico: holarthritic
Holismo: holism
Holístico: holistic
Hólmio: holmium (Ho)
Holoacárdia: holoacardius
Holo-ACP sintase: holo-ACP synthase
Holoacrania: holoacrania
Holoanencefalia: holoanencephaly
Holoblástico: holoblastic
Holocarboxilase sintetase: holocarboxylase synthetase
Holocefálico: holocephalic
Holocorda: holocord
Holócrino: holocrine
Holodiastólico: holodiastolic
Holoendêmico: holoendemic
Holoenzima: holoenzyme
Holofítico: holophytic
Hologastrosquise: hologastroschisis
Hologínico: hologynic
Holografia: holography
Holograma: hologram
Holomastigota: holomastigote
Holometábolo: holometabolous
Holomiântica (infecção): holomiantic (infection)
Holomorfose: holomorphosis
Holoprosencefalia: holoprosencephaly
Holoproteína: holoprotein
Holorraquísquise: holorachischisis
Holosídio: holoside
Holossistólico: holosystolic
Holotelencefalia: holotelencephaly
Holotríquio: holotrichous
Holoturinas: holothurins
Holozóico: holozoic
Homalocéfalo: homalocephalous
Homalúria: homaluria
Homatropina: homatropine
Homeométrico: homeometric
Homeomorfo: homeomorphous
Homeopata: homeopath, homeopathist
Homeopatia: homeopathy
Homeopático: homeopathic
Homeoplasia: homeoplasia, homoioplasia
Homeoplásico: homeoplastic
Homeorrese: homeorrhesis
Homeose: homeosis
Homeostasia: homeostasis
Homeostático: homeostatic
Homeoterapêutico: homeotherapeutic
Homeoterapia: homeotherapy, homeotherapeutics

Homeotérmico: hematherm, hemathermal, hemathermous, hematothermal, homeothermal, homeothermic, homoiothermal, warm-blooded
Homeotermo: homeotherm
Homeótico: homeotic
Homeotípico: homeotypical
Homergia: homergy
Homicida: homicidal
Homicídio: homicide
Homoarginina: homoarginine (Har)
Homoaxial: homaxial
Homobiotina: homobiotin
Homoblástico: homoblastic
Homocárion: homokaryon
Homocariótico: homokaryotic
Homocarnosina: homocarnosine
Homocarnosinose: homocarnosinosis
Homocêntrico: homocentric
Homoceratoplastia: homokeratoplasty
Homocisteína: homocysteine (Hcy)
Homocistina: homocystine
Homocistinemia: homocystinemia
Homocistinúria: homocystinuria
Homocitotrópico: homocytotropic
Homocitrulinúria: homocitrullinuria
Homocládico: homocladic
Homócrono: homochronous
Homodonte: homodont
Homódromo: homodromous
Homoenxerto: homograft
Homoerotismo: homoerotism, homoeroticism
Homófilo: homophil
Homofobia: homophobia
Homófonos: homophenes
Homogamético: homogametic
Homogamia: homogamy
Homogeinização: homogenization
Homogeinizar: homogenize
Homogeneizado: homogenate
Homogêneo: homogeneous
Homogênese: homogenesis
Homogenia: homogeny
Homogênico: homogenous
Homogentisato 1,2-dioxigenase: homogentisate 1,2-dioxygenase
Homoglicana: homoglycan
Homolateral: homolateral
Homolipídios: homolipids
Homólise: homolysis
Homolisina: homolysin
Homologia: homology
Homólogo: homolog, homologous, homologue
Homomórfico: homomorphic
Homônimo: homonymous
Homonomia: homonomy
Homônomo: homonomous
Homonuclear: homonuclear
Homoplásico: homoplastic

Homopolímero: homopolymer
Homopolímero de cloreteno: chlorethene homopolymer
Homoprolina: homoproline
Homorgânico: homorganic
Homoscedasticidade: homoscedasticity
Homossalato: homosalate
Homosserina: homoserine
Homossexual: homosexual
Homossexualidade: homosexuality
4-homossulfanilamida: 4-homosulfanilamide
Homosteróide: homosteroid
D-homosteróide: D-homosteroid
Homotálico: homothallic
Homotérmico: homothermal
Homotípico: homotypic, homotypical
Homotipo: homotype
Homotônico: homotonic
Homotópico: homotopic
Homotransplante: homotransplantation
Homotrópico: homotroppic
Homozigosidade: homozygosity, homozygosis
Homozigoto: homozygote, homozygous
Homozóico: homozoic
Homúnculo: homunculus
Hordenina: hordenine
Hordéolo: hordeolum
Horizontal: horizontalis
Horizonte(s) de desenvolvimento de Streeter: Streeter developmental horizon(s)
Hórmese: hormesis
Hórmio: hormion
Hormogonal: hormogonal
Hormonal: hormonal
Hormônio: hormone
Hormônio luteínico: luteohormone
Hormonogênese: hormonogenesis
Hormonogênico: hormonogenic
Hormonopoese: hormonopoiesis
Hormonopoético: hormonopoietic
Hormonoprivo: hormonoprivia
Hormonoterapia: hormonotherapy
Horóptero: horopter
Horripilação: horripilation
Horror: horror
Hortelã: spearmint
Hortelã-pimenta: peppermint
Hospedeiro: host
Hospital: hospital
Hospitalista: hospitalist
Hospitalização: hospitalization
Hóstia: wafer
Humina: humin
Humor: humor, **gen.** humoris, mood, temper
Humoral: humoral
Humoralismo: humoralism, humorism

Humorismo: fluidism
Humulina: humulin

I

Iacona: yaqona
Iangona: yanggona
Iatralíptica: iatraliptics
Iatralíptico: iatraliptic
Iátrico: iatric
Iatrofísica: iatrophysics
Iatrofísico: iatrophysical, iatrophysicist
Iatrogênico: iatrogenic
Iatrologia: iatrology
Iatromatemático: iatromathematical
Iatromecânico: iatromechanical
Iatroquímica: iatrochemistry
Iatroquímico: iatrochemical, iatrochemist
Iatrotécnica: iatrotechnique
Ibogaína: ibogaine
Ibuprofeno: ibuprofen
Icor: ichor
Icoremia: ichoremia
Icoróide: ichoroid
Icoroso: ichorous
Icorréia: ichorrhea
Icorremia: ichorrhemia
Icosaédrico: icosahedral
Icossomas: iccosomes
Ictal: ictal
Ictamol: ichthammol
Icterícia: icterus, jaundice
Ictérico: icteric
Icteroanemia: icteroanemia
Icterogênico: icterogenic
Íctero-hematúrico: icterohematuric
Íctero-hemoglobinúria: icterohemoglobinuria
Icteróide: icteroid
Ictioacantotoxismo: ichthyoacanthotoxism
Ictiófago: ichthyophagous
Ictiofobia: ichthyophobia
Ictio-hemotoxina: ichthyohemotoxin
Ictio-hemotoxismo: ichthyohemotoxism
Ictióide: ichthyoid
Ictiose: ichthyosis, sauriasis
Ictiosismo: ichthyism, ichthyismus
Ictiossarcotoxina: ichthyosarcotoxin
Ictiossarcotoxismo: ichthyosarcotoxism
Ictiótico: ichthyotic
Ictiotóxico: ichthyotoxicon
Ictiotoxicologia: ichthyotoxicology
Ictiotoxina: ichthyootoxin, ichthyotoxin
Ictiotoxismo: ichthyotoxism
Ictômetro: ictometer

Ictus: ictus
Id: id
Idade: age
Ideação: ideation
Ideacional: ideational
Ideal: ideal
Ideal do eu: ego-ideal
Idéia: idea
Idéia fixa: idée fixe
Identidade: identity
Identificação: identification
Identificação psicossexual: psychogender
Ideocinético: ideokinetic
Ideofobia: ideophobia
Ideologia: ideology
Ideomoção: ideomotion
Ideomotor: ideomotor
Idioaglutinina: idioagglutinin
Idiodinâmico: idiodynamic
Idiofrênico: idiophrenic
Idiogênese: idiogenesis
Idioglossia: idioglossia
Idioglótico: idioglottic
Idiográfico: idiographic
Idiograma: idiogram
Idio-heteroaglutinina: idioheteroagglutinin
Idio-heterolisina: idioheterolysin
Idio-hipnotismo: idiohypnotism
Idioisoaglutinina: idioisoagglutinin
Idioisolisina: idioisolysin
Idiolalia: idiolalia
Idiolisina: idiolysin
Idiomuscular: idiomuscular
Idionodal: idionodal
Idiopatético: idiopathetic
Idiopatia: idiopathy
Idiopático: idiopathic
Idiopsicológico: idiopsychologic
Idiorreflexo: idioreflex
Idiossincrasia: idiosyncrasy
Idiossincrásico: idiosyncratic
Idiossoma: idiosome
Idiota: moron
Idiota-prodígio: idiot-prodigy, idiot-savant
Idiotipo: idiotype
Idiótopo: idiotope
Idiotrófico: idiotrophic
Idiotrópico: idiotropic
Idioventricular: idioventricular
Iditol: iditol
Idoxuridina: idoxuridine (IDU)
Iduronato: iduronate
Iersiniose: yersiniosis
Ignipuntura: ignipuncture
Ignotina: ignotine
Ikota: ikota
Ileadelfo: ileadelphus
Ileal: ileac, ileal
Ilectomia: ileectomy
Ileíte: ileitis
Íleo: ileum
Íleo paralítico: ileus
Ileocecal: ileocecal
Ileoceco: ileocecum
Ileococecocistoplastia: ileocecocystoplasty

Ileocecostomia: ileocecostomy
Ileocistoplastia: ileocystoplasty
Ileocólico: ileocolic
Ileocolite: ileocolitis
Ileocolônico: ileocolonic
Ileocolostomia: ileocolostomy
Ileoentectropia: ileoentectropy
Ileoileostomia: ileoileostomy
Ileojejunite: ileojejunitis
Ileopexia: ileopexy
Ileoproctostomia: ileoproctostomy
Ileorrafia: ileorrhaphy
Ileorretostomia: ileorectostomy
Ileossigmoidostomia: ileosigmoidostomy
Ileostomia: ileostomy
Ileotomia: ileotomy
Ileotransversostomia: ileotransversostomy
Ilha: island
Ilhota: islet
Ilíaco: iliac, iliacus
Iliadelfo: iliadelphus
Ilídios: ylides
Ilinição: illinition
Ílio: ilium, **pl.** ilia
Iliococcígeo: iliococcygeal
Iliocolotomia: iliocolotomy
Iliocostal: iliocostal, iliocostalis
Iliofemoral: iliofemoral
Iliofemoroplastia: iliofemoroplasty
Ílio-hipogástrico: iliohypogastric
Ilioinguinal: ilioinguinal
Ilioisquiático: iliosciatic
Iliolombar: iliolumbar
Iliópago: iliopagus
Iliopectíneo: iliopectineal
Iliopélvico: iliopelvic
Iliospinhal: iliospinal
Iliossacro: iliosacral
Iliotibial: iliotibial
Iliotoracopago: iliothoracopagus
Iliotrocantérico: iliotrochanteric
Ilioxifópago: ilioxiphopagus
Iluminação: illumination
Iluminismo: illuminism
Ilusão: delusion, illusion
Ilusório: illusional
Imagem: image, scan
Imaginação: imagery
Imaginário: imaginal
Imago: imago, **pl.** imagines
Imbecil: imbecile
Imbricação: imbrication
Imbricar: imbricate, imbricated
Imediatamente: statim
Imedicável: immedicable
Imersão: immersion
Imida: imide
Imidazol: imidazole
Imidazolil: imidazolyl
4-imidazolona-5-propionato: 4-imidazolone-5-propionate
Imidodipeptidase: imidodipeptidase
Imidodipeptidúria: imidodipeptiduria
Imidol: imidole

Iminazolil: iminazolyl
Iminoácidos: imino acids
Iminocarbonil: iminocarbonyl
Iminodipeptidase: iminodipeptidase
Iminoglicinúria: iminoglycinuria
Imino-hidrolases: iminohydrolases
Iminostilbenos: iminostilbenes
Imipenem: imipenem
Imiscível: immiscible
Imissão: immission
Imitância: immittance
Imitar ou simular: mimic
Immunoblot, immunoblotting: immunoblot, immunoblotting
Imo: imus
Imobilização: immobilization, splinting
Imobilizar: immobilize
Imortalização: immortalization
IMP-aspartato ligase: IMP-aspartate ligase
Impacção: impaction
Impactado: impacted
Impacto: impact
Impedância: impedance
Impelir: subduce, subduct
Impercepção: imperception
Imperfuração: imperforation
Imperfurado: imperforate
Impermeante: impermeant
Impermeável: impermeable
Impersistência: impersistence
Impérvio: impervious
Impetiginização: impetiginization
Impetiginoso: impetiginous
Impetigo: impetigo
Ímpeto: impetus
Implantação: implantation
Implante: implant
Implante tríplice: triplant
Implosão: implosion
Imponderabilidade: weightlessness
Impotência: impotence, impotency
Impregnação: impregnation
Impregnar: impregnate
Impressão: impressio, impression, **pl.** impressiones
Impressão de polegar: thumbprinting
Impressão digital: fingerprint
Impressão digital genética: footprinting
Imprinting: imprinting
Impromidina: impromidine
Impróspero: unthrifty
Impulsão: impulsion
Impulsivo: impulsive
Impulso: driving, impulse
Imune: immune
Imunidade: immunity
Imunidade por infecção: infection-immunity
Imunifaciente: immunifacient
Imunização: immunization
Imunizar: immunize

Imunoadjuvante: immunoadjuvant
Imunoaglutinação: immunoagglutination
Imunobiologia: immunobiology
Imunoblasto: immunoblast
Imunócito: immunocyte
Imunocitoaderência: immunocytoadherence
Imunocitoquímica: immunocytochemistry
Imunocompetência: immunocompetence
Imunocompetente: immunocompetent
Imunocomplexo: immunocomplex
Imunocomprometido: immunocompromised
Imunoconglutinina: immunoconglutinin
Imunodeficiência: immunodeficiency
Imunodeficiente: immunodeficient
Imunodepressor: immunodepressant, immunodepressor
Imunodiagnóstico: immunodiagnosis
Imunodifusão: immunodiffusion
Imunoeletroforese: immunoelectrophoresis
Imunoematologia: immunohematology
Imunoensaio: immunoassay
Imunoferritina: immunoferritin
Imunofilinas: immunophilins
Imunofluorescência: immunofluorescence
Imunogenética: immunogenetics
Imunogenicidade: immunogenicity
Imunogênico: immunogenic
Imunógeno: immunogen
Imunoglobulina: immunoglobulin (Ig)
Imunointensificador: immunoenhancer
Imunoistoquímica: immunohistochemistry
Imunolocalização: immunolocalization
Imunologia: immunology
Imunologista: immunologist
Imunomodulador: immunomodulatory
Imunopatologia: immunopathology
Imunopotenciação: immunopotentiation
Imunopotencializador: immunopotentiator
Imunoprecipitação: immunoprecipitation
Imunoquímica: immunochemistry
Imunorreação: immunoreaction
Imunorreativo: immunoreactive

Imunosseleção: immunoselection
Imunossimpatectomia: immunosympathectomy
Imunossorvente: immunosorbent
Imunossupressão: immunosuppression
Imunossupressivo: immunosuppressive
Imunossupressor: immunosuppressant
Imunoterapia: immunotherapy
Imunotolerância: immunotolerance
Imunotransfusão: immunotransfusion
Imunovigilância: immunosurveillance
In extremis: in extremis
In situ: in situ
In vitro: in vitro
In vivo: in vivo
Inação: inaction
Inácia: ignatia
Inadaptação: dysadaptation
Inalação: inhalation, snuff
Inalação de cola: glue-sniffing
Inalador: inhaler
Inalante: inhalant
Inalar: inhale
Inanição: inanition, starvation
Inanimado: inanimate
Inaparent: inapparent
Inapetência: inappetence
Inarticulado: inarticulate
Inatenção: inattention
Inativação: inactivation
Inativação do X: X-inactivation
Inativador da anafilatoxina: anaphylatoxin inactivator
Inativar: inactivate
Inatividade elétrica cerebral: electrocerebral inactivity
Inato: inborn, innate
Incapacidade: disability
Incapaz: crippled
Incendiarismo: incendiarism
Incenso: thus
Incentivo: incentive
Incesto: incest
Incestuoso: incestuous
Incicloducção: incycloduction
Incicloforia: incyclophoria
Inciclotropia: incyclotropia
Incidência: incidence, view
Incidentaloma: incidentaloma
Incidente: incident
Incisal: incisal
Incisão: incision
Incisar: incise
Incisivo: incisive, incisor
Incisura: crena, **pl.** crenae; incisura, **pl.** incisurae; incisure, notch
Inclinação: dip, inclinatio, inclination, **pl.** inclinationes; slope, tilt
Inclinação da cabeça: head-tilt
Inclinômetro: inclinometer
Incluído: imbed

Inclusão: enclave, inclusion
Incoerente: incoherent
Incompatibilidade: incompatibility
Incompatível: incompatible
Incompetência: incompetence, incompetency
Inconsciência: unconsciousness
Inconsciente: unconscious
Inconstante: inconstant
Incontinência: incontinence, incontinentia
Incontinente: incontinent
Incoordenação: incoordination
Incorporação: incorporation
Increção: incretion
Incremento: increment
Incretina: incretin
Incrustação: incrustation, inlay
Incrustar: embed
Incubação: incubation
Incubadora: incubator
Incubo: incubus
Incudal: incudal
Incudectomia: incudectomy
Incudiforme: incudiform
Incudoestapedial: incudostapedial
Incudomaleal: incudomalleal
Incurável: incurable
Indanedionas: indanediones
Indecíduo: indeciduate
Indenização: indenization
Indentação: indentation
Independência: independence
Indicação: indication
Indicador: indicant, indicator
Indicana: indican
Indicanidrose: indicanidrosis
Indicanúria: indicanuria
Índice: index, **gen.** indicis, **pl.** indices, indexes
Índice de Cálculo da Linha Marginal: Marginal Line Calculus Index (MLC)
Índice de Higiene Oral: Oral Hygiene Index (OHI)
Índice de Placa: Plaque Index
Índice de Röhrer: Röhrer index
Índice Gengival: Gingival Index (GI)
Índice Gengivoperiodontal: Gingival-Periodontal Index (GPI)
Índice Periodontal de Russell: Russell Periodontal Index
Índice respiratório: spiro-index
Índice Simplificado de Higiene Oral: Simplified Oral Hygiene Index (OHI-S)
Índice Superficial de Cálculo (ISC): Calculus Surface Index (CSI)
Indiferenciado: undifferentiated
Indígena: indigenous
Indigestão: indigestion
Índigo: indigo
Índigo-azul: indigo blue
Índigo-carmim: indigo carmine
Indigotina: indigotin

Glossário

Indigoúria: indigouria, indiguria
Índio: indium (In)
Índio-111 (In^{111}): indium-111 (^{111}In)
Índio-113m (In^{113m}): indium-113m (^{113m}In)
Indisposição: indisposition
Individuação: individuation
Indocibina: indocybin
Indofenol oxidase: indophenol oxidase
Indofenolase: indophenolase
Indol: indole
Indolacetúria: indolaceturia
Indolamina: indolamine
Indolente: indolent
Indolil: indolyl
Indológeno: indologenous
Indolúria: indoluria
Indometacina: indomethacin
Indoramina: indoramin
Indoxil: indoxyl
Indoxilúria: indoxyluria
Indução: induction
Indulina: indulin
Indulinófilo: indulinophil, indulinophile
Induração: induration
Indurado: indurated, indurative
α-L-iduronidase: α-L-iduronidase
Indúsio: indusium, **pl.** indusia
Indutância: inductance (L)
Indutor: inducer, inductor
Indutório: inductorium
Indutotermia: inductothermy
Indutotermo: inductotherm
Induzir: induce
Ineal: inial
Inebriamento: inebriation
Inebriante: inebriant
Inércia: inertia
Inerente: inherent
Inerte: inert
Inervação: innervation
Infância: childhood
Infanticida: infanticide
Infantil: infantile
Infantilismo: infantilism
Infartação: infarction
Infarto: infarct
Infecção: infection
Infecciosa: infectious
Infecciosidade: infectiosity, infectiousness
Infectante: infective
Infectar: infect
Infectividade: infectivity
Infecundidade: infecundity
Inferência: inference
Inferior: inferior, lower
Inferioridade: inferiority
Infertilidade: infertility
Infestação: infestation
Infestar: infest
Infibulação: infibulation
Infiltração: infiltration
Infiltrar: infiltrate
Infinito: infinity
Inflação: inflation

Inflamação: inflammation
Inflamatório: inflammatory
Inflamável: flammable, inflammable
Inflator: inflator
Inflexão: inflection, inflexion
Influenza: influenza
Informática: informatics
Informoferos: informofers
Informossomas: informosomes
Infra-axilar: infraaxillary
Infracardíaco: infracardiac
Infracerebral: infracerebral
Infraclavicular: infraclavicular
Infracortical: infracortical
Infracostal: infracostal
Infracotilóide: infracotyloid
Infracrista: infracristal
Infradental: infradentale
Infradiafragmático: infradiaphragmatic
Infradução: deorsumduction, infraduction
Infra-escapular: infrascapular
Infra-espinal: infraspinatus, infraspinous
Infra-esplênico: infrasplenic
Infra-esternal: infrasternal
Infraglenóide: infraglenoid
Infraglótico: infraglottic
Infra-hepático: infrahepatic
Infra-hióide: infrahyoid
Inframamário: inframammary
Inframamilar: inframamillary
Inframandibular: inframandibular
Inframarginal: inframarginal
Inframaxilar: inframaxillary
Infranadante: infranatant
Infra-oclusão: infraclusion, infraocclusion
Infra-orbitário: infraorbital
Infrapatelar: infrapatellar
Infraprotrusão: infrabulge
Infrapsíquico: infrapsychic
Infra-regulação: down-regulation
Infra-sônico: infrasonic
Infra-subespecífico: infrasubspecific
Infratemporal: infratemporal
Infratonsilar: infratonsillar
Infratorácico: infrathoracic
Infratroclear: infratrochlear
Infra-umbilical: infraumbilical
Infravermelho: infrared (IR, ir)
Infraversão: infraversion
Infundibular: infundibular
Infundibulectomia: infundibulectomy
Infundibuliforme: infundibuliform
Infundibulina: infundibulin
Infundíbulo: infundibulum, **pl.** infundibula
Infundibuloma: infundibuloma
Infundibulopélvico: infundibulopelvic
Infundibulovariano: infundibulo-ovarian
Infusão: infusion

Infusível: infusible
Infusório: infusorian
Infusórios: Infusoria
Ingestão: ingesta, ingestion
Ingestivo: ingestive
Inglês gestual: manual English
Ingravescente: ingravescent
Inguinal: inguinal
Inguinocrural: inguinocrural
Inguinodinia: inguinodynia
Inguinolabial: inguinolabial
Inguinoperitoneal: inguinoperitoneal
Inguinoscrotal: inguinoscrotal
Ingurgitamento: engorgement
Iníaco: iniac
Inial: iniad
Inibição: inhibition
Inibidor: inhibitor
Inibidores da serina protease: serpins
Inibina: inhibin
Inibir: inhibit
Inibitina: inhibitine
Inibitório: inhibitory
Iniciador: primer, starter
Início: initiation
Iniencefalia: iniencephaly
Ínio: inion
Iniópago: iniopagus
Iniopsia: iniops
Inite: initis
Injeção: injection
Injetado: injected
Injetar: inject
Injetável: injectable
Injetor: injector
Inocente: innocent
Inoculabilidade: inoculability
Inoculação: inoculation
Inocular: inoculate
Inoculável: inoculable
Inóculo: inoculum
Inócuo: innocuous, innoxious
Inominado: anonyma, innominatal, innominate
Inopéctico: inopectic
Inoperável: inoperable
Inopexia: inopexia
Inorgânico: inorganic
Inosamina: inosamine
Inoscopia: inoscopy
Inose: inose
Inosemia: inosemia
Inosina: inosine (I, Ino)
Inosina 5′-difosfato (IDP): inosine 5′-diphosphate (IDP)
Inosina 5′-monofosfato (IMP): inosine 5′-monophosphate (IMP)
Inosina 5′-trifosfato (ITP): inosine 5′-triphosphate (ITP)
Inosina pranobex: inosine pranobex
Inosinato: inosinate
Inosinicase: inosinicase
Inosinil: inosinyl
Inosita: inosite
Inositídeo: inositide
Inositol: inositol
Inositúria: inosituria

Inosúria: inosuria
Inotrópico: inotropic
Inquérito: inquest
Inquilino: inquiline
Insalubre: insalubrious, peccant
Insanidade: insanity
Insano: insane
Insaturado: unsaturated
Inscrição: inscriptio, inscription
Insectário: insectarium
Insegurança: insecurity
Inseminação: insemination, semination
Inseminoma: seminoma
Inseminomatoso: seminomatous
Insensível: insensible
Inserção: insert, insertion
Inseticida: insecticide
Insetífugo: insectifuge
Insetívoro: insectivorous
Insetos: Insecta
Insetos parasitas: vermin
Insidioso: insidious
Insinuação: engagement
Insolação: insolation, sunstroke
Insolúvel: insoluble
Insone: insomniac
Insônia: insomnia, sleeplessness
Inspeção: inspection
Inspersão: inspersion
Inspiração: inspiration
Inspirar: inspire
Inspiratório: inspiratory
Inspirômetro: inspirometer
Inspissação: inspissation
Inspissador: inspissator
Inspissar: inspissate
Instabilidade: instability
Instar: instar
Instilação: instillation
Instilador: instillator
Instintivo: instinctive, instinctual
Instinto: instinct
Instrumentação: instrumentation
Instrumentário: instrumentarium
Insudato: insudate
Insuficiência: failure, insufficiency
Insuflação: insufflation
Insuflador: insufflator
Insuflar: insufflate
Ínsula: insula, **gen. e pl.** insulae
Insular: insular
Insulina: insulin
Insulinemia: insulinemia
Insulinogênese: insulinogenesis
Insulinogênico: insulinogenic, insulogenic
Insulinoma: insulinoma
Insulite: insulitis
Insulto: insult
Insuscetibilidade: insusceptibility
Integração: integration, mainstreaming
Integral: integral
Integridade: integrity

Integrinas: integrins
Integumentar: integumentary
Integumento: integument
Integumento comum: integumentum commune
Inteiro: entire
Intelectualização: intellectualization
Inteligência: intelligence
Intemperança: intemperance
Intenção: intention
Intensidade: intensity
Intensificação imune: immunoenhancement
Intensificador de imagem: image intensifier
Intensificadores: enhancers
Intensivo: intensive
Interação: interaction
Interacinar: interacinar, interacinous
Interações medicamentosas: drug interactions
Interalveolar: interalveolar
Interanular: interannular
Interaritenóide: interarytenoid
Interarticular: interarticular
Interastérico: interasteric
Interatrial: interatrial
Interaural: interaural
Interauricular: interauricular
Intercadência: intercadence
Intercadente: intercadent
Intercalação: intercalation
Intercalado: intercalated
Intercalar: intercalary
Intercanalicular: intercanalicular
Intercapilar: intercapillary
Intercarotídeo: intercarotic, intercarotid
Intercarpal: intercarpal
Intercartilaginoso: intercartilaginous
Intercavernoso: intercavernous
Intercelular: intercellular
Intercentral: intercentral
Intercerebral: intercerebral
Intercílio: intercilium
Intercinese: interkinesis
Interclavicular: interclavicular
Intercoccígeo: intercoccygeal
Intercolunar: intercolumnar
Intercondilar: intercondylar, (intercondylic, intercondyloid)
Intercondral: interchondral
Interconversão: interconversion
Intercorporal: interbody
Intercorrente: intercurrent
Intercostal: intercostal
Intercostoumeral: intercostohumeral, intercostohumeralis
Intercricotireotomia: intercricothyrotomy
Intercrinas: intercrines
Intercristal: intercristal
Intercrural: intercrural
Intercurso: intercourse
Intercúspide: intercusping

Intercuspidiano: intercuspation
Intercutaneomucoso: intercutaneomucous
Interdeferencial: interdeferential
Interdental: interdental
Interdentário: interdentium
Interdição: commitment
Interdigitação: interdigitation
Interdigital: interdigital
Interdígito: interdigit
Interdisciplinar: interdisciplinary
Interditável: certifiable
Interescapular: interscapular
Interescápulo: interscapulum
Interespaço: interspace
Interespinal: interspinal, interspinalis, interspinous
Interface: interface
Interfacial: interfacial
Interfalângico: interphalangeal
Interfascicular: interfascicular
Interfase: interphase
Interfemoral: interfemoral
Interferência: interference
Interferometria: interferometry
Interferômetro: interferometer
Interferon: interferon (IFN)
Interferon-β2: interferon-β2
Interfibrilar: interfibrillar, interfibrillary
Interfibroso: interfibrous
Interfilamentoso: interfilamentous
Interfilético: interphyletic
Interfrontal: interfrontal
Interganglionar: interganglionic
Intergênico: intergenal
Intergiral: intergyral
Interglobular: interglobular
Interglúteo: intergluteal
Intergonial: intergonial
Inter-hemisférico: interhemicerebral
Interictal: interictal
Interimplantação: interplanting
Interimplante: interplant
Interior: interior
Interisquiático: interischiadic, intersciatic
Interlamelar: interlamellar
Interleucina: interleukin
Interleucina humana recombinante 11: rhIL-11
Interleucina-1 (IL-1): interleukin-1 (IL-1)
Interleucina-2 (IL-2): interleukin-2 (IL-2)
Interleucina-3 (IL-3): interleukin-3 (IL-3)
Interleucina-4 (IL-4): interleukin-4 (IL-4)
Interleucina-5 (IL-5): interleukin-5 (IL-5)
Interleucina-6 (IL-6): interleukin-6 (IL-6)
Interleucina-7 (IL-7): interleukin-7 (IL-7)

Interleucina-8 (IL-8): interleukin-8 (IL-8)
Interleucina-9 (IL-9): interleukin-9 (IL-9)
Interleucina-10 (IL-10): interleukin-10 (IL-10)
Interleucina-11 (IL-11): interleukin-11 (IL-11)
Interleucina-12 (IL-12): interleukin-12 (IL-12)
Interleucina-13 (IL-13): interleukin-13 (IL-13)
Interleucina-14 (IL-14): interleukin-14 (IL-14)
Interleucina-15 (IL-15): interleukin-15 (IL-15)
Interleucina-16 (IL-16): interleukin-16 (IL-16)
Interleucina-17 (IL-17): interleukin-17 (IL-17)
Interleucina-18 (IL-18): interleukin-18 (IL-18)
Interlobar: interlobar
Interlobite: interlobitis
Interlobular: interlobular
Intermaleolar: intermalleolar
Intermamário: intermammary
Intermamilar: intermammillary
Intermaxilar: intermaxilla, intermaxillary
Intermediário: intermediary, intermediate, mediate
Intermedina: intermedin
Intermédio: intermedius
Intermediolateral: intermediolateral
Intermembranoso: intermembranous
Intermeníngeo: intermeningeal
Intermenstrual: intermenstrual
Intermetacarpal: intermetacarpal
Intermetamérico: intermetameric
Intermetatarsal: intermetatarsal
Intermetatarso: intermetatarseum
Intermissão: intermission
Intermitência: intermittence, intermittency
Intermitente: intermittent
Intermuscular: intermuscular
Internalização: internalization
Internasal: internarial, internasal
Interneuromérico: interneuromeric
Interneurônios: interneurons
Internista: internist
Interno: internal, interne, internus
Internodal: internodal
Internodo: internode
Internuclear: internuclear
Internuncial: internuncial
Interoceptivo: interoceptive
Interoceptor: interoceptor
Interoclusal: interocclusal
Interolivar: interolivary
Interorbitário: interorbital
Interósseo: interosseal, interosseous, interosseus, **pl.** interossei

Interpalpebral: interpalpebral
Interpapilar: intergemmal
Interparietal: interparietal
Interparoxístico: interparoxysmal
Interpedicular: interpediculate
Interpeduncular: interpeduncular
Interpessoal: interpersonal
Interpretação: interpretation
Interproximal: interproximal
Interpúbico: interpubic
Interpupilar: interpupillary
Inter-radial: interradial
Inter-renal: interrenal
Interromper: intermit
Interrupção respiratória: breath-holding
Interseção: intersectio, **pl.** intersectiones
Intersecção: intersection
Intersegmentar: intersegmental
Interseptal: interseptal
Intersepto: interseptum
Interseptovalvular: interseptovalvular
Intersexual: intersexual
Intersexualidade: intersexuality
Intersticial: interstitial
Interstício: interstice, **pl.** interstices, interstitium
Intertalâmico: interthalamic
Intertarsal: intertarsal
Intertransversal: intertransversalis
Intertransverso: intertransverse
Intertriginoso: intertriginous
Intertrigo: intertrigo
Intertrocantérico: intertrochanteric
Intertubular: intertubular
Interureteral: interureteral
Interuretérico: interureteric
Intervalo: interval
Intervascular: intervascular
Intervenção: intervention
Interventricular: interventricular
Intervertebral: intervertebral
Interviloso: intervillous
Intestinal: intestinal
Intestino: bowel, gut, intestine, intestinum, **pl.** intestina
Intestino anterior: foregut, headgut
Intestino médio: midgut
Intestino posterior: end-gut, hindgut
Intestino terminal: tailgut
Intestinotoxina: intestinotoxin
Íntima: intima, intimal
Intimite: intimitis
Intolerância: intolerance
Intorção: intorsion
Intoxicação: intoxation, intoxication
Intoxicante: intoxicant
Intra-abdominal: intraabdominal
Intra-acinoso: intraacinous
Intra-adenóide: intraadenoidal

Glossário

Intra-arterial: intraarterial
Intra-articular: intraarticular
Intra-atrial: intraatrial
Intra-aural: intraaural
Intra-auricular: intraauricular
Intrabrônquico: intrabronchial
Intrabucal: intrabuccal
Intracanalicular: intracanalicular
Intracapsular: intracapsular
Intracardíaco: intracardiac, intracordal
Intracárpico: intracarpal
Intracartilaginoso: intracartilaginous
Intracateter: intracatheter
Intracavitário: intracavitary
Intracelíaco: intracelial
Intracelular: intracellular
Intracerebelar: intracerebellar
Intracerebral: intracerebral
Intracerebroventricular: intracerebroventricular
Intracervical: intracervical
Intracisternal: intracisternal
Intracístico: intracystic
Intracólico: intracolic
Intracoronal: intracoronal
Intracorporal: intracorporeal
Intracorpuscular: intracorpuscular
Intracostal: intracostal
Intracraniano: intracranial
Intrácrino: intracrine
Intracutâneo: intracutaneous
Intradérmico: intradermal, intradermic
Intraducto: intraduct
Intradural: intradural
Intra-embrionário: intraembryonic
Intra-epidérmico: intraepidermal
Intra-epifisário: intraepiphysial
Intra-epitelial: intraepithelial
Intra-escrotal: intrascrotal
Intra-espinal: intraspinal
Intra-esplênico: intrasplenic
Intra-estromal: intrastromal
Intrafaradização: intrafaradization
Intrafascicular: intrafascicular
Intrafebril: intrafebrile
Intrafilamentar: intrafilar
Intrafusal: intrafusal
Intragalvanização: intragalvanization
Intragástrico: intragastric, introgastric
Intragênico: intragenal
Intragiral: intragyral
Intraglandular: intraglandular
Intraglobular: intraglobular
Intra-hepático: intrahepatic
Intra-hióide: intrahyoid
Intralaríngeo: intralaryngeal
Intraligamentoso: intraligamentous
Intralobar: intralobar
Intralobular: intralobular

Intralocular: intralocular
Intraluminal: intraluminal
Intramedular: intramedullary
Intramembranoso: intramembranous
Intrameníngeo: intrameningeal
Intramiocárdico: intramyocardial
Intramiométrico: intramyometrial
Intramitocondrial: intramitochondrial
Intramolecular: intramolecular
Intramural: intramural
Intramuscular: intramuscular (I.M., i.m.)
Intranasal: intranasal
Intranatal: intranatal
Intraneural: intraneural
Intranuclear: intranuclear
Intra-ocular: intraocular
Intra-oral: intraoral
Intra-orbitário: intraorbital
Intra-ósseo: intraosseous, intraosteal
Intra-ovariano: intraovarian
Intra-ovular: intraovular
Intrapapilar: intragemmal
Intraparietal: intraparietal
Intraparto: intrapartum
Intrapélvico: intrapelvic
Intrapericárdico: intrapericardiac, intrapericardial
Intraperitoneal: intraperitoneal (I.P., i.p.)
Intrapessoal: intrapersonal
Intrapial: intrapial
Intrapirético: intrapyretic
Intrapleural: intrapleural
Intrapontino: intrapontine
Intraprostático: intraprostatic
Intraprotoplasmático: intraprotoplasmic
Intrapsíquico: intrapsychic
Intrapulmonar: intrapulmonary
Intra-raquidiano: intrarrhachidian, intrarachidian
Intra-renal: intrarenal
Intra-retal: intrarectal
Intra-retiniano: intraretinal
Intra-sinovial: intrasynovial
Intratarsal: intratarsal
Intratável: intractable
Intratecal: intrathecal
Intratimpânico: intratympanic
Intratonsilar: intratonsillar
Intratorácico: intrathoracic
Intratubário: intratubal
Intratubular: intratubular
Intra-uterino: intrauterine
Intravascular: intravascular
Intravenoso: intravenous (I.V., i.v.)
Intraventricular: intraventricular (I-V)
Intravesical: intravesical
Intravitelino: intravitelline
Intravítreo: intravitreous
Intrínseco: intrinsic

Introflexão: introflection, introflexion
Intróito: introitus
Introjeção: introjection
Introjetado: introject
Intromissão: intromission
Intromitente: intromittent
Intron: intron
Introspecção: introspection
Introspectivo: introspective
Introssuscepção: introsusception
Introversão: introversion
Introvertido: introvert
Intubação: intubation
Intubador: introducer, intubator
Intubar: intubate
Intumescência: intumescentia, oncoides
Intumescente: intumescent
Intumescer: intumesce
Intumescimento: intumescence
Intussuscepção: intussusception
Intussusceptivo: intussusceptive
Intussuscepto: intussusceptum
Intussuscipiente: intussuscipiens
Inulase: inulase
Inulina: alant starch, inulin (In)
Inulinase: inulinase
Inulol: inulol
Inunção: inunction
Invaginação: invagination
Invaginador: invaginator
Invaginar: invaginate, vaginate
Invalidez: invalidism
Inválido: invalid
Invasão: invasion
Invasina: invasin
Invasivo: invasive
Inveja: envy
Inventário: inventory
Inversão: inversion
Inversor: invertor
Invertase: invertase
Invertebrado: invertebrate
Invertebrados: Invertebrata
Invertido: invert
Invertina: invertin
Inveterado: inveterate
Inviscação: inviscation
Involução: devolution, involution
Involucrina: involucrin
Invólucro: envelope, involucre, involucrum, **pl.** involucra
Involuntário: involuntary
Involutivo: involutional
Iodamida: iodamide
Iodar: iodinate
Iodato: iodate
Iodeto: iodide
Iodeto de caseína: caseo-iodine
Iodeto de dimetil tubocurarina: dimethyl tubocurarine iodide
Iodeto de ditiazanina: dithiazanine iodide
Iodeto de ecotiofato: echothiophate iodide
Iodeto de estilbázio: stilbazium iodide

Iodeto de metocurina: metocurine iodide
Iodeto de tetrametilamônio: tetramethylammonium iodide
Iodeto mercuroso: mercurous iodide
Iodeto vermelho de mercúrio: mercuric iodide, red
Iódico: iodic
Iodimetria: iodimetry
Iodinase: iodinase
Iodipamida: iodipamide
Iodismo: iodism
Iodixanol: iodixanol
Iodizar: iodize
Iodo: iodine (I)
Iodo-123 (I^{123}): iodine-123 (^{123}I)
Iodo-125 (I^{125}): iodine-125 (^{125}I)
Iodo-127 (I^{127}): iodine-127 (^{127}I)
Iodo-131 (I^{131}): iodine-131 (^{131}I)
Iodo-132 (I^{132}): iodine-132 (^{132}I)
Iodoacetamida: iodoacetamide
Iodocaseína: iodocasein
Iodocloroidroxiquina: iodochlorhydroxyquin, iodochlorohydroxyquinoline
Iodoclorol: iodochlorol
Iododermia: iododerma
Iodofendilato: iodophendylate
Iodofilia: iodophilia
Iodófilo: iodinophil, iodinophile, iodinophilous
Iodofórmio: iodoform
Iodóforo: iodophor
Iodoftaleína: iodophthalein
Iodoglobulina: iodoglobulin
Iodoipurato sódico: iodohippurate sodium
Iodometamato sódico: iodomethamate sodium
Iodometria: iodometry
Iodométrico: iodometric
Iodopiraceto: iodopyracet
3-iodo-1,2-propanediol: 3-iodo-1,2-propanediol
γ-iodopropilenoglicol: γ-iodopropyleneglycol
Iodopropilidenoglicerol: iodopropylideneglycerol
Iodoproteínas: iodoproteins
Iodopsina: iodopsin
Iodoquinol: iodoquinol
Iodoterapia: iodotherapy
Iodotironinas: iodothyronines
Iodotirosina: iodotyrosine
Iodoxamato de meglumina: iodoxamate meglumine
Iodúria: ioduria
Ioexol: iohexol
Iofendilato: iophendylate
Iofobia: iophobia
Ioimbina: yohimbine
Iômetro: iometer
Íon: ion
Íon dipolar: zwitterionic
Íon-grama: gram-ion
Iônico: ionic
Iônio: ionium
Ionização: ionization
Ionizar: ionize
Ionoferograma: ionopherogram

Ionoforese: ionophoresis
Ionoforético: ionophoretic
Ionóforo: ionophore
Ionograma: ionogram
Ionona: ionone
Íons dipolares: amphions
Iontoforese: iontophoresis
Iontoforético: iontophoretic
Iontoterapia: iontotherapy
Iopamidol: iopamidol
Iopentol: iopentol
Iopromida: iopromide
Iota: iota (ι)
Iotacismo: iotacism
Iotiouracil sódico: iothiouracil sodium
Iotrol: iotrol
Iotrolan: iotrolan
Ioversol: ioversol
Ioxaglato: ioxaglate
Ioxilan: ioxilan
Ioxitalamato: ioxithalamate
Ipeca: ipecac
Ipecacuanha: ipecacuanha
Ipodato: ipodate
Ipoméia: ipomea, morning glory
Ipratrópio: ipratropium
Iproniazida: iproniazid
Iproveratril: iproveratril
Ipsiliforme: ypsiliform
Ipsilóide: upsiloid
Ípsilon: upsilon
Ipsilateral: ipsilateral
Irial: iridal, iridial, iridian, iridic
Iridectomia: iridectomy
Iridênclise: iridencleisis
Irideremia: irideremia
Iridescente: iridescent
Iridese: iridesis
Iridina: iridin
Irídio: iridium (Ir)
Iridoavulsão: iridoavulsion
Iridocele: iridocele
Iridociclectomia: iridocyclectomy
Iridociclite: iridocyclitis
Iridociclocoroidite: iridocyclochoroiditis
Iridocinético: iridokinetic
Iridocistectomia: iridocystectomy
Iridocoloboma: iridocoloboma
Iridocorneano: iridocorneal
Iridocoroidite: iridochoroiditis
Iridodiagnóstico: iridodiagnosis
Iridodiálise: iridodialysis
Iridodilatador: iridodilator
Iridodonese: iridodonesis
Iridoesclerotomia: iridosclerotomy
Iridologia: iridology
Iridomalacia: iridomalacia
Iridomesodiálise: iridomesodialysis
Iridomotor: iridomotor
Iridoparalisia: iridoparalysis
Iridopatia: iridopathy
Iridoplegia: iridoplegia
Iridoptose: iridoptosis
Iridorrexia: iridorrhexis
Iridosquise: iridoschisis
Iridotomia: iridotomy
Iridovírus: *Iridovirus*
Irigenina: irigenin
Íris: irides, iris, **pl.** irides; orris
Irisina: irisin
Irite: iritis
Irítico: iritic
Irmã: sister
Irmãos: sib, sibling, sibship
Irracional: irrational
Irradiação: irradiation
Irradiar: irradiate
Irredutível: irreducible
Irregular: erose
Irrespirável: irrespirable
Irresponsabilidade: irresponsibility
Irreversível: irreversible
Irrigação: irrigation
Irrigador: irrigator
Irrigar: irrigate
Irritabilidade: irritability
Irritação: irritation
Irritante: irritant
Irritativo: irritative
Irritável: irritable
Irrupção: irruption
Irruptivo: irruptive
Isauxese: isauxesis
Iscoquimia: ischochymia
Iscurético: ischuretic
Iscúria: ischuria
Isento de carreador: carrier-free
Isetionato: isethionate
Isetionato de dibromopropamidina: dibromopropamidine isethionate
Isetionato de hexamidina: hexamidine isethionate
Isetionato de hidroxiestilbamidina: hydroxystilbamidine isethionate
Isetionato de pentamidina: pentamidine isethionate
Isoaglutinação: isoagglutination
Isoaglutinina: isoagglutinin
Isoaglutinógeno: isoagglutinogen
Isoalelo: isoallele
Isoaloxazina: isoalloxazine
Isoamila: isoamyl
Isoamilase: isoamylase
Isoaminila: isoaminile
Isoandrosterona: isoandrosterone
Isoanticorpo: isoantibody
Isobárico: isobaric
Isóbaro: isobar
Isobornil tiocianoacetato: isobornyl thiocyanoacetate
Isobutano: isobutane
Isobuteína: isobuteine
Isocapnia: isocapnia
Isocelular: isocellular
Isocianato: isocyanate
Isocianeto: isocyanide
Isocitolisina: isocytolysin
Isocitrase: isocitrase, isocitratase
Isocitrato: isocitrate
Isocitritase: isocitritase
Isóclina: isocline
Isoconazol: isoconazole
Isocoria: isocoria
Isocórico: isochoric
Isocórtex: isocortex
Isocromático: isochromatic, isochrous
Isocromatófilo: isochromatophil, isochromatophile
Isocromossoma: isochromosome
Isocronismo: isochronia
Isócrono: isochronous
Isodactilia: isodactylism
Isodenso: isodense
Isodesmosina: isodesmosine
Isodinâmico: isodynamic
Isodinamogênico: isodynamogenic
Isodose: isodose
Isodulcita: isodulcit
Isoemaglutinação: isohemagglutination
Isoemaglutinina: isohemagglutinin
Isoemólise: isohemolysis
Isoemolisina: isohemolysin
Isoenergético: isoenergetic
Isoenxerto: isograft
Isoenzima: isoenzyme
Isoeritrólise: isoerythrolysis
Isofagia: isophagy
Isofluorofato: isofluorphate
Isoflurano: isoflurane
Isogameta: isogamete
Isogamia: isogamy
Isogênico: isogeneic, isogenic, isogenous
Isogentibiose: isogentiobiose
Isoglutamina: isoglutamine
Isognato: isognathous
Isoídrico: isohydric
Isoidrúria: isohydruria
Isoimunização: isoimmunization
Isolador: insulator
Isolamento: insulation, isolation
Isolar: insulate, isolate
Isolécito: isolecithal
Isoleucila: isoleucyl
Isoleucina: isoleucine (I)
Isoleucoaglutinina: isoleukoagglutinin
Isólise: isolysis
Isolisina: isolysin
Isolítico: isolytic
Isólogo: isologous
Isomaltase: isomaltase
Isomastigota: isomastigote
Isomerase: isomerase
Isomérico: isomeric
Isomerismo: isomerism
Isomerização: isomerization
Isômero: isomer, isomerous
Isometadona: isomethadone
Isometepteno: isometheptene
Isométrico: isometric
Isometropia: isometropia
Isomórfico: isomorphic
Isomorfismo: isomorphism
Isomorfo: isomorphous
Isonaftol: isonaphthol
Isoncótico: isoncotic
Isoniazida (INH): isoniazid
Isonitrila: isonitrile
Isonitrosoacetona: isonitrosoacetone
Isopatia: isopathy
Isopentenilpirofosfato: isopentenylpyrophosphate
Isopentila: isopentyl
Isopeptídeo: isopeptide
Isopícnico: isopyknic
Isopirocalciferol: isopyrocalciferol
Isoplassontes: isoplassonts
Isoplástico: isoplastic
Isopleta: isopleth
Isopotencial: isopotential
Isoprecipitina: isoprecipitin
Isoprenilação: isoprenylation
Isopreno: isoprene
Isoprenóides: isoprenoids
Isopropanol: isopropanol
Isopropilcarbinol: isopropylcarbinol
Isopropiltiogalactosídeo: isopropylthiogalactoside (iPrSGal, IPTG)
Isóptero: isopter
Isoquinolina: isoquinoline
Isorréia: isorrhea
Isorriboflavina: isoriboflavin
Isosbéstico: isosbestic
Isosmótico: isoosmotic, isosmotic
Isosporíase: isosporiasis
Isosquisômero: isoschizomer
Isossensibilizar: isosensitize
Isossexual: isosexual
Isossorbida: isosorbide
Isostenúria: isosthenuria
Isosterismo: isosstery
Isóstero: isosstere
Isotérmico: isothermal
Isotiocianato de fluoresceína: fluorescein isothiocyanate (FITC)
Isotiocianato: isothiocyanate
Isotipendil: isothipendyl
Isotípico: isotypic
Isotipo: isotype
Isotonia: isotonia
Isotonicidade: isotonicity
Isotônico: isotonic
Isotono: isotone
Isotópico: isotopic
Isótopo: isotope
Isotransplante: isotransplantation
Isotretinoína: isotretinoin
Isotrópico: isotropic, isotropous
Isovaleril-CoA: isovaleryl-CoA
Isovaleril coenzima A: isovalerylcoenzyme A
Isovaltina: isovalthine
Isovolume: isovolume
Isovolumétrico: isovolumetric, isovolumic
Isozima: isozyme
Isquemia: ischemia

Isquêmico: ischemic
Isquese: ischesis
Isquialgia: ischialgia
Isquiático: ischiadic, ischiadicus, ischial, ischiatic
Ísquio: ischium, gen. ischii, pl. ischia
Isquioanal: ischioanal
Isquiobulbar: ischiobulbar
Isquiocapsular: ischiocapsular
Isquiocavernoso: ischiocavernosus, ischiocavernous
Isquiocele: ischiocele
Isquiococcígeo: ischiococcygeal, ischiococcygeus
Isquiodinia: ischiodynia
Isquiofemoral: ischiofemoral
Isquiofibular: ischiofibular
Isquiômelo: ischiomelus
Isquionite: ischionitis
Isquiópago: ischiopagus
Isquioperineal: ischioperineal
Isquiopúbico: ischiopubic
Isquiorretal: ischiorectal
Isquiossacral: ischiosacral
Isquiotibial: ischiotibial
Isquiotoracópago: ischiothoracopagus
Isquiovaginal: ischiovaginal
Isquiovertebral: ischiovertebral
Istmectomia: isthmectomy
Ístmico: isthmic, isthmian
Istmo: isthmus, pl. isthmi, isthmuses
Istmoparalisia: isthmoparalysis
Istmoplegia: isthmoplegia
Iter: iter
Iteral: iteral
Itérbio: ytterbium (Yb)
Itiocola: ichthyocolla
Ítrio: yttrium (Y)
Ítrio-90: yttrium-90
Ivermectina: ivermectin
Ixodíase: ixodiasis
Ixódico: ixodic
Ixodídeo: ixodid

J

Já desejado: déjà voulu
Já visto: déjà vu
Jacksoniano: jacksonian
Jalapa: jalap
Janela: fenestra, pl. fenestrae; window
Janícipite: janiceps
Jargão: jargon
Jato: gusher, jet
Jatrofa: *Jatropha*
Jejunal: jejunal
Jejunectomia: jejunectomy
Jejunite: jejunitis
Jejuno: jejunum
Jejunocolostomia: jejunocolostomy
Jejunoileal: jejunoileal
Jejunoileíte: jejunoileitis
Jejunoileostomia: jejunoileostomy
Jejunojejunostomia: jejunojejunostomy
Jejunoplastia: jejunoplasty
Jejunostomia: jejunostomy
Jejunotomia: jejunotomy
Joanete: bunion
Joelho: geniculum, pl. genicula; genu, gen. genus, pl. genua; knee
Joelho recurvado: back-knee
Joelho valgo: knock-knee
Joelho varo: bandy-leg, bow-b, bowleg
Jogo: game
Jonina: johnin
Joule: joule (J)
Jugal: jugal
Jugo: jugum, pl. juga; yoke
Jugomaxilar: jugomaxillary
Jugular: jugular
Junção: junctio, junction, juncture
Junguiano: jungian
Junta médica: consultation
Juramento: oath
Juramento de Hipócrates: Hippocratic Oath
Justácrina: juxtacrine
Justaepifisário: juxtaepiphysial
Justaglomerular: juxtaglomerular
Justalocórtex: juxtallocortex
Justamedular: juxtamedullary
Justaposição: juxtaposition
Justiça: justice

K

Kawa kawa: methysticum
Kernicterus: kernicterus
Khat: Catha edulis
Konzo: konzo
Koro: koro, shook jong
Kra-kra: craw-craw
Kuru: kuru
Kwashiorkor: kwashiorkor

L

Lã: lana, gen. e pl. lanae; wool
Lã de madeira: wood wool
Labiação: lipping
Labial: labial
Labialismo: labialism
Labialmente: labially
Lábil: labile
Labilidade: lability
Lábio: labium, gen. labii, pl. labia; labrum, pl. labra; lip
Lábio leporino: harelip
Labiocervical: labiocervical
Labioclinação: labioclination
Labiocolocação: labioplacement
Labiodental: labiodental
Labiogengival: labiogingival
Labioglossofaríngeo: labioglossopharyngeal
Labioglossolaríngeo: labioglossolaryngeal
Labiomentual: labiomental
Labionasal: labionasal
Labiopalatino: labiopalatine
Labioplastia: labioplasty
Labioversão: labioversion
Labirintectomia: labyrinthectomy
Labiríntico: labyrinthine
Labirintite: labyrinthitis
Labirinto: labyrinth, labyrinthus, maze
Labirintotomia: labyrinthotomy
Labítomo: labitome
Laboratório: laboratory
Laboratorista: laboratorian
Laca: lacca
Lacase: laccase
Laceração: laceration, tear
Lacerado: lacerated
Lacerável: lacerable
Lacerto: lacertus
Lacíneas da trompa: laciniae tubae
Lacrimal: lachrymal, lacrimal
Lacrimatório: lacrimatory
Lacrimejamento: lacrimation
Lacrimejante: lacrimator
Lacrimotomia: lacrimotomy
Lactação: lactation
Lactacidemia: lactacidemia
Lactacidose: lactacidosis
Lactacional: lactational
Lactalbumina: lactalbumin
Lactamase: lactamase
β-lactamase: β-lactamase
β-lactâmico: β-lactam
Lactância: infancy
Lactase: lactase
Lactato: lactate
Lactato 2-monoxigenase: lactate 2-mono-oxygenase
Lactato de amrinona: amrinone lactate
Lactato de ciclizina: cyclizine lactate
Lactato de esqualamina: squalamine lactate
Lactato de etacridina: acrinol, ethacridine lactate
Lactato desidrogenase: lactic acid dehydrogenase
Lactato ferroso: ferrous lactate
Lactenina: lactenin
Lactente: infant
Lácteo: lacteal
Lactescente: lactescent
Lactífero: lactiferous
Lactífugo: lactifugal, lactifuge
Lactígeno: lactigenous
α-lactil-tiamina pirofosfato: α-lactyl-thiamin pyrophosphate
Lactimorbo: lactimorbus
Lactinado: lactinated
Lactobacilo: lactobacillus
Lactobacilos: lactobacilli
Lactobezoar: lactobezoar
Lactobutirômetro: lactobutyrometer
Lactocele: lactocele
Lactócrito: lactocrit
Lactocromo: lactochrome
Lactodensímetro: lactodensimeter
Lactoferrina: lactoferrin
Lactoflavina: lactoflavin
Lactogênese: lactogenesis
Lactogênico: lactogenic
Lactogênio: lactogen
Lactoglobulina: lactoglobulin
Lactoilglutationa liase: lactoylglutathione lyase
Lactômetro: lactometer
Lactona: lactone
Lactonase: lactonase
Lactoperoxidase: lactoperoxidase
Lactoproteína: lactoprotein
Lactorréia: lactorrhea
Lactoscópio: lactoscope
Lactose: lactose
Lactosúria: lactosuria
Lactoterapia: lactotherapy
Lactotrófico: lactotrophic
Lactotropina: lactotropin
Lactovegetariano: lactovegetarian
Lactulose: lactulose
Lacuna: lacuna, pl. lacunae
Lacunar: lacunar
Lacúnula: lacunule
Lado: latus, gen. lateris, pl. latera; side
Laetrila: laetrile
Lagarta: caterpillar
Lago: lacus, pl. lacus; lake
Lagoftalmia: lagophthalmia, lagophthalmos
Lagomorfo: lagomorph
Lágrima: tear
Laliatria: laliatry
Laliofobia: laliophobia
Lalognose: lalognosis
Laloplegia: laloplegia
Laloquezia: lalochezia
Lama: sludge
Lambda: lambda
Lambdacismo: lambdacism
Lambdóide: lambdoid
Lamblíase: lambliasis
Lamela: lamella, pl. lamellae
Lamelado: lamellate, lamellated
Lamelar: lamellar
Lamelipódio: lamellipodium, pl. lamellipodia
Lâmina: lamina, pl. laminae; plate, slide
Lâmina do teto: roofplate
Lâmina supracorióide da esclera: suprachoroidea
Laminação: lamination
Laminado: laminated
Laminar: laminar
Laminária: laminaria
Laminarina: laminarin
Lâminas beta: beta sheets
Laminectomia: laminectomy
Laminina: laminin

Laminite: laminitis
Laminografia: laminagraphy, laminography
Laminógrafo: laminagraph
Laminograma: laminagram
Laminotomia: laminotomy
Lamínula: coverslip
Lamotrigina: lamotrigine
Lâmpada: lamp
Lâmpada de fenda: slitlamp
L-α-narcotina: L-α-narcotine
Lanatosídeo D: lanatoside D
Lanatosídeos A, B e C: lanatosides A, B e C
Lancamicina: lankamycin
Lanceta: lancet
Lancetar: lance
Lancinante: lancinating
Lanolina: lanolin
Lanosterol: lanosterol
Lantânico: lanthanic
Lantanídeos: lanthanides
Lantânio: lanthanum (La)
Lantionina: lanthionine
Lanugo: lanugo
Laparoendoscópico: laparoendoscopic
Laparogastroscopia: laparogastroscopy
Laparomiosite: laparomyositis
Laparorrafia: laparorrhaphy
Laparoscopia: laparoscopy
Laparoscópio: laparoscope
Laparotomia: laparotomy
Laranja: orange
Laranja acridina: acridine orange
Laranja de metila: methyl orange
Laranja ou orange G: orange G
Laranja-vitória: Victoria orange
Largura: width
Largura de banda: bandwidth
Laringe: larynx, **pl.** larynges
Laringectomia: laryngectomy
Laringectomizado: laryngectomee
Laríngeo: laryngeal
Laringismo: laryngismus
Laringite: laryngitis
Laringítico: laryngitic
Laringocele: laryngocele
Laringofaringectomia: laryngopharyngectomy
Laringofaríngeo: laryngopharyngeal
Laringofaringite: laryngopharyngitis
Laringofissura: laryngofissure
Laringoftise: laryngophthisis
Laringografia: laryngography
Laringógrafo: laryngograph
Laringologia: laryngology
Laringomalacia: laryngomalacia
Laringoparalisia: laryngoparalysis
Laringoplastia: laryngoplasty
Laringoplegia: laryngoplegia
Laringoptose: laryngoptosis
Laringoscopia: laryngoscopy
Laringoscópico: laryngoscopic
Laringoscópio: laryngoscope
Laringoscopista: laryngoscopist
Laringospasmo: laryngospasm
Laringostenose: laryngostenosis
Laringostomia: laryngostomy
Laringostroboscópio: laryngostroboscope
Laringotomia: laryngotomy
Laringotraqueal: laryngotracheal
Laringotraqueíte: laryngotracheitis
Laringotraqueobronquite: laryngotracheobronchitis
Laringotraqueoplastia: laryngotracheoplasty
Larva: grub, larva, **pl.** larvae; maggot
Larvado: larvaceous, larvate
Larvário: larval
Larvicida: larvicidal, larvicide
Larvifágico: larviphagic
Larvíparo: larviparous
Lasca: chip
Laser: laser
Lassitude: lassitude
Latência: abeyance, latency
Latência do nitrogênio: nitrogen lag
Latente: latent
Lateral: lateral, lateralis
Lateralidade: laterality
Lateralização: lateralization
Lateroabdominal: lateroabdominal
Laterodesvio: laterodeviation
Laterodução: lateroduction
Lateroflexão: lateriflexion, lateriflection, lateroflexion, lateroflection
Lateroposição: lateroposition
Lateropulsão: lateropulsion
Laterotorção: laterotorsion
Laterotrusão: laterotrusion
Lateroversão: lateroversion
Látex: latex
Laticacidemia: lactic acidemia
Látigo: lactic
Latirismo: lathyrism
Latirógeno: lathyrogen
Laudanina: laudanine
Láudano: laudanum
Laudanosina: laudanosine
Laurêncio: lawrencium (Lr, Lw)
Lavado: lavage
Lavagem cerebral: brainwashing
Lavagem gástrica: gastrolavage
Laxação: laxation
Laxativo: laxative
Lazareto: lazaret, lazaretto
Lecanora: crottle, cudbear
Lecítico: lecithal
Lecitina: lecithin
Lecitina-colesterol aciltransferase: lecithin-cholesterol acyltransferase (LCAT)
Lecitinase: lecithinase
Lecitoblasto: lecithoblast
Lecitoproteína: lecithoprotein
Lectina: lectin
Legionelose: legionellosis
Legumina: legumin
Leguminívoro: leguminivorous
Lei: law
Lei de Nasse: Nasse law
Lei de Vogel: Vogel law
Lei do tudo-ou-nada: all or none
Leidigarca: leydigarche
Leiomiofibroma: leiomyofibroma
Leiomioma: leiomyoma
Leiomiomatose: leiomyomatosis
Leiomiomectomia: leiomyomectomy
Leiomiossarcoma: leiomyosarcoma
Leishmânia: leishmania, **pl.** leishmaniae
Leishmaniose: leishmaniasis, leishmaniosis
Leishmanóide: leishmanoid
Leite: lac, **gen.** lactis, milk
Leito: bed
Leitura: reading
Leitura da mente: mind-reading
Lembrança: recall
Lemnisco: fillet, lemniscus, **pl.** lemnisci
Lemoblasto: lemmoblast
Lemócito: lemmocyte
Lêndea: nit
Lenitivo: lenitive
Lensectomia: lensectomy
Lensômetro: lensometer, vertometer
Lensopatia: lensopathy
Lente: lens
Lente esferocilíndrica: spherocylinder
Lente intra-ocular protética: prosthetophacos
Lenticone: lenticonus
Lenticular: lenticular
Lentículo: lenticulus, **pl.** lenticuli
Lentículo-estriado: lenticulostriate
Lentículo-óptico: lenticulo-optic
Lenticulopapular: lenticulopapular
Lenticulotalâmico: lenticulothalamic
Lentiforme: lentiform
Lentiginose: lentiginosis
Lentiglobo: lentiglobus
Lentigo: lentigo, **pl.** lentigines
Lentilha: coquille
Lentogênico: lentogenic
Lentual: lentula, lentulo
Leontíase: leontiasis
Lepídico: lepidic
Lepidópteros: Lepidoptera
Lepotrix: lepothrix
Lepra: leprosy
Leprechaunismo: leprechaunism
Lépride: leprid
Leproma: leproma
Lepromatoso: lepromatous
Lepromina: lepromin
Leprosário: leprosarium, leprosery
Leproso: leper, leprotic, leprous
Leprostático: leprostatic
Leptandra: leptandra
Leptina: leptin
Leptocefalia: leptocephaly
Leptocéfalo: leptocephalous
Leptócito: leptocyte
Leptocitose: leptocytosis
Leptocromático: leptochromatic
Leptodactiloso: leptodactylous
Leptofonia: leptophonia
Leptofônico: leptophonic
Leptomeníngeo: leptomeningeal
Leptomeninges: leptomeninges, leptomeninx, **sing.** leptomeninx
Leptomeningite: leptomeningitis
Leptômero: leptomere
Leptomônada: leptomonad
Leptonema: leptonema
Leptopodia: leptopodia
Leptoprosopia: leptoprosopia
Leptoprosópico: leptoprosopic
Leptorrino: leptorrhine
Leptoscópio: leptoscope
Leptospira: leptospire
Leptospirose: leptospirosis
Leptospirúria: leptospiruria
Leptossômico: leptosomatic, leptosomic
Leptóteno: leptotene
Leptotricose: leptothricosis
Lergotrila: lergotrile
Lesão: damage, injury, lesion
Lesão de Lohlein-Baehr: Lohlein-Baehr lesion
Lesar: injure
Lesbianismo: lesbianism
Lésbica: lesbian
***l*-estercobilinogênio:** *l*-stercobilinogen
Letal: lethal
Letalidade: lethality
Letargia: lethargy
Leucaférese: leukapheresis
Leucanemia: leukanemia
Leucemia: leukemia
Leucêmico: leukemic
Leucêmide: leukemid
Leucemogênese: leukemogenesis
Leucemogênico: leukemogenic
Leucemógeno: leukemogen
Leucemóide: leukemoid
Leucina: leucin, leucine (L, Leu), leukin
Leucinose: leucinosis
Leucinúria: leucinuria
Leucoaglutinina: leukoagglutinin
Leucoarmina: leucoharmine
Leucobilina: leukobilin
Leucoblasto: leukoblast
Leucoblastose: leukoblastosis
Leucocidina: leukocidin
Leucocinética: leukokinetics

Leucocinético: leukokinetic
Leucocitaxia: leukocytaxia, leukocytaxis
Leucocitemia: leukocythemia
Leucocítico: leukocytal, leukocytic
Leucócito: leukocyte
Leucocitoblasto: leukocytoblast
Leucocitoclasia: leukocytoclasis
Leucocitogênese: leukocytogenesis
Leucocitóide: leukocytoid
Leucocitólise: leukocytolysis
Leucocitolisina: leukocytolysin
Leucocitolítico: leukocytolytic
Leucocitoma: leukocytoma
Leucocitômetro: leukocytometer
Leucocitopenia: leukocytopenia
Leucocitoplania: leukocytoplania
Leucocitopoese: leukocytopoiesis
Leucocitose: leukocytosis
Leucocitotático: leukocytactic, leukocytotactic
Leucocitotaxia: leukocytotaxia
Leucocitotoxina: leukocytotoxin
Leucocitúria: leukocyturia
Leucocloroma: leukochloroma
Leucocoria: leukocoria, leukokoria
Leucocraurose: leukokraurosis
Leucoderma: leukoderma, leukopathia, leukopathy
Leucodermatoso: leukodermatous
Leucodistrofia: leukodystrophia, leukodystrophy
Leucodontia: leukodontia
Leucoencefalite: leukoencephalitis
Leucoencefalopatia: leukoencephalopathy
Leucoeritroblastose: leukoerythroblastosis
Leucolina: leucoline
Leucólise: leukolysis
Leucolisina: leukolysin
Leucolítico: leukolytic
Leucoma: leukoma
Leucomatoso: leukomatous
Leucometileno azul: leucomethylene blue
Leucomielite: leukomyelitis
Leucomielopatia: leukomyelopathy
Leucon: leukon
Leuconecrose: leukonecrosis
Leuconíquia: leukonychia
Leucopedese: leukopedesis
Leucopenia: leukopenia
Leucopênico: leukopenic
Leucoplaquia: leukoplakia
Leucopoese: leukopoiesis
Leucopoético: leukopoietic
Leucoprotease: leukoprotease
Leucorragia: leukorrhagia
Leucorréia: leukorrhea
Leucorreico: leukorrheal

Leucorriboflavina: leukoriboflavin
Leucotático: leukotactic
Leucotaxia: leukotaxia, leukotaxis
Leucotaxina: leukotaxine
Leucotomia: leukotomy
Leucótomo: leukotome
Leucotoxina: leukotoxin
Leucotrienos: leukotrienes (LT)
Leucotríquia: leukotrichia
Leucovorina: leucovorin
Leuencefalina: leuenkephalin
Leupeptina: leupeptin
Levamisol: levamisole
Levano: levan
Levanossacarase: levansucrase
Levantador: levator
Levantamento: survey
Levarterenol: levarterenol
Leve: mitis
Levedura: yeast
Levocardia: levocardia
Levocardiograma: levocardiogram
Levocarnitina: levocarnitine
Levociclodução: levocycloduction
Levoclinação: levoclination
Levodopa: levodopa
Levodução: levoduction
Levofacetoperano: levophacetoperane
Levofobia: levophobia
Levoforme: levoform
Levógiro: levogyrate, levogyrous
Levoglicose: levoglucose
Levograma: levogram
Levonordefrina: levonordefrin
Levorrotação: levorotation
Levorrotatório: levorotatory
Levotorção: levotorsion
Levoversão: levoversion
Levulano: levulan
Levulina: levulin
Levulinato: levulinate
Levulosano: levulosan
Levulose: levulose
Levulosemia: levulosemia
Levulosúria: levulosuria
Lewisita: lewisite
Léxico: lexical
Liase: lyase
Liase hialurônica: hyaluronic lyase
Liberador: liberator
Liberinas: liberins
Liberomotor: liberomotor
Libertar: deliver
Libidinização: libidinization
Libidinoso: libidinous
Libido: libido
Libra: pound
Licantropia: lycanthropy
Licoctonina: lycoctonine
Licófora: lycophora
Licopenemia: lycopenemia
Licopeno: lycopene
Licoperdonose: lycoperdonosis
Licopódio: lycopodium

Licor: liqueur
Lidoflazina: lidoflazine
Lienectomia: lienectomy
Lienomedular: lienomedullary
Lienomielógeno: lienomyelogenous
Lienopancreático: lienopancreatic
Lienorrenal: lienorenal
Lienteria: lientery
Lientérico: lienteric
Liga: alloy
Ligação: bond, bonding, ligation, link, linkage
Ligação ao X: Y-linkage
Ligação cruzada: cross-link
Ligado: linked
Ligado ao X: X-linked
Ligador: linker
Ligadura: ligature
Ligamento: ligament, ligamentum, **pl.** ligamenta
Ligamentopexia: ligamentopexis, ligamentopexy
Ligamentoso: ligamentous
Ligandina: ligandin
Ligante: ligand
Ligar: bind, ligate
Ligase: ligase
Ligase do ácido graxo de cadeia longa-CoA: long-chain fatty acid-CoA ligase
Lígneo: ligneous
Lignina: lignin
Lima: file
Limão: lemon, limon, gen. limonis
Límbico: limbic
Limbo: limbus, **pl.** limbi
Límen: limen, **pl.** limina
Limiar: limes (L), liminal, threshold
Liminômetro: liminometer
Limitado: bound
Limite: cutpoint, limit
Limnologia: limnology
Limpeza: cleaning
Lincomicina: lincomycin
Lindano: lindane
Linear: linear
Linearidade: linearity
Linestrenol: lynestrenol
Linfa: lymph, lympha
Linfadenectomia: lymphadenectomy
Linfadenite: lymphadenitis
Linfadenografia: lymphadenography
Linfadenóide: lymphadenoid
Linfadenoma: lymphadenoma
Linfadenopatia: lymphadenopathy
Linfadenose: lymphadenosis
Linfadenovariz: lymphadenovarix
Linfaférese: lymphapheresis
Linfagogo: lymphagogue
Linfangeíte: lymphangeitis
Linfangial: lymphangial
Linfangiectasia: lymphangiectasis, lymphangiectasia

Linfangiectásico: lymphangiectatic
Linfangiectomia: lymphangiectomy
Linfângio: lymphangion
Linfangioendotelioma: lymphangioendothelioma
Linfangioflebite: lymphangiophlebitis
Linfangiografia: lymphangiography
Linfangioliomiomatose: lymphangioleiomyomatosis
Linfangiologia: lymphangiology
Linfangioma: lymphangioma
Linfangiomatoso: lymphangiomatous
Linfangiomiomatose: lymphangiomyomatosis
Linfangioplastia: lymphangioplasty
Linfangiossarcoma: lymphangiosarcoma
Linfangiotomia: lymphangiotomy
Linfangite: lymphangiitis, lymphangitis
Linfático: lymphatic
Linfáticos: lymphatics
Linfaticostomia: lymphaticostomy
Linfatite: lymphatitis
Linfatólise: lymphatolysis
Linfatolítico: lymphatolytic
Linfatologia: lymphatology
Linfectasia: lymphectasia
Linfedema: lymphedema
Linfemia: lymphemia
Linfização: limphization
Linfoblástico: lymphoblastic
Linfoblasto: lymphoblast
Linfoblastoma: lymphoblastoma
Linfoblastose: lymphoblastosis
Linfocele: lymphocele
Linfocerastismo: lymphocerastism
Linfocinas: lymphokine
Linfocinese: lymphokinesis
Linfocinesia: lymphocinesis, lymphocinesia
Linfocintigrafia: lymphoscintigraphy
Linfocitemia: lymphocythemia
Linfocítico: lymphocytic
Linfócito: lymphocyte
Linfocitoblasto: lymphocytoblast
Linfocitoférese: lymphocytapheresis
Linfocitoma: lymphocytoma
Linfocitopenia: lymphocytopenia
Linfocitopoese: lymphocytopoiesis
Linfocitose: lymphocytosis
Linfoderma: lymphoderma
Linfoducto: lymphoduct
Linfoestase: lymphostasis
Linfogênese: lymphogenesis
Linfogênico: lymphogenic
Linfógeno: lymphogenous

Linfografia: lymphography
Linfogranuloma: lymphogranuloma
Linfogranulomatose: lymphogranulomatosis
Linfo-histiocitose: lymphohistiocytosis
Linfóide: lymphoid
Linfoidectomia: lymphoidectomy
Linfoidócito: lymphoidocyte
Linfoleucócito: lympholeukocyte
Linfologia: lymphology
Linfoma: lymphoma
Linfomatóide: lymphomatoid
Linfomatose: lymphomatosis
Linfomatoso: lymphomatous
Linfonodo: lymph node, lymphaden, lymphoglandula, lymphonodus, nodus lymphaticus, **pl.** nodi lymphatici; nodus lymphoideus, **pl.** nodi lymphoidei
Linfopatia: lymphopathia, lymphopathy
Linfopenia: lymphopenia
Linfoplasmaférese: lymphoplasmapheresis
Linfopoese: lymphopoiesis
Linfopoético: lymphopoietic
Linforragia: lymphorrhagia
Linforréia: lymphorrhea
Linforreticulose: lymphoreticulosis
Linforróida: lymphorrhoid
Linfose: lymphosis
Linfotaxia: lymphotaxis
Linfotoxicidade: lymphotoxicity
Linfotoxina: lymphotoxin
Linfotrofia: lymphotrophy
Linfúria: lymphuria
Língua: lingua, **gen. e pl.** linguae; tongue
Língua presa: tongue-tie
Linguagem: language
Lingual: lingual
Linguatulíase: linguatuliasis
Lingüiforme: linguiform
Língula: lingula, **pl.** lingulae
Lingular: lingular
Lingulectomia: lingulectomy
Linguoclinação: linguoclination
Linguoclusal: linguo-occlusal
Linguoclusão: linguoclusion
Linguodistal: linguodistal
Linguogengival: linguogingival
Linguopapilite: linguopapillitis
Linguoversão: linguoversion
Linha: line, linea, **gen. e pl.** lineae
Linha de Correra: Correra line
Linha de frente: front
Linha de Ohngren: Ohngren line
Linha de Sydney: Sydney line
Linhagem: lineage
Linimento: liniment
Linina: linin
Linite: linitis

Linoleato: linoleate
Lioenzima: lyoenzyme
Liofílico: lyophilic
Liofilização: lyophilization
Liófilo: lyophil, lyophile
Liofóbico: lyophobic
Liófobo: lyophobe
Liólise: lyolysis
Lionização: lyonization
Liosorção: lyosorption
Liótrico: leiotrichous
Liotrópico: lyotropic
Lipancreatina: lipancreatin
Liparocele: liparocele
Lipase: lipase
Lipectomia: lipectomy
Lipedema: lipedema
Lipemia: lipemia
Lipêmico: lipemic
Lipidemia: lipidemia
Lipídio: lipid
Lipidolítico: lipidolytic
Lipidose: lipidosis, **pl.** lipidoses
Lipoamida: lipoamide
Lipoamida desidrogenase: lipoamide dehydrogenase
Lipoamida redutase: lipoamide reductase (NADH)
Lipoartrite: lipoarthritis
Lipoato: lipoate
Lipoato-acetiltransferase: lipoate acetyltransferase
Lipoatrofia: lipoatrophia, lipoatrophy
Lipoblasto: lipoblast
Lipoblastoma: lipoblastoma
Lipoblastomatose: lipoblastomatosis
Lipocardíaco: lipocardiac
Lipocatabólico: lipocatabolic
Lipocera: lipocere
Lipoceratoso: lipoceratous
Lipócito: lipocyte
Lipoclase: lipoclasis
Lipoclástico: lipoclastic
Lipocôndrias: lipochondria
Lipocondrodistrofia: lipochondrodystrophy
Lipócrito: lipocrit
Lipocromo: lipochrome
Lipodermóide: lipodermoid
Lipodiérese: lipodieresis
Lipodistrofia: lipodystrophia, lipodystrophy
Lipoedema: lipoedema
Lipoemia: lipohemia
Lipoescultura: liposuctioning
Lipofagia: lipophagy
Lipofágico: lipophagic
Lipófago: lipophage
Lipofanerose: lipophanerosis
Lipofecção: lipofection
Lipofectina: lipofectin
Lipófero: lipoferous
Lipofibroma: lipofibroma
Lipofílico: lipophilic
Lipófilo: lipophil
Lipofosfodiesterase I: lipophosphodiesterase I
Lipofosfodiesterase II: lipophosphodiesterase II

Lipofuscina: lipofuscin
Lipofuscinose: lipofuscinosis
Lipogênese: lipogenesis
Lipogênico: lipogenic, lipogenous
Lipogranuloma: lipogranuloma
Lipogranulomatose: lipogranulomatosis
Lipóide: lipoid
Lipoidemia: lipoidemia
Lipoidose: lipoidosis
Lipoil: lipoyl
Lipoil desidrogenase: lipoyl dehydrogenase
Lipoinjeção: lipoinjection
Lipolipoidose: lipolipoidosis
Lipólise: lipolysis
Lipolítico: lipolytic
Lipoma: lipoma
Lipomatóide: lipomatoid
Lipomatose: lipomatosis
Lipomatoso: lipomatous
Lipomeningocele: lipomeningocele
Lipomucopolissacaridose: lipomucopolysaccharidosis
Liponucleoproteínas: liponucleoproteins
Lipopenia: lipopenia
Lipopênico: lipopenic
Lipopeptídeo: lipopeptid, lipopeptide
Lipopolissacarídeo: lipopolysaccharide (LPS)
Lipoproteína: lipoprotein
Lipoproteína lipase: lipoprotein lipase
Lipose: liposis
Lipositol: lipositol
Lipossarcoma: liposarcoma
Lipossolúvel: liposoluble
Lipossoma: liposome
Lipossucção: liposuction
Lipotrofia: lipotrophy
Lipotrófico: lipotrophic
Lipotropia: lipotropy
Lipotrópico: lipotropic
Lipotropina: lipotropin
Lipovacina: lipovaccine
Lipovitelina: lipovitellin
Lipoxenia: lipoxeny
Lipoxênico: lipoxenous
Lipoxidase: lipoxidase
Lipoxigenase: lipoxygenase
Lipressina: lypressin
Lipúria: lipuria
Lipúrico: lipuric
Liquefação: liquefaction
Liquefaciente: liquefacient
Liquefativo: liquefactive
Líquen: lichen
Liquenificação: lichenification
Liquenina: lichenin
Liquenóide: lichenoid
Líquido: liquid (l), liquor, **gen.** liquoris, **pl.** liquores
Líquido de montagem de Farrant: Farrant mounting fluid
Líquido sinovial: synovia
Liquorréia: liquorrhea

Lira: lyra
Lisado: lysate
Lisar: lyse, lyze
Lise: lysis
Lisemia: lysemia
Lisergamida: lysergamide
Lisergida: lysergide
Lisergol: lysergol
Lisil: lysyl (K)
Lisil-bradicinina: lysyl-bradykinin
Lisina: lysin, lysine (K, Lys)
8-lisina vasopressina: 8-lysine vasopressin
Lisinemia: lysinemia
Lisínio: lysinium
Lisinogênico: lysinogenic
Lisinogênio: lysinogen
Lisinopril: lisinopril
Lisinúria: lysinuria
Lisocefalina: lysocephalin
Lisocinase: lysokinase
Lisoestafina: lysostaphin
Lisofosfatidilcolina: lysophosphatidylcholine
Lisofosfatidilserina: lysophosphatidylserine
Lisofosfolipase: lysophospholipase
Lisogênese: lysogenesis
Lisogenia: lysogeny
Lisogenicidade: lysogenicity
Lisogênico: lysogenic
Lisogenização: lysogenization
Lisógeno: lysogen
Lisolecitina: lysolecithin
Lisolecitinase: lysolecithinase
Lisossoma: lysosome
Lisótipo: lysotype
Lisozima: lysozyme
Lissamina rodamina B 200: lissamine rhodamine B 200
Lissencefalia: lissencephalia, lissencephaly
Lissencefálico: lissencephalic
Lissótrico: lissotrichic, lissotrichous
Listeriose: listeriosis
Listerismo: listerism
Lisurida: lisuride
Litagogo: lithagogue
Litargírio: litharge
Litectomia: lithectomy
Literatura: literature
Litíase: lithiasis
Lítico: lytic
Lítio: lithium (Li)
Litmo: litmus
Litocélifo: lithokelyphos
Litocelifopédio: lithokelyphopedion, lithokelyphopedium
Litoclasto: lithoclast
Litogênese: lithogenesis, lithogeny
Litogênico: lithogenic, lithogenous
Litóide: lithoid
Litolábio: bilabe, litholabe
Litolapaxia: litholapaxy
Litólise: litholysis

Glossário

Litolítico: litholytic
Litólito: litholyte
Litômilo: lithomyl
Litonefrite: lithonephritis
Litopédio: lithopedion, lithopedium
Litotomia: lithotomy
Litotomista: lithotomist
Litótomo: lithotome
Litotrese: lithotresis
Litotripsia: lithotripsy, lithotrity
Litotríptico: lithotriptic
Litotriptor: lithotriptor
Litotriptoscopia: lithotriptoscopy
Litótrito: lithotrite
Litótrofo: lithotroph
Litro: liter (L, l)
Liturese: lithuresis
Litúria: lithuria
Livedo: livedo
Livedóide: livedoid
Livetina: livetin
Lividez: lividity
Lívido: livid
Livor: livor
Lixitol: lyxitol
Lixívia: lixivium, lye
Lixiviação: leaching
Lixoflavina: lyxoflavin
Lixose: lyxose
Lixulose: lyxulose
Lobado: lobate, lobose, lobous
Lobar: lobar
Lobectomia: lobectomy
Lobélia: lobelia
Lobelina: lobeline, lobelin
Lobite: lobitis
Lobo: lobe, lobus, **gen. e pl.** lobi
Lobomicose: lobomycosis
Lobopódio: lobopodium, **pl.** lobopodia
Lobotomia: lobotomy
Lobulado: lobulate, lobulated
Lobular: lobular
Lóbulo: lobule, lobulus, **gen. e pl.** lobuli
Lóbulo semilunar inferior: crus II
Lóbulo semilunar superior: crus I
Local: local, site
Localização: localization
Localizado: localized
Localizador: locator
Loção: lotion, wash
Locomotivo: locomotive
Locomotor: locomotor, locomotorial, locomotorium, locomotory
Locos: loci
Loculação: loculation
Loculado: loculate
Locular: locular
Lóculo: loculus, **pl.** loculi
Lofentanil: lofentanil
Lofodonte: lophodont
Lofotríquio: lophotrichate, lophotrichous
Logaritmo: logarithm

Logetronografia: logetronography
Logoespasmo: logospasm
Logopedia: logopedia, logopedics
Logorréia: logorrhea, polyphrasia
Logoterapia: logotherapy
Loíase: loiasis
Lolismo: loliism
Lombar: lumbar
Lombarização: lumbarization
Lombo: lumbus, **gen. e pl.** lumbi
Lomboabdominal: lumboabdominal
Lombocostal: lumbocostal
Lomboilíaco: lumboiliac
Lomboinguinal: lumboinguinal
Lombossacro: lumbosacral
Lombovariano: lumbo-ovarian
Lombrical: lumbrical, lumbricalis
Lombricida: lumbricidal, lumbricide
Lombricóide: lumbricoid, lumbricus
Lombricose: lumbricosis
Lomustina: lomustine
Longevidade: longevity
Longitipo: longitype
Longitudinal: longitudinal, longitudinalis
Lopremona: lopremone
Loquial: lochial
Loquiometro: lochiometra
Loquiorragia: lochiorrhagia
Loquiorréia: lochiorrhea
Lóquios: lochia
Lorazepam: lorazepam
Lorcainida: lorcainide
Lordoescoliose: lordoscoliosis
Lordose: lordosis
Lordótico: lordotic
Louco: mad
Loucura: lunacy, madness
Louvável: laudable
Lovastatina: lovastatin
Loxapina: loxapine
Loxocelismo: loxoscelism
Lucensomicina: lucensomycin
Lucidez: lucidity
Lúcido: lucid
Luciferases: luciferases
Luciferinas: luciferins
Lucífugo: lucifugal
Lucimicina: lucimycin
Lucípeto: lucipetal
Lues: lues
Luético: luetic
Luliberina: luliberin
Lumbago: lumbago
Lumícromo: lumichrome
Lumiflavina: lumiflavin
Luminal: luminal, luminalis
Luminância: luminance
Luminescência: luminescence
Luminífero: luminiferous
Luminóforo: luminophore
Luminoso: luminous
Lumirodopsina: lumirhodopsin
Lumisterol: lumisterol

Lunar: lunar
Lunático: lunatic
Lunatomalacia: lunatomalacia
Lúnula: lunula, **pl.** lunulae, lunule, selene unguium
Lupa: loupe
Lupinidina: lupinidine
Lupinose: lupinosis
Lupóide: lupoid
Lupulina: lupulin
Lúpulo: hops, humulus
Lúpus: lupus
Lura: lura
Lural: lural
Lusitropia: lusitropy
Lusitrópico: lusitropic
Lutécio: lutecium, lutetium (Lu)
Luteína: lutein
Luteinização: luteinization
Luteinizar: luteinize
Luteinoma: luteinoma
Lúteo: luteal, luteus
Luteogênico: luteogenic
Luteol: luteol, luteole
Luteolina: luteolin
Luteólise: luteolysis
Luteolisina: luteolysin
Luteolítico: luteolytic
Luteoma: luteoma
Luteotrópico: luteotropic, luteotrophic
Lutropina: lutropin
Lututrina: lututrin
Luva: gauntlet
Lux: candle-meter, lux (lx), meter-candle
Luxação: dislocatio, dislocation, luxatio, luxation
Luxar: dislocate
Luxo: luxus
Luz: light, lumen, **pl.** lumina, lumens

M

Má absorção: malabsorption
Má aparência: dyschroia, dyschroa
Má assimilação: malassimilation
Má digestão: maldigestion
Má emissão: malemission
Má erupção: maleruption
Má interdigitação: malinterdigitation
Má oclusão: malocclusion
Má rotação: malrotation
Maca: stretcher
Macaco: macaque
Macaco-de-rosca: jackscrew
Maceração: insuccation, maceration
Macerar: macerate
Machadinha: hatchet
Macho: male
Macicez: dullness, dulness
Maclurina: maclurin
Maconha: marihuana

Macroadenoma: macroadenoma
Macroamilase: macroamylase
Macroamilasemia: macroamylasemia
Macrobactéria: macrobacterium
Macróbio: macrobiote
Macrobiose: macrobiosis
Macrobiótica: macrobiotics
Macrobiótico: macrobiotic
Macroblasto: macroblast
Macroblefaria: macroblepharon
Macrobraquia: macrobrachia
Macrocardia: macrocardia
Macrocefalia: macrocephaly, macrocephalia
Macrocefálico: macrocephalic, macrocephalous
Macrocisto: macrocyst
Macrocitemia: macrocythemia
Macrócito: macrocyte
Macrocitose: macrocytosis
Macrocnemia: macrocnemia
Macrococo: macrococcus
Macrocólon: macrocolon
Macroconídio: macroconidium, **pl.** macroconidia
Macrocórnea: macrocornea
Macrocrânio: macrocranium
Macrocrioglobulina: macrocryoglobulin
Macrocrioglobulinemia: macrocryoglobulinemia
Macrodactilia: macrodactylia, macrodactylism, macrodactyly
Macrodistrofia lipomatosa: macrodystrophia lipomatosa
Macrodonte: macrodont
Macrodontia: macrodontia, macrodontism
Macroelementos: macroelements
Macroencefalia: macrencephaly, macrencephalia
Macroencéfalo: macroencephalon
Macroeritroblasto: macroerythroblast
Macroeritrócito: macroerythrocyte
Macroesplâncnico: macrosplanchnic
Macroestesia: macroesthesia
Macrófago: macrophage
Macrofagócito: macrophagocyte
Macroftalmia: macrophthalmia
Macrogameta: macrogamete
Macrogametócito: macrogametocyte
Macrogamia: macrogamy
Macrogamonte: macrogamont
Macrogastria: macrogastria
Macrogenitossomia: macrogenitosomia
Macrogiria: macrogyria
Macróglia: macroglia
Macroglobulinas: macroglobulins
Macroglobulinemia: macroglobulinemia

Macroglossia: macroglossia
Macrognatia: macrognathia
Macrografia: macrography
Macroleucoblasto: macroleukoblast
Macrolídeo: macrolide
Macrolídeos: macrolides
Macromastia: macromastia, macromazia
Macromelanossoma: macromelanosome
Macromelia: macromelia
Macrômero: macromere
Macromerozoíta: macromerozoite
Macromieloblasto: macromyeloblast
Macrominerais: macrominerals
Macromolécula: macromolecule
Macromonócito: macromonocyte
Macroniquia: macronychia
Macronormoblasto: macronormoblast
Macronormocromoblasto: macronormochromoblast
Macronúcleo: macronucleus
Macronutrientes: macronutrients
Macroorquidismo: macroorchidism
Macroparasita: macroparasite
Macropatologia: macropathology
Macropênis: macropenis, macrophallus
Macropodia: macropodia
Macropolícito: macropolycyte
Macropromielócito: macropromyelocyte
Macroprosopia: macroprosopia
Macroprosópico: macroprosopous
Macropsia: macropsia
Macroquilia: macrocheilia, macrochilia, macrolabia
Macroquilomícron: macrochylomicron
Macroquímica: macrochemistry
Macroquiria: macrocheiria, macrochiria
Macrorrinia: macrorhinia
Macroscelia: macroscelia
Macroscopia: macroscopy
Macroscópico: gross, macroscopic
Macrose: macrosis
Macrosmático: macrosmatic
Macrosporo: macrospore
Macrossigmóide: macrosigmoid
Macrossomia: macrosomia
Macrostereognosia: macrostereognosis
Macrostomia: macrostomia
Macrotia: macrotia
Macrótomo: macrotome
Mácula: macula, **pl.** maculae; macule, spot, tache
Macular: macular, maculate
Maculocerebral: maculocerebral

Maculoeritematosa: maculoerythematous
Maculopápula: maculopapule
Maculopatia: maculopathy
Madarose: madarosis
Madeira da laranjeira: orange wood
Maduro: mature
Maduromicose: maduromycosis
Mafenida: mafenide
Má-formação: malformation
Magaldrato: magaldrate
Magistral: magistral
Magma: magma
Magnésia: magnesia
Magnésio: magnesium (Mg)
Magnético: magnetic
Magnetismo: magnetism
Magneto: magnet
Magnetocardiografia: magnetocardiography
Magnetoencefalografia: magnetoencephalography
Magnetoencefalograma: magnetoencephalogram (MEG)
Magnetômetro: magnetometer
Magnéton: magneton
Magnetoterapia: magnetotherapy
Magnitude: magnitude
Magno: magnus
Magnocelular: magnocellular
Maior: major
Mal: mal, malum
Mal das montanhas: soroche
Mal do rei: king's evil
Malacia: malacia
Malácico: malacic
Malacoplaquia: malacoplakia, malakoplakia
Malacose: malacosis
Malacótico: malacotic
Maláctico: malactic
Malagma: malagma
Malar: mala, malar
Malária: malaria
Malária crônica: limnemia
Malárico: malarial
Malariologia: malariology
Malarioso: malarious
Malarioterapia: malariotherapy
Malation: malathion
Malato: malate
Malaxação: malaxation
Maleato de acetofenazina: acetophenazine maleate
Maleato de azatadina: azatadine maleate
Maleato de bromofeniramina: brompheniramine maleate
Maleato de carbinoxamina: carbinoxamine maleate
Maleato de carfenazina: carphenazine maleate
Maleato de clorfeniramina: chlorpheniramine maleate
Maleato de dexbronfeniramina: dexbrompheniramine maleate
Maleato de dexclorfeniramina: dexchlorpheniramine maleate

Maleato de dimetindeno: dimethindene maleate
Maleato de enalapril: enalapril maleate
Maleato de feniramina: pheniramine maleate
Maleato de mepiramina: mepyramine maleate
Maleato de metilergometrina: methylergometrine maleate
Maleato de metilergonovina: methylergonovine maleate
Maleato de metisergida: methysergide maleate
Maleato de nomifensina: nomifensine maleate
Maleato de perexilina: perhexiline maleate
Maleato de pirilamina: pyrilamine maleate
Maleato de profempiridamina: prophenpyridamine maleate
Maleato de tietilperazina: thiethylperazine maleate
Maleato de timolol: timolol maleate
Maleável: malleable
Malebrina: mallebrin
Maleilacetoacetato: maleylacetoacetate
Maleoincudal: malleoincudal
Maleolar: malleolar
Maléolo: malleolus, **pl.** malleoli
Maleotomia: malleotomy
Mal-estar: malaise
Malignidade: malignancy
Maligno: malignant
Malonato: malonate
Malonato semi-aldeído: malonate semialdehyde
Malonil: malonyl
Malonil-CoA: malonyl-CoA
Malonilcoenzima A: malonylcoenzyme A
Maloniluréia: malonylurea
Maltase: maltase
Malte: malt
Maltobiose: maltobiose
Maltose: maltose
Maltotetrose: maltotetrose
Mama: mamma, **gen. e pl.** mammae
Mamalgia: mammalgia
Mamão: papaw, papaya, pawpaw
Mamário: mammary
Mamectomia: mammectomy
Mamelão: mamelon
Mamelonação: mamelonation
Mamelonado: mamelonated
Mamífero: mammal
Mamiforme: mammiform
Mamilado: mammillate
Mamilar: mammillare, mammillary
Mamiliforme: mammilliform
Mamilite: mammillitis
Mamilo: mammilla, **pl.** mammillae; nipple, teat, thele
Mamiloplastia: mammillaplasty

Mamiloso: mammilation
Mamografia: mammography
Mamograma: mammogram
Mamona: castor bean
Mamoplastia: mammaplasty, mammoplasty
Mamose: mammose
Mamossomatotrofo: mammosomatotroph
Mamotomia: mammotomy
Mamotrofo: mammotroph
Mamotrópico: mammotropic, mammotrophic
Mamotropina: mammotropin, mammotrophin
Maná: manna
Mananas: mannans
Mancha: blot, mottle, patch
Mandelato: mandelate
Mandelitropina: mandelytropine
Mandíbula: jaw, manddibulum, mandible, mandibula, **pl.** mandibulae; submaxilla
Mandibular: mandibular, submaxillary
Mandibulectomia: mandibulectomy
Mandibulofacial: mandibulofacial
Mandibulofaríngeo: mandibulopharyngeal
Mandibulo-oculofacial: mandibulo-oculofacial
Mandrágora: mandragora, mandrake
Mandril: mandrel, mandril, mandrill, mandrin
Maneirismo: mannerism
Manequim: manikin
Manganês: manganese (Mn), manganum
Mangânico: manganic
Manganoso: manganous
Manguito: cuff
Mania: mania
Maníaco: maniac, maniacal, manic, manicky
Maníaco-depressivo: manic-depressive
Manifalange: maniphalanx
Manifestação: manifestation
Manita: mannite
Manitol: mannitol
Manjerona: marjoram
Manobra: maneuver
Manodinamômetro: manudynamometer
Manoeptulose: mannoheptulose
D-*mano*-heptulose: D-*manno*-heptulose
Manometria: manometry
Manométrico: manometric
Manômetro: manometer
Manomustina: mannomustine
Manoproteínas: mannoproteins
Manosamina: mannosamine
Manosanas: mannosans
Manoscopia: manoscopy
Manose: mannose (Man)

Glossário

Manose-1-fosfato guaniliiltransferase: mannose-1-phosphate guanylyltransferase (GDP)
Manosefosfato isomerase: mannosephosphate isomerase
Manosidases: mannosidases
Manosídeo: mannoside
Manosidose: mannosidosis
Mansoneliase: mansonelliasis
Mansonelose: mansonellosis
Mantenedor: maintainer
Mantenedor de espaço: regainer
Manto: mantle
Manúbrio: manubrium, **pl.** manubria
Manutenção: maintenance
Mão: hand, main, manus, **gen. e pl.** manus
Mão em garra: clawhand
Mão torta: clubhand
Mapa: map
Mapeamento: mapping
Mapina: mappine
Maprotilina: maprotiline
Máquina: machine
Marântico: marantic
Marásmico: marasmic
Marasmo: marasmus
Marasmóide: marasmoid
Marca: mark
Marca de nascimento: birthmark
Marcação: targeting
Marcador: marker, tag
Marcadores de DNA: DNA markers
Marcapasso: pace-maker
Marcar: label
Marcha: gait
Marcha de passos altos: steppage
Maré: tide
Marenostrina: marenostrin
Marfanóide: marfanoid
Margarida-dos-campos: daisy
Margem: border, brim, edge, margin, margo, **gen.** marginis, **pl.** margines; rim
Marginação: margination
Marginal: marginal
Marinobufotoxina: marinobufotoxin
Mariposia: mariposia
Marmelo: quince
Marmoreado: marmorated
Marmota: marmot
Marroio-branco, marroio-comum: horehound, hoarhound
Marsupial: marsupial
Marsupialização: marsupialization
Marsúpio: marsupium
Martelo: hammer, malleus, **gen. e pl.** mallei
Maruim: gnat
Mascaliperidrose: maschalyperidrosis
Máscara: mask
Mascarado: masked
Mascaramento: masking

Masculinidade: masculinity
Masculinização: masculinization
Masculinizar: masculinize
Masculino: masculine, masculinus
Masoquismo: masochism
Masoquista: masochist
Massa: bulkage, mass (m), massa, **gen. e pl.** massae
Massa pilular: pill mass
Massa semifluida: slurry
Massagem: massage
Massagista: masseur, masseuse
Masseter: masseter
Massoterapia: massotherapy
Mastadenite: mastadenitis
Mastadenoma: mastadenoma
Mastalgia: mastalgia
Mastatrofia: mastatrophy, mastatrophia
Mastauxe: mastauxe
Mastectomia: mastectomy
Mastigação: mastication
Mastigar: masticate
Mastigatório: masticatory
Mastigota: mastigote
Mástique: mastic, mastich, mastiche
Mastite: mastitis
Mastoccipital: mastoccipital
Mastócito: labrocyte, mastocyte
Mastocitogênese: mastocytogenesis
Mastocitoma: mastocytoma
Mastocitose: mastocytosis
Mastodinia: mastodynia
Mastoescamoso: mastosquamous
Mastóide: mastoid, mastoidale
Mastoidectomia: mastoidectomy
Mastóideo: mastoidal
Mastoidite: mastoiditis
Mastoncose: mastoncus
Masto-occipital: masto-occipital
Mastoparietal: mastoparietal
Mastopatia: mastopathy
Mastopexia: mastopexy
Mastoplasia: mastoplasia
Mastoplastia: mastoplasty
Mastoptose: mastoptosis
Mastorragia: mastorrhagia
Mastossiringe: mastosyrinx
Mastotomia: mastotomy
Masturbação: masturbation
Masturbar: masturbate
Máter: mater
Matéria: materia, matter
Material: material
Maternidade: maternity
Materno: maternal
Matraz: matrass
Matricial: matrical, matricial
Matricídio: matricide
Matrilinear: matrilineal
Matriz: matrix, **pl.** matrices
Matriz da unha: onychostroma
Maturação: maturation
Maturidade: maturity

Maxila: maxilla, **gen. e pl.** maxillae
Maxilar: maxillary
Maxilectomia: maxillectomy
Maxilite: maxillitis
Maxilodental: maxillodental
Maxilofacial: maxillofacial
Maxilojugal: maxillojugal
Maxilomandibular: maxillomandibular
Maxilopalatino: maxillopalatine
Maxilotomia: maxillotomy
Maxiloturbinal: maxilloturbinal
Máximo: maximum
Mazamorra: mazamorra
Mazindol: mazindol
m-cloral: *m*-chloral
m-cresol: *m*-cresol
Meatal: meatal
Meato: meatus, **pl.** meatus
Meatômetro: meatometer
Meatoplastia: meatoplasty
Meatorrafia: meatorrhaphy
Meatoscopia: meatoscopy
Meatoscópio: meatoscope
Meatotomia: meatotomy
Meatótomo: meatotome
Mebanazina: mebanazine
Mebendazol: mebendazole
Mebrofenidramina: mebrophenhydramine
Mebutamato: mebutamate
Mecânica: mechanics
Mecânico: mechanical
Mecanismo: mechanism
Mecanismo dentário: dental engine
Mecanocardiografia: mechanocardiography
Mecanócito: mechanocyte
Mecanofobia: mechanophobia
Mecanorreceptor: mechanicoreceptor, mechanoreceptor
Mecanorreflexo: mechanoreflex
Mecanoterapia: mechanotherapy
Mecha: mèche
Mecismo: mecism
Meclastina: meclastine
Meclofenamato sódico: meclofenamate sodium
Meclofenoxato: meclofenoxate
Mecômetro: mecometer
Meconato: meconate
Meconina: meconin
Mecônio: meconium
Meconiorréia: meconiorrhea
Medfalam: medfalan
Medfalan: medphalan
Média: average, mean, media
Mediação: mediation
Mediador: mediator
Medial: mediad, medial, medialis
Medialização: medialization
Mediano: median, medianus
Mediastinal: mediastinal
Mediastinite: mediastinitis
Mediastino: mediastinum

Mediastinografia: mediastinography
Mediastinopericardite: mediastinopericarditis
Mediastinoscopia: mediastinoscopy
Mediastinoscópio: mediastinoscope
Mediastinotomia: mediastinotomy
Medicação: medication
Medicado: medicated
Medicador: medicator
Medicamento: medicament, medicine
Medicamentoso: medicamentosus
Medicar: medicate
Medicável: medicable
Medicefálico: medicephalic
Medicina: physic
Medicinal: medicinal
Médico: healer, medical, physician
Médico-biológico: medicobiologic, medicobiological
Médico-físico: medicophysical
Médico-legal: medicolegal
Médico-mecânico: medicomechanical
Medida: measurement
Medida da lente de Genebra: Geneva lens measure
Medidas de tendência central: measures of central tendency
Medidor: gage
Medidor de Boley: Boley gauge
Médio: medius, middle
Mediocarpal: mediocarpal
Mediodente: mediodens
Mediodorsal: mediodorsal
Mediolateral: mediolateral
Mediolécito: medialecithal
Medionecrose: medionecrosis
Médio-occipital: mediooccipital
Mediotarsal: mediotarsal
Mediotrusão: mediotrusion
Medir: measure
Meditação transcendental (MT): transcendental meditation (TM)
Medrilamina: medrylamine
Medrisona: medrysone
Medrogestona: medrogestone
Medula: medulla, **pl.** medullae; pith
Medula oblonga: oblongata
Medula óssea: marrow
Medulação: medullation
Medulado: medullated
Medular: medullar, medullary
Medulectomia: medullectomy
Medulização: medullization
Meduloartrite: medulloarthritis
Meduloblastoma: medulloblastoma
Meduloepitelioma: medulloepithelioma
Medulomioblastoma: medullomyoblastoma

Medusa: jellyfish
Mefenesina: mephenesin
Mefenitoína: mephenytoin
Mefentermina: mephentermine
Mefexamida: mefexamide
Mefítico: mephitic
Mefloquina: mefloquine
Mefobarbital: mephobarbital
Megabactéria: megabacterium
Megabexiga: megalocystis
Megacalicose: megacalycosis
Megacarioblasto: megacaryoblast, megakaryoblast
Megacariócito: megacaryocyte, megakaryocyte
Megacefalia: megacephalia, megacephaly
Megacefálico: megacephalic
Megacéfalo: megacephalous
Megaciclo: megacycle
Megacinas: megacins
Megacisto: megacystis
Megacoco: megacoccus, **pl.** megacocci
Megacolo: megacolon
Megadina: megadyne
Megadolicocolo: megadolichocolon
Megaesôfago: megaesophagus
Megaesporo: megaspore
Megagameta: megagamete
Megahertz: megahertz (MHz)
Megalécito: megalecithal
Megalgia: megalgia
Megaloblasto: megaloblast
Megalocardia: megacardia, megalocardia
Megalocariócito: megalokaryocyte
Megalocefalia: megalocephaly, megalocephalia
Megalocitemia: megalocythemia
Megalócito: megalocyte
Megalocitose: megalocytosis
Megalocórnea: megalocornea
Megalodactilia: megadactyly, megadactylia, megadactylism, megalodactylia, megalodactylism, megalodactyly
Megalodonte: megadont, megalodont
Megalodontia: megalodontia
Megalodontismo: megadontism
Megaloencefalia: megaloencephaly
Megaloencefálico: megaloencephalic
Megaloencéfalo: megaloencephalon
Megaloesplâncnico: megalosplanchnic
Megaloftalmo: megalophthalmos
Megalogastria: megalogastria
Megaloglossia: megaloglossia
Megalognatia: megagnathia
Megalografia: megalographia
Megalomania: megalomania
Megalomaníaco: megalomaniac

Megalomelia: megalomelia
Megalopodia: megalopodia
Megaloquiria: megalocheiria, megalochiria
Megalosporo: megalospore
Megalossindactilia: megalosyndactyly, megalosyndactylia
Megaloureter: megaloureter
Megalouretra: megalourethra
Megamerozoíta: megamerozoite
Meganúcleo: meganucleus
Megapoetina: megapoietin
Megaprosopia: megaprosopia
Megaprosópico: megaprosopous
Megarreto: megarectum
Megassemo: megaseme
Megassigmóide: megasigmoid
Megassomia: megasomia
Megatrombócito: megathrombocyte
Megaureter: megaureter
Megavolt: megavolt
Megavoltagem: megavoltage
Meglitinidas: meglitinides
Meglumina: meglumine
Megoftalmo: megophthalmus
Megohm: megohm
Megoxicito: megoxycyte, megoxyphil, megoxyphile
Meia-lua: demilune, half-moon
Meia-luva: demigauntlet
Meia-vida: half-life
Meibomiano: meibomian
Meibomite: meibomitis, meibomianitis
Meimendro: henbane, nightshade
Meio: environment, medium, **pl.** media; milieu
Meio-hapteno: half-hapten
Meiose: meiosis
Meio-tempo: half-time
Meiótico: meiotic
Mel: honey, mel
Melagra: melagra
Melalgia: melalgia
Melancolia: melancholia, melancholy
Melancólico: melancholic
Melanemia: melanemia
Melanífero: melaniferous
Melanina: melanin
Melanismo: melanism
Melanoacantoma: melanoacanthoma
Melanoameloblastoma: melanoameloblastoma
Melanoblasto: melanoblast
Melanoceratose: melanokeratosis
Melanócito: melanocyte
Melanocitoma: melanocytoma
Melanodendrócito: melanodendrocyte
Melanodermatite: melanodermatitis
Melanodermia: melanoderma
Melanófago: melanophage
Melanóforo: melanophore

Melanogenemia: melanogenemia
Melanogênese: melanogenesis
Melanogênio: melanogen
Melanoglossia: melanoglossia
Melanóide: melanoid
Melanoleucodermia: melanoleukoderma
Melanoliberina: melanoliberin
Melanoma: melanoma
Melanomatose: melanomatosis
Melanoníquia: melanonychia
Melanopatia: melanopathy
Melanoplaquia: melanoplakia
Melanoproteína: melanoprotein
Melanorragia: melanorrhagia
Melanorréia: melanorrhea
Melanose: melanosis
Melanossoma: melanosome
Melanostatina: melanostatin
Melanótico: melanotic
Melanotonina: melanotonin
Melanotríquio: melanotrichous
Melanotrofo: melanotroph
Melanotropina: melanotrophin, melanotropin
Melanúria: melanuria
Melanúrico: melanuric
Melarsoprol: melarsoprol
Melasma: melasma
Melatonina: melatonin
Melena: melena
Melenêmese: melenemesis
Meletina: meletin
Melfalan: melphalan
Melhoria: amelioration
Melibiase: melibiase
Melibiose: melibiose
Melicéris: melicera, meliceris
Melioidose: melioidosis
Melissa: melissa
Melissofobia: melissophobia
Melite: melitis
Melitina: melittin
Melito: mellitum, **gen.** melliti, **pl.** mellita
Melitose: melitose
Melitriose: melitriose
Melodídimo: melodidymus
Melomania: melomania
Melomelia: melomelia
Meloplastia: meloplasty
Melorreostose: melorheostosis
Melosquise: meloschisis
Melotia: melotia
Membrana: membrana, **gen. e pl.** membranae, membrane
Membrana timpânica: drum, drumhead
Membranáceo: membranaceous
Membranectomia: membranectomy
Membranela: membranelle
Membraniforme: membraniform
Membranocartilaginoso: membranocartilaginous
Membranóide: membranoid
Membranoso: membranate, membranous

Membro: member, membrum, **pl.** membra
Memória: memory, mneme
Menacma: menacme
Menadiona: menadione
Menaftona: menaphthone
Menaquina: menaquinone (MK, MQ)
Menaquinona-6: menaquinone-6 (MK-6)
Menaquinona-7: menaquinone-7 (MK-7)
Menarca: menarche
Menárquico: menarcheal, menarchial
Mendelévio: mendelevium (Md)
Mendeliano: mendelian
Mendelismo: mendelism
Mendelização: mendelizing
Meninge: meninx, **gen.** meningis, **pl.** meninges
Meníngeo: meningeal
Meningeocortical: meningeocortical
Meningeorrafia: meningeorrhaphy
Meningioangiomatose: meningioangiomatosis
Meningioma: meningioma
Meningiomatose: meningiomatosis
Meningismo: meningism
Meningite: meningitis, **pl.** meningitides
Meningítico: meningitic
Meningocele: meningocele
Meningócito: meningocyte
Meningococcemia: meningococcemia
Meningococo: meningococcus, **pl.** meningococci
Meningocortical: meningocortical
Meningoencefalite: meningoencephalitis
Meningoencefalocele: meningoencephalocele
Meningoencefalomielite: meningoencephalomyelitis
Meningoencefalopatia: meningoencephalopathy
Meningomielite: meningomyelitis
Meningomielocele: meningomyelocele
Meningoosteoflebite: meningo-osteophlebitis
Meningorradicular: meningoradicular
Meningorradiculite: meningoradiculitis
Meningorragia: meningorrhagia
Meningorraquidiano: meningorrhachidian
Meningose: meningosis
Meningovascular: meningovascular
Meningúria: meninguria
Meniscectomia: meniscectomy
Meniscite: meniscitis

Menisco: meniscus, **pl.** menisci
Meniscopexia: meniscopexy
Meniscorrafia: meniscorrhaphy
Meniscótomo: meniscotome
Menocelidose: menocelis
Menofania: menophania
Menometrorragia: menometrorrhagia
Menopausa: menopause
Menopáusico: menopausal
Menor: minor
Menorragia: menorrhagia
Menorralgia: menorrhalgia
Menotropinas: menotropins
Menoúria: menouria
Menoxenia: menoxenia
Mensageiro: messenger
Mensal: mensual
Menstruação: menses, menstruation
Menstrual: menstrual
Menstruante: menstruant
Menstruar: menstruate
Mênstruo: menstruum, **pl.** menstrua
Mensuração: mensuration
Menta: mint
Mental: mental
Mentalidade: mentality
Mentano: menthane
Mente: mind
Mento: menton, mentum, **gen.** menti
Mentol: menthol
Mentolabial: mentolabialis
Mentoniano: genial, genian
Mentoplastia: mentoplasty
Mepirapona: mepyrapone
Meprobamato: meprobamate
Meptazinol: meptazinol
Meralgia: meralgia
Meralurida: meralluride
Merbromina: merbromin
Mercaptal: mercaptal
Mercaptana: mercaptan
Mercaptoetanol: mercaptoethanol
2-mercaptoetanol: 2-mercaptoethanol
β-mercaptoetanol: β-mercaptoethanol
Mercaptol: mercaptol
3-mercaptolactato: 3-mercaptolactate
Mercaptolactato-cisteína dissulfidúria: mercaptolactate-cysteine disulfiduria
Mercaptomerina sódica: mercaptomerin sodium
3-mercaptopiruvato: 3-mercaptopyruvate
6-mercaptopurina: 6-mercaptopurine (Shy)
Mercocresóis: mercocresols
Mercumatilina: mercumatilin
Mercuramida: mercuramide
Mercurial: mercurial
Mercurialente: mercurialentis
Mercurialismo: mercurialism
Mercúrico: mercuric

Mercúrio: mercury (Hg), quicksilver
Mercurocromo: mercurochrome
Mercurofeno: mercurophen
Mercurofilina sódica: mercurophylline sodium
Mercuroso: mercurous
Mereprina: mereprine
Merfalan: merphalan
Meridiano: meridian, meridianus, **pl.** meridiani
Meridional: meridional
Merisporo: merispore
Meristemático: meristematic
Merístico: meristic
Meroacrania: meroacrania
Meroanencefalia: meroanencephaly
Merócrino: merocrine
Merodiastólico: merodiastolic
Merogástrula: merogastrula
Merogênese: merogenesis
Merogenético: merogenetic, merogenic
Merogonia: merogony
Meromelia: meromelia
Meromicrossomia: meromicrosomia
Meromiosina: meromyosin
Meronte: meront
Merorraquisquise: merorachischisis, merorrhachischisis
Merosmia: merosmia
Merosporângio: merosporangium
Merossistólico: merosystolic
Merotomia: merotomy
Merozigoto: merozygote
Merozoíta: merozoite
Mersalil: mersalyl
Mesamebóide: mesameboid
Mesangial: mesangial
Mesângio: mesangium
Mesângio extraglomerular: polkissen of Zimmermann
Mesaortite: mesaortitis
Mesaraico: mesareic, mesaraic
Mesarterite: mesarteritis
Mesaticefálico: mesaticephalic
Mesatipélico: mesatipellic, mesatipelvic
Mesaxônio: mesaxon
Mescalina: mescaline
Mesectoderma: mesectoderm
Mesencefálico: mesencephalic
Mesencefalite: mesencephalitis
Mesencéfalo: mesencephalon, midbrain
Mesencefalotomia: mesencephalotomy
Mesênquima: mesenchyma, mesenchyme
Mesenquimatoso: mesenchymal
Mesenquimoma: mesenchymoma
Mesentérico: mesenteric
Mesentério: mesenterium, mesentery

Mesenteríolo: mesenteriolum
Mesenteriopexia: mesenteriopexy
Mesenteriorrafia: mesenteriorrhaphy
Mesenteriplicatura: mesenteriplication
Mesenterite: mesenteritis
Mesêntero: mesenteron
Mesial: mesad, mesiad
Mesilato de benzotropina: benztropine mesylate
Mesilato de bitolterol: bitolterol mesylate
Mesilato de deferoxamina: deferoxamine mesylate
Mesilato de desferrioxamina: desferrioxamine mesylate
Mesilato de diidroergotoxina: dihydroergotoxine mesylate
Mesilato de dimetotiazina: dimethothiazine mesylate
Mesilato de fentolamina: phentolamine mesylate
Mesilato de fonazina: fonazine mesylate
Mesilato de pergolida: pergolide mesylate
Mesiobucal: mesiobuccal
Mesiobucoclusal: mesiobucco-occlusal
Mesiobucopulpar: mesiobuccopulpal
Mesiocervical: mesiocervical
Mesioclusal: mesio-occlusal
Mesioclusão: mesioclusion, mesio-occlusion
Mesiodente: mesiodens
Mesiodeslocamento: mesioplacement
Mesiodistal: mesiodistal
Mesiodistoclusal: mesiodistocclusal (MOD)
Mesiogengival: mesiogingival
Mesiognático: mesiognathic
Mesioincisal: mesioincisal
Mesiolabial: mesiolabial
Mesiolingual: mesiolingual
Mesiolinguoclusal: mesiolinguo-occlusal
Mesiolinguopulpar: mesiolinguopulpal
Mesiopulpar: mesiopulpal
Mesioversão: mesioversion
Mesmerismo: mesmerism
Mesmerizar: mesmerize
Mesoapêndice: mesoappendix
Mesobilano: mesobilane
Mesobileno: mesobilene, mesobilene-β
Mesobilirrubina: mesobilirubin
Mesobilirrubinogênio: mesobilirubinogen
Mesobiliviolina: mesobiliviolin
Mesoblastema: mesoblastema
Mesoblastêmico: mesoblastemic
Mesoblástico: mesoblastic
Mesoblasto: mesoblast
Mesocardia: mesocardia
Mesocárdio: mesocardium, **pl.** mesocardia

Mesocarpal: mesocarpal, midcarpal
Mesoccipital: midoccipital
Mesocecal: mesocecal
Mesoceco: mesocecum
Mesocefálico: mesocephalic
Mesocéfalo: mesocephalous
Meso-cistina: *meso*-cystine
Mesocólico: mesocolic
Mesocolo: mesocolon
Mesocolopexia: mesocolopexy
Mesocoloplicatura: mesocoloplication
Mesocórdio: mesocord
Mesocuneiforme: mesocuneiform
Mesoderma: mesoderm
Mesodérmico: mesodermal, mesodermic
Mesodiastólico: mesodiastolic
Mesodonte: mesodont
Mesoduodenal: mesoduodenal
Mesoduodeno: mesoduodenum
Mesoenteríolo: mesoenteriolum
Mesoepidídimo: mesoepididymis
Mesoesterno: midsternum
Mesofílico: mesophilic
Mesófilo: mesophil, mesophile
Mesoflebite: mesophlebitis
Mesofragma: mesophragma
Mesófrio: mesophryon
Mesogástrico: mesogastric
Mesogástrio: mesogaster, mesogastrium
Mesogênico: mesogenic
Mesóglia: mesoglia
Mesoglúteo: mesogluteal
Mesognático: mesognathic, mesognathous
Mesognátio: mesognathion
Mesográcil: midgracile
Mesoíleo: mesoileum
Meso-inositol: *meso*-inositol
Mesojejuno: mesojejunum
Mesolinfócito: mesolymphocyte
Mesolobo: mesolobus
Mesomelia: mesomelia
Mesomélico: mesomelic
Mesomenstrual: midmenstrual
Mesomérico: mesomeric
Mesomerismo: mesomerism
Mesômero: mesomere
Mesométrio: mesometrium
Mesomórfico: mediotype, mesomorphic
Mesomorfo: mesomorph
Meson: meson
Mesonéfrico: mesonephric
Mesonefro: mesonephros, **pl.** mesonephroi
Mesonefroma: mesonephroma
Mesoneurite: mesoneuritis
Mesontomorfo: meso-ontomorph
Mesopexia: mesopexy
Mesópico: mesopic
Mesopneumônio: mesopneumonium
Mesoporfirinas: mesoporphyrins

Mesoprosópico: mesoprosopic
Mesopulmão: mesopulmonum
Mesórquico: mesorchial
Mesórquio: mesorchium
Mesorrafia: mesorrhaphy
Mesorreto: mesorectum
Mesorríneo: mesorrhine
Mesoscópio: mesoscope
Mesossalpinge: mesosalpinx
Mesossema: mesoseme
Mesossigmóide: mesosigmoid
Mesossigmoidite: mesosigmoiditis
Mesossigmoidopexia: mesosigmoidopexy
Mesossistólico: mesosystolic
Mesossomático: mesosomatous
Mesossomia: mesosomia
Mesossomo: mesosome
Mesostênio: mesostenium
Mesosterno: mesosternum
Mesotarsal: midtarsal
Mesotársico: mesotarsal
Mesotelial: mesothelial
Mesotélio: mesothelium, **pl.** mesothelia
Mesotelioma: mesothelioma
Mesotendão: mesotendon
Mesotendíneo: mesotendineum
Mesotímpano: mesotympanum
Mesotório: mesothorium
Mesotrópico: mesotropic
Mesourânico: mesouranic
Mesovário: mesoarium, mesovarium, **pl.** mesovaria
Messulfeno: mesulphen
Mestanolona: mestanolone
Mestenediol: mestenediol
Mestranol: mestranol
Mesurânico: mesuranic
Metaanálise: metaanalysis
Metabase: metabasis
Metabiose: metabiosis
Metabólico: metabolic
Metabolímetro: metabolimeter
Metabolina: metabolin
Metabolismo: metabolism
Metabólito: metabolite
Metabolizar: metabolize
Metacarpal: metacarpal
Metacarpectomia: metacarpectomy
Metacarpo: metacarpus, **pl.** metacarpi
Metacarpofalângico: metacarpophalangeal
Metacêntrico: metacentric
Metacercária: metacercaria, **pl.** metacercariae
Metacestódeo: metacestode
Metacinesia: metakinesis, metakinesia
Metacloral: metachloral
Metacone: metacone
Metaconídio: metaconid
Metacontraste: metacontrast
Metacônulo: metaconule
Metacresol: metacresol
Metacriptozoíta: metacryptozoite

Metacromagem: metachroming
Metacromasia: metachromasia
Metacromático: metachromatic
Metacromatismo: metachromatism
Metacromófilo: metachromophil, metachromophile
Metacrônico: metachronous
Metacrose: metachrosis
Metade: dim, moiety
Metadisenteria: metadysentery
Metaestável: metastable
Metaestro: metestrus, metestrum
Metaestrôngilo: metastrongyle
Metáfase: metaphase
Metafisário: metaphysial, metaphyseal
Metáfise: metaphysis, pl. metaphyses
Metafisite: metaphysitis
Metaictérico: metaicteric
Metainfeccioso: metainfective
Metal: metal (M)
Metal coloidal: electrosol
Metaldeído: metaldehyde
Metalenestril: methallenestril
Metálico: metallic
Metalocianeto: metallocyanide
Metaloenzima: metalloenzyme
Metalofilia: metallophilia
Metaloflavodesidrogenase: metalloflavodehydrogenase
Metaloflavoenzima: metalloflavoenzyme
Metaloflavoproteína: metalloflavoprotein
Metalofobia: metallophobia
Metalóide: metalloid
Metaloporfirina: metalloporphyrin
Metaloproteína: metalloprotein
Metaloproteinase: metalloproteinase
Metalotioneína: metallothionein
Metaluético: metaluetic
Metamérico: metamer, metameric
Metamerismo: metamerism
Metâmero: metamere
Metamielócito: metamyelocyte
Metamorfopsia: metamorphopsia
Metamorfose: allaxis, metamorphosis
Metamorfótico: metamorphotic
Metampirona: methampyrone
Metandienona: methandienone
Metandriol: methandriol
Metandrostenolona: methandrostenolone
Metanéfrico: metanephric
Metanefrina: metanephrine
Metanefro: metanephros, **pl.** metanephroi
Metanefrogênico: metanephrogenic, metanephrogenous
Metaneutrófilo: metaneutrophil, metaneutrophile
Metano: methane

Metanógeno: methanogen
Metanol: methanol
Metapirético: metapyretic
Metapirileno: methapyrilene
Metapirocatecase: metapyrocatechase
Metaplasia: metaplasia, metaplasis
Metaplásico: metaplastic
Metaplexo: metaplexus
Metapófise: metapophysis
Metaporo: metapore
Metaproteína: metaprotein
Metapsicologia: metapsychology
Metaqualona: methaqualone
Metarbital: metharbital
Metargeno: methargen
***meta*-rodopsina I, *meta*-rodopsina II, *meta*-rodopsina III:** *meta*-rhodopsin I, *meta*-rhodopsin II, *meta*-rhodopsin III
Metarrodopsina: metarhodopsin
Metarrubricito: metarubricyte
Metarteríola: metarteriole
Metassífilis: metasyphilis
Metassifilítico: metasyphilitic
Metástase: metastasis, **pl.** metastases; secondaries
Metastático: metastatic
Metastatizar: metastasize
Metatálamo: metathalamus
Metatarsal: metatarsal
Metatarsalgia: metatarsalgia
Metatarsectomia: metatarsectomy
Metatarso: metatarsus, **pl.** metatarsi
Metatarsofalângico: metatarsophalangeal
Metátese: metathesis
Metatípico: metatypical
Metatrófico: metatrophic
Metatrofo: metatroph
Metatrópico: metatropic
Metaxalona: metaxalone
Metazolamida: methazolamide
Metazoonose: metazoonosis
Metemalbumina: methemalbumin
Metemalbuminemia: methemalbuminemia
Metemioglobina: methemyoglobin (metMb)
Metemoglobina: methemoglobin (metHb)
Metemoglobinemia: methemoglobinemia
Metemoglobinúria: methemoglobinuria
Metenamina: methenamine
Metenamina de prata: methenamine-silver
Metencefálico: metencephalic
Metencefalina: metenkephalin
Metencéfalo: metencephalon
Meteno: methene
Meteorismo: meteorism
Meteoropatia: meteoropathy

Meteorotrópico: meteorotropic
Metergolina: metergoline, methergoline
Metformina: metformin
Meticilina sódica: methicillin sodium
Meticlotiazida: methyclothiazide
Metil sulfato de bevônio: bevonium methyl sulfate
Metila: methyl (Me)
Metilação: methylation
2-metilacetoacetil-CoA tiolase: 2-methylacetoacetyl-CoA thiolase
Metilar: methylate
Metilbenzeno: methylbenzene
Metilbrometo de anisotropina: anisotropine methylbromide
Metilbrometo de pipenzolato: pipenzolate methylbromide
Metil-CCNU: methyl-CCNU
Metilcelulose: methylcellulose
Metilcinase: methylkinase
5-metilcitosina: 5-methylcytosine
Metilcitrato: methylcitrat
Metilclorofórmio: methylchloroform
Metilcobalamina: methylcobalamin
3-metilcolantreno, 20-metilcolantreno: 3-methylcholanthrene, 20-methylcholanthrene
3-metilcrotonil-CoA: 3-methylcrotonyl-CoA
Metildicloroarsina: methyldichloroarsine (MD)
Metildopa: methyldopa
Metileno: methylene
3,4-metilenodioximetanfetamina: 3,4-methylenedioxymethamphetamine
Metilenofílico: methylenophilic, methylenophilous
Metilenófilo: methylenophil, methylenophile
Metilexanoamina: methylhexaneamine
Metilglioxal: methylglyoxal
Metilglioxalase: methylglyoxalase
Metilglucamina: methylglucamine
3-metilglutacônico acidúria: 3-methylglutaconic aciduria
3-metilglutaconil-CoA hidratase: 3-methylglutaconyl-CoA hydratase
Metilmalonil-CoA: methylmalonyl-CoA
Metilmercúrio: methylmercury
Metilmorfina: methylmorphine
Metilol: methylol
Metilose: methylose
Metilparabeno: methylparaben
Metilpentose: methylpentose
Metilprednisolona: methylprednisolone

Glossário

5-metilresorcinol: 5-methylresorcinol
Metilsulfato de difemanil: diphemanil methylsulfate
Metilsulfato de pentapipério: pentapiperium methylsulfate
Metilsulfato de piribenzil: pyribenzyl methyl sulfate
Metilsulfato de poldina: poldine methylsulfate
Metiltestosterona: methyltestosterone
17α-metiltestosterona: 17α-methyltestosterone
Metiltioadenosina: methylthioadenosine
Metiltiouracil: methylthiouracil
Metiltocol: methyltocol
Metiltransferase: methyltransferase
Metilxantinas: methylxanthines
Metimazol: methimazole
Metiodal sódico: methiodal sodium
Metiodida do ácido nicotino-hidroxâmico: nicotinehydroxamic acid methiodide
Metionina: methionine (Met, M)
Metiprilona: methyprylon, methyprylone
Metirapona: metyrapone
Metirosina: metyrosine
Metisazona: methisazone
Metitural: methitural
Metocarbamol: methocarbamol
Metocloreto de prociclidina: procyclidine methochloride
Metodismo: methodism
Método: method
Método de Abell-Kendall: Abell-Kendall method
Método de Wilson: Wilson method
Metodologia: methodology
Metoexital sódico: methohexital sodium
Metofenazina: methophenazine
Metofolina: methopholine
Metolazona: metolazone
Metópago: metopagus
Metópico: metopic
Metopismo: metopism
Metopoplastia: metopoplasty
Metoposcopia: metoposcopy
Metopterina: methopterin
Metorfinano: methorphinan
Metosserpidina: methoserpidine
Metossulfato de trimetídio: trimethidium methosulfate
Metossuximida: methsuximide
Metotrexato: methotrexate
Metotrimeprazina: methotrimeprazine
Metoxenia: metoxeny
Metóxeno: metoxenous
Metoxicloro: methoxychlor
Metoxiflurano: methoxyflurane
Metoxil: methoxyl
5-metoxindol-3-acetato: 5-methoxyindole-3-acetate

Metoxissaleno: methoxsalen
5-metoxitriptamina: 5-methoxytryptamine
Metratonia: metratonia
Métrico: metric
Metrifonato: metrifonate
Metriocefálico: metriocephalic
Metrite: metritis
Metrizamida: metrizamide
Metrizoato sódico: metrizoate sodium
Metro: meter (m)
Metrócito: metrocyte
Metrodinamômetro: metrodynamometer
Metrodinia: metrodynia
Metroestenose: metrostenosis
Metroflebite: metrophlebitis
Metrolinfangite: metrolymphangitis
Metronidazol: metronidazole
Metronoscópio: metronoscope
Metropatia: metropathia, metropathy
Metropático: metropathic
Metroperitonite: metroperitonitis
Metroplastia: metroplasty
Metrorragia: metrorrhagia
Metrorréia: metrorrhea
Metrossalpingite: metrosalpingitis
Metrostaxe: metrostaxis
Metrotomia: metrotomy
Mevalonato: mevalonate
Mevalônico acidúria: mevalonic aciduria
Mevastatina: mevastatin
Mevinolina: mevinolin
Mexenona: mexenone
Mexiletina: mexiletine
Mezlocilina sódica: mezlocillin sodium
Mialgia: myalgia
Miastenia: myasthenia
Miastênico: myasthenic
Miatonia: myatonia, myatony
Miatrofia: myatrophy
Mibefradil: mibefradil
Micatose: micatosis
Micção: miction, micturition, urination
Micela: micelle
Micelar: micellar
Miceliano: mycelian
Micélio: mycelium, pl. mycelia
Micelióide: mycelioid
Micetismo: mycetism, mycetismus
Miceto: mycete
Micetogenético: mycetogenetic, mycetogenic
Micetógeno: mycetogenous
Micetoma: mycetoma
Micobactérias: mycobacteria
Micobacteriose: mycobacteriosis
Micobactina: mycobactin
Micodermatite: mycodermatitis
Micófago: mycophage

Micogastrite: mycogastritis
Micol: mykol
Micologia: mycology
Micologista: mycologist
Micoplasma: mycoplasma, pl. mycoplasmata
Micose: mycosis, pl. mycoses
Micostático: mycostatic
Micosteróis: mycosterols
Micótico: mycotic
Micotoxicose: mycotoxicosis
Micotoxina: mycotoxin
Micovírus: mycovirus
Microabscesso: microabscess
Microadenoma: microadenoma
Microaeróbio: microaerobion
Microaerófilo: microaerophil, microaerophile, microaerophilic, microaerophilous
Microaerossol: microaerosol
Microagulha: microneedle
Microalbuminúria: microalbuminuria
Microanálise: microanalysis
Microanastomose: microanastomosis
Microanatomia: microanatomy
Microanatomista: microanatomist
Microaneurisma: microaneurysm
Microangiografia: microangiography
Microangiopatia: microangiopathy
Microangioscopia: microangioscopy
Microarteriografia: microarteriography
Microatelectasia: microatelectasis
Microbalança: microbalance
Microbiano: microbial, microbic
Microbicida: microbicidal, microbicide
Micróbio: microbe
Microbiologia: microbiology
Microbiológico: microbiologic
Microbiologista: microbiologist
Microbiótico: microbiotic
Microbismo: microbism
Microblasto: microblast
Microbléfaro: microblepharia, microblepharism, microblepharon
Microbraquia: microbrachia
Microcalcificações: microcalcifications
Microcardia: microcardia
Microcefalia: microcephalia, microcephaly
Microcefálico: microcephalic
Microcefalismo: microcephalism
Microcéfalo: microcephalous
Microcentro: microcentrum
Microcida: microcide
Microcinematografia: microcinematography

Microcintigrafia: microscintigraphy
Microcirculação: microcirculation
Microcirurgia: microsurgery
Microcirúrgico: micrurgical
Microcisto: microcyst
Microcitemia: microcythemia
Micrócito: microcyte
Microcitose: microcytosis
Micrococo: micrococcus, pl. micrococci
Microcolite: microcolitis
Microcolo: microcolon
Microcolônia: microcclony
Microconídio: microconidium, pl. microconidia
Microcoria: microcoria
Microcórnea: microcornea
Microcorpo: microbody
Microcoulomb: microcoulomb (μC)
Microcristalino: microcrystalline
Microcurie: microcurie (μCi)
Microdactilia: microdactylia, microdactyly
Microdáctilo: microdactylous
Microdiálise: microdialysis
Microdisgenesia: microdysgenesia
Microdissecção: microdissection
Microdonte: microdont
Microdontia: microdontia, microdontism
Microdose: microdose
Microdrepanocitose: microdrepanocytosis
Microelementos: microelements
Microeletrodo: microelectrode
Microencefalia: micrencephalia, micrencephaly, microencephaly
Microencéfalo: micrencephalous
Microepatia: microhepatia
Microeritrócito: microerythrocyte
Microesferocitose: microspherocytosis
Microespectrofotometria: microspectrophotometry
Microespectroscópio: microspectroscope
Microesplâncnico: microsplanchnic
Microeterogeneidade: microheterogeneity
Microevolução: microevolution
Micrófago: microphage
Microfagócito: microphagocyte
Microfalo: microphallus
Microfibrila: microfibril
Microfilamento: microfilament
Microfilaremia: microfilaremia
Microfilária: microfilaria, pl. microfilariae
Microfilme: microfilm
Microflora: microflora
Microfobia: microphobia
Microfone: microphone
Microfonia: microphonia, microphony

Microfonoscópio: microphonoscope
Microfotografia: microphotograph
Microftalmia: microphthalmia, microphthalmos
Microgameta: microgamete
Microgametócito: microgametocyte
Microgamia: microgamy
Microgamonte: microgamont
Microgastria: microgastria
Microgenia: microgenia
Microgenitalismo: microgenitalism
Microgiria: microgyria
Micróglia: microglia
Microgliácito: microgliacyte
Microglioma: microglioma
Microgliomatose: microgliomatosis
Microgliose: microgliosis
Microglobulina: microglobulin
Microglossia: microglossia
Micrognatia: micrognathia
Micrografia: micrography
Micrógrafo: micrograph
Micrograma: microgram (μg, γ)
Microhm: microhm ($\mu\Omega$)
Microincineração: microincineration
Microincisão: microincision
Microinjetor: microinjector
Microinvasão: microinvasion
Microkatal: microkatal
Microleucoblasto: microleukoblast
Microlitíase: microlithiasis
Micrólito: microlith
Microlitro: microliter (μl, μL)
Micrologia: micrology
Micromanipulação: micromanipulation
Micromanipulador: micromanipulator
Micromazia: micromazia
Micromelia: micromelia
Micrômero: micromere
Micromerozoíta: micromerozoite
Micrometástase: micrometastasis
Micrometastático: micrometastatic
Micrometria: micrometry
Micrômetro: micrometer (μm)
Micromicrograma: micromicrogram ($\mu\mu g$)
Micromielia: micromyelia
Micromieloblasto: micromyeloblast
Microminerais: microminerals
Micromol: micromole (μmol)
Micromolar: micromolar ($\mu mol/L$)
Micromotoscópio: micromotoscope
Mícron: micron (μ)
Micronema: microneme
Micrônico: micronic
Microníquia: micronychia

Micronistagmo: micronystagmus
Micronodular: micronodular
Micronúcleo: micronucleus
Micronutrientes: micronutrients
Micro-ohm: micro-ohm
Microondas: microwaves
Microparasita: microparasite
Micropatologia: micropathology
Micropênis: micropenis
Micrópila: micropyle
Micropipeta: micropipette, micropipet
Microplania: microplania
Microplasia: microplasia
Micropletismografia: microplethysmography
Micropodia: micropodia
Microporo: micropore
Micropromielócito: micropromyelocyte
Microprosopia: microprosopia
Micropsia: micropsia
Micropunção: micropuncture
Microquilia: microcheilia, microchilia
Microquimatoterapia: microkymatotherapy
Microquimerismo: microchimerism
Microquímica: microchemistry
Microquiria: microcheiria, microchiria
Microrganismo: microorganism
Microrradiografia: microradiography
Microrrefratômetro: microrefractometer
Microrrespirômetro: microrespirometer
Microscopia: microscopy
Microscópico: microscopic, microscopical
Microscópio: microscope
Microscópio de Rheinberg: Rheinberg microscope
Microsfera: microsphere
Microsfigmia: microsphygmy, microsphyxia
Microsídeos: microsides
Microsmático: microsmatic
Microsplenia: microsplenia
Microsporídios: microsporidia
Microsporidiose: microsporidiasis, microsporidiosis, microsporidiasis
Microssacadas: microsaccades
Microssema: microseme
Microsseringa: microsyringe
Microssolda: microwelding
Microssoma: microsome
Microssomia: microsomia
Microstetofone: microstethophone
Microstetoscópio: microstethoscope
Microstomia: microstomia
Microtelia: microthelia
Microtia: microtia
Microtomia: microtomy

Micrótomo: microtome
Microtonômetro: microtonometer
Microtropia: microtropia
Microtúbulo: microtubule
Microvesícula: microvesicle
Microvilosidade: microvillus, pl. microvilli
Microvolt: microvolt (μv)
Microxífilo: microxyphil
Microzoário: microzoon
Micuim: harvest bug
Midaleína: mydaleine
Midatoxina: mydatoxin
Midríase: mydriasis
Midriático: mydriatic
Miectomia: myectomy
Miectopia: myectopy, myectopia
Mielapoplexia: myelapoplexy
Mielatelia: myelatelia
Mielauxe: myelauxe
Mielemia: myelemia
Mielencéfalo: myelencephalon
Miélico: myelic
Mielina: myelin
Mielínico: myelinic
Mielinização: myelination, myelinization
Mielinizado: myelinated
Mielinoclasia: myelinoclasis
Mielinogênese: myelinogenesis
Mielinólise: myelinolysis
Mielinopatia: myelinopathy
Mielite: myelitis
Mielítico: myelitic
Mieloarquitetônico: myeloarchitectonics
Mieloblastemia: myeloblastemia
Mieloblasto: myeloblast
Mieloblastoma: myeloblastoma
Mieloblastose: myeloblastosis
Mielocatexia: myelokathexis
Mielocele: myelocele
Mielocístico: myelocystic
Mielocisto: myelocyst
Mielocistocele: myelocystocele
Mielocistomeningocele: myelocystomeningocele
Mielocitemia: myelocythemia
Mielocítico: myelocytic
Mielócito: medullocell, myelocyte
Mielocitoma: myelocytoma
Mielocitomatose: myelocytomatosis
Mielocitose: myelocytosis
Mielodiástase: myelodiastasis
Mielodisplasia: myelodysplasia
Mielofibrose: myelofibrosis
Mielogênese: myelogenesis
Mielogênico: myelogenetic, myelogenic
Mielógeno: myelogenous
Mielogônio: myelogone, myelogonium
Mielografia: myelography
Mielograma: myelogram
Mielóico: myeloic
Mielóide: myeloid
Mieloidose: myeloidosis
Mieloleucemia: myeloleukemia

Mielolinfócito: myelolymphocyte
Mielolipoma: myelolipoma
Mielólise: myelolysis
Mieloma: myeloma
Mielomalacia: myelomalacia
Mielomatose: myelomatosis
Mielomeningocele: myelomeningocele
Mielômero: myelomere
Mielomonócito: myelomonocyte
Mieloneurite: myeloneuritis
Mielônico: myelonic
Mieloparalisia: myeloparalysis
Mielopatia: myelopathy
Mielopático: myelopathic
Mieloperoxidase: myeloperoxidase
Mielópeto: myelopetal
Mieloplasto: myeloplast
Mieloplegia: myeloplegia
Mielopoese: myelopoiesis
Mielopoético: myelopoietic
Mieloproliferativo: myeloproliferative
Mielorradiculite: myeloradiculitis
Mielorradiculodisplasia: myeloradiculodysplasia
Mielorradiculopatia: myeloradiculopathy
Mielorradiculopolineurite: myeloradiculopolyneuronitis
Mielorrafia: myelorrhaphy
Mielorragia: myelorrhagia
Mielosclerose: myelosclerosis
Mielose: myelosis
Mielospôngio: myelospongium
Mielosquise: myeloschisis
Mielossífilis: myelosyphilis
Mielotísica: myelophthisis
Mielotísico: myelophthisic
Mielotomia: myelotomy
Mielótomo: myelotome
Mielotomografia: myelotomography
Mielotóxico: myelotoxic
Mientérico: myenteric
Miênteron: myenteron
Miestesia: myesthesia, myoesthesis, myoesthesia
Mifepristona: mifepristone, RU-486
Miíase: myiasis
Milabris: mylabris
Milfose: milphosis
Miliampere: milliampere (ma, mA)
Miliar: miliary
Miliária: miliaria
Milibar: millibar
Milicurie: millicurie (mc, mCi)
Miliequivalente: milliequivalent (mEq, meq)
Miligrama: milligram (mg)
Mililambert: millilambert
Mililitro: milliliter
Milímetro: millimeter (mm)
Milimícron: bicron, millimicron (mμ)
Milimol: millimole (mmol)

Miliosmol: milliosmole
Milípede: millipede
Milissegundo (ms): millisecond (ms, msec)
Milium colóide: colloid milium
Milivolt: millivolt (mV)
Milo-hióideo: mylohyoid, mylohyoideus
Milrinona: milrinone
Mimação: mimmation
Mimese: mimesis
Mimético: mimetic
Mineral: mineral
Mineralização: mineralization
Mineralocorticóide: mineralocoid, mineralocorticoid
Mineralotrópico: mineralotropic
Mingau: gruel
Minilaparotomia: minilaparotomy
Minimiosina: minimyosin
Mínimo: minim (m), minimum
Minitoracotomia: minithoracotomy
Minociclina: minocycline
Minoxidil: minoxidil
Mioadenilato desaminase: myoadenylate deaminase
Mioalbumina: myoalbumin
Mioarquitetônico: myoarchitectonic
Mioatrofia: myoatrophy
Mioblástico: myoblastic
Mioblasto: myoblast
Mioblastoma: myoblastoma
Miobradia: myobradia
Miocárdico: myocardial
Miocárdio: myocardium, **pl.** myocardia
Miocardiógrafo: myocardiograph
Miocardiopatia: cardiomyopathy, myocardiopathy
Miocardioplastia: cardiomyoplasty
Miocardiorrafia: myocardiorrhaphy
Miocardiotomia: cardiomyotomy
Miocardite: myocarditis
Miocardítico: myocarditic
Miocele: myocele
Miocelialgia: myocelialgia
Miocelite: myocelitis
Miocelulite: myocellulitis
Miocerose: myocerosis, myokerosis
Miocinase: myokinase
Miocinesímetro: myocinesimeter, myokinesimeter
Miócito: myocyte
Miocitólise: myocytolysis
Miocitoma: myocytoma
Mioclonia: myoclonia
Mioclônico: myoclonic

Mioclônus: myoclonus
Mioclônus múltiplo: polyclonia
Miocolpite: myocolpitis
Miocrismo: myocrismus
Miocromo: myochrome
Miocronoscópio: myochronoscope
Miocutâneo: myocutaneous
Miodegeneração: myodegeneration
Miodemia: myodemia
Miodérmico: myodermal
Miodiástase: myodiastasis
Miodídimo: miodidymus, miodymus
Miodinamia: myodynamia
Miodinâmica: myodynamics
Miodinamômetro: myodynamometer
Miodinia: myodynia
Miodistonia: myodystony
Miodistrofia: myodystrophy, myodystrophia
Mioedema: mounding, myoedema, myoidema
Mioelástico: myoelastic
Mioelétrico: myoelectric
Mioendocardite: myoendocarditis
Mioepitelial: myoepithelial
Mioepitélio: myoepithelium
Mioepitelioma: myoepithelioma
Mioesferulose: myospherulosis
Mioespasmo: myospasm, myospasmus
Mioestenômetro: myosthenometer
Mioestroma: myostroma
Miofascial: myofascial
Miofascite: myofascitis
Miofibrila: myofibril, myofibrilla, **pl.** myofibrillae
Miofibrilar: myofibrillar
Miofibroblasto: myofibroblast
Miofibroma: myofibroma
Miofibromatose: myofibromatosis
Miofibrose: myofibrosis
Miofibrosite: myofibrositis
Miofilamentos: myofilaments
Miofone: myophone
Miofosforilase: myophosphorylase
Miofuncional: myofunctional
Miogênese: myogenesis
Miogênico: myogenetic, myogenic, myogenous
Miógeno: myogen
Mioglobina: myoglobin (Mb, MbCO, MbO$_2$), myohemoglobin
Mioglobinúria: myoglobinuria
Mioglobulina: myoglobulin
Mioglobulinúria: myoglobulinuria
Miognato: myognathus
Miografia: myography
Miográfico: myographic
Miógrafo: myograph
Miograma: myogram
Mióide: myoid

Mioinositol: myoinositol
Mio-inositol: *myo*-inositol
Mioisquemia: myoischemia
Miolécito: miolecithal
Miolema: myolemma
Miolipoma: myolipoma
Miólise: myolysis
Miologia: myologia, myology
Miologista: myologist
Mioma: myoma
Miomalacia: myomalacia
Miomatoso: myomatous
Miomectomia: myomectomy
Miomelanose: myomelanosis
Miômero: myomere
Miometrial: myometrial
Miométrio: myometrium
Miometrite: myometritis
Miômetro: myometer
Miomitocôndria: myomitochondrion, **pl.** myomitochondria
Miomotomia: myomotomy
Mion: myon
Mionecrose: myonecrosis
Mionema: myoneme
Mioneural: myoneural
Mioneuroma: myoneuroma
Mionimia: myonymy
Miopatia: myopathy
Miopático: myopathic
Miopericardite: myopericarditis
Mioperitonite: myoperitonitis
Miopia: myopia (M), nearsightedness, shortsightedness
Miópico: myopic (M)
Mioplasma: myoplasm
Mioplastia: myoplasty
Mioplástico: myoplastic
Miopo: miopus
Miopolar: myopolar
Miopragia: miopragia
Mioproteína: myoprotein
Mioquimia: myokymia
Miorrafia: myorrhaphy
Miorrexe: myorrhexis
Miosclerose: myosclerosis
Miose: miosis
Miosina: myosin
Miosinogênio: myosinogen
Miosinose: myosinose
Miosite: myositis
Miosítico: myositic
Miossalpinge: myosalpinx
Miossalpingite: myosalpingitis
Miossarcoma: myosarcoma
Miossepto: myocomma, **pl.** myocommata, myoseptum
Miostromina: myostromin
Miotasia: myotasis
Miotático: myotactic, myotatic
Miotenosite: myotenositis
Miotenotomia: myotenotomy
Miotérmico: myothermic
Miótico: miotic
Miotomia: myotomy
Miótomo: myotome
Miotonia: myotonia
Miotônico: myotonic

Miotonóide: myotonoid
Miotônus: myotone, myotonus, myotony
Miotrofia: myotrophy
Miotubo: myotube
Miotúbulo: myotubule
Mira: mire
Miracídio: miracidium, **pl.** miracidia
Mirex: mirex
Mirica: myrica
Miricina: myricin
Miringe: myringa, myrinx
Miringectomia: myringgectomy
Miringite: myringitis
Miringodermatite: myringodermatitis
Miringoestapediopexia: myringostapediopexy
Miringoplastia: myringoplasty
Miringosclerose: myringosclerosis
Miringotomia: myringotomy
Miringótomo: myringotome
Miristato de isopropila: isopropyl myristate
Miristicina: myristicin
Mirmécia: myrmecia
Mirosinase: myrosinase
Mirra: myrrh
Misandria: misandry
Misantropia: misanthropy
Miscigenação: miscegenation
Miscível: miscible
Misofilia: mysophilia
Misofobia: mysophobia
Misogamia: misogamy
Misoginia: misogyny
Misopedia: misopedia, misopedy
Misoprostol: misoprostol
Mistura: confounding, mixing, mixture
Mistura de Basham: Basham mixture
Mitacismo: mytacism
Mitigar: mitigate
Mitocôndria: mitochondrion, **pl.** mitochondria
Mitocondrial: mitochondrial
Mitogênese: mitogenesis
Mitogenético: mitogenetic
Mitogênico: mitogenic
Mitógeno: mitogen
Mitomicina: mitomycin
Mitoplasto: mitoplast
Mitose: mitosis, **pl.** mitoses
Mitotano: mitotane
Mitótico: mitotic
Mitral: mitral
Mitralização: mitralization
Mitramicina: mithramycin, mitramycin
Mitridatismo: mithridatism
Mivacúrio: mivacurium
Mixadenite labial: myxadenitis labialis
Mixastenia: myxasthenia
Mixedema: myxedema
Mixedematóide: myxedematoid
Mixedematoso: myxedematous

Mixemia: myxemia
Mixócito: myxocyte
Mixocondrofibrossarcoma: myxochondrofibrosarcoma
Mixocondroma: myxochondroma
Mixofibroma: myxofibroma
Mixofibrossarcoma: myxofibrosarcoma
Mixóide: myxoid
Mixolipoma: myxolipoma
Mixoma: myxoma
Mixomatose: myxomatosis
Mixomatoso: myxomatous
Mixomiceto: myxomycete
Mixoneuroma: myxoneuroma
Mixopapiloma: myxopapilloma
Mixopoese: myxopoiesis
Mixossarcoma: myxosarcoma
Mixotrofia: mixotrophy
Mixovírus: myxovirus
Mnemismo: mnemism
Mnemônica: mnemonics
Mnemônico: mnemenic, mnemic, mnemonic
Mobilização: mobilization
Mobilizar: mobilize
Moda: mode
Modalidade: modality
Modelagem: modeling, molding
Modelagem de tecido: tissue-trimming
Modelo: model
Modelo de Adair-Koshland-Némethy-Filmer: Adair-Koshland-Némethy-Filmer model (AKNF)
Modelo KNF: KNF model
Modificação: change, modification
Modificador: modifier
Modíolo: modiolus, **pl.** modioli
Modo B: B-mode
Modo M: M-mode
Modo M: TM-mode
Modulação: modulation
Modulador: modulator
Módulo: modulus
Mofebutazona: mofebutazone
Mofo: mold
Mogiartria: mogiarthria
Mogifonia: mogiphonia
Mogilalia: mogilalia
Molal: molal
Molalidade: molality (m)
Molar: molar
Molaridade: molarity (M, M)
Molariforme: molariform
Moldagem: moulage
Moldagem periférica: muscletrimming
Molde: cast, die, mould, templete
Molécula: molecule
Molécula-grama: gram-molecule
Molecular: molecular
Molecularidade: molecularity
Molibdato: molybdate
Molibdênico: molybdenic, molybdenous
Molibdênio: molybdenum (Mo)
Molibdênio-99: molybdenum-99 (^{99}Mo)
Molíbdico: molybdic
Molibdoenzimas: molybdoenzymes
Molibdoflavo-proteínas: molybdoflavoproteins
Molibdopterina: molybdopterin
Molibdoso: molybdous
Molilalia: molilalia
Molímen: molimen
Molismofobia: molysmophobia
Molusco: mollusc, molluscum, mollusk
Momento: moment
Momismo: momism
Mônada: monad
Monamida: monamide
Monamina: monamine
Monaminúria: monaminuria
Monarda: monarda
Monarticular: monarticular
Monártrico: monarthric
Monartrite: monarthritis
Monáster: monaster
Monaural: monaural
Monestro: monestrous
Mongólico: mongolian
Moniletrix: monilethrix
Monilial: monilial
Moniliase: moniliasis
Moniliforme: moniliform
Monismo: monism
Monístico: monistic
Monitor: monitor
Monitorização: monitoring
Monoacilglicerol: monoacylglycerol
Monoamelia: monoamelia
Monoamida: monoamide
Monoamina: monoamine
Monoamina oxidase: monoamine oxidase (MAO)
Monoaminérgico: monoaminergic
Monoaminúria: monoaminuria
Monoamniótico: monoamniotic
Monoassociado: monoassociated
Monoatômico: monatomic
Monoauxotrofo: monoauxotroph
Monoaxônico: monaxonic
Monobactâmico: monobactam
Monobásico: monobasic
Monobenzona: monobenzone
Monoblasto: monoblast
Monobráquio: monobrachius
Monobromato: monobromated, monobrominated
Monocamadas: monolayers
Monocardíaco: monocardian
Monocéfalo: monocephalus
Monocina: monokine
Monocistrônico: monocistronic
Monócito: monocyte
Monocitopenia: monocytopenia
Monocitose: monocytosis
Monoclínico: monoclinic
Monoclonal: monoclonal
Monoclorfenamida: monochlorphenamide
Monocorial: monochorial
Monocoriônico: monochorionic
Monocrânio: monocranius
Monocróico: monochroic
Monocromador: monochromator
Monocromasia: monochromasia, monochromasy
Monocromático: monochromatic
Monocromatismo: monochromatism
Monocromatófilo: monochromatophil, monochromatophile
Monocrômico: monochromic
Monocromófilo: monochromophil, monochromophile
Monocrótico: monocrotic
Monocrotismo: monocrotism
Monoctanoína: monooctanoin
Monocular: monocular
Monóculo: monocle, monoculus
Monodactilia: monodactyly, monodactylism
Monodisperso: monodisperse
Monoestrático: monostratal
Monoetanolamina: monoethanolamine
Monofagismo: monophagism
Monofasia: monophasia
Monofásico: monophasic
Monofenol monoxigenase: monophenol monooxygenase
Monofenol oxidase: monophenol oxidase
Monofilético: monophyletic
Monofiletismo: monophyletism
Monofiodonte: monophyodont
Monofobia: monophobia
3',5'-monofosfato cíclico de adenosina (AMPc): adenosine 3',5'-cyclic monophosphate (cAMP)
5'-monofosfato de guanosina: guanosine 5'-monophosphate
Monoftalmia: monophthalmos
Monoftalmo: monophthalmus
Monogamético: monogametic
Monogamia: monogamy
Monogênese: monogenesis
Monogenético: monogenetic, monogenous
Monogênico: monogenic
Monogerminal: monogerminal
Monoglicerídeo: monoglyceride
Monografia: monograph
Monoideísmo: monoideism
Monoidratado: monohydrated
Monoídrico: monohydric
Monoinfecção: monoinfection
Monoiodotirosina (MIT): monoiodotyrosine (MIT)
Monoisonitrosoacetona: monoisonitrosoacetone
Monolocular: monolocular
Monomania: monomania
Monomaníaco: monomaniac
Monomastigota: monomastigote
Monomélico: monomelic
Monomérico: monomeric
Monômero: monomer
Monometálico: monometallic
Monomicrobiano: monomicrobic
Monomioplegia: monomyoplegia
Monomiosite: monomyositis
Monomolecular: monomolecular
Monomorfo: monomorphic
Mononema: mononeme
Mononeural: mononeural, mononeuric
Mononeurite múltipla: mononeuritis multiplex
Mononeuropatia: mononeuropathy
Monônfalo: monomphalus
Mononuclear: mononuclear
Mononucleose: mononucleosis
Mononucleotídeo: mononucleotide
Mononucleotídeo de nicotinamida (NMN): nicotinamide mononucleotide (NMN)
Monoparesia: monoparesis
Monoparestesia: monoparesthesia
Monopatia: monopathy
Monopático: monopathic
Monope: monops
Monopenia: monopenia
Monoplasmático: monoplasmatic
Monoplástico: monoplastic
Monoplasto: monoplast
Monoplegia: monoplegia
Monoplóide: monoploid
Monopodia: monopodia
Monoptíquico: monoptychial
Monorquia: monorchia
Monorquídico: monorchidic, monorchid
Monorquidismo: monorchidism
Monorquismo: monorchism
Monorrecidiva: monorecidive
Monorrínico: monorhinic
Monóscelo: monoscelous
Monoscenismo: monoscenism
Monose: monose
Monospermia: monospermy
Monossacarídeo: monosaccharide
Monossifílide: monosyphilide
Monossináptico: monosynaptic
Monossintomático: monosymptomatic
Monossomia: monosomia, monosomy
Monossômico: monosomic, monosomous
Monossubstituído: monosubstituted
Monostoma: monostome
Monostótico: monostotic
Monotermia: monothermia

Monoterpenos: monoterpenes
Monotioglicerol: monothioglycerol
Monótoco: monotocous
Monotremo: monotreme
Monotríquio: monotrichate, monotrichous
Monovalência: monovalence, monovalency
Monovalente: monovalent
Monoxeno: monoxenous
Monóxido: monoxide
Monóxido de chumbo: massicot
Monóxido de dinitrogênio: dinitrogen monoxide
Monoxigenases: monooxygenases
Monozigótico: monozygotic, monozygous
Monozóico: monozoic
Monstro: monster
Monstro-de-gila: Gila monster
Montagem: mounting
Montar: mount
Monte: mons, **gen.** montis, **pl.** montes
Montelucaste sódico (MSD): montelukast sodium
Montículo: monticulus, **pl.** monticuli
Morbidade: morbidity
Mórbido: morbid
Morbífico: morbific
Morbígeno: morbigenous
Morbilidade: morbility
Morbiliforme: morbilliform
Morbo: morbus
Morcego: bat
Mordente: mordant
Morder: bite
Mordida cruzada: crossbite
Mordiscar: moriscatio
Morféia: morphea
Morfema: morpheme
Morfina: morphine
Morfofisiologia: morphophysiology
Morfogênese: morphogenesis
Morfogenético: morphogenetic
Morfologia: morphology
Morfológico: morphologic
Morfometria: morphometry
Morfométrico: morphometric
Morfon: morphon
Morfose: morphosis
Morfossíntese: morphosynthesis
Morfotipo: morphotype
Morgan: morgan (M)
Morgue: morgue
Moria: moria
Moribundo: moribund
Morina: morin
Mormo: glanders
Moroxidina: moroxydine
Morruato de sódio: morrhuate sodium
Morsolo: morsulus
Mortal: mortal
Mortalidade: mortality
Morte: death, mors, **gen.** mortis
Mortificação: mortification

Morto: dead
Mortuário: mortuary
Mórula: morula
Morulação: morulation
Morulóide: moruloid
Mosaicismo: mosaicism
Mosaico: mosaic
Mosca: fly
Mosca-de-estábulo: *Stomoxys calcitrans*
Mosca do berne: botfly
Mosca-doméstica: housefly
Moscas-dos-olhos: *Hippelates*
Moscas varejeiras: fleshflies
Moscas volantes: muscae volitantes
Mosqueamento: mottling
Mosquito: mosquito, **pl.** mosquitoes
Mosquito-pólvora: midge, sandfly
Mostarda: mustard
Mosto: must
Mostrador: dial
Motilidade: motility
Motilina: motilin
Motivação: motivation
Motivo: motive
Motômetro: motormeter
Motoneurônio: motoneuron
Motor: motor, motorial
Móvel: motile
Movimento: motion, movement
Moxa: moxa
Moxabustão: moxibustion
Moxalactam: moxalactam
Moxissilita: moxisylyte
Mucase: mucase
Mucicarmina: mucicarmine
Múcide: mucid
Muciemateína: mucihematein
Mucífero: muciferous
Mucificação: mucification
Muciforme: muciform
Mucígeno: mucigenous
Mucilagem: mucilage
Mucilaginoso: mucilaginous
Mucina: mucin
Mucinase: mucinase
Mucinemia: mucinemia
Mucinogênio: mucinogen
Mucinóide: mucinoid
Mucinolítico: mucinolytic
Mucinose: mucinosis
Mucinoso: mucinous
Mucinúria: mucinuria
Mucíparo: muciparous
Mucite: mucitis
Muco: mucus
Mucocele: mucocele
Mucociliar: mucociliary
Mucoclase: mucoclasis
Mucocolite: mucocolitis
Mucocolpo: mucocolpos
Mucocutâneo: mucocutaneous
Mucoenterite: mucoenteritis
Mucoepidermóide: mucoepidermoid
Mucoglobulina: mucoglobulin
Mucóide: mucoid

Mucolipidose: mucolipidosis, **pl.** mucolipidoses
Mucólise: mucolysis
Mucolítico: mucolytic
Mucomembranoso: mucomembranous
Mucopeptídeo: mucopeptide
Mucoperiosteal: mucoperiosteal
Mucoperiósteo: mucoperiosteum
Mucopolissacaridase: mucopolysaccharidase
Mucopolissacarídeo: mucopolysaccharide
Mucopolissacaridose: mucopolysaccharidosis, **pl.** mucopolysaccharidoses
Mucopolissacaridúria: mucopolysacchariduria
Mucoproteína: mucoprotein
Mucopurulento: mucopurulent, puromucous
Mucopus: mucopus, mycopus
Mucormicose: mucormycosis
Mucosa: mucosa
Mucoso: mucosal, mucous
Mucossanguíneo: mucosanguineous, mucosanguinolent
Mucossectomia: mucosectomy
Mucosseroso: mucoserous
Mucostático: mucostatic
Mucoviscidose: mucoviscidosis
Mucro: mucro, **pl.** mucrones
Mucron: mucron
Mucronado: mucronate
Muda: molt, moult
Mudança: shift, switching
Mudança de classe: class switch
Mudança de função: metergasia
Mudo: mute
Muleta: crutch
Mülleriano: müllerian
Multiangular: multangular
Multiarticular: multiarticular
Multibacilar: multibacillary
Multicapsular: multicapsular
Multicelular: multicellular
Multicolinearidade: multicollinearity
Multicuspidado: multicuspidate
Multicúspide: multicuspid
Multienzimático: multienzyme
Multifetação: multifetation
Multífido: multifid, multifidus
Multifocal: multifocal
Multiforme: multiform, protean
Multiglandular: multiglandular
Multigrávida: multigravida
Multiinfecção: multi-infection
Multilobar: multilobar, multilobate, multilobed
Multilobular: multilobular
Multilocal: multilocal
Multilocular: multilocular
Multinodal: multinodal
Multinodular: multinodular, multinodulate
Multinuclear: multinuclear, multinucleate
Multinucleose: multinucleosis

Multípara: multipara
Multiparidade: multiparity
Multíparo: multiparous
Multiplicador de contracorrente: countercurrent multiplier
Múltiplo: multiple
Multipolar: multipolar
Multirradicular: multirooted
Multirrotação: multirotation
Multissináptico: multisynaptic
Multissubstrato: multisubstrate
Multivalência, polivalência: multivalence, multivalency
Multivalente: multivalent
Mumificação: mummification
Mural: mural
Muramidase: muramidase
Mureínas: mureins
Murexida: murexide
Muriático: muriatic, muriatic acid
Muriato: muriate
Muriforme: muriform
Murino: murine
Muromonab-CD3: muromonab-CD3
Muscarina: muscarine
Muscarínico: muscarinic
Muscarinismo: muscarinism
Muscicida: muscicide
Muscimol: muscimol
Muscona: muscone
Musculamina: musculamine
Muscular: muscular, muscularis
Muscularidade: muscularity
Musculatura: musculature
Músculo: muscle, musculus, **gen. e pl.** musculi
Músculo antitrágico: antitragicus
Músculo constritor inferior da faringe: laryngopharyngeus
Músculo longuíssimo da cabeça: trachelalis
Músculo mental: mentalis
Músculo palatofaríngeo: palatopharyngeus
Músculo tarsal: tarsalis
Músculo temporal: temporalis
Músculo vasto intermédio: crureus
Musculoaponeurótico: musculoaponeurotic
Musculocutâneo: musculocutaneous
Musculoespiral: musculospiral
Músculo-esquelético: musculoskeletal
Músculofrênico: musculophrenic
Musculomembranáceo: musculomembranous
Musculotendíneo: musculotendinous
Musculotrópico: musculotropic
Musgo: moss
Musicoterapia: musicotherapy
Mussitação: mussitation
Mutação: mutation

Mutacismo: mutacism
Mutagênese: mutagenesis
Mutagênico: mutagen, mutagenic
Mutante: mutant
Mutarrotação: mutarotation
Mutarrotase: mutarotase
Mutase: mutase
Muteína: mutein
Mutilação: mutilation
Mutilar: maim
Mutismo: mutism
Muton: muton
Mutualismo: mutualism
Mutualista: mutualist
Mutuca: gadfly, horse-fly

N

N-acetilaspartato: N-acetylaspartate
N-acetilglicosamina: N-acetylglucosamine
N-acetilglutamato: N-acetylglutamate (NAG)
N^1-**acetilsulfanilamida:** N^1-acetylsulfanilamide
N^4-**acetilsulfanilamida:** N^4-acetylsulfanilamide
N-acilesfingosina: N-acylsphingosine
Nabilona: nabilone
Nacarado: nacreous
$NAD(P)^+$ **nucleosidase:** $NAD(P)^+$ nucleosidase
Nádegas: breech, buttocks, clunes, nates
Nadida: nadide
Nadir: nadir
Nadolol: nadolol
Nafato de cefamandol: cefamandole nafate
Nafcilina: nafcillin
Nafta: naphtha
Naftaleno: naphthalene
Naftalenol: naphthalenol
Naftalina: naphthalin
Naftil: naphthyl
α-naftiltiouréia: α-naphthylthiourea (ANTU)
Naftol: naphthol
Naftolato: naphtholate
Naftoquinona: naphthoquinone
Nagana: nagana
N-alilonormorfina: N-allylnormorphine
Nalorfina: nalorphine
Naltrexona: naltrexone
Nandrolona: nandrolone
Nanismo: dwarfism, nanism
Nanocefalia: nanocephalia, nanocephaly
Nanocéfalo, nanocefálico: nanocephalous, nanocephalic
Nanocormia: nanocormia
Nanoftalmia: nanophthalmia, nanophthalmos
Nanograma: nanogram (ng)

Nanokatal: nanokatal (nkat)
Nanomelia: nanomelia
Nanômetro: nanometer (nm)
Nanta: Nanta
Nanukayami: nanukayami
Não-alelo: nonallele
Não-cariogênico: noncariogenic
Não-celular: noncellular
Não-comedogênico: noncomedogenic
Não-comercial: nonproprietary name
Não-cromógenos: nonchromogens
Não-disjunção: nondisjunction
Não-eletrólito: nonelectrolyte
Não-estriado: unstriated
Não-estrogênico: nonestrogenic, nonoestrogenic
Não-fisiológico: unphysiologic
Não-imune: nonimmune
Não-imunidade: nonimmunity
Não-infeccioso: noninfectious
Não-invasivo: noninvasive
Não-iônico: nonionic
Não-maleficência: nonmaleficence
Não-medulado: nonmedullated
Não-mielinizado: nonmyelinated
Não-neoplásico: nonneoplastic
Não-nucleado: non-nucleated
Não-oclusão: nonocclusion
Não-oficial: unofficial
Não-paramétrico: nonparametric
Não-penetrância: nonpenetrance
Não-proteogênico: nonproteogenic
Não-reajuste do nodo sinoatrial: nonreset nodus sinuatrialis
Não-rotação: nonrotation
Não-sanitário: unsanitary
Não-saponificável: nonsaponifiable
Não-secretor: nonsecretor
Não-secretório: asecretory
Não-união: nonunion
Não-uterotrópico: nonuterotropic
Não-valente: nonvalent
Não-vascular: nonvascular
Não-verbal: nonverbal
Não-viável: nonviable
Napex: napex
Napier: napier
Naproxeno: naproxen
Napsilato: napsylate
Napsilato de dextropropoxifeno: dextropropoxyphene napsylate
Napsilato de levopropoxifeno: levopropoxyphene napsylate
Napsilato de propoxifeno: propoxyphene napsylate
Narceína: narceine
Narcisismo: narcissism
Narcoanálise: narcoanalysis
Narco-hipnia: narcohypnia

Narco-hipnose: narcohypnosis
Narcolepsia: narcolepsy
Narcoléptico: narcoleptic
Narcose: narcosis
Narcossíntese: narcosynthesis
Narcoterapia: narcotherapy
Narcótico: narcotic
Narcotismo: narcotism
Narina: naris, **pl.** nares; nostril
Nariz: nose
Nasal: nasal, rhinal
Nascente: nascent
Nascido vivo: livebirth, live birth
Násio: nasion
Nasioiníaco: nasioiniac
Nasoantral: nasoantral
Nasociliar: nasociliary
Nasofaringe: nasopharynx
Nasofaríngeo: nasopharyngeal
Nasofaringolaringoscópio: nasopharyngolaryngoscope
Nasofaringoscopia: nasopharyngoscopy
Nasofaringoscópio: nasopharyngoscope
Nasofrontal: nasofrontal
Nasogástrico: nasogastric
Nasolabial: nasolabial
Nasolacrimal: nasolacrimal
Naso-oral: nasooral
Nasopalatino: nasopalatine
Nasorrostral: nasorostral
Nasossinusite: nasosinusitis
Natal: natal
Natalidade: natality
Natamicina: natamycin
Natimorto: stillborn
Natremia, natriemia: natremia, natriemia
Natriférico: natriferic
Natriurese: natriuresis
Natriurético: natriuretic
Naturopata: naturopath
Naturopatia: naturopathy
Naturopático: naturopathic
Naupatia: naupathia
Náusea: nausea, nauseate, sicchasia
Nauseado: nauseated
Nauseante: nauseant
Nauseoso: nauseous
Navícula: navicula
N-carboxianidridos: N-carboxyanhydrides
N-carboxiuréia: N-carboxyurea
n-decano: n-decane
N,N-dimetiltriptamina: N,N-dimethyltryptamine (DMT)
Neartrose: nearthrosis
Nebramicina: nebramycin
Nébula: nebula (nebul.), **pl.** nebulae
Nebularina: nebularine
Nebulina: nebulin
Nebulização: nebulization
Nebulizador: nebulizer
Nebulizar: nebulize
Necatoríase: necatoriasis
Necessidade: requirement
Necrectomia: necrectomy
Necrobacilose: necrobacillosis

Necrobiose: necrobiosis
Necrobiótico: necrobiotic
Necrocitose: necrocytosis
Necrófago: necrophagous
Necrofilia: necrophilia, necrophilism
Necrófilo: necrophilous
Necrofobia: necrophobia
Necrogênico: necrogenic
Necrógeno: necrogenous
Necrogranulomatoso: necrogranulomatous
Necrólise: necrolysis
Necrologia: necrology
Necrologista: necrologist
Necromania: necromania
Necrômetro: necrometer
Necroparasita: necroparasite
Necropatia: necropathy
Necropsia: autopsy, necropsy
Necrosar: necrose
Necroscopia: necroscopy
Necrose: necrosis
Necrospermia: necrospermia
Necrossadismo: necrosadism
Necrossectomia: necrosectomy
Necrosteose: necrosteon, necrosteosis
Necrótico: necrotic
Necrotomia: necrotomy
Nefelometria: nephelometry
Nefelômetro: nephelometer
Nefralgia: nephralgia
Nefrálgico: nephralgic
Nefrectomia: nephrectomy
Nefredema: nephredema
Nefrelcose: nephrelcosis
Néfrico: nephric
Nefrídio: nephridium, **pl.** nephridia
Nefrite: nephritis, **pl.** nephritides
Nefrítico: nephritic
Nefritogênico: nephritogenic
Nefroblastema: nephroblastema
Nefroblastoma: nephroblastoma
Nefrocalcinose: nephrocalcinosis
Nefrocapsectomia: nephrocapsectomy
Nefrocardíaco: nephrocardiac
Nefrocele: nephrocele
Nefrocistose: nephrocystosis
Nefrogenético, nefrogênico: nephrogenetic, nephrogenic
Nefrógeno: nephrogenous
Nefrografia: nephrography
Nefrograma: nephrogram
Nefróide: nephroid
Nefrólise: nephrolysis
Nefrolisina: nephrolysin
Nefrolitíase: nephrolithiasis
Nefrolítico: nephrolytic
Nefrólito: nephrolith
Nefrolitotomia: nephrolithotomy
Nefrologia: nephrology
Nefroma: nephroma
Nefromalacia: nephromalacia
Nefromegalia: nephromegaly
Nefrômero: nephromere
Néfron: nephron

Glossário

Nefropatia: nephropathia, nephropathy
Nefropático: nephropathic
Nefropexia: nephropexy
Nefropiose: nephropyosis
Nefroptose: nephroptosis, nephroptosia
Nefrorrafia: nephrorrhaphy
Nefrosclerose: nephrosclerosis
Nefrosclerótico: nephrosclerotic
Nefroscópio: nephroscope
Nefrose: nephrosis
Nefrostograma: nephrostogram
Nefróstoma: nephrostoma, nephrostome
Nefrostomia: nephrostomy
Nefrótico: nephrotic
Nefrotísica: nephrophthisis
Nefrotomia: nephrotomy
Nefrotômico: nephrotomic
Nefrótomo: nephrotome
Nefrotomografia: nephrotomography
Nefrotomograma: nephrotomogram
Nefrotoxicidade: nephrotoxicity
Nefrotóxico: nephrotoxic
Nefrotoxina: nephrotoxin
Nefrotrófico: nephrotrophic
Nefrotrópico: nephrotropic
Nefrotuberculose: nephrotuberculosis
Nefroureterectomia: nephroureterectomy
Nefroureterectasia: nephroureterectasis
Nefroureterocistectomia: nephroureterocystectomy
Negação: denial, negation
Negativismo: negativism
Negativo: negative
Negatron: negatron
Negra: nigra
Negro de amida 10B: amido black 10B
Neisseria: neisseria, **pl.** neisseriae
Nematelminto: nemathelminth, roundworm
Nematização: nematization
Nematoblasto: nematoblast
Nematocida: nematicidal, nematocidal, nematicide, nematocide
Nematocisto: cnida, **pl.** cnidae; cnidocyst, nematocyst
Nematódeo: nematode, threadworm
Nematodíase: nematodiasis
Nematóide: nematoid
Nematologia: nematology
Nematologista: nematologist
Nematospermia: nematospermia
Neo-adjuvante: neoadjuvant
Neo-antígenos: neoantigens
Neo-arsfenamina: neoarsphenamine
Neo-artrose: neoarthrosis
Neobexiga: neobladder
Neobiogênese: neobiogenesis
Neoblástico: neoblastic

Neocerebelo: neocerebellum
Neocincofeno: neocinchophen
Neocinético: neokinetic
Neocistostomia: neocystostomy
Neocórtex: neocortex
Neodímio: neodymium (Nd)
Neoencéfalo: neencephalon
Neo-encéfalo: neoencephalon
Neofetal: neofetal
Neofeto: neofetus
Neofobia: neophobia
Neoformação: neoformation
Neogênese: neogenesis
Neogenético: neogenetic
Neolalismo: neolallism
Neologismo: neologism
Neomorfo, neomorfismo: neomorph, neomorphism
Néon, neônio: neon (Ne)
Neonatal: neonatal
Neonato: neonate
Neonatologia: neonatology
Neonatologista: neonatologist
Neoneurotização: neoneurotization
Neopálio: neopallium
Neopiritiamina: neopyrithiamin
Neoplasia: neoplasia
Neoplásico: neoplastic
Neoplasma: neoplasm
Neopterina: neopterin
Neoquimiotripsinogênio: neochymotrypsinogen
Neorretinal b: neoretinal b
Neorretineno B: neoretinene B
Neostigmina: neostigmine
Neostomia: neostomy
Neostriado: neostriatum
Neotálamo: neothalamus
Neotenia: neoteny
Neotirosina: neotyrosine
Neovascularização: neovascularization
Neper: neper (Np)
Neral: neral
Neriína: nerine
Nervimovimento: nervimotion
Nervino: nervine
Nervo: nerve, nervus, **gen. e pl.** nervi
Nervomotilidade: nervimotility
Nervona: nervone
Nervosismo: nervousness
Nervoso: nervous
Nesidiectomia: nesidiectomy
Nesidioblasto: nesidioblast
Nesidioblastose: nesidioblastosis
Nesselerizar: nesslerize
Netúnio: neptunium (Np)
Neural: neural
Neuralgia: neuralgia
Neuralgia de Sluder: Sluder neuralgia
Neurálgico: neuralgic
Neuralgiforme: neuralgiform
Neuramebímetro: neuramebimeter
Neuraminidase: neuraminidase
α_2-neuraminoglicoproteína: α_2-neuraminoglycoprotein
Neuranagênese: neuranagenesis

Neurapófise: neurapophysis
Neurapraxia: neurapraxia
Neurarquia: neurarchy
Neurastenia: neurasthenia
Neurastênico: neurasthenic
Neuraxônio, neuroaxônio: neuraxon, neuraxone
Neurectasia: neurectasis, neurectasia, neurectasy
Neurectomia: neurectomy
Neurectopia: neurectopia, neurectopy
Neurepitélio: neurepithelium
Neuridina: neuridine
Neurilema: neurilemma
Neurilemoma: neurilemoma
Neurilidade: neurility
Neurimotilidade: neurimotility
Neurina: neurine
Neurinoma: neurinoma
Neurite: neuritis, **pl.** neuritides
Neurítico: neuritic
Neuroalergia: neuroallergy
Neuroanastomose: neuroanastomosis
Neuroanatomia: neuroanatomy
Neuroartropatia: neuroarthropathy
Neuroaumentativo neuroaugmentive
Neuroaumento: neuroaugmentation
Neurobiologia: neurobiology
Neurobiotaxia: neurobiotaxis
Neuroblasto: neuroblast
Neuroblastoma: neuroblastoma
Neuroborreliose: neuroborreliosis
Neurocardíaco: neurocardiac
Neurocele: neurocele
Neuroceratina: neurokeratin
Neurociência: neurosciences
Neurocirurgia: neurosurgery
Neurocirurgião: neurosurgeon
Neurócito: neurocyte
Neurocitólise: neurocytolysis
Neurocitoma: neurocytoma
Neurocladismo: neurocladism
Neurocoriorretinite: neurochorioretinitis
Neurocoroidite: neurochoroiditis
Neurocrânio: braincase, neurocranium
Neurocristopatia: neurocristopathy
Neurodendrito: neurodendrite
Neurodendro: neurodendron
Neurodermatite: neurodermatitis
Neurodinâmico: neurodynamic
Neurodinia: neurodynia
Neuroectoderma: neuroectoderm
Neuroectodérmico: neuroectodermal
Neuroectomia: neuroectomy
Neuroeixo: neuraxis
Neuroencefalomielopatia: neuroencephalomyelopathy

Neuroendócrino: neuroendocrine
Neuroendocrinologia: neuroendocrinology
Neuroepitelial: neuroepithelial
Neuroepitélio: neuroepithelium
Neuroesplâncnico: neurosplanchnic
Neuroespôngio: neurospongium
Neuroesteróide: neurosteroid
Neuroestimulador: neurostimulator
Neurofarmacologia: neuropharmacology
Neurofibra: neurofibra
Neurofibrila: neurofibril
Neurofibrilar: neurofibrillar
Neurofibroma: neurofibroma
Neurofibromatose: neurofibromatosis
Neurofilamento: neurofilament
Neurófilo: neurophilic
Neurofisinas: neurophysins
Neurofisiologia: neurophysiology
Neurofonia: neurophonia
Neuroftalmologia: neuro-ophthalmology
Neurogânglio: neuroganglion
Neurogástrico: neurogastric
Neurogênese: neurogenesis
Neurogênico, neurogenético: neurogenic, neurogenetic
Neurogênico: neurogenous
Neuróglia: neuroglia
Neuroglial: neuroglial, neurogliar
Neurogliócito: neurogliacyte
Neurogliomatose: neurogliomatosis
Neurografia: neurography
Neurograma: neurogram
Neuro-hemal: neurohemal
Neuro-hipofisário: neurohypophysial
Neuro-hipófise: neurohypophysis
Neuro-histologia: neurohistology
Neuro-hormônio: neurohormone
Neuróide: neuroid
Neurolema: neurolemma
Neuroleptanalgesia: neuroleptanalgesia
Neuroleptanestesia: neuroleptanesthesia
Neuroléptico: neuroleptic
Neurolinfa: neurolymph
Neurolinfomatose: neurolymphomatosis
Neurolingüística: neurolinguistics
Neurólise: neurolysis
Neurolisina: neurolysin
Neurolítico: neurolytic
Neurologia: neurology
Neurologista: neurologist
Neuroma: neuroma
Neuromalacia: neuromalacia
Neuromatose: neuromatosis

uromelanina: neuromelanin
uromeníngeo: euromeningeal
urômero: neuromere
uromiastenia: euromyasthenia
uromielite: neuromyelitis
uromimético: neuromimetic
uromiopatia: neuromyopathy
uromiosite: neuromyositis
uromotor: nervimotor, eurimotor
uromuscular: neuromuscular
uronal: neuronal
uroncologia: neurooncology
uronéfrico: neuronephric
uronevo: neuronevus
urônio: neuron, neurone
uronite: neuronitis
uronite vestibular: ubisagari, kubisagaru
uronixe: neuronyxis
uronofagia: neuronophagia, euronophagy
uronófago: neuronophage
uronopatia: neuronopathy
uroparalisia: neuroparalysis
uroparalítico: neuroparalytic
uropata: neuropath
uropatia: neuropathia, europathy
uropático: neuropathic
uropatogenia: europathogenesis
uropatologia: neuropathology
uropeptídeo: neuropeptide
urópilo: neuropil, neuropile
uroplasma: neuroplasm
uroplastia: neuroplasty
uroplégico: neuroplegic
uroplexo: neuroplexus
urópodos: neuropodia
uroporo: neuropore
uropraxia: neuropraxia
uropsicofarmacologia: europsychopharmacology
uropsicologia: europsychology
uropsicológico: europsychologic, europsychological
uropsicopatia: europsychopathy
uropsicopático: europsychopathic
uropsiquiatria: europsychiatry
uroquímica: neurochemistry
uroquitina: neurochitin
urorradiologia: europradiology
urorrafia: neurorrhaphy
urorrecidiva: neurorelapse
urorregulador: euroregulator
urorretinite: neuroretinitis
uroschwanoma: euroschwannoma
urose: neurosis, **pl.** neuroses
urossarcocleise: europsarcocleisis

Neurossarcoidose: neurosarcoidosis
Neurossarcoma: neurosarcoma
Neurossecreção: neurosecretion
Neurossecretor: neurosecretory
Neurossífilis: neurosyphilis
Neurossutura: neurosuture
Neurotaxia: neurotaxis
Neurotecoma: neurothekeoma
Neurotélio: neurothele
Neurotendinoso: neurotendinous
Neurotensão: neurotension
Neurotensina: neurotensin
Neuroterapêutica, neuroterapia: neurotherapeutics, neurotherapy
Neuroticismo: neuroticism
Neurótico: neurotic
Neurotização: neurotization
Neurotizar: neurotize
Neurotmese: neurotmesis
Neurotologia: neurootology
Neurotomia: neurotomy
Neurótomo: neurotome
Neurotônico: neurotonic
Neurotóxico: neurotoxic
Neurotoxina: neurotoxin
Neurotransmissão: neurotransmission
Neurotransmissor: neurotransmitter
Neurotrauma: neurotrauma
Neurotripsia: neurotripsy
Neurotrofia: neurotrophy
Neurotrófico: neurotrophic
Neurotropia, neurotropismo: neurotropy, neurotropism
Neurotrópico: neurotropic
Neurotrose: neurotrosis
Neurotúbulo: neurotubule
Neurovacina: neurovaccine
Neurovaricose, neurovaricosidade: neurovaricosis, neurovaricosity
Neurovascular: neurovascular
Neurovegetativo: neurovegetative
Neurovírus: neurovirus
Neurovisceral: neurovisceral
Neuroviscerolipidose familial: familial neuroviscerolipidosis
Nêurula: neurula, **pl.** neurulae
Neurulação: neurulation
Neutralização: neutralization
Neutralizar: neutralize
Neutro: neutral
Neutro de posterior: posterius
Neutroclusão: neutroclusion
Neutrofilia: neutrophilia
Neutrofílico: neutrophilic
Neutrófilo: neutrophil, neutrophile, neutrophilous
Neutrofilopenia: neutrophilopenia
Nêutron: neutron
Neutropenia: neutropenia
Neutrotaxia: neutrotaxis
Neve: snow

Nevo: mole, nevus, **pl.** nevi
Nevo achatado: spilus
Nevócito: nevocyte
Nevóide: nevoid
Nevoxantoendotelioma: nevoxanthoendothelioma
New berita: newberyite
Newton: newton (N)
Newton-metro: newtonmeter
Nexinas: nexins
Nexo: nexus, **pl.** nexus
N-formilcinurenina: N-formylkynurenine
N-formilmetionina: N-formylmethionine (fMet)
N^{10}-formiltetraidrofolato: N^{10}-formyltetrahydrofolate
N-formiminotetraidrofolato: N-formiminotetrahydrofolate
N^ω-fosfonocreatina: N^ω-phosphonocreatine
N-glicosídeo: N-glycoside
n-heptilpenicilina: n-heptylpenicillin
Niacina: niacin
Niacinamida: niacinamide
Nialamida: nialamide
Nicardipina: nicardipine
Nicho: niche
Niclosamida: niclosamide
Nicofuranose: nicofuranose
Nicotina: nicotine
Nicotinamida: nicotinamide
Nicotinamida adenina dinucleotídeo (NAD, NAD$^+$, NADH): nicotinamide adenine dinucleotide (NAD, NAD$^+$, NADH)
Nicotinato: nicotinate
Nicotínico: nicotinic
Nicotinomimético: nicotinomimetic
Nictação: nictation
Nictalgia: nyctalgia
Nictalopia: nyctalopia
Nictanopia: nyctanopia
Nictêmero: nycterohemeral, nyctohemeral
Nicterino: nycterine
Nictitação: nictitation
Nictofilia: nyctophilia
Nictofobia: nyctophobia
Nictúria: nycturia
Nicumalona: nicoumalone
Nidação: nidation
Nidal: nidal
Nidogene: nidogen
Nifedipina: nifedipine
Nifenazona: nifenazone
Nifuraldezona: nifuraldezone
Nifuratel: nifuratel
Nifuroxima: nifuroxime
Nigerose: nigerose
Nigricante: nigrities
Nigroestriatal: nigrostriatal
Nigrosina: nigrosin, nigrosine
Niilismo: nihilism
Nimodipina: nimodipine
Nimustina: nimustine
Ninfa: nymph, nympha, **pl.** nymphae

Ninfal: nymphal
Ninfectomia: nymphectomy
Ninfite: nymphitis
Ninfolabial: nympholabial
Ninfolepsia: nympholepsy
Ninfomania: nymphomania
Ninfomaníaca: nymphomaniac, nymphomaniacal
Ninfoncose: nymphoncus
Ninfotomia: nymphotomy
Ninhada: brood
Ninho, nicho: nest, nidus, **pl.** nidi
Ninidrina: ninhydrin
Nióbio: niobium (Nb)
Niovera: njovera
Níquel: nickel (Ni)
Niqueloplasmina: nickeloplasmin
Niquetamida: nikethamide
Niridazol: niridazole
Nisina: nisin
Nisoldipina: nisoldipine
Nistagmiforme: nystagmiform
Nistagmo: nystagmic, nystagmus
Nistagmografia: nystagmography
Nistagmógrafo: nystagmograph
Nistagmograma: nystagmogram
Nistagmóide: nystagmoid
Nistatina: nystatin
Niton: niton
Nitrato: nitrate
Nitrato de butoconazol: butoconazole nitrate
Nitrato de isobutila: isobutyl nitrite
Nitrato de miconazol: miconazole nitrate
Nitrato de peroxiacetil: peroxyacetyl nitrate
Nitrato de prata: lunar caustic
Nitrato de propatila: propatyl nitrate
Nitrato fenilmercúrico: phenylmercuric nitrate
Nitrazepam: nitrazepam
Nitrendipina: nitrendipine
Nitreto: nitride
Nitridação: nitridation
Nitrificação: nitrification
Nitrila: nitrile, nitryl
Nitrito: nitrite
Nitritúria: nitrituria
Nitro: niter
Nitrocelulose: nitrocellulose
Nitroclorofórmio: nitrochloroform
Nitrofenilsulfenil: nitrophenylsulfenyl (Nps)
Nitrofuranos: nitrofurans
Nitrofurantoína: nitrofurantoin
Nitrofurazona: nitrofurazone
Nitrogenase: nitrogenase
Nitrogênio: nitrogen (N)
Nitrogênio-13 (N^{13}): nitrogen-13 (^{13}N)
Nitrogênio-14 (N^{14}): nitrogen-14 (^{14}N)
Nitrogênio-15 (N^{15}): nitrogen-15 (^{15}N)

Glossário

Nitrogenoso: nitrogenous
Nitroglicerina: nitroglycerin
Nitromanitol: nitromannitol
Nitromersol: nitromersol
Nitrômetro: nitrometer
Nítron: nitron
Nitroprussiato: nitroprusside
Nitrosaminas: nitrosamines
Nitrosil: nitrosyl
Nitroso: nitrous
Nitrosouréia: nitrosourea
Nitroxi: nitroxy
Nitroxila: nitroxyl
Nitroxolina: nitroxoline
Nível: level
Nível de corte: tomolevel
Nizatidina: nizatidine
N^5,N^{10}-meteniltetraidrofolato: N^5,N^{10}-methenyltetrahydrofolate
N-metilcarnosina: N-methylcarnosine
N^5,N^{10}-metilenotetraidrofolato redutase: N^5,N^{10}-methylenetetrahydrofolate reductase
N-metilglucamina: N-methylglucamine
N-metilistidina: N-methylhistidine
N^5-metiltetraidrofolato: N^5-methyltetrahydrofolate
Nó: knob, knot, nodus, **pl.** nodi
Nó AV: AV node
Nó dos dedos: knuckle
Nó sinoatrial: atrionector
NO sintase: NO synthase
Nó vital: noeud vital
Nobélio (No): nobelium (No)
Nocardia: nocardia, **pl.** nocardiae
Nocardíase: nocardiasis
Nocardioforme: nocardioform
Nocardiose: nocardiosis
Nocaute: knock-out
Nocebo: nocebo
Nociceptivo: nociceptive
Nociceptor: nociceptor
Nocifensor: nocifensor
Nocivo: noxious
Noctalbuminúria: noctalbuminuria
Noctifobia: noctiphobia
Noctógrafo: noctograph
Noctúria: nocturia
Nodal: nodal
Nodo: node
Nodos: nodi
Nodoso: nodose
Nodulação: nodulation
Nodulectomia: lumpectomy
Nódulo: nodule, nodulus, **pl.** noduli
Nódulo dos ordenhadores: pseudocowpox
Noemático: noematic
Noese: noesis
Noético: noetic
Noma: noma
Nome comercial: proprietary name
Nome genérico: generic name

Nome semi-sistemático: semisystematic name
Nome semitrivial: semitrivial name
Nome sistemático: systematic name
Nomenclatura: nomenclature
Nomografia: nomograph
Nomograma: nomogram
Nomotético: nomothetic
Nomotópico: nomotopic
Nonapeptídeo: nonapeptide
Nonose: nonose
Nonoxinol 9: nonoxynol 9
Nordazepam: nordazepam
Norepinefrina: noradrenaline, norepinephrine
Noresteróides: norsteroids
Noretandrolona: norethandrolone
Noretindrona: norethindrone
Noretinodrel: norethynodrel
Noretisterona: norethisterone
Norfloxacina: norfloxacin
Norgestrel: norgestrel
Norleucina: norleucine (Nle)
Norma: norm
Normal: normal (N)
Normalização: normalization
Normalizar: normalize
Normativo: normative
Normeperidina: normeperidine
Normetadona: normethadone
Normetanefrina: normetanephrine
Normobárico: normobaric
Normoblasto: normoblast
Normoblastose: normoblastosis
Normocapnia: normocapnia
Normocefálico: normocephalic
Normócito: normocyte
Normocitose: normorcytosis
Normocromia: normochromia
Normocrômico: normochromic
Normoeritrócito: normoerythrocyte
Normoglicemia: normoglycemia
Normoglicêmico: normoglycemic
Normopotassemia, normocaliemia: normokalemia, normokaliemia
Normostenúria: normosthenuria
Normotenso: normotensive
Normotermia: normothermia
Normotônico: normotonic
Normotopia: normotopia
Normotópico: normotopic
Normovolemia: normovolemia
Normoxia: normoxia
Norpipanona: norpipanone
Norsimpatol: norsympatol
Norsinefrina: norsynephrine
Noscapina: noscapine
Nosematose: nosematosis
Nosetiologia: nosetiology
Nosoacusia: nosoacusis
Nosocomial: nosocomial
Nosoctonografia: nosochthonography
Nosofilia: nosophilia

Nosófito: nosophyte
Nosofobia: nosophobia
Nosogênese, nosogenia: nosogenesis, nosogeny
Nosogênico: nosogenic
Nosogeografia: nosogeography
Nosografia: nosography
Nosográfico: nosographic
Nosologia: nosology
Nosológico: nosologic
Nosomania: nosomania
Nosometria: nosometry
Nosomicose: nosomycosis
Nosonomia: nosonomy
Nosopoético: nosopoietic
Nosotaxia: nosotaxy
Nosotóxico: nosotoxic
Nosotoxicose: nosotoxicosis
Nosotoxina: nosotoxin
Nosotropia: nosotrophy
Nosotrópico: nosotropic
Nostalgia: nostalgia
Nostofobia: nostophobia
Nostomania: nostomania
Nostro: nostrum
Notal: notal
Notancefalia: notancephalia
Notanencefalia: notanencephalia
Notatina: notatin
Notencefalocele: notencephalocele
Notocorda: notochord
Notocordal: notochordal
Noturno: nocturnal
Nous: nous
Novobiocina: novobiocin
Noxa: noxa
Noxitiolina: noxythiolin
Noz de areca: betel nut
Noz-de-galha: galla, nutgall
Noz-moscada: myristica, nutmeg
Noz-vômica: nux vomica
N-sulfanililacetamida: N-sulfanilylacetamide
N-sulfanililbenzamida: N-sulfanilylbenzamide
N^ε-trimetilisina: N^ε-trimethyllysine
Nubécula: nubecula
Nuca: nape, nucha
Nucal: nuchal
Nucleação: nucleation
Nucleado: nucleated
Nuclear: nuclear
Nuclease: nuclease
Nucleato: nucleate
Nucleiforme: nucleiform
Núcleo: core, nucleus, **pl.** nuclei
Núcleo denteado do cerebelo: dentatum
Núcleo do fastígio: fastigatum
Núcleo lentiforme: lenticula
Nucleocapsídeo: nucleocapsid
Nucleoesqueleto: nucleoskeleton
Nucleofilamentos: nucleofilaments
Nucleofílico: nucleophilic
Nucleófilo: nucleophil, nucleophile

Nucleofosfatases: nucleophosphatases
Núcleo-histona: nucleohistone
Nucleóide: nucleoid
Nucleolar: nucleolar
Nucleoliforme: nucleoliform
Nucléolo: nucleolus, **pl.** nucleoli
Nucleolóide: nucleoloid
Nucleolonema: nucleolonema
Nucleomicrossoma: nucleomicrosome
Nucleon: nucleon
Nucleoplasma: nucleoplasm
Nucleoplasmina: nucleoplasmin
Nucleoproteína: nucleoprotein
Nucleoquilema: nucleochylema
Nucleoquimo: nucleochyme
Nucleorretículo: nucleoreticulum
Nucleorrexe: nucleorrhexis
Nucleosidases: nucleosidases
Nucleosídeo: nucleoside (Nuc, N)
Nucleosídeo difosfato cinase: nucleoside diphosphate kinase
Nucleossoma: nucleosome
Nucleotidases: nucleotidases
Nucleotídeo: nucleotide
Nucleotidiltransferases: nucleotidyltransferases
Nucleotoxina: nucleotoxin
Nuclídeo: nuclide
Nuligrávida: nulligravida
Nulípara: nonparous, nullipara, nulliparous
Nuliparidade: nulliparity
Numênico: noumenal
Número: number
Número da dibucaína: dibucaine number (DN)
Número de ondas: wavenumber (σ)
Número de Polenské: Polenské number
Número do fluoreto: fluoride number
Numiforme: nummiform
Numulação: nummulation
Numular: nummular
Nutação: nutation
Nutrição: nutrition
Nutriente: nutrient
Nutrílitos: nutrilites
Nutritivo: nutritive

O

O-acetilcarnitina: O-acetylcarnitine
Obelíaco: obeliac
Obélio: obelion
Obesidade: obesity
Obeso: obese
Óbex: obex
Objetivo: goal, objective
Objeto: object
Obliquidade: obliquity

Oblíquo: oblique, obliquus
Obliteração: obliteration
Obnubilação: obnubilation
Obrigatório: obligate
Observador: observer
Obsessão: obsession
Obsessivo-compulsivo: obsessive-compulsive
Obsolescência: obsolescence
Obstetra: obstetrician
Obstetrícia: obstetrics (OB)
Obstétrico: obstetric, obstetrical
Obstinado: obstinate
Obstipação: obstipation
Obstrução: obstruction
Obstrutivo: obstruent
Obtundir: obtund
Obturação: filling, obturation
Obturador: obturator, packer, plugger
Obtusão: obtusion
Obtuso: dull, obtuse
Occipício: occiput, gen. occipitis
Occipital: occipital, occipitalis
Occipitalização: occipitalization
Occipitoatlóide: occipitoatloid
Occipitoaxial: occipitoaxial, occipitoaxoid
Occipitobregmático: occipitobregmatic
Occipitofacial: occipitofacial
Occipitofrontal: occipitofrontal, occipitofrontalis
Occipitomastóide: occipitomastoid
Occipitomentual: occipitomental
Occipitoparietal: occipitoparietal
Occipitotalâmico: occipitothalamic
Occipitotemporal: occipitotemporal
Ocelo: eyespot, ocellus, pl. ocelli
Ocitocina: ocytocin, oxytocin (OXT)
Oclofobia: ochlophobia
***o*-clorobenzalmalononitrilo:** *o*-chlorobenzalmalononitrile
***o*-clorofenol:** *o*-chlorophenol
Ocluir: occlude
Oclusal: occlusal
Oclusão: occlusion
Oclusivo: occlusive
Oclusômetro: occlusometer
Oclusor: occluder
Oco: hollow
Ocratoxina: ochratoxin
Ocrilato: ocrylate
Ocrodermia: ochrodermia
Ocrômetro: ochrometer
Ocronose: ochronosis
Ocronótico: ochronotic
Octã: octan
Octafluoropropano: octafluoropropane
Octametil pirofosforamida: octamethyl pyrophosphoramide (OMPA)
Octamilamina: octamylamine
Octanoato: octanoate
Octanoil-CoA sintetase: octanoyl-CoA synthetase
Octapeptídeo: octapeptide
Octaploidia: octaploidy
Octapressina: octapressin
Octavalente: octad, octavalent
Octilfenoxi polietoxietanol: octylphenoxy polyethoxyethanol
Octilgalato: octyl gallate
Octopamina: octopamine
Octose: octose
Octoxinol: octoxynol
Octulose: octulose
Ocular: eyepiece, ocular
Oculista: oculist, optician
Oculística: opticianry
Oculoauriculovertebral: oculoauriculovertebral
Oculocardíaco: oculocardiac
Oculocerebrorrenal: oculocerebrorenal
Oculocutâneo: oculocutaneous
Oculodentodigital: oculodentodigital
Oculodérmico: oculodermal
Oculodinia: oculodynia
Oculofacial: oculofacial
Oculogiria: oculogyria
Oculogírico: oculogyric
Oculografia: oculography
Oculomandibulodiscefalia: oculomandibulodyscephaly
Oculomotor: oculomotor, oculomotorius
Oculonasal: oculonasal
Oculopatia: oculopathy
Oculopletismografia: oculoplethysmography
Oculopneumopletismografia: oculopneumoplethysmography
Oculopupilar: ocuulopupillary
Óculos: eyeglasses, glasses, oculi
Óculos de proteção: goggle
Oculossimpático: oculosympathetic
Oculovertebral: oculovertebral
Oculozigomático: oculozygomatic
Oculto: occult
***o*-difenolase:** *o*-diphenolase
Odinacusia: odynacusis
Odinofagia: odynophagia
Odinofonia: odynophonia
Odogênese: odogenesis
Odontalgia: odontalgia, toothache
Odontálgico: odontalgic
Odontectomia: odontectomy
Odonterismo: odonterism
Odontíase: odontiasis
Odontinóide: odontinoid
Odontite: odontitis
Odontoameloblastoma: odontoameloblastoma
Odontoblasto: odontoblast
Odontoblastoma: odontoblastoma
Odontoclasto: odontoclast
Odontodinia: odontodynia
Odontodisplasia: odontodysplasia
Odontofobia: odontophobia
Odontogênese: odontogenesis
Odontogenia: odontogeny
Odontóide: odontoid
Odontólise: odontolysis
Odontologia: dentistry, odontology
Odontoloxia: odontoloxia, odontoloxy
Odontoma: odontoma
Odontoneuralgia: odontoneuralgia
Odontonomia: odontonomy
Odontonosologia: odontonosology
Odontoparalaxe: odontoparallaxis
Odontopatia: odontopathy
Odontoplastia: odontoplasty
Odontoprise: odontoprisis
Odontoptose: odontoptosis
Odontorragia: odontorrhagia
Odontoscopia: odontoscopy
Odontoscópio: odontoscope
Odontose: odontosis
Odontosquismo: odontoschism
Odontoterapia: odontotherapy
Odontotomia: odontotomy
Odor: odor
Odorante: odorant
Odoratismo: odoratism
Odorífero: odoriferous, odorous
Odorigrafia: odorography
Odorimetria: odorimetry
Odorímetro: odorimeter
Odorivecção: odorivection
Ofegar: pant
Ofíase: ophiasis
Oficial: official
Oficinal: officinal
Ofidíase: ophidiasis
Ofidiofobia: ophidiophobia
Ofídios: Ophidia
Ofidismo: ophidism
***O*-fosfosserina:** *O*-phosphoserine
Ófrio: ophryon
Ofriogênese: ophryogenes
Ofriose: ophryosis
Ofrite: ophritis, ophryitis
***o*-ftalaldeído:** *o*-phthalaldehyde
Oftalmalgia: ophthalmalgia
Oftalmia: ophthalmia
Oftálmico: ophthalmic
Oftalmodinamometria: ophthalmodynamometry
Oftalmodinamômetro: ophthalmodynamometer
Oftalmolito: ophthalmolith
Oftalmologia: ophthalmology
Oftalmologista: ophthalmologist
Oftalmomalacia: ophthalmomalacia
Oftalmomelanose: ophthalmomelanosis
Oftalmômetro: ophthalmometer
Oftalmomicose: ophthalmomycosis
Oftalmomiíase: ophthalmomyiasis
Oftalmopatia: ophthalmopathy
Oftalmoplegia: ophthalmoplegia
Oftalmoplégico: ophthamoplegic
Oftalmoscopia: ophthalmoscopy
Oftalmoscópico: ophthalmoscopic
Oftalmoscópio: ophthalmoscope
Oftalmótropo: ophthalmotrope
Oftalmovascular: ophthalmovascular
Ofuscação: obfuscation
Ofuscamento: dazzling, glare
Ohmamperímetro: ohmammeter
Ohmômetro: ohmmeter
Oídio: oidium, pl. oidia
Oitavo nervo craniano: octavus
Olamina: olamine
Olamina de piroxicam: piroxicam olamine
Oleaginosa: oleaginous
Oleandro: oleander
Oleato: oleate
Oleato de mercúrio: mercuric oleate
Olécrano: olecranon
Olefina: olefin
Oleil-CoA: oleyl-CoA
Oleil-coenzima A: oleyl-coenzyme A
Oleína: olein
Óleo: oil
Óleo canforado: camphorated oil
Óleo cloroiodado: chloriodized oil
Óleo de açafroa: safflower oil
Óleo de ajovan: ajowan oil
Óleo de ajowan: ptychotis oil
Óleo de alcatrão de bétula: birch tar oil
Óleo de alecrim: rosemary oil
Óleo de amêndoa: almond oil
Óleo de amendoim: arachis oil, peanut oil
Óleo de cade: cade oil
Óleo de cajepute: cajeput oil, cajuput oil
Óleo de canela: cinnamon oil
Óleo de cássia: cassia oil
Óleo de cedro: cedar wood oil
Óleo de chaulmogra: chaulmoogra oil
Óleo de colza: rapeseed oil
Óleo de cravo: clove oil
Óleo de cróton: croton oil
Óleo de endro: dill oil
Óleo de estragão: estragon oil
Óleo de faia: beech oil
Óleo de fígado de bacalhau: cod liver oil
Óleo de fígado de hipogloso: halibut liver oil
Óleo de fígado de tubarão: shark liver oil
Óleo de folha de cedro: cedar leaf oil

Óleo de gaultéria: checkerberry oil, gaultheria oil, wintergreen oil
Óleo de gergelim: benne oil, gingili oil
Óleo de germe de trigo: wheat germ oil
Óleo de ginocárdia: gynocardia oil
Óleo de hidnocarpo: hydnocarpus oil
Óleo de manjerona: origanum oil
Óleo de milho: corn oil, maise oil
Óleo de mostarda: mustard oil
Óleo de noz-moscada: nutmeg oil
Óleo de percomorfo: percomorph oil
Óleo de pimenta: allspice oil
Óleo de rícino: castor oil
Óleo de rosa: attar of rose, otto of rose
Óleo de sândalo: sandalwood oil, santal oil
Óleo de semente de algodão: cottonseed oil
Óleo de semente de damasco: apricot kernel oil
Óleo de semente de girassol: sunflower seed oil
Óleo de semente de pêssego: peach kernel oil
Óleo de sésamo ou de gergelim: teel oil
Óleo de tarragona: tarragon oil
Óleo de terebintina: oleum terebinthinae, turpentine oil
Óleo etiodado: ethiodized oil
Óleo iodado: iodized oil
Óleo mineral: mineral oil
Óleo pérsico: persic oil
Oleogomenol: oleogomenol
Oleogranuloma: oleogranuloma
Oleoma: oleoma
Oleômetro: oleometer
Oleopalmitato: oleopalmitate
Oleorresina: oleoresin
Oleoso: oleosus
Oleoso ou gorduroso: fatty
Oleostearato: oleostearate
Oleoterapia: eleotherapy, oleotherapy
Oleovitamina: oleovitamin
Olfação: olfaction, osmesis
Olfatia: olfactie, olfacty
Olfato: osphresis
Olfatofobia: olfactophobia
Olfatologia: olfactology
Olfatometria: olfactometry
Olfatômetro: olfactometer
Olfatório: olfactory, osmatic
Olhar fixo: stare
Olho: eye, oculus, **gen. e pl.** oculi
Olíbano: olibanum
Oligâmnio: oligamnios
Oligemia: oligemia
Oligêmico: oligemic
Oligidria: olighidria, oligidria
Oligo: oligo

Oligo-α-1,6-glicosidase: oligo-α-1,6-glucosidase
Oligoâmnio: oligoamnios
Oligocístico: oligocystic
Oligocolia: oligocholia
Oligodactilia: oligodactyly, oligodactylia
Oligodendria: oligodendria
Oligodendroblasto: oligodendroblast
Oligodendroblastoma: oligodendroblastoma
Oligodendrócito: oligodendrocyte
Oligodendróglia: oligodendroglia
Oligodendroglioma: oligodendroglioma
Oligodinâmico: oligodynamic
Oligodipsia: oligodipsia
Oligodontia: oligodontia
Oligofrenia: oligophrenia
Oligogalactia: oligogalactia
Oligoglicanorramificante glicosiltransferase: oligoglucan-branching glycosyltransferase
Oligoidrâmnio: oligohydramnios
Oligoidrúria: oligohydruria
Oligolécito: oligolecithal
Oligomenorréia: oligomenorrhea
Oligômero: oligomer
Oligomórfico: oligomorphic
Oligonefrônico: oligonephronic
Oligonucleotídeo: oligonucleotide
Oligopepsia: oligopepsia
Oligoplásico: oligoplastic
Oligopnéia: oligopnea
Oligoptialismo: oligoptyalism
Oligoquilia: oligochylia
Oligoquimia: oligochymia
Oligoria: oligoria
Oligospermia: oligospermia, oligospermatism
Oligossacarídeo: oligosaccharide
Oligossialia: oligosialia
Oligossináptico: oligosynaptic
Oligossintomático: oligosymptomatic
Oligotimia: oligothymia
Oligotricose: oligotrichosis
Oligotriquia: oligotrichia
Oligotrofia: oligotrophia, oligotrophy
Oligozoospermia: oligozoospermatism, oligozoospermia
Oligúria: oliguria
Oliva: oliva, **pl.** olivae; olive
Olivar: olivary
Olivífugo: olivifugal
Olivípeto: olivipetal
Olivococlear: olivocochlear
Olivopontocerebelar: olivopontocerebellar
Olofonia: olophonia
Ololiúqui: ololiuqui

Ombro: shoulder
Ombrofobia: ombrophobia
Omental: omental
Omentectomia: omentectomy, omentumectomy
Omentite: omentitis
Omento: omentum, **pl.** omenta
Omento maior: pileus
Omento menor: omentulum
Omentofixação: omentofixation
Omentopexia: omentopexy
Omentoplastia: omentoplasty
Omentorrafia: omentorrhaphy
Omentovólvulo: omentovolvulus
Omeprazol: omeprazole
Omoclavicular: omoclavicular
Omofagia: omophagia
Omo-hióideo: omohyoid
Omotireóideo: omothyroid
OMP-descarboxilase: OMP decarboxylase
OMP pirofosforilase: OMP pyrophosphorylase
Onça: ounce (oz.)
Onça líquida: fluidounce
Oncocercíase: onchocerciasis
Oncocercídeo: onchocercid
Oncocercoma: onchocercoma
Oncocercose: onchocercosis, volvulosis
Oncócito: oncocyte
Oncocitoma: oncocytoma
Oncofetal: oncofetal
Oncogene: oncogene
Oncogênese: oncogenesis
Oncogênico: oncogenic, oncogenous
Oncografia: oncography
Oncógrafo: oncograph
Oncólise: oncolysis
Oncolítico: oncolytic
Oncologia: oncology
Oncologista: oncologist
Oncometria: oncometry
Oncométrico: oncometric
Oncômetro: oncometer
Oncose: oncosis
Oncosfera: oncosphere
Oncostatina M: oncostatin M
Oncoterapia: oncotherapy
Oncótico: oncotic
Oncotomia: oncotomy
Oncotrópico: oncotropic
Oncovírus: oncovirus
Onda: wave
Ondansetron: ondansetron
Ondina: Ondine
Ondulado: undulate
Ondulipódio: undulipodium, **pl.** undulipodia
Onfalectomia: omphalectomy
Onfalelcose: omphalelcosis
Onfálico: omphalic
Onfalite: omphalitis
Onfaloangiópago: omphaloangiopagus
Onfalocele: omphalocele
Onfaloentérico: omphaloenteric
Onfaloespinhoso: omphalospinous

Onfaloflebite: omphalophlebitis
Onfalomesentérico: omphalomesenteric
Onfalópago: omphalopagus
Onfalorragia: omphalorrhagia
Onfalorréia: omphalorrhea
Onfalorrexe: omphalorrhexis
Onfalosito: omphalosite
Onfalotomia: omphalotomy
Onfalotripsia: omphalotripsy
Onfalovesical: omphalovesical
Onicalgia: onychalgia
Onicatrofia: onychatrophia, onychatrophy
Onicauxe: onychauxis
Onicoclase: onychoclasis
Onicocriptose: onychocryptosis
Onicodistrofia: onychodystrophy
Onicoeteropia: onychoheterotopia
Onicofagia: onychophagy, onychophagia
Onicofose: onychophosis
Onicógrafo: onychograph
Onicogripose: onychogryposis
Onicóide: onychoid
Onicólise: onycholysis
Onicologia: onychology
Onicomadese: onychomadesis
Onicomalacia: onychomalacia
Onicomicose: onychomycosis
Onicopatia: onychopathy
Onicopatologia: onychopathology
Onicoptose: onychoptosis
Onicorrexia: onychorrhexis
Onicose: onychosis
Onicosquizia: onychoschizia
Onicotilomania: onychotillomania
Onicotomia: onychotomy
Onicotrofia: onychotrophy
Oniomania: oniomania
Oniquectomia: onychectomy
Oníquia: onychia
Onírico: oneiric, oniric
Onirismo: oneirism
Onirocrítico: oneirocritical
Onirodinia: oneirodynia
Onirofrenia: oneirophrenia
Onirologia: oneirology
Onívoro: omnivorous
Onomatofobia: onomatophobia
Onomatomania: onomatomania
Onomatopoese: onomatopoiesis
Ontogênese: ontogenesis
Ontogenético: ontogenetic, ontogenic
Ontogenia: ontogeny
Ontologia: ontology
Oocineto: ookinete
Oocisto: oocyst
Oofagia: oophagia, oophagy
Ooforalgia: oophoralgia
Ooforectomia: oophorectomy
Ooforite: oophoritis
Oóforo: oophoron
Ooforocistectomia: oophorocystectomy

Ooforocistose: oophorocystosis
Ooforopatia: oophoropathy
Ooforopexia: oophoropexy
Ooforoplastia: oophoroplasty
Oofororrafia: oophororrhaphy
Oofororragia: oophorrhagia
Ooforossalpingectomia: oophorosalpingectomy
Ooforossalpingite: oophorosalpingitis
Ooforotomia: oophorotomy
Oolema: oolemma
Oomicose: oomycosis
Ooplasma: ooplasm
Oosporângio: oosporangium
Oosporo: oospore
Oossoma: oosome
Ooteca: ootheca
Oótide: ootid
Oótipo: ootype
Opacidade: opacity
Opacificação: opacification
Opaco: opaque
Opalescente: opalescent
Operação: operation
Operador: operator
Operar: operate
Operatório: operative
Operável: operable
Operculado: operculated
Opercular: opercular
Operculite: operculitis
Opérculo: operculum, **gen.** operculi, **pl.** opercula
Opéron: operon
Opiáceo: opiate
Opianil: opianyl
Opianina: opianine
Opilativo: oppilative
Opina: opine
Ópio: opium
Opiocortina: opiocortin
Opióide: opioid
Opiomelanocortina: opiomelanocortin
Opistenar: opisthenar
Opístio: opisthion
Opistiobasial: opisthiobasial
Opistionasal: opisthionasial
Opistomastigota: opisthomastigote
Opistoquilia: opisthocheilia, opisthochilia
Opistorquíase: opisthorchiasis
Opistorquídeo: opisthorchid
Opistótico: opisthotic
Opistotônico: opisthotonic
Opistótono: opisthotonos, opisthotonus
Opistotonóide: opisthotonoid
Opobálsamo: opobalsamum
Opodídimo: opodidymus
Oponente: opponens
Oportunista: opportunistic
Oposição: opposure
Opsina: opsin
Opsinogênio: opsinogen
Opsiúria: opsiuria
Opsoclono: opsoclonus
Opsogênio: opsogen
Opsomania: opsomania

Opsônico: opsonic
Opsonina: opsonin
Opsonização: opsonization
Opsonocitofágico: opsonocytophagic
Opsonofilia: opsonophilia
Opsonofílico: opsonophilic
Opsonometria: opsonometry
Óptica: optics
Óptico: optic, optical
Opticociliar: opticociliary
Opticopupilar: opticopupillary
Optocinético: optokinetic
Optometria: optometry
Optometrista: optometrist
Optômetro: optometer
Optomiômetro: optomyometer
Optótipos: optotypes, test types
Oral: oral
Oralidade: orality
Orbicular: orbicular, orbicularis
Orbículo ciliar: orbiculus ciliaris
Órbita: orbit, orbita, **gen.** orbitae
Orbital: orbital
Orbitoesfenóide: orbitosphenoid
Orbitografia: orbitography
Orbitonasal: orbitonasal
Orbitonometria: orbitonometry
Orbitonômetro: orbitonometer
Orbitópago: orbitopagus
Orbitopatia: orbitopathy
Orbitotomia: orbitotomy
Orceína: orcein
Orcinol: orcin, orcinol
Ordem: order
Ordenada: ordinate
Ordenado: ordered
Ordenhar: strip
Oréctico: orectic
Orelha: auris (a, a, aur), **pl.** aures; ear, pinna, **pl.** pinnae
Orelha pendente: lop-ear
Orexia: orexia
Orexígeno: orexigenic
Orf: orf, soremouth
Órfão: orphan
Organela: organelle
Organicismo: organicism
Organicista: organicist
Orgânico: organic
Organismo: organism
Organização: organization
Organizador: organizer
Organizar: organize
Organoaxial: organoaxial
Organoférrico: organoferric
Organofilia: organophilicity
Organofílico: organophilic
Organofosforados: organophosphates
Organogel: organogel
Organogênese: organogenesis
Organogenético: organogenetic, organogenic
Organogenia: organogeny
Organografia: organography
Organóide: organoid
Organoléptico: organoleptic
Organologia: organology
Organomegalia: organomegaly

Organomercurial: organomercurial
Organometálico: organometallic
Organonimia: organonymy
Organonomia: organonomy
Organopatia: organopathy
Organopexia: organopexy, organopexia
Organossol: organosol
Organotaxia: organotaxis
Organoterapia: organotherapy
Organotrófico: organotrophic
Organotropia: organotropy
Organotrópico: organotropic
Organotropismo: organotropism
Órgão: organ, organon, organum, **pl.** organa
Órgão-específico: organ-specific
Orgasmo: orgasm
Orgástico: orgasmic, orgastic
Oricenina: orycenin
Orientação: orientation
Orifício: trema
Origem: origin
Ornitina: ornithine (Orn)
Ornitinemia: ornithinemia
Ornitinúria: ornithinuria
Ornitose: ornithosis
Orodigitofacial: orodigitofacial
Orofacial: orofacial
Orofaringe: oropharynx
Orofaríngeo: oropharyngeal, pharyngo-oral
Orolingual: orolingual
Oronasal: oronasal
Orosomucóide: orosomucoid
Orotato: orotate (Oro)
Orotidilato: orotidylate (OMP)
Orotidina: orotidine (O, Ord)
Orotidinúria: orotidinuria
Orquialgia: orchalgia, orchialgia
Orquicoréia: orchichorea
Orquidectomia: orchidectomy
Orquídico: orchidic
Orquidômetro: orchidometer
Orquidopexia: orchidopexy
Orquidoptose: orchidoptosis
Orquidorrafia: orchidorraphy
Orquiectomia: orchectomy, orchiectomy
Orquiepididimite: orchiepididymitis
Orquiocele: orchiocele
Orquiodinia: orchiodynia
Orquioncose: orchioncus
Orquioneuralgia: orchioneuralgia
Orquiopatia: orchiopathy
Orquiopexia: orchiopexy
Orquioplastia: orchioplasty
Orquiorrafia: orchiorrhaphy
Orquioterapia: orchiotherapy
Orquiotomia: orchiotomy, orchotomy
Orquite: orchiditis, orchitis
Orquítico: orchitic
Órtese: cast brace, orthesis, orthosis, **pl.** orthoses
Ortoácido: orthoacid

Ortocaína: orthocaine
Ortocefálico: orthocephalic
Ortocéfalo: orthocephalous
Ortoceratologia: orthokeratology
Ortoceratose: orthokeratosis
Ortocinética: orthokinetics
Ortocitose: orthocytosis
Ortocrasia: orthocrasia
Ortocromático: orthochromatic
Ortocromófilo: orthochromophil, orthochromophile
Ortodentina: orthodentin
Ortodeoxia: orthodeoxia
Ortodigitismo: orthodigita
Ortodontia: orthodontia, orthodontics
Ortodontista: orthodontist
Ortodrômico: orthodromic
Ortoestereoscópio: orthostereoscope
Ortoforia: orthophoria
Ortofórico: orthophoric
Ortofosfato: orthophosphate
Ortofrenia: orthophrenia
Ortogênese: orthogenesis
Ortogênica: orthogenics
Ortogênico: orthogenic
Ortognático: orthognathic, orthognathous
Ortognatismo: orthognathia
Ortógrado: orthograde
Ortomecânico: orthomechanical
Ortomecanoterapia: orthomechanotherapy
Ortomélico: orthomelic
Ortômetro: orthometer
Ortomolecular: orthomolecular
Ortopedia: orthopaedics, orthopedics
Ortopédico: orthopaedic, orthopedic
Ortopedista: orthopaedist, orthopedist
Ortopercussão: orthopercussion
Ortopnéia: orthopnea
Ortopneico: orthopneic
Ortoprótese: orthoprosthesis
Ortopsiquiatria: orthopsychiatry
Ortóptica: orthetics, orthoptics
Ortoscópio: orthoscope
Ortostático: orthostatic
Ortotanasia: orthothanasia
Ortotolidina: orthotolidine
Ortótono: orthotonos, orthotonus
Ortotópico: orthotopic
Ortotrópico: orthotropic
Ortovoltagem: orthovoltage
Osazona: osazone
Oscilação: bobbing, oscillation, wobble
Oscilador: oscillator
Oscilografia: oscillography
Oscilógrafo: oscillograph
Oscilometria: oscillometry
Oscilométrico: oscillometric
Oscilômetro: oscillometer
Oscilopsia: oscillopsia

Glossário

Osciloscópio: oscilloscope
Ósculo: osculum, **pl.** oscula
Osfresiofilia: osphresiophilia
Osfresiofobia: osphresiophobia
Osfresiologia: osphresiology
Osfresiológico: osphresiologic
Osfrético: osphretic
Osmato: osmate
Ósmica: osmics
Osmicação: osmication, osmification
Ósmio: osmium (Os)
Osmiófilo: osmiophilic
Osmiofóbico: osmiophobic
Osmoceptor: osmoceptor
Osmodisforia: osmodysphoria
Osmófilo: osmophil, osmophilic
Osmofobia: osmophobia
Osmóforo: osmophore
Osmograma: osmogram
Osmol: osmole
Osmolalidade: osmolality
Osmolar: osmolar
Osmolaridade: osmolarity
Osmologia: osmology
Osmometria: osmometry
Osmômetro: osmometer
Osmorreceptor: osmoreceptor
Osmorregulador: osmoregulatory
Osmose: osmosis
Osmosidade: osmosity
Osmoterapia: osmotherapy
Osmótico: osmotic
Osqueoplastia: oscheoplasty
Ósseo: osseous, osteal
Osseomucina: osseomucin
Osseomucóide: osseomucoid
Ossicular: ossicular
Ossiculectomia: ossiculectomy
Ossículo: bonelet, ossicle, ossiculum, **pl.** ossicula
Ossiculotomia: ossiculotomy
Ossífero: ossiferous
Ossificação: ossification
Ossificar: ossify
Ossiforme: ossiform
Osso: bone, os, **gen.** ossis, **pl.** ossa
Osso piramidal: pyramidal, pyramidale
Osso tibial posterior (sesamóide): tibiale posticum
Ostealgia: ostealgia
Osteanáfise: osteanaphysis
Osteanagênese: osteanagenesis
Ostectomia: ostectomy, osteoectomy
Osteína: ostein, osteine
Osteíte: osteitis, ostitis
Osteítico: osteitic, ostitic
Ostemia: ostemia
Ostempiese: ostempyesis
Osteoalisterese: osteohalisteresis
Osteoanagênese: osteoanagenesis
Osteoartrite: arthrosis, osteoarthritis
Osteoartropatia: osteoarthropathy
Osteoartrose: osteoarthrosis

Osteoblástico: osteoblastic
Osteoblasto: osteoblast, osteoplast
Osteoblastoma: osteoblastoma
Osteocalcina: osteocalcin
Osteocartilaginoso: osseocartilaginous, osteocartilaginous
Osteocistoma: osteocystoma
Osteócito: osteocyte
Osteoclasia: osteoclasis, osteoclasia
Osteoclástico: osteoclastic
Osteoclasto: osteoclast, osteophage
Osteoclastoma: osteoclastoma
Osteocondrite: osteochondritis
Osteocondrodisplasia: osteochondrodysplasia
Osteocondrodistrofia: osteochondrodystrophy
Osteocondrodistrofia deformante: osteochondrodystrophia deformans
Osteocondroma: osteochondroma
Osteocondromatose: osteochondromatosis
Osteocondrose: osteochondrosis
Osteocondroso: osteochondrous
Osteocondrossarcoma: osteochondrosarcoma
Osteocrânio: osteocranium
Osteodentina: osteodentin
Osteodermatopecilose: osteodermatopoikilosis
Osteodesmose: osteodesmosis
Osteodiástase: osteodiastasis
Osteodinia: osteodynia
Osteodisplasia: osteodysplasty
Osteodistrofia: osteodystrophia, osteodystrophy
Osteoepífise: osteoepiphysis
Osteoesclerótico: osteosclerotic
Osteoespongioma: osteospongioma
Osteoesteatoma: osteosteatoma
Osteofibroma: osteofibroma
Osteofibrose: osteofibrosis
Osteófito: osteophyte
Osteoflebite: osteophlebitis
Osteogênese: osteogenesis, osteogeny
Osteogênico: osteogenic, osteogenetic, osteogenous
Osteógeno: osteogen
Osteografia: osteography
Osteóide: osteoid
Osteoipertrofia: osteohypertrophy
Osteolipocondroma: osteolipochondroma
Osteólise: osteolysis
Osteolítico: osteolytic
Osteologia: osteologia, osteology
Osteologista: osteologist
Osteoma: osteoma
Osteomalacia: osteomalacia
Osteomalácico: osteomalacic

Osteomatóide: osteomatoid
Osteômero: osteomere
Osteometria: osteometry
Osteomielite: osteomyelitis
Osteomielodisplasia: osteomyelodysplasia
Ósteon: osteon, osteone
Osteoncose: osteoncus
Osteonecrose: osteonecrosis
Osteonectina: osteonectin
Osteopatia: osteopathia, osteopathy, osteosis
Osteopático: osteopathic
Osteopatologia: osteopathology
Osteopecilose: osteopoikilosis
Osteopenia: osteopenia
Osteoperiostite: osteoperiostitis
Osteopetrose: osteopetrosis
Osteopetrótico: osteopetrotic
Osteoplaca: osteoplaque
Osteoplásico: osteoplastic
Osteoplastia: osteoplasty
Osteoponina: osteoponin
Osteopontina: osteopontin
Osteoporose: osteoporosis
Osteoporótico: osteoporotic
Osteoprotegerina: osteoprotegerin
Osteorradiologia: osteoradiology
Osteorradiologista: osteoradiologist
Osteorradionecrose: osteoradionecrosis
Osteorrafia: osteorrhaphy, osteosuture
Osteosclerose: osteosclerosis
Osteose: ostosis
Osteossarcoma: osteosarcoma
Osteossíntese: osteosynthesis
Osteotimpânico: osteotympanic
Osteotomia: osteotomy
Osteótomo: osteotome
Osteótribo: osteotribe
Osteótrito: osteotrite
Osteotrofia: osteotrophy
Osteotrombose: osteothrombosis
Ostial: ostial
Óstio: orifice, orificium, **pl.** orificia; ostium, **pl.** ostia
Ostomia: ostomy
Ostomizado: ostomate
Ostráceo: ostraceous
Ostreotoxismo: ostreotoxism
O-succinil-homosserina (tiol)-liase: O-succinylhomoserine (thiol)-lyase
Otalgia: earache, otalgia
Ótico: otic
Otimismo: optimism
Otite: otitis
Otítico: otitic
Otoacústico: otoacoustic
Otobiose: otobiosis
Otocefalia: otocephaly
Otocerebrite: otocerebritis
Otocisto: otocyst
Otocraniano: otocranial
Otocrânio: otocranium
Otodético: otodectic

Otodinia: otodynia
Otoencefalite: otoencephalitis
Otoespongiose: otospongiosis
Otofaríngeo: otopharyngeal
Otogênico: otogenic, otogenous
Otolaringologia: otolaryngology
Otolaringologista: otolaryngologist
Otólito: otoliths, otolites
Otólitos: otoconia, **sing.** otoconium; sagitta
Otologia: otology
Otológico: otologic
Otologista: otologist
Otomicose: otomycosis
Otomucormicose: otomucormycosis
Otoneuralgia: otoneuralgia
Otopalatodigital: otopalatodigital
Otopatia: otopathy
Otoplastia: otoplasty
Otorréia: otorrhea
Otorrinolaringologia: otorhinolaryngology
Otosclerose: otosclerosis
Otoscopia: otoscopy
Otoscópio: otoscope
Otosteal: otosteal
Ototoxicidade: ototoxicity
Ototóxico: ototoxic
Ouabagenina: ouabagenin
Ouabaína: ouabain
Ouro: aurum
Ouro (Au): gold (Au)
Ouro coloidal radioativo: radiogold colloid
Ouvir: hear
Ovalbumina: ovalbumin
Ovalocitose: ovalocytosis
Ovarialgia: ovarialgia
Ovariano: ovarian
Ovariectomia: ovariectomy
Ovário: ovarium, **pl.** ovaria; ovary
Ovariocele: ovariocele
Ovariocentese: ovariocentesis
Ovariodisneuria: ovariodysneuria
Ovariogênico: ovariogenic
Ovariolítico: ovariolytic
Ovariopatia: ovariopathy
Ovariorrexe: ovariorrhexis
Ovariossalpingectomia: ovariosalpingectomy
Ovariossalpingite: ovariosalpingitis
Ovariostomia: ovariostomy
Ovariotomia: ovariotomy
Ovarite: ovaritis
Ovicida: ovicidal
Oviductal: oviducal, oviductal
Ovífero: oviferous
Oviforme: oviform
Ovigênese: ovigenesis
Ovigênico: ovigenetic, ovigenic
Ovígeno: ovigenous
Ovígero: ovigerous
Ovino: ovine
Oviparidade: oviparity

Ovíparo: oviparous
Oviposição: oviposition
Ovipositor: ovipositor
Ovo: egg, ovum, **gen.** ovi, **pl.** ova
Ovocinese: ookinesis, ookinesia
Ovócito: oocyte, ovocyte
Ovoflavina: ovoflavin
Ovogênese: oogenesis, ovogenesis
Ovogenético: oogenetic
Ovogênico: oogenic, oogenous
Ovoglobulina: ovoglobulin
Ovogônia: oogonium, **pl.** oogonia
Ovóide: ovoid
Ovolarvíparo: ovolarviparous
Ovomucina: ovomucin
Ovomucóide: ovomucoid
Ovoplasma: ovoplasm
Ovotestículo: ovotestis
Ovotransferrina: ovotransferrin
Ovovivíparo: ovoviviparous
Ovulação: ovulation
Ovular: ovular
Ovulatório: ovulatory
Óvulo: ovule, ovulum, **pl.** ovula
Ovulocíclico: ovulocyclic
Oxacilina sódica: oxacillin sodium
Oxafenamida: oxaphenamide
Oxalaldeído: oxalaldehyde
Oxalato: oxalate
Oxalemia: oxalemia
Oxalil: oxalyl
Oxaliluréia: oxalylurea
Oxaloacetato transacetase: oxaloacetate transacetase
Oxalose: oxalosis
Oxalossuccínico carboxilase: oxalosuccinic carboxylase
Oxalouréia: oxalourea
Oxalúria: oxaluria
Oxamniquina: oxamniquine
Oxanamida: oxanamide
Oxandrolona: oxandrolone
Oxazepam: oxazepam
Oxazina: oxazin
Oxazol: oxazole
Oxazolidinedionas: oxazolidinediones
Oxazolidinonas: oxazolidinones
Oxeladina: oxeladin
Oxiacóia: oxyacoia, oxyakoia
Oxiafia: oxyaphia
Oxibarbitúricos: oxybarbiturates
Oxibenzona: oxybenzone
Oxibiotina: oxybiotin
Oxicalorímetro: oxycalorimeter
Oxicefalia: oxycephalia, oxycephaly
Oxicefálico: oxycephalic, oxycephalous
Oxicelulose: oxycellulose
Oxicloreto: oxychloride
Oxicodona: oxycodone
Oxiconazol: oxiconazole
11-oxicorticóides: 11-oxycorticoids
Oxicromático: oxychromatic
Oxicromatina: oxychromatin

Oxidação: oxidation
Oxidante: oxidant, oxidative
Oxidar: oxidize
Oxidase: oxidase
Óxido: oxide
Óxido amarelo de mercúrio: mercuric oxide, yellow
Óxido de antimônio: antimonous oxide
Óxido de arsênico: arsenous oxide
Óxido de estanho: stannic oxide
Óxido de etileno: oxirane
Óxido de zircônio: zirconium oxide
Óxido férrico: ferric oxide
Óxido nítrico (NO): nitric oxide (NO)
Óxido nitroso: nitrous oxide
Óxido sulfúrico: sulfuric oxide
Óxido sulfuroso: sulfurous oxide
Óxido vermelho de mercúrio: mercuric oxide, red
Oxiemoglobina: oxyhemoglobin (HbO_2)
Oxifembutazona: oxyphenbutazone
Oxifílico: oxyphilic
Oxifonia: oxyphonia
Oxigenação: oxygenation
Oxigenador de bomba: pump-oxygenator
Oxigenar: oxygenate, oxygenize
Oxigenase: oxygenase
Oxigênico: oxygenic
Oxigênio: oxygen (O)
Oxigênio-15: oxygen-15 (^{15}O)
Oxigênio-16: oxygen-16 (^{16}O)
Oxigênio-17: oxygen-17 (^{17}O)
Oxigênio-18: oxygen-18 (^{18}O)
Oxiiodeto: oxyiodide
Oxiluciferina: oxyluciferin
Oxima: oxime
Oximesterona: oxymesterone
Oximetolona: oxymetholone
Oximetria: oximetry
Oxímetro: oximeter
Oximioglobina: oxymyoglobin (MbO_2)
Oxinervona: oxynervone
Oxíntico: oxyntic
Oxipertina: oxypertine
Oxipoligelatina: oxypolygelatin
Oxipurina: oxypurine
Oxipurinol: oxypurinol
Oxirredução: oxidation-reduction
Oxirredutase: oxidoreductase
Oxirregmia: oxyrygmia
Oxirrino: oxyrhine
Oxitalano: oxytalan
Oxitetraciclina: oxytetracycline
Oxitiamina: oxythiamin
Oxitocia: oxytocia
Oxitócico: oxytocic
Oxitrifilina: oxtriphylline
Oxiuricida: oxyuricide
Oxiurídeo: oxyurid
Oxiúro: pinworm, seatworm

3-oxoácido-CoA transferase: 3-oxoacid-CoA transferase
3-oxoacil-ACP redutase: 3-oxoacyl-ACP reductase
3-oxoacil-ACP sintase: 3-oxoacyl-ACP synthase
17-oxoesteróides: 17-oxosteroids
2-oxoglutarato desidrogenase: 2-oxoglutarate dehydrogenase
Oxolamina: oxolamine
5-oxoprolina: 5-oxoproline (Glp)
4-oxoprolina redutase: 4-oxoproline reductase
5-oxoprolinase: 5-oxoprolinase
5-oxoprolinúria: 5-oxoprolinuria
Oxotremorina: oxotremorine
Ozena: ozena
Ozenoso: ozenous
Ozocerita: ozocerite, ozokerite
Ozonador: ozonator
Ozonide: ozonide
Ozônio: ozone
Ozonioscópio: ozonoscope
Ozonólise: ozonolysis
Ozonômetro: ozonometer
Ozostomia: ozostomia

P

P congênita: P congenitale
P mitral: P mitrale
P *pulmonale*: P *pulmonale*
p,p′-diclorodifenilmetilcarbinol: p,p′-dichlorodiphenyl methyl carbinol (DMC)
Pabular: pabular
Pábulo: pabulum
Paciente: patient
Paciente externo: outpatient
Paciniano: pacinian
Paclitaxel: paclitaxel
Padiola: litter
Padrão: pattern, standard
Padrão de bandas: banding
Padronização: standardization
Pagético: pagetic
Pagetóide: pagetoid
Pagofagia: pagophagia
Paixão: passion
Paládio: palladium (Pd)
Palanestesia: pallanesthesia
Palatiforme: palatiform
Palatinase: palatinase
Palatino: palatal, palatine
Palatinose: palatinose
Palatite: palatitis
Palato: palate, palatum, **pl.** palati
Palatofaríngeo: palatopharyngeal
Palatofaringoplastia: palatopharyngoplasty
Palatofaringorrafia: palatopharyngorrhaphy
Palatoglosso: palatoglossal
Palatognato: palatognathous
Palatógrafo: palatograph
Palatograma: palatogram

Palatomaxilar: palatomaxillary
Palatomiógrafo: palatomyograph
Palatonasal: palatonasal
Palatoplastia: palatoplasty
Palatoplegia: palatoplegia
Palatorrafia: palatorrhaphy, velosynthesis
Palatosquise: palatoschisis
Palencéfalo: paleencephalon
Paleocerebelo: paleocerebellum
Paleocinético: paleokinetic
Paleocórtex: paleocortex
Paleoestriado: paleostriatal, paleostriatum
Paleopatologia: paleopathology
Paleotálamo: paleothalamus
Palestesia: pallesthesia
Palestésico: pallesthetic
Paliar: palliate
Paliativo: palliative
Paliçada: palisade
Palicinesia: palikinesia, palicinesia
Palidectomia: pallidectomy
Palidez: pallor
Pálido: pallidal
Palidoamigdalotomia: pallidoamygdalotomy
Palidotomia: pallidotomy
Palíndrome: palindrome
Palindromia: palindromia
Palindrômico: palindromic
Palma: palm, palma, **pl.** palmae
Palma da mão ou da sola do pé: vola
Palmar: palmar, palmaris
Palmelina: palmellin
Palmitaldeído: palmitaldehyde
Palmitato: palmitate
Palmitato de ascorbila: ascorbyl palmitate
Palmitina: palmitin
Palmoscopia: palmoscopy
Palpação: palpation
Palpar: palpate
Palpável: palpable
Pálpebra: blepharon, eyelid, lid, palpebra, **pl.** palpebrae
Palpebrado: palpebrate
Palpebral: palpebral
Palpitação: palpitation, trepidatio cordis
Palpitação cardíaca: palpitatio cordis
Palustre: paludal
Pamaquina: pamaquine
***p*-aminopropiofenona:** *p*-aminopropiophenone (PAPP)
Pamoato: pamoate
Pamoato de cicloguanil: cycloguanil pamoate
Pamoato de pirantel: pyrantel pamoate
Pamoato de pirvínio: pyrvinium pamoate
Pampiniforme: pampiniform
Pampinocele: pampinocele
Panacéia: panacea
Pan-aglutinável: panagglutinable

Pan-aglutininas: panagglutinins
Pan-angeíte: panangiitis
Panarício: felon, whitlow
Pan-arterite: panarteritis
Pan-artrite: panarthritis
Pan-atrofia: panatrophy, pantatrophia, pantatrophy
Pan-blástico: panblastic
Pan-bronquiolite: panbronchiolitis
Pancardite: pancarditis
Pancitopenia: pancytopenia
Pancolectomia: pancolectomy
Pâncreas: pancreas, **pl.** pancreata
Pancreatalgia: pancreatalgia
Pancreatectomia: pancreatectomy, pancreectomy
Pancreatenfraxe: pancreatemphraxis
Pancreático: pancreatic
Pancreaticoduodenal: pancreaticoduodenal
Pancreatite: pancreatitis
Pancreatocolecistostomia: pancreatocholecystostomy
Pancreatoduodenectomia: pancreaticoduodenectomy, pancreatoduodenectomy
Pancreatoduodenostomia: pancreatoduodenostomy
Pancreatogastrostomia: pancreatogastrostomy
Pancreatogênico: pancreatogenic, pancreatogenous
Pancreatografia: pancreatography
Pancreatojejunostomia: pancreatojejunostomy
Pancreatólise: pancreatolysis
Pancreatolitectomia: pancreatolithectomy
Pancreatolitíase: pancreatolithiasis
Pancreatolítico: pancreatolytic
Pancreatólito: pancreatolith
Pancreatolitotomia: pancreatolithotomy
Pancreatomegalia: pancreatomegaly
Pancreatopatia: pancreatopathy, pancreopathy
Pancreatopeptidase E: pancreatopeptidase E
Pancreatotomia: pancreatomy, pancreatotomy
Pancreatrópico: pancreatropic
Pancrelipase: pancrelipase
Pancreólito: pancreolith
Pancreozimina: pancreozymin
Pandemicidade: pandemicity
Pandêmico: pandemic
Pandiculação: pandiculation
Panencefalite: panencephalitis
Pan-endoscópio: panendoscope
Pan-esclerose: pansclerosis
Pan-espermia: panspermia, panspermatism

Pan-esporoblástico: pansporoblastic
Pan-esporoblasto: pansporoblast
Panestesia: panesthesia
Panfobia: panphobia
Pan-hidrômetro: panhydrometer
Pan-hiperemia: panhyperemia
Pan-hipopituitarismo: panhypopituitarism (PHP)
Pânico: panic
Paniculectomia: panniculectomy
Paniculite: panniculitis
Panículo: panniculus, **pl.** panniculi
Panidrose: panhidrosis, panidrosis
Pan-imunidade: panimmunity
Pan-mieloftise: panmyelophthisis
Panmielose: panmyelosis
Pan-mixia: panmixis
Pan-oftalmite: panophthalmitis
Pan-óptico: panoptic
Pan-osteíte: panosteitis
Pan-otite: panotitis
Pano: pannus, **pl.** panni
Pansinusite: pansinuitis, pansinusitis
Pansistólico: pansystolic
Pantafobia: pantaphobia
Pantalgia: pantalgia
Pantamórfico: pantamorphic
Pantamorfismo: pantamorphia
Pantanencefalia: pantanencephaly, pantanencephalia
Pantenol: panthenol
Panteteína: pantetheine
Pantetina: pantethine
Pantoato: pantoate
Pantógrafo: pantograph
Pantoil: pantoyl
Pantoiltaurina: pantoyltaurine
Pantomografia: pantomography
Pantomógrafo: pantomograph
Pantomograma: pantomogram
Pantomórfico: pantomorphic
Pantomorfismo: pantomorphia
Pantonina: pantonine
Pantoscópico: pantoscopic
Pantotenato: pantothenate
Pantotenil: pantothenyl
Papa: pap
Papaína: papayotin
Papaína, papainase: papain, papainase
Papaverina: papaverine
Papel: paper, role
Papila: papilla, **pl.** papillae
Papilar: papillary, papillate
Papilectomia: papillectomy
Papiledema: papilledema
Papilífero: papilliferous
Papiliforme: papilliform
Papilite: papillitis
Papiloadenocistoma: papilloadenocystoma

Papilocarcinoma: papillocarcinoma
Papiloma: papilloma
Papilomatose: papillomatosis
Papilomatoso: papillomatous
Papilomavírus humano: human papillomavirus (HPV)
Papilorretinite: papilloretinitis
Papilotomia: papillotomy
Papiráceo: papyraceous
Papoula: poppy
Papovavírus: papovavirus
Pápula: papule
Papular: papular
Papuloeritematoso: papuloerythematous
Papuloescamoso: papulosquamous
Papulopústula: papulopustule
Papulopustular: papulopustular
Papulose: papulosis
Papulovesícula: papulovesicle
Papulovesicular: papulovesicular
Paquiblefarose: pachyblepharon
Paquicefalia: pachycephalia, pachycephaly
Paquicefálico: pachycephalic, pachycephalous
Paquicolia: pachycholia
Paquicromático: pachychromatic
Paquidactilia: pachydactylia, pachydactyly
Paquidáctilo: pachydactylous
Paquidermia: pachyderma, pachydermatosis
Paquidermodactilia: pachydermodactyly
Paquidermoperiostose: pachydermoperiostosis
Paquigiria: pachygyria
Paquiglossia: pachyglossia
Paquignático: pachygnathous
Paquileptomeningite: pachyleptomeningitis
Paquimeninge: pachymeninx
Paquimeningite: pachymeningitis
Paquimeningopatia: pachymeningopathy
Paquímetro: pachometer, pachymeter
Paquinema: pachynema
Paquinse: pachynsis
Paquíntico: pachyntic
Paquioníquia: pachyonychia
Paquiotia: pachyotia
Paquiperiostite: pachyperiostitis
Paquiperitonite: pachyperitonitis
Paquipleurite: pachypleuritis
Paquípode: pachypodous
Paquiquilia: pachycheilia, pachychilia
Paquiquimia: pachychymia
Paquissomia: pachysomia
Paquíteno: pachytene
Paquivaginalite: pachyvaginalitis
Paquivaginite: pachyvaginitis

Par: pair, par
Para-actinomicose: para-actinomycosis
Para-apendicite: para-appendicitis
Parabiose: parabiosis
Parabiótico: parabiotic
Parabulia: parabulia
Paracantoma: paracanthoma
Paracantose: paracanthosis
Paracapacismo: parakappacism
Paracarmim: paracarmine
Paracaseína: paracasein
Paracenestesia: paracenesthesia
Paracentese: paracentesis
Paracentésico: paracentetic
Paracentral: paracentral
Paraceratose: parakeratosis
Paracervical: paracervical
Paracérvice: paracervix
Paracetaldeído: paracetaldehyde
Paracetamol: paracetamol
Paraciese: paracyesis
Paracinesia: paracinesia, paracinesis, parakinesia, parakinesis
Paracístico: paracystic
Paracístio: paracystium
Paracistite: paracystitis
Paracítico: paracytic
Paraclorofenol: parachlorophenol
Paracmástico: paracmastic
Paracme: paracmasis, paracme
Paracoccidioidina: paracoccidioidin
Paracoccidioidomicose: paracoccidioidomycosis
Paracólera: paracholera
Paracolite: paracolitis
Paracolpite: paracolpitis
Paracolpo: paracolpium
Paracone: paracone
Paracônide: paraconid
Paracordal: parachordal
Paracórtex: paracortex
Parácrino: paracrine
Paracromia: parachroma
Paracusia: paracousis, paracusis, paracusia
Parada: standstill
Paradenite: paradenitis
Paradental: paradental
Paradídimo: paradidymis, **pl.** paradidymides
Paradipsia: paradipsia
Paradoxo: paradox
Paraescarlatina: parascarlatina
Paraesternal: parasternal
Parafasia: paraphasia
Parafásico: paraphasic
Parafia: paraphia
Parafilia: paraphilia
Parafimose: paraphimosis
Parafina: paraffin
Parafinoma: paraffinoma
Parafisário: paraphysial, paraphyseal
Paráfise: paraphysis, **pl.** paraphyses

Paraflagelado: paraflagellate
Paraflagelo: paraflagellum, **pl.** paraflagella
Paraflóculo ventral: paraflocculus ventralis, ventral paraflocculus
Parafolicular: parafollicular
Parafonia: paraphonia
Paraformaldeído: paraformaldehyde
Parafrasia: paraphrasia
Parafucsina: parafuchsin
Parafuso: screw
Paragamacismo: paragammacism
Paragânglio: paraganglion, **pl.** paraganglia
Paraganglioma: paraganglioma
Paragenital: paragenital
Parageusia: parageusia
Paragêusico: parageusic
Paragnato: paragnathus
Paragonimíase: paragonimiasis
Paragonorreico: paragonorrheal
Paragrafia: paragraphia
Paragramatismo: paragrammatism
Para-hepático: parahepatic
Para-hidrose: parahidrosis
Para-hipófise: parahypophysis
Para-hormônio: parahormone
Paraláctico: parallactic
Paralalia: paralalia
Paralambdacismo: paralambdacism
Paralaxe: parallax
Paraldeído: paraldehyde
Paralelismo: parallelism
Paralelômetro: parallelometer
Paralepra: paraleprosis
Paralepsia: paralepsy
Paralérgico: parallergic
Paralexia: paralexia
Paralgesia: paralgesia
Paralgia: paralgia
Paralipofobia: paralipophobia
Paralisar: paralyze
Paralisia: paralysis, **pl.** paralyses
Paralisia agitante: trembles
Paralisia ou paresia: palsy
Paralítico: paralytic
Paralogia, paralogismo: paralogia, paralogism, paralogy
Paramagnético: paramagnetic
Paramagnetismo: paramagnetism
Paramastigota: paramastigote
Paramastóide: paramastoid
Paramediano: paramedian
Paramédico: paramedic, paramedical
Paramenia: paramenia
Paramesial: paramesial
Paramesonéfrico: paramesonephric
Parametadiona: parametadione
Parametasona: paramethasone
Parametrial: parametrial
Paramétrico: parametric

Parametrio: parametrium, **pl.** parametria
Parametrite: parametritis
Parametrítico: parametritic
Parâmetro: parameter
Paramiloidose: paramyloidosis
Paramimia: paramimia
Paramioclônus múltiplo: paramyoclonus multiplex
Paramiotonia: paramyotonia
Paramiotônus: paramyotonus
Paramnésia: paramnesia
Paramolar: paramolar
Paramorfina: paramorphine
Paramusia: paramusia
Paranalgesia: paranalgesia
Paranasal: paranasal
Paranéfrico: paranephric
Paraneoplasia: paraneoplasia
Paraneoplásico: paraneoplastic
Paranestesia: paranesthesia
Paraneurônio: paraneurone
Paranfistomíase: paramphistomiasis
Paranóia: paranoia
Paranóico: paranoiac
Paranóide: paranoid
Paranomia: paranomia
Paranuclear: paranuclear, paranucleate
Paranúcleo: paranucleus
Paranucléolo: paranucleolus
Paraoccipital: paroccipital
Paraolfatório: parolfactory
Paraolivar: parolivary
Paraonfálico: paraomphalic
Paraonfalocele: paromphalocele
Paraooforite: paroophoritis
Paraoóforo: paroöphoron
Paraoral: paraoral
Paraorquidia: parorchidium
Paraovariano: paraovarian
Paraoxon: paraoxon
Parapancreático: parapancreatic
Paraparesia: paraparesis
Paraparético: paraparetic
Parapedese: parapedesis
Paraperitoneal: paraperitoneal
Parapeste: parapestis
Parapineal: parapineal
Paraplasma: paraplasm
Paraplástico: paraplastic
Paraplegia: paraplegia
Paraplégico: paraplegic
Parapraxia: parapraxia
Paraproctite: paraproctitis
Paraprostatite: paraprostatitis
Paraproteína: paraprotein
Paraproteinemia: paraproteinemia
Parapsicologia: parapsychology
Parapsoríase: parapsoriasis
Paraquat: paraquat
Paraquimosina: parachymosin
Parar: arrest
Pararama: pararama
Pararrenal: pararenal
Pararretal: pararectal
Pararritmia: pararrhythmia
Pararrosanilina: pararosanilin
Pararrotacismo: pararhotacism

Parasita: parasite
Parasitar: parasitize
Parasitário: parasitic
Parasitemia: parasitemia
Parasiticida: parasiticidal, parasiticide
Parasitismo: parasitism
Parasitocenose: parasitocenose
Parasitofobia: parasitophobia
Parasitogênese: parasitogenesis
Parasitogênico: parasitogenic
Parasitóide: parasitoid
Parasitologia: parasitology
Parasitologista: parasitologist
Parasitoma: parasitome
Parasitose: parasitosis
Parasitotropia: parasitotropy
Parasitotrópico: parasitotropic
Parasitotropismo: parasitotropism
Parassacral: parasacral
Parassalpingite: parasalpingitis
Parassexualidade: parasexuality
Parassífilis: parasyphilis
Parassifilítico: parasyphilitic
Parassifilose: parasyphilosis
Parassigmatismo: parasigmatism
Parassimpático: parasympathetic
Parassimpaticolítico: parasympatholytic
Parassimpaticomimético: parasympathomimetic
Parassimpaticotonia: parasympathotonia
Parassinapse: parasynapsis
Parassinovite: parasynovitis
Parassinusal: parasinoidal
Parassístole: parasystole
Parassonia: parasomnia
Parassubículo: parasubiculum
Parastasia: parastasis
Parataxia: parataxia, parataxis
Paratáxico: parataxic
Paratendão: paratenon
Paratênese: paratenesis
Paraterminal: paraterminal
Paratiflite: paratyphlitis
Paratimia: parathymia
Paration: parathion
Paratireóide: parathyroid
Paratireoidectomia: parathyroidectomy
Paratireotrófico: parathyrotropic, parathyrotrophic
Paratopo: paratope
Paratormônio: parathormone, parathyrin
Paratricose: paratrichosis
Paratripsia: paratripsis
Paratrófico: paratrophic
Paraumbilical: paraumbilical, parumbilical
Parauretral: paraurethral
Paravacínia: paravaccinia
Paravaginal: paravaginal
Paravaginite: paravaginitis
Paravalvular: paravalvular
Paravenoso: paravenous

Paravertebral: paravertebral
Paravesical: paravesical
Paraxial: paraxial
Paraxônio: paraxon
Parazoário: parazoon
Pareamento cromossômico: chromosome pairing
Parede: paries, **gen.** parietis, **pl.** parietes; wall
Paregórico: paregoric
Pareletronômico: parelectronomic
Parencefalia: parencephalia
Parencefalite: parencephalitis
Parencéfalo: parencephalous
Parencefalocele: parencephalocele
Parênquima: parenchyma
Parenquimatite: parenchymatitis
Parenquimatoso: parenchymal, parenchymatous
Parente de sangue: blood relative
Parenteral: parenteral
Parentes: kindred
Parentesco: kinship
Parepicele: parepicele
Parepidídimo: parepididymis
Parepitimia: parepithymia
Pareretise: parerethisis
Paresia: paresis
Parestesia: paraesthesia, paresthesia
Parestésico: paresthetic
Parético: paretic
Paridade: parity
Parido: parous
Paridrose: paridrosis
Parietal: parietal
Parietoescamoso: parietosquamosal
Parietoesfenóide: parietosphenoid
Parietoesplâncnico: parietosplanchnic
Parietofrontal: parietofrontal
Parietografia: parietography
Parietomastóide: parietomastoid
Parietoocipital: parietooccipital
Parietotemporal: parietotemporal
Parietovisceral: parietovisceral
Parkinsoniano: parkinsonian
Parkinsonismo: parkinsonism
Parodinia: parodynia
Parodontite: parodontitis
Paroníquia: paronychia, perionychia
Parorexia: parorexia
Parorquia: parorchis
Parosfresia: parosphresia
Parosmia: parosmia
Parosteal: parosteal
Parosteíte: parosteitis, parostitis
Parosteose: parosteosis, parostosis
Parótico: parotic
Parótida: parotid
Parotidectomia: parotidectomy

Glossário

Parotidite: parotiditis, parotitis
Parotidoauricular: parotidoauricularis
Parotina: parotin
Parovárico: parovarian
Parovário: parovarium
Parovariotomia: parovariotomy
Parovarite: parovaritis
Paroxipropiona: paroxypropione
Paroxismo: paroxysm
Paroxístico: paroxysmal
Parreira-brava: pareira
Parricídio: parricide
Parte laríngea da faringe: laryngopharynx
Parte: pars, **pl.** partes; part, piece
Parteira: midwife
Parteiro: accoucheur
Partenofobia: parthenophobia
Partenogênese: parthenogenesis
Partícula: particle
Particulado: particulate
Particulados: particulates
Parto: accouchement, birth, birthing, childbirth, delivery, parturition
Partograma: partogram
Parturiente: parturient
Parturifaciente: parturifacient
Parúlia: parulis, **pl.** parulides
Parurese: paruresis
Parvalbumina: parvalbumin
Parvocelular: parvocellular
Parvolina: parvoline
Párvulo: parvule
Pascal: pascal (Pa)
Paspalismo: paspalism
Passagem: passage
Passiflora: passiflora
Passividade: passivism, passivity
Passivo: passive
Pasta: pasta, **gen. e pl.** pastae; paste
Pasteurela: pasteurella, **pl.** pasteurellae
Pasteurelose: pasteurellosis
Pasteurização: pasteurization
Pasteurizador: pasteurizer
Pasteurizar: pasteurize
Pastilha: lozenge, pastil, pastille
Patágio: patagium, **pl.** patagia
Patela: kneecap, patella, **gen. e pl.** patellae
Patelar: patellar
Patelectomia: patellectomy
Pateliforme: patelliform
Pátema: pathema
Patente azul V: leuco patent blue
Patergia: pathergy
Patético: pathetic
Patoamina: pathoamine
Patocidina: pathocidin
Patóclise: pathoclisis
Patocrinia: pathocrinia
Patodontia: pathodontia
Patofobia: pathophobia
Patofórmico: pathoformic
Patogenia: pathogenesis, pathogeny

Patogenicidade: pathogenicity
Patogênico: pathogenic, pathogenetic
Patógeno: pathogen
Patognomia: pathognomy
Patognomônico: pathognomonic
Patognóstico: pathognostic
Patologia: pathology
Patológico: pathologic, pathological
Patologista: pathologist
Patometria: pathometry
Patométrico: pathometric
Patomimese: pathomimesis, pathomimicry
Patomiose: pathomiosis
Patomorfismo: pathomorphism
Patonomia: pathonomia, pathonomy
Patopoese: pathopoiesis
Patose: pathosis
Patotropismo: pathotropism
Patricida: patricide
Patrilinear: patrilineal
Patulina: patulin
Pauciarticular: pauciarticular
Paucibacilar: paucibacillary
Paucissináptico: paucisynaptic
Pausa: pause
***p*-cloral:** *p*-chloral
***p*-clorofenol:** *p*-chlorophenol
***p*-cloromercuribenzoato:** *p*-chloromercuribenzoate (PCMB, *p*CMB, *p*-CMB)
P-dextrocardíaco: P-dextrocardiale
Pé: foot, pes, **gen.** pedis, **pl.** pedes
Pé caído: footdrop
Pé em garra: clawfoot
Pé fetal: footling
Pé ígneo: ignipedites
Pé plano: flatfoot
Pé torto: clubfoot
Peça terminal: end-piece
Pecatifobia: peccatiphobia
Pechblenda: pitchblende
Pecilocina: pecilocin
Peciloicose: paeciloycosis
Pecilotérmico: hematocryal
**Peciloterm
o:** allotherm
Peciolado: petiolate, petiolated, petioled
Pecíolo: petiole, petiolus
Pectase: pectase
Pécten: pecten
Pectenite: pectenitis
Pectenose: pectenosis
Péctico: pectic
Pectina: pectin
Pectinado: pectinate
Pectinase: pectinase
Pectíneo: pectineal, pectineus
Pectinesterase: pectinesterase
Pectiniforme: pectiniform
Pectinoso: pectous
Pectização: pectization
Pectoralgia: pectoralgia
Pectorilóquia: pectoriloquy
Pectorofonia: pectorophony
Pectose: pectose

Pedal: pedal
Pedatrofia: pedatrophia, pedatrophy
Pederasta: pederast
Pederastia: pederasty
Pedese: pedesis
Pediatra: pediatrician, pediatrist
Pediatria: pediatrics, pediatry
Pediátrico: pediatric
Pedicelação: pedicellation
Pedicelo: pedicel
Pediculado: pedicellate, pediculate, pedunculate
Pedicular: pedicular
Pediculicida: antipedicular, pediculicide
Pedículo: pedicle, pediculus, **pl.** pediculi; stalk
Pediculofobia: pediculophobia, phthiriophobia
Pediculose: pediculosis
Pediculoso: lousy, pediculous
Pedicuro: pedicure
Pediofobia: pediophobia
Pedodinamômetro: pedodynamometer
Pedodontia: pedodontia, pedodontics
Pedodontista: pedodontist
Pedofilia: pedophilia
Pedófilo: pedophilic
Pedogênese: pedogenesis
Pedografia: pedography
Pedógrafo: pedograph
Pedograma: pedogram
Pedômetro: pedometer
Pedomorfismo: pedomorphism
Pedra-pomes: pumice
Pedra-sabão: soapstone
Peduncular: peduncular
Pedúnculo: peduncle, pedunculus, **pl.** pedunculi
Pedunculotomia: pedunculotomy
Pega: grasp, take
Peiote: pellote, peyote, peyotl
Peito: breast, pectus, **gen.** pectoris, **pl.** pectora
Peitoral: pectoral
Pelada: pelade
Pelagra: maidism, mayidism, pellagra
Pelagróide: pellagroid
Pelagroso: pellagrous
Pele: skin
Pele anserina: gooseflesh
Pé-libra: foot-pound
Película: pellicle
Pelicular: pellicular, pelliculous
Peliose: peliosis
Pelma: pelmatic
Pelmatograma: pelmatogram
Pêlo: fur, hair, pilus, **pl.** pili
Pêlo púbico: pubes
Peloterapia: pelopathy, pelotherapy
Pelta: pelta
Peltação: peltation
Pelúcido: pellucid

Pelve: pelvis, **pl.** pelves
Pelve maior: justo major
Pelve menor: justo minor
Pelvicefalografia: pelvicephalography, pelvocephalography
Pelvicefalometria: pelvicephalometry
Pélvico: pelvic
Pelviespondilite ossificante: pelvospondylitis ossificans
Pelvifixação: pelvifixation
Pelvilitotomia: pelvilithotomy
Pelvimetria: pelvimetry
Pelvioscopia: pelvioscopy
Pelviperitonite: pelvioperitonitis, pelviperitonitis
Pelviplastia: pelvioplasty
Pelviscopia: pelvoscopy
Pelviscópio: pelviscope
Pelvissacra: pelvisacral
Pelvitermo: pelvitherm
Pelviureterografia: pelviureterography
Pemolina: pemoline
Pempidina: pempidine
Penectomia: penectomy
Peneira: sieve
Penetração: breakthrough, penetration
Penetrância: penetrance
Penetrar: penetrate
Penetrômetro: penetrometer
Pênfigo: pemphigus
Penfigóide: pemphigoid
Peniafobia: peniaphobia
Peniano: penial, penile
Penicilamina: penicillamine
Penicilanato: penicillanate
Penicilar: penicillary
Penicilato: penicillate
Penicilina: penicilin
Penicilinase: penicillinase
Penicilinato: penicillinate
Peniciliose: penicilliosis
Penicilo: penicillus, **pl.** penicilli
Peniciloil polilisina: peniciloyl polylysine
Penicina: penicin
Peniforme: pennate, penniform
Penina: penin
Pênis: penis, **pl.** penes
Penisquise: penischisis
Penoescrotal: penoscrotal
Penotomia: penotomy
Pensamento: thinking, thought
Pentabásico: pentabasic
Pentaclorofenol: pentachlorophenol
Pentadáctilo: pentadactyl, pentadactyle
Pentaeritritol: pentaerythritol
Pentagastrina: pentagastrin
Pentalogia: pentalogy
Pentâmero: pentamer
Pentapeptídeo: pentapeptide
Pentaquina: pentaquine
Pentastomíase: pentastomiasis
Pentatômico: pentatomic
Pentavalente: pentavalent

Pentazocina: pentazocine
Pentetato trissódico de cálcio: pentetate trisodium calcium
Pentifilina: pentifylline
Pentil: pentyl
Pentilenotetrazol: pentylenetetrazol
Pentitol: pentitol
Pentobarbital: pentobarbital
Penton: penton
Pentosana: pentosan
Pentose: pentose
Pentostatina: pentostatin
Pentosúria: pentosuria
Pentóxido: pentoxide
Pentoxifilina: pentoxifylline
Pentulose: pentulose
Penumbra: penumbra
Peplo: peplos
Peplômero: peplomer
Pé-poundal: foot-poundal
Pepsina: pepsin
Pepsinar: pepsinate
Pepsinífero: pepsiniferous
Pepsinogênico: pepsinogenous
Pepsinogênio: pepsinogen
Pepsinúria: pepsinuria
Pepstatina: pepstatin
Péptico: pepsic, peptic
Peptidase: peptidase
Peptídeo: peptide
Peptídeo C: C-peptide
Peptidérgico: peptidergic
Peptidil dipeptidase A: peptidyl dipeptidase A
Peptidiltransferase: peptidyltransferase
Peptidoglicano: peptidoglycan
Peptidóide: peptidoid
Peptidolítico: peptidolytic
Peptização: peptization
Peptocrinina: peptocrinine
Peptogênico: peptogenic, peptogenous
Peptóide: peptoid
Peptolídeo: peptolide
Peptólise: peptolysis
Peptolítico: peptolytic
Peptona: peptone
Peptônico: peptonic
Peptonização: peptonization
Pequeno: parvus
Peracéfalo: peracephalus
Perácido: peracid
Peragudo: peracute
Peratodinia: peratodynia
Peraxilar: peraxillary
Perazina: perazine
Percentil: percentile
Percepção: perception, sensing
Perceptividade: perceptivity
Perceptivo: perceptive
Percepto: percept
Perceptório: perceptorium
Percevejo: bedbug, bug
Percolação: percolation
Percolador: percolator
Percussão: percussion
Percussor: percussor
Percutâneo: percutaneous
Percutir: percuss

Perda: bereavement
Perencefalia: perencephaly
Perfeccionismo: perfectionism
Perfenazina: perphenazine
Perfil: profile
Perflação: perflation
Perflubron: perflubron
Perforina: perforin
Perfrigeração: perfrigeration
Perfundir: perfuse
Perfuração: perforation, tresis
Perfurado: perforated
Perfurador: perforator
Perfurante: perforans
Perfurar: drill
Perfusado: perfusate
Perfusão: perfusion
Periacinoso: periacinal, periacinous
Periadenite: periadenitis
Perianal: perianal
Periangeíte: periangitis
Periangiocolite: periangiocholitis
Periaórtico: periaortic
Periaortite: periaortitis
Periapendicite: periappendicitis
Periapendicular: periappendicular
Periapical: periapical
Periápice: periapex
Periarterial: periarterial
Periarterite: periarteritis
Periarticular: periarticular
Periártrico: periarthric
Periartrite: periarthritis
Periatrial: periatrial
Periauricular: periauricular, periconchal
Periaxial: periaxial
Periaxilar: periaxillary
Periaxonal: periaxonal
Periblasto: periblast
Peribrônquico: peribronchial
Peribronquiolar: peribronchiolar
Peribronquiolite: peribronchiolitis
Peribronquite: peribronchitis
Peribucal: peribuccal
Peribulbar: peribulbar
Pericanalicular: pericanalicular
Pericardectomia: pericardectomy
Pericárdico: pericardiac, pericardial
Pericardiectomia: pericardiectomy
Pericárdio: pericardium, **pl.** pericardia
Pericardiocentese: pericardicentesis, pericardiocentesis
Pericardiofrênico: pericardiophrenic
Pericardiologia: pericardiology
Pericardioperitoneal: pericardioperitoneal
Pericardiopleural: pericardiopleural

Pericardiorrafia: pericardiorrhaphy
Pericardiostomia: pericardiostomy
Pericardiotomia: pericardiotomy, pericardotomy
Pericardite: pericarditis
Pericardítico: pericarditic
Pericário: perikaryon, **pl.** perikarya
Pericecal: pericecal
Pericelular: pericellular, pericytial
Pericemental: pericemental
Pericentral: pericentral
Pericerático: perikeratic
Periciazina: pericyazine
Pericimo: perikymata, **sing.** perikyma
Pericístico: pericystic
Pericistite: pericystitis
Pericisto: pericystium
Pericito: pericyte
Pericolangite: pericholangitis
Pericólico: pericolic
Pericolite: pericolitis, pericolonitis
Pericolpite: pericolpitis
Pericondral: perichondral, perichondrial
Pericôndrio: perichondrium
Pericondrite: perichondritis
Pericórdio: perichord
Pericorioidal: perichoroidal
Pericórneo: pericorneal
Pericoronal: pericoronal
Pericoronite: pericoronitis
Pericranial: pericranial
Pericrânio: pericranium
Pericranite: pericranitis
Pericromo: perichrome
Peridental: peridental
Peridente: peridens
Peridentite: peridentitis
Periderme: periderm, periderma
Peridérmico: peridermal, peridermic
Peridésmico: peridesmic
Peridesmite: peridesmitis
Peridesmo: peridesmium
Perididimite: perididymitis
Perídio: peridium
Peridiverticulite: peridiverticulitis
Peridrociclopenta[a]fenantreno: perhydrocyclopenta[a]phenanthrene
Periduodenite: periduodenitis
Peridural: peridural
Periencefalite: periencephalitis
Perientérico: perienteric
Perienterite: perienteritis
Periepático: perihepatic
Periepatite: perihepatitis
Periependimário: periependymal
Perierniário: perihernial
Periesofágico: periesophageal
Periesofagite: periesophagitis
Periespermatite: perispermatitis
Perifaríngeo: peripharyngeal

Periferia: periphery
Periférico: peripheral, peripheralis
Periferina: peripherin
Periferocentral: peripherocentral
Periflebite: periphlebitis
Periflebítico: periphlebitic
Perifocal: perifocal
Perifolicular: perifollicular
Perifoliculite: perifolliculitis
Periganglionar: periganglionic
Perigástrico: perigastric
Perigastrite: perigastritis
Perigemal: perigemmal
Periglandulite: periglandulitis
Periglote: periglottis
Periglótico: periglottic
Perijejunite: perijejunitis
Perilabirintite: perilabyrinthitis
Perilaríngeo: perilaryngeal
Perilenticular: perilenticular
Periligamentar: periligamentous
Perilinfa: perilymph, perilympha
Perilinfangial: perilymphangial
Perilinfangite: perilymphangitis
Perilinfático: perilymphatic
Perimeningite: perimeningitis
Perimenopausa: perimenopause
Perimetria: perimetry
Perimétrico: perimetric
Perimétrio: perimetrium, **pl.** perimetria
Perimetrite: perimetritis
Perimetrítico: perimetritic
Perímetro: perimeter
Perimielite: perimyelitis
Perimielo: perimyelis
Perimilólise: perimolysis
Perimiocardite: perimyocarditis
Perimiosite: perimyositis
Perimisial: perimysial
Perimisiite: perimysiitis, perimysitis
Perimísio: perimysium, **pl.** perimysia
Perimplantoclasia: peri-implantoclasia
Perinatal: perinatal
Perinato: perinate
Perinatologia: perinatology
Perinatologista: perinatologist
Perineal: perineal
Perinéfrico: perinephrial, perinephric
Perinefrite: perinephritis
Perinefro: perinephrium, **pl.** perinephria
Períneo: perineum, **pl.** perinea
Perineocele: perineocele
Perineoescrotal: perineoscrotal
Perineômetro: perineometer
Perineoplastia: perineoplasty
Perineorrafia: perineorrhaphy
Perineossíntese: perineosynthesis
Perineostomia: perineostomy
Perineotomia: perineotomy
Perineovaginal: perineovaginal

Perineural: perineural, perineurial
Perineurite: perineuritis
Perineuro: perineurium, **pl.** perineuria
Perinuclear: perinuclear
Periocular: periocular
Periodato: periodate
Periodicidade: periodicity
Periódico: periodic
Período: period
Periodontal: periodontal
Periodontia: periodontics
Periodontista: periodontist
Periodontite: periodontitis
Periodonto: paradentium, parodontium, peridentium, periodontium, **pl.** periodontia
Periodontoclasia: periodontoclasia
Periodontólise: periodontolysis
Periodontose: periodontosis
Perioftálmico: periophthalmic
Perioftalmite: periophthalmitis
Perionfálico: periomphalic
Perioníquio: perionychium, **pl.** perionychia, perionyx
Periooforite: perioophoritis
Perioforossalpingite: perioophorosalpingitis
Perioperatório: paraoperative, perioperative
Perioral: perioral
Periórbita: periorbit, periorbita
Periorbital: periorbital
Periorquite: periorchitis
Periosteal: periosteal
Periosteíte: periosteitis
Periósteo: periost, periosteous, periosteum, **pl.** periostea
Periosteófito: periosteophyte
Periosteoma: periosteoma
Periosteomedulite: periosteomedullitis
Periosteomielite: periosteomyelitis
Periosteopatia: periosteopathy
Periosteose: periosteosis
Periosteosteíte: periostosteitis
Periosteotomia: periosteotomy, periostotomy
Periosteótomo: periosteotome
Periostite: periostitis
Periostoma: periostoma
Periostose: periostosis, **pl.** periostoses
Periostótomo: periostotome
Periótico: periotic
Periovarite: periovaritis
Periovular: periovular
Peripancreatite: peripancreatitis
Peripapilar: peripapillary
Peripaquimeningite: peripachymeningitis
Peripatético: peripatetic
Peripeniano: peripenial
Peripileflebite: peripylephlebitis
Peripílico: peripylic
Peripilórico: peripyloric
Periplasma: periplasm
Periplocina: periplocin

Peripoese: peripolesis
Peripolar: peripolar
Periporite: periporitis
Periporta: periportal
Peripróctico: periproctic
Periproctite: periproctitis
Periprostático: periprostatic
Periprostatite: periprostatitis
Perirrenal: perirenal
Perirretal: perirectal
Perirretite: perirectitis
Perirrinal: perirhinal
Perirrizoclasia: perirhizoclasia
Periscópico: periscopic
Perisplâncnico: perisplanchnic
Perisplancnite: perisplanchnitis
Perisplênico: perisplenic
Perisplenite: perisplenitis
Perispondílico: perispondylic
Perispondilite: perispondylitis
Perissalpinge: perisalpinx
Perissalpingite: perisalpingitis
Perissalpingoovarite: perisalpingoovaritis
Perissigmoidite: perisigmoiditis
Perissinovial: perisynovial
Perissinusal: perisinuous
Perissistólico: perisystolic
Peristalse: peristalsis
Peristáltico: peristaltic
Peristasia: peristasis
Perístole: peristole
Peristólico: peristolic
Perístoma: peristoma, peristome
Peristomático: peristomal, peristomatous
Peristrumoso: peristrumous
Peritécio: perithecium, **pl.** perithecia
Peritectomia: peritectomy
Peritélio: perithelium, **pl.** perithelia
Peritendão: peritenon
Peritendíneo: peritendineum, **pl.** peritendinea
Peritendinite: peritendinitis, peritenontitis
Peritíflico: perityphlic
Peritiflite: perityphlitis
Peritireoidite: perithyroiditis
Perito: coroner
Peritomia: peritomy
Peritomista: peritomist
Peritoneal: peritoneal
Peritonealgia: peritonealgia
Peritoneocentese: peritoneocentesis
Peritoneoclise: peritoneoclysis
Peritoneopatia: peritoneopathy
Peritoneopericárdico: peritoneopericardial
Peritoneopexia: peritoneopexy
Peritoneoplastia: peritoneoplasty
Peritoneoscopia: peritoneoscopy, ventroscopy
Peritoneoscópio: peritoneoscope
Peritoneotomia: peritoneotomy
Peritônio: peritoneum, **pl.** peritonea
Peritonite: peritonitis

Peritonsilar: peritonsillar
Peritonsilite: peritonsillitis
Peritorácico: perithoracic
Peritraqueal: peritracheal
Peritríquio: peritrichal, peritrichate, peritrichic, peritrichous
Peritrocantérico: peritrochanteric
Periumbilical: periumbilical
Periungueal: periungual
Periureteral: periureteral, periureteric
Periureterite: periureteritis
Periuretral: periurethral
Periuretrite: periurethritis
Periuterino: periuterine
Periuvular: periuvular
Perivaginite: perivaginitis
Perivascular: perivascular
Perivasculite: perivasculitis
Perivenoso: perivenous
Perivertebral: perivertebral
Perivesical: perivesical
Perivisceral: perivisceral
Periviscerite: perivisceritis
Perivitelino: perivitelline
Perkinismo: perkinism
Perlaboração: working through
Perlasso: pearl-ash
Perlèche: perlèche
Perlingual: perlingual
Permanganato: permanganate
Permeabilidade: permeability
Permeação: permeation
Permear: permeate
Permease: permease
Permeável: patent, permeable
Permissão: allowance
Permuta: crossing-over, crossover
Permutador catiônico: cation exchanger
Permutador de ânion: anion exchanger
Perna: crus, **gen.** cruris, **pl.** crura; leg
Perniciosiforme: perniciosiform
Pernicioso: pernicious
Pérnio: chilblain
Perniose: perniosis
Perobráquio: perobrachius
Perocéfalo: perocephalus
Perodactilia: perodactyly, perodactylia
Perogênio: perogen
Pérola: pearl
Pérola de esmalte: enameloma
Peromelia: peromelia, peromely
Perópode: peropus
Peroquiro: perochirus
Peroral: peroral
Perosplancnia: perosplanchnia
Perósseo: perosseous
Peroxidases: peroxidases
Peróxido: peroxide
Peroxila: peroxyl
Peroxissoma: peroxisome
Persal: persalt
Perseveração: perseveration
Persistência: persistence

Persistente: persister
Personalidade: personality
Persuasão: persuasion
Persulfato: persulfate
Persulfeto: persulfide
Pertactina: pertactin
Pertecnetato: pertechnetate
Perturbação: derangement
Pervaporação: perstillation, pervaporation
Perversão: perversion
Pervertido: pervert, perverted
Pervinca: *Vinca rosea*
Pérvio: pervious
Pesar: grief
Pescoço: neck
Pescovegetariano: pescovegetarian
Peso: weight
Pesquisa: research
Pessário: pessary
Pessimismo: pessimism
Pessoas-ano: person-years
Peste: pest, pestilence, pestis, plague
Pesticemia: pesticemia
Pesticida: pesticide
Pestífero: pestiferous
Pestilencial: pestilential
Petéquias: petechiae, **sing.** petechia
Petequial: petechial
Petidina: pethidine
Petrificação: petrifaction
Petroccipital: petroccipital, petrooccipital
Petroescamoso: petrosquamosal, petrosquamous
Petroesfenóide: petrosphenoid
Petroestafilino: petrostaphylinus
Petrofaríngeo: petropharyngeus
Petrolato: petrolatum
Petróleo: coal oil, petroleum
Petromastóide: petromastoid
Petrosa: petrosa, **pl.** petrosae
Petrosite: petrositis, petrousitis
Petroso: petrosal, petrous
Petrosomastóide: petrosomastoid
Petrossalpingoestafilino: petrosalpingostaphylinus
Pé-vela: footcandle
Pexia: pexis
Pexina: pexin
Pexinogênio: pexinogen
P-glicoproteína: P-glycoprotein
***p*-hidroxifenilacetato:** *p*-hydroxyphenylacetate
***p*-hidroxifenilactato:** *p*-hydroxyphenyllactate
***p*-hidroxifenilpiruvato:** *p*-hydroxyphenylpyruvate
Pi: pi
Pia-aracnite: pia-arachnitis
Pia-aracnóide: pia-arachnoid, piarachnoid
Pial: pial
Pia-máter: pia, pia mater
Piartrose: pyarthrosis
Pica: pica

Piche: pitch
Pícnico: pyknic
Picnodisostose: pyknodysostosis
Picnoepilepsia, picnolepsia: pyknoepilepsy, pyknolepsy
Picnofrasia: pyknophrasia
Picnolepsia: pyknolepsy
Picnomorfo: pyknomorphous
Picnose: pyknosis
Picnótico: pyknotic
Pico: peak
Picograma: picogram (pg)
Picokatal: picokatal (pkat)
Picômetro: picometer (pm)
Picomol: picomole (pmol)
Picornavírus: picornavirus
Picrato: picrate
Picrilo: picryl
Picrocarmim: picrocarmine
Picroformol: picroformol
Picronigrosina: picronigrosin
Picrotoxina: picrotoxin
Picrotoxinina: picrotoxinin
Pictografia: pictograph
Piebaldismo: piebaldism, piebaldness
Piedra: piedra
Pielectasia: pyelectasis, pyelectasia
Pielite: pyelitis
Pielítico: pyelitic
Pielocalicial: pyelocaliceal, pyelocalyceal
Pielocaliectasia: pyelocaliectasis
Pielocistite: pyelocystitis
Pielofluoroscopia: pyelofluoroscopy
Pielografia: pyelography
Pielograma: pyelogram
Pielolinfático: pyelolymphatic
Pielolitotomia: pelviolithotomy, pyelolithotomy
Pielonefrite: pyelonephritis
Pielonefrose: pyelonephrosis
Pieloplastia: pyeloplasty
Pieloplicatura: pyeloplication
Pieloscopia: pyeloscopy
Pielostomia: pyelostomy
Pielotomia: pyelotomy
Pieloureterectasia: pyeloureterectasis
Pieloureterografia: pyeloureterography
Pielovenoso: pyelovenous
Piêmese: pyemesis
Piemia: pyemia
Piêmico: pyemic
Piencéfalo: pyencephalus
Piese: pyesis
Piezoeletricidade: piezoelectricity
Piezoelétrico: piezoelectric
Piezogênico: piezogenic
Piezômetro: piesimeter, piesometer, piezometer
Piezoquímica: piezochemistry
Pigalgia: pygalgia
Pigmalionismo: pygmalionism
Pigmentação: pigmentation
Pigmentado: pigmented
Pigmentar: pigmentary

Pigmento: pigment
Pigmento negro: pigmentum nigrum
Pigmentolisina: pigmentolysin
Pigmeu: pigmy, pygmy
Pigoamorfo: pygoamorphus
Pigodídimo: pygodidymus
Pigômelo: pygomelus
Pigópago: pygopagus
Pilão: pestle
Pilar: pillar
Pileflebite: pylephlebitis
Piletromboflebite: pylethrombophlebitis
Piletrombose: pylethrombosis
Pilha: pile
Pilimicção: pilimiction
Pilina: pilin
Pilocarpina: pilocarpine
Pilocarpo: pilocarpus
Pilocístico: pilocystic
Piloereção: piloerection
Pilomatrixoma: pilomatrixoma
Pilomotor: pilomotor
Pilonidal: pilonidal
Piloralgia: pyloralgia
Pilorectomia: pylorectomy
Pilórico: pyloric
Piloriestenose: pyloristenosis
Pilorite: pyloritis
Piloro: pylorus, **pl.** pylori
Piloroduodenite: pyloroduodenitis
Pilorogastrectomia: pylorogastrectomy
Piloromiotomia: pyloromyotomy
Piloroplastia: pyloroplasty
Piloroptose: pyloroptosis, pyloroptosia
Pilorospasmo: pylorospasm
Pilorostenose: pylorostenosis
Pilorostomia: pylorostomy
Pilorotomia: pylorotomy
Pilose: pilosis
Piloso: pilar, pilary, pilose
Pilossebáceo: pilosebaceous
Pílula: pill, pilula, **gen. e pl.** pilulae
Pilular: pilular
Pimaricina: pimaricin
Pimelorréia: pimelorrhea
Pimelortopnéia: pimelorthopnea
Pimenta: pimenta, pimento
Pimenta negra: piper
Pimozida: pimozide
Pinacianol: pinacyanol
Pinça: clamp
Pinça saca-bocado: rongeur
Pinçamento: pincement
Pinçar: pinch
Pindolol: pindolol
Pineal: pineal
Pinealectomia: pinealectomy
Pinealócito: pinealocyte
Pinealoma: pinealoma
Pinealopatia: pinealopathy
Pineoblastoma: pineoblastoma
Pineocitoma: pineocytoma
Pinguécula: pinguecula, pinguicula

Pingue-pongue: ping-pong
Pinheiro: pine
Piniforme: piniform
Pinípede: pinniped
Pino: dowel, pin
Pinócito: pinocyte
Pinocitose: pinocytosis
Pinossoma: pinosome
Pinta: azul, pint, pinta
Píntides: pintids
Piocéfalo: pyocephalus
Piocele: pyocele
Piociânico: pyocyanic
Piocianogênico: pyocyanogenic
Piocianolisina: pyocyanolysin
Piocina: pyocin
Piocisto: pyocyst, pyocystis
Piócito: pyocyte
Piococo: pyococcus
Piocolpo: pyocolpos
Piocolpocele: pyocolpocele
Piodermite: pyoderma
Pioemia: pyohemia
Pioemotórax: pyohemothorax
Piofisométrio: pyophysometra
Piogênese: pyogenesis
Piogênico: pyogenic, pyogenetic, pyogenous
Piógeno: pyogen
Pióide: pyoid
Piolho: louse, **pl.** lice
Piometra: pyometra
Piometrite: pyometritis
Piomiosite: pyomyositis
Piomiosite tropical: bungpagga, lambo lambo
Pionefrite: pyonephritis
Pionefrolitíase: pyonephrolithiasis
Pionefrose: pyonephrosis
Pio-ovário: pyo-ovarium
Piopericárdio: pyopericardium
Piopericardite: pyopericarditis
Pioperitônio: pyocelia, pyoperitoneum
Pioperitonite: pyoperitonitis
Piopielectasia: pyopyelectasis
Piopneumocolecistite: pyopneumocholecystitis
Piopneumoepatite: pyopneumohepatitis
Piopneumopericárdio: pyopneumopericardium
Piopneumoperitônio: pyopneumoperitoneum
Piopneumoperitonite: pyopneumoperitonitis
Piopneumotórax: pyopneumothorax
Piopoese: pyopoiesis
Piopoético: pyopoietic
Pioquezia: pyochezia
Piorréia: pyorrhea
Piortopnéia: pyorthopnea
Piose: pyosis
Piosemia: pyosemia
Piospermia: pyospermia
Piossalpinge: pyosalpinx
Piossalpingite: pyosalpingitis
Piossalpingo-ooforite: pyosalpingo-oophoritis

Piossepticemia: pyosepticemia
Piostático: pyostatic
Piostomatite: pyostomatitis
Piotórax: pyothorax
Pioúraco: pyourachus
Pioureter: pyoureter
Pipamazina: pipamazine
Pipamperona: pipamperone
Pipazetato: pipazethate
Pipecurônio: pipecuronium
Piperacilina sódica: piperacillin sodium
Piperazina: piperazine
Piperazina acefilina: acefylline piperazine
Piperidina: piperidine
Pipeta: pipette, pipet
Pipobromano: pipobroman
Pipossulfano: piposulfan
Piprinidrinato: piprinhydrinate
Pipsila: pipsyl (Ips)
Piracina: pyracin
Piramidal: triquetrum
Pirâmide: pyramid, pyramis, **pl.** pyramides
Piramidotomia: pyramidotomy
Piramina: pyramin, pyramine
Pirano: pyran
Piranona: pyranone
Piranose: pyranose
Pirazinamida: pyrazinamide
Pirazolona: pyrazolone
Pirbuterol: pirbuterol
Pirenemia: pyrenemia
Pirenóide: pyrenoid
Pirenzepina: pirenzepine
Piretanida: piretanide
Pirético: pyrectic, pyretic
Piretogênese: pyretogenesis
Piretogenético: pyretogenetic, pyretogenic
Piretogênico: pyretogenous
Piretógeno: pyretogen
Piretoterapia: pyretotherapy
Piretrinas: pyrethrins
Píretro: pyrethrum
Piretróides: pyrethroids
Piretrolona: pyrethrolone
Pirexia: pyrexia
Piréxico: pyrexial
Pirexiofobia: pyrexiophobia
Piribedil: piribedil
Piridina: pyridine
Piridínio: pyridinium
Piridinolina: pyridinoline
Piridofilina: pyridofylline
Piridoxal: pyridoxal
Piridoxamina: pyridoxamine
Piridoxamina-fosfato oxidase: pyridoxamine-phosphate oxidase
Piridoxina: pyridoxine
Piridoxina 4-desidrogenase: pyridoxine 4-dehydrogenase
Piriforme: piriform, pyriform
Pirimetamina: pyrimethamine
Pirimidina: pyrimidine (Pyr)
Pirina: pyrin
Piritiamina: pyrithiamin
Pirocalciferol: pyrocalciferol

Pirocatecase: pyrocatechase
Pirocatecol: pyrocatechol
Pirocatequina: pyrocatechin
Pirofobia: pyrophobia
Pirofosfatase: pyrophosphatase
Pirofosfato: pyrophosphate (PP, PP_i)
Pirofosfato de farnesil: farnesyl pyrophosphate
Pirofosfato de geranil: geranyl pyrophosphate
Pirofosfato de geranilgeranil: geranylgeranyl pyrophosphate
Pirofosfato de lipotiamida: lipothiamide pyrophosphate
Pirofosfocinases: pyrophosphokinases
Pirofosforilases: pyrophosphorylases
Pirofosfotransferases: pyrophosphotransferases
Pirogalol: pyrogallol
Pirogalolftaleína: pyrogallolphthalein
Pirogênico: pyrogenic
Pirogênio: pyrogen
Piroglobulinas: pyroglobulins
Pirolenhoso: pyroligneous
Pirólise: pyrolysis
Piromania: pyromania
Piromaníaco: pyromaniac
Piromena: piromen, pyromen
Pirômetro: pyrometer
Pirona: pyrone
Pironina: pyronin
Pironinofilia: pyroninophilia
Piroplasmose: piroplasmosis
Piropoiquilocitose: pyropoikilocytosis
Piroscópio: pyroscope
Pirose: heartburn, pyrosis
Piroterapia: pyrotherapy
Pirótico: pyrotic
Pirotoxina: pyrotoxin
Piroxilina: pyroxylin
Pirprofeno: pirprofen
Pirrol: pyrrole
Pirrolase: pyrrolase
Pirrolidina: pyrrolidine
Pirrolidina-2-carboxilato: pyrrolidine-2-carboxylate
Pirrolidona-5-carboxilato: pyrrolidone-5-carboxylate
Pirrolina: pyrroline
1-pirrolina-5-carboxilato desidrogenase: 1-pyrroline-5-carboxylate dehydrogenase
Pirrolina-2-carboxilato redutase: pyrroline-2-carboxylate reductase
Pirrolina-5-carboxilato redutase: pyrroline-5-carboxylate reductase
Piruvaldoxina: pyruvaldoxine
Piruvato: pyruvate
6-piruvoiltetraidropterina sintase: 6-pyruvoyltetrahydropterin synthase (6-PTS)
Piscadela: palpebration
Piscar: blink, nictitate, wink

Pisiforme: pisiform
Pitecóide: pithecoid
Pitiríase: pityriasis
Pitiríase liquenóide crônica: pityriasis lichenoides chronica
Pitogênese: pythogenesis
Pitogênico: pythogenic, pythogenous
Pituícito: pituicyte
Pituicitoma: pituicytoma
Pituíta: pituita
Pituitária: pituitarium, pituitary
Pituitarismo: pituitarism
Pituitoso: pituitous
Piúria: pyuria
Pivalato: pivalate
Pivô: abutment, pivot
Pixel: pixel
Placa: plaque, scute, scutum, **pl.** scuta
Placa básica: baseplate
Placa de mordida: biteplate, biteplane
Placa lingual: linguoplate
Placa terminal: endplate, end-plate
Placalbumina: plakalbumin
Placebo: placebo
Placenta: placenta
Placentação: placentation
Placentário: placental
Placentite: placentitis
Placentoma: placentoma
Placentoterapia: placentotherapy
Placóide: placode
Plagiocefalia: plagiocephalism, plagiocephaly
Plagiocefálico: plagiocephalic, plagiocephalous
Plâncton: plankton
Planctônico: planktonic
Planigrafia: planigraphy
Planimetria: planimetry
Planímetro: planimeter
Planitórax: planithorax
Plano: plane, planum, **pl.** plana
Plano médio: midplane
Planocelular: planocellular
Planocôncavo: planoconcave
Planoconvexo: planoconvex
Planografia: planography
Planomania: planomania
Planovalgo: planovalgus
Planta: pelma, planta, **gen. e pl.** plantae; sole, wort
Plantar: plantar, plantaris
Plantígrado: plantigrade
Plânula: planula, **pl.** planulae
Planúria: planuria
Plaqueamento: plating
Plaqueta: platelet
Plaquetoférese: plateletpheresis
Plaquinas: plakins
Plasma: plasm, plasma
Plasmacininas: plasmakinins
Plasmacitoblasto: plasmacytoblast
Plasmacitoma: plasmacytoma
Plasmácrito: plasmacrit
Plasmaférese: plasmapheresis

Plasmaferético: plasmapheretic
Plasmagene: plasmagene
Plasmais: plasmals
Plasmalema: plasmalemma
Plasmalogênios: plasmalogens
Plasmalógenos: phosphoglyceracetals
Plasmático: plasmatic
Plasmatogamia: plasmatogamy
Plásmico: plasmic
Plasmídeo: paragene, plasmid
Plasmina: plasmin
Plasminocinase: plasminokinase
Plasminogênio: plasminogen
Plasminoplastina: plasminoplastin
Plasmoblasto: plasmablast
Plasmocinina: plasmokinin
Plasmócito: plasmacyte
Plasmocitose: plasmacytosis
Plasmodial: plasmodial
Plasmódio: plasmodium, **pl.** plasmodia
Plasmodiotrofoblasto: plasmodiotrophoblast
Plasmogamia: plasmogamy
Plasmogênio: plasmogen
Plasmolema: plasmolemma
Plasmolisar: plasmolyze
Plasmólise: plasmolysis
Plasmolítico: plasmolytic
Plasmônio: plasmon
Plasmorrexe: plasmorrhexis
Plasmosina: plasmosin
Plasmosquise: plasmoschisis
Plasmótipo: plasmotype
Plasmotomia: plasmotomy
Plasmotrópico: plasmotropic
Plasmotropismo: plasmotropism
Plasmozima: plasmozyme
Plasteína: plastein
Plasticidade: plasticity
Plástico: plastic
Plastídio: plastid
Plastocromenol-8: plastochromenol-8
Plastocromonal-3, plastocromonal E_3: plastochromanol-3, plastochromanol E_3
Plastogamia: plastogamy
Plastoquinona: plastoquinone (PQ)
Plastoquinona-9, plastoquinona E_9: plastoquinone-9 (PQ-9), plastoquinone E_9
Plastrom: plastron
Plataforma de força: force platform
Platelminto: flatworm, platyhelminth
Platibasia: platybasia
Platicefalia: platycephaly
Platicnemia: platycnemia, platycnemism
Platicnêmico: platycnemic
Platicrânia: platycrania
Platiglosso: platyglossal

Platiiérico: platyhieric
Platimérico: platymeric
Platimorfia: platymorphia
Platina: platinum (Pt)
Platínico: platinic
Platinoso: platinous
Platiopia: platyopia
Platiópico: platyopic
Platipélico: platypellic
Platipelóide: platypelloid
Platipnéia: platypnea
Platirrinia: platyrrhiny
Platirrino: platyrrhine
Platisma: platysma, **pl.** platysmas, platysmata
Platispondilia: platyspondylia, platyspondylisis
Platistencefalia: platystencephaly
Platô: plateau
Plectrídio: plectridium
Pleiotropia: pleiotropy, pleiotropia
Pleiotrópico: pleiotropic
Pleocitose: pleocytosis
Pleocromia: pleochroism, pleochromatism
Pleocrômico: pleochroic, pleochromatic
Pleomastia, pleomazia: pleomastia, pleomazia
Pleomorfismo: pleomorphism
Pleomorfo: pleomorphic, pleomorphous
Pleonasmo: pleonasm
Pleonosteose: pleonosteosis
Pleóptica: pleoptics
Pleoptóforo: pleoptophor
Pleotrópico: polyphenic
Plerocercóide: plerocercoid
Plesiomórfico: plesiomorphic
Plesiomorfismo: plesiomorphism
Plesiomorfo: plesiomorphous
Plessestesia: plessesthesia
Plessimétrico: plessimetric
Plessímetro: plessimeter
Plessor: plessor
Pletismografia: plethysmography
Pletismógrafo: plethysmograph
Pletismometria: plethysmometry
Pletora: plethora
Pletórico: plethoric
Pleura: pleura, **gen. e pl.** pleurae
Pleural: pleural
Pleuralgia: pleuralgia
Pleurapófise: pleurapophysis
Pleurectomia: pleurectomy
Pleurisia: pleurisy
Pleurite: pleuritis
Pleurítico: pleuritic
Pleuritogênico: pleuritogenous
Pleurocele: pleurocele
Pleurocentese: pleuracentesis, pleurocentesis
Pleurocentro: pleurocentrum
Pleuróclise: pleuroclysis
Pleurodese: pleurodesis

Pleurodinia: pleurodynia
Pleurogênico: pleurogenic, pleurogenous
Pleurografia: pleurography
Pleuro-hepatite: pleurohepatitis
Pleurólise: pleurolysis
Pleurólito: pleurolith
Pleuropericárdico: pleuropericardial
Pleuropericardite: pleuropericarditis
Pleuroperitoneal: pleuroperitoneal
Pleuropneumectomia: pleuropneumonectomy
Pleuropulmonar: pleuropulmonary
Pleuroscopia: pleuroscopy
Pleurotifóide: pleurotyphoid
Pleurotomia: pleurotomy
Pleurovisceral: pleurovisceral
Plexectomia: plexectomy
Plexiforme: plexiform
Plexímetro: pleximeter
Plexite: plexitis
Plexo: plexus, **pl.** plexus, plexuses
Plexogênico: plexogenic
Plexômetro: plexometer
Plexopatia: plexopathy
Plexor: plexor
Plicatura: plication
Plicotomia: plicotomy
Ploidia: ploidy
Plosivo: plosive
Plumbagem: plombage
Plúmbico: plumbic
Plumbismo: plumbism
Plumoso: plumose
Pluricausal: pluricausal
Pluriglandular: pluriglandular
Plurilocular: plurilocular
Plurinuclear: plurinuclear
Pluripotente, pluripotencial: pluripotent, pluripotential
Plurirresistente: pluriresistant
Plutomania: plutomania
Plutônio: plutonium (Pu)
Plutonismo: plutonism
***p*-mercuribenzoato:** *p*-mercuribenzoate
Pneumartrografia: pneumarthrography, pneumoarthrography
Pneumartrograma: pneumarthrogram
Pneumartrose: pneumarthrosis
Pneumatemia: pneumatohemia
Pneumática: pneumatics
Pneumático: pneumatic
Pneumatismo: pneumatism
Pneumatistas: pneumatists
Pneumatização: pneumatization
Pneumatizado: pneumatized
Pneumatocardia: pneumatocardia
Pneumatocele: pneumatocele
Pneumatoentérico: pneumatoenteric
Pneumatômetro: pneumatometer

Pneumatórraque: pneumatorrhachis
Pneumatoscópio: pneumatoscope
Pneumatose: pneumatosis
Pneumatúria: pneumaturia
Pneumectomia: pulmonectomy
Pneumobulbar: pneumobulbar
Pneumocéfalo: pneumocephalus
Pneumocele: pneumocele
Pneumocentese: pneumocentesis, pneumonocentesis
Pneumocistografia: pneumocystography
Pneumocistose: pneumocystosis
Pneumócito: pneumocyte, pneumonocyte
Pneumococcemia: pneumococcemia
Pneumococcida: pneumococcidal
Pneumocócico: pneumococcal, pneumonococcal
Pneumococo: pneumococcus, **pl.** pneumococci; pneumonococcus
Pneumocócólise: pneumococcolysis
Pneumococose: pneumococcosis
Pneumococosúria: pneumococcosuria
Pneumocolecistite: pneumocholecystitis
Pneumocolo: pneumocolon
Pneumoconiose: pneumoconiosis, pneumokoniosis, **pl.** pneumoconioses; pneumonoconiosis, pneumonokoniosis
Pneumocrânio: pneumocranium
Pneumoderma: pneumoderma
Pneumodinâmica: pneumodynamics
Pneumoemia: pneumohemia
Pneumoemotórax: pneumohemothorax
Pneumoempiema: pneumoempyema
Pneumoencefalografia: pneumoencephalography
Pneumoencefalograma: pneumoencephalogram
Pneumofagia: pneumophagia
Pneumogástrico: pneumogastric
Pneumogastrografia: pneumogastrography
Pneumografia: pneumography
Pneumógrafo: pneumograph
Pneumograma: pneumogram
Pneumoidrometria: pneumohydrometra
Pneumoidropericárdio: pneumohydropericardium
Pneumoidroperitônio: pneumohydroperitoneum
Pneumoidrotórax: pneumohydrothorax
Pneumoipodermia: pneumohypoderma

Pneumólise: pneumolysis
Pneumolitíase: pneumolithiasis
Pneumólito: pneumolith
Pneumologia: pneumology
Pneumomalacia: pneumomalacia
Pneumomassagem: pneumomassage
Pneumomediastino: pneumomediastinum
Pneumomelanose: pneumomelanosis, pneumonomelanosis
Pneumomicose: pneumomycosis
Pneumomielografia: pneumomyelography
Pneumonectomia: pneumonectomy
Pneumonia: pneumonia
Pneumônico: pneumonic
Pneumonite: pneumonitis, pulmonitis
Pneumonocele: pneumonocele
Pneumo-orbitografia: pneumo-orbitography
Pneumopatia: pneumonopathy
Pneumopericárdio: pneumopericardium
Pneumoperitônio: pneumoperitoneum
Pneumoperitonite: pneumoperitonitis
Pneumopexia: pneumonopexy, pneumopexy
Pneumopielografia: pneumopyelography
Pneumopleurite: pneumonopleuritis, pneumopleuritis
Pneumorradiografia: pneumoradiography, pneumoroentgenography
Pneumorrafia: pneumonorrhaphy
Pneumorraque: pneumorrhachis
Pneumorressecção: pneumoresection
Pneumorretroperitônio: pneumoretroperitoneum
Pneumoscópio: pneumoscope
Pneumotacógrafo: pneumotachograph
Pneumotacograma: pneumotachogram
Pneumotacômetro: pneumotachometer
Pneumotermomassagem: pneumothermomassage
Pneumótipo: pneumatype
Pneumotomia: pneumonotomy, pneumotomy
Pneumotórax: pneumothorax
Pneumoventrículo: pneumoventricle
Pnigofobia: pnigophobia
Pó: powder
Poção: potion
Podagra: podagra
Podalgia: podalgia
Podálico: podalic

Podartrite: podarthritis
Pododema: pododema
Podiatra: podiatrist, podiatry
Podiátrico: podiatric
Podismo: podismus
Podite: poditis
Podobromidrose: podobromidrosis
Podócito: podocyte
Pododinamômetro: pododynamometer
Pododinia: pododynia
Podofilina: podophyllin
Podofilo: May apple, podophyllum
Podofilotoxina: podophyllotoxin
Podofilox: podofilox
Podógrafo: podograph
Podograma: podogram
Podolito: dahllite
Podólito: podolite
Podologia: podology
Podólogo: podologist
Podomecanoterapia: podomechanotherapy
Podômetro: podometer
Podospasmo: podospasm, podospasmus
Pogoníase: pogoniasis
Pogônio: pogonion
Poiquiloblasto: poikiloblast
Poiquilócito: poikilocyte
Poiquilocitose: poikilocythemia, poikilocytosis
Poiquilodentose: poikilodentosis
Poiquilodermia: poikiloderma
Poiquilotermia: poikilothermy, poikilothermism
Poiquilotérmico; pecilotérmico: poikilothermic, poikilothermal, poikilothermous
Poiquilotermo: poikilotherm
Poiquilotimia: poikilothymia
Poiquilotrombócito: poikilothrombocyte
Poise: poise (P)
Polacidipsia: pollakidipsia
Polaciúria: pollakiuria
Polar: polar
Polaridade: polarity
Polarimetria: polarimetry
Polarímetro: polarimeter
Polariscopia: polariscopy
Polariscópico: polariscopic
Polariscópio: polariscope
Polarização: polarization
Polarizador: polarizer
Polarizar: polarize
Polarografia: polarography
Polegar: pollex, **gen.** pollicis, **pl.** pollices; thumb
Pólen: pollen
Polenose: pollenosis, pollinosis
Poli(aminoácidos): poly(amino acids)
Poli(U): poly(U)
Poliácido: polyacid
Poliacrilamida: polyacrylamide
Poliadenilação: polyadenylation
Poliadenite: polyadenitis

Poliadenopatia: polyadenopathy
Poliadenose: polyadenosis
Poliadenoso: polyadenous
Poliálcool: polyalcohol
Polialelismo: polyallelism
Poliamina: polyamine
Poliangeíte: polyangiitis
Poliânion: polyanion
Poliarterite: polyarteritis
Poliarticular: polyarthric, polyarticular
Poliartrite: polyarthritis
Poliauxotrófico: polyauxotroph
Poliavitaminose: polyavitaminosis
Polibásico: polybasic
Poliblenia: polyblennia
Policarbófilo: polycarbophil
Policariócito: polykaryocyte
Policêntrico: polycentric
Policiese: polycyesis
Policístico: polycystic
Policistrônico: polycistronic
Policitemia: polycythemia
Policização: pollicization
Policlínico: polyclinic
Policlonal: polyclonal
Policondrite: polychondritis
Policoria: polycoria
Policromasia: polychromasia
Policromático: polychromatic
Policromatócito: polychromatocyte
Policromatofilia: polychromatophilia, polychromophilia
Policromatófilo: polychromatophil, polychromatophile, polychromatophilic, polychromophil
Policromatose: polychromatosis
Policromemia: polychromemia
Policromia: polychromia
Policrótico: polycrotic
Policrotismo: polycrotism
Polidactilia: polydactylism, polydactyly
Polidáctilo: polydactylous
Polidipsia: polydipsia
Polidispersóide: polydispersoid
Polidisplasia: polydysplasia
Polidistrofia: polydystrophy
Polidistrófico: polydystrophic
Polidontia: polydentia, polyodontia
Polidor: burnisher
Poliédrico: polyhedral
Poliembrionia: polyembryony
Poliendocrinopatia: polyendocrinopathy
Polieno: polyene
Poliérgico: polyergic
Poliespermia, polispermia: polyspermia, polyspermism
Poliestesia: polyesthesia
Poliestro: polyestrous
Polietilenoglicóis: polyethylene glycols (PEGs)
Poliexoses: polyhexoses
Polifagia: polyphagia

Polifálico: polyphallic
Polifarmácia: polypharmacy
Polifenol oxidase: polyphenol oxidase
Polifilético: polyphyletic
Polifiletismo: polyphyletism
Polifiodonte: polyphyodont
Polifobia: polyphobia
Polifosforilase: polyphosphorylase
Polifrutose: polyfructose
Poligalactia: polygalactia
Poligalacturonase: polygalacturonase
Poliganglionar: polyganglionic
Poligene: polygene
Poligênico: polygenic
Poligiria: polygyria
Poliglactina 910: polyglactin 910
Poliglandular: polyglandular
Poli-β-glucosaminidase: poly-β-glucosaminidase
Poliglutamato: polyglutamate
Polignato: polygnathus
Polígrafo: polygraph
Poliíbrido: polyhybrid
Poliidrâmnio: polyhydramnios
Poliídrico: polyhydric
Poliidrose: polyhidrosis
Poliipermenorréia: polyhypermenorrhea
Poliipomenorréia: polyhypomenorrhea
Poliisoprenóides: polyisoprenoids
Poliisoprenos: polyisoprenes
Polilactosaminas: polylactosamines
Poliléptico: polyleptic
Polilogia: polylogia
Polimastia: multimammae, polymastia
Polimastigota: polymastigote
Polimegetismo: polymegethism
Polimelia: polymelia
Polimenorréia: polymenorrhea
Polimento: milling-in, polishing
Polimerase: polymerase
Polimerase α: polymerase α
Polimerase β: polymerase β
Polimerase γ: polymerase γ
Polimeria: polymerria
Polimérico: polymeric
Polimerização: polymerization
Polimerizar: polymerize
Polímero: polymer
Polimetacarpalismo: polymetacarpalia, polymetacarpalism
Polimetatarsalismo: polymetatarsalia, polymetatarsalism
Polimialgia: polymyalgia
Polimicrolipomatose: polymicrolipomatosis
Polimioclônus: polymyoclonus
Polimiosite: polymyositis
Polimixina: polymyxin
Polimórfico: polymorphic
Polimorfismo: polymorphism

Polimorfo: polymorph, polymorphous
Polimorfocelular: polymorphocellular
Polimorfonuclear: polymorphonuclear
Polinésico: polynesic
Polineural: polyneural
Polineuralgia: polyneuralgia
Polineurite: polyneuritis
Polineuronite: polyneuronitis
Polineuropatia: polyneuropathy
Polinoxilina: polynoxylin
Polinuclear, polinucleado: polynuclear, polynucleate
Polinucleose: polynucleosis
Polinucleotidases: polynucleotidases
Polinucleotídeo: polynucleotide
Polinucleotídeo metilases: polynucleotide methylases
Pólio: polio
Polioclástico: polioclastic
Poliodistrofia: poliodystrophia, poliodystrophy
Polioencefalite: polioencephalitis
Polioencefalomeningomielite: polioencephalomeningomyelitis
Polioencefalomielite: polioencephalomyelitis
Polioencefalopatia: polioencephalopathy
Poliol: polyol
Poliomielite: poliomyelitis
Poliomieloencefalite: poliomyeloencephalitis
Poliomielopatia: poliomyelopathy
Polioncose: polyoncosis, polyonchosis
Polioníquia: polyonychia, polyunguia
Poliopia: polyopia, polyopsia
Poliorquia; poliorquidismo: polyorchism, polyorchidism
Poliose: poliosis
Poliostótico: polyostotic
Poliotia: polyotia
Poliovírus: poliovirus
Poliovular: polyovular
Poliovulatório: polyovulatory
Polipapiloma: polypapilloma
Polipatia: polypathia
Polipectomia: polypectomy
Polipeptídeo: polypeptide
Polipiforme: polypiform
Poliplásico: polyplastic
Poliplóide: polyploid
Poliploidia: polyploidy
Polipnéia: polypnea
Pólipo: polyp, polypus, **pl.** polypi
Polinucleotídeo: polynucleotide
Pólipo fibroso: fibropolypus
Polipodia: polypodia
Polipóide: polypoid
Polipose: polyposis
Poliposia: polyposia
Poliposo: polypous

Polipótomo: polypotome
Polipótrito: polypotrite
Polipragmasia: polypragmasy
Poliprenóis: polyprenols
Poliquilia: polychylia
Poliquiria: polycheiria, polychiria
Polirradiculite: polyradiculitis
Polirradiculomiopatia: polyradiculomyopathy
Polirradiculoneuropatia: polyradiculoneuropathy
Polirradiculopatia: polyradiculopathy
Polirréia: polyrrhea
Polirribonucleotídeo nucleotidiltransferase: polyribonucleotide nucleotidyltransferase
Polirribossomas: polyribosomes
Poliscelia: polyscelia
Poliscópio: polyscope
Polispermia: polyspermy
Polisplenia: polyasplenia, polysplenia
Polissacarídeo: polysaccharide
Polisserosite: polyserositis
Polissimbraquidactilia: polysymbrachydactyly
Polissináptico: polysynaptic
Polissindactilia: polysyndactyly
Polissinusite: polysinusitis
Polissomas: polysomes
Polissomia: polysomia, polysomy
Polissômico: polysomic
Polissonografia: polysomnography
Polissonograma: polysomnogram
Polissorbato 80: polysorbate 80
Polissuspensóide: polysuspensoid
Polistiquia: polystichia
Politelia: polythelia
Politendinite: polytendinitis
Politenização: polytenization
Politeno: polytene
Politerpenos: polyterpenes
Politiazida: polythiazide
Polítoco: polytocous
Politomografia: polytomography
Politricose: polytrichosis
Politriquia: polytrichia
Politrópico: polytrophic
Poliúria: polyuria
Poliuronidas: polyuronides
Polivalente: multipartial, polyvalent
Polividona: polyvidone
Polivinil: polyvinyl
Polivinilpirrolidona: polyvinylpyrrolidone (PVP)
Polizigótico: polyzygotic
Polizóico: polyzoic
Pólo: pole, polus, **pl.** poli
Polócito: polocyte
Polônio: polonium (Po)
Poloxalcol: poloxalkol
Poloxaleno: poloxalene

Polpa: pulp
Polpação: pulpifaction
Poluente: pollutant
Poluição: pollution
Pomada: pomade, pomatum, salve
Pomada oftálmica: oculentum, **pl.** oculenta
Pomo-de-adão: Adam's apple
Ponderância ventricular: ventricular ponderance
Ponfólige: pompholyx
Ponofobia: ponophobia
Ponógrafo: ponograph
Ponose: ponos
Ponta: spike, tip
Pontada: twinge
Ponte: bridge, pons, **pl.** pontes
Ponte dentária: bridge-work
Pôntico: pontic
Pontículo: ponticulus
Pontilhado: punctate, stippling
Pontino: pontile, pontine
Ponto: point, punctum, **gen.** puncti, **pl.** puncta
Ponto auricular: auriculare, **pl.** auricularia
Ponto de ruptura: breakpoint
Ponto jugal: jugale
Ponto oral: orale
Pontocerebelo: pontocerebellum
Poplíteo: popliteal, popliteus
População: population
Porção: portio, **pl.** portiones; portion
Porção ectópica: socia
Porcelana: porcelain
Porencefalia: porencephalia, porencephaly
Porencefálico: porencephalic, porencephalous
Porencefalite: porencephalitis
Porfina: porphin, porphine
Porfiria: porphyria
Porfirina: porphyrin
Porfirina férrica: ferriporphyrin
Porfirina ferrosa: ferroporphyrin
Porfirinas: porphyrins
Porfirinogênios: porphyrinogens
Porfirinopatia: porphyrinopathy
Porfirinúria: porphyrinuria
Porfirismo: porphyrism
Porfirização: porphyrization
Porfirúria: porphyruria
Porfobilina: porphobilin
Porfobilinogênio: porphobilinogen (PBG)
Porinas: porins
Pório: porion, **pl.** poria
Poriomania: poriomania
Pornolagnia: pornolagnia
Poro: pore, porus, **pl.** pori
Porocefalíase: porocephaliasis
Porocefalose: porocephalosis
Poroceratose: porokeratosis
Poroconídio: poroconidium
Poroma: poroma
Porosidade: porosis, **pl.** poroses; porosity
Poroso: porotic, porous

Porosporo: porospore
Porquinho-da-índia: guinea pig
Porta: port, porta, **pl.** portae
Porta-agulha: needle-holder, needle-carrier, needle-driver
Portador: carrier
Portal: portal
Porta-objetiva: nosepiece
Portiplexo: portiplexus
Portobilioarterial: portobilioarterial
Portocava: portacaval
Portoenterostomia: portoenterostomy
Portografia: portography
Portograma: portogram
Portossistêmico: portosystemic
Portovenografia: portovenography
Pós-acetabular: postacetabular
Pós-adolescência: postadolescence
Pós-anal: postanal
Pós-anestésico: postanesthetic
Pós-apoplético: postapoplectic
Pós-axial: postaxial
Pós-braquial: postbrachial
Pós-cardinal: postcardinal
Pós-carga: afterload
Pós-central: postcentral
Pós-clavicular: postclavicular
Pós-coital: postcoital
Pós-coito: postcoitus
Pós-contração: aftercontraction
Pós-cordial: postcordial
Pós-coroa: postcrown
Pós-corrente: aftercurrent
Pós-costal: postcostal
Pós-cromação: postchroming
Pós-cromagem: afterchroming
Pós-descarga: afterdischarge
Pós-diastólico: postdiastolic
Pós-dicrótico: postdicrotic
Pós-diftérítico: postdiphtheritic
Pós-dormital: postdormital
Pós-dórmito: postdormitum
Pós-douração: aftergilding
Pós-ductal: postductal
Pós-encefalítico: postencephalitic
Pós-epiléptico: postepileptic
Pós-escapular: postscapular
Pós-escarlatina: postscarlatinal
Pós-esfígmico: postsphygmic
Pós-esofágico: postesophageal
Pós-esplênico: postsplenic
Pós-estro: postestrus, postestrum
Pós-faríngeo: postpharyngeal
Pós-febril: postfebrile
Pós-ganglionar: postganglionic
Pós-hemiplégico: posthemiplegic
Pós-hemorrágico: posthemorrhagic
Pós-hepático: posthepatic
Pós-hióide: posthyoid
Pós-hipnótico: posthypnotic
Posição: lie, position
Posição anormal: malposition
Posicionador: positioner

Pós-ictal: postictal
Pós-imagem: afterimage
Pós-impressão: afterimpression
Pós-influenza: postinfluenzal
Pós-isquiático: postischial
Positivo: positive
Pósitron: positron (β^+)
Pós-maduro: postmature
Pós-malárico: postmalarial
Pós-mastóide: postmastoid
Pós-mediano: postmedian
Pós-mediastinal: postmediastinal
Pós-mediastino: postmediastinum
Pós-menopausa: postmenopausal
Pós-mínimo: postminimus
Pós-movimento: aftermovement
Pós-nasal: postnasal
Pós-natal: postnatal
Pós-necrótico: postnecrotic
Pós-neurítico: postneuritic
Pós-ocular: postocular
Posologia: posology
Posológico: posologic
Pós-operatório: postoperative
Pós-oral: postoral
Pós-orbital: postorbital
Pós-palatino: postpalatine
Pós-paralítico: postparalytic
Pós-parto: postpartum
Pós-percepção: afterperception
Pós-picnótico: postpyknotic
Pós-pneumônico: postpneumonic
Pós-potencial: afterpotential
Pós-prandial: postprandial
Pós-puberal: postpuberal, postpubertal
Pós-puberdade: postpuberty
Pós-pubescente: postpubescent
Pós-rolândico: postrolandic
Pós-sacral: postsacral
Pós-sináptico: postsynaptic
Pós-tarsal: posttarsal
Póstero-anterior: posteroanterior
Póstero-externo: posteroexternal
Póstero-interno: posterointernal
Póstero-lateral: posterolateral
Póstero-medial: posteromedial
Póstero-mediano: posteromedian
Póstero-oclusão: posteroclusion
Póstero-parietal: posteroparietal
Póstero-superior: posterosuperior
Póstero-temporal: posterotemporal
Postetomia: posthetomy
Pós-tibial: posttibial
Pós-tifóide: posttyphoid
Postioplastia: posthioplasty
Postite: posthitis
Postólito: postholith
Pós-tradução: posttranslational
Pós-transcricional: posttranscriptional
Pós-transverso: posttransverse
Pós-traumático: posttraumatic

Postulado: postulate
Postura: posture
Postural: postural
Posturografia: posturography
Pós-ulnar: postcubital
Pós-uterino: postuterine
Pós-vacinal: postvaccinal
Pós-valvar, pós-valvular: postvalvar, postvalvular
Potamofobia: potamophobia
Potassa: potash
Potássico: potassic
Potássio: kalium (K), potassium (K)
Potássio-39: potassium-39 (^{39}K)
Potássio-40: potassium-40 (^{40}K)
Potássio-42: potassium-42 (^{42}K)
Potássio-43: potassium-43 (^{43}K)
Potável: potable
Potência: potency, power
Potencial: potential
Potencialização: potentiation
Potencializador: potentiator
Potencializador B da bradicinina: bradykinin potentiator B
Potenciômetro: potentiometer
Potente: potent
Poundal: poundal
Povidona: povidone
Povidona-iodo: povidone-iodine
Poxvírus: poxvirus
Pragmática: pragmatics
Pragmatismo: pragmatism
2-pralidoxima: 2-pralidoxime (2-PAM)
Prancheta: planchet
Prandial: prandial
Prantear: mourn
Praseodímio: praseodymium (Pr)
Prata: argentum, **gen.** argenti, silver (Ag)
Prateleira: ledge, shelf
Prática: practice
Prato: dish
Pravastatina: pravastatin
Praxiologia: praxiology
Práxis: praxis
Prazepam: prazepam
Praziquantel: praziquantel
Pré-agônico: preagonal
Pré-albumina: prealbumin
Pré-anal: preanal
Pré-anestésico: preanesthetic
Pré-anti-séptico: preantiseptic
Pré-aórtico: preaortic
Pré-asséptico: preaseptic
Pré-auricular: preauricular
Pré-axial: preaxial
Pré-calciferol: precalciferol
Pré-calicreína: prekallikrein
Pré-câncer: precancer
Pré-canceroso: precancerous
Pré-capilar: precapillary
Pré-cardíaco: precardiac
Pré-cardinal: precardinal
Pré-carga: preload
Pré-cartilagem: precartilage
Precauções: precautions
Precauções Universais: Universal Precautions

Pré-central: precentral
Precipitação: precipitation
Precipitante: precipitant
Precipitar: precipitate
Precipitável: precipitable
Precipitina: precipitin
Precipitinogênio: precipitinogen, precipitogen
Precipitinogenóide: precipitinogenoid
Precipitóforo: precipitophore
Precipitóide: precipitoid
Precisão: precision
Pré-clínico: preclinical
Precoce: precocious
Precocidade: precocity
Precognição: precognition
Pré-consciência: foreconscious
Pré-consciente: preconscious
Pré-convulsivo: preconvulsive
Pré-cordal: prechordal
Precordial: precordial
Precordialgia: precordialgia
Precórdio: antecardium, precordium
Precórdios: precordia
Pré-costal: precostal
Pré-crítico: precritical
Pré-cromagem: prechroming
Pré-cuneal: precuneal
Pré-cúneo: precuneus
Precursor: precursor
Precursor da angiotensina: angiotensin precursor
Pré-dentina: predentin
Pré-diabetes: prediabetes
Pré-diástole: prediastole
Pré-diastólico: prediastolic
Pré-dicrótico: predicrotic
Pré-digestão: predigestion
Predispor: predispose
Predisposição: predisposition
Prednilideno: prednylidene
Prednisolona: prednisolone
Prednisona: prednisone
Pré-ductal: preductal
Pré-eclâmpsia: preeclampsia
Preensão: prehension
Preênsil: prehensile
Pré-epiglótico: preepiglottic
Pré-eruptivo: preeruptive
Pré-esfenóide: presphenoid
Pré-esfígmico: presphygmic
Pré-espinal: prespinal
Pré-espondilolistese: prespondylolisthesis
Pré-esterno: presternum
Pré-excitação: preexcitation
Preferência sexual: sexual preference
Pré-formação: preformation
Pré-frontal: prefrontal
Prega: crease, fold, plica, **gen. e pl.** plicae
Prega de Sydney: Sydney crease
Pré-ganglionar: preganglionic
Pregnanediol: pregnanediol
Pregnanediona: pregnanedione
Pregnanetriol: pregnanetriol
Pregnano: pregnane

Pregneninolona: pregneninolone
Pregneno: pregnene
Pregnenolona: pregnenolone
Pregueado: plicate
Pré-hálux: prehallux
Pré-helicino: prehelicine
Pré-hióide: prehyoid
Pré-hormônio: prehormone
Pré-ictal: preictal
Pré-indução: preinduction
Pré-lacrimal: prelacrimal
Pré-laríngeo: prelaryngeal
Pré-leptóteno: preleptotene
Pré-leucemia: preleukemia
Pré-límbico: prelimbic
Preliminares: foreplay
Prelúdio: forepleasure
Pré-maligno: premalignant
Pré-maníaco: premaniacal
Prematuridade: prematurity
Prematuro: premature
Pré-maxila: premaxilla
Pré-maxilar: premaxillary
Pré-medicação: premedication
Pré-melanossoma: premelanosome
Pré-menstrual: premenstrual
Pré-mieloblasto: premyeloblast
Pré-mielócito: premyelocyte
Pré-mitocôndria: premitochondria
Pré-molar: premolar
Pré-monócito: premonocyte
Pré-mórbido: premorbid
Premunição: premunition
Premunitivo: premunitive
Pré-narina: prenaris, **pl.** prenares
Pré-natal: antenatal, prenatal
Pré-neoplásico: preneoplastic
Prenil: prenyl
Prenilação: prenylation
Prenilamina: prenylamine
Pré-operatório: preoperative
Pré-óptico: preoptic
Pré-oral: preoral
Pré-osteoblasto: preosteoblast
Pré-oxigenação: preoxygenation
Pré-palatino: prepalatal
Preparo: preparation
Pré-parturiente: preparturient
Pré-patelar: prepatellar
Pré-peritoneal: preperitoneal
Pré-pilórico: prepyloric
Pré-placentário: preplacental
Preponderância: preponderance
Pré-potencial: prepotential
Pré-pró-colágeno: preprocollagen
Pré-pró-insulina: preproinsulin
Pré-pró-proteína: preproprotein
Pré-proteína: preprotein
Pré-psicótico: prepsychotic
Pré-púbere: prepuberal, prepubertal
Pré-pubescente: prepubescent
Prepucial: preputial
Prepúcio: foreskin, prepuce, preputium, **pl.** preputia
Prepuciotomia: preputiotomy

Pré-reduzido: prereduced
Pré-renal: prerenal
Pré-retal: prerectal
Pré-retiniano: preretinal
Presa: fang
Pré-sacral: presacral
Presbiacusia: presbyacousia, presbyacusis, presbyacusia, presbycusis
Presbiastasia: presbyastasis
Presbiatria: presbyatrics
Presbiopia: presbyopia (Pr)
Presbiópico: presbyopic
Prescrever: prescribe
Prescrição: prescription
Pré-senil: presenile
Pré-senilidade: presenility
Preservativo: condom
Pré-sináptico: presynaptic
Pré-sístole: presystole
Pré-sistólico: presystolic
Pré-somito: presomite
Pressão: pressure (P, *P*)
Pressão sanguínea: piesis
Pressor: pressor
Pressorreceptivo: pressoreceptive, pressosensitive
Pressorreceptor: pressoreceptor
Pressossensibilidade: pressosensitivity
Pré-supurativo: presuppurative
Pré-tarsal: pretarsal
Pré-tectal: pretecta
Pré-teto: pretectum
Pré-tibial: pretibial
Pré-timpânico: pretympanic
Pré-tireóideo: prethyroid, prethyroideal, prethyroidean
Pré-traqueal: pretracheal
Pré-tremático: pretrematic
Prevalência: prevalence
Preventivo: preventive
Pré-vertebral: prevertebral
Pré-vesical: prevesical
Pré-zona: prezone
Priapismo: priapism
Príapo: priapus
Primário: primal, primary
Primase: dnaG, primase
Primata: primate
Primazia: primacy
Primeiro: primus
Primeiros socorros: first aid
Primidona: primidone
Primigrávida: primigravida
Primípara: primipara, primiparous
Primiparidade: primiparity
Primitivo: primitive
Primito: primite
Primordial: primordial
Primórdio: anlage, **pl.** anlagen, primordium
Primossoma: primosome
Prímula: primula
Primulina: primulin
Principal: princeps, **pl.** principes
Princípio: principle
Príon: prion
Prisma: prism, prisma, **pl.** prismata

Prismático: prismatic
Privação: deprivation
Privacidade: privacy
Pró-acelerina: proaccelerin
Pró-acrosina: proacrosin
Pró-acrossômico: proacrosomal
Proal: proal
Pró-âmnion: proamnion
Pró-ativador: proactivator
Probabilidade: likelihood, probability (P)
Pró-bacteriófago: probacteriophage
Probando: proband, propositus, **pl.** propositi
Probenecida: probenecid
Probilifuscinas: probilifuscins
Probiose: probiosis
Probiótico: probiotic
Problema: problem
Probóscide: proboscis, **pl.** proboscides, proboscises
Probucol: probucol
Procapsídeo: procapsid
Procarboxipeptidase: procarboxypeptidase
Pró-carcinógenos: procarcinogens
Procariota: procaryote, prokaryote
Procariótico: procaryotic, prokaryotic
Procatarse: procatarxis
Procatártico: procatarctic
Procedimento: procedure
Procedimento de Damus-Kaye-Stancel: Damus-Kaye-Stancel procedure
Procefálico: procephalic
Procélico: procelous
Procentríolo: procentriole
Procercóide: procercoid
Processador: processor
Processamento: processing
Processo: process, processus, **pl.** processus
Processamento de dados ou informações: data processing
Processo lenticular da bigorna: orbiculare
Processo xifóide: metasternum
Procidência: procidentia
Proclorperazina: prochlorperazine
Pró-colágeno: procollagen
Procondral: prochondral
Pró-convertina: proconvertin
Procordal: prochordal
Procriação: procreation
Procriador: procreative
Procriar: procreate
Proctalgia: proctalgia
Proctatresia: proctatresia
Proctectasia: proctectasia
Proctectomia: proctectomy
Proctite: proctitis
Proctocele: proctocele
Proctocistocele: proctocystocele
Proctocistoplastia: proctocystoplasty

Proctocistotomia: proctocystotomy
Proctoclise: proctoclysis
Proctococcipexia: proctococcypexy
Proctocolectomia: proctocolectomy
Proctocolite: proctocolitis
Proctocolonoscopia: proctocolonoscopy
Proctocolpoplastia: proctocolpoplasty
Proctodeal: proctodeal
Proctodinia: proctodynia
Proctódio: proctodeum, **pl.** proctodea
Proctoespasmo: proctospasm
Proctoestenose: proctostenosis
Proctofobia: proctophobia
Proctologia: proctology
Proctológico: proctologic
Proctologista: proctologist
Proctoparalisia: proctoparalysis
Proctoperineoplasias: proctoperineoplasty
Proctopexia: proctopexy
Proctoplastia: proctoplasty
Proctoplegia: proctoplegia
Proctopólipo: proctopolypus
Proctoptose: proctoptosia, proctoptosis
Proctorrafia: proctorrhaphy
Proctorragia: proctorrhagia
Proctorréia: proctorrhea
Proctoscopia: proctoscopy
Proctoscópio: proctoscope
Proctossigmóide: proctosigmoid
Proctossigmoidectomia: proctosigmoidectomy
Proctossigmoidite: proctosigmoiditis
Proctossigmoidoscopia: proctosigmoidoscopy
Proctossigmoidoscópio: proctosigmoidoscope
Proctostasia: proctostasis
Proctostato: proctostat
Proctostomia: proctostomy
Proctotomia: proctotomy
Proctótomo: proctotome
Proctotresia: proctotresia
Proctovalvotomia: proctovalvotomy
Procumbente: procumbent
Procurvação: procurvation
Prodigiosina: prodigiosin
Pró-droga: prodrug
Prodrômico: prodromal, prodromic, prodromous, proemial
Pródromo: prodrome, prodromus, **pl.** prodromi
Produtivo: productive
Produto: product
Pró-elastase: proelastase
Proeminência: hillock, prominence, prominentia, **pl.** prominentiae
Proeminente: prominens
Proencefalina: proenkephalin
Proenzima: proenzyme

Proeritroblasto: proerythroblast
Proeritrócito: proerythrocyte
Proescólex: proscolex
Proestro: proestrum, proestrus
Proestrogênio: proestrogen
Profago: prophage
Prófase: prophase
Pró-fibrinolisina: profibrinolysin
Profilactina: profilactin
Profilático: prophylactic
Profilaxia: prophylaxis, **pl.** prophylaxes
Profilina: profilin
Profilômetro: profilometer
Profissional: practitioner
Proformifeno: proformiphen
Profunda: profunda
Profundidade: depth
Profundo: deep, profundus
Profusão: profusion
Progabida: progabide
Progastrina: progastrin
Progênie: progeny
Progenital: progenitalis
Progenitor: progenitor
Progeria: progeria
Progestacional: progestational
Progesterona: progesterone
Progestina: progestin
Progestógeno: progestogen
Proglote: proglottid, proglottis, **pl.** proglottides
Prognatia: progenia
Prognático: prognathic, prognathous
Prognatismo: prognathism
Prognosticador: prognostician
Prognosticar: prognose, prognosticate
Prognóstico: prognosis, prognostic
Progonoma: progonoma
Prógrado: prograde
Programa: program
Programação: programming
Progranulócito: progranulocyte
Progressivo: progressive
Progresso: progress
Pró-hormônio: prohormone
Pró-insulina: proinsulin
Projeção: projection
Projeto Genoma Humano: Human Genome Initiative, Human Genome Project
Prolabial: prolabial
Prolábio: prolabium
Prolactina: prolactin (PRL)
Prolactinoma: prolactinoma
Prolaminas: prolamines
Prolapsar: prolapse
Prolectivo: prolective
Prolepse: prolepsis
Proléptico: proleptic
Proleucócito: proleukocyte
Prolidase: prolidase
Proliferação: proliferation
Proliferar: proliferate
Proliferativo: proliferative, proliferous
Prolífico: prolific

Prolígero: proligerous
Prolil: prolyl (Pro, prolyl)
Prolilglicina dipeptidase: prolylglycine dipeptidase
Prolina: proline (Pro)
Prolinase: prolinase
Promastigota: promastigote
Promécio: promethium (Pm)
Promegaloblasto: promegaloblast
Prometáfase: prometaphase
Promielócito: promyelocyte
Promitocôndria: promitochondria
Promoção: promotion
Promonócito: promonocyte
Promontório: promontorium, **pl.** promontoria; promontory
Promotor: promoter
Pronação: pronation
Pronador: pronator
Pronar: pronate
Pronefro: forekidney, pronephros, **pl.** pronephroi
Proninfa: protonymph
Prono: prone
Pronógrado: pronograde
Pronômetro: pronometer
Pronormoblasto: pronormoblast
Prontuário: record
Pronúcleo: pronucleus, **pl.** pronuclei
Pró-opiomelanocortina: proopiomelanocortin (POMC)
Pró-ótico: prootic
Pró-oxidantes: pro-oxidants
Propafenona: propafenone
Propagação: propagation
Propagar: propagate
Propagativo: propagative
Propalinal: propalinal
Propamidina: propamidine
Propanidida: propanidid
Propano: propane
Propanoíla: propanoyl
Propanol: propanol
1,2,3-propanotriol: 1,2,3-propanetriol
Propenil: propenyl
Propeno: propene
Propenso a acidentes: accident-prone
Propepsina: propepsin
Propeptona: propeptone
Properdina: properdin
Properitoneal: properitoneal
Propicilina: propicillin
Propil: propyl (Pr)
Propilcarbinol: propylcarbinol
Propileno: propylene
Propilexedrina: propylhexedrine
Propiliodona: propyliodone
Propilparabeno: propylparaben
Propiltiouracil: propylthiouracil (PTU)
Propiocortina: propiocortin
Propiolactona: propiolactone
Propionato: propionate
Propionato de clobetasol: clobetasol propionate

Propionato de dromostanolona: dromostanolone propionate
Propionil: propionyl
Propionil-CoA: propionyl-CoA
Propionilglicina: propionylglycine
Propiromazina: propyromazine
Proplasia: proplasia
Proplasmócito: proplasmacyte
Propofol: propofol
Próprio: self
Propriocepção: proprioception
Proprioceptivo: proprioceptive
Proprioceptor: proprioceptor
Propriospinal: propriospinal
Proproteínas: proproteins
Proptômetro: proptometer
Proptose: proptosis
Proptótico: proptotic
Propulsão: propulsion
Proquilia: procheilia, prochilia
Proquimosina: prochymosin
Proquiral: prochiral
Proquiralidade: prochirality
Pró-renina: prorennin
Pró-rubricito: prorubricyte
Proscilaridina: proscillaridin
Pró-secretina: prosecretin
Prosencéfalo: forebrain, proencephalon, prosencephalon
Prosodêmico: prosodemic
Prosódia: prosody
Prosopagnosia: prosopagnosia
Prosópago: prosopagus, prosopopagus
Prosopectasia: prosopectasia
Prosoplasia: prosoplasia
Prosopoanosquise: prosopoanoschisis
Prosoposquise: prosoposchisis
Prosopotoracópago: prosopothoracopagus
Prostaciclina: prostacyclin
Prostaglandina: prostaglandin (PG)
Prostanóides: prostanoids
Próstata: prostata, prostate
Prostatalgia: prostatalgia
Prostatectomia: prostatectomy
Prostático: prostatic
Prostaticovesical: prostaticovesical
Prostatismo: prostatism
Prostatite: prostatitis
Prostatocistite: prostatocystitis
Prostatodinia: prostatodynia
Prostatólito: prostatolith
Prostatolitotomia: prostatolithotomy
Prostatomegalia: prostatomegaly
Prostatorréia: prostatorrhea
Prostatotomia: prostatomy, prostatotomy
Prostatovesiculectomia: prostatoseminalvesiculectomy, prostatovesiculectomy
Prostatovesiculite: prostatovesiculitis
Prosternação: prosternation

Próstio: prostheon, prosthion
Prostoceratoplastia: prosthokeratoplasty
Prostodontia: prosthodontia, prosthodontics
Prostodontista: prosthodontist
Prostração: prostration
Protactínio: proactinium, protactinium (Pa)
Protalbumose: protalbumose
Protamina: protamine
Protaminase: protaminase
Protanomalia: protanomaly
Protanopia: protanopia
Protease: protease
Proteção: protection
Proteína: protein (p)
Proteináceo: proteinaceous
Proteinase: proteinase
Proteinogênico: proteinogenic
Proteinóides: proteinoids
Proteinose: proteinosis
Proteinúria: proteinuria
Proteoclástico: proteoclastic
Proteogênico: proteogenic
Proteoglicano I: proteoglycan I
Proteoglicanos: proteoglycans
Proteolipídios: proteolipids
Proteólise: proteolysis
Proteolítico: proteolytic
Proteometabólico: proteometabolic
Proteometabolismo: proteometabolism
Proteopepsia: proteopepsis
Proteopético: proteopectic, proteopexic
Proteopexia: proteopexis
Proteose: proteose
Proteossoma: proteosome
Prótese: prosthesis, **pl.** prostheses
Prótese dentária híbrida: overdenture
Prótese simples: pylon
Protético: denturist, prosthetic, prosthetist
Protetor: protector
Protetor de boca: mouth guard
Protetor solar: sunscreen
Prótio: protium
Protipendil: prothipendyl
Protirelina: protirelin
Protista: protist
Proto-actínio: protoactinium
Protoalbumose: protoalbumose
Protoalcalóide: protoalkaloid
Protobiologia: protobiology
Protocolo: protocol
Protocone: protocone
Protoconídeo: protoconid
Protocoproporfiria: protocoproporphyria
Protoderma: protoderm
Protodiastólico: protodiastolic
Protoduodeno: protoduodenum
Protoeritrócito: protoerythrocyte
Protoesporo: protospore
Protofilamento: protofilament

Protogonoplasma: protogonoplasm
Protoleucócito: protoleukocyte
Protolisado: protolysate
Protomérito: primerite
Protomerito: protomerite
Protômero: protomer
Protometrócito: protometrocyte
Próton: proton (p)
Protoncogene: protooncogene
Protoneurônio: protoneuron
Protopático: protopathic
Protopectina: protopectin
Protopianoma: protopianoma
Protoplasma: protoplasm
Protoplasmático, protoplásmico: protoplasmatic, protoplasmic
Protoplasmólise: protoplasmolysis
Protoplasto: protoplast
Protoporfiria: protoporphyria
Protoporfirina férrica: ferriprotoporphyrin
Protoporfirina ferrosa: ferroprotoporphyrin
Protoporfirina tipo III: protoporphyrin type III
Protoporfirinogênio tipo III: protoporphyrinogen type III
Protoproteose: protoproteose
Protossal: protosalt
Protossulfato: protosulfate
Protostoma: protostoma, protostome
Prototáxico: prototaxic
Prototecose: protothecosis
Protótipo: prototype
Prototrófico: prototrophic
Prototrofismo: prototrophism
Prototrofo: prototroph
Protoveratrina A e B: protoveratrine A and B
Protovértebra: protovertebra
Protovertebral: protovertebral
Protóxido: protoxide
Protozoário: protozoal, protozoan, protozoon, **pl.** protozoa
Protozoíase: protozoiasis
Protozoicida: protozoicide
Protozoófago: protozoophage
Protozoologia: protozoology
Protozoólogo: protozoologist
Protração: protraction
Protrair: protrude
Protrator: protractor
Protrombase: prothrombase
Protrombina: prothrombin
Protrombinase: prothrombinase
Protrombinogênio: prothrombinogen
Protrombinopenia: prothrombinopenia
Protrombocinase: prothrombokinase
Protrusão: protrusion
Protrusão do acetábulo: protrusio acetabuli

Protuberância: protuberance, protuberantia
Pró-uroquinase: prourokinase
Prova de Chick-Martin: Chick-Martin test
Prova delta: Δ check
Provértebra: provertebra
Provírus: provirus
Provitamina: provitamin
Proxêmica: proxemics
Proximal: mesial, proximad, proximal, proximalis
Próximo: proximate
Proximoataxia: proximoataxia
Proximobucal: proximobuccal
Proximolabial: proximolabial
Proximolingual: proximolingual
Prozigose: prozygosis
Prozona: prozone
Prurido: itch, itching, pruritus
Pruriginoso: pruritic
Prurigo: prurigo
Prussiato: prussiate
Psamocarcinoma: psammocarcinoma
Psamoma: psammoma
Psamomatoso: psammomatous
Pselismo: psellism
Pseudacromegalia: pseudacromegaly
Pseudagrafia: pseudagraphia
Pseudalesqueríase: pseudallescheriasis
Pseudartrose: pseudarthrosis
Pseudestesia: pseudoesthesia
Pseudo-acantose nigricante: pseudoacanthosis nigricans
Pseudo-acéfalo: pseudoacephalus
Pseudo-acondroplasia: pseudoachondroplasia
Pseudo-actinomicose: pseudoactinomycosis
Pseudo-aglutinação: pseudoagglutination
Pseudo-agrafia: pseudoagraphia
Pseudo-agramatismo: pseudoagrammatism
Pseudo-ainhum: pseudo-ainhum
Pseudo-albuminúria: pseudalbuminuria, pseudoalbuminuria
Pseudo-alcalóides: pseudoalkaloids
Pseudo-alélico: pseudoallelic
Pseudo-alelismo: pseudoallelism
Pseudo-alopecia areata: pseudo-alopecia areata
Pseudo-anafilático: pseudoanaphylactic
Pseudo-anafilaxia: pseudoanaphylaxis
Pseudo-anemia: pseudoanemia
Pseudo-aneurisma: pseudoaneurysm
Pseudo-angina: pseudangina, pseudoangina
Pseudo-anodontia: pseudoanodontia

Pseudo-anquilose: pseudankylosis
Pseudo-apendicite: pseudoappendicitis
Pseudo-apraxia: pseudoapraxia
Pseudo-artrose: pseudoarthrosis
Pseudo-autenticidade: pseudoauthenticity
Pseudobacilo: pseudobacillus
Pseudobactéria: pseudobacterium
Pseudobolsa: pseudopocket
Pseudobulbar: pseudobulbar
Pseudocancro: pseudochancre
Pseudocartilagem: pseudocartilage
Pseudocartilaginoso: pseudocartilaginous
Pseudocefalocele: pseudocephalocele
Pseudocele: pseudocele
Pseudoceloma: pseudocelom
Pseudociese: pseudocyesis
Pseudocilindro: pseudocast
Pseudocilindróide: pseudocylindroid
Pseudocirrose: pseudocirrhosis
Pseudocisto: pseudocyst
Pseudoclônus: pseudoclonus
Pseudocoarctação: pseudocoarctation
Pseudocolinesterase: pseudocholinesterase
Pseudocolóide: pseudocolloid
Pseudocolusão: pseudocollusion
Pseudocoma: pseudocoma
Pseudoconvulsão: pseudoseizure
Pseudocoréia: pseudochorea
Pseudocoxalgia: pseudocoxalgia
Pseudocriptorquismo: pseudocryptorchism
Pseudocrise: pseudocrisis
Pseudocromestesia: pseudochromesthesia
Pseudocromidrose: pseudochromidrosis, pseudochromhidrosis
Pseudocrupe: pseudocroup
Pseudocumeno: pseudocumene
Pseudocumol: pseudocumol
Pseudodeciduose: pseudodeciduosis
Pseudodemência: pseudodementia
Pseudodextrocardia: pseudodextrocardia
Pseudodiabetes: pseudodiabetes
Pseudodiastólico: pseudodiastolic
Pseudodifteria: pseudodiphtheria
Pseudodigitoxina: pseudodigitoxin
Pseudodipsia: pseudodipsia
Pseudodisenteria: pseudodysentery
Pseudodivertículo: pseudodiverticulum
Pseudodominância: pseudodominance

Pseudodominante: quasidominant
Pseudo-erisipela: pseudoerysipelas
Pseudo-escarlatina: pseudoscarlatina
Pseudo-esclerose: pseudosclerosis
Pseudo-esfoliação: pseudoexfoliation
Pseudo-estesia: pseudesthesia
Pseudo-estrabismo: pseudostrabismus
Pseudofacodonese: pseudophakodonesis
Pseudofacos: pseudophacos
Pseudofaquia: pseudophakia
Pseudofilídeo: pseudophyllid
Pseudoflutuação: pseudofluctuation
Pseudofoliculite: pseudofolliculitis
Pseudofotestesia: pseudophotesthesia
Pseudofratura: pseudofracture
Pseudofrutose: pseudofructose, psicose
Pseudogânglio: pseudoganglion
Pseudogene: pseudogene
Pseudogeusestesia: pseudogeusesthesia
Pseudogeusia: pseudogeusia
Pseudoginecomastia: pseudogynecomastia
Pseudoglioma: pseudoglioma
Pseudoglobulina: pseudoglobulin
Pseudoglomérulo: pseudoglomerulus
Pseudoglucosazona: pseudoglucosazone
Pseudogota: pseudogout
Pseudogravidez: pseudopregnancy
Pseudo-helminto: pseudelminth
Pseudo-hematúria: pseudohematuria
Pseudo-hemoptise: pseudohemoptysis
Pseudo-hermafrodita: pseudohermaphrodite
Pseudo-hermafroditismo: pseudohermaphroditism
Pseudo-hérnia: pseudohernia
Pseudo-heterotopia: pseudoheterotopia
Pseudo-hidrocefalia: pseudohydrocephaly
Pseudo-hidronefrose: pseudohydronephrosis
Pseudo-hifa: pseudohypha
Pseudo-hipercalemia: pseudohyperkalemia
Pseudo-hiperparatireoidismo: pseudohyperparathyroidism
Pseudo-hipertelorismo: pseudohypertelorism
Pseudo-hipertrofia: pseudohypertrophy
Pseudo-hipertrófico: pseudohypertrophic

Pseudo-hiponatremia: pseudohyponatremia
Pseudo-hipoparatireoidismo: pseudohypoparathyroidism
Pseudo-icterícia: pseudoicterus, pseudojaundice
Pseudo-íleo: pseudoileus
Pseudo-infarto: pseudoinfarction
Pseudo-*influenza*: pseudoinfluenza
Pseudo-intraligamentar: pseudointraligamentous
Pseudo-isocromático: pseudoisochromatic
Pseudo-isoenzimas: pseudoisoenzymes
Pseudolêndea: pseudonit
Pseudolinfócito: pseudolymphocyte
Pseudolinfoma: pseudolymphoma
Pseudolipoma: pseudolipoma
Pseudolisogenia: pseudolysogeny
Pseudolisogênico: pseudolysogenic
Pseudolitíase: pseudolithiasis
Pseudologia: pseudologia
Pseudomalignidade: pseudomalignancy
Pseudomama: pseudomamma
Pseudomania: pseudomania
Pseudomasturbação: pseudomasturbation
Pseudomegacolo: pseudomegacolon
Pseudomelanose: pseudomelanosis
Pseudomembrana: pseudomembrane
Pseudomeningite: pseudomeningitis
Pseudomenstruação: pseudomenstruation
Pseudometaplasia: pseudometaplasia
Pseudomicélio: pseudomycelium
Pseudomiopia: pseudomyopia
Pseudomixoma: pseudomyxoma
Pseudomnésia: pseudomnesia
Pseudomônada: pseudomonad
Pseudomoniletrix: pseudomonilethrix
Pseudomonomolecular: pseudomonomolecular
Pseudomorfo: pseudomorph
Pseudomormo: pseudoglanders
Pseudonarcótico: pseudonarcotic
Pseudoneoplasia: pseudoneoplasm
Pseudoneuroma: pseudoneuroma
Pseudo-osteomalacia: pseudo-osteomalacia
Pseudo-osteomalácico: pseudo-osteomalacic
Pseudopapiledema: pseudopapilledema

Pseudoparalisia: pseudoparalysis
Pseudoparaplegia: pseudoparaplegia
Pseudoparasita: pseudoparasite
Pseudoparênquima: pseudoparenchyma
Pseudoparesia: pseudoparesis
Pseudopelada: pseudopelade
Pseudopericardite: pseudopericarditis
Pseudoperoxidase: pseudoperoxidase
Pseudoplaqueta: pseudoplatelet
Pseudópode: pseudopod, pseudopodium, **pl.** pseudopodia
Pseudopolidistrofia: pseudopolydystrophy
Pseudopólipo: pseudopolyp
Pseudoporfiria: pseudoporphyria
Pseudoprognatismo: pseudoprognathism
Pseudopterígio: pseudopterygium
Pseudoptose: pseudoptosis
Pseudopuberdade: pseudopuberty
Pseudoqueratina: pseudokeratin
Pseudoquiloso: pseudochylous
Pseudo-raquitismo: pseudorickets
Pseudo-reação: pseudoreaction
Pseudo-réplica: pseudoreplica
Pseudo-retinite pigmentosa: pseudoretinitis pigmentosa
Pseudo-reumatismo: pseudorheumatism
Pseudo-roseta: pseudorosette
Pseudo-rubéola: pseudorubella
Pseudo-sarcoma: pseudosarcoma
Pseudosmia: pseudosmia
Pseudostoma: pseudostoma
Pseudotabes: pseudotabes
Pseudotronco arterial: pseudotruncus arteriosus
Pseudotubérculo: pseudotubercle
Pseudotuberculose: pseudotuberculosis
Pseudotumor: pseudotumor
Pseudo-unimolecular: pseudounimolecular
Pseudo-uridina: pseudouridine (Ψ, Q)
Pseudovacúolo: pseudovacuole
Pseudovaríola: pseudosmallpox, pseudovariola
Pseudovitamina: pseudovitamin
Pseudovômito: pseudovomiting
Pseudoxantoma elástico: pseudoxanthoma elasticum
Psi: psi
Psicalgia: psychalgalia, psychalgia
Psicanálise: psychoanalysis
Psicanalista: psychoanalyst
Psicanalítico: psychoanalytic
Psicanopsia: psychanopsia
Psicataxia: psychataxia

Psicoacústica: psychoacoustics
Psicoalergia: psychoallergy
Psicoativo: psychoactive
Psicoauditivo: psychoauditory
Psicobiologia: psychobiology
Psicocatarse: psychocatharsis
Psicocinese, psicocinesia: psychokinesis, psychokinesia
Psicocirurgia: psychosurgery
Psicocromestesia: psychochromesthesia
Psicocromo: psychochrome
Psicodélico: psychedelic
Psicodiagnóstico: psychodiagnosis
Psicodinâmica: psychodynamics
Psicodometria: psychodometry
Psicodrama: psychodrama
Psicoendocrinologia: psychoendocrinology
Psicoestimulante: psychormic, psychostimulant
Psicoexploração: psychoexploration
Psicofarmacologia: psychopharmacology
Psicofármacos: psychopharmaceuticals
Psicofísica: psychophysics
Psicofísico: psychophysical
Psicofisiologia: psychophysiology
Psicofisiológico: psychophysiologic
Psicogalvânico: psychogalvanic
Psicogalvanômetro: psychogalvanometer
Psicogênese: psychogenesis
Psicogenia: psychogeny
Psicogênico, psicogenético: psychogenic, psychogenetic
Psicogêusico: psychogeusic
Psicogógico: psychogogic
Psicografia: psychography
Psicográfico: psychographic
Psico-história: psychohistory
Psicolingüística: psycholinguistics
Psicologia: psychology
Psicologia médica: medicopsychology
Psicológico: psychologic, psychological
Psicólogo: psychologist
Psicometria: psychometrics, psychometry
Psicomotor: psychomotor
Psiconeuroimunologia: psychoneuroimmunology
Psiconeurose: psychoneurosis
Psiconeurótico: psychoneurotic
Psiconocivo: psychonoxious
Psiconomia: psychonomy
Psiconômico: psychonomic
Psiconosologia: psychonosology
Psico-oncologia: psycho-oncology
Psicopata: psychopath
Psicopatia: psychopathy
Psicopático: psychopathic

Glossário

Psicopatologia: psychopathology
Psicopatologista: psychopathologist
Psicoprofilaxia: psychoprophylaxis
Psicorrelaxamento: psychorelaxation
Psicose: psychosis, **pl.** psychoses
Psicosina: psychosine
Psicossensorial: psychosensory, psychosensorial
Psicossexual: psychosexual
Psicossíntese: psychosynthesis
Psicossocial: psychosocial
Psicossomático: psychosomatic
Psicotécnica: psychotechnics
Psicoterapeuta: psychotherapist
Psicoterapêutica: psychotherapeutics
Psicoterapêutico: psychotherapeutic
Psicoterapia: psychotherapy
Psicótico: psychotic
Psicotogênico: psychotogenic
Psicotógeno: psychotogen
Psicotomimético: psychosomimetic, psychotomimetic
Psicotrópico: psychotropic
Psicroalgia: psychroalgia
Psicroestesia: psychroesthesia
Psicrofílico: psychrophilic
Psicrófilo: psychrophile, psychrophil
Psicrofobia: psychrophobia
Psicróforo: psychrophore
Psicrometria: psychrometry
Psicrômetro: psychrometer
Psílio hidrófilo mucilóide: psyllium hydrophilic mucilloid
Psilocibina: psilocybin
Psilocina: psilocin
Psilose: psilosis
Psilótico: psilotic
Psilotina: psilothin
P-sinistrocardíaca: P-sinistrocardiale
Psique: psyche
Psiquiatra: psychiatrist
Psiquiatria: psychiatrics, psychiatry
Psiquiátrico: psychiatric
Psíquico: psychic, psychical
Psiquismo: psychism
Psitacina: psittacine
Psitacose: psittacosis
Psoas: psoas
Psomofagia: psomophagia, psomophagy
Psoraleno: psoralen
Psorenterite: psorenteritis
Psoríase: psoriasis
Psoriasiforme: psoriasiform
Psoriático: psoriatic
p-**sulfamilacetanilida:** *p*-sulfamylacetanilide
Ptármico: ptarmic
p-**terfenil:** *p*-terphenyl
Pteridina: pteridine
Pterígio: pterygium

Pterigóide: pterygoid
Pterigomandibular: pterygomandibular
Pterigomaxilar: pterygomaxillare, pterygomaxillary
Pterigopalatino: pterygopalatine
Pterina: pterin
Ptério: pterion
Pteropterina: pteropterin
Ptialagogo: ptyalagogue
Ptialectasia: ptyalectasis
Ptialina: ptyalin
Ptialismo: ptyalism
Ptialocele: ptyalocele
Ptialografia: ptyalography
Ptialolitíase: ptyalolithiasis
Ptialólito: ptyalolith
Ptialolitotomia: ptyalolithotomy
Ptiócrino: ptyocrinous
Ptomaína: ptomaine
Ptomainemia: ptomainemia
Ptomatina: ptomatine
Ptomatropina: ptomatropine
Ptose: ptosis, **pl.** ptoses
Ptótico: ptosed, ptotic
Pubarca: pubarche
Puberal: puberal, pubertal
Puberdade: puberty
Pubescência: pubescence
Pubescente: pubescent
Púbico: pubic
Pubiotomia: pubiotomy
Púbis: pubis
Pubocapsular: pubocapsular
Pubococcígeo: pubococcygeal
Pubofemoral: pubofemoral
Puboprostático: puboprostatic
Puborretal: puborectal
Pubovesical: pubovesical
Pudendo: pudendal, pudendum, **pl.** pudenda; pudic
Puérpera: puerpera, **pl.** puerperae
Puerperal: puerperal, puerperant
Puerpério: puerperium, **pl.** puerperia
Pulga: flea
Pulicida: pulicicide, pulicide
Pulmão: lung, pulmo, **gen.** pulmonis, **pl.** pulmones
Pulmólito: pulmolith
Pulmonar: pulmonary, pulmoniç
Pulpa: pulpa
Pulpalgia: pulpalgia
Pulpar: pulpal
Pulpectomia: pulpectomy
Pulpiforme: pulpiform
Pulpite: pulpitis
Pulpodontia: pulpodontia
Pulposo: pulposus, pulpy
Pulpotomia: pulpotomy
Pulsação: pulsation
Pulsador: pulsator
Pulsão: drive, pulsion
Pulsar: pulsate, throb
Pulsátil: pulsatile
Pulselo: pulsellum
Pulsímetro: pulsimeter, pulsometer
Pulso: pulse, pulsus

Pultáceo: pultaceous
Pululação: pullulation
Pululanase: pullulanase
Pulular: pullulate
Pulverização: poudrage, pulverization
Pulverizar: pulverize
Pulverulento: pulverulent
Pulvinado: pulvinate
Pulvinar: pulvinar
Punção: nyxis
Puncionar: puncture, tap
Pungente: pungent
Punho: carpus, **gen. e pl.** carpi, manchette, wrist
Puntiforme: punctiform
Pupa: pupa, **pl.** pupae
Pupila: pupil (p), pupilla, **pl.** pupillae
Pupiloestatômetro: pupillostatometer
Pupilografia: pupillography
Pupilometria: pupillometry
Pupilômetro: pupillometer
Pupilomotor: pupillomotor
Pupíparo: pupiparous
Pureza: purity
Purgação: purgation
Purgar: purge
Purgativo: purgative
Puriforme: puriform
Purina: purine (Pur)
Purinemia: purinemia
Puro: pure
Puromicina: puromycin
Púrpura: purple, purpura
Púrpura de bromocresol: bromcresol purple
Púrpura de Ruhemann: Ruhemann purple
Purpúrico: purpuric
Purpurina: purpurin
Purpurinúria: purpurinuria
Purulência: purulence, purulency
Purulento: purulent
Purulóide: puruloid
Pus: pus
Pústula: pock, pustule
Pustulação: pustulation
Pustulante: pustulant
Pustular: pustular
Pustulocrustáceo: pustulocrustaceous
Pustulose: pustulosis
Putame: putamen
Putrefação: putrefaction
Putrefativo: putrefactive
Putrefazer: putrefy
Putrescência: putrescence
Putrescente: putrescent
Putrescina: putrescine
Pútrido: putrid

Q

Qat: khat
Quadrado: quadrate
Quadrado latino: Latin square

Quadrados mínimos: least squares
Quadrangular: quadrangular
Quadrantanopsia: quadrantanopia
Quadrante: quadrant
Quadribásico: quadribasic
Quadríceps: quadriceps
Quadricepsplastia: quadricepsplasty
Quadricúspide: quadricuspid
Quadridigitado: quadridigitate
Quadrigêmeo: quadrigeminal, quadrigeminum, quadrigeminus
Quadrigeminismo: quadrigeminy
Quadril: hip
Quadriparesia: quadriparesis
Quadriplegia: quadriplegia
Quadriplégico: quadriplegic
Quadripolar: quadripolar
Quadrissecção: quadrisection
Quadrisseccionar: quadrisect, quartisect
Quadritubercular: quadritubercular
Quadrivalente: quadrivalent
Quadro: table
Quadrúpede: quadruped
Quádruplo: quadruplet
Quantil: quantile
Quantum: quantum, **pl.** quanta
Quarentena: quarantine
Quark: quark
Quartã: quartan
Quarto: quart
Quartzo: quartz
Quassação: quassation
Quássia: Picrasma, quassia
Quaternário: quaternary (Q)
Quazepam: quazepam
Quebracho: quebracho
Quebraquina: quebrachine
Queda d'água: waterfall
Queda do pé: dropfoot
Queilalgia: cheilalgia, chilalgia
Queilectomia: cheilectomy, chilectomy
Queilectropia: cheilectropion, chilectropion
Quêilion: cheilion
Queilite: cheilitis, chilitis
Queilognatoglossosquise: cheilognathoglossoschisis
Queima: fire
Queimadura solar: sunburn
Queimar: burn
Queixa: complaint
Queixo: chin
Queixoso: querulent
Quelação: chelation
Quelar: chelate
Queléctomo: kelectome
Quelícera: chelicera, **pl.** chelicerae
Quelina: khellin
Quelóide: cheloid, keloid
Queloidose: keloidosis
Quelossomia: kelosomia
Quemose: chemosis
Quemótico: chemotic

Quenodiol: chenodiol
Quenopódio: chenopodium
Queratina: keratin
Queratinases: keratinases
Queratinização: keratinization
Queratinizado: keratinized
Quercetina: quercetin
Querco: quercus
Quérion: kerion
Querosene: kerosene
Querubismo: cherubism
Questionário: questionnaire
Qui: chi
Quiasma: chiasm, chiasma, **pl.** chiasmata
Quiasmapexia: chiasmapexy
Quiasmático: chiasmatic
Quiescente: quiescent
Quiláceo: chylaqueous
Quilangioma: chylangioma
Quilemia: chylemia
Quilidrose: chylidrosis
Quilífero: chyliferous
Quilificação: chylifaction, chylification
Quilificativo: chylifactive
Quiliforme: chyliform
Quilo: chyle
Quilobase: kilobase (kb)
Quilocaloria: kilocalorie (kcal)
Quilocele: chylocele
Quilociclos: kilocycle (kc)
Quilocisto: chylocyst
Quilofagia: cheilophagia, chilophagia
Quilofórico: chylophoric
Quilognatopalatosquise: cheilognathopalatoschisis
Quilognatouranosquise: cheilognathouranoschisis
Quilograma: kilogram (kg)
Quilograma-metro: kilogram-meter
Quilohertz: kilohertz
Quilojoule: kilojoule
Quilomastigíase: chilomastigiasis
Quilomastose: chilomastosis
Quilomediastino: chylomediastinum
Quilomícron: chylomicron, **pl.** chylomicra, chylomicrons
Quilomicronemia: chylomicronemia
Quiloohm: kilohm
Quilopericárdio: chylopericardium
Quiloperitônio: chyloperitoneum
Quiloplastia: cheiloplasty
Quilopleura: chylopleura
Quilopneumotórax: chylopneumothorax
Quilopodíase: chilopodiasis
Quilopoese: chylopoiesis
Quilopoético: chylopoietic
Quilorrafia: cheilorrhaphy
Quilorréia: chylorrhea
Quilose: cheilosis, chilosis, chylosis
Quiloso: chylous

Quilotomia: cheilotomy
Quilotórax: chylothorax
Quilovolt: kilovolt (kv)
Quilovoltímetro: kilovoltmeter
Quilúria: chyluria
Quimase: chymase
Quimera: chimera
Quimérico: chimeric
Quimerismo: chimerism
Quimiatria: chemiatry
Química: chemistry
Químico: chemical, chemist
Quimificação: chymification
Quimioatrativos: chemoattractants
Quimioautotrófico: chemoautotrophic
Quimioautótrofo: chemoautotroph
Quimiobiodinâmica: chemobiodynamics
Quimiocautério: chemicocautery, chemocautery
Quimioceptor: chemoceptor
Quimiocinas: chemokines
Quimiocinese: chemokinesis
Quimiocinético: chemokinetic
Quimiocirurgia: chemosurgery
Quimiodectoma: chemodectoma
Quimiodectomatose: chemodectomatosis
Quimiodiferenciação: chemodifferentiation
Quimioesfoliação: chemexfoliation
Quimioeterotrófico: chemoheterotrophic
Quimioeterótrofo: chemoheterotroph
Quimioimunologia: chemoimmunology
Quimiólise: chemolysis
Quimiolitotrofia: chemolithotrophy
Quimiolitotrófico: chemolithotrophic
Quimiolitótrofo: chemolithotroph
Quimioluminescência: chemiluminescence, chemoluminescence
Quimionucleólise: chemonucleolysis
Quimioorganotrófico: chemoorganotrophic
Quimioorganótrofo: chemoorganotroph
Quimiopalidectomia: chemopallidectomy
Quimiopalidotalamectomia: chemopallidothalamectomy
Quimiopalidotomia: chemopallidotomy
Quimiopercepção: chemosensation
Quimioprevenção: chemoprevention
Quimioprofilaxia: chemoprophylaxis
Quimiorrecepção: chemoreception

Quimiorreceptivo: chemoreceptive
Quimiorreceptor: chemoreceptor
Quimiorreflexo: chemoreflex
Quimiorresistência: chemoresistance
Quimiorresposta: chemoresponse
Quimiosmose: chemosmosis
Quimiossensível: chemosensitive
Quimiossíntese: chemosynthesis
Quimiossoroterapia: chemoserotherapy
Quimiostato: chemostat
Quimiotalamectomia: chemothalamectomy
Quimiotalamotomia: chemothalamotomy
Quimiotático: chemotactic
Quimiotaxia: chemiotaxis, chemotaxis
Quimioterapêutica: chemotherapeutics
Quimioterapêutico: chemotherapeutic
Quimioterapia: chemotherapy
Quimiotransmissor: chemotransmitter
Quimiótrofo: chemotroph
Quimiotropismo: chemotropism
Quimo: chyme, chymus
Quimografia: kymography
Quimógrafo: kymograph
Quimograma: kymogram
Quimopapaína: chymopapain
Quimopoese: chymopoiesis
Quimorréia: chymorrhea
Quimoscópio: kymoscope
Quimosina: chymosin
Quimosinogênio: chymosinogen
Quimoso: chymous
Quimostatina: chymostatin
Quimotripsina: chymotrypsin
Quimotripsinogênio: chymotrypsinogen
Quina: quina
Quinaquina: quinaquina
Quinato: quinate
Quinazolinas: quinazolines
Quinestradiol: quinestradiol, quinestradol
Quinestrol: quinestrol
Quinetazona: quinethazone
Quinidina: quinidine
Quinidrona: quinhydrone
Quinina: quinine
Quininismo: quininism
Quiniofon: chiniofon
Quinol: quinol
Quinoleína: chinoleine
Quinolina: quinoline
Quinolinol: quinolinol
Quinolizidinas: quinolizidines
Quinologia: quinology
Quinolonas: quinolones
Quinona: quinone
Quinovose: quinovose
Qüinqüedigitado: quinquedigitate

Qüinqüetubercular: quinquetubercular
Qüinqüevalente: quinquevalent
Quinquina: quinquina
Quintã: quintan
Quíntuplo: quintuplet
Quinurrenina: kynurenine
Quinurreninase: kynureninase
Quion: kion
Qui-quadrado: chi-square
Quiralgia: cheiralgia
Quiralidade: chirality
Quirartrite: cheirarthritis, chirarthritis
Quirocinestesia: cheirokinesthesia, chirokinesthesia
Quirocinestésico: cheirokinesthetic
Quiroespasmo: cheirospasm, chirospasm
Quirognóstico: cheirognostic, chirognostic
Quirologia: cheirology, chirology
Quiromegalia: cheiromegaly, chiromegaly
Quiropodalgia: cheiropodalgia, chiropodalgia
Quiropodia: chiropody
Quiropodista: chiropodist
Quiroponfólix: cheiropompholyx, chiropompholyx
Quiroprático: chiropractic, chiropractor
Quiroscópio: chiroscope
Quisqualato: quisqualate
Quitina: chitin
Quitinase: chitinase
Quitinoso: chitinous
Quitobiose: chitobiose
Quitosamina: chitosamine
Quociente: quotient
Quotidiano: quotidian

R

Rã: frog
Rabarberona: rhabarberone
Rabditiforme: rhabditiform
Rabdócito: rhabdocyte
Rabdoesfíncter: rhabdosphincter
Rabdofobia: rhabdophobia
Rabdóide: rhabdoid
Rabdomioblasto: rhabdomyoblast
Rabdomiólise: rhabdomyolysis
Rabdomioma: rhabdomyoma
Rabdomiossarcoma: rhabdomyosarcoma
Rabdossarcoma: rhabdosarcoma
Rabdovírus: rhabdovirus
Racefemina: racefemine
Racemase: racemase
Racemato: racemate

Glossário

Racêmico: racemic (r)
Racemização: racemization
Racemoso: racemose
Racional: rational
Racionalização: rationalization
Rad: rad
Radectomia: radectomy
Radiabilidade: radiability
Radiação: radiatio, **pl.** radiationes, radiation
Radiação X: x-radiation
Radial: radial, radialis
Radiano: radian (rad)
Radiante: radiant
Radiar(-se): radiate
Radiável: radiable
Radical: radical
Radicotomia: radicotomy
Radícula: radicle, radicula
Radiculalgia: radiculalgia
Radicular: radicular
Radículas: rootlets
Radiculectomia: radiculectomy
Radiculite: radiculitis
Radiculoganglionite: radiculoganglionitis
Radiculomeningomielite: radiculomeningomyelitis
Radiculomielopatia: radiculomyelopathy
Radiculoneuropatia: radiculoneuropathy
Radiculopatia: radiculopathy
Radiectomia: radiectomy
Radífero: radiferous
Rádio: radium (Ra), radius, **gen. e pl.** radii
Radioatividade: radioactivity
Radioativo: radioactive
Radioautografia: radioautography
Radioautograma: radioautogram
Radiobicipital: radiobicipital
Radiobiologia: radiobiology
Radiocálcio: radiocalcium
Radiocarbono: radiocarbon
Radiocardiografia: radiocardiography
Radiocardiograma: radiocardiogram
Radiocarpal: radiocarpal
Radiocefalopelvimetria: radiocephalpelvimetry
Radiochumbo: radiolead
Radiocineangiocardiografia: radiocineangiocardiography
Radiocineangiografia: radiocineangiography
Radiocinematografia: radiocinematography
Radiocirurgia: radiosurgery
Radiocloro: radiochlorine
Radiocobalto: radiocobalt
Radiocolangiografia: radiocholangiography
Radiocolecistografia: radiocholecystography
Radiocurável: radiocurable
Radiodensidade: radiodensity
Radiodenso: radiodense
Radiodermatite: radiodermatitis
Radiodiagnóstico: radiodiagnosis
Radiodigital: radiodigital
Radioelemento: radioelement
Radioeletrofisiologia: radioelectrophysiology
Radioeletrofisiólografo: radioelectrophysiograph
Radioeletrofisiolograma: radioelectrophysiogram
Radioenxofre: radiosulfur
Radioepitelite: radioepithelitis
Radioestereoscopia: radiostereoscopy
Radioestrôncio: radiostrontium
Radiofármaco: radiopharmaceutical
Radioferro: radioiron
Radiofobia: radiophobia
Radiofósforo: radiophosphorus
Radiofreqüência: radiofrequency
Radiogálio: radiogallium
Radiogênese: radiogenesis
Radiogênico: radiogenic
Radiografia: radiograph, radiography, roentgenography
Radiograma: radiogram
Radioimunidade: radioimmunity
Radioimunodifusão: radioimmunodiffusion
Radioimunoeletroforese: radioimmunoelectrophoresis
Radioimunoensaio: radioimmunoassay (RIA)
Radioimunoprecipitação: radioimmunoprecipitation (RIP)
Radioiodado: radioiodinated
Radioiodo: radioiodine
Radioisótopo: radioisotope
Radiolesão: radiolesion
Radioligante: radioligand
Radíolo: radiolus
Radiologia: radiology
Radiológico: radiologic, radiological
Radiologista: radiologist, roentgenologist
Radiomarcado: radiolabeled
Radiômetro: radiometer
Radiomicrômetro: radiomicrometer
Radiomimético: radiomimetic
Radiomuscular: radiomuscular
Radionecrose: radionecrosis
Radioneurite: radioneuritis
Radionitrogênio: radionitrogen
Radionuclídeo: radionuclide
Radiopacidade: radiopacity
Radiopaco: radiopaque
Radiopalmar: radiopalmar
Radiopatologia: radiopathology
Radiopelvimetria: radiopelvimetry
Radiopílula: radiopill
Radiopotássio: radiopotassium
Radioprotetor: radioprotectant
Radioquímica: radiochemistry
Radiorreceptor: radioreceptor
Radiorresistente: radioresistant
Radioscopia: radioscopy
Radiossensibilidade: radiosensitivity
Radiossensibilização: radiosensitization
Radiossensibilizador: radiosensitizer
Radiossensível: radiosensitive
Radiossódio: radiosodium
Radiotelemetria: radiotelemetry
Radioterapeuta: radiotherapist
Radioterapêutica: radiotherapeutics
Radioterapêutico: radiotherapeutic
Radioterapia: radiotherapy
Radiotermia: radiothermy
Radiotireoidectomia: radiothyroidectomy
Radiotiroxina: radiothyroxin
Radiotoxemia: radiotoxemia
Radiotraçador: radiotracer
Radiotransparência: radiolucency
Radiotransparente: radiolucent, radiotransparent
Radiotrópico: radiotropic
Radioulnar: radioulnar
Radioumeral: radiohumeral
Radisectomia: radisectomy
Radônio: radon (Rn)
Rafania: raphania, rhaphania
Rafe: raphe, rhaphe
Rafinose: gossypose, raffinose
Rágades: rhagades
Ragadiforme: rhagadiform
Railietiníase: raillietiniasis
Raio: ray
Raio X: x-ray
Raios: radii
Raiva: rabies, rage
Raivoso: rabid
Raiz: radix, **gen.** radicis, **pl.** radices; root
Raiz de altéia: marshmallow root
Raiz de angélica: angelica root
Raiz de genciana: gentian root
Raiz seca de *Ipomoea orizabensis*: orizaba jalap root
Raloxifeno: raloxifene
Ramicina: ramycin
Ramicotomia: ramicotomy
Ramificação: branching, ramification
Ramificar: ramify
Ramissecção: ramisection
Ramite: ramitis
L-ramnose: L-rhamnose (Rha)
Ramnosídeo: rhamnoside
Ramnoxantina: rhamnoxanthin
Ramo: branch, ramus, **pl.** rami
Ramoso: ramose, ramous
Rampa: ramp
Râmulo: ramulus, **pl.** ramuli; twig
Rancidez: rancidity
Rancidificar: rancidify
Rançoso: rancid
Randomização: randomization
Rangido: crunch
Ranino: ranine
Ranitidina: ranitidine
Rânula: ranula
Ranular: ranular
Raque: rachis, **pl.** rachides, rachises
Raquial: rachial
Raquicentese: rachicentesis
Raquidiano: rachidial, rachidian
Raquilise: rachilysis
Raquiocentese: rachiocentesis
Raquiópago: rachiopagus
Raquioplegia: rachioplegia
Raquioquise: rachiochysis
Raquiotomia: rachiotomy
Raquiótomo: rachiotome
Raquípago: rachipagus
Raquisquise: rachischisis
Raquisquise total: araphia
Raquítico: rachitic, rickety
Raquitismo: rachitis, rachitism, rickets
Raquitogênico: rachitogenic
Raquítomo: rachitome
Rarefação: rarefaction
Rarefazer: rarefy
Rasceta: rasceta
Rasoura: spoke-shave
Raspado: scrape, scraping
Raspador: scaler
Raspagem: scaling
Rastreamento de ligador: linker scanning
Rato: rat
Rayl: rayl
Razão: ratio
Reabilitação: rehabilitation
Reabsorção: resorption
Reabsorver: resorb
Reação: reaction
Reação autolítica de Yorke: Yorke autolytic reaction
Reação cruzada: cross-matching
Reação de Fernandez: Fernandez reaction
Reação de Nadi: Nadi reaction
Reação de Sakaguchi: Sakaguchi reaction
Reação leucemóide: leukemoid reaction
Reagente: reactant
Reagente de Lloyd: Lloyd reagent
Reagente de Mandelin: Mandelin reagent
Reagente de Marme: Marme reagent
Reagente de Marquis: Marquis reagent
Reagente de Mecke: Mecke reagent
Reagente de Rosenthaler-Turk: Rosenthaler-Turk reagent
Reagente de Schaer: Schaer reagent

Reagente de Scheibler: Scheibler reagent
Reagina: reagin
Reagínico: reaginic
Reagir: react
Reajuste do nó sinoatrial: reset nodus sinuatrialis
Realce: enhancement
Realidade: reality
Reaprendizado: relearning
Reaquecimento: rewarming
Rearranjo: rearrangement
Rearranjo de exons: exon shuffle
Reatância: reactance (X)
Reativação: reactivation
Reativador da colinesterase: cholinesterase reactivator
Reativar: reactivate
Reatividade: reactivity
Reativo: reagent
Rebaixo: undercut
Rebordo: flange
Recaída: relapse
Recalcificação: recalcification
Recanalização: recanalization
Recapitulação: recapitulation
Receita médica: recipe (℞)
Recém-nascido: newborn
Receptáculo: receptaculum, **pl.** receptacula
Receptivo: receptive
Receptor: ceptor, receiver, receptor, recipient
Receptossomas: receptosomes
Recessão: recession
Recessividade: recessitivity
Recessivo: recessive
Recesso: bay, recess, recessus, **pl.** recessus
Rechaçável: ballottable
Rechaço: ballottement
Recidiva: recidivation
Recidivante: relapsing
Recidividade: recidivism
Recidivista: recidivist
Reciprocação: reciprocation
Recirculação: recirculation
Recolocação: replacement
Recombinação: recombination
Recombinante: recombinant
Recompensa: reward
Récon: recon
Reconstituição: reconstitution
Reconstrução: reconstruction
Recorrência: recurrence
Recorrente: recurrent
Recorte: scalloping
Recrudescência: recrudescence
Recrudescente: recrudescent
Recrutamento: recruitment
Recumbente: recumbent
Recuperação: recovery, recuperation, retrieval
Recuperar: recuperate
Recurvação: recurvation
Rede: meshwork, net, network, rete, **pl.** retia
Rede fibrosa: feltwork
Rédia: redia, **pl.** rediae

Rediferenciação: redifferentiation
Redox: redox
Redução: reduction
Redundância: redundancy
Reduplicação: reduplication
Redutase: reductase
Redutível: reducible
Redutor: reductant
Reduviídeo: reduvid, reduviid
Reduzir: reduce
Reembasar: rebase, reline
Reentrada: reentry
Reestenose: restenosis
Refeição: meal, refection
Refinar: refine
Refletância: reflectance
Refletir: reflect
Refletor: reflector
Reflexão: reflection
Reflexo: jerk, reflex
Reflexo de alimentação: fressreflex
Reflexo de Chodzko: Chodzko reflex
Reflexo de Phillipson: Phillipson reflex
Reflexo de Weingrow: Weingrow reflex
Reflexófilo: reflexophil, reflexophile
Reflexogênico: reflexogenic
Reflexógeno: reflexogenous
Reflexógrafo: reflexograph
Reflexologia: reflexology
Reflexômetro: reflexometer
Reflexoterapia: reflexotherapy
Refluxo: reflux
Reforço: booster, bracing, reinforcement, reinforcer
Reformatar: reformat
Refração: refraction
Refracionista: refractionist
Refracionômetro: refractionometer
Refrangível: refrangible
Refratar: refract
Refratário: refractory
Refratável: refractable
Refratividade: refractivity
Refrativo: refractive
Refratometria: refractometry
Refratômetro: refractometer
Refratura: refracture
Refrigeração: refrigeration
Refrigerante: refrigerant
Refringência: refringency
Refringente: refringent
Regeneração: regeneration
Regenerar: regenerate
Região: regio, region, **gen.** regionis, **pl.** regiones
Regime: regimen
Regional: regional
Registro: recording, register, registration
Registro clínico: charting
Registro interoclusão: checkbite
Regma: rhegma

Regmatógeno: rhegmatogenous
Rego: spillway
Rego lacrimal: rivus lacrimalis
Regra: rule
Regra de Cowling: Cowling rule
Regra de Goriaew: Goriaew rule
Regressão: regression
Regressivo: regressive
Régua: ruler
Regulação: regulation
Regulador: regulator
Régulon: regulon
Regurgitação: regurgitation
Regurgitante: regurgitant
Regurgitar: regurgitate
Reidratação: rehydration
Reimplantação: reimplantation, replantation
Reimplantar: replant
Reinalação: rebreathing
Reinervação: reinnervation
Reinfecção: reinfection
Reino: kingdom
Reinoculação: reinoculation
Reinserção: reattachment
Reintegração: redintegration, reintegration
Reinterpretação: reenactment
Reinversão: reinversion
Rejeição: rejection
Rejuvenescimento: rejuvenescence
Relação: rapport, relation
Relacionamento: relationship
Relativo a: rhonchal, rhonchial
Relaxamento: relaxation
Relaxante: relaxant
Relaxar: relax
Relaxina: relaxin, releasin
Remediador: remedial
Remediável: remediable
Remédio: remedy
Remineralização: remineralization
Reminiscência: reminiscence
Remissão: remission
Remitência: remittence
Remitente: remittent
Remitir: remit
Remoção: disimpaction
Remoção do tálus: astragalectomy
Remodelagem: remodeling
Renal: renal
Renase: rennase
Renaturação: renaturation
Rendimento: yield
Renículo: reniculus, **pl.** reniculi
Reniforme: reniform
Renina: renin, rennin
Reninismo primário: primary reninism
Reninogênio: renninogen, rennogen
Rênio: rhenium (Re)
Reniportal: reniportal
Renocardíaco: renicardiac
Renocutâneo: renicutaneous
Renogástrico: renogastric

Renogênico: renogenic
Renografia: renography
Renograma: renogram
Renointestinal: renointestinal
Renomegalia: renomegaly
Renopatia: renopathy
Renoprivo: renoprival
Renopulmonar: renopulmonary
Renotrófico: renotrophic
Renotrofina: renotrophin
Renotrópico: renotropic
Renotropina: renotropin
Renovação: turnover
Renovar: refresh
Renovascular: renovascular
Renúnculo: renunculus
Reóbase: rheobase
Reobásico: rheobasic
Reocardiografia: rheocardiography
Reocrisidina: rheochrysidin
Reoencefalografia: rheoencephalography
Reoencefalograma: rheoencephalogram
Reograma: rheogram
Reologia: rheology
Reologista: rheologist
Reometria: rheometry
Reômetro: rheometer
Reopexia: rheopexy
Reostato: rheostat
Reostose: rheostosis
Reotaxia: rheotaxis
Reotropismo: rheotropism
Reparação: repair
Repelente: repellent
Reperfusão: refusion
Repetição: rehearsal
Repetição invertida: inverted repeat
Réplica: replica
Replicação: replication
Replicador: replicator
Replicar: replicate
Replicase: replicase
Réplicon: replicon
Repolarização: repolarization
Reposição: repositio, reposition
Reposicionamento: repositioning
Repositor: repositor
Representação: acting out, representation
Repressão: repression
Repressor: repressor
Reprimido: repressed
Reprodução: reproduction
Reprodutibilidade: reproducibility
Reprodutivo: reproductive
Reptilase: reptilase
Repulsão: repulsion
Repululação: repullulation
Resazurina: resazurin
Rescinamina: rescinnamine
Reserpina: reserpine
Reserva: reserve
Reservatório: reservoir
Residente: house officer, intern, resident

Glossário

Residual: residual
Resíduo: residue, residuum, **pl.** residua, debris
Resiliência: resilience
Resina: resin
Resinas: resines
Resinatos: resinates
Resinóide: resinoid
Resinóis: resinols
Resinoso: resinous
Resistência: fastness, hardiness, resistance
Resistente ao iodo: iodinefast
Resistividade: resistivity
Resistor: resistor
Resolução: resolution
Resolvase: resolvase
Resolvente: resolvent
Resolver: resolve
Resorcina: resorcin
Resorcinol: resorcinol
Resorcinolftaleína: resorcinolphthalein
Respiração: breath, breathing, pneusis, respiration
Respirador: respirator, ventilator
Respirar: respire
Respiratório: respiratory
Respirável: respirable
Respirômetro: respirometer
Resposta: response
Ressalto: overhang
Ressecar: resect
Ressecável: resectable
Ressecção: resection
Ressectoscópio: resectoscope
Ressoador: resonator
Ressonância: resonance
Ressuscitação: resuscitation
Ressuscitar: resuscitate
Restauração: restoration
Restaurativo: restorative
Restiforme: restiform
Restítopo: restitope
Restituição: restitution
Resto: remnant
Restocitemia: rhestocythemia
Restrição: restriction
Retal: rectal
Retalgia: rectalgia
Retalho: flap
Retardado: retardate
Retardador: retarder
Retardamento: retardation
Retardo: lagging
Retectomia: rectectomy
Retenção: retention
Retenção de ar: airtrapping
Retentor: retainer
Reticulação: reticulation
Reticular: retial, reticular, reticulated
Reticulina: reticulin
Retículo: reticulum, **pl.** reticula
Retículo de difração: diffraction grating
Reticulócito: reticulocyte
Reticulocitopenia: reticulocytopenia
Reticulocitose: reticulocytosis

Reticuloendotelial: reticuloendothelial
Reticuloendotélio: reticuloendothelium
Reticuloendotelioma: reticuloendothelioma
Reticuloespinal: reticulospinal
Retículo-histiocitoma: reticulohistiocytoma
Retículo-histiocitose: reticulohistiocytosis
Reticulóide: reticuloid
Reticulopenia: reticulopenia
Reticuloperitélio: retoperithelium
Reticulose: reticulosis
Reticulotomia: reticulotomy
Retificador: rectifier
Retificar: rectify
Retiforme: retiform
Retina: optomeninx, retina
Retináculo: retinaculum, **gen.** retinaculi, **pl.** retinacula
Retinaldeído: retinaldehyde
Retinectomia: retinectomy
Retineno: retinene
Retineno-1: retinene-1
Retineno-2: retinene-2
Retiniano: retinal
Retinite: retinitis
Retinoblastoma: retinoblastoma
Retinocorióide: retinochoroid
Retinocorioidite: retinochoroiditis
Retinodiálise: retinodialysis
Retinóide: retinoid
Retinóides: retinoids
Retinol: retinol
Retinopapilite: retinopapillitis
Retinopatia: retinopathy
Retinopexia: retinopexy
Retinopiese: retinopiesis
Retinoscopia: retinoscopy, skiascopy
Retinoscópio: retinoscope
Retinosquise: retinoschisis
Retinotomia: retinotomy
Retite: rectitis
Reto: rectum, **pl.** rectums, recta
Retoabdominal: rectoabdominal
Retocele: rectocele
Retóclise: rectoclysis
Retococcígeo: rectococcygeal
Retococcipexia: rectococcypexy
Retocolite: rectocolitis
Retoestenose: rectostenosis
Retofobia: rectophobia
Retoperineal: rectoperineal
Retoperineorrafia: rectoperineorrhaphy
Retopexia: rectopexy
Retoplastia: rectoplasty
Retorno: return
Retorrafia: rectorrhaphy
Retorta: retort
Retoscopia: rectoscopy
Retoscópio: rectoscope
Retossigmóide: rectosigmoid
Retostomia: rectostomy
Retotomia: rectotomy
Retótomo: rectotome

Retouretral: rectourethral
Retouterino: rectouterine
Retovaginal: rectovaginal
Retovesical: rectovesical
Retovestibular: rectovestibular
Retração: retraction
Retrair: retract
Retrátil: retractile
Retrator: retractor
Retroalimentação: feedback
Retroauricular: retroauricular
Retrobucal: retrobuccal
Retrobulbar: retrobulbar
Retrocalcaneobursite: retrocalcaneobursitis
Retrocecal: retrocecal
Retrocervical: retrocervical, retrocollic
Retrocessão: retrocession
Retrocesso: backtracking
Retrocólico: retrocolic
Retrocondução: retroconduction
Retrocursivo: retrocursive
Retrodeslocamento: retrodisplacement
Retrodesvio: retrodeviation
Retrodifusão: backscatter
Retroesofágico: retroesophageal
Retroespondilolistese: retrospondylolisthesis
Retroesternal: retrosternal
Retroesteróide: retrosteroid
Retrofaringe: retropharynx
Retrofaríngeo: retropharyngeal
Retrofletido: retroflected, retroflexed
Retroflexão: retroflection, retroflexion
Retrognático: retrognathic
Retrognatismo: retrognathism
Retrógrado: retrograde
Retrografia: retrography
Retrogressão: retrogression
Retroinibição: retroinhibition
Retroiridiano: retroiridian
Retrojeção: retrojection
Retrojetor: retrojector
Retrolenticular: retrolental, retrolenticular
Retrolingual: retrolingual
Retromamário: retromammary
Retromandibular: retromandibular
Retromastóideo: retromastoid
Retromolar: retromolar
Retromorfose: retromorphosis
Retronasal: retronasal
Retroobturação: retrofilling
Retrooclusão: retroclusion
Retroocular: retro-ocular
Retroperitoneal: retroperitoneal
Retroperitônio: retroperitoneum
Retroperitonite: retroperitonitis
Retroplacentário: retroplacental
Retroplasia: retroplasia
Retroposição: retroposition
Retroposon: retroposon
Retroposto: retroposed
Retroprojetor: overhead projector
Retropúbico: retropubic

Retropulsão: retropulsion
Retrospecção: retrospection
Retrospectivo: retrospective
Retrotarsal: retrotarsal
Retrouterino: retrouterine
Retroversão: retroversion
Retroversoflexão: retroversioflexion
Retrovertido: retroverted
Retrovírus: retrovirus
Retrusão: retrusion
Reuma: rheum
Reumatalgia: rheumatalgia
Reumático: rheumatic
Reumátide: rheumatid
Reumatismal: rheumatismal
Reumatismo: rheumatism
Reumatóide: rheumatoid
Reumatologia: rheumatology
Reumatologista: rheumatologist
Revacinação: revaccination
Revascularização: revascularization
Revelador: developer
Revelar: develop
Reverberação: reverberation
Reversão: reversal, reversion
Reversão sorológica: seroreversion
Reversível: reversible
Revertente: revertant
Revestimento: facing, investing, investment, liner, lining
Revisão: proofreading, review
Revivescência: revivescence
Revivificação: revivification
Revulsão: derivation, revulsion
rhe: rhe
Rianodina: ryanodine
Ribavirina: ribavirin
α-ribazole: α-ribazole
Ribitila: ribityl
Ribitol: ribitol
Ribo-2-hexulose: ribo-2-hexulose
Riboflavina: flavin, flavine, riboflavin, riboflavine
Riboforinas: ribophorins
Ribofuranose: ribofuranose
9-β-D-ribofuranosiladenina: 9-β-D-ribofuranosyladenine
1-β-D-ribofuranosilcitosina: 1-β-D-ribofuranosylcytosine
9-β-D-ribofuranosilguanina: 9-β-D-ribofuranosylguanine
9-β-D-ribofuranosilpurina: 9-β-D-ribofuranosylpurine
Ribofuranosiltimina: ribofuranosylthymine
1-β-D-ribofuranosiluracila: 1-β-D-ribofuranosyluracil
Ribonuclease: ribonuclease (RNase)
Ribonuclease (Bacillus subtilis): ribonuclease (Bacillus subtilis)
Ribonuclease (pancreática): ribonuclease (pancreatic)
Ribonucleinase: ribonucleinase

Ribonucleoproteína: ribonucleoprotein (RNP)
Ribonucleosídeo: ribonucleoside
Ribonucleotídeo: ribonucleotide
Ribopiranose: ribopyranose
Ribose: ribose (Rib)
Ribose-5-fosfato: ribose-5-phosphate
Ribosídeo: riboside
Ribosila: ribosyl
Ribosilação: ribosylation
1-ribosilorotato: 1-ribosylorotate
Ribosilpurina: ribosylpurine
Ribosiltimidina: ribosylthymidine
Ribossoma: ribosome
Ribosúria: ribosuria
Ribotídeo: ribotide
Ribotídeo de 5-formamidoimidazol-4-carboximida: 5-formamidoimidazole-4-carboximide ribotide
Ribotídeo de *N*-formilglicinamida: *N*-formylglycinamide ribotide (FGAR)
Ribotimidina: ribothymidine (T, Thd)
Ribovírus: ribovirus
Ribozima: ribozyme
Ribulose: ribulose
Ribulose-1,5-difosfato carboxilase: ribulose-1,5-bisphosphate carboxylase
Ribulose-fosfato-3-epimerase: ribulose-phosphate 3-epimerase
Ricina: ricin
Ricinismo: ricinism
Ricinoleato: ricinoleate
Rifamicina: rifamycin, rifomycin
Rifampicina: rifampicin
Rifampina: rifampin
Rigidez: rigidity, rigor
Riluzol: riluzole
Rim: kidney, nephros, ren, **gen.** renis, **pl.** renes
Rim de Rose-Bradford: Rose-Bradford kidney
Rima: rima, **gen. e pl.** rimae
Rimantadina: rimantadine
Rimoso: rimose
Rímula: rimula
Rinalgia: rhinalgia
Rinedema: rhinedema
Rinencefalia: rhinocephaly, rhinocephalia
Rinencefálico: rhinencephalic
Rinencéfalo: rhinencephalon, smell-brain
Rinenquise: rhinenchysis
Rínio: rhinion
Rinite: rhinitis
Rinoanemômetro: rhinoanemometer
Rinocele: rhinocele
Rinocifose: rhinokyphosis
Rinodimia: rhinodymia
Rinodinia: rhinodynia

Rinoestenose: rhinocleisis
Rinoestrose: rhinoestrosis
Rinofaringe: rhinopharynx
Rinofaríngeo: rhinopharyngeal
Rinofaringolito: rhinopharyngolith
Rinofima: rhinophyma, rum-blossom
Rinofonia: rhinophonia
Rinógeno: rhinogenous
Rinolalia: rhinism, rhinolalia
Rinolitíase: rhinolithiasis
Rinolito: rhinolite, rhinolith
Rinologia: rhinology
Rinológico: rhinologic
Rinologista: rhinologist
Rinomanometria: rhinomanometry
Rinomanômetro: rhinomanometer
Rinonecrose: rhinonecrosis
Rinopatia: rhinopathy
Rinoplastia: rhinoplasty
Rinopneumonite: rhinopneumonitis
Rinorréia: rhinorrhea
Rinoscleroma: rhinoscleroma
Rinoscopia: rhinoscopy
Rinoscópico: rhinoscopic
Rinoscópio: rhinoscope
Rinosporidiose: rhinosporidiosis
Rinossalpingite: rhinosalpingitis
Rinossinusite: rhinosinusitis
Rinostenose: rhinostenosis
Rinotomia: rhinotomy
Rinotraqueíte: rhinotracheitis
Rinovírus: rhinovirus
Ripário: riparian
Riparofobia: rhypophobia
Riquetsial: rickettsial
Riquetsiose: rickettsiosis
Riquetsiose variceliforme: rickettsialpox
Riquetsiostático: rickettsiostatic
Riscar: scribe
Risco: risk
Riso: risus
Riso sardônico: sardonic grin
Risório: risorius
Ristocetina: ristocetin
Rítide: rhytide
Ritidectomia: rhytidectomy
Ritidoplastia: rhytidoplasty
Ritidose: rhytidosis
Ritmo: rhythm
Ritodrina: ritodrine
Ritual: ritual
Rivalidade: rivalry
Riziforme: riziform
Rizóide: rhizoid
Rizoma: rhizome
Rizomelia: rhizomelia
Rizomélico: rhizomelic
Rizomeningomielite: rhizomeningomyelitis
Rizoplasto: rhizoplast
Rizopterina: rhizopterin
Rizotomia: rhizotomy
RNA de transferência: transfer-RNA

RNA mensageiro: messenger RNA (mRNA)
Robótico: robotic
Robustez: robustness
Rocela: archil
Rocelina: orchella, orchil, roccellin
Roda: wheel
Roda de Burlew: Burlew wheel
Rodamina B: rhodamine B
Rodanato: rhodanate
Rodanese: rhodanese
Rodenticida: rodenticide
Rodeose: rhodeose
Rodina: rhodin
Ródio: rhodium (Rh)
Rodofilático: rhodophylactic
Rodofilaxia: rhodophylaxis
Rodogênese: rhodogenesis
Rodopsina: rhodopsin
Roentgencimografia: roentgenkymography
Roentgencimógrafo: roentgenkymograph
Roentgencimograma: roentgenkymogram
Roentgenógrafo: roentgenograph
Roentgenograma: roentgenogram
Roentgenometria: roentgenometry
Roentgenômetro: roentgenometer
Roentgenoscopia: roentgenoscopy
Roentgenoscópio: roentgenoscope
Roentgenoterapia: roentgenotherapy
Rofeocitose: rhopheocytosis
Rolândico: rolandic
Rolitetraciclina: rolitetracycline
Rolo: roll
Romã: granatum, pomegranate
Rombencéfalo: hindbrain, rhombencephalon
Rômbico: rhombic
Romboatlóide: rhomboatloideus
Rombocele: rhombocele
Rombóide: rhomboid, rhomboidal, rhomboideus
Rombômero: rhombomere
Rompimento: brisement
Ronco: rhonchus, **pl.** rhonchi; snore
Ronronar: purr
Ropalocitose: ropalocytosis
Roptria: rhoptry, **pl.** rhoptries
Rosa: rose
Rosa bengala: rose bengal
Rosácea: rosacea
Rosanilina: rosanilin
Rosaprostol: rosaprostol
Rosário: rosary
Roséola: roseola
Roseta: rosette
Rostelo: rostellum
Rostrado: rostrate
Rostral: rostral, rostralis
Rostriforme: rostriform
Rostro: rostrum, **pl.** rostra, rostrums

Rotação: rotation
Rotação para trás: derotation
Rotacismo: rhotacism
Rotador: rotator
Rotador medial: intortor
Rotamase: rotamase
Rotâmero: rotamer
Rotâmetro: rotameter
Rotavírus: rotavirus
Rotenona: rotenone
Rotoescoliose: rotoscoliosis
Rotoxamina: rotoxamine
Roubo: steal
Rouco: hoarse
Roupa antichoque: antishock garment
Rouquidão: hoarseness
Rubefação: rubefaction
Rubefaciente: rubefacient
Rubelina: rubellin
Rubéola: röteln, roetheln, rubella
Rubeose: rubeosis
Rubescente: rubescent
Rubídio: rubidium (Rb)
Rubidomicina (daunorrubicina): rubidomycin (daunorubicin)
Rubina S, rubina: rubin S, rubine
Rubor: blush, flare, flush, rubor
Rubratoxina: rubratoxin
Rubredoxinas: rubredoxins
Rubriblasto: rubriblast
Rubrica: rubric
Rubricito: rubricyte
Rubrospinal: rubrospinal
Rudimentar: rudimentary
Rudimento: rudiment, rudimentum, **pl.** rudimenta
Rufo: erythristic, ruff
Ruga: ruga, **pl.** rugae; wrinkle
Ruga cutânea: chytide
Rugina: raspatory
Rugosidade: rugosity
Rugoso: rough, rugose, rugous
Ruibarbo: rhubarb
Ruído: bruit, noise
Ruivo: rufous
Rum: rum
Ruminação: rumination
Ruminante: ruminant
Ruminativo: ruminative
Rupia: rupia
Rupióide: rupioid
Ruptura: abruption, break
Rutênio: ruthenium (Ru)
Rutidose: rutidosis
Rutina: rutin
Rutinose: rutinose
Rutinosídeo: rutoside

S

Sabão: soap
Sabor: flavor
Saborear: taste
Sabugueiro: elder, elder flowers
Sabuloso: sabulous
Saburra: saburra, sordes
Saburrento: saburral

Saca-bocado: punch
Sacada: saccade
Sacádico: saccadic
Sacarase: saccharase, sucrase
Sacarato: saccharate, sucrate
Sacarefidrose: saccharephidrosis
Sacárico: saccharic
Sacárides: saccharides
Sacarífero: sacchariferous
Sacarificação: saccharification
Sacarificar: saccharify
Sacarímetro: saccharimeter
Sacarina: saccharin
Sacarino: saccharine
Sacarolítico: saccharolytic
Sacarometabólico: saccharometabolic
Sacarometabolismo: saccharometabolism
Sacarômetro: saccharometer
Sacaropina: saccharopine
Sacaropinúria: saccharopinuria
Sacarose: saccharose, sucrose
Sacarose α-D-glicoidrolase: sucrose α-D-glucohydrolase
Sacarosemia: sucrosemia
Sacarosúria: sucrosuria
Saciedade: satiation
Saciforme: sacciform
Saco: sac, saccus, **pl.** sacci
Sacral: sacral
Sacralgia: sacralgia
Sacralização: sacralization
Sacrectomia: sacrectomy
Sacro: sacrum, **pl.** sacra
Sacrociático: sacrosciatic
Sacrococcígeo: sacrococcygeal, sacrococcygeus
Sacrodinia: sacrodynia
Sacroespinal: sacrospinal
Sacroilíaco: sacroiliac
Sacroiliíte: sacroiliitis
Sacrolombar: sacrolumbalis, sacrolumbar
Sacrotomia: sacrotomy
Sacrovertebral: sacrovertebral
Sacudir: succuss
Saculação: sacculation
Sacular: saccate, saccular, sacculated
Sáculo: saccule, sacculus, **pl.** sacculi
Saculocolear: sacculocochlear
S-adenosil-L-homocisteína: S-adenosyl-L-homocysteine
Sádico: sadist, sadistic
Sadio: healthy
Sadismo: sadism
Sadomasoquismo: sadomasochism
Safena: saphena
Safenectomia: saphenectomy
Safeno: saphenous
Safismo: sapphism
Safranina O: safranin O
Safranófilo: safranophil, safranophile
Safrol: safrole
Sagital: sagittal, sagittalis
Saída: exitus

Sais de sulfônio: sulfonium salts
Sal: sal, **pl.** sales, salt
Sal básico: subsalt
Sal ósseo: bone-salt
Sala de dissecção: prosectorium
Sala de recuperação: recovery room
Salada de palavras: word salad
Salbutamol: salbutamol
Salgueiro: willow
Salicil: salicyl
Salicilado: salicylated
Salicilamida: salicylamide
Salicilanilida: salicylanilide
Salicilato: sallicylate
Salicilato de carbazocromo: carbazochrome salicylate
Salicilato de mentila: menthyl salicylate
Salicilato de mercúrio: mercuric salicylate
Salicilato de metila: methyl salicylate
Salicilazossulfapiridina: salicylazosulfapyridine
Salicilismo: salicylism
Salicina: salicin
Saliência: salient
Salificar: salify
Salificável: salifiable
Saligenina, saligenol: saligenin, saligenol
Salímetro: salimeter
Salino: saline
Salinômetro: salinometer
Salitre: saltpeter
Saliva: saliva, spittle
Salivação: salivation
Salivador: salivator
Salivante: salivant
Salivar: salivary, salivate
Salivolitíase: salivolithiasis
Salmonelose: salmonellosis
Salpinge: salpinx, **pl.** salpinges
Salpingectomia: salpingectomy
Salpingiano: salpingian
Salpingioma: salpingioma
Salpingite: salpingitis
Salpingítico: salpingitic
Salpingocele: salpingocele
Salpingociese: salpingocyesis
Salpingofaríngeo: salpingopharyngeal, salpingopharyngeus
Salpingografia: salpingography
Salpingólise: salpingolysis
Salpingoneostomia: salpingoneostomy
Salpingo-ooforectomia: laparosalpingo-oophorectomy, salpingo-oophorectomy, tubo-ovariectomy
Salpingo-ooforite: salpingo-oophoritis, tubo-ovaritis
Salpingo-ooforocele: salpingo-oophorocele
Salpingo-ovariectomia: salpingo-ovariectomy

Salpingoperitonite: salpingoperitonitis
Salpingopexia: salpingopexy
Salpingoplastia: salpingoplasty
Salpingorrafia: salpingorrhaphy
Salpingorragia: salpingorrhagia
Salpingoscopia: salpingoscopy
Salpingostomia: salpingostomy
Salpingotomia: salpingotomy
Salsalato: salsalate
Salsaparrilha: sarsaparilla
Saltada: saltation
Saltatório: saltatory
Salterial: psalterial
Saltério: psalterium, **pl.** psalteria
Salubre: salubrious
Salurese: saluresis
Salurético: saluretic
Salutar: salutary, sanitary
Salva: volley
Sálvia: sage, salvia
Samandarina: samandarine
Samário: samarium (Sm)
Sambuco: sambucus
Sanativo: sanative, sanatory
Sanatório: salutarium, sanatorium
Saneamento: sanitation
Sangramento: bleeding
Sangramento nasal: nosebleed
Sangrante: bleeder
Sangrar: bleed, leeching
Sangria: bloodletting
Sangue: blood
Sanguessuga: leech
Sanguifaciente: sanguifacient
Sanguífero: sanguiferous
Sanguificação: sanguification
Sanguinarina: sanguinarine
Sanguíneo: sanguine, sanguineous
Sanguinolento: sanguinolent
Sanguinopurulento: sanguinopurulent
Sanguívoro: sanguivorous
Sanidade: sanity
Sânie: sanies
Saniopurulento: saniopurulent
Sanioso: sanious
Saniosseroso: sanioserous
Sanitarista: sanitarian
Sanitização: sanitization
Santonina: santonin
São: sane
Sapogenina: sapogenin
Saponáceo: saponaceous
Saponificação: saponification
Saponificar: saponify
Saponinas: saponins
Sapremia: sapremia
Sapróbico: saprobic
Sapróbio: saprobe
Saprodontia: saprodontia
Saprófilo: saprophilous
Saprófita: saprophyte
Saprofítico: saprophytic
Saprogênico, sapógeno: saprogen, saprogenic, saprogenous
Saprozóico: saprozoic
Saprozoonose: saprozoonosis

Sarampo: measles, morbilli, rubeola
Sarcina: sarcine
α-sarcina: α-sarcin
Sarcoblasto: sarcoblast
Sarcode: sarcode
Sarcóglia: sarcoglia
Sarcóide: sarcoid
Sarcoidose: sarcoidosis
Sarcolema: sarcolemma
Sarcolêmico: sarcolemmal, sarcolemmic, sarcolemmous
Sarcolisina: sarcolysine
Sarcologia: sarcology
Sarcoma: sarcoma
Sarcomatóide: sarcomatoid
Sarcomatose: sarcomatosis
Sarcomatoso: sarcomatous
Sarcômero: sarcomere
Sarconema: sarconeme
Sarcoplasma: sarcoplasm
Sarcoplásmico: sarcoplasmic
Sarcoplasto: sarcoplast
Sarcopoético: sarcopoietic
Sarcóptico: sarcoptic
Sarcoptídeo: sarcoptid
Sarcose: sarcosis
Sarcosina: sarcosine (Sar)
Sarcosinemia: sarcosinemia
Sarcoso: sarcous
Sarcossistose: sarcocystosis
Sarcossoma: sarcosome
Sarcostose: sarcostosis
Sarcótico: sarcotic
Sarcotripsia: sarcotripsy
Sarcotúbulos: sarcotubules
Sarda: freckle
Sargramostima: sargramostim
Sarina: sarin
Sarna: mange
Sartório: sartorius
Sassafrás: sassafras
Satélite: satellite
Satelitose: satellitosis
Satiríase: satyriasis
Satirismo: satyrism
Saturação: saturation
Saturar: saturate
Saturnino: saturnine
Saturnismo: saturnism
Saudação alérgica: allergic salute
Saúde: health
Saxitoxina: saxitoxin
Schwanoma: schwannoma
Schwanose: schwannosis
Sebáceo: sebaceous, sebaceus
Sebiagogo: sebiagogic
Sebífero: sebiferous
Sebíparo: sebiparous
Sebo: sebum, sevum, suet, tallow
Seborréia: seborrhea
Seborreico: seborrheic
Secante: siccant
Secção: sectio, section, **pl.** sectiones
Secção média: midsection
Secobarbital: secobarbital
Secreção: secretion
Secreções: secreta

Secretagogo: secretagogue, secretogogue
Secretar: secrete
Secretase: secretase
Secretina: oxykrinin, secretin
Secretomotor: secretomotor, secretomotory
Secretor: secretor, secretory
Séctil: sectile
Secundina: afterbirth
Secundinas: secundina, **pl.** secundinae, secundines
Secundípara: secundigravida, secundipara
Seda: silk
Sedação: sedation
Sedar: sedate
Sedativo: sedative
Sede: thirst
Sedenho: seton
Sedimentação: sedimentation
Sedimentador: sedimentator
Sedimentar: sedimentate
Sedimento: sediment, sedimentum
Sedimentômetro: sedimentometer
Sedoeptulose: sedoheptulose
Segmentação: segmentation
Segmentador: segmenter
Segmentar: segmental
Segmentectomia: segmentectomy
Segmento: segment, segmentum, **pl.** segmenta
Segregação: segregation
Segregador: segregator
Seguro: insurance.
Seio: sinus, **pl.** sinus, sinuses
Seiva: sap
Sela: saddle, sella
Selafobia: selaphobia
Selante: sealant
Selar: sellar
Seleção: selection
Selectina: selectin
Selegilina: selegiline
Selênio: selenium (Se)
Selenocisteína: selenocysteine
Selenodonte: selenodont
Selenometionina: selenomethionine
Selo: seal
Semântica: semantics
Sêmen: semen, **pl.** semina, semens
Semente: seed
Semente de aipo: celery seed
Semente de linho: linseed
Semente de painço: millet seed
Semente de psílio: psyllium seed
Semente do linho, linhaça: flaxseed
Sementes de ipoméia: morning glory seeds
Semi-aldeído: semialdehyde
δ-semialdeído aminoadípico sintase: aminoadipic δ-semialdehyde synthase
Semi-aldeído de metilmalonato: methylmalonate semialdehyde

Semicanal: semicanal, semicanalis, **pl.** semicanales
Semicartilaginoso: semicartilaginous
Semicircular: semicircular
Semicoma: semicoma
Semicomatoso: semicomatose
Semicondutor: semiconductor
Semiconsciente: semiconscious
Semiconservador: semiconservative
Semicrista: semicrista
Semidecussação: semidecussation
Semi-espinal: semispinal
Semiflexão: semiflexion
Semilunar: lunate, semilunar, semilunare
Semilunar (osso): lunare
Semimembranáceo: semimembranosus, semimembranous
Seminal: seminal
Seminífero: seminiferous
Seminormal: seminormal (N/2)
Semiopático: semiopathic, semeiopathic
Semi-orbicular: semiorbicular
Semiose: semiosis, semeiosis
Semiótica: semiotics, semeiotics
Semiótico: semiotic, semeiotic
Semipenado: semipennate
Semipeniforme: demipenniform, semipenniform
Semipermeável: semipermeable
Semipronação: semipronation
Semiprono: semiprone
Semiquinona: semiquinone
Semi-sintético: semisynthetic
Semi-sulco: semisulcus
Semi-supinação: semisupination
Semi-supino: semisupine
Semitendinoso: semitendinosus, semitendinous
Semiterçã: semitertian
Semivalente: semivalent
Semustina: semustine
Senciente: sentient
Sene: senna
Seneciose: seneciosis
Sênega: senega
Senescência: insenescence, senescence
Senescente: senescent
Senil: senile
Senilidade: senility
Senosídeo A, senosídeo B: sennoside A, sennoside B
Sensação: sensation
Sensação de mordedura: odaxesmus
Sensação tardia: aftersensation
Sensibilidade: sensibility, sensitivity
Sensibilização: sensitization
Sensibilizador: sensitizer
Sensibilizar: sensitize
Sensífero: sensiferous
Sensígeno: sensigenous

Sensímetro: sensimeter
Sensitivo: sensitive
Sensitometria: sensitometry
Sensível: sensible
Sensomobilidade: sensomobility
Sensomotor: sensomotor
Sensomóvel: sensomobile
Sensor: sensor
Sensorial: sensorial, sensory
Sensoriglandular: sensoriglandular
Sensorimotor: sensorimotor
Sensorimuscular: sensorimuscular
Sensório: sensorium, **pl.** sensoria, sensoriums
Sensorivascular: sensorivascular
Sensorivasomotor: sensorivasomotor
Sensual: sensual
Sensualidade: sensuality
Sensualismo: sensualism
Sentido: sense
Sentido incorreto: missense
Sentimento: feeling, sentiment
Sentissecção: sentisection
Separação: hersage, separation
Separador: separator
Sepse, sépsis: sepsis, **pl.** sepses
Septã: septan
Septado: septate
Septal: septal
Septectomia: septectomy
Septicemia: septicemia
Septicemia tifóidea: typhosepsis
Septicêmico: septicemic
Séptico: septic
Septicopiemia: septicopyemia
Septicopiêmico: septicopyemic
Septivalente: septivalent
Septo: dissepiment, septum, gen. septi, **pl.** septa
Septodermoplastia: septodermoplasty
Septomarginal: septomarginal
Septonasal: septonasal
Septoplastia: septoplasty
Septorrinoplastia: septorhinoplasty
Septostomia: septostomy
Séptulo: septulum, **pl.** septula
Seqüela: sequela, **pl.** sequelae
Seqüência: sequence
Seqüencial: sequential
Seqüenciamento: sequencing
Seqüestração: sequestration
Seqüestrectomia: sequestrectomy, sequestrotomy
Seqüestro: sequestrum, **pl.** sequestra
Sequoiose: sequoiosis
Série: series, **pl.** series
Seril: seryl
Serina: serine (S, Ser)
Seringa: syringe
Sério: grave
Seriografia: seriography
Seriógrafo: seriograph
Serioscopia: serioscopy

Serocístico: serocystic
Serocolite: serocolitis
Serofibrinoso: serofibrinous
Serofibroso: serofibrous
Seroma: seroma
Seromembranoso: seromembranous
Seromiotomia: seromyotomy
Seromucóide: seromucoid
Seromucoso: seromucous
Serorresistente: serofast
Serosamucina: serosamucin
Serosidade: serosity
Serosite: serositis
Seroso: serous
Serossanguíneo: serosanguineous
Serosseroso: seroserous
Serossinovial: serosynovial
Serossinovite: serosynovitis
Serotaxia: serotaxis
Seroterapia: serotherapy
Serotino: serotina
Serotonina: serotonin
Serotoninérgico: serotonergic
Serozima: serozyme
Serpentária: serpentaria, snakeroot
Serpente: snake
Serpiginoso: serpiginous
Serra: saw
Serração: serration
Serreado: serrate, serrated
Serrilhado: serrulate, serrulated
Sertralina: sertraline
Servente: ancillary, diener
Serviços protéticos: denture service
Servidor: mainframe
Servomecanismo: servomechanism
Sésamo: sesame
Sesamóide: sesamoid
Sesquiidratos: sesquihydrates
Sesquiterpenos: sesquiterpenes
Séssil: sessile
Sesterterpenos: sesterterpenes
Setáceo: setaceous
Setífero: setiferous
Setígero: setigerous
Setoranopia: sectoranopia
Setorial: sectorial
Sevoflurano: sevoflurane
Sexdigital: sedigitate, sexdigitate
Sexo: sex
Sexologia: sexology
Sextã: sextan
Sexual: sexual
Sexualidade: sexuality
Sexualização: sexualization
Sezão: ague
Shigelose: shigellosis
Sialadenite: sialadenitis
Sialadenotrópico: sialadenotropic
Sialagogo: sialagogue
Sialectasia: sialectasis
Sialêmese: sialemesis, sialemesia
Siálico: sialic

Sialidase: sialidase
Sialidose: sialidosis
Sialina: sialine
Sialismo: sialism, sialismus
Sialoadenectomia: sialoadenectomy
Sialoadenite: sialoadenitis
Sialoadenotomia: sialoadenotomy
Sialoaerofagia: sialoaerophagy
Sialoangiectasia: sialoangiectasis
Sialoangiite: sialoangiitis
Sialocele: sialocele
Sialodocoplastia: sialodochoplasty
Sialodoquite: sialodochitis
Sialoestenose: sialostenosis
Sialógeno: sialogenous
Sialoglicoesfingolipídio: sialoglycosphingolipid
Sialogogo: sialogogue
Sialografia: sialography
Sialograma: sialogram
Sialolitíase: sialolithiasis
Sialólito: sialolith
Sialolitotomia: sialolithotomy
Sialometaplasia: sialometaplasia
Sialometria: sialometry
Sialorréia: sialorrhea
Sialose: sialosis
Sialosquese: sialoschesis
Sialossemiologia: sialosemiology, sialosemeiology
Sibilante: sibilant
Sibilo: sibilus, wheeze, whistle
Sicativo: siccative
Sicoestável: siccostabile, siccostable
Sicolábil: siccolabile
Sicose: sycosis
Sideração: sideration
Sideroblasto: sideroblast
Siderócito: siderocyte
Siderófago: siderophage
Siderofibrose: siderofibrosis
Siderofilinas: siderophilins
Siderófilo: siderophil, siderophile, siderophilous
Sideróforo: siderophore
Siderógeno: siderogenous
Sideropenia: sideropenia
Sideropênico: sideropenic
Siderose: siderosis
Siderossilicose: siderosilicosis
Siderótico: siderotic
Siemens: mho, siemens (S)
Sievert: sievert (Sv)
Sifão: siphon
Sifilemia: syphilemia
Sifílide: syphilid
Sifilimetria: syphilimetry
Sífilis: syphilis
Sifilítico: syphilitic
Sifilodermia: syphiloderm, syphiloderma
Sifilóide: syphiloid
Sifilologia: syphilology
Sifilologista: syphilologist
Sifiloma: syphiloma

Sifonagem: siphonage
Sigilo: confidentiality
Sigma: sigma
Sigmatismo: sigmatism
Sigmóide: sigmoid
Sigmoidectomia: sigmoidectomy
Sigmoidicidade: sigmoidicity
Sigmoidite: sigmoiditis
Sigmoidopexia: sigmoidopexy
Sigmoidoproctostomia: sigmoidoproctostomy
Sigmoidorretostomia: sigmoidorectostomy
Sigmoidoscopia: sigmoidoscopy
Sigmoidoscópio: sigmoidoscope
Sigmoidostomia: sigmoidostomy
Sigmoidotomia: sigmoidotomy
Sigmoscópio: sigmoscope
Significância estatística: statistical significance
Significante: significant
Sildenafil: sildenafil
Silêncio eletrocerebral: electrocerebral silence (ECS)
Silencioso: silent
Sílica: silica
Sílica da oliva: siliqua olivae
Silicato: silicate
Silicatose: silicatosis
Silícico: silicic
Silício: siliceous, silicon (Si)
Silicoantracose: silicoanthracosis
Silicofluoreto: silicofluoride
Silicone: silicone
Silicoproteinose: silicoproteinosis
Silicose: pneumosilicosis, silicosis
Silicoso: silicious
Silicossiderose: silicosiderosis
Silicotuberculose: silicotuberculosis
Silvático: sylvatic
Silviano: sylvian
Silvol: silvol
Simbalofone: symballophone
Simbionte: symbion, symbiont
Simbiose: symbiosis
Simbiota: symbiote
Simbiótico: symbiotic
Simbléfaro: symblepharon
Simbolia: symbolia
Simbolismo: symbolism
Simbolização: symbolization
Símbolo: symbol
Símbolos de teste: test symbols
Simbraquidactilia: symbrachydactyly
Simelia: symmelia
Simeticona: simethicone
Simetria: symmetry
Simpatectomia: sympathectomy, sympathetectomy
Simpatetoblasto: sympathetoblast
Simpatia: sympathy

Simpaticectomia: sympathicectomy
Simpático: sympathetic, sympathic
Simpaticoblasto: sympathicoblast
Simpaticoneurite: sympathiconeuritis
Simpaticopatia: sympathicopathy
Simpaticotonia: sympathicotonia
Simpaticotônico: sympathicotonic
Simpaticotripsia: sympathicotripsy
Simpatina: sympathin
Simpatismo: sympathism
Simpatizante: sympathizer
Simpatoadrenal: sympathoadrenal
Simpatoblasto: sympathoblast
Simpatogonia: sympathogonia
Simpatolítico: sympatholytic
Simpatomimético: sympathomimetic
Simperitoneal: symperitoneal
Simplasmático: symplasmatic
Simplasto: symplast
Simples: simple
Simpodia: sympodia, sympus
Simpolidactilia: synpolydactyly
Simportador: symporter
Simporte: symport
Simptose: symptosis
Simulação: malingering, simulation
Simulador: malingerer, simulator
Simular: malinger
Simultagnosia: simultagnosia
Simultanagnosia: simultanagnosia
Sinadelfo: synadelphus
Sinaforreceptores: synaphoceptors
Sinal: sign
Sinal de Cantelli: Cantelli sign
Sinal de Hoagland: Hoagland sign
Sinal de Metenier: Metenier sign
Sinal de Mirchamp: Mirchamp sign
Sinal de Romberg: rombergism
Sinal de Toma: Toma sign
Sinanamorfo: synanamorph
Sinanastomose: synanastomosis
Sinandrogênico: synandrogenic
Sinantema: synanthem, synanthema
Sinapse: synapse, pl. synapses; synapsis
Sinapsina I: synapsin I
Sináptico: synaptic
Sinaptofisina: synaptophysin
Sinaptologia: synaptology
Sinaptossoma: synaptosome
Sinartrodia: synarthrodia
Sinartrodial: synarthrodial
Sinartrófise: synarthrophysis

Sinartrose: synarthrosis, pl. synarthroses
Sincalídeo: sincalide
Sincanto: syncanthus
Sincário: syncaryon, synkaryon
Sincefalia: syncephaly
Sincéfalo: syncephalus
Sincianina: syncyanin
Sincicial: syncytial
Sincício: syncytium, pl. syncytia
Sinciciotrofoblasto: syncytiotrophoblast
Sincinese: syncinesis
Sincinesia: synkinesis
Sincinético: synkinetic
Sincipital: sincipital
Sincipúcio: sinciput, pl. sincipita, sinciputs
Sinclinal: synclinal
Sinclítico: synclitic
Sinclitismo: synclitism
Sincondrose: synchondrosis, pl. synchondroses
Sincondroseotomia: synchondroseotomy
Sincondrotomia: synchondrotomy
Sincopal: syncopal
Síncope: syncope
Sincópico: syncopic
Sincorial: synchorial
Sincreção: syncretio
Sincronia: synchronia, synchrony
Sincrônico: synchronic, synchronous
Sincronismo: synchronism
Síncrono: cross-sectional
Síncrotron: synchrotron
Sindactilia: syndactylia, syndactylism, syndactyly
Sindáctilo: syndactyl, syndactyle, syndactylous
Sindeína: syndein
Sindesmectomia: syndesmectomy
Sindesmite: syndesmitis
Sindesmocorial: syndesmochorial
Sindesmodial: syndesmodial
Sindesmófito: syndesmophyte
Sindesmografia: syndesmography
Sindesmologia: syndesmologia, syndesmology
Sindesmose: syndesmosis, pl. syndesmoses
Sindesmótico: syndesmotic
Síndrome: syndrome
Síndrome de Landau-Kleffner: Landau-Kleffner syndrome
Síndrome de Turcot: Turcot syndrome
Sindrômico: syndromic
Sinecótomo: synechotome
Sinectenterotomia: synectenterotomy
Sinematina B: synnematin B
Sinencefalocele: synencephalocele

Sinenxerto: syngraft
Sinéquia: synechia, **pl.** synechiae
Sinequiotomia: synechiotomy
Sinérese: syneresis
Sinergia: synergia, synergy
Sinérgico: synergetic, synergic, synergistic
Sinergismo: synergism
Sinergista: synergist
Sinestesia: synesthesia
Sinestesialgia: synesthesialgia
Sinfalangismo: symphalangism, symphalangy
Sínfise: symphysis, **gen.** symphyses
Sinfisial: symphysial, symphyseal
Sinfísico: symphysic
Sinfísio: symphysion
Sinfisiotomia: symphysiotomy, symphyseotomy
Sinfisiótomo: symphysiotome, symphyseotome
Singamia: syngamy
Singênese: syngenesis
Singenético: syngenetic
Singênico: syngeneic, syngenic
Singnatia: syngnathia
Singulto: singultus
Singultoso: singultous
Sinidrose: synidrosis
Sinigrase, sinigrinase: sinigrase, sinigrinase
Sinistralidade: sinistrality
Sinistro: sinister, sinistrad, sinistral, sinistrous
Sinistrocardia: sinistrocardia
Sinistrocerebral: sinistrocerebral
Sinistrocular: sinistrocular
Sinistrógiro: sinistrogyration
Sinistrômano: sinistromanual
Sinistromanual: left-handed
Sinistropedal: left-footed, sinistropedal
Sinistrorrotação: sinistrorotation
Sinistrorso: sinistrorse
Sinistrotorção: sinistrotorsion
Sinizese: synizesis
Sinoatrial: sinoatrial, sinuatrial (S-A)
Sinofre: synophrys
Sinoftalmia: synophthalmia, synophthalmus
Sinografia: sinography
Sinônimo: synonym
Sinoníquia: synonychia
Sinoptófaro: synoptophore
Sinopulmonar: sinopulmonary
Sinorquidismo: synorchidism, synorchism
Sinósqueo: synoscheos
Sinosteologia: synosteology
Sinostose: synosteosis, synostosis
Sinostótico: synostotic
Sinotia: synotia
Sinovaginal: sinovaginal

Sinovectomia: synovectomy
Sinóvia: synovium
Sinovial: synovial
Sinovíparo: synoviparous
Sinovite: synovitis
Sinquilia: syncheilia, synchilia
Sinquiria: syncheiria, synchiria
Sínquise: synchysis
Sintalidade: syntality
Sintase: synthase
Sintática: syntactics
Sintaxe: syntexis
Sintênico: syntenic
Sintenismo: synteny
Sintérmico: synthermal
Síntese: synthesis, **pl.** syntheses
Sintetase: synthetase
Sintético: syntectic, synthetic
Sintetizar: synthesize
Sintoma: symptom
Sintoma de Bolognini: Bolognini symptom
Sintomático: symptomatic
Sintomatolítico: symptomatolytic, symptomolytic
Sintomatologia: symptomatology
Sintônico: syntonic
Sintórax: synthorax
Sintrofismo: syntrophism
Sintrofoblasto: syntrophoblast
Sintropia: syntropy
Sintrópico: syntropic
Sinusite: sinusitis
Sinusoidal: sinusoidal
Sinusóide: sinusoid
Sinusotomia: sinusotomy
Sinvastatina: simvastatin
Sinzima: synzyme
Sireniforme: sireniform
Sirenomelia: sirenomelia
Siríase: siriasis
Sirigmo: syrigmus
Siringadenoso: syringadenosus
Siringe: syrinx, **pl.** syringes
Siringectomia: syringectomy
Siríngico: syringeal
Siringite: syringitis
Siringoadenoma: syringadenoma, syringoadenoma
Siringobulbia: syringobulbia
Siringocarcinoma: syringocarcinoma
Siringocele: syringocele
Siringocistadenoma: syringocystadenoma
Siringocistoma: syringocystoma
Siringoencefalomielia: syringoencephalomyelia
Siringóide: syringoid
Siringoma: syringoma
Siringomeningocele: syringomeningocele
Siringomielia: siringomyelus, syringomyelia
Siringomielocele: syringomyelocele
Siringopontia: syringopontia
Siringotomia: syringotomy

Siringótomo: syringotome
Sirosingopina: syrosingopine
Sismocardiograma: seismocardiogram
Sismoterapia: seismotherapy, sismostherapy
Sissarcódico: syssarcotic
Sissarcose: syssarcosis
Sissarcósico: syssarcosic
Sistema: system, systema
Sistema Internacional de Unidades: Système International d'Unités
Sistemático: systematic
Sistematização: systematization
Sistêmico: systemic
Sistemóide: systemoid
Sístole: systole
Sistólico: systolic
Sistolômetro: systolometer
Sistrema: systremma
Sítio: situs
Sítio de policlonagem: polylinker
Sitostano: sitostane
β-sitosterol: β-sitosterol
Sitosterolemia: sitosterolemia
Sitotaxia: sitotaxis
Sitotoxina: sitotoxin
Sitotoxismo: sitotoxism
Sitotropismo: sitotropism
Situação: situation
Sizígia: syzygium, syzygy
Sizigial: syzygial
Sizigiologia: syzygiology
Skodaico: skodaic
S-nitroso hemoglobina: S-nitrosohemoglobin
Sobrecarga: load, loading
Sobreenxerto: overgrafting
Sobrefechamento: overclosure
Sobremordida: overbite
Sobrenadante: supernatant
Sobrescrito: superscription
Sobretom: overtone
Sobrevida: survival
Socaloína: socaloin
Socialização: socialization
Socioacusia: socioacusis
Sociocêntrico: sociocentric
Sociocentrismo: sociocentrism
Sociocosmo: sociocosm
Sociogênese: sociogenesis
Sociograma: sociogram
Sócio-médico: sociomedical
Sociometria: sociometry
Sociopata: sociopath
Sociopatia: sociopathy
Soda: soda
Sódico: sodic
Sódio: natrium (Na), sodium (Na)
Sódio-24: sodium-24 (^{24}Na)
Sodoku: sodoku
Sodomia: sodomy
Sodomita: sodomist, sodomite
Sofismar: sophisticate
Soforetina: sophoretin
Soja: soja, soya, soybean
Sokosho: sokosho

Sol: sol
Solação: solation
Solanáceo: solanaceous
Solanocromeno: solanochromene
Solapsona: solapsone
Solassulfona: solasulfone
Solda: solder
Soldadura: brazing
Soldagem: soldering
Solenóide: solenoid
Solenopsina A: solenopsin A
Sóleo: soleus
Solidismo: solidism
Solidista: solidist
Solidístico: solidistic
Sólido: solid, solidus
Sólido de cor: color solid
Solípede: soliped
Solipsismo: solipsism
Solubilidade: solubility
Solução: solutio, solution (sol., soln.)
Solução de Hanks: Hanks solution
Solução diferenciadora de Gallego: Gallego differentiating solution
Soluço, singulto: hiccup, hiccough, singultation
Soluços: thumps
Soluto: solute
Solúvel: soluble
Solvatação: solvation
Solvato: solvate
Solvente: solvent
Solvólise: solvolysis
Som: sound
Som secundário: aftersound
Soma: soma
Somação: summation
Somastenia: somasthenia
Somatagnosia: somatagnosia
Somatalgia: somatalgia
Somatastenia: somatasthenia
Somatestesia: somatesthesia
Somatestético: somatesthetic
Somático: somatic
Somaticoesplâncnico: somaticosplanchnic
Somaticovisceral: somaticovisceral
Somatista: somatist
Somatização: somatization
Somatocrinina: somatocrinin
Somatocromo: somatochrome
Somatofrenia: somatophrenia
Somatogênico: somatogenic
Somatoliberina: somatoliberin
Somatologia: somatology
Somatomamotropina: somatomammotropin
Somatomedina: somatomedin
Somatomedinas: somatomedins
Somatometria: somatometry
Somatópago: somatopagus
Somatopatia: somatopathy
Somatopático: somatopathic
Somatopausa: somatopause
Somatoplasma: somatoplasm
Somatopleura: somatopleure

Glossário

Somatoprotética: somatoprosthetics
Somatopsicose: somatopsychosis
Somatopsíquico: somatopsychic
Somatoscopia: somatoscopy
Somatossensorial: somatosensory
Somatossexual: somatosexual
Somatostatina: somatostatin
Somatostatinoma: somatostatinoma
Somatoterapia: somatotherapy
Somatotipo: somatotype
Somatotipologia: somatotypology
Somatotopagnose: somatotopagnosis
Somatotopia: somatotopy
Somatotópico: somatotopic
Somatotrófico: somatotrophic
Somatotrofo: somatotroph
Somatotrópico: somatotropic
Somatotropina: somatotropin
Somatotropos: somatotropes
Somatrem: somatrem
Somatropina: somatropin
Somestesia: somesthesia
Somito: somite
Sonambulismo: sleepwalking, somnambulance, somnambulism
Sonâmbulo: sleepwalker, somnambulist
Sonda: probe
Sonda interligada de Davis: Davis interlocking sound
Sone: sone
Sonho: dream
Sônico: sonic
Sonifaciente: somnifacient
Sonífero: somniferous
Sonífico: somnific
Soniloquência: somniloquence, somniloquism
Soniloquia: somniloquy
Soniloquismo: sleeptalking
Soniloquista: somniloquist
Sono: sleep
Sonografia: sonography
Sonógrafo: sonograph, sonographer
Sonograma: sonogram
Sonolência: drowsiness, sleepiness, somnolence, somnolency, somnolentia
Sonolento: somnolent, somnolescent
Sonomicrômetro: sonomicrometer
Sonomotor: sonomotor
Sonoquímica: sonochemistry
Sonotransparente: sonolucent
Sopor: sopor
Soporífero: soporiferous
Soporífico: soporific
Soporoso: soporose, soporous
Soprador de fragmentos: chip-blower
Sopro: murmur, souffle

Sopro de Cole-Cecil: Cole-Cecil murmur
Soral: serumal
Sorbina: sorbin
Sorbinose: sorbinose
Sorbitan: sorbitan
Sorbitol: sorbite, sorbitol
D-sorbitol-6-fosfato desidrogenase: D-sorbitol-6-phosphate dehydrogenase
Sorbitose: sorbitose
L-sorbose: L-sorbose
Soro: serum, **pl.** serums, sera; whey
Soro de leite: buttermilk
Soroalbumina: seralbumin
Soroconversão: seroconversion
Sorodiagnóstico: serodiagnosis
Soroenterite: seroenteritis
Soroepidemiologia: seroepidemiology
Sorogrupo: serogroup
Sorologia: serology
Sorológico: serologic
Soronegativo: seronegative
Soropositivo: seropositive
Soropurulento: seropurulent
Soropus: seropus
Soro-resistente: serum-fast
Sorotipo: serotype
Sorovacinação: serovaccination
Sorovariante: serovar
S-sulfocisteína: S-sulfocysteine
Statcoulomb: statcoulomb
Statfarad: statfarad
Stathenry: stathenry
Stat-volt: statvolt
Stokes: stokes
Suarda: suint
Subabdominal: subabdominal
Subabdominoperitoneal: subabdominoperitoneal
Subacetato: subacetate
Subacromial: subacromial
Subagudo: subacute
Subalimentação: subalimentation
Subanal: subanal
Subaórtico: subaortic
Subapical: subapical
Subaponeurótico: subaponeurotic
Subaracnóide: subarachnoid
Subareolar: subareolar
Subarqueado: subarcuate
Subatômico: subatomic
Subaural: subaural
Subauricular: subauricular
Subaxial: subaxial
Subaxilar: subaxillary
Sub-basal: subbasal
Sub-braquicefálico: subbrachycephalic
Subcalcarino: subcalcarine
Subcapsular: subcapsular
Subcarbonato: subcarbonate
Subcardinal: subcardinal
Subcartilaginoso: subcartilaginous
Subcecal: subcecal
Subcelular: subcellular

Subcepção: subception
Subclasse: subclass
Subclavicular: subclavicular
Subclávio: subclavian, subclavius
Subclínico: subclinical
Subclonagem: subcloning
Subcloreto: subchloride
Subcolateral: subcollateral
Subcondral: subchondral
Subconjuntival: subconjunctival
Subconjuntivite: subconjunctivitis
Subconsciência: subconsciousness
Subconsciente: subconscious
Subcoracóide: subcoracoid
Subcorar: understain
Subcorioidal: subchoroidal
Subcoriônico: subchorionic
Subcórtex: subcortex
Subcortical: subcortical
Subcostal: subcostal
Subcostalgia: subcostalgia
Subcostoesternal: subcostosternal
Subcraniano: subcranial
Subcrepitação: subcrepitation
Subcrepitante: subcrepitant
Subcultura: subculture
Subcurativo: subcurative
Subcutâneo: subcutaneous (sc., SQ)
Subcuticular: subcuticular
Subdeltóide: subdeltoid
Subdentário: subdental
Subdiafragmático: subdiaphragmatic
Subdorsal: subdorsal
Subdural: subdural
Subendimário: subendymal
Subendocárdico: subendocardial
Subendotelial: subendothelial
Subendotélio: subendothelium
Subenovelamento: underwinding
Subependimário: subependymal
Subependimoma: subependymoma
Subepidérmico: subepidermal, subepidermic
Subepitelial: subepithelial
Subepitélio: subepithelium
Suberose: suberosis
Subescapular: subscapular, subscapularis
Subescleral: subscleral
Subesclerótico: subsclerotic
Subespinal: subspinale
Subespinhoso: subspinous
Subesternal: substernal
Subesternomastóideo: substernomastoid
Subestrutura: substructure
Subfamília: subfamily
Subfaríngeo: subpharyngeal
Subfascial: subfascial
Subfertilidade: subfertility

Subfilo: subphylum
Subfissura: subfissure
Subfólio: subfolium
Subfrênico: subphrenic
Subgalato: subgallate
Subgênero: subgenus
Subgengival: subgingival
Subglenóide: subglenoid
Subglosso: subglossal
Subglótico: subglottic
Subgranular: subgranular
Sub-hepático: subhepatic
Sub-hialóide: subhyaloid
Sub-hióide: subhyoid, subhyoidean
Subictérico: subicteric
Subicular: subicular
Subículo: subiculum, **pl.** subicula
Subilíaco: subiliac
Subílio: subilium
Subimpulso: undershoot
Subinfecção: subinfection
Subinflamatório: subinflammatory
Subíntimo: subintimal
Subintrante: subintrant
Subinvolução: subinvolution
Subiodeto: subiodide
Subjacente: subjacent
Subjetivo: subjective
Subjugal: subjugal
Subletal: sublethal
Subleucemia: subleukemia
Sublimação: sublimation
Sublimar: sublimate, sublime
Sublime: sublimis
Subliminal: subliminal
Sublingual: sublingual
Sublobular: sublobular
Sublombar: sublumbar
Subluminal: subluminal
Subluxação: semiluxation, subluxation
Submamário: submammary
Submandibular: submandibular
Submarginal: submarginal
Submedial, submediano: submedial, submedian
Submembranoso: submembranous
Submental: submental
Submergido: submerged
Submetacêntrico: submetacentric
Submicrônico: submicronic
Submicroscópico: submicroscopic
Submorfo: submorphous
Submucosa: submucosa
Submucoso: submucous
Subnarcótico: subnarcotic
Subnasal: subnasal
Subnásio: subnasion
Subneural: subneural
Subnitrato: subnitrate
Subnormal: subnormal
Subnormalidade: subnormality
Subnotocordal: subnotochordal
Subnúcleo: subnucleus

Subnutrição: undernutrition
Suboccipital: suboccipital
Suborbitário: suborbital
Subordem: suborder
Subótimo: suboptimal
Suboxidação: suboxidation
Subóxido: suboxide
Subparietal: subparietal
Subpatelar: subpatellar
Subpeitoral: subpectoral
Subpelviperitoneal: subpelviperitoneal
Subpercepção: undersensing
Subpericárdico: subpericardial
Subperiósteo: subperiosteal
Subperitoneal: subperitoneal
Subperitoneoabdominal: subperitoneoabdominal
Subperitoneopélvico: subperitoneopelvic
Subpetroso: subpetrosal
Subpial: subpial
Subpiramidal: subpyramidal
Subplacentário: subplacental
Subplatina: substage
Subpleural: subpleural
Subprepucial: subpreputial
Subpúbico: subpubic
Subpulmonar: subpulmonary
Sub-reino: subkingdom
Sub-retiniano: subretinal
Subsartorial: subsartorial
Subserosa: subserosa
Subseroso: subserous, subserosal
Substância: substance, substantia, **pl.** substantiae
Substância branca: alba
Substância cinzenta: grey matter
Substituição: substitution
Substituto: locum tenens, substitute, surrogate
Substrato: substrate (S), substratum
Subsulfato: subsulfate
Subtalâmico: subthalamic
Subtálamo: subthalamus
Subtalar: subastragalar
Subtarsal: subtarsal
Subtentorial: subtentorial
Subterminal: subterminal
Subtetânico: subtetanic
Subtilisina: subtilisin
Subtilopeptidase: subtilopeptidase
Subtimpânico: subtympanic
Subtireóideo: subthyroideus
Subtração: subtraction
Subtrapezial: subtrapezial
Subtribo: subtribe
Subtrocantérico: subtrochanteric
Subtroclear: subtrochlear
Subtuberal: subtuberal
Subumbilical: subumbilical
Subungueal: subungual, subunguial
Subunidade: subunit
Suburetral: suburethral

Subvaginal: subvaginal
Subvalvar: subvalvar, subvalvular
Subvertebral: subvertebral
Subvigília: subwaking
Subviril: subvirile
Subvírion: subvirion
Subvítreo: subvitrinal
Subzigomático: subzygomatic
Subzonal: subzonal
Sucagogo: succagogue
Sucção: suction
Succinato: succinate
Succinato de doxilamina: doxylamine succinate
Succinato ferroso: ferrous succinate
Succinato semialdeído: succinate semialdehyde
Succinil acetona: succinylacetone
Succinil-CoA: succinyl-CoA
Succinil-CoA ligase: succinyl-CoA ligase
Succinil-coenzima A: succinyl-coenzyme A
Succinilcolina: succinylcholine
Succinildicolina: succinyldicholine
Succinilsulfatiazol: succinylsulfathiazole
Succinimida: succinimide
Succissulfona iminodietanol: succisulfone iminodiethanol
Sucedâneo: succedaneous, succedaneum
Suco: juice
Suco de cereja: cherry juice
Sucorréia: succorrhea
Sucralfato: sucralfate
Súcubo: succubus
Sucussão: succussion
Sudação: sudation
Sudâmina: sudamen, **pl.** sudamina
Sudanofilia: sudanophilia
Sudanofílico: sudanophilic
Sudanofóbico: sudanophobic
Sudomotor: sudomotor
Sudorese: sudoresis, sweating
Sudorífero: sudoriferous
Sudorífico: sudorific
Sudorômetro: sudorometer
Sufocação: suffocation
Sufocar: suffocate
Sufusão: suffusion
Sugar: suck
Sugestão: suggestion
Sugestibilidade: suggestibility
Sugestionável: suggestible
Sugestivo: suggestive
Sugilação: suggillation
Suicídio: suicide
Suicidologia: suicidology
Suíno: porcine
Sujeira: soil
Sulbactam: sulbactam
Sulbetina: sulbentine
Sulcado: sulcate
Sulciforme: sulciform

Sulco: furrow, groove, sulcus, **gen. e pl.** sulci
Súlculo: sulculus, **pl.** sulculi
Sulfa: sulfa
Sulfabenzamida: sulfabenzamide
Sulfacetamida: sulfacetamide
Sulfácido: sulfacid
Sulfacitina: sulfacytine
Sulfadiazina: sulfadiazine
Sulfadimetoxina: sulfadimethoxine
Sulfadimidina: sulfadimidine
Sulfadoxina: sulfadoxine
Sulfaetidol: sulfaethidole
Sulfafenazol: sulfaphenazole
Sulfafurazol: sulfafurazole
Sulfaguanidina: sulfaguanidine
Sulfaguinidina: sulfaguine
Sulfaleno: sulfalene
Sulfamerazina: sulfamerazine
Sulfametazina: sulfamethazine
Sulfametizol: sulfamethizole
Sulfametoxazol: sulfamethoxazole
Sulfametoxidiazina: sulfamethoxydiazine
Sulfametoxipiridazina: sulfamethoxypyridazine
Sulfâmetro: sulfameter
Sulfamoxol: sulfamoxole
Sulfanilamida: sulfanilamide
Sulfapirazina: sulfapyrazine
Sulfapiridina: sulfapyridine
Sulfassalazina: sulfasalazine
Sulfatase: sulfatase
Sulfatiazol: sulfathiazole
Sulfatidatos: sulfatidates
Sulfatidos: sulfatides
Sulfatidose: sulfatidosis
Sulfatização: sulfation
Sulfato: sulfate
Sulfato de amicacina: amikacin sulfate
Sulfato de betanidina: betanidine sulfate, bethanidine sulfate
Sulfato de bleomicina: bleomycin sulfate
Sulfato de butacaína: butacaine sulfate
Sulfato de capreomicina: capreomycin sulfate
Sulfato de cobre: cupric sulfate
Sulfato de *d*-anfetamina: *d*-amphetamine sulfate
Sulfato de debrisoquina: debrisoquine sulfate
Sulfato de dextroanfetamina: dextroamphetamine sulfate
Sulfato de dibutolina: dibutoline sulfate
Sulfato de dimetila: dimethyl sulfate
Sulfato de fenelzina: phenelzine sulfate
Sulfato de guanaclina: guanacline sulfate
Sulfato de guanadrel: guanadrel sulfate

Sulfato de guanetidina: guanethidine sulfate
Sulfato de guanocloro: guanochlor sulfate
Sulfato de guanoxano: guanoxan sulfate
Sulfato de heparana: heparan sulfate
Sulfato de heparitina: heparitin sulfate
Sulfato de hidroxicloroquina: hydroxychloroquine sulfate
Sulfato de isoprenalina: isoprenaline sulfate
Sulfato de isoproterenol: isoproterenol sulfate
Sulfato de metaproterenol: metaproterenol sulfate
Sulfato de neomicina: neomycin sulfate
Sulfato de netilmicina: netilmicin sulfate
Sulfato de orciprenalina: orciprenaline sulfate
Sulfato de paromomicina: paromomycin sulfate
Sulfato de queratano: keratan sulfate
Sulfato de sisomicina: sisomicin sulfate
Sulfato de terbutalina: terbutaline sulfate
Sulfato de tranilcipromina: tranylcypromine sulfate
Sulfato de vimblastina: vinblastine sulfate
Sulfato de vincristina: leurocristine, vincristine sulfate
Sulfato férrico: ferric sulfate
Sulfato férrico de amônio: ferric ammonium citrate ammonium sulfate
Sulfato ferroso: ferrous sulfate
Sulfemetemoglobina: sulfmethemoglobin
Sulfemoglobina: sulfhemoglobin
Sulfemoglobinemia: sulfhemoglobinemia
Sulfeto: sulfide, sulfuret
Sulficinase: sulfikinase
Sulfidrato: sulfhydrate, sulfydrate
Sulfidrila: sulfhydryl (SH)
Sulfimpirazona: sulfinpyrazone
Sulfisomidina: sulfisomidine
Sulfissoxazol: sulfisoxazole
Sulfito: sulfite
Sulfitúria: sulfituria
Sulfoácido: sulfoacid
3-sulfoalanina: 3-sulfoalanine
Sulfobromoftaleína sódica: sulfobromophthalein sodium
Sulfocianato: sulfocyanate
Sulfocinase: sulfokinase
3-sulfogalactosilceramida: 3-sulfogalactosylceramide
Sulfogel: sulfogel
Sulfoidrato: sulfohydrate
Sulfólise: sulfolysis

Sulfometato sódico de colistina: cholistine sulphomethate sodium
Sulfomixina sódica: sulfomyxin sodium
Sulfomucina: sulfomucin
Sulfona: sulfone
Sulfonamidas: sulfonamides
Sulfonato: sulfonate
Sulfonato de vermelho-escarlate: scarlet red sulfonate
Sulfoniluréias: sulfonylureas
Sulfoproteína: sulfoprotein
6-sulfoquinovosil diacilglicerol: 6-sulfoquinovosyl diacylglycerol
Sulformetoxina: sulformethoxine
Sulforrodamina B: sulforhodamine B
Sulfossol: sulfosol
Sulfossuccinato cálcico de dioctila: dioctyl calcium sulfosuccinate
Sulfossuccinato sódico de dioctila: dioctyl sodium sulfosuccinate
Sulfotransferase: sulfotransferase
Sulfóxido: sulfoxide
Sulfóxido de dimetila: dimethyl sulfoxide (DMSO)
Sulfoxilato de fenarsona: phenarsone sulfoxylate
Sulfoxona sódica: sulfoxone sodium
Sulfúrico: sulfuric
Sulfuril: sulfuryl
Sulfuroso: sulfurous
Sulindac: sulindac
Sulisobenzona: sulisobenzone
Sulpirida: sulpiride
Sultiame: sulthiame
Suor: sudor, sweat
Superabdução: superabduction
Superacidez: superacidity
Superagudo: superacute
Superalimentação: superalimentation, suralimentation
Superantígeno: superantigen
Superatividade: superactivity
Supercílio: eyebrow, supercilium, pl. supercilia
Supercompensação: overcompensation
Superdeterminação: overdetermination
Superdicrótico: superdicrotic
Superdistensão: superdistention
Superdominância: overdominance
Superdominante: overdominant
Superego: superego
Superenrolamento: superhelicity
Supererupção: overeruption
Superespiral: supercoiling
Superestímulo: overdrive
Superestrutura: superstructure
Superexcitação: superexcitation
Superextensão: superextension
Superfetação: superfetation
Superficial: superficial, superficialis
Superfície: surface
Superflexão: superflexion
Superfundir: superfuse
Superfusão: superfusion
Supergorduroso: superfatted
Superidratação: overhydration
Superimpregnação: superimpregnation
Superinduzir: superinduce
Superinfecção: superinfection
Superinvolução: superinvolution
Superior: superior
Superlactação: superlactation
Supermedial: supermedial
Supermotilidade: supermotility
Supernutrição: supernutrition
Súpero-lateral: superolateral
Superovulação: superovulation
Superóxido: superoxide
Superparasita: superparasite
Superparasitismo: superparasitism
Superpetroso: superpetrosal
Superposição: overlap
Superposição horizontal: overjet, overjut
Supersaturar: supersaturate
Supersônico: supersonic
Supertensão: supertension
Supervoltagem: supervoltage
Supinação: supination
Supinador: supinator
Supinar: supinate
Supino: supine
Suporte: brace, supporter
Suporte angulado: bracket
Suporte básico de vida: basic life support
Suposição: assumption
Supositório: suppository
Supra-acromial: superacromial, supra-acromial
Supra-anal: superanal, supra-anal
Supra-auricular: supra-auricular
Supra-axilar: supra-axillary
Suprabucal: suprabuccal
Supracardinal: supracardinal
Supracerebelar: supracerebellar
Supracerebral: supracerebral
Supraciliar: superciliary, supraciliary
Supraclavicular: supraclavicular, supraclavicularis
Supracondilar: supracondylar
Supracondilóide: supracondyloid
Supracorióide: suprachoroid
Supracostal: supracostal
Supracotilóide: supracotyloid
Supradiafragmático: supradiaphragmatic
Supradução: supraduction
Supra-epicondilar: supraepicondylar
Supra-escapular: suprascapular
Supra-escleral: suprascleral
Supra-espinal: supraspinal, supraspinalis, supraspinatus, supraspinous
Supra-estapedial: suprastapedial
Supra-esternal: suprasternal
Suprafisiológico: supraphysiologic, supraphysiological
Supraglenóide: supraglenoid
Supraglótico: supraglottic
Supraglotite: supraglottitis
Supra-hepático: suprahepatic
Supra-hióideo: suprahyoid
Supra-inguinal: suprainguinal
Supra-intestinal: supraintestinal
Supraliminal: supraliminal
Supralombar: supralumbar
Supramaleolar: supramalleolar
Supramamário: supramammary
Supramandibular: supramandibular
Supramarginal: supramarginal
Supramastóideo: supramastoid
Supramaxilar: supramaxillary
Supramental: supramental, supramentale
Supranasal: supranasal
Supraneural: supraneural
Supranuclear: supranuclear
Supranumerário: supernumerary
Supra-oclusão: supraocclusion
Supra-orbital: supraorbital
Supra-orbitomeatal: supraorbitomeatal
Suprapatelar: suprapatellar
Suprapélvico: suprapelvic
Suprapúbico: suprapubic
Supra-regulação: up-regulation
Supra-renal: suprarenal, surrenal
Supra-selar: suprasellar
Supra-silviano: suprasylvian
Supra-sinfisário: suprasymphysary
Supratemporal: supratemporal
Supratentorial: supratentorial
Supratimpânico: supratympanic
Supratonsilar: supratonsillar
Supratorácico: suprathoracic
Supratroclear: supratrochlear
Supravaginal: supravaginal
Supravalvar: supravalvar, supravalvular
Supraventricular: supraventricular
Supraversão: supraversion
Supressão: suppression, withdrawal
Supressor: suppressor
Suprofeno: suprofen
Supuração: suppuration
Supurar: fester, suppurate
Supurativo: suppurant, suppurative
Sural: sural
Suramina sódica: suramin sodium
Surdez: deafness
Surdo: deaf
Surfactante: surfactant
Sursundução: sursumduction
Sursunversão: sursumversion
Suscetibilidade: susceptibility
Suspensão: suspension
Suspensóide: suspensoid
Suspensor: suspensory
Suspiro: sigh
Sussurrar: whisper
Sussurro: susurrus
Sustentacular: sustentacular
Sustentáculo: sustentaculum, pl. sustentacula
Sutura: sutura, pl. suturae; suture
Sutura plana: harmonia
Sutura por planos: terrace
Sutural: sutural
Suturar: stitch
Suturectomia: suturectomy
Suxametônio: suxamethonium

T

Tabaco: tobacco
Tabanídeo: tabanid
Tabaqueira: snuffbox
Tabaqueira anatômica: anatomic snuffbox, tabatière anatomique
Tabardilho: tabardillo
Tabela: chart
Tabela de crescimento de Tanner: Tanner growth chart
Tabes: tabes
Tabescência: tabescence
Tabescente: tabescent
Tabético: tabetic
Tabetiforme: tabetiform
Tábido: tabic, tabid
Tablatura: tablature
Tablete: tablet, tabule
Tabu: taboo, tabu
Tabular: tabular
Taça: poculum
Tacografia: tachography
Tacógrafo: tachograph
Tacograma: tachogram
Tacômetro: tachometer
Tacrina: tacrine
Tactômetro: tactometer
Tafofilia: taphophilia
Tafofobia: taphophobia
Tagatose: tagatose
Tagliacotiano: tagliacotian
Takadiastase: Taka-diastase
Talalgia: talalgia
Talamectomia: thalamectomy
Talâmico: thalamic
Tálamo: thalamus, pl. thalami
Talamocortical: thalamocortical
Talamoencefálico: thalamencephalic
Talamoencéfalo: thalamencephalon

Talamolenticular: thalamolenticular
Talamotomia: thalamotomy
Talar: astragalar, talar
Talassemia: thalassemia, thalassanemia
Talassofobia: thalassophobia
Talassoposia: thalassoposia
Talassoterapia: thalassotherapy
Talco: talc, talcum
Talcose: talcosis
Talião: talion
Tálico: thallic
Talidomida: thalidomide
Tálio: thallium (TI)
Tálipe: talipes
Talipédico: talipedic
Talo: thalus
Talocalcâneo: astragalocalcanean, calcaneoastragaloid, talocalcaneal, talocalcanean
Talocrural: talocrural
Talofibular: astragalofibular, talofibular
Talófito: thallophyte
Talonavicular: astragaloscaphoid, talonavicular, taloscaphoid
Talose: talose
Talotibial: astragalotibial, talotibial
Talotoxicose: thallotoxicosis
Tálus: talus, **gen.** tali
Tamarindo: tamarind
Tambor: tambour
Tampão: buffer, plug, tampon
Tamponamento: packing, tamponade, tamponage, tamponing, tamponment
Tanacetol: tanacetol, tanacetone
Tanase: tannase
Tanato: tannate
Tanatobiológico: thanatobiologic
Tanatofídios: thanatophidia
Tanatofobia: thanatophobia
Tanatofórico: thanatophoric
Tanatognomônico: thanatognomonic
Tanatografia: thanatography
Tanatóide: thanatoid
Tanatologia: thanatology
Tanatomania: thanatomania
Tánatos: thanatos
Tanchagem: plantago
Tangencialidade: tangentiality
Tanicito: tanycyte
Tânico: tannic
Tanifonia: tanyphonia
Tanil acetato: tannylacetate
Tanino: tannin
Tanque: tank
Tântalo: tantalum (Ta)
Tapete: tapetum, **pl.** tapeta
Tapetocorioidal: tapetochoroidal
Tapetorretiniano: tapetoretinal
Tapetorretinopatia: tapetoretinopathy
Tapinocefalia: tapinocephaly

Tapinocefálico: tapinocephalic
Tapioca: tapioca
Tapotagem: tapotement, tapping
Taquiarritmia: tachyarrhythmia
Taquiauxese: tachyauxesis
Taquicardia: polycardia, tachycardia, tachysystole
Taquicardíaco: tachycardiac
Taquicárdico: tachycardic
Taquicinina: tachykinin
Taquicrótico: tachycrotic
Taquiestimulação: tachypacing
Taquifilaxia: tachyphylaxis
Taquipnéia: tachypnea
Taquirritmia: tachyrhythmia
Taquisterol: tachysterol
Taquistoscópio: tachistoscope
Taquizoíta: tachyzoite
Tarantismo: tarantism
Tarântula: tarantula
Taraxaco: taraxacum
Tardio: tardive
Targretina: targretin
Tarsal: tarsal, tarsale, **pl.** tarsalia
Tarsalgia: tarsalgia
Tarsectomia: tarsectomy
Tarsectopia: tarsectopia, tarsectopy
Tarsite: tarsitis
Tarso: tarsus
Tarsoclasia: tarsoclasia, tarsoclasis
Tarsofalângico: tarsophalangeal
Tarsomalacia: tarsomalacia
Tarsomegalia: tarsomegaly
Tarsometatarsal: tarsometatarsal
Tarso-orbital: tarso-orbital
Tarsorrafia: tarsorhaphy
Tarsotarsal: tarsotarsal
Tarsotibial: tarsotibial
Tarsotomia: tarsotomy
Tartamudear: stammer, stutter
Tartamudez: stammering, stuttering
Tartarado: tartrated
Tartarato: tartrate
Tartarato de butorfanol: butorphanol tartrate
Tartarato de dextromoramida: dextromoramide tartrate
Tartarato de diidrocodeína: dihydrocodeine tartrate
Tartarato de dimetacrina: dimetacrine tartrate
Tartarato de dimetilpiperazina: dimethylpiperazine tartrate
Tartarato de fempentermina: phenpentermine tartrate
Tartarato de fendimetrazina: phendimetrazine tartrate
Tartarato de fenindamina: phenindamine tartrate
Tartarato de hidramitrazina: hydramitrazine tartrate
Tartarato de levalorfano: levallorphan tartrate
Tartarato de levorfanol: levorphanol tartrate

Tartarato de metoprolol: metoprolol tartrate
Tartarato de nicotinil: nicotinyl tartrate
Tartarato de pentolínio: pentolinium tartrate
Tartarato de trimeprazina: trimeprazine tartrate
Tártaro: tartar
Tartrazina: tartrazine
Tátil: tactile
Tatuagem: tattoo
Taumatropia: thaumatropy
Taurina: taurine
Taurocolato: taurocholate
Taurodontismo: taurodontism
Tauromérico: tauromeric
Tautomerismo: tautomerism
Taxa: rate
Taxanos: taxanes
Taxia: taxis
Táxon: taxon, **pl.** taxa
Taxonomia: taxonomy
Taxonômico: taxonomic
t-**butoxicarbonila:** *t*-butoxycarbonyl (BOC, *t*-BOC, Boc)
Tebaico: thebaic
Tebaína: thebaine
Tebutato: tebutate
Teca: theca, **pl.** thecae; thèque
Tecal: thecal
Tecido: textus, tissue
Tecido adiposo: fat
Tecido subcutâneo: subcutis
Tecidual: tissular
Teclotiazida: teclothiazide
Tecnécio: technetium (Tc)
Tecnécio-99: technetium-99 (^{99}Tc)
Tecnécio-99m (Tc^{99m}): technetium-99m (^{99m}Tc)
Técnica: technic, technique
Técnica da janela cutânea de Rebuck: Rebuck skin window technique
Técnico: technical, technician
Técnico em radiografia: radiographer
Tecnocause: technocausis
Tecnologia: technology
Tecnólogo: technologist
Tecodonte: thecodont
Tecoma: thecoma
Tecomatose: thecomatosis
Tectônico: tectonic
Tectonologia: tectology
Tectorial: tectorial
Teflurano: teflurane
Tefrilômetro: tephrylometer
Tefromalacia: tephromalacia
Tegme; teto: tegmen, **gen.** tegminis, **pl.** tegmina
Tegmentar: tegmental
Tegmento: tegmentum, **pl.** tegmenta
Tegmentotomia: tegmentotomy
Tegumentar, tegumentário: tegumental, tegumentary
Tegumento: tegument
Teia: web

Teia de aranha: spider-burst
Teicopsia: teichopsia
Teinismo, teísmo: theinism, theism, theaism
Tela: screen, tela, **gen. e pl.** telae
Telalgia: telalgia
Telangiectasia: telangiectasia, telangiectasis, **pl.** telangiectases
Telangiectásico: telangiectatic
Telangiectóides: telangiectodes
Telângio: telangion
Telangioma: telangioma
Telangiose: telangiosis
Telarca: thelarche
Telazíase: thelaziasis
Tele: *tele*
Telecanto: telecanthus
Telecardiofone: telecardiophone
Telecardiograma: telecardiogram
Telecobalto: telecobalt
Telediagnóstico: telediagnosis
Telediastólico: telediastolic
Teleletrocardiograma: telelectrocardiogram
Telemetria: telemetry
Telêmetro: telemeter
Telencefálico: telencephalic
Telencefalização: telencephalization
Telencéfalo: endbrain, telencephalon
Teleologia: teleology
Teleomitose: teleomitosis
Teleomorfo: teleomorph
Teleonomia: teleonomy
Teleonômico: teleonomic
Teleopsia: teleopsia
Teleorgânico: teleorganic
Telepatia: telepathy
Telepatina: telepathine
Telergia: telergy
Telerrádio: teleradium
Telerradiografia: teleradiography, teleroentgenography, teleroentgentherapy
Telerradiologia: teleradiology
Telerreceptor: telereceptor
Telescópio: telescope
Telese: telesis
Telessistólico: telesystolic
Teleterapia: teletherapy
Télio: thelium, **pl.** thelia
Telocinesia: telokinesia
Telodendro: end-brush, telodendron
Telófase: telophase
Telógeno: telogen
Telóglia: teloglia
Telognose: telognosis
Telolécito: telolecithal
Telomerase: telomerase
Telômero: telomere
Telopeptídio: telopeptide
Telorragia: thelorrhagia
Telotismo: telotism
Telúrico: telluric
Telúrio: tellurium (Te)
Telurismo: tellurism
Temazepam: temazepam

Temor: fear
Temperado: temperate
Temperamento: temperament
Temperança: temperance
Temperar: anneal
Temperatura: temperature
Tempestade: storm
Tempo: time (t)
Tempoestável: tempostabile, tempostable
Tempolábil: tempolabile
Têmpora: temple
Temporal: temporal
Temporário: fugitive
Temporesfenóide: temporosphenoid
Temporoauricular: temporoauricular
Temporoccipital: temporo-occipital
Têmporo-hióideo: temporohyoid
Temporomandibular: temporomandibular
Temporomaxilar: temporomaxillary
Temporoparietal: temporoparietal
Temporopontino: temporopontine
Temporozigomático: temporomalar, temporozygomatic
Tenacidade: tenacity
Tenáculo: tenaculum, **pl.** tenacula
Tenaldina: thenaldine
Tenalgia: tenalgia
Tenar: thenal, thenar
Tenaz: tenacious
Tenazes: tweezers
Tenda cirúrgica: turunda, **pl.** turundae
Tendão: sinew, tendo, tendon, **gen.** tendinis, **pl.** tendines
Tendenciosidade: bias
Tendíneo: tendinous
Tendinite: tendinitis, tendonitis, tenontitis
Tendinoplastia: tendinoplasty
Tendinossutura: tendinosuture
Tendões do jarrete: hamstring
Tendomucina: tendomucin, tendomucoid
Tenectomia: tenectomy, tenonectomy
Tenésmico: tenesmic
Tenesmo: tenesmus
Tênia: taenia, tapeworm, tenia, **pl.** teniae
Teníase: taeniasis, teniasis
Tenicida: teniacide, tenicide
Tenídio: taeniid
Teniforme: teniform
Tenífugo: teniafuge, tenifugal, tenifuge
Tenil: thenyl
Tenióide: taenioid, tenioid
Teníola: teniola
Tenodese: tenodesis

Tenodinia: tenodynia
Tenófito: tenophyte
Tenofonia: tendophony, tenophony
Tenólise: tendolysis, tenolysis
Tenomioplastia: tenomyoplasty
Tenomiotomia: tenomyotomy
Tenonite: tenonitis
Tenontografia: tenontography
Tenontologia: tenontology
Tenontomioplastia: tenontomyoplasty
Tenontomiotomia: tenontomyotomy
Tenontoplastia: tenontoplasty
Tenontoplástico: tenontoplastic
Tenoplastia: tenoplasty
Tenoplástico: tenoplastic
Tenorrafia: tenorrhaphy
Tenorreceptor: tenoreceptor
Tenossinovectomia: tenosynovectomy
Tenossinovite: tendosynovitis, tendovaginitis, tenosynovitis
Tenossuspensão: tenosuspension
Tenossutura: tenosuture
Tenostose: tenostosis
Tenotomia: tendotomy, tenotomy
Tenotomia aquiléia: achillotenotomy
Tenovaginal: tendovaginal
Tenovaginite: tenovaginitis
Tensão: tension
Tensiômetro: tensiometer
Tenso: tense
Tensoativo: surface-active
Tensor: tensor, **pl.** tensores
Tenta: tent
Tentáculo: tentacle
Tentativa e erro: trial and error
Tentorial: tentorial
Tentório: tentorium, **pl.** tentoria
Teobroma: theobroma
Teobromina: theobromine
Teoclato de prometazina: promethazine theoclate
Teofilina: theophylline
Teofobia: theophobia
Teomania: theomania
Teorema: theorem
Teoria: theory
Teoterapia: theotherapy
Teprotídio: teprotide
Terapeuta: therapeutist, therapist
Terapêutica: therapeusis, therapeutics
Terapêutico: therapeutic
Terapia: therapia, therapy
Terapia protética: prosthetics
Terático: teratic
Teratismo: teratism
Teratoblastoma: teratoblastoma
Teratocarcinoma: teratocarcinoma
Teratofobia: teratophobia
Teratogênese: teratogenesis
Teratogenicidade: teratogenicity

Teratogênico: teratogenic, teratogenetic
Teratógeno: teratogen
Teratóide: teratoid
Teratologia: teratology
Teratológico: teratologic
Teratoma: teratoma
Teratomatoso: teratomatous
Teratose: teratosis
Teratospermia: teratospermia
Teratozoospermia: teratozoospermia
Térbio: terbium (Tb)
terc-butiloxicarbonila: tert-butyloxycarbonyl (tBoc)
Terça: tertian
Terciarismo: tertiarism, tertiarismus
Terçol: sty, stye, **pl.** sties, styes
Terebeno: terebene
Terebintina: terebinthine, turpentine
Terebintinato: terebinthinate
Terebintinismo: terebinthinism
Terebração: terebration
Terebrante: terebrant, terebrating
Terencéfalo: therencephalous
Terfenadina: terfenadine
Tergal: tergal
Tergo: tergum
Teríaca: theriaca
Teriaga: treacle
Teriomorfismo: theriomorphism
Termacogênese: thermacogenesis
Termal: thermal
Termalgesia: thermalgesia
Termalgia: thermalgia
Termanalgesia: thermanalgesia
Termanestesia: thermanesthesia
Termatologia: thermatology
Termelômetro: thermelometer
Termestesia: thermesthesia
Termestesiômetro: thermesthesiometer
Terminação: ending, terminatio, **pl.** terminationes, termination
Terminações axônicas: end-feet, pieds terminaux
Terminal: terminal
Término: terminus, **pl.** termini
Termistor: thermistor
Termo: term
Termoacidófilos: thermoacidophiles
Termoalgesia: thermoalgesia
Termoanalgesia: thermoanalgesia
Termoanestesia: thermoanesthesia
Termocauterectomia: thermocauterectomy
Termocautério: thermocautery
Termoceratoplastia: thermokeratoplasty
Termocoagulação: thermocoagulation
Termocorrente: thermocurrent
Termocróico: thermochroic

Termocroísmo: thermochroism
Termocrose: thermochrose, thermochrosis
Termocrosia: thermochrosy
Termodifusão: thermodiffusion
Termodiluição: thermodilution
Termodinâmica: thermodynamics
Termodúrico: thermoduric
Termoeletricidade: thermoelectricity
Termoelétrico: thermoelectric
Termoestável: heat-stable
Termoestesia: thermoesthesia
Termoestesiômetro: thermoesthesiometer
Termoexcitatório: thermoexcitory
Termofílico: thermophilic, thermophylic
Termófilo: thermophile, thermophil
Termofixo: thermoset
Termofobia: thermophobia
Termóforo: thermophore
Termogênese: thermogenesis
Termogenético: thermogenetic, thermogenic
Termogênica: thermogenics
Termogênico: thermogenous
Termogenina: thermogenin
Termografia: thermography
Termógrafo: thermograph
Termograma: thermogram
Termoinibitório: thermoinhibitory
Termointegrador: thermointegrator
Termoiperalgesia: thermohyperalgesia
Termoiperestesia: thermohyperesthesia
Termoipestesia: thermohypesthesia
Termoipoestesia: thermohypoesthesia
Termojunção: thermojunction
Termolábil: heat-labile, thermolabile
Termólise: thermolysis
Termolítico: thermolytic
Termologia: thermology
Termomassagem: thermomassage
Termometria: thermometry
Termométrico: thermometric
Termômetro: thermometer
Termoneurose: thermoneurosis
Termônio: termone
Termonuclear: thermonuclear
Termopar: thermocouple
Termopenetração: thermopenetration
Termopilha: thermopile
Termoplacentografia: thermoplacentography
Termoplasma: thermoplasma, **pl.** thermoplasmata
Termoplástico: thermoplastic
Termoplegia: heatstroke, thermoplegia

Termoquímica: thermochemistry
Termorreceptor: thermoreceptor
Termorregulação: thermoregulation
Termorregulador: thermoregulator
Termoscópio: thermoscope
Termossistáltico: thermosystaltic
Termossistaltismo: thermosystaltism
Termostato: thermostat
Termostável: thermostabile, thermostable
Termosterese: thermosteresis
Termotático: thermotactic, thermotaxic
Termotaxia: thermotaxis
Termoterapia: thermotherapy
Termótica: thermotics
Termótico: thermotic
Termotonômetro: thermotonometer
Termotropismo: thermotropism
Ternário: ternary
Teróide: theroid
Terologia: therology
Teróxido: teroxide
Terpeno: terpene
Terpina: terpin
Terpineol: terpineol
Terpinol: terpinol
Terra: earth
Terra japonesa: terra japonica
Territorialidade: territoriality
Terror noturno: night terror, pavor nocturnus
Tesaurismose: thesaurismosis
Tesaurismótico: thesaurismotic
Tesaurose: thesaurosis
Tese: thesis, **pl.** theses
Tesla: tesla (T)
Tesoura: shears
Testa: brow, testa
Testalgia: testalgia
Testar: test
Teste: testing
Teste de Betke-Kleihauer: Betke-Kleihauer test
Teste de Harris e Ray: Harris and Ray test
Teste de Kurzrok-Ratner: Kurzrok-Ratner test
Teste de Quinlan: Quinlan test
Teste de redução do corante de Motulsky: Motulsky dye reduction test
Teste de Rimini: Rimini test
Teste de Ropes: Ropes test
Teste de Schaffer: Schaffer test
Teste de Stenger: Stenger test
Testectomia: testectomy
Testicular: testicular
Testículo: orchis, **pl.** orchises; testicle, testiculus, testis, **pl.** testes
Testiforme: textiform
Testite: testitis
Testóide: testoid

Testolactona: testolactone
Testosterona: testosterone
Testotoxicose: testotoxicosis
Tetania: tetany
Tetânico: tetanic
Tetaniforme: tetaniform
Tetanígeno: tetanigenous
Tetanismo: tetanism
Tetanização: tetanization
Tetanizar: tetanize
Tétano: tetanus
Tetanóide: tetanoid
Tetanolisina: tetanolysin
Tetanômetro: tetanometer
Tetanomotor: tetanomotor
Tetanospasmina: tetanospasmin
Tetanotoxina: tetanotoxin
Tetinas: thetins
Teto: plafond, roof, tectum, **pl.** tecta
Tetospinal: tectospinal
Tetrabásico: tetrabasic
Tetrabenazina: tetrabenazine
Tetrabráquio: tetrabrachius
Tetrabromofenolftaleína sódica: tetrabromophenolphthalein sodium
Tetraciclina: tetracycline
Tetraclormetiazida: tetrachlormethiazide
Tetracloroetano: cellon, tetrachloroethane
Tetracloroetileno: tetrachlorethylene, tetrachloroethylene
Tetraclorometano: tetrachloromethane
Tetracoco: tetracoccus, **pl.** tetracocci
Tetracosactida: tetracosactide, tetracosactin
Tetracrótico: tetracrotic
Tetracúspide: tetracuspid
Tetradáctilo: tetradactyl
Tétrade: tetrad
Tetrádico: tetradic
Tetraetil pirofosfato: tetraethyl pyrophosphate (TEPP)
Tetraetilmonotionopirofosfato: tetraethylmonothionopyrophosphate
Tetrafocomelia: tetraphocomelia
Tetragastrina: tetragastrin
Tetrágono: tetragon, tetragonum, tetragonus
Tetraídrico: tetrahydric
Tetraidrocanabinol: tetrahydrocannabinol (THC)
5,6,7,8-tetraidrofolato desidrogenase: 5,6,7,8-tetrahydrofolate dehydrogenase
Tetraidrofolato metiltransferase: tetrahydrofolate methyltransferase
Tetraiodofenolftaleína sódica: tetraiodophenolphthalein sodium
Tetralogia: tetralogy
Tetramastia: tetramastia

Tetramastigota: tetramastigote
Tetramasto: tetramastous
Tetramelia: tetra-amelia
Tetrâmelo: tetramelus
Tetramérico: tetrameric, tetramerous
Tetrametildiarsina: tetramethyldiarsine
Tetrametilputrescina: tetramethylputrescine
Tetranitrato de eritritil: erythrityl tetranitrate
Tetranitrato de pentaeritritol: pentaerythritol tetranitrate
Tetranitrol: tetranitrol
Tetranucleotídio: tetranucleotide
Tetraoto: tetraotus
Tetraparesia: tetraparesis
Tetrapeptídio: tetrapeptide
Tetraperomelia: tetraperomelia
Tetrapirrol: tetrapyrrole
Tetraplegia: tetraplegia
Tetraplégico: tetraplegic
Tetraplóide: tetraploid
Tetrápode: tetrapus
Tetráquiro: tetrachirus
Tetráscelo: tetrascelus
Tetrassacarídio: tetrasaccharide
Tetrassômico: tetrasomic
Tetráster: tetraster
Tetrastiquíase: tetrastichiasis
Tetraterpenos: tetraterpenes
Tetratômico: tetratomic
Tetravalente: tetravalent
Tetrazol: tetrazole
Tetrazólio: tetrazolium
Tetrodotoxina: tetrodotoxin (TTX)
Tetrose: tetrose
Tetroto: tetrotus
Tetróxido: tetroxide
Textura: texture
Textural: textural
Therm: therm
Thogotovírus: Thogotoviruses
Tiabendazol: thiabendazole
Tiabutazida: thiabutazide
Tiacetazona: thiacetazone
Tialbarbital: thialbarbital
Tiambutosina: thiambutosine
Tiamilal sódico: thiamylal sodium
Tiamina: thiamin, thiamine
Tiaminase: thiaminase
Tianfenicol: thiamphenicol
Tiazidas: thiazides
Tiazina: thiazin
Tiazolidinedionas: thiazolidinediones
Tiazolsulfona: thiazolsulfone
Tibamato: tybamate
Tíbia: shank, tibia, **gen. e pl.** tibiae
Tibial: tibial, tibialis
Tibiocalcâneo: tibiocalcanean
Tibiofascial: tibiofascialis
Tibiofemoral: tibiofemoral
Tibiofibular: peroneotibial, tibiofibular, tibioperoneal

Tibionavicular: tibionavicular, tibioscaphoid
Tibiotarsal: tibiotarsal
Ticarcilina dissódica: ticarcillin disodium
Ticolubante: ticolubant
Ticosteróide: secosteroid
Tiel: thiel
Tiemia: thiemia
Tienamicina: thienamycin
Tienil: thienyl
Tienilalanina: thienylalanine
Tifínia: typhinia
Tiflectasia: typhlectasis
Tiflectomia: typhlectomy
Tiflenterite: typhlenteritis
Tiflite: typhlitis
Tiflodiclidite: typhlodicliditis
Tifloempiema: typhloempyema
Tifloenterite: typhloenteritis
Tiflolitíase: typhlolithiasis
Tiflomegalia: typhlomegaly
Tiflopexia: typhlopexy, typhlopexia
Tiflorrafia: typhlorrhaphy
Tiflose: typhlosis
Tiflostomia: typhlostomy
Tiflotomia: typhlotomy
Tifo: typhus
Tifóide: typhoid, typhoidal
Tifolisina: typholysin
Tifomania: typhomania
Tifoso: typhous
Tiglato: tiglate
Tiglil-CoA: tiglyl-CoA
Tiglil-coenzima A: tiglyl-coenzyme A
Tigmestesia: thigmesthesia
Tigmotaxia: thigmotaxis
Tigmotropismo: thigmotropism
Tigróide: tigroid
Tigrólise: tigrolysis
Tilectomia: tylectomy
Tílio: tylion, **pl.** tylia
Tiloma: tyloma
Tilorona: tilorone
Tilose: tylosis, **pl.** tyloses
Tiloxapol: tyloxapol
Timazolina: tymazoline
Timbre: timbre
Timectomia: thymectomy
Timelcose: thymelcosis
Timerosal: thimerosal
Tímico: thymic
Timicolinfático: thymicolymphatic
Timidilato sintase: thymidylate synthase
Timidina: thymidine (dThd)
Timidina 5′-difosfato: thymidine 5′diphosphate (dTDP)
Timidina 5′-monofosfato: thymidine 5′-monophosphate (dTMP)
Timidina 5′-trifosfato: thymidine 5′-triphosphate (dTTP)
Timina: thymin, thymine (Thy)
Timinúria: thyminuria
Timite: thymitis

Timo: thymus, **pl.** thymi, thymuses
Timocinético: thymokinetic
Timócito: thymocyte
Timogênico: thymogenic
Timol: thymol
Timoma: thymoma
Timonuclease: thymonuclease
Timopoetina: thymopoietin
Timoprivo: thymoprival, thymoprivic, thymoprivous
Timosina: thymosin
Timoxamina: thymoxamine
Timpanectomia: tympanectomy
Timpania: tympania
Timpanicidade: tympanicity
Timpânico: tympanal, tympanic, tympanous
Timpanismo: tympanism, tympanites, tympany
Timpanite: tympanitis
Timpanítico: tympanitic
Tímpano: eardrum, tympanum, **pl.** tympana, tympanums
Timpanocentese: tympanocentesis
Timpanoescamoso: tympanosquamosal
Timpanoeustaquiano: tympanoeustachian
Timpanofonia: tympanophonia, tympanophony
Timpanograma: tympanogram
Timpanomandibular: tympanomandibular
Timpanomastoidectomia: tympanomastoidectomy
Timpanomastóideo: tympanomastoid
Timpanomastoidite: tympanomastoiditis
Timpanometria: tympanometry
Timpanoplastia: tympanoplasty
Timpanosclerose: tympanosclerosis
Timpanostapédico: tympanostapedial
Timpanostomia: tympanostomy
Timpanotemporal: tympanotemporal
Timpanotomia: tympanotomy
Tindalização: tyndallization
Tingibilidade: tingibility
Tingível: tinctable, tingible
Tinha: ringworm, serpigo, tinea
Tinidazol: tinidazole
Tinido: tinnitus
Tintorial: tinctorial
Tintura: paint, tinction, tinctura, **gen. e pl.** tincturae; tincture
Tioácido: thioacid
Tioálcool: thioalcohol
Tioamida: thioamide
Tioato: thioate
Tiobarbitúricos: thiobarbiturates
Tiocarbamida: thiocarbamide
Tiocarlida: thiocarlide
Tiocianato: thiocyanate
Tiocinase: thiokinase

Tiocinase (tioquinase) succínica: succinic thiokinase
Tioconazol: tioconazole
Tiocromo: thiochrome
Tiodepsipeptídio: thiodepsipeptide
Tiodifenilamina: thiodiphenylamine
Tioéster: thioester
Tioesterase: thioesterase
Tioésteres: thioesters
Tioetanolamina acetiltransferase: thioethanolamine acetyltransferase
Tioéter: thioether
Tiofenicol: thiophenicol
Tiofeno: thiophene
Tioflavina S: thioflavine S
Tioflavina T: thioflavin T
Tioforase acetoacetilsuccínica: acetoacetyl-succinic thiophorase
Tiofurano: thiofuran
Tioglicerol: thioglycerol
Tioglicolato: thioglycolate, thioglycollate
Tioglicosidase: thioglucosidase
Tioguanina: thioguanine
Tiol: thiol, thiole
Tiolase: thiolase
Tiolesterase: thiolesterase
Tiólise: thiolysis
Tiolistidilbetaína: thiolhistidylbetaine
Tioltransacetilase A: thioltransacetylase A
Tiomersal: thiomersal
Tiomersalato: thiomersalate
Tiometiladenosina: thiomethyladenosine
β-tionase: β-thionase
Tioneína: thionein, thioneine
Tiônico: thionic
Tionina: thionine
Tiopental sódico: thiopental sodium
Tioproperazina: thioproperazine
Tiorredoxina: thioredoxin
Tiosemicarbazida: thiosemicarbazide
Tiosemicarbazona: thiosemicarbazone
Tiossulfato: thiosulfate
Tiotepa: thiotepa
Tiotixeno: thiothixene
Tiotransacetilase B: thiotransacetylase B
2-tiouracil: 2-thiouracil
4-tiouracil: 4-thiouracil
Tiouréia: thiourea
Tioxanteno: thioxanthene
Tioxolona: thioxolone
Tipagem: typing
Tipo: type, typus
Tipo sangüíneo: blood type
Tipóia: sling
Tique: tic
Tique facial: palmus, **pl.** palmi
Tiramina: tyramine

Tiraminase: tyraminase
Tiranismo: tyrannism
Tirêmese: tyremesis
Tireoadenite: thyroadenitis
Tireoaplasia: thyroaplasia
Tireoaritenóideo: thyroarytenoid
Tireocalcitonina: thyrocalcitonin
Tireocardíaco: thyrocardiac
Tireocele: thyrocele
Tireocervical: thyrocervical
Tireocolóide: thyrocolloid
Tireoepiglótico: thyroepiglottic
Tireofaríngeo: thyropharyngeal
Tireofissura: thyrofissure
Tireogênico: thyrogenic, thyrogenous
Tireoglobulina: thyroglobulin
Tireoglosso: thyroglossal
Tíreo-hióideo: thyrohyoid
Tireóide: thyroid, thyroidea
Tireoidectomia: thyroidectomy
Tireoidismo: thyroidism
Tireoidite: thyroiditis
Tireoidologia: thyroidology
Tireoidotomia: thyroidotomy
Tireointoxicação: thyrointoxication
Tireolaríngeo: thyrolaryngeal
Tireoliberina: thyroliberin
Tireolingual: thyrolingual
Tireolítico: thyrolytic
Tireomegalia: thyromegaly
Tireopalatino: thyropalatine
Tireoparatireoidectomia: thyroparathyroidectomy
Tireopatia: thyropathy
Tireoperoxidase: thyroperoxidase
Tireoplastia: thyroplasty
Tireoprivia: thyroprivia
Tireoprivo: thyroprival, thyroprivic, thyroprivous
Tireoproteína: thyroprotein
Tireoptose: thyroptosis
Tireotomia: thyrotomy
Tireotóxico: thyrotoxic
Tireotoxicose: thyrotoxicosis
Tireotoxina: thyrotoxin
Tireotrófico: thyrotrophic
Tireotrofina: thyrotrophin
Tireotrofo: thyrotroph
Tireotrópico: thyrotropic
Tireotropina: thyrotropin
Tirocetonúria: tyroketonuria
Tirocidina: tyrocidin, tyrocidine
Tirocinase: tyrosinase
β-tirocinase: β-tyrosinase
Tirógeno: tyrogenous
Tiróide: tyroid
Tiroma: tyroma
Tironina: thyronine
Tiropanoato sódico: tyropanoate sodium
Tirose: tyrosis
Tirosilúria: tyrosyluria
Tirosina: tyrosine (Tyr, Y)
Tirosinemia: tyrosinemia
Tirosinose: tyrosinosis
Tirosinúria: tyrosinuria

Tirotoxina: thyroxine (T_4), thyroxin
Tirotoxismo: tyrotoxism
Tirotricina: tyrothricin
Tisiologista: phthisiologist
Titânio: titanium (Ti)
Titilação: titillation
Titina: titin
Titubeação: titubation
Titulação: titration
Titulante: titrant
Titular: titrate
Título: titer
Tixolábil: thixolabile
Tixotrópico: thixotropic
Tobramicina: tobramycin
Tococromanol-3: tocochromanol-3
Tocodinágrafo: tocodynagraph
Tocodinamômetro: tocodynamometer
Tocoferilquinona: tocopherylquinone
Tocoferol: tocopherol (T)
α-tocoferol: α-tocopherol (α-T)
β-tocoferol: β-tocopherol (β-T)
γ-tocoferol: γ-tocopherol (γ-T)
Tocoferolquinona: tocopherolquinone (TQ)
Tocofobia: tocophobia
Tocografia: tocography
Tocógrafo: tocograph
Tocol: tocol
Tocolítico: tocolytic
Tocologia: tocology
Tocômetro: tocometer
Tocoquinona: tocoquinone
Tocotrienol: tocotrienol
Tocotrienolquinona: tocotrienolquinone
Tofáceo: tophaceous
Tofo: tophus, **pl.** tophi
Togavírus: togavirus
Tolazamida: tolazamide
Tolbutamida: tolbutamide
Tolciclamida: tolcyclamide
Tolerância: tolerance
Tolerância G: g-tolerance
Tolerante: tolerant
Tolerogênico: tolerogenic
Tolerógeno: tolerogen
Tolexamida: tolhexamide
Tolil: tolyl
Tolmetina: tolmetin
Tolnaftato: tolnaftate
Tolpropamina: tolpropamine
Tolueno: toluene
Toluidina: toluidine
Toluoil: toluoyl
Toluol: toluol
Tom: tone
Tomilho: thyme
Tomografia: stratigraphy, tomography
Tomógrafo: tomograph
Tomograma: tomogram
Tomomania: tomomania
Tonafasia: tonaphasia
Tonalidade: hue, tint
Toner: toner
Tonicidade: tonicity

Tônico: tonic
Tônico-clônico: tonicoclonic
Tonina: tonin
Tonitrofobia: tonitrophobia
Tonoclônico: tonoclonic
Tonofanto: tonophant
Tonofibrila: tenofibril, tonofibril
Tonofilamento: tonofilament
Tonografia: tonography
Tonógrafo: tonograph
Tonometria: tonometry
Tonômetro: tonometer
Tonoplasto: tonoplast
Tonoscilógrafo: tonoscillograph
Tonotópico: tonotopic
Tonotrópico: tonotropic
Tonsila: tonsil, tonsilla, **pl.** tonsillae
Tonsilar: tonsilar, tonsillary
Tonsilectomia: tonsillectomy
Tonsilite: tonsillitis
Tonsilólito: tonsillolith, tonsilolith
Tonsilopatia: tonsillopathy
Tonsilotomia: tonsillotomy
Tonsilótomo: tonsillotome
Tonteira: dizziness
Tônus: tonus
Topagnose: topagnosis
Topestesia: topesthesia
Tópico: topical
Tópicos: topica
Topístico: topistic
Topoanestesia: topoanesthesia
Topofilaxia: topophylaxis
Topofobia: topophobia
Topognose: topognosis, topognosia
Topogômetro: topogometer
Topografia: topography
Topoisomerase: topoisomerase
Topologia: topology
Toponarcose: toponarcosis
Toponimia: toponymy
Topônimo: toponym
Topopatogenia: topopathogenesis
Topotecana: topotecan
Toque: taction, touch
Toracalgia: thoracalgia
Toracentese: thoracentesis
Torácico: thoracal, thoracic
Torácico-abdominal: thoracicoabdominal
Torácico-acromial: thoracicoacromial
Torácico-humeral: thoracicohumeral
Toracoabdominal: thoracoabdominal
Toracoacromial: thoracoacromial
Toracocelosquise: thoracoceloschisis
Toracocentese: thoracocentesis
Toracocilose: thoracocyllosis
Toracocirtose: thoracocyrtosis
Toracodelfo: thoracodelphus, thoradelphus
Toracodinia: thoracodynia

Toracodorsal: thoracodorsal
Toracogastrosquise: thoracogastroschisis
Toracolaparotomia: thoracolaparotomy
Toracólise: thoracolysis
Toracolombar: thoracolumbar
Toracômelo: thoracomelus
Toracômetro: thoracometer
Toracomiodinia: thoracomyodynia
Toracópago: thoracopagus
Toracoparacéfalo: thoracoparacephalus
Toracopatia: thoracopathy
Toracoplastia: thoracoplasty
Toracopneumoplastia: thoracopneumoplasty
Toracoscopia: thoracoscopy
Toracoscópio: thoracoscope
Toracosquise: thoracoschisis
Toracostenose: thoracostenosis
Toracosternotomia: thoracosternotomy
Toracostomia: thoracostomy
Toracotomia: thoracotomy
Tórax: chest, thorax, **gen.** thoracis, **pl.** thoraces
Tórax em funil: trichterbrust
Torção: torsion
Torcedura: kink
Torcicolar: torticollar
Torcicolo: torticollis, wryneck
Torcionômetro: torsionometer
Torcipelve: tortipelvis
Torcular de Herófilo: torcular herophili
Tórico: toric
Tório: thorium (Th)
Torniquete: tourniquet
Torno mecânico: lathe
Tornozelo: ankle
Toro: elevation, torus, **pl.** tori
Toroso: torose, torous
Torpente: torpent
Tórpido: torpid
Torpor: torpor
Torque: torque (T)
Torr: torr
Torrefação: torrefaction
Torrefazer: torrefy
Torsade de pointes: torsade de pointes
Torsiversão: torsiversion
Torso: torso
Torsoclusão: torsoclusion
Tortuoso: tortuous
Tórulo: torulus, **pl.** toruli
Tosil: tosyl
Tosilato: tosylate
Tosilato de bretílio: bretylium tosylate
Tosilato de itramina: itramin tosylate
Tosse: cough, tussis
Tosse seca: tussiculation
Totem: totem
Totemismo: totemism
Totemístico: totemistic
Totipotência: totipotency, totipotence

Totipotente, totipotencial: totipotent, totipotential
Touca: headgear
Toxafeno: toxaphene
Toxanemia: toxanemia
Toxemia: toxemia
Toxêmico: toxemic
Toxicemia: toxicemia
Toxicidade: toxicity
Tóxico: toxic, toxicant
Toxicofobia: toxicophobia
Toxicogênico: toxicogenic
Toxicóide: toxicoid
Toxicologia: toxicology
Toxicológico: toxicologic
Toxicologista: toxicologist
Toxicopático: toxicopathic
Toxicose: toxicosis
Toxiferinas: toxiferines
Toxífero: toxiferous
Toxifobia: toxiphobia
Toxigenicidade: toxigenicity
Toxigênico: toxigenic
Toxina: toxin
Toxínico: toxinic
Toxinogenicidade: toxinogenicity
Toxinogênico: toxinogenic
Toxinologia: toxinology
Toxinose: toxinosis
Toxisterol: toxisterol
Toxoalbuminas: toxalbumins
Toxocaríase: toxocariasis
Toxófilo: toxophil, toxophile
Toxóforo: toxophore, toxophorous
Toxóide: toxoid
Toxona: toxon, toxone
Toxonema: toxoneme
Toxonose: toxonosis
Toxopirimidina: toxopyrimidine
Toxoplasmose: toxoplasmosis
Trabalho: work
Trabalho de parteira: midwifery
Trabalho de parto: labor
Trabécula: trabecula, **gen. e pl.** trabeculae
Trabeculação: trabeculation
Trabeculado: trabeculate
Trabecular: trabecular
Trabeculectomia: trabeculectomy
Trabeculoplastia: trabeculoplasty
Trabeculotomia: trabeculotomy
Traçado: draw-sheet, tracing
Traçador: tracer
Tração: traction, tug, tugging
Traço: trace, trait
Tracoma: trachoma
Tracomatoso: trachomatous
Tradução: translation
Tragacanto: tragacanth, tragacantha
Tragal: tragal
Trágico: tragicus
Trágio: tragion
Trago: antilobium, tragus, **pl.** tragi

Tragofonia: tragophonia, tragophony
Tragomascalia: tragomaschalia
Traje: suit
Trajeto: path
Tramadol: tramadol
Tranqüilizante: tranquilizer
Transação: transaction
Transacetilação: transacetylation
Transacetilase: transacetylase
Transacilação: transacylation
Transacilases: transacylases
Transaldolação: transaldolation
Transaldolase: transaldolase
Transamidação: transamidation
Transamidinação: transamidination
Transamidinases: transamidinases
Transaminação: transamination
Transaminase glutâmico aspártica: glutamic-aspartic transaminase
Transaminase glutâmico oxaloacética (TGO): glutamic-oxaloacetic transaminase (GOT)
Transaminase glutâmico pirúvica (TGP): glutamic-pyruvic transaminase (GPT)
Transaminase glutâmico-oxaloacética sérica (TGO): serumglutamic-oxaloacetic transaminase (SGOT)
Transaminase glutâmico-pirúvica sérica (TGP): serum glutamic-pyruvic transaminase (SGPT)
Transaminases: transaminases
Transaudiente: transaudient
Transcapsidação: transcapsidation
Transcarbamoilação: transcarbamoylation
Transcarbamoilases: transcarbamoylases
Transcarboxilases: transcarboxylases
Transcetolação: transketolation
Transcetolase: transketolase
Transcitose: transcytosis
Transcobalaminas: transcobalamins
Transcondilar: transcondylar
Transcortical: transcortical
Transcortina: transcortin
Transcrição: transcription
Transcricionista médico: medical transcriptionist
Transcriptase: transcriptase
Transcutâneo: transcutaneous
Transdérmico: transdermic
Transdução: transduction
Transducina: transducin
Transdutante: transductant
Transdutor: transducer
Transduzir: transduce
Transe: trance

Transecção: transection, transsection
Transegmentar: transsegmental
Transeptal: transseptal
Transesfenoidal: transsphenoidal
Transetmoidal: transethmoidal
Transexual: transsexual
Transexualismo: transsexualism
Transfecção: transfection
Transferases: transferases
Transferência: transfer, transference
Transferência de carga: charge transfer
Transferrina: transferrin
Transfixação: transfixion
Transformação: transformation
Transformada: transform
Transformante: transformant
Transfosfatases: transphosphatases
Transfosforilação: transphosphorylation
Transfosforilases: transphosphorylases
Transfundir: transfuse
Transfusão: transfusion
Transgene: transgene
Transgênese: transgenesis
Transgênico: transgenic
Transglicosidação: transglycosidation
Transglicosilase: transglucosylase, transglycosylase
Transglótico: transglottic
Transglutaminase: transglutaminase
Trans-hiatal: transhiatal
Transição: transition
Transicional: transitional
Transilíaco: transiliac
Transiluminação: transillumination
Transináptico: transsynaptic
Transinsular: transinsular
Transiquiático: transischiac
Transístmico: transisthmian
Trânsito: trafficking
Transitório: transient
Transjunção: trans-splicing
Translocação: translocation
Translúcido: translucent
Transmembrana: transmembrane
Transmetilação: transmethylation
Transmetilase: transmethylase
Transmigração: transmigration
Transmissão: transmission
Transmissível: communicable, transmissible
Transmural: transmural
Transmutação: transmutation
Transocular: transocular
Transonância: transonance
Transônico: transonic
Transparietal: transparietal
Transpeptidação: transpeptidation

Transpeptidase: transpeptidase
Transperitoneal: transperitoneal
Transpiração: perspiration, transpiration
Transpirar: transpire
Transpirável: transpirable
Transplacentário: transplacental
Transplantar: transplant, transplantar
Transplante: transplantation
Transpleural: transpleural
Transpor: transpose
Transporte: carry-over, transport
Transporte bidirecional: shuttle
Transposase: transposase
Transposição: transposition
Transposon: transposon
Trans-retinal: *trans*-retinal
Transretinal total: all-*trans*-retinal
Transtalâmico: transthalamic
Transtentorial: transtentorial
Transtermia: transthermia
Transtiretina: transthyretin
Transtorácico: transthoracic
Transtoracotomia: transthoracotomy
Transtorno: disorder
Transudação: transudation
Transudar: transude
Transudato: transudate
Transulfuração: transsulfuration
Transulfurase: transsulfurase, transulfurase
Transureteroureterostomia: transureteroureterostomy (TUU)
Transuretral: transurethral
Transvaalina: transvaalin
Transvaginal: transvaginal
Transvector: transvector
Transversal: transversalis
Transversão: transversion
Transversectomia: transversectomy
Transverso: transverse, transversus
Transversocostal: transversocostal
Transverso-espinais: transversospinales
Transversouretral: transversourethralis
Transvestismo: transvestism, transvestitism
Trapezial: trapezial
Trapeziforme: trapeziform
Trapézio: trapezium, **pl.** trapezia; trapeziums, trapezius
Trapeziometacarpal: trapeziometacarpal
Trapezóide: trapezoid
Trapidil: trapidil
Traqueal: tracheal, trachealis
Traquealgia: trachealgia
Traquéia: trachea, **pl.** tracheae; windpipe
Traqueíte: tracheitis, trachitis

Traquelectomia: trachelectomy
Traquelematoma: trachelematoma
Traqueliano: trachelian
Traquelismo: trachelism, trachelismus
Traquelite: trachelitis
Traquelo: trachelos
Traqueloccipital: tracheloccipitalis
Traquelocele: trachelocele
Traquelomastóideo: trachelomastoid
Traquelopano: trachelopanus
Traquelopexia: trachelopexia, trachelopexy
Traqueloplastia: tracheloplasty
Traquelorrafia: trachelorrhaphy
Traquelosquise: tracheloschisis
Traquelotomia: trachelotomy
Traqueoaerocele: tracheoaerocele
Traqueobiliar: tracheobiliary
Traqueobroncomegalia: tracheobronchomegaly
Traqueobroncoscopia: tracheobronchoscopy
Traqueobronqueopatia osteoplásica: tracheobroncheopathia osteoplastica
Traqueobrônquico: tracheobronchial
Traqueobronquite: tracheobronchitis
Traqueocele: tracheocele
Traqueoesofágico: tracheoesophageal
Traqueofaríngeo: tracheopharyngeal
Traqueofonia: tracheophony
Traqueofonose: tracheophonesis
Traqueolaríngeo: tracheolaryngeal
Traqueomalacia: tracheomalacia
Traqueomegalia: tracheomegaly
Traqueopatia: tracheopathia, tracheopathy
Traqueoplastia: tracheoplasty
Traqueorragia: tracheorrhagia
Traqueoscopia: tracheoscopy
Traqueoscópico: tracheoscopic
Traqueoscópio: tracheoscope
Traqueósquise: tracheoschisis
Traqueostenose: tracheostenosis
Traqueostoma: tracheostoma
Traqueostomia: tracheostomy
Traqueotomia: tracheotomy
Traqueótomo: tracheotome
Traquicromático: trachychromatic
Traquifonia: trachyphonia
Traquioníquia: trachyonychia
Tratamento: treatment
Tratar: treat
Tratelo: tractellum, **pl.** tractella
Trato: tract, tractus
Trator: tractor

Tratotomia: tractotomy
Traumático: traumatic
Traumatismo: trauma, **pl.** traumata, traumas; traumatism
Traumatizar: traumatize
Traumatologia: traumatology
Traumatonose: traumatonesis
Traumatopatia: traumatopathy
Traumatopira: traumatopyra
Traumatopnéia: traumatopnea
Traumatosepse: traumatosepsis
Traumatoterapia: traumatotherapy
Trava: lock
Travestido: transvestite
Travestismo: cross-dressing
Treala: trehala
Trealase: trehalase
Trealose: mycose, trehalose
Trefócito: trephocyte
Treinamento: training
Treliça: lattice
Tremacamra: tremacamra
Trematódeo: fluke, trematode, trematoid
Trematódeo digenético: *Prosthogonimus macrorchis*
Tremedeira: shakes
Tremelóide: tremelloid, tremellose
Tremógrafo: tremograph
Tremograma: tremogram, tremorgram
Tremolábil: tremolabile
Tremor: shiver, trembling, tremor
Tremor de frio ou de medo: shivering
Tremores da cabeça: head-nodding
Tremorina: tremorine
Tremostável: tremostable
Trêmulo: tremulous
Treonina: threonine (T, Thr)
Treose: threose
Trepanação: trepanation, trephination
Trépano: burr, trephine
Trepidação: trepidation
Treponema: treponeme
Treponematose: treponematosis
Treponemíase: treponemiasis
Treponemicida: treponemicidal
Tretinoína: tretinoin
Trevo aquático: bogbean
Trevo d'água: menyanthes
Triacetilglicerol: triacetylglycerol
Triaceliloleandomicina: triacetyloleandomycin
Triacetina: triacetin
Triacilglicerol: triacylglycerol
Tríade: triad
Triagem: triage
Triamelia: tri-amelia
Triancinolona: triamcinolone
Triangular: triangularis
Triângulo: triangle, triangulum
Triângulo de Burger: Burger triangle
Triângulo de cor: collor triangle

Triantereno: triamterene
Triazolam: triazolam
Triazologuanina: triazologuanine
Tribásico: tribasic
Tribasilar: tribasilar
Tribo: tribe
Tribologia: tribology
Triboluminescência: triboluminescence
Tribraquia: tribrachia
Tribráquio: tribrachius
Tribromsalan: tribromsalan
Tributirase: tributyrase
Tributirilglicerol: tributyrylglycerol
Tributirina: tributyrin
Tributirinase: tributyrinase
Tricalgia: trichalgia
Tricângio: trichangion
Tricatrofia: trichatrophia
Tricauxe: trichauxis
Tricéfalo: tricephalus
Tríceps: triceps
Tricetopurina: triketopurine
Tricipital: tricipital
Triclofenol piperazina: triclofenol piperazine
Triclofos: triclofos
Tricloral: trichloral
Tricloreto: trichloride
Triclorfon: trichlorfon
Tricloridrato de sedoxantrona: sedoxantrone trihydrochloride
Triclormetiazida: trichlormethiazide
Triclormetina: trichlormethine
Tricloroetano: trichloroethane
Tricloroetanol: trichloroethanol
Tricloroeteno: trichloroethene
Tricloroetileno: trichloroethylene
Triclorofenol: trichlorophenol
Triclorofluorometano: trichlorofluoromethane
Triclorometano: trichloromethane
Tricloromonofluorometano: trichloromonofluoromethane
Tricocisto: trichocyst
Tricodinia: trichodynia
Tricodiscoma: trichodiscoma
Tricodistrofia: trichodystrophy
Tricoepitelioma: trichoepithelioma
Tricoestesia: trichoesthesia
Tricofagia: trichophagia, trichophagy
Tricofítico: trichophytic
Tricofitobezoar: trichophytobezoar
Tricofitose: trichophytosis
Tricofobia: trichophobia
Tricofoliculoma: trichofolliculoma
Tricógeno: trichogen
Tricoglossia: trichoglossia
Tricoialina: trichohyalin
Tricóide: trichoid
Tricolemoma: tricholemmoma
Tricologia: trichology
Tricoma: trichoma
Tricomatose: trichomatosis
Tricomegalia: trichomegaly
Tricomicetose: trichomycetosis
Tricomicose: trichomycosis
Tricomonacida: trichomonacide
Tricomônade: trichomonad
Tricomoníase: trichomoniasis
Triconodose: trichonodosis
Triconose: trichonosis
Tricopatia: trichopathy
Tricopático: trichopathic
Tricopatofobia: trichopathophobia
Tricopoliodistrofia: trichopoliodystrophy
Tricopoliose: trichopoliosis
Tricoptilose: trichoptilosis
Tricorne: tricorn, tricornute
Tricorrexe: trichorrhexis
Tricose: trichosis
Tricosomatoso: trichosomatous
Tricosporonose: trichosporonosis
Tricosporose: trichosporosis
Tricosquise: trichoschisis
Tricostase espinhosa: trichostasis spinulosa
Tricostrôngilo: trichostrongyle
Tricostrongilose: trichostrongylosis
Tricotilomania: trichotillomania
Tricotiodistrofia: trichothiodystrophy
Tricotomia: trichotomy
Tricotoxina: trichotoxin
Tricotrofia: trichotrophy
Tricresol: tricresol
Tricróico: trichroic
Tricroísmo: trichroism
Tricromático: trichromatic
Tricromatismo: trichromatism
Tricrômato: trichromat
Tricromatopsia: trichromatopsia
Tricrômico: trichromic
Tricromo: trichrome
Tricrótico: tricrotic
Tricrotismo: tricrotism
Tricroto: tricrotous
Tricuríase: trichuriasis
Tricúspide: tricuspid, tricuspidal, tricuspidate
Tridáctilo: tridactylous, tridigitate
Tridentado: tridentate
Tridente: trident
Tridérmico: tridermic
Tridermoma: tridermoma
Tridimita: tridymite
Trídimo: tridymus
Trielcon: trielcon
Trietanolamina: triethanolamine
Trietilenofosforamida: triethylenephosphoramide (TEPA)
Trietilenoglicol: triethylene glycol
Trietilenomelamina: triethylenemelamine (TEM)
Trietilenotiofosforamida: triethylenethiophosphoramide
Trietiliodeto de galamina: gallamine triethiodide
Triexosilceramida: trihexosylceramide
Trifacial: trifacial
Trífido: trifid
Trifluoroacetil: trifluoroacetyl
2,2,2-trifluoroetilvinil: 2,2,2-trifluoroethylvinyl
5-trifluorometildesoxiuridina: 5-trifluoromethyldeoxyuridine
Trifluridina: trifluridine
Trifocal: trifocal
5′-trifosfato de citidina: cytidine 5′-triphosphate (CTP)
5′-trifosfato de guanosina: guanosine 5′-triphosphate (GTP)
Trifurcação: trifurcation
Trigástrico: trigastric
Trigêmeo: trigeminus
Trigeminal: trigeminal
Trigeminismo: trigeminy
Trigenolina: trigenolline
Triglicerídio: triglyceride
Trigonal: trigonal
Trigonelina: trigonelline
Trigônide: trigonid
Trigonite: trigonitis
Trígono: trigone, trigonum, pl. trigona
Trigonocefalia: trigonocephaly
Trigonocefálico: trigonocephalic
Trigonocéfalo: copperhead
Tríbrido: trihybrid
Triídrico: trihydric
Triidroxiestrina: trihydroxyestrin
Triiniódimo: triiniodymus
Triiodeto: triiodide
Triiodometano: triiodomethane
3,5,3′-triiodotironina (TITh, T₃): 3,5,3′-triiodothyronine (TITh, T₃)
Trilábio: trilabe
Trilaminar: trilaminar
Trilateral: trilateral
Trilobado: trilobate, trilobed
Trilocular: trilocular
Trilogia: trilogy
Trilostano: trilostane
Trimastigota: trimastigote
Trímero: trimer
Trimestre: trimester
Trimetadiona: trimethadione
Trimetazidina: trimetazidine
Trimetilamina: trimethylamine
Trimetilaminúria: trimethylaminuria
Trimetilcarbinol: trimethylcarbinol
Trimetileno: trimethylene
Trimetiletileno: trimethylethylene
Trimetilomelamina: trimethylomelamine
Trimetoprima: trimethoprim
Trimetoprima-sulfametoxazol: trimethoprim-sulfamethoxazole
Trimetozina: trimetozine
Trimetrexato: trimetrexate
Trimipramina: trimipramine
Trimolecular: termolecular
Trimórfico: trimorphic, trimorphous
Trimorfismo: trimorphism
Trinitrocelulose: trinitrocellulose
Trinitroglicerina: trinitroglycerin
Trinitrotolueno: trinitrotoluene (TNT)
Trinitrotoluol: trinitrotoluol
Trinucleotídio: trinucleotide
Triocinase: triokinase
Trioftalamo: triophthalmos
Triol: triol
Trioleína: triolein
Triorquismo: triorchism
Triortocresil fosfato: triorthocresyl phosphate (TOCP)
Triose: triose
Triose fosfato isomerase: triosephosphate isomerase
Triosecinase: triosekinase
Trioto: triotus
Trióxido: trioxide
Trioximetileno: trioxymethylene
Trioxsaleno: trioxsalen
Tripalangia: triphalangia
Tripalmitina: tripalmitin
Tripanicida: trypanicidal, trypanicide
Tripanide: trypanid
Tripanocida: trypanocidal, trypanocide
Tripanossoma: trypanosome
Tripanossomatídeo: trypanosomatid
Tripanossomíase: trypanosomiasis
Tripanossomíase rodesiense: kaodzera
Tripanossomicida: trypanosomicide
Tripanossômico: trypanosomic
Tripanossomide: trypanosomid
Tripanossomose: trypanosomosis
Triparanol: triparanol
Triparsamida: tryparsamide
Tripeptidases: tripeptidases
Tripeptídio: tripeptide
Triplegia: triplegia
Trípleto: triplet
Triploblástico: triploblastic
Triplóide: triploid
Triploidia: triploidy
Triplopia: triplopia
Trípode: tripod
Tripodia: tripodia
Tripomastigota: trypomastigote
Triprosopo: triprosopus
Tripse: tripsis
Tripsina: trypsin
Tripsinogênio: protrypsin, trypsinogen, trypsogen

Triptamina: tryptamine
Triptamina-estrofantidina: tryptamine-strophanthidin
Tríptico: tryptic
Triptofanase: tryptophanase
Triptofano: tryptophan (Trp, W)
Triptofanúria: tryptophanuria
Triptona: tryptone
Triptonemia: tryptonemia
Tríquetro: triquetrous
Triquíase: trichiasis
Triquilemoma: trichilemmoma
Triquina: trichina, **pl.** trichinae
Triquinelíase: trichinelliasis
Triquinelose: trichinellosis
Triquiníase: trichiniasis
Triquinífero: trichiniferous
Triquinização: trichinization
Triquinoscópio: trichinoscope
Triquinose: trichinosis
Triquinoso: trichinous
Tríquio: trichion
Triquite: trichite
Trirradiado: triradial, triradiate
Trirrádio: triradius
Tris(hidroximetil)aminometano: tris(hydroxymethyl)aminomethane (Tris)
Tris(hidroximetil)metilamina: tris(hydroxymethyl)methylamine (Tris)
Triscaidecafobia: triskaidekaphobia
Trísmico: trismic
Trismo: lockjaw, trismus
Trismóide: trismoid
Trisplâncnico: trisplanchnic
Trissacarídio: trisaccharide
Trissomia: trisomy
Trissômico: trisomic
Trissulcado: trisulcate
Tristearina: tristearin
Trístíquia: tristichia
Tritanomalia: tritanomaly
Tritanopia: tritanopia
Triterpenos: triterpenes
Tritiado: tritiated
Tritíceo: triticeous, triticeum
Triticeoglosso: triticeoglossus
Tritil: trityl
Trítio: tritium (T, *t*)
Tritubercular: tritubercular
Trituração: trituration
Triturar: triturate
Triturável: triturable
Trivalência: trivalence, trivalency
Trivalente: trivalent
Trivalvar: trivalve
Trizonal: trizonal
tRNA isoaceptor: isoacceptor tRNA
Troca: exchange
Troca de ânion: anion exchange
Troca de cátions: cation exchange
Troca iônica: ion exchange
Trocador de filmes: film changer
Trocador de íons: ion exchanger

Trocanter: trochanter
Trocanter menor: trochantin
Trocantérico: trochanterian, trochanteric
Trocanterplastia: trochanterplasty
Trocarte: trocar
Trocisco: troche, trochiscus (troch), **pl.** trochisci
Tróclea: pulley, trochlea, **pl.** trochleae
Troclear: trochlear, trochlearis
Trocleiforme: trochleariform, trochleiform
Trococardia: trochocardia
Trocóide: trochoid
Trocorizocardia: trochorizocardia
Trofectoderma: trophectoderm
Troficidade: trophicity
Trófico: trophic
Trofismo: trophism
Trofoblástico: trophoblastic
Trofoblastina: trophoblastin
Trofoblasto: trophoblast
Trofócito: trophocyte
Trofocromatina: trophochromatin
Trofocromídios: trophochromidia
Trofoderma: trophoderm
Trofodermatoneurose: trophodermatoneurosis
Trofodinâmica: trophodynamics
Trofoneurose: trophoneurosis
Trofoneurótico: trophoneurotic
Trofonúcleo: trophonucleus
Trofoplasto: trophoplast
Trofospongia: trophospongia
Trofotaxia: trophotaxis
Trofotrópico: trophotropic
Trofotropismo: trophotropism
Trofozoíta: trophozoite
Troglitazona: troglitazone
Trolamina: trolamine
Troland: troland
Troleandomicina: troleandomycin
Trombase: thrombase
Trombastenia: thrombasthenia, thromboasthenia
Trombectomia: thrombectomy
Trombiculíase: trombiculiasis
Trombiculídeo: trombiculid
Trombina: thrombin
Trombinogênese: thrombinogenesis
Trombinogênio: thrombinogen
Trombo: thrombus, **pl.** thrombi
Tromboangeíte: thromboangiitis
Tromboarterite: thromboarteritis
Tromboblasto: thromboblast
Trombocatilisina: thrombokatilysin
Trombocinase: thrombokinase
Trombocisto: thrombocyst, thrombocystis
Trombocitastenia: thrombocytasthenia

Trombocitemia: thrombocythemia
Trombocitina: thrombocytin
Trombócito: thrombocyte
Trombocitopatia: thrombocytopathy
Trombocitopenia: thrombocytopenia
Trombocitopoese: thrombocytopoiesis
Trombocitose: thrombocytosis
Tromboclástico: thromboclastic
Tromboelastógrafo: thromboelastograph
Tromboelastograma: thromboelastogram
Tromboembolectomia: thromboembolectomy
Tromboembolia: thromboembolism
Tromboendarterectomia: thromboendarterectomy
Tromboendocardite: thromboendocarditis
Trombofilia: thrombophilia
Tromboflebite: thrombophlebitis
Trombogene: thrombogene
Trombogênico: thrombogenic
Trombogênio: thrombogen
Tromboide: thromboid
Trombólico: thrombolic
Trombolinfangite: thrombolymphangitis
Trombólise: thrombolysis
Trombolítico: thrombolytic
Trômbolo: thrombolus
Trombomodulina: thrombomodulin
Trômbon: thrombon
Trombonecrose: thrombonecrosis
Trombopatia: thrombopathy
Trombopenia: thrombopenia
Tromboplastídio: thromboplastid
Tromboplastina: thromboplastin
Tromboplastinogênio: thromboplastinogen
Trombopoese: thrombopoiesis
Trombopoetina: thrombopoietin
Trombosado: thrombosed
Trombose: thrombosis, **pl.** thromboses
Trombosina: thrombosin
Trombostasia: thrombostasis
Trombostenina: thrombosthenin
Trombótico: thrombotic
Trombotonina: thrombotonin
Tromboxano: thromboxane
Tromboxanos: thromboxanes
Trombozima: thrombozyme
Trometamina: trometamine
Trona: trona
Tronco: stem, truncus, **gen. e pl.** trunci; trunk
Tronco encefálico: braistem, brain stem
Troncular: truncal

Tropano: tropane
Tropato: tropate
Tropeína: tropeine
Tropentano: tropentane
Tropeolinas: tropeolins
Tropia: tropia
Tropicamida: tropicamide
Tropina: tropine
Tropismo: tropism
Tropocolágeno: tropocollagen
Tropoelastina: tropoelastin
Tropômetro: tropometer
Tropomiosina: tropomyosin
Troponina: troponin
Troxerutina: troxerutin
Troxidona: troxidone
Truncado: truncate
Trusão: trusion
Tsé-tsé: tsetse
Tuamino-heptano: tuaminoheptane
Tuba: tuba, **gen. e pl.** tubae
Tuba auditiva: otosalpinx
Tuba uterina: oviduct
Tubagem: tubage
Tubário: tubal
Tubectomia: tubectomy
Túber: tuber, **pl.** tubera
Tuberculação: tuberculation
Tubercular: tubercular, tuberculated
Tubercúlide: tuberculid
Tuberculina: tuberculin
Tuberculite: tuberculitis
Tubérculo: tubercle, tuberculum, **pl.** tubercula
Tuberculocele: tuberculocele
Tuberculocida: tuberculocidal
Tuberculoderma: tuberculoderma
Tuberculofibróide: tuberculofibroid
Tuberculóide: tuberculoid
Tuberculoma: tuberculoma
Tuberculoproteína: tuberculoprotein
Tuberculoquimioterápico: tuberculochemotherapeutic
Tuberculose (TB): tuberculosis (TB)
Tuberculoso: tuberculous
Tuberculostático: tuberculostatic
Tuberculostato: tuberculostat
Tuberífero: tuberiferous
Tuberosidade: tuberositas, tuberosity
Tuberoso: tuberose, tuberous
Tubo: tube, tubus, **pl.** tubi
Tubo graduado: graduate
Tuboabdominal: tuboabdominal
Tuboligamentoso: tuboligamentous
Tuboperitoneal: tuboperitoneal
Tuboplastia: tuboplasty
Tubos brônquicos: bronchia
Tubotimpânico: tubotympanic, tubotympanal
Tubotorção: tubatorsion, tubotorsion
Tubouterino: tubouterine

Tubovaginal: tubovaginal
Tubovárico: tubo-ovarian
Tubuladura: tubulature
Tubular: tubular
Tubuliforme: tubuliform
Tubulina: tubulin
Tubulização: tubulization
Túbulo: tubule, tubulus, **pl.** tubuli
Tubulocisto: tubulocyst
Tubulodermóide: tubulodermoid
Tubuloneogênese: tubuloneogenesis
Tubulorracemoso: tubuloracemose
Tubulorrexe: tubulorrhexis
Tubuloso: tubulose, tubulous
Tufo: tuft
Tuftsina: tuftsin
Tuia: thuja, thuya
Tujol: thujol, thuyol, thuyone
Tujona: thujone
Tularemia: tularemia
Túlio: thulium (Tm)
Tumefação: swelling, tumefaction, tumentia
Tumefaciente: tumefacient
Tumefazer: tumefy
Tumefeito: tumorous
Tumescência: tumescence
Tumescente: tumescent
Túmido: tumid
Tumor: tumor
Tumor de Landschutz: Landschutz tumor
Tumoricida: tumoricidal
Tumorigênese: tumorigenesis
Tumorigênico: tumorigenic
Túnel: tunnel
Tungíase: tungiasis
Tungstato: tungstate
Tungstênio: tungsten (W)
Túnica: tunic, tunica, **pl.** tunicae
Túnica albugínea do testículo: perididymis
Túnica conjuntiva: conjunctiva, **pl.** conjunctivae
Túnica dartos: dartos
Túnica serosa: serosa
Turanose: turanose
Turbidez: turbidity
Turbidimetria: turbidimetry
Turbidimétrico: turbidimetric
Turbidímetro: turbidimeter
Turbinado: turbinated
Turbinal: turbinal
Turbinectomia: turbinectomy
Turbinotomia: turbinotomy
Turbinótomo: turbinotome
Turbulência: turbulence
Turgescência: turgescence
Turgescente: turgescent
Túrgido: turgid
Turgor: turgor
Turricefalia: turricephaly
Turvo: turbid
Tussicular: tussicular
Tussígeno: tussigenic
Tussivo: tussal

U

Ubiidroquinona: ubihydroquinone
Ubiquinol: ubiquinol (QH_2, H_2Q)
Ubiquinona: ubiquinone
Ubiquinona-6: ubiquinone-6 ($-Q_6$)
Ubiquinona-10: ubiquinone-10 ($-Q_{10}$)
Ubiquitina: ubiquitin
Ucambina: ukambin
UDP galactose: UDPgalactose
UDPgalactose 4-epimerase: UDPgalactose 4-epimerase
UDPglicose: UDPglucose
UDPglicose 4-epimerase: UDPglucose 4-epimerase
UDPglicose-hexose-1-fosfato uridililtransferase: UDPglucose-hexose-1-phosphate uridylyltransferase
UDPglicuronato-bilirrubina glicuronosídio glicuronosil transferase: UDPglucuronate-bilirubinglucuronoside glucuronosyltransferase
UDPglicuronato-bilirrubina glicuronosil transferase: UDPglucuronate-bilirubin glucuronosyltransferase
UDP-N-acetilglucosamina:enzima lisossômica N-acetilglicosaminil-1-fosfotransferase: UDP-N-acetylglucosamine:lysosomalenzyme N-acetylglucosaminyl-1-phosphotransferase
UDPxilose: UDPxylose
Úlcera: ulcer, ulcus, **pl.** ulcera
Úlcera de decúbito: bedsore
Ulceração: ulceration
Ulcerado: ulcerated
Ulcerante: exulcerans
Ulcerar: ulcerate
Ulcerativo: ulcerative
Ulcerogênico: ulcerogenic
Ulceroglandular: ulceroglandular
Ulceromembranoso: ulceromembranous
Ulegiria: ulegyria
Uleritema: ulerythema
Ulex européia: ulex europaeus
Ulna: ulna, **gen. e pl.** ulnae
Ulnar: cubital, ulnad, ulnar, ulnaris
Ulnocarpal: ulnocarpal
Ulnorradial: ulnoradial
Ulóide: uloid
Ulótrico: ulotrichous
Ultimobranquial: ultimobranchial
Ultra-acústica: ultrasonics
Ultrabraquicefálico: ultrabrachycephalic
Ultracentrífuga: ultracentrifuge
Ultracentrifugação: ultracentrifugation
Ultracitóstomo: ultracytostome
Ultradiano: ultradian
Ultradolicocefálico: ultradolichocephalic
Ultra-estrutura: ultrastructure
Ultrafiltração: ultrafiltration
Ultrafiltro: ultrafilter
Ultraligadura: ultraligation
Ultramicroscópico: ultramicroscopic
Ultramicroscópio: ultramicroscope
Ultramicrotomia: ultramicrotomy
Ultramicrótomo: ultramicrotome
Ultramotividade: ultromotivity
Ultrapassagem: overshoot
Ultra-som: ultrasound
Ultra-sônico: ultrasonic
Ultra-sonocirurgia: ultrasonosurgery
Ultra-sonografia: ultrasonography
Ultra-sonografista: ultrasonographer
Ultra-sonógrafo: ultrasonograph
Ultra-sonograma: ultrasonogram
Ultratermo: ultratherm
Ultravioleta: ultraviolet
Ululação: ululation
Umbigo: belly button, navel, umbilicus, **pl.** umbilici; umbo, **gen.** umbonis, **pl.** umbones
Umbilicação: umbilication
Umbilicado; em forma de umbigo: umbilicate, umbilicated
Umbilical: umbilical
Umectação: humectation
Umectante: humectant
Umeral: humeral
Úmero: humerus, **gen. e pl.** humeri
Umeroescapular: humeroscapular
Umerorradial: humeroradial
Umeroulnar: humeroulnar
Umidade: humidity
Úmido: damp
UMP sintase: UMP synthase
Uncal: uncal
Unção: unction
Unciforme: unciform, unciforme
Uncinado: uncinate, uncinatum
Uncinaríase: uncinariasis
Uncipressão: uncipressure
Unco: uncus, **pl.** unci
Uncovertebral: uncovertebral
Undecilenato: undecylenate
Undina: undine
Ungueal: ungual
Ungüento: unguent
Ungüícula: unguiculus
Ungüiculado: unguiculate
Ungüiculados: Unguiculata
Ungüinal: unguinal
Ungulado: ungulate
Ungulados: Ungulata
Ungulígrado: unguligrade
Unha: nail, onyx, unguis, **pl.** ungues
Unha (dos dedos da mão): fingernail
Unha (dos dedos do pé): toe-nail
União: union
Uniarticular: uniarticular
Uniaxial: uniaxial
Unibasal: unibasal
Unicameral: unicameral, unicamerate
Unicelular: unicellular
Unicentral: unicentral
Unicorne: unicorn
Unicórneo: unicornous
Unicúspide: unicuspid, unicuspidate
Unidade: unit (U)
Unidade de Fishman-Lerner: Fishman-Lerner unit
Unifamilial: unifamilial
Uniflagelado: uniflagellate
Uniforme: uniform
Unigerminal: unigerminal
Uniglandular: uniglandular
Unilaminar; unilaminado: unilaminar, unilaminate
Unilateral: unilateral
Unilobar: unilobar
Unilocal: unilocal
Unilocular: unilocular
Unimolecular: unimolecular
Uninuclear; uninucleado: uninuclear, uninucleate
Uniocular: uniocular
Unioval; uniovular: unioval, uniovular
Unipenado: unipennate
Unipolar: unipolar
Uniportador: uniporter
Uniporte: uniport
Unipotente: unipotent
Unisseptado: uniseptate
Univalência: univalence, univalency
Univalente: univalent
Untuoso: unctuous
Untura: uncture
Uracal: urachal
Uracil: uracil (Ura, U)
Úraco: urachus
Uramustina: uramustine
Uranil: uranyl
Uranina: uranin
Uraninita: uraninite
Urânio: uranium (U)
Uranisco: uraniscus
Urancisconite: uranisconitis
Uraniscoplastia: uraniscoplasty
Uraniscorrafia: uraniscorrhaphy
Uranoplastia: uranoplasty
Uranorrafia: uranorrhaphy
Uranosquise: uranoschisis
Uranostafiloplastia: uranostaphyloplasty
Uranostafilorrafia: uranostaphylorrhaphy
Uranostafilosquise: uranostaphyloschisis

Uranovelosquise: uranoveloschisis
Urapidil: urapidil
Uraroma: uraroma
Urartrite: urarthritis
Uratemia: uratemia
Uraterribonucleotídio fosforilase: urateribonucleotide phosphorylase
Urático: uratic
Urato: urate
Uratólise: uratolysis
Uratolítico: uratolytic
Uratoma: uratoma
Uratose: uratosis
Uratúria: uraturia
Urceiforme: urceiform
Urceolado: urceolate
Ureagênese: ureagenesis
Urease: urease
Uredema: uredema
Uréia: urea
Ureico: ureal, ureic
Ureído: ureide
3-ureidoidantoína: 3-ureidohydantoin
Urelcose: urelcosis
Uremia: uremia
Urêmico: uremic
Uremigênico: uremigenic
Ureopoiese: ureapoiesis
Ureotelia: ureotelia
Ureotélico: ureotelic
Ureotelo: ureotele
Ureritrina: urerythrin
Urese: uresis
Uresiestesia: uresiesthesia
Uretana; uretano: urethan, urethane
Ureter: ureter
Ureteral: ureteral
Ureteralgia: ureteralgia
Ureterectasia: ureterectasia
Ureterectomia: ureterectomy
Uretérico: ureteric
Ureterite: ureteritis
Ureterocalicostomia: ureterocalicostomy
Ureterocele: ureterocele
Ureterocelorrafia: ureterocelorraphy
Ureterocistoplastia: ureterocystoplasty
Ureterocistoscópio: uretercystoscope, ureterocystoscope
Ureterocistostomia: ureterocystostomy
Ureterocólico: ureterocolic
Ureterocolostomia: ureterocolostomy
Ureteroentérico: ureteroenteric
Ureteroenterostomia: ureteroenterostomy
Ureteroestenose: ureterostenosis
Ureterografia: ureterography
Ureteroidronefrose: ureterohydronephrosis
Ureteroileoneocistostomia: ureteroileoneocystostomy

Ureteroileostomia: ureteroileostomy
Ureterólise: ureterolysis
Ureterolitíase: ureterolithiasis
Ureterolitotomia: ureterolithotomy
Ureteronefrectomia: ureteronephrectomy
Ureteroneocistostomia: ureteroneocystostomy
Ureteropatia: ureteropathy
Ureteropielite: ureteropyelitis
Ureteropielografia: ureteropyelography
Ureteropieloplastia: ureteropyeloplasty
Ureteropielostomia: ureteropyelostomy
Ureteropiose: ureteropyosis
Ureteroplastia: ureteroplasty
Ureteroproctostomia: ureteroproctostomy
Ureterorrafia: ureterorrhaphy
Ureterorragia: ureterorrhagia
Ureterorretostomia: ureterorectostomy
Ureteroscópio: ureteroscope
Ureterossigmóide: ureterosigmoid
Ureterossigmoidostomia: ureterosigmoidostomy
Ureterostomia: ureterostomy
Ureterotomia: ureterotomy
Ureterotrigonoenterostomia: ureterotrigonoenterostomy
Ureteroureteral: ureteroureteral
Ureteroureterostomia: ureteroureterostomy
Ureterovesical: ureterovesical
Ureterovesicostomia: ureterovesicostomy
Uretra: urethra
Uretral: urethral
Uretralgia: urethralgia
Uretrectomia: urethrectomy
Uretremorragia: urethremorrhagia
Uretrismo; uretrospasmo: urethrism, urethrismus
Uretrite: urethritis
Uretrobulbar: urethrobulbar
Uretrocele: urethrocele
Uretrocistometria: urethrocystometry
Uretrocistometrografia: urethrocystometrography
Uretrocistopexia: urethrocystopexy
Uretrodinia: urethrodynia
Uretroestenose: urethrostenosis
Uretrografia: urethrography
Uretrômetro: urethrometer
Uretropeniano: urethropenile
Uretroperineal: urethroperineal
Uretroperineoescrotal: urethroperineoscrotal
Uretropexia: urethropexy
Uretroplastia: urethroplasty
Uretroprostático: urethroprostatic
Uretrorrafia: urethrorrhaphy

Uretrorragia: urethrorrhagia
Uretrorréia: urethrorrhea
Uretrorretal: urethrorectal
Uretroscopia: urethroscopy
Uretroscópico: urethroscopic
Uretroscópio: urethroscope
Uretrospasmo: urethrospasm
Uretrostaxe: urethrostaxis
Uretrostomia: urethrostomy
Uretrotomia: urethrotomy
Uretrótomo: urethrotome
Uretrovaginal: urethrovaginal
Uretrovesical: urethrovesical
Uretrovesicopexia: urethrovesicopexy
Urgência: urgency
Urgínea: urginea
Uricase: uricase
Úrico: uric
Uricólise: uricolysis
Uricolítico: uricolytic
Uricossoma: uricosome
Uricosúria: uricosuria
Uricosúrico: uricosuric
Uricotelia: uricotelia
Uricotélico: uricotelic
Uricotelo: uricotele
Uridiltransferase: uridyltransferase
Uridina: uridine (Urd)
Uridina difosfogalactose: uridine diphosphogalactose (UDPGal)
Uridina difosfoglicose: uridine diphosphoglucose (UDPG, UDPGlc)
Uridina difosfoxilose: uridine diphosphoxylose
Uridrose: uridrosis
Uriestesia: uriesthesia
Urina: urine
Urinálise: urinalysis
Urinar: micturate, urinate
Urinário: urinary
Urinífero: uriniferous
Urinífico: urinific
Uriníparo: uriniparous
Urinogenital: urinogenital
Urinógeno: urinogenous
Urinol: urinal
Urinoma: urinoma
Urinometria: urinometry
Urinômetro: urinometer
Urinoscopia: urinoscopy
Urinoso: urinous
Urinossexual: urinosexual
Uriposia: uriposia
Uroamoníaco: uroammoniac
Uroantelona: uroanthelone
Urobilina: urobilin
Urobilina IXα: urobilin IXα
Urobilinemia: urobilinemia
Urobilinogênio: urobilinogen
Urobilinogênio IXα: urobilinogen IXα
Urobilinúria: urobilinuria
Urocanase: urocanase
Urocanate: urocanate
Urocanicase: urocanicase
Urocele: urocele
Urocianina: urocyanin

Urocianogênio: urocyanogen
Urocianose: urocyanosis
Urocístico: urocystic
Urocisto: urocyst, urocystis
Urocrise: urocrisia, urocrisis
Urocromo: urochrome
Urocromogênio: urochromogen
Urodinâmica: urodynamics
Urodinia: urodynia
Uroematina: urohematin
Uroematoporfirina: urohematoporphyrin
Uroenterona: uroenterone
Uroeparina: uroheparin
Uroeritrina: uroerythrin
Uroespectrina: urospectrin
Urofânico: urophanic
Urofeína: urophein
Uroflavina: uroflavin
Urofluxômetro: uroflowmeter
Urofolitropina: urofollitropin
Urofuscoematina: urofuscohematin
Urogastrona: urogastrone
Urogenital: urogenital
Urógeno: urogenous
Uroglaucina: uroglaucin
Urogonadotrofina: urogonadotropin
Urografia: urography
Urograma: urogram
Urogravímetro: urogravimeter
Uroipertensina: urohypertensin
Urolagnia: urolagnia
Urolitíase: urolithiasis
Urolítico: urolithic
Urólito: urolith
Urolitologia: urolithology
Urologia: urology
Urológico: urologic, urological
Urologista: urologist
Uroluteína: urolutein
Uromelanina: uromelanin
Urômetro: urometer
Uronco: uroncus
Uronoscopia: uronoscopy
Uropatia: uropathy
Uropoese: uropoiesis
Uropoético: uropoietic
Uroporfirina: uroporphyrin
Uroporfirinogênio: uroporphyrinogen
Uropsamo: uropsammus
Uropterina: uropterin
Uropurpurina: uropurpurin
Uroquera: urocheras
Uroquesia: urochesia
Uroquinase: urokinase
Urorradiologia: uroradiology
Urorretal: urorectal
Urorroseína: urorosein
Urorrubina: urorubin
Urorrubroematina: urorubrohematin
Uroscopia: uroscopy
Uroscópico: uroscopic
Urosquese: uroschesis
Urossemiologia: urosemiology
Urossepsina: urosepsin
Urossépsis: urosepsis
Urotélio: urothelium

Urotion: urothion
Urotórax: urothorax
Uroxantina: uroxanthin
Uroxina: uroxin
Ursodiol: ursodiol
Urticação: urtication
Urticante: urticant
Urticar: urticate
Urticária: hives, urticaria
Urticariáceo: urticarial
Urtiga: nettle, urtica
Urtiga-do-mar: sea nettle
Urushiol: urushiol
Ustilaginismo: ustilaginism
Ustulação: ustulation
Usurpação: usurpation
Uta: uta
Uterino: uterine
Útero: metra, uterus, **pl.** uteri; womb
Uteroabdominal: uteroabdominal
Uterocervical: uterocervical
Uterocistostomia: uterocystostomy
Uteroglobina: uteroglobin
Uteroglobina-aducina: uteroglobin-adducin
Uterólito: uterolith
Uterômetro: uterometer
Útero-ovariano: utero-ovarian
Uteroparietal: uteroparietal
Uteropélvico: uteropelvic
Uteropexia: uteropexy
Uteroplacentário: uteroplacental
Uteroplastia: uteroplasty
Uteroscopia: uteroscopy
Uteroscópio: uteroscope
Uterossacral: uterosacral
Uterossalpingografia: uterosalpingography
Uterotomia: uterotomy
Uterotônico: uterotonic
Uterotrópico: uterotropic
Uterotubário: uterotubal
Uterotubografia: uterotubography
Uterovaginal: uterovaginal
Uteroventral: uteroventral
Uteroverdina: uteroverdine
Uterovesical: uterovesical
Utilidade: utility
Utricular: utricular
Utriculite: utriculitis
Utrículo: utricle, utriculus, **pl.** utriculi
Utriculossacular: utriculosaccular
Utriforme: utriform
Uva-ursina: uva ursi
Úvea: uvea
Uveal: uveal
Uveíte: uveitis, **pl.** uveitides
Uveítico: uveitic
Uveoencefalite: uveoencephalitis
Uveoesclerite: uveoscleritis
Uviforme: uvaeformis, uviform
Uviol: uviol
Uviômetro: uviometer

Uviorresistente: uviofast, uvioresistant
Uviossensível: uviosensitive
Uvitex 2B: uvitex 2B
Uvomorulina: uvomorulin
Úvula: uvula, **pl.** uvuli
Uvular: uvular, uvularis
Uvulectomia: uvulectomy
Uvulite: uvulitis
Uvulopalatofaringoplastia: uvulopalatopharyngoplasty
Uvulopalatoplastia: uvulopalatoplasty
Uvuloptose: uvulaptosis, uvuloptosis
Uvulotomia: uvulotomy
Uvulótomo: uvulatome, uvulotome

V

V. máx: V-max
Vaca: cow
Vacina: vaccina, vaccine, vaccinum
Vacinação: vaccination
Vacinador: vaccinator, vaccinist
Vacinal: vaccinal
Vacinar: vaccinate
Vacínia: vaccinia
Vacinial: vaccinial
Vaciniforme: vacciniform
Vacinização: vaccinization
Vacinógeno: vaccinogen, vaccinogenous
Vacinóide: vaccinoid
Vacinostilo: vaccinostyle
Vácuo: vacuum
Vacuolação: vacuolation
Vacuolado: vacuolate, vacuolated
Vacuolar: vacuolar
Vacuolização: vacuolization
Vacúolo: vacuole
Vacuoma: vacuome
Vagal: vagal
Vagectomia: vagectomy
Vagido uterino: vagitus uterinus
Vagina: vagina, **gen. e pl.** vaginae
Vaginal: vaginal
Vaginectomia: vaginectomy
Vaginismo: vaginism, vaginismus
Vaginite: vaginitis, **pl.** vaginitides
Vaginoabdominal: vaginoabdominal
Vaginocele: vaginocele
Vaginodinia: vaginodynia
Vaginofixação: vaginofixation
Vagino-histerectomia: vaginohysterectomy
Vaginolabial: vaginolabial
Vaginomicose: vaginomycosis
Vaginopatia: vaginopathy
Vaginoperineal: vaginoperineal

Vaginoperineoplastia: vaginoperineoplasty
Vaginoperineorrafia: vaginoperineorrhaphy
Vaginoperineotomia: vaginoperineotomy
Vaginoperitoneal: vaginoperitoneal
Vaginopexia: vaginapexy, vaginopexy
Vaginoplastia: vaginoplasty
Vaginoscopia: vaginoscopy
Vaginose: vaginosis
Vaginotomia: vaginotomy
Vaginovesical: vaginovesical
Vaginovulvar: vaginovulvar
Vago: vagus, **gen. e pl.** vagi
Vagoacessório: vagoaccessorius
Vagoglossofaríngeo: vagoglossopharyngeal
Vagólise: vagolysis
Vagolítico: vagolytic
Vagomimético: vagomimetic
Vagotomia: vagotomy
Vagotonia: vagotonia
Vagotônico: vagotonic
Vagotrópico: vagotropic
Vagovagal: vagovagal
Valado: vallate
Vale: vallum, **pl.** valla
Valécula: vallecula, **pl.** valleculae; valley, vallis
Valência: valence, valency
Valente: valent
Valepotriatos: valepotriates
Valerato: valerate
Valeriana: valerian, vandal root
Valerianato: valerianate
Valetudinarianismo: valetudinarianism
Valetudinário: valetudinarian
Valgo: valgus
Valgóide: valgoid
Validação: validation
Validade: validity
Válido: valid
Valil: valyl (Val, V)
Valina: valine (Val, V)
Valinomicina: valinomycin
Valmetamida: valmethamide
Valnoctamida: valnoctamide
Valóide: valoid
Valor: value
Valva: valva, **pl.** valvae; valve
Valvado: valvate
Valvar: valval, valvar
Valviforme: valviform
Valvoplastia: valvoplasty
Valvotomia: valvotomy
Válvula: valvula, **pl.** valvulae; valvule
Valvular: valvular
Valvulite: valvulitis
Valvuloplastia: valvuloplasty
Valvulotomia: valvulotomy
Valvulótomo: valvulotome
Vanadato: vanadate
Vanádio: vanadium (V)
Vancomicina: vancomycin
Vanilato: vanillate
Vanilina: vanillin

Vanilismo: vanillism
Vapor: vapor
Vaporização: vaporization
Vaporizador: vaporizer
Vaporizar: vaporize
Vaportórax: vaporthorax
Vapoterapia: vapotherapy
Varejeira: blowfly
Variabilidade: variability
Variação: range, variation
Variação de humor: mood swing
Variância: variance
Variante: variant
Variável: variable, variate
Varicação: varication
Varicela: chickenpox, varicella
Varicelação: varicellation
Variceliforme: varicelliform
Varicelóide: varicelloid
Variciforme: variciform
Varicobléfaro: varicoblepharon
Varicocele: varicocele
Varicocelectomia: varicocelectomy
Varicoflebite: varicophlebitis
Varicografia: varicography
Varicóide: varicoid
Varicônfalo: varicomphalus
Varicose: varicosis, **pl.** varicoses
Varicosidade: varicosity
Varicoso: variceal, varicose
Varicotomia: varicotomy
Varícula: varicula, varicule
Variegação: variegation
Varíola: smallpox, variola
Varíola do macaco: monkeypox
Varíola verrucosa: wartpox
Variolação: variolation
Variolar: variolar
Variólico: variolic
Varioliforme: varioliform
Variolização: variolization
Variolóide: varioloid
Varioloso: variolous
Variolovacina: variolovaccine
Variz, varizes: varix, **pl.** varices
Varo: varus
Varredura: scanning, sweep
Vasal: vasal
Vascolejo: clapotage, clapotement
Vascular: vascular
Vascularidade: vascularity
Vascularização: vascularization
Vascularizado: vascularized
Vasculatura: vasculature
Vasculite: vasculitis
Vásculo: vasculum, **pl.** vascula
Vasculocardíaco: vasculocardiac
Vásculo-emocional: emotiovascular
Vasculogênese: vasculogenesis
Vasculomielinopatia: vasculomyelinopathy
Vasculomotor: vasculomotor
Vasculopatia: vasculopathy
Vasectomia: vasectomy
Vaselina: petroleum jelly
Vasiformação: vasifaction

Vasiformador: vasifactive
Vasiforme: vasiform
Vasite: vasitis
Vaso: vas, **gen.** vasis, **pl.** vasa, **gen. e pl.** vasorum; vessel
Vaso sangüíneo: blood vessel
Vasoativo: vasoactive
Vasoconstrição: vasoconstriction
Vasoconstritivo: vasoconstrictive
Vasoconstritor: vasoconstrictor
Vasodentina: vasodentin
Vasodepressão: vasodepression
Vasodepressor: vasodepressor
Vasodilatação: vasodilatation, vasodilation
Vasodilatador: vasodilative, vasodilator
Vasoepididimostomia: vasoepididymostomy
Vasoespasmo: vasospasm
Vasoespástico: vasospastic
Vasoestimulante: vasostimulant
Vasoformação: vasoformation
Vasoformador: vasofactive, vasoformative
Vasogânglio: vasoganglion
Vasografia: vasography
Vasoinibidor: vasoinhibitor
Vasoinibitório: vasoinhibitory
Vasolábil: vasolabile
Vasoligadura: vasoligation
Vasomotor: vasomotor
Vasomotricidade: vasomotion
Vasoneuropatia: vasoneuropathy
Vasoparalisia: vasoparalysis
Vasoparesia: vasoparesis
Vasopressina: vasopressin (VP)
Vasopressor: vasopressor
Vasopunção: vasopuncture
Vasorquidostomia: vaso-orchidostomy
Vasorreflexo: vasoreflex
Vasorrelaxamento: vasorelaxation
Vasos: vasa
Vasossensorial: vasosensory
Vasostomia: vasostomy
Vasotocina: vasotocin
Vasotomia: vasosection, vasotomy
Vasotonia: vasotonia
Vasotônico: vasotonic
Vasotrófico: vasotrophic
Vasotrombina: vasothrombin
Vasotrópico: vasotropic
Vasovagal: vasovagal
Vasovasostomia: vasovasostomy
Vasovesiculectomia: vasovesiculectomy
Vasto: vastus
Vastomia: vastomy
Vazão: issue
Vecção: vection
Vegetação: vegetation
Vegetal: vegetable, vegetal
Vegetalidade: vegetality

Vegetarianismo: vegetarianism
Vegetariano: vegetarian
Vegetativo: vegetative
Vegetoanimal: vegetoanimal
Veia: vein, vena, **gen. e pl.** venae
Veia cava inferior: postcava
Veia cava superior: precava
Veia emissária: emissarium
Veículo: vehicle
Vela: bougie, candle, candle-power
Velame: velamen, **pl.** velamina; velamentum, **pl.** velamenta
Velamentoso: velamentous
Velames: velamina
Velar: velar
Velas de Maloney: Maloney bougies
Veliforme: veliform
Velo: vellus
Velocidade: speed, velocity (v)
Velofaríngeo: velopharyngeal
Venação: venation
Venado: veined
Veneno: bane, poison, venom
Venenosidade: venenosity
Venenoso: poisonous, venenous
Venenossalivar: venenosalivary, venomosalivary
Venéreo: venereal
Venereofobia: venereophobia
Venereologia: venereology
Venina: venin
Venipuntura: venipuncture
Venissecção: venesection
Venocavografia: venacavography
Venóclise: venoclysis
Venofibrose: venofibrosis
Venografia: venography
Venograma: venogram
Venomotor: venomotor
Venoperitoneostomia: venoperitoneostomy
Venopressor: venopressor
Venosclerose: venosclerosis
Venosidade: venosity
Venoso: venose, venous
Venossinusal: venosinal
Venostase: venostasis
Venostato: venostat
Venostomia: venostomy
Venotomia: venotomy
Venovenostomia: venovenostomy
Ventilação: ventilation
Ventilar: ventilate
Ventral: ventral, ventralis
Ventre: belly
Ventricoso: ventricose
Ventricular: ventricular, ventricularis
Ventricularização: ventricularization
Ventriculectomia: ventriculectomy
Ventriculite: ventriculitis
Ventrículo: ventricle
Ventriculoatrial: ventriculoatrial

Ventriculocisternostomia: ventriculocisternostomy
Ventriculofásico: ventriculophasic
Ventriculografia: ventriculography
Ventriculomastoidostomia: ventriculomastoidostomy
Ventriculoplastia: ventriculoplasty
Ventriculopuntura: ventriculopuncture
Ventriculoscopia: ventriculoscopy
Ventriculossubaracnóideo: ventriculosubarachnoid
Ventriculostomia: ventriculostomy
Ventriculotomia: ventriculotomy
Ventridução: ventriduction
Ventrodorsal: ventrodorsad
Ventroinguinal: ventroinguinal
Ventrolateral: ventrolateral
Ventromediano: ventromedian
Vênula: veinlet, venula, **pl.** venulae; venule
Venular: venular
Venuloso: venulous
Verapamil: verapamil
Veratridina: veratridine
Veratrina: veratrine
Verbigeração: verbigeration
Verbomania: verbomania
Verde: green
Verde brilhante: brilliant green
Verde de bromocresol: bromcresol green, bromocresol green
Verde de etila: ethyl green
Verde de indocianina: indocyanine green
Verde de malaquita: malachite green
Verde de metila: methyl green
Verde-claro SF amarelado: light green SF yellowish
Verde-guiné B: guinea green B
Verdeperoxidase: verdoperoxidase
Verdete: verdigris
Verdoglobina: verdoglobin
Verga: virga
Vergão: welt, wheal
Vergência: vergence
Verme: vermis, **pl.** vermes; worm
Vermelhão: vermilion
Vermelhidão temporária da pele: rubedo
Vermelho: red
Vermelho ácido 87: acid red 87
Vermelho ácido 91: acid red 91
Vermelho cresol: cresol red
Vermelho de amidonaftol: amidonaphthol red
Vermelho de clorfenol: chlorphenol red
Vermelho de Darrow: Darrow red
Vermelho de metila: methyl red

Vermelho de quinaldina: quinaldine red
Vermelho de rutênio: ruthenium red.
Vermelho de toluileno: toluylene red
Vermelho tripano: trypan red
Vermelho vital: vital red
Vermelho vital brilhante: brilliant vital red
Vermelho-alaranjado: turkey red
Vermelho-Congo: Congo red
Vermelho-cromo: chrome red
Vermelho-escarlate de Biebrich: Biebrich scarlet red
Vermelho-escarlate medicinal: medicinal scarlet red
Vermes pulmonares: lungworms
Vermicida: vermicidal, vermicide
Vermiculação: vermiculation
Vermicular: vermicular
Vermículo: vermicule, vermiculose, vermiculous, vermiculus
Vermiforme: vermiform
Vermífugo: vermifugal, vermifuge
Vermilionectomia: vermilionectomy
Verminação: vermination
Verminose: invermination
Verminoso: verminal, verminous
Verniz: veneer, vernix
Verniz (dentário): varnish (dental)
Verruciforme: verruciform
Verrucose: verrucosis
Verrucoso: verrucose, verrucous, warty
Verruga: verruca, **pl.** verrucae, verruga, wart
Versão: version
Versicolor: versicolor
Vértebra: vertebra, **gen. e pl.** vertebrae
Vertebrado: vertebrate, vertebrated
Vertebral: vertebral
Vertebrectomia: vertebrectomy
Vertebroarterial: vertebroarterial
Vertebrocondral: vertebrochondral
Vertebrocostal: vertebrocostal
Vertebrofemoral: vertebrofemoral
Vertebroilíaco: vertebroiliac
Vertebrossacral: vertebrosacral, vertebrosternal
Vertical: vertical, verticalis
Vértice: vertex, **pl.** vertices
Verticilado: verticillate, whorled
Verticilo: verticil
Verticomentual: verticomental
Vertigem: vertigo
Vertiginoso: vertiginous

Vesaliano: vesalianum
Vesicação: vesication
Vesical: vesical
Vesicante: vesicant
Vesicar: vesicate
Vesicoabdominal: vesicoabdominal
Vesicobolhosa: vesicobullous
Vesicocervical: vesicocervical
Vesicoclise: vesicoclysis
Vesicoespinal: vesicospinal
Vesicointestinal: vesicointestinal
Vesicoprostático: vesicoprostatic
Vesicopúbico: vesicopubic
Vesicopústula: vesicopustule
Vesicopustular: vesicopustular
Vesicorretal: vesicorectal
Vesicorretostomia: vesicorectostomy
Vesicossigmóide: vesicosigmoid
Vesicossigmoidostomia: vesicosigmoidostomy
Vesicostomia: vesicostomy
Vesicotomia: vesicotomy
Vesicoumbilical: vesicoumbilical
Vesicoureteral: vesicoureteral
Vesicouretral: vesicourethral
Vesicouterino: vesicouterine
Vesicouterovaginal: vesicouterovaginal
Vesicovaginal: vesicovaginal
Vesicovaginorretal: vesicovaginorectal
Vesicovisceral: vesicovisceral
Vesícula: blister, vesicle, vesicula, **gen. e pl.** vesiculae
Vesícula biliar: cholecyst, cholecystis, gallbladder
Vesiculação: blistering, vesiculation
Vesiculado: vesiculate
Vesicular: vesicular
Vesiculectomia: vesiculectomy
Vesiculite: vesiculitis
Vesiculobrônquico: vesiculobronchial
Vesiculocavernoso: vesiculocavernous
Vesiculografia: vesiculography
Vesiculopapular: vesiculopapular
Vesiculoprostatite: vesiculoprostatitis
Vesiculotimpânica: vesiculotympanic
Vesiculotomia: vesiculotomy
Vesiculotubular: vesiculotubular
Veste pneumática antichoque: pneumatic antishock garment
Vestibulado: vestibulate
Vestibular: vestibular, vestibularis
Vestibulite: vestibulitis
Vestíbulo: vestibule, vestibulum, **pl.** vestibula
Vestibulocerebelo: archeocerebellum
Vestibulococlear: vestibulocochlear
Vestibuloespinal: vestibulospinal
Vestibulopatia: vestibulopathy
Vestibuloplastia: vestibuloplasty
Vestibulotomia: vestibulotomy
Vestibulouretral: vestibulourethral
Vestigial: vestigial
Vestígio: vestige, vestigium, **pl.** vestigia
Vesuvina: vesuvin
Veterinário: veterinarian, veterinary
Vetor: vector
Vetorcardiografia: vectorcardiography
Vetorcardiograma: vectorcardiogram
Vetorial: vectorial
Véu: veil, velum, **pl.** vela
Via: pathway, via, **pl.** viae
Viabilidade: viability
Viável: viable
Vibesato: vibesate
Víbora: viper
Vibração: bruissement, vibration
Vibrador: vibrator
Vibratório: vibrative, vibratory
Vibrião: vibrio
Vibriose: vibriosis, **pl.** vibrioses
Vibrissa: vibrissa, **pl. e gen.** vibrissae
Vibrissal: vibrissal
Vibrocardiograma: vibrocardiogram
Vibromassageador: vibromasseur
Vibroterapêutica: vibrotherapeutics
Vicariante: vicarious
Vicina: vicine
Vida: life
Vidarabina: vidarabine
Videoceratoscópio: videokeratoscope
Videoendoscopia: videoendoscopy
Videoendoscópio: videoendoscope
Vidiano: vidian
Vidro: glass
Viga: beam
Vigabatrina: vigabatrin
Vigilambulismo: vigilambulism
Vigilância: surveillance, vigilance
Vigília: vigil
Vilina: villin
Vilite: villitis
Vilo: villus, **pl.** villi
Vilosidade: villosity
Vilosite: villositis
Viloso: villose, villous
Vimentina: vimentin
Vinagre: acetum, **pl.** aceta; vinegar
Vincaleucoblastina: vincaleucoblastine
Vinculina: vinculin
Vínculo: vinculum, **pl.** vincula
Vindesina: vindesine
Vinho: wine
Vinhoso: vinous
Vínico: vinic
Vinil: vinyl
Vinilbenzeno: vinyl benzene
Vinileno: ethenylene, vinylene
Vinilideno: vinylidene
Violáceo: violaceous
Violência doméstica: domestic violence
Violeta: violet
Violeta de genciana: gentian violet
Violeta de Lauth: Lauth violet
Violeta de metila: methyl violet
Viomicina: viomycin
Viosterol: viosterol
Vipoma: VIPoma
Viraginidade: viraginity
Viral: viral
Viremia: viremia
Virgem: virgin
Virginal: virginal
Virgindade: maidenhead, virginity
Virgofrenia: virgophrenia
Viricida: viricidal, viricide
Viril: virile
Virilescência: virilescence
Virilha: groin, inguen
Virilidade: virility
Virilismo: virilism
Virilização: virilization
Virilizante: virilizing
Vírion: virion
Viripotente: viripotent
Viróide: viroid
Virola: ferrule
Virologia: virology
Virologista: virologist
Viropexia: viropexis
Virucida: virucidal, virucide
Virucopria: virucopria
Virulência: virulence
Virulento: virulent
Virulífero: viruliferous
Virúria: viruria
Vírus: virus, **pl.** viruses
Vírus Coxsackie: coxsackievirus
Vírus da poliomielite: poliovirus hominis
Vírus ECHO: echovirus
Vírus ECHO 28: Echovirus 28
Virus herpes simples: Simplexvirus
Vírus influenza: Influenza virus
Virusóide: virusoid
Visão: sight, vision
Viscância: viscance
Víscera: viscus, **pl.** viscera, vitals
Visceral: visceral
Visceralgia: visceralgia
Viscerimotor: viscerimotor
Viscerocrânio: viscerocranium
Visceroesquelético: visceroskeletal
Visceroesqueleto: visceroskeleton
Viscerogênico: viscerogenic
Viscerógrafo: viscerograph
Visceroinibitório: visceroinhibitory
Visceromegalia: visceromegaly
Visceromotor: visceromotor
Visceroparietal: visceroparietal
Visceroperitoneal: visceroperitoneal
Visceropleural: visceropleural
Visceroptose: visceroptosis, visceroptosia
Viscerossensorial: viscerosensory
Viscerossomático: viscerosomatic
Viscerotomia: viscerotomy
Viscerótomo: viscerotome
Viscerotonia: viscerotonia
Viscerotrófico: viscerotrophic
Viscerotrópico: viscerotropic
Viscidez: viscidity
Víscido: viscid
Viscidose: viscidosis
Visco: mistletoe, viscum
Viscoelasticidade: viscoelasticity
Viscômetro: viscometer
Viscosidade: viscosity
Viscosimetria: viscosimetry
Viscosímetro: viscosimeter
Viscoso: viscous
Viscotoxinas: viscotoxins
Visual: visual
Visualizar: visualize
Visuoauditivo: visuoauditory
Visuoespacial: visuospatial
Visuognose: visuognosis
Visuomotor: visuomotor
Visuopsíquico: visuopsychic
Visuoscópio: visuscope
Visuossensorial: visuosensory
Vital: vital
Vitalidade: vitality
Vitalismo: vitalism
Vitalístico: vitalistic
Vitalizar: vitalize
Vitalômetro: vitalometer
Vitamina: vitamin
Vitamina A: axerophthol
Vitelário: vitellarium
Viteliforme: vitelliform
Vitelina: ovovitellin, vitellin
Vitelino: vitelline
Vitelo: vitellus, yolk
Vitelogênese: vitellogenesis
Vitelogenina: vitellogenin
Viteloluteína: vitellolutein
Vitelorrubina: vitellorubin
Vitiliginoso: vitiliginous
Vitiligo: vitiligo, **pl.** vitiligines
Vitrectomia: vitrectomy
Vitreína: vitrein
Vitreíte: vitreitis
Vítreo: vitreous
Vitreodentina: vitreodentin
Vitreorretinal: vitreoretinal

Vitreorretinopatia: vitreoretinopathy
Vitrificação: vitrification
Vitriol: vitriol
Vitríolo verde: copperas
Vitronectina: vitronectin
Vitrosina: vitrosin
Viveiro: vivarium, **pl.** vivaria
Vividiálise: vividialysis
Vividifusão: vividiffusion
Vivificação: vivification
Viviparidade: viviparity
Vivíparo: viviparous
Vivipercepção: viviperception
Vivissecção: vivisection
Vivisseccionar: vivisect
Vivisseccionista, vivissector: vivisectionist, vivisector
Vocal: vocal
Volar: volar, volaris
Volátil: volatile (vol.)
Volatilização: volatilization
Volatilizar: volatilize
Volfrâmio: wolfram, wolframium
Volição: volition
Volicional: volitional
Volt: volt (v, V)
Voltagem: voltage
Voltaico: voltaic
Voltaísmo: voltaism
Voltâmetro: voltameter
Voltampère: voltampere
Voltímetro: voltmeter
Volume: volume (V, V)
Volumenômetro: volumenometer
Volumétrico: volumetric
Volumômetro: volumometer
Voluntário: voluntary
Voluptuoso: voluptuous
Volutina: volutin
Voluto: volute
Vólvulo: volvulus
Vômer: vomer, **gen.** vomeris
Vomeriano: vomerine
Vomerobasilar: vomerobasilar
Vomeronasal: vomeronasal
Vomitação: vomition
Vomitar: vomit
Vômito: vomiting, vomitus
Vórtice: vortex, **pl.** vortices, whorl
Vorticoso: vorticose
Voyeurismo: voyeurism
Voz: voice, vox
Voz glotalizada: vocal fry
Vulgar: vulgaris
Vulsela: volsella, vulsella, vulsellum
Vulva: cunnus, vulva, **pl.** vulvae
Vulvar: vulvar, vulval
Vulvectomia: vulvectomy
Vulvismo: vulvismus
Vulvite: vulvitis
Vulvocrural: vulvocrural
Vulvodinia: vulvodynia
Vulvouterino: vulvouterine
Vulvovaginal: vulvovaginal
Vulvovaginite: vulvovaginitis
V-Y-plastia: V-Y plasty

W

Walleriano: wallerian
Warfarin sódico: warfarin sodium
Wassermann-resistente: Wassermann-fast
Weddellita: weddellite
Weismanismo: weismannism
Whewellita: whewellite
W-plastia: W-plasty
Wrightina: wrightine
Wuchereríase: wuchereriasis

X

Xantelasma: xanthelasma
Xantematina: xanthematin
Xantemia: xanthemia
Xanteno: xanthene
Xântico: xanthic
Xantil: xanthyl
Xantílico: xanthylic
Xantina: xanthine (Xan)
Xantinol niacinato, xantinol nicotinato: xanthinol niacinate, xanthinol nicotinate
Xantinúria: xanthinuria
Xantismo: xanthism
Xantiúria: xanthiuria
Xantoastrocitoma: xanthoastrocytoma
Xantocromático: xanthochromatic
Xantocromia: xanthochromia
Xantocrômico: xanthochromic
Xantoderma: xanthoderma
Xantodonte: xanthodont
Xantofila: xanthophyll
Xantogranuloma: xanthogranuloma
Xantogranulomatoso: xanthogranulomatous
Xantoma: xanthoma
Xantomatose: xanthomatosis
Xantoproteico: xanthoproteic
Xantoproteína: xanthoprotein
Xantopsia: xanthopsia
Xantopucina: xanthopuccine
Xantose: xanthosis
Xantosina: xanthosine (X, Xao)
Xantoso amarelado: xanthous
Xantúria: xanthuria
Xarope: sirup, syrup, syrupus (syr)
Xaroposo: syrupy
Xemilofibam: xemilofiban
Xenil: xenyl
Xenobiótico: xenobiotic
Xenodiagnóstico: xenodiagnosis
Xenoenxerto: xenograft
Xenofobia: xenophobia
Xenofonia: xenophonia
Xenogênico: xenogeneic, xenogenic
Xenógeno: xenogenous
Xenônio: xenon (Xe)
Xenônio-133 (Xe^{133}): xenon-133 (^{133}Xe)
Xenoparasita: xenoparasite
Xerântico: xerantic
Xerasia: xerasia
Xerodermia: xeroderma
Xerofagia: xerophagia, xerophagy
Xeroftalmia: xerophthalmia, xerophthalmus
Xerografia: xerography
Xerograma: xerogram
Xeroma: xeroma
Xeromamografia: xeromammography
Xeromenia: xeromenia
Xeromicteria: xeromycteria
Xeroquilia: xerochilia
Xerorradiografia: xeroradiography
Xerorradiograma: xeroradiograph
Xerose: xerosis
Xerostomia: xerostomia
Xerótico: xerotic
Xerotripsia: xerotripsis
Xifocostal: xiphocostal
Xifodinia: xiphodynia
Xifoesternal: xiphisternal
Xifoesterno: xiphisternum
Xifoidalgia: xiphoidalgia
Xifóide: gladiate, xiphoid
Xifoidite: xiphoiditis
Xifópago: xiphopagus
Xilazina: xylazine
Xileno: xylene
Xilenol: xylenol
Xilidina: xylidine
Xilil: xylyl
Xilileno: xylylene
Xilitol: xylitol
Xilitol desidrogenase: xylitol dehydrogenase
Xilobiose: xylobiose
Xilocetose: xyloketose
Xiloidina: xyloidin
Xilol: xylol
Xilopiranose: xylopyranose
Xilose: xylose (Xy, Xyl)
Xilulose: xylulose
L-xilulosúria: L-xylulosuria
Xisma: xysma

Y

Yin-yang: yin-yang

Z

Zafirlukast: zafirlukast
Zanamivir: zanamivir
Zeatina: zeatin
Zeaxantina: zeaxanthin
Zeaxantol: zeaxanthol
Zeína: zein
Zelofobia: zelophobia
Zelotipia: zelotypia
Zeolita: zeolite
Zeoscópio: zeoscope
Zero: zero
Zeta: zeta
Zetácrito: zetacrit
Zetaproteína: zetaprotein
Zeumatografia: zeugmatography
Zidovudina: zidovudine
Zigal: zygal
Zigapofisário: zygapophysial, zygapophyseal
Zigapófise: zygapophysis, **pl.** zygapophyses
Zígio: zygion
Zigoma: zygoma
Zigomático: zygomatic
Zigomaticoauricular: zygomaticoauricular, zygomaticoauricularis
Zigomaticoesfenóide: zygomaticosphenoid
Zigomaticofacial: zygomaticofacial
Zigomaticofrontal: zygomaticofrontal
Zigomaticomaxilar: zygomaticomaxillary
Zigomaticoorbital: zygomatico-orbital
Zigomaticotemporal: zygomaticotemporal
Zigomaxilar: zygomaxillare, zygomaxillary
Zigomicetos: Zygomycetes
Zigomicose: zygomycosis
Zígon: zygon
Zigonema: zygonema
Zigopódio: zygopodium
Zigose: zygosis
Zigosidade: zygosity
Zigosperma: zygosperm
Zigosporo: zygospore
Zigossindactilia: zygosyndactyly
Zigóteno: zygotene
Zigótico: zygotic
Zigoto: zygote
Zigotoblasto: zygotoblast
Zigotômero: zygotomere
Zimase: zymase
Zimbro: juniper
Zimódemo: zymodeme
Zimogênese: zymogenesis
Zimogênico: zymogenic
Zimogênio: zymogen
Zimógeno: zymogenous
Zimograma: zymogram
Zimosan: zymosan
Zimoscópio: zymoscope
Zimosterol: zymosterol
Zincífero: zinciferous
Zinco: zinc (Zn)
Zinco-65 (Zn^{65}): zinc-65 (^{65}Zn)
Zincóide: zincoid
Zircônio: zirconium (Zr)
Zixina: zyxin

Zoantropia: zoanthropy
Zoantrópico: zoanthropic
Zoético: zoetic
Zóico: zoic
Zoíta: zoite
Zolpidem: zolpidem
Zomepirac sódico: zomepirac sodium
Zona: zona, **pl.** zonae; zone
Zonado: zonate
Zonagem: zoning
Zonal: zonal
Zonar: zonary
Zonestesia: zonesthesia
Zonoesqueleto: zonoskeleton
Zonografia: zonography
Zônula: zonula, **pl.** zonulae; zonule

Zonular: zonular
Zonulite: zonulitis
Zonulólise: zonulolysis, zonulysis
Zooantroponose: zooanthroponosis
Zooblasto: zooblast
Zoocromo: zoochrome
Zoodérmico: zoodermic
Zooenxerto: zoograft
Zooenxerto: zoografting
Zooerastia: zooerastia
Zoófago: zoophagous
Zoofilia: zoophilia
Zoofílico: zoophilic
Zoofilismo: zoophilism
Zoófilo: zoophile
Zoófito: zoophyte

Zoofobia: zoophobia
Zoofulvina: zoofulvin
Zoogênese: zoogenesis
Zoogeografia: zoogeography
Zoogléia: zooglea
Zoogonia: zoogony
Zoógono: zoogonous
Zoóide: zooid
Zoolagnia: zoolagnia
Zoolito: zoolite, zoolith
Zoologia: zoology
Zoologista: zoologist
Zoom: zoom
Zoomania: zoomania
Zoonose: zoonosis
Zoonótico: zoonotic
Zooparasita: zooparasite
Zoopatologia: zoopathology

Zooplastia: zooplasty
Zoosmose: zoosmosis
Zoospermia: zoospermia
Zoossadismo: zoosadism
Zoosterol: zoosterol
Zootecnia: zootechnics
Zoótico: zootic
Zootoxina: zootoxin
Zootrófico: zootrophic
Zorrubicina: zorubicin
Zoster: zoster
Zosteriforme: zosteriform
Zosteróide: zosteroid
Zoxazolamina: zoxazolamine
Z-plastia: Z-plasty
Zumbido: hum
Zwitterions: zwitterions

Serviços de impressão e acabamento
executados, a partir de filmes fornecidos,
nas oficinas gráficas da EDITORA SANTUÁRIO
Fone: (0XX12) 565-2140 - Fax (0XX12) 565-2141
http://www.redemptor.com.br - Aparecida-SP

O Dicionário Médico Stedman à Primeira Vista

O dicionário Stedman é organizado em um formato de entradas principais e subentradas. As subentradas tanto definirão as entradas como serão uma referência para o termo escolhido, onde aparece a definição.

Letras maiúsculas são usadas para as entradas principais com numerosas subentradas

CELL

Indica que existe uma ilustração do termo

Pronúncia em inglês

cell (sel). **1.** Célula; a menor unidade de estrutura viva capaz de existência independente, composta de uma massa de protoplasma encerrada por membrana e contendo um núcleo ou nucleóide. As células são muito variáveis e especializadas em estrutura e função, embora todas devam, em algum estágio, replicar proteínas e ácidos nucleicos, utilizar energia e reproduzir-se. **2.** Uma pequena cavidade fechada ou parcialmente fechada; um compartimento ou receptáculo oco. **3.** Um recipiente de vidro, cerâmica ou outro material sólido dentro do qual ocorrem reações químicas, gerando eletricidade, ou são colocadas soluções para ensaios fotométricos. [L. *cella*, despensa, câmara] — **Entrada principal**

— **Etimologia**

A palavra principal está abreviada nas subentradas

anaplastic c., c. anaplásica; **(1)** uma célula que voltou a um estado embrionário; **(2)** uma c. indiferenciada característica de neoplasias malignas. — **Subentradas**

acid c., c. ácida. SIN *parietal c.* — **Entrada principal com definição**

exudation c., c. de exsudação. SIN *exudation corpuscle.*

Em locuções ou expressões, encontre a definição na palavra em itálico

T helper c.'s (Th), células T auxiliares; subgrupo de linfócitos que secretam várias citocinas reguladoras da resposta imune: *subgrupo 1*, que sintetizam gama interferon e interleucina 2 e estão envolvidas na imunidade celular; *subgrupo 2*, que sintetizam interleucinas 4, 5, 10, e estão envolvidas na síntese de imunoglobulina.

cel'lulae ethmoida'les [TA], células etmoidais. SIN *ethmoid cells*, em *cell*. — ***Terminologia Anatomica*; procure a definição do termo no sinônimo em inglês**

Abreviatura

TERMINOLOGIA ANATOMICA

ethmoid c.'s, células etmoidais; células aéreas etmoidais; evaginações da mucosa dos meatos médio e superior da cavidade nasal para o labirinto etmoidal, formando múltiplos pequenos seios paranasais; são subdivididas em seios etmoidais anterior, médio e posterior. VER anterior ethmoidal c.'s, middle ethmoidal c.'s, posterior ethmoidal c.'s. SIN cellulae ethmoidales [TA], ethmoid air c.'s [TA], ethmoidal c.'s [TA], antra ethmoidalia, ethmoidal sinuses, sinus ethmoidales.

As barras azuis iniciam e finalizam os Termos de Alta Importância

TERMOS DE ALTA IMPORTÂNCIA
Entradas muito importantes para a prática da medicina e para a saúde mundial

car·ci·no·ma (CA), pl. **car·ci·no·mas, car·ci·no·ma·ta** (kar-si-nō'mă, -măz). Carcinoma; qualquer dos vários tipos de neoplasias malignas derivadas das células epiteliais, principalmente glandulares (adenocarcinoma) ou escamosos (c. de células escamosas); o tipo de câncer mais comum. [G. *karkinōma*, de *karkinos*, câncer, + *-oma*, tumor]

CÓDIGO

♻ Formas Combinantes	✮ Termo oficial alternativo para a *Terminologia Anatomica*
ℹ Indica que o termo é ilustrado, ver Índice de Ilustrações	[MIM] Mendelian Inheritance in Man
SIN Sinônimo	
Cf. Comparar, confrontar	I.C. Índice de Corantes
[NA] *Nomina Anatomica*	
[TA] *Terminologia Anatomica*	Termo de Alta Importância